BLOOD

PRINCIPLES AND PRACTICE OF HEMATOLOGY

SECOND EDITION

BLOOD

PRINCIPLES AND PRACTICE OF HEMATOLOGY

SECOND EDITION

Robert I. Handin, MD
PROFESSOR OF MEDICINE
HARVARD MEDICAL SCHOOL
EXECUTIVE VICE CHAIRMAN
DEPARTMENT OF MEDICINE
CO-DIRECTOR, HEMATOLOGY DIVISION
BRIGHAM AND WOMEN'S HOSPITAL
BOSTON, MASSACHUSETTS

Samuel E. Lux IV, MD
ROBERT A. STRANAHAN PROFESSOR OF PEDIATRICS
HARVARD MEDICAL SCHOOL
CHIEF, DIVISION OF HEMATOLOGY/ONCOLOGY
CHILDREN'S HOSPITAL BOSTON
ASSOCIATE IN PEDIATRICS
DEPARTMENT OF PEDIATRIC ONCOLOGY
DANA-FARBER CANCER INSTITUTE
BOSTON, MASSACHUSETTS

Thomas P. Stossel, MD
ELLISON-AMERICAN CANCER SOCIETY PROFESSOR OF MEDICINE
HARVARD MEDICAL SCHOOL
CO-DIRECTOR, HEMATOLOGY DIVISION
BRIGHAM AND WOMEN'S HOSPITAL
BOSTON, MASSACHUSETTS

WITH 120 CONTRIBUTING AUTHORS

Illustrated by Joy Marlowe and Wendy Beth Jackelow

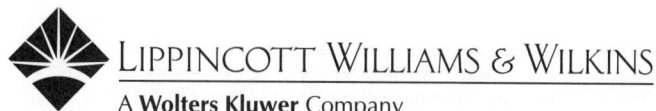

LIPPINCOTT WILLIAMS & WILKINS
A **Wolters Kluwer** Company
Philadelphia · Baltimore · New York · London
Buenos Aires · Hong Kong · Sydney · Tokyo

Acquisitions Editor: Jonathan W. Pine, Jr.
Developmental Editor: Keith Donnellan
Supervising Editor: Steven P. Martin
Production Editors: Lucinda Myers Ewing, Silverchair Science + Communications;
Amanda Waltman Yanovitch, Silverchair Science + Communications
Manufacturing Manager: Tim Reynolds
Cover Designer: Christine Jenny
Compositor: Silverchair Science + Communications
Printer: Quebecor World-Versailles

© 2003 by LIPPINCOTT WILLIAMS & WILKINS
530 Walnut Street
Philadelphia, PA 19106 USA
LWW.com

Printed in the USA
First edition published in 1995

Library of Congress Cataloging-in-Publication Data
Blood : principles and practice of hematology / [edited by] Robert I. Handin, Samuel E.
Lux, Thomas P. Stossel.-- 2nd ed.
    p. ; cm.
    Includes bibliographical references and index.
    ISBN 0-7817-1993-3
    1. Hematology. 2. Blood--Diseases. I. Handin, Robert I. II. Lux, Samuel E. III.
Stossel, Thomas P.
    [DNLM: 1. Hematologic Diseases. 2. Hematology. WH 120 B656 2002]
RC636 B575 2002
616.1'5--dc21

                                                        2002067539

Care has been taken to confirm the accuracy of the information presented and to describe generally
accepted practices. However, the authors, editors, and publisher are not responsible for errors or
omissions or for any consequences from application of the information in this book and make no
warranty, expressed or implied, with respect to the currency, completeness, or accuracy of the contents of the publication. Application of this information in a particular situation remains the professional responsibility of the practitioner.

The authors, editors, and publisher have exerted every effort to ensure that drug selection and
dosage set forth in this text are in accordance with current recommendations and practice at the
time of publication. However, in view of ongoing research, changes in government regulations,
and the constant flow of information relating to drug therapy and drug reactions, the reader is
urged to check the package insert for each drug for any change in indications and dosage and for
added warnings and precautions. This is particularly important when the recommended agent is
a new or infrequently employed drug.

Some drugs and medical devices presented in this publication have Food and Drug Administration (FDA) clearance for limited use in restricted research settings. It is the responsibility of
health care providers to ascertain the FDA status of each drug or device planned for use in their
clinical practice.

10 9 8 7 6 5 4 3 2 1

We dedicate this book to Marcia, Kathryn, and Kerry.
R.I.H., S.E.L., T.P.S.

Contents

Contributing Authors

Blanche P. Alter, MD, MPH
Expert, Clinical Genetics Branch
Division of Cancer Epidemiology and
Genetics
National Cancer Institute
Rockville, Maryland

Kenneth C. Anderson, MD
Professor of Medicine
Harvard Medical School
Department of Clinical Oncology
Dana-Farber Cancer Institute
Boston, Massachusetts

Nancy C. Andrews, MD, PhD
Associate Professor of Pediatrics
Harvard Medical School
Associate Investigator
Howard Hughes Medical Institute
Division of Hematology/Oncology
Children's Hospital Boston
Department of Pediatric Oncology
Dana-Farber Cancer Institute
Boston, Massachusetts

Joseph H. Antin, MD
Associate Professor of Medicine
Harvard Medical School
Brigham and Women's Hospital
Chief, Adult Oncology Stem Cell
Transplant Program
Dana-Farber Cancer Institute
Boston, Massachusetts

Robert J. Arceci, MD, PhD
Director and King Fahd Professor of
Pediatric Oncology
The Sidney Kimmel Comprehensive
Cancer Center at Johns Hopkins
Professor of Oncology and Pediatrics
Johns Hopkins University School of Medicine
Baltimore, Maryland

Robert A. S. Ariëns, PhD
Senior Lecturer
Academic Unit of Molecular Vascular
Medicine
University of Leeds Medical School
Leeds, United Kingdom

James O. Armitage, MD
Dean of the College of Medicine
University of Nebraska Medical Center
Omaha, Nebraska

Jon C. Aster, MD, PhD
Associate Professor
Harvard Medical School
Department of Pathology
Brigham and Women's Hospital
Boston, Massachusetts

Bernard M. Babior, MD, PhD
Professor and Head, Division of Biochemistry

Department of Molecular and Experimental
Medicine
The Scripps Research Institute
La Jolla, California

Kenneth A. Bauer, MD
Associate Professor
Department of Medicine
Harvard Medical School
Boston, Massachusetts
Veterans Affairs Boston Healthcare
System
West Roxbury, Massachusetts

Charles L. Bennett, MD, PhD
Professor
Department of Medicine
Northwestern University Medical School
Associate Director, Veterans Affairs Mid-
west Center for Health Services and Policy
Research
Associate Director, Veterans Affairs Chi-
cago Healthcare System, Lakeside Division
Chicago, Illinois

Joel S. Bennett, MD
Professor
Department of Medicine
Division of Hematology/Oncology
University of Pennsylvania School of
Medicine
Philadelphia, Pennsylvania

Barbara E. Bierer, MD
Professor of Medicine
Harvard Medical School
Dana-Farber Cancer Institute
Boston, Massachusetts

R. Gregory Bociek, MD, MSc
Assistant Professor
Department of Medicine
University of Nebraska Medical Center
Omaha, Nebraska

Francisco A. Bonilla, MD, PhD
Assistant Professor of Pediatrics
Harvard Medical School
Children's Hospital Boston
Boston, Massachusetts

Lawrence F. Brass, MD, PhD
Professor of Medicine and Pharmacology
Department of Medicine
University of Pennsylvania School of
Medicine
Philadelphia, Pennsylvania

Carlo Brugnara, MD
Professor of Pathology
Harvard Medical School
Department of Laboratory Medicine
Children's Hospital Boston
Boston, Massachusetts

H. Franklin Bunn, MD
Professor
Department of Medicine
Harvard Medical School
Hematology Division
Brigham and Women's Hospital
Boston, Massachusetts

George P. Canellos, MD, DSc(Hon), FRCP
William Rosenberg Professor
Department of Medicine
Harvard Medical School
Dana-Farber Cancer Institute
Boston, Massachusetts

Ralph Carmel, MD
Director of Research
Department of Medicine
New York Methodist Hospital
Brooklyn, New York
Professor of Medicine
Joan and Sanford I. Weill Medical College
of Cornell University
New York, New York

Bruce A. Chabner, MD
Professor of Medicine
Harvard Medical School
Massachusetts General Hospital
Boston, Massachusetts

Désiré Collen, MD, PhD
Professor of Medicine
Center for Molecular and Vascular Biology
University of Leuven
Campus Gasthuisberg
Leuven, Belgium

Laurence M. Corash, MD
Professor
Department of Laboratory Medicine
University of California, San Francisco,
School of Medicine
San Francisco, California

Mark A. Crowther, MD, MSc
Associate Professor of Medicine
McMaster University Faculty of Health
Sciences
Hamilton, Ontario, Canada

Paola S. Dal Cin, PhD
Associate Professor
Department of Pathology
Harvard Medical School
Brigham and Women's Hospital
Boston, Massachusetts

David C. Dale, MD
Professor
Department of Medicine
University of Washington School of
Medicine
Seattle, Washington

Alan D. D'Andrea, MD
Professor of Pediatrics
Harvard Medical School
Department of Pediatric Oncology
Dana-Farber Cancer Institute
Division of Pediatric Hematology/Oncology
Children's Hospital Boston
Boston, Massachusetts

Cynthia E. Dunbar, MD
Section Chief, Hematology Branch
National Heart, Lung, and Blood
Institute
Bethesda, Maryland

Stefan W. Eber, MD
Professor of Medicine
Department of Pediatric Hematology,
Immunology, Oncology, and Bone Marrow
Transplantation
Universitäts-Kinderklinik
Zurich, Switzerland

Joan E. Etzell, MD
Assistant Clinical Professor
Department of Laboratory Medicine
University of California, San Francisco,
School of Medicine
San Francisco, California

Bruce M. Ewenstein, MD, PhD
Assistant Professor of Medicine
Harvard Medical School
Boston, Massachusetts
Global Medical Director
Hemophilia Therapies
Baxter Bioscience
Glendale, California

Stefan Faderl, MD
Assistant Professor of Medicine
Department of Leukemia
University of Texas M. D. Anderson Cancer
Center
Houston, Texas

Judith A. Ferry, MD
Associate Professor
Department of Pathology
Harvard Medical School
Massachusetts General Hospital
Boston, Massachusetts

Mark D. Fleming, MD, DPhil
Assistant Professor
Department of Pathology
Harvard Medical School
Children's Hospital Boston
Boston, Massachusetts

Kenneth A. Foon, MD
Clinical Professor of Medicine
Division of Oncology
Stanford University School of Medicine
Stanford, California
Director, Clinical Development of
Oncology
Abgenix Inc.
Fremont, California

Bernard G. Forget, MD
Professor of Medicine and Genetics
Department of Internal Medicine
Yale University School of Medicine
New Haven, Connecticut

Jonathan W. Friedberg, MD
Assistant Professor of Medicine

James P. Wilmot Cancer Center
University of Rochester School of Medicine
and Dentistry
Rochester, New York

Barbara C. Furie, PhD
Professor of Medicine
Harvard Medical School
Chief, Division of Hemostasis and
Thrombosis
Beth Israel Deaconess Medical Center
Boston, Massachusetts

Bruce Furie, MD
Professor of Medicine
Center for Hemostasis and Thrombosis
Harvard Medical School
Boston, Massachusetts

Patrick G. Gallagher, MD
Associate Professor
Department of Pediatrics
Division of Neonatal-Perinatal Medicine
Yale University School of Medicine
Attending Physician
Yale-New Haven Hospital
New Haven, Connecticut

Stephen J. Galli, MD
Mary Hewitt Loveless, MD, Professor
Professor of Pathology, Microbiology, and
Immunology
Department of Pathology
Stanford University School of Medicine
Stanford, California

Guillermo Garcia-Manero, MD
Assistant Professor of Medicine
Department of Leukemia
University of Texas M. D. Anderson Cancer
Center
Houston, Texas

Raif S. Geha, MD
Prince Turki bin Abdul Aziz Al-Saud
Professor of Pediatrics
Harvard Medical School
Chief, Division of Immunology
Children's Hospital Boston
Boston, Massachusetts

Gary E. Gilbert, MD
Assistant Professor
Department of Medicine
Harvard Medical School
Hematology Division
Brigham and Women's Hospital
Boston, Massachusetts
Veterans Affairs Boston Healthcare
System
West Roxbury, Massachusetts

D. Gary Gilliland, MD, PhD
Associate Professor of Medicine
Harvard Medical School
Hematology Division
Brigham and Women's Hospital
Boston, Massachusetts

Jeffrey S. Ginsberg, MD, FRCPC
Professor
Department of Medicine
McMaster University Faculty of Health
Sciences
Hamilton, Ontario, Canada

Gregory A. Grabowski, MD
Professor of Pediatrics

Division and Program in Human Genetics
Children's Hospital Medical Center
Cincinnati, Ohio

Peter J. Grant, MD
Professor and Head of Academic Unit of
Molecular Vascular Medicine
Department of Medicine
Leeds, United Kingdom

Charles S. Greenberg, MD
Professor
Departments of Medicine and Pathology
Duke University School of Medicine
Durham, North Carolina

Robert I. Handin, MD
Professor of Medicine
Harvard Medical School
Executive Vice Chairman
Department of Medicine
Co-Director, Hematology Division
Brigham and Women's Hospital
Boston, Massachusetts

John A. Hansen, MD
Professor of Medicine
University of Washington School of Medicine
Fred Hutchinson Cancer Research Center
Seattle, Washington

Nancy Lee Harris, MD
Austin L. Vickery, Jr., Professor of
Pathology
Department of Pathology
Massachusetts General Hospital
Boston, Massachusetts

John H. Hartwig, PhD
Associate Professor of Medicine
Harvard Medical School
Hematology Division
Brigham and Women's Hospital
Boston, Massachusetts

Joseph E. Italiano, Jr., PhD
Instructor
Department of Medicine
Hematology Division
Brigham and Women's Hospital
Boston, Massachusetts

Chad T. Jacobsen, MD
Fellow
Division of Pediatric Hematology–Oncology
Department of Pediatrics
University Hospitals of Cleveland
Cleveland, Ohio

Mark L. Kahn, MD
Assistant Professor
Department of Medicine/Cardiology
University of Pennsylvania School of
Medicine
Philadelphia, Pennsylvania

Hagop M. Kantarjian, MD
Professor and Chairman
Department of Leukemia
University of Texas M. D. Anderson Cancer
Center
Houston, Texas

Allen P. Kaplan, MD
Professor of Medicine
Medical University of South Carolina
College of Medicine
Charleston, South Carolina

John G. Kelton, MD
Professor
Department of Medicine
McMaster University Faculty of Health
Sciences
Hamilton, Ontario, Canada

Nancy A. Kernan, MD
Member, Memorial Hospital
Department of Pediatrics
Memorial Sloan-Kettering Cancer
Center
New York, New York

Jeffery L. Kutok, MD, PhD
Assistant Professor
Department of Pathology
Harvard Medical School
Brigham and Women's Hospital
Boston, Massachusetts

David J. Kwiatkowski, MD, PhD
Associate Professor
Department of Medicine
Harvard Medical School
Brigham and Women's Hospital
Boston, Massachusetts

Thung-S. Lai, PhD
Assistant Research Professor
Department of Medicine
Division of Hematology
Duke University Medical Center
Durham, North Carolina

Marcel Levi, MD, PhD
Professor of Medicine
Department of Internal Medicine
Academic Medical Center
Amsterdam, The Netherlands

Roger H. Lijnen, PhD
Professor of Biochemistry
Department of Molecular and
Cardiovascular Research
University of Leuven
Campus Gasthuisberg
Leuven, Belgium

W. Conrad Liles, MD, PhD
Associate Professor of Medicine
Adjunct Associate Professor of Pathology
Departments of Medicine and Pathology
University of Washington School of
Medicine
Seattle, Washington

Stuart E. Lind, MD
Professor of Medicine and Pathology
University of Oklahoma Health Sciences
Center
Oklahoma City, Oklahoma

Samuel E. Lux IV, MD
Robert A. Stranahan Professor of Pediatrics
Harvard Medical School
Chief, Division of Hematology/Oncology
Children's Hospital Boston
Associate in Pediatrics
Department of Pediatric Oncology
Dana-Farber Cancer Institute
Boston, Massachusetts

Lucio Luzzatto, MD, PhD
Scientific Director
Instituto Nazionale per la Ricerca Sul
Cancro (IST)
Genova, Italy

Peter W. Marks, MD, PhD
Instructor in Medicine
Harvard Medical School
Hematology Division
Brigham and Women's Hospital
Boston, Massachusetts

Maria Paola Martelli, MD, PhD
Dipartimento di Biotecnologie Cellulari e
Ematologia
Sezione di Ematologia
University of Rome "La Sapienza"

Jeffrey McCullough, MD
Professor and Variety Club Chair
Department of Laboratory Medicine and
Pathology
University of Minnesota Medical School—
Minneapolis
Minneapolis, Minnesota

Eric M. Mickelson, BS
Staff Scientist
Human Immunogenetics Program
Fred Hutchinson Cancer Research Center
Seattle, Washington

Kenneth B. Miller, MD
Professor of Medicine
Tufts University School of Medicine
Director of Bone Marrow Transplantation
Department of Medicine
Division of Hematology/Oncology
Tufts-New England Medical Center
Boston, Massachusetts

Cynthia C. Morton, PhD
William Lambert Richardson Professor of
Obstetrics, Gynecology, and Reproductive
Biology
Professor of Pathology
Departments of Obstetrics, Gynecology,
and Reproductive Biology and Pathology
Brigham and Women's Hospital
Boston, Massachusetts

Hamza Mujagic, MS, MD, PhD
Visiting Scholar
Division of Hematology/Oncology
Massachusetts General Hospital
Boston, Massachusetts

Ronald L. Nagel, MD
Irving D. Karpas Professor of Medicine
Professor of Physiology and Biophysics
Head, Division of Hematology
Department of Medicine
Albert Einstein College of Medicine
Bronx, New York

Mohandas Narla, DSc
Vice President for Research
New York Blood Center
New York, New York

Rosario Notaro, MD
Laboratory of Human Molecular Genetics
Instituto Nazionale per la Ricerca Sul
Cancro (IST)
Genova, Italy

Nancy F. Olivieri, MD, FRCPC
Professor of Pediatrics and Medicine
Program Head of Hemoglobinopathies
University of Toronto Faculty of
Medicine
The Hospital for Sick Children
Toronto, Ontario, Canada

Effie W. Petersdorf, MD
Associate Professor
Department of Medicine
Division of Medical Oncology
Fred Hutchinson Cancer Research Center
Seattle, Washington

Orah S. Platt, MD
Professor of Pediatrics
Harvard Medical School
Chair, Department of Laboratory Medicine
Children's Hospital Boston
Boston, Massachusetts

Mortimer Poncz, MD
Professor
Department of Pediatrics
Children's Hospital of Philadelphia
Philadelphia, Pennsylvania

Thomas A. Puchalski, PharmD
Research Fellow in Medicine
Department of Hematology/Oncology
Harvard Medical School
Massachusetts General Hospital
Boston, Massachusetts

Paul G. Richardson, MD
Instructor in Medicine
Division of Hematologic Oncology
Department of Adult Oncology
Harvard Medical School
Dana-Farber Cancer Institute
Boston, Massachusetts

David S. Rosenblatt, MDCM
Professor
Departments of Human Genetics, Medi-
cine, and Pediatrics
McGill University Faculty of Medicine
McGill University Health Centre
Montreal, Quebec, Canada

Daniel Rosenblum, MD
Clinical Assistant Professor
Department of Hematology–Oncology
Georgetown University School of Medicine
Washington, D.C.

Wendell F. Rosse, MD
Florence McAlister Professor Emeritus of
Medicine
Division of Hematology and Medical
Oncology and Transplantation
Duke University Medical Center
Durham, North Carolina

David A. Roth, MD
Assistant Professor of Medicine
Center for Hemostasis and Thrombosis
Research
Harvard Medical School
Beth Israel Deaconess Medical Center
Boston, Massachusetts

Malek M. Safa, MD
Assistant Professor of Medicine
Department of Internal Medicine
Division of Hematology/Oncology
University of Cincinnati College of Medicine
The Barrett Cancer Center
Cincinnati, Ohio

Stephen E. Sallan, MD
Professor of Pediatrics
Harvard Medical School
Chief of Pediatric Clinical Oncology and
Chief of Staff

Dana-Farber Cancer Institute
Boston, Massachusetts

Shigeru Sassa, MD, PhD
Medical Director
Yamanouchi Pharmaceutical Co., Ltd.
Tokyo, Japan

David T. Scadden, MD
Associate Professor of Medicine
Harvard Medical School
Massachusetts General Hospital
Boston, Massachusetts

Shigeki Shibahara, MD, PhD
Professor of Molecular Biology
Department of Molecular Biology and
Applied Physiology
Tohoku University School of Medicine
Sendai, Japan

Akiko Shimamura, MD, PhD
Instructor of Pediatrics
Harvard Medical School
Department of Pediatric Oncology
Dana-Farber Cancer Institute
Division of Hematology/Oncology
Children's Hospital Boston
Boston, Massachusetts

Susan B. Shurin, MD
Professor of Pediatrics
Department of Pediatric Hematology/
Oncology
Rainbow Babies and Children's Hospital
Cleveland, Ohio

Colin Sieff, MD
Associate Professor of Pediatrics
Harvard Medical School
Department of Pediatric Oncology
Dana-Farber Cancer Institute
Division of Hematology/Oncology
Children's Hospital Boston
Boston, Massachusetts

Michael Silverberg, PhD
Associate Professor
Department of Medicine
State University of New York at Stony
Brook
Stony Brook Health Sciences Center
Stony Brook, New York

Lewis B. Silverman, MD
Assistant Professor of Pediatrics
Harvard Medical School
Department of Pediatric Oncology
Dana-Farber Cancer Institute
Division of Pediatric Hematology/
Oncology
Children's Hospital Boston
Boston, Massachusetts

Arthur T. Skarin, MD
Associate Professor of Medicine
Department of Adult Oncology
Harvard Medical School
Dana-Farber Cancer Institute
Boston, Massachusetts

Jerry L. Spivak, MD
Professor of Medicine and Oncology
Department of Medicine
Johns Hopkins University School of
Medicine
Baltimore, Maryland

Thomas P. Stossel, MD
Ellison-American Cancer Society
Professor of Medicine
Harvard Medical School
Co-Director, Hematology Division
Brigham and Women's Hospital
Boston, Massachusetts

Jeffrey G. Supko, PhD
Assistant Professor of Medicine
Department of Hematology/Oncology
Harvard Medical School
Massachusetts General Hospital
Boston, Massachusetts

Martin S. Tallman, MD
Professor of Medicine
Division of Hematology/Oncology
Northwestern University Medical School
Chicago, Illinois

Moshe Talpaz, MD
Chairman and Professor of Medicine
Department of Bioimmunotherapy
University of Texas M. D. Anderson Cancer
Center
Houston, Texas

Hugo ten Cate, MD, PhD
Professor of Internal Medicine
Department of Biochemistry
Cardiovascular Research Institute Maastricht
Maastricht University
Professor of Internal Medicine
Department of Internal Medicine
Academic Hospital Maastricht
Maastricht, The Netherlands

Mindy Tsai, DMSc
Senior Research Scientist
Department of Pathology
Stanford University School of Medicine
Stanford, California

Erik C. M. van Gorp, MD, PhD
Department of Internal Medicine
Slotervaart Hospital
Amsterdam, The Netherlands

Thomas J. Vulliamy, PhD
Honorary Lecturer
Department of Haematology
Imperial College of Science, Technology
and Medicine
Hammersmith Hospital
London, United Kingdom

Loren D. Walensky, MD, PhD
Fellow in Hematology/Oncology
Children's Hospital Boston
Department of Pediatric Oncology
Dana-Farber Cancer Institute
Boston, Massachusetts

Theodore E. Warkentin, MD, FRCPC
Professor
Department of Pathology and Molecular
Medicine
Professor
Department of Medicine
McMaster University Faculty of Health
Sciences
Hamilton Regional Laboratory Medicine
Program
Hamilton Health Sciences Corporation,
Hamilton General Site
Hamilton, Ontario, Canada

John W. Weisel, PhD
Professor
Department of Cell and Developmental
Biology
University of Pennsylvania School of
Medicine
Philadelphia, Pennsylvania

Peter F. Weller, MD, FACP
Professor of Medicine
Harvard Medical School
Chief, Division of Allergy and Inflammation
Co-Chief of Infectious Diseases
Vice-Chair of Medicine for Research
Beth Israel Deaconess Medical Center
Boston, Massachusetts

Gilbert C. White, MD
John C. Parker Professor of Medicine and
Pharmacology
Department of Medicine and Pharmacology
University of North Carolina at Chapel Hill
School of Medicine
Chapel Hill, North Carolina

David A. Williams, MD
Associate Chair for Translational Research
Cincinnati Children's Hospital Medical
Center
Beatrice C. Lampkin Chair and Professor of
Pediatrics
Department of Pediatrics
University of Cincinnati College of Medicine
Director, Division of Experimental
Hematology
Cincinnati Children's Hospital Research
Foundation
Cincinnati, Ohio

Neal S. Young, MD
Chief, Hematology Branch
National Heart, Lung, and Blood
Institute
Bethesda, Maryland

Hagop Youssoufian, MD
Adjunct Associate Professor
Department of Molecular and Human
Genetics
Baylor College of Medicine
Houston, Texas
Director of Clinical Discovery
Bristol-Myers Squibb Co.
Princeton, New Jersey

Andrew X. Zhu, MD, PhD
Assistant in Medicine
Department of Hematology/Oncology
Massachusetts General Hospital
Boston, Massachusetts

Leonard I. Zon, MD
Grousbeck Professor of Pediatrics
Harvard Medical School
Investigator
Howard Hughes Medical Institute
Division of Hematology/Oncology
Children's Hospital Boston
Department of Pediatric Oncology
Dana-Farber Cancer Institute
Boston, Massachusetts

Jeffrey I. Zwicker, MD
Clinical Fellow
Department of Hematology/Oncology
Beth Israel Deaconess Medical Center
Boston, Massachusetts

Preface

We embarked on the publication of *Blood: Principles and Practice of Hematology* a number of years ago. Our vision was to provide our readers with a readable, up-to-date, and comprehensive reference textbook covering virtually all aspects of hematology. We hoped that clinicians caring for patients with blood disorders, educators and scientists with interests in hematology, as well as students, house staff, and fellows seeking information about blood and its disorders would use our textbook. We hoped to be all things to all men and women interested in hematology. Since its publication, we have received nice notes and comments from colleagues and strangers commenting on the high quality and usefulness of the book, which pleased us greatly. One colleague who was asked to review the literature on an obscure congenital anemia told us he could not find a single reference beyond those already cited in the book. Another colleague, who is a busy practitioner, told us that, of the three hematology texts on his shelf, ours was his personal favorite. The enthusiastic reception accorded the first edition was the best reward we could have received for the collective efforts of the editors, authors, and our publisher.

As we began to prepare for the second edition, we faced two large issues. First, there were dazzling changes in many aspects of clinical and research hematology that had to be added to an already substantial book. Second, the means of communicating information had changed, and rapid electronic publication of journal materials and reviews, a proliferation of Web sites devoted to disseminating medical information, and the development of instantly updatable "ebooks" were predicted to curtail the publication of traditional books like ours. We debated the merits of radically changing the format and abandoning a conventional print publication but decided, in the end, to publish another print edition for the following reason: Although we all spend much more time online seeking information, there is still something uniquely satisfying and rewarding about turning the pages of a book. Knowing that some distant server has the collected wisdom of hematology on its tapes and hard drives and that it can be electronically searched is not quite the same as reaching for a familiar, dog-eared book and flipping through its pages. So, at the outset, the second edition of our textbook, written for the same audience as the first, looks very much like its predecessor—large, comprehensive, and, we hope, well written and carefully edited. We anticipate that you, our readers, share our love of books and will want to own copies for your personal and professional libraries.

However, we are not Luddites, so we have added electronic enhancements to the basic book. Each book has an accompanying CD-ROM that is searchable and can be used on a personal computer. We are also exploring an online site for updates between editions and, perhaps, for an updatable version of the parent book. We hope that you, the reader, find the book useful and enjoyable. We hope you derive as much pleasure from reading it as we have in putting it together.

Robert I. Handin, MD
Samuel E. Lux IV, MD
Thomas P. Stossel, MD

The Editors

Acknowledgments

As always, we are in awe of the considerable skills of our talented authors, who have summarized and interpreted this complex field in a single text. We are indebted to Linda Lyster, who quietly but firmly kept the editors and authors on track during the long process of revising the book. Thanks are also due to Joyce Patterson and Karen Vengerow for their administrative assistance and to Joy Marlowe and Wendy Beth Jackelow for their wonderful illustrations. We also appreciate the support of our publisher, Lippincott Williams & Wilkins, and particularly of our project editor, Keith Donnellan, who has worked with us on each of the many steps needed to publish this book and has displayed diplomacy and patience—alternately pushing, prodding, and stepping back, as needed. Most important, we are grateful to you, our readers, who we hope will find the book as useful to read as we have found it to write and edit.

R.I.H.
S.E.L.
T.P.S.

PART 1

Fundamentals of Hematology: Tools of the Trade

CHAPTER 1

Consultation in Hematology

Daniel Rosenblum

WHAT EXACTLY IS HEMATOLOGY?

To hematologists, defining hematology as "the study of blood and blood-forming organs" seems much too limiting because the field is in constant flux. Over the past century, hematologists have studied the effects of blood metabolites in the skin, bone marrow, and brain; of iron storage on liver, pancreas, and heart; of monoclonal protein disorders on kidney, bone, and eye; and of essential bone marrow nutrients on the gastrointestinal tract and neurologic function. To probe the structure and function of the components of the blood and to search for causes of blood disorders, hematologists have exploited many scientific disciplines and invaded the territory of most of the other specialties in medicine.

One acknowledgment of innovative investigations in hematology is the array of Nobel prizes in physiology and medicine that has been awarded for studies related to blood and bone marrow (Table 1-1). It is noteworthy that during the last 20 years, eight of the prizes have been awarded for work in this area. Innovation is a hallmark of research in hematology. Shown in Table 1-2 are examples of some other pioneering steps taken by hematologists.

An explosion of information in hematology followed the pioneering steps. For example, bone marrow transplantation, first used for aplastic anemia, is now used for a variety of diseases including bone marrow malignancies, bone marrow failure, nonhematologic malignancy, thalassemia, lipid storage, and autoimmune diseases. Hundreds of aberrant red cell proteins have been discovered, including over 500 hemoglobin (Hgb) variants, 65 glucose-6-phosphate dehydrogenase (G6PD)

variants, and variants of other glycolytic enzymes. Dozens of chromosomal changes have been identified, including translocations, transpositions, and breaks; many are highly specific for disease entities, and some have therapeutic and prognostic significance. Indeed, "basic" scientific discoveries have led to ingenious therapeutic innovations, including growth factors (erythropoietin, colony stimulating factors, and thrombopoietin), all-*trans*-retinoic acid for acute promyelocytic leukemia, clopidogrel to block platelet participation in arterial occlusion, and a specific tyrosine kinase inhibitor to suppress chronic myelogenous leukemia.

Besides being a remarkably innovative field, advances in hematology laboratories and clinical research have had broad impact on other fields. Research in thrombosis and hemostasis has broad implications for surgery, cardiology, pulmonology, neurology, and gastroenterology. Research on immunocytes forms the core of immunology and rheumatology. Studies on the growth factors and microendocrine systems involving benign and malignant cells and their supporting structures have affected many other areas of medicine. The scope of hematology is limited only by the human imagination.

CONSULTATION IN HEMATOLOGY

In addition to being a scientific discipline, hematology is a consultant subspecialty of internal medicine and pediatrics. Hematologists provide consultations in the following areas: (a) benign and malignant disorders of stem cells, bone marrow, blood, and lymph nodes; (b) disorders of development, proliferation, sur-

TABLE 1-1. Nobel Prizes Related to Hematology (Blood, Blood Cells, or Blood Cell Products)

Year	Recipients	Related Research
1930	Karl Landsteiner	ABO system
1934	George Minot, William Murphy, George Whipple	Liver therapy for anemia
1943	Henrik Dam, E.A. Doisy	Purification of vitamin K
1966	Peyton Rous	(Avian) leukemia virus
1974	Christian de Duve	Lysosomes (granules in white blood cells)
1975	David Baltimore, Renato Dulbecco, Howard Temin	Reverse transcriptase (led to understanding of acquired immunodeficiency syndrome and viral lymphomas)
1980	Baruj Benacerraf, Jean Dausset, George Snell	HLA antigen system
1982	Sune K. Bergström, Bengt I. Samuelsson, John R. Vane	Prostaglandins (leukotrienes, thromboxanes)
1987	Susumu Tonegawa	Structure of antibodies
1988	Gertrude Elion, George Hitchings	6-Mercaptopurine (leukemia therapy)
1990	E. Donnall Thomas	Bone marrow transplantation
1992	Edmond Fischer, Edwin Krebs	Reversible protein phosphorylation (tyrosine kinase in chronic myelogenous leukemia)
1994	Alfred G. Gilman	Signal transduction (mutations in leukemic cells)
1996	Peter C. Doherty, Rolf M. Zinkernagel	Immune recognition (lymphocytes)

vival, and function of white cells, red cells, and platelets; (c) disorders of hemostasis; (d) transfusion of blood components; and (e) bone marrow transplantation. Although many hematologists devote a majority of their attention to the care of patients with nonhematologic malignancies (medical oncology), all hematologists are expected to consult on, diagnose, and treat patients with relatively less common hematologic diseases.

Unlike primary care doctors, hematologists generally function as specialists who respond to requests (i.e., *referrals*) to use their expertise to solve problems that have previously been addressed by other physicians. Thus, instead of performing an initial history and physical examination, they are expected to begin a process that will help provide the answers to the questions that prompted the referral. This process is called *consultation* and is the core topic of this chapter.

With rare exceptions (1), little has been written about the formalities of medical consultation. Hematologists usually develop consultation skills by imitating their mentors or by trial and error. In preparing the second edition of this text, we sought advice on providing consultation from 40 hematologists from academic institutions and private practice. We generalized elements from each of them and combined this knowledge with our joint experience of providing consultations for over three decades. We adapted the information into a structure used by nonphysician consultants (2).

Because people in addition to the patient with the illness seek help from consultants, the generic word *client* is used to refer to all persons seeking advice. However, because of long use and convenience, the term *patient* is used interchangeably when the client is the one with the illness in question. To avoid identification errors, it is useful to include the patient's full name and date of birth or Social Security number on each page of all records. An institutional record number is a helpful addition but should not be used as a substitute because of the risk of error. In addition to patients, it is important to identify other important clients associated with the patient who may play a major role in the interaction. Medical information and decisions about pediatric patients, especially adolescents, should be shared with parents, legal guardians, and/or caretakers, who are often the principal clients seeking the consultant's expert advice. Adult patients often prefer to have another adult participate in medical decision-making, particularly when the problem is complex or life-threatening. All of these individuals should be regarded as clients, fully informed of the consultant's opinions, and educated by the consultant to a level at which they can understand the implications of the information and intelligently participate in the decision-making process.

The principal clients may be other physicians, whose referrals are requests for advice and not an offer to transfer responsibility for evaluation and management. Some referring physicians may send patients with questions in hand, others speak directly to specialists without allowing them to see their patients (i.e., "curbstone consultations"). In both cases, the referring doctors are seeking direct responses to specific ques-

TABLE 1-2. Pioneering Advances in Medicine Primarily Related to Blood and Blood Diseases

Innovation or Discovery	Related Area
Splenectomy for hemorrhage	Idiopathic thrombocytopenic purpura
Curative radiation therapy	Hodgkin's disease
Cytotoxic therapy for malignancy	Leukemia
Purine antagonists	Leukemia
Amino acid substitution causes hereditary disease in humans	Valine for glutamic acid causes sickle cell anemia
Chromosome translocation causes acquired disease	Philadelphia chromosome causes chronic myelogenous leukemia
Enzyme defect causes chemical sensitivity	Glucose-6-phosphate dehydrogenase deficiency causes favism and pamaquine sensitivity
Hereditary defects in the regulation of protein synthesis cause disease	Thalassemia
Malignant cell populations are monoclonal	Myeloma
Pathologic protein–protein interactions in disease	Blood coagulation
Human surface antigens	ABO system in red cells, HLA antigen system
Identification of a defective carrier protein system in disease	Pernicious anemia
Protein inhibition as a form of treatment	Anticoagulant therapy
Vitamin inhibition as a form of treatment	Anticoagulant therapy
Amino acid substitution causes hypercoagulable state	Factor V Leiden

tions. Consultants should develop a comfortable method of addressing these requests that minimizes the risk of error and recognizes the importance of the relationship between primary physicians and their patients.

If the patient has had previous care, the documents that describe it may have a major bearing on the consultation. Referring physicians and patients should be encouraged to provide relevant information, especially laboratory test results and reports of imaging studies, to the specialist. A summary cover letter can be a valuable aid, especially if the data are complex. The consultant needs to know what treatments have been tried, the name of each medication, the dose, the duration of therapy, and the outcomes. Ideally, this information should be tabulated and provided before the first contact with the consultant.

It may become apparent that the consultant is expected to assume the role of treating physician. Specialty management offers advantages, particularly when the problems are either rare or complex. Common and simple problems may best be managed by primary care physicians, with appropriate guidance from the specialist.

Hematologists should confirm their plans with patients and referring physicians when they assume responsibility for evaluation and management to clarify responsibility and elicit mutual consent. Such discussions should be held whether the planned transitions are prompted by client expectations or circumstances of the illnesses.

Experienced consultants take extra steps to greet and receive new clients personally, expressing warmth, caring, and concern for their well-being. Many patients are terrified by the mere fact of being referred to a hematologist. Some fear the diseases we treat, particularly acute leukemia, and others are anxious because of the confusion that preceded the referral. Their rationality may be overwhelmed by extremes of emotion resulting in outbursts of anger, anxiety, and grief, or they may mask their feelings by denial, particularly if their disease is fatal and time is short (3,4). Although trust may be difficult to establish, sincere caring and unhurried gentleness can have enduring beneficial effects.

Once the client has been identified, the consultation can begin. At the outset and in all subsequent steps, consultants should aim to inform and assist their clients at the same time that they are gathering and assessing data, drawing conclusions, and making recommendations. Consultants should begin by informing clients about themselves. They may do so by means of a brochure, certificates on the wall, or an oral statement. Clients develop increased trust if they learn details that confirm their consultant's competence. Information to supply includes the following: name of the training program, Hematology Board certification, membership in the American Society of Hematology, institutional and private practice affiliations, research achievements, participation in clinical trials and centers of excellence, and other special interests.

Communication is essential to consultation. Consultants should assure patients and referring physicians that they will provide oral and written responses to their questions. They should anticipate their need for access by providing telephone numbers on a calling card, describing coverage arrangements, and identifying members of the office staff who can respond to emergencies by telephone. Consultants should respond promptly when called. They should introduce their clients to key staff members and give them a walking tour of the facility. Such measures establish trust, increase the value of the consultation, and encourage compliance.

Communication depends on effective listening (5). For several minutes, consultants should listen to patients without interrupting them, using body language to show interest and receptivity. During this period, consultants should observe their patients'

language, behaviors, sophistication, emotional control, and organizational skills. The language of a patient's initial statement can guide a consultant's style of communication. Typically, it includes words and gestures that indicate the extent of the patient's desire to be informed of medical details, to take control or yield it, and to participate in the decision-making process or avoid it. It often includes messages about personal priorities, self-image, pain, anxiety, hope, and despair. The language reflects educational level, clinical competence, and access to background information. Consultants should adapt their language and style of communication to their patients' level of comfort.

To resolve confusion about the purpose of the consultation, consultants may initiate a discussion with a statement intended to focus the attention on the principal issues. The statement might begin with, "As I understand it, the reason for the consultation is. . . ." Clients should be encouraged to respond with corrections. The process advances mutual understanding of the purpose of the visit.

What is happening during the first several minutes of the interview is the negotiation of a working relationship or contract. Impatient consultants who sweep past contract negotiation fail to develop maximally effective working partnerships with their clients.

During contract negotiation, clients are likely to ask the questions that are of the most importance to them. These questions, like the "chief complaint" of a primary history, should be accorded respect by consultants. Even if precise answers are not attainable, consultants should record the questions and revisit them. During contract negotiation, clients also reveal the role they expect their consultants to play. Some clients may wish their consultants to become treating physicians. Others may wish to retain responsibility for decision-making and implementation of treatment regimens. Acceptability, trust, and compliance are all supported by recognition and incorporation of the clients' wishes for autonomy; consultants may offer opinions regarding the advisability of maintaining autonomy, but they must leave decisions about it to the clients.

During contract negotiation, consultants can make statements defining their ability and willingness to meet their clients' expectations. The consultant may specify the time available for the visit, the expected length of treatment, the opportunities to work with other health care providers or to include alternative medicine in the regimen, and the contributions expected from the client (physical, mental, and financial). Consultants may wish to specify an acceptable level of patient autonomy. It is important that the consultant make quite clear the services that will not be provided. If precise statements are difficult to make, the consultant can roughly outline the arrangements, including an agenda for the day's activities.

Whatever level of autonomy clients maintain, they continue to expect consultants to be helpful. To be perceived as helpful, consultants must respond to their clients' agendas. Unless consultants respond to their clients' questions and perceived needs, the clients may be distinctly disappointed, even if their consultants listen thoughtfully, address the major clinical issues, and make clear recommendations. The task for consultants, then, is to learn what their clients' questions and expectations are as soon as possible and to begin working on them.

It is also important in the initial phases of the contract to establish the terms of an enduring relationship, to establish trust, to make clear the consultant's willingness to listen and respond, and to provide the client with a route of access. Even clients planning no more than a single visit may be advised, when appropriate, to maintain contact with the consultant.

A consultation differs from a primary history and physical examination. Consultations are requested by physicians who have encountered problems while evaluating their patients' complaints. The patients may not always have symptoms or complaints related to the problems for which they are referred. For example, consultation might be requested for asymptomatic lymphocytosis discovered during an evaluation for hypertension. Hematologists can be more helpful consultants when they identify the referring doctors' questions and address them. A clear statement of the problems guides the consultant in collecting data, formulating an assessment, and articulating a response to the clients' questions.

If the client is referred because of a problem or an abnormal laboratory finding without having received an evaluation by another physician, an initial history and physical examination are needed in addition to a consultation for the special problem. The consultant may choose to do the initial history and physical or to refer the client to a primary care physician.

Particular care should be taken in developing responses to rare or complex problems. Consultants should openly discuss their plans for evaluation and management, making their range of competence and limitations clear. In the course of a career, consultants are likely to see problems that are extremely rare, even unique, or complex to a level which challenges our current knowledge in hematology. Rare and complex problems present opportunities for consultants to excel in linking patients with experienced authorities and investigators.

Client access to information has had a major impact on the shape, content, and duration of many hematology consultations. Some of the information comes from sources not ordinarily used by hematologists (e.g., family and friends, lay publications, Web sites, chat rooms, support groups, and patient advocacy groups). Some of this information derives from authoritative sources. In response to client questions, consultants are challenged to review the information and comment on it.

Urgent problems often demand urgent solutions. If the patient is acutely ill, the consultant may address the urgent problems with appropriate tests and treatments before proceeding to a detailed history. A hematologist should expect to respond quickly when asked to see an immunocompromised patient with an infection or any patient with uncontrolled hemorrhage, acute thrombosis, complex coagulation disorders, thrombotic thrombocytopenic purpura, acute leukemia, markedly abnormal laboratory values, acute chest syndrome complicating sickle cell anemia (SCA), hypercalcemia with multiple myeloma, or therapeutic misadventures such as tumor lysis syndrome.

The hematology consultant should plan for emergencies by becoming familiar with local facilities which can provide specialized blood products and medications and laboratories which can perform specialized tests.

APPROACH TO HISTORY TAKING IN HEMATOLOGY

When taking histories, hematologists focus their attention on the problems they intend to resolve. They gather enough information to avoid errors. Some problems require only a brief history and no physical examination. Others require an expanded history and physical examination, particularly if the hematologist is planning to provide direct care or the illness is complex.

In taking the history of a patient with a hematologic problem, hematologists think about the characteristics of blood as detailed in Table 1-3. They proceed with a mind open to possibilities, think in terms of clinical patterns, and create a prioritized list of diagnoses based on the patient's history. They suspend judgment until confirmatory data has been obtained. For example, if the patient is a young woman with a microcytic

---

TABLE 1-3. Characteristics of Blood to Consider When Taking a History

Rapid growth of component cells
Limited survival of cells, limited half-life of proteins
Characteristics of distribution in the circulatory system and tissues
Vulnerability to stress on the host
Liquidity, leakage, coagulability
Trauma, sequestration, and antibodies
Migration through and interaction with other organs
Accessibility to iatrogenic manipulation
Changes caused by dysfunction of other organs, especially liver and kidney
Genetic influences, long lists of familial disorders
Susceptibility to mutation after exposure to ionizing radiation and chemotherapy

---

anemia, the hematologist should avoid a presumption that her anemia is due to iron deficiency caused by blood loss without considering other possible causes of microcytic anemia, such as thalassemia minor.

Asking patients and their families to recall highly specific information can be challenging for them. It is important to create a relaxing, reassuring, nonjudgmental, and pleasant environment to soothe anxiety before the process begins and to offer continued reassurance as communication continues.

Diagnoses are sometimes made by sophisticated detective work, revealing details about the patient's habits. Aggressive exercise is sometimes a cause of traumatic hemolysis. Storage of clothes in mothballs (naphthalene) can induce hemolysis in G6PD deficiency. Sniffing glue fumes can induce aplastic anemia. Exposure to cats can cause lymphadenopathy and cat-scratch disease. Travel to tropical areas can be followed by malaria or schistosomiasis; travelers to Cape Cod occasionally acquire babesiosis. Exposure to benzene through work or home activities can lead to aplastic anemia or acute leukemia. Industrial exposure to heavy metals such as arsenic, arsine, copper (used in smelting, alloy production, fertilizers, and pesticides), and lead and zinc (used in making pottery and producing batteries) can cause aplastic anemia, sideroblastic anemia, hemolytic anemia, thrombocytopenia, and eosinophilia. Splenectomy can be followed by bizarre peripheral blood cell morphology.

The triad of glycosuria, cirrhosis, and hyperpigmentation of the skin is a sign of advanced hemochromatosis. The triad has become relatively rare because of increased screening for saturated iron stores and notification of potentially affected family members. Early manifestations of hemochromatosis include fatigue, arthralgia, erectile dysfunction, and cardiac abnormalities. Even when another hematologic diagnosis seems likely, it is important to keep hemochromatosis in mind, because it is the most prevalent monoallelic genetic disease in U.S. whites (6). With a gene frequency of 0.056, the frequency of heterozygotes in the United States is 0.104 and of homozygotes is 0.003. Africans have an increased risk of hereditary hemochromatosis based on a different gene (see Chapter 46 for a detailed discussion).

Medical history can provide clues to linked events such as previous hematologic diagnoses, pregnancy-related hematologic disease, previous exposure to sensitizing agents, transfusion history, and episodes of bleeding. For example, autoimmune thrombocytopenia may precede or follow autoimmune hemolytic anemia by weeks to years. After high-dose chemotherapy and autologous bone marrow transplantation, a group of 230 patients was observed to have a 12% risk of myelodysplasia and acute leukemia (7).

Medications can cause a variety of hematologic disorders, including hemorrhage and anemia, bone marrow suppression,

TABLE 1-4. Hematologic Disorders Associated with Alcohol Consumption

Macrocytic anemia
Gastrointestinal hemorrhage
Iron deficiency anemia
Folic acid deficiency
Anemia of chronic disease
Hypersplenism
Coagulation factor deficiency
Neutropenia
Thrombocytopenia
Thrombocytosis
Bone marrow failure

immune blood cell lysis, nonimmune hemolysis, platelet dysfunction, methemoglobinemia, and altered susceptibility to hematinics and anticoagulants. Phenytoin can cause lymphadenopathy. G6PD deficiency can cause hemolysis after exposure to many medications. Neutropenia is a side effect of radiation therapy and many classes of medications, especially antibiotics, anticonvulsants, antihistamines, antimalarials, antithyroid agents, cardiovascular agents, diuretics, antineoplastics, and phenothiazines. Severe deficiency of B-complex vitamins, iron, or protein can cause bone marrow failure. Warfarin therapy is antagonized by ingestion of vitamin K–rich food (especially brussels sprouts, broccoli, and spinach) and enhanced by antibiotics that suppress bacterial flora. Indeed, warfarin therapy is affected either positively or negatively by dozens of medications. Iron deficiency anemia has been associated with ingestion of clay, pica in children, and hunger for ice (i.e., pagophagia). A detailed dietary history and a complete list of all nonprescription additives may help resolve the patient's hematologic problem. Hematologically active agents may be among the ingredients of brand name medications. For example, salicylates are included in more than 60 nonprescription formulations [8]. Alcohol exposure deserves special emphasis. Chronic alcohol consumption can result in a broad variety of blood disorders (Table 1-4).

Fever, chills, sweats, and weight loss are "B" symptoms of lymphoma that worsen the prognosis. Itching, especially after a hot shower or bath, is a troublesome symptom of polycythemia vera. Advanced myeloma may be accompanied by pathologic fractures and chronic back pain. Paroxysmal nocturnal hemoglobinuria can cause mysterious pains, thrombotic episodes, and dark urine. Hematologic causes of spontaneous abortion include α-thalassemia, "lupus anticoagulant," and other thrombotic disorders. The risk of infection is increased after splenectomy and in acquired immunodeficiency syndrome (AIDS), myeloma, chronic lymphocytic leukemia (CLL), neutropenia, Wiskott-Aldrich syndrome, Kostmann's congenital agranulocytosis, and combined immunodeficiency syndrome. Some infections are typically related to specific hematologic disorders. SCA increases the risk of salmonella osteomyelitis [9]. Individuals with lymphocytic dysfunction, especially AIDS [10] and hairy cell leukemia [11], are unusually susceptible to disseminated *Mycobacterium avium*-intracellulare. Hodgkin's disease increases the risk of herpes zoster. Hemochromatosis increases susceptibility to a variety of agents, including potentially fatal *Vibrio vulnificus* infection, acquired by eating raw shellfish [12]. Deferoxamine, a chelating agent used to remove excess iron from patients with hemochromatosis, can increase susceptibility to zygomycosis (i.e., mucormycosis).

Some hematologic disorders are linked to other disorders: Autoimmune thrombocytopenia and autoimmune hemolytic anemia are associated with systemic lupus erythematosus and CLL; pure red cell aplasia is associated with myasthenia gravis

and thymoma. Polycythemia vera is linked to myelofibrosis. Aplastic anemia, paroxysmal nocturnal hemoglobinuria, and myelodysplasia are linked to acute leukemia.

Past blood tests can establish or eliminate a pattern of progression of a hematologic abnormality. Sources in addition to records from other physicians may include life insurance physicals, employment screening, health fairs, and blood banks. Therapeutic phlebotomies and transfusions help to quantify iron loss or gain (approximately 250 mg of iron/pint of blood). Transfusions also increase the risk of transmission of bloodborne diseases, hepatitis, and AIDS and sensitization to blood products.

After taking an initial history, hematologists may seek additional information that they should ask patients to provide. Patients should be encouraged to keep records of personal observations of fever, bleeding episodes, exposures, ingestion of medications, and responses to treatment. Quantitation of menstrual blood loss, normally less than 80 cc/cycle [13], is often difficult. A variety of questions may help the patient to approximate a description of the volume of blood loss, such as asking about the number, size, and degree of soaking of the pads or tampons, the number of days of heavy bleeding, and the number of cycles per year. Women may find it easier to estimate the size of blood clots than the volume of menstrual flow.

Ethnic background may provide a clue to genetically determined diseases. Thalassemia is found in Mediterranean and Asian populations. G6PD deficiency, Gaucher's disease, and factor XI deficiency are more common in Ashkenazi Jews. SCA is concentrated in people of African origin.

Heredity plays a prominent role in hematology. Multigenerational genealogic charts simplify analysis of genetic traits. The broad spectrum of hereditary hematologic diseases is represented in Table 1-5.

While taking the history, the hematologist forms hypotheses regarding the diagnosis and makes selective decisions about the path of further inquiry. For example, the combination of thrombocytopenia with anemia or leukopenia prompts consideration of bone marrow failure involving more than one cell line or infiltration. Isolated thrombocytopenia, on the contrary, suggests extramedullary platelet destruction or isolated megakaryocyte dysplasia and prompts the hematologist to focus on a different set of potentially causative agents. The rare—but lethal—thrombotic thrombocytopenic purpura should be kept in mind. It is often associated with fever, renal failure, neurologic changes, and microangiopathic hemolytic anemia and infrequently with visible thrombosis or purpura.

Specific historical information sharpens diagnostic accuracy and improves treatment of coagulopathies. A history of thrombosis with associated pregnancy or the use of oral contraceptives suggests the possibility of a heritable disorder (factor V Leiden, protein-S or -C deficiency). These disorders increase the risk of thrombosis and pulmonary embolism associated with estrogen therapy. A history of mucous membrane and joint bleeding is typical of hemophilia. A history of troublesome bleeding after surgery, trauma, and minor injuries predicts future risks with surgery and prompts laboratory investigation for exposure to platelet antagonists, inherited or acquired platelet disorders, thrombocytopenia, von Willebrand's disease, and factor XI deficiency. Information about previous treatment, inhibitors, and exposures can point the way to effective therapeutic choices.

PHYSICAL EXAMINATION

Physical findings characteristic of hematologic diseases are discussed in the chapters related to those diseases. A "complete" physical examination should be done on every patient referred

TABLE 1-5. Hereditary Hematologic Diseases

Category	Diseases
Erythrocyte shape	Hereditary spherocytosis, hereditary stomatocytosis, hereditary elliptocytosis, hereditary xerocytosis
Erythrocyte enzymes	Glycolytic enzymes (e.g., glucose-6-phosphate dehydrogenase)
Hemoglobinopathies	Sickle cell anemia, Hgb C, etc.
Hgb synthesis	α-Thalassemia, β-thalassemia
Iron metabolism	Hemochromatosis, atransferrinemia, etc.
Malignancy	Acute lymphoblastic leukemia of childhood (associated with Down's syndrome, Bloom's syndrome, Fanconi's anemia, ataxia telangiectasia, hereditary immunoglobulin A deficiency, and Wiskott-Aldrich syndrome); increased risk in siblings, especially monozygotic twins
Leukocyte quantity	Hereditary neutropenia, hereditary neutrophilia
Leukocyte function	Chédiak-Higashi syndrome, chronic granulomatous disease, familial erythrophagocytic lymphohistiocytosis, leukocyte adhesion deficiency, lysosomal storage disease (Gaucher's, Niemann-Pick, Tay-Sachs), myeloperoxidase deficiency, specific granule deficiency
Coagulation disorders	Congenital dysfibrinogenemia, factor deficiency (V, VIII, IX, XI, XIII), plasminogen deficiency, protein-C or -S deficiency, factor V Leiden, von Willebrand's disease
Platelet disorders	Bernard-Soulier syndrome, Glanzmann's thrombasthenia, Scott's syndrome, neonatal thrombocytopenia
Others	Hereditary amyloidosis, porphyria, primary immunodeficiency

Hgb, hemoglobin.

for consultation. However, if a complete physical examination has recently been performed, some hematologists believe that it need not be repeated. Because of their significance to hematologists, special attention is directed to the lymph nodes, spleen, integument, and neurologic system.

LYMPH NODES

Judging the malignant potential of enlarged lymph nodes in adults is a frequent challenge for the hematology consultant, as the differential diagnosis is lengthy and complex (Table 1-6). Size, anatomic distribution, texture, tenderness, and number contribute to the clinical appraisal and should be assessed. A drawing or table can provide a rapid, shorthand device for recording the findings. The hematologist should examine the tonsils, anterior and posterior cervical, supraclavicular, axillary, epitrochlear, inguinal, and popliteal nodes. Tender, localized nodes are typically found after an acute infection and usually regress within weeks. Prominent, generalized lymphadenopathy occurs with infectious mononucleosis, toxoplasmosis, systemic lupus erythematosus, and mixed connective tissue disease, as well as with CLL and lymphoma. Anatomic location of enlarged lymph nodes may point to a probable pathologic diagnosis (Fig. 1-1), especially in children. Even if malignancy is considered unlikely, it should be excluded in individuals with a massive lymphadenopathy or a single node greater than 2 cm (Fig. 1-2). Nodes smaller than 1 cm, particularly if they are in the neck or groin region, are usually benign. Biopsy is often favored for nodes 1 to 2 cm unaccompanied by an obvious cause, although malignancy is unlikely. A retrospective chart review of asymptomatic lymphadenopathy in a large family practice (14) found no cases of malignancy in its patients, 0.5% of whom had lymphadenopathy and 0.22% of whom had nodes greater than 1 cm. Slap and others reported that biopsy of nodes greater than 2 cm yielded a diagnosis of granulomatous disease or malignancy in 71% of their patients (15). Unexplained lymphadenopathy in the neck of an adult should prompt ear, nose, and throat panendoscopy and imaging studies of the head, neck, and chest.

The history may help to decide the malignant potential of lymph nodes. It is useful to ask about exposures to trauma, cat scratch, and drugs (especially phenytoin); travel; sexual exposures; evidence of infection; and time spent in a rural environment. Early biopsy is appropriate if the lymph node is greater than 2 cm, has measurably grown, feels rubbery, is located in a suspicious place such as the supraclavicular fossa, or is among several suspicious nodes. Biopsy can be deferred if the node is less than 2 cm, is tender or fluctuant, appears to be associated with an infection, or is localized to an area often associated with inflammation, such as the anterior cervical triangle or inguinal area. If a biopsy is deferred, however, the physician should remeasure the node at 2- or 3-month intervals and examine the other lymph node–bearing regions each time. A biopsy is indicated if the node enlarges or if further unexplained lymphadenopathy occurs.

Asymptomatic, small nodes in children are most often benign. In a retrospective study of 239 children undergoing

TABLE 1-6. Differential Diagnosis of Lymphadenopathy

Reactive diseases
  Infectious
    Bacterial: streptococcal, staphylococcal, tuberculosis, chancroid, leprosy, tularemia
    Viral: Epstein-Barr virus, cytomegalovirus, human immunodeficiency virus, measles
    Spirochetal: syphilis
    Mycotic: blastomycosis, histoplasmosis
    Other: toxoplasmosis, cat-scratch fever
  Dermatopathic
    Reactive lymphadenopathy
    Lymphoma cutis (Sézary's syndrome)
  Inflammatory
    Sarcoidosis
    Systemic lupus erythematosus
    Rheumatoid arthritis
    Serum sickness
    Berylliosis
  Metabolic
    Hyperthyroidism
    Addison's disease
    Hypopituitarism
  Storage diseases
    Gaucher's disease
    Lipidoses
  Drugs
    Diphenylhydantoin
  Other
    Castleman's disease
Malignant diseases
  Primary hematologic
    Hodgkin's disease
    Non-Hodgkin's lymphoma
    Chronic lymphocytic leukemia
    Acute leukemia (chloroma)
  Metastatic malignancy

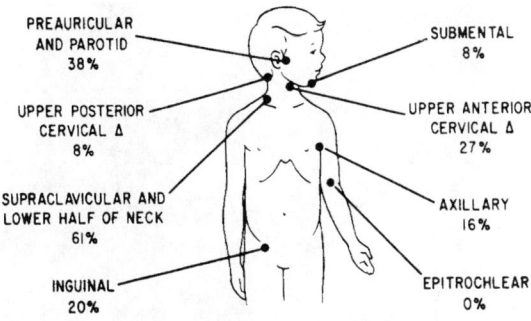

Figure 1-1. Lymphadenopathy by site. Percentage at each site of adenopathy is diagnostic yield for that location. High yield from supraclavicular adenopathy was due to Hodgkin's disease, whereas that in upper cervical and preauricular areas was due to atypical mycobacteria. Δ, change. (From Knight PJ, Mulne AF, Vassy LE. When is lymph node biopsy indicated in children with enlarged peripheral nodes? *Pediatrics* 1982;69:391, with permission.)

peripheral lymph node biopsy, a histologic or microbiologic diagnosis was obtained in only 41% of cases (16). Reactive hyperplasia (52%), granulomatous disease (32%), and neoplasia (13%) were the most common diagnoses. Location was important. Supraclavicular and lower neck nodes were pathologic in 61%, whereas only 8% of superior posterior cervical nodes were pathologic.

Nodal pain after alcohol consumption has been reported in up to 7% of patients with Hodgkin's disease (17). Rapid growth of stable lymph nodes in low-grade lymphoma signals a transformation to high-grade lymphoma (Richter's syndrome). Phenytoin and other drugs can induce benign, reversible lymphadenopathy. On occasion, however, phenytoin-induced lymphadenopathy can become malignant (18).

SPLEEN

Although primary hematologic diseases can cause splenomegaly, nonhematologic causes are more common (Table 1-7). Important hematologic diseases that cause splenomegaly include a wide variety of hereditary and acquired hemolytic anemias, myeloproliferative disorders, Hodgkin's disease, lymphomas, paraproteinemias, and leukemias. Splenomegaly can also be caused by storage diseases (e.g., Gaucher's disease and Niemann-Pick disease), metastatic malignancy, cysts, and abscesses. Not all enlarged spleens are pathologic. Palpable

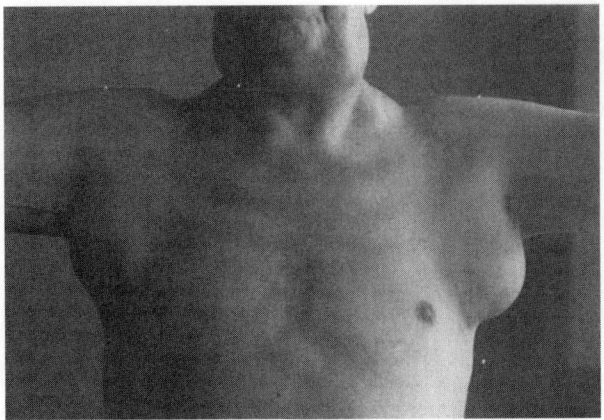

Figure 1-2. Malignant adenopathy of lymphoma. The nodes are larger than 2 cm in diameter, multiple, rubbery, and nontender. (See Color Fig. 1-2.)

TABLE 1-7. Differential Diagnosis of Splenomegaly

Infectious diseases
  Infectious mononucleosis
  Cytomegalovirus
  Human immunodeficiency virus infection
  Toxoplasmosis
  Viral hepatitis
  Salmonellosis
  Relapsing fever
  Tularemia
  Syphilis
  Malaria
  Subacute bacterial endocarditis
  Tuberculosis
  Schistosomiasis
Inflammatory diseases
  Felty's syndrome
  Systemic lupus erythematosus
  Rheumatic fever
  Serum sickness
  Sarcoid
Congestive diseases
  Intrahepatic
    Cirrhosis
    Venoocclusive disease
    Congenital hepatic fibrosis
  Portal vein obstruction
  Splenic vein obstruction
  Hepatic vein occlusion (Budd-Chiari syndrome)
  Congestive heart failure
Primary hematologic diseases
  Acquired and hereditary hemolytic disorders, enzymopathies, hemoglobinopathies, autoimmune hemolytic anemia
  Polycythemia vera
  Myeloid metaplasia with myelofibrosis
  Primary thrombocytosis
  Chronic myelogenous leukemia
  Chronic lymphocytic leukemia
  Acute leukemia
  Lymphoma (Hodgkin's and non-Hodgkin's)
  Hairy cell leukemia
Storage diseases
  Gaucher's disease
  Niemann-Pick disease
Miscellaneous conditions
  Tropical splenomegaly
  Primary splenic hyperplasia
  Metastatic cancer (especially melanoma)

spleen tips were reported in 3% of "healthy" college freshmen (19). Because splenic rupture has occasionally been reported, caution is advised when palpating a tender spleen or one that has rapidly enlarged.

Splenic size can be assessed by percussion, palpation, and diagnostic imaging devices. Palpation is performed with the patient relaxed in the supine position. The examiner (preferably seated) should feel with the fingertips and a flat, relaxed hand (slightly flexed at the wrist), beginning in the lower abdomen and proceeding to the left costal margin. If an edge is felt, it should be measured with respect to anatomic landmarks. Palpation in the right lateral decubitus position does not increase the sensitivity (20). If both percussion and palpation are positive, the examination is reported to have a 46% sensitivity and a 97% specificity, especially in lean patients (20). However, a newly discovered left upper quadrant mass is not always a spleen. Left upper quadrant sonography and/or abdominal computed tomographic scan can be used to measure splenic size and to exclude sarcomas and other cancers, enlarged kidneys, pancreatic pseudocysts, and other causes of a left upper quadrant mass.

Massive splenic enlargement deserves special attention. The spleen may be more than 5 kg and extend into the pelvis or the right lower quadrant. Unless care is taken in palpation, such

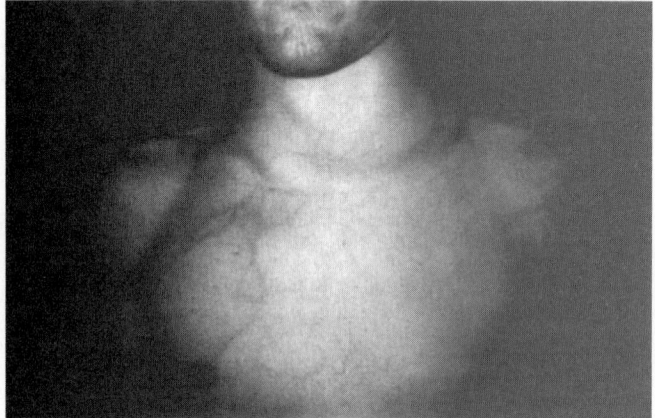

Figure 1-3. Venous engorgement secondary to superior vena cava obstruction. (See Color Fig. 1-3.)

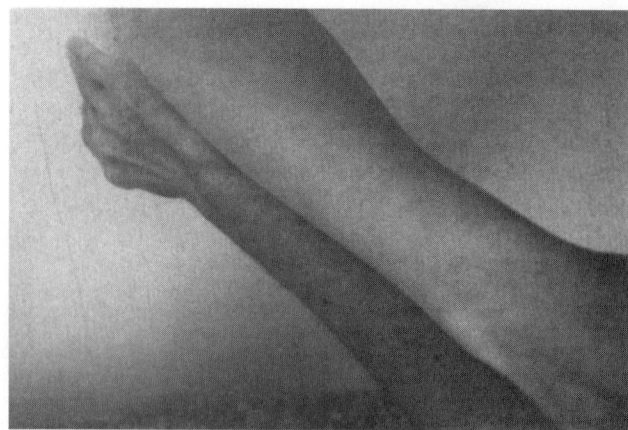

Figure 1-4. Slate gray discoloration of the skin of a patient with hemachromatosis, compared with normal coloration. (See Color Fig. 1-4.)

spleens may be missed, much to the chagrin of the examiner. Massive splenic enlargement may cause left upper quadrant discomfort or pain, left shoulder ache, and early satiety. The latter is caused by pressure of the spleen on the stomach and can lead to anorexia and significant weight loss. These effects are largely mechanical and are generally associated with spleens weighing more than 1 kg (normal spleens range from 100 to 250 g). The mechanical symptoms may be relieved by therapies that reduce the splenic bulk and may require urgent attention in distressed patients.

INTEGUMENT

Anemia can cause pallor when the Hgb is less than 8 g/dL. However, pale people may not be anemic, and anemic people may not be pale. Pallor can be caused by vasoconstriction, hypovolemia, and hypotension due to bleeding or nonhematologic causes such as panic, medications, dehydration, and circulatory collapse. Pallor due to severe anemia (Hgb <5 g/dL) can be confirmed by finding pale, palpebral conjunctivae and lack

of color in the palmar creases. A ruddy face is seen in some patients with polycythemia vera, but it is not a specific sign.

Superior vena cava obstruction (Fig. 1-3) is marked by isolated plethora of the face and upper chest associated with suffused conjunctivae and distended veins (including the sublingual veins). It is usually caused by a large mediastinal mass. Up to 4% of patients with non-Hodgkin's lymphomas present with the superior vena cava syndrome (21). Slate gray or silvery skin can be seen with advanced hemochromatosis (Fig. 1-4).

Examination of the skin and mucous membranes is essential to the evaluation of patients with bleeding disorders. Heavy bleeding confined to a single site suggests a localized problem, whereas bleeding from several sites suggests a coagulation disorder. *Petechiae*, characteristic of platelet disorders, are painless, 1- to 2-mm, reddish-purple, nontender, flat lesions, which often appear in clusters on the shins of patients with platelet dysfunction or moderate to severe thrombocytopenia (< 50×10^9/L) (Fig. 1-5). Petechiae do not blanch when viewed through a piece of glass pressed against the skin. Bright red lesions smaller than 1 mm are not petechiae. Petechiae can be seen in the absence of

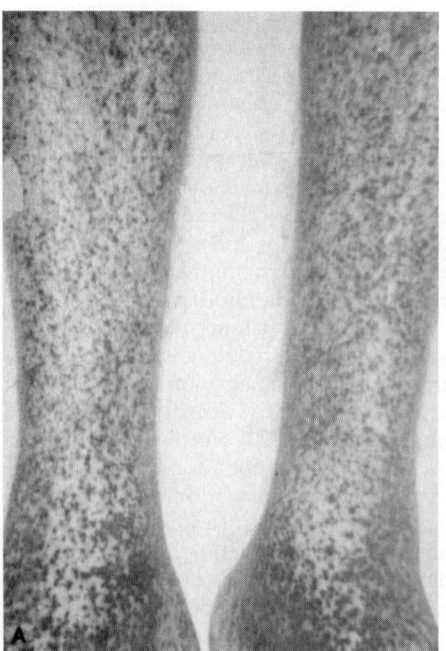
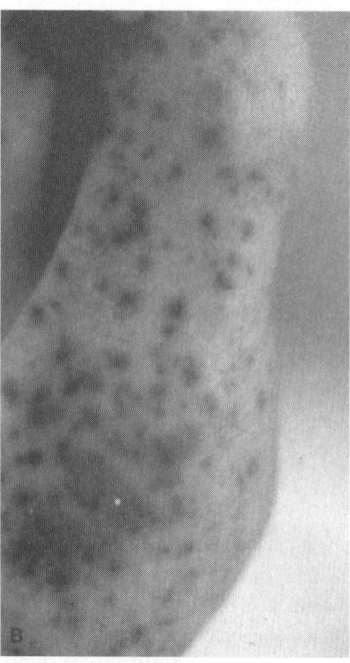

Figure 1-5. A: Showers of petechiae and purpura on the legs of a thrombocytopenic patient. **B:** Close-up of same patient. (See Color Fig. 1-5.)

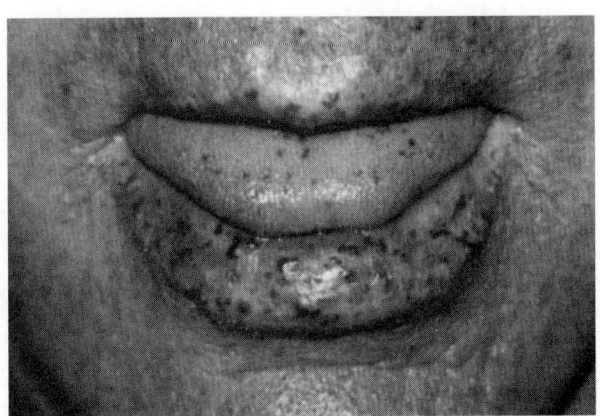

Figure 1-6. Mucosal telangiectasias in a patient with Rendu-Osler-Weber disease. (See Color Fig. 1-6.)

thrombocytopenia in patients with Waldenström's macroglobulinemia and myeloma.

An *ecchymosis* is a nonpalpable, painless, subcutaneous collection of blood larger than several millimeters. It may be red, blue, or purple. As the Hgb is degraded, it changes colors (green, yellow, brown). Senile purpura is a descriptive name for ecchymoses on the extensor surfaces of the forearm and dorsum of the hand in individuals with aging or thin skin. It is caused by rupture of fragile cutaneous vessels and is relatively harmless. Multiple ecchymoses in untraumatized areas suggest a coagulopathy. In contrast to an ecchymosis, a hematoma is a palpable, often painful subcutaneous collection of blood. Extravasated blood often diffuses into adjacent tissues (e.g.,

from the nose to the periorbital tissues) or dissects its way to a more dependent site (e.g., from the upper leg to the foot). The depth declines exponentially as the area expands. A hematoma measuring more than 30 cm in diameter suggests a massive internal bleed. *Telangiectasias* are dilated capillary clusters. They can appear as red macules, papules, or spiders. They blanch when pressed under a piece of glass. Telangiectasias around and in the mouth are a sign of hereditary telangiectasia (Rendu-Osler-Weber disease), a condition associated with internal bleeding and chronic iron deficiency (Fig. 1-6).

The skin and mucous membranes are often sites of infection in immunocompromised patients. Patients suspected of severe neutropenia or acute leukemia should be carefully examined, but the examination should be gentle, avoiding even mild trauma, deferring an internal rectal examination but including inspection and palpation of the perianal area. Oral sores and infiltrations, purulent nasal and sinus infections, abscesses, and cellulitis may establish a cause of fever or reveal unsuspected candidiasis. Acute monocytic leukemia is the acute leukemic variant most likely to be associated with skin infiltration (leukemia cutis) (22). The lesions are small, painless, nonpruritic, raised nodules that are salmon or pinkish purple (Fig. 1-7). Purplish subcutaneous lesions and massive infiltration are also associated with acute leukemia. Twenty percent of patients with CLL have pathologic skin changes, including macules, nodules, diffuse erythroderma, and bullous pemphigoid (23), an exaggerated response to insect bites (Fig. 1-8), and a potentially fatal necrotizing reaction after live viral vaccinations. Over 40% of patients with juvenile chronic myelogenous leukemia have skin lesions, including xanthomas, café-au-lait spots, and erythematous maculopapules.

Pruritus exacerbated by hot bathing is considered pathognomonic of polycythemia vera. Pruritus occurs in 12% of patients

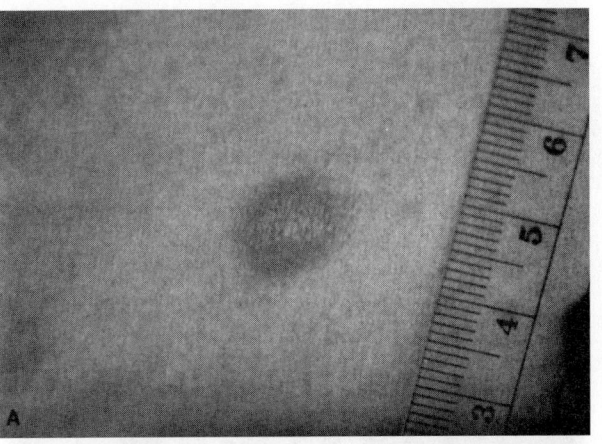

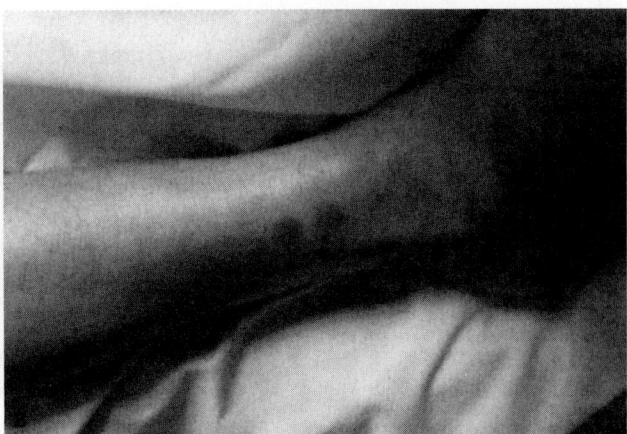

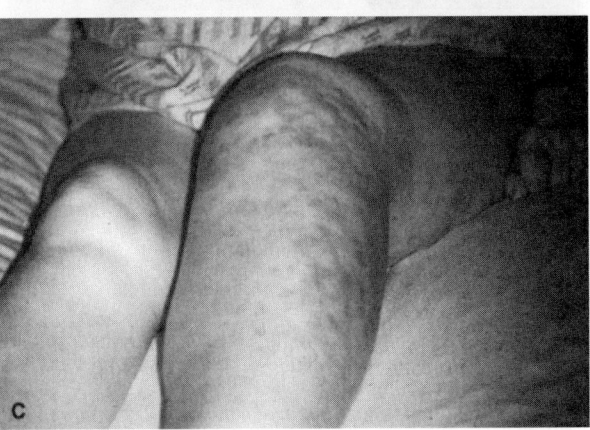

Figure 1-7. Leukemia cutis. **A:** Small salmon-colored nodules. **B:** Larger purplish subcutaneous lesions. **C:** Massive cutaneous infiltration by leukemia. (See Color Fig. 1-7.)

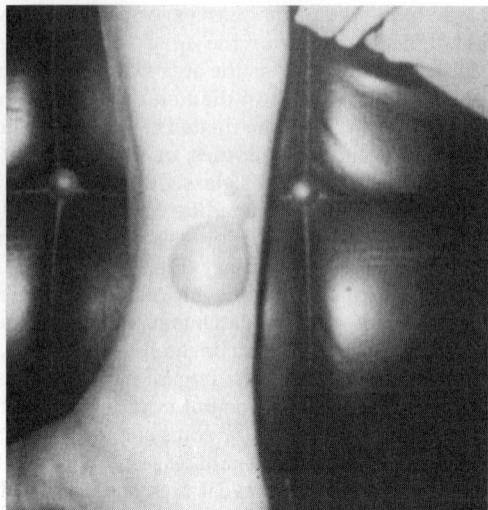

Figure 1-8. Exaggerated response to mosquito bite in a patient with chronic lymphocytic leukemia. (See Color Fig. 1-8.)

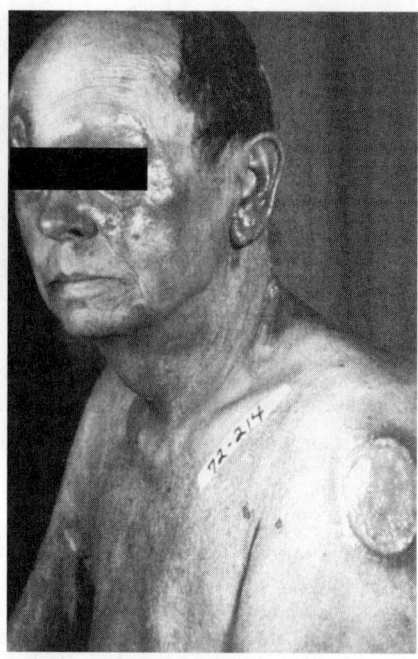

Figure 1-10. Mycosis fungoides. Note plaques and ulcerative nodules. (See Color Fig. 1-10.)

with Hodgkin's disease (24) and may worsen as the disease progresses. Intense pruritus with excoriation may precede the diagnosis. Cutaneous involvement with leukemia or lymphoma takes many forms. The red man syndrome (i.e., *l'homme rouge*) is a diffuse, intensely pruritic eczematoid eruption characterizing Sézary's syndrome. As cutaneous lymphoma becomes more severe, hyperkeratosis with painful fissuring and leonine facies appears (25) (Fig. 1-9). The later stages of the T-cell lymphoproliferative process, mycosis fungoides, are marked by serpentine scaling plaques and ulcerated nodules (Fig. 1-10). In contrast, rapidly evolving nonpruritic subcutaneous nodules are typical

of human T-cell lymphotrophic virus type 1–associated adult T-cell leukemia-lymphoma (26) (Fig. 1-11).

Cutaneous manifestations of hairy cell leukemia are underrecognized. Eight percent of patients develop erythematous papules over their extremities, trunks, and palms (27). Cutaneous vasculitis is rarer (28). Rashes are seen in 45% of patients

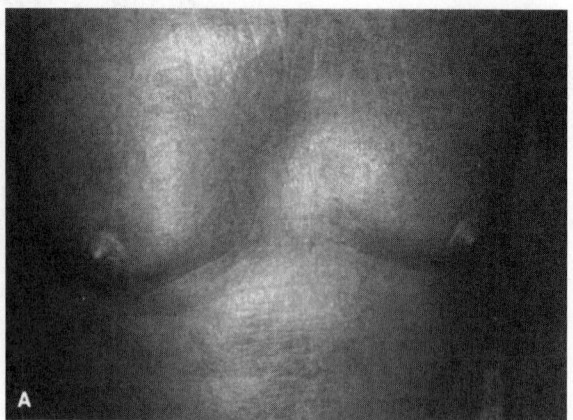

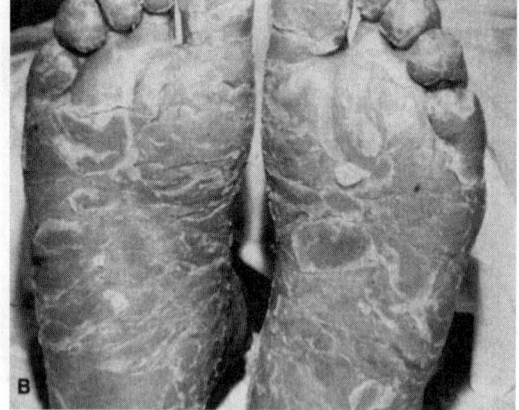

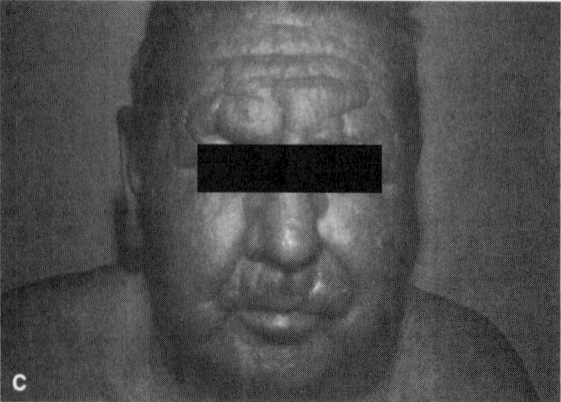

Figure 1-9. Sézary's syndrome. **A:** *L'homme rouge.* **B:** Hyperkeratosis with fissuring. **C:** Leonine facies. (See Color Fig. 1-9.) (From Wieselthier JS, Koh HK. Sézary's syndrome: diagnosis, prognosis and critical review of treatment options. *J Am Acad Dermatol* 1990;22:381, with permission.)

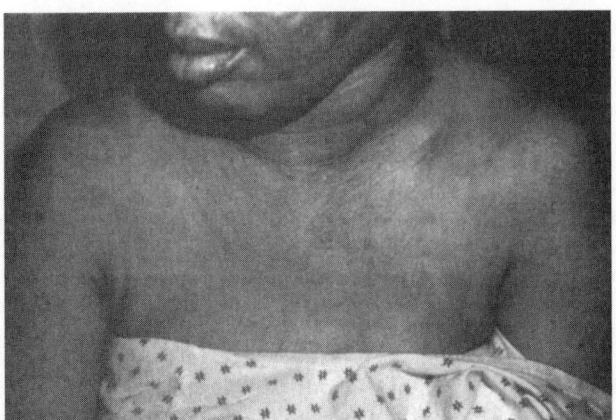

Figure 1-11. Erythematous, nonpruritic nodular infiltrate in a patient with adult T-cell leukemia-lymphoma. (See Color Fig. 1-11.)

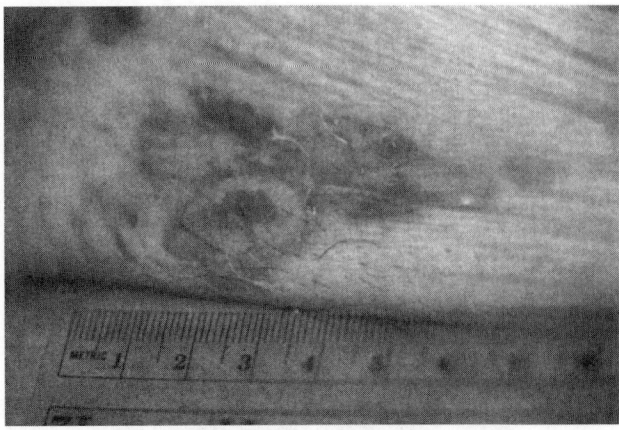

Figure 1-13. Necrosis of the skin after warfarin administration in a patient with protein-C deficiency. (See Color Fig. 1-13.)

with angioimmunoblastic lymphadenopathy with dysproteinemia. Some have nonspecific maculopapular eruptions; others have severe urticaria (29). Intense pruritus, skin nodules, and dermatographism typify urticaria pigmentosa, the cutaneous form of systemic mastocytosis (Fig. 1-12).

Recognition of the early dermal manifestations of adverse reactions to anticoagulant therapy may help prevent more severe sequelae. In excess of 10 million people are estimated to be receiving anticoagulants, making rare adverse reactions more common than many other hematologic diseases.

Warfarin-induced skin necrosis begins as a central erythematous macule on the extremities, trunk, breast, or penis (30) (Fig. 1-13). Unless promptly treated, it can rapidly progress to a purpuric, and then necrotic, lesion. It is a consequence of transient hypercoagulability seen shortly after starting warfarin in susceptible individuals, including some with protein-C or protein-S deficiency. Urgent treatment is indicated, including cessation of warfarin, administration of heparin and vitamin K, and possible administration of protein C. Dermal changes may herald heparin-induced thrombocytopenia (31), another severe complication of anticoagulant therapy. The findings range from small erythematous papules to large areas of dermal necrosis occurring 5 or more days after starting heparin and may precede the

thrombocytopenia. Heparin should be discontinued immediately. Argatroban has been used as a suitable alternative (32).

Skin biopsy often provides pathologic information essential to the diagnosis of a variety of premalignant and malignant disorders involving lymphocytes, including cutaneous T-cell lymphoma, which can be an insidious masquerader. A biopsy can be of help in resolving other confusing hematologic problems associated with a rash, such as neutrophilic dermatosis (Sweet's syndrome) (Fig. 1-14), intravascular lymphoma, and the histiocytoses. Discoloration, bullae, and chronic scarring are found in porphyria cutanea tarda. Several forms of porphyria are characterized by photosensitivity, which causes cutaneous bullae or vesicles (Fig. 1-15). Ankle ulcers associated with SCA (Fig. 1-16) and Hgb S–α-thalassemia require intervention.

NERVOUS SYSTEM

Disorders of the nervous system may be initial manifestations or sequelae of a wide variety of hematologic disorders, including hemorrhagic states, hypercoagulability, anemias (especially cobalamin deficiency and SCA), erythrocytosis, neutropenia, blastic leukemia, thrombocytopenia, thrombocytosis, lymphoma,

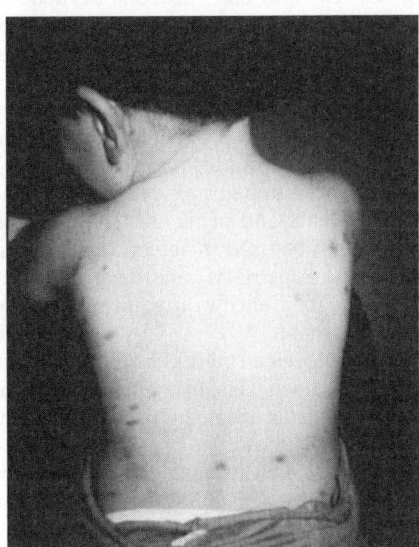

Figure 1-12. Multiple reddish-brown nodules in a patient with urticaria pigmentosa. (See Color Fig. 1-12.)

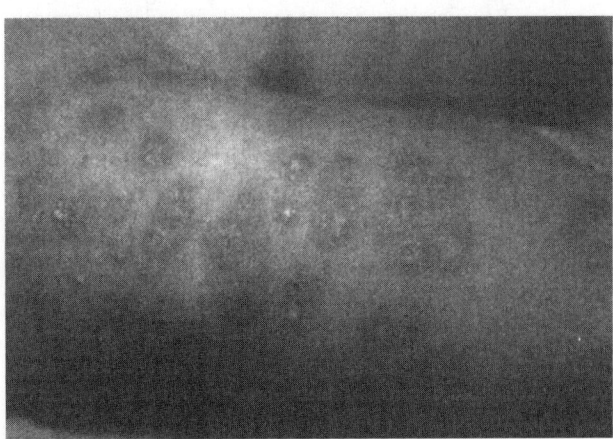

Figure 1-14. Patient with Sweet's syndrome. (See Color Fig. 1-14.) (From Dover JS. Case records of the Massachusetts General Hospital. Weekly clinicopathological exercises. Case 30-1990. A 47-year-old man with a rash, fever, and headaches. *N Engl J Med* 1990;323:254, with permission.)

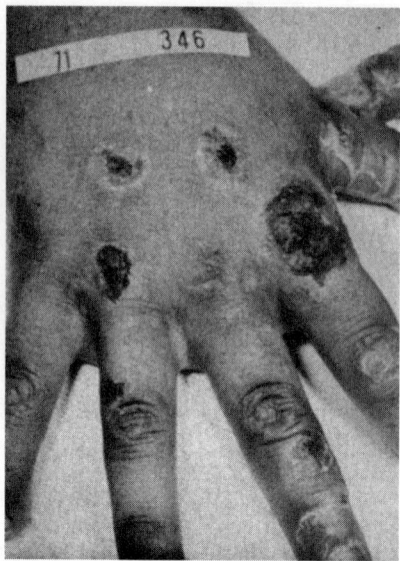

Figure 1-15. Necrotic ulcerations in a patient with erythropoietic porphyria. (See Color Fig. 1-15.)

myeloma, macroglobulinemia, immunodeficiency, myelodysplasia, and extramedullary hematopoiesis associated with myeloproliferative disorders.

Disorders of mentation are a common consequence of hematologic disorders. Because dementia may impair physician-patient communication, an assessment of the patient's mental status is advisable. The efficient, standardized Mini-Mental State examination is the most widely used method in the United States (33). It provides a standard of comparison for later evaluation (34). The value of the test is controversial in some settings, because age, education, language barriers, anxiety, and hearing and vision impairments can alter the results.

Neurologic disorders, including dementia (35), have been increasingly linked to cobalamin deficiency in recent decades. Rarely seen today are the classic neurologic changes of severe cobalamin deficiency, posterior column myelopathy resulting in ataxia, and loss of vibration and position sense.

Acute alterations in mentation due to intracranial hemorrhage constitute a medical emergency. Hematologic causes of intracranial hemorrhage include a hereditary or acquired hemostatic defect, thrombocytopenia, and polycythemia vera, or exposure to an anticoagulant, thrombolytic agent, or platelet antagonist. Because they can exacerbate bleeding from other

causes, these disorders deserve consideration even when another diagnosis, such as head trauma, has been made. Occlusion of large cerebral vessels can occur as a result of thrombosis associated with polycythemia vera, essential thrombocytosis, and SCA. Up to 7% of children with SCA have strokes. Reversible cerebral dysfunction caused by microvascular hemostasis and sludging occurs with acute lymphoblastosis ($>100 \times 10^9/L$), paraproteinemia sufficient to cause hyperviscosity, and polycythemia with a hematocrit greater than 45%. Left untreated, such patients are at risk of permanent neurologic sequelae. Cerebral venous thrombosis, a rare phenomenon, should prompt consideration of paroxysmal nocturnal hemoglobinuria.

Lymphoma in the central nervous system (CNS) occurs in 10% of patients with non-Hodgkin's lymphoma and 20% of patients who have AIDS or organ transplants (36,37). Initial manifestations may be changes in mentation, seizures, or cranial nerve palsies. Patients with non-Hodgkin's lymphomas involving facial structures, especially the nasal area, are at a particularly high risk of developing subsequent CNS lymphoma. A high index of suspicion, early examination of the cerebrospinal fluid by microscopy and flow cytometry, and contrast-enhanced magnetic resonance imaging of the brain aid in diagnosis.

Sweet's syndrome (i.e., neutrophilic dermatosis), a rare, protean disorder associated with skin infiltrations, fever, and involvement of a variety of organs, can cause neurologic and psychiatric disorders. It is most often associated with hematologic malignancies, especially myelodysplastic syndromes.

Thrombotic thrombocytopenic purpura is easy to miss, but important to recognize, as a cause of neurologic changes. The patient may have mild or moderate thrombocytopenia and no clinical evidence of thrombosis or purpura. It should be suspected in a patient with otherwise unexplained acute confusion, headache, focal neurologic defects, or coma, particularly if associated with microangiopathic hemolytic anemia. Other described features include fever, abdominal pain, hematuria, proteinuria, mild renal insufficiency, cardiac arrhythmias, congestive heart failure, and pulmonary edema. Free plasma Hgb and elevated lactate dehydrogenase help to establish the diagnosis. Therapeutic interventions (such as plasma exchange) have been known to restore a decerebrate patient to a normal neurologic state (personal observation).

Lymphoma and myeloma are important considerations in the evaluation of back pain and may coexist with degenerative arthritis, disc disease, and osteoporosis. Because the onset of malignancy can be insidious, lymphoma and myeloma should be considered in all patients with back pain. Unusual severity and progression after treatment for benign disease are clues that a relatively less common hematologic malignancy might be present. A contrast-enhanced magnetic resonance image of the spine is a sensitive screening test for malignancy. To exclude lymphoma, a computed tomographic scan of the abdomen is a valuable adjunct. Serum and urine electrophoresis and immunoelectrophoresis can be used to screen for myeloma. Electrophoresis should be routinely considered in patients with osteoporosis, as the incidence of myeloma is between 20 and $35/10^5$ in elderly women.

Chloromas and masses formed as a result of extramedullary hematopoiesis (e.g., in thalassemia and myeloid metaplasia) can compress CNS structures (including the pituitary) and peripheral nerves. They should be considered in the differential diagnosis of localized CNS disorders. Peripheral nerve involvement is a key component of POEMS (an acronym for *p*olyneuropathy, *o*rganomegaly, *e*ndocrinopathy, *m*yeloma, and *s*kin changes) syndrome, an often sclerotic variant of myeloma (38). Myeloma can also cause nerve damage as a result of compression by a plasmacytoma, infiltration by tumor cells, or autoim-

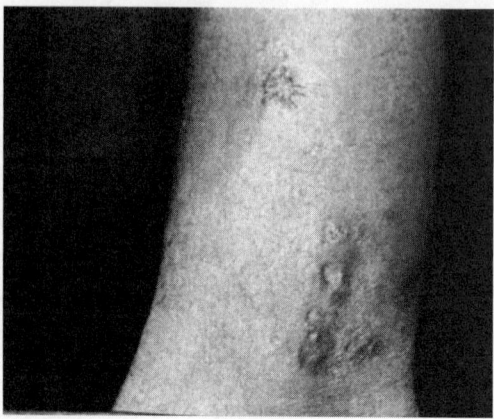

Figure 1-16. Scars with hyperpigmented borders due to recurrent ulceration in a patient with sickle cell anemia. (See Color Fig. 1-16.)

mune damage from paraprotein. Amyloid deposition can cause carpal tunnel syndrome.

DATA COLLECTION AND ANALYSIS

Consultants should seek the most efficient means of resolving clinical problems, simultaneously avoiding errors of omission and excess. Simply stated, consultants are expected to provide factual foundations for their opinions without squandering resources. Because a hematologic evaluation depends on laboratory values, consultants usually personally examine blood and bone marrow specimens and verify that specialized testing has been performed under rigorous conditions. The value and efficiency of the consultation is improved by the use of high standards. Poor data lead to misdiagnoses and mistreatment. To maintain high quality, it is critically important to conduct a personal review of previously examined pathology material, especially bone marrow and lymph nodes, enlisting the aid of regional experts in hematopathology when appropriate.

The decision to perform a bone marrow examination should be made carefully. The indications are addressed in detail in Chapter 3, Examination of the Bone Marrow. Consultants should be prepared to assess the benefits of performing the procedure, to anticipate the kinds of data that will be derived from it, and to suggest that it be deferred unless it has a measurable value for their patients.

CONCLUSIONS (CLINICAL IMPRESSIONS)

Clients expect to be answered thoughtfully, comprehensively, promptly, and clearly. The expectations can be onerous when the consultant lacks data and time and the clients lack communication skills. The difficulty of the task should not deter consultants from striving to satisfy their clients' expectations.

Open dialog is a process that may ease the burden if initiated early in the course of communication. Rather than wait until all data have been assembled, the consultant presents interim conclusions or "clinical impressions" based on the information available to that point and defines a plan to be used to resolve uncertain issues. Communication is improved by using a transparently logical process for establishing diagnoses and selecting treatments. When the diagnosis is uncertain, a differential diagnosis should be presented, with the options listed in order of declining likelihood and a plan for resolving clinically significant issues.

Each diagnosis should be stated using generally accepted terminology. Doing so can be a challenge when a single entity is called by different names. Consultants should base their selection of diagnostic terms on currently accepted authoritative sources. For example, patients referred with a paraprotein may initially be told that they have a *monoclonal gammopathy*. If no evidence of malignancy is found after evaluation, the consultant should then apply the term *monoclonal gammopathy of unknown significance*. On the contrary, if the evidence supports it, the diagnostic term *myeloma* may be used. In each case, the consultant should make clear what evidence has been used to support the use of the term. The significance of the diagnostic term is clearer when qualifying terms are used [e.g., monoclonal gammopathy of unknown significance (immunoglobulin A [IgA], kappa, 0.3 g/dL) or myeloma (Durie-Salmon stage IIIB, IgG, lambda, 8.0 g/dL, Hgb 7.5 g/dL, Cr 3.0)].

Diagnostic modifiers clarify the logic of the consultant's recommendations. For example, if the term *myelodysplastic syndrome* is followed by *(refractory anemia)*, the consultant has identified an indolent and slowly progressive disorder that justifies a "watch and wait" recommendation. An alternate modifier, *(refractory anemia with excess of blasts)*, an unstable disorder that often converts to acute leukemia, would probably be followed by a discussion of the risks and benefits of selected interventions.

Two aphorisms apply to consultations: "Brevity is the soul of wit" (39) and "Trust the man who hesitates in his speech and is quick and steady in action, but beware of long arguments and long beards" (40).

Answers to the clients' questions should follow the diagnosis. Some consultants prefer to list the questions and follow them with their suggested answers. The statements should be brief. References should be provided if requested. Literature reviews are generally more appropriate in discussions with colleagues than they are in consultation notes. Carefully worded handouts may be useful for patients and families.

Diagnosis is an art. It involves logic, pattern recognition, and intuition. Success at diagnosis depends greatly on skill at data accumulation and analysis. It also requires a readiness to admit fallibility and restart the process when essential elements do not fit. It is valuable to develop a logical framework for approaching diagnosis in hematology and to avoid self-humiliation and guilt when the system produces the "wrong" answers. If the framework is used properly, the diagnostic impressions can be stated in a way that enables active thinking to continue as the clinical pattern emerges. A flexible mind is a great asset.

RECOMMENDATIONS

At regular intervals, consultants should advise their clients regarding planned evaluations and suggested therapeutic interventions. Even if the consultant does all of the evaluation and management, the referring doctor should be kept informed. The consultant's plan may include a list of options together with the risks and benefits, costs, and feasibility of exercising them. For example, if a bone marrow transplantation is a recommended option, the consultant should outline the protocol to be used and describe a suitable donor source, the short- and long-term procedure-related morbidity and mortality, the estimated costs, and the means of paying for them. If the recommended treatment is novel or investigational, a copy of the protocol should be provided and informed consent should be obtained in compliance with the local Institutional Review Board.

Information expected to be of high emotional impact should be communicated to patients and their companions in an appropriate environment, including comfortable seating, a soothing milieu, and privacy (41,42). Consultants may expect to lead such discussions, but they should be alert to their clients' alternative agendas. Today, many patients wish to exercise leadership in the development of evaluation and treatment plans. Some are not content to confine their participation to the overall design and major decisions, but clearly wish to choose the therapeutic agents, doses, and monitoring intervals themselves. Communication is more effective if active dialog is maintained. Patients and companions with unresolved questions or piquant anxiety may comprehend and retain information better if they are allowed to determine the pace and content of the discussion. Indeed, moments of silence associated with compassionate body language can be a powerful way of expressing empathy and improving understanding.

Many consultants welcome opportunities to educate their clients. They avail themselves of teaching aids such as charts, diagrams, drawings, and models. They use feedback to identify areas of confusion. They adjust their language and tempo to adapt to their audience. They provide handouts to supplement

TABLE 1-8. Required Elements in a Consultation Note

Identification of the patient, full name, date of birth, Social Security number. Institutional identification number (optional).

Identification of the referring physician.

Identification of the consultant, date of consultation, time of day.

Means of communicating with consultant (usually on letterhead) to include address, telephone number, fax, e-mail address, answering service (hospital consultants should leave pager numbers).

Reason for consultation, including client's questions.

History of the problems that prompted consultation.

Selected, relevant elements of current history, past medical history, social history, family history, physical examination, imaging study results, and laboratory data.

List of prescription and nonprescription medications and alternative therapies, including dosages, frequency, and duration of therapy.

Assessment (clinical impression)
  Diagnosis
  Stage or severity modifiers
  Data that justify the diagnosis (optional)

Answers to the client's questions

Recommendations, including (a) type, frequency, and intended use of laboratory tests and imaging studies and (b) treatments, including dosage, frequency, duration, and parameters for monitoring.

Follow-up consultations should include results of interventions, interval history.

their oral descriptions. Some send their patients copies of their consultation notes. The notes should be carefully written, because clients scrutinize them.

The consultation note or letter should include the salient elements emphasized in this chapter (Table 1-8). The content of the communication depends on the complexity of the problem. Indeed, problems that are easily solved usually merit succinct letters. To avoid prolixity, the letter should be no more than two pages, although it is more work to write less.

OUTCOMES

Consultants should monitor outcomes. Parameters to measure include morbidity and mortality, complete and partial remission rate, quality of life, and length of survival. Consultants should monitor their own patient records and those of referred patients under the care of other physicians.

REFERENCES

1. Goldman L, Lee T, Rudd P. Ten commandments for effective consultations. *Arch Intern Med* 1983;143:1753.
2. Ulschak FL. *Consultation skills for health care professionals.* San Francisco, CA: Jossey-Bass, 1990.
3. Harpham WS. *Diagnosis cancer. Your guide through the first few months.* New York: WW Norton & Co., 1992.
4. Rosenblum D. *A time to hear, a time to help. Listening to people with cancer.* New York: The Free Press, 1993.
5. Matthews DA, Suchman AL, Branch WT Jr. Making "connexions": enhancing the therapeutic potential of patient-clinician relationships. *Ann Intern Med* 1993;118:973.
6. Andrews ND. Medical progress: disorders of iron metabolism. *N Engl J Med* 1999;341:1986.
7. Micallef INM, Lillington DM, Apostolidis J, et al. Therapy related myelodysplasia and acute myelogenous leukemia after high-dose therapy with autologous progenitor-cell support for lymphoid malignancies. *J Clin Oncol* 2000;18:947.
8. *Drug facts and comparisons 2000 Edition.* St Louis: Wolters Kluwer Co., 2000.
9. Ortiz-Neu C, Marr JS, Cherubin CE, et al. Bone and joint infections due to salmonella. *J Infect Dis* 1978;138:820.
10. Horsburgh CR Jr, Selik RM. The epidemiology of disseminated nontuberculous mycobacterial infection in the acquired immunodeficiency syndrome (AIDS). *Am Rev Respir Dis* 1989;139:4.
11. Weinstein RA, Golomb HM, Grumet G, et al. Hairy cell leukemia: association with disseminated atypical mycobacterial infection. *Cancer* 1981;48:380.
12. Barton JC, McDonnell SM, Adams PC, et al. Management of hemochromatosis. *Ann Intern Med* 1998;129:932.
13. Ryan KJ, Dunaif AE, Barbieri RL, et al. *Kistner's gynecology and women's health,* 7th ed. St. Louis: Mosby–Year Book, 1999.
14. Allhiser JN, McKnight TA, Shank JC. Lymphadenopathy in a family practice. *J Fam Pract* 1981;12:27.
15. Slap GB, Connor JL, Wigton RS, et al. Validation of a model to identify young patients for lymph node biopsy. *JAMA* 1986;255(20):2768.
16. Knight PJ, Mulne AF, Vassy LE. When is lymph node biopsy indicated in children with enlarged peripheral nodes? *Pediatrics* 1982;69:391.
17. Atkinson K, Austin DE, McElwain TJ, et al. Alcohol pain in Hodgkin's disease. *Cancer* 1976;37:895.
18. Li FP, Willard DR, Goodman R, et al. Malignant lymphoma after diphenylhydantoin (dilantin) therapy. *Cancer* 1975;36:1359.
19. McIntyre OR, et al. Palpable spleens in college freshmen. *Arch Int Med* 1967;66:301.
20. Barkun AN, Camus M, Green L, et al. The bedside assessment of splenic enlargement. *Am J Med* 1991;91:512.
21. Perez-Soler R, McLaughlin P, Velasquez WS, et al. Clinical features and results of management of superior vena cava syndrome secondary to lymphoma. *J Clin Oncol* 1984;2:260.
22. Tobelem G, Jacquillat C, Chastang C, et al. Acute monoblastic leukemia: a clinical and biologic study of 74 cases. *Blood* 1980;55:71.
23. Dreizen S, McCredie KB, Keating MJ, et al. Leukemia-associated skin infiltrates. *Postgrad Med* 1989;85:45.
24. Gobbi PG, Cavalli C, Gendarini A, et al. Reevaluation of prognostic significance of symptoms in Hodgkin's disease. *Cancer* 1985;56:2874.
25. Wieselthier JS, Koh HK. Sézary's syndrome: diagnosis, prognosis and critical review of treatment options. *J Am Acad Dermatol* 1990;22:381.
26. Kuefler PR, Bunn PA Jr. Adult T cell leukemias/lymphoma. *Clin Haematol* 1986;15:695.
27. Arai E, Ikeda S, Itoh S, et al. Specific skin lesions as the presenting symptom of hairy cell leukemia. *Am J Clin Pathol* 1988;90:459.
28. Farcet JP, Weschsler J, Wirquin V, et al. Vasculitis in hairy cell leukemia. *Arch Intern Med* 1987;147:660.
29. Steinberg AD, Seldin MF, Jaffe ES, et al. NIH conference. Angioimmunoblastic lymphadenopathy with dysproteinemia. *Ann Intern Med* 1988;108:575.
30. Bauer KA. Coumarin-induced skin necrosis. *Arch Dermatol* 1993;129:766.
31. Kelton JG, Warkentin TE. Heparin-induced thrombocytopenia: diagnosis, natural history, and treatment options. *Postgrad Med* 1998;103[Suppl 12]:169.
32. Messmore HL Jr. Heparin-induced thrombocytopenia: historical review. *Clin Appl Thromb Hemost* 1999;5[Suppl 1]:S2.
33. Folstein MF, Folstein SE, McHugh PR. "Mini-mental state." A practical method for grading the cognitive state of patients for the clinician. *J Psychiatr Res* 1975;12:189.
34. Tangalos EG, Smith GE, Ivnik RJ, et al. The Mini-Mental State Examination in general medical practice: clinical utility and acceptance. *Mayo Clin Proc* 1996; 71:829.
35. Carmel R, Karnaze DS, Weiner JM. Neurologic abnormalities in cobalamin deficiency are associated with higher cobalamin "analogue" values than are hematologic abnormalities. *J Lab Clin Med* 1988;111:57.
36. Flinn IW, Ambinder RF. AIDS primary central nervous system lymphoma. *Curr Opin Oncol* 1996;8:373.
37. Cote TR, Manns A, Hardy CR, et al. Epidemiology of brain lymphoma among people with or without acquired immunodeficiency syndrome. *J Natl Cancer Inst* 1996;88:675.
38. Miralles GD, O'Fallon JR, Talley NJ. Plasma-cell dyscrasia with polyneuropathy. The spectrum of POEMS syndrome. *N Engl J Med* 1992;327:1919.
39. Shakespeare W. *Hamlet,* II:2.
40. Santayana G. On the British character. *Soliloquies in England and later soliloquies.* London: Constable and Co., Ltd, 1922.
41. Rosenblum D. Listening to people with cancer. *Semin Oncol* 1994;21:701.
42. Buckman R. *How to break bad news. A guide for health care professionals.* Baltimore: The Johns Hopkins University Press, 1992:223.

CHAPTER 2

Laboratory Hematology: Methods for the Analysis of Blood

Joan E. Etzell and Laurence M. Corash

Enumeration and qualitative classification of the various cell types in blood present a complicated challenge because of the intrinsic nature of blood. First, blood is a complex suspension of cells in plasma protein. The plasma protein fraction is coagulable, and the process of coagulation may alter the form and quantity of the cellular fraction. Second, blood and its constituents are relatively labile and require immediate processing. Third, some cellular components occur at low frequencies, which presents further problems in achieving adequate measurement precision. Finally, there are substantial variations among and within individuals because of sex, age, and ethnicity, which complicate the definition of the normal reference range for interpreting results from single samples. However, current analytic methods have overcome many of these problems, and the analysis of blood is rapid and cost-effective. In fact, this technology has probably led to overuse because the cost is low. The technology of blood analysis continues to evolve at a rapid pace, and physicians, particularly those in the field of hematology, require an ongoing understanding of it to make the best use of the information.

SAMPLE COLLECTION AND PREPARATION

Virtually all samples for analysis of blood cells or their constituents, such as hemoglobin, are collected in tubes containing potassium or sodium salts of ethylenediaminetetraacetic acid (EDTA). An avid calcium chelator, EDTA serves as an effective anticoagulant to inhibit activation of the coagulation system and production of fibrin clots. Samples with clots are not suitable for analysis of cellular components. Usually, blood samples are collected in evacuated blood drawing tubes to produce a final EDTA concentration of 4.5 mmol/L. Blood drawn under these conditions is generally stable at room temperature for 24 hours without significant deterioration in the quality or quantity of the different cell classes. Platelet concentrations in EDTA-anticoagulated whole blood are more stable with storage at 4°C, but lower temperatures result in reduction of leukocyte counts and morphologic integrity. In most clinical laboratories, blood samples are retained at room temperatures (20° to 24°C) for 24 hours and discarded.

Under certain circumstances, blood for analysis of cellular constituents may be drawn into sodium citrate or heparin. One volume of sodium citrate (3.2% or 3.8%) is diluted with nine volumes of whole blood; this ratio produces a dilution error that must be corrected after blood cell enumeration. Citrated samples may be useful for platelet counting when persistent platelet–leukocyte satellitism is observed on peripheral smears prepared from EDTA blood samples. This phenomenon is mediated by agglutinins—either immunoglobulin (Ig) G or IgM, which may be calcium dependent (1–3). Although platelet–leukocyte satellitism appears to be an *in vitro* phenomenon, it can result in spurious thrombocytopenia or pseudo-thrombocytopenia due to platelet agglutination or leukocyte adherence during sample processing. Citrated blood samples may also be useful for platelet counting when patient samples show repeated platelet clumping when drawn into EDTA.

Heparin can be used as an anticoagulant without introducing a dilution error; unfortunately, it causes platelet and leukocyte agglutination, which interferes with cell enumeration accuracy. For these reasons, citrate and heparin are not routinely used for blood sample collection. Oxalate, previously used as an anticoagulant, is no longer in common use. Tubes for blood drawing may be prepared (rather than purchased) by placing 0.5 mL of a 100 mmol/L EDTA solution in a dry tube to which 10 mL of whole blood is added.

Red Blood Cell, Platelet, and Leukocyte Morphology

Blood smears can be prepared directly from fingerstick samples or from anticoagulated blood tubes. Either 22-mm square coverslips or standard glass microscope slides (25 mm × 75 mm × 1 mm) may be used. Full-sized glass microscope slides offer the advantage that they can be conveniently stained in automated staining devices, whereas coverslips can be stained manually only. Blood smears prepared by either method should result in a thin blood film with a portion of the smear in which the red blood cells (RBCs) are evenly distributed with adequate preservation of central pallor (Fig. 2-1). The area containing singly distributed RBCs with well-preserved central pallor is the best region to examine RBC, leukocyte, and platelet morphology (Fig. 2-2). Blood smears also may be prepared using automated centrifugal spinner devices that provide excellent morphology (4). Although the thick portions or the feathered edge of blood smears contain more leukocytes, they generally distort cellular features, which can lead to serious errors in interpreting the maturity of nuclear chromatin patterns.

Blood smears should be thoroughly air-dried without heating before staining. Morphologic analysis is best accomplished with polychrome-stained smears using a variety of different

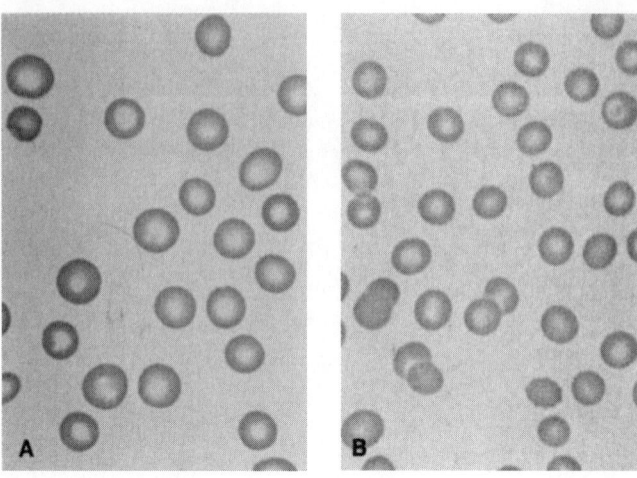

Figure 2-1. Thin peripheral blood smear from a newborn infant **(A)** and an adult **(B)**. Note the adequate preservation of central pallor. The mean corpuscular volume of the newborn blood is 108 fL, whereas that of the adult blood is 92 fL. This difference is not perceptible on the peripheral smear. (See Color Fig. 2-1.)

stains that are eosin–methylene blue combinations in methyl alcohol—Wright, Giemsa, or Romanowsky (5). Automated staining devices offer the advantage of greater uniformity of staining conditions with considerable savings in labor.

Microscopic Reticulocyte Enumeration

Reticulocytes, newly released RBCs containing RNA, also may be enumerated using peripheral smears prepared after RBCs have been incubated with supravital dyes such as new methylene blue or brilliant cresyl blue. These dyes precipitate intracellular RNA and allow identification of reticulocytes (6). Reticulocyte counting requires the preparation of thin smears on which reticulocytes containing a blue precipitate can be detected. The amount of reticulum or precipitate varies in reticulocytes of different maturation states (Fig. 2-3). Younger reticulocytes exhibit larger and denser precipitates. Reticulocytes may also be enumerated by flow cytometry using fluorescent dyes that bind to RNA. This automated counting technique allows evaluation of a larger number of red cells, resulting in better accuracy and precision. These two reticulocyte enumeration techniques are discussed in more detail in the section Reticulocyte Enumeration.

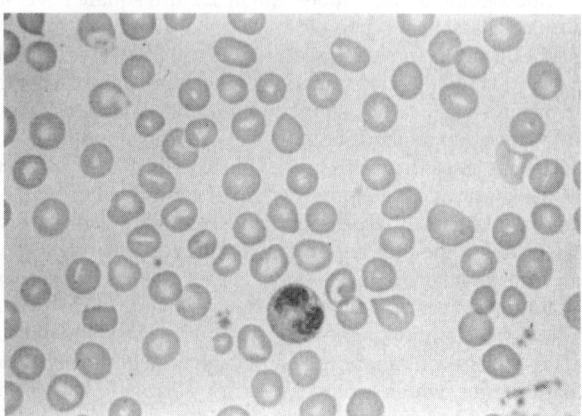

Figure 2-2. Peripheral smear with adequate preservation of central pallor. Platelets and a single polymorphonuclear leukocyte are present. Red blood cells vary in size and shape. (See Color Fig. 2-2.)

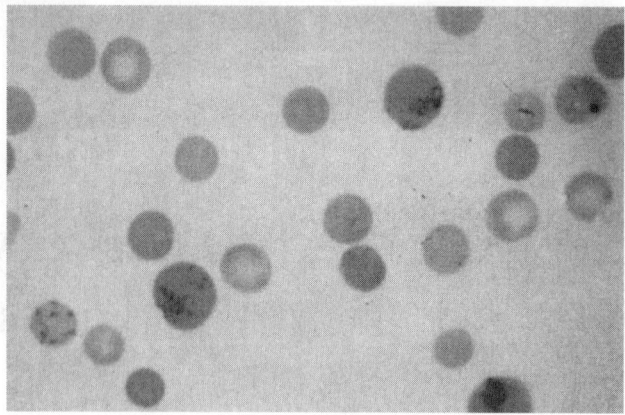

Figure 2-3. Reticulocyte preparation using new methylene blue. Precipitated RNA of varying sizes can be seen in the different cells.

Detection of Fetal Hemoglobin

Detection of fetal hemoglobin (hemoglobin F) in individual RBCs is useful to establish the diagnosis of fetal–maternal transfusion and to evaluate hemoglobin F content in patients with thalassemias or hemoglobinopathies. The modified Kleihauer-Betke technique is easily adaptable to the clinical laboratory (7). This method is described in the National Committee for Clinical Laboratory Standards (NCCLS) proposed guideline for fetal red cell detection (8). Thin blood smears are prepared and fixed with 80% ethanol. The fixed slides are then exposed to an acid–citrate solution at pH 3.2 to elute hemoglobin A, followed by erythrocin B or similar eosin counterstain. Cells containing hemoglobin A appear as pale ghosts, whereas cells with hemoglobin F stain pink (Fig. 2-4). Fetal cells demonstrate uniform bright pink staining, as do cells from most patients who are homozygous for hereditary persistence of hemoglobin F. Blood from hereditary persistence of hemoglobin F heterozygotes usually demonstrates variation in cell staining intensity, as do samples from heterozygotes for β-thalassemia and δβ-thalassemia.

The acid elution technique appears well suited to evaluate samples for fetal–maternal transfusion, but it lacks sensitivity for detection of small amounts of hemoglobin F. Mollison (9) has described the use of a formula to calculate the volume of a fetal–maternal transfusion for the estimation of Rh_O (D)

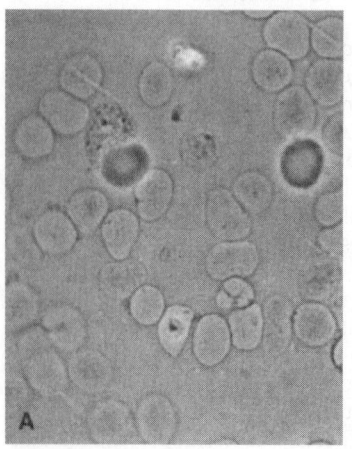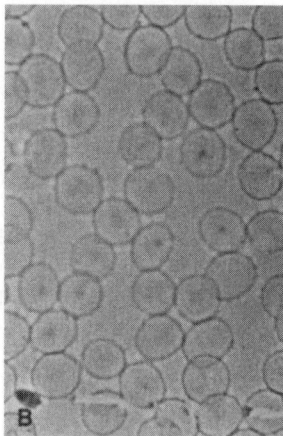

Figure 2-4. Detection of fetal hemoglobin using the Kleihauer-Betke acid elution technique. Cells containing fetal hemoglobin are stained pink, and cells containing hemoglobin A appear as pale ghosts. Note the presence of two hemoglobin F cells in a sample of maternal blood **(A)** and the absence of hemoglobin F cells in an adult man's control sample **(B)**.

immune globulin dosage based on the relative ratio of fetal to maternal cells.

Hemoglobin F also may be detected by immunofluorescence microscopy using monoclonal antibodies to the F-specific γ-chain (10,11). Wood et al. (11) used a purified antihemoglobin F polyclonal antibody conjugated to fluorescein isothiocyanate (FITC) to measure the incidence of cells containing hemoglobin F in normal white and black subjects. Normal black subjects had an average of 2.8% ± SD 1.6% F cells, and normal white subjects had an average of 2.6% ± SD 1% F cells. The combined average was 2.7%, with a range of 0.5% to 7.0%. Wood et al. (11) also concluded that the fluorescence test was much more sensitive than the acid elution technique for the detection of small amounts of hemoglobin F, but they noted that the immunofluorescence technique was less satisfactory than the acid elution technique for samples with more than 30% fetal cells.

Allen et al. (12) have reported the use of a two-color technique with monoclonal antibodies against the β- and γ-chains of hemoglobin to establish the absence of β-chains in antenatal samples for the diagnosis of β-thalassemia. Fetal blood samples were obtained, and cytocentrifuge preparations of the RBCs were fixed and treated with a combination of anti–β-chain and anti–γ-chain monoclonal reagents. Monoclonal antibody to γ-chain was detected with rhodanine-conjugated goat antimouse Ig, and biotin-conjugated anti–β-chain was detected with an avidin–fluorescein isothiocyanate conjugate. The dual labeling technique permitted the identification of fetal cells followed by selective examination of these cells for the simultaneous weak expression of β-chain product. Contaminating maternal cells, which stain intensely for β-chains, can easily be avoided. Sensitivity was equal to that obtained with radioisotopic β/γ-chain ratio synthesis studies (12).

Recently, flow cytometric methods have been developed to detect cells containing hemoglobin F to quantitate fetal–maternal bleeding, diagnose β-thalassemia, or quantitate hemoglobin F–containing cells in sickle cell anemia (13–16). In these procedures, red cells are fixed with glutaraldehyde or formaldehyde and permeabilized with Triton X-100 or sodium dodecyl sulfate. Cells are incubated with FITC-labeled monoclonal antibody to hemoglobin F or the hemoglobin γ-chain and analyzed by flow cytometry. Flow cytometric evaluation of hemoglobin F has shown good correlation with high-pressure liquid chromatography methods (13,14), the Kleihauer-Betke acid elution technique (15), and immunofluorescence microscopy (16). In addition, flow cytometry provides better precision [coefficient of variation (CV) <15%] than the acid elution technique (15) because a larger number of red cells can be evaluated. For fetal maternal hemorrhage with Rhesus factor incompatibility, a monoclonal anti-D antibody may be used; this technique provides accurate quantitation of fetal–maternal hemorrhage greater than 1 mL (17).

Detection of Heinz Bodies

Heinz bodies are membrane-bound mixed disulfides of denatured hemoglobin and erythrocyte membrane proteins (18). They may be seen in association with unstable hemoglobins or in disorders in which the ability of the cell to maintain hemoglobin in a reduced state is impaired—for example, glucose-6-phosphate dehydrogenase deficiency. Spontaneously formed Heinz bodies may be seen on peripheral blood smears after staining with rhodanile blue dye (19). In contrast with other dyes such as new methylene blue, rhodanile blue has the advantages of not staining reticulocytes and not causing oxidative damage. Heinz bodies are not visible in the peripheral blood of most patients with unstable hemoglobin, especially if splenic function is intact (20). Alternatively, blood samples can be treated with an oxidant agent, acetylphenylhydrazine, then

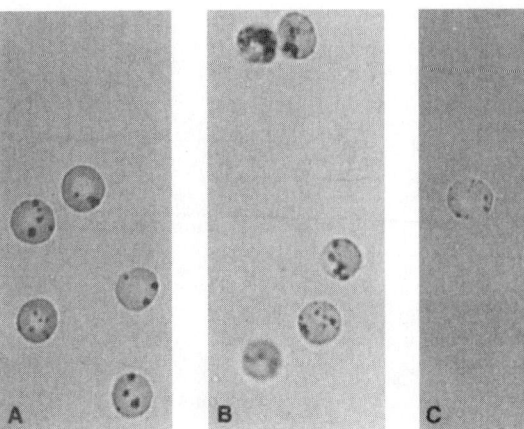

Figure 2-5. Heinz body preparation after treatment of normal red blood cells (RBCs) **(A,C)** and G6PD-deficient RBCs **(B)** with acetylphenylhydrazine and methyl violet stain. Normal RBCs develop a limited number (no more than three) of small Heinz bodies per cell. In contrast, G6PD-deficient cells **(B)** develop more than four Heinz bodies per cell, which are generally large.

stained and examined for the presence of Heinz bodies. Methyl violet may be used in place of rhodanile blue for the demonstration of Heinz bodies (Fig. 2-5).

The isopropanol solubility test is a sensitive technique to demonstrate the presence of an unstable hemoglobin (21). A small volume of hemolysate is added to a tube containing a mixture of isopropanol and buffer. If unstable hemoglobin is present, a flocculent precipitate forms. This simple method appears to have a high level of sensitivity for detecting unstable hemoglobin molecules.

Nomarski Optics

Whole blood may be collected into buffered glutaraldehyde solution and examined using Nomarski optics with an interference phase contrast microscope to visualize the cell surface (22). As little as one drop of fresh blood may be added to 0.5 mL of buffered glutaraldehyde solution, then held for examination at a later time. With intact splenic function, the RBC surface appears uniform and smooth. If splenic function is impaired, the RBC surface contains numerous small pocks and craters (22,23). The proportion of pocked or cratered RBCs can be determined and used as an index of splenic function (22). Although the presence of Howell-Jolly bodies (Fig. 2-6) also indicates asplenia or splenic hypofunction, the reliability of this index is reduced by their relative sparseness (22).

Cytochemistry

A number of cytochemical stains may be performed on air-dried peripheral blood smears to aid specific identification of abnormal cells and to provide additional diagnostic information about normal-appearing peripheral blood cells.

LEUKOCYTE ALKALINE PHOSPHATASE

Leukocyte alkaline phosphatase (LAP) is an enzyme present in the specific granules of myelocytes and more mature cells of the myeloid lineage. The LAP stain of peripheral blood smears may be used in the evaluation of patients with leukocytosis to aid discrimination of chronic myelogenous leukemia (CML) from granulocytic leukocytosis (leukemoid reactions) as well as evaluation of paroxysmal nocturnal hemoglobinuria. However, more specific assays have been developed for the diagnosis of these disorders; thus, the LAP stain is now infrequently used. Reverse-

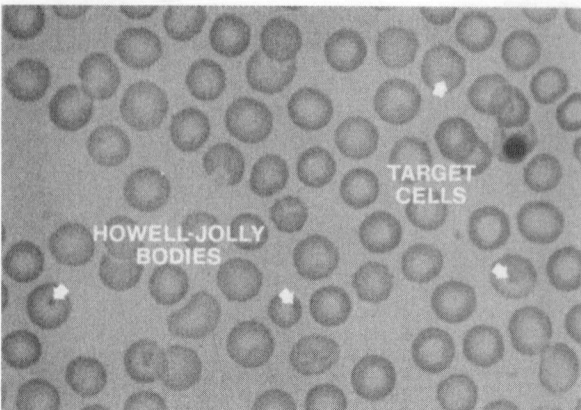

Figure 2-6. Peripheral blood smear from an infant with congenital asplenia. Note the presence of increased numbers of target cells *(arrows)* and the small round darkly staining cellular inclusions [Howell-Jolly bodies *(arrows)*]. A nucleated red blood cell is also present in the field. The Howell-Jolly bodies represent retained nuclear material that has not been removed because of lack of splenic function. (See Color Fig. 2-6.)

transcription polymerase chain reaction (RT-PCR) is used to detect the bcr–abl fusion transcript of CML, whereas flow cytometry allows identification of the abnormalities seen in paroxysmal nocturnal hemoglobinuria. The LAP stain is best performed on fresh fingerstick peripheral blood smears without use of EDTA, which inhibits LAP activity. Slides are fixed in citrate–acetone solution, and staining is achieved using naphthyl phosphate as a substrate for the enzyme, with formation of an insoluble reaction product using either diazonium salt or fast blue salt as a capture agent (24,25). Smears are counterstained with hematoxylin to facilitate identification of neutrophils, and positive cells contain either pink or blue granules, depending on the capture agent (Fig. 2-7). After staining, 100 mature neutrophils and band forms are counted, and each cell is scored from 0 to 4+ according to the staining intensity. A total LAP score is obtained by summing the products of the numbers of cells in each staining class multiplied by the class intensity score. Although a maximum score of 400 is possible, the normal range is approximately 11 to 95. Due to subjective interobserver variation, each laboratory should establish its own normal range.

MYELOPEROXIDASE

Myeloperoxidase (MPO) is an enzyme present in the primary granules of myeloid and monocytic lineage cells. Myeloid cells

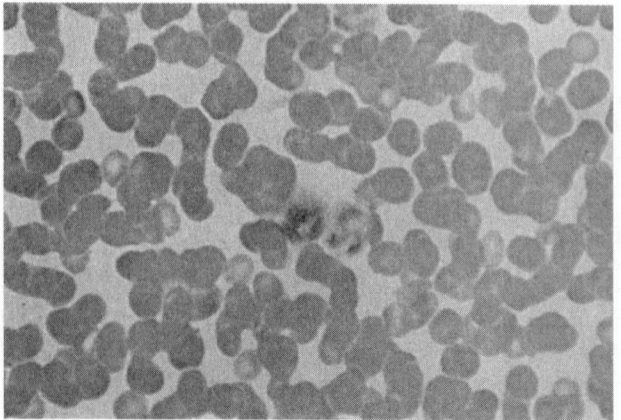

Figure 2-7. Leukocyte alkaline phosphatase stain. Note the presence of variable numbers of dark blue granules in the cytoplasm of two mature polymorphonuclear leukocytes. (See Color Fig. 2-7.)

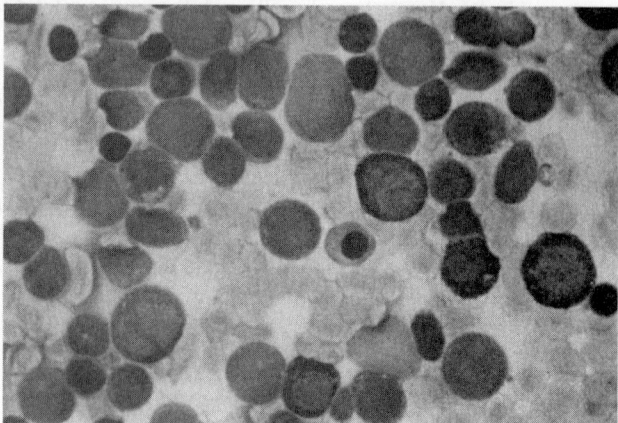

Figure 2-8. Myeloperoxidase stain. Granules containing myeloperoxidase stain an intense red-orange. Some cells contain only a few positive granules, and others are intensely positive. (See Color Fig. 2-8.)

exhibit greater staining intensity than monocytic cells, eosinophils are intensely positive, basophils are weakly positive, and lymphocytes are negative. Staining to detect MPO activity may be performed on EDTA-anticoagulated specimens after fixation in paraformaldehyde–acetone fixative. Alcohol fixation inhibits peroxidase activity. Hydrogen peroxide is used as the substrate for the endogenous MPO enzyme with 3-amino-9-ethyl carbazole as a capture agent for liberated oxygen radicals (26). Stained smears are counterstained with hematoxylin to facilitate identification of cells. The nuclei are stained pale blue, and the peroxidase reaction product is bright red (Fig. 2-8). Although a normal blood sample is stained in parallel as a control, quality control of the staining procedure is best ensured by identification of a few positive cells in the patient sample. Failure to identify any positive cells should raise questions about the validity of the stain. Congenital or acquired MPO deficiency may be demonstrated by low-intensity staining or by the complete absence of MPO staining in recognizable mature polymorphonuclear cells. Immunohistochemical staining using an antibody against MPO also is a useful technique. This staining method does not rely on a functional MPO enzyme within the cells of interest as the cytochemical stain does and thus may be positive in some cases in which the cytochemical stain is negative.

CHLORACETATE ESTERASE

Chloracetate esterase is an enzyme present in the primary granules of myeloid cells but not monocytic cells. This enzyme also is present in normal mast cells as well as those associated with mast cell disease. It is not present in normal eosinophils or basophils. Chloracetate esterase activity increases with cellular maturation and may not be present in myeloid blasts. This stain may be useful to determine the lineage of abnormal or dysplastic cells in the peripheral blood. Acquired chloracetate esterase deficiency may be seen in association with the myelodysplastic syndromes. Eosinophils associated with acute myelomonocytic leukemia with inversion of chromosome 16 demonstrate chloracetate esterase activity in contrast to that seen in normal eosinophils (27,28). Either α-naphthol chloracetate or naphthol AS-D chloracetate may be used as the substrate for chloracetate esterase with a hematoxylin counterstain (29). The reaction product is captured with pararosaniline to form a red precipitate (Fig. 2-9). The presence of a positive internal control cell confirms that the chloracetate esterase reaction is working properly. The chloracetate esterase stain may also be used in paraffin-embedded biopsy material, in which case it is commonly referred to as the *Leder stain.*

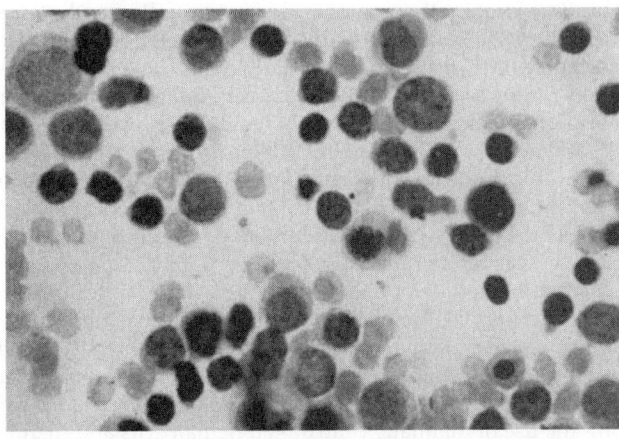

Figure 2-9. Chloracetate esterase stain. Two immature band neutrophil cells demonstrate intense cytoplasmic staining. (See Color Fig. 2-9.)

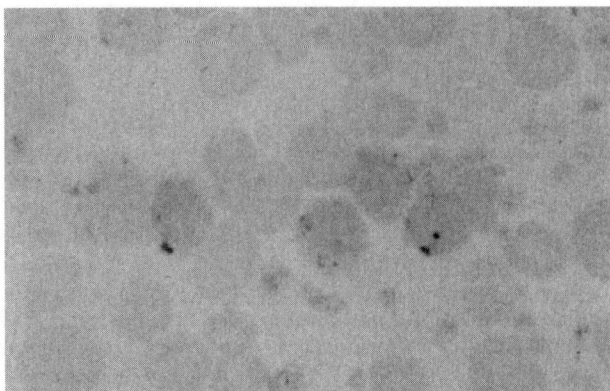

Figure 2-11. Tartrate-resistant acid phosphatase stain. Abnormal lymphoid cells from a patient with leukemic reticuloendotheliosis (hairy cell leukemia) are stained with acid phosphatase in the presence of tartrate. (See Color Fig. 2-11.)

NONSPECIFIC ESTERASE

Nonspecific esterase activity may be used as a marker for monocytes, although other cells express variably low levels of activity. Several different substrates may be used for this reaction: α-naphthyl acetate, naphthol AS-D acetate, or α-naphthyl butyrate. The last produces an intense red color after coupling with pararosaniline (Fig. 2-10). The butyrate substrate is less sensitive but more specific than the acetate substrates. Myeloid lineage cells do not contain nonspecific esterase activity; lymphocytes and megakaryocytes may stain weakly, whereas tissue macrophages stain brightly (30). The nonspecific esterase stain is useful in monocytic leukemias and in discrimination of monocytes from abnormal T lymphocytes (Sézary cells), both of which have convoluted nuclei.

TARTRATE-RESISTANT ACID PHOSPHATASE

Tartrate-resistant isoenzyme 5 of acid phosphatase (TRAP) activity is useful for identification of the abnormal cell of hairy cell leukemia (31). Lymphoid cells, monocytes, megakaryocytes, macrophages, nucleated erythroid cells, and myeloid cells stain variably for acid phosphatase activity in the absence of tartrate, but only the abnormal cells of hairy cell leukemia or other rare lymphomas stain in the presence of tartrate, an inhibitor of most acid phosphatase isoenzymes (32).

Naphthol AS-BI phosphoric acid is used as the substrate with fast garnet as a capture agent and hematoxylin counterstain. This stain may be difficult to interpret and requires the use of

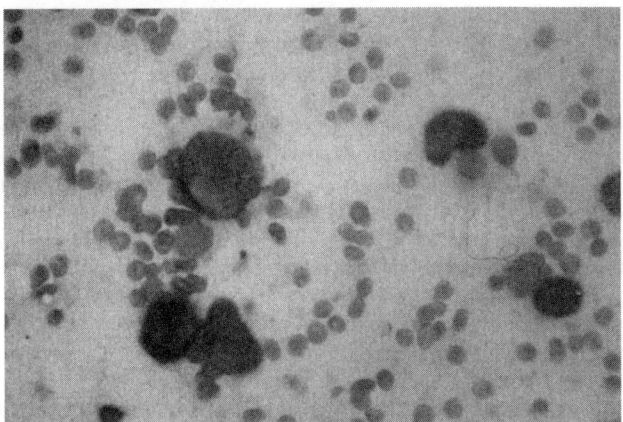

Figure 2-10. Nonspecific esterase stain. The butyrate substrate was used to demonstrate a positive reaction in this case of acute monoblastic leukemia (French-American-British M-5a). (See Color Fig. 2-10.)

careful controls. Positive cells are identified by the presence of bright red granules (Fig. 2-11). Fresh fingerstick smears are preferred, but fresh peripheral smears made from EDTA-anticoagulated blood may be used. Control slides obtained from similar specimens without tartrate should demonstrate platelet and granulocyte staining as well as lymphoid cell staining. After incubation with tartrate, platelets and granulocytes should not stain. Normal lymphoid cells show a marked reduction in activity but may not be completely negative. The lymphoid cells of hairy cell leukemia continue to stain strongly in the presence of tartrate. The TRAP stain is difficult to interpret and is less frequently used since the advent of immunophenotyping by flow cytometry. Hairy cell leukemia shows a characteristic immunophenotype, notably a monoclonal B-cell population (positive for CD19, CD20, and CD22) with strong expression of CD11c and CD25 and expression of CD103. Although these immunophenotypic findings are not entirely specific for the diagnosis of hairy cell leukemia, the presence of characteristic cellular morphology and flow cytometric surface antigen staining intensity allows a diagnosis of hairy cell leukemia.

A number of other cytochemical stains have been used for identification of abnormal cells, but they are no longer commonly used because they lack specificity or because they have been replaced by better techniques. Sudan black staining for identification of myeloid cells has been largely replaced by MPO staining because of improved counterstaining with the MPO technique. Because the periodic acid–Schiff reagent stains glycogen in a wide variety of cells, it has largely been replaced by more specific cytochemical markers to identify abnormal cells. β-Glucuronidase activity also is present in a wide range of lymphoid and myeloid cells and has limited usefulness for evaluation of abnormal cells.

COMPLETE BLOOD CELL COUNT

Red Blood Cell Counting

The complete blood count (CBC), the most commonly ordered test, consists of the following components: leukocyte (white blood cell) count, erythrocyte (RBC) count, mean corpuscular hemoglobin (MCH), mean corpuscular volume (MCV), MCH concentration (MCHC), and hematocrit or packed cell volume. Depending on the methods used, these properties may be either directly measured or calculated from other measured values. Each of these parameters may be measured by manual techniques; except for the hematocrit, manual methods have largely disappeared from the routine laboratory. Automated methodology using available instrumentation offers vastly improved precision over the older manual methods, and it has the potential to provide more information than the manual methods.

As new instrumentation and techniques for performance of laboratory tests are introduced into the clinical laboratory, physicians who use the laboratory may seek guidelines to evaluate the performance of those tests. During the evaluation of new tests, the laboratory performs comparisons with either existing methods or reference methods. Calibration methods for hemoglobin, hematocrit, and cell counting are described (33,34). In addition, when new tests or methods are introduced, normal range studies consisting of at least 100 normal subjects should be completed and the reference range for the test established.

Physicians will want to know about the linearity of the test over the dynamic range of patient samples that they may submit. This information should be available from the clinical laboratory before the test is introduced. The most important characteristics of a test are precision and accuracy. Test accuracy is usually assessed through the use of calibrated reference materials, but in the hematology laboratory, the only calibrated reference materials available are hemoglobin standards. Commercial cell suspensions may serve as control materials to ensure that instruments are operating within specified limits, but they do not constitute calibrated reference materials that can be used to assess accuracy.

Precision can be assessed by determining the CV for a series of replicate samples—usually 20. The CV equals the SD divided by the mean for the series of replicate results. As a general rule, a CV of less than 5% for a test is considered acceptable. For many measurements in hematology, CVs of less than 2% can be achieved. For certain tests, such as the reticulocyte count, CVs of 9% to 10% may be the best that can be obtained. Many other quality control procedures are used in the clinical laboratory to ensure correct instrument operation on a daily basis, but this information is rarely of value to the clinical hematologist unless the laboratory indicates that a specific test is out of the normal control range. Knowledge of the reference range for a test and the precision of the test at various levels of measurement provides the clinician with an understanding of the operating characteristics of the test. In the following sections this information is presented in tabular form for the various tests under discussion.

Manual Red Blood Cell Counting

Manual RBC counting with dilution pipettes, counting chambers, and the microscope has virtually disappeared from the clinical laboratory; descriptions of these methods are available in reference texts (35). These manual techniques have been replaced by automated flow cytometric instruments, which examine far greater numbers of cells and have improved precision over the entire clinically relevant dynamic range. Modern reference methods for RBC counting rely on the use of single-channel or multichannel electric impedance counting instruments. The only manual methods regularly used in clinical laboratories are hematocrit and hemoglobin measurements.

Manual Hemoglobin and Hematocrit Determinations

Manual hemoglobinometry serves as a reference method for calibration of automated instruments and as an alternative method when interfering substances prevent automated hemoglobinometry. The NCCLS has published an approved procedure for manual measurement of hemoglobin using the cyanmethemoglobin method (36). This method depends on the conversion of hemoglobin to a cyanmethemoglobin derivative followed by measurement of the absorbance at 540-nm–wavelength light. The absorbance of this solution is proportional to the hemoglobin concentration according to the Lambert-Beer law. The molar absorption coefficient of cyanmethemoglobin is well characterized, and accurate measurement of hemoglobin concentrations is achievable in the routine hematology laboratory. Hemoglobin concentration is expressed in grams per liter or grams per deciliter and may be converted to millimoles per liter by multiplying the concentration of grams per deciliter by 0.621.

Manual hemoglobinometry is useful when interfering substances such as lipids or abnormal leukocytes cause turbidity so that automated optic hemoglobinometry cannot be performed. Excessively high leukocyte counts also may interfere with accurate RBC counting and automated hemoglobinometry, necessitating the use of manually centrifuged hematocrits and manual hemoglobin measurement.

Manual hematocrit determinations—that is, measurement of packed RBC volume—are frequently used to assess RBC mass. The performance of manual hematocrit requires the use of calibrated centrifuges to ensure uniform cell packing, standard microcapillary tubes, and an acceptable reading device. The NCCLS has published recommended guidelines for the microhematocrit method (37). The manual hematocrit method is frequently used to provide accurate measurement of the packed cell volume when automated methods provide spurious results because of problems with RBC deformability, interfering leukocytes, or plasma proteins.

Automated Methods

Two basic technologies are used for routine measurement of the CBC components: electric impedance and light scatter. The former is the older technology and has proven its value through many years of use. With this methodology, blood is aspirated into the system, and the sample stream is split. One portion is used for hemoglobinometry, one portion for RBC counting, and one portion for leukocyte counting. Hemoglobinometry is accomplished after cell lysis by chemical conversion of hemoglobin to a single form, most often cyanmethemoglobin, followed by measurement of the hemoglobin concentration by absorbance spectrophotometry. This highly precise technique provides replicate measurements with a CV for replicate samples, within-batch samples, and between-batch samples of 1% or less (38). Failure of cells to lyse completely because of abnormal hemoglobin, such as hemoglobin AC, or because of hyperosmolar plasma, as in uremia, interferes with hemoglobin measurement.

Red blood cell counting and size analysis are performed by passing the RBCs singly through a small direct current (Fig. 2-12A), which generates a small pulse due to a temporary increase in impedance. The height of the pulse is proportional to cell volume and provides information about cell number and cell volume. Pulses that pass through the orifice in a path other than central generate a pulse that is distorted and not a true reflection of cell volume (Fig. 2-12B and C). This problem has been resolved by the use of hydrodynamic focusing to force all cells through the central path of the sensing orifice. As for measurement of hemoglobin, the precision of these measurements is excellent, with replicate sample CVs of less than 1% (38).

MCH, MCHC, and hematocrit are not directly measured by electric impedance systems but are derived by calculation from the directly measured parameters of hemoglobin, RBC count, and RBC volume. These parameters are calculated from the following formulas:

$$MCH = \text{hemoglobin (g/L)/RBC } (10^6/\mu L)$$

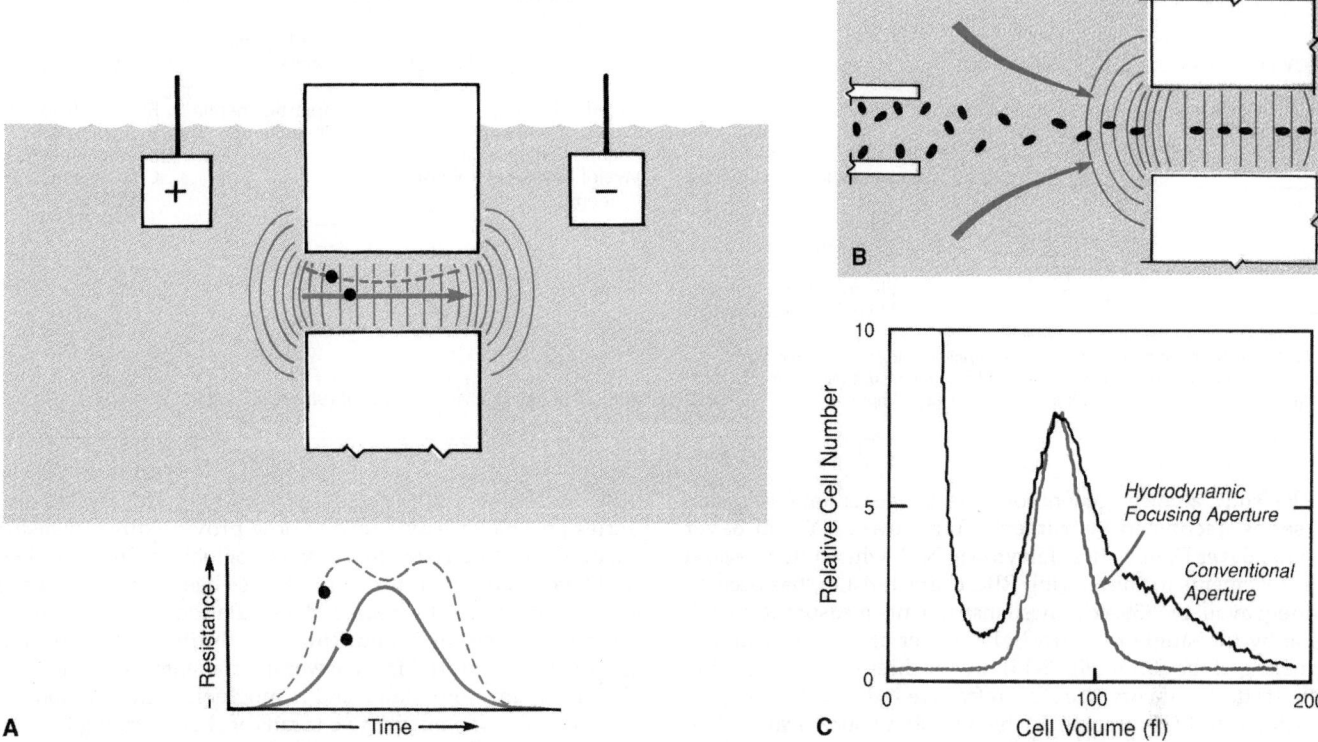

Figure 2-12. A: Electric impedance cell counting. Cells are diluted in an isosmolar conducting solution and drawn through an orifice to which a small electric field has been applied. As the cell passes through the orifice, it generates resistance, measured as pulse height, which is proportional to the cell volume. The width of the pulse is proportional to the time it takes the cell to traverse the orifice. The solid line represents the pulse generated by cells that follow a central path through the orifice, and the broken line indicates the pulse for cells that do not follow a central path through the orifice. **B:** Hydrodynamic focusing. Cells that do not pass through the center of the orifice generate an aberrant pulse and spurious volume signature. Hydrodynamic focusing uses a surrounding sheath fluid stream to force the particles through a center path in the orifice so that all cells take the same trajectory through the volume sensor. **C:** Effects of hydrodynamic focusing on cell volume. Cells that pass through the orifice aberrantly under conventional flow conditions give rise to a volume distribution that is broader than that obtained under hydrodynamic focusing conditions, in which cells pass through the center of the orifice. Hydrodynamic focusing provides a more accurate measurement of the red blood cell volume distribution. (Adapted from Haynes JL. Principles of flow cytometry. *Cytometry* 1988;9[Suppl 3]:7–17.)

$$MCHC = \text{hemoglobin (g/dL)/hematocrit (\%)}$$

$$\text{Hematocrit} = \text{MCV (fL)} \times \text{RBC} \ (10^6/\mu L)$$

Although precision of the MCV measurement is excellent with replicate samples, abnormalities of membrane deformability or cellular hemoglobin concentration may lead to inaccurate MCV measurements with subsequent inaccuracies of the calculated indices (38,39).

More recently, new versions of these instruments provide histograms of the RBC volume distribution in addition to the numeric measure of central tendency in the form of the MCV (Fig. 2-13). This format provides information about subpopulations of abnormal cells and also provides a measure of dispersion for the RBC volume distribution, the red cell distribution width (RDW). The RDW is the CV of the RBC volume distribution expressed as a percentage. Combined with the volume distribution, the RDW provides information about variation in cell size (anisocytosis) and is more sensitive than microscopic examination of the smear for detection of abnormal RBC subpopulations. These new parameters have been used to improve the diagnosis of anemia based on a bifunctional algorithm using MCV and RDW (40). Although this algorithm may not be sensitive for all cases, it does provide a useful approach to the diagnosis of anemia (41) (Table 2-1).

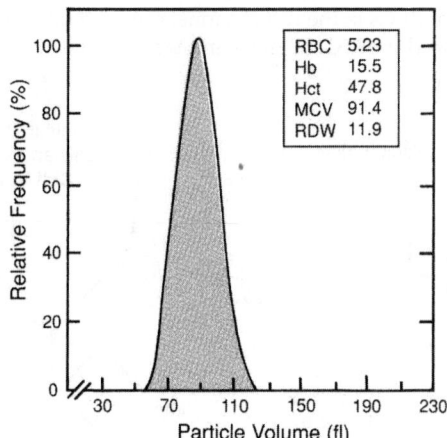

Figure 2-13. Red blood cell (RBC) volume distribution obtained with a Coulter-type electric impedance instrument. Cell number, expressed as relative frequency, is indicated on the y-axis, and cell volume is indicated on the x-axis. Mean corpuscular volume (MCV) and red cell distribution width (RDW), a measure of the dispersion of the volume distribution curve, are computed and reported. Hb, hemoglobin; Hct, hematocrit. (Adapted from Bessman JD. *Automated blood counts and differentials: a practical guide.* Baltimore: Johns Hopkins University Press, 1986.)

TABLE 2-1. Classification of Anemia Based on Red Cell Mean Corpuscular Volume (MCV) and Red Cell Distribution Width (RDW)

MCV Low, RDW Normal	MCV Low, RDW High	MCV Normal, RDW Normal	MCV Normal, RDW High	MCV High, RDW Normal	MCV High, RDW High
Heterozygous thalassemia	Iron deficiency	Normal	Mixed deficiency	Aplastic anemia	Folate deficiency
Chronic disease	S-β-thalassemia	Chronic disease	Early iron or folate deficiency	Preleukemia	B$_{12}$ deficiency
—	Hemoglobin H	Chronic liver disease	Anemic hemoglobinopathy	—	Immune hemolysis
—	Fragmentation	Hemoglobinopathy trait (S, C)	Myelofibrosis, sideroblastic anemia	—	Cold agglutinins CLL[a]
—	—	Transfusion	—	—	—
—	—	Chemotherapy	—	—	—
—	—	CLL, CML	—	—	—
—	—	Hemorrhage	—	—	—
—	—	Hereditary spherocytosis	—	—	—

CLL, chronic lymphocytic leukemia; CML, chronic myelogenous leukemia.
[a]Because of inclusion of leukocytes in the red cell volume distribution in CLL.
Data from Bessman JD, Gilmer PR Jr, Gardner FH, et al. Improved classification of anemias by MCV and RDW. *Am J Clin Pathol* 1983;80:322–326.

Recently, a newer generation of instrumentation (Technicon H series, Technicon Instruments, Tarrytown, NY, and Bayer Advia, Bayer Diagnostics, Tarrytown, NY), which offers several improvements for measuring RBC characteristics, has become widely available (39,42). These instruments measure RBC volume by low-angle forward light scatter after isovolumetric sphering of the RBCs (Fig. 2-14). Under these conditions, using Mie scattering theory, the RBC refractive index is directly proportional to the intracellular hemoglobin concentration (43) (Fig. 2-15). Thus, corpuscular hemoglobin concentration (CHC) may now be measured directly, and the distribution of CHC, measures of central tendency of MCHC, and the dispersion of this distribution may be measured (Fig. 2-16). The dispersion of the CHC distribution is termed the *hemoglobin distribution width* and is the CV expressed as a percentage for this distribution. More important, inspection of the CHC distribution (Fig. 2-16) provides an excellent means of detecting subpopulations of cells with abnormal hemoglobin concentrations—for example, dehydrated cells associated with sickle cell anemia (39).

The direct measurement of MCHC represents an improvement over earlier electric impedance systems, in which the automated MCHC did not agree well with manual determinations (39) (Fig. 2-17). The lack of agreement was due to poor deformability of RBCs with MCHC levels above 36 g/dL. Sphering of RBCs in the RBC channel resolved this problem and has improved the MCHC measurement as a means of assessing RBC hydration and internal viscosity (39). The Technicon H series and Bayer Advia format now provide direct measurement of four RBC characteristics: hemoglobin, volume, number, and hemoglobin concentration. Because hemoglobin concentration can be precisely measured, calculation of the hematocrit from measured MCV and RBC is of limited value and may gradually be removed from newer instruments. Combined with the histograms for volume and hemoglobin concentration, this information offers an effective means of characterizing RBC disorders and of detecting conditions such as cold agglutinins, which may affect the measurement of RBC properties (41).

AUTOMATED LEUKOCYTE COUNT

As for RBC counting methods, manual leukocyte counts have virtually disappeared from practice in modern clinical laboratories. Manual leukocyte counts performed with dilution pipettes and calibrated counting chambers exhibited CVs ranging from 10% to 20% for normal leukocyte counts, and at lower levels, the CV was increased further. Semiautomated or fully automated electric impedance leukocyte counting offers the advantages of greater precision and efficiency than achieved with older, manual methods. Automated leukocyte counting relies on lysis of RBCs in the leukocyte channel with either subsequent electric impedance or optic detection of intact leukocytes (Fig. 2-12A).

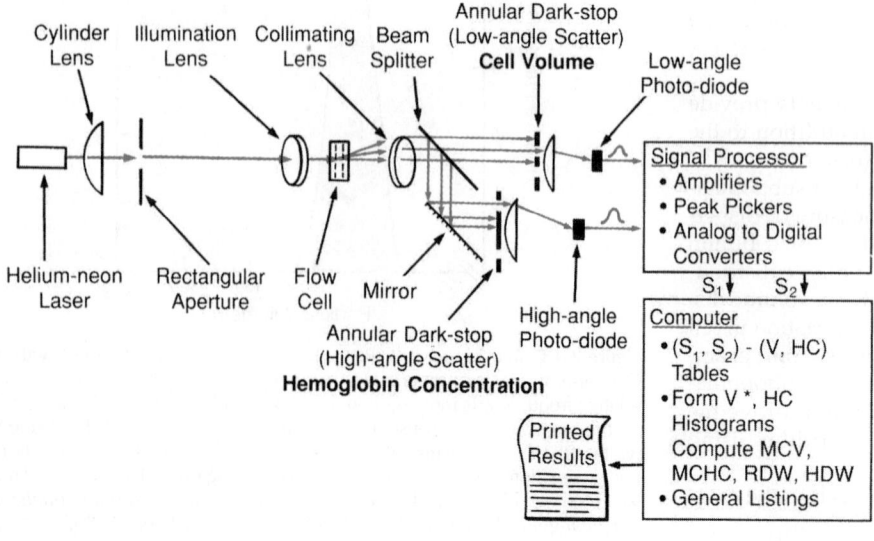

Figure 2-14. Schematic representation of the red blood cell (RBC) channel of the Technicon H*1 instrument. Five thousand to 10,000 RBCs are sphered and drawn through a flow cell with simultaneous measurement of low-angle (2-degree to 3-degree) scatter and high-angle (5-degree to 15-degree) scatter. Low-angle scatter is used as a measure of cell volume (V), and high-angle scatter is used to measure hemoglobin concentration (HC). HDW, hemoglobin distribution width; MCHC, mean corpuscular hemoglobin concentration; MCV, mean corpuscular volume; RDW, red cell distribution width. (Adapted from Mohandas N, Kim YR, Tycko DH, et al. Accurate and independent measurement of volume and hemoglobin concentration of individual RBCs by laser light scattering. *Blood* 1986;68:506–513.)

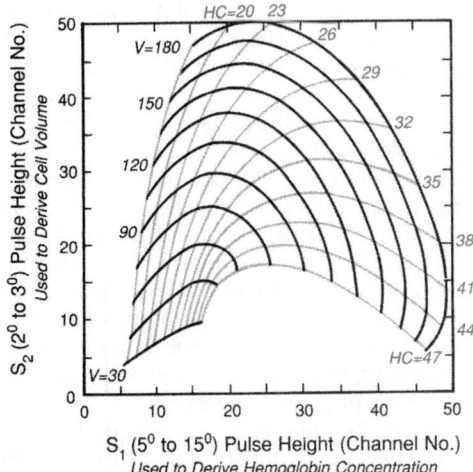

Figure 2-15. Bivariant mapping of red blood cell volume and hemoglobin concentration. The results from the Technicon H*1 red blood cell channel are represented as a bivariant scatter plot of cell volume (V, y-axis) and cell hemoglobin concentration (HC, x-axis). (Adapted from Mohandas N, Kim YR, Tycko DH, et al. Accurate and independent measurement of volume and hemoglobin concentration of individual red cells by laser light scattering. *Blood* 1986;68:506–513.)

Leukocyte counts ranging from 2.1 to 26 × 10^9/L demonstrate CVs from 1.7% to 3.1% for replicate samples, within-batch samples, and between-batch samples using electric impedance methods (38). Optic-based instruments exhibit within-run CVs ranging from 6.2% to 0.7% for leukocyte counts ranging from 0.8 to 44 × 10^9/L (42).

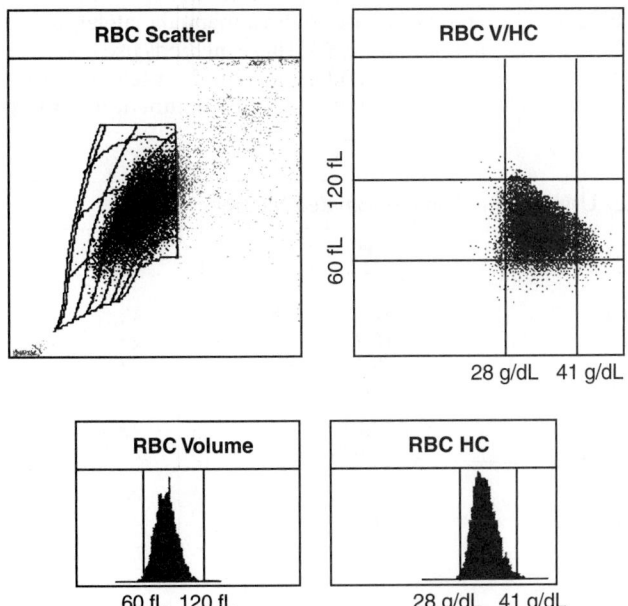

Figure 2-16. Analysis of the Bayer Advia 120 red blood cell (RBC) channel. Data from this channel are presented in three different plots. The bivariant scatter plot provides a cluster analysis of the abnormal cell populations, which may exhibit variation in volume (V) or hemoglobin concentration (HC). The volume distribution is reduced to a single parameter histogram from which mean corpuscular volume and the coefficient of variation, a measure of red cell distribution width, are computed. The hemoglobin concentration distribution is also reduced to a single parameter histogram with computation of mean corpuscular HC and the coefficient of variation of that distribution, which is referred to as the *hemoglobin distribution width*. The hemoglobin distribution width provides an estimate of the variation in hemoglobin concentration among the RBC population.

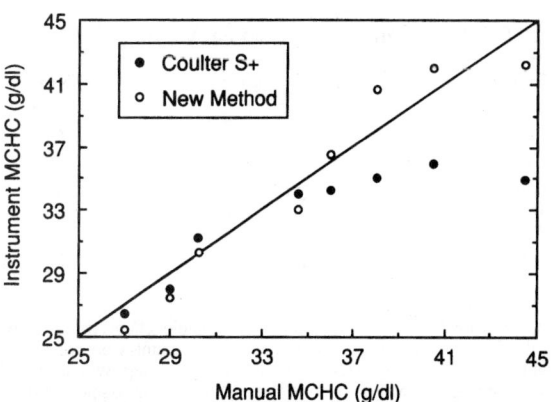

Figure 2-17. Comparison of mean corpuscular hemoglobin concentration (MCHC) determined with manual or automated methods. The MCHC of a series of samples was compared using manual methods, the Coulter S Plus, and the Technicon H*1 (new method). Good agreement over the entire range of MCHC values was obtained between the manual and electrooptic Technicon H*1 methods. In contrast, at higher manual MCHC values, the electric impedance Coulter S Plus MCHC values were lower than the manual values. (Adapted from Mohandas N, Kim YR, Tycko DH, et al. Accurate and independent measurement of volume and hemoglobin concentration of individual RBCs by laser light scattering. *Blood* 1986;68:506–513.)

PLATELET COUNTING

Manual Platelet Counting

The only method of manual platelet counting widely used at this time is the phase microscopic chamber counting method (44). This method is still the reference method in many laboratories, although its precision limitations are well understood. For platelet counts within the normal range, CVs in the range of 11% to 16.6% have been reported (44,45). Many laboratories use a peripheral blood smear estimating technique as a rapid means of verifying questionable platelet counts obtained with automated methods (46,47). With a standard wedge peripheral smear stained with polychrome stain under 1000× oil magnification, the number of platelets in ten fields is enumerated in the area of the smear where RBCs are evenly distributed, with good preservation of central pallor. The number of platelets per ten fields is multiplied by 2000 to obtain an estimate of the absolute platelet count per microliter of whole blood (46). If wide-field oculars are used instead of standard oculars, only eight 1000× fields are counted (46).

For either optic system, the agreement between the electric impedance counts and the slide estimates is reasonable (r = 0.98 to 0.96). Nosanchuk et al. (46) observed a CV of 50% by slide estimate for a platelet count of 27,000/μL established by an automated electric impedance technique. For automated platelet counts ranging from 65,000 to 100,000/μL, the CV of the slide estimates varied from 20% to 23%; the CV declined to 9% to 15% for platelet counts ranging from 163,000 to 590,000/μL. Thus, slide estimate provides a reliable means to verify the approximate range of automated platelet counts.

The platelet count is frequently used to decide whether to transfuse platelets prophylactically. Historically, the transfusion threshold value has been 20,000/μL (48,49), but more recent data suggest that a lower threshold (5000 to 15,000/μL) may be more appropriate (50–53). Pretransfusion and posttransfusion platelet counts should be obtained to determine whether an acceptable increment has been achieved. Thus, the precision of platelet counts in this range and the confidence with which a platelet count of 20,000/μL can be distinguished from a count of 30,000/μL is a relevant issue. Based on the studies of Nosan-

TABLE 2-2. Within-Run Precision at Varying Platelet Levels[a]

Platelet Level[b]	CV Impedance[c]	CV Optic[d]
13	8.2	7.7
29	4.4	8.9
45	3.0	5.7
100	2.0	2.3
255	1.5	2.2
415	1.5	1.5
700	2.7	1.8

CV, coefficient of variation.
[a]Comparison of within-run precision for varying platelet counts using two whole blood platelet counting instruments. Twenty replicate counts were performed at each platelet level ($\times 10^9$/L), and the CV, expressed as a percentage, was determined.
[b]Random samples ranging from 13×10^9/L to 700×10^9/L were selected and counted using standard automated whole blood platelet counting instruments.
[c]Coulter S Plus II (Coulter Electronics, Hialeah, FL).
[d]Technicon H*1 (Technicon Instruments Corp., Tarrytown, NY).
Data from Bollinger PB, Drewinko B, Brailas CD, et al. The Technicon H*1—an automated hematology analyzer for today and tomorrow. *Am J Clin Pathol* 1987;87:71–78.

chuk et al. (46), the slide estimate technique is not sufficiently precise for platelet counts below 65,000/µL.

Automated Platelet Counting

Most current blood counting instruments also offer a whole blood platelet count using either an electric impedance or electrooptic detection system (42,54,55). The degree of precision for both types of instruments is comparable over a wide range of platelet counts (Table 2-2). The precision of newer instrumentation is superior to that obtained with earlier instruments or phase contrast platelet counts, as demonstrated in the study by Wertz and Koepke (56) (Table 2-3). Data from this study provide information about the accuracy of phase contrast platelet counts performed by a group of qualified hematology laboratories.

Information is limited about the ability of automated platelet counting methods to discriminate among varying degrees of severe thrombocytopenia around the critical threshold for platelet transfusion. With the advent of more precise particle counters, the precision of the platelet count at low levels (Table 2-4) has improved so that platelet counts of 10,000/µL can be discriminated from those of 20,000/µL in most cases.

Both impedance and optic platelet methods rely on particle size to count platelets. Thus, particles of similar size, such as red cell or white cell fragments, may interfere with the platelet count and result in overestimation of the platelet count by the impedance and optic automated methods. Conversely, impedance methods often use a fixed upper limit for the particle size threshold, resulting in underestimation of the platelet count in patients with large or giant platelets.

More recently, automated optic methods have been introduced that use two angles of light scatter to identify the platelet population. The new-generation Bayer Advia instrument uses platelet methodology similar to the red cell analysis in the Technicon and Bayer instruments. Low-angle light scatter (2 to 3 degrees), a parameter measuring particle volume, and high-angle light scatter (5 to 15 degrees), a measure of refractive index, are used to delineate the platelet population. The Abbott Cell-Dyn 4000 uses two different angles of optic light scatter, 7 degrees and 90 degrees, to provide an optic platelet count. When these two-dimensional optic methods are compared with immunologic antibody staining methods, they show better correlation than impedance methods (57–59). Data to date are limited, but these two-dimensional optic methods also may allow better discrimination between platelets and other interfering particles of similar size, such as red cell or white cell fragments.

Flow cytometric immunologic methods have recently been developed for counting platelets, and it has been proposed that this procedure replace phase contrast manual platelet counts as the reference method (57,60,61). These methods use fluorescent-labeled monoclonal antibodies specific for platelet antigens, such as CD41a, CD42b, and CD61, in conjunction with optic

TABLE 2-3. Estimation of Platelet Count Accuracy Using Manual and Automated Methods[a]

Method	Labs, n[b]	Mean Count[c] ($\times 10^9$/L)	SD[d]	CV[e]
Light microscopy				
Ammonium oxalate	58	104.4	35.2	33.7
Unopette[f]	810	82.7	18.2	22.0
Crystal violet	34	100.6	29.1	28.9
Other[g]	120	109.6	34.1	31.1
Phase contrast microscopy				
Ammonium oxalate	99	104.4	27.7	26.6
Unopette[f]	383	84.3	21.6	25.6
Automated methods				
Thrombocounter[h]	197	77.8	34.4	44.2
Model ZBI[h]	61	87.4	31.7	36.3
Model FN or F[h]	109	76.6	39.4	51.5
Autocounter[i]	52	120.6	26.7	22.2
MK-4HC[j]	43	95.8	9.7	10.1

CV, coefficient of variation; SD, standard deviation.
[a]Based on a College of American Pathologists Comprehensive Hematology Survey (1976) in which a calibrated standard platelet suspension was sent to participating laboratories for blinded counting. Results of this survey were reported by Wertz and Koepke (56). The target value of the prepared standard was 91.52×10^9/L with a SD of 1.13×10^9/L and a CV of 1.2% based on 56 replicate counts using the Coulter Model Z particle counter.
[b]Within each methodologic class.
[c]For all laboratories within a designated methodologic class.
[d]SD for the designated method.
[e]CV of each method among different laboratories.
[f]Becton Dickinson.
[g]Method not specified.
[h]Coulter Electronics.
[i]Technicon Instruments Corp.
[j]J.T. Baker Co.

TABLE 2-4. Within-Run Precision of Very Low Platelet Counts[a]

Mean Count[b]	SD[c]	CV[d]	2-SD Range[e]
Coulter S Plus IV			
2.0	0.4	20.3	1.2–2.8
8.0	1.8	22.9	4.4–11.6
10.0	0.9	8.5	8.2–11.8
13.0	0.9	6.7	11.2–14.8
16.0	1.8	11.1	12.4–19.6
19.0	1.5	7.7	16.0–22.0
Technicon H*1			
6.0	0.6	9.8	4.8–7.2
12.0	0.8	6.9	10.4–13.6
13.0	1.1	8.6	10.8–15.2
14.0	1.6	11.2	10.9–17.1
18.0	1.2	6.4	15.6–20.4
18.0	1.8	9.8	14.4–21.5

CV, coefficient of variation; SD, standard deviation.
[a]Unpublished data, L Corash, 1993. Random blood samples from patients with severe thrombocytopenia were selected, and five replicate counts were performed using two whole blood platelet counting instruments: Coulter S Plus IV (Coulter Electronics, Hialeah, FL) and Technicon H*1 (Technicon Instruments Corp., Tarrytown, NY).
[b]Represents the average platelet (×10⁹/L) based on five replicate analyses within a single run.
[c]SD of the mean platelet count.
[d]CV for the five replicate platelet counts.
[e]Indicated for each sample.

light scatter characteristics to identify the platelet population. Platelets are then enumerated by comparison to calibrated reference beads of a known concentration or by derivation of a ratio of platelet events to red blood cell events. The CV ranges from 5.6% at a platelet count of 10×10^9/L (60) to 10% at 1.1×10^9/L (61). At platelet counts less than 100×10^9/L, the flow cytometric immunologic platelet counting method correlates better with dual-angle optic counters than with impedance methods (57). An immunologic method using a monoclonal antibody for CD61, platelet glycoprotein IIIa, has been automated and implemented on the Abbott Cell-Dyn 4000. This method shows good correlation with phase microscopy counts ($R^2 = 0.97$), has a CV of 2.89% at platelet counts less than 50×10^9/L (62), and may be somewhat superior to optic and impedance methods at low platelet counts (62,63).

Common Sources of Error

Errors in measurement of the RBC count, hemoglobin, leukocyte count, platelet count, and RBC indices may arise because of abnormalities intrinsic to the sample rather than because of instrument or operator error. Cornbleet (64) has summarized the sources of these errors (Table 2-5).

Measurement of Platelet Volume

Physicians and laboratory technologists have long been cognizant of the variation in platelet size on routine peripheral blood smears. Although the biologic significance of platelet volume heterogeneity remains controversial, effort has continued in the measurement of platelet size as a diagnostic test to evaluate patients with either thrombocytopenia or thrombocytosis (65–68). Several investigators have reported that microscopic measurement of platelet size on smears may provide useful diagnostic information (69–71). Microscopic measurement of platelet size has never been widely adopted because of the technical difficulties, labor-intensive methodology, and a time-dependent effect of EDTA anticoagulant on platelet volume (71). With the advent of electric impedance measurement of blood cell num-

bers and volume and the ability to count and size platelets in whole blood samples, measurement of platelet volume has become a more feasible test. This practice rapidly expanded with the widespread availability of platelet volume measurement on highly automated hematology instruments in clinical laboratories (72,73). Mean platelet volume (MPV) measurement is routinely available in most clinical laboratories, but controversy about its diagnostic usefulness persists. Current laboratory instrumentation measures platelet volume distribution from EDTA-anticoagulated whole blood samples by either electric impedance or electrooptic methods. With both techniques, platelet volume has been observed to vary with time of exposure to anticoagulant (74–78). With electric impedance instruments, platelet volume in EDTA-anticoagulated whole blood increases over time (74–76). The greatest increase occurs in the first 2 hours, followed by a slower but progressive increase of up to 50% of baseline compared with that found in citrated blood, in which platelet volume is stable (76,78). In contrast, platelet volume in EDTA-anticoagulated blood may either increase or decrease with time when measured by electrooptic techniques (77). Although the rate of anticoagulant-induced change in platelet volume may decrease with time, the effect is highly variable over a period of several hours. Within the confines of the clinical laboratory's operating conditions, it appears impossible to measure platelet volumes accurately in all samples under routine blood collection and sample processing conditions.

Levin and Bessman (74) reported an inverse but nonlinear relation between platelet volume and platelet number with EDTA samples from normal subjects. Thompson et al. (75) observed an inverse linear relation between platelet volume and number in a second study of normal subjects using citrated blood. The study by Levin and Bessman (74) was performed with EDTA-anticoagulated samples in which platelet volumes may not have been adequately stabilized, whereas the study by Thompson (75) was performed with stabilized samples. In light of these divergent studies, it is not clear how to define a normal range for the relation between platelet volume and number in the routine clinical laboratory when sample stability and the interval between collection and analysis are highly variable.

Generally there is greater interest in measurement of MPV in thrombocytopenic samples. The observation of an increased MPV in association with thrombocytopenia is usually interpreted to indicate that thrombopoiesis is stimulated (69,74,79). When MPV is normal in the face of thrombocytopenia, thrombopoiesis is assumed to be impaired. Although Bessman et al. (79) have obtained MPV values for thrombocytopenic patients with routine instrumentation, others have been unable to obtain a reliable measurement of platelet volume with routine laboratory instrumentation (80,81), possibly partly due to the limited volume measuring range of the automated instruments and to the markedly decreased signal to noise ratio with thrombocytopenic samples. An additional problem in thrombocytopenic samples is that a relatively small number of nonplatelet particles such as red cell or white cell fragments may result in significant interference with the MPV if these particles are included in the platelet population. Niethammer and Forman (82) have suggested that the highest peak of the platelet volume distribution curve may better discriminate increased platelet destruction from decreased platelet production in patients with thrombocytopenia. In contrast with most clinical conditions associated with thrombocytopenia, platelets in Wiskott-Aldrich syndrome are typically small (83), and platelet sizing may be useful in this situation.

Platelet volume measurements in patients with thrombocytosis have been inconsistent and nonreproducible when repeated in different laboratories. In reactive thrombocytosis, MPV has been reported as normal (80,84), decreased (85), or

TABLE 2-5. Potential Causes of Erroneous Results with Automated Cell Counters

Parameter	Causes of Spurious Increase	Causes of Spurious Decrease
WBC count	Cryoproteins Heparin Paraproteins Nucleated RBCs Platelet clumping Incomplete red cell lysis	Clotting Smudge cells Uremia + immunosuppressants
RBC count	Cryoproteins Giant platelets WBC count >50,000/μL	Autoagglutination Clotting *In vitro* hemolysis Microcytic RBCs
Hemoglobin	Carboxyhemoglobin >10% Cryoproteins *In vivo* hemolysis Heparin WBC count >50,000/μL Hyperbilirubinemia Lipemia Paraproteins	Clotting Sulfhemoglobin (?)
Hematocrit (automated)	Cryoproteins Giant platelets WBC count >50,000/μL Hyperglycemia (>600 mg/dL)	Autoagglutination Clotting *In vitro* hemolysis Microcytic RBCs
Hematocrit (microhematocrit)	Hyponatremia Plasma trapping	Excess EDTA *In vitro* hemolysis Hypernatremia
MCV	Autoagglutination WBC count >50,000/μL Hyperglycemia Reduced RBC deformability	Cryoproteins Giant platelets *In vitro* hemolysis Microcytic RBCs Swollen RBCs
MCHC	Autoagglutination Clotting *In vitro* hemolysis Spuriously high hemoglobin Spuriously low hematocrit	WBC count >50,000/μL Spuriously low hemoglobin Spuriously high hematocrit
Platelets	Cryoproteins Hemolysis Microcytic RBCs RBC inclusions WBC fragments	Clotting Giant platelets Heparin Platelet clumping Platelet satellitosis

EDTA, ethylenediaminetetraacetic acid; MCHC, mean corpuscular hemoglobin concentration; MCV, mean corpuscular volume; RBC, red blood cell; WBC, white blood cell.
Adapted from Cornbleet J. Spurious results from automated hematology counters. *Lab Med* 1983;14:509–514.

even increased in a small proportion of patients with benign hematologic diseases (74). In myeloproliferative disorders, MPV has been normal in some studies (80,84) and increased in a proportion of patients in other studies (74,86). Osselaer et al. (68) showed a higher median MPV in myeloproliferative disorders than in reactive thrombocytosis. However, there was significant overlap in the individual values from the two groups; thus, this parameter was not useful in distinguishing reactive thrombocytosis from a myeloproliferative process.

LEUKOCYTE DIFFERENTIAL

Manual Methods

The microscopic manual differential has been the traditional means of classifying the five basic leukocyte classes: neutrophils, lymphocytes, monocytes, eosinophils, and basophils. In most laboratories, this technique requires the preparation of a thin, air-dried wedge smear stained with a polychrome stain (discussed in the section Red Blood Cell, Platelet, and Leukocyte Morphology). A reference method for the manual microscopic leukocyte differential has been recommended (87). Under these guidelines, two examiners perform a 200-cell dif-

ferential on two different wedge smears prepared from a single venous blood sample anticoagulated with EDTA. The results are calculated from the pooled 400-cell differential count. Normal range reference data are determined by performing 400-cell differential counts on a population of at least 100 normal subjects (adults without evidence of disease) (87). The previous reference method, proposed by the NCCLS in 1984 (88), was similar to the present recommendations except that 200-cell differential counts were performed on four slides and results based on the pooled 800-cell differential count. These guidelines have been used in some studies as the reference method.

A typical set of reference data is illustrated in the study by Koepke et al. (89) (Table 2-6). Common practice in the busy routine hematology laboratory is to perform a single 100-cell differential count (54). Previously, results of leukocyte differentials have been reported as relative frequencies of leukocyte subclasses expressed as percentages. More recently, the calculation of absolute values for each leukocyte class has been encouraged, and most automated instruments now report absolute values expressed as the number of cells per microliter of whole blood. The use of absolute values has made definition of the normal range more precise.

Errors in performance of the leukocyte differential have been classified as either distributional or morphologic. Studies to examine the frequency of these types of errors have been con-

TABLE 2-6. Reference Ranges for the Differential Leukocyte Count in Adults[a]

Cell Type	Proportional Count (%)[b]	Absolute Count (×10⁹/L)[c]
Segmented neutrophil	37–80	2.0–6.93
Band neutrophil	0–12	0–0.87
Normal lymphocyte	10–50	0.6–3.44
Variant lymphocyte	0–8.5	0–0.66
Monocyte	0–12	0.03–0.90
Eosinophil	0–9.5	0–0.67
Basophil	0–2.5	0–0.20

[a]Using the 1984 National Committee for Clinical Laboratory Standards H20 T reference method requiring an 800-cell manual differential (88). Differentials were performed on 114 normal adult subjects with normal complete blood cell count, normal total leukocyte count, and no recent infections.
[b]Of the total leukocyte population. The central 95th percentile range is indicated.
[c]Calculated from the total leukocyte count (method unspecified). The central 95th percentile for the total leukocyte count was 4.6 × 10⁹/L to 10.2 × 10⁹/L.

ducted and will continue to be performed and compared with the reference method as new leukocyte differential techniques evolve. Koepke et al. (89) have reported a comparison of the routine 100-cell differential with the original 800-cell differential NCCLS reference method (88) for detection of a number of diseases in which either distributional or morphologic leukocyte abnormalities exist (Table 2-7).

The sensitivity of the routine differential for detection of a myeloid left shift or monocytosis is low, and specific definitions for the band form and the variant lymphocyte have been published in an effort to improve interlaboratory performance of routine leukocyte differentials (90,91). The band cell has been defined as having "a nucleus that could be described as a curve or coiled band, no matter how marked the indentation, if it does not completely segment the nucleus into lobes connected by a filament" (92).

TABLE 2-7. Sensitivity of the Routine Leukocyte Differential in Detecting Distributional and Morphologic Abnormalities[a]

Referee Finding	n[b]	Agreement (%)	False-Normal (%)	False-Abnormal (%)
Normal	18	91	—	9
Distributional abnormalities				
Granulocytosis	9	96	4	—
Left shift	19	34	66	—
Lymphocytosis	4	100	—	—
Monocytosis	6	80	20	—
Eosinophilia	5	72	18	—
Agranulocytosis	3	100	—	—
Morphologic abnormalities				
Variant lymphocytosis	10	64	36	—
Erythrocyte precursors	15	81	19	—
Leukocyte blasts	10	91	2	7

[a]National Committee for Clinical Laboratory Standards 800-cell differential reference method (1984) (88) and routine 100-cell leukocyte differentials were performed for a series of slides obtained from patients with the following disorders: acute inflammation, acute allergic reaction, viral infection, acute leukemia, severe anemia or myelophthisic anemia, and aplastic anemia. Five laboratories performed a single routine 100-cell differential on each abnormal slide. The incidences of agreement, false-normal, and false-abnormal results between the routine 100-cell differential and the reference method are expressed as a percentage. Distributional abnormalities indicate differences in the relative proportions of normal cells, and morphologic abnormalities indicate errors in the identification of abnormal cells.
[b]The number of cases evaluated for each abnormality is indicated.
Data from Koepke JA, Dotson MA, Shifman MA, et al. A critical evaluation of the manual/visual differential leukocyte counting method. *Blood Cells* 1985;11:173–181.

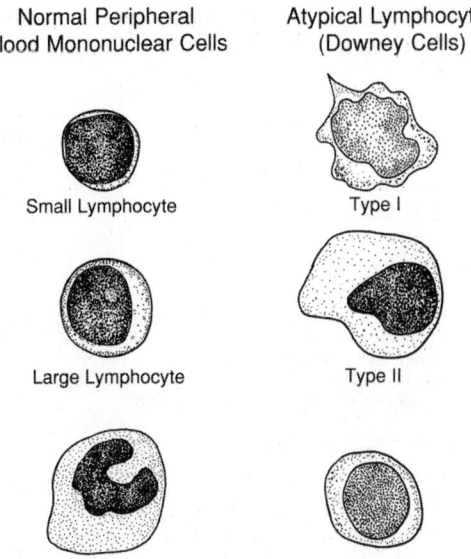

Figure 2-18. Schematic representation of the morphology of normal and atypical or variant lymphocytes. (Adapted from Sun NCJ. *Hematology: an atlas and diagnostic guide.* Philadelphia: WB Saunders, 1983.)

Identification of atypical or variant lymphocytes has been troublesome because of variation in the morphologic definition of these cells by microscopists. Normal lymphocytes may be small or large, with dense nuclear chromatin and sparse azurophilic cytoplasmic granules. Normal large lymphocytes exhibit more cytoplasm than the small cell, which is typified by a scant rim of cytoplasm. Variant lymphocytes, frequently associated with viral infections, are characterized by increased size, greater cytoplasmic area, basophilia, nuclear convolutions, and nuclear chromatin that is less dense than that of normal cells but not as fine as that found in lymphoblasts (Figs. 2-18 and 2-19). Some variant cells may appear similar to plasma cells; these are referred to as *plasmacytoid lymphocytes* or *stimulated lymphocytes.* The latter functional designation is derived from the similarity of these variant lymphocytes to cells in stimulated cultures. Nuclear shape may become kidneylike, in contrast to the round configuration of normal lymphocytes. Variant lymphocytes may contain nucleoli. The sensitivity for detection of variant lymphocytes and erythroid precursors is suboptimal, whereas the detection of highly abnormal cells (blasts) is reasonable. The NCCLS

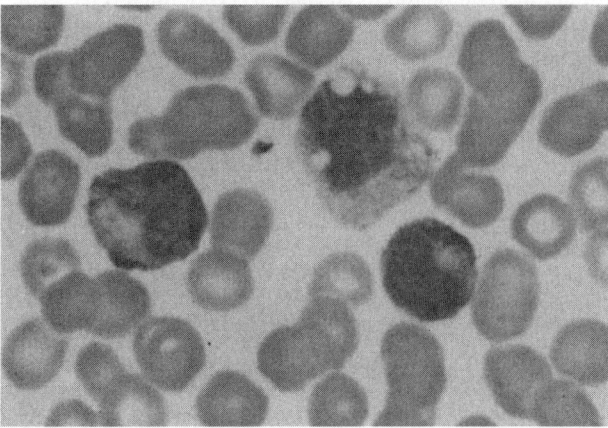

Figure 2-19. Examples of variant lymphocytes obtained from the blood of a patient with infectious mononucleosis. Large mononuclear cells with open nuclear chromatin can be seen. (See Color Fig. 2-19.)

TABLE 2-8. Correlation between the Reference Method and the Routine Differential for Detection of Different Leukocytes[a]

Cell Type	Slope	r
Segmented neutrophil	0.88	0.87
Band neutrophil	0.53	0.67
Normal lymphocyte	0.85	0.73
Variant lymphocyte	0.35	0.30
Monocyte	0.56	0.41
Eosinophil	0.90	0.83
Basophil	0.58	0.32

[a]The National Committee for Clinical Laboratory Standards 800-cell differential reference method (1984) (88) was compared with the routine 100-cell differential for detection of different leukocyte cell classes.
Data from Koepke JA, et al. A critical evaluation of the manual/visual differential leukocyte counting method. *Blood Cells* 1985;11:173–181.

standard concluded that new leukocyte differential methods should correlate with the 400-cell reference method (87).

Two critical points in the evaluation process are detection of abnormal proportions of the normal leukocytes (distributional abnormalities) and detection of abnormal cells (morphologic abnormalities). The routine 100-cell manual differential was found comparable with the NCCLS 800-cell differential reference method (Table 2-8). Thus, new techniques can reliably detect infrequent cell classes such as monocytes, variant lymphocytes, and basophils.

Electric Impedance

With improvement in flow cytometric technology, automated leukocyte differential cell counters have become widely available to the routine clinical hematology laboratory. A number of instruments that perform a two-part, three-part, or five-part automated differential are in common use (Table 2-9). These instruments use a variety of technologies to subclassify leukocytes and have been compared with the manual differential technique using the NCCLS standard (87,88). The three-part differential using electric impedance technology to discriminate granulocytes, lymphocytes, and mononuclear cells has gained widespread acceptance because of its availability in combination with CBC and platelet count capacity in an economical format. RBCs are hemolyzed with a reagent system, which leaves leukocytes intact and detectable by electric impedance. Approximately 10,000 to 20,000 leukocytes are examined, and a single parameter histogram with relative and absolute quantitative enumeration of the three cell classes is generated (Fig. 2-20).

Most studies on the impedance three-part differential instruments have been performed on the original Coulter S Plus IV. This analyzer is no longer available, but one might expect similar characteristics with other impedance instruments. The Coulter S Plus IV has been evaluated using the NCCLS standard, and a reference range for the normal three-part differential has been established (93) (Table 2-10). Comparison of precision between the reference method and the Coulter S Plus IV demonstrated one order of magnitude improvement in precision using the instrument (93). The accuracy of the Coulter S Plus IV has been compared with a well-accepted reference method, the 400-cell manual differential. Of 252 patient samples with a wide range of both distributional and morphologic abnormalities, 188 were abnormal by the reference method. Only 1.6% of those that failed were not detected by the automated technique. Of 185 samples that could be analyzed, 97% were flagged as having either abnormal morphology or distribution, and 3% could not be detected. For 64 normal samples, 12.5% were flagged, representing false-positive results. The posi-

tive predictive value for this patient population was 95.8%, the negative predictive value was 91.8%, and the overall test efficiency was 94.8% (93). If both distributional and morphologic abnormalities are evaluated in a combined manner, the rates decline slightly, but overall test efficiency remains high (87.6%). The absence of morphologic flags and distributional abnormalities, when compared with the reference range, confirms with a high degree of probability that the specimen is normal.

In another study using a large number of abnormal samples, the precision and efficiency of the Coulter S Plus IV three-part differential were evaluated (94). Thirty-nine percent of samples generated review flags. The automated counter flagged lymphocyte and monocytic abnormalities more accurately than granulocytic changes. This study emphasized that the mononuclear population should not be equated with the monocyte fraction determined by manual differential (94). Among the nonflagged samples, 7.6% did not agree with the result obtained from manual differential. The major sources of error were leukopenia, monocytosis, and lymphoblastosis. The lack of agreement of leukopenic samples may have been caused by poor results obtained with the manual method as a result of distributional abnormalities (94).

The sensitivity and specificity in this large study, in which samples were defined by a routine manual differential, were informative about the relative value of the three-part differential in a clinical laboratory setting (Table 2-11). Both sensitivity and specificity were suboptimal, and 39% of samples would have required microscopic review based on morphologic abnormalities without consideration of distributional abnormalities. The precision of the distributional measurements for both granulocytes and lymphocytes was acceptable. Thus, in an inpatient setting, the three-part differential would appear to require a high rate of microscopic review with less than optimal sensitivity.

Cytochemical Leukocyte Differential

Another leukocyte differential technology that evolved considerably over the past several decades is the cytochemical differential. The current version of this approach is used on the Bayer Technicon H series (H-6000, H*1, H*2, and H*3) and the Bayer Advia 120 instruments (Bayer Diagnostics). These instruments are based on an earlier five-part cytochemical differential instrument, the Technicon D-90 (95). The Bayer Technicon H series instruments and Bayer Advia provide a five-part differential based on light scatter and peroxidase cytochemical staining for detection of granulocytes and monocytes (42,96,97). The H-6000 instrument detects immature granulocytes through elevated peroxidase activity, the high peroxidase (HPX) fraction. The H-6000 (Fig. 2-21) contains a discrete cytochemical basophil channel that has been replaced with a noncytochemical technique on the newer H*1, H*2, H*3, and Advia instruments (Fig. 2-22). Although many of the studies regarding leukocyte differential have been performed on the earlier H*1 instrument, similar results might be expected with the H*2, H*3, and Advia instruments because the methodology is essentially the same.

Simultaneous measurement of cell size by forward-angle light scatter and peroxidase staining of individual cells is used to classify cells as lymphocytes, large unstained cells, monocytes, neutrophils, and eosinophils. Basophils are enumerated in a separate channel in which cells are exposed to an acid buffer and lysing reagent, which cause the cytoplasm to be removed from all leukocytes except basophils (97). In addition, with this technology, nuclear contour is examined by forward- and side-angle light scatter in this channel, and a lobularity index (LI) is calculated. This index is used to detect immature cells that have a low LI because of reduced nuclear segmentation.

TABLE 2-9. Automated Leukocyte Differential Instruments

Manufacturer	Model	Method	Result
Abbott	Cell-Dyn 1700	Impedance	Granulocytes Mid range[c] Lymphocytes
ABX	Micros 60	Impedance	Granulocytes Monocytes Lymphocytes
Bayer	Advia 60	Impedance	Granulocytes Monocytes Lymphocytes
Beckman Coulter	A[c] T Series	Impedance	Granulocytes Mononuclear cells Lymphocytes
Abbott	Cell-Dyn 3700	Light scatter	Granulocytes Monocytes Lymphocytes Eosinophils Basophils
Abbott	Cell-Dyn 4000	Light scatter Fluorescence	Granulocytes Monocytes Lymphocytes Eosinophils Basophils
ABX	Pentra 60 and 120	Cytochemistry[a] Impedance Light absorbance	Granulocytes Monocytes Lymphocytes Atypical lymphocytes Eosinophils Basophils Large immature cells
Bayer	Advia 120	Cytochemistry[b] Light scatter	Granulocytes Monocytes Lymphocytes Eosinophils Basophils Large unstained cells[d]
Beckman Coulter	MAXM, STKS, GenS	Impedance Conductivity Light scatter	Granulocytes Monocytes Lymphocytes Eosinophils Basophils
Sysmex	SF-3000	Light scatter	Granulocytes Monocytes Lymphocytes Eosinophils Basophils
Sysmex	SE-9000 SE-9500	Radio frequency Impedance Selective lysing agents	Granulocytes Monocytes Lymphocytes Eosinophils Basophils

[a]Cytochemistry consists of Eosinofix, a specific reagent for staining eosinophil granules.
[b]Cytochemistry consists of peroxidase staining for the detection of granulocytes and monocytes.
[c]Mid range consists predominantly of monocytes but may include small proportions of other cells.
[d]Cells that are peroxidase-negative with cell volume greater than that of normal lymphocytes. This class may include variant lymphocytes, peroxidase-negative dysplastic or immature monocytes, peroxidase-negative granulocytes, and peroxidase-negative blasts.

These instruments offer the advantage of a complete five-part differential with precise monocyte, eosinophil, and basophil measurements. There is a remarkable degree of consistency in the five-part cytochemical differential normal ranges determined in different populations (98–100). The H*1 has shown good correlation with manual reference methods for neutrophils, lymphocytes, monocytes, and eosinophils (101–103) and performs well in recognizing basophils (102,103).

Several studies have examined the precision of the H*1 and H*2 instruments with respect to the total leukocyte count and the leukocyte subclasses (Table 2-12). Precision of the total leukocyte count is excellent even at low levels, and the precision for the infrequent cell classes is superior to that obtainable with manual techniques. The precision in leukopenic patients is important in

the treatment of this group because of the risk associated with profound neutropenia. Kinsey and Watts (104) compared the Technicon H*1 absolute neutrophil count with the routine 100-cell microscopic differential and demonstrated good agreement ($r = 0.9$) for absolute counts ranging from less than 100 to 800/µL. The H*1 instrument has limited sensitivity in detecting band neutrophils through the left shift flagging algorithm (105). For microscopic band counts below 11%, the sensitivity was 76% (106). Prospective evaluation of a group of patients with documented appendicitis using the H*1 differential demonstrated the following sensitivities: 79% in detecting left shift, 82% in detecting absolute neutrophilia, and 91% in detecting leukocytosis (106).

Bentley et al. (107) examined the sensitivity of the routine 100-cell microscopic band count in comparison with a 200-cell

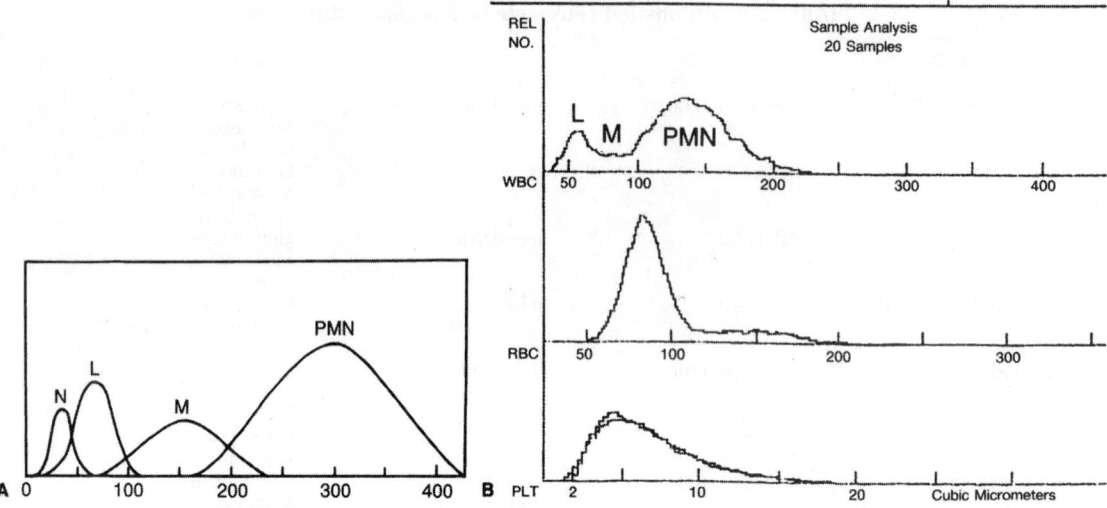

Figure 2-20. Electric impedance red blood cell (RBC) volume, platelet volume, and leukocyte differential distribution. **A:** Schematic representation of the volume distribution of nucleated RBCs (N), lymphocytes (L), mononuclear cells (M), and polymorphonuclear leukocytes (PMN). **B:** An example of the leukocyte differential volume distribution (WBC), RBC volume distribution, and platelet volume distribution (PLT) obtained using the Coulter S Plus IV instrument.

microscopic differential, the H-6000 differential including the HPX flag, and the H*1 differential including the LI and left shift flags in patients with positive blood cultures. The routine microscopic band count had poor sensitivity (30.4%) for detection of bacteremic patients, whereas the automated tests had the following sensitivities: absolute neutrophils, 66.1%; HPX, 61.6%; LI, 49.1%; and left shift flag, 71.4%. The diagnostic sensitivity could be further improved by using pairs of these tests.

Bentley et al. (96) compared the H*2 to the NCCLS leukocyte differential reference method (87) for detecting quantitative and qualitative leukocyte abnormalities (Table 2-13). This instrument appeared similar to the Coulter STKS, Abbott Cell-Dyn 3000, and Sysmex NE-8000 in their study. Fernández-Castro and Viloria (108) investigated the detection of blasts by the H*1 in a pediatric patient population. In their study, all patients with a blast count greater than 5% were detected by morphologic flags on the instrument,

whereas 2.2% (five samples) of samples with less than 5% blasts resulted in no morphologic instrument flag. The cytochemical peroxidase channel also has been useful in distinguishing acute myelogenous leukemias (AMLs) from acute lymphoblastic leukemias (ALLs) (109–111), although traditional slide or flow cytometric methods of MPO detection are necessary for definitive diagnosis.

Volumetric Impedance, Conductivity, and Light Scatter

More recently, a new technology that uses a combination of volumetric impedance, high-frequency electromagnetic energy, and

TABLE 2-10. Three-Part Leukocyte Differential Reference Range[a]

Cell Type	Mean[b]	Lower[c]	Upper[c]
144 normal subjects			
Lymphocyte	2.4	1.2	3.5
Mononuclear	0.4	0.1	0.6
Granulocyte	4.2	1.4	7.0
200 outpatients without hematologic disease[d]			
Lymphocyte		1.1	4.6
Mononuclear[e]		0.3	0.8
Granulocyte[f]		2.3	8.4

[a]Based on data from a normal range study using 144 adult subjects defined as normal by the National Committee for Clinical Laboratory Standards reference method (93) and 200 outpatients without hematologic disease (Duncan KL, Gottfried EL. Utility of the three-part leukocyte differential count. *Am J Clin Pathol* 1987;88:308–313). Each sample was analyzed four times, and the data were averaged.
[b]Values are expressed as absolute numbers of cells ×10⁹/L whole blood.
[c]Lower and upper limits of the normal reference range encompassing 2 standard deviations about the mean are indicated.
[d]The lower and upper limits of the central 95% confidence interval determined by nonparametric methods are indicated.
[e]Monocytes, variant lymphocytes, blasts, progranulocytes, plasma cells, and abnormal lymphocytes.
[f]Mature neutrophils, eosinophils, and basophils.

TABLE 2-11. Specificity and Sensitivity of the Three-Part Differential[a]

Category	Flagged	Unflagged	Total[b]
Abnormal[c]	81.7%[d]	18.3%[e]	229 (23.9%)[f]
Normal	26.3%[g]	73.7%[h]	760 (76.1%)[i]
Total[j]	387	602	989

[a]From a study that examined the ability of the three-part differential to detect morphologic abnormalities. Samples were analyzed using the S Plus IV differential counter and classified as flagged or unflagged using manufacturer criteria. Whether a sample was flagged or unflagged did not indicate whether it was abnormal or normal. Each sample also was examined with a 100-cell or 200-cell microscopic differential.
[b]Total number of samples and relative proportion expressed as a percentage for each category.
[c]Defined by manual 100-cell or 200-cell microscopic differential as containing detectable nucleated erythrocytes, blasts, promyelocytes, lymphoma cells, more than 5% basophils, more than 5% myelocytes, more than 5% metamyelocytes, more than 10% eosinophils, more than 10% reactive lymphocytes. In contrast, normal samples were defined as all other samples, and distributional abnormalities were not used to define normal and abnormal samples.
[d]True-positive samples, a measure of sensitivity.
[e]False-negative samples.
[f]Fraction of abnormal samples, a measure of prevalence.
[g]False-positive samples for morphologic abnormalities.
[h]True-negative samples, a measure of specificity.
[i]Fraction of normal samples.
[j]Total number of samples in each category.
Adapted from Cornbleet J, Kessinger S. Evaluation of Coulter S-Plus three-part differential in population with a high prevalence of abnormalities. *Am J Clin Pathol* 1985;84:620–626.

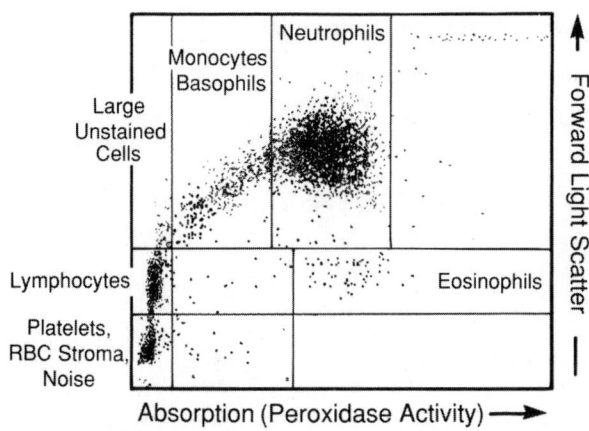

Figure 2-21. Bivariant scatter analysis of five-part cytochemical differential using the Technicon H-6000 instrument. The *y*-axis indicates forward scatter, an index of cell size. The *x*-axis represents peroxidase activity, measured by absorbance. The location of the different cell classes is indicated. Basophils are also counted in a discrete basophil channel, not shown on this diagram. RBC, red blood cell. (Adapted from Breakall ES, Marchand A, Marcus R, et al. Comparison of performance for leukocyte differential counting of the Technicon H-6000 system with a manual reference method using the NCCLS standard. *Blood Cells* 1985;11:257–279.)

light scatter [volume–conductivity–scatter (VCS)] has been introduced to provide a five-part leukocyte differential (Fig. 2-23). This technology is used by the Beckman-Coulter MAXM, STKS, and GenS instruments. Approximately 8000 leukocytes are examined during differential analysis. These instruments use impedance to determine cell volume, a high-frequency electromagnetic probe to determine conductivity, a measure of internal cellular constituents, and median-angle light scatter to determine cell-surface characteristics, morphology, and granulation. Conductivity is particularly useful in distinguishing cells of similar size such as lymphocytes and basophils. Studies with instruments using the VCS system have documented its precision (Table 2-14). Only the basophil measurements consistently had a high CV in comparison with those of the H*1 system. Several studies have investigated the ability of the STKS and GenS to provide screening for leukocyte abnormalities, and the results have been somewhat variable (Table 2-13). In general, the agreement between the instruments and the NCCLS reference method (87) is reasonable. However, with strict definitions of morphologic abnormalities, such as that used by Bentley et al. (96), which included the presence of any degree of neutrophilic left shift or presence of variant lymphocytes, the false-negative rate may be significant. For minor morphologic abnormalities, this discrepancy may have little clinical impact. For the presence of blasts, these instruments

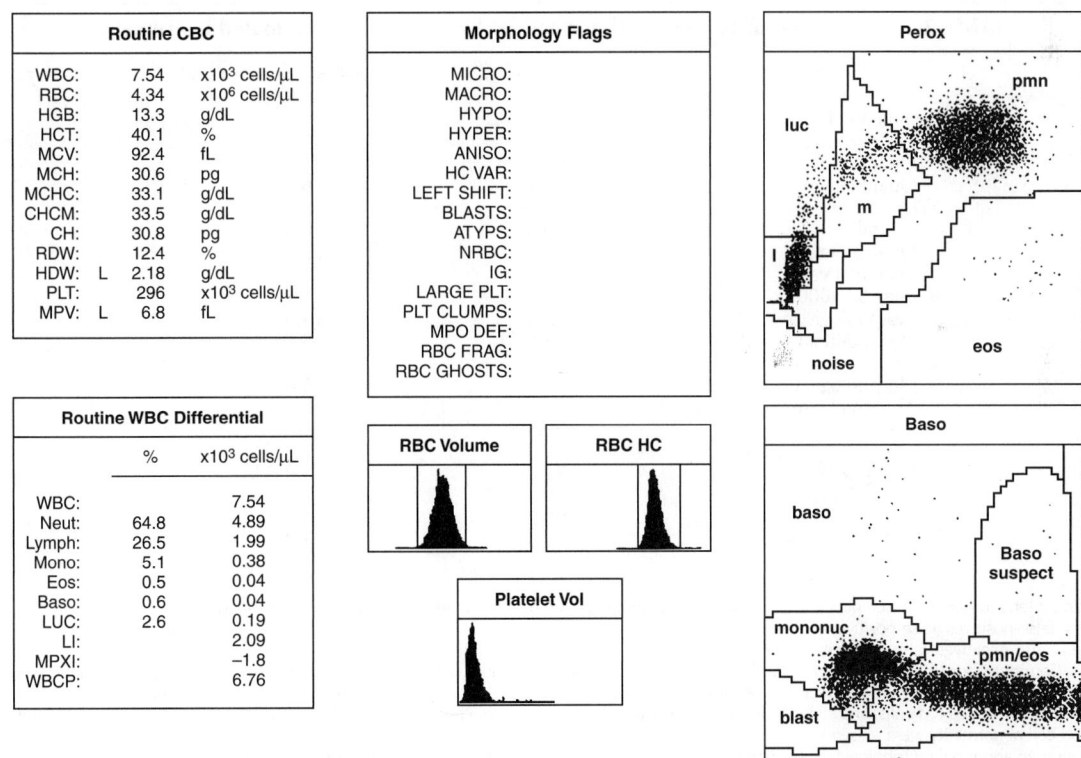

Figure 2-22. Results and histogram display for a complete blood cell count (CBC), platelet (PLT) count, and five-part differential obtained on the Bayer Advia 120 system. Two channels are used to perform the differential: the peroxidase channel (perox) and the basophil channel (baso). The results from both channels are presented as bivariant scatter plots. In the peroxidase channel, the *y*-axis indicates cell size measured by forward light scatter, and the *x*-axis represents peroxidase activity measured by absorbance. In the basophil channel, the *y*-axis represents cell size by forward light scatter, and the *x*-axis represents nuclear lobularity measured by wide-angle light scatter. Respective cell classes are indicated as follows: baso, basophils; eos, eosinophils; l, lymphocytes; luc, large unstained cells; m, monocytes; mononuc, mononuclear cells; and pmn, polymorphonuclear leukocytes. CH, corpuscular hemoglobin content; CHCM, cellular hemoglobin concentration, mean; HCT, hematocrit; HDW, hemoglobin distribution width; HGB, hemoglobin; IG, immature granulocytes; LI, lobularity index; MCH, mean corpuscular hemoglobin; MCHC, mean corpuscular hemoglobin concentration; MCV, mean corpuscular volume; MPO, myeloperoxidase; MPV, mean platelet volume; MPXI, mean peroxidase index; RBC, red blood cell; RDW, red cell distribution width; WBCP, white blood cell peroxidase.

TABLE 2-12. Precision of the Five-Part Cytochemical Leukocyte Differential[a]

Study	Total[b]	Neutrophils	Lymphocytes	Monocytes	Eosinophils	Basophils	LUCs[c]
Kershaw (38)[d]	(2.1) 3.1%[e]	—	—	—	—	—	—
	(7.4) 2.3%	—	—	—	—	—	—
	(26.0) 1.3%	—	—	—	—	—	—
Bollinger (42)[f]	(0.8) 4.9%	—	—	—	—	—	—
	(1.1) 3.2%	—	—	—	—	—	—
	(2.2) 3.2%	—	—	—	—	—	—
	(5.0) 2.1%	—	—	—	—	—	—
	(8.0) 2.1%	—	—	—	—	—	—
	(12.0) 1.8%	—	—	—	—	—	—
	(25.0) 1.5%	—	—	—	—	—	—
	(44.0) 1.0%	—	—	—	—	—	—
Wenz (105)[g]	(12.7) 1.3%	(2.78) 3.7%	(2.12) 1.8%	(0.35) 3.1%	(0.22) 8.2%	(0.05) 16%	(0.15) 11%
Bentley (96)[h]	—	1.27%	1.38%	1.96%	7.62%	6.67%	15.20%

LUCs, large unstained cells.
[a]Absolute cell counts ($\times 10^9$/L) are indicated in parentheses, and the coefficient of variation is expressed as a percentage.
[b]Total leukocyte count ($\times 10^9$/L).
[c]Large unstained cells are defined as peroxidase-negative with cell volume by forward scatter greater than small lymphocytes.
[d]From ten replicate samples within a single run.
[e]Absolute cell counts $\times 10^9$/L are in parentheses.
[f]From 20 replicate determinations within a single run.
[g]From within-run studies; number of replicates not indicated.
[h]Determined by performing 20 replicate analyses on the H*2 using at least three different samples.

TABLE 2-13. Detection of Leukocyte Abnormalities by Flagging on Automated Instruments[a]

Study	Instrument	Agreement (%)	False-Positive Rate (%)[b]	False-Negative Rate (%)[c]
Bentley (96)[d]	Technicon H*2			
	Overall	68.6	35.4	28.2
	Qualitative	62.2	31.7	48.7
	Quantitative	81.2	16.5	22.4
	STKS			
	Overall	70.8	27.8	30.4
	Qualitative	64.3	27.9	49.6
	Quantitative	82.5	13.1	24.6
Buttarello (295)[e]	Sysmex SE-9000			
	Morphologic (n = 337)	75.7	14.5	33.9
	Distributional (n = 280)	89.6	35.1	6.6
Picard (112)[f]	GenS			
	Morphologically normal	73.2	26.8	NA
	Abnormal lymphocytes	80.0	NA	20.0
	Immature granulocytes	96.5	NA	3.5
	Promyelocytes/blasts	96.3	NA	3.7
Vives-Corrons (115)[g]	Cell-Dyn 3500	71.6	33.0	15.0
Fournier (114)[h]	Cell-Dyn 3500			
	Blasts	90.2	9.0	15.0
	Immature granulocytes	75.3	24.0	28.0

NA, not available.
[a]Studies use different criteria to define a discrepancy with the manual method; thus, the results are not directly comparable. See specific criteria as defined below.
[b]False-positive rate = false-positives/(false-positives + true-negatives).
[c]False-negative rate = false-negatives/(false-negatives + true-positives).
[d]Using the National Committee for Clinical Laboratory Standards leukocyte differential procedure as the reference standard (87). A total of 322 samples were analyzed on the Bayer Technicon H*2, and 325 samples were analyzed on the Coulter STKS. Reference manual qualitative abnormalities included: neutrophil left shift and presence of immature granulocytes, blasts, nucleated red cells, and atypical or variant lymphocytes. Samples were considered qualitatively abnormal on the instrument if one or more flags indicating a white blood cell abnormality were present.
[e]Samples were considered abnormal morphologically by manual methods if bands >7%, metamyelocytes or myelocytes >1%, blasts >0%, atypical lymphocytes >4%, or erythroblasts >1%. Samples were considered morphologically abnormal on the Sysmex SE-9000 if differential count was incomplete, there was a generic flag on total white blood cell count or a given subpopulation, or there was a morphologic flag for nucleated cells. Distribution abnormality was considered present if at least one leukocyte subpopulation was outside reference intervals. Of the 58 false-negative morphologic abnormalities in this study, 44 had distributional abnormalities that would have prompted manual slide review. The other 14 cases included five with bands >7%, six with variant lymphocytes >4%, and three with atypical lymphocytes.
[f]Using the National Committee for Clinical Laboratory Standards leukocyte differential procedure as the reference standard (87). Study included 127 samples without morphologic abnormalities, 15 samples with abnormal lymphocytes, 29 samples with immature granulocytes, and 27 samples with promyelocytes/blasts. Samples were considered abnormal by the instrument if any suspect flag was present.
[g]Study included 190 samples. Blood smears were manually classified as abnormal if band >6%, myelocytes or metamyelocytes or promyelocytes >2%, atypical or immature or abnormal lymphocytes >5%, blasts >1%, or nucleated red blood cells >2%. Samples were considered abnormal by the instrument if one or more flags indicating an abnormality of the leukocyte population were positive.
[h]Study based on 439 samples obtained from normal adults, newborns, infants, children, and patients with hematologic disease or solid tumors. Instrument false-positive results were defined by the presence of an analyzer flag indicating the presence of abnormal cells that were not identified by microscopy. Instrument false-negative results were defined by the absence of flags when abnormal cells were identified by microscopy. Reference microscopy was performed by two independent observers to a total count of 400 cells.

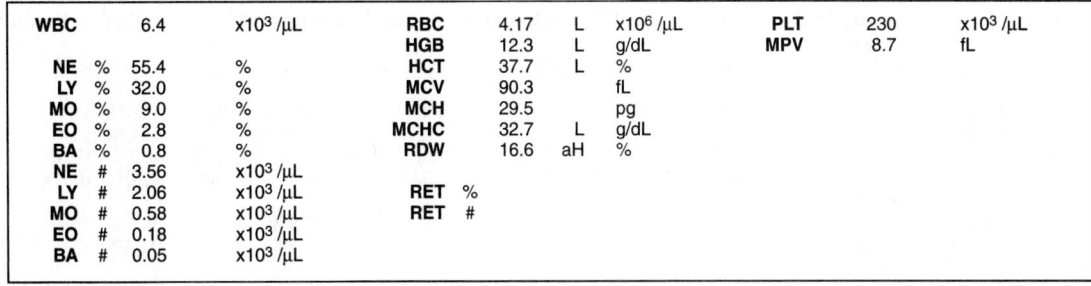

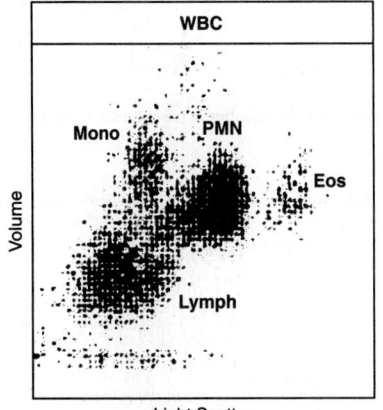

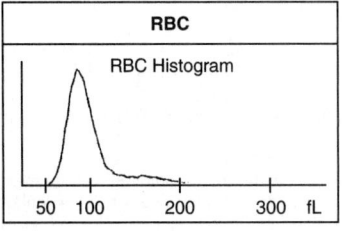

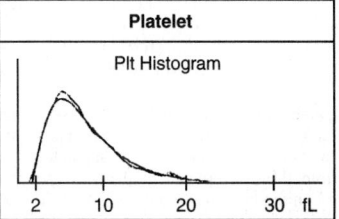

Figure 2-23. Results and histogram display for complete blood cell count, platelet (PLT) count, and differential on the Beckman-Coulter GenS instrument. The white blood cell (WBC) differential is based on volumetric impedance, electromagnetic conductivity, and light scatter. In the two-dimensional display above, the x-axis indicates rotated light scatter, which provides information about cellular complexity. The y-axis indicates cell volume by electric impedance. On the instrument display, a three-dimensional cube may be viewed that includes a z-axis representing electromagnetic conductivity. BA, basophils; Eos, eosinophils; HCT, hematocrit; HGB, hemoglobin; LY, lymphocytes; MCH, mean corpuscular hemoglobin; MCHC, mean corpuscular hemoglobin concentration; MCV, mean corpuscular volume; MO, monocytes; MPV, mean platelet volume; NE, neutrophils; PMN, polymorphonuclear leukocytes; RBC, red blood cell; RDW, red cell distribution width; RET, reticulocytes.

provide acceptable sensitivity. The GenS identified an abnormality in 96.3% of cases with promyelocytes or blasts in the study by Picard et al. (112). The STKS identified more than 90% of AML and ALL cases by generating a blast flag or other leukocyte suspect flag, and 109 (99%) of 110 when other instrument parameters routinely included as criteria for manual slide review, such as cytopenias or increased RDW, were used (113).

The Sysmex NE and SE series (Sysmex Corp. of America, Long Grove, IL) use low-frequency direct current (impedance) and high-frequency or radio frequency energy to perform a five-part differential. The eosinophils and basophils are measured in separate channels using direct current and cell-specific lysing reagents. The SE series (SE-9000 and SE-9500) also includes an immature cell information channel for measuring immature cells. In this channel, detergent reagents result in differential lysis of leukocytes, with mature cells completely lysed, whereas immature cells are only partially lysed based on their degree of immaturity. The immature cell information scatterplot contains regions for left shift, immature granulocytes, and blasts. The precision of the Sysmex SE-9000 is comparable with that of the Beckman-Coulter VCS instruments (Table 2-14), whereas the Bayer Technicon H*1 shows better basophil precision. Data on the ability of the Sysmex SE-9000 to detect abnormal samples appropriately are provided in Table 2-13.

In addition to the combined use of impedance (low-frequency current) and conductivity (high-frequency current or radio frequency) technology, systems based on light scatter alone for leukocyte differential are also available (Abbott Cell-Dyn Series,

Abbott Diagnostics, Abbott Park, IL). The Cell-Dyn 3200, 3500, and 3700 use a small helium–neon laser to evaluate individual cells in a sample stream that is hydrodynamically focused. Four different measurements are obtained to provide a five-part differential: 0-degree light scatter (size), 10-degree light scatter (complexity), 90-degree light scatter (lobularity), and 90-degree depolarized light scatter (granularity). In comparison with the NCCLS manual reference method (87), the Cell-Dyn 3500 provided excellent correlation for enumeration of neutrophils ($r = 0.974$), eosinophils ($r = 0.880$), and lymphocytes ($r = 0.967$) and reasonable correlation for monocytes ($r = 0.628$) and basophils ($r = 0.410$) (114). Other studies have obtained similar results (115,116). In leukopenic samples, correlation with the manual method was excellent for neutrophils ($r = 0.889$), lymphocytes ($r = 0.925$), and monocytes ($r = 0.926$) but somewhat lower for eosinophils ($r = 0.377$) and basophils ($r = 0.346$) (114). The Cell-Dyn 3500 also shows excellent correlation with the Technicon H*2 cytochemical method for classification of neutrophils ($r = 0.989$), lymphocytes ($r = 0.975$), monocytes ($r = 0.811$), and eosinophils ($r = 0.993$) but a lower correlation for basophils ($r = 0.224$) (115). This instrument has precision similar to the Beckman-Coulter and Sysmex instruments (Table 2-14). Data on the instrument's ability to detect abnormal samples appropriately are shown in Table 2-13.

The newest Cell-Dyn instrument, the Cell-Dyn 4000, also uses light scatter, with similar 0-degree, 7-degree, 90-degree, and 90-degree depolarized light scatter measurements to perform the leukocyte differential (Fig. 2-24). The precision is similar to that of other instruments (Table 2-14). The Cell-Dyn 4000

TABLE 2-14. Precision of the Leukocyte Differential Using Impedance, Conductivity, and Light Scatter Methodologies[a]

Study	Instrument	Total	Neutrophils	Lymphocytes	Monocytes	Eosinophils	Basophils
Barnard (296)[b]	Coulter VCS	—	(59.3%) 1.2%	(29.1%) 3.3%	(8.9%) 5.7%	(2.4%) 4.3%	(0.3%) 121.5%
Bentley (96)[c]	STKS	1.67%	0.71%	3.35%	7.55%	43.80%	40.00%
Picard (112)[d]	GenS	(2.35) 1.4%	(60.0%) 1.17%	(29.6%) 2.08%	(8.9%) 1.72%	(0.7%) 12.5%	(0.8%) 12.2%
		(8.83) 1.07%	(66.9%) 0.71%	(26.6%) 1.45%	(4.1%) 6.36%	(2.0%) 10.6%	(0.4%) 21.6%
Buttarello (295)[e]	Sysmex SE-9000						
	Samples overall	—	3.35%	4.25%	7.9%	9.5%	44.2%
	Leukopenic samples	—	5.4%	7.0%	7.7%	16.0%	58.4%
Vives-Corrons (115)[f]	Cell-Dyn 3500						
	Within batch	1.87%	2.14%	4.42%	11.52%	18.70%	32.00%
	Between batch	1.94%	2.14%	4.40%	11.53%	18.80%	32.00%
Grimaldi (297)[g]	Cell-Dyn 4000						
	Within batch	2.44%	1.32%	1.55%	3.80%	3.32%	24.80%
	Between batch	2.47%	1.34%	1.53%	3.93%	4.90%	21.33%

[a]For total leukocyte count, the number in parentheses represents absolute cell counts ($\times 10^9$/L). For the individual cell types, the number in parentheses represents cell proportion in %. The coefficient of variation is expressed as a percentage.
[b]From within-run studies on triplicates of 21 separate samples on the Coulter VCS.
[c]Precision determined by 20 replicate analyses of a single sample on the Beckman Coulter STKS instrument.
[d]Study performed on the Beckman Coulter GenS. Values obtained from two samples, one with a low leukocyte count and one with a normal leukocyte count. Precision determined by ten replicate analyses of each sample.
[e]Imprecision calculated on duplicate analysis on all samples without instrument flags (n = 264) and separately on 35 leukopenic samples.
[f]Imprecision calculated on 20 samples in triplicate run three times.
[g]Based on 20 samples in triplicate in two batches on the same day.

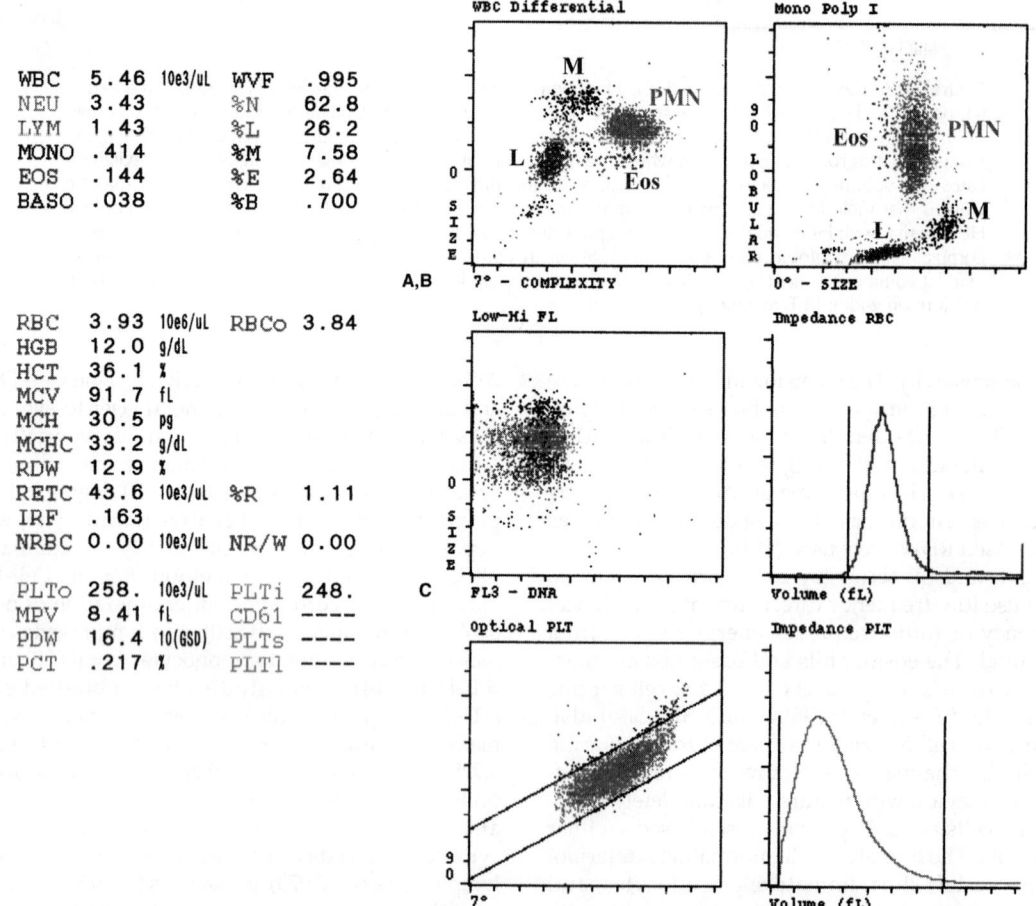

Figure 2-24. Results and histogram display from the Abbott Cell-Dyn 4000. **A,B:** The white blood cell (WBC) differential is based on 0-degree, 7-degree, and 90-degree light scatter characteristics. Cell classes are indicated as follows: Eos, eosinophils; L, lymphocytes; M, monocytes; and PMN, neutrophils. **C:** Histogram plotting cell size (y-axis) and fluorescence due to a DNA binding dye on the x-axis. If nonviable leukocytes or nucleated red cells are present, the cell populations are shifted to the right. BASO, basophils; HCT, hematocrit; HGB, hemoglobin; IRF, immature reticulocyte fraction; MCH, mean corpuscular hemoglobin; MCHC, mean corpuscular hemoglobin concentration; MCV, mean corpuscular volume; MPV, mean platelet volume; PCT, platelet "crit"; PDW, platelet distribution width; PLT, platelet; RBC, red blood cell; RDW, red cell distribution width; RETC, reticulocyte count; WVF, WBC viability fraction. (See Color Fig. 2-24.)

uses an argon ion laser; in addition to the routine light scatter, it has incorporated fluorescent DNA binding dye technology to identify nucleated red cells and nonviable leukocytes. Correlation of the instrument nucleated red blood cell count and manual counts was excellent ($r = 0.984$) (117). Because nucleated red cells can interfere with the total white blood cell count and leukocyte differential, this instrument may provide more accurate data in some patient populations, such as neonates, in whom nucleated red cells are frequently seen.

RETICULOCYTE ENUMERATION

Manual Methods

Enumeration of reticulocytes is the simplest and perhaps best means of evaluating the effectiveness of RBC production. Under conditions of normal hematopoiesis, newly produced RBCs, *reticulocytes*, constitute 1% to 2% of the peripheral RBC population. A common test to determine the concentration of reticulocytes in peripheral blood uses supravital stains to precipitate intracellular RNA, the distinguishing feature of reticulocytes. After staining, thin smears are prepared, and the percentage of reticulocytes in the RBC population is determined by light microscopy. The NCCLS has published a standard in which a reticulocyte is defined as an RBC containing two or more dots of precipitated RNA (118). Normal values for the reticulocyte concentration in adults are reported to be 0.5% to 1.5% (24,000 to 84,000 reticulocytes/µL) (35).

The raw or uncorrected reticulocyte count may be adjusted for the degree of anemia and the degree of reticulocyte immaturity and expressed as the reticulocyte index (119). Correction for the level of anemia is derived from an empiric formula in which the raw reticulocyte count is multiplied by the packed cell volume divided by 45 to provide a corrected reticulocyte percentage (119). This correction also may be performed by determining the absolute number of reticulocytes per microliter of whole blood. This calculation is accomplished by multiplying the reticulocyte percentage by the absolute RBC count. If erythropoiesis is stimulated, the normal reticulocyte maturation time decreases, and the corrected reticulocyte count is again adjusted to correct for the prolonged circulation of immature, or shift, reticulocytes.

Hillman and Finch (119) have described an approximate correction factor of 2 based on an assumed halving of the maturation time with stimulated RBC production. This correction may be more precisely calculated using correction factors based on the assumed lifespan of the reticulocyte reflected in the degree of anemia as measured by the hematocrit or packed cell volume (PCV). For example, with a PCV of 45%, the lifespan is estimated to be 1 day, and no correction is required. With progressive reduction of the PCV, the reticulocyte lifespan in the peripheral circulation is prolonged, and the corrected count is divided by the appropriate factor to provide a corrected reticulocyte index: if the PCV is 35%, divide by 1.5; if the PCV is 25%, divide by 2; if the PCV is 15%, divide by 3.

Typically, 1000 RBCs are examined, and the number of reticulocytes is determined. Alternative methods using field reduction devices have been introduced to shorten counting time (120). Both the precision and the accuracy of this manual technique are suboptimal and have been subjects of considerable study (121,122). Where R is the reticulocyte count expressed as a percentage and N is the number of RBCs counted to determine the reticulocyte count, the 95% confidence interval (CI) for a reticulocyte count can be expressed as follows

$$R \pm 2\sqrt{(R(100-R))/N}$$

Several specific analytic factors that contribute to the imprecision and inaccuracy of the microscopic reticulocyte count have been identified. The most important factors are interobserver variation in identification of reticulocytes and variation in counting techniques. Several studies have examined the precision of reticulocyte counting with overall CVs of 20% to 25% (123–127) and with CVs as high as 46.05% for manual methods with normal-range reticulocyte counts (121) and 70.78% for decreased reticulocyte counts (128).

Automated Methods

Standardization of reticulocyte count specimen preparation and counting techniques have been under study, and significant improvement has been achieved using flow cytometry and automated hematology analyzers. Flow cytometric methods use fluorescent dyes that selectively bind to intracellular RNA present in reticulocytes but not in mature RBCs. Some automated hematology analyzers also use fluorescent RNA binding dyes, whereas others use supravital stains that bind RNA and rely on light absorbance or scatter to quantify the reticulocyte population. These techniques are advantageous because of greater sample size, easier data collection techniques, and improved analytic methods.

Theoretically, the use of a larger sample size with automated reticulocyte enumeration should result in greater precision than that obtained with the manual technique. The 95% CI around an average reticulocyte count may be calculated. For a count of 1% obtained from a manual 1000-cell count, the CI will be 0.4% to 1.6%; thus, with 95% certainty, the true percentage of reticulocytes will lie in this range. For an automated reticulocyte count in which 10,000 cells are counted, the 95% CI will be reduced to 0.8% to 1.2%, with an approximate CV of 20%.

Several fluorescent dyes have been described for use in fluorescent reticulocyte enumeration assays and have been widely used to develop fluorescence-activated flow cytometric reticulocyte enumeration assays: acridine orange (129–131), pyronin Y (132,133), thioflavin T (134–136), cyanine dye $DiOC_1$ (137), ethidium bromide (138,139), thiazole orange (TO) (7,126,127,138–147), and auramine O (124,139,144,146–149). Currently, TO and auramine O are the most commonly used fluorescent dyes. TO is advantageous because it does not require precise incubation times, has an excitation maximum (480 nm) that matches the optimum wavelength of argon lasers (488 nm), and has a higher quantum yield than other reticulocyte dyes when bound to RNA. Auramine O is used in the Sysmex dedicated reticulocyte count flow cytometric systems. The Abbott Cell-Dyn 4000 hematology analyzer and Abx Pentra 120 Retic use a proprietary fluorescent RNA binding dye and a proprietary formulation of thiazole orange, respectively, for reticulocyte enumeration.

Both the normal range for the fluorescent reticulocyte count in adults with normal erythropoiesis and the sensitivity of this technique in patients with abnormal erythropoiesis have been examined. Normal-range data are presented in Table 2-15, with manual and flow cytometric methods showing acceptable correlation ($r > 0.80$) in most studies (124–127,144,146–148). Normal-range data are roughly comparable for the manual and various flow cytometric studies, although the fluorescence techniques generally yield reticulocyte levels that are slightly higher than those observed with the manual technique. The Sysmex flow cytometric systems dedicated to reticulocyte counting generally show a narrower reference range than the other flow cytometry methods, with the reference range similar to that of the manual methods.

In addition to fluorescent methods, supravital staining of RNA has been added to several automated hematology analyzers to enumerate reticulocytes. The Abbott Cell-Dyn 3500 and the Beckman Coulter STKS, MAXM, and GenS use new methylene

TABLE 2-15. Reticulocyte Reference Ranges

Method	Reference Range (%)	Reference Range ×10⁹/L
Manual[a]	—	24.0–84.0
Manual (new methylene blue)[b]	0.40–2.30	NR
Manual (brilliant cresyl blue)[c]	0.35–2.35	16.0–116.0
Sysmex R-1000	0.60–1.85[c]	28.0–85.0[c]
	0.15–1.25[d]	24.6–62.6[d]
Flow cytometry thiazole orange	0.48–2.64[e]	19.7–123.7[e]
	1.6–4.0[f]	NR[f]
	NR	35.0–133.0
Flow cytometry thioflavin T	NR	32.5–133.0
Technicon-Miles H3[c]	0.65–2.3	35.1–112.0
Abbott Cell-Dyn 3500[g]	0.72–2.18	37.7–104.0

NR, not reported.

[a]Data from Morris M, Davey F. *Basic examination of blood: clinical diagnosis and management by laboratory methods*, 19th ed. Philadelphia: WB Saunders, 1996:549–593.

[b]Data from Buttarello M, Bulian P, Pra MD, et al. Reticulocyte quantification by Coulter MAXM VCS (volume, conductivity, light scatter) technology. *Clin Chem* 1996;42:1930–1937.

[c]Data from Buttarello M, Bulian P, Venudo A, et al. Laboratory evaluation of the Miles H.3 automated reticulocyte counter: a comparative study with manual reference method and Sysmex R-1000. *Arch Pathol Lab Med* 1995;119:1141–1148; reference range 95%.

[d]Data from Kojima K, Niri M, Setoguchi K, et al. An automated optoelectronic reticulocyte counter. *Am J Clin Pathol* 1989;92:57–61.

[e]Data from Lofsness KG, Kohnke ML, Geier NA. Evaluation of automated reticulocyte counts and their reliability in the presence of Howell-Jolly bodies. *Am J Clin Pathol* 1994;101:85–90; reference range expressed as mean ± 2 standard deviations.

[f]Data from Davis BH, Bigelow NC. Flow cytometric reticulocyte quantification using thiazole orange provides clinically useful reticulocyte maturity index. *Arch Pathol Lab Med* 1989;113:684–689; reference range expressed as mean ± 2 standard deviations.

[g]Data from Grotto HZ, Vigoritto AC, Noronha JF, et al. Immature reticulocyte fraction as a criterion for marrow engraftment: evaluation of a semi-automated reticulocyte counting method. *Clin Lab Haematol* 1999;21:285–287.

blue staining. Reticulocytes are distinguished from other red cells by light scatter characteristics with the Cell-Dyn 3500 and by VCS characteristics with the Beckman-Coulter instruments. The Technicon-Miles H3 and Bayer Advia use oxazine 750, a basic nucleic acid binding dye, in conjunction with low-angle light scatter (correlated to cell size), high-angle light scatter (correlated to hemoglobin concentration), and light absorbance (correlated to staining intensity) to define the reticulocyte population. The reference ranges for these methods appear similar to those of the fluorescent flow cytometry assays (Table 2-15).

The CV for the automated techniques is superior to the previously published values for the manual technique (121), whether the reticulocyte concentration is low, normal, or high (124,128,135,138,142,146,150,151). Generally, for the automated methods, the CVs are approximately 10% to 20% for a low reticulocyte count, 3% to 16% for a normal count, and 2% to 10% for a high reticulocyte count (124,125,128,139,144,151,152). The sample size of the automated techniques is much greater than that of the manual technique. Therefore, according to the binomial distribution (153), the 95% CI for a reticulocyte count, in which the total number of cells enumerated is 10,000 rather than 1000 as in the manual technique, is narrower.

A study of the normal range of reticulocytes in newborn infants also was performed with the thioflavin T method (134). Previous studies (154) using manual techniques demonstrated that newborn infants have a greater reticulocyte concentration than adults. Fluorescent reticulocyte counts were performed on blood samples obtained 2 hours after birth from 176 newborn infants with normal hematocrits, normal birth weights, 5-minute APGAR scores of 7 or higher, and gestational ages of 38 to 42 weeks. The median reticulocyte concentration for this

TABLE 2-16. Absolute Reticulocyte Concentration Distribution for 176 Normal Newborn Infants Determined by the Thioflavin T Fluorescent Technique

Parameter	Reticulocyte Count[a]
Minimum value	48.0
Maximum value	358.3
Mean value	131.4
Median value	124.9
Geometric mean	125.5

[a]Expressed × 1000/μL whole blood. The interval from 2.5% to 97.5% of the cumulative frequency distribution is 65 × 10³/μL to 230 × 10³/μL.

population was greater than that of the normal adult population, and the range was correspondingly shifted (Table 2-16). The fluorescent reticulocyte count levels were consistent with the previously reported manually determined values during the first 5 days of life in normal, full-term infants (154). The computed range of reticulocytes for healthy full-term newborn infants was 65,000 to 230,000/μL of whole blood using the fluorescence technique.

In another study to examine the effect of sex on reticulocyte levels, the median value for males was 56,500/μL and for females was 49,100/μL. The 95% CI was similar for both sexes. Comparable sex-biased values also were observed using auramine O (K. Fujimoto, *personal communication*, 1990) and TO (126).

The sensitivity of the fluorescent reticulocyte count in states of abnormal erythropoiesis was determined by examining the reticulocyte concentration in blood from patients with clinical evidence of bone marrow failure or in patients with disorders associated with increased RBC destruction with intact bone marrow function (Table 2-17). Patients with bone marrow failure consistently had subnormal reticulocyte levels (138). In contrast, 20 of 24 patients with documented increased RBC destruction had increased reticulocyte levels, and only 4 of 20 had levels within the normal range. These patients may have had ineffective erythropoiesis as well as increased RBC destruction (155).

Several factors that may interfere with the accuracy of flow cytometric reticulocyte counting have been noted. Many of the fluorescent dyes bind nucleic acid nonspecifically and thus stain not only RNA but also DNA. Nucleated red cells and white cells can usually be excluded from analysis based on fluorescence, which is much greater than that of reticulocytes. However, staining of DNA can result in significant interference in asplenic or hyposplenic patients with appreciable numbers of circulating Howell-Jolly bodies (126,156,157), and this interference is

TABLE 2-17. Thioflavin T Fluorescent Reticulocyte Count and Hemoglobin Concentration in Patients with Abnormal Erythropoiesis[a]

Erythropoiesis	Hemoglobin Concentration	Reticulocytes
Decreased	9.3	16.6
Range	7.6–13.1	0.4–42.3
Increased	11.1	241.5
Range	7.8–15.8	99.8–465.4
Normal	14.0	81.3
Range	12.0–16.0	32.5–133.0

[a]The median value for the hemoglobin concentration in g/dL and the reticulocyte concentration × 1000/μL whole blood are indicated. A total of 24 subjects with the clinical diagnosis of decreased red blood cell production and 24 subjects with the clinical diagnosis of increased red blood cell production were evaluated.

roughly proportional to the number of Howell-Jolly bodies present (126). The nucleic acid of intracellular malarial parasites also has been reported to interfere with fluorescence reticulocyte measurement (158). In addition to interference of the reticulocyte count by cells containing DNA, red cells with precipitated hemoglobin (Heinz bodies) may show increased intrinsic autofluorescence compared to normal red cells. This autofluorescence may result in a spuriously elevated reticulocyte count (159,160). Examination of the instrument histogram usually shows a pattern suggesting the presence of an interfering substance, and a manual reticulocyte count can be performed.

Because the intensity of fluorescence, light absorbance, or light scatter as measured by the automated count is proportional to the RNA content, the automated techniques provide information on the maturation stages of reticulocytes in the peripheral circulation (132,142,144–146,161–163). By using fluorescence staining methods, the reticulocyte fractions have been arbitrarily divided into a low-fluorescence reticulocyte fraction, a medium-fluorescence reticulocyte fraction, and a high-fluorescence reticulocyte fraction, with similar categories for methods using light scatter or absorbance to identify reticulocytes. There have been several definitions proposed for the reticulocyte maturity index, including an RNA index or content (143) and the highly immature reticulocyte fraction (145). More recently, the term *immature reticulocyte fraction* (IRF) has been proposed to define reticulocytes with the highest fluorescence intensity (164), and this value is usually calculated using both the high-fluorescence reticulocyte fraction and medium-fluorescence reticulocyte fraction as a fraction of total reticulocytes.

Although studies have used different definitions for immature reticulocytes, most have shown that the immature reticulocyte count is an early indicator of marrow engraftment after transplantation (143,163,165–169) and marrow recovery after intensive chemotherapy for acute leukemia (170,171). The detection of immature reticulocytes usually precedes an absolute neutrophil count of greater than 0.5×10^9/L by several days (143,163,165–169). Newer CBC analyzers can reliably detect neutrophil counts as low as 0.2×10^9/L. Additional studies comparing the IRF to this neutrophil threshold will be useful to determine whether this reticulocyte parameter is an earlier indicator of engraftment or marrow recovery than the neutrophil count alone.

The clinical utility of identifying immature reticulocytes in patients with anemia is not currently well defined. Davis et al. (162) in their series of 413 anemic patients showed only a weak correlation between reticulocyte maturity index and hemoglobin, hematocrit, reticulocyte percentage, and absolute reticulocyte count (ARC), with only slightly stronger correlations with erythropoietin levels ($r^2 = 0.181$) and transferrin receptor levels ($r^2 = 0.191$). Chang and Kass (161) showed a weak correlation of IRF with ARC ($r^2 = 0.18$, $p = .0001$) and reticulocyte production index ($r^2 = 0.15$, $p = .0001$), an index defined before automated reticulocyte counting to account for earlier release of reticulocytes from the marrow in patients with anemia (119,172,173). In their series, specimens with a normal or a subnormal ARC and an IRF less than 0.23 were associated with disorders of decreased erythropoietic activity, such as renal insufficiency. In contrast, samples with normal or subnormal ARC and IRF of 0.23 or higher were associated with various underlying conditions, including acute infection, iron deficiency, sickle cell disease with crisis, pregnancy, human immunodeficiency virus (HIV) infection, and myelodysplastic syndromes. Although these results suggest that the IRF may be useful to discriminate etiologic differences in patients with anemia, the data are currently insufficient to subclassify the etiology of these anemias adequately.

EXAMINATION OF PERIPHERAL BLOOD BY FLOW CYTOMETRIC IMMUNOPHENOTYPING

Rapid progress in the development of flow cytometric immunophenotyping instruments, fluorochromes, and fluorochrome-conjugated monoclonal antibodies directed against blood cell surface antigens has revolutionized the analysis of peripheral blood. The combined use of these technologies is termed *immunophenotypic analysis*, and it has become commonplace in many hematology laboratories. This technology has been used to improve the identification of abnormal cells and to quantify and assess the function of normal cells. The most widespread use has been in the diagnosis of hematopoietic malignancies—lymphoma and leukemia—and in the analysis of cellular constituents of the immune system. Flow cytometric analysis also has been used to measure cellular function (174) and to quantify cellular DNA content (175). The latter application may be useful for identifying neoplastic cells and providing prognostic information about malignant cell populations. These techniques are most useful in conjunction with morphologic and functional analytic methods.

Peripheral blood may be examined using flow cytometric methods based on identification of cell-surface antigens, cytoplasmic or nuclear antigens, internal organelle structure, or DNA content. Greatest use has been made of cell-surface antigen analysis with monoclonal antibodies directed against defined surface proteins. More recently, detection of cytoplasmic and nuclear proteins also has become common practice. The wide array of monoclonal antibodies initially gave rise to a confusing nomenclature, which has been unified under the cluster designation, or CD, system (Table 2-18). To denote surface and cytoplasmic antigen expression, *s* and *c* are frequently used, respectively, before the CD designation (e.g., sCD22, cCD3). Some antibodies are specific for a single cell type or lineage, whereas others may be expressed on several cell types. Combinations of several antibodies are used to improve specificity.

Instrumentation

The current generation of flow cytometric analyzers uses air-cooled argon ion lasers to generate light scatter and fluorescence emission characteristics of individual cells. In some instruments, an additional helium–neon or red diode laser is available, allowing the use of additional fluorochromes. Argon lasers produce excitation at 488 nm, whereas helium–neon and red diode lasers produce excitation at 633 nm. The light scatter characteristics define physical properties of cells, such as cell size determined by forward-angle light scatter, and cytoplasmic complexity (e.g., granulation or vacuolization) determined by side-angle light scatter. These light scatter characteristics are useful in selecting the cell population of interest for further evaluation. Fluorescent DNA binding dyes or fluorescent labeled antibodies are then used to determine DNA content, or antigen expression inside or on the surface of individual cells.

Cells in suspension are aspirated from a sample tube and passed individually through the path of the laser beam. Emitted light from individual cells is given off and passed through a series of filters and dichroic mirrors that isolate defined wavelengths. These light signals are collected by photomultiplier tubes and converted to digital signals for computer analysis (Fig. 2-25). For each individual cell, multiple data points are stored, including forward light scatter (cell size), side-angle light scatter (complexity), and information resulting from excitation of up to four fluorochromes. The resulting data for the entire cell suspension are displayed for a single parameter as a histogram (Fig. 2-26) or for two parameters at a time in a dot plot or contour plot format (Fig. 2-27).

TABLE 2-18. Membrane and Intracellular Antigens Identified by Monoclonal Antibodies[a]

Antigen	Cell Lineage	Neoplasm	Comments
CD1a	Thymocytes, dendritic reticulum cells, Langerhans' cells	Lymphoblastic lymphoma, Langerhans' cell histiocytosis	—
CD2	T, NK	T, NK, some AML	—
CD3	T	T	T receptor, cCD3ε present in NK
CD4	Helper T, M	Lymphoblastic and peripheral T, AML	MHC class II coreceptor
CD5	T, B subset	T, B CLL, mantle cell lymphoma	—
CD7	T, NK, early myeloid	T, NK, some AML	Lost in some mature T tumors (e.g., mycosis fungoides/ATLL)
CD8	Cytotoxic and suppressor T, NK	Cytotoxic and suppressor T, NK	—
CD10	Early B, follicular center B, mature G	B-precursor ALL, follicular center cell lymphoma, Burkitt lymphoma	Common acute lymphoblastic leukemia antigen
CD11c	M, G, NK	Weak on many hematopoietic malignancies, strong on hairy cell leukemia	—
CD13	G, M	Most AML (except M6b and M7), some ALL	—
CD14	M, G weak	Monocytic leukemias	Endotoxin receptor
CD15	G, M	AML, R-S	—
CD16	NK, mature G	NK, mature G	—
CD19	B	Precursor-B lymphoblastic, most B lymphomas	—
CD20	B	B lymphomas, variable or weak in ALL	—
CD21	Mantle and marginal B, FDC	FDC neoplasms, some B tumors	—
CD22	B	Most B lymphomas and precursor-B ALL	Weak surface expression in ALL and CLL
CD23	Act B, Eo, M, FDC	B tumors, moderate expression in CLL	IgE Fc receptor
CD25	Act T, Act B, M, NK	Hairy cell and ATLL	Interleukin-2 receptor
CD30	Act T, Act B	ALCL, R-S, other large cell lymphomas	Growth factor receptor
CD33	G, M	Most AML, may be dim in ALL	—
CD34	Stem cells, endothelial cells	Primitive leukemias	Sialomucin, not lineage-specific
CD36	Plt, M, fetal RBC	AML M-4, M-5, some M-6	GpIIIb
CD38	PC, lymphoid progenitors	Plasma cell tumors, weak in many others	—
CD41	Meg, Plt	AML M-7	GpIIb
CD42b	Meg, Plt	Some AML M-7	GpIb
CD43	T, Act B, G, M, PC	Most CLL and mantle cell, some other low-grade B, AML	Leukosialin
CD45	Panleukocyte	Most hematopoietic malignancies	Leukocyte common antigen
CD45RA	B	Most B malignancies	Not lineage-specific
CD45RO	Memory T, M, G	Most T malignancies	Not lineage-specific
CD55	All hematopoietic	—	Decay accelerating factor useful in PNH
CD56	NK	NK, some AMLs, some MM	NCAM, also present in neuroendocrine tumors
CD57	T subset, NK subset	—	—
CD59	Many hematopoietic cells	—	Membrane inhibitor of reactive lysis, useful in PNH
CD61	Meg, Plt	AML M-7	GpIIIA
CD64	G, M	Monocytic leukemias bright	FcγR1 receptor
CDw65	G, M	Some AMLs	
CD71	E, L precursors, proliferating cells	Many hematopoietic neoplasms	Transferrin receptor
CD79a	B, PC	B lymphomas (cytoplasmic)	—
CD99	Immature L	ALL, Ewing's sarcoma, other childhood small round blue cell tumors	—
CD103	Intraepithelial L	Hairy cell leukemia	—
CD117	Progenitor cells, MC	Many AMLs	c-kit
CD138	PC	MM	—
HLA-DR	B, Act T, M, myeloid precursors	Many AML (except promyelocytic), B-lineage ALL, some T-lineage ALL	MHC class II
MPO	G, M	Many AML	Myeloperoxidase
Terminal deoxynucleotidyl transferase	L precursors	Precursor ALL, some primitive AML	Terminal deoxynucleotidyl transferase
Surface Ig	Mature B	CLL, ALL L3, B lymphomas	—
Cytoplasmic Ig	PC	MM, lymphoplasmacytoid lymphoma	—
Glycophorin A	E, RBC	AML M-6	—
FMC-7	B	B (not CLL)	—

Act B, activated B cell; Act T, activated T cell; ALCL, anaplastic large cell lymphoma; ALL, acute lymphoblastic leukemia; AML, acute myelogenous leukemia; ATLL, adult T-cell leukemia/lymphoma; B, B cell; CLL, chronic lymphocytic leukemia; E, erythroblast; Eo, eosinophil; FDC, follicular dendritic cell; G, granulocyte; Gp, glycoprotein; Ig, immunoglobulin; L, lymphocyte; M, monocyte; MC, mast cell; Meg, megakaryocyte; MHC, major histocompatibility complex; MM, multiple myeloma; MPO, myeloperoxidase; NCAM, neuronal cell adhesion molecule; NK, natural killer cell; PC, plasma cell; Plt, platelet; PNH, paroxysmal nocturnal hemoglobinuria; RBC, red blood cell; R-S, Reed-Sternberg cell; T, T cell; TCR, T cell receptor.

[a]AML subtypes drawn from the French-American-British classification system.

Data from Borowitz M, Silberman M. *Cases in flow cytometry.* Interactive CD-ROM. Charlottesville, VA: Carden Jennings Publishing Co, 1999; and Knowles D. Immunophenotypic markers useful in the diagnosis and classification of hematopoietic neoplasms. In: Knowles D, ed. *Neoplastic hematopathology,* 2nd ed. Philadelphia: Lippincott Williams & Wilkins, 2001:93–226.

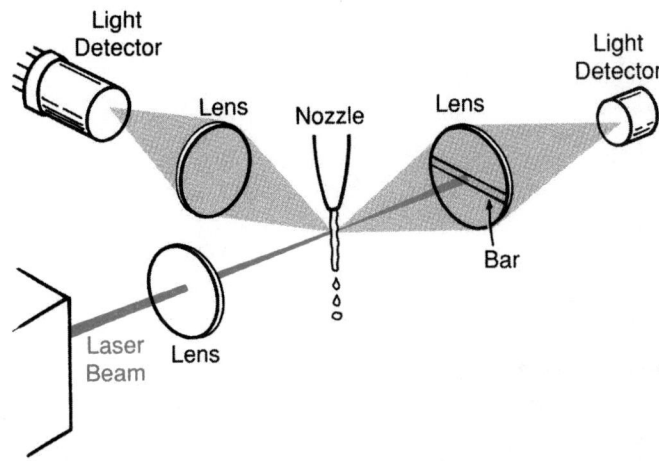

Figure 2-25. Diagram of a fluorescence-activated cell analyzer. A laser beam is focused on a particle stream; a forward scatter, a side scatter, and two fluorescence detectors are available to measure two-color emissions and light scatter.

Defined cell populations of interest may be selected using light scatter or immunophenotypic characteristics in a process known as *gating* (Fig. 2-28). Historically, gating has been performed using forward and side light scatter characteristics. Generally, lymphocytes and blasts have low forward and side light scatter, mono-

cytes high forward scatter and moderate side scatter, and granulocytes moderate to high forward scatter and high side scatter (Fig. 2-28B). Although neoplastic cells may have unique light scatter characteristics, often there is overlap with normal cell populations. Selective gating on cells of interest can be improved in many cases by using a combination of side-angle light scatter and leukocyte common antigen (CD45) expression to gate the cell population of interest (176). Neoplastic hematopoietic cells often have weaker CD45 expression than normal cells; thus, this gating technique may allow better separation of neoplastic cells from the background normal cell population (Fig. 2-28A). Once the patient's disease phenotype is defined, the sensitivity of the technique for detecting minimal residual disease can be enhanced by gating using cell lineage–specific antigens such as CD19 in precursor–B-cell ALL. Within a single-cell suspension, multiple populations may be defined by gating and each population examined for expression of selected cell-surface proteins using fluorochrome-conjugated antibodies. Current flow cytometric techniques most commonly label a cell suspension with three or four antibodies labeled with different fluorochromes, and data are most often expressed in a dot plot format or contour plot format. The use of argon ion lasers is advantageous because multiple fluorochromes with different emission spectra may be excited with 488-nm light.

The fluorescent staining intensity of all cell populations is heterogeneous. An important aspect of this type of cell analysis is determination of the threshold to divide negative from positive events. This determination is frequently accomplished by stain-

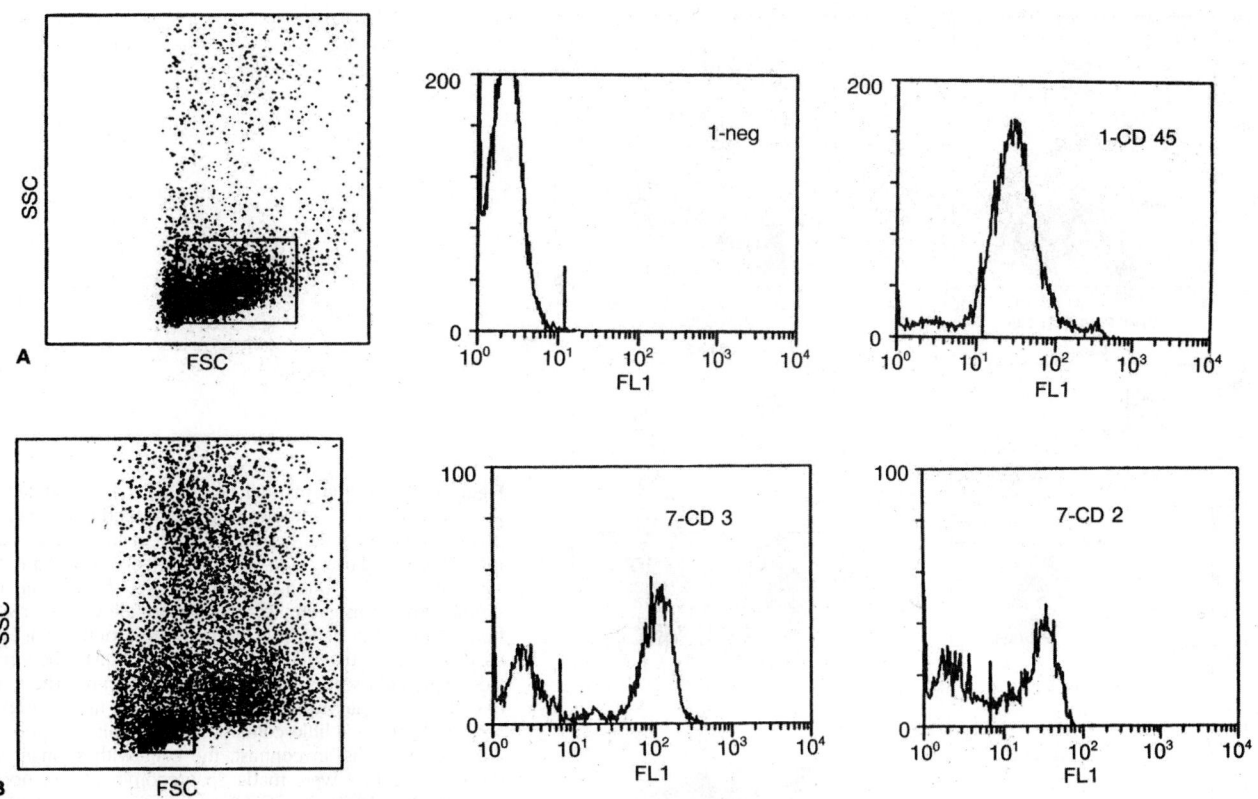

Figure 2-26. Data output from a fluorescence-activated analyzer. **A:** The analysis of peripheral blood from a patient with acute lymphoblastic leukemia. A bivariant dot plot of forward scatter (FSC) versus side scatter (SSC) demonstrates a well-defined blast population outlined by the gating box (*left*). The other panels represent a negatively stained control and a positively stained sample for the CD45 antigen. The vertical line in the negative control sample at the edge of the distribution defines the negative–positive threshold. In the positively stained sample, 95% of the cells lie above the threshold and are defined as positively stained. **B:** An analysis in which a homogeneous blast population could not be well defined. The gating box was set around a presumed abnormal cell population, but subsequent analysis with CD3 and CD2 demonstrates two cell populations.

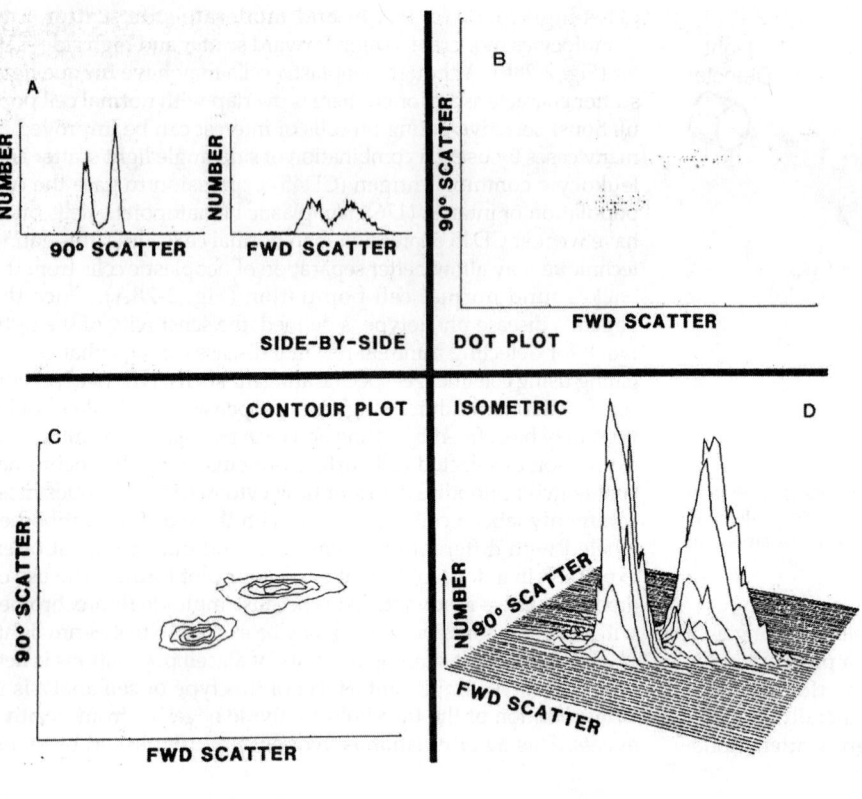

Figure 2-27. Data presentation for two different parameters. **A:** Single-parameter analysis for right angle (90-degree) scatter and forward (FWD) scatter. The data are presented as frequency histograms for each property. **B:** Bivariate analysis of both 90-degree and FWD scatter presented as a dot or scatter plot. Two cell populations are present; one exhibits greater 90-degree scatter and FWD scatter. **C:** Representation of the data from **(B)** as a contour plot. **D:** Representation of the data from **(B)** as an isometric plot so that the cell number in each population can be examined simultaneously.

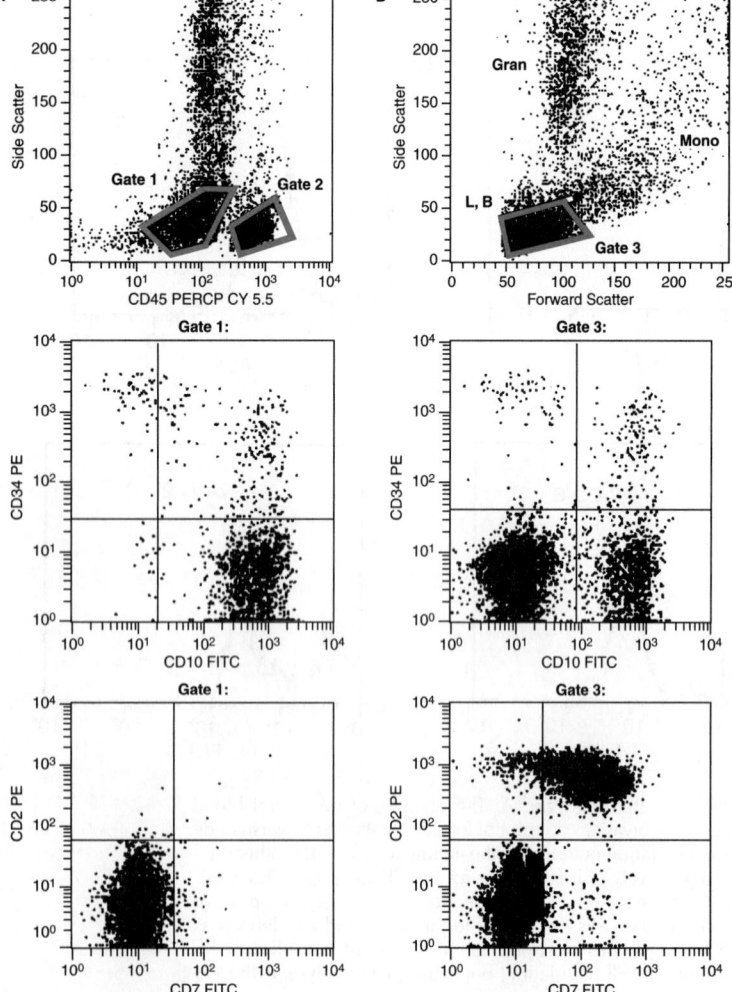

Figure 2-28. Histograms demonstrating gating strategies in flow cytometry. These studies were performed in a patient with precursor–B-cell acute lymphoblastic leukemia (ALL). **A:** Gating is performed using side light scatter (complexity) and CD45 staining intensity. Often, abnormal cells show weak CD45 staining; thus, this gating technique often allows better separation of abnormal cells from normal background cells. In this case of acute leukemia, gate 1 contains blasts showing low side-angle light scatter and weak CD45 staining. The majority of cells in this gate express CD10, a frequent finding in precursor-B ALL. There is little contamination of this cell population with normal cells. In contrast, the cells with stronger CD45 staining in gate 2 were made up predominantly of normal T lymphocytes expressing CD2 and CD7 (data not shown). **B:** Historically, gating has been performed using forward (cell size) and side (complexity) light scatter characteristics. Cell classes are indicated as follows: B, blasts; Gran, granulocytes; L, lymphocytes; Mono, monocytes. In the region where the blast population would be expected (gate 3), there is a mixture of CD10-expressing blasts and normal T lymphocytes expressing CD2 and CD7. FITC, fluorescein isothiocyanate; PE, phycoerythrin; PERCP CY5.5, peridinin chlorophyll protein cyanine 5.5.

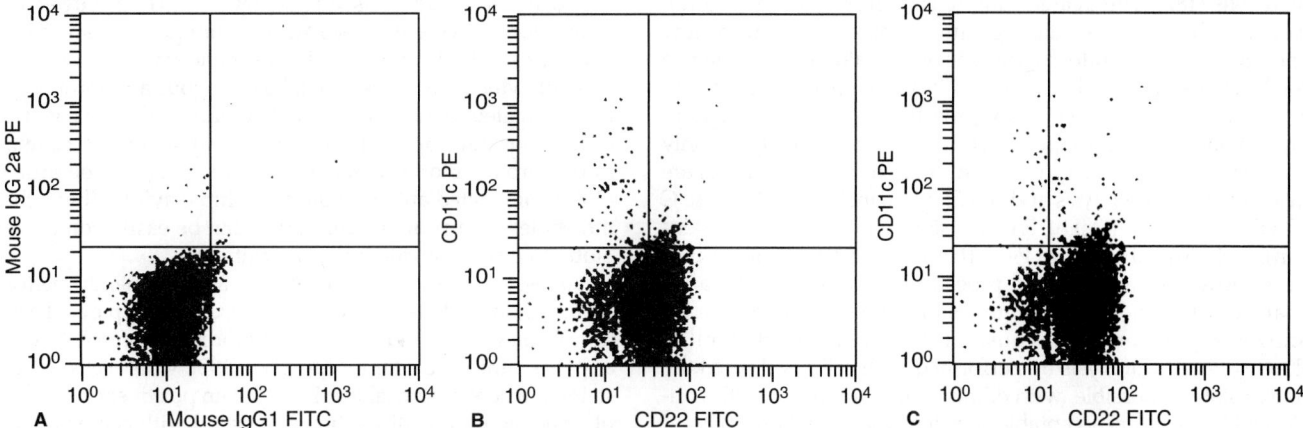

Figure 2-29. Flow cytometry histogram data in acute lymphoblastic leukemia showing weak expression of CD22. **A:** Negative control tube containing mouse immunoglobulin (Ig) G1 and IgG2a subtype antibodies that do not recognize human antigens. **B:** CD22 data (x-axis) showing a slight shift to the right of the population compatible with weak antigen expression. The proportion of cells considered positive with the quadrant marker remaining in the position determined by the negative control is 56%. **C:** The vertical quadrant marker has been moved to delineate the population considered to have weak antigen expression. The proportion of cells now considered positive is 94%. FITC, fluorescein isothiocyanate; PE, phycoerythrin.

ing one aliquot of the cell suspension with an irrelevant antibody (negatively stained) and the other with the antibody of interest (positively stained) (Fig. 2-26). A threshold is set at the upper end of the fluorescent distribution of the negatively stained suspension, and all events with fluorescent intensity beyond that threshold in the positively stained sample are classified as positive events. There is no agreement about a criterion for considering a marker positive; some investigators have used 10% as the critical level (177), whereas others have chosen 20% (178–180). However, there is currently consensus that a strict percent-positive approach is not appropriate for the analysis of neoplasia (181). Percent positive is only informative if the gated cell population includes only cells of interest or if the antigen intensity distribution allows clear separation of positive and negative events. Rather than setting a strict threshold to define positive cells, it is more useful to compare the positively stained sample with the negative control to determine whether there is a cell population that shows a shift in fluorescence intensity (Fig. 2-29). If there is a significant shift in fluorescence intensity, the marker can qualitatively be considered positive. However, if the expression of an antigen is weak, it may be difficult to distinguish weakly positive from negative populations. Most methods rely on arbitrary criteria to make this distinction. Fortunately, interpretation of a flow cytometric study is based rarely on weak positive expression of a single antigen. Sometimes use of a different fluorochrome antibody conjugate may aid in defining the presence of a weakly positive cell population. When antibodies to antigens expressed by normal cells are used to identify a malignant or abnormal cell population, it is important to select the abnormal cell population for analysis carefully. If the abnormal cell population cannot be adequately segregated or identified, successful analysis may not be performed. Immunophenotyping also can be achieved with fluorescent microscopy or immunohistochemistry, but most workers think that flow cytometric techniques are superior (182).

Flow cytometry can examine greater numbers of cells and provide more objective classification criteria than microscopic methods. Flow cytometry is a more sensitive technique to detect infrequent cell subpopulations because large numbers of cells can be examined more rapidly with flow cytometry than with microscopy. Additionally, the capacity to collect data in list mode for subsequent analysis greatly enhances the value and versatility of this technique. The United States–Canadian Consensus recommendations on flow cytometry provide detailed information regarding standardization and validation of laboratory procedures, selection of antibody combinations, data analysis and interpretation, and medical indications (181,183–185).

Sample Preparation

Peripheral blood samples and bone marrow aspirate samples are suitable for immunophenotyping using flow cytometry in conjunction with fluorescent-labeled monoclonal antibodies. Samples are usually collected in EDTA anticoagulant, which provides specimen stability up to 30 hours (186). Heparin or acid citrate dextrose may be used to prolong the stability period of the sample up to 48 hours (186). Blood samples require simple preparatory steps to remove erythrocytes and to stain nucleated cells.

Several approaches are used for the preparation of peripheral blood samples for fluorescence-activated flow cytometric analysis (187). Before sample preparation, air-dried smears should be prepared and stained with polychrome stain to provide a morphologic analysis of the cells in the sample. In addition, a leukocyte count should be performed to facilitate calculation of cell recoveries after preparation. At the completion of all preparative and staining procedures, a cytocentrifuge slide of the final cell suspension should be made so that the morphologic characteristics of the sample can be reviewed.

The preferred method to remove erythrocytes is a red cell lysis procedure, which can be performed before or after staining with monoclonal antibodies (183,187). Whole blood samples may be directly stained with fluorescent reagents, followed by lysis of erythrocytes with buffered ammonium chloride (187) or hypotonic saline. This method is simple and limits the number of tube transfers. If the frequency of abnormal cells is low and large numbers of normal cells remain, data analysis requires highly selective gating to identify the population of interest and to exclude residual normal elements. Excess ammonium chloride must be removed immediately because it produces leukocyte damage with lysis that will affect light scatter and the ability to identify cell subpopulations. In rare cases, a fragile neoplastic cell population may be lost with routine lysis procedures and may require more gentle lysis reagents to preserve cellular integrity. Alternatively, erythrocytes may be lysed first with ammonium chloride, followed by washing and antibody staining of the residual nucleated cells (187). The treated sample is then stained with monoclonal antibodies. After staining, samples may be fixed using low concentrations of paraformaldehyde or formaldehyde to stabilize the labeled antigens. This step permits batch analysis of samples at later times. In addition, this approach allows the use of a preparation and hold technique, in which samples are analyzed only if additional data are required. A number of commercial kits are available for red cell lysis and cell fixation, including OptiLyse C (Coulter), Uti-Lyse (Dako), FACS Lysing solution (Becton Dickinson), and LF-1000 Lyse and Flow (Harlan Sera-Lab, United Kingdom). Any lysis and fixation procedure may alter light scatter characteristics and may sometimes provide variable results for antigen expression (188). Thus, it is recommended that initial flow cytometric analysis be performed with cells as close to the native state as possible, with elimination of erythroid cells considered the minimal acceptable specimen manipulation (183).

A third preparatory method uses partial purification of leukocytes with simple density gradient centrifugation (183,187). Whole blood is diluted with buffer, layered over Ficoll-Hypaque solution (1.077 g/mL), and centrifuged (400g for 30 minutes). During centrifugation, lymphocytes and monocytes collect at the interface, and this mononuclear leukocyte fraction may be isolated. The theory behind density gradient separation assumes that the cells of interest and normal lymphocytes will sediment similarly, an assumption that may not always be true. Thus, multiple layers of the density gradient may need to be evaluated to find the cells of interest (183). Some platelet contamination is present, and the sample must be washed to remove excess Ficoll-Hypaque solution. Other density gradient media systems such as albumin or the convenient Leuco-Prep system also may be used to isolate leukocyte fractions. These isolation methods can sometimes result in selective loss of the cell population of interest (189,190).

If intracellular or nuclear antigens are of interest, cells must also be fixed and permeabilized. Usually fixation with paraformaldehyde (191) is performed after removal of red cells by lysis or by density gradient methods. To detect antigens that may be denatured by cross-linking fixatives such as paraformaldehyde, ethanol or methanol may be used instead. These alcohols also solubilize lipids, resulting in simultaneous cellular permeabilization. Detergents such as Tween-20 or alcohols are used in conjunction with paraformaldehyde to permeabilize cells (191). The concentration of fixation and permeabilization reagents usually needs to be adjusted for the specific antigen of interest. A number of fixation and permeabilization commercial kits are now available, including FACS Brand (Becton Dickinson), Optilyse B (Immunotech), Ortho PermeaFix (Ortho Diagnostic Systems), and Fix & Perm (An der Grub and Caltag).

Cell staining is accomplished with either a single-step direct technique or a two-step indirect method. The direct method uses monoclonal antibodies conjugated to fluorochromes. The most commonly used fluorochromes are FITC and phycoerythrin (PE); the former emits in the green region, and the latter emits in the red region. More recently, with the advent of three-color and four-color flow cytometry, peridinin chlorophyll-A protein, allophycocyanin, and Cy-5 have been used as additional "colors" in the clinical laboratory. FITC, PE, and peridinin chlorophyll-A protein require excitation at 488 nm by an argon laser, whereas allophycocyanin and Cy-5 require excitation at 633 nm by a helium–neon or red diode laser (183). In addition to these single fluorochromes, tandem conjugates of two distinctly different fluorochromes have been developed. These conjugates are comprised of donor and acceptor fluorochromes that rely on transfer of energy such that excitation occurs at 488 nm and results in an emission spectrum greater than 630 nm. The donor fluorochrome is most commonly PE, the acceptor either Texas red or Cy-5. Combinations of these

fluorochromes may be used to achieve two-color, three-color, or four-color analyses. The two-stage technique uses an unlabeled primary antibody followed by a secondary color developing reagent, which may consist of a heterologous antiimmunoglobulin conjugated to a fluorochrome or biotin. If a biotin conjugate is used, color development is achieved with an avidin-conjugated fluorochrome. Biotin conjugates are advantageous because each biotin conjugated antibody binds multiple avidin–fluorochrome molecules, and primary antibodies can be easily conjugated to biotin to provide greater reagent flexibility.

Assessment of sample viability is also frequently performed because nonviable cells may compromise phenotypic analysis. The sample may be stained with a DNA binding fluorescent dye, such as propidium iodide, for this purpose (192). Viable cells will not be stained, whereas nonviable cells will stain positively because cytoplasmic membrane disruption associated with cell death allows entry of the dye. In a sample with poor viability, a DNA binding dye may be used in the same aliquots with cell-surface markers to allow gating, which excludes the nonviable cells.

Immunophenotyping of Acute Leukemia

Immunophenotypic analysis of peripheral blood is frequently used in the diagnosis of suspected acute leukemia. Although bone marrow cell suspensions may be a more homogeneous source of abnormal cells, with sufficient numbers of abnormal cells in the peripheral blood, this material may be useful. Griffin et al. (178) compared the results of immunophenotypic analysis on paired samples of peripheral blood and bone marrow from 31 patients with acute myeloblastic leukemia and observed no major differences in diagnostic sensitivity between these two different sources. Peripheral blood is especially useful when an adequate bone marrow sample cannot be obtained. Although immunophenotypic analysis may be of great value, its usefulness is enhanced when used in conjunction with morphology and cytochemistry.

The cytochemical stains of greatest use are MPO, chloracetate esterase, and butyrate or nonspecific esterase. Morphologic analysis of suspected acute leukemias is enhanced by obtaining a paraffin or plastic-embedded biopsy section on initiation of the workup (193). As the diagnostic evaluation evolves, this material can be used to perform multiple cytochemical and immunohistochemical analyses for comparison with the flow cytometric immunophenotypic results. This option is especially advantageous because the flow cytometric method does not permit individual cell identification. Identification of individual cells is helpful when abnormal cells may be admixed with reactive normal hematopoietic elements. Final interpretation of flow cytometric data is frequently improved by correlation of morphologic and cytochemical information with immunophenotypic analysis.

ACUTE LYMPHOBLASTIC LEUKEMIA

Immunophenotypic analysis has been extensively used to classify suspected lymphoid malignancies, including ALL. If the blasts are MPO-negative, the diagnosis of acute lymphoid leukemia should be strongly entertained, although the lack of peroxidase activity is not conclusive proof of lymphoid lineage. A panel of immunophenotypic markers may be used to confirm lymphoid lineage and then to subclassify the abnormal cells as either T-cell or B-cell lineage. The frequency of lymphoid antigen expression in ALL is provided in Table 2-19. This lineage information may be used to determine therapy and to provide a prognosis.

Stewart et al. (184) in the United States–Canadian Consensus recommendations have outlined the antigens of greatest interest in evaluation of acute leukemias (Table 2-20). These antigens

TABLE 2-19. Lymphoid Antigen Expression in Acute Lymphoblastic Leukemia[a]

Phenotype (Cases, n)[b]	CD2	CD3	CD4	CD5	CD7	CD8	CD10	CD19	CD20	Terminal Deoxynucleotidyl Transferase
Precursor-B cell, adult (132)	1.7	0	0	3	0.9	0	83.7	100	46.8	98
Precursor-B cell, pediatric (39)	0	6	9	0	3	0	92	100	37	97
B cell, adult (5)	0	0	0	0	0	0	75	100	100	0
Precursor-T cell, adult (28)	86	68	30	96	100	54	12	0	0	96
Precursor-T cell, pediatric (6)	100	67	50	100	100	67	20	0	0	50

[a]Expression of each antigen is given in %.
[b]Not all cases were studied for all antigens.
Adapted from Khalidi HS, Chang KL, Medeiros LJ, et al. Acute lymphoblastic leukemia: survey of immunophenotype, French-American-British classification, frequency of myeloid antigen expression, and karyotypic abnormalities in 210 pediatric and adult cases. *Am J Clin Pathol* 1999;111:467–476.

are primarily present on the cell surface, but permeabilization techniques allow evaluation of nuclear and cytoplasmic antigens, such as terminal deoxynucleotidyl transferase (TdT), cCD22, and cCD3, as well.

Immunologic marker studies have resulted in subclassification of B-lineage ALL (194–196) (Table 2-21) in an attempt to define biologically different diseases. This subclassification scheme includes two immature B-cell forms (precursor-B and pre-B) and mature B-cell ALL [French-American-British classification (FAB) L-3]. The latter is uncommon and is distinguished by the presence of surface immunoglobulin and lack of TdT. B-precursor ALL is thought to have a more favorable prognosis in children (194,197) and adults (196), with prognosis worsening as the phenotype matures. However, some studies have failed to document a difference in prognosis between the immature phenotypes (precursor-B and pre-B) (198,199). In some series, the less favorable prognosis of pre-B ALL is attributed to an increased incidence of the t(1;19) translocation (200,201), an unfavorable cytogenetic finding. Although it is accepted that the mature B-cell phenotype should be a separate diagnostic category, subclassification of the immature phenotypes (B-precursor and pre-B) is currently not widely used. The proposed World Health Organization (WHO) classification (202) does not distinguish these immature B-cell subtypes and

includes B-precursor and pre-B in the category of precursor–B-cell lymphoblastic leukemia or lymphoma.

T-lineage ALL must be distinguished from B-lineage ALL for therapeutic and prognostic purposes. Historically, childhood T-lineage ALL has carried a worse prognosis than B-lineage ALL (203–205); however, with newer intensive chemotherapeutic regimens, T-lineage ALL in children has a prognosis similar to B-lineage leukemia (206). Subclassification of T-cell ALL has been attempted, with conflicting results. Some studies in childhood ALL suggest that the less mature phenotypes respond less well to induction chemotherapy (204) and have poorer overall survival (206), although this finding is not universal. At this time, subclassification of T-lineage ALL is not routinely performed. Currently in adults, T-lineage ALL has a better prognosis than B-lineage disease (198,207,208), and expression of six or more T-cell antigens has been associated with longer survival than expression of three or fewer (208).

Individual antigens have also been studied for their relationship with prognosis, but again, results have been conflicting. CD34, a stem cell marker, has been associated with a more favorable prognosis in children with B-lineage ALL (209–211), although a more recent study has failed to confirm this finding (180). The opposite appears true in adult B-lineage ALL, in which CD34 expression has been associated with other adverse clinical prognostic factors (212) and shorter survival (208). The independent significance of this finding is unclear because this phenotypic group includes a higher proportion of patients with unfavorable cytogenetics, namely t(9;22) and t(4;11). The presence of CD10 has been shown to be favorable in ALL overall (199,213), T-lineage ALL (198,203,205,213,214), and childhood B-lineage ALL (215,216). However, if infants younger than 1 year are excluded, CD10 is not predictive of prognosis in childhood B-lineage ALL (180,194,217). The increased incidence of t(4;11) in infants may account for this finding because this cytogenetic abnormality is unfavorable and is associated with CD10 negative disease. Borowitz et al. (180) have shown by quantitative flow cytometry that stronger CD45 and CD20 staining intensity is associated with a poorer outcome in childhood B-precursor ALL independent of previously reported prognostic factors. Although studies suggest that some individual phenotypic markers may aid in prognosis in ALL, the independent prognostic significance of such findings is not yet well established.

In addition to the lymphoid antigens, a subset of lymphoid leukemia cells expresses myeloid antigens, most frequently CD13 or CD33 (Table 2-22). Myeloid antigen expression in adult ALL has been suggested to be associated with a poorer prognosis (179), but with more recent intensive chemotherapy and the effective exclusion of AML M-0 by immunophenotyping, no prognostic difference is seen in ALL coexpressing myeloid antigens in children (218,219) or adults (208).

TABLE 2-20. Cellular Antigens Useful in the Diagnosis and Classification of Acute Leukemia

B Lineage	T Lineage	Myeloid	Other
Core antigens			
CD19	CD2	CD13	CD34 (stem cell)
κ	CD5	CD14	HLA-DR
λ	CD7	CD33	CD10 (common acute lymphoblastic leukemia antigen)
Supplemental antigens			
CD20	CD1a	CD15	CD16
s/cCD22	s/cCD3	CD41	CD38
	CD4	CD42b	CD71
	CD8	CD61	CD117
		CD64	Terminal deoxynucleotidyl transferase
		Myeloperoxidase	
		Glycophorin A	

s/c, surface/cytoplasmic.
Adapted from Stewart CC, Behm FG, Carey JL, et al. U.S.-Canadian Consensus recommendations on the immunophenotypic analysis of hematologic neoplasia by flow cytometry: selection of antibody combinations. *Cytometry* 1997;30:231–235.

TABLE 2-21.   Immunologic Classification of Acute Lymphoblastic Leukemia

Classification	Phenotype	Incidence	Comments
Early pre-B or B-precursor	CD19, CD20$^{-/+}$, CD10, CD34, TdT	60–70% childhood, 50% adults	t(9;22); CD10$^-$ subtype associated with 11q23 rearrangement
Pre-B	CD19, CD20$^{+/-}$, CD10, CD34$^-$, cIgM, Tdt$^{+/-}$	20–25% childhood, 20% of all ALL	—
B cell	CD19, CD20, CD22, CD10$^{+/-}$, CD34$^-$, Tdt$^-$, sIg	2–5% of ALL	Equivalent to Burkitt lymphoma
T cell	CD1, CD2, cCD3, CD5, CD7, dual CD4/CD8, C10$^{+/-}$, CD34$^{-/+}$, Tdt	15% childhood, 25% adult	—

ALL, acute lymphoblastic leukemia; Ig, immunoglobulin; Tdt, terminal deoxynucleotidyl transferase.
Data from Pui CH, Behm FG, Crist WM. Clinical and biologic relevance of immunologic marker studies in childhood acute lymphoblastic leukemia. *Blood* 1993;82:343–362; Jennings CD, Foon KA. Recent advances in flow cytometry: application to the diagnosis of hematologic malignancy. *Blood* 1997;90:2863–2892; and Copelan EA, McGuire EA. The biology and treatment of acute lymphoblastic leukemia in adults. *Blood* 1995;85:1151–1168.

Flow cytometry is also increasingly being used for detection of minimal residual disease in patients with ALL. This technique allows for identification of one neoplastic cell for every 10^2 to 10^4 background cells. Flow cytometry is most useful in this situation when leukemic cells have a phenotype different from normal hematopoietic cells. This difference may be aberrant expression of antigens from other lineages, asynchronous expression of antigens not usually expressed at the same time during normal cellular maturation, or a difference in staining intensity from normal cells. Distinct leukemia-associated immunophenotypes can currently be identified in approximately 90% of ALL cases (220–222) using an extensive multiparameter flow cytometry panel. Minimal residual disease can be detected in nearly all T-cell ALL cases using CD3 or CD5 in conjunction with TdT or CD34. B-cell precursor ALL poses more difficulty because the phenotype in these cases is often similar to that of normal B-cell precursors in the marrow known as *hematogones*. If an extensive antibody panel is used, a leukemia-associated immunophenotype can be identified in 85% of B-cell precursor ALL cases (222). Patients with detectable minimal residual disease by flow cytometry have significantly higher rates of relapse (223–225). Van Dongen et al. (223) in their series of 240 childhood ALL patients tested at various time points demonstrated a relapse rate of 3% to 15% in patients without detectable disease, compared with 39% to 86% in patients in whom minimal disease was identified. Coustan-Smith et al. (224) studied 195 children with ALL for minimal residual disease at the end of induction therapy and at weeks 14, 32, and 56. At all points, detection of residual disease was associated with a higher 5-year incidence of relapse. Relapse rates in those with

detectable disease were 43%, 69%, 86%, and 51% when tested after induction, at week 14, at week 32, and at week 56, respectively, compared with 10%, 10%, 14%, and 12% in those patients without detectable disease. In addition, patients with 1% or more residual leukemic cells at the end of induction, standard-risk ALL patients with 0.1% or more leukemic cells after induction, and patients with 0.1% or more leukemic cells at week 14 had a particularly high relapse rate (72%, 91%, and 83%, respectively). These studies document the utility of flow cytometry for detection of minimal residual disease in ALL. Flow cytometry provides independent prognostic information that may be useful in therapeutic decisions.

ACUTE MYELOID LEUKEMIA

Immunophenotypic analysis also may be used to classify AML in selected cases. Cytochemical stains such as MPO, chloracetate esterase, and butyrate esterase correctly identify the lineage in most cases. In rare circumstances, cytochemical stains may be either negative or inadequate, and immunophenotypic analysis will be of use. Immunophenotyping is particularly useful in minimally differentiated AML (FAB M-0) and acute megakaryoblastic leukemia (FAB M-7).

The presence of MPO can also be determined by flow cytometry using cellular permeabilization techniques. Flow cytometry in this setting is advantageous because the ability to detect the enzyme does not depend on a functional enzyme as in the cytochemical techniques. Nguyen et al. (226) demonstrated concordance with cytochemical methods in 27 of 30 cases. The discordant cases included an AML M-0 and two AML M-5a, all of which were positive for MPO by flow cytometry and negative

TABLE 2-22.   CD45, CD34, HLA-DR, and Nonlymphoid Antigen Expression in Acute Lymphoblastic Leukemia[a]

Phenotype (Cases, n)[b]	CD2	CD11c	CD13	CD14	CD15	CD33	CD36	CD117	CD34	CD56	CD61	Glycophorin A	HLA-DR
Precursor-B cell, adult (132)	87	4	21.3	0	16	30.1	8	0	77.4	0	0	16	97
Precursor-B cell, pediatric (39)	84	0	35	0	22	23	8	0	76	13	0	14	97
B cell, adult (5)	100	0	0	0	0	0	0	0	0	0	0	0	100
T cell, adult (28)	100	0	17	4	14	11	12	0	30	11	12	12	29
T cell, pediatric (6)	100	ND	0	0	0	20	ND	ND	40	ND	ND	ND	40
Total acute lymphoblastic leukemia (210)	88.9	2	23.0	0.5	16.6	25.3	8	0	69.2	6	2	14	87.9

ND, not defined.
[a]Expression of each antigen is given in %.
[b]Not all cases were studied for all antigens.
Adapted from Khalidi HS, Chang KL, Medeiros LJ, et al. Acute lymphoblastic leukemia: survey of immunophenotype, French-American-British classification, frequency of myeloid antigen expression, and karyotypic abnormalities in 210 pediatric and adult cases. *Am J Clin Pathol* 1999;111:467–476.

TABLE 2-23. Proposed World Health Organization Classification of Acute Leukemias

Class	French-American-British Subtype
Precursor–B-cell neoplasm	
Precursor-B lymphoblastic leukemia/lymphoma (precursor–B-cell acute lymphoblastic leukemia)	
Mature (peripheral B-cell) neoplasms	
Burkitt lymphoma/Burkitt leukemia	
Precursor–T-cell neoplasm	
Precursor-T lymphoblastic lymphoma/leukemia (precursor–T-cell acute lymphoblastic leukemia)	
AMLs	
I. AMLs with recurrent cytogenetic translocations	
AML with t(8;21)(q22;q22)	
Acute promyelocytic leukemia [AML with t(15;17)(q22;q11-12) and variants]	AML M-3
AML with abnormal bone marrow eosinophils [inv(16)(p13q22) or t(16;16)(p13;q22)]	
AML with 11q23 (MLL) abnormalities	
II. AML with multilineage dysplasia	
With previous myelodysplastic syndrome	
Without previous myelodysplastic syndrome	
III. AML and myelodysplastic syndrome, therapy-related	
Alkylating agent-related	
Epipodophyllotoxin-related (some may be lymphoid)	
Other types	
IV. AML not otherwise categorized	
AML minimally differentiated	AML M-0
AML without maturation	AML M-1
AML with maturation	AML M-2
Acute myelomonocytic leukemia	AML M-4
Acute monoblastic and monocytic leukemia	AML M-5
Acute erythroid leukemia	AML M-6
Acute megakaryocytic leukemia	AML M-7
Acute basophilic leukemia	
Acute panmyelosis with myelofibrosis	

AML, acute myeloid leukemia.
Adapted from Harris NL, Jaffe ES, Diebold J, et al. The World Health Organization classification of neoplastic diseases of the hematopoietic and lymphoid tissues: report of the Clinical Advisory Committee meeting, Airlie House, Virginia, November, 1997. *Ann Oncol* 1999;10:1419–1432.

TABLE 2-24. Antigen Expression in Acute Myelogenous Leukemia[a]

Antigens	Expression (%)
Nonlymphoid	
CD45	97.2
CD4	48.1
CD11c	87.6
CD13	94.3
CD14	16.0
CD15	74.3
CD33	95.3
CD36	59.0
Glycophorin A	6.7
CD117	64.2
CD56	29.2
CD61	21.2
HLA-DR	84.9
CD34	58.5
Myeloperoxidase	83.0
Lymphoid	
CD2	7.5
CD3	6.7
CD5	4.8
CD7	16.0
CD10	2.9
CD19	9.8
CD20	17.0

[a]A total of 106 cases studied, including 7 M-0, 15 M-1, 21 M-2, 7 M-3, 11 M-4, 5 M-4eos, 3 M-5a, 6 M-5b, 2 M-6, 1 M-7, 17 myelodysplastic syndromes/acute myelogenous leukemia, and 11 acute myelogenous leukemia, not otherwise specified.
Adapted from Khalidi HS, Medeiros LJ, Chang KL, et al. The immunophenotype of adult acute myeloid leukemia: high frequency of lymphoid antigen expression and comparison of immunophenotype, French-American-British classification, and karyotypic abnormalities. *Am J Clin Pathol* 1998;109:211–220.

by cytochemical techniques. This study suggests flow cytometry may be more sensitive in the detection of MPO than cytochemistry. The four ALL cases in their study were negative for MPO, as were 24 cases described by García Vela et al. (227), although other investigators have shown weak MPO positivity in 1 (16.7%) of 6 (228), 6 (20%) of 29 (229), and 7 (70%) of 10 (230) ALL cases. These discrepancies could be caused by the specific reagents used in the various studies.

The WHO has recently proposed a new classification scheme for AML (Table 2-23). In addition to subtypes based on differentiation characteristics as in the FAB system, this classification includes AMLs with recurrent cytogenetic abnormalities, AML with associated multilineage dysplasia, and AML secondary to previous therapy. All these factors have been shown to have prognostic importance. Thus, morphology, clinical characteristics, and cytogenetics also are necessary for classification of AML.

The United States–Canadian Consensus recommendations for antibody selection in evaluation of acute leukemias are listed in Table 2-20. The frequency of nonlymphoid and lymphoid antigen expression in AML is listed in Table 2-24. Based on myeloid antigen expression, only minimally differentiated AML (AML M-0), acute erythroid leukemia (AML M-6), and acute megakaryocytic leukemia (AML M-7) can be reliably classified

by immunophenotypic means. Minimally differentiated AML is negative for MPO and requires phenotypic documentation of the presence of myeloid antigens to distinguish it from ALL. The erythroid component of acute erythroid leukemia is often positive for glycophorin A, whereas acute megakaryocytic leukemia is frequently positive for CD41, CD61, or both. Acute promyelocytic leukemia (AML M-3) is also noted to have a characteristic phenotype, namely positivity for CD13, CD33, or both; CD9 positivity; absent to low expression of CD34; and absent HLA-DR expression. However, Exner et al. (231) recently suggested that the microgranular variant of acute promyelocytic leukemia may be a more phenotypically heterogeneous disease. Although immunophenotyping can provide useful information, morphology and cytochemistry are still essential for diagnosis and subclassification of AML.

Several studies have investigated the prognostic value of immunophenotyping in AML and have shown conflicting results (178,232–243); thus, immunophenotyping is not routinely used in AML for prognostic purposes. Recently, Legrand et al. (244) showed in their series of 177 cases that those cases having a *panmyeloid* phenotype, defined as expression of MPO, CD13, CD33, CDw65, and CD117, have better disease-free survival and overall survival than those expressing fewer than all five antigens. Further studies are necessary to delineate the role of immunophenotyping in prognosis for AML.

Investigations regarding the use of flow cytometry for detection of minimal residual disease in AML are ongoing. Leukemic blasts show aberrant phenotypes in approximately 70% to 85% of cases (245–247), allowing them to be distinguished from normal myeloid blasts in the bone marrow. Unfortunately, the phenotype of AML is often heterogeneous, with several phenotypically distinct blast populations present at diagnosis (245,247), requiring the use of multiple antibody combinations at follow-up. Sievers et al. (248) showed that detection of minimal residual disease in pediatric AML in first remission predicted earlier relapse (median, 153 days versus 413 days), although relapse rates were high in both groups of patients (13 of 14 patients with detectable disease and 9 of 11 without evidence of residual disease). San Miguel et al. (245) investigated minimal residual disease in 53 AML patients using an extensive phenotyping panel and found that greater than 5×10^{-3} residual cells (5 per 1000 normal cells) at first remission predicted a higher rate of relapse, 67%, compared with 20% in patients with fewer than this threshold. At the end of intensification chemotherapy, 69% of patients with greater than 2 $\times 10^{-3}$ leukemic cells relapsed compared with 32% with fewer leukemic cells. In contrast, Venditti et al. (249) in their series of 56 AML patients found no difference in relapse rate when detecting minimal residual disease after induction therapy. In their study, a threshold of 3.5×10^{-4} was most predictive of relapse after consolidation, with 77% with detectable disease levels above this threshold relapsing, compared with 17% below this cut-off. The differences in these studies may be caused by the specific chemotherapeutic regimens used. It appears flow cytometry is useful in detecting minimal residual disease in AML, but the optimal time for testing and level of detectable disease predicting prognosis have not been determined.

Recently, multidrug resistance protein 1 (MDR1, also known as *P-glycoprotein*) has been identified in AML and myelodysplastic syndromes and is associated with chemotherapy resistance to a variety of unrelated agents and a poor prognosis. MDR1 is seen in a higher proportion of elderly patients with AML (71%) (250) in comparison to younger individuals (35%) (251) and may at least partially account for the poor prognosis in this age group. A variety of MDR1 modulators, such as verapamil and cyclosporine A, have been identified that can reverse the MDR1-mediated chemotherapy resistance *in vitro* and *in vivo*; thus, it may be clinically important to recognize leukemias expressing this protein. Flow cytometric methods have been developed to assess the surface expression of MDR1 and functional activity of this protein in AML. Often, three-color immunophenotyping methods using monoclonal antibodies to MDR1, CD34, and CD33 or other leukemia-specific antigens are used to detect the presence of the MDR1 protein on the myeloid blast population (244,250,251). In addition to antigen expression, functional assays have also been developed that, in most cases, correlate with the presence or absence of the protein. However, it has been recognized that some cases with antigen expression may not demonstrate molecule efflux, whereas some cases lacking MDR1 may be positive by functional studies (252), suggesting more than one protein plays a role in this process. In the functional efflux flow cytometric assays, cells are incubated with a fluorescent dye such as $Di(OC)_2$ or rhodamine 123, which is taken up by the cells. Next the cells are resuspended and incubated in fresh dye-free media with or without an MDR1 modulator such as cyclosporin A. Cells are then examined by flow cytometry, with those cells having a functional multidrug resistance protein extruding the dye and showing a lesser degree of fluorescence. Comparison of cells incubated with and without the MDR1 modulator allows determination of a functional drug resistance protein. Most studies have shown a correlation of both MDR1 expression and function with a poor outcome in AML and myelodysplastic syndromes (250,251,253,254), although some studies have failed to demonstrate that protein expression alone is a sufficient prognostic indicator (244). Other drug resistance proteins have also been identified, including multidrug resistance–associated protein 1 and lung resistance protein, but these proteins may not be significant predictors of patient outcome (251); further studies are necessary to elucidate their role in drug resistance in AML.

TABLE 2-25. Scoring System for the Definition of Biphenotypic Acute Leukemias[a]

Points	B Lineage	T Lineage	Myeloid Lineage
2	CD79a	CD3(c/s)	Antimyeloperoxidase (antilysozyme)[b]
	cIgM	Anti–T-cell receptor	
	cCD22		
1	CD19	CD2	CD13
	CD10	CD5	CD33
	CD20	CD8	CDw65
		CD10	
0.5	TdT	TdT	CD14
	CD24	CD7	CD15
		CD1a	CD64
			CD117

c, cytoplasmic; IgM, immunoglobulin M; s, surface; TdT, terminal deoxynucleotidyl transferase.
[a]Biphenotypic acute leukemia is defined by scores greater than 2 for the myeloid and one lymphoid lineage.
[b]Specificity being assessed.
Adapted from Bene MC, Castoldi G, Knapp W, et al. Proposals for the immunological classification of acute leukemias. European Group for the Immunological Characterization of Leukemias (EGIL). *Leukemia* 1995;9:1783–1786.

MIXED LINEAGE ACUTE LEUKEMIA

Rarely, acute leukemia cells express sufficient characteristics of more than one cell lineage, suggesting that the blasts are derived from more than one lineage. Such cases are frequently referred to as *mixed lineage* or *biphenotypic leukemias*. A number of scoring systems have been developed to unify the diagnostic criteria for this diagnosis, although no single scheme is universally used at this time. Most of the systems give different levels of lineage importance to a variety of commonly studied antigens, with the most lineage-specific carrying the most weight. One such system, proposed by the European Group for the Immunological Characterization of Leukemias (255), is shown in Table 2-25.

CHRONIC MYELOGENOUS LEUKEMIA, ACCELERATED PHASE, AND BLAST CRISIS

During the accelerated and blast crisis phases of CML, the peripheral blood contains increased numbers of blast cells. If these cells are present in sufficient numbers, they may be classified using immunophenotypic analysis. CML is a stem cell disorder, and accelerated phase or blast crisis may be of myeloid or precursor-B lymphoid lineage. Staining for MPO is useful in diagnosis of myeloid blast crisis, but MPO is detected by cytochemical methods in only 33% to 40% of myeloid blast crises. Thus, immunophenotyping by flow cytometry is required in a significant proportion of cases to document cell lineage. The incidence of myeloid and precursor–B-cell blast crisis has been reported in several studies (256–258). Myeloid blast crisis accounts for approximately 50% to 65% of cases, whereas precursor-B lineage is noted in 20% to 35% of cases. In addition, mixed lineage blast crisis is seen in approximately 10% of cases (257). Immunophenotypic classification may be helpful in detection of lymphoid blast crisis that appears to be more responsive to therapy than other forms, and this information may aid in decisions about bone marrow transplantation.

Chronic Leukemia and Lymphoma

When sufficient numbers of abnormal cells are present in the peripheral blood, flow cytometric immunophenotypic analysis may be of benefit in diagnosis (Table 2-26). The United States–Canadian Consensus recommendations for antibody selection in

TABLE 2-26. B-Cell Lymphoproliferative Disorders

Disorder	sIg	cIg	DR	CD5	CD10	CD19	CD20	CD22	CD23	CD11c	CD25	CD43	FMC7	Comments
CLL/SLL	Weak IgM and IgD	−/+	+	+	−	+	+ weak	− to weak	+	+/−	+/−	+	−	CD23⁻ in 10%
LPL	Usu IgM	+	−	−	−	+	+	+	−	−/+	−/+	+/−	+	
MCL	Mod IgM > IgD	+	+	+	−	+	+	+	−	−	−	+	+	CD23⁺ in 15%
FCL	Bright IgM +/− IgD>IgG >IgA	−	+	−	+/−	+	+	+	+/−	−	−	−	+	
MZL and associ- ated lym- phomas	Mod IgM > IgG > IgA	+ (40 %)	+	−	−	+	+	+	−	+/−	−	−/+	+	CD103⁻; SLVL: CD25⁻/⁺
HCL	IgM +/− IgM, IgD, or IgA	−	+	−	−	+	+	+	−	+	+	NR	+	CD103⁺

CLL/SLL, chronic lymphocytic leukemia/small lymphocytic lymphoma; DR, HLA-DR; FCL, follicular lymphoma; HCL, hairy cell leukemia; Ig, immunoglobulin; LPL, lymphoplasma-cytic lymphoma; MCL, mantle cell lymphoma; Mod, moderate; MZL, marginal zone lymphoma; NR, not reported; SLVL, splenic lymphoma with villous lymphocytes; Usu, usually. See references 195, 260, and 302.

lymphoproliferative diseases are listed in Table 2-27. Disorders with sufficient numbers of abnormal cells in the peripheral blood include those that typically present as leukemia, such as chronic lymphocytic leukemia and hairy cell leukemia, as well as a number of low-grade to intermediate-grade lymphomas that frequently demonstrate peripheral blood involvement. A positive flow cytometric study in peripheral blood has been shown to correlate with bone marrow involvement in the low-grade lymphomas (259). The scope of this chapter does not allow discussion of all lymphoproliferative disorders and focuses on those entities in which phenotyping of peripheral blood is most often useful.

Immunophenotypic analysis is usually not necessary for providing either a diagnosis or a prognosis for patients with chronic lymphocytic leukemia (CLL). Generally, the diagnosis of CLL is based on the clinical findings, persistent lymphocytosis, and characteristic cellular morphology. The cells of CLL are usually small, mature lymphocytes with round nuclei, coarse nuclear chromatin, scant cytoplasm, and inconspicuous nucleoli. Prolymphocytes are usually also present but account for less

TABLE 2-27. Antigens Useful in the Identification and Classification of Lymphoproliferative Disease in Blood and Bone Marrow

Core	Supplemental
CD3	CD2
CD4	CD11c
CD5	CD16
CD7	CD22
CD8	CD23
CD10	CD25
CD19	CD56
CD20	CD57
CD45	CD38
κ	FMC7
λ	BB4
	TCRαβ
	TCRγδ

TCR, T-cell receptor.
Adapted from Stewart CC, Behm FG, Carey JL, et al. U.S.-Canadian Consensus recommendations on the immunophenotypic analysis of hematologic neoplasia by flow cytometry: selection of antibody combinations. *Cytometry* 1997;30:231–235.

than 10% of lymphocytes. Flow immunophenotyping is most useful in cases with an atypical clinical presentation or unusual cellular morphology to distinguish CLL from other lymphoproliferative disorders presenting with peripheral blood involvement. The abnormal lymphocytes of CLL exhibit low-intensity surface IgD or IgM, surface light-chain restriction, and concomitant anomalous expression of CD5 and B-cell–associated antigens (CD19, CD20, CD79a, and CD43) (195,260,261). CLL can usually be distinguished from mantle cell lymphoma, the other B-cell lymphoproliferative disorder that characteristically expresses CD5, by weaker surface immunoglobulin expression, the presence of CD23, and the lack of FMC7 expression (261,262). In addition, cyclin D1 expression can be identified in mantle cell lymphoma by immunohistochemistry, whereas only rare cases of CLL show expression of this protein (263).

In contrast to CLL, *de novo* B-lineage prolymphocytic leukemia (PLL) is characterized by strong expression of surface immunoglobulin staining, absent expression of CD5, and expression of CD22. The cells in PLL also have a lower nuclear to cytoplasmic ratio, with finer nuclear chromatin and prominent nucleoli. *De novo* PLL may be difficult to distinguish from prolymphocytic transformation of CLL if appropriate clinical history is not available. In prolymphocytic transformation of CLL, the cells may have phenotypic characteristics similar to those of CLL, such as CD5 expression and weak sIg (195), but the distinction can be made in most cases based on morphology.

Lymphoplasmacytic lymphoma is a partially differentiated B-cell neoplasm associated with the clinical syndrome of Waldenström's macroglobulinemia. Morphologically, this neoplasm consists of small lymphocytes, plasmacytoid lymphocytes, and plasma cells. Plasmacytoid differentiation is also seen in other B-cell lymphoproliferative disorders, including CLL, mantle cell lymphoma, follicular lymphoma, and marginal zone lymphomas. It is currently recommended that such cases be classified according to their major features, with the term *lymphoplasmacytic lymphoma* reserved for cases without features of these other lymphoproliferative disorders (260). Lymphoplasmacytic lymphoma expresses surface and cytoplasmic immunoglobulin, usually of the IgM type, and the B-cell markers CD19, CD20, CD22, and CD79a; in contrast with CLL, it is negative for CD5. In some cases, expression of CD38, an antigen present on plasma cells, is also seen (261).

Multiple myeloma may be associated rarely with significant numbers of circulating plasma cells, in which case it is referred to as *plasma cell leukemia*. Generally, the diagnosis of plasma cell leukemia is made if plasma cells account for more than 20% of circulating white cells or their absolute number is greater than $2 \times 10^9/L$. Plasma cells represent terminal differentiation of B cells and at this stage usually show weak or absent expression of leukocyte common antigen (CD45) and have lost the pan–B-cell markers CD19, CD20, and CD22, although in some cases, CD19 (195) or CD79a (260) may be present. Plasma cells do not express surface immunoglobulin, although cytoplasmic immunoglobulin is present and can be detected by flow cytometry using cellular permeabilization techniques. CD38 is a useful antigen for detection of normal and neoplastic plasma cells, but one must be cautious in interpretation of this antigen as it is nonspecific and may be seen on other tumors. Thus, it is most useful when correlated with morphology. CD56 also is useful in evaluation of plasma cells, as it is not present on normal plasma cells but is seen in more than half the cases of multiple myeloma (195,260).

Hairy cell leukemia is an uncommon B-cell lymphoproliferative disorder characterized by pancytopenia, splenomegaly, and bone marrow infiltration. Circulating cells are seen that are small to medium in size with an oval nucleus, slightly open nuclear chromatin, and abundant pale cytoplasm with cytoplasmic projections on smear preparations. In some cases, only a few neoplastic cells are present in the peripheral blood, making a morphologic diagnosis difficult. TRAP staining is a useful morphologic tool because it is usually positive in hairy cell leukemia. However, this stain is technically difficult and may be negative in rare cases. In addition, TRAP positivity has been documented in rare cases of other lymphoproliferative disorders (32). Flow cytometric immunophenotyping is useful because hairy cell leukemia demonstrates a characteristic phenotype, namely a light-chain–restricted B cell with strong expression of CD11c and CD25, the interleukin-2 receptor (264,265), and expression of CD103, the mucosal lymphocyte antigen. CD103 appears to be the most useful marker in distinguishing hairy cell leukemia from other B-lineage leukemias (195,260,265,266). Expression of single antigens is not specific for the diagnosis of hairy cell leukemia, and caution should be exercised when interpreting phenotypic results. However, the aggregate phenotype of antigen expression in conjunction with morphologic findings allows a diagnosis of hairy cell leukemia in most cases. However, the hairy cell leukemia variant subgroup and splenic marginal zone lymphoma, in particular splenic lymphoma with villous lymphocytes, share some morphologic and immunophenotypic characteristics with hairy cell leukemia and should be considered in the differential diagnosis. In contrast with typical hairy cell leukemia, the hairy cell variant usually presents with leukocytosis characterized by circulating lymphocytes with prominent nucleoli and cells lacking expression of CD25 (267,268).

Splenic marginal zone lymphoma with and without villous lymphocytes is a distinct form of lymphoma that differs morphologically and clinically from extranodal marginal zone lymphoma of the mucosa-associated lymphoid tissue type and from nodal marginal zone lymphoma. Patients with splenic marginal zone lymphoma have splenomegaly with bone marrow and peripheral blood involvement but usually lack lymphadenopathy. Splenic marginal zone lymphoma with villous lymphocytes may resemble hairy cell leukemia morphologically and immunophenotypically, with approximately one-half of cases expressing CD11c and 25% expressing CD25 (269). Few cases express all three antigens (CD11c, CD25, CD103) typically seen in hairy cell leukemia (269,270).

Follicular lymphomas usually present with diffuse lymphadenopathy, but bone marrow involvement is common, and occasionally circulating cells are identified in the peripheral blood. These B-cell lymphomas are made up of centrocytes (cleaved follicle center cells) and centroblasts (large noncleaved cells). The cells circulating in the peripheral blood are most often centrocytes, which are small with scant cytoplasm, coarse chromatin, nuclear indentations, and inconspicuous nucleoli. Phenotypically, the neoplastic cells express light-chain–restricted surface immunoglobulin and pan–B-cell markers with coexpression of CD10 in approximately 60% of cases (265).

Flow cytometric immunophenotyping also is useful in the T-cell and natural killer (NK)-cell leukemias and lymphomas (Table 2-28). Unfortunately, a clonal marker equivalent to light-chain restriction in B-cell processes is not available for evaluation by flow cytometry in these malignancies. Diagnosis of malignancy is dependent on morphologic findings or the documentation of antigen expression patterns not seen in normal cells. In T-cell malignancies, clonal rearrangements of the T-cell receptor (TCR) can often be demonstrated by molecular methods, but no similar clonal marker is available at this time for the evaluation of NK-cell populations. Several T-cell and NK-cell malignancies show peripheral blood involvement. These disorders, by WHO classification, include T-cell prolymphocytic leukemia, T-cell granular lymphocytic leukemia, aggressive NK-cell leukemia, mycosis fungoides/Sézary's syndrome, adult T-cell lymphoma or leukemia, and hepatosplenic γδ T-cell lymphoma.

The morphologic features of these T-cell and NK-cell malignancies show significant overlap, and immunophenotyping is necessary to distinguish T-cell from NK-cell lineage, a distinction which has prognostic importance. The confirmation of T-cell lineage requires demonstration of surface CD3 (the TCR) or a clonal TCR gene rearrangement by molecular methods. Other phenotypic features may be similar. For example, T and NK cells both express CD2 and CD7, and T-cell malignancies may coexpress NK-associated antigens such as CD16, CD56, and CD57. In addition, NK-cell neoplasms may express the ε-chain

TABLE 2-28. Selected T-Cell and Natural Killer–Cell Lymphoproliferative Disorders

Disorder	CD2	sCD3	CD4	CD5	CD7	CD8	CD25	CD16	CD56	CD57	Comments
T-PLL	+	+	+	+	+	−	−	−	−	NR	~20% CD4+CD8+, rare CD8+
LGL-T	+	+	−	−	−	+	−	+	−	+/−	—
Aggressive natural killer leukemia	+	−	−	NR	NR	+/−	−	+	+/−	−	Epstein-Barr virus + in some cases
Mycosis fungoides/SS	+	+	+	+	−/+	−	−	−	−	NR	One third CD7+, rare CD25+
Adult T-cell leukemia/ lymphoma	+	+	+	+	−	−	+	−	−	NR	Rare CD8+
HS γδ T-cell lymphoma	+	+	−	−/+	−/+	−/+	—	+/−	+/−	−	—

HS, hepatosplenic; LGL-T, large granular lymphocytic leukemia, T cell; NR, not reported; SS, Sézary's syndrome; T-PLL, T cell prolymphocytic leukemia.
See references 195, 260, and 302.

of CD3 in the cytoplasm, which can be detected by immunohistochemistry on paraffin-embedded tissue.

Proliferation of large granular lymphocytes may be of either T-cell or NK-cell lineage. T-cell granular lymphocytic leukemia is more common, representing approximately 85% of cases (271). This disease is seen most often in the elderly, presents with infections related to neutropenia, and is associated with rheumatoid arthritis in 25% of cases (271). The abnormal cell phenotype is that of a cytotoxic T-cell with expression of the NK-associated antigens CD16 and CD57, and the diagnosis is established by demonstrating a TCR gene rearrangement. However, oligoclonal expansions of cells with a similar phenotype may be seen in normal individuals (271). NK-lineage proliferations of large granular lymphocytes can be divided into two categories: aggressive NK-cell leukemia and chronic NK lymphocytosis, an entity that likely represents a reactive process. In comparison with T-cell granular lymphocytic leukemia, aggressive NK-cell leukemia may show more morphologic atypia (272) and in some cases is associated with Epstein-Barr virus infection (271,272). Aggressive NK-cell leukemia differs from T-cell granular lymphocytic leukemia in that it lacks surface CD3 and typically expresses CD16 and CD56 and lacks CD57 (195,271).

Mycosis fungoides/Sézary's syndrome is a T-cell neoplasm with skin infiltration and variable peripheral blood involvement. The neoplastic cells are characterized by marked nuclear irregularity with a cerebriform appearance. In the past, this morphologic feature was the cornerstone for diagnosis, with morphologic techniques developed to detect this characteristic (273). More recently, flow cytometry has been used to examine peripheral blood in patients with cutaneous mycosis fungoides. The usual phenotype is that of a T-helper lymphocyte expressing CD4, with approximately two-thirds of cases lacking CD7 (260). A normal subset of T-helper lymphocytes has a similar phenotype, and caution must be exercised in interpreting phenotypic results. In our laboratory, T-helper lymphocytes (CD4+) lacking CD7 may represent up to 13% of total lymphocytes in normal individuals. In ambiguous cases, demonstration of a clonal TCR rearrangement by molecular methods may be useful. Adult T-cell lymphoma/leukemia, a disorder associated with human T-cell leukemia virus type 1 infection, is also made up of lymphocytes with nuclear irregularities and a T-helper phenotype lacking CD7. Most cases of adult T-cell lymphoma/leukemia express intense CD25, whereas only rare cases of mycosis fungoides/Sézary's syndrome express this antigen.

Hepatosplenic γδ T-cell lymphoma usually presents in young adults, with a male predominance, marked hepatosplenomegaly, systemic symptoms, and pancytopenia. Lymphadenopathy is rare, and peripheral blood involvement is seen in some cases. This lymphoma is comprised of a monotonous population of medium-size cells that infiltrate liver, spleen, and bone marrow in a sinusoidal pattern. In contrast with most other T-cell malignancies, most cases of hepatosplenic T-cell lymphoma express the γδ TCR, although recently, cases expressing the αβ TCR have also been described (274). By flow cytometry, most cases express the T-cell antigens CD2, CD3, and CD7 and are negative for CD4, CD5, and CD8. In addition, the NK-cell markers CD16 and CD56 are frequently expressed, whereas CD57 is usually absent (275).

Paroxysmal Nocturnal Hemoglobinuria

Paroxysmal nocturnal hemoglobinuria (PNH) is a hematopoietic stem cell disorder characterized by complement-mediated hemolytic anemia, thrombosis, and bone marrow failure. The stem cells of PNH have a mutation in the pig-a gene, resulting in a deficiency of a glycophosphatidylinositol (GPI) anchor protein that attaches many proteins to the cell membrane. Red cells show increased susceptibility to complement-mediated lysis due to

loss of decay accelerating factor (CD55) and membrane inhibitor of reactive lysis (CD59). A number of other cell-surface antigens also are lost, including the endotoxin receptor (CD14) and CD16.

The Ham test, or sucrose lysis test, was used in the past to make a diagnosis of PNH. However, the absence of cell-surface proteins on the red cells of these patients makes flow cytometry an ideal diagnostic tool. Flow cytometry is commonly used to evaluate CD55 and CD59 on red blood cells. Red cells are most often gated by forward and side light scatter characteristics. Usually only a single monoclonal antibody is added to each sample aliquot because multiple antibodies may result in red cell agglutination, but at least two red cell surface proteins should be evaluated in separate aliquots in each case, as a rare hereditary deficiency may result in isolated loss of CD55 or CD59. Cells are then classified as type I (normal), type II (partial deficiency), and type III (complete deficiency). Often the population of abnormal red cells is relatively small because they are selectively lost by complement-mediated lysis. Evaluation of red cells should be performed on a sample before blood transfusion because transfusion may make it more difficult to identify a small population of abnormal red cells.

More recently, techniques have been developed to define the phenotype of granulocytes in PNH using monoclonal antibodies against CD16, CD55, and CD59. Gating is best achieved using side light scatter and a non–GPI-linked protein such as CD45 or CD33 to identify neutrophils. If CD16 is used, care must be taken to exclude eosinophils, as they are negative for CD16. In addition, polymorphism of CD16 may not be detected by some of the antibodies. The granulocyte clone of PNH is usually proportionally larger than the red cell clone. As with evaluation of red cells, it is important to evaluate more than one GPI-linked protein in granulocytes.

A flow cytometric technique has been developed using fluorescent aerolysin (276), a protein that selectively binds to GPI anchors. This technique can be used on a variety of cell types and shows increased sensitivity over CD59 in detection of abnormal granulocytes and monocytes.

Stem Cell Enumeration

With the advent of bone marrow transplantation, multiple methods have been devised to predict engraftment potential of transplanted hematopoietic cells. The absolute mononuclear cell count has been a useful indicator in bone marrow harvests (277,278), but this technique is not sufficient for peripheral blood stem cell collections because of the variable numbers of progenitor cells in harvests. Clonogenic assays such as those detecting granulocyte-macrophage colony-forming units have been used to predict engraftment potential, but the interval necessary for such studies is a serious limitation. More recently, flow cytometric methods for detection of CD34 have been developed. CD34 is a hematopoietic stem cell marker restricted to progenitors of all lineages and thus is a useful antigen for this purpose. Most studies have found a correlation between flow cytometry for CD34 and colony-forming assays (279). Peripheral stem cell collection after mobilization results in a relatively low proportion of CD34-positive cells, ranging from 0.1% to 8%, necessitating the need for a highly accurate method of quantitative measurement. Several methods have been developed and are reviewed by Gratama et al. (279). These methods rely on light scatter characteristics, CD45 staining intensity, and CD34 staining to quantify the progenitor cell population of interest.

Immunodeficiency

Flow cytometric immunophenotypic analysis has enhanced the ability of clinicians to evaluate patients with immunodeficiency

TABLE 2-29. Immunophenotypic Analysis of Primary Immunodeficiency Disorders

Disorder	B Cells	T Cells	Natural Killer Cells
Severe combined immunodeficiency	Variable mature B cells (CD19, CD20, CD21)	3 T-cell phenotypes: CD2⁻, CD3⁻, CD4⁻, CD8⁻; CD2⁻, CD3⁻, CD4⁻, CD8⁻, CD38⁺, transferrin receptor⁺; CD3⁺, CD4⁺, CD8⁺, CD38⁺	Variable CD16, CD56
Adenosine deaminase deficiency	Absent	Absent	—
Bare lymphocyte syndrome	Normal, ↑sIgD⁺, sIgM⁺	Normal numbers; CD2⁺, CD3⁺, CD4⁺ are CD45R⁺ (virgin T cells); CD8⁺ are CD28⁺ (cytotoxic phenotype)	—
X-linked hypogammaglobulinemia	Mature cells absent; immature cells present	Normal numbers; virgin T-cell phenotype, CD4:CD8 normal	—
Common variable immunodeficiency	Normal numbers	Normal numbers; CD2⁺, CD3⁺, CD4⁺(5/9)ᵃ ↓, CD4:CD8 often ↓	—
Selective IgA deficiency	Normal numbers; most sIgA⁺ are sIgD⁺ sIgM⁺	Normal numbers; CD2⁺, CD3⁺	—
DiGeorge syndrome	Normal numbers	↓CD3⁺, CD8⁺ often ↓	—
Wiskott-Aldrich syndrome	Decreased numbers	↓CD3⁺, ↓CD2⁺	—

Ig, immunoglobulin; ↑, increased; ↓, decreased.
ᵃ5/9 is a monoclonal antibody identifying a subset of CD4⁺ cells in which all helper function is present.
Adapted from Nicholson JKA. Use of flow cytometry in the evaluation and diagnosis of primary and secondary immunodeficiency diseases. *Arch Pathol Lab Med* 1989;113:598–605.

disorders (Table 2-29); immunophenotype and function may not always be well correlated (280). Patients with severe combined immunodeficiency (SCID) exhibit several different patterns. According to the classification of Reinherz et al. (281), one group lacked expression of mature T-cell antigens (CD2, CD3, CD4, CD8) and an immature antigen (CD38). A second group lacked mature T cells but had some immature CD38-bearing cells. The third group had cells that coexpressed mature antigens (CD3, CD4, CD8) and immature antigens as well. SCID patients appear to exhibit variable numbers of B cells with surface immunoglobulin or mature B-cell antigens (CD19, CD20, CD21), but these cells apparently do not synthesize Ig in a normal manner. Another subset of SCID patients have adenosine deaminase deficiency associated with reduced numbers of either T or B lymphocytes so that immunologic studies are not informative (280). Linch and Levinsky (282) have suggested that flow cytometric analysis of fetal blood samples is useful in the prenatal diagnosis of SCID.

Other rare syndromes also may be defined using flow cytometric studies, and the development of new antibodies and direct conjugates with fluorochromes enhances the ability to perform dual-label studies to define further the cell phenotypes associated with these syndromes. A number of the primary immunodeficiency syndromes have been studied with immunophenotypic analysis, and the results are best summarized from the work of Nicholson (280) (Table 2-29).

Acquired immunodeficiency may be associated with acute viral infections such as cytomegalovirus or chronic viral infections (e.g., HIV). Viral infections generally result in an increased frequency of CD8⁺ cells in the peripheral blood. HIV infection is characterized by coexpression of immature antigens such as CD38 on the CD8⁺ cells and a decrease in CD4 cells (280). Precise measurement of CD4 cell concentrations in peripheral blood of patients with acquired immunodeficiency–related syndromes is an important diagnostic step in clinical assessment. Koepke and Landay (283) have emphasized the importance of obtaining precise absolute lymphocyte counts. Use of a combination of an automated total leukocyte count and the relative lymphocyte frequency derived from a 100-cell routine microscopic differential does not provide adequate precision to calculate the absolute lymphocyte count. Automated three-part and five-part leukocyte differential counters are capable of enumerating lymphocytes with a CV of less than 5%, an acceptable level for calculating the number of CD4 cells. The absolute lymphocyte concentration may then be used in conjunction with immu-

nophenotypic analysis to estimate absolute concentrations of lymphocyte subsets. Most laboratories use the pan–T-cell antigen CD3 in conjunction with CD4 and CD8 to quantitate T-cell subpopulations, as well as CD19, which is a pan–B-cell marker; and CD16, CD56, or both, which are NK-cell markers.

MOLECULAR DIAGNOSTIC METHODS

In recent years, molecular genetic methods have become increasingly important in the diagnosis, prognosis, and monitoring of hematopoietic malignancies. Several excellent reviews have been written on this topic (284–286). Molecular techniques allow identification of clonal cell populations or specific chromosomal changes and provide tools for monitoring minimal residual disease. These techniques are advantageous because they can detect small abnormalities not identified by routine cytogenetic analysis, do not require viable cells capable of division, can be performed in a short time (2 to 4 days), and have the sensitivity to detect as few as 0.001% to 1% abnormal cells among a normal cell population. Currently, the most commonly used techniques in the clinical laboratory are PCR, RT-PCR, Southern blot analysis, and fluorescence *in situ* hybridization. These techniques may be performed on peripheral blood, bone marrow aspirate or biopsy material, and tissue biopsies.

Polymerase Chain Reaction

PCR is a nucleic acid amplification technique commonly used in the diagnosis and monitoring of leukemias and lymphomas. PCR is performed with a single tube containing sample DNA, two short oligonucleotides referred to as *primers*, a heat-stable DNA polymerase, individual nucleotides, and a buffer containing magnesium chloride. Knowledge of the nucleic acid sequence of the disease-specific genetic locus is required so that oligonucleotide primers, usually 15 to 20 nucleotides in length, may be designed that flank the region of interest. Usually primers are chosen so that the amplified product is less than 500 base pairs for fresh material and less than 200 base pairs if paraffin-embedded tissue is to be used. The reaction mixture is added to the tube and undergoes a repetitive sequence of three steps: DNA denaturation, primer annealing, and primer extension (Fig. 2-30). These steps require specific, temperature-controlled conditions that are achieved by placing the tube in a heat block,

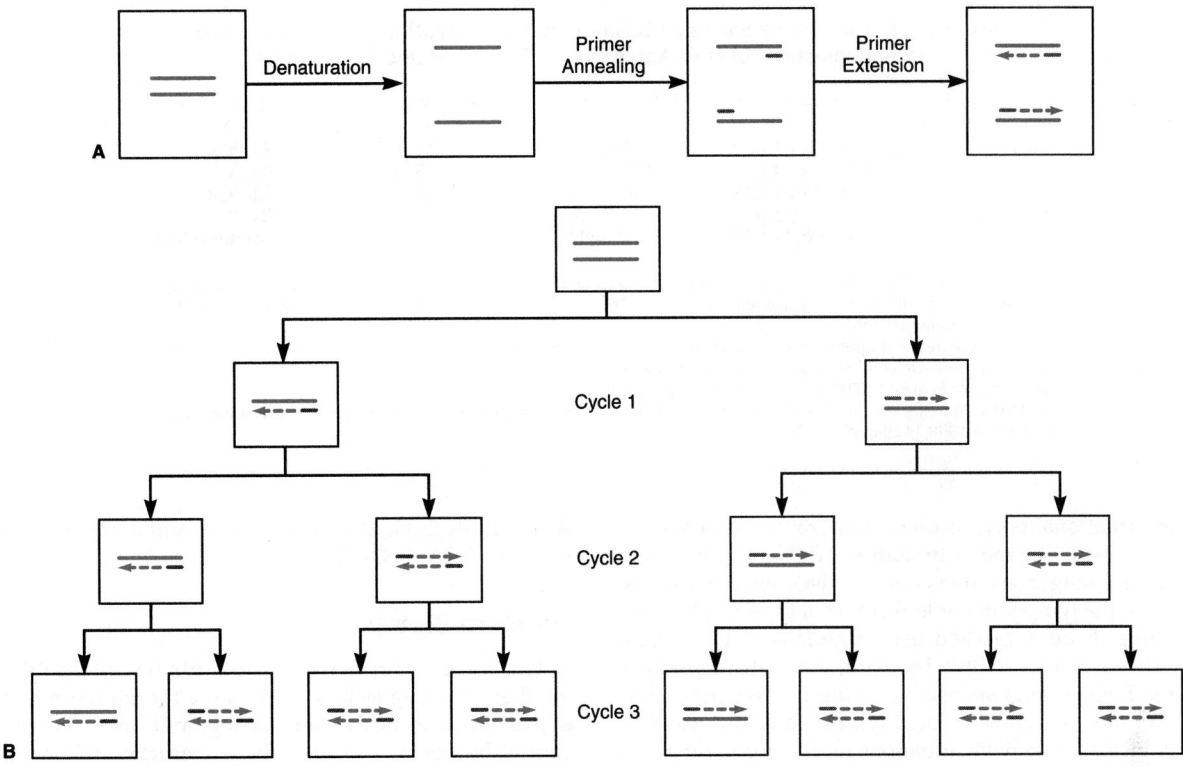

Figure 2-30. Polymerase chain reaction. **A:** A typical polymerase chain reaction cycle includes three steps: DNA denaturation, primer annealing, and primer extension. **B:** With each cycle, the number of copies of the DNA of interest doubles.

which rapidly alters temperature repetitively for 25 to 40 cycles. With each cycle, doubling of the target DNA occurs, resulting in a several million–fold increase of the abnormal disease-specific DNA sequence of interest. After amplification, the DNA may be analyzed by gel electrophoresis with ethidium bromide staining, which allows detection of the abnormal DNA product of the size expected based on the distance between primers. Gel electrophoresis may be combined with probe hybridization or a number of colorimetric, fluorescent, or chemiluminescent detection systems.

Conventional PCR is most commonly used for detection of antigen receptor gene rearrangements to document B-lymphocyte or T-lymphocyte clonal expansion or clonality. The loci analyzed for B-cell and T-cell clonality are those that rearrange earliest in B-lymphocyte and T-lymphocyte ontogeny, namely the Ig heavy chain (IgH) and the TCR-γ, respectively. The antigen receptor genes contain numerous variable regions and several

joining and constant segments in the germline configuration. In addition, several diversity regions are present in the IgH, TCR-β, and TCR-δ genes in the germline configuration. Rearrangement occurs to bring variable, diversity, and joining segments together with variable numbers of different nucleotides inserted at the junctions by TdT. PCR methods use variable-specific and joining-specific or consensus primers to amplify the DNA segments of interest. In a polyclonal lymphocyte population, different numbers of nucleotides will be added with each individual rearrangement, resulting in a smear of different size DNA fragments by gel electrophoresis after PCR. In a clonal cell population, the rearrangement includes the same number of added nucleotides in each cell, resulting in a sharp band on gel electrophoresis after PCR amplification. Additional method modifications may enhance the sensitivity and specificity of detection by including sequence analysis of DNA products, denaturing-gradient gel electrophoresis (287), single-

TABLE 2-30. Common Recurring Chromosomal Translocations in Myeloid Leukemia Amenable to Routine Molecular Analysis[a]

Disease	Translocation	Genes Involved	Frequency (%)[b]	Preferred Method
AML-M2	t(8;21)(q22;q22)	AML1-ETO	30	RT-PCR
AML-M3	t(15;17)(q22;q11–12)	PML-RARα	100	RT-PCR
AML-M4Eo	inv(16)(p13;q22)	CBFβ-MYH11	100	RT-PCR
AML-M4/M5	t(11;19)(q23;p13)	MLL-ENL	25	RT-PCR
AML-M5	t(9;11)(p21;q23)	MLL-AF9	40	RT-PCR
CML	t(9;22)(q34;q11)	BCR-ABL	100	RT-PCR

AML, acute myeloid leukemia; BCR, breakpoint cluster region; CBF, core binding factor; CML, chronic myelogenous leukemia; MLL, mixed lineage leukemia gene; MYH11, myosin heavy-chain gene; PML, promyelocytic leukemia; RAR, retinoic acid receptor; RT-PCR, reverse-transcription polymerase chain reaction.
[a]Each specific translocation involving MLL is best documented with a specific RT-PCR assay. Alternatively, a single Southern blot analysis may be used to detect essentially all (more than 35) translocations affecting MLL.
[b]Approximate frequency per disease category. Reported frequencies may vary depending on detection method used.
Adapted with minor modifications from Bagg A, Kallakury BV. Molecular pathology of leukemia and lymphoma. *Am J Clin Pathol* 1999;112[Suppl 1]:S76–S92.

TABLE 2-31. Common Recurring Chromosomal Translocations in B-Lineage Acute Lymphoblastic Leukemia Amenable to Routine Molecular Analysis

Disease	Translocation	Genes Involved	Frequency (%)[a]	Preferred Method
Precursor-B ALL	t(12;21)(p13;q22)	TEL-AML1	25	RT-PCR
	t(9;22)(q34;q11)	BCR-ABL	5–25[b]	RT-PCR
	t(4;11)(q21;q23)	MLL-AF4	10[c]	RT-PCR
Pre-B-ALL	t(1;19)(q23;p13)	E2A-PBX1	25	RT-PCR
B-ALL	t(8;14)(q24;q32)	MYC-IgH	75	Southern blot

ALL, acute lymphoblastic leukemia; AML, acute myeloid leukemia; BCR, breakpoint cluster region; IgH, immunoglobulin heavy chain; MLL, mixed lineage leukemia gene; MYC, c-MYC protooncogene; RT-PCR, reverse-transcription polymerase chain reaction.
[a]Approximate frequency per disease category. Reported frequencies may vary depending on detection method used.
[b]Lower frequency in children; higher frequency in adults.
[c]Much higher frequency (70%) in infantile acute leukemia.
Adapted with minor modifications from Bagg A, Kallakury BV. Molecular pathology of leukemia and lymphoma. *Am J Clin Pathol* 1999;112[Suppl 1]:S76–S92.

strand conformational polymorphism (288,289), and heteroduplex analysis (290). The major limitation of PCR amplification for the IgH rearrangement detection is false-negative results, depending on the lymphoma or leukemia subtype and the specific PCR amplification method used. The false-negative rate can be reduced to 10% to 30% by using two sets of primers (291). Some B-cell malignancies, including the follicular lymphomas and the mucosa-associated lymphoid tissue lymphomas, show increased somatic mutations or deletions within the IgH gene and are thus less amenable to PCR amplification. False-negative results are rarely a problem in CLL and mantle cell lymphoma. PCR amplification to detect the TCR-λ rearrangement is able to detect clonality in 70% to 80% of T-cell malignancies (292–294). This technique may also be limited by false-positive results because of the more limited junctional diversity.

The usefulness of conventional DNA-based PCR amplification is limited in many chromosomal translocations because the breakpoints span large intronic sequences, making it difficult to detect all breakpoints with a simple PCR assay. This limitation can be overcome by amplification of RNA using RT-PCR because intronic sequences are spliced out during the normal synthesis and processing of messenger RNA. Messenger RNA is initially reverse transcribed by reverse transcriptase into complementary DNA, which is followed by conventional PCR. This technique is commonly used in translocations associated with

AML (Table 2-30), ALL (Tables 2-31 and 2-33), and some lymphomas (Table 2-32).

Southern Blot

Polymerase chain reaction methods have largely replaced Southern blotting techniques because the Southern blot is more expensive, technically demanding, and time consuming, and cannot be performed reliably on paraffin-embedded tissue. However, the Southern technique is still useful in some situations in which PCR methods are not optimal, such as translocations with multiple partners (e.g., bcl-6), or in which there is lack of breakpoint clustering (e.g., c-myc) (Tables 2-31, 2-32, and 2-33). The Southern technique also is used as a second method for analysis of IgH and TCR rearrangements because PCR may be limited by false-negative or false-positive results. In the Southern blot technique (Fig. 2-31), restriction endonucleases are used to cleave DNA at sequence-specific sites. The DNA fragments are then electrophoresed on an agarose gel and transferred to a nylon membrane. This membrane blot is hybridized with a radioactive or chemiluminescent DNA probe that is complementary to the DNA sequence of interest. The labeled blot is then exposed to x-ray film that is then developed to reveal the sites of hybridization. The expected size of the normal DNA fragments can be predicted from the genomic DNA sequence and restriction enzyme sequence-specific cleavage sites. For

TABLE 2-32. Common Recurring Chromosomal Translocations in Non-Hodgkin's Lymphoma Amenable to Molecular Analysis

Disease	Translocation	Genes Involved	Frequency (%)[a]	Preferred Method
B cell				
Follicle center cell	t(14;18)(q32;q21)	IgH-BCL2	90	PCR
Burkitt	t(8;14)(q24;q32)	MYC-IgH	75	Southern blot[b]
	t(2;8)(q12;q24)	Igκ-MYC	16	Southern blot[b]
	t(8;22)(q24;q11)	MYC-Igλ	9	Southern blot[b]
Mantle cell	t(11;14)(q13;q32)	CCND1-IgH	70	PCR
Lymphoplasmacytic	t(9;14)(p13;q32)	PAX5-IgH	50	[c]
Diffuse large cell	t(3q27)	BCL6	40	Southern blot[b]
Marginal zone	t(11;18)(q21;q21)	API2-MLT	35	[c]
T cell				
Anaplastic large cell	t(2;5)(p23;q35)	NPM-ALK	35	RT-PCR

ALK, anaplastic lymphoma kinase; API2, apoptosis inhibitor-2; CCND1, cyclin D1 gene; Ig, immunoglobulin; IgH, immunoglobulin heavy chain; MLT, MALT lymphoma-associated translocation; MYC, c-MYC protooncogene; NPM, nucleophosmin; PCR, DNA-based polymerase chain reaction; RT-PCR, reverse-transcription polymerase chain reaction.
[a]Approximate frequency per disease category. Reported frequencies may vary depending on the detection method used.
[b]Advocated when there are either multiple translocation partners (BCL6) or lack of breakpoint clustering (MYC), precluding design of simple or single assays. Fluorescence *in situ* hybridization may also be used.
[c]Optimal detection method not yet established.
Adapted with minor modifications from Bagg A, Kallakury BV. Molecular pathology of leukemia and lymphoma. *Am J Clin Pathol* 1999;112[Suppl 1]:S76–S92.

TABLE 2-33. Recurring Translocations in T-Lineage Acute Lymphoblastic Leukemia Amenable to Molecular Analysis

Translocation	Genes Involved	Approximate Incidence (%)	Molecular Detection
t(8;14)(q24;q11)	c-MYC–TCRα/δ	2	FISH
t(10;14)(q24;q11)[a]	HOX11-TCRα/δ	5–10	Southern blot
t(11;14)(p15;q11)[a]	LMO1-TCRα/δ	1	Southern blot
t(11;14)(p13;q11)[a]	LMO2-TCRα/δ	5–10	Southern blot
t(1;14)(p32;q11)[a]	TAL1-TCRα/δ	1–3	Southern blot
inv(14)(q11;q32)	TCL1-TCRα/δ	<1	FISH

FISH, fluorescence *in situ* hybridization; TCR, T-cell receptor.
[a]Variant translocations have been described; only the most commonly involved TCR locus is included.
Adapted from Macintyre EA, Delabesse E. Molecular approaches to the diagnosis and evaluation of lymphoid malignancies. *Semin Hematol* 1999;36:373–389.

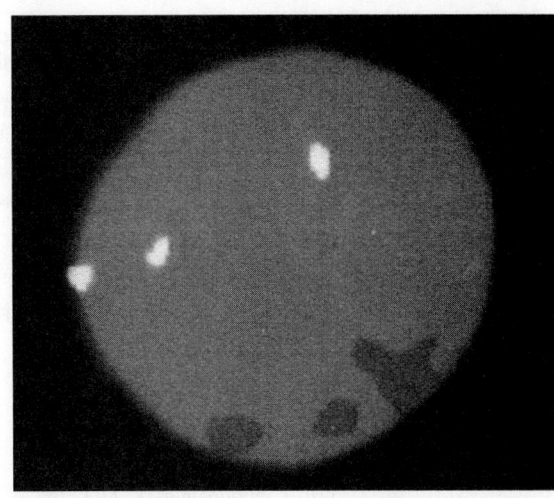

Figure 2-32. Fluorescence *in situ* hybridization using centromeric probes for chromosomes 6 (red) and 21 (green) in a pediatric patient with acute lymphoblastic leukemia. The leukemia shows trisomy for chromosomes 6 and 21. (See Color Fig. 2-32.) (Photograph courtesy of Dr. K. Richkind, Genzyme Genetics, Santa Fe, NM.)

IgH or TCR rearrangements, a distinct band separate from the germline band is identified in clonal cell populations. For translocations, a DNA fragment different in size from that expected in normal genomic DNA is seen.

Fluorescence *in Situ* Hybridization

Fluorescence *in situ* hybridization is a technique that uses fluorescent-labeled DNA probes to characterize chromosomal regions of interest. In comparison to routine cytogenetics, this technique is advantageous because it does not require dividing cells, allows a larger number of cells to be analyzed, and is able to detect smaller genetic abnormalities. The probe may be a DNA clone specific for a defined region of a particular chromosome, or chromosome-specific DNA that allows whole chromosome painting. The probe is hybridized to the cells of interest and visualized using a fluorescent microscope. Numeric alter-

ations (e.g., monosomy or trisomy) may be readily identified in interphase cells using chromosome-specific centromeric probes (Fig. 2-32). With metaphase spreads, translocations may be identified using painting probes from the two chromosomes involved or using gene-specific probes for the loci involved in the translocation. Gene-specific probes are advantageous because they also may be used for analysis of interphase cells. Usually, gene-specific probes for both loci involved in a translocation result in a fusion of signals from the two loci, indicating a translocation. Alternatively, a probe may be used that spans the translocation breakpoint. If the translocation is present, the

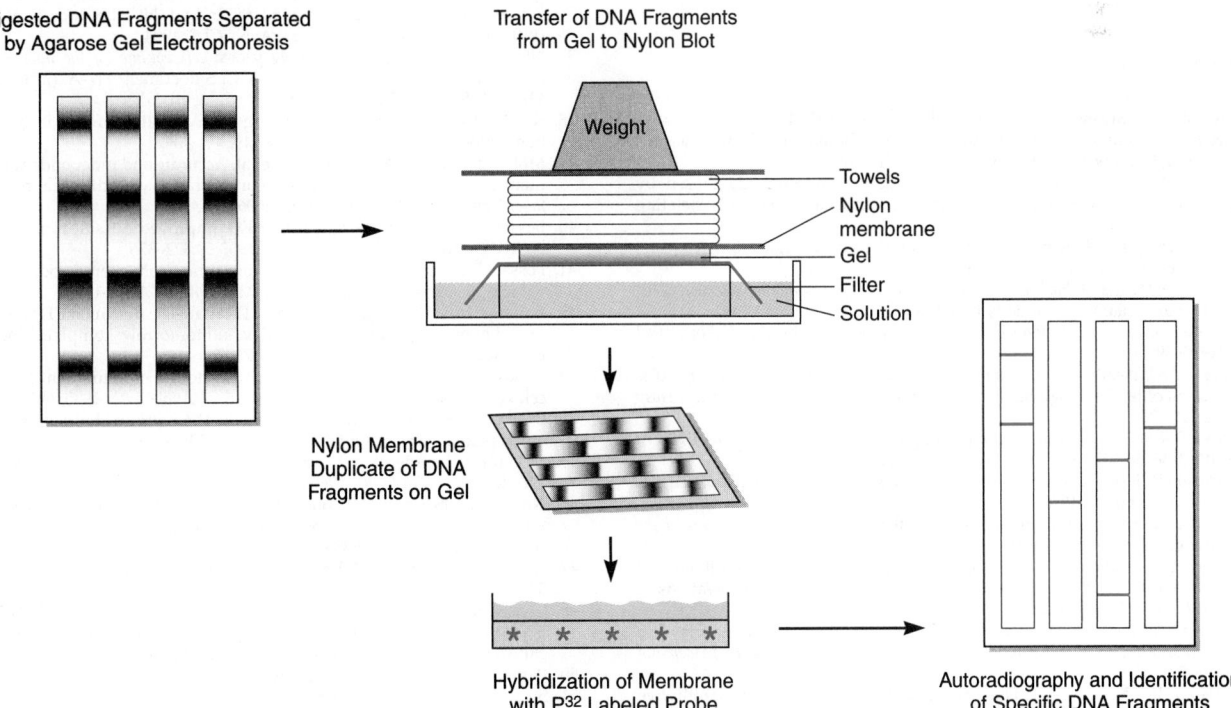

Digested DNA Fragments Separated by Agarose Gel Electrophoresis

Transfer of DNA Fragments from Gel to Nylon Blot

Weight

Towels
Nylon membrane
Gel
Filter
Solution

Nylon Membrane Duplicate of DNA Fragments on Gel

Hybridization of Membrane with P32 Labeled Probe

Autoradiography and Identification of Specific DNA Fragments

Figure 2-31. Southern blot technique.

TABLE 2-34. Recurring Abnormalities in Hematopoietic Malignancies Detected by Fluorescence *In Situ* Hybridization

Disease	Abnormality	Potential Gene Probe
Chronic myeloid leukemia	t(9;22)(q34;q11)	ABL, BCR
Myelodysplastic syndrome/AML	−5, −7, +8	Chromosome-specific
AML[a]		
AML M-2	t(8;21)(q22;q22)	ETO, AML1
AML M-3, M-3V	t(15;17)(q22;q11–12)	PML, RARα
AML M-4eos	inv(16)(p13;q22) or t(16;16)(p13;q22)	MYH11, CBFβ
AML M-4, M-5	t(9;11)(p22;q23)	AF9, MLL
	11q23 abnormalities	MLL
Acute lymphoblastic leukemia		
Precursor B	t(12;21)(p12;q22)	TEL, AML1
	t(9;22)(q34;q11)	ABL; BCR
	11q23 abnormalities	MLL
B cell	t(8;14)(q24;q32)	c-MYC, IgH
Precursor T	t(8;14)(q24;q11)	c-MYC, TCRα/δ
	inv(14)(q11;q32)	TCL1, TCRα/δ
Non-Hodgkin's lymphoma		
Follicular, diffuse large cell	t(14;18)(q32;q21)	IgH, BCL2
Diffuse large cell	t(3;14)(q27;q32)	BCL6, IgH
Mantle cell lymphoma	t(11;14)(q13;q32)	BCL1, IgH
Burkitt lymphoma	t(8;14)(q24;q32)	c-MYC, IgH
Lymphoplasmacytic	t(9;14)(p13;q32)	PAX5, IgH

AML, acute myeloid leukemia; BCR, breakpoint cluster region; CBF, core binding factor; IgH, immunoglobulin heavy chain; MLL, mixed-lineage leukemia gene; MYH11, myosin heavy-chain gene; PML, promyelocytic leukemia; RAR, retinoic acid receptor; TCR, T-cell receptor.
[a]AML subtypes according to French-American-British classification.

probe is split, resulting in three fluorescent signals, one from the normal chromosome and two from the probe split by the translocation. Fluorescence *in situ* hybridization analysis may be a useful alternative or addition to routine cytogenetics in CML, myelodysplasia, acute leukemia, and lymphoma (Table 2-34).

REFERENCES

1. Kjeldsberg C, Swanson J. Platelet satellitism. *Blood* 1974;43:831–836.
2. Greipp PR, Gralnick H. Platelet to leukocyte adherence phenomena associated with thrombocytopenia. *Blood* 1976;47:513–521.
3. Onder O, Weinstein A, Hoyer LW. Pseudothrombocytopenia caused by platelet agglutinins that are reactive in blood anticoagulated with chelating agents. *Blood* 1980;56:177–182.
4. Ingram M, Minter F. Semiautomatic preparations of coverglass blood smears using a centrifugal device. *Am J Clin Pathol* 1969;51:214.
5. Nelson D, Morris M. *Basic methodology: clinical diagnosis and management*, 17th ed. Philadelphia: WB Saunders, 1984:578–625.
6. Brecher G. New methylene blue as a reticulocyte stain. *Am J Clin Pathol* 1949;19:895–896.
7. Shepard M, Weatherall D, Conley C. Semiquantitative estimation of the distribution of fetal hemoglobin in red cell populations. *Bull Johns Hopkins Hosp* 1962;110:293.
8. NCCLS. *Fetal red cell detection: proposed guideline*. NCCLS document H52-P (ISBN 1-56238-402-3). Wayne, PA: NCCLS, 2000.
9. Mollison P. *Blood transfusion in clinical medicine*, 7th ed. Oxford: Blackwell Scientific Publications, 1983.
10. Tomoda Y. Demonstration of foetal erythrocytes by immunofluorescent staining. *Nature* 1964;202:910.
11. Wood W, Stamatoyannopoulos G, Lim G, et al. F-cells in the adult: normal values and levels in individuals with hereditary and acquired elevations of Hb F. *Blood* 1975;46:671–682.
12. Allen C, Weeseratne H, Gale R, et al. The use of monoclonal antibodies UCHβ and UCH for the antenatal diagnosis of β-thalassemia. *Br J Haematol* 1987;65:199–203.
13. Navenot JM, Merghoub T, Ducrocq R, et al. New method for quantitative determination of fetal hemoglobin-containing red blood cells by flow cytometry: application to sickle-cell disease. *Cytometry* 1998;32:186–190.
14. Campbell TA, Ware RE, Mason M. Detection of hemoglobin variants in erythrocytes by flow cytometry. *Cytometry* 1999;35:242–248.
15. Davis BH, Olsen J, Bigelow NC, et al. Detection of fetal red cells in fetomaternal hemorrhage using a fetal hemoglobin monoclonal antibody by flow cytometry. *Transfusion* 1998;38:749–756.
16. Chen JC, Bigelow N, Davis BH. Proposed flow cytometric reference method for the determination of erythroid F-cell counts. *Cytometry* 2000;42:239–246.
17. Lloyd-Evans P, Kumpel BM, Bromelow I, et al. Use of a directly conjugated monoclonal anti-D (BRAD-3) for quantification of fetomaternal hemorrhage by flow cytometry. *Transfusion* 1996;36:432–437.
18. Sears DA, Friedman JM, White DR. Binding of intracellular protein to the erythrocyte membrane during incubation: the production of Heinz bodies. *J Lab Clin Med* 1975;86:722–732.
19. Simpson CF, Carlisle JW, Mallard L. Rhodanile blue: a rapid and selective stain for Heinz bodies. *Stain Technol* 1970;45:221–223.
20. Zinkham WH, Winslow RM. Unstable hemoglobins: influence of environment on phenotypic expression of a genetic disorder. *Medicine* 1989;68:309–320.
21. Carrell RW, Kay R. A simple method for the detection of unstable haemoglobins. *Br J Haematol* 1972;23:615–619.
22. Pearson HA, Johnston D, Smith KA. The born-again spleen: return of splenic function after splenectomy for trauma. *N Engl J Med* 1978;298:1389–1392.
23. Holroyde CP, Oski FA, Gardner FH. The "pocked" erythrocyte: red-cell surface alterations in reticuloendothelial immaturity of the neonate. *N Engl J Med* 1969;281:516–520.
24. Kaplow L. Cytochemistry of leukocyte alkaline phosphatase: use of complex naphthol as phosphatase in azo dye-coupling techniques. *Am J Clin Pathol* 1963;39:430–449.
25. Kaplow L. Leukocyte alkaline phosphatase cytochemistry: application and methods. *Ann N Y Acad Sci* 1968;155.
26. Kaplow L. Substitute for benzidine in myeloperoxidase stain. *J Clin Pathol* 1975;63:451.
27. Liso V, Troccoli G, Specchia G, et al. Cytochemical "normal" and "abnormal" eosinophils in acute leukemias. *Am J Hematol* 1977;2:123–131.
28. Le Beau MM, Larson RA, Bitter MA, et al. Association of an inversion of chromosome 16 with abnormal marrow eosinophils in acute myelomonocytic leukemia: a unique cytogenetic-clinicopathological association. *N Engl J Med* 1983;309:630–636.
29. Yam LT, Li CY, Crosby WH. Cytochemical identification of monocytes and granulocytes. *Am J Clin Pathol* 1971;55:283–290.
30. Li CY, Lam KW, Yam LT. Esterases in human leukocytes. *J Histochem Cytochem* 1973;21:1–12.
31. Yam LT, Li CY, Lam KW. Tartrate-resistant acid phosphatase isoenzyme in the reticulum cells of leukemic reticuloendotheliosis. *N Engl J Med* 1971;284:357–360.
32. Neiman RS, Sullivan AL, Jaffe R. Malignant lymphoma simulating leukemic reticuloendotheliosis: a clinicopathologic study of ten cases. *Cancer* 1979;43:329–342.
33. Gilmer PR Jr, Williams LJ, Koepke JA, et al. Calibration methods for automated hematology instruments. *Am J Clin Pathol* 1977;68[Suppl 1]:185–190.
34. Gilmer PR Jr, Williams LJ. The status of methods of calibration in hematology. *Am J Clin Pathol* 1980;74[Suppl 4]:600–605.
35. Morris M, Davey F. *Basic examination of blood: clinical diagnosis and management by laboratory methods*, 19th ed. Philadelphia: WB Saunders, 1996:549–593.
36. NCCLS. *Reference and selected procedures for the quantitative determination of hemoglobin in blood: approved standard*, 2nd ed. NCCLS document H15-A2 (ISBN 1-56238-237-3). Villanova, PA: NCCLS, 1994.
37. NCCLS. *Procedure for determining packed cell volume by the microhematocrit method: approved standard*, 3rd ed. NCCLS document H7-A2(ISBN 1-56238-413-9). Villanova, PA: NCCLS, 2000.
38. Kershaw GW, Robin H, Kronenberg H. Evaluation of the Technicon H-1 hematology analyser. *Pathology* 1987;19:305–309.
39. Mohandas N, Kim YR, Tycko DH, et al. Accurate and independent measurement of volume and hemoglobin concentration of individual red cells by laser light scattering. *Blood* 1986;68:506–513.
40. Bessman JD, Gilmer PR Jr, Gardner FH. Improved classification of anemias by MCV and RDW. *Am J Clin Pathol* 1983;80:322–326.
41. Fossat C, David M, Harle JR, et al. New parameters in erythrocyte counting: value of histograms. *Arch Pathol Lab Med* 1987;111:1150–1154.
42. Bollinger PB, Drewinko B, Brailas CD, et al. The Technicon H*1—an automated hematology analyzer for today and tomorrow: complete blood count parameters. *Am J Clin Pathol* 1987;87:71–78.
43. Tycko DH, et al. Flow-cytometric light scattering measurement of red blood cell volume and hemoglobin concentration. *Appl Optics* 1985;24:1355–1365.
44. Brecher G, Schneiderman M, Cronkite E. The reproducibility and constancy of the platelet count. *Am J Clin Pathol* 1953;23:15–26.
45. Bull BS, Schneiderman M, Brecher G. Platelet counts with the Coulter counter. *Am J Clin Pathol* 1965;44:678–688.
46. Nosanchuk JS, Chang J, Bennett JM. The analytic basis for the use of platelet estimates from peripheral blood smears: laboratory and clinical applications. *Am J Clin Pathol* 1978;69:383–387.
47. Abbey AP, Belliveau RR. Enumeration of platelets. *Am J Clin Pathol* 1978;69:55–56.
48. Consensus Conference. Platelet transfusion therapy. *JAMA* 1987;257:1777–1780.
49. Murphy S, Litwin S, Herring LM, et al. Indications for platelet transfusion in children with acute leukemia. *Am J Hematol* 1982;12:347–356.
50. Patten E. Blood component therapy for cancer patients. *Tex Med* 1985;81:31–34.
51. Strauss R. The risks of thrombocytopenia and the standard uses of platelet transfusions. *Plasma Ther Transfus Technol* 1986;7:279–285.
52. Rebulla P, Finazzi G, Marangoni F, et al. The threshold for prophylactic platelet transfusions in adults with acute myeloid leukemia. Gruppo Italiano Malattie Ematologiche Maligne dell'Adulto. *N Engl J Med* 1997;337:1870–1875.

53. Heckman KD, Weiner GJ, Davis CS, et al. Randomized study of prophylactic platelet transfusion threshold during induction therapy for adult acute leukemia: 10,000/microL versus 20,000/microL. *J Clin Oncol* 1997;15:1143–1149.
54. Payne BA, Pierre RV, Lee WK. Evaluation of the Toa E-5000 automated hematology analyzer. *Am J Clin Pathol* 1987;88:51–57.
55. Kickler TS. Clinical analyzers: advances in automated cell counting. *Anal Chem* 1999;71:363R–365R.
56. Wertz RK, Koepke JA. A critical analysis of platelet counting methods. *Am J Clin Pathol* 1977;68[Suppl 1]:195–201.
57. Harrison P, Horton A, Grant D, et al. Immunoplatelet counting: a proposed new reference procedure. *Br J Haematol* 2000;108:228–235.
58. Ault KA. Platelet counting: is there room for improvement. *Lab Hematol* 1996;2:139–143.
59. Ault KA, et al. Implementation of the immunological platelet count on a haematology analyser, the Abbott CELL-DYN 4000. *Lab Hematol* 1997;3:125–128.
60. Dickerhoff R, Von Ruecker A. Enumeration of platelets by multiparameter flow cytometry using platelet-specific antibodies and fluorescent reference particles. *Clin Lab Haematol* 1995;17:163–172.
61. Kunz D, Hoffkes H, Kunz WS, et al. Standardized flow cytometric method for the accurate determination of platelet counts in patients with severe thrombocytopenia. *Cytometry* 2000;42:284–289.
62. Gill JE, Davis KA, Cowart WJ, et al. A rapid and accurate closed-tube immunoassay for platelets on an automated hematology analyzer. *Am J Clin Pathol* 2000;114:47–56.
63. Kunz D, Kunz WS, Scott CS, et al. Automated CD61 immunoplatelet analysis of thrombocytopenic samples. *Br J Haematol* 2001;112:584–592.
64. Cornbleet J. Spurious results from automated hematology counters. *Lab Med* 1983;14:509–514.
65. Corash L. Platelet density heterogeneity [Letter]. *Blood* 1985;65:779–780.
66. Martin JF, Trowbridge EA. Platelet density heterogeneity [Letter]. *Blood* 1985;65:779–781.
67. Bath PM, Butterworth RJ. Platelet size: measurement, physiology and vascular disease. *Blood Coagul Fibrinolysis* 1996;7:157–161.
68. Osselaer JC, Jamart J, Scheiff JM. Platelet distribution width for differential diagnosis of thrombocytosis. *Clin Chem* 1997;43[6 Pt 1]:1072–1076.
69. Garg SK, Amorosi EL, Karpatkin S. Use of the megathrombocyte as an index of megakaryocyte number. *N Engl J Med* 1971;284:11–17.
70. Kraytman M. Platelet size in thrombocytopenias and thrombocytosis of various origin. *Blood* 1973;41:587–598.
71. Zeigler Z, Murphy S, Gardner FH. Microscopic platelet size and morphology in various hematologic disorders. *Blood* 1978;51:479–486.
72. Rowan RM, Fraser C, Gray JH, et al. The Coulter Counter Model S Plus—the shape of things to come. *Clin Lab Haematol* 1979;1:29–40.
73. Giles C. The platelet count and mean platelet volume. *Br J Haematol* 1981;48:31–37.
74. Levin J, Bessman JD. The inverse relation between platelet volume and platelet number: abnormalities in hematologic disease and evidence that platelet size does not correlate with platelet age. *J Lab Clin Med* 1983;101:295–307.
75. Thompson CB, Diaz DD, Quinn PG, et al. The role of anticoagulation in the measurement of platelet volumes. *Am J Clin Pathol* 1983;80:327–332.
76. Threatte GA, Adrados C, Ebbe S, et al. Mean platelet volume: the need for a reference method. *Am J Clin Pathol* 1984;81:769–772.
77. Lippi U, Schinella M, Modena N, et al. Unpredictable effects of K3 EDTA on mean platelet volume. *Am J Clin Pathol* 1987;87:391–393.
78. O'Malley T, Ludlam CA, Fox KA, et al. Measurement of platelet volume using a variety of different anticoagulant and antiplatelet mixtures. *Blood Coagul Fibrinolysis* 1996;7:431–436.
79. Bessman JD, Gilmer PR, Gardner FH. Use of mean platelet volume improves detection of platelet disorders. *Blood Cells* 1985;11:127–135.
80. Corash L. Platelet sizing: techniques, biological significance, and clinical applications. *Curr Top Hematol* 1983;4:99–122.
81. Corash L, Shafer B, Blaese RM. Platelet-associated immunoglobulin, platelet size, and the effect of splenectomy in the Wiskott-Aldrich syndrome. *Blood* 1985;65:1439–1443.
82. Niethammer AG, Forman EN. Use of the platelet histogram maximum in evaluating thrombocytopenia. *Am J Hematol* 1999;60:19–23.
83. Ochs HD, Slichter SJ, Harker LA, et al. The Wiskott-Aldrich syndrome: studies of lymphocytes, granulocytes, and platelets. *Blood* 1980;55:243–252.
84. Small BM, Bettigole RE. Diagnosis of myeloproliferative disease by analysis of the platelet volume distribution. *Am J Clin Pathol* 1981;76:685–691.
85. Friedhoff AJ, Miller JC, Karpatkin S. Heterogeneity of human platelets. VII. Platelet monoamine oxidase activity in normals and patients with autoimmune thrombocytopenic purpura and reactive thrombocytosis: its relationship to platelet protein density. *Blood* 1978;51:317–323.
86. Bessman JD, Williams LJ, Gilmer PR Jr. Platelet size in health and hematologic disease. *Am J Clin Pathol* 1982;78:150–153.
87. NCCLS. *Reference leukocyte differential count (proportional) and evaluation of instrumental methods: approved standard.* NCCLS document H20-A (ISBN 1-56238-131-8). Villanova, PA: NCCLS, 1992.
88. NCCLS. *Tentative standard H20-T: leukocyte differential counting.* Villanova, PA: NCCLS, 1984.
89. Koepke JA, Dotson MA, Shifman MA. A critical evaluation of the manual/visual differential leukocyte counting method. *Blood Cells* 1985;11:173–186.
90. Koepke JA. Standardization of the manual leukocyte differential leukocyte count. *Lab Med* 1980;11:371–375.
91. College of American Pathologists Hematology and Clinical Microscopy Committee. *Color atlas of hematology and illustrated field guide based on proficiency testing.* Glassy ER, ed. Northfield, IL: College of American Pathologists, 1998.
92. Mathay K, Koepke JA. The clinical usefulness of segmented vs. stab: neutrophil criteria for differential leukocyte counts. *Am J Clin Pathol* 1974;61:947–958.
93. Richardson-Jones A, Hellman R, Twedt D. The Coulter Counter leukocyte differential. *Blood Cells* 1985;11:203–240.
94. Cornbleet J, Kessinger S. Evaluation of Coulter S-Plus three-part differential in population with a high prevalence of abnormalities. *Am J Clin Pathol* 1985;84:620–626.
95. Corash L. Automated leukocyte differential analysis by flow cytochemistry. *Lab Med* 1983;14:503–508.
96. Bentley SA, Johnson A, Bishop CA. A parallel evaluation of four automated hematology analyzers. *Am J Clin Pathol* 1993;100:626–632.
97. De Cresce R. The Technicon H*1: a discrete, fully automated complete blood count differential analyzer. *Lab Med* 1986;17:17–21.
98. Breakell ES, Marchand A, Marcus R, et al. Comparison of performance for leukocyte differential counting of the Technicon H6000 system with a manual reference method using the NCCLS standard. *Blood Cells* 1985;11:257–279.
99. Swaanenburg JC, Rutten WP, Holdrinet AC, et al. The determination of reference values for hematologic parameters using results obtained from patient populations. *Am J Clin Pathol* 1987;88:182–191.
100. Ross DW, Bentley SA. Evaluation of an automated hematology system (Technicon H-1). *Arch Pathol Lab Med* 1986;110:803–808.
101. Buttarello M, Gadotti M, Lorenz C, et al. Evaluation of four automated hematology analyzers: a comparative study of differential counts (imprecision and inaccuracy). *Am J Clin Pathol* 1992;97:345–352.
102. Warner BA, Reardon DM, Marshall DP. Automated haematology analysers: a four-way comparison. *Med Lab Sci* 1990;47:285–296.
103. Burns ER, Lampasso J, Kowatch N, et al. Performance characteristics of state-of-the-art hematology analyzers. *Clin Lab Sci* 1992;5:181–185.
104. Kinsey SE, Watts MJ. Accurate automated leucocyte differential counts despite profound leucopenia. *J Clin Pathol* 1988;41:1236–1239.
105. Wenz B, Ramirez MA, Burns ER. The H*1 hematology analyzer: its performance characteristics and value in the diagnosis of infectious disease. *Arch Pathol Lab Med* 1987;111:521–524.
106. Banez EI, Bacaling JH. An evaluation of the Technicon H-1 automated hematology analyzer in detecting peripheral blood changes in acute inflammation. *Arch Pathol Lab Med* 1988;112:885–888.
107. Bentley SA, Pegram MD, Ross DW. Diagnosis of infective and inflammatory disorders by flow cytometric analysis of blood neutrophils. *Am J Clin Pathol* 1987;88:177–181.
108. Fernández-Castro M, Viloria A. Utility of the Technicon H-1 flags in the detection of peripheral blood blast cells of paediatric acute leukaemia patients. *Acta Haematol* 1995;93:9–12.
109. Krause JR, Costello RT, Krause J, et al. Use of the Technicon H-1 in the characterization of leukemias. *Arch Pathol Lab Med* 1988;112:889–894.
110. Penchansky L, Krause J. Flow cytochemical study of acute leukemia of childhood with the Technicon H*1. *Lab Med* 1991;22:184.
111. Tsakona CP, Kinsey SE, Goldstone AH. Use of flow cytochemistry via the H*1 in FAB identification of acute leukaemias. *Acta Haematol* 1992;88:72–77.
112. Picard F, Giquel C, Marnet L, et al. Preliminary evaluation of the new hematology analyzer COULTER GEN-S in a university hospital. *Clin Chem Lab Med* 1999;37:681–686.
113. Hoyer JD, Fisher CP, Soppa VM, et al. Detection and classification of acute leukemia by the Coulter STKS hematology analyzer. *Am J Clin Pathol* 1996;106:352–358.
114. Fournier M, Gireau A, Chretien MC, et al. Laboratory evaluation of the Abbott Cell DYN 3500 5-part differential. *Am J Clin Pathol* 1996;105:286–292.
115. Vives-Corrons JL, Besson I, Jou JM, et al. Evaluation of the Abbott Cell-DYN 3500 hematology analyzer in university hospital. *Am J Clin Pathol* 1996;105:553–559.
116. Chow EY, Leung KK. Evaluating the CELL-DYN 3500 haematology analyser in an acute general hospital. *Clin Lab Haematol* 1996;18:187–193.
117. Kim YR, Yee M, Metha S, et al. Simultaneous differentiation and quantitation of erythroblasts and white blood cells on a high throughput clinical haematology analyser. *Clin Lab Haematol* 1998;20:21–29.
118. NCCLS. *Methods for reticulocyte counting (flow cytometry and supravital dyes): approved guideline.* Wayne, PA: National Committee for Clinical Laboratory Standards (NCCLS), 1997.
119. Hillman RS, Finch CA. The misused reticulocyte. *Br J Haematol* 1969;17:313–315.
120. Brecher G, Schneiderman M. A time-saving device for the counting of reticulocytes. *Am J Clin Pathol* 1950;20:1079–1083.
121. Savage RA, Skoog DP, Rabinovitch A. Analytic inaccuracy and imprecision in reticulocyte counting: a preliminary report from the College of American Pathologists Reticulocyte Project. *Blood Cells* 1985;11:97–112.
122. Peebles DA, Hochberg A, Clarke TD. Analysis of manual reticulocyte counting. *Am J Clin Pathol* 1981;76:713–717.
123. Davies JI, Smyth MS, Martin JH. Automated reticulocyte counting: evaluation of the Coulter STKS haematology analyser reticulocyte counting function. *Clin Lab Haematol* 1997;19:89–92.
124. Buttarello M, Bulian P, Venudo A, et al. Laboratory evaluation of the Miles H.3 automated reticulocyte counter: a comparative study with manual reference method and Sysmex R-1000. *Arch Pathol Lab Med* 1995;119:1141–1148.
125. Buttarello M, Bulian P, Pra MD, et al. Reticulocyte quantification by Coulter MAXM VCS (volume, conductivity, light scatter) technology. *Clin Chem* 1996;42:1930–1937.
126. Lofsness KG, Kohnke ML, Geier NA. Evaluation of automated reticulocyte counts and their reliability in the presence of Howell-Jolly bodies. *Am J Clin Pathol* 1994;101:85–90.

127. Ferguson DJ, Lee SF, Gordon PA. Evaluation of reticulocyte counts by flow cytometry in a routine laboratory. *Am J Hematol* 1990;33:13–17.

128. Yu PH, So CC, Wong KF, et al. Automated reticulocyte counting—an evaluation of GEN-S, Cell-Dyn 3500 and Cell-Dyn 4000. [Letter] *Clin Lab Haematol* 1999;21:145–147.

129. Seligman PA, Allen RH, Kirchanski SJ, et al. Automated analysis of reticulocytes using fluorescent staining with both acridine orange and an immunofluorescence technique. *Am J Hematol* 1983;14:57–66.

130. Schmitz FJ, Werner E. Optimization of flow-cytometric discrimination between reticulocytes and erythrocytes. *Cytometry* 1986;7:439–444.

131. Wearne A, Robin H, Joshua DE, et al. Automated enumeration of reticulocytes using acridine orange. *Pathology* 1985;17:75–77.

132. Tanke HJ, Rothbarth PH, Vossen JM, et al. Flow cytometry of reticulocytes applied to clinical hematology. *Blood* 1983;61:1091–1097.

133. Tanke HJ, Nieuwenhuis IA, Koper GJ, et al. Flow cytometry of human reticulocytes based on RNA fluorescence. *Cytometry* 1981;1:313–320.

134. Corash L, Rheinschmidt M, Lieu S, et al. Fluorescence-activated flow cytometry in the hematology clinical laboratory. *Cytometry Suppl* 1988;3:60–64.

135. Metzger DK, Charache S. Flow cytometric reticulocyte counting with thioflavin T in a clinical hematology laboratory. *Arch Pathol Lab Med* 1987;111:540–544.

136. Sage BH Jr, O'Connell JP, Mercolino TJ. A rapid, vital staining procedure for flow cytometric analysis of human reticulocytes. *Cytometry* 1983;4:222–227.

137. Jacobberger JW, Horan PK, Hare JD. Flow cytometric analysis of blood cells stained with the cyanine dye DiOC1[3]: reticulocyte quantification. *Cytometry* 1984;5:589–600.

138. Corash L, et al. Enumeration of reticulocytes using fluorescence-activated flow cytometry. *Pathol Immunopathol Res* 1988;7:381–394.

139. Davis BH, Bigelow NC, Koepke JA, et al. Flow cytometric reticulocyte analysis: multiinstitutional interlaboratory correlation study. *Am J Clin Pathol* 1994;102:468–477.

140. Lee LG, Chen CH, Chiu LA. Thiazole orange: a new dye for reticulocyte analysis. *Cytometry* 1986;7:508–517.

141. Carter JM, McSweeney PA, Wakem PJ, et al. Counting reticulocytes by flow cytometry: use of thiazole orange. *Clin Lab Haematol* 1989;11:267–271.

142. Davis BH, Bigelow NC. Flow cytometric reticulocyte quantification using thiazole orange provides clinically useful reticulocyte maturity index. *Arch Pathol Lab Med* 1989;113:684–689.

143. Davis BH, Bigelow N, Ball ED, et al. Utility of flow cytometric reticulocyte quantification as a predictor of engraftment in autologous bone marrow transplantation. *Am J Hematol* 1989;32.81–87.

144. Lacombe F, Lacoste L, Vial JP, et al. Automated reticulocyte counting and immature reticulocyte fraction measurement: comparison of ABX PENTRA 120 Retic, Sysmex R-2000, flow cytometry, and manual counts. *Am J Clin Pathol* 1999;112:677–686.

145. Davis BH, DiCorato M, Bigelow NC, et al. Proposal for standardization of flow cytometric reticulocyte maturity index (RMI) measurements. *Cytometry* 1993;14:318–326.

146. Davis B, Bigelow N, Van Hove L. Immature reticulocyte fraction (IRF) and reticulocyte counts: comparison of CELL-DYN 4000, Sysmex R-3000, thiazole flow cytometry, and manual counts. *Lab Hematol* 1996;2:144–150.

147. Villamor N, Kirsch A, Huhn D, et al. Interference of blood leucocytes in the measurements of immature red cells (reticulocytes) by two different (semi-) automated flow-cytometry technologies. *Clin Lab Haematol* 1996;18:89–94.

148. Kojima K, Niri M, Setoguchi K, et al. An automated optoelectronic reticulocyte counter. *Am J Clin Pathol* 1989;92:57–61.

149. Tichelli A, Gratwohl A, Driessen A, et al. Evaluation of the Sysmex R-1000: an automated reticulocyte analyzer. *Am J Clin Pathol* 1990;93:70–78.

150. Hamilton JL, Pollard Y, Grant D, et al. Evaluation of a semi-automated reticulocyte counting method using the Coulter STKS-2A blood cell counter. *Clin Lab Haematol* 1995;17:145–149.

151. Rudensky B. Comparison of a semi-automated new Coulter methylene blue method with fluorescence flow cytometry in reticulocyte counting. *Scand J Clin Lab Invest* 1997;57:291–296.

152. d'Onofrio G, Kim YR, Schulze S, et al. Evaluation of the Abbott Cell Dyn 4000 automated fluorescent reticulocyte measurements: comparison with manual, FACScan and Sysmex R1000 methods. *Clin Lab Haematol* 1997;19:253–260.

153. Greenberg ER, Beck JR. The effects of sample size on reticulocyte counting and stool examination: the binomial and Poisson distributions in laboratory medicine. *Arch Pathol Lab Med* 1984;108:396–398.

154. Matoth Y, Zaizov R, Varsano I. Postnatal changes in some red cell parameters. *Acta Paediatr Scand* 1971;60:317–323.

155. Conley CL, Lippman SM, Ness PM, et al. Autoimmune hemolytic anemia with reticulocytopenia and erythroid marrow. *N Engl J Med* 1982;306:281–286.

156. van Houte AJ, Bartels PC, Schoorl M, et al. Methodology-dependent variations in reticulocyte counts using a manual and two different flow cytometric procedures. *Eur J Clin Chem Clin Biochem* 1994;32:859–863.

157. Pappas AA, Owens RB, Flick JT. Reticulocyte counting by flow cytometry: a comparison with manual methods. *Ann Clin Lab Sci* 1992;22:125–132.

158. Hoffmann JJ, Pennings JM. Pseudo-reticulocytosis as a result of malaria parasites. *Clin Lab Haematol* 1999;21:257–260.

159. Español I, Pedro C, Remacha AF. Heinz bodies interfere with automated reticulocyte counts. *Haematologica* 1999;84:373–374.

160. Hinchliffe RF. Errors in automated reticulocyte counts due to Heinz bodies. *J Clin Pathol* 1993;46:878–879.

161. Chang CC, Kass L. Clinical significance of immature reticulocyte fraction determined by automated reticulocyte counting. *Am J Clin Pathol* 1997;108:69–73.

162. Davis BH, Ornvold K, Bigelow NC. Flow cytometric reticulocyte maturity index: a useful laboratory parameter of erythropoietic activity in anemia. *Cytometry* 1995;22:35–39.

163. Grotto HZ, Vigoritto AC, Noronha JF, et al. Immature reticulocyte fraction as a criterion for marrow engraftment: evaluation of a semi-automated reticulocyte counting method. *Clin Lab Haematol* 1999;21:285–287.

164. Davis BH. Immature reticulocyte fraction (IRF): by any name, a useful clinical parameter of erythropoietic activity. *Lab Hematol* 1996;2:2–8.

165. Davies SV, Cavill I, Bentley N, et al. Evaluation of erythropoiesis after bone marrow transplantation: quantitative reticulocyte counting. *Br J Haematol* 1992;81:12–17.

166. Kanold J, Bezou MJ, Coulet M, et al. Evaluation of erythropoietic/hematopoietic reconstitution after BMT by highly fluorescent reticulocyte counts compares favorably with traditional peripheral blood cell counting. *Bone Marrow Transplant* 1993;11:313–318.

167. Greinix HT, Linkesch W, Keil F, et al. Early detection of hematopoietic engraftment after bone marrow and peripheral blood stem cell transplantation by highly fluorescent reticulocyte counts. *Bone Marrow Transplant* 1994;14:307–313.

168. Santamaria A, Martino R, Bellido M, et al. Reticulocyte recovery is faster in allogeneic and autologous peripheral blood stem cell transplantation than in bone marrow transplantation [Letter]. *Eur J Haematol* 1997;58:362–364.

169. George P, Wyre RM, Bruty SJ, et al. Automated immature reticulocyte counts are early markers of engraftment following autologous PBSC transplantation in patients with lymphoma. *J Hematother Stem Cell Res* 2000;9:219–223.

170. Kuse R, Foures C, Jou JM, et al. Automated reticulocyte counting for monitoring patients on chemotherapy for acute leukaemias and malignant lymphomas. *Clin Lab Haematol* 1996;18[Suppl 1]:39–43.

171. Kuse R. The appearance of reticulocytes with medium or high RNA content is a sensitive indicator of beginning granulocyte recovery after aplasiogenic cytostatic drug therapy in patients with AML. *Ann Hematol* 1993;66:213–214.

172. Hillman RS, Finch CA. Erythropoiesis: normal and abnormal. *Semin Hematol* 1967;4:327–336.

173. Hillman RS. Characteristics of marrow production and reticulocyte maturation in normal man in response to anemia. *J Clin Invest* 1969;48:443–453.

174. Stelzer GT. Analysis of leukocyte function by flow cytometric techniques. *Cytometry Suppl* 1988;3:52–59.

175. Coon JS, Landay AL, Weinstein RS. Advances in flow cytometry for diagnostic pathology. *Lab Invest* 1987;57:453–479.

176. Borowitz MJ, Guenther KL, Shults KE, et al. Immunophenotyping of acute leukemia by flow cytometric analysis: use of CD45 and right-angle light scatter to gate on leukemic blasts in three-color analysis. *Am J Clin Pathol* 1993;100:534–540.

177. Chan LC, Pegram SM, Greaves MF. Contribution of immunophenotype to the classification and differential diagnosis of acute leukaemia. *Lancet* 1985;1:475–479.

178. Griffin JD, Davis R, Nelson DA, et al. Use of surface marker analysis to predict outcome of adult acute myeloblastic leukemia. *Blood* 1986;68:1232–1241.

179. Sobol RE, Mick R, Royston I, et al. Clinical importance of myeloid antigen expression in adult acute lymphoblastic leukemia. *N Engl J Med* 1987;316:1111–1117.

180. Borowitz MJ, Shuster J, Carroll AJ, et al. Prognostic significance of fluorescence intensity of surface marker expression in childhood B-precursor acute lymphoblastic leukemia: a Pediatric Oncology Group study. *Blood* 1997;89:3960–3966.

181. Borowitz MJ, Bray R, Gascoyne R, et al. U.S.-Canadian Consensus recommendations on the immunophenotypic analysis of hematologic neoplasia by flow cytometry: data analysis and interpretation. *Cytometry* 1997;30:236–244.

182. Sobol RE, Bloomfield CD, Royston I. Immunophenotyping in the diagnosis and classification of acute lymphoblastic leukemia. *Clin Lab Med* 1988;8:151–162.

183. Stelzer GT, Marti G, Hurley A, et al. U.S.-Canadian Consensus recommendations on the immunophenotypic analysis of hematologic neoplasia by flow cytometry: standardization and validation of laboratory procedures. *Cytometry* 1997;30:214–230.

184. Stewart CC, Behm FG, Carey JL, et al. U.S.-Canadian Consensus recommendations on the immunophenotypic analysis of hematologic neoplasia by flow cytometry: selection of antibody combinations. *Cytometry* 1997;30:231–235.

185. Davis BH, Foucar K, Szczarkowski W, et al. U.S.-Canadian Consensus recommendations on the immunophenotypic analysis of hematologic neoplasia by flow cytometry: medical indications. *Cytometry* 1997;30:249–263.

186. Kidd PG, Nicholson JKA. Immunophenotyping by flow cytometry. In: Rose N, Conway de Macario E, Folds J, et al., eds. *Manual of clinical laboratory immunology*, 5th ed. Washington, DC: American Society of Microbiology Press, 1997:229–244.

187. Jackson A, Warner N. Preparation, staining, and analysis by flow cytometry of peripheral blood leukocyte. In: Rose N, Friedman H, Fahey J, eds. *Manual of clinical laboratory immunology*, 3rd ed. Washington, DC: American Society for Microbiology, 1986:226–235.

188. Macey MG, McCarthy DA, Milne T, et al. Comparative study of five commercial reagents for preparing normal and leukaemic lymphocytes for immunophenotypic analysis by flow cytometry. *Cytometry* 1999;38:153–160.

189. De Paoli P, Villalta D, Battistin S, et al. Selective loss of OKT8 lymphocytes on density gradient centrifugation separation of blood mononuclear cells. *J Immunol Methods* 1983;61:259–260.

190. Renzi P, Ginns LC. Analysis of T-cell subsets in normal adults: comparison of whole blood lysis technique to Ficoll-Hypaque separation by flow cytometry. *J Immunol Methods* 1987;98:53–56.

191. Holmes K, et al. *Current protocols in immunology*. New York: John Wiley and Sons, 1995.

192. Sasaki DT, Dumas SE, Engleman EG. Discrimination of viable and non-viable cells using propidium iodide in two color immunofluorescence. *Cytometry* 1987;8:413–420.
193. Beckstead JH, Halverson PS, Ries CA, et al. Enzyme histochemistry and immunohistochemistry on biopsy specimens of pathologic human bone marrow. *Blood* 1981;57:1088–1098.
194. Pui CH, Behm FG, Crist WM. Clinical and biologic relevance of immunologic marker studies in childhood acute lymphoblastic leukemia. *Blood* 1993;82:343–362.
195. Jennings CD, Foon KA. Recent advances in flow cytometry: application to the diagnosis of hematologic malignancy. *Blood* 1997;90:2863–2892.
196. Copelan EA, McGuire EA. The biology and treatment of acute lymphoblastic leukemia in adults. *Blood* 1995;85:1151–1168.
197. Crist W, Boyett J, Jackson J, et al. Prognostic importance of the pre-B-cell immunophenotype and other presenting features in B-lineage childhood acute lymphoblastic leukemia: a Pediatric Oncology Group study. *Blood* 1989;74:1252–1259.
198. Boucheix C, David B, Sebban C, et al. Immunophenotype of adult acute lymphoblastic leukemia, clinical parameters, and outcome: an analysis of a prospective trial including 562 tested patients (LALA87). French Group on Therapy for Adult Acute Lymphoblastic Leukemia. *Blood* 1994;84:1603–1612.
199. Hann IM, Richards SM, Eden OB, et al. Analysis of the immunophenotype of children treated on the Medical Research Council United Kingdom Acute Lymphoblastic Leukaemia Trial XI (MRC UKALLXI). Medical Research Council Childhood Leukaemia Working Party. *Leukemia* 1998;12:1249–1255.
200. Crist WM, Carroll AJ, Shuster JJ, et al. Poor prognosis of children with pre-B acute lymphoblastic leukemia is associated with the t(1;19)(q23;p13): a Pediatric Oncology Group study. *Blood* 1990;76:117–122.
201. Raimondi SC, Behm FG, Roberson PK, et al. Cytogenetics of pre-B-cell acute lymphoblastic leukemia with emphasis on prognostic implications of the t(1;19). *J Clin Oncol* 1990;8:1380–1388.
202. Harris NL, Jaffe ES, Diebold J, et al. The World Health Organization classification of neoplastic diseases of the hematopoietic and lymphoid tissues: report of the Clinical Advisory Committee meeting, Airlie House, Virginia, November, 1997. *Ann Oncol* 1999;10:1419–1432.
203. Shuster JJ, Falletta JM, Pullen DJ. Prognostic factors in childhood T-cell acute lymphoblastic leukemia: a Pediatric Oncology Group study. *Blood* 1990;75:166–173.
204. Crist WM, Shuster JJ, Falletta J, et al. Clinical features and outcome in childhood T-cell leukemia-lymphoma according to stage of thymocyte differentiation: a Pediatric Oncology Group study. *Blood* 1988;72:1891–1897.
205. Dowell BL, Borowitz MJ, Boyett JM, et al. Immunologic and clinicopathologic features of common acute lymphoblastic leukemia antigen-positive childhood T-cell leukemia: a Pediatric Oncology Group study. *Cancer* 1987;59:2020–2026.
206. Uckun FM, Sensel MG, Sun L, et al. Biology and treatment of childhood T-lineage acute lymphoblastic leukemia. *Blood* 1998;91:735–746.
207. Larson RA, Dodge RK, Burns CP, et al. A five-drug remission induction regimen with intensive consolidation for adults with acute lymphoblastic leukemia: cancer and leukemia group B study 8811. *Blood* 1995;85:2025–2037.
208. Czuczman MS, Dodge RK, Stewart CC, et al. Value of immunophenotype in intensively treated adult acute lymphoblastic leukemia: cancer and leukemia Group B study 8364. *Blood* 1999;93:3931–3939.
209. Pui CH, Hancock ML, Head DR, et al. Clinical significance of CD34 expression in childhood acute lymphoblastic leukemia. *Blood* 1993;82:889–894.
210. Borowitz MJ, Shuster JJ, Civin CI, et al. Prognostic significance of CD34 expression in childhood B-precursor acute lymphocytic leukemia: a Pediatric Oncology Group study. *J Clin Oncol* 1990;8:1389–1398.
211. Uckun FM, Sather H, Gaynon P, et al. Prognostic significance of the CD10+CD19+CD34+ B-progenitor immunophenotype in children with acute lymphoblastic leukemia: a report from the Children's Cancer Group. *Leuk Lymphoma* 1997;27:445–457.
212. Thomas X, Archimbaud E, Charrin C, et al. CD34 expression is associated with major adverse prognostic factors in adult acute lymphoblastic leukemia. *Leukemia* 1995;9:249–253.
213. Gómez E, San Miguel JF, Gonzalez M, et al. The value of the immunological subtypes and individual markers compared to classical parameters in the prognosis of acute lymphoblastic leukemia. *Hematol Oncol* 1991;9:33–42.
214. Pui CH, Rivera GK, Hancock ML, et al. Clinical significance of CD10 expression in childhood acute lymphoblastic leukemia. *Leukemia* 1993;7:35–40.
215. Sallan SE, Ritz J, Pesando J, et al. Cell surface antigens: prognostic implications in childhood acute lymphoblastic leukemia. *Blood* 1980;55:395–402.
216. Pui CH, Williams DL, Raimondi SC, et al. Unfavorable presenting clinical and laboratory features are associated with CALLA-negative non-T, non-B lymphoblastic leukemia in children. *Leuk Res* 1986;10:1287–1292.
217. Consolini R, Legitimo A, Rondelli R, et al. Clinical relevance of CD10 expression in childhood ALL. The Italian Association for Pediatric Hematology and Oncology (AIEOP). *Haematologica* 1998;83:967–973.
218. Pui CH, Behm FG, Singh B, et al. Myeloid-associated antigen expression lacks prognostic value in childhood acute lymphoblastic leukemia treated with intensive multiagent chemotherapy. *Blood* 1990;75:198–202.
219. Putti MC, Rondelli R, Concito MG, et al. Expression of myeloid markers lacks prognostic impact in children treated for acute lymphoblastic leukemia: Italian experience in AIEOP-ALL 88-91 studies. *Blood* 1998;92:795–801.
220. Griesinger F, Piro-Noack M, Kaib N, et al. Leukaemia-associated immunophenotypes (LAIP) are observed in 90% of adult and childhood acute lymphoblastic leukaemia: detection in remission marrow predicts outcome. *Br J Haematol* 1999;105:241–255.
221. García Vela JA, Monteserin MC, Delgado I, et al. Aberrant immunophenotypes detected by flow cytometry in acute lymphoblastic leukemia. *Leuk Lymphoma* 2000;36:275–284.
222. Campana D, Coustan-Smith E. Detection of minimal residual disease in acute leukemia by flow cytometry. *Cytometry* 1999;38:139–152.
223. van Dongen JJ, Seriu T, Panzer-Grumayer ER, et al. Prognostic value of minimal residual disease in acute lymphoblastic leukaemia in childhood. *Lancet* 1998;352:1731–1738.
224. Coustan-Smith E, Sancho J, Hancock ML, et al. Clinical importance of minimal residual disease in childhood acute lymphoblastic leukemia. *Blood* 2000;96:2691–2696.
225. Coustan-Smith E, Behm FG, Sanchez J, et al. Immunological detection of minimal residual disease in children with acute lymphoblastic leukaemia. *Lancet* 1998;351:550–554.
226. Nguyen PL, Olszak I, Harris NL, et al. Myeloperoxidase detection by three-color flow cytometry and by enzyme cytochemistry in the classification of acute leukemia. *Am J Clin Pathol* 1998;110:163–169.
227. García Vela JA, Delgado I, Oña F. Myeloperoxidase detection by three-color flow cytometry in acute lymphoblastic leukemia [Letter]. *Am J Clin Pathol* 1999;112:122–124.
228. Drach D, Drach J, Glassl H, et al. Flow cytometric detection of cytoplasmic antigens in acute leukemias: implications for lineage assignment. *Leuk Res* 1993;17:455–461.
229. Nakase K, Sartor M, Bradstock. Detection of myeloperoxidase by flow cytometry in acute leukemia. *Cytometry* 1998;34:198–202.
230. Farahat N, van der Plas D, Praxedes M, et al. Demonstration of cytoplasmic and nuclear antigens in acute leukaemia using flow cytometry. *J Clin Pathol* 1994;47:843–849.
231. Exner M, Thalhammer R, Kapiotis S, et al. The "typical" immunophenotype of acute promyelocytic leukemia (APL-M3): does it prove true for the M3-variant? *Cytometry* 1999;42:106–109.
232. Bradstock K, Matthews J, Benson E, et al. Prognostic value of immunophenotyping in acute myeloid leukemia. Australian Leukaemia Study Group. *Blood* 1994;84:1220–1225.
233. Campos L, Guyotat D, Archimbaud E, et al. Surface marker expression in adult acute myeloid leukaemia: correlations with initial characteristics, morphology and response to therapy. *Br J Haematol* 1989;72:161–166.
234. Creutzig U, Harbott J, Sperling C, et al. Clinical significance of surface antigen expression in children with acute myeloid leukemia: results of study AML-BFM-87. *Blood* 1995;86:3097–3108.
235. de Nully Brown P, Jurlander J, Pedersen-Bjergaard J, et al. The prognostic significance of chromosomal analysis and immunophenotyping in 117 patients with de novo acute myeloid leukemia. *Leuk Res* 1997;21:985–995.
236. Del Poeta G, Stasi R, Venditti A, et al. Prognostic value of cell marker analysis in de novo acute myeloid leukemia. *Leukemia* 1994;8:388–394.
237. Kita K, Miwa H, Nakase K, et al. Clinical importance of CD7 expression in acute myelocytic leukemia. The Japan Cooperative Group of Leukemia/Lymphoma. *Blood* 1993;81:2399–2405.
238. Lee EJ, Yang J, Leavitt RD, et al. The significance of CD34 and TdT determinations in patients with untreated de novo acute myeloid leukemia. *Leukemia* 1992;6:1203–1209.
239. Schwartz S, Heinecke A, Zimmermann M, et al. Expression of the C-kit receptor (CD117) is a feature of almost all subtypes of de novo acute myeloblastic leukemia (AML), including cytogenetically good-risk AML, and lacks prognostic significance. *Leuk Lymphoma* 1999;34:85–94.
240. Schwarzinger I, Valent P, Koller U, et al. Prognostic significance of surface marker expression on blasts of patients with de novo acute myeloblastic leukemia. *J Clin Oncol* 1990;8:423–430.
241. Solary E, Casasnovas RO, Campos L, et al. Surface markers in adult acute myeloblastic leukemia: correlation of CD19+, CD34+ and CD14+/DR– phenotypes with shorter survival. Groupe d'Etude Immunologique des Leucémies (GEIL). *Leukemia* 1992;6:393–399.
242. Sperling C, Buchner T, Creutzig U, et al. Clinical, morphologic, cytogenetic and prognostic implications of CD34 expression in childhood and adult de novo AML. *Leuk Lymphoma* 1995;17:417–426.
243. Venditti A, Del Poeta G, Buccisano F, et al. Prognostic relevance of the expression of Tdt and CD7 in 335 cases of acute myeloid leukemia. *Leukemia* 1998;12:1056–1063.
244. Legrand O, Perrot JY, Baudard M, et al. The immunophenotype of 177 adults with acute myeloid leukemia: proposal of a prognostic score. *Blood* 2000;96:870–877.
245. San Miguel JF, Martinez A, Macedo A, et al. Immunophenotyping investigation of minimal residual disease is a useful approach for predicting relapse in acute myeloid leukemia patients. *Blood* 1997;90:2465–2470.
246. Reading CL, Estey EH, Huh YO, et al. Expression of unusual immunophenotype combinations in acute myelogenous leukemia. *Blood* 1993;81:3083–3090.
247. Macedo A, Orfao A, Gonzalez M, et al. Immunological detection of blast cell subpopulations in acute myeloblastic leukemia at diagnosis: implications for minimal residual disease studies. *Leukemia* 1995;9:993–998.
248. Sievers EL, Lange BJ, Buckley JD, et al. Prediction of relapse of pediatric acute myeloid leukemia by use of multidimensional flow cytometry. *J Natl Cancer Inst* 1996;88:1483–1488.
249. Venditti A, Buccisano F, Del Poeta G, et al. Level of minimal residual disease after consolidation therapy predicts outcome in acute myeloid leukemia. *Blood* 2000;96:3948–3952.
250. Leith CP, Kopecky KJ, Godwin J, et al. Acute myeloid leukemia in the elderly: assessment of multidrug resistance (MDR1) and cytogenetics distinguishes biologic subgroups with remarkably distinct responses to standard

chemotherapy: a Southwest Oncology Group study. *Blood* 1997;89:3323–3329.

251. Leith CP, Kopecky KJ, Chen IM, et al. Frequency and clinical significance of the expression of the multidrug resistance proteins MDR1/P-glycoprotein, MRP1, and LRP in acute myeloid leukemia: a Southwest Oncology Group study. *Blood* 1999;94:1086–1099.

252. Leith CP, Chen IM, Kopecky KJ, et al. Correlation of multidrug resistance (MDR1) protein expression with functional dye/drug efflux in acute myeloid leukemia by multiparameter flow cytometry: identification of discordant MDR–/efflux+ and MDR1+/efflux– cases. *Blood* 1995;86:2329–2342.

253. Willman CL. The prognostic significance of the expression and function of multidrug resistance transporter proteins in acute myeloid leukemia: studies of the Southwest Oncology Group Leukemia Research Program. *Semin Hematol* 1997;34[Suppl 5]:25–33.

254. Wattel E, Solary E, Hecquet B, et al. Quinine improves results of intensive chemotherapy (IC) in myelodysplastic syndromes (MDS) expressing P-glycoprotein (PGP). Updated results of a randomized study. Groupe Français des Myélodysplasies (GFM) and Groupe GOELAMS. *Adv Exp Med Biol* 1999;457:35–46.

255. Bene MC, Castoldi G, Knapp W, et al. Proposals for the immunological classification of acute leukemias. European Group for the Immunological Characterization of Leukemias (EGIL). *Leukemia* 1995;9:1783–1786.

256. Adachi K, Okumura M, Tanimoto M, et al. Analysis of immunophenotype, genotype, and lineage fidelity in blastic transformation of chronic myelogenous leukemia: a study of 20 cases. *J Lab Clin Med* 1988;111:125–132.

257. Nair C, Chopra H, Shinde S, et al. Immunophenotype and ultrastructural studies in blast crisis of chronic myeloid leukemia. *Leuk Lymphoma* 1995;19:309–313.

258. Khalidi HS, Brynes RK, Medeiros LJ, et al. The immunophenotype of blast transformation of chronic myelogenous leukemia: a high frequency of mixed lineage phenotype in "lymphoid" blasts and a comparison of morphologic, immunophenotypic, and molecular findings. *Mod Pathol* 1998;11:1211–1221.

259. Hanson CA, Kurtin PJ, Katzmann JA, et al. Immunophenotypic analysis of peripheral blood and bone marrow in the staging of B-cell malignant lymphoma. *Blood* 1999;94:3889–3896.

260. Harris NL, Jaffe ES, Stein H, et al. A revised European-American classification of lymphoid neoplasms: a proposal from the International Lymphoma Study Group. *Blood* 1994;84:1361–1392.

261. Frizzera G, Wu CD, Inghirami G. The usefulness of immunophenotypic and genotypic studies in the diagnosis and classification of hematopoietic and lymphoid neoplasms: an update. *Am J Clin Pathol* 1999;111[Suppl 1]:S13–S39.

262. Kilo MN, Dorfman DM. The utility of flow cytometric immunophenotypic analysis in the distinction of small lymphocytic lymphoma/chronic lymphocytic leukemia from mantle cell lymphoma. *Am J Clin Pathol* 1996;105:451–457.

263. Yang WI, Zukerberg LR, Motokura T, et al. Cyclin D1 (Bcl-1, PRAD1) protein expression in low-grade B-cell lymphomas and reactive hyperplasia. *Am J Pathol* 1994;145:86–96.

264. Robbins BA, Ellison DJ, Spinosa JC, et al. Diagnostic application of two-color flow cytometry in 161 cases of hairy cell leukemia. *Blood* 1993;82:1277–1287.

265. Tbakhi A, Edinger M, Myles J, et al. Flow cytometric immunophenotyping of non-Hodgkin's lymphomas and related disorders. *Cytometry* 1996;25:113–124.

266. DiGiuseppe JA, Borowitz MJ. Clinical utility of flow cytometry in the chronic lymphoid leukemias. *Semin Oncol* 1998;25:6–10.

267. Yamaguchi M, Machii T, Shibayama H, et al. Immunophenotypic features and configuration of immunoglobulin genes in hairy cell leukemia-Japanese variant. *Leukemia* 1996;10:1390–1394.

268. de Totero D, Tazzari PL, Lauria F, et al. Phenotypic analysis of hairy cell leukemia: "variant" cases express the interleukin-2 receptor beta chain, but not the alpha chain (CD25). *Blood* 1993;82:528–535.

269. Matutes E, Morilla R, Owusu-Ankomah K, et al. The immunophenotype of splenic lymphoma with villous lymphocytes and its relevance to the differential diagnosis with other B-cell disorders. *Blood* 1994;83:1558–1562.

270. Matutes E, Morilla R, Owusu-Ankomah K, et al. The immunophenotype of hairy cell leukemia (HCL). Proposal for a scoring system to distinguish HCL from B-cell disorders with hairy or villous lymphocytes. *Leuk Lymphoma* 1994;14[Suppl 1]:57–61.

271. Lamy T, Loughran TP Jr. Current concepts: large granular lymphocyte leukemia. *Blood Rev* 1999;13:230–240.

272. Kinney MC. The role of morphologic features, phenotype, genotype, and anatomic site in defining extranodal T-cell or NK-cell neoplasms. *Am J Clin Pathol* 1999;111[Suppl 1]:S104–S118.

273. Fletcher V, Zackheim HS, Beckstead JH. Circulating Sézary cells: a new preparatory method for their identification and enumeration. *Arch Pathol Lab Med* 1984;108:954–958.

274. Macon W, et al. Hepatosplenic αβ T-cell lymphomas: a report of four cases with features similar to hepatosplenic γδ T-cell lymphomas. *Mod Pathol* 1998;11:135a(abst).

275. Weidmann E. Hepatosplenic T cell lymphoma: a review on 45 cases since the first report describing the disease as a distinct lymphoma entity in 1990. *Leukemia* 2000;14:991–997.

276. Brodsky RA, Mukhina GL, Li S, et al. Improved detection and characterization of paroxysmal nocturnal hemoglobinuria using fluorescent aerolysin. *Am J Clin Pathol* 2000;114:459–466.

277. Mehta J, Powles R, Treleaven J, et al. Number of nucleated cells infused during allogeneic and autologous bone marrow transplantation: an important modifiable factor influencing outcome [Letter]. *Blood* 1997;90:3808–3810.

278. Sierra J, Storer B, Hansen JA, et al. Transplantation of marrow cells from unrelated donors for treatment of high-risk acute leukemia: the effect of leukemic burden, donor HLA-matching, and marrow cell dose. *Blood* 1997;89:4226–4235.

279. Gratama JW, Orfao A, Barnett D, et al. Flow cytometric enumeration of CD34+ hematopoietic stem and progenitor cells. European Working Group on Clinical Cell Analysis. *Cytometry* 1998;34:128–142.

280. Nicholson JK. Use of flow cytometry in the evaluation and diagnosis of primary and secondary immunodeficiency diseases. *Arch Pathol Lab Med* 1989;113:598–605.

281. Reinherz EL, Cooper MD, Schlossman SF, et al. Abnormalities of T cell maturation and regulation in human beings with immunodeficiency disorders. *J Clin Invest* 1981;68:699–705.

282. Linch DC, Levinsky RJ. Prenatal diagnosis of immunodeficiency disorders. *Br Med Bull* 1983;39:399–404.

283. Koepke JA, Landay AL. Precision and accuracy of absolute lymphocyte counts. *Clin Immunol Immunopathol* 1989;52:19–27.

284. Bagg A, Kallakury BV. Molecular pathology of leukemia and lymphoma. *Am J Clin Pathol* 1999;112[Suppl 1]:S76–S92.

285. Willman CL. Molecular evaluation of acute myeloid leukemias. *Semin Hematol* 1999;36:390–400.

286. Macintyre EA, Delabesse E. Molecular approaches to the diagnosis and evaluation of lymphoid malignancies. *Semin Hematol* 1999;36:373–389.

287. Tierens A, Lozano MD, Wichert R, et al. High-resolution analysis of immunoglobulin heavy-chain gene rearrangements using denaturing gradient gel electrophoresis. *Diagn Mol Pathol* 1996;5:159–165.

288. Guitart J, Kaul K. A new polymerase chain reaction-based method for the detection of T-cell clonality in patients with possible cutaneous T-cell lymphoma. *Arch Dermatol* 1999;135:158–162.

289. Baruchel A, Cayuela JM, MacIntyre E, et al. Assessment of clonal evolution at Ig/TCR loci in acute lymphoblastic leukaemia by single-strand conformation polymorphism studies and highly resolutive PCR derived methods: implication for a general strategy of minimal residual disease detection. *Br J Haematol* 1995;90:85–93.

290. Bottaro M, Berti E, Biondi A, et al. Heteroduplex analysis of T-cell receptor gamma gene rearrangements for diagnosis and monitoring of cutaneous T-cell lymphomas. *Blood* 1994;83:3271–3278.

291. Aubin J, Davi F, Nguyen-Salomon F, et al. Description of a novel FR1 IgH PCR strategy and its comparison with three other strategies for the detection of clonality in B cell malignancies. *Leukemia* 1995;9:471–479.

292. Diss TC, Watts M, Pan LX, et al. The polymerase chain reaction in the demonstration of monoclonality in T cell lymphomas. *J Clin Pathol* 1995;48:1045–1050.

293. Slack DN, McCarthy KP, Wiedemann LM, et al. Evaluation of sensitivity, specificity, and reproducibility of an optimized method for detecting clonal rearrangements of immunoglobulin and T-cell receptor genes in formalin-fixed, paraffin-embedded sections. *Diagn Mol Pathol* 1993;2:223–232.

294. McCarthy KP, Sloane JP, Kabarowski JH, et al. A simplified method of detection of clonal rearrangements of the T-cell receptor-gamma chain gene. *Diagn Mol Pathol* 1992;1:173–179.

295. Buttarello M, Bulian P, Temporin V, et al. Sysmex SE-9000 hematology analyzer: performance evaluation on leukocyte differential counts using an NCCLS H20-A protocol. National Committee for Clinical Laboratory Standards. *Am J Clin Pathol* 1997;108:674–686.

296. Barnard DF, Barnard SA, Carter AB, et al. An evaluation of the Coulter VCS differential counter. *Clin Lab Haematol* 1989;11:255–266.

297. Grimaldi E, Scopacasa F. Evaluation of the Abbott CELL-DYN 4000 hematology analyzer. *Am J Clin Pathol* 2000;113:497–505.

298. Borowitz M, Silberman M. *Cases in flow cytometry.* Interactive CD-ROM. Charlottesville, VA: Carden Jennings Publishing Co. 1999.

299. Knowles D. Immunophenotypic markers useful in the diagnosis and classification of hematopoietic neoplasms. In: Knowles D, ed. *Neoplastic hematopathology*, 2nd ed. Philadelphia: Lippincott Williams & Wilkins, 2001:93–226.

300. Khalidi HS, Chang KL, Medeiros LJ, et al. Acute lymphoblastic leukemia: survey of immunophenotype, French-American-British classification, frequency of myeloid antigen expression, and karyotypic abnormalities in 210 pediatric and adult cases. *Am J Clin Pathol* 1999;111:467–476.

301. Khalidi HS, Medeiros LJ, Chang KL, et al. The immunophenotype of adult acute myeloid leukemia: high frequency of lymphoid antigen expression and comparison of immunophenotype, French-American-British classification, and karyotypic abnormalities. *Am J Clin Pathol* 1998;109:211–220.

302. Foucar K. Chronic lymphoid leukemias and lymphoproliferative disorders. *Mod Pathol* 1999;12:141–150.

303. Haynes JL. Principles of flow cytometry. *Cytometry* 1988;9[Suppl 3]:7–17.

304. Bessman JD. *Automated blood counts and differentials: a practical guide.* Baltimore: Johns Hopkins University Press, 1986.

305. Sun NCJ. *Hematology: an atlas and diagnostic guide.* Philadelphia: WB Saunders, 1983.

306. Breakall ES, Marchand A, Marcus R, et al. Comparison of performance for leukocyte differential counting of the Technicon H-6000 system with a manual reference method using the NCCLS standard. *Blood Cells* 1985;11:257–279.

CHAPTER 3

Examination of the Bone Marrow

Mark D. Fleming, Jeffery L. Kutok, and Arthur T. Skarin

Ever since the role of bone marrow in blood cell production was described in 1868, this organ has been examined intensively by anatomists, pathologists, hematologists, and oncologists (1). As techniques to sample the marrow *in vivo* emerged, observation of the process of blood formation became a reality (2). Few organs are as accessible to sampling as the bone marrow. In concert with review of the peripheral blood smear, a bone marrow examination provides much of the attainable information regarding the status of the hematopoietic system. Although aspiration and biopsy of the marrow are technically simple procedures, samples can be processed by increasingly sophisticated methods, including flow cytometry, immunohistochemistry, cytogenetics, and molecular diagnostics, to yield more information than morphology alone can provide. This chapter reviews these methods and offers a standard procedure to obtain, process, and report bone marrow specimens.

INDICATIONS FOR BONE MARROW EXAMINATION

The decision to perform a bone marrow examination is based on the assumption that relevant data will be obtained and that the attendant risks of the procedure are acceptable. Although the risks of marrow sampling are few (see Complications), the probability of useful information being garnered for specific cases is difficult to estimate. Retrospective estimates are flawed by sampling biases; specific prospective series are largely lacking, even for common marrow diseases, except when generated as part of treatment protocols for hematologic and nonhematologic malignancies. Because meaningful pretest probabilities are unavailable, current suggestions represent the collective opinions of clinicians and pathologists, even though complete agreement is lacking (3–5). Situations in which bone marrow examination is regularly performed are listed in Table 3-1.

TECHNICAL ASPECTS

Instruments

A variety of needles are available for aspiration or biopsy of the bone marrow (6). Simple needles with obturators, such as the Osgood or Rosenthal needles, suffice for aspiration alone. The Illinois sternal puncture needle, although similar in design to the latter, is equipped with a guard to prevent traversing the adult sternum completely (Fig. 3-1). The Jamshidi-Swaim needle yields biopsy specimens with well-preserved architecture and can be used for obtaining bone marrow aspirates and biopsies through the same needle (7). Disposable Jamshidi needles are now in common use (Fig. 3-2). Several newer instruments, including the Islam needle, are equipped with a core-securing device to prevent the biopsy from slipping out of the needle during the process of extraction (8).

Sites for Aspiration and Biopsy

The choice of a site for bone marrow aspiration or biopsy is dependent on several factors, such as age, weight, marrow distribution, patient status, and physician experience. The normal adult skeleton contains approximately 1500 g of marrow, 40% of which is concentrated in the pelvis (9) (Table 3-2). For this reason, and because of the fact that it is easily identified and sampled, the posterior iliac crest is the preferred site to obtain marrow in most patients. In obese patients, whose landmarks are obliterated by flank fat, and whose posterior iliac spines lie too deep beneath the skin, the anterior iliac spine may be used. Sampling is not significantly discordant between these two sites (9). In infants and small children, a variety of other sites for aspiration are potentially available, including the proximal tibia and the femur (Table 3-3). Similar to biopsy in adults, the posterior iliac crest is the preferred site for needle biopsy in infants, but one may also be obtained from the anterior iliac crest or the proximal tibia (10).

Procedure for Bone Marrow Aspiration

The bone marrow aspiration procedure and its possible complications should be explained fully to the patient, and documentation of consent should be entered in the patient's medical record. The following equipment should be assembled:

- Biopsy needle
- Aspiration needle
- Ten to 15 glass slides or square coverslips
- 5-mL bottle of fixative

TABLE 3-1. Indications for Bone Marrow Examination

Primary indications
  Anemia, leukopenia, or thrombocytopenia of uncertain etiology
  Pancytopenia
  Leukoerythroblastosis
  Unexplained erythroid or myeloid precursors present on the peripheral blood smear
  Unexplained teardrop erythrocytes on the peripheral blood smear
  Lymphoma staging
  Evaluation of myeloproliferative and myelodysplastic disorders
  Evaluation of paraproteinemia or paraproteinuria
  Diagnosis of lipid storage disorders
  Monitoring of response to therapy in leukemia or lymphoma
  Staging of nonhematopoietic malignancies in tumors commonly metastatic to bone, or when bone marrow metastases are clinically suspected
Secondary indications
  Suspected iron deficiency
  Evaluation of granulomatous and fungal infections
  Fever of unknown origin

- Ethylenediaminetetraacetic acid (EDTA) anticoagulant tubes
- Preservative-free sodium heparin anticoagulant
- Syringes (10 mL) and needles (25 and 20 gauge)
- Lidocaine hydrochloride
- Sterile surgical blade
- Gauze pads
- Povidone-iodine solution
- Sterile gloves

Pretreatment with antianxiety medications is generally not required in adults. For the extremely anxious adult patient, 2 to 5 mg of diazepam can be administered parenterally 15 to 20 minutes before the procedure. By contrast, in children, sedation or even general anesthesia is usually required (11). For the posterior iliac spine approach, the patient should be in the prone position or on one side with the legs slightly bent (Fig. 3-3). In either position, patient comfort facilitates maximal cooperation.

The posterior iliac spine is located and marked as shown in Figure 3-3. In thinner patients, the posterior iliac spine can be palpated as a bony prominence that is superior and approximately three fingerbreadths lateral to the intergluteal cleft. The skin overlying its upper aspect may be dimpled. The area is cleansed thoroughly with a povidone-iodine solution and wiped dry. The overlying skin is anesthetized with intradermal lidocaine hydrochloride using a 25-gauge needle. With a larger needle (20 gauge), the skin is pierced and the needle advanced to the periosteum. An area approximately 1 cm in diameter should be anesthetized by withdrawing and redirecting the needle several times. The needle tip should be firmly planted in

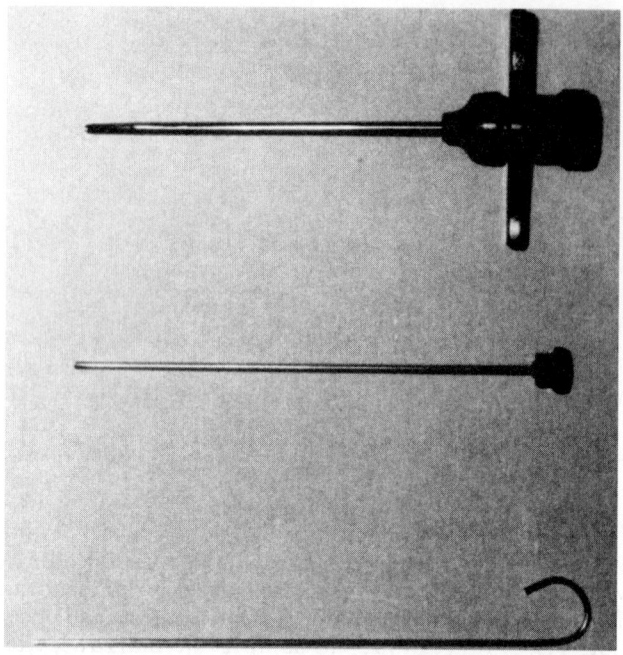

Figure 3-2. Disposable Jamshidi needle **(top)**. Obturator **(middle)**. Stylet **(bottom)**.

the bone, as the anesthetic is injected under pressure. Allow several minutes for the anesthetic to take effect.

A small skin incision may be made with a surgical blade at the site of injection. The bone marrow needle, with its obturator fixed in place, is pushed through the skin and twisted several times in a clockwise-counterclockwise fashion while downward pressure is exerted, until the solid surface of the periosteum is reached. Because of the curvature of the posterior iliac spine, the needle should be directed cephalad, toward the anterior iliac spine (Fig. 3-4). Using similar clockwise-counterclockwise rotations, the needle is advanced through the periosteum and cortex until firmly in place. The operator may sense a sudden lack of resistance as the softer trabecular bone is entered. The stylet is removed, and a 10-mL syringe is attached to the anchored needle. By swiftly withdrawing the plunger, negative pressure is created and approximately 0.5 mL of marrow is collected. A sharp, fleeting pain as the marrow is aspirated is a reliable sign that the marrow cavity was entered successfully (12). Aspirated marrow may then be used to prepare direct smears or anticoagulated for processing in the laboratory (see Processing of Specimens).

TABLE 3-2. Marrow Distribution in the Adult

Site	Marrow Weight (g)	Red Marrow Weight (g)	Red Marrow Total (%)
Head	182.2	136.6	13.1
Upper limb girdle	115.5	86.7	8.3
Sternum	39.0	23.4	2.3
Ribs	206.8	82.6	7.9
Cervical vertebrae	47.4	35.8	3.4
Thoracic vertebrae	197.0	147.9	14.1
Lumbar vertebrae	152.2	114.1	10.9
Sacrum	194.0	145.6	13.9
Lower limb girdle	363.6	273.0	26.1
Total	**1497.7**	**1045.7**	**100.0**

Adapted from Ellis RB. The distribution of active marrow in the adult. *Phys Med Biol* 1961;5:255.

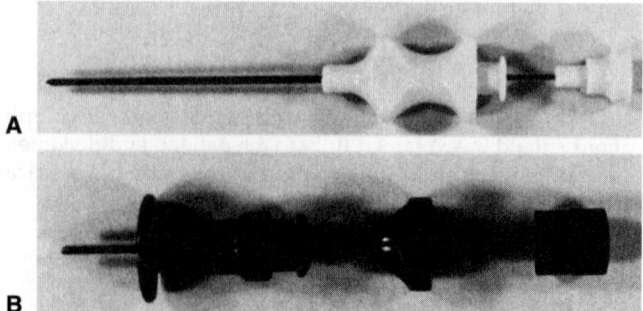

Figure 3-1. Aspiration needles. Disposable Rosenthal needle **(A)**. Illinois needle with guard **(B)**.

TABLE 3-3. Sites for Bone Marrow Aspiration

Site	Age When Practical
Tibia	Birth to 12 mo
Femur	Birth to 12 mo
Anterior iliac crest	Any age
Posterior iliac crest	Any age
Vertebral spinous process	2 yr and older
Sternum	6 mo[a] and older

[a]Only when supervised.
From Pochedly C. How to perform bone marrow puncture in small children. *Clin Pediatr (Phila)* 1969;8:705.

When marrow cannot be aspirated after three or four attempts from one site (a dry tap), touch preparations should be made by gently imprinting a glass slide or coverslip on the biopsy specimen. Alternatively, additional punctures may be made at the same or other sites. A dry tap may be due to several reasons, the most common being a failure to enter the marrow cavity. However, marrow may be inaspirable in other situations, such as sites involved by metastatic carcinoma; certain lymphoproliferative disorders, including hairy cell leukemia; fatty replacement, as in aplastic anemia; or marrow fibrosis, as in some chronic myeloproliferative disorders.

PROCEDURE FOR BONE MARROW BIOPSY

Patient positioning and preparation for a biopsy is the same as for aspiration. After aspiration is completed, the needle is removed and directed to an anesthetized area adjacent to the aspiration site to avoid introducing aspiration artifact in the biopsy. The stylet is locked in place, and the needle ensemble is advanced through the cortical bone using alternating clockwise and counterclockwise rotations until it is firmly anchored. The stylet is then removed, and the needle advanced to a depth of 2 to 3 cm. The size of the core can be approximated by carefully reinserting the obturator until some resistance is encountered and estimating the length that protrudes beyond the proximal end of the shaft of the needle. To loosen the core from its bony moorings, the needle is rotated in place while it is gently jiggled, then slowly removed with alternating rotary motions. The most common reason for failure to obtain a biopsy specimen is that the core is left in place while the needle is being withdrawn. After the core is obtained, the bone marrow biopsy is dislodged onto a clean glass slide by inserting the probe into the distal, tapered end of the biopsy needle. At this point, touch

preparations may be made, and the biopsy specimen may be placed in a container of the fixative of choice and submitted for preparation of paraffin-embedded sections. Ideally, biopsy samples should be at least 2 cm in length (7).

Biopsy versus Aspiration

Whether bone marrow biopsy augments the diagnostic yield of the aspirate is controversial and, in large part, depends on the ultimate diagnosis. An accurate interpretation of published data comparing the two requires attention to the methods of preparation and evaluation of samples, the adequacy of either specimen, and the most likely diagnoses to be confirmed or excluded. Furthermore, because the quality of biopsy histology varies so greatly from laboratory to laboratory, the value of the biopsy relative to the aspirate may differ significantly at any one institution compared to another. These caveats notwithstanding, several large series have concluded that the bone marrow biopsy increases the diagnostic accuracy of the aspirate by approximately 10%. This is particularly true in cases of disseminated granulomas, myelofibrosis, aplastic anemia, metastatic carcinoma, metabolic bone disease, lymphoma, and vasculitis (6,7,13,14). The procedures tend to be complementary in diagnosing acute leukemia, chronic lymphocytic leukemia, and chronic myelogenous leukemia (CML). The biopsy may also illuminate important pathology even in instances in which aspiration alone traditionally has been indicated, such as in megaloblastic anemias, microcytic or normocytic anemias, neutropenias, and thrombocytopenias (15). Given this, a cogent argument can be made to perform an aspirate and biopsy in all cases, even though indications for each have been suggested and clearly overlap (16). All would agree, however, that a biopsy is indicated after a dry tap (17).

Complications

Complications of both bone marrow aspiration and biopsy are rare. The infection rate in one large series of bone marrow biopsies was only 0.14%, in spite of the fact that many procedures were performed in neutropenic patients (18). Although its specific incidence is unknown, hemorrhage is uncommon even in severely thrombocytopenic patients if the procedure is performed carefully and a pressure dressing is applied after the procedure (15). In patients with very low platelet counts, evidence of bleeding such as petechiae, or platelet dysfunction, prophylactic platelet transfusions can be considered. Some authors believe that patients with hemophilia and other coagulopathies should receive factor replacement before a bone marrow examination (19), whereas others simply advise cautious

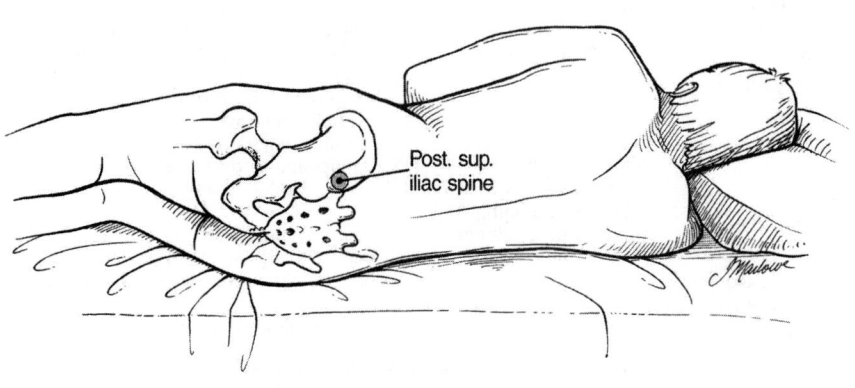

Figure 3-3. Positioning of patient on side. The prone position may also be used.

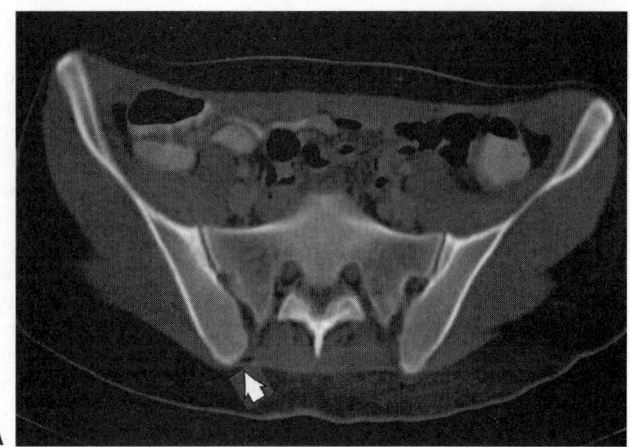
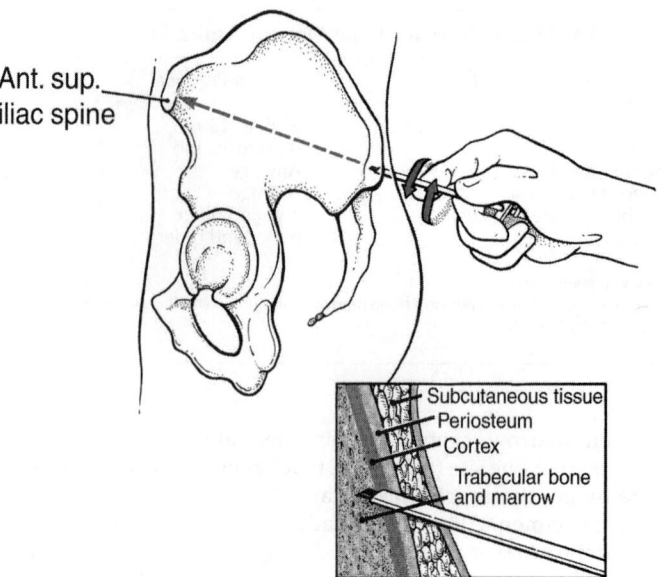

Ant. sup.
iliac spine

Subcutaneous tissue
Periosteum
Cortex
Trabecular bone
and marrow

A   B

Figure 3-4. A: Posterior view of posterior iliac crest biopsy and aspiration site (*arrow*). **B:** Lateral view of direction of needle insertion.

technique. Therapeutic systemic anticoagulation should also not be viewed as an absolute contraindication to bone marrow sampling. Rather, in this case, the urgency of the bone marrow procedure should be weighed against the risk of suspending anticoagulation for several days, at which time the procedure can be performed. In sum, if marrow aspiration and biopsy are deemed necessary in a patient with a hemorrhagic disorder, they may proceed after an assessment of the risks and benefits of not pretreating the patient.

Sternal aspiration is associated with more severe complications than iliac aspiration; 15 fatalities were reported in the literature before 1964, and most were due to myocardial or aortic lacerations (20). In most institutions, sternal aspiration is no longer routinely performed. However, the sternum may be the most accessible site in severely obese patients or in patients on mechanical ventilators. Biopsies should not be performed using a sternal approach.

PROCESSING OF SPECIMENS

Modern hematology and pathology laboratories are equipped to perform a wide array of diagnostic procedures. As the number of options for special testing increases, the practitioner must be cognizant of how to prepare these specimens to take full advantage of the available tests, to maximize diagnostic information, and to provide important prognostic and therapy-related data. A thorough sense of the nature of the clinical problem is essential before obtaining the bone marrow sample to obtain, prepare, and distribute specimens appropriately.

Bone Marrow Aspirate Processing

Several options exist for the preparation of aspirate-derived marrow material (Table 3-4). A well-stained, air-dried smear remains the best means of evaluating the cytology of the bone marrow elements. To prepare a smear, liquid marrow is first discharged onto the upper end of a glass slide held at a slant to allow excess peripheral blood to run off. The marrow particles are smeared over the slide by laying a second slide over the first and gently pulling laterally without exerting direct pressure,

the weight of the second slide being sufficient to disaggregate the hematopoietic elements from the particles (Fig. 3-5). Alternatively, marrow particles can be picked up from the inclined slide with the corner of a coverslip and smeared across a second coverslip. Gentle pressure is applied while smearing the marrow to disperse the particles and to avoid undue morphologic distortion. A marrow sample may also be promptly anticoagulated in EDTA for additional smears to be prepared later in the laboratory, but smears free of anticoagulant typically result in better cytologic detail. Heparin-anticoagulated aspirate material is not suitable for morphologic preparations due to artifacts introduced by the anticoagulant (16).

The fluid nature of the marrow aspirate makes it particularly useful for a wide variety of special procedures, including cytogenetics, flow cytometry, and molecular diagnostic studies (Table 3-4). Therefore, an additional 5 to 10 mL of anticoagulated mar-

TABLE 3-4. Processing of Bone Marrow Aspirates

Desired Test[a]	Requirement
Wright-Giemsa stain	Air-dried direct or EDTA-anticoagulated smears; air-dried touch preparations
Hematoxylin and eosin stain	Histologic clot or particle sections
Iron stain	Air-dried smear, fat layer from buffy coat; histologic clot or particle sections
Histochemical stains	Air-dried or buffy coat smears; air-dried touch preparations
Immunohistochemical stains	Air-dried smears or cytospins; histologic clot or particle sections
Cytogenetics or FISH	Heparin-anticoagulated sample
Flow cytometry	EDTA-anticoagulated sample
DNA/RNA for PCR or Southern blotting	EDTA-anticoagulated sample
Microbiologic cultures	Sterile tube without anticoagulant
Electron microscopy	Anticoagulated aspirate or aspirate directly deposited into electron microscopy fixative

EDTA, ethylenediaminetetraacetic acid; FISH, fluorescence *in situ* hybridization; PCR, polymerase chain reaction.
[a]In general, 1 to 2 mL of sample is sufficient for most procedures; however, this amount and the anticoagulant may vary among laboratories.

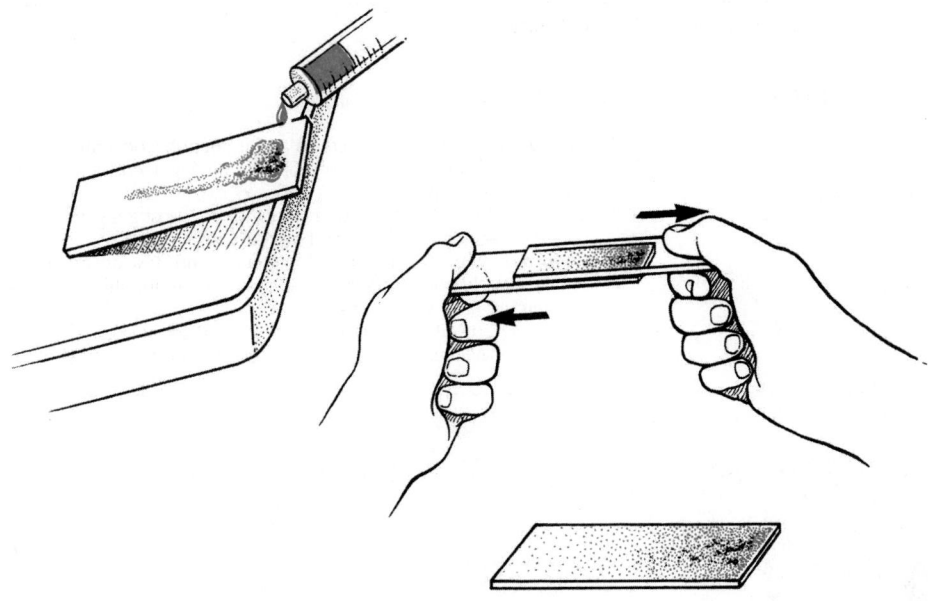

Figure 3-5. Preparation of bone marrow smears. The slides or coverslips are pulled laterally without downward pressure.

row should be obtained routinely and distributed for special procedures if they are required. EDTA-anticoagulated marrow may be stored for several days, if necessary, and distributed for special procedures after Wright-Giemsa (W-G) stained preparations have been reviewed. Cytogenetics and other procedures that require viable cells are, however, best processed immediately from samples anticoagulated with preservative-free sodium heparin.

Aspirate-derived bone marrow is also useful for the generation of histologic sections, known as *particle* or *clot preparations*. Particle sections are prepared from anticoagulated marrow particles concentrated by one of several filtration methods (21–23). After a cell pellet is obtained, the concentrated particles are placed in fixative, embedded in paraffin, and sectioned in a manner similar to that for a core biopsy specimen (see Bone Marrow Biopsy Processing). Clot preparations differ only in that the aspirated marrow is deposited directly into fixative solution. These fixed aspirate preparations retain the architectural organization of the marrow without the need for decalcification, which may impede other studies such as immunohistochemistry (see Immunohistochemical Stains).

Finally, anticoagulated marrow aspirates may be treated with Ficoll-paque or discontinuous Percoll gradients to separate and concentrate bone marrow fractions (24). The resulting cellular layer or "buffy coat" can be used for smear preparations. This technique is most useful in the morphologic evaluation of hypoplastic marrows, but may also be used to prepare cells for flow cytometric studies.

Bone Marrow Biopsy Processing

Examination of the bone marrow core biopsy specimen provides valuable information regarding the spatial relationships of the various marrow elements, the overall marrow cellularity, and the presence of cohesive cellular components that are often inaspirable. The biopsy is most commonly used for histologic sections, but may be used for a variety of other procedures if prepared correctly (Table 3-5). The steps involved in the processing of bone marrow biopsies for paraffin embedding and sectioning include (a) thorough fixation and decalcification; (b) dehydration, clearing, and paraffin infiltration and embedding; and (c) sectioning and staining (25).

There are several fixatives available for bone marrow core biopsy specimens (Table 3-6). Mercury-based fixatives (e.g., B5 and Zenker's acetic) provide the best cytologic detail, but strict

regulations concerning the proper disposal of these reagents make routine use costly and cumbersome. Buffered formaldehyde solutions (formalin) are less expensive and easier to use; however, the need for additional decalcifying steps, often in a hydrochloric acid solution, typically results in both a loss of cytologic detail and a loss of reactivity in immunohistochemical studies. Zenker's acetic fixative has the advantage of providing superior cytologic detail and mild decalcification, but certain commonly used antibodies do not react well in Zenker's acetic-fixed tissue (e.g., L26/CD20). Bouin's solution also gives good cytologic detail and uses acetic acid as a decalcification agent, but does not contain mercury. However, Bouin-fixed tissue may become too brittle to process easily if left long enough to ensure thorough decalcification. Given these considerations, each laboratory must weigh the relative advantages and disadvantages of these fixatives and decalcifying agents, and tailor their use to suit the needs of their clinical practice.

To circumvent decalcification altogether, bone marrow biopsies may be processed for plastic embedding (26). Although this technique affords excellent cytologic detail, available staining procedures are restricted, and it requires equipment and techniques not otherwise routinely used in most histology laboratories.

Touch preparations of the bone marrow biopsy should be prepared routinely before fixation and may be used in place of aspirate smears for essentially any application. In addition, in

TABLE 3-5. Processing of Bone Marrow Biopsies

Desired Test	Requirement
Giemsa stain	Paraffin-embedded section
Hematoxylin and eosin stain	Paraffin-embedded section
Reticulin, iron, and microbio- logic stains	Paraffin-embedded section
Immunohistochemical stain	Paraffin-embedded section or cry- ostat section
FISH	Paraffin-embedded section or dis- aggregated unfixed sample
Flow cytometry	Disaggregated unfixed sample
DNA for PCR	Paraffin-embedded section or unfixed core biopsy
Microbiologic cultures	Sterile unfixed core biopsy

FISH, fluorescence *in situ* hybridization; PCR, polymerase chain reaction.

TABLE 3-6. Comparison of Bone Marrow Biopsy Fixatives

Fixative	Composition	Additional Decalcification Required	Comment
Formalin	10% phosphate buffered formalin (3.7% formaldehyde)	Yes	Compatible with most special stains and immunohistochemical procedures. Less nuclear detail; use of decalcifying agents affects histology and antigenicity.
B5	Mercuric chloride, sodium acetate, formaldehyde	Yes	Excellent cytologic detail, good preservation for most antigens. Requires decalcifying agent and mercury disposal.
Zenker's acetic	Potassium dichromate, mercuric chloride, acetic acid	No	Rapid fixation with excellent histologic detail and slow decalcification. Relatively poor antigen preservation for immunohistochemistry. Mercury disposal required.
Bouin's solution	Picric acid, acetic acid, formaldehyde	No	Sharp cytologic detail with slow decalcification. Picric acid can degrade DNA and may interfere with polymerase chain reaction studies.

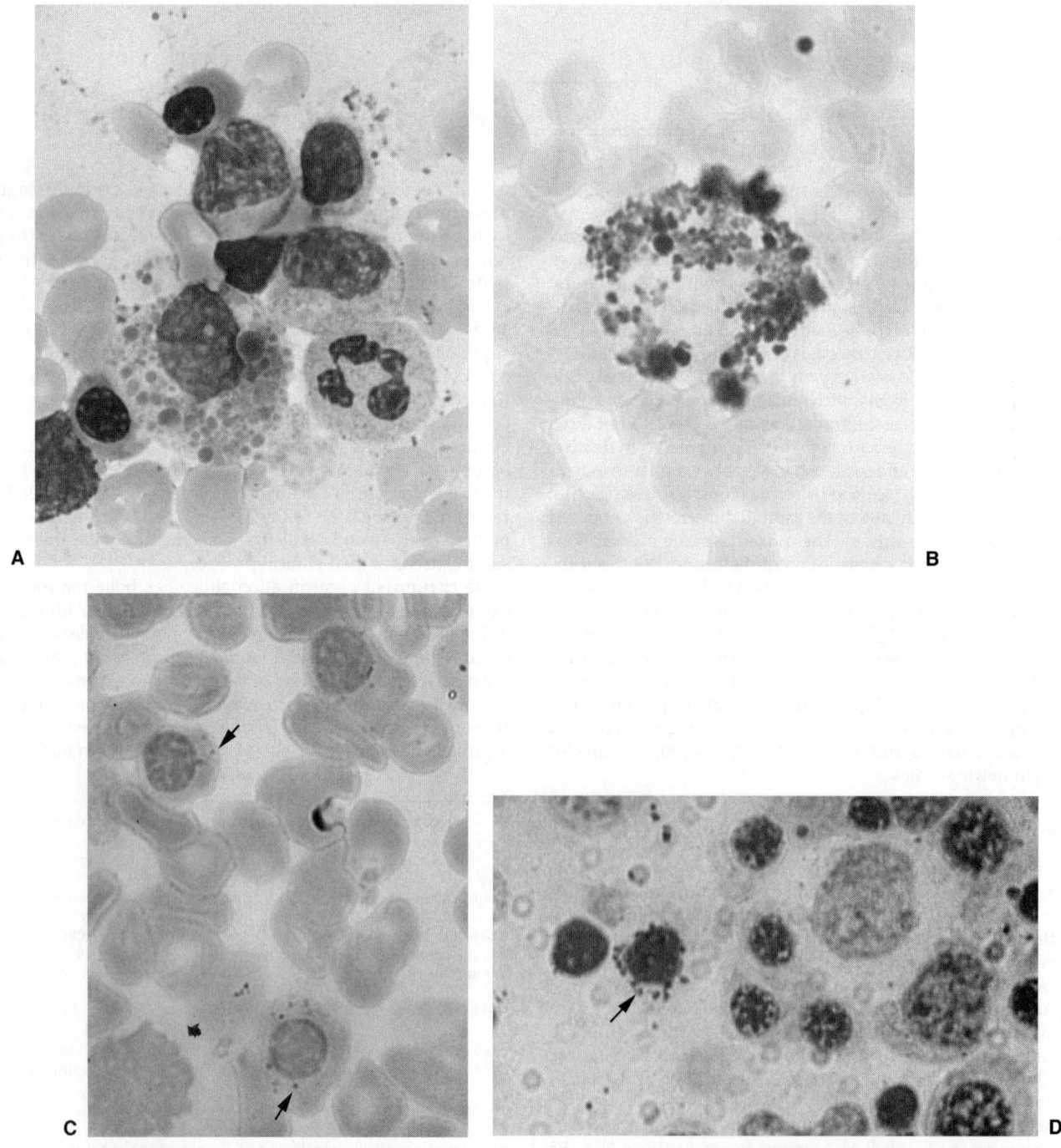

Figure 3-6. Siderophage (Wright-Giemsa, aspirate) **(A)**, siderophage **(B)**, sideroblast **(C)** (*arrows*), and ringed sideroblasts **(D)** (*arrow*). **B–D**: Prussian blue aspirates. **A–D**: ×1000. (See Color Fig. 3-6.)

cases in which an aspirate smear or adequate touch preparation cannot be obtained, but cytologic preparations are essential to the diagnosis, portions of the core biopsy can be mechanically disaggregated with surgical blades. The resulting cell suspension is used for conventional and histochemical stains, cytogenetics, and flow cytometric studies.

In summary, a complete bone marrow sample should include the following:

- Eight to ten air-dried smears prepared from unanticoagulated marrow on glass slides or square coverslips
- One or two air-dried touch preparations on glass slides or square coverslips
- Several milliliters of EDTA-anticoagulated marrow for additional aspirate smears
- Several milliliters of EDTA-anticoagulated marrow for additional studies as required (e.g., flow cytometry or molecular diagnostics)
- Several milliliters of sodium heparin–anticoagulated marrow for cytogenetics as required
- Bone marrow biopsy in fixative

ROUTINE AND SPECIAL HISTOCHEMICAL STAINS

Wright-Giemsa and Giemsa

The W-G stain is the most commonly used stain for aspirate smear specimens. It contains a combination of acidic and basic dyes that produce color reactions characteristic of different cellular components. The basic dye component stains acid tissue components such as DNA and RNA blue (basophilic), whereas the acidic dye component stains most proteins red or pink (acidophilic). The appearance of specific hematopoietic cell lineages on the W-G stain is discussed below. In bone marrow tissue sections, a largely similar staining pattern can be seen with a Giemsa stain (27). This stain is superior to routine hematoxylin and eosin (H&E) staining, providing good nuclear and cytoplasmic detail and excellent differential staining between cells of myeloid and erythroid origin.

Iron Stain

The evaluation of marrow iron stores is useful in the differential diagnosis of anemia. The Prussian blue or Perls' stain is used to identify ferric iron loosely bound in protein complexes such as ferritin and hemosiderin; iron that is strongly bound, as in heme, does not react (28). An acid solution of potassium ferrocyanide reacts with ferric ions to yield a characteristic, insoluble, bright blue pigment called *Prussian blue* (Fig. 3-6). For best results, the stain is applied to air-dried smear preparations, as iron may leach out in some of the acidic fixatives and decalcification solutions. Nonetheless, iron is still demonstrable in bone marrow specimens that are fixed overnight in Zenker's solution with 3% acetic acid (25). The fatty layer obtained from buffy coat preparations is also an excellent substrate for iron staining.

Storage iron in macrophages may be present as a diffuse cytoplasmic blush or as variably coarse cytoplasmic granules apparent at a low to moderate magnification. A crude scale designates marrow storage iron as absent or markedly decreased, present, or increased, and it is prone to observational error. A more quantitative appraisal of marrow iron can be determined after examining fifty or more oil immersion fields (Table 3-7) (29). In addition to macrophage iron, in iron-replete normal marrows, as many as 40% of erythroid precursors (sideroblasts) contain one to several small, often peripherally placed iron

TABLE 3-7. Bone Marrow Iron Quantification

Score	Criteria
0	No iron observed
Trace	Rare intracellular iron granules
1+	Iron granules seen, but fewer than normal
2+	Normal iron content (iron granules present in 10% or more of fields)
3+	Considerable amounts of iron in every field
4+	Considerable degree of iron excess

Adapted from Beutler E, Robson MJ, Buttenwieser E. A comparison of the plasma iron, iron-binding capacity, sternal marrow iron and other methods in the clinical evaluation of iron stores. *Ann Intern Med* 1958;48:60.

granules apparent only under oil immersion, which represent iron in ferritin (30). Siderocytes, which are mature, anucleated erythrocytes containing stainable iron granules, are rarely observed in normal marrow preparations, but may be seen in patients with sideroblastic anemias. In the sideroblastic anemias, iron accumulates within mitochondria, yielding multiple (usually more than six), relatively large iron granules distributed in a perinuclear pattern, forming the ringed sideroblast (31) (Fig. 3-6).

Reticulin Stain

Paraffin-embedded sections of the bone marrow biopsy can be impregnated with silver to demonstrate reticulin and/or collagen fibers that are increased in primary and secondary myelofibrotic states. Using this method, the reticulin fibers stain black to deep purple. Mature collagen fibers (type 1) stain brown, whereas immature collagen fibers (types 3 and 4) stain black. One example of bone marrow reticulin quantitation is demonstrated in Table 3-8 (32).

Histochemical Stains

Histochemical stains take advantage of the specific enzymatic and cytochemical properties of each of the bone marrow lineages (33). Aspirate smears, or touch or buffy coat preparations, are generally used for this purpose. Histochemical stains, together with morphologic and immunophenotypic features, continue to play a major role in lineage identification and leukemia classification. The specificities of these stains for identifying individual cell types are listed in Table 3-9, and the stains themselves are represented in Figure 3-7.

TABLE 3-8. Bone Marrow Reticulin Quantification

Score	Criteria
0	No reticulin fibers demonstrable
Normal	Perivascular and occasional fine individual fibers only
1+	Occasional fine individual fibers, plus foci of fine fiber network
2+	Fine fiber network throughout most of the section, no coarse fibers demonstrated
3+	Diffuse fiber network with scattered thick, coarse fibers but no true collagen (negative trichrome stain)
4+	Diffuse, often coarse, fiber network with areas of collagenization (positive trichrome stain)

Adapted from Bauermeister DE. Quantitation of bone marrow reticulin—a normal range. *Am J Clin Pathol* 1971;56:24–31.

TABLE 3-9. Histochemical Stains

Stain	Positive Cell Types
Myeloperoxidase (MPO)	Neutrophils
	Eosinophils
Sudan Black B (SBB)	Neutrophils
	Eosinophils
	Basophils
	Monocytes (few granules)
Specific esterase (SE)	
Naphthol AS-D chloracetate esterase (CAE/ Leder)	Neutrophils
	Mast cells
Nonspecific esterase (NSE)	
α-Naphthyl acetate esterase	Monocytes and macrophages (inhibited by sodium fluoride)
	Megakaryocytes
α-Naphthyl butyrate esterase	Monocytes and macrophages
	Megakaryocytes (weak)
Periodic acid-Schiff (PAS)	Neutrophils (diffuse granular pattern)
	Monocytes (few granules)
	Lymphoblasts in acute lymphoblastic leukemia (perinuclear, coarse, block-like granular pattern)
	Erythroleukemia (chunky positivity in blasts and erythroid precursors)

SPECIAL PROCEDURES

Immunohistochemical Stains

Over the past several decades, there have been dramatic advances in immunodiagnostic methods that have had substantial impact on all aspects of laboratory medicine. This is especially true in the study of hematologic diseases, by which intensive research efforts have led to an understanding of the protein expression changes that occur during the differentiation of myeloid (34), lymphoid (35,36), and erythroid cells. This work has resulted in the development of a large panel of specific monoclonal or polyclonal antibodies directed against cellular antigens that are present in normal and neoplastic states (Table 3-10).

Immunohistochemistry is based on the principle that antibodies bound to their cognate antigens can be detected by a colorimetric enzyme-substrate reaction using an enzyme-conjugated secondary antibody. The most widely used detection systems are peroxidase based and involve the peroxidase-antiperoxidase and the avidin-biotin complex methods (37,38). In the bone marrow, the presence of endogenous peroxidase in erythrocytes and granulocytes may limit their usefulness. This problem can be minimized by substituting alkaline phosphatase for peroxidase as in the alkaline phosphatase–antialkaline phosphatase method (39–41).

In most laboratories, the use of immunohistochemistry in the evaluation of bone marrow specimens has become as routine as the use of any other special stain. However, as mentioned previously, the fixation and decalcification methods necessary for the preparation of bone marrow biopsies can result in the loss of antigenic immunoreactivity. This processing limits the number of antibodies useful in examining paraffin-embedded bone marrow biopsy specimens. The use of unfixed, air-dried aspirate smears or cytospin preparations can greatly expand the repertoire of antibodies available for this purpose. The major clinical applications for immunohistochemistry in bone marrow samples include the determination of the immunophenotype of a lymphomatous or leukemic infiltrate, the quantification of bone marrow involvement by an infiltrative process, the assessment of clonality using antiimmunoglobulin light chain antibodies in plasma cell dyscrasias, and the identification of histologically inapparent metastatic tumor deposits (Fig. 3-8).

Flow Cytometry

Flow cytometry is a laser-based technology that measures a variety of characteristics from a single biological particle. The applications of flow cytometry are diverse and include the analysis of membrane, cytoplasmic, and nuclear antigens. However, for most hematologic conditions, it is the evaluation of the membrane antigens that is the most diagnostically relevant (42,43). Anticoagulated bone marrow aspirate cell suspensions are first incubated with panels of monoclonal antibodies conjugated to fluorescent dyes that bind specific cell-surface proteins (44). Next, a fluid stream of single cells is generated and passed through a beam of laser light from an excitation source. The scattered light or emitted fluorescence that results is then measured for each individual particle as it passes through a series of photodetectors. Finally, computer software analyzes and stores the data. The resulting immunophenotypic profile is particularly well suited for the subclassification of acute leukemias, the determination of clonality by light chain expression in lymphoid neoplasms, the subclassification of lymphoid neoplasms, and the detection of minimal residual disease. Special techniques for examining intracellular antigens have been developed that allow for the detection of nuclear and cytoplasmic antigens, including terminal deoxynucleotidyl transferase (45,46), cytoplasmic immunoglobulin (47), and myeloperoxidase (48). In addition, fluorescent dyes, such as propidium iodide, that bind nucleic acid can be used for the determination of DNA content and for the quantitation of reticulocytes (49). There are many advantages to flow cytometric technology over other forms of antigen detection. In particular, flow cytometry allows for the rapid, simultaneous analysis of multiple markers in a cell population and permits characterization of unique subpopulations by recording and analyzing data obtained from individual cells.

Antibodies directed against the antigens listed in Table 3-10 are routinely used in the identification and classification of myeloid and lymphoid leukemias and T-cell and B-cell lymphomas in most flow cytometry and immunohistochemistry laboratories.

Cytogenetic and Molecular Diagnostic Techniques

The level of understanding of the molecular basis of disease is currently greater for hematologic malignancies than for any other type of cancer. This understanding has led to significant changes in the identification and classification of myeloid and lymphoid neoplasms (50,51). Molecular diagnostic strategies using the polymerase chain reaction (PCR) or Southern blot hybridization are now routinely used to determine clonality in both B- and T-lymphoid proliferations. In addition, specific cytogenetic abnormalities, present in both lymphoid and myeloid disorders, can be identified by Giemsa banding, fluorescence in situ hybridization (FISH) or PCR techniques. Additional marrow aspirate material should be routinely taken for cytogenetic and/ or molecular diagnostic analysis in all myeloid abnormalities (e.g., chronic myeloproliferative disorders, acute leukemias, myelodysplastic syndromes) and in lymphoid neoplasms in cases in which clonality must be established or specific abnormalities will aid in classification, including the t(8;14) in Burkitt lymphoma, the t(11;14) in mantle cell lymphoma, and the t(14;18) in follicular lymphoma. Table 3-11 lists the most commonly used molecular diagnostic tests available in clinical reference laboratories.

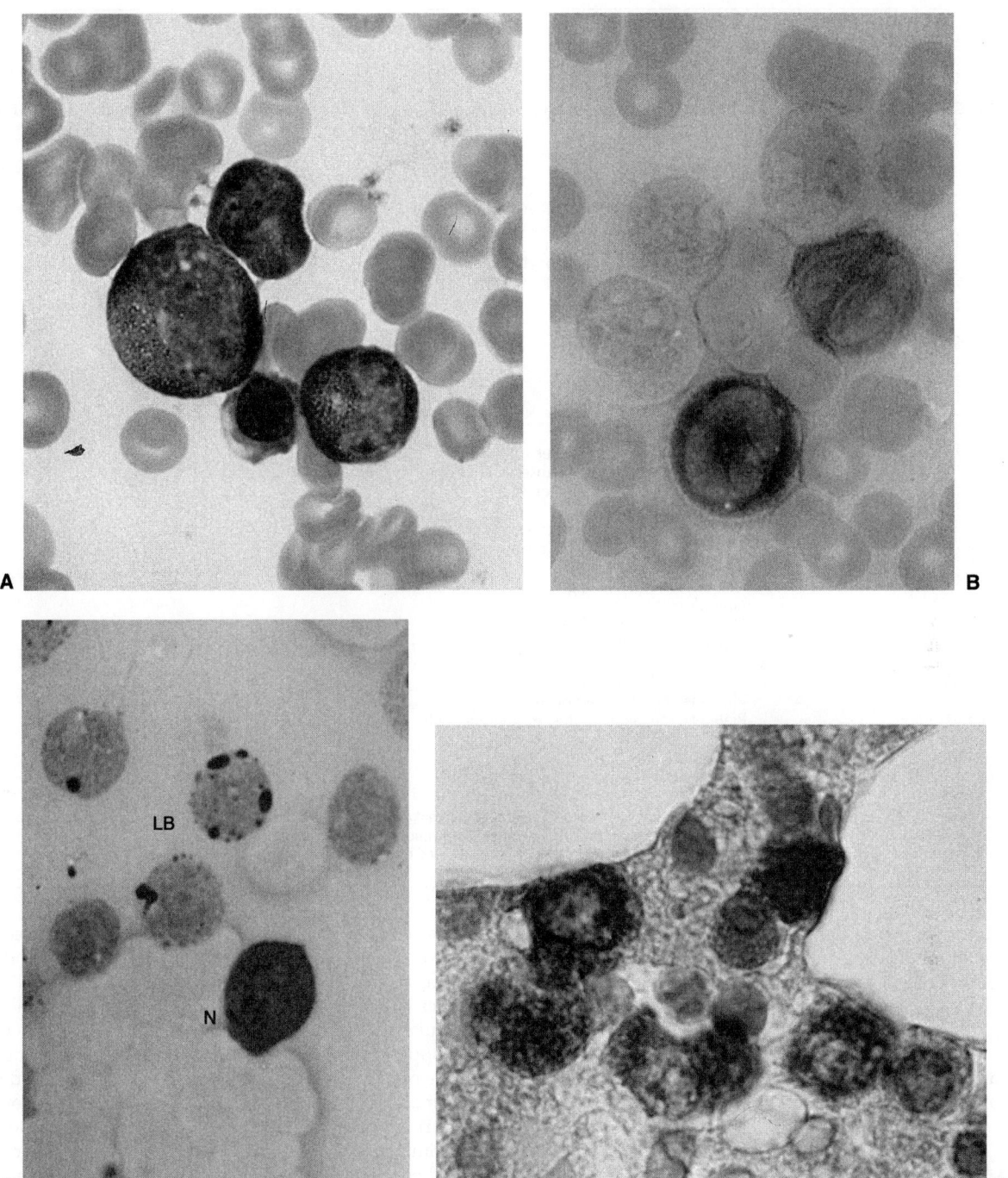

Figure 3-7. Histochemical stains. Granulocytes and myeloblasts positive for myeloperoxidase (myeloperoxidase; aspirate) **(A)**. Monocyte precursors positive for nonspecific esterase (nonspecific esterase; aspirate) **(B)**. Diffuse positivity of neutrophil (N) and block positivity of lymphoblast (LB) on periodic acid-Schiff stain (periodic acid-Schiff; aspirate) **(C)**. Neutrophilic myeloid precursors positive for chloroacetate esterase (chloroacetate esterase; biopsy) **(D)**. **A–D:** ×1000. (See Color Fig. 3-7.)

MORPHOLOGIC EXAMINATION OF BONE MARROW

Evaluation of Specimens

Regardless of the clinical indication for obtaining a bone marrow sample, evaluation of the aspirate and biopsy specimens should be approached in a systematic manner, including assessments of cellularity, hematopoietic constituents, accessory marrow elements, and infiltrating cells. Because of the rapidity with which W-G stain smears can be prepared compared to paraffin-embedded tissue sections, initial impressions of the sample are typically based on the aspirate smear. The aspirate also offers cytologic detail superior to even the best bone marrow tissue sections. Nonetheless, examination of the biopsy provides essential information such as a more quantitative assessment of marrow cellularity, detail of the marrow architecture, and the possibility of examining marrows that are not aspirable or aspirates that are technically unsatisfactory. Many excellent atlases and other texts devoted solely to normal and abnormal bone

TABLE 3-10. Selected Flow Cytometric and Immunohistochemical Markers

Antigen or CD Group	Reactivity in Hematopoietic Cells	Flow Cytometry	Immunohistochemistry Unfixed	Immunohistochemistry Fixed
Hematopoietic				
CD45	Leukocytes	+	+	+
TdT	B- and T-lymphoblasts	+	+	+
B-lymphoid				
CD20	B-lymphocytes	+	+	+
CD19	B-lymphocytes	+	+	–
CD79a	B lymphoblasts, B lymphocytes, plasma cells	–	–	+
CD10	B-lymphocyte subsets, granulocytes	+	+	+
CD23	B-lymphocytes subsets	+	+	+
Surface Ig	Mature B-lymphocytes	+	+	+/–
Cytoplasmic Ig	Plasma cells	–/+	+	+
CD138	Plasma cells	+	+	+
T-lymphoid				
CD2	T-lymphocytes	+	+	+
CD3	T-lymphocytes	+	+	+
CD5	T-lymphocytes	+	+	+
CD4	T-lymphocyte helper subset	+	+	+/–
CD8	T-lymphocyte cytotoxic subset	+	+	+
CD1a	Thymocytes, Langerhans' cells	–	+	+
Myelomonocytic				
CD33	CFU-GEMM to promyelocytes, monocytes	+	–	–
CD13	CFU-GM to granulocytes, monocytes	+	–	–
CD14	Monocytes	+	–	–
CD68	Monocytes, macrophages	–	+	+
CD15	Granulocytes	+	+	+
Myeloperoxidase	Neutrophils, eosinophils	+	+	+
Lysozyme	Myelomonocytic cells	–	+	+
Megakaryocytic				
CD41 (GPIIb/IIIa)	Platelets and megakaryocytes	+	+	–
CD42	Platelets and megakaryocytes	+	+	–
von Willebrand factor	Platelets, megakaryocytes, endothelial cells	–	+	+
Erythroid				
Glycophorin A	Red blood cells and precursors	+	+	+
Hemoglobin	Red blood cells and precursors	–	+	+

CD, cluster designation; CFU-GEMM, colony-forming unit granulocyte-erythroid-macrophage-megakaryocyte; CFU-GM, colony-forming unit granulocyte-monocyte; cIg, cytoplasmic immunoglobulin; sIg, surface immunoglobulin; GP, glycoprotein; TdT, terminal deoxynucleotidyl transferase.
NOTE: Immunohistochemical techniques vary greatly among laboratories. The most commonly used or technically feasible applications are indicated by a "+".

marrow morphology are available (52–54). The following offers a brief description of the evaluation of normal bone marrow and a method to report aspirate and biopsy findings.

Cellularity

The cellularity and composition of the marrow varies with age. The marrow of the newborn is devoid of fat. After birth, red

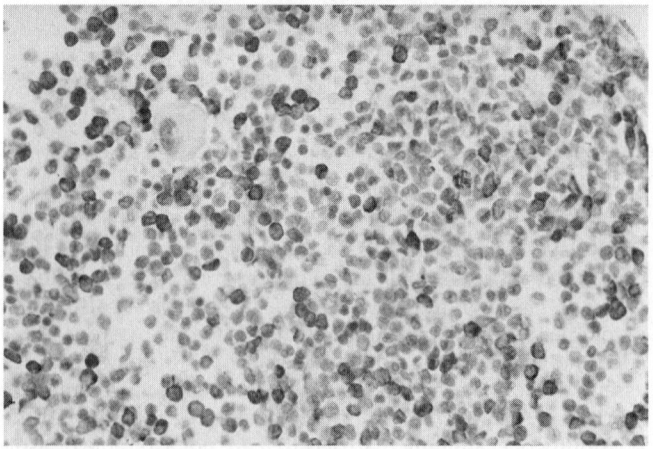

Figure 3-8. Immunohistochemical staining for CD34 in a case of acute myelogenous leukemia with 35% blasts (CD34; biopsy; ×200). (See Color Fig. 3-8.)

marrow containing hematopoietic elements is replaced by fatty, nonhematopoietic, yellow marrow beginning in the distal extremities and proceeding centripetally. In the adult, hematopoietically active marrow is concentrated in the axial skeleton, particularly in the skull, sternum, ribs, spine, and pelvis. In general, approximately 80% of marrow is cellular during the first decade of life, declining to 50% in a 30-year-old and decreasing further after a person reaches 70 years (55). Thus, a normocellular marrow for an adult is taken as 50% cellularity and 50% fat.

Estimation of cellularity on a W-G–stained aspirate smear should be viewed as a qualitative, rather than quantitative, measure. Smears should be scanned at low magnification to identify marrow spicules (Fig. 3-9), which are clumps of tissue composed of marrow fat, stroma, and hematopoietic elements. Sites where lipid droplets have been removed by processing appear as oval staining voids within the spicule. In hypercellular marrows, these areas are reduced, whereas in hypocellular marrows, they are more pronounced and the stromal elements of the spicule may stand out in the absence of hematopoietic cells. Extremely hypocellular spicules can be distinguished from aspirated subcutaneous fat by the presence of occasional immature hematopoietic elements admixed with lymphocytes, mast cells, plasma cells, and histiocytes, the latter of which may contain hemosiderin pigment. An impression of hypercellularity may be appreciated on samples that lack spicules but contain large sheets of hematopoietic cells, as is often the case in acute leukemias, chronic myeloproliferative disorders, or in young children, in whom it is a normal finding. Conversely, designation of a specimen as hypo-

TABLE 3-11. Molecular Diagnostic Tests in Hematopoietic Malignancies

Cytogenetics
  Karyotyping
  Fluorescence *in situ* hybridization
      t(14;18) (*BCL2*/IgH) in follicular lymphoma
      t(11;14) (*BCL1*/IgH) in mantle cell lymphoma
      t(9;22) (*BCR/ABL*) in CML and ALL
      t(15;17) (*PML/RARα*) in APML
      t(12;21) (*TEL/AML1*) in pre–B-cell ALL
      t(8;21) (*AML1/ETO*) in AML-M2
      inv(16) (CBFβ/MYH11) in AML-M4Eo
      (11q23) (*MLL*) rearrangements in acute leukemia
      monosomies or trisomies
      X, Y sex chromosomes for donor chimerism post–bone marrow
          transplantation
Southern blotting
  Immunoglobulin heavy (IgH) and κ– and λ–light chain rearrangements
  T-cell receptor β- and γ-chain gene rearrangements
  EBV clonality in EBV-associated lymphoproliferations
  t(14;18) (*BCL2*/IgH) in follicular lymphoma
Polymerase chain reaction
  Immunoglobulin heavy chain (IgH) rearrangements
  T-cell receptor γ-chain gene rearrangements
  t(14;18) (*BCL2*/IgH) in follicular lymphoma
  t(9;22) (*BCR/ABL*) in CML and ALL
  t(15;17) (*PML/RARα*) in APML
  t(12;21) (*TEL/AML1*) in pre–B-cell ALL

ALL, acute lymphoblastic leukemia; AML, acute myelogenous leukemia; APML, acute promyelocytic leukemia; CML, chronic myelogenous leukemia; EBV, Epstein-Barr virus; M4Eo, acute myelomonocytic leukemia with marrow eosinophilia.

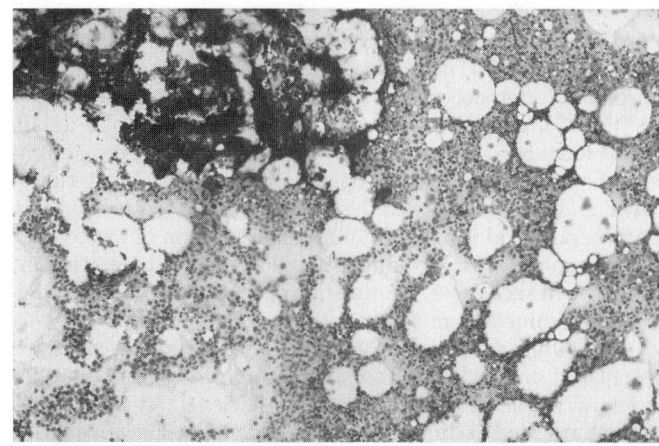

Figure 3-9. Normocellular bone marrow aspirate (Wright-Giemsa; aspirate; ×200). (See Color Fig. 3-9.)

cellular requires the presence of spicules. Only when marrow hypocellularity is severe can cellularity be recognized reproducibly as abnormal (56). Aspicular specimens diluted by blood can be distinguished from peripheral blood by the presence of nucleated erythroid precursors and immature myeloid elements.

Cellularity is better assessed on bone marrow biopsies, where it can be viewed as a semiquantitative assessment in an individual specimen (Fig. 3-10). However, the density of hematopoietic activity may vary from site to site and even within a single specimen (55,57). Intraspecimen variation commonly occurs in the setting of hypoproliferative disorders and in the recovery period after intensive chemotherapy. Overall, cellularity should be estimated as a percentage of the space between bone trabeculae and reported either as percent cellularity or percent fat.

Differential Count

In most cases, examination of two or three well-prepared W-G–stained aspirate smears is sufficient for each specimen. The samples should be scanned at low power to identify well-spread, well-preserved representative areas to perform a differ-

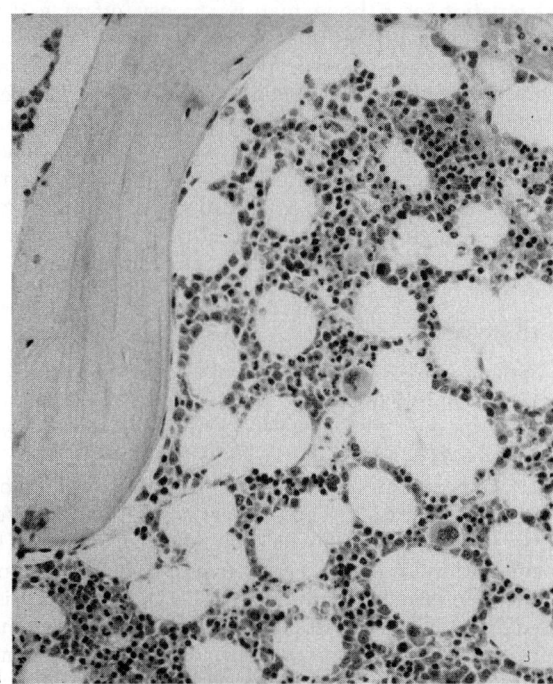

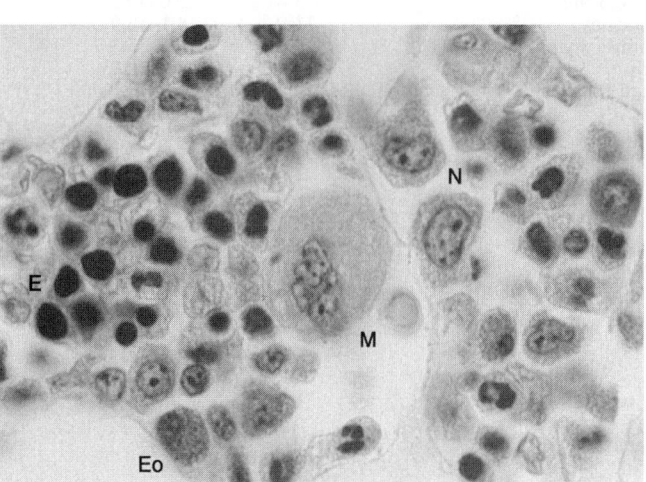

Figure 3-10. Normal bone marrow biopsy, showing distribution of hematopoietic cells, fat, and trabecular bone: erythroid precursors (E), neutrophil precursors (N), eosinophil precursor (Eo), megakaryocyte (M). [Giemsa; biopsies; ×250 **(A)** and ×1000 **(B)**.] (See Color Fig. 3-10.)

ential count. The extreme edges of the smear should be avoided, as larger cells, such as blasts, often accumulate there. In addition, an artifact that imparts a more immature appearance to the chromatin often occurs at the edge. Blood or excess cellularity in "thick" areas of the smear may also obscure cellular detail. Areas ideal for differential counting often occur at the periphery of spicules. Here, the cells are often in a confluent monolayer, and the proximity to the spicule ensures that dilution by peripheral blood is at a minimum. Enumeration of the cellular components in dilute specimens should be viewed with circumspection. In such cases, examination of a touch preparation may provide a more accurate count.

For routine purposes, a 200-cell differential count enumerating blasts, myeloid precursors, erythroid precursors, lymphocytes, and other cells as necessary, is sufficient. Megakaryocytes are not included in differential counts due to their relative rarity. Individual cases in which a more accurate, quantitative assessment of the cellular composition is desired require a more extensive differential count. Examples in which a more extensive differential count may be of use include infiltrative diseases, such as multiple myeloma and chronic lymphocytic leukemia, in which marrow involvement may be variable from area to area. Adaptations for individual disease processes, such as counting basophils when CML is a diagnostic consideration, can also be incorporated. Normal differential counts for adults are listed in Table 3-12.

In addition to focusing the observer's attention on the characteristics of individual cells, the differential count provides a means to calculate the myeloid to erythroid (M:E) ratio. In normal adults, the M:E ratio is typically 3:1–4:1. Marrows in which this ratio is significantly lower are said to have a relative erythroid hyperplasia, and those in which it is higher are said to have a relative myeloid hyperplasia. In addition to estimating the M:E ratio, rough determination of an absolute lineage hyperplasia or hypoplasia may be made on a bone marrow biopsy, which normalizes for cellularity. The M:E ratio may be slightly higher in the normal infant and child.

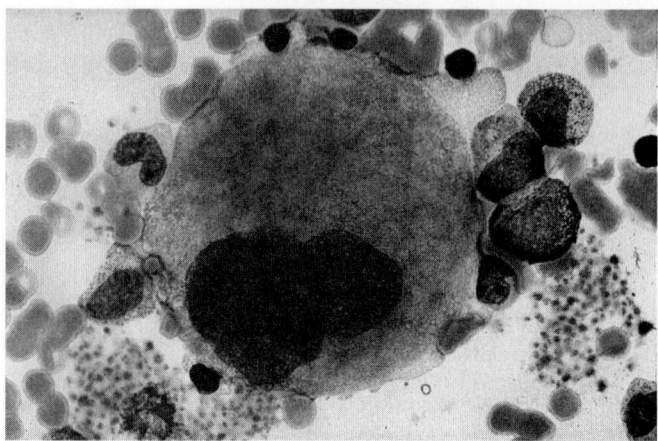

Figure 3-11. Megakaryocyte (Wright-Giemsa; aspirate; ×1000). (See Color Fig. 3-11.)

Megakaryocytes

By virtue of their size, megakaryocytes are easily recognized from low power. They are the largest of the hematopoietic cells, ranging in size from 35 to 150 μm (Figs. 3-9 to 3-11). Their most distinctive feature is their highly variable nuclear lobation, in which the nuclear lobes appear to be superimposed on one another. The cytoplasm is filled with indistinct fine violet granules, which resemble the central "granulomere" portion of platelets in the peripheral blood. Quantification of megakaryocytes on smears is inexact. Three or four megakaryocytes per low-power (4×) microscopic field is typical. Gross increases in megakaryocyte numbers can be appreciated; however, decreases are often difficult to discern. Megakaryocytes do not disaggregate well and may remain embedded within spicules. For that reason, the spicules themselves should be examined closely for megakaryocytes. Furthermore, the absence of megakaryocytes on specimens that lack spicules, even if they are otherwise quite cellular, should be interpreted with caution.

Examination of a bone marrow biopsy offers a distinct advantage over aspirates in the quantification of megakaryocytes. In a biopsy, megakaryocytes can be enumerated on a per-unit-area basis, independent of the variability of spicule density or disaggregation. Generally speaking, two to four megakaryocytes per 40× high-power field can be considered normal. An assessment of increased or decreased numbers can be made with reference to this norm. In addition, clustering of megakaryocytes, which may be associated with disease processes such as myeloproliferative disorders, can be appreciated.

Granulocytes

Cells of the neutrophilic lineage are the most abundant cells in the marrow, comprising nearly 60% of the cellularity in adults. Myeloid maturation is characterized by a progressive decrease in cell size beyond the promyelocyte stage, increasing nuclear complexity and chromatin condensation, and the acquisition of lineage-specific granules. The earliest recognizable myeloid precursor is the myeloblast, which is a relatively large cell (14–18 μm) with a round nucleus, evenly distributed fine chromatin, and one to several distinct nucleoli (Fig. 3-12). The nucleus is surrounded by a thin rim of basophilic (blue) cytoplasm that may or may not contain several granules. Physiologically normal myeloblasts are rare in resting marrows, but are more abundant in recovering marrows after chemotherapy. The promyelocyte is the largest of the granulocyte precursors (up to 25 μm) and can

TABLE 3-12. Differential Counts of Bone Marrow Aspirates from 20 Normal Adults

Cell Type	Mean (%)	Range (%)
Neutrophil series	56.0	45.1–66.5
Myeloblasts	1.0	0.5–1.8
Promyelocytes	3.4	2.6–4.6
Myelocytes	11.9	8.1–16.9
Metamyelocytes	18.0	9.8–25.3
Bands	11.0	8.5–20.8
Mature neutrophils	10.7	8.0–16.0
Eosinophil series	3.2	1.2–6.2
Eosinophilic myelocytes	0.9	0.3–1.9
Eosinophilic metamyelocytes	1.4	0.3–2.3
Eosinophilic bands	1.0	0.3–2.7
Mature eosinophils	0.9	0.1–1.7
Basophil series	<0.1	0.0–0.2
Erythroid series	21.5	14.2–30.4
Proerythroblasts	0.6	0.2–1.4
Basophilic erythroblasts	2.0	0.7–3.7
Polychromatophilic erythroblasts	12.4	12.2–24.2
Orthochromatic erythroblasts	6.5	2.0–22.7
Lymphocytes	15.8	10.8–22.7
Monocytes	1.8	0.2–2.8
Plasma cells	1.8	0.2–2.2
Histiocytes/reticulum cells	0.3	0.0–0.5
Megakaryocytes	<0.1	0.0–0.2

From Jandl JH. *Blood: textbook of hematology.* Boston: Little, Brown and Company, 1987:27.

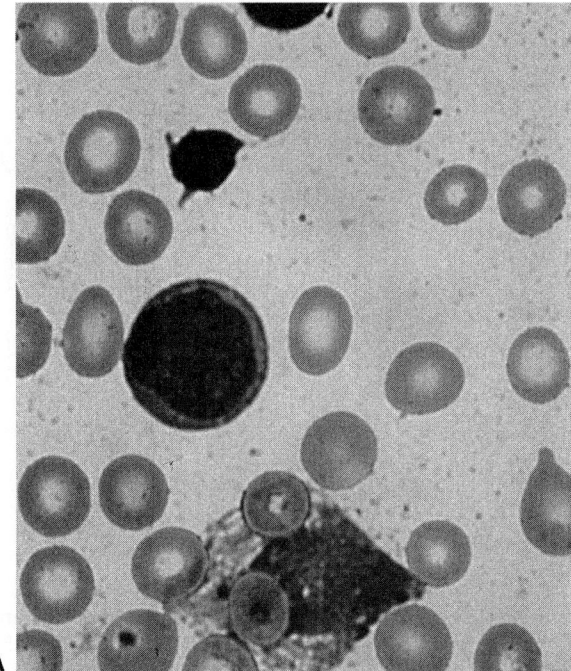

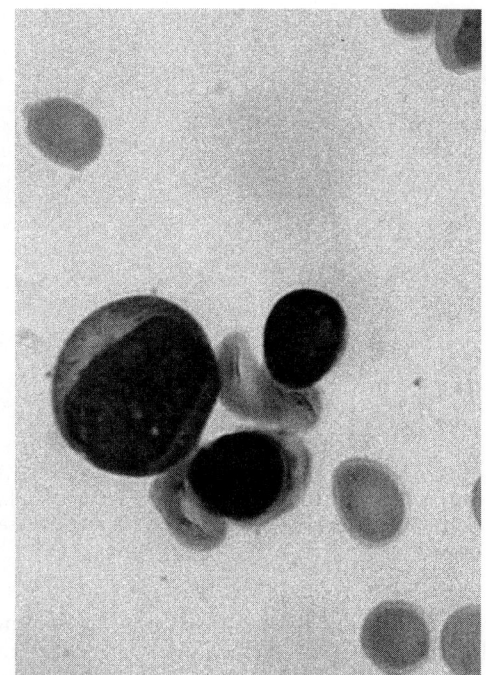

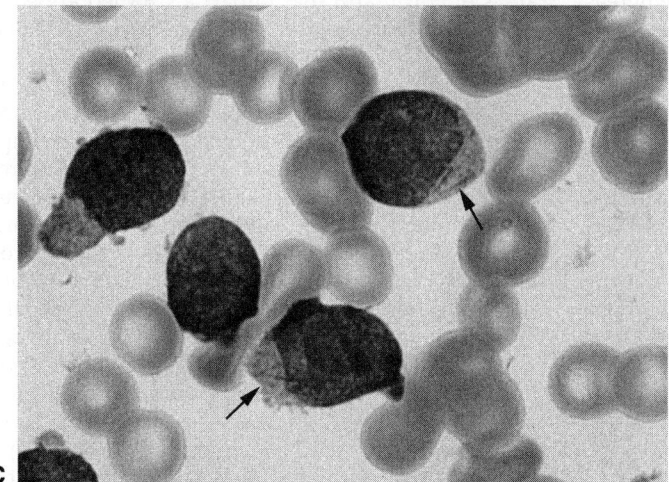

Figure 3-12. Myeloblasts in normal **(A, B)** and neoplastic **(C)** marrows. Note Auer rods (*arrows*). (Wright-Giemsa; aspirates; ×1000.) (See Color Fig. 3-12.)

be easily distinguished from a blast by the presence of numerous, coarse, deeply purple (azurophilic) primary granules in the cytoplasm that often appear to overlie the nucleus (Fig. 3-13). Compared to the myeloblast, the promyelocyte cytoplasm is more abundant and slightly redder (acidophilic), the nuclear chromatin more condensed, and, if present, the nucleoli less distinct. At the myelocyte stage, the chromatin is coarser and the nucleus is slightly oblong and often minimally indented by a perinuclear area of pallor (Fig. 3-14). The characteristic feature of the myelocyte, however, is the presence of granules specific for the neutrophilic, eosinophilic, or basophilic lineages. Neutrophilic granules stain poorly with W-G and may be very pale red or cast in relief by pale-pink cytoplasmic background. In comparison, eosinophilic and basophilic granules are relatively large and distinctly orange-red and dark blue, respectively. Neutrophilic and eosinophilic myelocytes are common in normal marrows; however, the detection of substantial basophil precursors is unusual and is typically associated with primary bone marrow diseases, particularly myeloproliferative disorders. Maturation from the myelocyte stage to the mature granulocyte is characterized by further indentation of the nucleus and

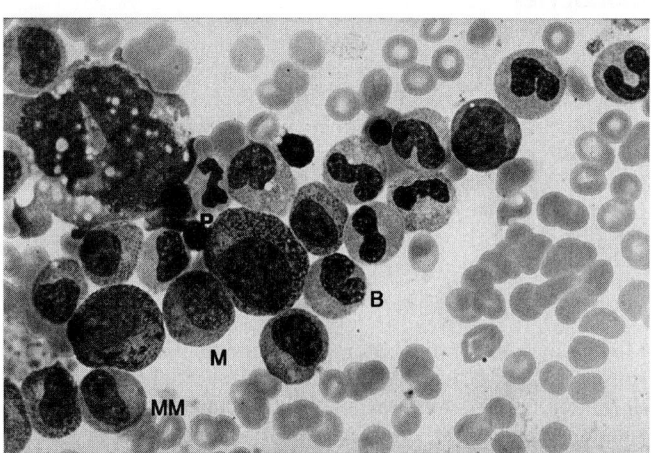

Figure 3-13. Neutrophilic maturation: promyelocyte (P), neutrophilic myelocyte (M), neutrophilic metamyelocyte (MM), band neutrophil (B). (Wright-Giemsa; aspirate; ×1000.) (See Color Fig. 3-13.)

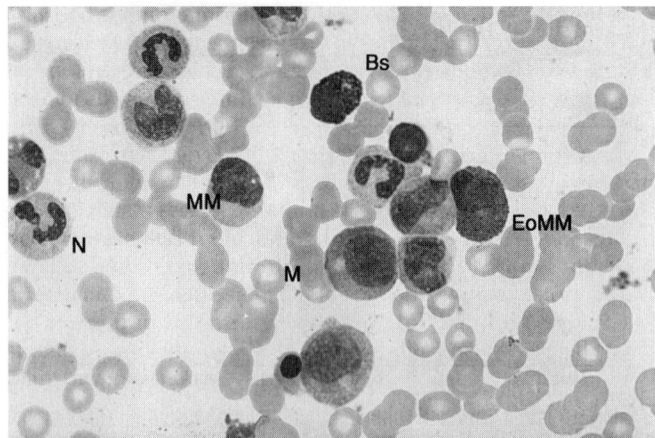

Figure 3-14. Myeloid maturation: neutrophilic myelocyte (M), neutrophilic metamyelocyte (MM), band neutrophil (B), segmented neutrophil (N), eosinophilic metamyelocyte (EoMM), basophil (Bs). (Wright-Giemsa; aspirate; ×1000.) (See Color Fig. 3-14.)

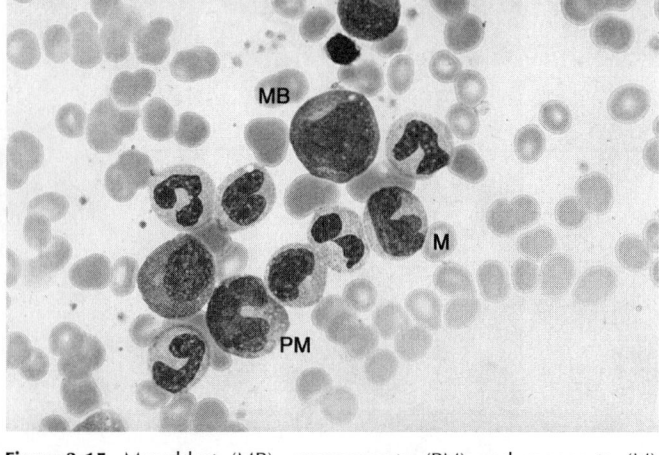

Figure 3-15. Monoblast (MB), promonocyte (PM) and monocyte (M) (Wright-Giemsa; aspirate; ×1000.) (See Color Fig. 3-15.)

condensation of the chromatin, dissipation of the few remaining primary granules, and segmentation of the nucleus into distinct lobes (Fig. 3-14). Mature neutrophils typically have three or four nuclear lobes separated by thin chromatin strands, whereas mature eosinophils typically have two and sometimes three nuclear lobes.

As the marrow is both a maturation and storage compartment for granulocytes, mature neutrophils and band forms may constitute nearly half of the myeloid cellularity. Marrows in which metamyelocytes and earlier forms are expanded and begin to predominate in the myeloid compartment are referred to as *left shifted*, similar to the situation in which bands and earlier forms appear in the peripheral blood.

In bone marrow biopsies, the earliest myeloid precursors tend to be localized adjacent to bone trabeculae, with maturation occurring radially outward. On tissue sections, the Giemsa stain is particularly useful for distinguishing the granular components of cells (Fig. 3-10). Promyelocytic granules stain purple, neutrophilic granules pale pink, eosinophilic granules deep red, and mast cell granules reddish purple. Basophilic granules are destroyed in processing, and basophils cannot be distinguished in routinely processed and stained biopsies.

Monocytes

Monocyte precursors represent 1% to 2% of the marrow cellularity. Occasionally, very early monocyte precursors compatible with monoblasts may be identified. Promonocytes are large mononuclear cells with indistinct nucleoli, abundant and deeply basophilic cytoplasm, and several small cytoplasmic granules (Fig. 3-15). As these cells mature, the nucleus develops a folded, polyploid shape, with smooth nuclear contours and grayish cytoplasm that may contain a few small granules or vacuoles.

Erythroid Precursors

Morphologic erythroid maturation proceeds with a progressive diminution in cell size, coarsening and eventual complete condensation of the chromatin, and hemoglobinization of the cytoplasm, eventuating in enucleation. The earliest erythroid precursor is the proerythroblast (pronormoblast or erythroblast), which is a large cell (15 to 20 μm) with a round nucleus, fine chromatin, and one to several indistinct nucleoli that may appear to abut one another (Fig. 3-16). The scant cytoplasm is a

characteristic deep blue and agranular, and it often has a shallow area of perinuclear pallor. Basophilic erythroblasts (basophilic normoblasts) are smaller cells with finely condensed areas of chromatin that impart a stippled appearance to the nucleus. Their cytoplasm is only slightly paler blue than that of the proerythroblast. The chromatin of polychromatophilic normoblasts is condensed into dense aggregates interposed between areas of clarity. By this time, the cell has begun to produce substantial amounts of hemoglobin, which imparts a paler blue to gray appearance to the cytoplasm. Polychromatophilic erythroblasts are the most numerous erythroid precursors in the marrow. The orthochromatic erythroblast (orthochromatic normoblast) may have a nucleus with small, clear chromatin windows, but by and large, the nucleus is homogenous. At this point in differentiation, the cytoplasm is decidedly red. Cells very late in maturation have the cytoplasm of a reticulocyte.

On the biopsy, later erythroid precursors are readily identified by perfectly round, densely staining nuclei and scant cytoplasm (Fig. 3-10). Early erythroblasts can be difficult to distinguish from early myeloid precursors on a biopsy, but they are characterized by round vesicular nuclei that often have elongated or bar-shaped nucleoli. Like myeloid precursors, erythroid precursors tend to be nonrandomly distributed in the

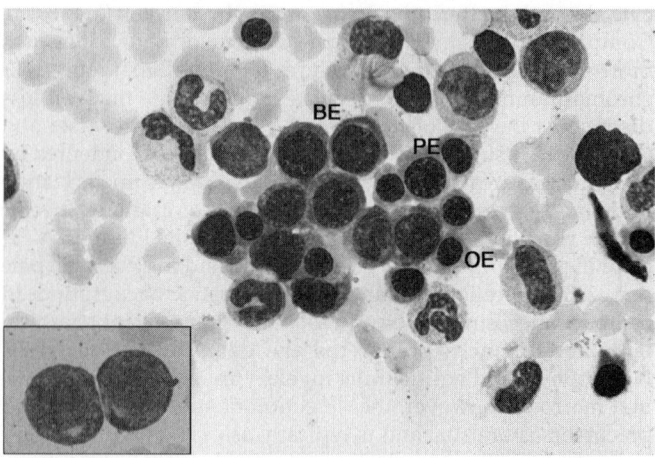

Figure 3-16. Erythroid maturation: proerythroblasts **(inset)**, basophilic erythroblast (BE), polychromatophilic erythroblasts (PE), and orthochromatic erythroblasts (OE) (Wright-Giemsa; aspirate; ×1000.) (See Color Fig. 3-16.)

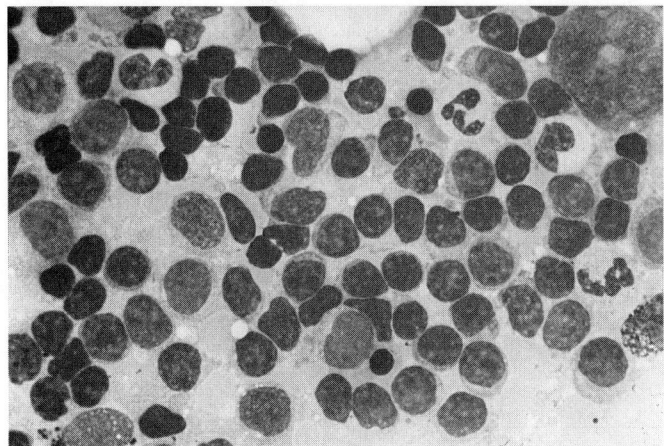

Figure 3-17. Reactive lymphoid aggregate (Wright-Giemsa; aspirate; ×1000). (See Color Fig. 3-17.)

marrow and are typically located away from the trabeculae in clusters, termed *erythroid islands*, in which the late precursors are often located at the periphery. In some cases, these erythroid islands may be appreciated on aspirate smears as weakly cohesive clusters of erythroid precursors.

Lymphocytes and Plasma Cells

The percent and morphology of normal lymphocytes in the marrow is variable and highly dependent on the age of the patient from whom the sample is obtained. Mature lymphocytes constitute approximately 15% of marrow cellularity in the adult. Small lymphoid cells with round to ovoid nuclei, coarsely clumped to streaky chromatin, and very scant cytoplasm predominate (Fig. 3-17). Occasional larger cells with more ample pale-blue cytoplasm, often containing several small granules, termed *large granular lymphocytes*, may be seen. In infants and young children, lymphocytes may constitute

30% to 50% of the marrow cellularity. Characteristically, a subpopulation of lymphocytes in young children is somewhat larger and has finer, immature-appearing chromatin and a small amount of basophilic cytoplasm. These cells are often referred to as *"immature" lymphocytes* or *hematogones*, and they likely represent functionally normal lymphoid precursors, but distinction from malignant lymphoblasts may be difficult in some cases.

Lymphoid aggregates are a common finding in bone marrow particle sections in older adults, among whom they may be seen in up to 47% of patients (mean age, 71.9 years) without lymphoproliferative disorders (58). The frequency of marrow lymphoid aggregates is lower in younger age groups. The prevalence of these aggregates in older individuals may lead to uncertainty in the histologic diagnosis of minimal involvement by low-grade lymphoproliferative disorders such as chronic lymphocytic leukemia (59). Benign lymphoid aggregates are typically located around marrow arterioles and often contain a mixed population of small and occasional large lymphocytes, macrophages, plasma cells, and mast cells. Secondary follicles may be present. Despite their frequency on tissue sections, it is relatively uncommon to appreciate distinct nonneoplastic lymphoid aggregates on bone marrow aspirate smears.

Plasma cells are a minor component (<2%) of the marrow cellularity; however, their numbers may increase significantly in chronic inflammatory conditions, among other disorders. Plasma cell morphology can vary greatly. The typical plasma cell is an oblong cell with a round, eccentrically placed nucleus with clumped chromatin, a distinct area of pallor directly adjacent to the nucleus, a so-called perinuclear hoff, and otherwise-uniform lavender (amphophilic) cytoplasm with smooth borders (Fig. 3-18). Occasional cells with very abundant cytoplasm, or ruffled cytoplasm with red-tinged edges, may be present. Multinuclearity, although often associated with malignant plasma cells, may be seen in reactive conditions. Plasma cells tend to be located at the periphery of blood vessels and are consequently often found within the stromal spicule on aspirate smears.

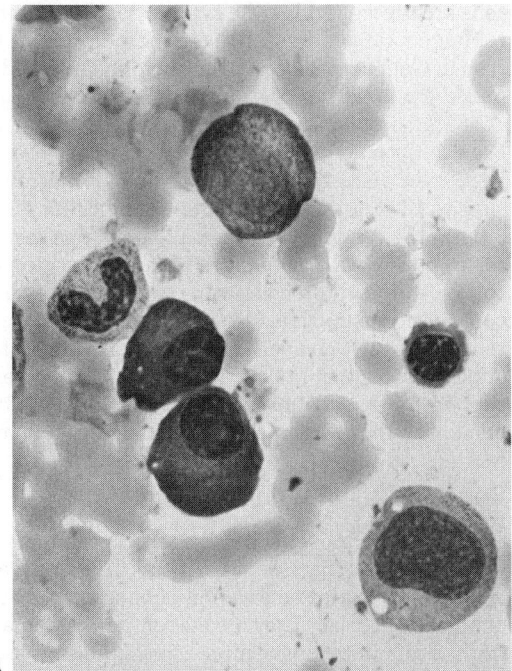 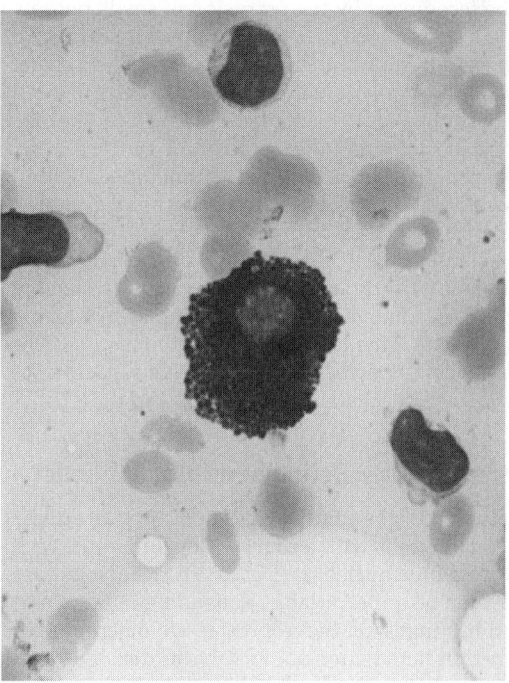

Figure 3-18. Plasma cells **(A)** and mast cell **(B)** (Wright-Giemsa; aspirates; ×1000). (See Color Fig. 3-18.)

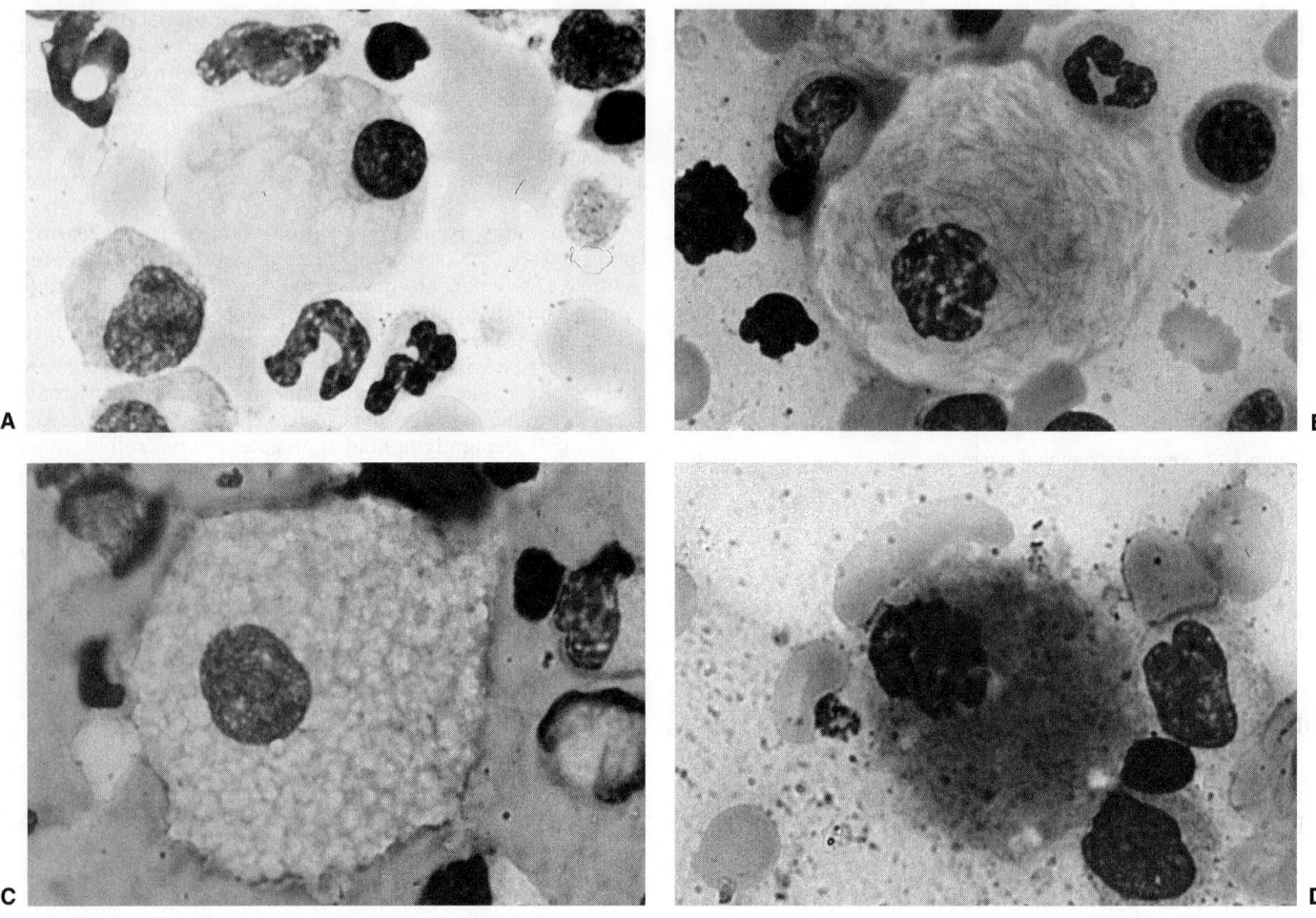

Figure 3-19. Histiocytes/macrophages: histiocyte **(A)**, Gaucher cell **(B)**, Niemann-Pick cell **(C)**, sea-blue histiocyte **(D)** (Wright-Giemsa; aspirates; ×1000). (See Color Fig. 3-19.)

Mast Cells

Mast cells can be recognized by the profusion of small, densely packed, dark-purple granules that occupy the cytoplasm and may obscure the small, round nucleus (Fig. 3-18). Their shape can vary from round to polygonal to spindled. They are often confused with basophils, but can be distinguished by the size and quality of the granules and the shape of the nucleus. They disaggregate poorly and are most often identified deep within aspirated spicules. Mast cell granules, unlike basophil granules, are resistant to routine histologic processing, and on Giemsa-stained sections, mast cell cytoplasm is purple-red and finely granular. Mast cells are ordinarily an inconspicuous marrow occupant; however, in some disorders, including bone marrow failure syndromes and some low-grade lymphomas, particularly lymphoplasmacytic lymphoma (Waldenström's macroglobulinemia), they may be particularly prominent.

Macrophages and Other Reticuloendothelial Cells

Macrophages, also known as *reticulum cells* or *histiocytes*, appear in the marrow as large cells with a round or oval nucleus, with a single, round, pale-blue nucleolus (Fig. 3-19). The appearance of the cytoplasm can be quite variable, depending in large part on what the cell has ingested. Siderophages are macrophages containing iron-rich hemosiderin and ferritin derived from effete cells, particularly red blood cells. Hemosiderin pigment is coarsely granular and rusty brown on both biopsies and aspi-

rates and stains dark blue with the Perls' or Prussian blue stain (Fig. 3-6). Intact red blood cells and nucleated hematopoietic cells are present within the cytoplasm of macrophages in erythrophagocytic and hemophagocytic syndromes. Gaucher cells, seen in Gaucher's disease, are macrophages filled with uncatabolized glucocerebrosides, imparting a pale-staining, streaky, or "crinkled tissue paper" appearance to the cytoplasm (Fig. 3-19). Pseudo-Gaucher cells with a similar cytologic appearance may be seen in diseases associated with high marrow cell turnover, such as CML. Macrophages in Niemann-Pick disease and some other inherited lipidoses have a foamy appearance due to accumulated lipids. Macrophages with foamy cytoplasm are also a common finding in chemotherapy-ablated marrows. Ceroid-containing histiocytes (sea blue histiocytes) are mononuclear cells containing coarsely granular, peroxidized fatty acids that appear blue-green in both W-G–stained aspirates and Giemsa-stained tissue sections. These histiocytes may be observed in persons with the lipidoses, CML, or acute leukemia.

Bone and Its Cellular Constituents

The bone cells most likely to be seen in aspirates are osteoclasts and osteoblasts (Figs. 3-20 and 3-21). These cells are responsible for the growth and remodeling of bone and lie at the periphery of bone trabeculae. They are evident rarely in marrow aspirates from adults, and may be more conspicuous in association with a variety of pathologic conditions, including metastatic solid tumors, or as a repair reaction after prior biopsies. By contrast,

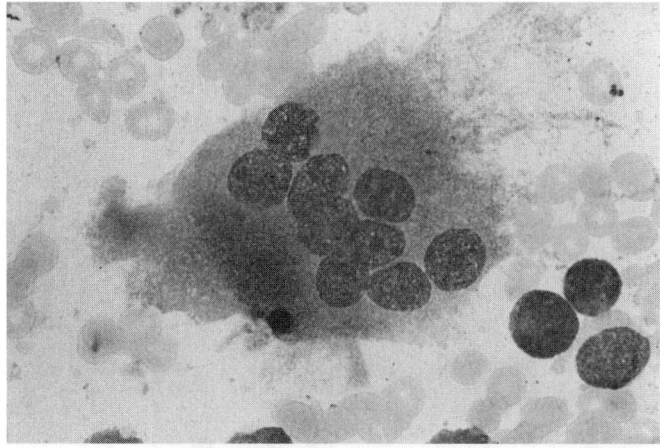

Figure 3-20. Osteoclast (Wright-Giemsa; aspirate; ×1000). (See Color Fig. 3-20.)

in growing children, osteoclasts and osteoblasts are a relatively common finding due to the fact that the biopsy and aspirate procedures must transgress the growth plate to reach the marrow cavity.

Osteoclasts are huge (up to 100 μm), multinucleated cells (Fig. 3-20). They can be mistaken for megakaryocytes, but can be distinguished by the appearance of their nuclei. An osteoclast nucleus resembles that of a histiocyte in being uniformly round to oval and having one indistinct, bluish nucleolus. In contrast to megakaryocytes, the nuclei are distinct, not lobated, and usually do not overlie one another. The cytoplasm of an osteoclast is pale and is interspersed with fine, purplish-red granules.

Osteoblasts are intermediate-sized cells (up to 30 μm) with eccentric nuclei, often closely apposed to the cytoplasmic border (Fig. 3-21). The cytoplasm is pale bluish gray, agranular, and may contain an area of pallor that is discontiguous with the nucleus. Osteoblasts tend to be aspirated in loose clusters and can be mistaken for metastatic carcinoma or for plasma cells.

Bone marrow biopsies also sample the bone itself, which should not be overlooked. In patients who have undergone autotransplantation or have had multiple previous biopsies, healing biopsy sites are a common finding. Bone changes characteristic of renal osteodystrophy or Paget's disease may be seen in a rare specimen. Irregular, thickened bone trabeculae are typical of agnogenic myeloid metaplasia with myelofibrosis,

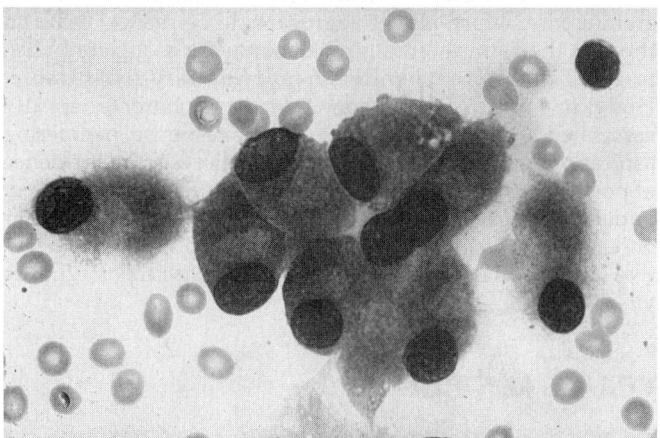

Figure 3-21. Osteoblasts (Wright-Giemsa; aspirate; ×1000). (See Color Fig. 3-21.)

and they may aid in the distinction between other myeloproliferative disorders with marrow fibrosis. Distortion of bone architecture may also signal the presence of metastatic tumor in an adjacent area, even though the tumor itself may not be evident in the section.

EVALUATION OF SPECIAL CONDITIONS

Bone Marrow Necrosis

Necrosis of normal hematopoietic elements with gelatinous transformation has been described in patients with anorexia nervosa, involuntary starvation, and acquired immunodeficiency syndrome, among other disorders (60). Fat necrosis occurs in infarcts, fracture sites, malignancy, and pancreatitis. Sheets of necrotic tumor occupying the marrow cavity are most often seen in Burkitt lymphoma, lymphoblastic leukemia, and acute myelogenous leukemia, and occasionally seen in metastatic solid tumors (61).

Granulomas and Bone Marrow Infections

Granulomas are aggregates of macrophages, often admixed with lymphocytes and plasma cells. They are essentially only seen on biopsies, and are rarely appreciated on aspirate smears. Granulomas composed of tight clusters of macrophages with abundant, dense, pink cytoplasm are known as *epithelioid granulomas* and may or may not be associated with central necrosis. Epithelioid granulomas may be seen in a variety of infectious, inflammatory, and malignant processes, including tuberculosis, leprosy, lymphogranuloma venereum, tularemia, cat-scratch disease, syphilis, infectious mononucleosis, brucellosis, histoplasmosis, sarcoidosis, non-Hodgkin's lymphomas, Hodgkin's disease, and other malignancies (62). In some cases, these bone marrow granulomas are paraneoplastic or epiphenomena, and do not necessarily imply marrow involvement by the disorder. Conversely, granulomas may not be evident in immunocompromised patients with marrow involvement by infectious organisms that typically evoke a granulomatous response. For example, of patients with *Mycobacterium avium*-intracellulare cultured from bone marrow biopsy specimens, over 50% do not exhibit granulomas (63).

Bone marrow culture is useful for the diagnosis of certain granulomatous infections, particularly histoplasmosis. Most studies reveal a high yield of histoplasmosis on bone marrow culture ranging from 25% to 70%. In 30% to 80% of cases of histoplasmosis not confirmed by marrow fungal stains, the marrow culture is positive. The yield of bone marrow culture in patients with miliary tuberculosis is variable (15% to 55%) and is complimentary to the liver biopsy in establishing the diagnosis (64–66).

Although of low yield, bone marrow sampling in patients with fever of undetermined origin is justifiable. In most cases, peripheral blood abnormalities prompt examination of the marrow, but even when lacking, blind biopsies may be worth performing. In approximately 10% of cases, marrow sampling establishes the diagnosis, most commonly hematologic malignancies (21%) or tuberculosis (5%) (67). In patients with acquired immunodeficiency syndrome, bone marrow biopsy, aspiration, and culture are commonly used in the evaluation of fever of undetermined origin (68,69).

Lipogranulomas, which are not associated with infection, are aggregates of fat-laden macrophages, plasma cells, lymphocytes, and mast cells. They are quite common, being present in nearly 10% of bone marrow biopsies (70), but their clinical significance is unclear.

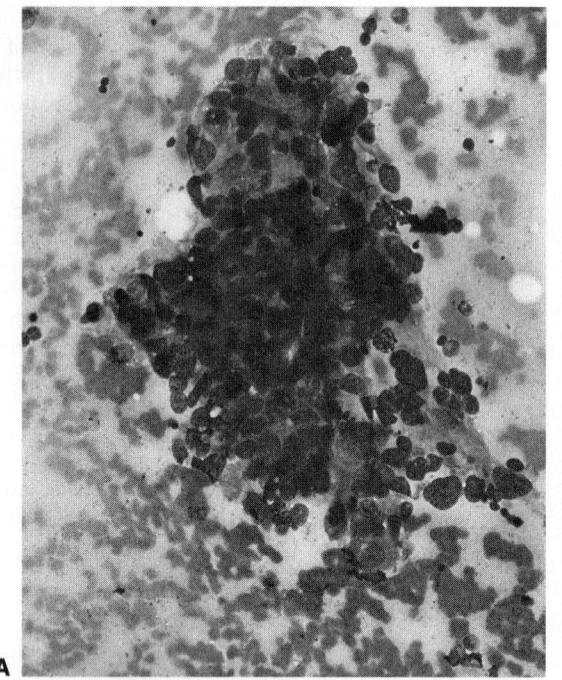
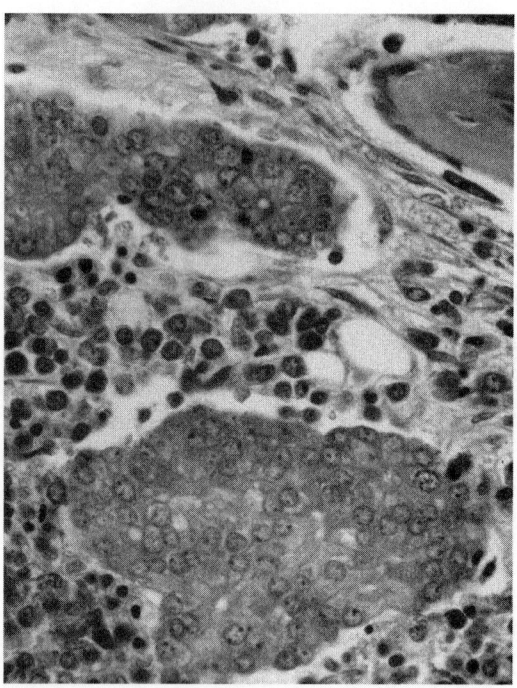

Figure 3-22. Metastatic prostate carcinoma aspirate (Wright-Giemsa; aspirate; ×400) **(A)** and biopsy (Giemsa; biopsy; ×400) **(B)**. (See Color Fig. 3-22.)

Metastatic Tumors in Adults

As a test for identifying cancer metastases, bone marrow sampling is diagnostic in 15% to 25% of patients with nonhematologic tumors (71). It should be reserved for patients with signs of marrow invasion (e.g., leukoerythroblastosis or unexplained cytopenias), for those in whom a positive finding would significantly alter treatment, and for patients with malignancies commonly metastatic to the bone marrow, such as small cell carcinoma of the lung, breast cancer, prostate cancer, and some sarcomas. Blind bone marrow biopsy as an attempt to establish a diagnosis of malignancy in a patient with constitutional symptoms is of low yield unless some objective evidence of disease exists (e.g., hypercalcemia, elevated alkaline phosphatase). In a large series of bone marrow biopsies reviewed retrospectively, only 11% were of specific diagnostic value. Of these, only 1.7% established the diagnosis of metastatic carcinoma (6).

Carcinoma metastatic to the bone marrow is most easily seen in histologic sections, but may be present on aspirate smears (Fig. 3-22). Because of the stromal fibrosis engendered by many metastatic tumors seen in adults, a dry tap may be obtained, or tumor cells may not themselves be aspirable. In these cases and in others with significant marrow fibrosis, a touch preparation may be invaluable (72,73). Aspirate or touch preparations should be viewed under low power, because metastatic carcinoma cells are almost always larger than all hematopoietic elements other than megakaryocytes, and they most often occur in clumps. Because of their size, they may also be distributed at the periphery of the smear. Common artifacts simulating tumor cells in marrow aspirates include megakaryocytic nuclei, platelet aggregates, and clusters of erythroblasts (74).

On biopsies, tumor cells may be inconspicuous compared to the surrounding stromal reaction that frequently accompanies metastatic carcinoma. Some tumors may be difficult to appreciate due to the relative paucity of stromal response or their small size. For example, the coordinate use of immunohistochemistry for cytokeratin in patients with metastatic lobular carcinoma of the breast significantly increases the detection of small tumor deposits (75,76).

Metastatic Pediatric Solid Tumors

Bone marrow aspiration and biopsy are complementary procedures in the workup for metastases in children with solid tumors. In one series of children with nonhematologic malignancies, the bone marrow biopsy was positive in 45%, and in slightly more than 50% of these, the aspirate was nondiagnostic. Conversely, the aspirate was positive in 55% of cases when the biopsy was negative, and in 21%, both the biopsy and the aspirate were diagnostic (77).

Lymphoma Staging

As a staging procedure, bone marrow biopsy is important for patients with non-Hodgkin's lymphoma, regardless of initial stage. Positive results are obtained nearly twice as often on biopsies compared to smears, in the absence of ancillary tests such as flow cytometry (78). Bilateral sampling increases the yield by approximately 20% over unilateral biopsies (79). The sensitivity of the biopsy is likely related to the preservation of architecture, which allows aggregates to be recognized, and the fact that lymphoid aggregates may be associated with reticulin fibers that render them relatively inaspirable. Hodgkin's disease in the bone marrow is characteristically associated with a dense, fibrohistiocytic response, hampering aspiration. In patients with Hodgkin's disease, the incidence of positive bone marrows is stage related. From 12% to 25% of patients with stage III disease are upstaged to stage IV after bone marrow biopsy, even though initial aspirates were negative (80,81). Bilateral biopsies further increase the diagnostic yield (79).

RESULTS REPORTING

The bone marrow report should be presented in an orderly and consistent manner to provide the optimal amount of information from the study. The organization should convey the fact

TABLE 3-13. Bone Marrow Results Reporting

Bone marrow biopsy	
Technical quality	Size/fragmentation/aspiration or crush artifacts/hemorrhage
Cellularity	Reported as % cellularity or % fat Normo/hyper/hypocellular for age
M:E	>/< 3:1–4:1
Erythroid morphology	Maturation/full/limited/megaloblastic/ left shifted Dyserythropoiesis
Myeloid morphology	Maturation/full/limited/left shifted Increased eosinophils or other lineages Dysmyelopoiesis
Blasts	Numerical estimation/clustering
Megakaryocytes	Normal/increased/decreased/clustering Dysmegakaryocytopoiesis
Lymphocytes and plasma cells	Lymphoid aggregates/infiltrates Plasma cell aggregates/infiltrates
Histiocytes and other cells	Storage cells and other histiocytes Granulomas/metastatic tumor
Stromal background	Fibrosis, reticulin stain
Hemosiderin	Hemosiderin, iron stain
Bone	Osteoblastic and osteoclastic activity Bone trabecular architecture
Immunohistochemical stains	—
Bone marrow aspirate	
Technical quality	Dilute/spicules present or absent/touch preparation only
Cellularity	Normal/increased/decreased
Megakaryocytes	Normal/increased/decreased Dysmegakaryocytopoiesis
M:E	>/< 3:1–4:1
Differential count	—
Blasts	Myeloid/lymphoid
Myeloid	Maturation/full/limited/left shifted Increased eosinophils, basophils, or monocytes Dysmyelopoiesis
Erythroid	Maturation/full/limited/megaloblastic/ left shifted Dyserythropoiesis
Lymphocytes	Cellular atypia
Plasma cells	Cellular atypia
Other cells	Storage cells and other histiocytes Metastatic tumor
Iron stain	Storage iron/ringed sideroblasts
Histochemical stains	MPO, NSE, CAE/SE, PAS, SBB
Peripheral blood smear	—
Flow cytometry	—
Cytogenetics	—
Molecular diagnostics	—
Diagnosis	—

CAE/SE, chloracetate esterase/specific esterase; M:E, myeloid to erythroid ratio; MPO, myeloperoxidase; NSE, nonspecific esterase; PAS, periodic acid-Schiff; SBB, Sudan black B.
Adapted from a protocol from Dr. Geraldine Pinkus, Brigham and Women's Hospital, Boston, MA.

that the specimens were reviewed in a systematic manner and synthesized into a diagnosis that is pertinent to the clinical question being posed. Although flow cytometry, cytogenetic, and molecular diagnostic results may not be available at the time of the report, they should be considered in rendering a diagnosis whenever possible. Table 3-13 contains a checklist for reviewing and reporting marrow specimens.

BONE MARROW IMAGING

The bone marrow may be imaged by one of several methods, including scintigraphy, computed tomography (CT), and magnetic resonance imaging (MRI).

Scintigraphy uses an isotope to yield a direct physiologic assessment of hematopoiesis or the reticuloendothelial system (RES) and an indirect evaluation of total marrow function by surveying surrounding osseous structures. For erythropoietic marrow imaging, radiolabeled iron (^{52}Fe) is the prototypic tracer used (82). Technetium-99m (^{99m}Tc) sulfur colloid is infused for imaging the RES. Although erythropoietic marrow and the RES can be imaged individually, distribution of the isotope in each case is similar. Indirect imaging assesses bone remodeling using the labeled colloid ^{99m}Tc diphosphonate. Radioiron and colloid isotopes provide equally sensitive studies, but lack of anatomic detail and low specificity are drawbacks of scintigraphy in general (83).

Images produced by CT occur as an x-ray beam is attenuated by marrow elements of varying electron densities. Fatty marrow generates low-density images, whereas hematopoietic marrow and trabecular bone yield higher-density images with positive Hounsfield values. Thus, the appearance of CTs are location dependent and should be compared with contralateral views. CT provides excellent anatomic detail: Trabecular bone is well defined, and some separation of fatty and hematopoietic marrow can be made (84).

MRI generates the most detailed radiologic evaluation of all bone marrow elements. The biophysical differences of bone marrow tissues resulting in variations in MRI scans include proton density and T1 and T2 relaxation times (85). Although spin-echo sequences with T1- and T2-weighted images are used frequently, newer approaches are under investigation (86,87).

Yellow marrow produces a signal similar to that of subcutaneous fat, whereas red marrow is hypodense in comparison (88). In sites with increased red marrow fractions, such as the spine, the signal intensity is lower than in locations predominantly populated with fatty marrow (distal skeleton). As conversion of red to yellow marrow proceeds with age, focal replacement with fat is demonstrated as bright spots on T1 images (89). Bony trabeculae appear as bands of low-signal intensity on short– and long repetition time–echo delay sequences.

MRI reliably can identify infiltrative lesions in the marrow, but is unable to delineate tissue histology, and the appearances of images overlap for benign and malignant processes (90). Specific patterns for leukemic infiltration as well as marrow alterations after chemotherapy or radiotherapy are being described, and thus, MRI may evolve as a useful means of monitoring marrow changes in these patients (91). It is useful in staging malignancies that have a high predilection to spread to bone marrow, including high-grade lymphomas (particularly Burkitt lymphoma), carcinomas (especially breast, prostate, and small cell lung carcinoma), and certain pediatric tumors (Ewing's sarcoma and neuroblastoma). Bone marrow involvement in these malignancies may extend into the spinal canal and cause cord compression (Fig. 3-23). In conditions resulting in myeloid depletion, the MRI signal pattern is characteristic of fatty marrow, although signal intensity varies with the clinical condition. MRI is highly sensitive for demonstrating bone marrow ischemia (92), and bone marrow edema results in signals on short-repetition time–echo delay sequence images commensurate with the degree of increase in tissue water (93).

Positron emission tomography scanning using the glucose analog ^{18}F-2-fluoro-2-deoxy-D-glucose is quite reliable in detecting bone, bone marrow, and other sites of metastatic tumor spread. Most malignancies have a higher rate of glucose consumption than resting cells accounting for the spectroscopic differentiation of tumor cells. Presently, the high cost of a dedicated positron emission tomography scanner prohibits its usage in routine staging of most malignancies; but as the cost

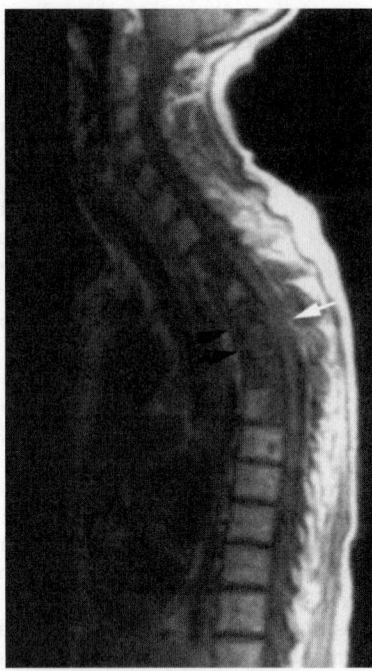

Figure 3-23. T1-weighted sagittal magnetic resonance imaging scan of the upper spine. Normal marrow appears white due to the high fat content, whereas the marrow in several vertebral bodies appears black due to replacement by metastatic lung carcinoma (*black arrows*). The tumor extends into the spinal cord at T3 and is associated with cord displacement and compression (*white arrow*).

decreases and comparative studies with other staging procedures are conducted, its use will likely increase (94).

REFERENCES

1. Neumann E. Ueber die beduetung des knochenmarks fur die Blutbilding. *Centralblatt Med Wiss* 1868;6:689.
2. Damashek W. Biopsy of the sternal bone marrow. *Am J Med Sci* 1935;190:617.
3. Frankel S, Reitman S, Sonnenwirth AC. *Gradwohl's clinical laboratory methods and diagnosis.* St. Louis: Mosby, 1970.
4. Miale JB. *Laboratory medicine: hematology.* St. Louis: Mosby, 1972.
5. Sonnenwirth AC, Jarett L. *Gradwohl's clinical laboratory methods and diagnosis.* St. Louis: Mosby, 1980.
6. Ellis LD, Wallace NJ, Westerman MP. Needle biopsy of bone and marrow. *Arch Intern Med* 1964;114:213.
7. Jamshidi K, Swaim WR. Bone marrow biopsy with unaltered architecture: a new biopsy device. *J Lab Clin Med* 1971;77:335–342.
8. Islam A. A new bone marrow biopsy needle with core securing device. *J Clin Pathol* 1982;35:359–364.
9. Ellis RB. The distribution of active marrow in the adult. *Phys Med Biol* 1961;5:255.
10. Pochedly C. How to perform marrow puncture in small children. *Clin Pediatr (Phila)* 1969;8:705.
11. Lowrie L, Weiss AH, Lacombe C. The pediatric sedation unit: a mechanism for pediatric sedation. *Pediatrics* 1998;102:E30.
12. Colvin BT. How to biopsy the marrow. *Br J Hosp Med* 1980;24:176–178.
13. Grann V, Pool JL, Mayer K. Comparative study of bone marrow aspiration and biopsy in patients with neoplastic disease. *Cancer* 1966;19:1898–1900.
14. Bearden JD, Ratkin GA, Coltman CA. Comparison of the diagnostic value of bone marrow biopsy and bone marrow aspiration in neoplastic disease. *J Clin Pathol* 1974;27:738–740.
15. Bemis EL. Bone marrow examination. *Postgrad Med* 1970;48:49–52.
16. Brynes RK, McKenna RW, Sundberg RD. Bone marrow aspiration and trephine biopsy. An approach to a thorough study. *Am J Clin Pathol* 1978;70:753–759.
17. Navone R, Colombano MT. Histopathological trephine biopsy findings in cases of 'dry tap' bone marrow aspirations. *Appl Pathol* 1984;2:264–271.
18. Gilbert EH, Earle JD, Glatstein E, et al. Indium bone marrow scintigraphy as an aid in selecting marrow biopsy sites for the evaluation of marrow elements in patients with lymphoma. *Cancer* 1976;38:1560–1567.
19. Bird AR, Jacobs P. Trephine biopsy of the bone marrow. *S Afr Med J* 1983;64:271–276.
20. Garnier H, Reynier J, Dimopoulos F. A propos des accidents de la ponction sternale. *Ann Chir* 1964;67:373.
21. Rywlin AM, Marvan P, Robinson MJ. A simple technique for the preparation of bone marrow smears and sections. *Am J Clin Pathol* 1970;53:389–393.
22. Liao KT. The superiority of histologic sections of aspirated bone marrow in malignant lymphomas. A review of 1,124 examinations. *Cancer* 1971;27:618–628.
23. Cetto GL, Iannucci A, Perini A, et al. Bone marrow evaluation: the relative merits of particle sections and smear preparations. *Appl Pathol* 1983;1:181–193.
24. Ellis WM, Georgiou GM, Roberton DM, et al. The use of discontinuous Percoll gradients to separate populations of cells from human bone marrow and peripheral blood. *J Immunol Methods* 1984;66:9–16.
25. Carson FL. *Histotechnology: a self instructional text.* Chicago: ASCP Press, 1997.
26. Moosavi H, Lichtman MA, Donnelly JA, et al. Plastic–embedded human marrow biopsy specimens: improved histochemical methods. *Arch Pathol Lab Med* 1981;105:269–273.
27. Cramer AD, Rogers ER, Parker JW, et al. The Giemsa stain for tissue sections: an improved method. *Am J Clin Pathol* 1973;60:148–156.
28. Gomori G. Microtechnical demonstration of iron. *Am J Pathol* 1936;12:655.
29. Beutler E, Robson MJ, Buttenwieser E. A comparison of the plasma iron, iron-binding capacity, sternal marrow iron and other methods in the clinical evaluation of iron stores. *Ann Intern Med* 1958;48:60.
30. Kaplan E, Zuelzer WW, Mouriquand C. Sideroblasts: a study of stainable nonhemoglobin iron in marrow normoblasts. *Blood* 1954;9.
31. Cartwright GE, Deiss A. Sideroblasts, siderocytes, and sideroblastic anemia. *N Engl J Med* 1975;292:185–193.
32. Bauermeister DE. Quantitation of bone marrow reticulin—a normal range. *Am J Clin Pathol* 1971;56:24–31.
33. Hayhoe FGJ, Quaglino D. *Haematological cytochemistry.* Edinburgh, U.K.: Churchill Livingstone, 1988.
34. Freedman AS, Nadler LM. Cell surface markers in hematologic malignancies. *Semin Oncol* 1987;14:193–212.
35. Volger LB. Bone marrow B cell development. *Clin Haematol* 1982;11:509.
36. Romain PL, Schlossman SF. Human T lymphocyte subsets. Functional heterogeneity and surface recognition structures. *J Clin Invest* 1984;74:1559–1565.
37. Sternberger LA, Hardy PH Jr, Cuculis JJ, et al. The unlabeled antibody enzyme method of immunohistochemistry: preparation and properties of soluble antigen-antibody complex (horseradish peroxidase-antihorseradish peroxidase) and its use in identification of spirochetes. *J Histochem Cytochem* 1970;18:315–333.
38. Hsu SM, Raine L, Fanger H. A comparative study of the peroxidase-antiperoxidase method and an avidin-biotin complex method for studying polypeptide hormones with radioimmunoassay antibodies. *Am J Clin Pathol* 1981;75:734–738.
39. Moir DJ, Ghosh AK, Abdulaziz Z, et al. Immunoenzymatic staining of haematological samples with monoclonal antibodies. *Br J Haematol* 1983;55:395–410.
40. Cordell JL, Falini B, Erber WN, et al. Immunoenzymatic labeling of monoclonal antibodies using immune complexes of alkaline phosphatase and monoclonal anti-alkaline phosphatase (APAAP complexes). *J Histochem Cytochem* 1984;32:219–229.
41. Neumann MP, de Solas I, Parkin JL, et al. Monoclonal antibody study of Philadelphia chromosome-positive blastic leukemias using the alkaline phosphatase anti-alkaline phosphatase (APAAP) technic. *Am J Clin Pathol* 1986;85:564–572.
42. Jennings CD, Foon KA. Recent advances in flow cytometry: application to the diagnosis of hematologic malignancy. *Blood* 1997;90:2863–2892.
43. Sullivan JG, Wiggers TB. Immunophenotyping leukemias: the new force in hematology. *Clin Lab Sci* 2000;13:117–122.
44. Steinkamp JA. Flow cytometry. *Rev Sci Instrum* 1984;55:1375.
45. Syrjala MT, Tiirikainen M, Jansson SE, et al. Flow cytometric analysis of terminal deoxynucleotidyl transferase. A simplified method. *Am J Clin Pathol* 1993;99:298–303.
46. Roma AO, Kutok JL, Shaheen G, et al. A novel, rapid, multiparametric approach for flow cytometric analysis of intranuclear terminal deoxynucleotidyl transferase. *Am J Clin Pathol* 1999;112:343–348.
47. Groenveld K, te Marvelde JG, van den Beemd MW, et al. Flow cytometric detection of intracellular antigens for immunophenotyping of normal and malignant leukocytes. *Leukemia* 1996;10:1383–1389.
48. Nguyen PL, Olszak I, Harris NL, et al. Myeloperoxidase detection by three-color flow cytometry and by enzyme cytochemistry in the classification of acute leukemia. *Am J Clin Pathol* 1998;110:163–169.
49. Davis BH, Bigelow NC. Flow cytometric reticulocyte quantification using thiazole orange provides clinically useful reticulocyte maturity index. *Arch Pathol Lab Med* 1989;113:684–689.
50. Harris NL, Jaffe ES, Diebold J, et al. World Health Organization classification of neoplastic diseases of the hematopoietic and lymphoid tissues: report of the Clinical Advisory Committee meeting-Airlie House, Virginia, November 1997. *J Clin Oncol* 1999;17:3835–3849.
51. Jaffe ES, Harris NL, Stein H, et al. Pathology and genetics of tumours of the haematopoietic and lymphoid tissues. In: *World Health Organization Classification of Tumours.* Lyon: IARC Press, 2001;1–352.
52. Kapff CT, Jandl JH. *Blood: atlas and sourcebook of hematology.* Boston: Little Brown, 1981.
53. Zucker-Franklin D, Greaves MF, Grossi CE, et al. *Atlas of blood cells: function and pathology.* Philadelphia: Lea & Febiger, 1981.
54. Wickramasinghe SN. Bone marrow. In: Sternberg SS, ed. *Histology for pathologists.* New York: Raven Press, 1992:1–31.

55. Hartsock RJ, Smith EB, Petty CS. Normal variations with aging of the amount of hematopoietic tissue in bone marrow from the anterior iliac crest. *Am J Clin Pathol* 1965;43:326.

56. Morley A, Blake J. Observer error in histological assessment of marrow hypocellularity. *J Clin Pathol* 1975;28:104–108.

57. Rywlin AM. *Histopathology of the bone marrow.* Boston: Little Brown, 1976.

58. Rywlin AM, Ortega RS, Dominguez CJ. Lymphoid nodules of bone marrow: normal and abnormal. *Blood* 1974;43:389–400.

59. Faulkner-Jones BE, Howie AJ, Boughton BJ, et al. Lymphoid aggregates in bone marrow: study of eventual outcome. *J Clin Pathol* 1988;41:768–775.

60. Smith RR, Spivak JL. Marrow cell necrosis in anorexia nervosa and involuntary starvation. *Br J Haematol* 1985;60:525–530.

61. Conrad ME. Bone marrow necrosis. *J Intensive Care Med* 1995;10:171–178.

62. Peace G. Granulomatous lesions in bone marrow. *Blood* 1956;11:720.

63. Cohen RJ, Samoszuk MK, Busch D, et al. Occult infections with M. intracellulare in bone-marrow biopsy specimens from patients with AIDS. *N Engl J Med* 1983;308:1475–1476.

64. Sarosi GA, Voth DW, Dahl BA, et al. Disseminated histoplasmosis: results of long-term follow-up. A center for disease control cooperative mycoses study. *Ann Intern Med* 1971;75:511–516.

65. Smith JW, Utz JP. Progressive disseminated histoplasmosis. A prospective study of 26 patients. *Ann Intern Med* 1972;76:557–565.

66. Bodem CR, Hamory BH, Taylor HM, et al. Granulomatous bone marrow disease. A review of the literature and clinicopathologic analysis of 58 cases. *Medicine (Baltimore)* 1983;62:372–383.

67. Larson EB, Featherstone HJ, Petersdorf RG. Fever of undetermined origin: diagnosis and follow-up of 105 cases, 1970–1980. *Medicine (Baltimore)* 1982;61:269–292.

68. Ciaudo M, Doco-Lecompte T, Guettier C, et al. Revisited indications for bone marrow examinations in HIV-infected patients. *Eur J Haematol* 1994;53:168–174.

69. Benito N, Nunez A, de Gorgolas M, et al. Bone marrow biopsy in the diagnosis of fever of unknown origin in patients with acquired immunodeficiency syndrome. *Arch Intern Med* 1997;157:1577–1580.

70. Rywlin AM, Ortega R. Lipid granulomas of the bone marrow. *Am J Clin Pathol* 1972;57:457–462.

71. Garrett TJ, Gee TS, Lieberman PH, et al. The role of bone marrow aspiration and biopsy in detecting marrow involvement by nonhematologic malignancies. *Cancer* 1976;38:2401–2403.

72. Engeset A, Nesheim A, Sokolowski J. Incidence of 'dry tap' on bone marrow aspirations in lymphomas and carcinomas. Diagnostic value of the small material in the needle. *Scand J Haematol* 1979;22:417–422.

73. James LP, Stass SA, Schumacher HR. Value of imprint preparations of bone marrow biopsies in hematologic diagnosis. *Cancer* 1980;46:173–177.

74. Vernon SE. Clumping of erythroblasts simulating a metastatic neoplasm. *Arch Pathol Lab Med* 1985;109:569–570.

75. Bitter MA, Fiorito D, Corkill ME, et al. Bone marrow involvement by lobular carcinoma of the breast cannot be identified reliably by routine histological examination alone. *Hum Pathol* 1994;25:781–788.

76. Lyda MH, Tetef M, Carter NH, et al. Keratin immunohistochemistry detects clinically significant metastases in bone marrow biopsy specimens in women with lobular breast carcinoma. *Am J Surg Pathol* 2000;24:1593–1599.

77. Penchansky L. Bone marrow biopsy in the metastatic work-up of solid tumors in children. *Cancer* 1984;54:1447–1448.

78. Vinciguerra V, Silver RT. The importance of bone marrow biopsy in the staging of patients with lymphosarcoma. *Blood* 1973;41:913–920.

79. Brunning RD, Bloomfield CD, McKenna RW, et al. Bilateral trephine bone marrow biopsies in lymphoma and other neoplastic diseases. *Ann Intern Med* 1975;82:365–366.

80. Webb DI, Ubogy G, Silver RT. Importance of bone marrow biopsy in the clinical staging of Hodgkin's disease. *Cancer* 1970;26:313–317.

81. Han T, Stutzman L, Rogue AL. Bone marrow biopsy in Hodgkin's disease and other neoplastic diseases. *JAMA* 1971;217:1239–1241.

82. Fordham EW, Ali A. Radionuclide imaging of bone marrow. *Semin Hematol* 1981;18:222–239.

83. Datz FL, Taylor A. The clinical use of radionuclide bone marrow imaging. *Semin Nucl Med* 1985;15:239–259.

84. Genant HK, Wilson JS, Bovill EG, et al. Computed tomography of the musculoskeletal system. *J Bone Joint Surg Am* 1980;62:1088–1101.

85. Mitchell DG, Burk DL, Vinitski S, et al. The biophysical basis of tissue contrast in extracranial MR imaging. *AJR Am J Roentgenol* 1987;149:831–837.

86. Hendrick RE, Kneeland JB, Stark DD. Maximizing signal-to-noise and contrast-to-noise ratios in FLASH imaging. *Magn Reson Imaging* 1987;5:117–127.

87. Winkler ML, Ortendahl DA, Mills TC, et al. Characteristics of partial flip angle and gradient reversal MR imaging. *Radiology* 1988;166:17–26.

88. Wismer GL, Rosen BR, Buxton R, et al. Chemical shift imaging of bone marrow: preliminary experience. *AJR Am J Roentgenol* 1985;145:1031–1037.

89. Hajek PC, Baker LL, Goobar JE, et al. Focal fat deposition in axial bone marrow: MR characteristics. *Radiology* 1987;162:245–249.

90. Nyman R, Rehn S, Glimelius B, et al. Magnetic resonance imaging in diffuse malignant bone marrow diseases. *Acta Radiol* 1987;28:199–205.

91. McKinstry CS, Steiner RE, Young AT, et al. Bone marrow in leukemia and aplastic anemia: MR imaging before, during, and after treatment. *Radiology* 1987;162:701–707.

92. Beltran J, Herman LJ, Burk JM, et al. Femoral head avascular necrosis: MR imaging with clinical-pathologic and radionuclide correlation. *Radiology* 1988;166:215–220.

93. Vogler JB, Murphy WA. Bone marrow imaging. *Radiology* 1988;168:679–693.

94. Oehr P, Ruhlmann J, Biersack HJ. FDG-PET in clinical oncology: review of the literature and report of one institution's experience. *J Investig Med* 1999;47:452–461.

CHAPTER 4

Molecular Genetics and Genomics for the Hematologist

Hagop Youssoufian

Over the past several decades, molecular genetics has revolutionized our ability to analyze gene structure, expression, and function in the context of human disease. Although originally available only in a few elite laboratories, molecular genetic methods are now widely accessible and routinely applied to a variety of biomedical problems. Hematology has consistently been at the forefront of these developments. The end of the twentieth century also witnessed the marvelous achievements of the Human Genome Project, and with breathtaking speed, the technology and philosophy of genomics have begun to permeate every aspect of scientific inquiry and medical practice. In this chapter, general principles and methods of molecular genetics and genomics relevant to hematology are described. Additional background on cell and molecular biology and protocols on recombinant DNA technology can be found elsewhere (1–3).

Variation is the essence of genetics, and DNA is its ultimate reservoir. Variation may be viewed either as neutral *polymorphism* or pathogenic *mutation*. Although historically variant traits were identified using functional or protein-based assays, the relative simplicity of recombinant DNA technology and the possibility of establishing a direct link between phenotype and genotype have made many of the former approaches obsolete. For example, if a structurally abnormal protein is found in association with a clinical disorder, analysis of the gene encoding the mutant protein provides the most fundamental demonstration of the underlying molecular pathology. One of the earliest successes of the molecular genetic approach was the demonstration that a single nucleotide substitution in the β-globin gene that gives rise to sickle cell disease can be detected by a simple molecular technique.

With recombinant DNA methods, genes and their products may be produced in virtually unlimited quantities for functional studies and clinical applications. Moreover, normal and mutant genes can be readily introduced into cells and animals and their physiologic effects determined. Therefore, it should come as no surprise that recombinant DNA methods have profoundly advanced our understanding of cellular physiology, the pathobiology of disease, and the design of new therapeutic reagents. More recently, genomic technology has transformed the more traditional and reductionist study of individual genes into one that is integrated and global in character.

COMPLEXITY AND ORGANIZATION OF THE HUMAN GENOME

The flow of genetic information is primarily from DNA to messenger RNA (mRNA) to protein. DNA is a linear polymer of two interwoven chains (double helix) composed of four monomeric units, the deoxyribonucleotides (also called *nucleotides* or *bases*) adenine (A), cytosine (C), guanine (G), and thymine (T). Because of strict pairing rules of A to T and G to C, the sequence of the two strands is complementary.

Genetic information is present in both nuclei and mitochondria of eukaryotic cells, and mutations in both genomes can result in human disorders. The mitochondrial genome is circular and compact. Mutations in mitochondrial DNA have been associated with certain hematopoietic disorders, such as Pearson syndrome. However, most of our understanding of genomic organization, regulation, and function has focused on the cell nucleus. Unlike the mitochondrial genome, the nuclear genome is much larger and organized into linear arrays of DNA polymers, as well as proteins. The highest order of assembly of genomic DNA is its packaging with nucleoproteins into chromosomes (see Chapter 5 for a discussion of cytogenetics). The astounding complexity of the genome is attributed partly to its large size: The haploid genome contains approximately 3×10^9 nucleotides, or 3000 megabases (Mb). Although a precise number cannot yet be assigned, the human genome is believed to harbor approximately 50,000 to 100,000 genes.

Most nuclear genes are considerably larger than the precursor mRNAs (Fig. 4-1). This was first demonstrated for genes of animal viruses and soon thereafter for mouse β-globin and immunoglobulin genes. The additional sequences, called *intervening sequences* or *introns,* interrupt split genes into two or more units. Although the precise role and function of introns is obscure, it has been noted that they often subdivide the coding regions, or *exons,* of genes into structural blocks that correspond to functional domains of proteins. Such an arrangement may provide a mechanism by which exons have been shuffled during evolution to produce new proteins from preexisting units.

Several modifications accompany the transcription of eukaryotic DNA into RNA. Unlike mature mRNA, the primary transcript of the eukaryotic gene, called *heterogeneous nuclear RNA* (hnRNA), contains introns that are removed during RNA processing (splicing), so that the interrupted exons are joined

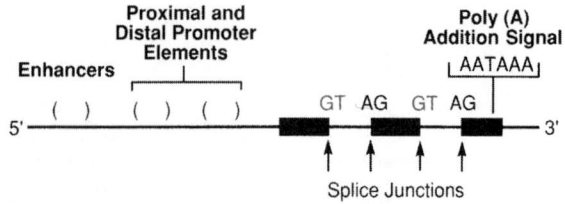

Figure 4-1. Schematic diagram of a prototypical eukaryotic gene illustrating the exons (*black boxes*), introns (*solid lines* connecting exons), splice junctions within introns (GT, AG), 5' regulatory elements, and a 3' polyadenylation site.

precisely and assembled into mature mRNA. Short-sequence motifs containing the dinucleotides GT and AG mark the beginning and end, respectively, of introns. Sequence motifs near the 3' end of the gene direct processing and polyadenylation of mRNA and may influence its stability. Mutations in this region have been observed in human disorders, such as one type of thrombophilia caused by a mutation in the 3' untranslated region of the prothrombin gene that enhances mRNA survival and thereby elevates the steady state level of prothrombin in plasma (see Chapter 31). Frequently, different mRNAs can be produced from the same hnRNA by differential splicing of exons (alternative splicing) or by differential use of the 3' polyadenylation sites. The pattern of splicing may be regulated by cell-specific factors, and the resulting protein products may have cell-specific functions.

Other DNA motifs, called *cis elements*, can be found within or near coding sequences and serve important regulatory functions. Promoter elements required for transcription are usually located just upstream of the site at which mRNA synthesis is initiated. Promoters often include short-sequence motifs, which are recognized by sequence-specific, DNA-binding proteins located within the nucleus. The activity of a promoter is established through the combined action of both ubiquitous and cell-specific nuclear proteins (4). Aside from promoters, *cis* elements located considerably upstream, downstream, or within genes may also play major roles in regulating gene expression, including cell type–specific transcription. Although such DNA elements, called *enhancers*, have no intrinsic promoter function, they often augment transcription from linked promoters. Moreover, DNA regions far removed from a gene may be responsible for activating entire chromosomal domains that may contain a cluster of related genes. A classic example is the locus control region of β-globin (see Chapter 49). Thus, the interplay of *cis* elements with nuclear proteins generates the exquisite and complex regulation of eukaryotic genes during normal growth and differentiation. The activation of the β-globin locus during the switch from embryonic to adult erythropoiesis uses many of these mechanisms.

Finally, the processed mRNA is transported to the cytoplasm and translated on ribosomes to polypeptides. Because the genetic code is degenerate, most amino acids can be specified by several codons that vary at their third position. Akin to transcription, specific structural elements regulate the initiation and efficiency of translation. In conjunction with several proteins called *initiation factors*, the ribosomal 40S subunit binds to a methylated structure at the 5' end of the mRNA, the *cap site*. This protein complex then migrates down the chain and scans for an initiator AUG codon (which encodes methionine). On finding an appropriate AUG, the 60S ribosome joins the complex to commence protein synthesis. The sequence context of the AUG is critical for recognition by the complex. In practice, the *Kozak sequence*—a consensus sequence around the AUG frequently found in proven initiation codons—is used to assign the beginning of a polypeptide sequence in a complementary DNA (cDNA). Other sequences in the 5' untranslated region of mRNA can form stem-loop structures by intramolecular bonding and influence the efficiency of translation. Translational control has been studied most intensively in genes that govern iron metabolism. Mutations in several genes that alter the translational efficiency of mRNA have been associated with hematologic disorders, including familial thrombocythemia (mutation of the thrombopoietin gene) and hyperferritinemia/cataract syndrome (mutation of the ferritin gene) (5).

MOLECULAR CLONING

The study of individual genes frequently begins with methods to purify and enrich DNA for further analysis. *Cloning* is the process by which a DNA molecule is joined to another DNA molecule (vector) that can propagate autonomously in a microbial host, usually a bacterium. An indispensable tool of molecular cloning is the *restriction endonuclease* (also called *restriction enzyme*; Fig. 4-2). These bacterial enzymes cleave double-stranded DNA at or near specific recognition sequences. Many restriction enzymes can generate staggered DNA ends with short, single-stranded regions (sticky ends), which facilitates the joining of unrelated, but similarly digested, DNA molecules. After annealing, these ends may be joined covalently by another enzyme, DNA ligase. Thus, restriction enzymes provide the essential reagents by which DNA may be reproducibly cleaved to smaller subunits and then recombined with other DNA fragments to create recombinant molecules.

Numerous vectors have been developed for gene cloning. The choice of vector depends on several considerations, including the size of the desired DNA fragment and the ability to be expressed in a particular host cell; different regulatory elements are required for expression of the same gene in bacteria or in

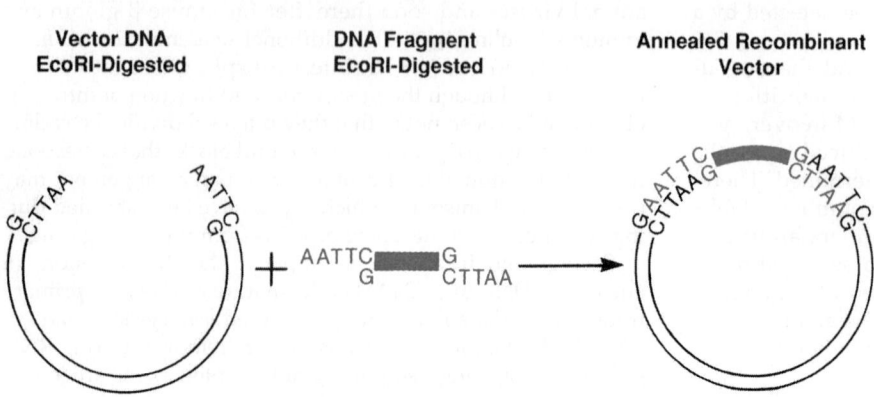

Vector DNA
EcoRI-Digested

DNA Fragment
EcoRI-Digested

Annealed Recombinant
Vector

Figure 4-2. Cleavage and rejoining of DNA at a restriction site. The restriction enzyme EcoRI recognizes and cleaves the double-stranded oligonucleotide sequence 5'-GAATTC-3', generating single-stranded sticky ends. Cleavage of a hypothetic plasmid or bacteriophage vector at a suitable EcoRI recognition site with this enzyme would allow the annealing of an unrelated DNA fragment that contains complementary, EcoRI-generated sticky ends. The two ends of the annealed DNA fragments can be joined covalently with DNA ligase, resulting in a new recombinant vector.

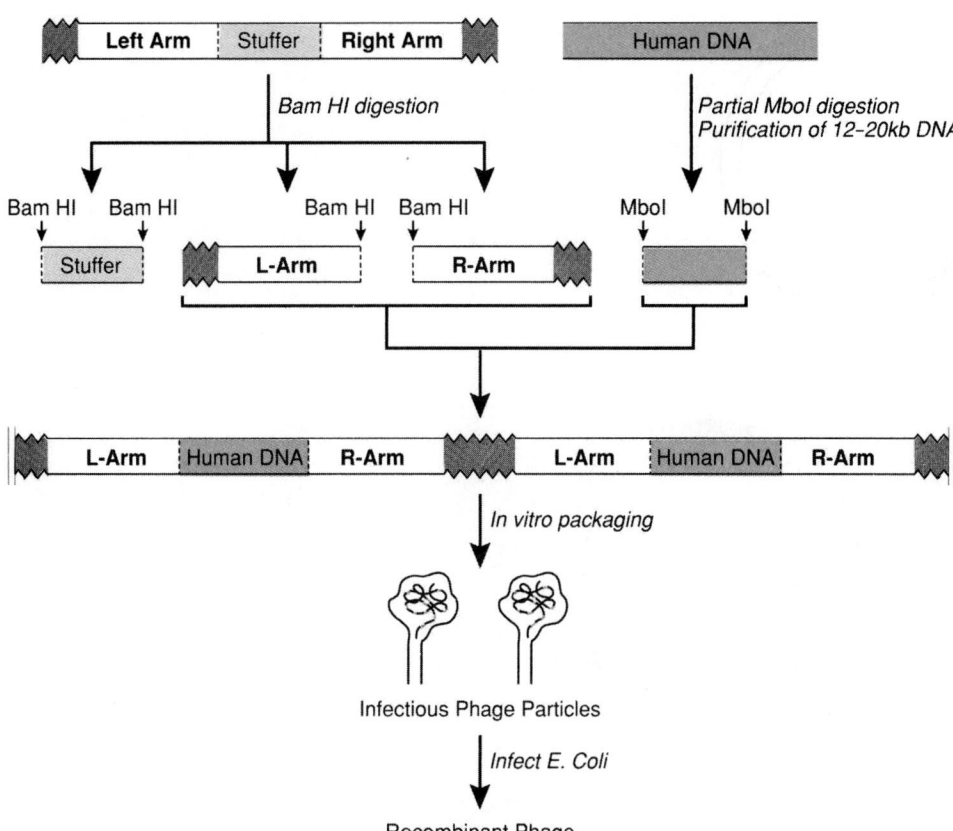

Figure 4-3. Cloning of genomic DNA in bacteriophage λ vectors. The cloning of human genomic DNA into bacteriophage λ vectors begins by cleavage of the vector and human DNAs with restriction enzymes that result in compatible sticky ends. In this example, the recognition sequence of MboI (5'-GATC-3') is a subset of the recognition sequence of BamHI (5'-GGATCC-3'). Ligation of the two types of DNA fragments into a recombinant molecule and its packaging into infectious bacteriophage particles are accomplished by the incubation of the DNA ligation mixture with extracts of bacteriophage proteins. The resulting recombinant virions are now capable of infecting suitable bacterial hosts. Typically, the infected bacteria are plated on nutrient agar plates, and plaques are generated in the bacterial lawn after lysis of the bacterial host cells by phage particles.

hematopoietic cells. The sizes of DNA fragments that can be cloned into vectors range from short molecules (a few hundred to several thousand nucleotides) to very large ones (approximately 1 Mb). Among the most convenient and widely used vectors for the cloning of mammalian genes has been the bacteriophage λ (Fig. 4-3). This virus, approximately 50 kilobases (kb) in length, infects and propagates efficiently in *Escherichia coli*. Because the central region of the bacteriophage is expendable, foreign DNA sequences can be inserted between the phage arms, which can then be reconstituted into infectious virions *in vitro*. After infection of a bacterial lawn, these recombinant phages lyse the host cells and generate plaques. Each plaque represents the lytic activity of a single bacterium.

Because the mammalian genome is complex, the cloning of moderately large genomic DNA segments is experimentally advantageous, as it reduces the number of independent recombinant clones needed to encompass the genome completely. A collection of independent clones estimated to include virtually all genes expressed in a particular tissue is often referred to as a *library*. The screening of a library encompassing a large number of plaques can be completed in a matter of a few days. The screening process typically uses radiolabeled DNA fragments generated either from a previously cloned segment or from chemically synthesized DNA. Phage DNA, transferred by adsorption to filters, is denatured *in situ* and allowed to anneal (or hybridize) to a complementary DNA strand of the labeled probe. On average, each bacteriophage can accommodate up to approximately 20 kb of foreign DNA. The generation of essentially random DNA fragments of this size from genomic DNA permits the construction of a *genomic library*. Approximately 50,000 independent clones in a library can be considered to represent the equivalent of a complete genome. Advances in the isolation of specific chromosomes by microdissection, fluorescence-activated sorting, and somatic cell

hybrids have made possible the construction of chromosome-specific genomic libraries (6).

Plasmids are closed, circular, double-stranded DNA molecules that are most often used for cloning smaller DNA fragments and for the manipulation of cloned DNA segments (Fig. 4-4). Plasmids contain an origin of replication to allow maintenance of the vector at high copy numbers in the bacterial host, a selectable marker (usually an antibiotic-resistance gene) to facilitate identification of bacterial clones harboring the plasmid, and restriction enzyme sites to which DNA fragments may be fused (or ligated). In general, DNA fragments of less than 20 kb are conveniently carried and manipulated in these vectors.

Strategies for the cloning of large segments of DNA rely on yet another set of vectors. *Cosmids* share features of both bacteriophages and plasmids and can accommodate DNA molecules of roughly 40 to 50 kb in length (7). Additional vectors in this category include the P1 bacteriophage, which can accommodate approximately 75- to 100-kb fragments; bacterial artificial chromosomes (BACs), which can accommodate approximately 300 kb inserts; and yeast artificial chromosomes (YACs), which have the largest known capacity for cloning and can accommodate inserts of approximately 1 Mb (8). Each of these vectors is adapted from microorganisms and exploits key regulatory sequences for replication and propagation in the host cells. For example, YACs contain segments of yeast chromosomes, such as centromeric sequences, which allow autonomous replication of the recombinant vectors in yeast. The analysis of inserts in these vectors is not always a straightforward exercise. Genomic rearrangements, deletions, or chimeric molecules can be found with reasonable frequency, particularly in YACs, which necessitate comparisons with uncloned genomic DNA. Nevertheless, these technical advances have formed the cornerstone of modern positional cloning and genomic strategies.

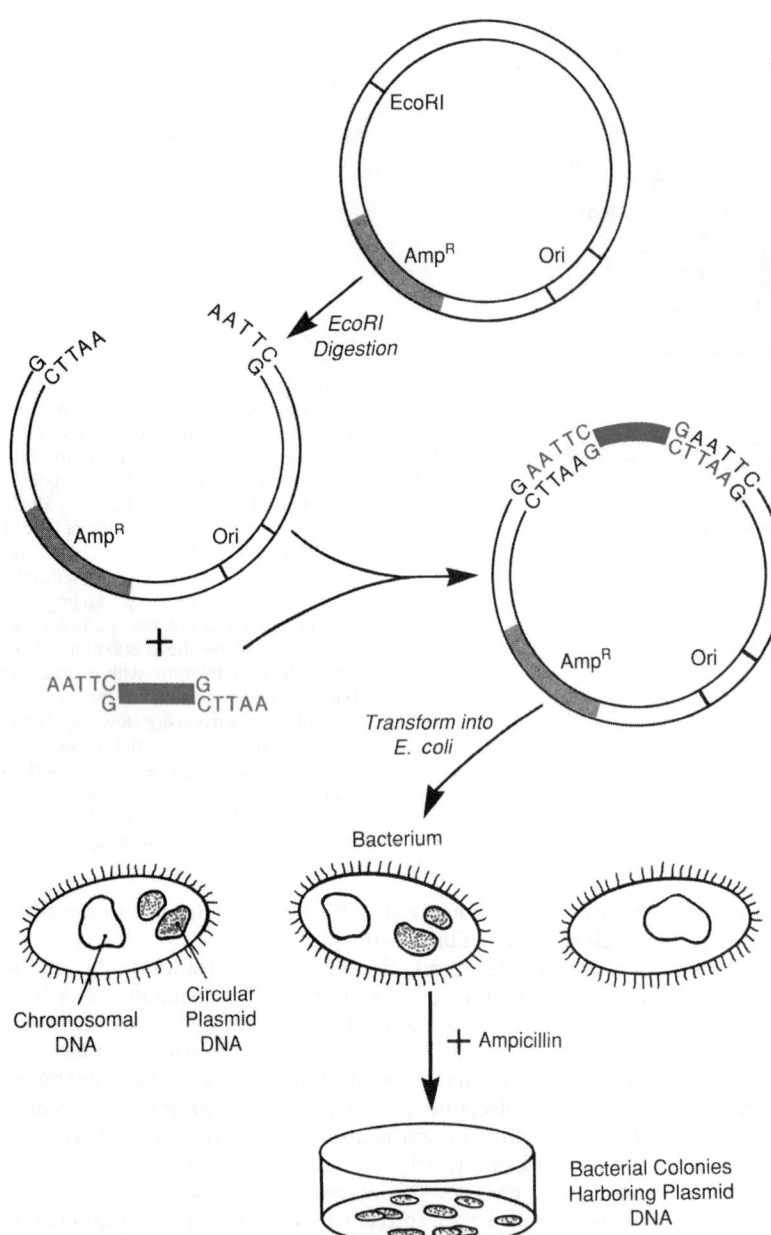

Figure 4-4. The closed circular plasmid vector carries a bacterial origin of DNA replication (Ori), and it encodes an ampicillin resistance gene (Amp). The vector also contains an EcoRI site in a nonessential region, which is cleaved to allow the insertion of foreign DNA sequences that have matching EcoRI ends. Suitable strains of bacteria can be rendered competent to accept foreign DNA sequences by pretreating them with calcium chloride or other chemicals. Incubation of plasmid DNA with competent bacteria leads to the transformation of a fraction of the host bacteria. The circular plasmid DNA replicates autonomously, and bacteria harboring plasmids may be selected by growth on nutrient agar plates containing ampicillin.

Because only a subset of genomic DNA is ultimately transcribed into mRNA, the cloning of mRNA or its complementary copy, known as *cDNA*, presents another strategy by which reagents for, and specific information about, particular genes may be obtained. cDNAs may be generated *in vitro* by copying mRNAs with reverse transcriptase, the RNA-dependent DNA polymerase. Subsequent modifications of the cDNA termini facilitate cloning into plasmid or bacteriophage vectors. Similar to genomic libraries, a collection of cDNA clones derived from a particular tissue is referred to as a *cDNA library*.

Identification of Recombinant Clones

Several strategies have been developed to identify a specific clone among numerous recombinant clones in genomic or cDNA libraries. In practice, the approach chosen depends on the abundance of the clone in the library, the nature of the gene product, and the reagents available to the investigator. If a desired clone is thought to be highly abundant in a cDNA library, it may be sufficient to isolate a few clones at random and characterize each one

by DNA sequencing. For example, because β-globin and immunoglobulin are by far the predominant proteins in reticulocytes and plasma cells, respectively, the isolation and sequencing of a handful of random clones from the corresponding cDNA libraries is likely to yield the desired clones. However, the abundance of many cDNAs is far lower than that in these examples, necessitating the use of other strategies.

Identification by Homology

The most common screening approach uses nucleic acid hybridization. For example, if a cDNA clone for a specific mRNA has been previously isolated, but not the corresponding genomic clone, the cDNA may be radiolabeled and used as a probe to identify the desired gene within a bacteriophage library (9). Variations on this theme are also useful in the identification of related but nonidentical genes or cDNAs: If such homologous genes are sought, reduced stringency (usually lower temperature or higher salt concentration) of hybridization and washing of the bound probe may permit their isolation. In addition, information obtained from a protein sequence can be used to design short, synthetic DNA molecules (oligonucleotides) that can subsequently be used as hybridization probes. Because of the degenerate nature of the genetic code, several oligonucleotide probes differing at the third coding position may need to be designed and used simultaneously to isolate the most homologous sequence.

Identification by Function

In the absence of any structural data on a protein of interest, antisera or other protein reagents can help. Antisera may be used to identify proteins and their cDNAs in bacteria infected with a bacteriophage cDNA library. The bacteriophage vector encodes a fusion protein, consisting of the *E. coli* β-galactosidase and a library of cDNAs from cells of interest. If a specific antibody recognizes epitopes present only in the fusion protein, cDNA clones may be identified accurately, with few false-positives (10). After isolation of a segment of the desired cDNA, nucleic acid hybridization may be used to recover additional related or even full-length cDNA clones. Because intracellular proteins frequently interact with other proteins *in vivo*, it is also possible to identify the genes of such interacting partners by a variety of methods. These include purification of the protein complex, microsequencing, and cloning of the genes encoding the interacting proteins. However, one of the most versatile is a genetic strategy called the *yeast two-hybrid method*. It relies on the transcriptional activation of promoters through the interaction of two proteins, the test protein (called *bait*) and the hitherto unknown protein (called *prey*). The activation of the promoter in turn activates reporter genes, such as β-galactosidase, in the yeast cells, which indicates that both bait and prey are present together in the yeast cell. It is then relatively straightforward to recover the plasmid encoding the prey and analyze it by DNA sequencing. Note that this method does not require protein microsequencing. cDNA libraries especially suitable for yeast two-hybrid analysis have been constructed from a variety of cells and tissues, including hematopoietic cells.

In a general strategy referred to as *expression cloning*, a cDNA or genomic clone is isolated by taking advantage of particular biological functions. (This is a somewhat artificial classification: Cloning by yeast two-hybrid or immunoscreening can also be considered as expression cloning.) Thus, if a biological assay exists for a protein, such as a hematopoietic cytokine, transfection of a cell that does not ordinarily express the cytokine with an appropriate cDNA library results in a few cells that synthesize and secrete the cytokine in the culture medium. The assay of the tissue culture medium then marks the subgroup of transfected cells responsible for this activity. It then becomes possible to recover the corresponding cDNA from those cells. The success of this method depends on the sensitivity and reliability of the bioassay. Many cDNAs that encode hematopoietic growth factors (11) or receptors have also been isolated by expression of appropriate cDNA or genomic libraries in heterologous cells (e.g., fibroblasts, COS cells [monkey kidney cells]), followed by detection of the growth factor in the media or the receptor on the cell surface by the binding of the radiolabeled ligand.

Introduction of total genomic DNA directly into mammalian cells may also be used to identify DNA fragments that confer phenotypic alterations to the host cells. Early examples of this strategy centered on the identification of dominant-acting oncogenes, which can lead to malignant transformation of suitable host cells (12). Other prominent examples relevant to hematology include cloning of the transferrin receptor gene (13) and the genes that mediate variable (diversity) junction (V(D)J) recombination in B and T cells (14).

Identification by Position

The ability to map disease loci on chromosomes by DNA linkage analysis constitutes the first step of positional cloning (15). The disease gene locus is narrowed further by taking advantage of polymorphic DNA markers (see Spectrum of Mutations and Polymorphisms). Candidate cDNAs from the critical region of interest are then analyzed for mutations in affected individuals. Positional cloning allows the identification of disease genes without prior knowledge of protein or nucleic acid sequences and without the need for antisera or functional assays.

ANALYTICAL METHODS FOR DNA AND RNA

The ability to detect DNA alterations facilitates various types of studies, including carrier detection in families at risk for genetic disorders, prenatal diagnosis, and large association studies in human populations, as well as the development of prognostic factors such as those associated with malignancies (e.g., the molecular assessment of minimal residual disease). In practice, different strategies are required to identify gross and subtle alterations, although, not uncommonly, these strategies can also be used in tandem.

Two classic procedures, known as *Southern blot* and *Northern blot* analyses, have been widely used to characterize the molecular structure of DNA and RNA, respectively (Fig. 4-5). In Southern transfer, DNA fragments generated by restriction enzymes are separated on agarose gels by electrophoresis and then transferred and immobilized onto nitrocellulose or nylon membranes. Specific sequences can be identified by incubation of the membranes with radioactive DNA probes. Thus, it is possible to identify a single gene or a portion thereof within the complex milieu of total genomic DNA. Although the presence or absence of a specific fragment can be ascertained in this fashion, the size of the detected fragment also provides valuable data regarding the position of restriction enzyme cleavage sites that flank a DNA segment. With use of a variety of restriction enzyme digests, a physical map of a DNA region may be constructed. Whereas conventional Southern blot analysis is best suited for study of DNA fragments 20 kb or less in length, long-range mapping methods, such as pulsed-field gel electrophoresis, allow the resolution of substantially larger DNA fragments (16). Thus, restriction maps of chromosomes may be constructed. The long-range mapping techniques bridge an important gap between Southern analysis and cytogenetic analysis.

Northern blot analysis is similar in principle to Southern analysis, except that the substrate for electrophoresis is RNA, and no prior enzymatic manipulation is required. This method provides information on the size and abundance of RNA transcripts and is especially useful in revealing the tissue distribution of particular mRNAs in tissue or cell samples. RNA structure and expression may also be evaluated more precisely by various nuclease procedures (S1 nuclease and ribonuclease mapping methods), in which a radiolabeled DNA or RNA strand is hybridized to mRNA, and mismatched regions are removed by enzymatic digestion (1–3). Examination of the fragments of these protected probes provides information on the abundance and organization of the mRNA. Efforts are also being made to increase the throughput of RNA analysis by using microarray technology (see Functional Genomics).

More than any other technique, the polymerase chain reaction (PCR) (17) has revolutionized the analysis of gene structure and function (Fig. 4-6). PCR requires synthetic primers flanking a target DNA and heat-resistant DNA polymerases. The amount of target DNA can be exceedingly small. Using three

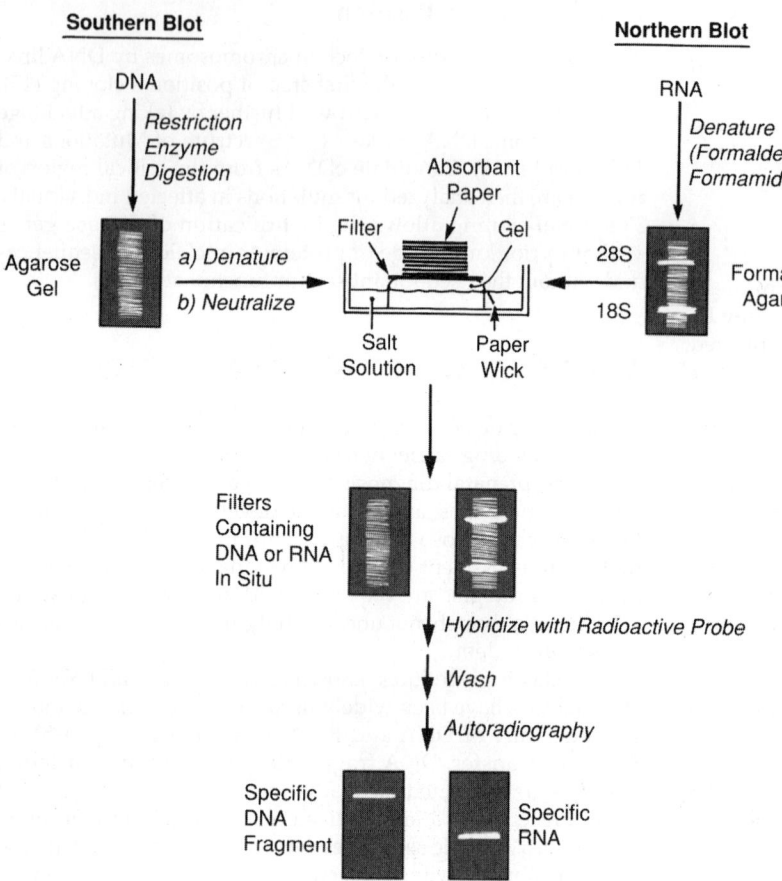

Figure 4-5. Schematic illustrations of Southern and Northern blot procedures. In the Southern blot procedure, DNA is cleaved with restriction enzymes, subjected to electrophoresis on agarose gels, and denatured with sodium hydroxide to yield single-stranded fragments *in situ*. In the Northern blot procedure, strong denaturants are used to disrupt intramolecular secondary structure formation as well as to prevent degradation of RNA. The RNA is subjected to electrophoresis on agarose gels in the presence of formaldehyde. Further transfer and hybridization steps for the two procedures are similar. Binding of denatured DNA or RNA to filters (nitrocellulose or nylon) is generally accomplished by capillary transfer procedures, whereby the nucleic acids are eluted from the gel by the upward movement of buffer. Filters containing immobilized DNA or RNA can now be hybridized with radioactive probes and subjected to autoradiography.

basic steps (denaturation of double-stranded DNA, annealing of the synthetic primers to their homologous sequences, and extension of the primer sequence by DNA polymerase), the targeted DNA segment can be amplified over 1 million times to yield abundant material for cloning, as well as for direct analysis by techniques such as restriction enzyme analysis, blot hybridization, and DNA sequencing. The method is exquisitely sensitive and versatile, and modifications in buffer composition or time of extension greatly extend its capabilities.

The precise techniques used for detection of a mutation depend on the particular situation at hand. Often, Southern blot analysis may be the first step, especially if gross structural alterations, such as gene deletions, are anticipated. Increasingly, PCR is being applied for detection of mutations, particularly in the identification and characterization of single or few nucleotide alterations, for which Southern blotting is generally insensitive. Although PCR-generated fragments may be sequenced without further manipulations, it is often desirable to delimit the region of mutation within an otherwise-large gene before sequencing. Two popular methods include denaturing gradient gel electrophoresis and single-stranded conformational polymorphism. Denaturing gradient gel electrophoresis exploits the sequence-dependent melting behavior of double helical DNA as it migrates through an increasing concentration of denaturant. In practice, PCR-amplified DNA is subjected to electrophoresis on polyacrylamide gels containing a gradient of a denaturant, usually formamide. Strand separation occurs at a particular concentration of denaturant, and single base differences between otherwise-identical fragments alter the critical point of denaturation of the two strands, resulting in a differential pattern of migration (18). Single-stranded conformational polymorphism is based on the observation that single-stranded

DNA fragments adapt unique conformations by intramolecular interactions, and it is technically easier (19). The PCR-amplified DNA fragments are denatured to single strands and then fractionated on nondenaturing gels. During migration, the single-stranded fragments assume different confirmations, resulting in differences in electrophoretic mobility. Heteroduplexes can also be detected and cleaved by certain chemicals, such as hydroxylamine and osmium tetroxide, which forms the basis of the chemical cleavage method. Finally, physicochemical techniques, such as denaturing high-performance liquid chromatography and mass spectrometry, are becoming increasingly popular in high-throughput mutation surveys. These methods have greatly simplified the screening for single base alterations in DNA.

As the primary amino acid sequence defines a protein, the nucleotide sequence defines DNA. Two elegant methods, the dideoxy-chain termination procedure (20) and the chemical degradation method (21), permit rapid and highly accurate determination of DNA sequence. The former and more popular method uses DNA polymerase to synthesize DNA from cloned templates in the presence of dideoxynucleoside triphosphates; these bases halt chain elongation when incorporated into DNA. Four reactions are carried out on each template, each using a different chain terminator that corresponds to each of the four bases. The resulting series of fragments can then be displayed by size on long polyacrylamide gels. Automated versions of this protocol using fluorescent dyes coupled with computerized databases of nucleotide sequences have been the engines of the genome project.

The primary nucleotide sequence of a gene or a cDNA provides a substantial database for further analysis. The coding potential of cDNA immediately predicts the amino acid

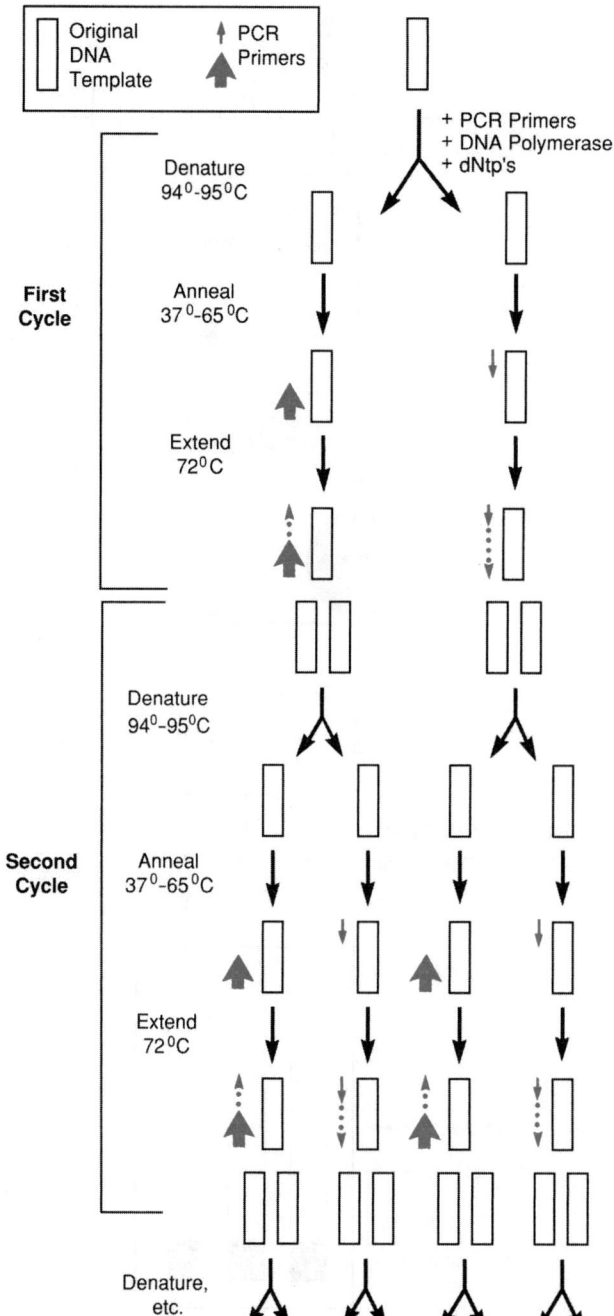

Figure 4-6. The polymerase chain reaction (PCR) amplification. PCR involves the successive repetition of three core steps—denaturation, annealing, and extension. In the first step, the double-stranded DNA template is denatured at high temperature. While the temperature is decreased, the denatured strands that have remained free in solution anneal to extension primers, a pair of synthetic oligonucleotides complementary to one or the other strand of the template. Because the primers are present in large excess relative to the DNA template, the formation of primer–template complex is favored over the reassociation of the two strands at lower temperatures. Finally, the primer is extended in a 5'-to-3' direction by DNA polymerase. A set of these three steps is called a *cycle.* Repetition of this cycle 20 or 30 times in an automated apparatus causes an exponential increase in the amount of the nascent product. dNtps, deoxyribonucleotide triphosphates.

sequence of the encoded protein and may suggest possible functions by identifying relationships to previously described polypeptides. From such comparisons, domains of proteins may also be placed into gene families and thereby suggest additional functional and evolutionary relationships.

SPECTRUM OF MUTATIONS AND POLYMORPHISMS

Differences in the structure of a particular region of DNA among individuals may reflect either functionally neutral polymorphism or altered structure, or expression of the encoded protein product. These alterations may take various forms and include deletions or insertions of nucleotides, as well as single base substitutions. Deletions, insertions, or inversions of larger DNA segments may cause either gross alterations that are detected by molecular or cytogenetic techniques or more subtle alterations that are detected principally by sensitive molecular techniques (see Analytical Methods for DNA and RNA). Frequently, single nucleotide changes lead to defective function of a gene or protein. A common mechanism of generating single base substitution is by spontaneous deamination of 5-methylcytosine at CpG dinucleotides, resulting in C-to-T changes. Whatever the mechanism, the effects of single base changes on the expression or function of the encoded protein can be dramatic. A classic example is the A-to-T change in the sixth codon of the β-globin gene that results in the substitution of valine for glutamic acid. The altered solubility of the mutant hemoglobin leads to the clinical sequelae of sickle cell anemia. A single base change may also result in a stop signal for translation (termed a *nonsense mutation*). The encoded protein is therefore truncated and frequently unstable. Nonsense mutations have been documented in some forms of β-thalassemia, as well as in many other disorders. Nucleotide changes in the conserved sequences near the junctions of exons and intervening sequences often lead to deleterious effects on RNA processing, as is also evident in various forms of thalassemia (22). Finally, single nucleotide mutations may adversely affect promoter function or 3' mRNA processing.

Single base changes also result in functionally neutral polymorphisms. A common form of DNA polymorphism is termed *restriction fragment length polymorphism*, which is generated by single nucleotide substitutions at every few hundred base-pair intervals in the genome that result in the creation or loss of a restriction endonuclease cleavage site. Restriction fragment length polymorphisms have provided invaluable genetic markers within families and populations and led to the generation of gene maps for linkage analysis. Repetitive DNA sequences have also been used with great success to construct physical maps or identify variations among individuals. Minisatellites, also called *variable number of tandem repeats*, are composed of tandem arrays of a core unit that includes ten nucleotides or more, in which the number of units in different alleles is highly variable. The distribution of minisatellites is biased toward the ends of chromosomes, the telomeres. Perhaps the most versatile and informative polymorphisms are microsatellites, or short tandem repeats, which are composed of tandem repeats of mononucleotides, dinucleotides, trinucleotides, and tetranucleotides (e.g., dinucleotide repeat GTGTGT). Most recently, single nucleotide polymorphisms, called *SNPs*, have surfaced as potentially useful guideposts in the human genome. It has been estimated that the human genome contains one SNP at every 30- to 100-kb interval of DNA, and one of the goals of the genome project is to identify such SNPs and create high-density maps that can then be used in various association studies (23). The number of copies of a particular DNA fragment containing such markers may be estimated by comparison with control DNA samples. For an autosomal gene, the deletion of a single copy would be expected to result in reduction of the signal intensity by half. Additional copies of a gene, perhaps acquired through gene amplification, which often is associated with malignancy, may be similarly detected by an increase in band intensity.

FROM STRUCTURE TO FUNCTION: AN OVERVIEW

Cloning and sequencing of a gene is merely the first step in molecular genetics. It is often desirable to understand the physical organization, transcriptional activity, protein product (if any), and the effect of mutations in a particular gene. A number of the more commonly encountered techniques are reviewed.

Introduction of Cloned DNA into Cells

If it were not for methods to assess the function of cloned genes and their products, assignment of specific functions to different genetic domains or the consequences of particular mutations on gene function would remain an inferential exercise. Numerous approaches are now available for the expression of cloned DNA in either prokaryotic or eukaryotic cells, particularly bacteria, yeast, and mammalian cells. Each system has its advantages and drawbacks. For example, although it would be possible to express the gene for CD34 in bacteria and obtain large amounts of protein, the inability of bacteria to glycosylate the protein may be a significant shortcoming. If such a modification is important for protein function, an alternative system must be chosen.

Transfection is the introduction of recombinant genes or genomic DNA into mammalian cells. The use of certain chemical agents (including diethylaminoethanol dextran, calcium phosphate, and polyethylene glycol) and liposomes can greatly enhance the efficiency of transfection. A special category of transfection that uses viral vectors (e.g., retroviruses, adenoviruses, and vaccinia viruses) is called *transduction*. In addition, DNA, as well as other macromolecules, may be introduced directly into individual cells by microinjection. A versatile strategy used to insert recombinant DNA or other macromolecules into cells is electroporation (24). This method uses high-voltage electric discharge, which generates transient pores in the cell membrane and facilitates the entry of macromolecules. For certain cell types in which chemical transfection methods are either ineffective or toxic, electroporation serves as an efficient substitute. It is currently the method of choice in many laboratories for transfection of hematopoietic cells.

By choosing appropriate transfection strategies and cell lines, recombinant genes may be expressed in mammalian cells either over many cell generations in pure cellular clones or for a period of a few days among a pool of positive and negative cells; these two approaches are referred to as *stable* and *transient expression*, respectively. Two mammalian cell culture systems that illustrate some of the differences between stable and transient transfection and allow for overexpression of recombinant genes deserve mention. These are Chinese hamster ovary (CHO) and COS cells. For unknown reasons, CHO cells can amplify stably integrated genes of dihydrofolate reductase (DHFR). CHO cells that are deficient in DHFR can be cotransfected with a DHFR-containing plasmid and a second plasmid containing the gene of interest. Interestingly, the test gene integrates close to the DHFR gene, which is subsequently amplified by growing these cells in increasing concentrations of methotrexate. Cell lines that carry over 1000 copies of the gene-DHFR unit can be generated (25). Stable clones of CHO cells that express erythropoietin and coagulation factors have been invaluable for generating large amounts of these recombinant proteins for patient care. COS cells, derived from African green monkey kidney cells, are transformed with a defective mutant of simian vacuolating virus 40 (SV40) and express high levels of the SV40 large tumor (large T) antigen. After binding to the sequence-specific origin of replication on the viral genome, the large T antigen initiates high levels of viral DNA replication. This property of the large T antigen has been exploited by cloning the SV40 origin of replication into plasmid vectors.

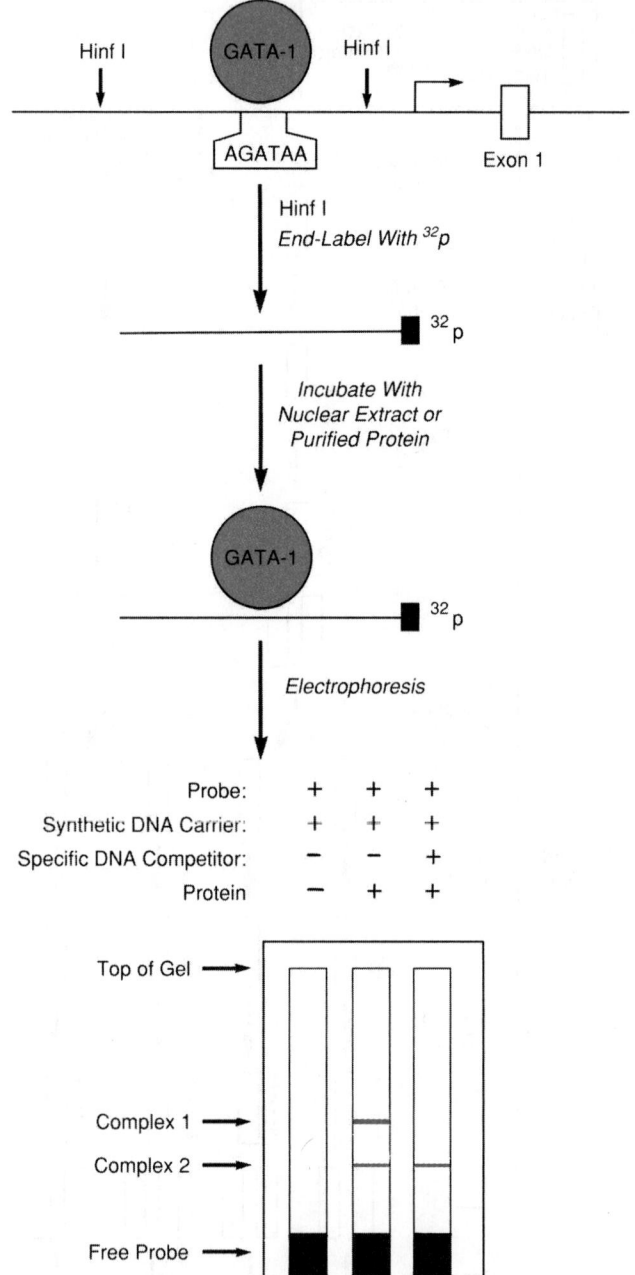

Figure 4-7. Schematic diagram of gel mobility retardation assay. A DNA fragment obtained by cleavage of the 5' regulatory region of an erythroid-specific gene with the restriction enzyme HinfI is used as a probe to identify proteins that bind to this region. This restriction fragment contains the nucleotide sequence AGATAA, which constitutes the binding site for the hematopoietic transcription factor GATA-1. Incubation of the radiolabeled HinfI fragment with a protein source containing GATA-1 allows the formation of a noncovalent complex between GATA-1 and its target sequence on the DNA. Formation of the protein-DNA complex is then detected by electrophoresis of the mixture on relatively porous, nondenaturing acrylamide gels. Migration of the bound complex relative to the free probe is detected as slow-moving bands (complexes 1 and 2) by autoradiography. To ascertain the specificity of interaction between GATA-1 and its target sequence, appropriate competitor DNA fragments are included in the incubation mixture. Addition of a nonradiolabeled HinfI fragment competes for binding of GATA-1 and thus abolishes the complex (complex 1), whereas the addition of an unrelated DNA fragment that lacks the GATA-1 binding site does not disturb the specific complex. The bent arrow indicates the transcriptional start site.

The recombinant plasmids can be replicated autonomously to very high numbers in COS cells under the influence of the large T antigen. Transfection of COS cells with recombinant plasmid DNA is usually performed with the diethylaminoethanol-dextran method. Two or three days after transfection, 10% to 20% of the cells express the cDNA at sufficiently high levels to allow detection with sensitive bioassays or immunoassays. This system has been widely used to clone and transiently express a variety of molecules of importance in hematology (11).

In recent years, there has been an explosion of information on the characterization of regulatory *cis* elements and the proteins, called *trans-acting factors*, that interact with them. In addition to histone and nonhistone proteins, nucleoproteins also include *trans*-acting factors that may play critical roles in determining transcriptional activity. Two complementary approaches are used to delineate such interactions. In the first approach, the function of *cis* elements containing candidate promoters or enhancers is assessed by linking them to unrelated reporter genes encoding easily detectable proteins, such as chloramphenicol acetyltransferase, β-galactosidase, and green fluorescent protein. The resultant recombinant constructs are transfected into appropriate cell lines, and the presence or absence of *cis* regulatory elements is inferred from the activity or level of the reporter protein. This type of analysis can also be performed in the context of the whole animal by generation of transgenic mice bearing reporter constructs (see Creating New Animal Models of Disease). A second approach relies on the physical and biochemical characterization of *trans*-acting factors. Perhaps the most basic method used to characterize protein-DNA interactions is the gel mobility retardation assay (also called *gel shift* or *band retardation*). In this assay (Fig. 4-7), a radiolabeled DNA fragment spanning a putative transcriptional regulatory element (e.g., a promoter or an enhancer) is incubated with a protein extract from an appropriate tissue source, and the DNA-protein mixture is subjected to electrophoresis. The difference in migration through the gel between the protein-DNA complex and the unbound DNA can be a clue to specific binding (2,3). These protein-DNA interactions can be further refined by footprinting techniques, which delineate specific nucleotide residues that are in contact with the protein, and ultimately by more sophisticated biophysical techniques, including nuclear magnetic resonance.

Altering Structure on Demand

Methods of site-directed mutagenesis allow a more complete analysis of the function of cloned cDNAs. These methods include the introduction of simple deletions and insertions when convenient restriction sites are available in the gene of interest. Other methods of introducing deletions use exonucleases that digest DNA processively from one end. More commonly, such restriction sites are not available, and in any case it is often desirable to insert, delete, or substitute single base pairs at critical regions of a cDNA that are not accessible to DNA-modifying enzymes. Many of these strategies take advantage of mutant synthetic oligonucleotides to create single base mismatches. A popular method uses uracil incorporation into a single-stranded DNA template, use of the uracil-containing template to synthesize a complementary strand *in vitro* in the presence of a mutant oligonucleotide primer, and selection against the original strand that contains uracil *in vivo*, leaving only the strand that has incorporated the mutant oligonucleotide for propagation (2,3) (Fig. 4-8).

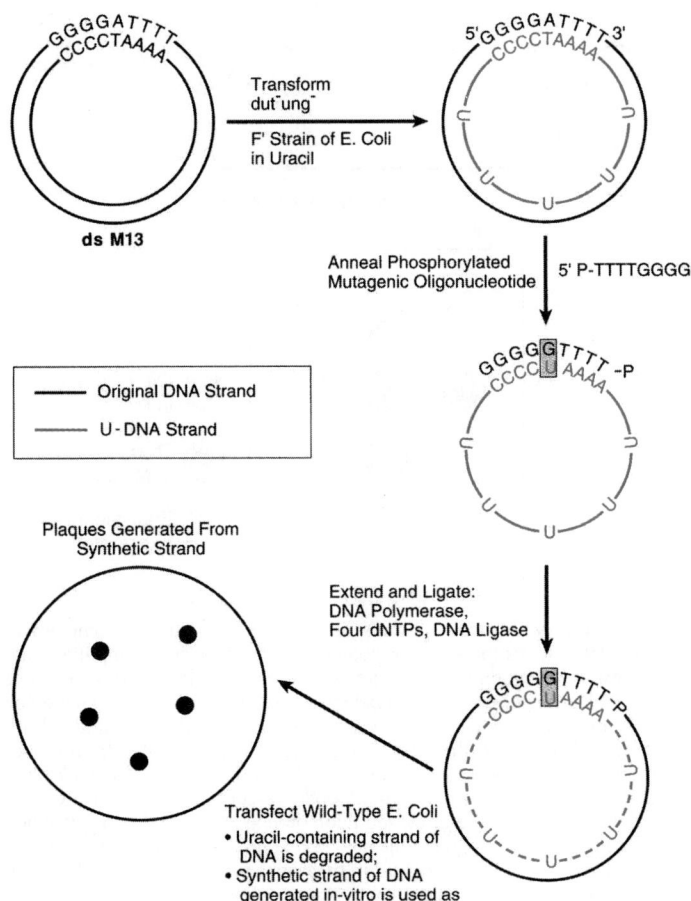

Figure 4-8. A strategy of site-directed mutagenesis. A strain of *Escherichia coli* that is deficient in deoxyuracil triphosphatase (dUTPase) and uracil-*N*-glycosylase, called dut⁻ and ung⁻, accumulates dUTP and is unable to remove misincorporated uracil from DNA. When a recombinant M13 bacteriophage is grown in such a strain in the presence of uracil, a fraction of thymine residues are replaced by uracil. Uracil-substituted, single-stranded M13 bacteriophage particles are extruded from the *E. coli,* which are used *in vitro* as templates for DNA synthesis in the presence of mutant oligonucleotides. The nascent DNA chain contains the mutant oligonucleotide and thymine, but no uracil. Transformation of wild-type *E. coli* with this DNA results in the replication of the uracil-free strand and destruction of the uracil-containing strand. dNTP, deoxyribonucleotide triphosphate.

GENOMIC MEDICINE

The term *genomics* was conceived in 1986 in conjunction with the launch of a new journal bearing this name (26). It has since become a part of the common parlance, spawned many exciting technologies, and brought new perspectives to biomedicine. Genomics—the study of genomes—espouses a global and integrative philosophy, favoring the forest over the trees. It may be useful to subdivide genomics into structural and functional components, although these are often intertwined. The former, consisting of the construction of genetic and physical maps and culminating in the sequencing of the human genome, is essentially complete and ready for finishing touches by blending the existing and new polymorphic maps with the finished human genome sequence. Functional genomics uses the road map provided by structural genomics and attempts to couple it with normal and abnormal physiology. Together, these strategies are widely expected to revolutionize predictive genetic testing, the identification of novel genetic targets for drugs, and the monitoring of therapeutic interventions.

Structural Genomics

The most polymorphic DNA markers in widespread use are microsatellites. Hundreds of microsatellites have been mapped to specific regions of the genome, and DNA sequences flanking these polymorphic sites have been characterized. This has allowed the detection of length polymorphisms throughout the genome by PCR. The availability of microsatellite reference maps is extremely useful for mapping of disease genes using genome-wide screening with closely spaced markers. In due course, because of their greater frequency in the genome and the potential for creating maps of higher density, SNPs may well supplant microsatellites as the preferred markers for genotyping. A "rough draft" of the complete human genome is now available online, and publication of the complete genome is imminent.

Structural genomics has also enhanced our understanding of the mutational basis of human disorders. Large genomic rearrangements leading to deletions, duplication, or inversions can occur by unequal crossing over and homologous recombination. A critical requirement is the presence of large tracts of uninterrupted sequence identity (often >95%) in the parental genes. Such tracts have been recognized in several regions of the genome, and disorders attributable to these mechanisms have been termed *genomic disorders* (27). The hematology literature is replete with illustrative case studies. For example, recombination between tandem repeats of the α-globin genes separated by approximately 4 kb gives rise to the most common form of α-thalassemia. Similarly, a large genomic inversion accounts for the most common form of severe hemophilia A. In this case, a gene of unknown function that resides in intron 22 of the factor VIII gene is separated from two additional copies 500 kb away on the X chromosome that are present in an inverted configuration. Intramolecular recombination between the intronic copy and either of the two inverted copies leads to the inversion of exons 1 through 22 of the factor VIII gene (see Chapter 38). These mechanisms are also likely to apply to acquired disorders, such as chemotherapy-related malignancies.

Functional Genomics

Functional genomics is an evolving concept. The next decade may witness many more applications of structural genomics

that are not immediately apparent to us. Nevertheless, one of the major current goals of functional genomics is to assign function to the cloned genes. This is a challenging task and frequently requires input from biochemistry and cell biology, as well as comparative genomics. Indeed, at least two-thirds of the genes in the yeast or fruit fly genome have not yet been assigned specific functions. This figure is likely to be much more modest for the human genome.

Another goal is the ability to generate molecular profiles of cells by simultaneous monitoring of the expression of the entire genome during various physiologic states. The technique, called *transcriptional profiling*, uses high-density arrays (or microarrays) consisting of multiple rows and columns of nucleic acids on glass slides (28), which are either spotted by robots either as plasmids or PCR fragments or synthesized *in situ* using oligonucleotides (Fig. 4-9). Next, RNAs isolated from two different sources (e.g., normal and leukemic lymphocytes) are labeled with different fluorescent nucleotides during reverse transcription to cDNAs. The two cDNA probes are then mixed and hybridized to the microarray. After scanning the slides, the relative expression of each gene in the two cell types can be quantified by the ratio of the two fluorescent signals. A parallel effort in proteomics is under way to facilitate the molecular profiling of proteins. Therefore, global differences in RNA or protein expression can be determined relatively expeditiously. These technologies are increasingly being applied to the classification of leukemias and lymphomas, the discovery of

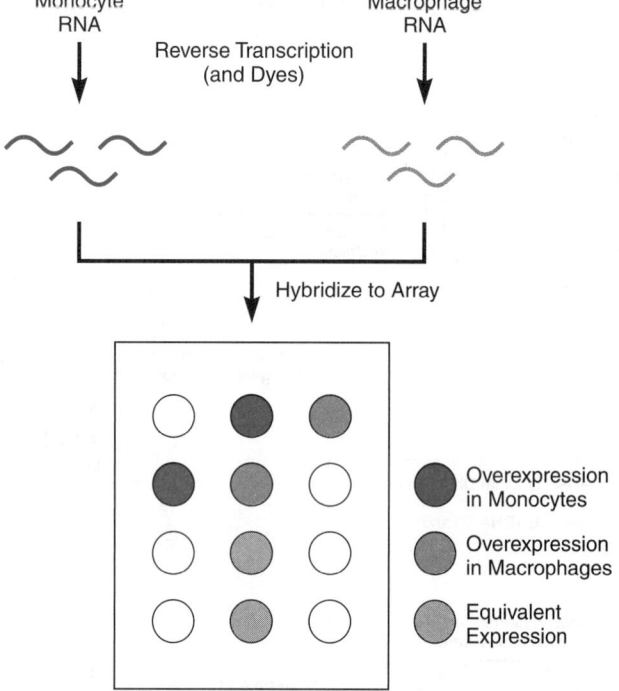

Figure 4-9. Microarrays for transcriptional profiling. Known complementary DNA clones (plasmids or polymerase chain reaction–amplified fragments) or oligonucleotides are spotted onto glass slides. Relative differences in gene expression between two cell types can be assessed by labeling RNA from each source with fluorescent nucleotides and hybridizing the mixture to the array. For example, RNA harvested from monocytes and macrophages are labeled with red (Cy3) (shown as dark blue) and green (Cy5) (shown as light blue) fluorescent dyes, respectively. After cohybridization to the array, the fluorescence is detected and quantified by a scanner. A red signal indicates overexpression in monocytes, a green signal indicates overexpression in macrophages, a yellow signal (shown as gray) indicates equivalent levels of expression, and a blank signal suggests lack of expression in both cell types.

new genetic and metabolic pathways that are disturbed in different hematologic disorders, and the effect of drugs or toxins on cell physiology.

Bioinformatics

No discussion of molecular genetics and genomics can be complete without paying homage to the impact of computer science on gene discovery and analysis. Computer-assisted predictions of protein structures, search for homologous sequences either in the same genome or in the genome of model organisms (e.g., yeast or fruit fly), and search for potential drug targets have become indispensable extensions of the wet lab. A popular set of software programs for DNA sequence comparisons is the Basic Local Alignment Search Tool (BLAST), which is currently maintained by the National Center for Biotechnology Informa-

tion (NCBI). It can be accessed by laboratory investigators through www.ncbi.nlm.nih.gov.

CREATING NEW ANIMAL MODELS OF DISEASE

The introduction of foreign DNA sequences into the germline of mice and generation of transgenic mouse strains has facilitated the study of gene structure and function in the context of the whole organism and led to the generation of animal models of disease (Fig. 4-10) (29). Transgenic mice have been particularly useful in delineating *cis* regulatory sequences required for tissue and temporal-specific gene expression. The major experimental approaches are (a) microinjection of cloned DNA into the pronucleus, (b) infection of embryos with retroviral vectors (insertional mutagens) to create mutant phenotypes, (c) transfer of genetic

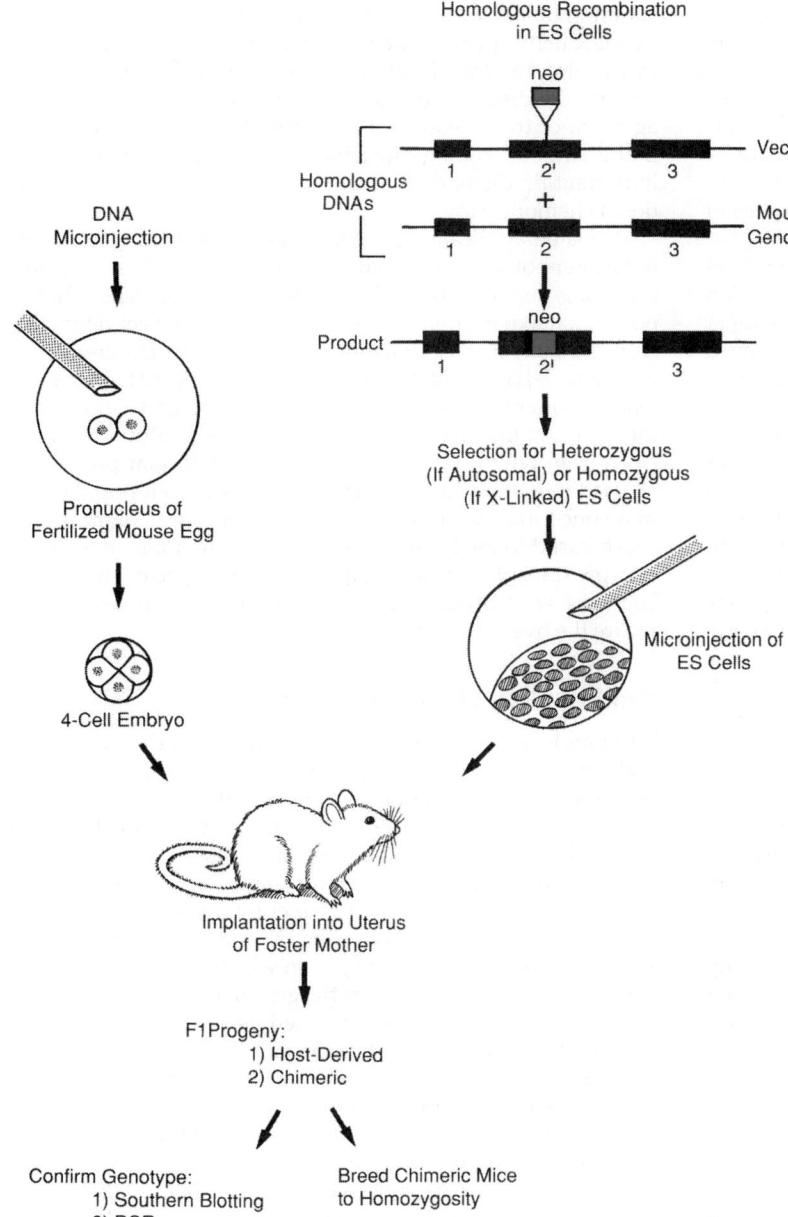

Figure 4-10. Manipulation of the mouse genome. The most widely used technique for creating transgenic mice involves the microinjection of cloned DNA into the pronucleus of a one-cell fertilized mouse egg. The DNA integrates randomly in the mouse genome. A second technique initially uses embryonic stem cells as a target for foreign DNA, which is usually introduced by electroporation. The vector contains a selection marker (neo) that is inserted in a part of a gene that is otherwise homologous to sequences on the mouse genome. The selection marker disrupts the normal coding region of the gene. Recombination of vector DNA with the homologous mouse genomic locus substitutes the new inactive allele bearing the insertion for the endogenous functional one. Selection for recombinant embryonic stem (ES) cells is accomplished by a variety of strategies conferring drug resistance. The embryo is implanted into the uterus of a foster mother (whose genotype is irrelevant). The foster mother gives birth to either chimeric offspring or those that are host derived. Male chimeras are then mated to breed the new genotype to homozygosity. Polymerase chain reaction (PCR) and Southern analysis are used most frequently to screen for integration of the foreign DNA.

sequences to hematopoietic stem cells via retroviruses, and (d) transfer of DNA or retroviruses into embryonic stem cells and subsequent injection into blastocysts to generate chimeric mice.

The value of transgenic mice to modern science cannot be overemphasized. To date, numerous normal or mutant genes have been introduced into the mouse germline to generate mice with anemias, lymphomas, and models of bone marrow failure. The effects of oncogenes, hematopoietic transcription factors, cytokines, and their receptors on specific tissues have been evaluated by restricted expression in transgenic mice with tissue-specific promoters. In addition, cooperative interactions between two or more oncogenes at the onset or progression of cancer have been studied in transgenic mouse models. Other molecules of importance to hematology have also been introduced into the mouse germline. For example, the generation of a line of transgenic mice expressing the human multidrug-resistance gene (MDR1) in various cell lineages of the bone marrow (30) has been used to assess the activity of chemotherapeutic agents.

Infection of hematopoietic stem cells by viral vectors (usually retroviruses and lentiviruses), followed by adoptive transfer into immunodeficient mice, has also been used to create murine models of human disease. For example, to understand the evolution and pathogenesis of chronic myelogenous leukemia (CML), recombinant retroviruses that encode the hybrid *bcr-abl* gene are used to infect hematopoietic stem cells *in vitro*. This is followed by transplantation of irradiated mice with the modified stem cells (31). The observation that CML may be recapitulated in mice by adoptive transfer of bone marrow cells highlights the use of such models for fundamental studies of pathobiology and for evaluation of novel therapeutics.

Another particularly exciting technology is the development of mouse embryonic stem (ES) cells as targets for gene introduction and modification (Fig. 4-10). ES cells are derived from the inner cell mass of the embryo. With the use of feeder layers, conditioned media, or leukemia inhibitory factor, ES cells may be maintained in tissue culture in an undifferentiated state. On injection into blastocysts, ES cells contribute to the host embryo, ultimately giving rise to chimeric mice. Under optimal conditions, these cells also contribute to the germline. Breeding of the chimeric mice can lead to germline transmission of genes introduced into the cultured ES cells. Because ES cells can be transfected and are proficient in homologous recombination, directed modifications of endogenous mouse genes may be achieved. Ultimately, mice homozygous for a directed mutation or modification can be produced by a series of matings. The power and potential of this approach are immense. For example, it is now possible in principle to generate animal models for many of the inherited, single-gene disorders of man. As the molecular basis of specific disorders is dissected by molecular genetics, efforts can be made to produce similar conditions in mice. Although the phenotype of a genetic disorder in mice may often be similar to that in humans, this is not always the case. For example, mice with inactivated Fanconi's anemia genes fail to develop pancytopenia despite being highly sensitive to cross-linkers, the *sine qua non* of the disease. It is possible that other genes in the mouse genome modify the phenotype. Genetic modifiers can alter the penetrance or expressivity of many genetic disorders. The availability of classic as well as attenuated phenotypes of human disorders in mouse models will be useful for basic and translational studies.

APPLICATIONS OF RECOMBINANT DNA TECHNOLOGY IN HEMATOLOGY

The development of recombinant DNA methods has profoundly influenced the practice of hematology. The identifica-

tion of specific gene mutations in hematologic disorders such as thalassemia has caused significant reductions in the incidence of births of affected persons, partly because of the successful application of molecular diagnostic techniques. The following selected examples illustrate some of the techniques and strategies discussed in the preceding sections.

Diagnosis of Inherited and Acquired Disorders

A classic example of tailoring a test for a specific mutation is in the molecular analysis of sickle cell anemia. It is fortuitous that the sickle mutation abolishes a recognition site in the β-globin gene for the restriction enzyme Mst II, altering the sizes of genomic fragments generated by digestion of total DNA. With Southern blotting or PCR, carriers of sickle cell disease and sickle homozygotes may be readily and accurately distinguished from normal individuals and used to identify fetuses at risk for the disorder.

Many hematologic malignancies, such as CML, are characterized by specific chromosomal translocations. Because translocations frequently involve particular DNA sequences and common breakpoints, it is possible to identify such alterations by PCR using primers flanking the breakpoints. Aside from identifying the translocations at the molecular level and confirming the disease, such approaches can also guide the management of the disease. For example, the detection of a single malignant cell among more than 10^6 normal cells may be an important predictor of outcome and suggest the need for additional chemotherapy.

A related application is in the assessment of clonality within heterogeneous cell populations. For lymphoid cells, clonal expansion suggests the proliferation of malignant cells, whereas polyclonal expansion is generally thought to reflect nonmalignant changes, such as inflammatory conditions. Differentiation of B- and T-lymphoid cells is accompanied by a stage-specific rearrangement of the immunoglobulin genes and T-cell receptor genes, respectively. As a result, Southern blot analysis of DNA from lymphoid cells with suitable molecular probes can be used to detect clonal expansion of specific cell populations. In a conceptually similar strategy, polymorphic markers can also be used to establish the origin of cells after allogeneic bone marrow transplantation and quantify the degree of chimerism. Together with other findings, such information can help to secure the overall clinical assessment.

Identification of Disease Genes

If the molecular pathogenesis of an inherited disorder is not understood and the deficient protein product is unavailable for analysis, positional cloning can come to the rescue. Assuming that appropriate pedigrees can be found, polymorphic DNA markers closely linked to a particular disease locus may be tracked within families at risk for the disorder. The chromosomal locus may be narrowed further by fine mapping or with the use of patient samples bearing DNA rearrangements, such as translocations. After the region in which the gene is thought to reside is narrowed sufficiently, genomic fragments derived from this "critical" region are used as probes to search for expressed sequences. Identification of mRNAs that show either quantitative or qualitative abnormalities further implicates the gene in the disease process, but the ultimate proof requires a demonstration of intragenic mutations. One of the first examples of this approach involved the characterization of the X-linked form of chronic granulomatous disease, an inherited disorder of phagocyte function. A more recent example is the HFE gene mutated in hereditary hemochromatosis (see Chapter 47).

Molecular Pathology of Hematologic Disorders

The thalassemia syndromes have long been known to result from a quantitative imbalance of globin chains. One of the contributions of molecular genetics was the demonstration that the thalassemias are caused by a wide spectrum of genetic mutations (22). As such, the thalassemias represent an example of genetic heterogeneity, which can be due to either multiple different mutations in the same gene (as in β-globin mutations and β-thalassemia) or mutations in several distinct genes that give rise to the same phenotype (e.g., mutations in at least seven distinct genes cause Fanconi's anemia). As more is learned about the molecular pathogenesis of inherited disorders, it is becoming increasingly clear that genetically homogeneous disorders, such as sickle cell anemia, represent the exceptions rather than the rule.

The hypercoagulable state can also be regarded as an example of genetic heterogeneity. Until a few years ago, the cause of hypercoagulability could be determined in only a small fraction of patients. A series of discoveries has led to the identification of several major genetic risk factors for this disorder. A point mutation that changes arginine at position 506 of factor V to glutamine is the basis of factor V Leiden (32). The mutant protein resists proteolysis by activated protein C. Another point mutation in the 3' end of the prothrombin gene (G20210A) leads to elevated antigen and activity levels of prothrombin (33). Together, these mutations in the heterozygous state account for 18% to 26% of the cases of thrombophilia in unselected white patients compared with 8% in the asymptomatic population. The ability to detect these point mutations by simple oligonucleotide hybridization techniques not only establishes the diagnosis in individual patients but also facilitates large-scale epidemiological studies.

Impact on Treatment of Hematologic Disorders

Recombinant DNA technology provides new products for direct administration to patients. Recombinant hematopoietic growth factors have profoundly changed the practice of hematology. Erythropoietin and granulocyte colony-stimulating factor are now a part of the armamentarium of chronic anemia of renal disease and neutropenia, respectively. Recombinant factor VIII is widely used to treat inherited coagulation disorders. Aside from replacement therapy, efforts are also under way to influence gene expression *in vivo* in an effort to correct inherited disorders. For example, to reduce the severity of sickle cell anemia or thalassemia, a number of pharmacologic agents are being tested for their ability to augment fetal hemoglobin production. Based on the association of lower levels of gene activity with methylation of cytosine residues in DNA, 5'-azacytidine, a drug that leads to demethylation, was tested for its effects on fetal hemoglobin production in patients with sickle cell anemia or thalassemia. Although the precise mechanism of action of this drug *in vivo* is controversial, it produces a substantial increase in fetal hemoglobin. A variety of other cytotoxic agents, such as hydroxyurea, also appear to exert a similar effect on fetal hemoglobin production *in vivo*. A knowledge of the precise molecular targets of these drugs and their effect on transcription may lead to the identification of other small molecules that have greater potency and selectivity.

Modification of the Hematopoietic Genetic Program

The ability to introduce genes into mammalian cells and the burgeoning knowledge of the molecular mechanisms of cell survival and apoptosis makes it possible to regulate the proliferation of hematopoietic stem or progenitor cells by genetic manipulation. For example, forced up-regulation of telomerase activity in hematopoietic stem cells might be expected to immortalize these cells and increase their proliferative potential. Such strategies may be useful in certain disease states, such as myelodysplastic syndromes, characterized by depletion of the stem cell pool. Thus, it might be possible to replete the stem cell pool of these patients by transfection of rare hematopoietic stem cells with the cDNA for the catalytic component of telomerase or with antiapoptotic genes.

Advances in Gene Therapy

Experience with the isolation of genes and their reintroduction into cells has paved the way for the permanent correction of a deficiency state in cells by gene therapy. The primary approach is to target the somatic cells of an affected person (somatic gene therapy), rather than the germ cells, with viral vectors as well as chemical or liposomal preparations or by direct injection of naked DNA. Many of the current therapeutic trials involve the use of viral vectors, including retroviruses, lentiviruses, adenoviruses, and adenoassociated viruses. In all of these cases, the endogenous mutant gene is left unaltered. Because precise correction of a mutant gene *in situ* in the chromosome would ensure appropriate regulation of expression throughout cellular differentiation, it would be preferable to use targeted methods of gene insertion or modification. However, at present, the efficiency of homologous recombination in human cells is too low to contemplate its use in clinical settings.

Currently, somatic gene therapy is being attempted for a number of severe or life-threatening disorders for which current medical management is unsatisfactory. For example, for the hemophilias, gene transfer could afford continuous protection and obviate the need for potentially hazardous factor infusions. Hemophilia B appears to be particularly amenable to gene therapy. The relatively small size of factor IX, its ability to be expressed in a variety of cell types, the availability of both mouse and dog models for preclinical testing, and the need for relatively modest expression levels to achieve correction of the coagulopathy make it one of the most promising candidates for gene therapy. Most of the studies to date have used adenoassociated virus vectors directed to the liver or the skeletal muscle. These advances notwithstanding, many problems still must be solved before gene therapy enters the mainstream of hematology therapeutics. Chief among them is the host immune response to the virus and all therapeutic products.

Pluripotent stem cells are also highly attractive targets for gene therapy. Transfer of new genetic material into stem cells ensures its presence in more differentiated progenitors. The infusion of genetically modified cells of the affected patient, rather than stem cells from a histocompatible donor, is akin to autologous bone marrow transplantation. In this regard, the extensive clinical experience in bone marrow transplantation provides invaluable lessons for reconstitution of the hematopoietic system by infusion of the donor cells and management of the host after transplantation (34). As stated previously, preclinical testing for safety and efficacy can be greatly facilitated by the availability of animal models, and considerable progress has been made in the use of retroviruses for gene transfer into pluripotent hematopoietic stem cells of mice. However, retroviruses cannot transduce nondividing cells, such as pluripotent stem cells. Lentiviruses are more successful in this regard, partly because of their ability of deliver viral proteins to the nucleus without the need for nuclear membrane breakdown. In addition, infection of sufficient numbers of stem cells by recombinant viruses and adequate expression of the therapeutic genes in stem cells and their progeny remain formidable technical problems. Attempts are under way to optimize gene expression and enrich stem cell preparations for more efficient infection. Some of these lessons are already being put to the test. The use of recombinant lentiviruses encoding the human β-globin gene along with large segments of its locus control region has been reported to give long-term and high-level expression of human β-globin in β-thalassemic heterozygous mice (35).

Additional examples of hematologic disorders that may be amenable to gene therapy include severe combined immunodeficiency, metabolic storage disorders, and Fanconi's anemia. While the search for more effective vectors and for site-directed correction of mutant genes continues, the recent demonstrations of cellular and clinical amelioration of severe combined immunodeficiency in human patients by a retroviral vector (36) bodes well for the future of gene therapy.

CONCLUSION

This brief survey is intended to illustrate the range and breadth of molecular genetic and genomic concepts and technology. Although it is impossible to communicate the full sense of excitement and promise of molecular genetics, it should be apparent that these ideas and methods are now integral parts of modern hematology. Specific hypotheses may be tested with genetic and molecular approaches, and new experimental strategies for treatment may be evaluated in a logical and systematic manner. Hematology has been at the forefront of application of molecular genetics to medical science. This tradition will likely continue in full force in the future.

REFERENCES

1. Watson JD, Gilman M, Witkowski J, et al. *Recombinant DNA*, 2nd ed. New York: WH Freeman, 1992.
2. Ausubel FM, Brent R, Kingston RE, et al. *Current protocols in molecular biology*. New York: John Wiley & Sons, 1995.
3. Dracopoli NC, Haines JL, Korf BR, et al. *Current protocols in human genetics*. New York: John Wiley & Sons, 1995.
4. Semenza GL. *Transcription factors and human disease*. New York: Oxford University Press, 1998.
5. Cazzola M, Skoda RC. Translational pathophysiology: a novel molecular mechanism of human disease. *Blood* 2000;95:3280.
6. Meltzer PS, Guan X-Y, Burgess A, et al. Rapid generation of region specific probes by chromosome microdissection and their application. *Nat Genet* 1992;1:24.
7. Collins J, Hohn B. Cosmids: a type of plasmid gene-cloning vector that is packageable in vitro in bacteriophage lambda heads. *Proc Natl Acad Sci U S A* 1978;75:4242.
8. Burke DT, Carle GF, Olson MV. Cloning of large segments of exogenous DNA into yeast by means of artificial chromosome vectors. *Science* 1987;236:806.
9. Benton WD, Davis RW. Screening λgt recombinant clones by hybridization to single plaques in situ. *Science* 1977;196:180.
10. Young RA, Davis RW. Efficient isolation of genes by using antibody probes. *Proc Natl Acad Sci U S A* 1983;80:1194.
11. Wong GG, Witek J, Temple PA. Human GM-CSF: molecular cloning of the complementary DNA and purification of the recombinant protein. *Science* 1985;228:810.
12. Goldfarb M, Shimizu K, Perucho M, et al. Isolation and preliminary characterization of a human transforming gene from T24 bladder carcinoma cells. *Nature* 1982;296:404.
13. Kühn LC, McClelland A, Ruddle FH. Gene transfer expression and molecular cloning of the human transferrin receptor gene. *Cell* 1984;37:95.
14. Schatz DG, Oettinger MA, Baltimore D. The V(D)J recombination activating gene, RAG-1. *Cell* 1989;59:1035.
15. Collins FS. Positional cloning: let's not call it reverse anymore. *Nat Genet* 1992;1:3.
16. Chu G, Vollrath D, Davis RW. Separation of large DNA molecules by contour-clamped homogeneous electric fields. *Science* 1986;234:1582.
17. Saiki R, Gelfand D, Stoffel S, et al. Primer-directed enzymatic amplification of DNA with a thermostable DNA polymerase. *Science* 1988;239:487.
18. Lerman LS, Silverstein K. Computational simulation of DNA melting and its application to denaturing gradient gel electrophoresis. *Methods Enzymol* 1987;155:482.
19. Orita M, Suzuki Y, Sekiya T, et al. Rapid and sensitive detection of point mutations and DNA polymorphisms using the polymerase chain reaction. *Genomics* 1989;5:874.
20. Sanger F, Nicklen S, Coulson AR. DNA sequencing with chain-terminating inhibitors. *Proc Natl Acad Sci U S A* 1977;74:5463.
21. Maxam AM, Gilbert W. A new method for sequencing DNA. *Proc Natl Acad Sci U S A* 1977;74:560.
22. Orkin SH, Kazazian HH Jr. The mutation and polymorphism of the human β-globin gene and its surrounding DNA. *Annu Rev Genet* 1984;18:131.
23. McCarthy JJ, Hilfiker R. The use of single-nucleotide polymorphism maps in pharmacogenomics. *Nat Biotechnol* 2000;18:505.
24. Potter H. Review. Electroporation in biology: methods, applications, and instrumentation. *Anal Biochem* 1988;174:361.
25. Kaufman RJ. Strategies for obtaining high level expression in mammalian cells. *Technique* 1990;2:221.
26. Anonymous. Genomics: structural and functional studies of genomes. *Genomics* 1997;45:244.
27. Lupski JR. Genomic disorders: structural features of the genome can lead to DNA rearrangements and human disease traits. *Trends Genet* 1998;14:417.
28. Lockhart DJ, Winzeler EA. Genomics, gene expression and DNA arrays. *Nature* 2000;405:827.
29. Jaenisch R. Transgenic animsals. *Science* 1988;240:1468.
30. Galski H, Sullivan M, Willingham MC, et al. Expression of a human multidrug-resistance cDNA (MDR1) in the bone marrow of transgenic mice: resistance to daunomycin-induced leukopenia. *Mol Cell Biol* 1989;9:4357.
31. Daley GQ, Van Etten RA, Baltimore D. Induction of chronic myelogenous leukemia in mice by the P210$^{bcr/abl}$ gene of the Philadelphia chromosome. *Science* 1990;247:824.
32. Bertina RM, Koeleman BPC, Koster T, et al. Mutations in blood coagulation factor V associated with resistance to activated protein C. *Nature* 1994;369:64.
33. Poort SR, Rosendaal FR, Reitsma PH, et al. A common genetic variation in the 3'-untranslated region of the prothrombin gene is associated with elevated prothrombin levels and an increase in venous thrombosis. *Blood* 1996;88:3698.
34. Sorrentino BP, Nienhius AW. The hematopoietic system as a target for gene therapy. In: Friedmann T. *Development of gene therapy*. New York: Cold Spring Harbor Laboratory Press, 1999.
35. May C, Rivella S, Callegari J, et al. Therapeutic haemoglobin synthesis in beta-thalassaemic mice expressing lentivirus-encoded human beta-globin. *Nature* 2000;406:82.
36. Cavazzana-Calvo M, Hacein-Bey S, de Saint Basile G, et al. Gene therapy of human severe combined immunodeficiency (SCID)-X1 disease. *Science* 2000;288:669.

CHAPTER 5

Cytogenetics for the Hematologist

Paola S. Dal Cin and Cynthia C. Morton

Cytogenetics is the area of biology that deals with the study of chromosomes. In the past decade, this discipline has witnessed remarkable developments with significant scientific contributions of relevance to the field of hematology (1). Cytogenetics is an integral part of the clinical practice of hematology, in addition to its traditional descriptive role in dysmorphology, reproductive medicine, and prenatal diagnosis. Recurring chromosomal abnormalities are important prognostic indicators for the hematologist (2). Beyond the clinical relevance of cytogenetic studies in diagnosis, prognosis, and treatment, this science has been used widely in gene mapping and in the identification of genes, and, in numerous examples, has led to the cloning of genes responsible for specific diseases. Identification of genes involved in neoplastic hematologic disorders has contributed to an elucidation of the biology of hematopoiesis, and the functional consequences of genetic changes have led to a new era of targeted drug therapy.

ORGANIZATION OF HUMAN CHROMOSOMES AND METHODS OF STUDY

The human chromosome is a complex structure that consists of approximately equal amounts of DNA, histone and non-histone proteins, and a minor amount of RNA. A single helix of DNA is bound on each end by a structure known as a telomere. Each normal human chromosome has one centromere. The centromere is the site at which the kinetochore forms for attachment of the mitotic spindle, which is required for proper movement of the chromosome during cell division. The centromere divides the chromosome into two arms. In human chromosomes, the position of the centromere is either central (metacentric), distal (acrocentric), or somewhere in between (submetacentric), providing a useful landmark in the identification of a particular chromosome (Fig. 5-1). The two arms of the human chromosome are identified as *p* (petite) for the short arm and *q* for the long arm.

Human chromosomes vary in size, with the largest chromosome designated number 1. In 1956, Tjio and Levan (3) determined that there are a total of 46 chromosomes: 22 pairs of autosomes and one pair of sex chromosomes. With the exception of pairs 21 and 22, the numeric designation reflects the size of the chromosome (e.g., chromosome 4 is the fourth largest chromosome). Although chromosome 21 is smaller than chromosome 22, this inconsistency in nomenclature has been perpetuated to avoid confusion owing to historic references to Down's syndrome as trisomy 21. Before development of banding techniques that provide unequivocal identification of each

chromosome, the size and position of the centromere were used to place chromosomes into groups. Although infrequently used today to refer to a particular chromosome, the groupings still are useful in instances in which banding may be inadequate to identify precisely the chromosome in question. The groups are as follows: A (1 to 3), B (4 to 5), C (6 to 12 and X), D (13 to 15), E (16 to 18), F (19 to 20), and G (21 to 22 and Y) (Fig. 5-2).

A karyotype is a display of chromosomes from largest to smallest (with the exception of pairs 21 and 22) with chromosomes oriented so that the p arm is on top. In the human species, the female is the homogametic sex, and a normal female karyotype is designated 46,XX; the male is the heterogametic sex, and a normal male karyotype is described as 46,XY (Fig. 5-2). Excluding chromosomal abnormalities and variants, karyotypes of two unrelated males or females may appear virtually identical; furthermore, excluding sex chromosomes, karyotypes of males and females are indistinguishable.

Chromosome Analysis

Most cytogenetic analyses are performed on chromosomes that are in metaphase of mitosis because, at this stage of the cell cycle, the chromatin is highly condensed and the chromosomes are individually distinguishable. Special studies to investigate a particular region of a chromosome may require less condensed chromosomes, such as those found in prometaphase. The most frequently used tissues for cytogenetic evaluation of hematologic disorders are bone marrow, peripheral blood lymphocytes, and lymph nodes. The process of preparing chromosomes for analysis is known as a harvest.

Chromosomes are harvested either directly from the tissue or after short-term culture. In hematologic malignancies, adequate metaphases can be obtained from direct harvests of lymph nodes, 24-hour cultures, and cultures of several days with mitogens for chronic lymphoid proliferations. With the exception of chronic lymphoid proliferations, mitogens such as phytohemagglutinin or pokeweed are not added to cultures to promote cell growth, as the neoplastic cells are dividing spontaneously. In all cases, dividing cells must be arrested during mitosis, usually by the addition of colchicine to the culture. Colchicine functions to destroy the mitotic spindle and collect the cells in metaphase. After incubation in colchicine, the harvest proceeds with a hypotonic treatment, ordinarily 0.075 mol potassium chloride or 0.8% sodium citrate, which serves to swell the cells. Several rounds of fixation in methanol-acetic acid (3:1) complete the harvest. Metaphases will now be ready to be dropped onto slides. Prepa-

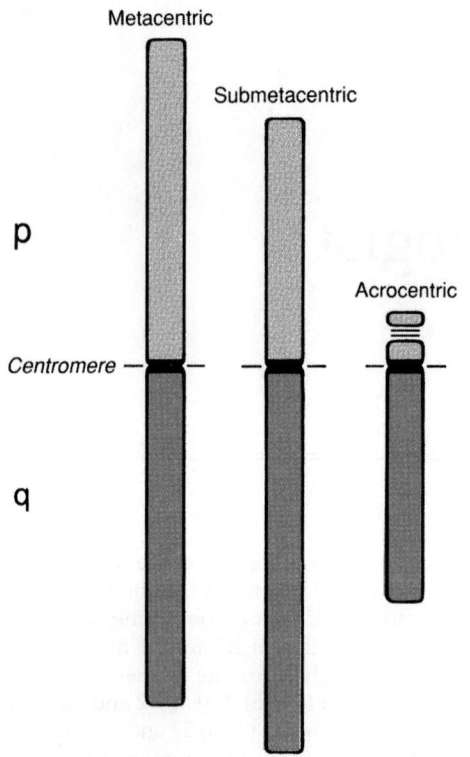

Figure 5-1. Schematic diagram of prototypic human chromosomes demonstrating metacentric, submetacentric, and acrocentric chromosomes. p, short arm; q, long arm.

ration of slides following the harvest is one of the most critical steps in obtaining quality material for analysis. Factors that influence surface tension such as temperature and humidity are doubtless crucial variables in slide making.

Banding Techniques

Many different banding techniques are used routinely in cytogenetics laboratories. Several of the most popular techniques are G-banding (4,5), Q-banding (6), and R-banding (7–9) (Fig. 5-3); the most frequently used method is G-banding (Fig. 5-2). Although various methods for producing a G-banded karyotype exist, a popular technique uses proteolytic digestion of chromosomes with trypsin followed by staining in Giemsa. A pattern of alternating light and dark bands is produced, enabling identification of each chromosome pair by bright field microscopy. Investigations of chromosome banding patterns with antinucleotide antibodies indicate that light G bands are predominantly GC rich and that dark G bands are AT rich (10). Light bands are believed to contain more euchromatin, DNA that is replicated early in S phase of the cell cycle and is transcribed. In contrast, dark bands are thought to be composed largely of heterochromatin, DNA that is more condensed and late replicating. In general, clinical laboratories perform banding techniques on chromosomes in mid-metaphase, at which time 350 to 400 bands can be resolved.

Idiograms and Chromosome Nomenclature

An idiogram is a schematic standardized karyotype that is derived from measured band sizes. The idiogram and chromo-

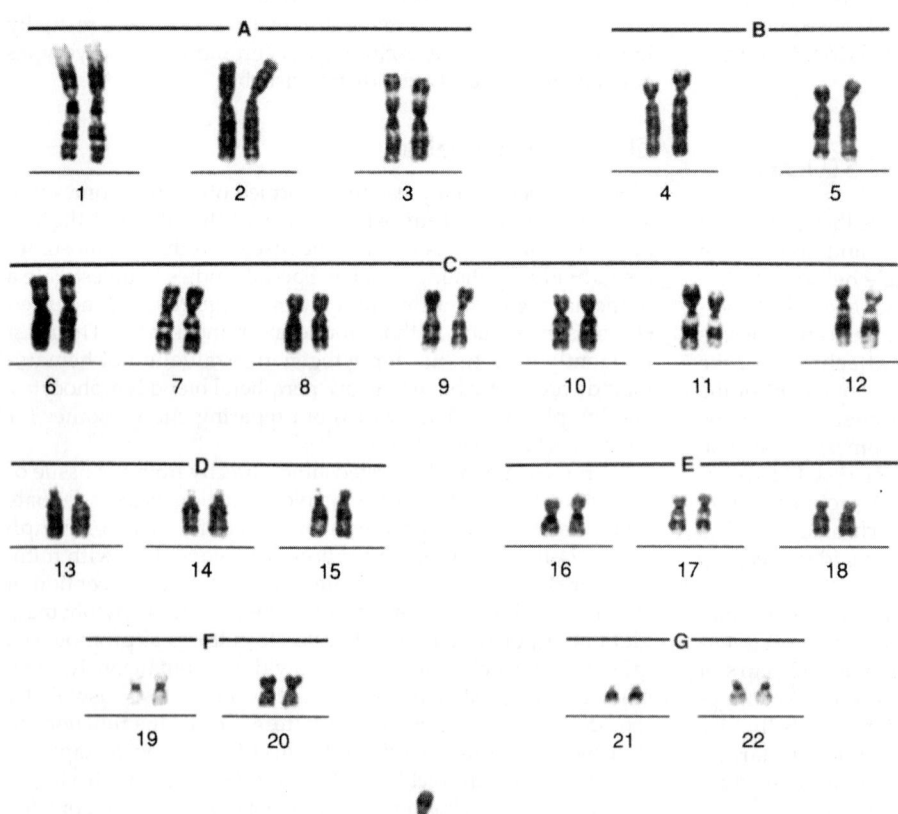

Figure 5-2. A representative normal human male GTG-banded karyotype, 46,XY. Designations of the subgroups of chromosomes (**A–G**) are indicated above the chromosomes; the X chromosome is placed in the C group and the Y chromosome in the G group.

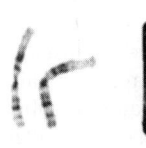 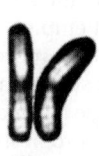 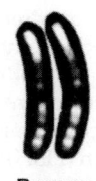 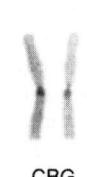 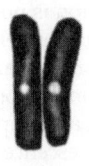 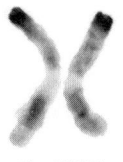

GTG   QFQ   Reverse   CBG   DA/DAPI   Rx-FISH

Figure 5-3. Chromosome 1 shown after various banding techniques: GTG, QFQ, reverse, CBG, DA/DAPI, and cross-species color banding (Rx-fluorescence *in situ* hybridization). (See Color Fig. 5-3.)

some nomenclature have been designed by an international committee that has met periodically since 1960 (the Denver Report) to establish uniform language for describing chromosome bands and chromosomal aberrations (11). Chromosome regions are subdivided into bands and, at higher resolution, into subbands. For example, the designation 14q32 indicates chromosome 14, the long arm, region 3, band 2. On the idiogram, chromosome bands are numbered in an ascending fashion from centromere to telomere on each arm of the chromosome.

Owing to the increase in the amount and variety of data on chromosome aberrations associated with neoplasia, terminology was needed for describing acquired aberrations. A supplement, *Guidelines for Cancer Cytogenetics* (12), was published in 1991 to address nomenclature for cytogenetic abnormalities that was not adequately covered in the 1985 International System for Human Cytogenetic Nomenclature (ISCN) (13). A fairly sophisticated set of rules governs the description of chromosomal abnormalities; the current version of the nomenclature was revised in 1995 (14). The ISCN convention is to specify first the total number of chromosomes followed by the sex chromosomes (e.g., the normal male karyotype is given as 46,XY). The autosomes are indicated only when an aberration or variant is present. In the description of a karyotype with chromosomal abnormalities, sex chromosome aberrations are given first, followed by abnormalities of the autosomes listed in numeric order irrespective of the type of aberration. A comma separates each abnormality. Aberrations are considered in two categories, numeric or structural. Numeric changes include either gain (+) or loss (–) of chromosomes (e.g., a female with trisomy 21 may be designated as 47,XX,+21; a male with loss of the Y chromosome is described as 45,X,–Y). Gain of an entire set or sets of chromosomes is indicated as 69,XXY for a male triploid or 92,XXXX for a female tetraploid. Structural changes include the following: translocation (t), in which chromatin is exchanged between two or more chromosomes; inversion (inv), in which chromatin is repositioned within a chromosome arm (paracentric) or between the p and q arms, thus involving the centromere (pericentric); deletion (del), in which there is a net loss of chromatin; duplication (dup), in which addition of chromatin occurs; and derivative chromosome (der), in which one or more rearrangements within a single chromosome occurs (e.g., the unbalanced segregant of a translocation). An abbreviated list of symbols used to designate chromosomal abnormalities in cancer cytogenetics is given in Table 5-1. The chromosome(s) involved in a structural change is specified in parentheses directly following the symbol identifying the type of rearrangement [e.g., inversion of chromosome 2 is given as inv(2) and a translocation between chromosomes 9 and 22 as t(9;22)]. In all structural changes, the location of any given chromosome break is specified by the chromosome band in which that break has occurred [e.g., t(9;22)(q34;q11.2) describes a balanced translocation between the q34 band of chromosome 9 and the q11.2 band of chromosome 22] (Fig. 5-4).

Chromosomal aberrations are considered to be either constitutional (i.e., present in all cells in the body) or acquired (i.e., occurring in a particular tissue or stem cell). Acquired abnormalities are those associated largely with cancer development and tumor progression. Our understanding of the cause of these acquired rear-

rangements is still limited, but the association of specific rearrangements in particular disorders is well documented. Acquired genomic alterations fall into two groups: those that are considered to be primary changes and most useful diagnostically, and those that are additional and likely reflect evolution of the neoplasm. A simple view of the potential biologic implications of primary versus additional rearrangements is that the primary rearrangement establishes a proliferative advantage for the tumor stem cell, whereas additional rearrangements may enable the tumor to invade and metastasize in the host. [Note: In this chapter, the term "secondary" is used to describe a leukemia that occurs after therapy; these leukemias are also referred to as "therapy-related" leukemias. Secondary is not used to indicate chromosomal aberrations that are found in association with the

TABLE 5-1. Partial List of Symbols and Abbreviated Terms Used in Cancer Cytogenetics (14)

Symbol	Definition
add	Additional material of unknown origin
brackets, square [ ]	Used to indicate clone size and number of cells with a clonal abnormality
c	Constitutional anomaly
comma (,)	Separates chromosome numbers, sex chromosomes, and chromosomal abnormalities
cp	Composite karyotype
dash (-)	Interval, uncertain breakpoint localization
del	Deletion
der	Derivative chromosome
dic	Dicentric chromosome
dmin	Double minute chromosome
dup	Duplication
hsr	Homogeneously staining region
i	Isochromosome
idem	Used to denote the stemline karyotype in subclones
ider	Isoderivative chromosome
idic	Isodicentric chromosome
inc	Incomplete karyotype
ins	Insertion
inv	Inversion
mar	Marker chromosome
minus (–)	Loss
ml	Mainline
multiplication sign (×)	Denotes multiple copies of diploid clones or rearranged chromosomes
or	Alternative interpretation
p	Short arm of chromosome
p10	Short arm part of the centromere
parentheses ( )	Surrounds structurally altered chromosome(s) and breakpoints
plus (+)	Gain
q	Long arm of chromosome
q10	Long arm part of the centromere
question mark (?)	Questionable identification of a chromosome or structure
r	Ring chromosome
semicolon (;)	Separates chromosomes and bands in structural rearrangements involving more than one chromosome
sl	Stemline
slant line (/)	Separates clones
t	Translocation
tas	Telomeric association
underline	Distinguishes homologous chromosomes

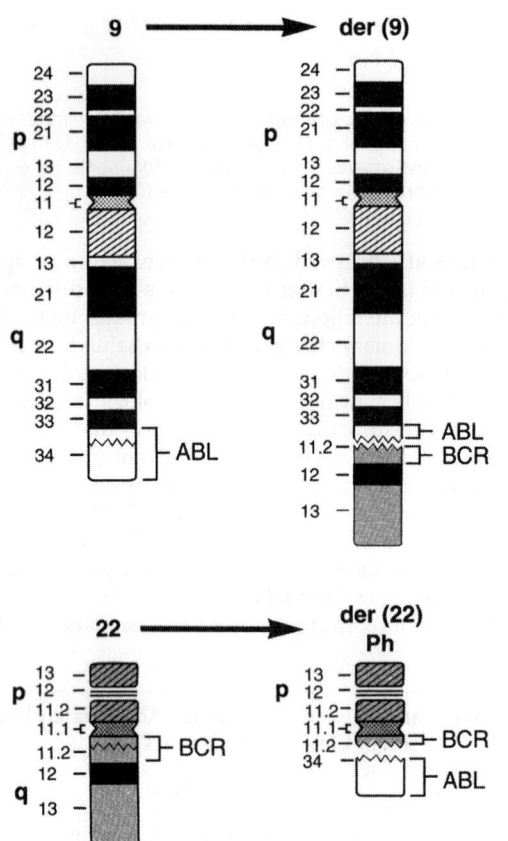

Figure 5-4. Ideogram of GTG-banded chromosomes 9 and 22 and derivative (der) chromosomes 9 and 22, demonstrating the t(9;22)(q34;q11.2) translocation as seen in chronic myelogenous leukemia, resulting in the *BCR/ABL* fusion. p, short arm; Ph, Philadelphia chromosome; q, long arm.

evolution of disease; these aberrations are known as "additional" anomalies, as described above. Also, the term *de novo* (and not primary) is used to describe a leukemia that has arisen without any preceding therapy, such as prior chemotherapy for a solid tumor.]

A clone is defined as a cell population derived from a single progenitor. A number of cells having the same chromosomal abnormality is inferred to be of clonal origin. A clone is not necessarily completely homogeneous, because subclones may be derived during evolution of the malignancy. To be recognized as a clonal abnormality, the same structural abnormality or gain of a chromosome must be observed in at least two cells; for a missing chromosome, at least three cells with the numeric change must be detected to be designated as a clone. A general rule in cancer cytogenetics is that only clonal chromosomal abnormalities should be reported. If nonclonal aberrations are reported from a chromosome analysis, then they must be clearly indicated distinct from the clonal aberration and not written in the formal description of the karyotype. Interpretation of the importance of nonclonal abnormalities will depend on the number of metaphase cells analyzed, the nature of the aberration, the culture type, and the time in culture before harvest. Assessment of the significance of nonclonal abnormalities may be limited by the number of metaphases analyzed (as the mitotic activity may vary from one specimen to another), by the type of malignancy, and due to medical treatment of the patient. An alternative method of study may be warranted that does not require dividing cells, such as *in situ* hybridization, to evaluate further the relevance of a nonclonal aberration.

A normal karyotype is not an infrequent finding in a hematologic malignancy and is not an indication that a neoplastic prolif-

eration is not present. Rather, it may reflect the lack of detection of tumor cells by the cytogenetic method employed. Owing to improvements in cytogenetic methodology, more experience among cytogeneticists in the detection of structural abnormalities, and improvement in molecular biologic techniques [notably fluorescence *in situ* hybridization (FISH)], a progressively smaller percentage of normal karyotypes is being reported from hematologic malignancies. The recognition that some characteristic rearrangements (e.g., translocations involving exchanges of telomeric regions or regions of chromosomes with similar G-banding patterns) are cryptic by conventional cytogenetic methods has mandated the use of molecular methods for a complete analysis. Well known among this category of aberrations is a frequent translocation in childhood acute leukemia involving the *TEL(ETV6)* gene at 12p12-p13 and the *acute myeloid leukemia (AML)* 1 gene at 21q22 (15,16). [The nomenclature used to describe human genes in this chapter will be either the primary name as assigned by the Human Gene Nomenclature Committee (http://www.gene.ucl.ac.uk/nomenclature), an alias for the Human Gene Nomenclature Committee gene name (http://www.gdb.org), or a combination thereof, such as *TEL(ETV6)*.]

Molecular Techniques in Cancer Cytogenetics

The poor quality of metaphases, low mitotic index, poor growth in culture, and complexity and stability of chromosomal rearrangements in neoplastic specimens can be problematic in conventional karyotyping. For these and other reasons, the analyzable metaphases may not necessarily be representative of the *in vivo* situation. These confounding technical and biologic issues can lead to incomplete results, with chromosomal aberrations remaining unidentified. Molecular methods have revolutionized cytogenetic studies, providing a means to detect efficiently a particular aberration in both dividing and nondividing cells. Specifically, FISH technology overcomes many difficulties in analyses, including increasing the sensitivity of achieving a diagnosis in certain disorders, bypassing the culturing process and requirement for dividing cells, and decreasing the reporting time. However, in contrast to conventional cytogenetic analysis in which the presence of virtually all chromosomal abnormalities can be visualized, FISH is a targeted approach that requires *a priori* knowledge of a suspected aberration. Multicolor FISH methods (e.g., spectral karyotyping, multicolor FISH, and cross-species color banding), can readily reveal complex chromosomal rearrangements in a single hybridization experiment, but their successful application also depends on the availability of a sufficient number of evaluable mitoses. Comparative genomic hybridization (CGH), a variation of the FISH method, is independent of the quality of mitoses or dividing cells. This method provides an approach for the genome-wide definition of chromosomal aberrations in complex karyotypes and makes possible detection of genomic imbalances in a population of cells at a resolution of approximately 10 megabases (Mb). Most recently, its application to the microarray platform permits detection of chromosomal gains and losses in spotted genomic clones (i.e., BACs) at the 100-kilobase (kb) level. No doubt, as CGH to microarrays becomes widely available, it is likely to be the next most important technological improvement in clinical cytogenetics. CGH is not particularly helpful in identifying characteristic chromosomal rearrangements (i.e., translocations or inversions) that can serve as critical parameters for the classification in many human leukemias and lymphomas; such rearrangements typically are not associated with sizable loss or gain of chromatin and thus are not detectable by CGH. However, genomic imbalances may be found in hematologic neoplasms and are considered in most cases to be additional chromosomal changes associated with tumor progression, ultimately correlating with clinical parameters and of prognostic relevance (17). CGH would be applicable in identifying such aneuploidies, if desired.

Fluorescence *In Situ* Hybridization

Among the advantages of chromosomal *in situ* hybridization is that a rather precise chromosomal assignment can be determined in a relatively short time frame. The two different approaches to this technique are isotopic (18,19) and nonisotopic or FISH (20,21). Probes are labeled with radionucleotides (in the isotopic method) or with biotin or digoxigenin (in the nonisotopic method) and are then hybridized to slides on which metaphase chromosomes have been prepared and denatured. Following hybridization and washing, slides are dipped in photographic emulsion for detection of radionucleotide signal; alternatively, slides may be incubated with avidin conjugated to a fluorescent dye, such as fluorescein, or streptavidin conjugated with peroxidase for detection of biotinylated probes. Metaphases are analyzed and scored for hybridization to a particular chromosomal region over the background hybridization to other chromosomes.

Although isotopic methods were popular for single gene mapping in the 1980s, the use of fluorescent methods has replaced isotopic *in situ* hybridization. This methodologic change is due in part to rapid detection of signal (i.e., within hours as compared to days or weeks for autoradiography), simple and reliable performance, abundance of commercially available probes, and to obviating the need to deal with use and disposal of radionucleotides. FISH analysis has provided a considerably increased ability to identify chromosomal regions, reveal cryptic abnormalities, describe complex chromosomal rearrangements, and detect chromosomal rearrangements in interphase nuclei from nondividing cells, including paraffin-embedded fixed tissues. It must be emphasized that the performance of the FISH assay, including reproducibility, specificity, and sensitivity, must be established within each laboratory for each probe using appropriate tissue samples before performing testing of clinical specimens. The complementary use of cytogenetic analysis and FISH has provided a remarkably powerful tool for cancer cytogenetics. Included in the ISCN 1995 report is nomenclature for describing the results of FISH studies (Table 5-2).

A variety of different types of probes are used to detect chromosomal abnormalities by FISH (22) (Fig. 5-5). Some of the first probes to be developed commercially were those that identify a specific chromosome structure; a well-known example of this type are those that recognize the centromeres of human chromosomes (i.e., alpha- and beta-satellite sequences). Alpha satellite probes have been developed that hybridize to a single chromosome. These probes hybridize to multiple copies of a 171 base pair (bp)–repeat unit present at the centromeres of human chromosomes, resulting in a very bright fluorescent signal in metaphase and interphase cells. In diploid cells, two signals are present, representing the two chromosome homologs. Detection of monosomy, trisomy, and other aneuploidies is particularly suitable with this type of centromere-specific probe, especially in interphase nuclei. FISH with alpha-satellite probes derived from the X and Y chromosomes provides a rapid tool to assess the outcome of a sex-mismatched bone marrow transplant (Fig. 5-6). However, the ability of FISH to detect aneuploidy in a small percentage of a cell population (e.g., to assess minimal residual disease) is limited owing to hybridization inefficiencies and false background signals. The finding of monosomy due to technical artifact can vary from 3% to 9% of all nucleated cells (23).

TABLE 5-2. Partial List of Symbols and Abbreviated Terms Used for *In Situ* Hybridization (14)

Symbol	Definition
amp	Amplified signal
con	Connected signals (signals are adjacent)
dim	Diminished signal intensity
double plus (++)	Duplication on a specific chromosome
enh	Enhanced signal intensity
ish	*In situ* hybridization; when used without a prefix applies to chromosomes (usually metaphase or prometaphase) of dividing cells
minus (–)	Absent from a specific chromosome
multiplication sign (×)	Precedes the number of signals seen
mv	Moved signal (signal moved from original location)
nuc ish	Nuclear or interphase *in situ* hybridization
pcp	Partial chromosome paint (hybridization with probe mixtures prepared from partial chromosome scrapings, contigs, etc.)
period (.)	Separates cytogenetic observations from results of *in situ* hybridization
plus (+)	Present on a specific chromosome
rev ish	Reverse *in situ* hybridization, including comparative genomic *in situ* hybridization
semicolon (;)	Probes on different derivative chromosomes
sep	Separated signals (signals are separated)
sp	Split signal (single copy probe signal maps to more than one location)
st	Stationary signal (signal remaining in original location)
wcp	Whole chromosome paint

Another type of probe hybridizes to multiple chromosomal sequences located on a particular chromosome; such probes are known as *chromosome painting probes* (Fig. 5-5). These probes may be developed from DNA libraries derived from flow-sorted human chromosomes or from DNA amplified from human monochromosomal somatic cell hybrids (24). Hybridization results in the fluorescent staining, or painting, of the entire chromosome. These probes are available for each of the human chromosomes and are particularly useful for identifying chromosomes involved in rearrangements generally not visible by standard banding analysis. Painting probes are not as useful in the analysis of interphase cells because the signal domains are large and diffuse compared to the hybridization of probes developed to specific chromosomal regions.

A third type of FISH probe hybridizes to unique locus-specific DNA sequences. These probes are usually genomic clones (but may be cDNAs) and vary in size from approximately 1 kb to hundreds of kb. Recurrent rearrangements can be identified in metaphase or interphase cells using genomic probes derived from the breakpoints (25). In most clinical cytogenetics laboratories, the detection of chromosomal abnormalities is limited to probes that are commercially available, although laboratories may develop probes considered to be "home-brew" reagents for special studies. Early limitations in the inability to distinguish more than one target sequence at a time are now overcome by new hybridization protocols that allow simultaneous detection of several target sequences using different fluorochromes (26). Several different diagnostic schemes are possible, dependent on selection of the DNA sequences for the probes. One of the first generation of probes to detect a breakpoint was that for the t(15;17)(q22;q21) APL rearrangement involving the promyelocytic leukemia (*PML*)/retinoic acid receptor-α (*RARA*) genes, and is known as a single fusion probe. Sequences from *PML* are present in one probe that is detected as a red signal, and sequences from *RARA* are detected as a green signal. In a normal cell, two green and two red signals are visualized. In a cell with a

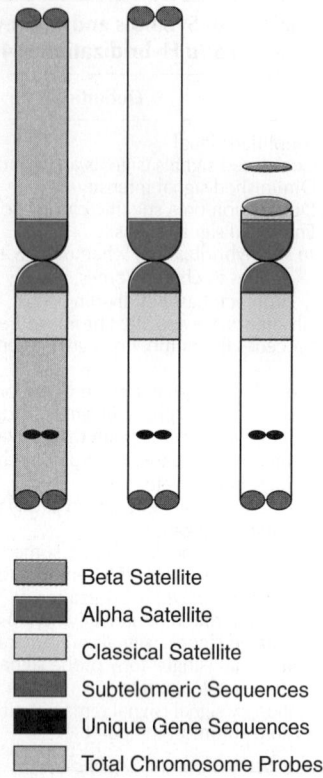

Beta Satellite

Alpha Satellite

Classical Satellite

Subtelomeric Sequences

Unique Gene Sequences

Total Chromosome Probes

Figure 5-5. Schematic diagram of the different types of probes commonly used in fluorescence *in situ* hybridization, including alpha, beta, and classical satellite probes, whole chromosome "painting" probes, and locus-specific probes (subtelomeric and other unique sequences).

typical t(15;17), one red and one green signal represent the normal copies of chromosomes 15 and 17, respectively, and the yellow signal indicates the juxtaposition of *PML* and *RARA* sequences in the der(15) (Fig. 5-7A). Some loss of sensitivity of detection of a true *PML/RARA* fusion results from the stochastic positioning of these sequences in a cell. An improvement in the technology for detection of chimeric genes has been made by

using a DNA sequence for one of the genes that would be split in the rearrangement; for example, a cell with a typical t(9;22)(q34;q11.2) observed commonly in chronic myelogenous leukemia (CML) would show one green signal for breakpoint cluster region (*BCR*) and two red signals for *ABL*, one on the normal 9 and one on the der(9), and a yellow fusion signal (Fig. 5-7B). This *extra-signal probe* makes it possible to discriminate cells potentially representing false positives owing to the requirement to have the extra red signal from *ABL*. Yet another variation on this theme is the selection of DNA sequences for probes that span both heavy chain gene (*IGH*) and *BCL2* genes such that a cell with a t(14;18)(q32;q21) is detectable by two yellow fusion signals present on both the der(14) and der(18) chromosomes; such probes are known as *dual fusion probes* (Fig. 5-7C). Finally, another method is to use DNA probes from the same locus differentially labeled that give a single color signal on normal chromosomes (e.g., yellow), and two colors (e.g., red and green) when a chromosomal rearrangement such as a translocation occurs between them (Fig. 5-7D). This type of probe is referred to as a *break-apart probe* and is especially useful for detecting chromosomal rearrangements of genes such as mixed-lineage leukemia (*MLL*) for which there are multiple partner chromosomes.

It is important to consider the limitations of FISH (27) and to recognize when alternative molecular methods may be of greater use. Reverse-transcriptase polymerase chain reaction (RT-PCR) assay is used to detect many fusion genes and is generally the method of choice for monitoring clinical responses to therapy and detecting minimal residual disease; its sensitivity varies from 10^{-4} to 10^{-6}. In contrast, the sensitivity of FISH to detect the t(9;22) was determined to be 10^{-3} (28). Nonetheless, each method has its limitations, and caution is necessary in interpreting RT-PCR results for the detection of specific translocation products in minimal residual disease studies. For example, it has been reported that in AML cases with a t(8;21) or inv(16), RT-PCR often detects the respective chimeric transcripts even when patients are in remission (29). Similarly, the presence of the *E2A/PBX1* product at the end of consolidation therapy does not necessarily predict relapse in acute lymphoblastic leukemia (ALL) patients with a t(1;19) (30). In the following sections of this chapter is a review of some of the subtypes of leukemias and lymphomas that are associated with recurrent chromosomal abnormalities.

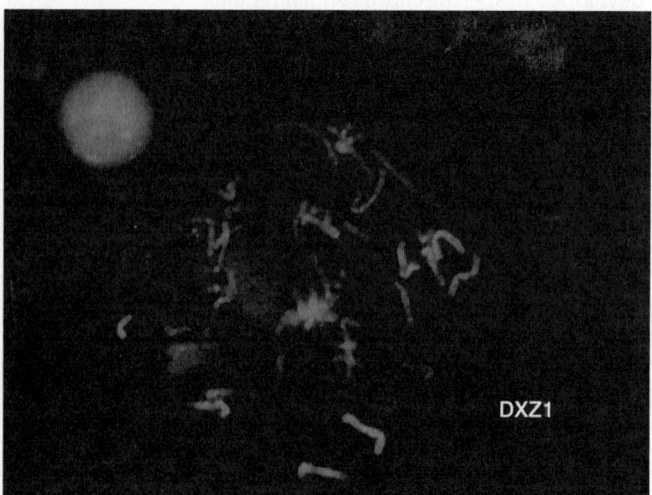
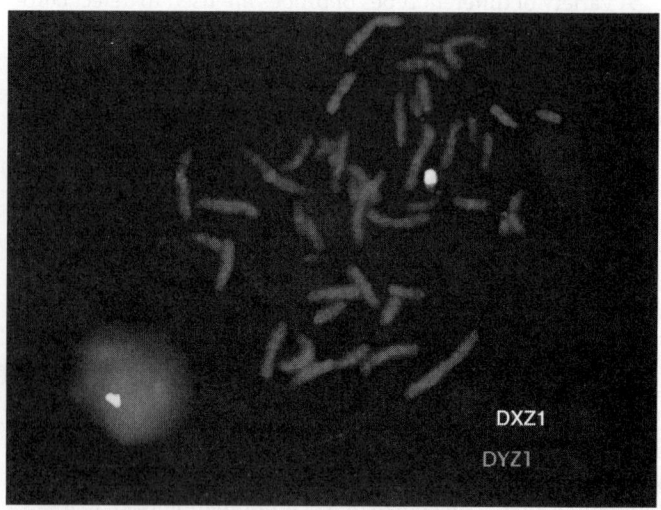

A

B

Figure 5-6. Interphase nuclei hybridized with probes for the X and Y chromosomes reveal disomy for the X chromosome (i.e., two red signals), designated nuc ish Xcen(DXZ1x2) **(A)** and monosomy for both the X and the Y chromosomes (i.e., one red and one green signal), designated nuc ish Xcen(DXZ1x1),Yq11.2(DYZ1x1) **(B)**. (See Color Fig. 5-6.)

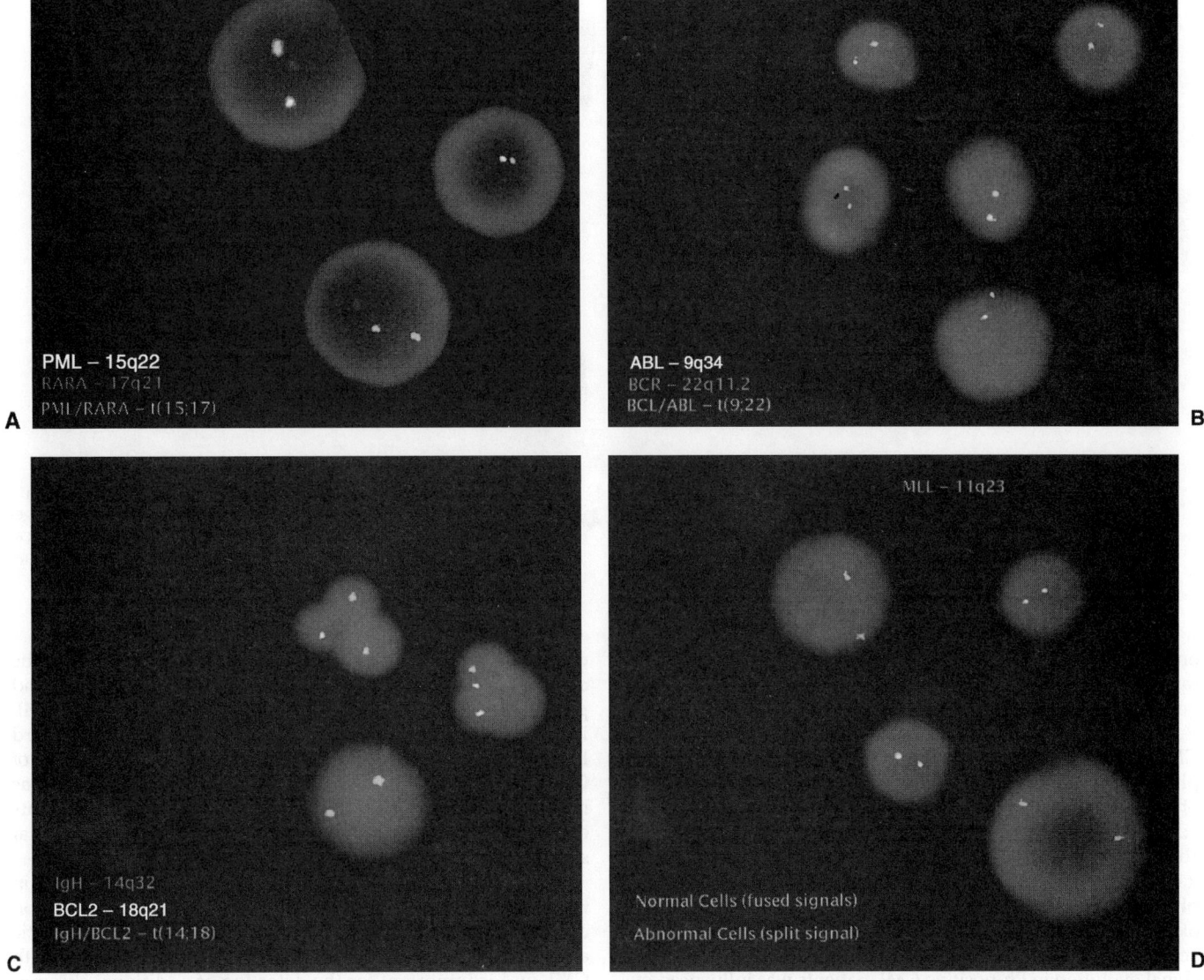

Figure 5-7. Locus-specific probes reveal recurrent breakpoints by fluorescence *in situ* hybridization. A single fusion probe is shown in **(A)** for detection of the *PML/RARA* fusion from a t(15;17)(q22;q21); this result is described as nuc ish 15q22(PMLx2),17q21(RARAx2)(PML con RARAx1). The *BCR/ABL* fusion from a t(9;22)(q34;q11.2) is detected by an extra-signal probe in **(B)**; this result is described as nuc ish 9q34(ABLx2),22q12(BCRx2)(ABL con BCRx1). A dual fusion probe is visualized in **(C)** for an *IGH/BCL2* fusion from a t(14;18)(q32;q21); this result is described as nuc ish 14q32(IGHx2)(IGH con BCL2x1),18q21(BCL2x2)(BCL2 con IGHx1). A break-apart probe reveals a rearrangement in the *MLL* gene **(D)**; this result is described as nuc ish 11q23(MLLx2)(5'MLL sep 3'MLLx1). (See Color Fig. 5-7.)

MYELOPROLIFERATIVE DISORDERS

Among the myeloproliferative disorders (MPDs), the prototype is CML; the other accepted entities by the World Health Organization (WHO) classification (31) are essential thrombocythemia (ET), polycythemia vera (PV), chronic neutrophilic leukemia, and idiopathic myelofibrosis.

Chronic Myelogenous Leukemia and the Philadelphia Chromosome

CML has the distinction of being the first human malignant disease for which a consistent chromosomal rearrangement was identified (32). In 1960, Nowell and colleagues (33) reported their observation of an unusually small chromosome in leukemic cells of two males with CML. Originally considered to be a

shorter Y chromosome, observation of the same abnormality in leukemic cells of female patients with CML suggested that this chromosome was a member of the G group (either a 21 or 22) (34). The chromosome was designated the Philadelphia (Ph) chromosome (after the location of the laboratory in which it was first discovered) and is now recognized as a diagnostic criterion in CML. Following introduction of banding methods, the Ph chromosome was identified as a deleted chromosome 22 (22q–) (35,36); this rearrangement was further elucidated by Rowley in 1973 to be a reciprocal translocation between the long arms of chromosomes 9 and 22, t(9;22)(q34;q11.2) (32) (Fig. 5-8).

Although the t(9;22) is the most common rearrangement producing the Ph chromosome, approximately 5% of Ph rearrangements are variant translocations, in which a third (or more) chromosome is involved besides chromosomes 9 and 22. However, a consistent translocation of *ABL* to a rather limited region

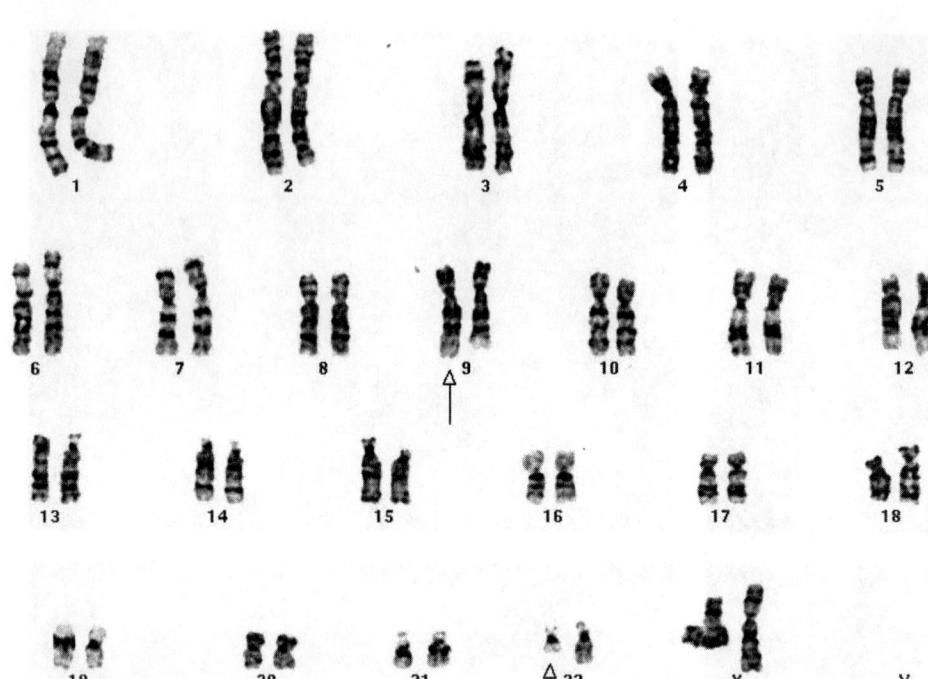

Figure 5-8. GTG-banded karyotype from a male with a diagnosis of chronic myelogenous leukemia. The characteristic translocation involving the long arms of chromosomes 9 and 22 is seen, and the karyotype is described as 46,XX,t(9;22)(q34;q11.2).

on chromosome 22, known as *BCR*, is present. Variant Ph rearrangements are thought to have the same diagnostic and prognostic implications as the simple (9;22) translocation.

During transition to the accelerated and blast phases of CML, which can be either myeloid (70% of patients) or lymphoid (30% of patients), additional chromosome changes are often seen including an extra Ph chromosome and either an additional chromosome 8, an extra chromosome 17, or an isochromosome for 17q (37). Trisomy 8 is the most common, and i(17)(q10) occurs almost exclusively in the myeloid type blast phase. These additional changes are consistent with the notion of tumor progression and may precede the clinically evident acute phase by several months. Retrospectively, the survival in clonal evolution in Ph-positive CML patients was influenced by the presence of a chromosome 17 abnormality, the percentage of abnormal metaphases, and the time of clonal evolution (38). Additional Ph chromosomes, generated by duplication of the original Ph chromosome due to nondisjunction, have been found in up to 3% of CML patients in the chronic phase, but in 16% to 32% of patients in the blast phase (39). However, a very high frequency of a second *BCR/ABL* fusion signal has been reported in patients with advanced disease (40).

The molecular consequence of the t(9;22) is the creation of a chimeric *BCR/ABL* gene that is transcribed into a *BCR/ABL* fusion messenger RNA and the resultant 210-kd protein, which is a constitutively active cytoplasmic tyrosine kinase. The *ABL* gene has 11 exons, spans approximately 230 kb, and encodes a nonreceptor tyrosine kinase of 145 kd (41). The rearrangements in *ABL* usually occur 5' of exon 2. As a consequence, *ABL* exons 2 to 11 are transposed into the major breakpoint cluster region (M-bcr), which extends over 5.8 kb of the *BCR* gene on chromosome 22 between exons 12 and 16.

A cytogenetically identical t(9;22) is also found in ALL (adult and children); however, the majority of the breaks on chromosome 22 fall 5' of the M-bcr within a smaller segment (10 kb) in the first intron, referred to as the minor breakpoint cluster region (m-bcr) (42). A smaller BCR-ABL fusion protein of 190 kd is the product. Approximately 50% to 70% of adult ALL express p190, whereas the remaining express p210. In childhood ALL, p210 is more fre-

quently expressed. However, both *BCR/ABL* transcripts can be detected in Ph-positive ALL patients. Coexpression of p190 and p210 transcripts has also been demonstrated in patients with CML in the chronic phase and on α-interferon therapy (43). A third large BCR-ABL fusion protein of 230 kd was found in a group of CML patients with an unusually low white cell count classified as having neutrophilic CML (44). In these cases, 22q breakpoints occur outside other major and minor *BCR* regions, occasionally at sites 3' to the M-bcr region, in the μ-BCR region.

Most data suggest that the *BCR/ABL* hybrid gene is involved in the pathogenesis of CML (45,46); however, *BCR/ABL* expression can be detected in some healthy individuals (47). Cytogenetic analysis reveals the Ph chromosome in 90% of the patients with CML and is important for the detection of additional chromosomal abnormalities that herald a blast crisis. FISH, using *ABL* and *BCR* probes labeled in differently colored fluorophores, and RT-PCR are commonly performed to detect a *BCR/ABL* fusion and for monitoring patients who are receiving therapy (48) (Fig. 5-7B).

A specific inhibitor of the BCR/ABL tyrosine kinase, STI571 (or Gleevec) is a relatively new drug that has achieved striking preliminary results in treating CML and ALL patients with Ph chromosome (49,50). STI571 functions through competitive inhibition at the adenosine triphosphate–binding site of the BCR/ABL protein, thus preventing phosphorylation. The effect is arrest of growth or apoptosis in hematopoietic cells that express *BCR/ABL*, without an effect on normal cells (51,52).

PH-NEGATIVE BUT *BCR/ABL*-POSITIVE CHRONIC MYELOGENOUS LEUKEMIA

Between 5% and 10% of CML cases are Ph chromosome–negative. Of these, approximately 5% are Ph-negative but *BCR/ABL*-positive, detected by FISH, Southern blot, or RT-PCR. In most cases, the *BCR/ABL* fusion gene is on chromosome 22 (Fig. 5-9). Two mechanisms have been postulated to explain how the molecular *BCR/ABL* event develops without the cytogenetic finding: (a) a double translocation mechanism, in which a second translocation occurs between the derivative chromosomes 9 and 22 (53), or (b) a small fragment of the 9q34 region inserted into the middle of the *BCR* gene (54). The disease, therapeutic

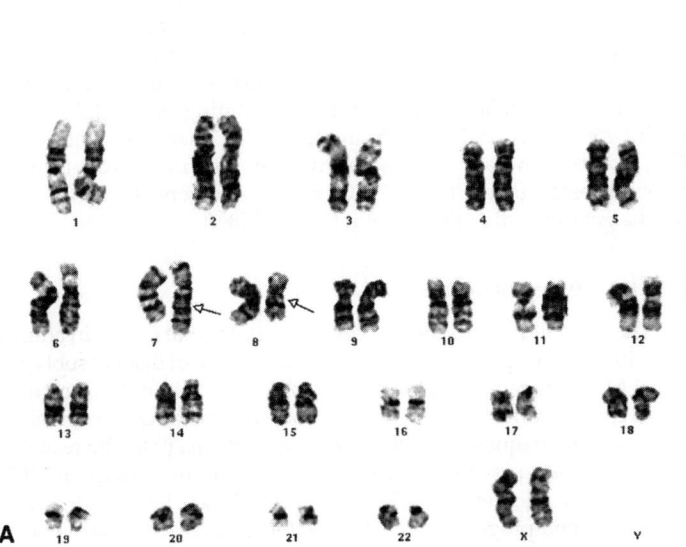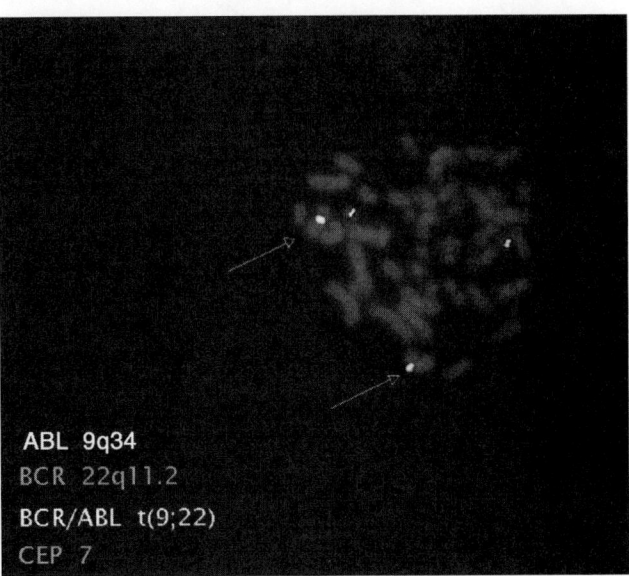

ABL 9q34
BCR 22q11.2
BCR/ABL t(9;22)
CEP 7

A   B

Figure 5-9. GTG-banded karyotype from a patient with chronic myelogenous leukemia who is Philadelphia-negative but *BCR/ABL*-positive due to a cryptic rearrangement. Conventional cytogenetic analysis shown in **(A)** reveals a 46,XX,t(7;8)(q22;q13), and fluorescence *in situ* hybridization studies reveal a *BCR/ABL* fusion in one copy of chromosome 22 and a deletion of *ABL* sequences on the der(9) detectable by the extra-signal probe for *ABL* that spans the breakpoint in *ABL* **(B)**. This karyotype is described as 46,XY,t(7;8)(q22;q13).ish 9q34(ABLx1),22q11(BCRx2)(ABL con BCRx1). (See Color Fig. 5-9B.)

response, and outcome of these patients are indistinguishable from those of individuals with Ph-positive CML (55).

However, there are a few reports of Ph-negative cases with a *BCR/ABL* fusion gene signal on chromosome 9 (56,57). A "reverse" *BCR/ABL* fusion mechanism has been suggested to occur on chromosome 9. It consists of a typical 9;22 rearrangement followed by a reverse translocation that restores apparent cytogenetic normality with a shift of the *BCR/ABL* fusion gene (53). These cases are postulated to have a worse prognosis than those with the typical *BCR/ABL* fusion gene on chromosome 22 (58).

A deletion of the region proximal to the rearranged *ABL* gene on 9q has been found in a group of CML Ph-positive patients with resistance to interferon therapy and a poor prognosis (59) (Fig. 5-9). The phenomenon of the 9q deletion was found to be consistent through the course of the disease, suggesting that the 9q deletion is not acquired during disease progression (60).

PH-NEGATIVE AND *BCR/ABL*-NEGATIVE CHRONIC MYELOGENOUS LEUKEMIA

No evidence of either t(9;22)(q34;q11.2) or a *BCR/ABL* fusion gene has been reported in 5% of CML cases indistinguishable from *BCR/ABL*-positive patients in terms of clinical and laboratory findings. The majority present with atypical, heterogeneous clinical features and have a relatively poor prognosis compared with *BCR/ABL*-positive cases (61,62). The molecular pathogenesis of these BCR/ABL-negative MPDs is poorly understood principally because most cases show a normal karyotype or only numeric chromosomal changes, of which the most common are –Y, +8, and –7. However, occasionally an acquired chromosomal translocation is observed. A distinct MPD is associated with specific translocations involving the chromosome region 8p11-12 (63). The biphenotypic features of these MPDs strongly suggest that the genetic abnormality occurs in the hematopoietic stem cells. The gene involved is the fibroblast growth factor receptor 1 (*FGFR1*), which is fused to one of three different partners at 6q27, 9q32-34, or 13q12 (64). The t(6;8)(q27;p11) results in a fusion between *FGFR1* and *FOP* genes

(65), whereas in the t(8;13)(p11;q12), the partner gene is the *FIM* gene (also called *RAMP* or *ZNF198*) (66). It is particularly striking that another tyrosine kinase is deregulated in a few MPD translocations involving 5q33, which contains the gene encoding the platelet-derived growth factor β receptor (*PDGFBR*), namely t(5;12)(q33;p13) with a *PDGFBR/TEL* fusion gene (67), t(5;7)(q33;q11) with a *PDGFBR/HIP1* fusion gene (68), and t(5;10)(q33;q21) with a *PDGFBR/H4* fusion gene (69). Remarkably, very similar clinical pictures are seen in patients who have primary deregulation of disease with *PDGFBR* involvement. Deletions of regions of several chromosomes, such as del(12p), del(13q), del(5q), and del(7q), have been reported in some patients, but these deletions are more frequently associated with myelodysplastic syndromes (MDSs) (70).

Essential Thrombocythemia

Approximately 5% of 170 patients with ET, cytogenetically reviewed in the Third International Workshop (1980), had chromosomally abnormal clones, but no specific abnormalities could be identified. With progression of disease, further chromosomal abnormalities, such as trisomies 8 and 9, may occur (71–73).

Polycythemia Vera

Chromosomal abnormalities are encountered in 20% to 30% of the PV patients (74). Cytogenetic aberrations are more common when transformation to acute leukemia occurs. Some cytogenetic changes are found more commonly than others and include dup(1q), del(20q), +9, and +8 (75–77). Deletion of the long arm of chromosome 20, del(20q), is often associated with PV but is also found in patients with different MPDs and can occur in other MDSs (78). Until 1992, it was interpreted as a terminal deletion at 20q11. Subsequent FISH mapping studies supported the hypothesis of an interstitial deletion affecting 20q11 to q13, with molecular heterogeneity at the breakpoint sites (79–81). Recently, chromosome 20 deletions in myeloid malignancies were defined by FISH and microsatellite analysis, with a reduction of the common deleted region in MPD of 2.7 Mb, in MDS/AML of 2.6 Mb, and in a combined "myeloid" overlapping region of 1.7 Mb—too small to be cytogenetically visible. These data identify a set of genes and are both positional and expression candidates for the target gene on 20q (82).

Chronic Neutrophilic Leukemia

Chronic neutrophilic leukemia is a rare myeloproliferative disease. There is no Ph chromosome or *BCR/ABL* fusion gene.

Idiopathic Myelofibrosis

No specific chromosomal aberrations have been identified in idiopathic myelofibrosis.

MYELOPROLIFERATIVE/ MYELODYSPLASTIC DISEASES

These diseases, at the time of the initial presentation, showed some features of chronic MPD and others as MDS. Chronic myelomonocytic leukemia (CMML), atypical chronic myeloid leukemia, and juvenile myelomonocytic leukemia (JMML) are merely variations of the same disease process; however, there are sufficient differences to warrant their separation in a classification scheme (31). Clonal chromosomal aberrations are found in 40% to 80% of cases, but none is specific. There is no Ph chromosome or *BCR/ABL* fusion gene. Structural abnormalities of 12p13 and 8p11 have been described in CMML, of 5q33 in atypical chronic myeloid leukemia and monosomy 7 in JMML.

MYELODYSPLASTIC SYNDROMES

MDSs predominate in elderly patients and are associated with a high risk of progression to AML. They were classified by the French-American-British (FAB) classification into five groups: refractory anemia (RA), RA with ringed sideroblasts, RA with excess of blasts, RA with excess of blasts in transformation, and CMML (83). However, in the proposed WHO classification of neoplastic disease, there are several changes in classification (31).

Clonal chromosomal aberrations are found in 30% to 50% of *de novo* MDSs and in 80% of secondary MDS (sMDS). None of the chromosomal aberrations encountered in MDS are specific for MDS but can also be found in AML or MPDs. However, a predominance of total or partial chromosomal loss, a relatively high incidence of gains, and the rarity of translocations (except of sMDS) are characteristic of these disorders. The most frequent cytogenetic abnormalities (at least 50% of the MDS) involve deletions of all or part of chromosomes, resulting in the loss of genetic material coding for tumor-suppressor genes (84,85). Deletions of 5q are the most frequent, followed by del (20q), del (11q), and del(7q), whereas del(13q) is found less often.

5q Deletions

Deletions of the long (q) arm of chromosome 5 are generally interstitial, with a proximal breakpoint between bands 5q13 and 5q22 and a distal breakpoint between bands 5q32 and 5q35. The type of deletion is often correlated with clinical features. For example, the most common type of deletion, del(5)(q13q33), found in 40% of cases, is predominant in females, shares clinical features with the 5q– syndrome, and carries a relatively good prognosis (86). Efforts are still in progress to determine the molecular event in 5q dele-

tions because of the highly complex and heterogeneous genetic features that result from deletion of the 5q3 region, suggesting that more than one gene is responsible. Many growth factors and growth factor receptors have been localized to 5q31-q33, such as granulocyte-macrophage colony-stimulating factor (GM-CSF), interleukin (IL)-3, IL-4, IL-5, and IL-9 (87). Other genes within the same region have also been investigated [i.e., *ERG1* tumor-suppressor gene; *CDC25C*, a G2 checkpoint gene (88), *FMS*, and the gene encoding the receptor for *CSF1* (89)].

The 5q– Syndrome

The 5q– syndrome is an uncommon disorder that occurs in adults, with a female predominance. It is associated with distinct subtypes of MDS, characterized by RA, interstitial deletion of the long arm of chromosome 5 (q12q32) as the sole chromosomal abnormality, and a low frequency of progression to leukemia (90). The relationship of the 5q– syndrome with the other types of 5q deletion MDS is unclear. However, the 5q– syndrome is associated with a relatively good prognosis in contrast to the generally poor survival of patients with the other 5q– MDS.

7q Deletions

In 80% of cases with chromosome 7 involvement, deletions of the long arm occur mainly in two important regions: proximal breakpoints in 7q11-q22 and distal breakpoints in 7q31-q36. In the remaining cases, deletions are observed in the 7q32-q33 region (91). The smallest overlapping region deleted is 7q22, which contains genes that are involved in DNA repair mechanisms (i.e., *EPO*, *PLANH1*, and *ASNS*). Their role in the pathogenesis of MDS is still unclear.

17p Deletions

Unbalanced translocation of chromosome 17 often can result in 17p deletion, such as t(5;17)(p11;p11), t(7;17)(p11;p11), or i(17)(q10). Generally, it is associated with other chromosomal abnormalities. A particular type of dysgranulopoiesis, combining pseudo–Pelger-Huët hypolobulation of the nucleus and small vacuoles in neutrophils, is often seen. Of interest, the same type of dysgranulopoiesis is seen in CML in blast crisis exhibiting an i(17)(q10) (92). These patients usually have point mutations in *TP53* with a poor response to chemotherapy and short survival (93).

12p Deletions

Multiple karyotypic changes are more common than *de novo* disorders with a 12p deletion as the sole aberration. These deletions are usually interstitial between p11 and p13, and both *TEL(ETV6)* and *CDKN1B* genes are generally deleted (94). However, FISH studies have revealed that some of these deletions have hidden rearrangements of *TEL(ETV6)*. Although the t(5;12)(q33;p13) was first described in patients with CMML, it has been observed in other MDS types, frequently associated with eosinophilia and monocytosis (95,96). The translocation results in a fusion transcript between *TEL(ETV6)* at 12p13 and *PDGFBR* at 5q33 (67). Variant translocations involving chromosomal regions such as 3q26, 5q31, 6p21, and 10q24 have been described, and new fusion partners of *TEL(ETV6)* have been identified in MDS (97).

Monosomy 7

Monosomy 7 is frequently observed as an isolated chromosomal aberration in adults younger than 50 years of age (98), whereas in older patients it is associated with other chromosomal abnormalities. It can be readily detected by FISH analysis (99). It is the most frequent chromosomal change seen, as the sole abnormality in MDS children younger than 4 years of age. Monosomy 7 syndrome occurs predominantly in boys with splenomegaly, thrombocytopenia, and a poor prognosis, and may not be readily distinguished from JMML, which also shows monosomy 7 in 25% of the cases (100). Monosomy 7 is also found in childhood preleukemic disorders that may evolve to MDS and AML, such as Fanconi's anemia, Kostmann's syndrome, Shwachman-Diamond syndrome, neurofibromatosis type I, and a rare type of so-called familial myelodysplasia (101).

Therapy-Related Myelodysplastic Syndromes

Generally, therapy-related (t) MDSs are much more aggressive clinically than de novo MDSs. Multiple cytogenetic anomalies are present, mostly involving chromosomes 5 (–5/5q–) and 7 (–7/7q–) (102). Translocations (balanced or unbalanced) are rare in MDS, unless associated with topoisomerase II activators (103,104). Patients with either t-AML or t-MDS who received high doses of epipodophyllotoxin usually exhibited balanced translocations most frequently involving either 11q23 or 21q22, where the *MLL* and *AML1* genes are located, respectively (105). In addition, other balanced translocations, such as inv(16), t(8;16), t(15;17), and t(6;9) have also been observed.

Some MLL breakpoints map to preferred sites for topoisomerase II cleavage *in vitro* (106). The 3' portion of the MLL bcr is one of these sites (107), and in one series of t-AML patients, MLL breakpoints mapped close to this site (108). Recently, a new target gene in t-MDS/AML, *NUP98*, in chromosome band 11p15 has been implicated because of its recurrent involvement in several different chromosomal rearrangements, such as inv(11)(p15q22), t(11;17)(p15;q21), t(11;12)(p15;p13), t(7;11)(p15;p15), t(11;20) (p15;q11), t(2;11)(q31;p15), and t(4;11)(q21;p15) (109). The mechanisms that underlie these translocations are unclear. A role of DNA topoisomerase II in the generation of the 11p15 translocations has been suggested because of the finding of 4-bp microduplications at the breakpoints of both derivative chromosomes (109), implying that these translocations were initiated by a 4-bp staggered DNA break as it occurs *in vitro* (110).

Rearrangements of 3q26

Generally, patients with this anomaly have received prior therapy with an alkylating agent for an unrelated disease, with poor response to chemotherapy and short survival. Dysmegakaryopoiesis is present in 90% of cases carrying an inv(3)(q21q26) or t(3;3)(q21;q36). An activated or inappropriate expression of the *EVI1* oncogene located at 3q26 is observed. However, *EVI1* is also activated in 30% of MDS without 3q rearrangements (111). Patients with a t(3;21)(q26;q22) usually exhibit thrombocytopenia. This translocation has also been observed in CML and leads to a fusion between *EVI1* at 3q26 and *AML1* at 21q22 (112). The involved genes in the t(3;5)(q25;q34) are *MLF1* and *NPA*, respectively (113).

Other Structural Rearrangements and Numeric Changes

A typical structural rearrangement involving chromosome X, idic (X)(q13), has been observed in patients with sideroblastic anemia with or without ring sideroblasts (114). Unbalanced translocations leading to partial monosomy or trisomy often involve chromosomes 1, 5, 7, and 17. Several unbalanced translocations involving the long arm of chromosome 1, resulting in partial trisomy 1q have been described: der(1;7)(q10;p10), der(1;15)(q10;q10), der(1;16)(q10;p10), der(Y;1)(q12;q10), and der(1;18)(q10;q10) (115).

Among numeric changes, trisomy 8 is the most frequent chromosome gain, observed either alone or with other chromosomal abnormalities. Less common trisomies are trisomy 6 (116), trisomy 13 (117), trisomy 15 (118), and trisomy 21 (119).

ACUTE MYELOGENOUS LEUKEMIA

AML is the most extensively cytogenetically analyzed hematopoietic disorder. Although the cytogenetic pattern of AML is heterogeneous, chromosomal aberrations have been shown to constitute indices of diagnostic and prognostic importance. Nonetheless, a significant number of AML patients have been found to have normal karyotypes. Improvements in cytogenetic methodology, the increased level of experience in the detection of structural aberrations, and the introduction of molecular genetic techniques (e.g., FISH, Southern blot analysis, and RT-PCR) have decreased the percentage of normal karyotypes. However, in some patients, the finding of a normal karyotype is a genuine phenomenon rather than a technical failure. Significant proportions of patients with AML display only one cytogenetic aberration, and a high proportion of these sole abnormalities have been seen recurrently. Such leukemia-specific changes (i.e., primary changes) are believed to play an important role in leukemia pathogenesis. Many genes within or adjacent to translocation breakpoints have been cloned, and it has become clear that most of them encode transcription factors. Abnormal protein products of fusion genes created by translocations or inversions dysregulate proliferation, differentiation, or programmed cell death (apoptosis) of blood cell precursors.

The most common classification system for AML, the FAB classification, is primarily based on cellular morphology and immunology (120) and includes the following: acute myelocytic/myeloblastic leukemia (M1, M2), acute PML (M3), and its microgranular variant (M3 variant), acute myelomonocytic leukemia (M4), and M4 with eosinophilia (M4Eo), acute monocytic leukemia (M5), erythroleukemia (M6), and acute megakaryoblastic leukemia (M7). Revised criteria allowed for a more precise distinction between M1 (without cellular maturation) and M2 (with cellular maturation), between M5a (with a high percentage of poorly differentiated cells) and M5b (with relatively well-differentiated monocytic cells), and for the recognition of minimally differentiated AML (M0) (121). Recently, the WHO classification has applied the principles of the Revised European-American Classification of Lymphoid Neoplasms (REAL) classification (122) to myeloid diseases, integrating genetic and clinical features with morphology, cytochemistry, and immunophenotype (31). One of the major modifications of the FAB classification is the reduction in percentage of blasts (i.e., 30% to 20%) for a diagnosis of AML. Four major categories were recognized: AML with recurrent cytogenetic translocations; AML with multilineage dysplasia; AML and MDSs, therapy-related; and AML, not otherwise categorized (31).

Cytogenetic studies are viewed as an integral part of most acute leukemia protocols because of the relationship of specific chromosomal abnormalities to morphologic, classification, and prognostic significance. Some chromosomal aberrations have an association with well-defined types; however, other abnormalities appear to be more common in subgroups of morphologic-related types of leukemias but lack specificity. An association between recurrent chromosomal abnormalities and morphologic subgroups of FAB-type AML has been demonstrated, and many of the genes involved in the aberrations have been identified (Table 5-3). This section emphasizes certain aberrations that occur frequently and the molecular events that underlie the chromosomal changes.

TABLE 5-3. Nonrandom Chromosomal Aberrations and Gene(s) Involved in French-American-British (FAB) Subtypes of Acute Myeloid Leukemia

Abnormality	FAB	Gene(s) Involved
inv(3)(q21q26) or t(3;3)(q21;q26)[a]	M1–M7	RPN1/EVI1
+4	M1, M2, M4	Unknown
+11	M1, M2	MLL
t(9;22)(q34;q11.2)	M1, M2	ABL/BCR
+8	M1, M4, M5	Unknown
t(8;21)(q22;q22)	M1, M2	ETO/AML1
t(6;9)(p23;q34)	M2, M4	DEK/CAN
t(7;11)(p15;p15)	M2	HOX49/NUP98
t(16;21)(p11;q22)	M1, M2, M5, M7	TLS(FUS)/AML1
t(1;11)(q23;p15)	M2	PMX1/NUP98
t(15;17)(q22;q21)	M3	PML/RARA
t(5;17)(q34;q21)	M3, variant	NPM/RARA
t(11;17)(q23;q21)	M3, variant	PLZF/RARA
t(11;17)(q13;q21)	M3, variant	NUMA/RARA
inv(16)(p13q22) or t(16;16)	M4Eo	MYH11/CBFB
t(11;V)(q23;V)[b]	M4, M5	MLL/V[b]
t(10;11)(p12-p14;q14-q21)	M5	AF10/CALM
t(8;16)(p11.2;p13.3)	M5b	MOZ/CBP
inv(8)(p11.2q13)	M0, M1, M5	MOZ/TIF2
t(8;22)(p11.2q13)	M5	MOZ/EP300
t(1;22)(p13;q13)[c]	M7	OTT/MAL

[a]Change also seen in myelodysplastic syndromes.
[b]V denotes various chromosomes, breakpoints, and genes participating in translocations with chromosome 11 at band q23.
[c]Translocation observed almost exclusively in children.

t(8;21)(q22;q22), with or without additional changes, occurs almost exclusively in the M2 FAB subgroup (Fig. 5-10A). Loss of the Y chromosome and interstitial deletion of the long arm of chromosome 9 (9q–) are the most frequent additional changes. This translocation is associated with an excellent rate of remission when compared to patients with other forms of AML, including M2 with other chromosomal aberrations. However, this favorable prognosis of t(8;21) appears to be compromised by the clinically unique presentation as granulocytic sarcoma at diagnosis (123). Molecular characterization of the t(8;21) has shown the involvement of *AML1* (also referred to as *CBFA2*) at 21q22 and *ETO* (for *e*ight *t*wenty-*o*ne), also known as *MTG8/CDR*, at 8q22 (124–126). As result of the t(8;21), the amino-terminal DNA-binding domain of *AML*, a critical regulator of normal hematopoiesis, becomes fused with the carboxy-terminus of *ETO*, a zinc finger protein of unknown function. Variant chromosomal rearrangements, such as complex translocations involving a third chromosome in addition to chromosomes 8 and 21 (called three-way translocations) are also being described. They also have an *AML1/ETO* fusion gene, identified either by detection of *AML1/ETO* fusion transcripts using RT-PCR, or by FISH analysis demonstrating co-localization of *AML1* and *ETO* on the rearranged chromosome 8 at q22. The "simple" variant involves either the chromosome band 8q22 or 21q22 with a chromosome other than its usual partner (127). The clinicobiologic features of AML-M2 patients with these "simple variants" are similar to those of AML-M2 patients with the classic t(8;21); however, molecular investigations revealed either a hidden three-way translocation in some cases (128), or no *AML1/ETO* fusion transcript, suggesting the presence of a fusion gene between *ETO* or *AML1* and an unidentified gene (129).

t(15;17)(q22;q21) is observed only in the M3 type and its variant form M3v, with trisomy 8 as an additional change in almost one-third of patients (Fig. 5-10B). The exact chromosomal location of breakpoints in the t(15;17) has been the subject of some disagreement. Various investigators have reported all bands from 15q22 to 15q26 and 17q11 to 17q25. Most recent studies

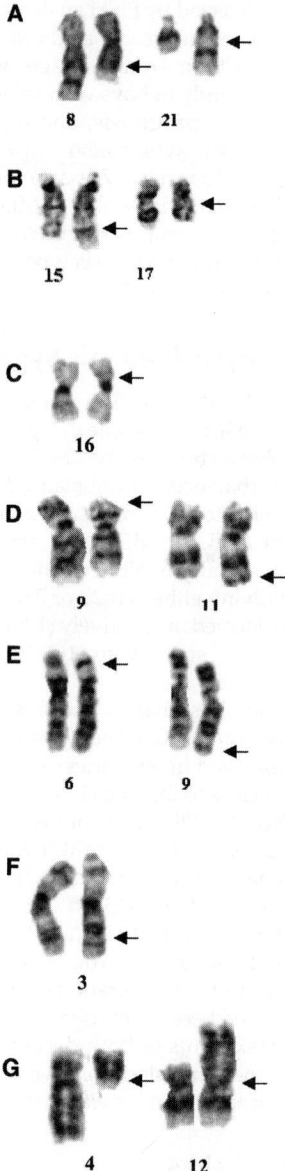

Figure 5-10. Partial karyotypes from GTG-banded metaphase cells depicting recurrent chromosomal rearrangements observed in malignant myeloid diseases: t(8;21)(q22;q22) in AML-M2 **(A)**, t(15;17)(q22;q21) in AML-M3 **(B)**, inv(16)(p13q22) in AML-M4Eo **(C)**, t(9;11)(p22;q23) in AML-M5 **(D)**, t(6;9)(p21-22;q34) in AML-M2 or M4 **(E)**, inv(3)(q21q26) **(F)**, and t(4;12)(q12;p13) **(G)**.

described the breakpoints as band 15q24, but the bands on 17q have ranged from q12 to q21 (130). A few variant translocations have been found: t(5;17)(q32;q21), t(11;17)(q13;q21), and t(11;17)(q23;q21). The t(15;17) results from the fusion of the *PML* gene on 15q22 with *RARA* on 17q21 (131,132). The result is formation of two functional chimeric genes: *PML/RARA* (found in almost all patients) and *RARA/PML* (found in approximately 70% to 80% of patients) (133). Although breakpoints of 17q invariably occur in the second intron of *RARA*, three different genomic breakpoints may occur in *PML*, referred to as *bcr3* or *s* (short) form of the fusion transcript, *bcr1* or *l* (long) form, and *bcr 2* or *V* (variable) form (134). *PML* has been shown to function as a tumor-suppressor (135). *RARA* has differentiation-promoting and growth-suppressing activities and is essential for normal hematopoiesis (136). The aberrant *PML/RARA* fusion protein acts as a dominant negative inhibitor of both wild-type

PML and *RARA* alleles through the formation of heterodimers with *PML* or other retinoic acid-binding proteins. The critical role of the *PML/RARA* fusion protein in APL leukemogenesis has been demonstrated through the creation of a transgenic mouse that developed a myeloproliferative disorder (137).

APL was the first human leukemia treated successfully with a differentiation agent, all-*trans*-retinoic acid (ATRA) (138). However, APL cells ultimately develop resistance to retinoic acid, and patients treated with it alone experience relapses. Therefore, ATRA therapy must be followed by conventional chemotherapy in APL patients with the classic t(15;17) and either variant, t(5;17)(q32;q21) or t(11;17)(q13;q21). In both instances, *RARA* is disrupted as in the t(15;17) and translocated with the gene *NPM* (nucleophosmin) on chromosome 5q32 or *NUMA* (nuclear mitotic apparatus) on chromosome 11q13 (139,140). In contrast, patients with t(11;17)(q23;q21), resulting in fusion of *PLZF* (promyelocytic leukemia zinc finger) and *RARA* genes, failed to achieve complete remission after standard chemotherapy or ATRA (141).

inv(16)(p13q22), t(16;16)(p13;q22) or del(16)(q22) is invariably associated with M4Eo (Fig. 5-10C). However, these changes have been reported in M4 and M2 (142,143). Genes involved in the inv(16) have been identified to be within *CBFB* (core-binding factor β) on 16q, the human homolog of a mouse subunit of a heterodimeric transcription factor regulating genes expressed in T cells, and *MYH11* on 16p, a smooth muscle myosin heavy chain gene (144). The molecular heterogeneity of the fusion transcripts is due to variable genomic breakpoints in both the *CBFB* and *MYH11* genes and alternative splicing (144). The most common is type A, fusing *CBFB* nucleotide 495 with *MYH11* nucleotide 1921, which occurs in more than 90% of AML cases with inv(16) or t(16;16). At least seven other types of fusion transcripts (from B to H) have been reported. By conventional cytogenetics, the inv(16) may be overlooked when metaphase cells are suboptimal, and additional screening by FISH should be performed. The presence of trisomy 22 as an apparent sole abnormality in M4 is an indication of the possible presence of a hidden inv(16) (145).

Rearrangements of band 11q23 have been seen in all FAB subtypes but predominantly in patients with M4 or M5 (Fig. 5-10D). A gene that is the human homolog of the *Drosophila* trithorax gene located at 11q23 (*MLL* gene, also known as *ALL1*, *HRX*, and *HTRX1*) has been found to be rearranged in acute myeloid and lymphoid leukemias (146–149). In a recent study of leukemias with *MLL* translocations analyzed by transcriptional profiling, it was reported that differences in gene expression patterns are robust enough to classify leukemias as MLL, ALL, or AML (150). Translocation breakpoints cluster in an 8.5-kb region of *MLL* between exons 5 and 11 and fuse the amino-terminal region of MLL, containing the AT-hook and methyltransferase domains, to a variety of partner proteins. More than 30 different partner genes for *MLL* have been discovered. However, not all reciprocal partners have been identified; thus, Southern blot analysis or FISH must be employed to evaluate *MLL* for evidence of rearrangement (151). In most studies, structural abnormalities involving band 11q23 have been associated with an unfavorable clinical outcome, except for patients with a t(9;11)(p22;q23) (152). *MLL* has been found to be amplified in double minutes, homogeneously staining regions, and ring chromosomes in cases with complex karyotypic abnormalities; the clinical phenotype is similar, though it includes later age at presentation, an aggressive course with poor response to therapy, and short survival (153). 11q23 abnormalities have been reported in acute leukemia in children and young adults, as well as in therapy-induced AML cases, particularly those due to topoisomerase II exposure (104,154).

t(9;22)(q34;q11.2), Ph chromosome, the hallmark of CML, may also occur in acute leukemia (Fig. 5-8). In AML, it is rare

and appears predominantly in M1. The fusion protein observed is 190 kd from rearrangements in the m-bcr, as most frequently observed in ALL.

t(6;9)(p21-22;q34) is mostly seen in M2 or M4, and there is a strong but not absolute association with an increase in bone marrow basophilia (Fig. 5-10E). It is reported in young adults, and the prognosis is unfavorable. The translocation breakpoint at 9q34 is at the same cytologic site as that of the breakpoint in the t(9;22) seen in CML, but not the same on a molecular level. Interestingly, basophilia is also a common finding in CML. The breakpoints on chromosome 6 occur in one intron of the *DEK* gene, and rearrangements in chromosome 9 reside some 360 kb downstream of *ABL* in a large intron of the *CAN* gene (155). The *DEK/CAN* fusion protein is suspected to be involved in the control of DNA transcription (155).

Several structural *rearrangements of the long arm of chromosome 3* have been described, including t(1;3)(p36;q21), inv(3)(q21q26), t(3;3)(q21;q26), and ins(5;3)(q14;q21q26) (Fig. 5-10F). These rearrangements have been identified in all AML subtypes (except M3) and in a few patients with MDS. The oncogenic effect of involvement of 3q21 and 3q26 regions is unclear, because the molecular breakpoints in these regions are heterogeneous. Three genes have been implicated in 3q26: *EAP*, *EVI1*, and *MDS1* (112,156). It has been suggested that on 3q21 the ribophorin I gene causes the activation of *EVI1* in the inv/t(3;3) (157) and *MEL1* in the t(1;3)(p36;q21) (158).

Recurrent cytogenetic *abnormalities of the 8p11-12 region* are associated with either M4 or M5. The t(8;16)(p11.2;p13.3) is essentially confined to the M5b type and is associated with young age (younger than 17 years), hepatosplenomegaly, and marked erythrophagocytosis. This translocation has been shown to fuse the *MOZ* gene at 8p11.2 and the *CBP* gene at 16p13.3 (159). In the inv(8)(p11.2q13), *MOZ* is fused with the *TIF2* gene at 8q13 (160). In the t(8;22)(p11.2;q13), *MOZ* is fused to *EP300*, the adenovirus E1A-associated protein p300 gene (161).

The *TEL(ETV6) gene*, located at 12p13, is frequently involved in chromosomal translocations in different human malignancies; 35 different chromosome bands have been found to be involved, and 13 partner genes cloned (162) (Fig. 5-10G). Several partner genes have been identified in AML translocations, including *ARNT* (1q21), *ARG* (1q25), *MDS1* (3q26), *BTL* (4q11), *PDGFRB* (5q33), *CDX2* (13q12), *TRKC* (15q25), *AML1* (21q22), and *MN1* (22q11).

Translocations involving 11p15 have been reported in patients with both de novo and t-AML and MDS. The gene involved is *NUP98*, and several partner genes have been identified (163).

Besides the above well-defined structural changes, there is a series of *numeric changes* in AML. Trisomy 8 is the most common chromosomal abnormality seen, occurring as either the sole aberration or as an additional change. It is not associated with a specific FAB type but is found most frequently in M1, M4, and M5. It is generally associated with a poor or intermediate prognosis. FISH studies for detection of +8 must be applied in samples where +8 is considered to be a nonclonal cytogenetic aberration to establish its exact frequency. Trisomy 4 as the sole chromosomal abnormality is mostly associated with M4 and M2 as a de novo or secondary leukemia. The prognostic significance is not yet clear, but it is possibly poor. Other trisomies and double minutes can be seen in addition to trisomy 4. Trisomy 11 is the only recurrent numeric change associated with a specific molecular defect [i.e., partial tandem duplication of *MLL(ALL1)* located at 11q23]. Moreover, it has been demonstrated that this gene rearrangement is present on only one of the three chromosomes 11, as well as on only one of the two chromosomes 11 in some karyotypically normal patients. These findings suggest that +11 is not crucial for the *MLL(ALL1)*-associated leukemo-

TABLE 5-4. Nonrandom Additional Aberrations Associated with Selected Primary Structural Abnormalities in Acute Myeloid Leukemia

Primary Aberration	Additional Aberration[a]
t(1;3)(p36;q21)	del(5q)
der(1;7)(q10;p10)	+8
inv(3)(q21q26)	−7, del(5q)
t(6;9)(p23;q34)	+8, +13
t(8;21)(q22;q22)	−Y, −X, del(9q)
t(9;11)(p22;q23)	+8
t(9;22)(q34;q11.2)	+8, −7, +Ph, +19
t(15;17)(q22;q21)	+8
inv(16)(p13q22)	+22, +8
t(16;21)(p11;q22)	+10

[a]The most common additional aberration is specified first.

genesis effect (164,165). Trisomy 21 is often observed in infants and in AML M7 type.

Additional Changes in Acute Myeloid Leukemia

Chromosomal changes that are present (in addition to the primary changes) at diagnosis or at relapse are called additional changes. These changes are less specific, but they are nonrandom (Table 5-4); however, the clinical significance is largely unexplored. Unlike primary changes, common additional changes are almost exclusively unbalanced; that is, they result in a gain or loss of genetic material (i.e., trisomy, monosomy, deletions, and unbalanced translocations). Frequent additional aberrations are −7, +8, and +21, and relatively less commonly seen are 5q−, −5, 7q−, 9q−, and der(16)t(1;16)(q12-23;q12-q24). Recent findings suggest that the acquisition of additional aberrations may depend on the type of the primary aberration. Trisomy 22 is the most common additional abnormality in patients with inv(16) (145). Loss of the Y and X chromosomes and the presence of 9q− are most frequently observed in patients with t(8;21)(q22;q22) (166).

Secondary Acute Myeloid Leukemia

Secondary AML (sAML) is a general term referring to an AML resulting from treatment with cytotoxic drugs or radiotherapy, or from exposure to environmental toxic agents. The rate of chromosomal abnormalities is higher than in primary AML. These abnormalities are rarely seen in primary AML. The most common aberrations are −5/5q− and −7/7q−, which are often present in the same clone. Other abnormalities involve 3q, 11q, 12p, 17p, and 21q. Complex and hypodiploid karyotypes are also a common feature. Cytogenetically, sAML is very similar to sMDS, with some correlation between the cytogenetic abnormalities and the type of exposure. Monosomy 7 is more common in patients exposed to cytostatic chemotherapy; 5q− is associated with exposure to ionizing radiation; etoposides induce 11q23 abnormalities; aberrations of 17p, 16q22, and 11q+ are documented in exposure to pesticides and organic solvents (167). Overall, the prognosis of sAML is poor.

Acute Myeloid Leukemia in Children

Chromosomal aberrations found at diagnosis in childhood AML are similar to those found in young adults, although their incidence varies with the age of the child. Monosomy 7 is found in approximately 5% to 7% of children with AML without any particular association with FAB type. The prognosis of these cases remains dismal, with a rapidly progressive course and poor response to conventional chemotherapy (100). Other numeric

changes (seen as the sole chromosomal abnormality) involving chromosomes 4, 9, 10, 11, 13, 21, and 22 are observed but rare. Approximately 50% of AML involves structural chromosomal aberrations; the most common are t(8;21), t(15;17), inv(16), and t(9;11), which are associated with a relatively good prognosis. A poor prognosis can be predicted with a complex karyotype, uncommon translocations [i.e., t(1;22), t(6;9), t(8;16)], or translocations involving MLL (168). Molecular studies have shown that MLL is rearranged more frequently than revealed by cytogenetic analysis (169). Therefore, Southern blotting or FISH analyses are more informative than cytogenetics for detecting MLL rearrangements than RT-PCR, because there are numerous 11q23 partners. Most pediatric patients with an MLL rearrangement are classified as M4 or M5. In contrast with the findings in ALL, 11q23 translocations in AML do not appear to confer an adverse prognosis. Some studies claim that patients with a t(9;11) have a better outcome than those carrying a different 11q23 aberration (170), as observed in adults (152). However, other studies showed no prognostic differences among AML pediatric patients with 11q23 rearrangements. Other rarely observed chromosomal rearrangements have been reported: (a) 3q abnormalities involving 3q26 [i.e., inv(3), t(3;3), t(3;21), ins(3;3)]; (b) t(6;9)(p23;q34), mostly in young adults; (c) 8p11 abnormalities [i.e., t(8;16)(p11.2;p13.3) accompanied by erythrophagocytosis and associated with young age at diagnosis and a poor outcome (171), t(8;9)(p11;q13), and t(8;22)(p11;q13) (172,173)]; (d) t(3;5)(q25.1;q34) with a fusion gene between MFL1 and MPM, associated with an unfavorable prognosis (174); (e) t(5;11)(q35;p15.5) associated with del(5q), with breakpoints between the NPM1 and fms-related tyrosine kinase 4 (FLT4) genes at 5q35 and the Harvey ras-1-related gene complex (HRC) and the radixin pseudogene (RDPX1) at 11p15.5 (175); and (f) t(16;21)(p11;q22), fusing TLS/FUS at 16p11 with ERG at 22q22 (176).

Secondary leukemia is a serious complication in children initially treated for ALL with epipodophyllotoxins (i.e., teniposide and etoposide), drugs that target DNA topoisomerase II (177). In general, these therapy-related leukemias are of the M4 or M5 types, with characteristic MLL rearrangements. The most frequent chromosome partners described are 9p22, 19p13.1, 19p13.3, 21q22, 16p13.3, and 22q13. Molecular studies have shown that the MLL breakpoints are the same in secondary as in de novo 11q23 acute leukemia (178,179).

Leukemia in Infants

Fourteen percent of pediatric AMLs occur in infancy (younger than 1 year of age), and the frequency of MLL rearrangements is very high (168,180). The most frequently observed translocations are t(9;11)(p22;q23), t(11;19)(q23;p13.1), and t(11;19)(q23;p13.3), but several other partners can be involved including 1q21, 2p21, 6q27, 10p11, or 17q25 (181). Also, it has been suggested that specific chemical exposure of the fetus during pregnancy may cause MLL fusions (182). Translocation (1;22)(p13;q13) is a rare nonrandom specific rearrangement associated with AML-M7 in infants and children of 3 years of age or younger (183). Genes involved in this translocation have recently been identified as OTT (for one-twenty-two) and MAL (megakaryocytic acute leukemia) on chromosomes 1 and 22, respectively. A cryptic t(7;12)(q36;p13) was recently associated with infants younger than 20 months of age at diagnosis and the presence of additional copies of chromosomes 19 or 8. This translocation involves the TEL(ETV6) gene, but the partner gene remains to be identified (184).

Trisomy 21 in neonates can be either constitutional (i.e., associated with Down's syndrome) or acquired. In the acquired cases, the trisomy is only found in mitogen-unstimulated blood or bone marrow, and this transient myeloproliferative disorder is called *transient abnormal myelopoiesis* (185). It resolves in most of the cases without antileukemic therapy; however, there is a risk of developing AML (megakaryoblastic type). Of note, children with Down's syndrome have a high risk of leukemia (20- to 30-fold that of chromosomally normal children).

ACUTE LYMPHOBLASTIC LEUKEMIA

By far, the most commonly used morphologic classification of the acute leukemias is the FAB system, in which three types of ALL are recognized: L1, L2, and L3 (186). The proposed WHO classification of lymphoid neoplasms adopts the REAL, and the morphologic classification of ALL is supplanted by an immunologic classification (122). The B- and T-cell neoplasms are stratified into precursors or lymphoblastic neoplasms (ALL and lymphoblastic lymphoma), and mature (peripheral) B- and T-cell neoplasms. Therefore, the FAB terms (L1, L2, and L3) were no longer relevant. There was a consensus that the precursor neoplasms presenting as solid tumors and those presenting with marrow and blood involvement are biologically the same disease but with different clinical presentations. Most precursor lymphoid neoplasms present as leukemia, and thus, it was agreed that the classification should retain the term *ALL* for the leukemic phase of precursor neoplasms of B and T types. Technical improvements and the development of FISH techniques have allowed important advances in the cytogenetic analysis of ALLs. Recurring cytogenetic abnormalities and new genes have provided prognostic and diagnostic insights into ALL, especially in childhood types.

Although chromosomal abnormalities of ALL are basically identical in childhood and adult patients, there are differences in their incidence and the prognostic implications for some of these abnormalities in the two groups. More than 90% of ALL children achieve complete remission with conventional therapy (187). In contrast, in adults, the prognosis is less favorable, with fewer than 40% of patients being long-term event-free survivors (188,189). To improve recognition of high- and low-risk subsets of patients, several molecular techniques (i.e., FISH and RT-PCR) have made it possible to detect the precise chromosomal and molecular defects. In this section, the most important chromosomal aberrations in childhood and adult ALL and their clinical relevance are summarized.

Childhood Acute Lymphoblastic Leukemia

ALL is the most common pediatric malignancy, accounting for approximately 25% to 30% of all types of childhood neoplasms. Remarkably, the prognosis of children with ALL has improved over the last two decades (187).

Hyperdiploidy with greater than 50 chromosomes is a chromosomal aberration found in 25% to 30% of ALL of children, but rarely in adults. These patients almost invariably have precursor B-cell ALL, usually common acute lymphoid leukemia antigen–positive. Chromosomes 4, 6, 10, 14, 17, 18, and X are usually trisomic (Fig. 5-11A). Two extra copies of chromosome 21 are frequently reported (190). Such patients can expect cure rates exceeding 80% to 90% (191). However, some heterogeneity is recognized in this group, as patients with chromosome numbers in the range of 51 to 56 have a less favorable outcome than those with 56 to 67 chromosomes (190). The presence of additional structural aberrations [i.e., dup(1q)] confers a less favorable outcome (192). A less favorable course also is expected in patients with *near-triploid or near-tetraploid karyotypes* (193). Patients with 47 to 50 chromosomes, often with additional structural abnormalities, have an unfavorable prognosis (194). A very poor prognosis is associated with a near haploid (less than 30 chromosomes) karyotype (Fig. 5-11B) (195) that may be underdiagnosed when masked by a coexisting hyperdiploid line; this situation has to be distinguished from the common good-prognosis hyperdiploid ALL (196).

The most common structural abnormalities in childhood B-cell ALL closely correlate with specific immunologic subgroups and are summarized with the corresponding gene rearrangements in Table 5-5. The *t(12;21)(p13;q22)* is the most frequent structural chromosomal abnormality in pediatric B-cell ALL and seems to correlate with a favorable outcome (197,198). The t(12;21) was originally considered as a rare abnormality because the translocation is cryptic, but it is now identified readily by FISH analysis (Fig. 5-12A) (15). This translocation fuses the genes *TEL(ETV6)* at 12p13 (between exons 5 and 6) and *AML1* at 21q22 (between exons 1 and 2, or 2 and 3) (199). Remarkably, there is frequently loss of the normal *TEL* gene, which is not involved in the translocation, suggesting a possible role of *TEL* as a tumor-suppressor gene (Fig. 5-12B) (200). Several chromosomal partners other than 21q22 have been involved in 12p13 translocations. Although some of the partner genes, such as *STL* (6q23), *JAK2* (9p24), and *ABL* (9q34), have been identified, others have not yet been isolated (201). Chromosome 21

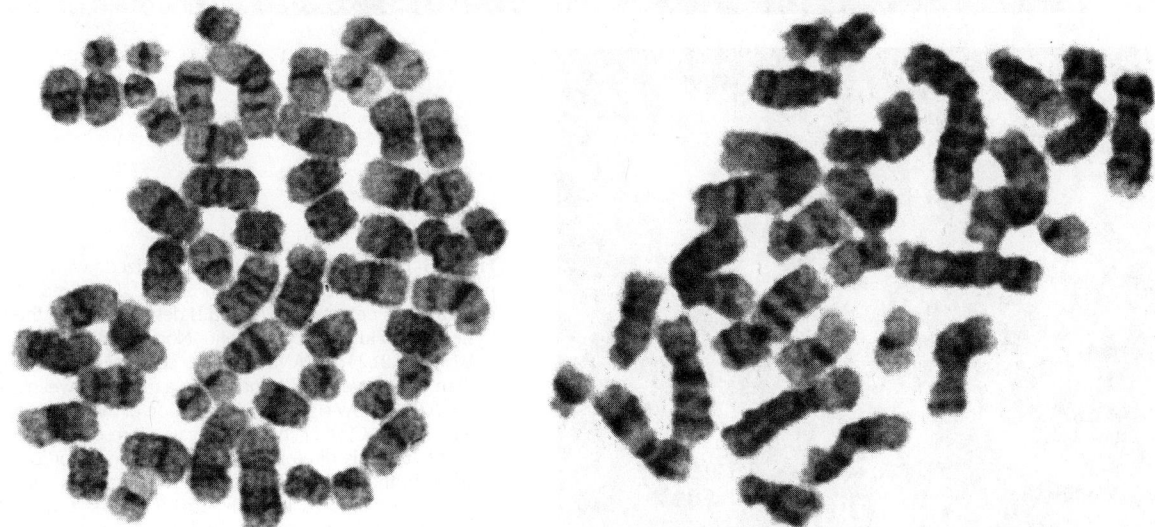

A   **B**

Figure 5-11. GTG-banded hyperdiploid **(A)** and near-haploid **(B)** metaphase spreads from patients with acute lymphoblastic leukemia.

TABLE 5-5. Recurrent Chromosomal Abnormalities and Gene Rearrangements in Childhood B-Lineage Acute Lymphoblastic Leukemia (ALL)

Chromosomal Abnormality	Gene Involved	Diagnosis	Prognosis
t(1;11)(p32;q23)	MLL/AF1P	Pro-B ALL	Poor
t(4;11)(q21;q23)	MLL/AF4	Pro-B ALL	Poor
t(11;19)(q23;p13.3)	MLL/ENL	Pro-B ALL	Poor
t(17;19)(q21;p13)	HLF/E2A	Pro-B ALL	Poor
Hyperdiploid (>50)	—	Common ALL/pre-B	Good
t(5;14)(q31;q32)	IL3/IGH	Common ALL/pre-B	Poor
t(9;22)(q34;q11)	BCR/ABL	Common ALL/pre-B	Poor
t(12;21)(p13;q22)	TEL/AML1	Common ALL/pre-B	Good(?)
t(1;19)(q23;p13)	PBX1/E2A	Pre-B ALL	Intermediate–good
t(8;14)(q24;q32)	MYC/IGH	B-ALL	Good
t(2;8)(p12;q24)	IGK/MYC	B-ALL	Good
t(8;22)(q24;q11)	MYC/IGL	B-ALL	Good

abnormalities with *AML1* amplification have been recently reported to occur in B-cell ALL (Fig. 5-12C) (202).

The *t(1;19)(q23;p13)* can be present in children with pre–B-cell ALL, but it is also observed in common ALL. It is detected as the balanced form in two-thirds of cases but may also be found in an unbalanced state [i.e., two normal chromosomes 1, one normal chromosome 19, and a der(19)t(1;19)]. However, there are no differences correlated with clinical features of the patients (203). Moreover, the t(1;19) has not only been described as a primary change, but it is often reported as an additional aberration. At the molecular level, this translocation fuses two genes, *E2A* at 19p13 and *PBX1* at 1q23 (204). The t(1;19) was once associated with a poor prognosis, but in recent years, the introduction of more intensive therapy has improved the outcome of patients with this translocation. The improvement in outcome seems to be restricted to the more common unbalanced der(19)t(1;19) subgroup, whereas the rarer balanced t(1;19) remains an adverse prognostic factor (205).

The *t(17;19)(q21;p13)* is a rare chromosomal abnormality that occurs in adolescents with a pro-B immunophenotype ALL and is frequently associated with hypercalcemia and disseminated intravascular coagulation at diagnosis (206). Genes involved are *E2A* at 19p13 and the bZIP transcription factor gene *HLF* at 17q21 (207).

The *t(8;14)(q24;q32)* was first described in 1972 in B-cell lymphoma (208), but it can be found in 5% of all childhood ALL with a mature B-cell leukemia (L3 morphology) with a predominance of male gender, frequent extramedullary disease, and central nervous system involvement (209). In addition to the t(8;14), two variants are known: t(2;8)(q12;q24) and t(8;22)(q24;q11) (Fig. 5-13). Many of these translocations are believed to result from errors in the normal process of recombination that accompanies immunoglobulin gene rearrangements during B-cell development. In all three translocations, the *MYC* gene at 8q24 is rearranged with an immunoglob-

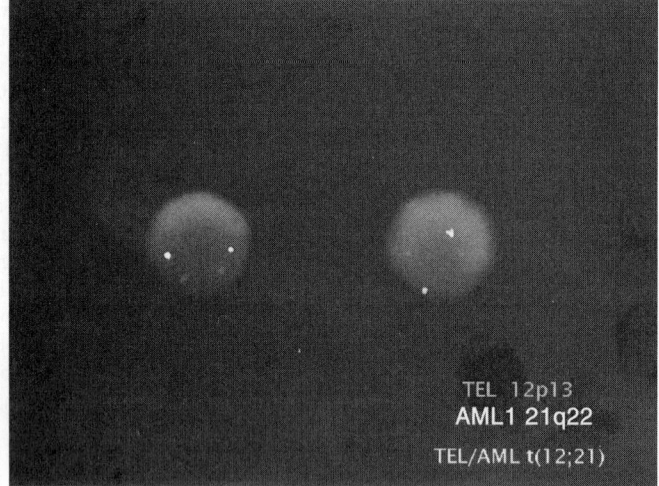

A

TEL 12p13
AML1 21q22

TEL/AML t(12;21)

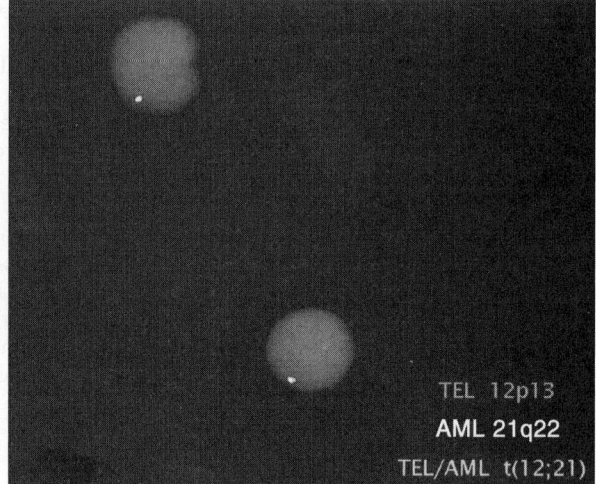

TEL 12p13

AML 21q22

TEL/AML t(12;21)   B

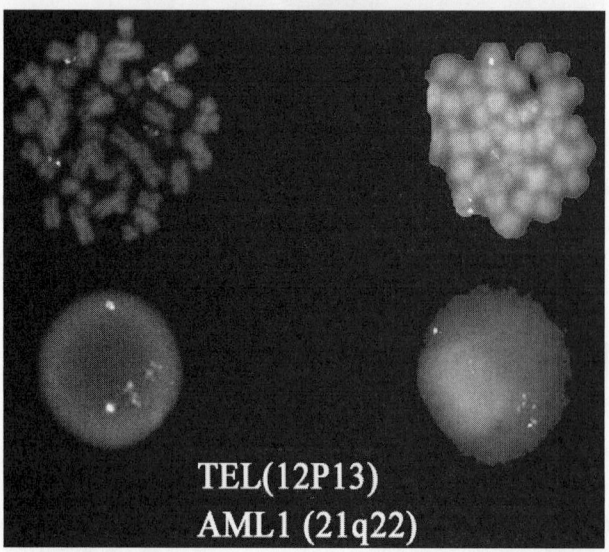

TEL(12P13)

AML1 (21q22)

C

Figure 5-12. Interphase nuclei hybridized with the *TEL/AML1* probe: *TEL* is indicated in green and *AML1* in red. A typical rearrangement is detected in (**A**) and is described using the International System for Human Cytogenetic Nomenclature 1995 as nuc ish 12p13(TELx2),21q22(AML1x2)(TEL con AML1x1). A hybridization pattern is observed in (**B**), indicating a fusion between chromosomes 12 and 21 (yellow signal) and a deletion of the other copy of *TEL* (no green signal). One of the red signals representing the translocated copy of *AML1* is diminished in size due to a portion of the probe residing in the fusion signal. This fluorescence *in situ* hybridization result is described as nuc ish 12p13(TELx1), 21q22(AML1x2)(TEL con AML1x1). In (**C**), multiple red signals are present, representing amplification of *AML1*, and this finding is described as nuc ish 21q22(AML1amp). (See Color Fig. 5-12.)

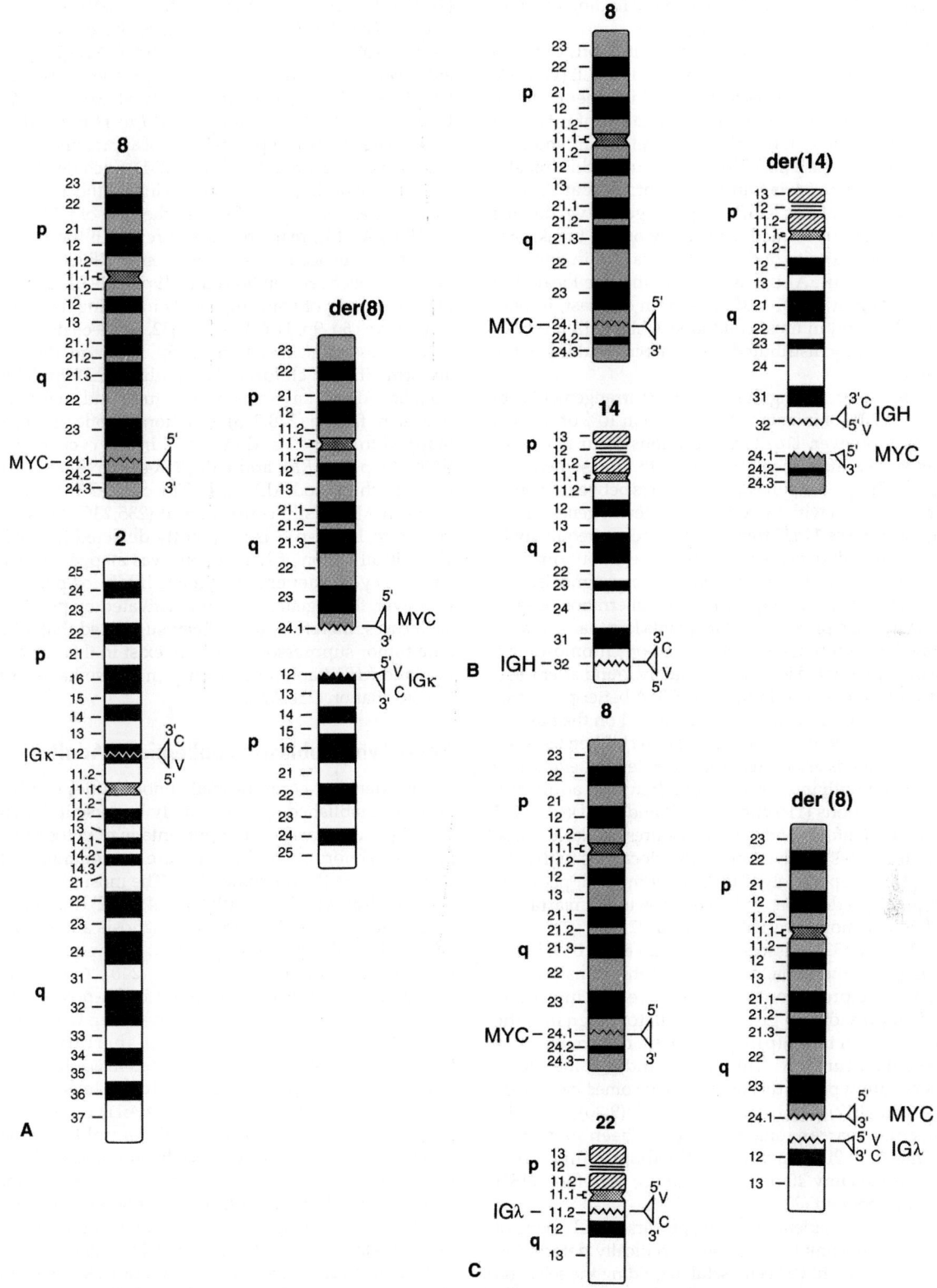

Figure 5-13. Characteristic translocations seen in Burkitt lymphoma: variant, t(2;8)(p11;q24) **(A)**; classic, t(8;14)(q24;q32) **(B)**; and t(8;22)(q24;q11) **(C)**. der, derivative; IGH, heavy chain gene; IGκ, kappa light chain gene; IGλ, lambda light chain gene; p, short arm; q, long arm. (Adapted from Rowley JD. Biological implications of consistent chromosome rearrangements in leukemia and lymphoma. *Cancer Res* 1984;44:3159.)

ulin gene, namely the *IGH* gene at 14q32, the kappa light chain gene (*IGK*) at 2p12, or the lambda light chain gene (*IGL*) at 22q11. The break at 8q24 occurs upstream or in the 5' region of *MYC* in the t(8;14) and 3' of *MYC* in the variant t(2;8) and t(8;22), but all three translocations lead to deregulated expression of *MYC*. A subset of patients has been reported to show the classic t(8;14) associated with mature B-cell ALL but with an immunophenotype more consistent with immature B-cell ALL (210). In such cases, a search for a cryptic t(12;21) should be pursued based on the finding of its co-occurrence with a *MYC* translocation (211).

The *t(9;22)(q34;q11.2)* was first described in CML but was subsequently found in 3% to 5% of children with ALL (Fig. 5-4) (212). This translocation appears to be found in older children suffering from common ALL, is never seen in infants, and seems to correlate with a high white blood cell count and central nervous system disease (213,214). As a result of this translocation, *ABL*, located at 9q34, is translocated into *BCR* at 22q11.2, resulting in formation of a *BCR/ABL* chimeric gene. Two distinct fusion transcripts can be formed, depending on the breakpoint within *BCR*. In the majority of the CML cases and in approximately one-half of adult ALLs, the breakpoints are located in the M-bcr, resulting in the 210-kd protein. In contrast, in one-half of adult ALLs and in most childhood ALLs with a t(9;22), breakpoints are usually distributed in the m-bcr, resulting in the 190-kd protein.

11q23 abnormalities resulting in *MLL* gene rearrangements are present in 60% to 70% of infants with ALL and in 10% of cases in older children. Moreover, 11q23 translocations occur in 80% of secondary leukemias after chemotherapy with topoisomerase II inhibitors (215). The gene involved, *MLL*, breaks between exons 5 and 11 and can be fused with more than 30 different genes. However, only a few of these 11q23 translocations occur frequently in childhood ALL, and all patients with one of these abnormalities have very similar clinical features and a poor prognosis. The most common is the t(4;11)(q21;q23), a specific aberration of early (pro)-B ALL that is also predominant in infants less than 1 year of age. This translocation fuses *MLL* with *AF4* on chromosome 4 (216) and in therapy-related leukemia is mainly found after treatment with a topoisomerase II inhibitor (217). A better prognosis subset of *MLL*-positive patients can be identified on the basis of age and immunophenotype. Thus, the t(4;11) in children between 1 and 10 years of age is associated with an extended event-free survival compared with infants, older children, and adult ALL (218). The translocations (11;19)(q23;p13.3) and (X;11)(q13;q23) are mostly found in infants with clinical features similar to those with a t(4;11); the genes involved in the translocations with *MLL* are *ENL* and *AFX*, respectively (219,220). Of interest, pediatric ALL cases with 11q23 deletions or inversions without rearrangement of *MLL* have a more favorable prognosis (221).

A rare *t(5;14)(q31;q32)* is associated with an early B-cell phenotype and hypereosinophilia. As a result of this translocation, *IGH* is joined to the promotor of *IL3*, which results in overexpression of *IL3*, providing a growth-stimulatory signal to the leukemic cells (222). A t(5;15)(p15;q11-q13) is a recurring abnormality of a B-cell precursor ALL in children under 12 months of age (223). Very rare types of dicentric chromosomes have been reported (i.e., dic(9;12)(p11-12;p11-13) and dic(9;20)(p?3;q11), but no molecular rearrangements have yet been identified (224,225). The dic(9;20) is a very subtle abnormality, often appearing as monosomy 20 or deletion of 9p; therefore, FISH analysis is recommended (226).

In contrast to the experience of B-cell precursor ALL, none of the recurring chromosomal aberrations specifically detected in children with *T-cell ALL* have been useful in guiding the selection of therapy (227,228). Nonrandom translocations preferentially occur in the T-cell receptor (*TCR*) loci at 7q34 (*TCRB*) and 14q11 (*TCRA* and *TCRD*), and less frequently in *TCRG* at 7p15. Like the translocations identified in B-cell ALL and Burkitt lymphoma (BL), these translocations in T-ALL appear to result from errors in the normal recombination process involved in the generation of functional antigen receptors (229). The most frequent abnormalities of T-ALL involve the *TCRA* and *TCRD* genes in 14q11. Several chromosomal partners have been described to be fused with 14q11, among them 1p32 (*TAL1*), 8q24 (*MYC*), 10q24

(*HOX11*), 11p13 (*LMOZ1/RBTN2*), 11p15 (*LMOZ2/RBTN1*), and 21q22 (*BHLHB1*) (230). Most of these translocations [i.e., t(10;14)(q24;q11), t(11;14)(p13;q11) and t(8;14)(q24;q11)] juxtapose enhancer elements responsible for expression of *TCRD* next to different genes, leading to their deregulated expression. Of interest is the t(1;14)(p32;q11), which joins *TAL1* to *TCRD*; *TAL1* expression is associated with a cryptic deletion of approximately 90 kb within a gene, *SCL*, situated 5' of *TAL1* (231). Such deletions are much more frequent than translocations in childhood ALL and can be easily recognized by RT-PCR. In the case of t(7;9)(q34;q34) and t(7;19)(q34;p13), rearrangements result in the production of a potentially oncogenic fusion between *TCRB* and *TAN1* and *LYL1* genes, respectively, on 9q34 and 19p13 (204,232). In addition, a high frequency of rearrangements involving non-T-cell–specific loci, such as 6q, 9p, 11q23, and 14q32, has been described (228).

Chromosomal deletions on 6q, 9p, 12p, and 19p are common abnormalities in childhood and adult ALL. 9p deletions have been linked to unfavorable risk features and an increased risk of treatment failure (228,233). Deletions of one or more genes, all mapped to 9p21-22 and involved in cell cycle regulation, p16 (*INK4A*), p14 (*ARF*), and p15 (*INK4B*) have been described to occur in childhood ALL (234). The clinical importance of these genes in ALL is still controversial (235,236). Loss of heterozygosity on 12p12-p13 is frequently detected in pediatric ALL. The critical region of 12 deletions was mapped near *TEL(ETV6)* and the cyclin-dependent kinase inhibitor p27 (*KIP1*) (237). However, these genes are not inactivated by point mutation in such cases; therefore, it has been suggested that a third candidate tumor-suppressor gene may exist in this region, although *TEL* and *KIP1* haploinsufficiency may also have a role in ALL transformation (238,239).

Acute Lymphoblastic Leukemia in Adults

The incidence of chromosomal abnormalities in adult ALL can only be established approximately because it depends on the technique used and on the percentage of cytogenetic failures. Numeric abnormalities in adults are not common and have less of an effect on the outcome (215). The most frequent translocation in adult ALL is the t(9;22)(q34;q11.2). Patients with a Ph chromosome have the poorest prognosis among the different adult ALL subtypes, independent of the localization of the breakpoint within the *BCR* region (240). Additional chromosomal abnormalities are frequent in Ph-positive adult ALL, with hyperdiploid karyotypes correlating with a better prognosis than monosomy 7 and 9p aberrations (241). The t(1;19)(q23;p13) has also been detected in adult ALL and associated with a poor prognosis. In adults, deletions of 11q23 or translocations of 11q23 other than t(4;11) carry the same poor prognosis as t(4;11) (242). 12p abnormalities in adult ALL, where the t(12;21) is rare, have been associated with a good prognosis (243). There are no clear-cut data on the incidence of deletions in adult ALL. Deletions of 6q are a common abnormality but are not specific for ALL. No significant increase in rates of relapse was noted for the *INK4A* and *ARF* deletions at 9p21-22 in adults (215). Methylation of *INK4B* has been associated with a poor outcome in adults (244).

B-CELL ACUTE LYMPHOBLASTIC LEUKEMIA INVOLVING 14Q32

The t(8;14)(q24;q32) and its variants, t(2;8) and t(8;22), are very common translocations among the Burkitt type of ALL (FAB-L3). The prognosis has improved with newer therapy protocols. A rare t(5;14)(q31;q32) resulting in the inactivation of *IL3* has also been reported in association with eosinophilia (245). The t(14;18)(q32;q21) has generally been associated with follicular lymphoma (FL). However, it also may be associated with ALL without evidence of previous FL and indicates a poor prognosis (246). A series of translocations involving TCR loci at 14q11, 7q34-q35, and 7p15 have been described, but these translocations are uncommon in adult T-ALL. Also, the *TAL1* gene is rarely involved in adult ALL (247).

LYMPHOPROLIFERATIVE DISORDERS

Non-Hodgkin's lymphoma (NHL) in adults has been the subject of a number of different pathologic classifications. In the early 1970s, lymphoid cells were found to have surface antigens or receptors useful for identifying the lineage of both normal and neoplastic cells. This new information, applied to the classification of lymphomas, led to the Kiel classification, published in final form in 1974 (248) and updated in 1988 (249). The Kiel classification became widely used in Europe but did not achieve general acceptance in the United States. An International Lymphoma Study Group adopted a new approach to lymphoma classification. A combination of morphology, immunophenotypes, genetic features, and clinical features were used to define each disease entity. Because this classification represented a revision of current and prior European and American lymphoma classifications, it was called the REAL (250) classification. Most recently, the WHO adopted the REAL classification for lymphoid neoplasms (122). This classification recognized three major groups (with multiple subsets): B-cell NHL, T/natural killer (NK) NHL, and Hodgkin's disease (HD).

The importance of cytogenetics in differentiating the various forms of lymphoma has been documented over the past decades, and, in addition, cytogenetic analysis has led to the discovery of many important genes involved in cell cycle control and apoptosis. Many of the cytogenetic abnormalities observed in lymphoid neoplasms are translocations involving the following: the immunoglobulin heavy-chain genes (*IGH* at 14q32) and, less commonly, the kappa and lambda light-chain genes (*IGK* at 2p11 and *IGL* at 22q11, respectively) in B-cell NHL; and the T-cell receptor loci (*TCRA* at 14q11, *TCRB* at 7q35, *TCRG* at 7p15 and *TCRD* at 14q11) in T-cell NHL. Overall, these translocations tend to show a high degree of association with specific NHL subsets.

B-Cell Neoplasms

Chromosomal translocations involving immunoglobulin (Ig) loci are frequently observed in B-cell malignancies, with the exception of B-cell precursor acute lymphoblastic leukemia (see ALL section) and B-cell chronic lymphocytic leukemia, where Ig translocations are infrequent. The most common translocations in NHL involve *IGH* at 14q32.3. IGH translocations are implicated in the pathogenesis of B-cell lymphoma via the dysregulation of oncogenes located at the partner chromosome band (i.e., *BCL1* (11q13), *BCL2* (18q21), *BCL6(LAZ3)*(3q27), *PAX5* (9p13), and *MYC* (8q24) (251). Such specific rearrangements correlate with certain subtypes of lymphoma, showing distinct pathologic, immunophenotypic, and clinical features, and may correlate with the prognosis of B-cell lymphoma (252). Standard cytogenetic techniques are not always successful for the detection of such abnormalities, particularly in the presence of complex karyotypes and poor-quality metaphases obtained from lymph node cultures. FISH analysis often supplements cytogenetic analysis to detect the 14q32.3 translocations in such cases, as well as in interphase nuclei from tumor cells obtained from flow cytometry or paraffin-embedded sections (253).

The involvement of *IGH* in most of the B-cell lymphoma translocations implies that they arise as a result of errors in intragenic V(D)J or "switch" recombination. The *IGH* breakpoints in t(11;14) in mantle cell lymphoma, t(14;18) in FL, and t(8;14) in endemic BL occur in the *IGH* D–J region with the insertion of variable length nontemplated "N" sequences at the junctions, indicating that these translocations may arise due to errors of V(D)J recombination in B-cell precursors (pro-B/pre-B cell) (254). However, the majority of *IGH* rearrangements occur within the "switch region," suggesting their origin in germinal center B cells (255). Recurrent chromosomal abnormalities and the genes deregulated in lymphoproliferative disorders are summarized in this section. Some of the abnormalities are discussed in more detail because of their diagnostic and prognostic significance.

B-CHRONIC LYMPHOCYTIC LEUKEMIA/ SMALL LYMPHOCYTIC LYMPHOMA

B-CLL is a low-grade lymphoma (leukemia) arising from circulating CD5/CD23 peripheral B cells. Clonal chromosomal abnormalities are detected in almost one-half of patients with CLL using conventional cytogenetic analysis after B-cell mitogen stimulation *in vitro*, such as lipopolysaccharide, tetradecanoyl phorbol acetate, IL-4, or molecular techniques with FISH on interphase cells (256–258). A complex karyotype is found in approximately 12% of CLL cases and is known to be adverse prognostically. Trisomy 12 and 13q– are the most common chromosomal abnormalities. Interestingly, these abnormalities are found together less frequently than expected from their individual frequencies. The prevalence of trisomy 12 by routine karyotyping averages around 10%, whereas FISH of interphase nuclei generally yields a frequency of approximately 20%, presumably due to the suboptimal mitotic stimulation of the tumor cells. Trisomy 12 is usually present in only a proportion of the leukemic cells, and it has been frequently interpreted as a secondary event (259). Although numerous studies link trisomy 12 in CLL with atypical lymphocyte morphology and higher clinical stage (260), the independent prognostic significance remains debatable. Structural abnormalities, mostly deletions, at or near 13q14, are cytologically visible in approximately 10% of CLL cases. These deletions are usually interstitial and in the vicinity of the retinoblastoma gene (261,262). Deletions in this area are seen in a much higher percentage (approximately 50%) of patients by FISH with a trend toward longer treatment-free survival than those without this abnormality (263). Deletions of 11q22-q23 occur in approximately 5% of CLL cases by conventional analyses and in 17% to 20% of cases by FISH. An 11q deletion is more likely to occur in cases with "classic" CLL morphology and immunophenotype and is associated with higher stage, more rapid disease progression and, perhaps, shortened survival (264). *TP53* deletions have been associated with complex karyotypes and 17p abnormalities (11% of CLL cases); these cases fall in an adverse prognostic category (265). FISH analysis for *TP53* deletions could be considered for those cases with an unsuccessful chromosome analysis (266).

Translocations affecting immunoglobulin genes involving diverse chromosome partners have also been reported. However, recurrence of such translocations is infrequent, with the exception of t(14;19)(q32;q13) and t(11;14)((q13;q32) (267,268). The t(14;19)(q32;q13) is associated with a young age of presentation (younger than 40 years) and a poor prognosis. As a result of this translocation, *BCL3* (at 19q13) is overexpressed (269). The t(11;14)(q13;q32) is found in a wide variety of B-cell malignancies; a consequence of the translocation is the overexpression of cyclin D1 (*PRAD1* or *BCL1*), a D-type cyclin involved in control of the cell cycle (270).

B-CELL PROLYMPHOCYTIC LEUKEMIA

B-cell prolymphocytic leukemia is a rare distinct leukemia of mature B cells. Complex hyperdiploid karyotypes with several chromosomal abnormalities have been described, including t(11;14)(q13;q32) and deletions of 11q23 and 13q14 (271,272).

PLASMA CELL MYELOMA/PLASMACYTOMA

Cytogenetic investigations in multiple myeloma (MM) are difficult because of the low proliferation rate of plasma cells. Recently, the detection of abnormal karyotypes at diagnosis has increased because of improving culture methods for myeloma cell growth, with long-term culture (5 to 6 days) and the addition of cytokines such as GM-CSF and IL-3, IL-4, and IL-6 (273). However, chromosomal abnormalities can be demonstrated in almost every patient with MM (newly diagnosed as well as treated and relapsing patients) with FISH analysis (274,275). Structural rearrangements of 14q32.3 may be easily missed without FISH analysis (276,277). Cryptic translocations appear to be prevalent in myeloma [i.e., t(4;14)(p16;q32) and t(6;14)(p25;q32)], which are difficult to detect by cytogenetic analysis due to the telomeric position of the breakpoints on both chromosomes. New partner chromosomal regions have also been identified; however, only a few genes involved in these new translocations are known (278). *NUM1/IRF4* and *MAF* are involved in t(6;14)(p25;q32) and t(14;16)(q32;q23), respectively, and they are overexpressed as a consequence of the translocation (279,280). The effects of t(4;14)(p16;q32) are unusual because they lead to the apparent deregulation of the *FGFR3* and *WHSCH1/MMSET* genes, which are closely associated on 4p16.3 (281,282). The presence of *IGH/MMSET* hybrid transcripts detectable by RT-PCR is particularly important because FISH is the only valid means for the detection of this cryptic translocation (283). The t(11;14)(q13;q32) is the most frequent translocation involving *IGH* (278), and an association between its presence in MM and an especially aggressive disease association has been suggested (284). Overexpression of cyclin D1 has been found in MM carrying a t(11;14), and breakpoints in 11q13 are scattered over a relatively large area, encompassing the cyclin D1 region (285). Although monosomy 13 or deletion of 13q are frequently observed by karyotyping, FISH analysis detects a higher percentage of 13q14 deletion in MM patients (286–288). Moreover, it has been demonstrated that the presence of this deletion is the most independent variable associated with inferior clinical outcome after conventional-dose chemotherapy (289).

HAIRY CELL LEUKEMIA

Although there are a limited number of hairy cell leukemia cases cytogenetically investigated, multiple unrelated or partially related abnormal clones have been described. The detected aberrations include those typically seen in B-cell lymphoma (i.e.,+3, +12, 6q–, 11q–, 14q–, and 14q32+), but also rather distinctive abnormalities of several other chromosomes (290). An overrepresented region of chromosome 5, 5q13-q31, has been observed using CGH (291).

LYMPHOPLASMACYTIC LYMPHOMA/ WALDENSTRÖM'S MACROGLOBULINEMIA

Approximately 50% of lymphoplasmacytic lymphoma, a low-grade B-cell lymphoma, shows a t(9;14)(p13;q32) and rearrangement of *PAX5* (292).

EXTRANODAL MARGINAL ZONE LYMPHOMA OF MUCOSA-ASSOCIATED LYMPHOID TISSUE

The chromosomal abnormalities observed in extranodal marginal zone lymphoma of mucosa-associated lymphoid tissue, a low-grade lymphoma, tend to be simple. Trisomy 3 (or trisomy 3q) is the most frequent numeric chromosome change, whereas t(11;18)(q21;q21) represents the most frequent structural abnormality (293). The genes rearranged in this translocation are the apoptosis inhibitor gene *API2*, also known as *cIAP2, HIP1*, and *MIHC*, and a novel gene, named *MLT*, respectively (294). Interestingly, another apoptosis regulating gene (with an amino-terminal CARD domain similar to *API2*), designated *BCL10*, has been found to be involved in the recurrent chromosomal abnormality t(1;14)(p22;q32) (295,296). However, its precise role in lymphomagenesis is presently controversial (297,298). Other chromosomal aberrations include trisomies of chromosomes 7, 12, and 18, and rearrangements of regions 1p34 and 1q21 (299). High-grade tumors exhibit complex karyotypes, with t(8;14)(q24;q32) being the only recurrent translocation (300).

SPLENIC MARGINAL ZONE LYMPHOMA (+/– VILLOUS LYMPHOCYTES)

The most recurrent chromosomal abnormality in splenic marginal zone lymphoma, often as the sole change, is a del(7)(q23) (301,302). Other chromosomal rearrangements have been reported, such as trisomy 3/3q, +18, rearrangements of 1p34, 1q21, and 8q. Of interest is the fact that these changes have been observed in marginal zone B-cell lymphomas of different sites (303). In splenic lymphoma with villous lymphocytes, the most common finding is t(11;14)(q13;q32) (304). However, the possibility that these cases represent examples of mucosa-associated lymphoid tissue has not been excluded.

NODULAR MARGINAL ZONE B-CELL LYMPHOMA (+/– MONOCYTOID B CELLS)

Cytogenetic data on nodular marginal zone B-cell lymphoma are limited. However, the chromosome changes (trisomy 3/3q, +18, 1p34, and 1q21 rearrangements) are similar to those described in other mucosa-associated lymphoid tissue lymphomas (303,305).

FOLLICULAR LYMPHOMA

More than 75% of FL cases show a t(14;18)(q32;q21). This translocation juxtaposes *BCL2* (one of a family of proteins involved in the regulation of apoptosis) at 18q21.3, with an *IGH* joining region at 14q32. *BCL2* breakpoints tend to cluster either to the 2.8-kb M-bcr (located in the non-coding portion of exon 3) or in the more distal cluster region. Breakpoints on chromosome 14 are relatively constant, clustering at or near the 5' end of one of the six J segments, usually J5 or J6 (306). The result is deregulated expression of the BCL2 protein, leading to prolongation of cell survival through inhibition of apoptosis. Almost all cases display secondary chromosomal aberrations at initial diagnosis; their influence on disease progression has not been fully determined (307). Deletions of the long arm of chromosome 6 are the most frequent secondary aberration (308). The presence of a t(8;14)(q24;q32) in association with t(14;18) has been also reported (309). All reported patients with dual translocations have had a poor clinical outcome despite aggressive therapy. Rearrangement of *MYC* is thought to be the cause of the transformation of low-grade FL to high-grade lymphoma or leukemia (310). The t(8;14)(q24;q32) has also been reported in the absence of the 14;18 translocation. In these cases, the t(8;14) was clearly distinct from that seen in BL and other high-grade lymphomas. Molecular analysis did not demonstrate any rearrangements or point mutations of *MYC*, and the patients had an indolent clinical course (311). Translocations involving 3q27 with rearrangements of *BCL6(LAZ3)* have also been documented in 6% to 13% of FL, with or without the presence of a t(14;18) (312–314).

MANTLE CELL LYMPHOMA

The characteristic chromosomal change of mantle cell lymphoma is the t(11;14)(q13;q32), which juxtaposes the cyclin D1(*CCND1/PRAD1/BCL1*) locus to the immunoglobulin gene sequences and leads to deregulation of cyclin D1 (315). Additional multiple karyotypic changes involving deletions of 1p, 6q, 11q, 13q, and 17p are frequently encountered (316,317).

DIFFUSE LARGE B-CELL LYMPHOMA

The most frequent chromosomal abnormalities are t(3;14)(q27;q32), t(8;14)(q24;q32), and t(14;18)(q21;q32), which together make up approximately 50% of all diffuse large B-cell lymphomas. In these translocations, expression of *BCL6(LAZ3)*(3q27), *MYC* (8q24), and *BCL2* (18q21) is deregulated as a result of their juxtaposition to *IGH*. Rearrangements of *BCL6(LAZ3)* involve not only loci of immunoglobulin genes, 14q32, 2p12, and 22q11, but also a variety of other loci (i.e., 1p32, 1p34, 3p14, 6q23, 12p13, 14q11, and 16p13.3); some of these sites have remained uncharacterized (313,318,319).

BURKITT LYMPHOMA

BL is characterized by translocations involving *MYC*, the most common being t(8;14)(q24;q32), and less commonly t(2;8)(p12;q24) and t(8;22)(q24;q11). Immunoglobulin genes for IGH, IGK, and IGL reside at 14q32, 2p12, and 22q11, respectively, while *MYC* is located at 8q24. Juxtaposition of *MYC* next to immunoglobulin genes leads to overexpression of *MYC*, the major event in the pathogenesis of BL. Depending on the clinical form of the disease, distinct patterns of rearrangements can occur at the molecular level. Breakpoints in *MYC* differ in endemic and sporadic forms of BL (320). In endemic BL, the breaks are generally 5' to *MYC* exon 1, and the 3' border of exon 1 is frequently mutated, whereas in the sporadic form, *MYC* generally breaks within exon 1 or intron 1. In either case, the coding region remains intact, whereas the regulatory region of exon 1 is either lost or disrupted by somatic mutations. These mechanisms lead to overexpression of functionally active Myc protein. Breakpoints within *IGH* are also different in endemic and sporadic forms. In endemic BL, the breaks occur within the joining segments of *IGH*, suggesting a translocation that occurred during primary rearrangement of the antibody locus. In contrast, in sporadic BL, breakpoints cluster within the switch region, indicating that the translocation occurred while the locus was undergoing an isotope switch. Therefore, the t(8;14) occurs in the early pre–B-cell precursor in the endemic BL, whereas in the sporadic form, the translocation occurs in a mature B-cell precursor that has already rearranged its antibody genes and undergone a secondary heavy chain isotype rearrangement.

T-Cell and Natural Killer Cell Neoplasms

T-cell lymphoma represents 12% to 30% of all NHLs, depending to some extent on the geographic region. They have not been extensively studied except for anaplastic large cell lymphoma.

ANAPLASTIC LARGE CELL LYMPHOMA, T-CELL/NULL CELL

Ki-1 (CD30)–positive anaplastic large cell lymphoma (ALCL) constitutes approximately 5% of all NHL but accounts for 30% to 40% of pediatric large cell lymphomas (321). The most common chromosomal aberration is a t(2;5)(p23;q35), leading to fusion of a tyrosine kinase gene, anaplastic lymphoma kinase (*ALK*), to the *NPM* gene, respectively, which results in aberrant expression of the Alk protein (322). Because Alk protein is not expressed in normal lymphocytes, monoclonal and polyclonal anti-Alk antibodies have been widely used to detect *NPM/ALK*-positive ALCL (323,324). However, Alk immunostaining is observed in the cytoplasm and nucleus in some cases, but only in the cytoplasm in other cases, suggesting that *ALK* may become activated through fusion with other translocation partners unassociated with nuclear transport (325,326). The finding of several variant translocations supports this suggestion [i.e., t(1;2)(q25;p23), t(2;3)(p23;q21), and inv(2)(p23q35)] (327). Retrospective analyses of a large series of ALCL by Alk immunostaining have established that Alk-positive ALCL occurs often extranodally in significantly younger patients and has a markedly better clinical outcome as compared to Alk-negative patients (326,328).

T-CELL PROLYMPHOCYTIC LEUKEMIA

Complex karyotypes characterize T-cell prolymphocytic leukemia, but inv(14)(q11q32), t(14;14)(q11;q32), and abnormalities of chromosome 8 are the most frequent chromosomal abnormalities encountered (329). Recurrent deletions of 12p13 have also been reported by FISH analysis (330). Missense mutations at the ataxia-telangiectasia gene (*ATM*) located at 11q23 have been reported (331,332).

NATURAL KILLER CELL LYMPHOMA/LEUKEMIA

Little is known about the cytogenetic characteristics of NK-cell lymphomas and leukemias, which are uncommon lymphoid disorders often associated with Epstein-Barr virus infection. Although no specific recurrent chromosomal aberrations have been reported, deletions of the long arm of chromosome 6 appear to be the most common abnormality (333).

ADULT T-CELL LYMPHOMA/LEUKEMIA

Virtually every case of adult T-cell lymphoma/leukemia exhibits clonal chromosomal abnormalities, with rearrangements of 14q32 or 14q11 and 6q deletions being the most frequent aberrations (334).

HEPATOSPLENIC γ/δ T-CELL LYMPHOMA

Isochromosome 7q, i(7)(q10), and trisomy 8 have been reported by different groups as recurrent cytogenetic findings in hepatosplenic γ/δ T-cell lymphoma, a rare, aggressive entity occurring most frequently in young men (335,336).

MYCOSIS FUNGOIDES/SÉZARY'S SYNDROME

Nonclonal chromosomal aberrations are frequently observed in mycosis fungoides, whereas hyperdiploidy and near-tetraploid karyotypes with rearrangements of several chromosomes are usually present in Sézary's syndrome (337).

PERIPHERAL T-CELL LYMPHOMA, NOT OTHERWISE CHARACTERIZED

In peripheral T-cell lymphoma, not otherwise characterized, correlations between chromosomal abnormalities and histology are still difficult due to the paucity of published series and the use of various histologic classifications, as well as failure to take the immunologic phenotype into account. Clonal chromosomal rearrangements are more frequent and complex in high-grade lesions (338,339).

ANGIOIMMUNOBLASTIC T-CELL LYMPHOMA

In angioimmunoblastic T-cell lymphoma, a high frequency of cytogenetically unrelated clones and single-cell aberrations have been reported, far exceeding the frequency in malignant lymphoma in general (340). Overall, by combining interphase and metaphase cytogenetics, the most frequent nonrandom chromosomal aberrations observed are +3, +5, and +X (341).

Hodgkin's Disease

Successful cytogenetic studies in HD are rare, mainly because of difficulties in obtaining a sufficient number of mitoses from Reed-Sternberg cells. No chromosomal changes typical for this disorder have been described, except for hyperdiploidy. However, the chromosome bands more frequently involved in HD belong to the list of well-established breakpoints in lymphoid malignancies (342). Combination of immunophenotype with cytogenetic analysis, and recently with FISH, has been helpful in attributing hyperdiploid karyotypes to Reed-Sternberg cells (338,341,343).

PERSPECTIVE

Although much has been learned about the relationship between chromosomal rearrangement and human cancer, much remains to be known about how these genomic alterations effect cellular changes that promote altered growth and proliferation. The initiating and subsequent events in chromosomal rearrangement have yet to be elucidated fully.

Molecular cloning has permitted dissection of translocation breakpoints, initially in B- and T-cell neoplasms, in which immunoglobulin and T-cell receptor genes provided a landmark from which to isolate largely unknown genes. The characterization of previously unknown sequences identified in this way continues, and the role of these genes in normal growth and development must be studied to interpret alterations that accompany tumorigenesis.

Ultimately, a more complete understanding of the precise contribution of genes to deregulated cellular growth will doubtless enhance our knowledge of the processes that control normal cellular growth and will contribute to new approaches for the diagnosis and treatment of cancer.

ACKNOWLEDGMENT

Drs. Dal Cin and Morton express their sincere appreciation and gratitude to Dr. Avery Sandberg for his review of this chapter.

REFERENCES

1. Mitelman F, Johansson B, Mertens F, eds. Mitelman Database of Chromosome Aberrations in Cancer; 2002. Available at: http://cgap.nci.nih.gov/Chromosomes/Mitelman.
2. Grimwade D, Walker H, Oliver F, et al. The importance of diagnostic cytogenetics on outcome in AML: analysis of 1,612 patients entered into the MRC AML 10 trial. The Medical Research Council Adult and Children's Leukaemia Working Parties. *Blood* 1998;92(7):2322–2333.
3. Tjio JH, Levan A. The chromosome number of man. *Hereditas* 1956;42:1–6.
4. Seabright M. A rapid banding technique for human chromosomes. *Lancet* 1971;2(7731):971–972.
5. Drets ME, Shaw MW. Specific banding patterns of human chromosomes. *Proc Natl Acad Sci U S A* 1971;68(9):2073–2077.
6. Caspersson T, Lomakka G, Zech L. The 24 fluorescence patterns of the human metaphase chromosomes—distinguishing characters and variability. *Hereditas* 1972;67(1):89–102.
7. Sehested J. A simple method for R banding of human chromosomes, showing a pH-dependent connection between R and G bands. *Humangenetik* 1974;21(1):55–58.
8. Sahar E, Latt SA. Enhancement of banding patterns in human metaphase chromosomes by energy transfer. *Proc Natl Acad Sci U S A* 1978;75(11):5650–5654.
9. Schweizer D. Simultaneous fluorescent staining of R bands and specific heterochromatic regions (DA-DAPI bands) in human chromosomes. *Cytogenet Cell Genet* 1980;27(2–3):190–193.
10. Schreck RR, Warburton D, Miller OJ, et al. Chromosome structure as revealed by a combined chemical and immunochemical procedure. *Proc Natl Acad Sci U S A* 1973;70(3):804–807.
11. Denver Conference. A proposed standard system of nomenclature of human mitotic chromosomes. *Lancet* 1960;i:1063–1065.
12. Mitelman F, ed. *Guidelines for cancer cytogenetics.* Basel: Karger, 1991.
13. An International System for Human Cytogenetic Nomenclature (1985) ISCN 1985. Report of the Standing Committee on Human Cytogenetic Nomenclature. *Birth Defects: Original Article Series* 1985;21(1):1–117.
14. *An International System for Human Cytogenetic Nomenclature* (1995). Basel: Karger, 1995.
15. Romana SP, Le Coniat M, Berger R. t(12;21): a new recurrent translocation in acute lymphoblastic leukemia. *Genes Chromosomes Cancer* 1994;9(3):186–191.
16. Raimondi SC, Williams DL, Callihan T, et al. Nonrandom involvement of the 12p12 breakpoint in chromosome abnormalities of childhood acute lymphoblastic leukemia. *Blood* 1986;68(1):69–75.
17. Johansson B, Mertens F, Mitelman F. Primary vs. secondary neoplasia-associated chromosomal abnormalities—balanced rearrangements vs. genomic imbalances? *Genes Chromosomes Cancer* 1996;16(3):155–163.
18. Harper ME, Saunders GF. Localization of single copy DNA sequences of G-banded human chromosomes by in situ hybridization. *Chromosoma* 1981;83(3):431–439.
19. Morton CC, Kirsch IR, Taub R, et al. Localization of the beta-globin gene by chromosomal in situ hybridization. *Am J Hum Genet* 1984;36(3):576–585.
20. Van Prooijen-Knegt AC, Van Hoek JF, Bauman JG, et al. In situ hybridization of DNA sequences in human metaphase chromosomes visualized by an indirect fluorescent immunocytochemical procedure. *Exp Cell Res* 1982; 141(2):397–407.
21. Pinkel D, Straume T, Gray JW. Cytogenetic analysis using quantitative, high-sensitivity, fluorescence hybridization. *Proc Natl Acad Sci U S A* 1986;83(9):2934–2938.
22. Yung JF. New FISH probes—the end in sight. *Nat Genet* 1996;14(1):10–12.
23. Poddighe PJ, Moesker O, Smeets D, et al. Interphase cytogenetics of hematological cancer: comparison of classical karyotyping and in situ hybridization using a panel of eleven chromosome specific DNA probes. *Cancer Res* 1991;51(7):1959–1967.
24. Pinkel D, Landegent J, Collins C, et al. Fluorescence in situ hybridization with human chromosome-specific libraries: detection of trisomy 21 and translocations of chromosome 4. *Proc Natl Acad Sci U S A* 1988;85(23):9138–9142.
25. Tkachuk DC, Westbrook CA, Andreeff M, et al. Detection of bcr-abl fusion in chronic myelogeneous leukemia by in situ hybridization. *Science* 1990; 250(4980):559–562.
26. Nederlof PM, van der Flier S, Wiegant J, et al. Multiple fluorescence in situ hybridization. *Cytometry* 1990;11(1):126–131.
27. Gozzetti A, Le Beau MM. Fluorescence in situ hybridization: uses and limitations. *Semin Hematol* 2000;37(4):320–333.
28. Dewald GW, Wyatt WA, Juneau AL, et al. Highly sensitive fluorescence in situ hybridization method to detect double BCR/ABL fusion and monitor response to therapy in chronic myeloid leukemia. *Blood* 1998;91(9):3357–3365.
29. Jurlander J, Caligiuri MA, Ruutu T, et al. Persistence of the AML1/ETO fusion transcript in patients treated with allogeneic bone marrow transplantation for t(8;21) leukemia. *Blood* 1996;88(6):2183–2191.
30. Hunger SP, Fall MZ, Camitta BM, et al. E2A-PBX1 chimeric transcript status at end of consolidation is not predictive of treatment outcome in childhood acute lymphoblastic leukemias with a t(1;19)(q23;p13): a Pediatric Oncology Group study. *Blood* 1998;91(3):1021–1028.
31. Jaffe ES, Harris NL, Stein H, Vardiman JW. *World Health Organization classification of tumors. Pathology and genetics of tumours of haematopoietic and lymphoid tissues.* Lyon: IARC Press, 2001.
32. Rowley JD. Letter: A new consistent chromosomal abnormality in chronic myelogenous leukaemia identified by quinacrine fluorescence and Giemsa staining. *Nature* 1973;243(5405):290–293.
33. Nowell PC, Hungerford DA. A minute chromosome in human chronic granulocytic leukemia. *Science* 1960;132:1497.
34. Baikie AG, Court Brown WM, Jacobs PA. Chromosome studies in leukaemia. *Lancet* 1960;1:168.
35. Caspersson T, Gahrton G, Lindsten J, Zech L. Identification of the Philadelphia chromosome as a number 22 by quinacrine mustard fluorescence analysis. *Exp Cell Res* 1970;63(1):238–240.
36. O'Riordan ML, Robinson JA, Buckton KE, Evans HJ. Distinguishing between the chromosomes involved in Down's syndrome (trisomy 21) and chronic myeloid leukaemia (Ph1) by fluorescence. *Nature* 1971;230(5290):167–168.
37. Mitelman F. The cytogenetic scenario of chronic myeloid leukemia. *Leuk Lymphoma* 1993;11(Suppl 1):11–15.
38. Majlis A, Smith TL, Talpaz M, et al. Significance of cytogenetic clonal evolution in chronic myelogenous leukemia. *J Clin Oncol* 1996;14(1):196–203.
39. Cervantes F, Rozman M, Rosell J, et al. A study of prognostic factors in blast crisis of Philadelphia chromosome-positive chronic myelogenous leukaemia. *Br J Haematol* 1990;76(1):27–32.
40. Cabot GP, Bentz M, Scholl C, et al. High incidence of a second BCR-ABL fusion in chronic myeloid leukemia revealed by interphase cytogenetic analysis on blood and bone marrow smears. *Cancer Genet Cytogenet* 1996;87(2):107–111.
41. Kurzrock R, Gutterman JU, Talpaz M. The molecular genetics of Philadelphia chromosome-positive leukemias. *N Engl J Med* 1988;319(15):990–998.
42. Kurzrock R, Shtalrid M, Romero P, et al. A novel c-abl protein product in Philadelphia-positive acute lymphoblastic leukaemia. *Nature* 1987;325(6105): 631–635.
43. van Rhee F, Hochhaus A, Lin F, et al. p190 BCR-ABL mRNA is expressed at low levels in p210-positive chronic myeloid and acute lymphoblastic leukemias. *Blood* 1996;87(12):5213–5217.
44. Pane F, Frigeri F, Sindona M, et al. Neutrophilic-chronic myeloid leukemia: a distinct disease with a specific molecular marker (BCR/ABL with C3/A2 junction). [see comments]. [erratum appears in *Blood* 1997 Jun 1;89(11): 4244]. *Blood* 1996;88(7):2410–2414.

45. Daley GQ, Van Etten RA, Baltimore D. Induction of chronic myelogenous leukemia in mice by the P210bcr/abl gene of the Philadelphia chromosome. *Science* 1990;247(4944):824–830.
46. Elefanty AG, Hariharan IK, Cory S. bcr-abl, the hallmark of chronic myeloid leukaemia in man, induces multiple haemopoietic neoplasms in mice. *EMBO J* 1990;9(4):1069–1078.
47. Biernaux C, Loos M, Sels A, et al. Detection of major bcr-abl gene expression at a very low level in blood cells of some healthy individuals. *Blood* 1995;86(8):3118–3122.
48. Yee K, Anglin P, Keating A. Molecular approaches to the detection and monitoring of chronic myeloid leukemia: theory and practice. *Blood Rev* 1999;13(2):105–126.
49. Druker BJ, Sawyers CL, Kantarjian H, et al. Activity of a specific inhibitor of the BCR-ABL tyrosine kinase in the blast crisis of chronic myeloid leukemia and acute lymphoblastic leukemia with the Philadelphia chromosome. [see comments]. *N Engl J Med* 2001;344(14):1038–1042.
50. Druker BJ, Talpaz M, Resta DJ, et al. Efficacy and safety of a specific inhibitor of the BCR-ABL tyrosine kinase in chronic myeloid leukemia. [see comments]. *N Engl J Med* 2001;344(14):1031–1037.
51. Deininger MW, Goldman JM, Lydon N, Melo JV. The tyrosine kinase inhibitor CGP57148B selectively inhibits the growth of BCR-ABL-positive cells. *Blood* 1997;90(9):3691–3698.
52. Gambacorti-Passerini C, le Coutre P, Mologni L, et al. Inhibition of the ABL kinase activity blocks the proliferation of BCR/ABL+ leukemic cells and induces apoptosis. *Blood Cells Mol Dis* 1997;23(3):380–394.
53. Inazawa J, Nishigaki H, Takahira H, et al. Rejoining between 9q+ and Philadelphia chromosomes results in normal-looking chromosomes 9 and 22 in Ph1-negative chronic myelocytic leukemia. *Hum Genet* 1989;83(2):115–118.
54. Nishigaki H, Misawa S, Inazawa J, Abe T. Absence in Ph-negative, M-BCR rearrangement-positive chronic myelogenous leukemia of linkage between 5' ABL and 3' M-BCR sequences in Philadelphia translocation. *Leukemia* 1992;6(5):385–392.
55. Cortes JE, Talpaz M, Beran M, et al. Philadelphia chromosome-negative chronic myelogenous leukemia with rearrangement of the breakpoint cluster region. Long-term follow-up results. *Cancer* 1995;75(2):464–470.
56. Hagemeijer A, Buijs A, Smit E, et al. Translocation of BCR to chromosome 9: a new cytogenetic variant detected by FISH in two Ph-negative, BCR-positive patients with chronic myeloid leukemia. *Genes Chromosomes Cancer* 1993;8(4):237–245.
57. Nacheva E, Holloway T, Brown K, et al. Philadelphia-negative chronic myeloid leukaemia: detection by FISH of BCR-ABL fusion gene localized either to chromosome 9 or chromosome 22. *Br J Haematol* 1994;87(2):409–412.
58. Aurich J, Dastugue N, Duchayne E, et al. Location of the BCR-ABL fusion gene on the 9q34 band in two cases of Ph-positive chronic myeloid leukemia. *Genes Chromosomes Cancer* 1997;20(2):148–154.
59. Sinclair PB, Nacheva EP, Leversha M, et al. Large deletions at the t(9;22) breakpoint are common and may identify a poor-prognosis subgroup of patients with chronic myeloid leukemia. *Blood* 2000;95(3):738–743.
60. Cohen N, Rozenfeld-Granot G, Hardan I, et al. Subgroup of patients with Philadelphia-positive chronic myelogenous leukemia characterized by a deletion of 9q proximal to ABL gene: expression profiling, resistance to interferon therapy, and poor prognosis. *Cancer Genet Cytogenet* 2001;128(2):114–119.
61. Kantarjian HM, Shtalrid M, Kurzrock R, et al. Significance and correlations of molecular analysis results in patients with Philadelphia chromosome-negative chronic myelogenous leukemia and chronic myelomonocytic leukemia. *Am J Med* 1988;85(5):639–644.
62. Martiat P, Michaux JL, Rodhain J. Philadelphia-negative (Ph-) chronic myeloid leukemia (CML): comparison with Ph+ CML and chronic myelomonocytic leukemia. The Groupe Francais de Cytogenetique Haematologique. *Blood* 1991;78(1):205–211.
63. Macdonald D, Aguiar RC, Mason PJ, et al. A new myeloproliferative disorder associated with chromosomal translocations involving 8p11: a review. *Leukemia* 1995;9(10):1628–1630.
64. Chaffanet M, Popovici C, Leroux D, et al. t(6;8), t(8;9) and t(8;13) translocations associated with stem cell myeloproliferative disorders have close or identical breakpoints in chromosome region 8p11-12. *Oncogene* 1998;16(7):945–949.
65. Popovici C, Zhang B, Gregoire MJ, et al. The t(6;8)(q27;p11) translocation in a stem cell myeloproliferative disorder fuses a novel gene, FOP, to fibroblast growth factor receptor 1. *Blood* 1999;93(4):1381–1389.
66. Popovici C, Adelaide J, Ollendorff V, et al. Fibroblast growth factor receptor 1 is fused to FIM in stem-cell myeloproliferative disorder with t(8;13). *Proc Natl Acad Sci U S A* 1998;95(10):5712–5717.
67. Golub TR, Barker GF, Lovett M, Gilliland DG. Fusion of PDGF receptor beta to a novel ets-like gene, tel, in chronic myelomonocytic leukemia with t(5;12) chromosomal translocation. *Cell* 1994;77(2):307–316.
68. Ross TS, Bernard OA, Berger R, Gilliland DG. Fusion of Huntingtin interacting protein 1 to platelet-derived growth factor beta receptor (PDGFbetaR) in chronic myelomonocytic leukemia with t(5;7)(q33;q11.2). *Blood* 1998;91(12):4419–4426.
69. Kulkarni S, Heath C, Parker S, et al. Fusion of H4/D10S170 to the platelet-derived growth factor receptor beta in BCR-ABL-negative myeloproliferative disorders with a t(5;10)(q33;q21). *Cancer Res* 2000;60(13):3592–3598.
70. Dewald GW, Wright PI. Chromosome abnormalities in the myeloproliferative disorders. *Semin Oncol* 1995;22(4):341–354.
71. Elis A, Amiel A, Manor Y, et al. The detection of trisomies 8 and 9 in patients with essential thrombocytosis by fluorescence in situ hybridization. *Cancer Genet Cytogenet* 1996;92(1):14–17.
72. Sterkers Y, Preudhomme C, Lai JL, et al. Acute myeloid leukemia and myelodysplastic syndromes following essential thrombocythemia treated with hydroxyurea: high proportion of cases with 17p deletion. *Blood* 1998;91(2):616–622.
73. Uozumi K, Ohno N, Shimotakahara S, et al. Trisomy 8 in essential thrombocythemia in leukemic transformation. *Cancer Genet Cytogenet* 2000;116(1):84–86.
74. Third International Workshop on Chromosomes in Leukemia. *Cancer Genet Cytogenet* 1981;4:95–142.
75. Berger R, Bernheim A, Flandrin G, et al. Cytogenetic studies on acute non-lymphocytic leukemias following polycythemia vera. *Cancer Genet Cytogenet* 1984;11(4):441–451.
76. Diez-Martin JL, Graham DL, Petitt RM, Dewald GW. Chromosome studies in 104 patients with polycythemia vera. *Mayo Clin Proc* 1991;66(3):287–299.
77. Swolin B, Weinfeld A, Westin J. A prospective long-term cytogenetic study in polycythemia vera in relation to treatment and clinical course. *Blood* 1988;72(2):386–395.
78. Aatola M, Armstrong E, Teerenhovi L, Borgstrom GH. Clinical significance of the del(20q) chromosome in hematologic disorders. *Cancer Genet Cytogenet* 1992;62(1):75–80.
79. Roulston D, Espinosa R III, Stoffel M, et al. Molecular genetics of myeloid leukemia: identification of the commonly deleted segment of chromosome 20. *Blood* 1993;82(11):3424–3429.
80. Rao PN, Hayworth-Hodge R, Carroll AJ, et al. Further definition of 20q deletion in myeloid leukemia using fluorescence in situ hybridization. *Blood* 1994;84(8):2821–2823.
81. Nacheva E, Holloway T, Carter N, et al. Characterization of 20q deletions in patients with myeloproliferative disorders or myelodysplastic syndromes. *Cancer Genet Cytogenet* 1995;80(2):87–94.
82. Bench AJ, Nacheva EP, Hood TL, et al. Chromosome 20 deletions in myeloid malignancies: reduction of the common deleted region, generation of a PAC/BAC contig and identification of candidate genes. UK Cancer Cytogenetics Group (UKCCG). *Oncogene* 2000;19(34):3902–3913.
83. Bennett JM, Catovsky D, Daniel MT, et al. Proposals for the classification of the myelodysplastic syndromes. *Br J Haematol* 1982;51(2):189–199.
84. Fenaux P, Morel P, Lai JL. Cytogenetics of myelodysplastic syndromes. *Semin Hematol* 1996;33(2):127–138.
85. Mecucci C. Molecular features of primary MDS with cytogenetic changes. *Leuk Res* 1998;22(4):293–302.
86. Pedersen B. 5q-: pathogenetic importance of the common deleted region and clinical consequences of the entire deleted segment. *Anticancer Res* 1993;13(5C):1913–1916.
87. Boultwood J, Lewis S, Wainscoat JS. The 5q-syndrome. *Blood* 1994;84(10):3253–3260.
88. Zhao N, Stoffel A, Wang PW, et al. Molecular delineation of the smallest commonly deleted region of chromosome 5 in malignant myeloid diseases to 1-1.5 Mb and preparation of a PAC-based physical map. *Proc Natl Acad Sci U S A* 1997;94(13):6948–6953.
89. Jaju RJ, Boultwood J, Oliver FJ, et al. Molecular cytogenetic delineation of the critical deleted region in the 5q- syndrome. *Genes Chromosomes Cancer* 1998;22(3): 251–256.
90. Van den Berghe H, Cassiman JJ, David G, et al. Distinct haematological disorder with deletion of long arm of no. 5 chromosome. *Nature* 1974;251(5474):437–438.
91. Le Beau MM, Espinosa R, Davis EM, et al. Cytogenetic and molecular delineation of a region of chromosome 7 commonly deleted in malignant myeloid diseases. *Blood* 1996;88(6):1930–1935.
92. Sessarego M, Ajmar F. Correlation between acquired pseudo-Pelger-Huet anomaly and involvement of chromosome 17 in chronic myeloid leukemia. *Cancer Genet Cytogenet* 1987;25(2):265–270.
93. Lai JL, Preudhomme C, Zandecki M, et al. Myelodysplastic syndromes and acute myeloid leukemia with 17p deletion. An entity characterized by specific dysgranulopoiesis and a high incidence of P53 mutations. *Leukemia* 1995;9(3):370–381.
94. Sato Y, Suto Y, Pietenpol J, et al. TEL and KIP1 define the smallest region of deletions on 12p13 in hematopoietic malignancies. *Blood* 1995;86(4):1525–1533.
95. Lerza R, Castello G, Sessarego M, et al. Myelodysplastic syndrome associated with increased bone marrow fibrosis and translocation (5;12)(q33;p12.3). *Br J Haematol* 1992;82(2):476–477.
96. Wessels JW, Fibbe WE, van der Keur D, et al. t(5;12)(q31;p12). A clinical entity with features of both myeloid leukemia and chronic myelomonocytic leukemia. *Cancer Genet Cytogenet* 1993;65(1):7–11.
97. Yagasaki F, Jinnai I, Yoshida S, et al. Fusion of TEL/ETV6 to a novel ACS2 in myelodysplastic syndrome and acute myelogenous leukemia with t(5;12)(q31;p13). *Genes Chromosomes Cancer* 1999;26(3):192–202.
98. Fenaux P, Preudhomme C, Helene Estienne M, et al. De novo myelodysplastic syndromes in adults aged 50 or less. A report on 37 cases. *Leuk Res* 1990;14(11–12):1053–1059.
99. Flactif M, Lai JL, Preudhomme C, Fenaux P. Fluorescence in situ hybridization improves the detection of monosomy 7 in myelodysplastic syndromes. *Leukemia* 1994;8(6):1012–1018.
100. Luna-Fineman S, Shannon KM, Lange BJ. Childhood monosomy 7: epidemiology, biology, and mechanistic implications. *Blood* 1995;85(8):1985–1999.

101. Luna-Fineman S, Shannon KM, Atwater SK, et al. Myelodysplastic and myeloproliferative disorders of childhood: a study of 167 patients. *Blood* 1999;93(2):459–466.
102. Park DJ, Koeffler HP. Therapy-related myelodysplastic syndromes. *Semin Hematol* 1996;33(3):256–273.
103. Karp JE, Smith MA. The molecular pathogenesis of treatment-induced (secondary) leukemias: foundations for treatment and prevention. *Semin Oncol* 1997;24(1):103–113.
104. Felix CA. Secondary leukemias induced by topoisomerase-targeted drugs. *Biochim Biophys Acta* 1998;1400(1–3):233–255.
105. Pedersen-Bjergaard J, Philip P. Balanced translocations involving chromosome bands 11q23 and 21q22 are highly characteristic of myelodysplasia and leukemia following therapy with cytostatic agents targeting at DNA-topoisomerase II. *Blood* 1991;78(4):1147–1148.
106. Felix CA, Lange BJ, Hosler MR, et al. Chromosome band 11q23 translocation breakpoints are DNA topoisomerase II cleavage sites. *Cancer Res* 1995;55(19):4287–4292.
107. Aplan PD, Chervinsky DS, Stanulla M, et al. Site-specific DNA cleavage within the MLL breakpoint cluster region induced by topoisomerase II inhibitors. [see comments]. *Blood* 1996;87(7):2649–2658.
108. Broeker PL, Super HG, Thirman MJ, et al. Distribution of 11q23 breakpoints within the MLL breakpoint cluster region in de novo acute leukemia and in treatment-related acute myeloid leukemia: correlation with scaffold attachment regions and topoisomerase II consensus binding sites. *Blood* 1996;87(5):1912–1922.
109. Ahuja HG, Felix CA, Aplan PD. Potential role for DNA topoisomerase II poisons in the generation of t(11;20)(p15;q11) translocations. *Genes Chromosomes Cancer* 2000;29(1):96–105.
110. Ripley LS. Deletion and duplication sequences induced in CHO cells by teniposide (VM-26), a topoisomerase II targeting drug, can be explained by the processing of DNA nicks produced by the drug-topoisomerase interaction. *Mutat Res* 1994;312(2):67–78.
111. Russell M, List A, Greenberg P, et al. Expression of EVI1 in myelodysplastic syndromes and other hematologic malignancies without 3q26 translocations. *Blood* 1994;84(4):1243–1248.
112. Nucifora G, Begy CR, Erickson P, et al. The 3;21 translocation in myelodysplasia results in a fusion transcript between the AML1 gene and the gene for EAP, a highly conserved protein associated with the Epstein-Barr virus small RNA EBER 1. *Proc Natl Acad Sci U S A* 1993;90(16):7784–7788.
113. Yoneda-Kato N, Look AT, Kirstein MN, et al. The t(3;5)(q25.1;q34) of myelodysplastic syndrome and acute myeloid leukemia produces a novel fusion gene, NPM-MLF1. *Oncogene* 1996;12(2):265–275.
114. Dewald GW, Brecher M, Travis LB, et al. Twenty-six patients with hematologic disorders and X chromosome abnormalities. Frequent idic(X)(q13) chromosomes and Xq13 anomalies associated with pathologic ringed sideroblasts. *Cancer Genet Cytogenet* 1989;42(2):173–185.
115. Wan TS, Ma SK, Au WY, et al. Derivative (1;18)(q10;q10): a recurrent and novel unbalanced translocation involving 1q in myeloid disorders. *Cancer Genet Cytogenet* 2001;128(1):35–38.
116. La Starza R, Matteucci C, Crescenzi B, et al. Trisomy 6 is the hallmark of a dysplastic clone in bone marrow aplasia. *Cancer Genet Cytogenet* 1998;105(1):55–59.
117. Michaux L, Zeller W, Deneys V, et al. Trisomy 13 in myeloid malignancies: clinical, morphologic and immunologic correlations and characterization by combined immunophenotyping and interphase fluorescence in situ hybridization (FISH). *Blood* 1996;88:372a.
118. Baumgartner BJ, Shurafa M, Terebelo H, et al. Trisomy 15, sex chromosome loss, and hematological malignancy. *Cancer Genet Cytogenet* 2000;117(2):132–135.
119. Wan TS, Au WY, Chan JC, et al. Trisomy 21 as the sole acquired karyotypic abnormality in acute myeloid leukemia and myelodysplastic syndrome. *Leuk Res* 1999;23(11):1079–1083.
120. Bennett JM, Catovsky D, Daniel MT, et al. Proposed revised criteria for the classification of acute myeloid leukemia. A report of the French-American-British Cooperative Group. *Ann Intern Med* 1985;103(4):620–625.
121. Bennett JM, Catovsky D, Daniel MT, et al. Proposal for the recognition of minimally differentiated acute myeloid leukaemia (AML-MO). [see comments]. *Br J Haematol* 1991;78(3):325–329.
122. Harris NL, Jaffe ES, Diebold J, et al. The World Health Organization classification of neoplastic diseases of the haematopoietic and lymphoid tissues: Report of the Clinical Advisory Committee Meeting, Airlie House, Virginia, November 1997. [see comments]. *Histopathology* 2000;36(1):69–86.
123. Byrd JC, Weiss RB, Arthur DC, et al. Extramedullary leukemia adversely affects hematologic complete remission rate and overall survival in patients with t(8;21)(q22;q22): results from *Cancer* and *Leukemia* Group B 8461. *J Clin Oncol* 1997;15(2):466–475.
124. Gao J, Erickson P, Gardiner K, et al. Isolation of a yeast artificial chromosome spanning the 8;21 translocation breakpoint t(8;21)(q22;q22.3) in acute myelogenous leukemia. *Proc Natl Acad Sci U S A* 1991;88(11):4882–4886.
125. Miyoshi H, Shimizu K, Kozu T, et al. t(8;21) breakpoints on chromosome 21 in acute myeloid leukemia are clustered within a limited region of a single gene, AML1. *Proc Natl Acad Sci U S A* 1991;88(23):10431–10434.
126. Erickson P, Gao J, Chang KS, et al. Identification of breakpoints in t(8;21) acute myelogenous leukemia and isolation of a fusion transcript, AML1/ETO, with similarity to Drosophila segmentation gene, runt. *Blood* 1992;80(7):1825–1831.
127. Minamihisamatsu M, Ishihara T. Translocation (8;21) and its variants in acute nonlymphocytic leukemia. The relative importance of chromosomes 8 and 21 to the genesis of the disease. *Cancer Genet Cytogenet* 1988;33(2):161–173.
128. Xue Y, Yu F, Xin Y, et al. t(8;20)(q22;p13): a novel variant translocation of t(8;21) in acute myeloblastic leukaemia. *Br J Haematol* 1997;98(3):733–735.
129. Xue Y, Lu D, Yuan YZ, et al. A rare variant translocation t(3;8)(q29;q22) without AML1/ETO fusion transcript in a case of oligoblastic leukemia. *Leuk Res* 1998;22(11):1015–1019.
130. Stock AD, Dennis TR, Spallone PA. Precise localization by microdissection/reverse ISH and FISH of the t(15;17)(q24;q21.1) chromosomal breakpoints associated with acute promyelocytic leukemia. *Cancer Genet Cytogenet* 2000;119(1):15–17.
131. de The H, Chomienne C, Lanotte M, et al. The t(15;17) translocation of acute promyelocytic leukaemia fuses the retinoic acid receptor alpha gene to a novel transcribed locus. *Nature* 1990;347(6293):558–561.
132. Kakizuka A, Miller WH, Umesono K, et al. Chromosomal translocation t(15;17) in human acute promyelocytic leukemia fuses RAR alpha with a novel putative transcription factor, PML. *Cell* 1991;66(4):663–674.
133. Grimwade D, Howe K, Langabeer S, et al. Establishing the presence of the t(15;17) in suspected acute promyelocytic leukaemia: cytogenetic, molecular and PML immunofluorescence assessment of patients entered into the M.R.C. ATRA trial. M.R.C. Adult Leukaemia Working Party. *Br J Haematol* 1996;94(3):557–573.
134. Gallagher RE, Li YP, Rao S, et al. Characterization of acute promyelocytic leukemia cases with PML-RAR alpha break/fusion sites in PML exon 6: identification of a subgroup with decreased in vitro responsiveness to all-trans retinoic acid. *Blood* 1995;86(4):1540–1547.
135. Wang ZG, Delva L, Gaboli M, et al. Role of PML in cell growth and the retinoic acid pathway. *Science* 1998;279(5356):1547–1551.
136. Chen Z, Tong JH, Dong S, et al. Retinoic acid regulatory pathways, chromosomal translocations, and acute promyelocytic leukemia. [see comments]. *Genes Chromosomes Cancer* 1996;15(3):147–156.
137. He LZ, Tribioli C, Rivi R, et al. Acute leukemia with promyelocytic features in PML/RARalpha transgenic mice. *Proc Natl Acad Sci U S A* 1997;94(10):5302–5307.
138. Tallman MS, Andersen JW, Schiffer CA, et al. All-trans-retinoic acid in acute promyelocytic leukemia. [see comments]. [erratum appears in *N Engl J Med* 1997;337(22):1639]. *N Engl J Med* 1997;337(15):1021–1028.
139. Redner RL, Rush EA, Faas S, et al. The t(5;17) variant of acute promyelocytic leukemia expresses a nucleophosmin-retinoic acid receptor fusion. *Blood* 1996;87(3):882–886.
140. Wells RA, Hummel JL, De Koven A, et al. A new variant translocation in acute promyelocytic leukaemia: molecular characterization and clinical correlation. *Leukemia* 1996;10(4):735–740.
141. Licht JD, Chomienne C, Goy A, et al. Clinical and molecular characterization of a rare syndrome of acute promyelocytic leukemia associated with translocation (11;17). *Blood* 1995;85(4):1083–1094.
142. Betts DR, Rohatiner AZ, Evans ML, et al. Abnormalities of chromosome 16q in myeloid malignancy: 14 new cases and a review of the literature. *Leukemia* 1992;6(12):1250–1256.
143. Marlton P, Keating M, Kantarjian H, et al. Cytogenetic and clinical correlates in AML patients with abnormalities of chromosome 16. *Leukemia* 1995;9(6):965–971.
144. Liu PP, Hajra A, Wijmenga C, Collins FS. Molecular pathogenesis of the chromosome 16 inversion in the M4Eo subtype of acute myeloid leukemia. [see comments]. [erratum appears in *Blood* 1997;89(5):1842]. *Blood* 1995;85(9):2289–2302.
145. Grois N, Nowotny H, Tyl E, et al. Is trisomy 22 in acute myeloid leukemia a primary abnormality or only a secondary change associated with inversion 16? *Cancer Genet Cytogenet* 1989;43(1):119–129.
146. Ziemin-van der Poel S, McCabe NR, Gill HJ, et al. Identification of a gene, MLL, that spans the breakpoint in 11q23 translocations associated with human leukemias. [erratum appears in *Proc Natl Acad Sci U S A* 1992;89(9):4220]. *Proc Natl Acad Sci U S A* 1991;88(23):10735–10739.
147. Tkachuk DC, Kohler S, Cleary ML. Involvement of a homolog of Drosophila trithorax by 11q23 chromosomal translocations in acute leukemias. *Cell* 1992;71(4):691–700.
148. Djabali M, Selleri L, Parry P, et al. A trithorax-like gene is interrupted by chromosome 11q23 translocations in acute leukaemias. [erratum appears in *Nat Genet* 1993;4(4):431]. *Nat Genet* 1992;2(2):113–118.
149. Gu Y, Cimino G, Alder H, et al. The (4;11)(q21;q23) chromosome translocations in acute leukemias involve the VDJ recombinase. *Proc Natl Acad Sci U S A* 1992;89(21):10464–10468.
150. Armstrong SA, Staunton JE, Silverman LB, et al. MLL translocations specify a distinct gene expression profile that distinguishes a unique leukemia. *Nat Genet* 2002;30(1):41–47.
151. van der Burg M, Beverloo HB, Langerak AW, et al. Rapid and sensitive detection of all types of MLL gene translocations with a single FISH probe set. *Leukemia* 1999;13(12):2107–2113.
152. Mrozek K, Heinonen K, Lawrence D, et al. Adult patients with de novo acute myeloid leukemia and t(9; 11)(p22; q23) have a superior outcome to patients with other translocations involving band 11q23: a cancer and leukemia group B study. *Blood* 1997;90(11):4532–4538.
153. Michaux L, Wlodarska I, Stul M, et al. MLL amplification in myeloid leukemias: A study of 14 cases with multiple copies of 11q23. *Genes Chromosomes Cancer* 2000;29(1):40–47.

154. Andersen MK, Johansson B, Larsen SO, Pedersen-Bjergaard J. Chromosomal abnormalities in secondary MDS and AML. Relationship to drugs and radiation with specific emphasis on the balanced rearrangements. *Haematologica* 1998;83(6):483–488.

155. von Lindern M, Fornerod M, van Baal S, et al. The translocation (6;9), associated with a specific subtype of acute myeloid leukemia, results in the fusion of two genes, dek and can, and the expression of a chimeric, leukemia-specific dek-can mRNA. *Mol Cell Biol* 1992;12(4):1687–1697.

156. Morishita K, Parganas E, William CL, et al. Activation of EVI1 gene expression in human acute myelogenous leukemias by translocations spanning 300-400 kilobases on chromosome band 3q26. *Proc Natl Acad Sci U S A* 1992;89(9):3937–3941.

157. Suzukawa K, Parganas E, Gajjar A, et al. Identification of a breakpoint cluster region 3' of the ribophorin I gene at 3q21 associated with the transcriptional activation of the EVI1 gene in acute myelogenous leukemias with inv(3)(q21q26). *Blood* 1994;84(8):2681–2688.

158. Mochizuki N, Shimizu S, Nagasawa T, et al. A novel gene, MEL1, mapped to 1p36.3 is highly homologous to the MDS1/EVI1 gene and is transcriptionally activated in t(1;3)(p36;q21)-positive leukemia cells. *Blood* 2000;96(9):3209–3214.

159. Aguiar RC, Chase A, Coulthard S, et al. Abnormalities of chromosome band 8p11 in leukemia: two clinical syndromes can be distinguished on the basis of MOZ involvement. *Blood* 1997;90(8):3130–3135.

160. Carapeti M, Aguiar RC, Goldman JM, Cross NC. A novel fusion between MOZ and the nuclear receptor coactivator TIF2 in acute myeloid leukemia. *Blood* 1998;91(9):3127–3133.

161. Chaffanet M, Gressin L, Preudhomme C, et al. MOZ is fused to p300 in an acute monocytic leukemia with t(8;22). *Genes Chromosomes Cancer* 2000;28(2):138–144.

162. Odero MD, Carlson K, Calasanz MJ, et al. Identification of new translocations involving ETV6 in hematologic malignancies by fluorescence in situ hybridization and spectral karyotyping. *Genes Chromosomes Cancer* 2001;31(2):134–142.

163. Ahuja HG, Popplewell L, Tcheurekdjian L, Slovak ML. NUP98 gene rearrangements and the clonal evolution of chronic myelogenous leukemia. *Genes Chromosomes Cancer* 2001;30(4):410–415.

164. Caligiuri MA, Strout MP, Schichman SA, et al. Partial tandem duplication of ALL1 as a recurrent molecular defect in acute myeloid leukemia with trisomy 11. *Cancer Res* 1996;56(6):1418–1425.

165. Caligiuri MA, Strout MP, Oberkircher AR, et al. The partial tandem duplication of ALL1 in acute myeloid leukemia with normal cytogenetics or trisomy 11 is restricted to one chromosome. *Proc Natl Acad Sci U S A* 1997;94(8):3899–3902.

166. Schoch C, Haase D, Haferlach T, et al. Fifty-one patients with acute myeloid leukemia and translocation t(8;21)(q22;q22): an additional deletion in 9q is an adverse prognostic factor. *Leukemia* 1996;10(8):1288–1295.

167. Cuneo A, Fagioli F, Pazzi I, et al. Morphologic, immunologic and cytogenetic studies in acute myeloid leukemia following occupational exposure to pesticides and organic solvents. *Leuk Res* 1992;16(8):789–796.

168. Pui CH, Ribeiro RC, Campana D, et al. Prognostic factors in the acute lymphoid and myeloid leukemias of infants. *Leukemia* 1996;10(6):952–956.

169. Martinez-Climent JA, Thirman MJ, Espinosa R III, et al. Detection of 11q23/MLL rearrangements in infant leukemias with fluorescence in situ hybridization and molecular analysis. *Leukemia* 1995;9(8):1299–1304.

170. Martinez-Climent JA, Espinosa R, Thirman MJ, et al. Abnormalities of chromosome band 11q23 and the MLL gene in pediatric myelomonocytic and monoblastic leukemias. Identification of the t(9;11) as an indicator of long survival. *J Pediatr Hematol Oncol* 1995;17(4):277–283.

171. Bernstein R, Pinto MR, Spector I, Macdougall LG. A unique 8;16 translocation in two infants with poorly differentiated monoblastic leukemia. *Cancer Genet Cytogenet* 1987;24(2):213–220.

172. Stark B, Resnitzky P, Jeison M, et al. A distinct subtype of M4/M5 acute myeloblastic leukemia (AML) associated with t(8;16)(p11:p13), in a patient with the variant t(8;19)(p11:q13)—case report and review of the literature. *Leuk Res* 1995;19(6):367–379.

173. Lai JL, Zandecki M, Fenaux P, et al. Acute monocytic leukemia with (8;22)(p11;q13) translocation. Involvement of 8p11 as in classical t(8;16)(p11;p13). *Cancer Genet Cytogenet* 1992;60(2):180–182.

174. Raimondi SC, Dube ID, Valentine MB, et al. Clinicopathologic manifestations and breakpoints of the t(3;5) in patients with acute nonlymphocytic leukemia. *Leukemia* 1989;3(1):42–47.

175. Jaju RJ, Haas OA, Neat M, et al. A new recurrent translocation, t(5;11)(q35;p15.5), associated with del(5q) in childhood acute myeloid leukemia. The UK *Cancer Cytogenetics Group (UKCCG). Blood* 1999;94(2):773–780.

176. Kong XT, Ida K, Ichikawa H, et al. Consistent detection of TLS/FUS-ERG chimeric transcripts in acute myeloid leukemia with t(16;21)(p11;q22) and identification of a novel transcript. *Blood* 1997;90(3):1192–1199.

177. Pui CH, Behm FG, Raimondi SC, et al. Secondary acute myeloid leukemia in children treated for acute lymphoid leukemia. [see comments]. *N Engl J Med* 1989;321(3):136–142.

178. Domer PH, Head DR, Renganathan N, et al. Molecular analysis of 13 cases of MLL/11q23 secondary acute leukemia and identification of topoisomerase II consensus-binding sequences near the chromosomal breakpoint of a secondary leukemia with the t(4;11). *Leukemia* 1995;9(8):1305–1312.

179. Cimino G, Rapanotti MC, Biondi A, et al. Infant acute leukemias show the same biased distribution of ALL1 gene breaks as topoisomerase II related secondary acute leukemias. *Cancer Res* 1997;57(14):2879–2883.

180. Sorensen PH, Chen CS, Smith FO, et al. Molecular rearrangements of the MLL gene are present in most cases of infant acute myeloid leukemia and are strongly correlated with monocytic or myelomonocytic phenotypes. *J Clin Invest* 1994;93(1):429–437.

181. Mercher T, Busson-Le Coniat M, Khac FN, et al. Recurrence of OTT-MAL fusion in t(1;22) of infant AML-M7. *Genes Chromosomes Cancer* 2002;33(1):22–28.

182. Alexander FE, Patheal SL, Biondi A, et al. Transplacental chemical exposure and risk of infant leukemia with MLL gene fusion. *Cancer Res* 2001;61(6):2542–2546.

183. Bernstein J, Dastugue N, Haas OA, et al. Nineteen cases of the t(1;22)(p13;q13) acute megakaryoblastic leukaemia of infants/children and a review of 39 cases: report from a t(1;22) study group. *Leukemia* 2000;14(1):216–218.

184. Tosi S, Harbott J, Teigler-Schlegel A, et al. t(7;12)(q36;p13), a new recurrent translocation involving ETV6 in infant leukemia. *Genes Chromosomes Cancer* 2000; 29(4):325–332.

185. Homans AC, Verissimo AM, Vlacha V. Transient abnormal myelopoiesis of infancy associated with trisomy 21. [see comments]. *Am J Pediatr Hematol Oncol* 1993;15(4):392–399.

186. Bennett JM, Catovsky D, Daniel MT, et al. Proposals for the classification of the acute leukaemias. French-American-British (FAB) co-operative group. *Br J Haematol* 1976;33(4):451–458.

187. Pui CH, Evans WE. Acute lymphoblastic leukemia. *N Engl J Med* 1998;339(9):605–615.

188. Hoelzer D, Thiel E, Ludwig WD, et al. The German multicentre trials for treatment of acute lymphoblastic leukemia in adults. The German Adult ALL Study Group. *Leukemia* 1992;6(Suppl 2):175–177.

189. Hoelzer D, Ludwig WD, Thiel E, et al. Improved outcome in adult B-cell acute lymphoblastic leukemia. *Blood* 1996;87(2):495–508.

190. Raimondi SC, Pui CH, Hancock ML, et al. Heterogeneity of hyperdiploid (51–67) childhood acute lymphoblastic leukemia. *Leukemia* 1996;10(2):213–224.

191. Trueworthy R, Shuster J, Look T, et al. Ploidy of lymphoblasts is the strongest predictor of treatment outcome in B-progenitor cell acute lymphoblastic leukemia of childhood: a Pediatric Oncology Group study. *J Clin Oncol* 1992; 10(4):606–613.

192. Pui CH, Raimondi SC, Dodge RK, et al. Prognostic importance of structural chromosomal abnormalities in children with hyperdiploid (greater than 50 chromosomes) acute lymphoblastic leukemia. *Blood* 1989;73(7):1963–1967.

193. Pui CH, Carroll AJ, Head D, et al. Near-triploid and near-tetraploid acute lymphoblastic leukemia of childhood. *Blood* 1990;76(3):590–596.

194. Raimondi SC, Roberson PK, Pui CH, et al. Hyperdiploid (47–50) acute lymphoblastic leukemia in children. *Blood* 1992;79(12):3245–3252.

195. Pui CH, Carroll AJ, Raimondi SC, et al. Clinical presentation, karyotypic characterization, and treatment outcome of childhood acute lymphoblastic leukemia with a near-haploid or hypodiploid less than 45 line. *Blood* 1990; 75(5):1170–1177.

196. Stark B, Jeison M, Gobuzov R, et al. Near haploid childhood acute lymphoblastic leukemia masked by hyperdiploid line: detection by fluorescence in situ hybridization. *Cancer Genet Cytogenet* 2001;128(2):108–113.

197. Rubnitz JE, Downing JR, Pui CH, et al. TEL gene rearrangement in acute lymphoblastic leukemia: a new genetic marker with prognostic significance. *J Clin Oncol* 1997;15(3):1150–1157.

198. Rubnitz JE, Shuster JJ, Land VJ, et al. Case-control study suggests a favorable impact of TEL rearrangement in patients with B-lineage acute lymphoblastic leukemia treated with antimetabolite-based therapy: a Pediatric Oncology Group study. *Blood* 1997;89(4):1143–1146.

199. Golub TR, McLean T, Stegmaier K, et al. The TEL gene and human leukemia. *Biochim Biophys Acta* 1996;1288(1):M7–M10.

200. Raynaud S, Cave H, Baens M, et al. The 12;21 translocation involving TEL and deletion of the other TEL allele: two frequently associated alterations found in childhood acute lymphoblastic leukemia. *Blood* 1996;87(7):2891–2899.

201. Rubnitz JE, Pui CH, Downing JR. The role of TEL fusion genes in pediatric leukemias. *Leukemia* 1999;13(1):6–13.

202. Busson-Le Coniat M, Nguyen Khac F, Daniel MT, et al. Chromosome 21 abnormalities with AML1 amplification in acute lymphoblastic leukemia. *Genes Chromosomes Cancer* 2001;32(3):244–249.

203. Pui CH, Raimondi SC, Hancock ML, et al. Immunologic, cytogenetic, and clinical characterization of childhood acute lymphoblastic leukemia with the t(1;19) (q23; p13) or its derivative. *J Clin Oncol* 1994;12(12):2601–2606.

204. Mellentin JD, Smith SD, Cleary ML. lyl-1, a novel gene altered by chromosomal translocation in T cell leukemia, codes for a protein with a helix-loop-helix DNA binding motif. *Cell* 1989;58(1):77–83.

205. Uckun FM, Sensel MG, Sather HN, et al. Clinical significance of translocation t(1;19) in childhood acute lymphoblastic leukemia in the context of contemporary therapies: a report from the Children's *Cancer* Group. *J Clin Oncol* 1998;16(2):527–535.

206. Raimondi SC, Privitera E, Williams DL, et al. New recurring chromosomal translocations in childhood acute lymphoblastic leukemia. *Blood* 1991;77(9):2016–2022.

207. Inaba T, Inukai T, Yoshihara T, et al. Reversal of apoptosis by the leukaemia-associated E2A-HLF chimaeric transcription factor. *Nature* 1996;382(6591):541–544.

208. Manolov G, Manolova Y. Marker band in one chromosome 14 from Burkitt lymphomas. *Nature* 1972;237(5349):33–34.

209. Lange BJ, Raimondi SC, Heerema N, et al. Pediatric leukemia/lymphoma with t(8;14)(q24;q11). *Leukemia* 1992;6(7):613–618.

210. Navid F, Mosijczuk AD, Head DR, et al. Acute lymphoblastic leukemia with the (8;14)(q24;q32) translocation and FAB L3 morphology associated with a B-precursor immunophenotype: the Pediatric Oncology Group experience. *Leukemia* 1999;13(1):135–141.

211. Loh ML, Samson Y, Motte E, et al. Translocation (2;8)(p12;q24) associated with a cryptic t(12;21)(p13;q22) TEL/AML1 gene rearrangement in a child with acute lymphoblastic leukemia. *Cancer Genet Cytogenet* 2000;122(2):79–82.

212. van Biervliet JP, van Hemel J, Geurts K, et al. Letter: Philadelphia chromosome in acute lymphocytic leukaemia. *Lancet* 1975;2(7935):617.

213. Ribeiro RC, Abromowitch M, Raimondi SC, et al. Clinical and biologic hallmarks of the Philadelphia chromosome in childhood acute lymphoblastic leukemia. *Blood* 1987;70(4):948–953.

214. Crist W, Carroll A, Shuster J, et al. Philadelphia chromosome positive childhood acute lymphoblastic leukemia: clinical and cytogenetic characteristics and treatment outcome. A Pediatric Oncology Group study. *Blood* 1990; 76 (3):489–494.

215. Faderl S, Kantarjian HM, Talpaz M, Estrov Z. Clinical significance of cytogenetic abnormalities in adult acute lymphoblastic leukemia. *Blood* 1998;91 (11):3995–4019.

216. Hilden JM, Kersey JH. The MLL (11q23) and AF-4 (4q21) genes disrupted in t(4;11) acute leukemia: molecular and clinical studies. *Leuk Lymphoma* 1994;14 (3–4):189–195.

217. Borkhardt A, Repp R, Schlieben S. Molecular genetics detection of chromosomal abnormalities at 11q23 in patients with de novo and secondary acute leukemia. In: Buchner T, Hiddemann W, eds. *Acute leukemia. VI. Prognostic factors and treatment strategies.* New York: Springer Verlag, 1997:107–110.

218. Uckun FM, Herman-Hatten K, Crotty ML, et al. Clinical significance of MLL-AF4 fusion transcript expression in the absence of a cytogenetically detectable t(4;11)(q21;q23) chromosomal translocation. *Blood* 1998;92(3):810–821.

219. Rubnitz JE, Behm FG, Curcio-Brint AM, et al. Molecular analysis of t(11;19) breakpoints in childhood acute leukemias. *Blood* 1996;87(11):4804–4808.

220. Borkhardt A, Repp R, Haas OA, et al. Cloning and characterization of AFX, the gene that fuses to MLL in acute leukemias with a t(X;11)(q13;q23). *Oncogene* 1997;14(2):195–202.

221. Raimondi SC, Frestedt JL, Pui CH, et al. Acute lymphoblastic leukemias with deletion of 11q23 or a novel inversion (11)(p13q23) lack MLL gene rearrangements and have favorable clinical features. *Blood* 1995;86(5):1881–1886.

222. Meeker TC, Hardy D, Willman C, et al. Activation of the interleukin-3 gene by chromosome translocation in acute lymphocytic leukemia with eosinophilia. [see comments]. *Blood* 1990;76(2):285–289.

223. Heerema NA, Arthur DC, Sather H, et al. Cytogenetic features of infants less than 12 months of age at diagnosis of acute lymphoblastic leukemia: impact of the 11q23 breakpoint on outcome: a report of the Childrens Cancer Group. *Blood* 1994;83(8):2274–2284.

224. Behrendt H, Charrin C, Gibbons B, et al. Dicentric (9;12) in acute lymphocytic leukemia and other hematological malignancies: report from a dic(9;12) study group. *Leukemia* 1995;9(1):102–106.

225. Slater R, Smit E, Kroes W, et al. A non-random chromosome abnormality found in precursor-B lineage acute lymphoblastic leukaemia: dic(9;20)(p1?3;q11). *Leukemia* 1995;9(10):1613–1619.

226. Heerema NA, Maben KD, Bernstein J, et al. Dicentric (9;20)(p11;q11) identified by fluorescence in situ hybridization in four pediatric acute lymphoblastic leukemia patients. *Cancer Genet Cytogenet* 1996;92(2):111–115.

227. Raimondi SC, Behm FG, Roberson PK, et al. Cytogenetics of childhood T-cell leukemia. *Blood* 1988;72(5):1560–1566.

228. Heerema NA, Sather HN, Sensel MG, et al. Frequency and clinical significance of cytogenetic abnormalities in pediatric T-lineage acute lymphoblastic leukemia: a report from the Children's Cancer Group. *J Clin Oncol* 1998;16 (4):1270–1278.

229. McKeithan TW, Shima EA, Le Beau MM, et al. Molecular cloning of the breakpoint junction of a human chromosomal 8;14 translocation involving the T-cell receptor alpha-chain gene and sequences on the 3' side of MYC. *Proc Natl Acad Sci U S A* 1986;83(17):6636–6640.

230. Hwang LY, Baer RJ. The role of chromosome translocations in T cell acute leukemia. *Curr Opin Immunol* 1995;7(5):659–664.

231. Begley CG, Green AR. The SCL gene: from case report to critical hematopoietic regulator. *Blood* 1999;93(9):2760–2770.

232. Ellisen LW, Bird J, West DC, et al. TAN-1, the human homolog of the Drosophila notch gene, is broken by chromosomal translocations in T lymphoblastic neoplasms. *Cell* 1991;66(4):649–661.

233. Chilcote RR, Brown E, Rowley JD. Lymphoblastic leukemia with lymphomatous features associated with abnormalities of the short arm of chromosome 9. *N Engl J Med* 1985;313(5):286–291.

234. Okuda T, Shurtleff SA, Valentine MB, et al. Frequent deletion of p16INK4a/MTS1 and p15INK4b/MTS2 in pediatric acute lymphoblastic leukemia. *Blood* 1995;85(9):2321–2330.

235. Drexler HG. Review of alterations of the cyclin-dependent kinase inhibitor INK4 family genes p15, p16, p18 and p19 in human leukemia-lymphoma cells. *Leukemia* 1998;12(6):845–859.

236. Maloney KW, McGavran L, Odom LF, Hunger SP. Acquisition of p16(INK4A) and p15(INK4B) gene abnormalities between initial diagnosis and relapse in children with acute lymphoblastic leukemia. *Blood* 1999;93 (7):2380–2385.

237. Aissani B, Bonan C, Baccichet A, Sinnett D. Childhood acute lymphoblastic leukemia: is there a tumor suppressor gene in chromosome 12p12.3? *Leuk Lymphoma* 1999;34(3–4):231–239.

238. Stegmaier K, Pendse S, Barker GF, et al. Frequent loss of heterozygosity at the TEL gene locus in acute lymphoblastic leukemia of childhood. *Blood* 1995;86(1):38–44.

239. Komuro H, Valentine MB, Rubnitz JE, et al. p27KIP1 deletions in childhood acute lymphoblastic leukemia. *Neoplasia* 1999;1(3):253–261.

240. Kantarjian HM, Talpaz M, Dhingra K, et al. Significance of the P210 versus P190 molecular abnormalities in adults with Philadelphia chromosome-positive acute leukemia. *Blood* 1991;78(9):2411–2418.

241. Rieder H, Ludwig WD, Gassmann W, et al. Prognostic significance of additional chromosome abnormalities in adult patients with Philadelphia chromosome positive acute lymphoblastic leukaemia. *Br J Haematol* 1996;95(4): 678–691.

242. Cytogenetic abnormalities in adult acute lymphoblastic leukemia: correlations with hematologic findings outcome. A Collaborative Study of the Group Francais de Cytogenetique Hematologique. [erratum appears in *Blood* 1996;88(7):2818]. *Blood* 1996;87(8):3135–3142.

243. Secker-Walker LM, Prentice HG, Durrant J, et al. Cytogenetics adds independent prognostic information in adults with acute lymphoblastic leukaemia on MRC trial UKALL XA. MRC Adult Leukaemia Working Party. [see comments]. *Br J Haematol* 1997;96(3):601–610.

244. Wong IH, Ng MH, Huang DP, Lee JC. Aberrant p15 promoter methylation in adult and childhood acute leukemias of nearly all morphologic subtypes: potential prognostic implications. [see comments]. *Blood* 2000;95(6):1942–1949.

245. Fishel RS, Farnen JP, Hanson CA, et al. Acute lymphoblastic leukemia with eosinophilia. *Medicine* 1990;69(4):232–243.

246. Kramer MH, Raghoebier S, Beverstock GC, et al. De novo acute B-cell leukemia with translocation t(14;18): an entity with a poor prognosis. *Leukemia* 1991;5(6):473–478.

247. Stock W, Westbrook CA, Sher DA, et al. Low incidence of TAL1 gene rearrangements in adult acute lymphoblastic leukemia: A cancer and leukemia group B study (8762). *Clin Cancer Res* 1995;1(4):459–463.

248. Gerard-Marchant R. [Current nosologic concepts in malignant non-Hodgkin lymphomas]. *Ann Anat Pathol (Paris)* 1974;19(2):149–162.

249. Stansfeld AG, Diebold J, Noel H, et al. Updated Kiel classification for lymphomas. [erratum appears in *Lancet* 1988 Feb 13;1(8581):372]. *Lancet* 1988; 1(8580):292–293.

250. Harris NL, Jaffe ES, Stein H, et al. A revised European-American classification of lymphoid neoplasms: a proposal from the International Lymphoma Study Group. [see comments]. *Blood* 1994;84(5):1361–1392.

251. Willis TG, Dyer MJ. The role of immunoglobulin translocations in the pathogenesis of B-cell malignancies. *Blood* 2000;96(3):808–822.

252. Chaganti RS, Nanjangud G, Schmidt H, Teruya-Feldstein J. Recurring chromosomal abnormalities in non-Hodgkin's lymphoma: biologic and clinical significance. *Semin Hematol* 2000;37(4):396–411.

253. Tamura A, Miura I, Iida S, et al. Interphase detection of immunoglobulin heavy chain gene translocations with specific oncogene loci in 173 patients with B-cell lymphoma. *Cancer Genet Cytogenet* 2001;129(1):1–9.

254. Haluska FG, Tsujimoto Y, Croce CM. Oncogene activation by chromosome translocation in human malignancy. *Annu Rev Genet* 1987;21:321–345.

255. Han S, Dillon SR, Zheng B, et al. V(D)J recombinase activity in a subset of germinal center B lymphocytes. *Science* 1997;278(5336):301–305.

256. Crossen PE. Genes and chromosomes in chronic B-cell leukemia. *Cancer Genet Cytogenet* 1997;94(1):44–51.

257. Juliusson G, Merup M. Cytogenetics in chronic lymphocytic leukemia. *Semin Oncol* 1998;25(1):19–26.

258. Dohner H, Stilgenbauer S, Dohner K, et al. Chromosome aberrations in B-cell chronic lymphocytic leukemia: reassessment based on molecular cytogenetic analysis. *J Mol Med* 1999;77(2):266–281.

259. Garcia-Marco J, Matutes E, Morilla R, et al. Trisomy 12 in B-cell chronic lymphocytic leukaemia: assessment of lineage restriction by simultaneous analysis of immunophenotype and genotype in interphase cells by fluorescence in situ hybridization. *Br J Haematol* 1994;87(1):44–50.

260. Matutes E, Oscier D, Garcia-Marco J, et al. Trisomy 12 defines a group of CLL with atypical morphology: correlation between cytogenetic, clinical and laboratory features in 544 patients. *Br J Haematol* 1996;92(2):382–388.

261. Hawthorn LA, Chapman R, Oscier D, Cowell JK. The consistent 13q14 translocation breakpoint seen in chronic B-cell leukaemia (BCLL) involves deletion of the D13S25 locus which lies distal to the retinoblastoma predisposition gene. *Oncogene* 1993;8(6):1415–1419.

262. Liu Y, Corcoran M, Rasool O, et al. Cloning of two candidate tumor suppressor genes within a 10 kb region on chromosome 13q14, frequently deleted in chronic lymphocytic leukemia. *Oncogene* 1997;15(20):2463–2473.

263. Juliusson G, Oscier DG, Fitchett M, et al. Prognostic subgroups in B-cell chronic lymphocytic leukemia defined by specific chromosomal abnormalities. *N Engl J Med* 1990;323(11):720–724.

264. Dohner H, Stilgenbauer S, James MR, et al. 11q deletions identify a new subset of B-cell chronic lymphocytic leukemia characterized by extensive nodal involvement and inferior prognosis. *Blood* 1997;89(7):2516–2522.

265. Shaw GR, Kronberger DL. TP53 deletions but not trisomy 12 are adverse in B-cell lymphoproliferative disorders. *Cancer Genet Cytogenet* 2000;119(2):146–154.

266. Dohner H, Stilgenbauer S, Benner A, et al. Genomic aberrations and survival in chronic lymphocytic leukemia. *N Engl J Med* 2000;343(26):1910–1916.

267. Michaux L, Dierlamm J, Wlodarska I, et al. t(14;19)/BCL3 rearrangements in lymphoproliferative disorders: a review of 23 cases. *Cancer Genet Cytogenet* 1997;94(1):36–43.

268. Cuneo A, Balboni M, Piva N, et al. Atypical chronic lymphocytic leukaemia with t(11;14)(q13;q32): karyotype evolution and prolymphocytic transformation. *Br J Haematol* 1995;90(2):409–416.

269. McKeithan TW, Rowley JD, Shows TB, Diaz MO. Cloning of the chromosome translocation breakpoint junction of the t(14;19) in chronic lymphocytic leukemia. *Proc Natl Acad Sci U S A* 1987;84(24):9257–9260.

270. Bosch F, Jares P, Campo E, et al. PRAD-1/cyclin D1 gene overexpression in chronic lymphoproliferative disorders: a highly specific marker of mantle cell lymphoma. *Blood* 1994;84(8):2726–2732.

271. Brito-Babapulle V, Pittman S, Melo JV, et al. Cytogenetic studies on prolymphocytic leukemia. 1. B-cell prolymphocytic leukemia. *Hematol Pathol* 1987;1(1):27–33.

272. Lens D, Matutes E, Catovsky D, Coignet LJ. Frequent deletions at 11q23 and 13q14 in B cell prolymphocytic leukemia (B-PLL). *Leukemia* 2000;14(3):427–430.

273. Hernandez JM, Gutierrez NC, Almeida J, et al. IL-4 improves the detection of cytogenetic abnormalities in multiple myeloma and increases the proportion of clonally abnormal metaphases. *Br J Haematol* 1998;103(1):163–167.

274. Drach J, Schuster J, Nowotny H, et al. Multiple myeloma: high incidence of chromosomal aneuploidy as detected by interphase fluorescence in situ hybridization. *Cancer Res* 1995;55(17):3854–3859.

275. Tabernero D, San Miguel JF, Garcia-Sanz M, et al. Incidence of chromosome numeric changes in multiple myeloma: fluorescence in situ hybridization analysis using 15 chromosome-specific probes. *Am J Pathol* 1996;149(1):153–161.

276. Nishida K, Tamura A, Nakazawa N, et al. The Ig heavy chain gene is frequently involved in chromosomal translocations in multiple myeloma and plasma cell leukemia as detected by in situ hybridization. *Blood* 1997;90(2):526–534.

277. Kuipers J, Vaandrager JW, Weghuis DO, et al. Fluorescence in situ hybridization analysis shows the frequent occurrence of 14q32.3 rearrangements with involvement of immunoglobulin switch regions in myeloma cell lines. *Cancer Genet Cytogenet* 1999;109(2):99–107.

278. Avet-Loiseau H, Brigaudeau C, Morineau N, et al. High incidence of cryptic translocations involving the Ig heavy chain gene in multiple myeloma, as shown by fluorescence in situ hybridization. *Genes Chromosomes Cancer* 1999;24(1):9–15.

279. Iida S, Rao PH, Butler M, et al. Deregulation of MUM1/IRF4 by chromosomal translocation in multiple myeloma. *Nat Genet* 1997;17(2):226–230.

280. Chesi M, Bergsagel PL, Shonukan OO, et al. Frequent dysregulation of the c-maf proto-oncogene at 16q23 by translocation to an Ig locus in multiple myeloma. *Blood* 1998;91(12):4457–4463.

281. Richelda R, Ronchetti D, Baldini L, et al. A novel chromosomal translocation t(4;14)(p16.3;q32) in multiple myeloma involves the fibroblast growth-factor receptor 3 gene. *Blood* 1997;90(10):4062–4070.

282. Chesi M, Nardini E, Lim RS, et al. The t(4;14) translocation in myeloma dysregulates both FGFR3 and a novel gene, MMSET, resulting in IgH/MMSET hybrid transcripts. *Blood* 1998;92(9):3025–3034.

283. Malgeri U, Baldini L, Perfetti V, et al. Detection of t(4;14)(p16.3;q32) chromosomal translocation in multiple myeloma by reverse transcription-polymerase chain reaction analysis of IGH-MMSET fusion transcripts. *Cancer Res* 2000;60(15):4058–4061.

284. Tricot G, Barlogie B, Jagannath S, et al. Poor prognosis in multiple myeloma is associated only with partial or complete deletions of chromosome 13 or abnormalities involving 11q and not with other karyotype abnormalities. *Blood* 1995;86(11):4250–4256.

285. Ronchetti D, Finelli P, Richelda R, et al. Molecular analysis of 11q13 breakpoints in multiple myeloma. *Blood* 1999;93(4):1330–1337.

286. Tricot G, Sawyer JR, Jagannath S, et al. Unique role of cytogenetics in the prognosis of patients with myeloma receiving high-dose therapy and autotransplants. *J Clin Oncol* 1997;15(7):2659–2666.

287. Seong C, Delasalle K, Hayes K, et al. Prognostic value of cytogenetics in multiple myeloma. *Br J Haematol* 1998;101(1):189–194.

288. Perez-Simon JA, Garcia-Sanz R, Tabernero MD, et al. Prognostic value of numeric chromosome aberrations in multiple myeloma: A FISH analysis of 15 different chromosomes. *Blood* 1998;91(9):3366–3371.

289. Zojer N, Konigsberg R, Ackermann J, et al. Deletion of 13q14 remains an independent adverse prognostic variable in multiple myeloma despite its frequent detection by interphase fluorescence in situ hybridization. *Blood* 2000;95(6):1925–1930.

290. Haglund U, Juliusson G, Stellan B, et al. Hairy cell leukemia is characterized by clonal chromosome abnormalities clustered to specific regions. *Blood* 1994;83(9):2637–2645.

291. Dierlamm J, Stefanova M, Wlodarska I, et al. Chromosomal gains and losses are uncommon in hairy cell leukemia: a study based on comparative genomic hybridization and interphase fluorescence in situ hybridization. *Cancer Genet Cytogenet* 2001;128(2):164–167.

292. Iida S, Rao PH, Ueda R, et al. Chromosomal rearrangement of the PAX-5 locus in lymphoplasmacytic lymphoma with t(9;14)(p13;q32). *Leuk Lymphoma* 1999;34(1–2):25–33.

293. Rosenwald A, Ott G, Stilgenbauer S, et al. Exclusive detection of the t(11;18)(q21;q21) in extranodal marginal zone B cell lymphomas (MZBL) of MALT type in contrast to other MZBL and extranodal large B cell lymphomas. *Am J Pathol* 1999;155(6):1817–1821.

294. Dierlamm J, Baens M, Wlodarska I, et al. The apoptosis inhibitor gene API2 and a novel 18q gene, MLT, are recurrently rearranged in the t(11;18)(q21;q21)p6ssociated with mucosa-associated lymphoid tissue lymphomas. *Blood* 1999;93(11):3601–3609.

295. Willis TG, Jadayel DM, Du MQ, et al. Bcl10 is involved in t(1;14)(p22;q32) of MALT B cell lymphoma and mutated in multiple tumor types. *Cell* 1999;96(1):35–45.

296. Zhang Q, Siebert R, Yan M, et al. Inactivating mutations and overexpression of BCL10, a caspase recruitment domain-containing gene, in MALT lymphoma with t(1;14)(p22;q32). *Nat Genet* 1999;22(1):63–68.

297. Dyer MJ. Bcl10 mutations in malignancy. *Br J Cancer* 1999;80(10):1491.

298. Fakruddin JM, Chaganti RS, Murty VV. Lack of BCL10 mutations in germ cell tumors and B cell lymphomas. *Cell* 1999;97(6):683–4; discussion 686–688.

299. Dierlamm J, Wlodarska I, Michaux L, et al. Genetic abnormalities in marginal zone B-cell lymphoma. *Hematol Oncol* 2000;18(1):1–13.

300. Ott G, Katzenberger T, Greiner A, et al. The t(11;18)(q21;q21) chromosome translocation is a frequent and specific aberration in low-grade but not high-grade malignant non-Hodgkin's lymphomas of the mucosa-associated lymphoid tissue (MALT-) type. *Cancer Res* 1997;57(18):3944–3948.

301. Sole F, Woessner S, Florensa L, et al. Frequent involvement of chromosomes 1, 3, 7 and 8 in splenic marginal zone B-cell lymphoma. *Br J Haematol* 1997;98(2):446–449.

302. Mateo M, Mollejo M, Villuendas R, et al. 7q31-32 allelic loss is a frequent finding in splenic marginal zone lymphoma. *Am J Pathol* 1999;154(5):1583–1589.

303. Dierlamm J, Pittaluga S, Wlodarska I, et al. Marginal zone B-cell lymphomas of different sites share similar cytogenetic and morphologic features. *Blood* 1996;87(1):299–307.

304. Troussard X, Mauvieux L, Radford-Weiss I, et al. Genetic analysis of splenic lymphoma with villous lymphocytes: a Groupe Francais d'Hematologie Cellulaire (GFHC) study. *Br J Haematol* 1998;101(4):712–721.

305. Dierlamm J, Michaux L, Wlodarska I, et al. Trisomy 3 in marginal zone B-cell lymphoma: a study based on cytogenetic analysis and fluorescence in situ hybridization. *Br J Haematol* 1996;93(1):242–249.

306. Knutsen T. Cytogenetic mechanisms in the pathogenesis and progression of follicular lymphoma. *Cancer Surv* 1997;30:163–192.

307. Horsman DE, Connors JM, Pantzar T, et al. Analysis of secondary chromosomal alterations in 165 cases of follicular lymphoma with t(14;18). *Genes Chromosomes Cancer* 2001;30(4):375–382.

308. Offit K, Parsa NZ, Gaidano G, et al. 6q deletions define distinct clinicopathologic subsets of non-Hodgkin's lymphoma. *Blood* 1993;82(7):2157–2162.

309. Karsan A, Gascoyne RD, Coupland RW, et al. Combination of t(14;18) and a Burkitt's type translocation in B-cell malignancies. *Leuk Lymphoma* 1993;10(6):433–441.

310. Yano T, Jaffe ES, Longo DL, et al. MYC rearrangements in histologically progressed follicular lymphomas. *Blood* 1992;80(3):758–767.

311. Ladanyi M, Offit K, Parsa NZ, et al. Follicular lymphoma with t(8;14)(q24;q32): a distinct clinical and molecular subset of t(8;14)-bearing lymphomas. *Blood* 1992;79(8):2124–2130.

312. Bastard C, Deweindt C, Kerckaert JP, et al. LAZ3 rearrangements in non-Hodgkin's lymphoma: correlation with histology, immunophenotype, karyotype, and clinical outcome in 217 patients. *Blood* 1994;83(9):2423–2427.

313. Wlodarska I, Mecucci C, Stul M, et al. Fluorescence in situ hybridization identifies new chromosomal changes involving 3q27 in non-Hodgkin's lymphomas with BCL6/LAZ3 rearrangement. *Genes Chromosomes Cancer* 1995;14(1):1–7.

314. Chaganti SR, Chen W, Parsa N, et al. Involvement of BCL6 in chromosomal aberrations affecting band 3q27 in B-cell non-Hodgkin lymphoma. *Genes Chromosomes Cancer* 1998;23(4):323–327.

315. Rosenberg CL, Wong E, Petty EM, et al. PRAD1, a candidate BCL1 oncogene: mapping and expression in centrocytic lymphoma. *Proc Natl Acad Sci U S A* 1991;88(21):9638–9642.

316. Cuneo A, Bigoni R, Rigolin GM, et al. Cytogenetic profile of lymphoma of follicle mantle lineage: correlation with clinicobiologic features. *Blood* 1999;93(4):1372–1380.

317. Bentz M, Plesch A, Bullinger L, et al. t(11;14)-positive mantle cell lymphomas exhibit complex karyotypes and share similarities with B-cell chronic lymphocytic leukemia. *Genes Chromosomes Cancer* 2000;27(3):285–294.

318. Chaganti SR, Rao PH, Chen W, et al. Deregulation of BCL6 in non-Hodgkin lymphoma by insertion of IGH sequences in complex translocations involving band 3q27. *Genes Chromosomes Cancer* 1998;23(4):328–336.

319. Cigudosa JC, Parsa NZ, Louie DC, et al. Cytogenetic analysis of 363 consecutively ascertained diffuse large B-cell lymphomas. *Genes Chromosomes Cancer* 1999;25(2):123–133.

320. Pelicci PG, Knowles DM II, Magrath I, et al. Chromosomal breakpoints and structural alterations of the c-myc locus differ in endemic and sporadic forms of Burkitt lymphoma. *Proc Natl Acad Sci U S A* 1986;83(9):2984–2988.

321. Sandlund JT, Pui CH, Roberts WM, et al. Clinicopathologic features and treatment outcome of children with large-cell lymphoma and the t(2;5)(p23;q35). *Blood* 1994;84(8):2467–2471.

322. Morris SW, Kirstein MN, Valentine MB, et al. Fusion of a kinase gene, ALK, to a nucleolar protein gene, NPM, in non-Hodgkin's lymphoma. *Science* 1994;263(5151):1281–1284.

323. Pulford K, Lamant L, Morris SW, et al. Detection of anaplastic lymphoma kinase (ALK) and nucleolar protein nucleophosmin (NPM)-ALK proteins in normal and neoplastic cells with the monoclonal antibody ALK1. *Blood* 1997;89(4):1394–1404.

324. Hutchison RE, Banki K, Shuster JJ, et al. Use of an anti-ALK antibody in the characterization of anaplastic large-cell lymphoma of childhood. *Ann Oncol* 1997;8(Suppl 1):37–42.

325. Benharroch D, Meguerian-Bedoyan Z, Lamant L, et al. ALK-positive lymphoma: a single disease with a broad spectrum of morphology. *Blood* 1998;91(6):2076–2084.

326. Falini B, Pileri S, Zinzani PL, et al. ALK+ lymphoma: clinico-pathological findings and outcome. *Blood* 1999;93(8):2697–2706.

327. Colleoni GW, Bridge JA, Garicochea B, et al. ATIC-ALK: A novel variant ALK gene fusion in anaplastic large cell lymphoma resulting from the recurrent cryptic chromosomal inversion, inv(2)(p23q35). *Am J Pathol* 2000;156(3):781–789.

328. Gascoyne RD, Aoun P, Wu D, et al. Prognostic significance of anaplastic lymphoma kinase (ALK) protein expression in adults with anaplastic large cell lymphoma. *Blood* 1999;93(11):3913–3921.

329. Maljaei SH, Brito-Babapulle V, Hiorns LR, et al. Abnormalities of chromosomes 8, 11, 14, and X in T-prolymphocytic leukemia studied by fluorescence in situ hybridization. *Cancer Genet Cytogenet* 1998;103(2):110–116.

330. Hetet G, Dastot H, Baens M, et al. Recurrent molecular deletion of the 12p13 region, centromeric to ETV6/TEL, in T-cell prolymphocytic leukemia. *Hematol J* 2000;1:42–47.

331. Vorechovsky I, Luo L, Dyer MJ, et al. Clustering of missense mutations in the ataxia-telangiectasia gene in a sporadic T-cell leukaemia. *Nat Genet* 1997;17(1):96–99.

332. Yuille MA, Coignet LJ, Abraham SM, et al. ATM is usually rearranged in T-cell prolymphocytic leukaemia. *Oncogene* 1998;16(6):789–796.

333. Wong KF, Zhang YM, Chan JK. Cytogenetic abnormalities in natural killer cell lymphoma/leukaemia—is there a consistent pattern? *Leuk Lymphoma* 1999;34(3–4):241–250.

334. Kamada N, Sakurai M, Miyamoto K, et al. Chromosome abnormalities in adult T-cell leukemia/lymphoma: a karyotype review committee report. *Cancer Res* 1992;52(6):1481–1493.

335. Jonveaux P, Daniel MT, Martel V, et al. Isochromosome 7q and trisomy 8 are consistent primary, non-random chromosomal abnormalities associated with hepatosplenic T gamma/delta lymphoma. *Leukemia* 1996;10(9):1453–1455.

336. Coventry S, Punnett HH, Tomczak EZ, et al. Consistency of isochromosome 7q and trisomy 8 in hepatosplenic gammadelta T-cell lymphoma: detection by fluorescence in situ hybridization of a splenic touch-preparation from a pediatric patient. *Pediatr Dev Pathol* 1999;2(5):478–483.

337. Thangavelu M, Finn WG, Yelavarthi KK, et al. Recurring structural chromosome abnormalities in peripheral blood lymphocytes of patients with mycosis fungoides/Sezary syndrome. *Blood* 1997;89(9):3371–3377.

338. Schlegelberger B, Himmler A, Godde E, et al. Cytogenetic findings in peripheral T-cell lymphomas as a basis for distinguishing low-grade and high-grade lymphomas. *Blood* 1994;83(2):505–511.

339. Lepretre S, Buchonnet G, Stamatoullas A, et al. Chromosome abnormalities in peripheral T-cell lymphoma. *Cancer Genet Cytogenet* 2000;117(1):71–79.

340. Heim S, Mitelman F. Cytogenetically unrelated clones in hematological neoplasms. *Leukemia* 1989;3(1):6–8.

341. Schlegelberger B, Zhang Y, Weber-Matthiesen K, et al. Detection of aberrant clones in nearly all cases of angioimmunoblastic lymphadenopathy with dysproteinemia-type T-cell lymphoma by combined interphase and metaphase cytogenetics. *Blood* 1994;84(8):2640–2648.

342. Falzetti D, Crescenzi B, Matteuci C, et al. Genomic instability and recurrent breakpoints are main cytogenetic findings in Hodgkin's disease. *Haematologica* 1999;84(4):298–305.

343. Nolte M, Werner M, von Wasielewski R, et al. Detection of numeric karyotype changes in the giant cells of Hodgkin's lymphomas by a combination of FISH and immunohistochemistry applied to paraffin sections. *Histochem Cell Biol* 1996;105(5):401–404.

CHAPTER 6

Molecular Basis of Oncology

David J. Kwiatkowski

The development of a malignancy in the human occurs with rare exception as the culmination of a series of genetic and epigenetic events. These events, which include mutation, changes in expression, and, in many cases, loss of significant amounts of genetic material, typically occur during a substantial period of time and are usually completely unrecognizable by patient and physician until a full-blown carcinoma or other malignancy becomes evident. Human cancer development is characterized by broad themes but with specific molecular details, which are often tissue- and tumor-type specific. The vast amount of molecular information learned about cancer in the past 20 years, which continues to expand, can produce a state of bewilderment in the casual or novice reader. It sometimes appears as though nearly all of the approximately 30,000 genes in the genome participate in one way or another in cancer development. This overwhelming amount of molecular detail can both obscure the broad principles of malignant development and severely diminish the appetite of the reader who is initially interested in understanding cancer pathogenesis.

This chapter begins with a review of some of the critical experiments that laid the foundation for our current understanding of cancer development. This is done to introduce important concepts for all readers and to provide a familiar background for older readers seeking an update on this subject. Eight essential features of malignant pathogenesis (1) are then presented, which together explain the molecular basis of oncology. For each of these essential features important aspects are discussed, but we cannot be comprehensive in either subject material or literature references owing to space limitations. Normal physiology as well as the derangements that occur in malignant cells, and potential therapeutic avenues are considered. Throughout this chapter, the focus is on epithelial malignancies given their collective predominant importance to the public health of the North American population.

EARLY STUDIES ENABLING MOLECULAR ONCOLOGY AND THE DISCOVERY OF DOMINANT-ACTING ONCOGENES

The delineation of hallmark pathologic findings to distinguish normal tissues from malignant tissues was an early first step in our understanding of cancer that enabled subsequent molecular advances. The pathologic features recognizable in malignant tumors include the overall pattern of growth and

the appearance of individual tumor cells. Tumor cells generally have an increased nuclear/cytoplasmic ratio, clumping of chromatin, unusual mitotic figures, and major alterations in cytoplasmic organization and the contacts that occur between cells. They also display unordered growth that extends beyond normal tissue boundaries with invasion into other tissues and organs.

A major advance in our understanding of malignant development occurred when chromosome identification became possible through specialized preparative methods and staining techniques. This provided early insight into the genetic changes that occur in malignancies and had immediate relevance to the field of hematologic malignancies with the identification of the Philadelphia chromosome in samples from patients with chronic myeloid leukemia (2). Further extensive discussion of cytogenetics in hematology and oncology is given in Chapter 5.

Further analysis of cancer was greatly facilitated by the development of culture techniques, which enabled the study of cancer cells *in vitro* using methods of genetics, biochemistry, and cell biology. This was a critical step, as it provided a means to bypass the many limitations of studying cancer development *in vivo* either in patients or in animal model systems. Although this was a critical advance, the analysis of cells in tissue culture has profound limitations that have taken years of study to illuminate and may yet confound some of our understanding of cancer pathogenesis. For example, when malignant cells are cultured, typical survival rates are on the order of 1 in 1000 to 1 in 1,000,000 cells. Thus, most malignant cells die in the process, and an extremely selective pressure to adapt to tissue culture conditions is enforced. The consequences of this selection are often a distorted picture of the characteristics of malignant cells.

A major discovery based on the use of genetics and cultured cancer cells was the identification of ras, the first human oncogene (3). Although several oncogenes had been identified earlier in oncogenic viruses of animals, this was a major breakthrough in our understanding of human cancer pathogenesis. Transfer of an activated ras oncogene into the appropriate recipient cell (a cultured mouse fibroblast) converts that cell from a relatively benign state to a so-called transformed state. The *transformed state* means that the cell no longer requires the same concentration of serum or specific growth factors to grow, can grow to a higher culture density, and can grow up into a colony from one or a few cells within an agarose gel on the tissue culture plate.

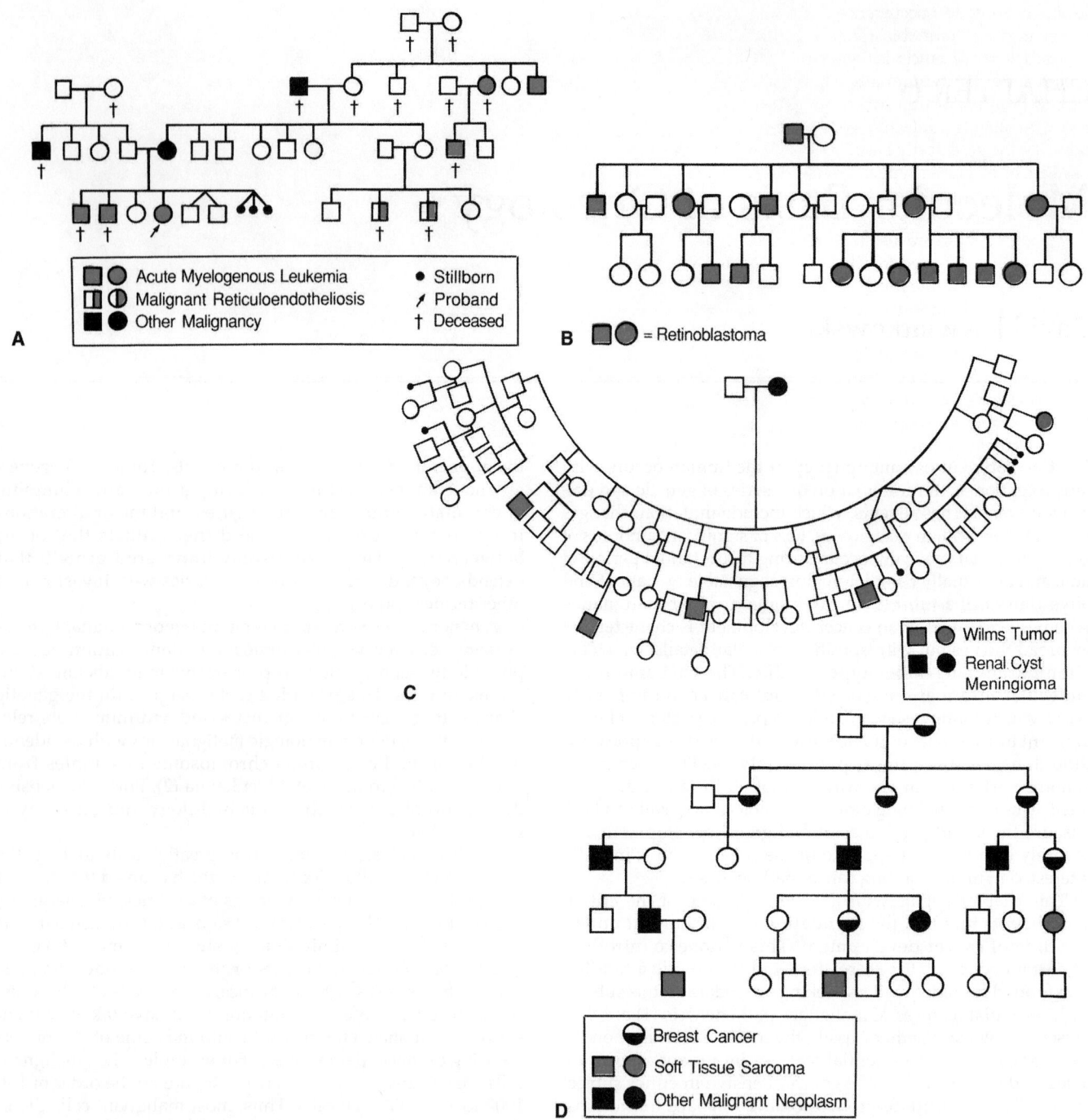

Figure 6-1. Examples of "cancer families." Pedigrees are shown for families with a high frequency of acute myelogenous leukemia **(A)**, retinoblastoma **(B)**, Wilms' tumor **(C)**, and breast and other cancers **(D)**.

Finally and most important, injection of transformed cells into nude mice will cause formation of a tumor.

CANCER FAMILIES AND THE DISCOVERY OF TUMOR-SUPPRESSOR GENES

Some of the earliest evidence for the importance of genetic factors in the pathogenesis of cancer was the delineation of families by astute clinicians in which cancer, usually restricted in distribution to one or a few organs, occurred at much higher rates than in the general population (4) (Fig. 6-1). These so-called cancer families have been identified for almost every type of cancer, although they are much more common for certain types than others. In some cases, these familial aggregations of cancer are likely to be due to shared environmental or dietary factors or even by chance alone. However, in many cases, the familial aggregation is so striking and occurs in a pattern consistent with autosomal-dominant inheritance that a genetic basis is strongly implicated.

Cancer families vary from one to another in several clinical respects (Fig. 6-1). First, in some cases, such as the hereditary nonpolyposis colorectal cancer syndrome, patients are predisposed to development of many different forms of cancer (including colorectal, gastric, and endometrial) that also occur relatively frequently in the general population. In other cancer families, cancer is limited in occurrence to a single rather unusual organ. For example, in retinoblastoma (Fig. 6-1B), the predominant site for occurrence of cancer is the retina, with an increase in osteosarcoma and other tumors much later in life. Secondly, the cancer risk in families of this sort may be as high as nearly 100% in those carrying the defective gene in some cases, whereas in other families, the genetically based risk is less than 10% (Fig. 6-1C). In families of this latter type, a genetic component may still be evident based on consideration of the rarity of the neoplasm in the general population (e.g., familial Wilms' tumor).

However, there are also features common to nearly all cancer families. First, affected family members will have multiple primary cancers at a rate much higher than that of the general population. Second, tumors will occur at an earlier age of onset than in the general population. Theoretical considerations, originally presented by Knudsen in 1971, led to the hypothesis that these observations could fit a model in which a single allele (or copy) of a gene was mutated in members of cancer families (5). Inheritance of this mutant copy would be transmitted in an autosomal-dominant pattern and could explain the accelerated rate of carcinogenesis, because this single mutation would place the individual one step further along the path toward cancer development than other individuals in the general population.

At approximately the same time as this work was proceeding, a series of studies using techniques of somatic cell genetics also explored the genetic basis of cancer. These studies nicely complemented the previously mentioned familial studies. The principal technique in somatic cell genetics is to fuse together two different types of cells in tissue culture and observe the characteristics of the resulting hybrids. Further, as hybrids are grown in tissue culture over time, they tend to lose components from each of the two genomes that were brought together, typically in the form of loss of an entire chromosome, and a correlation can be made between the characteristics of the hybrid derivatives and which parts of the two genomes that were originally put together are retained. This approach was used to investigate the basis of the malignant potential of cancer-derived cell lines. Henry Harris and associates observed that when highly malignant mouse cells were fused with normal mouse embryo cells, the resulting hybrids had a low malignant potential and would not form tumors when injected into mice (6). However, after tissue culture for multiple passages, clonal derivatives of the initial hybrids would regain full malignant potential. It was possible to correlate the malignant potential of the derived clones with which chromosomes were retained from the normal mouse embryo cells used in the original cell fusion. The conclusion was drawn that the presence of certain wild-type genes on normal chromosomes that had been introduced from the normal cells were able to block the malignant phenotype.

Such genes that can block the malignant phenotype are therefore called *tumor-suppressor genes*. Because the malignant phenotype could be suppressed by a single copy of a normal cellular gene, it was deduced that this characteristic was a recessive trait. Nearly all tumor cell lines are inhibited by hybrid formation with normal cells, suggesting that the loss of such tumor-suppressor genes is an essential pathogenic feature of nearly all tumors. Although it became possible to introduce single chromosomes and their fragments into malignant cells to refine the localization of potential tumor-suppressor genes, it proved difficult to use these methods to complete the final goal of gene identification.

In contrast, detailed analysis of cancer families, using techniques of genetic linkage analysis and complemented by steady progress in the development of genomic reagents for mapping and gene identification as part of the Human Genome Project, enabled the identification and characterization of a substantial number of tumor-suppressor genes (Table 6-1). We now review

TABLE 6-1. Tumor-Suppressor Genes

Gene Symbol	Syndrome	Cancer Types[a]
APC	Adenomatous polyposis coli	Colorectal, pancreatic, desmoid, hepatoblastoma
BRCA1	Familial breast/ovarian cancer	Breast, ovarian
BRCA2	Familial breast/ovarian cancer	Breast, ovarian, pancreatic, gallbladder, bile duct
CDH1	Familial gastric carcinoma	Gastric
CDKN2A	Familial melanoma	Melanoma
CYLD	Familial cylindromatosis	Cylindromas
EXT1	Multiple exostoses	Exostoses, osteosarcoma
EXT2	Multiple exostoses	Exostoses, osteosarcoma
CDKN1C	Beckwith-Wiedemann syndrome	Wilms' tumor, rhabdomyosarcoma
STK11	Peutz-Jeghers syndrome	Jejunal hamartomas, ovarian, testicular, pancreatic
MEN1	Multiple endocrine neoplasia type 1	Parathyroid/pituitary adenoma, islet cell, carcinoid tumors
MLH1	Familial nonpolyposis colorectal cancer	Colorectal, endometrial, ureter, small intestine
MSH2	Familial nonpolyposis colorectal cancer	Colorectal, endometrial, ureter, small intestine
MSH6	Familial nonpolyposis colorectal cancer	Colorectal, endometrial, ureter, small intestine
NF1	Neurofibromatosis type 1	Neurofibroma, glioma
NF2	Neurofibromatosis type 2	Meningioma, acoustic neuroma
PMS1	Familial nonpolyposis colorectal cancer	Colorectal, endometrial, ureter, small intestine
PMS2	Familial nonpolyposis colorectal cancer	Colorectal, endometrial, ureter, small intestine
PRKAR1A	Carney complex	Myxoma, endocrine tumors
PTCH	Nevoid basal cell carcinoma syndrome	Basal cell carcinoma, medulloblastoma
PTEN	Cowden disease	Hamartomas, glioma, prostate, endometrial, breast
RB1	Familial retinoblastoma	Retinoblastoma, sarcomas, breast, lung
RET	Multiple endocrine neoplasia type 2	Medullary thyroid, pheochromocytoma, parathyroid adenoma
SDHD	Familial paraganglioma	Paraganglioma
MADH4	Juvenile polyposis	Gastrointestinal polyps, colorectal, pancreatic
SMARCB1	Rhabdoid predisposition syndrome	Malignant rhabdoid tumors
P53	Li-Fraumeni syndrome	Sarcoma, adrenocortical, breast, glioma, leukemia
TSC1	Tuberous sclerosis	Hamartomas, renal cell
TSC2	Tuberous sclerosis	Hamartomas, renal cell
VHL	von Hippel-Lindau syndrome	Renal cell, hemangioma, pheochromocytoma
WT1	Familial Wilms' tumor	Wilms' tumor

[a]Organs listed are those where cancer develops, unless otherwise noted.

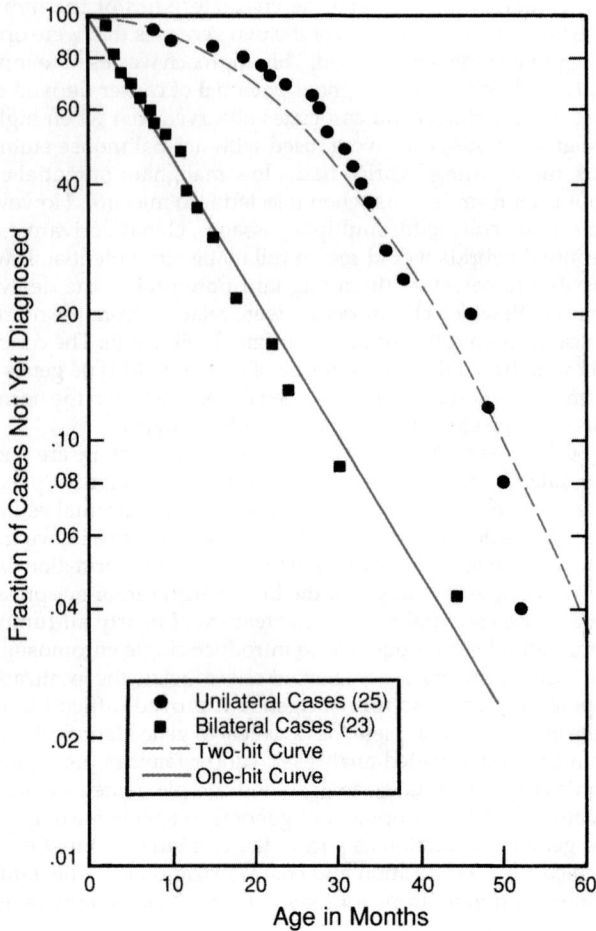

Figure 6-2. Comparison between the predicted and actual incidence of retinoblastoma using a two-hit model for unilateral cases and a one-hit model for bilateral cases. (Adapted from Knudson AG Jr. Mutation and cancer: statistical study of retinoblastoma. *Proc Natl Acad Sci U S A* 1971;68:820–823.)

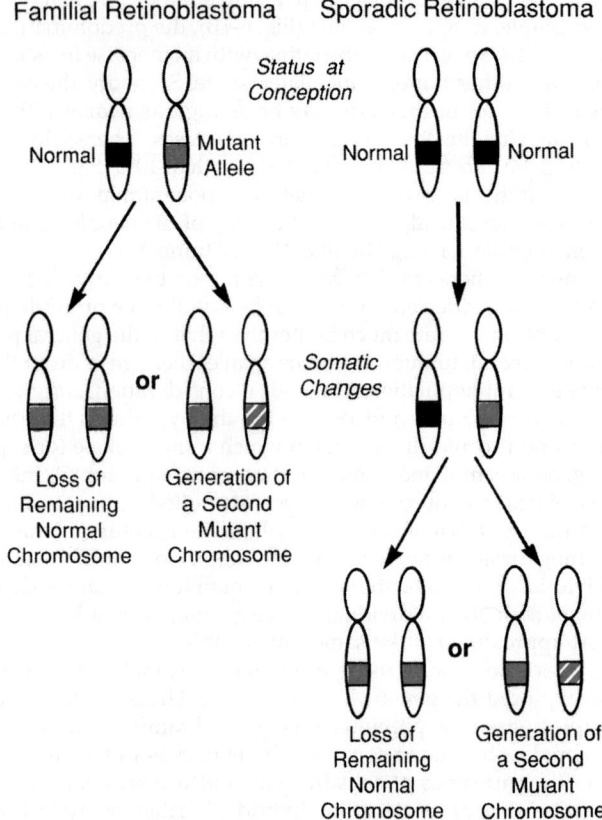

Figure 6-3. The two-hit model for development of retinoblastoma. Patients with familial retinoblastoma start with one mutant allele (the first hit) and require only one further change (the second hit) per cell to develop retinoblastoma. Patients with sporadic retinoblastoma must have two hits within the same cell, affecting both alleles, to inactivate both copies of the retinoblastoma gene.

the discovery of the first characterized tumor-suppressor gene, the retinoblastoma gene.

Retinoblastoma was the first tumor suspected to arise from the inactivation of a growth-suppressor gene. The incidence of retinoblastoma in the general population is less than 1 in 40,000, with a median age of onset of 3 years. Patients with hereditary retinoblastoma typically develop two to five tumors, counting both eyes, and have a younger age at diagnosis than patients with nonhereditary retinoblastoma. Long before the identification of the retinoblastoma gene and based on statistical analysis of the data on the frequency of occurrence of retinoblastoma in hereditary and sporadic cases, Knudson proposed a model in which sporadic retinoblastomas occurred as the result of two mutational events, and hereditary cases occurred as the result of a single mutational event (5) (Figs. 6-2 and 6-3). These calculations were, of course, in stark contrast to the situation with the development of the usual adult malignancies, in which a similar statistical analysis leads to a calculation that multiple (three to seven) mutational events are necessary for carcinogenesis.

Efforts to identify the retinoblastoma gene used two complementary approaches. First, retinoblastomas were analyzed by cytogenetics to look for chromosomal regions that were consistently deleted. These studies provided the insight that deletions of a small region of chromosome 13, band q14.1, were consistently seen in retinoblastomas (7). This led to the suspicion that in retinoblastomas, a germline mutational event

in one copy of the retinoblastoma gene on 13q14.1 was complemented by a second hit event in which loss of the second copy of the retinoblastoma gene on the other chromosome occurred. This second hit event would result in a loss of a substantial portion of chromosome 13q, which could be seen by cytogenetic methods.

Construction of a library of DNA fragments from chromosome 13 permitted identification of a set of DNA markers that could be used to identify *polymorphisms*, or random differences in the DNA sequence occurring naturally on chromosome 13. One such chromosome 13 fragment was found to be completely absent in several retinoblastomas. This observation suggested that this fragment was likely to be located close to the critical retinoblastoma gene that was deleted in both copies of chromosome 13 in these tumors. Further experiments were then performed to identify genes that were located near this particular DNA fragment. A sizable gene was discovered nearby that was expressed in normal retinal cells but was absent in some retinoblastomas. Further study indicated that small chromosomal deletions within this gene were also seen in some retinoblastoma samples and had occurred in the germline of some patients with hereditary retinoblastoma. The fact that such intragenic deletions could affect this gene and not any of the nearby genes suggested that it was the bona fide retinoblastoma gene (8). Further study confirmed the critical role of this gene in the pathogenesis of hereditary and sporadic retinoblastoma, and molecular studies have confirmed the important role of this gene and protein in normal cell cycle control.

INTRODUCTION TO THE HALLMARK FEATURES OF THE MALIGNANT CELL

In the following sections, we delineate seven hallmark features of the malignant cell (1). These are

1. Self-sufficiency in growth capacity
2. Cell cycle deregulation
3. Apoptosis evasion
4. Limitless replicative potential
5. Angiogenesis acquisition
6. Metastasis competence
7. Mutation aquisition and genome instability

Self-Sufficiency in Growth Capacity

Cancer cells have an acquired independence in growth capacity. This characteristic is in strong contrast to the requirement of normal cells for mitogenic growth signals to transit from a normal quiescent state into a state of active proliferation.

This critical difference between normal and cancer cells was first observed in some of the earliest experimental investigation into the basis of malignancy. Normal mesenchymal and epithelial cells require a proper surface and diffusible growth factors to be cultured *in vitro*. In many cases, tissue culture dishes must be coated with an extracellular matrix (ECM) constituent (e.g., fibronectin or collagen) to enable the growth of normal cells. In other cases, it has proven extremely difficult to get normal cells from some tissues to grow in culture, although continuing investigation has led to identification of growth factors that permit at least short-term cultures to be established. Fetal calf serum at concentrations of 10% to 20% is typically used to stimulate the growth of these cells, as it was found early on empirically to be the best growth stimulant, owing to the fact that it contains a relatively high concentration of multiple growth factors that can stimulate cell growth. Cancer cells are typically easier to grow than normal cells, though this is not always the case and may relate to the interaction between cancer cells and stromal cells (see further below). Nonetheless, most cancer cells can be cultured *in vitro* without special coating of culture dishes and at reduced concentrations of growth factors compared to normal cells. Indeed, a number of cancers regularly generate cultures in which the cells are only weakly adherent to the substratum, reflecting complex changes in the expression of cell surface proteins that mediate cell–substrate and cell–cell interaction.

This difference in growth capacity between cancer and normal cells was also one of the first features of the malignant cell to be defined at the molecular level by experimental means. Dominant oncogenes directly affect this growth capacity. As above, *ras* was the first dominant oncogene discovered and directly influences the growth self-sufficiency of a cultured fibroblast cell line, NIH3T3 cells. Further studies have defined a large number of genes whose protein products are elements of, or interact with, a central growth signaling pathway used by all cells (1, 9–12).

CENTRAL SIGNALING PATHWAY FOR REGULATION OF CELL GROWTH

Signaling, in the cellular context, is a term used to describe methods by which information is transmitted from one cellular compartment to another. In the case of growth control, for example, extracellular signals, such as growth factors, are capable of causing a cell to undergo cell division. There must be a mechanism for transmitting the growth signal from the cell exterior to the nucleus, where many events must take place to permit the final outcome of cell division.

Intensive study of the biochemical basis of this process, with a strong influence from work cataloguing and comparing the differences between normal and cancer cells, has led to the definition of a central or core growth signaling pathway, which runs from the cell exterior to the nucleus. One feature of this signaling pathway that makes its description complicated is that it is not a linear series of interacting proteins. Rather, there are multiple interactions, so-called cross-talk, at nearly every level (13). Another aspect of this pathway is that of redundancy. Many genes and proteins in the pathway are members of multigene families in which several genes produce products whose structures and functions are similar to varying degrees. Members of such families usually, but not always, have some unique property that helps to explain this partial redundancy.

GROWTH FACTORS AND THEIR RECEPTORS

Cells express a large number of surface proteins that can interact with external molecules, including soluble diffusible proteins, such as cytokines, and insoluble proteins making up the ECM. These surface proteins occur in several different types and include those proteins that form contacts with adjacent cells (including gap and tight junctions); integrins, which can bind to external ligands and have some signaling capability (14); and ion channels, which control the flux of electrolytes into and out of cells. A last and most important class of surface protein, from the point of view of this discussion, is growth factor receptors (Fig. 6-4A). Growth factor receptors consist of an extracellular domain, which is usually glycosylated (added sugar groups) and can bind to external ligands; a short transmembrane peptide domain, which consists of hydrophobic amino acids and serves to anchor the protein in a fixed position in the membrane; and an intracellular domain. Because growth factor receptors are confined to a single dimension (the surface) of the three-dimensional cell, they are often expressed at relatively low levels, less than 1000 receptors per cell.

Most growth factor receptors have an important property: When activated by growth factor binding externally, the intracellular domain acquires a property termed *intrinsic protein tyrosine kinase activity* (15). This means that the intracellular portion of the activated growth factor receptor has the ability to catalyze the transfer of a phosphate group from adenosine triphosphate (ATP) to the hydroxyl groups on tyrosine amino acid residues present in its intracellular domain and in other proteins. Growth factor receptors usually occur as single polypeptide chains ("monomers") which, in response to external ligand binding, are induced to undergo pairwise association ("dimerization"), which leads to activation of the kinase domains (Fig. 6-4B). However, in the case of the insulin receptor family of receptor tyrosine kinases, the receptor is always present in a dimerized state, but the tyrosine kinase activity is nonetheless activated by the binding of a ligand (16).

Cytokines such as erythropoietin and interferon also activate surface receptors through a binding interaction. However, their receptors lack an intracellular domain with tyrosine kinase activity. Instead, receptors for these cytokines bind to members of the Jak family of nonreceptor tyrosine kinases in response to external ligand binding (17). The mechanism of activation by these cytokines is otherwise similar to that of the growth factors described above.

Growth factor receptors that undergo dimerization during activation include the following: the epidermal growth factor (EGF) receptor, the transforming growth factor (TGF)-α receptor, the insulin and insulinlike growth factor receptors, the colony-stimulating factor receptor, and the platelet-derived growth factor (PDGF) receptor (18). The dimerization process plays a critical role in the activation of these receptors and

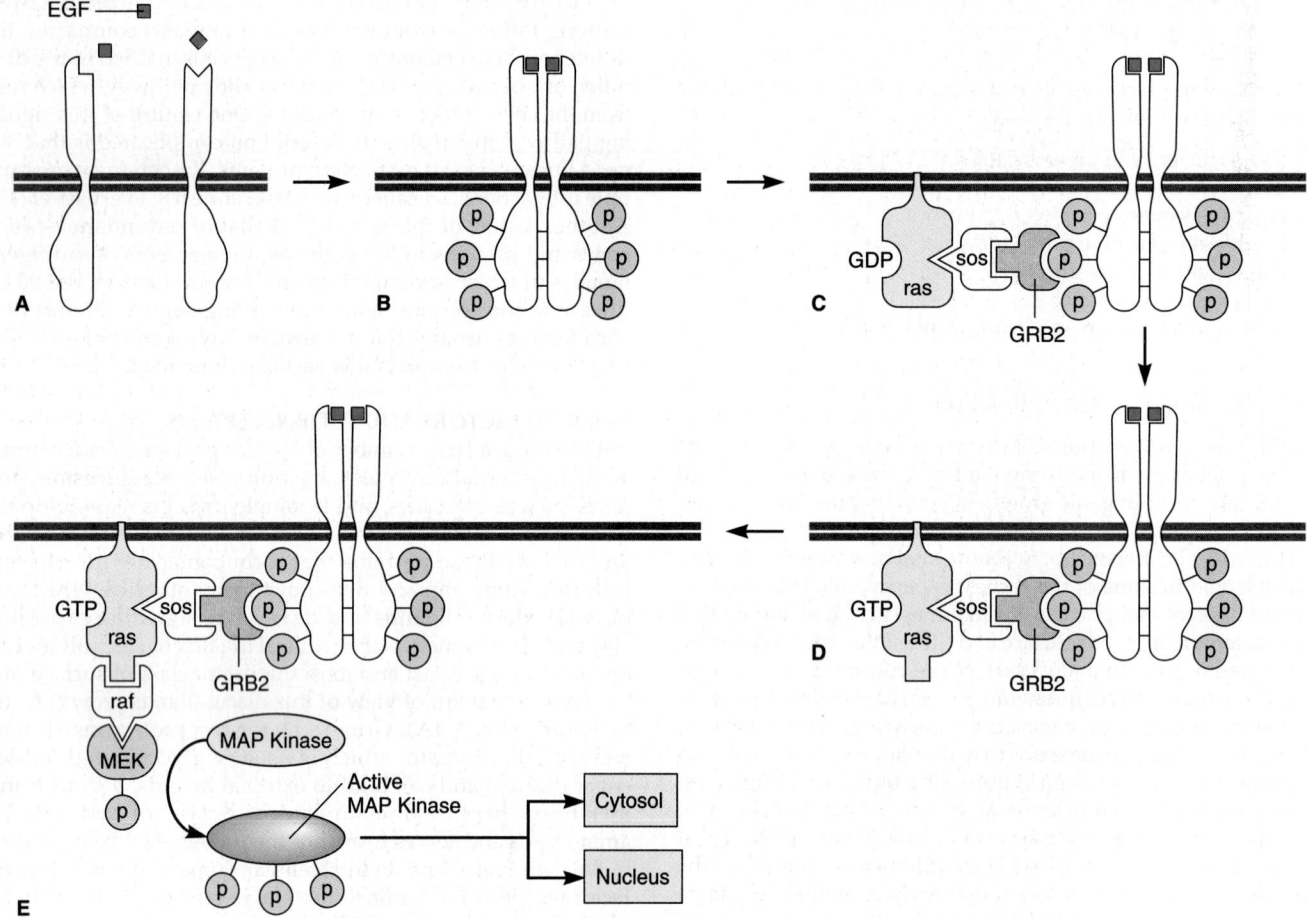

Figure 6-4. The central pathway for signaling of cell growth. Growth factors, such as epidermal growth factor (EGF), interact with their receptors to induce dimerization and activation of the tyrosine kinase domain **(A)**, leading to phosphorylation and dimerization of the receptor (p) **(B)**. These phosphate groups lead to formation of a molecular assembly of the adaptor proteins GRB2 and sos, which recruit ras and induce it to exchange guanosine diphosphate (GDP) for guanosine triphosphate (GTP) **(C,D)**. GTP-ras then is active at binding to the raf kinase, which then binds to the MEK kinase and phosphorylates it. Phosphorylated MEK can then phosphorylate the MAP kinase at both serine and tyrosine residues, putting it in an active conformation. Active MAP kinase then disseminates the growth signal to other cytoplasmic proteins and also enters the nucleus to effect growth by phosphorylation of other critical substrates **(E)**.

appears to stimulate receptor phosphorylation by a simple *trans*-acting proximity mechanism (19). The kinase activity of these receptors provides a mechanism for transmission of growth signal within the cell to other proteins that are also phosphorylated by the activated receptor.

Growth factors and their receptors provide the first potential mechanisms by which cancer cells can acquire self-sufficiency in growth capacity (20). Some cancer cells begin to synthesize and secrete growth factors to which they can then respond. This creates a positive feedback loop called *autocrine stimulation*. This mechanism is used by several different types of human cancers, including glioblastomas, which produce PDGF; some sarcomas, which produce TGF-α; and small cell lung cancer, which produces bombesin and other growth factors. Receptor overexpression or sensitization is a second mechanism used by cancer cells to become self-sufficient in cell growth (21). Although not proven to be critical for cancer cell growth in every case, EGF receptor overexpression commonly occurs in stomach, brain, breast, and lung cancer; a close relative of the EGF receptor, the HER2/neu receptor, is overexpressed in many stomach and breast cancers and in some lung cancers. The importance of this

mechanism in growth stimulation is underscored by recent clinical successes using an antibody against HER2/neu in the treatment of breast cancer.

RAS–MAP KINASE CIRCUIT

In addition to phosphorylating and activating other proteins, activated, phosphorylated growth factor receptors bind to several proteins to transmit positive growth signals toward the cell nucleus. A so-called adaptor protein, Grb2 binds to many activated receptors at their sites of phosphorylation through a domain termed the *SH2 domain* (named after the oncogenic nonreceptor tyrosine kinase src, which also contains this domain) (Fig. 6-4C). Grb2 binds to the protein Sos through another domain, the SH3 domain of Grb2. These binding associations illustrate a common theme in many proteins—that of modular domain organization (22). A protein will often consist of several domains capable of binding individually to other proteins, providing opportunity for dissemination of signal from one protein to several others as well as cross-talk and interaction with other signaling proteins and pathways. Grb2 and Sos may also be recruited indirectly to activated receptors through intermediary modular linker proteins, such as Shc and IRS1.

The binding of Sos to Grb2-activated receptor brings Sos close to the plasma membrane and provides access by Sos to the small G protein ras. Sos has an important activity on ras—that of stimulating nucleotide exchange by ras (Fig. 6-4C, D). Ras is a member of a large family of small proteins that bind to guanosine diphosphate (GDP) or guanosine triphosphate (GTP) (23,24). When bound to GDP, these proteins are in an "off" configuration. When bound to GTP, ras molecules are in an "on" configuration, ready to transmit growth activation signals onward to the nucleus. All ras proteins are posttranslationally modified by prenylation, which results in the addition of a lipid group to a conserved cysteine near the C-terminus of the protein. Some forms of ras also have additional lipid groups added, and the effect of these lipid additions is that ras is permanently anchored in the membranes of the cell. Thus, when Sos is recruited to the cell membrane by binding to Grb2, it is in close proximity to ras. The lipid modification of ras is one molecular target in malignant cells that is being approached clinically at present, using compounds that inhibit farnesyltransferase, the enzyme responsible for this modification.

Sos is a representative member of one class of proteins that regulate ras activation—the guanine nucleotide exchange factors. A second important class of proteins that affect ras activation are the GTPase activating proteins (GAPs). There are two major GAPs for ras, p120GAP and neurofibromin (25). Although these proteins enhance the rate of conversion of GTP to GDP in the ras·GTP complex and thereby tend to extinguish positive signals emanating from ras·GTP, it also appears that they can transmit signals from ras to other cellular proteins. Neurofibromin is the product of the NF1 gene, mutation in which causes the human tumor-suppressor gene syndrome neurofibromatosis type 1. Neurofibromatosis type 1 patients develop many neurofibromas and are at increased risk for myeloid, mesodermal, and nervous system malignancies. These clinical observations illustrate the importance of these GAPs in limiting positive growth signals that involve the ras GTPase.

Activated ras·GTP interacts with several "effector" proteins to transmit the signal forward and stimulates several intracellular processes. Foremost among ras·GTP binding partners is Raf, an intracellular kinase (Fig. 6-4E). Raf is activated by ras binding, and phosphorylates MEK kinase at a serine residue. MEK then phosphorylates MAPK on threonine and tyrosine residues, leading to its activation. MAPK then phosphorylates a number of cytoplasmic substrates, including receptor tyrosine kinases and Sos, to amplify the growth-promoting signal. In addition, MAPK is translocated to the nucleus, where it phosphorylates and activates transcription factors.

Other ras binding partners include phosphoinositide 3-kinase, discussed further below, and several other proteins that also have roles in signal transduction. There are three major members of the ras family that participate in this growth signaling pathway: N-ras, K-ras, and H-ras. These ras isoforms differ in their ability to activate raf versus other important downstream effectors of ras signaling.

The major importance of ras in cell growth signaling and its participation in malignant development is underscored by the observation that ras mutations are seen in approximately 25% of all carcinomas and hematologic malignancies (26). In some types of cancer, ras mutations are seen in over 50% of tumors (e.g., colon and pancreas). Nonetheless, ras mutations are not seen uniformly in any cancer cell type. In addition, the genetic or expression abnormality that compensates for a lack of ras mutation in these tumors is completely unknown.

LIPID SIGNALING CIRCUITS RADIATING OUTWARD FROM RECEPTOR ACTIVATION

Activation of many growth factor receptor kinases leads to rapid stimulation of phosphoinositide metabolism and generation of multiple second messengers. Phospholipase Cγ (PLCγ) binds to activated receptors through its SH2 domain, leading to its phosphorylation and activation (27). Activated PLCγ hydrolyzes phosphatidyl inositol (4,5) bisphosphate [PI(4,5)P2] to form two lipid second messenger molecules, diacylglycerol and inositol(1,4,5)P3 (IP3). IP3 binds to intracellular receptors to stimulate the release of Ca^{2+} from intracellular stores. Ca^{2+} has multiple effects including binding to calmodulin, which can then activate a number of additional protein kinases. Diacylglycerol and Ca^{2+} also bind to the protein kinase C (PKC) family of serine-threonine kinases. These protein kinases can phosphorylate additional substrates, including transcription factors.

Phosphoinositide 3-kinase (PI3K) is also activated during growth signaling by two mechanisms (28). First, PI3K can bind directly to phosphorylated receptor tyrosine kinases. This interaction is mediated by an SH2 domain present in the regulatory subunit of PI3K. Second, the regulatory subunit can bind directly to ras·GTP (Fig. 6-5). Binding of the regulatory subunit of PI3K activates the catalytic subunit of PI3K, which generates the second messengers phosphatidyl inositol (3,4)

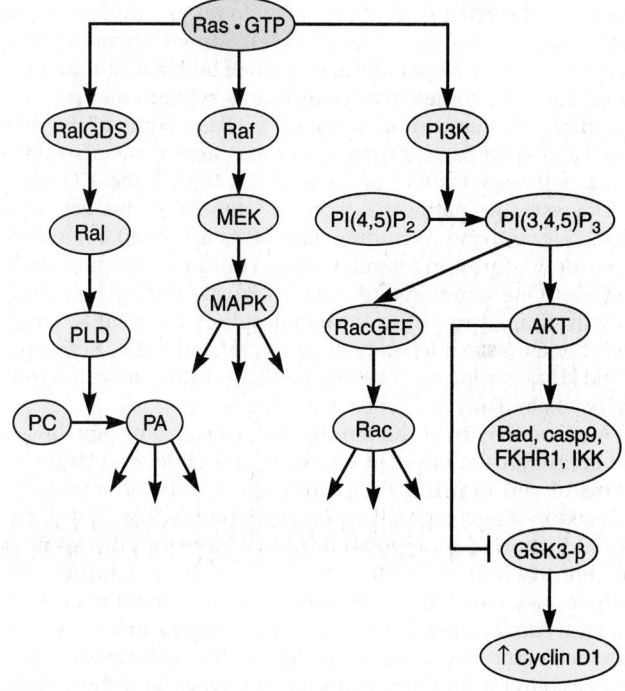

Figure 6-5. Multiple branching pathways emanate from activated ras. In addition to stimulating the central MAP kinase (MAPK) pathway for cell growth, ras also activates at least two other important pathways. On the left, ras activates the exchange protein ralGDS, which activates the ral guanosine triphosphate(GTP)ase. Ral·GTP activates phospholipase D (PLD), which converts phosphatidyl choline (PC) to phosphatidic acid (PA), which has many diverse effects on cell growth. On the right, ras activates the phosphoinositide 3-kinase (PI3K), which converts phosphatidylinositide(4,5)bisphosphate [PI(4,5)P2] to phosphatidylinositide(3,4,5)trisphosphate [PI(3,4,5)P3]. PI(3,4,5)P3 has diverse effects as well, but one effect is the stimulation of the kinase AKT. Activated AKT phosphorylates several proteins, such as Bad, Caspase-9 (casp9), FKHR1, and IKK, all of which serve to inhibit apoptosis. AKT also phosphorylates the GSK3-β kinase, leading to increased levels of cyclin D1. PI(3,4,5)P3 also stimulates exchange factors with the rac GTPase, leading to activation of rac, which is involved in both cell motility and growth signaling.

bisphosphate [PI(3,4)P2] and phosphatidyl inositol (3,4,5) tris-phosphate [PI(3,4,5)P3]. PI(3,4,5)P3 mediates the membrane localization and activation of a number of other signaling proteins (29). Some of these, such as AKT and its substrate the transcription factor FKHR1, have important roles in regulation of apoptosis and are discussed further later in this chapter. Others are the docking proteins Grp1 and Gab1 and phospholipase Cγ1. PI3K activation is also important in the generation of H2O2 that occurs in response to growth factor stimulation, which is another second messenger that serves to transmit and eventually regulate the positive growth signal (30).

RALGDS AND RHO AS DOWNSTREAM EFFECTORS OF RAS

In addition to the raf-MAPK circuit and PI3K pathway, ras activates a family of exchange factors for other members of the ras family of small GTPases, including ralGDS, RGL, and RGL2/Rlf (Fig. 6-5). These proteins serve to activate the ral GTPase (increasing levels of ral·GTP) but also may have other direct functions in transmission of growth stimulatory signals. Ral·GTP interacts with phospholipase D (PLD) to increase its activity. PLD catalyzes the conversion of phosphatidylcholine to phosphatidic acid, which has additional diverse signaling effects.

The rho family of GTPases is a subfamily of the ras superfamily, which consists of cdc42, rac, and rho. Rho proteins also undergo cyclic binding of GTP and GDP. Rho GTPases participate in growth signaling in several different ways with separate and parallel mechanisms of activation to ras and divergent and convergent signaling pathways (12). Some transmembrane receptors lead to the parallel activation of both ras and rho family GTPases. In some circumstances, ras activation appears to lead directly to activation of the rac GTPase. Some of the guanine nucleotide exchange factors that act on ras also have domains that are capable of causing activation of rho GTPases.

Downstream pathways that are stimulated by activated cdc42, rac, and rho (including each of its isoforms) have some common features and some features unique to each of these GTPases. One common target is PAK kinase. PAK can augment growth stimulatory pathways by phosphorylating MEK, which serves to enhance interaction between raf and MEK. Activation of rho kinases appears to be required for positive growth signaling by ras in many cell types.

A major activity of rho family proteins is that of signaling to the actin cytoskeleton for orchestration of several different forms of cell motility (12). Common to all of the motility induced by these proteins is the formation of focal adhesions and induction of actin polymerization. However, the forms of the motility induced differ for each protein. In addition, the pathways by which these proteins lead to cell motility also differ, with cdc42 acting through the ARP complex to induce actin polymerization, rac being dependent on the actin-severing protein gelsolin for its activity in some cell types, and rho activating a rho kinase, which leads to activation of protein elements needed for actomyosin contraction.

CONTROL OF GROWTH SIGNALING PATHWAYS AND CELL SPECIFICITY

Several mechanisms exist within cells to limit or degrade growth-stimulatory signals. Growth factor stimulation of many receptors leads to rapid endocytosis (internalization into membrane-bound structures within the cell) and eventual degradation by lysosomal enzymes. One oncogenic protein, Cbl, appears to accelerate this process by acting as a docking protein that enhances contact between activated receptor and elements of the proteasome, a protein-degration complex. A second mechanism occurs through activation of PKC. Although PKC does some positive growth signaling, it can also phosphorylate receptors at serine and threonine residues, which reduces their tyrosine kinase activity, limiting their signaling capability. A third mechanism for control of growth stimulatory signals is protein tyrosine phosphatases (PTPs) (31). PTPs serve to negatively regulate growth factor receptor signaling by removing phosphate groups from tyrosine residues. Application of inhibitors of PTP to cells results in activation of many growth factor receptors, indicating their general importance in growth control.

We have considered only primary aspects of growth factor signaling in cells, yet the complexity of this signaling network is easily evident. Additional complexity enters the system when one considers that cell adhesion can also influence growth signaling by receptors and that additional parallel pathways for stimulation of cell growth exist, which we have not yet discussed, including G protein–coupled receptors and the TGF-β family of cytokines and their receptors. This leads to a compelling question: How are all of these growth factor signals integrated and processed by the cell into decisions regarding growth? This area of signal integration and global analysis is complex, methods for analysis are difficult, and it is likely that much further investigation is required for better understanding. One element that is clearly critical in signal integration is the precise repertoire of expressed proteins. The cell's expression pattern is likely influenced by the developmental stage of the organ, tissue, and cell. This expression repertoire will determine what the level of expression of all elements of the growth circuit are, including growth factor receptors, docking proteins, lipases, other kinases, and GTPases. This will clearly have an important influence on the cellular response to external signals.

Cell Cycle Deregulation

The eventual outcome of the complex processes described above that control and initiate cell growth is a decision by the cell as to whether it should replicate its DNA and undergo cell division. Although events at the cell surface and within the cytoplasm are extremely important in this process, the regulation and mechanics of these ultimate steps occur within the cell nucleus. Study of the cell cycle in a variety of organisms, including mammals and yeast, has yielded an intricate map of the expression, regulation, and molecular functions of the essential cell cycle proteins. In this section, we review these essential molecular players and attempt to indicate how these protein elements are deregulated or dysfunctional in the malignant cell. Although one might think that direct genetic (or epigenetic) assault on the regulation of the cell cycle might not be necessary in a cell with sufficient mutation and activation of cytoplasmic growth stimulatory signaling, this is not the case. Cell cycle checkpoints exist to monitor and control positive growth signals. Several examples are known in which excessive growth stimulatory signals (e.g., expression of a mutated ras oncogene) lead to cell cycle checkpoint activation and growth arrest in otherwise normal cells.

CELL CYCLE

The are four phases to the active cell cycle and one quiescent phase, G_0 (32) (Fig. 6-6). The majority of cells in the body reside in G_0, performing various functions but without any activity indicative of growth. Cells exit G_0 when stimulated by growth signals and enter the phase known as G_1. During G_1, cells undergo a number of steps that are preparatory for entry into the synthetic or S phase. Late during this period, cells pass through an instant in time termed the *restriction point*. After that time, they are committed to DNA synthesis and cell division, and no external growth factors or other signals are required for completion of the process. During S phase, chromosomes are replicated, and dur-

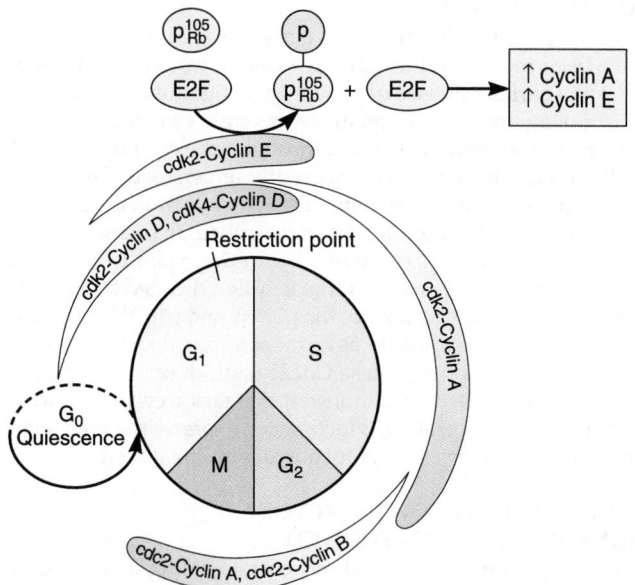

Figure 6-6. A model for the cell cycle and the actions of cyclin-dependent kinase (cdk)-cyclin complexes. Five phases of the cell cycle—G_0, G_1, S, G_2, M—are shown. The width of the bands indicates the relative amounts of the various cdk-cyclin complexes, which are generated during different phases of the cell cycle. Cdk2 and cdk4 are most important during the G_1 phase when cells respond to initial growth signals and prepare for DNA synthesis. A major effect of the cdk2 and cdk4 complexes is the phosphorylation of the retinoblastoma protein, p105Rb, which becomes inactive for binding to the transcription factor E2F. Free E2F then induces expression of a number of genes required for S phase, including production of both G_1 and S phase cyclins.

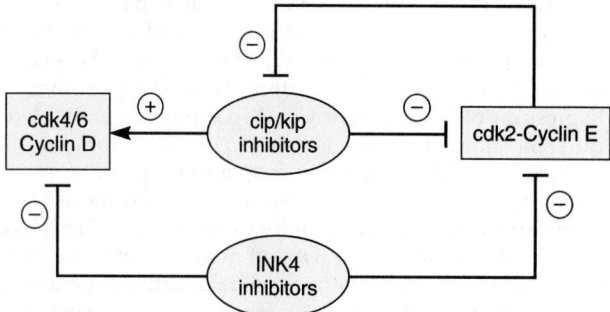

Figure 6-7. A model for the actions of two classes of cyclin-dependent kinase (cdk) inhibitors, the cip/kip family and the INK4 family. Cip/kip inhibitors have positive effects on cdk4 and cdk6 but negative effects on cdk2. As G_1 progresses, cdk2-cyclin E levels increase, leading to reduction in cip/kip protein levels, and accelerating progression to S phase.

ing G_2, preparation is made for mitosis. M (for mitosis) phase concludes the process with segregation of chromosomes to each of the daughter cells as well as *cytokinesis*, the process of separation of the cytoplasm between the two daughter cells.

G_1 CYCLINS AND CYCLIN-DEPENDENT KINASES

Cyclin-dependent kinases (cdks) are the critical proteins that regulate transition among the parts of the cell cycle (32) (Fig. 6-6). These kinases are active only when they have a bound cofactor—a cyclin. Passage through the restriction point and initiation of S phase is dependent on two sets of cdks, the cyclin D– and cyclin E–dependent kinases. The three D-type cyclins (D1, D2, and D3) interact with cdk4 and cdk6 to yield six possible combinations, each of which can drive the appropriate cell type forward from G_1 into S phase. Cyclins are short-lived unstable proteins whose level of expression varies greatly during the cell cycle. A major endpoint of cytoplasmic growth signaling is to increase cyclin D levels. In contrast, cdk4 and cdk6 are relatively long-lived proteins.

Formation of the cyclin D–cdk4/cdk6 complex activates its kinase activity, and a primary target is the Rb protein, a product of the retinoblastoma gene. Phosphorylation of Rb by the cdks has the effect of dissociating Rb from complexes that serve to inhibit DNA synthesis, particularly the E2F transcription factor (33). Rb binding to E2F not only inhibits the transcriptional activity of E2F, but the Rb-E2F complex still binds to E2F DNA binding sites and actively represses transcription of E2F-regulated genes. In addition, Rb may inhibit transcription by E2F through binding and recruitment of histone deacetylases and SWI/SNF chromatin-remodeling complexes to the DNA binding sites that E2F recognizes. Thus, inhibition of Rb activity leads to activation of transcription of the many target genes of E2F, including genes that regulate DNA metabolism, cyclin E,

and cyclin A. Cyclin E forms a complex with cdk2, which becomes activated, and cdk2 further phosphorylates Rb, serving to reinforce Rb inactivation. This occurrence also explains how growth factor signaling is no longer necessary after the restriction point, when cyclin E and A expression is high enough to maintain Rb inactivation without cdk4 and cdk6.

Cyclin D expression, like that of cyclin E and A, increases in response to growth stimulatory signals from the cytoplasm, including those derived from the ras-MAPK pathway. In addition, stimulation of PI3K during growth leads to activation of AKT, which leads to inactivation of the glycogen synthase kinase 3β (GSK3β). When not phosphorylated by AKT, GSK3-β phosphorylates cyclin D1, which leads to nuclear export and degradation (34). The cyclin D1 gene is activated or overexpressed in several different types of human cancer. It is activated by chromosomal translocation in parathyroid adenoma cells. Overexpression of cyclin D1 is seen in esophageal, colorectal, breast, and lung cancer. In many cases, overexpression is achieved by amplification of the genomic region containing the native cyclin D1 gene. Thus, increasing cyclin D1 expression is one method by which cancers are able to push the cell cycle regulatory system toward unregulated growth.

CDK INHIBITORS: THE CIP/KIP FAMILY

The next protein element serving a regulatory function in the cell cycle is a group of inhibitors of cdk2 that is termed the *Cip/Kip family* (32) (Fig. 6-7). This family includes p21[Cip1], p27[Kip1], and p57[Kip2]. These inhibitors serve a complex role in regulation of the cell cycle. First, they bind to cyclin D–cdk4/cdk6 complexes but do not inhibit their kinase activity, rather, they enhance it. Second, they bind to cyclin E–cdk2 complexes and have a purely inhibitory effect on cdk2 kinase activity. Therefore, in quiescent nongrowing cells, Cip/Kip cdk inhibitors serve to reduce further any cdk2 activity. When growth signaling begins, levels of cyclin D–cdk4/cdk6 increase and bind tightly to Cip/Kip cdk inhibitors, releasing cdk2 for activation by cyclin E as the cell approaches the restriction point. Active cyclin E–cdk2 phosphorylates p27[Kip1], leading to its degradation in proteasomes, so that there is a positive feedback loop leading to increased cyclin E–cdk2 activity and cell cycle progression. Indicative of a complex role for p27[Kip1] in cell cycle regulation is the observation that this gene displays an unusual dose-response in tumorigenesis. Both mice that are null for p27[Kip1] and those with one deleted and one normal copy of the gene have increased rates of neoplasia when treated with tumor induction regimens. Mice that are heterozygous at the p27[Kip1] gene also do not display loss of expression of the remaining normal allele. Lowered but not absent levels of p27^{Kip1} are seen in a variety of forms of cancer in humans and are associated with poorer prognosis in patients with breast cancer. This is also consistent with a dose response effect of p27^{Kip1} expression.

Expression of the different Cip/Kip inhibitors is regulated by different stimuli (35). The expression of p21^{Cip}, for example, is increased by p53 expression in response to several forms of DNA damage and is a primary mechanism for the induction of cell cycle arrest by p53. Mice null for expression of p21^{Cip1} have normal development and are without marked tumor predisposition. However, when the appropriate additional genetic or environmental measures are applied to these mice, accelerated tumorigenesis is seen.

CDK INHIBITORS: THE INK4 FAMILY
A second major class of genes and proteins that have cdk inhibitor activity are the INK4 proteins (32) (Fig. 6-7). There are four different INK4 genes and encoded proteins: the INK4a–d genes and their respective proteins p16^{INK4a}, p15^{INK4b}, p18^{INK4c}, and p19^{INK4d}. The INK4a and INK4b genes are located near one another on the short arm of chromosome 9, whereas the other two genes are at other chromosomal sites. The importance of these genes (particularly INK4a and INK4b) to cell cycle progression is reflected by the common occurrence of heterozygous loss of all of chromosome 9p in many types of human cancer and the occurrence of smaller homozygous deletions affecting these specific genes.

INK4 proteins bind cdk4/cdk6 in binary complexes, releasing Cip/Kip proteins for interaction with cyclin E–cdk2. This has the effect of augmenting cell cycle arrest effects and is dependent on a functional Rb gene or protein. A functional unphosphorylated Rb protein, the result of efficient cdk inhibition by the INK4 family and the Cip/Kip family, is effective in binding to E2F thereby suppressing E2F transcriptional activity. If Rb is absent or mutated, then E2F transcription proceeds, leading to high levels of cyclin E–cdk2 kinase activity, which can override the effects of both INK4 and Cip/Kip cdk inhibitors. This model emphasizes the critical importance of Rb in cell cycle regulation in what has been termed the *Rb pathway* (32).

Molecular studies in patients and their tumors strongly support the importance of these proteins in this model of cell cycle regulation. The INK4a gene is mutated in a proportion of families in which risk for development of melanoma and other tumors occurs. In these patients, loss of the second normal allele follows the classic Knudsen model of tumor-suppressor gene inactivation. In sporadic human cancers, a reciprocal relationship between INK4a and retinoblastoma gene inactivation has been seen. In small cell lung cancer, approximately 90% of tumors have lost Rb expression, and the remainder has INK4a inactivation by deletion or cyclin D amplification (36). Interestingly, in non–small cell lung cancer, the majority has inactivation of the INK4a gene by some combination of single allele loss, homozygous deletion, or promoter hypermethylation, whereas a minority has inactivation of the Rb gene.

In addition, some tumors are known in which the INK4b gene is inactivated by hypermethylation of its promoter region, including hematopoietic malignancies, suggesting it is also an important molecular target whose elimination facilitates tumor growth (37). At present, there is little evidence of a critical role for the other INK genes in the pathogenesis of human cancer. Similarly, in the mouse, deletions of either INK4a or INK4b lead to predisposition of tumorigenesis, whereas deletions of INK4c or INK4d have milder phenotypes. Overall, the INK4 genes are involved in one way or another in many forms of human cancer, leading to the conclusion that the Rb pathway is a critical target for inactivation in the pathogenesis of human cancer.

MYC ONCOPROTEINS
The myc gene family consists of c-myc and N-myc. These genes have been recognized as having a role in cancer development from the earliest phases of cancer investigation. In contrast to most oncogenes, activation of the myc genes is nearly always driven by overexpression, often through gene amplification, and their mechanism of action is only partly understood. Direct modulation of expression or activity of several key proteins in the cell cycle by myc expression has been described. Expression of myc increases the kinase activity of cdk2 in the cyclin E–cdk2 complex, leading to an increase in transcription directed by E2F. Myc also antagonizes the activity of the p27^{Kip1} and p16^{INK4a} cdk inhibitors. Myc also acts directly as a transcriptional factor, inducing expression of the phosphatase Cdc25a, which serves to enhance the activity of cdks, the E2F transcription factor, cyclin D, and Id2 (38). Id2 is nuclear protein, which, when expressed at high levels, binds to and sequesters Rb, functionally inactivating it.

TRANSFORMING GROWTH FACTOR-β SIGNALING AND THE CELL CYCLE
The TGF-β family of external receptor signaling molecules has an important and complex role in cancer pathogenesis (39,40). This signaling pathway affects cell cycle kinetics and progression, and therefore is discussed in this section. TGF-β factors act by assembling receptor complexes that activate the "SMAD" family of transcription factors by phosphorylation. Regulation of activation of TGF-β receptors by TGF-β factors is complex in that many soluble proteins can bind to TGF-β factors, limiting their access to TGF-β receptors. Smad proteins reside in the cytoplasm, but after phosphorylation by activated TGF-β receptors, they translocate to the nucleus where they influence transcription by interacting with DNA-binding cofactors and transcriptional coactivators and corepressors.

Inhibition of cell proliferation is a major function of the TGF-β signaling pathway in epithelial, endothelial, hematopoietic, neural, and mesenchymal cells. This is accomplished in two major ways: inhibition of cdk activity and down-regulation of myc. One direct effect of TGF-β is increasing the expression of p15^{INK4b} and to a lesser extent that of p21^{CIP1}. Down-regulation of the expression of myc has diverse complementary effects enhancing cell growth blockade.

Inactivation of the TGF-β signaling pathway occurs in the majority of pancreatic and colon cancers. Inactivating mutations in type II TGF-β receptors occur in most colon and gastric carcinomas in which microsatellite instability develops by alteration of a polyadenine repeat sequence within the receptor's coding region (41). Mutations in the SMAD proteins also occur in cancer. The Smad4 gene is the target of biallelic loss in approximately one-half of pancreatic cancers and one-third of colon cancers. Repression of expression of the TGF-β receptors is also a common event in malignant cells.

P53-ARF-MDM2 PATHWAY
The p53 gene is commonly mutated in human cancer and plays an intimate if indirect role in cell cycle regulation (32). It also has important activity in apoptosis, which is discussed in detail in the next section. Here, we focus on the role of the p53 gene in the cell cycle and its interaction with two other proteins: ARF and Mdm2 (42) (Fig. 6-8).

p53 is a nuclear phosphorylated protein that has a critical activity in response to cell signals, including growth stimulatory signals, in which it directs decisions to proceed either into cell cycle arrest or apoptosis. p53 protein acts in a tetrameric complex as a transcription factor. In normal unstimulated cells, p53 protein levels are low because of the activity of the Mdm2 gene. Mdm2 binds to the transactivation domain of p53-blocking p53-depen-

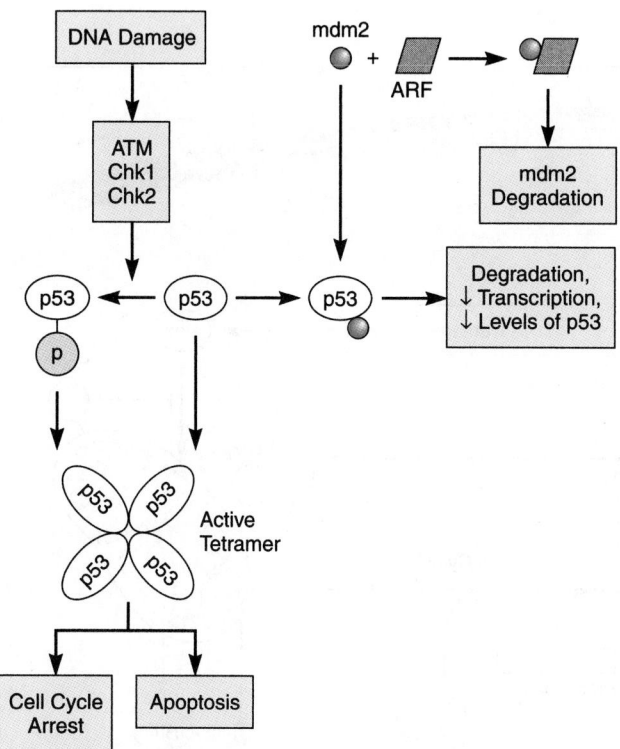

Figure 6-8. A model for the interaction between ARF, MDM2, and p53. In normal quiescent and growing cells, levels of MDM2 are sufficient for it to bind to p53, leading to its sequestration and destruction. In response to abnormal growth signals, ARF expression is induced, and ARF binds to MDM2, leading to its destruction. Sufficient p53 is then free to form tetramers and lead to cell cycle arrest or apoptosis. Alternatively, DNA damage leads to induction of a DNA damage response pathway in which the ATM, Chk1, or Chk2 kinases phosphorylate p53, blocking binding to MDM2 and leading to accumulation of p53.

dent gene expression, blocks p53 transcription, ubiquinates p53, and enhances p53 export from the nucleus for degradation in the proteasome. Mdm2 expression is regulated in part by p53 so that expression of p53 leads to Mdm2 expression, serving to terminate p53 expression by a feedback mechanism.

ARF is the third protein element in this pathway. ARF is a small protein that acts to antagonize the effects of Mdm2 on p53 function in several ways: It sequesters Mdm2 from the nucleoplasm in the nucleolus, blocks Mdm2 ubiquitinization of p53, and also blocks Mdm2-based nuclear export and degradation of p53. ARF expression is activated by abnormal growth signals, including high-level myc expression and activated ras, leading to p53 expression and cell cycle arrest or apoptosis. In cells lacking p53, there is a failure of this mechanism, leading to continued growth of premalignant or malignant cells. Similarly, cells that lack ARF are also unable to undergo growth arrest.

Interestingly, the ARF protein is encoded by the same gene that encodes p16[INK4a] (43). Such parsimony is extremely unusual in the human genome. Two distinct promoters are used to drive transcription for each of the two proteins, and the coding regions of the two genes overlap but are in different reading frames. The close functional connection between ARF and p53 is illustrated by the fact that mice that are null for either protein have a similar phenotype with rapid development of lymphomas, carcinomas, and sarcomas in several sites, although the ARF-null mice survive much longer than the p53-null mice.

The importance of the p53-ARF-Mdm2 pathway is also illustrated by the frequency of genetic and epigenetic events affecting one member of this trio. As above, mutation of the p16[INK4a] gene occurs in a substantial fraction of human cancers through deletion or hypermethylation of the promoter region, and in many cases, these events also extinguish expression of the ARF transcript. p53 mutations are among the most common in human cancer, affecting over 50% of all cancer cases. Alteration of Mdm2 occurs less frequently in human cancer, but gene amplification occurs in approximately 20% of soft tissue sarcomas, leading to overexpression (42). In addition, genetic events affecting this pathway tend to occur in a complementary fashion.

CYCLINS AND KINASES IN THE S, G_2, AND M PHASES

Cyclin A binds to and activates the cdk2 and cdc2 kinases, which are required at the start of S phase and at the G_2-M transition. Cyclin B associates with the cdc2 kinase, which is required for M phase onset and completion. Cancer-related mutations or disruptions of these genes and proteins have not been described.

Apoptosis Evasion

Apoptosis, or programmed cell death, is a somewhat orderly and predictable process, highly conserved evolutionarily, for the termination and destruction of cells that are unwanted by multicellular organisms. Although recognized morphologically for decades by some histopathologists, apoptosis was recognized as an important physiologic process only in the past decade. Histologic and morphologic hallmarks of apoptosis include ruffling and blebbing of the peripheral cell cytoplasm as well as nuclear changes. One characteristic result of apoptosis is the cleavage of DNA into small fragments that are multiples of 180 base pairs, the so-called nucleosomal ladder. Induction of apoptosis is one means by which mammals can eliminate cells that have incurred mutations that cause deregulation of normal growth control. Thus, disruption of this normal physiologic pathway is a common occurrence during cancer development.

In this section, we consider the normal pathways by which apoptosis induction occurs, the essential protein components, and the role of the p53 gene. We also examine the ways in which malignant cells have been able to subvert these pathways to enhance their survival.

CASPASES: A PROTEASE CASCADE FOR THE INDUCTION OF APOPTOSIS

A protein element of critical importance in apoptosis is a set of intracellular proteases termed *caspases* (44–46). Over 12 caspases are known to exist, of which six or seven play important roles in apoptosis. They contain active site cysteine residues and cleave proteins at aspartic acid residues, but they require a specific recognition motif of three amino acid residues just in front of the aspartic acid. Caspases occur in cells in an inactive "pro" state and are typically activated in a cascade pathway that is similar to the clotting cascade, leading to digestion and activation of caspase-3, the major "effector" caspase (Fig. 6-9). Although activated caspase-3 and other effector caspases can cleave many different proteins, there appear to be just a few substrates that are of critical importance. One of the major substrates for caspases during apoptosis is a protein called *ICAD*, whose basal function in the absence of apoptosis is to bind to and inactivate caspase-activated DNAse (CAD). Caspase digestion of ICAD releases CAD, which then enters the nucleus and cleaves DNA to generate the nucleosomal ladder of DNA fragments. Other critical substrates include nuclear lamins, the essential structural component of the nuclear membrane, whose digestion contributes to nuclear shrinking and budding during apoptosis; fodrin and gelsolin, cytoskeletal proteins whose deregulation by digestion leads to partial disassembly of the actin cytoskeleton; and PAK2, the

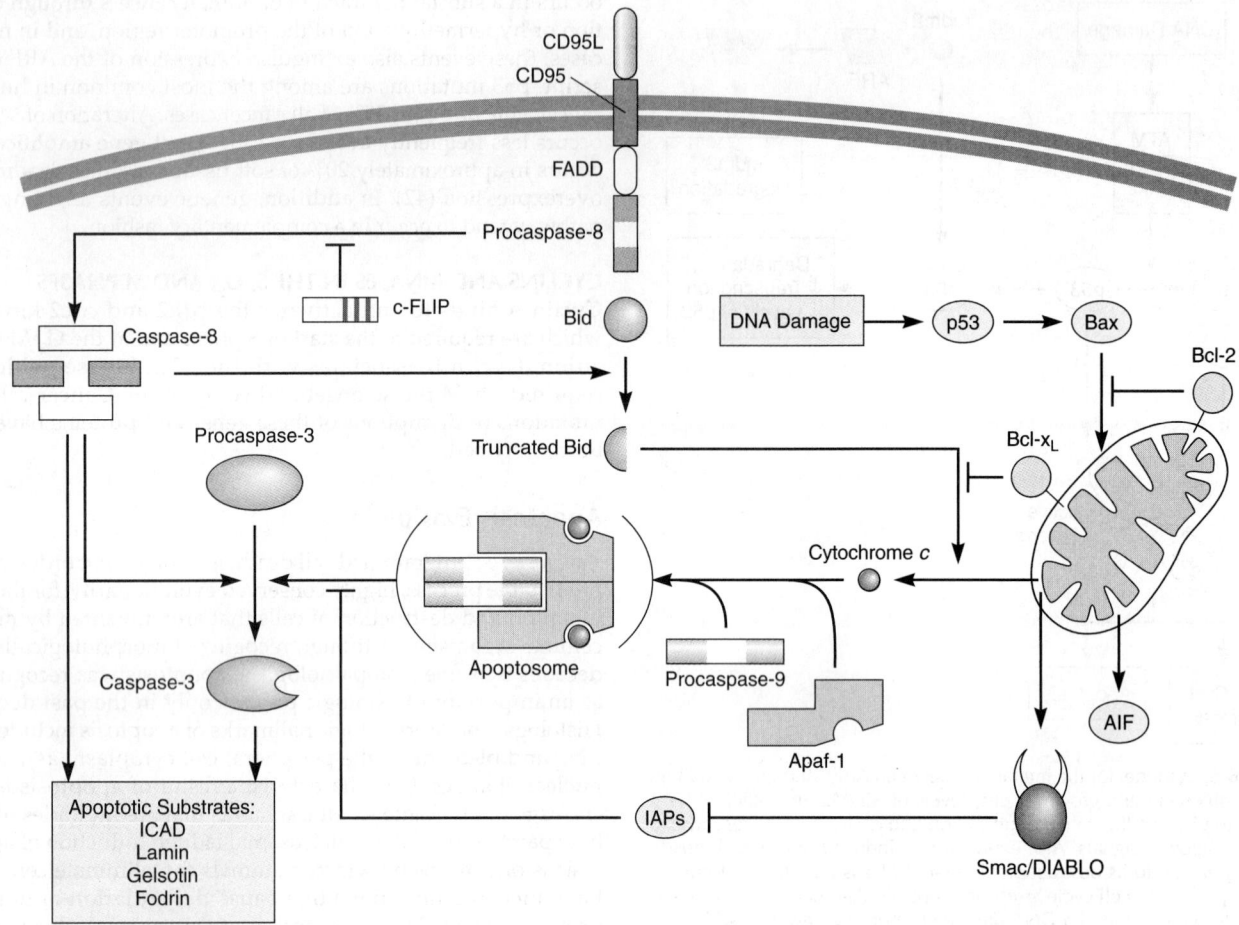

Figure 6-9. A model of intracellular events occurring during apoptosis. Activation of the death receptor pathway is shown at the top, with CD95L engaging the CD95 receptor, leading to formation of a large complex including FADD, and cleavage and activation of procaspase-8. c-FLIP, a nonfunctional caspase homologue can retard caspase-8 activation. Activation of the mitochondrial pathway by DNA damage and other stimuli is shown on the right. Pro- and antiapoptotic bcl-2 family members (at times modified by cleavage or phosphorylation) on the surface of the mitochondria determine the release of cytochrome C, AIF, and other components. Cytochrome C binds to Apaf-1, adenosine triphosphate or deoxyadenosine triphosphate, and procaspase-9 in the apoptosome, leading to generation of caspase-9. Both caspase-8 and caspase-9 converge on activation of caspase-3, which can then cleave many intracellular substrates shown in the box at lower left. (Adapted from Hengartner MO. The biochemistry of apoptosis. *Nature* 2000;407:770–776, with permission.)

kinase effector of rac, which, when cleaved, also contributes to the ruffling and blebbing of cytoplasm in apoptotic cells.

INITIATION OF APOPTOSIS: DEATH RECEPTORS AND MITOCHONDRIA

There are two major pathways for the induction of apoptosis. The first is the death-receptor pathway (Fig. 6-9). Fas and tumor necrosis factor are two important examples of initiators of the death-receptor pathway. Fas ligand engages the fas receptor and leads to recruitment of the adaptor protein FADD, which contains a death effector domain (DED). The DED domain of FADD then binds to a similar DED domain present in procaspase-8. Through clustering of activated fas receptor, high local concentrations of procaspase-8 are achieved, and it is believed that the low cleavage activity of the proenzyme is sufficient to initiate some cleavage and activation of caspase-8, which then rapidly accelerates into full induction of apoptosis. This model of activation of caspase-8 is known as the *induced proximity model* (47).

The other major pathway for induction of apoptosis is the mitochondrial pathway, which is both more complex and less understood. Procaspase-9 is the caspase that is activated in this

pathway, and in distinction to other caspases, cleavage of the pro domain does not enhance its proteolytic activity substantially. Instead, caspase-9 is activated by binding to two protein cofactors, Apaf-1 and cytochrome C, as well as deoxyATP or ATP. Cytochrome C release from the mitochondria is the crucial regulatory step in the activation of this pathway. These three proteins and possibly others assemble into a large complex that is likely to contain multiple copies of each of these proteins and has been termed the *apoptosome*, the engine of apoptosis emanating from the mitochondria (48). Release of mitochondrial contents to initiate formation of the apoptosome occurs under complex regulation by the bcl-2 family of proteins (see below).

Both caspase-8 and caspase-9 in the apoptosome then converge in the activation of caspase-3 and other effector caspases, leading to cleavage of the major substrates, morphologic changes, and apoptosis completion in the form of cell death.

BCL-2 FAMILY MEMBERS AND REGULATION OF MITOCHONDRIAL ACTIVATION

Bcl-2 is a gene whose expression is up-regulated by chromosomal translocation in follicular B-cell lymphoma, and bcl-2 is the founding member of a family of proteins with a role in the regulation of the induction of the mitochondrial pathway of apoptosis. There are three subgroups to the bcl-2 protein family (49). The first subgroup, subgroup I, includes members bcl-2, bcl-x_L, and bcl-w. All of these proteins contain four conserved domains (BH1–BH4), and these proteins all have antiapoptotic activity. The second subgroup, subgroup II, contains proteins with proapoptotic activity: Bax, Bak, and Bok. They share three domains with subgroup I members but are missing the N-terminal BH4 domain. Subgroup III includes a more diverse set of proteins with structural homology limited to the BH3 domain of bcl-2. Members of subgroup III include Bad, Bik, Blk, Hrk/DP5, Bid, Bim, and Noxa; these proteins also have proapoptotic activity.

Subgroup I and II members of the bcl-2 proteins contain hydrophobic C-terminal domains, which allow the proteins to reside in the outer membrane of the mitochondrion, projecting into the cytoplasm. All of these proteins also occur in the cell as dimers, and heterodimerization is common; for example, one molecule of bcl-2 may be bound to one molecule of Bax. The relative expression of all of the subgroup I versus subgroup II proteins appears to be an important determinant of the proapoptotic versus antiapoptotic stance of an individual cell (50).

The mechanism by which bcl-2 members regulate cytochrome C exit from the mitochondrion are debated. The most likely mechanism is that in which proapoptotic Bax and Bak proteins oligomerize into large complexes that insert into the mitochondrial membrane, creating a channel through which mitochondrial contents may exit. Alternatively, Bax subfamily members may interact with other mitochondrial outer membrane proteins to form channels; the voltage-dependent anion channel is one major possibility.

Many subgroup III proteins are expressed at relatively high levels in many cell types and are subject to activation and modulation by posttranslational modification (51). Bid is cleaved by caspase-8, and the cleaved product tBid interacts with Bax on the surface of the mitochondrion to cause release of mitochondrial contents (52). This provides a mechanism for cross-talk between the death receptor and mitochondrial pathways of apoptosis induction. Bad is phosphorylated by several kinases to cause its release from bcl-2 and other subgroup I family members, resulting in enhancement of their function (see PI3K, AKT, and PTEN Pathway and Apoptosis).

Cytochrome C release is a common but not quite universal event during apoptosis, suggesting that it has critical importance in the process in most cases. However, it is not the only molecule released from the mitochondrion that has proapoptotic effects. AIF is a flavoprotein that is also released from the mitochondrion with strong but poorly understood proapoptotic effects. Smac/DIABLO (see further below) and significant amounts of procaspases, including caspase-2, -3, and -9, also reside in the mitochondrion.

Bcl-2 expression has been seen in a large number of carcinomas and other tumor types in addition to follicular lymphoma and has a complex relationship to prognosis and response to therapy (53). In diffuse large cell lymphoma, bcl-2 expression is a significant independent predictor of reduced response to chemotherapy and shorter survival. In contrast, in breast and colon cancer, bcl-2 expression is associated with favorable clinicopathologic features and improved disease-free and overall survival. This also appears to be the case in other epithelial malignancies. Alteration in Bax expression may partially explain these observations. Bax appears to be a target of mutational inactivation in colon and gastric carcinoma, as well as some hematologic malignancies, through a polyG tract in its coding region, which is frequently mutated. The balance between bcl-2 and Bax expression may be the most critical determinant of apoptosis predisposition through the mitochondrial pathway.

NEGATIVE REGULATION OF APOPTOSIS

From the preceding discussion, it would appear that all cells are poised to undergo apoptosis and that random activation of a few molecules of caspase-8 might be all that is required for initiation of an irreversible process leading to cell death. However, there are several proteins and protein complexes that are known as inhibitors of apoptosis (IAPs): XIAP, c-IAP1, c-IAP2, and survivin. These proteins will bind irreversibly to activated caspases, particularly caspase-3, blocking their caspase activity, and in some cases, accelerating their degradation in the proteasome. Thus, high-level expression of IAPs is a mechanism for a cell to be relatively resistant to apoptosis. However, there is another level of control in favor of apoptosis in the form of Smac/DIABLO (54,55). This protein is released from mitochondria by the Bax subfamily proteins and binds to IAP proteins (at least XIAP), neutralizing their antiapoptotic activity. Thus, Smac/DIABLO ensures that apoptosis will proceed, particularly when mitochondrial rupture accompanies apoptosis.

Survivin is expressed in normal fetal but not adult differentiated tissues (53). However, it is consistently expressed in nearly all malignant cell lines and primary carcinomas, which is consistent with an important role in apoptosis evasion by tumors.

PHOSPHOINOSITIDE 3-KINASE, AKT, AND PTEN PATHWAY AND APOPTOSIS

In addition to its role in growth factor signaling, PI3K plays an important role in avoidance of apoptosis through stimulation of the AKT kinase (56) (Fig. 6-5). AKT kinase is one member of a small family of kinases that binds to phosphatidylinositol-3-phosphate lipids generated by activated PI3K. Other kinases (PDK1) in this family also bind to these lipids and phosphorylate AKT within its activation loop to cause its activation. Activated AKT then phosphorylates multiple protein substrates that are relevant to apoptosis. For example, both Bad and caspase-8 are phosphorylated, rendering them inactive in sequestration of subgroup I bcl-2 members and in protease activity, respectively. The third participant in this pathway, PTEN, has phosphatase activity that is specific for the 3 position of phosphatidylinositol-3-phosphates. Thus, the normal role of PTEN is to degrade lipid products derived from PI3K to prevent or limit AKT activation.

The importance of this pathway in regulation of apoptosis and tumorigenesis is amply demonstrated by several clinical molecular studies. Mutations in PTEN cause the rare autosomal-dominant tumor-suppressor gene syndrome Cowden disease, in which patients develop a variety of benign tumors and have a 40% lifetime incidence of breast cancer. Tumors from these patients show deletion of the normal PTEN allele consistent with a two-hit mechanism. Inactivation of PTEN by combined mutation and allele loss has also been found in 30% of gliomas, and is common in prostate and endometrial cancers. In addition, tumor cell lines deficient in PTEN have a high level of AKT activation as judged by phosphorylation, and this is reversed by replacement of active PTEN (57).

P53 AND APOPTOSIS

The p53 gene has important roles in the cellular response to growth overstimulation and DNA damage. This response requires some decision making on the part of the cell as to whether simple cell cycle arrest or, alternatively, apoptosis occurs (58,59). Extensive DNA damage tends to induce apoptosis through activation of the checkpoint (see Genome Instability). Checkpoint activation induces activation of several kinases, including the DNA-dependent protein kinase, ATM,

Chk1, and Chk2. All of these kinases phosphorylate p53 protein in a region near its N-terminus close to where the MDM2 protein binds to p53 (Fig. 6-8). This phosphorylation thus blocks the binding of p53 to MDM2, leading to stabilization of p53 expression, and permitting p53 to act as a transcription factor. p53 influences transcription of several genes that are proapoptotic, including Bax, Noxa, p53AIP1, and Pidd. Some of the activity of p53 in transcription is mediated by the transcription factor nuclear factor-κB (NF-κB), whose expression is crucial for full p53 apoptosis induction (60). Noxa interacts with bcl-2 to neutralize its antiapoptotic activity, whereas the functions of p53AIP1 and Pidd are less certain. The mechanism of cell choice to proceed with apoptosis as opposed to simple cell cycle arrest is not certain but appears to depend partly on the level of expression of p53. Lower levels of expression cause cell cycle arrest, whereas higher levels lead to apoptosis.

EVASION OF APOPTOSIS BY THE MALIGNANT CELL

The complexity of the pathways of apoptosis provide ample opportunity for subversion and evasion by the malignant cell. As discussed above, p53 mutations, expression of bcl-2, inactivation of Bax, inactivation of PTEN, and expression of survivin are all commonly seen in a variety of human cancers, and it is likely that each contributes to evasion of apoptosis by the malignant cell. In addition, lung and colon carcinomas commonly express a nonsignaling decoy receptor for fas ligand that circumvents proapoptotic signaling through fas receptor. It is likely that other mechanisms are also used by tumor cells to avoid untimely cell death, but are as yet unrecognized.

Limitless Replicative Potential

Cancer cells have the ability to maintain their chromosome ends (telomeres) over multiple generations by an evolutionarily conserved mechanism that is not operative in the majority of normal differentiated adult tissues. This characteristic appears to be a crucial component of the set of acquired abilities that are necessary for human cancer development. Although this ability interacts in ways with some of the pathways discussed in the above sections, it has unique aspects, and therefore is discussed in detail here.

TELOMERES AND TELOMERASE

Telomeres are specialized nucleoprotein structures that are present at the ends of all human chromosomes (61–64). They exist as a resolution to a problem known as the *end replication problem*, which is a consequence of the linear, noncircular nature of human chromosomes. Because DNA polymerases are able to replicate single-stranded DNA in one (5' to 3') direction only, if a specialized mechanism did not exist whereby the end of the DNA molecule could be maintained, chromosome ends would shorten by 50 to 100 base pairs per cell division. Eventually, chromosome ends would erode into genes that happened to reside near the ends of chromosomes. In addition, the eroded ends would stimulate cell cycle arrest or aberrant chromosomal end joinings (see further below). Progressive chromosomal end shortening has been observed in many human somatic tissues on extended culture *in vitro*, consistent with the attrition rate noted above.

Human telomeres consist of several hundred to a few thousand tandem repeats of the DNA sequence TTAGGG (63). This sequence is typically present in a length equivalent to 2- to 20-kilobase pairs of DNA. Although the majority of the telomere is normal double-stranded DNA, the tip end consists of a 3' overhang of approximately 150 bases. This single-stranded end piece folds back on the remainder of the chromosomal end, forming a unique structure called the *t loop*.

Telomere maintenance in human embryonic and certain other actively dividing somatic cells is achieved by a large nucleoprotein complex termed *telomerase* (63). Two components have been identified within telomerase thus far that are essential for its activity. The first is an RNA component, hTER, that serves as the template for the addition of TTAGGG repeats to the end of the telomere. The second is the catalytic subunit, hTERT, which has RNA-dependent transcriptase (reverse transcriptase) activity. hTER is expressed widely in all embryonic and adult tissues. However, most human somatic cells lack telomerase activity and do not express hTERT. On the other hand, human cancers most often do express hTERT and have telomerase activity.

LINK BETWEEN TELOMERASE AND CANCER

Circumstantial evidence suggests that telomerase expression is an important characteristic of human cancers (63). Approximately 90% of human cancers express telomerase, in contrast to the normal tissues from which they are derived. In addition, when human cells are transformed by artifical means (oncogenic viruses) *in vitro*, they typically acquire telomerase activity. Although the telomeres of these malignant cell lines are often shorter than those seen in normal human cells, they appear to be sufficient to permit normal chromosomal end replication and stability.

However, not all human cancers express telomerase. In some cases, telomeres are maintained in the absence of telomerase using a mechanism that has been termed *alternate telomere maintenance* (ALT). In cells using this mechanism, telomeres have different structural features from telomeres present in normal cells, but they nevertheless appear to function normally during chromosome replication. The biochemistry of this ALT pathway of telomere function is not understood, but it appears to account for the distinct minority of human cancers. Nonetheless, it is of concern for potential escape from the effects of telomerase inhibition approaches being developed for treatment of cancer.

TELOMERASE AS A CRITICAL COMPONENT FOR HUMAN CELL IMMORTALIZATION

The observation that most cultured human cells lack telomerase and undergo progressive telomere shortening led to the hypothesis that telomeres may act as a mitotic clock. In the most recent elaboration of this model, once telomeres shorten to a critical length, they have a tendency to become recognized as being "uncapped" (61) (Fig. 6-10). Although telomere shortening is a progressive process, owing to the heterogeneity in the size of telomeres in cells at the start of culture, and variation in the extent of telomere erosion with each cell division, uncapping of telomeres is viewed as a stochastic process. Thus, growing cells will develop uncapped ends at a variable rate. When uncapping occurs, this elicits recognition by a nucleoprotein complex of enzymes that responds to DNA damage, because the uncapped end of a chromosome has the same physical appearance as a double-strand break in a chromosome. In the normal cell, this elicits cell cycle arrest while the cell attempts to repair the apparent damage. Thus, after a limited number of cell divisions, all normal cells in a population without telomerase will eventually become arrested due to production of uncapped telomeres.

This model is supported by the observation that cultured cells will continue to grow for only a limited number of divisions before becoming senescent (failing to grow further) despite delivery of growth factors and other conditions favorable for growth. Moreover, introduction of hTERT expression by artificial means (transfection) is able to prevent telomere shortening as well as the onset of senescence in these cultures (62).

Importantly, these normal human cells in which hTERT has been expressed are not malignant. They do not grow in the

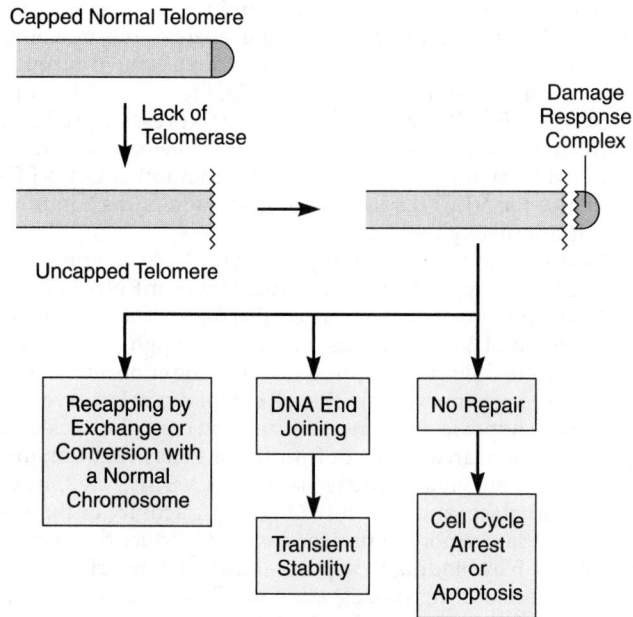

Figure 6-10. A model for the function of a capped chromosome. A normal capped chromosome is shown at top. In response to a reduction in levels of telomerase, chromosome ends become uncapped by erosion of the TTAGGG repeat and are recognized by a DNA damage response complex as being abnormal. This elicits one of three responses: (a) The uncapped end is repaired by exchange or conversion with a normal capped chromosome end, (b) nonhomologous end joining occurs with another uncapped chromosome end (to provide transient stability), or (c) cell cycle arrest or apoptosis occurs.

absence of normal growth factors, and they respond normally to DNA damage, high-density conditions, and other treatments. They will not form tumors in nude mice. Thus, telomerase expression appears to be independent of other cancer-related mechanisms for circumvention of cell growth and cell cycle control mechanisms.

Recently, further compelling evidence for the importance of telomerase expression as an independent and necessary factor for cancer development has been reported (65). Introduction of three defined genetic elements was shown to be necessary and sufficient for the complete tumorigenic conversion of normal human fibroblast and epithelial cells. The three elements were the simian virus 40 large T oncoprotein, which binds to and inactivates both p53 and Rb; a mutated, activated ras gene (H-ras); and the hTERT subunit of telomerase. All three of these genetic elements were required for the tumorigenic conversion of the cells as assessed by tumor formation in nude mice. Other studies served to exclude the possibility that additional genetic effects were required that occurred stochastically in the manipulated cells. The simian virus 40 large T oncoprotein is an important element in this process that achieves two significant effects: blocking the cell cycle arrest functions of p53 and Rb. Nonetheless, this experiment serves to emphasize the limited number of genetic changes absolutely required for malignant development in the human and the important role of telomerase in the process.

TELOMERE STUDIES IN THE MOUSE

Generation of a mouse that is deficient in telomerase by deletion of the TERT gene has provided an opportunity for analysis of the critical *in vivo* functions of telomerase (66,67). As predicted, the cells of these mice develop progressive telomere shortening that begins to cause significant clinical problems only after several

generations have elapsed and telomeres have become critically shortened. Of greatest interest was the tumor predisposition of these mice. Mice lacking TERT developed tumors spontaneously at an accelerated rate compared to age-matched wild-type controls. However, the tumors developed only in older mice (age >1 year), suggesting that the telomerase effect was modest. Nonetheless, the tumors contained chromosomes that had undergone end-to-end fusion events (robertsonian chromosomes) consistent with the results of telomere erosion.

Lack of telomerase in mice also displayed an interaction with partial or complete deletion of the p53 gene. In these mice, there was a modest acceleration of the rate of tumor development compared to mice with p53 mutation alone. However, the majority of the p53 heterozygous telomerase-deficient mice developed epithelial cancers. This is in contrast to p53 heterozygous mice, which usually develop greater than 90% lymphomas and sarcomas. Moreover, these carcinomas demonstrated a variety of aberrant chromosomes, including those derived from nonreciprocal translocations, end-to-end fusions, and more complex chromosomal events. These chromosomal abnormalities are rare in the usual lymphomas and sarcomas of p53 heterozygous mice. The observations suggest that the lack of telomerase and shortened telomeres in epithelial cells lead to a higher rate of chromosomal aberrances, which interact with the lack of p53 to lead to greatly accelerated epithelial carcinogenesis. The observation is also important because the majority of human epithelial cancers display complex chromosomal karyotypes that are similar to those noted in the p53 heterozygous telomerase null mice. In all, the observations suggest that epithelial carcinogenesis in humans may proceed through an early phase in which telomerase is absent and telomeres are quite short, leading to complex chromosomal translocations to accelerate the process of transformation but then followed by expression of telomerase to achieve some level of genomic stability.

CLINICAL APPLICATION

Treatment strategies that target telomerase are in their infancy, so there is as yet limited clinical support for the concept that telomerase represents an ideal tumor Achilles heel. Our discussion indicates the prevalence of telomerase expression in malignant cancers and cell lines, as well as the likely untoward effects of telomerase inhibition on telomere function and cell survival. The issues in translating this research to clinical practice relate to how well telomerase can be inhibited; how quickly the effects might be seen in cancer cells *in vivo*, that is, how long a period of treatment is required before seeing telomere erosion and significant cell cycle effects; and the side effects due to inhibition of telomerase in normal cells. At present, there is evidence that telomerase inhibition may be an effective therapeutic intervention (68,69), but further study is required.

Angiogenesis Acquisition

The development of angiogenesis within a solid tumor has long been recognized as an important necessary step in human carcinogenesis (70,71). In recent years, the molecular steps involved in angiogenesis have been identified, inhibitors with several different mechanisms of action have been developed, and clinical trials of these compounds are now under way.

TUMORS REQUIRE OXYGEN FOR GROWTH

All mammalian cells require oxygen for growth and survival and are therefore located within 200 μm of blood vessels under normal conditions—which is the diffusion limit for oxygen in solid and aqueous substances (70,71). During embryonic development, formation of new blood vessels occurs by two means.

Vasculogenesis is the formation of blood vessels *de novo* from precursor cells called *angioblasts*, which cluster and organize to form rudimentary vascular channels. Once a primary vascular system is developed, new capillaries develop from preexisting capillaries by sprouting from their sides or by splitting (intussusception), and both of these processes are termed *angiogenesis*.

Tumors are generally thought to begin their development without angiogenesis, and this leads to a size limitation of approximately 1 mm in diameter owing to the diffusion limit of oxygen. Indeed, it is thought that many tumors of this size may exist in the body and remain dormant, that is to say, clinically insignificant, for many years. Within such microtumors, there may be continuing cell division on the outer surface which is compensated by continuing cell death, possibly by apoptosis, within the hypoxic interior.

Further development of such microtumors is dependent on turning the "angiogenic switch" to the "on" position (70,71). This is a matter of changing the balance of angiogenic factors from being predominantly antiangiogenic to predominantly proangiogenic. However, it has also been shown in mouse model systems that tumors can co-opt the normal vasculature of an organ to their own advantage to achieve growth beyond 1-mm diameter (72). In these circumstances, the tumor growth is limited by the normal vascular structure and other anatomic limitations, so that again at some later point, angiogenesis must occur to permit the tumor to expand further.

Events which may favor the turning on of the angiogenic switch are not completely understood (73). They include factors that are common to many tumors but appear to be insufficient on their own, such as hypoxia, acidosis, hypoglycemia, and mechanical stress. Infiltrating immune and inflammatory cells may also be important, as are genetic mutations, including many of those already described (e.g., p53 inactivation), which result in a shift to angiogenesis.

An important observation is that the vasculature induced within cancers is abnormal. Tumor vessels are typically disorganized at every level of inspection (fractal theory has been applied to their study) (74) and are tortuous and dilated, with uneven diameter and excessive branching and shunts (75). Tumors may have regions of overabundant vessel supply and relative regions of insufficient supply, and the overabundant regions may be predisposed to spontaneous hemorrhage. In addition, tumor vessels often lack perivascular cells so that normal vascular responses are perturbed or absent. Further, vessel walls are not always formed by a homogeneous layer of endothelial cells, so in some cases, tumor cells form part or all of a vessel wall. Finally, even when present, endothelial cells in tumor vessel walls can be characterized as leaky in that they have large numbers of openings, widened junctions between cells, and a discontinuous basement membrane.

ANGIOGENIC FACTORS

Angiogenic factors are soluble factors that have the ability to induce angiogenesis (70,71). Because both sprouting and splitting forms of angiogenesis require endothelial cell growth, angiogenic factors are always endothelial cell growth factors. There are two major families of angiogenic factors: the vascular endothelial growth factor (VEGF) family and the angiopoietin (Ang) family, as well as an assortment of other soluble factors that have nonexclusive proangiogenic activity. Regulation of endothelial cell growth is similar to that described for cells in general in the first section.

VEGF is the major inducer of angiogenesis produced by malignant cells and is the major growth factor regulating endothelial cell growth (70,71). It is a member of a family including VEGF-B, VEGF-C, VEGF-D, and VEGF-E. VEGF is the most crit-

ical member of this family during embryonic angiogenesis because ablation of even a single VEGF allele results in embryonic lethality in the mouse. There are three known receptor tyrosine kinases that bind VEGFs: VEGFR-1, VEGFR-2, and VEGFR-3. VEGFR-1 and VEGFR-2 are expressed predominantly in the blood vascular endothelium, whereas VEGFR-3 is restricted in expression to the lymphatic endothelium. VEGF stimulates the VEGFR's leading to activation of ras and other growth stimulating pathways.

Expression of VEGF messenger RNA (mRNA) and protein is increased by hypoxia *in vitro*, and VEGF mRNA is often increased in regions of tumor necrosis (70,71). The mechanism of regulation of VEGF expression occurs through the action of hypoxia-inducible transcription factors. Under normal conditions, these proteins reside in the cell cytoplasm at low levels. In response to hypoxia, they are stabilized and enter the nucleus to influence the transcription of multiple genes that enhance hypoxic cell survival directly, as well as VEGF, Ang2, nitric oxide synthetase, and PDGF-B. One major activity of the von Hippel-Lindau tumor-suppressor gene is to reduce the production of VEGF by binding to hypoxia-inducible transcription factors and accelerating its degradation. This explains the high level of angiogenesis associated with tumors occurring in von Hippel-Lindau syndrome.

The angiopoietin family of proteins consists of four members (Ang1, Ang2, Ang3, and Ang4) that bind to a single receptor, called *Tie-2* (70,71). Roles for these proteins and the receptor are well defined in normal angiogenesis, but their function during tumor-induced angiogenesis appears complex. Ang2 and Ang3 are inhibitors of the Tie-2 receptor and angiogenesis, and Ang2 is expressed at sites of tumor angiogenesis. The Tie signaling pathway appears to be particularly important in the regulation of vessel size and in cell–cell contact within and surrounding capillaries.

Several other less specific growth factors also have effects on endothelial cells, including basic fibroblast growth factor (FGF), TGF-β, the ephrin family of ligands, and the Delta family of Notch ligands.

ANGIOGENIC INHIBITORS

Multiple types of angiogenic inhibitors have been discovered, including angiostatin, endostatin, antithrombin III, thrombospondin-1, and interferon-α/β. Endostatin is a proteolytic fragment of collagen XVIII, a component of the ECM. Angiostatin is a proteolytic fragment of plasmin, an element of the blood clotting system. The precise mechanisms of action of these compounds are uncertain, which hinders a search for smaller molecules with similar activity.

ANGIOGENESIS AND METASTASIS

Metastasis is a complex process that is discussed in detail in the following section. However, there is an intricate relationship between angiogenesis and metastasis which we now consider.

Angiogenesis generally and the vascular density of tumors in particular have been shown to be associated with tumor metastasis (76). This association has been quantified in the form of a relationship between frequency of metastasis and vessel density within tumor sections. A correlation between these two processes makes sense for several reasons. First, VEGF and βFGF secreted by tumor cells induce the expression of both plasminogen activator and collagenases, which contribute to ECM destruction to enhance metastasis. Second, the capillaries, which are produced by tumor angiogenesis, are typically disordered and leaky, permitting tumor cells to enter the circulation. Third, incipient micrometastases require angiogenesis for growth.

In addition, induction of the lymphatic branch of angiogenesis by expression of VEGF-C by tumor cells and interaction with

VEGFR-3 will lead to lymphatic vessel proliferation. Such lymphatic vessels may have the same aberrant growth pattern seen in the primary angiogenic response, leading to entrance into lymphatics of tumor cells and providing a pathway for lymphatic metastasis, usually the earliest form of metastasis in human cancer.

CLINICAL TRIALS OF ANTIANGIOGENESIS AGENTS
Therapeutic approaches to limit or reverse angiogenesis within tumors are by far the most developed molecular strategy for the therapy of cancer. Nonetheless, they are still at an early stage and of unproven benefit. The approach is attractive for several reasons. First, as described, angiogenesis is crucial for cancer development and growth. Second, unlike tumor cells, which are genetically unstable, heterogeneous, and capable of adaptation to a variety of therapeutic strategies, endothelial cells are not mutant and are the primary target of antiangiogenic treatments. Third, the endothelium receives the full dose of administered drug without limitations of drug delivery.

However, there are also several limitations to this therapeutic approach. Because many cancers are already large and metastatic at the time of their discovery, antiangiogenic therapies will have to reduce existing vasculature as well as limit formation of new vessels to be effective. Second, the potential for adaptation by human cancers should not be underestimated. It is quite possible that cancer cells will respond to one form of antiangiogenic attack by elaboration of secondary and tertiary methods of inducing and stabilizing vessels using different angiogenic circuits. In addition, because these therapies appear likely to induce tumor dormancy only and not complete eradication, long-term therapy may be required with potential for serious long-term side effects.

Nonetheless, in murine models, several compounds have been shown to be effective (77). Such treatments in mice are effective whether given early on during tumor development or at later time points in which regression of large end-stage cancer was achieved.

The compounds that are currently in clinical trials include: TNP470, a small molecule inhibitor of endothelial cell proliferation; angiostatin and endostatin; thalidomide, which inhibits endothelial cell growth by unknown mechanisms; squalamine, an extract of shark liver that inhibits the sodium-hydrogen exchanger, NHE3; SU5416 and SU6668, small compounds that block VEGF signaling; and an antiVEGF antibody (http://cancertrials.nci.nih.gov/news/angio/table.html).

Metastasis Competence
Nearly all epithelial cancers develop metastases during the course of disease, and these lesions make a substantial contribution to patient morbidity and mortality. If metastases could be prevented or eliminated, most epithelial cancers could be treated surgically with good results. Thus, metastasis is an important clinical problem that is a crucial aspect of malignant development. Many years of investigation have led to a good understanding of the basic principles of metastatic development, and increasingly, the molecular details of these principles are being understood.

METASTATIC CASCADE: SURVIVAL OF THE FITTEST
Six critical steps must occur for cancer cells to be successful at development of metastasis, each of which requires different tumor cell characteristics (78). The requirement for multiple independent steps may help to partially explain why metastasis is not an even more common clinical problem. All of these steps occur subsequent to the acquisition of angiogenesis for two important reasons. First, without angiogenic development,

tumors remain too small to have any statistical chance of completing the six steps. Second, the disordered vasculature that is part of tumor angiogenesis greatly enhances the chances of the malignant cell completing the first two steps.

The first step is *local invasion*. This is the ability of the tumor cell to invade host stroma and gain access to the circulation. The disordered vascular architecture in cancers that have acquired angiogenesis, including thin walls, being lined directly by tumor cells in some regions, and lack of a basement membrane, all facilitate this process. Nonetheless, tumor cell motility and invasive ability are required for the cells to enter the circulation. The second step is *detachment and embolization*. Single or clumps of tumor cells must then detach from the interior of the vessel and embolize through the circulation. This achievement may actually conflict in some ways with the invasion step in that motility and invasion require good surface attachment, whereas embolization requires release. The third step is *survival* in the circulation. This step is nontrivial in that even malignant, transformed cells will grow better when attached to a substrate and cannot survive buffeted about in the vascular environment indefinitely. The fourth step is *arrest*. Tumor cells within the circulation must arrest within the capillary bed of a distant organ by adhering either to capillary endothelial cells or to small regions of exposed basement membrane. Specialized mechanisms exist for each variety of normal blood cell (granulocytes, lymphocytes, and platelets) to achieve adherence at specific sites. A similar mechanism must apply to tumor cells unless simple mechanical obstruction is sufficient owing to the size of the tumor aggregate present in the circulation. The fifth step is *extravasation*. This is the reverse of the first step and is likely to require similar cellular properties of motility and invasive capacity. The sixth step is that of *proliferation*. Within the new organ, the metastatic cell or cell aggregate must be able to grow and develop into a colony. Although this might seem relatively simple, the different composition of the new organ in terms of cellular content and ECM may have strong growth inhibitory effects that terminate or limit the growth of metastasis at this stage. Such incipient metastases would then go unrecognized and have no clinical relevance.

The importance of tumor cell intracellular architecture, motility, and invasive ability on metastasis has led to intense investigation of these properties of malignant cells. As usual, these studies have benefited from a deep and progressing understanding of the general subject of cell organization and motility with the field of cell biology.

TUMOR CELL INTRACELLULAR ORGANIZATION, MOTILITY, AND INVASION
Malignant transformation of cells is characterized by dramatic changes in cell shape and intracellular organization that affect the internal architecture of the cell known as the *cytoskeleton* (79). The cytoskeleton consists of three primary structural elements that determine the overall shape of the cell, which are regulated in their disposition and arrangement by a large number of associated proteins, including both intracellular and transmembrane proteins. These three primary elements are microtubules, intermediate filaments, and actin microfilaments. All three of these structural elements are capable of dynamic changes between existence in cells in the form of single subunit monomers and organization into extended polymerized rodlike structures. The actin filament architecture in cells has the most important role in the determination of the overall structure and motile and invasive capacity of cells and is typically greatly altered in malignant cells. Several protein elements that interact with actin are reduced in expression in malignant cells, including some tropomyosin isoforms, gelsolin, α-actinin, and vinculin. Studies in which reexpression of these proteins in malignant cells has served to reduce

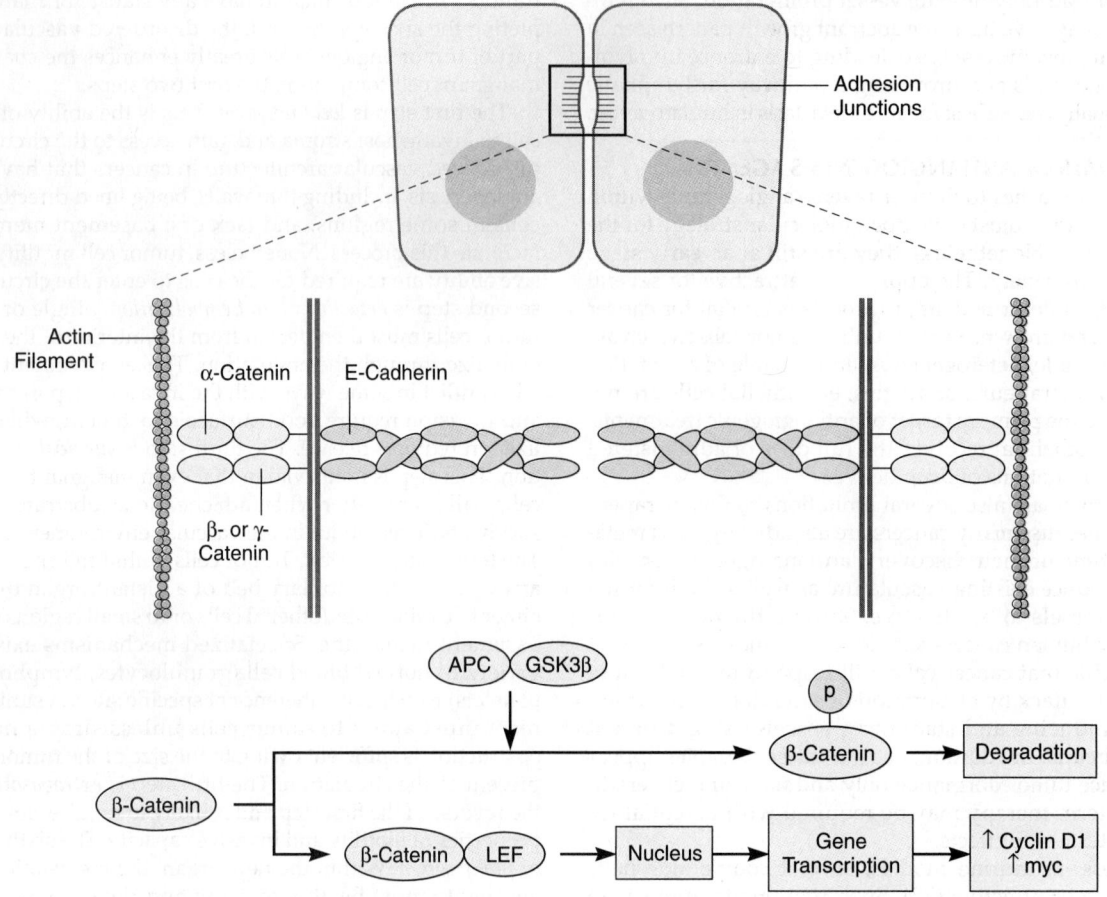

Figure 6-11. Cadherins and catenins in adhesion junctions and signaling. In normal epithelial cells, E-cadherin forms an extracellular bridge between cells, which connects to α-, β-, and γ-catenins and the actin filament architecture within the cell. The adenomatous polyposis coli (APC) and glycogen synthase kinase 3β (GSK3β) complex phosphorylates free β-catenin, leading to its degradation. In cells lacking APC, this does not occur, and free β-catenin can bind to LEF, which translocates to the nucleus to transmit positive growth signaling.

malignant potential have confirmed the importance of these expression changes. In addition, the protein merlin, which is encoded by the gene that causes neurofibromatosis type 2, a tumor-suppressor gene syndrome in which patients are predisposed to development of schwannomas and meningioma, also binds to actin and links it to the plasma membrane of the cell.

Cell structure and motile events are regulated by a group of GTP-binding proteins that are related to the ras family. This rho GTPase family includes cdc42, rac, and rho and serves to transmit motility signals derived from external ligands through receptors to the actin cytoskeleton. Expression of the rho GTPase has been shown to be necessary and sufficient for generation of lung metastasis in a mouse model after tail vein injection (80).

CADHERIN-CATENIN SIGNALING IN TUMORIGENESIS AND METASTASIS

Connections between the actin cytoskeleton and transmembrane proteins are particularly important in the morphologic organization of epithelial cells (Fig. 6-11). Normal epithelial cells *in vivo* form tight contacts with adjacent cells through structures known as *adhesion junctions* (also called *zonula adherens*). These structures are a critical element in the barrier function that epithelial cell layers perform in preventing absorption or passage of materials from external locations through the epithelial boundary layer. A major protein component of the adhesion junction is the cadherin family of transmembrane

glycosylated proteins (81). E-cadherin is the major cadherin isoform expressed in epithelial cells. E-cadherin contains a large extracellular domain which displays Ca^{2+}-dependent self-dimerization capability. Structural studies have shown that E-cadherin begins as an unordered structure that becomes a rigid rodlike structure in response to Ca^{2+} binding, which is then capable of first *cis* dimerization with a second E-cadherin protein on the same cell, followed by *trans* dimerization with E-cadherin expressed on a neighboring cell. This combination of *cis* and *trans* interactions leads to the forming of a strong extended region of E-cadherin binding between adjacent epithelial cells in a model known as the *zipper hypothesis*.

Cadherins are linked through their intracellular domains to a complex of proteins called *catenins*, including α-catenin, β-catenin, and γ-catenin/plakoglobin. The catenin complexes are connected with the actin cytoskeleton to reinforce the structural organization of both external and internal cell components. This complete structural assembly—E-cadherin–catenin complex-actin microfilament system—appears to be extremely important in the organization of epithelial cell layers throughout the body and is uniformly disrupted in epithelial cancers. For example, reduction or loss of expression of E-cadherin has been documented in a high proportion of all epithelial malignancies and typically correlates with the degree of differentiation of the tumor.

In addition, E-cadherin–catenin organization is deregulated by signaling through the EGF receptor (EGFR). As noted above, EGF signaling is amplified by receptor overexpression in several types of epithelial cancers. In addition to its role in growth signaling, activated EGFR can directly phosphorylate both E-cadherin and catenins, which leads to their dissociation from the normal E-cadherin–catenin complexes. This also leads to production of free β-catenin, which has other important activities (see below). A number of growth factors isolated from malignant cells also activate receptor-based pathways, which lead to similar disruption of E-cadherin–catenin complexes. As a counterbalancing factor, signaling through some members of the rho family of GTPases, which are downstream of ras during growth factor stimulation, leads to inhibition of a protein called *IQGAP1*, which serves to enhance E-cadherin–catenin complex interaction and stability (82).

The protein product of the adenomatous polyposis coli gene (APC) also has an important role in the formation of E-cadherin complexes and maintenance of normal epithelial shape (83). APC normally forms a complex with a specific kinase, GSK3β, and other proteins that can bind to and phosphorylate free β-catenin. This has the effect of enhancing the degradation of free, noncomplexed β-catenin. In colon cancers that occur in patients with the APC syndrome and other nonhereditary forms of colon cancer, the APC gene is commonly mutated or inactivated. This has the effect of eliminating this mechanism for elimination of β-catenin.

Free β-catenin has a remarkable additional property: It can form a complex with transcription factors called LEF. The β-catenin–LEF complex enters the nucleus where the LEF protein is active in transcription of a set of genes that are important in maintaining positive cell growth signaling and survival. LEF increases expression of the myc gene and the cyclin D1 gene.

Direct mutation of the genes involved in this pathway have been identified in some cancers. E-cadherin is a direct target for mutation in some forms of gastric and breast carcinoma, and its expression is reduced by hypermethylation in other cancers. There is also a hereditary diffuse gastric cancer syndrome in which there is high predisposition to development of a distinctive form of gastric cancer, in which there are germline mutations in the E-cadherin gene (84).

EXTRACELLULAR MATRIX AND MATRIX METALLOPROTEINASES

The ECM is composed of structural molecules, including collagen, proteoglycans, and glycoproteins. It is a critical structural component of all organs and tissues, and is required for normal development. As cancers develop, ECM boundaries are both degraded and violated repeatedly by malignant cells. Several classes of proteins are capable of degrading the ECM, but the family with greatest importance in this activity in most malignant cells is the matrix metalloproteinases (MMPs) family (85).

MMPs are a large family of related proteins, all of which contain a conserved catalytic domain whose activity is dependent on the presence of Zn^{2+}. Most MMPs are secreted enzymes, but cell-surface–bound forms have also been identified. Secreted MMPs must be activated through removal of a prodomain and are also regulated by inhibitors that are called *tissue-specific inhibitors of matrix-metalloproteinases* (TIMPs). MMPs can proteolytically digest all of the elements that make up the ECM.

Much evidence has been obtained to indicate that MMP expression is an important attribute of the malignant cell that contributes to metastasis formation (85,86). MMP expression was first identified in a transformed cell line in which its level of expression was greatly increased. MMP levels have been found to be a prognostic factor in several different types of cancer. Overexpression of MMP-3 increases the invasive properties of breast epithelial cells, whereas application of TIMPs to invasion assays leads to a reduction in invasion and metastasis in cultured cell assays. MMP expression has also been recognized as important in the earliest phases of tumor growth, in which ECM degradation is helpful to reduce structural restraints to progressive growth. MMP expression also is important in the development of angiogenesis, presumably contributing to the tissue remodeling that is required for effective vascular development. In addition, tumor cells can induce expression of MMPs in adjacent stromal cells to enhance their further development.

Proteolytic cleavage of ECM components by MMPs also results in the release of signaling components, which are embedded in the ECM and can contribute to tumor development. For example, MMP-3 can cleave the molecule decorin, which will release TGF-β from the matrix, leading to growth stimulation in the tumor cells and enhancement of angiogenesis. In addition, MMPs have the ability to cleave other substrates near tumor cells, potentially altering cell–cell and cell-matrix connections by, for example, cleaving integrins and E-cadherin.

These multiple actions of MMPs during cancer cell growth have led to vigorous investigation of the potential benefit of MMP inhibitors in mouse model studies and several trials in cancer patients, some of which are ongoing (85). MMPs would appear to be an ideal target because they are not required for most normal organ functions, and therefore, side effects should be limited. However, clinical trials of MMP inhibitors have been complicated by the development of connective tissue and joint pains, presumably reflecting normal MMP function in these organs. Trials in mice have shown activity for a number of different types of tumors with MMP inhibitors, but also indicate that they are most effective for early lesions in halting further development. Clinical trials in patients have focused on metastatic disease patients, for obvious reasons, but with little evidence for benefit so far.

SEED AND SOIL HYPOTHESIS: ZIP-CODING FOR METASTASES?

The nonrandom nature of metastasis has been recognized for over 100 years. Although the draining of lymph nodes is the major avenue for metastasis for many cancers, hematogenous spread is also frequent and at times occurs in a manner that suggests that there is tissue-specific tropism. The concept that certain cancer cells (the seed) might have a specific affinity for the certain host cells or organ environments (the soil) was an hypothesis put forward in 1889 by Paget (87). This model has been validated by studies in mice in which organ tropism of metastases has been shown and could be enhanced by serial culture of cells migrating to specific sites. The molecular basis of this organ tropism remains largely unknown, but it may relate to organ-specific growth factors or the influence of the organ environment on the invasive phenotype of the cells.

It is also possible that tumor cells bear surface receptors that enhance their localization from the circulation to the endothelial cells of certain organs. In an extension of this concept, peptide sequences have been identified that will bind selectively to the endothelial cells present in a tumor (88). This observation has promise in the site-specific delivery of antineoplastic drugs.

NEGATIVE REGULATORS OF METASTASIS

A series of genes or regions within the human genome have been identified that appear to serve as negative regulators of metastasis (89). The best characterized of these genes is the nm23 gene (90). This gene was identified by comparison of gene expression between cell lines with low and high metastatic potential in mouse model experiments. Subsequently, reduction of nm23 expression has been found in most but not all metastatic cancers. Moreover, gene transfer of nm23 into a number of highly metastatic cell lines can revert their metastatic potential. The mechanism of action of nm23 in producing this effect is uncertain. The protein has been shown to have nucleoside diphosphate kinase activity.

One other gene with this activity, KAI1, has been identified. The hope is that through understanding the biochemical activity of these gene products, inhibitors could be developed that would reduce cancer metastasis.

Mutation Acquisition and Genome Instability

The discussion so far has highlighted the many ways in which cancer cells differ from their normal counterparts. In many cases, these differences are based on mutation within the cancer cell genome, whereas in other cases, the differences are based on changes in protein expression that reflect epigenetic changes (see further below).

Given the importance of accretion of mutations to neoplastic development and progression, in this section we consider the normal physiologic mechanisms by which cells respond to and correct mutation, and how these are deranged in cancer cells. We also consider the mechanisms and derangements that occur in epigenetic mechanisms of alteration of gene expression.

SINGLE BASE SUBSTITUTION MUTATIONS
Although there is considerable variance by gene in the types of mutation that are seen in human genetic disease and cancer, point mutations in general are by far the largest contributor to new human mutations (91). Point mutation activation or inactivation is also common for certain genes involved in neoplastic development (e.g., ras and p53), although not all.

Point mutations can affect each of the four nucleotides in the genome, and examples of conversion to each of the other three nucleotides are known. However, the CpG dinucleotide is a frequent target for mutation in human genes (it accounts for 29% of all point mutations) during cancer development, which relates to the occurrence of methylation on the C residues of CpG sequence (91) (see Epigenetic Silencing of Transcription). Methylcytosine can be converted by spontaneous deamination to the exact structure of thymine. Thymine-guanosine mismatches cannot be resolved precisely by error-correcting protein complexes because each base appears to be perfectly correct. Thus, either one or the other base is chosen as the template base. If the thymine base is chosen, then the guanosine base is replaced, and mutation occurs. One effect of this process over evolutionary timescales is that the frequency of CpG dinucleotides in the genome is approximately one-fifth that predicted by the relative proportions of C and G residues.

The mechanism by which point mutations occur, apart from that described for CpG sequences, is poorly understood and has the usual difficulties associated with studying extremely rare events. Overall, the frequency and types of germline point mutation in the human genome match well with those seen in *in vitro* reactions using a major human DNA polymerase, polymerase β. This suggests that a substantial proportion of the point mutations that occur are due to misincorporation of bases during DNA replication (91,92).

However, there is considerable evidence associating exposure to certain chemical compounds (e.g., tobacco smoke) with the development of cancer in certain organ systems (e.g., the lung), arguing strongly that environmental exposure to carcinogenic compounds is a causative factor in cancer development. Moreover, formation of DNA adducts between compounds present in tobacco smoke (benzo[a]pyrene) and certain nucleotides within the p53 gene has been directly documented (93). These same nucleotides are those that are common sites for mutation in the p53 gene in lung cancers, directly implicating benzo[a]pyrene as the proximate carcinogen for lung cancer development.

The mechanism by which carcinogens produce mutation is, however, indirect (94). Most carcinogens present in tobacco smoke, including benzo[a]pyrene, are organic molecules, which are not directly chemically reactive with DNA. Instead, as part of the normal biochemical processing of exogenous substances for excretion, they are modified in two phases. The first phase is that of activation, in which members of the P450 family of enzymes add hydroxyl groups, forming compounds that contain epoxide and phenolic groups. The second phase is conjugation by glutathione S-transferases and related enzymes, in which glucuronide or sulfate groups are added to the hydroxyl groups, creating compounds which may be excreted in the bile or urine. The epoxide and phenolic products of the first phase are chemically reactive and can form DNA adducts. This, clearly, can lead to mutation when normal error-correcting mechanisms fail. These studies have also led to the concept that individuals who have strong first phase activity and reduced second phase activity, for genetic or other reasons, might be at increased risk for development of carcinogen-related cancers. Considerable investigation has led to some support for this hypothesis, as there is considerable genetic variation in the genes that perform these functions, but further validation in large cohorts of patients is required (94). In addition, twin studies of risk for lung cancer development has produced weak results, arguing against an important genetic component.

INSERTION AND DELETION MUTATIONS AND THE MISMATCH REPAIR COMPLEX
Insertion and deletion mutations, in which small numbers of bases (<20) are either deleted or added to a gene's sequence, are also common causes of human genetic disease (91). The vast majority of these mutations occur at short direct repeats by a mechanism termed *slipped strand mispairing* (95). A direct repeat is a nucleotide sequence in which a string of bases is directly repeated. For example, the GT dinucleotide sequence may be repeated three times, as in the sequence CAGTGTGTCC. These short repeats are common within the coding region of all genes as well as elsewhere in the genome. During replication of such a sequence, it is possible for the newly synthesized strand to slip forward or back on the opposing template single strand, resulting in the deletion or addition, respectively, of one copy of the GT repeat sequence.

A greatly increased tendency for insertion and deletion mutations at repetitive DNA sequences has been recognized in a subset of tumors arising in the colon, stomach, lung, ovary, breast, and other sites (96). This phenomenon has been called RER+ for replication error, as well as MIN or MSI for microsatellite instability. Microsatellites are tracts of repeated sequences (>5 repeats) for which the core unit is 1 to 5 bases in length. They occur frequently and are distributed throughout the genome. The most common of these is the GT/CA repeat, which occurs in runs of greater than ten repeats over 30,000 times in the genome. Tumors that are RER+ have alterations in the lengths of the repeats at many microsatellite sequences in the genome and also have relatively frequent, but less common, mutation at shorter repeat sequences. These tumors thus have a profound form of genomic instability that can mutate many genes.

A subset of patients with tumors that are RER+ have an inherited predisposition toward development of this type of tumor. These patients have the hereditary nonpolyposis coli cancer (HNPCC) syndrome, which is characterized by autosomal-dominant transmission of predisposition to cancer in the colon, endometrium, stomach, small intestine, and ureter at rates four to 22 times that of the normal population (97).

Germline mutations, which cause the HNPCC syndrome, may involve any of the following genes: hMSH2, hMLH1, hMSH6, hPMS1, and hPMS2 (97). The first two of these genes account for the majority of mutations. The protein products of these genes form a DNA mismatch repair complex, which resides in the nucleus and whose function is to identify sites of DNA mismatch, including single-base mismatches and small deletions and insertions. Typically, these mismatches are generated during DNA replication, and most are corrected by the DNA polymerase itself before involvement by the DNA mismatch repair complex. When activated, the mismatch repair complex recognizes the correct error-free strand of the DNA heteroduplex, and bases are excised from the mismatched newly synthesized strand. Subsequently, additional enzymes are recruited to the site of damage, including exonucleases, helicases, polymerases, and ligases to effect the repair (98).

The HNPCC syndrome occurs as an autosomal-dominant trait, following the classic Knudsen model described earlier. Individuals with this syndrome have a mutation in one copy of one of the mismatch repair genes (e.g., hMSH2). In somatic tissues, second-hit events occur in the other normal copy of hMSH2, which result in the complete loss of the protein, inactivation of the mismatch repair function, and RER+ features.

Many colon cancers are RER+ without an indication that the patient has the HNPCC syndrome (97). In some of these cases, inactivating somatic mutations have been identified in both copies of one of the mismatch repair genes, but more commonly, epigenetic silencing of hMLH1 has occurred (see further below) (99). RER+ cancers have a pathogenesis that appears distinct from that of nonRER+ colon cancers, with infrequent aneuploidy and gross chromosomal changes. Instead, RER+ cancers have increased rates of mutation at short repeat sequences throughout the genome. Two common targets for mutation in these tumors have been identified: the type II TGF-β receptor gene, and the proapoptotic gene Bax. Both are inactivated by mutation of a direct repeat present within the coding region.

EPIGENETIC SILENCING OF GENE TRANSCRIPTION

DNA methylation at CpG sequences does not affect the base pairing, but the methyl groups protrude into the major groove of the double helix, where their presence can be detected by a variety of DNA binding proteins (100). DNA methylation is used within the promoter elements of genes (regions generally upstream of the transcription initiation site) to mark genes for transcriptional silencing—that is, to turn off their expression. This method of regulation of transcription is used in a variety of normal cell and developmental settings. For example, the inactive X chromosome present in female cells sustains extensive CpG methylation to silence nearly all of the genes present on that chromosome.

The mechanism by which CpG methylation causes transcriptional silencing is not entirely clear, and there is even thought that methylation may represent a signature of a transcriptionally repressed region rather than being a causative factor. One mechanism that does occur is the binding of a transcriptional repressor, MeCP2 (101). MeCP2 binds to methylated DNA independent of the specific sequence present but with increasing affinity as the frequency of methylcytosine residues increases in a genomic region. MeCP2 binding leads to recruitment of a complex that acts to inhibit transcription. One of the mechanisms by which transcription is repressed is the deacetylation (removal of acetyl groups) from the histone molecules in the region of the methyl-C residues. This covalent modification of this essential protein component of the nucleosome directly influences how transcriptionally active the region will be. In addition, the DNA methyltransferase enzymes themselves often occur in a complex with the enzymes that contain histone deacetylases (102). Thus, both methylation and histone deacetylation may occur simultaneously, consistent with methylation being a marker for rather than a cause of silencing.

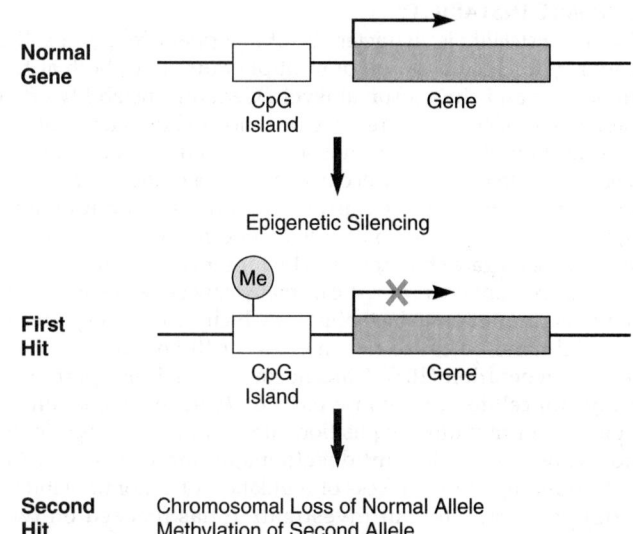

Figure 6-12. A model for epigenetic silencing of tumor-suppressor genes. A normal gene is shown at top. Epigenetic silencing occurs at one allele of the gene by methylation (Me) of the C residues at CpG sites within the CpG island adjacent to the transcriptional start site, thereby blocking transcription. A second hit occurs by chromosomal loss of the second allele (as in Fig. 6-3) or hypermethylation of the second allele to completely inactivate the gene.

CpG islands are GC- and CpG-rich regions of the genome, typically 500–1000 bases in length, that are often found near the promoter (transcriptional control) region of many widely expressed genes (Fig. 6-12). Apart from the X chromosome and certain imprinted genes, CpG islands near genes are not methylated in normal somatic tissues. Whenever cells are cultured in vivo, however, widespread CpG island methylation occurs. Moreover, widespread and aberrant methylation of CpG islands also occurs in neoplastic tissues (103). Because this change correlates with a reduction in expression of the genes associated with the individual CpG islands, and there is no mutational event occurring, this occurrence has been termed epigenetic silencing of gene transcription.

Epigenetic transcriptional silencing has considerable importance, as it provides a mechanism for the inactivation of genes that have tumor-suppressor or growth-limiting activity. In hereditary cancer syndromes, epigenetic silencing appears to be a rare cause of loss of expression of the wild-type allele; loss of heterozygosity or point mutation appear to be much more common. In sporadic cancers, epigenetic silencing is much more common and often affects several genes, suggesting that there is a global deregulation with widespread de novo methylation. The positive growth benefits to the developing malignant cell are that inactivation of multiple growth-limiting genes can occur at once. A major example of this phenomenon is in the subset of RER+ nonhereditary colorectal cancers in which mismatch-repair function has been lost (99), as indicated above. In most of these tumors, the RER+ phenotype has developed through methylation of the CpG island promoter region of the hMLH1 gene.

CpG island methylation has been shown to occur in the earliest stages of neoplastic development in Wilms' tumor by analysis of preneoplastic lesions adjacent to resected tumors (104). In addition, the importance of this phenomenon in tumor development has been clearly shown in mouse models. Mice that have a heterozygous defective allele in the APC gene (APC$^{Min/+}$) when interbred with mice that have a single null allele for a DNA methyl transferase gene display a markedly reduced rate of colonic polyp formation compared to APC$^{Min/+}$ mice, consistent with a direct benefit from the reduced occurrence of CpG methylation (105).

GENOMIC INSTABILITY

Genomic instability is characteristic of malignant cells and is the tendency for accumulation of multiple mutations, both at the single base and chromosomal levels. Genomic instability often leads to *aneuploidy*, the presence of abnormal total amounts of DNA and numbers of chromosomes per cell. Aneuploidy has been shown to be an early occurrence in most cancers arising in the uterine cervix, breast, prostate, lung, urothelium, and esophagus and appears to be due to a permanent defect in the ability to segregate chromosomes by tumor cells (106).

An important characteristic of many cancer cells with aneuploidy is chromosomal instability, in which there is missegregation of chromosomes at a rate in excess of 10^{-2} per chromosome per cell generation (107). Chromosomal instability permits a malignant cell to rapidly lose parts of its genome, enabling a rapid rate of mutation acquisition and evolution further down the pathway of malignant development and metastasis. An understanding of the process of regulation of genomic stability is not yet complete, but investigation has focused on two aspects of the malignant cell. The first is the mechanism of chromosomal instability. The second is normal pathways by which cells repair double-stranded breaks in the genome and how these might be disrupted in malignant cells.

The occurrence of chromosomal instability seems likely to reflect derangement in the mitotic machinery, which leads to proper chromosome segregation (106). This machinery is complex, and thus, multiple subunits are potential targets for disruption by mutation or other means. In the mitotic cell, the centrosomes or spindle poles are sites at which microtubules nucleate and from which the mitotic spindle is regulated. *Microtubules* are the structural elements along which the chromosomes migrate during mitosis. Chromosome condensation must occur, and they must attach to the kinetochores, which form the attachment to the microtubule spindles. Molecular motors then cause migration of the chromosomes to the centrosomes. Nearly all of these components, but particularly the microtubules and the centrosomes, are potential targets for defects that can contribute to chromosome missegregation and aneuploidy.

Recent progress has occurred in understanding the normal mechanisms by which cells detect and respond to double-stranded breaks in DNA (108,109). Such breaks occur spontaneously, and if not repaired properly, they have the potential to lead to chromosomal translocations and missegregation. The importance of this pathway has also been highlighted by the involvement of several genes with genetically defined roles in cancer development.

Proteins involved in the maintenance of genome stability have been categorized into those that have sensor functions, transducer functions, and effector functions. Sensor proteins and complexes are those that are responsible for detection of DNA damage. The identity of the sensor proteins is not certain, but candidates include the protein poly (ADP-ribose) polymerase and DNA-dependent protein kinase. It is also possible that several proteins in a large complex named BASC (BRCA1-associated genome-surveillance complex) that contains the product of the BRCA1 and ataxia-telangiectasia genes, several genome surveillance proteins with homologs in yeast, the Bloom's helicase protein, and some mismatch repair proteins (products of the hMSH2, hMSH6, and hMLH2 genes), are the main sensors (110).

The result of recruitment of the sensor proteins to double-stranded breaks is the activation of the ATM and ATR kinases (108). ATM is the product of the ataxia-telangiectasia gene, and ATR is a structural relative. Activated ATM and ATR kinases phosphorylate the Chk1 and Chk2 kinases. These kinases then effect a block in cell cycle progression and enable a repair response. Ultimately, either the double-strand break is repaired properly, or, in normal cells, an apoptotic response is elicited, and the cell dies.

Double-strand breaks can be repaired by either of two processes (108,109). First, nonhomologous end joining can occur. In this repair pathway, there is no template for the repair of the break. Rather, the two disconnected DNA ends are joined after the nucleotide sequence is blunted, and insertion of up to several bases occurs. Thus, nonhomologous end joining always results in some degree of mutation. The second pathway of double-strand break repair is through homologous recombination. This depends on the presence of a second normal copy of the chromosome to serve as the guide and involves a complex of proteins including helicases, ligases, and a repair protein complex.

REFERENCES

1. Hanahan D, Weinberg RA. The hallmarks of cancer. *Cell* 2000;100:57–70.
2. Nowell PC, Hungerford DA. A minute chromosome in human chronic granulocytic leukemia. *Science* 1960;132:1497.
3. Tabin CJ, Bradley SM, Bargmann CI, et al. Mechanism of activation of a human oncogene. *Nature* 1982;300:143–149.
4. Lynch HT, Krush AJ, Larsen AL. Heredity and multiple primary malignant neoplasms: six cancer families. *Am J Med Sci* 1967;254:322–329.
5. Knudson AG Jr. Mutation and cancer: statistical study of retinoblastoma. *Proc Natl Acad Sci U S A* 1971;68:820–823.
6. Harris H, Miller OJ, Klein G, et al. Suppression of malignancy by cell fusion. *Nature* 1969;223:363–368.
7. Yunis JJ, Ramsay N. Retinoblastoma and subband deletion of chromosome 13. *Am J Dis Child* 1978;132:161–163.
8. Friend SH, Bernards R, Rogelj S, et al. A human DNA segment with properties of the gene that predisposes to retinoblastoma and osteosarcoma. *Nature* 1986;323:643–646.
9. Rebollo A, Martinez AC. Ras proteins: recent advances and new functions. *Blood* 1999;94:2971–2980.
10. Shields JM, Pruitt K, McFall A, et al. Understanding Ras: "it ain't over 'til it's over." *Trends Cell Biol* 2000;10:147–154.
11. Schlessinger J. New roles for Src kinases in control of cell survival and angiogenesis. *Cell* 2000;100:293–296.
12. Bar-Sagi D, Hall A. Ras and Rho GTPases: a family reunion. *Cell* 2000;103:227–238.
13. Hunter T. Oncoprotein networks. *Cell* 1997;88:333–346.
14. Lukashev ME, Werb Z. ECM signaling: orchestrating cell behaviour and misbehaviour. *Trends Cell Biol* 1998;8:437–441.
15. Ullrich A, Schlessinger J. Signal transduction by receptors with tyrosine kinase activity. *Cell* 1990;61:203–212.
16. Jiang G, Hunter T. Receptor signaling: when dimerization is not enough. *Curr Biol* 1999;9:R568–R571.
17. Darnell JE Jr, Kerr IM, Stark GR. Jak-STAT pathways and transcriptional activation in response to IFNs and other extracellular signaling proteins. *Science* 1994;264:1415–1421.
18. Lemmon MA, Schlessinger J. Regulation of signal transduction and signal diversity by receptor oligomerization. *Trends Biochem Sci* 1994;19:459–463.
19. Hubbard SR, Mohammadi M, Schlessinger J. Autoregulatory mechanisms in protein-tyrosine kinases. *J Biol Chem* 1998;273:11987–11990.
20. Yarden Y, Ullrich A. Growth factor receptor tyrosine kinases. *Annu Rev Biochem* 1988;57:443–464.
21. Slamon DJ, Clark GM, Wong SG, et al. Human breast cancer: correlation of relapse and survival with amplification of the HER-2/neu oncogene. *Science* 1987;235:177–182.
22. Pawson T, Scott JD. Signaling through scaffold, anchoring, and adaptor proteins. *Science* 1997;278:2075–2080.
23. Rommel C, Hafen E. Ras—a versatile cellular switch. *Curr Opin Genet Dev* 1998;8:412–418.
24. Medema RH, Bos JL. The role of p21ras in receptor tyrosine kinase signaling. *Crit Rev Oncog* 1993;4:615–661.
25. Cichowski K, Jacks T. NF1 tumor suppressor gene function: narrowing the GAP. *Cell* 2001;104:593–604.
26. Ellis CA, Clark G. The importance of being K-Ras. *Cell Signal* 2000;12:425–434.
27. Rebecchi MJ, Pentyala SN. Structure, function, and control of phosphoinositide-specific phospholipase C. *Physiol Rev* 2000;80:1291–1335.
28. Rameh LE, Cantley LC. The role of phosphoinositide 3-kinase lipid products in cell function. *J Biol Chem* 1999;274:8347–8350.
29. Czech MP. PIP2 and PIP3: complex roles at the cell surface. *Cell* 2000;100:603–606.
30. Bae YS, Sung JY, Kim OS, et al. Platelet-derived growth factor-induced H(2)O(2) production requires the activation of phosphatidylinositol 3-kinase. *J Biol Chem* 2000;275:10531–10531.
31. Camps M, Nichols A, Arkinstall S. Dual specificity phosphatases: a gene family for control of MAP kinase function. *Faseb J* 2000;14:6–16.
32. Sherr CJ. The Pezcoller lecture: cancer cell cycles revisited. *Cancer Res* 2000;60:3689–3695.
33. Harbour JW, Dean DC. Rb function in cell-cycle regulation and apoptosis. *Nat Cell Biol* 2000;2:E65–E67.

34. Diehl JA, Cheng M, Roussel MF, Sherr CJ. Glycogen synthase kinase-3beta regulates cyclin D1 proteolysis and subcellular localization. *Genes Dev* 1998;12:3499–3511.

35. Malumbres M, Ortega S, Barbacid M. Genetic analysis of mammalian cyclin-dependent kinases and their inhibitors. *Biol Chem* 2000;381:827–838.

36. Shapiro GI, Edwards CD, Kobzik L, et al. Reciprocal Rb inactivation and p16INK4 expression in primary lung cancers and cell lines. *Cancer Res* 1995;55:505–509.

37. Ruas M, Peters G. The p16INK4a/CDKN2A tumor suppressor and its relatives. *Biochim Biophys Acta* 1998;1378:F115–F177.

38. Lasorella A, Noseda M, Beyna M, Iavarone A. Id2 is a retinoblastoma protein target and mediates signaling by Myc oncoproteins. *Nature* 2000;407:592–598.

39. Massague J, Blain SW, Lo RS. TGFbeta signaling in growth control, cancer, and heritable disorders. *Cell* 2000;103:295–309.

40. de Caestecker MP, Piek E, Roberts AB. Role of transforming growth factor-beta signaling in cancer. *Natl Cancer Inst* 2000;92:1388–1402.

41. Markowitz S, Wang J, Myeroff L, et al. Inactivation of the type II TGF-beta receptor in colon cancer cells with microsatellite instability. *Science* 1995;268:1336–1338.

42. Momand J, Wu HH, Dasgupta G. MDM2—master regulator of the p53 tumor suppressor protein. *Gene* 2000;242:15–29.

43. Chin L, Pomerantz J, DePinho RA. The INK4a/ARF tumor suppressor: one gene—two products—two pathways. *Trends Biochem Sci* 1998;23:291–296.

44. Nicholson DW. Caspase structure, proteolytic substrates, and function during apoptotic cell death. *Cell Death Differ* 1999;6:1028–1042.

45. Hengartner MO. The biochemistry of apoptosis. *Nature* 2000;407:770–776.

46. Green DR. Apoptotic pathways: paper wraps stone blunts scissors. *Cell* 2000;102:1–4.

47. Salvesen GS, Dixit VM. Caspase activation: the induced-proximity model. *Proc Natl Acad Sci U S A* 1999;96:10964–10967.

48. Cain K, Bratton SB, Langlais C, et al. Apaf-1 oligomerizes into biologically active approximately 700-kDa and inactive approximately 1.4-MDa apoptosome complexes. *J Biol Chem* 2000;275:6067–6070.

49. Antonsson B, Martinou JC. The Bcl-2 protein family. *Exp Cell Res* 2000;256:50–57.

50. Zhang L, Yu J, Park BH, et al. Role of BAX in the apoptotic response to anti-cancer agents. *Science* 2000;290:989–992.

51. Huang DC, Strasser A. BH3-Only proteins—essential initiators of apoptotic cell death. *Cell* 2000;103:839–842.

52. Li H, Zhu H, Xu CJ, Yuan J. Cleavage of BID by caspase 8 mediates the mitochondrial damage in the Fas pathway of apoptosis. *Cell* 1998;94:491–501.

53. Jaattela M. Escaping cell death: survival proteins in cancer. *Exp Cell Res* 1999;248:30–43.

54. Verhagen AM, Ekert PG, Pakusch M, et al. Identification of DIABLO, a mammalian protein that promotes apoptosis by binding to and antagonizing IAP proteins. *Cell* 2000;102:43–53.

55. Du C, Fang M, Li Y, et al. Smac, a mitochondrial protein that promotes cytochrome c-dependent caspase activation by eliminating IAP inhibition. *Cell* 2000;102:1–210.

56. Cantley LC, Neel BG. New insights into tumor suppression: PTEN suppresses tumor formation by restraining the phosphoinositide 3-kinase/AKT pathway. *Proc Natl Acad Sci U S A* 1999;96:4240–4245.

57. Di Cristofano A, Pandolfi PP. The multiple roles of PTEN in tumor suppression. *Cell* 2000;100:387–390.

58. Vogelstein B, Lane D, Levine AJ. Surfing the p53 network. *Nature* 2000;408:307–310.

59. Vousden KH. p53: Death star. *Cell* 2000;103:691–694.

60. Ryan KM, Ernst MK, Rice NR, Vousden KH. Role of NF-kappaB in p53-mediated programmed cell death. *Nature* 2000;404:892–897.

61. Blackburn EH. Telomere states and cell fates. *Nature* 2000;408:53–56.

62. Artandi SE, DePinho RA. A critical role for telomeres in suppressing and facilitating carcinogenesis. *Curr Opin Genet Dev* 2000;10:39–46.

63. Oulton R, Harrington L. Telomeres, telomerase, and cancer: life on the edge of genomic stability. *Curr Opin Oncol* 2000;12:74–81.

64. Sherr CJ, DePinho RA. Cellular senescence: mitotic clock or culture shock? *Cell* 2000;102:407–410.

65. Hahn WC, Counter CM, Lundberg AS, et al. Creation of human tumour cells with defined genetic elements. *Nature* 1999;400:464–468.

66. Lee HW, Blasco MA, Gottlieb GJ, et al. Essential role of mouse telomerase in highly proliferative organs. *Nature* 1998;392:569–574.

67. Artandi SE, Chang S, Lee SL, et al. Telomere dysfunction promotes non-reciprocal translocations and epithelial cancers in mice. *Nature* 2000;406:641–645.

68. Zhang X, Mar V, Zhou W, et al. Telomere shortening and apoptosis in telomerase-inhibited human tumor cells. *Genes Dev* 1999;13:2388–2399.

69. Hahn WC, Stewart SA, Brooks MW, et al. Inhibition of telomerase limits the growth of human cancer cells. *Nat Med* 1999;5:1164–1170.

70. Carmeliet P, Jain RK. Angiogenesis in cancer and other diseases. *Nature* 2000;407:249–257.

71. Saaristo A, Karpanen T, Alitalo K. Mechanisms of angiogenesis and their use in the inhibition of tumor growth and metastasis. *Oncogene* 2000;19:6122–6129.

72. Holash J, Maisonpierre PC, Compton D, et al. Vessel cooption, regression, and growth in tumors mediated by angiopoietins and VEGF. *Science* 1999;284:1994–1998.

73. Kerbel RS. Tumor angiogenesis: past, present and the near future. *Carcinogenesis* 2000;21:505–515.

74. Gazit Y, Baish JW, Safabakhsh N, et al. Fractal characteristics of tumor vascular architecture during tumor growth and regression. *Microcirculation* 1997;4:395–402.

75. Helmlinger G, Yuan F, Dellian M, Jain RK. Interstitial pH and pO2 gradients in solid tumors *in vivo*: high-resolution measurements reveal a lack of correlation. *Nat Med* 1997;3:177–182.

76. Weidner N, Semple JP, Welch WR, Folkman J. Tumor angiogenesis and metastasis—correlation in invasive breast carcinoma. *N Engl J Med* 1991;324:1–8.

77. Bergers G, Javaherian K, Lo KM, et al. Effects of angiogenesis inhibitors on multistage carcinogenesis in mice. *Science* 1999;284:808–812.

78. Gutman M, Fidler IJ. Biology of human colon cancer metastasis. *World J Surg* 1995;19:226–234.

79. Ben-Ze'ev A. Cytoskeletal and adhesion proteins as tumor suppressors. *Curr Opin Cell Biol* 1997;9:99–108.

80. Clark EA, Golub TR, Lander ES, Hynes RO. Genomic analysis of metastasis reveals an essential role for RhoC. *Nature* 2000;406:532–535.

81. Behrens J. Cadherins and catenins: role in signal transduction and tumor progression. *Cancer Metastasis Rev* 1999;18:15–30.

82. Kuroda S, Fukata M, Nakagawa M, et al. Role of IQGAP1, a target of the small GTPases Cdc42 and Rac1, in regulation of E-cadherin-mediated cell–cell adhesion. *Science* 1998;281:832–835.

83. Beavon IR. The E-cadherin-catenin complex in tumour metastasis: structure, function and regulation. *Eur J Cancer* 2000;36:1607–1620.

84. Guilford P, Hopkins J, Harraway J, et al. E-cadherin germline mutations in familial gastric cancer. *Nature* 1998;392:402–405.

85. McCawley LJ, Matrisian LM. Matrix metalloproteinases: multifunctional contributors to tumor progression. *Mol Med Today* 2000;6:149–156.

86. Sternlicht MD, Bissell MJ, Werb Z. The matrix metalloproteinase stromelysin-1 acts as a natural mammary tumor promoter. *Oncogene* 2000;19:1102–1113.

87. Paget S. The distribution of secondary growths in cancer of the breast. *Cancer Metastasis Rev* 1989;8:98–101.

88. Arap W, Pasqualini R, Ruoslahti E. Cancer treatment by targeted drug delivery to tumor vasculature in a mouse model. *Science* 1998;279:377–380.

89. Yoshida BA, Sokoloff MM, Welch DR, Rinker-Schaeffer CW. Metastasis-suppressor genes: a review and perspective on an emerging field. *J Natl Cancer Inst* 2000;92:1717–1730.

90. Steeg PS, Bevilacqua G, Kopper L, et al. Evidence for a novel gene associated with low tumor metastatic potential. *J Natl Cancer Inst* 1988;80:200–204.

91. Cooper DN, Krawczak M, Antonarakis S. The nature and mechanisms of human gene mutation. In: Vogelstein B, Kinzler AW, eds. *The genetic basis of human cancer*. New York: McGraw-Hill, 1998: 65–94.

92. Kunkel TA, Alexander PS. The base substitution fidelity of eucaryotic DNA polymerases. Mispairing frequencies, site preferences, insertion preferences, and base substitution by dislocation. *J Biol Chem* 1986;261:160–166.

93. Denissenko MF, Pao A, Tang M, Pfeifer GP. Preferential formation of benzo[a]pyrene adducts at lung cancer mutational hotspots in P53. *Science* 1996;274:430–432.

94. Hecht SS. Tobacco smoke carcinogens and lung cancer. *J Natl Cancer Inst* 1999;91:1194–1210.

95. Streisinger G, Okada Y, Emrich J, et al. Frameshift mutations and the genetic code. *Cold Spring Harb Symp Quant Biol* 1966;31:77–84.

96. Ionov Y, Peinado MA, Malkhosyan S, et al. Ubiquitous somatic mutations in simple repeated sequences reveal a new mechanism for colonic carcinogenesis. *Nature* 1993;363:558–561.

97. Lynch HT, de la Chapelle A. Genetic susceptibility to non-polyposis colorectal cancer. *J Med Genet* 1999;36:801–818.

98. Fishel R, Kolodner RD. Identification of mismatch repair genes and their role in the development of cancer. *Curr Opin Genet Dev* 1995;5:382–395.

99. Herman JG, Umar A, Polyak K, et al. Incidence and functional consequences of hMLH1 promoter hypermethylation in colorectal carcinoma. *Proc Natl Acad Sci U S A* 1998;95:6870–6875.

100. Jones PA, Laird PW. Cancer epigenetics comes of age. *Nat Genet* 1999;21:163–167.

101. Nan X, Ng HH, Johnson CA, et al. Transcriptional repression by the methyl-CpG-binding protein MeCP2 involves a histone deacetylase complex. *Nature* 1998;393:386–389.

102. Rountree MR, Bachman KE, Baylin SB. DNMT1 binds HDAC2 and a new co-repressor, DMAP1, to form a complex at replication foci. *Nat Genet* 2000;25:269–277.

103. Baylin SB, Herman JG, Graff JR, et al. Alterations in DNA methylation: a fundamental aspect of neoplasia. *Adv Cancer Res* 1998;72:141–196.

104. Moulton T, Crenshaw T, Hao Y, et al. Epigenetic lesions at the H19 locus in Wilms' tumour patients. *Nat Genet* 1994;7:440–447.

105. Laird PW, Jackson-Grusby L, Fazeli A, et al. Suppression of intestinal neoplasia by DNA hypomethylation. *Cell* 1995;81:197–205.

106. Pihan GA, Doxsey SJ. The mitotic machinery as a source of genetic instability in cancer. *Semin Cancer Biol* 1999;9:289–302.

107. Lengauer C, Kinzler KW, Vogelstein B. Genetic instability in colorectal cancers. *Nature* 1997;386:623–627.

108. Zhou BB, Elledge SJ. The DNA damage response: putting checkpoints in perspective. *Nature* 2000;408:433–439.

109. Rich T, Allen RL, Wyllie AH. Defying death after DNA damage. *Nature* 2000;407:777–783.

110. Wang Y, Cortez D, Yazdi P, et al. BASC, a super complex of BRCA1-associated proteins involved in the recognition and repair of aberrant DNA structures. *Genes Dev* 2000;14:927–939.

PART 2

Hematopoietic System

CHAPTER 7

Hematopoiesis

David A. Williams, H. Franklin Bunn, Colin Sieff, and Leonard I. Zon

The formed elements of the blood together with the stem and progenitor cells that give rise to these functional cells play a vital role in the normal functioning of a healthy person. Certain characteristics of the hematopoietic tissue are clearly different from those of other vital organs and are important in the understanding of normal and abnormal hematopoiesis. These differences include the short lifespan of most functional cells of the hematopoietic system, the multiplicity of cell types required for normal hematopoietic functioning, and the wide dispersion of cells performing specific hematopoietic functions throughout the body. Although exceptions exist in the lymphoid compartment, the lifespan of most hematopoietic cells is extremely short—from hours to a few months. The short lifespan requires the continuous production of enormous numbers of cells to replace these lost and generally postmitotic cells. Estimates of 10^{10} red blood cells (RBCs) and 10^8 to 10^9 white blood cells produced per hour demonstrate the numbers involved but belie the complexity of the hematopoietic system, because the final number of circulating cells is maintained within strict limits.

The physiologic functioning of the hematopoietic system also requires that the bone marrow be capable of responding quickly to the need for additional cells of any lineage. Also, despite the requirements for massive production of differentiated cells, stem cells must be maintained in adequate numbers (a process termed *self-renewal*) to provide input progenitor cells constantly throughout the person's lifetime.

Delineation of the relations of different cells in this complex system has been made possible by exemplary research by a number of investigators working in the field of experimental hematology.* Careful study of staining and morphologic characteristics of bone marrow and blood cells by hematologists over the last 50 years has

produced a relatively clear idea of the maturational sequence during precursor cell differentiation. Development by Till and McCulloch (1) of an *in vivo* stem cell assay, the colony-forming unit-spleen (CFU-S) assay (discussed in the section Stem Cell Compartment), in the early 1960s led to an enormous growth of knowledge about stem cell self-renewal and proliferation. Shortly thereafter, the development of *in vitro* clonogenic culture systems for hematopoietic progenitor cells by Pluznik and Sachs (2) and Bradley and Metcalf (3) led to new understanding of growth factor requirements for hematopoietic cell differentiation. These discoveries ultimately led to the molecular cloning of multiple cytokines and their receptors, which affect hematopoietic cell proliferation and differentiation (4,5). An insightful personal history of the last several decades of research in experimental hematology has recently been published (6).

Description of an *in vitro* culture system that allowed continuous proliferation and differentiation of hematopoietic cells in long-term bone marrow cultures by Dexter et al. (7) provided new insights into the role of the hematopoietic microenvironment in the physiology of hematopoietic stem cells and the requirement for direct cell–cell contact in hematopoiesis. Knowledge gained from these and many other studies provides some general concepts about hematopoiesis. More recently, the use of homologous recombination to generate mice deficient in specific proteins has contributed unparalleled understanding of *in vivo* requirements for blood production (8).

FUNCTIONAL RELATIONS IN HEMATOPOIETIC CELL DIFFERENTIATION

The hematopoietic system can be envisioned as a continuum of functional compartments (Fig. 7-1). In general, the more primitive

---

*For a concise review of previous studies in experimental hematology as they relate to current understanding of hematopoiesis, see reference 374.

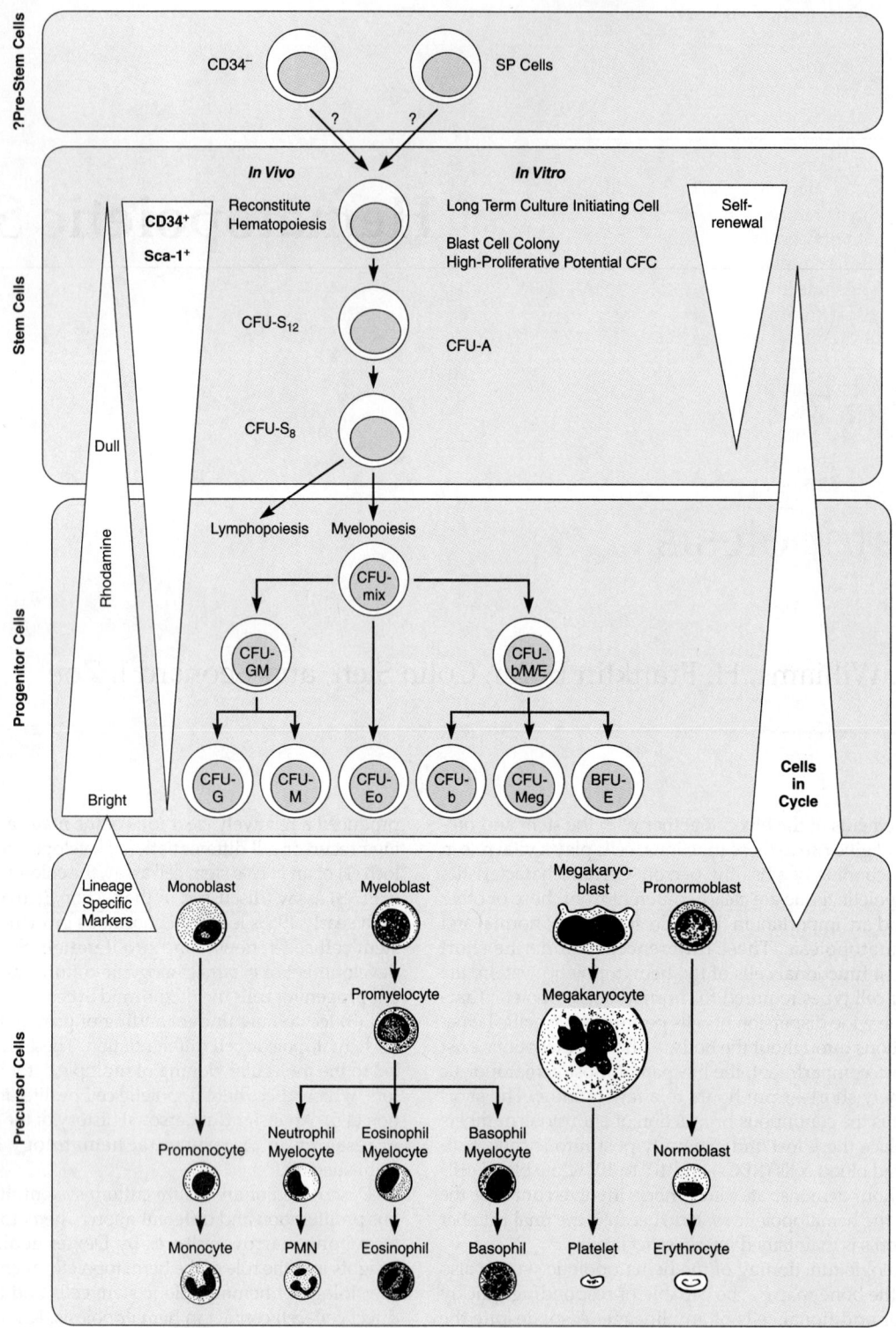

Figure 7-1. Schematic view of some general properties and assays for the heterogeneous cells that make up the stem cell and progenitor cell compartments. As indicated on the diagram, cells capable of permanently reconstituting *in vivo* hematopoiesis are separable from cells that give rise to day 12 colony-forming unit-spleen (CFU-S), but the precise developmental stage of *in vitro* long-term culture-initiating cells and blast cell colony progenitors is not established. The recent identification of so-called SP cells and CD34⁻ cells is diagrammatically shown, but the physiologic relevance of these cells is currently unknown. In the progenitor compartment, mixed colonies of almost all myeloid lineage combinations have been described. The basophil-megakaryocyte-erythroid progenitor (CFU-b/M/E) is inferred from the restricted lineage expression of the transcription factor GATA-1 to cells of these lineages (716). The precursor cell compartment shows the morphologically recognizable cells of the hematopoietic organs. BFU-E, erythroid burst-forming unit; CFC, colony-forming cell; CFU-A, type A colony-forming unit; CFU-Eo, eosinophil colony-forming unit; CFU-G, granulocyte colony-forming unit; CFU-GM, granulocyte-macrophage colony-forming unit; CFU-Meg, megakaryocyte colony-forming unit; CFU-Mix, mixed-lineage colony-forming unit; PMN, polymorphonuclear neutrophil.

stem cell compartment is made up of rare pluripotent stem cells with high self-renewal capacity, the capacity to give rise to all cell lineages, and a low incidence of mitotically active cells (9). The self-renewal capacity of the stem cell compartment must be maintained throughout the lifespan of the individual, and through a process termed *commitment*, these cells also are constantly capable of providing more differentiated cells into the next compartment.

Transition to the *progenitor compartment* is characterized by some restriction in differentiation and proliferative capacity. This compartment is composed mostly of unipotent progenitor cells, with some bipotent and rare multipotent progenitors. These progenitor cells demonstrate little, if any, self-renewal capacity and are more numerous and mitotically more active than stem cells. In contrast, cells in the most differentiated *precursor compartment* make up most cells in the bone marrow, have no self-renewal capacity, are unipotent, and are mostly in active cell cycle. These precursor cells exhibit well-described nuclear and cytoplasmic morphology during the final steps of differentiation into functional cells. Because of the large quantity of precursor cells, considerable amplification of cell numbers occurs in this compartment.

In sum, early cells have the capacity to give rise to large numbers of progeny cells on a clonal basis through expansion during differentiation. These principles are not only salient to normal hematopoietic cell biology but are also important when considering pathologic conditions of the blood.

ONTOGENY OF HEMATOPOIESIS

The development of hematopoiesis during gestation is characterized in mammalian systems by sequential change in the major anatomic site of blood cell formation and by multiple changes in the blood cells themselves. Although best studied in relation to globin gene expression, these changes affect all aspects of hematopoietic cell biology. In the progressive developmental differences seen in hematopoietic cells during ontogeny, it is unclear what role programmed changes in hematopoietic cell gene expression play compared with local environmental inductive signals.

The site or sites of origin of hematopoietic cells in the developing embryo of mammals are now controversial. Although some studies have demonstrated hematopoietic activity in the aorta-gonad-mesonephros (AGM) region of the embryo, older and other recent studies implicate the fetal yolk sac as the origin of blood formation (10,11). During early embryogenesis, cells (termed *hemangioblasts*) located in the extraembryonic mesoderm and allantois undergo rapid proliferation at the site of the future blood islands (Fig. 7-2). This induction occurs in response to unknown signals but may require participation of the visceral yolk sac endoderm, a highly secretory cell layer located immediately adjacent to the mesoderm cells (12,13) (Fig. 7-3). These changes occur at days 7.5 through 8.5 *postcoitus* in mice, the best studied mammalian model of fetal hematopoiesis, and at approximately 16 days of development in humans. Recent studies have implicated vascular endothelial growth factor (VEGF), its receptor flk-1 (14), bone morphogenetic protein-4 (BMP-4) (15,16), fibroblast growth factor, and hedgehog as key regulators of early hematopoiesis (15,16).

During further development, hemangioblasts segregate into peripheral cells destined to become vascular endothelial cells, and round mononuclear cells located centrally and destined to become primitive hematopoietic cells (17,18) (Fig. 7-3, inset). The collection of cells, referred to as *blood islands*, subsequently is connected to similar islands, forming the circulatory and blood systems of the developing embryo. Although little is known about the yolk sac phase of hematopoiesis, several studies show clear differences between these cells and cells derived later in embryo-

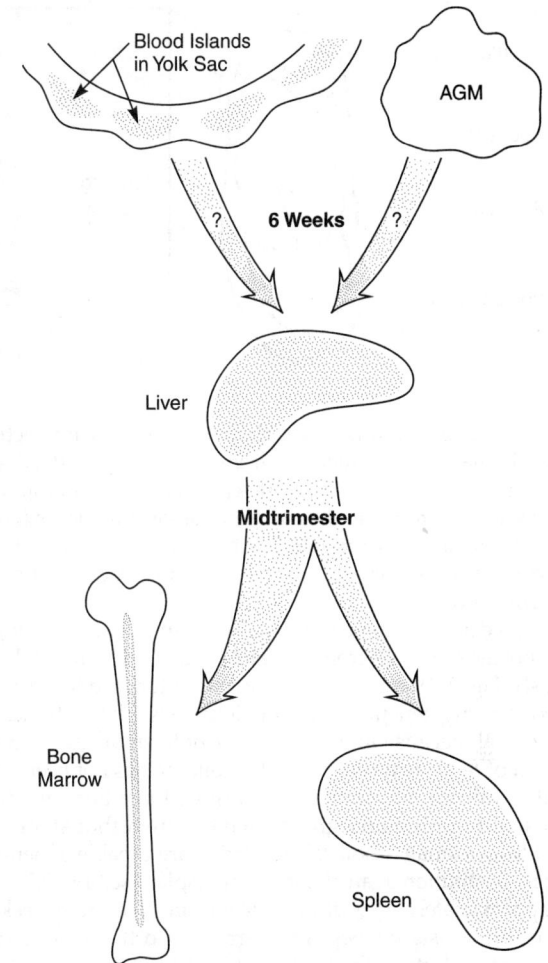

Figure 7-2. Ontogeny of hematopoiesis: schematic representation of the anatomic locations of hematopoiesis in the developing fetus. Hematopoiesis begins in blood islands located in extraembryonic tissues (fetal yolk sac) in the first trimester or in the aorto-gonad-mesnenophros (AGM) region (or both) (Fig. 7-3). At approximately 6 weeks of gestation, hematopoiesis occurs predominantly in the fetal liver. Beginning at midterm, the medullary cavity gradually replaces the fetal liver as the main site of hematopoiesis. In some species, such as the mouse, the spleen is a major site of hematopoiesis in the adult.

genesis in the fetal liver or neonatal or adult bone marrow. Differentiation is predominantly (completely in the mouse) limited to erythroid cells (19–21), although pluripotent cells are present (10). Yolk sac cells appear to have an altered sensitivity to the hormone erythropoietin (EPO), because studies in the mouse and sheep suggest an increased sensitivity to EPO or lack of dependence on EPO altogether for RBC formation (22–24).

Yolk sac erythroid cells are macrocytic, and most retain nuclei that exhibit a coarse chromatin pattern (25,26). Yolk sac stem cells exhibit a higher proliferative index compared with adult stem cells (24,27,28). Although differentiation is severely restricted to erythroid cells *in situ*, murine fetal yolk sac stem cells are capable of multilineage differentiation and can effect full reconstitution when injected into lethally irradiated adult recipients (10). In addition, studies by Micklem et al. (29) and Moore and Metcalf (10) show that stem cells located in the yolk sac are capable of extended serial transplantation in irradiated adult syngeneic recipients, data that suggest that these stem cells have higher self-renewal capacity than stem cells derived from adult bone marrow. However, some studies suggest that fetal yolk sac stem cells are not efficient in engrafting and reconstituting adult recipients with

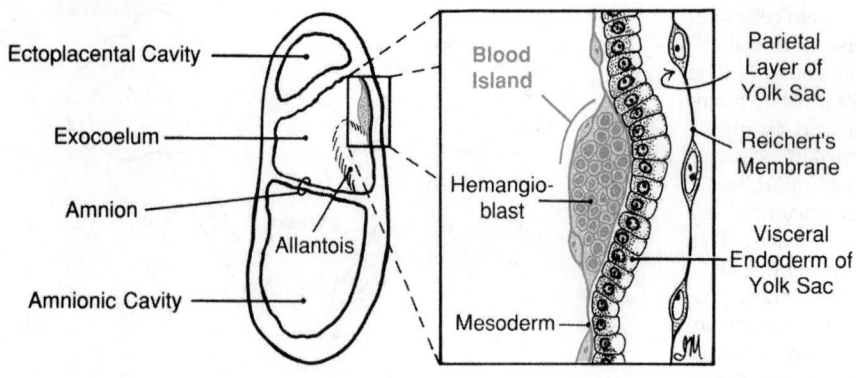

Ectoplacental Cavity

Exocoelum

Amnion

Allantois

Amnionic Cavity

Blood Island

Hemangio- blast

Mesoderm

Parietal Layer of Yolk Sac

Reichert's Membrane

Visceral Endoderm of Yolk Sac

Figure 7-3. Schematic view of yolk sac hematopoiesis in the mouse at approximately 7 days of gestation. Blood islands form in the yolk sac mesoderm and allantois. The yolk sac mesoderm contains multipotent progenitors, termed *hemangioblasts,* that differentiate into endothelial cells lining the blood islands, and primitive hematopoietic stem and progenitor cells. The visceral endoderm of the yolk sac forms an epithelium directly opposed to the mesoderm.

intrinsic (although yet unknown) changes caused by interactions with the hematopoietic microenvironment (11,30). Indeed, evidence suggests that the first adult-repopulating hematopoietic stem cells actually reside in the paraaortic splanchnopleure/AGM region (31). Finally, it is possible that both yolk sac cells and cells derived from the AGM are capable of giving rise to definitive adult hematopoiesis (32).

Definitive adult hematopoiesis appears to arise by seeding of hematopoietic stem cells from the fetal circulation to the fetal liver (10,33,34) (Fig. 7-2). It is generally accepted that the liver anlage does not directly generate hematopoietic cells. These studies are controversial, because in avian and tadpole embryos, a similar migration of fetal stem cells from the yolk sac has not been demonstrated (35,36). No such observations have been made in humans, although many groups have shown that stem cells derived from human umbilical circulation are capable of hematopoietic reconstitution in an allogeneic transplant setting (37–39).

At approximately $10^{1/2}$ days postcoitus in mice and 6 weeks in humans, blood islands begin to regress, and the major site of hematopoiesis shifts to the fetal liver (10,39–42). There is a large increase in the absolute numbers of hematopoietic cells during this stage of development (43). In humans and mice, this change is accompanied by a switch in globin chain production in developing red blood cells from primitive to fetal globins (fetal to adult in mice). Hematopoietic cell differentiation continues to be restricted predominantly to the erythroid lineage (21,44,45), although a large number of myeloid progenitors are present in the fetal liver (44,46,47). RBCs produced in the fetal liver are smaller than those produced during primitive yolk sac erythropoiesis. Erythroid cell nuclear structure also more closely resembles normoblasts of adult bone marrow, and the site of hematopoiesis is predominantly extravascular (41,48,49). Markers of primitive hematopoietic cells in yolk sac and AGM, as well as fetal liver, include c-kit, CD34, AA41, and possibly the β_2-integrin Mac-1 (11,50–52).

Other differences between the hematopoietic cells developing in human fetal liver and the adult cells are expression of i surface antigen (versus I antigen) and low levels of the enzyme carbonic anhydrase, a prominent nonhemoglobin protein of RBCs (53,54). These fetal characteristics are sometimes seen in adult life during episodes of hematopoietic stress, such as bone marrow failure and posttransplantation reconstitution.

The relation of developing blood cells to stromal or parenchymal hepatic elements during this early phase of hematopoiesis is largely unstudied. Medlock and Haar (55) and Medlock et al. (56) have reported an orderly morphologic transition from prehepatocytes, apparently secreting reticulum and forming a three-dimensional supporting network for hematopoietic cells, to uniform epithelial cells with evidence of high secretory activity characteristic of the differentiated phenotype of the mature hepatocyte. The full expression of an epithelial cell phenotype coincides with the cessation of hematopoiesis in the fetal liver as the bone marrow medullary cavity becomes the major source of blood cells. Although

hematopoietic differentiation in the fetal liver is restricted predominantly to erythroid cells, circulating platelets and granulocytes are seen; evidence suggests, at least in the murine system, that pre-B lymphocytes are present in the liver environment (56,57). At the time of transition of the anatomic site of hematopoiesis in the mouse from the yolk sac to the fetal liver, an abrupt switch in globin from fetal (EI, EII, EIII) to adult (α_2 and β_2) occurs (20,58). During human embryonic development, embryonic α-like ζ and β-like ε globin chains are expressed. These lead to the production of Hb Gower-2 ($\alpha_2\varepsilon_2$), Hb Gower-1 (ε_4), and Hb Portland ($\zeta_2\alpha_2$). These embryonic hemoglobins are detected until approximately 9 weeks of gestation in the human. From late in the first trimester, the majority of hemoglobin in the developing embryo is HbF ($\alpha_2\gamma_2$). By the end of the first trimester in human fetuses, the major hemoglobin produced in fetal RBCs is derived from γ-gene expression (HbF) (59).* During the midtrimester, hematopoietic cells are also seen in lymph nodes, thymus, and bone marrow space (60,61).

The final anatomic site of hematopoiesis during ontogeny is the medullary cavity of bone in humans and the medullary cavity and spleen in mice (Fig. 7-2). Although human hematopoietic cells can be seen in the medullary cavity space by 8 to 9 weeks, this site becomes the major site of hematopoiesis at approximately 5 months of gestation (60). Although little erythropoiesis is observed in the medullary cavity of mice and rats until after birth (61), differentiation occurs along all lineages within the medullary cavity of human fetuses. By the final trimester, all available medullary space is filled with hematopoietic cells. The medullary cavity of the fetus has little capacity to respond to stress and relies on reactivation of hematopoietic cell production by the liver and cell production in the spleen (extramedullary hematopoiesis) to respond to requirements for additional formed elements during stress (62,63).

Later in childhood and adult life, the medullary cavity can respond to similar stress by expansion into fatty marrow, and the incidence of extramedullary hematopoiesis is markedly reduced (63). Thus, blood cell formation proceeds through multiple anatomic sites and displays characteristic changes in gene expression during fetal development. The microenvironment and growth factor requirements for hematopoiesis and specific changes in expression of the major gene studied (globin) during fetal development are described here.

PHYSIOLOGIC CHANGES AFTER BIRTH

Major changes in erythropoiesis accompany the transition from intrauterine to newborn hematopoiesis. During the last trimester of fetal life, medullary hematopoiesis reaches a stable level with little capacity for expanded cell production without the recruitment of extramedullary sites (62,63). At the time of birth, erythropoietic activity rapidly declines, as evidenced by decreased reticulocyte

---

*For an extensive review of hemoglobin switching, see Chapter 48 or reference 61a.

counts, falling hemoglobin concentration, and decreased bone marrow cellularity noted in newborn infants (64–67). The fall in RBC production and a shortened half-life of fetal erythrocytes lead to a physiologic hemoglobin nadir at approximately 2 to 3 months of age in the full-term infant and as early as 4 weeks in the premature infant (68).

Coincident with the fall in hemoglobin is a gradual lowering of oxygen affinity with a shift to the right in the oxygen dissociation curve, resulting both from replacement of fetal hemoglobin with adult hemoglobin and from an increase in erythrocyte 2,3-diphosphoglycerate (2,3-DPG) (69–71). This increase in 2,3-DPG increases the oxygen delivery capacity of erythrocytes of newborn infants as the hemoglobin falls; therefore, the level of hemoglobin must be interpreted in the light of both oxygen delivery and oxygen use. The transition from fetal to adult erythropoiesis appears to be a closely regulated multifactorial system allowing replacement of erythroid cells suited for oxygen delivery in the intrauterine environment with erythroid cells suited for oxygen delivery in postnatal life (72).

The level of fetal hemoglobin gradually falls over the first year after birth, maintaining a low but detectable level in most persons throughout adult life (73). Conditions associated with erythroid stress as well as mutations around the γ-gene and β-gene loci (such as hereditary persistence of fetal hemoglobin) are associated with elevation of fetal hemoglobin levels in childhood and adult life (74–79). The physiologic nadir of hemoglobin of approximately 11 g of hemoglobin in the full-term infant is generally attained at approximately 3 months of age. The nadir is reached earlier in the premature infant and is generally 1 to 2 g less than in full-term infants (9 to 10 g hemoglobin).

Despite the relative hypoplasia of erythroid production during the first months of postnatal life, newborn bone marrow is capable of responding to anemic stress (80). Infants born after intrauterine hypoxic episodes demonstrate elevated cord blood EPO levels, and congenital hemolytic anemias are associated with elevated EPO levels in the amniotic fluid and increased reticulocytes and nucleated RBCs in the peripheral blood (81,82). Infants with significant ongoing hemolysis occasionally appear to be incapable of sustained compensation during the first 3 to 4 months of life. In addition, some premature infants demonstrate low concentrations of EPO; inadequate production of EPO has been postulated to underlie the anemia seen in these infants (83–86). Therefore, RBC transfusion requirements for hemolysis and anemia during this period do not predict chronic transfusion dependence. The use of recombinant human EPO for the treatment of anemia in very-low-birth-weight infants has been under study (86–88) (discussed in the section Erythropoietin: Clinical Indications). Studies of myeloid growth factors in neonatal neutropenia associated with stress, sepsis, or both are also under way (89,90) [reviewed in Frenck and Shannon (91)].

STEM CELL COMPARTMENT

Pluripotent Stem Cells Retain the Capacity for Self-Renewal and Maintain Hematopoiesis by Clonal Proliferation

Arising from embryonic totipotential stem cells, pluripotent hematopoietic stem cells, which reside within hematopoietic tissues, are responsible for maintenance of blood formation throughout the lifetime of the individual. The traditional view holds that these hematopoietic stem cells are committed only to blood formation and that the key to sustained hematopoiesis is self-renewal of these cells. Recent observations by multiple investigators using a number of different experimental models suggest that the functional potential of hematopoietic stem cells may not be restricted to blood

and that these cells may, under some circumstances, give rise to other (nonblood) cell types, a property termed *plasticity* (discussed in the section Stem Cell Plasticity). The presence of hematopoietic stem cells in mice was first indicated by experiments performed by Jacobson et al. (92), who showed that mice could be protected from the effects of whole-body irradiation if the spleen was exteriorized and excluded from the radiation field. Furthermore, the continued presence of the unirradiated spleen was unnecessary. It could be removed as little as 1 hour after irradiation and still show the effect on improved survival (93). That this protective effect was cell-mediated rather than noncellular was demonstrated by the observation that injected spleen cells could initiate recovery and reestablish hematopoiesis in irradiated animals (94). The essential defining characteristic of the most immature stem cells is thus the ability to *repopulate both the immune and hematopoietic lineages* after transfer; in mice, these cells show no decline in repopulating ability with age (95–97).

Although these repopulation experiments showed the functional importance of stem cells, Till and McCulloch (1) recognized that the colonies that formed in the spleens of lethally irradiated mice after injection of bone marrow cells were stem cell-derived, and the following method became available for quantitating stem cells: CFU-S colonies are obtained by injecting a limited number of bone marrow cells intravenously into a heavily irradiated, syngeneic recipient mouse. After 8 to 14 days, the spleens are harvested and can be fixed (for counting or histologic analysis), or the individual spleen colonies can be dissected and analyzed further.

The cells that give rise to these colonies are designated *CFU-Ss*. The splenic colonies contain erythroid, phagocytic, or megakaryocyte progenitors and precursors, and spleen colonies that appear late (day 14 or CFU-S$_{14}$) also contain stem cells that can form additional spleen colonies of differentiated progeny when infused into a second irradiated recipient (98,99). Analysis of individual CFU-S–derived spleen colonies demonstrates heterogeneity from colony to colony with respect to their content of new CFU-Ss (98,100,101). Most colonies contain few CFU-Ss, whereas some contain large numbers. Experiments with karyotypically marked cells or retroviral-tagged cells have shown that cells that make up CFU-S–derived spleen colonies are of *clonal* origin. Under steady-state conditions, no more than 20% to 30% of CFU-Ss are in cycle during a 3-hour exposure to high-dose ^{3}H-thymidine or in hydroxyurea suicide experiments, although strain variations have been documented (102–104).

Stem cells are extremely rare. The incidence of reconstituting stem cells is estimated at 1 to 2.5 per 100,000 injected nucleated marrow cells (based on comparative repopulation methods and variabilities using the binomial formula) to 1 per 10,000 transplanted cells (based on limiting dilution analysis) (105–107). Stem cells can repopulate both the myeloid and the lymphoid systems. This ability has been demonstrated by the use of radiation-induced chromosome markers; by injection of fetal mice with mixtures of cells distinguishable by differences in hemoglobin, isoenzyme, and immunoglobulin types; and by analysis of the progeny of cells marked by unique retroviral integration sites (108,109).

In sum, the spleen colony technique was used to establish several fundamental properties of hematopoietic stem cells: their ability to generate clonally derived populations of maturing cells, their extensive capacity for self-renewal, their multipotential capacity, and the fact that most of these cells are not in cell cycle.

Purification of Stem Cells

Application of the CFU-S assay and analysis of hematopoietic stem cells generally have been hindered by the low incidence of stem cells in the hematopoietic population and the lack of reagents to identify stem cells. Considerable work by many investigators has led to the ability to enrich stem cells. Murine hematopoietic stem cells can be highly purified by density gradient centrifugation and by labeling with antibodies, lectins, or intracellular dyes (or combinations of these) followed by separation using fluorescence-activated cell sorting, immunopanning, or immunomagnetic bead separation (110). Immunologic characteristics that define murine stem cell populations include weak expression of Thy-1; expression of antigens defined by Qa-m7, Sca-1 (Ly6), and the receptor tyrosine kinase c-kit; and lack of expression of lineage markers, such as B220, Mac-1, Gr-1, CD3, CD4, CD8, and Ter119. Using the combination of lineage depletion and selection of Thy-1$^+$ and Sca-1$^+$ cells by fluorescence-activated cell sorting, Spangrude et al. (111) purified murine stem cells such that as few as 30 cells could reconstitute half of lethally irradiated syngeneic recipients. The immunophenotypic characterization of putative primitive human hematopoietic stem cells has defined Thy-1 and CD34 as critical antigens (112). More recently, the monoclonal antibody AC133 has been reported to identify primitive human hematopoietic cells (113).

Bertoncello et al. (114,115) used antibodies to the Qa-m7 antigen and immunomagnetic bead separation to purify a primitive murine hematopoietic cell population, termed *high proliferative potential colony-forming cells* (HPP-CFCs). HPP-CFCs give rise to macroscopically visible (larger than 5 mm) *in vitro* colonies. Although HPP-CFCs are considered by some to be the equivalent of the reconstituting stem cell (116), more recent data suggest that reconstituting stem cells show only some characteristics of HPP-CFCs. In these studies, up to 30% of the purified cell populations were HPP-CFCs. Visser et al. (117) and Visser and deVries (118) used combinations of density gradient centrifugation and labeling with wheat germ agglutinin and rhodamine 123 dye to purify stem cells capable of 30-day radioprotection after transplantation into lethally irradiated syngeneic murine recipients. Studies in humans and nonhuman primates have used similar purification schemes and the CD34 antigen to enrich partially for stem cells (119–121). Radioprotection of primates with CD34$^+$ selected cells has been achieved, although definitive proof of multilineage reconstitution with these cells has not been shown (33,121).

More recent studies have provided evidence that CD34$^-$ cells have the capacity to reconstitute hematopoiesis in multiple species (Fig. 7-1). A CD34$^-$ negative murine stem cell with full engrafting capacity was first defined by Nakauchi et al. (122). Subsequent work by Dick et al. (123) demonstrated a human CD34$^-$ cell derived from umbilical cord blood with reconstitution capacity, albeit with a very low frequency, in nonobese diabetic/severe combined immunodeficient (NOD/SCID) xenograft studies in mice (123). Supporting findings using human CD34$^-$ lineage marker–negative bone marrow cells have been reported in fetal sheep xenografts (124). Lack of CD34 expression was also noted on engrafting cells derived by purification using Hoechst dye exclusion, so-called side population, or SP, cells described by Goodell et al. (125). Initially defined in murine bone marrow cells by flow analysis, SP cells have now been identified in rat, pig, primate, and human bone marrow. These studies demonstrate that cells not expressing CD34 can engraft and reconstitute hematopoiesis *in vivo*, but the physiologic relevance of these cells in normal steady-state hematopoiesis or, importantly, in the posttransplant setting has not yet been determined.

Indeed, the expression of CD34 has now been shown to be variable and can be induced by experimental manipulation (126). Further, it appears that the exclusion of dyes and toxins, presumably by membrane pumps, that is responsible for the SP population phenotype may vary in activity during ontogeny, and that *in vitro* culture of cells can lead to the induced expression of CD34$^-$. In all of these studies, the frequency of CD34$^-$ (or SP) is quite low, and accurate quantitation of the repopulating capacity of these cell populations is less well defined. For instance, Bhatia et al.

(123) estimated reconstitution using CD34$^-$ cells at approximately 100-fold less frequency in NOD/SCID mice compared with CD34$^+$ cells. These studies present potential questions about the current practice of using CD34$^+$-enriched cell populations for transplantation purposes. Although long-term stable engraftment in humans has been seen with CD34$^+$ cells, to date, the technology used assures contamination with non-CD34–expressing cells. However, as the selection technology improves, at least a theoretic risk exists that long-term engraftment may be deficient when highly enriched CD34$^+$ populations are used. Thus, the relevance of CD34$^-$ and SP cells remains unknown, and further study is required to define the role of these cells, if any, in transplant biology and hematopoietic ontogeny.

Stem Cell Plasticity

As noted, recent experimental observations have challenged the long-held belief that stem cells residing in somatic tissues are restricted to differentiate into those cells making up that specific tissue (for reviews, see 127 and 128). Experiments have suggested the ability of cells within muscle to give rise to blood cells (129), the ability of purified hematopoietic stem cells to give rise to muscle (130–132), the ability of brain stem cells to give rise to blood cells (133), and the ability of transplanted bone marrow to participate in the repair of damaged myocardium (134). Although these results are biologically intriguing, the implications and therapeutic potential of such "transdifferentiated" cells remain unknown and are the subject of intense scrutiny. Skepticism remains because most studies have not yet adequately shown functional properties of derived cells and because the frequency of cells capable of "changing" differentiation pathways appears very low (130).

Heterogeneity of Stem Cells

The results of CFU-S and other studies have led to refinements in the assignment of primitive cells in the stem cell compartment and to the realization that the stem cell compartment is heterogeneous (135) (Fig. 7-1). The stem cell compartment may be observed as a continuum of three broad classes of stem cells with respect to self-renewal and proliferative capacities (9,136–138). The most primitive stem cell has extensive self-renewal and proliferative capacity and is likely to be responsible for long-term reconstitution of the hematopoietic system after bone marrow transplantation. Less primitive cells, represented by stem cells that give rise to spleen colonies 12 to 14 days after injection into irradiated recipients (CFU-S$_{12}$), exhibit less self-renewal and proliferative capacity and are generally limited to myeloid differentiation (98). The least primitive stem cell compartment, represented by stem cells that give rise to spleen colonies 6 to 8 days after transplantation (CFU-S$_8$), have limited self-renewal and proliferative capacities and may represent cells more restricted to erythroid differentiation (98,139). The relation between this last group of stem cells and progenitor cells that give rise to mixed lineage colonies *in vitro* (CFU-GEMM or CFU-Mix) and colonies of primitive blast cells capable of forming additional colonies after replating is at this point unresolved.

Other *in vitro* assays have been described that measure cells with properties similar to CFU-S$_{12}$, such as the HPP-CFC (136) and the type A colony-forming units (CFU-As) (140), which are present at the same frequency, have similar density and cycling characteristics, and respond to growth factors in a similar fashion when compared with *in vivo* CFU-S$_{12}$. Additional assays for primitive human hematopoietic cells involve engraftment of human cell populations in immunocompromised mice or fetal sheep (xenograft assays). The most widely used of these assays involves infusion of human hematopoietic cells into NOD/SCID mice, which lack T/B and natural killer (NK) lymphocyte function (141). Human cells capable of establishing hematopoiesis in these mice are termed *SCID repopulating cells* (SRCs). The relationship of SRCs to human reconstituting hematopoietic stem cells is not clear, but retrovirus marking studies suggest that these two cell types might be closely related (142). These considerations are of clinical relevance, because any manipulations of human bone marrow before allogeneic or autologous transplantation require preservation of the most primitive stem cell compartment. In addition, some applications may depend on expansion of less primitive progenitor cells that may be responsible for short-term engraftment. Morphologically, stem cells appear to be medium-sized mononuclear cells with large nuclei, prominent nucleoli, and basophilic cytoplasm devoid of granules.

For obvious reasons, examination of human stem cells *in vivo* has been impossible using the murine techniques described. Antin et al. (143) have reported microscopic, multilineage hematopoietic colonies in the spleens of humans after bone marrow transplantation. In murine transplantation studies and in human xenograft studies, some evidence exists for short-term repopulating cells that appear distinct, at least functionally, from long-term reconstituting hematopoietic stem cells (139,144–147). Both human and murine stem cells can form colonies in semisolid media. Several such assays have been established, but the relation of the cells that form *in vitro* colonies in these assays to pluripotent stem cells with extensive self-renewal capacity or even short-term engraftment is still not clear (Fig. 7-1).

Cultures initiated on bone marrow stromal cells (termed *Dexter cultures*) have been modified to include rigorous limiting dilution analysis (so-called long-term culture-initiating cell assay) or to quantify nests of primitive cells that develop within the stroma with time (*cobblestone assays*) (148–150). These *in vitro*–based assays attempt to provide quantitative and functional readouts for primitive hematopoietic stem cells.

Multipotent progenitor cells can be assayed by their ability to form colonies of maturing granulocytes, erythrocytes, monocytes, and megakaryocytes (CFU-GEMM) when immobilized in a semisolid medium (either methylcellulose or agar) and stimulated with the appropriate hematopoietic growth factors (151,152). The relation of this cell to the cell or cells detected by the CFU-S assay is not certain: Similarities in sedimentation velocities, proliferative states, differentiation potentials, and self-renewal properties suggest that they may represent overlapping populations. Reconstitution of hematopoiesis in irradiated recipients and CFU-S–derived spleen colonies can be obtained after exposure of bone marrow *ex vivo* to 4-hydroperoxycyclophosphamide, but this treatment renders CFU-GEMM undetectable and indicates that CFU-GEMMs do not contain cells with reconstituting capacity (153,154). Studies have also identified a unique type of *in vitro* colony (CFU-Blast) that contains small numbers of blast cells with higher self-renewal and differentiating capacity than CFU-GEMM (155). Murine and, to a lesser extent, human stem cells can be cultured for prolonged periods *in vitro* in a culture system that provides direct stem cell contact with stromal cells as first described by Dexter et al. (7) (discussed in the section Hematopoietic Microenvironment).

Clonal Succession, or the Continuous Proliferation of Pluripotent Stem Cells: a Favorite Poem

Two stem cells, call them Abraham and Moses
In their first-class compartment, filled with roses
Feeding on royal jelly, one supposes
And ask the question, fateful for each stem
"When should I next divide," says A to M,
"Will both of me become like two of them?"

"These things" said Moses after solemn pause
"Must be determined by almighty cause
And not by chance. We must define our laws."
And swiftly consummating that mitotic burst,
Knowing that two of them must be dispersed,
Two Abrahams were fractionally first
And pushed both Moses through the compartment door
Saying as they did so "What a tedious bore!
Why should they think we need to have a law?"

—H.E.M. Kay (156)

The hypothesis that a series of stem cells may contribute clones successively to maintain hematopoiesis throughout the lifespan of an individual was first advanced by Kay (157). Support for this hypothesis comes from transplant studies of recipients of small numbers of bone marrow cells (158,159) and from experiments in which mixtures of fetal liver cells from different inbred mouse strains were introduced into *dominant white spotting* (W)-mutant fetuses. W-mutants exhibit a genetically determined deficiency of hematopoietic stem cells as well as germ cells and melanocytes (see below). Long-term monitoring in these mice showed clonal dominance followed by decline of cells of particular genotypes (160).

The use of retroviral-mediated gene transfer to mark hematopoietic stem cells has lent strong support to this hypothesis. Analysis of the viral integration patterns at intervals after transplantation has documented concurrent contributions of small numbers of stem cells to hematopoiesis, with changing patterns over time (108,161,162). However, these results may also reflect the limited number of stem cells marked or transplanted or may be affected by the transplant procedure itself. These conclusions are not supported by the work of Harrison et al. (106), who measured variances at successive intervals in recipients of marrow mixtures from two congenic donors. The pattern of contributions by each congenic donor observed in these studies suggests that the transplanted stem cells continuously produce descendants (106). If 10 to 20 clones are contributing to hematopoiesis simultaneously, however, even with clonal succession, variances might be expected to be minimized between two alloenzymes at sequential samplings.

Furthermore, a recent longer-term analysis of viral integration patterns in multiple lineage progeny of stem cells transplanted into mice shows that integration patterns are unstable initially, then stabilize and maintain a consistent pattern over many months (108). Reports using sensitive polymerase chain reaction amplification in primate and human studies also suggest much larger numbers of stem and progenitor cells contributing to active hematopoiesis (163,164). It is not possible to determine whether the immediate progeny of the transplanted (and retrovirally marked) stem cells might not all still have self-renewal capacity and subsequently contribute to hematopoiesis successively. Such clones would carry the same integration marker. Differences in stem cell behavior may also be genetically determined, at least in part. Homeobox genes have been implicated in stem cell function [reviewed by Lansdorp (165)].

Thus, the hypothesis of clonal succession remains somewhat controversial, and studies of human transplant recipients not using retrovirus marking suggest that clonal succession is not observed in posttransplantation hematopoiesis (166).

Influence of Drugs on Cycling of Hematopoietic Stem Cells

Although the factors that control the decision of a stem cell to undergo either self-renewal or commitment to differentiation down one of the alternate lineage pathways are poorly understood, the cell cycle status of stem cells can be influenced in a number of ways. Thus, the proportion of stem cells in cycle can be increased by exposure to agents that act through β-adrenergic or cholinergic mechanisms, suggesting that specific receptors may exist on the surface of these cells; these agents may stimulate proliferation through adenylate cyclase, cyclic AMP, and cyclic GMP, respectively (167–169). In addition, *in vivo* stem cells clearly respond to factors elicited by damage to the hematopoietic compartment. For instance, sublethal doses of chemotherapy or irradiation administered to mice result in increased cycling activity of surviving stem cells. *In vitro*, although studies reporting expansion of reconstituting stem cells remain somewhat controversial, primitive progenitor cells can clearly be induced to enter active division by exposure to some cytokines and growth factors.

Hematopoietic Growth Factors and Stem Cell Function

Hematopoietic growth factors also appear to influence at least some classes of stem cells. Whereas interleukin (IL)-3 is necessary for blast cell colony formation, IL-6, granulocyte colony-stimulating factor (G-CSF), and IL-11 appear to decrease the time interval until blast cell colonies begin to proliferate in culture (170–174). In addition, recent studies with retroviral vectors have shown that preincubation of bone marrow cells with IL-3, IL-6, stem cell factor, and fetal liver tyrosine kinase 3 ligand (Flt3L) increase the efficiency of gene transduction of the reconstituting hematopoietic stem cell (175,176). Such gene insertions require the stem cells to be actively cycling, and these studies provide indirect evidence for the potential roles of several growth factors in stem cell survival. Studies using long-term marrow cultures suggest an important role for transforming growth factor-β (TGF-β) in regulating stem cell cycle activity (177).

The isolation of the kit ligand or stem cell factor and its receptor, encoded by the c-kit protooncogene, has provided unique insight into two mouse mutants known for many years to have abnormal stem cell function. The two murine mutations that have been characterized in some detail are the *steel (Sl)* and *W* mutations (Fig. 7-4). *Sl* encodes stem cell factor (SCF), whereas *W* encodes c-kit. Because SCF appears to be a critical protein in the hematopoietic microenvironment, these mutants are discussed in more detail later in this chapter.

The *Sl* gene encodes a protein that exists in both membrane and secreted forms (178–180). Thus, it is likely that the SCF plays a role in stromal cell–stem cell interactions. The biologic properties of the SCF *in vitro* are characterized by lack of colony-stimulating activity alone but marked synergy with many of the colony-stimulating factors (CSFs) specific for different cell lineages. SCF appears particularly important in the development of the erythroid lineage and mast cells.

Stochastic Nature of Stem Cell Commitment

Two models have been proposed to explain the mechanisms that influence the choice of stem cells between self-renewal and commitment (181–183). A stochastic model was proposed by Till et al. (183). In this model, self-renewal or differentiation is considered to occur in a random or stochastic manner, dictated only by a certain probability. Because no extrinsic source of stem cells exists, under steady-state conditions, the overall probability of stem cell division resulting in self-renewal must be 0.5; probabilities lesser or greater than this value would lead to progressive stem cell depletion (aplasia) or expansion (leukemia), respectively.

The commitment of stem cells could occur symmetrically, in which case overall, half the stem cells would divide to produce

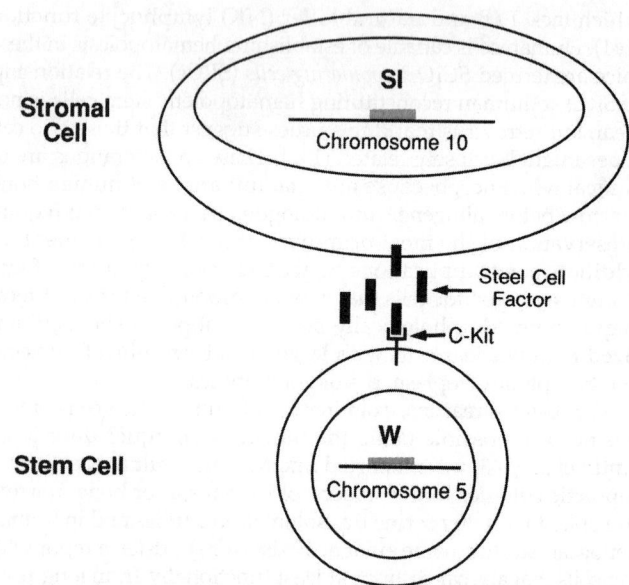

Figure 7-4. *Dominant white spotting (W)* and *Steel (Sl)* gene products. The protooncogene c-kit maps to the murine *W* locus, and its product, a tyrosine kinase cell-surface receptor, is abnormal in numerous mutations of this gene; this leads to abnormalities of hematopoietic stem cells. The *Sl* gene encodes the ligand for c-kit, otherwise known as *stem cell factor* or *Steel factor*. Mutations at the locus lead to abnormal function of the hematopoietic microenvironment.

progeny, with both progenitors entering a differentiation pathway, whereas half the stem cells would generate progeny that were both stem cells (165). Alternatively, asymmetric division would give rise to one stem cell and one cell committed to differentiate. Analysis of single cells from blast cell colonies has shown that hematopoietic cells can divide asymmetrically; these micromanipulated single cells give rise to colonies that account for almost all possible lineage combinations (184). These data provide strong support for a stochastic mechanism to explain both commitment and restriction of differentiation potential. Differentiation of single blast cells into mature cells occurs in these methylcellulose cultures in the absence of an intact microenvironment. A source of hematopoietic growth factor is obligatory, as is the case for all colonies grown in semisolid media.

Although these random events occur with a given probability, it must be possible for that probability to be altered. For example, during the regeneration of hematopoietic tissues after injury by radiation or cytotoxic drugs, the probability of generating stem cells must increase. How this probability is altered is one of the outstanding unanswered questions in hematopoiesis.

A contrasting model proposed by Trentin et al. (181) postulated that the hematopoietic microenvironment was inductive (HIM), based on the observation that differentiation within a single spleen colony was variegated and geographically determined (182). Erythroid HIMs predominate in murine spleen, whereas granulocytic HIMs predominate in bone marrow. Transfer experiments showed that granulocytic cells predominated in the CFU-S–derived spleen colonies arising at junctional regions of bone marrow fragments implanted in spleen, whereas erythroid cells predominated in the splenic portion of the same colony. A major drawback for this model comes from an analysis of progenitors within these colonies. No correlations were observed between mature cells and their respective committed progenitors (185).

The preponderance of differentiating cells of one type or other within colonies thus appears to result from later events.

The nature of these events has not been established, but possibilities include the release of short-range lineage-specific factors by stromal cells, or perhaps the display of such growth factor molecules on the surface of their cell membranes. The Dexter culture system also lends powerful support to an essential role of stromal cells for stem cell survival, because the concentration of stem cells is highest within the adherent stromal layer itself (186,187). This and other observations related to the morphology of the focal development of hematopoietic islands attached to adherent cells have led to the postulate that hematopoietic stem cells reside within stromal cell "niches" that play a vital role in supporting stem cell survival, perhaps by intimate cell contact (188). *In vivo*, it appears that the most primitive stem cells reside in the region of the medullary cavity closest to the periosteal bone (182).

In sum, it appears likely that two types of control can affect stem cell regulation. At one level is control by stromal cells and, possibly, adhesion itself, perhaps primarily on stem cell survival but also on their response to humoral factors. At a second level are the humoral growth factors, which appear to affect stem cells but probably have a greater effect on committed maturing progenitors and precursors.

PROGENITOR CELL COMPARTMENT

The progeny of differentiating stem cells include cells committed to develop into the mature cells of a single lineage. These committed progenitors are characterized by loss of self-renewal capacity and by less potential for multilineage differentiation compared with stem cells. Most of the progenitors that can be analyzed in semisolid cultures are unipotent, and over time they can clonally generate colonies composed of 50 to 100,000 mature cells (2,3). Similar to stem cells, progenitors show marked heterogeneity within any given lineage. It is convenient to distinguish different progenitor classes based on their proliferative capacity and responsiveness to growth factors. This is probably an artificial classification because a continuum most likely exists *in vivo*, with the most immature progenitors merging with stem cells and the most mature progenitors merging with recognizable precursors.

Progenitors are assayed by their capacity to form colonies *in vitro*, and the original technique involved immobilization of a single cell suspension of bone marrow cells in a serum-enriched medium that contained a source of CSF, usually conditioned medium from cell lines, and was rendered semisolid by the addition of agar (2,3,189). Subsequent modifications to this technique include the use of methylcellulose or agarose in place of agar, the addition of highly purified recombinant CSFs in place of conditioned media, and purification of the progenitor cells. The time required for a progenitor cell to develop into a colony of mature cells depends on both species and stage of differentiation. Mature and immature murine progenitors take approximately 2 and 7 to 10 days, respectively, whereas the analogous human progenitors require 7 and 14 days, respectively. The most mature progenitor-derived colonies are the first to develop into small colonies or clusters in culture, whereas the more immature progenitors take longer to mature and develop into bigger colonies.

Within this continuum, conventional classifications include immature erythroid burst-forming units (BFU-Es), large multisubunit colonies of normoblasts that derive their name from their characteristic "burst-like" morphologic appearance in culture, and more mature single-subunit erythroid colony-forming units (CFU-Es); and immature granulocyte-macrophage, granulocyte, macrophage, or eosinophil colony-forming units (CFU-

GM, CFU-G, CFU-M, CFU-Eo) (more than 40 cells) or more mature clusters (less than 40 cells); in some culture systems, progenitors of the basophil mast cell and megakaryocyte lineages can be identified (CFU-Mast, CFU-MK). The frequency of progenitor varies with the source of cells and also depends on the number and concentration of growth factors. In murine and human bone marrow, myeloid progenitors are present at a frequency of approximately 1 per 10^3 cells.

PRECURSOR CELL COMPARTMENT

Most cells in the bone marrow of a healthy person are recognizable precursor cells of the myeloid or erythroid cell compartments: 60% to 70% of these cells are myeloid precursors, 20% to 30% are erythroid precursors, and the remaining 10% include lymphocytes, plasma cells, macrophages, and the very rare stem and progenitor cells discussed. In addition, normally, 4 to 5 megakaryocytes are found per 1000 nucleated bone marrow cells. The normal ratio of myeloid to erythroid precursors ranges from 3:1 to 3.5:1. Alterations in these numbers are difficult to determine with bone marrow aspirate samples because of variations in dilution of peripheral blood. Bone marrow biopsy is the preferred method of quantitation of the relative incidence of precursor types. Specific alterations in the precursor populations are discussed in chapters describing various pathologic conditions.

As previously discussed, the bone marrow of newborn infants is characteristically very cellular and devoid of fat cells (62,63). Erythroid precursors make up most marrow cells, and immediately after birth, the number of erythroid cells and the total cellularity of the marrow cavity begin to decline (65). Cellularity may decline by as much as 75% in the first 2 weeks of life, but gradually increases thereafter to a maximum at 3 months. (The physiologic nadir of erythroid cells in the newborn was discussed in the section Physiologic Changes after Birth.) Thus, in the newborn, the typical myeloid to erythroid ratio is not seen until approximately 1 month of age; the ratio is 1.2:1 on the first day of life and varies from 4:1 to 6:1 during the next 2 weeks. This dramatic reversal coincides with the diminished erythroid activity typical of the first 3 months of infancy (64,66). In addition, infant bone marrows are characterized by a large percentage of lymphocytes (the percentage can reach as high as 50% in the first year of life) (67). The relative lymphocytosis generally persists for the first 4 to 5 years and is accompanied by a lymphocytosis in the peripheral blood.

MATURATION OF THE ERYTHROID LINEAGE

As seen on standard Wright-Giemsa staining at the light microscope level, the normal differentiation of RBCs occurs in well-defined stages. The first identifiable and also the largest precursor of the erythroid lineage is the pronormoblast. The cell diameter is 14 to 19 µm, and the nucleus is large, oval, and homogeneously staining (violet) with indistinct nucleoli. The cytoplasm is darkly basophilic with lighter staining areas (hyaloplasm) usually near the nucleus, reflecting the position of the Golgi and lipid-containing mitochondria. Maturation to the basophilic normoblast is accompanied by reduction in cell size and pronounced changes in the nuclear chromatin structure. The basophilic normoblast is 12 to 17 µm in diameter with basophilic cytoplasm, and the nuclear chromatin shows a coarsening and prominent clumping leading to descriptions of a spoked wheel or cartwheel appearance. Nucleoli are generally not seen. The polychromatic normoblast is nearly the same size as the basophilic normoblast. The accumulation of hemoglobin is now seen by the presence of less basophilic and muddy gray cytoplasm. As the normoblast matures, the nucleus shows further condensation. The last nucleated RBC precursor is the orthochromatic normoblast. The cell now approaches the diameter of a reticulocyte (8 to 12 μm), and the eosinophilic staining cytoplasm contains nearly a full amount of hemoglobin. The nucleus is now fully condensed and pyknotic.

Extrusion of the nucleus results in the *reticulocyte,* a cell slightly larger than a fully mature erythrocyte. The reticulocyte is characterized by the presence of a fine granular or reticular network of ribosomal RNA observed with supravital stains such as cresyl blue or methylene blue. Such cells are present in small quantities in the peripheral blood of normal persons but are increased in response to stress on the erythroid lineage, such as hemolysis or blood loss. *Stress reticulocytes* are prematurely released into the peripheral blood, where cellular maturation continues. Stress reticulocytes are larger in diameter than reticulocytes normally found in the peripheral blood, and their cytoplasm is more basophilic.

Other morphologic indications of stress erythropoiesis are polychromatophilia (violet tinting seen with Wright-Giemsa staining) and basophilic stippling (blue or black stippling diffusely distributed throughout the cell). Both are the result of RNA-containing remnants that stain in the cytoplasm of the erythrocyte. The premature destruction of erythroid precursors in the medullary cavity, termed *ineffective erythropoiesis,* is accompanied by elevation of serum lactate dehydrogenase, decreased levels of haptoglobin, slight elevation of the reticulocyte count (2% to 4%), and the occasional appearance of nucleated erythrocytes in the peripheral blood. The destruction of erythrocyte precursors in the medullary cavity normally involves less than 10% of the developing cells, but loss of much larger numbers of cells is seen in β-thalassemia, in several rare congenital anemias such as the congenital dyserythropoietic anemias, and certain acquired disorders, particularly megaloblastic anemias and myelodysplasia.

The final stage of erythroid maturation is the erythrocyte. The cell is a biconcave, relatively flat, nonnucleated disk 7 to 8 μm in diameter. The normal survival of the mature erythrocyte is 100 to 120 days.

LEUKOCYTE DIFFERENTIATION

Leukocytes that circulate in the peripheral blood are divided into those of the myeloid, monocyte-macrophage, and lymphocytic lineages. The differentiation and function of the lymphocytic lineage are discussed in Chapter 18. Four distinct granule populations are seen in the myeloid and monocyte lineages and distinguish these cells morphologically during differentiation. Azurophilic granules are present in cells of both lineages, stain pink with Romanovsky dyes, and contain myeloperoxidase, acid phosphatase, basic cationic protein, and other hydrolases. Eosinophilic granules are conspicuous reddish orange, and basophilic granules are intensely blue. Specific neutrophilic granules do not stain intensely with standard Wright-Giemsa stains.

MYELOID DIFFERENTIATION

The earliest identifiable cell of the myeloid lineage is the myeloblast. The cell is approximately 12 to 14 μm in diameter, with a round or oval nucleus and basophilic cytoplasm that lacks granules. Nuclear chromatin is fine, and one to five nucleoli are easily visible. The nucleus often stains reddish. Promyelocytes are the largest and most common of the primitive myeloid precursors. Promyelocytes are variable in nuclear shape, with less prominent nucleoli and chromatin of medium density, which is more coarse than that of the myeloblast. The cytoplasm is deeply basophilic and contains variable numbers of peroxidase-positive granules. These granules can overlie the nucleus, vary in color from deep red to blue, and distinguish the promyelocyte from the myeloblast. Myelocytes are characterized by round to oval nuclei with characteristic nuclear indentations, indistinct nucleoli, and unevenly stained, coarse chromatin structure.

The cytoplasm stains pale gray-brown or pink-brown, with numerous specific granules covering the nucleus and throughout the cytoplasm, except in a clear area near the nuclear indentation (centrosphere), which represents the Golgi apparatus. The myelocyte is also characterized by the first appearance of specific granules and is the last cell capable of division during myeloid differentiation. The metamyelocyte, band neutrophil, and segmented neutrophil show progressive condensation and restriction of the nucleus. The metamyelocyte exhibits a characterized bean-shaped nucleus, the band neutrophil exhibits a horseshoe-shaped or S-shaped nuclear structure without recognizable constrictions, and the segmented neutrophil shows the characteristic nuclear segmentations for which it is named that divide the nucleus into two to five lobes. These myeloid forms exhibit similar cytoplasmic characteristics to the myelocyte without the centrosphere and with progressive reduction in overall cell size. An additional nuclear lobule in the shape of a drumstick is present in 10% to 12% of segmented neutrophils of females, morphologic documentation of random inactivation of one of the two X-chromosomes.

Maturation of the eosinophil and basophil follows the same morphologic steps as that of the neutrophil until the appearance of specific granules. The eosinophil exhibits a bilobed nucleus, with the basophilic cytoplasm filled with prominent orange-red granules. Basophils have less segmentation of the nucleus and cytoplasm that is sparsely filled with deeply staining blue to purple metachromatic granules. The granules often obscure the nucleus and cytoplasm, which stains pink to reddish pink and frequently exhibits vacuoles. The incidence of these last two cell types in the peripheral blood of normal persons is 1% to 4% and 0% to 0.5%, respectively.

MONOCYTE DIFFERENTIATION

The earliest cell of the monocyte-macrophage lineage is difficult to distinguish from the myeloblast. The cell is 12 to 18 μm in diameter, with a round or oval nucleus that is frequently convoluted. The chromatin is fine, and nucleoli are variably present. The cytoplasm is basophilic with a grayish cast and, although devoid of granules, may contain vacuoles. Blunt pseudopodia are sometimes present. The naphthol-AS0 acetate esterase reaction is positive and inhibited by fluoride. The promonocyte is a large cell with an indented nucleus exhibiting fine chromatin and a single nucleolus. The cytoplasm stains light blue with azurophilic granules and a small centrosphere. The monocyte is the largest cell present in the peripheral blood and measures 13 to 20 μm in diameter. The nucleus is large and lobulated or bean-shaped with coarse nuclear chromatin, lacks nucleoli, and is often eccentric in location. The cytoplasm stains a characteristic smoke blue with azurophilic granules. The chromatin structure of the monocyte is less clumped and the cytoplasm more gray than the lymphocyte—characteristics which, along with nuclear convolutions, help to distinguish these cells from moderately sized lymphocytes in the peripheral blood.

Blunt pseudopodia provide another helpful distinguishing characteristic. Monocytes usually make up 5% to 10% of the peripheral blood leukocytes. Egress of monocytes from the blood into tissues is associated with increased cell size and larger, lighter-staining nuclei. These cells, termed *macrophages* or *histiocytes*, are phagocytic and mobile, and intracellular debris and pseudopodia are often present.

MEGAKARYOCYTES

Morphologic differentiation of platelet-forming cells is different from that of either erythroid or leukocytic cell lineages. Distinct morphologic maturational steps and divisions do not take place, replaced by the process of *polyploidization.* In this process, successive nuclear divisions without concomitant cytoplasmic divisions lead to megakaryocytes with 1 to 32 nuclei representing 2N to 64N nuclear content. The first identifiable cell in this lineage is the megakaryoblast, a distinctly large cell with a high nuclear to cytoplasmic ratio. The nucleus shows variable chromatin coarseness and may contain nucleoli. The nuclear shape varies, but the nucleus frequently displays convolutions or deep furrows. The cytoplasm stains basophilic, does not contain granules, and may exhibit fraying at the cytoplasmic membrane. Some megakaryoblasts may contain multiple nuclei. The promegakaryocyte exhibits lobulated nuclear structure without nucleoli and with coarse chromatin structure. The cytoplasm is basophilic with azurophilic granules adjacent to the nucleus, and formed platelets are seen on the cytoplasmic cell surface.

Occasionally, the presence of other cells apparently within the cytoplasm (emperipolesis) of the promegakaryocyte is noted; the mechanism leading to this occurrence is unknown. Mature megakaryocytes are the largest hematopoietic cells of the bone marrow. The nucleus is lobulated and exhibits coarse and clumped chromatin. Nuclear number varies from eight diploid nuclei (65% of marrow megakaryocytes) to four nuclei (10% of marrow megakaryocytes). The cytoplasm is basophilic with numerous azurophilic granules. Platelets can be seen at the periphery of the cytoplasm and attached to the cell membrane. Megakaryocytes constitute less than 1.0% of cells in the medullary cavity in normal persons.

HEMATOPOIETIC MICROENVIRONMENT

Hematopoiesis occurs within a complex environment in the medullary cavity in mammals (7,181,190). The spatial arrangements in the medullary cavity are nonrandom and have been studied in some detail *in situ* and experimentally (191–193). Branches of the central longitudinal artery traverse the space between the interior of the bone and the cortex, either joining directly to venous sinuses or communicating indirectly by means of the Haversian canals in the bony cortex (194) (Fig. 7-5). These vascular connections, now moving toward the interior of the medullary cavity, separate groups of developing hematopoietic cells into so-called hematopoietic cords (195). Within the

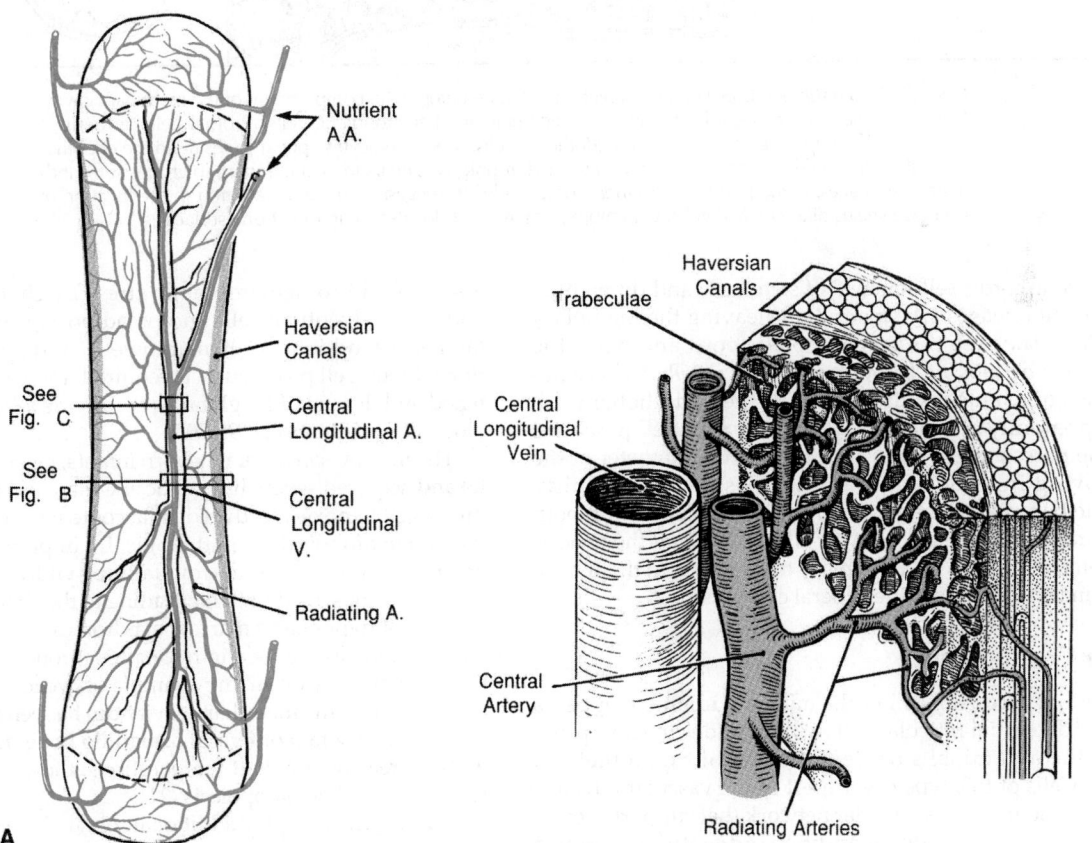

Figure 7-5. Hematopoietic microenvironment in the medullary cavity. **A:** Schematic representation of longitudinal cross section of a long bone. **B:** Schematic depiction of a sagittal cross-section of the medullary cavity. Nutrient arteries feed the bone after entering the medullary space and giving rise to the central longitudinal artery. Progressive branches of this artery (radiating arteries) cross the medullary space toward the outside of the bone, connecting directly with hematopoietic sinuses or indirectly with cords through Haversian canals. Hematopoietic cells leaving the medullary cavity collect in venous sinuses, enter the central longitudinal vein, and then enter the general circulation. (*continued*)

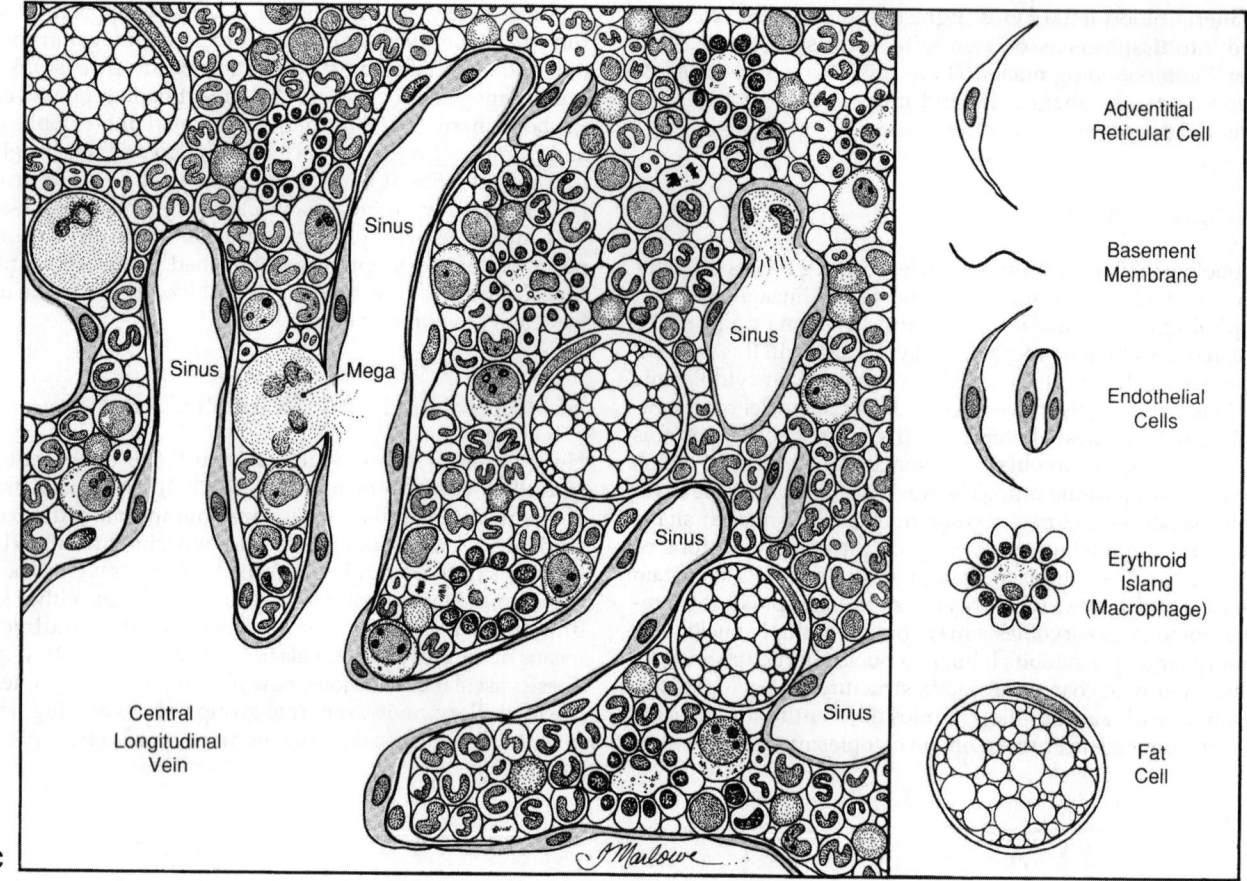

Figure 7-5. (continued) C: Schematic depiction of the hematopoietic compartment of the medullary cavity. Hematopoiesis occurs in cords composed of differentiating hematopoietic cells, stromal cells, adventitial reticular cells, adipocytes (fat cells), and endothelial cells. Megakaryocytes appear to reside in the endothelial cell walls, shedding platelets into the sinus. Erythropoiesis appears to occur, in part, in groups surrounding macrophages, termed *erythroid islands*. Some evidence suggests structured variation in the location of primitive versus differentiated cells, with more primitive cells located nearer the bone surface.

hematopoietic cords, self-renewal of stem cells and differentiation along all lineages take place. Cells leaving the medullary cavity must traverse the hematopoietic cord and enter the venous sinus by moving through endothelial cells.* This complex series of events involves pores in the endothelial wall, which apparently are located near, but not at, cell junctions (196). The pores are generally smaller than the diameter of the cells moving into the sinus, and increased deformability appears to be a characteristic of more differentiated cells in both the erythroid and myeloid lineages (194,197). From the venous sinus, hematopoietic cells are rapidly transported to the central longitudinal vein and into the general circulation.

Cellular Constituents

An important accessory cell of the microenvironment appears to be the adventitial reticular cell, which resides in close proximity to the abluminal surface of the venous endothelium (198,199). Cells of this type cover most of the vascular adventitial surface and provide a reticular network that supports developing hematopoietic cells. In addition, adventitial cells and preadipocytes may play an active role in hematopoiesis by direct cell contact or local secretion of cytokines or other growth-regulating proteins (200–206). It appears that such cells

also respond to hematopoietic stress by changes in volume. Although adventitial cells and preadipocytes normally contain fat and extend into the hematopoietic cord space, when additional blood cell production is required, these cells become flattened and devoid of fat globules to provide additional space for blood cell production (198,207).

The marrow cavity of newborn infants, persons with congenital and acquired severe hemolytic anemias, and those exposed to prolonged hypoxia is reduced in fat content (208,209). In contrast, when hematopoiesis is pathologically impaired, as in aplastic anemia or other bone marrow failure syndromes, the marrow cavity becomes filled with fat, leading to the characteristic yellow marrow of hypoplastic marrow syndromes (198,210). These fatty changes can also be seen in mice after chronic RBC transfusions (209). A naturally occurring example of cyclic changes in adipocyte content of the medullary cavity can be seen in the armadillo. The medullary fat content of armadillo bone marrow increases with decreasing ambient temperatures; these changes correlate with decreased hematopoiesis (211).

Adipocytes may play additional roles in hematopoiesis as reservoirs for lipids needed in cell metabolism during proliferation (212,213). Medullary adipocytes demonstrate characteristics similar to both white adipocyte (lipid-containing cells involved in lipid and energy metabolism) and brown adipocyte (lipid-containing cells involved in heat production) tissues (203). During starvation, white adipocyte tissue is rapidly depleted, whereas fat in the bone marrow is spared. Insulin appears to be

---

*For a complete review of the architecture of the medullary cavity, see Chapter 14, Bone Marrow, in reference 197a.

required for differentiation of white adipocyte cells; these cells exhibit lipogenic responses to insulin treatment. In contrast, bone marrow adipocytes appear to differentiate in response to glucocorticoids and do not respond to insulin (214). During prolonged starvation, bone marrow fat cells are depleted, and the marrow cavity is replaced by a gelatinous tissue (215,216). Finally, the increasing fat content seen in long bones of older children and adults is associated with decreased limb temperatures compared with those of neonates and infants (62,63). Thus, marrow adipocytes are not clearly classified as either white or brown adipocyte tissue.

Hematopoietic Organization in the Medullary Sinus

At the cellular level, the hematopoietic sinus also displays some organization, although the significance of this organization remains unknown. Most prominently, megakaryocytes are located adjacent to the vascular endothelium, usually occupying space in the vascular wall. From this location, platelets are shed directly into the venous sinus, reducing any requirements for cell movement on the part of the megakaryocyte. Developing erythrocytes often occur in groups termed *erythroblastic islands* around bone marrow macrophages (198,200,217,218). Megakaryocytes tend to occur near vascular endothelial cells, and groups of myeloid cells, B lymphoid cells, and stromal cells appear to cluster (219). Studies by several groups show that hematopoietic stem and progenitor cells reside in distinct locations within the medullary cavity.

Hematopoietic stem cells with less proliferative activity tend to reside at the periphery of hematopoietic cords in the subcortical space (191,192,220). In contrast, stem cells with higher proliferative activity and myeloid progenitor cells reside toward the middle of the hematopoietic sinus. Lord et al. (191) have also observed nonrandom localization of erythroid progenitors in the murine femoral medullary cavity. Such spatial arrangements may reflect the general flow of cells toward the venous sinus during differentiation or may relate to specific cellular interactions with membrane proteins or extracellular matrix proteins of stromal cells making up the hematopoietic microenvironment.

The hematopoietic microenvironment probably provides more than passive structural support for hematopoietic cells during proliferation and differentiation. For instance, the spleen environment in the mouse appears particularly suited for erythroid differentiation, whereas the medullary cavity supports granulocytic differentiation (181). As noted, studies by Wolff and Trentin (182) show effects of specific microenvironments on stem cell differentiation. Femoral shafts placed in spleen pulp give rise to hematopoietic colonies located at the junction of the femur and spleen environments with a geographic distribution of differentiated cells. In these experiments, differentiation within a clonally derived hematopoietic colony was myeloid within the marrow environment and erythroid within the spleen environment. Based on these and other observations, Curry and Trentin (98) proposed that specific locations provide an inductive microenvironment for stem cell proliferation and differentiation.

As previously noted, differentiation within the yolk sac and fetal liver microenvironments is severely restricted to the erythroid lineage. The molecular and biochemical bases for the microenvironment regulation of differentiation are not yet known.

In Vitro Cultures Recapitulate the Hematopoietic Microenvironment

The development of an *in vitro* culture system that mimics the hematopoietic microenvironment has significantly aided the study of hematopoietic stem cell–microenvironment interac-

tions (Fig. 7-6). First described by Dexter et al. (7) and later modified by Greenberger (214), these cultures are made up of a complex adherent cell population containing endothelial cells, fibroblasts, macrophages, and preadipocytes.* The cultures are created by forcing a large inoculum of medullary cavity cells into flasks with media containing prescreened horse serum (later modified to include hydrocortisone; Fig. 7-6). Cultures are maintained in high CO_2 at low temperatures (33°C) and depopulated of 50% to 70% of nonadherent cells and media at weekly feedings of fresh media. These culture conditions encourage the growth of the adherent cell population, which matures over approximately 3 weeks.

Hematopoiesis occurs within the adherent cell population, and on the surface of the adherent cells, hematopoietic cells are continuously shed into the overlying media (200,221). Large groups of round, refractile cells, termed *hematopoietic islands* or *cobblestone areas*, are present within the adherent cell population and contain stem and progenitor cells (222). In sharp contrast to other cell culture systems, hematopoietic stem cells are maintained for several months *in vitro*, and stem cells harvested from such cultures maintain the ability to reconstitute fully the hematopoietic tissues of lethally irradiated recipients.

In many culture systems, maintenance of the stem cell population in such cultures requires direct stem cell–stromal cell contact, because conditioned media from such cultures do not support the survival of stem cells *in vitro* (223,224). Hellman et al. (158) and other researchers have demonstrated that stem cells present in such cultures exhibit structured variation in self-renewal capacity (186,187,225). Stem cells present in the adherent cell layer demonstrate considerably more self-renewal capacity than stem cells present in the nonadherent media overlying the cultures. These observations support the stem cell "niche" hypothesis proposed by Schofield (188) that direct contact of hematopoietic stem cells with the microenvironment maintains stem cell characteristics (226). It is proposed that loss of direct stem cell contact with the microenvironment is accompanied by exposure of the stem cell to differentiation pressures with concomitant loss of self-renewal capacity. On the other hand, adhesion has been shown to limit the cycling activity of primitive hematopoietic cells, providing one potential mechanism for the maintenance of the primitive phenotype (227).

The contribution of individual adherent cell types in long-term marrow cultures to the maintenance of stem cells is not known but is the focus of active research. Roles of the hematopoietic microenvironment in hematopoiesis have been proposed to involve direct communication of stromal with stem cells through tight cell-to-cell contact (228); co-localization of growth factors and stem cells at the point of cell contact or prevention of growth factor degradation by binding of these cytokines to extracellular matrix proteins (229,230); and secretion of stromal-derived growth-regulating factors (231,232), including inhibitors of DNA synthesis (233).

Long-term cultures, as originally described by Dexter et al. (7), provide an excellent model for myeloid differentiation. Full maturation to granulocytes and macrophages takes place in the cultures, whereas the relative concentration of myeloid compartments (stem, progenitor, precursor, differentiated cell) reflects normal hematopoiesis (234). Further modification of long-term marrow culture conditions by elimination of horse serum and hydrocortisone leads to proliferation of pre-B lymphocytes as described by Whitlock and Witte (190) and Whitlock et al. (235). Several groups have modified long-term cultures to allow full erythroid differentiation by including a

---

*For a wonderful review of the historical background of our understanding of the hematopoietic microenvironment, see reference 220a.

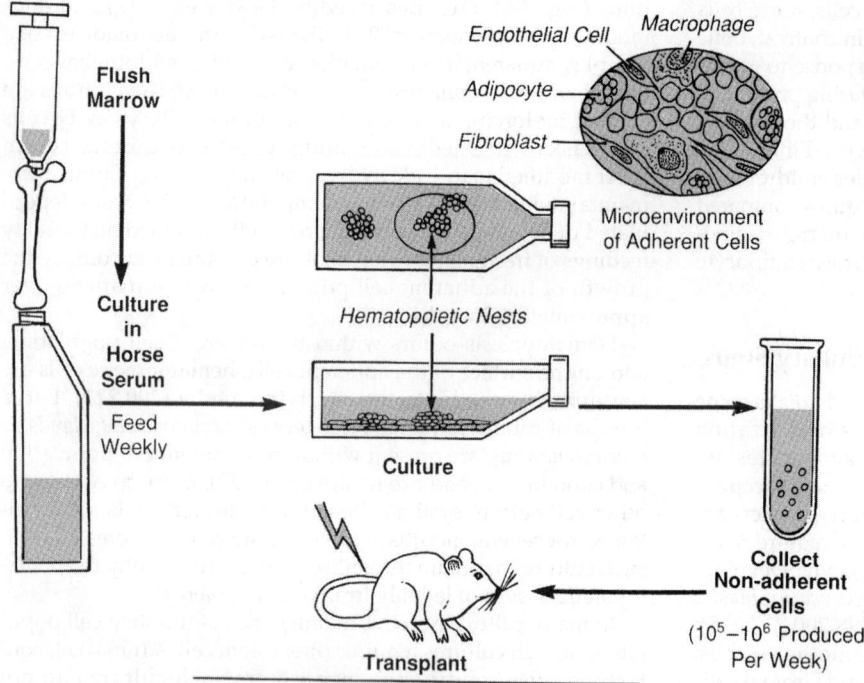

Myeloid Cultures:
- Adipocytes apparent in 2–3 weeks
- CFU-S, CFU-GM present for 2–4 months
- BFU-E present for 2 months

Lymphoid Cultures:
- Eliminate horse serum & hydrocortisone
- Pre-B cells produced (B220$^+$, IgM$_{cyt}^+$)

Erythroid Cultures:
- Source of Epo, mouse serum
- Feed twice weekly
- Erythroid precursors make up 70% of nucleated cells

Figure 7-6. *In vitro* analysis of the hematopoietic microenvironment using long-term marrow (Dexter) cultures. Bone marrow is flushed from the marrow cavity and allowed to establish an adherent layer composed of endothelial cells, macrophages, adipocytes, and fibroblasts. Within this stromal layer, hematopoietic nests of actively proliferating stem and progenitor cells enlarge. Hematopoietic cells, including stem and progenitor cells, are shed into the supernatant, which can be harvested and used to rescue lethally irradiated transplant recipients. Such cultures can be modified to yield myeloid, lymphoid, and erythroid elements. BFU-E, erythroid burst-forming unit; CFU-GM, granulocyte-macrophage colony-forming unit; CFU-S, colony-forming unit-spleen; Epo, erythropoietin; Ig, immunoglobulin.

small amount of fetal calf serum, feeding more frequently, and including EPO in the cultures (236–239).

Long-term cultures have also been useful in the study of human hematopoiesis with several modifications of the techniques used in murine cultures as described (240). Autologous marrow transplants from long-term cultures have led to successful, but transient, engraftment of normal stem cells in persons with myeloid leukemias (241,242). Human long-term marrow cultures appear morphologically distinct, lacking the classic cobblestone areas seen in rodent cultures. In addition, stem cells are maintained *in vitro* for considerably shorter times (usually less than 2 months) in human cultures compared with several months in murine cultures (243). The basis of these differences is not yet understood.*

STROMAL CELLS PLAY A CRITICAL ROLE IN HEMATOPOIESIS

The complexity of long-term marrow cultures has hindered some areas of hematopoietic research, specifically the study of stem cell–stromal cell interactions.† Several laboratories have

now established immortalized stromal cell lines from long-term marrow cultures (206,223,224,244–248).

Many stromal cell lines support the maintenance of myeloid and lymphoid progenitors *in vitro* for several weeks (206,224,244,245,247,249–252). In addition, a few lines have been shown to support primitive myeloid stem cells (CFU-S$_{12}$) for extended periods; these lines effectively replace a complex long-term marrow culture in this regard (206,223,224,251). One immortalized stromal cell line has been shown by male-female transplantation to support the maintenance of long-term reconstituting and multipotential stem cells in murine cultures for up to 3 weeks *in vitro* (224). Similarly, stromal cell lines have been shown to support the proliferation of pre-B lymphocytes under conditions similar to those established by Whitlock et al. (247) and Hunt et al. (244) for long-term lymphocyte cultures (223). Conditioned media from stromal cell lines contain a variety of known hematopoietic growth factors but cannot support the maintenance of primitive stem cells in culture (202,205,231,246,253–259). The maintenance of stem and progenitor populations in stromal long-term cultures depends on direct hematopoietic cell–stromal cell contact and therefore closely mimics the stem cell maintenance in traditional long-term marrow cultures (260). Established stromal cell lines appear to represent a heterogeneous group of adherent cells (261).

Although the appearance of adipocytes in murine long-term marrow cultures is temporally related to increased hematopoietic activity, several stromal cell lines that support progenitor cell proliferation do not appear to be adipocytic. In general, the

---

*For an extensive review of all aspects of long-term bone marrow cultures and the hematopoietic microenvironment, see reference 243a.
†A summary of stromal cells and hematopoiesis is contained in reference 243.

preadipocyte phenotype appears to correlate with support of myeloid hematopoiesis *in vitro* (7,262). In contrast, support of lymphopoiesis appears to be related to the capacity of stromal cell lines to accumulate fat globules (262). Gimble et al. (201,263) have shown that several stromal cell lines respond to inducing agents such as dexamethasone, hydrocortisone, and methyl-isobutylxanthine by accumulation of triglycerides and cholesterol esters and increased expression of adipocyte-specific enzymes (adipocyte P2, adipsin, lipoprotein lipase). Stromal cell lines also appear heterogeneous with respect to expression of extracellular matrix and intermediate filament proteins (261).

Many stromal cell lines capable of supporting the proliferation of myeloid progenitor cells are characterized by production of the endothelial proteins laminin and type IV collagen as well as fibronectin (264,265). Fibroblast-like stromal cell lines appear less capable of supporting hematopoiesis in murine cultures and are characterized by expression of collagens type I and III (206,261,266–268). A primate stromal cell line recently described expresses collagens type I, III, and V and supports progenitor cells capable of giving rise to both myeloid and mixed colonies for up to 3 weeks *in vitro* (231). Therefore, it remains unclear whether key stromal cell types in long-term marrow cultures differ in rodent and other species (including human).

Stromal Cells Produce a Variety of Growth-Regulatory Molecules

Stromal cell lines also differ considerably with respect to production of hematopoietic growth factors (264,269).* Some of these differences may be explained by experimental techniques, because more sensitive assays for growth factor production, such as polymerase chain reaction RNA analysis, have more recently been applied to the analysis of stromal cell lines. Stromal cell lines have been demonstrated to produce IL-6, IL-7, G-CSF, granulocyte-macrophage CSF (GM-CSF), TGF-β, macrophage CSF (M-CSF), SCF, Flt3L, and IL-1, either constitutively or after induction with IL-1 or other inducing agents (264,270). The induction of growth factor production may play an important role in the microenvironment regulation of hematopoiesis. Cashman et al. (255) used IL-1, platelet-derived growth factor (PDGF), TGF-β, and IL-2; Billips et al. (254) used IL-1 and IL-4 to demonstrate induction of stromal cell cytokine production.

In addition, long-term marrow cultures and some stromal cell lines have been shown to inhibit hematopoietic differentiation and stem cell DNA synthesis. Several groups have partially characterized proteins that have apparent negative regulatory roles in hematopoiesis (271–273). Toksoz et al. (233) reported that conditioned media from long-term marrow cultures contain a molecule that prevents the entry of primitive myeloid hematopoietic stem cells (CFU-S$_{12}$) into S phase as measured by thymidine suicide. A protein with similar characteristics has recently been defined and molecularly cloned from a macrophage cell line (269). This protein, termed *stem cell inhibitor*, is identical to a previously characterized chemokine, termed *macrophage inflammatory protein-1-α* (MIP-1α) (274). Biologic activities of stem cell inhibitor/MIP-1α suggest that it is an important regulator of stem cell proliferation and may have therapeutic applications in protecting stem cells from cycle-specific chemotherapeutic agents. However, clinical development of MIP-1α specifically and chemokines in general has been slow.†

Zipori et al. (262) and Zipori (275) have demonstrated that hematopoietic cells adherent to stromal cells fail to differentiate into macroscopic colonies of differentiated cell types even in the presence of exogenous CSFs. In addition, Verfaillie and Burroughs (276) have demonstrated that adhesion of stem and progenitor cells via integrin receptors also prevents cells from entering active division. Thus, it appears that direct cell contact between hematopoietic stem cells and stromal cells can restrict differentiation of stem cells in some culture systems. Zipori et al. (262) and Zipori (275) have also identified a membrane-associated glycoprotein, restrictin-P, which specifically inhibits the growth of the plasmacytoma cell line MPC-11 (277). These studies emphasize the differences between short-term progenitor cultures, in which CSFs are added, hematopoiesis is of short duration, and differentiation predominates, and long-term stromal-associated cultures in which stem cells are maintained for extended periods.

A major goal of research is understanding these differences. Because the only *in vitro* system in which stem cells with full reconstitution capacity are maintained for prolonged periods involves direct stem cell–stromal cell contact, the hematopoietic microenvironment is likely to play a critical role, either directly or indirectly, in hematopoietic stem cell biology.

The hematopoietic microenvironment may also be important in pathologic conditions affecting hematopoiesis. Murine mutants of bone marrow failure, such as the *Sl* mutants, exhibit characteristics attributable to defective microenvironments, including the hematopoietic microenvironment (Fig. 7-4) (278–280).††

Phenotypically, *Sl* and the better characterized *W* mutant are black-eyed white mice with multiple cellular defects (281). Careful study has revealed defects in all hematopoietic lineages (282,283). Affected mouse mutants at these loci have a severe macrocytic anemia associated with increased radiation sensitivity, deficiency of mast cells and other blood lineages, lack of coat pigmentation, and sterility. Although phenotypically similar, these mutations map to different chromosomes (*W* to chromosome 5, *Sl* to chromosome 10) and have distinct hematologic characteristics (281). Best characterized at the molecular level, the *W* mutation appears to result in a functional deficiency of primitive hematopoietic progenitor and stem cells. Transplantation of normal bone marrow into compound heterozygote (deficient) *W*/*W-viable (v)* recipients completely corrects the hematopoietic abnormalities, whereas transplantation of *W* bone marrow into lethally irradiated normal mice fails to reconstitute hematopoiesis (278).

The *W* gene has been shown to be allelic with the c-kit protooncogene, which is known to be a member of the tyrosine kinase receptor family that includes receptors for CSF-1 and PDGF. Several variants of the *dominant white spotting* mutant have been shown to be phenotypic expressions of specific molecular mutations of the c-kit protooncogene (284,285), and the severity of the phenotypic changes associated with specific alleles correlates with the degree of functional impairment of kinase activity (286).

In contrast, the *steel* mutation affects the function of the cells of the microenvironment. Compound *Sl/Sl-dickie (d)* bone marrow cells are capable of reconstituting hematopoiesis in irradiated normal mice, whereas transplantation of normal bone marrow into *Sl/Sl^d* animals fails to cure the defect (287). A deeper insight into the molecular nature of this mutant was provided by the purification of a factor that can stimulate mast cell proliferation and the growth of mouse bone marrow previously treated with 5-fluorouracil (the resulting cells are enriched for primitive stem cells but depleted of mature progenitors) (288,289). This factor, termed *stem cell factor* (also *mast cell growth factor*, *kit ligand*, or *steel factor*), was purified and its complemen-

---

*For a review of stromal cells and hematopoiesis, see reference 203.
†For a more complete review of negative regulators in hematopoiesis, see reference 274a.

††For a wonderful historical background, see reference 281.

tary DNA (cDNA) cloned (178,290,291). Labeling studies with the purified recombinant protein demonstrate that it is the ligand for the c-kit receptor (288,289,291).

Administration of the factor to Sl/Sl^d mice corrects their macrocytic anemia and repairs their mast cell deficiency locally at the injection site. The gene maps to the *steel* locus on chromosome 10 (292–294). Confirmation for the hypothesis that stem cell factor is encoded by the *steel* gene comes from Southern analysis of DNA obtained from stromal lines from normal and *Sl/Sl* homozygotes (the *Sl* mutation, unlike the commonly studied Sl^d mutation, is a homozygous embryonic lethal). These studies reveal that the coding sequences of the *steel* gene locus are completely deleted from the genome of homozygous (*Sl/Sl*) steel mice (294). Less severe mutations at the *Sl* locus such as Sl^d are associated with smaller deletions at the *Sl* locus (293). The hematopoietic abnormalities of the *Sl* animal are not cured by transplantation of congenic normal marrow, but the anemia can be partially improved by transplantation of intact spleens into the peritoneal cavity, an observation that has led several investigators to postulate that the mutation responsible for the hematologic abnormalities resides in the hematopoietic microenvironment (279,280,287,295). In support of this view, Dexter and Moore (296) have demonstrated that long-term marrow cultures from *Sl* mice do not support hematopoietic cells from normal congenic mice *in vitro*. Several laboratories have reported the cloning of the gene product of the *Sl* mutation and characterized the molecular basis of several of the known *Sl* mutations (178,290,292–294,297).

The product of the *Sl* gene has now been shown to be a 28-kd to 35-kd growth factor, with a leader sequence, a transmembrane domain, and a differentially spliced exon including a proteolytic cleavage site (178,288,289). The protein product can thus be membrane-bound or secreted, although the physiologic role of these different forms is not clear. Flanagan et al. (180) have demonstrated that the *steel-dickie* (Sl^d) allele, which is known to be a nonlethal *Sl* mutation, is encoded by a *Sl* gene with a deletion of the transmembrane domain. The resulting protein is secreted and biologically active. This observation suggests that the membrane-bound form of the *Sl* gene product may play an important role in hematopoiesis. The *Sl* gene product is now known to be the ligand for the c-kit protooncogene (288,292,294). The *dominant white spotting* mutation is known to be allelic with this tyrosine kinase receptor family member (284,285).

Although no congenital human bone marrow failure syndrome has been shown to be due to a microenvironment defect, the failure of bone marrow transplant engraftment in some patients with aplastic anemia suggests that such abnormalities may exist. The use of newer molecular methods, growth-regulatory probes, and more powerful genetic approaches to study affected kindreds may define abnormalities in the hematopoietic microenvironment associated with some congenital bone marrow failure syndromes. Interestingly, mutations of c-kit in humans are associated in the heterozygous state with piebaldism. No individuals homozygous for c-kit mutations have been described, suggesting the possibility of embryonic lethality in humans.*

FACTORS REGULATING THE EGRESS OF HEMATOPOIETIC CELLS FROM THE BONE MARROW

The movement of cells from the medullary cavity into the bloodstream has been studied in most detail using radiolabeled iron to monitor the development and release of erythroid cells.

Classic ferrokinetic studies show that after initial uptake of ^{59}Fe in the bone marrow, newly synthesized erythrocytes are released into the bloodstream in 4 to 6 days (299). The generation time of proliferating erythroid precursors (pronormoblasts, basophilic and polychromatophilic normoblasts) normally averages approximately 24 hours at each stage of maturation (300,301). Nondividing erythroid precursors (orthochromatophilic normoblasts and reticulocytes) reside in the medullary space for approximately 48 hours (302). Normal maturation includes an average of four divisions and the generation of 8 to 16 cells from each pronormoblast. The maturation time can be shortened during stress by one of several mechanisms.

Commonly regarded as a critical mechanism in the erythroid compartment response to stress, erythrocytes can exit the medullary cavity prematurely after having skipped some divisions. These cells maintain primitive characteristics, such as macrocytosis, elevated fetal hemoglobin, and persistence of i (versus I) antigen on the cell surface (303). In addition, erythrocyte maturation time may be shortened by decreasing the duration of each mitosis or by decreasing the maturation time of nondividing erythrocyte precursors (304). Finally, RBC mass may be elevated by increasing the number of erythrocytes actually entering the bloodstream.

The last mechanism could result either from less destruction of RBC precursors (*ineffective erythropoiesis*) in the medullary cavity (normally approximately 10%) or from an expansion in the number of primitive cells entering the erythroid maturational sequence (305). The latter appears to be the usual mechanism of expansion of the erythroid compartment during times of increased requirement for RBCs as a result of chronic hemolysis or blood loss.

In vitro studies have begun to elucidate the molecular basis for the movement of erythroid cells out of the medullary cavity. Patel and Lodish (306) have demonstrated that an erythroid cell line (murine erythroleukemia cells) binds specifically to the extracellular matrix protein fibronectin and that loss of adhesion to fibronectin occurs during induced differentiation of these cells. Subsequent studies demonstrated that binding to fibronectin involves a specific peptide in the fibronectin molecule, Arg-Gly-Asp-Ser (RGDS), and this interaction is mediated by a β_1 integrin receptor on the surface of erythrocytes, $\alpha_5\beta_{1-5}$, a member of the integrin supergene family of receptors (307). Loss of adhesion of differentiating erythrocytes is associated with loss of this receptor at the reticulocyte stage of development (307). It is interesting that the efficiency of enucleation of murine erythroleukemia cells in response to inducers of differentiation is improved dramatically by differentiation on a fibronectin matrix (308).

A greater understanding of the molecular basis of cell adhesion, particularly as it relates to leukocyte–endothelial interactions, has also begun to elucidate some of the mechanisms involved in leukocyte trafficking (309,310). Egress of leukocytes from the blood to sites of inflammation appears to involve sequential interactions with several cell adhesion molecules. Leukocytes first appear to tether and roll on endothelial cells via one of several selectin proteins. Selectins are Ca^{2+}-dependent glycoproteins that mediate sheer-resistant adhesion to specific carbohydrate ligands. Selectins involved in leukocyte–endothelial interactions are P (platelet)-selectin, E (endothelial)-selectin, and L (leukocyte)-selectin. Subsequent to tethering via selectins, firm adhesion of cells to endothelium occurs via activated integrin receptors. Integrins are type I membrane glycoproteins that consist of α and β subunits and are involved in cell–cell and cell–matrix interactions (311). Several integrins are expressed on hematopoietic stem and progenitor cells, but β_1 integrins appear particularly important. Specifically, both $\alpha_4\beta_1$ and $\alpha_5\beta_1$ integrins are expressed and appear functional on primitive murine and

---

*A more complete review of these interesting mutants can be found in reference 298.

human hematopoietic stem cells (312–317). The ligand for $\alpha_5\beta_1$, the Arg-Gly-Asp-Ser tetra peptide, is contained within the extracellular matrix protein fibronectin (318), which is expressed throughout the bone marrow cavity (319). The integrin $\alpha_4\beta_1$ has at least two ligands: the carboxy-terminal IIICS domain of fibronectin containing the CS-1 sequence (320) and the vascular cell adhesion molecule-1, which is expressed by bone marrow stromal cells and vascular endothelial cells. Adhesion of primitive hematopoietic cells appears to be mediated by both $\alpha_4\beta_1$ and $\alpha_5\beta_1$ integrins *in vitro*. Blocking of homing *in vitro* has been demonstrated by antibody to β_1 integrins (312), and antibodies to the α_4 integrin subunit have been shown to dislodge progenitor cells from the marrow into the blood (316,317). In addition, expression of β_1 integrin receptor is necessary for homing of primitive cells to the fetal liver and bone marrow, as demonstrated with genetic methods (321). Selectins also appear to mediate stem cell adhesion and may affect stem cell function (322).

These studies demonstrate the role of integrin receptors in adhesion in the bone marrow and, in the case of $\alpha_4\beta_1$, imply a role in mobilization. However, mobilization of stem and progenitor cells into the blood is incompletely understood. Recent experiments suggest that the release of neutrophil granules and subsequent digestion of matrix by granule enzymes play a role in cytokine (i.e., G-CSF)-induced mobilization (323). However, it is possible that mobilization in response to a different agonist (such as IL-8 or chemotherapy) may rely on different underlying mechanisms. Even less well understood is the role of stem and progenitor cell migration. Certain cytokines, termed *chemokines*, clearly stimulate stem and progenitor cell migration *in vitro* (324). However, it is unclear what relation *in vitro* migration of stem and progenitor cells has to *in vivo* mobilization (325). One recent study does show that a genetic alteration in stem cells—mutation of the Rho GTPase Rac2—reduces adhesion via $\alpha_4\beta_1$, increases migration *in vitro* in response to chemokines, and increases the frequency of stem and progenitor cells in the blood at baseline and with mobilization (326).

Similar molecular studies have not yet elucidated the mechanisms responsible for the release of differentiated myeloid cells from the medullary cavity. It is clear that the medullary compartment consists of both a mitotic pool (myeloblasts, promyelocytes, myelocytes) and a storage pool of granulocyte precursors (metamyelocytes and band forms) and granulocytes. Stress and pharmacologic administration of steroids produce a large mobilization of granulocytes into the peripheral blood. The storage pool in the medullary cavity is significantly larger than the peripheral blood pool of granulocytes (estimated at 500,000/µL and 10,000/µL, respectively, except in newborn infants, in whom marrow reserves of these cells appear to be limited) (327,328).

Tritiated thymidine studies have demonstrated that the maturation time for cells of the neutrophil series is approximately 8 days. These studies are in good agreement with the response of patients with neutropenia to administration of the late-acting cytokine G-CSF as well as the recovery of neutrophil counts after administration of cytotoxic chemotherapy (329–331). The peripheral blood pool of granulocytes is composed of both circulating and marginated compartments of cells, with a distribution of approximately half in each compartment (332,333). Administration of epinephrine and stress-related endogenous release of cortisol induce rapid demargination of neutrophils, with subsequent doubling of the peripheral leukocyte counts within 30 minutes (332).

Studies have demonstrated at least some of the basic mechanisms involved in the egress of leukocytes from the bloodstream into sites of inflammation. Neutrophils are present in the bloodstream for a relatively short time, probably less than 12 hours. As noted, neutrophils initially interact with the endothelial wall of blood vessels by means of a group of related proteins, termed *selectins*. Subsequently, leukocyte membrane proteins that belong to the integrin family of heterodimeric receptors mediate firm adhesion. The members of this family include LFA-1 (CD11a), Mo1 (also known as *Mac-1*) (CD11b), and p150,95 (CD11c). Persons with congenital absence of these receptors (CD11/CD18 leukocyte glycoprotein deficiency) suffer from recurrent infections because of the inability of neutrophils to egress from the bloodstream into sites of inflammation (among other abnormalities) (334). All three receptors share a common β-subunit (CD18) (335), and the molecular defect in at least some affected kindreds has been described by several investigators to be the lack of expression of this β-subunit, with secondary instability of each of the α-subunits (336–339).

Similar interactions appear to control the movement of lymphocytes between the bloodstream and specific effector organs such as peripheral lymph nodes and Peyer's patches of the gut (340). Lymphocyte interactions appear to include not only the integrin family of receptors but also receptors related to the immunoglobulin supergene family and selectin interactions (340).

Although not as well studied, the homing of hematopoietic stem cells to the microenvironment is partially characterized (341). Aizawa and Tavassoli (342,343) have shown that adhesion of hematopoietic stem cells to stromal cells of long-term marrow cultures *in vitro* and homing of stem cells to the spleen *in vivo* can be blocked by synthetic proteins containing mannosyl and galactosyl (but not fucosyl) lectins. The native proteins and receptors responsible for this interaction are unknown. Williams et al. (312) and Verfaillie et al. (344) have shown that hematopoietic stem and progenitor cells interact with the C-terminal heparin binding domain of fibronectin. This interaction appears to involve the $\alpha_4\beta_1$ integrin receptor and the CS-1 amino acid sequence in fibronectin or the second ligand for $\alpha_4\beta_1$ expressed on endothelium, vascular cell adhesion molecule-1. Therefore, stem cells are likely to interact with the microenvironment through multiple ligands and receptors, a situation similar to the homing of lymphocytes to specific environments that specialize in immune function.

Pores can be observed in the endothelial lining of the venous sinuses of the bone marrow, but it is not clear whether these are permanent features of the surface or whether they are present in response to specific signals from departing cells. In addition, areas of marked attenuation of the endothelial cell thickness have also been observed in scanning electron micrographs (345). Apparently, cells departing from the hematopoietic cord must deform to a considerable degree to gain entry into the venous sinus. These observations, along with physical measurements of cell deformability, have led to the theory that increasing deformability associated with differentiation in both the erythroid and myeloid lineages is an important component of the normal physiology of hematopoietic cell egress from the medullary cavity space (194,346–348).

Two other mechanisms may contribute to the movement of cells from the medullary cavity into the circulation. One group has shown that a factor or factors in neutropenic serum can stimulate the release of neutrophils from the bone marrow (349,350). This increase in neutrophil release is not endotoxin related and is not a reflection of demargination, and the factor appears distinct from molecules that have a proliferative effect on myeloid precursors. Some evidence suggests that attenuation of the adventitial cover over the sinuses is reduced after endotoxin administration, which may allow more rapid egress of hematopoietic cells (351). Distinct factors may be involved in the release of each cell type from the marrow cavity, but few data are available. Some evidence suggests that EPO may act as a releasing factor for reticulocytes (352). Finally, the presence of changes in the blood flow to the medullary cavity has been postulated to play a role in blood cell release, but little experimental evidence has been published in support of this theory (194).

HEMATOPOIETIC GROWTH FACTORS

Perhaps more than any other advances in understanding hematopoiesis, the identification and cloning of proteins that affect hematopoietic cell survival, growth, and differentiation (termed *cytokines* and *growth factors*) have impacted clinical hematology and cancer care. Effects of these proteins are mediated through specific receptors on hematopoietic cells. The cytokine receptors form a family of single-membrane spanning receptors (type I) characterized by structural motives (Fig. 7-7). One example germane to stem cells, the interaction of stem cell factor with the receptor tyrosine kinase c-kit, has already been described. Clinical use of two cytokines, erythropoietin and granulocyte colony-stimulating factor (discussed in Chapter 59), has become widespread. This section provides a general introduction of growth factor biology, highlights the work on erythropoietin and erythropoietin receptor (EPOR) signaling to illustrate the complexity of this family of proteins, and briefly covers other cytokines.

The proliferation, differentiation, and survival of immature hematopoietic progenitor cells is sustained by the hematopoietic growth factors (Table 7-1). In addition to their effect on immature cells, these factors also influence the survival and function of mature cells. The nomenclature of the hematopoietic growth factors may appear confusing and unsatisfactory to the uninitiated, but remember that the original names were operationally derived. Thus, the first factors to be described derived their names as *colony-stimulating factors* from the *in vitro* observation that they stimulate progenitor cells to form colonies of recognizable maturing cells; prefixes are used to denote the cell type in the mature colonies, such as G-CSF for granulocyte CSF. Another large group of factors, the interleukins, derived their names initially from their cellular sources as well as their actions on leukocytes. Recent additions to the family have been given a sequential IL numeric notation.

During the 1980s and 1990s, the genes for multiple murine and human hematopoietic growth factors were cloned. This ability led to the production and purification of the respective recombinant proteins. The advances afforded by molecular methods have allowed intensive investigations of the actions of purified CSFs, their cellular origins, and their regulatory mechanisms, whereas the availability of large quantities of highly purified CSFs such as GM-CSF, G-CSF, M-CSF, EPO, and thrombopoietin (TPO) led to preclinical and clinical evaluation of their effectiveness *in vivo*.

Types of Hematopoietic Growth Factors

The development of semisolid colony-forming assays for progenitor cells of all the hematopoietic lineages provided the means to distinguish several colony-stimulating activities that were present both in media conditioned by different murine and human cell types and in human urine. Separative protein chemistry applied to large volumes of starting material led to the purification of murine M-CSF, GM-CSF, G-CSF, and IL-3 (353). Human urine yielded M-CSF (354) and EPO (355), and a human bladder carcinoma cell line was used to purify human G-CSF (356).

In general, four classes of hematopoietic growth factors (HGFs) can be distinguished. IL-3 and GM-CSF are multilin-

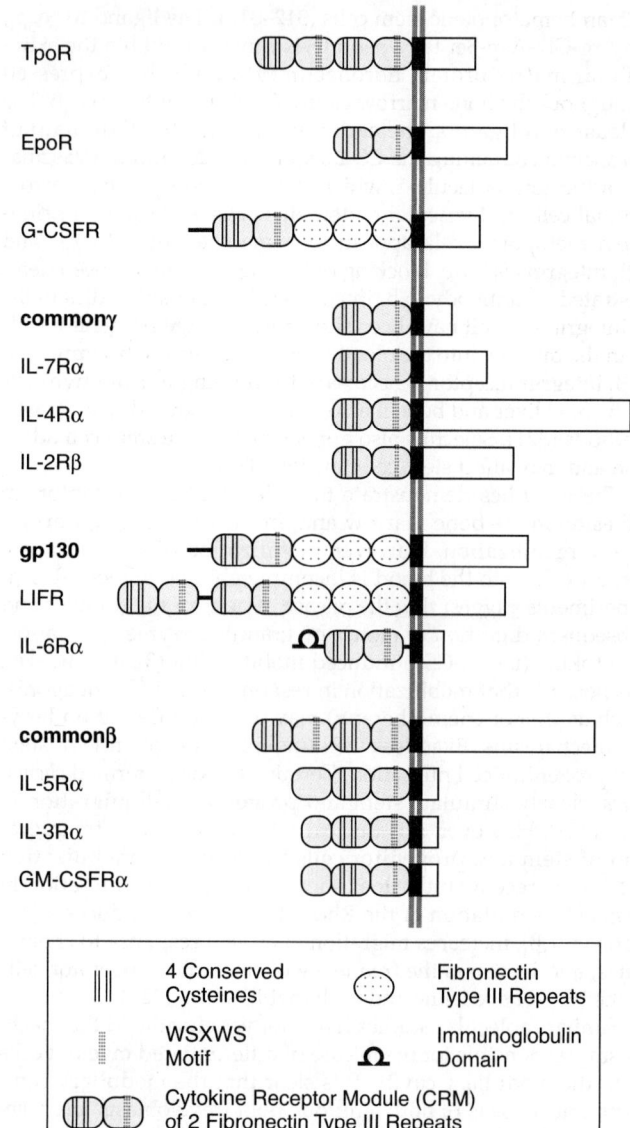

Figure 7-7. Hematopoietic growth factor receptor family. The extracellular domains are all characterized by one or two regions, the cytokine receptor modules (CRMs) that comprise two fibronectin type III–like domains; the first contains four conserved cysteines and the second a tryptophan-serine-x-tryptophan-serine (WSXWS) motif. Unique features: the interleukin (IL)-6 receptor contains an immunoglobulin-like domain; the granulocyte colony-stimulating factor receptor (G-CSFR) contains three additional fibronectin type III–like repeats. The intracellular domains show less homology. Serine and proline residues are enriched in the cytoplasmic domains of several members, such as the IL-2, IL-3, IL-4, IL-7, and erythropoietin receptors (EpoRs). GM-CSFR, granulocyte-macrophage colony-stimulating factor receptor; LIFR, leukemia inhibitory factor receptor; TpoR, thrombopoietin receptor.

eage HGFs and stimulate the survival, proliferation, and differentiation of a broad range of progenitors, including cells with stem cell properties. In contrast, G-CSF, M-CSF, IL-5, EPO, and TPO are lineage-specific and stimulate the proliferation and differentiation of more mature granulocyte, monocyte, eosinophil, erythroid, and megakaryocyte progenitor cells, respectively. Both sets of factors influence mature cell function, and the pattern of responsive cells for each CSF broadly coincides with the lineages of the less mature cells affected by each factor. Two other early acting HGFs, *steel* factor or SCF and Flt3L (357–359), are important for the survival

TABLE 7-1. Human Hematopoietic Growth Factors

Factor	Synonym	Chromosome	RNA, kb	Protein, kd Core	Glycosylated	Biologic Activities Progenitors	Mature Cells
IL-3	Multi-CSF	5q23–31	1.0	15.4	15–30	All CFCs	Eosinophil, baso-phil
GM-CSF	CSFα	5q23–31	0.8	14.4	14–34	All CFCs	Neutrophil, mono-cyte, eosinophil
G-CSF	CSFβ	17q11.2–21	1.6	18.6	20	CFU-G	Neutrophil
M-CSF	CSF-I	1p13–21	4.0	26	70–90 (35–45 dimer)	CFU-M	Monocyte
			1.6	16	40–50 (20–25 dimer)		
EPO	—	7q11–22	1.6	18.4	34–39	BFU-E CFU-E	
IL-5	EDF BCGF-II TRF	5q31	13.2	15.0	46	CFU-Eo	
IL-6	BSF2, IFNα$_2$, Hemo-poietin-1	7p15	1.3	20.8	26	Synergistic with IL-3 or SF on blast CFC	
IL-1α (p15)	—	2q13		31.0	17	Induces HGF pro-duction	
IL-1β (p17)	—	2q13–21	1.6	31.0	17	—	
IL-4	BSF1	5q23.2–31.2	0.6	17.5	15–19	Synergistic with EPO, G-CSF, M-CSF on pro-genitors	
IL-8	Neutrophil attractant protein	4q12–13	1.6	11.1	—	—	Neutrophil chemo-taxis
IL-9	—	5q31.1	0.6	15.9	20–30	BFU-E	
IL-10	Mouse cyto-kine synthe-sis inhibitory factor	1q31–32	1.6	20.5	17–21	—	Inhibits synthesis of IFN-γ
IL-11	—	19q13.3–13.4	2.3	21.4	—	Synergistic with IL-3 or SF on blast CFC	
IL-12A	—	3p12–13.2	1.0	24.9	35 ⎱ 75	Supports stem cells (with SF and IL-3)	Induces IFN-γ
IL-12B	—	5q31.1–33.1	2.3	37.2	40 ⎰ (dimer)		
IL-13	—	5q23–31	1.3	14.3	12–14	—	Increases monocyte and B-cell CD23 and class II anti-gen expression; increases Ig syn-thesis
SF	Mast cell growth fac-tor; stem cell factor	12	5.4–6.5	20	—	Synergistic with IL-3, GM-CSF, G-CSF, EPO on blast CFC and progenitors	

BFU-E, erythroid burst-forming unit; CFC, colony-forming cell; CFU, colony-forming unit; CFU-E, erythroid colony-forming unit; CFU-Eo, eosinophil colony-forming unit; CFU-G, granulocyte colony-forming unit; CFU-M, monocyte-macrophage colony-forming unit; EPO, erythropoietin; G-CSF, granulocyte colony-stimulating factor; GM-CSF, granulocyte-macrophage colony-stimulating factor; HGF, hematopoietic growth factor; IFN, interferon; Ig, immunoglobulin; IL, interleukin; M-CSF, monocyte colony-stimulating factor; SF, Steel factor.

of stem cell populations and also act synergistically with many other HGFs. Stem cells and progenitors may also be stimulated by three other synergistic interleukins, IL-1, IL-6, and IL-11, but the actions of these factors may be indirect or may require the presence of other cytokines. Recent data show that three other ligand–receptor interactions may affect stem cell self-renewal, perhaps synergistically. These are Notch receptors, activated by the ligands Delta, Jagged 1 and Jagged 2; Sonic hedgehog, acting through Patched and Smoothened receptors; and Wnt, which activates Frizzled and lipoprotein receptor–related protein pathways.

Several CSFs may have roles outside the hematopoietic system. GM-CSF and G-CSF influence the migration and prolifera-tion of endothelial cells (360). High-affinity binding sites for both CSFs are present on these cells. M-CSF acts on tropho-blasts, and production of M-CSF by uterine cells increases markedly during gestation (361,362). Placental cells express c-*fms* (the M-CSF receptor) (363) and low-affinity GM-CSF recep-tors (364). Finally, murine neurons and astrocytes express IL-3 messenger RNA (mRNA) by Northern and *in situ* hybridization analysis (365).

Several recent reviews have detailed the steps in the isola-tion of the hematopoietic growth factor genes (4,5,366,367). Some general comments follow, together with a brief summary. Two approaches were taken to identify cDNAs for these genes. The first was the classic route by which, for example, the human G-CSF, M-CSF, and EPO proteins were purified, part of their amino acid sequence determined, and oligonucleotide probes constructed to screen appropriate cDNA libraries (368–371). The CSFs are present in minute concentrations in most starting materials, and for several CSFs, purification has been very difficult. The second approach obviated the obstacle of CSF purification in a novel manner: GM-CSF and IL-3 cDNA libraries were constructed from suitable human cell lines; pools of cDNAs from the library were then introduced into "high expression" vectors and directly expressed in mammalian cell lines after transfection. Because of the potency of these CSFs, the gene products of the cDNA pools could be screened in sensitive bioassays and the single cDNA isolated by sib selection (372,373).

Hematopoietic Growth Factor Receptors

Membrane receptors for five murine hematopoietic growth factors have been characterized using iodinated, purified, natural or recombinant preparations (367,374). Consistent with the lack of structural homology among the growth factors is the existence of distinct receptors for each factor, which range in size from 50 to 160 kd. Distribution of receptors within the hematopoietic system is restricted to undifferentiated and maturing cells of the appropriate target cell lineages. Because progenitor cells respond to more than one factor, overlap in receptor expression occurs. The number of IL-3, GM-CSF, G-CSF, and EPO receptors per cell is strikingly low (1000 sites per cell), whereas M-CSF receptors are present at 10,000 sites per monocyte.

In all cases, affinity of a receptor for its ligand is high, with dissociation constants usually in the picomolar range. Stimulation of target cells can occur at concentrations of factor orders of magnitude lower than the equilibrium constant at which 50% of receptors are occupied; therefore, low receptor occupancy is apparently sufficient to produce biologic effects. Although the four murine CSFs do not cross-compete for binding at 0°C, 21°C, or 37°C, IL-3 inhibits binding of GM-CSF, G-CSF, and M-CSF to murine bone marrow cells, and GM-CSF inhibits binding of G-CSF and M-CSF (375). Metcalf et al. have suggested that this hierarchic down-modulation results in activation of the modulated receptor without binding ligand, and the model provides an intriguing explanation for the correlation between the pattern of down-regulation and the biologic activity of IL-3 and GM-CSF.

Expression cloning strategies were successfully applied to isolate the cDNAs that encode the human or murine IL-1, IL-6, EPO, GM-CSF, IL-3, IL-4, IL-7, and G-CSF receptors (364,376–385). Although the IL-1 receptor has three extracellular immunoglobulin-like domains and appears to be a member of the immunoglobulin superfamily, the IL-6, EPO, GM-CSF, IL-3, IL-4, IL-7, and G-CSF receptors are distinct (Fig. 7-7). They show features that are analogous to the (p70 to p75) β-chain of the IL-2 receptor (386) and to the prolactin and growth hormone receptors (387–389). These polypeptides share a number of features as a group and show no apparent homology to other known receptors, but they are all type 1 membrane glycoproteins with extracellular N-termini and single transmembrane domains. They contrast with c-kit (discussed previously), *c-fms*, and *Flt3*, which are class III receptor tyrosine kinases (Fig. 7-8).

The major homology lies in the extracellular domain, which is characterized by conserved extracellular regions called *cytokine receptor modules* that comprise two fibronectin type III-like domains; four conserved cysteine residues mark the N-terminal domain, and a Trp-Ser-X-Trp-Ser (WSXWS, where X is any amino acid) motif characterizes the C-terminal domain (usually just external to the plasma membrane) (Figs. 7-7,7-8). The IL-6

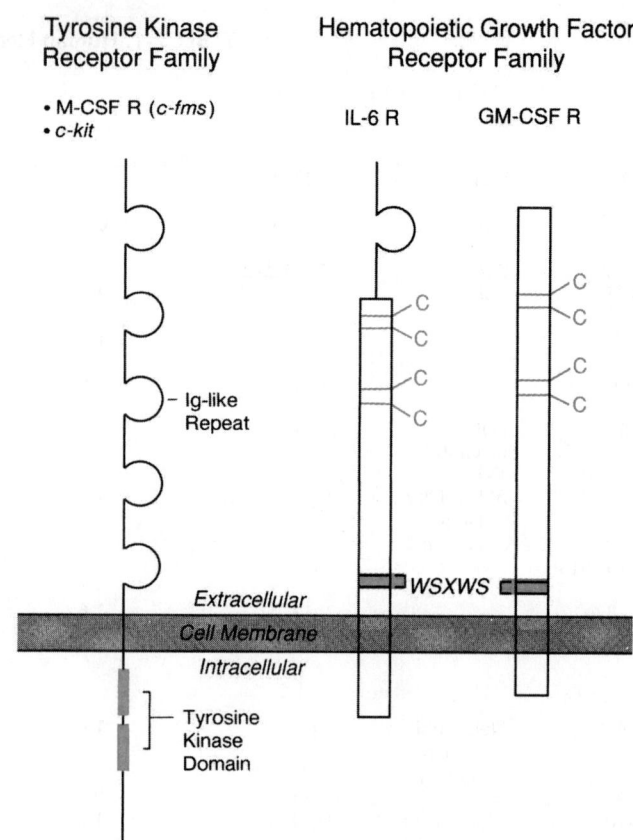

Figure 7-8. Hematopoietic growth factor receptors. Two other important hematopoietic growth factor receptors, c-*kit* and the macrophage colony-stimulating factor (M-CSF) receptor, c-*fms*, are structurally distinct from the receptor family shown in Fig. 7-7, represented here by the granulocyte-macrophage colony-stimulating factor (GM-CSF) and interleukin (IL)-6 receptors. M-CSF (c-*fms*) and c-*kit* are type III tyrosine kinase cell-surface receptors; their extracellular domains are characterized by five immunoglobulin-like repeats, whereas the cytoplasmic regions contain a tyrosine kinase domain separated by an insert. Ig, immunoglobulin.

receptor has both these structural features, but it differs from the other members in that it has one N-terminal immunoglobulin-like domain, and the WSXWS motif is located slightly more proximally (377). The cytoplasmic regions of the receptor family show much less homology, although there are similarities between the IL-2β chain and the EPO receptor. The length of the cytoplasmic domains varies from 54 amino acids (GM-CSF receptor) to 568 amino acids (IL-4 receptor). Furthermore, IL-2, IL-3, IL-4, IL-7, EPO, and an isoform of the GM-CSF receptor (390) are rich in serines and prolines. The mechanisms by which ligand binding induces a cell signal remains to be determined in many cases and is reviewed in more detail below.

An interesting feature of the cytokine receptor family is that the conserved extracellular structural features are mirrored in conserved structural features of their ligands as well. For example, G-CSF (391) and IL-6 are characterized by four α-helices that fold in a tertiary structure of antiparallel cylinders connected by interhelical loops (Fig. 7-9). This common tertiary structure is based on the radiographic structure of IL-2 (392) and of growth hormone–growth hormone receptor complex (393). Mutational studies of growth hormone receptors suggest that the exposed surface of helix D (394) forms the receptor binding site. The cytokine receptors in turn share conserved motifs that provide spatial constraints for tertiary folding (395). The data are consistent with a model in which two clusters of

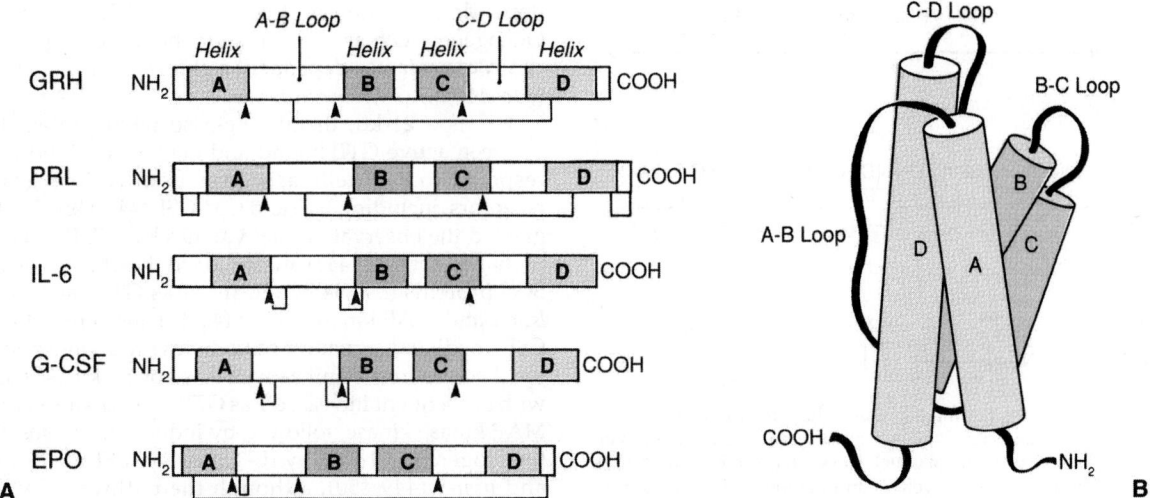

Figure 7-9. Secondary and tertiary structure prediction for a group of gonadotropin-releasing hormone (GRH)–like cytokines. **A:** Location of secondary structural elements in the human sequences for GRH, prolactin (PRL), erythropoietin (EPO), interleukin (IL)-6, and granulocyte colony-stimulating factor (G-CSF). The four helices from the GRH x-ray structure (322) are labeled A–D; loops between helices are appropriately named. Known disulfide bridge connections are marked. Gene exon boundaries have been mapped onto the respective protein sequences by arrowheads. An IL-6 variant lacking the amino-terminal 28 residues is bioactive (323). This deletion would effectively shorten IL-6 helix A but would not affect the overall fold or predicted recognition helix D. **B:** Drawing of the GRH fold (322), emphasizing the helix bundle core and loop connectivity. The exposed surface of helix D is thought to play an important role in receptor binding. (Adapted from Bazan JF. Hemopoietic receptors and helical cytokines. *Immunol Today* 1990;11:350.)

antiparallel β-strands are separated by a V-shaped trough that is formed by a hydrophobic hinge region (the WSXWS loop; Fig. 7-10). This trough may constitute the binding region.

GENERAL CONCEPTS IN GROWTH FACTOR RECEPTOR SIGNALING

Much is known about the precise cascade of intracellular events initiated by the binding of growth factors to their cell-surface receptors. It has recently been shown that the β common component of the IL-3/GM-CSF receptor is tyrosine phosphorylated after IL-3 or GM-CSF stimulation (396,397). Evidence has also strongly implicated Jak2 in IL-3 signaling (398). There are four Janus tyrosine kinases (JAKs): JAK1, JAK2, JAK3, and TYK2 (399–401) (Fig. 7-11). These kinases act through a group of transcription factors called *STATs* for *signal transduction and activator of transcription* (402). On ligand stimulation of cytokines, JAK becomes phosphorylated (403). There is a KEYY motif in the activation loop of JAKs that leads to autophosphorylation (404), and JAK kinases become associated with cytokine receptors (405). When activated JAK phosphorylates the receptors, STAT is recruited and binds through its SH2 domain (406–408). Phosphorylated STAT proteins can homodimerize and heterodimerize and bind to the phosphorylated tyrosine in the C-terminal domain of each STAT molecule. The dimerized STAT molecules enter the nucleus and bind DNA, where they activate or repress transcription (402,409–411). Activated JAK-STAT pathways are countered by phosphatases.

JAK1 knock-outs lead to perinatal lethality and defective lymphoid development (412). Erythropoietin signaling leads to rapid phosphorylation of JAK2 (403) and the activation of STATs (Fig. 7-11). A knock-out of the JAK2 kinase leads to an anemia predominantly of definitive erythropoiesis, very similar to that of the erythropoietin receptor, strongly suggesting that JAK2 acts downstream of the erythropoietin receptor (413,414). JAK2 knock-out cells also do not respond to thrombopoietin, IL-3, and GM-CSF. Fibroblasts from the knock-out line do not

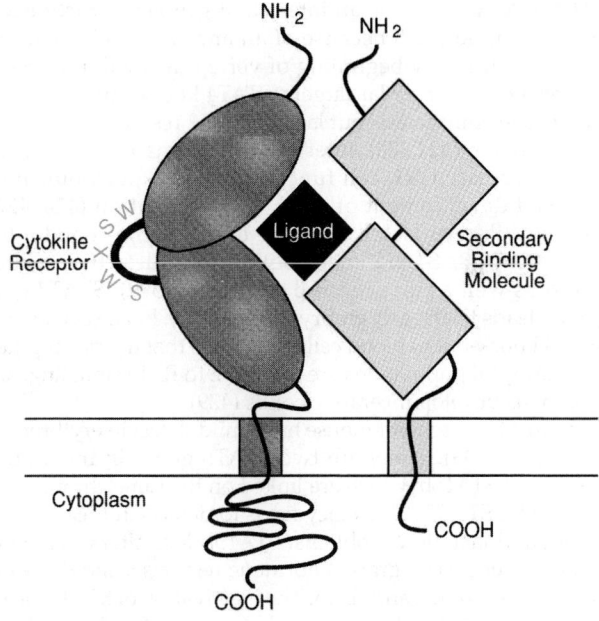

Figure 7-10. Tertiary folding of β-strands in receptor domains. Predicted configuration of a canonical receptor binding segment on the cell surface. The linked domains pack with barrel axes at an angle so as to create a V-shaped trough lined by β-sheet surfaces; these converge on a hydrophobic hinge region with a proximal WSXWS loop. Linked to a transmembrane helix and a nonspecific cytoplasmic tail, the receptor is shown docked to a cytokine ligand (*black diamond*). In addition, the receptor–cytokine complex interacts with a secondary binding molecule that recognizes the free surface of bound cytokine as well as selected receptor loops distal from the pocket. In this case, the bilobed accessory molecule is analogous to the interleukin-2 receptor 55-kd chain or the common β-chain of the granulocyte-macrophage colony-stimulating factor and interleukin-3 receptors. (Adapted from Bazan JF. Structural design and molecular evolution of a cytokine receptor superfamily. *Proc Natl Acad Sci U S A* 1990;87:6934–6938.)

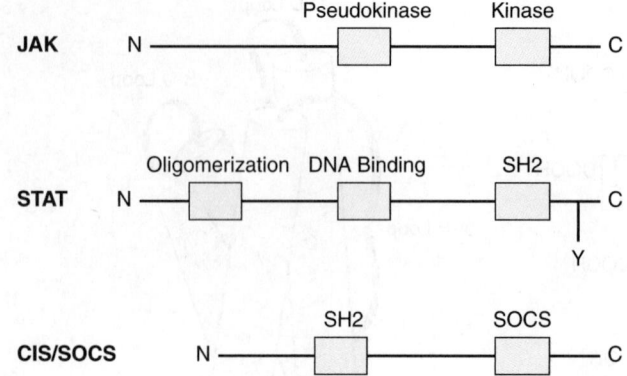

Figure 7-11. Structure of signaling molecules that are critical for normal hematopoiesis. The Janus kinases (JAKs) consist of an N-terminal domain and two kinaselike domains, one of which lacks kinase activity. The STATs contain a DNA binding motif as well as an oligomerization domain. In addition, they have an SH2 binding domain. The CIS/SOCS genes contain an SH2 binding domain as well as a SOCS box.

respond to γ-interferon. Adjacent to the BOX1 of the erythropoietin receptor is a tryptophan 282, which forms a docking site for the transcription factor JAK2. JAK3 deficiency is observed in some patients with immunodeficiency and is autosomal-recessive (415). JAK3 knock-out mice have a small thymus and spleen, similar to the IL-7 receptor knock-out (416–418). Tel-JAK chimeric genes have been found in lymphoid and myeloid leukemias (419,420).

The STAT genes have an interesting genomic structure and are often paired (421) because of an ancient duplication that occurred at the very beginning of vertebrate evolution. STAT proteins induce particular targets. STAT4 knock-outs show normal myeloerythropoiesis but lack the IL-12 response in the TH1 cell population (422,423). Interferon-γ responses decrease, and there is decreased NK cell function. STAT6 knock-outs have decreased development of their TH2 population (424–426). STAT1 knock-outs lack a response to interferon-α and interferon-β (427,428). STAT2 knock-outs are also defective in interferon-α as well as interferon-β responses (399). STAT3 gene deletion leads to an early embryonic lethality, but a specific conditional knock-out in blood cells illustrates that the macrophage and neutrophil populations are defective to IL-10 signaling, and the animals develop ulcerative colitis (429).

The STAT5 knock-out mouse has a mild defect in erythropoiesis (428,430–433). There are two STAT5 genes in the mouse, STAT5a and STAT5b, which are linked on the same chromosome with STAT3. STAT5a deficiency leads to defects in breast development and lactation problems. STAT5b loss alters liver gene expression, decreases growth hormone response, and decreases NK responses to IL-2 and IL-15. The inactivation of STAT5a leads to no hematopoietic phenotype, whereas the STAT5b knock-out mouse may have a slight anemia. Double knock-out of STAT5a and STAT5b results in a mild anemia that was subsequently found to be due to inadequate antiapoptotic signaling through bcl-x (434). Recent studies have demonstrated that a mild anemia occurs in these mice that is likely due to a decreased response to erythropoietin. STAT5 stimulates IL-2 receptor expression and associates with the T-cell receptor (435). Constitutive STAT5 in a hematopoietic cell line confers IL-3 independence, and target genes for STAT5 have been implicated, including the PIM1 gene, bcl-xl, and c-myc (436).

Evidence that tyrosine phosphorylation is important for cell proliferation comes from the observation that the introduction of the EGF receptor, a known tyrosine kinase, into an IL-3–

dependent cell line can convert it to EGF dependence (437). Oncogenes such as v-fms or v-src that encode tyrosine kinases can convert factor-dependent cell lines to factor independence (438–440).

Ras is a 21-kd, membrane-associated protein that cycles between active GTP-bound and inactive GDP-bound forms in response to extracellular signals from various growth factor receptors, including IL-3 and GM-CSF (441,442). Excitement has greeted the observation that vav has Ras GDP/GTP nucleotide exchange activity (443) analogous to the *Drosophila* and murine SOS proteins (444,445), and that Ras GTP can associate with Raf-1 and MAP kinase kinase (446). Thus, a possible IL-3/GM-CSF–mediated signaling cascade involves phosphorylation of the β common subunit as well as tyrosine kinases such as vav, with subsequent increased Ras GTP and activation of Raf-1, and MAP kinase kinase, followed by induction of c-fos. Other protooncogenes induced by IL-3 and GM-CSF are c-myc (447,448) and pim-1 (449,450), although the pathways by which this occurs have not been established.

Some growth factors and receptors can activate phosphatidyl inositol–specific phospholipase C with subsequent diacylglycerol-mediated protein kinase C (PKC) activation and increased inositol triphosphate–mediated intracellular calcium. Activation of PKC has been reported in response to IL-3 in factor-dependent cell lines and in macrophages, whereas other studies have failed to document enhanced enzyme activity (451–453).

PHOSPHATASES

Phosphatases are also involved in cytokine signaling. There are several phosphatases, including shp1 and shp2. Shp1 is also known as sh2ptp1, hcp, or ptpt1c. It binds to the SH2 domain in the C-terminus of the erythropoietin receptor (454). Shp2 attenuates the erythropoietin signal (455). These phosphatases are thought to be regulators of erythropoiesis by binding to the erythropoietin receptor and dampening levels of erythropoiesis. In the absence of these factors, signaling through the erythropoietin receptor is amplified.

Phosphorylated STAT proteins are down-regulated by the phosphatase (455–459) as well as by the ubiquitin pathway (460). The STATs require phosphorylation on serine for activation, and there are also MAP kinase sites. The *shp1* gene is in lymphoid and myeloid cells. Mutation in *shp1* leads to the *motheaten* mouse, which has an autoimmune disorder (461). There is M-CSF independent proliferation of macrophages and decreased erythroid cells. *Shp2* knock-outs have deficiencies in mesoderm patterning (462). Ship is an inositol pyrophosphatase (463). It negatively regulates the signaling kinases PI3K and AKT. The homozygote mutants are viable and fertile but have a myeloproliferative disorder (464). Lymphoid and late erythroid cells have decreased levels of SOCS proteins.

SOCS GENES

The CIS and SOCS genes are suppressors of cytokine signaling proteins (465) (Fig. 7-11). SOCS genes bind to JAKs. The first member of this family, known as CIS (466), has an SH2 domain and a CH domain (also known as a *SOCS box*) (467,468). The function of these two domains remains to be determined, but there is some evidence that the SH2 domain can bind to JAKs and the CH domain can bind to elongins B and C. Elongins can target these factors for degradation by the ubiquitin-mediated proteasome. STAT5 activates the CIS promoter (469). CIS associates with the tyrosine 401 of the erythropoietin receptor at one of the major sites where STAT5 binds (470). SOCS1 has been shown to be an immediate early response gene induced by IL-2, IL-3, and erythropoietin (465). Overexpression of SOCS1 inhibits STAT activation and function. SOCS1 is also associated with receptor tyrosine kinases and negatively regulates mitogenesis (471). The SOCS1 knock-out is similar to mice that have been administered γ-interferon: There is decreased thymus size, fatty infiltration in the liver, and embryonic lethality, and the lymphocytes have an accelerated apoptosis (472–475). When the SOCS1 knock-out is mated to the immunodeficient *rag2* knock-out or γ-interferon–deficient animals, embryonic lethality is rescued. Therefore, SOCS1 deficiency leads to a hypersensitivity to γ-interferon. SOCS3 leads to an erythrocytosis; thereby, it is hypothesized to regulate fetal liver hematopoiesis negatively (476). CIS1, SOCS1, and SOCS3 each inhibit erythropoietin, prolactin, growth hormone, IL-2, and IL-3–induced proliferation (477). These genes may inhibit JAKs and associate with the receptors or could lead to a degradation of JAK proteins.

OTHER KINASES

We are learning a tremendous amount about other factors that participate in the erythropoietic process. The lyn kinase is required for erythropoietin-induced differentiation in J2E cells (478). It has been shown that lyn associates with SH2 binding sites at tyrosine 464 and 479 of the membrane proximal domain of the erythropoietin receptor. However, gene-targeting experiments do not indicate that lyn is required for normal erythropoiesis (479,480). The serine threonine kinase PI3K binds to tyrosine 479, and this binding is independent of STAT5 or RAS signaling (481). *erk2* is part of the MAP kinase pathways and certainly is involved in cytokine receptor signaling. Signaling through the erythropoietic receptor protects against apoptosis of erythroid cells. This antiapoptotic effect is thought to occur via the action of bcl-xl, whose expression depends on STAT5 (431). AP1 is also induced by erythropoietin signaling, including c-JUN and JUNb. The oncogene BCR-ABL can regulate the signal directed by the erythropoietin receptor and can rescue progenitor formation in erythropoietin receptor knock-out animals. BCR-ABL is thought to work through the serine kinases PI3K and AKT in other cell types, suggesting that these PI3K and AKT pathways may be involved in erythropoiesis.

The erythropoietin receptor is also able to activate members of the MAP kinase pathway. This includes the proliferative signal through *erk1* and *erk2* and a stress-activated signal through the JNK1 and *p38* pathways. It is possible that the proliferative signal is directed through *erk1*; however, the significance of activation of the stress-activated MAP kinase pathways remains to be determined.

ERYTHROPOIESIS

The regulation of the proliferation and maturation of erythroid progenitors depends on interaction with a number of growth factors. EPO is essential for the terminal maturation of erythroid cells. Its major effect appears to be at the level of the CFU-E during adult erythropoiesis, and recombinant preparations (482) are as effective as the natural hormone (483,484). These progenitors do not require burst-promoting activity (BPA) (245,485) in the form of IL-3 or GM-CSF, and their dependence on EPO is emphasized by the observation that they will not survive *in vitro* in the absence of EPO. Because most CFU-Es are in cycle, their survival in the presence of EPO is probably tightly linked to

their proliferation and differentiation to mature erythrocytes. EPO also acts on a subset of presumptive mature BFU-Es, which also require EPO for survival and terminal maturation.

A second subset of BFU-Es, presumably less mature, survives EPO deprivation if BPA is present, either as IL-3 or GM-CSF. When EPO is added to these cultures on day 3, these BFU-Es form typical colonies (482). Similar results are obtained in serum-deprived methylcellulose cultures in which the usual 30% fetal calf serum is substituted by BSA-adsorbed cholesterol, iron-saturated transferrin, and insulin (486). Under serum-deprived culture conditions, the combination of IL-3 and GM-CSF results in more BFU-Es than either factor alone when EPO is added on day 3.

The *kit* ligand—also termed *steel factor* (SF), *stem cell factor*, or *mast cell growth factor*—has been shown to have marked synergistic effects on BFU-E cultured in the presence of EPO (290). Alone, it has no colony-forming ability. Progenitors obtained from human fetal liver and cultured in serum-free conditions differ in their requirements for BPA and EPO (45,487). Whereas adult BFU-Es require IL-3 or GM-CSF and EPO for the development of maximal BFU-E colony number and size, embryonic BFU-Es require only EPO for maximal BFU-E cloning efficiency; the addition of IL-3 or GM-CSF increases BFU-E size but not number. These results suggest that EPO receptors are expressed at an earlier stage of erythroid maturation in fetal cells and that, during ontogeny, expression of the EPO receptor becomes restricted to a subset of mature BFU-Es and CFU-Es. During fetal development, the EPO receptor may be expressed by even more immature myeloid-erythroid progenitors such as CFU-Mix.

Newborn infants with severe Rh hemolytic disease and very high EPO levels are born with neutropenia and thrombocytopenia (488). *In vitro*, high concentrations of EPO reduce the number of CFU-GM colonies and decrease the number of granulocytes per colony, with newborn cells more sensitive to this effect than progenitors from adults (489). The effect does not appear to result from crowding in the culture dishes, because cord blood cells are plated at low density.

In sum, the data are consistent with the hypothesis that the fetal EPO receptor is expressed on bipotent progenitor cells and can influence the subsequent maturation of these cells.

Factors distinct from the classic CSFs may positively regulate erythropoiesis, either directly or indirectly. Limiting dilution studies of highly purified CFU-E in serum-free culture show that insulin and insulin-like growth factor I act directly on these cells (490). The presence of EPO is essential in these studies, which contrast with earlier murine studies of unfractionated cells in which CFU-Es respond to IGF-1 or insulin in the absence of EPO (491). Another factor that enhances both BFU-E and CFU-E colony formation is activin. This protein dimer, also known as *follicle-stimulating hormone-releasing protein*, appears to have a lineage-specific effect on erythropoiesis that is indirect, because removal of monocytes or T lymphocytes abrogates its effect (492). Activin has been identified as the factor produced by vegetal cells during blastogenesis that induces animal ectodermal cells to form primary mesoderm (493).

Negative Regulation of Erythropoiesis

Observations that subsets of lymphocytes with an immunologic suppressor phenotype isolated from normal subjects can inhibit erythroid activity *in vitro* (494–496) correlate with reports of patients with a variety of disorders in whom anemia or granulocytopenia is associated with an expansion of certain T-lymphocyte populations (497–501). In the rare disorder T lymphocytosis with cytopenia (502), *in vitro* suppression of erythropoiesis has been correlated with the expansion of a T-lymphocyte population that may be the counterpart of the hematopoietic suppressor cells isolated from normal peripheral blood.

The phenotype of these cells has been described in detail (496,502). The cell is a large granular lymphocyte that is both E rosette–positive and T8 (classic suppressor phenotype)-positive. Suppressor T cells may also be involved in some cases of aplastic anemia (503,504) or neutropenia (505) without an underlying immunologic disorder or an overt T-cell proliferation. Exactly how such suppressor T cells interact with hematopoietic progenitors and what surface antigens are "seen" by the suppressors is uncertain. Evidence supports the concept that suppression of erythroid colony expression *in vitro* is regulated by T cells and may be genetically restricted (496,503). Cell–cell interactions in immunologic systems have been well characterized with regard to surface determinants that allow for cellular recognition. That certain phenotypes of T cells "recognize" distinct classes of histocompatibility antigens on immunologic cell surfaces has been well described (506). Thus, the observation that hematopoietic progenitors have a unique distribution of class II histocompatibility antigens on their cell surface suggests a role for these antigens in the cell–cell interactions that regulate hematopoietic differentiation (507–510).

T cells may also inhibit erythropoiesis in a non–HLA-restricted fashion by the production of inhibitory cytokines. Some lymphokines may inhibit erythropoiesis *in vitro* by a complex lymphokine cascade. Activation of T cells by the T-cell antigen receptor CD3 results in cell-surface expression of the IL-2 receptor α-chain (p55) and the acquisition of IL-2 responsiveness (511). IL-2 inhibits BFU-Es in the presence of these IL-2 receptor–positive cells, possibly by inducing their release of interferon-γ; CD2 can serve as an alternative pathway of T-cell activation and may do so through binding to its ligand LFA-3 on antigen-presenting cells. Blockade of CD2 with monoclonal antibody leads to abrogation of IL-2/interferon-γ–mediated BFU-E suppression (512). These data are difficult to reconcile with the observation that IL-2 incubation of PMA/calcium ionophore-activated CD4+ T cells leads to marked expansion of IL-3 and GM-CSF mRNA-positive cells by *in situ* hybridization (513). Most CD4+ T cells express CD28 as well, and evidence suggests that IL-3 production is restricted to CD28+ T cells (514). It is thus paradoxic that both potent stimulating and inhibitory lymphokines can be produced by activating T cells through the same pathway.

Tumor necrosis factor (TNF) also suppresses erythropoiesis *in vitro* (515,516). The injection of peritoneal macrophages into Friend murine leukemia virus–infected animals results in rapid but transient resolution of the massive erythroid hyperplasia associated with this disease, possibly due to elaboration by macrophages of IL-1α, which does not suppress erythropoiesis itself but acts by the induction of TNF. This effect is reversed by EPO (517). A more detailed review of erythropoietin and the erythropoietin receptor follows.

ERYTHROPOIETIN

Erythropoietin is *primus inter pares* among the hematopoietic growth factors. It was the first discovered and characterized. Moreover, its biologic functions and clinical relevance are better understood in comparison to any of the other cytokines. EPO is produced primarily in the kidney and, to a lesser extent, in the liver in response to hypoxia (518,519). It circulates in the plasma until it binds to specific receptors located primarily on erythroid progenitor cells, enabling them to proliferate and differentiate into red blood cells (Fig. 7-12). Thus, EPO, like thrombopoietin, functions as a true hormone.

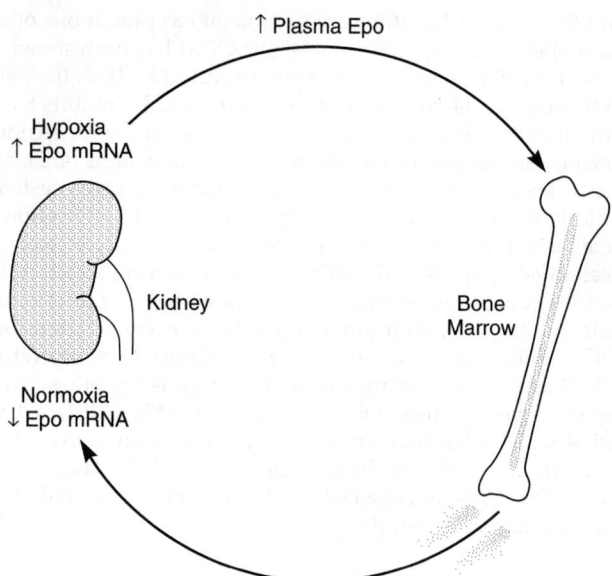

Figure 7-12. Feedback loop responsible for the regulation of erythropoiesis. Epo, erythropoietin; mRNA, messenger RNA.

Historical Perspective

In 1906, Carnot and Deflandre (520) reported that injection of serum from anemic rabbits made normal rabbits polycythemic. Because these experiments were difficult to reproduce, the concept of an erythropoietic hormone was regarded with skepticism over the next 4 decades, until Krumdieck (521), Erslev (522), and Erslev et al. (523) demonstrated dose-dependent increases in reticulocytes after the administration of anemic plasma to rabbits. At approximately the same time, Reissmann (524), using parabiotic rats, observed enhanced red cell production in both animals when only one was subjected to hypoxia. The subsequent development of accurate and reliable bioassays provided unequivocal evidence that this hormone, designated *erythropoietin*, was elevated in the plasma and urine of humans and experimental animals subjected to various types of hypoxia. In anemic patients, the levels of EPO correlated inversely with the red cell mass. Despite considerable effort, attempts at purification were elusive until 1977, when Miyake et al. (525) were able to isolate approximately 10 mg of homogeneous human EPO and subsequently determined the partial amino acid sequence. This achievement enabled the isolation of genomic and cDNA clones of human (526,527) and mouse (528,529) EPO. The production of large amounts of recombinant human EPO not only has provided experimental hematologists with a critically important reagent but also has given the clinician a safe and effective means of treating anemias, particularly anemia due to chronic renal failure (530,531) (Chapters 56 and 59).

Properties of Erythropoietin

Human erythropoietin is a 34-kd glycoprotein containing approximately 40% carbohydrate. The initial translation product of 193 residues is converted to 166 by the removal of an N-terminal signal peptide. The mature protein contains two disulfide bonds, only one of which is important for function. Complex N-linked glycosylation takes place on three asparagine residues. In addition, there is one O-linked glycosylation site. Thorough structural analyses show that recombinant EPO expressed in mammalian cells is similar in carbohydrate sequence to the native protein (532). X-ray diffraction analysis reveals that EPO, like other cytokines, folds into a four α-helical bundle structure. The three-dimensional structures of the hematopoietic growth factors are discussed elsewhere in the chapter.

In a variety of experimental animals, circulating EPO has a plasma half-life of several hours. Renal clearance accounts for only a small fraction of the plasma turnover. The molecule circulates in plasma until it finds high-affinity (approximately 200 to 5000 pM) receptors present in small numbers (approximately 100 to 700/cell) on the surface of erythroid precursor cells in the bone marrow (14–16). Ligand binding results in proliferation of erythroid cells as well as induction of terminal differentiation. In humans, the hematopoietic role of EPO appears to be restricted to the erythron, whereas in the mouse, EPO stimulates megakaryocyte proliferation and maturation as well (533).

Sites of Erythropoietin Production

The classic experiments of Jacobsen et al. (534) provided early and convincing evidence that the kidney is the primary site of EPO production (Fig. 7-12). Realizing that renal cortical blood flow closely matches oxygen consumption, Erslev et al. (535) proposed that the proximal tubule is the ideal location for EPO production. Subsequently, *in situ* hybridization studies with ^{35}S-labeled *EPO* RNA (536,537) or DNA (538) probes on kidney tissue from anemic mice revealed *EPO* mRNA in peritubular interstitial cells. The number of these cells expressing *EPO* mRNA increased with decreasing hematocrit (539). The demonstration of 5'-ectonucleotidase in EPO-producing cells suggests that they are likely to be fibroblasts (540,541), a conclusion supported by observations on a line of transgenic mice in which the SV40 T-antigen gene was fortuitously integrated into the endogenous *EPO* locus by homologous recombination. Expression of the SV40 T antigen permitted immunohistochemical identification of the EPO-producing cells to be the fibroblast-like type I interstitial cells.

During fetal development, EPO is primarily produced in the liver, with a switch to the kidney shortly after birth (542,543). The signals regulating this change are poorly understood. In the liver, blood from the portal triads becomes depleted of oxygen as it flows toward the central vein. Consequently, in both normal mice and in those expressing the human *EPO* transgene, EPO is produced at the site of lowest oxygen tension, near the central vein (537), in hepatocytes as well as nonparenchymal cells (537,544) subsequently shown to be Ito cells (545).

Small amounts of EPO are also produced in the lung, spleen, brain, and testis of rats (546,547). The discovery that both *EPO* mRNA and EPO protein are expressed in erythroid progenitors (548,549) has raised the intriguing possibility that tonic low-level erythropoiesis may be supported by autocrine stimulation, whereas circulating (hormonal) EPO provides a more robust stimulus to erythropoiesis during hypoxic stress.

Of further interest is the demonstration of both EPO and EPO receptors in the brain (546,550–552). Oxygen-regulated expression of *EPO* has been observed in astrocytes both *in vitro* (550,552) and *in vivo* (546,552), suggesting the possibility of a paracrine function for EPO in neural tissue. Administration of EPO has been shown to protect against experimental brain injury *in vivo* (553,554).

Investigation of the molecular basis of *EPO* gene regulation has been greatly facilitated by the discovery that the human hepatoma cell lines Hep3B and HepG2 produce significant amounts of EPO constitutively, with marked induction in response to hypoxia and cobalt (555). The magnitude and time course of the induction of *EPO* mRNA parallel EPO protein production. This regulation is primarily at the level of transcription but may also involve mRNA stability.

Regulation of the Erythropoietin Gene

Tissue-specific expression of the EPO gene and its induction by hypoxia are dependent on far upstream cis elements and an enhancer element downstream of the polyadenylation signal. Transgenic mice experiments indicate the presence of an element or elements between 0.4 and 6 kb 5' of the promoter that suppress promiscuous expression, and an element or elements 9.5 and 14 kb upstream that are necessary for kidney-specific expression (556–559). The 3' enhancer binds to two transcription factors, hypoxia-inducible factor (HIF) and the nuclear receptor HNF-4. As shown in Figure 7-13, these two DNA binding proteins interact with the transcriptional coactivator p300/CREB binding protein (CBP), triggering transcriptional activation.

Hypoxia-Inducible Factor 1

Hypoxic induction of EPO as well as a number of other physiologically relevant genes such as VEGF depends in large part on the transcription factor, HIF-1. HIF is activated in cells exposed to hypoxia, cobalt, or iron chelators, enabling it to bind to a con-

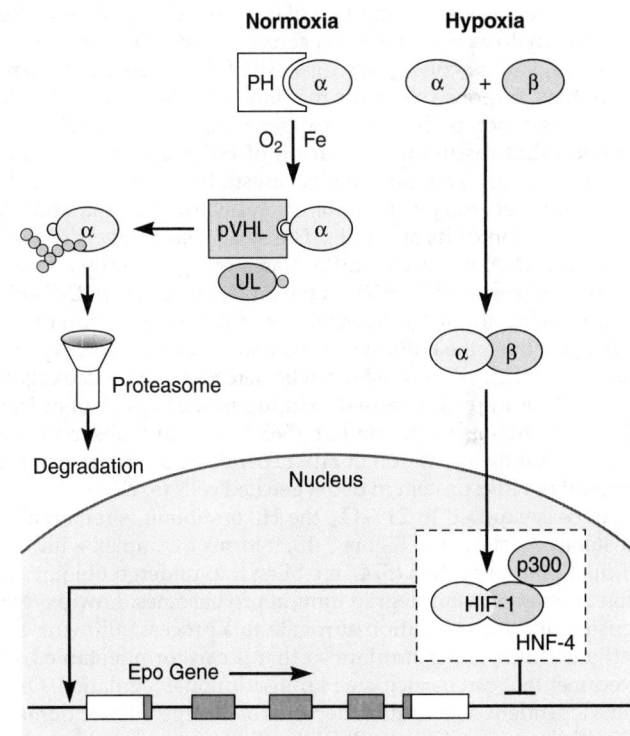

Figure 7-13. Assembly of transcription factors on the 3' enhancer of the erythropoietin (Epo) gene (*5' and 3' untranslated exons depicted as rectangles and the coding regions shown in black*). In hypoxic cells, the hypoxia-inducible factor (HIF) 1 heterodimer is transferred to the nucleus and binds to a HIF binding consensus sequence on the enhancer. Downstream of this site, the nuclear receptor HNF-4 binds constitutively to tandem repeat hormone response elements. HIF-1 and HNF-4 bind to the transcriptional activator p300, thereby initiating Epo gene expression. In contrast, when cells are exposed to higher oxygen tension, this enhanceosome cannot assemble because the HIF-1α subunit is rapidly degraded. A HIF-1α–specific prolyl hydroxylase (PH) serves as the oxygen sensor. In the presence of a threshold level of oxygen and iron, PH catalytically hydroxylates two specific proline residues on HIF-1α. This structural modification allows HIF-1α to bind to von Hippel-Lindau protein (pVHL), which in turn enables the ubiquitin ligase system (UL) to attach ubiquitin molecules (*small blue circles*) covalently to HIF-1α. This process targets HIF-1α to the proteasome, where it is rapidly degraded.

sensus sequence (5'-TACGTGCT-3') first identified in the EPO 3' enhancer (560) (Fig. 7-13). Wang and Semenza showed that HIF is a heterodimer composed of 120-kd α-subunits and 91- to 94-kd β-subunits (561). Molecular cloning (562) revealed that both subunits are basic helix-loop-helix proteins in the PAS family of transcription factors. HIFα is a novel protein,* whereas HIFβ is the previously cloned and characterized aryl hydrocarbon receptor nuclear translocator (ARNT) (562).

HIF activity can be induced by hypoxia in a wide variety of cells, as demonstrated both by gel mobility shift experiments (563) and by transfections of a reporter gene containing an HIF sequence or sequences (564). HIF activation, irrespective of stimulus, depends on *de novo* protein synthesis (565) and is markedly affected by inhibitors of protein kinases and phosphatases (566–568), suggesting that phosphorylation is involved. A heuristic prototype of the functional importance of phosphorylation in hypoxia-induced transcription can be found in nitrogen-fixing bacteria, *Rhizobium*, whose oxygen sensor is a heme protein containing a protein kinase domain (568,569).

OXYGEN SENSING AND HYPOXIA-INDUCIBLE FACTOR ACTIVATION

The EPO gene is the prototype of a growing number of physiologically important genes that are up-regulated by hypoxia. Others include those encoding vascular endothelial growth factor, tyrosine hydroxylase, heme oxygenase 1, inducible nitric oxide synthase, and glycolytic enzymes. All of these genes and many more have response elements that bind HIF. Moreover, all cells share a common pathway for oxygen sensing and signal transduction that results in activation of HIF during periods of hypoxia. To understand the mechanism by which HIF is activated, it is necessary to monitor carefully how hypoxia impacts the expression of its subunits. The steady-state levels of both HIF-1α mRNA and ARNT mRNA are not significantly affected by oxygen tension (570–572). At the protein level, the ARNT subunit remains abundant irrespective of the oxygenation of the cell. In contrast, the HIFα subunit cannot be detected on oxygenated cells (572). HIFα protein can be detected only in deoxygenated cells or in those exposed to inducers such as cobalt or iron chelators that also activate HIF (565,573). These observations suggest that the activation of HIF depends on an increase in the amount of HIFα protein in deoxygenated cells (572).

In cells exposed to 21% O_2, the HIFα subunit is remarkably unstable. As shown in Figure 7-13, it forms a complex with von Hippel-Lindau protein (574), enabling it to undergo ubiquitination and subsequent degradation in proteasomes. Low oxygen tension and iron chelation abrogate this process, allowing the HIFα subunit to accumulate so that it can form a stable heterodimer that can participate in transcriptional regulation. Oxygen-dependent degradation depends on a large interior domain in HIFα that contains two PEST (proline, glutamic acid, serine, threonine)-rich regions (575). When this element is deleted, the protein is stable and capable of transactivation, even in oxygenated cells. A recent series of elegant studies have shown that in the presence of a threshold level of oxygen, two specific proline residues within the oxygen-dependent degradation domain are hydroxylated (576–579). As depicted in Figure 7-13 (see also Fig. 56-3), this posttranslational modification is necessary and sufficient for the binding of HIFα to the von Hippel-Lindau protein, enabling HIFα to be ubiquitinated and targeted to the protea-

some. There is now convincing evidence that the oxygen sensor for this pathway is an HIFα-specific prolyl hydroxylase (580). Like the classic collagen prolyl hydroxylase, this enzyme uses oxygen as a substrate and iron, ascorbate, and α-ketoglutarate as cofactors. The activation of HIF by iron chelation and by certain transition metals such as cobalt can be explained by the removal or the displacement of iron from the reaction center.

Downstream from the HIF binding site, the EPO 3' enhancer contains two tandem consensus steroid hormone response elements separated by 2 bp (Fig. 7-13). Mutations at these hexanucleotides either abolish or markedly inhibit hypoxic induction of reporter genes (565,581–583). Nuclear proteins from a variety of cells in both normoxia and hypoxia bind strongly to these tandem repeats (565,581). Hormones whose biologic actions depend on binding to nuclear receptors had no effect on the hypoxic induction of a reporter gene containing the EPO promoter and EPO enhancer (581). These negative results suggested that the response elements in the EPO enhancer interact with an orphan nuclear receptor—that is, a DNA binding protein that shares structural homology with hormone-binding nuclear receptors but lacks a known ligand. The orphan receptor HNF-4 appears to play a critical role in EPO gene regulation (583). The expression of HNF-4 is limited to renal cortex and liver, sites of EPO production, and also intestine. The binding of HNF-4 to the EPO enhancer contributes importantly both to the high level induction of the EPO gene and to tissue specificity.

P300

As shown in Figure 7-13, the C-terminal portion of HIFα binds specifically to p300 (584), a general transcriptional activator that participates in a number of biologic functions such as induction of tissue-specific expression, regulation of cell cycle, and stimulation of differentiation pathways. This very large protein, which is closely homologous to CBP, does not bind to DNA but does interact with a number of other proteins, including HNF-4 and other nuclear receptors. Hypoxic induction of endogenous EPO mRNA as well as an EPO-reporter gene was inhibited by E1A, a viral protein that can bind to p300/CBP and abrogates transcriptional coactivation. Moreover, overexpression of p300 enhanced hypoxic induction. Thus, as depicted in Figure 7-13, the HIF heterodimer, activated by hypoxia, participates in a macromolecular assembly with p300 (or a related family member) and with HNF-4 to transduce a signal to the EPO promoter, enabling activation of transcription. It is very likely that such a combinatorial process applies to other genes induced by hypoxia.

Regulation of Erythropoietin Messenger RNA Stability

Enhanced transcription accounts for most but not all of the hypoxic induction of the EPO gene. In Hep3B cells, nuclear run-on experiments revealed approximately a tenfold increase in transcription of EPO mRNA during exposure to 1% O_2 in the setting of a 50-fold to 100-fold increase in the steady-state level of EPO mRNA (585). This observation raises the issue of whether the hypoxic induction of EPO expression is also regulated at the level of mRNA stability. There is circumstantial evidence that this may be the case. In two other physiologically relevant genes, tyrosine hydroxylase (TH) (586,587) and VEGF (588), approximately 50% of the enhanced gene expression in response to hypoxia is due to increased mRNA stability. For both genes, specific mRNA binding proteins have been demonstrated in cytosolic extracts of hypoxic cells (589,590). In comparison to TH and VEGF, much less is known about posttranscriptional regulation of the EPO gene. Two proteins of

---

*Subsequently, two additional isoforms of HIFα have been discovered. The original, designated HIF-1α, is expressed in nearly all cells, whereas HIF-2α or E-PAS has a more limited range of tissue expression. Both are regulated by oxygen as described and are referred to in this chapter as HIFα. Very little is known about the third isoform, HIF-3α.

70 kd and 135 kd have been shown to bind specifically to the 3' untranslated region of EPO mRNA. The binding of these proteins was not affected by changes in oxygen tension (591) but may be subject to redox control (592). Thus, in contrast to TH and VEGF, there is no convincing evidence to date that the half-life of EPO mRNA is prolonged by hypoxia.

Structure of the Ligand-Binding Domain of the Erythropoietin Receptor

Erythroid progenitors respond to the hormone erythropoietin. The proliferative and antiapoptotic signals directed by erythropoietin are the result of signaling by a ligand–receptor interaction. The erythropoietin receptor includes extracellular cystine motifs, a WSXWS box in the extracellular domain, a single transmembrane domain, and a cytoplasmic signaling domain that includes docking sites for transducing molecules (395,593). The erythropoietin receptor requires homodimerization for function. There is a single hormone to two receptor monomers, and the two surfaces of ligand contact binding sites (594–596). Erythropoietin mimetic peptides (EMPs) and erythropoietin work similarly (594). Erythropoietin binders (ERBs) are obtained in a peptide display library experiment and have the characteristics of CXXGWVGXCXXW (595,597). The thrombopoietin receptor is the cytokine receptor most similar to EPOR (598–600). Thrombopoietin receptor mimetics do not resemble EPOR mimetics (596). The crystal structure of the EPOR has been solved with the EMP peptide bound to the extracellular domain of the receptor (595). The EMP binds to two ERBs as a peptide dimer, producing a two to two ratio. The receptor looks like two fibronectin type III domains aligned at approximately 90 degrees to each other. The complex is held together by ligand receptor interactions, and there is a high-affinity as well as a low-affinity surface. In the unligated form, the receptor adopts an open, scissorlike configuration. Ligand binding brings the cytoplasmic domains closer together so that JAK2 (see later section on JAKs and STATs) can associate with the receptor. The membrane proximal domain of the erythropoietin receptor contains a hydrophobic motif that is α-helical. This is required for activated JAK2 to induce phosphorylation of erythropoietin. The function of the WSXWS box is thought to occur at the level of dimerization, but it may occur at a protein interface to allow other receptor subunits to interact. The erythropoietin receptor apparently does not have any other subunits.

An arginine 129 to cysteine mutation constitutively activates the erythropoietin receptor signaling apparatus (601). This activation is thought to be due to increased ability of the mutant forms to homooligomerize (602,603). This mutant provides a unique tool for understanding cytokine signaling. Other members of the cytokine receptor family are constitutively active, including a truncation of the N-terminus of the c-mpl gene, the thrombopoietin receptor (604). In the mouse system, a Friend virus glycoprotein, gp55, is capable of dimerizing with the erythropoietin receptor through its transmembrane domain, allowing constitutive activation of the receptor (605,606).

Other cytokine receptor superfamily members have multiple subunits, including α-chains, β-chains, γ-chains, and δ-chains. For instance, the IL-2 receptor has an α-chain that is not a member of the superfamily and encodes a single transmembrane protein (607,608). The β-chain and γ-chain are members of the cytokine receptor superfamily. It is the γ-chain that is required for signaling. With the GM-CSF receptor complex (609,610), it is the α-chain that is the binding domain and the β-chain is the signal transducer. The hydrophobic transmembrane domains of cytokine receptor families are highly conserved and are thus thought to be areas of interaction with other signaling factors and receptors.

Intracellular Domains of the Erythropoietin Receptor

Mutagenesis analysis has been performed for the erythropoietin receptor, describing domains that are critical to signal transduction (611). C-terminal truncation of the erythropoietin receptor leads to a receptor that is highly expressed on the cell surface, perhaps tenfold more than wild-type, and allows increased proliferation (612). Mutations in human patients from an Olympic swimming family have demonstrated a polycythemia phenotype with increased exercise capacity (613). Some other mutations in the erythropoietin receptor apparently lead to polycythemia in several families (614–616). Investigators are using knock-in technology to create more mutants to test the models of their hyperactive receptors.

Juxtaposed to the transmembrane domain is a region called the *proliferation box*. Activation of *myc* occurs through this box (617). The erythropoietin receptor C-terminus is riddled with tyrosine moieties that are docking sites for signal transduction factors. Each of these pathways leads to activation of signals, and the sum is to allow cell survival of the lineage. The erythropoietin receptor knock-out mouse has no definitive erythropoiesis (618–620). Three independent groups have performed a targeted disruption of the erythropoietin receptor, each confirming that erythropoietin receptor function is required for normal definitive hematopoiesis. The animals die at 12.5 days and have an embryonic anemia. Surprisingly, the primitive hematopoietic program is normal. Embryonic red cells mature normally in the absence of erythropoietin. In addition, the progenitor numbers of BFU-E and CFU-E are normal in a fetal liver of an erythropoietin receptor knock-out. Retroviral transduction of cells with a retrovirus encoding the wild-type copy of erythropoietin receptor rescues erythropoiesis in progenitor assays. The erythropoietin receptor signaling domain is not so special with regard to these proliferation and antiapoptotic pathways. Thrombopoietin stimulation of fetal liver cells can also rescue fetal liver hematopoiesis *in vitro* (620). Thus, the progenitor number is not affected, but the maturation and survival of progenitors are affected by erythropoietin receptor signaling. The availability of the retroviral transduction assay has allowed the investigation of signaling factors that may participate downstream of erythropoietin (618,621). In particular, retroviral transduction of the prolactin receptor (622) and stimulation of cells with prolactin rescue fetal liver erythropoiesis *in vitro*, as does expression of BCR-ABL (623). This finding demonstrates that the cytokine receptor activation is not necessarily instructive as a result of the erythropoietin receptor, but rather provides the signals necessary for maintenance or survival of the lineage.

Impact of Erythropoietin Production on Clinical Disorders

In a variety of clinical settings, anemia can be caused by underproduction of EPO, whereas erythrocytosis can result from overproduction.

UNDERPRODUCTION OF ERYTHROPOIETIN

Patients with renal failure generally develop severe anemia, owing in part to suppression of erythropoiesis from a buildup of metabolic wastes and in part to a moderate reduction in red cell lifespan. However, the most important contributor to the anemia of uremia is insufficient EPO production (624,625). The degree of anemia correlates roughly with the extent of renal functional impairment. In renal failure due to a wide variety of causes, insufficient EPO production results either from direct damage to EPO-producing cells in the kidney or from the suppression of EPO production by inflammatory cytokines.

Patients with inflammatory disorders have inappropriately low levels of plasma erythropoietin. Examples include rheumatoid arthritis (626), cancer (627), and acquired immunodeficiency syndrome (AIDS) (628). It is likely that inflammatory cytokines suppress *EPO* gene expression in these disorders. In human hepatoma cell lines and isolated perfused rat kidneys, the inflammatory cytokines TNF-α and IL-1 suppress EPO production (629,630).

Exposure to certain metals may result in disordered structure and function of the renal proximal tubule, resulting in suppression of EPO production out of proportion to impairment in global renal function. Such a pathogenetic process is likely the basis for the marked anemia often encountered in cancer patients who have been treated with *cis*-platinum or individuals suffering from chronic cadmium intoxication (631,632).

OVERPRODUCTION OF ERYTHROPOIETIN

Various forms of chronic arterial hypoxemia often result in erythrocytosis owing to overexpression of erythropoietin expression. Table 7-2 presents a pathophysiologic scheme for classifying the different causes of erythrocytosis. The highest documented hematocrit levels have been observed in patients with right to left cardiac shunts. The erythropoietic response in patients with hypoxemia due to chronic obstructive pulmonary disease is variable, depending in part on whether there is coexisting infection, which, as explained, can suppress erythropoietin expression.

Increased oxygen affinity of red cells causes impaired delivery of oxygen to tissues and therefore hypoxia at the cellular level, which triggers increased EPO expression and therefore secondary erythrocytosis (633). Such a "shift to the left" in the oxyhemoglobin dissociation curve can be caused by mutations in α-globin or β-globin subunits or in certain red cell enzymes. Deficiency in cytochrome b5 reductase causes congenital methemoglobinemia and mild erythrocytosis. A more pronounced increase in red cell mass has been reported in very rare families with deficiency of bisphosphoglycerate mutase, the enzyme responsible for the buildup of high levels of red cell 2,3-bisphosphoglycerate, a critical modulator of intracellular hemoglobin function (634). Individuals with mutations causing left-shifted O_2-binding curves are generally asymptomatic because impaired oxygen delivery is balanced by increased oxygen carrying capacity.

Occasional individuals have chronic elevations of plasma EPO not due to hypoxemia, increased oxygen affinity, or tumor.

TABLE 7-2. Differential Diagnosis of Polycythemia (Erythrocytosis)

I. Primary (autonomous) erythrocytosis (low EPO production)
  A. Polycythemia rubra vera
  B. Mutants of the EPO receptor
II. Secondary erythrocytosis (increased EPO production)
  A. Inappropriate
    1. EPO-producing tumors
      a. Renal cell carcinoma
      b. Hepatoma
      c. von Hippel-Lindau syndrome
    2. Chuvash polycythemia
  B. Appropriate (hypoxia)
    1. High altitude
    2. Pulmonary disease
    3. Cardiac right to left shunt
    4. Abnormal hemoglobin function
      a. Methemoglobinemia
      b. CO-hemoglobinemia (heavy smoking?)
      c. Increased fetal hemoglobin
      d. Hemoglobin mutant—high O_2 affinity

EPO, erythropoietin.

A number of families with congenital polycythemia have been encountered in Chuvashia, a circumscribed region in the Russian Federation in which there may have been inbreeding and there is a high likelihood of a founder effect (635). The erythrocytosis (mean hemoglobin levels of 23 g/dL and hematocrit of 67%) follows an autosomal-recessive pattern of inheritance. Affected individuals have elevated erythropoietin levels and increased incidence of thrombotic and hemorrhagic complications as well as varicose veins and clubbing. Furthermore, the genetic mutation is not linked to either the *EPO* or EPOR genes. In fact, recent studies indicate that affected individuals are homozygous for a missense mutation at the C-terminus of the von Hippel-Lindau protein (636). It is curious how significantly this mutation differs in phenotype from those associated with von Hippel-Lindau syndrome.

Erythrocytosis due to overproduction of EPO can be encountered in various neoplasms, particularly those arising in kidney, liver, and cerebellum—organs that are physiologic sites of erythropoietin expression. In particular, secondary erythrocytosis occurs in patients with renal carcinomas, Wilms' tumor, hepatomas, and cerebellar hemangioblastomas (518). In some cases, the tumor cells secrete EPO. In other cases, the surrounding normal kidney or liver tissue secretes EPO, presumably because of local ischemia.

Highly vascular renal and central nervous system tumors can arise in families and sporadically due to mutations in the von Hippel-Lindau gene. This protein is required for the oxygen-dependent degradation of HIFα. Inactivating mutations lead to constitutive activation of HIF and therefore overexpression of HIF-responsive genes (637,638), particularly VEGF, which causes the tumors to be highly vascular. In a subset of affected individuals (approximately 15%), overexpression of EPO leads to erythrocytosis.

Although not strictly a neoplasm, polycythemia vera is a clonal hematopoietic stem cell disorder associated with enhanced erythroid proliferation despite low levels of plasma EPO. Much less commonly, erythrocytosis combined with low plasma EPO levels is encountered in families with activating mutations of the EPO receptor (633).

Erythropoietin (Therapy)

One of the most important benefits of the revolution in recombinant DNA technology is the capability for high-level expression of purified proteins for use in clinical medicine. Of all such products currently in use, recombinant human erythropoietin (rhEPO) is the most successful in terms of number of patients being treated, commercial revenue generated, and a remarkably high quotient of efficacy over toxicity.

BIOLOGIC RESPONSE

In keeping with its role as an erythroid-specific cytokine, the primary indication for rhEPO therapy is anemia. As explained earlier in this chapter, in most patients with anemia, the production of erythropoietin, as reflected by plasma levels, increases markedly in proportion to the decrement in red cell mass. However, erythropoietin production is markedly impaired in patients with renal failure and modestly blunted in patients with chronic inflammation. Therefore, it is understandable that rhEPO treatment is most predictably effective in these disorders. In general, a patient whose plasma erythropoietin level is lower than expected for the degree of anemia (see Appendix 37) is more likely to respond to treatment (639). Response to treatment also depends on the patient's iron status. In those who have inadequate iron stores, the reticulocytes induced by rhEPO treatment have decreased hemoglobin content and concentration (640,641). Accordingly, iron supplementation is required to achieve a full therapeutic response (530). The primary goal of treatment is, of course, an increase in red cell mass. In addition, early in treatment patients may benefit from the induction of a cohort of young red cells rich in 2,3-bisphosphoglycerate, which lowers the affinity of hemoglobin for oxygen, enhancing oxygen delivery to tissues (642,643).

Although erythropoietin is generally regarded as erythroid cell-specific, it has other biologic effects. In patients with renal failure, rhEPO treatment induces a modest, clinically insignificant increase in platelet count and ameliorates pruritus, presumably by inhibiting the production of histamine in mast cells (644). rhEPO therapy also has measurable, although modest, nonhematologic effects, including enhancement of testosterone production in Leydig cells (645) and, perhaps, stimulation of pituitary ACTH and FSH (645).

These nonerythroid effects notwithstanding, rhEPO, when administered properly, has virtually no discernible side effects or toxicity. However, a very rare complication of treatment is the development of anti-EPO antibodies that cross-react with the patient's endogenous erythropoietin, resulting in the development of severe aregenerative anemia (646–648).

ADMINISTRATION

The *in vivo* turnover of rhEPO circulating in the plasma is similar to that of endogenous EPO, with a $T_{1/2}$ of approximately 5 hours. When rhEPO is administered intravenously to a patient deficient in erythropoietin, the plasma concentration falls exponentially from a very high initial value to subtherapeutic levels 18 to 24 hours later. In contrast, when the same dose of rhEPO is given by subcutaneous injection, the hormone enters the circulation slowly, allowing therapeutic levels to persist in the circulation for several days (649–651). Thus, the subcutaneous route is more efficient and cost-effective than intravenous therapy and has the additional advantage that routine administration does not require skilled medical personnel. Most patients are treated with subcutaneous rhEPO three times a week. Although the treatment is relatively simple and well tolerated, it is expensive and inconvenient. These problems may be lessened by the development of a hyperglycosylated rhEPO that has a considerably longer half-life in the circulation (652), enabling a lower dose to be given less frequently.

The ideal way to obviate the need for frequent injections of rhEPO is to develop a safe and effective form of gene therapy that would allow sustained and controlled production of erythropoietin. Robust increases in plasma erythropoietin levels have been achieved in experimental animals by transfer of EPO-expressing retrovirus (653), replication defective adenoviruses (654–656), and adeno-associated virus (657). Alternatively, effective expression of erythropoietin can also be achieved by injection of naked plasmid DNA into either muscle (658,659) or skin (660). Repeated injections would be required for maintenance therapy. Challenges implicit in the clinical application of either viral vectors or plasmid DNA include safety and the need for long-term and regulated expression of erythropoietin. One way to achieve physiologically appropriate levels of hormone is by inclusion of a drug-dependent element in the promoter driving the EPO gene (657). Optimal physiologic regulation would require that the gene contain functional oxygen-dependent regulatory elements, as discussed earlier in this chapter.

CLINICAL INDICATIONS

Anemia of Renal Insufficiency. By far the most frequent and effective use of rhEPO worldwide is in patients with kidney failure in whom anemia is due primarily to insufficient erythro-

poietin production (530,661). The response to treatment is prompt and sustained provided that adequate iron stores are maintained. Therapy is very well tolerated provided that the patient's hematocrit is kept in the mid to high 30s. In most patients with renal failure, relatively low doses (50 to 150 U/kg thrice weekly) are required to achieve this objective. Overtreatment with rhEPO may result in worsening hypertension along with increased risk for developing thrombosis of vascular access (662) as well as life-threatening cardiovascular and cerebrovascular complications (663,664). Properly treated patients enjoy significant improvement in quality of life, including less fatigue and depression as well as enhanced appetite, exercise tolerance, and sexual performance (665–667).

Anemia of Chronic Inflammation. Patients with cancer, chronic infections, and connective tissue disorders commonly have a mild to moderate anemia (see Chapter 56). As discussed in the section Biologic Response, levels of plasma erythropoietin in these patients are generally lower that that expected for the degree of anemia. Those patients in whom the anemia is more pronounced and therefore a cause of clinical symptoms may benefit from treatment with rhEPO (626). The U.S. Food and Drug Administration has approved the use of rhEPO in patients with AIDS and cancer. The former group may develop severe, often transfusion-dependent anemia, particularly if they are treated with antiviral medication. In those who have relatively low levels of plasma erythropoietin, rhEPO treatment significantly reduces the need for red cell transfusions (668). Treatment of cancer patients with rhEPO results in a significant improvement in anemia, although higher doses are required than in patients with renal failure (627,669). Those who respond to therapy have improved quality of life (670). Most oncologists agree that only a subset of cancer patients are appropriate candidates for rhEPO therapy. Those whose chemotherapy regimens include *cis*-platinum are particularly likely to benefit from treatment because these patients often have more marked anemia owing to the drug's nephrotoxicity and impairment of renal production of erythropoietin (671–673). The indication for rhEPO therapy is even less clear in patients with other disorders of chronic inflammation. In those with rheumatoid disease, therapy generally induces modest increments in hematocrit (674–676). Because of other limitations that beset these patients, it is difficult to assess how rhEPO therapy impacts their overall clinical course.

Primary Bone Marrow Disorders. Anemia is a common and often dominant feature in disorders of hematopoiesis. Elderly individuals commonly develop refractory anemia due to myelodysplasia. Only a small fraction of these patients respond to treatment with rhEPO alone. However, when rhEPO is given in combination with G-CSF, the fraction of responders increases to respectable levels approximating 35% (677–679). Those with sideroblastic anemia have an even better response rate. Occasional patients with aplastic anemia also respond to the combination rhEPO and G-CSF (678–680). Some of these patients achieve trilineage recovery. Anemia is also a common problem in patients with multiple myeloma whether or not they have associated renal disease. The majority of myeloma patients treated with rhEPO achieve a significant improvement in red cell mass (>2 g/dL hemoglobin) (681–683). In patients who undergo allogeneic bone marrow transplantation for hematologic malignancies, treatment with rhEPO hastens the rate of erythropoietic recovery (684–686). In all of these bone marrow disorders, high doses of rhEPO (100-300 U/kg/day) are required. As with other types of anemia, the patients most likely to respond are those whose levels of plasma erythropoietin are lower than that predicted by the degree of anemia.

Other Clinical Applications of Recombinant Human Erythropoietin. In certain unusual clinical situations, red cell transfusions may be urgently needed yet not feasible. For example, occasional patients develop alloantibodies, either against a broad array of common antigens or against a public antigen, that preclude successful matching of donor red cells. Some patients may for religious reasons refuse to accept blood transfusion. In these settings, the administration of rhEPO along with parenteral iron supplementation may be life-saving.

Even though blood transfusions in developed nations have reached a remarkably high level of safety, many patients are reluctant to accept blood from an unknown donor. In response to this concern, there is increasing interest in the use of autologous transfusions, particularly for elective surgery. The preoperative administration of rhEPO and iron enables patients to tolerate more extensive preoperative phlebotomy (687–690). Moreover, these autologous units have a significantly higher hemoglobin level. The administration of rhEPO in the perioperative setting may also be effective in ameliorating blood loss anemia from major surgery and in reducing the need for postoperative red cell transfusions (691,692).

Infants born prematurely develop often severe anemia owing to inadequate endogenous erythropoietin production (693). When low-birth-weight infants are treated with rhEPO during the first 6 weeks of life, there is a significant decrease in the need for blood transfusions (694–696).

Because the administration of rhEPO effectively raises the level of fetal hemoglobin in primates (697), it has been proposed for the treatment of sickle cell disease and β-thalassemia. Initial studies suggested that rhEPO stimulated fetal hemoglobin production in SS patients (698), but the results of subsequent clinical studies have been conflicting (699–701). Although some patients with β-thalassemia respond to rhEPO therapy with increased hemoglobin levels (702,703), they tend to be those with milder disease (thalassemia intermedia).

MYELOPOIESIS

Murine IL-3 stimulates a broad spectrum of myeloid progenitor cells, including pluripotent stem cells, granulocyte or macrophage colony-forming cells or units (CFU-GM, CFU-G, CFU-M), BFU-E, eosinophil CFUs (CFU-Eo), megakaryocyte CFUs (CFU-MK), and mast cells. As its name implies, GM-CSF was initially shown to be more restricted as a stimulus of the proliferation and development of CFU-GM. Murine studies with purified or recombinant factor have shown that it also stimulates the initial proliferation of other progenitors such as BFU-E (353). The other murine factors, G-CSF and M-CSF, are more restricted and predominantly stimulate CFU-G and CFU-M, respectively (704,705).

With the possible exception of GM-CSF, the activities of the human CSFs are similar to those of the corresponding murine factors. Because of the lack of an assay for human pluripotent stem cells that is analogous to the murine CFU-S spleen colony assay, it is difficult to compare results in the two species. Both IL-3 and GM-CSF affect a similar broad spectrum of human myeloid progenitor cells, including CFU-GEMM, CFU-GM, CFU-G, CFU-M, and CFU-Eo. In full serum cultures, IL-3 and GM-CSF alone stimulate the formation of colonies derived from CFU-GM, CFU-G, CFU-M, and CFU-Eo. Data from serum-free cultures suggest that in the presence of IL-3 or GM-CSF alone, myeloid colony formation is much reduced, and that optimal CFU-G or CFU-M proliferation requires the addition of G-CSF or M-CSF, respectively, to the cultures (486,706). Even in serum-replete conditions, IL-3 acts additively or synergistically with

G-CSF to induce more granulocyte colony formation than is observed with either factor alone (707). The serum-free studies may have important implications for the use of combinations of CSFs *in vivo*, and it is apparent that the use of such culture conditions may provide further insight into the *in vitro* activities of the different factors.

In addition to their effects on progenitor differentiation, the CSFs induce a variety of functional changes in mature cells. GM-CSF inhibits polymorphonuclear neutrophil migration under agarose (708), induces antibody-dependent cytotoxicity (ADCC) for human target cells (709), and increases neutrophil phagocytic activity (710). Some of these functional changes may be related to a GM-CSF–induced increase in the cell-surface expression of a family of antigens that function as cell-adhesion molecules (711). The increase in antigen expression is rapid and is associated with increased aggregation of neutrophils; both are maximal at the migration inhibitory concentration of 500 pmol/L, and granulocyte–granulocyte adhesion can be inhibited by an antigen-specific monoclonal antibody. GM-CSF also acts as a potent stimulus of eosinophil ADCC, superoxide production, and phagocytosis (712).

Granulocyte colony-stimulating factor acts as a potent stimulus of neutrophil superoxide production, ADCC, and phagocytosis (713), whereas M-CSF activates mature macrophages (714) and enhances macrophage cytotoxicity.

The actions of the CSFs on mature cells apparently parallel their spectrum of activity on immature progenitors. Murine IL-3, in contrast to human IL-3, activates neutrophil function. The explanation for this difference lies in the observation that murine IL-3 neutrophils express the IL-3 receptor (715), whereas this receptor is undetectable on the surface of human neutrophils.

SPECIFIC GROWTH FACTORS

Interleukin-3

BIOCHEMICAL CHARACTERIZATION AND MOLECULAR BIOLOGY

Media conditioned by the murine WEHI-3B myelomonocytic cell line or by activated T lymphocytes contain multiple biologic activities that include mast cell growth factor activity, multipotential colony-stimulating activity, burst-promoting activity, 20α steroid dehydrogenase-inducing activity, and *Thy*-1 antigen-inducing activity. Biochemical purification of a 28-kd glycoprotein from WEHI-3B–conditioned medium (716) or from activated T lymphocytes (717) showed that these activities were all properties of this single protein, named *IL-3*. cDNA clones (718,719) encode a 15.5-kd secreted protein (140 amino acids) after cleavage of the signal peptide. However, native murine IL-3 is considerably larger, a monomer of 23 to 32 kd, as a result of glycosylation.

Four N-glycosylation sites are predicted from the sequence, and variable glycosylation probably accounts for this broad range of molecular weights. Thus, approximately 30% to 50% of the molecular weight is carbohydrate. However, the carbohydrate is unnecessary for the *in vitro* or *in vivo* actions of the protein, because bacterially synthesized IL-3 is fully active.

The cDNA clone for primate IL-3 was isolated by expression screening of a library made from a gibbon T-lymphoblast cell line (373). This cDNA clone was used to obtain the human gene, and analysis of the gibbon and human recombinant proteins shows that they differ in only 11 amino acid positions. The human IL-3 gene encodes a 152–amino acid precursor that is N-terminally modified to yield a 133–amino acid mature protein that has one internal disulfide bridge. The human and murine genes have similar structures (5 exons) and show nucleotide homology that is greater in the 5' and 3' noncoding regions (59%) than in the coding regions (49%); the proteins are 29% homologous. Biologic activity is not maintained by the human protein on murine cells.

INTERLEUKIN-3 AND GRANULOCYTE-MACROPHAGE COLONY-STIMULATING FACTOR ARE COORDINATELY REGULATED IN LYMPHOCYTES

Little is known about the levels of production of any of the CSFs or interleukins under steady-state conditions. Levels in normal mice are very low or undetectable, and it has been difficult to detect CSFs in long-term bone marrow cultures. Part of the difficulty may lie in the fact that the hematopoietic growth factors act at picomolar concentrations and thus may function under steady-state conditions at very low concentrations. Another possibility is that GM-CSF and IL-3 may be sequestered by glycosaminoglycans and heparan sulfate in the extracellular matrix (230).

Injection of bacterial endotoxin into mice results in a rapid but small rise of GM-CSF in the serum (353). This finding contrasts with the inability to detect an increase in IL-3 and a marked rise in G-CSF, M-CSF, IL-5, and IL-6. All murine tissues contain extractable growth factors (353), suggesting that synthesis of the CSFs may occur in cells common to all organs, such as fibroblasts, endothelial cells, lymphocytes, and macrophages. Many human organs are capable of synthesizing CSFs, and bioactivity assays on medium conditioned by purified cell populations have documented CSF production by T lymphocytes (494,720,721), monocytes (722–725), endothelial cells (726,727), and fibroblasts (Fig. 7-14).

Identification of the specific factors produced by these cells has come from mRNA analysis of different purified cell populations, cell lines, or tumors. Phytohemagglutinin-stimulated blood mononuclear cells (made up of monocytes and lymphocytes) contain both GM-CSF and IL-3 mRNAs. Furthermore, phorbol ester–stimulated T-cell clones and T-cell/NK cell fractions isolated from mononuclear cell preparations are the only hematopoietic cell sources that are IL-3 mRNA-positive (728). *In situ* hybridization studies of purified lymphocytic subsets indicate that CD4, CD8, and NK fractions are positive for GM-CSF and IL-3 mRNA (513). Only a small subset of T lymphocytes become GM-CSF–positive or IL-3–positive after stimulation with phorbol ester and a calcium ionophore ionomycin (10% and 1%, respec-

tively) (513). This fraction can be increased approximately five-fold by preincubation with IL-2.

A number of conserved elements in the promoter region of the CSF genes may bind nuclear factors that regulate transcriptional activity. The IL-3 promoter contains several *cis*-acting sequences that play both positive and negative roles in transcription (729). Although the CK-1 and CK-2 elements of the GM-CSF promoter (see text that follows) are conserved in the IL-3 promoter, they do not appear to play a role in transcription. Two adjacent motifs that are homologous to the cAMP response element and the "OCT-1" element (in the IL-2 promoter) are important for positive regulation in transient transfection assays in the gibbon T-cell line, MLA-144, as is a more distal AP-1 site. A transcriptional repressor lies between these two elements (729).

INTERLEUKIN-3 RECEPTORS

Murine IL-3 binds to both low-affinity and high-affinity receptors (730). High-affinity receptors for IL-3 are present on human eosinophils, monocytes, and some cell lines (731). Cross-linking with human (166) IL-3 shows at least two bands of net molecular weight 135 and 70 kd (732), whereas similar murine studies show complexes of 140, 120, and 60 to 70 kd. A murine cDNA clone that encodes an IL-3 binding protein (AIC2A) was recently isolated from an IL-3–dependent mast cell line, MC/9 (379). The mature AIC2A protein has 856 amino acids, with an external domain of 417 amino acids, a transmembrane region of 26 amino acids, and a cytoplasmic domain of 413 amino acids that lacks a tyrosine kinase consensus sequence.

Cross-linking studies with transfected L cells show complexes of 160, 140, and 90 kd, in agreement with the bands seen in the parental MC/9 cell line. Transfected L cells bind IL-3 with low affinity (18 nM) and do not internalize IL-3 in response to ligand binding. The IL-3 receptor belongs to the new family of hematopoietic growth factor receptors but, unlike the other members, has a duplication of the conserved extracellular cysteines and the WSXWS motif. A second cDNA (AIC2B) that encodes an 896–amino acid protein was also isolated from MC/9 cells (733). It has 91% amino acid homology with AIC2A, but Southern analysis indicates that the proteins are encoded by two genes. After transfection into fibroblasts, AIC2B was expressed at the cell surface as determined by antibody binding, but it did not bind IL-3. Coexpression of both proteins does not alter the affinity of IL-3 binding. The roles of these polypep-

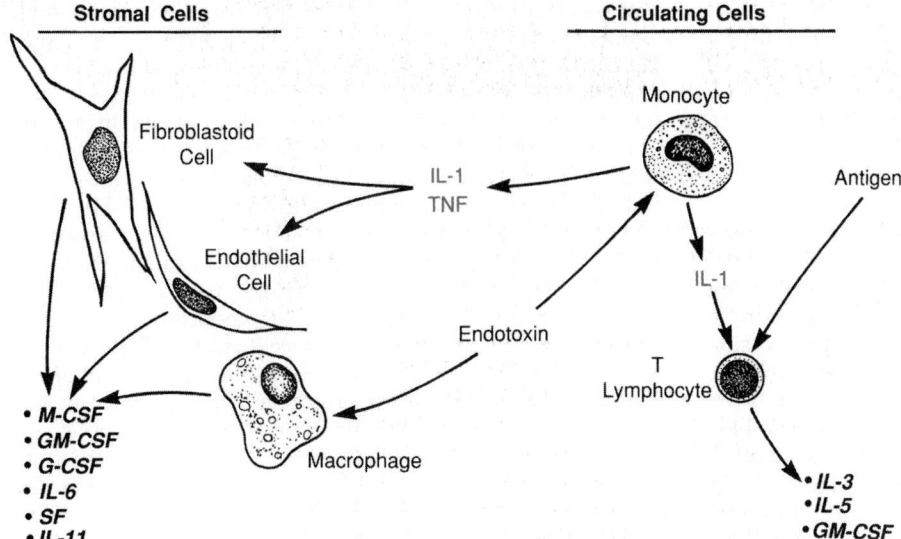

Figure 7-14. Major cytokine sources. Cells of the bone marrow microenvironment, such as macrophages, endothelial cells, and reticular fibroblastoid cells, produce macrophage colony-stimulating factor (M-CSF), granulocyte-macrophage colony-stimulating factor (GM-CSF), granulocyte colony-stimulating factor (G-CSF), interleukin (IL)-6, IL-11, and probably *Steel* factor (SF) after induction with endotoxin or IL-1 or tumor necrosis factor (TNF). The cellular sources of SF have not yet been precisely determined, but SF is produced by fibroblasts. T cells produce IL-3, GM-CSF, and IL-5 in response to antigenic and IL-1 stimulation.

tides in murine hematopoiesis have been clarified. AIC2A was used to isolate a cDNA (IL-3α) that binds murine IL-3 with low affinity but, when coexpressed with either AIC2A or AIC2B, confers high-affinity IL-3 binding (734). As mentioned, the GM-CSF, IL-3, and IL-5 receptors share subunits. There are two common subunits called α and β. There is a low-affinity receptor that is specific to each cytokine, whereas the α receptor has no binding capacity but is part of a high-affinity receptor binding site (410,735,736). The human receptor uses only the β common (βc) chain. These mouse receptors are 56% identical to human receptors and 91% identical to each other (737). The β_{IL-3} receptor does not form part of the high-affinity receptor for IL-5 or GM-CSF but does form a complex with IL-3 (734). The βc and IL-3 receptors are closely linked on mouse chromosome 15, suggesting a tandem duplication of recent origin (738). The βc knock-out leads to alveolar proteinosis, similar to the GM-CSF knock-out phenotype (737,739). Eosinophils are decreased and lack the normal response to parasites. The β_{IL-3} knock-out cell still responds to IL-3 and shows a completely normal phenotype, likely due to redundancy with IL-3 binding to βc.

AIC2B also acts as a *common β polypeptide* for the murine GM-CSF receptor α and IL-5 receptor α-chains and confers high-affinity binding of GM-CSF and IL-5 when coexpressed with those α-chains, respectively (734,740). A human polypeptide whose cDNA was isolated through its homology to these IL-3 receptors plays an important role in high-affinity GM-CSF binding when coexpressed with human GM-CSF receptor α (discussed in the section Granulocyte-Macrophage Colony-Stimulating Factor). This β common cDNA was used to isolate a human cDNA that encodes a low-affinity, IL-3–binding polypeptide (IL-3 receptor α). When β common and IL-3 receptor α are coexpressed, high-affinity IL-3 binding is observed. Although it serves as the high-affinity converter for the IL-5 receptor α (735,736), β common does not itself bind GM-CSF, IL-3, or IL-5.

IL-3 induces rapid and transient phosphorylation of a variety of cellular substrates in factor-dependent cell lines. These include proteins of 160, 140, 95, 90, 70, 55, and 38 kd in a variety of cell lines (741–744). The proteins of 140, 90, 70, 55, and 38 kd are phosphorylated on tyrosine. The identity of some of these proteins has been determined. Proteins that are tyrosine phosphorylated in response to IL-3 binding and may be components of a signaling pathway include van (397), c-*fes* (745), and mitogen-activated protein kinase (MAPK) (746,747). The tyrosine kinase responsible for ligand-induced receptor phosphorylation could be lyn (748,749), fyn (749), or c-*fes*. One candidate is phosphatidyl inositol kinase (750). Another candidate is c-*raf*, a serine/threonine kinase that is phosphorylated in response to IL-3 in some murine cell lines (751).

Granulocyte-Macrophage Colony-Stimulating Factor

BIOCHEMICAL CHARACTERIZATION AND MOLECULAR BIOLOGY

Complementary cDNA clones for murine GM-CSF were isolated after an amino acid sequence was obtained from partial purification of the murine protein (752). Clones containing cDNAs for human GM-CSF were isolated by constructing a cDNA library from the M-07 leukemia cell line in an expression vector and by directly screening transfected monkey COS cells for transient expression of GM-CSF (372). The human DNA sequence contains a single open reading frame encoding a 144–amino acid precursor protein. In an analogous fashion to other secreted proteins, 17 amino acids are cleaved from the N-terminal sequence to yield a mature protein of 127 amino acids. Murine and human GM-CSF are only 56% homologous, and the

proteins do not cross-react. Purification of both natural and recombinant human GM-CSF (rhGM-CSF) to homogeneity yields identical proteins, which are heterogeneous when analyzed by sodium dodecyl sulfate-polyacrylamide gel electrophoresis, migrating with an apparent molecular mass of 14 to 35 kd (372). This is due to variable glycosylation; the sequence contains two potential N-linked (asparagine) glycosylation sites, and zero, one, or two asparagines may be occupied by oligosaccharides (753).

The degree of occupancy appears to affect function. The most heavily glycosylated form of the molecule is not as active *in vitro* but is cleared much more slowly *in vivo* from the circulation than the nonglycosylated form. This finding may have important implications in the choice of bacteria (nonglycosylated) or mammalian/yeast cells (glycosylated) as expression systems for producing recombinant GM-CSF for therapy. The explanation for the difference in bioactivity of the two forms may be related to affinity of the ligand for its cell-surface receptor. The glycosylated form of GM-CSF has a lower affinity than the nonglycosylated molecule, which is accounted for by differences in the kinetic association rate (754).

The amino acid sequence of murine GM-CSF predicts two α-helices close to the N-terminus (positions 13 to 27 and 31 to 46). These appear to be required for biologic activity, because introduction of a helix-breaking glycine residue markedly reduces the activity of the molecule (755). The receptor binding site of human GM-CSF has been mapped to regions between residues 38 and 48 as well as between 94 and 111 by chimeric mouse–human hybrid analysis and by mapping with monoclonal antibodies (756,757). These two regions may lie adjacent to each other in the tertiary structure of the molecule.

Although human IL-3 and GM-CSF are distinct at the gene sequence level, these molecules demonstrate a number of similarities. Like GM-CSF, IL-3 has two potential N-linked glycosylation sites, and polyacrylamide gel analysis of the recombinant protein expressed in mammalian cells shows a similar range of molecular weights (14 to 28 kd). More intriguing are the *in situ* hybridization and somatic cell hybrid analyses that map the IL-3 and GM-CSF genes within 10 kb of each other on the long arm of chromosome 5 [5q23-q32 (758,759); Fig. 7-15]. The 5' noncoding regions contain similar eukaryotic promoter elements (760–762), and the 3' noncoding regions both contain a sequence rich in adenine-thymidine base pairs that is an important determinant of RNA instability (763). Finally, the genes appear to be coordinately regulated in T lymphocytes. Despite these similarities, only T lymphocytes produce both CSFs; other mesenchymal cells that produce GM-CSF do not produce IL-3 (see later discussion).

REGULATION OF GRANULOCYTE-MACROPHAGE COLONY-STIMULATING FACTOR PRODUCTION

Endothelial cells (764–766) and lung, skin, and fetal liver fibroblasts (765,767) accumulate GM-CSF mRNA after induction with IL-1 or TNF, whereas monocytes accumulate GM-CSF mRNA after stimulation with endotoxin (766) (Fig. 7-14).

Because monocytes produce IL-1 in response to endotoxin (768), this cell type may perform a central role in inducing increased hematopoiesis during stress by producing growth factors and, perhaps more importantly, by producing IL-1 and TNF. Together with antigen, IL-1 may induce circulating T lymphocytes to produce both GM-CSF and IL-3. Removal of T lymphocytes from bone marrow before allogeneic bone marrow transplantation to prevent graft-versus-host disease therefore could deplete the marrow of a cell critical for proliferation of the transplanted pluripotent stem cells. Monocyte-derived IL-1, TNF, or both may also induce bone marrow stromal cell populations to produce GM-CSF (769). This possibility is consistent with published evidence dem-

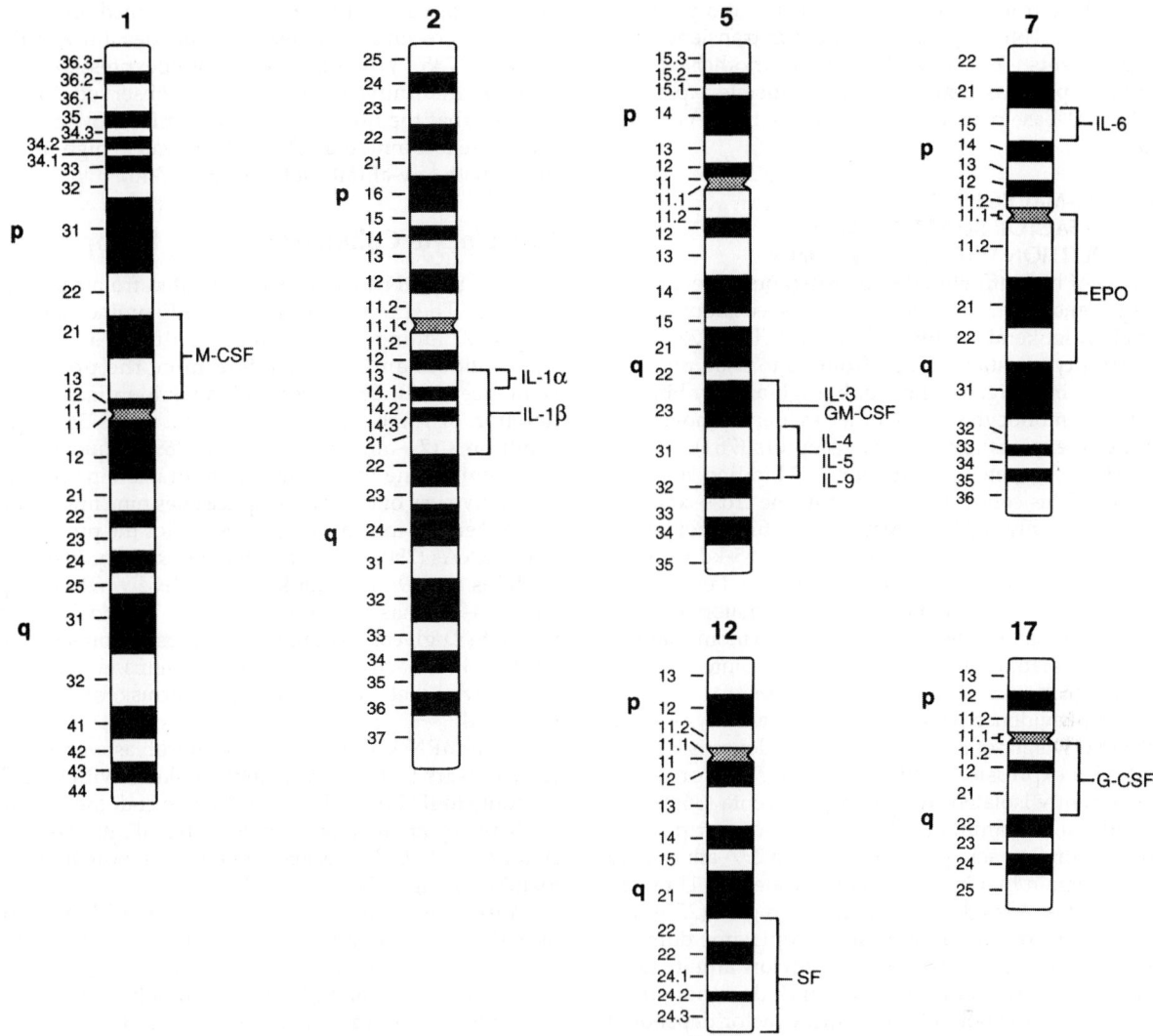

Figure 7-15. Chromosome locations of some hematopoietic growth factor genes. Schematic representation of the chromosomes on which the indicated hematopoietic growth factor genes have been mapped. *In situ* hybridization and hybrid analysis were used in most cases to localize the genes to a particular banded region of each chromosome. EPO, erythropoietin; G-CSF, granulocyte colony-stimulating factor; GM-CSF, granulocyte-macrophage colony-stimulating factor; IL, interleukin; M-CSF, macrophage colony-stimulating factor; SF, Steel factor.

onstrating the ability of "monokines" present in monocyte-conditioned medium to induce endothelial (770,771), fibroblast (772), and T-lymphocyte (773) production of burst-promoting and colony-stimulating activities.

The mechanism by which mesenchymal cells accumulate GM-CSF mRNA is poorly understood. Studies on lung fibroblasts suggest several different mechanisms. Messenger RNA accumulation after exposure to sodium fluoride indicates that a G protein may be involved (774). The response to tumor promoters such as 12-O-tetradecanoylphorbol-13-acetate suggests that PKC is also a stimulatory signal. Another potent stimulator of GM-CSF mRNA accumulation is ouabain, which blocks the Na^+-K^+-ATPase pump and results in elevation of Na^+ and Ca^{2+}. Further studies with Ca ionophores suggest that the increased Ca^{2+} is important for GM-CSF mRNA accumulation. Finally, TNF-stimulated increases of GM-CSF mRNA appear to require neither PKC nor Ca^{2+}; therefore, this potential physiologic regulator operates through an as yet undefined mechanism.

The induction of expression in fibroblasts and endothelial cells is mediated by increased mRNA stability (775) and

increased transcriptional activity (775,776). In contrast, the accumulation of GM-CSF mRNA in murine peritoneal macrophages after exposure to endotoxin is not associated with increased transcription but results from message stabilization (777). This stabilization requires the synthesis of new protein that prevents RNA degradation, possibly by interaction with an AU-rich sequence that is present in the 3' untranslated region of many transiently expressed genes, including GM-CSF, IL-1, IL-2, IL-3, G-CSF, interferon-α, interferon-β, interferon-γ, TNF, and protooncogenes such as c-*fos*, c-*myc*, c-*sis*, and c-*myb* (763). Murine macrophages also accumulate GM-CSF mRNA after other events that may occur during inflammation such as phagocytosis and adherence in the presence of fibronectin (777).

Different elements identified in the GM-CSF promoter may play a tissue-specific or inducer-specific role. For example, two elements termed *CK-1* and *CK-2* (–96 to –75) were found to bind two distinct nuclear factors (NF-GMa and NF-GMb) (760). Although gel shift assays show that NF-GMb is induced by phorbol esters in the bladder carcinoma cell line 5637, NF-GMa is constitutively produced in these cells. In contrast, NF-GMa is inducible by TNF-α in embryonic fibroblasts, and the CK-1 sequence acts as a TNF-responsive element in transient transfection experiments (761). T-cell lines show another pattern, with binding of proteins associated with inducible expression localized to a 90–base pair region close to the mRNA cap site (–53 to +37) (762).

GRANULOCYTE-MACROPHAGE COLONY-STIMULATING FACTOR RECEPTORS AND CROSS-COMPETITION WITH INTERLEUKIN-3

Low numbers of high-affinity GM-CSF receptors are expressed by mature polymorphonuclear neutrophils, by eosinophils, and by the myeloid leukemic cell lines KG1 and HL60 (778–780). Reported affinity constants range from 15 to 1000 pmol/L. Although some investigators note only high-affinity binding sites on human monocytes (780), other evidence shows that monocytes also express low-affinity receptors (781). At 4°C, human GM-CSF competes partially for IL-3 binding, and vice versa (731,782). This contrasts with the murine cross-competition, which occurs only at 37°C. Cross-linking studies with radiolabeled GM-CSF have shown either a single 85-kd receptor (780) or several bands of 135, 100, and 80 kd (783). Low-affinity GM-CSF receptors are present on several nonhematopoietic cell lines (784,785). These include non–small cell carcinoma, adenocarcinoma, and squamous lung carcinoma, gastrointestinal carcinoma, osteosarcoma, and choriocarcinoma lines.

Cross-linking evidence shows that the low-affinity receptor has a molecular weight of 80 kd (786); this evidence is in good agreement with expression studies with the receptor whose cDNA was recently isolated from human placenta (364). This cDNA encodes a 400–amino acid (45-kd) precursor protein. The mature 378–amino acid polypeptide has a 297–amino acid extracellular domain that is heavily glycosylated on 11 potential N-linkage sites. A single transmembrane region (27 amino acids) is followed by a 54–amino acid cytoplasmic domain. The transfected receptor binds GM-CSF with low affinity (K_d 2 to 8 nmol/L) and binds only GM-CSF; IL-3 does not cross-compete. After introduction into the murine factor-dependent cell line FDC-P1, the receptor confers human GM-CSF dependence (787).

Recently, a second isoform of the human GM-CSF receptor (α_2) was isolated from the factor-dependent cell line M-07 (390). This cDNA encodes a polypeptide that is identical with the placental form (GM-CSF receptor α_1) in its extracellular and transmembrane domains. The intracellular domain is slightly longer (64 vs. 54 amino acids) and is identical with GM-CSF receptor α_1 in its proximal portion. An alternate splice results in a polypeptide that diverges completely from GM-CSF receptor α_1 in the distal cytoplasmic region. The divergent sequence is rich in serine, a residue that has been implicated in the function of the IL-2 receptor β. Both isoforms are expressed in bone marrow and placental cells, but expression of GM-CSF receptor α_2 is approximately 20 times lower. Like GM-CSF receptor α_1, GM-CSF receptor α_2 also binds GM-CSF with low affinity (K_d <4 nmol/L) and confers human GM-CSF dependence to FDC-P1 cells.

High-affinity binding may be restricted to hematopoietic cells, and only on hematopoietic cells is the 135-kd band seen (786). Recently, a human cDNA that is homologous to the murine AIC2B was isolated (788). It encodes a cell-surface protein that binds neither IL-3 nor GM-CSF, but when cotransfected into COS cells with GM-CSF receptor α_1, high-affinity binding is observed. These data suggest that at least two GM-CSF cell-surface binding proteins exist—an α-chain of 80 kd that may be expressed as more than one isoform, and a β-chain (β common) of approximately 135 kd. Recent data also suggest the existence of a secreted form of the low-affinity receptor that

lacks the transmembrane region (789). Furthermore, a cDNA clone was recently isolated that encodes a low-affinity IL-3 receptor (735). When this gene was coexpressed with β common, high-affinity IL-3 binding was observed. These results indicate that the human GM-CSF and IL-3 low-affinity receptors share a common β-subunit that confers high-affinity binding on both low-affinity subunits (Fig. 7-16).

Granulocyte Colony-Stimulating Factor

Two G-CSF cDNA clones were isolated from different tumor cell lines. The first clone encodes a 207–amino acid protein, of which 177 amino acids compose mature G-CSF, whereas 30 hydrophobic amino acids determine the probable leader sequence (368). The second clone is identical apart from a deletion of three amino acids at positions 36 to 38, which results in a 174–amino acid protein (369). Sequence analysis of a genomic clone that expresses both proteins indicates that alternative use of two donor splice sites nine nucleotides apart at the 5' end of intron 2 is responsible for the production of the two mRNAs (790). The predicted molecular masses of the two proteins are 19 and 18.6 kd, respectively, whereas purified native G-CSF has a molecular mass of 19.6 kd. This difference is due to O-glycosylation; no N-glycosylation sites exist. Differences in bioactivity of the two proteins may exist, but it is not known whether two analogous forms of native G-CSF are produced.

GCSF mRNA accumulation in fibroblasts and endothelial cells appears to be coordinately regulated with GM-CSF after exposure to IL-1 or TNF-α (764–767). In endothelial cells, this is mediated by an increase in transcriptional rate (776). Monocyte synthesis of G-CSF appears to depend on induction with endotoxin (766) (Fig. 7-14).

Murine and human G-CSF receptor cDNA clones were recently isolated that bind G-CSF with high affinity, similar to the native receptor (K_d 100 to 500 pmol/L) (383,384). The murine receptor is an 812–amino acid polypeptide (90,814 daltons) with an extracellular domain of 601 amino acids, 24 hydrophobic transmembrane amino acids, and a cytoplasmic domain of 187 amino acids. One part (amino acids 95 to 317) of the extracellular domain of the G-CSF receptor is homologous to other members of the hematopoietic growth factor family. Another part (amino acids 375 to 601) is homologous to chicken contactin, a neuronal cell-surface glycoprotein that plays a role in cellular communication between neural cells (791). Contactin is homologous to fibronectin type III, and it is possible that this part of G-CSF receptor acts as a cell-adhesion protein.

Macrophage Colony-Stimulating Factor

Because of two alternative splice sites and extensive posttranslational modification, the biosynthesis of M-CSF is much more complex (Fig. 7-17). The M-CSF gene is 21 kb in length and is composed of ten exons (792). Exons 1 to 8 contain the coding sequence, and exons 9 and 10 contain 3' untranslated sequence. The first reported cDNA, isolated from a library made from a phorbol myristate acetate–stimulated pancreatic tumor cell line, encodes a 1.6-kb mRNA (370). This is translated into a 26-kd precursor that undergoes N-terminal (32 residue leader sequence) and C-terminal processing to yield a mature subunit of approximately 145 amino acids (16 kd). Analysis of a cDNA that represents the more common 4-kb mRNA shows that this form of message results from alternative splicing during transcription, leading to an in-frame insertion of 894 nucleotides (793). The transcript also has a larger 3' noncoding region which, unlike the

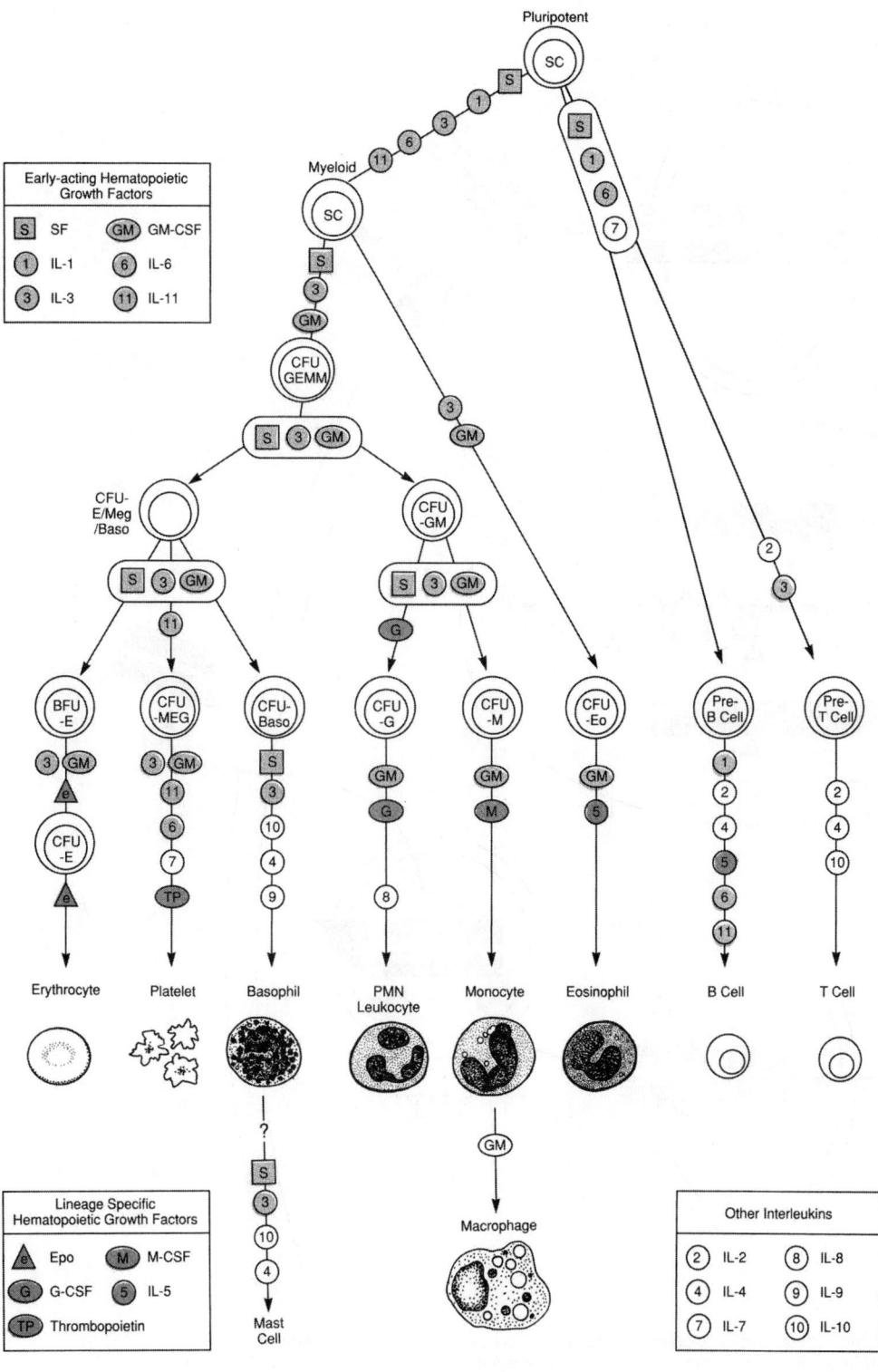

Figure 7-16. Major cytokine actions. The predominant actions of the different cytokines are indicated schematically. Interleukin (IL)-3 and granulocyte-macrophage colony-stimulating factor (GM-CSF) act broadly on most progenitor cells. IL-3, together with Steel factor (SF) and IL-6, acts on more primitive cells than GM-CSF. The other cytokines are shown on the lineage pathways to which their actions are restricted. BFU-E, erythroid burst-forming unit; CFU-Eo, eosinophil colony-forming unit; CFU-G, granulocyte colony-forming unit; CFU-GM, granulocyte-macrophage colony-forming unit; CFU-M, macrophage colony-forming unit; G-CSF, granulocyte colony-stimulating factor; M-CSF, macrophage colony-stimulating factor.

untranslated region of the shorter mRNA, contains an AU-rich region that is associated with RNA instability (763). This mRNA produces a primary translation product of 61 kd that contains an extra 298 residues. Identical N-terminal processing (32 amino acids) and more extensive C-terminal processing (294 residues) yield a mature protein of 223 amino acids (26 kd). Both the 16-kd and 26-kd forms of M-CSF are N-glycosylated to yield monomers of 20 to 25 kd and 35 to 45 kd, respectively. M-CSF exists as a dimer, and the monomers thus yield two forms of CSF, 40-kd to 50-kd and 70-kd to 90-kd glycoproteins, respectively. Native M-

CSFs of both sizes have been purified (794–796). However, it is not yet clear whether the smaller protein, purified from human urine, results from biosynthesis of the 1.6-kb mRNA or from proteolysis of the large molecule. The common 75–amino acid C-terminal sequence contains a 23–amino acid hydrophobic region, which suggests transmembrane insertion. This finding is consistent with evidence that membrane and secretory forms of M-CSF may exist (797–799). The membrane-bound form may be derived from the 1.6-kb cDNA, because the latter lacks an intracellular proteolytic cleavage site encoded in the 5' portion of exon 6. This

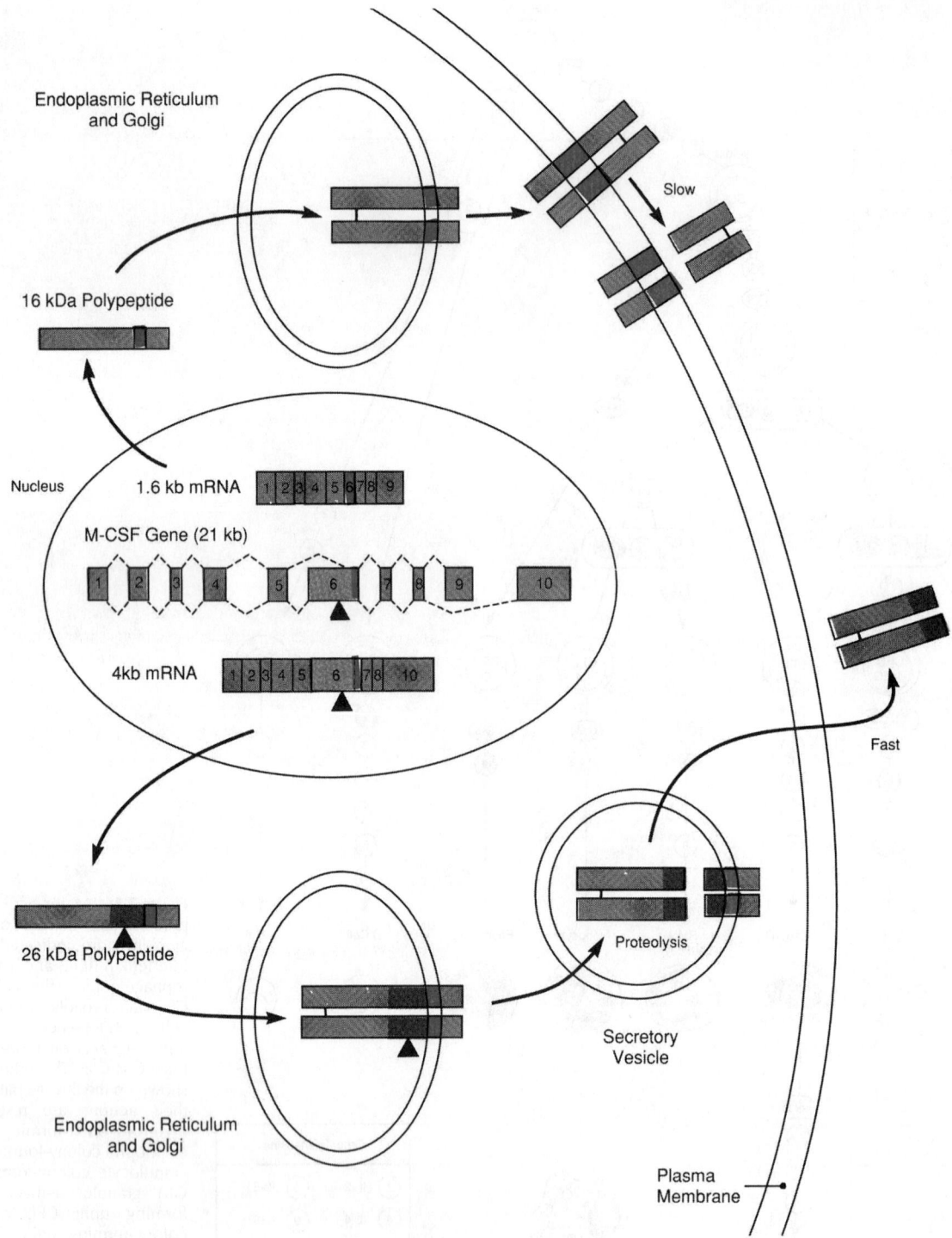

Figure 7-17. Biosynthesis of macrophage colony-stimulating factor (M-CSF). Four M-CSF complementary DNAs have been isolated. Two are illustrated here to show biosynthesis of the cell surface and soluble forms of M-CSF. The genome comprises ten exons. The 4-kb messenger RNA (mRNA) is encoded by exons 1 to 8 and 10, whereas the 1.6-kb mRNA is encoded by exons 1 to 9, with differential splicing of exon 6 that includes the loss of a sequence that encodes an intracellular proteolytic cleavage site (*arrowhead in exon 6*). The protein product of the 4-kb mRNA is cleaved at this intracellular proteolytic cleavage site in the secretory vesicle, which results in rapid secretion of M-CSF. The 1.6-kb mRNA is expressed on the cell surface and slowly released by extracellular proteolytic cleavage.

is present in the 4-kb cDNA and leads to rapid secretion after cleavage within the Golgi apparatus.

Evidence suggests that uninduced monocytes, fibroblasts, and endothelial cells contain M-CSF mRNA (766). Other investigators report, however, that phorbol myristate acetate, interferon-γ, and

GM-CSF induce M-CSF accumulation in monocytes (800–802), whereas IL-1 and TNF have the same effect in endothelial cells (776). Fetal calf serum can induce M-CSF mRNA accumulation in monocytes, and it is possible that this led to "constitutive" production in this cell type.

MACROPHAGE COLONY-STIMULATING FACTOR RECEPTOR

The interaction of M-CSF with its receptor on bone marrow macrophages has been studied. At 37°C, bone marrow macrophages internalize labeled CSF (803). Recent evidence shows that the major mechanism of clearance of M-CSF in mice occurs through binding and internalization of circulating M-CSF by liver and splenic macrophages (804). In contrast to the family of hematopoietic growth factor receptors outlined, the M-CSF or CSF-1 receptor, encoded by the c-*fms* protooncogene, is a member of the family of receptors that exhibits ligand-induced tyrosine phosphorylation (805). Evidence that c-*fms* and the M-CSF receptors are identical comes from the observations that the proteins are of similar size (165 kd) and exhibit tyrosine kinase activity; an antibody to c-*fms* precipitates a protein that is phosphorylated on tyrosine in the presence of purified M-CSF, and [^{125}I] M-CSF can be recovered from immunoprecipitates of receptor-membrane extracts (806). This family of receptors includes the PDGF, insulin, EGF, and c-*kit* receptors (Fig. 7-8). The PDGF-β isoform shares a high degree of amino acid sequence homology with the M-CSF receptor (807), and analysis of genomic clones shows that the two genes are juxtaposed in a head to tail tandem array, with less than 0.5 kb between the polyadenylation signal of the PDGF receptor β-gene and exon 1 of c-*fms* (808). Presumably, the two genes were divided by duplication of an ancestral gene and subsequent divergence. Each gene is approximately 60 kb long, and transcription is initiated in a tissue-specific manner. Exon 1, which specifies untranslated sequence, is transcribed in placental trophoblasts. In contrast, monocyte transcription is initiated from exon 2, which encodes the signal peptide and is separated by a 26-kb intron from exon 1. The mature human M-CSF receptor is an integral transmembrane glycoprotein 972 amino acids long (809). The 512–amino acid extracellular domain is organized into five immunoglobulin-like regions, and a 25–amino acid transmembrane region separates it from the 435–amino acid intracellular domain that contains the tyrosine kinase activity. The latter is separated into two regions by a 72–amino acid "kinase insert." During biosynthesis of the M-CSF receptor, asparagine-linked glycosylation of a 105-kd precursor protein results in a mature glycoprotein of 150 kd.

MACROPHAGE COLONY-STIMULATING FACTOR–MEDIATED SIGNAL TRANSDUCTION

Macrophage colony-stimulating factor binding rapidly up-regulates receptor protein tyrosine kinase activity, probably through transphosphorylation of the receptor itself by aggregation of M-CSF receptor subunits (Fig. 7-18). Tyrosine (denoted by the letter Y in the single amino acid code letter) phosphorylation has been mapped to three sites, two within the kinase insert (Y699 and Y708) and one in the C-terminal kinase consensus sequence (Y809). Evidence suggests that the M-CSF receptor is linked through a pertussis toxin-sensitive G-protein to activation of PKC (474). PDGF-β binds to and phosphorylates phospholipase C-γ, an enzyme that cleaves phosphatidyl inositol 4,5-bisphosphate to yield inositol 1,4,5-trisphosphate and 1,2-diacylglycerol, which in turn mobilize calcium and activate PKC, respectively. Phospholipase C-γ does not appear to be a substrate of the activated M-CSF receptor (810). However, recent evidence shows that M-CSF activation of PKC is mediated by a phosphatidylcholine-specific phospholipase C that catalyzes the formation of 1,2-diacylglycerol and phosphoryl choline (811). After stimulation with M-CSF, the M-CSF receptor also binds to a novel phosphatidylinositol-3-kinase. The association requires tyrosine kinase activity and is triggered by receptor phosphorylation on tyrosine; mutants that lack kinase function show reduced phosphatidylinositol-3-kinase activity (812).

Several tyrosine-phosphorylated proteins can be detected in macrophages after M-CSF treatment, but none of these polypeptides has been characterized in detail. A possible role for the c-*ras* gene product, p21 ras, is suggested by the observation that microinjected monoclonal antibodies to this protein inhibit the proliferation of fibroblasts transformed by v-*fms*, the M-CSF receptor (813). Another protooncogene product, c-*raf*, is a serine/threonine kinase and is also phosphorylated after stimulation of fibroblasts by PDGF or their transformation by v-*fms* (814).

TRANSFORMATION BY V-*FMS*

v-*fms* is the oncogene of the McDonough strain of feline sarcoma virus, and expression at the cell surface is required for transformation (813). The virus was first isolated from a feline fibrosarcoma (815), and fibroblast cell lines are transformed with the highest efficiency (805). Because fibroblasts secrete M-CSF (816) and the v-*fms* product appears to contain an almost complete extracellular domain, it is possible that transformation of fibroblasts depends on ligand binding and transduction of a signal through a functional receptor in a cell that does not normally require M-CSF for growth. However, simian virus 40-immortalized macrophages that are CSF-1–dependent do not secrete or express CSF-1. They can be rendered CSF-1–independent after introduction of the v-*fms* gene (438). The C-terminal end of v-*fms* differs from c-*fms* in that 40 amino acids of c-*fms* are replaced by 11 unrelated residues in the v-*fms* product (809). This change results in constitutive autophosphorylation of v-*fms*, contrasting with c-*fms*, in which autophosphorylation is enhanced by CSF-1. This suggests that the factor independence induced by v-*fms* expression in macrophages is due to unregulated kinase activity that provides growth stimulation in the absence of ligand. v-*fms* has not been implicated in naturally occurring hematopoietic neoplasms *in vivo*. However, bone marrow infected with helper-free virus containing v-*fms* can be engrafted into irradiated mice. Spleen cells that contain the integrated provirus can be transplanted into irradiated secondary recipients, some of which develop erythroleukemias or B-cell lymphomas (817). These data are of considerable interest and provide more evidence linking oncogenes and growth factors. Other examples include v-*erb* B, which encodes a protein that is a truncated form of the epidermal growth factor receptor (818), and c-*sis*, which encodes for a polypeptide chain of PDGF (819).

Interleukin-1

IL-1 is a monocyte–macrophage product with two distinct polypeptides, IL-1α and IL-1β. The two forms have identical biologic properties, mediated by binding to the same receptor (820,821).

MOLECULAR STRUCTURE AND BIOSYNTHESIS

Both forms of IL-1 have been cloned and are encoded by seven exons that share 45% nucleotide homology (822–825). Both proteins are synthesized as 31-kd precursors. They lack signal peptides, and the precursor forms, which are found in the cytosolic and liposomal fractions, are released from lysosomes by the action of serine proteases (826). Forms of 31 and 22 kd remain associated with the monocyte cell membrane, whereas 31-kd and 17-kd forms, as well as several small polypeptides of 11, 4, and 2 kd, are secreted (827). Evidence exists that in human monocytes, the precursor forms of IL-1α remain primarily cell-associated, whereas both the precursor forms and the mature 17-kd forms of IL-1β are released (828). Furthermore, the IL-1 receptor binds the precursor form of IL-1α but not IL-1β, suggesting that the biologic activity associated with the larger, 31-kd form is due to the IL-1α precursor (829).

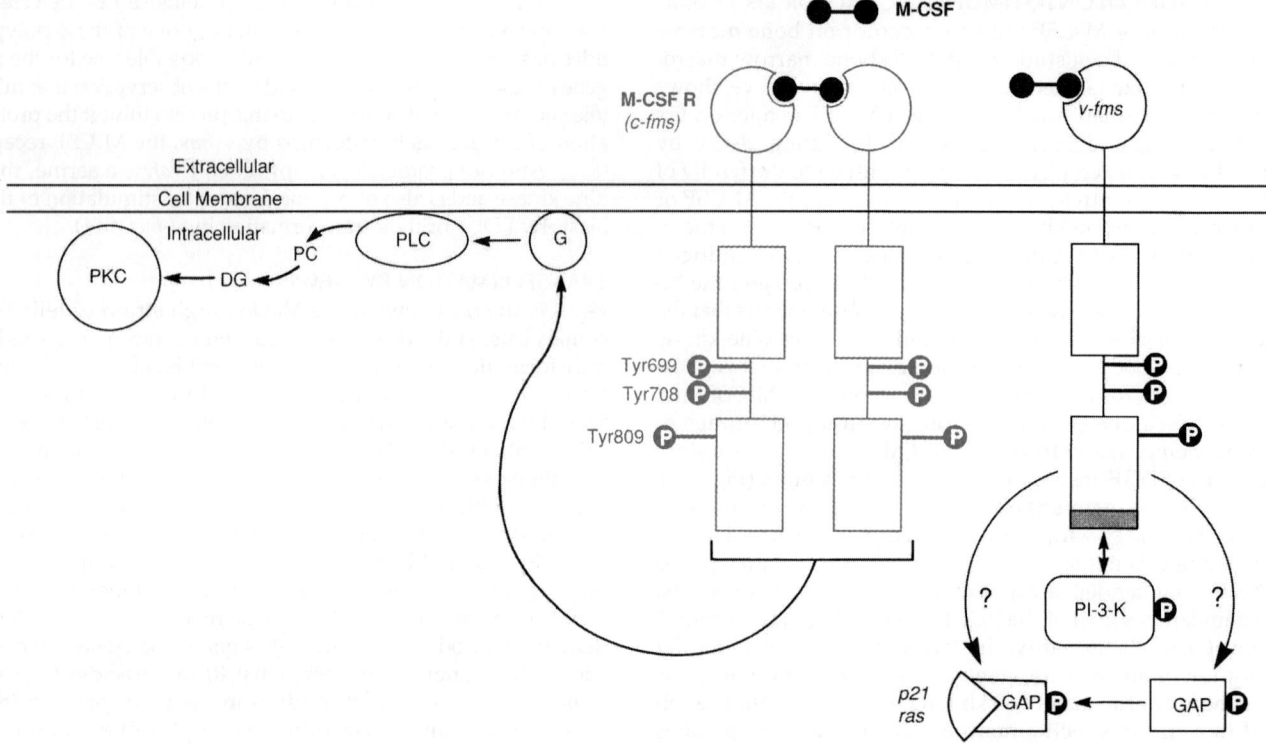

Figure 7-18. Signal transduction by macrophage colony-stimulating factor (M-CSF). M-CSF binds to its receptor and up-regulates receptor protein tyrosine kinase (PTK) activity. By analogy with other receptors of this class, dimerization probably occurs, followed by autophosphorylation or transphosphorylation of the receptor at tyrosines 699, 708, and 809. Activation of receptor PTK activity leads to phosphorylation of heterologous substrates within seconds of M-CSF stimulation, causing membrane ruffling and vacuolization, increased Na^+/H^+ exchange resulting in cytoplasmic alkalization, increased hexose transport, and induction of genes such as c-fos. The pathways involved in these effects and the protein substrates activated by receptor PTK activity have not yet been identified, but some clues exist. The oncogene v-fms has a number of potent mutations and is distinct in its C-terminus from c-fms. Transformation of cells by v-fms induces phosphorylation of the c-raf protooncogene, itself a serine-threonine protein kinase. Also, antibodies to the c-ras gene product (p21 ras) inhibit growth of v-fms–transformed cells by an unknown mechanism. p21 ras requires bound GTP for its activity. v-fms could therefore inhibit GTPase-accelerating protein (GAP), a protein that accelerates the p21 ras-mediated hydrolysis of GTP to GDP and thus decreases p21 ras activity. Alternatively, the receptor might increase p21 ras activity by another mechanism. A novel phosphatidyl inositol-3' kinase (PI-3-K) physically associates with v-fms. Last, activation of protein kinase C (PKC) may occur through receptor-mediated activation of a G protein (G) specific for phosphatidylcholine (PC). M-CSF stimulation of monocytes is associated with hydrolysis of PC to phosphorylcholine and diacylglycerol (DG) by phospholipase C (PLC). DG, in turn, stimulates PKC.

IL-1α is produced by blood monocytes and a wide variety of tissue macrophages, including pulmonary alveolar, splenic, and peritoneal macrophages and Kupffer's cells. It is also produced by nonphagocytic cells such as fibroblasts, endothelial cells, smooth muscle cells, astrocytes, and epithelial cells from skin, cornea, gingiva, and thymus. A prime stimulus for production is endotoxin, but other microbial products, plant lectins, immune complexes, complement components, and antigens also induce IL-1. Regulation by IL-1 itself and positive and negative regulation by other cytokines is complex and may also be important. IL-1 induces IL-1 production by monocytes, smooth muscle cells, and endothelial cells (830,831). IL-1 also induces interferon-γ production, which suppresses IL-1–induced IL-1 production but augments production induced by endotoxin (832). Prostaglandin E_2 and IL-6 also suppress IL-1 production, whereas TNF acts as a positive stimulus.

INTERLEUKIN-1 RECEPTOR

The murine IL-1 receptor was cloned from T cells, and the cDNA product binds IL-1α and IL-1β in a manner indistinguishable from the native low-affinity (>500 pmol/L) receptor

(376). The 319–amino acid extracellular domain of the receptor contains seven potential N-linked glycosylation sites. Treatment of the IL-1 receptor with N-glycanase removes the carbohydrate chain and reduces the size of the receptor from 80 to 62 kd, close to the predicted size of 64.6 kd. The extracellular region is followed by a 21–amino acid hydrophobic transmembrane region, then a 217–amino acid intracellular domain. The IL-1 receptor belongs to the immunoglobulin (Ig) gene superfamily, and the extracellular portion is organized into three Ig domains. This organization is similar to that of the extracellular domain of some tyrosine kinase receptor family members such as the fibroblast growth factor receptor [three Ig-like domains and the M-CSF and PDGF receptors (five Ig-like domains); Fig. 7-8] but is distinct in that the intracellular region does not contain sequences typical of tyrosine kinases or of tyrosine kinase acceptor sites. The sequence His-His-Ser-Arg-Arg (amino acids 429 to 433) resembles a PKC acceptor site.

Another polypeptide or polypeptides may be involved in IL-1 binding. High-affinity binding (K_d 5 to 15 pmol/L) occurs on a variety of cells, and bands distinct from the predicted 80-kd binding protein have been seen in cross-linking studies (833–

835). In view of the unknown mechanism by which the IL-1 receptor transduces its signal, it is likely that, similar to the IL-6 and IL-2 receptors, other polypeptides are involved in both high-affinity binding and signal transmission.

BIOLOGIC ACTIVITIES

IL-1α has been shown to be identical with a factor called *hemopoietin 1*, which was purified from HBT 5637 cell line-conditioned medium (836,837). This protein, termed *synergistic factor* (116), does not stimulate colony formation alone; it acts synergistically with M-CSF to induce the formation of large macrophage colonies from primitive colony-forming cells with high proliferative potential, which are enriched in bone marrow obtained from 5-fluorouracil–treated mice (HPP-CFC). The data suggest that primitive cells responsive to IL-1 and M-CSF proliferate and differentiate into cells responsive to IL-3 and M-CSF and subsequently to cells responsive to M-CSF alone (838,839). The synergistic effects of IL-1 are evident when bone marrow cells are plated at low density (500 cells per 35-mm plate), suggesting that its action is direct. IL-1α and IL-1β are now known to be potent inducers of GM-CSF, G-CSF, and IL-6 production by mesenchymal cells, and it is possible that the IL-1 effects are mediated indirectly by induction of known or as yet unidentified hematopoietic growth factors.

IL-1 given *in vivo* to mice before lethal whole-body irradiation has a marked radioprotective effect, which results from accelerated hematopoietic recovery (840). Suboptimal doses that are nonradioprotective achieve optimal radioprotection when combined with GM-CSF (841). These results have been extended to protection from the myelosuppressive effects of 5FU, in which case IL-1α acts synergistically with G-CSF (842) and cyclophosphamide (843). Administration of IL-1β for short periods of time (2 and 7 days) to primates after 5FU is myelostimulatory. In contrast, IL-1 given for longer periods (14 days) is ineffective, partly because of the release of TNF-α (844).

Interleukin-4

Several other interleukins may act synergistically with the CSFs on hematopoietic progenitors. IL-4 (B-cell stimulatory factor 1) is a B-lymphocyte proliferation and activation factor that is also a growth factor for mast cells and T lymphocytes. cDNAs for murine and human IL-4 were isolated (719,845,846). The human factor is a glycoprotein of 153 amino acids. Its effects are mediated by binding to a single class of high-affinity specific cell-surface receptors. cDNA clones for murine and human IL-4 receptor were recently isolated and encode a 140-kd membrane glycoprotein (380,381). Two independent clones isolated from two murine cDNA libraries encode a soluble form of the IL-4 receptor (381). The expressed cDNA is secreted, and the soluble receptor binds IL-4. Although a native secreted receptor has not been identified, a cDNA that encodes a soluble form of the IL-7 receptor has also been found (382), and soluble IL-6 receptor has been identified in urine (847). These results raise the possibility that secreted forms of growth factor receptors may play a physiologic role in the regulation of factor action.

Evidence suggests that IL-4 may act as a costimulant with EPO, G-CSF, and possibly M-CSF to increase erythroid, granulocyte, and macrophage colony numbers; paradoxically, it may inhibit IL-3 effects on less mature progenitors (848,849).

Interleukin-5

IL-5 (eosinophil differentiation factor or B-cell growth factor II) is a 46-kd glycoprotein that, like M-CSF, exists as a dimer of two identical subunits. It was identified as a factor with biologic activities both on eosinophils and their precursors (850) and on B lymphocytes. cDNA clones for both murine (851) and human IL-5 (852) have been isolated.

Murine IL-5 induces eosinophil differentiation and acts as a proliferative and differentiating stimulus for B cells. It enhances IgA synthesis in lipopolysaccharide-stimulated B cells. Human recombinant IL-5 stimulates the development of eosinophil colonies from human bone marrow. The effect of IL-5 is lineage-specific, and it does not produce as many eosinophil colonies as IL-3 or GM-CSF when tested on unenriched bone marrow mononuclear cells in serum-replete cultures (853). IL-5 has an additive, not synergistic, effect on eosinophil colonies and appears to stimulate a more mature subset of progenitors than IL-3 or GM-CSF (853). The appearance of eosinophils in the blood of rodents infected with the nematode *Nippostrongylus brasiliensis* is completely blocked by injection of monoclonal antibody to IL-5 (854), indicating that IL-5 is important for eosinophilia *in vivo*. In contrast, the IgE response in these animals is unaffected by antibody to IL-5 but is prevented by antibodies to IL-4 (855).

Interleukin-6

MOLECULAR CLONING AND PROTEIN STRUCTURE

The isolation of cDNA clones for IL-6 illustrates the power of the molecular approach to the study of growth factors with broad spectra of biologic activities. A factor that stimulates antibody production by B cells (BSF2) and the differentiation of B cells into antibody-producing cells (BCDF) was purified and its cDNA cloned (856). The sequence of this cDNA was identical to that of three others cloned at approximately the same time: interferon-β₂ (857), 26-kd protein (858), and hybridoma/plasmacytoma growth factor (859).

The protein consists of 184 amino acids with two potential N-glycosylation sites and four cysteine residues that are completely conserved between mouse and human proteins. IL-6 has significant homology to G-CSF, both at the amino acid level (four conserved cysteines) and at the level of gene organization (857).

REGULATION OF INTERLEUKIN-6 PRODUCTION

IL-6 is produced by a variety of mesenchymal cells of hematopoietic origin (T cells, B cells, monocytes) and nonhematopoietic origin (fibroblasts, endothelial cells, bone marrow stroma, keratinocytes, astrocytes, mesangial cells). T-cell production is induced by mitogens or by antigen in the presence of macrophages (860). Lipopolysaccharide enhances IL-6 production by monocytes, whereas lipopolysaccharide, IL-1, TNF, and PDGF induce fibroblast mRNA accumulation (Fig. 7-14) (859).

INTERLEUKIN-6 RECEPTOR

The cDNA for the IL-6 receptor was cloned using high-level COS expression (377). In contrast to other members of the hematopoietic growth factor receptor family, the 468–amino acid IL-6 receptor is characterized by a 90–amino acid N-terminal immunoglobulin-like domain which, like the IL-1, PDGF, and M-CSF receptors, belongs to the C2 set of the immunoglobulin superfamily. The molecular weight of the receptor is 80 kd, and ligand binding induces the association of this polypeptide with a 130-kd membrane protein that is responsible for signal transduction (861).

INTERLEUKIN-6 AND LYMPHOCYTIC PROLIFERATIVE DISEASE

IL-6 has been implicated in the pathogenesis of several diseases. It appears to be an autocrine growth factor for human myeloma cells (862). Myeloma cells produce and respond *in vitro* to IL-6, and growth *in vitro* can be inhibited by antibodies to IL-6. Responsiveness to IL-6 is characteristic of early-stage but not late-stage myeloma, suggesting that autocrine stimulation of these cells may be an early event.

Castleman's disease is characterized by fever, anemia, hypergammaglobulinemia, and increased acute-phase proteins in association with benign hyperplastic lymphadenopathy (863). Germinal center B cells produce large amounts of IL-6, and dramatic clinical improvement occurs after surgical excision of involved nodes. Thus, abnormal regulation of IL-6 expression could be important in the pathogenesis of this disease.

BIOLOGIC ACTIVITIES

IL-6 induces B cells to mature into antibody-secreting cells. Like IL-3, it acts as a permissive factor for blast cell colony proliferation in cultures of marrow from 5FU-treated mice and in human enriched progenitor cell cultures as well. In combination with IL-3, IL-6 reduces the period during which the blast cells begin to divide to form colonies, suggesting that it influences stem cell cycling (170).

Interleukin-7

IL-7 is a 25-kd glycoprotein that was originally defined by its ability to stimulate the proliferation of murine pre-B lymphocytes (B220+, sIg–) in long-term cultures (864). The murine (232) and human (865) cDNAs have been cloned. The factor binds to two classes of cell-surface receptors with low and high affinity. Both murine and human cDNAs for the IL-7 receptor were isolated (382) and when expressed in COS cells encode a polypeptide that binds IL-7 with low and high affinity. Several human cDNA clones were isolated that encode a secreted form of the receptor (382).

Interleukin-8

IL-8 was first identified as a small peptide (72 amino acids) that is secreted by monocytes in response to lipopolysaccharide and both activates and attracts polymorphonuclear neutrophils (866). Recombinant human IL-8 increases expression of CD11b/CD18 and CD11c/CD18 on human polymorphonuclear neutrophils and stimulates CD11b/CD18 binding activity, suggesting that IL-8 may promote leukocyte adhesion and recruit polymorphonuclear neutrophils to sites of tissue inflammation (867,868). Endothelial cells secrete IL-8 in response to IL-1, TNF, or lipopolysaccharide, and at nanomolar concentrations, IL-8 inhibits neutrophil adhesion to cytokine-activated endothelial cells (869).

Interleukin-9

IL-9 is a novel growth factor that was cloned from a human T-cell leukemia virus-transformed cell line (870). The cDNA encodes a 144–amino acid protein (predicted size, 16 kd) with four potential sites for asparagine-linked glycosylation. The secreted protein is variably glycosylated and ranges from 20 to 30 kd. The sequence is homologous with a newly identified murine growth factor for helper T-cell clones designated *T-cell growth factor P40* (871).

Recombinant human IL-9 acts selectively on BFU-E in cultures of enriched blood progenitors supplemented with EPO (872). Large, diffuse, late-maturing BFU-E were observed, suggesting an action on an early immature progenitor. IL-9 is not as effective as IL-3 or GM-CSF in inducing BFU-E in the presence of EPO but appears to be more selective.

Interleukin-10

IL-10 (mouse cytokine synthesis inhibitory factor) is a 17-kd to 21-kd protein that inhibits the synthesis of interferon-γ and other cytokines produced by stimulated murine T-helper 1 (T_H1) clones. The cDNA was isolated from a murine T_H2 clone and contains a 178-amino acid open reading frame with an 18–amino acid hydrophobic signal sequence (873). IL-10 is closely related to a gene in the Epstein-Barr virus genome, BCRFI, and it is likely that at some time the virus is captured with the cytokine gene. Because T_H1 clones secrete both IL-2 and interferon-γ and preferentially induce delayed-type hypersensitivity and macrophage activation, it is possible that Epstein-Barr virus exploits the biologic activity of IL-10 to suppress the immune response in the host.

Interleukin-11

IL-11 is a novel cytokine that was cloned by expression of a plasmacytoma stimulatory factor from an immortalized primate stromal cell line (874). The cDNA contains a 597-nucleotide open reading frame that encodes a 199–amino acid polypeptide. The first 17 to 20 amino acids are hydrophobic and resemble a leader sequence. Sodium dodecyl sulfate-polyacrylamide gel electrophoresis analysis of transfected COS cell supernatants shows a 21-kd species, consistent with the molecular mass expected for a 180–amino acid secreted protein. The protein lacks cysteine residues and a consensus sequence for asparagine-linked carbohydrate. The primate sequence shares 97% nucleotide identity with the human cDNA (874).

IL-11 enhances the formation of immunoglobulin-secreting B cells, and enhances IL-3 stimulated megakaryocyte colony formation. Its actions are therefore similar to those of IL-6 and IL-7, although there is no sequence homology to either gene. Evidence indicates that it also acts synergistically with IL-3 to shorten the G_0 period of blast cell colony progenitors (172).

Interleukin-12

IL-12 is a 75-kd protein with two subunits of 40 and 35 kd (p40 and p35) that are encoded by distinct genes on two different chromosomes. The p40 subunit is related to the extracellular domain of the IL-6 receptor, whereas p35 is distantly related to IL-6 itself. The complex does not signal through gp130. The p40 subunit is expressed mainly by monocytes, macrophages, and B cells, whereas p35 is more widely expressed. IL-12 induces interferon-γ expression in T and NK cells. The recombinant protein also supports hematopoietic stem cell development in combination with SF and IL-3 and is an important regulator of T_H1 cell development (875).

Interleukin-13

IL-13 is a 12-kd, 113–amino acid protein that was recently cloned from murine T_H2 and human helper T cells (876–878).The gene maps to human chromosome 5q23-31 close to the IL-4 gene (879), and the protein has limited homology (20% to 25%) to IL-4. IL-13 acts on monocytes and B cells in a manner somewhat similar to IL-4. On human monocytes, it increases adherence by inducing expression of CD23 and major histocompatibility complex class II antigens (878) and inhibits antibody-dependent cytotoxicity and lipopolysaccharide-induced cytokine release (880). Both alone and synergistically with IL-2, it increases large granular lymphocytic interferon-γ synthesis (880). On human B cells, it increases CD23, major histocompatibility complex class II, CD72, and surface IgM expression and increases B-cell proliferation and synthesis of IgE, IgG, and IgM (878,881). It competes weakly with IL-4 for binding to its receptor, suggesting that the two receptors share a common β-subunit.

Other Cytokine Receptors

INTERLEUKIN-2 RECEPTOR

The IL-2 receptor is composed of at least three individual chains (607,608). There is an α receptor that has low affinity and does not bear resemblance to other cytokine receptors. It is transiently expressed on pro-B cells (882) and on CD3–, 4–, and 8– immature T cells (883–885). The knock-out of this chain shows that it is not involved in signaling (886). The α and γ receptors resemble the cytokine receptor superfamily (887,888). The β receptor is shared with the IL-15 receptor and signals through its tail. It is expressed on fetal and adult thymocytes, in αβ cells, and in a small number of mature αβ cells in the postnatal thymus (889–891). The γ receptor is shared by the IL-4, IL-7, IL-9, and IL-15 receptors (892–896). The IL-2 receptor β-chain knock-out shows normal T and B cells (889). Hypersplenism occurs, and inflammatory bowel disease ensues. The phenotype of the γ-chain knock-out is very similar to that of the IL-7 knock-out mouse (897,898), which blocks B-cell lymphopoiesis at the pro–B cell stage. There are no detectable NK cells, whereas the IL-7 knock-out has NK cells. The IL-7 receptor knock-out has a decrease in splenic and lymph node cellularity (899). The cellularity in the thymus is decreased 10-fold to 10,000-fold. Thus, the different subunits of the IL-2 receptor have distinct roles in the immune system.

MEGAKARYOPOIESIS

The cloning of TPO has greatly clarified our understanding of the regulation of megakaryocytopoiesis (900). Before the discovery of TPO, several factors (901), including IL-3 (902), IL-6 (903), IL-11 (904), kit ligand (905,906) and even erythropoietin (907–909), were shown to stimulate megakaryocytopoiesis and thrombopoiesis *in vitro* and *in vivo*. IL-11 has even entered clinical trials (910). IL-3, IL-6, and IL-11 engage heterodimeric receptors of the β common (IL-3R) and gp130 families (IL-6R and IL-11R). Kit ligand engages a receptor of the intracellular domain, which expresses tyrosine kinase activity on ligand binding. As already emphasized, ligand engagements of these receptor families are known to induce early multipotent progenitors to proliferate and even differentiate toward lineage-specific progenitors, and kit ligand, IL-3, and IL-11 participate in the induction of the proliferation and differentiation of lineage-specific progenitors. Hence, all of the hematopoietic growth factors mentioned except erythropoietin can contribute collectively to what is known biologically as *megakaryocyte colony-stimulating activity* (meg-CSA) (908). Erythropoietin is probably not a functional component of meg-CSA. It induces only slight megakaryocyte differentiation and only at enormous concentrations (911). It probably does so because the developing erythroid progenitor passes through a stage of trilineage restriction that includes erythroid, megakaryocytic, and basophil potential (912) and because, as mentioned, erythropoietin and thrombopoietin share structural homology.

Meg-CSA is therefore a "soup" of growth factors that transduce three of the four classes of receptors that drive hematopoietic differentiation (901). Three of these are the familiar β common, tyrosine kinase, and gp130 families. All of these receptors, when engaged, drive early progenitor proliferation and partial differentiation to more mature progenitors, but the final steps of lineage committed mature progenitor development into recognizable marrow precursors require a lineage-specific growth factor—G-CSF for the granulocyte, M-CSF for the macrophage, IL-5 for the eosinophil, and erythropoietin for the erythrocyte.

The discovery of TPO provides the final step of understanding of megakaryocytopoiesis because this factor, and probably no other, actually induces lineage-restricted megakaryocyte progenitor proliferation, differentiation of those committed progenitors to megakaryoblasts, and, finally, differentiation of megakaryoblasts to the megakaryocytes that in turn produce platelets. However, this finding in no way implies that other meg-CSA components may not be useful in the therapy of hypoplastic thrombocytopenias. As emphasized, circulating TPO levels are high in those conditions, just as EPO levels are elevated in the erythroid hypoplasias. Administration of high doses of EPO is usually of little benefit in the latter conditions. TPO may be just as unsuccessful in certain megakaryocyte hypoplasias because those conditions are often associated with severe depletion of lineage-specific or multipotent progenitors. One or more of the growth factors that compose meg-CSA, such as IL-11, may be more useful in such circumstances. Clinical trials now in progress will decide that issue.

THROMBOPOIETIN

In 1993, Methia et al. (913) performed what proved to be a critically important experiment. They demonstrated that exposure of CD34– positive progenitor cells in culture to oligonucleotides that were antisense to c-mpl, a protooncogene, inhibited the ability of these cells to form megakaryocyte but not other hematopoietic colonies. This experiment, formed in the laboratory of Francoise Wendling, had its roots in Wendling's 1986 description of mpl, an oncogenic viral complex that produces a murine myeloproliferative and, ultimately, leukemic disease (914). Four years later, Wendling's group cloned the virus and demonstrated that a gene transduced by the virus might be a cytokine receptor and was responsible for the transforming function (604). Two years later, another French group, including one member of Wendling's laboratory, cloned the human homolog of mpl and demonstrated that it is a member of the hematopoietic growth factor receptor superfamily. The physiologic ligand for this receptor was as yet unknown (915,916).

Wendling's 1993 experiment strongly suggested that the unknown ligand might be the long-sought TPO, and in 1994, several laboratories cloned or purified and sequenced the all-important growth factor (598,600,917,918), and important physiologic studies of TPO were launched, particularly by Kaushansky (900) and his co-workers. As mentioned, the TPO gene is localized on the long arm of chromosome three. It contains five exons, the boundaries of which line up precisely with those of the EPO gene. The gene enjoys widespread tissue expression, including liver, kidney, smooth muscle, endothelial cells, and fibroblasts. Thus, TPO is produced at the site of hematopoiesis. Therefore, although its activity is increased in the blood during episodes of thrombopenia, it does not necessarily function as a hormone, because it is produced directly at the site of thrombopoiesis. In this sense, it differs from erythropoietin, which is not produced at all in marrow stroma. It is likely that the level of production of TPO is quite constant in all tissues. The blood levels may increase in thrombopenic states merely because circulating platelets and tissue megakaryocytes sop up the growth factor and carry it out of the circulation (919,920). This theory has received support from observations in mice with disruption of the murine transcription factor gene called NF-E2 (921); although these animals are thrombocytopenic, they have an increase in megakaryocyte mass and no increase in serum TPO levels (R. Shivdasani, S. Orkin, and F. de Sauvage, *unpublished observations*).

As reviewed by Kaushansky (900), the TPO molecule is considerably longer than the other hematopoietic growth factor polypeptides. Its 5' half bears 23% sequence homology to erythropoietin, whereas the 3' half bears no structural homology to any cytokine and may be removed by a proteolytic mechanism. Indeed, removal of this half does not ablate physiologic function. The resemblance of the 5' domain of the molecule to erythropoietin may explain the synergy of thrombopoietin and erythropoietin in megakaryocyte colony formation and platelet production (900,901). It is well recognized that splenectomized individuals with persistent anemia usually have significant thrombocytosis, and many individuals with red cell aplasia and high EPO levels also have thrombocytosis and megakaryocytosis.

The function of TPO has been studied carefully *in vivo* and *in vitro*. Although some of the *in vitro* experiments can be criticized because it is very difficult to achieve conditions in which only one factor at a time is studied, the model of megakaryocytosis discussed in the section Megakaryocytes has been loosely confirmed (900). Lineage-specific, CD34⁻-positive meg progenitors bear receptors for SF, IL-3, IL-11, and TPO, the four major classes of hematopoietic cytokine receptors. Maximal meg colony formation probably requires signaling by all four receptors, but TPO is absolutely required for the final stages of meg maturation, including maximal ploidy and cytoplasmic volume and, therefore, platelet production.

Early therapeutic trials of TPO in mice have shown that TPO is species-specific. Treatment of mice with murine TPO induces massive thrombocytosis, whereas human TPO is much less active in these animals. More importantly, TPO is active in reducing the platelet nadir in mice and in primates rendered thrombopenic by chemotherapy or radiation. Whether it will be superior to IL-11 in this regard will likely depend on the extent of the progenitor depletion that occurs in human diseases. For example, repeated doses of chemotherapy in patients with cancer may so reduce the progenitor pool that drugs that induce proliferation of progenitors such as IL-3 or IL-11 may be more effective than TPO or may be required in addition to TPO for maximal restoration of megakaryocyte development.

CIRCULATING PLATELETS

The differential diagnosis of thrombocytopenia rests first on evaluation of platelet morphology. In conditions in which megakaryocytopoiesis is accelerated, circulating platelet volume (and usually diameter) is increased. The reasons for this shift in volume are disputed. Some claim that young platelets are larger than old platelets (922). Others suggest that large megakaryocytes give rise to large platelets (923). Neither explanation satisfies all experimental and clinical conditions, but in general, thrombocytopenia secondary to increased destruction of platelets is associated with platelets of large volume, and thrombocytopenia related to decreased production of platelets is associated with platelets of normal size. There are major exceptions to this rule. Patients with hyposplenism tend to have large platelets in their blood, whether thrombopoiesis is increased or not, and patients with primary abnormalities of platelet function, such as Wiskott-Aldrich syndrome or Bernard-Soulier syndrome, have platelet sizes that bear no relationship to platelet production. Thrombopoietin increases platelet production by increasing both the number and size of individual megakaryocytes. Although TPO is probably solely responsible for the later stages of recognizable megakaryocyte differentiation and proliferation

of megakaryocyte progenitors, its function depends, at least in part, on the additional stimulation of megakaryocyte progenitors (and probably early megakaryocytes as well) with other growth factors, including IL-3, IL-11, and SF. As discussed in the section Megakaryopoiesis, these last growth factors contribute, in combination, to what is known as *meg-CSA*.

DOWN-REGULATION OF MEGAKARYOCYTES

Great uncertainty exists about possible down-regulation of megakaryocytes. Platelet factor 4 seems to down-regulate colony formation *in vitro*, which, if active *in vivo*, would provide an interesting feedback loop (924). Transforming growth factor β is also a potent inhibitor *in vitro* (925). NK cells, thought by some (but not many) to be general suppressors of hematopoiesis *in vitro*, actually enhance megakaryocyte colony formation *in vitro* (926). When an antibody to NK cells is given intraperitoneally in massive doses to mice, it abolishes the formation of colonies of megakaryocytes that can be grown in culture from murine marrow. This finding suggests that NK cells may actually play a stimulating role *in vivo* (927). These interesting studies are subject to varying interpretations.

GENE LOCALIZATION OF THE HEMATOPOIETIC GROWTH FACTORS AND THEIR RECEPTORS

The genes for GM-CSF, IL-3, IL-4, IL-5, and the M-CSF receptor c-*fms* have been mapped to the long arm of chromosome 5 (928–931) (Fig. 7-15, Table 7-1). Both endothelial cell growth factor and the receptor for PDGF have also been mapped to this region. G-CSF and EPO have been mapped to chromosomes 17 and 7, respectively (932–934), and M-CSF has been assigned to chromosome 1. A proportion of patients with either refractory anemia or acute myeloblastic leukemia have an interstitial deletion of the long arm of chromosome 5 (5q-); these cases appear always to show a critical deletion of bands 5q21 to 32. IL-3 and GM-CSF are deleted in every case, and c-*fms* is usually deleted as well. How this deletion bears on the pathogenesis of the myeloproliferative disorder in these patients is unknown. Abnormal function of one of the hematopoietic growth factors or growth factor receptors is one possibility; loss of one allele of an as yet unidentified suppressor gene is also possible.

The genes for several hematopoietic growth factor receptors have recently been mapped. The EPO receptor gene maps to chromosome 19pter-q12 (935). The GM-CSF receptor α-chain gene maps to the pseudoautosomal region of the X and Y chromosomes (936), and the IL-5 receptor α-gene maps to chromosome 3p24-26 (936). The β common gene maps to chromosome 22q12-2q13.1 (937).

TRANSCRIPTION FACTORS INVOLVED IN HEMATOPOIESIS AND STEM CELL PRODUCTION

The regulation of hematopoiesis involves the activation of cell-specific receptors, which transduces signals for proliferation and survival. For example, the erythropoietin receptor is specifically expressed by erythroid cells, and ligand activation of this receptor triggers the proliferation of erythroid cells. It has long been hypothesized that the events regulating lineage commitment of the erythroid lineage would also be controlled directly by the erythropoietin receptor. Several experiments have recently addressed this notion. First, the erythropoietin receptor could be replaced with a different receptor. The prolactin receptor can be introduced into EPOR-deficient hematopoietic cells, and stimulation with prolactin leads to the production of erythroid progenitors (938). In addition, the thrombopoietin receptor, which shows structural similarity with erythropoietin, can stimulate the production of erythroid progenitors in the absence of the EPOR (260). Finally, activation of downstream signaling molecules such as BCR-abl (939) in the absence of erythropoietin receptors still can lead to erythroid colonies. Thus, there is nothing distinct about the signaling of the erythropoietin receptor to indicate a major role for lineage commitment or differentiation.

The processes of lineage commitment and differentiation are coupled to intrinsic properties of the hematopoietic cell rather than exogenous signals. Combinatorial codes of cell-specific and ubiquitous nuclear transcription factors have been found to control cell fate and maturation (940). Early in the field of transcription factor biology, it was thought that single lineage-restrictive transcription factors controlled the production of each lineage. In other words, a red cell–specific transcription factor could be responsible for generating the erythroid lineage, and a white cell–specific factor controlled myeloid development. There might be competition for erythroid and myeloid transcription factors at the progenitor level. In fact, this general concept may be true, but evidence strongly suggests that combinations of transcription factors are required for the full maturation of each lineage.

As the growth factor field began to mature and define many exogenous regulators of hematopoiesis, the transcription factor field blossomed with a similar level of detail. This section reviews some of the major transcription factors involved in hematopoiesis. It is not meant to be an exhaustive listing of all the transcription factors involved in hematopoiesis.

GATA-1

In the mid 1980s, *cis*-regulatory elements in promoters and enhancers were found to be critical for blood gene expression. Several elements in hematopoietic tissues have been defined, particularly in the erythroid lineage. A GATA site was found in almost every erythroid-specific promoter and enhancer, including the globin genes, porphobilinogen deaminase, and other heme biosynthetic proteins (941–943). The mutation of these GATA sites led to a decreased transcriptional activity, suggesting that the factor that bound to GATA was a critical regulator of the erythroid lineage and might be a commitment factor. The factor that bound to GATA was isolated and called *GATA-1* (944,945). GATA-1 contains two zinc fingers that are required for DNA binding. The transcription factor was found to be expressed specifically in hematopoietic cells. The finding of GATA-1 in erythroid lineage meant that a single factor could be critical for the regulation of a blood lineage; however, GATA-1 was subsequently found to be expressed also by megakaryocytes, mast cells, and eosinophils, suggesting that it had a role in these other lineages (912,946–948).

Targeted gene disruption of GATA-1 led to a severe embryonic anemia (949). Blood cells were present and committed to the erythroid lineage, but the cells underwent programmed cell death at the proerythroblast stage (950). This finding suggested additional factors that regulated erythroid lineage commitment. The GATA-1 knock-out mouse not only had difficulty with erythropoiesis but also had trouble making platelets (951,952). This was a relatively late block in megakaryocyte differentiation compared to the early block in erythropoiesis.

GATA-1 is a member of a superfamily of transcription factors that now includes six factors in the vertebrate (953). GATA-1, GATA-2, and GATA-3 are expressed in hematopoietic cells, whereas GATA-4, GATA-5, and GATA-6 are expressed in endo-

derm derivatives as well as in the heart (954). Gene targeting experiments of GATA-2 demonstrated it to be required for hematopoietic cell proliferation (955). The animals are anemic and have a lower number of blood cells but still have erythroid commitment and full differentiation of the lineage. It is possible that GATA-1 and GATA-2 have redundant roles. Gene expression analysis demonstrated that GATA-2 is expressed extremely early in stem cells and is down-regulated as erythroid differentiation occurs (956). As maturation occurs, GATA-1 is expressed in the erythroid lineage, and GATA-1 is then down-regulated in maturing erythroid cells. GATA-3 is expressed in T cells and has been shown to be critically required for the development of T-cell lineage (953,957,958). When GATA-3 –/– ES cells are injected into immunodeficient rag2 deficient blastocysts, there is no contribution of GATA-3 –/– cells to the T-cell lineage in the resulting chimeric animal. In addition, GATA-3 is required for the commitment of T_H2 cells at a later stage of T-cell differentiation. Based on the knock-out phenotype, GATA-2 and GATA-3 are also required for the function of other tissues such as the brain and the kidney.

GATA-1 functions together with a cofactor called *FOG-1* (959,960). FOG-1 contains nine zinc fingers, but a subset of fingers binds to GATA-1 at the N-terminal finger. Targeting gene disruption of FOG-1 leads to an embryonic anemia reminiscent of GATA-1 deficiency (961). Thus, FOG-1 and GATA-1 appear to work coordinately to regulate the erythroid program. There is some evidence that FOG-1 can also act as a repressor of blood formation (962). Patients with mutations in the FOG-1 interacting domain of GATA-1 have congenital dyserythropoiesis and thrombocytopenia (963), strongly suggesting that the activity of FOG-1 and GATA-1 are critical for the regulation of both platelet and erythroid development. This suggestion is consistent with the mouse knock-out in which FOG-1 has an early defect in megakaryopoiesis with barely any platelets or megakaryocytes (961). FOG-1 is also a member of a family that includes FOG-2, a gene product required for myocardial and gut development (964). Thus, the GATA and FOG factors are important families of transcription factors that have been shown to regulate organ formation.

SCL

SCL is a basic helix-loop-helix transcription factor that was originally isolated as a chromosomal translocation in T-cell acute lymphocytic leukemia patients (965–967). The gene is physically translocated in roughly 5% of all T-cell acute lymphocytic leukemias, but it is found to be misregulated in as many as 75% to 95% of the cases. SCL is expressed by early stem cell populations and continues to be expressed in many hematopoietic lineages, including erythroid, myeloid, and mast cell lineages (968). It is not expressed in normal T cells. However, because most T-cell acute lymphocytic leukemia patients express the SCL gene, it is apparent that there is an oncogenic mechanism to maintain or up-regulate SCL expression in these leukemias. An understanding of the factors that control SCL expression may therefore elucidate the mechanism of T-cell leukemia.

SCL has been shown to heterodimerize with a ubiquitous member of the basic helix-loop-helix family called E2A (969–973). This heterodimer of SCL and E2A binds the site CAXXTG (called an *E box*). Surprisingly, despite the cell-specific expression of SCL in the hematopoietic system, there are no E box sites that have been found critically important in normal hematopoietic gene expression. The one example of a potential site is in the c-kit promoter, where there is an E box site adjacent to a GATA motif (974). Experiments in cell lines have demonstrated that these sites are critically required for c-kit expression on the cell surface. This result has yet to be confirmed *in vivo* but indicates the potential of SCL and E12 to act as transcriptional regulators for the hematopoietic programs.

SCL is expressed in stem cells during development in several species, including zebrafish (975,976), *Xenopus* (977), chickens (978), and mammals. It serves as one of the earliest markers of hemangioblasts that are fated to become hematopoietic cells. Embryonic stem cells can be differentiated *in vitro* to hematopoietic lineages during both primitive and definitive hematopoiesis. Gene targeting experiments of SCL in mice have demonstrated that it is critically required for normal hematopoiesis (979,980). SCL knock-out embryos have a severe embryonic anemia at day 9.5. Other tissues are also affected in the SCL knock-out embryos in addition to the defect in progenitor production. *In vitro* differentiation of SCL-deficient embryonic stem cells demonstrates that early markers of hematopoiesis such as GATA-2 and LMO2 are expressed (981). In contrast, GATA-1 and heme-biosynthetic enzymes are not expressed. This finding suggests that the next stage of hematopoietic differentiation after stem cell production is affected.

The role of SCL in early hemangioblast development has also been studied using another assay for the differentiation of embryonic stem cells (982,983). During early embryonic stem cell differentiation *in vitro*, embryoid bodies are formed. These embryoid bodies can be disrupted and plated, and blast colonies form. These blast colonies represent hemangioblasts based on gene expression and on blood and endothelial potential in replating assays. SCL mutant ES cells have difficulties making the blast cell colonies. An examination of gene expression of these blast colonies demonstrates that SCL gene expression correlates with the genesis of blast colonies. These experiments suggest that SCL is an excellent marker of hemangioblast development and that the SCL gene is required for hemangioblast production *in vivo*.

SCL is not expressed in normal T cells; however, SCL is required for stem cells to differentiate into T cells. In chimeric mouse experiments, embryonic stem cells deficient in SCL do not contribute to the T-cell lineage in immunodeficient rag2 –/– host animals (984). This finding strongly suggests that SCL deficiency leads to an early stem cell block that prevents early differentiation to the lymphoid lineage.

SCL is sufficient to induce hematopoietic stem cells during embryogenesis (975–977). The zebrafish and *Xenopus* SCL orthologs were isolated and used in overexpression experiments during early embryogenesis. Xenopus SCL overexpression led to the induction of hematopoietic cells from ectoderm, demonstrating that SCL has the capacity to specify hematopoietic mesoderm. In addition, the SCL gene in zebrafish was shown to convert kidney mesoderm into hematopoietic mesoderm, demonstrating formally that SCL is both necessary and sufficient to induce hematopoietic cells during development.

SCL is also expressed in the blood vessel lineage. It marks distinct hemangioblast populations and angioblast populations during embryogenesis. The zebrafish mutant *cloche* fails to make blood or blood vessels and also has a severe decrease in SCL expression. Forced SCL expression in *cloche* mutants can rescue both hematopoiesis and vasculogenesis (976). These results demonstrate that SCL can induce blood production during embryogenesis, but also indicates a role during vasculogenesis. The SCL knock-out embryos were found to have a major defect in angiogenesis on the yolk sac (985). Therefore, similar to *cloche*, the SCL has a role not only in blood production but also in blood vessel production. Structure–function experiments performed in the zebrafish *cloche* mutant as well as in SCL deficient murine embryonic stem cells have surprisingly demonstrated that the DNA binding domain of SCL is not required for its activity to rescue hematopoiesis or angiogenesis (986).

LMO2

LMO2 (LIM only 2) is a protein that was originally isolated as a chromosomal translocation in T-cell acute lymphocytic leukemias (987). The LIM domain consists of cysteines that resemble a zinc finger, and this domain is thought to help with the interaction of other proteins. The LMO2 gene is also specifically expressed in early blood stem cell populations during embryogenesis (988,989). Later in development, it is rather widely expressed. Gene targeting of LMO2 demonstrated that it is critically required for hematopoietic stem cell differentiation, similar to SCL, suggesting that these genes may act together to regulate the early hematopoietic program (990). SCL and LMO2 were found to bind to each other using coimmunoprecipitation analysis and are thought to associate *in vivo* (991). During normal T-cell development, LMO2 is not expressed; however, in T-cell acute lymphocytic leukemias, LMO2 is up-regulated. The factors that control both SCL and LMO2 expression may therefore be important for understanding leukemogenesis. LMO2 is a transcription factor of the LIM family, and there are other factors that specifically bind these domains. One of those factors, LDB1 (LIM domain binding protein 1), was found in a complex with LMO2 (992). This transcription factor holocomplex also includes SCL, E2A, and LDB1 (971). Incubation of nuclear extracts with DNA containing a GATA site linked to an E box site demonstrated that GATA-1 can be part of this SCL complex. Still, there is no physiologic documentation of such cooperation *in vivo*. The transcription factor FOG-1 does not seem to be part of the transcription factor holocomplex, suggesting some specificity of the involved factors.

Is there evidence that the factors work together? The LMO2 gene was isolated in *Xenopus* (988) and was shown to have similar expression to SCL. In addition, LMO2 on its own can induce hematopoietic mesoderm from naïve ectoderm, suggesting it is also involved in the specification of this tissue. Forced expression of SCL and LMO2 together leads to a synergistic activation of the blood program and turns the entire embryo into a large blood island. This synergistic activity strongly supports the concept that the transcription factor holocomplex is involved in the specification of the early blood cells of the embryo.

AML1

The observations that there are multiple waves of hematopoiesis during development has been substantiated by targeted gene disruptions of several protooncogenes in murine ES cells. The AML1 gene was originally isolated as a chromosomal translocation in acute myelogenous leukemia patients (993–1000). The gene encodes a transcription factor with a runt domain. In *Drosophila*, runt is involved in the specification of particular organs. During definitive hematopoiesis in the ventral wall of the dorsal aorta, AML is specifically expressed by the hemogenic endothelial cells (1001,1002). This expression was documented using a knock-in of a marker, lacZ. AML expression precedes the expression of blood-specific markers such as CD45 or c-myb. AML1 is required for the transition of hemogenic endothelial cells to hematopoietic stem cells. Cell sorting experiments for hematopoietic stem cells in the marrow based on AML1 expression have found that AML1 expression is a hallmark of the stem cell population (1003). The current model is that AML can lead to specification of fetal and adult blood stem cells.

The AML1 gene normally is expressed specifically in endothelial and hematopoietic cells as well as in the brain (1004). AML1 functions with CBFβ, a transcription factor that participates in the ability of AML1 to bind to DNA and to transactivate promoters

(995,1005). It is interesting that chromosomal translocation partners in leukemia are often involved in normal hematopoiesis. Leukemic translocations involving CBFβ have also been found (1006,1007). A knock-out of CBFβ leads to a severe embryonic anemia reminiscent of that in the AML1 knock-out. Thus, CBFβ, the partner of AML1, similarly controls definitive hematopoiesis. The knock-out of AML1 shows a complete lack of definitive hematopoiesis, and the animals ultimately die of anemia. There is a secondary effect on the endothelial cells, particularly in parts of the central nervous system in which bleeding has been observed. Most of vasculogenesis on the yolk sac is unaffected, and primitive erythropoiesis is normal, even though AML is expressed in the primitive lineage cells (1001,1004,1008,1009). Thus, the AML knock-out illustrates that the two lineages, primitive and definitive hematopoietic cells, are distinct from the perspective of genetic program.

C-myb

C-myb is a protooncogene and leads to viral myeloblastosis in avian species (1010). C-myb contains a tryptophan motif, which is a novel binding domain found in many metazoans. C-myb is broadly expressed, but is highly expressed in hematopoietic stem cells (1011). Expression of c-myb correlates to the proliferation of cell populations. In the ventral wall of the dorsal aorta, c-myb expression defines the developing stem cells (1012–1014). C-myb was one of the first protooncogenes to be studied by gene targeting, and this study demonstrated a severe fetal anemia (1015), indicating that c-myb was critically required for definitive hematopoiesis. However, primitive hematopoiesis was normal. An analysis of the c-myb knock-out embryos demonstrated the critical requirement of c-myb for fetal liver hematopoiesis as well as for the development of the stem cell population in the AGM. This finding suggests that c-myb is required for a subsequent differentiation of the AML-expressing cells (1016–1018).

Pu.1

The transcription factor Pu.1 (or Spi-1) is an ets-related transcription factor. It was originally isolated as an activator of myeloid-specific gene expression and also as a factor regulating globin transcription (1019,1020). Pu.1 is expressed in most hematopoietic cell lineages, and ets sites have been found in several hematopoietic-specific promoters. Two laboratories performed targeted gene disruption of the Pu.1 locus and demonstrated that it is critically required for fetal liver hematopoiesis (1021,1022). However, primitive hematopoiesis occurs in a normal manner. Pu.1 is also expressed in the ventral wall of the developing dorsal aorta, suggesting that the stem cell population is involved (1002). The knock-out of Pu.1 lacks all definitive cells, both in the embryo and in the adult, establishing that this is another critical factor for definitive hematopoiesis.

Recent studies have defined the progenitor population as being GATA-1–expressing and Pu.1-expressing. GATA-1 drives progenitors to the erythroid lineage, whereas Pu.1 expression stimulates the development of the myeloid lineage (1023–1026). There is competition between the two factors for the commitment of the individual lineages. Interestingly, Pu.1 and GATA-1 have been shown to interact specifically, and they regulate their opposing functions through this direct interaction.

tel-1

The tel-1 transcription factor is an ets-related transcription factor that is important in leukemogenesis (1027). There are several Tel fusion proteins, including Tel/AML1 and Tel/Jak2, and these form potent oncogenes that lead to the genesis of leukemia (419,1028). Tel has been found to be critically required for normal adult hematopoiesis based on gene-targeting experiments in mice. The tel knock-out embryos have normal embryonic and fetal blood production but lack adult hematopoiesis (1029). Tel is thought to control the homing of hematopoietic progenitors and stem cells to the marrow. Despite this, fetal liver hematopoiesis is normal, demonstrating that there is no intrinsic defect in the fetal stem cell populations.

EKLF

Miller and Bieker (1030) and Bieker and Southwood (1031) described the factor EKLF, a Krüppel-like zinc finger protein that is involved in β-globin production (1030,1031). EKLF was isolated by a strategy to look for genes induced during the differentiation of murine-erythroleukemia cells. It was subsequently found to be specifically expressed in the red cell lineage, both in the primitive and definitive adult blood populations. EKLF binds a CACCC motif present in many of the erythroid-specific promoters. There is differential binding of particular CACCC sites, and one favored site is the β-globin CACCC site. The β-globin CACCC site that binds EKLF is required for normal activation of globin transcription. Further, EKLF knock-out animals fail to express adult β-globin at normal levels, suggesting a role in globin switching (1032–1035). Mating of a transgene for the β-globin gene demonstrates rescue of anemia of the EKLF knock-out mouse, suggesting that EKLF plays a prominent role in hemoglobin switching (1036). Despite EKLF being expressed in the primitive erythroid cells, there is no apparent defect in yolk sac hematopoiesis in the EKLF knock-out embryos.

C/EBP Proteins

Granulocytic differentiation is controlled by the C/EBP factors. C/EBPα is specifically expressed in the myeloid lineages of the hematopoietic system, although it is expressed in other tissues (1037–1040). The promoters for the cytokine and growth factor receptors contain sites for C/EBP, including the G-CSF receptor (G-CSFR) (1041). The C/EBP mouse knock-out does not make myeloid cells, including granulocytes and monocytes (1042). In contrast, erythroid and lymphoid elements are present in normal numbers. There is a selective loss of CFU-G progenitors, but the CFU-GM progenitors are normal. This finding is thought to be due to the absence of G-CSFR and mirrors the Pu.1 knock-out, in which GM-CSFRα and M-CSFR expression is absent. The C/EBPα knock-out mice also have a defect in IL-6 signaling, perhaps due to lower expression of IL-6Rα expression (1043). Using retroviral transduction, forced expression of the G-CSFR or the IL-6Rα partially corrects the myeloid defect in the C/EBP knock-out, and restoration of both receptors leads to a better rescue. Other targets for C/EBP are likely to exist besides the receptors.

C/EBPε is another member of the family that is specifically expressed in myeloid cells, and it is also expressed in lymphoid populations (1044). The knock-out of C/EBPε demonstrates a maturation arrest at the metamyelocyte stage (1045–1047), leading to function defects in the resulting myeloid cells and a difficulty dealing with infection. It appears that there is a selective deficiency of particular granule proteins that leads to this defect.

REFERENCES

1. Till JE, McCulloch EA. A direct measurement of the radiation sensitivity of normal mouse bone marrow cells. *Radiat Res* 1961;14:213–222.
2. Pluznik DH, Sachs L. The cloning of normal "mast" cells in tissue cultures. *J Cell Comp Physiol* 1965;66:319–324.

3. Bradley TR, Metcalf D. The growth of mouse bone marrow cells in vitro. *Aust J Exp Biol Med Sci* 1966;44:287–293.

4. Clark SC, Kamen R. The human hematopoietic colony-stimulating factors. *Science* 1987;236:1229–1237.

5. Metcalf D. The molecular biology and functions of the granulocyte-macrophage colony-stimulating factors. *Blood* 1986;67:257–267.

6. Metcalf D. *Summon up the blood: in dogged pursuit of the blood cell regulators.* Miamisburg, Ohio: Alpha Med Press, 2000.

7. Dexter TM, Allen TD, Lajtha LG. Conditions controlling the proliferation of haemopoietic stem cells in vitro. *J Cell Physiol* 1976;91:335–344.

8. Orkin SH. GATA-binding transcription factors in hematopoietic cells. *Blood* 1992;80:575–581.

9. Botnick LE, Hannon EC, Hellman S. Nature of the hematopoietic stem cell compartment and its proliferative potential. *Blood Cells* 1979;5:195–206.

10. Moore MA, Metcalf D. Ontogeny of the haemopoietic system: yolk sac origin of in vivo and in vitro colony forming cells in the developing mouse embryo. *Br J Haematol* 1970;18:279–296.

11. Yoder MC, Hiatt K, Dutt P, et al. Characterization of definitive lymphohematopoietic stem cells in the day 9 murine yolk sac. *Immunity* 1997;7:335–344.

12. Miura Y, Wilt FH. Tissue interaction and the formation of the first erythroblasts of the chick embryo. *Dev Biol* 1969;19:201–211.

13. Haar JL, Ackerman GA. A phase and electron microscopic study of vasculogenesis and erythropoiesis in the yolk sac of the mouse. *Anat Rec* 1970;170:199–224.

14. Shalaby F, Ho J, Stanford WL, et al. A requirement for Flk1 in primitive and definitive hematopoiesis and vasculogenesis. *Cell* 1997;89:981–990.

15. Bhatia M, Bonnet D, Wu D, et al. Bone morphogenetic proteins regulate the developmental program of human hematopoietic stem cells. *J Exp Med* 1999;189:1139–1148.

16. Zon LI. Self-renewal versus differentiation, a job for the mighty morphogens. *Nat Immunol* 2001;2:142–143.

17. Edmonds RH. Areas of attachment between developing blood cells. *J Ultrastruct Res* 1964;11:577–580.

18. Edmunds RH. Electron microscopy of erythropoiesis in the avian yolk sac. *Anat Rec* 1966;154:785–805.

19. Russell ES, Bernstein SE. Blood and blood formation. In: Green EL, ed. *Biology of the laboratory mouse*, 2nd ed. New York: McGraw–Hill, 1966:351–372.

20. Barker JE. Development of the mouse hematopoietic system, I: types of hemoglobin produced in embryonic yolk sac and liver. *Dev Biol* 1968;18:14–18.

21. Kelemen E, Calvo W, Fliedner TM. *Atlas of human hematopoietic development.* Berlin: Springer-Verlag, 1979.

22. Roodman GD, Zanjani ED. Endogenous erythroid colony forming cells in fetal and newborn sheep. *J Lab Clin Med* 1979;94:699–707.

23. Rich IN, Kubanek B. The ontogeny of erythropoiesis in the mouse detected by the erythroid colony-forming technique, II: transition in erythropoietin sensitivity during development. *J Embryol Exp Morphol* 1980;58:143–155.

24. Peschle C, Migliaccio AR, Migliaccio G, et al. Identification and characterization of three classes of erythroid progenitors in human fetal liver. *Blood* 1981;58:565–572.

25. Block M. An experimental analysis of hematopoiesis in the rat yolk sac. *Anat Rec* 1946;96:289–311.

26. Bethlenfalvay NC, Block M. Fetal erythropoiesis: maturation in megaloblastic (yolk sac) erythropoiesis in the C 57 B1–6J mouse. *Acta Haematol* 1970;44:240–245.

27. Weinberg S, Stohlman F Jr. Growth of mouse yolk sac cells cultured in vitro. *Br J Haematol* 1976;32:543–555.

28. Weinberg SR, Stohlman F Jr. Factors regulating yolk sac hematopoiesis in diffusion chambers: various types of sera, cyclophosphamide, irradiation and long-term culture. *J Exp Hematol* 1977;5:374–384.

29. Micklem HS, Ford CE, Evans EP, et al. Competitive in vivo proliferation of fetal and adult haematopoietic cells in lethally irradiated mice. *J Cell Physiol* 1972;79:293–298.

30. Matsuoka S, Tsuji K, Hisakawa H, et al. Generation of definitive hematopoietic stem cells from murine early yolk sac and paraaortic splanchnopleures by aorta-gonad-mesonephros region-derived stromal cells. *Blood* 2001;98:6–12.

31. Muller AM, Medvinsky A, Strouboulis J, et al. Development of hematopoietic stem cell activity in the mouse embryo. *Immunity* 1994;1:291–301.

32. Godin I, Dieterlen-Lievre F, Cumano A. Emergence of multipotent hemopoietic cells in the yolk sac and paraaortic splanchnopleura in mouse embryos, beginning at 8.5 days postcoitus. *Proc Natl Acad Sci U S A* 1995;92:773–777.

33. Weissman I, Papaioannou V, Gardner R. Fetal hematopoietic origins of the adult hematolymphoid system. In: Clarkson B, Marks PA, Till JE, eds. *Differentiation of normal and neoplastic hematopoietic cells.* Cold Spring Harbor: Cold Spring Harbor Laboratory, 1978:371–387.

34. Moore MA, Owen JJ. Hypothesis: stem-cell migration in developing myeloid and lymphoid systems. *Lancet* 1967;September:658–659.

35. Dieterien-Lievre F. On the origin of haemopoietic stem cells in the avian embryo: an experimental approach. *J Embryol Exp Morphol* 1975;33:607–619.

36. Hollyfield JG. The origin of erythroblasts in Rana pipiens tadpoles. *Dev Biol* 1966;14:461–480.

37. Linch DC, Brent L. Marrow transplantation: can cord blood be used? *Nature* 1989;340:676.

38. Gluckman E, Broxmeyer HE, Auerbach AD, et al. Hematopoietic reconstitution in a patient with Fanconi's anemia by means of umbilical-cord blood from an HLA-identical sibling. *N Engl J Med* 1989;321:1174–1178.

39. Thomas DB, Yoffey JM. Human foetal haematopoiesis. *Br J Haematol* 1964;10:193–197.

40. Rifkind RA, Chui D, Epler H. An ultrastructural study of early morphogenetic events during the establishment of foetal hepatic erythropoiesis. *J Cell Biol* 1969;40:343–365.

41. Jones RO. Ultrastructural analysis of hepatic haematopoiesis in the foetal mouse. *J Anat* 1970;107:301–314.

42. Hahn IM, Bodger MP, Hoffbrand AV. Development of pluripotent hematopoietic progenitor cells in the human fetus. *Blood* 1983;62:118–123.

43. Morrison SJ, Hemmati HD, Wandycz AM, et al. The purification and characterization of fetal liver hematopoietic stem cells. *Proc Natl Acad Sci U S A* 1995;92:10302–10306.

44. Slaper-Cortenback I, Ploemacher R, Lowenberg B. Different stimulative effects of human bone marrow and fetal liver stromal cells on erythropoiesis in long-term culture. *Blood* 1987;69:135–139.

45. Migliaccio AR, Migliaccio G. Human embryonic hemopoiesis: control mechanisms underlying progenitor differentiation *in vitro*. *Dev Biol* 1988;125:127–134.

46. Barak Y, Karov Y, Levin S, et al. Granulocyte-macrophage colonies in cultures of human fetal liver cells: morphologic and ultrastructural analysis of proliferation and differentiation. *J Exp Hematol* 1980;8:837.

47. Symann M, Quesenberry P, Fontebuoni A, et al. Fetal hemopoiesis in diffusion chamber cultures, II: cell proliferation and differentiation. *Nouv Rev Fr Hematol* 1976;16:321–328.

48. Ackerman GA, Grasso JA, Knouff RA. Erythropoiesis in the mammalian embryonic liver as revealed by electron microscopy. *Lab Invest* 1961;10:787–796.

49. Grasso JA, Swift H, Ackerman GA. Observations on the development of erythrocytes in mammalian fetal liver. *J Cell Biol* 1962;14:235–254.

50. Sanchez MJ, Holmes A, Miles C, et al. Characterization of the first definitive hematopoietic stem cells in the AGM and liver of the mouse embryo. *Immunity* 1996;5:513–525.

51. Jordan CT, McKearn JP, Lemischka IR. Cellular and developmental properties of fetal hematopoietic stem cells. *Cell* 1990;61:953–963.

52. Ikuta K, Kina T, MacNeil I, et al. A developmental switch in thymic lymphocyte maturation potential occurs at the level of hematopoietic stem cells. *Cell* 1990;62:863–874.

53. Marsh WL. Anti-i: a cold antibody defining the Ii relationship in human red cells. *Br J Haematol* 1961;7:200–209.

54. Weatherall DJ, McIntyre PA. Developmental and acquired variations in erythrocyte carbonic anhydrase isozymes. *Br J Haematol* 1967;13:106–114.

55. Medlock ES, Haar JL. The liver hemopoietic environment, I: developing hepatocytes and their role in fetal hemopoiesis. *Anat Rec* 1983;207:31–41.

56. Medlock ES, Landreth KS, Kincade PW. Putative B lymphocyte lineage precursor cells in early murine embryos. *Dev Comp Immunol* 1984;8:887–894.

57. Denis KA, Treiman LJ, St Claire JI, et al. Long-term cultures of murine fetal liver retain very early B lymphoid phenotype. *J Exp Med* 1984;160:1087–1101.

58. Craig ML, Russell EL. A developmental change in hemoglobins correlated with an embryonic red cell population in the mouse. *Dev Biol* 1964;10:191–201.

59. Karlsson S, Nienhuis AW. Developmental regulation of human globin genes. *Ann Rev Biochem* 1985;54:1071.

60. Rosenberg M. Fetal hematopoiesis: case report. *Blood* 1969;33:66–78.

61. Metcalf D, Moore MAS. Embryonic aspects of haemopoiesis. In: Neuberger A, Tatum EL, eds. *Frontiers of biology.* Amsterdam: North Holland Publishing; 1971:172–271.

61a. Stamatoyannopoulos G, Neinhuis A. Hemoglobin switching. In: Stamatoyannopoulos G, Neinhuis A, Leder P, et al., eds. *The molecular basis of blood diseases.* Philadelphia: WB Saunders, 1987.

62. Hudson G. Bone-marrow volume in the human foetus and newborn. *Br J Haematol* 1965;11:446–452.

63. Custer RP, Ahlfeldt FE. Studies on the structure and function of bone marrow, II: variations in cellularity in various bones with advancing years of life and their relative response to stimuli. *J Lab Clin Med* 1932;17:960–962.

64. Garby L, Sjolin S, Viulle JC. Studies on erythrokinetics in infancy, III: disappearance from plasma and red cell uptake of radioactive iron injected intravenously. *Acta Paediat* 1963;52:537.

65. Glaser K, Limarzi LR, Poncher HG. Cellular composition of the bone marrow in normal infants and children. *Pediatrics* 1950;6:789.

66. Siep M. The reticulocyte level and the erythrocyte production judged from reticulocyte studies in newborn infants during the first week of life. *Acta Paediatr* 1955;44:355.

67. Sturgeon P. Volumetric and microscopic pattern of bone marrow in normal infants and children, II: cytologic pattern. *J Pediatr* 1951;7:642.

68. Pearson HA. Life-span of the fetal red blood cell. *J Pediatr* 1967;70:166–171.

69. Delivoria-Papadopoulos M, Roncevic NP, Oski FA. Postnatal changes in oxygen transport of term, premature, and sick infants: the role of red cell 2, 3-diphosphoglycerate and adult hemoglobin. *Pediatr Res* 1971;5:235–245.

70. Bunn HF, Kitchen H. Hemoglobin function in the horse: the role of 2,3-diphosphoglycerate in modifying the oxygen affinity of maternal and fetal blood. *Blood* 1973;42:471.

71. Dhindsa DA, Hoversland AS, Templeton JW. Postnatal changes in oxygen affinity and concentrations of 2,3-diphosphoglycerate in dog blood. *Biol Neonate* 1972;20:226.

72. Bunn HF, Forget BG. Animal hemoglobins. In: Dyson J, ed. *Hemoglobin: molecular, genetic and clinical aspects*, 1st ed. Philadelphia: WB Saunders, 1986:126–168.

73. Huehns ER, Beaven GH. Developmental changes in human haemoglobins. *Clin Dev Med* 1971;37:175–203.

74. Dover GJ, Boyer SH, Bell WR. Microscopic method for assaying F cell production: illustrative changes during infancy and in aplastic anemia. *Blood* 1978;52:664.

75. Collins FS, Boehm CD, Waber PG, et al. Concordance of a point mutation 5' to the G gamma globin gene with G gamma beta +: hereditary persistence of fetal hemoglobin in the black population. *Blood* 1984;64:1292–1296.

76. Gilman JG, Huisman TH. DNA sequence variation associated with elevated fetal G gamma-globin production. *Blood* 1985;66:783–787.

77. Collins FS, Metherall JE, Yamakawa M, et al. A point mutation in the A gamma-globin gene promoter in Greek hereditary persistence of fetal haemoglobin. *Nature* 1985;313:325–326.

78. Gelinas R, Endlich B, Pfeiffer C, et al. G to A substitution at the distal CCAAT box of the A gamma-globin gene in Greek hereditary persistence of fetal haemoglobin. *Nature* 1985;313:323–325.

79. Giglioni B, Casini C, Mantovani R, et al. A molecular study of a family with Greek hereditary persistence of fetal hemoglobin and beta-thalassemia. *EMBO J* 1984;3:2641.

80. Oski FA. Clinical implications of the oxyhemoglobin dissociation curve in the neonatal period. *Crit Care Med* 1979;7:412.

81. Halvorsen S. Plasma erythropoietic levels in cord blood and in blood during the first week of life. *Acta Paediatr Scand* 1963;52:425.

82. Gilmour JR. Erythroblastosis fetalis. *Arch Dis Child* 1944;19:1.

83. Ross MP, Christensen RD, Rothstein G, et al. A randomized trial to develop criteria for administering erythrocyte transfusions to anemic preterm infants 1 to 3 months of age. *J Perinatol* 1989;9:246–253.

84. Stockman JA III, Graeber JE, Clark DA, et al. Anemia of prematurity: determinants of the erythropoietin response. *J Pediatr* 1984;105:786–792.

85. Brown MS, Garcia JF, Phibbs RH, et al. Decreased response of plasma immunoreactive erythropoietin to "available oxygen" in anemia of prematurity. *J Pediatr* 1984;105:793–798.

86. Christensen RD. Recombinant erythropoietic growth factors as an alternative to erythrocyte transfusion for patients with "anemia of prematurity." *J Pediatr* 1989;83:793–796.

87. Halperin DS, Wacker P, Lacourt G, et al. Effects of recombinant human erythropoietin in infants with the anemia of prematurity: a pilot study. *J Pediatr* 1990;116:779–786.

88. Donato H, Vain N, Rendo P, et al. Effect of early versus late administration of human recombinant erythropoietin on transfusion requirements in premature infants: results of a randomized, placebo-controlled, multicenter trial. *Pediatrics* 2000;105:1066–1072.

89. Sreenan C, Osiovich H. Myeloid colony-stimulating factors: use in the newborn. *Arch Pediatr Adolesc Med* 1999;153:984–988.

90. Bilgin K, Yaramis A, Haspolat K, et al. A randomized trial of granulocyte-macrophage colony-stimulating factor in neonates with sepsis and neutropenia. *Pediatrics* 2001;107:36–41.

91. Frenck RW Jr, Shannon KM. Hematopoietic growth factors in pediatrics. *Curr Opin Pediatr* 1993;5:94–102.

92. Jacobson LO, Marks EK, Gaston EO, et al. Role of the spleen in radiation injury. *Proc Soc Exp Biol Med* 1949;70:7440–7442.

93. Jacobson LO, Simmons EL, Marks EK, et al. Further studies on recovery from radiation injury. *J Lab Clin Med* 1951;37:683–697.

94. Ford CE, Hamerton JL, Barnes DWH, et al. Cytological identification of radiation chimeras. *Nature* 1956;177:452–454.

95. Ogden DA, Micklem HS. The fate of serially transplanted bone marrow cell populations from young and old donors. *Transplantation* 1976;22:287–293.

96. Harrison DE, Astle CM, Delaittre JA. Loss of proliferative capacity in immunohemopoietic stem cells caused by serial transplantation rather than aging. *J Exp Med* 1978;147:1526–1531.

97. Harrison DE, Astle CM. Loss of stem cell repopulating ability upon transplantation: effects of donor age, cell number, and transplantation procedure. *J Exp Med* 1982;156:1767–1779.

98. Curry JL, Trentin JJ. Hemopoietic spleen colony studies, I: growth and differentiation. *Dev Biol* 1967;15:395–413.

99. Juraskova V, Tkadlecek L. Character of primary and secondary colonies of haematopoiesis in the spleen of irradiated mice. *Nature* 1965;206:951–952.

100. Siminovitch L, Till JE, McCulloch EA. The distribution of colony-forming cells among spleen colonies. *J Cell Comp Physiol* 1963;62:327–336.

101. Lewis JP, Trobaugh FE. Haematopoietic stem cells. *Nature* 1964;204:589–590.

102. Becker AJ, McCulloch EA, Siminovitch L, et al. The effect of differing demands for blood cell production on DNA synthesis by hemopoietic colony-forming cells of mice. *Blood* 1965;26:296–308.

103. VanZant G, Eldridge PW, Behringer RR, et al. Genetic control of hematopoietic kinetics revealed by analyses of allophenic mice and stem cell suicide. *Cell* 1983;35:639–645.

104. Necas E, Znojil V, Frindel E. Thymidine suicide and hydroxyurea kill ratios accurately reflect the proliferative status of stem cells (CFU–S). *Exp Hematol* 1989;17:53–55.

105. Micklem HS, Lennon JE, Ansell JD, et al. Numbers and dispersion of repopulating chimeras as functions of cell dose. *Exp Hematol* 1987;15:251–257.

106. Harrison DE, Astle CM, Lerner C. Number and continuous proliferative pattern of transplanted primitive immunohematopoietic stem cells. *Proc Natl Acad Sci U S A* 1988;85:822–826.

107. Boggs DR, Boggs SS, Saxe DR, et al. Hematopoietic stem cells with high proliferative potential. *J Clin Invest* 1982;70:242–253.

108. Lemischka IR, Raulet DH, Mulligan RC. Developmental potential and dynamic behavior of hematopoietic stem cells. *Cell* 1986;45:917–927.

109. Wu AM, Till JE, Siminovitch L, et al. A cytological study of the capacity for differentiation of normal hematopoietic colony-forming cells. *J Cell Physiol* 1967;69:177.

110. Visser JW, VanBekkum DW. Purification of pluripotent hemopoietic stem cells: past and present. *J Exp Hematol* 1990;18:248–256.

111. Spangrude GJ, Heimfeld S, Weissman IL. Purification and characterization of mouse hematopoietic stem cells. *Science* 1988;241:58–62.

112. Uchida N, Weissman IL. Searching for hematopoietic stem cells: evidence that Thy-1.1lo Lin- Sca-1+ cells are the only stem cells in C57BL/Ka-Thy1.1 bone marrow. *J Exp Med* 1992;175:175–184.

113. Miraglia S, Godfrey W, Yin AH, et al. A novel five-transmembrane hematopoietic stem cell antigen: isolation, characterization, and molecular cloning. *Blood* 1997;90:5013–5021.

114. Bertoncello I, Bartelmez SH, Bradley TR, et al. Increased Qa-m7 antigen expression is characteristic of primitive hemopoietic progenitors in regenerating marrow. *J Immunol* 1987;139:1096–1103.

115. Bertoncello I, Bartelmez SH, Bradley TR, et al. Isolation and analysis of primitive hemopoietic progenitor cells on the basis of differential expression of Qa-m7 antigen. *J Immunol* 1986;136:3219–3224.

116. Bradley TR, Hodgson GS. Detection of primitive macrophage progenitor cells in mouse bone marrow. *Blood* 1979;54:1446–1450.

117. Visser JW, Bauman JG, Mulder AH, et al. Isolation of murine pluripotent hemopoietic stem cells. *J Exp Med* 1984;59:1576–1590.

118. Visser JW, deVries P. Isolation of spleen-colony forming cells (CFU–S) using wheat germ agglutinin and rhodamine 123 labeling. *Blood Cells* 1988;14:369–384.

119. Civin CI, Strauss LC, Brovall C, et al. Antigenic analysis of hematopoiesis, III: a hematopoietic progenitor cell surface antigen defined by a monoclonal antibody raised against KG-1a cells. *J Immunol* 1984;133:157–165.

120. Tindle RW, Nichols RAB, Chan L, et al. A novel monoclonal antibody BI-3C5 recognizes myeloblasts and non-B non-T lymphoblasts in acute leukemias and CGL blast crises, and reacts with immature cells in normal bone marrow. *Leuk Res* 1985;9:1.

121. Berenson RJ, Andrews RG, Bensinger WI, et al. Antigen CD 34+ marrow cells engraft lethally irradiated baboons. *J Clin Invest* 1988;81:951–955.

122. Osawa M, Hanada KI, Hamada H, et al. Long-term lymphohematopoietic reconstitution by a single CD34-low/negative hematopoietic stem cell. *Science* 1996;273:242–245.

123. Bhatia M, Bonnet D, Murdoch B, et al. A newly discovered class of human hematopoietic cells with SCID-repopulating activity. *Nat Med* 1998;4:1038–1045.

124. Zanjani ED, Almeida-Porada G, Livingston AG, et al. Human bone marrow CD34- cells engraft in vivo and undergo multilineage expression that includes giving rise to CD34+ cells. *Exp Hematol* 1998;26:353–360.

125. Goodell MA, Rosenzweig M, Kim H, et al. Dye efflux studies suggest that hematopoietic stem cells expressing low or undetectable levels of CD34 antigen exist in multiple species. *Nat Med* 1997;3:1337–1345.

126. Sato T, Laver JH, Ogawa M. Reversible expression of CD34 by murine hematopoietic stem cells. *Blood* 1999;94:2548–2554.

127. Lemischka I. The power of stem cells reconsidered? *Proc Natl Acad Sci U S A* 1999;96:14193–14195.

128. Anderson DJ, Gage FH, Weissman IL. Can stem cells cross lineage boundaries? *Nat Med* 2001;7:393–395.

129. Jackson KA, Mi T, Goodell MA. Hematopoietic potential of stem cells isolated from murine skeletal muscle. *Proc Natl Acad Sci U S A* 1999;96:14482–14486.

130. Makino S, Fukuda K, Miyoshi S, et al. Cardiomyocytes can be generated from marrow stromal cells in vitro. *J Clin Invest* 1999;103:697–705.

131. Ferrari G, Cusella-De Angelis G, Coletta M, et al. Muscle regeneration by bone marrow-derived myogenic progenitors [published erratum appears in *Science* 1998;281:923]. *Science* 1998;279:1528–1530.

132. Gussoni E, Soneoka Y, Strickland CD, et al. Dystrophin expression in the mdx mouse restored by stem cell transplantation. *Nature* 1999;401:390–394.

133. Bjornson CR, Rietze RL, Reynolds BA, et al. Turning brain into blood: a hematopoietic fate adopted by adult neural stem cells in vivo. *Science* 1999;283:534–537.

134. Orlic D, Kajstura J, Chimenti S, et al. Bone marrow cells regenerate infarcted myocardium. *Nature* 2001;410:701–705.

135. Lajtha LG. Stem cell concepts. *Differentiation* 1979;14:23–34.

136. Hodgson GS, Bradley TR. Properties of haematopoietic stem cells surviving 5-fluorouracil treatment: evidence for a pre-CFU-S cell? *Nature* 1979;281:381–382.

137. Botnick LE, Hannon EC, Obbagy J, et al. The variation of hematopoietic stem cell self–renewal capacity as a function of age: further evidence for heterogenicity of the stem cell compartment. *Blood* 1982;60:268–271.

138. Mauch P, Botnick LE, Hannon EC, et al. Decline in bone marrow proliferative capacity as a function of age. *Blood* 1982;60:245–252.

139. Magli MC, Iscove NN, Odartchenko N. Transient nature of early haematopoietic spleen colonies. *Nature* 1982;295:527–529.

140. Eckmann L, Freshney M, Wright EG, et al. A novel in vitro assay for murine haematopoietic stem cells. *Br J Cancer* 1988;58:36–40.

141. Kamel-Reid S, Dick JE. Engraftment of immune-deficient mice with human hematopoietic stem cells. *Science* 1988;242:1706–1709.

142. Larochelle A, Vormoor J, Hanenberg H, et al. Identification of primitive human hematopoietic cells capable of repopulating NOD/SCID mouse bone marrow: implications for gene therapy. *Nat Med* 1996;2:1329–1337.

143. Antin JH, Weinberg DS, Rappeport JM. Evidence that pluripotential stem cells form splenic colonies in humans after marrow transplantation. *Transplantation* 1985;39:102–105.

144. Jones RJ, Wagner JE, Celano P, et al. Separation of pluripotent haematopoietic stem cells from spleen colony-forming cells. *Nature* 1990;347:188–189.

145. Glimm H, Eisterer W, Lee K, et al. Previously undetected human hematopoietic cell populations with short-term repopulating activity selectively engraft NOD/SCID-beta2 microglobulin-null mice. *J Clin Invest* 2001;107:199–206.

146. Morrison SJ, Weissman IL. The long-term repopulating subset of hematopoietic stem cells is deterministic and isolatable by phenotype. *J Immunol* 1994;1:661–673.

147. Guenechea G, Gan OI, Dorrell C, et al. Distinct classes of human stem cells that differ in proliferative and self-renewal potential. *Nat Immunol* 2001;2:75–82.

148. Sutherland HJ, Eaves CJ, Eaves AC, et al. Characterization and partial purification of human marrow cells capable of initiating long-term hematopoiesis in vitro. *Blood* 1989;74:1563–1570.

149. Ploemacher RE, van der Sluijs JP, Voerman SA, et al. An in vitro limiting-dilution assay of long-term repopulating hematopoietic stem cells in the mouse. *Blood* 1989;74:2755–2763.

150. Breems DA, Blokland EA, Neben S, et al. Frequency analysis of human primitive haematopoietic stem cell subsets using a cobblestone area forming cell assay. *Leukemia* 1994;8:1095–1104.

151. Fauser AA, Messner HA. Proliferative state of human pluripotent hemopoietic progenitors (CFU-GEMM) in normal individuals and under regenerative conditions after bone marrow transplantation. *Blood* 1979;54:1197–1200.

152. Fauser AA, Messner HA. Granuloerythropoietic colonies in human bone marrow, peripheral blood, and cord blood. *Blood* 1978;52:1243–1248.

153. Porcellini A, Manna A, Talevi N, et al. Effect of two cyclophosphamide derivatives on hemopoietic progenitor cells and pluripotential stem cells. *J Exp Hematol* 1984;12:863–866.

154. Yeager AM, Kaizer H, Santos GW, et al. Autologous bone marrow transplantation in patients with acute nonlymphocytic leukemia, using ex vivo marrow treatment with 4-hydroperoxycyclophosphamide. *N Engl J Med* 1986;315:141–147.

155. Hara H, Ogawa M. Murine hemopoietic colonies in culture containing normoblasts, macrophages, and megakaryocytes. *Am J Hematol* 1978;4:23–34.

156. Kay HE. Stem-Cells: a poem. *Blut* 1983;46:183.

157. Kay HE. Hypothesis: how many cell-generations? *Lancet* 1965;August:418–419.

158. Hellman S, Botnick LE, Hannon EC, et al. Proliferative capacity of murine hematopoietic stem cells. *Proc Natl Acad Sci U S A* 1978;75:490–494.

159. Micklem HS, Ansell JD, Wayman JE, et al. The clonal organization of hematopoiesis in the mouse. *Prog Immunol V* 1983;5:633–640.

160. Mintz B, Anthony K, Litwin S. Monoclonal derivation of mouse myeloid and lymphoid lineages from totipotent hematopoietic stem cells experimentally transplanted in fetal hosts. *Proc Natl Acad Sci U S A* 1984;81:7835–7839.

161. Chapel B, Hawley R, Covarrusias L, et al. Clonal contributions of small numbers of retrovirally marked hematopoietic stem cells engrafted in unirradiated W/W mice. *Proc Natl Acad Sci U S A* 1989;86:4564–4569.

162. Keller G, Snodgrass R. Life span of multipotential hematopoietic stem cells in vivo. *J Exp Med* 1990;171:1407–1418.

163. Schmidt M, Hoffmann G, Wissler M, et al. Detection and direct genomic sequencing of multiple rare unknown flanking DNA in highly complex samples. *Hum Gene Ther* 2001;12:743–749.

164. Lemischka IR, Jordan CT. The return of clonal marking sheds new light on human hematopoietic stem cells. *Nat Immunol* 2001;2:11–12.

165. Lansdorp P. Self-renewal of stem cells. *Biol Blood Marrow Transplant* 1997;3:171–178.

166. Nash R, Storb R, Neiman P. Polyclonal reconstitution of human marrow after allogeneic bone marrow transplantation. *Blood* 1988;72:2031–2037.

167. Byron JW. Comparison of the action of 3H-leucine and hydroxyurea on testosterone-treated hemopoietic stem cells. *Blood* 1972;40:198.

168. Byron JW. Manipulation of the cell cycle of the hemopoietic stem cell. *J Exp Hematol* 1975;3:44–53.

169. Byron JW. Drug receptors and the haematopoietic stem cell. *Nature* 1973;241:152.

170. Ikebuchi K, Wong GG, Clark SC, et al. Interleukin-6 enhancement of interleukin-3-dependent proliferation of multipotential hemopoietic progenitors. *Proc Natl Acad Sci U S A* 1987;84:9035–9039.

171. Ikebuchi K, Clark SC, Ihle JW, et al. Granulocyte colony stimulating factor enhances interleukin-3-dependent proliferation of multipotential hemopoietic progenitors. *Proc Natl Acad Sci U S A* 1988;85:3445–3449.

172. Musashi M, Yang Y-C, Paul SR, et al. Direct and synergistic effects of interleukin 11 on murine hematopoiesis in culture. *Proc Natl Acad Sci U S A* 1991;88:765–769.

173. Leary AG, Ikebuchi K, Hirai Y, et al. Synergism between interleukin-6 and interleukin-3 in supporting proliferation of human hematopoietic stem cells: comparison with interleukin-1a. *Blood* 1988;71:1759–1763.

174. Tsuji K, Lyman SD, Sudo T, et al. Enhancement of murine hematopoiesis by synergistic interactions between steel factor (ligand for *c-kit*), interleukin-11, and other early acting factors in culture. *Blood* 1992;79:2855–2860.

175. Lim B, Apperley JF, Orkin SH, et al. Long-term expression of human adenosine deaminase in mice transplanted with retrovirus-infected hematopoietic stem cells. *Proc Natl Acad Sci U S A* 1989;86:8892–8896.

176. Bodine DM, Karlsson S, Nienhuis AW. Combination of interleukins 3 and 6 preserves stem cell function in culture and enhances retrovirus-mediated gene transfer into hematopoietic stem cells. *Proc Natl Acad Sci U S A* 1989;86:8897–8901.

177. Eaves CJ, Cashman JD, Kay RJ, et al. Mechanisms that regulate the cell cycle status of very primitive hematopoietic cells in long-term human marrow cultures, II: analysis of positive and negative regulators produced by stromal cells within the adherent layer. *Blood* 1991;78:110–117.

178. Anderson DM, Lyman SD, Baird A, et al. Molecular cloning of mast cell growth factor: a hematopoietin that is active in both membrane bound and soluble forms. *Cell* 1990;63:235–243.

179. Flanagan JG, Leder P. The kit ligand: a cell surface molecule altered in steel mutant fibroblasts. *Cell* 1990;63:185–194.

180. Flanagan JG, Chan DC, Leder P. Transmembrane form of the kit ligand growth factor is determined by alternative splicing and is missing in the *Sl^d* mutant. *Cell* 1991;64:1025–1035.

181. Trentin JJ, Curry JC, Wolf N, et al. Factors controlling stem cell differentiation and proliferation: the hematopoietic inductive microenvironment (HIM): the proliferation and spread of neoplastic cells. *M.D. Anderson Hospital 21st annual symposium on fundamental cancer research*, 21st ed. Baltimore: Williams & Wilkins, 1967:713.

182. Wolff NS, Trentin JJ. Hemopoietic colony studies, V: effect of hemopoietic organ stroma on differentiation of pluripotent stem cells. *J Exp Med* 1968;127:205–214.

183. Till JE, McCulloch EA, Siminovich L. A stochastic model of stem cell proliferation based on growth of spleen colony-forming cells. *Proc Natl Acad Sci U S A* 1964;51:29–36.

184. Suda T, Suda J, Ogawa M. Disparate differentiation in mouse hemopoietic colonies derived from paired progenitors. *Proc Natl Acad Sci U S A* 1984;81:2520–2524.

185. Gregory CJ, McCulloch EA, Till JE. Repressed growth of C57BL marrow in hybrid hosts reversed by antisera directed against non-H-2 alloantigens. *Transplantation* 1972;13:138–141.

186. Coulombel L, Eaves AC, Eaves CJ. Enzymatic treatment of long-term human marrow cultures reveals the preferential location of primitive hemopoietic progenitors in the adherent layer. *Blood* 1983;62:291–297.

187. Mauch P, Greenberger JS, Botnick L, et al. Evidence for structured variation in self renewal capacity within long term bone marrow cultures. *Proc Natl Acad Sci U S A* 1980;77:2927–2930.

188. Schofield R. The relationship between the spleen colony-forming cell and the haemopoietic stem cell: a hypothesis. *Blood Cells* 1978;4:7–25.

189. Metcalf D, Moore MAS. Colony-stimulating factor (CSF). In: Neuberger A, Tatum EL, eds. *Frontiers of biology: haemopoietic cells*. Amsterdam: North-Holland Publishing, 1971:399–403.

190. Whitlock CA, Witte ON. Long term culture of B lymphocytes and their precursors from murine marrow. *Proc Natl Acad Sci U S A* 1982;79:3608–3612.

191. Lord BI, Testa AG, Hendry JH. The relative spatial distributions of CFUs and CFUs in the normal mouse femur. *Blood* 1975;46:65–72.

192. Lambertsen RH, Weiss LA. A model of intramedullary hematopoietic microenvironments based on stereologic study of the distribution of endocloned marrow colonies. *Blood* 1984;63:287–297.

193. Frassoni F, Testa NG, Lord BI. The relative spatial distribution of erythroid progenitor cells (BFUe and CFUe) in the normal mouse femur. *Cell Tissue Kinet* 1982;15:447–445.

194. Lichtman MA, Chamberlain JK, Weed RI, et al. The regulation of the release of granulocytes from normal marrow. In: Greenwalt TJ, Jamieson GA, eds. *The granulocyte: function and clinical utilization*, 13th ed. New York: Alan R. Liss, 1977:53–75.

195. Weiss L, Chen L-T. The organization of hematopoietic cords and vascular sinuses in bone marrow. *Blood Cells* 1975;1:617.

196. Campbell FR. Ultrastructural studies of transmural migration of blood cells in the bone marrow of rats, mice and guinea pigs. *Am J Anat* 1972;135:521–536.

197. Lichtman MA. The ultrastructure of the hemopoietic environment of the marrow: a review. *J Exp Hematol* 1981;9:391–410.

197a. Weiss L. *Cell and tissue biology: a textbook of histology*, 6th ed. Baltimore: Urban & Scharzenberg, 1988.

198. Weiss L. The hematopoietic microenvironment of the bone marrow: an ultrastructural study of the stroma in rats. *Anat Rec* 1976;186:161.

199. Shaklai M, Tavassoli M. Cellular relationship in the rat bone marrow studied by freeze fracture and lanthanum impregnation thin-sectioning electron microscopy. *J Ultrastruct Res* 1979;69:343–361.

200. Allen TD, Dexter TM. Long term bone marrow cultures: an ultrastructural review. *Scan Electron Microsc* 1983;4:1851–1866.

201. Gimble JM, Dorheim M-A, Cheng Q, et al. Response of bone marrow stromal cells to adipogenic antagonists. *Mol Cell Biol* 1989;57:4587–4595.

202. Iscove NN, Fagg B, Keller G. A soluble activity from adherent marrow cells cooperates with IL-3 in stimulating growth of pluripotential hematopoietic precursors. *Blood* 1988;71:953–957.

203. Gimble JM. The function of adipocytes in the bone marrow stroma. *New Biol* 1990;2:304–312.

204. Tavassoli M. Marrow adipose cells and hemopoiesis: an interpretative review. *J Exp Hematol* 1984;12:139–146.

205. Hines DL. Lipid accumulation and production of colony-stimulating activity by the 266AD cell line derived from mouse bone marrow. *Blood* 1983;61:397–402.

206. Kodama H-A, Sudo H, Koyama H, et al. In vitro hemopoiesis within a microenvironment created by MC3T3-G2/PA6 preadipocytes. *J Cell Physiol* 1984;118:233–240.

207. Tavassoli M. Marrow adipose cells: histochemical identification of labile and stable components. *Arch Pathol Lab Med* 1976;100:16.

208. Weiss L. The structure of bone marrow: functional interrelationships of vascular hematopoietic compartments in experimental hemolytic anemia. *J Morphol* 1965;117:467–481.

209. Brookoff D, Weiss L. Adipocyte development and the loss of erythropoietic capacity in the bone marrow of mice after sustained hypertransfusion. *Blood* 1982;60:1337–1344.

210. Islam A. Do bone marrow fat cells or their precursors have a pathogenic role in idiopathic anaemia? *Med Hypotheses* 1988;25:209–217.

211. Weiss LP, Wislocki GB. Seasonal variations in hematopoiesis in the dermal bones of the nine-banded armadillo. *Anat Rec* 1956;126:143–163.

212. Hussain MM, Mahley RW, Boyles JK, et al. Chylomicron-chylomicron remnant clearance by liver and bone marrow in rabbits. *J Biol Chem* 1989;264:9571–9582.

213. Hussian MM, Mahley RW, Boyles JK, et al. Chylomicron metabolism: chylomicron uptake by bone marrow in different animal species. *J Biol Chem* 1989;264:17931–17938.

214. Greenberger JS. Sensitivity of corticosteroid-dependent insulin-resistant lipogenesis in marrow preadipocytes of obese-diabetic (db/db) mice. *Nature* 1978;275:752–754.

215. Bathija A, Davis S, Trubowitz S. Bone marrow adipose tissue: response to acute starvation. *Am J Hematol* 1979;6:191–198.

216. Tavassoli M, Eastlund DT, Yam LT, et al. Gelatinous transformation of bone marrow in prolonged self-induced starvation. *Scand J Haematol* 1976;16:311–319.

217. Besis M, Breton-Gorius J. Nouvelles observations: sur l'îlot erythroblastique et la rhopheocytose de la ferritine. *Rev Hematol* 1959;14:165–175.

218. Crocker PR, Gordon S. Isolation and characterization of resident stromal macrophages and hematopoietic cell clusters from mouse bone marrow. *J Exp Med* 1985;162:993–1014.

219. Kincade PW, Lee G, Pietrangeli CE, et al. Cells and molecules that regulate B lymphopoiesis in bone marrow. *Annu Rev Immunol* 1989;7:111–143.

220. Lord BI, Hendry JH. The distribution of haemopoietic colony-forming units in the mouse femur and its modification by x-rays. *Br J Radiol* 1972;45:110.

220a. Trentin JJ. Hemopoietic microenvironments, historical perspectives, status, and projections. In: Tavassoli M, ed. *Handbook of the hemopoietic microenvironment*. Clifton, NJ: Humana Press, 1989.

221. Roberts RA, Spooncer E, Parkinson EK, et al. Metabolically inactive 3T3 cells can substitute for marrow stromal cells to promote the proliferation and development of multipotent haemopoietic stem cells. *J Cell Physiol* 1987;132:203–214.

222. Dexter TM, Spooncer F, Simmons P, et al. Long-term marrow culture: an overview of techniques and experience. In: Wright DG, Greenberger JS, eds. *Long-term bone marrow culture*, 18th ed. Kroc Foundation Series. New York: Alan R. Liss, 1984:57–96.

223. Williams DA, Rosenblatt MF, Beier DR, et al. Generation of murine stromal cell lines supporting hematopoietic stem cell proliferation by use of recombinant retrovirus vectors encoding simian virus 40 large T antigen. *Mol Cell Biol* 1988;8:3864–3871.

224. Rios M, Williams DA. Systematic analysis of the ability of stromal cell lines derived from different murine adult tissues to support maintenance of hematopoietic stem cells in vitro. *J Cell Physiol* 1990;145:434–443.

225. Goodman R, Grate H, Hannon E, et al. Hematopoietic stem cells: effect of preirradiation, bleeding, and erythropoietin on thrombopoietic differentiation. *Blood* 1977;49:253–261.

226. Gordon MY, Greaves MF. Physiological mechanisms of stem cell regulation in bone marrow transplantation and haemopoiesis. *Bone Marrow Transplant* 1989;4:335–338.

227. Hurley RW, McCarthy JB, Verfaillie CM. Direct adhesion to bone marrow stroma via fibronectin receptors inhibits hematopoietic progenitor proliferation. *J Clin Invest* 1995;96:511–519.

228. Dexter TM, Spooncer E, Varga J, et al. Stromal cells and diffusible factors in the regulation of haemopoietic cell development. In: Killman S-A, Cronkite EP, Muller-Berat CN, eds. *Haemopoietic stem cells*. Copenhagen: Munksgaard, 1983:303–318.

229. Gordon MY, Riley GP, Watt SM, et al. Compartmentalization of a haemopoietic growth factor (GM-CSF) by glycosaminoglycans in the bone marrow microenvironment. *Nature* 1987;326:403–405.

230. Roberts R, Gallagher J, Spooncer E, et al. Heparin sulphate bound growth factors: a mechanism for stromal cell mediated haemopoiesis. *Nature* 1988;332:376–378.

231. Paul SR, Yang Y-C, Donahue RE, et al. Stromal cell-associated hematopoiesis immortalization and characterization of a primate bone marrow-derived stromal cell line. *Blood* 1991;77:1723–1733.

232. Namen AE, Lupton S, Hjerrild K, et al. Stimulation of B-cell progenitors by cloned murine interleukin-7. *Nature* 1988;333:571–573.

233. Toksoz D, Dexter TM, Lord BI, et al. The regulation of hematopoiesis in long-term bone marrow cultures, II: stimulation and inhibition of stem cell proliferation. *Blood* 1980;55:931–936.

234. Allen TD, Dexter TM. Cellular interrelationships during in vitro granulopoiesis. *Differentiation* 1976;6:191–194.

235. Whitlock CA, Robertson D, Witte ON. Murine B cell lymphopoiesis in long term culture. *J Immunol Methods* 1984;67:353–369.

236. Dexter TM, Testa NG, Allen TD, et al. Molecular and cell biologic aspects of erythropoiesis in long-term bone marrow cultures. *Blood* 1981;58:699–707.

237. Eliason JF, Testa NG, Dexter TM. Erythropoietin-stimulated erythropoiesis in long term bone marrow culture. *Nature* 1979;281:382–384.

238. Corey CA, DeSilva A, Williams DA. Erythropoiesis in murine long term marrow cultures following transfer of the erythropoietic cDNA into marrow stromal cells. *J Exp Hematol* 1990;18:201–204.

239. Oddos T, Nacol-Lizard S, Blanchet JP. Erythropoiesis in murine long-term bone-marrow cell cultures: dependence on erythropoietin and endogenous production of an erythropoietic stimulating activity. *J Cell Physiol* 1987;133:72–78.

240. Gartner S, Kaplan HS. Long-term culture of human bone marrow cells. *Proc Natl Acad Sci U S A* 1980;77:4756–4759.

241. Chang J, Coutino L, Morgenster G, et al. Reconstitution of haematopoietic system with autologous marrow taken during relapse of acute myeloblastic leukemia and grown in long-term culture. *Lancet* 1986;1:294–295.

242. Coulombel L, Kalousek DK, Eaves CJ, et al. Long term marrow culture reveals chromosomally normal hematopoietic progenitor cells in patients with Philadelphia chromosome positive chronic myelogenous leukemia. *N Engl J Med* 1983;308:1493–1498.

243. Singer JW. Studies with human long-term marrow cultures. In: Wright DG, Greenberger JS, eds. *Long-term bone marrow culture*, 18th ed. New York: Alan R. Liss, 1984:235–242.

243a. Tavassoli M, ed. *Handbook of the hemopoietic microenvironment*. Clifton, NJ: Humana Press, 1989.

244. Hunt P, Robertson D, Weiss D, et al. A single bone-marrow derived stromal cell type supports the in vitro growth of early lymphoid and myeloid cells. *Cell* 1987;48:997–1007.

245. Li CL, Johnson GR. Stimulation of multipotential, erythroid and other murine haematopoietic progenitor cells by adherent cell lines in the absence of detectable multi-CSF (IL3). *Nature* 1985;316:633–636.

246. Rennick D, Yang G, Gemmell L, et al. Control of hemopoiesis by a bone marrow stromal cell clone: lipopolysaccharide- and interleukin-1-inducible production of colony-stimulating factors. *Blood* 1987;69:682–691.

247. Whitlock CA, Tidmarsh GF, Muller-Sieburg C, et al. Bone marrow stromal cell lines with lymphopoietic activity express high levels of a pre-B neoplasia-associated molecule. *Cell* 1987;48:1009–1021.

248. Thiemann FT, Moore KA, Smogorzewska EM, et al. The murine stromal cell line AFT024 acts specifically on human CD34+CD38- progenitors to maintain primitive function and immunophenotype in vitro. *Exp Hematol* 1998;26:612–619.

249. Singer JW, Charbord P, Keating A, et al. Simian virus 40-transformed adherent cells from human long-term marrow cultures: cloned cell lines produce cells with stromal and hematopoietic characteristics. *Blood* 1987;70:464–474.

250. Harigaya K, Handa H. Generation of functional clonal cell lines from human bone marrow stroma. *Proc Natl Acad Sci U S A* 1985;82:3477–3480.

251. Moore JO, Dodge RK, Amrein PC, et al. Granulocyte-colony stimulating factor (filgrastim) accelerates granulocyte recovery after intensive postremission chemotherapy for acute myeloid leukemia with aziridinyl benzoquinone and mitoxantrone: Cancer and Leukemia Group B study 9022. *Blood* 1997;89:780–788.

252. Cornelissen JJ, Wognum AW, Ploemacher RE, et al. Efficient long-term maintenance of chronic myeloid leukemic cobblestone area forming cells on a murine stromal cell line. *Leukemia* 1997;11:126–133.

253. Slack JL, Nemunaitis J, Andrews DF III, et al. Regulation of cytokine and growth factor gene expression in human bone marrow stromal cells transformed with simian virus 40. *Blood* 1990;75:2319–2327.

254. Billips LG, Petitte D, Landreth S. Bone marrow stromal cell regulation of B lymphopoiesis: interleukin-1 (IL-1) and IL-4 regulate stromal cell support of pre-B cell production in vitro. *Blood* 1990;75:611–619.

255. Cashman JD, Eaves AC, Raines EW, et al. Mechanisms that regulate the cell cycle status of very primitive hematopoietic cells in long-term human marrow cultures, I: stimulatory role of a variety of mesenchymal cell activators and inhibitory role of TGF-beta. *Blood* 1990;75:96–101.

256. Godard CM, Augery YL, Ginsbourg M, et al. Established cell lines of mouse marrow adherent cells producing differentiation factor(s) for the granulocyte-macrophage lineage. *In Vitro* 1983;19:897–902.

257. Song ZX, Shadduck RK, Innes DJ Jr, et al. Hematopoietic factor production by a cell line (TC-1) derived from adherent murine marrow cells. *Blood* 1985;66:273–281.

258. Harigaya K, Cronkite EP, Miller ME, et al. Murine bone marrow cell line producing colony-stimulating factor. *Proc Natl Acad Sci U S A* 1981;78:6963–6966.

259. Lanotte M, Metcalf D, Dexter TM. Production of monocyte/macrophage colony-stimulating factor by preadipocyte cell lines derived from murine marrow stroma. *J Cell Physiol* 1982;112:123–127.

260. Breems DA, Blokland EA, Siebel KE, et al. Stroma-contact prevents loss of hematopoietic stem cell quality during ex vivo expansion of CD34+ mobilized peripheral blood stem cells. *Blood* 1998;91:111–117.

261. Zipori D, Duksin D, Tamir M, et al. Cultured mouse marrow stromal cell lines, II: distinct subtypes differing in morphology, collagen types, myelopoietic factors, and leukemic cell growth modulating activities. *J Cell Physiol* 1985;122:81–90.

262. Zipori D, Kalai M, Tamir M. Restrictins: stromal cell associated factors that control cell organization in hemopoietic tissues. *Nat Immun Cell Growth Regul* 1988;7:185–192.

263. Gimble JM, Dorheim M-A, Cheng Q, et al. Adipogenesis in a murine bone marrow stromal cell line capable of supporting B lineage lymphocyte growth

and proliferation: biochemical and molecular characterization. *Eur J Immunol* 1990;20:379–387.

264. Zipori D. Cultured stromal cell lines from hemopoietic tissues. In: Tavassoli M, ed. *Handbook of the hematopoietic microenvironment*, 1st ed. Clifton, NJ: Humana Press, 1989:287–333.

265. Perkins S, Fleischman RA. Stromal cell progeny of murine bone marrow fibroblast colony-forming units are clonal endothelial-like cells that express collagen IV and laminin. *Blood* 1990;75:620–625.

266. Zipori D, Toledo J, von der Mark K. Phenotypic heterogeneity among stromal cell lines from mouse bone marrow disclosed in their extracellular matrix composition and interactions with normal and leukemic cells. *Blood* 1985;66:447–455.

267. Zipori D, Friedman A, Tamir M, et al. Cultured mouse marrow cell lines: interactions between fibroblastoid cells and monocytes. *J Cell Physiol* 1984;118:143–152.

268. Garnett HM, Harigaya K, Cronkite EP. Influence of a fibroblastoid cell line derived from murine bone marrow (H-1 cells) on stem cell proliferation. *Proc Soc Exp Biol Med* 1984;175:70–73.

269. Graham GJ, Wright EG, Hewick R, et al. Identification and characterization of an inhibitor of haemopoietic stem cell proliferation. *Nature* 1990;344:442–444.

270. Gimble JM, Pietrangeli C, Henley A, et al. Characterization of murine bone marrow and spleen-derived stromal cells: analysis of leukocyte marker and growth factor mRNA transcript levels. *Blood* 1989;74:303–311.

271. Pojda Z, Dexter TM, Lord BI. Production of a multipotential cell (CFU-S) proliferation inhibitor by various populations of mouse and human macrophages. *Br J Haematol* 1988;68:153–157.

272. Lenfant M, Wdzieczak-Bakala J, Guittet E, et al. Inhibitor of hematopoietic pluripotent stem cell proliferation: purification and determination of its structure. *Proc Natl Acad Sci U S A* 1989;86:779–782.

273. Pragnell IB, Wright EG, Lorimore SA, et al. The effect of stem cell proliferation regulators demonstrated with an in vitro assay. *Blood* 1988;72:196–201.

274. Wolpe SD, Cerami A. Macrophage inflammatory proteins 1 and 2: members of a novel superfamily of cytokines. *FASEB J* 1989;3:2565–2573.

274a. Broxmeyer H. Negative regulators of hematopoiesis. In: Wright D, Greenberger J, eds. *Long-term bone marrow culture: present experience and future possibilities*. New York: Alan R. Liss, 1984.

275. Zipori D. Stromal cells from the bone marrow: evidence for a restrictive role in regulation of hemopoiesis. *Eur J Haematol* 1989;42:225–232.

276. Verfaillie CM, Burroughs JM. Negative feedback regulation by direct stroma-progenitor contact of human CD34+/DR– progenitor proliferation. *Blood* 1992;80:22a.

277. Zipori D, Tamir M, Toledo J, et al. Differentiation stage and lineage-specific inhibitor from the stroma of mouse bone marrow that restricts lymphoma cell growth. *Proc Natl Acad Sci U S A* 1986;83:4547–4551.

278. Bernstein SE, Russell ES, Keighley G. Two hereditary mouse anemias (*Sl/Sl^d* and *W/W^v*) deficient in response to erythropoietin. *Ann N Y Acad Sci* 1968;149:475–485.

279. Altus MS, Bernstein SE, Russell ES, et al. Defect extrinsic to stem cells in spleens of *steel* anemic mice. *Proc Soc Exp Biol Med* 1971;138:985–988.

280. Fried W, Chamberlin W, Knospe WH, et al. Studies on the defective haematopoietic microenvironment of *Sl/Sl^d* mice. *Br J Haematol* 1973;24:643–650.

281. Russell ES. Hereditary anemias of the mouse: a review for geneticists. *Adv Genet* 1979;20:357–459.

282. Ruscetti FW, Boggs DR, Torok BJ, et al. Reduced blood and marrow neutrophils and granulocytic colony-forming cells in S1/S1d mice. *Proc Soc Exp Biol Med* 1976;152:398–402.

283. Ebbe S, Phalen E, Stohlman F Jr. Abnormalities of megakaryocytes in *Sl/Sl^d* mice. *Blood* 1973;42:865–871.

284. Chabot B, Stephenson DA, Chapman VM, et al. The proto-oncogene *c-kit* encoding a transmembrane tyrosine kinase receptor maps to the mouse W locus. *Nature* 1988;335:88–89.

285. Geissler EN, Ryan MA, Housman DE. The *dominant-white spotting (W)* locus of the mouse encodes the *c-kit* proto-oncogene. *Cell* 1988;55:185–192.

286. Reith AD, Rottapel R, Giddens E, et al. W mutant mice with mild or severe developmental defects contain distinct point mutations in the kinase domain of the c-kit receptor. *Genes Dev* 1990;4:390–400.

287. McCulloch EA, Siminovitch L, Till JE, et al. The cellular basis of the genetically determined hemopoietic defect in anemic mice of genotype *Sl-Sl^d*. *Blood* 1965;26:399–410.

288. Williams DE, Eisenman J, Baird A, et al. Identification of a ligand for the c-kit proto-oncogene. *Cell* 1990;63:167–174.

289. Zsebo KM, Wypych J, McNiece IK, et al. Identification, purification, and biological characterization of hematopoietic stem cell factor from buffalo rat liver-conditioned medium. *Cell* 1990;63:195–201.

290. Martin FH, Suggs SV, Langley KE, et al. Primary structure and functional expression of rat and human stem cell factor DNAs. *Cell* 1990;63:203–211.

291. Nocka K, Buck J, Levi E, et al. Candidate ligand for the *c-kit* transmembrane kinase receptor: KL, a fibroblast derived growth factor stimulates mast cells and erythroid progenitors. *EMBO J* 1990;9:3287–3294.

292. Huang E, Nocka K, Beier DR, et al. The hematopoietic growth factor KL is encoded at the *Sl* locus and is the ligand of the *c-kit* receptor, the gene product of the *W* locus. *Cell* 1990;63:225–233.

293. Copeland NG, Gilbert DJ, Cho BC, et al. Mast cell growth factor maps near the steel locus on mouse chromosome 10 and is deleted in a number of steel alleles. *Cell* 1990;63:175–183.

294. Zsebo KM, Williams DA, Geissler EN, et al. Stem cell factor is encoded at the *Sl* locus of the mouse and is the ligand for the c-kit tyrosine kinase receptor. *Cell* 1990;63:213–224.

295. Bernstein SE. Tissue transplantation as an analytic and therapeutic tool in hereditary anemias. *Am J Surg* 1970;119:448–451.

296. Dexter TM, Moore MA. In vitro duplication and "cure" of haemopoietic defects in genetically anaemic mice. *Nature* 1977;269:412–414.

297. Witte ON. Steel locus defines new multipotent growth factor. *Cell* 1990;63:5–6.

298. Williams DA. *Dominant white spotting* and *steel mutants* in hematopoiesis. In: Zon L, ed. *Hematopoiesis*. New York: Oxford University Press, 2001:647–662.

299. Botwell TH, Callender S, Mallett B, et al. Study of erythropoiesis using tracer quantities of radioactive iron. *Br J Haematol* 1956;2:1–16.

300. Donohoe DM, Reiff RH, Hanson ML, et al. Quantitative measurement of the erythrocytic and granulocytic cells of the marrow and blood. *J Clin Invest* 1958;37:1571–1576.

301. Lajtha LG, Gilbert CW, Guzman EE. Kinetics of haematopoietic colony growth. *Br J Haematol* 1971;20:343.

302. Hillman RS, Finch CA. Erythropoiesis: normal and abnormal. *Semin Hematol* 1967;4:327–336.

303. Hillman RS, Giblett ER. Red cell membrane alteration associated with "marrow stress." *J Clin Invest* 1965;44:1730.

304. Hanna IR, Spicer SS, Green WB, et al. Shortening of the cell-cycle time of erythroid precursors in response to anaemia. *Br J Haematol* 1969;16:381.

305. Eaves CJ, Eaves AC. Erythroid progenitor cell numbers in human marrow—implications for regulation. *J Exp Hematol* 1979;7:54.

306. Patel VP, Lodish HF. Loss of adhesion of murine erythroleukemia cells to fibronectin during erythroid differentiation. *Science* 1984;224:996–998.

307. Patel VP, Lodish HF. The fibronectin receptor on mammalian erythroid precursor cells: characterization and developmental regulation. *J Cell Biol* 1986;102:449–456.

308. Patel VP, Lodish HF. A fibronectin matrix is required for differentiation of murine erythroleukemia cells into reticulocytes. *J Cell Biol* 1987;105:3105–3118.

309. Springer TA. Adhesion receptors of the immune system. *Nature* 1990;346:425–434.

310. Butcher EC. Leukocyte-endothelial cell recognition: three (or more) steps to specificity and diversity. *Cell* 1991;67:1033–1036.

311. Hynes RO. Integrins: versatility, modulation, and signaling in cell adhesion. *Cell* 1992;69:11–25.

312. Williams DA, Rios M, Stephens C, et al. Interactions of primitive hematopoietic stem cells with the hematopoietic microenvironment: role of fibronectin and VLA-4 integrin. *Nature* 1991;352:438–441.

313. Verfaillie CM, McCarthy JB, McGlave PB. Differentiation of primitive human multipotent hematopoietic progenitors into single lineage clonogenic progenitors is accompanied by alterations in their interaction with fibronectin. *J Exp Med* 1991;174:693–703.

314. Simmons PJ, Masinovsky B, Longenecker BM, et al. Vascular cell adhesion molecule-1 expressed by bone marrow stromal cells mediates the binding of hematopoietic progenitor cells. *Blood* 1992;80:388–395.

315. Teixido J, Parker CM, Kassner PD, et al. Functional and structural analysis of VLA-4 integrin alpha 4 subunit cleavage. *J Biol Chem* 1992;267:1786–1791.

316. Papayannopoulou T, Nakamoto B. Peripheralization of hemopoietic progenitors in primates treated with anti-VLA4 integrin. *Proc Natl Acad Sci U S A* 1993;90:9374–9378.

317. Papayannopoulou T, Craddock C, Nakamoto B, et al. The VLA4/VCAM-1 adhesion pathway defines contrasting mechanisms of lodgement of transplanted murine hemopoietic progenitors between bone marrow and spleen. *Proc Natl Acad Sci U S A* 1995;92:9647–9651.

318. Hemler ME. VLA proteins in the integrin family: structures, functions, and their role on leukocytes. *Annu Rev Immunol* 1990;8:365–400.

319. Yoder MC, Williams DA. Matrix molecule interactions with hematopoietic stem cells. *Exp Hematol* 1995;23:961–967.

320. Mould AP, Humphries MJ. Identification of a novel recognition sequence for the integrin 4 1 in the COOH-terminal heparin-binding domain of fibronectin. *EMBO J* 1991;10:4089–4095.

321. Potocnik AJ, Brakebusch C, Fassler R. Fetal and adult hematopoietic stem cells require beta1 integrin function for colonizing fetal liver, spleen, and bone marrow. *Immunity* 2000;12:653–663.

322. Levesque J, Zannettino A, Pudney M, et al. PSGL-1 mediated adhesion of human hematopoietic progenitors to P-selectin results in suppression of hematopoiesis. *Immunity* 1999;11:369–378.

323. Pruijt JF, Willemze R, Fibbe WE. Mechanisms underlying hematopoietic stem cell mobilization induced by the CXC chemokine interleukin-8. *Curr Opin Hematol* 1999;6:152–158.

324. Aiuti A, Webb IJ, Bleul C, et al. The chemokine SDF-1 is a chemoattractant for human CD34+ hematopoietic progenitor cells and provides a new mechanism to explain the mobilization of CD34+ progenitors to peripheral blood. *J Exp Med* 1997;185:111–120.

325. Mohle R, Bautz F, Rafii S, et al. Regulation of transendothelial migration of hematopoietic progenitor cells. *Ann N Y Acad Sci* 1999;872:176–185, discussion 185–186.

326. Yang FC, Atkinson SJ, Gu Y, et al. Rac and Cdc42 GTPases control hematopoietic stem cell shape, adhesion, migration, and mobilization. *Proc Natl Acad Sci U S A* 2001;98:5614–5618.

327. Baehner RL. Disorders of leukocytes leading to recurrent infection. *Pediatr Clin North Am* 1972;19:935–956.

328. Cartwright GE, Athens JW, Wintrobe MM. The kinetics of granulopoiesis in normal man. *Blood* 1964;24:780.
329. Cronkite EP, Fliedner TM. Granulocytopoiesis. *N Engl J Med* 1964;270:1347.
330. Morstyn G, Cambell L, Souza LM, et al. Effect of granulocyte colony stimulating factor on neutropenia induced by cytotoxic chemotherapy. *Lancet* 1988;1:667–672.
331. Glaspy JA, Golde DW. Clinical applications of the myeloid growth factors. *Semin Hematol* 1989;26:14–17.
332. Athens JW, Raab SO, Haab OP, et al. Leukokinetic studies, III: the distribution of granulocytes in the blood of normal subjects. *J Clin Invest* 1961;40:159.
333. Craddock GG Jr, Perry S, Ventzke LE, et al. Evaluation of marrow granulocyte reserves in normal and disease states. *Blood* 1960;15:840.
334. Todd RF, Freyer DR. The CD11/CD18 leukocyte glycoprotein deficiency. In: Curnutte JT, ed. *Hematology/oncology clinics of North America*. Philadelphia: WB Saunders, 1988:13–31.
335. Sanchez-Madrid F, Nagy JA, Robbins E, et al. A human leukocyte differentiation antigen family with distinct alpha-subunits and a common beta-subunit: the lymphocyte function-associated antigen (LFA-1), the C3bi complement receptor (OKM1/Mac-1), and the p150,95 molecule. *J Exp Med* 1983;158:1785–1803.
336. Dana N, Todd RF III, Pitt J, et al. Deficiency of a surface membrane glycoprotein (Mo1) in man. *J Clin Invest* 1984;73:153.
337. Arnaout MA, Spits H, Terhorst C, et al. Deficiency of a leukocyte surface glycoprotein (LFA-1) in two patients with Mo1 deficiency: effects of cell activation on Mo1/LFA-1 surface expression in normal and deficient leukocytes. *J Clin Invest* 1984;74:1291.
338. Beatty PG, Ochs HD, Harlan JM, et al. Absence of monoclonal-antibody defined protein complex in a boy with abnormal leukocyte function. *Lancet* 1984;1:535.
339. Springer TA, Thompson WS, Miller LJ, et al. Inherited deficiency of the Mac-1, LFA-1, p150-95 glycoprotein family and its molecular basis. *J Exp Med* 1986;160:1901–1918.
340. Gallatin M, St John TP, Siegelman M, et al. Lymphocyte homing receptors. *Cell* 1986;44:673–680.
341. Gordon MY. Annotation: adhesive properties of haemopoietic stem cells. *Br J Haematol* 1988;68:149–151.
342. Aizawa S, Tavassoli M. Marrow uptake of galactosyl-containing neoglycoproteins: implications in stem cell homing. *J Exp Hematol* 1988;16:811–813.
343. Aizawa S, Tavassoli M. Interaction of murine granulocyte-macrophage progenitors and supporting stroma involves a recognition mechanism with galactosyl and mannosyl specificities. *J Clin Invest* 1987;80:1698–1705.
344. Verfaillie C, McCarthy J, McGlave P. Differentiation of primitive human lin-34+DR-hematopoietic progenitors is accompanied by transition of adhesion from the heparin-binding domain to the cell-binding domain of fibronectin (FN). *Blood* 1992;76:10–125a.
345. De Bruyn PPH, Michelson S, Thomas TB. The migration of blood cells of the bone marrow through the sinusoidal wall. *J Morphol* 1971;133:417–437.
346. Lichtman MA. Cellular deformability during maturation of the myeloblast: possible role in marrow egress. *N Engl J Med* 1970;283:943–948.
347. Lichtman MA, Weed RI. Alteration of the cell periphery during granulocyte maturation: relationship to cell function. *Blood* 1972;39:301–316.
348. Lichtman MA, Weed RI. Peripheral cytoplasmic characteristics of leukocytes in monocytic leukemia: relationship to clinical manifestations. *Blood* 1972;40:52–61.
349. Boggs DR, Cartwright GE, Wintrobe MM. Neutrophilia-inducing activity in plasma of dogs recovering from drug induced myelotoxicity. *Am J Physiol* 1966;211:51–60.
350. Boggs DR, Marsh JC, Chervenick PA, et al. Neutrophil releasing activity in plasma of normal human subjects injected with endotoxin. *Proc Soc Exp Biol Med* 1968;127:689–693.
351. Weiss L. Transmural cellular passage in vascular sinuses of rat bone marrow. *Blood* 1970;36:189.
352. Chamberlain JK, Leblond PF, Weed RI. Reduction of adventital cell cover: an early direct effect of erythropoietin on bone marrow ultrastructure. *Blood Cells* 1975;1:655–674.
353. Metcalf D. *The hemopoietic growth factors*. Amsterdam: Elsevier Science, 1984.
354. Das SK, Stanley ER, Guilbert LJ, et al. Human colony-stimulating factor (CSF-1) radioimmunoassay: resolution of three subclasses of human colony-stimulating factors. *Blood* 1981;58:630–641.
355. Miyake T, Kung CK, Goldwasser E. Purification of human erythropoietin. *J Biol Chem* 1977;252:5558–5564.
356. Welte K, Platzer E, Lu L, et al. Purification and biochemical characterization of human pluripotent hematopoietic colony stimulating factor. *Proc Natl Acad Sci U S A* 1985;82:1526–1530.
357. Lyman SD, James L, Johnson L, et al. Cloning of the human homologue of the murine flt3 ligand: a growth factor for early hematopoietic progenitor cells. *Blood* 1994;83:2795–2801.
358. Lyman SD, James L, Vanden Bos T, et al. Molecular cloning of a ligand for the flt3/flk-2 tyrosine kinase receptor: a proliferative factor for primitive hematopoietic cells. *Cell* 1993;75:1157–1167.
359. Hannum C, Culpepper J, Campbell D, et al. Ligand for FLT3/FLK2 receptor tyrosine kinase regulates growth of haematopoietic stem cells and is encoded by variant RNAs. *Nature* 1994;368:643–648.
360. Bussolino F, Wang JM, Defilippi P, et al. Granulocyte- and granulocyte-macrophage-colony stimulating factors induce human endothelial cells to migrate and proliferate. *Nature* 1989;337:471–473.
361. Athanassakis I, Bleackley RC, Paetkau V, et al. The immunostimulatory effect of T cells and T cell lymphokines on murine fetally derived placental cells. *J Immunol* 1987;138:37–44.
362. Pollard JW, Bartocci A, Arceci R, et al. Apparent role of the macrophage growth factors, CSF-1, in placental development. *Nature* 1987;330:484–486.
363. Arceci RJ, Shanahan F, Stanley ER, et al. Temporal expression and location of colony-stimulating factor 1 (SCF-1) and its receptor in the female reproductive tract are consistent with CSF-1-regulated placental development. *Proc Natl Acad Sci U S A* 1989;86:8818–8822.
364. Gearing DP, King JA, Gough NM, et al. Expression cloning of a receptor for human granulocyte-macrophage colony-stimulating factor. *EMBO J* 1989;8:3667–3676.
365. Farrar WL, Vinocour M, Hill JM. In situ hybridization histochemistry localization of interleukin-3 mRNA in mouse brain. *Blood* 1989;73:137–140.
366. Sieff CA. Hematopoietic growth factors. *J Clin Invest* 1987;79:1549–1557.
367. Nicola NA. Hemopoietic cell growth factors and their receptors. *Annu Rev Biochem* 1989;58:45–77.
368. Nagata S, Tsuchiya M, Asano S, et al. Molecular cloning and expression of cDNA for human granulocyte colony-stimulating factor. *Nature* 1986;319:415–418.
369. Souza LM, Boone TC, Gabrilove J, et al. Recombinant human granulocyte colony-stimulating factor: effects on normal and leukemic myeloid cells. *Science* 1986;232:61–65.
370. Kawasaki ES, Ladner MB, Wang AM, et al. Molecular cloning of a complimentary DNA encoding human macrophage-specific colony-stimulating factor (CFS-1). *Science* 1985;230:291–296.
371. Jacobs KC, Shoemaker C, Rudersdorf R, et al. Isolation and characterization of genomic and cDNA clones of human erythropoietin. *Nature* 1985;313:806–810.
372. Wong GG, Witek JS, Temple PA, et al. Human GM-CSF: molecular cloning of the complementary DNA and purification of the natural and recombinant proteins. *Science* 1985;228:810–815.
373. Yang Y-C, Ciarletta AB, Temple PA, et al. Human IL-3 (Multi-CSF): identification by expression cloning of a novel hematopoietic growth factor related to murine IL-3. *Cell* 1986;47:3–10.
374. Metcalf D. *The molecular control of blood cells*. Cambridge, MA: Harvard University Press, 1988.
375. Walker F, Nicola NA, Metcalf D, et al. Hierarchical down-modulation of hemopoietic growth factor receptors. *Cell* 1985;43:269–276.
376. Sims JE, March CJ, Cosman D, et al. cDNA expression cloning of the IL-1 receptor, a member of the immunoglobulin superfamily. *Science* 1988;241:585–589.
377. Yamasaki K, Taga T, Hirata Y, et al. Expression of the human interleukin-6 (BSF-2/IFNbeta 2) receptor. *Science* 1988;241:825–828.
378. D'Andrea AD, Lodish HF, Wong GG. Expression cloning of the murine erythropoietin receptor. *Cell* 1989;57:277–285.
379. Itoh N, Yonehara S, Schreurs J, et al. Cloning of an interleukin-3 receptor gene: a member of a distinct receptor gene family. *Science* 1990;247:324–327.
380. Idzerda RL, March CL, Mosley B, et al. Human interleukin 4 receptor confers biological responsiveness and defines a novel receptor superfamily. *J Exp Med* 1990;171:861–873.
381. Mosley B, Beckmann MP, March CJ, et al. The murine interleukin-4 receptor: molecular cloning and characterization of secreted and membrane bound forms. *Cell* 1989;59:335–348.
382. Goodwin R, Friend D, Ziegler SF, et al. Cloning of the human and murine interleukin-7 receptors: demonstration of a soluble form and homology to a new receptor superfamily. *Cell* 1990;60:941–951.
383. Fukunaga R, Ishizaka-Ikeda E, Seto Y, et al. Expression cloning of a receptor for murine granulocyte colony-stimulating factor. *Cell* 1990;61:341–350.
384. Fukunaga R, Seto Y, Mizushima S, et al. Three different mRNAs encoding human granulocyte colony-stimulating factor receptor. *Proc Natl Acad Sci U S A* 1990;87:8702–8706.
385. Cosman D, Lyman SD, Idzerda RL, et al. A new cytokine receptor superfamily. *Trends Biochem Sci* 1990;15:265–270.
386. Hatakeyama M, Tsudo M, Minamoto S, et al. Interleukin-2 receptor beta chain gene: generation of three receptor forms by cloned human alpha and beta chain cDNA's. *Science* 1989;244:551–556.
387. Leung DW, Spencer SA, Cachianes G, et al. Growth hormone receptor and serum binding protein: purification, cloning and expression. *Nature* 1987;330:537–543.
388. Boutin J-M, Jolicoeur C, Okamura H, et al. Cloning and expression of the rat prolactin receptor, a member of the growth hormone/prolactin receptor gene family. *Cell* 1988;53:69–77.
389. Edery M, Jolicoeur C, Levi-Meyrueis C, et al. Identification and sequence analysis of a second form of prolactin receptor by molecular cloning of complementary DNA from rabbit mammary gland. *Proc Natl Acad Sci U S A* 1989;86:2112–2116.
390. Crosier KE, Wong GG, Mathey-Prevot B, et al. A functional isoform of the human granulocyte-macrophage colony-stimulating factor receptor contains a unique cytoplasmic domain. *Proc Natl Acad Sci U S A* 1991;88:7744.
391. Lu HS, Boone TC, Souza LM, et al. Disulfide and secondary structures of recombinant human granulocyte colony stimulating factor. *Arch Biochem Biophys* 1989;268:81–92.
392. Brandhuber BJ, Boone T, Kenney WC, et al. Three-dimensional structure of interleukin-2. *Science* 1987;238:1707–1709.
393. de Vos AM, Ultsch M, Kossiakoff AA. Human growth hormone and extracellular domain of its receptor: crystal structure of the complex. *Science* 1992;255:306–312.

394. Cunningham BC, Wells JA. High-resolution epitope mapping of hGH-receptor interactions by alanine-scanning mutagenesis. *Science* 1989;244:1081–1085.

395. Bazan JF. Structural design and molecular evolution of a cytokine receptor superfamily. *Proc Natl Acad Sci U S A* 1990;87:6934–6938.

396. Sakamaki K, Miyajima I, Kitamura T, et al. Critical cytoplasmic domains of the common beta subunit of the human GM-CSF, IL-3 and IL-5 receptors for growth signal transduction and tyrosine phosphorylation. *EMBO J* 1992;11:3541–3549.

397. Mui A-F, Cutler R, Alai M, et al. Steel factor and interleukin-3 stimulate the tyrosine phosphorylation of p95vav in hematopoietic cell lines. *Exp Hematol* 1992;20:752(abst).

398. Silvennoinen O, Witthuhn BA, Quelle FW, et al. Structure of the murine Jak2 protein-tyrosine kinase and its role in interleukin 3 signal transduction. *Proc Natl Acad Sci U S A* 1993;90:8429–8433.

399. Ward AC, Touw I, Yoshimura A. The Jak-Stat pathway in normal and perturbed hematopoiesis. *Blood* 2000;95:19–29.

400. Nosaka T, Kitamura T. Janus kinases (JAKs) and signal transducers and activators of transcription (STATs) in hematopoietic cells. *Int J Hematol* 1999; 71:309.

401. Imada K, Leonard WJ. The Jak-STAT pathway. *Mol Immunol* 2000;37:1–11.

402. Darnell JE Jr, Kerr IM, Stark GR. Jak-STAT pathways and transcriptional activation in response to IFNs and other extracellular signaling proteins. *Science* 1994;264:1415–1421.

403. Witthuhn BA, Quelle FW, Silvennoinen O, et al. JAK2 associates with the erythropoietin receptor and is tyrosine phosphorylated and activated following stimulation with erythropoietin. *Cell* 1993;74:227–236.

404. Feng J, Witthuhn BA, Matsuda T, et al. Activation of Jak2 catalytic activity requires phosphorylation of Y1007 in the kinase activation loop. *Mol Cell Biol* 1997;17:2497–2501.

405. Murakami M, Narazaki M, Hibi M, et al. Critical cytoplasmic region of the interleukin 6 signal transducer gp130 is conserved in the cytokine receptor family. *Proc Natl Acad Sci U S A* 1991;88:11349–11353.

406. Shuai K, Horvath CM, Huang LH, et al. Interferon activation of the transcription factor Stat91 involves dimerization through SH2-phosphotyrosyl peptide interactions. *Cell* 1994;76:821–828.

407. Heim MH, Kerr IM, Stark GR, et al. Contribution of STAT SH2 groups to specific interferon signaling by the Jak-STAT pathway. *Science* 1995;267:1347–1349.

408. Stahl N, Farruggella TJ, Boulton TG, et al. Choice of STATs and other substrates specified by modular tyrosine-based motifs in cytokine receptors. *Science* 1995;267:1349–1353.

409. Lamb P, Seidel HM, Haslam J, et al. STAT protein complexes activated by interferon-gamma and gp130 signaling molecules differ in their sequence preferences and transcriptional induction properties. *Nucleic Acids Res* 1995; 23:3283–3289.

410. Seidel HM, Milocco LH, Lamb P, et al. Spacing of palindromic half sites as a determinant of selective STAT (signal transducers and activators of transcription) DNA binding and transcriptional activity. *Proc Natl Acad Sci U S A* 1995;92:3041–3045.

411. Decker T, Kovarik P, Meinke A. GAS elements: a few nucleotides with a major impact on cytokine-induced gene expression. *J Interferon Cytokine Res* 1997;17:121–134.

412. Rodig SJ, Meraz MA, White JM, et al. Disruption of the Jak1 gene demonstrates obligatory and nonredundant roles of the Jaks in cytokine-induced biologic responses. *Cell* 1998;93:373–383.

413. Neubauer H, Cumano A, Muller M, et al. Jak2 deficiency defines an essential developmental checkpoint in definitive hematopoiesis. *Cell* 1998;93:397–409.

414. Parganas E, Wang D, Stravopodis D, et al. Jak2 is essential for signaling through a variety of cytokine receptors. *Cell* 1998;93:385–395.

415. Noguchi M, Yi H, Rosenblatt HM, et al. Interleukin-2 receptor gamma chain mutation results in X-linked severe combined immunodeficiency in humans. *Cell* 1993;73:147–157.

416. Thomis DC, Gurniak CB, Tivol E, et al. Defects in B lymphocyte maturation and T lymphocyte activation in mice lacking Jak3. *Science* 1995;270:794–797.

417. Nosaka T, van Deursen JM, Tripp RA, et al. Defective lymphoid development in mice lacking Jak3. *Science* 1995;270:800–802.

418. Park SY, Saijo K, Takahashi T, et al. Developmental defects of lymphoid cells in Jak3 kinase-deficient mice. *Immunity* 1995;3:771–782.

419. Lacronique V, Boureux A, Valle VD, et al. A TEL-JAK2 fusion protein with constitutive kinase activity in human leukemia. *Science* 1997;278:1309–1312.

420. Peeters P, Raynaud SD, Cools J, et al. Fusion of TEL, the ETS-variant gene 6 (ETV6), to the receptor-associated kinase JAK2 as a result of t(9;12) in a lymphoid and t(9;15;12) in a myeloid leukemia. *Blood* 1997;90:2535–2540.

421. Copeland NG, Gilbert DJ, Schindler C, et al. Distribution of the mammalian Stat gene family in mouse chromosomes. *Genomics* 1995;29:225–228.

422. Thierfelder WE, van Deursen JM, Yamamoto K, et al. Requirement for Stat4 in interleukin-12-mediated responses of natural killer and T cells. *Nature* 1996;382:171–174.

423. Kaplan MH, Sun YL, Hoey T, et al. Impaired IL-12 responses and enhanced development of Th2 cells in Stat4-deficient mice. *Nature* 1996;382:174–177.

424. Takeda K, Tanaka T, Shi W, et al. Essential role of Stat6 in IL-4 signalling. *Nature* 1996;380:627–630.

425. Kaplan MH, Schindler U, Smiley ST, et al. Stat6 is required for mediating responses to IL-4 and for development of Th2 cells. *Immunity* 1996;4:313–319.

426. Shimoda K, van Deursen J, Sangster MY, et al. Lack of IL-4-induced Th2 response and IgE class switching in mice with disrupted Stat6 gene. *Nature* 1996;380:630–633.

427. Meraz MA, White JM, Sheehan KC, et al. Targeted disruption of the Stat1 gene in mice reveals unexpected physiologic specificity in the JAK-STAT signaling pathway. *Cell* 1996;84:431–442.

428. Teglund S, McKay C, Schuetz E, et al. Stat5a and Stat5b proteins have essential and nonessential, or redundant, roles in cytokine responses. *Cell* 1998;93:841–850.

429. Takeda K, Noguchi K, Shi W, et al. Targeted disruption of the mouse Stat3 gene leads to early embryonic lethality. *Proc Natl Acad Sci U S A* 1997;94:3801–3804.

430. Moriggl R, Topham DJ, Teglund S, et al. Stat5 is essential for IL-2-induced cell cycle progression of peripheral T cells. *Immunity* 1999;10:249–259.

431. Socolovsky M, Fallon AE, Wang S, et al. Fetal anemia and apoptosis of red cell progenitors in Stat5a-/-5b-/- mice: a direct role for Stat5 in Bcl-X(L) induction. *Cell* 1999;98:181–191.

432. Feldman GM, Rosenthal LA, Liu X, et al. STAT5A-deficient mice demonstrate a defect in granulocyte-macrophage colony-stimulating factor-induced proliferation and gene expression. *Blood* 1997;90:1768–1776.

433. Imada K, Bloom ET, Nakajima H, et al. Stat5b is essential for natural killer cell-mediated proliferation and cytolytic activity. *J Exp Med* 1998;188:2067–2074.

434. Socolovsky M, Nam H, Fleming MD, et al. Ineffective erythropoiesis in Stat5a(−/−)5b(−/−) mice due to decreased survival of early erythroblasts. *Blood* 2001;98:3261–3273.

435. Nakajima H, Liu XW, Wynshaw-Boris A, et al. An indirect effect of Stat5a in IL-2-induced proliferation: a critical role for Stat5a in IL-2-mediated IL-2 receptor alpha chain induction. *Immunity* 1997;7:691–701.

436. Nosaka T, Kawashima T, Misawa K, et al. STAT5 as a molecular regulator of proliferation, differentiation and apoptosis in hematopoietic cells. *EMBO J* 1999;18:4754–4765.

437. Pierce JH, Ruggiero M, Fleming TP, et al. Signal transduction through the EGF receptor transfected in IL-3-dependent hematopoietic cells. *Science* 1988;239:628–631.

438. Wheeler EF, Rettenmeier CW, Look AT, et al. The v-fms oncogene induces factor independence and tumorigenicity in CSF-1 dependent macrophage cell line. *Nature* 1986;324:377–380.

439. Wheeler EF, Askew D, May S, et al. The v-fms oncogene induces factor–independent growth and transformation of the interleukin-3-dependent myeloid cell line FDC-P1. *Mol Cell Biol* 1987;7:1673–1680.

440. Watson JD, Jenkins DR, Eszes M, et al. Effect of granulocyte-macrophage colony-stimulating factor and interleukin 3 on the v-src oncogene. *J Immunol* 1988;140:501–507.

441. Satoh T, Nakafuku M, Miyajima A, et al. Involvement of ras p21 protein in signal-transduction pathways from interleukin 2, interleukin 3, and granulocyte/macrophage colony-stimulating factor, but not from interleukin 4. *Proc Natl Acad Sci U S A* 1991;88:3314–3318.

442. Duronio V, Welham MJ, Abraham S, et al. p21ras activation via hemopoietin receptors and c-kit requires tyrosine kinase activity but not tyrosine phosphorylation of p21ras GTPase-activating protein. *Proc Natl Acad Sci U S A* 1992;89:1587–1591.

443. Gulbins E, Coggeshall KM, Baier G, et al. Tyrosine kinase-stimulated guanine nucleotide exchange activity of vav in T cell activation. *Science* 1993;260: 822–825.

444. McCormick F. Signal transduction: how receptors turn Ras on [News, comment]. *Nature* 1993;363:15–16.

445. Feig LA. The many roads that lead to Ras. *Science* 1993;260:767–768.

446. Moodie SA, Willumsen BM, Weber MJ, et al. Complexes of Ras.GTP with Raf-1 and mitogen-activated protein kinase kinase. *Science* 1993;260:1658–1661.

447. McColl SR, DiPersio JF, Caon AC, et al. Involvement of tyrosine kinases in the activation of human peripheral blood neutrophils by granulocyte-macrophage colony-stimulating factor. *Blood* 1991;78:1842–1852.

448. Schwartz EL, Chamberlin H, Brechbuhl AB. Regulation of c-myc expression by granulocyte-macrophage colony-stimulating factor in human leukemia cells. *Blood* 1991;77:2716–2723.

449. Berns A. Tumorigenesis in transgenic mice: identification and characterization of synergizing oncogenes. *J Cell Biochem* 1991;47:130–135.

450. Lilly M, Le T, Holland P, et al. Sustained expression of the pim-1 kinase is specifically induced in myeloid cells by cytokines whose receptors are structurally related. *Oncogene* 1992;7:727–732.

451. Farrar WL, Thomas TP, Anderson WB. Altered cytosol/membrane enzyme redistribution on interleukin-3 activation of protein kinase C. *Nature* 1985; 315:235–237.

452. Whetton AD, Monk PN, Consalvey SD, et al. Interleukin 3 stimulates proliferation via protein kinase C activation without increasing inositol lipid turnover. *Proc Natl Acad Sci U S A* 1988;85:3284–3288.

453. Whetton AD, Monk PN, Consalvey SD, et al. The haematopoietic growth factors interleukin 3 and colony stimulating factor-1 stimulate proliferation but do not induce inositol lipid breakdown in murine bone-marrow-derived macrophages. *EMBO J* 1986;5:3281–3286.

454. Klingmuller U, Wu H, Hsiao JG, et al. Identification of a novel pathway important for proliferation and differentiation of primary erythroid progenitors. *Proc Natl Acad Sci U S A* 1997;94:3016–3021.

455. You M, Yu DH, Feng GS. Shp-2 tyrosine phosphatase functions as a negative regulator of the interferon-stimulated Jak/STAT pathway. *Mol Cell Biol* 1999;19:2416–2424.

456. Klingmuller U, Lorenz U, Cantley LC, et al. Specific recruitment of SH-PTP1 to the erythropoietin receptor causes inactivation of JAK2 and termination of proliferative signals. *Cell* 1995;80:729–738.

457. Fuhrer DK, Feng GS, Yang YC. Syp associates with gp130 and Janus kinase 2 in response to interleukin-11 in 3T3-L1 mouse preadipocytes. *J Biol Chem* 1995;270:24826–24830.

458. Jiao H, Berrada K, Yang W, et al. Direct association with and dephosphorylation of Jak2 kinase by the SH2-domain-containing protein tyrosine phosphatase SHP-1. *Mol Cell Biol* 1996;16:6985–6992.

459. Carpenter LR, Farruggella TJ, Symes A, et al. Enhancing leptin response by preventing SH2-containing phosphatase 2 interaction with Ob receptor. *Proc Natl Acad Sci U S A* 1998;95:6061–6066.

460. Zhang JG, Farley A, Nicholson SE, et al. The conserved SOCS box motif in suppressors of cytokine signaling binds to elongins B and C and may couple bound proteins to proteasomal degradation. *Proc Natl Acad Sci U S A* 1999;96:2071–2076.

461. Shultz LD, Schweitzer PA, Rajan TV, et al. Mutations at the murine motheaten locus are within the hematopoietic cell protein-tyrosine phosphatase (Hcph) gene. *Cell* 1993;73:1445–1454.

462. Saxton TM, Pawson T. Morphogenetic movements at gastrulation require the SH2 tyrosine phosphatase Shp2. *Proc Natl Acad Sci U S A* 1999;96:3790–3795.

463. Liu L, Damen JE, Cutler RL, et al. Multiple cytokines stimulate the binding of a common 145-kilodalton protein to Shc at the Grb2 recognition site of Shc. *Mol Cell Biol* 1994;14:6926–6935.

464. Helgason CD, Damen JE, Rosten P, et al. Targeted disruption of SHIP leads to hemopoietic perturbations, lung pathology, and a shortened life span. *Genes Dev* 1998;12:1610–1620.

465. Krebs DL, Hilton DJ. SOCS: physiological suppressors of cytokine signaling. *J Cell Sci* 2000;113:2813–2819.

466. Yoshimura A, Ohkubo T, Kiguchi T, et al. A novel cytokine-inducible gene CIS encodes an SH2-containing protein that binds to tyrosine-phosphorylated interleukin 3 and erythropoietin receptors. *EMBO J* 1995;14:2816–2826.

467. Starr R, Willson TA, Viney EM, et al. A family of cytokine-inducible inhibitors of signaling. *Nature* 1997;387:917–928.

468. Hilton D, Richardson R, Alexander W, et al. Twenty proteins containing a C-terminal SOCS box form five structural classes. *Proc Natl Acad Sci U S A* 1998;95:114–119.

469. Matsumoto A, Masuhara M, Mitsui K, et al. CIS, a cytokine inducible SH2 protein, is a target of the JAK-STAT5 pathway and modulates STAT5 activation. *Blood* 1997;89:3148–3154.

470. Endo TA, Masuhara M, Yokouchi M, et al. A new protein containing an SH2 domain that inhibits JAK kinases. *Nature* 1997;387:921–924.

471. De Sepulveda P, Okkenhaug K, Rose JL, et al. Socs1 binds to multiple signalling proteins and suppresses steel factor-dependent proliferation. *EMBO J* 1999;18:904–915.

472. Starr R, Metcalf D, Elefanty AG, et al. Liver degeneration and lymphoid deficiencies in mice lacking suppressor of cytokine signaling-1. *Proc Natl Acad Sci U S A* 1998;95:14395–14399.

473. Naka T, Matsumoto T, Narazaki M, et al. Accelerated apoptosis of lymphocytes by augmented induction of Bax in SSI-1 (STAT-induced STAT inhibitor-1) deficient mice. *Proc Natl Acad Sci U S A* 1998;95:15577–15582.

474. Alexander WS, Starr R, Fenner JE, et al. SOCS1 is a critical inhibitor of interferon gamma signaling and prevents the potentially fatal neonatal actions of this cytokine. *Cell* 1999;98:597–608.

475. Marine JC, Topham DJ, McKay C, et al. SOCS1 deficiency causes a lymphocyte-dependent perinatal lethality. *Cell* 1999;98:609–616.

476. Marine JC, McKay C, Wang D, et al. SOCS3 is essential in the regulation of fetal liver erythropoiesis. *Cell* 1999;98:617–627.

477. Cohney SJ, Sanden D, Cacalano NA, et al. SOCS-3 is tyrosine phosphorylated in response to interleukin-2 and suppresses STAT5 phosphorylation and lymphocyte proliferation. *Mol Cell Biol* 1999;19:4980–4988.

478. Tilbrook PA, Ingley E, Williams JH, et al. Lyn tyrosine kinase is essential for erythropoietin-induced differentiation of J2E erythroid cells. *EMBO J* 1997;16:1610–1619.

479. Hibbs ML, Tarlinton DM, Armes J, et al. Multiple defects in the immune system of Lyn-deficient mice, culminating in autoimmune disease. *Cell* 1995;83:301–311.

480. Nishizumi H, Taniuchi I, Yamanashi Y, et al. Impaired proliferation of peripheral B cells and indication of autoimmune disease in lyn-deficient mice. *Immunity* 1995;3:549–560.

481. Damen JE, Cutler RL, Jiao H, et al. Phosphorylation of tyrosine 503 in the erythropoietin receptor (EpR) is essential for binding the P85 subunit of phosphatidylinositol (PI) 3-kinase and for EpR-associated PI 3-kinase activity. *J Biol Chem* 1995;270:23402–23408.

482. Sieff CA, Emerson SG, Mufson A, et al. Dependence of highly enriched human bone marrow progenitors on hemopoietic growth factors and their response to recombinant erythropoietin. *J Clin Invest* 1986;77:74–81.

483. Eaves CJ, Eaves AC. Erythropoietin (Ep) dose-response curves for three classes of erythroid progenitors in normal human marrow and in patients with polycythemia vera. *Blood* 1978;52:1196–1210.

484. Eaves AC, Eaves CJ. Erythropoiesis in culture. *J Clin Haematol* 1984;13:371–391.

485. Iscove NN. Erythropoietin-dependent stimulation of early erythropoiesis in adult bone marrow cultures by conditioned media from lectin stimulated mouse spleen cells. In: Golde DW, Cline MJ, Metcalf D, et al., eds. *Hematopoietic cell differentiation*. New York: Academic Press, 1978:37–52.

486. Sieff CA, Ekern SC, Nathan DG, et al. Combinations of recombinant colony-stimulating factors are required for optimal hematopoietic differentiation in serum-deprived culture. *Blood* 1989;73:688–693.

487. Valtieri M, Gabbianelli M, Pelosi E, et al. Erythropoietin alone induces erythroid burst formation by human embryonic but not adult BFU-E in unicellular serum-free culture. *Blood* 1989;74:460–470.

488. Koenig JM, Christensen RD. Neutropenia and thrombocytopenia in infants with Rh hemolytic disease. *J Pediatr* 1989;114:625–631.

489. Christensen RD, Koenig JM, Viskochil DH, et al. Down-modulation of neutrophil production by erythropoietin in human hematopoietic clones. *Blood* 1989;74:817–822.

490. Sawada K, Krantz SB, Dessypris EN, et al. Human colony-forming units-erythroid do not require accessory cells, but do require direct interaction with insulin-like growth factor I and/or insulin for erythroid development. *J Clin Invest* 1989;83:1701–1709.

491. Kurtz A, Jelkmann W. Insulin stimulates erythroid colony formation independently of erythropoietin. *Br J Haematol* 1983;53:311–316.

492. Yu J, Shao L, Vaughan J, et al. Characterization of the potentiation effect of activin on human erythroid colony formation in vitro. *Blood* 1989;73:952–960.

493. Smith JC, Price BM, van Nimmen K, et al. Identification of a potent Xenopus mesoderm-inducing factor as a homologue of activin A. *Nature* 1990;345:729–731.

494. Mangan KF, Chikkappa G, Sieler LZ, et al. Regulation of human blood erythroid burst-forming unit (BFU-E) proliferation by T lymphocyte subpopulations defined by Fc receptors and monoclonal antibodies. *Blood* 1982;59:990–996.

495. Torok-Storb BJ, Martin PJ, Hansen JA. Regulation of in vitro erythropoiesis by normal T cells: evidence for two T cell subsets with opposing functions. *Blood* 1981;58:171–174.

496. Lipton JM, Nadler LM, Canellos GP, et al. Evidence for genetic restriction in the suppression of erythropoiesis by a unique subset of T lymphocytes in man. *J Clin Invest* 1983;72:694–706.

497. Hoffman R, Kopel SD, Hsu SD, et al. T cell chronic lymphocytic leukemia: presence in bone marrow and peripheral blood of cells that suppress erythropoiesis *in vitro. Blood* 1978;52:255–260.

498. Bagby GC Jr. T lymphocytes involved in inhibition of granulopoiesis in two neutropenic patients are of the cytotoxic/suppressor (T3+T8+) subset. *J Clin Invest* 1981;68:1597–1600.

499. Abdou JI, NaPombejara C, Balentine L, et al. Suppressor cell-mediated neutropenia in Felty's syndrome. *J Clin Invest* 1978;61:738–743.

500. Sugimoto M, Wakabayashi Y, Shiokawa Y, et al. Effect of peripheral blood lymphocytes from systemic lupus erythematosus patients on human bone marrow granulocyte precursor cells (colony-forming units in culture). *Stem Cells* 1982;2:164–176.

501. Bom-van Noorloos AA, Pegels JG, van Oeers HJ, et al. Proliferation of T8 cells with killer-cell activity in two patients with neutropenia and recurrent infections. *N Engl J Med* 1980;302:933–937.

502. Linch DC, Cawley JC, MacDonald SM, et al. Acquired pure red cell aplasia associated with an increase of T cells bearing receptors for the Fc of IgG. *Acta Haematol* 1981;65:270–274.

503. Torok-Storb BJ, Sieff C, Storb R, et al. In vitro tests for distinguishing possible immune-mediated aplastic anemia from transfusion-induced sensitization. *Blood* 1980;55:211–217.

504. Bacigalupo AM, Podesta M, Mingari MC, et al. Immune suppression of hematopoiesis in aplastic anemia: activity of T lymphocytes. *J Immunol* 1980;125:1449–1453.

505. Linch DC, Cawley JC, Worman CP, et al. Abnormalities of T-cell subsets in patients with neutropenia and an excess of lymphocytes in the bone marrow. *Br J Haematol* 1981;48:137–145.

506. Krensky AM, Reiss CS, Mier JW, et al. Long-term human cytolytic T-cell lines allospecific for HLA-DR6 antigen are OKT4+. *Proc Natl Acad Sci U S A* 1982;79:2365–2369.

507. Falkenburg JH, Jansen J, van der Vaart-Duinkerken N, et al. Polymorphic and monomorphic HLA-DR determinants on human hematopoietic progenitor cells. *Blood* 1984;63:1125–1132.

508. Sieff C, Bicknell D, Cain G, et al. Changes in cell surface antigen expression during hemopoietic differentiation. *Blood* 1982;60:703–713.

509. Greaves MF, Katz FE, Myers CD, et al. Selective expression of cell surface antigens on human haematopoietic progenitor cells. In: Palek J, ed. *Hematopoietic stem cell physiology*. New York: Alan R. Liss, 1985:301.

510. Sparrow RL, Williams N. The pattern of HLA-DR and HLA-DQ antigen expression on clonable subpopulations of human myeloid progenitor cells. *Blood* 1986;67:379–384.

511. Burdach SEG, Levitt LJ. Receptor-specific inhibition of bone marrow erythropoiesis by recombinant DNA-derived interleukin-2. *Blood* 1987;69:1368–1375.

512. Burdach S, Shatsky M, Wagenhorst B, et al. The T-cell CD2 determinant mediates inhibition of erythropoiesis by the lymphokine cascade. *Blood* 1988;72:770–775.

513. Wimperis JZ, Niemeyer CM, Sieff CA, et al. Granulocyte-macrophage colony-stimulating factor and interleukin 3 mRNAs are produced by a small fraction of blood mononuclear cells. *Blood* 1989;74:1525–1530.

514. Guba SC, Stella G, Turka LA, et al. Regulation of interleukin 3 gene induction in normal human T cells. *J Clin Invest* 1989;84:1701–1706.

515. Roodman DC, Bird A, Hutzler D, et al. Tumor necrosis factor-alpha and hematopoietic progenitors: effects of tumor necrosis factor on the growth of erythroid progenitors CFU-E and BFU-E and the hematopoietic cell lines K562, HL60, and HEL cells. *J Exp Hematol* 1987;15:928–935.

516. Broxmeyer HE, Williams DE, Lu L, et al. The suppressive influences of human tumor necrosis factor on bone marrow hematopoietic progenitor

cells from normal donors and patients with leukemia: synergism of tumor necrosis factor and interferon-gamma. *J Immunol* 1986;136:4487.

517. Furmanski P, Johnson CS. Macrophage control of normal and leukemic erythropoiesis: identification of the macrophage-derived erythroid suppressing activity as interleukin-1 and the mediator of its in vivo action as tumor necrosis factor. *Blood* 1990;75:2328–2334.

518. Jelkmann W. Erythropoietin: structure, control of production, and function. *Physiol Rev* 1992;72:449–489.

519. Semenza GL. Regulation of erythropoietin production. *Hematol Oncol Clin North Am* 1994;8:863–884.

520. Carnot P, Deflandre C. Sur l'activite hemopoietique des differents organeau au cours de la regeneration du sang. *C R Searces Acad Sci* 1906;143:432–435.

521. Krumdieck N. Erythropoietic substance in the serum of anemic animals. *Proc Soc Exp Biol Med* 1943;54:14–17.

522. Erslev A. In vitro production of erythropoietin by kidneys perfused with a serum free solution. *Blood* 1974;44:77–85.

523. Erslev AJ, Lavietes PH, Wagenen GV. Erythropoietic stimulation induced by "anemic serum." *Proc Soc Exp Biol Med* 1953;83:548–550.

524. Reissmann KR. Studies on the mechanism of erythropoietic stimulation in parabiotic rats during hypoxia. *Blood* 1950;5.

525. Miyake T, Kung CK, Goldwasser E. Purification of human erythropoietin. *J Biol Chem* 1977;252:5558–5564.

526. Jacobs K, Shoemaker C, Rudersdorf R, et al. Isolation and characterization of genomic and cDNA clones of human erythropoietin. *Nature* 1985;313:806–810.

527. Lin FK, Suggs S, Lin CH, et al. Cloning and expression of the human erythropoietin gene. *Proc Natl Acad Sci U S A* 1985;82:7580–7584.

528. McDonald J, Lin FK, Goldwasser E. Cloning, sequencing and evolutionary analysis of the mouse erythropoietin gene. *Mol Cell Biol* 1986;6:842–848.

529. Shoemaker CB, Mitsock LD. Murine erythropoietin gene: cloning, expression, and human gene homology. *Mol Cell Biol* 1986;6:849–858.

530. Eschbach J, Ergie J, Downing M, et al. Correction of the anemia of endstage renal disease with recombinant human erythropoietin. *N Engl J Med* 1987;316:73–78.

531. Winearls C, Oliver D, Pippard M, et al. Effect of human erythropoietin derived from recombinant DNA on the anemia of patients maintained on chronic hemodialysis. *Lancet* 1986;2:1175–1181.

532. Sasaki H, Bothner B, Dell A, et al. Carbohydrate structure of erythropoietin expressed in Chinese hamster ovary cells by a human erythropoietin cDNA. *J Biol Chem* 1987;262:12059–12076.

533. Clark DA, Dessypris EN. Effects of recombinant erythropoietin on murine megakaryocytic colony formation in vitro. *J Lab Clin Med* 1986;108:423–429.

534. Jacobsen LO, Goldwasser E, Fried W, et al. Role of the kidney in erythropoiesis. *Nature* 1957;179:633–634.

535. Erslev AJ, Caro J, Besarab A. Why the kidney? *Nephron* 1985;41:213–216.

536. Koury ST, Bondurant MC, Koury MJ. Localization of erythropoietin synthesizing cells in murine kidneys by in situ hybridization. *Blood* 1988;71:524–527.

537. Koury ST, Bondurant MC, Koury MJ, et al. Localization of cells producing erythropoietin in murine liver by in situ hybridization. *Blood* 1991;77:2497–2503.

538. Lacombe C, DaSilva J-L, Bruneval P, et al. Peritubular cells are the site of erythropoietin synthesis in the murine hypoxic kidney. *J Clin Invest* 1988;81:620–623.

539. Koury ST, Koury MJ, Bondurant MC, et al. Quantitation of erythropoietin-producing cells in kidneys of mice by in situ hybridization: correlation with hematocrit, renal erythropoietin mRNA, and serum erythropoietin concentration. *Blood* 1989;74:645–651.

540. Bachmann S, Hir ML, Eckardt KU. Co-localization of erythropoietin mRNA and ecto-5'-nucleotidase immunoreactivity in peritubular cells of rat renal cortex indicates that fibroblasts produce erythropoietin. *J Histochem Cytochem* 1993;41:335–341.

541. Maxwell PH, Osmond MK, Pugh CW, et al. Identification of the renal erythropoietin-producing cells using transgenic mice. *Kidney Int* 1993;44:1149–1162.

542. Zanjani ED, Poster J, Burlington H, et al. Liver as the site of Epo formation in the fetus. *J Lab Clin Med* 1977;89:640–644.

543. Dame C, Fahnenstich H, Hofmann PF, et al. Erythropoietin mRNA expression in human fetal and neonatal tissues. *Blood* 1998;92:3218–3225.

544. Schuster SJ, Koury ST, Bohrer M, et al. Cellular sites of extrarenal and renal erythropoietin production in anemic rats. *Br J Haematol* 1992;81:153–159.

545. Maxwell PH, Ferguson DJP, Osmond MK, et al. Expression of a homologously recombined erythropoietin-SV40 T antigen fusion gene in mouse liver: evidence for erythropoietin production by Ito cells. *Blood* 1994;84:1823–1830.

546. Tan CC, Eckardt K-U, Ratcliffe PJ. Organ distribution of erythropoietin messenger RNA in normal and uremic rats. *Kidney Int* 1991;40:69–76.

547. Fandrey J, Bunn HF. In vivo and in vitro regulation of erythropoietin mRNA: measurement by competitive polymerase chain reaction. *Blood* 1993;81:617–623.

548. Hermine O, Beru N, Pech N, et al. An autocrine role for erythropoietin in mouse hematopoietic cell differentiation. *Blood* 1991;78:2253.

549. Stopka T, Zivny JH, Stopkova P, et al. Human hematopoietic progenitors express erythropoietin. *Blood* 1998;91:3766–3773.

550. Masuda S, Okano M, Yamagishi K, et al. A novel site of erythropoietin production: oxygen-dependent production in cultured rat astrocytes. *J Biol Chem* 1994;269:19488–19493.

551. Digicaylioglu M, Bichet S, Marti HH, et al. Localization of specific erythropoietin binding sites in defined areas of the mouse brain. *Proc Natl Acad Sci U S A* 1995;92:3717–3720.

552. Marti HH, Wenger RH, Rivas LA, et al. Erythropoietin gene expression in human, monkey and murine brain. *Eur J Neurosci* 1996;8:666–676.

553. Sakanaka M, Wen TC, Matsuda S, et al. In vivo evidence that erythropoietin protects neurons from ischemic damage. *Proc Natl Acad Sci U S A* 1998;95:4635–4640.

554. Brines ML, Ghezzi P, Keenan S, et al. Erythropoietin crosses the blood–brain barrier to protect against experimental brain injury. *Proc Natl Acad Sci U S A* 2000;97:10526–10531.

555. Goldberg MA, Glass GA, Cunningham JM, et al. The regulated expression of erythropoietin by two human hepatoma cell lines. *Proc Natl Acad Sci U S A* 1987;84:7972–7976.

556. Semenza GL, Dureza RC, Traystman MD, et al. Human erythropoietin gene expression in transgenic mice: multiple transcription initiation sites and cis-acting regulatory elements. *Mol Cell Biol* 1990;10:930–938.

557. Semenza GL, Traystman M, Gearhart JD, et al. Polycythemia in transgenic mice expressing the human erythropoietin gene. *Proc Natl Acad Sci U S A* 1989;86:2301–2305.

558. Semenza GL, Koury ST, Nejfelt MK, et al. Cell-type-specific and hypoxia-inducible expression of the human erythropoietin gene in transgenic mice. *Proc Natl Acad Sci U S A* 1991;88:8725–8729.

559. Madan A, Lin C, Hatch SL, et al. Regulated basal, inducible, and tissue-specific human erythropoietin gene expression in transgenic mice requires multiple cis DNA sequences. *Blood* 1995;85:2735–2741.

560. Semenza GL, Nejfelt MK, Chi SM, et al. Hypoxia-inducible nuclear factors bind to an enhancer element located 3' to the human erythropoietin gene. *Proc Natl Acad Sci U S A* 1991;88:5680–5684.

561. Wang GL, Semenza GL. Purification and characterization of hypoxia-inducible factor-1. *J Biol Chem* 1995;270:1230–1237.

562. Hoffman EC, Reyes H, Chu F-F, et al. Cloning of a factor required for activity of the Ah (dioxin) receptor. *Science* 1991;252:954–958.

563. Wang GL, Semenza GL. General involvement of hypoxia-inducible factor 1 in transcriptional response to hypoxia. *Proc Natl Acad Sci U S A* 1993;90:4304–4308.

564. Maxwell PH, Pugh CW, Ratcliffe PJ. Inducible operation of the erythropoietin 3' enhancer in multiple cell lines: evidence for a widespread oxygen-sensing mechanism. *Proc Natl Acad Sci U S A* 1993;90:2423–2427.

565. Semenza GL, Wang GL. A nuclear factor induced by hypoxia via de novo protein synthesis binds to the human erythropoietin gene enhancer at a site required for transcriptional activation. *Mol Cell Biol* 1992;12:5447–5454.

566. Wang GL, Jiang B-H, Semenza GL. Effect of protein kinase and phosphatase inhibitors on expression of hypoxia-inducible factor 1. *Biochem Biophys Res Commun* 1995;216:669–675.

567. Wang GL, Semenza GL. Characterization of hypoxia-inducible factor 1 and regulation of DNA binding activity by hypoxia. *J Biol Chem* 1993;268:21513–21518.

568. Gilles-Gonzalez MA, Ditta GS, Helinski DR. A haemoprotein with kinase activity encoded by the oxygen sensor of Rhizobium meliloti. *Nature* 1991;350:170–172.

569. Gilles-Gonzalez MA, Gonzalez G, Perutz MF, et al. Heme-based sensors exemplified by the kinase FixL, are a new class of heme protein with distinctive ligand binding and autoxidation. *Biochemistry* 1994;33:8067–8073.

570. Wood SM, Gleadle JM, Pugh CW, et al. The role of the aryl hydrocarbon receptor nuclear translocator (ARNT) in hypoxic induction of gene expression. *J Biol Chem* 1996;269:15117–15123.

571. Gradin K, McGuire J, Wenger RH, et al. Functional interference between hypoxia and dioxin signal transduction pathways: competition for recruitment of the Arnt transcription factor. *Mol Cell Biol* 1996;16:5221–5231.

572. Huang LE, Arany Z, Livingston DM, et al. Activation of hypoxia-inducible transcription factor depends primarily upon redox-sensitive stabilization of its alpha subunit. *J Biol Chem* 1996;271:32253–32259.

573. Wang GL, Semenza GL. Desferrioxamine induces erythropoietin gene expression and hypoxia-inducible factor 1 DNA-binding activity: implications for models of hypoxia signal transduction. *Blood* 1993;82:3610–3615.

574. Maxwell PH, Wiesener MS, Chang G-W, et al. The tumor suppressor protein VHL targets hypoxia-inducible factors for oxygen-dependent proteolysis. *Nature* 1999;399:271–275.

575. Huang LE, Gu J, Schau M, et al. Regulation of hypoxia-inducible factor 1a is mediated by an oxygen-dependent degradation domain via the ubiquitin-proteasome pathway. *Proc Natl Acad Sci U S A* 1998;95:7987–7992.

576. Ivan M, Kondo K, Yang H, et al. Proline hydroxylation targets HIF for destruction by the von Hippel-Lindau protein: implications for O_2 sensing. *Science* 2001 (in press).

577. Jaakkola P, Mole DR, Tian Y-M, et al. Oxygen-regulated modification by enzymatic prolyl hydroxylation targets HIF-a to the von Hippel-Lindau ubiquitylation complex. *Science* 2001 (in press).

578. Yu F, White SB, Zhao Q, et al. HIF-1alpha binding to VHL is regulated by stimulus-sensitive proline hydroxylation. *Proc Natl Acad Sci U S A* 2001;98:9630–9635.

579. Masson N, Willam C, Maxwell PH, et al. Independent function of two destruction domains in hypoxia-inducible factor-alpha chains activated by prolyl hydroxylation. *EMBO J* 2001;20:5197–5206.

580. Epstein AC, Gleadle JM, McNeill LA, et al. C. elegans EGL-9 and mammalian homologs define a family of dioxygenases that regulate HIF by prolyl hydroxylation. *Cell* 2001;107:43–54.

581. Blanchard KL, Acquaviva AM, Galson DL, et al. Hypoxic induction of the human erythropoietin gene: cooperation between the promoter and

enhancer, each of which contains steroid receptor response elements. *Mol Cell Biol* 1992;12:5373–5385.

582. Pugh CW, Ebert BL, Ebrahim O, et al. Characterisation of functional domains within the mouse erythropoietin 3' enhancer conveying oxygen-regulated responses in different cell lines. *Biochem Biophys Acta* 1994;1217:297–306.

583. Galson DL, Tsuchiya T, Tendler DS, et al. The orphan receptor hepatic nuclear factor 4 functions as a transcriptional activator for tissue-specific and hypoxia-specific erythropoietin gene expression and is antagonized by EAR3/COUP-TF1. *Mol Cell Biol* 1995;15:2135–2144.

584. Arany Z, Huang LE, Eckner R, et al. Participation by the p300/CBP family of proteins in the cellular response to hypoxia. *Proc Natl Acad Sci U S A* 1996;93:12969–12973.

585. Goldberg M, Gaut CC, Bunn HF. Erythropoietin mRNA levels are governed by both the rate of gene transcription and post-transcriptional events. *Blood* 1991;77:271–277.

586. Czyzyk-Krzeska MF, Furnari BA, Lawson EE, et al. Hypoxia increases rate of transcription and stability of tyrosine hydroxylase mRNA in pheochromocytoma (PC12) cells. *J Biol Chem* 1994;269:760–764.

587. Czyzyk-Krzeska MF, Dominski Z, Kole R, et al. Hypoxia stimulates binding of the cytoplasmic protein to a pyrimidine-rich sequence in the 3'-untranslated region of rat tyrosine hydroxylase mRNA. *J Biol Chem* 1994;269:9940–9945.

588. Levy AP, Levy NS, Goldberg MA. Post-translational regulation of vascular endothelial growth factor by hypoxia. *J Biol Chem* 1996;271:2746–2753.

589. Czyzyk-Krzeska MF, Beresh JE. Characterization of the hypoxia-inducible protein binding site within the pyrimidine-rich tract in the 3'-untranslated region of the tyrosine hydroxylase mRNA. *J Biol Chem* 1996;271:3293–3299.

590. Levy NS, Chung S, Furneaux H, et al. Hypoxic stabilization of vascular endothelial growth factor mRNA by the RNA-binding protein HuR. *J Biol Chem* 1998;273:6417–6423.

591. Rondon IJ, MacMillan LA, Beckman BS, et al. Hypoxia upregulates the activity of a novel erythropoietin mRNA binding protein. *J Biol Chem* 1991;266:16594–16598.

592. Rondon IJ, Scandurro AB, Wilson RB, et al. Changes in redox affect the activity of erythropoietin RNA binding protein. *FEBS Lett* 1995;359:267–270.

593. D'Andrea A, Lodish H, Wong G. Expression cloning of the murine erythropoietin receptor. *Cell* 1989;57:277–285.

594. Livnah O, Stura EA, Johnson DL, et al. Functional mimicry of a protein hormone by a peptide agonist: the EPO receptor complex at 2.8 A. *Science* 1996;273:464–471.

595. Wrighton NC, Farrell FX, Chang R, et al. Small peptides as potent mimetics of the protein hormone erythropoietin. *Science* 1996;273:458–464.

596. Wilson IA, Jolliffe LK. The structure, organization, activation and plasticity of the erythropoietin receptor. *Curr Opin Struct Biol* 1999;9:696–704.

597. McConnell SJ, Dinh T, Le MH, et al. Isolation of erythropoietin receptor agonist peptides using evolved phage libraries. *Biol Chem* 1998;379:1279–1286.

598. Lok S, Kaushansky K, Holly RD, et al. Cloning and expression of murine thrombopoietin cDNA and stimulation of platelet production *in vivo. Nature* 1994;369:565.

599. de Sauvage FJ, Hass PE, Spencer SD, et al. Stimulation of megakaryocytopoiesis and thrombopoiesis by the c-Mpl ligand. *Nature* 1994;369:533.

600. Bartley TD, Bogenberger J, Hint P, et al. Identification and cloning of a megakaryocyte growth and development factor that is a ligand for the cytokine receptor Mpl. *Cell* 1994;77:1117–1124.

601. Yoshimura A, Longmore G, Lodish HF. Point mutation in the exoplasmic domain of the erythropoietin receptor resulting in hormone-independent activation and tumorigenicity. *Nature* 1990;348:647–649.

602. Miura O, Ihle JN. Dimer- and oligomerization of the erythropoietin receptor by disulfide bond formation and significance of the region near the WSXWS motif in intracellular transport. *Arch Biochem Biophys* 1993;306:200–208.

603. Watowich S, Yoshimura A, Longmore G, et al. Homodimerization and constitutive activity of the erythropoietin receptor. *Proc Natl Acad Sci U S A* 1992;89:2140–2144.

604. Souyri M, Vigon I, Penciolelli JF, et al. A putative truncated cytokine receptor gene transduced by the myeloproliferative leukemia virus immortalizes hematopoietic progenitors. *Cell* 1990;63:1137–1147.

605. Li J-P, D'Andrea AD, Lodish HF, et al. Activation of cell growth by binding of Friend spleen focus-forming virus gp55 glycoprotein to the erythropoietin receptor. *Nature* 1990;343:762–764.

606. Zon LI, Moreau JF, Koo JW, et al. The erythropoietin receptor transmembrane region is necessary for activation by the Friend spleen focus-forming virus gp55 glycoprotein. *Mol Cell Biol* 1992;12:2949–2957.

607. Hunig T, Schimpl A. The IL-2 deficiency syndrome: a lethal disease caused by abnormal lymphocyte survival. In: Durum SK, Muegge S, eds. *Cytokine knockouts.* Totowa, NJ: Humana Press, 1998.

608. Nelson BH, Willerford DM. Biology of the interleukin-2 receptor. *Adv Immunol* 1998;70:1–81.

609. Okuda K, Foster R, Griffin JD. Signaling domains of the beta c chain of the GM-CSF/IL-3/IL-5 receptor. *Ann N Y Acad Sci* 1999;872:305–312, discussion 312–303.

610. D'Andrea RJ, Gonda TJ. A model for assembly and activation of the GM-CSF, IL-3 and IL-5 receptors: insights from activated mutants of the common beta subunit. *Exp Hematol* 2000;28:231–243.

611. Constantinescu SN, Ghaffari S, Lodish HF. The erythropoietin receptor: structure, activation and intracellular signal transduction. *Trends Endocrinol Metab* 1999;10:18–23.

612. D'Andrea AD, Yoshimura A, Youssoufian H, et al. The cytoplasmic region of the erythropoietin receptor contains nonoverlapping positive and negative growth-regulatory domains. *Mol Cell Biol* 1991;11:1980–1987.

613. de la Chapelle A, Traskelin AL, Juvonen E. Truncated erythropoietin receptor causes dominantly inherited benign human erythrocytosis. *Proc Natl Acad Sci U S A* 1993;90:4495–4499.

614. Goyal RK, Longmore GD. Abnormalities of cytokine receptor signalling contributing to diseases of red blood cell production. *Ann Med* 1999;31:208–216.

615. Kralovics R, Indrak K, Stopka T, et al. Two new EPO receptor mutations: truncated EPO receptors are most frequently associated with primary familial and congenital polycythemias. *Blood* 1997;90:2057–2061.

616. Arcasoy MO, Degar BA, Harris KW, et al. Familial erythrocytosis associated with a short deletion in the erythropoietin receptor gene. *Blood* 1997;89:4628–4635.

617. Joneja B, Wojchowski DM. Mitogenic signaling and inhibition of apoptosis via the erythropoietin receptor Box-1 domain. *J Biol Chem* 1997;272:11176–11184.

618. Wu H, Liu X, Jaenisch R, et al. Generation of committed erythroid BFU-E and CFU-E progenitors does not require erythropoietin or the erythropoietin receptor. *Cell* 1995;83:59–67.

619. Lin CS, Lim SK, D'Agati V, et al. Differential effects of an erythropoietin receptor gene disruption on primitive and definitive erythropoiesis. *Genes Dev* 1996;10:154–164.

620. Kieran MW, Perkins AC, Orkin SH, et al. Thrombopoietin rescues in vitro erythroid colony formation from mouse embryos lacking the erythropoietin receptor. *Proc Natl Acad Sci U S A* 1996;93:9126–9131.

621. Constantinescu SN, Huang LJ, Nam H, et al. The erythropoietin receptor cytosolic juxtamembrane domain contains an essential, precisely oriented, hydrophobic motif. *Mol Cell* 2001;7:377–385.

622. Socolovsky M, Dusanter-Fourt I, Lodish HF. The prolactin receptor and severely truncated erythropoietin receptors support differentiation of erythroid progenitors. *J Biol Chem* 1997;272:14009–14012.

623. Ghaffari S, Wu H, Gerlach M, et al. BCR-ABL and v-SRC tyrosine kinase oncoproteins support normal erythroid development in erythropoietin receptor-deficient progenitor cells. *Proc Natl Acad Sci U S A* 1999;96:13186–13190.

624. Caro J, Brown S, Miller O, et al. Erythropoietin levels in uremic nephric and anephric patients. *J Lab Clin Med* 1979;93:449–458.

625. Cotes PM. Physiological studies of erythropoietin in plasma. In: Jelkmann W, Gross AJ, eds. *Erythropoietin.* Berlin: Springer, 1989:57–79.

626. Means JRT. Clinical application of recombinant erythropoietin in the anemia of chronic disease. *Hematol Oncol Clin North Am* 1994;8:933–944.

627. Spivak JL. Recombinant human erythropoietin and the anemia of cancer [Editorial]. *Blood* 1994;84:997–1004.

628. Fischl M, Galpin JE, Levine JD, et al. Recombinant human erythropoietin for patients with AIDS treated with zidovudine. *N Engl J Med* 1990;322:1488–1493.

629. Faquin WC, Schneider TJ, Goldberg MA. Effect of inflammatory cytokines on hypoxia-induced erythropoietin production. *Blood* 1992;79:1987–1994.

630. Jelkmann W, Pagel WH, Wolff M, et al. Monokines inhibiting erythropoietin production in human hepatoma cultures and in isolated perfused rat kidneys. *Life Sci* 1992;50:301–308.

631. Horiguchi H, Kayama F, Oguma E, et al. Cadmium and platinum suppression of erythropoietin production in cell culture. *Blood* 2000;96:3743–3747.

632. Horiguchi H, Teranishi H, Niiya K, et al. Hypoproduction of erythropoietin contributes to anemia in chronic cadmium intoxication: clinical study on Itai-itai disease in Japan. *Arch Toxicol* 1994;68:632–636.

633. Prchal JF, Prchal JT. Molecular basis for polycythemia. *Curr Opin Hematol* 1999;6:100–109.

634. Rosa R, Prehu M-O, Beuzard Y, et al. The first case of a complete deficiency of diphosphoglycerate mutase in human erythrocytes. *J Clin Invest* 1978;62:907.

635. Sergeyeva A, Gordeuk VR, Tokarev YN, et al. Congenital polycythemia in Chuvashia. *Blood* 1997;89:2148–2154.

636. Ang SO, Chen H, Stockton DW, et al. Von Hippel Lindau protein, Chuvash polycythemia and oxygen sensing. *Blood* 2001;98:748a.

637. Gnarra JR, Zhou S, Merrill MJ, et al. Post-transcriptional regulation of vascular endothelial growth factor mRNA by the product of the VHL tumor suppressor gene. *Proc Natl Acad Sci U S A* 1996;93:10589–10594.

638. Iliopoulos O, Levy AP, Jiang C, et al. Negative regulation of hypoxia-inducible genes by the von Hippel-Lindau protein. *Proc Natl Acad Sci U S A* 1996;93:10595–10599.

639. Ludwig H, Fritz E, Leitgeb C, et al. Prediction of response to erythropoietin treatment in chronic anemia of cancer. *Blood* 1994;84:1056–1063.

640. Major A, Mathez-Loic F, Rohling R, et al. The effect of intravenous iron on the reticulocyte response to recombinant human erythropoietin. *Br J Haematol* 1997;98:292–294.

641. Cazzola M, Mercuriali F, Brugnara C. Use of recombinant human erythropoietin outside the setting of uremia. *Blood* 1997;89:4248–4267.

642. Linde T, Sandhagen B, Bratteby LE, et al. Reduced oxygen affinity contributes to improved oxygen releasing capacity during erythropoietin treatment of renal anaemia. *Nephrol Dial Transplant* 1993;8:524–529.

643. Brunet P, Berland Y, Merzouk T, et al. Effect of recombinant human erythropoietin treatment in uremic patients on oxygen affinity of hemoglobin. *Nephron* 1994;66:147–152.

644. De Marchi S, Cecchin E, Villalta D, et al. Relief of pruritus and decreases in plasma histamine concentrations during erythropoietin therapy in patients with uremia. *N Engl J Med* 1992;326:969–974.

645. Foresta C, Mioni R, Bordon P, et al. Erythropoietin stimulates testosterone production in man. *J Clin Endocrinol Metab* 1994;78:753–756.

646. Garcia JE, Senent C, Pascual C, et al. Anaphylactic reaction to recombinant human erythropoietin [Letter]. *Nephron* 1993;65:636–637.

647. Montagnac R, Boffa GA, Schillinger F, et al. Sensitization to recombinant human erythropoietin in a woman under hemodialysis [Letter]. *Presse Med* 1992;21:84–85.

648. Peces R, de la Torre M, Alcazar R, et al. Antibodies against recombinant human erythropoietin in a patient with erythropoietin-resistant anemia [Letter]. *N Engl J Med* 1996;335:523–524.

649. McMahon FG, Vargas R, Ryan M, et al. Pharmacokinetics and effects of recombinant human erythropoietin after intravenous and subcutaneous injections in healthy volunteers. *Blood* 1990;76:1718–1722.

650. Nielson OJ. Pharmacokinetics of recombinant human erythropoietin in chronic hemodialysis patients. *Pharmacol Toxicol* 1990;66:83–86.

651. Kaufman JS, Reda DJ, Fye CL, et al. Subcutaneous compared with intravenous epoetin in patients receiving hemodialysis. Department of Veterans Affairs Cooperative Study Group on Erythropoietin in Hemodialysis Patients. *N Engl J Med* 1998;339:578–583.

652. Elliott SG, Lorenzini T, Strickland T, et al. Rational design of a novel erythropoiesis stimulating protein (Aranesp): a super-sialiated molecule with increased biological activity. *Blood* 2000;96:82a.

653. Villeval JL, Rouyer-Fessard P, Blumenfeld N, et al. Retrovirus-mediated transfer of the erythropoietin gene in hematopoietic cells improves the erythrocyte phenotype in murine beta-thalassemia. *Blood* 1994;84:928–933.

654. Tripathy SK, Goldwasser E, Lu MM, et al. Stable delivery of physiologic levels of recombinant erythropoietin to the systemic circulation by intramuscular injection of replication-defective adenovirus. *Proc Natl Acad Sci U S A* 1994;91:11557–11561.

655. Setoguchi Y, Danel C, Crystal RG. Stimulation of erythropoiesis by in vivo gene therapy: physiologic consequences of transfer of the human erythropoietin gene to experimental animals using an adenovirus vector. *Blood* 1994;84:2946–2953.

656. Svensson EC, Black HB, Dugger DL, et al. Long-term erythropoietin expression in rodents and non-human primates following intramuscular injection of a replication-defective adenoviral vector. *Hum Gene Ther* 1997;8:1797–1806.

657. Bohl D, Salvetti A, Moullier P, et al. Control of erythropoietin delivery by doxycycline in mice after intramuscular injection of adeno-associated vector. *Blood* 1998;92:1512–1517.

658. Tripathy SK, Svensson EC, Black HB, et al. Long-term expression of erythropoietin in the systemic circulation of mice after intramuscular injection of a plasmid DNA vector. *Proc Natl Acad Sci U S A* 1996;93:10876–10880.

659. Rizzuto G, Cappelletti M, Maione D, et al. Efficient and regulated erythropoietin production by naked DNA injection and muscle electroporation. *Proc Natl Acad Sci U S A* 1999;96:6417–6422.

660. Klinman DM, Conover J, Leiden JM, et al. Safe and effective regulation of hematocrit by gene gun administration of an erythropoietin-encoding DNA plasmid. *Hum Gene Ther* 1999;10:659–665.

661. Winearls EC, Oliver DO, Pippard MI, et al. Effect of human erythropoietin derived from recombinant DNA on the anaemia of patients maintained by chronic haemodialysis. *Lancet* 1986;2:1175.

662. Muirhead N. Erythropoietin is a cause of access thrombosis. *Semin Dial* 1993; 6:184–188.

663. Raine AE. Hypertension, blood viscosity, and cardiovascular morbidity in renal failure: implications of erythropoietin therapy. *Lancet* 1988;1:97–100.

664. Besarab A, Bolton WK, Browne JK, et al. The effects of normal as compared with low hematocrit values in patients with cardiac disease who are receiving hemodialysis and epoetin. *N Engl J Med* 1998;339:584–590.

665. Mayer G, Thum J, Cada EM, et al. Working capacity is increased following recombinant human erythropoietin treatment. *Kidney Int* 1988;34:525–528.

666. Evans RW, Rader B, Manninen DL. The quality of life of hemodialysis recipients treated with recombinant human erythropoietin. Cooperative Multicenter EPO Clinical Trial Group. *JAMA* 1990;263:825–830.

667. Canadian Erythropoietin Study Group. Association between recombinant human erythropoietin and quality of life and exercise capacity of patients receiving haemodialysis. *BMJ* 1990;300:573–578.

668. Fischl M, Galpin JE, Levine JD, et al. Recombinant human erythropoietin for patients with AIDS treated with zidovudine. *N Engl J Med* 1990;322:1488–1493.

669. Henry DH, Abels RI. Recombinant human erythropoietin in the treatment of cancer and chemotherapy-induced anemia: results of double-blind and open-label follow-up studies. *Semin Oncol* 1994;21:21–28.

670. Demetri GD, Kris M, Wade J, et al. Quality-of-life benefit in chemotherapy patients treated with epoetin alfa is independent of disease response or tumor type: results from a prospective community oncology study. Procrit Study Group. *J Clin Oncol* 1998;16:3412–3425.

671. Matsumoto T, Endoh K, Kamisango K, et al. Effect of recombinant human erythropoietin on anticancer drug-induced anaemia. *Br J Haematol* 1990;75:463–468.

672. Bray GL, Reaman GH. Erythropoietin deficiency: a complication of cisplatin therapy and its treatment with recombinant human erythropoietin. *Am J Pediatr Hematol Oncol* 1991;13:426–430.

673. Markman M, Reichman B, Hakes T, et al. The use of recombinant human erythropoietin to prevent carboplatin-induced anemia. *Gynecol Oncol* 1993; 49:172–176.

674. Means RT, Olsen NJ, Krantz SB, et al. Treatment of the anemia of rheumatoid arthritis with recombinant human erythropoietin: clinical and in vitro studies. *Arthritis Rheum* 1989;32:638–642.

675. Pincus T, Olsen NJ, Russell IJ, et al. Multicenter study of recombinant human erythropoietin in correction of anemia in rheumatoid arthritis. *Am J Med* 1990;89:161–168.

676. Murphy EA, Bell AL, Wojtulewski J, et al. Study of erythropoietin in treatment of anaemia in patients with rheumatoid arthritis. *BMJ* 1994;309:1337–1338.

677. Negrin RS, Stein R, Vardiman J, et al. Treatment of the anemia of myelodysplastic syndromes using recombinant human granulocyte colony-stimulating factor in combination with erythropoietin. *Blood* 1993;82:737–743.

678. Bessho M, Jinnai I, Hirashima K, et al. Trilineage recovery by combination therapy with recombinant human granulocyte colony-stimulating factor and erythropoietin in patients with aplastic anemia and refractory anemia. *Stem Cells* 1994;12:604–615.

679. Negrin RS, Stein R, Doherty K, et al. Maintenance treatment of the anemia of myelodysplastic syndromes with recombinant human granulocyte colony-stimulating factor and erythropoietin: evidence for in vivo synergy. *Blood* 1996;87:4076–4081.

680. Kurzrock R, Talpaz M, Gutterman JU. Very low doses of GM-CSF administered alone or with erythropoietin in aplastic anemia. *Am J Med* 1992;93:41–48.

681. Ludwig H, Fritz E, Kotzmann H, et al. Erythropoietin treatment of anemia associated with multiple myeloma. *N Engl J Med* 1990;322:1693–1699.

682. Barlogie B, Beck T. Recombinant human erythropoietin and the anemia of multiple myeloma. *Stem Cells* 1993;11:88–94.

683. Osterborg A, Boogaerts MA, Cimino R, et al. Recombinant human erythropoietin in transfusion-dependent anemic patients with multiple myeloma and non-Hodgkin's lymphoma—a randomized multicenter study. The European Study Group of Erythropoietin (Epoetin Beta) Treatment in Multiple Myeloma and Non-Hodgkin's Lymphoma. *Blood* 1996;87:2675–2682.

684. Link H, Brune T, Hubner G, et al. Effect of recombinant human erythropoietin after allogenic bone marrow transplantation. *Ann Hematol* 1993;67:169–173.

685. Mitus AJ, Antin JH, Rutherford CJ, et al. Use of recombinant human erythropoietin in allogeneic bone marrow transplant donor/recipient pairs. *Blood* 1994;83:1952–1957.

686. Link H, Boogaerts MA, Fauser AA, et al. A controlled trial of recombinant human erythropoietin after bone marrow transplantation. *Blood* 1994;84: 3327–3335.

687. Goodnough LT, Rudnick S, Price TH, et al. Increased preoperative collection of autologous blood with recombinant human erythropoietin therapy. *N Engl J Med* 1989;321:1163–1168.

688. Biesma DH, Kraaijenhagen RJ, Dalmulder J, et al. Recombinant human erythropoietin in autologous blood donors: a dose-finding study. *Br J Haematol* 1994;86:30–35.

689. Mercuriali F, Gualtieri G, Sinigaglia L, et al. Use of recombinant human erythropoietin to assist autologous blood donation by anemic rheumatoid arthritis patients undergoing major orthopedic surgery. *Transfusion* 1994;34:501–506.

690. Sowade O, Warnke H, Scigalla P, et al. Avoidance of allogeneic blood transfusions by treatment with epoetin beta (recombinant human erythropoietin) in patients undergoing open-heart surgery. *Blood* 1997;89:411–418.

691. Canadian Orthopedic Perioperative Erythropoietin Study Group. Effectiveness of perioperative recombinant human erythropoietin in elective hip replacement. *Lancet* 1993;341:1227–1232.

692. Rutherford CJ, Schneider TJ, Dempsey H, et al. Efficacy of different dosing regimens for recombinant human erythropoietin in a simulated perisurgical setting: the importance of iron availability in optimizing response. *Am J Med* 1994;96:139–145.

693. Shannon KM, Naylor GS, Torkildson JC, et al. Circulating erythroid progenitors in the anemia of prematurity. *N Engl J Med* 1987;317:728–733.

694. Soubasi V, Kremenopoulos G, Diamandi E, et al. In which neonates does early recombinant human erythropoietin treatment prevent anemia of prematurity? Results of a randomized, controlled study. *Pediatr Res* 1993;34:675–679.

695. Meyer MP, Meyer JH, Commerford A, et al. Recombinant human erythropoietin in the treatment of the anemia of prematurity: results of a double-blind, placebo-controlled study. *Pediatrics* 1994;93:918–923.

696. Maier RF, Obladen M, Scigalla P, et al. The effect of Epoetin beta (recombinant human erythropoietin) on the need for transfusion in very-low-birth-weight infants. *N Engl J Med* 1994;330:1173–1178.

697. al-Khatti A, Veith RW, Papayannopoulou T, et al. Stimulation of fetal hemoglobin synthesis by erythropoietin in baboons. *N Engl J Med* 1987;317:415.

698. al-Khatti A, Umemura T, Clow J, et al. Erythropoietin stimulates F-reticulocyte formation in sickle cell anemia. *Trans Assoc Am Physicians* 1988;101:54–59.

699. Goldberg MA, Brugnara C, Dover GJ, et al. Treatment of sickle cell anemia with hydroxyurea and erythropoietin. *N Engl J Med* 1990;323:366–372.

700. Rodgers GP, Dover GJ, Uyesaka N, et al. Augmentation by erythropoietin of fetal hemoglobin response to hydroxyurea in sickle cell patients. *N Engl J Med* 1993;328:73–79.

701. Nagel RL, Vichinsky E, Shah M, et al. F reticulocyte response in sickle cell anemia treated with recombinant human erythropoietin: a double-blind study. *Blood* 1993;81:9–14.

702. Rachmilewitz EA, Aker M. The role of recombinant human erythropoietin in the treatment of thalassemia. *Ann N Y Acad Sci* 1998;850:129–138.

703. Nisli G, Kavakli K, Aydinok Y, et al. Recombinant erythropoietin trial in children with transfusion-dependent homozygous beta-thalassemia. *Acta Haematol* 1997;98:199–203.

704. Metcalf D, Stanley ER. Haematological effects in mice of partially purified colony stimulating factor (CSF) prepared from human urine. *Br J Haematol* 1971;21:481–492.

705. Metcalf D, Nicola NA. Proliferative effects of purified granulocyte colony-stimulating factor (G-CSF) on normal mouse hematopoietic cells. *J Cell Physiol* 1983;116:198–206.

706. Sonoda Y, Yang Y-C, Wong GG, et al. Analysis in serum-free culture of the targets of recombinant human hemopoietic growth factors: interleukin 3 and granulocyte-macrophage colony-stimulating factor are specific for early developmental stages. *Proc Natl Acad Sci U S A* 1988;85:4360–4364.

707. Sieff CA, Niemeyer CM, Nathan DG, et al. Stimulation of human hematopoietic colony formation by recombinant gibbon multi-colony-stimulating factor or interleukin 3. *J Clin Invest* 1987;80:818–823.

708. Gasson JC, Weisbart RH, Kaufman SE, et al. Purified human granulocyte-macrophage colony–stimulating factor: direct action on neutrophils. *Science* 1984;226:1339–1342.

709. Weisbarat RH, Golde DW, Clark SC, et al. Human granulocyte-macrophage colony-stimulating factor is a neutrophil activator. *Nature* 1985;314:361–363.

710. Metcalf D, Begley CG, Johnson GR. Biologic properties in vitro of a recombinant human granulocyte-macrophage colony-stimulating factor. *Blood* 1986;67:37–45.

711. Arnaout MA, Wang EA, Clark SC, et al. Human recombinant granulocyte macrophage colony-stimulating factor increases cell to cell adhesion and surface expression of adhesion promoting surface glycoproteins on mature granulocytes. *J Clin Invest* 1986;78:597–601.

712. Lopez AF, To LB, Yang Y-C, et al. Stimulation of proliferation, differentiation, and function of human cells by primate interleukin 3. *Proc Natl Acad Sci U S A* 1987;84:2761–2765.

713. Lopez AF, Nicola NA, Burgess AW, et al. Activation of granulocyte cytotoxic function by purified mouse colony stimulating factors. *J Immunol* 1983;131:2983–2988.

714. Hamilton JA, Stanley ER, Burgess AW, et al. Stimulation of macrophage plasminogen activator activity by colony-stimulating factors. *J Cell Physiol* 1980;103:435–445.

715. Nicola NA, Metcalf D. Binding of iodinated multipotential colony-stimulating factor (interleukin-3) to murine bone marrow cells. *J Cell Physiol* 1986;128:180–188.

716. Ihle JN, Keller J, Henderson L, et al. Procedures for the purification of interleukin 3 to homogeneity. *J Immunol* 1982;129:2431–2436.

717. Cutler RL, Metcalf D, Nicola NA, et al. Purification of a multipotential colony-stimulating factor from pokeweed mitogen-stimulated mouse spleen cell conditioned medium. *J Biol Chem* 1985;260:6579–6587.

718. Fung MC, Hapel AJ, Yuner S, et al. Molecular cloning for cDNA for murine interleukin-3. *Nature* 1984;307:233–237.

719. Yokota T, Lee T, Rennick D, et al. Isolation and characterization of a mouse cDNA clone that expresses mast-cell growth factor activity in monkey cells. *Proc Natl Acad Sci U S A* 1984;81:1070–1074.

720. Cline MJ, Golde DW. Production of colony stimulating activity by human lymphocytes. *Nature* 1974;248:703–704.

721. Nathan DG, Chess L, Hillman DG, et al. Human erythroid burst-forming unit: T-cell requirement for proliferation in vitro. *J Exp Med* 1978;147:324–339.

722. Chervenick PA, LoBuglio AF. Human blood monocytes: stimulation of granulocyte and mononuclear colony formation *in vitro*. *Science* 1972;178:164–166.

723. Golde DW, Cline MJ. Identification of colony-stimulating cells in human peripheral blood. *J Clin Invest* 1972;51:2981–2983.

724. Zuckerman KS. Human erythroid burst-forming units: growth in vitro is dependent on monocytes but not T lymphocytes. *J Clin Invest* 1981;67:702–709.

725. Reid CP, Batista LC, Chanarin I. Erythroid colony growth in vitro from human peripheral blood null cells: evidence for regulation by T lymphocytes and monocytes. *Br J Haematol* 1981;48:155–164.

726. Knudson S, Mortenson BT. Growth stimulation of human bone marrow cells in agar culture by vascular cells. *Blood* 1975;46:937–943.

727. Quesenberry PJ, Gimbrone MA. Vascular endothelium as a regulator of granulopoiesis: production of colony stimulating activity by cultured human endothelial cells. *Blood* 1980;56:1060–1067.

728. Niemeyer CM, Sieff CA, Mathey-Prevot B, et al. Interleukin 3 (IL-3) is produced only by activated human T-lymphocytes. *Blood* 1987;73:945–951.

729. Mathey-Prevot B, Andrews NC, Murphy HS, et al. Positive and negative elements regulate human interleukin 3 expression. *Proc Natl Acad Sci U S A* 1990;87:5046–5050.

730. Schreurs J, Arai K, Miyajima A. Evidence for a low-affinity interleukin-3 receptor. *Growth Factors* 1990;2:221–234.

731. Park LW, Friend D, Price V, et al. Heterogeneity in human interleukin-3 receptors. *J Biol Chem* 1989;264:5420–5427.

732. Kuwaki T, Kitamura T, Tojo A, et al. Characterization of human interleukin-3 receptors on a multi-factor-dependent cell line. *Biochem Biophys Res Commun* 1989;161:16–22.

733. Gorman DM, Itoh N, Kitamura T, et al. Cloning and expression of a gene encoding an interleukin 3 receptor-like protein: identification of another member of the cytokine receptor gene family. *Proc Natl Acad Sci U S A* 1990;87:5459–5463.

734. Hara T, Miyajima A. Two distinct functional high affinity receptors for mouse interleukin-3 (IL-3). *EMBO J* 1992;11:1875–1884.

735. Kitamura T, Sato N, Arai K, et al. Expression cloning of the human IL-3 receptor cDNA reveals a shared beta subunit for the human IL-3 and GM-CSF receptors. *Cell* 1991;66:1165–1174.

736. Tavernier J, Devos R, Cornelis S, et al. A human high affinity interleukin-5 receptor (IL5R) is composed of an IL5-specific alpha chain and a beta chain shared with the receptor for GM-CSF. *Cell* 1991;66:1175–1184.

737. Nishinakamura R, Miyajima A, Mee PJ, et al. Hematopoiesis in mice lacking the entire granulocyte-macrophage colony-stimulating factor/interleukin-3/interleukin-5 functions. *Blood* 1996;88:2458–2464.

738. Gorman DM, Itoh N, Jenkins NA, et al. Chromosomal localization and organization of the murine genes encoding the beta subunits (AIC2A and AIC2B) of the interleukin 3, granulocyte/macrophage colony-stimulating factor, and interleukin 5 receptors. *J Biol Chem* 1992;267:15842–15848.

739. Nishinakamura R, Nakayama N, Hirabayashi Y, et al. Mice deficient for the IL-3/GM-CSF/IL-5 beta c receptor exhibit lung pathology and impaired immune response, while beta IL3 receptor-deficient mice are normal. *Immunity* 1995;2:211–222.

740. Devos R, Plaetinck G, Van der Heyden J, et al. Molecular basis of a high affinity murine interleukin-5 receptor. *EMBO J* 1991;10:2133–2137.

741. Morla AO, Schreurs J, Miyajima A, et al. Hematopoietic growth factors activate the tyrosine phosphorylation of distinct sets of proteins in interleukin-3-dependent murine cell lines. *Mol Cell Biol* 1988;8:2214–2218.

742. Isfort RJ, Stevens D, May WS, et al. Interleukin 3 binds to a 140-kDa phospho-tyrosine-containing cell surface protein. *Proc Natl Acad Sci U S A* 1988;85:7982–7986.

743. Isfort R, Huhn RD, Frackelton AR, et al. Stimulation of factor-dependent myeloid cell lines with interleukin 3 induces tyrosine phosphorylation of several cellular substrates. *J Biol Chem* 1988;263:19203–19209.

744. Sorensen PH, Mui AL-F, Murphy SC, et al. Interleukin-3, GM-CSF, and TPA induce distinct phosphorylation events in an interleukin-3-dependent multi-potential cell line. *Blood* 1989;73:406–418.

745. Hanazono Y, Chiba S, Sasaki K, et al. c-fps/fes protein-tyrosine kinase is implicated in a signaling pathway triggered by granulocyte-macrophage colony-stimulating factor and interleukin-3. *EMBO J* 1993;12:1641–1646.

746. Okuda K, Sanghera J, Pelech SL, et al. Granulocyte-macrophage colony-stimulating factor, interleukin-3, and steel factor induce rapid tyrosine phosphorylation of p42 and p44 MAP kinase. *Blood* 1992;79:2880–2887.

747. Welham MJ, Duronio V, Sanghera JS, et al. Multiple hemopoietic growth factors stimulate activation of mitogen-activated protein kinase family members. *J Immunol* 1992;149:1683–1693.

748. Torigoe T, O'Connor R, Santoli D, et al. Interleukin-3 regulates the activity of the LYN protein-tyrosine kinase in myeloid-committed leukemic cell lines. *Blood* 1992;80:617–624.

749. Kobayashi N, Kono T, Hatakeyama M, et al. Functional coupling of the src-family protein tyrosine kinases p59fyn and p53/56lyn with the interleukin 2 receptor: implications for redundancy and pleiotropism in cytokine signal transduction. *Proc Natl Acad Sci U S A* 1993;90:4201–4205.

750. Kaplan DR, Whitman M, Schaffhausen B, et al. Common elements in growth factor stimulation and oncogenic transformation: 85 kd phosphoprotein and phosphatidylinositol kinase activity. *Cell* 1987;50:1021–1029.

751. Carroll MP, Clark-Lewis I, Rapp UR, et al. Interleukin-3 and granulocyte-macrophage colony-stimulating factor mediate rapid phosphorylation and activation of cytosolic c-raf. *J Biol Chem* 1990;265:19812–19817.

752. Gough N, Gough J, Metcalf D, et al. Molecular cloning of cDNA encoding a murine haematopoietic growth regulator, granulocyte-macrophage. *Nature* 1984;309:763–767.

753. Donahue RE, Wang EA, Kaufman RJ, et al. Effects of N-linked carbohydrate on the in vivo properties of human GM-CSF. *Cold Spring Harb Symp Quant Biol* 1986;51:685–692.

754. Cebon J, Nicola N, Ward M, et al. Granulocyte-macrophage colony stimulating factor from human lymphocytes. *J Biol Chem* 1990;265:4483–4491.

755. Gough NM, Grail D, Gearing DP, et al. Mutagenesis of murine granulocyte/macrophage colony-stimulating factors reveals critical residues near the N terminus. *Eur J Biochem* 1987;169:353–358.

756. Kaushansky K, Shoemaker SG, Alfaro S, et al. Hematopoietic activity of granulocyte/macrophage colony-stimulating factor is dependent upon two distinct regions of the molecule: functional analysis based upon the activities of interspecies hybrid growth factors. *Proc Natl Acad Sci U S A* 1989;86:1213–1217.

757. Brown CB, Hart CE, Curtis DM, et al. Two neutralizing monoclonal antibodies against human granulocyte-macrophage colony-stimulating factor recognize the receptor binding domain of the molecule. *J Immunol* 1990;144:2184–2189.

758. Yang Y-C, Kovacic S, Kriz R, et al. The human genes for GM-CSF and IL 3 are closely linked in tandem on chromosome 5. *Blood* 1988;71:958–961.

759. Yang Y-C, Clark SC. Molecular cloning for interleukin 3. *Lymphokines* 1991;15:375–391.

760. Shannon MF, Gamble JR, Vadas MA. Nuclear proteins interacting with the promoter region of the human granulocyte/macrophage colony-stimulating factor gene. *Proc Natl Acad Sci U S A* 1988;85:674–678.

761. Shannon MF, Pell LM, Lenardo MJ, et al. A novel tumor necrosis factor-responsive transcription factor which recognized a regulatory element in hemopoietic growth factor genes. *Mol Cell Biol* 1990;10:2950–2959.

762. Nimer SD, Morita EA, Martis MJ, et al. Characterization of the human granulocyte-macrophage colony-stimulating factor promoter region by genetic

analysis: correlation with DNase I footprinting. *Mol Cell Biol* 1988;8:1979–1984.

763. Shaw G, Kamen R. A conserved AU sequence from the 3' untranslated region of GM-CSF mRNA mediates selective mRNA degradation. *Cell* 1986;46:659–667.

764. Broudy VC, Kaushansky K, Segal GM, et al. Tumor necrosis factor type alpha stimulates human endothelial cells to produce granulocyte/macrophage colony-stimulating factor. *Proc Natl Acad Sci U S A* 1986;83:7467–7471.

765. Munker R, Gasson J, Ogawa M, et al. Recombinant human TNF induces production of granulocyte-monocyte colony-stimulating factor. *Nature* 1986;323:79–82.

766. Sieff CA, Tsai S, Faller DV. Interleukin 1 induces cultured human endothelial cell production of granulocyte-macrophage colony stimulating factor. *J Clin Invest* 1987;79:48–51.

767. Yang Y-C, Tsai S, Wong GG, et al. Production of colony-stimulating factors by interleukin-1-induced human stromal cells. *J Cell Physiol* 1988;134:292–296.

768. Dinarello CA. Interleukin 1 and the pathogenesis of the acute-phase response. *N Engl J Med* 1984;311:1413–1418.

769. Broudy VC, Zuckerman KS, Jetmalani S, et al. Monocytes stimulate fibroblastoid bone marrow stromal cells to produce multilineage hematopoietic growth factors. *Blood* 1986;68:530–534.

770. Bagby GC, McCall E, Bergstrom KA, et al. A monokine regulates colony–stimulating activity production by vascular endothelial cells. *Blood* 1983;62:663–668.

771. Zuckerman KS, Bagby GC, McCall E, et al. A monokine stimulates the production of human erythroid burst-promoting activity by endothelial cells *in vitro*. *J Clin Invest* 1985;75:722–725.

772. Bagby GC, McCall E, Layman DL. Regulation of colony stimulating activity production: interactions of fibroblasts, mononuclear phagocytes, and lactoferrin. *J Clin Invest* 1983;71:340–344.

773. Bagby GC, Rigas VD, Bennett RM, et al. Interaction of lactoferrin, monocytes, and T lymphocyte subsets in the regulation of steady-state granulopoiesis *in vitro*. *J Clin Invest* 1981;68:56–63.

774. Yamato K, El-Hajjaoui Z, Kuo JF, et al. Granulocyte-macrophage colony-stimulating factor: signals for its mRNA accumulation. *Blood* 1989;74:1314–1320.

775. Koeffler HP, Gasson J, Tobler A. Transcriptional and posttranscriptional modulation of myeloid colony-stimulating factor expression by tumor necrosis factor and other agents. *Mol Cell Biol* 1988;8:3432–3438.

776. Seelentag WK, Mermod J-J, Montesano R, et al. Additive effects of interleukin 1 and tumor necrosis factor alpha on the accumulation of the three granulocyte and macrophage colony-stimulating factor mRNAs in human endothelial cells. *EMBO J* 1987;6:2261–2265.

777. Thorens B, Mermod J-J, Vassalli P. Phagocytosis and inflammatory stimuli induce GM-CSF mRNA in macrophages through posttranscriptional regulation. *Cell* 1987;48:671–679.

778. Gasson JC, Kaufman SE, Weisbart RH, et al. High-affinity binding of granulocyte-macrophage colony-stimulating factor to normal and leukemic human myeloid cells. *Proc Natl Acad Sci U S A* 1986;83:669–673.

779. Park LW, Friend D, Gillis S, et al. Characterization of the cell surface receptor for human granulocyte/macrophage colony-stimulating factor. *J Exp Med* 1986;164:251–262.

780. DiPersio J, Billing P, Kaufman S, et al. Characterization of the human granulocyte-macrophage colony-stimulating factor receptor. *J Biol Chem* 1988;263:1834–1841.

781. Sieff CA, Kannourakis G. Interleukin-3 and granulocyte-macrophage colony-stimulating factor are synergistic and interact at the cell surface. In: Abraham NG, Kowalinka G, Sachs L, et al., eds. *Molecular biology of hematopoiesis*. Andover: Intercept, 1991.

782. Gesner TG, Mufson RA, Norton CR, et al. Specific binding, internalization, and degradation of human recombinant interleukin-3 by cells of the acute myelogenous leukemia line, KG-1. *J Cell Physiol* 1988;136:493–499.

783. Chiba S, Tojo A, Kitamura T, et al. Characterization and molecular features of the cell surface receptor for human granulocyte-macrophage colony-stimulating factor. *Leukemia* 1990;4:29–36.

784. Baldwin GC, Gasson JC, Kaufman SE, et al. Nonhematopoietic tumor cells express functional GM-CSF receptors. *Blood* 1989;73:1033–1037.

785. Miyagawa K, Chiba S, Shibuya K, et al. Frequent expression of receptors for granulocyte-macrophage colony-stimulating factor on human nonhematopoietic tumor cell lines. *J Cell Physiol* 1990;143:483–487.

786. Chiba S, Shibuya K, Piao Y-F, et al. Identification and cellular distribution of distinct proteins forming human GM-CSF receptor. *Cell Regul* 1990;1:327–335.

787. Metcalf D, Nicola NA, Gearing DP, et al. Low-affinity placenta-derived receptors for human granulocyte-macrophage colony-stimulating factor can deliver a proliferative signal to murine hematopoietic cells. *Proc Natl Acad Sci U S A* 1990;87:4670–4674.

788. Hayashida K, Kitamura T, Gorman DM, et al. Molecular cloning of a second subunit of the receptor for human granulocyte-macrophage colony-stimulating factor (GM-CSF): reconstitution of a high-affinity GM-CSF receptor. *Proc Natl Acad Sci U S A* 1990;87:9655–9659.

789. Ashworth A, Kraft A. Cloning of a potentially soluble receptor for human GM-CSF. *Nucleic Acids Res* 1990;18:7178.

790. Nagata S, Tsuchiya M, Asano S, et al. The chromosomal gene structure and two mRNAs for human granulocyte colony-stimulating factor. *EMBO J* 1986;5:575–581.

791. Ranscht B, Dours MT. Sequence of contactin, a 130-kD glycoprotein concentrated in areas of interneuronal contact, defines a new member of the immuno-globulin supergene family in the nervous system. *J Cell Biol* 1988;107:1561–1573.

792. Ladner MB, Martin GA, Noble JA, et al. Human CSF-1: gene structure and alternative splicing of mRNA precursors. *EMBO J* 1987;6:2693–2698.

793. Wong GG, Temple PA, Leary AC, et al. Human CSF-1: molecular cloning and expression of a 4kb cDNA encoding the human urinary protein. *Science* 1987;235:1504–1508.

794. Stanley ER, Heard PM. Factors regulating macrophage production and growth: purification and some properties of the colony stimulating factor from medium conditioned by mouse L-cells. *J Biol Chem* 1977;252:4305–4312.

795. Stanley ER, Hansen G, Woodcock J, et al. Colony stimulating factor and the regulation of granulopoiesis and macrophage production. *Fed Proc* 1975;34:2272–2278.

796. Motoyoshi K, Suda T, Kusumoto K, et al. Granulocyte-macrophage colony-stimulating and binding activities of purified human urinary colony-stimulating factor to murine and human bone marrow cells. *Blood* 1982;60:1378–1386.

797. Cifone M, Defendi V. Cyclic expression of a growth conditioning factor (MGF) on the cell surface. *Nature* 1974;252:151.

798. Stanley ER, Cifone M, Heard PM, et al. Factors regulating macrophage production and growth: identity of colony-stimulating factor and macrophage growth factor. *J Exp Med* 1976;143:631–647.

799. Rettenmier CW, Roussel MF, Ashman RA, et al. Synthesis of membrane-bound colony-stimulating factor 1 (CSF-1) and down modulation of CSF-1 receptors in NIH 3T3 cells transformed by cotransfection of the human CSF-1 and c-fms (CSF-1 receptor) genes. *Mol Cell Biol* 1987;7:2378–2387.

800. Horiguchi J, Warren MK, Ralph P, et al. Expression of the macrophage specific colony-stimulating factor (CSF-1) during human monocyte differentiation. *Biochem Biophys Res Commun* 1986;141:924–930.

801. Rambaldi A, Young DG, Griffin JD. Expression of the M-CSF (CSF-1) gene by human monocytes. *Blood* 1987;69:1409–1413.

802. Ralph R, Warren MK, Lee MT, et al. Inducible production of human macrophage growth factor, CSF-1. *Blood* 1986;68:633–639.

803. Guilbert LJ, Stanley ER. The interaction of 125I-colony-stimulating factor-1 with bone marrow-derived macrophages. *J Biol Chem* 1986;261:4024–4032.

804. Bartocci A, Mastrogiannis DS, Migliorati G, et al. Macrophages specifically regulate the concentration of their own growth factor in the circulation. *Proc Natl Acad Sci U S A* 1987;84:6179–6183.

805. Sherr CJ. Colony-stimulating factor-1 receptor. *Blood* 1990;75:1–12.

806. Sherr CJ, Rettenmier CW, Sacca R, et al. The c-fms proto-oncogene product is related to the receptor for the mononuclear phagocytic growth factor CSF-1. *Cell* 1985;41:665–676.

807. Yarden Y, Escobedo JA, Kuang W-J, et al. Structure of the receptor for platelet-derived growth factor helps define a family of closely related growth factor receptors. *Nature* 1986;323:226–232.

808. Roberts WM, Look AT, Moussel MF, et al. Tandem linkage of human CSF-1 receptor (c-fms) and PDGF receptor genes. *Cell* 1988;55:655–661.

809. Coussens L, Van Beveren C, Smith D, et al. Structural alteration of viral homologue of receptor proto-oncogene fms at carboxy terminus. *Nature* 1986;320:277–280.

810. Downing JR, Margolis BL, Zilberstein A, et al. Phospholipase C-gamma, a substrate for PDGF receptor kinase, is not phosphorylated on tyrosine during the mitogenic response to CSF-1. *EMBO J* 1989;8:3345–3350.

811. Imamura K, Dianoux A, Nakamura T, et al. Colony-stimulating factor 1 activates protein kinase C in human monocytes. *EMBO J* 1990:2423–2429.

812. Shurtleff SA, Downing JR, Rock CO, et al. Structural features of the colony-stimulating factor 1 receptor that affect its association with phosphatidylinositol 3-kinase. *EMBO J* 1990:2415–2421.

813. Roussel MF, Rettenmier CW, Look AT, et al. Cell surface expression of v-fms-coded glycoproteins is required for transformation. *Mol Cell Biol* 1984;4:1999–2009.

814. Morrison DK, Kaplan DR, Rapp U, et al. Signal transduction from membrane to cytoplasm: growth factors and membrane-bound oncogene products increase Raf-1 phosphorylation and associated protein kinase activity. *Proc Natl Acad Sci U S A* 1988;85:8855–8859.

815. McDonough SK, Larsen S, Brodey RS, et al. A transmissible feline fibrosarcoma of viral origin. *Cancer Res* 1971;31:953–956.

816. Tushinski RJ, Oliver IT, Guilbert LJ, et al. Survival of mononuclear phagocytes depends on a lineage-specific growth factor that the differentiated cells selectively destroy. *Cell* 1982;28:71–81.

817. Heard J-M, Roussel MF, Rettenmier CW, et al. Multilineage hematopoietic disorders induced by transplantation of bone marrow cells expressing the v-fms oncogene. *Cell* 1987;51:663–673.

818. Downward J, Yarden Y, Mayes E, et al. Close similarity of epiderma, growth factor receptor and v-erb-B oncogene protein sequences. *Nature* 1984;307:521–527.

819. Waterfield MD, Scrace GT, Whittle N, et al. Platelet-derived growth factor is structurally related to the putative transforming protein p28sis of simian sarcoma virus. *Nature* 1983;304:35–39.

820. Dinarello CA, Cannon JG, Mier JW, et al. Multiple biological activities of human recombinant interleukin 1. *J Clin Invest* 1986;77:1734–1739.

821. Schindler R, Dinarello CA. Interleukin 1. In: Habenicht A, ed. *Growth factors, differentiation factors, and cytokines*. Berlin: Springer-Verlag, 1990:85–102.

822. Lomedico PT, Gubler U, Hellmann CP, et al. Cloning and expression of murine interleukin-1 cDNA in Escherichia coli. *Nature* 1984;312:458–462.

823. Furitani Y, Notake M, Fukui T, et al. Complete nucleotide sequence of the gene for human interleukin-1 alpha. *Nucleic Acids Res* 1986;14:3167–3179.

824. Auron PE, Webb AC, Rosenwasser LJ, et al. Nucleotide sequence of human monocyte interleukin 1 precursor cDNA. *Proc Natl Acad Sci U S A* 1984;81:7907–7911.

825. Clark BD, Collins KL, Gandy MS, et al. Genomic sequence for human proin-terleukin 1 beta: possible evolution from a reverse transcribed prointerleukin 1 alpha gene. *Nucleic Acids Res* 1986;14:7897–7914.

826. Bakouche O, Brown DC, Lachman L. Subcellular localization of human monocyte interleukin 1: evidence for an inactive precursor molecule and a possible mechanism for IL 1 release. *J Immunol* 1987;138:4249–4255.

827. Auron PE, Warner SJC, Webb AC, et al. Studies on the molecular nature of human interleukin 1. *J Immunol* 1987;138:1447–1456.

828. Hazuda DJ, Lee JC, Young PR. The kinetics of interleukin 1 secretion from activated monocytes: differences between interleukin 1-alpha and interleu-kin 1-beta. *J Biol Chem* 1988;263:8473–8479.

829. Mosley B, Urdal DL, Prickett KS, et al. The interleukin-1 receptor binds the human interleukin-1-alpha precursor but not the interleukin-1-beta precur-sor. *J Biol Chem* 1987;262:2941–2944.

830. Warner SJ, Auger KR, Libby P. Human interleukin 1 induces interleukin 1 gene expression in human vascular smooth muscle cells. *J Exp Med* 1987;165:1316–1331.

831. Warner SJ, Auger KR, Libby P. Interleukin 1 induces interleukin 1, II: recom-binant human interleukin 1 induces interleukin 1 production by adult human vascular endothelial cells. *J Immunol* 1987;139:1911–1917.

832. Ghezzi P, Dinarello CA. IL-1 induces IL-1, III: specific inhibition of IL-1 pro-duction by IFN-gamma. *J Immunol* 1988;140:4238–4244.

833. Bird TA, Gearing AJ, Saklatvala J. Murine interleukin-1 receptor: differences in binding properties between thymoblastic and thymoma cells and evidence for a two-chain receptor model. *FEBS Lett* 1987;225:21–26.

834. Bird TA, Saklatvala J. Identification of a common class of high affinity recep-tors for both types of porcine interleukin-1 on connective tissue cells. *Nature* 1986;324:263–266.

835. Kroggel R, Martin M, Pingoud V, et al. Two-chain structure of the interleukin 1 receptor. *FEBS Lett* 1988;229:59–62.

836. Mochizuki DY, Eisenman JR, Conlon PJ, et al. Interleukin 1 regulates hema-topoietic activity, a role previously ascribed to hemopoietin 1. *Proc Natl Acad Sci U S A* 1987;84:5267–5271.

837. Jubinsky PT, Stanley ER. Purification of hemopoietin-1, a multilineage hemopoietic growth factor. *Proc Natl Acad Sci U S A* 1985;82:2764–2768.

838. Bartelmez SH, Stanley ER. Synergism between hemopoietic growth factors (HGFs) detected by their effects on cells bearing receptors for a lineage spe-cific HGF: assay of hemopoietin-1. *J Cell Physiol* 1985;122:370–378.

839. McNiece IK, Bradley TR, Kriegler AB, et al. Subpopulations of mouse bone marrow high-proliferative-potential colony-forming cells. *J Exp Hematol* 1986;14:856–860.

840. Neta R, Douches S, Oppenheim JJ. Interleukin-1 is a radioprotector. *J Immu-nol* 1986;136:2483–2485.

841. Neta R, Oppenheim JJ, Douches SD. Interdependence of the radioprotective effects of human recombinant interleukin 1-alpha, tumor necrosis factor alpha, granulocyte colony-stimulating factor, and murine recombinant gran-ulocyte-macrophage colony-stimulating factor. *J Immunol* 1988;140:108–111.

842. Moore MA, Warren DJ. Synergy of interleukin 1 and granulocyte colony-stimulating factor: *in vivo* stimulation of stem-cell recovery and hematopoi-etic regeneration following 5-fluorouracil treatment of mice. *Proc Natl Acad Sci U S A* 1987;84:7134–7138.

843. Stork L, Barczuk L, Kissinger M, et al. Interleukin-1 accelerates murine granulo-cyte recovery following treatment with cyclophosphamide. *Blood* 1989;73:938–944.

844. Gasparetto C, Laver J, Abboud M, et al. Effects of interleukin-1 on hemato-poietic progenitors: evidence of stimulatory and inhibitory activities in a pri-mate model. *Blood* 1989;74:547–550.

845. Noma Y, Sideras P, Naito T, et al. Cloning of cDNA encoding the murine IgG1 induction factor by a novel strategy using SP6 promoter. *Nature* 1986;319:640–646.

846. Yokoto T, Otsuka T, Mossman T. Isolation and characterization of a human interleukin cDNA clone, homologous to mouse B-cell-stimulatory factor 1, that expresses B-cell and T-cell-stimulating activities. *Proc Natl Acad Sci U S A* 1986;83:5894–5898.

847. Novick D, Engelmann H, Wallach D, et al. Soluble cytokine receptors are present in normal human urine. *J Exp Med* 1989;170:1409–1414.

848. Peschel C, Paul WE, Ohara J, et al. Effects of B cell stimulatory factor-1/inter-leukin 4 on hematopoietic progenitor cells. *Blood* 1987;70:254–263.

849. Broxmeyer HE, Lu L, Cooper S, et al. Synergistic effects of purified recombinant human and murine B cell growth factor-1/IL-4 on colony formation in vitro by hematopoietic progenitor cells: multiple actions. *J Immunol* 1988;141:3852–3862.

850. Sanderson CJ, Warren DJ, Strath M. Identification of a lymphokine that stim-ulates eosinophil differentiation in vitro. *J Exp Med* 1985;162:60–74.

851. Kinashi T, Harada N, Severinson E, et al. Cloning of complementary DNA encoding T cell replacing factor and identity with B-cell growth factor II. *Nature* 1986;324:70–73.

852. Azuma C, Tanabe T, Konishi M, et al. Cloning of cDNA for human T-cell replacing factor (interleukin-5) and comparison with the murine homologue. *Nucleic Acids Res* 1986;14:9149–9158.

853. Clutterbuck EJ, Hirst EMA, Sanderson CJ. Human interleukin-5 (IL-5) regu-lates the production of eosinophils in human bone marrow cultures: com-parison and interaction with IL-1, IL-3, IL-6, and GMCSF. *Blood* 1989;73:1504–1512.

854. Coffman RL, Seymour BWP, Hudak S, et al. Antibody to interleukin-5 inhib-its helminth-induced eosinophilia in mice. *Science* 1989;245:308–310.

855. Sieff CA, Emerson SG, Donahue RE, et al. Human recombinant granulocyte-macrophage colony-stimulating factor: a multilineage hematopoietin. *Sci-ence* 1985;230:1171–1173.

856. Hirano T, Yasukawa K, Harada H, et al. Complementary DNA for a novel human interleukin (BSF-2) that induces B lymphocytes to produce immuno-globulin. *Nature* 1986;324:73–76.

857. Zilberstein A, Ruggieri R, Korn JH, et al. Structure and expression of cDNA and genes for human interferon-beta-2, a distinct species inducible by growth-stimulatory cytokines. *EMBO J* 1986;5:2529–2537.

858. Haegeman G, Content J, Volkaert G, et al. Structural analysis of the sequence coding for an inducible 26-kDa protein in human fibroblasts. *Eur J Biochem* 1986;159:625–632.

859. Van Damme J, Opdenakker G, Simpson RJ, et al. Identification of the human 26-kD protein, interferon-beta2 (IFN-beta2), as a B cell hybridoma/plas-mocytoma growth factor induced by interleukin 1 and tumor necrosis factor. *J Exp Med* 1987;165:914–919.

860. Horii Y, Muraguchi A, Suematsu S, et al. Regulation of BSF-2/IL-6 produc-tion by human mononuclear cells. Macrophage-dependent synthesis of BSF-2/IL-6 by T cells. *J Immunol* 1988;141:1529.

861. Taga T, Masahiko H, Hirata Y, et al. Interleukin-6 triggers the association of its receptor with a possible signal transducer, gp130. *Cell* 1989;58:573–581.

862. Kawano M, Hirano T, Matsuda T, et al. Autocrine generation and require-ment of BSF-2/IL-6 for human multiple myelomas. *Nature* 1988;332:83–85.

863. Castleman B, Iverson L, Menendez VP. Localized mediastinal lymph node hyperplasia resembling thymoma. *Cancer* 1956;9:822–830.

864. Namen AE, Schmierer AE, March CJ, et al. B cell precursor growth-promot-ing activity. *J Exp Med* 1988;167:988–1002.

865. Goodwin RG, Lupton S, Schmierer A, et al. Human interleukin 7: molecular cloning and growth factor activity on human and murine B-lineage cells. *Proc Natl Acad Sci U S A* 1989;86:302–306.

866. Baggiolini M, Walz A, Kunkel SL. Neutrophil-activating peptide-1/interleu-kin 8, a novel cytokine that activates neutrophils. *J Clin Invest* 1989;84:1045–1049.

867. Schmid J, Weissmann C. Induction of mRNA for a serine protease and a beta-thromboglobulin-like protein in mitogen-stimulated human leuko-cytes. *J Immunol* 1987;139:250–256.

868. Detmers PA, Lo SK, Olsen-Egbert E, et al. Neutrophil-activating protein 1/ interleukin 8 stimulates the binding activity of the leukocyte adhesion recep-tor CD11b/CD18 on human neutrophils. *J Exp Med* 1990;171:1155–1162.

869. Gimbrone MA, Obin MS, Brock AF, et al. Endothelial interleukin-8: a novel inhibitor of leukocyte-endothelial interactions. *Science* 1989;246:1601–1603.

870. Yang Y-C, Ricciardi S, Ciarletta A, et al. Expression cloning of a cDNA encod-ing novel human hematopoietic growth factor: human homologue of murine T-cell growth factor P40. *Blood* 1989;74:1880–1884.

871. Van Snick J, Goethals A, Renauld J-C, et al. Cloning and characterization of a cDNA for a new mouse T cell growth factor (P40). *J Exp Med* 1989;169:363–368.

872. Donahue RE, Yang Y-C, Clark SC. Human P40 T-cell growth factor (interleu-kin-9) supports erythroid colony formation. *Blood* 1990;75:2271–2275.

873. Moore KW, Vieira P, Fiorentino DF, et al. Homology of cytokine synthesis inhibitory factor (IL-10) to the Epstein-Barr virus gene BCRFI. *Science* 1990;248:1230–1234.

874. Paul SR, Bennett F, Calvetti JA, et al. Molecular cloning of a cDNA encoding interleukin 11, a novel stromal cell-derived lymphopoietic and hematopoi-etic cytokine. *Proc Natl Acad Sci U S A* 1990;87:7512–7516.

875. Clark S. *Interleukin-12: a heterodimeric cytokine with multiple biologic activities.* 8th Symposium. Basil, Switzerland: 1993.

876. Cherwinski HM, Schumacher JH, Brown KD, et al. Two types of mouse helper T cell clone, III: further differences in lymphokine synthesis between Th1 and Th2 clones revealed by RNA hybridization, functionally monospe-cific bioassays, and monoclonal antibodies. *J Exp Med* 1987;166:1229–1244.

877. Brown KD, Zurawski SM, Mosmann TR, et al. A family of small inducible proteins secreted by leukocytes are members of a new superfamily that includes leukocyte and fibroblast-derived inflammatory agents, growth fac-tors, and indicators of various activation processes. *J Immunol* 1989;142:679–687.

878. McKenzie AN, Culpepper JA, de Waal Malefyt R, et al. Interleukin 13, a T-cell-derived cytokine that regulates human monocyte and B-cell function. *Proc Natl Acad Sci U S A* 1993;90:3735–3739.

879. Morgan JG, Dolganov GM, Robbins SE, et al. The selective isolation of novel cDNAs encoded by the regions surrounding the human interleukin 4 and 5 genes. *Nucleic Acids Res* 1992;20:5173–5179.

880. Minty A, Chalon P, Derocq JM, et al. Interleukin-13 is a new human lymphokine regulating inflammatory and immune responses. *Nature* 1993;362:248–250.

881. Punnonen J, Aversa G, Cocks BG, et al. Interleukin 13 induces interleukin 4-independent IgG4 and IgE synthesis and CD23 expression by human B cells. *Proc Natl Acad Sci U S A* 1993;90:3730–3734.

882. Rolink A, Grawunder U, Winkler TH, et al. IL-2 receptor alpha chain (CD25, TAC) expression defines a crucial stage in pre-B cell development. *Int Immu-nol* 1994;6:1257–1264.

883. Takacs L, Osawa H, Diamantstein T. Detection and localization by the mono-clonal anti-interleukin 2 receptor antibody AMT-13 of IL 2 receptor-bearing cells in the developing thymus of the mouse embryo and in the thymus of cortisone-treated mice. *Eur J Immunol* 1984;14:1152–1156.

884. Raulet DH. Expression and function of interleukin-2 receptors on immature thymocytes. *Nature* 1985;314:101–103.

885. Ceredig R, Lowenthal JW, Nabholz M, et al. Expression of interleukin-2 receptors as a differentiation marker on intrathymic stem cells. *Nature* 1985;314:98–100.

886. Willerford DM, Chen J, Ferry JA, et al. Interleukin-2 receptor alpha chain regulates the size and content of the peripheral lymphoid compartment. *Immunity* 1995;3:521–530.

887. Giri JG, Ahdieh M, Eisenman J, et al. Utilization of the beta and gamma chains of the IL-2 receptor by the novel cytokine IL-15. *EMBO J* 1994;13:2822–2830.

888. Grabstein KH, Eisenman J, Shanebeck K, et al. Cloning of a T cell growth factor that interacts with the beta chain of the interleukin-2 receptor. *Science* 1994;264:965–968.

889. Suzuki H, Kundig TM, Furlonger C, et al. Deregulated T cell activation and autoimmunity in mice lacking interleukin-2 receptor beta. *Science* 1995;268:1472–1476.

890. Tanaka T, Takeuchi Y, Shiohara T, et al. In utero treatment with monoclonal antibody to IL-2 receptor beta-chain completely abrogates development of Thy-1+ dendritic epidermal cells. *Int Immunol* 1992;4:487–491.

891. Takeuchi Y, Tanaka T, Hamamura K, et al. Expression and role of interleukin-2 receptor beta chain on CD4-CD8- T cell receptor alpha beta+ cells [Corrected]. *Eur J Immunol* 1992;22:2929–2935.

892. Kondo M, Takeshita T, Ishii N, et al. Sharing of the interleukin-2 (IL-2) receptor gamma chain between receptors for IL-2 and IL-4. *Science* 1993;262:1874–1877.

893. Kondo M, Takeshita T, Higuchi M, et al. Functional participation of the IL-2 receptor gamma chain in IL-7 receptor complexes. *Science* 1994;263:1453–1454.

894. Russell SM, Keegan AD, Harada N, et al. Interleukin-2 receptor gamma chain: a functional component of the interleukin-4 receptor. *Science* 1993;262:1880–1883.

895. Noguchi M, Nakamura Y, Russell SM, et al. Interleukin-2 receptor gamma chain: a functional component of the interleukin-7 receptor. *Science* 1993;262:1877–1880.

896. Russell SM, Johnston JA, Noguchi M, et al. Interaction of IL-2R beta and gamma c chains with Jak1 and Jak3: implications for XSCID and XCID. *Science* 1994;266:1042–1045.

897. von Freeden-Jeffry U, Moore TA, et al. IL-7 knockout mice and the generation of lymphocytes. In: Durum SK, Muegge S, eds. *Cytokine knockouts.* Totowa, NJ: Humana Press, 1998.

898. von Freeden-Jeffry U, Vieira P, Lucian LA, et al. Lymphopenia in interleukin (IL)-7 gene-deleted mice identifies IL-7 as a nonredundant cytokine. *J Exp Med* 1995;181:1519–1526.

899. He YW, Malek TR. Interleukin-7 receptor alpha is essential for the development of gamma delta + T cells, but not natural killer cells. *J Exp Med* 1996;184:289–293.

900. Kaushansky K. Thrombopoietin: the primary regulator of platelet production. *Blood* 1995;86:419–431.

901. Debili N, Masse JM, Katz A, et al. Effects of the recombinant hematopoietic growth factors interleukin-3, interleukin-6, stem cell factor, and leukemia inhibitory factor on the megakaryocytic differentiation of CD34+ cells. *Blood* 1993;82:84–95.

902. Guinan EC, Lee YS, Lopez KD, et al. Effects of interleukin-3 and granulocyte-macrophage colony-stimulating factor on thrombopoiesis in congenital amegakaryocytic thrombocytopenia. *Blood* 1993;81:1691–1698.

903. Hill RJ, Warren MK, Stenberg P, et al. Stimulation of megakaryocytopoiesis in mice by human recombinant interleukin-6. *Blood* 1991;77:42–48.

904. Neben S, Turner K. The biology of interleukin 11. *Stem Cells* 1993;11[Suppl 2]:156–162.

905. Broudy VC, Lin NL, Kaushansky K. Thrombopoietin (c-mpl ligand) acts synergistically with erythropoietin, stem cell factor, and interleukin-11 to enhance murine megakaryocyte colony growth and increases megakaryocyte ploidy in vitro. *Blood* 1995;85:1719–1726.

906. Briddell RA, Bruno E, Cooper RJ, et al. Effect of c-kit ligand on the in vitro human megakaryocytopoiesis. *Blood* 1991;78:2854–2859.

907. Ishibashi T, Koziol JA, Burstein SA. Human recombinant erythropoietin promotes differentiation of murine megakaryocytes in vitro. *J Clin Invest* 1987;79:286–289.

908. McDonald TP, Sullivan PS. Megakaryocytic and erythrocytic cell lines share a common precursor cell. *Exp Hematol* 1993;21:1316–1320.

909. Longmore GD, Pharr P, Neumann D, et al. Both megakaryocytopoiesis and erythropoiesis are induced in mice infected with a retrovirus expressing an oncogenic erythropoietin receptor. *Blood* 1993;82:2386–2395.

910. Tepler I, Elias L, Smith W II, et al. A randomized placebo-controlled trial of recombinant human interleukin-11 in cancer patients with severe thrombocytopenia due to chemotherapy. *Blood* 1996;87:3607–3614.

911. McDonald TP, Cottrell MB, Clift RE, et al. High doses of recombinant erythropoietin stimulate platelet production in mice. *J Exp Hematol* 1987;15:719–721.

912. Martin DI, Zon LI, Mutter IS, et al. Expression of an erythroid transcription factor in megakaryocytic and mast cell lineages. *Nature* 1990;344:444.

913. Methia N, Louache F, Vainchenker W, et al. Oligodeoxynucleotides antisense to the proto-oncogene c-mpl specifically inhibit in vitro megakaryocytopoiesis. *Blood* 1993;82:1395–1401.

914. Wendling F, Varlet P, Charon M, et al. MPLV: a retrovirus complex inducing an acute myeloproliferative leukemic disorder in adult mice. *Virology* 1986;149:242–246.

915. Cosman D. The hematopoietin receptor superfamily. *Cytokine* 1993;5:95–106.

916. Vigon I, Mornon JP, Cocault L, et al. Molecular cloning and characterization of MPL, the human homolog of the v-mpl oncogene: identification of a member of the hematopoietic growth factor receptor superfamily. *Proc Natl Acad Sci U S A* 1992;89:5640–5644.

917. Kato T, Ogami K, Shimada Y, et al. Purification and characterization of thrombopoietin. *J Biochem (Tokyo)* 1995;118:229–236.

918. Kuter DJ, Beeler DL, Rosenberg RD. The purification of megapoietin: a physiological regulator of megakaryocyte growth and platelet production. *Proc Natl Acad Sci U S A* 1994;91:11104.

919. Emmons RV, Reid DM, Cohen RL, et al. Human thrombopoietin levels are high when thrombocytopenia is due to megakaryocyte deficiency and low when due to increased platelet destruction. *Blood* 1996;87:4068–4071.

920. Kuter DJ, Rosenberg RD. The reciprocal relationship of thrombopoietin (c-Mpl ligand) to changes in the platelet mass during busulfan-induced thrombocytopenia in the rabbit. *Blood* 1995;85:2720–2730.

921. Shivdasani RA, Rosenblatt MF, Zucker-Franklin D, et al. Transcription factor NF-E2 is required for platelet formation independent of the actions of thrombopoietin/MGDF in megakaryocyte development. *Cell* 1995;81:695–704.

922. Karpatkin S. Heterogeneity of human platelets, I: metabolic and kinetic evidence suggestive of young and old platelets. *J Clin Invest* 1969;48:1073–1082.

923. Paulus JM, Breton-Gorius J. Platelets, production, function, transfusion, and storage. In: Baldini MG, Ebbe S, eds. *Megakaryocyte ultrastructure and ploidy in human macrothrombocytosis.* New York: Grune & Stratton, 1974.

924. Gewirtz AM, Calabretta B, Rucinksi B, et al. Inhibition of human megakaryocytopoiesis in vitro by platelet factor 4 (PF4) and a synthetic COOH-terminal PF4 peptide. *J Clin Invest* 1989;83:1477–1486.

925. Ishibashi T, Miller SL, Burstein SA. Type beta transforming growth factor is a potent inhibitor of murine megakaryocytopoiesis in vitro. *Blood* 1987;69:1737–1741.

926. Gewirtz AM, Zu WY, Mangan KF. Role of natural killer cells, in comparison with T lymphocytes and monocytes, in the regulation of normal human megakaryocytopoiesis in vitro. *J Immunol* 1987;139:2915–2924.

927. Pantel K, Nakeff A. Differential effect of natural killer cells on modulating CFU-meg and BFU-E proliferation *in situ. J Exp Hematol* 1989;17:1017–1021.

928. Huebner K, Isobe M, Croce CM, et al. The human gene encoding GM–CSF is at 5q21-q32, the chromosome region deleted in the 5q-anomaly. *Science* 1985;230:1282–1285.

929. LeBeau MM, Epstein ND, O'Brien SJ, et al. The interleukin 3 gene is located on human chromosome 5 and is deleted in myeloid leukaemias with a deletion of 5q. *Proc Natl Acad Sci U S A* 1987;84:5913–5917.

930. Pettenati MJ, LeBeau MM, Lemons RS, et al. Assignment of CSF-1 to 5q33.1: evidence for clustering of genes regulating hematopoiesis and for their involvement in the deletion of the long arm of chromosome 5 in myeloid disorders. *Proc Natl Acad Sci U S A* 1987;84:2970–2974.

931. LeBeau MM, Westbrook CA, Diaz MO, et al. Evidence for the involvement of GM-CSF and FMS in the deletion (5q) in myeloid disorders. *Science* 1987;231:984–987.

932. Watkins PC, Eddy R, Hoffman N, et al. Regional assignment of the erythropoietin gene to human chromosome region 7pter – q22. *Cytogenet Cell Genet* 1986;42:214–218.

933. Law ML, Cai G-Y, Lin F-K, et al. Chromosomal assignment of the human erythropoietin gene and its DNA polymorphism. *Proc Natl Acad Sci U S A* 1986;83:6920–6924.

934. Simmers RN, Webber LM, Shannon MF, et al. Localization of the G–CSF gene on chromosome 17 proximal to the breakpoint in the t (15;17) in acute promyelocytic leukemia. *Blood* 1987;70:330–332.

935. Budarf M, Huebner K, Emanuel B, et al. Assignment of the erythropoietin receptor (EPOR) gene to mouse chromosome 9 and human chromosome 19. *Genomics* 1990;8:575–578.

936. Isobe M, Kumura Y, Murata Y, et al. Localization of the gene encoding the alpha subunit of human interleukin-5 receptor (IL5RA) to chromosome region 3p24-3p26. *Genomics* 1992;14:755–758.

937. Shen Y, Baker E, Callen DF, et al. Localization of the human GM-CSF receptor beta chain gene (CSF2RB) to chromosome 22q12.2→q13.1. *Cytogenet Cell Genet* 1992;61:175–177.

938. Socolovsky M, Fallon AE, Lodish HF. The prolactin receptor rescues EpoR-/- erythroid progenitors and replaces EpoR in a synergistic interaction with c-kit. *Blood* 1998;92:1491–1496.

939. Ghaffari S, Kitidis C, Fleming MD, et al. Erythropoiesis in the absence of janus-kinase 2: BCR-ABL induces red cell formation in JAK2(-/-) hematopoietic progenitors. *Blood* 2001;98:2948–2957.

940. Cantor AB, Orkin SH. Hematopoietic development: a balancing act. *Curr Opin Genet Dev* 2001;11:513–519.

941. Evans T, Reitman M, Felsenfeld G. An erythrocyte-specific DNA-binding factor recognizes a regulatory sequence common to all chicken globin genes. *Proc Natl Acad Sci U S A* 1988;85:5976–5980.

942. Martin DI, Tsai SF, Orkin SH. Increased gamma-globin expression in a nondeletion HPFH mediated by an erythroid-specific DNA-binding factor. *Nature* 1989;338:435–438.

943. Eleouet JF, Romeo PH. CCACC-binding or simian-virus-40-protein-1-binding proteins cooperate with human GATA-1 to direct erythroid-specific transcription and to mediate 5' hypersensitive site 2 sensitivity of a TATA-less promoter. *Eur J Biochem* 1993;212:763–770.

944. Tsai SF, Martin DI, Zon LI, et al. Cloning of cDNA for the major DNA-binding protein of the erythroid lineage through expression in mammalian cells. *Nature* 1989;339:446–451.

945. Evans T, Felsenfeld G. The erythroid-specific transcription factor Eryf1: a new finger protein. *Cell* 1989;58:877–885.

946. Romeo PH, Prandini MH, Joulin V, et al. Megakaryocytic and erythrocytic lineages share specific transcription factors. *Nature* 1990;344:447–449.

947. Zon LI, Yamaguchi Y, Yee K, et al. Expression of mRNA for the GATA-binding proteins in human eosinophils and basophils: potential role in gene transcription. *Blood* 1993;81:3234–3241.

948. Zon LI, Gurish MF, Stevens RL, et al. GATA-binding transcription factors in mast cells regulate the promoter of the mast cell carboxypeptidase A gene. *J Biol Chem* 1991;266:22948–22953.

949. Perry L, Simon MC, Robertson E, et al. Erythroid differentiation in chimeric mice blocked by a targeted mutation in the gene for transcription factor GATA-1. *Nature* 1991;349:257.

950. Weiss MJ, Orkin SH. Transcription factor GATA-1 permits survival and maturation of erythroid precursors by preventing apoptosis. *Proc Natl Acad Sci U S A* 1995;92:9623–9627.

951. Vyas P, Ault K, Jackson CW, et al. Consequences of GATA-1 deficiency in megakaryocytes and platelets. *Blood* 1999;93:2867–2875.

952. Shivdasani RA, Fujiwara Y, McDevitt MA, et al. A lineage-selective knockout establishes the critical role of transcription factor GATA-1 in megakaryocyte growth and platelet development. *EMBO J* 1997;16:3965–3973.

953. Yamamoto M, Ko LJ, Leonard MW, et al. Activity and tissue-specific expression of the transcription factor NF-E1 multigene family. *Genes Dev* 1990;4:1650–1662.

954. Arceci RJ, King AA, Simon MC, et al. Mouse GATA-4: a retinoic acid-inducible GATA-binding transcription factor expressed in endodermally derived tissues and heart. *Mol Cell Biol* 1993;13:2235–2246.

955. Tsai F-Y, Keller G, Kuo FC, et al. An early haematopoietic defect in mice lacking the transcription factor GATA-2. *Nature* 1994;371:221–226.

956. Zon LI, Mather C, Burgess S, et al. Expression of GATA-binding proteins during embryonic development in Xenopus laevis. *Proc Natl Acad Sci U S A* 1991;88:10642–10646.

957. Zheng W, Flavell RA. The transcription factor GATA-3 is necessary and sufficient for Th2 cytokine gene expression in CD4 T cells. *Cell* 1997;89:587–596.

958. Ting CN, Olson MC, Barton KP, et al. Transcription factor GATA-3 is required for development of the T-cell lineage. *Nature* 1996;384:474–478.

959. Tsang AP, Visvader JE, Turner CA, et al. FOG, a multitype zinc finger protein, acts as a cofactor for transcription factor GATA-1 in erythroid and megakaryocytic differentiation. *Cell* 1997;90:109–119.

960. Crispino JD, Lodish MB, MacKay JP, et al. Use of altered specificity mutants to probe a specific protein-protein interaction in differentiation: the GATA-1:FOG complex. *Mol Cell* 1999;3:219–228.

961. Tsang AP, Fujiwara Y, Hom DB, et al. Failure of megakaryopoiesis and arrested erythropoiesis in mice lacking the GATA-1 transcriptional cofactor FOG. *Genes Dev* 1998;12:1176–1188.

962. Deconinck AE, Mead PE, Tevosian SG, et al. FOG acts as a repressor of red blood cell development in Xenopus. *Development* 2000;127:2031–2040.

963. Nichols KE, Crispino JD, Poncz M, et al. Familial dyserythropoietic anaemia and thrombocytopenia due to an inherited mutation in GATA1. *Nat Genet* 2000;24:266–270.

964. Tevosian SG, Deconinck AE, Cantor AB, et al. FOG-2: A novel GATA-family cofactor related to multitype zinc-finger proteins Friend of GATA-1 and U-shaped. *Proc Natl Acad Sci U S A* 1999;96:950–955.

965. Begley CG, Aplan PD, Davey MP, et al. Chromosomal translocation in a human leukemic stem-cell line disrupts the T-cell antigen receptor delta-chain diversity region and results in a previously unreported fusion transcript. *Proc Natl Acad Sci U S A* 1989;86:2031–2035.

966. Xia Y, Brown L, Tsan JT, et al. The translocation (1;14)(p34;q11) in human T-cell leukemia: chromosome breakage 25 kilobase pairs downstream of the TAL1 protooncogene. *Genes Chromosomes Cancer* 1992;4:211–216.

967. Begley CG, Green AR. The SCL gene: from case report to critical hematopoietic regulator. *Blood* 1999;93:2760–2770.

968. Visvader J, Begley CG, Adams JM. Differential expression of the LYL, SCL and E2A helix-loop-helix genes within the hemopoietic system. *Oncogene* 1991;6:187–194.

969. Voronova AF, Lee F. The E2A and tal-1 helix-loop-helix proteins associate in vivo and are modulated by Id proteins during interleukin 6-induced myeloid differentiation. *Proc Natl Acad Sci U S A* 1994;91:5952–5956.

970. Condorelli G, Vitelli L, Valtieri M, et al. Coordinate expression and developmental role of Id2 protein and TAL1/E2A heterodimer in erythroid progenitor differentiation. *Blood* 1995;86:164–175.

971. Wadman IA, Osada H, Grutz GG, et al. The LIM-only protein Lmo2 is a bridging molecule assembling an erythroid, DNA-binding complex which includes the TAL1, E47, GATA-1 and Ldb1/NLI proteins. *EMBO J* 1997;16:3145–3157.

972. Vitelli L, Condorelli G, Lulli V, et al. A pentamer transcriptional complex including tal-1 and retinoblastoma protein downmodulates c-kit expression in normal erythroblasts. *Mol Cell Biol* 2000;20:5330–5342.

973. Hsu HL, Wadman I, Baer R. Formation of in vivo complexes between the TAL1 and E2A polypeptides of leukemic T cells. *Proc Natl Acad Sci U S A* 1994;91:3181–3185.

974. Krosl G, He G, Lefrancois M, et al. Transcription factor SCL is required for c-kit expression and c-Kit function in hemopoietic cells. *J Exp Med* 1998;188:439–450.

975. Gering M, Rodaway AR, Gottgens B, et al. The SCL gene specifies haemangioblast development from early mesoderm. *EMBO J* 1998;17:4029–4045.

976. Liao EC, Paw BH, Oates AC, et al. SCL/Tal-1 transcription factor acts downstream of cloche to specify hematopoietic and vascular progenitors in zebrafish. *Genes Dev* 1998;12:621–626.

977. Mead PE, Kelley CM, Hahn PS, et al. SCL specifies hematopoietic mesoderm in Xenopus embryos. *Development* 1998;125:2611–2620.

978. Goodwin G, MacGregor A, Zhu J, et al. Molecular cloning of the chicken SCL cDNA. *Nucleic Acids Res* 1992;20:368.

979. Robb L, Elwood NJ, Elefanty AG, et al. The scl gene product is required for the generation of all hematopoietic lineages in the adult mouse. *EMBO J* 1996;15:4123–4129.

980. Shivdasani RA, Mayer EL, Orkin SH. Absence of blood formation in mice lacking the T-cell leukemia oncoprotein tal-1/SCL. *Nature* 1995;373:432.

981. Elefanty AG, Robb L, Birner R, et al. Hematopoietic-specific genes are not induced during in vitro differentiation of scl-null embryonic stem cells. *Blood* 1997;90:1435–1447.

982. Robertson SM, Kennedy M, Shannon JM, et al. A transitional stage in the commitment of mesoderm to hematopoiesis requiring the transcription factor SCL/tal-1. *Development* 2000;127:2447–2459.

983. Faloon P, Arentson E, Kazarov A, et al. Basic fibroblast growth factor positively regulates hematopoietic development. *Development* 2000;127:1931–1941.

984. Porcher C, Swat W, Rockwell K, et al. The T cell leukemia oncoprotein SCL/tal-1 is essential for development of all hematopoietic lineages. *Cell* 1996; 86:47–57.

985. Visvader JE, Fujiwara Y, Orkin SH. Unsuspected role for the T-cell leukemia protein SCL/tal-1 in vascular development. *Genes Dev* 1998;12:473–479.

986. Porcher C, Liao EC, Fujiwara Y, et al. Specification of hematopoietic and vascular development by the bHLH transcription factor SCL without direct DNA binding. *Development* 1999;126:4603–4615.

987. Royer-Pokora B, Loos U, Ludwig WD. TTG-2, a new gene encoding a cysteine-rich protein with the LIM motif, is overexpressed in acute T-cell leukaemia with the t(11;14)(p13;q11). *Oncogene* 1991;6:1887–1893.

988. Mead PE, Deconinck AE, Huber TL, et al. Primitive erythropoiesis in the Xenopus embryo: the synergistic role of LMO-2, SCL and GATA-binding proteins. *Development* 2001;128:2301–2308.

989. Thompson MA, Ransom DG, Pratt SJ, et al. The cloche and spadetail genes differentially affect hematopoiesis and vasculogenesis. *Dev Biol* 1998;197:248–269.

990. Warren AJ, Colledge WH, Carlton MB, et al. The oncogenic cysteine–rich LIM domain protein rbtn2 is essential for erythroid development. *Cell* 1994;78:45–57.

991. Valge-Archer VE, Osada H, Warren AJ, et al. The LIM protein RBTN2 and the basic helix-loop-helix protein TAL1 are present in a complex in erythroid cells. *Proc Natl Acad Sci U S A* 1994;91:8617–8621.

992. Visvader JE, Mao X, Fujiwara Y, et al. The LIM-domain binding protein Ldb1 and its partner LMO2 act as negative regulators of erythroid differentiation. *Proc Natl Acad Sci U S A* 1997;94:13707–13712.

993. Erickson P, Gao J, Chang KS, et al. Identification of breakpoints in t(8;21) acute myelogenous leukemia and isolation of a fusion transcript, AML1/ETO, with similarity to Drosophila segmentation gene, runt. *Blood* 1992;80:1825–1831.

994. Tighe JE, Daga A, Calabi F. Translocation breakpoints are clustered on both chromosome 8 and chromosome 21 in the t(8;21) of acute myeloid leukemia. *Blood* 1993;81:592–596.

995. Speck NA. Core binding factor and its role in normal hematopoietic development. *Curr Opin Hematol* 2001;8:192–196.

996. Ogawa E, Maruyama M, Kagoshima H, et al. PEBP2/PEA2 represents a family of transcription factors homologous to the products of the Drosophila runt gene and the human AML1 gene. *Proc Natl Acad Sci U S A* 1993;90:6859–6863.

997. Miyoshi H, Kozu T, Shimizu K, et al. The t(8;21) translocation in acute myeloid leukemia results in production of an AML1-MTG8 fusion transcript. *EMBO J* 1993;12:2715–2721.

998. Meyers S, Downing JR, Hiebert SW. Identification of AML-1 and the (8;21) translocation protein (AML-1/ETO) as sequence-specific DNA-binding proteins: the runt homology domain is required for DNA binding and protein-protein interactions. *Mol Cell Biol* 1993;13:6336–6345.

999. Song WJ, Sullivan MG, Legare RD, et al. Haploinsufficiency of CBFA2 causes familial thrombocytopenia with propensity to develop acute myelogenous leukaemia. *Nat Genet* 1999;23:166–175.

1000. Pepling ME, Gergen JP. Conservation and function of the transcriptional regulatory protein Runt. *Proc Natl Acad Sci U S A* 1995;92:9087–9091.

1001. North T, Gu TL, Stacy T, et al. Cbfa2 is required for the formation of intra-aortic hematopoietic clusters. *Development* 1999;126:2563–2575.

1002. Okada H, Watanabe T, Niki M, et al. AML1(−/−) embryos do not express certain hematopoiesis-related gene transcripts including those of the PU.1 gene. *Oncogene* 1998;17:2287–2293.

1003. Cai Z, de Bruijn M, Ma X, et al. Haploinsufficiency of AML1 affects the temporal and spatial generation of hematopoietic stem cells in the mouse embryo. *Immunity* 2000;13:423–431.

1004. Wang Q, Stacy T, Binder M, et al. Disruption of the Cbfa2 gene causes necrosis and hemorrhaging in the central nervous system and blocks definitive hematopoiesis. *Proc Natl Acad Sci U S A* 1996;93:3444–3449.

1005. Wang Q, Stacy T, Miller JD, et al. The CBFbeta subunit is essential for CBFalpha2 (AML1) function in vivo. *Cell* 1996;87:697–708.

1006. Castilla LH, Wijmenga C, Wang Q, et al. Failure of embryonic hematopoiesis and lethal hemorrhages in mouse embryos heterozygous for a knocked-in leukemia gene CBFB-MYH11. *Cell* 1996;87:687–696.

1007. Niki M, Okada H, Takano H, et al. Hematopoiesis in the fetal liver is impaired by targeted mutagenesis of a gene encoding a non-DNA binding subunit of the transcription factor, polyomavirus enhancer binding protein 2/core binding factor. *Proc Natl Acad Sci U S A* 1997;94:5697–5702.

1008. Okuda T, van Deursen J, Hiebert SW, et al. AML1, the target of multiple chromosomal translocations in human leukemia, is essential for normal fetal liver hematopoiesis. *Cell* 1996;84:321–330.

1009. Yergeau DA, Hetherington CJ, Wang Q, et al. Embryonic lethality and impairment of haematopoiesis in mice heterozygous for an AML1-ETO fusion gene. *Nat Genet* 1997;15:303–306.

1010. Beug H, Hayman MJ, Graf T. Myeloblasts transformed by the avian acute leukemia virus E26 are hormone-dependent for growth and for the expression of a putative myb-containing protein, p135 E26. *EMBO J* 1982;1:1069–1073.

1011. Slamon DJ, Shimotohno K, Cline MJ, et al. Antigens encoded by the 3'-terminal region of human T-cell leukemia virus: evidence for a functional gene. *Science* 1984;226:57–64.

1012. Mukouyama Y, Chiba N, Hara T, et al. The AML1 transcription factor functions to develop and maintain hematogenic precursor cells in the embryonic aorta-gonad-mesonephros region. *Dev Biol* 2000;220:27–36.

1013. Mukouyama Y, Chiba N, Mucenski ML, et al. Hematopoietic cells in cultures of the murine embryonic aorta-gonad-mesonephros region are induced by c-Myb. *Curr Biol* 1999;9:833–836.

1014. Vandenbunder B, Pardanaud L, Jaffredo T, et al. Complementary patterns of expression of c-ets 1, c-myb and c-myc in the blood-forming system of the chick embryo. *Development* 1989;107:265–274.

1015. Mucenski ML, McLain K, Kier AB, et al. A functional c-myb gene is required for normal murine fetal hepatic hematopoiesis. *Cell* 1991;65:677–689.

1016. Sumner R, Crawford A, Mucenski M, et al. Initiation of adult myelopoiesis can occur in the absence of c-Myb whereas subsequent development is strictly dependent on the transcription factor. *Oncogene* 2000;19:3335–3342.

1017. Clarke D, Vegiopoulos A, Crawford A, et al. In vitro differentiation of c-myb(−/−) ES cells reveals that the colony forming capacity of unilineage macrophage precursors and myeloid progenitor commitment are c-Myb independent. *Oncogene* 2000;19:3343–3351.

1018. Krause DS, Mucenski ML, Lawler AM, et al. CD34 expression by embryonic hematopoietic and endothelial cells does not require c-Myb. *Exp Hematol* 1998;26:1086–1092.

1019. DeKoter RP, Singh H. Regulation of B lymphocyte and macrophage development by graded expression of PU.1. *Science* 2000;288:1439–1441.

1020. Galson DL, Hensold JO, Bishop TR, et al. Mouse beta-globin DNA-binding protein B1 is identical to a proto-oncogene, the transcription factor Spi-1/PU.1, and is restricted in expression to hematopoietic cells and the testis. *Mol Cell Biol* 1993;13:2929–2941.

1021. Scott EW, Simon MC, Anatasi J, et al. Requirement of transcription factor PU.1 in the development of multiple hematopoietic lineages. *Science* 1994;265:1573.

1022. Henkel GW, McKercher SR, Yamamoto H, et al. PU.1 but not ets-2 is essential for macrophage development from embryonic stem cells. *Blood* 1996;88:2917–2926.

1023. Rekhtman N, Radparvar F, Evans T, et al. Direct interaction of hematopoietic transcription factors PU.1 and GATA-1: functional antagonism in erythroid cells. *Genes Dev* 1999;13:1398–1411.

1024. Zhang P, Behre G, Pan J, et al. Negative cross-talk between hematopoietic regulators: GATA proteins repress PU.1. *Proc Natl Acad Sci U S A* 1999;96:8705–8710.

1025. Zhang P, Zhang X, Iwama A, et al. PU.1 inhibits GATA-1 function and erythroid differentiation by blocking GATA-1 DNA binding. *Blood* 2000;96:2641–2648.

1026. Nerlov C, Querfurth E, Kulessa H, et al. GATA-1 interacts with the myeloid PU.1 transcription factor and represses PU.1-dependent transcription. *Blood* 2000;95:2543–2551.

1027. Golub TR, Barker GF, Lovett M, et al. Fusion of PDGF receptor beta to a novel ets-like gene, tel, in chronic myelomonocytic leukemia with t(5;12) chromosomal translocation. *Cell* 1994;77:307–316.

1028. Golub TR, Barker GF, Bohlander SK, et al. Fusion of the TEL gene on 12p13 to the AML1 gene on 21q22 in acute lymphoblastic leukemia. *Proc Natl Acad Sci U S A* 1995;92:4917–4921.

1029. Wang LC, Swat W, Fujiwara Y, et al. The TEL/ETV6 gene is required specifically for hematopoiesis in the bone marrow. *Genes Dev* 1998;12:2392–2402.

1030. Miller IJ, Bieker JJ. A novel, erythroid cell-specific murine transcription factor that binds to the CACCC element and is related to the Kruppel family of nuclear proteins. *Mol Cell Biol* 1993;13:2776–2786.

1031. Bieker JJ, Southwood CM. The erythroid Kruppel-like factor transactivation domain is a critical component for cell-specific inducibility of a beta-globin promoter. *Mol Cell Biol* 1995;15:852–860.

1032. Wijgerde M, Gribnau J, Trimborn T, et al. The role of EKLF in human beta-globin gene competition. *Genes Dev* 1996;10:2894–2902.

1033. Lim SK, Bieker JJ, Lin CS, et al. A shortened life span of EKLF−/− adult erythrocytes, due to a deficiency of beta-globin chains, is ameliorated by human gamma-globin chains. *Blood* 1997;90:1291–1299.

1034. Perkins AC, Gaensler KM, Orkin SH. Silencing of human fetal globin expression is impaired in the absence of the adult beta-globin gene activator protein EKLF. *Proc Natl Acad Sci U S A* 1996;93:12267–12271.

1035. Guy LG, Mei Q, Perkins AC, et al. Erythroid Kruppel-like factor is essential for beta-globin gene expression even in absence of gene competition, but is not sufficient to induce the switch from gamma-globin to beta-globin gene expression. *Blood* 1998;91:2259–2263.

1036. Perkins AC, Peterson KR, Stamatoyannopoulos G, et al. Fetal expression of a human Agamma globin transgene rescues globin chain imbalance but not hemolysis in EKLF null mouse embryos. *Blood* 2000;95:1827–1833.

1037. Hohaus S, Petrovick MS, Voso MT, et al. PU.1 (Spi-1) and C/EBP alpha regulate expression of the granulocyte-macrophage colony-stimulating factor receptor alpha gene. *Mol Cell Biol* 1995;15:5830–5845.

1038. Zhang DE, Hohaus S, Voso MT, et al. Function of PU.1 (Spi-1), C/EBP, and AML1 in early myelopoiesis: regulation of multiple myeloid CSF receptor promoters. *Curr Top Microbiol Immunol* 1996;211:137–147.

1039. Zhang DE, Hetherington CJ, Meyers S, et al. CCAAT enhancer-binding protein (C/EBP) and AML1 (CBF alpha2) synergistically activate the macrophage colony-stimulating factor receptor promoter. *Mol Cell Biol* 1996;16:1231–1240.

1040. Ford AM, Bennett CA, Healy LE, et al. Regulation of the myeloperoxidase enhancer binding proteins Pu1, C-EBP alpha, -beta, and -delta during granulocyte-lineage specification. *Proc Natl Acad Sci U S A* 1996;93:10838–10843.

1041. Smith LT, Hohaus S, Gonzalez DA, et al. PU.1 (Spi-1) and C/EBP alpha regulate the granulocyte colony-stimulating factor receptor promoter in myeloid cells. *Blood* 1996;88:1234–1247.

1042. Zhang DE, Zhang P, Wang ND, et al. Absence of granulocyte colony-stimulating factor signaling and neutrophil development in CCAAT enhancer binding protein alpha-deficient mice. *Proc Natl Acad Sci U S A* 1997;94:569–574.

1043. Zhang P, Iwama A, Datta MW, et al. Upregulation of interleukin 6 and granulocyte colony-stimulating factor receptors by transcription factor CCAAT enhancer binding protein alpha (C/EBP alpha) is critical for granulopoiesis. *J Exp Med* 1998;188:1173–1184.

1044. Morosetti R, Park DJ, Chumakov AM, et al. A novel, myeloid transcription factor, C/EBP epsilon, is upregulated during granulocytic, but not monocytic, differentiation. *Blood* 1997;90:2591–2600.

1045. Yamanaka R, Barlow C, Lekstrom-Himes J, et al. Impaired granulopoiesis, myelodysplasia, and early lethality in CCAAT/enhancer binding protein epsilon-deficient mice. *Proc Natl Acad Sci U S A* 1997;94:13187–13192.

1046. Lekstrom-Himes J, Xanthopoulos KG. CCAAT/enhancer binding protein epsilon is critical for effective neutrophil-mediated response to inflammatory challenge. *Blood* 1999;93:3096–3105.

1047. Kubota T, Kawano S, Chih DY, et al. Representational difference analysis using myeloid cells from C/EBP epsilon deletional mice. *Blood* 2000;96:3953–3957.

CHAPTER 8

Inherited Bone Marrow Failure Syndromes

Blanche P. Alter and Alan D. D'Andrea

Constitutional aplastic anemia was defined by O'Gorman Hughes (1) as "chronic bone marrow failure associated with other features, such as congenital anomalies, a familial incidence, or thrombocytopenia at birth." In fact, he was referring to *inherited aplastic anemia*. Patients with constitutional aplastic anemia are genetically at risk for bone marrow failure, which may be expressed at birth (and therefore congenital), but it often develops later. O'Gorman Hughes further divided constitutional aplastic anemia into three types by using terminology that is confusing and no longer relevant. We refer to each disorder by its eponym, until more specific information becomes available, and to the entire group as the *inherited bone marrow failure syndromes*, so as to distinguish them from acquired aplastic anemia.

We can sometimes identify homozygotes for autosomal-recessive types of inherited bone marrow failure syndromes (or hemizygotes for X-linked disorders) by phenotype, although we cannot easily identify heterozygotes except by inference from family studies or by mutation analysis in disorders and in families in which the mutation is known. Inherited bone marrow failure is probably more common than published reports indicate, because the phenotype may range from severely abnormal to entirely normal (see the section Inheritance and Environment). In this section, we discuss the classic phenotypes in the major inherited bone marrow failure syndromes and emphasize the variation within each category. Some of this variation may result from the inadvertent inclusion of patients with congenital but not inherited phenotypes that resemble the genetic conditions (phenotypes), because until recently there was no specific diagnostic test for most of the disorders.

The incidence of inherited marrow failure is difficult to ascertain from the literature. Among 134 patients with all types of aplastic anemia who were seen at the Children's Hospital Medical Center in Boston from 1958 to 1977, 40 patients appeared to have inherited disorders (2) (Fig. 8-1). Twenty-six patients had Fanconi's anemia (all diagnosed in the era before testing of chromosome breakage), four patients developed aplastic anemia after amegakaryocytic thrombocytopenia, and ten patients had familial aplastic anemia without physical or cytogenetic evidence for Fanconi's anemia. In 21 years at the Prince of Wales Hospital in Australia (1964 to 1984), 12 of 34 patients were found to have inherited syndromes, including eight patients with Fanconi's anemia (3).

In our earlier analysis of the literature, we found that approximately 25% of cases of childhood aplastic anemia were diagnosed as inherited, which is probably an underestimate (4). The genetic syndromes must be considered carefully in patients of any age with aplastic anemia, because the prognosis, treatment, and approach to bone marrow transplantation (BMT) and potential gene therapy are different when the hematologic disorder is inherited rather than acquired. More detailed reviews of the inherited bone marrow failure syndromes can be found elsewhere (5,6).

PANCYTOPENIAS

Fanconi's Anemia

Fanconi's anemia was first described by Fanconi (7) in 1927 in three brothers with pancytopenia combined with physical

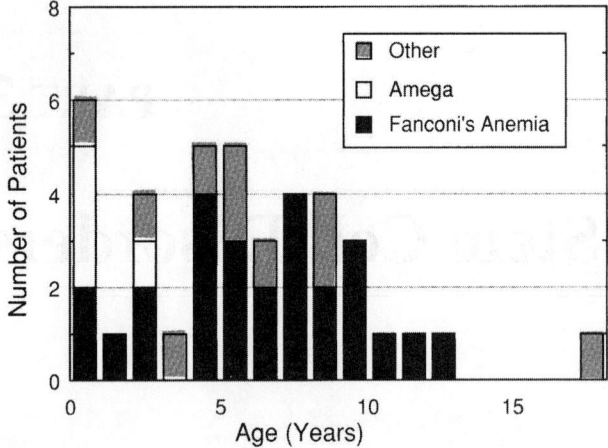

Figure 8-1. Age at diagnosis of inherited aplastic anemia in 40 patients who were seen at the Children's Hospital Medical Center, Boston, from 1958 to 1970. Twenty-six patients had Fanconi's anemia, four patients had amega-karyocytic thrombocytopenia (Amega) and developed aplastic anemia, and ten patients (in six families) had other familial bone marrow failure syndromes. (Adapted from Alter BP, Potter NU, Li FP. Classification and aetiology of the aplastic anaemias. *Clin Haematol* 1978;7:431–465.)

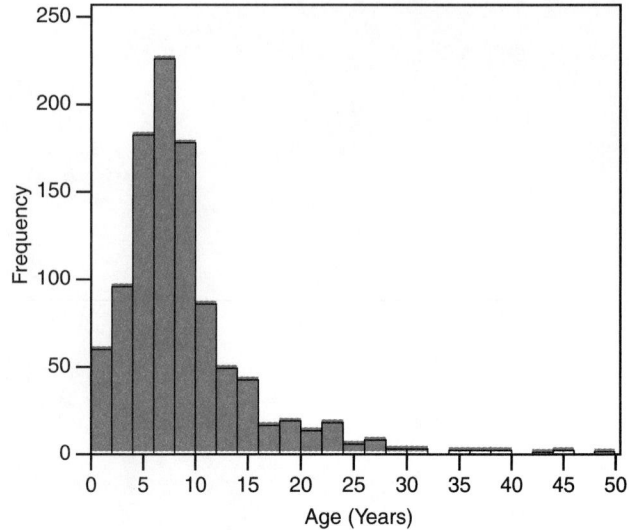

Figure 8-2. Age at diagnosis in approximately 1200 cases of Fanconi's anemia that were published from 1927 to 2000.

abnormalities. The anemia was macrocytic and thus was called *pernizioisiforme*, despite no further evidence for megaloblastic anemia. Uehlinger (8) then reported a similar patient with aplastic anemia and abnormalities of the thumb and kidney, and Fanconi (9) indicated that Naegeli had suggested in 1931 that familial aplastic anemia plus congenital anomalies should be called *Fanconi's anemia*.

The diagnosis of Fanconi's anemia is based on the finding of characteristic chromosomal breaks in cells that are cultured with a clastogenic agent and is confirmed by complementation or mutation analysis (see the section Cellular Phenotype). The patient's physical appearance may be normal, and he or she may or may not have aplastic anemia. More than 1200 cases of Fanconi's anemia have been mentioned in the literature with sufficient detail for many of the analyses that are described in this section (Table 8-1). The male to female ratio is 1.2:1.0, which is consistent with autosomal-recessive inheritance. Patients have been reported from more than 60 countries and represent all ethnic and racial groups, including whites, blacks, Asians, Native Americans, and persons from India. Figure 8-2 shows the distribution of ages at diagnosis.

TABLE 8-1. Fanconi's Anemia Literature

	All Patients
Number of cases	1206
Male to female ratio	1.24:1.00
Male age at diagnosis (in yr)	
Mean	8.1
Median	6.5
Range	0–48
Female age at diagnosis (in yr)	
Mean	9
Median	8
Range	0–48
Number of males ≤ 1 yr of age	27 (4%)
Number of females ≤1 yr of age	16 (3%)
Number of males ≥16 yr of age	57 (9%)
Number of females ≥16 yr of age	47 (9%)
Percent of patients who were reported deceased	38
Projected median survival (in yr)	20

Although diagnoses were usually made when aplastic anemia was detected, some diagnoses were made in nonanemic siblings. More recently, diagnoses have also been made after cytogenetic studies in patients with physical anomalies and normal blood counts. The median age at diagnosis in males and females was 6.5 and 8 years of age, respectively. Although the majority of the patients were younger than 15 years of age at the time of the diagnosis of Fanconi's anemia, 4% were diagnosed between birth and 1 year of age, and less than half of those patients had hematologic manifestations at the time of diagnosis. Twenty-seven patients were male, and 16 patients were female. Thus, Fanconi's anemia cannot be excluded as the cause of aplastic anemia in the first year of life, because "the patient is too young." At the other end of the age spectrum, 9% of patients were diagnosed at 16 years of age or older. Fifty-seven patients were male, and 47 patients were female. The proportion of patients with Fanconi's anemia who are adults is undoubtedly underestimated. Inherited aplastic anemia is not usually considered in an adult with aplastic anemia, with or without characteristic physical findings. Testing for chromosome breakage is required to identify Fanconi's anemia as the cause of the aplasia, but it is usually not performed for adult patients.

PHYSICAL EXAMINATION

The first patients were diagnosed with Fanconi's anemia because of the combination of aplastic anemia and physical anomalies or because of other family members with aplastic anemia or anomalies, or both. This bias in the literature may have contributed to the perception that patients must have physical anomalies for this diagnosis. The more recent tests for chromosome breakage and for specific genotypes have led to diagnoses in older patients and in those without overt birth defects. Patients with characteristic anomalies are often diagnosed without hematologic involvement.

Overall, approximately 25% of the literature cases had no anomalies, whereas 11% had only short stature or skin pigmentary changes, or both. The frequencies of the more common birth defects are summarized in Table 8-2. Physical abnormalities occurred more frequently in the patients who were diagnosed in infancy than in those who were diagnosed as adults, with the exception of short stature and café-au-lait spots. Figure

TABLE 8-2. Physical Abnormalities in Fanconi's Anemia

Abnormality	All Patients	Age at Diagnosis	
		≤1 Yr of Age	≥16 Yr of Age
Number of cases	1206	43 (4%)	104 (9%)
Skin pigment or café-au-lait spots, or both	55	37	61
Short stature	51	47	57
Upper limbs	43	63	39
Abnormal gonads, male	32	37	44
Abnormal gonads, female	3	50	6
Head	26	37	18
Eyes	23	33	24
Renal	21	42	19
Birth weight ≤ 2500 g	11	47	8
Developmental disability	11	5	8
Ears, hearing decreased	9	23	11
Legs	8	16	7
Cardiopulmonary	6	16	5
Gastrointestinal	5	28	6
No anomalies	25	16	23
Short stature or skin pigment, or both	11	5	19

NOTE: All values, except those in the "Number of cases" row, are percentages.

8-3 shows a boy with almost all the classic anomalies that are seen in patients with Fanconi's anemia. The breadth of anomalies is wide, and some patients clearly have none.

The abnormalities in Fanconi's anemia are listed in detail in Table 8-3. The most common finding is skin hyperpigmentation, a generalized brown melanin-like darkening that is most prominent on the trunk, neck, and intertriginous areas and that becomes more obvious with age. Children who are affected are often thought to have a permanent suntan. Café-au-lait spots are common, alone or combined with hyperpigmentation, and

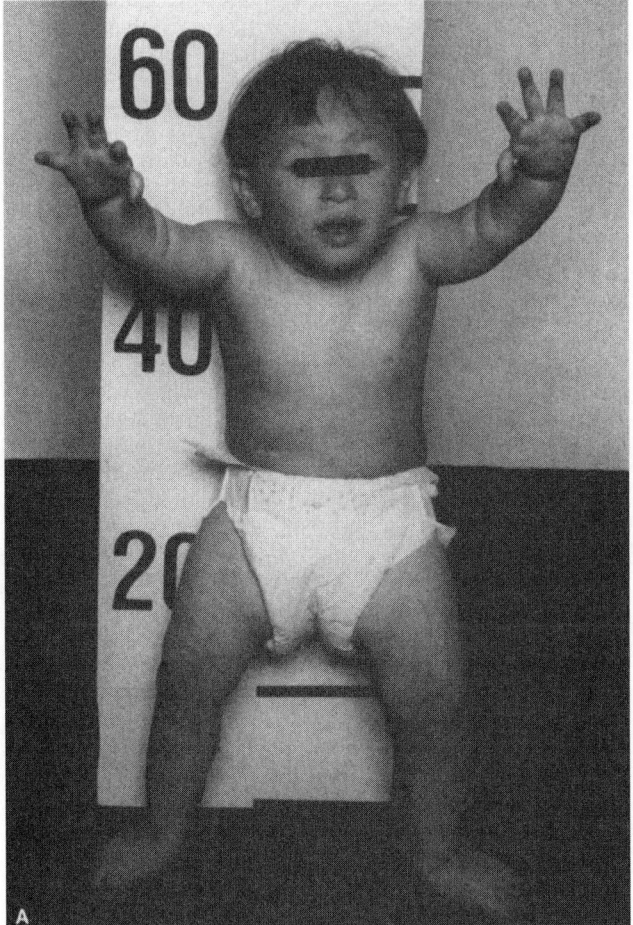
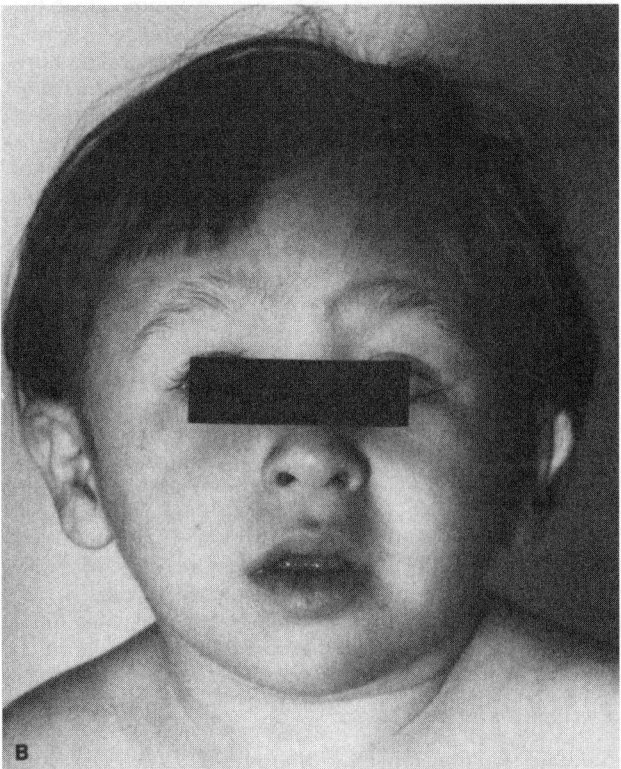

Figure 8-3. Three-year-old boy with Fanconi's anemia, with several phenotypic features. **A:** Front view. **B:** Face. (*continued*)

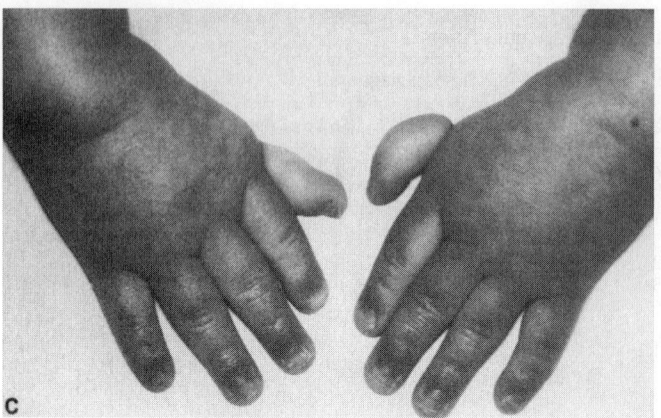
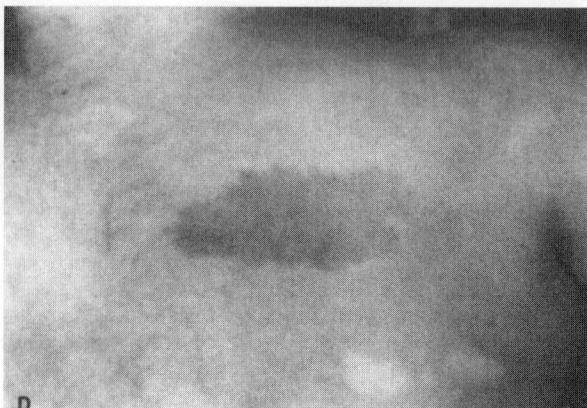

Figure 8-3. (continued) C: Hands. **D:** The back of the right shoulder. Features to be noted are short stature, thumbs attached by threads, microcephaly, broad nasal base, epicanthal folds, micrognathia, and café-au-lait spot with hypopigmented areas beneath.

hypopigmented areas are also seen. The number and size of these pigment changes increases with age (10). Café-au-lait spots may actually be more common than hyperpigmentation, but many case reports do not differentiate between them (11).

Microsomia, which is manifested by short stature and small delicate features, was often the presenting complaint before the development of hematologic problems. Many patients did not eat or grow well in the early years. Upper limb abnormalities, particularly absence or hypoplasia of thumbs, were reported in more than one-half of patients. Absent or hypoplastic radii were always associated with absent or hypoplastic thumbs [unlike thrombocytopenia-absent radius (TAR) syndrome, in which the thumbs are always present despite the absence of the radii]. Supernumerary, bifid thumbs and thumbs that were attached only by threads were also common. Flattening of the thenar eminence and weakness of radial pulses are subtle but common findings in our own experience, and are more common than the literature reflects.

The next most common physical problem involves the genitalia in one-third of male patients, with underdevelopment or undescended testes, or both. Abnormal gonadal development was commented on in only 3% of females, although abnormalities in menses and early menopause were also mentioned in a few instances.

Abnormally shaped heads were reported in 25% of patients with Fanconi's anemia, with most having microcephaly. The facies are often characteristic (Fig. 8-3). Neck anomalies lead to the perception of short or webbed necks, and spine anomalies also occur. The most common abnormalities of the eyes are microphthalmia and strabismus, as well as epicanthal folds, hypertelorism, and ptosis. Ear problems, including deafness as well as structural abnormalities of the external or middle ear, occur in approximately 10% of patients.

Renal defects, most often ectopic, pelvic, or horseshoe kidneys, as well as absent or hypoplastic kidneys, are found in more than 20% of Fanconi's anemia patients. Most of the renal problems are structural, although functional defects that result in reflux or infections can occur. The incidence of renal structural abnormalities may actually be higher than is cited here, because many patients do not have imaging studies performed.

Several abnormalities were described in fewer than 10% of the reports. These include low birth weight (particularly in those who were diagnosed in infancy), developmental delay, defects that involve the lower limbs, congenital heart disease, and gastrointestinal anomalies. Some of the feeding difficulties of infants with Fanconi's anemia might be due to undocu-

mented gastrointestinal abnormalities. The incidence and types of anomalies are similar in both sexes.

Auerbach et al. (12) used a stepwise multivariate analysis of the first 162 patients in the International Fanconi Anemia Registry (IFAR) to develop a scoring system that discriminated between patients with clastogenic stress-induced chromosome breakage [using diepoxybutane (DEB)] and those without chromosome breakage. One point each is added for microphthalmia, birthmarks, genitourinary abnormalities, growth retardation, thrombocytopenia, and the absence of radius or thumb, or both. One point is subtracted for learning disabilities, and one point is subtracted for other skeletal abnormalities. Higher scores mean that the probability of Fanconi's anemia is increased. This system was developed before the use of complementation or mutation analysis to confirm the diagnosis of Fanconi's anemia.

The terms *constitutional aplastic anemia type II* and *Estren-Dameshek aplastic anemia* were used to describe patients who have familial aplastic anemia but lack anomalies. The original paper by Estren and Dameshek (13) described two such families. In fact, two of the patients did have undescended testes. Li and Potter (14) reinvestigated one of these families and discovered that a second cousin, whose parents were both cousins of the original parents, had typical Fanconi's anemia. Now that chromosome breakage and molecular testing are available, patients whose anemia might have been called *Estren-Dameshek* can be correctly diagnosed as Fanconi's anemia. Many patients who were reported in the literature were entirely normal or had only short stature or changes in skin pigment.

Further evidence that the Estren-Dameshek patients belong to the Fanconi's anemia spectrum is provided by the IFAR data (12). In that registry, the diagnosis of Fanconi's anemia was made only when clastogenic stress-induced chromosome breaks were found, independent of physical appearance and family history (although many of the physically and hematologically normal children were tested only because of a positive family history). Thirty percent of the Fanconi's anemia group had aplastic anemia without anomalies, and 7% had neither. Two smaller studies of affected siblings of probands showed that at least 25% of those who were affected lacked anomalies (15,16). Fanconi's anemia is considered to include a spectrum of physical findings, which range from totally normal to the extreme of all the problems that were previously listed.

INHERITANCE AND ENVIRONMENT

Fanconi's anemia is clearly inherited in an autosomal-recessive pattern, despite the apparent slight preponderance in the

TABLE 8-3. Specific Types of Anomalies in Fanconi's Anemia Patients

Skin
  Generalized hyperpigmentation on trunk, neck, and intertriginous areas; café-au-lait spots; hypopigmented areas
Body
  Short stature, delicate features
Upper limbs
  Thumbs—absent or hypoplastic, supernumerary, bifid, rudimentary, short, low set, attached by a thread, triphalangeal, tubular, stiff, and hyperextensible
  Radii—absent or hypoplastic (only with abnormal thumbs); absent or weak pulse
  Hands—clinodactyly; hypoplastic thenar eminence; six fingers; absent first metacarpal; enlarged, abnormal fingers; short fingers
  Ulnae—dysplastic
Gonads
  Males—hypogenitalia; undescended testes; hypospadias; abnormal, absent testis; atrophic testes; azoospermia; phimosis; abnormal urethra; micropenis; delayed development
  Females—hypogenitalia; bicornuate uterus; abnormality, aplasia of uterus and vagina; atresia of uterus, vagina, and ovary
Other skeletal anomalies
  Head and face—microcephaly, hydrocephalus, micrognathia, peculiar face, bird face, flat head, frontal bossing, scaphocephaly, sloped forehead, choanal atresia
  Neck—Sprengel's deformity, short, low hairline, webbed
  Spine—spina bifida (thoracic, lumbar, cervical, occult sacral), scoliosis, abnormal ribs, sacrococcygeal sinus, Klippel-Feil syndrome, vertebral anomalies, extra vertebrae
Eyes
  Small, strabismus, epicanthal folds, hypertelorism, ptosis, slanted, cataracts, astigmatism, blindness, epiphora, nystagmus, proptosis, small iris
Ears
  Deaf (usually conductive), abnormal shape, atresia, dysplasia, low set, large, small, infections, abnormal middle ear, absent drum, dimples, rotated, canal stenosis
Kidneys
  Ectopic or pelvic, abnormality, horseshoe, hypoplastic or dysplastic, absent, hydronephrosis or hydroureter, infections, duplicated, rotated, reflux, hyperplasia, no function, abnormal artery
Gastrointestinal system
  High arch palate, atresia (esophagus, duodenum, jejunum), imperforate anus, tracheoesophageal fistula, Meckel's diverticulum, umbilical hernia, hypoplastic uvula, abnormal biliary ducts, megacolon, abdominal diastasis, Budd-Chiari syndrome
Lower limbs
  Feet—toe syndactyly, abnormal toes, flat feet, short toes, clubfoot, six toes, supernumerary toe
  Legs—congenital hip dislocation, Perthes' disease, coxa vara, abnormal femur, thigh osteoma, abnormal legs
Cardiopulmonary system
  Patent ductus arteriosus, ventricular septal defect, abnormality, peripheral pulmonic stenosis, aortic stenosis, coarctation, absent lung lobes, vascular malformation, aortic atheromas, atrial septal defect, tetralogy of Fallot, pseudotruncus, hypoplastic aorta, abnormal pulmonary drainage, double aortic arch, cardiac myopathy
Other anomalies
  Slow development, hyperreflexia, Bell's palsy, central nervous system arterial malformation, stenosis of the internal carotid, small pituitary

NOTE: Abnormalities are listed in approximate order of occurrence within each category.
Reproduced from Young NS, Alter BP. *Aplastic anemia: acquired and inherited.* Philadelphia: WB Saunders, 1994:410, with permission.

literature of males who are affected (Table 8-1). In a large study, 30% of families had two children who were affected, and consanguinity was found in 10% (17). The literature reports include 90 families with consanguinity, 325 families with affected siblings, and ten families with affected cousins. Mothers of Fanconi's anemia patients appear to have an unusual number of miscarriages (30 noted in the literature), and some of those fetuses were found to have significant phys-

ical anomalies. Rogatko and Auerbach (18) confirmed a monogenic autosomal-recessive pattern by segregation analysis of the 86 cases in the report of Schroeder et al. (17) and of 88 affected persons in the IFAR.

The heterozygote incidence may be 1 in 300 persons in the United States and approximately 1 in 100 Afrikaans in South Africa and Ashkenazi Jews, owing to separate founder effects (17,19,20). Physical abnormalities were reported in a few parents, suggesting phenotypic changes in heterozygotes (21–23). Others have suggested that relatives of persons with Fanconi's anemia (possible heterozygotes) have an increased incidence of congenital malformations, particularly genitourinary and hand malformations (24). Some siblings had characteristic physical abnormalities without hematologic disease (25–28). (These children may subsequently have developed aplastic anemia.) Some families have children with pancytopenia and normal physical examinations in addition to children with classic malformations (29–31). A family was described in 1944 with one child who had typical Fanconi's anemia and his brother who had paroxysmal nocturnal hemoglobinuria, developed lung cancer, and was proven to have Fanconi's anemia in 1987 by DEB-induced chromosome breakage (32) (E. C. Gordon-Smith, *personal communication*). A cousin, who was related maternally and paternally to the family, died of leukemia. These variations may reflect incomplete expression of the homozygous state or may occur in heterozygotes. Most of the reports predated stress-induced chromosome breakage studies. The varied expression may indicate allelic but different genetic mutations, interacting mutant genes, or the influence of the environment on the Fanconi's anemia phenotype.

Patients with Fanconi's anemia can now be diagnosed by chromosome breakage or genetic studies before the onset of hematologic or malignant complications [preanemic phase (33–37)]. There are several advantages to presymptomatic diagnoses. Patients can be told to avoid drugs and other agents that have been implicated in the development of acquired aplastic anemia. Prospective analysis leads to a determination of the actual incidences of aplastic anemia, leukemia, and other malignancies. Factors that lead to the development of these complications (second hits) may be identified. Early recognition of Fanconi's anemia in a family may be used for choices regarding family planning.

The environment has been invoked to explain the aplastic anemia in some cases. In one family with three Fanconi's anemia homozygotes (38), one sister died of aplastic anemia at 16 years of age (according to another sister, she had been treating skin infections with coal tar). The other two sisters, who were proven to be Fanconi's anemia homozygotes by DEB-induced chromosome breakage, despite only mild hypoplastic anemia more than 20 years later, developed myelodysplastic syndrome (MDS) and oral cancers in their 30s and 40s, respectively (B. P. Alter, *unpublished data*, 1997). Aplastic anemia developed in some Fanconi's anemia patients after viral illnesses, hepatitis, and tuberculosis (30,31,39,40). Cases of Fanconi's anemia have been reported in which the patient received chloramphenicol before the onset of aplastic anemia (21,41–44). These infectious or drug-related cases suggest a role for the environment in the development of bone marrow failure. Reports of other families in whom siblings had the onset of pancytopenia at the same age suggest additional genetic components (17,39,45,46). Thus, the exact roles of genetics and environment are not yet clarified.

LABORATORY FINDINGS
The blood counts of patients often reveal thrombocytopenia or leukopenia before pancytopenia, which is usually mild or mod-

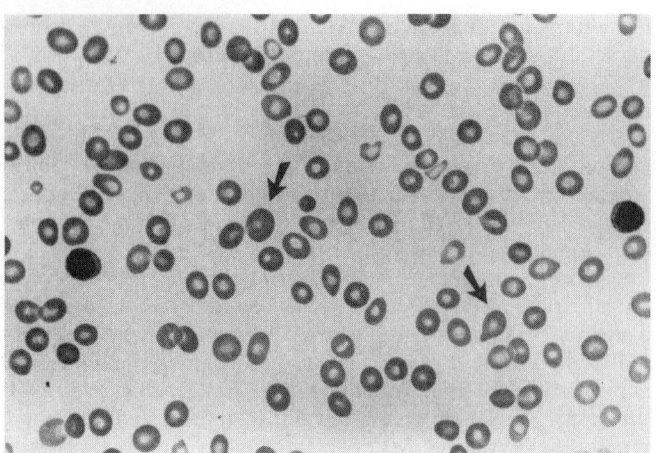

Figure 8-4. Peripheral blood from a patient with Fanconi's anemia. Note anisocytosis, macrocytes (*arrows*), thrombocytopenia, and neutropenia. (Courtesy of Dr. Gail Wolfe. From Alter BP. The bone marrow failure syndromes. In: Nathan DG, Oski FA, eds. *Hematology of infancy and childhood*, 3rd ed. Philadelphia: WB Saunders, 1987:159–241, with permission.)

erate initially; severe aplasia eventually develops in most cases. Even in the Fanconi's anemia patient with normal blood counts (the preanemic, or the treatment-responsive patient), erythrocytes are macrocytic, with mean cell volumes (MCVs) that are usually greater than 100 fL. The blood smear shows large red blood cells (RBCs) with mild poikilocytosis and anisocytosis, as well as a paucity of platelets and leukocytes, if the numbers of these components are reduced (Fig. 8-4). Eventually, all three cell lines may fail.

At the aplastic stage, the bone marrow is hypocellular and fatty, with few hematopoietic elements and a relative increase, which is identical with that found in the marrow of patients with acquired aplasia, in lymphocytes, reticulum cells, mast cells, and plasma cells. In early Fanconi's anemia, areas of hypercellular marrow may be evident, but these disappear as aplasia progresses (9).

Erythropoiesis in the Fanconi's anemia patient is characterized as stress erythropoiesis and is associated with the production of erythrocytes with fetal characteristics, as in patients who have acquired aplastic anemia—spontaneously or after marrow transplantation—during recovery (47,48). The features of this fetal-like erythropoiesis, which occurs during stress and is present in preanemic, anemic, and remission-stage Fanconi's anemia patients, include macrocytosis, increased fetal hemoglobin (HbF) (by alkali denaturation and Kleihauer-Betke acid elution), and presence of the i antigen. These features have also helped to identify nonanemic, affected siblings of known patients. The HbF is distributed unevenly, not clonally, and no concordance of the various fetal-like features exists at the level of single cells (49). The level of HbF or degree of macrocytosis does not provide any prognostic information.

RBC lifespan may be slightly short, but hemolysis is not a major component of the anemia. Some patients with apparently short RBC lifespan may have had blood loss that was associated with thrombocytopenia. Ferrokinetic studies suggest that most patients have a component of ineffective erythropoiesis in addition to relative marrow failure. Dyserythropoiesis was noted in the marrow erythroblasts in some cases, with fragmentation and multinuclearity (21,40,50). Bone marrow imaging with technetium-99m sulfur colloid showed paradoxical and irregular tracer distribution in Fanconi's anemia that was distinct from the uniform reduction seen in acquired aplastic anemia

(51). This may be related to the varied and irregular onset of aplasia in Fanconi's anemia patients. RBC enzymes have been decreased, increased, or normal in several contradictory studies (37,52–54); the variable results may reflect the heterogeneity of Fanconi's anemia.

The small stature of Fanconi's anemia patients was ascribed to growth hormone (GH) deficiency in 22 patients in whom GH was reported to be measured (39,55–71), whereas six patients were found not to be GH deficient (59,72–74). Treatment with GH led to increased growth without hematologic improvement in 12 of 15 GH-deficient patients. In some families, GH deficiency and Fanconi's anemia segregated independently (64,65). In a study of patients in the IFAR (self-selected for participation, and perhaps biased toward short stature), 44% of patients had a subnormal GH response to stimulation, and 36% of patients were hypothyroid (75). Three patients were treated with recombinant GH, one of whom died from acute myelogenous leukemia. It is thought that the frequency of leukemia in patients with other risk factors that predispose them to leukemia is probably not increased further by GH treatment (76,77), although the use of GH replacement in Fanconi's anemia still warrants careful consideration.

Chromosome Breakage. The characteristic laboratory finding consists of chromosome aberrations, which are seen most easily in metaphase preparations of phytohemagglutinin-stimulated, cultured, peripheral blood lymphocytes. These reveal breaks, gaps, rearrangements, exchanges, and endoreduplications (Fig. 8-5), which are seen in less than 10% of the cells from normal persons but in much higher proportions in cells from Fanconi's anemia homozygotes (78–84). These features are seen infrequently in direct preparations of bone marrow cells, perhaps because cells with significant abnormalities may divide slowly or may not survive *in vivo* (81,85–87). Cultured skin fibroblasts also have abnormal chromosomes (79,80,82). It is thought that the spontaneous aberrations that are seen in cultured blood lymphocytes or fibroblasts may be artifacts of culture that are induced by unknown factors in the medium. Because marrow studies are usually direct or cultured only briefly, these artifacts may not appear. The abnormal lymphocyte chromosomes have no relation to any hematologic findings, and variations in the proportions of abnormal cells or in the number of breaks per cell do not correlate with the clinical course. Furthermore, spontaneous breaks are sometimes absent in bona fide Fanconi's anemia cases (12). Similar spontaneous chromosomal changes have been reported in Bloom's syndrome and ataxia-telangiectasia (88).

Cells from Fanconi's anemia patients are sensitive to oncogenic agents, such as simian virus 40 viral transformation (89), ionizing radiation (90), and alkylating agents (91). These agents damage DNA and produce significantly increased numbers of chromosomal aberrations in Fanconi's anemia cells. The chemicals that are used in several laboratories include DEB, nitrogen mustard, mitomycin C (MMC), cyclophosphamide, and platinum compounds (91–96). Homozygotes are diagnosed based on an amplification of several times the rate of chromosomal aberrations, compared to the baseline spontaneous rate. The cited agents do not result in increased breakage in the cells of patients with non-Fanconi's anemia chromosome breakage syndromes. In addition, cells of patients with Bloom's syndrome show increased sister chromatid exchange after treatment with 5-bromodeoxyuridine, whereas Fanconi's anemia patients' cells do not (97). The chromosome breakage rate in Fanconi's anemia heterozygotes overlaps with the normal range and is not diagnostic of the carrier state.

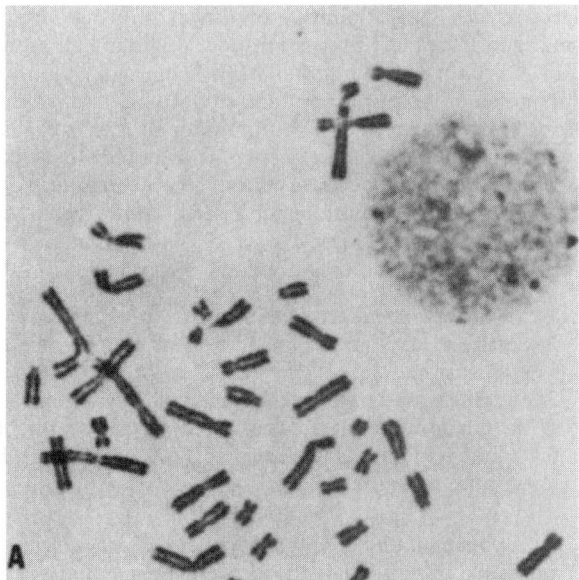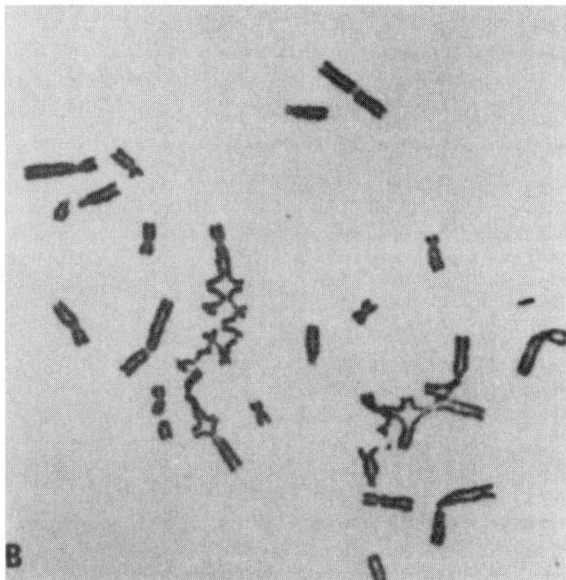

Figure 8-5. Cytogenetic findings in a patient with Fanconi's anemia. **A:** No clastogen. **B:** After culture with diepoxybutane. (From Auerbach AD, Adler B, Chaganti RS. Prenatal and postnatal diagnosis and carrier detection of Fanconi anemia by a cytogenetic method. *Pediatrics* 1981;67:128–135, with permission.)

Although most patients had multiple chromatid breaks and exchanges in most of their peripheral blood lymphocytes, 10% of the patients reported by Auerbach and Alter (98) had breaks in only 10% to 40% of their DEB-treated lymphocytes. Clonal results have been reported by others as well (99). These patients can be diagnosed, because the number of breaks per cell with breaks is still high. In addition, fibroblasts show breaks in a consistent and nonclonal manner. Molecular explanations have now been provided for some of these cases of somatic mosaicism (see the section Somatic Mosaicism in Fanconi's Anemia).

Another approach to the diagnosis of Fanconi's anemia through the use of alkylating agents involves flow cytometry rather than a count of chromosomal aberrations. Treated cells fail to divide, but undergo DNA replication and accumulate in the G_2 phase of the cell cycle, where they are detected because of the increased amount of DNA per cell (100–104).

Prenatal diagnosis has been performed by examination of fetal amniotic fluid cells or chorionic villus specimens (CVS) for increased chromosome breaks (98,105,106). In one series, 14 samples were obtained by CVS, three of which had increased spontaneous and DEB-induced breaks (98). In the same series, 7 of 46 fetuses that were studied by amniocentesis also had increased breaks by both assays. One false-negative was obtained by CVS, with no confirmatory amniocentesis sample. In the positive cases, the cultured cells also grew more slowly. Three cases were also examined using fetal blood that was obtained prenatally, primarily (107) or to confirm an abnormal CVS or amniotic fluid result (108,109). Of the affected cases, only three had physical anomalies, which further supports the suggestion that a large proportion of Fanconi's anemia homozygotes do not have malformations. Spontaneous and clastogenic stress tests also suggested Fanconi's anemia prenatally in two cases in which the fetuses were not known to be at risk for Fanconi's anemia but in which cytogenetic studies were performed for other reasons (108,110). Prenatal testing can be done by mutation analysis in appropriate families (see the section Cellular Phenotype).

The laboratory evaluation of patients in whom Fanconi's anemia is suspected should include complete blood counts, RBC size analysis, and HbF measurement. Skeletal radio-graphs and renal ultrasonography are useful. The usual diagnostic test ascertains chromosome breakage rates after clastogenic stress. This test has identified Fanconi's anemia homozygosity as the reason for physical anomalies in patients who were not anemic at the time (33–35) and led to the diagnosis of Fanconi's anemia in patients with aplastic anemia who lacked malformations (105,111).

PATHOPHYSIOLOGY

The relationship between birth defects, hematopoietic failure, increased risk of malignancies, chromosome breakage, and DNA repair remains to be elucidated. *In utero*, the development of hematopoiesis and the organs that are most frequently abnormal in Fanconi's anemia occurs at approximately the same time (at 25 to 34 days of gestation), and a common toxic insult has been invoked (46). The Fanconi's anemia genotype may make homozygotes more susceptible to agents that can cause acquired aplastic anemia in normal persons. The oncogenic compounds that damage DNA *in vitro* may also be toxic *in vivo*.

Cellular Phenotype. Fanconi's anemia cells have several other cellular phenotypic abnormalities, which are summarized in Table 8-4, in addition to cross-link sensitivity; a detailed description of these studies is beyond the scope of this chapter. Many of these cellular assays have been performed on cells from multiple complementation groups (see section on Complementation Groups). Accordingly, it remains unclear whether these cellular abnormalities correspond to all Fanconi's anemia complementation groups or to only a subset. Most of the abnormalities that are described for Fanconi's anemia cells may be epiphenomena and may not relate directly to the primary cellular defect in each complementation group. A true understanding of the primary cellular defect in Fanconi's anemia, such as DNA repair, cell cycle regulation, or prevention of apoptosis, may ultimately result from studies of cloned proteins (see the section Fanconi's Anemia Genes).

Several lines of evidence suggest that Fanconi's anemia cells have an underlying molecular defect in cell cycle regulation. First, the cells display a cell cycle arrest with 4N DNA content that is enhanced by treatment with chemical cross-

TABLE 8-4. Cellular Abnormalities in Fanconi's Anemia

Feature	References
Spontaneous chromosome breaks	78–84
Sensitivity to cross-linking agents	91–96
Prolongation of G_2 phase of cell cycle	100,112
Sensitivity to O_2	
Poor growth at ambient O_2	113
Overproduction of O_2 radicals	114
Deficient O_2 radical defense	115
Deficiency in superoxide dismutase	116,117
Sensitivity to ionizing radiation during G_2	118
Overproduction of tumor necrosis factor-α	119
Direct defects in DNA repair	
Accumulation of DNA adducts	120
Defective repair of DNA cross-links	121
Hypermutability (by deletion)	122
Increased apoptosis	123–125
Abnormal induction of p53	124,126
Intrinsic stem cell defect	
Decreased colony growth in vitro	127–133
Decreased gonadal stem cell survival	134

Adapted from D'Andrea AD, Grompe M. Molecular biology of Fanconi anemia: implications for diagnosis and therapy. *Blood* 1997;90:1725–1736.

linking agents (100,112). Second, the cell cycle arrest and reduced proliferation of Fanconi's anemia cells can be partially corrected by overexpression of a protein called *SPHAR*, a member of the cyclin family of proteins (136). Third, caffeine abrogates the G_2 arrest of Fanconi's anemia cells (124). Consistent with these results, caffeine constitutively activates the cyclin-dependent kinase cdc2 and overrides a normal G_2 cell cycle checkpoint in Fanconi's anemia cells. Finally, the FANCC protein (see below) binds to cdc2, suggesting that the Fanconi's anemia complex may be a substrate or modulator of the cyclin B–cdc2 complex (137).

Fanconi's anemia cells also have an underlying defect in DNA repair. The cells are sensitive to DNA cross-linking agents and ionizing radiation, which suggests a specific defect in the repair of cross-linked DNA or double-strand breaks (138). DNA damage results in a hyperactive p53 response, which suggests the presence of defective repair yet intact checkpoint activities (124). Fanconi's anemia cells also have a defect in the fidelity of nonhomologous end joining and an increased rate of homologous recombination (139–141). Based on these extensive phenotypic defects, it has been hypothesized that Fanconi's anemia results from an underlying molecular defect in cell cycle regulation or DNA repair.

Hematopoietic Defects. Decreased bone marrow short-term and long-term hematopoietic growth was observed by several

groups (127–133). Colony growth was improved but not normalized in some cultures with added stem cell factor (SCF) (131). Production of interleukin (IL)-6 and granulocyte-macrophage colony-stimulating factor (GM-CSF) was decreased in long-term cultures (142). Although one report suggested that nonanemic patients had decreased colonies in vitro (129), we found a relation between erythroid colony growth and hematologic status in vivo, with better growth in those patients whose blood counts were closer to normal (130). From this, we developed a clinical hematologic classification scheme:

1. Severe aplastic anemia on transfusions.
2. Severe aplastic anemia on androgens, but not responsive on transfusion.
3. Severe or moderate aplasia, responsive to androgens.
4. Severe or moderate aplasia, about to start treatment.
5. Stable, with mild cytopenias, high MCV, and high HbF.
6. Normal hematology.

Complementation Groups. Hybrid cells that were formed from Fanconi's anemia and normal cells resulted in correction of the Fanconi's anemia breakage (143–147). Other cell fusion studies that used cell lines from a variety of Fanconi's anemia patients led to the demonstration of at least two complementation groups, which involved at least nine patients (145–147), although only a single group was found in five Japanese patients (148). Duckworth-Rysiecki et al. also found two complementation groups (144).

At least eight distinct complementation groups (A, B, C, D1, D2, E, F, G) have now been identified using somatic cell fusion techniques and complementation of MMC sensitivity in fused hybrid cells (149–151). These complementation groups are shown in Table 8-5. Several approaches are now available for the rapid diagnosis and assignment of complementation groups to patients (see the section Implications for Diagnosis and Complementation Group). Some differences in the clinical severity of Fanconi's anemia are also now apparent, when comparing different complementation groups or specific mutations within a complementation group. In particular, null mutations appear to be more severe than those mutations that lead to an altered protein (152).

Fanconi's Anemia Genes. Using functional complementation of the eight Fanconi's anemia groups, six genes have now been cloned: FANCA, FANCC, FANCD2, FANCE, FANCF, and FANCG (153–158). The FANCA and FANCD2 genes were also cloned by a positional approach (155,159). The FANCG gene is homologous to the previously described XRCC9 gene (160). The FANCD complementation group is genetically heterogeneous, with at least two genes (FANCD1 and FANCD2) in this group (155). Characteristics of the six cloned genes are summarized in

TABLE 8-5. Fanconi's Anemia Complementation Groups and Genes

Gene	Locus	Genomic DNA (kb)	Complementary DNA (kb)	Exons	Protein (kd)	Amino Acids	Percent of Patients
FANCA	16q24.3	80	5.5	43	163	1455	Approximately 70
FANCB	N/A	—	—	—	—	—	Rare
FANCC	9q22.3	80	1.8	14	63	558	Approximately 10
FANCD1	13q12.3	70	11.4	27	384	3418	Rare
FANCD2	3p25.3	80	4.4	44	162	1451	Rare
FANCE	6p21-22	15	1.6	10	60	536	Approximately 10
FANCF	11p15	—	1.1	1	42	374	Rare
FANCG	9p13	—	2.5	14	70	622	Approximately 10

N/A, not available, not mapped or cloned.

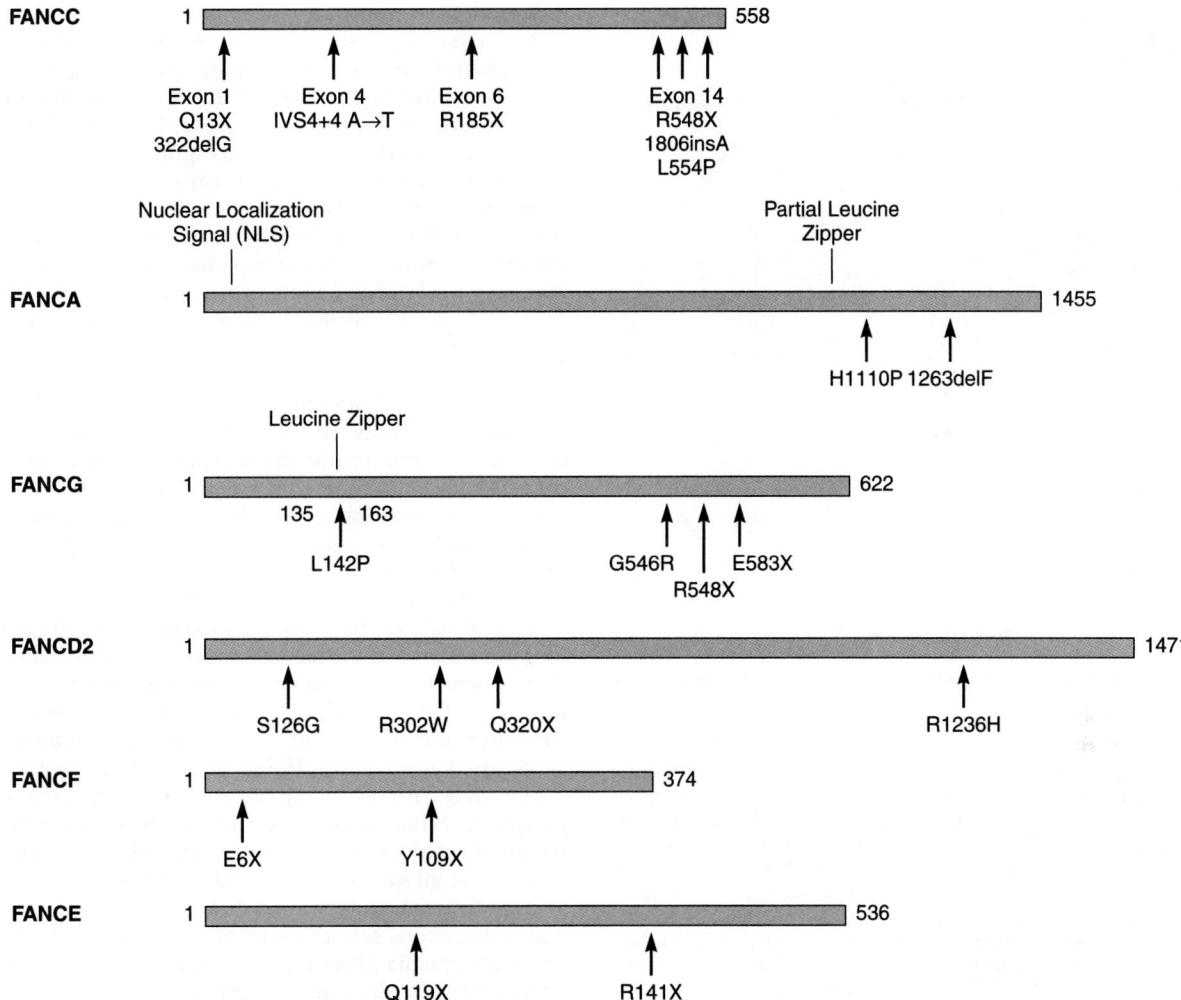

Figure 8-6. Schematic representation of the six cloned Fanconi's anemia proteins. A few patient-derived mutations are indicated. These mutations were identified by systematic mutational analysis of the FANCC (154,161,162), FANCA (163,164), and FANCG genes (165). Fewer patient-derived mutations have been detected for the FANCE (156), FANCF (157), and FANCD2 (155) genes.

Table 8-5. The availability of these gene sequences and their encoded proteins has substantially altered the diagnostic and subtyping approach to the disease.

Five of the seven cloned Fanconi's anemia proteins have little or no homology to other known proteins in genetic databases (Fig. 8-6). However, absence of any one of these proteins, by biallelic mutation of the corresponding gene, results in the common clinical and cellular abnormalities in Fanconi's anemia. Accordingly, it was suggested that these six proteins interact in a common biochemical pathway (166), and recent studies have demonstrated that this hypothesis may be correct (Fig. 8-7). Several of the proteins (including FANCA, FANCC, FANCE, FANCF, and FANCG) appear to be subunits of a large multisubunit protein complex in the nucleus of normal cells (157,167–173). This protein complex appears to be a ubiquitin ligase, which is capable of modifying the downstream, Fanconi's anemia protein, FANCD2 (174). Alternatively, the FA complex may regulate the activity of a ubiquitin ligase. When a normal cell is exposed to DNA damage, the Fanconi's anemia protein complex modifies the FANCD2 protein by monoubiquitination, thereby targeting this protein to DNA repair foci within the nucleus. Ubiquitin is a 76 amino-acid peptide that is added posttranslationally to

regulated proteins. Monoubiquitination of the FANCD2 protein does not alter the stability of the protein but instead appears to direct its translocation to the DNA repair foci in the nucleus. Interestingly, these DNA repair foci contain other proteins that are known to be involved in DNA repair, such as BRCA1, RAD51, and NBS (174–176). The recent discovery (176a) that FANCD1 is caused by bialleleic mutations on BRCA2 links the Fanconi genes, BRCA1, and BRCA2 in a common pathway. Moreover, other recent evidence (176b) links the Fanconi anemia and ataxia telangiectasia pathways. The ATM (ataxia telongiectasia mutated) gene encodes an ionizing radiation–activated kinase that phosphorylates the FANCD2 protein, which is monoubiquitinated by the FANC (A, C, E, F, and G) protein complex. Loss of any of the proteins in the Fanconi pathway leads to spontaneous chromosome breakage, which is increased by cellular exposure to MMC or DEB. These studies suggest that the six cloned Fanconi's anemia proteins interact in a novel biochemical pathway that is activated in response to DNA damage. Disruption of this pathway leads to the characteristic clinical and cellular abnormalities that are observed in Fanconi's anemia. Whether there are other functions of the Fanconi's anemia proteins outside the context of this biochemical pathway remains unknown.

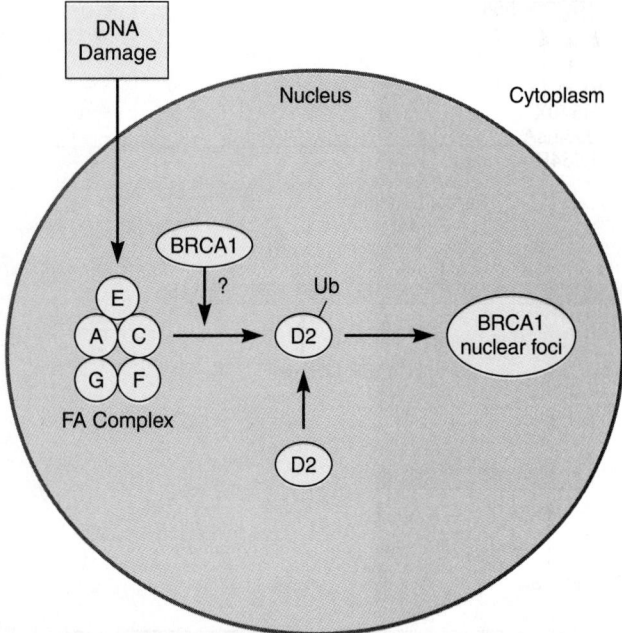

Figure 8-7. Interaction of the FA proteins in a cellular pathway. The FA proteins (A, C, E, F, and G) bind in a functional nuclear complex. This multisubunit complex appears to function as an enzyme. On activation of this complex by DNA damage, the complex enzymatically modifies (monoubiquitinates) the downstream D2 protein. The activated D2 protein is thereby targeted to nuclear foci that are required for DNA repair. These foci contain many proteins (i.e., BRCA1, NBS, RAD51) that are known to play a role in DNA repair and in the maintenance of chromosome stability. Defects in BRCA2 are observed in FANCD1. The role of BRCA2 in this pathway is uncertain. Disruption of the FA pathway leads to the characteristic cellular and clinical abnormalities that are observed in Fanconi's anemia. (Adapted from Garcia-Higuera I, Taniguchi T, Ganesan S, et al. Interaction of the Fanconi anemia proteins and BRCA1 in a common pathway. *Mol Cell* 2001;7:1–20, with permission.)

Implications for Diagnosis and Complementation Group.
Several studies have provided mutational analysis of patients, including those patients in group C (162,177), group A (163,178), and group G (165). While FANCC is a relatively rare group (Table 8-5), there is a common mutant allele for FANCC, IVS4+4 A to T, which is prevalent in Ashkenazi Jews (162), with a carrier frequency of approximately 0.9% in this population (20). FANCA is the most common group. The FANCA gene is large, encompassing 43 exons, and there are a wide range of mutant alleles, thereby making direct mutational screening of FANCA patients costly and inefficient. There is an increased frequency of group G in the German population, as it is associated with a German mutant allele (165). In some ethnic backgrounds, Fanconi's anemia can be diagnosed by direct mutational screening of specific founder mutations.

Knowledge of the specific genotype of a patient is often informative. For instance, for FANCC, the IVS4+4 A to T mutant allele is associated with a more severe phenotype, whereas the delG322 mutation may have a relatively mild phenotype (179). Disease severity may also depend on genetic background, however, as Japanese patients with the IVS4+4 A to T mutation have a comparatively mild phenotype (180).

Although direct mutational screening is not always practical, complementation group assignment is relatively easy and cost effective. Cell lines and primary cells from known Fanconi's anemia patients can be subtyped by using a combination of retroviral complementation with the six cloned Fanconi's anemia complementary DNAs (cDNAs) and by immunoblotting with antisera that are specific to the six proteins (181). Complementation analysis suggests that FANCA patients have a relatively mild phenotype, compared to patients in group C or group G (152). Group typing may be useful in predicting disease severity or in guiding the relative urgency of risky clinical interventions, such as unrelated BMT. Group assignment is a necessary precondition for the use of gene therapy (135).

Because the six cloned FA proteins appear to interact in a common pathway (Fig. 8-7), it is theoretically possible to screen the downstream events in this pathway (i.e., the monoubiquitination of the FANCD2 protein) as a measure of the integrity of the pathway. Whether such a screening test will replace the DEB test for Fanconi's anemia diagnosis remains unknown.

Somatic Mosaicism in Fanconi's Anemia. The phenomenon of somatic reversion for Fanconi's anemia has recently been described. Somatic reversion results when a mutant gene reverts to a wild-type gene (or to a functionally wild-type gene), thus encoding a functional Fanconi's anemia protein. Reverted cells have a selective growth advantage over mutant cells. Approximately 15% of Fanconi's anemia patients have somatic mosaicism in their peripheral blood (182,183). A mixture of MMC-sensitive and MMC-resistant cells is found in these samples. Mitotic recombination or compensatory frameshifts were shown to be molecular mechanisms of somatic reversion (184). Somatic mosaicism may make the diagnosis of Fanconi's anemia difficult, because of false-negative chromosome breakage studies. If Fanconi's anemia is strongly suspected in a patient, despite inconclusive breakage studies in peripheral blood, a definitive test can be performed by chromosome breakage studies of primary skin fibroblasts or by direct Fanconi's anemia gene mutational screening.

The high percentage of patients with somatic mosaicism indicates a strong selective advantage for cells that have lost the Fanconi's anemia phenotype. In principle, if the somatic reversion occurs in a pluripotent hematopoietic progenitor cell, then these corrected cells could give rise to clonal repopulation of the bone marrow. This raises the possibility that gene therapy in Fanconi's anemia may be aided by *in vivo* selection. At this time it is unclear whether any special physiologic circumstances are required for this selection to occur. The high incidence of somatic reversion also suggests that many mutant Fanconi's anemia genes have frameshift mutations. These mutations may be "corrected" by new mutations that correct the open reading frame of the Fanconi's anemia gene.

Somatic mosaicism may also cause some complications for Fanconi's anemia patients, especially if the reversion occurs in a more differentiated T lymphocyte. A high incidence of graft rejection has been noted in BMT of mosaic patients (185). Because of their increased sensitivity to bifunctional alkylating agents, Fanconi's anemia patients typically receive a much less aggressive ablative treatment before BMT. If the recipient patient has somatic mosaicism (particularly in T cells), some endogenous cells may be resistant to the ablative regimen and may cause graft rejection. Further studies are required to confirm this hypothesis.

Gene Therapy for Fanconi's Anemia. For gene therapy, bone marrow from a Fanconi's anemia patient of known group can be harvested, transduced *ex vivo* with a retroviral or adenoviral construct that contains the corresponding wild-type cDNA, and reinfused into the recipient. In principle, the genetically corrected stem cells and early progenitor cells should have a selective advantage *in vivo*, which allows for a clonal or oligoclonal reengraftment of the bone marrow and a reconstitution of normal hematopoiesis. The restoration of the Fanconi's anemia pathway by retroviral transduction of the missing functional Fanconi's anemia protein may provide a convenient screening test for the efficacy of gene therapy *in vitro* (Fig. 8-7). Studies that evaluated clinical gene therapy protocols for Fanconi's anemia have been described (186).

Mouse models have provided a useful, albeit nonideal, model for Fanconi's anemia gene therapy. At present, there are FANCC and FANCA knock-out mouse models for Fanconi's anemia (134,187,188), all of which exhibit a "partial" phenotype. These mice have normal development and organogenesis and no obvious cancer predisposition, but they all have decreased fertility. Although the baseline hematopoiesis of the mouse models is relatively normal (189,190), the primary FANCC (–/–) cells undergo enhanced chromosome breakage and decreased survival on exposure to MMC. Systematic comparisons of primary bone marrow cells from FANCC (–/–) and FANCC (+/+) mice were performed (191). In a competitive repopulation assay in an irradiated, normal mouse model, FANCC (+/+) cells selectively outgrew FANCC (–/–) cells, especially on serial transplantation. When wild-type bone marrow cells were transplanted into an unconditioned FANCC (–/–) recipient, the wild-type cells displayed a growth advantage that was enhanced with MMC conditioning *in vivo*. In other studies, FANCC (–/–) mice were shown to have decreased numbers of CD34$^+$ cells, which suggests a defect in the differentiation of CD34$^-$ to CD34$^+$ cells (191,192).

Gene therapy for Fanconi's anemia has several theoretical advantages over conventional therapies. Fanconi's anemia cells that have been corrected by retroviral transduction have a survival advantage over untransduced cells. Retroviral transduction of FANCC or FANCA cDNA improves the clonogenic survival of human FANCC or FANCA mutant bone marrow cells (193,194) or murine FANCC (–/–) bone marrow cells (186). Taken together, these studies suggest that a gene therapy approach to Fanconi's anemia could potentially result in a competitive advantage of corrected cells and an *in vivo* correction of hematopoiesis. Moreover, this competitive engraftment could be enhanced by MMC administration *in vivo* (191). This is also supported by the observation that the FANCC transgene was only detectable in a patient who was given transduced CD34$^+$ cells after radiation therapy for a concurrent malignancy (186). The frequent finding of somatic mosaicism of peripheral blood lymphocytes from Fanconi's anemia patients further supports a model of *in vivo* selection of corrected cells. In addition, constitutive overexpression of the Fanconi's anemia proteins does not have deleterious effects on hematopoietic cell growth or colony formation. In fact, a transgenic mouse expressing FANCC constitutively has a slight increase in colony-forming unit–erythrocyte (CFU-E) colony cells. Also, Fanconi's anemia cell lines that are complemented with the FANCA, FANCG, and FANCC cDNA and express high levels of the corresponding Fanconi's anemia protein have normal growth in culture.

Despite these theoretical advantages, gene therapy for Fanconi's anemia also carries various disadvantages and risks. Gene therapy is limited by the relatively poor retroviral transduction efficiency of hematopoietic stem cells with existing retroviral and lentiviral supernatants. Functional complementation with the FANCC cDNA could theoretically "rescue" a premalignant cell and thereby enhance leukemic transformation for the Fanconi's anemia patient. This may be a higher risk for a patient with a stable chromosomal (clonal) abnormality of the bone marrow cells. Expression of the FANCC cDNA in a differentiated lymphocyte could potentially create T-cell mosaicism of the recipient. T-cell mosaicism may decrease the success of bone marrow engraftment, if a patient requires a subsequent unrelated donor bone marrow transplant. Expression of an exogenous Fanconi's anemia protein after gene therapy could theoretically result in an immune response to the foreign antigen and, subsequently, in graft rejection.

Preimplantation Genetic Diagnosis for Fanconi's Anemia. Through preimplantation genetic diagnosis (PGD), parents of a known Fanconi's anemia patient with a known group and genotype can use *in vitro* fertilization to generate multiple sibling embryos. By polymerase chain reaction amplification analysis of cells that are obtained from these embryos, the embryos can be tested and screened for HLA type (to ensure that the sibling embryo is a match for the affected child) and for the Fanconi's anemia mutations that are carried in the family (to ensure that the sibling embryo does not have disease). PGD has been successfully performed for other genetic diseases, including cystic fibrosis (58) and Lesch-Nyhan syndrome (195,196). More recently, PGD was used successfully for a family with a known FANCC mutation. After the birth of a normal sibling, the cord blood can be used for transplantation of the older child who is affected. PGD has been limited by the reduced viability of reimplanted embryos after genetic analysis *ex vivo* and by the absolute requirement for accurate detection of the two mutant Fanconi's anemia alleles that are carried in the family. As stated previously, it is often difficult to detect the precise mutation in the Fanconi's anemia gene by direct mutational analysis, and it is difficult to distinguish true pathogenic missense mutations from benign base pair polymorphisms.

Implications for Cancer Diagnostics. Because biallelic germline mutations in a Fanconi's anemia gene result in cancer susceptibility in Fanconi's anemia patients, it is possible that acquired (somatic) mutations in Fanconi's anemia genes may also be oncogenic. A systematic screening of the Fanconi's anemia pathway in tumors from cancer patients from the general (non-Fanconi's anemia) population is therefore warranted (Fig. 8-7). For instance, somatic mutation of an upstream Fanconi's anemia gene may result in loss of a functional Fanconi's anemia pathway and subsequent chromosome instability. Chromosome instability is a common feature of cancer progression. Whether specific Fanconi's anemia groups or mutant alleles within a specific group predispose to a specific cancer remains untested.

PROGNOSIS

In the past, when patients were diagnosed because they had already developed aplastic anemia, and when the only treatment was RBC transfusions, 80% of patients were reported to die within 2 years (197). Almost all patients died within 4 years, with only rare long-term survivals (198,199). Because diagnoses can now be made before the onset of clinically significant hematologic or malignant symptoms, survival from the time of diagnosis is longer. More reliable information should eventually emerge from prospective data, in which a large proportion of patients are identified who have no symptoms.

The cumulative survival of Fanconi's anemia patients in the literature is shown in Figure 8-8. In the entire group, the median predicted cumulative survival is 20 years of age. However, cases reported in the 1990s had a predicted median survival of 30 years of age. Those patients who were 1 year of age or younger had a median survival of 5 years of age, and those who were 16 years of age or older when Fanconi's anemia was diagnosed had a median predicted survival of 30 years of age.

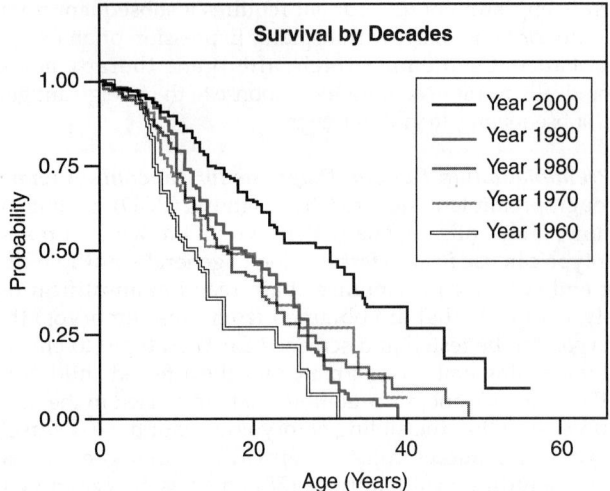

Figure 8-8. Kaplan-Meier plot of cumulative survival in Fanconi's anemia patients. Time is shown as age in years. Lines represent 118 cases that were reported from 1927 to 1960, 117 cases from 1961 to 1970, 254 cases from 1971 to 1980, 314 cases from 1981 to 1990, and 331 cases from 1991 to 2000. The differences are significant.

Older Patients. Older Fanconi's anemia men may be small, with underdeveloped genitalia and abnormalities in spermatogenesis (200). There are four Fanconi's anemia men who are reported to have fathered children (17,201,202); they represent less than 5% of men who have reached 16 years of age. This percentage may be due to underreporting, as well as decreased fertility, which has been noted by several patients (B. P. Alter, *unpublished data*).

Older women with Fanconi's anemia have irregular menses and early menopause (72,79,201,203). At least 20 Fanconi's anemia patients were reported to have been pregnant; 30 pregnancies have resulted in 21 living infants (36,79,201,203–213). Pregnancies occurred at a median age of 23 years (with a range from 18 to 34 years of age). Transfusions were often necessary because of worsening of maternal anemia, and cesarean sections were performed in six cases because of failure of labor to progress. There were eight miscarriages and four cases of preeclampsia. Nine of the women required RBC transfusions during their pregnancies, and six women required platelets. None of the mothers died during pregnancy, but ten women died at a median age of 32 years (with a range from 26 to 45 years of age), with seven women dying from cancer (see the section Complications) and three women dying from complications of pancytopenia.

TREATMENT

Androgen Therapy. Shahidi and Diamond (214) reported the use of androgens in 1959, with improvement in the first six patients. The response rate was noted to be 75% in the series by Sanchez-Medal (215) and Najean (216). As with any new therapy, initial enthusiasm must give way to reality, and the response rate is now estimated at closer to 50%. The first sign of response is a rise in the reticulocyte count, followed by a rise in hemoglobin (Hgb) within 1 to 2 months. The white blood cell count is somewhat slower, and the platelet response, usually incomplete, may take 6 to 12 months.

Only a few patients were reported to successfully discontinue androgen therapy (often at the time of puberty) and maintain their blood counts (37,128,205,217–224). Many patients eventually become refractory to the androgen with which

they are treated, and changing to another androgen only occasionally succeeds in buying more time for the patient. Some of the complications that are described in the following discussion develop in older patients, in whom androgens may have prolonged life sufficiently for these complications to appear, or they may have contributed to these developments.

Although some reports suggest that androgens alone are as effective as androgens that are combined with corticosteroids, the general recommendation is for a combination of androgens and corticosteroids (216). The growth acceleration of androgens may be counterbalanced by the growth retardation of the corticosteroids (225). In addition, corticosteroids may decrease bleeding at a given platelet count, perhaps by promoting vascular stability (226). The most frequently used androgen is oxymetholone, an oral 17-alkylated androgen, at 2 to 5 mg/kg/day. When prednisone is also given, it is at 5 to 10 mg every other day. If an injectable androgen is desired because of decreased risk of hepatotoxicity, the usual form is nandrolone decanoate, 1 to 2 mg/kg/week, injected intramuscularly, with ice packs and pressure applied to prevent hematomas.

Potential side effects of androgens are obstructive liver disease, peliosis hepatis, and liver tumors. Patients who receive androgens should be monitored frequently with liver chemistries and ultrasonography. If a response occurs, the drug should be tapered slowly but probably not discontinued entirely. The only group of patients in whom discontinuation has been considered routinely are those from South Africa, who may be a genetically distinct Fanconi's anemia variant (227). In most experiences elsewhere, relapses ensue when androgens are stopped, and subsequent remissions on the same or different preparations are sometimes elusive. Although an attenuated androgen, such as danazol, has theoretical appeal because of reduced side effects, there is some concern about its hematopoietic effectiveness. There are only two reports of its use in Fanconi's anemia, with a response in one patient (228,229).

Indications for androgens depend on the degree of cytopenia, not solely on the knowledge that the patient has Fanconi's anemia. One or more of Hgb below 8 g/dL, platelets less than 30,000/μL, or a neutrophil count of less than 500/μL may warrant treatment.

Hematopoietic Stem Cell Transplantation. Reconstitution of Fanconi's anemia patients with allogeneic hematopoietic stem cells offers the potential of a cure for the aplastic anemia and perhaps cure or prevention of leukemia. However, it does not prevent and may even accelerate the appearance of other malignancies (see section Solid Tumors). More than 200 transplants have been performed worldwide, with survival from HLA-matched siblings almost double that of alternative donors (Fig. 8-9). Although the majority of the reported transplants were from bone marrow, the use of cord blood is increasing, and mobilized peripheral blood may be considered.

The outcome was poor in the first marrow transplants from HLA-matched siblings using the standard aplastic anemia cyclophosphamide regimen of 100 to 200 mg/kg given over 3 to 4 days (230,231). Several studies showed that a metabolite of cyclophosphamide is toxic to DNA, which explains the clinical symptoms of severe mucositis with intestinal malabsorption and hemorrhages, fluid retention, cardiac failure, and hemorrhagic cystitis (92,232,233). Gluckman then introduced a modified protocol, using a total cyclophosphamide dose of 20 mg/kg, divided over 4 days, plus 5 Gy of thoracoabdominal radiation (138,233). This protocol became standard and has a cumulative survival probability of approximately 70% (234,235). The

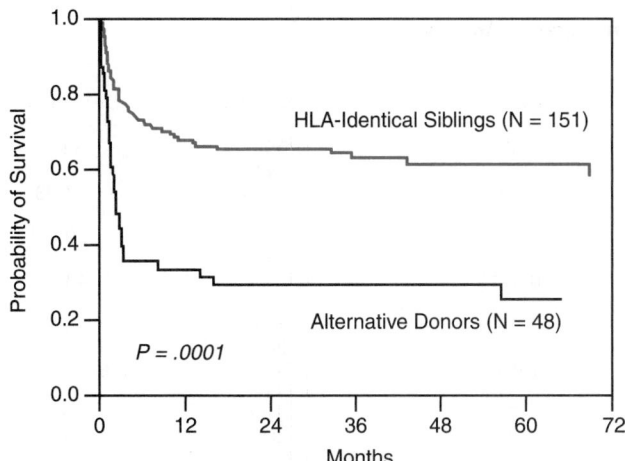

Figure 8-9. Kaplan-Meier plot of cumulative survival after bone marrow transplantation for patients with Fanconi's anemia. Time is shown as months from transplantation. One-hundred and fifty-one patients were transplanted from HLA-identical siblings. Forty-eight patients had alternative donors. (From Gluckman E, Auerbach AD, Horowitz MM, et al. Bone marrow transplantation for Fanconi anemia. *Blood* 1995;86:2856–2862, with permission.)

best predictor of survival was a low number of transfusions before transplant. Recently, nonmyeloablative regimens have shown promise, using fludarabine combined with low-dose cyclophosphamide, for related and unrelated donor transplants (236,237). One concern is that there may be incomplete mixed chimerism, with residual Fanconi's anemia cells that might have a malignant potential.

The preferred donors for Fanconi's anemia transplantations are HLA-matched siblings, who need to be screened with thorough physical examinations, complete blood counts (including examination of the RBC, MCV, and HbF), and cytogenetic studies for chromosome breakage, baseline and after culture, with a clastogenic stress agent, such as DEB. Mutation analysis should be offered in families with known mutations. In more than one case, the donor turned out to have Fanconi's anemia that had not been diagnosed before transplantation (238). Parents have an unexpectedly high rate of HLA identity with Fanconi's anemia patients, only partly accounted for by consanguinity, and may serve as marrow donors (239,240).

In many instances, no HLA-compatible sibling is found who can be a marrow donor. Alternative donors include parents (who may be only haploidentical), other relatives, or unrelated adult donors; the cumulative survival is approximately 30% (234,241). Persons with such transplants are particularly at risk for rejection or graft-versus-host disease. A review from the European group registry suggested that T-cell depletion reduced acute graft-versus-host disease but increased the risk of graft failure, thus leading to no net improvement in survival (241). They reported predictors of worse outcome, including extensive malformations, positive cytomegalovirus serology, prior treatment with androgens (which may have been correlated with abnormal liver function), and female donors. Matched unrelated donors were better than mismatched related donors (235).

Because umbilical cord blood contains hematopoietic progenitor cells, investigators proposed cryopreservation of these cells from a non-Fanconi's anemia sibling who is diagnosed *in utero*, to use for later transplantation (242). Fetal cells are obtained by chorionic villus sampling or amniocentesis, tested for Fanconi's anemia homozygosity by using clastogen-induced chromosome breakage tests or mutation analysis (see the section Cellular Phe-

notype), and HLA typed by serologic and molecular methods. Several cases have now been done, with good results when the donor was related to the patient (228,243). Results from cases that use unrelated cord donors are not nearly as good as those obtained in cases in which the donors are siblings (235,244). An extreme example of the use of placental blood for transplant is the pregnancy that results from PGD and implantation of one or more unaffected, HLA-matched blastocysts (see the section Preimplantation Genetic Diagnosis for Fanconi's Anemia).

The incidence of malignancies is increased in Fanconi's anemia patients (see the section Complications). It is clear that BMT does not reduce this risk (except for hematologic malignancies); in fact, the cytoreductive therapy and radiation may increase it. Cancer of the tongue has been reported in several transplanted patients (see the section Solid Tumors).

Indications for transplant depend on the type of donor. Those with an HLA-matched sibling donor might be considered for transplant when their cytopenias require intervention (e.g., Hgb <8 g/dL, platelets <30,000/μL, and absolute neutrophil count <500/μL). Those for whom an alternative donor is the only option might benefit from androgens, granulocyte colony-stimulating factor (G-CSF), and even supportive care. Only those with leukemia or unmanageable cytopenias from aplastic anemia or MDS might be candidates for unrelated or mismatched transplants.

Other Treatment. *Supportive care* must be provided, as it should for any patient with aplastic anemia. ε-Aminocaproic acid may be used for symptomatic bleeding, at a dose of 0.1 g/kg every 6 hours orally (245). No family member should be used as a blood product donor, until it is decided that a transplant will not be done (even from an unrelated donor) to decrease the chance of sensitization. Washed or leukofiltered RBCs should be used to reduce the risk of reactions and HLA sensitization from white cells. The possibility of marrow transplantation must be considered early in the course of the patient's anemia. Although the use of androgens and transfusions does not preclude transplantation, the best results are seen in those whose medical complications are minimal. Drugs and chemicals that may be implicated as causal in acquired aplastic anemia should be avoided. In addition, medications or substances that interfere with platelet function (such as aspirin, some antihistamines, nonsteroidal antiinflammatory drugs, glycerol guaiacolate, vitamin E, and cod liver oil) should not be given to thrombocytopenic patients. If a severe allergic reaction occurs during a blood transfusion, diphenhydramine (Benadryl) can be used acutely.

Splenectomy has no apparent role in the management of Fanconi's anemia. More than 40 cases were reported to have had this procedure with no apparent long-term benefit. In some patients, transient improvement of pancytopenia occurred, but it was at a time when the bone marrow was not yet hypocellular.

Immunotherapy has no theoretical or factual basis. Although use of high-dose methylprednisolone (246) was reported rarely in Fanconi's anemia, there are unreported instances of several patients in whom this agent or antithymocyte globulin as well as cyclosporin A was used without success (B. P. Alter, *unpublished data*). In fact, approximately 10% of adults who failed to respond to any of these approaches were shown subsequently by clastogenic stress-induced chromosome breakage studies to have previously undiagnosed Fanconi's anemia (A. D. Auerbach and N. S. Young, *unpublished data*).

Lithium was reported to improve the blood counts in two of five Fanconi's anemia patients, presumably those whose marrow reserve was still present (248).

Hematopoietic growth factors may have a limited role in the future management of Fanconi's anemia patients. GM-CSF was

TABLE 8-6. Complications in Fanconi's Anemia

	All Patients	Leukemia	Myelodysplastic Syndrome	Solid Tumor	Liver Tumor
Number of cases	1206	103	74	59	34
Percent of total	100	8.5	6.1	4.9	2.8
Male to female ratio	1.24	1.51	1.06	0.37	1.43
Age at diagnosis of Fanconi's anemia (yr)					
Mean	8.4	10.4	11.5	13.2	9.4
Median	7	9	9.5	9.5	7
Range	0–48	0.13–28	0.3–43	0.1–44	3–48
Age at complication (yr)					
Mean	—	14.5	15.9	23.4	16.1
Median	—	13.8	14	26	13
Range	—	0.13–29	1.8–43	0.3–45	6–48
Number of reported deceased	455	73	37	35	27
Percent of reported deceased	38%	71%	50%	59%	79%
Projected median survival (yr)	20	16	22	31	14

found to produce transient increases in neutrophil counts without effects on Hgb or platelets and without induction of acute leukemia or cytogenetic clones at up to 15 months (249,250). Results were similar with G-CSF, which also increased neutrophils but did not impact on Hgb or platelets (251,252). However, clonal cytogenetics (including monosomy 7 in three cases) or increased myeloblasts, or both, were observed in 4 out of 16 patients during or after G-CSF treatment. These complications may be manifestations of the natural history of Fanconi's anemia (see the section Complications). The use of G-CSF or GM-CSF should be restricted to patients with severe neutropenia and risk of serious infections and should be monitored with frequent blood counts, bone marrow examinations, and bone marrow cytogenetic studies.

COMPLICATIONS

The *in vitro* data regarding defects in DNA repair and cellular damage in Fanconi's anemia suggest that it might be a premalignant condition, which is borne out by the *in vivo* observations. Approximately 200 cases have been reported with leukemia or solid tumors—an overall incidence of approximately 15%. Because this incidence reflects biased reporting of interesting cases, the true figure may differ from this estimate. More than 100 patients were reported with leukemia, more than 30 were reported with liver tumors, and approximately 60 were reported with other cancers (Table 8-6). German observed that cancer in Fanconi's anemia patients has been reported only since the mid 1960s and suggested that androgen therapy,

which began in the early 1960s, allowed patients to survive long enough to develop the malignancy for which they were at risk (253). He also suggested that androgens might be implicated in the cause of these malignancies. Many patients who never received androgens developed leukemia or cancer, however, and, thus, the role of androgens is not relevant except, perhaps, for liver tumors.

The finding of a single gene for Fanconi's anemia (heterozygosity) was thought to be sufficient to confer a risk of malignancy. Garriga and Crosby (254) reported an increased incidence of leukemia in Fanconi's anemia families, and Swift (239,255) found a predisposition to cancer in heterozygotes. Subsequently, these analyses were extended from the original eight families to 25 families by Swift et al. (256) and to nine families by Potter et al. (257); neither study found an increase in cancer in Fanconi's anemia families. [Another disorder that was thought to be present at increased incidence in Fanconi's anemia heterozygotes is diabetes mellitus (258,259).] The earlier and perhaps erroneous conclusions regarding cancer were attributed to small numbers, incorrect assignment of Fanconi's anemia heterozygotes, and biased selection. The cancer risk of heterozygotes should be clarified in the near future, because heterozygote status can be confirmed with mutation analysis.

Leukemia. Leukemia has been reported in more than 100 cases, representing almost 10% of Fanconi's anemia patients in the literature (Table 8-7 and Fig. 8-10). In a single series of 44 patients, nine patients developed leukemia (20%), and five

TABLE 8-7. Leukemia in Fanconi's Anemia

Leukemia	Male	Female	All Patients	References
Acute lymphocytic leukemia	3	2	5	67,262–265
AML, unspecified	23	14	37	21,217,224,236,260,266–286
AML M1, acute myelocytic, without maturation	1	1	2	287,288
AML M2, acute myelocytic, with maturation	2	2	4	279,289,290
AML M3, acute promyelocytic	0	0	0	—
AML M4, acute myelomonocytic	12	8	20	17,81,84,291–305
AML M5, acute monocytic	6	4	10	40,284,306–312
AML M6, erythroleukemia	5	2	7	59,87,217,309,313,314
AML M7, acute megakaryocytic	1	0	1	315
AML, acute nonlymphocytic	1	5	6	243,312,316–318
Other acute leukemia	8	3	11	17,43,86,260,311,319–322
Total	62	41	103	—

AML, acute myeloid leukemia.

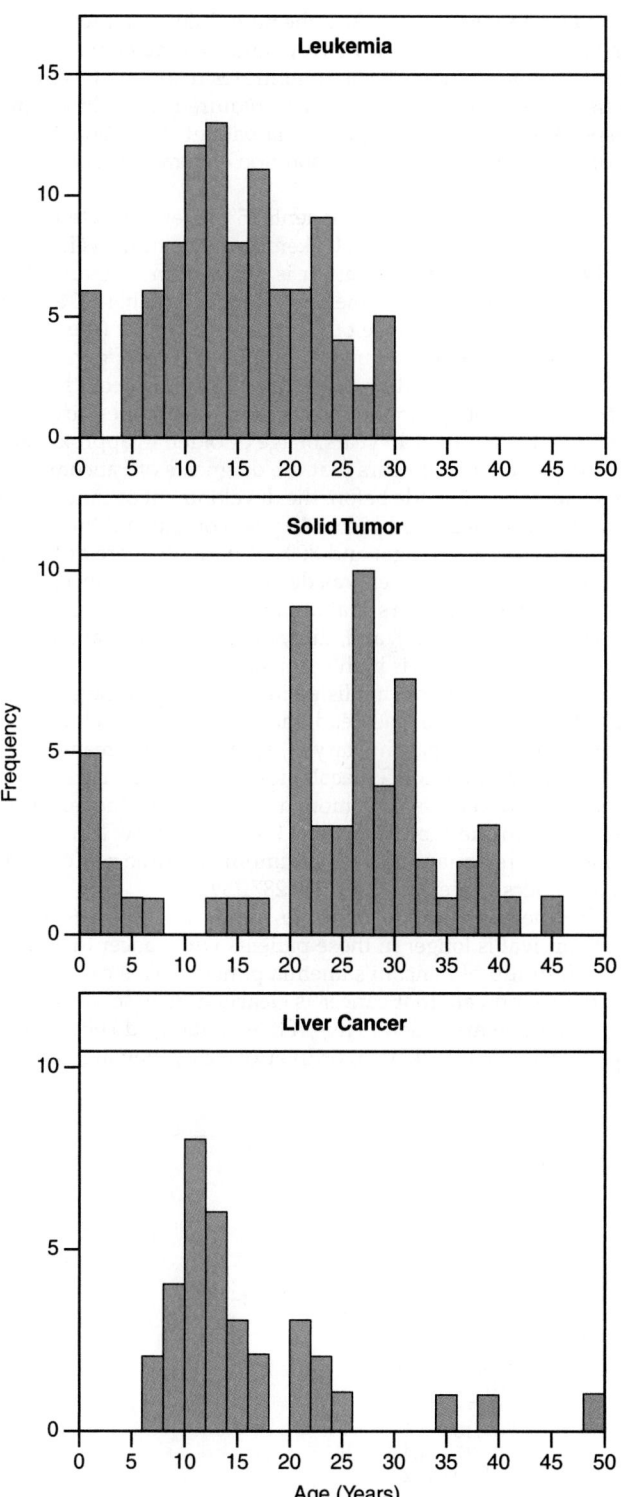

Figure 8-10. Age at diagnosis of cancer in Fanconi's anemia in 94 patients with leukemia, 60 patients with solid tumors, and 28 patients with liver tumors. Age at complication was not reported for all patients with those diagnoses.

are an unlikely cause of leukemia. At least two patients presented with acute myelomonocytic leukemia, and they were treated with bone marrow transplants. They developed toxicity from the preparation, and the diagnosis of Fanconi's anemia was made retrospectively, after they were found to have increased chromosome breakage (261).

The characteristics of patients with Fanconi's anemia and leukemia are compared to the characteristics of the total group and those with other malignancies in Table 8-6. The male to female ratio is 1.5:1.0. The diagnosis of Fanconi's anemia was made at a median age of 9 years in those who eventually developed leukemia, which is significantly older than the diagnosis at a median of 7 years of age in those who did not develop leukemia. Leukemia was diagnosed at a median of 14 years of age (with a range from 0.1 to 29.0 years of age). Sixteen patients were over 16 years of age at the time of diagnosis of Fanconi's anemia, and, in ten of these patients, Fanconi's anemia was first diagnosed when the patients presented with leukemia.

Because the most common leukemia in children is lymphocytic, it is noteworthy that, until 1989, all leukemias reported in Fanconi's anemia were myeloid. Five cases of acute lymphocytic leukemia (ALL) have now been reported, although most of the leukemias are myeloid (Table 8-7). Because several patients were discussed in more than one publication, the number of literature reports of patients with Fanconi's anemia and leukemia probably exceeds the actual number of cases. Five patients with leukemia had coincidental hepatic tumors, which were usually discovered at postmortem examination (221,271,280,293,319,323).

Treatment of the leukemia was less than satisfactory, and deaths usually occurred within the first 2 months after diagnosis. Fanconi's anemia patients with leukemia are exquisitely sensitive to the toxic effects of chemotherapy, as predicted by the previous discussion regarding agents that increase damage to DNA. The combination of the forms of leukemia that are difficult to treat in anyone (e.g., myeloid), abnormal DNA repair, and a lack of marrow reserve does not afford a good prognosis. The only apparent long-term remission that has been reported is one of 9 years in duration (304,305,315; K. J. Roozendaal, *personal communication*, 1989). One 2-year survivor after reduced-dosage chemotherapy subsequently succumbed to varicella (92; A. D. Auerbach, *personal communication*). The median survival age for patients with leukemia is 16 years of age, which is younger than the survival age for Fanconi's anemia patients without leukemia. Seventy-five percent of patients with leukemia died at the time of the reports, and further follow-up was not available for most of the other patients. Although bone marrow transplant offers a theoretical cure for the leukemia of patients with Fanconi's anemia, these patients are usually very ill, and only a few have survived (243,290).

Will all patients develop leukemia if they do not succumb to aplastic anemia first? Probably not, because the development of leukemia appears to reach a plateau by age 30, whereas the older patients have the additional risk of solid tumors. Only long-term prospective studies can answer this question definitively.

Myelodysplastic Syndrome. Patients with Fanconi's anemia may develop syndromes that are variably called *myelodysplastic, refractory anemia,* or *preleukemia.* Some conditions evolve into full-blown leukemia; other patients die in their preleukemic phase, or their conditions are reported before further developments ensue. The risk of MDS was between 11% and 34% in cross-sectional studies (251,260,324,325). Although more than one-half of the cases of leukemia in Fanconi's anemia have cytogenetic clones, it has not been shown that the presence of a clone in the absence of leukemia means that leukemia is inevitable. A cytogenetic clone is included in the French-American-British classification of MDS

more patients were preleukemic (260). In 25% of those patients with leukemia, the diagnosis of Fanconi's anemia was made only during the evaluation for leukemia. Approximately one-third of the patients had received androgens, which indicates the severity of preexisting aplastic anemia. Because two-thirds of those with leukemia had not received androgens, androgens

(326), and specific clones impact on the prognosis of MDS in the general population (327). However, application of these criteria to MDS in Fanconi's anemia may not be appropriate. Until recently, most of the reported cases had MDS diagnosed because of dysplastic marrow morphology or the presence of a clone, or both. In a systematic analysis in which clonality was considered independently of morphologic MDS, we found that one-half of the patients with adequate cytogenetic preparations had a clone, and clonal variation that included disappearance was common (325). One-third of the patients had morphologic MDS, and, thus, there were patients with cytogenetic clones who did not have MDS by other criteria. Poor outcome correlated with MDS, not with the presence of a clone. Patients with clones have survived for more than 12 years without the development of leukemia or died from cytopenic but nonmalignant complications of MDS. No consistent pattern was found in the involved chromosomes, although chromosomes 1 and 7 were more common than others; partial or complete deletions, translocations, and marker chromosomes were found. Details of the cytogenetic findings can be found elsewhere (279,283,325,328). Less than 10% of the Fanconi's anemia patients reported with leukemia had documented MDS; in those with prior MDS, the emergence of leukemia was within 1.5 years. The relevance of clonal cytogenetics may become more apparent when methods that are more sensitive than classic banding are widely used, such as fluorescence *in situ* hybridization (329).

The relation between morphologic MDS, cytogenetic clones, and acute myelogenous leukemia (AML) is not entirely clear, and remains the topic of active investigation. Because the age of the patient at diagnosis of Fanconi's anemia, complication (MDS or AML), and death is older in those with MDS than it is those with AML, it is not immediately apparent that all MDS become AML (Table 8-6). For this reason, it is not recommended that a bone marrow transplant be offered to the Fanconi's anemia patient who has a clone without other clinical indications of a need for transplant.

Three Fanconi's anemia patients were reported with Sweet's syndrome [acute neutrophilic infiltration of skin, which is asso-

ciated with malignancy 20% of the time (330)]. All three patients had myelodysplastic bone marrow, and two had clonal chromosomal abnormalities. The skin infiltrates responded to prednisone, but sustained treatment was required. This differs from responses in non-Fanconi's anemia patients with Sweet's syndrome, in which permanent resolution of symptoms occurs.

Solid Tumors. Fifty-nine patients (5%) were reported with a total of 70 cancers other than leukemia or liver tumors (Tables 8-6 and 8-8). The group with cancer is different in several features from the entire Fanconi's anemia population (Table 8-6 and Fig. 8-10). The preponderance of women with cancer (the male to female ratio is 0.4) is owing to the prevalence of gynecologic malignancies. The median age at diagnosis of Fanconi's anemia was 9.5 years of age in the cancer group, with one-third of the patients diagnosed at 16 years of age or older. In approximately 20% of patients, it appears that the diagnosis of Fanconi's anemia had not been made before the development of cancer. Eight tumors were diagnosed before 10 years of age, but the median age was 26 years of age, and 80% of patients were at least 20 years of age when cancer was detected. The usual median age for the types of cancers that are seen in Fanconi's anemia is approximately 65 (331), and, thus, their occurrence at a median age of 26 years of age is highly unusual.

The types of tumors are listed in Table 8-8. The largest number of tumors was in the head and neck region, including the tongue, gingiva, pharynx, larynx, epiglottis, and mandible, as well as the esophagus. Gynecologic cancers, particularly vulvar and cervical, were also common in women. The other areas that are listed in the table occurred less frequently. Most of the tumors were squamous cell carcinomas. Three patients had solid tumors as well as AML (269,287,289).

The median survivals that are shown in Table 8-6 suggest that survival is longer in those patients with cancer than in the overall group of Fanconi's anemia patients. This can be interpreted to indicate that cancer is clearly a disease of the older Fanconi's anemia patient. Thus, if these patients do not die from aplastic anemia, leukemia, or liver disease, they are at a high

TABLE 8-8. Solid Tumors in Fanconi's Anemia

Type	Male	Female	All Patients	References
Nonhepatic				
Oropharynx	10	12	22	201,207,221,268,293,307,332–347
Esophagus	1	8	9	44,204,332,348–354
Vulva and anus	—	4	4	79,299,334,355
Vulva	—	5	5	338,356–358
Anus	—	2	2	201,359
Cervix	—	3	3	269,355,356
Brain	1	3	4	287,360,361
Skin (nonmelanoma)	0	5	5	201,279,284,359,362
Breast	—	4	4	201,206,222,229
Lung	2	0	2	17,182
Lymphoma	1	1	2	363,364
Gastric	2	0	2	365,366
Renal	0	3	3	201,209,360,367
Colon	0	1	1	299
Osteogenic sarcoma	0	1	1	368
Retinoblastoma	0	1	1	289
Total cancers	17	53	70	—
Total patients	16	43	59	—
Hepatic				
Adenoma	6	5	11	211,319,369–375
Hepatoma	14	8	22	73,205,221,268,271,280,293,323, 344,350,376–390
Not stated	0	1	1	211,372
Total liver tumors	20	14	34	—

risk for a solid tumor. The predicted median survival age for patients with solid tumors is 31 years of age, at which age more than 75% of the total group of Fanconi's anemia patients have already died. Survival is short after the diagnosis of a malignancy. Treatment of most of these tumors is difficult because of increased toxicity from chemotherapy or radiation therapy, and surgery is recommended whenever possible. More than one-half of the patients had died by the time that they were reported.

Tumors that occurred after bone marrow transplant were not included in the previous analyses, because transplant itself may be a risk factor for solid tumors. At least eight patients (four men, four women) were reported (some of them more than once) with tongue cancer after marrow transplant (188,211,391–398); five had died at the time of the reports. The tumors were diagnosed at 3 to 15 years after transplant in patients between 11 and 33 years of age. The incidence of solid tumors after transplant, specifically in Fanconi's anemia, is not known, because there is no clear denominator. Among more than 1000 long-term survivors who were transplanted for all hematologic indications in the European Blood and Marrow Transplantation Registry, the actuarial incidence of malignant neoplasms was 13% at 15 years, and oral or esophageal cancers were increased tenfold compared to the general population in the Danish and German Cancer Registries (399). Thus, it would appear that the combination of Fanconi's anemia and transplant might have an even higher risk.

Liver Tumors. Hepatic tumors were reported in 34 patients (3%). The male to female ratio of 1.4:1.0 and median age at diagnosis of Fanconi's anemia of 7 years (Table 8-6) indicate that this group is not different from the overall group. The median age at which the liver tumors were detected was 13 years of age, although the range was wide and encompassed the oldest patients (Fig. 8-10). Because only one patient did not have antecedent androgen treatment, it might be argued that androgen treatment increases the risk of liver tumors in Fanconi's anemia patients. Hepatocellular carcinomas were twice as common as adenomas (Table 8-8), although the former were not overtly malignant in that they did not metastasize or invade, and they were often not associated with an increase in serum α-fetoprotein. One patient also had tongue cancer (344), one had esophageal cancer (350), and five had leukemia (221,271,280,293,319,323). The liver tumors were often found at postmortem examination. In general, patients with liver tumors, whether adenomas or hepatomas, did not die from their liver tumors but from other malignancies or complications of bone marrow failure. Discontinuation of androgens, alone or combined with BMT, often led to resolution of the tumors (205,372). Peliosis hepatis also reversed when androgens were stopped. Surgical removal of tumors was undertaken occasionally.

Summary of Malignancy in Fanconi's Anemia. The risk of the development of leukemia, a liver tumor, or a solid tumor in Fanconi's anemia patients totals greater than 15% in the literature, although the true frequency may be obscured by overreporting. It is an important risk, particularly in older patients, because the average age at which malignancies are diagnosed is beyond the age of survival of many Fanconi's anemia patients. Prolongation of survival by a combination of androgens, better supportive care, and stem cell transplantation (and gene therapy, in the future) may lead to more time for malignancies to appear and may even increase the risk of cancer (399a,399b). In addition, Fanconi's anemia may now be diagnosed by chromosome breakage or mutation analysis in patients with characteristic cancers but without any other stigmata of Fanconi's anemia. Concerns about the development of cancer in older patients cannot be used as contraindications for aggressive management, such as stem cell transplantation. However, cytoreductive chemotherapy and irradiation may themselves increase the risk of malignancies. To some degree, aplastic anemia may soon be considered to be the least of the problems of the Fanconi's anemia patient.

Dyskeratosis Congenita

Dyskeratosis congenita, also known as *Zinsser-Cole-Engman syndrome*, which is named after the first physicians who described these patients, is a rare form of ectodermal dysplasia, with a 40% to 50% frequency of aplastic anemia and a 10% to 15% frequency of cancer. The diagnostic triad consists of dermatologic manifestations and nail dystrophies that usually begin in the first decade of life, and leukoplakia that begins in the second decade of life; all of these conditions become more extreme with increasing age (Fig. 8-11). Aplastic anemia usually develops in the second decade of life, and cancer develops in the third and fourth decades of life.

INHERITANCE AND ENVIRONMENT
More than 275 cases of dyskeratosis congenita have been reported as case reports with data that could be analyzed on an individual basis, many of which are summarized elsewhere (400,401). Dokal reviewed the 148 members of the Dyskeratosis

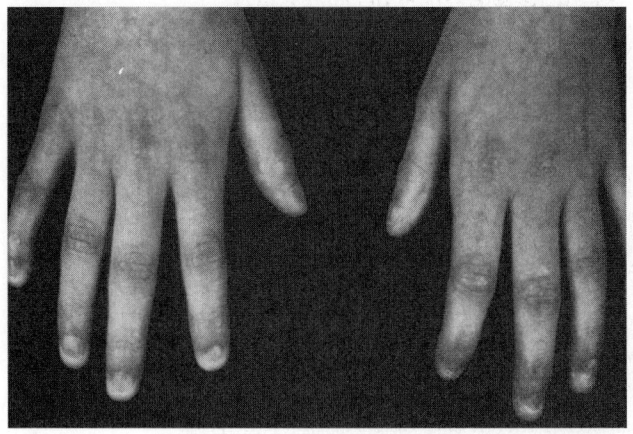
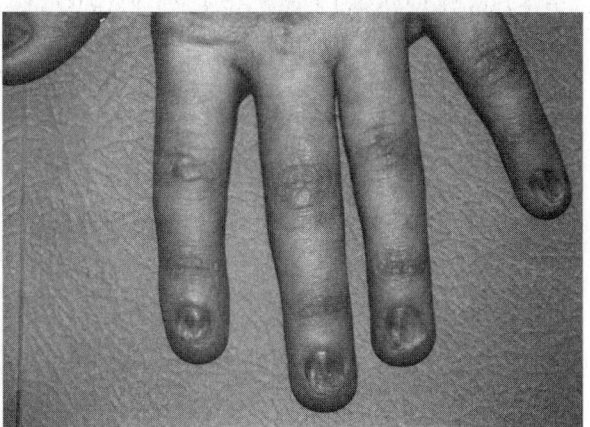

Figure 8-11. A–D: Dystrophic fingernails in dyskeratosis congenita. (From Alter BP, Drachtman RA. Dyskeratosis congenita: nails and hands. *Am J Hematol* 1998;58:298, with permission.) (*continued*)

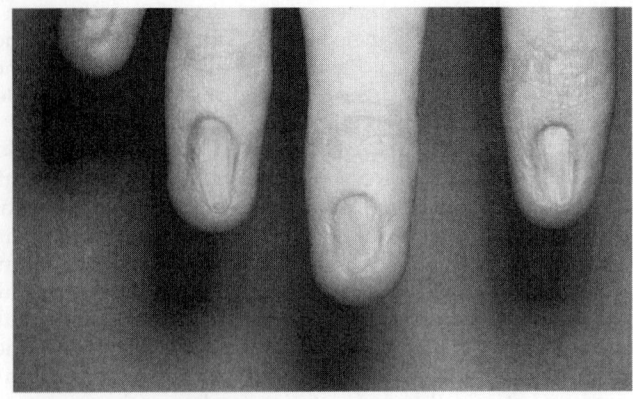
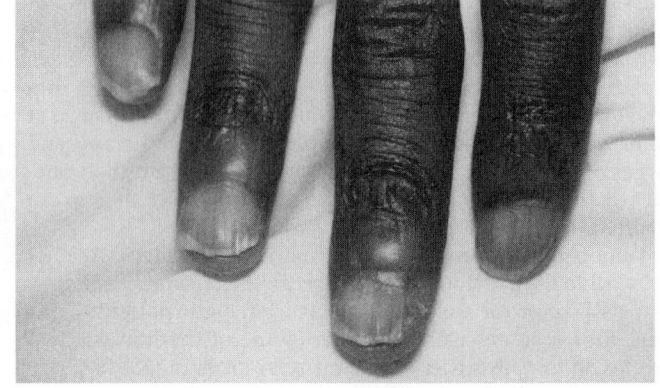

C   D

Figure 8-11. (*continued*)

Congenita Registry (DCR) that was established at Hammersmith Hospital (402). Although the impression is that dyskeratosis congenita is an X-linked disorder, the male to female ratio is 4.5:1.0 in the literature cases and 3.9:1.0 in the DCR (Table 8-9).

Presumed X-linked recessive: More than 200 males have been reported as single cases or from families with males only. More than 30 males were in sibships, with an additional seven families with uncles and nephews and five families with maternal cousins.

Possible autosomal recessive: Forty-four patients were sporadic females or males and females in sibships. Seven families had affected children who were the products of consanguineous marriages. There is an excess of females in this category, because sporadic males could not be distinguished from X-linked males.

Possible autosomal dominant: Thirty cases were in families in which the transmission appeared to be dominant, with two or more generations involved. The sex ratio is approximately 1 in this group.

The families that appear to be autosomal recessive or dominant might be X-linked with inactivation of the normal X chromosome and variable levels of expression, but it is more likely that the dyskeratosis congenita phenotype may be due to more

than one gene. Similarly, the presumably X-linked male group may contain autosomal-recessive patients who happen to be male, as well as new mutation dominants. These possibilities may explain the apparent preponderance of females in the autosomal groups. The X-linked recessive group can be defined more specifically using Xq28 restriction fragment-length polymorphisms (403) and mutation analyses (see the section Pathophysiology) (402). No ethnic and sex association was found; blacks have been reported in all groups, and Asians have been reported in the X-linked and autosomal-recessive groups.

Tables 8-9 through 8-12 compare the findings in the three groups. In comparison to the X-linked recessive males, the autosomal-dominant patients appear to be milder, with a lower frequency of all the components in the diagnostic triad and a lower rate of serious complications. The autosomal-recessive group resembles the X-linked males, although there may be a higher frequency of aplastic anemia in the autosomal-recessive patients.

The age at diagnosis of dyskeratosis congenita in the three groups is depicted in Figure 8-12. The ages may be inappropriately skewed to the high side, because, in many cases, the only age available was that given at the time of the report. The

TABLE 8-9. Dyskeratosis Congenita Literature

Characteristic	X-linked and Sporadic Male	Autosomal Recessive	Autosomal Dominant
Number of cases	200	44	30
Male/female	200/0	10/34	14/16
Ratio	—	0.29	0.88
Age at diagnosis (or report) (yr)			
Mean	18.2	14.9	30
Median	15	13	25
Range	0.3–68	1.2–42	7–58
Age at presentation of nail changes (yr)			
Mean	8.5	5.8	9.5
Median	8	5	7
Range	0–34	0–15	7–17
Age at presentation of skin pigmentation (yr)			
Mean	9.4	7.1	13.1
Median	9	4	13
Range	0–30	0–29	7–18
Age at presentation of leukoplakia (yr)			
Mean	12.6	9	15.3
Median	10	7	17
Range	0.7–43	2–25	12–17

NOTE: Compiled from individual case reports, not including the Dyskeratosis Congenita Registry summary (402). Physical features were not always reported.

TABLE 8-10. Physical Abnormalities in Dyskeratosis Congenita

Characteristic	X-linked and Sporadic Male	Autosomal Recessive	Autosomal Dominant
Number of cases	200	44	30
Skin pigmentation	92	86	67
Nail dystrophy	90	39	13
Leukoplakia	68	68	33
Eye abnormalities	40	43	13
Teeth abnormalities	19	30	10
Developmental delay	15	16	0
Skeletal anomalies	11	25	7
Short stature	13	23	3
Hyperhidrosis	11	9	7
Hair loss	14	30	23
Urinary tract abnormalities	8	5	3
Gastrointestinal abnormalities	13	23	7
Other conditions	10	23	10
Gonadal anomalies	4	9	3

NOTE: Physical features were not always reported. Numbers are percent of cases except in top row, where they are total numbers.

TABLE 8-11. Complications in Dyskeratosis Congenita

	X-linked and Sporadic Male	Autosomal Recessive	Autosomal Dominant
Number of cases	200	44	30
Male to female ratio	—	0.29	0.88
Age at time of diagnosis (or report) (yr)			
Mean	18.2	14.9	30
Median	15	13	25
Range	0.3–68	1.2–42	7–58
Aplastic anemia			
Number of cases (%)	72 (36)	26 (59)	1 (3)
Age at diagnosis (yr)			
Mean	13.3	13.7	16
Median	10.5	11	16
Range	1–41	2–45	16
Cancer			
Number of cases (%)	35 (13)	6 (14)	2 (7)
Age at diagnosis (yr)			
Mean	30.4	27.8	30
Median	29	24.5	30
Range	13–68	21–42	17, 43
Deceased			
Number of cases (%)	60 (30)	12 (27)	1 (3)
Age at diagnosis (yr)			
Mean	21.2	21.2	39
Median	19.5	22.5	39
Range	2–70	5–34	39
Projected median	33	34	—

TABLE 8-12. Cancer in Dyskeratosis Congenita

Type	X-linked and Sporadic Male	Autosomal Recessive Male	Autosomal Recessive Female	Autosomal Dominant Male	Autosomal Dominant Female	All Patients	References[a]
Oropharyngeal	12	0	4	0	1	17	402,419,435–445
Gastrointestinal	12	0	0	0	0	12	402,410,420,435,439,446–455
Myelodysplastic syndrome	4	0	0	0	0	4	402,452
Skin	3	1	0	1	0	5	402,456–460
Hodgkin's disease	2	0	0	0	0	2	461,462
Bronchial	0	2	0	0	0	2	402,463
Pancreatic	0	1	0	0	0	1	402,461
Liver	1	0	0	0	0	1	464
Cervical and vaginal	0	0	1	0	0	1	465
Total cancers	37	1	5	1	1	45	—
Total patients	35	1	5	1	1	43	—

[a]Some cases were cited in more than one reference.

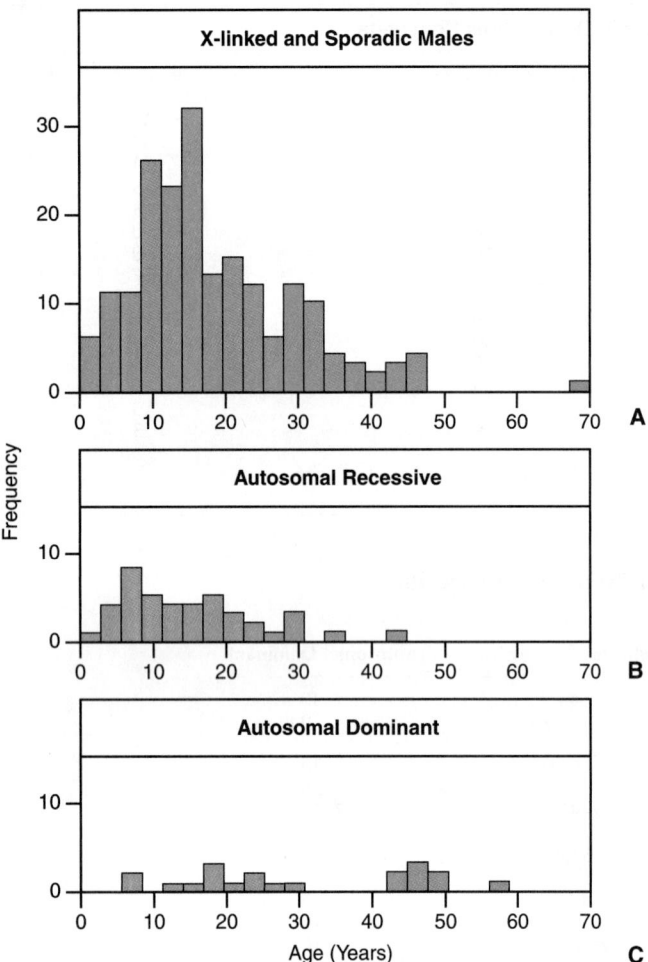

Figure 8-12. Age at diagnosis of dyskeratosis congenita in more than 250 published cases from 1910 to 2000. **A:** Two hundred X-linked and sporadic males. **B:** Forty-four autosomal-recessive patients. **C:** Thirty autosomal-dominant patients.

median age was 15 years of age for X-linked and sporadic males, 13 years of age for autosomal recessives, and 25 years of age for autosomal dominants, thus distinguishing the latter group again. The ages at the development of the components of the diagnostic triad are summarized in Table 8-9. All findings occurred earlier in the autosomal-recessive patients than in the other categories. All three components of the diagnostic triad were reported in more than 70% of the X-linked and autosomal-recessive patients and in 50% of the dominant cases.

PHYSICAL EXAMINATION

The major skin finding in patients with dyskeratosis congenita is lacy, reticulated hyperpigmentation, with dark, grayish macules on an atrophic and sometimes hypopigmented background, which involves the face, neck, shoulders, and trunk. These changes become more dramatic with increasing age. The dystrophic nail changes (hands and feet) include small nail plates, which may develop longitudinal ridging and then may become hypoplastic and eventually disappear. Leukoplakia involves the oral and other mucous membrane surfaces.

Several other systems are also involved (Table 8-10). The eyes are affected in approximately 40% of the patients, most often with epiphora (excessive tearing) due to blocked lacrimal ducts or blepharitis, as well as cataracts, a lack of eyelashes, conjunctivitis, ectropion, abnormal fundi, glaucoma, strabis-

mus, and ulcers. Many patients have poor dentition, with multiple caries and early loss of all teeth. Skeletal abnormalities include osteoporosis, frequent fractures, aseptic necroses (all but one of the latter eight patients had received prednisone), and scoliosis. Several patients have intracranial calcifications. Approximately 15% of the patients are short, slender, delicate, or asthenic in appearance. Hyperhidrosis of palms and soles is common. Early hair thinning or loss and premature graying were also reported. Urinary tract involvement was primarily mucosal, with meatal and urethral stenosis, phimosis, hypospadias, pyelonephritis, penile leukoplakia, and one horseshoe kidney reported. Gastrointestinal problems include esophageal stenosis, diverticula, spasm, duodenal ulcer, anal leukoplakia, bifid uvula, and umbilical hernia. Male hypogonadism with hypoplastic testes was reported in a few cases, similar to Fanconi's anemia. One woman had a vaginal constriction, one had vulvar leukoplakia, and one had a hysterectomy. Four women apparently had successful pregnancies. Other rare reports include deafness, absent eardrum, bird face, cardiac disease, Dandy-Walker deformity, cholesteatoma, and microcephaly.

Because of the coincidence of skin abnormalities, aplastic anemia, and malignancies, dyskeratosis congenita has sometimes been confused or compared with Fanconi's anemia (404–409). In fact, in one series of five Fanconi's anemia patients, one patient probably had dyskeratosis congenita and not Fanconi's anemia (199). The genetics and physical abnormalities of patients with Fanconi's anemia and dyskeratosis congenita are actually quite different; although the same systems may be involved, the types of anomalies are characteristic. In addition, aplastic anemia usually occurs earlier in Fanconi's anemia than in dyskeratosis congenita. These disorders should not be confused clinically and can be distinguished definitively by analysis of chromosome breakage after clastogenic stress or by mutation analyses.

APLASTIC ANEMIA

Thirty-six percent of the X-linked male dyskeratosis congenita patients and 59% of the autosomal-recessive patients were reported to develop aplastic anemia at a median age of 11 years (Table 8-11). Aplastic anemia was rare in the autosomal-dominant patients. In many cases, hematologic symptoms preceded the diagnosis of dyskeratosis congenita, although, in retrospect, the physical abnormalities of dyskeratosis congenita had been present for several years. In the younger patients, hematologic changes may have occurred before the appearance of the dyskeratosis congenita triad. The frequency of bone marrow failure was much higher in the Hammersmith DCR cases, in which it occurred in 86% of the 118 men, with an actuarial probability of 94% by 40 years of age (402). This difference may be related to biased referrals of patients with severe hematologic involvement.

LABORATORY FINDINGS

Blood Counts. Thrombocytopenia or anemia, or both, are the initial signs in most patients who ultimately develop aplastic anemia. Macrocytosis and elevated HbF are common manifestations of stress erythropoiesis, even in patients without pancytopenia. Bone marrow aspirates may be hypercellular at first, and several patients were initially thought to have hypersplenism. Decreased megakaryocytes, hypocellularity, and aplasia eventually ensue. Ferrokinetic studies are consistent with aplastic anemia (406,407,410). A few patients had decreased immunoglobulins (Igs) or decreased cellular immunity, but this has been inconsistent (411).

Chromosome Breakage. Chromosome breakage was studied in several patients. In a few patients, baseline breakage was apparently increased, but the data from many patients and, particularly, from controls were often not cited. Breakage studies were normal in most patients, including those who were examined with DEB, MMC, or nitrogen mustard. Patients with dyskeratosis congenita probably do not have increased breakage in lymphocytes, particularly with clastogenic stress, and can be differentiated from those with Fanconi's anemia on this basis. However, cultured fibroblasts develop chromosomal rearrangements, which suggests that dyskeratosis congenita may be considered a chromosomal instability disorder (412).

Hematopoietic Cultures. Hematopoietic cultures have been performed in a few instances of patients with dyskeratosis congenita. In all patients, the numbers of progenitors were reduced or there were none. All these patients were studied when they already had hematologic symptoms (127,413–419). Addition of GM-CSF increased colony numbers (418), as did SCF (131). Long-term cultures were also defective in dyskeratosis congenita (420).

PATHOPHYSIOLOGY

Dyskeratosis congenita is inherited in a predominantly X-linked pattern, but there are families with apparently autosomal-recessive inheritance, as well as others with dominant inheritance. The autosomal recessives might have X-linked inheritance with lyonization and variable expression in males and females. The more compelling explanation is that there are at least three dyskeratosis congenita genes. Patients with dyskeratosis congenita have a genetic risk for bone marrow failure, but an environmental factor may be required for its manifestation. At least one patient received chloramphenicol before the development of pancytopenia (421).

The X-linked gene was localized to Xq28 with restriction fragment-length polymorphisms (403,422). Subsequently, genetic linkage and XCIP (X chromosome inactivation pattern) analysis narrowed the region to only 1.4 Mb (423). One of the 28 positional gene candidates in this region was found to have a 3'

deletion in one patient, and missense mutations were found in others, thus allowing identification of the dyskeratosis congenita gene, DKC1 (424,425). Verification of DC as the causative gene in the disease came from the identification of multiple missense mutations in the open reading frame (402,426,427). Because the gene is highly conserved with genes in other lower eukaryotes, the distinction between true missense mutations and benign polymorphisms is readily apparent.

The DKC1 gene is composed of 15 exons that span 15 kilobases (kb), and the cDNA is 2.5 kb. The corresponding protein, dyskerin, is 514 amino acids in size, with a predicted molecular weight of 57 kd. A mutational screen of dyskeratosis congenita patients and patients with a related syndrome, Hoyeraal-Hreidarsson, led to the recognition of a wide range of mutations (Fig. 8-13). Because most of these are missense mutations, it is likely that they encode mutant proteins with partial activity. True null mutations in the DC gene may be lethal (402).

The cellular function of dyskerin remains unclear. The protein contains multiple phosphorylation sites and a carboxy-terminal lysine-rich repeat domain. Dyskerin is the ortholog of rat NAP57 and yeast CBF5, suggesting that this protein may function in ribosomal RNA biogenesis and in the assembly of ribosomes (424,428). Consistent with this hypothesis are studies that showed that dyskerin localizes to the nucleolus of mammalian cells. Taken together, these data suggest that dyskerin plays a role in ribosomal assembly and, therefore, indirectly in protein translation and in cell survival. The two tissues that are most highly affected in dyskeratosis congenita (skin epithelium and bone marrow) have a high turnover in adults, suggesting that dyskerin plays a role in survival of cells with a high proliferative capacity.

Although Fanconi's anemia cells have a characteristic cellular phenotype (i.e., sensitivity to DNA cross-linkers), dyskeratosis congenita cells have no consistent phenotype, which makes complementation studies and functional assessment of mutations more difficult. One study found that dyskerin binds to

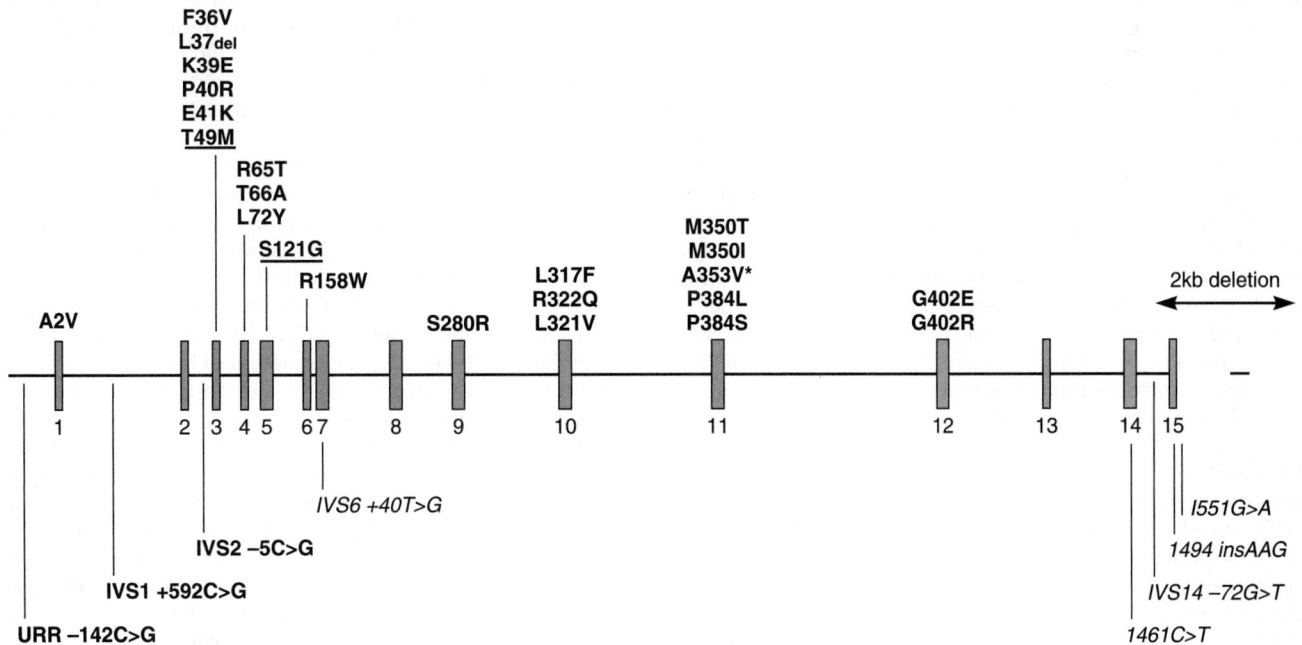

Figure 8-13. Mutations in the DKC1 gene. Schematic representation of the 15 exons with patient-derived mutations *(bold)* and polymorphisms *(italics).* Asterisk indicates the A353V mutation that has recurred in 17 different families. Underlined mutations were found in patients with the Hoyeraal-Hreidarsson syndrome. kb, kilobase. (Modified from Dokal I. Dyskeratosis congenita in all its forms. *Br J Haematol* 2000;110:768–779, with permission.)

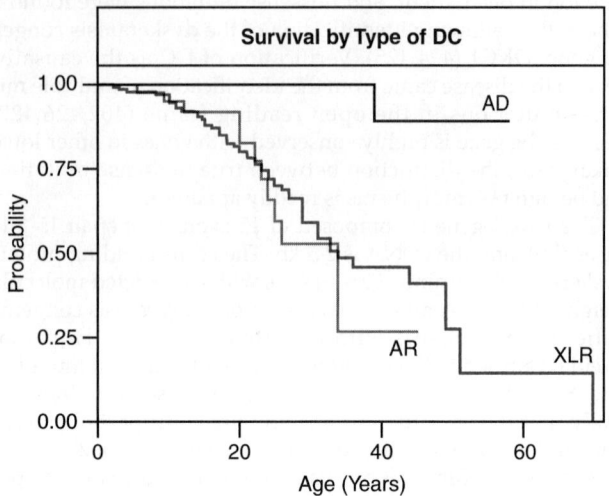

Figure 8-14. Kaplan-Meier plot of cumulative survival in dyskeratosis congenita (DC). Time is shown as age in years. AD, 20 autosomal-dominant patients; AR, 42 autosomal-recessive patients; XLR, 195 X-linked and sporadic males. The differences are significant.

telomerase and therefore may play a role in telomere length maintenance (429). Peripheral blood cells of patients with X-linked dyskeratosis congenita have much shorter telomeres than those in normal cells (430). This is especially interesting, because accelerated telomere shortening is associated with murine carcinomas (431) and may therefore be relevant to the development of squamous cell carcinomas in dyskeratosis congenita (see the section Cancer).

The cloning of the DKC1 gene has important implications for the diagnosis of dyskeratosis congenita and related syndromes. The clinical abnormalities are variable from patient to patient in severity and age of onset. However, pulmonary disease, myelodysplasia, and malignancy may develop in the older patients who survive or avoid the complications of early bone marrow failure.

Mutational screening of the DKC1 gene is warranted in any patient with clinical signs that are consistent with the disease, although considerable disease heterogeneity is evident. In the related syndrome, the *Hoyeraal-Hreidarsson syndrome*, patients have a severe multisystem disorder that is characterized by microcephaly, cerebellar hypoplasia, growth retardation, immunodeficiency, and aplastic anemia. This syndrome was found to result from unique missense mutations in the DKC1 gene (432–434). Based on these new findings, mutational screening of the DKC1 gene should be considered in any patient with severe clinical phenotypes who has some of the features of dyskeratosis congenita or Hoyeraal-Hreidarsson syndrome, even if he or she does not have the more classic signs of dyskeratosis congenita, such as skin and nail changes.

PROGNOSIS

The prognosis is poor in dyskeratosis congenita. One-third of the X-linked and sporadic male patients and of the autosomal-recessive patients died by the time of the reports, at an actuarial median age of 34 and 26 years of age, respectively (Fig. 8-14). More than one-half of the deaths were due to complications of aplastic anemia, such as infection or hemorrhage. Unsuccessful bone marrow transplants and cancer were responsible for most of the rest of the poor outcomes (see the section Cancer). Dokal suggested that patients with dyskeratosis congenita have a predisposition to endothelial activation and damage, based on the observation of increased levels of von Willebrand's factor and

pulmonary complications in several patients, including some complications that occurred posttransplant (402).

CANCER

Cancers were reported in 35 X-linked males, six autosomal-recessive patients (one male, five females), and one male and one female who were in the autosomal-dominant group (Tables 8-11 and 8-12). This summary includes the cases that were reported by Dokal (402), and, thus, there may be inadvertent duplicate reporting. At least two patients had two or more tumors. The majority of the tumors were squamous cell carcinomas. The sites were similar to those reported in patients with Fanconi's anemia (Table 8-8) and involve areas that are known to be abnormal in dyskeratosis congenita, such as mucous membranes and the gastrointestinal tract. The median age for cancer was similar in all three types of dyskeratosis congenita and was approximately 30 years of age, with a range from 13 to 68 years of age, which is substantially higher than the median age of 11 years for the development of aplastic anemia (Table 8-11). Among those who developed cancer, the predicted median survival is 36 years of age. In contrast to Fanconi's anemia patients, only a rare patient with dyskeratosis congenita has been reported to have leukemia or MDS.

TREATMENT

Treatment for the aplastic anemia of dyskeratosis congenita is similar to that for Fanconi's anemia. Almost 40 patients were reported to receive *androgens*, usually combined with prednisone, as described earlier for Fanconi's anemia, and approximately 50% of patients responded, a similar response rate to that seen in Fanconi's anemia. As in Fanconi's anemia, responses are not cures, and androgens must be maintained; subsequent failures do ensue. *Splenectomies* were reported in at least eight male patients, with only temporary improvements. *Supportive care* with RBC and platelet transfusions, antibiotics, and ε-aminocaproic acid (466) should all be provided when indicated clinically. There are no reports on the use of antilymphocyte globulin or cyclosporin A, but these agents would not be expected to work (one of our patients received these at another institution without response) (400).

Hematopoietic growth factors were used in a small number of cases, mostly for brief intervals in which only neutrophil responses were documented. GM-CSF was effective in two patients (467,468), IL-3 was effective for one of three patients (469), and G-CSF was effective for three patients (470–472). All of those were X-linked or sporadic male cases. We treated one man from an autosomal-recessive family with G-CSF for more than 1 year [with erythropoietin (EPO) for the last 10 months] with an excellent neutrophil response and a 6-month improvement in Hgb and platelets (473). Unfortunately, severe aplastic anemia recurred despite continuation of both cytokines. Nevertheless, the combination of G-CSF and EPO might warrant additional long-term trials.

BMT was reported in 20 X-linked or sporadic males (452,460,470,474–483), with six survivors (30%) when reported. Four of seven autosomal-recessive patients (57%) were alive when reported (460,475,484–488). Causes of deaths included acute and chronic graft-versus-host disease, infections, venooclusive disease of the liver at as long as 7 years after transplantation, and pulmonary fibrosis at up to 20 years. Some patients developed a mucositis syndrome that was similar to that seen in Fanconi's anemia patients who received standard levels of cyclophosphamide preparation. Most of the dyskeratosis congenita patients were prepared for transplant with standard cyclophosphamide plus irradiation. The long-term prognosis for most patients after transplant is poor, with actuarial median

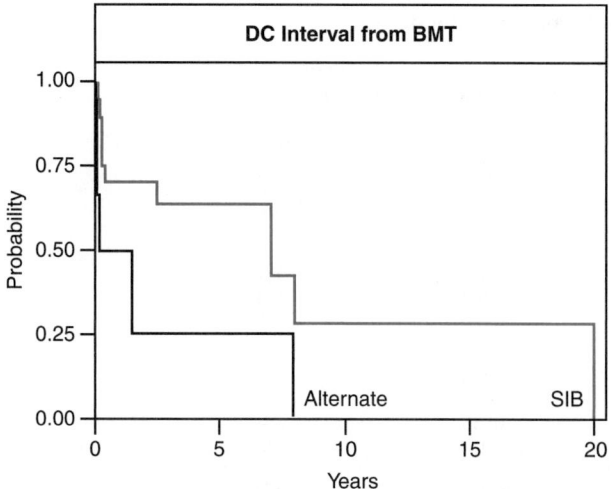

Figure 8-15. Kaplan-Meier plot of cumulative survival after bone marrow transplantation (BMT) for patients with dyskeratosis congenita (DC). Time is shown as years from transplantation. One patient was unsuccessfully transplanted from a brother with DC (not shown). The difference between sibling and alternate donors is not significant. Alternate, seven patients were transplanted from alternate donors; SIB, 20 patients were transplanted from HLA-identical siblings.

survivals of 7 years for those with HLA-matched sibling donors, and 1.5 years for the five cases in which alternate donors were used (Fig. 8-15). The median survivals were 8 years for the autosomal-recessive patients, and 1.5 years for the X-linked and sporadic men.

Transplantation in dyskeratosis congenita patients must thus be approached with caution. In addition, because the physical features of dyskeratosis congenita may appear late or may be subtle, potential donors who may in fact be affected with dyskeratosis congenita may be difficult to detect unless they have an identifiable mutation. Finally, we can speculate that, as in Fanconi's anemia, marrow transplantation does not reduce (and may increase) the risk of development of tumors. None have been reported so far, perhaps because the long-term survival after transplant has been short, and the number of patients who have undergone transplants is small.

Disorders That Are Related to Dyskeratosis Congenita

As mentioned previously in the discussion of the DKC1 gene (see the section Pathophysiology), a small number of male patients has been described under the rubric of *Hoyeraal-Hreidarsson syndrome*. The patients are small, with intrauterine growth retardation, microcephaly, cerebellar hypoplasia, developmental delay, progressive pancytopenia, and immunodeficiencies, and the inheritance appears to be X-linked. Recent studies of three patients identified mutations in the DKC1 gene (432,489). Seven of the 11 patients died from infectious or hemorrhagic complications of aplastic anemia, and the oldest survivor was 5 years of age and was 3 years of age after an unrelated bone marrow transplant.

An even more rare disorder, *Revesz syndrome*, has been reported in four cases, and one of the authors is aware of two more (486,490,491; B. P. Alter, *unpublished data*, 1999). There were three males and three females, and the characteristic findings include intrauterine growth retardation, cerebellar hypoplasia, and microcephaly. The patients have features of dyskeratosis congenita, such as dystrophic nails, oral leukoplakia, sparse

hair, and reticular skin pigmentation, as well as bone marrow failure in four of the six patients. However, the unique feature of these patients is bilateral exudative retinopathy, which was called *Coats' retinopathy*, but which resembles Norrie's disease (492). No germline mutations were found in the DKC1 gene or the Norrie's gene in one of our patients, however, and the genetic basis of this syndrome remains unclear. A major concern is the combination of thrombocytopenia and hemorrhagic retinopathy, and it is recommended that platelet transfusions be provided for unresponsive thrombocytopenia to decrease further retinal hemorrhages. All patients, who were younger than 4 years of age when reported, were alive, although Revesz's original patient subsequently died (T. Revesz, *personal communication*, 1999).

Still another disorder with overlap with those disorders that were previously mentioned is the *ataxia-pancytopenia syndrome*, which was first described by Li et al. (493,494) in a family with ataxia in the father and all five children. Two brothers died with aplastic anemia, one with acute myeloblastic leukemia, and one with acute myelomonocytic leukemia. The only surviving sibling was a 19-year-old girl with mild anemia. A second family was reported by Daghistani et al. (495) in which the mother, her son, and her daughter had ataxia; the son had pancytopenia and monosomy 7 and developed acute myeloblastic leukemia. There are a small number of additional case reports of families or sporadic cases with men and women with ataxia, cerebellar atrophy, microcephaly, tongue ulcers, immunodeficiencies, and aplastic anemia or leukemia (496–499); none of these cases had monosomy 7. Eight of the 15 patients died between 3 and 10 years of age; four died from leukemia, and four died from complications of aplastic anemia. Treatment of pancytopenia with prednisone was effective in one case (497), whereas antithymocyte globulin, cyclosporine, and G-CSF were ineffective on another (496), and prednisone plus danazol were also ineffective (498).

Shwachman-Diamond Syndrome

The Shwachman-Diamond (Bodian Shwachman) syndrome consists of exocrine pancreatic insufficiency plus neutropenia (500–502). More than 300 cases have been reported (Table 8-13). Signs of pancreatic insufficiency, usually apparent in infancy, are diarrhea, malabsorption, steatorrhea, and failure to thrive. Neutropenia is identified early as part of the general workup or because of skin infections or pneumonia. Additional hematologic problems develop in 40% of patients, such as anemia, thrombocytopenia, and pancytopenia. Occasionally anemia or thrombocytopenia is the initial hematologic problem. The ratio of males to females is 1.6:1.0. Segregation analysis provides evidence that the inheritance is autosomal recessive, although reports of consanguinity are rare (503). Shwachman-Diamond syndrome has been reported in all racial groups, with no ethnic propensity. Pregnancies and birth histories of patients are uneventful, although more than 10% of patients had low birth weight. One Shwachman-Diamond patient was reported who had a successful pregnancy, during which her white blood cell count rose slightly, her absolute neutrophil count doubled from her usual range of less than 2000/μL to approximately 4000/μL, and her platelets dropped from more than 120,000/μL to less than 110,000/μL. She required a caesarean section for cephalopelvic disproportion, which perhaps was related to her small stature. However, there were no major complications from her Shwachman-Diamond syndrome (504).

The most prominent physical findings are related to malnourishment, including short stature in more than one-half of patients, protuberant abdomen, and low weight. Forty percent of patients had radiographic evidence for metaphyseal dysosto-

TABLE 8-13. Shwachman-Diamond Syndrome Literature

	All Patients	Cytopenias	No Anemia or Thrombocytopenia
Number of cases (%)	336	134 (40)	202 (60)
Male/female	196/121	79/53	117/68
Ratio	1.6	1.5	1.7
Number with metaphyseal dysostosis (%)	124 (37)	51 (38)	73 (36)
Age at malabsorption			
Mean	1.1	1.0	1.1
Median	0.3	0.3	0.3
Range	0–16	0–16	0–16
Age at marrow failure			
Mean	—	7.5	—
Median	—	3	—
Range	—	0–35	—
Number with mental retardation (%)	33 (10)	20 (15)	13 (6)
Number with abnormal physical examination (%)	43 (13)	18 (13)	25 (12)
Leukemia			
Number of cases (%)	23 (7)	10 (7)	13 (6)
Male/female	19/1	9/1	10/0
Age at diagnosis (yr)			
Mean	17.6	11.5	24.3
Median	14	7.8	23.5
Range	1.8–43	1.8–38	6–43
MDS			
Number of cases (%)	30 (9)	5 (4)	25 (12)
Male/female	15/11	3/2	12/9
Age at diagnosis (yr)			
Mean	10.3	7.6	10.8
Median	8.1	7.5	8.1
Range	2–42	3.5–12	2–42
MDS clone alone	5	—	—
Died	2	—	—
MDS morphology alone	6	—	—
Died	4	—	—
Deceased			
Number of cases (%)	68 (20)	32 (24)	36 (18)
Male/female	37/25	20/12	17/13
Age at death (yr)			
Mean	7.6	8.2	7.1
Median	3.3	5.3	0.9
Range	0.3–43	0.4–35	0.3–43
Projected median age for all patients (yr)	35	25	37
Leukemia	14	—	—
MDS	16	—	—

MDS, myelodysplastic syndrome.

sis. Ten percent had mental retardation, and 1.5% had microcephaly. Several had an ichthyotic skin rash. Rare physical anomalies include hypertelorism, retinitis pigmentosa, toe or finger syndactyly, cleft palate, dental dysplasia, ptosis, strabismus, short neck, coxa valga, and skin pigmentation.

The combination of pancreatic dysfunction plus bone marrow failure was noted by Ozsoylu and Argun (505), who found decreased duodenal trypsin in patients with acquired aplastic anemia or Fanconi's anemia. Those patients did not have symptomatic malabsorption. In addition, patients with Shwachman-Diamond syndrome have decreased amylase and lipase, as well as trypsin.

LABORATORY FINDINGS

By definition, all patients with Shwachman-Diamond syndrome have neutropenia (neutrophils below 1500/μL on more than one occasion). It may be chronic, intermittent, or cyclic and is usually noted early in childhood. Thirty percent of patients were reported to have two involved lineages, and 10% had all three lineages involved. Pancytopenia occurred at a median age of 3 years (with a range from 0 to 35 years of age). There are a few reports of defects in neutrophil mobility, but this is an inconsistent finding (506–509).

Bone marrow examination shows myeloid hypocellularity or maturation arrest. The erythroid series is normal or hyperplastic. HbF levels are often elevated, even without anemia, which suggests hematopoietic stress (510). Igs are occasionally decreased. Hepatic dysfunction and fibrosis have also been noted. Chromosomes are normal, and no increased breakage is found after clastogenic stress.

Pancreatic insufficiency is documented by the demonstration of low or absent duodenal trypsin, amylase, and lipase. Less invasive than duodenal incubation, serum trypsinogen was shown to be low in young patients, although it does increase with age and is associated with improvement in absorption (511). Other methods for demonstration of pancreatic insufficiency include ultrasound or imaging studies that demonstrate a fatty pancreas. Patients do not have cystic fibrosis, and sweat chloride levels are normal.

PATHOPHYSIOLOGY

The inheritance of Shwachman-Diamond syndrome is autosomal recessive (503). Although the exocrine pancreas and bone marrow hematopoiesis develop at approximately the same time during gestation, familial cases, as well as Shwachman-Diamond syndrome in only one of a pair of twins argue against an intrauterine insult as the cause (512). Culture of bone marrow progenitors shows decreased colony-forming units granulocyte-macrophage (CFU-GM) and CFU-E in most patients, which suggests a stem cell deficit. No evidence is found for humoral or cellular inhibitors of granulopoiesis. Shwachman-Diamond syndrome thus resembles other inherited bone marrow failure disorders, with reduced numbers of hematopoietic progenitor cells.

The gene for Shwachman-Diamond syndrome has been mapped to the centromere of chromosome 7, and, so far, the data are consistent with a single locus with several different mutations (513).

THERAPY AND OUTCOME

Malabsorption responds to treatment with oral pancreatic enzymes. Infections are treated with the appropriate antibiotics and may decrease with age. Supportive care should be provided, with transfusions for anemia and platelets for thrombocytopenia. Corticosteroids or androgens, or both, were used in approximately a dozen patients, with hematologic improvement in one-half. The neutropenia does respond to G-CSF (514). Among 12 patients who were reported to receive G-CSF, four developed mildly dysplastic bone marrows with clonal cytogenetics (see the following section, Myelodysplastic Syndrome).

Evolution to pancytopenia or leukemia are the major hematologic complications. Deaths were reported in 24% of the group with cytopenias, 18% of those with only neutropenia, and 70% of those with leukemia (Table 8-13). The projected median survival age for the entire group is 35 years of age; the median survival is 25 years of age for those with cytopenias, 14 years of age for those with leukemia, and 37 years of age for those without hematologic complications. Those without these complications reach a plateau of almost 80% survival by the late teenage years (Fig. 8-16). The reported deaths were usually due to infection, bleeding, or leukemia.

More than 20 patients had a bone marrow transplant; one-half received bone marrow from sibling donors, and one-half received

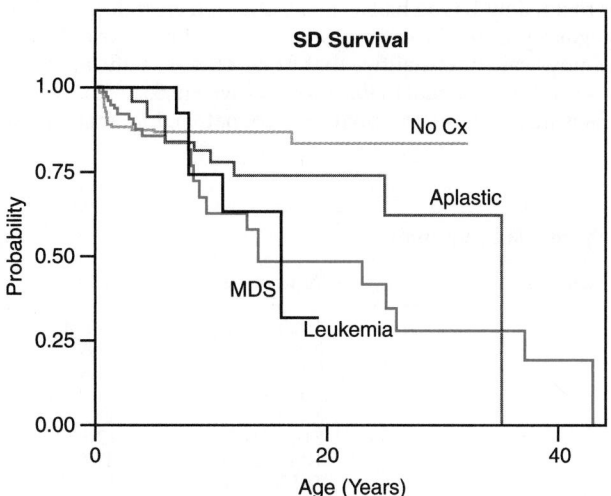

Figure 8-16. Kaplan-Meier plot of cumulative survival in Shwachman-Diamond (SD) syndrome. The differences between curves are significant. Aplastic, 94 patients with aplastic anemia; Leukemia, 18 patients with leukemia; MDS, 16 patients with myelodysplastic syndrome; No Cx, 156 patients with no hematologic complications.

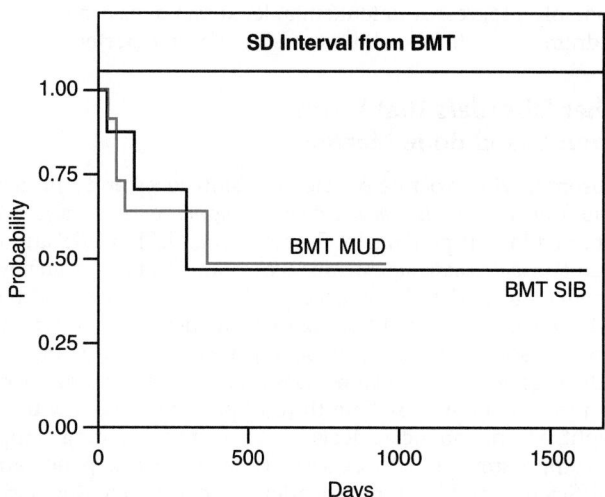

Figure 8-17. Kaplan-Meier plot of cumulative survival after bone marrow transplantation (BMT) for patients with Shwachman-Diamond (SD) syndrome. Time is shown as days from transplantation. The differences are not significant. MUD, 12 patients had matched, unrelated donors; SIB, seven patients were transplanted from HLA-identical siblings.

marrow from alternative donors (515–531). The outcomes were similar, with an absolute mortality of approximately 50% from either type of donor, projected median survivals of approximately 1 year, and plateaus at 47% survival (Fig. 8-17). Deaths after transplant were from complications of marrow transplant, including cyclophosphamide cardiotoxicity, or from leukemia. As with other inherited bone marrow failure disorders, cases may have been reported because of severity or complications (e.g., leukemia), and Shwachman-Diamond syndrome may be milder than it would appear from the literature.

Leukemia. Twenty-three patients, all male except one, developed leukemia (7%) at a median of 14 years of age (with a range from 2 to 43 years of age). Five patients had acute lymphoblastic leukemia, 17 had acute megaloblastic leukemia (four M1, two M2, three M4, three M5, five M6) and one had juvenile chronic myelocytic leukemia (500,502,519–521,524,526,529,532–541). Ten patients had prior histories of cytopenias, whereas 13 patients did not. Seventy percent died at a median age of 14 years for the total leukemic group; the median age of death was 8 years of age for those with prior cytopenias and 24 years of age for those without cytopenias.

Myelodysplastic Syndrome. Thirty patients had MDS, of whom eight developed leukemia and are included in the analyses that were previously mentioned (519–522,524–528,530,533,540,542–546). Unlike leukemia, the male to female ratio in MDS was similar to the ratio in all Shwachman-Diamond patients. MDS was more frequent in those without cytopenias. The median age was 8 years (with a range from 2 to 42 years of age). The projected median age at death for those with MDS was 16 years of age (Fig. 8-16).

Five of the 30 patients had marrow cytogenetic clones without morphologic evidence of MDS. Clones included monosomy 7 with t(6;13), t(4;7) and deletion 7 in patients who had received G-CSF, as well as monosomy 7 in three patients, isochromosome 7q in 11 patients, der(7) in three, and other clones in five other patients, all of whom did not receive G-CSF. Chromosome 7 was involved in a total of 22 patients.

Shwachman-Diamond syndrome thus resembles many of the other inherited bone marrow failure syndromes in that it has a malignant propensity. Although it is not clear that MDS inevitably progresses to leukemia, leukemia does occur in the syndrome. To date, no solid tumors have been reported.

Other Disorders That Involve Pancreas and Bone Marrow

A disorder with exocrine pancreatic insufficiency and *refractory sideroblastic anemia with vacuolization of bone marrow precursors* was identified in four patients by Pearson et al. (547) in 1979 and is called *Pearson's syndrome*. Anemia was more significant than neutropenia, myeloid and erythroid precursors had vacuoles, and there were ringed sideroblasts. Since then, there have been more than 70 cases reported. The male to female ratio is 0.7, and the median age at detection of anemia is 2 months (with a range from birth to 7 years of age). One-third of patients have low birth weight, and metabolic acidosis is a frequent presenting symptom. Approximately 30% of patients have exocrine pancreatic insufficiency, and insulin-dependent diabetes often develops. Liver and renal failure ensue, and contribute to the metabolic problems. The anemia requires transfusions, although there may be some response to EPO and to G-CSF for neutropenia. The anemia may improve in more than one-third of the patients, at a median of 2 years of age (with a range from 3 months to 10 years of age). One-half of the cases died from acidosis, renal or liver failure, sepsis, and heart block when they were reported; the patients usually did not die from bone marrow failure.

The molecular basis for this syndrome was found to be large deletions of mitochondrial DNA (548). The features of the syndrome that are consistent with a mitochondrial disorder include the involvement of multiple tissues, the paradox of ringed sideroblasts (a problem of iron loading rather than of heme synthesis) and macrocytic anemia, and severe and usually fatal metabolic acidosis (549). Mitochondrial DNA is cytoplasmic, inherited maternally, and heteroplasmic at the mitochondrial, cellular, and organ levels. Each cell has many mitochondria, which may have normal and mutant DNA within the mitochondrion and within the cell, and the proportion of cells with mutant mitochondria varies from organ to organ. Thus, the clinical problems are highly variable from organ to organ, patient to patient, and time to time. The size of the DNA deletion and the presence or absence of duplications and rearrangements does not correlate with the clinical course (550). Those who survive often develop Kearns-Sayre syndrome (progressive ophthalmoplegia, pigmentary retinopathy, cardiac conduction defect, hearing loss, and endocrinopathies), in which the same mitochondrial deletions have been found; patients whose first diagnosis is Kearns-Sayre syndrome usually do not have a preceding marrow failure phase (551).

Patients with *cartilage hair hypoplasia* have an autosomal-recessive disorder with metaphyseal dysostosis, short stature, and characteristic fine hair (552). Approximately 80% of 108 Finnish patients had mild macrocytic anemia, which was severe in 16% of those patients. Lymphopenia was detected in 65% of patients, and neutropenia was detected in 25%, but pancreatic insufficiency was rare. The incidence of malignancy was increased by sevenfold and included Hodgkin's disease in two patients, non-Hodgkin's lymphoma in three patients, melanosis progonoma (retinoblastic teratoma) of the testis in one patient, one vocal cord squamous cell carcinoma, and three cases of basal cell carcinoma (552–555). The gene was mapped to 9p13 in 1994, and mutations were recently found in the RNA component of RNase MRP (556,557). Disruption of the MRP gene may interfere with cell cycle control, but this mechanism is currently speculative.

Amegakaryocytic Thrombocytopenia

A small number of patients present with thrombocytopenia, usually in infancy, and subsequently develop aplastic anemia. This was called type III constitutional aplastic anemia by O'Gorman Hughes (295), but the term *megakaryocytic thrombocytopenia* is more descriptive. Although the differential diagnosis of neonatal thrombocytopenia is lengthy, the entity to be discussed here excludes those conditions with increased bone marrow megakaryocytes as well as those that are due to congenital infection (particularly viral, such as rubella). Immune thrombocytopenias are also not included, despite the occasional development of amegakaryocytosis, which is presumably due to the reactivity of antiplatelet antibodies with megakaryocytes (558). In addition, TAR syndrome is discussed later, because it represents a pure single cytopenia. Fanconi's anemia, which can begin with thrombocytopenia, was already discussed. Finally, children with associated trisomies, such as trisomy 13 and 18, have also been excluded. Various syndromes that are associated with inherited thrombocytopenias are listed in Table 8-14. The accepted cases of amegakaryocytic thrombocytopenia are summarized in Table 8-15, with separate analyses of those with normal appearances and those with congenital anomalies.

More than 50 patients were reported with normal physical appearance, in whom thrombocytopenia occurred primarily early in the first year of life, with absent or reduced bone marrow megakaryocytes (1,6,559–561). The male to female ratio was approximately 1. One-half as many children were described with amegakaryocytic thrombocytopenia in the first year of life who had physical abnormalities that fit no other specific syndrome; the sex ratio was equal in this group as well (6,562,563). The birth defects included microcephaly, micrognathia, intracranial struc-

---

TABLE 8-14. Inherited Thrombocytopenia Syndromes

Disorder	Genetics	Chromosome	Gene
Amegakaryocytic thrombocytopenia, no birth defects	AR	1p34	c-mpl
Amegakaryocytic thrombocytopenia, with birth defects	AR	N/A	N/A
Thrombocytopenia—absent radii syndrome	AR	N/A	N/A
X-linked macrothrombocytopenia	X-linked	Xp11.23	GATA-1
Hoyeraal-Hreidarsson syndrome	X-linked	Xq28	DC1
Familial platelet disorder—acute myelocytic leukemia	AD	21q22.1-.2	CBFA2
Familial dominant thrombocytopenia	AD	10p11.2-12	THC2
Amegakaryocytic thrombocytopenia, with radioulnar synostosis	AD	7p15-p14.2	HOXA11
Trisomy 13	Nondisjunction	Trisomy 13	—
Trisomy 18	Nondisjunction	Trisomy 18	—
Jacobsen syndrome	11q monosomy, partial deletion	11q23	N/A

AD, autosomal dominant; AR, autosomal recessive; N/A, not available.

TABLE 8-15. Amegakaryocytic Thrombocytopenia Literature

	No Anomalies	Anomalies	Patients
Number of cases	52	20	72
Male/female	27/24	11/8	38/32
Ratio	1.1	1.4	1.1
Age at diagnosis (d)			
Mean	301	49	237
Median	40	0	6
Range	0–3285	0–365	0–3285
Aplastic anemia			
Number of cases (%)	25 (48)	3 (15)	28 (39)
Age at diagnosis (yr)			
Mean	3.4	3.5	3.4
Median	3	2.3	2.9
Range	0.4–12.5	2.2–6	0.4–12.5
Leukemia and preleukemia, number of cases (%)	2 (4)	0	2 (3)
Deceased			
Number of cases (%)	17 (33)	13 (65)	30 (42)
Age at death (yr)			
Mean	5.5	2.4	4.2
Median	4	0.5	2.8
Range	0.01–21.00	0–10	0–21
Projected median age	9	2.7	7

tural anomalies, congenital heart disease, failure to thrive, and developmental delays. Some of the specific cases with cerebellar atrophy were recently shown to belong to the Hoyeraal-Hreidarsson syndrome, with mutations in the DKC1 gene that is mutant in dyskeratosis congenita (see the section Dyskeratosis Congenita). The physical findings in some patients resembled those that are seen in Fanconi's anemia, and the diagnosis of Fanconi's anemia cannot be excluded retrospectively from the reports. The inheritance may be autosomal recessive, because some families had affected siblings or consanguinity, or both.

In both groups, the pregnancies and deliveries were essentially unremarkable, although the frequency of spontaneous abortions was 10%. Low birth weight was recorded in 25% of patients with normal appearance and in almost one-half of those with birth defects. The presentation was usually due to bleeding in the skin, mucous membranes, or gastrointestinal tract. Evolution to aplastic anemia was reported in almost one-half of the patients, primarily in those without birth defects.

LABORATORY FINDINGS

The initial abnormality is thrombocytopenia, with normal white blood cell counts and Hgb levels. Reported platelet counts ranged from 0/μL to 88,000/μL at diagnosis, white blood cell counts were normal, and Hgbs were low only after bleeding had occurred. Macrocytosis, as well as increased HbF and i antigen, suggested a broader level of marrow failure. One 5-year-old boy with amegakaryocytic thrombocytopenia had increased MCV and HbF but had not yet developed aplastic anemia (564). Bone marrow cellularity is normal until aplastic anemia appears, except for markedly decreased or absent megakaryocytes; those that are present are small and apparently inactive. Homologous platelet survival is normal, because the defect is underproduction not increased destruction (565). Peripheral blood chromosomes do not show the increased breaks that are characteristic of Fanconi's anemia.

Prenatal diagnosis is possible by means of platelet counts in fetal blood that is obtained during the midtrimester. Mibashan and Millar (566) examined three fetuses who were at risk and detected thrombocytopenia in one fetus. Because the gene has now been cloned (see Pathophysiology), molecular diagnosis should be possible.

PATHOPHYSIOLOGY

The thrombocytopenia is apparently due to a defect in production, because megakaryocytes are decreased or absent. After pancytopenia develops, hematopoietic progenitor cells are decreased or absent (127,561,567,568). Thrombocytopenia may be the first sign of aplastic anemia in many conditions, although this group is distinguished by the relatively long duration before pancytopenia. Serum levels of thrombopoietin (TPO), IL-11, and IL-6 were elevated, which is related to megakaryocytic deficiency (569,570). Cultures did not respond to added TPO, and the expression of c-mpl RNA was impaired (571).

The gene that is involved in amegakaryocytic thrombocytopenia is the receptor for TPO, which is encoded by the c-mpl gene. Mutations in c-mpl have been reported in at least 15 patients, all of whom are without birth defects (560,561,572,573).

OUTCOME

Aplastic anemia developed in almost one-half the patients, at a median of 3 years of age, the oldest was 12 years of age. One-half of the patients in whom aplastic anemia developed died from bleeding or infection. One-half of those without aplastic anemia died also from central nervous system or gastrointestinal hemorrhages. Two-thirds of the deaths were in cases that were described before 1980, and systematic platelet support was not reported. The predicted median survival is 9 years of age in those without birth defects and younger than 3 years of age in those with physical anomalies, and the actual median ages at reported deaths were 4 and 0.5 years of age. The oldest patient in the former group died at 21 years of age, and the oldest patient in the latter group died at 10 years of age.

One male with normal physical appearance had amegakaryocytic thrombocytopenia from birth, developed aplastic anemia at 5 years of age, responded poorly to androgens plus steroids, and evolved further into acute myelomonocytic leukemia at 16 years of age, with death at 17 years of age (295; N. Potter and B. P. Alter, *unpublished data*). A female patient had thrombocytopenia at 2 months of age, pancytopenia at 5 months of age, and a preleukemic picture with abnormalities that involved chromosome 19 (M. B. Harris, V. Najfeld, M. A. Weiner, et al., *unpublished data*, 1984). Thus, amegakaryocytic thrombocytopenia

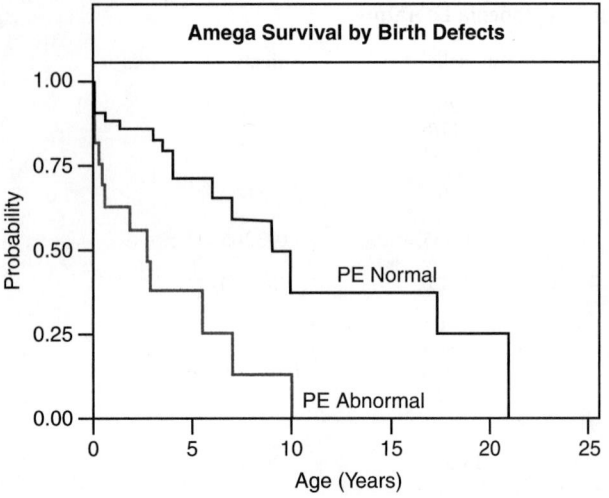

Figure 8-18. Kaplan-Meier plot of cumulative survival in amegakaryo-cytic thrombocytopenia (Amega). Patients with only thrombocytopenia and those with aplastic anemia are pooled, because the numbers are small. Outcomes were not available for all patients. The differences are significant. PE abnormal, 16 patients with birth defects; PE normal, 42 patients without birth defects.

may also be one of the marrow failure syndromes with a propensity to malignancy.

TREATMENT

Steroids alone were not effective in the treatment of amegakaryocytic thrombocytopenia. Steroids plus androgens resulted in temporary or partial responses in a few patients. Splenectomies were performed in four patients without effect. Figure 8-18 shows the survival curves for patients without and patients with anomalies. We can speculate that platelet support might prevent early deaths from thrombocytopenia, but the rate of evolution to aplastic anemia might then be higher. Hematopoietic growth factors that stimulate platelet production might be considered when they become available. Guinan et al. (559) did show a platelet response to IL-3 but not to GM-CSF in five patients in a phase I and II trial, and Taylor et al. (563) reported slight responses in two out of six patients with PIXY321 (GM-CSF and IL-3 fusion protein), but neither of these agents is currently available.

Fifteen patients were treated with BMT; ten of the transplants were from HLA-matched siblings, and five were from unrelated donors, two of which were cord bloods. All of these patients were in the group without birth defects, and all but one patient survived (4,243,561,574–576). Thus, stem cell transplant has the potential to cure thrombocytopenia and prevent the development of aplastic anemia or leukemia.

Familial Marrow Dysfunction

Several families have been reported with various combinations of physical and immunologic abnormalities, in which hematopoietic defects and often leukemia have occurred. The ages at the development of hematologic manifestations vary from childhood to adulthood, and the inheritance patterns have been of all types. Some of the families have anomalies that resemble but in fact differ from those described in Fanconi's anemia. One group, the Estren-Dameshek familial aplastic patients, has been reclassified as Fanconi's anemia. Another group of patients has anomalies that resemble those that are seen in Fanconi's anemia patients, but the group does not have Fanconi's anemia. Other patients fit into known genetic syndromes, such as Brachmann-de Lange, Dubowitz's, Seckel's, and Down's syndromes, and are discussed separately. Several patients with physical anomalies and aplasia are sporadic.

Some patients inherited their disease in an autosomal-dominant manner. The *IVIC syndrome*, which is named for the initials of the institution that first reported it (Instituto Venezolano de Investigaçiones Cientificas), is characterized by radial ray hypoplasia, with absent thumbs or hypoplastic radial carpal bones, hearing impairment, strabismus, imperforate anus, and thrombocytopenia. The physical anomalies were noted in 24 members of five generations in the first family, in two children and their father in the second family, and in a mother and son in the third family that was reported (577–579). Mild thrombocytopenia and leukocytosis appeared before 50 years of age in 13 persons in the first family. The incidence of hematologic abnormalities is unknown, because many patients are still young. Baseline chromosome breakage was normal. Despite the lack of complete aplastic anemia, the physical findings resemble those that are seen in Fanconi's anemia. It has been suggested that this syndrome be renamed *oculootoradial syndrome* (580).

The *WT syndrome* was named after the initials of the first (and, so far, the only) two families who have been reported (581). Twelve patients were described, with three generations in one family and five generations in the other family. They had radial-ulnar hypoplasia, abnormal thumbs, short fingers, fifth-finger clinodactyly, pancytopenia or thrombocytopenia, and leukemia. Baseline chromosomes were normal without increased breakage. As in the IVIC syndrome, the physical findings in the WT syndrome were subtly different from those in Fanconi's anemia. The authors suggested that several cases of atypical Fanconi's anemia might be WT syndrome instead. Chromosome studies after clastogenic stress should help to sort out this confusion.

A family was described with dominant bone marrow failure, acute nonlymphocytic leukemia, hyperpigmented skin, warts, immune dysfunction, and multiple spontaneous abortions (582). DEB-induced chromosome breakage was not increased. This disorder resembles Fanconi's anemia clinically but not genetically.

Aufderheide (583) reported a five-generation family with 14 members who developed mild to profound single cytopenias or pancytopenia by the third decade of life. Vascular occlusions were also present in nine members of this family. One patient had chromosome breaks in 20% of his cells, but his father, who also had aplastic anemia, had normal chromosomes. Kato et al. (584) reported a mother with aplastic anemia and her son with adult-onset neutropenia and thrombocytopenia.

Dokal et al. (585) reported two families with dominantly inherited proximal fusion of the radius and ulna. Among the 16 cases with this anomaly, four cases had adult-onset aplastic anemia or leukemia. Two families were noted recently in which the fathers had radioulnar synostosis and their children had synostosis plus amegakaryocytic thrombocytopenia, which was cured by stem cell transplantation; germline mutations were identified in HOXA11, a gene that is involved in bone morphogenesis (586).

The syndrome of cerebellar ataxia and pancytopenia was discussed previously in the section Dyskeratosis Congenita.

In a report on 19 members of eight families with acquired aplastic anemia, four families with nine patients had a vertical pattern, with a parent or aunt or uncle who also had aplasia (587). These could be due to common environmental factors or to a genetic propensity for bone marrow failure.

Autosomal-recessive inheritance is the apparent pattern in several other families. Abels and Reed (588) reported two brothers who had short stature and macrocytosis and who developed pancytopenia at approximately 10 years of age. One brother had immune deficiency and multiple cutaneous squamous and basal cell carcinomas. He also had oral telangiectasias and neck and chest poikiloderma, but these findings were insufficient to diagnose dyskeratosis congenita. Because the patients were both male, the inheritance might also have been X-linked recessive.

Another family with associated immune disorders and hematopoietic failures was described by Linsk et al. (589). Four of six siblings from a consanguineous marriage had pure red cell aplasia or neutropenia, or both, as well as unusual crystalloid structures that were demonstrated in the neutrophils by electron microscopy. Chitambar et al. (590) described 8 of 14 members in one generation of a large maternal kindred in which aplastic anemia, acute nonlymphocytic leukemia, and monosomy 7 were found. This association of aplasia and leukemia was also noted in families with possible X-linked recessive inheritance. In the Scandinavian report on acquired aplastic anemia with multiple family members (587), ten patients in four families belonged to sibships.

Monosomy 7 was also a feature in the family that was discussed by Chitambar et al. (590). A sporadic patient with ataxia and hypoplastic anemia was described by Samad et al. (591). This 16-year-old man had Friedreich's ataxia, short stature, hypogonadism, and hyperreflexia. His macrocytic anemia responded to testosterone. Peripheral blood but not marrow chromosomes showed baseline increased breakage.

A clearly X-linked family was presented by Li et al. (592), in which eight males in three generations had adult-onset pancytopenia, acute myelogenous leukemia, light chain disease, or ALL (one case).

Another X-linked syndrome with hematopoietic complications is the *X-linked lymphoproliferative syndrome*, to which more than 25 kindreds belong (593). At least 17 of these boys developed fatal aplastic anemia during or before malignant infectious mononucleosis. Other components of this syndrome include hypoproliferative disorders, agranulocytosis, and hypogammaglobulinemia, as well as proliferative disorders that are associated with the Epstein-Barr virus, including American Burkitt lymphoma, immunoblastic B-cell sarcoma, plasmacytoma, and fatal mononucleosis. The disease is caused by a defect in the SH2DIA (SH2-domain 1A) gene at Xq25 (594,594a,594b). This gene, also called SAP for SLAM (signaling lymphocyte activation molecule)-associated protein, helps regulate T-cell activation during immune responses.

There are also reports of sporadic cases with aplastic anemia and physical abnormalities. One patient and a set of twins had anomalies that were similar to those that are seen in patients with Fanconi's anemia, and increased baseline chromosome breaks were seen in one patient (595,596). This case did not have increased breakage after clastogenic stress (A. D. Auerbach, *personal communication*). In a larger series of cases that were reported to the IFAR, 11 children had aplastic anemia and anomalies, and their chromosome breakage was not increased by DEB (597). It is probable that many cases that were called *Fanconi's anemia* in the older literature and are included in our own analyses did not have Fanconi's anemia. Only modern testing with DEB or MMC can help to properly categorize all of these cases.

Also, there are cases that do not fit into any categories. Two adult siblings had thrombocytopenia (not pancytopenia) and a robertsonian translocation (t13;14), although six other patients with the translocation did not have hematologic problems (598). In three of the eight families with 19 members with aplastic anemia, who were previously cited (587), anemia might have been related to drugs. In other reports, four families had more than one patient with chloramphenicol-related aplastic anemia (599–601). Two families had siblings with aplastic anemia after hepatitis (602,603). Gold, methyprylon (piperidine), and idiopathic aplastic anemia also have each been reported in sets of siblings (604–606). A mother and child pair with idiopathic aplastic anemia was also reported (607).

Thus, aplastic anemia might be associated with familial (genetic) predisposition to specific adverse environments. In some cases, physical abnormalities may call attention to the possibly inherited nature of the condition. The familial and inherited marrow failure syndromes are clearly heterogeneous, with a large variety of phenotypes and all the possible inheritance patterns. It remains for future investigations to elucidate the relevant genetic and environmental factors.

LABORATORY FINDINGS

The patients in this heterogeneous group with familial marrow dysfunction have variable degrees of pancytopenia, macrocytosis, elevated HbF, and hypocellular bone marrow. Families with additional findings, such as immune deficiencies, novel chromosomes, or monosomy 7, may be distinguishable from those with nonfamilial disorders, but those with familial disease without characteristic findings are more difficult to diagnose. Baseline chromosome breakage is usually normal in the non-Fanconi's anemia familial cases, but examination with clastogenic agents is required for definitive distinction. The numbers of hematopoietic stem cells are also reduced, but this too is nondiagnostic (567).

PATHOPHYSIOLOGY

The combination of genetic and environmental factors is essentially unique to each of the types of cases that are outlined in this section on familial marrow dysfunctions. The inheritance patterns are of all types. At the hematopoietic level, the defects may be multiple, because some of the patients have only single cytopenias. Thus, the pluripotent or committed progenitor cells may be defective.

THERAPY AND OUTCOME

Several of the patients that were described previously were treated with transfusions, antilymphocyte globulin, or androgens, with some limited success. Because each case is practically unique, no guidelines can be established, except to suggest that androgens might be more effective than immunosuppression. Because immune dysfunction is part of some of the syndromes, even that statement is overly simplistic. In general, the drug and supportive care should be the same as the treatment that was described previously for patients with Fanconi's anemia or acquired aplastic anemia. Although BMT cannot be dismissed out of hand, it is risky, because related donors may have the same condition. In several families, aplastic anemia is just the first step to preleukemia and leukemia. Overall, the prognosis for familial bone marrow failure is not good.

Down's Syndrome

Trisomy 21, or Down's syndrome, is often associated with a neonatal transient myeloproliferative syndrome and, later, with an increased risk of leukemia (608). A few patients have been reported with aplastic anemia. A 17-year-old boy had idiopathic aplastic anemia and trisomy 21 and apparently responded to androgen treatment (609). Vetrella et al. (610) described a newborn with trisomy 21, cystic fibrosis, and amegakaryocytic thrombocytopenia, who died at 49 days of age, with pancytopenia shortly before death. A 12-year-old boy developed aplastic anemia that was unresponsive to androgens and died within 10 weeks of diagnosis (611); another patient was mentioned with aplastic anemia at 19 months, who appeared to respond to androgens (612). A fifth case was published in which a patient developed aplastic anemia at 9 months of age and died at 26 months of age with gastroenteritis (613). Although bone marrow was generally hypocellular in these patients, the last case had increased numbers of CFU-GM, apparently with cellular and serum inhibitors of hematopoiesis. The few patients with trisomy 21 who developed aplastic anemia raise the question of whether this is a true association or merely coincidence.

Dubowitz's Syndrome

A rare, apparently autosomal-recessive condition in which aplastic anemia has occurred is Dubowitz's syndrome. In a review of 141 cases, hematologic and malignant complications were noted in 12 (614). The major features are intrauterine and postnatal growth retardation, microcephaly, moderate mental retardation, hyperactivity, eczema, and facial anomalies, such as hypertelorism, epicanthal folds, blepharophimosis, broad nose, and abnormal ears. Six patients had aplastic anemia, two had leukopenia, and one each had acute lymphoblastic leukemia, non-Hodgkin's lymphoma, malignant lymphoma, and neuroblastoma. Thus, approximately 10% of the patients with Dubowitz's syndrome have had hematopoietic or oncologic problems. This is another syndrome with growth defects that are associated with hematopoietic disorders and malignancies.

Seckel's Syndrome

Another rare, autosomal-recessive condition in which aplastic anemia has been reported is Seckel's syndrome. Although more than 60 patients have been published as having this syndrome, it may be an overused term that is applied to a heterogeneous group of microcephalic dwarfs; thus, the true number is not clear. The stringent definition includes severe intrauterine and postnatal growth retardation, severe microcephaly, severe mental retardation, the typical face with receding forehead and chin, antimongoloid slant of palpebral fissures, prominently curved nose, relatively large eyes and teeth, highly arched palate, hirsutism, and clinodactyly (615).

Among the group with Seckel's syndrome, at least 10% of patients developed aplastic anemia (616–620), although two patients also had hypersplenism (617). One-half of those patients died from sepsis during childhood. All received transfusions, and androgen treatment was ineffective. One patient died 2 weeks after BMT, whereas another was cured (620). Fanconi's anemia was considered in all cases, because the patients were small, microcephalic, and retarded and had pancytopenia. In fact, the patients with Seckel's syndrome are much smaller and more severely microcephalic and retarded than those with Fanconi's anemia. Chromosome studies were normal in two of the patients with aplastic anemia. Endogenous breakage was increased in one patient and further increased with MMC in the sibling of that patient, but the diagnosis of Fanconi's anemia could not be firmly established. Another patient with aplastic anemia had increased spontaneous and MMC-induced breakage in fibroblasts and lymphocytes (621). Two patients who did not have aplastic anemia had normal chromosomes, by the criteria of endogenous breakage, as well as SCEs (622). One patient was reported to develop AML at 26 years of age (623). Seckel's syndrome is another autosomal-recessive syndrome with growth retardation, a small but real risk of aplastic anemia, and, perhaps, leukemia. There is probably no association with increased chromosome breakage. The genes that are responsible for Seckel's syndrome have not been identified, but there is no evidence that Seckel's syndrome patients have mutations in FA genes (624).

SINGLE CYTOPENIAS: RED BLOOD CELLS

Diamond-Blackfan Anemia

The first descriptions of red cell aplasia in infancy consisted of two cases that were reported by Josephs (625) in 1936 and four cases that were reported by Diamond and Blackfan (626) in 1938. A variety of synonyms and eponyms have been used: congenital hypoplastic anemia, chronic congenital aregenerative anemia, erythrogenesis imperfecta, chronic idiopathic erythroblastopenia with aplastic anemia (type Josephs-Diamond-Blackfan), and Diamond-Blackfan anemia (DBA). Diamond and Blackfan used the term *congenital hypoplastic anemia* because they thought the disorder differed from complete aplastic anemia only in degree. The term *hypoplastic* is now used when marrow depression (pancytopenia) is only partial; thus, the term is not appropriate for a single cytopenia. Erythrogenesis imperfecta is probably the most descriptive appellation, but now the commonly used term is *DBA*.

The following are diagnostic criteria for DBA:

- Normochromic, usually macrocytic but occasionally normocytic, anemia that develops early in childhood
- Reticulocytopenia
- Normocellular bone marrow with selective deficiency of red-cell precursors
- Normal or slightly decreased leukocyte counts
- Normal or often increased platelet counts

These criteria clearly differentiate DBA from aplastic anemia, but may not always distinguish it from transient erythroblastopenia of childhood (TEC) (see the section Transient Erythroblastopenia of Childhood).

More than 700 cases of DBA have been reported in case reports, and many of the references are cited in previous reviews (4,627–629). Additionally, there are almost 500 cases that are summarized in large series, although many of these patients may also have been subjects in individual case reports (131,630–633). The ages at which DBA was diagnosed (or the first transfusion or treatment initiated) are shown in Figure 8-19 and summarized in Table 8-16. Boys were slightly younger than girls (with medians of 2 and 3 months of age). Ten percent of patients were severely anemic at birth, with severe anemia presenting in 25% by 1 month of age, 50% by 3 months of age, 75% by 6 months of age, and 90% by 18 months of age. Five percent of patients were diagnosed between 1.5 and 2.5 years of age, 3% before 6 years of age, and another 2% between 6 and 68 years of age. The male to female ratio is 1.1:1. Most of the reports from almost 50 countries are of white patients, but DBA has been described in blacks, Asians, and Indians.

A dozen cases presented in patients who were older than 6 years of age. A 34-year-old man with anemia had an anemic daughter who was diagnosed at 6 years of age, and, subsequently, a grandson was diagnosed with classic DBA (634,635). A female who was diagnosed as anemic at 16 years of age had a son who was diagnosed at 9 months of age (636). The paternal grandfather in a family in which four males were diagnosed in three generations was diagnosed at 20 years of age (637). One male was diagnosed at 9 years of age in a large consanguineous family in which seven members were affected in one generation, of whom five were male siblings and two were male and female cousins (638). Two women, who were 25 and 64 years of age, had long-standing anemia that responded to prednisone, were of short stature, and had other findings that are typical of DBA, including webbed necks and thenar atrophy (639). Two additional males were diagnosed at 7 and 22 years of age (640), and three females were diagnosed at 11, 13, and 35 years of age (630,640–642).

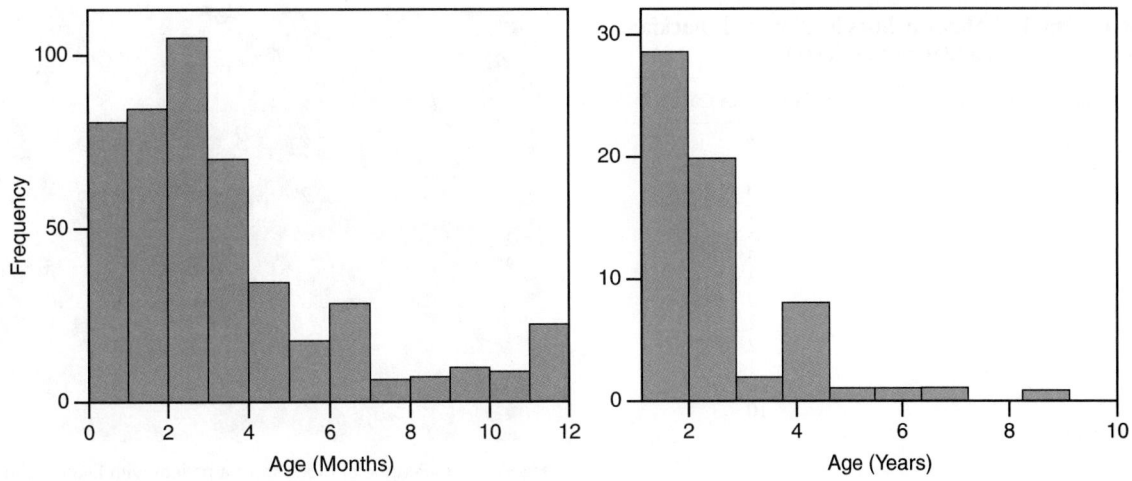

Figure 8-19. Age at onset of anemia in approximately 550 published cases with Diamond-Blackfan anemia. Note the scale on the abscissa is in months on the left, for those between 0 and 12 months of age, and in years on the right, for those between 1 and 10 years of age. Not shown are nine patients who were between 11 and 64 years of age at diagnosis.

INHERITANCE AND ENVIRONMENT

The inheritance of DBA appears to have more than a single pattern. There were more than 30 families with *dominant* disease that involved parent-child transmission. The carrier parent often had a history of anemia, although, in some cases, the parent only had increased HbF or macrocytosis, or both, without significant anemia. The ratio of males to females in the dominant group was approximately 1. The incidence of physical abnormalities was lower, and the clinical course was generally milder than it was in the overall DBA population. A large series that was reported by Willig et al. (643,644) had 33 families with classic DBA in at least two generations. Twenty-one of 154 sporadic cases had a first-degree relative with anemia, increased MCV, or increased red-cell adenosine deaminase (ADA) (see the section Laboratory Findings), and these relatives had the same DBA gene mutation as the proband in their family, which suggests that some "sporadic" cases may be autosomal dominant.

Another 30 families might be construed as *recessive*, because, apparently, there were affected siblings and normal parents, consanguinity, or affected cousins. In addition to one set of male twins in a sibship with three affected males (645), a set of affected identical twins has also been reported (646). The incidence of anomalies was actually slightly higher in the recessives than in the overall group, but the anemia was milder and more responsive. The inheritance in the apparently recessive families might be dominant with variable expression, but that is less likely, because there are several families with consanguinity. Removal of all of the patients in families leaves several hundreds of cases that are apparently sporadic, which suggests that DBA occurs as a new mutation or as an acquired disease or that penetrance is extremely variable.

Several patients were the products of problem pregnancies, which suggests that they had congenitally acquired marrow failure. The pregnancy problems include preeclampsia, toxemia, rashes, premature placental separation, hemorrhage, spotting, and positive tests for syphilis. Exposures during pregnancy include diethylstilbestrol, x-rays, chlorothiazide, reserpine, thyroid hormone, prednisone, phenylbutazone, chloramphenicol, and anagyrine. A few mothers had previous spontaneous abortions or miscarriages. Seven percent of the patients weighed 2500 g or less at birth, but only 14 patients were born at less than 36 weeks gestation, and, thus, most

were small for gestational age (intrauterine growth retardation). The low birth weight might reflect pregnancy problems or poor growth that is intrinsic to DBA itself.

The anemia in patients with DBA was often noted at birth or during infancy. Jaundice due to hemolytic disease of the newborn from Rh or ABO blood group incompatibility occurred occasionally and led to prolonged anemia that became chronic (647) or that sometimes resolved after a few months (648). A few patients had antecedent illnesses such as diarrhea, respiratory infections, urinary tract infections, measles, or mumps, or a smallpox vaccination. One child was treated with chloramphenicol (649). In most patients, the illness was more likely to be due to the anemia or to be unrelated than to be the cause of the anemia. The signs of anemia were usually pallor, lethargy, irritability, and heart failure.

PHYSICAL EXAMINATION

Physical abnormalities were described in more than 160 patients (25%) (Table 8-17). Abnormalities of the head and

TABLE 8-16. Diamond-Blackfan Anemia Literature

	All Patients
Number of cases	705
Male/female	332/313
Ratio	1.1
Male age at diagnosis (mo)	
Mean	9.6
Median	2.0
Range	0–408
Female age at diagnosis (mo)	
Mean	14.2
Median	3.0
Range	0–768
Number of male patients older than 1 year of age	29 (9%)
Number of female patients older than 1 year of age	39 (12%)
Deceased	
Number of cases	90 (13%)
Age at death (yr)	
Mean	11.5
Median	8.8
Range	0–65
Projected median age	43

TABLE 8-17. Physical Abnormalities in Diamond-Blackfan Anemia (Percent of Cases)

Abnormality	Percent of Cases
Birthweight ≤2500 g	7
Head, face, palate	7
Upper limbs	8
Short	12
Eyes	5
Renal	4
Neck	3
Hypogonads	2
Retardation	2
Cardiopulmonary	2
Nose	1
Other skeletal	4
Other	10
At least one anomaly[a]	25
Short stature alone	3

[a]Not including low birth weight or short stature. Many patients had more than one abnormality. Physical descriptions were available for 650 patients.

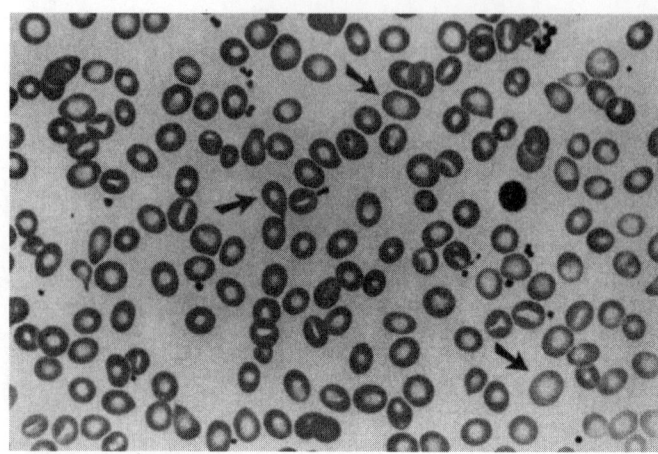

Figure 8-20. Peripheral blood from a patient with Diamond-Blackfan anemia. Note anisocytosis with microcytosis and macrocytosis, as well as teardrop erythrocytes *(arrows)*. (Courtesy of Dr. Gail Wolfe. From Alter BP. The bone marrow failure syndromes. In: Nathan DG, Oski FA, eds. *Hematology of infancy and childhood*, 3rd ed. Philadelphia: WB Saunders, 1987:159–241, with permission.)

face were common. The typical face was described by Cathie (650) as "tow-colored hair, snub nose, thick upper lips, rather wide set eyes, and an intelligent expression" and was observed in many of the children, who resemble each other more than they do their own family members. Cleft lip and palate were noted. Other findings include micrognathia, microcephaly or macrocephaly, macroglossia, wide fontanelle, and dysmorphic features.

Upper limbs, particularly thumbs, are often abnormal. In our experience, the most common features are subtle flattening of the thenar eminences and weakness of radial pulses. Other radial hand anomalies are also common. Triphalangeal thumbs were noted in 22 patients who were otherwise similar to the total group of patients. Although this association was initially separated by some into the *Aase syndrome* (651), it is probably an inappropriate example of splitting rather than lumping patients into groups according to their abnormalities (652). Fourteen patients had duplicated thumbs, and 13 had otherwise abnormal thumbs, such as absent or subluxed thumbs. Thumb anomalies may be unilateral or bilateral. The presence of abnormal thumbs does not predict the course of the anemia.

Another common finding in DBA patients is short stature. Because many patients have received corticosteroids, it is often difficult to identify genetic short stature, but it was seen in more than 10% of the patients. There were four reports of dwarfism, including achondroplasia (653,654), metaphyseal dysostosis (655), and cartilage hair hypoplasia (655). Short or webbed necks were reported in 3% of patients, including both Klippel-Feil syndrome (fused cervical vertebrae) and Sprengel's deformity (elevation of the scapula). A Turnerlike phenotype was sometimes mentioned.

Five percent of patients had eye anomalies, most frequently hypertelorism, as well as blue sclerae, glaucoma, epicanthal folds, microphthalmos, cataracts, and strabismus. Kidney abnormalities, including horseshoe, duplicated, and absent kidney, were also noted in a few patients. Male hypogonadism was noted in 2%, and 2% of patients were retarded. Lower limb problems included dislocated hips, achondroplasia, and clubfoot. Congenital heart disease of all kinds was seen occasionally. The presence of anomalies serves more to confirm the diagnosis of DBA than to provide any prognosis regarding the course of the disease.

LABORATORY FINDINGS

All patients with DBA are anemic by definition. Hgb levels at birth show a range of 2.6 to 14.8 g/dL, with a median of 7 g/dL. In approximately 60 infants who were diagnosed with DBA between birth and 2 months of age, the median Hgb was 4 g/dL, with a range from 1.5 to 10.0 g/dL. In those who were diagnosed later, the Hgb was also usually in the 4 g/dL range. Macrocytosis was almost uniform, and reticulocytes were usually absent. Figure 8-20 shows a representative blood film, with anisocytosis, macrocytosis, and an occasional teardrop.

White-cell counts are generally normal in DBA patients, although counts sometimes decrease with the person's age. Values of 5000/μL or less were found at some time in 20% of patients, and values of less than 3000/μL were found in 5%. Two heavily transfused older patients developed significant neutropenia (N. S. Young, *unpublished data*). Platelet counts are also usually normal, although 25% of patients had at least one count that was less than 150,000/μL, and 20% had one count that was greater than 400,000/μL. Buchanan et al. (656) noted elevated platelets in 50% of 38 patients and decreased platelets in 25% on at least one occasion. They found that platelet function was normal.

HbF is usually increased and is distributed heterogeneously (Fig. 8-21), which indicates that the patients do not have a single clone of completely fetal cells. The proportion of Gγ to Aγ plus Gγ is greater than 50%, which is similar to that found in fetal RBCs. The titer of red cell–membrane i antigen is also increased, as in fetuses, whereas the adult counterpart, I antigen, remains at adult levels. These fetal-like erythrocyte features are seen in newly diagnosed patients, patients who respond to corticosteroids, and patients in spontaneous remissions. They are not unique to patients who are affected with DBA, but they are characteristic of the stress erythropoiesis that is seen in any type of bone marrow failure (47,48).

Bone marrow examination by aspiration or biopsy shows normal cellularity, myeloid cells, and megakaryocytes. Lymphocytes are often increased (this is seen even in normal infants; most of the marrow tests are done in infants with DBA) and were initially thought to be hematogones (657). Eosinophilia is occasional (658). Three patterns of erythroid development were described by Bernard et al. (659):

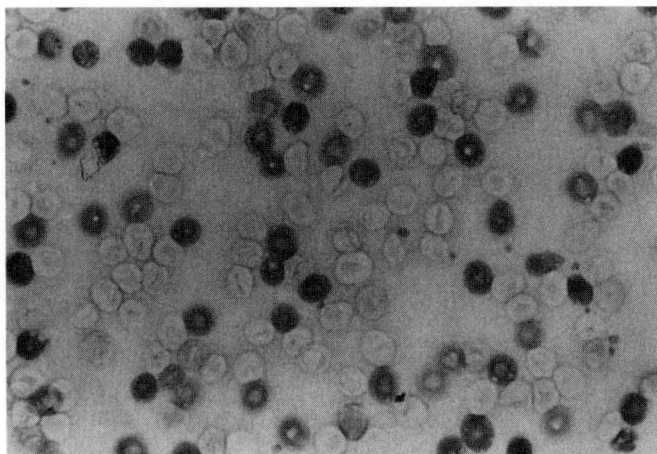

Figure 8-21. Kleihauer-Betke acid elution study of blood from a patient with Diamond-Blackfan anemia, showing the heterogeneous distribution of the fetal hemoglobin. (Courtesy of Dr. Gail Wolfe. From Alter BP. The bone marrow failure syndromes. In: Nathan DG, Oski FA, eds. *Hematology of infancy and childhood*, 3rd ed. Philadelphia: WB Saunders, 1987:159–241, with permission.)

- Erythroid hypoplasia or total aplasia is seen in 90% of patients with DBA (Fig. 8-22). The only erythroid precursors in some patients are immature proerythroblasts.
- Five percent of cases have normal numbers and maturation of erythroblasts.
- The remaining 5% of patients have erythroid hyperplasia, but this is present with a maturation arrest and increased numbers of immature precursors.

Despite the variable bone marrow picture, all DBA patients have reticulocytopenia. Thus, a few patients must have ineffective erythropoiesis. Dyserythropoietic morphology has been seen occasionally (see section Congenital Dyserythropoietic Anemia). Ringed sideroblasts were noted rarely, then disappeared (660,661). Patients who receive many transfusions accumulate iron in the marrow (Fig. 8-22) and other organs.

Serum levels of iron, ferritin, folic acid, vitamin B$_{12}$, and EPO all are elevated, and DBA is not due to a deficiency of any of the normal hematinic agents (662). DBA patients do not have antibodies to EPO. Routine urinalysis is normal. It was once thought that an abnormality in tryptophan metabolism occurs (663,664), but other investigators failed to confirm this (665). Hypocalcemia was reported only once (666), and mild hypogammaglobulinemia was noted in several patients (627,659,667,668). These parameters are normal in many other patients. Low numbers of T lymphocytes and a reduction in the ratio of helper to suppressor T cells were reported by Finlay et al. (669), but abnormalities of T-cell function were not observed. Ferrokinetic studies showed the delay in plasma iron clearance and low RBC utilization that were expected in aplastic anemia (659,666,670). Autologous RBC survival times were slightly shortened (627,671), and haptoglobins were low in three patients (627,672), which suggests a mild hemolytic anemia.

Patients with DBA have negative direct antiglobulin (Coombs') tests, and their disease is not due to RBC autoantibodies, although alloantibodies may develop after many transfusions. Results of bone marrow cultures and erythropoietic inhibitor assays are described in the section Pathophysiology.

Abnormalities were observed in RBC enzymes and involved purine or pyrimidine metabolism. Giblett et al. (673) described a patient with atypical DBA who also had lymphopenia and nucleoside phosphorylase deficiency; other patients had normal nucleoside phosphorylase levels (674,675). Increased levels of the pyrimidine enzymes orotate phosphoribosyl transferase and orotidine monophosphate decarboxylase (ODC) were reported in five patients in one study (675), and increased ODC was reported in five of ten patients in another study (676). ODC is an age-dependent enzyme that is increased in cord blood cells, and the elevation is consistent with the presence of young, fetal-like erythrocytes.

Glader et al. (674) and Glader and Backer (676,677) have observed increased RBC *ADA* in 26 of 29 DBA patients. ADA, a critical enzyme in the purine salvage pathway, is not elevated in erythrocytes from cord blood or in patients with hemolytic or other aplastic anemias. ADA was also elevated in 2 of 12 DBA parents (674). Whitehouse et al. (678) found an increase in ADA in 9 of 19 patients and in 2 of 15 relatives. The significance of ADA is not clear, because it is also increased in some children with acute lymphoblastic leukemia, and thus may indicate disordered erythropoiesis that is distinct from fetal-like erythropoiesis (677). Increased ADA does help to distinguish DBA from TEC (see the section Transient Erythro-

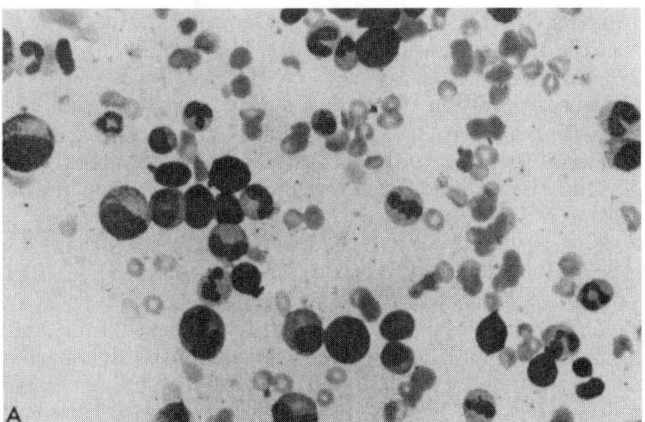 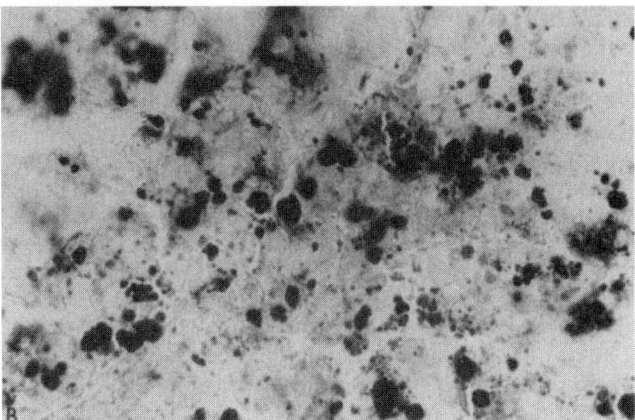

Figure 8-22. A: Bone marrow aspirate from a patient with Diamond-Blackfan anemia, showing normal cellularity with erythroid hypoplasia. **B:** Iron stain of bone marrow aspirate from a 2-year-old child with transfusion-dependent Diamond-Blackfan anemia. (Courtesy of Dr. Gail Wolfe. From Alter BP. The bone marrow failure syndromes. In: Nathan DG, Oski FA, eds. *Hematology of infancy and childhood*, 3rd ed. Philadelphia: WB Saunders, 1987:159–241, with permission.)

blastopenia of Childhood). As mentioned previously, some otherwise normal parents of classic DBA patients have elevated ADA and a mutant DBA gene, which is supportive of a dominant inheritance pattern in those families (643,644).

Chromosomes are normal in most patients with DBA (627). Rare abnormalities include an achromatic area in chromosome 1 (666), a pericentric inversion in one patient (679), enlargement of chromosome 16 in three of six patients (680), and breaks and endoreduplication of chromosome 16 (681). One patient had increased spontaneous and x-ray–induced chromosome breakage, without increased breakage due to MMC (682). Others showed no increased breakage to DEB (683,684). Sister chromatid exchange is normal. Chromosome breakage studies are not informative, except to distinguish DBA from Fanconi's anemia. However, several patients were identified with translocations or rearrangements that permitted mapping and cloning of the first DBA gene (see the section Diamond-Blackfan Anemia Genes).

A small number of patients with clinical DBA were found to have parvovirus DNA in their marrow. Three patients who had documented, second-trimester, intrauterine infections did not respond to intravenous Ig therapy (685). One patient died from respiratory failure at 9 months, whereas the other two patients remained transfusion-dependent. Three others whose marrows contained parvovirus DNA at the time of their diagnosis of DBA underwent spontaneous remissions after steroid treatment for 2 months, 3 years, and 9 years (686).

Prenatal Diagnosis. One fetus in a family with two DBA children had an apparently high-output cardiac failure when it was studied with two-dimensional fetal Doppler echocardiography, (687) although the reliability of this test has been questioned (681). Ultrasound may be used to detect cardiomegaly and effusions from hydropic anemic fetuses, and intrauterine transfusions might be offered (688,689). The possibilities of increased fetal erythrocyte ADA or decreased fetal blood erythroid burst-forming units (BFU-E) have not been examined. Prenatal gene mutation analyses might also be considered (see the section Diamond-Blackfan Anemia Genes).

PATHOPHYSIOLOGY

Erythropoiesis. DBA may have more than a single basis, because the genetics and the phenotypes appear to be multiple. Most *in vitro* studies of the erythropoietic defect have been limited to small numbers of patients. Different results may be related to true variability of the disease. The general consensus is that the erythroid progenitor cell is intrinsically abnormal. The major erythropoietic hormone, EPO, is increased in DBA patients to levels that are higher than expected for a given degree of anemia (662).

A few of the early patients appeared to have RBC alloantibodies (647,648,690,691). These patients had neonatal jaundice and ABO or Rh incompatibility; anemia persisted longer than expected, or bona fide DBA was eventually diagnosed. Antibody specificity may have extended to erythroblasts or progenitors, or blood group sensitization may have been a real but unrelated episode. Blood group incompatibility was not found to be significant in a large number of patients (628).

Cellular inhibitors were proposed by Hoffman et al. (692), but one of those patients was later studied by Nathan et al. (693), who were unable to detect inhibitory lymphocytes when HLA-identical marrow was used as the target population. Another patient was found to have normal erythroid

progenitors and no cellular inhibitors (694). Nathan et al. (695) found no inhibition of normal or autologous marrow CFU-E by the lymphocytes in four transfusion-dependent patients and no inhibition of normal or patient blood BFU-E by the lymphocytes of eight patients, who ranged from transfusion-dependent to those with steroid-independent remissions. They demonstrated that patient T cells were actually stimulatory to normal-blood null-cell BFU-E, as are normal T cells (696).

Cumulative evidence indicates that the erythroid stem cell is abnormal in DBA. Cultures of bone marrow and blood mononuclear cells in plasma clot or methylcellulose showed reduced numbers of CFU-E or BFU-E in more than 50 patients, and normal numbers in approximately 12 patients (697). Patients with normal quantities of progenitors may have been younger and untreated. It was suggested that those patients who subsequently responded to prednisone had better erythroid growth *in vitro*. Addition of steroids *in vitro* was also found to increase erythropoiesis in a few studies (695,698).

Several studies suggested that DBA erythroid progenitor cells required unusually high concentrations of EPO (695,699–702). These EPO studies used crude EPO, which may have contained other erythroid growth-promoting factors. Lipton et al. (701) demonstrated increased EPO sensitivity in DBA bone marrow cultures to which a source of burst-promoting activity (BPA) was added; this suggested that BPA might act directly on the progenitor cell and not through accessory cell mediation (702). Halperin et al. (699) found that IL-3 increased the size and number of marrow BFU-E. The earlier suggestion that DBA erythroid progenitor cells were insensitive to EPO may have reflected a specific insensitivity to BPA or to IL-3. The protective role of EPO was supported by the observation by Perdahl et al. that the hormone was required to prevent accelerated apoptosis (703). Dianzani et al. (704) showed that there were no mutations in the receptor for erythropoietin and also that there was no pathogenetic role for IL-9 or for the 5q hematopoietic cluster (705).

Another candidate ligand-receptor set is SCF and its receptor, c-kit, which are mutant in Steel and W mice that have a macrocytic anemia. *In vitro* addition of SCF to bone marrow BFU-E cultures resulted in increased colony numbers in the majority of DBA studies (131,640,706). However, mutations were not found in SCF or c-kit genes (707–709), and SCF gene expression was normal (710,711). In addition, treatment of both Steel and W mice with prednisone in doses that are comparable to those that are effective in DBA patients did not improve the anemia of the mice (712).

Diamond-Blackfan Anemia Genes. The identification of DBA genes has relied on the mapping of DBA loci through large kindreds. The first clue to localization of a gene at 19q13 was provided by one patient with a reciprocal X;19 translocation (713) and three patients with microdeletion syndromes that involved 19q13.2 (714–717). The translocation breakpoint occurred within the gene for ribosomal protein S19 (718). Approximately 25% of unrelated DBA patients were shown to have mutations in this gene, including nonsense, frameshift, splice site, or missense mutations (Fig. 8-23). Only one of the two RPS19 alleles was mutated in the DBA patients, which suggested that the disease results from haploinsufficiency at this genetic locus. Presumably, biallelic mutation of the RPS19 gene would be lethal. How a 50% reduction in a ribosomal subunit can cause the developmental abnormalities of DBA remains unknown. A decrease in function of this ribosomal subunit may result in impaired protein translation. This

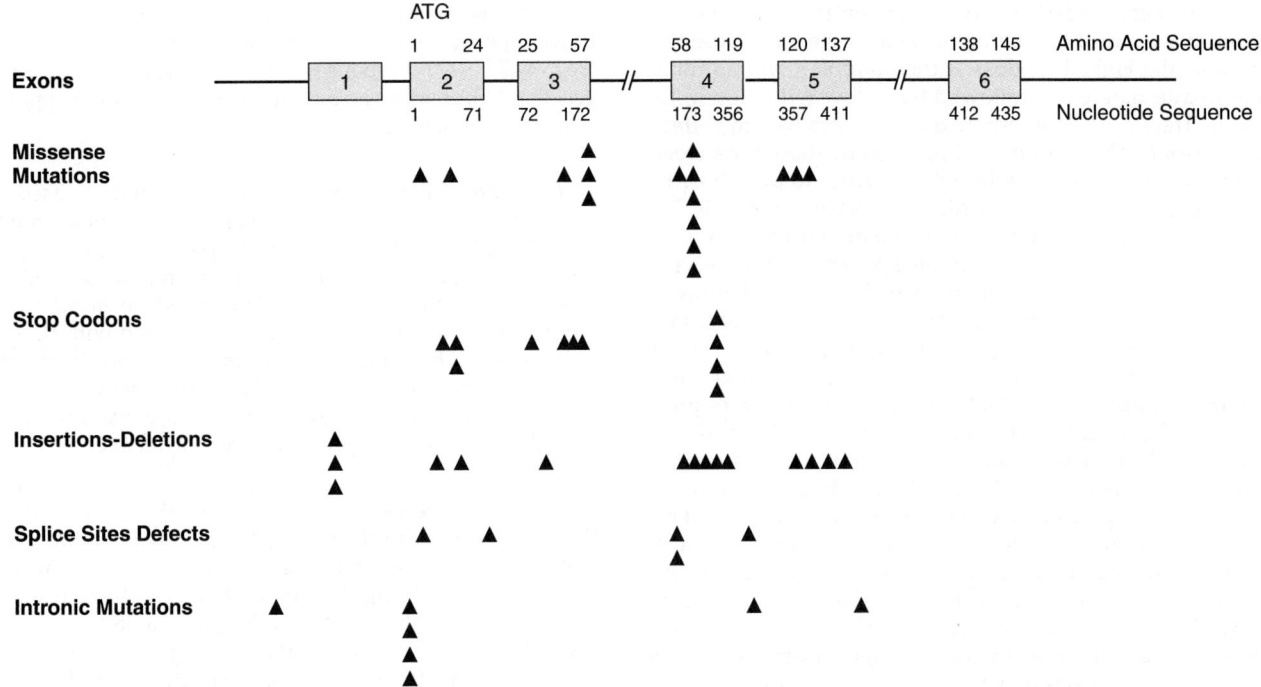

Figure 8-23. Point mutations in RPS19, one of the Diamond-Blackfan anemia genes. The positions of single nucleotide substitutions or small deletions or insertions in the RPS19 gene, which are found in DBA patients, are indicated along the six exons of the RPS19 gene. (From Willig T, Draptchinskaia N, Dianzani I, et al. Mutations in ribosomal protein S19 gene and Diamond Blackfan anemia: wide variations in phenotypic expression. *Blood* 1999;94:4294–4306, with permission.)

impairment may be most evident in specific cell lineages, such as the erythrocyte lineage.

Another DBA genetic locus was recently identified at chromosome 8p23.2-p22, and evidence was obtained for at least a third gene (719). In that study of 38 families, 47% mapped to 8p, 34% to 19q, and the remaining 18% to neither of those loci. No ribosomal subunit genes map to the 8p region, which suggests that the DBA gene at this locus may have an alternative function.

The cloning of DBA genes has diagnostic implications. Some DBA patients have clinical findings that resemble those that are seen in Fanconi's anemia, although DBA patients differ in that the anemia may respond to corticosteroid therapy. Genetic diagnoses may serve to identify the patient as DBA, if the Fanconi's anemia testing is inconclusive. At this time, the only specific test that can be offered to suspected DBA patients is mutational analysis of the RPS19 genetic locus (720). One "common" mutant allele has been identified, which allows for direct screening of this polymorphic site (644).

THERAPY AND OUTCOME

Transfusions. The only treatment that was initially available for DBA patients was transfusions, without which affected children died of anemia (625). This remains the mainstay of the steroid-resistant patient. White-cell free-packed RBCs are given every 3 to 6 weeks, as needed, to keep the Hgb at a level higher than 6 g/dL. Careful cross-matching for minor blood groups is usually done only when alloantibodies develop from sensitization. The major complication from transfusions is hemosiderosis. This was the cause of death in at least 20% of the more than 50 patients for whom the cause of death was stated. The side effects of iron overload in DBA are identical with those that are seen in thalassemia major, including diabetes, cardiac failure, liver disease, growth failure, and failure to enter puberty. These complications do not develop as rapidly in DBA patients as they do in thalassemia patients, in whom there is the added complication of a hemolytic, rather than an aplastic, anemia. Chelation of iron with subcutaneous deferoxamine should begin soon after the patients have begun a chronic transfusion program, as they are shown to have increased iron stores. Although an oral chelator is under development, its use is not advised in DBA because of the risk of neutropenia (721–723).

Splenectomy. Splenectomy was reported in approximately 40 patients, with no apparent benefit except in those who had hypersplenism that was related to transfusions. Fifty percent of the splenectomized patients were reported to have died, and at least one-half of those deaths were due to infections. Splenectomy is not usually recommended today.

Corticosteroids. Gasser first proposed the treatment of DBA patients with steroids, based on his observations of transient erythroblastopenia in patients with transient allergic disorders and of eosinophils in the bone marrow of DBA patients (658,724). The first drugs were cortisone or adrenocorticotropic hormone (725), but prednisone and prednisolone have become the drugs of choice. Twelve of 22 patients responded in the first series by Allen and Diamond (726). The current recommendation is prednisone, 2 mg/kg/day, in three or four divided doses. Reticulocytes usually appear within 1 to 2 weeks. Some of the erythropoiesis is apparently ineffective, because a sustained rise in Hgb may not occur for several weeks, although it usually appears within 1 month. The high divided-dose protocol is maintained until the Hgb reaches 10 g/dL. It is then tapered slowly, by sequential removal of the divided doses, until the patient is on a single daily dose that maintains the Hgb. This dose is then doubled and administered on alternate days, followed by a slow reduction in the amount. Treatment on alternate days reduces the side effects of the steroids. One group used prednisone daily for a week, followed by 1 to 2 weeks without any drug, to permit better growth (670), but this protocol did not work in our hands. The alternate-day dose depends on the patient and varies from as low as 1 mg to more than 40 mg; some patients are sensitive to small doses, as well as to small changes in dose. Failure to remit with the previously outlined prednisone protocol may be an indication for a trial of 4 to 6 mg/kg/day or a trial of prednisolone or dexamethasone. Any medications that might be marrow suppressive or that affect the metabolism of prednisone, such as phenytoin or phenobarbital, should be discontinued. Steroid remissions have occurred in patients after 10 years of transfusions (627,649,727); thus, a history of transfusions should not preclude an adequate trial of steroids that are combined with iron chelation, as needed. Steroid side effects include growth retardation in more than one-half the patients (628) and osteoporosis, aseptic necroses of femoral or humoral heads, weight gain, cushingoid appearance, hypertension, diabetes, fluid retention, gastric ulcers, cataracts, and glaucoma. These side effects may be sufficiently serious to warrant switching to a transfusion program, despite hematologic response.

There are several patterns of response to steroids:

- Rapid response, followed by steroid-independent remission (less than 5%).
- Intermittent response (approximately 5%).
- Response, followed by steroid dependence (60%). As many as 20% of these patients may eventually be able to maintain their Hgb levels without steroids.
- Steroid response and dependence, followed by later failure to respond to the same or higher doses (5%).
- Requirement for large daily doses, which usually means resuming transfusions because of the steroid side effects (less than 5%).
- No response (30% to 40%). Overall, steroid nonresponders, high-dose responders, or subsequent failures make up almost 50% of cases.

In general, 15% to 25% of patients may eventually have a hematologic remission that is unrelated to their treatment or response to treatment (728).

Several other therapeutic approaches also have been attempted. Androgens (see the section Fanconi's Anemia) were reported in more than 50 patients, with apparent response in only three patients. Immunosuppressive drugs were given to a few patients. 6-Mercaptopurine was used successfully in one patient (729) and unsuccessfully in another (730). Two patients had transient reticulocytosis after administration of cyclophosphamide and antilymphocyte globulin (731) (N. S. Young, *unpublished data*), whereas others had no response to cyclophosphamide (730,732,733). Vincristine has also been ineffective (731,733,734). Ozsoylu (735) suggested that high doses of intravenous methylprednisolone are effective, as was described previously for severe acquired aplastic anemia.

Cyclosporin A. Cyclosporin A treatment was reported in 29 patients. It permitted the elimination of prednisone in only three patients (736–739), but it did result in lower doses of prednisone in another 13 patients (740–746). However, some of these responses were only transient. Twelve patients did not respond to cyclosporin A alone or when it was combined with prednisone (742,744,745,747). Responses to immunosuppressive agents suggest that DBA may be an autoimmune disease, but supportive *in vitro* data are lacking.

Cytokines. EPO treatment seemed reasonable, based on the *in vitro* data that suggest response to high doses of the hormone. In a total of ten patients, doses of up to 200 U/kg/day for as long as 5 months had no impact on erythropoiesis (748,749).

IL-3 was also a good candidate based on *in vitro* studies. Approximately 100 DBA patients were treated with IL-3 in five studies, with the achievement of independence from transfusions and steroids in 10% (630,750–753). However, side effects included serious allergic responses, fevers, chills, and deep vein thromboses, and this agent is no longer available.

Hematopoietic Stem Cell Transplant. BMT is an option for those patients who do not respond to reasonable doses of steroids. Almost 40 patients have been transplanted from HLA-matched sibling donors, with a 75% absolute survival. Eight cases had alternative donors, with a 38% absolute survival. Their ages at transplantation ranged from 1 to 31 years of age and 1 to 18 years of age, respectively, and most were steroid nonresponders or had relapsed on steroids and had received transfusions. The survivals plateau at 76% and 43%, respectively, with exclusion of the last death, which was from metastatic osteosarcoma that developed after the transplant, in the group with alternative donors (Fig. 8-24). The results for marrow donors were similar to those for cord donors, with respective actuarial survivals of 59% and 63%. The Diamond-Blackfan Anemia Registry reported an actuarial survival of 88%, when sibling donors were used, and 28% with the alternative donors (728). It should be noted that they include one patient who had late-onset osteogenic sarcoma and who was originally reported by Giri et al. (754). The results suggest that DBA may be cured by hematopoietic stem cell transplant.

Reported deaths after transplant were related to interstitial pneumonitis, graft rejection, graft-versus-host disease, and

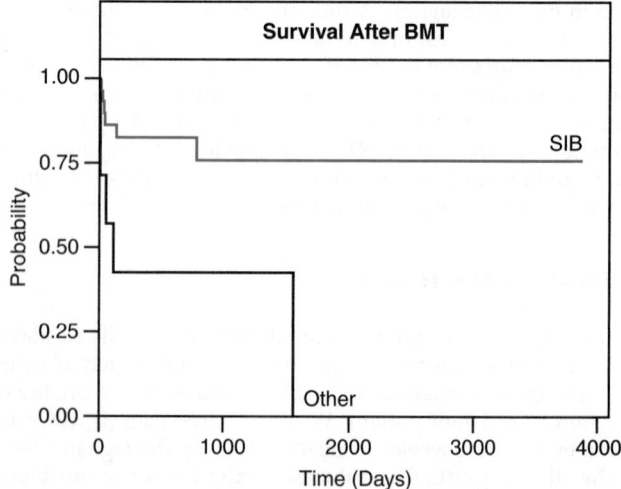

Figure 8-24. Kaplan-Meier plot of cumulative survival in Diamond-Blackfan anemia after bone marrow transplantation (BMT). Time is shown as time after BMT in days. Other, 3 matched unrelated donor marrows, 3 matched unrelated donor cords, 1 mother, 1 grand uncle; SIB, 38 patients with a sibling donor.

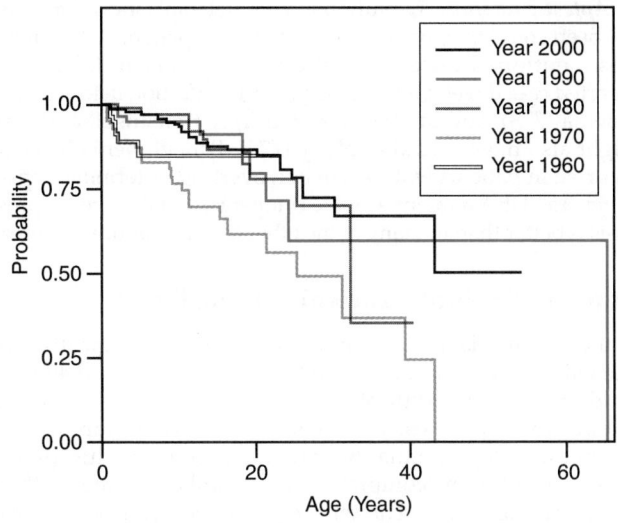

Figure 8-25. Kaplan-Meier plot of cumulative survival in Diamond-Blackfan anemia. Time is shown as age in years, because most cases are diagnosed in infancy. Lines represent 78 cases reported from 1936 to 1960, 113 cases from 1961 to 1970, 90 cases from 1971 to 1980, 115 cases from 1981 to 1990, and 309 cases from 1991 to 2000. The differences are significant.

venoocclusive disease in the sibling group and graft-versus-host disease, sepsis, Epstein-Barr virus lymphoma in donor cells, and venoocclusive disease in the alternative donor group. The decision for transplantation in DBA is not easy, because perhaps 20% of patients may eventually have a remission. In general, stem cell transplants are more successful in young, relatively untransfused (and unsensitized) patients; thus, the decision to undergo transplant sometimes must be made before a potential remission may occur. As in other genetic diseases, DBA must be ruled out in the donors.

Survival Data. The *survival data* on more than 600 patients that were reported in the literature are shown in Figure 8-25. Patients who are reported in more recent years have a cumulative survival that is better than those who were reported initially, reflecting the effect of steroid treatment and better

programs for transfusion and chelation. The projected median survival for all patients is 43 years of age. Almost 100 patients were reported to have died (13%) at a median of 6 years of age in the entire group (Table 8-16). The most common causes of death were complications of iron overload and pneumonia or sepsis. Other deaths were due to BMT complications, leukemia, cancer, renal disease, anesthesia, pulmonary emboli, and undefined central nervous system disorders.

The quality of life is good for most patients. The spontaneous remitters and the steroid responders who can be maintained on low doses live essentially normal lives. Those who must be transfused can receive chelation therapy, as do patients with thalassemia major. The future of hematopoietic stem cell transplants lies in cautious optimism, with improvements needed for those for whom alternative donors are needed. Gene therapy may also become available as that technology is developed and as the genes become identified.

Pregnancy. Many DBA patients have grown to adulthood and had children. Among 25 reported DBA females who had 29 pregnancies, 12 babies were normal, and 16 had DBA; there was one miscarriage (504). In the Boston series of 76 DBA patients, five men and three women had 13 children, three of whom had DBA (631). Pregnancy is undoubtedly underreported, except in the context of dominant inheritance. From the limited information that is available, there appears to be temporary worsening of anemia during pregnancy in almost one-half of the cases, perhaps due to marrow suppression by estrogens. We advised maintenance of maternal Hgb at a level greater than 8 to 9 g/dL to avoid maternal anemia that might lead to intrauterine growth retardation, preterm delivery, or fetal distress (504). Seven of the 28 deliveries required cesarean sections, owing to fetal anemia, toxemia, and failure of labor to progress.

COMPLICATIONS

Leukemia. Leukemia was reported in ten patients (Table 8-18). One girl had a spontaneous remission of DBA at 5 years of age, developed ALL at 13 years of age, and, after complete remission of the ALL, she was free from both conditions at 17 years of age (755; G. Schaison, *personal communication*, 1982). Nine patients

TABLE 8-18. Cancer in Diamond-Blackfan Anemia

Type	Male	Female	Unknown	All Patients	References
Leukemia					
Acute lymphoblastic	0	1	0	1	759
Acute myeloblastic[a]	5	2	2	9	276,631,733,757,758,760–762
MDS[b]	2	0	0	2	760,764
Total leukemia + MDS	7	3	2	12	—
Osteogenic sarcoma	2	3	0	5	632,754,763,764
Sarcoma, soft tissue	1	0	0	1	764
Breast	—	2	0	2	632,765
Hodgkin's disease	2	0	0	2	632,766,767
Non-Hodgkin's lymphoma	0	1	0	1	768
Hepatoma	2	0	0	2	769,770
Colon	0	1	0	1	764
Fibrohistiocytoma	1	0	0	1	771
Stomach cancer	1	0	0	1	770
Melanoma	0	1	0	1	631
Total solid tumors	9	8	0	17	—

MDS, myelodysplastic syndrome.
[a]One patient had MDS that developed into acute myeloid leukemia within 1 year.
[b]MDS is not considered cancer in these analyses. Some cases were reported more than once. No patient had more than one cancer.

had various forms of AML. These included two patients who were from the original series of Diamond et al. (756) and who had intermittent remissions of DBA but died of acute myeloblastic leukemia at 31 and 43 years of age (757; F. H. Gardner, *unpublished data*, 1984). One patient had received radiation to his thymus and long bones to stimulate the bone marrow. A girl whose DBA treatment included cyclophosphamide died of acute promyelocytic leukemia at 13 years of age (733). One boy developed acute megakaryoblastic leukemia at 14 months of age; it is possible that his anemia from 2 months of age was really a long preleukemic phase (758). Potential extenuating circumstances were less apparent for the other cases. The majority of the patients died from their leukemia. Janov et al. (631) calculated the relative risk of leukemia to be 200-fold.

Myelodysplastic Syndrome. One patient had MDS that developed into AML within one year, whereas two others had MDS at the time of the reports and died from complications of bone marrow failure (760,764).

Solid Tumors. Seventeen patients with DBA developed nonhematologic neoplasms (Table 8-18). The most common were sarcomas, including five osteogenic and one soft-tissue sarcoma. There were two Hodgkin's and one non-Hodgkin's lymphoma, two breast cancers, and one each of colon, fibrohistiocytoma, gastric, and melanoma cancers. Two patients also developed hepatomas, one of whom had transfusional iron overload, and the other had received androgens. Although a formal risk ratio cannot be determined from literature case series, DBA can be classified in the premalignant category in which many of the bone marrow failure syndromes now appear to belong.

Aplastic Anemia. Evolution to complete aplastic anemia has not been convincingly documented in DBA patients, although it was mentioned once without details by Najean (772). One reported case developed cytomegalovirus infection before pancytopenia (773), and another was multiply transfused and thus might also have a viral etiology (774). Pancytopenia has also occurred in patients with severe iron overload or terminal sepsis. In general, DBA remains a single cytopenia, and the overall prognosis is better than in many of the other marrow failure disorders.

Transient Erythroblastopenia of Childhood

Acute erythroblastopenia in previously hematologically normal children was first described by Gasser (724) in 1949 in 12 children in whom erythroblastopenia followed toxic, allergic, or infectious episodes. These children recovered rapidly and did not develop anemia. Baar then studied RBC lifespan in an 8-year-old with "complete transient aplasia of the erythropoietic tissue" (775). The term *erythroblastopenia of childhood* was first used by Wranne in 1970 to describe four cases with temporary red cell aplasia (776). More than 500 cases have been reported since 1970, as detailed case reports and as series of cases without individual data (5,6,697). TEC is defined as peripheral blood reticulocytopenia, usually with anemia and with bone marrow erythroblastopenia and normal white blood cell and platelet counts, and is temporary in duration. Some of the younger patients with TEC were sometimes initially thought to have DBA; Table 8-19 lists several features that distinguish the two conditions.

The male to female ratio is 1.3:1 among those with TEC. It is an acquired condition and occurs at a median of 23 months of

TABLE 8-19. Comparison of Diamond-Blackfan Anemia and Transient Erythroblastopenia of Childhood

	Diamond-Blackfan Anemia	Transient Erythroblastopenia of Childhood
Number of reported cases	>700	>500
Male/female	1.1	1.3
Age at diagnosis (mo)		
Mean	11	26
Median	3	23
Range	0–768	1–192
Patients older than 1 yr of age at diagnosis	12%	84%
Etiology	Genetic	Acquired
Antecedent history	None	Viral illness
Physical examination abnormal	25%	0%
Laboratory		
Hemoglobin g/dL	1.2–14.8	2.2–12.5
White blood cells <5000/μL	15%	20%
Platelets >400,000/μL	20%	45%
Red blood cell adenosine deaminase	Increased	Normal
Mean cell volume increased at diagnosis	80%	5%
During recovery	100%	90%
In remission	100%	0%
Fetal hemoglobin increased at diagnosis	100%	20%
During recovery	100%	100%
In remission	85%	0%
i Antigen increased	100%	20%
During recovery	100%	60%
In remission	90%	0%

Adapted from Alter BP. The bone marrow failure syndromes. In: Nathan DG, Oski FA, eds. *Hematology of infancy and childhood*, 3rd ed. Philadelphia: WB Saunders, 1987:159–241; and Link MP, Alter BP. Fetal erythropoiesis during recovery from transient erythroblastopenia of childhood (TEC). *Pediatr Res* 1981;15:1036–1039.

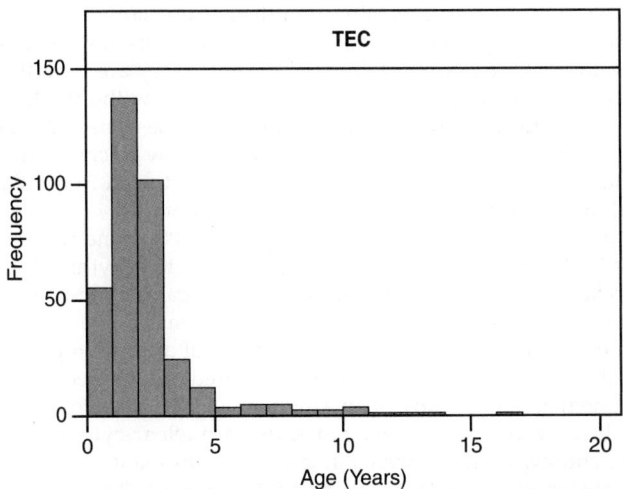

Figure 8-26. Age at diagnosis in more than 500 published cases with transient erythroblastopenia of childhood (TEC). Compare this figure with Figure 8-19 for Diamond-Blackfan anemia.

age (Fig. 8-26). More than 80% of patients who were studied were older than 1 year of age, compared to only approximately 10% of those with DBA in the same age range (compare Figs. 8-19 and 8-26). Only 10% of TEC patients were older than 3 years of age, and only four patients were older than 10 years of age; the oldest was 16 years of age.

The presenting symptom of TEC was pallor in a previously normal child, in whom prior normal blood counts were sometimes available. More than one-half of patients gave a history of a preceding illness (the median time interval between the prior illness and TEC presentation was 1 month, with a range of 0 to 4 months), which was usually viral—upper respiratory or gastrointestinal. Because these illnesses are common in young children, their relevance is difficult to ascertain, although a viral cause of the aplasia is appealing (see the section Pathophysiology). A few children had neurologic manifestations of anemia: seizures, breath holding, or transient ischemic attacks (777–785). Drug or toxin exposure included piperazine, aspirin, sulfonamides, valproic acid, phenytoin, and phenobarbital (782,786–790).

Familial TEC has been recorded rarely. Identical and fraternal twins had simultaneous onset of anemia (787,791,792). Four pairs of siblings had TEC at similar ages, but 2 to 3 years apart in onset (792,793). In these familial cases, TEC might have been caused by the same viral or environmental factor, combined with a genetic propensity. TEC has been reported from 17 countries, and cases have included blacks, Hispanics, and Japanese. Most of the reports have been from temperate climates.

TEC is somewhat seasonal, with the largest numbers of cases from the Northern Hemisphere occurring between October and January. However, the number of cases with this information is sufficiently small that monthly variations may be due to chance alone. At a given center, clusters may be due to specific local viral epidemics. Until the putative etiologic virus is identified, the cause remains speculative.

Physical examinations in TEC patients are normal except for pallor, and findings relate to anemia, such as tachycardia. The anemia is of gradual onset; thus, the pallor often is not noticed by parents until the anemia is profound.

LABORATORY FINDINGS

Hgb levels ranged from 2.2 to 12.5 g/dL, with a median of 5.6 g/dL. Reticulocytes were less than 1% in most of the children.

White blood cell counts were generally normal, but the absolute neutrophil count was less than 1000/µL in approximately 6% of the patients, and thrombocytopenia of less than 100,000/µL was reported in approximately 5%, some of whom were also neutropenic. It is possible that whatever suppresses the erythroid series may affect all cell lines in a few patients. Twenty percent had white blood counts greater than 10,000/µL, which perhaps is associated with intercurrent infections, although one patient did have true leukoerythroblastosis, perhaps due to marrow stimulation by hypoxia (794). Platelet counts greater than 400,000/µL were noted in almost one-half the patients, which is more than the proportion of DBA children with increased platelet counts. The MCVs were usually normal for age, with mean and median of 80 fL, although the range was from 62 to 112 fL. HbF levels also were usually normal, although the range was from 0.2% to 9.2%. A suggestion from one small study that blood group A patients predominate (759) was not borne out in another small study (795). Bone marrow examinations showed significant to profound erythroblastopenia in more than 90% of patients. In those in whom erythroblasts were seen, a maturation arrest was often present. Marrow lymphocytes were frequently elevated and led to the incorrect diagnosis of acute leukemia in at least one case (796). The 5% to 10% of patients with reticulocytosis or erythroid hyperplasia at presentation presumably had begun to recover without the benefit of medical attention.

Several erythrocyte characteristics may distinguish TEC from DBA. Wang and Mentzer (797) pointed out that the RBCs in TEC were adult or normal for age in MCV, HbF, i antigen, and RBC enzyme levels. In DBA, these parameters were more fetal-like. This distinction, which is based on normal versus fetal-like features, is only relevant to the reticulocytopenic patient at the time of diagnosis. During recovery from TEC, the RBCs have the features of stress erythropoiesis and are identical with those seen during any bone marrow recovery. This transient cohort of fetal-like erythrocytes can be detected as soon as the first reticulocytes appear, using a sensitive immunologic assay for F-reticulocytes (798,799). As Link and Alter (795) documented, this cohort of fetal-like erythrocytes then evolves again into normal RBCs. Thus, interpretation of fetal-like features depends on the stage of the disorder, and the ultimate distinction between TEC and DBA may be clear only from the outcome. Macrocytosis, elevated HbF, and reticulocytopenia, as well as marrow erythroblastopenia, in a child younger than 1 year of age most likely indicate DBA. Elevated RBC ADA is found in DBA and not in TEC (677).

PATHOPHYSIOLOGY

A viral cause for TEC is most likely. The history of an antecedent (usually viral) illness that presents 2 months before TEC is intriguing. Suppression of erythropoiesis in a normal person would require symptom duration of 1 to 2 months to be manifest as symptomatic anemia. It is not clear why recovery would then occur within another month. If the cause is viral, the time course of the development of specific antibodies would be relevant. The prime suspect is parvovirus. However, almost 50 cases have been analyzed individually or by one laboratory for parvovirus antibody, but only 20% of cases were found to have antibody, and causality remains to be proven. Because parvovirus inhibits the growth of CFU-E, it is logical that this particular virus leads to aplasia in patients with shortened RBC survival due to hemolytic anemia. Its role in those with previously normal erythropoiesis has not yet been proven and requires sensitive assays for antigen or for parvoviral DNA.

Several groups have investigated the erythropoietic defect in TEC. Levels of EPO are high (800). Erythroid progenitor cell cultures have provided a wide variety of results. A consensus of all of the culture studies is difficult to reach, because not all parameters were examined in all patients. Probably one-half of all cases of TEC have reduced erythroid progenitor cell numbers. More than one-half of cases have serum inhibitors in autologous or allogeneic cultures, usually IgG. Inhibitory mononuclear cells may be present in one-fourth of cases. No patients had serum and cellular inhibitors, but few were examined for both (697). TEC may be due to an as yet unknown virus, which may infect CFU-E and not be cleared until specific antibodies develop to the virus. In some cases, a specific IgG may be directed against epitopes on erythroid progenitors themselves, thus inhibiting growth of autologous or allogeneic erythroid colonies. Recovery in these cases might require antiidiotype antibodies.

THERAPY AND OUTCOME

As indicated by the name of this disorder, TEC is transient, and all patients recover. Recurrent TEC was observed only twice and occurred within 1 year (800,801). Most patients show signs of recovery within the first month after diagnosis, and 5% to 10% of patients have already begun to recover when they are first seen. The longest interval to recovery without recurrence was 8 months, and only nine patients took more than 4 months to recover. No treatment was necessary for approximately one-half of the patients for whom the clinical course was described. In most patients, the nadir Hgb was reached by the time they were seen. More than one transfusion was needed in less than 10% of patients. Prednisone was administered to 10% to 20% of patients, but reticulocytes appeared within 1 day in many patients, a phenomenon that is almost certainly unrelated to the treatment.

Our recommendation for TEC is watchful waiting, with transfusion only when anemia leads to cardiovascular compromise. These children tolerate their anemia extremely well, because it has developed gradually, and it is often the cardiovascular status of the physician rather than the patient that leads to transfusion. Prednisone, anabolic steroids, and other immunosuppressive therapies have no apparent role in the management of TEC. The prognosis is excellent, and the distinction from DBA is simple in retrospect (Table 8-19).

Congenital Dyserythropoietic Anemia

Dyserythropoiesis refers to ineffective, morphologically abnormal erythroid production. *Dysplastic* indicates qualitative abnormalities of the stem cell or the microenvironment. *Aplastic* refers to quantitative abnormalities of the same compartments. Although these congenital conditions are not, strictly speaking, bone marrow failure syndromes, they are inherited marrow disorders, which may result in anemia without reticulocytosis. Erythropoiesis is ineffective, because a discrepancy exists between erythroid output from marrow to circulation (anemia) and erythroid marrow content (erythroid hyperplasia), thus implying intramedullary destruction.

In healthy persons, approximately 1 in 1000 bone marrow erythroblasts is abnormal (802). Multinucleated erythroblasts and karyorrhexis are occasionally seen in megaloblastic anemia, iron deficiency, leukemia, and hemolytic anemia, and are indicative of bone marrow stress. The incidence of dyserythropoietic erythroblasts may be substantial in acquired or inherited aplastic anemia. In one study of aplastic anemia, 5% to 90% of erythroblasts were megaloblastic or showed nuclear-cytoplasmic asynchrony, 1% to 3% were binucleate, and as many as 5% had cytoplasmic connections or chromatin bridges (803). During recovery from BMT, all patients transiently had as many as 30% dyserythropoietic erythroblasts (804). These morphologic abnormalities are more extreme in congenital dyserythropoietic anemia (CDA) than in aplastic anemia or in marrow transplantation recovery.

All patients with CDA have anemia with insufficient reticulocytosis and ineffective erythropoiesis, and all ethnic groups are affected. The major types of CDA were described in detail in a book by Lewis and Verwilghen (805) in 1977 and are summarized in a recent review by Wickramasinghe (806). Table 8-20 outlines the major types:

Type I: macrocytosis, with bone marrow megaloblastoid changes and internuclear chromatin bridges between cells.

Type II: normocytosis or macrocytosis, with binucleated and multinucleated erythroblasts, pluripolar mitoses, and karyorrhexis.

Type III: macrocytosis, with erythroblastic multinuclearity of up to 12 nuclei (gigantoblasts).

Types I and III are diagnosed primarily by bone marrow morphology. Type II is characterized by positive reaction to some acidified normal sera [which is called *hereditary erythroblastic multinuclearity with a positive acidified serum (HEMPAS) test* (807)]. More than 50 additional cases have been reported that do not clearly fit into types I to III.

TYPE I

More than 100 cases of type I CDA have been reported [the first 20 cases were reported by Heimpel (808,809)]. The onset of anemia, jaundice, or both, ranges from infancy to old age, with a median age of onset of 10 years of age. The male to female ratio is

---

TABLE 8-20. Types of Congenital Dyserythropoietic Anemias

Feature	Type I	Type II	Type III
Reported cases	130	200	60
Male/female ratio	1.1	0.9	0.8
Anemia	Mild-moderate	Moderate	Mild-moderate
Red cell size	Macrocytic	Normo- or macrocytic	Macrocytic
Bone marrow erythroblasts	Megaloblastoid, binucleated (2–5%), chromatin bridges	Bi- and multinucleated (10–40%), karyorrhexis	Gigantoblasts (10–40%)
Inheritance	Recessive	Recessive	Dominant
Acid serum hemolysis	Negative	Positive	Negative
Anti-i reaction	Slight	Strong	Slight
Anti-I reaction	Slight	Strong	Slight
Effect of splenectomy (%)	50	96	100

1.1:1.0, and the inheritance is autosomal recessive. Consanguinity was reported in at least 15 families, and affected siblings or cousins were reported in almost 20. Physical examination may show icterus and splenomegaly, as well as brown skin pigmentation; a few patients had toe syndactyly or abnormal fingers.

The anemia is often mild, with a median Hgb of 9 g/dL and a range of 2 to 15 g/dL. Reticulocytes range from 1% to 7%. RBCs are macrocytic, with a median MCV of 100 fL and a range of 66 to 133 fL. The blood film shows anisocytosis, poikilocytosis, punctate basophilia, and occasional Cabot's rings. White blood cells and platelets are normal. Indirect bilirubin is elevated (1 to 4 mg/dL), as is serum lactate dehydrogenase, whereas haptoglobin is low and transferrin is saturated. Plasma iron turnover is as much as ten times the normal rate, and RBC utilization is reduced to less than 30%. RBC survival is slightly shortened, with a chromium-51 (^{51}Cr) half-life of 15 to 28 days (with a mean 21 days). Globin synthesis studies usually show non-α to α ratios of 1, although an imbalance of 0.5 to 0.7 was observed occasionally (810,811). Negative reactions are seen in the acidified serum test, and i antigen titer is usually in the adult low range, in contrast to that seen in type II CDA.

Bone marrow examination shows marked erythroid hyperplasia (812). The abnormalities are confined to the more mature erythroblasts and the polychromatophilic and orthochromatic series (Fig. 8-27). Nuclear maturation and cytoplasmic maturation are dissociated, and nuclei are immature and megaloblastoid. As many as 2% of erythroblasts are large cells with incomplete nuclear division, often with double nuclei in which one component is more mature than the other. As many as 2% of cells show thin chromatin bridges that connect the nuclei of two cells. Electron microscopy demonstrates widening of nuclear membrane pores in mature erythroblasts, with condensation, vacuolization, and disintegration of nuclear chromatin, with cytoplasmic penetrance. Structural changes are found in the nucleolus, microtubules, and siderotic material in the cytoplasm (812–814).

The defect in CDA is at the stem cell level. The numbers of CFU-E and BFU-E are normal, but the colonies contain a mixture of normal and abnormal cells, when they are examined by electron microscopy (815). This suggests that the abnormality is expressed variably in the mature progeny of each stem cell.

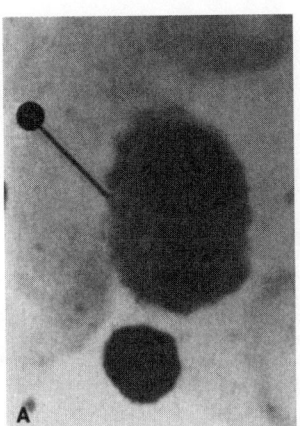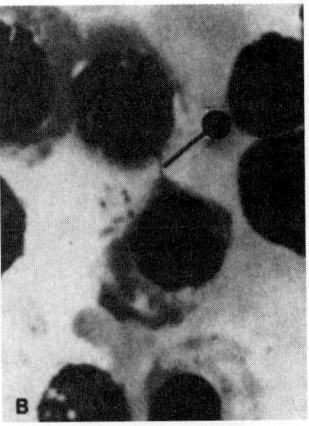

Figure 8-27. Bone marrow from a patient with congenital dyserythropoietic anemia type I. **A:** Dot and leader indicate binucleate erythroblast with nuclei of different sizes and maturity. **B:** Dot and leader indicate internuclear chromatin bridges that connect two erythroblasts. (From Lewis SM, Verwilghen RL, eds. *Dyserythropoiesis*. London: Academic Press, 1977, with permission.)

The gene for CDA I (CDAN1) was mapped in a large Israeli Bedouin kinship to chromosome 15q15.1-15.3 (816). However, several other unrelated patients of Lebanese and English origin did not have haplotypes that linked to this region, thus suggesting that there is genetic heterogeneity in CDA type I (817).

Treatment with the usual hematinics, such as vitamins, metals, and steroids, is without effect. A few transfusions were required in 20% of patients. Splenomegaly is common, but splenectomy (reported in 10% of cases) does not improve the anemia. Some patients develop gallstones from the hemolytic anemia. Hemosiderosis is the most important long-term complication because of increased intestinal absorption of iron, ineffective erythropoiesis, and mild hemolysis; phlebotomy or iron chelation with deferoxamine warrants consideration. Four of the patients were reported to have died, one at 10 years of age from complications of splenectomy, one at 84 years of age from old age, and two from persistent pulmonary hypertension in infancy (818,819).

The beneficial effect of interferon-α was discovered during treatment of a patient with CDA type I for posttransfusion chronic hepatitis C (820) and was confirmed in several other patients (821–823). A potential mechanism was suggested by the observation that Epstein-Barr virus transformed B lymphoblasts from patients with CDA type I produce less interferon-α *in vitro* than do normal cells (823). Addition of interferon-α to erythroid cultures improves the ultrastructural Swiss-cheese appearance of erythroblasts (824).

Successful bone marrow transplant was reported in one case, using a sibling donor (825).

TYPE II

Type II CDA, also known as *HEMPAS*, has been reported in approximately 200 patients. Many of the early cases were summarized by Verwilghen (826,827). More than two dozen cases were in sibships, and 11 cases were in families with consanguinity. The male to female ratio was 0.9:1, and the inheritance is autosomal recessive. Anemia is noted between infancy and adulthood, at a median of 14 years of age, and varies from mild to more severe anemia that requires regular transfusions. The median Hgb was 9.5 g/dL, and the range was from 3 to 15 g/dL. Jaundice, hepatosplenomegaly, and gallstones are more common in patients with type II CDA than in those with type I CDA.

Although anemia may be severe in patients with type II CDA, reticulocytosis is inadequate and averages 4%. RBCs are usually normochromic and normocytic, although macrocytosis has been observed; the median MCV is 94 fL, and the range is from 73 to 114 fL. The smear shows anisocytosis, poikilocytosis, teardrops, and basophilic stippling, all of which are nonspecific findings. The anemia and the RBC lifespan are worse in type II CDA than in type I CDA patients; the ^{51}Cr half-life averages 17 days (with a range from 7 to 31 days).

Electron microscopy shows an excess of endoplasmic reticulum parallel with the cell membrane, which leads to the appearance of a characteristic double membrane, or cistern, in late erythroblasts and some erythrocytes (813,814). Many patients with type II CDA also have bone marrow reticuloendothelial cells that resemble Gaucher cells, with birefringent, paraaminosalicylic acid–positive, needlelike inclusions. These inclusions may be the products of catabolism from the rapidly turning-over marrow erythroblasts. The marrow shows erythroid hyperplasia, with binucleated and multinucleated mature erythroblasts in 10% to 40% of the erythroid precursors (Fig. 8-28). The internuclear chromatin bridges of type I CDA are not seen, nor is the multinuclearity as extreme as is seen in type III CDA.

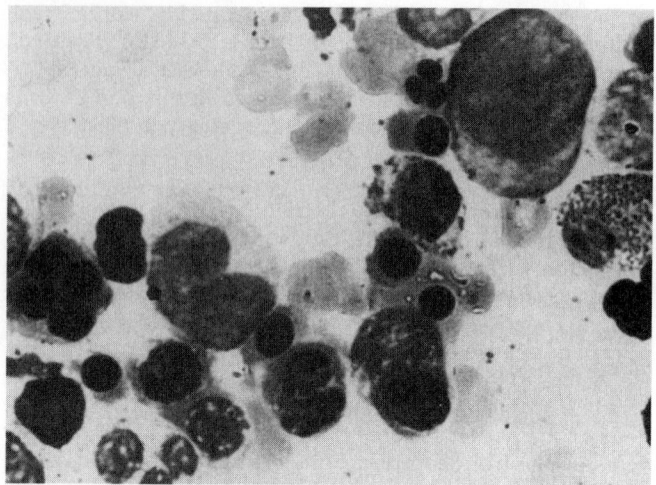

Figure 8-28. Bone marrow from a patient with congenital dyserythropoietic anemia type II, showing binucleated and multinucleated erythroblasts. (Courtesy of Dr. Gail Wolfe. From Alter BP. The bone marrow failure syndromes. In: Nathan DG, Oski FA, eds. *Hematology of infancy and childhood*, 3rd ed. Philadelphia: WB Saunders, 1987:159–241, with permission.)

The pathognomonic findings in HEMPAS are serologic (807,828,829). HEMPAS RBCs are lysed by approximately 30% of acidified sera from normal persons, but not by the patient's own serum. In contrast, in paroxysmal nocturnal hemoglobinuria, patient cells are lysed by acidified patient serum. In CDA type II, the RBCs have a specific HEMPAS antigen, and many normal sera contain an anti-HEMPAS IgM antibody. In some cases of type II CDA, up to 30 normal sera must be examined until a positive acidified test results; some were thought not to be type II CDA until this was obtained (830). HEMPAS erythrocytes are also distinct in that they are more strongly agglutinated with anti-i antibody than cells of newborn infants or of patients with stress erythropoiesis (831). Fluorescent labels demonstrated i antigen on all RBCs in HEMPAS. Heterozygotes also have increased expression of i antigen (807,832). HEMPAS RBCs also express increased amounts of I antigen. HEMPAS erythrocytes were shown by Rosse et al. (833) to bind a normal amount of complement C1, but more antibody and less C4 than normals. This causes binding of an excess of C3 and hemolysis. The RBC plasma membrane abnormality in HEMPAS is related to decreased N-glycan synthesis near the *N*-acetylglucosaminylphosphotransferase II and α-mannosidase II steps (834). Bands 3 and 4.5 lack glycosylation with lactosaminoglycans (835).

The number of erythroid progenitors is probably normal in marrow and blood. Although one study found only normal morphology of the erythroblasts that were produced in culture (836), other studies reported multinuclearity that was similar to that seen in the bone marrow (837,838). As in type I CDA, the defect in type II CDA is in the erythroid stem cell and is expressed variably in more mature erythroblasts.

One gene for CDA II (CDAN2) was localized to chromosome 20q11.2 by a genome-wide search using 12 Italian families and one French family (839). Further studies indicated that the majority of the Italian CDA type II patients linked to 20q11.2, but this was not due to a founder effect (840). Two other Italian families were not linked to this locus (841), and other patients were found to have mutations in the genes for α-mannosidase II (834). Thus CDA II has genetic heterogeneity.

Patients whose anemias are severe are supported by blood transfusions. Unlike in type I CDA, splenectomy is effective in approximately 70% of type II cases and leads to an increase in RBC lifespan and abrogation of transfusions. Iron accumulation, from transfusions and from increased intestinal absorption, is a major complication, even in untransfused patients. Phlebotomy and iron chelation have a definite role in the management of patients with type II CDA (842). Two of the patients died of hemochromatosis at 25 and 30 years of age.

Some of the phenotypic heterogeneity in CDA II could be related to coinherited Gilbert syndrome; serum bilirubin levels and gallstones were increased in patients with the homozygous A(TA)7TAA box variant of the UGT1A gene, which leads to reduced expression of uridine diphosphate glucuronosyl transferase (843). Similarly, iron overload was increased in a patient with CDA type II and hereditary hemochromatosis due to homozygous C282Y mutation in HFE (844).

TYPE III

Approximately 70 patients have been reported in 16 families with type III CDA (845,846). The male to female ratio was 0.8:1.0. Three families had apparently dominant CDA, whereas three had affected siblings, and one had consanguinity. The median age at diagnosis was 24 years of age, with a range from birth to old age, similar to that in types I and II CDA. Anemia is mild to moderate, and MCVs may be normal or increased (with a median 94 fL and a range from 79 to 135 fL). The bone marrow shows erythroid hyperplasia, with multinuclearity in 10% to 40% of erythroblasts, including some large gigantoblasts with up to 12 nuclei (Fig. 8-29). Hemolysis does not occur with acidified sera, and reactions with anti-i antigen are similar to those seen in stress erythropoiesis. RBC survival is slightly shortened, with a ^{51}Cr survival half-life of 21 days. The defect is in the stem cell, and *in vitro* culture results in colonies that contain normal and abnormal erythroblasts (847).

The gene for CDA III, CDAN3, was mapped to 15q21-25 in a large Swedish family that was the subject of many reports (848).

The need for transfusions or splenectomy is rare. As in the other CDAs, hemosiderosis is the major problem and resulted in the death of one patient who was 42 years of age. Members of the Swedish family have an increased risk of monoclonal gammopathy, myeloma, and ocular angioid streaks (849).

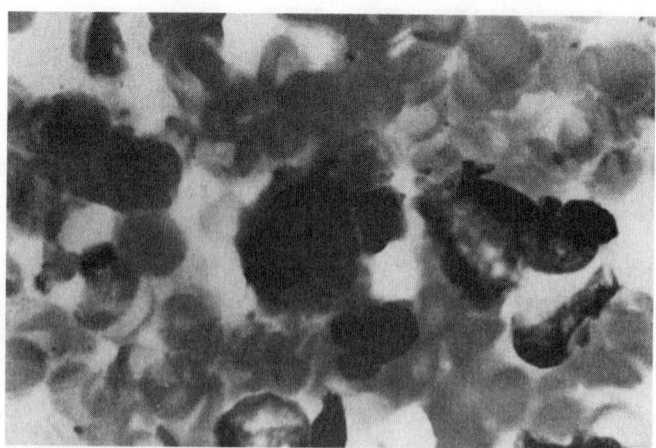

Figure 8-29. Bone marrow from a patient with congenital dyserythropoietic anemia type III, showing multinucleated erythroblast. (Courtesy of Dr. Gail Wolfe. From Alter BP. The bone marrow failure syndromes. In: Nathan DG, Oski FA, eds. *Hematology of infancy and childhood*, 3rd ed. Philadelphia: WB Saunders, 1987:159–241, with permission.)

VARIANTS

More than 50 patients have been reported with apparent CDA that does not conform to the types that were previously described (806). In rare cases, the bone marrow morphology resembled type II CDA, but the cases were classified as type IV CDA, because the acidified serum tests were negative, which might indicate only that an insufficient number of sera were examined. The level of i antigen was not increased. The inheritance was apparently dominant in one family; thus, at least some of these cases might indeed belong to a different type (850–854). Anemia was mild in all but one case and was diagnosed from infancy to adulthood. Binucleated erythroblasts made up 10% to 40% of the marrow erythroblasts. The clinical course was relatively benign in the reported cases, with splenectomy in only one.

Another group of patients was termed *CDA with thalassemia* (855–861). One family had dominant inheritance, and another family had three affected siblings. The age at diagnosis ranged from infancy to old age, the anemia was mild to moderate, MCVs ranged from microcytic to macrocytic, and multinuclearity was present in 25% to 35% of the erythroblasts. Tests with acidified sera were negative, and i antigen was positive in two of the three families. Globin chain synthesis was imbalanced, with β to α ratios of 0.5, which is similar to those seen in β-thalassemia trait. There may have been a coincidence of thalassemia trait and CDA, but two families were from ethnic groups without a high incidence of thalassemia.

Almost 40 other patients were reported with CDAs that are even more difficult to classify. Five families had an affected parent and child, two had consanguinity, and three had affected siblings. These cases all may represent different disorders. The proportion of binucleated or multinucleated erythroblasts was always low, less than 4%. In some, the morphology resembled type I CDA, with rare internuclear bridges, as well as type II CDA, with symmetric binuclearity, karyorrhexis, and even double membranes by electron microscopy. The ages at diagnosis of anemia ranged from birth to adulthood, and the anemia ranged from mild to severe. MCVs encompassed the entire spectrum. Acidified serum testing was usually negative, i antigen was variable, and RBC ^{51}Cr half-life ranged from 5 to 29 days. Splenectomy was reported in eight patients, with occasional efficacy. Erythroid cultures from one case demonstrated that multinuclearity was present in some cells in each colony, which indicates a stem cell disorder, as in the other CDAs (862). The clinical variability suggests that these cases may represent several types of CDA. Perhaps these patients are double heterozygotes, instead of homozygotes, for recessive CDA genes.

SINGLE CYTOPENIAS: WHITE BLOOD CELLS

Severe Congenital Neutropenia

Inherited isolated neutropenia was first recognized as a distinct entity in 1956 by Kostmann (863,864), who called it *infantile genetic agranulocytosis*. Other names for this condition are *severe chronic neutropenia*, and *severe congenital neutropenia (SCN)* (see Chapter 14 for a more complete discussion of neutropenia). The term *Kostmann's syndrome* might be reserved for patients in whom the inheritance is clearly autosomal recessive; most patients are autosomal dominants or sporadic new mutations. In this section, the term *SCN* is used for cases in which neutropenia is less than 200/μL, with severe pyogenic infections in infancy and a bone marrow myeloid arrest at the promyelocyte-myelocyte stage. More than 300 cases in the literature fit this description (Table 8-21). The male to female ratio is 1. Most of Kostmann's original 14 and subsequent ten

TABLE 8-21. Congenital Neutropenia Literature

	Reported on or before 1989	Reported after 1989	All Patients
Number of cases	128	178	306
Male/female	55/68	90/81	145/149
Ratio	0.8	1.1	1
Leukemia			
Number of cases (%)	3 (2)	23 (13)	26 (9)
Male/female	2/1	14/9	16/10
Age at diagnosis (yr)			
Mean	14	11.1	—
Median	14	12	—
Range	14–14	2–23	—
MDS[a]			
Number of cases (%)	0 (0)	13 (7)	13 (5)
Male/female	8/5	8/5	—
Age at diagnosis (yr)			
Mean	11.3	11.8	—
Median	11	11	—
Range	1–22	1–22	—
Deceased			
Number of cases (%)	67 (52)	15 (8)	82 (30)
Male/female	26/37	9/6	35/43
Age at death (yr)			
Mean	2.1	6.9	3
Median	0.7	3.3	0.8
Range	0.05–20	0.1–23	0.05–23
Projected median age for all patients (yr)	3	—	23
Leukemia	14	23	14.8
MDS	—	23	23

MDS, myelodysplastic syndrome.
[a]Includes four patients with bone marrow cytogenetic clones but without morphologic MDS.

cases were members of a large intermarried kinship in northern Sweden, which led to the suggestion that the inheritance is autosomal recessive (865). Cases have been reported in all ethnic groups, including blacks, Native Americans, and Asians. At least a dozen cases were in families with parental consanguinity, and more than 20 families had affected siblings. However, eight families appear to have dominant inheritance (866).

Age at presentation is young, with 50% of the patients symptomatic within the first month after birth and 90% symptomatic by 6 months of age. In fact, the few who were diagnosed later in life may not have had the same diagnosis. Birth weights are generally normal, as are physical examinations, except for signs of infection, such as skin abscesses.

LABORATORY FINDINGS

Neutropenia is extreme in these patients, although several infants had almost normal absolute neutrophil counts in the first week or two of life, which declined rapidly thereafter. The average absolute neutrophil count is less than 200/μL; many patients have total neutropenia. Eosinophils and monocytes are frequently high (as many as 50% monocytes in some patients), but these are not as effective as phagocytes as are neutrophils. Ig levels are also frequently increased. Congenital neutropenia is a single cytopenia, because the Hgbs are usually normal (with a mean level of 10 g/dL), and platelet counts are normal or even high. Bone marrow is cellular, with absent or markedly decreased myeloid precursors. When precursors are present, there is an arrest at the myelocyte or promyelocyte stage.

PATHOPHYSIOLOGY

Congenital neutropenia primarily affects the neutrophil series. Bone marrow cultures have decreased, increased, or, most often, normal numbers of colony-forming units (colony-forming unit culture). The colonies, which contain neutrophils in normal persons, that do grow in semisolid media have been reported rarely to contain neutrophils (867) or, more frequently, to contain eosinophils, monocytes, and abnormal or arrested myeloid precursors (868). A block in myeloid differentiation was also seen in long-term cultures from some patients (867). Thus, in some patients the *in vivo* defect in myeloid differentiation is apparent *in vitro*.

Recently linkage analysis in familial cases of autosomal-dominant cyclic neutropenia mapped the locus to 19p13.3 and identified mutations in the neutrophil elastase gene (ELA2) at that locus (869). The same group then showed that 22 of 25 patients with SCN had 18 different heterozygous mutations in ELA2 (870). The mutations in cyclic neutropenia cluster around the active site of the enzyme, whereas the mutations in SCN are on the opposite face. Thorough investigation of the mutant and wild-type proteins led to the conclusion that mutant ELA2 may act as a dominant negative inhibitor of the function of the normal enzyme (871).

THERAPY AND OUTCOME

The prognosis for patients with congenital neutropenia was poor in the era before G-CSF, with more than one-half of patients reported to have died at a median of 7 months of age, with a range of 2 weeks of age to 20 years of age. The Kaplan-Meier survival curve (Fig. 8-30) for this group indicates a projected median survival of 3 years of age, and only 10% of patients are long-term survivors. Most of the deaths were from sepsis or pneumonia. No cases evolved into aplastic anemia, which shows that congenital neutropenia is a true single cytopenia. Infections were treated with antibiotics, and many patients received prophylactic treatment. Lithium

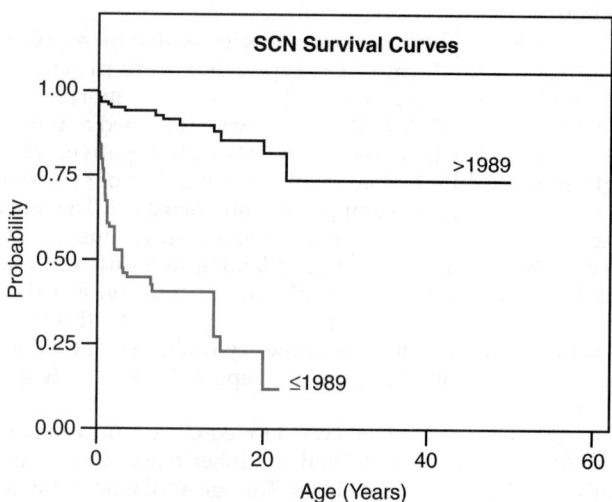

Figure 8-30. Kaplan-Meier plot of cumulative survival in severe congenital neutropenia (SCN). Time is shown as age in years. Lines represent 128 patients who were reported in the era before granulocyte colony-stimulating factor (before 1989) and 178 patients who were reported after granulocyte colony-stimulating factor (after 1989).

therapy was suggested because of its ability to raise white counts in hematologically normal persons, but it was relatively ineffective in congenital neutropenia (872,873). BMT cured one patient (874), but the graft was lost in another (875).

The most exciting therapeutic advance was the use of recombinant growth factors. Subcutaneous G-CSF is effective at raising neutrophil counts in children with congenital neutropenia in a dose-related manner. The factor must be administered chronically, but it seems to be without major short-term side effects (876,877). However, bone loss has been reported and warrants treatment (878,879).

Only 8% of the cases that have been reported since 1989 died, at a median of 3 years of age, with a range of 1 month of age to 23 years of age and a projected plateau of 75% survival at 23 years of age. Deaths still occur from sepsis. Since 1989, bone marrow transplant was reported in 19 patients, of whom five died from complications; most transplants were from alternative donors (880) (Fig. 8-31).

Prenatal diagnosis was considered early for congenital neutropenia, using fetal blood that was obtained in the middle trimester (881). However, the absolute neutrophil count is less than 200/μL in normal fetuses (882), and truly absolute neutropenia would be required to diagnose congenital neutropenia *in utero*. At this time, mutations in ELA2 might be sought *in utero*.

Leukemia. Before G-CSF, three patients developed acute monocytic leukemia, all at 14 years of age, and died at 4 to 6 months after diagnosis (883–885). One family was reported to have one child with congenital neutropenia and a sibling with acute lymphoblastic leukemia (886). Since the introduction of G-CSF, leukemia or MDS, or both, was observed in approximately 10% of the treated patients. In a large series reported from the Severe Chronic Neutropenia Registry in which leukemia and MDS were not analyzed separately, the frequency was 9% (887). In individual case reports, leukemia occurred in 13% of patients after 1989 and consisted mainly of AML that was not otherwise defined, acute myelomonocytic leukemia, and acute monocytic leukemia. MDS was reported in 7% of patients, and monosomy 7 clonality was noted in many

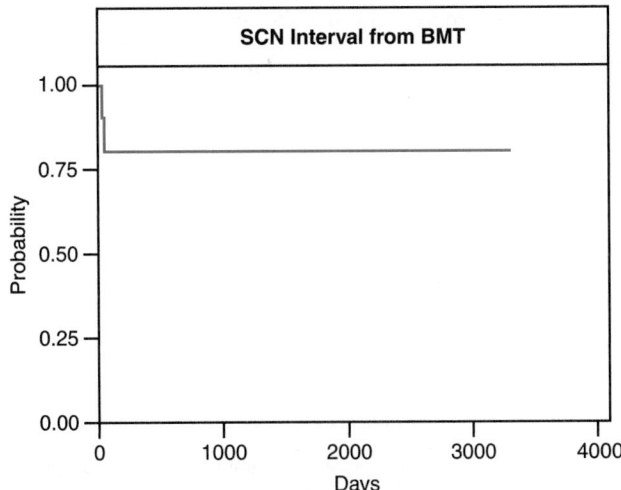

Figure 8-31. Kaplan-Meier plot of cumulative survival in six patients with severe congenital neutropenia (SCN) after bone marrow transplantation (BMT). Time is shown as the interval from BMT in days.

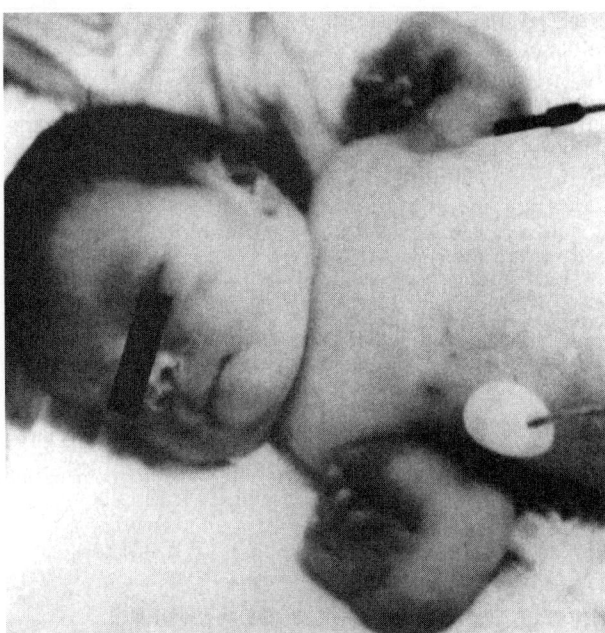

Figure 8-32. Newborn infant with thrombocytopenia–absent radius syndrome. Note that thumbs are present. (Courtesy of Dr. Jeffrey Lipton. From Alter BP. The bone marrow failure syndromes. In: Nathan DG, Oski FA, eds. *Hematology of infancy and childhood*, 3rd ed. Philadelphia: WB Saunders, 1987:159–241, with permission.)

patients with MDS and leukemia (887,888). Although the evolution to MDS or leukemia is worrisome, G-CSF has made a major contribution to the longevity of patients with congenital neutropenia.

Somatic mutations of one of the two alleles of the G-CSF receptor (G-CSF-R) have been described in several patients (889,890). The mutations generally result in loss of the carboxy terminal differentiation domain of the receptor. These truncated forms of the G-CSF-R are thought to have dominant activity, which results in increased cell growth without granulocyte differentiation. Importantly, because only somatic mutations in the G-CSF-R have been described, this gene is not the underlying genetic cause of congenital neutropenia. However, these somatic mutations may contribute to the transformation into acute myeloblastic leukemia (891) and have been identified before development of leukemia (892). The precise mechanism by which the truncated G-CSF-R acts dominantly over the endogenous wild-type allele remains unknown. The mutant receptor may have delayed internalization and down-regulation after ligand binding, resulting in a sustained proliferative signal. Such a strong proliferative drive may block the granulocyte differentiation signal that is generated from the wild-type G-CSF-R that is encoded by the normal allele (893).

A propensity for malignancy (leukemia) is seen in congenital neutropenia, as in many other bone marrow failure syndromes.

SINGLE CYTOPENIAS: PLATELETS

Thrombocytopenia with Absent Radii

TAR syndrome represents a true single cytopenia, with no reports of evolution to pancytopenia or malignancy. Comprehensive reviews are provided elsewhere (5,6,894–896). The patients are often diagnosed at birth, due to the combination of the characteristic physical appearance plus thrombocytopenia. The pathognomonic physical finding is bilateral absence of the radii, with thumbs present (Fig. 8-32). The presence of thumbs differentiates TAR from Fanconi's anemia (and from trisomy 18), in which thumbs are absent if radii are absent. Hemorrhagic manifestations in TAR patients are often also present at birth, with petechiae or bloody diarrhea, or both, apparent in 60% of

patients within the first week of life and in more than 95% of patients by 4 months of age.

Table 8-22 compares several features of TAR with Fanconi's anemia. The inheritance pattern in TAR is autosomal recessive, with several families reported with affected siblings and consanguinity reported in three families (897–899). The male to female ratio is 0.8:1.0. Two sets of identical twins had TAR (900,901), whereas only one of a pair of fraternal twins was affected (902). This finding is consistent with the cause being genetic rather than acquired. In most cases, parents of TAR patients are normal, and normal offspring of affected mothers have been reported (894,903). A few families involved more than one generation (aunts or uncles and nephews or nieces, with one example of parent-child transmission) or cousins (894,903–909), and one family had two affected half-siblings (910), suggesting that dominant (or perhaps pseudodominant) inheritance might be relevant in a few families. Although all ethnic groups are affected, including blacks, reports of Asians are rare; however, this may reflect a reporting, rather than a genetic, bias (911).

All TAR patients have absent radii, with thumbs present (Fig. 8-32). Most are affected bilaterally, with only five apparently bona fide cases in which the absent radius was unilateral, and the hematologic picture was typical (912–916). Short stature is common in TAR and Fanconi's anemia patients, but those with Fanconi's anemia are often smaller. The other hand abnormalities in TAR are shortening of the middle phalanx of the fifth finger, clinodactyly, occasional finger syndactyly, and, sometimes, hypoplasia of the thumbs. Additional abnormalities of the forearms may include absent ulnae or ulnar shortening or bowing in 40% of patients. Approximately one-third of patients have abnormal upper arms, with either short or absent humeri; the ulnar or humeral lesions are usually bilateral. Scapular hypoplasia and web necks further account for abnormal upper body appearances, along with micrognathia and occasional brachycephaly or microcephaly. Hypertelorism,

TABLE 8-22. Comparison of Thrombocytopenia–Absent Radius Syndrome and Fanconi's Anemia

Feature	Thrombocytopenia–Absent Radius Syndrome	Fanconi's Anemia
Number of reported cases	225	1200
Median age at diagnosis (yr)	0	8
Male to female ratio	0.8:1.0	1.2:1.0
Inheritance	Recessive	Recessive
Low birth weight (%)	9	11
Stature	Short	Short
Skeletal deformities		
Absent radii, thumbs present (%)	100	0
Hand anomalies (%)	40	43
Lower limbs (%)	37	8
Cardiac anomalies (%)	8	6
Skin		
Hemangiomas (%)	8	0
Pigmentation (%)	0	55
Blood	Thrombocytopenia	Pancytopenia
Marrow	Absent megakaryocytes	Aplastic
Marrow colonies decreased	Colony-forming unit megakaryocyte	Colony-forming unit granulocyte-macrophage, colony-forming unit erythroid
Fetal hemoglobin	Normal	Increased
Chromosome breaks	Absent	Present
Malignancies (%)	1	16
Reported deaths (%)	20	38
Projected median survival (yr)	—	20
Survival plateau	Approximately 75% at 4 yr	None

epicanthal folds, strabismus, and low-set ears are also seen, as are facial hemangiomas (in 10%).

The lower limbs are abnormal in 40% of patients. Abnormalities include deformed, subluxed, or hypoplastic knees (917); dislocated hips or patellae; and varus or valgus rotation at hips, knees, or feet. Short legs and absent tibiae or fibulae have been observed. Congenital heart disease (in 10% of patients) includes atrial or ventricular septal defects, tetralogy of Fallot, dextrocardia, and ectopia cordis. A few patients had gonadal anomalies, such as undescended testes, hypoplasia, unicornuate uterus, and vaginal atresia. Low birth weight was observed at term in 15% of the babies.

A major distinction of TAR from Fanconi's anemia is that, in Fanconi's anemia, thumbs are absent when radii are normal. In addition, TAR involves only thrombocytopenia, whereas Fanconi's anemia eventually develops pancytopenia. There are four reports of trisomy 18 with absent or hypoplastic radii or thrombocytopenia, or both (918–921), but they are distinguished by other characteristic anomalies, as well as the cytogenetic abnormality. Roberts' syndrome and SC phocomelia may have a similar phenotype (922,923). Other syndromes with radial anomalies are beyond the scope of this analysis.

Almost 20% of patients were reported to have bloody diarrhea in infancy, which was ascribed specifically to an allergy to cow's milk (894,914). Removal of milk from the diet alleviates that symptom and may perhaps lead to improvement of the thrombocytopenia.

LABORATORY FINDINGS

Platelet counts are less than 50,000/μL at the time of diagnosis in more than 75% of patients. Anemia is probably secondary to bleeding, and reticulocytosis is usually associated. Leukocytosis is a common finding, with white blood counts greater than 15,000/μL in more than 75% of those reported, greater than 20,000/μL in two-thirds of patients, and greater than 40,000/μL in one-third of infants. Levels of greater than 100,000/μL have been reported. More than 12 patients had immature myeloid precursors in the circulation, but none had true leukoerythroblastosis. This leukemoid reaction has been mistaken for congenital leukemia, but it is, in fact, transient and usually subsides during infancy. Splenomegaly

may occur due to extramedullary hematopoiesis, and eosinophilia is not uncommon. Bone marrow examinations show normal cellularity and normal or increased myeloid and erythroid cell lines, with absence of megakaryocytes in most patients and decreased, hypoplastic, or immature megakaryocytes in the rest.

Laboratory tests with normal results include MCV, HbF, and studies of chromosome breakage, spontaneous and with clastogenic stress, which distinguish TAR from Fanconi's anemia. Karyotypic analysis also distinguishes TAR from trisomy 18. Hypogammaglobulinemia was reported in one group of patients from Nigeria but has not been a general problem (912). Platelet size is normal, except in one report (924), and platelet function is generally normal (925–927), although abnormalities of platelet aggregation and storage pool defects were reported (924,928,929). Clinical symptoms are likely due to quantitative rather than qualitative defects.

PATHOPHYSIOLOGY

The inheritance pattern is most likely autosomal recessive, for a single or for more than one genetic defect, with a recurrence risk of one in four. TAR is one of several inherited hematologic conditions that are associated with radial ray anomalies (the others are Fanconi's anemia and DBA). In the case of TAR, only the platelet lineage is significantly affected. Cultures of hematopoietic progenitor cells indicate that the myeloid and erythroid lineages are normal (129,930–933). Although some studies found no growth of megakaryocytic progenitors (931–934), others found essentially normal numbers (935). A unique megakaryocyte colony-stimulating factor was increased in the plasma of one patient (934); this was probably TPO, which is elevated (936). Unlike amegakaryocytic thrombocytopenia (discussed previously in the section Amegakaryocytic Thrombocytopenia), the c-mpl gene is normal in TAR (937,938). However, because TAR is a true single cytopenia, without evolution to aplastic anemia or leukemia, the hematopoietic defect presumably involves only the megakaryocytic lineage.

THERAPY AND OUTCOME

Most infants with TAR have hemorrhagic manifestations, which they may outgrow after the first year of life. More than 40

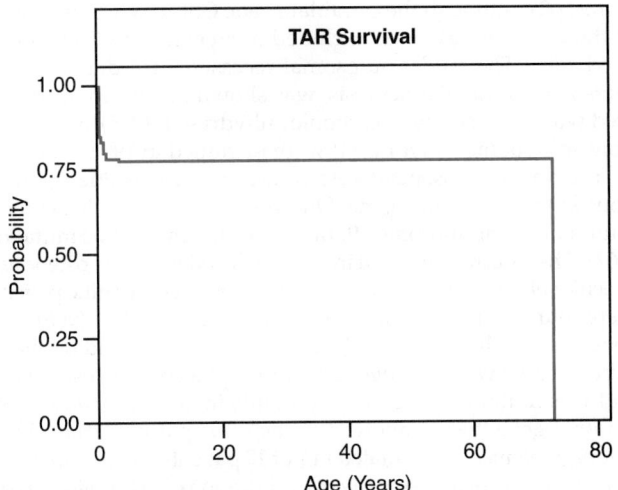

Figure 8-33. Kaplan-Meier plot of cumulative survival in thrombocytopenia–absent radius (TAR) syndrome. The plateau is approximately 75%, with the only death reported in a patient older than 4 years of age occurring in a 73-year-old patient with three different types of cancer.

Prenatal diagnosis was reported in more than two dozen cases. Absent radii may be diagnosed using radiography (943,944), ultrasonography (945), or fetoscopy (946,947). Because a few patients were reported with unilateral radial aplasia, both forearms must be examined. In one case, micrognathia was detected by ultrasonography (897). The diagnosis can be confirmed by a platelet count in fetal blood that is obtained by fetoscopy or cordocentesis (566,947,948). Seventy percent of the 28 fetuses studied so far were affected.

LEUKOERYTHROBLASTOSIS

Leukoerythroblastosis is the term that was suggested by Vaughan (949) in 1936 to describe "an anemia characterized by the presence in the peripheral blood of immature red cells and a few immature white cells of the myeloid series," that is, erythroblasts and leukoblasts. The RBCs are usually normochromic and normocytic, with poikilocytes, fragments, target cells, and teardrops. Giant platelets may also be seen. Leukoerythroblastosis must be distinguished from a *leukemoid reaction*, which is a reactive leukocytosis with an orderly progression of immature through mature myeloid cells. Another related term, *leukemic hiatus*, applies when the myeloid cells are immature and mature but without intermediate forms; thus, there is a gap or hiatus.

The disorders in which leukoerythroblastosis has been seen are outlined in Table 8-23, which is a composite of several large adult and pediatric series (950,951). The initial descriptions focused on the association with bone marrow invasion, particularly from metastatic solid tumors, hematologic malignancies, infections, or other marrow components, in which cells might be crowded out of the marrow prematurely (myelophthisis). Hypoxia from nonhematologic or hematologic causes might

deaths were reported (20%), 80% of which occurred in the first year of life. The projected survival curve is shown in Figure 8-33 and has a plateau of 75% survival by 4 years of age. Most deaths were from intracranial or gastrointestinal bleeding. The data cited here encompass 50 years of reports of TAR cases, many of whom received limited treatment. Patients who survive the perilous first year of life demonstrate an increase in platelet count to greater than 100,000/μL, which is adequate for the orthopedic surgical procedures that are needed for their arms and legs. Thrombocytopenia may recur during illnesses, but it usually is not severe. Dietary change may be helpful for those with milk allergy.

The most important therapy is platelet transfusions. These are provided during bleeding episodes or operations and are clearly indicated as prophylaxis for infants with severe symptomatic thrombocytopenia. Single donors should be used to reduce the risk of sensitization, and HLA-matched platelets can be obtained, if necessary. The platelet count should be maintained at more than 10,000 to 15,000/μL. The prediction is that the duration of this support is finite and short (less than 1 year). Other approaches have included splenectomy, corticosteroids, and androgens, all without apparent benefit. One adult showed a transient elevation of the platelet count after splenectomy (925). A small dose of prednisone might decrease the bleeding tendency at a given platelet count, and ε-aminocaproic acid may also be useful during bleeding episodes (see the section Treatment, in the section on Fanconi's anemia for details).

The leukemoid reaction and eosinophilia disappear during the first year of life in patients with TAR, although the high white-cell count has led to some infants being diagnosed with *congenital leukemia*. One patient was reported with acute lymphoblastic leukemia (939), one with stage D(S) neuroblastoma at birth who died at 3 months of age (940), and one who developed ileal adenocarcinoma at 67 year of age, ovarian cancer at 70 years of age, and bladder squamous cell carcinoma at 73 years of age (941).

Heroic treatments such as myelotoxic drugs or BMT are generally contraindicated, because spontaneous improvement occurs. One patient who had a life-threatening central nervous system hemorrhage was treated successfully by BMT (942). In general, this approach is excessive, and the prognosis for TAR patients is good.

TABLE 8-23. Conditions Associated with Leukoerythroblastosis

Marrow invasion
  Tumor
    Solid tumor with bone marrow metastases
    Lymphoma
    Hodgkin's disease
    Multiple myeloma
    Leukemia
    Neuroblastoma
    Preleukemia
  Infection
    Osteomyelitis
    Sepsis
    Tuberculosis
    Congenital
  Marrow components
    Osteopetrosis
    Storage disease
    Histiocytosis
    Vasculitis, including rheumatoid arthritis
Myeloproliferative disorders
  Polycythemia vera
  Myelofibrosis, myeloid metaplasia
  Down's syndrome, transient myeloproliferative disease
  Chronic myelogenous leukemia
  Erythroleukemia
  Thrombocythemia
Hematologic disease
  Erythroblastosis fetalis
  Pernicious anemia
  Thalassemia major
  Other hemolytic anemias
Hypoxia
  Cyanotic congenital heart disease
  Congestive heart failure
  Respiratory disease

also stimulate premature release of marrow cells. In myeloproliferative disorders, the premature release of nucleated cells might be related to the intrinsic abnormality of the cells. Diseases in which leukoerythroblastosis occurs are discussed in many other chapters in this book; this section is restricted to osteopetrosis.

Osteopetrosis

Osteopetrosis is a syndrome with three major forms: (a) infantile malignant autosomal recessive, (b) intermediate autosomal recessive, and (c) autosomal-dominant "marble bone disease," or Albers-Schönberg disease, which was first described in 1904 (952–954). The most severe form is diagnosed in infancy and early childhood, and is characterized by dense bones that fracture easily because of a defect in bone resorption. The patients have large heads, sclerotic bones, and hepatosplenomegaly, and they experience blindness, deafness, cranial nerve palsies, and pancytopenia. Many cases are familial, with a high degree of consanguinity. The disease may be severe *in utero*, because there is often a history of stillbirths and spontaneous abortions.

LABORATORY FINDINGS

The hematologic complications of osteopetrosis are severe, with components of leukoerythroblastosis including macrocytic anemia, reticulocytosis, teardrop RBCs, circulating erythroblasts, and leukocytosis with immature myeloid elements. One manifestation of the stress erythropoiesis that occurs is an increase in HbF (955). The marrow cavity is gradually narrowed by bone, and the diploic spaces are small. Bone marrow aspiration is difficult, and needles often break in attempts to penetrate the sclerotic bone. The marrow that remains is hypocellular and fibrotic. Osteoblasts, as well as osteoclasts, are increased (956). Hepatosplenomegaly develops because of extramedullary hematopoiesis. Hypersplenism follows and leads to thrombocytopenia, leukopenia, and hemolytic anemia due to extracorpuscular destruction of intrinsically normal erythrocytes (957).

PATHOPHYSIOLOGY

The osteoclasts are abnormal in osteopetrosis, as they are unable to resorb bone and produce the remodeling that occurs in normal bone. In experiments using osteopetrotic mice, Walker (958) showed that bone marrow or spleen cells from normal mice led to bone remodeling in osteopetrotic litter mates, and spleen cells from affected mice led to osteopetrosis in normal mice (959). Marrow transplantations that cured osteopetrosis and contained a cytoplasmic marker (giant lysosomes in Chédiak-Higashi mice) replaced recipient with donor osteoclasts (959). Similar studies using donors with defective erythropoiesis (W^e/W^v) indicated that the stem cell that gives rise to osteoclasts may be more primordial than the colony-forming unit spleen (960). Although osteopetrosis was cured and donor leukocytes and platelets were sustained, the defective donor erythrocytosis was replaced by the normal erythropoiesis of the recipient. Several laboratories have used *in vitro* studies to suggest that osteoclasts are derived from hematopoietic stem cells that are in the mononuclear light density fraction (961).

Hematopoiesis is intrinsically normal in osteopetrosis. The peripheral blood contains increased numbers of CFU-GM, BFU-E, and even CFU-E (normally found only in marrow), which may migrate from the crowded bone marrow cavity to sites of extramedullary hematopoiesis (962,963). Osteoclasts are numerically normal, morphologically normal or abnormal, and functionally abnormal.

Several genes have been found recently to be responsible for osteopetrosis. The autosomal-dominant form maps to chromosome 1p21, although the candidate gene CSF-1, which is mutant in the op/op mouse, was excluded in an extended Danish kindred (964). The milder autosomal-recessive disorder, in which there is renal tubular acidosis, was shown in 1985 to be associated with a deficiency of carbonic anhydrase II (965), and mutations in carbonic anhydrase II were identified in 1992 (966).

The severe autosomal-recessive osteopetrosis is due to mutations in more than one gene. One gene maps to 11q13, syntenic with mouse chromosome 19, the site of the murine oc mutation (967). The murine gene is Tcirg-1, which codes for the osteoclast-specific subunit of the vacuolar proton pump. Five of nine patients were found to have mutations in this gene, TCIRG1 (968). The gene is also called *OC116*, which is described as encoding the a3 subunit of the vacuolar adenosine triphosphatase from osteoclasts, and was mutant in five of ten patients in another study (969). Another gene that is involved in the same pathway, the CLC-7 chloride channel, was mutated in 1 of 12 patients and in mice (970). The disruption of the pathway of acidification of extracellular lysosome between osteoclasts and bone leads to a defect in bone degradation and severe osteopetrosis. Thus there are at least two genes that are responsible for the severe form of osteopetrosis.

THERAPY AND OUTCOME

Death usually occurs in infancy or early childhood in osteopetrosis patients; no patients have survived beyond 20 years of age. Most deaths are from the complications of bone marrow failure, infection, and hemorrhage. Circulating phagocytes, which may be derived from the same lineage as the osteoclasts, may function abnormally, leading to reduced host resistance to infection (971,972).

Symptomatic anemia and thrombocytopenia can be treated with transfusions of RBCs and platelets, although hypersplenism decreases the efficacy of such treatment. Splenectomy offers temporary improvement, but the rest of the reticuloendothelial system remains active and the primary bone disorder is not cured. Prednisone therapy was used in several patients, again with transient improvement, from decreased hypersplenism and reticuloendothelial suppression (971,973). Long-term therapy with interferon-γ was found to increase bone resorption and improve hematopoiesis, but did not provide a cure (974).

The only possible cure for osteopetrosis at this time is offered by BMT (975). More than 100 transplants have been done, with a 3-year probability of survival of 50% (976). In those situations in which a sex marker was found, the osteoclasts were of donor origin, whereas the osteoblasts remained host. Short-term follow-up indicated restoration of normal hematopoiesis, improvement of radiographic findings, and stabilization of physical changes. Long-term follow-up of nine Bedouin cases in a single center showed survival of four patients, with hematologic improvement but persistence of visual impairment (977), and, in another patient, progression of neurodegeneration after transplant with a 5/6 unrelated cord (978). Stem cell transplant must be done early, before the bony changes have encroached on hearing and vision.

Prenatal diagnosis by radiography was first performed in 1943 (979), although it was not always successful (980). More recently, increased bone density, fractures, macrocephaly, and hydrocephaly were detected by ultrasonography and confirmed by radiography (981,982). Linkage analysis was used in Bedouin families in which osteopetrosis was linked to 11q13; 3 of 12 patients were affected (983).

SUMMARY

The major inherited bone marrow failure disorders are summarized in Table 8-24. The diagnosis of acquired aplastic anemia

TABLE 8-24. Comparison of Inherited Bone Marrow Failure Syndromes

Feature	Fanconi's Anemia	Dyskeratosis Congenita	Shwachman-Diamond Syndrome	Amegakaryocytic Thrombocytopenia	Diamond-Blackfan Anemia	Severe Congenital Neutropenia	Thrombocytopenia–Absent Radius Syndrome
Number of cases	1200	275	340	75	700	300	225
Male to female ratio	1.2	4.5	1.6	1.1	1.1	1	0.8
Genetics	Autosomal recessive	X-linked, autosomal recessive and dominant	Autosomal recessive	Autosomal recessive	Autosomal recessive, dominant, or sporadic	Autosomal dominant and recessive	Autosomal recessive
Physical abnormalities (%)	~75	100	40	30	25	0	100
Hand and arm anomalies (%)	40	1	1	0	8	0	100
Median age at diagnosis of initial hematologic disease	8 yr	16 yr	<1 yr	~1 mo	2 mo	~1 mo	<1 wk
First hematologic manifestation	Pancytopenia	Pancytopenia	Neutropenia	Thrombocytopenia	Anemia	Neutropenia	Thrombocytopenia
Bone marrow	Aplastic	Aplastic	Hypocellular or myeloid arrest	Absent or small megakaryocytes	Erythroid hypoplasia	Promyelocyte arrest	Megakaryocytes absent or immature
Aplastic anemia (%)	>90	40	40	40	0	0	0
Leukemia (%)	9	0	7	3	1	9	0.4
Myelodysplastic syndrome (%)	6	1	9	0	0.3	5	0
Liver tumor (%)	3	0	0	0	0.3	0	0
Solid tumor (%)	5	14	0	0	2	0	0
Fetal hemoglobin	Increased	Increased	Increased	Increased	Increased	Normal	Normal
Chromosomes	Breaks increased with clastogens	Normal	Normal	Normal	Normal	Normal	Normal
Spontaneous remissions	Very rare	None	Very rare	None	15% to 25%	None	75%
Treatment; responses	Androgens; 50%, transient	Androgens; 50%, transient	Steroids or androgens; 50%, transient	None	Steroids; 60%, some transient	Granulocyte colony-stimulating factor; excellent	Platelets, as needed for <1 yr
Prognosis	Poor	Poor	Fair	Poor	Good	Good	Good
Prenatal diagnosis	Chromosomes, mutations	Mutations	Neutropenia	Thrombocytopenia, mutations	Anemia, adenosine deaminase, erythroid burst-forming unit, mutations	Neutropenia, mutations	Absent radii, thrombocytopenia
Projected median survival age	20 yr	33 yr	35 yr	7 yr	43 yr	23 yr	Older than 50 yr

should be made only after serious consideration of these inherited conditions. Physical anomalies may be absent, but family histories or specific tests (chromosome breakage or mutation analyses) may provide clues. The number of patients with each condition and the proportions with the cited complications *cannot* be construed as prevalence figures, because they are based on literature reports, not epidemiologic studies. Despite underreporting and underdiagnosis, the numbers do provide some perspective on these entities.

Most of the conditions that are discussed in this chapter and summarized in Table 8-24 are expressed in probable homozygotes (for autosomal recessives) or hemizygotes (X-linked), although a few are dominants. Because heterozygotes for recessive disorders cannot usually be identified (except as parents), patients with multiple bone marrow failure genes or those with apparently acquired diseases that may in fact be inherited cannot be defined at this time.

Treatment depends on diagnosis. Patients with pancytopenia due to Fanconi's anemia, dyskeratosis congenita, amegakaryocytic thrombocytopenia, or Shwachman-Diamond syndrome may respond to androgens. Those with Diamond-Blackfan anemia should receive corticosteroids, patients with SCN should receive G-CSF, and patients with TAR should receive platelets. BMT, particularly for those with Fanconi's anemia, requires modification of current preparative protocols; patients with DBA and TAR, which, respectively, may and do improve spontaneously, may not need transplantation at all.

In all cases in which transplantation is used, the donor must prove to be unaffected by the disease. Immunotherapy and growth factor treatment must be tailored for specific diseases. Risks of evolution of leukemia or other malignancies must be considered for all treatments, and those therapies with higher risk must be considered carefully in patients whose underlying condition is premalignant. Treatment of malignant complications is also difficult in inherited disorders in which abnormalities extend beyond hematopoietic tissues.

Prenatal diagnosis is possible for many of the inherited marrow failure disorders. Families at risk are usually identified through a proband, after which subsequent pregnancies may be monitored. Early diagnosis of an affected fetus may eventually permit treatment *in utero* or at birth. Diagnosis of a fetus that is not affected and is HLA-matched to the proband may provide placental blood for treatment by stem cell transplantation.

Much remains to be understood about the genetics, pathophysiology, and treatment of inherited and acquired aplastic anemia. This requires correct diagnoses, proper treatment, and careful follow-up. The prognoses for most of these disorders have improved with recent therapeutic advances, and it is anticipated that this improvement will accelerate with more knowledge of the specific molecular and cellular defects.

REFERENCES

1. O'Gorman Hughes DW. The varied pattern of aplastic anaemia in childhood. *Aust Paediatr J* 1966;2:228–236.
2. Alter BP, Potter NU, Li FP. Classification and aetiology of the aplastic anaemias. *Clin Haematol* 1978;7:431–465.
3. Windass B, Vowels MR, O'Gorman Hughes DW, et al. Aplastic anaemia in childhood: prognosis and approach to therapy. *Med J Aust* 1987;146:15–19.
4. Alter BP. The bone marrow failure syndromes. In: Nathan DG, Oski FA, eds. *Hematology of infancy and childhood*, 3rd ed. Philadelphia: WB Saunders, 1987:159–241.
5. Young NS, Alter BP. *Aplastic anemia: acquired and inherited*. Philadelphia: WB Saunders, 1994:410.
6. Alter BP, Young NS. The bone marrow failure syndromes. In: Nathan DG, Orkin SH, eds. *Hematology of infancy and childhood*. Philadelphia: WB Saunders, 1998:237–335.
7. Fanconi G. Familiare infantile perniziosaartige anamie (perniziöses blutbild und konstitution). *Jahrbuch fur Kinderheilkunde* 1927;117:257–289.
8. Uehlinger E. Konstitutionelle infantile (perniziosaartige) anamie. *Klin Wochenschr* 1929;32:1501–1503.
9. Fanconi G. Familial constitutional panmyelocytopathy, Fanconi's Anemia (F.A.). I. Clinical aspects. *Semin Hematol* 1967;4:233–240.
10. Shahidi NT. Fanconi anemia, dyskeratosis congenita, and WT syndrome. *Am J Med Genet* 1987;3[Suppl]:263–278.
11. Akar N, Gozdasoglu S. Spectrum of anomalies in Fanconi anaemia. *J Med Genet* 1984;21:75–76.
12. Auerbach AD, Rogatko A, Schroeder-Kurth TM. International Fanconi Anemia Registry: relation of clinical symptoms to diepoxybutane sensitivity. *Blood* 1989;73:391–396.
13. Estren S, Dameshek W. Familial hypoplastic anemia of childhood. Report of eight cases in two families with beneficial effect of splenectomy in one case. *Am J Dis Child* 1947;73:671–687.
14. Li FP, Potter NU. Classic Fanconi anemia in a family with hypoplastic anemia. *J Pediatr* 1978;92:943–944.
15. Glanz A, Fraser FC. Spectrum of anomalies in Fanconi anaemia. *J Med Genet* 1982;19:412–416.
16. Riley E, Caldwell R, Swift M. Comparison of clinical features in Fanconi anemia probands and their subsequently diagnosed siblings. *Am J Hum Genet* 1979;31:82A.
17. Schroeder TM, Tilgen D, Kruger J, et al. Formal genetics of Fanconi's anemia. *Hum Genet* 1976;32:257–288.
18. Rogatko A, Auerbach AD. Segregation analysis with uncertain ascertainment: application to Fanconi anemia. *Am J Hum Genet* 1988;42:889–897.
19. Rosendorff J, Bernstein R, Macdougall L, et al. Fanconi anemia: another disease of unusually high prevalence in the Afrikaans population of South Africa. *Am J Med Genet* 1987;27:793–797.
20. Verlander PC, Kaporis A, Liu Q, et al. Carrier frequency of the IVS4 + 4 A-T mutation of the Fanconi anemia gene FAC in the Ashkenazi Jewish population. *Blood* 1995;86:4034–4038.
21. Skikne BS, Lynch SR, Bezwoda WR, et al. Fanconi's anaemia, with special reference to erythrokinetic features. *S Afr Med J* 1978;53:43–50.
22. Altay C, Sevgi Y, Pirnar T. Fanconi's anemia in offspring of patient with congenital radial and carpal hypoplasia. *N Engl J Med* 1975;293:151–152.
23. Petridou M, Barrett AJ. Physical and laboratory characteristics of heterozygote carriers of the Fanconi aplasia gene. *Acta Paediatr Scand* 1990;79:1069–1074.
24. Welshimer K, Swift M. Congenital malformations and developmental disabilities in ataxia-telangiectasia, Fanconi anemia, and xeroderma pigmentosum families. *Am J Hum Genet* 1982;34:781–793.
25. Gershanik JJ, Morgan SK, Akers R. Fanconi's anemia in a neonate. *Acta Paediatr Scand* 1972;61:623–625.
26. Perkins J, Timson J, Emery AE. Clinical and chromosome studies in Fanconi's aplastic anaemia. *J Med Genet* 1969;6:28–33.
27. Reinhold JD, Neumark E, Lightwood R, et al. Familial hypoplastic anemia with congenital abnormalities (Fanconi's syndrome). *Blood* 1952;7:915–926.
28. O'Neill EM, Varadi S. Neonatal aplastic anaemia and Fanconi's anaemia. *Arch Dis Child* 1963;38:92–94.
29. Nilsson LR. Chronic pancytopenia with multiple congenital abnormalities (Fanconi's anaemia). *Acta Paediatr* 1960;49:518–529.
30. Cassimos C, Zannos L. Congenital hypoplastic anemia associated with multiple developmental defects (Fanconi's syndrome). *Am J Dis Child* 1952;84:347–350.
31. Beard ME, Young DE, Bateman CJ, et al. Fanconi's anaemia. *QJM* 1973;42:403–422.
32. Dacie JV, Gilpin A. Refractory anaemia (Fanconi type). Its incidence in three members of one family, with in one case a relationship to chronic haemolytic anaemia with nocturnal haemoglobinuria (Marchiafava-Micheli disease or 'nocturnal haemoglobinuria'). *Arch Dis Child* 1944;19:155–162.
33. Varela MA, Sternberg WH. Preanaemic state in Fanconi's anaemia. *Lancet* 1967;2:566–567.
34. Pignatti CB, Bianchi E, Polito E. Fanconi's anaemia in infancy: report of a case diagnosed in the preanaemic stage. *Helv Paediatr Acta* 1977;32:413–418.
35. McIntosh S, Breg WR, Lubiniecki AS. Fanconi's anemia. The preanemic phase. *Am J Pediatr Hematol Oncol* 1979;1:107–110.
36. Schroeder TM, Pohler E, Hufnagl HD, et al. Fanconi's anemia: terminal leukemia and "forme fruste" in one family. *Clin Genet* 1979;16:260–268.
37. Jalbert PP, Leger J, Bost M, et al. L'anemie de Fanconi: aspects cytogenetiques et biochimiques. A propos d'une famille. *Nouv Rev Fr Hematol* 1975;15:551–566.
38. Shahidi NT, Gerald PS, Diamond LK. Alkali-resistant hemoglobin in aplastic anemia of both acquired and congenital types. *N Engl J Med* 1962;266:117–120.
39. Jones R. Fanconi anemia: simultaneous onset of symptoms in two siblings. *J Pediatr* 1976;88:152.
40. De Vroede M, Feremans W, De Maertelaere-Laurent E, et al. Fanconi's anaemia. Simultaneous onset in 2 siblings and unusual cytological findings. *Scand J Haematol* 1982;28:431–440.
41. Silver HK, Blair WC, Kempe CH. Fanconi syndrome. Multiple congenital anomalies with hypoplastic anemia. *Am J Dis Child* 1952;83:14–25.
42. Voss R, Kohn G, Shaham M, et al. Prenatal diagnosis of Fanconi anemia. *Clin Genet* 1981;20:185–190.
43. Gotz M, Pichler E. Zur panmyelopathie im kindesalter. *Klin Paediatr* 1972;148:377–384.
44. Romero MG, Ortiz HC. Anemia de Fanconi. Respuesta a dosis bajas de anabolicos y asociacion con carcinoma de esofago. *Rev Invest Clin* 1984;36:353–356.

45. Schroeder TM, Drings P, Beilner P, et al. Clinical and cytogenetic observations during a six-year period in an adult with Fanconi's anaemia. *Blut* 1976;34:119–132.

46. Althoff H. Zur panmyelopathie fanconi als zustandsbild multipler abartungen. *Z Kinderheilk* 1953;72:267–292.

47. Alter BP. Fetal erythropoiesis in stress hematopoiesis. *Exp Hematol* 1979;7:200–209.

48. Alter BP. Fetal erythropoiesis in bone marrow failure syndromes. In: Stamatoyannopoulos G, Neinhuis AW, eds. *Cellular and molecular regulation of hemoglobin switching.* New York: Grune & Stratton, 1979;87–105.

49. Shepard MK, Weatherall DJ, Conley CL. Semi-quantitative estimation of the distribution of fetal hemoglobin in red cell populations. *Bull Johns Hopkins Hosp* 1962;110:293–310.

50. Dell'Orbo C, Arico M, Podesta A, et al. Fanconi's anemia: ultrastructural observations on erythroblasts. *Ultrastruct Pathol* 1983;4:145–150.

51. Chu JY, Ho JE, Monteleone PL, et al. Technetium colloid bone marrow imaging in Fanconi's anemia. *Pediatrics* 1979;64:635–639.

52. de Grouchy J, de Nava C, Marchand JC, et al. Etudes cytogenetique et biochimique de huit cas d'anemie de Fanconi. *Ann Genet* 1972;15:29–40.

53. Lohr GW, Waller HD, Anschutz F, et al. Hexokinasemangel in blutzellen bei einer sippe mit familiarer panmyelopathie (Typ Fanconi). *Klin Wochenschr* 1965;43:870–875.

54. Magnani M, Novelli G, Stocchi V, et al. Red blood cell hexokinase in Fanconi's anemia. *Acta Haematol* 1984;71:341–344.

55. Pochedly C, Colipp PJ, Wolman SR, et al. Fanconi's anemia with growth hormone deficiency. *J Pediatr* 1971;79:93–96.

56. Costin G, Kogut MD, Hyman CB, et al. Fanconi's anemia associated with isolated growth hormone (GH) deficiency. *Clin Res* 1972;20:253A.

57. Schonberg D. Plasma growth hormone in cerebral gigantism, Laurence-Moon-Bardet-Biedl syndrome, Bloom syndrome and Fanconi anemia. *Acta Paediatr Scand* 1973;62:111A.

58. Schettini P, Cavallo L. Deficit di ormone somatotropo nell'anemia di Fanconi. *Haematologica* 1988;58:800–802.

59. Prindull G, Jentsch E, Hansmann I. Fanconi's anaemia developing erythroleukaemia. *Scand J Haematol* 1979;23:59–63.

60. Zachmann M, Illig R, Prader A. Fanconi's anemia with isolated growth hormone deficiency. *J Pediatr* 1972;80:159–160.

61. Clarke WL, Weldon VV. Growth hormone deficiency and Fanconi anemia. *J Pediatr* 1975;86:814–815.

62. Gleadhill V, Bridges JM, Hadden DR. Fanconi's aplastic anaemia with short stature. Absence of response to human growth hormone. *Arch Dis Child* 1975;50:318–320.

63. Hayashi K, Schmid W. The rate of sister chromatid exchanges parallel to spontaneous chromosome breakage in Fanconi's anemia and to Trenimon-induced aberrations in human lymphocytes and fibroblasts. *Hum Genet* 1975;29:201–206.

64. Stubbe P, Prindull G. Fanconi's anemia. II. Are multiple endocrine insufficiencies a substantial part of the disease? *Acta Paediatr Scand* 1975;64:790–794.

65. Aynsley-Green A, Zachmann M, Werder EA, et al. Endocrine studies in Fanconi's anaemia. Report of 4 cases. *Arch Dis Child* 1978;53:126–131.

66. Nordan UZ, Humbert JR, MacGillivray MH, et al. Fanconi's anemia with growth hormone deficiency. *Am J Dis Child* 1979;133:291–293.

67. Wada E, Murata M, Watanabe S. Acute lymphoblastic leukemia following treatment by human growth hormone in a boy with possible preanemic Fanconi's anemia. *Jpn J Clin Oncol* 1989;19:36–39.

68. Standen GR, Hughes IA, Geddes AD, et al. Myelodysplastic syndrome with trisomy 8 in an adolescent with Fanconi anaemia and selective IgA deficiency. *Am J Hematol* 1989;31:280–283.

69. Cameron ES, Alleyne W, Charles W. Fanconi's aplastic anemia in two sisters in Trinidad and Tobago. *West Indian Med J* 1989;38:118–119.

70. Schoof E, Beck JD, Joenje H, et al. Growth hormone deficiency in one of two siblings with Fanconi's anaemia complementation group FA-D. *Growth Horm IGF Res* 2000;10:290–293.

71. Dupuis-Girod S, Gluckman E, Souberbielle JC, et al. Growth hormone deficiency caused by pituitary stalk interruption in Fanconi's anemia. *J Pediatr* 2001;138:129–133.

72. Berkovitz GD, Zinkham WH, Migeon CJ. Gonadal function in two siblings with Fanconi's anemia. *Horm Res* 1984;19:137–141.

73. Shapiro P, Ikeda RM, Ruebner BH, et al. Multiple hepatic tumors and peliosis hepatis in Fanconi's anemia treated with androgens. *Am J Dis Child* 1977;131:1104–1106.

74. Schiavulli E, Gabriele S. Anemia di Fanconi. *Minerva Pediatr* 1978;30:1251–1258.

75. Wajnrajch MP, Gertner JM, Huma Z, et al. Evaluation of growth and hormonal status in patients referred to the International Fanconi Anemia Registry. *Pediatrics* 2001;107:744–754.

76. Fisher DA, Job JC, Preece M, et al. Leukaemia in patients treated with growth hormone. *Lancet* 1988;1:1159–1160.

77. Blethen SL. Leukemia in children treated with growth hormone. *Trends Endocrinol Metab* 1998;9:367–370.

78. Schroeder TM, Anschutz F, Knopp A. Spontane chromosomenaberrationen bei familiarer panmyelopathie. *Humangenetik* 1964;1:194–196.

79. Swift MR, Hirschhorn K. Fanconi's anemia. Inherited susceptibility to chromosome breakage in various tissues. *Ann Intern Med* 1966;65:496–503.

80. Schmid W, Scharer K, Baumann T, et al. Chromosomenbruchigkeit bei der familiaren panmyelopathie (Typus Fanconi). *Schweiz Med Wochenschr* 1965;43:1461–1464.

81. Bloom GE, Warner S, Gerald PS, et al. Chromosome abnormalities in constitutional aplastic anemia. *N Engl J Med* 1966;274:8–14.

82. German J, Pugliatti Crippa L. Chromosomal breakage in diploid cell lines from Bloom's syndrome and Fanconi's anemia. *Ann Genet* 1966;9:143–154.

83. Bloom GE. Disorders of bone marrow production. *Pediatr Clin North Am* 1972;19:983–1008.

84. Gmyrek D, Witkowski R, Syllm-Rapoport I, et al. Chromosomal aberrations and abnormalities of red-cell metabolism in a case of Fanconi's anaemia before and after development of leukaemia. *Ger Med Mon* 1968;13:105–111.

85. Wolman SR, Swift M. Bone marrow chromosomes in Fanconi's anemia. *J Med Genet* 1972;9:473–474.

86. Shahid MJ, Khouri FP, Ballas SK. Fanconi's anaemia: report of a patient with significant chromosomal abnormalities in bone marrow cells. *J Med Genet* 1972;9:474–478.

87. Berger R, Bernheim A, Le Coniat M, et al. Chromosomal studies of leukemic and preleukemic Fanconi's anemia patients. Examples of acquired chromosomal amplification. *Hum Genet* 1980;56:59–62.

88. Schroeder TM, Kurth R. Spontaneous chromosomal breakage and high incidence of leukemia in inherited disease. *Blood* 1971;37:96–112.

89. Todaro GJ, Green H, Swift MR. Susceptibility of human diploid fibroblast strains to transformation by SV40 virus. *Science* 1966;153:1252–1254.

90. Higurashi M, Conen PE. In vitro chromosomal radiosensitivity in Fanconi's anemia. *Blood* 1971;38:336–342.

91. Sasaki MS, Tonomura A. A high susceptibility of Fanconi's anemia to chromosome breakage by DNA cross-linking agents. *Cancer Res* 1973;33:1829–1836.

92. Auerbach AD, Adler B, O'Reilly RJ, et al. Effect of procarbazine and cyclophosphamide on chromosome breakage in Fanconi anemia cells: relevance to bone marrow transplantation. *Cancer Genet Cytogenet* 1983;9:25–36.

93. Auerbach AD, Wolman SR. Susceptibility of Fanconi's anaemia fibroblasts to chromosome damage by carcinogens. *Nature* 1976;261:494–496.

94. Berger R, Bernheim A, Le Coniat M, et al. Nitrogen mustard-induced chromosome breakage: a tool for Fanconi's anemia diagnosis. *Cancer Genet Cytogenet* 1980;2:269–274.

95. Cervenka J, Arthur D, Yasis C. Mitomycin C test for diagnostic differentiation of idiopathic aplastic anemia and Fanconi anemia. *Pediatrics* 1981;67:119–127.

96. Poll EH, Arwert F, Joenje H, et al. Cytogenetic toxicity of antitumor platinum compound in Fanconi's anemia. *Hum Genet* 1982;61:228–230.

97. Chaganti RS, Schonberg S, German J. A many fold increase in sister chromatid exchanges in Bloom's syndrome lymphocytes. *Proc Natl Acad Sci U S A* 1974;71:4508–4512.

98. Auerbach AD, Alter BP. Prenatal and postnatal diagnosis of aplastic anemia. In: Alter BP, ed. *Methods in hematology: perinatal hematology.* Edinburgh, Scotland: Churchill Livingstone, 1989;225–251.

99. Arwert F, Kwee ML. Chromosomal breakage in response to cross-linking agents in the diagnosis of Fanconi anemia. In: Schroeder-Kurth TM, Auerbach AD, eds. *Fanconi anemia: clinical, cytogenetic and experimental aspects.* Berlin: Springer-Verlag, 1989;83–92.

100. Kaiser TN, Lojewski A, Dougherty C, et al. Flow cytometric characterization of the response of Fanconi's anemia cells to mitomycin C treatment. *Cytometry* 1982;2:291–297.

101. Miglierina R, Le Coniat M, Berger R. A simple diagnostic test for Fanconi anemia by flow cytometry. *Anal Cell Pathol* 1991;3:111–118.

102. Arkin S, Brodtman D, Alter BP, et al. A screening test for Fanconi anemia using flow cytometry. *Blood* 1993;82:176a.

103. Seyschab H, Friedl R, Sun Y, et al. Comparative evaluation of diepoxybutane sensitivity and cell cycle blockage in the diagnosis of Fanconi anemia. *Blood* 1995;85:2233–2237.

104. Heinrich MC, Hoatlin ME, Zigler AJ, et al. DNA cross-linker–induced G2/M arrest in group C Fanconi anemia lymphoblasts reflects normal checkpoint function. *Blood* 1998;91:275–287.

105. Auerbach AD, Sagi M, Adler B. Fanconi anemia: prenatal diagnosis in 30 fetuses at risk. *Pediatrics* 1985;76:794–800.

106. Auerbach AD, Liu Q, Ghosh R, et al. Prenatal identification of potential donors for umbilical cord blood transplantation for Fanconi anemia. *Transfusion* 1990;30:682–687.

107. Shipley J, Rodeck CH, Garrett C, et al. Mitomycin C induced chromosome damage in fetal blood cultures and prenatal diagnosis of Fanconi's anaemia. *Prenat Diagn* 1984;4:217–221.

108. Trunca C, Watson M, Auerbach A, et al. Prenatal diagnosis of Fanconi anemia in a fetus not known to be at risk. *Am J Hum Genet* 1984;36:198S.

109. Boue PJ, Deluchat C, Nicolas H, et al. Diagnostic prenatal des maladies geniques sur villosites choriales. *J Genet Hum* 1986;34:221–233.

110. Hirsch-Kauffmann M, Schweiger M, Wagner EF, et al. Deficiency of DNA ligase activity in Fanconi's anemia. *Hum Genet* 1978;45:25–32.

111. Cohen MM, Simpson SJ, Honig GR, et al. The identification of Fanconi anemia genotypes by clastogenic stress. *Am J Hum Genet* 1982;34:794–810.

112. Kubbies M, Schindler D, Hoehn H, et al. Endogenous blockage and delay of the chromosome cycle despite normal recruitment and growth phase explain poor proliferation and frequent endomitosis in Fanconi anemia cells. *Am J Hum Genet* 1985;37:1022–1030.

113. Schindler D, Hoehn H. Fanconi anemia mutation causes cellular susceptibility to ambient oxygen. *Am J Hum Genet* 1988;43:429–435.

114. Korkina LG, Samochatova EV, Maschan AA, et al. Release of active oxygen radicals by leukocytes of Fanconi anemia patients. *J Leukoc Biol* 1992;52:357–362.

115. Gille JJP, Wortelboer HM, Joenje H. Antioxidant status of Fanconi anemia fibroblasts. *Hum Genet* 1987;77:28–31.
116. Joenje H, Frants RR, Arwert F, et al. Erythrocyte superoxide dismutase deficiency in Fanconi's anaemia established by two independent methods of assay. *Scand J Clin Lab Invest* 1979;39:759–764.
117. Mavelli I, Ciriolo MR, Rotilio G, et al. Superoxide dismutase, glutathione peroxidase and catalase in oxidative hemolysis. A study of Fanconi's anemia erythrocytes. *Biochem Biophys Res Commun* 1982;106:286–290.
118. Bigelow SB, Rary JM, Bender MA. G2 chromosomal radiosensitivity in Fanconi's anemia. *Mutat Res* 1979;63:189–199.
119. Rosselli F, Sanceau J, Gluckman E, et al. Abnormal lymphokine production: a novel feature of the genetic disease Fanconi anemia. II. In vitro and in vivo spontaneous overproduction of tumor necrosis factor. *Blood* 1994;5:1216–1225.
120. Takeuchi T, Morimoto K. Increased formation of 8-hydroxydeoxyguanosine, an oxidative DNA damage, in lymphoblasts from Fanconi's anemia patients due to possible catalase deficiency. *Carcinogenesis* 1993;14:1115–1120.
121. Fujiwara Y, Tatsumi M, Sasaki MS. Cross-link repair in human cells and its possible defect in Fanconi's anemia cells. *J Mol Biol* 1977;113:635–649.
122. Papadopoulo D, Guillouf C, Mohrenweiser H, et al. Hypomutability in Fanconi anemia cells is associated with increased deletion frequency at the HPRT locus. *Proc Natl Acad Sci U S A* 1990;87:8383–8387.
123. Willingale-Theune J, Schweiger M, Hirsch-Kauffmann M, et al. Ultrastructure of Fanconi anemia fibroblasts. *J Cell Sci* 1989;93:651–665.
124. Kupfer GM, D'Andrea AD. The effect of the Fanconi anemia polypeptide, FAC, upon p53 induction and G2 checkpoint regulation. *Blood* 1996;88:1019–1025.
125. Wang J, Otsuki T, Youssoufian H, et al. Overexpression of the Fanconi anemia group C gene (FAC) protects hematopoietic progenitors from death induced by Fas-mediated apoptosis. *Cancer Res* 1998;58:3538–3541.
126. Rosselli F, Ridet A, Soussi T, et al. P53-dependent pathway of radio-induced apoptosis is altered in Fanconi anemia. *Oncogene* 1995;10:9–17.
127. Saunders EF, Freedman MH. Constitutional aplastic anaemia: defective haematopoietic stem cell growth in vitro. *Br J Haematol* 1978;40:277–287.
128. Daneshbod-Skibba G, Martin J, Shahidi NT. Myeloid and erythroid colony growth in non-anemic patients with Fanconi's anaemia. *Br J Haematol* 1980; 44:33–38.
129. Lui VK, Ragab AH, Findley HS, et al. Bone marrow cultures in children with Fanconi anemia and the TAR syndrome. *J Pediatr* 1977;91:952–954.
130. Alter BP, Knobloch ME, Weinberg RS. Erythropoiesis in Fanconi's anemia. *Blood* 1991;78:602–608.
131. Alter BP, Knobloch ME, He L, et al. Effect of stem cell factor on in vitro erythropoiesis in patients with bone marrow failure syndromes. *Blood* 1992;80: 3000–3008.
132. Stark R, Thierry D, Richard P, et al. Long-term bone marrow culture in Fanconi's anaemia. *Br J Haematol* 1993;83:554–559.
133. Martinez-Jaramillo G, Espinoza-Hernandez L, Benitez-Aranda H, et al. Long-term proliferation in vitro of hematopoietic progenitor cells from children with congenital bone marrow failure: effect of Rh GM-CSF and Rh EPO. *Eur J Haematol* 2000;64:173–181.
134. Whitney MA, Royle G, Low MJ, et al. Germ cell defects and hematopoietic hypersensitivity to gamma-interferon in mice with a targeted disruption of the Fanconi anemia C gene. *Blood* 1996;88:49–58.
135. D'Andrea AD, Grompe M. Molecular biology of Fanconi anemia: implications for diagnosis and therapy. *Blood* 1997;90:1725–1736.
136. Digweed M, Gunthert U, Schneider R, et al. Irreversible repression of DNA synthesis in Fanconi anemia cells is alleviated by the product of a novel cyclin-related gene. *Mol Cell Biol* 1995;15:305–314.
137. Kupfer GM, Yamashita T, Naf D, et al. The Fanconi anemia polypeptide, FAC, binds to the cyclin-dependent kinase, cdc2. *Blood* 1997;90:1047–1054.
138. Gluckman E, Devergie A, Dutreix J. Radiosensitivity in Fanconi anaemia: application to the conditioning regimen for bone marrow transplantation. *Br J Haematol* 1983;54:431–440.
139. Escarceller M, Buchwald M, Singleton BK, et al. Fanconi anemia C gene product plays a role in the fidelity of blunt DNA end-joining. *J Mol Biol* 1998;297:375–385.
140. Smith J, Andrau JC, Kallenbach S, et al. Abnormal rearrangements associated with V(D)J recombination in Fanconi anemia. *J Mol Biol* 1998;281:815–825.
141. Thyagarajan B, Campbell C. Elevated homologous recombination activity in Fanconi anemia fibroblasts. *J Biol Chem* 1997;272:23328–23333.
142. Stark R, Andre C, Thierry D, et al. The expression of cytokine and cytokine receptor genes in long-term bone marrow culture in congenital and acquired bone marrow hypoplasias. *Br J Haematol* 1993;83:560–566.
143. Yoshida MC. Suppression of spontaneous and mitomycin C-induced chromosome aberrations in Fanconi's anemia by cell fusion with human fibroblasts. *Hum Genet* 1980;55:223–226.
144. Duckworth-Rysiecki G, Cornish K, Clarke CA, et al. Identification of two complementation groups in Fanconi anemia. *Somatic Cell Mol Genet* 1985;11: 35–41.
145. Zakrzewski S, Sperling K. Genetic heterogeneity of Fanconi's anemia demonstrated by somatic cell hybrids. *Hum Genet* 1980;56:81–84.
146. Zakrzewski S, Sperling K. Analysis of heterogeneity in Fanconi's anemia patients of different ethnic origin. *Hum Genet* 1982;62:321–323.
147. Zakrzewski S, Koch M, Sperling K. Complementation studies between Fanconi's anemia cells with different DNA repair characteristics. *Hum Genet* 1983;64:55–57.
148. Yoshida MC. The absence of genetic heterogeneity in Fanconi's anemia in five patients demonstrated by somatic cell hybridization. *Cytogenet Cell Genet* 1982;32:329–330.
149. Buchwald M. Complementation groups: one or more per gene? *Nat Genet* 1995;11:228–230.
150. Joenje H, Oostra AB, Wijker M, et al. Evidence for at least eight Fanconi anemia genes. *Am J Hum Genet* 1997;61:940–944.
151. Joenje H, Levitus M, Waisfisz Q, et al. Complementation analysis in Fanconi anemia: assignment of the reference FA-H patient to group A. *Am J Hum Genet* 2000;67:759–762.
152. Faivre L, Guardiola P, Lewis C, et al. Association of complementation group and mutation type with clinical outcome in Fanconi anemia. *Blood* 2000;96:4064–4070.
153. Lo Ten Foe JR, Rooimans MA, Bosnoyan-Collins L, et al. Expression cloning of a cDNA for the major Fanconi anaemia gene, FAA. *Nat Genet* 1996;14:320–323.
154. Strathdee CA, Gavish H, Shannon WR, et al. Cloning of cDNAs for Fanconi's anaemia by functional complementation. *Nature* 1992;356:763–767.
155. Timmers C, Taniguchi T, Hejna J, et al. Positional cloning of a novel Fanconi anemia gene, FANCD2. *Mol Cell* 2001;7:241–248.
156. de Winter JP, Leveille F, van Berkel CGM, et al. Isolation of a cDNA representing the Fanconi anemia complementation group E gene. *Am J Hum Genet* 2000;67:1306–1308.
157. de Winter JP, Rooimans MA, van der Weel L, et al. The Fanconi anaemia gene FANCF encodes a novel protein with homology to ROM. *Nat Genet* 2000;24:15–16.
158. de Winter JP, Waisfisz Q, Rooimans MA, et al. The Fanconi anaemia group G gene FANCG is identical with XRCC9. *Nat Genet* 1998;20:281–283.
159. The Fanconi Anemia/Breast Cancer Consortium. Positional cloning of the Fanconi anaemia group A gene. *Nat Genet* 1996;14:324–328.
160. Liu N, Lamerdin JE, Tucker JD, et al. The human XRCC9 gene corrects chromosomal instability and mutagen sensitivities in CHO UV40 cells. *Proc Natl Acad Sci U S A* 1997;94:9232–9237.
161. Gibson RA, Ford D, Jansen S, et al. Genetic mapping of the FACC gene and linkage analysis in Fanconi anaemia families. *J Med Genet* 1994;31:868–871.
162. Whitney MA, Saito H, Jakobs PM, et al. A common mutation in the FACC gene causes Fanconi anemia in Ashkenazi Jews. *Nat Genet* 1993;4:202–205.
163. Levran O, Erlich T, Magdalena N, et al. Sequence variation in the Fanconi anemia gene FAA. *Proc Natl Acad Sci U S A* 1997;94:13051–13056.
164. Kupfer G, Naf D, Garcia-Higuera I, et al. A patient-derived mutant form of the Fanconi anemia protein, FANCA, is defective in nuclear accumulation. *Exp Hematol* 1999;27:587–593.
165. Demuth I, Wlodarski M, Tipping AJ, et al. Spectrum of mutations in the Fanconi anaemia group G gene, FANCG/XRCC9. *Eur J Hum Genet* 2000;8:861–868.
166. D'Andrea AD. Fanconi anaemia forges a novel pathway. *Nat Genet* 1996;14:240–242.
167. Yamashita T, Kupfer GM, Naf D, et al. The Fanconi anemia pathway requires FAA phosphorylation and FAA/FAC nuclear accumulation. *Proc Natl Acad Sci U S A* 1998;95:13085–13090.
168. Kupfer GM, Naf D, Suliman A, et al. The Fanconi anaemia proteins, FAA and FAG, interact to form a nuclear complex. *Nat Genet* 1997;17:487–490.
169. Garcia-Higuera I, Kuang Y, Naf D, et al. Fanconi anemia proteins FANCA, FANCC, and FANCG/XRCC9 interact in a functional nuclear complex. *Mol Cell Biol* 1999;19:4866–4873.
170. Garcia-Higuera I, D'Andrea AD. Regulated binding of the Fanconi anemia proteins, FANCA and FANCC. *Blood* 1999;93:1430–1432.
171. Garcia-Higuera I, Kuang Y, Hagan R, et al. Overexpression of the Fanconi anemia protein, FANCA, functionally complements a Fanconi anemia group H cell line. *Blood* 1999;94:414a.
172. Garcia-Higuera I, Kuang Y, Denham J, et al. The Fanconi anemia proteins FANCA and FANCG stabilize each other and promote the nuclear accumulation of the Fanconi anemia complex. *Blood* 2000;96:3224–3230.
173. Medhurst AL, Huber PAJ, Waisfisz Q, et al. Direct interactions of the five known Fanconi anaemia proteins suggest a common functional pathway. *Hum Mol Genet* 2001;10:423–429.
174. Garcia-Higuera I, Taniguchi T, Ganesan S, et al. Interaction of the Fanconi anemia proteins and BRCA1 in a common pathway. *Mol Cell* 2001;7:1–20.
175. Scully R, Chen J, Plug A, et al. Association of BRCA1 with rad51 in mitotic and meiotic cells. *Cell* 1997;88:265–275.
176. Wu X, Petrini JH, Heine WF, et al. Independence of R/M/N focus formation and the presence of intact BRCA1. *Science* 2000;289:11a.
176a. Howlett NG, Taniguchi T, Olson S, et al. Biallelic inactivation of BRCA2 in Fanconi anemia. *Science* 2202;297:606–609.
176b. Taniguchi T, Garcea-Higuera I, Xu B, et al. Covergence of the Fanconi anemia and ataxia telangiectasia signaling pathways. *Cell* 2002;109:459–472.
177. Verlander PC, Lin JD, Udono MU, et al. Mutation analysis of the Fanconi anemia gene FACC. *Am J Hum Genet* 1994;54:595–601.
178. Wijker M, Morgan NV, Herterich S, et al. Heterogeneous spectrum of mutations in the Fanconi anaemia group A gene. *Eur J Hum Genet* 1999;7:52–59.
179. Gillio AP, Verlander PC, Batish SD, et al. Phenotypic consequences of mutations in the Fanconi anemia FAC gene: an International Fanconi Anemia Registry study. *Blood* 1997;90:105–110.
180. Futaki M, Yamashita T, Yagasaki H, et al. The IVS4 +4 A to T mutation of the Fanconi anemia gene FANCC is not associated with a severe phenotype in Japanese patients. *Blood* 2000;95:1493–1498.
181. Pulsipher M, Kupfer GM, Naf D, et al. Subtyping analysis of Fanconi anemia by immunoblotting and retroviral gene transfer. *Mol Med* 1998;4:468–479.

182. Lo Ten Foe JR, Kwee ML, Rooimans MA, et al. Somatic mosaicism in Fanconi anemia: molecular basis and clinical significance. *Eur J Hum Genet* 1997; 5:137–148.

183. Gregory JJ Jr, Wagner JE, Verlander PC, et al. Somatic mosaicism in Fanconi anemia: evidence of genotypic reversion in lymphohematopoietic stem cells. *Proc Natl Acad Sci U S A* 2001;98:2532–2537.

184. Waisfisz Q, Morgan NV, Savino M, et al. Spontaneous functional correction of homozygous Fanconi anaemia alleles reveals novel mechanistic basis for reverse mosaicism. *Nat Genet* 1999;22:379–383.

185. MacMillan ML, Auerbach AD, DeFor TE, et al. Somatic lymphocyte mosaicism is predictive of graft failure (GF) in patients with Fanconi anemia (FA) transplanted with alternate donor hematopoietic cells. Paper presented at: 11th Annual International Fanconi Anemia Scientific Symposium; December 1999.

186. Mori PG, Priolo M, Lerone M, et al. Congenital hypoplastic anaemia in a patient with a new multiple congenital anomalies-mental retardation syndrome. *Am J Med Genet* 1999;87:36–39.

187. Chen M, Tomkins DJ, Querbach W, et al. Inactivation of Fac in mice produces inducible chromosomal instability and reduced fertility reminiscent of Fanconi anaemia. *Nat Genet* 1996;12:448–451.

188. Cheng NC, van de Vrugt HJ, van der Valk MA, et al. Mice with a targeted disruption of the Fanconi anemia homolog Fanca. *Hum Mol Genet* 2000; 9:1805–1811.

189. Haneline LS, Gobbett TA, Ramani R, et al. Loss of FancC function results in decreased hematopoietic stem cell repopulating ability. *Blood* 1999;94:1–8.

190. Battaile KP, Bateman RL, Mortimer D, et al. In vivo selection of wild-type hematopoietic stem cells in a murine model of Fanconi anemia. *Blood* 1999;94:2151–2158.

191. Carreau M, Gan OI, Liu L, et al. Hematopoietic compartment of Fanconi anemia group C null mice contains fewer lineage-negative CD34+ primitive cells and shows reduced reconstitution ability. *Exp Hematol* 1999;27:1667–1674.

192. Walsh CE, Grompe M, Vanin E, et al. A functionally active retrovirus vector for gene therapy in Fanconi anemia group C. *Blood* 1994;84:453–459.

193. Gush KA, Fu K, Grompe M, et al. Phenotypic correction of Fanconi anemia group C knockout mice. *Blood* 2000;95:700–704.

194. Fu KL, Lo Ten Foe JR, Joenje H, et al. Functional correction of Fanconi anemia group A hematopoietic cells by retroviral gene transfer. *Blood* 1997;90: 3296–3303.

195. Goossens V, Sermon K, Lissens W, et al. Clinical application of preimplantation genetic diagnosis for cystic fibrosis. *Prenat Diagn* 2000;20:571–581.

196. Ray PF, Harper JC, Ao A, et al. Successful preimplantation genetic diagnosis for sex linked Lesch-Nyhan syndrome using specific diagnosis. *Prenat Diagn* 1999;19:1237–1241.

197. Bernard J, Mathé G, Najean Y. Contribution á l'étude clinique et physiopathologique de la maladie de Fanconi. *Rev Franc Etudes Clin Biol* 1958;3:599–612.

198. Dawson JP. Congenital pancytopenia associated with multiple congenital anomalies (Fanconi type). *Pediatrics* 1955;15:325–333.

199. McDonald R, Goldschmidt B. Pancytopenia with congenital defects (Fanconi's anaemia). *Arch Dis Child* 1960;35:367–372.

200. Bargman GJ, Shahidi NT, Gilbert EF, et al. Studies of malformation syndromes of man XLVII: disappearance of spermatogonia in the Fanconi anemia syndrome. *Eur J Pediatr* 1977;125:163–168.

201. Alter BP, Frissora CL, Halperin DS, et al. Fanconi's anemia and pregnancy. *Br J Haematol* 1991;77:410–418.

202. Liu JM, Auerbach AD, Young NS. Fanconi anemia presenting unexpectedly in an adult kindred with no dysmorphic features. *Am J Med* 1991;91:555–557.

203. van Buchem FSP, Samsom N, Nieweg HO. Familial pancytopenia with congenital abnormalities (Fanconi's syndrome). *Acta Med Scand* 1954;149:19–29.

204. Esparza A, Thompson WR. Familial hypoplastic anemia with multiple congenital anomalies (Fanconi's syndrome)—report of three cases. *R I Med J* 1966;49:103–110.

205. Kew MC, Van Coller B, Prowse CM, et al. Occurrence of primary hepatocellular cancer and peliosis hepatis after treatment with androgenic steroids. *S Afr Med J* 1976;50:1233–1237.

206. Dosik H, Steier W, Lubiniecki A. Inherited aplastic anaemia with increased endoreduplications: a new syndrome or Fanconi's anaemia variant? *Br J Haematol* 1979;41:77–82.

207. Helmerhorst FM, Heaton DC, Crossen PE, et al. Familial thrombocytopenia associated with platelet autoantibodies and chromosome breakage. *Hum Genet* 1984;65:252–256.

208. Bauters F, Jouet JP, Lacroix D, et al. Maladie de Fanconi de revelation tardive en cours de grossesse. Etude cytogenetique. *Presse Med* 1984;13:2519–2520.

209. Carbone P, Barbata G, Mirto S, et al. Inherited aplastic anemia with abnormal clones in bone marrow and increased endoreduplication in peripheral lymphocytes. *Cancer Genet Cytogenet* 1984;13:259–266.

210. Zakut H, Lotan M, Virag I. Pregnancy in Fanconi's anemia. *Harefuah* 1984;107:238–239.

211. Flowers ME, Doney KC, Storb R, et al. Marrow transplantation for Fanconi anemia with or without leukemic transformation: an update of the Seattle experience. *Bone Marrow Transplant* 1992;9:167–173.

212. Seaward PG, Setzen R, Guidozzi F. Fanconi's anaemia in pregnancy: a case report. *S Afr Med J* 1990;78:691–692.

213. Koo WH, Knight LA, Ang PT. Fanconi's anaemia and recurrent squamous cell carcinoma of the oral cavity: a case report. *Ann Acad Med Singapore* 1996;25:289–292.

214. Shahidi NT, Diamond LK. Testosterone-induced remission in aplastic anemia. *Am J Dis Child* 1959;98:293–302.

215. Sanchez-Medal L. The hemopoietic action of androstanes. *Prog Hematol* 1971;7:111–136.

216. Najean Y. Androgen therapy in aplastic anaemia in childhood. In: *Congenital disorders of erythropoiesis, Ciba Foundation Symposium 37*. Amsterdam: Elsevier Science, 1976:354–363.

217. Meisner LF, Taher A, Shahidi NT. Chromosome changes and leukemic transformation in Fanconi's anemia. In: Hibino S, Takaku F, Shahidi NT, eds. *Aplastic anemia*. Tokyo: University of Tokyo Press, 1976:253–271.

218. Desposito F, Akatsuka J, Thatcher LG, et al. Bone marrow failure in pediatric patients. I. Cortisone and testosterone treatment. *J Pediatr* 1964;64:683–696.

219. McDonald R, Mibashan RS. Prolonged remission in Fanconi type anemia. *Helv Paediatr Acta* 1968;23:566–576.

220. Wasserman HP, Fry R, Cohn HJ. Fanconi's anaemia: cytogenetic studies in a family. *S Afr Med J* 1968;42:1162–1165.

221. Hirschman RJ, Schulman NR, Abuelo JG, et al. Chromosomal aberrations in two cases of inherited aplastic anemia with unusual clinical features. *Ann Intern Med* 1969;71:107–117.

222. Jacobs P, Karabus C. Fanconi's anemia. A family study with 20-year follow-up including associated breast pathology. *Cancer* 1984;54:1850–1853.

223. Rogers PC, Desai F, Karabus CD, et al. Presentation and outcome of 25 cases of Fanconi's anemia. *Am J Pediatr Hematol Oncol* 1989;11:141–145.

224. El Mauhoub M, Sudarshan G, Banerjee G, et al. Fanconi's anemia with associated acute nonlymphocytic leukemia. *Indian Pediatr* 1988;25:1124–1127.

225. Shahidi NT, Crigler JF Jr. Evaluation of growth and of endocrine systems in testosterone-corticosteroid-treated patients with aplastic anemia. *J Pediatr* 1967;70:233–242.

226. Kitchens CS. Amelioration of endothelial abnormalities by prednisone in experimental thrombocytopenia in the rabbit. *J Clin Invest* 1977;60:1129–1134.

227. Smith S, Marx MP, Jordan CJ, et al. Clinical aspects of a cluster of 42 patients in South Africa with Fanconi anemia. In: Schroeder-Kurth TM, Auerbach AD, Obe G, eds. *Fanconi anemia: clinical, cytogenetic and experimental aspects*. Berlin: Springer-Verlag, 1989:34–46.

228. Gluckman E, Broxmeyer HE, Auerbach AD, et al. Hematopoietic reconstitution in a patient with Fanconi's anemia by means of umbilical-cord blood from an HLA-identical sibling. *N Engl J Med* 1989;321:1174–1178.

229. Zatterale A, Calzone R, Renda S, et al. Identification and treatment of late onset Fanconi's anemia. *Haematologica* 1995;80:535–538.

230. Gluckman E, Devergie A, Schaison G, et al. Bone marrow transplantation in Fanconi anaemia. *Br J Haematol* 1980;45:557–564.

231. Zanis-Neto J, Ribeiro RC, Medeiros C, et al. Bone marrow transplantation for patients with Fanconi anemia: a study of 24 cases from a single institution. *Bone Marrow Transplant* 1995;15:293–298.

232. Berger R, Bernheim A, Gluckman E, et al. In vitro effect of cyclophosphamide metabolites on chromosomes of Fanconi anaemia patients. *Br J Haematol* 1980;45:565–568.

233. Gluckman E, Devergie A, Dutreix J. Bone marrow transplantation for Fanconi anemia. In: Schroeder-Kurth TM, Auerbach AD, Obe G, eds. *Fanconi anemia: clinical, cytogenetic and experimental aspects*. Berlin: Springer-Verlag, 1989:60–68.

234. Gluckman E, Auerbach AD, Horowitz MM, et al. Bone marrow transplantation for Fanconi anemia. *Blood* 1995;86:2856–2862.

235. Guardiola P, Socie G, Pasquini R, et al. Allogeneic stem cell transplantation of Fanconi anaemia. *Bone Marrow Transplant* 1998;21:S24–S27.

236. Kapelushnik J, Or R, Slavin S, et al. A fludarabine-based protocol for bone marrow transplantation in Fanconi's anemia. *Bone Marrow Transplant* 1997; 20:1109–1110.

237. Boulad F, Gillio A, Small TN, et al. Stem cell transplantation for the treatment of Fanconi anaemia using a fludarabine-based cytoreductive regimen and T-cell-depleted related HLA-mismatched peripheral blood stem cell grafts. *Br J Haematol* 2000;111:1153–1157.

238. Deeg HJ, Storb R, Thomas ED, et al. Fanconi's anemia treated by allogeneic marrow transplantation. *Blood* 1983;61:954–959.

239. Swift M. Malignant disease in heterozygous carriers. *Birth Defects Orig Artic Ser* 1976;12:133–144.

240. O'Reilly RJ, Pollack MS, Auerbach AD, et al. HLA histocompatibility between parent and affected child in Fanconi's anemia. *Pediatr Res* 1982; 16:210A.

241. Guardiola P, Pasquini R, Dokal I, et al. Outcome of 69 allogeneic stem cell transplantations for Fanconi anemia using HLA-matched unrelated donors: a study on behalf of the European Group for Blood and Marrow Transplantation. *Blood* 2000;95:422–429.

242. Broxmeyer HE, Douglas GW, Hangoc G, et al. Human umbilical cord blood as a potential source of transplantable hematopoietic stem/progenitor cells. *Proc Natl Acad Sci U S A* 1989;86:3828–3832.

243. Kurtzberg J, Laughlin M, Graham ML, et al. Placental blood as a source of hematopoietic stem cells for transplantation into unrelated recipients. *N Engl J Med* 1996;335:157–166.

244. Johnson FL. Placental blood transplantation and autologous banking—Caveat emptor. *J Pediatr Hematol Oncol* 1997;19:183–186.

245. Gardner FH, Helmer RE III. Aminocaproic acid. Use in control of hemorrhage in patients with amegakaryocytic thrombocytopenia. *JAMA* 1980; 243:35–37.

246. Ozsoylu S. Treatment of aplastic anemia. *J Pediatr* 1983;102:484.

247. Speck B, Gratwohl A, Nissen C, et al. Treatment of severe aplastic anaemia with antilymphocyte globulin or bone-marrow transplantation. *BMJ* 1981; 282:860–863.

248. Boggs DR, Joyce RA. The hematopoietic effects of lithium. *Semin Hematol* 1983;20:129–138.
249. Kemahli S, Canatan D, Uysal Z, et al. GM-CSF in the treatment of Fanconi's anaemia. *Br J Haematol* 1994;87:871–872.
250. Guinan EC, Lopez ED, Huhn RD, et al. Evaluation of granulocyte-macrophage colony-stimulating factor for treatment of pancytopenia in children with Fanconi anemia. *J Pediatr* 1994;124:144–150.
251. Rackoff WR, Orazi A, Robinson CA, et al. Prolonged administration of granulocyte colony-stimulating factor (Filgrastim) to patients with Fanconi anemia: a pilot study. *Blood* 1996;88:1588–1593.
252. Scagni P, Saracco P, Timeus F, et al. Use of recombinant granulocyte colony-stimulating factor in Fanconi's anemia. *Haematologica* 1998;83:432–437.
253. German J. Patterns of neoplasia associated with the chromosome-breakage syndromes. In: German J, ed. *Chromosome mutation and neoplasia.* New York: Alan R. Liss, 1983:97–134.
254. Garriga S, Crosby WH. The incidence of leukemia in families of patients with hypoplasia of the marrow. *Blood* 1959;24:1008–1014.
255. Swift M. Fanconi's anaemia in the genetics of neoplasia. *Nature* 1971;230:370–373.
256. Swift M, Caldwell RJ, Chase C. Reassessment of cancer predisposition of Fanconi anemia heterozygotes. *J Natl Cancer Inst* 1980;65:863–867.
257. Potter NU, Sarmousakis C, Li FP. Cancer in relatives of patients with aplastic anemia. *Cancer Genet Cytogenet* 1983;9:61–66.
258. Swift M, Sholman L, Gilmour D. Diabetes mellitus and the gene for Fanconi's anemia. *Science* 1972;178:308–310.
259. Morrell D, Chase CI, Kupper LL, et al. Diabetes mellitus in ataxia-telangiectasia, Fanconi anemia, xeroderma pigmentosum, common variable immune deficiency, and severe combined immune deficiency families. *Diabetes* 1986;35:143–147.
260. Schaison G, Leverger G, Yildiz C, et al. L'anemie de Fanconi. Frequence de l'evolution vers la leucemie. *Presse Med* 1983;12:1269–1274.
261. Gyger M, Perrault C, Belanger R, et al. Unsuspected Fanconi's anemia and bone marrow transplantation in cases of acute myelomonocytic leukemia. *N Engl J Med* 1989;321:120–121.
262. Ahmed OA, Al-Rimawi HS, Al-Rashid AA, et al. Fanconi's anemia with acute lymphoblastic leukaemia in a Bedouin girl. *Am Soc Hum Genet* 1989;45[Suppl]:14A.
263. Yetgin S, Tuncer M, Guler E, et al. Acute lymphoblastic leukemia in Fanconi's anemia. *Am J Hematol* 1994;45:94.
264. Tezcan I, Tuncer M, Uckan D, et al. Allogeneic bone marrow transplantation in Fanconi anemia from Turkey: a report of four cases. *Pediatr Transplant* 1998;2:236–239.
265. Sugita K, Taki T, Hayashi Y, et al. MLL-CBP fusion transcript in a therapy-related acute myeloid leukemia with the t(11;16)(q23;p13) which developed in an acute lymphoblastic leukemia patient with Fanconi anemia. *Genes Chromosomes Cancer* 2000;27:264–269.
266. Eldar M, Shoenfeld Y, Zaizov R, et al. Pulmonary alveolar proteinosis associated with Fanconi's anemia. *Respiration* 1979;38:177–179.
267. Perona G, Cetto GL, Bernardi F, et al. Fanconi's anaemia in adults: study of three families. *Haematologica* 1977;62:615–628.
268. Altay C, Alikasifoglu M, Kara A, et al. Analysis of 65 Turkish patients with congenital aplastic anemia: (Fanconi anemia and non-Fanconi anemia): Hacettepe experience. *Clin Genet* 1997;51:296–302.
269. Verbeek W, Haase D, Schoch C, et al. Induction of a hematological and cytogenetic remission in a patient with a myelodysplastic syndrome secondary to Fanconi's anemia employing the S-HAM regimen. *Ann Hematol* 1997;74:275–277.
270. Zawartka M, Restorff-Libiszowska H, Kowalski R, et al. Bialaczka szpikowa w prezebiegu anemii Fanconiego (AF). *Wiad Lek* 1976;29:145–151.
271. Perrimond H, Juhan-Vague I, Thevenieau D, et al. Evolution medullaire et hepatique apres androgenotherapie prolongee d'une anemie de Fanconi. *Nouv Rev Fr Hematol* 1977;18:228.
272. Van Gils JE, Mandel C, Van Weel-Sipman MH, et al. Acute leukemie bij Fanconi anemie. *Tijdschr Kindergeneeskd* 1987;55:68–72.
273. Submoke S, Kessacorn W. Fanconi's syndrome: presentation of a case of acute myeloblastic leukemia. *J Med Assoc Thai* 1985;68:480–484.
274. Barton JC, Parmley RT, Carroll AJ, et al. Preleukemia in Fanconi's anemia: hematopoietic cell multinuclearity, membrane duplication, and dysgranulogenesis. *J Submicrosc Cytol* 1987;19:355–364.
275. Tanzer J, Frocrain C, Desmarest MC. Anomalies du chromosome 1 dans 3 cas de leucemie compliquant une aplasie de Fanconi (FA). *Nouv Rev Franc D'Hematol* 1980;22:93.
276. Gardner FH. Unpublished, 1984.
277. Nowell P, Bergman G, Besa E, et al. Progressive preleukemia with a chromosomally abnormal clone in a kindred with the Estren-Dameshek variant of Fanconi's anemia. *Blood* 1984;64:1135–1138.
278. Woods WG, Nesbit ME, Buckley J, et al. Correlation of chromosome abnormalities with patient characteristics, histologic subtype, and induction success in children with acute nonlymphoblastic leukemia. *J Clin Oncol* 1985;3:3–11.
279. Maarek O, Jonveaux P, Le Coniat M, et al. Fanconi anemia and bone marrow clonal chromosome abnormalities. *Leukemia* 1996;10:1700–1704.
280. Obeid A, Hill FG, Harnden D, et al. Fanconi anemia: oxymetholone hepatic tumors, and chromosome aberrations associated with leukemic transition. *Cancer* 1980;46:1401–1404.
281. Auerbach AD, Weiner M, Warburton D, et al. Acute myeloid leukemia as the first hematologic manifestation of Fanconi anemia. *Am J Hematol* 1982;12:289–300.
282. Berger R, Bussel A, Schenmetzler C. Somatic segregation and Fanconi anemia. *Clin Genet* 1977;11:409–415.
283. Berger R, Le Coniat M. Cytogenetic studies in Fanconi anemia induced chromosomal breakage and cytogenetics. In: Schroeder-Kurth TM, Auerbach AD, Obe G, eds. *Fanconi anemia: clinical, cytogenetic and experimental aspects.* Berlin: Springer-Verlag, 1989:93–99.
284. Berger R, Le Coniat M, Schaison G. Chromosome abnormalities in bone marrow of Fanconi anemia patients. *Cancer Genet Cytogenet* 1993;65:47–50.
285. Alter BP, Scalise A, McCombs J, et al. Clonal chromosomal abnormalities in Fanconi's anemia: what do they really mean? *Br J Haematol* 1993;85:627–630.
286. Davies SM, Khan S, Wagner JE, et al. Unrelated donor bone marrow transplantation for Fanconi anemia. *Bone Marrow Transplant* 1996;17:43–47.
287. Griffin TC, Friedman DJ, Sanders JM, et al. Fanconi anemia complicated by acute myelogenous leukemia and malignant brain tumor. *Blood* 1992;80:382a.
288. Yoshida Y, Kawabata H, Anzai N. Cell biology and programmed cell death in MDS. *Leuk Res* 1994;18:5.
289. Gibbons B, Scott D, Hungerford JL, et al. Retinoblastoma in association with the chromosome breakage syndromes Fanconi's anaemia and Bloom's syndrome: clinical and cytogenetic findings. *Clin Genet* 1995;47:311–317.
290. Takizawa J, Kishi K, Moriyama Y, et al. Allogenic bone marrow transplantation for Fanconi's anemia with leukemic transformation from an HLA identical father. *Rinsho Ketsueki* 1995;36:615–620.
291. Manglani M, Muralidhar HP, Bhoyar A, et al. Leukemic transformation in Fanconi's anemia. *Indian Pediatrics* 1999;36:1054–1056.
292. Cowdell RH, Phizackerley PJ, Pyke DA. Constitutional anemia (Fanconi's syndrome) and leukemia in two brothers. *Blood* 1955;10:788–801.
293. Sarna G, Tomasulo P, Lotz MJ, et al. Multiple neoplasia in two siblings with a variant form of Fanconi's anemia. *Cancer* 1975;36:1029–1033.
294. Consarino C, Magro S, Dattilo A, et al. Acute leukemia in Fanconi's anemia. In: Department of Hematology Department of Hematology of University of Rome, eds. *Third International Symposium on Therapy of Acute Leukemias.* Rome: University of Rome, 1982:492.
295. O'Gorman Hughes DW. Aplastic anaemia in childhood. III. Constitutional aplastic anaemia and related cytopenias. *Med J Austr* 1974;1:519–526.
296. Dosik H, Hsu LY, Todaro GJ, et al. Leukemia in Fanconi's anemia: cytogenetic and tumor virus susceptibility studies. *Blood* 1970;36:341–352.
297. Stein AC, Blanck DM, Bennett AJ, et al. Acute myelomonocytic leukemia in a patient with Fanconi's anemia. *J Oral Surg* 1981;39:624–627.
298. Gyger M, Bonny Y, Forest L. Childhood monosomy 7 syndrome. *Am J Hematol* 1982;13:329–334.
299. Dosik H, Verma RS, Wilson C, et al. Fanconi's anemia and a familial stable chromosome abnormality in a family with multiple malignancies. *Blood* 1977;50:190a.
300. Kunze J. Estren-Dameshek-anamie mit myelomonocytarer leukamie (Subtyp der Fanconi-Anamie?). In: Spranger J, Tolksdorf M, eds. *Klinische genetik in der padiatrie.* Stuttgart, Germany: Thieme Medical Publishers, 1980:213–214.
301. Lux S. Unpublished data, 1984.
302. Bourgeois CA, Hill FG. Fanconi anemia leading to acute myelomonocytic leukemia. Cytogenetic studies. *Cancer* 1977;39:1163–1167.
303. Alimena G, Avvisati G, De Cuia MR, et al. Retrospective diagnosis of a Fanconi's anemia patient by diepoxybutane (DEB) test results in parents. *Haematologica* 1983;68:97–103.
304. Kwee ML, Poll EH, van de Kamp JJ, et al. Unusual response to bifunctional alkylating agents in a case of Fanconi anaemia. *Hum Genet* 1983;64:384–387.
305. Roozendaal KJ, Nelis KO. Leukaemia in a case of Fanconi's anaemia. *Clin Genet* 1981;25:208.
306. Ortega M, Caballin MR, Ortega JJ, et al. Follow-up by cytogenetic and fluorescence in situ hybridization analysis of allogeneic bone marrow transplantation in two children with Fanconi's anaemia in transformation. *Br J Haematol* 2000;111:329–333.
307. Ferti A, Panani A, Dervenoulas J, et al. Cytogenetic findings in a Fanconi anemia patient with AML. *Cancer Genet Cytogenet* 1996;90:182–183.
308. Sasaki MS. Fanconi's anemia. A condition possibly associated with a defective DNA repair. In: Hanawalt P, Friedberg EC, Fox CF, eds. *DNA repair mechanisms.* New York: Academic Press, 1978:675–684.
309. Meddeb B, Azzouz MM, Hafsia R, et al. Transformation en leucemie aigue de l'anemie de Fanconi: a propos de 2 cas dans une serie de 21 malades. *Tunis Med* 1986;64:755–759.
310. Ahuja HG, Advani SH, Gopal R, et al. Acute nonlymphoblastic leukemia in the first of three siblings affected with Fanconi's syndrome. *Am J Pediatr Hematol Oncol* 1986;8:347–349.
311. Gastearena J, Giralt M, Orue MT, et al. Fanconi's anemia. Clinical study of six cases. *Am J Pediatr Hematol Oncol* 1986;8:173–177.
312. Stivrins TJ, Davis RB, Sanger W, et al. Transformation of Fanconi's anemia to acute nonlymphocytic leukemia associated with emergence of monosomy 7. *Blood* 1984;64:173–176.
313. Villegas A, Aboin J, Alvarez-Sala JL, et al. Eritroleucemia en la evolucion de una anemia constitucional de Fanconi. *Sangre* 1983;28:225–226.
314. Rotzak R, Kaplinsky N, Chaki R, et al. Giant marker chromosome in Fanconi's anemia transforming into erythroleukemia in an adult. *Acta Haematol* 1982;67:214–216.
315. Dharmasena F, Catchpole M, Erber W, et al. Megakaryoblastic leukaemia and myelofibrosis complicating Fanconi anaemia. *Scand J Haematol* 1986;36:309–313.
316. Athale UH, Rao SR, Kadam PR, et al. Fanconi's anemia: a clinico-hematological and cytogenetic study. *Indian Pediatr* 1992;28:1003–1011.

317. Macdougall LG, Greeff MC, Rosendorff J, et al. Fanconi anemia in Black African children. *Am J Med Genet* 1990;36:408–413.

318. Russo CL, Zwerdling T. Letter to the editor: recognition of Fanconi's anemia eight years following treatment for acute nonlymphoblastic leukemia. *Am J Hematol* 1992;40:78–79.

319. Touraine RL, Bertrand Y, Foray P, et al. Hepatic tumours during androgen therapy in Fanconi anaemia. *Eur J Pediatr* 1993;152:691–693.

320. Sanchez MD, Cantoni AC, Alvarez BM, et al. Clinical and cytogenetic variability on twelve Fanconi anemia and its relationship with complementation group assignment. *Rev Invest Clin* 1999;51:273–283.

321. Hows JM, Chapple M, Marsh JC, et al. Bone marrow transplantation for Fanconi's anaemia: the Hammersmith experience 1977–1989. *Bone Marrow Transplant* 1989;4:629–634.

322. Hows JM. Unrelated donor bone marrow transplantation for severe aplastic anaemia and Fanconi's anaemia. *Bone Marrow Transplant* 1989;4[Suppl]:126–128.

323. Bessho F, Mizutani S, Hayashi Y, et al. Chronic myelomonocytic leukemia with chromosomal changes involving 1p36 and hepatocellular carcinoma in a case of Fanconi's anemia. *Eur J Haematol* 1989;42:492–495.

324. Butturini A, Gale RP, Verlander PC, et al. Hematologic abnormalities in Fanconi anemia: an International Fanconi Anemia Registry study. *Blood* 1994;84:1650–1655.

325. Alter BP, Caruso JP, Drachtman RA, et al. Fanconi's anemia: myelodysplasia as a predictor of outcome. *Cancer Genet Cytogenet* 2000;117:125–131.

326. Bennett JM, Catovsky D, Daniel MT, et al. Proposals for the classification of the myelodysplastic syndromes. *Br J Haematol* 1982;51:189–199.

327. Greenberg P, Cox C, LeBeau M, et al. International scoring system for evaluating prognosis in myelodysplastic syndromes. *Blood* 1997;89:2079–2088.

328. Alter BP. Fanconi's anemia and malignancies. *Am J Hematol* 1996;53:99–110.

329. Thurston VC, Ceperich TM, Vance GH, et al. Detection of monosomy 7 in bone marrow by fluorescence in situ hybridization. A study of Fanconi anemia patients and review of the literature. *Cancer Genet Cytogenet* 1999;109:154–160.

330. Baron F, Sybert VP, Andrews RG. Cutaneous and extracutaneous neutrophilic infiltrates (Sweet syndrome) in three patients with Fanconi anemia. *J Pediatr* 1989;115:726–729.

331. Ries LA, Kosary CL, Hankey BF, et al. *SEER cancer statistics review, 1973–1996.* Bethesda, MD: National Cancer Institute, 1999.

332. Nara N, Miyamoto T, Kurisu A, et al. Two siblings with Fanconi's anemia developing squamous cell carcinomas. *Rinshou Ketsueki* 1980;21:1944–1950.

333. McDonough ER. Fanconi anemia syndrome. *Arch Otolaryngol* 1970;92:284–285.

334. Swift M, Zimmerman D, McDonough ER. Squamous cell carcinomas in Fanconi's anemia. *JAMA* 1971;216:325–326.

335. Kozarek RA, Sanowski RA. Carcinoma of the esophagus associated with Fanconi's anemia. *J Clin Gastroenterol* 1981;3:171–174.

336. Vaitiekaitis AS, Grau WH. Squamous cell carcinoma of the mandible in Fanconi anemia: report of case. *J Oral Surg* 1980;38:372–373.

337. Schofield ID, Worth AT. Malignant mucosal change in Fanconi's anemia. *J Oral Surg* 1980;38:619–622.

338. Kennedy AW, Hart WR. Multiple squamous-cell carcinomas in Fanconi's anemia. *Cancer* 1982;50:811–814.

339. Kaplan MJ, Sabio H, Wanebo HJ, et al. Squamous cell carcinoma in the immunosuppressed patient: Fanconi's anemia. *Laryngoscope* 1985;95:771–775.

340. Fukuoka K, Nishikawa K, Mizumoto Y, et al. Fanconi's anemia with squamous cell carcinoma: a case report and a review of literature. *Jpn J Clin Hematol* 1989;30:1992–1996.

341. Snow DG, Campbell JB, Smallman LA. Fanconi's anaemia and post-cricoid carcinoma. *J Laryngol Otol* 1991;105:125–127.

342. Lustig JP, Lugassy G, Neder A, et al. Head and neck carcinoma in Fanconi's anaemia: report of a case and review of the literature. *Eur J Cancer* 1995;31:68–72.

343. Halvorson DJ, McKie V, McKie K, et al. Sickle cell disease and tonsillectomy. *Arch Otolaryngol Head Neck Surg* 1997;123:689–692.

344. Guy JT, Auslander MO. Androgenic steroids and hepatocellular carcinoma. *Lancet* 1973;1:148.

345. Reed K, Ravikumar TS, Gifford RR, et al. The association of Fanconi's anemia and squamous cell carcinoma. *Cancer* 1983;52:926–928.

346. Kozhevnikov BA, Khodorenko CA. Cancer of the mucous membrane of the left side of the mouth associated with congenital hypoplastic Fanconi's anemia in a 14-year-old boy. *Vestn Khir* 1986;136:105–106.

347. Doerr TD, Shibuya TY, Marks SC. Squamous cell carcinoma of the supraglottic larynx in a patient with Fanconi's anemia. *Otolaryngol Head Neck Surg* 1998;118:523–525.

348. Aho S. Clinical conferences. Case of Fanconi's anemia. *Kyobu Geka* 1980;33:397–399.

349. Rockelein G, Ulmer R, Kniewald A, et al. Osophaguskarzinom bei Fanconi-syndrom. *Pathologe* 1986;7:343–347.

350. Linares M, Pastor E, Gomez A, et al. Hepatocellular carcinoma and squamous cell carcinoma in a patient with Fanconi's anemia. *Ann Hematol* 1991;63:54–55.

351. Soravia C, Spilipoulos A. Carcinome épidermoïde de l'oesophage et anémie de Fanconi. *Schweiz Med Wochenschr* 1994;124:725–728.

352. Goluchova M, Urban O, Chalupa J. Spinocellular carcinoma in a patient with Fanconi's anemia. *Vnitr Lek* 1998;44:280–281.

353. Gendal ES, Mendelson DS, Janus CL, et al. Squamous cell carcinoma of the esophagus in Fanconi's anemia. *Dysphagia* 1988;2:178–179.

354. Sicular A, Fleshner PR, Cohen LB, et al. Fanconi's anemia and esophageal carcinoma. *Gullet* 1993;3:60–63.

355. Hersey P, Edwards A, Lewis R, et al. Deficient natural killer cell activity in a patient with Fanconi's anaemia and squamous cell carcinoma. Association with defect in interferon release. *Clin Exp Immunol* 1982;48:205–212.

356. Arnold WJ, King CR, Magrina J, et al. Squamous cell carcinoma of the vulva and Fanconi anemia. *Int J Gynaecol Obstet* 1980;18:395–397.

357. Ortonne JP, Jeune R, Coiffet J, et al. Squamous cell carcinomas in Fanconi's anemia. *Arch Dermatol* 1981;117:443–444.

358. Wilkinson EJ, Morgan LS, Friedrich EG Jr. Association of Fanconi's anemia and squamous-cell carcinoma of the lower female genital tract with condyloma acuminatum. A report of two cases. *J Reprod Med* 1984;29:447–453.

359. Lebbe C, Pinquier L, Rybojad M, et al. Fanconi's anaemia associated with multicentric Bowen's disease and decreased NK cytotoxicity. *Br J Dermatol* 1993;129:615–618.

360. de Chadarevian JP, Vekemans M, Bernstein M. Fanconi's anemia, medulloblastoma, Wilms' tumor, horseshoe kidney, and gonadal dysgenesis. *Arch Pathol Lab Med* 1985;109:367–369.

361. Alter BP, Tenner MS. Brain tumors in patients with Fanconi's anemia. *Arch Pediatr Adolesc Med* 1994;148:661–663.

362. Puligandla B, Stass SA, Schumacher HR, et al. Terminal deoxynucleotidyl transferase in Fanconi's anaemia. *Lancet* 1978;2:1263.

363. van Niekerk CH, Jordaan C, Badenhorst PN. Pancytopenia secondary to primary malignant lymphoma of bone marrow as the first hematologic manifestation of the Estren-Dameshek variant of Fanconi's anemia. *Am J Pediatr Hematol Oncol* 1987;9:344–349.

364. Goldsby RE, Perkins SL, Virshup DM, et al. Lymphoblastic lymphoma and excessive toxicity from chemotherapy: an unusual presentation for Fanconi anemia. *J Pediatr Hematol Oncol* 1999;21:240–243.

365. Hill LS, Dennis PM, Fairham SA. Adenocarcinoma of the stomach and Fanconi's anaemia. *Postgrad Med J* 1981;57:404.

366. Puig S, Ferrando J, Cervantes F, et al. Fanconi's anemia with cutaneous amyloidosis. *Arch Dermatol* 1993;129:788–789.

367. Ariffin H, Ariffin WA, Chan LI, et al. Wilms' tumour and Fanconi anaemia: an unusual association. *J Paediatr Child Health* 2000;36:196–198.

368. Levinson S, Vincent KA. Multifocal osteosarcoma in a patient with Fanconi anemia. *J Pediatr Hematol Oncol* 1997;19:251–253.

369. Mulvihill JJ, Ridolfi RL, Schultz FR, et al. Hepatic adenoma in Fanconi anemia treated with oxymetholone. *J Pediatr* 1975;87:122–124.

370. Corberand J, Pris J, Dutau G, et al. Association d'une maladie de Fanconi et d'une tumeur hepatique. Chez une malade soumise a un traitement androgenique au long cours. *Arch Fr Pediatr* 1975;32:275–283.

371. Resnick MB, Kozakewich HP, Perez-Atayde AR. Hepatic adenoma in the pediatric age group. Clinicopathological observations and assessment of cell proliferative activity. *Am J Surg Pathol* 1995;19:1181–1190.

372. Schmidt E, Deeg HJ, Storb R. Regression of androgen-related hepatic tumors in patients with Fanconi's anemia following marrow transplantation. *Transplantation* 1984;37:452–457.

373. Garel L, Kalifa G, Buriot D, et al. Multiple adenomas of the liver and Fanconi's anaemia. *Ann Radiol* 1980;24:53–54.

374. Farrell GC. Fanconi's familial hypoplastic anaemia with some unusual features. *Med J Aust* 1976;1:116–118.

375. Chandra RS, Kapur SP, Kelleher J, et al. Benign hepatocellular tumors in the young. A clinicopathologic spectrum. *Arch Pathol Lab Med* 1984;108:168–171.

376. LeBrun DP, Silver MM, Freedman MH, et al. Fibrolamellar carcinoma of the liver in a patient with Fanconi anemia. *Hum Pathol* 1991;22:396–398.

377. Ortega JJ, Olive T, Sanchez C, et al. Bone marrow transplant in Fanconi's anemia. Results in five patients. *Sangre* 1990;35:433–440.

378. Mokrohisky ST, Ambruso DR, Hathaway WE. Fulminant hepatic neoplasia after androgen therapy. *N Engl J Med* 1977;296:1411–1412.

379. Cattan D, Kalifat R, Wautier JL, et al. Maladie de Fanconi et cancer du foie. *Arch Fr Mal App Dig* 1974;63:41–48.

380. Abbondanzo SL, Manz HJ, Klappenbach RS, et al. Hepatocellular carcinoma in an 11-year-old girl with Fanconi's anemia. Report of a case and review of the literature. *Am J Pediatr Hematol Oncol* 1986;8:334–337.

381. Johnson FL, Feagler JR, Lerner KG, et al. Association of androgenic-anabolic steroid therapy with development of hepatocellular carcinoma. *Lancet* 1972;2:1273–1276.

382. Moldvay J, Schaff Z, Lapis K. Hepatocellular carcinoma in Fanconi's anemia treated with androgen and corticosteroid. *Zentralbl Pathol* 1991;137:167–170.

383. Recant L, Lacy P. Fanconi's anemia and hepatic cirrhosis. *Am J Med* 1965;39:464–475.

384. Cap J, Ondrus B, Danihel L. Focal nodular hyperplasia of the liver and hepatocellular carcinoma in children with Fanconi's anemia after long-term treatment with androgens. *Bratisl Lek Listy* 1983;79:73–81.

385. Port RB, Petasnick JP, Ranniger K. Angiographic demonstration of hepatoma in association with Fanconi's anemia. *AJR Am J Roentgenol* 1971;113:82–83.

386. Bernstein MS, Hunter RL, Yachnin S. Hepatoma and peliosis hepatis developing in a patient with Fanconi's anemia. *N Engl J Med* 1971;284:1135–1136.

387. Bagheri SA, Boyer JL. Peliosis hepatis associated with androgenic-anabolic steroid therapy. A severe form of hepatic injury. *Ann Intern Med* 1974;81:610–618.

388. Holder LE, Gnarra DJ, Lampkin BC, et al. Hepatoma associated with anabolic steroid therapy. *AJR Am J Roentgenol* 1975;124:638–642.

389. Sweeney EC, Evans DJ. Hepatic lesions in patients treated with synthetic anabolic steroids. *J Clin Pathol* 1976;29:626–633.

390. Evans DIK. Aplastic anaemia in childhood. In: Geary CG, ed. *Aplastic anaemia*. London: Bailliere Tindall, 1979:161–194.
391. Bradford CR, Hoffman HT, Wolf GT, et al. Squamous carcinoma of the head and neck in organ transplant recipients: possible role of oncogenic viruses. *Laryngoscope* 1990;100:190–194.
392. Millen FJ, Rainey MG, Hows JM, et al. Oral squamous cell carcinoma after allogeneic bone marrow transplantation for Fanconi anaemia. *Br J Haematol* 1997;99:410–414.
393. Jansisyanont P, Pazoki A, Ord RA. Squamous cell carcinoma of the tongue after bone marrow transplantation in a patient with Fanconi's anemia. *J Oral Maxillofac Surg* 2000;58:1454–1457.
394. Socie G, Henry-Amar M, Cosset JM, et al. Increased incidence of solid malignant tumors after bone marrow transplantation for severe aplastic anemia. *Blood* 1991;78:277–279.
395. Pierga JY, Socie G, Gluckman E, et al. Secondary solid malignant tumors occurring after bone marrow transplantation for severe aplastic anemia given thoraco-abdominal irradiation. *Radiother Oncol* 1994;30:55–58.
396. Murayama S, Manzo RP, Kirkpatrick DV, et al. Squamous cell carcinoma of the tongue associated with Fanconi's anemia: MR characteristics. *Pediatr Radiol* 1990;20:347.
397. Smith CH. The anemias of early infancy. Pathogenesis and diagnosis. *J Pediatr* 1940;16:375–395.
398. Somers GR, Tabrizi SN, Tiedemann K, et al. Squamous cell carcinoma of the tongue in a child with Fanconi anemia: a case report and review of the literature. *Pediatr Pathol Lab Med* 1994;15:597–607.
399. Kolb HJ, Socie G, Duell T, et al. Malignant neoplasms in long-term survivors of bone marrow transplantation. *Ann Intern Med* 1999;131:738–744.
399a. Alter B. Cancer in Fanconi's anemia, 1927–2001. *Cancer* 2003 (in press).
399b. Rosenberg PS, Greene MH, Alter BP. Cancer incidence in persons with Fanconi's anemia. *Blood* 2003 (in press).
400. Drachtman RA, Alter BP. Dyskeratosis congenita: clinical and genetic heterogeneity. Report of a new case and review of the literature. *Am J Pediatr Hematol Oncol* 1992;14:297–304.
401. Drachtman RA, Alter BP. Dyskeratosis congenita. *Dermatol Clin* 1995;13:33–39.
402. Dokal I. Dyskeratosis congenita in all its forms. *Br J Haematol* 2000;110:768–779.
403. Connor JM, Gatherer D, Gray FC, et al. Assignment of the gene for dyskeratosis congenita to Xq28. *Hum Genet* 1987;72:348–351.
404. Sirinavin C, Trowbridge AA. Dyskeratosis congenita: clinical features and genetic aspects. Report of a family and review of the literature. *J Med Genet* 1975;12:339–354.
405. Texier L, Maleville J. La symptomatologie cutanee de l'anemie perniciosiforme de Fanconi. Rapports avec la dyskeratose congenitale de Zinsser-Cole-Engman. *Ann Dermatol Syphiligraphie* 1963;90:553–568.
406. Steier W, Van Voolen GA, Selmanowitz VJ. Dyskeratosis congenita: relationship to Fanconi's anemia. *Blood* 1972;39:510–521.
407. Inoue S, Mekanik G, Mahallati M, et al. Dyskeratosis congenita with pancytopenia. Another constitutional anemia. *Am J Dis Child* 1973;126:389–396.
408. Korz R, Wienert V, Knechten H. Dyskeratosis congenita (Zinsser-Engman-Cole-Syndrom) und Fanconi-Anamie. *Hautarzt* 1982;33:112–114.
409. Schneider A, Mayer U, Gebhart E, et al. Clastogen-induced fragility may differentiate pancytopenia of congenital dyskeratosis from Fanconi anaemia. *Eur J Pediatr* 1988;145:37–39.
410. Jacobs P, Saxe N, Gordon W, et al. Dyskeratosis congenita. Haematologic, cytogenetic, and dermatologic studies. *Scand J Haematol* 1984;32:461–468.
411. Ortega JA, Swanson VL, Landing BH, et al. Congenital dyskeratosis. Zinsser-Engman-Cole syndrome with thymic dysplasia and aplastic anemia. *Am J Dis Child* 1972;124:701–704.
412. Dokal I, Luzzatto L. Dyskeratosis congenita is a chromosomal instability disorder. *Leuk Lymphoma* 1994;15:1–7.
413. Juneja HS, Elder FF, Gardner FH. Abnormality of platelet size and T-lymphocyte proliferation in an autosomal recessive form of dyskeratosis congenita. *Eur J Haematol* 1987;39:306–310.
414. Smith CM II, Ramsay NK, Branda R, et al. Response to androgens in the constitutional aplastic anemia of dyskeratosis congenita (DC). *Pediatr Res* 1979;13:441.
415. Hanada T, Abe T, Nakazawa M, et al. Bone marrow failure in dyskeratosis congenita. *Scand J Haematol* 1984;32:496–500.
416. Colvin BT, Baker H, Hibbin JA, et al. Haemopoietic progenitor cells in dyskeratosis congenita. *Br J Haematol* 1984;56:513–515.
417. Friedland M, Lutton JD, Spitzer R, et al. Dyskeratosis congenita with hypoplastic anemia: a stem cell defect. *Am J Hematol* 1985;20:85–87.
418. Michalevicz R, Baron S, Nordan U, et al. Granulocytic macrophage colony stimulating factor restores in vitro growth of granulocyte-macrophage bone marrow hematopoietic progenitors in dyskeratosis congenita. *Isr J Med Sci* 1989;25:193–195.
419. Misawa M, Haku Y, Ifuku H, et al. Pancytopenia. Dyskeratosis congenita. A case report of dyskeratosis congenita with pancytopenia in special reference to hemopoietic stem cells. *Rinsho Ketsueki* 1982;23:1222–1227.
420. Marsh JC, Will AJ, Hows JM, et al. "Stem cell" origin of the hematopoietic defect in dyskeratosis congenita. *Blood* 1992;79:3138–3144.
421. Georgouras K. Dyskeratosis congenita. *Aust J Dermatol* 1965;8:36–43.
422. Knight SW, Vulliamy TJ, Forni GL, et al. Fine mapping of the dyskeratosis congenita locus in Xq28. *J Med Genet* 1996;33:993–995.
423. Knight SW, Vulliamy TJ, Heiss NS, et al. 1.4 Mb candidate gene region for X linked dyskeratosis congenita defined by combined haplotype and X chromosome inactivation analysis. *J Med Genet* 1998;35:993–996.
424. Heiss NS, Knight SW, Vulliamy TJ, et al. X-linked dyskeratosis congenita is caused by mutations in a highly conserved gene with putative nucleolar functions. *Nat Genet* 1998;19:32–38.
425. Hassock S, Vetrie D, Giannelli F. Mapping and characterization of the X-linked dyskeratosis congenita (DKC) gene. *Genomics* 1999;55:21–27.
426. Knight SW, Heiss NS, Vulliamy TJ, et al. X-linked dyskeratosis congenita is predominantly caused by missense mutations in the DKC1 gene. *Am J Hum Genet* 1999;65:50–58.
427. Vulliamy TJ, Knight SW, Heiss NS. Dyskeratosis congenita caused by a 3' deletion: germline and somatic mosaicism in a female carrier. *Blood* 1999; 94:1254–1260.
428. Heiss NS, Bachner D, Salowsky R, et al. Gene structure and expression of the mouse dyskeratosis congenita gene, Dkc1. *Genomics* 2000;67:153–163.
429. Mitchell JR, Wood E, Collins K. A telomerase component is defective in the human disease dyskeratosis congenita. *Nature* 1999;402:551–555.
430. Vulliamy TJ, Knight SW, Mason PJ, et al. Very short telomeres in the peripheral blood of patients with X-linked and autosomal dyskeratosis congenita. *Blood Cell Mol Dis* 2001;27:353–357.
431. Artandi SE, Chang S, Lee SL, et al. Telomere dysfunction promotes non-reciprocal translocations and epithelial cancers in mice. *Nature* 2000;406:641–645.
432. Knight SW, Heiss NS, Vulliamy TJ, et al. Unexplained aplastic anaemia, immunodeficiency, and cerebellar hypoplasia (Hoyeraal-Hreidarsson syndrome) due to mutations in the dyskeratosis gene, DKC1. *Br J Haematol* 1999;107:335–339.
433. Yaghmai R, Kimyai-Asadi A, Rostamiani K, et al. Overlap of dyskeratosis congenita with the Hoyeraal-Hreidarsson syndrome. *J Pediatr* 2000;136:390–393.
434. Alter BP. Molecular medicine and bone marrow failure syndromes. *J Pediatr* 2000;136:275–276.
435. Cole HN, Cole HN, Lascheid WP. Dyskeratosis congenita. *Arch Dermatol* 1957;76:712–719.
436. Addison M, Rice MS. The association of dyskeratosis congenita and Fanconi's anaemia. *Med J Aust* 1965;1:797–799.
437. Krantz SB, Zaentz SD. Pure red cell aplasia. In: Gordon AS, Silber R, LoBue J, eds. *The year in hematology*. New York: Plenum Publishing, 1977:153–190.
438. Wasylyszyn J, Kryst L, Langner A. Dyskeratosis congenita (Zinsser-Engman-Cole). *Przeg Derm* 1974;61:687–691.
439. Camacho F, Moreno JC, Conejo-Mir JS, et al. Sindrome de Zinsser-Cole-Engman: disqueratosis congenita. *Med Cutan Ibero Lat Am* 1982;10:365–368.
440. Schmidt JB, Gebhart W. Zinsser-Engman-Cole-Syndrom. *Der Hautarzt* 1983; 34:286–287.
441. Anil S, Beena VT, Raji MA, et al. Oral squamous cell carcinoma in a case of dyskeratosis congenita. *Ann Dent* 1994;53:15–18.
442. Limmer RL, Zurowski SM, Swinfard RW, et al. Abnormal nails in a patient with severe anemia. *Arch Dermatol* 1997;133:97.
443. Lespinasse J, Bourrain JL, Blanc M. Dyskeratose congenitale ou dyskeratose de Zinsser-Cole-Engman. Un cas feminin probable. *Presse Med* 1988;17:1047.
444. Moretti S, Spallanzani A, Chiarugi A, et al. Oral carcinoma in a young man: a case of dyskeratosis congenita. *J Eur Acad Dermatol Venereol* 2000;14:123–125.
445. Hyodo M, Sadamoto A, Hinohira Y, et al. Tongue cancer as a complication of dyskeratosis congenita in a woman. *Am J Otolaryngol* 1999;20:405–407.
446. Garb J. Dyskeratosis congenita with pigmentation, dystrophia unguium, and leukoplakia oris. A follow-up report of two brothers. *Arch Dermatol* 1958;77:704–712.
447. Cannell H. Dyskeratosis congenita. *Br J Oral Surg* 1971;9:8–20.
448. Kubicz J. Syndroma Zinsser-Engman-Cole cum dyschromia extensiva corporis. *Pezegl Derm* 1970;57:239–242.
449. Schroeder TM, Hofbauer M. Letter: Dyskeratosis congenita Zinsser-Cole-Engman form with abnormal karyotype. *Dermatologica* 1975;151:316–319.
450. Lin TC, Lin CK, Lee JY, et al. X-linked dyskeratosis congenita with aplastic anemia: genetic and hematologic studies. *Chin Med J* 1989;43:57–62.
451. Kawaguchi K, Sakamaki H, Onozawa Y, et al. Dyskeratosis congenita (Zinsser-Cole-Engman syndrome). An autopsy case presenting with rectal carcinoma, non-cirrhotic hypertension, and *Pneumocystis carinii* pneumonia. *Virchows Archiv A Pathol Anat* 1990;417:247–253.
452. Dokal I, Bungey J, Williamson P, et al. Dyskeratosis congenita fibroblasts are abnormal and have unbalanced chromosomal rearrangements. *Blood* 1992; 80:3090–3096.
453. Chatura KR, Nadar S, Pulimood S, et al. Gastric carcinoma as a complication of dyskeratosis congenita in an adolescent boy. *Digest Dis Sci* 1996;41:2340–2342.
454. Herman TE, McAlister WH. Dyskeratosis congenita. *Pediatr Radiol* 1997;27:286.
455. Baselga E, Drolet BA, van Tuinen P, et al. Dyskeratosis congenita with linear areas of severe cutaneous involvement. *Am J Med Genet* 1998;75:492–496.
456. Auerbach AD, Lieblich LM, Ehrenbard L, et al. Dyskeratosis congenita: cytogenetic studies in a family with an unusual pattern of inheritance. *Am J Hum Genet* 1979;31:87A.
457. Costello MJ. Dyskeratosis congenita with superimposed prickle-cell epithelioma on the dorsal aspect of the left hand. *Arch Dermatol* 1957;75:451.
458. Auerbach AD, Adler B, Chaganti RS. Prenatal and postnatal diagnosis and carrier detection of Fanconi anemia by a cytogenetic method. *Pediatrics* 1981;67:128–135.
459. Kopysc Z, Jankowska-Skrzypek A, Bielniak J, et al. Zinsser-Engman-Cole syndrome (dyskeratosis congenita) in a 13-year-old boy. *Wiad Lek* 1988; 41:525–530.
460. Langston AA, Sanders JE, Deeg HJ, et al. Allogeneic marrow transplantation for aplastic anaemia associated with dyskeratosis congenita. *Br J Haematol* 1996;92:758–765.

461. Connor JM, Teague RH. Dyskeratosis congenita. Report of a large kindred. *Br J Dermatol* 1981;105:321–325.

462. Baykal C, Buyukbabani N, Kavak A. Dyskeratosis congenita associated with Hodgkin's disease. *Eur J Dermatol* 1998;8:385–387.

463. Morrison D, Rose EL, Smith AP, et al. Dyskeratosis congenita and nasopharyngeal atresia. *J Laryngol Otol* 1992;106:996–997.

464. Vanbiervliet P, Blockmans D, Bobbaers H. Dyskeratosis congenita and associated interstitial lung disease; a case report. *Acta Clin Belgica* 1998;53:198–202.

465. Sorrow JM, Hitch JM. Dyskeratosis congenita. *Arch Dermatol* 1963;88:340–347.

466. Woog JJ, Dortzbach RK, Wexler SA, et al. The role of aminocaproic acid in lacrimal surgery in dyskeratosis congenita. *Am J Ophthalmol* 1985;100:728–732.

467. Russo CL, Glader BE, Israel RJ, et al. Treatment of neutropenia associated with dyskeratosis congenita with granulocyte-macrophage colony-stimulating factor. *Lancet* 1990;336:751–752.

468. Putterman C, Safadi R, Zlotogora J, et al. Treatment of the hematological manifestations of dyskeratosis congenita. *Ann Hematol* 1993;66:209–212.

469. Gillio AP, Gabrilove JL. Cytokine treatment of inherited bone marrow failure syndromes. *Blood* 1993;81:1669–1674.

470. Pritchard SL, Junker AK. Positive response to granulocyte-colony-stimulating factor in dyskeratosis congenita before matched unrelated bone marrow transplantation. *Am J Pediatr Hematol Oncol* 1994;16:186–187.

471. Oehler L, Reiter E, Friedl J, et al. Effective stimulation of neutropoiesis with Rh G-CSF in dyskeratosis congenita: a case report. *Ann Hematol* 1994;69:325–327.

472. Yel L, Tezcan I, Sanal O, et al. Dyskeratosis congenita: unusual onset with isolated neutropenia at an early age. *Acta Paediatr Jpn* 1996;38:288–290.

473. Alter BP, Gardner FH, Hall RE. Treatment of dyskeratosis congenita with granulocyte colony-stimulating factor and erythropoietin. *Br J Haematol* 1997;97:309–311.

474. Lemarchand-Venencie F, Gluckman E, Devergie A, et al. Syndrome de Zinsser-Cole-Engmann. *Ann Dermatol Venereol (Paris)* 1982;109:783–784.

475. Mahmoud HK, Schaefer UW, Schmidt CG, et al. Marrow transplantation for pancytopenia in dyskeratosis congenita. *Blut* 1985;51:57–60.

476. Chessells J, Harper J. Bone marrow transplantation for dyskeratosis congenita. *Br J Haematol* 1992;81:314.

477. Berthou C, Devergie A, D'Agay MF, et al. Late vascular complications after bone marrow transplantation for dyskeratosis congenita. *Br J Haematol* 1991;79:335–344.

478. Forni G, Melevendi C, Jappelli S, et al. Dyskeratosis congenita: unusual presenting features within a kindred. *Pediatr Hematol Oncol* 1993;10:145–149.

479. Ivker RA, Woosley J, Resnick SD. Dyskeratosis congenita or chronic graft-versus-host disease? A diagnostic dilemma in a child eight years after bone marrow transplantation for aplastic anemia. *Pediatr Dermatol* 1993;10:362–365.

480. Storb R, Etzioni R, Anasetti C, et al. Cyclophosphamide combined with antithymocyte globulin in preparation for allogeneic marrow transplants in patients with aplastic anemia. *Blood* 1994;84:941–949.

481. Yabe M, Yabe H, Hattori K, et al. Fatal interstitial pulmonary disease in a patient with dyskeratosis congenita after allogeneic bone marrow transplantation. *Bone Marrow Transplant* 1997;19:389–392.

482. Rocha V, Devergie A, Socie G, et al. Unusual complications after bone marrow transplantation for dyskeratosis congenita. *Br J Haematol* 1998;103:243–248.

483. West CM, Ogden AK, Minniti C, et al. Unrelated placental/umbilical cord blood cell transplantation for dyskeratosis congenita. *Pediatr Res* 1999;45:154A.

484. Ling NS, Fenske NA, Julius RL, et al. Dyskeratosis congenita in a girl simulating chronic graft-versus-host disease. *Arch Dermatol* 1985;121:1424–1428.

485. Conter V, Johnson FL, Paolucci P, et al. Bone marrow transplantation for aplastic anemia associated with dyskeratosis congenita. *Am J Pediatr Hematol Oncol* 1988;10:99–102.

486. Kajtar P, Mehes K. Bilateral Coats retinopathy associated with aplastic anaemia and mild dyskeratotic signs. *Am J Med Genet* 1994;49:374–377.

487. Lau YL, Ha SY, Chan CF, et al. Bone marrow transplant for dyskeratosis congenita. *Br J Haematol* 1999;105:567–571.

488. Ghavamzadeh A, Alimoghadam K, Nasseri P, et al. Correction of bone marrow failure in dyskeratosis congenita by bone marrow transplantation. *Bone Marrow Transplant* 1999;23:299–301.

489. Gazda H, Lipton JM, Niemeyer CM, et al. Evidence for linkage of familial Diamond-Blackfan anemia to chromosome 8923.2-23.1 and for non-19q non-8p disease. *Blood* 1999;94:673a.

490. Tolmie JL, Browne BH, McGettrick PM, et al. A familial syndrome with Coats' reaction retinal angiomas, hair and nail defects and intracranial calcification. *Eye* 1988;2:297–303.

491. Revesz T, Fletcher S, Al-Gazali LI, et al. Bilateral retinopathy, aplastic anaemia, and central nervous system abnormalities: a new syndrome? *J Med Genet* 1992;29:673–675.

492. Berger W. Molecular dissection of Norrie disease. *Acta Anat (Basel)* 1998;162:95–100.

493. Li FP, Potter NU, Buchanan GR, et al. A family with acute leukemia, hypoplastic anemia and cerebellar ataxia. Association with bone marrow C-monosomy. *Am J Med* 1978;65:933–940.

494. Li FP, Hecht F, Kaiser-McCaw B, et al. Ataxia-pancytopenia: syndrome of cerebellar ataxia, hypoplastic anemia, monosomy 7, and acute myelogenous leukemia. *Cancer Genet Cytogenet* 1981;4:189–196.

495. Daghistani D, Curless R, Toledano SR, et al. Ataxia-pancytopenia and monosomy 7 syndrome. *J Pediatr* 1989;115:108–110.

496. Mahmood F, King MD, Smyth OP, et al. Familial cerebellar hypoplasia and pancytopenia without chromosomal breakages. *Neuropediatrics* 1998;29:302–306.

497. Gonzalez-Del Angel A, Cervera M, Gomez L, et al. Ataxia-pancytopenia syndrome. *Am J Med Genet* 2000;90:252–254.

498. Akaboshi S, Yoshimura M, Hara T, et al. A case of Hoyeraal-Hreidarsson syndrome: delayed myelination and hypoplasia of corpus callosum are other important signs. *Neuropediatrics* 2000;31:141–144.

499. Revy P, Busslinger M, Tashiro K, et al. A syndrome involving intrauterine growth retardation, microcephaly, cerebellar hypoplasia, B lymphocyte deficiency, and progressive pancytopenia. *Pediatrics* 2000;105:39.

500. Shwachman H, Diamond LK, Oski FA, et al. The syndrome of pancreatic insufficiency and bone marrow dysfunction. *J Pediatr* 1964;65:645–663.

501. Bodian M, Sheldon W, Lightwood R. Congenital hypoplasia of the exocrine pancreas. *Acta Paediatr* 1964;53:282–293.

502. Aggett PJ, Cavanagh NP, Matthew DJ, et al. Shwachman's syndrome. A review of 21 cases. *Arch Dis Child* 1980;55:331–347.

503. Ginzberg H, Shin J, Ellis L, et al. Segregation analysis in Shwachman-Diamond syndrome: evidence for recessive inheritance. *Am J Hum Genet* 2000;66:1413–1416.

504. Alter BP, Kumar M, Lockhart LL, et al. Pregnancy in bone marrow failure syndromes: Diamond-Blackfan anaemia and Shwachman-Diamond syndrome. *Br J Haematol* 1999;107:49–54.

505. Ozsoylu S, Argun G. Tryptic activity of the duodenal juice in aplastic anemia. *J Pediatr* 1967;70:60–64.

506. Thong YH. Impaired neutrophil kinesis in a patient with the Shwachman-Diamond syndrome. *Aust Paediatr J* 1978;14:34–37.

507. Aggett PJ, Harries JT, Harvey BA, et al. An inherited defect of neutrophil mobility in Shwachman syndrome. *J Pediatr* 1979;94:391–394.

508. Ruutu P, Savilahati E, Repo H, et al. Constant defect in neutrophil locomotion but with age decreasing susceptibility to infection in Shwachman syndrome. *Br J Haematol* 1984;70:502.

509. Repo H, Savilahti E, Leirisalo-Repo M. Aberrant phagocyte function in Shwachman syndrome. *Clin Exp Immunol* 1987;69:204–212.

510. Shwachman H, Holsclaw D. Some clinical observations on the Shwachman syndrome (pancreatic insufficiency and bone marrow hypoplasia). *Birth Defects Orig Artic Ser* 1972;8:46–49.

511. Ginzberg H, Shin J, Ellis L, et al. Shwachman syndrome. Phenotypic manifestations of sibling sets and isolated cases in a large patient cohort are similar. *J Pediatr* 1999;135:81–88.

512. Hudson E, Aldor T. Pancreatic insufficiency and neutropenia with associated immunoglobulin deficit. *Arch Intern Med* 1970;125:314–316.

513. Goobie S, Popovic M, Morrison J, et al. Shwachman-Diamond syndrome with exocrine pancreatic dysfunction and bone marrow failure maps to the centromeric region of chromosome 7. *Am J Hum Genet* 2001;68:1048–1054.

514. Dale DC, Bonilla MA, Davis MW, et al. A randomized controlled phase III trial of recombinant human granulocyte colony-stimulating factor (Filgrastim) for treatment of severe chronic neutropenia. *Blood* 1993;81:2496–2502.

515. Seymour JF, Escudier SM. Acute leukemia complicating bone marrow hypoplasia in an adult with Shwachman's syndrome. *Leuk Lymphoma* 1993;12:131–135.

516. Tsai PH, Sahdev I, Herry A, et al. Fatal cyclophosphamide induced congestive heart failure in a 10-year-old boy with Shwachman-Diamond syndrome and severe bone marrow failure treated with allogeneic bone marrow transplantation. *Am J Pediatr Hematol Oncol* 1989;12:472–476.

517. Barrios NJ, Kirkpatrick DV. Successful cyclosporin A treatment of aplastic anaemia in Shwachman-Diamond syndrome. *Br J Haematol* 1990;74:540–541.

518. Barrios N, Kirkpatrick D, Regueira O, et al. Bone marrow transplant in Shwachman-Diamond syndrome. *Br J Haematol* 1991;79:337–338.

519. Laporte JP, Lesage S, Portnoi MF, et al. Successful immunoadoptive therapy (IT) after allogeneic transplantation (BMT) for early relapse of myelodysplastic syndrome (MDS) in a Shwachman's Diamond syndrome (SD) patient. *Blood* 1995;86:954a.

520. Smith OP, Chan MY, Evans J, et al. Shwachman-Diamond syndrome and matched unrelated donor BMT. *Bone Marrow Transplant* 1995;16:717–718.

521. Smith O, Hann IM, Chessells JM, et al. Haematological abnormalities in Shwachman-Diamond syndrome. *Br J Haematol* 1996;94:279–284.

522. Bordigoni P. Bone marrow transplantation for inherited bone marrow failure syndromes. *Int J Pediatr Hem Oncol* 1995;2:441–452.

523. Bunin N, Leahey A, Dunn S. Related donor liver transplant for veno-occlusive disease following T-depleted unrelated donor bone marrow transplantation. *Transplantation* 1996;61:664–666.

524. Arseniev L, Diedrich H, Link H. Allogeneic bone marrow transplantation in a patient with Shwachman-Diamond syndrome. *Ann Hematol* 1996;72:83–84.

525. Davies SM, Wagner JE, Defor T, et al. Unrelated donor bone marrow transplantation for children and adolescents with aplastic anaemia or myelodysplasia. *Br J Haematol* 1997;96:749–756.

526. Dokal I, Rule S, Chen F, et al. Adult onset of acute myeloid leukaemia (M6) in patients with Shwachman-Diamond syndrome. *Br J Haematol* 1997;99:171–173.

527. Okcu F, Roberts WM, Chan KW. Bone marrow transplantation in Shwachman-Diamond syndrome: report of two cases and review of the literature. *Bone Marrow Transplant* 1998;21:849–851.

528. Faber J, Lauener R, Wick F, et al. Shwachman-Diamond syndrome: early bone marrow transplantation in a high risk patient and new clues to pathogenesis. *Eur J Pediatr* 1999;158:995–1000.

529. Cipolli M, D'Orazio C, Delmarco A, et al. Shwachman's syndrome: pathomorphosis and long-term outcome. *J Pediatr Gastroenterol Nutr* 1999;29:265–272.

530. Pratt N, Cunningham JJ, Sales M, et al. Do chromosome 7 abnormalities mandate bone marrow transplant in Shwachman-Diamond syndrome? *J Med Genet* 2000;37[Suppl]:S27.

531. Cesaro S, Guariso G, Calore E, et al. Successful unrelated bone marrow transplantation for Shwachman-Diamond syndrome. *Bone Marrow Transplant* 2001;27:97–99.

532. Nezeloff C, Watchi M. L'hypoplasie congenitale lipomateuse du pancreas exocrine chez l'enfant (deux observations et revue de la litterature). *Arch Fr Pediatr* 1961;18:1135–1172.

533. Huijgens PC, Van der Veen EA, Meijer S, et al. Syndrome of Shwachman and leukaemia. *Scand J Haematol* 1977;18:20–24.

534. Strevens MJ, Lilleyman JS, Williams RB. Shwachman's syndrome and acute lymphoblastic leukaemia. *BMJ* 1978;2:18.

535. Caselitz J, Kloppel G, Delling G, et al. Shwachman's syndrome and leukaemia. *Virchows Arch A Pathol Anat Histol* 1979;385:109–116.

536. Woods WG, Roloff JS, Lukens JN, et al. The occurrence of leukemia in patients with the Shwachman syndrome. *J Pediatr* 1981;99:425–428.

537. Woods WG, Krivit W, Lubin BH, et al. Aplastic anemia associated with the Shwachman syndrome. In vivo and in vitro observations. *Am J Pediatr Hematol Oncol* 1981;3:347–351.

538. Gretillat F, Delepine N, Taillard F, et al. Shwachman's syndrome transformed into leukaemia. *Presse Med* 1985;14:45.

539. MacMaster SA, Cummings TM. Computed tomography and ultrasonography findings for an adult with Shwachman syndrome and pancreatic lipomatosis. *Can Assoc Radiol J* 1993;44:301–303.

540. Passmore SJ, Hann IM, Stiller CA, et al. Pediatric myelodysplasia: a study of 68 children and a new prognostic scoring system. *Blood* 1995;85:1742–1750.

541. Spirito FR, Crescenzi B, Matteucci C, et al. Cytogenetic characterization of acute myeloid leukemia in Shwachman's syndrome. A case report. *Haematologica* 2000;85:1207–1210.

542. Maserati E, Minelli A, Olivieri C, et al. Isochromosome (7)(q10) in Shwachman syndrome without MDS/AML and role of chromosome 7 anomalies in myeloproliferative disorders. *Cancer Genet Cytogenet* 2000;121:167–171.

543. Kalra R, Dale D, Freedman M, et al. Monosomy 7 and activating RAS mutations accompany malignant transformation in patients with congenital neutropenia. *Blood* 1995;86:4579–4586.

544. Dror Y, Squire J, Durie P, et al. Malignant myeloid transformation with isochromosome 7q in Shwachman-Diamond syndrome. *Leukemia* 1998;12:1591–1595.

545. Sokolic RA, Ferguson W, Mark HF. Discordant detection of monosomy 7 by GTG-banding and FISH in a patient with Shwachman-Diamond syndrome without evidence of myelodysplastic syndrome or acute myelogenous leukemia. *Cancer Genet Cytogenet* 1999;115:106–113.

546. Howard J, Dunlop A, Kelly J, et al. Isochromosome 7q in two children with Shwachman-Diamond syndrome. *J Med Genet* 2000;37[Suppl]:235.

547. Pearson HA, Lobel JS, Kocoshis SA, et al. A new syndrome of refractory sideroblastic anemia with vacuolization of marrow precursors and exocrine pancreatic dysfunction. *J Pediatr* 1979;95:976–984.

548. Rotig A, Colonna M, Bonnefont JP, et al. Mitochondrial DNA deletion in Pearson's marrow/pancreas syndrome. *Lancet* 1989;1:902–903.

549. Pearson HA. The naming of a syndrome. *J Pediatr Hematol Oncol* 1997;19:271–273.

550. Rotig A, Bourgeron T, Chretien D, et al. Spectrum of mitochondrial DNA rearrangements in the Pearson marrow-pancreas syndrome. *Hum Molec Genet* 1995;4:1327–1330.

551. Kerr DS. Protean manifestations of mitochondrial diseases: a mini review. *J Pediatr Hematol Oncol* 1997;19:279–286.

552. Makitie O, Kaitila I. Cartilage-hair hypoplasia—clinical manifestations in 108 Finnish patients. *Eur J Pediatr* 1993;152:211–217.

553. Roberts MA, Arnold RM. Hodgkin's lymphoma in a child with cartilage-hair hypoplasia: case report. *Milit Med* 1984;149:280–281.

554. Gorlin RJ. Cartilage-hair-hypoplasia and Hodgkin disease. *Am J Med Genet* 1992;44:539.

555. Makitie O, Pukkala E, Teppo L, et al. Increased incidence of cancer in patients with cartilage-hair hypoplasia. *J Pediatr* 1999;134:315–318.

556. Sulisalo T, Francomano CA, Sistonen P, et al. High-resolution genetic mapping of the cartilage-hair hypoplasia (CHH) gene in Amish and Finnish families. *Genomics* 1994;20:347–353.

557. Ridanpaa M, van Eenennaam H, Pelin K, et al. Mutations in the RNA component of RNase MRP cause a pleiotropic human disease, cartilage-hair hypoplasia. *Cell* 2001;104:195–203.

558. Bizzaro N, Dianese G. Neonatal alloimmune amegakaryocytosis. *Vox Sang* 1988;54:112–114.

559. Guinan EC, Lee YS, Lopez KD, et al. Effects of interleukin-3 and granulocyte-macrophage colony-stimulating factor on thrombopoiesis in congenital amegakaryocytic thrombocytopenia. *Blood* 1993;81:1691–1698.

560. Van den Oudenrijn S, Bruin M, Folman CC, et al. Mutations in the thrombopoietin receptor, Mpl, in children with congenital amegakaryocytic thrombocytopenia. *Br J Haematol* 2000;110:441–448.

561. Ballmaier M, Germeshausen M, Schulze H, et al. C-mpl mutations are the cause of congenital amegakaryocytic thrombocytopenia. *Blood* 2001;97:139–146.

562. Gardner RJ, Morrison PS, Abbott GD. A syndrome of congenital thrombocytopenia with multiple malformations and neurologic dysfunction. *J Pediatr* 1983;102:600–602.

563. Taylor DS, Lee Y, Sieff CA, et al. Phase I/II trial of PIXY321 (granulocyte-macrophage colony stimulating factor/interleukin-3 fusion protein) for treatment of inherited and acquired marrow failure syndromes. *Br J Haematol* 1998;103:304–307.

564. Van Oostrom CG, Wilms RH. Congenital thrombocytopenia, associated with raised concentrations of haemoglobin F. *Helv Paediatr Acta* 1978;33:59–61.

565. Buchanan GR, Scher CS, Button LN, et al. Use of homologous platelet survival in the differential diagnosis of chronic thrombocytopenia in childhood. *Pediatrics* 1977;59:49–54.

566. Mibashan RS, Millar DS. Fetal haemophilia and allied bleeding disorders. *Br Med Bull* 1983;39:392–398.

567. Freedman MH. Congenital failure of hematopoiesis in the newborn infant. *Clin Perinatol* 1984;11:417–431.

568. Griffiths AD. Constitutional aplastic anaemia: a family with a new X-linked variety of amegakaryocytic thrombocytopenia. *J Med Genet* 1983;20:361–364.

569. Cremer M, Schulze H, Linthorst G, et al. Serum levels of thrombopoietin, IL-11, and IL-6 in pediatric thrombocytopenias. *Ann Hematol* 1999;78:401–407.

570. Mukai HY, Kojima H, Todokoro K, et al. Serum thrombopoietin (TPO) levels in patients with amegakaryocytic thrombocytopenia are much higher than those with immune thrombocytopenic purpura. *Thromb Haemost* 1996;76:675–678.

571. Muraoka K, Ishii E, Tsuji K, et al. Defective response to thrombopoietin and impaired expression of c-mpl mRNA of bone marrow cells in congenital amegakaryocytic thrombocytopenia. *Br J Haematol* 1997;96:287–292.

572. Ihara K, Ishii E, Eguchi M, et al. Identification of mutations in the c-mpl gene in congenital amegakaryocytic thrombocytopenia. *Proc Natl Acad Sci U S A* 1999;96:3132–3136.

573. Tonelli R, Scardovi AL, Pession A, et al. Compound heterozygosity for two different amino-acid substitution mutations in the thrombopoietin receptor (c-mpl gene) in congenital amegakaryocytic thrombocytopenia (CAMT). *Hum Genet* 2000;107:225–233.

574. Henter J, Winiarski J, Ljungman P, et al. Bone marrow transplantation in two children with congenital amegakaryocytic thrombocytopenia. *Bone Marrow Transplant* 1995;15:799–801.

575. Margolis D, Camitta B, Pietryga D, et al. Unrelated donor bone marrow transplantation to treat severe aplastic anaemia in children and young adults. *Br J Haematol* 1996;94:65–72.

576. MacMillan ML, Davies SM, Wagner JE, et al. Engraftment of unrelated donor stem cells in children with familial amegakaryocytic thrombocytopenia. *Bone Marrow Transplant* 1998;21:735–737.

577. Arias S, Penchaszadeh VB, Pinto-Cisternas J, et al. The IVIC syndrome: a new autosomal dominant complex pleiotropic syndrome with radial ray hypoplasia, hearing impairment, external ophthalmoplegia, and thrombocytopenia. *Am J Med Genet* 1980;6:25–59.

578. Sammito V, Motta D, Capodieci G, et al. IVIC syndrome: report of a second family. *Am J Med Genet* 1988;29:875–881.

579. Czeizel A, Goblyos P, Kodaj I. IVIC syndrome: report of a third family. *Am J Med Genet* 1989;32:282–283.

580. Neri G, Sammito V. Re: IVIC syndrome report by Czeizel et al. *Am J Med Genet* 1989;33:284.

581. Gonzalez CH, Durkin-Stamm MV, Geimer NF, et al. The WT syndrome: a "new" autosomal dominant pleiotropic trait of radial/ulnar hypoplasia with high risk of bone marrow failure and/or leukemia. *Birth Defects Orig Artic Ser* 1977;8:31–38.

582. Alter CL, Levine PH, Bennett J, et al. Dominantly transmitted hematologic dysfunction clinically similar to Fanconi's anemia. *Am J Hematol* 1989;32:241–247.

583. Aufderheide AC. Familial cytopenia and vascular disease: a newly recognized autosomal dominant condition. *Birth Defects Orig Artic Ser* 1972;8:63–68.

584. Kato J, Niitsu Y, Ishigaki S, et al. Chronic hypoplastic neutropenia. A case of familial occurrence of chronic hypoplastic neutropenia and aplastic anemia. *Rinsho Ketsueki* 1986;27:407–411.

585. Dokal I, Ganly P, Riebero I, et al. Late onset bone marrow failure associated with proximal fusion of radius and ulna: a new syndrome. *Br J Haematol* 1989;71:277–280.

586. Thompson AA, Nguyen LT. Amegakaryocytic thrombocytopenia and radio-ulnar synostosis are associated with HOXA11 mutation. *Nat Genet* 2000;26:397–398.

587. Sleijfer DT, Mulder NH, Niewig HO, et al. Acquired pancytopenia in relatives of patients with aplastic anaemia. *Acta Med Scand* 1980;207:397–402.

588. Abels D, Reed WB. Fanconi-like syndrome. Immunologic deficiency, pancytopenia, and cutaneous malignancies. *Arch Dermatol* 1973;107:419–423.

589. Linsk JA, Khoory MS, Meyers KR. Myeloid, erythroid, and immune system defects in a family. A new stem-cell disorder? *Ann Intern Med* 1975;82:659–662.

590. Chitambar CR, Robinson WA, Glode LM. Familial leukemia and aplastic anemia associated with monosomy 7. *Am J Med* 1983;75:756–762.

591. Samad FU, Engel E, Hartmann RC. Hypoplastic anemia, Friedreich's ataxia and chromosomal breakage: case report and review of similar disorders. *South Med J* 1973;66:135–140.

592. Li FP, Marchetto DJ, Vawter GR. Acute leukemia and preleukemia in eight males in a family: an X-linked disorder? *Am J Hematol* 1979;6:61–69.

593. Purtilo DT, Sakamoto K, Barnabei V, et al. Epstein-Barr virus-induced diseases in boys with the X-linked lymphoproliferative syndrome (XLP). Update on studies of the registry. *Am J Med* 1982;73:49–56.

594. Coffey AT, Brooksbank RA, Brandon O, et al. Host response to EBV infection in X-linked lymphoproliferative disease results from mutation in an SH2-domain encoding gene. *Nat Genet* 1998;20:129.

594a. Syos J, Wu C, Morra M, et al. The X-linked lymphoproliferative disease gene product of SAP regulates signals induced through the co-receptor SLAM. *Nature* 1998;395:462–469.

594b. Nichols KE, Harkin DP, Levitz S, et al. Inactivation mutation in an SH2 domain-encoding gene in X-linked lymphoproliferative syndrome. *Proc Natl Acad Sci U S A* 1998;95:13765–13770.

595. Sackey K, Sakati N, Aur RJ, et al. Multiple dysmorphic features and pancytopenia: a new syndrome. *Clin Genet* 1985;27:606–610.

596. Poole S, Smith AC, Hays T, et al. Fanconi anemia in monozygotic twin females. *Am J Hum Genet* 1988;43:65A.

597. Shaw JP, Marks J, Shen CC, et al. Anomalous and selective DNA mutations of the Old World monkey alpha-globin genes. *Proc Natl Acad Sci U S A* 1989;86:1312–1316.

598. Nowell P, Besa E, Emanuel B, et al. Two adult siblings with thrombocytopenia and a familial 13;14 translocation. *Cancer Genet Cytogenet* 1984;11:169–174.

599. Rosenthal RL, Blackman A. Bone-marrow hypoplasia following use of chloramphenicol eye drops. *JAMA* 1965;191:148–149.

600. Nora AH, Fernbach DJ. Acquired aplastic anemia in children. *Texas Med* 1969;65:38–43.

601. Nagao T, Mauer AM. Concordance for drug-induced aplastic anemia in identical twins. *N Engl J Med* 1969;281:7–11.

602. Boga M, Szemere PA. Infectious hepatitis and aplastic anaemia in two sisters. *Lancet* 1971;2:708.

603. Sears DA, George JN, Gold MS. Transient red blood cell aplasia in association with viral hepatitis. Occurrence four years apart in siblings. *Arch Intern Med* 1975;135:1585–1589.

604. Davidson LS, Davis LJ, Innes J. Studies in refractory anaemia. *Edinburgh Med J* 1943;50:355–377.

605. McLaren GD, Doukas MA, Muir WA. Methyprylon-induced bone marrow suppression in siblings. *JAMA* 1978;240:1744–1745.

606. Stolte JB. Familiare aplastische anamie. *Ned Tijdschr Geneeskd* 1948;92:4053–4055.

607. Keiser G. Erworbene panmyelopathien. *Schweiz Med Wochenschr* 1970;100:1938–1948.

608. Weinstein HJ. Congenital leukemia and the neonatal myeloproliferative disorders associated with Down's syndrome. *Clin Haematol* 1978;7:147–154.

609. Erdogan G, Aksoy M, Dincol K. A case of idiopathic aplastic anemia associated with trisomy 21 and partial endoreduplication. *Acta Haematol* 1967;37:137–142.

610. Vetrella M, Barthelmai W, Matsuda H. Kongenitale amegakaryocytare thrombocytopenie mit finaler pancytopenie bei trisomie 21 mit cystischer pankreasfibrose. *Z Kinderheilk* 1969;107:210–218.

611. Weinblatt ME, Higgins G, Ortega JA. Aplastic anemia in Down's syndrome. *Pediatrics* 1981;67:896–897.

612. McWilliams NB, Dunn NL. Aplastic anemia and Down's syndrome. *Pediatrics* 1982;69:501–502.

613. Hanukoglu A, Meytes D, Fried A, et al. Fatal aplastic anemia in a child with Down's syndrome. *Acta Paediatr Scand* 1987;76:539–543.

614. Tsukahara M, Opitz JM. Dubowitz syndrome: review of 141 cases including 36 previously unreported patients. *Am J Med Genet* 1996;63:277–289.

615. Majewski F, Goecke T. Studies of microcephalic primordial dwarfism I: approach to a delineation of the Seckel syndrome. *Am J Med Genet* 1982;12:7–21.

616. Upjohn C. Familial dwarfism associated with microcephaly, mental retardation and anaemia. *Proc Soc Med* 1955;48:334–335.

617. Seckel HP. *Bird-headed dwarfs*. Basel, Switzerland: S. Karger, 1960:241.

618. Lilleyman JS. Constitutional hypoplastic anemia associated with familial "bird-headed" dwarfism (Seckel syndrome). *Am J Pediatr Hematol Oncol* 1984;6:207–209.

619. Butler MG, Hall BD, Maclean RN, et al. Do some patients with Seckel syndrome have hematological problems and/or chromosome breakage? *Am J Med Genet* 1987;27:645–649.

620. Esperou-Bourdeau H, Leblanc T, Schaison G, et al. Aplastic anemia associated with "bird-headed" dwarfism (Seckel syndrome). *Nouv Rev Fr Hematol* 1993;35:99–100.

621. Woods CG, Leversha M, Rogers JG. Severe intrauterine growth retardation with increased mitomycin C sensitivity: a further chromosome breakage syndrome. *J Med Genet* 1995;32:301–305.

622. Cervenka J, Tsuchiya H, Ishiki T, et al. Seckel's dwarfism: analysis of chromosome breakage and sister chromatid exchanges. *Am J Dis Child* 1979;133:555–556.

623. Hayani A, Suarez CR, Molnar Z, et al. Acute myeloid leukaemia in a patient with Seckel syndrome. *J Med Genet* 1994;31:148–149.

624. Abou-Zahr F, Bejjani B, Kruyt FA, et al. Normal expression of the Fanconi anemia proteins FAA and FAC and sensitivity to mitomycin C in two patients with Seckel syndrome. *Am J Med Genet* 1999;83:388–391.

625. Josephs HW. Anaemia of infancy and early childhood. *Medicine* 1936;15:307–402.

626. Diamond LK, Blackfan KD. Hypoplastic anemia. *Am J Dis Child* 1938;56:464–467.

627. Alter BP. Childhood red cell aplasia. *Am J Pediatr Hematol Oncol* 1980;2:121–139.

628. Diamond LK, Wang WC, Alter BP. Congenital hypoplastic anemia. *Adv Pediatr* 1976;22:349–378.

629. Alter BP, Nathan DG. Red cell aplasia in children. *Arch Dis Child* 1979;54:263–267.

630. Ball SE, Tchernia G, Wranne L, et al. Is there a role for interleukin-3 in Diamond-Blackfan anaemia? Results of a European multicentre study. *Br J Haematol* 1995;91:313–318.

631. Janov AJ, Leong T, Nathan DG, et al. Diamond-Blackfan anemia. Natural history and sequelae of treatment. *Medicine* 1996;75:77–87.

632. Willig TN, Niemeyer CM, Leblanc T, et al. Identification of new prognosis factors from the clinical and epidemiologic analysis of a registry of 229 Diamond-Blackfan anemia patients. *Pediatr Res* 1999;46:553–561.

633. Ramenghi U, Garelli E, Valtolina S, et al. Diamond-Blackfan anaemia in the Italian population. *Br J Haematol* 1999;104:841–848.

634. Wallman IS. Hereditary red cell aplasia. *Med J Aust* 1956;2:488–490.

635. Gray P.H. Pure red-cell aplasia. Occurrence in three generations. *Med J Aust* 1982;1:519–521.

636. Neilson RF, Khokhar AA. Red cell aplasia in mother and son. *Clin Lab Haematol* 1991;13:224–225.

637. Gojic V, Van't Veer-Korthof ET, Bosch LJ, et al. Congenital hypoplastic anemia: another example of autosomal dominant transmission. *Am J Med Genet* 1994;50:87–89.

638. Madanat F, Arnaout M, Hasan A, et al. Red cell aplasia resembling Diamond-Blackfan anemia in seven children in a family. *Am J Pediatr Hematol Oncol* 1994;16:260–265.

639. Balaban EP, Buchanan GR, Graham. M., et al. Diamond-Blackfan syndrome in adult patients. *Am J Med* 1985;78:533–538.

640. Abkowitz JL, Sabo KM, Nakamoto B, et al. Diamond-Blackfan anemia: in vitro response of erythroid progenitors to the ligand for c-kit. *Blood* 1991;78:2198–2202.

641. Bastion Y, Campos L, Roubi N, et al. IL-3 increases marrow and peripheral erythroid precursors in chronic pure red cell aplasia presenting in childhood. *Br J Haematol* 1995;89:413–416.

642. Cetin M, Kara A, Gurgey A, et al. Congenital hypoplastic anemia in six patients: unusual association of short proximal phalanges with mild anemia. *Pediatr Hematol Oncol* 1995;12:153–158.

643. Willig TN, Perignon JL, Gustavsson P, et al. High adenosine deaminase level among healthy probands of Diamond Blackfan anemia (DBA) cosegregates with the DBA gene region on chromosome 19q13. *Blood* 1998;92:4422–4427.

644. Willig T, Draptchinskaia N, Dianzani I, et al. Mutations in ribosomal protein S19 gene and Diamond Blackfan anemia: wide variations in phenotypic expression. *Blood* 1999;94:4294–4306.

645. Bello A, Dorantes S, Alvarez-Amaya C. La anemia hipoplastica en la edad pediatrica. *Bol Med Hosp Infant Mex* 1983;40:718–723.

646. Waterkotte GW, McElfresh AE. Congenital pure red cell hypoplasia in identical twins. *Pediatrics* 1974;54:646–647.

647. Freedman MH. Diamond-Blackfan anemia. *Am J Pediatr Hematol Oncol* 1985;7:327–330.

648. Giblett ER, Varela JE, Finch CA. Damage of the bone marrow due to Rh antibody. *Pediatrics* 1956;17:37–44.

649. Schorr JB, Cohen ES, Schwarz A, et al. Hypoplastic anemia in childhood. *Jewish Mem Hosp Bull* 1962;6:126–136.

650. Cathie IA. Erythrogenesis imperfecta. *Arch Dis Child* 1950;25:313–324.

651. Aase JM, Smith DW. Congenital anemia and triphalangeal thumbs: a new syndrome. *J Pediatr* 1969;74:471–474.

652. Alter BP. Thumbs and anemia. *Pediatrics* 1978;62:613–614.

653. Sacrez R, Levy JM, Godar G, et al. Anemie de Blackfan-Diamond associee a des malformations multiples. *Med Infant* 1965;72:493–499.

654. O'Gorman Hughes DW. Hypoplastic anaemia in infancy and childhood: erythroid hypoplasia. *Arch Dis Child* 1961;36:349–361.

655. Harris RE, Baehner RL, Gleiser S, et al. Cartilage-hair hypoplasia, defective T-cell function, and Diamond-Blackfan anemia in an Amish child. *Am J Med Genet* 1981;8:291–297.

656. Buchanan GR, Alter BP, Holtkamp CA, et al. Platelet number and function in Diamond-Blackfan anemia. *Pediatrics* 1981;68:238–241.

657. Vogel P, Bassen FA. Sternal marrow of children in normal and in pathologic states. *Am J Dis Child* 1939;57:245–268.

658. Gasser C. Aplastische anamie (chronische erythroblastophthise) und cortison. *Schweiz Med Wochenschr* 1951;81:1241–1242.

659. Bernard J, Seligmann M, Chassigneux J, et al. Anemie de Blackfan-Diamond. *Nouv Rev Fr Hematol* 1962;2:721–739.

660. Boxer LA, Hussey L, Clarke TL. Sideroblastic anemia following congenital erythroid hypoplasia. *J Pediatr* 1971;79:681–683.

661. Girot R, Griscelli C. Erythroblastopenie a rechutes. A propos d'un cas suivi pendant 22 ans. *Nouv Rev Fr Hematol* 1977;18:555–562.

662. Hammond D, Shore N, Movassagli N. Production, utilization and excretion of erythropoietin. I. Chronic anemias. II. Aplastic crisis. III. Erythropoietic effects of normal plasma. *Ann N Y Acad Sci* 1968;149:516–526.

663. Altman KI, Miller G. A disturbance in tryptophan metabolism in congenital hypoplastic anaemia. *Nature* 1953;172:868.

664. Pearson HA, Cone TE Jr. Congenital hypoplastic anemia. *Pediatrics* 1957;19:192–200.

665. Price JM, Brown RR, Pfaffenbach EC, et al. Excretion of urinary tryptophan metabolites by patients with congenital hypoplastic anemia (Diamond-Blackfan syndrome). *J Lab Clin Med* 1970;75:316–324.

666. Tartaglia AP, Propp S, Amarose AP, et al. Chromosome abnormality and hypocalcemia in congenital erythroid hypoplasia (Blackfan-Diamond syndrome). *Am J Med* 1966;41:990–999.

667. Ogasawara T, Kasahara H, Watanabe T, et al. A case report of constitutional erythroid hypoplasia (Josephs-Blackfan-Diamond type) with immunodeficiency. *Shoni Shikagaku Zasshi* 1987;25:174–183.

668. Brookfield EG, Singh P. Congenital hypoplastic anemia associated with hypogammaglobulinemia. *J Pediatr* 1974;82:529–531.

669. Finlay JL, Shahidi NT, Horowitz S, et al. Lymphocyte dysfunction in congenital hypoplastic anemia. *J Clin Invest* 1982;70:619–626.

670. Sjolin S, Wranne L. Treatment of congenital hypoplastic anaemia with prednisone. *Scand J Haematol* 1970;7:63–72.

671. Feldges D, Schmidt R. Erythrogenesis imperfecta (Blackfan-Diamond-Anamie). *Schweiz Med Wochenschr* 1971;101:1813–1814.

672. Fondu P, Mandelbaum IM, Stryckmans PA, et al. Un cas d'erythroblastopenie de l'enfant a debut tardif. *Nouv Rev Fr Hematol* 1972;12:5–14.

673. Giblett ER, Ammann AJ, Wara DW, et al. Nucleoside-phosphorylase deficiency in a child with severely defective T-cell immunity and normal B-cell immunity. *Lancet* 1975;1:1010–1013.

674. Glader BE, Backer K, Diamond LK. Elevated erythrocyte adenosine deaminase activity in congenital hypoplastic anemia. *N Engl J Med* 1983;309:1486–1490.

675. Zielke HR, Ozand PT, Luddy RE, et al. Elevation of pyrimidine enzyme activities in the RBC of patients with congenital hypoplastic anaemia and their parents. *Br J Haematol* 1979;42:381–390.

676. Glader BE, Backer K. Comparative activity of erythrocyte adenosine deaminase and orotidine decarboxylase in Diamond-Blackfan anemia. *Am J Hematol* 1986;23:135–139.

677. Glader BE, Backer K. Elevated red cell adenosine deaminase activity: a marker of disordered erythropoiesis in Diamond-Blackfan anaemia and other haematologic diseases. *Br J Haematol* 1988;68:165–168.

678. Whitehouse DB, Hopkinson DA, Pilz AJ, et al. Adenosine deaminase activity in a series of 19 patients with the Diamond-Blackfan syndrome. *Adv Exp Med Biol* 1986;195:85–92.

679. Heyn R, Kurczynski E, Schmickel R. The association of Blackfan-Diamond syndrome, physical abnormalities, and an abnormality of chromosome 1. *J Pediatr* 1974;85:531–533.

680. Philippe N, Requin CH, Germain D. Etudes chromosomiques dans 6 cas d'anemie de Blackfan-Diamond. *Pediatrie* 1971;26:47–54.

681. Van der Mooren K. Fetal anemia. *Prenat Diagn* 1989;9:450.

682. Iskandar O, Jager MJ, Willenze R, et al. A case of pure red cell aplasia with high incidence of spontaneous chromosome breakage: a possible x-ray sensitive syndrome. *Hum Genet* 1980;55:337–340.

683. McFarland G, Say B, Carpenter NJ, et al. A condition resembling congenital hypoplastic anemia occurring in a mother and son. *Clin Pediatr* 1982;12:755–756.

684. Pfeiffer RA, Ambs E. The Aase syndrome: autosomal-recessive hereditary, connatal erythroid hypoplasia and triphalangeal thumbs. *Monatsschr Kinderheilkd* 1983;131:235–237.

685. Brown KE, Green SW, Antunez de Mayolo J, et al. Congenital anaemia after transplacental B19 parvovirus infection. *Lancet* 1994;343:895–896.

686. Heegaard ED, Hasle H, Clausen N, et al. Parvovirus B19 infection and Diamond-Blackfan anaemia. *Acta Paediat* 1996;85:299–302.

687. Visser GH, Desmedt MC, Meijboom EJ. Altered fetal cardiac flow patterns in pure red cell anaemia (the Blackfan-Diamond syndrome). *Prenat Diagn* 1988;8:525–529.

688. McLennan AC, Chitty LS, Rissik J, et al. Prenatal diagnosis of Blackfan-Diamond syndrome: case report and review of the literature. *Prenat Diagn* 1996;16:349–353.

689. Rogers BB, Bloom SL, Buchanan GR. Autosomal dominantly inherited Diamond Blackfan anemia resulting in nonimmune hydrops. *Obstet Gynecol* 1997;89:805–807.

690. Smith CH. Chronic congenital aregenerative anemia (pure red-cell anemia) associated with isoimmunization by the blood group factor A. *Blood* 1949;4:697–705.

691. Moody EA. Hypoplastic anemia following exchange transfusion for erythroblastosis fetalis associated with isoimmunization to blood group factor A. *J Pediatr* 1954;44:244–247.

692. Hoffman R, Zanjani ED, Vila J, et al. Diamond-Blackfan syndrome: lymphocyte-mediated suppression of erythropoiesis. *Science* 1976;193:899–900.

693. Nathan DG, Hillman DG, Breard J. The influence of T cells on erythropoiesis. In: Stamatoyannopoulos G, Nienhuis AW, eds. *Cellular and molecular regulation of hemoglobin switching.* New York: Grune & Stratton, 1979:291–304.

694. Harris RE, Baehner RL, Gleiser S, et al. Cartilage-hair hypoplasia, defective T-cell function, and Diamond-Blackfan anemia in an Amish child. *Am J Med Genet* 1981;8:291–297.

695. Nathan DG, Clarke BJ, Hillman DG, et al. Erythroid precursors in congenital hypoplastic (Diamond-Blackfan) anemia. *J Clin Invest* 1978;61:489–498.

696. Nathan DG, Hillman DG, Chess L, et al. Normal erythropoietic helper T cells in congenital hypoplastic (Diamond-Blackfan) anemia. *N Engl J Med* 1978;298:1049–1051.

697. Alter BP. Inherited bone marrow failure syndromes. In: Handin RI, Lux SE, Stossel TP, eds. *Blood: principles and practice of hematology.* Philadelphia: JB Lippincott Co, 1995:227–291.

698. Claustres M, Margueritte G, Sultan C. In vitro CFU-E and BFU-E responses to androgen in bone marrow from children with primary hypoproliferative anaemia—a possible therapeutic assay. *Eur J Pediatr* 1986;144:467–471.

699. Halperin DS, Estrov Z, Freedman MH. Diamond-Blackfan anemia: promotion of marrow erythropoiesis in vitro by recombinant interleukin-3. *Blood* 1989;73:1168–1174.

700. Chan HS, Saunders EF, Freedman MH. Diamond-Blackfan syndrome. I. Erythropoiesis in prednisone responsive and resistant disease. *Pediatr Res* 1982;16:474–476.

701. Lipton JM, Kudisch M, Gross R, et al. Defective erythroid progenitor differentiation system in congenital hypoplastic (Diamond-Blackfan) anemia. *Blood* 1986;67:962–968.

702. Tsai PH, Arkin S, Lipton JM. An intrinsic progenitor defect in Diamond-Blackfan anemia. *Br J Haematol* 1989;73:112–120.

703. Perdahl EB, Naprstek BL, Wallace WC, et al. Erythroid failure in Diamond-Blackfan anemia is characterized by apoptosis. *Blood* 1994;83:645–650.

704. Dianzani I, Garelli E, Dompe C, et al. Mutations in the erythropoietin receptor gene are not a common cause of Diamond-Blackfan anemia. *Blood* 1996;87:2568–2572.

705. Dianzani I, Garelli E, Crescenzio N, et al. Diamond-Blackfan anemia: expansion of erythroid progenitors in vitro by IL-9, but exclusion of a significant pathogenetic role for the IL-9 gene and the hematopoietic gene cluster on chromosome 5q. *Exp Hematol* 1997;25:1270–1277.

706. Sieff C, Guinan E. In vitro enhancement of erythropoiesis by steel factor in Diamond-Blackfan anemia and treatment of other congenital cytopenias with recombinant interleukin 3/granulocyte-macrophage colony stimulating factor. *Stem Cells* 1993;11:113–122.

707. Abkowitz JL, Broudy VC, Bennett LG, et al. Absence of abnormalities of c-kit or its ligand in two patients with Diamond-Blackfan anemia. *Blood* 1992;79:25–28.

708. Drachtman RA, Geissler EN, Alter BP. The SCF and c-kit genes in Diamond-Blackfan anemia. *Blood* 1992;79:2177–2178.

709. Spritz RA, Freedman MH. Lack of mutations of the MGF and KIT genes in Diamond-Blackfan anemia. *Blood* 1993;81:3165.

710. Sieff CA, Yokoyama CT, Zsebo KM, et al. The production of steel factor mRNA in Diamond-Blackfan anaemia long-term cultures and interactions of steel factor with erythropoietin and interleukin-3. *Br J Haematol* 1992;82:640–647.

711. McGuckin CP, Uhr MR, Liu M, et al. The use of recombinant SCF protein for rapid determination of c-kit expression in normal and abnormal erythropoiesis. *Eur J Haematol* 1996;57:72–78.

712. Alter BP, Gaston T, Lipton JM. Lack of effect of corticosteroids in W/WV and Sl/SlD mice: these mice are not a model for steroid-responsive Diamond-Blackfan anemia. *Eur J Haematol* 1993;50:275–278.

713. Gustavsson P, Skeppner G, Johansson B, et al. Diamond-Blackfan anaemia in a girl with a de novo balanced reciprocal X;19 translocation. *J Med Genet* 1997;34:779–782.

714. Cario H, Bode H, Gustavsson P, et al. A microdeletion syndrome due to a 3-Mb deletion on 19q13.2—Diamond-Blackfan anemia associated with macrocephaly, hypotonia, and psychomotor retardation. *Clin Genet* 1999;55:487–492.

715. Tentler D, Gustavsson P, Elinder G, et al. A microdeletion in 19q13.2 associated with mental retardation, skeletal malformations, and Diamond-Blackfan anaemia suggests a novel contiguous gene syndrome. *J Med Genet* 2000;37:128–131.

716. Gustavsson P, Garelli E, Draptchinskaia N, et al. Identification of microdeletions spanning the Diamond-Blackfan anemia locus on 19q13 and evidence for genetic heterogeneity. *Am J Hum Genet* 1998;63:1388–1395.

717. Gustavsson P, Willig TN, van Haeringen A, et al. Diamond-Blackfan anemia: genetic homogeneity for a gene on chromosome 19q13 restricted to 1.8 Mb. *Nat Genet* 1997;16:368–371.

718. Draptchinskaia N, Gustavsson P, Andersson B, et al. The gene encoding ribosomal protein S19 is mutated in Diamond-Blackfan anaemia. *Nat Genet* 1999;21:169–175.

719. Gazda H, Lipton JM, Willig TN, et al. Evidence for linkage of familial Diamond-Blackfan anemia to chromosome 8p23.3-p22 and for non-19q non-8p disease. *Blood* 2001;97:2145–2150.

720. Matsson H, Klar J, Draptchinskaia N, et al. Truncating ribosomal protein S19 mutations and variable clinical expression in Diamond-Blackfan anemia. *Hum Genet* 1999;105:496–500.

721. Hoffbrand AV, Bartlett AN, Veys PA, et al. Agranulocytosis and thrombocytopenia in patient with Blackfan-Diamond anaemia during oral chelator trial. *Lancet* 1989;2:457.

722. Alter BP. Agranulocytosis and thrombocytopenia, Blackfan-Diamond anaemia, and oral chelation. *Lancet* 1990;335:970.

723. Berdoukas V, Bentley P, Frost H, et al. Toxicity of oral iron chelator L1. *Lancet* 1993;341:1088.

724. Gasser C. Akute erythroblastopenie. *Schweiz Med Wochenschr* 1949;79:838–840.

725. Hill JM, Hunter RB. ACTH therapy in refractory anemias. In: Mote JR, ed. *Proceedings of the Second Clinical ACTH Conference, volume II—therapeutics.* New York: Blakiston, 1951:181–194.

726. Allen DM, Diamond LK. Congenital (erythroid) hypoplastic anemia. *Am J Dis Child* 1961;102:416–423.

727. Seaman AJ. Cobalt and cortisone therapy of chronic erythrocytic hypoplasia. *Am J Med* 1952;13:99.

728. Vlachos A, Federman N, Reyes-Haley C, et al. Diamond-Blackfan anaemia. Hematopoietic stem cell transplantation for Diamond Blackfan anemia: a report from the Diamond Blackfan Anemia Registry. *Bone Marrow Transplant* 2001;27:381–386.

729. Siegler J, Bognar I, Keleman K. Genesung einer isolierten chronischen erythrozytenaplasie wahrend einer behandlung mit 6-merkaptopurin. *Kinderaztl Prax* 1970;38:145–149.

730. Geller G, Krivit W, Zalusky R, et al. Lack of erythropoietic inhibitory effect of serum from patients with congenital pure red cell aplasia. *J Pediatr* 1975;86:198–201.

731. Marmont AM. Congenital hypoplastic anaemia refractory to corticosteroids but responding to cyclophosphamide and antilymphocytic globulin. Report

of a case having responded with a transitory wave of dyserythropoiesis. *Acta Haematol* 1978;60:90–99.

732. Altman AC, Gross S. Severe congenital hypoplastic anemia. Transmission from a healthy female to opposite sex step-siblings. *Am J Pediatr Hematol Oncol* 1983;5:99–101.

733. Krishnan EU, Wegner K, Garg SK. Congenital hypoplastic anemia terminating in acute promyelocytic leukemia. *Pediatrics* 1978;61:898–901.

734. August CS, King E, Githens JH, et al. Establishment of erythropoiesis following bone marrow transplantation in a patient with congenital hypoplastic anemia (Diamond-Blackfan syndrome). *Blood* 1976;48:491–498.

735. Ozsoylu S. High-dose intravenous corticosteroid treatment for patients with Diamond-Blackfan syndrome resistant or refractory to conventional treatment. *Am J Pediatr Hematol Oncol* 1988;10:217–223.

736. Williams DL, Mageed AS, Findley H, et al. Cyclosporine in the treatment of red cell aplasia. *Am J Pediatr Hematol Oncol* 1987;9:314–316.

737. Raghavachar A. Pure red cell aplasia: review of treatment and proposal for a treatment strategy. *Blut* 1990;61:47–51.

738. Gussetis ES, Peristeri J, Kitra V, et al. Clinical value of bone marrow cultures in childhood pure red aplasia. *J Pediatr Hematol Oncol* 1998;20:120–124.

739. Alessandri AJ, Rogers PC, Wadsworth LD, et al. Diamond-Blackfan anemia and cyclosporine therapy revisited. *J Pediatr Hematol Oncol* 2000;22:176–179.

740. Finlay JL, Shahidi NT. Cyclosporine A (CyA) induced remission in Diamond-Blackfan anemia (DBA). *Blood* 1984;64:104A.

741. Totterman TH, Nisell J, Killander A, et al. Successful treatment of pure red-cell aplasia with cyclosporin. *Lancet* 1984;2:693.

742. Peters C, Dover GJ, Casella JE, et al. Cyclosporine A (CSA) induces transient remissions in red cell aplasias. *Pediatr Res* 1986;20:285A.

743. Seip M, Zanussi GF. Cyclosporine in steroid-resistant Diamond-Blackfan anaemia. *Acta Paediatr Scand* 1988;77:464–466.

744. Leonard EM, Raefsky E, Griffith P, et al. Cyclosporine therapy of aplastic anaemia, congenital and acquired red cell aplasia. *Br J Haematol* 1989;72:278–284.

745. Splain J, Berman BW. Cyclosporin a treatment for Diamond-Blackfan anemia. *Am J Hematol* 1992;39:208–211.

746. Monteserin MC, Garcia Vela JA, Ona F, et al. Cyclosporin A for Diamond-Blackfan anemia: a new case. *Am J Hematol* 1993;42:406–407.

747. Bejaoui M, Fitouri Z, Sfar MT, et al. Failure of immunosuppressive therapy and high-dose intravenous immunoglobulins in four transfusion-dependent, steroid-unresponsive Blackfan-Diamond anemia patients. *Haematologica* 1993;78:38–39.

748. Niemeyer CM, Baumgarten E, Holldack J, et al. Treatment trial with recombinant human erythropoietin in children with congenital hypoplastic anemia. *Contrib Nephrol* 1991;88:276–280.

749. Fiorillo A, Poggi V, Migliorati R, et al. Letter to the editor: unresponsiveness to erythropoietin therapy in a case of Blackfan Diamond anemia. *Am J Hematol* 1991;37:65.

750. Dunbar CE, Smith DA, Kimball J, et al. Treatment of Diamond-Blackfan anaemia with haematopoietic growth factors, granulocyte-macrophage colony stimulating factor and interleukin 3: sustained remissions following IL-3. *Br J Haematol* 1991;79:316–321.

751. Gillio AP, Faulkner LB, Alter BP, et al. Treatment of Diamond-Blackfan anemia with recombinant human interleukin-3. *Blood* 1993;82:744–751.

752. Olivieri NF, Feig SA, Valentino L, et al. Failure of recombinant human interleukin-3 therapy to induce erythropoiesis in patients with refractory Diamond-Blackfan anemia. *Blood* 1994;83:2444–2450.

753. Bastion Y, Bordigoni P, Debre M, et al. Sustained response after recombinant interleukin-3 in Diamond Blackfan anemia. *Blood* 1994;83:617–619.

754. Giri N, Kang E, Tisdale JF, et al. Clinical and laboratory evidence for a trilineage haematopoietic defect in patients with refractory Diamond-Blackfan anaemia. *Br J Haematol* 2000;108:167–175.

755. D'Oelsnitz M, Vincent L, De Swarte M, et al. A propos d'un cas de leucemie aigue lymphoblastique survenue apres guerison d'une maladie de Blackfan-Diamond. *Arch Fr Pediatr* 1975;32:582.

756. Diamond LK, Allen DM, Magill FB. Congenital (erythroid) hypoplastic anemia. *Am J Dis Child* 1961;102:403–415.

757. Wasser JS, Yolken R, Miller DR, et al. Congenital hypoplastic anemia (Diamond-Blackfan syndrome) terminating in acute myelogenous leukemia. *Blood* 1978;51:991–995.

758. Basso G, Cocito MG, Rebuffi L, et al. Congenital hypoplastic anaemia developed in acute megakarioblastic leukaemia. *Helv Paediatr Acta* 1981;36:267–270.

759. Wegelius R, Weber TH. Transient erythroblastopenia in childhood. A study of 15 cases. *Acta Paediatr Scand* 1978;67:513–518.

760. Glader BE, Flam MS, Dahl GV, et al. Hematologic malignancies in Diamond Blackfan anemia. *Pediatr Res* 1990;27:142A.

761. Mori PG, Haupt R, Fugazza G, et al. Pentasomy 21 in leukemia complicating Diamond-Blackfan anemia. *Cancer Genet Cytogenet* 1992;63:70–72.

762. Haupt R, Dufour C, Dallorso S, et al. Diamond-Blackfan anemia and malignancy: a case report and a review of the literature. *Cancer* 1996;77:1961–1962.

763. Aquino VM, Buchanan GR. Osteogenic sarcoma in a child with transfusion-dependent Diamond-Blackfan anemia. *J Pediatr Hematol Oncol* 1996;18:230–232.

764. Lipton JM, Federman N, Khabbaze Y, et al. Osteogenic sarcoma associated with Diamond-Blackfan anemia: a report from the Diamond-Blackfan Anemia Registry. *J Pediatr Hematol Oncol* 2000;23:39–44.

765. Greinix HT, Storb R, Sanders JE, et al. Long-term survival and cure after marrow transplantation for congenital hypoplastic anemia (Diamond-Blackfan syndrome). *Br J Haematol* 1993;84:515–520.

766. Frappaz D, Richard O, Perrot S, et al. Maladie de Blackfan-Diamond et malignité: relations de cause à effet? *Pediatrie* 1992;47:535–540.

767. van Dijken PJ, Verwijs W. Diamond-Blackfan anemia and malignancy. A case report and review of the literature. *Cancer* 1995;76:517–520.

768. Hayashi AK, Kang YS, Smith BM. Non-Hodgkin's lymphoma in a patient with Diamond-Blackfan anemia. *AJR Am J Roentgenol* 1999;173:117–118.

769. Steinherz PG, Canale VC, Miller DR. Hepatocellular carcinoma, transfusion-induced hemochromatosis and congenital hypoplastic anemia (Blackfan-Diamond syndrome). *Am J Med* 1976;60:1032–1035.

770. Seip M. Malignant tumors in two patients with Diamond-Blackfan anemia treated with corticosteroids and androgens. *Pediatr Hematol Oncol* 1994;11:423–426.

771. Turcotte R, Bard C, Marton D, et al. Malignant fibrous histiocytoma in a patient with Blackfan-Diamond anemia. *Can Assoc Radiol* 1994;45:402–404.

772. Hardisty RM. Diamond-Blackfan anaemia. In: Ciba Foundation Symposium 37 (new series). *Congenital disorders of erythropoiesis*. Amsterdam: Elsevier Science, 1976:89–101.

773. Ladenstein R, Peters C, Minkov M, et al. A single centre experience with allogeneic stem cell transplantation for severe aplastic anaemia in childhood. *Klin Padiatr* 1997;209:201–208.

774. Rossbach H, Grana NH, Barbosa JL. Successful management of concomitant Diamond-Blackfan anaemia and aplastic anaemia with splenectomy. *Br J Haematol* 1999;106:569–570.

775. Baar HS. The life span of red blood corpuscles in erythronophthisis. *Acta Haematol* 1952;7:17–26.

776. Wranne L. Transient erythroblastopenia in infancy and childhood. *Scand J Haematol* 1970;7:76–81.

777. Young RS, Rannels E, Hilmo A, et al. Severe anemia in childhood presenting as transient ischemic attacks. *Stroke* 1983;14:622–623.

778. Michelson AD, Marshall PC. Transient neurological disorder associated with transient erythroblastopenia of childhood. *Am J Pediatr Hematol Oncol* 1987;9:161–163.

779. Beresford CH, Macfarlane SD. Temporal clustering of transient erythroblastopenia (cytopenia) of childhood. *Aust Paediatr J* 1987;23:351–354.

780. Elian JC, Frappaz D, Pozzetto B, et al. Transient erythroblastopenia of childhood presenting with echovirus 11 infection. *Acta Paediatr* 1993;62:492–494.

781. Hefelfinger DC. Simultaneous hyperphosphatasemia and erythroblastopenia of childhood. *Clin Pediatr* 1993;32:175–178.

782. Chabali R. Transient erythroblastopenia of childhood presenting with shock and metabolic acidosis. *Pediatr Emerg Care* 1994;10:278–280.

783. Colina KF, Abelson HT. Resolution of breath-holding spells with treatment of concomitant anemia. *J Pediatr* 1995;126:395–397.

784. Chan GC, Kanwar VS, Wilimas J. Transient erythroblastopenia of childhood associated with transient neurologic deficit: report of a case and review of the literature. *J Paediatr Child Health* 1998;34:299–301.

785. Tam DA, Rash FC. Breath-holding spells in a patient with transient erythroblastopenia of childhood. *J Pediatr* 1997;130:651–653.

786. Toogood IR, Speed IE, Cheney KC, et al. Idiopathic transient normocytic, normochromic anaemia of childhood. *Aust Paediatr J* 1978;14:28–33.

787. Labotka RJ, Maurer HS, Honig GR. Transient erythroblastopenia of childhood. Review of 17 cases, including a pair of identical twins. *Am J Dis Child* 1981;135:937–940.

788. Ritchie AK, Dainiak N, Hoffman R. Variable in vitro erythropoiesis in patients with transient erythroblastopenia of childhood. *Yale J Biol Med* 1985;58:1–8.

789. Schroder H. Transient erythroblastopenia in children. *Ugeskr Laeger* 1983;145:2140–2143.

790. Douchain F, Leborgne JM, Robin M, et al. Erythroblastopenie aigue par l'intolerance au dipropyl acetate de sodium. Premiere observation. *Nouv Press Med* 1980;9:1715–1716.

791. Glader BE. Diagnosis and management of red cell aplasia in children. *Hematol Oncol Clin North Am* 1987;1:431–447.

792. Skeppner G, Forestier E, Henter JI, et al. Transient red cell aplasia in siblings: a common environmental or a common hereditary factor? *Acta Paediatr* 1998;87:43–47.

793. Seip M. Transient erythroblastopenia in siblings. *Acta Paediatr Scand* 1982;71:689–690.

794. Mupanomunda O, Alter BP. Transient erythroblastopenia of childhood (TEC) presenting as leukoerythroblastic anemia. *J Pediatr Hem Oncol* 1997;19:165–167.

795. Link MP, Alter BP. Fetal erythropoiesis during recovery from transient erythroblastopenia of childhood (TEC). *Pediatr Res* 1981;15:1036–1039.

796. Gerrits GP, van Oostrom CG, de Vaan GAM. Severe anemia caused by transient erythroblastopenia in children (TEC). *Tijdschr Kindergeneeskd* 1982;50:97–105.

797. Wang WC, Mentzer WC. Differentiation of transient erythroblastopenia of childhood from congenital hypoplastic anemia. *J Pediatr* 1976;88:784–789.

798. Papayannopoulou T, Vichinsky E, Stamatoyannopoulos G. Fetal Hb production during acute erythroid expansion. I. Observations in patients with transient erythroblastopenia and post-phlebotomy. *Br J Haematol* 1980;44:535–546.

799. Dover GJ, Boyer SH, Zinkham WH. Production of erythrocytes that contain fetal hemoglobin in anemia. Transient in vivo changes. *J Clin Invest* 1979;63:173–176.

800. Lovric VA. Anaemia and temporary erythroblastopenia in children. A syndrome. *Aust Ann Med* 1970;1:34–39.

801. Freedman MH. 'Recurrent' erythroblastopenia of childhood. An IgM-mediated RBC aplasia. *Am J Dis Child* 1983;137:458–460.
802. Lewis SM, Verwilghen RL. Dyserythropoiesis: definition, diagnosis and assessment. In: Lewis SM, Verwilghen RL, eds. *Dyserythropoiesis*. London: Academic Press, 1977:3–20.
803. Frisch B, Lewis SM. The bone marrow in aplastic anaemia: diagnostic and prognostic features. *J Clin Pathol* 1974;27:231–241.
804. Rozman C, Feliu E, Granena A, et al. Transient dyserythropoiesis in repopulated human bone marrow following transplantation: an ultrastructural study. *Br J Haematol* 1982;50:63–73.
805. Lewis SM, Verwilghen RL, eds. *Dyserythropoiesis*. London: Academic Press, 1977:350.
806. Wickramasinghe SN. Congenital dyserythropoietic anaemias: clinical features, haematological morphology and new biochemical data. *Blood Rev* 1998;12:178–200.
807. Crookston JH, Crookston MC, Burnie KL, et al. Hereditary erythroblastic multinuclearity associated with a positive acidified-serum test: a type of congenital dyserythropoietic anaemia. *Br J Haematol* 1969;17:11–26.
808. Fayen WT, Harris JW. Thrombocytopenia with absent radii (the TAR syndrome). *Am J Med Sci* 1980;280:95–99.
809. Heimpel H. Congenital dyserythropoietic anaemia, type I. In: Lewis SM, Verwilghen RL, eds. *Dyserythropoiesis*. London: Academic Press, 1977:55–70.
810. Alloisio N, Jaccoud P, Dorleac E, et al. Alterations of globin chain synthesis and of red cell membrane proteins in congenital dyserythropoietic anemia I and II. *Pediatr Res* 1982;16:1016–1021.
811. Wickramasinghe SN, Pippard MJ. Studies of erythroblast function in congenital dyserythropoietic anaemia, type I: evidence of impaired DNA, RNA, and protein synthesis and unbalanced globin chain synthesis in ultrastructurally abnormal cells. *J Clin Pathol* 1986;39:881–890.
812. Heimpel H, Forteza-Vila J, Queisser W, et al. Electron and light microscopic study of the erythroblasts of patients with congenital dyserythropoietic anemia. *Blood* 1971;37:299–310.
813. Lewis SM, Frisch B. Congenital dyserythropoietic anaemias: electron microscopy. In: CIBA Foundation Symposium 37. *Congenital disorders of erythropoiesis*. Amsterdam: Elsevier Science, 1976:171–203.
814. Breton-Gorius J, Daniel MT, Clauvel JP, et al. Anomalies ultrastructurales des erythroblastes et des erythrocytes dans six cas de dyserythropoiese congenitale. *Nouv Rev Fr Hematol* 1973;13:23–50.
815. Vainchenker W, Guichard J, Bouguet J, et al. Congenital dyserythropoietic anaemia type I: absence of clonal expression in the nuclear abnormalities of cultured erythroblasts. *Br J Haematol* 1980;46:33–37.
816. Tamary H, Shalmon L, Shalev H, et al. Localization of the gene for congenital dyserythropoietic anemia type I to a <1-cM interval on chromosome 15q15.1-15.3. *Am J Hum Genet* 1998;62:1062–1069.
817. Hodges VM, Molloy GY, Wickramasinghe SN. Genetic heterogeneity of congenital dyserythropoietic anemia type I. *Blood* 1999;94:1139–1140.
818. Shalev H, Moser A, Kapelushnik J, et al. Congenital dyserythropoietic anemia type I presenting as persistent pulmonary hypertension of the newborn. *J Pediatr* 2000;136:553–555.
819. Kato K, Sugitani M, Kawataki M, et al. Congenital dyserythropoietic anemia type 1 with fetal onset of severe anemia. *J Pediatr Hematol Oncol* 2001;23:63–66.
820. Lavabre-Bertrand T, Blanc P, Navarro R, et al. Alpha-interferon therapy for congenital dyserythropoiesis type I. *Br J Haematol* 1995;89:929–932.
821. Virjee S, Hatton C. Congenital dyserthropoiesis type I and alpha-interferon therapy. *Br J Haematol* 1996;94:579–583.
822. Wickramasinghe SN. Response of CDA type I to alpha-interferon. *Eur J Haematol* 1997;58:121–123.
823. Wickramasinghe SN, Hasan R, Smythe J. Reduced interferon-alpha production by Epstein-Barr virus transformed B-lymphoblastoid cell lines and lectin-stimulated lymphocytes in congenital dyserythropoietic anaemia type I. *Br J Haematol* 1997;98:295–298.
824. Menike D, Wickramasinghe SN. Effects of four species of interferon-alpha on cultured erythroid progenitors from congenital dyserythropoietic anaemia type I. *Br J Haematol* 1998;103:825–830.
825. Ariffin WA, Karnaneedi S, Choo K, et al. Congenital dyserythropoietic anaemia: report of three cases. *J Paediatr Child Health* 1996;32:191–193.
826. Punt K, Borst-Eilers E, Nijessen JG. Congenital dyserythropoietic anaemia, type II (HEMPAS). In: Lewis SM, Verwilghen RL, eds. *Dyserythropoiesis*. London: Academic Press, 1977:71–81.
827. Verwilghen RL. Congenital dyserythropoietic anaemia type II (Hempas). In: CIBA Foundation Symposium 37. *Congenital disorders of erythropoiesis*. Amsterdam: Elsevier Science, 1976:151–170.
828. Crookston JH, Crookston M. Hereditary anemia with multinuclear erythroblasts (HEMPAS). *Birth Defects Orig Artic Ser* 1972;3:15–19.
829. Crookston JH, Crookston MC, Rosse WF. Red-cell abnormalities in HEMPAS (Hereditary erythroblastic multinuclearity with a positive acidified-serum test). *Br J Haematol* 1972;23:83–91.
830. Seip M, Skrede S, Bjerve K, et al. A case of variant congenital dyserythropoietic anemia revisited. *Scand J Haematol* 1982;28:278–280.
831. Giblett ER, Crookston MC. Agglutinability of red cells by anti-i in patients with thalassaemia major and other haematological disorders. *Nature* 1964; 201:1138–1139.
832. Enquist RW, Gockerman JP, Jenis EH, et al. Type II congenital dyserythropoietic anemia. *Ann Intern Med* 1972;77:371–376.
833. Rosse WF, Logue GL, Adams J, et al. Mechanisms of immune lysis of the red cells in hereditary erythroblastic multinuclearity with a positive acidified

834. Fukuda MN. HEMPAS. *Biochim Biophys Acta* 1999;1455:231–239.
835. Fukuda MN, Dell A, Scartezzini P. Primary defect of congenital dyserythropoietic anemia type II. Failure in glycosylation of erythrocyte lactosaminoglycan proteins caused by lowered N-acetylglucosaminyl transferase II. *J Biol Chem* 1987;262:7195–7206.
836. Tebbi K, Gross S. Absence of morphological abnormalities in marrow erythrocyte colonies (CFU-E) from a patient with HEMPAS-II. *J Lab Clin Med* 1978;91:797–801.
837. Vainchenker W, Guichard J, Breton-Gorius J. Morphological abnormalities in cultured erythroid colonies (BFU-E) from the blood of two patients with HEMPAS. *Br J Haematol* 1979;42:363–369.
838. Roodman GD, Clare CN, Mills G. Congenital dyserythropoietic anemia type II (CDA-II): chromosomal banding studies and adherent cell effects on erythroid colony (CFU-E) and burst (BFU-E) formation. *Br J Haematol* 1982; 50:499–507.
839. Gasparini P, del Giudice EM, Delaunay J, et al. Localization of the congenital dyserythropoietic anemia II locus to chromosome 20q11.2 by genome-wide search. *Am J Hum Genet* 1997;61:1112–1116.
840. Iolascon A, Servedio V, Carbone R, et al. Geographic distribution of CDA-II: did a founder effect operate in Southern Italy? *Haematologica* 2000;85:470–474.
841. Iolascon A, De Mattia D, Perrotta S, et al. Genetic heterogeneity of congenital dyserythropoietic anemia type II. *Blood* 1998;92:2593–2594.
842. Cazzola M, Barosi G, Bergamaschi G, et al. Iron loading in congenital dyserythropoietic anaemias and congenital sideroblastic anaemias. *Br J Haematol* 1983;54:649–654.
843. Perrotta S, del Giudice M, Carbone R, et al. Gilbert's syndrome accounts for the phenotypic variability of congenital dyserythropoietic anemia type II (CDA-II). *J Pediatr* 2000;136:556–559.
844. Fargion S, Valenti L, Fracanzani AL, et al. Hereditary hemochromatosis in a patient with congenital dyserythropoietic anemia. *Blood* 2000;96:3653–3655.
845. Wolff JA, Von Hofe FH. Familial erythroid multinuclearity. *Blood* 1951;6: 1274–1283.
846. Goudsmit R. Congenital dyserythropoietic anaemia, type III. In: Lewis SM, Verwilghen RL, eds. *Dyserythropoiesis*. London: Academic Press, 1977:83–92.
847. Vainchenker W, Breton-Gorius J, Guichard J, et al. Congenital dyserythropoietic anemia type III. Studies on erythroid differentiation of blood erythroid progenitor cells (BFUE) in vitro. *Exp Hematol* 1980;8:1057–1062.
848. Lind L, Sandstrom H, Wahlin A, et al. Localization of the gene for congenital dyserythropoietic anemia type III, CDAN3, to chromosome 15q21-q25. *Hum Mol Genet* 1995;4:109–112.
849. Sandstrom H, Wahlin A. Haematologica. Congenital dyserythropoietic anemia type III. *Haematologica* 2000;85:753–757.
850. McBride JA, Wilson WE, Baillie N. Congenital dyserythropoietic anaemia—type IV. *Blood* 1971;38:837.
851. Weatherly TL, Flannery EP, Doyle WF, et al. Congenital dyserythropoietic anemia (CDA) with increased red cell lipids. *Am J Med* 1974;57:912–919.
852. Benjamin JT, Rosse WF, Dalldorf FC, et al. Congenital dyserythropoietic anemia—type IV. *J Pediatr* 1975;87:210–216.
853. Bird AR, Karabus CD, Hartley PS. Type IV congenital dyserythropoietic anemia with an unusual response to splenectomy. *Am J Pediatr Hematol Oncol* 1985;7:196–199.
854. Wickramasinghe SN, Vora AJ, Will A, et al. Transfusion-dependent congenital dyserythropoietic anaemia with non-specific dysplastic changes in erythroblasts. *Eur J Haematol* 1998;60:140–142.
855. Weatherall DH, Clegg JB, Knox-Macaulay HH, et al. A genetically determined disorder with features both of thalassaemia and congenital dyserythropoietic anaemia. *Br J Haematol* 1973;24:681–702.
856. Hruby MA, Mason RG, Honig GR. Unbalanced globin chain synthesis in congenital dyserythropoietic anemia. *Blood* 1973;42:843–850.
857. Eldor A, Matzner Y, Kahane I, et al. Aberrant congenital dyserythropoietic anemia with negative acidified serum tests and features of thalassemia in a Kurdish family. *Isr J Med Sci* 1978;14:1138–1143.
858. Wickramasinghe SN, Illum N, Wimberley PD. Congenital dyserythropoietic anaemia with novel intra-erythroblastic and intra-erythrocytic inclusions. *Br J Haematol* 1991;79:322–330.
859. Tang W, Cai SP, Eng B, et al. Expression of embryonic zeta-globin and epsilon-globin chains in a 10-year-old girl with congenital anemia. *Blood* 1993;81: 1636–1640.
860. Dell'Orbo C, Marchi A, Quacci D. Ultrastructural findings of congenital dyserythropoietic sickle cell beta thal-associated anemia. *Histol Histopathol* 1992; 7:7–10.
861. Sansone G, Lupi L. An aberrant type of congenital dyserythropoietic anemia associated with a beta-thalassemia trait. *Ann Hematol* 1991;62:184–187.
862. Brochstein JA, Siena S, Weinberg RS, et al. Congenital dyserythropoietic anemia (CDA) with karyorrhexis. *Pediatr Res* 1985;19:258A.
863. Kostmann R. Infantile genetic agranulocytosis. A new recessive lethal disease in man. *Acta Paediatr Scand* 1956;45:1–78.
864. Kostmann R. Infantile genetic agranulocytosis. A review with presentation of ten new cases. *Acta Paediatr Scand* 1975;64:362–368.
865. Iselius L, Gustavson KH. Spatial distribution of the gene for infantile genetic agranulocytosis. *Hum Hered* 1984;34:358–363.
866. Briars GL, Parry HF, Ansari BM. Dominantly inherited severe congenital neutropenia. *J Infect* 1996;33:123–126.

867. Coulombel L, Morardet N, Veber F, et al. Granulopoietic differentiation in long-term bone marrow cultures from children with congenital neutropenia. *Am J Hematol* 1988;27:93–98.

868. Zucker-Franklin D, L'Esperance P, Good RA. Congenital neutropenia: an intrinsic cell defect demonstrated by electron microscopy of soft agar colonies. *Blood* 1977;49:425–436.

869. Horwitz M, Benson KF, Person RE, et al. Mutations in ELA2, encoding neutrophil elastase, define a 21-day biological clock in cyclic haematopoiesis. *Nat Genet* 1999;23:433–436.

870. Dale DC, Person RE, Bolyard AA, et al. Mutations in the gene encoding neutrophil elastase in congenital and cyclic neutropenia. *Blood* 2000;96:2317–2322.

871. Li F, Horwitz M. Characterization of mutant neutrophil elastase in severe congenital neutropenia. *J Biol Chem* 2001;276:14230–14241.

872. Barrett AJ. Clinical experience with lithium in aplastic anemia and congenital neutropenia. *Adv Exp Med Biol* 1980;127:305–320.

873. Chan HS, Freedman MH, Saunders EF. Lithium therapy of children with chronic neutropenia. *Am J Med* 1981;70:1073–1077.

874. Aldenhoff P, Waldenmaier C. Das TAR-Syndrom. In: Tolksdorf M, Spranranranranger J, eds. *Klinische genetik in der padiatrie.* Stuttgart, Germany: Thieme Medical Publishers, 1978:66–69.

875. O'Reilly RJ, Brochstein J, Dinsmore R, et al. Marrow transplantation for congenital disorders. *Semin Hematol* 1984;21:188–221.

876. Bonilla MA, Gillio AP, Ruggeiro M, et al. Effects of recombinant human granulocyte colony-stimulating factor on neutropenia in patients with congenital agranulocytosis. *N Engl J Med* 1989;320:1574–1580.

877. Welte K, Boxer LA. Severe chronic neutropenia: pathophysiology and therapy. *Semin Hematol* 1997;34:267–278.

878. Fewtrell MS, Kinsey SE, Williams DM, et al. Bone mineralization and turnover in children with congenital neutropenia, and its relationship to treatment with recombinant human granulocyte-colony stimulating factor. *Br J Haematol* 1997;97:7434–7736.

879. Yakisan E, Schirg E, Zeidler C, et al. High incidence of significant bone loss in patients with severe congenital neutropenia (Kostmann's syndrome). *J Pediatr* 1997;131:592–597.

880. Zeidler C, Welte K, Barak Y, et al. Stem cell transplantation in patients with severe congenital neutropenia without evidence of leukemic transformation. *Blood* 2000;95:1195–1198.

881. Cividalli G, Yarkoni S, Dar H, et al. Can infantile hereditary agranulocytosis be diagnosed prenatally? *Prenat Diagn* 1983;3:157–159.

882. Millar DS, Davis LR, Rodeck CH, et al. Normal blood cell values in the early mid-trimester fetus. *Prenat Diagn* 1985;5:367–373.

883. Gilman PA, Jackson DP, Guild HG. Congenital agranulocytosis: prolonged survival and terminal acute leukemia. *Blood* 1970;36:576–585.

884. Rosen RB, Kang SJ. Congenital agranulocytosis terminating in acute myelomonocytic leukemia. *J Pediatr* 1979;94:406–408.

885. Miller RW. Childhood cancer and congenital defects. A study of U.S. death certificates during the period 1960–1966. *Pediatr Res* 1969;3:389–397.

886. Lui V, Ragab AH, Findley H, et al. Infantile genetic agranulocytosis and acute lymphocytic leukemia in two sibs. *J Pediatr* 1978;92:1028.

887. Freedman MH, Bonilla MA, Fier C, et al. Myelodysplasia syndrome and acute myeloid leukemia in patients with congenital neutropenia receiving G-CSF therapy. *Blood* 2000;96:429–436.

888. Rosse WF. Epidemiology of PNH. *Lancet* 1996;348:560.

889. Dong F, Dale DC, Bonilla MA, et al. Mutations in the granulocyte colony-stimulating factor gene in patients with severe congenital neutropenia. *Leukemia* 1997;11:120–125.

890. Tidow N, Pilz C, Teichmann B, et al. Clinical relevance of point mutations in the cytoplasmic domain of the granulocyte colony-stimulating factor receptor gene in patients with severe congenital neutropenia. *Blood* 1997;89:2369–2375.

891. Hermans MH, Antonissen C, Ward AC, et al. Sustained receptor activation and hyperproliferation in response to granulocyte colony-stimulating factor (G-CSF) in mice with a severe congenital neutropenia/acute myeloid leukemia-derived mutation in the G-CSF receptor. *J Exp Med* 1999;189:683–691.

892. Tidow N, Pilz C, Kasper B, et al. Frequency of point mutations in the gene for the G-CSF receptor in patients with chronic neutropenia undergoing G-CSF therapy. *Stem Cells* 1997;15:113–120.

893. Ward AC, van Aesch YM, Schelen AM, et al. Defective internalization and sustained activation of truncated granulocyte colony-stimulating factor receptor found in severe congenital neutropenia/acute myeloid leukemia. *Blood* 1999;93:447–458.

894. Hall JG, Levin J, Kuhn JP, et al. Thrombocytopenia with absent radius (TAR). *Medicine* 1969;48:411–439.

895. Hall JG. Thrombocytopenia and absent radius (TAR) syndrome. *J Med Genet* 1987;24:79–83.

896. Hedberg VA, Lipton JM. Thrombocytopenia with absent radii. A review of 100 cases. *Am J Pediatr Hematol Oncol* 1988;10:51–64.

897. Shalev E, Weiner E, Feldman E, et al. Micrognathia-prenatal ultrasonographic diagnosis. *Int J Gynaecol Obstet* 1983;21:343–345.

898. Teufel M, Enders H, Dopfer R. Consanguinity in a Turkish family with thrombocytopenia with absent radii (TAR) syndrome. *Hum Genet* 1983;64:94–96.

899. Ceballos-Quintal JM, Pinto-Escalante D, Gongora-Biachi RA. TAR-like syndrome in a consanguineous Mayan girl. *Am J Med Genet* 1992;43:805–807.

900. Messen S, Vargas L, Garcia H, et al. Congenital thrombocytopenia and absent radius syndrome in identical twins. *Rev Child Pediatr* 1986;57:559–563.

901. Gounder DS, Ockelford PA, Pullon HW, et al. Clinical manifestations of the thrombocytopenia and absent radii (TAR) syndrome. *Aust N Z J Med* 1989;19:479–482.

902. Dodesini G, Frigerio G, Cocco E. La trombocitopenia congenita ipoplastica con aplasia bilaterale del radio. *Minerva Pediatr* 1979;31:1023–1046.

903. Turner RJ, Spencer RA, Miyazawa K. Successful cesarean section in a gravida with the thrombocytopenia with absent radius syndrome. A case report. *J Reprod Med* 1986;31:260–262.

904. Gross H, Groh C, Weippl G. Kongenitale hypoplastische thrombopenie mit radiusaplasie. Ein syndrom multipler abartungen. *Neue Oesterr Z Kinderheilk* 1956;1:574–582.

905. Edelberg SB, Cohn J, Brandt NJ. Congenital hypomegakaryocytic thrombocytopenia associated with bilateral absence of the radius—the TAR syndrome. Intra-family variation of the clinical picture. *Hum Hered* 1977;27:147–152.

906. Temtamy SA, McKusick VA. Radial defects with blood dyscrasias. In: Bergsma D, ed. *The genetics of hand malformations.* New York: Alan R. Liss, 1978:101–115.

907. Hays RM, Bartoshesky LE, Feingold M. New features of thrombocytopenia and absent radius syndrome. *Birth Defects Orig Artic Ser* 1982;18:115–121.

908. Ward RE, Bixler D, Provisor AJ, et al. Parent to child transmission of the thrombocytopenia absent radius (TAR) syndrome. *Am J Med Genet* 1986;2[Suppl]:207–214.

909. Schnur RE, Eunpu DL, Zackai EH. Thrombocytopenia with absent radius in a boy and his uncle. *Am J Med Genet* 1987;28:117–123.

910. Haarmann M, Lenz W, Petersen D. Radiusaplasie mit thrombocytopenie. *Ergeb Inn Med Kinderkeilkd* 1975;37:57–106.

911. Akatsuka J. Fanconi's anemia and radial aplasia-thrombocytopenia. *Nippon Rinsho* 1978;[Suppl]:1488–1489.

912. Adeyokunnu AA. Radial aplasia and amegakaryocytic thrombocytopenia (TAR syndrome) among Nigerian children. *Am J Dis Child* 1984;138:346–348.

913. Nilsson LR, Lundholm G. Congenital thrombocytopenia associated with aplasia of the radius. *Acta Paediatr* 1960;49:291–296.

914. Whitfield MF, Barr DG. Cow's milk allergy in the syndrome of thrombocytopenia with absent radius. *Arch Dis Child* 1976;51:337–343.

915. Fromm B, Niethard FU, Marquardt E. Thrombocytopenia and absent radius (TAR) syndrome. *Int Orthop* 1991;15:95–99.

916. Bajaj R, Jain M, Kasat L, et al. Tar syndrome with unilateral absent radius and associated esophageal atresia: a variant? *Indian J Pediatr* 1999;66:460–463.

917. Schoenecker PL, Cohn AK, Sedgwick WG, et al. Dysplasia of the knee associated with the syndrome of thrombocytopenia and absent radius. *J Bone Joint Surg* 1984;66:421–427.

918. Rabinowitz JG, Moseley JE, Mitty HA, et al. Trisomy 18, esophageal atresia, anomalies of the radius, and congenital hypoplastic thrombocytopenia. *Radiology* 1967;89:488–491.

919. Stoll C, Sacrez R, Willard D, et al. Un cas de trisomie 18 avec aplasie bilaterale du radius et thrombopenie. *Pediatrie* 1972;27:537–542.

920. Juif JG, Stoll C, Korn R. Thrombopenie hypoplasique congenitale avec aplasie du radius. *Arch Franc Ped* 1972;29:513–526.

921. Christodoulou C, Werner B. A girl with 18-trisomy and thrombocytopenia. *Acta Genet* 1967;17:77–80.

922. Waldenmaier C, Aldenhoff P, Klemm T. The Robert's syndrome. *Hum Genet* 1978;40:345–349.

923. Lenz W. Phenocopies. *J Med Genet* 1973;10:34–49.

924. Bessman JD, Harrison RL, Howard LC, et al. The megakaryocyte abnormality in thrombocytopenia-absent radius syndrome. *Blood* 1983;62[Suppl]:143a.

925. Armitage JO, Hoak JC, Elliott TE, et al. Syndrome of thrombocytopenia and absent radii: qualitatively normal platelets with remission following splenectomy. *Scand J Haematol* 1978;20:25–28.

926. Thevenieau D, Mattei JF, Juhan I, et al. Anomalies du membre superieur, thrombopenie et thrombopathie. A propos de trois observations. *Arch Franc Ped* 1978;35:631–640.

927. Giuffre L, Cammarata M, Corsello G, et al. Two new cases of thrombocytopenia absent radius (TAR) syndrome: clinical, genetic and nosologic features. *Klin Padiatri* 1988;200:10–14.

928. Sultan Y, Scrobohaci ML, Jeanneau C, et al. Anomalies de la lignee plaquettaire au cours du syndrome d'aplasie radiale avec thrombocytopenie. *Nouv Rev Franc Hematol* 1973;13:573–577.

929. Day HJ, Holmsen H. Platelet adenine nucleotide "storage pool deficiency" in thrombocytopenic absent radii syndrome. *JAMA* 1972;221:1053–1054.

930. Linch DC, Stewart JW, West C. Blood and bone marrow cultures in a case of thrombocytopenia with absent radii. *Clin Lab Haematol* 1982;4:313–317.

931. Homans AC, Cohen JL, Mazur EM. Defective megakaryocytopoiesis in the syndrome of thrombocytopenia with absent radii. *Br J Haematol* 1988;70:205–210.

932. Michalevicz R, Baron S, Burstein Y. Osteoclast-like cells grow in cultures of multipotent hematopoietic progenitors in thrombocytopenia and absent radii (TAR) syndrome. *Isr J Med Sci* 1988;24:42–45.

933. Akabutu J, Vergidis D, Poololak-Doiwidziak M, et al. Studies of hematopoietic progenitor cells in thrombocytopenia with absent radii (TAR) syndrome. *Blood* 1988;72[Suppl]:78a.

934. Kanz L, Kostjelniak E, Welte K. Colony-stimulating activity (CSA) unique for the megakaryocytic hemopoietic cell lineage present in the plasma of a patient with the syndrome of thrombocytopenia with absent radii (TAR). *Blood* 1989;74[Suppl]:248a.

935. De Alarcon PA, Graeve JLA, Levine RF, et al. Thrombocytopenia and absent radii syndrome: a defect in megakaryocyte maturation. *Blood* 1988;72[Suppl]:321a.

936. Ballmaier M, Schulze H, Cremer M, et al. Defective c-Mpl signaling in the syndrome of thrombocytopenia with absent radii. *Stem Cells* 1998;16:177–184.

937. Letestu R, Vitrat N, Masse A, et al. Existence of a differentiation blockage at the stage of a megakaryocyte precursor in the thrombocytopenia and absent radii (TAR) syndrome. *Blood* 2000;95:1633–1641.

938. Strippoli P, Savoia A, Iolascon A, et al. Mutational screening of thrombopoietin receptor (c-mpl) in patients with congenital thrombocytopenia and absent radii (TAR). *Br J Haematol* 1998;103:311–314.

939. Camitta BM, Rock A. Acute lymphoidic leukemia in a patient with thrombocytopenia/absent radii (TAR) syndrome. *Am J Pediatr Hematol Oncol* 1993;15:335–337.

940. Katzenstein HM, Bowman LC, Brodeur GM, et al. Prognostic significance of age, MYCN oncogene amplification, tumor cell ploidy, and histology in 110 infants with stage D(S) neuroblastoma: the Pediatric Oncology Group Experience—a Pediatric Oncology Group Study. *J Clin Oncol* 1998;16:2007–2017.

941. Symonds RP, Clark BJ, George WD, et al. Thrombocytopenia with absent radii (TAR) syndrome: a new increased cellular radiosensitivity syndrome. *Clin Oncol* 1995;7:56–58.

942. Brochstein JA, Shank B, Kernan NA, et al. Marrow transplantation for thrombocytopenia-absent radii syndrome. *J Pediatr* 1989;121:587–589.

943. Omenn GS, Figley MM, Graham CB, et al. Prospects for radiographic intrauterine diagnosis—the syndrome of thrombocytopenia with absent radii. *N Engl J Med* 1973;288:777–778.

944. Luthy DA, Hall JG, Graham CB. Prenatal diagnosis of thrombocytopenia with absent radii. *Clin Genet* 1979;15:495–499.

945. Hobbins JC, Bracken MB, Mahoney MJ. Diagnosis of fetal skeletal dysplasias with ultrasound. *Am J Obstet Gynecol* 1982;142:306–312.

946. Filkins K, Russo J, Bilinki I, et al. Prenatal diagnosis of thrombocytopenia absent radius syndrome using ultrasound and fetoscopy. *Prenat Diagn* 1984;4:139–142.

947. Labrune P, Pons JC, Khalil M, et al. Antenatal thrombocytopenia in three patients with TAR (thrombocytopenia with absent radii) syndrome. *Prenat Diagn* 1993;13:463–466.

948. Daffos F, Forestier F, Kaplan C, et al. Prenatal diagnosis and management of bleeding disorders with fetal blood sampling. *Am J Obstet Gynecol* 1988;158:939–946.

949. Vaughan JM. Leuco-erythroblastic anaemia. *J Pathol Bacteriol* 1936;42:541–564.

950. Weick JK, Hagedorn AB, Linman JW. Leukoerythroblastosis. Diagnostic and prognostic significance. *Mayo Clin Proc* 1974;49:110–113.

951. Sills RH, Hadley RA. The significance of nucleated red blood cells in the peripheral blood of children. *Am J Pediatr Hematol Oncol* 1983;5:173–177.

952. Albers-Schonberg H. Roentgenbilder einer seltenen Knochenerkrankung. *Munch Med Wochenschr* 1904;51:365.

953. Johnston CC Jr, Lavy N, Lord T, et al. Osteopetrosis. A clinical, genetic, metabolic, and morphologic study of the dominantly inherited, benign form. *Medicine* 1968;47:149–167.

954. Shapiro F. Osteopetrosis. Current clinical considerations. *Clin Orthop* 1993;294:34–44.

955. Schiliro G, Musumeci S, Pizzarelli G, et al. Fetal haemoglobin in early malignant osteopetrosis. *Br J Haematol* 1978;38:339–344.

956. Farber S, Vawter GF. Clinical pathological conference. *J Pediatr* 1965;67:133–143.

957. Sjolin S. Studies on osteopetrosis. II. Investigations concerning the nature of the anaemia. *Acta Paediatr* 1959;48:529–544.

958. Walker DG. Spleen cells transmit osteopetrosis in mice. *Science* 1975;190:785–787.

959. Ash P, Loutit JF, Townsend KM. Osteoclasts derived from haematopoietic stem cells. *Nature* 1980;283:669–670.

960. Marshall MJ, Nisbet NW, Menage J, et al. Tissue repopulation during cure of osteopetrotic (mi/mi) mice using normal and defective (W^e/W^v) bone marrow. *Exp Hematol* 1982;10:600–608.

961. Scheven BA, Visser JW, Nijweide PJ. In vitro osteoclast generation from different bone marrow fractions, including a highly enriched haematopoietic stem cell population. *Nature* 1986;321:79–81.

962. Ragab AH, Ducos R, Crist WM, et al. Granulopoiesis in osteopetrosis. *J Pediatr* 1975;87:422–424.

963. Marcus JR, Fibach E, Akrer M. Circulating myeloid and erythroid progenitor cells in malignant osteopetrosis. *Acta Haematol* 1982;67:185–189.

964. Van Hul W, Bollerslev J, Gram J, et al. Localization of a gene for autosomal dominant osteopetrosis (Albers-Schonberg disease) to chromosome 1p21. *Am J Hum Genet* 1996;61:363–369.

965. Sly WS, Whyte MP, Sundaram V, et al. Carbonic anhydrase II deficiency in 12 families with the autosomal recessive syndrome of osteopetrosis with renal tubular acidosis and cerebral calcification. *N Engl J Med* 1985;313:139–145.

966. Hu PY, Roth DE, Skaggs LA, et al. A splice junction mutation in intron 2 of the carbonic anhydrase II gene of osteopetrosis patients from Arabic countries. *Hum Mutat* 1992;1:288–292.

967. Heaney C, Shalev H, Elbedour K, et al. Human autosomal recessive osteopetrosis maps to 11q13, a position predicted by comparative mapping of the murine osteosclerosis (oc) mutation. *Hum Mol Genet* 1998;7:1407–1410.

968. Frattini A, Orchard PJ, Sobacchi C, et al. Defects in TCIRG1 subunit of the vacuolar proton pump are responsible for a subset of human autosomal recessive osteopetrosis. *Nat Genet* 2000;25:343–346.

969. Kornak U, Schulz A, Friedrich W, et al. Mutations in the a3 subunit of the vacuolar H+-ATPase cause infantile malignant osteopetrosis. *Hum Mol Genet* 2000;9:2059–2063.

970. Kornak U, Kasper D, Bosl MR, et al. Loss of the ClC-7 chloride channel leads to osteopetrosis in mice and man. *Cell* 2001;104:205–215.

971. Reeves J, Huffer W, August CS, et al. The hematopoietic effects of prednisone therapy in four infants with osteopetrosis. *J Pediatr* 1979;94:210–214.

972. Beard CJ, Key L, Newburger PE, et al. Neutrophil defect associated with malignant infantile osteopetrosis. *J Lab Clin Med* 1986;108:498–505.

973. Moe PJ, Skjaeveland A. Therapeutic studies in osteopetrosis. Report of 4 cases. *Acta Paediatr Scand* 1969;58:593–600.

974. Key LL, Rodriguiz RM, Willi SM, et al. Long-term treatment of osteopetrosis with recombinant human interferon gamma. *N Engl J Med* 1995;332:1594–1595.

975. Coccia PF, Krivit W, Cervenka J, et al. Successful bone-marrow transplantation for infantile malignant osteopetrosis. *N Engl J Med* 1980;302:701–708.

976. Fasth A, Porras O. Human malignant osteopetrosis: pathophysiology, management and the role of bone marrow transplantation. *Pediatr Transplant* 1999;3[Suppl]:102–107.

977. Kapelushnik J, Shalev C, Yaniv I, et al. Osteopetrosis: a single centre experience of stem cell transplantation and prenatal diagnosis. *Bone Marrow Transplant* 2001;27:129–132.

978. Locatelli F, Beluffi G, Giorgiani G, et al. Transplantation of cord blood progenitor cells can promote bone resorption in autosomal recessive osteopetrosis. *Bone Marrow Transplant* 1997;20:701–705.

979. Jenkinson EL, Pfisterer WH, Latteier KK, et al. A prenatal diagnosis of osteopetrosis. *AJR Am J Roentgenol* 1943;49:455–462.

980. Golbus MS, Koerper MA, Hall BD. Failure to diagnose osteopetrosis in utero. *Lancet* 1976;2:1246.

981. Khazen NE, Faverly D, Vamos E, et al. Lethal osteopetrosis with multiple fractures in utero. *Am J Med Genet* 1986;23:811–819.

982. Sen C, Madazli R, Aksoy F, et al. Antenatal diagnosis of lethal osteopetrosis. *Ultrasound Obstet Gynecol* 1995;5:278–280.

983. Shalev H, Mishori-Dery A, Kapelushnik J, et al. Prenatal diagnosis of malignant osteopetrosis in Bedouin families by linkage analysis. *Prenat Diagn* 2001;21:183–186.

CHAPTER 9

Acquired Bone Marrow Failure Syndromes

Neal S. Young and Akiko Shimamura

HISTORIC BACKGROUND

The medical study of bone marrow failure dates to 1888, when Paul Ehrlich (1) described a young woman with an explosive fatal illness marked by severe anemia, bleeding into the skin and retina, and high fever. The empty bone marrow and its devastating consequences for the patient have rightfully fascinated hematologists for a century, provoking an interest far out of proportion to the incidence of the disease. What other medical specialty is faced with the apparent disappearance of its organ of interest? The study of this disease has not lost its luster. Effective therapy is now available for most patients, but the implementation of curative regimens and the supportive care of the patient require high levels of technical competence and physician responsibility. In more recent times, we may be approaching an understanding of the basic mechanisms of marrow failure through the application of such disciplines as cell biology, immunology, virology, and toxicology.

Nosology

Bone marrow failure is characterized by a reduced bone marrow production of all three mature blood cell lineages that leads to peripheral blood pancytopenia. The combination of low blood cell counts and absent marrow precursor cells remains the essential feature of aplastic anemia and its relatives—pure red cell aplasia (PRCA), agranulocytosis, and amegakaryocytic thrombocytopenia. Aplastic anemia may be acquired or inherited. The causes are multiple, and natural histories are diverse.

Camitta and co-workers classified the severity of aplastic anemia to make possible the comparison of diverse groups of patients and different therapeutic approaches (2). Diagnosis of severe aplastic anemia requires that the patient have at least two of the following anomalies: a granulocyte count less than $500/\mu L$, a platelet count less than $20,000/\mu L$, and an absolute reticulocyte count less than or equal to $40 \times 10^9/L$. In addition, the bone marrow biopsy must contain less than 25% of the normal cellularity. *Very severe aplastic anemia* is further defined by a granulocyte count less than $200/\mu L$ (3). Mild or moderate aplastic anemia, sometimes called *hypoplastic anemia*, is distinguished from the severe form by the presence of mild or moderate cytopenias and more variable—but still deficient—bone marrow cellularity. These distinctions are more than semantic; they are critical for the prediction of outcome and the choice of therapy.

Differential Diagnosis of Pancytopenia

An empty bone marrow is usually obvious (Fig. 9-1). The workup of the pancytopenic patient should be focused on eliminating alternative diagnoses for which alternative curative therapies are available or for which treatments for aplastic anemia would be inappropriate. The most important and difficult choice of diagnoses in the pancytopenic patients rests among primary bone marrow diseases (Table 9-1). Several complicating factors should be recognized. In moderate aplastic anemia, only modest depression of marrow cellularity may be present. Bone marrow cellularity is imprecisely quantitated, sampling error is large, and "hot spots" of hematopoietic activity in an otherwise acellular specimen indicate heterogeneity in the pattern of cell loss. Chronic aplastic anemia can evolve into other hematologic diseases (see the section Complications of Immunosuppressive Therapy). Leukemia, dysplasia, and aplasia share etiologic risk factors (radiation, chemicals, and congenital chromosomal abnormalities). *Fanconi's anemia* is a genetic bone marrow failure syndrome that can present with aplastic anemia in the absence of other clinically overt stigmata of the disease. The diagnostic test for Fanconi's anemia is increased chromosomal breakage after exposure of the patient's cells to clastogenic agents such as diepoxybutane. Fanconi's anemia patients are exquisitely sensitive to DNA-damaging agents, and therapy must be tailored accordingly. Historically, paroxysmal nocturnal hemoglobinuria (PNH) may also present with pancytopenia and marrow aplasia, and it has been recently appreciated that there is enormous overlap between aplastic anemia and PNH (see the section Paroxysmal Nocturnal Hemoglobinuria). In some cases, separate pathophysiologic processes may be operating in a single patient who manifests more than a single disease [aplastic anemia and myelofibrosis (16), red blood cell (RBC) hypoplasia, myelodysplasia (17), and others] or shows a mixture of pathologic features on bone marrow examination.

The acute leukemias and myelodysplastic syndromes can atypically be associated with marrow hypocellularity and confused with aplastic anemia. The syndrome of hypoplastic or hypocellular acute leukemia has been estimated to account for 5% to 8% of acute nonlymphocytic leukemia (18,19). Acute lymphoblastic leukemia also can present as aplastic anemia in children (20) and adults (21). A significant proportion of patients with myelodysplasia also have hypocellular bone marrows (Chapter 11), and aplastic anemia and myelodysplasia are probably most often confused.

Pancytopenia can result from peripheral blood processes with relatively normal bone marrow function, but such syndromes usu-

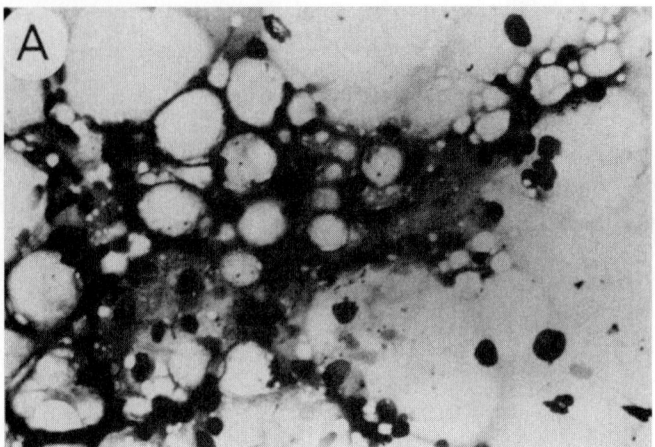
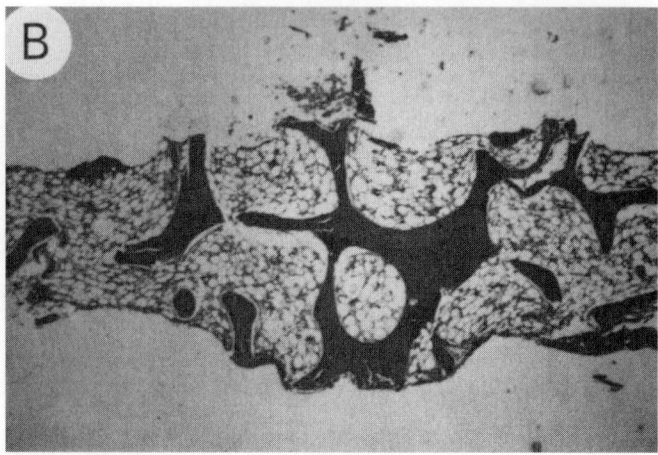

Figure 9-1. Bone marrow in aplastic anemia. Aspirate smear **(A)** and core biopsy **(B)** from a patient with severe aplastic anemia show residual stromal and lymphoid elements.

ally occur in an obvious clinical context as complications of nonhematologic primary disease. Pancytopenia is unlikely to be the presenting feature of hypersplenism in cirrhosis or of Evans's syndrome in systemic lupus erythematosus. Findings on physical examination may point strongly toward another diagnosis; for example, the patient with myelofibrosis usually has splenomegaly, whereas a patient with aplastic anemia rarely has a large spleen. Although B_{12} and folate deficiency have been reported to be associated with erythroid hypoplasia (22), it is rare. In general, the likelihood of confusion with other intrinsic bone marrow processes is not equal for all conditions. Therefore, before a bone marrow examination is performed, the list of possible diagnoses should be shortened by analyzing the patient's history and physical examination and by judging the probability of the alternative disorders.

The bone marrow examination is the ultimate basis for the diagnosis of most primary hematologic causes of pancytopenia. Both the aspirate smear and the biopsy must be examined to

arrive at an accurate diagnosis. Observation during the procedure itself may be helpful in the differential diagnosis; a fatty specimen can usually be aspirated without difficulty from a patient with aplastic anemia, and a true dry tap is more typical of the packed bone marrow seen in patients with chronic lymphocytic leukemia, hairy cell leukemia, and acute leukemia or the fibrotic marrow of myelofibrosis. The morphology of individual cells is better displayed on Wright-Giemsa stain of the aspirate smear, whereas the architecture of the marrow is seen on the biopsy section. A stained smear should be examined for the presence of characteristic individual cells or patterns of differentiation that point toward a specific diagnosis. Examination of the cells close to the spicules of a sparse aspirate smear may disclose a distinct population of leukemic blasts; or, the dysmorphic appearance of residual erythroid cells may more strongly suggest dysplasia than aplasia.

Cytogenetic analysis is also important because chromosomal analysis is usually normal in aplastic anemia patients and frequently abnormal in myelodysplasia patients (16,23,24). Lymphoid aggregates, nests of tumor cells, granulomas, and infectious particles may be visible only on the fixed biopsy specimen. An uncertain diagnosis jeopardizes not only the patient, who may be directed to an improper treatment, but also the integrity of clinical trials; in older hematologic studies, because of inadequate sampling and interpretation, diverse processes are often treated together, and inferences concerning natural history and therapeutic effects should be treated with caution by the modern reader.

TABLE 9-1. Differential Diagnosis of Pancytopenia

Pancytopenia with hypocellular bone marrow
    Acquired aplastic anemia
    Inherited aplastic anemia (Fanconi's anemia)
    Some myelodysplasia syndromes
    Rare aleukemic leukemia (acute myelogenous or lymphoblastic
     leukemia)
    Some acute lymphoblastic leukemia
    Some lymphomas of bone marrow
Pancytopenia with cellular bone marrow
    Myelodysplasia syndromes
    Paroxysmal nocturnal hemoglobinuria
    Myelofibrosis
    Some acute leukemia
    Myelophthisis
    Bone marrow lymphoma
    Hairy cell leukemia
Secondary to systemic diseases
    Systemic lupus erythematosus (4)
    Hypersplenism
    Vitamin B_{12}, folate deficiency [familial defect (5)]
    Overwhelming infection
    Alcohol
    Brucellosis (6)
    Sarcoidosis
    Tuberculosis (7–9)
Hypocellular bone marrow with or without cytopenia
    Q fever (10)
    Legionnaire's disease (11)
    Anorexia nervosa (12–14), starvation
    Mycobacteria (15)

APLASTIC ANEMIA

Aplastic anemia is the paradigm of bone marrow failure. The name encompasses heterogeneous disorders: the Chernobyl fireman with severe radiation damage, the child with infectious mononucleosis–associated aplasia who responds to immunosuppression, the adolescent presenting late with Fanconi's anemia. All affected persons exhibit the same pathology but suffer different disease processes. Patients with aplastic anemia are united by practical management considerations and also by apparently similar pathophysiologic mechanisms. These common features are stressed in this chapter.

Epidemiology

Results from the International Aplastic Anemia and Agranulocytosis Study indicate an annual incidence of aplastic anemia of two new cases/1 million population/year (25). This prospec-

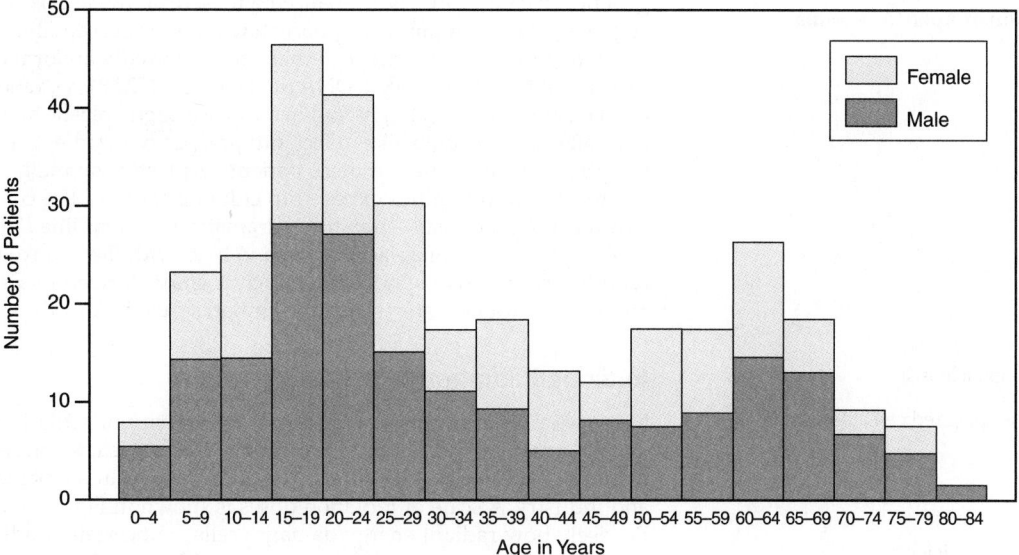

Figure 9-2. Distribution of age at diagnosis of more than 300 patients with an admitting diagnosis of severe aplastic anemia, seen at the Clinical Center of the National Institutes of Health between 1978 and 1998. (Reproduced with permission from Young NS. Acquired aplastic anemia. In: Young NS, ed. *Bone marrow failure syndromes.* Philadelphia: WB Saunders, 2000.)

tive study was conducted in Europe and Israel from 1980 to 1984. The study adhered to strict case definition criteria and required pathologic confirmation. By comparison, the incidences of acute myelogenous leukemia (AML) and multiple myeloma are approximately 35 and 27 cases/1 million people, respectively. Although an apparent increase in the incidence of aplastic anemia during the 1950s and 1960s was reported by some authors (26), more recent surveys show that the incidence has probably been stable in the past 20 years (27–29). Earlier studies may have been in error by inclusion of cases of pancytopenia secondary to cytostatic drug therapy or resulting from other diseases such as myelodysplasia. Figures of occurrence of aplastic anemia may be heavily influenced by the method of ascertainment and exclusion criteria (29,30). Few studies have included rigorous confirmation of the diagnosis by a hematologist's review of the chart and tissue. Until recently, chromosome analysis was infrequently performed in adults, and some cases of apparently acquired aplastic anemia almost certainly were misdiagnosed inherited aplastic anemia.

The incidence of aplastic anemia varies significantly with age. The incidence curve shows two peaks, with patients mainly presenting at 15 to 25 years of age or older than 60 years of age, and a trough in middle life (29,31) (Fig. 9-2). If inherited disease is included, a third peak appears in the first decade. Aplastic anemia occurs with equal frequency in both genders (27).

The most remarkable feature of the epidemiology of aplastic anemia is a large and unexplained geographic variation in its incidence. For years, physicians in the Orient and their foreign visitors have believed that aplastic anemia is far more common there than in the West (32). A nationwide survey in Japan in 1972 led to an estimate of *prevalence* (total number of cases in a population at a single time) of aplastic anemia of 31 to 48/1 million population (33). Two large population surveys in China arrived at similar estimates of 19 to 21/1 million people (34,35); for comparison, the prevalence of AML was 37/1 million people (Wang, Peoples' Hospital, Beijing, personal communication, 2000). Recent studies of the *incidence* (defined as the number of new cases in a population/year) of aplastic anemia in Thailand estimate an annual incidence of 4.0 to 5.6/million (36). Similarly elevated annual incidences have been reported for China (7.4/million) (37) and Malaysia (5/million) (38).

The explanation for the geographic variation in aplastic anemia is probably mainly environmental rather than genetic, because Japanese in Hawaii seem to have aplastic anemia at the same rate as Americans (39). [Conversely, American soldiers in the Pacific theater during World War II had a high incidence of aplastic anemia, attributed to use of quinacrine (40).] Chloramphenicol is a popular antibiotic in much of Asia, because of its efficacy and low cost, but reductions in its use have not been correlated with changes in incidence of aplastic anemia in Japan (41,42) or elsewhere (27,43), and no association was observed in the case control studies in Thailand (44). A case control study has shown relations to chemical exposures and exposures to viruses through blood transfusions, hepatitis, and occupation (45).

Clinical Associations and Pathogenesis

The importance of a classification scheme (Tables 9-2 and 9-3) is to assist in determining prognosis, therapy, and common features that can be related to pathogenesis. A too-strict division into categories can obscure important relations, the genetic basis for susceptibility to drugs or viruses, and common interactions with the immune system. Most patients have idiopathic disease of unknown cause, but for most clinical associations, the inductive mechanisms are uncertain. The determination of clinical association has generally been imprecise, and the basis for assigning patients in practice is the history: How closely is the patient questioned? How biased and repetitive are the inquiries? How conscientiously sought is a significant distant toxic exposure or how exaggerated is a brief episode? Patients with idiopathic and secondary disease require similar support and definitive therapies; with few exceptions, little basis exists for major differences in their clinical management.

Genetic Factors

Inherited forms of aplastic anemia are described in greater detail in Chapter 8. Patients with inherited aplastic anemia may present as adults. The expansion of diagnostic cytogenetic testing has revealed that many patients with Fanconi's anemia lack physical signs and, most important, may become pancytopenic well beyond childhood. The diagnosis of Fanconi's anemia, defined cytogenetically, should be pursued by chromosome analysis of peripheral blood cells in patients in middle life as well as in childhood. Approximately one-half of the patients with reported cases of dyskeratosis congenita have had aplastic anemia; typically, pancytopenia in this congenital disease does not appear until the third decade of life. Because

---

TABLE 9-2. Classification of Aplastic Anemia

Acquired aplastic anemia
  Secondary aplastic anemia
    Radiation
    Drugs and chemicals
      Regular effects
        Cytotoxic agents
        Benzene
      Idiosyncratic reactions
        Chloramphenicol
        Nonsteroidal antiinflammatories
        Antiepileptics
        Gold
        Other drugs and chemicals
    Viruses
      Epstein-Barr virus (infectious mononucleosis)
      Hepatitis (non-A, non-B, non-C)
      Parvovirus (transient aplastic crisis, pure red cell aplasia)
      Human immunodeficiency virus
    Immune diseases
      Eosinophilic fasciitis
      Hypoimmunoglobulinemia
      Thymoma and thymic carcinoma
      Graft-versus-host disease in immunodeficiency
    Pregnancy
  Idiopathic aplastic anemia
Inherited aplastic anemia
  Fanconi's anemia
  Dyskeratosis congenita
  Shwachman-Diamond syndrome
  Reticular dysgenesis
  Amegakaryocytic thrombocytopenia
  Other (familiar aplastic anemias)
  Preleukemia (monosomy 7 and others)
  Nonhematologic syndromes
  Down's, Dubowitz, Seckel syndromes

---

of its rarity, the association between the skin and blood disorders may be overlooked.

Genetic associations are suggested by the increased representation of certain HLA antigens [both class I (HLA-A2) and class II (HLA-DR2, HLA-DR4, HLA-DPw3)] among patients with acquired aplastic anemia (46–49). In Japanese patients, the class II haplotype DRB*1501 has been correlated with cyclosporin-responsive and cyclosporin-dependent disease (50). A recent study reports increased frequency of HLA-DR2 in patients with PNH and PNH/aplastic anemia syndrome (51). Genetic factors likely predispose rather than predetermine aplasia. Clinical evidence of pancytopenia in Fanconi's anemia patients commonly appears after a chemical exposure, although the chromosomal abnormalities are present from birth. Other, as yet undefined,

---

TABLE 9-3. Classification of the Single Cytopenias

Acquired Cytopenias	Inherited Cytopenias
Pure red cell aplasia	
Idiopathic	Diamond-Blackfan anemia
Drugs, toxins	
Immune	
Thymoma	
Transient erythroblastopenia of childhood	
Neutropenia	
Idiopathic	Kostmann's syndrome
Drugs, toxins	Shwachman-Diamond syndrome
	Reticular dysgenesis
Thrombocytopenia	
Idiopathic amegakaryocytic	Amegakaryocytic thrombocytopenia with absent radii
Drugs, toxins	

---

genetic variability in DNA repair enzymes, drug metabolizing enzymes, and the immune response may underlie susceptibility to inciting drugs and viruses. Perhaps the reportedly abnormal susceptibility of lymphocyte DNA to bleomycin (52,53), a strand breaker, and ultraviolet light (54) in adult acquired aplastic anemia reflects a Fanconi's-like defect, but prospective studies cannot easily be performed in these patients. Aplastic anemia has occurred within families exposed to chloramphenicol (55–57). One form of genetic susceptibility is dramatically exemplified by the high frequency of aplastic anemia in boys with the X-linked lymphoproliferative syndrome, which is characterized by an abnormal immune response to Epstein-Barr virus (EBV) (58).

Ionizing Radiation

Marrow aplasia is a major result of acute toxicity of radiation (59–61) from nuclear bomb explosions, fallout, reactor accidents, and accidental exposure to radiation sources in medicine and industry. A scale of radiation doses is shown in Figure 9-3. Precisely how radiant energy damages cells is uncertain. Radiant energy generates ions, peroxides, and free radicals, and radiation doses are defined in terms of ionization in tissue [1 gray (Gy) = absorbed energy equivalent to 1 J/kg unit mass; 1 Gy = 100 rad]. Large macromolecules, especially DNA, can be damaged (a) directly by large amounts of radiant energy that can rupture covalent bonds or (b) indirectly by interaction with highly charged and reactive small molecules resulting from ionization or free radical formation occurring in solution. With the singular exception of lymphocytes, a round of replication is required for radiation damage to become manifest. Mitotically active hematopoietic tissue is exquisitely sensitive to almost all types of radiation. In atomic bomb explosions, γ radiation has been the major effector of tissue damage, whereas α, β, γ, and neutron emissions all figure to variable degrees in civilian accidents. Bone marrow cells are probably most affected by high-energy γ rays, which penetrate the viscera, and secondarily by ingested or absorbed α and β particles (low-energy β particles burn but do not penetrate beyond the skin).

Chronic radiation is associated with many bone marrow diseases. Repeated exposures to low doses are less damaging to stromal cells, which may tolerate 40 to 50 Gy of fractionated radiation with some repair (59). Continuous low-dose γ radiation produces aplasia in approximately one-half of exposed dogs after a total dose of 20 Gy, with the survivors dying of granulocytic leukemia (62). Repeated low doses of radiation may be capable of damage to human bone marrow that initiates aplastic anemia, but the distinction of aplastic anemia from myelodysplasia in some of the older reports is not reliable.

Drugs and Chemicals

Drug or chemical exposure is the most frequently cited specific cause of aplastic anemia in both clinical series of patients and epidemiologic surveys (63–66). The agents cited vary with place and over time: Benzene and chloramphenicol have been replaced by antiepileptics and nonsteroidal antiinflammatory medications with changing patterns of industrial exposure and choice of medications (Table 9-4). Remarkably, aplastic anemia patients with a history of drug or toxin exposure have demographic and clinical characteristics, a similar prognosis, and equivalent responses to therapy that are identical to those of patients with idiopathic disease (67). Drug histories may be inadequate or chemical exposures unrecognized in patients with "idiopathic" disease, who may be genetically predisposed to exquisite drug susceptibility. On the other hand, the high percentage of patients in the clinical series with aplastic anemia

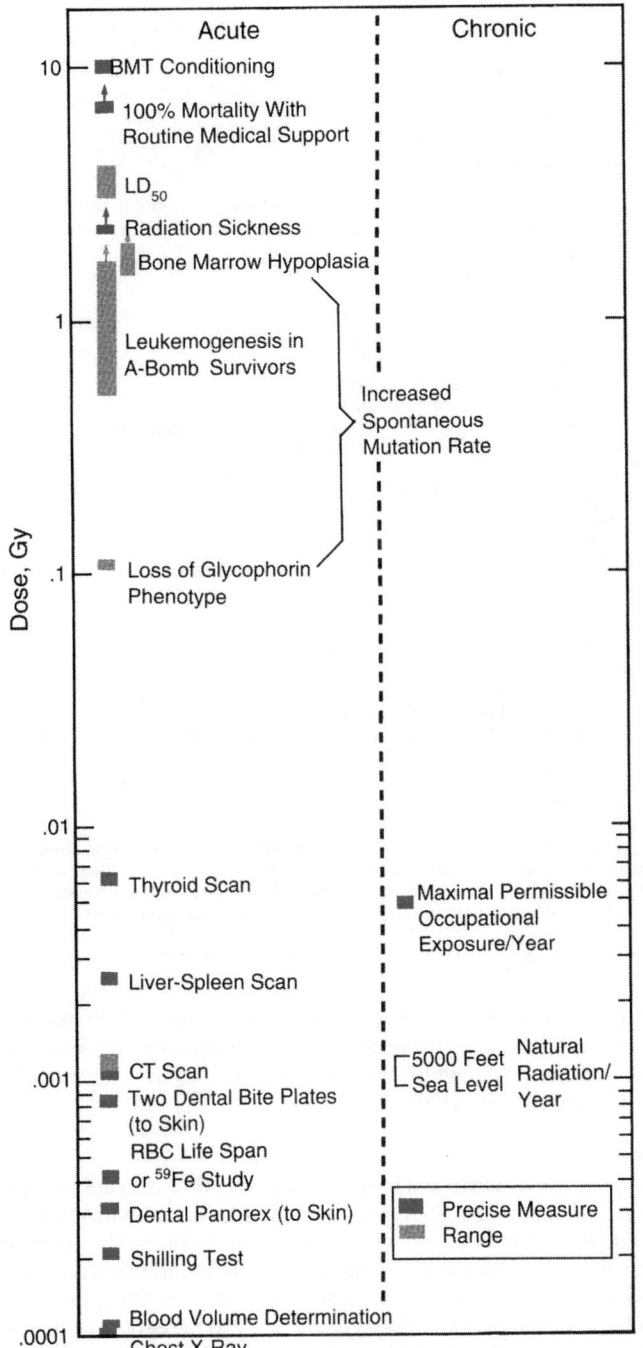

Figure 9-3. Scale of whole-body radiation doses. CT, computed tomography; ⁵⁹Fe, iron 59; LD₅₀, median lethal dose; RBC, red blood cell.

TABLE 9-4. Classification of Drugs and Chemicals Associated with Aplastic Anemia[a]

Agents that regularly produce marrow depression as major toxicity in commonly used doses or normal exposures

    Cytotoxic drugs used in cancer chemotherapy

    Benzene (less often, benzene-containing chemicals)

Agents probably associated with aplastic anemia but with a relatively low probability relative to their use

    Chloramphenicol

    Insecticides

    Antiprotozoals: aquinacrine and chloroquine (95–98)

    Nonsteroidal antiinflammatory drugs: phenylbutazone, indomethacin (105–108), ibuprofen (109), sulindac (110,111), aspirin (112,113)

    Anticonvulsants (117,118): hydantoins (119–123), carbamazepine (125–131), phenacemide (132)

    Gold [possibly, other heavy metals such as arsenic, bismuth (135–137), and mercury (140–142)]

    Sulfonamides as a class: some antibiotics (77,142,144–146), antithyroid drugs [methimazole (147–149), methylthiouracil (153), propylthiouracil (154)], antidiabetes drugs [tolbutamide (155–157), chlorpropamide (159,160)], carbonic anhydrase inhibitors [acetazolamide, methazolamide (161–165)]

    D-Penicillamine (167,168)

    Estrogens (in pregnancy and in high doses in animals)

Agents more rarely associated with aplastic anemia

    Antibiotics: streptomycin (69–71), tetracycline (72), methicillin (73), mebendazole (74), sulfonamides (75–78), trimethoprim/sulfamethoxazole (79,80), flucytosine (81,82)

    Antihistamines (83): cimetidine (84–86), ranitidine (87), chlorpheniramine (88,89)

    Sedative and tranquilizers: chlorpromazine (90–93), prochlorperazine (94), piperacetazine (99), chlordiazepoxide (100), meprobamate (101–103), methyprylon (104)

    Allopurinol (may potentiate marrow suppression by cytotoxic drugs) (114–116)

    Methyldopa (124)

    Quinidine (133,134)

    Lithium (138,139)

    Guanidine (143)

    Potassium perchlorate (150–152)

    Thiocyanate (158)

    Carbimazole (166)

[a]In the absence of references, see extended discussion in text. Citations are provided for archival interest and do not imply acceptance by the authors of a causal relation.

hypotheses, data of poor quality, absence of mechanism, and, especially, detection bias. In general, the link between drugs and adverse reactions is more often conditional or dubious than definitive or even probable (170). Case reports beget case reports, and patients with aplastic anemia are undoubtedly more closely questioned about potentially toxic exposures than patients with most other diseases. Interpretation of case reports is often confounded because many drugs are used in combination. The onset of marrow failure is notoriously difficult to date accurately and, therefore, to place temporally in relation to drug use; the delay in marrow disease after benzene use may be years or decades. Conversely, trivial case reports of drug use are virtually coincident with the onset of marrow failure. Authors are often explicit in incriminating an exposure only because there is no other blameworthy preceding event. Even the large, thorough, and expensive International Agranulocytosis and Aplastic Anemia Study has been faulted for biases in susceptibility, recall and interviewer, diagnostic suspicion, and choice of control group and exclusion (171).

Even confirmed associations do not establish causality, and some drugs may be preferentially used in a patient population that has an inherently high risk of marrow failure. Antibiotics may be prescribed for the first symptom of neutropenia or for the preceding causal viral infection. The platelet inhibitory effect of nonsteroidal antiinflammatory drugs may precipitate bleeding in an already thrombocytopenic patient. Some associa-

from a putative chemical cause may be a biased overestimate. Although approximately one-third of aplastic anemia patients studied by the European Cooperative Group had significant exposures, twice the percentage of control patients with other hematologic diseases had a similar history of drug exposure (68). Drug use or chemical exposure also did not figure significantly in a case control study of aplastic anemia (45).

Clear causal relations between drugs or chemicals and bone marrow failure have been established in only rare instances. The literature on idiosyncratic reactions is best approached with some skepticism. Many studies suffer from the lapses in scientific standards pointed out by Feinstein (169) in his criticism of epidemiologic studies of the "menace of daily life": lack of specific

tions, especially with drugs or chemicals in common use, are simply misconstrued. An example of error that is obvious in retrospect decades later is the association of aplastic anemia with glue sniffing; five of the six patients described in the initial report had sickle cell disease with transient aplastic crisis (TAC) (172), now recognized as resulting from parvovirus infection.

Aplastic anemia has been called "the most disabling, most frequently fatal, and, next to agranulocytosis, the most frequently reported of adverse reactions to drugs" (173). Quantitative estimates of risk are only approximate. In most retrospective studies, cases have been collected, drug use has been ascertained, and calculations have been based on the amount of drug produced and an average dose; each of these procedures is subject to error.

The conventional distinction between regular and idiosyncratic reactions is useful but not absolute. Many drugs associated idiosyncratically with aplastic anemia are linked more frequently with other forms of marrow suppression, such as agranulocytosis with phenylbutazone or gold, moderate neutropenia with antiepileptics, and reticulocytopenia with chloramphenicol. A low incidence of aplastic anemia may be a function of the doses commonly used in clinical practice; at very high doses, chloramphenicol, phenytoin, chlorpromazine, thiouracil, and methicillin all have been reported to occasionally produce reversible marrow depression in human subjects. *In vitro*, toxic drug effects can be demonstrated at high concentrations, which may be achieved in the rare patient with decreased renal or hepatic clearance or a specific drug metabolism defect. Presumably, many agents could be shown to affect marrow function at high doses if these were attainable without toxicity to other organ systems. Although it is a difficult point to prove, some dose-response relation probably exists even for idiosyncratic occurrences. Exquisitely small doses of drugs—a whiff of insecticide, an eyedrop of chloramphenicol—are unlikely to play a role in aplastic anemia (65); conversely, many case reports document administration of very large doses of drugs for use in the setting of hepatic or renal failure.

Dose-related and idiosyncratic marrow depression have been reported only rarely in the same person, but it is reasonable to assume that at least one mechanism responsible for rare drug reactions is a metabolic pathway that reproduces in the unusual individual the condition of excess drug administration (174). Similarly, the probability of developing aplastic anemia with a course of drugs may be a quantitative reflection of the number of genes for metabolic enzymes or histocompatibility types in the human population.

CYTOTOXIC CHEMOTHERAPY

Aplastic anemia is regularly produced by a chemically diverse group of drugs—the chemotherapeutic agents used in the treatment of cancer (175). Acute myelosuppression resulting from their use is usually dose dependent and predictable. These drugs have been selected for their antiproliferative effects on tumors, and their activity can be measured in tissue culture and animal models. Although virtually all chemotherapeutic drugs exert dose-dependent myelotoxicity, higher doses are not well correlated with late or irreversible damage to stem cells. Some agents, such as busulfan, at doses that cause relatively limited immediate reductions in stem cell numbers and self-renewal capacity, can cause profound late depression of bone marrow and reduce marrow regenerative capacity as measured in repopulation assays. In contrast, 5-fluorouracil and cyclophosphamide appear to spare the regenerating cell population, and long-term administration of cyclophosphamide in animals does not reduce the stem cell's ability to repopulate.

Late effects of chemotherapeutic agents are well documented in animal models of bone marrow failure such as the busulfan-treated mouse. The marrow of patients who have been

TABLE 9-5. Sources of Benzene Exposure

Industrial sources[a]
  Made as a byproduct
    Petrochemical plants
    Petroleum refineries
  Used in manufacture
    Drugs
    Chemicals (nitrobenzene, aniline, styrene, cumene, maleic anhydride, monochlorobenzene, dichlorobenzene, and phenol)
    Explosives
    Cements and adhesives
    Dyes
    Leathers and shoes
    Enamel
    Rubber and waterproof fabrics
    Lacquers, shellac, and paint thinners
    Bronzing, silvering, and gilding liquids
    Batteries, electroplating, lithography, and photography
    Dry cleaning
    Feather preparation
    Linoleum and celluloid
  Solvent
    Rubber
    Gum
    Resins
    Fats
    Alkaloids
    Grease
Household sources
  Solvent and solvent component
    Rubber solvent (1.5% benzene)
    Varnish maker and naphtha (0.1%), mineral spirits
    Stoddard solvent (0.1–0.7%)
  Gasoline storage and dispensing
  Cigarette smoke

[a]Listed are industries in which workers have been exposed or continue to be exposed to benzene and likely sources of benzene outside of industry (181a). Exposure is likely to be greater in open industries in which benzene is used for some secondary purpose than in closed-system industries in which benzene is produced.

subjected to chemotherapy is similarly damaged. Frank marrow failure in patients with chronic myelogenous leukemia, an uncommon occurrence, has been interpreted as a late effect of busulfan therapy (176).

BENZENE

Benzene is the chemical most convincingly linked to aplastic anemia by clinical and epidemiologic studies, with animal and *in vitro* data (177,178). Benzene myelotoxicity can be placed between the regular effects of chemotherapeutic agents and idiosyncratic drug reactions. Benzene is efficient enough at decreasing the white blood cell count to have been used briefly in the early treatment of leukemia; on the other hand, many workers have tolerated high doses in industry without developing aplastic anemia.

Enormous quantities of benzene are produced, used in industry, released into the atmosphere, and found in the household (64,179–181) (Table 9-5). Benzene is ubiquitous. Its low boiling point (80.1°C) and high vapor pressure ensure rapid evaporation, and fugitive industrial emissions add greatly to the biologic sources of ambient benzene. Inhaled benzene is rapidly absorbed into the body; uptake through mucous membranes and skin is relatively minor. Because of its low partition coefficient, benzene is concentrated in the fat of the bone marrow (182). Although the primary site of benzene metabolism is the liver, active metabolism also occurs in bone marrow (183,184). Water-soluble intermediate products such as phenols, hydroquinones, and catechols probably mediate toxicity (185–187). Benzene and its intermediate metabolites covalently and irreversibly bind to bone marrow DNA (188,189), inhibit DNA synthesis (190,191), and introduce DNA strand breaks (192).

Chromosomal abnormalities are produced by chronic administration in animals (191,193) and are present in benzene workers (194,195). The decrease in cell proliferation frequently measured *in vitro* could result from any number of indirect effects on cell function, such as irreversible protein binding (196,197), as well as from a direct action on DNA.

Leukopenia (198), thrombocytopenia (199), and anemia (200) each have been cited as the most common hematologic consequences of benzene; lymphocytopenia is also common. Other manifestations are macrocytosis, acquired Pelger-Huët anomaly, eosinophilia, basophilia, elevated fetal hemoglobin, and, less commonly, polycythemia, leukocytosis, thrombocytosis, and splenomegaly (198,201–203). The marrow of healthy workers is usually normocellular but may show moderate hypocellularity or hypercellularity (198); a hypercellular phase may precede complete aplasia in the course of benzene toxicity. The predictive value of abnormal blood counts is uncertain. Most workers with borderline values in one large clinic returned to normal, despite continued exposure to benzene (202); most workers with severe hematologic benzene poisoning completely recover (204,205). Chronic benzene exposure clearly increases the risk of AML (206–208) and a variety of lymphohematopoietic malignancies, including multiple myeloma (206,209–211). Aplastic anemia and acute leukemia have occurred in the same person (212). Both aplastic anemia and acute leukemia in benzene workers can manifest decades after exposure, but, similar to the effects of radiation, malignancy may be the more common late consequence. Cumulative benzene exposure has been statistically correlated with the risk of acute leukemia (206) and probably is an important variable for marrow failure (even short exposure to high doses can provoke blood changes) (213).

OTHER AROMATIC HYDROCARBONS

The common perception that other molecules resembling benzene in structure or containing a benzene ring also cause marrow suppression is not well supported by facts. Not all aromatic hydrocarbons share biologic activities. In contrast to benzene, neither the closely related alkylbenzenes (214) nor pure toluene and xylene (215,216) are marrow toxins. Often, an aromatic hydrocarbon has been implicated clinically only because no other apparent cause of aplastic anemia was found. For some substances, toxicity may be due to the presence of benzene itself, either as a contaminant in the synthesis of the molecule or in the petroleum distillates used to dissolve the product. Nevertheless, the total number of bone marrow failure cases reported is very small, considering the large populations exposed to this heterogeneous group of chemicals.

Case reports greatly outnumber series of patients, and only a few rigorous epidemiologic surveys have been performed. In the case of insecticides, for example, surveys of aplastic anemia patients directed toward causes have found 2% (68,217), 6% (218,219), and 9% (220) of cases associated with exposure. The significance of a handful of case reports in the context of vast use is questionable (221). A recent case control study did not confirm an association between household pesticide use and aplastic anemia in Thailand (222). The most frequently cited insecticides are chlordane (223–225) and lindane (225–229) or these products in combination with dichlorodiphenyltrichloroethane (225,229–231). Nevertheless, other surveys of pesticide makers or users (232–236) and farmers (237–240) have not shown an increased mortality rate from aplastic anemia, even though some of these workers have detectable blood levels of pesticide (241).

CHLORAMPHENICOL

Chloramphenicol was isolated from a Venezuelan *Streptomyces* sp. in 1947; the crystalline antibiotic was named *Chloromycetin*

because it contained chlorine and came from an actinomycete. The chemical structure of chloramphenicol contains a nitrobenzene ring, a unique property for a natural compound; its similarity to the structure of amidopyrine, a drug known to cause agranulocytosis, led to an early prediction of blood dyscrasias (242,243). Chloramphenicol was introduced into practice in 1949 and rapidly gained popularity because of its broad spectrum of antimicrobial activity and minimal gastrointestinal toxicity. The first published case of aplastic anemia associated with chloramphenicol appeared in 1950, followed by such an explosion of reports that the Food and Drug Administration was able to collect several hundred reports within a few years (244,245). A still remarkable feature of chloramphenicol was that, in contrast to most other agents associated with marrow suppression, pancytopenia, which is frequently fatal, was by far the most common hematologic toxicity encountered.

During the period of unrestrained use of chloramphenicol, it was considered the most common cause of aplastic anemia in the United States (217). Most affected patients died; a few survivors developed acute leukemia (246,247). Chloramphenicol use has been associated with leukemia independent of the occurrence of aplastic anemia (267). From 1949 to 1952, 47% of the 296 patients of aplastic anemia collected were associated with prior chloramphenicol use (245); from 1952 to 1954, after deservedly adverse publicity, 15% of 607 patients had prior exposure (244). Chloramphenicol use rebounded and continued to be the drug most frequently associated with aplastic anemia for several decades. In clinical series, chloramphenicol usually accounted for 20% to 30% of the total cases of aplastic anemia and one-half of the drug-associated cases; in epidemiologic surveys in California done in the early 1960s, chloramphenicol was associated with most of the drug-related cases of aplastic anemia (173,248).

With narrowing indications for the use of chloramphenicol, aplastic anemia associated with its use has almost disappeared. In 160 patients with acquired aplastic anemia admitted to the National Institutes of Health from 1978 to 1989, none had a history of chloramphenicol use. The International Agranulocytosis and Aplastic Anemia Study did not find chloramphenicol use in any of the 135 patients with aplastic anemia (249).

The perception that the introduction of chloramphenicol into the American market increased the number of cases of bone marrow failure (217,250) was only weakly supported by epidemiologic data (173). The decline in chloramphenicol use in Japan and Sweden has not been associated with a decrease in the incidence of aplastic anemia, and in regions where chloramphenicol continues to be widely used, aplastic anemia associated with its use is either infrequent [Hong Kong (251), Israel (252)] or may even have declined since its introduction [Colombia (253)]. An inference from these data is that chloramphenicol affected a subpopulation prone to drug effects on the bone marrow, with only the rapid introduction and popularity of the antibiotic leading to its recognition as a dramatic destructive agent. Genetic susceptibility is supported by the appearance of aplasia in family members treated with chloramphenicol (56,254). The dose-response relation of chloramphenicol and aplastic anemia has never been satisfactorily resolved. The early case collections and epidemiologic surveys stressed excessive dosage, often given in repeated or intermittent courses, and a high proportion of cases occurred among children (173,244,245,248,255). In a later collection of nearly 600 cases, most patients had received a dose of less than 10 g (57).

At the usual therapeutic doses, a stereotypical pattern of reversible alterations in erythropoiesis occurs in virtually every patient treated with chloramphenicol (256) (Table 9-6). Suppression of erythropoiesis is probably secondary to drug inhibition of mitochondrial protein synthesis, especially of heme synthesis

TABLE 9-6. Hematologic Toxicity from Chloramphenicol

	Reversible Toxicity	Aplastic Anemia
Incidence	Common	Rare
Blood	Reticulocytopenia progressing to anemia if treatment is prolonged; increased serum iron; occasional moderate leukopenia, thrombocytopenia	Pancytopenia, usually severe
Bone marrow appearance	Normal cellularity; decreased late erythroid cells, erythroblast nuclear/cytoplasmic vacuolization	Aplastic
Dose relation	Dose dependent	Either dose independent or greater drug sensitivity
Onset	With drug therapy	Several months after treatment
Symptoms	None (pallor with anemia)	Bleeding, infection, etc.
Outcome	Recovery	Usually fatal

enzymes such as ferrochelatase, which catalyzes the insertion of iron into protoporphyrin (257). Other enzymes inhibited include cytochrome oxidase, cytochrome b, and an adenosine triphosphatase (258). Vacuolization of erythroblasts represents mitochondria with condensed and fragmented matrices (259). Decreased iron use and reticulocytopenia may occur earlier in patients than in normal volunteers because of their increased erythropoietic activity (258,260). Suppression of erythropoiesis has not been correlated with the later occurrence of aplastic anemia (261). Chloramphenicol can inhibit hematopoietic colony formation, especially early erythroid (262–265), or diminish colony size (266), but usually at doses greater than that achieved in patients. Inhibition of marrow stromal cell proliferation (267) and production of growth factors (264) have also been reported. No consistent evidence shows abnormal marrow cell sensitivity to the drug in affected persons (268,269). Low chloramphenicol (266) and thiamphenicol (270) doses may actually stimulate colony-forming unit granulocyte-monocyte (CFU-GM)–derived colony formation; in the mouse, these doses may increase hematopoietic colony-forming and stem cell counts, either directly or in response to alterations in more mature marrow compartments. These results may account for the paradoxic stimulation of myelopoiesis observed in a single neutropenic patient (271). Chloramphenicol also suppresses some lymphocyte functions (272,273), and karyotype abnormalities involving C chromosomes have been described in a few cases of chloramphenicol-associated aplasia (274). Thiamphenicol, in which the paranitro group is substituted by a methylsulfonyl group, was originally thought to be an innocent relative of chloramphenicol, but it has been associated with at least six cases of irreversible aplastic anemia (275–277), a frequency of serious marrow failure that may be proportional to its use. Both chloramphenicol and thiamphenicol cause dose-related reversible suppression of erythropoiesis in patients and similarly inhibit hematopoietic colony formation (262).

No clear comprehensive theory exists for chloramphenicol's idiosyncratic hematologic toxicity regarding the precise toxic intermediates involved, the mechanisms of cellular damage, or the basis of rare individual susceptibility. Yunis (278) has shown that nitrosochloramphenicol [in which the paranitro group ($-NO_2$) has been reduced to the nitroso ($-NO$) form] can efficiently degrade isolated (279) and cellular DNA (280). However, the nitroso derivative is not made in the bone marrow and has a brief half-life. Dehydrochloramphenicol, another toxic

metabolite in culture and strand scission assays, is produced by gut bacteria (281); individual susceptibility is hypothesized to be caused by differences in intestinal bacteria, clearance of toxic metabolites, or hematopoietic cell sensitivity (278,281). Others have proposed that chloramphenicol toxicity is the result of covalent binding to cellular proteins of reactive oxidative metabolites, an oxalic acid derivative produced by cytochrome P-450–mediated oxidative dehalogenation or reduction to produce a chloramphenicol free radical and hydroxylamine intermediate, all capable of acylating proteins (282,283).

NONSTEROIDAL ANTIINFLAMMATORY DRUGS

It took far longer to associate phenylbutazone with aplastic anemia than it did for chloramphenicol (284). These drugs have been most frequently used in the treatment of rheumatic syndromes, and other therapies (gold and penicillamine) have also been associated with aplastic anemia in this group of patients. Neutropenia is far more common than pancytopenia as a hematologic toxicity of phenylbutazone (285).

Other nonsteroidal antiinflammatory drugs have been associated by occasional case reports with aplastic anemia, including aspirin, indomethacin, and ibuprofen (Table 9-4). Several large studies not only confirmed the risk of aplastic anemia with phenylbutazone but also identified even higher probabilities with some of the other nonsteroidal antiinflammatory drugs (25). Increased risk was suggested for drugs taken regularly for a prolonged period at high doses.

GOLD AND OTHER HEAVY METALS

Gold salts cause an extraordinarily high incidence of fatal adverse reactions, estimated at 1.6 in 10,000 prescriptions. Dose-dependent neutropenia is common, but several dozen cases of aplastic anemia have been reported (286,287). Gold was demonstrated in the bone marrow by electron microscopy in one case of aplastic anemia (288). Chelation therapy has not been helpful (289), but patients have been successfully treated with bone marrow transplantation (BMT) (290) and immunosuppression (291–293). High concentrations of gold salts inhibit hematopoietic colony formation *in vitro* (294); some evidence suggests a dose-response relation in patients, because high doses of gold have been associated with the development of blood dyscrasias in general and fatal pancytopenia, as opposed to transient neutropenia or thrombocytopenia (295).

The consistent leukopenic effect of inorganic arsenic once led to the use of potassium arsenite in the treatment of leukemia. Arsenic poisoning can result in neutropenia, anemia, and thrombocytopenia (296,297), with characteristic basophilic stippling as seen in lead poisoning. Organic arsenicals, originally used in the treatment of syphilis (arsphenamine) and now as antihelminthics (arsenamide), have also been associated with aplastic anemia (298), possibly because of the combined effect of the arsenic and benzene moieties. Bone marrow depression has been associated with other heavy metals, including bismuth and mercury.

Viruses

Temporary depression of blood counts, especially leukocytes and platelets, is frequent during common virus infections (299–301) (Table 9-7; Fig. 9-4). The role of viruses in more permanent forms of bone marrow failure has been recognized. Virus species of many different families are capable of infecting human bone marrow cells and inducing damage either by causing direct cytotoxicity or by invoking a host immune response. In contrast to drugs and chemicals, in which clinical associations are numerous but mechanisms are difficult to demonstrate in an

TABLE 9-7. Viruses That Infect Bone Marrow Cells

Virus Family	Animal Model	*In Vitro* Target	Human Disease
Parvovirus	FePV	FePV: hematopoietic progenitors, lymphocyte (300) B19: CFU-E, BFU-E (human) (302,303)	Transient aplastic crisis, pure red cell aplasia, nonimmune hydrops fetalis
Herpesvirus	Murine CMV (304)	CMV: fibroblast, hematopoietic progenitors (?) (305,306) EBV: lymphocytes, macrophage, BFU-E (?)	Post-BMT graft failure Infectious mononucleosis, aplastic anemia
Flavivirus	Bovine viral diarrhea (307)	Dengue: macrophage, hematopoietic progenitors (308)	Hematodepressive diseases, hepatitis C, aplastic anemia
Retrovirus	FeLV (309) FV	FeLV: BFU-E (310,311) FV: CFU-E HIV: macrophage/monocyte (312–317), megakaryocyte (318), marrow stroma cells (319) CFU-GM (?)	Acquired immunodeficiency syndrome

BFU-E, burst-forming unit erythroid; BMT, bone marrow transplantation; CFU-E, colony-forming unit erythroid; CFU-GM, colony-forming unit granulocyte-monocyte; CMV, cytomegalovirus; EBV, Epstein-Barr virus; FeLV, feline leukemia virus; FePV, feline parvovirus; FV, Friend virus; HIV, human immunodeficiency virus.

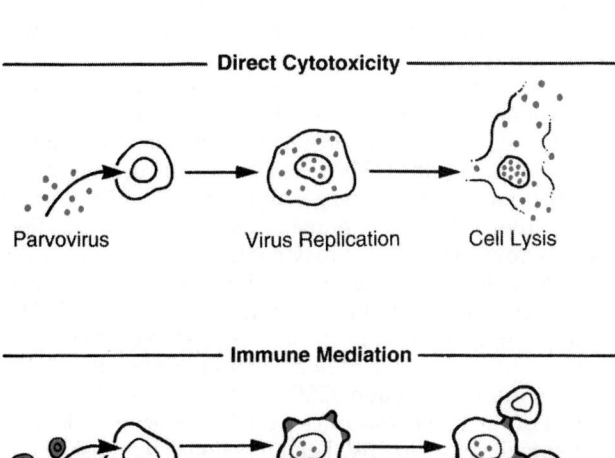

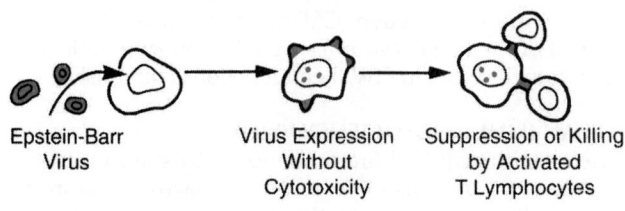

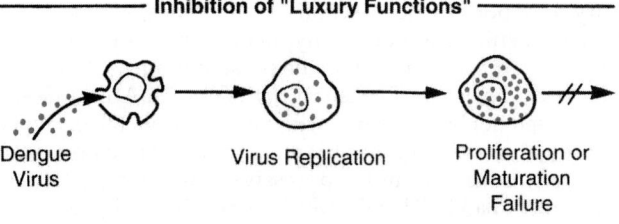

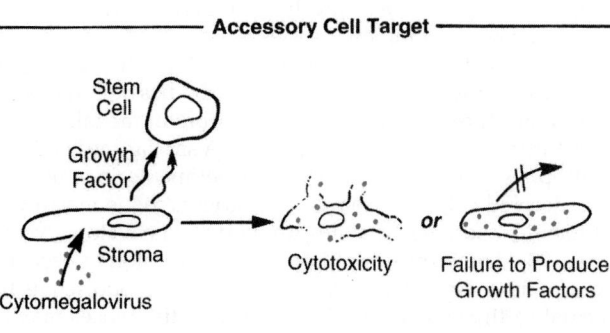

Figure 9-4. Mechanisms of virus-induced bone marrow failure.

individual patient, virus interactions with cells are readily produced *in vitro* and in animal models, whereas the presence of virus infection and its role in the patient require specific molecular and immunologic probes.

HEPATITIS AND FLAVIVIRUSES

Aplastic anemia may follow an episode of acute hepatitis (320–325). The association of hepatitis and aplastic anemia is not rare, and almost 200 cases could be collected in the literature to 1972 (326). As an identifiable clinical event, a prior episode of hepatitis is recognized in 2% to 5% of aplastic anemia patients in Western series (327). A previous episode of hepatitis was a significant risk factor in a case control study of aplastic anemia (45).

Hepatitis is frequently associated with mild blood count depression, but aplasia is a rare sequela, estimated to occur in less than 0.07% of total pediatric hepatitis cases (328) and less than 2.00% of non-A, non-B hepatitis cases (329–331). In patients with hepatic failure after non-A, non-B hepatitis, an astonishing 28% (9 of 32) developed aplastic anemia after liver transplantation (332,333). Posthepatitis aplastic anemia has not been associated with any of the known hepatitis viruses, including hepatitis viruses A, B, C, E, and G (334,335).

Hepatitis-associated aplastic anemia has several peculiar features (91,322,323,336). Bone marrow depression usually occurs just when the patient is recovering from acute liver inflammation, as judged by serum hepatic transaminase elevation, generally approximately 2 months from the episode of hepatitis. A large percentage of patients are male and young. Hepatitis confers a particularly poor prognosis on aplastic anemia patients. In Hagler's series of 174 cases, more than 90% of patients died within 1 year of diagnosis, and the average duration of survival was only 11 weeks from onset of pancytopenia (326). A history of hepatitis has been considered an indication for early BMT (336); patients have undergone successful transplantations (336–338), but some may also respond to antithymocyte globulin (ATG) (332,335). Aplastic anemia has occurred in some family members affected with hepatitis (339,340) and not in others (321); a genetic predisposition is suggested by the presence of HLA-B8 antigen in 6 of 11 cases (also associated with autoimmune hepatitis) (341). Blood count depression during the course of hepatitis is common, and the leukopenia, atypical lymphocytosis, erythroid macrocytosis, and thrombocytopenia mimic in milder form the hematologic changes of aplastic anemia. Much rarer reports of sequelae than severe aplastic anemia are transient pancytopenia (342,343), PRCA (340,344), agranulocytosis (345), and hypoplastic acute lymphocytic leukemia (346).

Inconsistent immune system changes have been reported. Hepatitis-associated aplastic anemia has been associated with generally diminished immune responsiveness, including decreased T-cell count and function and lower serum immunoglobulins (Igs), compared with idiopathic disease (347,348). Comparison with patients with hepatitis alone was not carried out. In contrast, others have reported heightened immune responsiveness, with more circulating activated suppressor T lymphocytes in children with hepatitis-associated aplasia (335,349,350), likely reflecting a cytotoxic lymphocyte response to the viral infection (see section Immune Suppression of Hematopoiesis). A serum sickness–like illness can occur during the course of hepatitis-associated aplastic anemia (331).

FLAVIVIRUSES

Flaviviruses are the etiologic agents of the arbovirus hemorrhagic fevers, dengue (Thai hematodepressive disease) (351,352), Russian spring-summer fever (353), South American hemorrhagic fever (354), Omsk hemorrhagic fever, and many others (355). These are acute infectious hematodepressive syndromes; in dengue, the neutrophil and platelet counts fall, often to very low levels, during the early viremic phase of illness, whereas immune events, probably secondary to cytokine release and reflected in atypical lymphocytosis, predominate during the second, shock phase of the disease. The bone marrow in dengue is hypocellular with an abnormal megakaryocyte appearance. Experimental inoculation of flaviviruses into human volunteers produced pancytopenia and marrow aplasia (356). Flaviviruses propagate efficiently in human bone marrow cultures and hematopoietic cell lines (308). Although not directly cytotoxic to marrow cells (308), dengue infection *in vitro* induces lymphocyte activation and release of cytokines such as interferon (IFN)-γ that suppress hematopoiesis (357) (see section Pathophysiology).

EPSTEIN-BARR VIRUS

Herpesviruses are large, genetically complex DNA viruses; two herpesviruses have been associated clinically and experimentally with bone marrow failure. Acute infection with EBV causes infectious mononucleosis, which has been rarely complicated by severe bone marrow failure. Agranulocytosis (358–360) and PRCA (361,362) have also been associated with EBV infection. Only nine cases of pancytopenia occurring shortly after infectious mononucleosis could be collected in 1981, and bone marrow hypocellularity was not documented in all. Some aplastic patients had spontaneous recoveries, others recovered with corticosteroid therapy, and some died (363). In our study, EBV was demonstrated by immunologic and molecular techniques in bone marrow cells of six patients with aplastic anemia (364). All patients had serologic evidence of recent infection or reactivation, but only two had a previous history of typical infectious mononucleosis, suggesting that the virus may be involved more frequently than inferred from the history alone, especially because a large number of primary EBV infections are unrecognized (364,365). After our observation of a sustained remission after acyclovir therapy in a young woman with aplastic anemia and herpes simplex infections, other patients with aplastic anemia have apparently responded to acyclovir therapy (366,367).

Suppressor T cells are activated during infectious mononucleosis (368) and may mediate hematopoietic failure. Lymphocyte suppression of hematopoiesis was shown in one patient with postmononucleosis aplastic anemia who responded to ATG therapy (369). An aberrant genetically determined immune response to the virus is suggested by the frequent mortality from bone marrow failure in boys with X-linked lymphoproliferative syndrome,

a familial syndrome characterized by various combinations of hypogammaglobulinemia, chronic or fatal acute infectious mononucleosis, B-cell lymphomas, and aplastic anemia (58).

The rare virus-associated hemophagocytic syndrome (see Chapters 30 and 56) is a related but clinically distinct syndrome that is also associated mainly with EBV infection (370). Here, the bone marrow is characterized by histiocytic hyperplasia and erythrocyte phagocytosis (although hematopoietic cell hypoplasia is also present), and the peripheral blood count depression is often associated with abnormalities of other organ systems, especially hepatosplenomegaly, lymphadenopathy, cutaneous eruptions, and pulmonary infiltrates (370–372). Hemophagocytosis is often observed on supravital stains of the marrow of patients with idiopathic aplastic anemia (373).

CYTOMEGALOVIRUS

Like EBV, cytomegalovirus (CMV) infection is common and usually benign in its effects. Even in immunosuppressed patients, CMV infection, as a result of either reactivation or new exposure, is not associated with a characteristic clinical syndrome (374). In the immunosuppressed bone marrow transplant patient, a second episode of marrow failure may follow CMV infection. In immunodeficient mice, murine CMV prevented bone marrow reconstitution despite the presence of stem cells, and cytotoxic (CD8+) lymphocytes protected animals against this lethal effect (304,375); virus can be demonstrated in thrombocytopenic mouse megakaryocytes (376). CMV promiscuously infects fibroblasts of many tissues, and its infection of bone marrow stromal cells may contribute to marrow failure (305). Some clinical isolates of CMV inhibited colony formation [both CFU-GM– and burst-forming unit erythroid (BFU-E)–derived], but no good correlation exists between these *in vitro* effects and the presence of neutropenia in the patient donor (306). As in EBV infection, CMV infection is associated with reversal of the helper/suppressor T-lymphocyte ratio, but in contrast to that seen in EBV, T-cell function is diminished (377).

HUMAN IMMUNODEFICIENCY VIRUS

Patients with acquired immunodeficiency syndrome (AIDS) often have cytopenias (378), but their marrow is more commonly cellular and dysplastic than empty. Although most patients have anemia and granulocytopenia and one-third have thrombocytopenia, many of these abnormalities may be secondary to opportunistic infections, medications, and neoplasms. Pancytopenia and marrow hypocellularity can occur (379). Marrow hypocellularity may be present in up to 20% of bone marrow biopsies performed in patients with AIDS (380–382), but it need not be associated with pancytopenia (379). Hypocellularity almost always has been reported in patients with concomitant infections and suppressive drug therapy (383,384); one patient had PNH (385). Much more frequently, blood count depression is associated with normal cellularity or hypercellularity (379,384,386), which is often dysplastic (383,384,387–389). Atypical lymphocytosis and lymphocytic infiltration of the bone marrow are common features.

Thrombocytopenia in patients with AIDS has been partly explained by the presence of platelet antibodies or immune complexes, but retroviral particles are visible in megakaryocytes from thrombocytopenic patients (318). A similar mechanism for neutrophils is supported by *in vitro* experiments, in which CFU-GM–derived colony formation by patients' bone marrow was inhibited by serum-containing antibodies to envelop glycoprotein (390). The numbers of hematopoietic colonies recovered from patients with AIDS have been variable, reported as both normal (390) and decreased (391). These differences may be a function of the balance between virus and antibody response in different patient populations or may reflect hematopoietic suppression by marrow infected with opportunistic organisms (392). Recent *in vitro* studies indicate that neither human immunodeficiency virus (HIV)-1 nor HIV-2 infects human CD34⁺ bone marrow cells (393). An immune mechanism of hematopoietic suppression has been inferred from *in vitro* studies of another pathogenic human retrovirus, HTLV-1 or the adult T-cell leukemia–lymphoma virus. Protease inhibitor therapy directed against HIV-1 modulates CD4⁺ T-cell activation and decreases susceptibility of CD4⁺ T cells to apoptosis (394). In a case of PRCA associated with HTLV-1 infection, T lymphocytes that suppressed BFU-E–derived progenitor growth were detected in colony culture experiments (392). A nonviral glycoprotein inhibitor of myelopoiesis was partially purified from supernatants of the bone marrow of patients with AIDS in one study (395).

OTHER VIRUSES
As an organ of actively proliferating cells accessible to the circulation, the bone marrow undoubtedly provides an attractive milieu for many types of viruses. Infection of human megakaryocytes has been inferred in congenital and acquired rubella (396–398), measles (399), and mumps (400), and it has been found after live attenuated measles vaccination (401) and demonstrated in varicella (chickenpox) (402) and in animals infected with CMV (376), Newcastle disease virus (403), encephalomyocarditis virus (404), and retrovirus-associated lymphomas (405). Aplastic anemia has been reported after influenza A infection (406).

Paroxysmal Nocturnal Hemoglobinuria
Aplastic anemia and PNH are clinically closely related syndromes (407–409). (See Chapter 10 for discussion of PNH.) During the course of PNH, pancytopenia is common, and approximately one-third of patients die of bone marrow failure. PNH is characterized by an increased sensitivity of erythrocytes to complement due to an inability to inactivate complement on the cell surface. Deficits were subsequently identified in specific membrane proteins, all of which shared a common structural feature—namely, the glycosylphosphatidylinositol (GPI) anchor linking these diverse proteins to the cell membrane. GPI binds covalently to specific carboxyl terminal protein sequences and attaches them to cell membrane phosphatidylinositol residues. The genetic defect in PNH is localized to the X-linked PIG-A (phosphatidylinositol glycan class A) gene whose product functions in the transfer of *N*-acetylglucosamine to phosphatidylinositol as an early step in GPI anchor formation.

The PNH defect can be detected by flow cytometry for the absence of GPI-anchored cell-surface proteins. Approximately 20% to 50% of patients presenting with aplastic anemia manifest the PNH cell phenotype on their granulocytes and erythrocytes by this assay (410–412). Detection of the PNH phenotype is more sensitive by flow cytometric analysis than by sucrose hemolysis or acid lysis tests (412). Flow cytometry can detect smaller numbers of abnormal cells and is not affected by prior red cell transfusion if neutrophils are assayed. The PNH defect may also appear during the course of otherwise typical aplastic anemia. PNH, like aplastic anemia, is also relatively common in Asia, where it is more frequently associated with aplastic anemia and less often with thromboses (413). Aplastic anemia-PNH patients can respond to immunosuppressive therapy. Severe combined immunodeficiency mice infused with bone marrow from PNH patients showed preferential engraftment with the PNH clones (414). Studies of hematopoiesis in these patients have not detected any selective proliferative advantage of the GPI-anchored protein-deficient hematopoietic clones (415). A subsequent study comparing *in vitro* proliferation of PIG-A(–)

and PIG-A(+) CD34 cells from PNH patients found a selective growth deficiency in the PIG-A(+) cell population rather than an advantage for the PIG-A mutant cells: Fas expression was elevated on the wild type compared with the GPI-deficient cells, suggesting increased resistance to apoptosis as one potential mechanism to explain these findings (416). The role of immune, proliferative, and survival mechanisms contributing to marrow aplasia remains a field of active investigation.

Immunologic Abnormalities
Aplastic anemia commonly occurs during the course of the rare syndrome eosinophilic fasciitis, a collagen vascular disease similar to scleroderma (417,418). Of the first 100 cases reported in the literature, nearly 10% had bone marrow failure. The rheumatologic symptoms of fasciitis respond to corticosteroids, but the associated aplastic anemia has a poor prognosis (417); some patients have responded to immunosuppression (419).

Aplastic anemia occasionally occurs in persons with hypogammaglobulinemia (420,421) (see Chapter 22) or in association with thymoma, thymic hyperplasia (422), or thymic carcinoma (423). In one case, suppressor T cells, already implicated in B-cell inhibition, were shown to suppress erythropoietic colony formation (424). Iatrogenic fatal aplastic anemia has been produced by the transfusion of competent lymphocytes into immunodeficient hosts (425–428).

Other than the specific and possibly pathophysiologic immunologic abnormalities to be described in the text that follows, immune system function is not severely impaired in most cases of aplastic anemia. Patients with aplastic anemia generally have normal Ig levels and normal antibody titers to common viral antigens (421,429–431). Approximately one-half of patients show skin test anergy to a common panel of antigens, but *in vitro* lymphocyte proliferation is normal (429). Monocytopenia and lymphocytopenia are responsible for reported specific abnormalities such as deficient differentiation of B cells on lectin stimulation (421) or lymphocyte proliferation that requires monocyte help (431). Aplastic patients do not behave clinically as if they were immunodeficient, and susceptibility to virus and protozoan organisms is related to immunosuppressive therapy.

Pathophysiology

HEMATOPOIETIC STEM CELLS
The most consistent laboratory finding in aplastic anemia is very low numbers of blood and bone marrow hematopoietic progenitor cells, including CFU-GM, BFU-E, colony-forming unit erythroid (CFU-E), and pluripotent colony-forming unit granulocyte-erythroid-macrophage-megakaryocyte. Although assays for human hematopoietic stem cells are limiting, the long-term culture-initiating cell has served as a surrogate estimate for this primitive cell. These cells are markedly reduced in both the marrow and blood of aplastic anemia patients (432,433). The CD34⁺ cell population, which includes the primitive hematopoietic cells, are greatly decreased in aplastic anemia (434–436). Decreased progenitors persist in patients long after successful treatment with BMT (437) or immunosuppression (438,439).

Several lines of evidence support the hypothesis that abnormalities in the hematopoietic stem cell may contribute to the development of aplastic anemia. Stem cell infusion from an identical twin donor without prior conditioning of the recipient is curative in approximately 50% of cases (440–443). These results are consistent with a primary underlying stem cell deficiency and argue against disorders of the bone marrow microenvironment as the cause of stem cell destruction, at least in a subset of patients. Low stem cell numbers persist even after hematologic recovery with immunosuppressive therapy (444). Blood cell parameters such as macrocytosis do not return to normal in many cases. The increased incidence of late clonal disorders such as PNH, myelodysplasia, and acute leukemia also points to an underlying stem cell disorder. Ball et al. reported significant telomere shortening in the leukocytes of aplastic anemia patients (445), raising the possibility that stem cell compromise of the telomere's probable role in stabilizing chromosome ends may play a role in marrow aplasia. A second study reported relatively normal telomere lengths in patients who responded to immunosuppression, whereas untreated or unresponsive patients showed significant telomere shortening (446). Whether telomere shortening represents a primary versus a secondary event in the genesis of aplastic anemia remains to be ascertained.

HEMATOPOIETIC STROMA AND GROWTH FACTORS

The hypothesis that bone marrow failure is a lesion of "soil" rather than "seed" (447) was based on several experimental observations: regeneration in isolated limbs after irradiation (discussed previously); defects of the sinusoidal vasculature in animals rejecting allogeneic bone marrow grafts; intrinsic differences in the ability of red and yellow, or predominantly fatty, marrow to support hematopoiesis after transplantation to extramedullary sites (448). Abnormal adipocyte proliferation, based on morphologic characteristics of fatty marrow in patients and controls, has even been proposed as the primary lesion in aplastic anemia (449). Direct evidence for a microenvironmental defect in aplastic patients has not been found in biochemical analysis of the composition of fat cells (450) or in ultrastructural studies of marrow microvasculature (451).

Bone marrow failure due to a stromal defect occurs in the Sl/Sl^d mouse (452,453) (see Chapter 7). In this disorder, a genetic defect of the Sl^d allele results in an anemia that is not corrected by stem cell infusion but is cured by spleen transplantation. The product of the Sl allele is stem cell factor, the ligand for c-kit (454–457). The presence of normal stem cells in Sl/Sl^d mice is shown by the ability of their spleen or bone marrow to cure W/W^v animals. Parallel results occur in long-term bone marrow cultures: Stroma of Sl/Sl^d animals does not support hematopoiesis by W/W^v cells, whereas W/W^v stroma supports hematopoiesis from Sl/Sl^d mice (458).

Evidence to date does not support a clear role for bone marrow stromal cell defects in the pathogenesis of aplastic anemia. After marrow transplantation, most stromal cell elements remain of host origin (459), yet these cells adequately support the donor's stem cells. In the laboratory, aplastic marrow usually provides normal adherent cell function in long-term or Dexter flask-type cultures; however, a patient's marrow is a poor source of clonogenic cells when grown on normal stroma, consistent with the defect in stem and progenitor cell numbers described earlier (460). Some investigators have reported low fibroblast colony formation in aplastic anemia (461), but this assay may not reflect stromal cell function.

Hematopoietic growth factor production and plasma levels are usually elevated rather than decreased in aplastic anemia patients (reviewed in 462). Circulating levels of erythropoietin, granulocyte colony-stimulating factor (G-CSF) and granulocyte-macrophage colony-stimulating factor (GM-CSF), thrombopoietin, and flt-3 ligand are elevated in patients with aplastic anemia. Stem cell factor levels have been reported to be low to normal. Levels of interleukin (IL)-1, produced by monocytes, are low in aplastic anemia. Therapeutic trials with these factors have not been successful (463), casting doubt on the pathophysiologic significance of deficiency of these factors.

A case of congenital hypoplastic anemia was imputed to a microenvironmental defect because erythroid colony formation was normal, whereas erythropoiesis by marrow fragments was depressed (464). Deficient burst-promoting activity by T lymphocytes in Diamond-Blackfan syndrome is also consistent with an accessory cell defect (465,466). In contrast, virtually all patients with aplastic anemia have markedly depressed hematopoietic colony formation with appropriate hematopoietic growth factor production. Although stromal cell function may be damaged or affected by viral pathogens or chemical toxins, it probably occurs in combination with effects on marrow stem cells, and marrow failure as a result of a specific stromal defect in acquired aplastic anemia probably occurs rarely, if at all.

IMMUNE SUPPRESSION OF HEMATOPOIESIS

Clinical observations provide a powerful impetus to the development of an immune theory of aplastic anemia. Mathé (467) first suggested an immune mechanism when he observed improvement in autologous bone marrow function after failed, mismatched BMT. His patients had been conditioned with antilymphocyte sera. Other cases were reported after cyclophosphamide conditioning (468–470). In one-half or more of syngeneic (twin) bone marrow transplants, simple infusion of stem cells is not sufficient to reconstitute hematopoiesis, and immunosuppressive conditioning of the host is required, suggesting some operational immunologic process (471). Approximately one-half of BMTs between syngeneic twins are not successful unless the host receives cytotoxic conditioning treatment (472), and marrow graft failure can occur even with adequate preparation (473). The laboratory data marshaled in support of an immune pathophysiology on the whole are persuasive of a lymphocyte-mediated process.

Aplasia often responds to treatment with antilymphocyte globulin (ALG)/ATG and/or cyclosporin without transplant. The antilymphocyte preparations contain heterogeneous mixtures of antibodies to lymphocytes and are clearly immunosuppressive as well as generally cytotoxic. They lead to rapid lymphopenia during and immediately after treatment, and reduced levels of activated lymphocytes persist for months. Cyclosporin exerts inhibitory T-cell effects and inhibits transcription of genes for cytokines including IL-2 and IFN-γ (474). The attribution of immune dysregulation as causal in aplastic anemia based on therapy must be tempered with caution because ATG and cyclosporin exert multiple effects in addition to immunosuppression. ATG is a complex mixture of diverse antibodies directed against a range of antigens, including signal transduction and adhesion molecules (475). The active component(s) of ATG in aplastic anemia have yet to be identified. Therapies with mixtures of monoclonal antibodies specific for human T cells have not been very effective in clinical trials to date (reviewed in 476). Furthermore, Igs can increase colony growth in normal, myelodysplastic syndrome (MDS), and aplastic anemia CD34$^+$ bone marrow cells in culture (477). ATG treatment also reduces the expression of Fas-Ag on aplastic anemia bone marrow CD34$^+$ cells (478). As cyclosporine is thought to be more specifically immunosuppressive than ATG, its efficacy further implicates T-cell mediation in the pathophysiology of aplastic anemia; however, cyclosporine therapy also has additional effects. Recent studies reporting ATG (479) or cyclosporin (480) to be effective in the treatment of myelodysplasia suggest either that these agents may exert effects on the bone marrow in addition to modulating immune function or that myelodysplastic processes may involve immune-mediated mechanisms (481).

LYMPHOCYTES

A role for immune dysregulation in aplastic anemia is supported by several studies of T-cell characteristics in aplastic anemia. T cells were first implicated by *in vitro* studies of an aplastic patient's bone marrow in mixing and depletion experiments. Hematopoietic colony formation occurred only after physical separation of myeloid cells from lymphocytes; colony formation was improved by addition of antilymphocyte serum; and the patient's bone marrow cells inhibited normal bone marrow colony formation. Confirmatory case reports followed (424,482–485), and in several larger series, inhibition was detected in most patients (486–488) or in a substantial minority (489–491). In other studies, only a minority of cases showed cellular suppression of hematopoiesis (492–494), and some efforts to identify inhibitory cells were completely unrewarding (495). In some patients, suppressor cell activity disappeared with successful therapy (496), but in others, it was present after hematologic improvement (487,497). Criticism of these studies came from workers in Seattle, who argued that prior transfusion of patients affected lymphocyte function measured *in vitro*. In humans, coculture inhibition was observed much more frequently in cells from patients who had been transfused and in coculture with histoincompatible marrow; only 3 of 16 untransfused patients inhibited HLA-compatible hematopoietic progenitors (498,499). Use of T-cell depletion was proposed to distinguish the transfusion effect; marrow BFU-E–derived colony formation was increased by this maneuver in 8 of 32 patients (500). However, other studies had used heavily transfused patients with diverse hematologic diseases as controls (486,501) or were based on the T-cell depletion assay (487,489). Of note, many reports studied T-cell characteristics of patients who had received treatment for aplastic anemia.

Analysis of cell-surface phenotypes further supported an immune-mediated pathogenesis for aplastic anemia. Lymphocytes with IgG receptors, Tγ+ cells, were reported in aplastic but not in normal bone marrow (502). Later, these cells were characterized phenotypically as *activated cytotoxic lymphocytes*—CD8+ T cells expressing the antigens HLA-DR and the receptor for IL-2; activated cytotoxic T cells circulate (503), but they may be present in the marrow when they are not detected in the blood (504). Cell clones of this phenotype have been isolated from patients, and *in vitro* they overproduce inhibitory cytokines (see below) and inhibit hematopoiesis (505–507). Altered T-helper and T-cytotoxic cell profiles have been reported in patients with aplastic anemia (508–510). Identification of a T-cell clone showing HLA-DRB1 0405–restricted cytotoxicity for hematopoietic cells has been reported in one patient with aplastic anemia (511). Studies of Vβ T-cell receptors have not found any general restriction of T-cell clonality or of dominant lymphocyte clones (512). Skewing of the CDR3 (complementarity determining region 3) of the Vβ region of the T-cell receptor, suggestive of clonal predominance, has been noted in a small group of cyclosporin-dependent patients (513). Furthermore, analysis of the CDR3 region of CD4 cells derived from five patients with aplastic anemia and an HLA-DR2 haplotype showed a high frequency of clones bearing identical CDR3 DNA sequences that were not found in normal controls (514). These results support a model of antigen-driven T-cell expansion underlying aplastic anemia, in which the number of pathogenic antigens is limited and shared among patients.

LYMPHOKINES

A new approach to the problem of immune cell suppression of hematopoiesis was initiated by Bacigalupo and colleagues (489). They generated suppressor cells from normal bone marrow by *in vitro* lectin stimulation; in comparison, the bone marrow cells of aplastic patients were spontaneously inhibitory, and their lymphocytes required only mild activation (515). In addition, the inhibitory activity was found in the supernatants of cultured cells (515). This soluble inhibitor ultimately was identified as IFN-γ. The IFNs as a class were known to be potent inhibitors of hematopoietic colony formation *in vitro* (516–520), in treated patients (521), and in animals (522). IFN-γ acts both directly on progenitors (523) and through accessory immune system cells (518). It also induces HLA-DR expression (524) (therefore, target cell recognition) and production of other inhibitors, such as tumor necrosis factor (TNF) (525,526) and lymphotoxin (527), and it increases the susceptibility of target cells to cytotoxic lymphocytes and natural killer cells (528). Coexpression of lymphokines is common (529), and, subsequently, lectin stimulation was shown to also release lymphotoxin (530), a molecule that acts synergistically with IFNs to suppress hematopoiesis (531–535). Other inhibitory cytokines, such as TNF (536) and macrophage inflammatory protein-1 (537,538), also are overexpressed in aplastic marrow. Both IFN and TNF directly and synergistically inhibit hematopoiesis *in vitro* (539). In long-term bone marrow culture, constitutive low-level expression of IFN-γ is sufficient to markedly reduce the output of both committed progenitor cells and long-term culture-initiating cells—the stem cell surrogate (540). Both IFN and TNF increase the potential for programmed cell death within the CD34+ compartment by increasing Fas antigen expression on target cells (541). (Fas antigen is a cell-surface molecule in the TNF receptor family; its activation signals apoptosis.) IFN-γ, TNF-α, or Fas-ligand may also modulate cytokine receptor expression on CD34+ bone marrow cells (542).

Lymphokine production *in vitro* was associated with acquisition of activation markers on the stimulated lymphocytes, with the receptor for interleukin-2 (IL-2R) appearing early and HLA-DR appearing late (516). *In vitro* inhibitory activity usually has been found in Fcγ-receptor–bearing cells (543), CD8+ (535,544,545), or nonhelper cells (546) and has been much less frequently localized to the subset of normal helper-inducer lymphocytes (CD4+) (547,548). The ability of normal activated lymphocytes to inhibit hematopoiesis can be demonstrated by other methods of activation, such as exposure to alloantigens in mixed lymphocyte culture (544,547) and in allogeneic spleen organ cultures (549), or by triggering of the CD3 antigen receptor complex with antibody (548). CD3 receptor activation leads to acquisition of the IL-2R, dependence for proliferation on IL-2, and IFN-γ mediation, at least in part, of BFU-E inhibition (550).

In measurements of specific lymphokines, IFN-γ was overproduced by mononuclear cells from aplastic patients (508), and production of IL-2 (551) and TNF (552) was also excessive *in vitro* (551). IFN-γ activity was present in sera, and antibodies to IFN-γ enhanced aplastic marrow progenitor growth (516). Patients can show inverted helper-inducer/suppressor-cytotoxic lymphocyte ratios in blood (508); a distinctive population of circulating activated lymphocytes was detected by the presence of CD8, HLA-DR, and the IL-2R on the cell surface using two-color flow cytometry (503). This population mediated suppression of hematopoiesis *in vitro* through lymphokine production. The expanded T-cell population in aplastic anemia was polyclonal by T-cell receptor rearrangement studies (553). These studies extended earlier reports implicating T8+ cells as mediators of myelopoietic suppression in isolated cases of neutropenia to aplastic anemia in general (554).

The functional importance of immunologic dysfunction has been suggested by the reduction in activated lymphocytes that followed successful immunosuppressive therapy with ATG (555) or cyclosporine (552). In a parallel investigation, CD8+ T-cell, IFN-γ–mediated immune suppression in nine patients disappeared after ATG treatment, and the presence of this cell population was correlated with the probability of improvement with immunosuppression (556). Lymphokine overproduction and lymphocyte activation are not related to prior blood transfusion (503,516,552).

History and Physical Examination

Most patients with aplastic anemia seek medical attention for symptoms, which may occur as a result of depression of any or all of the hematopoietic cell lines. Bleeding is the most alarming manifestation of pancytopenia and most frequently brings the patient to a doctor. Thrombocytopenia is usually not associated with massive bleeding. Instead, the patient reports easy bruising (ecchymoses) and red spots (petechiae) usually over dependent surfaces, bleeding gums with tooth brushing, and nosebleeds (epistaxis). Heavy menstrual flow or menorrhagia is common in menstruating women. In classic cases of PNH, dark red urine is reported, but visible bleeding from the genitourinary and gastrointestinal tracts is rare on presentation in patients with aplastic anemia. Massive hemorrhage from any organ does occur in aplastic anemia, but late in the course of the disease and generally in association with infections (especially invasive fungi), drug therapy (ulcerogenic corticosteroids), or traumatic therapeutic procedures (intravenous line placements).

The physiologic adaptation to a gradual reduction in hemoglobin concentration is usually good. The patient with the insidious onset of anemia may report fatigue, lassitude, shortness of breath, or ringing in the ears, but some persons can tolerate astonishingly low hemoglobins without effect. Angina precipitated by anemia may be a presenting symptom in the older patient. Even abrupt cessation of erythropoiesis leads only to a slow decline in hemoglobin (approximately 1 g/dL/week), but the presence, absence, or severity of anemia is not useful in judging the onset of disease because blood counts do not necessarily fall (or rise) concurrently.

Infection is not a common presenting symptom in patients newly diagnosed with aplastic anemia. The sore throat and fever of agranulocytosis are not observed frequently, presumably because other symptoms have appeared earlier in the patient with pancytopenia.

Except for specific complaints referable to the blood counts, most patients have no systemic symptoms; their sense of well-being is belied by the blood counts. Weight loss, persistent fever, and loss of appetite point to another diagnosis. Pain is unusual (557). A careful, persistent, and reiterative history often reveals exposure to implicated drugs or chemicals or a preceding viral infection, but for purposes of management, a history of blood diseases in other family members is most important.

Laboratory Features

PERIPHERAL BLOOD

In typical cases of aplastic anemia, all the blood cell counts are uniformly decreased. This simple finding indicates that cessation of bone marrow function is probably neither abrupt nor uniform among the hematopoietic cell lineages. (The presence of even small amounts of circulating blood elements also implies some degree of bone marrow function.) From the half-life in the circulation of granulocytes (approximately 6 to 12 hours), platelets (5 days), and erythrocytes (60 days), most patients would be expected to show neutropenia and thrombocytopenia, but anemia is common, and the granulocyte count often decreases during the first weeks of observation. The blood smear usually shows an obvious paucity of platelets and leukocytes but normal RBC morphology; toxic granulations may be present in the neutrophils. Automated cell counting frequently shows erythrocyte macrocytosis and a normal RBC distribution width, indicating little variation in RBC size (558).

Platelet size is normal and not increased, as it is in immune peripheral destruction, but the low platelet count may cause greater heterogeneity of size. The automated absolute reticulo-cyte count is greatly diminished. Prior transfusions obviously alter platelet, reticulocyte, and hemoglobin values. Most patients show a decrease in monocyte and lymphocyte counts as well as neutrophil numbers (559).

There is no characteristic pattern for other routine hematologic and clinical chemistry tests. Increased fetal hemoglobin concentrations (560) and i antigen (fetal) expression on erythrocytes (561), decreased erythrocyte membrane sialic acid content (562), and macrocytosis all may be evidence of stress erythrocytosis. Flow cytometry analysis for GPI-anchored protein-deficient erythrocyte and granulocyte populations offers a sensitive measure of patients with the aplastic anemia–paroxysmal nocturnal hemoglobinuria syndrome (407). The acidified serum (Ham) test detected less than one-half of such cases identified by flow cytometry (412). Folate, vitamin B_{12}, and erythropoietin levels are usually increased. Serum transaminases may be mildly elevated in patients with hepatitis-associated aplastic anemia.

BONE MARROW

The marrow must be assessed quantitatively and qualitatively for cellularity and morphology of residual cells. Both a bone marrow aspirate and biopsy (at least 1 cm long) should be obtained. Although the cellularity of aspirate smear and biopsy is correlated, dilution by sinusoidal blood often occurs, and the aspirate can be especially misleadingly hypocellular when the biopsy is hypercellular (563) or shows local areas of active hematopoiesis (84). Biopsy point counting (determination of numbers of cells in small grids) is the most accurate method of determining cellularity, but visual estimation is more frequently used (564). The lower limit of normal marrow cellularity is approximately 30%. In most aplastic patients, cellularity approaches 0%; in some, significant residual cellularity is present because of lymphocytosis; "hot pockets" of hematopoiesis may be present in a minority of patients (565). The marrow tends to contract centripetally with age and pathology, so in adults the sternal bone marrow is often more cellular than iliac crest sites (566).

The appearance of individual cells is best appreciated on Wright-Giemsa stain of the aspirate smear. In acellular specimens, the only cells visible usually are lymphocytes, plasma cells, stromal elements, and fibroblastoid and histiocytic cells. Dyserythropoiesis is common; usually the "megaloblastoid" features of macrocytosis and some nuclear-cytoplasmic maturation asynchrony, but sometimes more complex degenerative changes in nuclei and cytoplasm can be observed by light (567) and electron microscopy (567). These features are common to aplastic anemia and myelodysplasia, which may be difficult to distinguish prospectively (16). An increase in myeloblast count is not seen in patients with aplastic anemia and, if not evidence of aleukemic leukemia, may herald the evolution of leukemia from pancytopenia (568).

Bone marrow cytogenetics are typically normal for patients initially presenting with aplastic anemia. In contrast, cytogenetic abnormalities are frequently found in myelodysplastic bone marrows and may be helpful in distinguishing aplastic anemia from hypoplastic myelodysplasia. The subsequent development of clonal cytogenetic abnormalities represents a serious complication of aplastic anemia and is discussed later in this chapter.

Treatment

Severe aplastic anemia is a medical emergency. Severity is determined by the peripheral blood counts, the most common criteria being greatly reduced counts in two of three lineages: absolute neutrophil count less than 500/µL, platelet count less than 20,000/µL, and corrected reticulocyte count less than 1% (or an automated reticulocyte count less than 60,000/µL) (569).

TABLE 9-8. Allogeneic Bone Marrow Transplantation for Aplastic Anemia

Study (Reference)	Years of Study	Number	Age (Median) (yr)	Rejection/ Failure (%)	Chronic Graft-Versus- Host Disease (%)	Actual Survival (%)
Gluckman et al. (574)	1980–1989	107	5–46 (19)	3	35	68 ± 10 (at 5 yr)
Champlin et al. (575)	1984–1984	290	0.7–41.0 (19)	17	12	78 ± 10 (5 yr)
May et al. (576)	1984–1991	24	4–53	29	0	79 ± 8
Storb et al. (577)	1988–1993	39	2–52 (25)	5	34	92 (3 yr)[a]
Passweg et al. (578)	1988–1992	471	1–51 (20)	16	32	66 ± 6 (5 yr)
Reiter et al. (579)	1982–1996	20	17–37 (25)	0	53	95 (15 yr)
Storb et al. (580)	1988–1999	94	2–59 (26)	4	32	88 (6 yr)

[a]In an update, a total of 55 patients treated by the same regimen were reported to have 89% survival at 8 years (577a).
Revised from Young NS. Acquired aplastic anemia. In: Young NS, ed. *Bone marrow failure syndromes*. Philadelphia: WB Saunders Company, 2000:19.

The patient with severe aplastic anemia is at immediate risk for catastrophe if neutropenia and thrombocytopenia are carelessly regarded. In addition, there are advantages to rapid institution of definitive therapy. For example, early arrangement of histocompatibility testing can speed the appropriate patient to BMT, and tissue typing becomes more difficult if the leukocyte count later falls. Patients not seriously considered transplant candidates may receive unnecessary blood products, even transfusions from family members, which increase the risk of marrow graft rejection. Because of the delay in the hematologic response to immunosuppressive therapy, its institution before the complications of pancytopenia develop is also worthwhile.

BONE MARROW TRANSPLANTATION

Bone marrow was infused into an aplastic anemia patient as early as 1939 (570), and in the 1960s, several identical twins were successfully treated by infusion of syngeneic bone marrow (571). Subsequent definition of the human histocompatibility gene complex, development of immunosuppressive regimens, and improved support of severely pancytopenic patients led to more general application of this form of therapy. Stem cell transplant between identical twins in the absence of any conditioning regimen was curative in approximately 50% of cases (440–443). A recent study showed the highest long-term survival with identical twin transplants following an algorithm of initial transplant without conditioning followed by a subsequent

transplant with conditioning for any patients who did not engraft with the first transplant. None of the patients who did not respond to the first transplant died before receiving a second transplant, and they showed similar mortality to patients who received conditioning upfront (443).

Outcomes for HLA-matched allogeneic BMT have been reported by large registries, which combine the results of many contributing centers, or in single-center studies by the largest referral centers (572,573) (Table 9-8; Figs. 9-5, 9-6). Survival rates after HLA-identical sibling transplant have improved over time, in large part due to improvements in graft-versus-host disease (GVHD) prevention (578). From the most recent data reported to the International Bone Marrow Transplant Registry, among 1699 patients receiving HLA-identical sibling transplants for aplastic anemia between 1991 and 1997, the 5-year probabilities of survival (95% confidence intervals) were 75% ± 3% for patients up to 20 years of age, 68% ± 4% for patients between 21 and 39 years of age, and 35% ± 18% for patients older than 40 years of age. Survival data from single centers, while showing more variability, overlap with the 95% confidence intervals reported by the Registry (573). Patient age, duration of aplasia before transplant, prior transfusion history, and clinical status all affected survival rates. Survival was not affected by severity of aplasia.

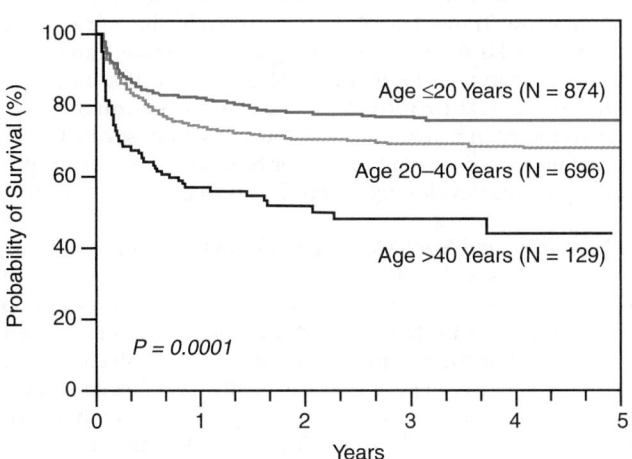

Figure 9-5. Probability of survival after HLA-identical sibling bone marrow transplants for aplastic anemia performed between 1991 and 1997 and reported to the International Bone Marrow Transplant Registry, by age. (Reproduced with permission from Horwitz MM. Current status of allogeneic bone marrow transplantation in acquired aplastic anemia. *Semin Hematol* 2000;37:37.)

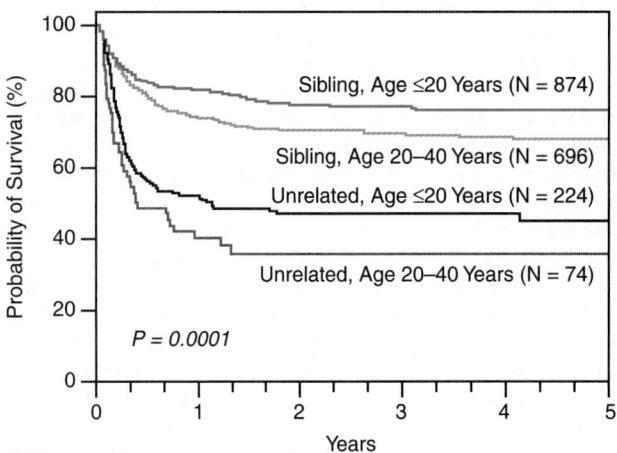

Figure 9-6. Probability of survival after HLA-identical sibling and unrelated donor bone marrow transplants for aplastic anemia performed between 1991 and 1997 and reported to the International Bone Marrow Transplant Registry, by age. Patients older than 40 years are excluded because few unrelated donor transplants have been performed in this population. (Reproduced with permission from Horwitz MM. Current status of allogeneic bone marrow transplantation in acquired aplastic anemia. *Semin Hematol* 2000;37:38.)

Graft Rejection. Graft rejection has been significantly higher for aplastic anemia patients as compared to transplants performed for leukemia. The more intensive conditioning regimens used to eradicate malignant disease may also more fully ablate the host immune system. Graft rejection may be underestimated because failure to engraft, which may have a similar mechanism, usually leads to an early death from infection. That graft rejection might be intrinsic to the pathophysiology of aplastic anemia has been suggested by the unexpectedly high percentage of failure in unprepared syngeneic transplants (440,441,581) even with adequate preconditioning (473). Mixed hematologic chimerism occurs commonly after transplantation in aplastic anemia, and persistence of donor lymphocytes is highly associated with graft rejection (30% vs. 5% in complete chimeras) (582). More rapid regeneration of bone marrow grafts has been observed in the presence of cyclosporine (583), and second grafts have been successful when ATG has been added to the conditioning regimen (584). Conversely, graft rejection can occur when cyclosporine is discontinued (585).

Successful engraftment requires that a sufficient number of hematopoietic stem cells be transplanted. An early study from the major transplant center at the University of Washington showed a correlation between the quantity of infused donor cells and graft acceptance (586). Hematopoietic stem cells circulate and can reconstitute hematopoietic function after ablation (587). A study comparing transplantation with G-CSF–mobilized peripheral blood stem cells versus bone marrow from HLA-identical relatives noted earlier engraftment using peripheral blood stem cells without significantly increasing the risk of GVHD (588).

Transfusion sensitization as a mechanism of graft failure was predicted from dog experiments, in which animals given as few as three transfusions rejected marrow from litter mates and transfusion sensitization of donor lymphocytes was predictive of graft acceptance (589,590). Graft rejection was observed in the first large trials of marrow transplantation in aplasia (586,591). Actuarial survival rate of 82% achieved in untransfused patients approximated that of identical twin transplants, with an incidence of graft rejection of only 10% (592). Better survival in patients without transfusions could also reflect the influence of other dependent variables, especially the absence of hemorrhage and infection in the patient who receives a transplant soon after diagnosis (593). Although approximately 80% of recipients receive transfusions before transplantation, the risk of graft rejection has progressively decreased since 1970 (594,595). This improvement in outcome has been credited, in part, to changes in blood product preparation, especially the routine use of leukocyte-free platelet and RBC transfusions and the strict avoidance of family members as donors (594). The influence of transfusion on graft rejection is relative and not absolute. In the International Bone Marrow Transplant Registry analysis, while untransfused patients had a low risk of rejection of approximately 5% and heavily transfused patients (more than 40 units) had a risk of greater than 25%, patients who received 1 to 40 units had an intermediate risk of approximately 15% for graft rejection (596); in the Seattle retrospective analysis, increased graft rejection was observed in patients who had received more than 10 units of erythrocytes or 40 or more units of platelets (594).

The influence of intensification of the immunosuppressive conditioning regimens on graft rejection in patients without transfusions is more of a problem. Graft rejection on the one hand and GVHD on the other behave as counterbalancing adverse consequences in protocol design. Frequently, protocols that are successful in improving graft acceptance result in greater GVHD. An example from a single institution is one early study in which addition of irradiation to cyclophosphamide

decreased the rejection rate from 42% to 0% but increased chronic GVHD from 17% to 48%. Combination conditioning chemotherapy (597,598), total body irradiation (599), and total lymphoid irradiation (600,601) all have improved graft acceptance in single-center studies, but they have not been shown to influence long-term survival in large retrospective analyses (596,602,603). Increased intensity of pretransplant conditioning regimens has been accompanied by significant decreases in graft rejection (3,604). The rate of successful second transplants in response to graft rejection has also improved (604). Bone marrow or stem cell transplantation is also discussed in depth in Chapter 60.

Graft-Versus-Host Disease. Donor mature T cells that recognize minor histocompatibility antigens mediate GVHD. Age is a major risk factor for GVHD, possibly because defective thymic function and lymphocyte maturation in older persons leads to inappropriate immune responses such as increased nonspecific suppressor activity and a deficiency of specific suppressor T cells. The reader is referred to Chapter 60 for a detailed discussion of this topic.

Although centers agree that age is correlated with GVHD and generally with a lower survival, there is less agreement as to an upper age limit for transplantation. The incidence of GVHD in the Seattle series showed a progressive increase with age (19% for patients 0 to 10 years, 46% at 11 to 30 years, and 90% in patients older than 31 years) (605). Several studies have suggested that the major difference in survival figures occurs at approximately 20 years of age. In the European Bone Marrow Transplant Group, a significant difference was observed in survival for those younger than 20 years (65%) compared with patients older than 20 years (56%), and there was no difference in survival for patients between 21 and 30 years and those 31 to 55 years (606). Young adults have fared better in other series. At University of California, Los Angeles (UCLA), the actuarial survival rate was 79% in patients younger than 20 years, 41% for those 21 to 35 years, and 20% for those older than 35 years (607). At Minnesota, survival of adults (median age, 27 years) was equivalent to children (median age, 10 years), although morbidity from severe GVHD was far more prevalent in the older patients (43% vs. 10%) (608). Studies of allogeneic transplantation of multiply transfused patients with severe aplastic anemia using a conditioning regimen combining cyclophosphamide with ATG (577) reported sustained engraftment in 96% of patients and 88% survival with a median follow-up time of 6 years (580). The International Bone Marrow Transplant Registry compared the efficacy over time of 1305 HLA-identical sibling bone marrow transplants performed between 1976 and 1992 and found that improvements in GVHD prophylaxis accounted for much of the improvements in 5-year survival. Mortality from severe GVDH has not improved substantially over time, although the proportion of patients developing severe GVHD has declined (609).

Nonsibling and Nonhistocompatible Donors. Approximately 70% of patients with aplastic anemia do not have histocompatible sibling donors. Alternative potential donors include phenotypically matched relatives, partially matched (mismatched) relatives, and histocompatible but unrelated volunteers. Haplotype sharing between parents occasionally has allowed successful transplantation between phenotypically matched (but genotypically mismatched) siblings (610,611), although long-term survival appears to be inferior to genotypically matched transplantations (612). Promising therapeutic regimens to minimize graft rejection and GVHD in matched unrelated transplants or mismatched transplants are discussed in Chapter 60. Survival after alternative donor transplants, although improving, has continued to be significantly lower than that achieved with matched HLA-identical sibling transplants for aplastic anemia (reviewed in 613) (Fig. 9-6). Umbilical cord blood has been used successfully as a source of hematopoietic stem cells for transplantation (614–618), and may facilitate HLA-mismatched transplantation. A retrospective study comparing HLA-identical sibling donor transplants with umbilical cord blood versus bone marrow as the source of hematopoietic stem cells reported lower rates of acute and chronic GVHD in patients receiving umbilical cord blood, although the rate of engraftment was also slower in these patients (619).

IMMUNOSUPPRESSIVE THERAPY

Antilymphocyte Sera. ATG or ALG, particularly in combination with additional agents, is an important therapy for aplastic anemia patients who do not receive BMTs (470). Both horse ATG (ATGAM, Upjohn) and rabbit ATG (SangStat) are approved by the U.S. Food and Drug Administration. In a study of ALG as a conditioning regimen for BMT, Mathé (467) noted clinical improvement in two aplastic anemia patients, at least one of whom was genotypically mismatched with the donor; other cases followed of autologous marrow reconstitution after infusion of incompatible bone marrow and preconditioning with ALG or cyclophosphamide, or both (467–469,620,621). In a collection of European patients treated with different antilymphocyte sera in a variety of dose regimens, sustained hematologic improvement occurred in 12 of 29 patients with severe aplastic anemia (41%), and the 1-year survival rate of the entire group was 55% (622). Skepticism greeted Mathé's original report and the early European studies, but the effectiveness of antilymphocyte sera has been repeatedly confirmed. Two important controlled trials were performed in the United States. In a combined center study, Swiss ALG was clearly superior to androgen treatment in a concurrent population and in historic controls; nearly 70% (20 of 29) of ALG-treated patients responded, compared with 18% (7 of 38) of androgen-treated patients, and the 1-year survival rate was 76% versus 22%, respectively (623). At UCLA, patients were randomly assigned to receive ATG or supportive care only; 11 of 12 treated patients (52%) responded hematologically, whereas there was no improvement over 3 months in an equal number of patients given supportive care (6 of 12 control patients later responded to ATG) (624). Patients with aplastic anemia of many suspected causes—including hepatitis-associated bone marrow failure (603,625) and gold-associated aplasia (290,626)—have responded to ATG.

Variability in patient populations, differences in the definition of hematologic response and the time at which a response is measured, and duplication of case material in the literature make an overall response rate difficult to approximate. The choice of specific criteria for improvement in aplastic anemia can include transfusion independence (which may be subjective and does not measure neutrophil improvement), blood counts (which are altered by transfusion and affected by error at the low rate range of reticulocyte and platelet determinations), and clinical assessments of improvement (627). Although the average time to improvement in neutrophil number (the only objective measure unaffected by transfusion) is 1 to 2 months (627) and to transfusion independence is approximately 2 to 3 months (628,629), continued improvement without further therapy commonly occurs after 3 months, and some patients may be true late responders [10% (624), 19% (628), and 35% (629) of responses occurred at 3 to 9 months] (Fig. 9-7). Some improvement in clinical status by 3 months is strongly correlated with long-term survival (627,630). Although the true response rate probably lies between 40% and 60%, reported remission rates for ATG and ALG have varied greatly, from low values of

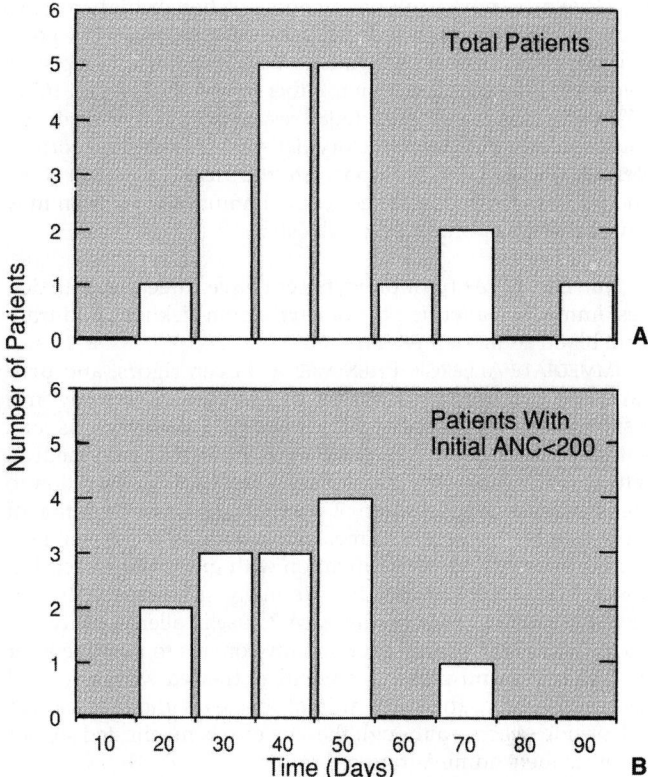

Figure 9-7. Time to response after treatment with antithymocyte globulin. **A:** Distribution of patients with severe aplastic anemia by time to achieve an increase in the absolute neutrophil count (ANC) of 1000/µL. **B:** Distribution of those patients with an initial ANC of less than 200/µL by time to achieve an ANC of 1000/µL. (After Young N, Griffith P, Brittain E, et al. A multicenter trial of anti-thymocyte globulin in aplastic anemia and related diseases. *Blood* 1988;72:1861.)

approximately 24% in severe disease (628) to extraordinarily high success rates approximating 85% (631,632). There is little statistical evidence for "inactive" lots of ATG or ALG or for variation in lymphocytotoxicity (633). Patient selection is important, because the likelihood of response to ALG has been correlated to disease severity (634), and, in particular, poor response rates have been measured in patients with "supersevere" disease, defined by an absolute neutrophil count of less than 200/µL (603). If they can survive the first month of therapy, severely neutropenic patients respond to ATG with the same probability as patients with higher neutrophil counts (627). Some centers or protocols may intentionally exclude patients who are too sick to tolerate treatment or who require an observation period that selects for the better prognosis cases.

The intensity of immunosuppression may be an important variable. In the National Heart, Lung, and Blood Institute trial that compared 10 days versus 28 days of ATG, a trend toward more rapid, frequent, and complete remissions was seen with the 28-day regimen, although there was no statistical difference in response rates (625). Horse serum administered beyond 10 days is given in the face of the host's immune response and rapid clearance of heterologous protein by the immune system; ATG's average half-time of 5.7 days is much shorter in the presence of anti–horse Ig (635). It is reasonable to administer equivalent doses of ATG or ALG by the schedule originally used in Europe—40 mg/kg/day for 4 days; horse Ig, both free and cell-bound, will have reached low levels in the circulation (636) by the time host IgG is circulating. A 4- to 5-day regimen is easier to administer, is associated with less serum sickness, and is as effective as a more prolonged course. Whether higher doses acutely administered would be more effective is a moot point that is unlikely to be tested. Patients have responded to repeated courses of immunosuppression, either repeated ALG [22% (634), 25% (631), 45% (637), 64% (638) response rate to the second course among initially refractory patients] or high-dose corticosteroids and ALG (27% response to the second therapy) (639), and patients treated with sequential immunosuppression may have better prospects of survival (640).

Side Effects. Antilymphocyte sera have three major toxicities: immediate allergic phenomena, serum sickness, and transient blood count depression.

IMMEDIATE ALLERGIC PHENOMENA. Fever, rigors, and urticaria are common on the first day or two of therapy and respond to antihistamines and meperidine. Anaphylaxis is rare, but its occurrence has been fatal even in the prepared medical setting (641). A positive immediate wheal and flare reaction to the epicutaneous application of the 50-mg/mL stock solution of ATG may be predictive of massive histamine release on systemic infusion, and desensitization with gradually increasing doses of ATG administered intradermally, subcutaneously, and then intravenously has permitted ATG use in allergic individuals (641). Skin tests only occasionally convert to positive after ATG therapy, and patients have been treated with a second course of ATG of the same animal species without increased risk of side effects—although the side effects manifested sooner on subsequent administration.

SERUM SICKNESS. The consequence of host production of antibody to horse protein, serum sickness occurs in almost all patients treated with ATG for 10 days or longer (642,643). Serum sickness usually begins 5 to 11 days after the first dose of horse Ig, and although usually a brief illness, symptoms can persist for weeks. Serum sickness is a pleomorphic syndrome, with prominent symptoms of fever, lassitude, a cutaneous maculopapular eruption, arthralgia and myalgia, and, less commonly, gastrointestinal and neurologic complaints. A serpiginous rash at the volardorsal border of the hands and feet is pathognomonic and precedes the full syndrome by approximately a day (Fig. 9-8). Although the urine sediment and creatine clearance may become transiently abnormal, frank azotemia is unusual. Severe serum sickness may include rhabdomyolysis and myocarditis. Corticosteroids are usually administered in moderate doses (1 mg/kg of prednisone or methylprednisolone) during the first 2 weeks to ameliorate serum sickness; they would not be expected to affect host antibody production (644) but may blunt the

inflammatory response. Serum sickness is much less frequent and less severe when horse Ig is administered over a shorter period of 4 or 5 days. Serum sickness correlates with the formation of circulating immune complexes and complement fixation; horse Ig can be demonstrated by immunofluorescence in affected skin, and immune complexes presumably are deposited in many organs (642). Hematologic recovery does not require the occurrence of serum sickness (645).

CYTOPENIAS. Neither ATG nor ALG is an immunologically specific reagent. The immunogen for ATG is normal human thymocytes, collected at pediatric cardiac surgery; for ALG, the immunogen is thoracic duct lymphocytes, collected during therapeutic cannulation. The immunized animals respond with production of antibodies that recognize a variety of human cell-surface antigens. Removal of antierythrocyte antibodies is a major limitation on commercial processing of horse sera, because the sera must be absorbed with erythrocyte stroma, derived from outdated human blood, and, often, residual human hemoglobin must be physically separated from the IgG fraction. Some batches of ALGs have been associated with positive antiglobulin tests in patients and, rarely, frank immune hemolytic anemia (305,646). ATG reacts with lymphocytes of all classes and also with cell-surface antigens present on granulocytes, platelets, thymocytes, and testicular cells, as well as with intracellular antigens of many human types (647). Decreased granulocyte and platelet numbers are common during the immediate period of ATG use.

ATG and ALG contain a heterogeneous mix of antibody specificities for lymphocytes, and direct binding and blocking studies have shown reactivity with antigens such as CD2, CD3, CD4, CD5, CD8, CD25 (the receptor for IL-2), and HLA-DR (312,633,648). Horse sera fix human complement efficiently, and all preparations are equally cytotoxic *in vitro*, with little difference between ATG and ALG or among lots for lymphocyte killing *in vitro* (633). Administration of ATG and ALG in patients results in rapid reduction in the number of circulating lymphocytes, usually to below 10% of starting values, and lymphocytopenia persists for several days after the last infusion. When lymphocyte numbers have returned to pretreatment values at 3 months, reductions in activated lymphocyte numbers in recovered patients persist (553,649). *In vitro* studies have observed inhibition of T-cell proliferation as well as reduced IL-2 and IFN-γ production and reduced IL-2 receptor expression in response to ALG (650). ATG also can induce Fas-mediated T-cell apoptosis (651).

As discussed in a previous section, ATG/ALG are crude antibody preparations, and the active component(s) have yet to

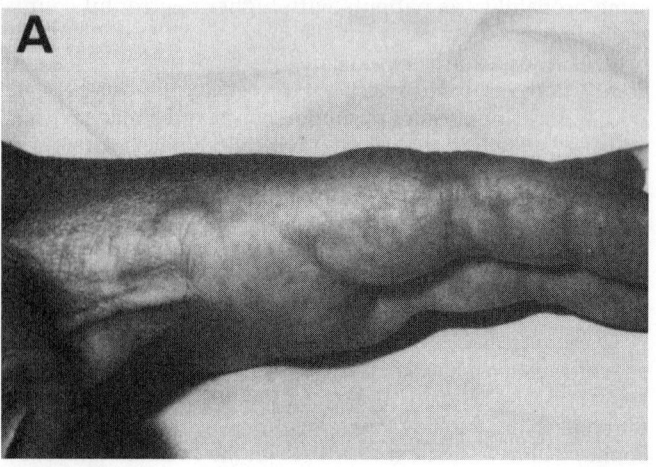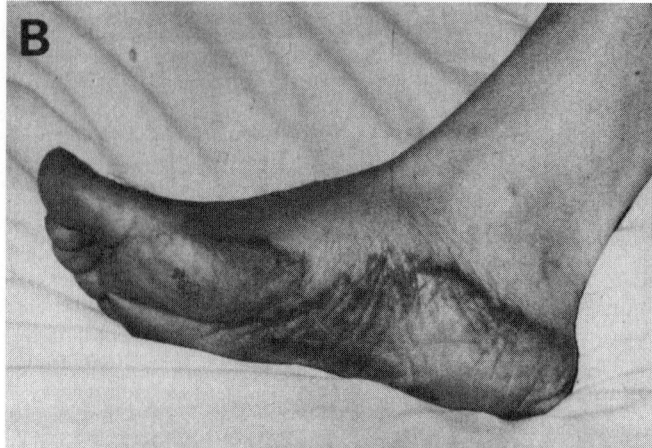

Figure 9-8. Serum sickness rash of the hand (**A**) and foot (**B**). If the patient has severe thrombocytopenia, petechiae may etch the serpiginous margin between volar and dorsal surfaces. (See Color Figure 9-8.)

be identified. In addition to its effects on the immune system, ATG can increase colony growth of cultured bone marrow cells (477) and reduces the expression of Fas-Ag on aplastic anemia bone marrow CD34+ cells (478). ATG also includes antibodies against a variety of signal transduction and cell adhesion molecules (475). Although ATG and monoclonal antibodies compete for the same antigenic binding sites *in vitro*, monoclonal antibodies directed to pan–T-cell specificities [as single agents (472) or in combination (652)] have not been effective in aplastic anemia, possibly because they are inadequately immunosuppressive. Naked antibody preparations have not found wide use in clinical practice, and even toxin-conjugated monoclonal antibodies that are potent *in vitro* may be without visible effect when injected into an animal.

In the absence of complement to effect lysis *in vitro*, ATG and ALG can stimulate lymphocyte function, suggesting the possibility that stimulations of hematopoiesis might be important in the therapeutic effect. ATG acts as a mitogen to stimulate lymphocyte proliferation, and it provokes both IL-2 and hematopoietic growth factor production by peripheral blood mononuclear cells; these effects are exaggerated for the cells of patients with aplastic anemia, perhaps reflecting their already activated status (653). T cells cloned after ALG stimulation produce GM-CSF or IL-3, and, less frequently, IL-2 and IFN-γ (654). Variation in stimulatory activity measured *in vitro* has been correlated with clinical response rates by some (655) but not others (653). In a mouse model, ATG increased circulating levels of colony-stimulating activity (656). ATG also binds directly to bone marrow precursor (647) and progenitor (657) cells. In normal marrow progenitor assays, ATG can stimulate erythroid colony formation (658) and growth of a peculiar, unusually mature type of myeloid colony—effects mediated at least partly through accessory T lymphocytes; direct action on myeloid precursor cells has been inferred by analogy from ATG induction of HL-60 leukemic cell differentiation (658).

Manipulation of bone marrow cultures *in vitro* before therapy might be expected to predict a response to therapy. In occasional cases, lymphocyte inhibitory activity disappeared after successful ATG therapy (659,660). Good correlations were reported between clinical response to immunosuppression and pretreatment improvement in hematopoietic colony formation after T-cell depletion (488), incubation of marrow with ALG (661), or in coculture assays (662), but these promising findings have not been confirmed in other studies (630,663–665).

Cyclosporine. Cyclosporine (or cyclosporin A), a fungal cyclical undecapeptide, is an effective immunosuppressive drug (666). Cyclosporine is not lymphocytotoxic, but it has highly specific inhibitory effects on T-lymphocyte function, inhibiting inducible gene transcription and preferentially affecting production of IL-2 and IFN-γ but not colony-stimulating factors. Cytotoxic T-cell activation of IL-2 receptors in response to lectins and alloantigens is prevented by cyclosporine. Cyclosporine has been successfully used in many autoimmune diseases. Shahidi and others (667–672) had success with cyclosporine in individual patients with aplastic anemia, many of whom had not responded to other therapies. These results were clouded by the frequent concomitant use of androgens. In a larger trial from South Africa (673), there was no response to cyclosporine given alone (six patients) or in combination with ALG (six patients); in other trials (674,675), only two of nine refractory aplastic patients improved. In one study (676), 22 patients who had not responded to ATG therapy were treated with cyclosporine alone or in combination with moderate doses of corticosteroids; eight patients responded, six to sustained transfusion independence and one who appeared to require continued cyclosporine

maintenance. Of the patients able to complete 3 months of treatment, more than one-half responded. Most patients showed some blood count increase during the first 3 months, but maximal effects were not seen until 6 months of cyclosporine therapy or even after discontinuation of the drug in some cases. No patients with absolute neutrophil counts of less than 200/μL responded. A major difference between the National Institutes of Health (NIH) protocol and previous regimens was the higher dose, 12 mg/kg/day for adults and 15 mg/kg/day for children, with adjustment based on plasma drug levels and side effects. In this study, none of the five patients treated for briefer periods before ATG therapy responded to cyclosporine, but a French cooperative study (677,678) randomly assigned severely aplastic patients to receive either ALG or cyclosporine as initial therapy, with apparently equivalent (but low) remission rates and survival.

In many cases, remissions have continued even after discontinuation of cyclosporine therapy. Some patients clearly experienced relapse when cyclosporine administration was discontinued and responded to its reinstitution (674,679) or required maintenance cyclosporine treatment (671,676). Optimal therapy requires periodic measurement of blood levels both to ensure adequately immunosuppressive levels and to avoid toxicity (666). Variability in cyclosporine metabolism, especially in children, may require serum levels to be determined every 2 weeks for dose adjustments (680). Cyclosporine toxicity is not minor. Hypertension, azotemia, hirsutism, and gingival hypertrophy are common, and increasing serum creatinine levels are an indication to lower the dose (666). Chronic, irreversible nephrotoxicity can occur with long-term exposure. Cyclosporine, especially in combination with corticosteroids, converts patients with aplastic anemia to temporary immunodeficiency and new susceptibility to unusual infectious agents; tuberculous pericarditis has been reported (681), and *Pneumocystis carinii* pneumonia, otherwise not seen in aplasia, can occur and be fatal. Unfortunately, and similar to the situation with ATG, clinical responses cannot be predicted by *in vitro* tests because cyclosporine does not increase progenitor growth *in vitro* (682).

Combination Immunosuppressive Therapy. The combination of ATG with cyclosporine is based on the clinical efficacy of each agent individually and on their separate and potentially complementary modes of action. A striking increase in the response rate to immunosuppression was observed in a cooperative German trial (683) in which patients treated initially with a combination of ALG and cyclosporine showed an 85% hematologic remission rate at 6 months compared with a rate of 50% in those treated with ALG alone, and cyclosporine appeared to increase the rapidity and extent of the responses. Subsequent trials confirm that their combination is more effective at inducing hematologic responses than either drug alone, with response rates generally around 70% to 80% and a 90% 5-year survival in those responding (684,685). Importantly, intensive immunosuppressive therapy has greatly improved the results of therapy in two groups notoriously refractory to ALG or ATG alone: patients with very severe disease and children. In the NIH Clinical Center trial (685), survival curves of those older and younger than 35 years of age were superimposable; also, there was no significant difference when the division was made at 20 years. A large ongoing study at the NIH, enrolling both children and adults, has found a response rate of 67% at 43 months and a 5-year actuarial survival rate of 70% (86% for responders and 16% for nonresponders) (686). The Gruppo Italiano Trapianti di Midolio Osseo/European Group for Blood and Marrow Transplantation (EBMT) study of 100 patients with severe aplastic anemia including children (median age 16 years) treated with ALG, cyclosporin A, prednisolone, and G-CSF found trilineage hematopoietic response in 77% after one or more courses of ALG (687).

ATG is typically given over a 4-day course followed by a 6- to 12-month course of cyclosporin. When cyclosporin is discontinued, blood counts should be especially closely monitored, and a decrease can often be treated with reinitiating the therapy. Some patients require continuous cyclosporin, and they should be maintained on the lowest effective dose. A review of ongoing trials by the German multicenter group and the NIH revealed that 29% and 14% of initial responders, respectively, required continuous treatment (686). The recurrence of frank pancytopenia generally requires a second course of ATG followed by full-dose cyclosporin. Patients treated with immunosuppressive therapy often continue to have subnormal counts, although levels are functionally adequate.

The addition of high-dose methylprednisolone (see the section Corticosteroids) to ALG has been associated with high response rates in some European trials [68% (631), 73% (632)] but not in other studies (688). Survival in the European Group for Bone Marrow Transplantation was the same for low- and high-dose methylprednisolone (603), and a retrospective analysis of published series has not shown any advantage for the high-dose regimen (470). Very high doses of corticosteroids can be associated with serious toxicity.

Relapse. Relapse is common after immunosuppressive therapy. The EBMT reported an actuarial risk of relapse at 35% at 14 years. Relapses were observed up to 10 years after treatment. Disease severity, age, sex, and etiology were not predictive of relapse. A short interval to response after initiation of therapy and a long interval from diagnosis to treatment correlated with an increased risk of relapse (689). A review of ongoing unpublished trials from the German multicenter group and the NIH shows an actuarial risk of relapse of 40% at 8.7 years or 43% at 5.0 years, respectively (686). The NIH study shows an apparent plateau at 64% between 7 and 10 years. Relapse has not significantly compromised survival in those patients who continue to respond to additional courses of immunosuppression.

Tichelli et al. studied the efficacy of repeated treatment with ALG for patients with severe aplastic anemia who either did not respond to an initial course of ALG or who experienced hematologic relapse (638). Transfusion independence was achieved in 63%, and survival probability was 52% ± 8% at 10 years. No differences were noted between patients retreated for nonresponse versus relapse. No increases in acute toxicity were noted with additional courses of ALG, although the timing of serum sickness tended to occur earlier after repeat ALG administration.

Complications of Immunosuppressive Therapy. Patients treated for aplastic anemia with immunosuppressive therapy have an increased risk of developing clonal hematopoietic disorders (reviewed in 690,691). In an analysis of 860 patients treated with immunosuppression, there were 19 cases of PNH, 11 cases of myelodysplasia, 15 cases of acute leukemia, 7 cases of solid tumors, and 1 case of non-Hodgkin's lymphoma (692). Of 748 patients treated with transplantation, nine malignancies were reported: two acute leukemias and seven solid tumors. The cumulative incidence of developing a malignant tumor at 10 years was 18.8% after immunosuppression and 3.1% after transplantation. A recent series of 122 NIH patients treated with immunosuppression showed a 33% actuarial risk of developing a clonal hematopoietic disorder at 10 years (31).

Significant telomere shortening has been observed in the leukocytes of aplastic anemia patients (445,446). Whether telomere shortening represents a primary versus a secondary event in the genesis of aplastic anemia remains to be ascertained.

IMMUNOSUPPRESSION VERSUS BONE MARROW TRANSPLANTATION

Antilymphocyte sera and BMT are alternative effective therapies for aplastic anemia. For the 25% of patients for whom a suitable HLA-identical sibling donor is available, the decision to treat with immunosuppression versus HLA-identical sibling stem cell transplant is based on a consideration of risks and benefits that vary depending mainly on patient age and neutrophil count. Both short- and long-term efficacy and side effects for each treatment must be carefully weighed. BMT is more expensive and riskier in the short term, but it is capable of restoring permanently normal hematopoiesis. Immunosuppression is cheaper and much less toxic, but it more often results in partial remission (470) or in gradual recovery (693) than prompt reconstitution of entirely normal blood counts. As discussed above, late complications of immunosuppressive therapy include relapse and the development of late clonal hematologic disorders and malignancies. BMT is also not without its late problems. A small number of patients may show late graft loss (605). Chronic thrombocytopenia occurred in 23% of patients who underwent transplants for diverse hematologic diseases (694). Acute leukemia has been reported to follow shortly on BMT for aplastic anemia (695). The conditioning drugs and radiation of the transplantation procedure produce their own delayed complications, including pulmonary disease, endocrine dysfunction and infertility, leukoencephalopathy, cataracts, and secondary malignancies (605,696).

A recent EBMT study of immunosuppressive therapy in patients aged 20 years and older showed that response to immunosuppression (62% at 12 months) was independent of age, but mortality increased with increasing age (697). Studies comparing BMT and immunosuppression in children have generally significantly favored stem cell transplant (Table 9-9). A recent report from the EBMT analyzed 1765 patients with aplastic anemia receiving initial treatment with either an HLA-identical sibling bone marrow transplant or immunosuppressive therapy (572). Analysis was performed on an "intent-to-treat" basis. Patients were aged 1 to 50 years and treated between 1974 and 1996. Five hundred eighty-three patients received HLA-identical sibling bone marrow transplant, and 1182 patients received immunosuppression. A comparison of immunosuppression versus bone marrow transplant in patients stratified by age and neutrophil count showed superior failure-free survival with bone marrow transplant for children regardless of their neutrophil count. The advantage of bone marrow transplant increased with increasing follow-up time, most likely due to the ongoing risks of late relapse and evolution to myelodysplasia and leukemia in the immunosuppression group. Children have a lower mortality with stem cell transplant and a longer posttreatment life expectancy, placing them at higher risk for late complications of immunosuppressive therapy than older adults. Thus, the recommendation of this group was to treat young patients (≤10 years) with HLA-identical sibling stem cell transplant when a suitable donor was available. Patients younger than 40 years of age with neutrophil counts <300/μL also did better with bone marrow transplant. Patients older than 40 years of age generally did better with immunosuppressive therapy. No clear advantage was apparent for either therapeutic option in patients between the ages of 20 and 40 with neutrophil counts >300/μL.

It is important to note that many patients in these studies of long-term outcomes were treated before the development of current immunosuppressive regimens containing both ATG and cyclosporin. Any differential long-term effects of

TABLE 9-9. Studies Comparing Bone Marrow Transplantation (BMT) to Immunosuppressive Therapy (IST)

Study, Year (Reference)	Population Age (yr)	BMT (No. of Patients)	Survival (2–15 yr) (%)	IST (No. of Patients)	Survival (2–15 yr) (%)	p
Speck, 1981 (629)	All ages	18	44	32	69	NS
Bayever, 1984 (698)	1–24	35	72	22	45	NS
Bacigalupo, 1988 (3)	1–50	218	63	291	61	NS
Halperin, 1989 (699)	Children	14	79	12	42	?
Locasciulli, 1990 (700)	Children	171	63	133	48	.002
Speck, 1990 (701)	All ages	34	50	111	71	NS
Paquette, 1995 (702)	Adults	55	72	155	45	NS
Lawlor, 1997 (703)	Children	9	75	18	92	NS
Doney, 1997 (704)	All ages	168	69	227	38	<.001
Gillio, 1997 (705)	1–20	25	75.6	23	73.8	NS
Fuhrer, 1998 (706)	Children	26	84	86	87	NS
Kojima, 2000 (707)	Children	37	97	63	55	<.0001
Fouladi, 2000 (708)	Children	26	96	20	70	?

No., number; NS, not significant.
Adapted from Bacigalupo A, Brand R, Oneto R, et al. Treatment of acquired severe aplastic anemia: bone marrow transplantation compared with immunosuppressive therapy—The European Group for Blood and Marrow Transplantation Experience. *Semin Hematol* 2000;37:75.

these more intensive immunosuppressive regimens remain to be ascertained.

ANDROGENS

Androgens no longer have a primary role in the management of aplastic anemia and are now used if first-line therapies are unavailable or unsuccessful. Testosterone was first successfully used by Shahidi and Diamond, who reported hematologic remissions in 9 of 17 children with acquired aplastic anemia and six of seven with hereditary aplasia (709). The Boston investigators noted the often prolonged duration of therapy required to response, the predictive value of residual marrow hematopoiesis, and occasional dependence of hematopoietic recovery on androgens (709,710). At that time, androgens represented the only effective therapy directed at underlying bone marrow failure in aplastic anemia, and they were widely used with good response rates in many clinics. Some centers, however, reported low numbers of remissions and no improvement in survival (711–715); one major retrospective analysis actually found poorer survival in androgen-treated patients (716).

The early androgen studies were uncontrolled, used different hormone preparations in different doses, lacked clearly defined endpoints, and described variable measures of success, from hematologic normalization to improvement in survival. An important flaw was selection bias. Although the clinical data are often inadequate for an accurate retrospective analysis, many series were composed of a large proportion of patients with moderate or chronic disease who could tolerate and survive a 3-month or longer treatment regimen and who constituted a disproportionate fraction of the androgen responders. The response rate to androgens has, in general, been lower in severe than in moderate disease [8% vs. 56% in one comparison (717)], and, in a large cooperative study of multiple androgens, only 20% of surviving patients had severe disease, compared with 58% in the initial group (718). In a randomized American trial that compared androgen therapy to BMT in patients with severe aplastic anemia (569), there was no difference in survival between patients without transplants who were treated with androgens and those who did not receive androgens. Three of 13 "untreated" patients (23%) appeared to go into remission, a figure no different from 11 of 50 patients (22%) treated with androgens who showed some degree of improvement.

Nevertheless, it would be unwise to discount androgen therapy in aplastic anemia for several reasons. First, 30% to 50% response rates (718), even if restricted to moderate or chronic disease, may represent the difference between transfusions and independence from continuous medical care. Second, some cases that would be classified retrospectively as severe have apparently responded to androgens, such as most of Shahidi's original series (709). Third, androgen dependence of hematologic recovery in some patients is strong evidence of a role of these agents in improving hematopoiesis (718–720). Fourth, androgen dose and type may be important variables. Some patients who had no response to conventional androgen therapy apparently responded to etiocholanolone, a 5β-metabolite androstane metabolite (721), and in European cooperative trials, significant differences in remission quality and survival were measured among androgens (fluoxymesterone greater than norethandrolone) and between high- and low-dose regimens (84). In some hands, treatment with etiocholanolone metabolites has resulted in remission and survival rates comparable to those with immunosuppression (722).

If they are used, androgens should be administered to patients who have not responded to immunosuppressive therapy. It should be anticipated that the hemoglobin response will be more impressive than improvement in granulocytes and, particularly, in platelets (718,723). An adequate trial is at least 3 months and possibly as long as 6 months at full doses. Androgen therapy has multiple toxic effects, especially virilization, hirsutism and acne, fluid retention, and psychologic alterations. Hepatotoxicity can occur with all preparations but is less frequent with parenteral preparations (724). The cholestatic pattern of liver function test abnormalities is usually reversible when androgens are discontinued, but the rare syndrome peliosis hepatis has been associated with androgen therapy (725). Children can tolerate high doses of androgens for more than a year without lasting effects on growth or maturation (726). Scintigraphy (727,728) and *in vitro* progenitor cultures have been proposed as predictors of clinical improvement (729).

The mechanism of action has been reviewed extensively by Gardner and Besa (730). Androgens have a variety of biologic effects (90,731), including several actions on hematopoiesis (91,728,732,733). High endogenous testosterone and the administration of testosterone correlate with higher hemoglobin levels and RBC mass as a result of androgenic stimulation of erythropoietin production by the kidney (92,93,734,735), and experiments with plethoric mice have suggested that the major erythropoietic effect of testosterone is exerted through this hormone (736–738). This is unlikely to be important in aplastic patients who produce abundant amounts of erythropoietin.

Androgens have direct effects on hematopoietic cells. Injection of mice with a variety of testosterone derivatives has increased granulocyte (739,740) and platelet (741) numbers as well as hemoglobin (92,742) and has accelerated recovery from irradiation (743) and chemotherapy (743,744). Androgens stimulate hematopoiesis in marrow suspension cultures (1056), in recovery of progenitor cells from treated animals (739,740,744) or suspension cultures (745), and when directly added to semisolid colony cultures (740,746–749). Testosterone is incorporated into the nuclei of rat bone marrow cells (750) and stimulates RNA metabolism (751), and an increase in the proportion of colony-forming unit stem cell in mitotic cycle has been observed with testosterone (752) and its 5β-metabolites (753,754). In a few experiments, androgens have also been implicated in increasing production of colony-stimulating factors by normal blood adherent cells (755) and in treated mice (756). Androgens have diverse, generally suppressive effects on the immune system (728), hypothesized to be an explanation for the heightened immune response and prevalence of autoimmune disease in female mice (757).

HEMATOPOIETIC GROWTH FACTORS

Although patients with aplastic anemia do not have a deficiency of most hematopoietic growth factors (see earlier), it was hypothesized that pharmacologic levels might stimulate hematopoiesis of one or more cell lines (reviewed in 463). Trials of GM-CSF (758–760), G-CSF (761,762), IL-3 (763–765), IL-1 (766), IL-6 (767), and stem cell factor (768) in aplastic anemia have been reported. The total number of patients treated in these protocols is not large. These studies do not support the use of growth factors as primary treatment for aplastic anemia. To date, no consistent benefit in terms of response rate or survival after the adjunctive use of growth factors in immunosuppressive regimens has been observed. A recent pediatric prospective randomized trial of G-CSF for aplastic anemia patients with neutrophil counts greater than 200/μL found no difference in the incidence of fever or infection with or without G-CSF (769). A few refractory patients have had responses to single or combined growth factors.

A major concern with G-CSF treatment of aplastic anemia patients is the potential risk of promoting the development or propagation of a dysplastic or malignant clone. A retrospective study of children with severe acquired aplastic anemia in Japan found that 11 out of 167 patients developed MDS/AML. Ten of the 11 cases showed monosomy 7. All 11 cases had received combination therapy with cyclosporin and G-CSF (770). It has been difficult to distinguish whether growth factor treatment is causally related to MDS/AML or whether growth factor therapy is initiated in response to the severity of the underlying bone marrow premalignant state. A recent study comparing 144 aplastic anemia patients on immunosuppressive therapy with or without G-CSF found that the risk of developing MDS/AML was similar between the two groups (771). In eight aplastic anemia patients who had developed MDS/AML, no mutations were detected in the cytoplasmic domain of the G-CSF receptor (772).

CORTICOSTEROIDS

Corticosteroids were used in the 1950s and 1960s in the treatment of aplastic anemia. These uncontrolled observations are now difficult to evaluate for many reasons: lack of objective criteria for classification and response, frequent combination of corticosteroids and androgens, an acknowledged preference to treat the most affected patients, and the limited availability of transfusion support. Bias is introduced because of the high proportion of patients with moderate disease and the mixing of acquired and inherited cases. Sporadically observed apparent remissions

(773,774) were not reproduced in more systematic surveys (267,775,776), and the general impression among experienced hematologists was that corticosteroids were without use in aplastic anemia (775,777–779) and might even be harmful (453,780).

More recently, large amounts of corticosteroids have been administered as intravenous boluses of 6-methylprednisolone. In a series of patients treated by the originators of this program, 15 of 39 patients (38%) responded (305,603,639). At first treatment, there was no difference on retrospective analysis in survival between patients treated with ALG and those treated with bolus methylprednisolone (781). There are several reasons, however, to prefer ATG or ALG as initial therapy. First, a high proportion of patients who did not respond to corticosteroid therapy subsequently remitted with ALG treatment (305,639). Second, these industrial doses of corticosteroids have great toxicity, especially metabolic (hypertension, hyperglycemia, volume overload, potassium wasting), infectious (an apparent increase in susceptibility to fungal disease and masking of fever), and psychiatric (psychosis); late aseptic necrosis of femoral and humeral heads also has occurred.

NEW THERAPIES

New therapeutic regimens are aimed at improving rates of hematologic response and minimizing acute and long-term complications of therapy (476). The current status of new agents is summarized below.

Cyclophosphamide. Administration of high doses of cyclophosphamide is an effective immunosuppressive therapy and is not myeloablative. Historically, a few patients who received high-dose cyclophosphamide as preparation for marrow transplant rejected their grafts and had autologous recovery. An early study of treatment with this drug without transplant indicated a complete response in seven of ten patients treated with 45 mg/kg/day for 4 days (782). Based on these results, a phase III prospective randomized trial compared high-dose cyclophosphamide plus cyclosporin to ATG plus cyclosporin as first-line therapy (783). The trial was terminated prematurely due to invasive fungal infections and three early deaths in the cyclophosphamide group (none in the ATG group). Responses at 6-month follow-up were seen in 6 of 13 (46%) patients treated with cyclophosphamide versus 9 of 12 (75%) patients treated with ATG.

New Immunosuppressive Therapies. Active investigation exploring the use of additional immunosuppressive agents in the treatment of aplastic anemia is ongoing. The following section discusses several promising agents currently under study.

The high affinity IL-2 receptor is present only on activated T cells and is required for T-cell activation and proliferation (784). An anti–IL-2 receptor monoclonal antibody, Daclizumab, has been approved for use in the prevention of renal transplant rejection. It is usually administered with cyclosporin and prednisone. The use of this agent for the treatment of aplastic anemia is currently under investigation in phase II trials.

Mycophenolate mofetil (MMF; Cell-Cept) is the prodrug of mycophenolic acid, which inhibits B- and T-cell proliferation through noncompetitive reversible inhibition of inosine monophosphate dehydrogenase, which is involved in the salvage pathway for guanine nucleotide synthesis (785). It has antifungal, antibacterial, antiviral, and immunosuppressive activity. MMF has been approved for prevention of renal transplant rejection. Although generally well tolerated, MMF's side effects include leukopenia and thrombocytopenia. Studies on MMF use in aplastic anemia are currently ongoing.

FK506 (tacrolimus; Prograf) has been effective in preventing organ transplant rejection, often in combination with other immunosuppressive agents. FK506 and cyclosporin are calcineurin inhibitors that decrease IL-2 production (786). FK506 and cyclosporin also share similar toxicity profiles. Given the similarities in action, it is not clear whether FK506 offers any advantage over cyclosporin, although their toxicity profiles are somewhat different.

Rapamycin (rapamune, sirolimus) inactivates the serine/threonine protein kinase p70 and is a potent inhibitor of IL-2–dependent T-cell proliferation (787,788). Although rapamycin is an effective drug for the prevention of solid organ transplant rejection, its myelosuppressive side effects may render it less useful for the treatment of aplastic anemia.

OTHER THERAPIES

Antiviral Therapy. Occasionally, patients treated by the authors and, subsequently, by others (364,365) improve after therapy with acyclovir, although the responses are temporary in most cases. Ig therapy is curative in patients with persistent B19 parvovirus infection (see the section Pure Red Cell Aplasia).

Plasmapheresis. To effectively remove Igs, plasmapheresis must be intensive and frequent (at least three times weekly); lymphocytopheresis that removes both soluble inhibitory factors and circulating lymphocytes should be most efficient in combination with cytotoxic chemotherapy to inhibit generation of new active cells. Lymphocytopheresis has only occasionally been successful in producing remissions in patients with aplastic anemia, although improvement was sustained in two cases in which it was combined with either prednisone or cyclophosphamide (789,790).

Splenectomy. A splenectomy was first performed for aplastic anemia in 1913. In a literature review up to 1957, 35 had been performed with benefit in 20; in 12 patients with marrow hypoplasia operated on at Walter Reed Army Hospital, six improved (791). Favorable results in individual patients were reported subsequently (773,775,777), and the operation has been used most recently in 26 patients in Basel to facilitate supportive care (631). Postoperative deaths can occur, usually from intraperitoneal hemorrhage or infection. Improvement is often slow and incomplete and therefore difficult to confidently accredit to the procedure. Some eminent hematologists have been skeptical of the usefulness of splenectomy in patients with severe depression of neutrophils and platelets (627,775). Although a modest decrease in RBC survival is seen in aplastic anemia, there is little other rationale for splenectomy, and the organs removed have almost invariably been normal in size and histology. Thus, despite some promising data, splenectomy has not been popular and, with many noninvasive medical alternatives available, is infrequently used.

Management of Bleeding

Bleeding is a common symptom in aplastic anemia, and death due to hemorrhage was frequent in the premodern era. Platelet transfusions can prevent and effectively treat bleeding during the period of definitive treatment with marrow transplantation or immunosuppression, and they can sustain a large minority of chronically thrombocytopenic patients for months or years; the effective use of platelet transfusions has been credited with a substantial improvement in survival in this disease (792). However, bleeding continues to complicate the management of serious infection, especially invasive fungal processes.

Platelets can be collected from individual units of blood or by apheresis; the latter method is preferred because it reduces antigenic exposure of the recipient. As defined by the American Association of Blood Banks (793), one platelet unit (from a single unit of blood) contains a minimum of 5.5×10^{10} platelets; an apheresis pack must contain at least 3×10^{11}, but efficient harvesting technique can net up to 6×10^{11}. A single unit of platelets should increase the platelet count in the recipient by 5000 to 10,000/μL. In patients with bone marrow failure, 56% of the platelets calculated to have been transfused can be recovered, and transfused platelets have survival of 5.2 ± 1.1 days. The slightly lower values in patients with marrow failure compared to normal recipients (65% recovery with 9.6 ± 0.6 days survival) have been thought to be secondary to vascular consumption, an obligatory interaction of platelets with endothelium, that removes a higher proportion of cells from the circulation of thrombocytopenic than normal persons (794).

Few studies of platelet therapy in aplastic anemia patients are available to guide transfusion practice, and transfusion principles have usually been extrapolated from studies in acute leukemia, often of childhood populations. Specific problems in aplastic anemia—the chronicity of disease, the absence of repeated intensive chemotherapy, and differences in immune system function—have not been addressed. Certain aspects of platelet transfusion therapy remain controversial, especially relating to prophylaxis and alloimmunization, and some common practices that are assumed to (and may well) be effective owe less to clinical trials than to the availability of large technologically advanced blood banks. For a general discussion of platelet transfusion therapy, the reader is referred to Chapter 57.

Early reports suggested that alloimmunization increased with time (795), but in other studies, approximately one-half of patients with leukemia did not become alloimmunized, regardless of the number of transfusions (796,797). Aplastic patients, who do not receive repetitive courses of chemotherapy and whose immune system is often activated, would be expected to be less tolerant of repeated antigen infusions than patients with leukemia receiving chemotherapy. In historic analyses of bone marrow failure patients receiving platelet transfusions, high percentages became immunized [66% (798) to 88% (799)]. In a retrospective analysis of aplastic anemia patients, clinical refractoriness was correlated with the number of previous platelet transfusions, but the percentage of refractory patients increased sharply only at more than 40 units and was not different in groups receiving 0 to 9 and 10 to 39 units (800). Measures to reduce the risk of allosensitization include the use of leukoreduced blood products and of the apheresis platelet units.

The level at which the risk of hemorrhage greatly increases has been debated. Certainly, many patients with chronic aplastic anemia and thrombocytopenia have little bleeding at platelet counts between 5000 and 20,000/μL. Prophylactic platelet transfusions at platelet counts below 5000 to 10,000/μL in stable outpatients with chronic severe aplastic anemia were feasible and safe in a recent study (801). Chronic platelet transfusions for aplastic anemia are not used as frequently as they are in leukemia, and they are usually given when there are symptoms of bleeding or if the patient is at increased bleeding risk (e.g., toddlers learning to walk, patients with hypertension while on cyclosporin, patients with fever and infection).

Commonsense measures to prevent bleeding include maintenance of dental hygiene to decrease gingival inflammation, avoidance of trauma, use of prophylactic stool softeners, control of hypertension, and avoidance of vasoconstrictive drugs (from pseudoephedrine to cocaine). Intramuscular injections can be administered to patients with thrombocytopenia if followed by 15 minutes of firm pressure. Topical Gelfoam, collagen, or thrombin may be useful to treat local oozing. Anterior nasal packing should be avoided because of the risk of infection. Antifibrinolytic agents such as aminocaproic acid and tranexamic acid may decrease bleeding episodes and the need for platelet and RBC transfusions (802,803). Amicar is inconvenient to administer because of the need for frequent dosing, variability in the optimal dosage, and gastrointestinal discomfort. The administration of low doses of prednisone (10 to 15 mg/day) to ameliorate bleeding has a very weak experimental basis. Improvement in endothelial cell thinning in rabbits (804) and humans (805) was observed, but the doses used in these studies were high (1 mg/kg); a change in the electron micrographic appearance of vessels has not been correlated with less bleeding, and the animal studies have not been reproducible (806).

Management of Infections

As with platelet transfusion therapy, few specific studies of infections in patients with aplastic anemia are available (559,811), and most recommendations are based on studies of neutropenia from chemotherapy (807–810). Duration is the major difference between the neutropenia of bone marrow failure and that induced by cytotoxic chemotherapy; severe granulocytopenia can persist for months and even years in patients with aplastic anemia. A second major dissimilarity is that neutropenia is part of a complex of problems in malignant disease. Immunosuppression is often an intrinsic feature of specific tumors or leukemias, and malignant tissue invasion, radical surgery, radiation therapy, and cytotoxic drug effects on mucosa and gut can directly compromise organ integrity. In aplastic anemia, in contrast, the immune system is activated and, with the exception of intravenous catheter placement, the integument is preserved. In patients with cancer, malignant progression remains a dominant cause of death; in our experience, most patients with aplastic anemia who do not respond to definitive therapy for their marrow failure die of infection. Studies of cancer patients have usually identified a "low-risk" category, determined by the relatively brief period of neutropenia; by this criteria, almost all unresponsive patients with aplastic anemia are "high risk."

Neutropenia increases susceptibility to bacterial infections. [In one study of a small number of aplastic anemia patients, monocytopenia was also correlated with infectious episodes (811).] In general, the number of infectious episodes correlates with the degree and duration of neutropenia. In an early classic study at the National Cancer Institute, 9% to 10% of days at granulocyte levels higher than 1500/μL were associated with proven infection, but this rose to 20% at granulocyte counts of 500 to 1000/μL, to 36% at 100 to 500/μL, and to 53% at less than 100 neutrophils/μL (812). Levels of extreme neutropenia, less than 100 neutrophils/μL, were associated with the most serious infections and high mortality rate (813). Susceptibility is so extremely high if the absolute neutrophil count is less than 200/μL that this value has been used to define a category of "supersevere" disease.

As severe granulocytopenia becomes prolonged, infection is inevitable (814). Neutropenia itself complicates the diagnosis of infection, because patients usually are unable to mount an inflammatory response. Minimal local inflammation around a catheter insertion site, mild tenderness and erythema rather than an obvious abscess in the perianal area, absence of a pulmonary infiltrate or sputum, and scanty white blood cells in the urine all represent the most subtle indicators of infection, if there are any signs at all (815). Bacteremia is present in only 20% of febrile neutropenic episodes, and in only approximately 40% can a microbiologic cause or localizing physical findings be identified (816). The ability to document sepsis or to locate the site of infection decreases with subsequent febrile episodes (817). There is no reliable method of distinguishing fever due to infection from a noninfectious cause.

Infection in neutropenia is caused by a relatively small number of common bacterial species: the gram-negative bacilli, *Escherichia coli*, *Klebsiella pneumoniae*, and *Pseudomonas aeruginosa*, and the gram-positive cocci, *Staphylococcus aureus* and *Staphylococcus epidermidis*, and some *Streptococcus* spp (808). Twenty years ago, gram-negative bacteremia and pneumonia had a fearsome reputation (818), whereas infections due to gram-positive organisms, which were generally extremely sensitive to the penicillin derivatives then available, were considered less serious. In the intervening decades, entirely new antibiotics and their aggressive and early use have greatly reduced the mortality of gram-negative infections, whereas the general prevalence of antibiotics and the use of indwelling catheters have caused a striking increase in gram-positive bacteria compared with gram-negative bacteria cultured from neutropenic patients (819–822).

In the individual patient, repeated treatment with antibiotics is associated with the emergence of resistant organisms, especially among the gram-negative bacteria (817), to cephalothins and some of the semisynthetic penicillins (816) and to fungal disease, presumably because of the altered microbial microenvironment of the host. The organisms that cause serious infection are almost always endogenous, originating from the patient's own gut, skin, oropharynx, and upper respiratory tract; this bacterial microenvironment is radically altered by illness and hospitalization (823). The rate of decrease of neutrophils may also be an important variable, and patients with chronic neutropenia may eventually tolerate their low white blood cells surprisingly well. Global immunosuppression, produced by conditioning for BMT in the treatment of GVHD, and with ATG and cyclosporine, is associated with unusual bacterial and fungal pathogens and with serious viral and protozoan infections (824).

FEVER IN THE NEUTROPENIC PATIENT

Fever is the cardinal symptom of sepsis in the neutropenic patient; even after thorough assessment, fever commonly is the only evidence of infection (825). Afebrile patients who have vague symptoms of sepsis (malaise, a sense of impending doom, mental disorientation) should also be seriously evaluated, especially if they are receiving corticosteroids (826). A patient with sepsis from a Hickman catheter may be asymptomatic. Initial assessment should include a pertinent history and physical examination, with special attention to the oral mucosa and perianal areas and to indwelling catheter sites. Microbial cultures of blood (including specimens obtained through catheters), urine, and sputum need to be obtained. The results of these investigations may be helpful in prescribing antibiotic therapy, but the decision to treat is not dependent on the results of any diagnostic tests. *If the absolute neutrophil count is less than 500/μL and infection is suspected, immediately begin broad-spectrum, parenteral antibacterial therapy.* Adherence to this principle usually prevents fatal overwhelming sepsis and seeding of organisms to tissues. Adoption of empirical antibiotic therapy has reduced the mortality rate from 80% (mainly because of gram-negative bacteria) to 10% to 40% overall (807,827). A discussion of specific antibiotic regimens is beyond the scope of this chapter. Specific organisms are isolated during only a minority of putative infectious episodes, but early discontinuation of antibiotics in persistently neutropenic patients is unwise.

Fungemia during an initial febrile episode is rare (816), but fungal infection becomes more likely with repeated courses of antibiotics. The frequency and rapidity of appearance of fungemia may be increasing because of the success of conventional antibiotic regimens and the prolongation of neutropenia from days to months (828,829).

Candida and *Aspergillus* account for almost all fungal disease in aplastic anemia patients. Colonization of the oropharynx and upper respiratory tract with fungus is common in patients receiving antibiotics. Fungal infection should be suspected when a neutropenic patient develops sinusitis, and routine nasal cultures may be helpful in predicting aspergillosis. *Candida* tends to disseminate and may be associated with septic cutaneous emboli (830) or a hepatosplenic syndrome with abdominal pain and rise in alkaline phosphatase level (831); *Candida* esophagitis also occurs (832). Aspergillosis usually localizes to the sinuses and lungs (829,833).

PREVENTION

About simple measures for prevention of infection, there is little dispute. Most important is hand washing, by the patient and by all medical personnel, because transmission of bacteria usually requires a human vector (807). The physical surroundings of a hospital ward should be well maintained to reduce nosocomial infection [two examples are the "miniepidemics" of legionellosis from water sources (834) and of aspergillosis from local construction activity] (835). Dental hygiene should be maintained and sources of infection removed with antibiotic and platelet prophylaxis (836). Nystatin oral rinses prevent thrush (837). In general, early attention to the signs of infection and good communication between patient and physician, especially after hospital discharge, can avert many of the catastrophic complications of initially minor infectious episodes.

Surveillance cultures can help document the acquisition of new gut bacteria and predict the species responsible for bacteremia (838,839), but their cost is high, and their value is controversial (839a). Most neutropenic patients receive broad-spectrum antibiotic therapy, regardless of the results of surveillance cultures. One exception is routine nasal culture for aspergillosis (840). Sterile diets, avoidance of fresh fruits and vegetables, and no flowers in the room are easy proscriptions but of similarly unproven practical value (841–843).

Red Blood Cell Transfusions and Hemochromatosis

Complete replacement of erythrocytes requires transfusion of approximately one unit of packed RBCs/week, usually given as two units every 2 weeks. There is no rationale for allowing a patient to suffer symptoms of anemia. After equilibrium is achieved, a constant amount of blood is required to maintain any hemoglobin concentration. With acclimation, fit individuals are usually not symptomatic at hemoglobin concentrations of more than 7 g/dL; patients with underlying cardiovascular disease should be maintained at a higher concentration, approximately 9 g/dL or more. In patients with anemia who are likely to remain dependent on erythrocyte transfusions, deferoxamine therapy is effective in chelating iron (844). Iron accumulation in critical organs, especially the heart, liver, and endocrine glands, can be prevented and sometimes reversed in the compliant patient who self-administers deferoxamine by subcutaneous infusion (844) or more aggressively by intravenous infusion (845). Iron chelation should be used in patients with unresponsive chronic anemia. As hemochromatotic damage to viscera begins after approximately 100 units of transfusion, a convenient starting time is after 50 to 100 units have been transfused or when the serum ferritin exceeds 500 ng/mL (usually 1 to 2 years after diagnosis) in a patient refractory to definitive therapy of aplastic anemia.

Spontaneous Recovery

Even minimal intervention, by modern standards, altered the natural history of bone marrow failure; a reading of the medical literature of the 1950s reveals the enormous impact of simple blood transfusions on the prospects of the patient with aplastic anemia. Certainly, spontaneous recovery was reported by physicians in the era predating even corticosteroid usage: a 9-year-old boy with severe symptoms of aplasia who was comatose for 2 weeks before recovery (846) and a 47-year-old woman with chloramphenicol-associated aplastic anemia whose severe pancytopenia persisted for 22 months before recovery (847). In most of the early clinical series, a small proportion of patients appeared to improve, sometimes to completely normal hematologic values, when supported only by RBC transfusions (848,849), and after the introduction of corticosteroids (217,773,774,850,851). In a series of pediatric patients treated mainly with transfusions, 14 of 33 achieved remission (852). These historic data are obscured by uncertainties in diagnosis, especially by the confounding influence of Fanconi's anemia and transient pancytopenias due to drug or toxin exposure, and by the inclusion of cases of myelodysplasia.

In those series in which blood counts of individual patients were published, it is clear that recovery usually occurred among patients who would now be classified as having moderate disease (at least 22 of 31 patients by the most conservative estimate in three series) (217,849,850). In a more recent study that randomized 21 patients to supportive care only, none improved during 3 months of observation (624). The fact that rare patients with aplastic anemia may recover even after years of severe pancytopenia is not an argument against therapy—rather, it is the opposite. Even in an era in which blood transfusions, corticosteroids, and penicillin constituted the entire armamentarium, the consensus of an eminent expert panel was "Never give up—at least almost never" (777).

PURE RED CELL APLASIA

PRCA is a rare disease; only a few hundred cases have been reported (853). PRCA shares many clinical associations and pathophysiologic mechanisms with aplastic anemia. In particular, a variety of inciting causes that activate a common immune response may result in identical pathology (Table 9-10). Although many cases of PRCA are idiopathic, a large proportion is associated with clinical immunologic abnormalities, and erythropoiesis may be suppressed by either humoral or cellular immune effectors or both. A variant of PRCA, transient erythroblastopenia of childhood (TEC), is discussed in detail in Chapter 8.

Clinical Features

Women are more commonly affected with PRCA than men, especially within the large subcategory of immune-mediated disease. For PRCA associated with thymoma, male/female ratios are 2:1 (927,928) or higher (929); male patients may also predominate in series in which PRCA is mainly associated with drugs or toxins (909) or with chronic lymphocytic leukemia (930). The mean age of onset in immune-mediated disease is approximately 60 years (879,928). There is no racial predisposition. Anemia, reticulocytopenia, and absent erythroid precursor cells define PRCA (931–934). The erythrocytes are usually normocytic or occasionally macrocytic. Neutrophil and platelet counts are normal, but neutropenia, thrombocytopenia, or full pancytopenia can develop. The bone marrow cellularity is normal and remarkable for the lack or paucity of recognizable erythroid cells. Marrow erythropoiesis can be monitored with Indium 935 scintigraphy (936). Cytogenetics are usually normal, and abnormal results of chromosome analysis suggest the possibility of myelodysplasia (937), including the 5q– syndrome (938). In children, PRCA may be acute and self-limited (TEC); in contrast, acquired disease in

TABLE 9-10. Clinical Classification of Pure Red Blood Cell Aplasia

Self-limited
    Transient erythroblastopenia of childhood
    Transient aplastic crisis of hemolysis (B19 parvovirus infection)
Fetal red blood cell aplasia
    Nonimmune hydrops fetalis (*in utero* B19 parvovirus infection)
Hereditary pure red cell aplasia
    Congenital pure red cell aplasia (Diamond-Blackfan syndrome)
Acquired pure red cell aplasia
    Thymoma (879,880,884,885)
    Lymphoid malignancies
        Chronic lymphocytic leukemia (see text)
        Malignant lymphoma (890–892)
        Malignant histiocytosis (893)
        Kaposi's sarcoma (895)
        Acute lymphocytic leukemia (897)
        Hodgkin's disease (899)
        Multiple myeloma (901)
    Other hematologic diseases
        Myelodysplasia (17)
        Chronic myelogenous leukemia (905)
        Myelofibrosis (908)
    Paraneoplastic to solid tumors (911,911a)
        Carcinoma of the bronchus, breast, stomach, thyroid, bile duct, and
            skin (853,912,913)
    Collagen vascular disease
        Systemic lupus erythematosus (914–916)
        Juvenile rheumatoid arthritis (917)
        Rheumatoid arthritis (918)
        Multiple endocrine gland insufficiency (919)
    Virus
        B19 parvovirus (920)
        Hepatitis (344,872,921)
        Adult T-cell leukemia virus (392)
        Epstein-Barr virus (922,923)
    Pregnancy (924–926)
    Drugs
        Probably causative associations
            Antiepileptics [diphenylhydantoin (854–861), carbamazepine
                (862), sodium dipropylacetate (863), sodium valproate (864)]
            Azathioprine (865–867)
            Chloramphenicol (see text) and thiamphenicol (868,869)
            Sulfonamides [salicylazosulfapyridine (870), Sulfathalidine (871),
                methazolamide (with hepatitis) (872), chlorpropamide (873–
                875), sulfathiazole (876,877), cotrimoxazole (878)]
            Isoniazid (856,881–883)
            Procainamide (175,883)
        Possibly coincidental associations
            Nonsteroidal antiinflammatory drugs [aminopyrine (886), phe-
                nylbutazone (887), fenoprofen (888,889), sulindac]
            Allopurinol (894)
            Halothane [and hepatitis (896)]
            D-penicillamine (898)
            Maloprin (dapsone and pyrimethamine) (900)
            Metolazone (902)
            Quinidine (133,903) and quinacrine
            Gold (904)
            Benzene (877) and benzene-containing compounds [pentachlo-
                rophenol (906), arsenicals (907), and insecticides (909,910)]
    Idiopathic

---

adults is almost always chronic. The clinical associations and, probably, the pathogenesis of the two diseases are different. Unless otherwise noted, the discussion here focuses on adult PRCA. TEC is covered in Chapter 8.

Clinical Associations

Most cases of PRCA are idiopathic, but a large number are associated with illnesses. The most interesting association is with thymoma (939), but the often-quoted 50% incidence of associated thymoma has been greatly exaggerated because of the propensity to report an unusual combination. The true percentage is probably closer to 10% (853,884,928). Conversely, approxi-

mately 5% of thymomas have been estimated to be associated with RBC aplasia (853). Thymoma can precede the onset of PRCA by many years, and PRCA may have its onset after removal of the tumor (940). The thymic mass is commonly composed of spindle cells and is usually benign (contained within the capsule), but the tumors can be malignant, locally invasive, and metastatic (879,884,885,941). In one large survey of published cases, 46 of 56 were well encapsulated (928). PRCA can complicate thymoma associated with several other autoimmune diseases such as myasthenia gravis (942,943), collagen vascular syndromes, and endocrine failure states (944). PRCA can occur with these syndromes individually or with associated thymoma. The association of thymoma and PRCA is most common in older women; its occurrence in childhood is extremely rare. The possibility of a mediastinal mass should be excluded in adult patients by computed tomography of the chest, which is far more sensitive than routine thoracic radiography (945).

PRCA in adults is also associated with other immunologic abnormalities, including myasthenia gravis (943), collagen vascular disorders (914,946–948), hypoimmunoglobulinemia (361,931,949), monoclonal gammopathy (950,951), anergy, and autoimmune hemolysis (934).

PRCA can accompany a variety of other neoplasms (911), most frequently lymphoid (930). The incidence of PRCA in chronic lymphocytic leukemia was estimated at 6% in one large series; PRCA may be present initially but more commonly appears several years after diagnosis (930). PRCA may also present in the setting of large granular lymphocyte leukemia (952). PRCA also can complicate other hematologic malignancies and nonthymic solid tumors. T-cell inhibition has been implicated in the pathophysiology of PRCA in lymphoproliferative disease; many of these same illnesses—or their therapy—are immunosuppressive and would be permissive for persistent parvovirus infection (see section Parvovirus).

Drugs have been associated with PRCA (853), most of which also are included in the black list for aplastic anemia treatment, but for only a few agents is there more than a single case report. Diphenylhydantoin is causally related to PRCA: Patients have developed marrow failure on drug rechallenge (855,953), and one patient has demonstrated a drug-dependent antibody that inhibited *in vitro* erythropoiesis (854).

Practically, it is most important to distinguish among PRCA that is (a) immunologically mediated (most idiopathic cases and those associated with thymoma, systemic lupus erythematosus, and chronic lymphocytic leukemia), (b) caused by primary bone marrow failure (myelodysplasia, myeloproliferative disease, cytogenetic abnormalities, and others), (c) secondary to persistent parvovirus infection, and (d) hereditary and presents in adulthood (954).

Pathogenesis and Pathophysiology

ANTIBODIES TO ERYTHROID PRECURSOR CELLS

A marrow-suppressing factor was first identified in a patient with PRCA, thymoma, and Hodgkin's disease (955). Antibody mediation of PRCA was proposed by Krantz and associates on the basis of observations in several patients: Their plasma contained an IgG that inhibited heme synthesis in suspension cultures of normal bone marrow cells (956,957) and in the presence of complement, lysed erythroblasts (958). Ig preparations from some patients were later shown to inhibit CFU-E–derived erythroid colony formation but not myeloid colony formation in the presence (959–961) or absence (962) of complement. The prevalence of antibody to erythroid precursor cells in PRCA is difficult to assess because of the limited number of patients and because of reporting bias; in a cooperative study, an antibody that inhibited erythropoiesis was found in 13 of 16 patients (870), but antibody generally has not been detected in patients with RBC aplasia secondary to lymphoma and other malignancies (930). A remarkable feature of the cytotoxic antibody in PRCA is its cross-species reactivity, including release of iron 59 from murine cells *in vitro*, inhibition of RBC production after injection into mice, and depletion of CFU-E in treated animals (although some inhibitors have been species specific) (870). The target antigen on erythroid precursor cells has not been identified. In some cases, erythropoiesis was inhibited by an antibody that bound directly to erythropoietin (963–967).

The strongest evidence of a pathogenic role for cytotoxic antibodies is their disappearance from the circulation of patients who respond to therapy, including antilymphocyte sera and immunosuppressive drugs (963), thymectomy (968), and plasmapheresis (969,970). In contrast, an Ig that specifically stained erythroblast nuclei, which was also found in patient plasma, often persisted despite effective therapy and hematologic improvement (969,971). It may represent a secondary antibody formed to the contents of lysed erythroblasts. Alloimmunized patients may have other antibodies directed to antigens on mature erythrocyte surfaces that can be distinguished from the characteristic inhibitor of erythropoiesis (961). In one case of PRCA and thymoma, a serum inhibitor of antigen-induced lymphocyte transformation was present (940); such an activity might account for defective production of erythropoietic factors by lymphocytes in some patients with PRCA (961). IgG inhibitors of erythropoiesis have also been documented in children with TEC (972).

CYTOTOXIC LYMPHOCYTES

T-cell inhibition of erythropoiesis is probably a more common mechanism of depression of RBC production than antibody formation (973). Lymphocyte inhibition may be particularly common in PRCA associated with chronic lymphocytic leukemia (930,974). T-cell inhibition of either CFU-E– or BFU-E–derived colony formation was present in eight of eight cases, whereas none showed a serum inhibitor of erythropoiesis (930); cells with the suppressor phenotype and function in erythropoietic colony culture were present in early, nonanemic stages of disease in a high percentage of patients (975). As in aplastic anemia, there may be an increased number of lymphocytes with receptors for IgG (T-γ cells) (976–978) or with the suppressor cell phenotype (CD8$^+$) (977–980), which inhibit erythroid colony formation by CFU-E and BFU-E. Genetic restriction of lymphocytic suppression of erythropoiesis by CD8$^+$, HLA-DR$^+$ lymphocytes was shown in one well-studied case (981). Clinical remission has been correlated with the disappearance of the suppressive population after immunosuppressive therapy or chemotherapy-induced remission of chronic lymphocytic leukemia (977–980,982). In some cases, the implicated population was a true suppressor cell, capable of inhibiting *in vitro* Ig synthesis as well as erythropoiesis (983,984).

Treatment

Approximately two-thirds of patients with PRCA respond to some form of immunosuppression, although trials of alternative forms of therapy may be necessary (985–987). Prednisone can induce remission in approximately 45% of cases, and the addition of a cytotoxic agent may improve the remission rate and lower the corticosteroid dose (986). Patients have responded to ATG (963,973,988,989) and cyclosporine (675,676,990,991), including cases refractory to steroids. One recent study reported responses to cyclosporin in 32 of 38 (82%) patients (992). Cytotoxic drug regimens include azathioprine (987), cyclophospha-

mide (987,993), and fludarabine (994); a 3- to 4-month trial is adequate. Relapse occurs in approximately one-half of the treated cases, and chronic cytotoxic chemotherapy may be required to maintain transfusion independence (995).

Plasmapheresis (969,970,996) and lymphocytopheresis (996) have been successful in inducing sustained remissions; in some patients, the clinical response has been correlated with removal of an antibody inhibitory to erythropoiesis *in vitro* (969,970). Splenectomy may sometimes be helpful (933,986). Some patients have responded to androgens (997), including three of three patients who responded to Danazol in one small series (998). Apparent responses have also been noted after high doses of intravenous Ig (991,999–1002). A small percentage of patients (approximately 15%) may have apparently spontaneous remissions (986). Patients with PRCA secondary to malignant disease can also respond to specific immunosuppressive therapy or cytotoxic chemotherapy (890,891,930,986,1003). A thymoma is necessarily removed for diagnosis and treatment of a possibly malignant chest mass, but the procedure probably benefits only a minority of patients. The percentage commonly quoted for remission of anemia after thymectomy is 30%, based on an analysis of the 9 of 26 patients who showed improvement (880); in three of these patients, remission occurred only with the postoperative addition of corticosteroids, and in three others no benefit was sustained. [It also is worth remembering that PRCA can occur years after removal of a thymoma (928).] Bone marrow transplant for refractory acquired PRCA in a 16-year-old patient conditioned with ATG and cyclophosphamide restored hematopoiesis even after reversion to autologous reconstitution at 2 years of follow-up (1004).

PRCA may be one of the few diseases in which hematopoietic colony cultures have clinical value in predicting response to treatment. Patients whose marrow contains CFU-E progenitors have a high probability of response to immunosuppression, whereas patients without detectable CFU-E—often cases secondary to myeloproliferative or malignant disease—have not responded (973,1005). These results confirm the earlier observation that a proliferative response in suspension culture to added erythropoietin predicts clinical improvement with therapy (956,957). In contrast, the presence of an antibody to erythroid progenitors in coculture does not correlate with responsiveness to immunosuppressive treatment, and antibodies are often undetectable in patients who behave clinically as if they have an autoimmune process (942,1005).

The obvious mainstay of therapy is RBC transfusion, and the same principles that were described earlier for the support of the patient with aplastic anemia should be applied here.

Parvovirus

Parvovirus B19 infection (Fig. 9-9) is a well established cause of both acute and chronic PRCA, and testing for this virus has become a routine part of the diagnostic workup (1006). The Parvoviridae, small single-stranded DNA viruses, are common animal pathogens. Feline panleukopenia virus was the first virus that was experimentally demonstrated to cause disease in animals; this virus infects cat hematopoietic and lymphocytic cells and causes fatal neutropenia (1007). The first parvovirus shown to cause human disease was only discovered in 1975 (1008). Acute infection with B19 parvovirus (named from the blood bank code for the donor from whom the virus was isolated) causes the childhood exanthem fifth disease (erythema infectiosum) (358,1009,1010). Children with fifth disease are usually not very ill, but the characteristic rash—the "slapped cheek" facial erythema and a lacy, reticular, evanescent maculopapular eruption over the trunk and proximal extremities—combined with

982. Hanada T, Abe T, Nakamura H, et al. Pure red cell aplasia: relationship between inhibitory activity of T cells to CFU-E and erythropoiesis. *Br J Haematol* 1984;58:107–113.

983. Nagasawa T, Abe T, Nakagawa T. Pure red cell aplasia and hypogammaglobulinemia associated with Tr-cell chronic lymphocytic leukemia. *Blood* 1981;57:1025–1031.

984. Shionoya S, Amano M, Imamura Y, et al. Suppressor T cell chronic lymphocytic leukaemia associated with red cell hypoplasia. *Scand J Haematol* 1984;33:231–238.

985. Gill PJ, Amare M, Larsen WE. Pure red cell aplasia: three cases responding to immunosuppression. *Am J Med Sci* 1977;273:213–219.

986. Clark DA, Dessypris EN, Krantz SB. Studies on pure red cell aplasia. XI. Results of immunosuppressive treatment of 37 patients. *Blood* 1984;63:277–286.

987. Firkin FC, Maher D. Cytotoxic immunosuppressive drug treatment strategy in pure red cell aplasia. *Eur J Haematol* 1988;41:212–217.

988. Krantz SB. Studies on red cell aplasia. 3. Treatment with horse antihuman thymocyte gamma globulin. *Blood* 1972;39:347–360.

989. Harris SI, Weinberg JB. Treatment of red cell aplasia with antithymocyte globulin: repeated inductions of complete remissions in two patients. *Am J Hematol* 1985;20:183–186.

990. Totterman TH, Nisell J, Killander A, et al. Successful treatment of pure red-cell aplasia with cyclosporin. *Lancet* 1984;2:693.

991. Katakkar SB. Cyclosporine and pure red cell aplasia. *Transplant Proc* 1988;20:314–316.

992. Mamiya S, Itoh T, Miura AB. Acquired pure red cell aplasia in Japan. *Eur J Haematol* 1997;59:199–205.

993. Yamada H, Mizoguchi H, Oshimi K. Cyclophosphamide therapy for pure red cell aplasia associated with granular lymphocyte-proliferative disorders. *Br J Haematol* 1997;97:392–399.

994. Lee T. Fludarabine therapy of pure red cell aplasia. *Blood* 1997;90[Suppl 1]:16b.

995. Zaentz SD, Krantz SB, Brown EB. Studies on pure red cell aplasia. Maintenance therapy with immunosuppressive drugs. *Br J Haematol* 1976;32:47–54.

996. Berlin G, Lieden G. Long-term remission of pure red cell aplasia after plasma exchange and lymphocytapheresis. *Scand J Haematol* 1986;36:121–122.

997. Change JC, Slutzker B, Lindsay N. Remission of pure red cell aplasia following oxymetholone therapy. *Am J Med Sci* 1978;275:345.

998. Lippman SM, Durie BG, Garewal HS, et al. Efficacy of danazol in pure red cell aplasia. *Am J Hematol* 1986;23:373–379.

999. Needleman SW. Durable remission of pure red cell aplasia after treatment with high-dose intravenous gammaglobulin and prednisone. *Am J Hematol* 1989;32:150–152.

1000. Etzioni A, Atias D, Pollack S, et al. Complete recovery of pure red cell aplasia by intramuscular gammaglobulin therapy in a child with hypoparathyroidism. *Am J Hematol* 1986;22:409–414.

1001. Katakkar SB. Pure red blood cell aplasia: response to intravenous immunoglobulins, a blocking antibody. *Arch Intern Med* 1986;146:2288.

1002. Larroche C, Mouthon L, Casadevall N, et al. Successful treatment of thymoma-associated pure red cell aplasia with intravenous immunoglobulins. *Eur J Haematol* 2000;65:74–76.

1003. Battle JD Jr, HJ, Hoffman GC. Prolonged erythroid aplasia in chronic lymphocytic leukemia: favorable response to adrenocortical steroids in four cases. [Letter]. *Ann Intern Med* 1963;58:731.

1004. Muller BU, Tichelli A, Passweg JR, et al. Successful treatment of refractory acquired pure red cell aplasia (PRCA) by allogeneic bone marrow transplantation. *Bone Marrow Transplant* 1999;23:1205–1207.

1005. Lacombe C, Casadevall N, Muller O, et al. Erythroid progenitors in adult chronic pure red cell aplasia: relationship of in vitro erythroid colonies to therapeutic response. *Blood* 1984;64:71–77.

1006. Anderson LJ, Young NS. Human parvovirus B19. In: *Monogr Virol* Vol. 20. Basel: Karger, 1997.

1007. Kurtzman GJ, Platanias L, Lustig L, et al. Feline parvovirus propagates in cat bone marrow cultures and inhibits hematopoietic colony formation in vitro. *Blood* 1989;74:71–81.

1008. Cossart YE, Field AM, Cant B, et al. Parvovirus-like particles in human sera. *Lancet* 1975;1:72.

1009. Ager E, Chin T, Poland J. Epidemic erythema infectiosum. *N Engl J Med* 1966;275:1326.

1010. Chorba T, Coccia P, Holman RC, et al. The role of parvovirus B19 in aplastic crisis and erythema infectiosum (fifth disease). *J Infect Dis* 1986;154:383–393.

1011. Reid DM, Reid TM, Brown T, et al. Human parvovirus-associated arthritis: a clinical and laboratory description. *Lancet* 1985;1:422–425.

1012. White DG, Woolf AD, Mortimer PP, et al. Human parvovirus arthropathy. *Lancet* 1985;1:419–421.

1013. Lyngar E. Samtidig optreden av anemisk kriser hos 3 barn i en familie med hemolytisk ikterus. *Nord Med* 1942;14:1246.

1014. Gasser C. Akute erythroblastopenie: 10 falle aplastischer erythroblastenkrisen mit riesenproerythroblasten bei allergisch-taxischen Zustandsbildern. *Helv Paediatr Acta* 1949;4:107.

1015. Owren P. Congenital hemolytic jaundice: the pathogenesis of the "hemolytic crisis." *Blood* 1948.

1016. Young N. Hematologic and hematopoietic consequences of B19 parvovirus infection. *Semin Hematol* 1988;25:159–172.

1017. Weiland HT, Salimans MM, Fibbe WE. Prolonged parvovirus B19 infection with severe anaemia in a bone marrow transplant recipient. [Letter]. *Br J Haematol* 1989;710:300.

1018. Lien-Keng K. Erythroblastopenia with giant pro-erythroblasts in kwashiorkor. *Blood* 1957;12:171.

1019. Zucker J, Tchernia G, Vuylsteke P, et al. Acute secondary and transitory erythroblastopenia in kwashiorkor under treatment. *Nouv Rev Fr Hematol* 1971;11:131–144.

1020. Pierce L, Rath C. Evidence for folic acid deficiency in the genesis of anemic sickle cell crisis. *Blood* 1962;20:19.

1021. Alperin J. Folic acid deficiency complicating sickle cell anemia. *Arch Intern Med* 1967;120:398.

1022. Broccia G, Dessalvi P. Acute pure red cell aplasia following bromosulphonphtalein injection in a patient with non Hodgkin lymphoma. *Haematologica* 1983;68:680–683.

1023. Choremis C, Megas H, Liaromati A, et al. Aplastic crisis in the course of infectious diseases: report of 10 cases. *Helv Paediatr Acta* 1961;2:134.

1024. Evans JP, Rossiter MA, Kumaran TO, et al. Human parvovirus aplasia: case due to cross infection in a ward. [Letter]. *BMJ (Clin Res Ed)* 1984;288:681.

1025. Shneerson JM, Mortimer PP, Vandervelde EM. Febrile illness due to a parvovirus. *BMJ* 1980;280:1580.

1026. Mortimer PP, Luban NL, Kelleher JF, et al. Transmission of serum parvovirus-like virus by clotting-factor concentrates. *Lancet* 1983;2:482–484.

1027. Lefrere JJ, Courouce AM, Bertrand Y, et al. Human parvovirus and aplastic crisis in chronic hemolytic anemias: a study of 24 observations. *Am J Hematol* 1986;23:271–275.

1028. McLellan NJ, Rutter N. Hereditary spherocytosis in sisters unmasked by parvovirus infection. *Postgrad Med J* 1987;63:49–50.

1029. Nunoue T, Koike T, Koike R, et al. Infection with human parvovirus (B19), aplasia of the bone marrow and a rash in hereditary spherocytosis. *J Infect* 1987;14:67–70.

1030. Kurtzman GJ, Gascon P, Caras M, et al. B19 parvovirus replicates in circulating cells of acutely infected patients. *Blood* 1988;71:1448–1454.

1031. Doran HM, Teall AJ. Neutropenia accompanying erythroid aplasia in human parvovirus infection. *Br J Haematol* 1988;69:287–288.

1032. Anderson MJ, Higgins PG, Davis LR, et al. Experimental parvoviral infection in humans. *J Infect Dis* 1985;152:257–265.

1033. Lefrere JJ, Got D. Peripheral thrombocytopenia in human parvovirus infection. *J Clin Pathol* 1987;40:469.

1034. Lefrere JJ, Courouce AM, Kaplan C. Parvovirus and idiopathic thrombocytopenic purpura. *Lancet* 1989;1:279.

1035. Conrad ME, Studdard H, Anderson LJ. Aplastic crisis in sickle cell disorders: bone marrow necrosis and human parvovirus infection. *Am J Med Sci* 1988;295:212–215.

1036. Pardoll DM, Rodeheffer RJ, Smith RR, et al. Aplastic crisis due to extensive bone marrow necrosis in sickle cell disease. *Arch Intern Med* 1982;142:2223–2225.

1037. Saunders PW, Reid MM, Cohen BJ. Human parvovirus induced cytopenias: a report of five cases. *Br J Haematol* 1986;63:407–410.

1038. Hanada T, Koike K, Takeya T, et al. Human parvovirus B19-induced transient pancytopenia in a child with hereditary spherocytosis. *Br J Haematol* 1988;70:113–115.

1039. Hamon MD, Newland AC, Anderson MJ. Severe aplastic anaemia after parvovirus infection in the absence of underlying haemolytic anaemia. *J Clin Pathol* 1988;41:1242.

1040. Tung J, Hadzic N, Layton M, et al. Bone marrow failure in children with acute liver failure. *J Pediatr Gastroenterol Nutr* 2000;31:557–561.

1041. Serjeant GR, Topley JM, Mason K, et al. Outbreak of aplastic crises in sickle cell anaemia associated with parvovirus-like agent. *Lancet* 1981;2:595–597.

1042. Saarinen UM, Chorba TL, Tattersall P, et al. Human parvovirus B19-induced epidemic acute red cell aplasia in patients with hereditary hemolytic anemia. *Blood* 1986;67:1411–1417.

1043. Lefrère J, Courouce AM, Bertrand Y, et al. Human parvovirus and aplastic crisis in chronic hemolytic anemias: a study of 24 observations. *Am J Hematol* 1986;23:271.

1044. Anderson MJ, Jones SE, Minson AC. Diagnosis of human parvovirus infection by dot-blot hybridization using cloned viral DNA. *J Med Virol* 1985;15:163–172.

1045. Clewley JP. Detection of human parvovirus using a molecularly cloned probe. *J Med Virol* 1985;15:173–181.

1046. Anderson LJ, Hurwitz ES. Human parvovirus B19 and pregnancy. *Clin Perinatol* 1988;15:273–286.

1047. Leads from the MMWR. Risks associated with human parvovirus B19 infection. *JAMA* 1989;261:1406–1408.

1048. Anand A, Gray ES, Brown T, et al. Human parvovirus infection in pregnancy and hydrops fetalis. *N Engl J Med* 1987;316:183–186.

1049. Cotmore SF, McKie VC, Anderson LJ, et al. Identification of the major structural and nonstructural proteins encoded by human parvovirus B19 and mapping of their genes by procaryotic expression of isolated genomic fragments. *J Virol* 1986;60:548–557.

1050. Porter HJ, Quantrill AM, Fleming KA. B19 parvovirus infection of myocardial cells. *Lancet* 1988;1:535.

1051. Schwarz TF, Roggendorf M, Hottentrager B, et al. Human parvovirus B19 infection in pregnancy. *Lancet* 1988;2:566.

1052. Frickhofen N, Young N. Persistent parvovirus B19 infections in humans. *Microb Pathog* 1989;7:319.

1053. Brown KE, Anderson SM, Young NS. Erythrocyte P antigen: cellular receptor for B19 parvovirus. *Science* 1993;262:114–117.

1054. Ozawa K, Kurtzman G, Young N. Replication of the B19 parvovirus in human bone marrow cell cultures. *Science* 1986;233:883–886.

1055. Kurtzman GJ, Ozawa K, Cohen B, et al. Chronic bone marrow failure due to persistent B19 parvovirus infection. *N Engl J Med* 1987;317:287–294.

1056. Kurtzman GJ, Cohen B, Meyers P, et al. Persistent B19 parvovirus infection as a cause of severe chronic anaemia in children with acute lymphocytic leukaemia. *Lancet* 1988;2:1159–1162.

1057. Ozawa K, Kurtzman G, Young N. Productive infection by B19 parvovirus of human erythroid bone marrow cells in vitro. *Blood* 1987;70:384–391.

1058. Yaegashi N, Shiraishi H, Takeshita T, et al. Propagation of human parvovirus B19 in primary culture of erythroid lineage cells derived from fetal liver. *J Virol* 1989;63:2422–2426.

1059. Young N, Harrison M, Moore J, et al. Direct demonstration of the human parvovirus in erythroid progenitor cells infected in vitro. *J Clin Invest* 1984;74:2024–2032.

1060. Ozawa K, Ayub J, Kajigaya S, et al. The gene encoding the nonstructural protein of B19 (human) parvovirus may be lethal in transfected cells. *J Virol* 1988;62:2884–2889.

1061. Kurtzman G, Frickhofen N, Kimball J, et al. Pure red-cell aplasia of 10 years' duration due to persistent parvovirus B19 infection and its cure with immunoglobulin therapy. *N Engl J Med* 1989;321:519–523.

1062. Corral D, Darras F, Jensen C, et al. Parvovirus B19 infection causing pure red cell aplasia in a recipient of pediatric donor kidneys. *Transplant* 1993;55:427–430.

1063. Nour B, Green M, Michaels M, et al. Parvovirus B19 in pediatric transplant patients. *Transplant* 1993;56:835–838.

1064. Frickhofen N, Abkowitz JL, Safford M, et al. Persistent B19 parvovirus infection in patients infected with human immunodeficiency virus type 1 (HIV-1): a treatable cause of anemia in AIDS. *Ann Intern Med* 1990;113:926–933.

1065. Berner YN, Berrebi A, Green L, et al. Erythroblastopenia in acquired immunodeficiency syndrome (AIDS). *Acta Haematol* 1983;70:273.

1066. Sallan SE, Buchanan GR. Selective erythroid aplasia during therapy for acute lymphoblastic leukemia. *Pediatrics* 1977;59:895–898.

1067. Conley CL, Lippman SM, Ness PM, et al. Autoimmune hemolytic anemia with reticulocytopenia and erythroid marrow. *N Engl J Med* 1982;306:281–286.

1068. Foy H, KA, MacDougall L. Pure red-cell aplasia in marasmus and kwashiorkor treated with riboflavine. *BMJ* 1961:937.

1069. Kurtzman GJ, Cohen BJ, Field AM, et al. Immune response to B19 parvovirus and an antibody defect in persistent viral infection. *J Clin Invest* 1989;84:1114–1123.

1070. Manoharan A, Williams NT, Sparrow R. Acquired amegakaryocytic thrombocytopenia: report of a case and review of literature. *QJM* 1989;70:243–252.

1071. Geissler D, Thaler J, Konwalinka G, et al. Progressive preleukemia presenting amegakaryocytic thrombocytopenic purpura: association of the 5q- syndrome with a decreased megakaryocytic colony formation and a defective production of Meg-CSF. *Leuk Res* 1987;11:731–737.

1072. Stoll DB, Blum S, Pasquale D, et al. Thrombocytopenia with decreased megakaryocytes. Evaluation and prognosis. *Ann Intern Med* 1981;94:170–175.

1073. Hallett JM, Martell RW, Sher C, et al. Amegakaryocytic thrombocytopenia with duplication of part of the long arm of chromosome 3. *Br J Haematol* 1989;71:291–292.

1074. Nieneltow M, Cooper M, Breg WR, et al. Evidence for the clonal origin of acquired hypomegakaryocytic thrombocytopenic purpura from a sex chromosome mosaic. *Cancer Genet Cytogenet* 1984;12:261–265.

1074a. Nagasawa T, Sakurai T, Kashiwagi H, et al. Cell-mediated amegakaryocytic thrombocytopenia associated with systemic lupus erythematosus. *Blood* 1986;67:479.

1074b. Subramanian VP. Thrombocytopenia and decreased megakaryocytes (letter). *Ann Intern Med* 1981;94:711.

1075. Slater LM, Katz J, Walter B, et al. Aplastic anemia occurring as amegakaryocytic thrombocytopenia with and without an inhibitor of granulopoiesis. *Am J Hematol* 1985;18:251–254.

1076. Iannelli S, Petrini MT. Acquired pure megakaryocytic aplasia in course of hepatitis in a patient with immune thrombocytopenic purpura. *Acta Haematol* 1984;72:355–356.

1077. Font J, Nomdedeu B, Martinez-Orozco F, et al. Amegakaryocytic thrombocytopenia and an analgesic. *Ann Intern Med* 1981;95:783.

1078. Lugassy G. Non-Hodgkin's lymphoma presenting with amegakaryocytic thrombocytopenic purpura. *Ann Hematol* 1996;73:41–42.

1079. Kouides PA, Rowe JM. Large granular lymphocyte leukemia presenting with both amegakaryocytic thrombocytopenic purpura and pure red cell aplasia: clinical course and response to immunosuppressive therapy. *Am J Hematol* 1995;49:232–236.

1080. Hoffman R, Bruno E, Elwell J, et al. Acquired amegakaryocytic thrombocytopenic purpura: a syndrome of diverse etiologies. *Blood* 1982;60:1173–1178.

1081. Milnes JP, Schofield KP, Low-Beer TS. Genetic haemochromatosis and thrombocytopenia. *Lancet* 1986;2:1336.

1082. Gewirtz AM, Sacchetti MK, Bien R, et al. Cell-mediated suppression of megakaryocytopoiesis in acquired amegakaryocytic thrombocytopenic purpura. *Blood* 1986;68:619–626.

1083. Hirsh EH, Vogler WR, McDonald TP, et al. Acquired hypomegakaryocytic thrombocytopenic purpura. Occurrence in a patient with absent thrombopoietic stimulating factor. *Arch Intern Med* 1980;140:721–723.

1084. Hoffman R, Briddell RA, van Besien K, et al. Acquired cyclic amegakaryocytic thrombocytopenia associated with an immunoglobulin blocking the action of granulocyte-macrophage colony-stimulating factor. *N Engl J Med* 1989;321:97–102.

1085. Worman CP, Mills KH, Linch DC, et al. A megakaryocytic thrombocytopenia associated with the excess of Leu 2a+ suppressor cells. *Scand J Haematol* 1982;28:215–219.

1086. Dharmasena F, Galton DA. Circulating blasts in acute myeloid leukaemia in remission. *Br J Haematol* 1986;63:211–213.

1087. Katai M, Aizawa T, Ohara N, et al. Acquired amegakaryocytic thrombocytopenic purpura with humoral inhibitory factor for megakaryocyte colony formation. *Intern Med* 1994;33:147–149.

1088. Khelif A, French M, Follea G, et al. Amegakaryocytic thrombocytopenic purpura treated with antithymocyte globulin. *Ann Intern Med* 1985;102:720.

1089. Faldt R. Remission of amegakaryocytic thrombocytopenia induced by antilymphocyte globulin (ALG). *Br J Haematol* 1986;63:205–207.

1090. Hill W, Landgraf R. Successful treatment of amegakaryocytic thrombocytopenic purpura with cyclosporine. *N Engl J Med* 1985;312:1060–1061.

1091. Peng CT, Kao LY, Tsai CH. Successful treatment with cyclosporin A in a child with acquired pure amegakaryocytic thrombocytopenic purpura. *Acta Paediatr* 1994;83:1222–1224.

1092. Telek B, Kiss A, Pecze K, et al. Cyclic idiopathic pure acquired amegakaryocytic thrombocytopenic purpura: a patient treated with cyclosporin A. *Br J Haematol* 1989;73:128–129.

1093. El Saghir NS, Geltman RL. Treatment of acquired amegakaryocytic thrombocytopenic purpura with cyclophosphamide. *Am J Med* 1986;81:139.

1094. Kayser W, Euler HH, Schmitz N, et al. Danazol in acquired amegakaryocytic thrombocytopenic purpura: a case report. *Blut* 1985;51:401–404.

1095. Lonial S, Bilodeau PA, Langston AA, et al. Acquired amegakaryocytic thrombocytopenia treated with allogeneic BMT: a case report and review of the literature. *Bone Marrow Transplant* 1999;24:1337–1341.

CHAPTER 10

Paroxysmal Nocturnal Hemoglobinuria

Lucio Luzzatto and Rosario Notaro

DEFINITION

Paroxysmal nocturnal hemoglobinuria (PNH) is a unique, nonmalignant, chronic clonal blood disorder. PNH is conventionally classified among hemolytic anemias, and the prominence of hemoglobinuria indicates that the hemolysis is largely intravascular; therefore, PNH has been traditionally and correctly classified as a hemolytic anemia (1–4). However, often the anemia is associated also with a decrease in neutrophils or platelets, or both, hinting to a broader pathology of the hematopoietic system; in fact, a component of bone marrow failure (BMF) is always present (5). In addition, patients with PNH are liable to the potentially devastating consequence of venous thrombosis, particularly in the veins of the portohepatic system. The triad of hemolytic anemia, pancytopenia, and thrombosis makes PNH a truly unique clinical syndrome (6,7).

EPIDEMIOLOGY

PNH is encountered in all populations throughout the world, and it can affect people of all ages and socioeconomic groups; however, it has never been reported as a congenital disease, and there is no report of family clustering (8). Thus, PNH is an acquired disease. There is little information on the population incidence of PNH; however, this is estimated to be five to ten times less than that of aplastic anemia (AA); thus, PNH is a rare disease, with a population frequency of 1/1 million to 1/100,000. There is no significant gender preference. It has been suggested that, like AA, PNH may be somewhat less rare in Southeast Asia and in the Far East (9,10).

PATHOGENESIS AND PATHOPHYSIOLOGY

Somatic Cell Mosaicism

A remarkable feature of patients with PNH, when compared with those who have hemolytic anemia due to some other intracorpuscular cause, is that not all their red cells participate in the hemolytic process; indeed, some of their red cells are qualitatively normal.* The most striking and biologically important evidence was that chromium 51–tagged red cells infused into normal recipients had a two-tiered survival curve (11,12). This and other findings led to the theory that PNH is a clonal disorder due to a somatic mutation (13). Direct experimental evidence

supporting this theory was obtained three decades ago in PNH patients who were heterozygous for the X-linked gene encoding glucose-6-phosphate dehydrogenase (14), as it was shown that all PNH cells expressed the same glucose-6-phosphate dehydrogenase allele.

Biochemical Abnormalities of Glycosyl Phosphatidyl Inositol–Linked Molecules

Serologic studies had suggested long ago that certain normal antigens were poorly expressed on the surface of PNH red cells (8,15–17). With the introduction of and the increasing use of flow cytometry (18,19), it was discovered that a bewildering multitude of membrane proteins (Table 10-1) is deficient in the abnormal population of blood cells of different lineages in patients with PNH (20). In most cases, there is no obvious similarity in the function of these proteins. Instead, they have a common structural element: namely, a phospholipid moiety; specifically, a glycosyl phosphatidyl inositol (GPI), which includes an ethanolamine that can form a peptide link with a C-terminal amino acid of certain proteins (21,22). Because this lipid is embedded in the lipid bilayer of the membrane, and it serves to retain the protein attached to the membrane, it is referred to as a *GPI anchor* (23,24). The fact that all GPI-linked proteins are deficient on the membrane of PNH cells suggested that the underlying defect might be in the complex biochemical pathway through which the GPI is synthesized in mammalian cells. Because deficiency of GPI-linked proteins is found in blood cells of all lineages (18,25,26) (Table 10-1), we must infer that the underlying somatic mutation is in a totipotent hematopoietic stem cell (HSC).

The somatic cell mosaicism in patients with PNH has made biochemical studies difficult, because patient material always consists of a mixture of both types of cells (27). However, a valid approach was to study cloned lymphoblastoid cell lines (LCL) that displayed the PNH phenotype obtained from PNH patients, and to use as controls LCLs with a normal phenotype obtained from the same patients (28). Comparative analysis of these two sets of cell lines revealed normal synthesis of phosphatidyl inositol but a failure to incorporate mannose or *N*-acetylglu-

---

*It is convenient to refer to the abnormal cells as *PNH cells*; the remaining cells do not have, by definition, the PNH phenotype. Because we will see that the remaining hematopoiesis in PNH patients is not normal, these cells should be called, strictly speaking, *non-PNH cells*. However, for the sake of brevity, they are often referred to as *normal cells*.

TABLE 10-1. Glycosyl Phosphatidyl Inositol (GPI)–Linked Molecules on Human Hematopoietic Cells

	Red Blood Cells	Granulocytes	Monocytes	Platelets	B Lymphocytes	T Lymphocytes	Natural Killer Lymphocytes	Hematopoietic Stem Cells
Complement regulators								
CD55 (DAF, Cromer antigen)	+	+	+	+	+	+	+	
CD59 (MIRL)	+	+	+	+	+	+	+	+
Adhesion molecules								
CD48		+	+		+	+	+	
CD58 (leukocyte function antigen-3)	+	a	a	a	a	a	a	
CD66b		+						
CD66c		+						
CD67		+						
GPI-80		+	+					
Enzymes								
Acetylcholinesterase (Yt antigen)	+							
Leukocyte alkaline phosphatase		+						
Monoadenosine diphosphate-ribosyl transferase		+				+		
DO (Dombroch/HG antigens)	+							
CD73					b	b		
CD157		+	+					
Receptors								
CD14			1					
CD16 (FcγRIII) (NA antigen)		+	b,c		+	b,c	b,c	
CD87 (urokinase plasminogen activator receptor)		+	+			+		
Others								
CD24		+			+			
CD52			+		+	+	+	
CD90						b		+
CDw108 (JMH antigen)	+				b	+		+
CD109 (Gov antigen)		+	+	b		b		+
NB1		+						
Prion protein	+	+	+	+	+	+	+	
GP500				+				

DAF, decay accelerating factor; MIRL, membrane inhibitor of reactive lysis.
[a] Present in both GPI-linked and transmembrane form.
[b] Expression only on activation or only in a cell subset.
[c] Present only in transmembrane form.
Adapted from Rosti V. The molecular basis of paroxysmal nocturnal hemoglobinuria. *Haematologica* 2000;85:82–87; and Bessler M, Schaefer A, Keller P. Paroxysmal nocturnal hemoglobinuria: insights from recent advances in molecular biology. *Transfus Med Rev* 2001;15:255–267.

cosamine (NAcGlcN), thus pinpointing a block at the level of the NAcGlcN transfer (29) (Fig. 10-1).

Molecular Genetics

Formal proof that the PNH abnormality is due to a genetic defect was obtained by somatic cell genetics. When a PNH LCL was fused with a non-PNH LCL and hybrid cell clones were isolated, these had a normal phenotype (30). This experiment proved that the PNH phenotype could be complemented, indicating that in the PNH cell it was due to a loss of function—in keeping, for instance, with an enzyme defect. At the same time, the experiment showed that the PNH phenotype was recessive, thus highlighting a paradox; namely, two successive genetic events would be needed to inactivate both alleles at the locus concerned, if autosomal. Because this is *a priori* very unlikely for a noninherited disease, it was inferred that the locus was on the X chromosome (30). Soon afterwards, the *PIG-A* gene (an acronym for phosphatidyl inositol gly-

can complementation group A) was isolated by expression cloning (31) [i.e., through its ability to restore the expression of GPI-anchored proteins on the surface of cells lacking those proteins, including those from PNH patients (32)]. *PIG-A* maps indeed to the short arm of the X chromosome on Xp22.1 (33) (Fig. 10-1). It became clear that acquired mutations of the *PIG-A* gene are responsible for PNH (32,34–36); to date, a total of 174 somatic mutations in the *PIG-A* gene have been identified by different investigators in more than 28 reports in 146 patients (37) (Fig. 10-2). Of these, 135 are such (large deletions, frameshifts, nonsense mutations) that we can predict complete functional inactivation of the *PIG-A* gene product (PIG-Ao); 35 are missense mutations; and 4 are small in frame deletions. These two groups presumably account for the existence in PNH patients of blood cells with a complete deficiency of GPI-anchored proteins (PNH III) or a partial deficiency (38,39) of GPI-anchored proteins (PNH II). The two types not infrequently coexist in the same patient (see Fig. 10-9B), indicating that two different clones are present.

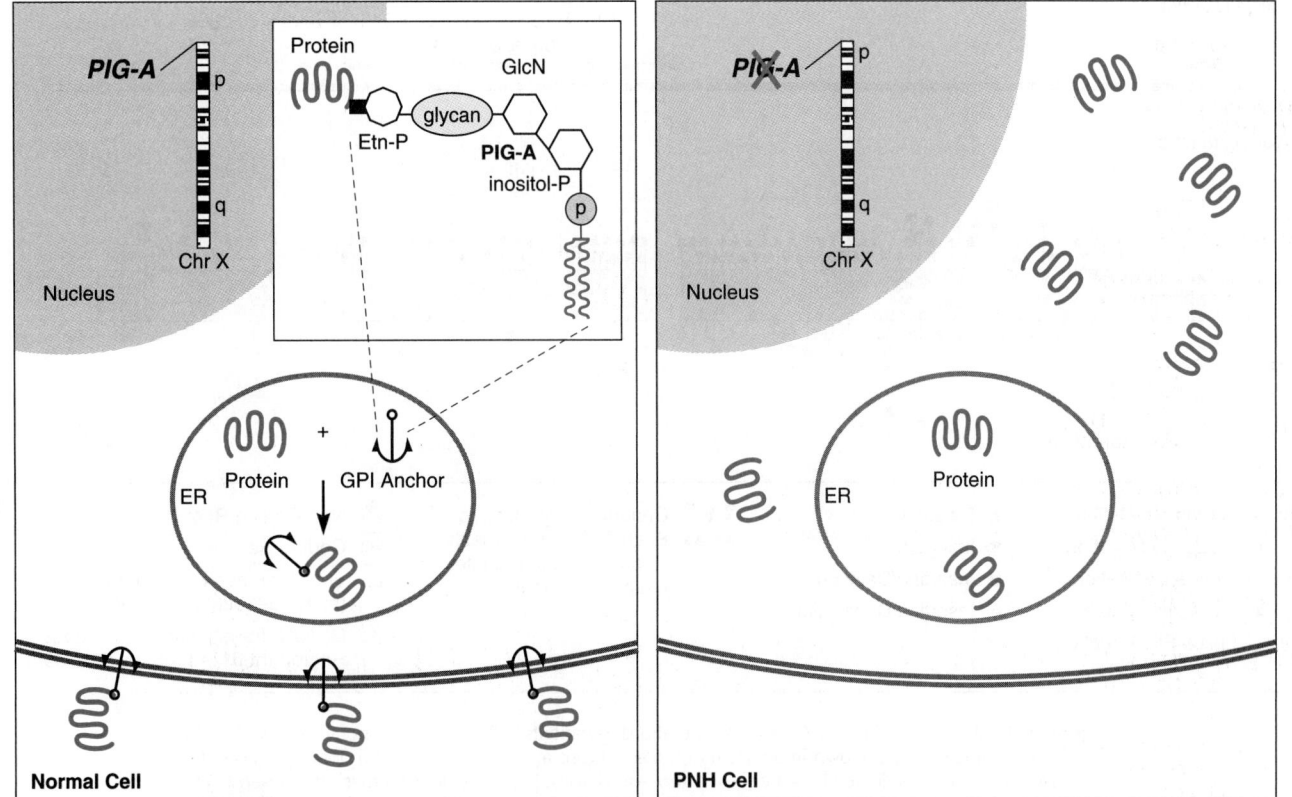

Figure 10-1. The molecular basis of the cellular abnormality in paroxysmal nocturnal hemoglobinuria (PNH). In a normal cell **(A)**, a complex biosynthetic pathway produces in the endoplasmic reticulum (ER) a glycophospholipid molecule **(inset)** called *glycosyl phosphatidyl inositol* (GPI). An early step in the biosynthetic pathway is catalyzed by an acetylglucosaminyl transferase: One of the subunits of this enzyme is encoded by the gene *PIG-A*, located on the short arm of the X chromosome (Chr X) (band Xp22). A number of cellular proteins become covalently linked to the GPI molecule that serves to convey and anchor them, as extracellular surface proteins, to the cell membrane. The PNH cell **(B)** has a mutation in the *PIG-A* gene, causing a serious defect in the acetylglucosaminyl transferase. This, in turn, causes a total or partial block in the synthesis of the GPI molecule. As a result, the proteins that require a GPI anchor are unable to become membrane-bound and will be lacking from the cell surface. (Modified from Karadimitris A, Luzzatto L. The cellular pathogenesis of paroxysmal nocturnal haemoglobinuria. *Leukemia* 2001;15:1148–1152.)

The predicted protein product of *PIG-A* consists of 484 amino acids. A hydrophobic region near the carboxyl terminus may be a transmembrane domain (amino acids 415 to 442). The hydrophilic carboxyl terminal region of 42 residues corresponds to the luminal domain of PIG-A. Watanabe et al. (40) have shown that PIG-A with three other proteins (PIG-H, PIG-C, and GPI1) constitutes a complex that mediates the first reaction step of the GPI anchor biosynthesis (i.e., the transfer of GlcNAc to phosphatidyl inositol) (41,42). The fact that PIG-A is part of an enzyme is in keeping with the fact that PNH mutations are recessive (43).

PIG-A mutations can be demonstrated in the blood cells of the majority of patients with PNH. Failure to find a mutation in the coding region of *PIG-A* in any individual patient is most likely due to technical reasons (44). However, there is a single known exception to the molecular basis of PNH being a *PIG-A* mutation. Yamashina et al. (45) have reported a patient with hemolytic anemia and thrombotic complications who had an isolated deficiency of CD59 but not of other GPI-linked proteins. Both parents had a partial deficiency of CD59, indicating that the patient was homozygous for a CD59 mutation. This patient provides genetic evidence that CD59 deficiency is sufficient to cause the PNH cellular phenotype. It is also still possible that, in rare cases, the PNH phenotype may arise through the mutation of both alleles of an autosomal gene encoding any of the proteins (other than PIG-A) that are required for the GPI biosynthetic pathway. The predominance of *PIG-A* mutations (over hypothetical mutations of such other genes) must be due to the fact that, because *PIG-A* is X-linked, an inactivating mutation (one-hit) directly causes the PNH phenotype.

Hemolysis

Unlike in autoimmune or alloimmune hemolytic anemia when normal red cells are attacked by an antibody, there is no specific antibody involved in PNH, because hemolysis is due to an intrinsic abnormality of the red cell. As a result, PNH red cells hemolyze whenever they are in the presence of activated complement (C), whether it is activated by an antibody (46) (e.g., anti-I, present at low titer in most normal people) or through the alternative pathway; for instance, this is performed *in vitro* by lowering pH, as in the acidified serum test (47), or by lowering ionic strength, as in the once-popular screening test called the *sucrose hemolysis test* (48), which should be probably regarded now as obsolete because it can give both false-positive and false-negative results (49). It took half a century before the biochemical basis for this peculiar hypersusceptibility to C was clarified. We now know that at least two GPI-linked membrane proteins, CD59 and

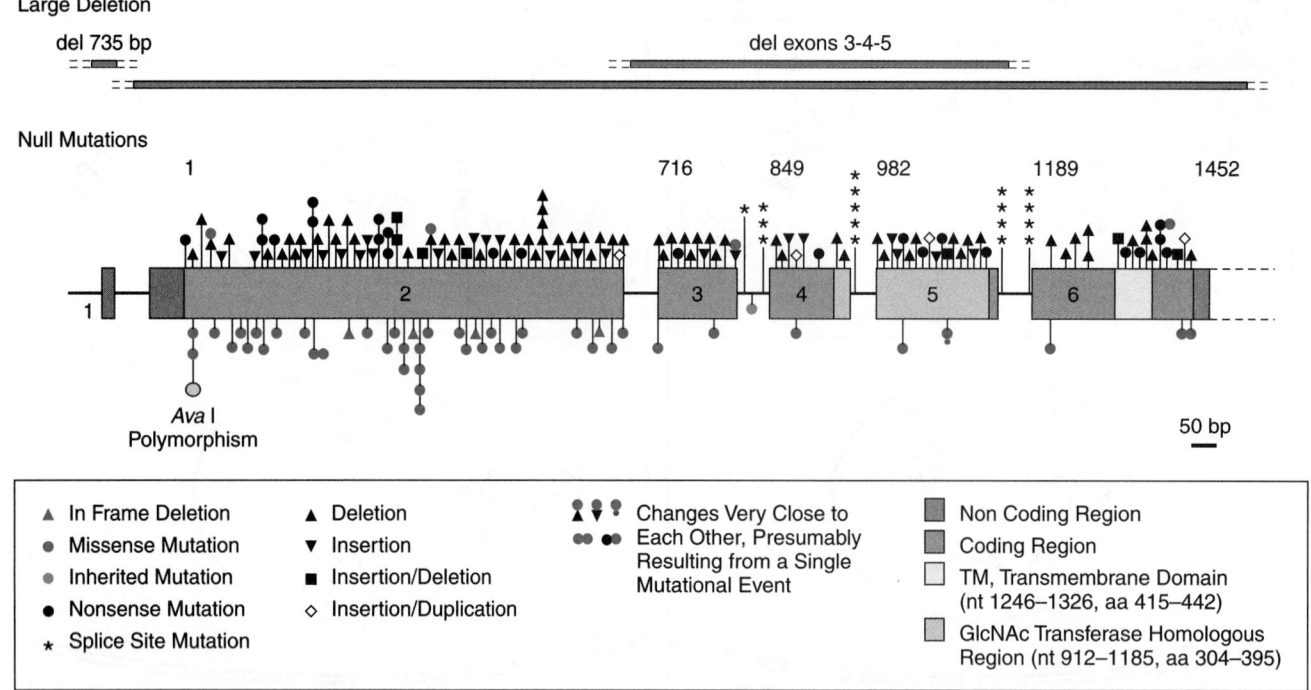

Figure 10-2. Structure of the *PIG-A* gene and mutations in patients with paroxysmal nocturnal hemoglobinuria. The coding region is shown in the form of boxes; introns are shown in the form of dashed lines (not drawn to scale). Nucleotide numbers are shown above the exons. Null mutations (frameshift, nonsense, and splicing) are indicated above the exons. Missense mutations and in-frame deletions are indicated below the exons. Each symbol represents one individual mutation. All mutations are somatic, except for the two shown in light blue. (Adapted from Luzzatto L, Nafa K. Genetics of PNH. In: Young NS, Moss J, eds. *Paroxysmal nocturnal hemoglobinuria and the GPI-linked proteins.* New York: Academic Press, 2000:21–47.)

CD55, protect cells—including normal red cells—against damage from the membrane attack complex of C (C5-C9). These proteins are severely deficient or completely absent from the membrane of PNH red cells (50) (Table 10-1). There is genetic evidence that the most critical of these is CD59 (45), a molecule that has been extensively characterized also in terms of its three-dimensional structure (51). CD59 specifically hinders the insertion into the membrane of C9 polymers (52–54) (Fig. 10-3).

Although the word *paroxysmal* is appropriately incorporated in the very name of PNH, it is important to appreciate that hemolysis is uniformly present: It is only its intensity that varies in time. CD59 deficiency offers a satisfactory explanation for chronic hemolysis in PNH: It also explains why the hemolysis is largely intravascular, and why it can be dramatically exacerbated in the course of a viral or bacterial infection, when antigen-antibody reactions associated with the infection cause bursts of C activation (7).

Thrombosis

Thrombosis is one of the most immediately life-threatening complications of PNH, and yet one of the least understood in its pathogenesis (55). In principle, we can envisage three sorts of mechanisms.

- Impaired fibrinolysis. The urokinase plasminogen activator receptor is a GPI-linked protein, and it is deficient in leukocytes belonging to the PNH clone (56). If leukocytes play a role in endogenous fibrinolysis, PNH leukocytes might be less efficient in this function due to their inability to bind urokinase. In addition, the levels of soluble urokinase plasminogen activator receptor (which may normally help to regulate urokinase activity) are significantly increased in PNH patients (57). This could result in reduced endogenous fibrinolysis. However, we must remember that tissue plasminogen activator is believed to be the main effector of the conversion of plasminogen to plasmin.

- Hypercoagulability. The coagulation cascade and, therefore, ultimately thrombin generation may become activated in PNH. For instance, the C5b-9 complex has been shown to induce release of platelet microparticles that express receptors for factor Va and exhibit prothrombinase (58) and "tenase" activity (59). It also has been held that intravascular hemolysis may release from red cell substances that have thromboplastin activity. However, in a series of 11 PNH patients, no abnormalities were seen in levels of thrombin/antithrombin complexes or in thrombin activation fragment F1.2 (60). We must also admit that thrombosis can occur in PNH patients even when they are fully "anticoagulated" with warfarin or hirudin, both of which would be expected to effectively prevent hypercoagulability through their effects on the "common coagulation pathway." Therefore, activated coagulation per se is not likely to be the main culprit for thrombosis in PNH.

- Hyperactivity of platelets. After treatment with C5b-9, PNH platelets undergo increased vesiculation and thrombin generation (61), and elevated levels of platelet-derived microparticles have been demonstrated in some PNH patients (62). The expression of activation markers is increased on the surface of platelets from PNH patients (60), probably because of abnormal C regulation, which may result in platelet activation (63,64). The lack of CD59 on the PNH platelet could lead to abnormal insertion of the C5b-9 complex in the platelet membrane, as is the case with the red cell.

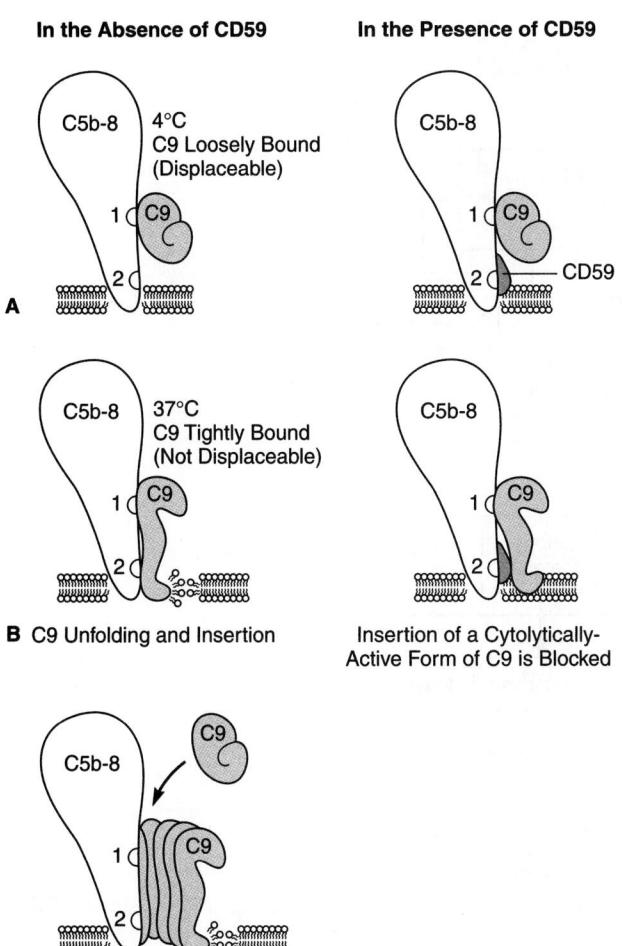

In the Absence of CD59 **In the Presence of CD59**

C5b-8 4°C / C9 Loosely Bound (Displaceable)

A

C5b-8 37°C / C9 Tightly Bound (Not Displaceable)

B C9 Unfolding and Insertion

Insertion of a Cytolytically-Active Form of C9 is Blocked

C Poly-C9

Figure 10-3. Role of CD59 in protecting red cells from the lytic action of complement (C). In this cartoon, the ovoidal body labeled C5b-8 represents the membrane attack complex, the final product that is formed when C is activated, whether through the classic or alternative activation pathway. As the first step in the lytic effector pathway (**A, right**), C5b-8 recruits a C9 monomer. The second step (**B, right**), the insertion of C9 into the lipid bilayer of the membrane, is now hindered by CD59, by virtue of the extracellular position of CD59, made possible by its glycosyl phosphatidyl inositol–linked structure. On the left, by contrast, the C9 monomer stretches into the lipid bilayer in the absence of CD59; this is followed by C9 polymerization (**C**), which produces real holes in the membrane, through which hemoglobin exits, ending up in complete lysis of the red cell. [Adapted from Meri S, Morgan BP, Davies A, et al. Human protectin (CD59), an 18,000–20,000 MW complement lysis restricting factor, inhibits C5b-8 catalysed insertion of C9 into lipid bilayers. *Immunology* 1990;71:1–9.]

Although all of these three factors may play a role in producing a thrombophilic state in PNH, it seems likely that the primary cause lies in the PNH platelets, which are abnormal precisely because they belong to the PNH clone. This theory is supported by the occurrence of cerebral infarction in a patient who did not have PNH but did have congenital CD59 deficiency and chronic hemolysis (65).

Bone Marrow Failure

The phrase *bone marrow failure* describes the functional consequence of aplastic anemia (AA), and there is a close association between PNH and AA. Patients with PNH and a hypoplastic marrow have been long referred to as having the "PNH-aplastic anemia syndrome" (66). Sometimes, patients with PNH become

increasingly pancytopenic and, in the end, have a clinical picture very similar to AA (67). More recently, PNH has been recognized with increasing frequency in patients with an original diagnosis of AA—whether or not they have been treated with antithymocyte globulin (ATG) (or antilymphocyte globulin) (68–74). Thus, an element of bone marrow failure (BMF) is probably present in all cases of PNH (75), and this may reflect a shared pathogenetic basis (76) (Fig. 10-4). AA is essentially an organ-specific autoimmune disease (77,78). In the peripheral blood and in the bone marrow of patients with AA, it is possible to find increased numbers of "activated" CD8+ T lymphocytes, which are able to inhibit the growth *in vitro* of both autologous and HLA-identical hematopoietic colonies (79). T lymphocytes might be implicated in causing AA in two ways. On one hand, by secreting interferon-γ (80,81) and tumor necrosis factor-α (82,83), they cause induction of Fas expression on CD34+ cells (84). On the other hand, cytotoxic T lymphocytes may ultimately cause apoptosis through Fas-FasL interaction (85) (although this sequence of events has not yet been conclusively demonstrated), leading to depletion of HSCs. The putative autoantigen that incites and serves as a target of the autoreactive cytotoxic T lymphocytes is not known. The strongest time-honored evidence for the immune basis of AA is that the majority of patients respond to immunosuppressive treatment (86–88). Recently, skewing of the T-cell receptor repertoire has been demonstrated in a subset of patients with AA by immunoscope analysis (89), and a detailed study conducted by the same approach has shown that one or several expanded T-cell clones are present in PNH patients three times more frequently than in control subjects (90) (Fig. 10-5).

Modeling the Pathogenesis of Paroxysmal Nocturnal Hemoglobinuria

Although PNH has elements of BMF, it is obviously different from AA because of its other prominent clinical features (hemolysis and thrombosis). One possible way to look at the pathophysiology of PNH is that it results precisely from the coexistence of BMF with a large *PIG-A* mutant clone (91). To explain the coexistence of these two components, we can surmise in principle three possibilities: (a) The PNH clone and BMF coexist by a sheer coincidence; (b) the PNH clone causes BMF; or (c) BMF favors the development or the expansion of the PNH clone (76). Because AA and PNH are both rare diseases, the first possibility can be discarded on statistical grounds as being too improbable. The second possibility is unlikely, because PNH often develops in patients originally experiencing AA, who, therefore, already had established BMF at a time when no PNH clone could be demonstrated. Thus, the third possibility seems the most likely, and it has recently obtained support through experimental findings in mice, as well as observations in humans (92).

Consequences of *PIG-A* Inactivation in Mice

By using the technique of conditional "knock-out," two groups have recently succeeded in producing mice that can be regarded as true models for human PNH (93,94). Indeed, the mice have two discrete populations of red cells, granulocytes, monocytes, and lymphocytes; in first approximation, the flow cytometry patterns are remarkably similar to those seen in patients with PNH. In addition, although the mice are not anemic, they do have evidence of hemolysis, and their red cells have increased susceptibility to C, with a positive Ham test (data on platelets and thrombosis are not yet available). Interestingly, the clinical course of the mice is very benign, and the proportion of PNH cells is remarkably stable, although these mice are born with a large

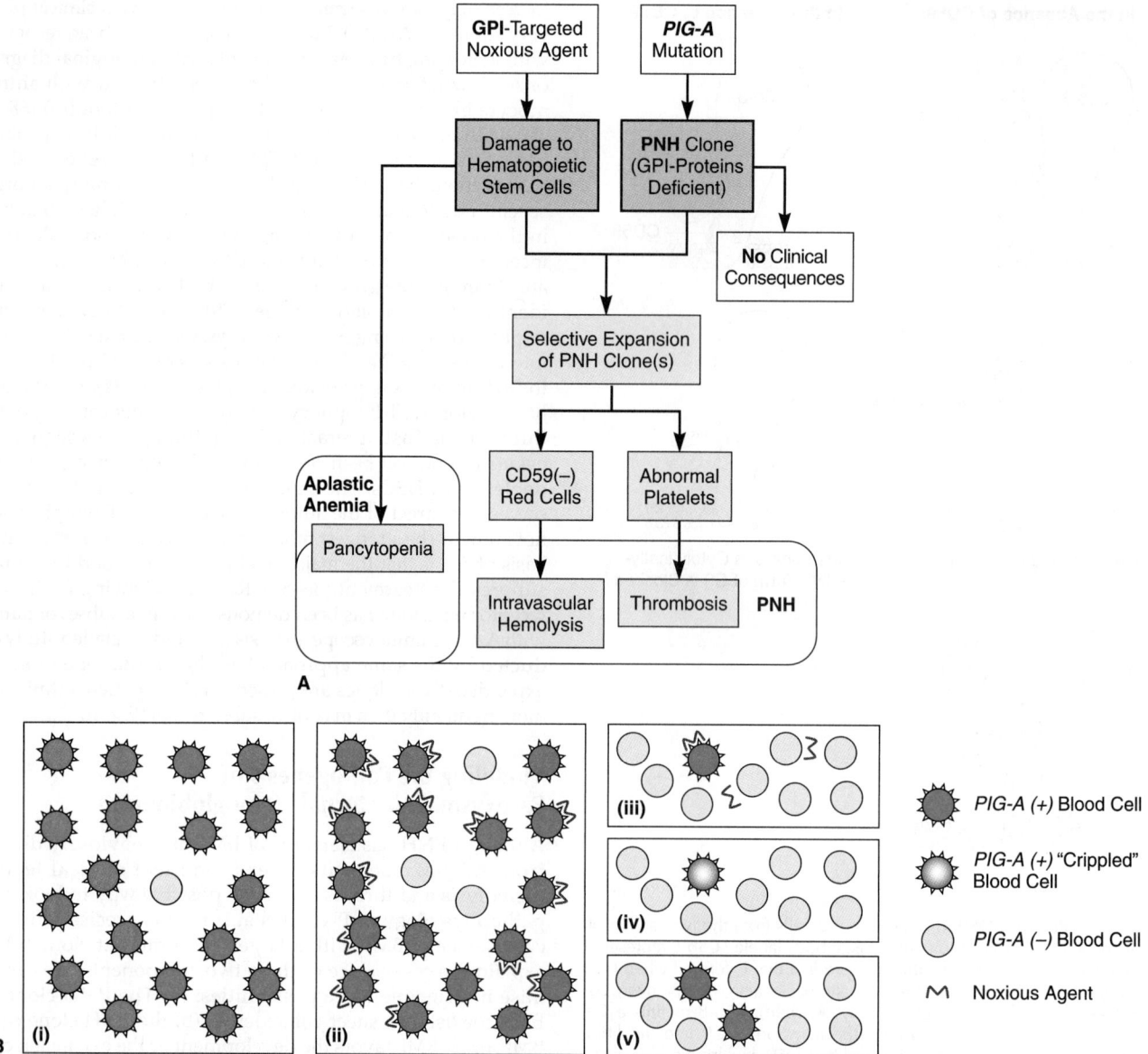

Figure 10-4. The dual pathogenesis of paroxysmal nocturnal hemoglobinuria (PNH). **A:** Two separate causal factors cooperate to produce the clinical picture of PNH. On one hand (*top right*), a *PIG-A* mutation produces a mutant clone, but this does not cause any clinical consequence per se. On the other hand (*top left*), a noxious agent that damages hematopoietic stem cells can cause aplastic anemia. If both events occur in the same patient—that is, a noxious agent damages only glycosyl phosphatidyl inositol (GPI)+ cells, and a GPI– clone exists as a result of a *PIG-A* mutation—then the clone selectively expands and causes PNH. Thus, of the PNH triad, pancytopenia is explained by the damage to hematopoietic stem cells; intravascular hemolysis and thrombosis result from the surface abnormalities of the PNH cells. **B:** The best candidate as a noxious agent that may have the ability to discriminate between GPI+ and GPI– cells is a set of autoreactive T cells that target a GPI-containing molecule. The left-hand panel (*i*) represents a normal bone marrow with a rare GPI– cell. The top right panel (*ii*) illustrates the process of selection. The three right-hand panels illustrate full-blown PNH; in (*iii*), the damage is still ongoing; in (*iv*), the damage has been done, and the remaining non-PNH stem cells are not competent for regenerating normal hematopoiesis; in (*v*), the damage is finished, and there are enough normal stem cells left to regenerate normal hematopoiesis. This last situation may underlie the spontaneous recovery that is seen in some patients after a long course of the disease.

number of preformed PNH cells (95). In humans, by contrast, before giving the clinical picture of PNH, the PNH cell population must have undergone substantial expansion, because it arises from a single mutant stem cell (95). Thus, these mice with *pig-a* mutant cells indeed have PNH cells, but they do not have clinical PNH; one possible reason is that they lack BMF, supporting the theory that this second factor, in addition to a *PIG-A* mutation, is needed to produce the human disease PNH.

Paroxysmal Nocturnal Hemoglobinuria Microclones in Humans and Clonal Selection

We have already mentioned that PNH III and PNH II can coexist in the same patient (38); indeed, by mutation analysis, it is not infrequent to find two or more clones in the same patient (9,44,96–99). In addition, small PNH clones have been detected in up to 50% of cases of bona fide AA (100). These findings are

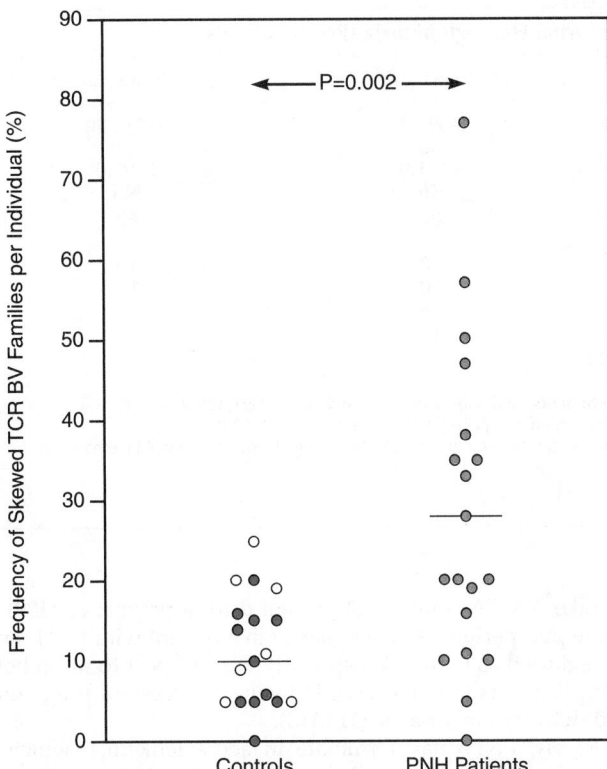

Figure 10-5. Evidence for abnormalities of the T-cell repertoire in paroxysmal nocturnal hemoglobinuria (PNH). Lymphocytes from PNH patients were subjected to "immunoscope" analysis, which consists in displaying the size distribution of the CDR3 region of the β-chain of the T-cell receptor (TCR) for each of the 24 β TCR families. The frequency of skewing in the distribution is much higher in PNH patients than in a control group consisting of normal subjects (*filled circles*) and of hemoglobinopathy patients who had received multiple blood transfusions (*empty circles*). BV, beta variable chain. (Reprinted from Karadimitris A, Manavalan JS, Thaler HT, et al. Abnormal T-cell repertoire is consistent with immune process underlying the pathogenesis of paroxysmal nocturnal hemoglobinuria. *Blood* 2000;96:2613–2620.)

strongly suggestive of the theory that these clones expand, simultaneously or in sequence, in response to a certain selective agent present in the patient's bone marrow environment. On the other hand, one can ask the complementary question: Is there evidence for PNH clones in normal people, and what is the fate of such clones? It has been shown recently that very small populations of PNH granulocytes and PNH erythrocytes are present in normal people, and these are probably generated simply by the "background" level of somatic mutations in the *PIG-A* gene (101). As in patients with PNH, missense, frameshifts, and nonsense mutations have been identified. Thus, *PIG-A* gene mutations are not sufficient for the development of PNH (101). The fact that these tiny PNH cell populations—which we could call *microclones*—do not expand clearly means that they do not have any growth advantage on their own. At the same time, this fact suggests that in PNH patients the same sort of clones may have expanded because an abnormal marrow environment gave them a relative advantage in growth or survival. We have suggested that the abnormal environment is produced by autoreactive T cells (90,102), and, recently, this theory has been corroborated by the finding of a unique association of T-cell large granular lymphocytic leukemia and PNH (103). In this condition, there is an expansion of natural killer–like T cells; interestingly, in mice, two proteins that bind to the NKG2D receptor of natural killer cells, REA-1 and H-60, are GPI-linked; it has been suggested that, by virtue of their absence from PNH

stem cells, these may escape from immune destruction (20). In addition, in PNH patients, non-PNH stem cells have a much higher level of Fas than PNH stem cells (104). Thus, non-PNH stem cells have a high rate of apoptosis and, therefore, are selectively destroyed under conditions in which there is an excess of Fas ligand.

Summary of Pathogenesis

Based on the above and other evidence (105,106), it is possible to formulate a coherent model for the pathogenesis of PNH (20,76,92) (Fig. 10-4), which explains at least most of its clinical and hematologic features, as follows.

1. PNH always coexists with BMF.
2. BMF is clinically obvious in patients who initially present with AA and then develop PNH. In patients who initially present with PNH, BMF may not be obvious because by the time of diagnosis, the PNH clone has expanded to the point where it provides a substantial proportion of the patient's hematopoiesis.
3. The PNH clone has a long but probably finite lifespan. If, by the time the PNH clone is exhausted, BMF has not recovered, the patient evolves clinically from PNH to AA. If, by the time the PNH clone is exhausted, BMF has recovered, the patient is "cured" of PNH.
4. A PNH clone arises through a *PIG-A* mutation in an HSC. Because there is only one active X-chromosome in each HSC, the mutated stem cell and its progeny acquire the PNH phenotype, and this can happen in any normal person. Cells with the PNH phenotype have no intrinsic growth advantage, and, therefore, PNH clones do not normally expand. As long as there is no BMF, clinical PNH does not develop.
5. The existence of a florid PNH clone while the rest of hematopoiesis is depressed suggests that the PNH clone can be spared selectively from the injury affecting the rest of the bone marrow.
6. To explain the previous point, we may surmise specifically that the damage to stem cells causing BMF is mediated through a GPI-linked surface molecule (102); in this case, the PNH cells lacking these molecules survive.
7. Thus, the very defect of the PNH clone may endow it with a relative survival or growth advantage in a patient with BMF. If the patient has such a clone, he or she presents with PNH; otherwise, he or she would present with overt AA. Thus, the development of PNH is conditional on a background of BMF.
8. A large PNH clone carries with it intravascular hemolysis and thrombosis—the "classic" manifestations of PNH.

CLINICAL FEATURES

The most common initial complaints in PNH are loss of energy and fatigue. In fact, anemia is a presenting feature in almost all cases (107): It may be from mild to very severe. Hemoglobinuria is reported on presentation by the patient's own initiative in only a minority of patients (Table 10-2); however, if specific questions are asked, or if serial urine specimens are collected and inspected, hemoglobinuria can be documented at some time in virtually all patients.

The most common physical findings in a patient with PNH in the steady state are pallor and jaundice; because hemolysis is largely intravascular, clinical jaundice is usually mild and may be absent. Particular attention ought to be devoted to examination of the abdomen: Tenderness may be elicited particularly by gentle to deep palpation, usually on the midline, more often above

TABLE 10-2. Clinical Features of Paroxysmal Nocturnal Hemoglobinuria (PNH) Patients

	Duke[a]	Hammersmith[b]	French Study Group[c]
Age (yr), range (mean)	3–21 (13)	16–75 (42)	6–82 (33)
Number of patients	26	80	220
Gender (female/male)	1/1	1.4/1.0	1.2/1.0
Hemoglobinuria at presentation (%)	15	26	NA
Neutropenia and/or thrombocytopenia at presentation (%)	73	80	60
Evidence of thrombosis at presentation (%)	12	18	19
Overall survival (yr)[d]	13.5	10	14.5
Aplastic anemia preceding PNH (%)	37	29	30
Spontaneous long-term remission (%)	0	15	NA

NA, not available.
[a]Data from Ware RE, Hall SE, Rosse WF. Paroxysmal nocturnal hemoglobinuria with onset in childhood and adolescence. *N Engl J Med* 1991;325:991–996.
[b]Data from Hillmen P, Lewis SM, Bessler M, et al. Natural history of paroxysmal nocturnal hemoglobinuria. *N Engl J Med* 1995;333:1253–1258.
[c]Data from Socie G, Mary JY, de Gramont A, et al. Paroxysmal nocturnal haemoglobinuria: long-term follow-up and prognostic factors. French Society of Haematology. *Lancet* 1996;348:573–577.
[d]Median overall survival estimated according to Kaplan-Meier.

than below the umbilicus. Most patients with PNH do not have hepatomegaly or splenomegaly: When the former is observed, it is highly indicative of hepatic vein thrombosis (Budd-Chiari syndrome); when the latter is observed, it is indicative of portal vein or splenic vein thrombosis. In a patient with Budd-Chiari syndrome, there may be also evidence of ascites. On questioning, it is not unusual to elicit a history of attacks of abdominal pain, which may last from hours to several days and may be associated with either diarrhea or constipation and, perhaps, with more intense hemoglobinuria. Recurrent dysphagia may also occur. In male patients, it may be appropriate to inquire about sexual activity, because erectile dysfunction may occur and may be a source of distress. Not infrequently, the anemia is associated with other cytopenias (Table 10-2). Therefore, the patient may report heavy menses, nosebleeds, or other hemorrhagic manifestations, and the patient may present with petechiae or with signs of infection.

Course and Complications

The natural history of PNH is that of a very chronic disorder, which may afflict the patient continuously for decades. Without treatment, the median survival is estimated to be approximately 10 years (67); in the past, the most common causes of death have been thrombosis or hemorrhage associated with severe thrombocytopenia. Sometimes, a PNH patient may become less hemolytic and more pancytopenic: This situation has been referred to as *spent PNH*; in practice, the patient has converted from PNH to AA. On the other hand, full spontaneous recovery from PNH has been documented (67).

Whether thrombosis is regarded as a complication or as part of the disease is a matter of semantics; it is estimated that [in the West as opposed to the Far East (55)], its cumulative frequency in PNH may be approximately 30% (55,108). The abdominal veins are by far the most common site, whereas deep vein thrombosis in the limbs is not very common. The most classic site is in the hepatic veins, causing Budd-Chiari syndrome, but the mesenteric vessels, the splenic vein, the portal vein, the renal veins, and the inferior vena cava may be also involved. Recurrent episodes of portal vein thrombosis may lead eventually to cavernous transformation of the portal vein or to portal hypertension, or both: This causes gastroesophageal varices, congestive splenomegaly, and, sometimes, hypersplenism, which may contribute to cytopenias. Next to abdominal veins, cranial veins rank second in terms of frequency of thrombosis: This can produce stroke. By contrast, arterial thrombosis is rare (Fig. 10-6).

Like AA, PNH may first present during pregnancy (109) or in the puerperium. Any pregnancy in a patient with PNH must be regarded as high risk, especially with respect to thrombotic complications (108,110,111). However, successful pregnancy and delivery are possible (112,113).

Rarely, PNH may terminate in acute leukemia, which is always acute myelogenous leukemia (AML). Although there is a significant literature on this ominous complication, it consists almost entirely of individual case reports. Therefore, the impression that this is a common event has been strongly influenced by a bias in publishing "interesting associations"; in fact, the risk of AML in PNH—although higher than in the general population—is probably less than 2% (114). Because PNH is a clonal disorder, one might presume that the transformation of PNH to AML is a good example of clonal evolution, and in some cases, this has been proved (115,116). However, in other cases, AML did not arise from within the PNH clone (114,117). Because AML can also emerge from AA, both PNH and AA must be regarded as conditions that are, although rarely, preleukemic. It appears that AML, for reasons on which we can for the

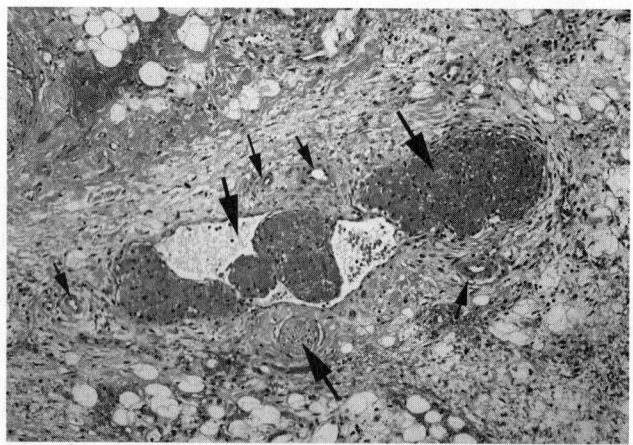

Figure 10-6. Histologic section from the large intestine of a 14-year-old girl who developed an acute abdomen and underwent resection of a portion of the descending colon, which had become necrotic after acute infarction. There is thrombus in practically all veins visible in the section (*thick arrows*). By contrast, arteries were unaffected (*thin arrows*). The patient had a history of anemia, thrombocytopenia, and jaundice, but the diagnosis of paroxysmal nocturnal hemoglobinuria was only made after this life-threatening episode.

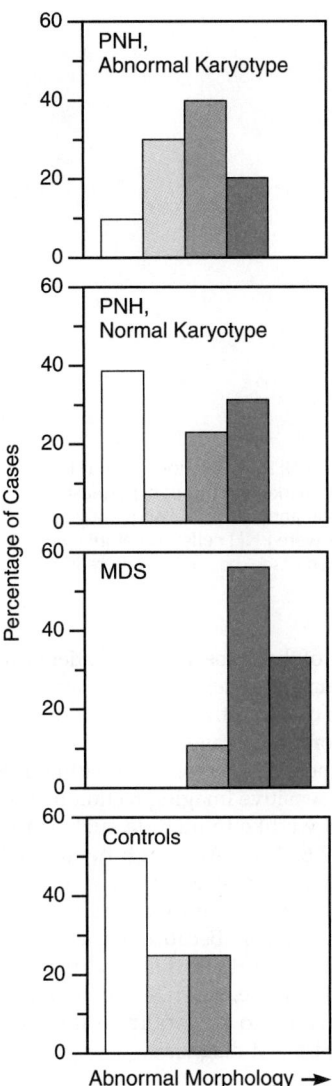

Figure 10-7. Morphologic abnormalities in the bone marrow of paroxysmal nocturnal hemoglobinuria (PNH) patients. Compared to normal controls, PNH patients have a significantly higher proportion of the type of changes that are currently classified as *myelodysplastic syndrome* (MDS): These changes are present, by definition, in all MDS patients. There is no significant difference in the extent of MDS changes in the marrows of PNH patients who also have clonal karyotypic abnormalities compared to PNH patients who do not have karyotypic abnormalities. These findings suggest that (a) these morphologic changes are part of PNH, and they do not justify an added diagnosis of MDS, and (b) the presence of a clonal karyotypic abnormality does not necessarily indicate a more ominous prognosis. (Modified from Araten DJ, Swirsky D, Karadimitris A, et al. Cytogenetic and morphological abnormalities in paroxysmal nocturnal haemoglobinuria. *Br J Haematol* 2001;115:360–368.)

moment only speculate, is more likely to develop in the damaged bone marrow that both conditions share (118,119).

Laboratory Investigations, Diagnosis, and Differential Diagnosis

The blood count shows, by definition, an anemia that may be mild to very severe and is associated with relative and usually absolute reticulocytosis. The blood smear may show anisocytosis; sometimes, the PNH red cell population is so much younger than the non-PNH red cell population that a bimodal size distribution may catch the eye (and may be obvious on the electronic

display). The mean corpuscular volume (MCV) is almost always elevated, in part on account of reticulocytosis; a normal MCV must raise the suspicion of superimposed iron deficiency. By contrast, poikilocytosis is conspicuous by its scarcity, especially by comparison to other hemolytic anemias (except, once again, if the patient has a superimposed iron deficiency). The neutrophils may range from normal to below 1000; the platelets may range from normal to below 20,000; the lymphocytes are usually normal, but there may be an increase in large granular lymphocytes. The bilirubin level is usually only moderately increased, in striking contrast to the lactic dehydrogenase level, which is often in the thousands, while haptoglobin is markedly decreased. It is desirable to include in the workup an assessment of the folic acid and iron status; with respect to the latter, it is better to rely on the transferrin saturation index than on the serum ferritin, because the latter may be spuriously elevated, thus masking iron deficiency. A bone marrow aspirate usually yields a cellular marrow with erythroid hyperplasia, which may be very marked. Not only the erythroid elements, but also those of other lineages (particularly megakaryocytes) may show morphologic abnormalities commonly referred to as the *myelodysplastic syndrome* (MDS) (Fig. 10-7). In fact, it has been reported recently that "MDS changes" in PNH are the rule rather than the exception (120), and, therefore, this finding must not be misconstrued as requiring a change of diagnosis. The eosinophils are normal, whereas basophils may be unusually prominent. The bone marrow trephine invariably confirms erythroid hyperplasia (Fig. 10-8A), but it proves often to be less cellular than might have been expected from the aspirate.

In most cases, the patient presents as a problem in the differential diagnosis of anemia, whether symptomatic or discovered incidentally (121). When a patient, who is otherwise well, reports noticing on waking up one morning that his or her urine was dark like Coca-Cola, it is difficult *not* to think of PNH. However, the patient may not notice or may not report this telltale sign and may simply complain of tiredness, or he or she may present with purpura or infection, thus leading us into a range of differential diagnosis. The combination that is most characteristic of PNH is the simultaneous presence of hemolysis and BMF; thus, a high reticulocytosis may stand out against the context of thrombocytopenia or neutropenia, or both. Once the suspicion of PNH is entertained, and if hemoglobinuria is demonstrated,* the differential diagnosis becomes drastically restricted from the array of all hemolytic anemias to the small number of those hemolytic anemias in which hemolysis is largely intravascular (Table 10-3). In the end, the diagnosis is clinched by using either the acidified serum test (Ham test) (122–124) or flow cytometry (19).

The Ham test is a time-honored method on which the diagnosis of PNH has relied for approximately half a century; it has been used mostly only as a qualitative test, but, when carried out carefully, it can produce also an accurate quantitation of the size of the PNH red cell population (49). Provided the controls are in order (these should include red cells from a patient with known PNH), the Ham test is very robust: There are no false-negative results. There are only two situations that may give rise to false-positive results. First, in congenital dyserythropoietic anemia type II, the Ham test is, by definition, positive—but only with a proportion of donor sera [those that contain "anti-HEMPAS" (*h*ereditary *e*rythroblastic *m*ultinuclearity with *p*ositive *a*cidified *s*erum)] and *not* with the patient's serum (125). Therefore, including an autologous serum control safeguards

---

*The differentiation between hematuria and hemoglobinuria may seem trivial; nevertheless, we have seen patients who have had extensive urologic investigations because the latter had been assumed to be the former.

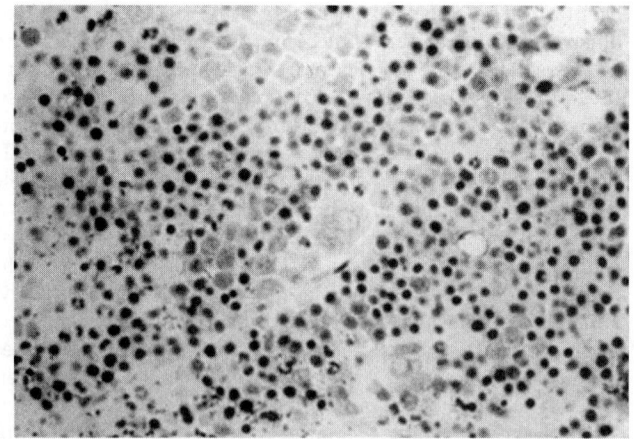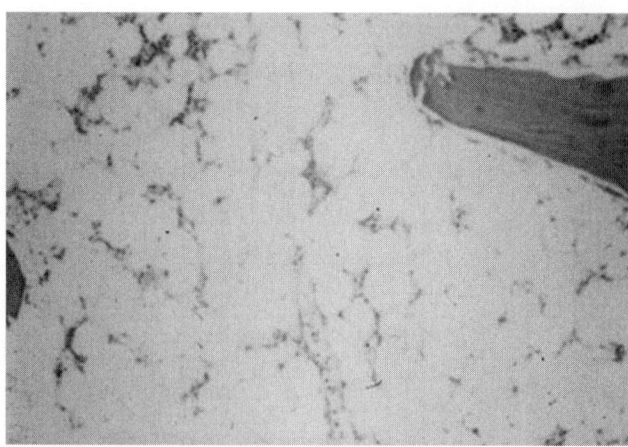

A   B

Figure 10-8. The bone marrow in paroxysmal nocturnal hemoglobinuria (PNH). **A:** Section from a 39-year-old man with florid hemolytic PNH, showing increased cellularity and marked erythroid hyperplasia. **B:** Section from a 30-year-old woman, initially diagnosed as having aplastic anemia but subsequently as having PNH. Note that in the patient in **(A)** approximately 95% of the cells were PNH cells. Therefore, we must realize that the non-PNH hematopoiesis is not very different in the two cases (i.e., in both there is a severe failure of normal hematopoiesis). (Courtesy of Dr. David Araten.)

against this rare possibility. Second, if the patient's red cells are already coated with an antibody, this may be lytic in the presence of C. Therefore, a direct Coombs' test ought to be carried out always parallel to a Ham test; when the former is positive, the latter becomes unreliable (and the likely diagnosis is autoimmune hemolytic anemia rather than PNH).

The introduction of flow cytometry has changed the picture considerably. A great asset of this technique is that it has made quantitation easier (19,126), as long as good antibodies and good controls are included and the gates are appropriately placed (Fig. 10-9). In addition, PNH II and PNH III cells can be well resolved (Fig. 10-9B). When flow cytometry data obtained with anti-CD59 are compared with Ham test data, the agreement is good with respect to PNH III red cells, whereas PNH II red cells are underestimated by the Ham test (49). Another consequence of the widespread use of flow cytometry is that it has increased the pickup rate of small PNH cell populations, which could have been missed (or dismissed as "background noise") when using the Ham test (127). A third advantage of flow cytometry is that one can test different cell types easily (Fig. 10-9A). In practice, quantitation of PNH red cells is most relevant to the rate of hemolysis, but it underestimates the size of the PNH clone, and the data are not meaningful after recent blood transfusion; quantitation of PNH granulocytes may be too sensitive (see below), but it provides a more reliable estimate of the size of PNH hematopoiesis, and it is not significantly influenced by blood transfusion (126).

Finally, one must be aware that sometimes the first presentation of PNH may be with signs and symptoms of thrombosis in a

deep vein in one of the limbs; in other patients, the first presentation may be recurrent attacks of severe abdominal pain, which may prove to be due to intraabdominal thrombosis; sometimes, there is already organ damage from previous thrombosis (in our experience, magnetic resonance venography (MRV) of the abdomen is the most sensitive imaging technique for abdominal vein thrombosis, and we like to include such a study as a baseline investigation) (7,67,128). Although hemoglobinuria does not cause renal damage per se, an attack of massive intravascular hemolysis may be associated with acute renal failure due to hypoxia and hypotension. Because of this potential multitude of clinical presentations of PNH, this condition has been called *the great impostor*. In practice, it is not uncommon to find that there has been a delay of 1 to 2 years from the onset of significant symptoms to the time of diagnosis.

Classification of Paroxysmal Nocturnal Hemoglobinuria

Although in principle the increased sensitivity of flow cytometry can be only an advantage, it does raise new questions; for instance, if a person has 9% PNH granulocytes and 2% PNH red cells, does that person have PNH? The question is of more than semantic importance, because these values are certainly abnormal (i.e., this person does have an expanded PNH clone). On the other hand, it is very unlikely that this person has a measurable increase in the rate of hemolysis, much less in hemoglobinuria; therefore, it does not seem reasonable or useful to label that person as having PNH. In practice, this issue is most likely

TABLE 10-3. Differential Diagnosis of Dark Urine

Different Sorts of Dark Urine	Causes	Additional Tests	Possible Diagnosis
Hematuria	Many	Clears on centrifugation	Mostly urinary tract pathology
Myoglobinuria	Rhabdomyolysis	Ultrafiltration; spectroscopy	March myoglobinuria
Hemoglobinuria	Intravascular hemolysis	Serology after blood transfusion	Incompatible blood transfusion
		Donath-Landsteiner antibody	Paroxysmal cold hemoglobinuria
		G6PD activity	G6PD deficiency
		Blood film for malaria parasites	"Blackwater fever"
		Ham; flow cytometry for CD59	Paroxysmal nocturnal hemoglobinuria

G6PD, glucose-6-phosphate dehydrogenase.

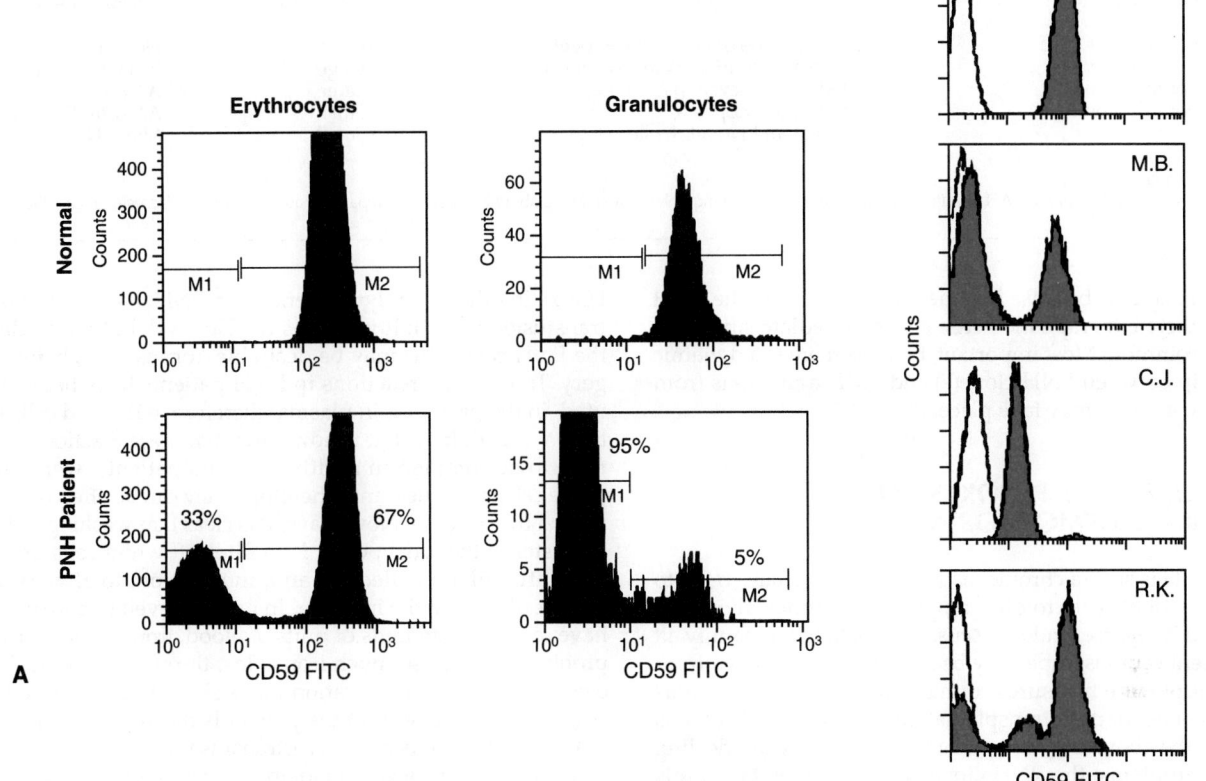

Figure 10-9. A: Flow cytometry analysis for the diagnosis of paroxysmal nocturnal hemoglobinuria (PNH). Normal blood cells (*top panels*) display a unimodal distribution when stained with anti-CD59. Blood cells from a PNH patient (*bottom panels*) display a bimodal distribution, from which the size of the PNH cell population is directly measured. Beware of flow cytometry reports that tend to list positive cells rather than negative cells. In the case of PNH, it is the negative cells that matter, and cells must not be classified as negative on the basis of an arbitrary cutoff point: It is the bimodal distribution that is diagnostic of PNH. The granulocyte histograms are more ragged simply because fewer events have been accumulated (the patient was actually neutropenic). Note that the normal cells in the PNH patient have the same fluorescence intensity as in the normal control. Characteristically, the proportion of PNH cells is much larger among granulocytes than among red cells (in this case, 95% and 33%, respectively). This difference is mainly due to the fact that PNH red cells have a much shorter survival time than normal red cells (12), and, therefore, they are underrepresented in peripheral blood compared to when they are released from the bone marrow. By contrast, there is no difference in survival between PNH granulocytes and normal granulocytes; therefore, the percentage of PNH granulocytes gives a much more accurate estimate of the proportion of hematopoiesis that stems from the PNH clone(s). **B:** Different patterns of PNH red cell populations in several PNH patients. The top panel is from a normal person. Patient M.B. has 57% red cells that lack CD59 completely (PNH III red cells). Patient C.J. has only 4% normal red cells: 96% of her red cells have a partial deficiency of CD59 (PNH II red cells), indicating that virtually her entire hematopoiesis is supported by a PNH clone with a missense mutation of *PIG-A*. In patient R.K., we see a trimodal distribution, indicating the coexistence, with normal red cells, of a PNH III clone (22%) and a PNH II clone (12%). In each panel, the isotypic negative control is shown in white. [Modified from Dacie JV, Lewis SM, Luzzatto L, et al. Laboratory methods used in the investigation of paroxysmal nocturnal haemoglobinuria (PNH). In: Dacie JV, Lewis SM, eds. *Practical haematology*, 8th ed. London: Churchill Livingstone, 1995:287–296.]

to come up in patients with AA who are tested by flow cytometry either as part of their initial diagnostic workup or during their follow-up [e.g., after treatment with antilymphocyte globulin (ATG) or other agents]. In our opinion, no useful purpose is served by changing the diagnosis from AA to PNH because a small PNH clone is present. One might wish to call this *lab PNH*, but if the patient is still pancytopenic, he or she needs to be treated for AA; the management may need to be different only if the patient develops *clinical* PNH. How well do these concepts fit the clinical reality of patients with PNH? This can be tested by considering, in each patient, the relative roles of the PNH clone(s) and of BMF in determining the clinical picture

(Table 10-4). At one end of the spectrum, we may find a patient in whom the PNH clone is so large that it masks BMF (almost) completely. The patient has signs and symptoms of brisk hemolysis and may have serious thrombotic complications but, apart from the anemia, the peripheral blood count is normal or near normal: The patient can be said to have "florid PNH." At the other end of the spectrum, we may find a patient who meets all criteria for severe AA and who is found (by sensitive analytic techniques) to also have a small proportion of GPI-negative cells in the blood. In such a patient, the presence of the PNH clone is not likely to significantly affect the clinical course, and, therefore, we prefer to designate the patient as having "AA

TABLE 10-4. Paroxysmal Nocturnal Hemoglobinuria (PNH): Clinical Heterogeneity and Proposed Terminology

Predominant Clinical Features	Blood Findings	Size of PNH Clone	Designation
Hemolysis ± thrombosis	Anemia; little or no other cytopenia	Large	Florid PNH
Hemolysis ± thrombosis	Anemia; mild to moderate other cytopenia(s)	Large	PNH, hypoplastic
Purpura and/or infection	Moderate to severe pancytopenia	Large	AA/PNH
Purpura and/or infection	Severe pancytopenia	Small	AA with PNH clone
Thrombosis	Normal; mild to moderate cytopenia(s)	Small	Mini-PNH

AA, aplastic anemia.
Adapted from Tremml G, Karadimitris A, Luzzatto L. Paroxysmal nocturnal hemoglobinuria: learning about PNH cells from patients and from mice. *Haematologica* 1998;1:12–20.

with a PNH clone," because it is the BMF rather than the PNH that must dictate therapeutic decisions. Intermediate situations are not uncommon. Most important, because there is a dynamic relationship between PNH clone(s) and BMF, transitions from one form to another may take place.

MANAGEMENT OF PAROXYSMAL NOCTURNAL HEMOGLOBINURIA

Because PNH is such a chronic disorder, it is important to get to know the patient well, to offer ample explanations about the disease and its course, and to discuss with patient and family all management options, especially because these may range from simple supportive measures to major interventions, such as allogeneic bone marrow transplantation (BMT) (Fig. 10-10). It is clear from the above that in a patient with PNH we are dealing with two problems: the PNH clone and BMF; inevitably, this must affect our approach to treatment (Fig. 10-4). Indeed, in first approximation, the management of patients we have called *AA with a PNH clone* does not differ significantly from that of patients with straightforward AA. By contrast, patients with "florid PNH" may present unique clinical problems, mainly massive hemolytic attacks and serious thrombotic complications. For these patients, the two extreme choices are radical treatment by BMT or supportive treatment only (of which red cell transfusions must often be a major component).

Supportive Treatment

Because in PNH there is a marked increase in erythropoiesis, folic acid supplementation (at least 3 mg/day) is mandatory throughout. Iron administration is indicated whenever the patient is severely anemic and iron deficient. Although time-honored anecdotes [dating back to Strübing in 1882! (129)] claim that iron administration can exacerbate hemolysis, this has never been documented; at any rate, we have seen hemoglobin (Hb) increments of up to 2 g/dL on iron repletion in PNH patients.

The use of blood transfusion is very important. As in every patient with anemia, it is not possible or desirable to set an arbitrary Hb level for administering transfusion; the decision must be based not only on that level, but also on other parameters: (a) rate of fall since the previous blood count, (b) objective clinical assessment, (c) subjective state of the patient, and (d) degree of physical exertion that is demanded by the patient to find the quality of life acceptable. In general, because of its chronic nature, the anemia in PNH is well tolerated. In the authors' experience, the variable degree of tolerance is epitomized at one extreme by a patient who plans his blood transfusions in relation to his performance in tennis singles and kayaking with his children and at the other extreme by a patient who declined postponing his skiing holiday when his Hb level was 6.2.

Unlike in other hemolytic anemias, in PNH, the effect of blood transfusion is dual: It increases the Hb level, but it also dilutes the PNH cells. This may be desirable, for instance, before surgery. Transfusion reactions in PNH patients have been attributed, in the past, to C in plasma; therefore, red blood cells used to be washed. In fact, it is now clear that these reactions, which used to be common in multitransfused patients, were due to white cell antibodies, and, therefore, they can be effectively prevented by filtration. Nowadays, it is clear that washing red cells is wasteful; the ideal policy is to filter off white cells immediately after blood collection and, in addition, to always use a white cell filter in the infusion. In general, even in patients who have received hundreds of units of blood, iron overload is not a problem, because so much iron is lost through the urine. However, the transferrin saturation index should be monitored; if it rises, it means either that the patient is turning from PNH into AA, or the patient is being overtransfused.

Erythropoietin levels tend to be very high in PNH (130); therefore, one would not expect it to be of help. However, there

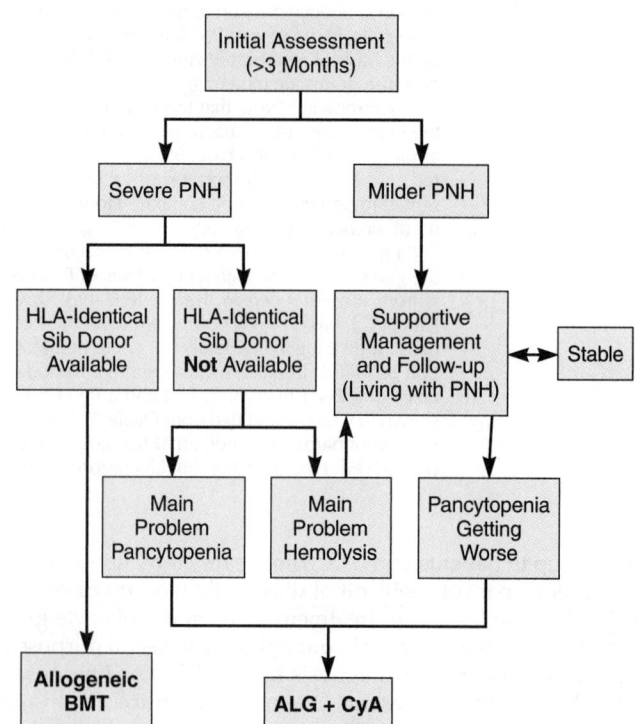

Figure 10-10. A self-explanatory algorithm for the management of paroxysmal nocturnal hemoglobinuria (PNH). It is always important to consider that PNH is a chronic disorder that may run its course over decades; therefore, both patient and doctor must be very patient. ALG, antilymphocyteglobulin; BMT, bone marrow transplantation; CyA, cyclosporin A.

are anecdotal reports that, at very high doses, erythropoietin may reduce or abolish blood transfusion requirement (131,132).

One of the most frustrating aspects of the management of PNH is that we do not yet have an effective way to control hemolysis in this condition. At the time when the differential diagnosis between PNH and autoimmune hemolytic anemia was being worked out and was still sometimes problematic, it was natural to experiment with corticosteroids in PNH (133), and today many patients are still being given prednisone (e.g., 20 mg on alternate days), sometimes for years. However, the basis of hemolysis in PNH is not autoimmune; it has not been proven that pharmacologic doses of prednisone reduce C-dependent hemolysis *in vitro*, and no longitudinal study has been published comparing *in vivo* hemolysis on and off prednisone. A short course of prednisone (0.5 to 1.0 mg/kg/day) may be helpful during an episode of severe exacerbation of hemolysis when it is suspected that it was triggered by an acute inflammatory process. On the other hand, the side effects of long-term prednisone include adrenal suppression, cushingoid features, changes in mood and affect, aseptic necrosis of the hip, and fungal infection—all of which we have seen in patients with PNH who had been on prednisone for months to years. Therefore, we think that this approach is contraindicated.

If a patient has had proven thrombosis, anticoagulant prophylaxis is imperative and should be continued for as long as the patient has PNH. Normally, this is performed with coumadin (warfarin), but a few patients have been on subcutaneous heparin; it remains to be seen whether this is advisable over a period of many years (67,128). The question of primary anticoagulant prophylaxis is unsolved (55). On one hand, one feels reluctant to subject every PNH patient to this additional burden, even before the patient had her or his first episode of thrombosis; on the other hand, PNH is probably the most vicious acquired thrombophilic state, and the first episode of thrombosis may be potentially devastating. One might be tempted to think that if a patient has had PNH for some time and no thrombosis, the risk is eliminated: This is probably true—but only after some 10 years. In practice, our policy is to carry out as baseline investigations a full thrombophilia screen, including antithrombin III, protein S, protein C, APC resistance, prothrombin G20210A, methylene tetrahydrofolate reductase, and the "lupus anticoagulant." Only if there is no evidence of thrombosis and all of these tests are normal/negative, do we withhold anticoagulant prophylaxis.

During an episode of abdominal vein thrombosis, thrombolytic therapy (134) with tissue plasminogen activator must be seriously considered because, although it is not free of risk (especially if the patient is thrombocytopenic), it may be highly effective, and it may prevent irreversible damage (135,136). Unlike with arterial thrombosis, tissue plasminogen activator is worth a trial of even several days and, perhaps, since the clinical onset of the thrombotic event.

In patients who have recurrent attacks of abdominal pain, it is important to establish and to customize an appropriate course of action. In most cases, we start with hydration by mouth and mild analgesics, but it is important to be in touch with the patient and to set a threshold for coming to clinic or admission to hospital, where parenteral fluids and more powerful analgesia, including opiates, may be required. Male patients with PNH who experience erectile dysfunction may benefit from administration of sildenafil, which must be done with caution.

Bone Marrow Transplantation

At the moment, BMT is the only approach to radical cure of PNH (137–141). This procedure has several modes of action: (a) elimination of the abnormal clone(s), (b) provision of normal HSCs, and (c) elimination of autoreactive immune cells. Unlike in leukemia, (a) is not the most important of the three; in PNH, (c) is probably the most important, and (b) is the necessary rescue.

The decision about BMT in PNH is difficult, as in all cases in which there is no perception of an immediate threat to life. A patient with florid PNH who may be at high risk of thrombosis, is transfusion dependent, and faces a 50% chance of being dead within 10 years (Fig. 10-11) may have both quality of life and lifespan restored to normal by BMT. At the other end of the spectrum, a patient who dies of a transplant-related complication may have life curtailed by years by virtue of having opted for BMT. For these reasons, one may be tempted to use delaying tactics (i.e., use supportive treatment only as long as the patient is reasonably well and proceed with BMT if the patient deteriorates). However, this attitude is not very rational, because the outcome of BMT is likely to be better if the procedure is carried out sooner rather than later; for instance, a patient who has developed a Budd-Chiari syndrome while waiting to decide would be now at a greater risk. [There is a single case report of successful BMT in a patient with PNH and Budd-Chiari syndrome, but this was a syngeneic transplant (142).] Broadly speaking, the results of BMT in PNH are similar to, but not as good as, those in AA. In a recent analysis of the European Group for Blood and Marrow Transplantation database, the most conspicuous difference between the two groups was that the interval between diagnosis and BMT was approximately five times longer in PNH than in AA (143), and this may well be a factor in producing less favorable results. On the other hand, in a recent small series (N = 7) from a single center, the 2-year disease-free survival has been 100% (144). Different conditioning regimens have been used. In a few instances, syngeneic BMT without conditioning failed (145): This supports the notion that intensive immunosuppression is absolutely required for the cure of PNH. On the other hand, it has been shown that

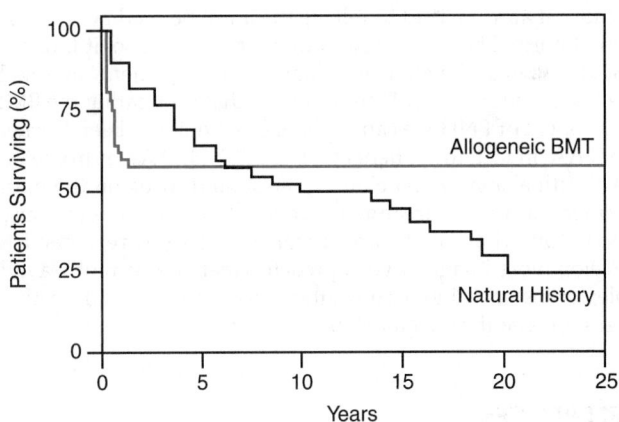

Figure 10-11. Long-term course of paroxysmal nocturnal hemoglobinuria (PNH). In the management of PNH, it is important to always consider that the patient may face decades of life with the disease. In a cohort of patients diagnosed between approximately 1950 and 1970, who received only supportive treatment, the median survival was approximately 8.5 years. By contrast, in a group of patients (compiled from the IBMTR) who received allogeneic bone marrow transplantation (BMT) from an HLA-identical sibling between 1976 and 1996, the disease-free survival was approximately 60%, and no patients were lost beyond 1.5 years from the BMT procedure. In a small recent series (144), the disease-free survival at 2 years was 100%. Note the plateau after 20 years in the natural history group: It appears that in the long run a proportion of patients may experience a spontaneous cure. (Modified from Araten DJ, Luzzatto L. Allogeneic bone marrow transplantation for paroxysmal nocturnal hemoglobinuria. *Haematologica* 2000;85:1–2.)

nonmyeloablative conditioning can be highly successful either from bone marrow stem cells (146) or peripheral stem cells (147): This indicates that complete removal of PNH cells at the time of BMT is not indispensable.

In practice, we think it is appropriate to offer BMT, as the only option that can produce a prompt definitive cure, to every young patient with PNH who has an HLA-identical sibling donor (Figs. 10-10 and 10-11). Not all patients want to take that option, and in our view, it is important to know the patient well to assess his or her motivation and to ensure we can provide the best assistance in reaching a decision. By contrast, the past record of BMT from unrelated donors in PNH is poor (141), and it must be still regarded as experimental in the treatment of this condition. Although recently three successful cases have been reported (148), it appears their clinical situation was more like AA than PNH.

Intensive Immunosuppressive Treatment

The protocol for intensive immunosuppressive treatment used for AA, consisting of ATG and high-dose methylprednisolone followed by cyclosporin A (149), is a valid treatment option, especially for patients with PNH who do not have an appropriate donor. The most compelling indication for this treatment is pancytopenia, especially if severe. Although no formal antilymphocyte globulin trial has been carried out, several case reports have been published (150–154), and probably even more patients so treated have not yet been published (155 and personal data, 2002). ATG treatment cannot be expected to influence the hemolytic process. Therefore, there may be little effect on the Hb level; response to treatment must be measured in terms of increase in neutrophils and platelets; a majority of patients respond in this way. In our experience, the most significant benefit is on the platelet count, and, therefore, we regard severe thrombocytopenia as the most common indication. We tend to continue cyclosporin A administration for 2 years, aiming to maintenance levels of 100 to 150 ng/mL. This type of treatment cannot be expected to eradicate the PNH clone, because it aims instead to relieve the immune-mediated inhibition of normal hematopoiesis; however, in doing so, it limits (if not eliminates) the abnormal marrow environment on which the PNH clone thrives. Thus, it is clear that for treating the BMF component of PNH we can capitalize on what has been learned from AA; in fact, for patients with the "PNH/AA syndrome" or "AA with a small PNH clone," one should focus on the management of AA. For treating the consequences of having a large PNH clone (hemolysis and thrombosis) we direly need to develop more imaginative approaches than are currently available; for instance, inhibition of the C cascade either at the activation step or at the effector step.

REFERENCES

1. Hijmans van den Bergh AA. Ictère hémolytique avec crises hémoglobinuriques: fragilité globulaire. *Rev Méd* 1911;31:63–69.
2. Marchiafava E, Nazari A. Nuovo contributo allo studio degli itteri cronici emolitici. Policlinico *Sez Med* 1911;18:241.
3. Hamburger LP, Bernstein A. Chronic hemolytic anemia with paroxysmal nocturnal hemoglobinuria. *Am J Med Sci* 1936;102:301–316.
4. Crosby WH. Paroxysmal nocturnal hemoglobinuria: relation of the clinical manifestations to underlying pathogenic mechanisms. *Blood* 1953;8:769–812.
5. Crosby WH. Paroxysmal nocturnal hemoglobinuria: plasma factors of the hemolytic system. *Blood* 1953;8:444–458.
6. Dacie JV, Lewis SM. Paroxysmal nocturnal haemoglobinuria: clinical manifestations, haematology, and nature of the disease. *Ser Haematol* 1972;5:3–23.
7. Dacie JV. Paroxysmal nocturnal haemoglobinuria. In: Dacie JV, ed. *The haemolytic anaemias: drug and chemical induced haemolytic anaemias, paroxysmal nocturnal haemoglobinuria, and haemolytic disease of the newborn*, vol. 5, 3rd ed. London: Churchill Livingstone, 1999:139–330.
8. De Sandre G, Ghiotto G, Mastella G. L'acetilcolinesterasi eritrocitaria. II. Rapporti con le malattie emolitiche. *Acta Med Patav* 1956;16:310.
9. Pramoonjago P, Pakdeesuwan K, Siripanyaphinyo U, et al. Genotypic, immunophenotypic and clinical features of Thai patients with paroxysmal nocturnal haemoglobinuria. *Br J Haematol* 1999;105:497–504.
10. Issaragrisil S. Epidemiology of aplastic anemia in Thailand. Thai Aplastic Anemia Study Group. *Int J Hematol* 1999;70:137–140.
11. Dacie JV, Mollison PL. Survival of transfused erythrocytes from a donor with nocturnal haemoglobinuria. *Lancet* 1949;i:390.
12. Lewis SM, Szur L, Dacie JV. The pattern of erythrocyte destruction in haemolytic anaemia, as studied with radioactive chromium. *Br J Haematol* 1960;6:122–139.
13. Dacie JV. Paroxysmal nocturnal haemoglobinuria. *Proc R Soc Med* 1963;56:587–596.
14. Oni SB, Osunkoya BO, Luzzatto L. Paroxysmal nocturnal hemoglobinuria: evidence for monoclonal origin of abnormal red cells. *Blood* 1970;36:145–152.
15. Auditore JV, Hartmann RC, Flexner JM, et al. The erythrocyte acetylcholinesterase enzyme in paroxysmal nocturnal hemoglobinuria. *Arch Pathol* 1960;69:534–540.
16. Nicholson-Weller A, March JP, Rosenfeld SI, et al. Affected erythrocytes of patients with paroxysmal nocturnal hemoglobinuria are deficient in the complement regulatory protein, decay accelerating factor. *Proc Natl Acad Sci U S A* 1983;80:5066–5070.
17. Sugarman J, Devine DV, Rosse WF. Structural and functional differences between decay-accelerating factor and red cell acetylcholinesterase. *Blood* 1986;68:680–684.
18. Nicholson-Weller A, Spicer DB, Austen KF. Deficiency of the complement regulatory protein, "decay-accelerating factor," on membranes of granulocytes, monocytes, and platelets in paroxysmal nocturnal hemoglobinuria. *N Engl J Med* 1985;312:1091–1097.
19. van der Schoot CE, Huizinga TW, van 't Veer-Korthof ET, et al. Deficiency of glycosyl-phosphatidylinositol-linked membrane glycoproteins of leukocytes in paroxysmal nocturnal haemoglobinuria, description of a new diagnostic cytofluorometric assay. *Blood* 1990;76:1853–1859.
20. Bessler M, Schaefer A, Keller P. Paroxysmal nocturnal haemoglobinuria: insights from recent advances in molecular biology. *Transfus Med Rev* 2001;15:255–267.
21. Low MG, Finean JB. Non-lytic release of acetylcholinesterase from erythrocytes by a phosphatidylinositol-specific phospholipase C. *FEBS Lett* 1977;82:143–146.
22. Davitz MA, Low MG, Nussenzweig V. Release of decay-accelerating factor (DAF) from the cell membrane by phosphatidylinositol-specific phospholipase C (PIPLC). Selective modification of a complement regulatory protein. *J Exp Med* 1986;163:1150–1161.
23. Ferguson MA, Low MG, Cross GA. Glycosyl-sn-1,2-dimyristylphosphatidylinositol is covalently linked to *Trypanosoma brucei* variant surface glycoprotein. *J Biol Chem* 1985;260:14547–14555.
24. Ferguson MA, Homans SW, Dwek RA, et al. Glycosyl-phosphatidylinositol moiety that anchors *Trypanosoma brucei* variant surface glycoprotein to the membrane. *Science* 1988;239:753–759.
25. Lewis SM, Dacie JV. Neutrophil (leucocyte) alkaline phosphatase in paroxysmal nocturnal haemoglobinuria. *Br J Haematol* 1965;11:549–556.
26. Aster RH, Enright SE. A platelet and granulocyte membrane defect in paroxysmal nocturnal hemoglobinuria: usefulness for the detection of platelet antibodies. *J Clin Invest* 1969;48:1199–1210.
27. Rotoli B, Robledo R, Scarpato N, et al. Two populations of erythroid cell progenitors in paroxysmal nocturnal hemoglobinuria. *Blood* 1984;64:847–851.
28. Hillmen P, Bessler M, Crawford DH, et al. Production and characterization of lymphoblastoid cell lines with the paroxysmal nocturnal hemoglobinuria phenotype. *Blood* 1993;81:193–199.
29. Hillmen P, Bessler M, Mason PJ, et al. Specific defect in N-acetylglucosamine incorporation in the biosynthesis of the glycosylphosphatidylinositol anchor in cloned cell lines from patients with paroxysmal nocturnal hemoglobinuria. *Proc Natl Acad Sci U S A* 1993;90:5272–5276.
30. Hillmen P, Bessler M, Luzzatto L. Paroxysmal nocturnal hemoglobinuria: correction of the abnormal phenotype by somatic cell hybridization. *Somatic Cell Genet* 1993;19:123–129.
31. Miyata T, Takeda J, Iida J, et al. The cloning of PIG-A, a component in the early step of GPI-anchor biosynthesis. *Science* 1993;259:1318–1320.
32. Bessler M, Mason PJ, Hillmen P, et al. Paroxysmal nocturnal haemoglobinuria (PNH) is caused by somatic mutations in the PIG-A gene. *Embo J* 1994;13:110–117.
33. Takeda J, Miyata T, Kawagoe K, et al. Deficiency of the GPI anchor caused by a somatic mutation of the PIG-A gene in paroxysmal nocturnal hemoglobinuria. *Cell* 1993;73:703–711.
34. Miyata T, Yamada N, Iida Y, et al. Abnormalities of PIG-A transcripts in granulocytes from patients with paroxysmal nocturnal hemoglobinuria. *N Engl J Med* 1994;330:249–255.
35. Ware RE, Rosse WF, Howard TA. Mutations within the Piga gene in patients with paroxysmal nocturnal hemoglobinuria. *Blood* 1994;83:2418–2422.
36. Nafa K, Mason PJ, Hillmen P, et al. Mutations in the PIG-A gene causing paroxysmal nocturnal hemoglobinuria are mainly of the frameshift type. *Blood* 1995;86:4650–4655.
37. Luzzatto L, Nafa K. Genetics of PNH. In: Young NS, Moss J, eds. *Paroxysmal nocturnal hemoglobinuria and the GPI-linked proteins*. New York: Academic Press, 2000:21–47.
38. Rosse WF, Adams JP, Thorpe AM. The population of cells in paroxysmal nocturnal haemoglobinuria of intermediate sensitivity to complement lysis: sig-

nificance and mechanism of increased immune lysis. *Br J Haematol* 1974;28: 181–190.

39. Rosse WF, Hoffman S, Campbell M, et al. The erythrocytes in paroxysmal nocturnal haemoglobinuria of intermediate sensitivity to complement lysis. *Br J Haematol* 1991;79:99–107.

40. Watanabe R, Inoue N, Westfall B, et al. The first step of glycosylphosphatidylinositol biosynthesis is mediated by a complex of PIG-A, PIG-H, PIG-C and GPI1. *Embo J* 1998;17:877–885.

41. Hirose S, Ravi L, Prince GM, et al. Synthesis of mannosylglucosaminylinositol phospholipids in normal but not paroxysmal nocturnal hemoglobinuria cells. *Proc Natl Acad Sci U S A* 1992;89:6025–6029.

42. Takahashi M, Takeda J, Hirose S, et al. Deficient biosynthesis of N-acetylglucosaminyl-phosphatidylinositol, the first intermediate of glycosyl phosphatidylinositol anchor biosynthesis, in cell lines established from patients with paroxysmal nocturnal hemoglobinuria. *J Exp Med* 1993;177:517–521.

43. Sevlever D, Chen R, Medof ME. Synthesis of GPI anchor. In: Young NS, Moss J, eds. *Paroxysmal nocturnal hemoglobinuria and the GPI-linked proteins*. New York: Academic Press, 2000:199–220.

44. Nafa K, Bessler M, Castro-Malaspina H, et al. The spectrum of somatic mutations in the PIG-A gene in paroxysmal nocturnal hemoglobinuria includes large deletions and small duplications. *Blood Cells Mol Dis* 1998;24:370–384.

45. Yamashina M, Ueda E, Kinoshita T, et al. Inherited complete deficiency of 20-kilodalton homologous restriction factor (CD59) as a cause of paroxysmal nocturnal hemoglobinuria. *N Engl J Med* 1990;323:1184–1189.

46. Rosse WF, Dacie JV. Immune lysis of normal human and paroxysmal nocturnal hemoglobinuria (PNH) red blood cells. I. The sensitivity of PNH red cells to lysis by complement and specific antibody. *J Clin Invest* 1966;45:736–748.

47. Ham TH, Dingle JH. Studies on destruction of red blood cells. II. Chronic hemolytic mechanism with special reference to serum complement. *J Clin Invest* 1938;18:657–672.

48. Hartmann RC, Jenkins DE. The "sugar-water" test for paroxysmal nocturnal hemoglobinuria. *N Engl J Med* 1966;275:155–157.

49. Dacie JV, Lewis SM, Luzzatto L, et al. Laboratory methods used in the investigation of paroxysmal nocturnal haemoglobinuria (PNH). In: Dacie JV, Lewis SM, eds. *Practical haematology*, 8th ed. London: Churchill Livingstone, 1995:287–296.

50. Parker CJ. Hemolysis in PNH. In: Young NS, Moss J, eds. *Paroxysmal nocturnal hemoglobinuria and the GPI-linked proteins*. New York: Academic Press, 2000:49–100.

51. Yu J, Abagyan R, Dong S, Gilbert A, et al. Mapping the active site of CD59. *J Exp Med* 1997;185:745–753.

52. Davies A, Simmons DL, Hale G, et al. CD59, an LY-6-like protein expressed in human lymphoid cells, regulates the action of the complement membrane attack complex on homologous cells. *J Exp Med* 1989;170:637–654.

53. Rosse WF. The control of complement activation by the blood cells in paroxysmal nocturnal hemoglobinuria. *Blood* 1986;67:268–269.

54. Meri S, Morgan BP, Davies A, et al. Human protectin (CD59), an 18,000-20,000 MW complement lysis restricting factor, inhibits C5b-8 catalysed insertion of C9 into lipid bilayers. *Immunology* 1990;71:1–9.

55. Sloand EM, Young NS. Thrombotic complication in PNH. In: Young NS, Moss J, eds. *Paroxysmal nocturnal hemoglobinuria and the GPI-linked proteins*. New York: Academic Press, 2000:101–112.

56. Plough M, Plesner T, Ronne E, et al. The receptor for urokinase-type plasminogen activator is deficient on peripheral blood leukocytes in patients with paroxysmal nocturnal hemoglobinuria. *Blood* 1992;79:1447–1455.

57. Ronne E, Pappot H, Grondahl-Hansen J, et al. The receptor for urokinase plasminogen activator is present in plasma from healthy donors and elevated in patients with paroxysmal nocturnal haemoglobinuria. *Br J Haematol* 1995;89:576–581.

58. Sims PJ, Faioni EM, Wiedmer T, et al. Complement proteins C5b-9 cause release of membrane vesicles from the platelet surface that are enriched in the membrane receptor for coagulation factor Va and express prothrombinase activity. *J Biol Chem* 1988;263:18205–18212.

59. Gilbert GE, Sims PJ, Wiedmer T, et al. Platelet-derived microparticles express high affinity receptors for factor VIII. *J Biol Chem* 1991;266:17261–17268.

60. Granlick HR, Vail M, McKeown LP, et al. Activated platelets in paroxysmal nocturnal haemoglobinuria. *Br J Haematol* 1995;91:697–702.

61. Wiedmer T, Hall SE, Ortel TL, et al. Complement-induced vesiculation and exposure of membrane prothrombinase sites in platelets of paroxysmal nocturnal hemoglobinuria. *Blood* 1993;82:1192–1196.

62. Hugel B, Socie G, Vu T, et al. Elevated levels of circulating procoagulant microparticles in patients with paroxysmal nocturnal hemoglobinuria and aplastic anemia. *Blood* 1999;93:3451–3456.

63. Zimmerman TS, Kolb WP. Human platelet-initiated formation and uptake of the C5-9 complex of human complement. *J Clin Invest* 1976;57:203–211.

64. Polley MJ, Nachman RL. Human complement in thrombin-mediated platelet function: uptake of the C5b-9 complex. *J Exp Med* 1979;150:633–645.

65. Shichishima T, Saitoh Y, Terasawa T, et al. Complement sensitivity of erythrocytes in a patient with inherited complete deficiency of CD59 or with the Inab phenotype. *Br J Haematol* 1999;104:303–306.

66. Lewis SM, Dacie JV. The aplastic anaemia–paroxysmal nocturnal haemoglobinuria syndrome. *Br J Haematol* 1967;13:236–251.

67. Hillmen P, Lewis SM, Bessler M, et al. Natural history of paroxysmal nocturnal hemoglobinuria. *N Engl J Med* 1995;333:1253–1258.

68. Ben-Bassat I, Brok-Simoni F, Ramot B. Complement-sensitive red cells in aplastic anemia. *Blood* 1975;46:357–361.

69. Najean Y, Haguenauer O. Long-term (5 to 20 years) evolution of nongrafted aplastic anemias. The Cooperative Group for the Study of Aplastic and Refractory Anemias. *Blood* 1990;76:2222–2228.

70. Schubert J, Vogt HG, Zielinska-Skowronek M, et al. Development of the glycosylphosphatidtylinositol-anchoring defect characteristic for paroxysmal nocturnal hemoglobinuria in patients with aplastic anemia. *Blood* 1994;83:2323–2328.

71. Tichelli A, Gratwohl A, Nissen C, et al. Late clonal complications in severe aplastic anemia. *Leuk Lymphoma* 1994;12:167–175.

72. Griscelli-Bennaceur A, Gluckman E, Scrobohaci ML, et al. Aplastic anemia and paroxysmal nocturnal hemoglobinuria: search for a pathogenetic link. *Blood* 1995;85:1354–1363.

73. Dunn DE, Tanawattanacharoen P, Boccuni P, et al. Paroxysmal nocturnal hemoglobinuria cells in patients with bone marrow failure syndromes. *Ann Intern Med* 1999;131:401–408.

74. Socie G, Rosenfeld S, Frickhofen N, et al. Late clonal diseases of treated aplastic anemia. *Semin Hematol* 2000;37:91–101.

75. Rotoli B, Robledo R, Luzzatto L. Decreased number of circulating BFU-Es in paroxysmal nocturnal hemoglobinuria. *Blood* 1982;60:157–159.

76. Rotoli B, Luzzatto L. Paroxysmal nocturnal hemoglobinuria. *Semin Hematol* 1989;26:201–207.

77. Marmont AM. The autoimmune myelopathies. *Acta Haematol* 1983;69:73–97.

78. Young NS, Maciejewski J. The pathophysiology of acquired aplastic anemia. *N Engl J Med* 1997;336:1365–1372.

79. Zoumbos NC, Gascon P, Djeu JY, et al. Circulating activated suppressor T lymphocytes in aplastic anemia. *N Engl J Med* 1985;312:257–265.

80. Zoumbos NC, Gascon P, Djeu JY, et al. Interferon is a mediator of hematopoietic suppression in aplastic anemia in vitro and possibly in vivo. *Proc Natl Acad Sci U S A* 1985;82:188–192.

81. Nistico A, Young NS. gamma-Interferon gene expression in the bone marrow of patients with aplastic anemia. *Ann Intern Med* 1994;120:463–469.

82. Hinterberger W, Adolf G, Aichinger G, et al. Further evidence for lymphokine overproduction in severe aplastic anemia. *Blood* 1988;72:266–272.

83. Miura A, Endo K, Sugawara T, et al. T cell-mediated inhibition of erythropoiesis in aplastic anaemia: the possible role of IFN-gamma and TNF-alpha. *Br J Haematol* 1991;78:442–449.

84. Maciejewski JP, Selleri C, Sato T, et al. Increased expression of Fas antigen on bone marrow CD34+ cells of patients with aplastic anaemia. *Br J Haematol* 1995;91:245–252.

85. Niho Y, Asano Y. Fas/Fas ligand and hematopoietic progenitor cells. *Curr Opin Hematol* 1998;5:163–165.

86. Speck B, Gratwohl A, Nissen C, et al. Treatment of severe aplastic anemia. *Exp Hematol* 1986;14:126–132.

87. Young N, Griffith P, Brittain E, et al. A multicenter trial of antithymocyte globulin in aplastic anemia and related diseases. *Blood* 1988;72:1861–1869.

88. Bacigalupo A, Bruno B, Saracco P, et al. Antilymphocyte globulin, cyclosporine, prednisolone, and granulocyte colony-stimulating factor for severe aplastic anemia: an update of the GITMO/EBMT study on 100 patients. European Group for Blood and Marrow Transplantation (EBMT) Working Party on Severe Aplastic Anemia and the Gruppo Italiano Trapianti di Midolio Osseo (GITMO). *Blood* 2000;95:1931–1934.

89. Zeng W, Nakao S, Takamatsu H, et al. Characterization of T-cell repertoire of the bone marrow in immune-mediated aplastic anemia: evidence for the involvement of antigen-driven T-cell response in cyclosporine-dependent aplastic anemia. *Blood* 1999;93:3008–3016.

90. Karadimitris A, Manavalan JS, Thaler HT, et al. Abnormal T-cell repertoire is consistent with immune process underlying the pathogenesis of paroxysmal nocturnal hemoglobinuria. *Blood* 2000;96:2613–2620.

91. Luzzatto L, Bessler M. The dual pathogenesis of paroxysmal nocturnal hemoglobinuria. *Curr Opin Hematol* 1996;3:101–110.

92. Luzzatto L, Bessler M, Rotoli B. Somatic mutations in paroxysmal nocturnal hemoglobinuria: a blessing in disguise? *Cell* 1997;88:1–4.

93. Murakami Y, Kinoshita T, Maeda Y, et al. Different roles of glycosylphosphatidylinositol in various hematopoietic cells as revealed by a mouse model of paroxysmal nocturnal hemoglobinuria. *Blood* 1999;94:2963–2970.

94. Tremml G, Dominguez C, Rosti V, et al. Increased sensitivity to complement and a decreased red blood cell life span in mice mosaic for a nonfunctional Piga gene. *Blood* 1999;94:2945–2954.

95. Luzzatto L. Paroxysmal murine hemoglobinuria(?): a model for human PNH. *Blood* 1999;94:2941–2944.

96. Bessler M, Mason P, Hillmen P, et al. Somatic mutations and cellular selection in paroxysmal nocturnal haemoglobinuria. *Lancet* 1994;343:951–953.

97. Yamada N, Miyata T, Maeda K, et al. Somatic mutations of the PIG-A gene found in Japanese patients with paroxysmal nocturnal hemoglobinuria. *Blood* 1995;85:885–892.

98. Endo M, Beatty PG, Vreeke TM, et al. Syngeneic bone marrow transplantation without conditioning in a patient with paroxysmal nocturnal hemoglobinuria: in vivo evidence that the mutant stem cells have a survival advantage. *Blood* 1996;88:742–750.

99. Nishimura J, Inoue N, Wada H, et al. A patient with paroxysmal nocturnal hemoglobinuria bearing four independent PIG-A mutant clones. *Blood* 1997; 89:3470–3476.

100. Schrezenmeier H, Hertenstein B, Wagner B, et al. A pathogenetic link between aplastic anemia and paroxysmal nocturnal hemoglobinuria is suggested by a high frequency of aplastic anemia patients with a deficiency of phosphatidylinositol glycan anchored proteins. *Exp Hematol* 1995;23:81–87.

101. Araten DJ, Nafa K, Pakdeesuwan K, et al. Clonal populations of hematopoietic cells with paroxysmal nocturnal hemoglobinuria genotype and phenotype are present in normal individuals. *Proc Natl Acad Sci U S A* 1999;96:5209–5214.
102. Karadimitris A, Luzzatto L. The cellular pathogenesis of paroxysmal nocturnal haemoglobinuria. *Leukemia* 2001;15:1148–1152.
103. Karadimitris A, Li K, Notaro R, et al. Association of clonal T-cell large granular lymphocyte disease and paroxysmal nocturnal hemoglobinuria (PNH): further evidence for a pathogenetic link between T cells, aplastic anaemia and PNH. *Br J Haematol* 2001;115:1–6.
104. Chen R, Nagarajan S, Prince GM, et al. Impaired growth and elevated fas receptor expression in PIGA(+) stem cells in primary paroxysmal nocturnal hemoglobinuria. *J Clin Invest* 2000;106:689–696.
105. Rosti V, Tremml G, Soares V, et al. Murine embryonic stem cells without pig-a gene activity are competent for hematopoiesis with the PNH phenotype but not for clonal expansion. *J Clin Invest* 1997;100:1028–1036.
106. Keller P, Payne JL, Tremml G, et al. FES-Cre targets phosphatidylinositol glycan class A (PIGA) inactivation to hematopoietic stem cells in the bone marrow. *J Exp Med* 2001;194:581–589.
107. Polli E, Sirchia G, Ferrone S, et al. *Emoglobinuria parossistica notturna. Revisione critica.* Milano: Edizioni Cilag-Chemie Italiana;1973.
108. Ray JG, Burows RF, Ginsberg JS, et al. Paroxysmal nocturnal hemoglobinuria and the risk of venous thrombosis: review and recommendations for management of the pregnant and nonpregnant patient. *Haemostasis* 2000;30:103–117.
109. Bais J, Pel M, von dem Borne A, et al. Pregnancy and paroxysmal nocturnal hemoglobinuria. *Eur J Obstet Gynecol Reprod Biol* 1994;53:211–214.
110. Frakes JT, Burmeister RE, Giliberti JJ. Pregnancy in a patient with paroxysmal nocturnal hemoglobinuria. *Obstet Gynecol* 1976;47:22S–24S.
111. Bais JM, Pel M. Late maternal mortality due to paroxysmal nocturnal hemoglobinuria and pregnancy. *Eur J Obstet Gynecol Reprod Biol* 1995;58:211.
112. Solal-Celigny P, Tertian G, Fernandez H, et al. Pregnancy and paroxysmal nocturnal hemoglobinuria. *Arch Intern Med* 1988;148:593–595.
113. Svigos JM, Norman J. Paroxysmal nocturnal haemoglobinuria and pregnancy. *Aust N Z J Obstet Gynaecol* 1994;34:104–106.
114. Harris JW, Koscick R, Lazarus HM, et al. Leukemia arising out of paroxysmal nocturnal hemoglobinuria. *Leuk Lymphoma* 1999;32:401–426.
115. Devine DV, Gluck WL, Rosse WF, et al. Acute myeloblastic leukemia in paroxysmal nocturnal hemoglobinuria. Evidence of evolution from the abnormal paroxysmal nocturnal hemoglobinuria clone. *J Clin Invest* 1987;79:314–317.
116. Nakahata J, Takahashi M, Fuse I, et al. Paroxysmal nocturnal hemoglobinuria with myelofibrosis: progression to acute myeloblastic leukemia. *Leuk Lymphoma* 1993;12:137–142.
117. Longo L, Bessler M, Beris P, et al. Myelodysplasia in a patient with pre-existing paroxysmal nocturnal haemoglobinuria: a clonal disease originating from within a clonal disease. *Br J Haematol* 1994;87:401–403.
118. Dameshek W. Riddle: what do aplastic anemia, paroxysmal nocturnal hemoglobinuria (PNH) and "hypoplastic" leukemia have in common? *Blood* 1967;30:251–254.
119. Young NS. The problem of clonality in aplastic anemia: Dr Dameshek's riddle, restated. *Blood* 1992;79:1385–1392.
120. Araten DJ, Luzzatto L. Allogeneic bone marrow transplantation for paroxysmal nocturnal hemoglobinuria. *Haematologica* 2000;85:1–2.
121. Rosse WF. Paroxysmal nocturnal hemoglobinuria. In: Handin RI, Lux SE, Stossel TP, eds. *Blood: principles and practice of hematology.* Philadelphia: Lippincott Williams & Wilkins,1995:367–376.
122. Ham TH. Chronic hemolytic anemia with paroxysmal nocturnal hemoglobinuria. A study of the mechanism of hemolysis in relation to acid-base equilibrium. *N Engl J Med* 1937;217:915–918.
123. Dacie JV. Diagnosis and mechanism of hemolysis in chronic hemolytic anemia with nocturnal hemoglobinuria. *Blood* 1949;4:1181–1195.
124. May JE, Rosse W, Frank MM. Paroxysmal nocturnal hemoglobinuria. Alternate-complement-pathway-mediated lysis induced by magnesium. *N Engl J Med* 1973;289:705–709.
125. Crookston JH, Crookston MC, et al. Red-cell abnormalities in HEMPAS (hereditary erythroblastic multinuclearity with a positive acidified-serum test). *Br J Haematol* 1972;23:[Suppl]:83–91.
126. Alfinito F, Del Vecchio L, Rocco S, et al. Blood cell flow cytometry in paroxysmal nocturnal hemoglobinuria: a tool for measuring the extent of the PNH clone. *Leukemia* 1996;10:1326–1330.
127. Araten DJ, Bessler M, McKenzie S, et al. Dynamics of hematopoiesis in paroxysmal nocturnal hemoglobinuria (PNH): no evidence for intrinsic growth advantage of PNH clones. *(submitted 2002)*
128. Socie G, Mary JY, de Gramont A, et al. Paroxysmal nocturnal haemoglobinuria: long-term follow-up and prognostic factors. French Society of Haematology. *Lancet* 1996;348:573–577.
129. Strübing P. Paroxysmale hämoglobinurie. *Dtsch Med Wocheschr* 1882;8:1–8.
130. McMullin MF, Hillmen P, Elder GE, et al. Serum erythropoietin levels in paroxysmal nocturnal haemoglobinuria: implications for therapy. *Br J Haematol* 1996;92:815–817.
131. Stebler C, Tichelli A, Dazzi H, et al. High-dose recombinant human erythropoietin for treatment of anemia in myelodysplastic syndromes and paroxysmal nocturnal haemoglobinuria: a pilot study. *Exp Hematol* 1990;18:1204–1208.
132. Astori C, Bonfichi M, Pagnucco G, et al. Treatment with recombinant human erythropoietin (rHuEpo) in a patient with paroxysmal nocturnal haemoglobinuria: evaluation of membrane proteins CD55 and CD59 with cytofluorometric assay. *Br J Haematol* 1997;97:586–588.
133. Rosse WF. Treatment of paroxysmal nocturnal hemoglobinuria. *Blood* 1982;60:20–23.
134. Sholar PW, Bell WR. Thrombolytic therapy for inferior vena cava thrombosis in paroxysmal nocturnal hemoglobinuria. *Ann Intern Med* 1985;103:539–541.
135. Kwan T, Hansard P. Recombinant tissue-plasminogen activator for acute Budd-Chiari syndrome secondary to paroxysmal nocturnal hemoglobinuria. *N Y State J Med* 1992;92:109–110.
136. McMullin MF, Hillmen P, Jackson J, et al. Tissue plasminogen activator for hepatic vein thrombosis in paroxysmal nocturnal haemoglobinuria. *J Intern Med* 1994;235:85–89.
137. Storb R, Evans RS, Thomas ED, et al. Paroxysmal nocturnal haemoglobinuria and refractory marrow failure treated by marrow transplantation. *Br J Haematol* 1973;24:743–750.
138. Szer J, Deeg HJ, Witherspoon RP, et al. Long-term survival after marrow transplantation for paroxysmal nocturnal hemoglobinuria with aplastic anemia. *Ann Intern Med* 1984;101:193–195.
139. Kawahara K, Witherspoon RP, Storb R. Marrow transplantation for paroxysmal nocturnal hemoglobinuria. *Am J Hematol* 1992;39:283–288.
140. Bemba M, Guardiola P, Garderet L, et al. Bone marrow transplantation for paroxysmal nocturnal haemoglobinuria. *Br J Haematol* 1999;105:366–368.
141. Saso R, Marsh J, Cevreska L, et al. Bone marrow transplants for paroxysmal nocturnal haemoglobinuria. *Br J Haematol* 1999;104:392–396.
142. Graham ML, Rosse WF, Halperin EC, et al. Resolution of Budd-Chiari syndrome following bone marrow transplantation for paroxysmal nocturnal haemoglobinuria. *Br J Haematol* 1996;92:707–710.
143. Bacigalupo A. Bone marrow transplantation for acquired severe aplastic anemia and PNH: diversities and similarities. Paroxysmal nocturnal hemoglobinuria (PNH) and related disorders: molecular aspects of pathogenesis. *Tokyo*, 2001.
144. Raiola AM, Van Lint MT, Lamparelli T, et al. Bone marrow transplantation for paroxysmal nocturnal haemoglobinuria. *Haematologica* 2000;85:59–62.
145. Nafa K, Bessler M, Deeg HJ, et al. New somatic mutation in the PIG-A gene emerges at relapse of paroxysmal nocturnal hemoglobinuria. *Blood* 1998;92:3422–3427.
146. Antin JH, Ginsburg D, Smith BR, et al. Bone marrow transplantation for paroxysmal nocturnal hemoglobinuria: eradication of the PNH clone and documentation of complete lymphohematopoietic engraftment. *Blood* 1985;66:1247–1250.
147. Suenaga K, Kanda Y, Niiya H, et al. Successful application of nonmyeloablative transplantation for paroxysmal nocturnal hemoglobinuria. *Exp Hematol* 2001;29:639–642.
148. Woodard P, Wang W, Pitts N, et al. Successful unrelated donor bone marrow transplantation for paroxysmal nocturnal hemoglobinuria. *Bone Marrow Transplant* 2001;27:589–592.
149. Frickhofen N, Kaltwasser JP, Schrezenmeier H, et al. Treatment of aplastic anemia with antilymphocyte globulin and methylprednisolone with or without cyclosporine. The German Aplastic Anemia Study Group. *N Engl J Med* 1991;324:1297–1304.
150. Nissen C, Wodnar-Filipowicz A, Slanicka Krieger MS, et al. Persistent growth impairment of bone marrow stroma after antilymphocyte globulin treatment for severe aplastic anaemia and its association with relapse. *Eur J Haematol* 1995;55:255–261.
151. van Kamp H, van Imhoff GW, de Wolf JT, et al. The effect of cyclosporine on haematological parameters in patients with paroxysmal nocturnal haemoglobinuria. *Br J Haematol* 1995;89:79–82.
152. Ebenbichler CF, Wurzner R, Sandhofer AD, et al. Anti-thymocyte globulin treatment of a patient for paroxysmal nocturnal haemoglobinuria-aplastic anaemia syndrome: complement activation and transient decrease of the PNH clone. *Immunobiology* 1996;196:513–521.
153. Stoppa AM, Vey N, Sainty D, et al. Correction of aplastic anaemia complicating paroxysmal nocturnal haemoglobinuria: absence of eradication of the PNH clone and dependence of response on cyclosporin A administration. *Br J Haematol* 1996;93:42–44.
154. Paquette RL, Yoshimura R, Veiseh C, et al. Clinical characteristics predict response to antithymocyte globulin in paroxysmal nocturnal haemoglobinuria. *Br J Haematol* 1997;96:92–97.
155. Rosse WF. Paroxysmal nocturnal hemoglobinuria. In: Hoffman R, Benz EJ Jr, Shattil SJ, et al, eds. *Hematology, basic principles and practice,* 2nd ed. New York: Churchill Livingstone, 1995:370–381.

CHAPTER 11

Myelodysplastic Syndromes

D. Gary Gilliland and Cynthia E. Dunbar

The myelodysplastic syndromes (MDSs) are a heterogeneous group of disorders characterized by inadequate and dysmorphic hematopoiesis. Varying degrees of reticulocytopenia, leukopenia, or thrombocytopenia may render patients dependent on red blood cell (RBC) transfusions and susceptible to infection or hemorrhage. Persons with MDS are also at high risk for evolution to acute leukemia. Central to consideration of these syndromes is the fact that they are clonal hematopoietic disorders. The progeny of a single myelodysplastic stem cell are able to dominate the bone marrow to the exclusion of their normal counterparts, despite an inability to maintain effective circulating cell populations. This property of clonality, along with demonstrations of cytogenetic abnormalities and mutations in cellular protooncogenes, has stimulated investigation of the myelodysplasias as prototypical premalignant processes.

Overlap of both clinical manifestations and biologic behavior of MDS with other hematologic disorders causes diagnostic confusion and invites errors in interpretation of pathophysiology (Fig. 11-1). Nutritional deficiencies are part of the differential diagnosis and must be excluded by clinical testing. Cytopenias are common to both aplastic anemia and MDS, and a minority of patients with MDS have hypocellular bone marrow. Dysmorphic features may be evident in the few residual bone marrow cells found in patients with aplastic anemia. Diagnostic distinction may be extremely difficult in the absence of a cytogenetic abnormality. In some patients with dysplastic marrow characteristics, monocytosis, neutrophilia, or thrombocytosis brings to mind a myeloproliferative syndrome.

Finally, the aforementioned frequent evolution to leukemia and the clonal nature of MDS emphasize the close relation of these disorders to acute myelogenous leukemia (AML). Despite this, MDSs have emerged as distinct clinical and morphologic entities deserving of clinical and laboratory investigation.

Our purpose in this chapter is to present a full account of the evolving knowledge about MDS (1–11). Their extensive array of clinical, morphologic, biochemical, and genetic abnormalities provides a rich but often confusing tableau for the clinical investigator and the practicing physician. It may not be clear whether a morphologic or laboratory abnormality is an essential element in the pathogenesis of MDS or an inconsequential result of a genetically unstable cellular environment. Furthermore, the clinician must balance a desire for therapy directed at an underlying pathogenetic mechanism with the realization that patients with MDS may be stable for long periods of time with only supportive care. Advances in understanding the regulation of hematopoiesis and the molecular genetics of DNA damage and repair should improve our ability to diagnose, treat, and perhaps prevent these disorders in the future.

HISTORY

The present conceptual framework for MDSs evolved gradually from two historically distinct areas of clinical investigation. During the 1920s and 1930s, a recognition of the nutritional requirements of hematopoietic cells emerged. Iron deficiency, pernicious anemia, and folate deficiency were identified and effectively treated, but many patients with chronic anemia failed to respond to these nutritional interventions. As assays were developed for quantitating iron, B_{12}, and folate, these refractory patients were found to have adequate levels of these substances. In 1938, Rhoads and Barker (12) described 60 patients with refractory anemia (RA), one-third of whom would have met the diagnostic criteria for MDS. Neutropenia and thrombocytopenia were noted in some of the patients, but progression to leukemia was not described. Subsequently, those with RA were better characterized with descriptions of specific dyserythropoietic features, such as ringed sideroblasts by Bjorkman (13) and the morphology of hypercellular bone marrows by Vilter and colleagues (14).

Investigators studying the acute leukemias noted that some patients had a chronic preleukemic phase characterized by cytopenias that preceded overt AML. In his 1949 paper, Hamilton-Paterson (15) suggested that the same dyshematopoietic factor was responsible for both the preceding cytopenias and the development of leukemia. Subsequent series contained descriptions of dysplastic bone marrow abnormalities in patients with preleukemia (16–19). Between 5% and 31% of patients with AML were found to have had a discernible preleukemic phase (19,20). By definition, the diagnosis of preleukemia was retrospective, made only after progression to acute leukemia. With the introduction of remission-inducing chemotherapy for AML, prospective identification of patients who would develop acute leukemia became of more than theoretical interest.

These two paths converged as investigators discussed and debated whether RA and preleukemic states were related

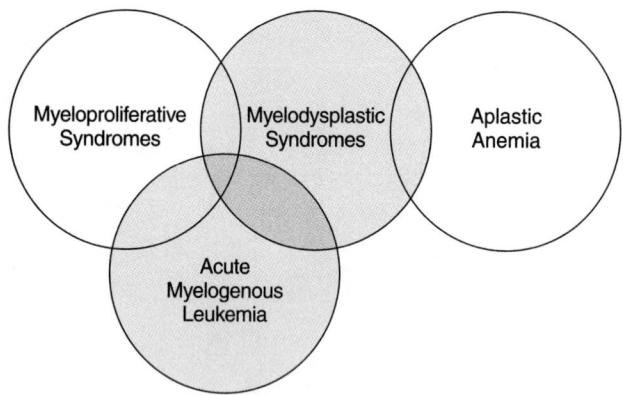

Figure 11-1. Venn diagram illustrating the interrelations among the myelodysplastic syndromes and several other hematologic disorders. Differentiation between hypocellular myelodysplastic syndromes and aplastic anemia may be difficult, and there is evolving evidence to suggest that there is overlap between these entities in some patients, as discussed in the text. Myelodysplastic syndromes can progress to acute myelogenous leukemia, and the transition may be indistinct (*overlapping areas*). Patients with chronic myelomonocytic leukemia, the monosomy 7 syndrome, or the 5q- syndrome share characteristics of both myelodysplastic syndromes and myeloproliferative syndromes, indicated by the overlap in the diagram.

TABLE 11-1. Morphologic Abnormalities of the Bone Marrow in Myelodysplasia

Abnormality	Incidence (%)
Lineage	
Dyserythropoiesis	73–100
Multinuclearity	
Intranuclear bridging	
Nuclear fragments and budding	
Megaloblastic changes	
Vacuolation	
Ringed sideroblasts	
Maturation arrest	
Dysmyelopoiesis	37–88
Giant primary granules	
Decreased primary granules	
Auer rods	
Decreased secondary granules	
Fragmented nuclei	
Maturation arrest	
Abnormal localization of immature myeloid precursors	
Dysmegakaryocytopoiesis	50–87
Micromegakaryocytes	
Decreased nuclear polyploidization	
Separated nuclei ("pawn ball")	
General features	
Cellularity	
Increased or normal	81–100
Decreased	0–19
Fibrosis	20–25

Data from references 60, 69, 76, 140, and 704.

(21,22). Dameshek (22) proposed that RA states were neoplastic because they lacked a consistent metabolic defect and were irreversibly progressive, with eventual replacement of normal marrow elements. Dreyfus and co-workers (23,24), Linman and Bagby (20), and Saarni and Linman (25) made the connection explicit in their careful descriptive studies.

The nomenclature and classifications applied to patients with RA and preleukemia became increasingly confusing. In an effort to provide uniform criteria for diagnosis and for clinical investigation, the French-American-British (FAB) Cooperative Group initially developed guidelines to separate patients with what they termed *MDSs* from patients with leukemia as part of their classification system for AML (26). In 1982, the same group focused on MDS more specifically and set forth a classification, defined nomenclature, and catalogued diagnostic morphologic features (27). By these criteria, most patients who had previously been given diagnoses of RA, idiopathic sideroblastic anemia, marrow dysplasia, preleukemia, oligoleukemia, smoldering leukemia, or chronic myelomonocytic leukemia (CMML) could be included in the MDS classification system.

The ability, gained during the past two decades, to cure or induce sustained remissions in several types of malignancies with aggressive chemotherapy or radiation therapy has also produced a new category of MDS (28–30). Long-term survivors of effectively treated neoplasms have an appreciable risk of developing cytopenias with trilineage marrow dysplasia. This hematologic disorder has been termed *therapy-related MDS* (t-MDS). Despite sharing many characteristics with primary MDS, t-MDS differs in many important respects and carries a more dismal prognosis with a higher risk of early progression to leukemia [therapy-related AML (t-AML)].

Most recently, a new World Health Organization (WHO) classification has been developed that incorporates several changes, including a separate category for refractory cytopenias with trilineage dysplasia, designation of refractory anemia with excess of blasts in transformation (RAEB-t) (>20%

bone marrow blasts) as AML, and recognition of CMML as an entity distinct from MDS (31).

BONE MARROW MORPHOLOGY

The diagnosis of MDS in a patient with anemia, neutropenia, or thrombocytopenia or all three depends on demonstrating characteristic dysmorphic features in the bone marrow. Indeed, the FAB classification and the more recent WHO modification is based almost entirely on abnormalities found in the bone marrow aspirate (7,27,31). Although often considered a diagnosis of exclusion, MDS can usually be recognized and differentiated from other hematologic disorders by thorough assessment of bone marrow morphology. Several comprehensive reviews of the bone marrow in MDS have been published, and the characteristic features are summarized in Table 11-1 (32–35).

Both a bone marrow aspirate and a biopsy should be obtained; cellular morphology and quantitation of myeloblasts can be done on an aspirate, but accurate assessment of cellularity and localization of immature precursors require biopsy sections (34,36,37). Definitive diagnostic evaluation of patients with MDS may require several separate samples because affected bone marrow may be distributed unevenly (38). If a bone marrow biopsy from the posterior iliac crest is hypocellular, adequate cells may often be obtained from a sternal aspirate.

Dyserythropoietic abnormalities include a dissociation between nuclear and cytoplasmic maturation and other megaloblastic characteristics (39) and bizarre nuclear configurations including binuclearity, nuclear bridging, and nuclear budding (40). Ringed sideroblasts, erythroblasts with at least five Prussian blue–staining iron granules encircling more than one-third

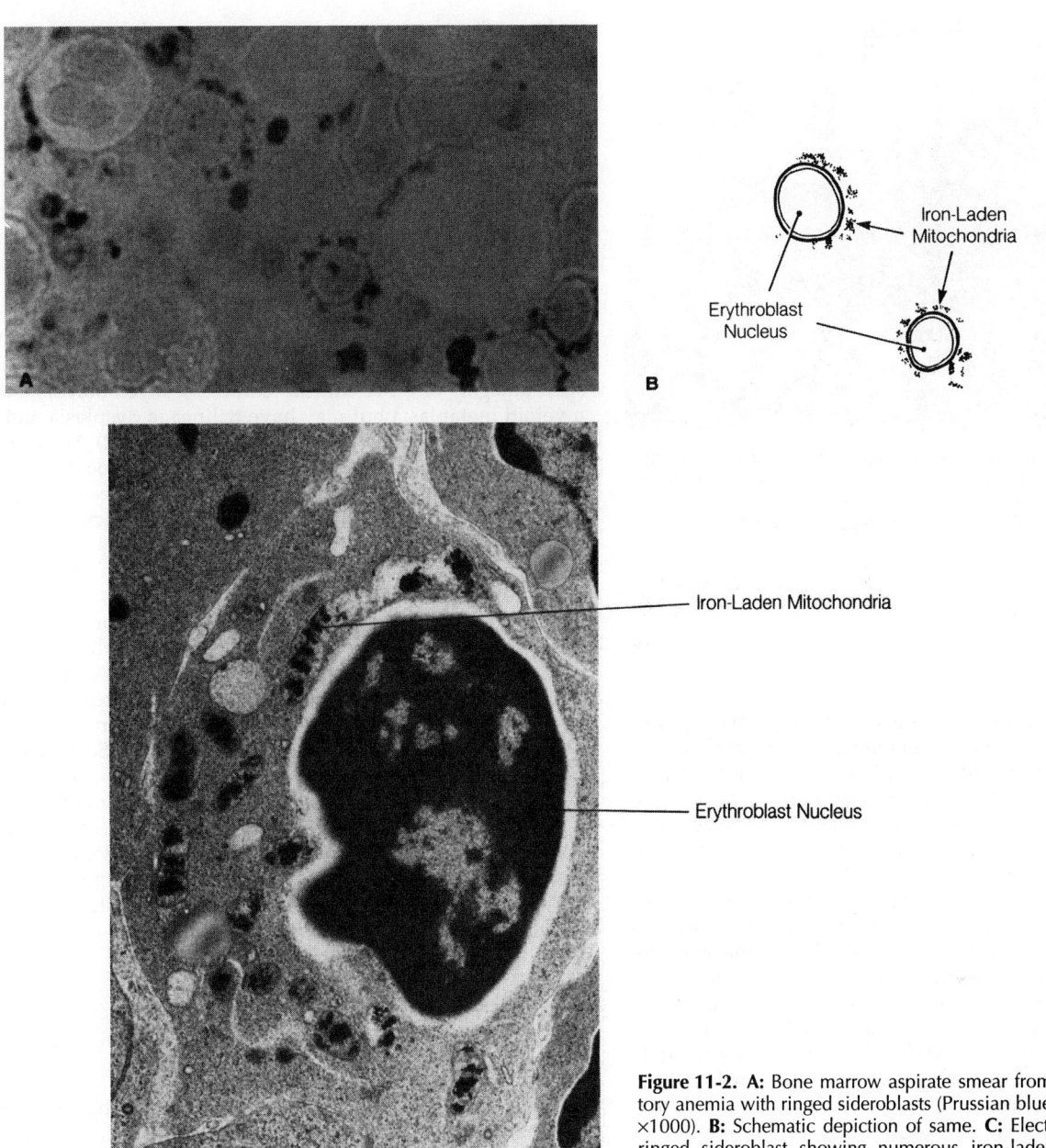

Figure 11-2. A: Bone marrow aspirate smear from patient with refractory anemia with ringed sideroblasts (Prussian blue stain, magnification ×1000). **B:** Schematic depiction of same. **C:** Electron micrograph of a ringed sideroblast showing numerous iron-laden mitochondria surrounding the nucleus (magnification ×11,000). (Adapted from Bottomley SS. Sideroblastic anaemia. *Clin Haematol* 1982;11:389.)

of the nucleus, are an important morphologic characteristic in MDS (41) (Fig. 11-2A). These cells were first described in 1956 by Bjorkman in the marrow of a patient with RA (13) and have been historically central to discussions on the nature and classification of MDS (21,22,27).

Thirty percent to 50% of normoblasts in the normal bone marrow contain iron granules detectable by light microscopy. These granules are small, located in the cytoplasm, and by electron microscopy are ferritin-iron aggregates (12,42,43). The number of these granules increases with either ineffective erythropoiesis or iron overload, as in thalassemia or pernicious anemia. In contrast, pathologic-ringed sideroblasts contain large perinuclear granules that have been shown, by electron microscopy, to be mitochondria enlarged and distorted by abnormal nonferritin iron deposition (44,45) (Fig. 11-2B). More than one-half of patients with all subtypes of MDS have an appreciable number of ringed sideroblasts (41).

Megakaryocytes have characteristic abnormalities in MDS (46). Absolute numbers of megakaryocytes may be increased, normal, or decreased, but individual cells often have defects in nuclear polyploidization and increased nuclear separation ("pawn ball" nuclei) (47). The most unusual megakaryocytes are small, with one or two round and widely separated nuclei and aberrant granulation (Fig. 11-3). These cells are most common in patients with the 5q- syndrome but can also be found in other patients with MDS (48). Anti–von Willebrand's factor antibodies may be used to stain biopsy sections to assist in the identification of megakaryocytes (49).

Abnormalities of myeloid maturation may be striking or subtle. A left shift toward more immature forms may be seen even without an actual excess of myeloblasts. Specific monoclonal antibodies may be useful in identifying immature myeloid cells that lack the typical morphologic characteristics (50). Both primary and secondary granulation are often decreased

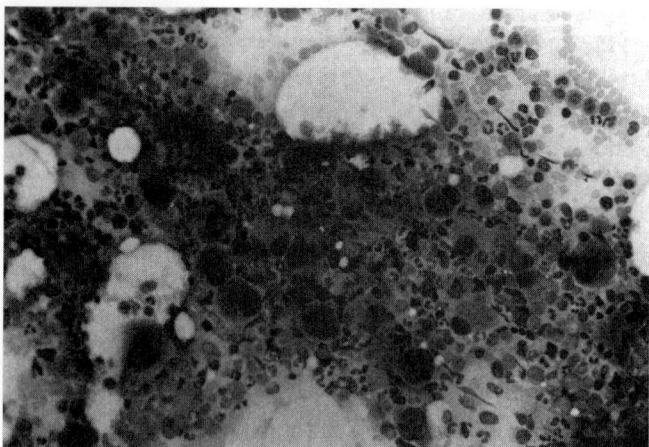

Figure 11-3. Bone marrow aspirate from a patient with refractory anemia and the 5q- syndrome. A large number of strikingly abnormal small and uninuclear megakaryocytes are characteristic of both the 5q- syndrome in particular and myelodysplastic syndromes in general (Wright's stain, magnification ×900).

and distributed abnormally within the cell. A lack of synchronization between nuclear and cellular maturation and granule formation is also observed. Some myeloid precursors stain with both specific and nonspecific esterases, suggesting infidelity between granulocytic and monocytic lineages (51).

The morphology and identification of myeloblasts is particularly pertinent to the FAB and WHO classification systems (27,31,52). Two types of myeloblasts are described on a Wright-Giemsa–stained aspirate; these differ primarily in their cytoplasmic characteristics (27). Type I myeloblasts are typical myeloblasts with high nuclear/cytoplasmic ratios, distinct nucleoli, uncondensed chromatin, and no cytoplasmic granules. Type II blasts may have a few primary azurophilic granules and lower nuclear/cytoplasmic ratios. Auer rods, elongated azurophilic inclusions resulting from fusion of primary granules, are found in the cells of 20% of patients with certain subtypes of MDS (53). Cells with eccentric nuclei, a well-developed Golgi apparatus (perinuclear clear zone), condensed chromatin, numerous granules, or a low nuclear/cytoplasmic ratio should be scored as promyelocytes instead of myeloblasts. The bone marrow blasts of most patients with MDS have immunochemical and cytochemical characteristics typical of myeloid or monocytoid blasts (54). Occasionally, the blasts exhibit features of the megakaryocytic or lymphoid lineage, supporting the concept that the basic defect in MDS is expressed at the level of the pluripotent stem cell (55,56).

Most characteristically, bone marrow cellularity is either increased or normal in patients with MDS (Table 11-1), but many studies have included patients with hypocellular bone marrows who have the typical morphologic and clinical characteristics of MDS. Recent reviews comparing patients with a hypocellular bone marrow with those with a hypercellular or normocellular bone marrow report similar biologic characteristics and prognosis (57–59). Myeloid/erythroid ratios are extremely heterogeneous but typically increased, except in the RA with ringed sideroblasts (RARS) subtypes in the FAB and WHO classification systems.

A significant increase in reticulin is seen in the bone marrow biopsies of 20% of patients with MDS (60,61). Patients with bone marrow fibrosis and MDS do not have significant splenomegaly or other clinical features of myelofibrosis with myeloid metaplasia but may have trilineage dysplasia and a prognosis similar to typical patients with MDS (62). Most such patients exhibit increased numbers of megakaryocytes, leading to speculation that excess fibrosis is due to release of fibroblast mitogens such as platelet-derived growth factor (PDGF) or transforming growth factor β (TGF-β) (62–64). Elevated levels of PDGF have been reported in the serum of patients with primary myelofibrosis (65).

The anatomic interrelations between hematopoietic precursors and the bone marrow stroma, particularly the interface between marrow and bone, may be disordered in patients with MDS. Such relations may be central to the regulation of normal hematopoiesis. First, stromal cells are an important source of various growth and inhibitory factors. Second, specific binding to stromal matrix proteins may also control the local concentration of growth factors (66–68). Tricot (37,69) was the first to call attention to abnormally localized immature precursors (ALIPs) in MDS patients. Myeloblasts and other immature forms are normally localized along the endosteal surface, but in many patients they form clusters (ALIPs) that are not contiguous with bony trabeculae.

CLASSIFICATION

French-American-British Classification

The diagnostic criteria and classification system for MDS proposed by the FAB Cooperative Group (7,27) became widely adopted, despite controversy over its morphologic emphasis and skepticism regarding its prognostic usefulness (10,70–73). The group reviewed morphologic features of bone marrow aspirates from 50 patients as well as clinical data, and they used the observations to define five subtypes of MDS (Table 11-2). (The qualitative morphologic abnormalities are summarized in Table 11-1.) The percentages of bone marrow and peripheral

TABLE 11-2. French-American-British Classification Criteria

Subtype	Abbreviation	Peripheral Blood	Bone Marrow
Refractory anemia	RA	Blasts <1%	Blasts <5%
Refractory anemia with ringed sideroblasts	RARS	Blasts <1%	Blasts <5%
Refractory anemia with excess of blasts	RAEB	Blasts 5%	Blasts 5–20%
Refractory anemia with excess of blasts in transformation	RAEBT	Blasts >5%	Blasts 20–30% or Auer rods
Chronic monomyelocytic leukemia	CMML	Monocytes 1 × 10⁹/L	Any of the above
Acute myeloid leukemia	AML	—	Blasts >30%

Bennett JM, Catovsky D, Daniel MT, et al. Proposals for the classification of the myelodysplastic syndromes. *Br J Haematol* 1982;51:189.

blood myeloblasts used to define categories are arbitrary and are not meant to imply separate biologic entities but to provide information that may be useful in assessing severity of disease and prognosis. The cut-off of 5% marrow myeloblasts used in FAB and other classification schemes derives from a study in which 1827 consecutive unselected bone marrow examinations were reviewed and a myeloblast percentage with respect to total nucleated marrow cells calculated. Patients (127 of 129) with more than 5% myeloblasts either had or later developed leukemia, and 127 of 136 patients who subsequently developed leukemia had previous marrows with greater than 5% myeloblasts (74).

The original FAB classification scheme defined subtypes by the percentage of myeloblasts in both bone marrow and peripheral blood (27) (Table 11-2). It has become clear that even patients with RA or RARS can have occasional circulating blasts that are not prognostically ominous (75,76). When a discrepancy exists between bone marrow and peripheral blood blast percentage FAB class, the marrow percentage should determine assignment. This problem rarely arises.

One difficulty in using the FAB classification scheme has been in calculating the myeloblast percentage in bone marrow specimens with an increased nucleated erythroid cell count. Some have suggested that the denominator should be total cells if the percentage of erythroid cells is less than 50% but that total myeloid cells should serve as the denominator if the erythroid component of the marrow exceeds 50% (7,77). For example, a marrow specimen with 80% erythroblasts and 20% myeloid cells including 10% myeloblasts would be classified as acute leukemia because the myeloblasts make up 50% of the myeloid component. This scheme gives some weight to the relative size of the erythroid component as an independent prognostic factor. More reasonable would be a consistent practice of expressing the percentage of myeloblasts with reference only to the total number of nonerythroid nucleated hematopoietic cells. Fortunately, this issue arises in few patients with MDS. Most patients with erythroid hyperplasia have RARS and few myeloblasts (76,78–80). Conversely, patients with prognostically unfavorable subtypes of MDS generally have a smaller marrow erythroid compartment.

In the original FAB classification system, patients with t-MDS were not placed in a separate category but into one of the five subtypes based on the usual criteria. It has become increasingly apparent that these patients behave differently from patients with primary MDS with respect to leukemic transformation and overall prognosis (7,70,81). Even patients presenting with a low percentage of bone marrow myeloblasts often have severe cytopenias and trilineage dysplasia and rapidly evolve into t-AML (82).

Most investigators found the FAB classification system to have useful prognostic applicability, with significantly longer survivals for patients with RA and RARS than for those with RA with excess of blasts (RAEB), RAEB-t, or CMML (75,83–86).

Another positive aspect of the FAB classification system for MDS was its functional continuity with the widely used FAB leukemia classification system (26). The FAB MDS nomenclature also allows for progression from one subtype to another over time. Several longitudinal studies found frequent progression from RA or RARS to RAEB, RAEB-t, or CMML, then to AML (76,87–89). In many ways, the subtypes can be considered as stages of disease rather than distinct entities.

The FAB classification system was also the focus of criticism and controversy (10,35,70–73). One problem has been semantic. Patients who present with isolated thrombocytopenia or neutropenia but with unambiguous morphologic or cytogenetic evidence for myelodysplasia fell into the subtype RA (89). It has been suggested that *refractory cytopenia* might be a preferable term (7). Another issue has been the classification of patients who fit criteria for more than one subtype, such as a patient with 20% ringed sideroblasts and 10% myeloblasts in the marrow. Prognostic predictions were more accurate in these cases when the patient is assigned to the subtype based on bone marrow myeloblast percentage (RAEB or RAEB-t) (75,86). This interpretation of the FAB guidelines has become standard.

The FAB recommendation to include any patient with marrow or circulating Auer rod–laden myeloblasts in RAEB-t was also controversial. In several small groups of patients, Auer rods were not associated with a worse prognosis or a higher risk of leukemic transformation than predicted by the overall myeloblast percentage (53,85,90). The issue deserves further investigation, but most investigators do not classify patients with Auer rods in RAEB-t unless they also have greater than 20% marrow myeloblasts.

The inclusion of the CMML subtype in the FAB system had also been criticized. Historically, patients with chronic disorders of the monocytoid lineage have been difficult to classify and characterize. Some investigators argued that CMML should be considered as a completely separate entity or should be included in the myeloproliferative syndrome (35,72). Most of these patients clearly have classic trilineage dysplastic marrows and other characteristic features of MDS. CMML patients frequently progress in and out of the CMML subtype to and from other FAB subtypes, supporting their inclusion into the MDS (76,88). Some confusion exists in the classification of patients with increased circulating monocytes and greater than 5% marrow myeloblasts. For prognostic purposes, inclusion of these patients in RAEB or RAEB-t has been preferred to inclusion in CMML (75,85,86,91).

World Health Organization Classification System

Because of these concerns, an alternative classification has recently been adopted that addresses some of the perceived deficiencies of the FAB classification system (31,52). As shown in Table 11-3, RA and RARS have been divided into two categories, each based on presence or absence of trilineage dysplasia. RA without dysplasia is defined as less than 5% bone marrow blasts and less than 15% ringed sideroblasts; RA with dysplasia is the same, but with greater than 10% dysplastic granulocytes and megakaryocytes. Similarly, RARS without dysplasia is defined as less than 5% blasts and greater than 15% ringed sideroblasts, whereas RARS with dysplasia is the same, with greater than 10% dysplastic granulocytes and megakaryocytes. The former categories of RAEB and RAEB-t have also been modified. RAEB is now two categories, with RAEB-I defined as 5% to 10% blasts, whereas RAEB-II is 11% to 19% blasts. RAEB-t, formerly defined as 20% to 30% bone marrow blasts, is now classified as AML, and CMML has been moved to a separate category of "myelodysplastic and myeloproliferative disorders."

The new classification system addresses some, but certainly not all, of the problems with the FAB classification system and adds several unusual twists. The recognition that 20% bone marrow blasts or higher should be characterized as AML would appear to be a step in the right direction. However, the categories of RA or RARS "without dysplasia" in a disease that is characterized by morphologic dysplasia would seem to be misnomers. The new system remains based almost entirely on morphologic findings, in part due to a lack of complete understanding of the genetic basis of MDS. It is not yet certain to what extent the WHO classification scheme will more accurately reflect clin-

TABLE 11-3. World Health Organization Classification System for Myelodysplastic Syndrome

Category	Peripheral Blood	Bone Marrow
1a. RA without dysplasia	Blasts <1%; monocytes <1000/mm^3	Blasts <5%; ringed sideroblasts <15%
1b. RA with dysplasia	Same + dysgranulocytes and/or giant platelets	Same + dysgranulocytes and/or dysmegakaryocytes
2a. RARS without dysplasia	Blasts <1%; monocytes <1000/mm^3	Blasts <5%; ≥15% ringed sideroblasts
2b. RARS with dysplasia	Same + dysgranulocytes and/or giant platelets	Same + dysgranulocytes and/or dysmegakaryocytes
3a. RAEB-I	Blasts 1–4%; monocytes <1000/mm^3	Blasts 5–10%
3b. RAEB-II	Blasts 5–19%; monocytes <1000/mm^3	Blasts 11–19%

RA, refractory anemia; RAEB, refractory anemia with excess blasts; RARS, refractory anemia with ringed sideroblasts.

ical outcome or response to therapy, if at all. As discussed below, this latter problem has been addressed through the new International Prognostic Scoring System (IPSS).

CLINICAL PRESENTATION

The MDSs are not common disorders in the general population, but most hematologists follow several such cases. The overall incidence is approximately 1/100,000 cases/year, with a median age at diagnosis of 65 to 70 years. The incidence increases dramatically over the age of 65 years, and may be as high as 20 to 50/100,000 in this age group. It has been estimated that there are approximately 1000 new pediatric and 12,000 new adult cases/year. MDS is thus among the most common hematologic malignancy in adults and occurs at an appreciable frequency in children (92). In addition, t-MDS has been more frequently observed as more intensive chemotherapy and radiation therapy have extended survival of patients with other underlying malignancies, as discussed in the section Therapy-Related Myelodysplasia.

Epidemiologic Characteristics

Table 11-4 summarizes data from several large studies on presenting characteristics of patients with MDS. MDS is primarily a disorder of the elderly (93,94), with a median onset in the seventh decade, although the syndrome may occur in any age group, including in the pediatric population (95–97). Five percent to 17% of children experience a myelodysplastic phase before the onset of AML, and similar or higher figures have been estimated for adults (19,95,98,99). There is a slight male predominance in all age groups. Few reports have been made of the familial occurrence of MDS (100–103). Initial clinical presen-

tation as children or young adults in these families has been typical, but Fanconi's anemia has not been rigorously excluded in every case.

Chronic exposure to low-dose radiation, especially radiopharmaceuticals that are taken up by the reticuloendothelial system, may increase the risk of MDS or AML (104–106). A pilot case control study reviewed the association between environmental and occupational exposures and MDS. They found that significantly more patients than controls had worked with ammonia, diesel fuel, or other petrochemicals (107). Significant benzene exposure may also be a risk factor (108). The development of MDS as a delayed complication of intensive chemotherapy or radiation (t-MDS) is discussed in the section Therapy-Related Myelodysplasia.

Several long-term follow-up studies of patients with aplastic anemia treated with antithymocyte globulin suggest an increased risk of subsequent MDS or AML (109–113). This increased risk has not been observed in bone marrow transplant recipients. In one study, the initial diagnosis of aplastic anemia may have been erroneous in some patients, because retrospective review of bone marrows obtained at initial presentation revealed trilineage dysplasia, fibrosis, and megakaryocytic hyperplasia (113). It is also possible that patients with recovered aplastic anemia are left with a greatly reduced number of stem cells, increasing the mutational stress on each stem cell and thus the risk of developing MDS (114). Abnormal cells that can escape immune surveillance may be selected for in the context of an abnormally active autoimmune response against hematopoietic cells in aplastic anemia (114). Several reports have also been cited of MDS in patients who had been in remission from AML (115,116). The patients had not received alkylating agents, making MDS secondary to chemotherapy unlikely. Perhaps a residual abnormal stem cell clone survived chemotherapy and gradually became dominant, with subsequent emergence of MDS.

TABLE 11-4. Clinical Characteristics of Myelodysplastic Syndrome Patients at Presentation

Study (and Ref)	Mean Age (yr)	Male:Female Ratio	Incidence			
			Splenomegaly	Anemia[a]	Thrombocytopenia[b]	Neutropenia[c]
Weisdorf (85)	70	100:0	25	83	28	36
Varela (536)	72	—	18	93	25	31
Mufti (91)	73	51:49	—	67	38	39
Oguma (458)	59	65:35	—	—	—	—
Sanz (140)	68	53:47	12	82	45	24
Tricot (531)	62	58:42	—	45	32	24
Kerkhofs (75)	73	50:50	—	85	—	—
Foucar (84)	68	52:48	12	—	—	—
Coiffier (60)	—	54:46	21	—	—	—

[a]Anemia: percentage of patients with hemoglobin below 12 g/dL.
[b]Thrombocytopenia: percentage of patients with platelet counts below 100,000/μL.
[c]Neutropenia: percentage of patients with neutrophil counts below 1500/μL.

The coincident occurrence of myeloma or other lymphopro-liferative disorders and MDS has been described more frequently (117–119). This may be due to the chance occurrence of two diseases that are more common in elderly patients, although some authors have made statistical arguments for a nonrandom association (117). No clonal markers were shown to be shared by both the dysplastic and the abnormal lymphoid clones in these patients. Perhaps impaired immune function associated with MDS, particularly decreased natural killer (NK) cell activity, could predispose to lymphoproliferative disorders (120,121).

Symptoms and Signs

Initial symptoms of MDSs are weakness or pallor secondary to anemia and, less frequently, bleeding or infection. Occasionally, patients complain of diffuse arthralgias. Intermittent fevers of unknown origin have also been reported (122). Approximately one-half of patients have no symptoms, with MDS being discovered during investigation of unrelated complaints or on a routine visit. Macrocytosis or mild anemia may be present for years before the development of more severe cytopenias that precipitate the diagnosis of MDS. Splenomegaly is found in approximately 20% of patients, most frequently in patients with CMML; hepatomegaly and lymphadenopathy are found less frequently. Physical examination rarely reveals any specific abnormalities. Several unusual dermatologic syndromes have been reported in association with MDS, including acute febrile neutrophilic dermatosis (Sweet's syndrome) (123,124), urticaria pigmentosa (125), and granulocytic sarcoma (126).

Hematologic Characteristics

The incidence of anemia, thrombocytopenia, and neutropenia in several large studies is shown in Table 11-4. Pancytopenia or bicytopenia is present in 20% to 35% of patients with MDS. Anemia is the most common isolated abnormality (30% to 35%), and isolated thrombocytopenia or neutropenia can occur in 1% to 9% of cases (38,60,127–129). Except in patients with CMML, a specific subtype of MDS, the total white count is usually normal or decreased. The granulocytic lineage is primarily affected, but reductions in total lymphocyte count can also occur. Patients with the 5q- syndrome can have thrombocytosis and, more rarely, neutrophilia (130).

Abnormalities of peripheral blood cell morphology are summarized in Table 11-5. Macrocytosis is common in patients with MDS but not universal (131,132). A distinctive dimorphic smear is often seen in patients with RARS, with both a hypochromic and microcytic population of cells, as well as a second macrocytic population. Decreased heme synthesis reduces hemoglobin production, and hypochromia results (133). Teardrops, RBC fragments, and nucleated RBCs are seen, especially in patients with increased marrow reticulin. Giant platelets are characteristic, and platelet granules may be sparse or increased in size. These platelet anomalies are most readily appreciated by electron microscopy (134,135). Granulocytes may manifest striking abnormalities, including a spectrum of nuclear variants such as hyposegmentation with a Pelger-Huët anomaly (136), unusual chromatin clumping and myelokathexis-like hypersegmentation (137–139), and abnormal granulation.

Occasional circulating myeloblasts can be detected in a large number of patients with MDS (75), and up to 10% of the differential count in RAEB-t patients can be myeloblasts without signaling progression to AML. A sudden increase in circulating myeloblasts should prompt a reexamination of the bone marrow. Generally, peripheral blast percentage changes in tandem

TABLE 11-5. Morphologic Abnormalities in the Peripheral Blood in Myelodysplastic Syndromes

Red cells
  Macrocytosis
  Dimorphism
  Anisopoikilocytosis
  Punctate basophilia
  Nucleated red blood cells
  Polychromasia
  Erythroblasts
White cells
  Hypogranulation
  Pelgeroid nuclei
  Hyposegmented or hypersegmented nuclei
  Ringed-shaped nuclei
  Döhle bodies
  Myeloblasts or other immature forms
Platelets
  Giant forms
  Hypogranulation
  Megakaryocyte fragments

with bone marrow blast percentage and is not an independent predictor of prognosis (76,140).

Laboratory Abnormalities

Blood chemistry analysis is often abnormal, but the findings are nonspecific. Ten percent to 40% of patients have elevated levels of lactate dehydrogenase, alkaline phosphatase, hepatic transaminases, uric acid, or bilirubin, but these abnormalities rarely help make the diagnosis. Vitamin B$_{12}$ levels are usually normal but may be elevated in patients with an expanded myeloid compartment. Serum and urine lysozyme (muramidase) may also be elevated in MDS, especially in CMML patients, presumably because of increased monocyte turnover (141). Because lysozyme levels may be elevated in many conditions, this test has little routine diagnostic usefulness (142,143).

Iron Metabolism

The finding of ringed sideroblasts is a characteristic feature of MDS. (What is known about metabolic abnormalities leading to iron deposition within mitochondria is summarized in the section Ringed Sideroblast Formation.) Directly relevant to clinical evaluation and care of patients with MDS is their predisposition to iron overload. They may have increased total body iron stores on presentation. Measurement of the serum iron, total iron-binding capacity, and ferritin is an essential part of the initial evaluation.

Patients with MDS may have received iron as empiric therapy for RA before accurate diagnosis. Furthermore, patients with a large but ineffective erythroid component in their bone marrow are predisposed to excess iron absorption. A strong positive correlation exists between the rate of iron turnover within the erythron and iron absorption independent of total-body iron stores (144). The mechanism of this relationship has not been established. The total iron absorbed, particularly in patients given empiric iron therapy, may be significant. Estimates suggest that 6% to 10% of the population may be heterozygous for primary hemochromatosis. The presence of such an abnormal gene in a patient with MDS undoubtedly enhances excess iron absorption. A possible nonrandom association has been suggested between the HLA A3 allele, which is closely linked to the primary hemochromatosis allele, and RARS, but this remains controversial (145–149).

The importance of evaluating iron stores on presentation is underscored by the fact that many patients require chronic transfusion therapy. Among those with the best prognoses are patients with ineffective erythropoiesis, who may present with high iron stores. Early institution of chelation therapy may be indicated to help avoid unnecessary morbidity and mortality.

SPECIFIC CLINICAL SYNDROMES

Lack of knowledge about the causes of MDS means that many of the clinical and morphologic delineations are arbitrary and may actually deter insight into pathogenesis and pathophysiology. In general, we have chosen to discuss MDSs collectively with respect to clinical features, pathophysiology, prognosis, and treatment. A large body of literature containing many important observations on several specific clinical syndromes exists and is summarized in this section.

Chronic Myelomonocytic Leukemia

Classification of patients with abnormal proliferation or differentiation of the monocytoid lineage has always been confusing. In their 1956 description of monocytic leukemias, Sinn and Dick (150) noted that a subset of patients with increased circulating monocytoid cell counts had a chronic course without inevitable progression to acute leukemia. Subsequent investigators reported that all hematopoietic lineages were frequently abnormal in these patients (151,152). In the 1970s, several carefully documented series of patients with these characteristics were described, and their disorder was termed *CMML* (141,153,154).

Usually, such patients were elderly (median age of 65 years) and presented with nonspecific symptoms. Sixty percent of patients had anemia or thrombocytopenia or both in addition to the characteristic peripheral blood monocytosis. Both circulating monocytes and granulocytes were found to have morphologic and functional abnormalities (155). The bone marrow exhibited trilineage dysplasia, with dyserythropoietic and dysmegakaryocytic features similar to those found in patients with preleukemic syndromes. Their bone marrows were uniformly hypercellular, with increased myeloid/erythroid ratios. Serum lysozyme concentration was almost always significantly elevated (142,156). Up to 60% of patients had polyclonal hypergammaglobulinemia, perhaps because of hyperstimulation of B cells by increased circulating activated monocytes (142).

The 1982 FAB classification system for myelodysplasia included CMML as a subclass (27). As noted above, some controversy has existed about classification of CMML as a myelodysplastic instead of as a myeloproliferative syndrome or as a separate entity (35,72). The trilineage dysplastic changes seen in these patients and the frequent evolution between CMML and other FAB subtypes seem to justify its inclusion in MDS (88,152,153). Diagnostic features that distinguish CMML from chronic myelogenous leukemia (CML) and AML are the lack of a Philadelphia chromosome, trilineage marrow dysplasia, and a less aggressive clinical course. Thus, the reclassification of CMML in the separate category of "myelodysplastic and myeloproliferative disease" by WHO criteria seems justified.

More is known about the pathophysiology of CMML than perhaps any of the MDS categories. At least five recurrent balanced reciprocal chromosomal translocations associated with the CMML phenotype have been cloned. Molecular cloning of these translocations has identified the t(5;12) TEL/PDGFβR, t(5;7) HIP1/PDGFβR, t(9;12) TEL/ABL, t(5;10) H4/PDGFβR, t(5;14) RAB5EP/PDGFβR, and t(9;12) TEL/JAK2 fusion proteins (157–166), respectively. Each translocation contains a tyrosine kinase domain [PDGFβ receptor (PDGFβR), ABL or JAK2] that is constitutively activated by the respective fusion partner. Consti-

tutive activation activates downstream signal transduction pathways and results in abnormal proliferation and survival of cells, with minimal effects on differentiation. Furthermore, expression of these fusions in primary murine bone marrow cells largely recapitulates the human disease phenotype of CMML and indicates that these fusion proteins are legitimate targets for therapeutic intervention (163,167). Gleevec (imatinib mesylate, STI571) was first identified as a potent PDGFβR inhibitor, and also inhibits the BCR/ABL fusion in CML. It is thus plausible that Gleevec may also have therapeutic efficacy in CMML patients (168) with constitutively activated PDGFβR or ABL fusion proteins. In fact, a recent report indicates activity of Gleevec in a patient with the RAB5EP/PDGFβR fusion activity (169), and responses to Gleevec have also been reported in abstract form in patients with CMML and the TEL/PDGFβR fusion (170). These observations provide a paradigm for molecularly targeted therapies of these disorders and suggest that a more detailed understanding of the molecular pathophysiology of MDS may lead to novel, rational therapeutic approaches.

5q- Syndrome

In 1974 and 1975, Van den Berghe and co-workers (171,172) described five patients with an acquired interstitial deletion of the long arm of chromosome 5 (5q-) and RA. The patients had severe macrocytic anemia, leukopenia, and normal or elevated platelet counts. Their bone marrows were hypercellular, with increased myeloblasts in some cases, and characteristic dysplastic, small, and uninuclear megakaryocytes. None of the original patients progressed to leukemia or had short survival times; thus, the authors suggested that these clinical findings portend a relatively good prognosis. They felt the association was specific and termed this constellation the *5q- syndrome*. Since that time, a great deal of interest has been generated in patients with this karyotypic abnormality and hematologic disease, especially after the discovery that the genes for several hematopoietic growth factors and their receptors were localized to the missing area of chromosome 5 (173–177). Several genes located in the deleted area of the 5q-, including IRF1, a putative tumor-suppressor gene, have been proposed as candidate genes in the pathogenesis of MDS. However, as yet no *bona fide* tumor-suppressor gene has been identified in MDS patients with 5q deletions. The syndrome in patients with the 5q- chromosome is similar to that found in other patients with primary MDS. Several larger studies have reported that many 5q- patients present with thrombocytopenia, along with anemia and neutropenia, and progression to AML has now been documented in many cases, even without evolution of additional cytogenetic abnormalities (178–180). The distinctive uninuclear or binuclear megakaryocytes, described by some authors as unique to patients with 5q- (48), can clearly be found in patients with dysplastic megakaryocytes and apparently normal chromosome 5 (174). The 5q- chromosomal abnormality has also been found in patients with a wide variety of other hematologic diseases, including AML, myeloproliferative syndromes, and t-MDS.

Inherited Myelodysplastic Syndromes

An inheritable syndrome, familial platelet disorder (FPD) with propensity to develop AML (FPD/AML syndrome) has many of the characteristics of an inherited myelodysplasia. The autosomal-dominant trait is characterized by thrombocytopenia with an "aspirinlike" platelet aggregation defect, by progressive dysplasia and pancytopenia with age with decreased hematopoietic colony-forming ability, and by progression to AML often associated with acquisition of secondary cytogenetic abnormalities (181,182). FPD/AML syndrome is caused by haploinsufficiency of the hematopoietic transcription factor AML1 (RUNX1) (183). These data indicate an important role for loss of function of hematopoietic transcription factors in the development of an MDS phenotype, and that loss of function of a single allele may be responsible for development of MDS. Thus, the search for a tumor-suppressor gene in commonly deleted regions in MDS, such as 5q, 7q, and 20q, should include assessment of haploid gene dosage.

Therapy-Related Myelodysplasia

The increased risk of acute leukemia in patients previously treated with cytotoxic chemotherapy for other conditions has been recognized for two decades. After investigators observed that t-AML was a panmyelosis accompanied by trilineage abnormalities, patients who had received chemotherapy began to be followed more closely and evaluated as soon as cytopenia, macrocytosis, or abnormal bone marrow morphology was detected (29). Most patients who develop t-AML have a detectable t-MDS phase (28,30). This realization has made risk assessment for these secondary hematologic syndromes more meaningful, because patients dying from complications of the cytopenias before developing actual t-AML are now generally included in epidemiologic surveys (184).

In recent large studies, patients with t-MDS account for up to 15% of total patients with MDS (60,84,185). The incidence of t-MDS and t-AML has increased because of the prolonged survivals (even cures) now attainable after aggressive chemotherapy and radiation therapy of tumors that were previously rapidly fatal. This unfortunate by-product of aggressive treatment, especially in young patients with curable tumors such as Hodgkin's lymphoma, has stimulated a reexamination of chemotherapy regimens in hopes of designing and implementing less mutagenic or carcinogenic combinations (186–188).

The primary tumors most frequently reported as preceding t-MDS or t-AML are Hodgkin's and non-Hodgkin's lymphomas, ovarian carcinoma, small cell lung cancer, multiple myeloma, breast cancer, and gastrointestinal tumors treated with adjuvant chemotherapy (28,184,189–198). Patients given alkylating agents for nonmalignant conditions such as rheumatoid arthritis or scleroderma are also at risk (199).

The risks of developing t-MDS or t-AML are disturbingly high: up to 13% at 10 years after aggressive Hodgkin's disease chemotherapy (200) and up to 14% at 4 years in one smaller study of patients treated intensively for small cell lung cancer (192). A 12-fold higher risk has been found in ovarian cancer patients treated with chemotherapy compared with that found in patients treated with surgery alone (194). The risk increases nonlinearly with duration and intensity of treatment. The highest risk occurs within the first 4 to 5 years after institution of chemotherapy or radiation therapy and reaches a plateau at 8 to 10 years (Fig. 11-4). The mean time to presentation with symptoms of t-MDS or t-AML from initial chemotherapy is 48 to 68 months (189,193,201–203).

Alkylating agents are strongly implicated, because aggressive chemotherapy regimens without an alkylating agent, such as those used for germ cell tumors or acute leukemias, do not increase the risk of t-MDS or t-AML (116,193,201,204,205). Alkylating agents are mutagenic and carcinogenic *in vitro* and in animal models (206). They interact directly and covalently with DNA, forming reactive intermediates that cross-link, break, and cause misreading of DNA strands. Agents such as methotrexate and vincristine, which do not directly interact with DNA, have not been shown to increase the risk of secondary neoplasms. It is not understood why agents such as cisplatin or daunorubicin,

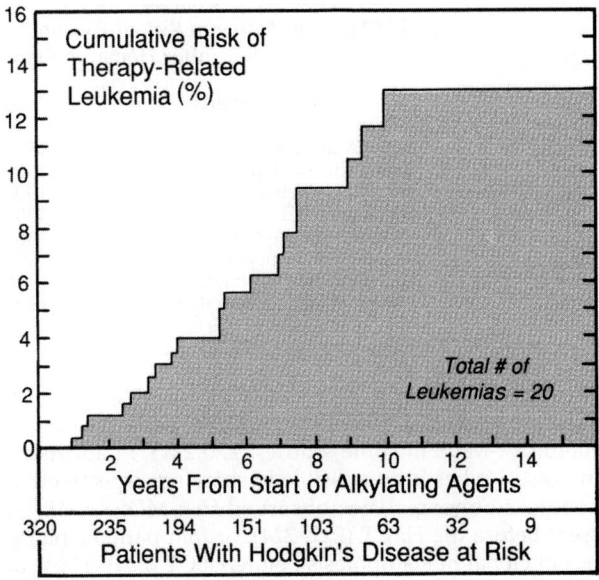

Figure 11-4. Kaplan-Meier plot of the cumulative risk of therapy-related myelodysplastic syndrome and acute myelogenous leukemia in a cohort of 320 patients up to 15 years after the start of alkylating agent chemotherapy for Hodgkin's disease. (Adapted from Pedersen-Bjergaard J, Larsen SO, Struck J, et al. Risk of therapy-related leukaemia and preleukaemia after Hodgkin's disease: relation to age, cumulative dose of alkylating agents, and time from chemotherapy. *Lancet* 1987;2:85.)

which do interact with DNA and cause strand breaks or conformational shifts, have not been associated with an appreciable rate of secondary tumors.

The link between external-beam radiation therapy and a higher risk of t-MDS or t-AML has been less clearly established. Some studies have failed to identify cases in patients treated with external-beam radiation therapy alone (28,190). Another reported a lower risk and a longer latency than after chemotherapy (202), whereas at least one other described several patients who had received external-beam radiation therapy alone and soon thereafter developed t-MDS. These patients had received extremely high radiation doses to the spine and pelvis (193). Chemotherapy, given in conjunction with external-beam radiation therapy, does not result in a higher risk than the same regimen of chemotherapy given alone (28,184,190,194,195).

Topoisomerase II inhibitors, such as epipodophyllotoxin [etoposide (VP-16)] are particularly potent in induction of t-MDS/AML. t-MDS/AML in this setting often involves abnormalities and rearrangements of the *MLL* gene on chromosome band 11q23 and may develop with shorter latencies than t-MDS induced by other agents (207). Etoposide may induce t-MDS/AML when given as therapy for underlying malignancy such as breast cancer (208) or pediatric acute lymphoblastic leukemia (209), or when given to mobilize stem cells in the context of hematopoietic stem cell transplantation (HSCT) (210).

Patients who undergo intensive therapy with HSCT have an increased risk of t-MDS/AML (211), in particular patients receiving HSCT for lymphoma (212–219) (Table 11-6). The actuarial risk ranges from 3% to as high as 24%, indicating that in some series, nearly one-fourth of all patients who survive their lymphoma after HSCT will develop the life-threatening complication of t-MDS/AML. The intensity of the conditioning regimen, especially one associated with whole-body irradiation, has been implicated in risk of t-MDS. However, an emerging literature suggests that the primary basis for increased risk may well be chemotherapy or radiation therapy received before HSCT. For example, prior therapy with high cumulative doses

TABLE 11-6. Actuarial Risk of Developing t-Myelodysplastic Syndrome/Acute Myelogenous Leukemia after Hematopoietic Stem Cell Transplantation for Lymphoma

Author/Institution	Year	Actuarial Risk %/Year	Reference
Miller/Minnesota	1996	14.5/4 yr	217
Bhatia/City of Hope	1996	13.5/6 yr	213
Darrington/Nebraska	1994	4/5 yr	214
Friedberg/DFCI	1999	19.8/10 yr	215
Pedersen-Bjergaard/Copenhagen	1997	24.3/3.6 yr	219
Andre/French Cooperative	1998	4.3/5 yr	212
Harrison/British Cooperative	1999	3.2/5 yr	216
Milligan/EMBT Cooperative	1999	4.6/5 yr	218

of alkylating agents is the most important risk factor for development of t-MDS in some studies (220,221). In addition, in many cases, it has been possible to show retrospectively that karyotypic abnormalities observed in t-MDS/AML were present before the HSCT (222–224), or that patients had evidence of clonal hematopoiesis before HSCT (225). These data suggest that early identification of suitable candidates for HSCT, and an effort to minimize alkylating agent therapy may be important to prevent t-MDS/AML.

Several clinical features of t-MDS should be emphasized. The mean age at presentation is approximately 10 years earlier than that seen in primary MDS (30,202). Occurrence of t-MDS in children is more common than primary MDS in this age group (226). Peripheral blood counts and cell morphology are similar to those found in primary MDS, except that severe pancytopenia is more common and increased numbers of basophils have been noted (29,189,202). Bone marrow cellularity is generally normal or increased, but 10% to 25% of patients have hypocellular bone marrows (201,202). The degree of trilineage dysplasia is often striking. Ringed sideroblasts can be found in appreciable numbers in up to 60% of t-MDS bone marrow samples (29,202).

The FAB, and likely the WHO, classification of patients with t-MDS is much less meaningful than in primary MDS. Even patients with less than 5% myeloblasts or large numbers of sideroblasts (RA or RARS) progress rapidly to AML or succumb to complications of severe cytopenias (82). Patients with t-MDS should always be separated from those with primary MDS in natural history studies and therapeutic trials, because their clinical course and prognosis are significantly different. Otherwise, results may be distorted, depending on the relative number of patients with t-MDS included. The new WHO classification does not delineate a separate category for t-MDS, even though there is a separate category for t-AML.

DIFFERENTIAL DIAGNOSIS

Few, if any, pathognomonic features are seen in myelodysplasia patients. Many patients must be followed for several months to determine whether their cytopenias have reversible or nonprogressive causes. Table 11-7 lists other possible causes of chronic cytopenias with an adequately cellular marrow, which should be excluded before making the diagnosis of MDS. The impressive macrocytosis and megaloblastic changes that often occur in MDS can strongly suggest B_{12} or folate deficiency, but serum levels or a Schilling test should be obtained before embarking on empiric vitamin replacement. During the regenerating recovery phase after marrow damage due to chemotherapy, alcohol, or benzene, many of the morphologic changes used to define MDS may be seen. Diagnosis of t-MDS should be made

only when cytopenia and marrow dysplasia are persistent or follow an initial period of full bone marrow recovery. Viral infection of erythroid precursors, such as with B19 parvovirus, can also produce bizarre erythroid dysplasia. Parvovirus infections should be excluded, especially in children or adults with immune deficiencies (227).

Ringed sideroblasts are not specific to MDS and do not by themselves imply that diagnosis. Table 11-8 gives a differential diagnosis of ringed sideroblasts. Several comprehensive review articles can be consulted for more detail (12,42). Reversible causes, such as drug- or alcohol-related marrow damage, should be ruled out and treated. A careful family history and hematologic workup are required to rule out hereditary sideroblastic anemia, especially in children presenting with isolated

---

TABLE 11-7. Differential Diagnosis of Chronic Cytopenias with Cellular Marrows

Nutritional conditions
    Vitamin B_{12} deficiency
    Folate deficiency
    Iron deficiency
Reversible marrow toxicity
    Alcohol
    Recovery phase from chemotherapy or irradiation
    Toxins or drugs
Anemia of chronic disease
    Renal failure
    Collagen vascular disease
    Chronic infection
Viral infection of marrow
    B19 parvovirus
    Human immunodeficiency virus
Neoplastic conditions
    Leukemia
    Nonleukemic tumor infiltration of marrow
    Paraneoplastic marrow suppression
Congenital or hereditary conditions
    Hereditary sideroblastic anemias
    Congenital dyserythropoietic anemias
    Fanconi's anemia
    Diamond-Blackfan syndrome
    Down's syndrome
    Shwachman syndrome
    Kostmann's syndrome
Myeloproliferative syndromes
    Polycythemia vera
    Essential thrombocythemia
    Chronic myelogenous leukemia
    Myelofibrosis with myeloid metaplasia
    Monosomy 7 syndrome
    Juvenile chronic myelogenous leukemia
Paroxysmal nocturnal hemoglobinuria
Hypersplenism
Myelodysplastic syndromes
    Primary idiopathic
    Therapy related

TABLE 11-8. Differential Diagnosis of Ringed Sideroblasts

Congenital
   Hereditary sideroblastic anemias
      X-linked (references 496–501)
      Autosomal (references 497, 498, 705–708)
Acquired
   Idiopathic (refractory anemia with ringed sideroblasts)
   Drug induced (reference 484)
      Isoniazid (reference 485)
      Other antituberculous drugs (reference 485)
      Chloramphenicol (reference 45)
      Zinc (reference 709)
   Ethanol induced (reference 484)

anemia and no dysplasia of nonerythroid lineages. Monomorphic, microcytic RBCs are also suggestive of hereditary rather than idiopathic acquired sideroblastic anemia.

Differentiation between aplastic anemia and MDS can be difficult in patients with a hypocellular bone marrow. A judgment regarding the degree of bone marrow dysplasia may be required. The finding of activated suppressor T lymphocytes in peripheral blood may support the diagnosis of aplastic anemia. Conversely, cytogenetic abnormalities of a clonal nature provide evidence that MDS is the correct diagnosis, although some patients with aplastic anemia have been reported with associated clonal cytogenetic abnormalities (228). Care should also be taken to identify patients with aleukemic leukemia who have a hypocellular bone marrow. If the myeloblast percentage is greater than 30%, such persons should be treated aggressively with chemotherapy (229). The distinction between aplastic anemia and MDS is further blurred by clinical observations indicating that some patients with aplastic anemia progress to MDS or AML, and, as discussed in the section Immunosuppressive Therapy, some patients diagnosed as having MDS respond to immunosuppressive therapies, such as antithymocyte globulin (ATG) (228,230–234) or cyclosporin A (235,236), which are more traditionally used to treat aplastic anemia.

Acquired or congenital hematologic diseases such as paroxysmal nocturnal hemoglobinuria, the myeloproliferative syndromes, Kostmann's syndrome, and Fanconi's anemia should not be classified as MDSs, even though statistically they carry an increased risk of leukemia and in that sense are preleukemic. This also applies to Down's syndrome and Bloom's syndrome. These disorders are not necessarily associated with hematologic abnormalities but are indeed associated with an increased risk of leukemia. MDS is rare in children who have not received chemotherapy; thus, careful family histories, chromosomal studies, and bone marrow examinations are required to exclude Diamond-Blackfan syndrome (pure RBC aplasia), congenital dyserythropoietic anemia, Fanconi's anemia, hereditary sideroblastic anemia, Shwachman syndrome, and other constitutive disorders in young patients with cytopenias.

PATHOGENETIC MECHANISMS

Of special consideration in the pathogenesis of MDSs is the fact that these are clonal disorders. Progeny of a single cell gain ascendancy in the bone marrow. Their selective advantage appears to derive from genetic mutations that free dysplastic cells from normal growth constraints and perturb their capacity for full maturation. An acquired or inherent genetic instability within the myelodysplastic clone appears to predispose to additional mutations, leading to the emergence of subclones and progressive evolution of the myelodysplastic process, initially manifesting as bone marrow dysfunction and ultimately as leukemia.

Clonal Nature

The primary evidence that MDS are clonal disorders is based on the fact that the two X chromosomes in female cells are structurally and functionally distinct. Early in embryonic development, one X chromosome in each somatic cell is randomly inactivated by mechanisms that include methylation of specific cytosine residues in DNA. If a female is heterozygous at a specific X-chromosome locus, each of the tissues is composed of cells expressing one or the other allele but not both. The best-known example is glucose-6-phosphate dehydrogenase (G6PD). In heterozygous women, the A and B isozymes of G6PD are present in roughly equal proportions in all tissues. Because X-chromosome inactivation occurs early in embryogenesis, the number of cells expressing either allele are approximately equal. If a population of cells in such a heterozygous individual is clonal, that is, they derive from a single somatic cell, it is composed of cells that are all producing the same isozyme (237).

In 1978, Prchal and co-workers (238) reported that a G6PD heterozygous woman with classic RARS expressed only one isozyme in platelets, RBCs, granulocytes, macrophages, B cells, and T cells. In this patient, RARS was shown to be a clonal disorder affecting a hematopoietic stem cell that became ascendant in all myeloid and lymphoid lineages. The observations of these researchers provided the first evidence of a common hematopoietic progenitor for myeloid and lymphoid cells in humans. Several other patients with MDS have since been shown to have clonal expression of G6PD, with a single isozyme present in all myeloid lineages, B cells, and Epstein-Barr virus (EBV)–immortalized B-cell lines, but not in T cells (239,240). This discrepancy in T-cell involvement among patients suggests that the myelodysplastic process could begin in progenitors or stem cells with varying T-lymphoid repopulating ability. Perhaps polyclonal, unaffected T cells persist for long periods in some patients.

Heterozygosity for G6PD is rare, limiting analysis of clonality in MDS to just a few patients. Recently, more general methods have been developed to investigate clonality. Many cytosine residues on the inactive X chromosome are methylated, whereas the corresponding residues on the active chromosome remain unmethylated. Several X-chromosome probes for restriction fragment length polymorphisms (RFLPs) have been identified. Using these probes, sequential digestion with two restriction enzymes can first identify female heterozygotes, then distinguish the activated from the inactivated X chromosome (241–243). This procedure is diagrammed in Figure 11-5. The first restriction enzyme distinguishes the maternally and paternally derived copies of the X-chromosome gene via an RFLP. The second enzyme is methylation-sensitive and distinguishes the active from the inactive copy of the gene via differential digestion patterns. Between 30% and 60% of women are heterozygotes for at least one of the presently available RFLP probes. This technique has already been used to demonstrate the monoclonal derivation of bone marrow and peripheral blood nucleated cells in seven of eight patients with MDS (244). More recently, sensitive assays for clonality based on X-inactivation have been developed using polymerase chain reaction (Fig. 11-5). The use of highly polymorphic triplet expansion repeat polymorphisms at the human androgen receptor locus on the X-chromosome renders nearly 90% of women informative for clonality analysis (225). In addition, coding polymorphisms in X-linked genes have allowed for clonality analysis based on expression rather than methylation status, which may have advantages in some clinical settings (245). Analysis using these approaches in larger numbers of patients has confirmed the clonal nature of MDS, and that in most cases the myeloid lineage is the primary lineage involved in MDS.

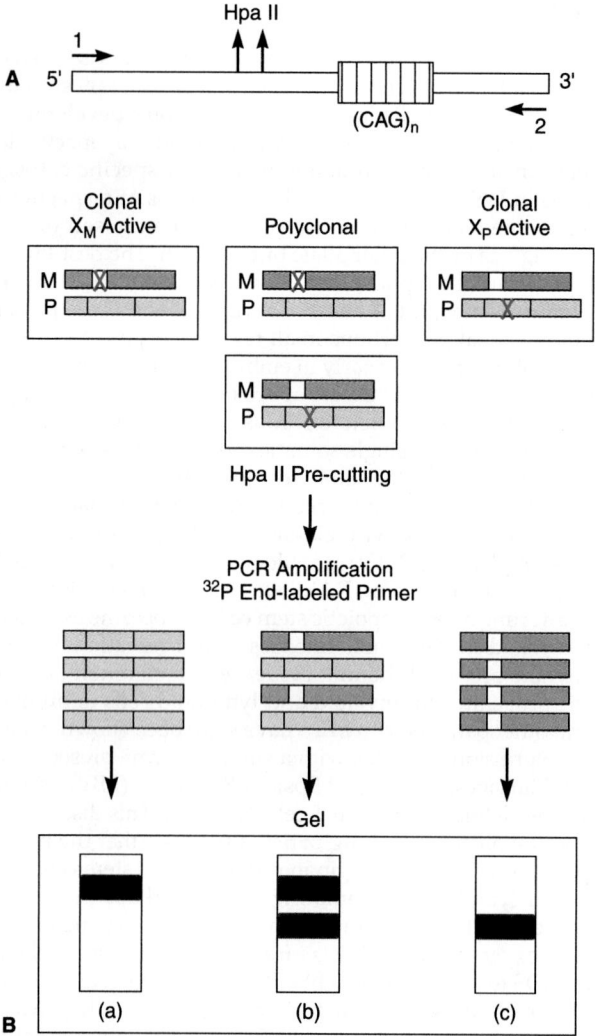

Figure 11-5. X-linked clonality assay at the human androgen receptor locus (HUMARA). **A:** Human androgen receptor locus on the X chromosome. Exon 1 contains a highly polymorphic CAG repeat with a heterozygosity frequency of greater than 90% in females. A site of differential methylation is 5' to the CAG repeat, and can be used to distinguish the active X allele and the inactive X allele. Within the differential methylation sites there are two restriction sites for the methylation sensitive restriction endonuclease Hpa II. Hpa II will cleave unmethylated, active X alleles, precluding amplification of these alleles by polymerase chain reaction (PCR) primers 1 and 2. **B:** The HUMARA clonality assay. DNA is digested with HpaII and amplified by PCR using ^{32}P end-labeled primers. In a polyclonal population of cells (b), both the maternal (M) and paternal (P) X alleles will be amplified and discriminated as two bands of different molecular weight on a denaturing polyacrylamide gel by the variable CAG repeat. In contrast, for a clonal population of cells [(a) or (c)], in which all cells are derived from a single common mutant progenitor cell, only the maternal or the paternal allele will be amplified, giving a single band.

Cytogenetic studies have also supported the concept of MDS as a clonal disorder of the pluripotent stem cell. The same specific chromosomal abnormalities have been identified in cells derived from either erythroid or myeloid colony-forming units (CFUs) grown *in vitro* from patients with MDS (246,247). EBV-immortalized B cells, but not T cells, from one patient had the same interstitial chromosomal deletion as bone marrow myeloid progenitor cells (248). One recent study provides some convincing evidence that, at least in patients with the 5q- syndrome, the defect is not present in lymphoid cells (248a).

In addition to the documentation of clonal markers in cells of multiple lineages, the transformation of MDS into several differ-

ent phenotypic varieties of acute leukemia provides evidence that the primary defect is at the level of the hematopoietic stem cell. Most patients with MDS who develop acute leukemia have typical AML that can be classified in the FAB scheme as M1 or M2; several instances of transformation to acute megakaryocytic leukemia (M7) (55,63) and several case reports documenting conversion to acute lymphocytic leukemia have been seen (55,249–252). One patient developed acute leukemia with two distinct populations of blast cells—one myeloid and one lymphoid (253)—and other patients have leukemic populations with lineage infidelity, the coexpression of markers or phenotypic characteristics normally not found coexisting in one cell (252).

Cytogenetic Abnormalities

Patients with MDS have frequently been found to have bone marrow cells with chromosomal abnormalities that are clonal, nonrandom, and prognostically informative (254–256a), although the exact role of most of these chromosomal changes in the pathogenesis of MDS is still uncertain. Using standard cytogenetic techniques (Chapter 5), 33% to 64% of patients with primary MDS have detectable abnormalities (257–268). Using higher-resolution techniques, Yunis and co-workers (269,270) found chromosomal abnormalities in 79% of patients with primary MDS. Specific abnormalities are not random: The most common are deletion of the long arm of chromosome 5 (5q-), monosomy 7 (7-), and trisomy 8 (+8). Recurrent chromosomal aberrations associated with MDS are summarized in Table 11-9 and include balanced reciprocal chromosomal translocations, unbalanced anomalies including deletions, and numerical abnormalities (271–276). The frequency of the more common cytogenetic abnormalities is indicated in Table 11-10 (277,278). A similar incidence (50%) and distribution of chromosomal changes have been reported in a small group of pediatric patients with MDS (279), except that abnormalities of chromosome 5 are much less common than in adults.

Deletion of the long arm of chromosome 5 (5q-) has been the most intensely studied chromosomal change associated with MDS for three reasons: (a) It is the most common chromosomal alteration found in association with MDS (269,277,278,280); (b) A 5q- syndrome, consisting of RA, thrombocytosis, and abnormal megakaryocyte morphology with a relatively good prognosis, has been reported; and (c) The genes for several hematopoietic growth factors and receptors have been mapped to the deleted region on chromosome 5. The 5q deletion is an acquired mutation, present in multipotent progenitor cells giving rise to both erythroid and granulocytic lineages (281), but not to fibroblasts or circulating T lymphocytes (171). The deletion is almost universally interstitial, with loss rather than translocation of the missing segment (130,282,283). The 5q- abnormality is also frequently reported in association with other hematologic disorders, including *de novo* and t-AML, acute lymphoblastic leukemia, polycythemia vera and other myeloproliferative syndromes, and pure RBC aplasia (130,180,284–287).

Several of the commonly detected abnormalities in MDS are also seen in patients with *de novo* AML, especially the elderly (288). This suggests a true biologic continuum between MDS and at least some types of AML. Furthermore, several of the translocations that are typically associated with AML, including t(8;21) with M2 AML, t(15;17) with M3 (promyelocytic) AML, t(9;22) with CML, as well as t(9;11) and inv(16) may also be associated with MDS, especially t-MDS (Table 11-9), further supporting a continuum between MDS and AML. No consistent associations between FAB subtypes of MDS and specific chromosomal abnormalities have yet been reported, although chromosomal changes are more common in patients with RAEB, RAEB-t, and CMML than in those with RARS or RA (263,268,289).

TABLE 11-9. Cytogenetic Abnormalities Associated with Myelodysplastic Syndrome

Balanced Structural Abnormalities	Unbalanced Structural Abnormalities	Numeric Abnormalities
t(1;3)(p36;q21)[a]	der(1;7)(q10;p10)[c]	-5^e
t(2;11)(p21;q23)[a]	dup(1)(q21-23q32-44)[a]	$+6^e$
t(3;21)(q26;q22)[b]	del(3)(p21-22)[b]	-7^f
inv(3)(q21q26)[b]	del(3)(q21-22)[a]	$+8^f$
t(3;3)(q21;q26)[a]	del(4)(q21-25q31-35)[a]	$+9^f$
t(5;12)(q23;p13)[a]	del(5)(q11-31q31-q35)[d]	$+11^f$
t(6;9)(p23;q34)[a]	dic(5;17)(q11-13;p11)[a]	$+14^f$
t(8;21)(q22;q22)[b]	del(6)(q13-24q23-27)[b]	$+19^f$
t(9;11)(p22;q23)[a]	del(7)(q11-34q22-36)[d]	$+21^f$
t(9;22)(q34;q11)[a]	i(7)(q10)[a]	$-X^e$
inv(16)(p13q22)[b]	i(8)(q10)[a]	$-Y^f$
	del(9)(q11-13q22)[b]	—
	del(11)(q13-23q23-25)[c]	—
	del(12)(p11-13)[c]	—

[a]Detected in five to ten patients.
[b]Detected in 11 to 25 patients.
[c]Detected in 26 to 100 patients.
[d]Detected in more than 100 patients.
[e]Detected as a sole abnormality in five to ten patients.
[f]Detected as a sole abnormality in more than ten patients.
Data from Mrozek K, Heinonen K, Bloomfield CD. Acute myeloid leukemia and myelodysplastic syndromes: clinical implications of cytogenetic abnormalities. *Adv Oncol* 2001;16(4):10–16.

The incidence of detectable cytogenetic abnormalities in patients with t-MDS is higher than in those with primary MDS—80% to 100% in several studies (29,193,201–203,290–292). Compared with that seen in other chromosomes, abnormalities of chromosome 5, chromosome 7, or both are relatively more common (50% to 95%) than in primary MDS. Changes in chromosomes 1, 3, 4, 12, 14, 17, 18, 19, and 21 have also been reported as being nonrandomly associated with t-MDS (193,201,291,293,294). Patients treated with chemotherapy but without active hematologic disease do not have these cytogenetic changes detectable in their marrows (290). Thus, detection of karyotypic changes may be of value for early diagnosis of t-MDS and could help to distinguish t-MDS from other causes of cytopenias in cancer patients, including relapse of the primary tumor with marrow suppression or infiltration.

Many investigators have performed serial karyotypes and have noted an association between progression of MDS, from RA or RARS to RAEB, RAEB-t, or frank AML, and new or additional chromosomal changes. In some cases, clonal evolution occurs as an initially abnormal clone acquires additional cytogenetic abnormalities (295–301); in others, several subclones with independent abnormalities have been shown to arise, coexist, and eventually either disappear or dominate (302–305). Even stronger correlations between new cytogenetic abnormalities and disease progression have been observed in t-MDS (193,201,203).

Adequate cytogenetic analysis of bone marrow or peripheral blood in MDS may be difficult because of low proliferation rates or absence of evaluable metaphases (254,263). Most investigators have cultured marrow cells for 12 to 72 hours in an attempt to increase yield; some have advocated synchronization procedures (269). Results may be skewed if an abnormal clone has a selective growth advantage or disadvantage in culture. Several studies have documented a difference in the number of or even presence of abnormal clones when bone marrow cells are assayed immediately after harvesting rather than after a period of *in vitro* culture (306–308).

Several other methods have been devised for assessing karyotype that do not depend on microscopic analysis of condensed chromosomes. The DNA content of cells can be measured by flow cytometry, which has been used to show that one-half of patients with MDS have aneuploidy of marrow cells (309). The advantages

of this method are that large numbers of cells can be analyzed easily and rapidly, without requiring *in vitro* proliferation. A disadvantage is an inability to detect balanced translocations and other pseudodiploid states. Direct DNA image cytometry on fixed cells shares with flow cytometry the advantage of not requiring mitotic cells, although allowing analysis of individual fixed cells on a slide and detection of small populations of abnormal cells (310). DNA probes specific for frequently altered chromosomal fragments can be used to assess cytogenetic changes in DNA harvested from fractionated MDS cell populations (311,312). DNA probes isolated from known chromosomal regions have also been useful for mapping breakpoints by pulsed field gel electrophoresis (313). Recent technologic advances have allowed for analysis of chromosomal translocations and abnormalities using fluorescence *in situ* hybridization with locus-specific probes, spectral karyotype analysis, comparative genomic hybridization, loss of heterozygosity analysis, and characterization of point mutations using DNA sequence analysis (314). These tests have increasing diagnostic value and have provided important new insights into the complexity of genomic rearrangements in MDS.

Mutations in Specific Genes

Substantial progress has been made in the past several years in elucidating the molecular genetics of MDS. MDS is a clonal disor-

TABLE 11-10. Incidence of Various Cytogenetic Abnormalities in Myelodysplastic Syndrome

Abnormality	Incidence (%)
Loss of all or part of chromosome 5	13
Loss of all or part of chromosome 7	5
Trisomy 8	5
Del(17p)	<1
Del(20q)	2
Loss of X or Y chromosome	2

Data from Greenberg P, Cox C, LeBeau MM, et al. International scoring system for evaluating prognosis in myelodysplastic syndromes. *Blood* 1997;89(6):2079–2088; and Heaney ML, Golde DW. Myelodysplasia. *N Engl J Med* 1999;340(21):1649–1660.

der typified by acquired somatic mutations as detailed below. Although much work remains, a spectrum of mutations has been identified over the past several years that can be causally implicated in pathogenesis of MDS and progression of MDS to AML.

RAS

The search for mutations of protooncogenes in the cells of patients with MDS has been focused thus far on the *RAS* gene family, Ha-, Ki-, and N-*RAS*. These genes encode 21-kd guanosine triphosphate (GTP)–binding proteins that localize to the inner surface of the plasma membrane and play an as-yet-undefined role in the transduction of signals from the cell surface (315). Overexpression of normal p21 protein can result in transformation of immortalized fibroblast cell lines, but transformation occurs with much lower levels of an altered activated p21 protein produced by *RAS* genes mutated at codons 12, 13, or 61. These abnormal p21 proteins have less intrinsic GTPase activity and may be locked in an activated, GTP-bound state.

An activated *RAS* gene was first found in DNA isolated from a human bladder tumor (316,317). Activated *RAS* genes have now been found in DNA isolated from many human tumors in up to 40% to 50% in AML, colon cancer, and adenocarcinoma of the lung (317). The high incidence of *RAS* mutations found in AML samples prompted investigators to screen bone marrow cells of patients with MDS with the hope of learning whether *RAS* mutations were an early event in the apparent multistep progression toward leukemia or a later event associated with actual leukemic transformation.

Activated *RAS* genes have been reported in bone marrow or peripheral blood samples of from 8% to 50% of patients with MDS, although in carefully conducted studies, the frequency in MDS has been estimated at 10% to 15% (244,318–326). Mutations in the N-*RAS* gene are most common, but activation of either of the other *RAS* genes has also been reported. No consistent association of *RAS* mutations with any one FAB subtype has been found, except that these mutations may be more common in patients with CMML (318,320). Mice that develop T-cell lymphomas secondary to alkylating agents have an extremely high incidence of activating *RAS* gene mutations in tumor DNA (327), but only one of nine patients with t-MDS secondary to chemotherapy was found to have these mutations (328). In several, a clear relation existed between *RAS* gene mutations and progression of MDS to leukemia. Such mutations are found in patients with indolent RA or RARS, and some investigators have not found them to predict more rapid progression to AML (318,319). However, in one recent study, N-*RAS* mutations were associated with a poor prognosis and an increased risk of progression to leukemia in patients with MDS (319a). Two patients in whom only a small percentage of bone marrow cells initially tested positive for a *RAS* mutation developed coincident increases in the percentage of cells with abnormal *RAS* genes and bone marrow myeloblasts (329). Another study reported significantly shorter survivals for patients with MDS with *RAS* mutations (326). RAS activation provides a proliferative or survival advantage to hematopoietic progenitors and is likely to contribute to the pathogenesis of MDS through this mechanism, although additional mutations may be required. Those MDS patients with activating mutations in RAS may be candidates for therapy with farnesyl transferase inhibitors (FTIs). As described below, FTIs inhibit RAS activity by inhibiting the farnesylation reaction required for targeting of RAS to the plasma membrane.

CHROMOSOMAL TRANSLOCATIONS INVOLVING TYROSINE KINASES

CMML may be associated with balanced reciprocal chromosomal translocations. As noted above, cloning and characterization of a number of these has demonstrated expression of fusion genes involving tyrosine kinases, including the TEL/PDGFβR, TEL/ABL, HIP1/PDGFβR, H4/PDGFβR, and RBTN/PDGFβR fusion proteins. In each case, the consequence of the fusion is oligomerization and constitutive activation of the kinase by the respective fusion partner, providing proliferative and survival signal to cells (157–166). Like BCR/ABL in CML, these constitutively activated tyrosine kinases activate a spectrum of downstream effectors of proliferation and survival, including the RAS/MAPK, PI3K/AKT, and STAT pathways. Each of these tyrosine kinases offers potential for therapeutic intervention through selective kinase inhibitors such as STI (571) that inhibit PDGFβR as well as ABL (169).

Activating Mutations in FLT3

As many as 35% of AML patients have mutations that constitutively activate FLT3 without requirement for chromosomal translocation. FLT3 may be activated by internal tandem duplication mutations in the juxtamembrane domain (FLT3-ITD), or by mutations in the activation loop of the tyrosine kinase domain, most often at position D835 (330–333). These mutations also activate the RAS/MAPK, PI3K, and STAT pathways and confer a proliferative advantage to hematopoietic cells in several contexts, including murine models of disease (334). The frequency of activating mutations in FLT3 has not been extensively studied in MDS, but is lower than in AML, with frequencies estimated in the 5% to 10% range (335). Mutation is more common in advanced stage MDS in transition to AML. As noted above, tyrosine kinases are attractive candidates for small molecule inhibitor therapy, such as STI571 to treat BCR/ABL positive CML. Several novel inhibitors have shown promising results in preclinical studies and are being tested in FLT3-positive MDS and AML patients in clinical trials (336–339).

Rearrangements and Mutations Involving Core Binding Factor

Core binding factor (CBF) is a heterodimeric transcription factor comprised of AML1 (RUNX1) and CBFβ subunits. The function is described in detail in Chapter 15, but, in brief, CBF is required for normal hematopoietic development (340). For example, knock-out mice that lack either AML1 or CBFβ have a complete lack of definitive hematopoiesis. AML1 and CBFβ are frequent targets of chromosomal translocations and mutation in AML, as well as in MDS, although the pattern and frequency of mutation are somewhat different. The consequence of all mutations that have been characterized thus far is loss of function of CBF. Thus, targeting of CBF would be expected to impair hematopoietic development. The available evidence in cell culture and murine models indicates that expression of CBF fusion genes, such as AML1/ETO, results in impaired hematopoietic development and may immortalize hematopoietic progenitors. However, although these mutations alone may be adequate to cause an MDS, additional mutations are required to cause AML (Chapter 15) (341,342).

AML1/EVI1 FUSION PROTEIN AND OVEREXPRESSION OF EVI1

EVI1 was originally identified as a site of viral integration in murine leukemias. It was subsequently shown to be involved in chromosomal translocations t(3;21) in MDS resulting in an AML1/EVI1 fusion gene. EVI1 may also be overexpressed as a consequence of other translocations, and a proportion of MDS cases demonstrate overexpression of EVI1 by unknown mechanisms. Although the mechanism of transformation mediated by

AML1/EVI1 is not fully understood, it appears to impair normal hematopoietic development through dominant negative interference with normal AML1 function. In this regard, it is similar to other fusion genes involving AML1 associated with AML (Chapter 15). In addition, AML1/EVI expression results in AML in murine models with a long latency, suggesting that additional mutations are required for transformation to AML (343–347).

LOSS OF FUNCTION OF AML1 BY POINT MUTATION

In addition to loss of function of AML1 as a consequence of chromosomal translocation, point mutations may inactivate AML1. Such mutations have been observed in inherited leukemia syndromes such as FPD/AML syndrome, as described in the section Inherited Myelodysplastic Syndrome (183), as well as in sporadic cases of MDS in approximately 3% to 5% of cases (348). In most cases of AML, mutations are biallelic (348); however, data from inherited MDS syndromes strongly indicate that loss of single copy may be sufficient to cause an MDS-like syndrome. These observations may have important implications for analysis of putative tumor-suppressor genes in MDS.

AML1/ETO AND CBFβ/SMMHC FUSION GENES

Although these are substantially more common in AML, collectively accounting for approximately 20% of adult AML, AML1/ETO, and CBFβSMMHC expression as a consequence of t(8;21) and inv(16), respectively, may be seen in MDS, especially in therapy-related disease. For more detail, see Chapter 15.

MLL/CBP and Other MLL Fusion Genes

More than 30 different translocations target the MLL locus on chromosome 11q23 in AML and MDS. Of these, the MLL/CBP fusion is most often associated with t-MDS (349), and as noted above, treatment with topoisomerase II inhibitors increases the risk of t-MDS associated with MLL gene rearrangements. The mechanism of transformation of the MLL/CBP fusion is not clear. In contrast with translocations involving transcription factors that bind to specific DNA sequences and transactivate or repress target genes, both MLL and CBP are transcriptional modulatory proteins that do not have any DNA binding specificity. MLL is thought to bind to the minor groove of DNA at promoters and facilitate association of transcription factors, and CBP is a transcriptional coactivator that is recruited by many transcription factors. Transduction of MLL/CBP into hematopoietic progenitors followed by transplantation into mice results in an MDS-like syndrome. However, development of AML requires a long latency of months, again suggesting that second mutations are required for transition to AML (350). Similar findings have been reported for the MLL-ELL and MLL/EML fusion genes (351–353). Although the t(9;11) giving rise to the MLL-AF9 fusion is more common in AML than MDS, analysis in murine models using "knock-in" targeting strategies also indicates requirement for second mutations (354,355).

PML/RARα

The promyelocytic leukemia/retinoic acid receptor α (PML/RARα) fusion is associated with t(15;17) in acute promyelocytic leukemia (APL) and is rarely observed in *de novo* MDS, but may be observed in cases of t-MDS. There is also ample evidence that the PML/RARα fusion alone is not sufficient to cause AML but must cooperate with additional mutations (356,357). Thus, PML/RARα joins a list of translocations and mutations involving transcription factors that result in impaired hematopoietic differentiation and may alone account for an MDS phenotype but require second mutation for progression to AML. For example, 40% of APL patients harbor activating mutations in FLT3, and FLT3-ITD and the PML/RARα fusion protein cooperate to cause AML in murine models (358). These observations have clinical relevance and indicate that some cases of MDS or AML may be responsive not only to all-*trans*-retinoic acid, but also to specific inhibitors of FLT3 (358).

5q, 7q, and 20q Deletions

Several models have been proposed to account for the association of acquired somatic cytogenetic changes with disordered hematopoiesis and increased risk of leukemia. These models are deletion of specific genes necessary for normal growth and differentiation with a resultant gene dosage effect, deletion of a tumor-suppressor gene with unmasking of a recessive abnormal allele on the homologous chromosome, and dysregulation of a protooncogene or alteration of its gene product due to abnormal juxtaposition of genetic information at the breakpoint. The 5q-, 7q-, and 20q- are among the more common deletions and have been observed in MDSs, t-MDS, t-AML, and in other hematologic disorders (130,180,284–287). The search for a pathogenetic link between these deletions and hematopoietic abnormalities has not yet been successful. The difficulties encountered are typical of the obstacles in trying to associate any specific chromosomal deletion with cancer pathogenesis.

Mapping the boundaries of the 5q deletion has generated conflicting results. High-resolution banding techniques localized the proximal breakpoint to q13.3 and the distal breakpoint to q33.1 in 15 of 15 patients with 5q- and MDS (283). Other reports have described patients with MDS with variations in both proximal and distal breakpoints (130,282,359). The breakpoints seem to be more variable in t-MDS and t-AML, but the critical shared deleted region is smaller (5q31) (193,359). Figure 11-6 shows the breakpoints compiled by one group of investigators on a large series of MDS, AML, t-MDS, t-AML, and 5q- syndrome patients. The variation in 5q deletion breakpoints has fostered the hypothesis that clinical abnormalities are caused by the loss of genes from a critical region rather than by the abnormal juxtaposition of genes at translocation junctions.

The long arm of chromosome 5 contains several genes relevant to hematopoiesis. Cells containing the 5q deletion are hemizygous for these genes. In 1985, the granulocyte-macrophage colony-stimulating factor (GM-CSF) gene and the *fms* protooncogene, which encodes the M-CSF receptor, were localized to within the deleted region (360–362). Other hematopoietic growth factors and their receptors have been mapped to this same region. These include M-CSF (363), interleukin-3 (IL-3) (364,365), IL-5 (359,366), and IL-4 (359,367,368), as well as the PDGFR (369,370), the $β_2$-adrenergic receptor (371), acidic fibroblast growth factor (372), a glucocorticoid receptor (373), CD14 (a myeloid membrane antigen) (374), a zinc-finger protein coregulated with the *fas* protooncogene (375), an ATX1 homolog (376,377), and the 5qNCA gene (378,379). Figure 11-6 diagrams the critical region deleted in patients with the 5q- syndrome, as well as patients with 5q deletions and other types of MDS or AML. The critically deleted region (CDR) on 5q31 has been further delimited, using loss of heterozygosity analysis with microsatellite markers to a region that is approximately 1.5 megabases. Predicted coding sequences and known genes in this region are being evaluated by mutational analysis (380–386). The analysis has been complicated by the suggestion that there may be more than one CDR on chromosome 5q in addition to 5q31, including a locus on 5q33 (377,387), and on 5q13 (388,389). Similar analysis has been used to delineate a CDR for chromosome 20q (390–394) and chromosome 7q (395,396).

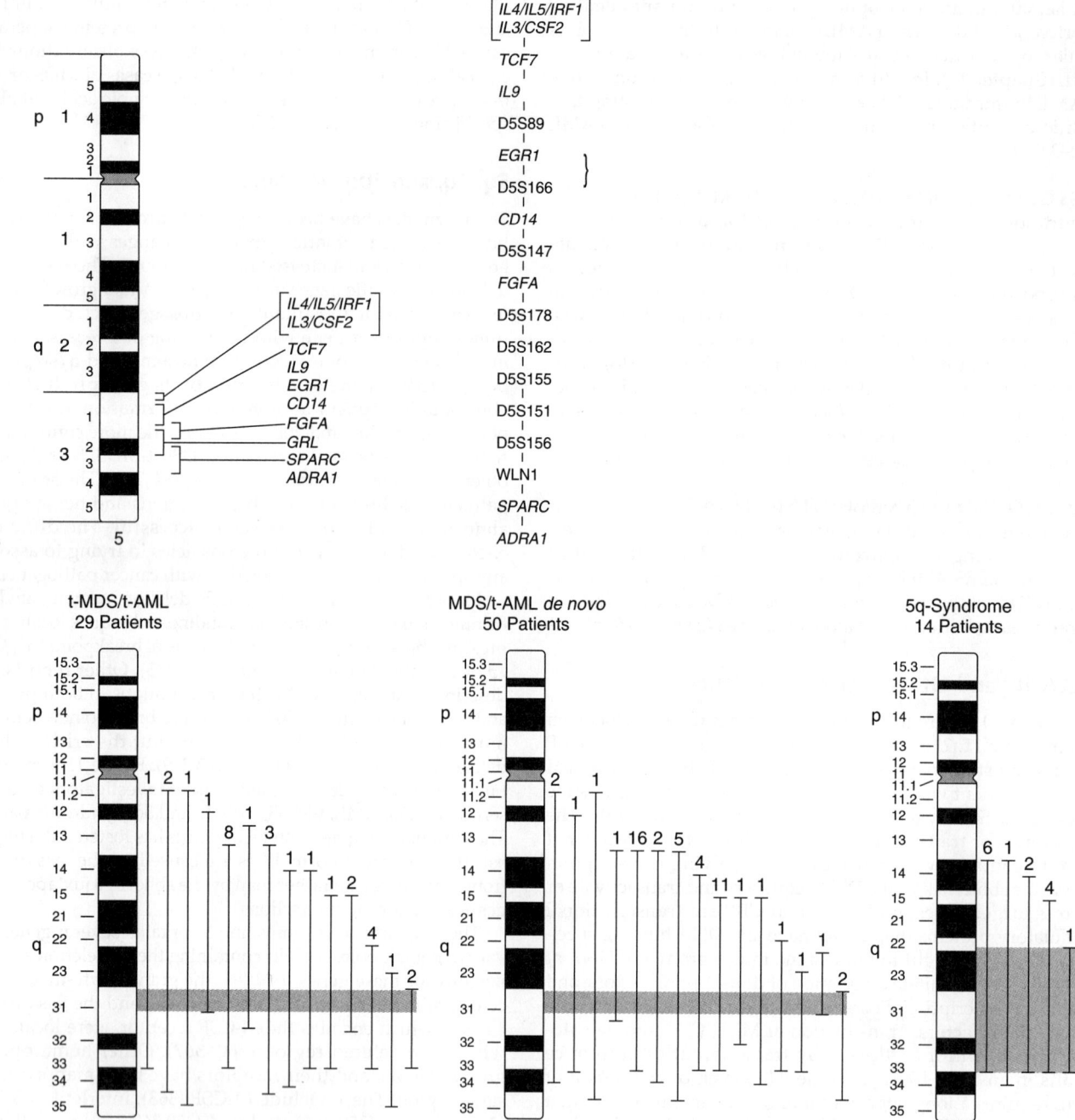

Figure 11-6. A: Schematic of the banding pattern of human chromosome 5, illustrating (*left*) the chromosomal localization and order of a spectrum of genes determined using fluorescence *in situ* hybridization, including the *IL4/IL5/IRF1, IL3/CSF2, TCF7, IL9, EGR1, CD14, FGFA, GRL, SPARC,* and *ADRA1* genes, and (*right*) the physical order of cosmid and phage clones and genes, and the relationship of loci on 5q to the critical region of 5q31 (brace). The CSF1 receptor (299) and the platelet-derived growth factor receptor (307,308) are located further toward the telomere, at band 5q33. **B:** Diagram of chromosome 5 illustrating the breakpoints of the interstitial deletions found in patients with therapy-related myelodysplastic syndrome or acute myelogenous leukemia (t-MDS/t-AML), *de novo* MDS or AML, and the 5q- syndrome. The vertical lines represent the regions that were deleted, and the numbers above these lines indicate the numbers of patients with each deletion. The horizontal lines indicate the critical region in each group—that is, the smallest overlapping region that was deleted in each of the patients. As noted in the text, additional critical deleted regions have been proposed in the bands 5q13 and 5q33 based on cytogenetic, fluorescence *in situ* hybridization, and loss of heterozygosity analysis in some patients with 5q deletion. (Courtesy of M. M. Le Beau, University of Chicago.)

Possible Role of Haploinsufficiency in Myelodysplastic Syndrome Associated with Deletions of 5q, 7q, and 20q

There has been an extensive effort to identify "classic" tumor-suppressor genes, as described above for Rb and p53, in which one copy of a gene is deleted, and the other is inactivated by point mutation or by epigenetic influences that result in decreased expression. However, even with the availability of the complete human genomic sequence and a working knowledge of all predicted coding sequences in the 5q, 7q, and 20q deleted regions, no gene has yet been identified that meets criteria for a classic tumor suppressor with loss of function of both alleles. These findings, and the observation that the inherited MDS-like syndrome FPD/AML can be caused by haploinsufficiency of AML1, suggests that assays for haploinsufficiency should be considered in the search for genes that may cause MDS. Although these models are difficult to test, efforts are ongoing to generate murine models of chromosomal deletion in several labs, and other vertebrate systems such as zebrafish may be useful because of the relative ease of generating haploid and gynogenetic diploid animals.

Other Genetic Abnormalities

Other abnormalities in MDS include consistent methylation of the p15 INK locus, a cyclin-dependent kinase inhibitor that is actively transcribed after TGF-β exposure (397). Methylation and altered expression of the locus may allow leukemic cells to escape inhibitory signals from the bone marrow microenvironment. In addition, in rare cases with 17p deletion, p53 loss of function mutations have been identified similar to those observed in solid tumors (398–401). However, microsatellite instability characteristic of solid tumors is rarely observed in MDS or in AML (402). Finally, there is emerging evidence that apoptosis is defective in MDS cells, as described in the section Pathophysiology, although

the molecular mechanisms for defects in apoptosis are not well understood (403–405). Only limited direct experimental data support genetic instability or aberrant DNA repair as causal mechanisms in MDS. MDS shares with Fanconi's syndrome, Bloom's syndrome, and ataxia telangiectasia a predisposition to leukemia or other hematologic malignancies. Patients with these disorders have been shown to have increased chromosomal breakage in response to ultraviolet light or chemical mutagens. Progress is being made toward identifying specific DNA repair defects in these disorders that produce an inability to withstand environmental mutagenic pressure (406–408). Preliminary reports of abnormalities of heterochromatin structure, sister chromatid exchange, and DNA repair after ultraviolet light mutagenesis in bone marrow cells from patients with MDS have been published (409–411). As more components of eukaryotic DNA repair pathways are defined, their function can be tested in patients with MDS and specific questions regarding underlying defects addressed.

Table 11-9 understates the genetic complexity of MDS. It is clear that point mutations in genes such as RAS, FLT3, and AML1 contribute to pathogenesis of MDS, and more mutations are likely to be identified with time. Deletions are particularly challenging problems to resolve at the genetic level, as are numerical abnormalities. However, significant progress has been made over the past several years. The majority of chromosomal translocations have been cloned, fusion genes identified and validated as targets in cell culture and murine models, and in some cases, molecularly targeted therapies are being developed.

Models for Evolution

One model that addresses many facets of the pathogenesis and biology of MDS is outlined in Figure 11-7. This model is based on a selection-driven process of carcinogenesis as outlined by Temin (412) and first suggested to us in the context of MDS by Dr. Alan Jacobs (*personal communication*, 1986). Implicit within

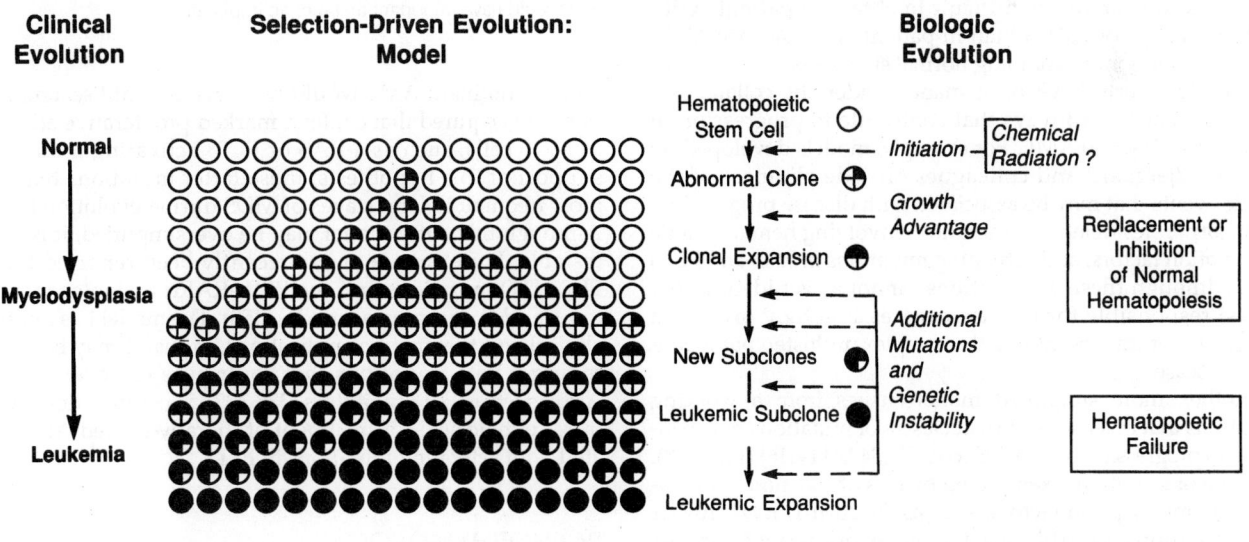

Figure 11-7. A model for the pathogenesis of the myelodysplastic syndromes. **A:** Representation of a selection-driven process of neoplasia. A cohort of cells is shown moving through time (for clarity, no increase in the total number of cells is shown). Each mutation is represented by a filled-in quadrant. A transformed, leukemic cell is completely filled in. Each mutated cell has a growth advantage over less mutated cells. Thus, mutant cells increase in relative quantity and are more likely to suffer further mutations. (Adapted from Temin HM. Evolution of cancer genes as a mutation-driven process. *Cancer Res* 1988;48:1698.) **B:** Representation of the possible corresponding events occurring in the development and progression of the myelodysplastic syndromes from an initial genetic insult to death from hematopoietic failure or leukemia. (Adapted from Jacobs A, Clark RE. Pathogenesis and clinical variations in the myelodysplastic syndromes. *Clin Haematol* 1986;15:928.)

this model is the infrequent occurrence of mutations that subtly enhance the growth properties of cells without rendering them fully neoplastic. Over time, gradual overgrowth occurs within the total population of cells possessing even a modest proliferative advantage. The occurrence of additional mutations is more likely within this expanding population, and gradually a mixture of competing subclones emerges within the population. This process of mutation and selective proliferation of an increasingly complex mixture of subclones and sub-subclones may go on indefinitely until the whole population of cells lacks sufficient maturational capacity to produce circulating blood elements in adequate numbers or until a subclonal population finally arises with frankly leukemic properties.

The model is supported by several of the biologic features of MDS. At any point in the evolution of the syndrome, the bone marrow may contain from one to several distinct subpopulations of cells, each derived from the original single hematopoietic stem cell, as well as ever-decreasing numbers of unaffected stem cells. Cytogenetic studies of MDS have documented the coexistence of subclones with unrelated karyotypic abnormalities (305,413), the accumulation over time of additional cytogenetic or point mutations in an already marked clone (267,295,296,298,299,329), and gradual replacement of one karyotypically marked subclone by another (302–304). Each subclone may contain an overlapping but distinct set of mutations that provide it with a selective growth advantage.

Emergence or loss of specific cytogenetic abnormalities or gene mutations may be caused by spontaneous competitive or therapy-induced shifts in subpopulations and need not call into question the relevance of a specific genetic change to the pathogenesis of MDS. Conversely, the disappearance of a specific cytogenetic abnormality need not reflect elimination of the entire dysplastic population of cells from the bone marrow but only that of the most actively proliferating and thus therapy-sensitive subclone. Therapy-induced remissions may be particularly difficult to achieve if the entire stem cell pool is occupied by dysplastic cells. This hypothesis is consistent with the fact that remissions are more difficult to obtain in patients with AML evolving from MDS than in patients with *de novo* AML, who may have some remaining normal stem cells.

Recently, efforts have been made to identify, collate, and order the genetic pathways that contribute to progression of disease from MDS to AML. For example, models developed by Pedersen-Bjergaard and colleagues provide glimpses of the genetic events that may be associated with disease progression, and incorporates deletions, mutations involving hematopoietic transcription factors, and activating mutations in RAS and FLT3 (335). Although these observations cannot as yet identify the gene(s) responsible for disease progression, they provide a framework for understanding the complex multistep pathogenesis of disease.

Another, more simplified model ensues from a working hypothesis that at least two broad classes of mutations may contribute to progression from MDS to AML (340,414–416) (Fig. 11-8). One type of mutation, exemplified by loss of function of hematopoietic transcription factors, such as the AML1/EVI1, AML1 point mutations, or MLL fusions, serves primarily to impair hematopoietic development and immortalize cells. There is experimental evidence to support the hypothesis that, for example, AML1/ETO alone is sufficient to cause an MDS-like syndrome in murine models and in cultured cells characterized by dysplastic growth and immortalization of hematopoietic progenitors (342). In this model, chromosomal deletions on 5q, 7q, or 20q would target one or more genes whose single gene dosage is sufficient to case an MDS-like syndrome due to loss of function of genes important in normal hematopoietic develop-

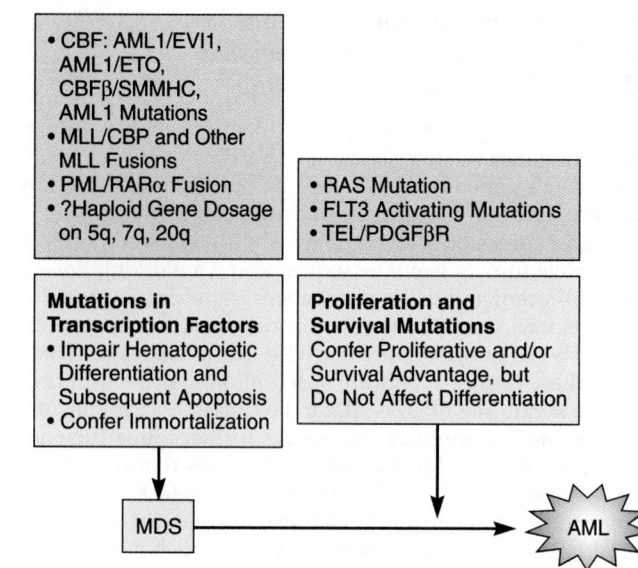

Figure 11-8. A model for progression of myelodysplastic syndrome (MDS) to acute myelogenous leukemia (AML). In this model, mutation first occurs in one of a broad class of genes that results in impaired hematopoietic differentiation and subsequent apoptosis of cells and confers an immortalization phenotype. There is evidence, for example, that AML1/ETO, which occurs frequently in AML and less commonly in MDS, can confer an MDS-like phenotype characterized by dysplastic growth and immortalization in murine hematopoietic progenitors. A similar effect is proposed for expression of the other fusions and point mutations. In each instance, there is evidence that these fusions impair differentiation, but are not sufficient to cause AML. This model further presupposes that, although the genes are not yet elucidated, the 5q, 7q, and 20q deletions cause MDS due to haploid dosage of one or more genes in the deleted interval, but still require additional second mutations for progression to AML. Acquisition of a second mutation that confers strong proliferative and/or survival advantage to cells results in progression to AML. Mutations in this class include activating mutants of RAS and FLT3. If this class of mutations occurs first, as for the TEL/PDGFβR fusion in CMML, then a myeloproliferative syndrome is observed first clinically. This model may be overly simplified, but is testable and would have important therapeutic implications.

ment. Fulminant AML would not develop until second mutations are acquired that confer a marked proliferative advantage to MDS cells, such as a RAS or FLT3 activating mutation. In support of this hypothesis, these latter mutations tend to be most frequent in later stages of MDS during evolution to AML. Although this latter model may be oversimplified, it is readily testable. For example, it has recently been reported that the FLT3-ITD mutations and the PML-RARα fusion cooperate to induce AML in a murine model (358). The model has important clinical and therapeutic applications, in that it may be possible to target both mutations that contribute to development of AML, such as FLT3 inhibitors (338,339), in combination with all-*trans*-retinoic acid for treatment of therapy-related APL associated with activating mutations in FLT3.

PATHOPHYSIOLOGY

Much effort has been devoted to characterizing the biologic and biochemical abnormalities of myelodysplastic hematopoietic cells. Recent advances in *in vitro* culture methodology and the isolation and characterization of hematopoietic growth factors and their receptors have stimulated attempts to define derangements in cellular proliferation and maturation. The myriad functional and biochemical abnormalities that presumably result from damage to the genome and disordered hematopoietic cell maturation are catalogued and their significance to the clinical manifestations of MDS is assessed.

Hematopoiesis

Techniques for growth of bone marrow progenitor cells in semisolid culture media have been developed over the past two decades and have proven invaluable to hematologic research (Chapter 7) (417).

Several facets of the pathophysiology of MDS can be analyzed with existing culture methodology. An understanding of the properties of hematopoietic progenitors that cause failure of blood cell formation is desired. Relevant parameters are number of progenitors, their capacity for maturation, their interaction with stromal elements and response to growth factors, and the existence of pathologic inhibitory mechanisms. Experiments have been performed to address each of these issues without yet providing simple answers.

Progenitor Growth

Granulocyte-macrophage CFUs (CFU-GM) are usually decreased in blood or bone marrow of patients with MDS (418–423). In addition, blocks in the differentiation of myeloid cells may be present (424–427). No strict correlations between colony growth patterns and FAB subclass exist (428), although patients in a transition phase to acute leukemia often develop increasingly abnormal colony growth characteristics. These patients have even fewer normal colonies with more small clusters and blast cell colonies than are characteristically found in cultures of leukemic marrow (429–431). Abnormally high cluster/colony ratios are also common in those with t-MDS (30).

Patients with CMML are an exception, because they often have increased or normal numbers of CFU-GM in their marrow (421). Additionally, GM colonies can be grown from many CMML patients without addition of the exogenous hematopoietic growth factors that are necessary to grow colonies from normal marrow (432,433).

Erythroid and megakaryocytic colony formation are also often abnormal in patients with MDS. The number of CFU-erythroid progenitors can be normal or increased, but the number of less mature burst-forming units–erythroid progenitor cells is generally profoundly decreased (418,419,421,434,435). Low numbers of CFU-megakaryocyte usually parallel decreased erythroid colony growth (434,436,437). Mixed colonies arising from multilineage progenitors were also decreased in one study (421). Patients with the 5q- abnormality and RA often have normal numbers of CFU-GM but profoundly decreased burst-forming units–erythroid (177,438).

The *in vitro* culture results may not fully reflect disordered hematopoiesis *in vivo*. Patients with absent CFU-GM growth may maintain adequate neutrophil counts (34), whereas cytogenetically abnormal progenitors can form both myeloid and erythroid colonies in culture (247,438,439). The proliferative capability of bone marrow precursors from all lineages as assessed *in vitro* by DNA synthesis or progression into S phase from G_1 is reduced (440–442). The ability of MDS progenitors to compete with normal progenitors *in vivo* also may not correlate with their *in vitro* behavior (306,308). Colony analysis of hematopoietic progenitors can help predict prognosis and plan therapy in some patients (30,423,430).

The response of MDS hematopoietic cells to growth factors may also be abnormal. In semisolid culture, CFU numbers can be increased or even normalized by the addition of higher than standard concentrations of growth factors (443–445). This increased requirement might result from down-regulated or poorly transducing receptors or from a relative deficiency of accessory cell-derived growth factors in cultures of MDS bone marrow (445). Most studies examining growth factor production by T cells or stromal cells from patients with MDS have shown normal production of hematopoietic growth factors (420,446,447).

Even less evidence is available for cell-mediated or humoral inhibition of normal hematopoiesis in patients with MDS. Both murine and human leukemic cells have been shown to secrete substances inhibitory to normal hematopoietic proliferation *in vitro* (448,449). Conflicting data exist regarding the presence of humoral factors that inhibit megakaryocytopoiesis in patients with MDS (436,450,451). One study reported NK cell inhibition of autologous CFU-GM in a small number of patients with MDS (452). Further investigation is required before the importance of inhibitory activities can be assessed.

Growth Factors

The possibility has been raised that patients with MDS do not respond to cytopenias *in vivo* by producing appropriately high concentrations of stimulatory hematopoietic growth factors. Several studies have reported much lower levels of megakaryocyte colony-stimulating activity than expected in the serum of patients with MDS and thrombocytopenia compared with that of patients with other causes for thrombocytopenia such as aplastic anemia (436,450,451). In general, serum erythropoietin (EPO) levels are elevated in patients with MDS, but not always to the extent predicted by the blood hemoglobin level (453). As in other situations in which the EPO response seems inappropriately blunted, such as in sickle cell anemia, anemia of chronic disease, or megaloblastic anemias, EPO production may be regulated by overall erythroid cellularity in the marrow as well as by blood oxygen–carrying capacity (454–457). Treatment with hematopoietic growth factors including EPO may have some rational basis if an impaired capacity for growth factor production is convincingly demonstrated.

Autocrine Mechanisms

Another intriguing possibility is that release from growth factor requirements allows affected MDS clones to gain dominance in the marrow. This mechanism seems potentially applicable when a dominant proliferative component is present, as in CMML patients, or during evolution to acute leukemia. CFU-GM, CFU-erythroid, and clusters that grow in culture without the addition of exogenous growth factors have been detected in the bone marrow of a small number of patients with MDS (418,436,447,458), with autonomous CFU-GM especially common in patients with CMML (432,433). Perhaps hyperresponsive progenitor cells can be stimulated by small amounts of growth factors present in the serum component of the culture media or secreted by accessory cells. Another possible explanation is that some MDS hematopoietic cells have dysregulated growth factor production. They may be able to abnormally produce and then respond to a particular factor (autocrine effects) or to stimulate or inhibit neighboring cells (paracrine effects).

The possibility that release from normal growth constraints by autocrine stimulation could be an important step in the development of neoplasia has been the focus of intense recent interest and experimentation (459,460). Blast cells from some patients with AML have been found to contain growth factor messenger RNA and to secrete a variety of factors. Several studies have demonstrated that antibodies that neutralize the secreted growth factors inhibit colony formation by these cells (460,461). A similar mechanism may contribute to dominance by abnormal clones or initiate progression to leukemia (462,463). Evidence is thus far lacking, except for a recent study that reported autocrine production of GM-CSF and IL-6 from cultured CMML marrow cells, with inhibition of colony formation by neutralizing antibodies to GM-CSF and IL-6 (432). The presence on bone marrow biopsy of ALIPs separated from the bony trabecular surface has suggested to some authors that these cells have become autonomous and are no longer dependent on stromally supplied growth factors (463).

It is unlikely that autocrine stimulation could be the sole or primary mechanism in MDS. Dysregulated production of several growth factors by hematopoietic progenitors has been shown in several animal models to lead to myeloproliferative states with preserved maturation (464–466). The defective maturation that is the hallmark of MDS probably results from another type of mutation.

Disordered Maturation of Hematopoietic Cells

Normal committed hematopoietic progenitors in each lineage experience a pathway of differentiation that culminates in mature, functional, nonmitotic cells. A myriad of biochemical and functional abnormalities within the cells of all lineages has been described in patients with MDS. An understanding of their incidence and functional consequences is an important goal because many patients with MDS die from infections or bleeding resulting at least partially from dysfunction of circulating cells. Damage to one or a few involved genes may result in disordered patterns of gene expression and thus cellular maturation and function. Observations of lineage infidelity and reversion to fetal cellular characteristics support this hypothesis. Specific biochemical defects might also arise if a mutation affected a normal allele at a locus that already harbored a defect on the opposite chromosome.

Abnormalities in Erythroid Cells

Erythroid activity in MDS bone marrow can vary widely from hypoplasia to hyperplasia with massively ineffective erythropoiesis (79). Many qualitative abnormalities have also been described, in some instances leading to hemolysis and worsening of anemia. Often, decreased activity is seen of RBC enzymes, including pyruvate kinase, phosphofructokinase, adenylate kinase, and diphosphoglycerate mutase or increases in the activities of 6-phosphogluconate dehydrogenase, and G6PD, hexokinase, aldolase, adenosine deaminase, and enolase (467–469). The patterns of enzyme alteration may vary among patients. Increased dihydrofolate reductase activity has been shown to persist to an abnormally late stage of erythroid development (470). Clinically significant hemolysis has been reported in association with a reduction in pyruvate kinase or an increase in adenosine deaminase activities (471–474).

Decreased expression of blood group antigens within the ABO group has been reported, probably resulting from decreased activity of the galactosyltransferases that add carbohydrate side chains to proteins on the RBC surface (469,475,476). In some cases, the i antigen (fetal) is expressed rather than the I antigen (adult). Fetal hemoglobin levels are elevated up to 5% to 37% of the total hemoglobin in RBCs from patients with MDS (477). In a few patients, acquired hemoglobin H (unstable tetramers of β-globin chains) has been detected (478–480). Decreased α-globin gene transcription can be shown in erythroid cells from these patients. The four α genes are intact, suggesting operation of a transacting mechanism.

Ringed Sideroblast Formation

Ringed sideroblasts are common in patients with MDS and can be detected in various quantities in all FAB subtypes (41). Over the past three decades, numerous attempts have been made to define the mechanism of ringed sideroblast formation and the connection between the presence of these cells and the underlying primary defects in MDS (12,42,43,145,481–484). An understanding of the pathogenesis of ringed sideroblasts in patients with MDS has been hampered in many investigations by the grouping together of the several different underlying conditions associated with ringed sideroblasts (Table 11-8).

Figure 11-9 shows diagrams of some of the steps iron takes between its arrival at an early erythroid cell and its incorporation into hemoglobin (these pathways are discussed in detail in Chapter 47). Heme synthesis intermediates are transported through the mitochondrial membrane at least twice, and several enzymatic steps occur within the mitochondria. Any hypothesis must account for normal or increased iron uptake into erythroid progenitors and abnormal accumulation within mitochondria, but decreased incorporation into heme, and thus into hemoglobin. At least three mechanisms for abnormal mitochondrial iron deposition in ringed sideroblasts and associated disordered erythropoiesis have been considered: (a) defects in the enzymes or cofactors of the heme synthetic pathway, (b) defects in the transport or processing of iron before it is incorporated into heme, (c) and generalized mitochondrial defects.

Interest in defects of the heme synthetic pathway enzymes or cofactors was generated by several observations. Pyridoxine after phosphorylation to pyridoxal phosphate is a cofactor for the enzyme δ-aminolevulinic acid synthase (ALA-S), which combines glycine and succinyl coenzyme A into ALA. In hepatic cells and less clearly in erythroid cells, this step is rate-limiting in heme synthesis. In some experimental animals, pyridoxine deficiency produces anemia and ringed sideroblast formation (368). Patients on isoniazid and other antituberculous drugs occasionally develop RARS, which disappear when the drugs are discontinued; the drug interferes with the transport of pyridoxine to the cells (42,484,485). At least a small percentage of patients with both acquired and hereditary sideroblastic anemia improve while on pharmacologic doses of pyridoxine (486,487).

ALA-S activity is decreased in bone marrow cells of some patients with either acquired or hereditary types of sideroblastic anemia (488–491). In several hereditary pyridoxine-responsive patients, the actual amount of ALA-S messenger RNA is low (492); in others, the ALA-S protein itself is abnormally sensitive to degradation by a mitochondrial protease (493,494). Further interest in this enzyme has been generated by the finding that although the hepatic isozyme gene is on chromosome 3 (495), the erythroid ALA-S gene is on the X chromosome (492). Most families with hereditary sideroblastic anemia exhibit an X-linked inheritance pattern, and mutations in ALA-S have been linked to hereditary sideroblastic anemia (496–502). Other enzymatic steps in the pathway—most frequently that of ferrochelatase (heme synthase)—have also been reported to be affected in at least some patients (489). Elevated levels of free erythrocyte protoporphyrin (FEP) result from blockage of the heme synthetic pathway at the ferrochelatase step (503,504).

Other evidence suggests that these enzyme defects are not the primary mechanisms for ringed sideroblast formation in RARS or in patients with MDS. In these patients, abnormal mitochondrial iron deposition can be detected in early erythroid precursors before initiation of heme synthesis (505). Lead inhibits heme synthesis enzymes, including ALA-S and ferrochelatase, but ringed sideroblasts are rare or nonexistent in the bone marrow of patients with lead poisoning (484). No evidence shows actual pyridoxine or pyridoxal phosphate deficiency in patients with MDS (506). In patients with erythropoietic porphyria, a specific defect in ferrochelatase activity is found. These patients have high levels of FEP and urine and stool porphyrins but do

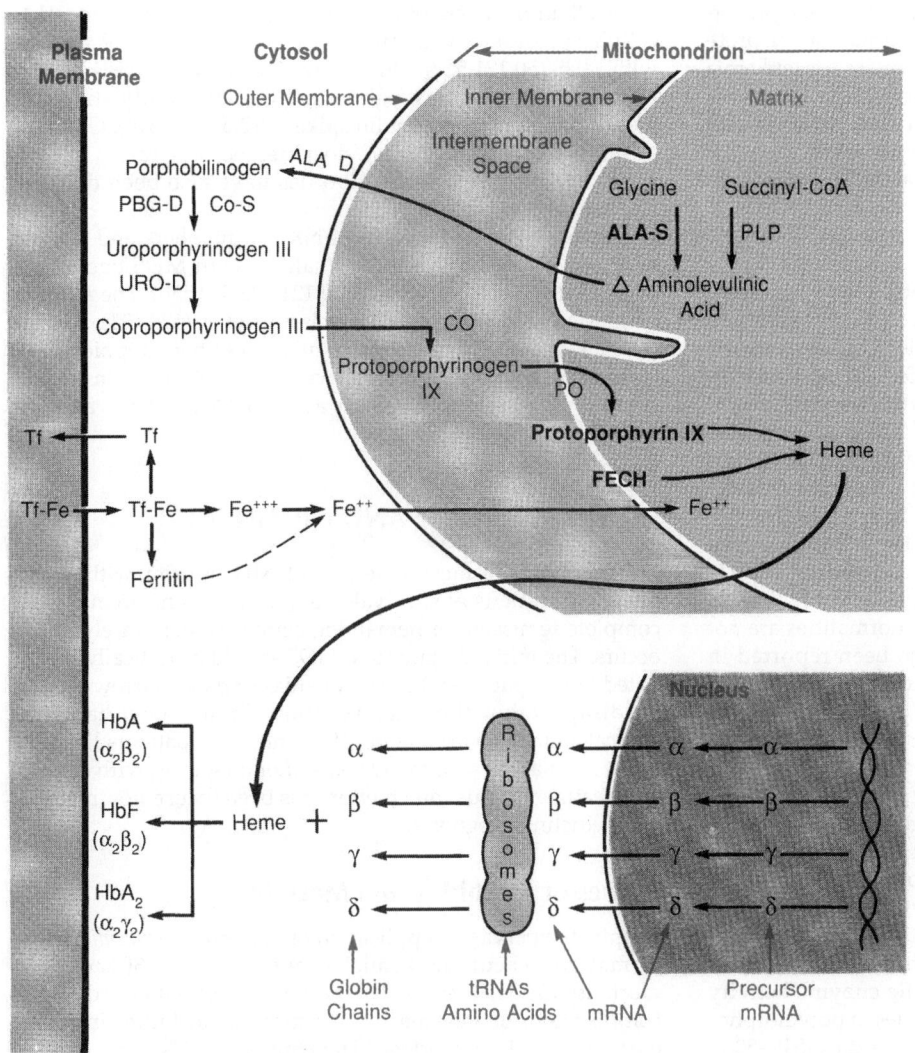

Figure 11-9. Pathways of heme synthesis. ALA D, δ-aminolevulinic acid dehydratase; ALA-S, δ-aminolevulinic acid synthase; CO, coproporphyrinogen oxidase; Co-S, uroporphyrinogen cosynthase; FECH, ferrochelatase; Hb, hemoglobin; mRNA, messenger RNA; PBG-D, porphobilinogen deaminase; PLP, pyridoxal phosphate; PO, protoporphyrinogen oxidase; Tf, transferrin; tRNA, transfer RNA; URO-D, uroporphyrinogen decarboxylase. (Courtesy of S. S. Bottomley, MD, University of Oklahoma.)

not develop ringed sideroblasts (507). A patient with RARS and high circulating levels of FEP was studied and found to have normal ALA-S and ferrochelatase activities but no photosensitivity or other signs of porphyria (503). At least two patients with RARS and high levels of FEP developed photosensitivity in conjunction with low ferrochelatase activity (504,508). Obviously, the situation is complicated and not yet well understood, even when patients with acquired and hereditary forms of sideroblastic anemias are carefully separated.

The second hypothesis involves primary defects of iron uptake or cellular processing. A small study found an association between RARS and the HLA A3 allele, which had previously been strongly linked to hemochromatosis (146). It was suggested that patients heterozygous for the hemachromatosis allele were in some way predisposed to developing ringed sideroblasts and RARS, but in larger series, this association was not borne out (147–149). Patients with iron overload from primary hemochromatosis or secondary hemosiderosis due to transfusion or ineffective erythropoiesis accumulate iron in normal ferritin storage granules but do not develop ringed sideroblasts.

Others have suggested that there is defective reduction of ferric iron (Fe^{3+}) to ferrous iron (Fe^{2+}), which is necessary before incorporation into heme can occur (42,484,503). An abnormal amount of Fe^{3+} could accumulate, damaging mitochondria via free radical formation, before precipitation as ferric phosphate (509). Feedback inhibition of iron uptake into cells may nor-

mally be controlled by intracellular heme concentration (484). If heme synthesis decreases, cells may continue to take up iron despite increased intracellular stores. By whatever mechanism, it is likely that abnormal iron deposition in mitochondria further disrupts the heme synthetic pathway and impairs erythropoiesis. Cellular iron deposition inhibits uroporphyrinogen decarboxylase (510). In fact, some patients with RARS or hereditary sideroblastic anemia have shown hematologic improvement with iron chelation or phlebotomy, presumably by interrupting this vicious cycle of iron deposition and further cellular damage (510–513).

The third hypothesis invokes a generalized mitochondrial defect. Aoki (514) demonstrated that the activities of many mitochondrial enzymes, including nonheme synthetic pathway enzymes, were decreased in patients with RARS, whereas ALA-S activity alone was decreased in patients with pyridoxine-responsive hereditary sideroblastic anemia. These defects were also detected in granulocytes from RARS patients, although not in lymphocytes. Secondary mitochondrial damage from iron deposition could be an explanation of generalized erythroid mitochondrial dysfunction, but the presence of defects in granulocyte mitochondria is difficult to explain except by a primary defect.

We do not yet know which, if any, of these hypotheses will explain the formation of ringed sideroblasts in patients with MDS. As with other functional and morphologic defects found in MDS cells, these abnormalities of the iron metabolic pathway may result from abnormal maturation of hematopoietic precursors. Processes leading to ringed sideroblast formation are probably secondary and not related to the propensity for leukemia seen in these patients. In contrast, hereditary sideroblastic anemias are not preleukemic or trilineage disorders; primary mechanisms in these anemias are much more likely to involve specific genetic defects in the heme synthetic pathway or iron transport.

Abnormalities in Platelets

Abnormalities of platelet function may contribute to the bleeding tendencies sometimes encountered even in patients with MDS with adequate platelet counts. Platelet granules may be sparse or abnormally large. In one study, 15 of 16 patients with MDS had giant dense granules that did not release their contents normally during platelet aggregation. The authors postulated that these granules arose through abnormal fusion of many smaller granules (134,135). Platelet adenosine diphosphate content and thromboxane A_2 activity are low in some patients with MDS (515). Responses to collagen and epinephrine can be blunted (128,515,516), and the bleeding time is increased in as many as one-half of patients with MDS, even with normal platelet counts (515). These abnormalities are not unique to patients with MDS, having also been reported in myeloproliferative syndromes, and are quite similar to those observed in affected individuals with FPD/AML syndrome.

Abnormalities in Myeloid Cells

As described earlier in this chapter, lineage infidelity of MDS granulocytes and monocytes, as assessed by surface marker and cytochemical phenotyping, is common (51,517). Tests of neutrophil function yield heterogeneous results, but in the most detailed study, 20 of 20 patients had at least one abnormality of chemotaxis, phagocytosis, adhesion, chemiluminescence, or microbicidal capacity of neutrophil-specific enzyme activity (518). The myeloperoxidase content of granules in polymorphonuclear leukocytes was low in a number of studies (519–522), but in vitro killing of Staphylococcus aureus or Candida albicans was not consistently impaired (519,520,522,523). Given the high mortality and morbidity rates due to infection in patients with MDS, neutrophil abnormalities may be significant in vivo.

Immune Dysfunction

The involvement of the lymphoid system in both the pathophysiology and the clinical manifestations of MDS has not been extensively investigated but could prove important. As noted previously in some studies, B lymphocytes, and less consistently T lymphocytes, are part of the abnormal affected clone in MDS (238–240,248,248a). Lymphoid cells are probably the primary source of many of the hematopoietic growth factors in vivo; the lack of normal factor production due to lymphoid dysfunction could be a mechanism for deranged hematopoiesis. It is also possible that disordered immune surveillance permits expansion of abnormal marrow clones. No experimental evidence exists for or against these hypotheses.

Immunophenotyping with monoclonal antibodies to cell-surface markers has documented pronounced decreases in T-cell count, specifically helper T4 cells, and a shift in the T4/T8 ratio (50,524–526). Some authors have suggested that the relative increase in T8 suppressor activity could inhibit both hematopoiesis and antibody production. These changes in T-cell populations might result from the primary disease or may be secondary to the multiple transfusions that most patients with MDS have received (526).

B-cell numbers are often decreased and antibody-dependent cellular cytotoxicity is impaired in some but not all patients with MDS (50,121,527). On the other hand, many patients with MDS have hypergammaglobulinemia; one study showed a monoclonal immunoglobulin spike in 12.5% (75,528). Coombs'-positive hemolysis has been documented only rarely in these patients, and other antoantibodies have also been detected (75,528).

Interest has also focused on NK cell numbers and activity, because NK activity is universally low in MDS because of decreased NK cell counts (50,120,121,525,529,530). The addition of interferon only partially corrects the defect (120,121). Because NK cells may be involved in regulation of hematopoiesis and seem to play a role in tumor surveillance, a decrease in NK-cell count could permit toleration of abnormal MDS clones and produce dyshematopoiesis.

CLINICAL COURSE AND PROGNOSIS

The prognosis for most patients with MDS is grim, with overall median durations of survival being only 2 years. Spontaneous complete remission or hematologic improvement rarely if ever occurs. The initial diagnosis of MDS should be critically reevaluated in any patient whose cytopenias or bone marrow dysplasia disappears without intervention. On the other hand, the clinical course is variable in MDS, and some patients live relatively normal lives for many years after diagnosis, with or without treatment. Thus, much effort has been focused on methods for predicting prognosis.

Causes of Morbidity and Mortality

Despite the pervasive application of the term preleukemia, transformation to acute leukemia accounts for only 30% of MDS mortality (60,84,85,185,531). Another 40% of patients die from complications of bone marrow dysfunction, including infection, bleeding, and iron overload. The remaining 30% of patients die from seemingly unrelated conditions, such as cardiovascular disease or nonhematologic malignancies. In fact, survival from the time of diagnosis of MDS is no worse or better in patients who develop leukemia than in those who do not (86,531,532). One possible explanation for this surprising finding is that patients with severe cytopenias die early from infection or bleeding, whereas those with less severe cytopenias survive longer, increasing the likelihood of progression to leukemia.

The most common infectious complications are bacterial in nature, in the lower respiratory tract, skin, and perineal area. Risk of infection is high even in patients with adequate numbers of neutrophils, presumably because of functional neutrophil impairment or generalized immune dysfunction (85,117,536). Likewise, bleeding in nonthrombocytopenic patients may occur because of platelet dysfunction so that platelet transfusions may be indicated before major surgery. The surprisingly high percentage of deaths attributed to causes with no known direct relation to MDS most likely reflects the advanced age of the affected population, but the chronic effects of anemia and immune dysfunction may contribute to second malignancies and cardiac mortality (85).

Parameters Predictive of Prognosis

The FAB classification system has prognostic usefulness (60,75,76,83,85,86,91,140,185,533,534). Table 11-11 summarizes the median survival after presentation and risk of progression to leukemia by FAB subtype in several large studies. Survival

TABLE 11-11. Prognosis in Myelodysplastic Syndromes

Study (and Reference Number)	Refractory Anemia	Refractory Anemia with Ringed Sideroblasts	Refractory Anemia with Excess Blasts	Refractory Anemia with Excess of Blasts in Transformation	Chronic Monomyelocytic Leukemia	Overall
Median survival in months from presentation by FAB subtype						
Kerkhofs (75)	50	60+	9	6	60+	47
Sanz (140)	26	34	9	5	12	15
Tricot (531)	46	53	28	11	23	15
Varela (536)	38	53	13	3	17	26
Foucar (84)	64	71	7	5	8	10
Coiffier (60)	102	131	26[a]	26[a]	28	53
Mufti (91)	32	76	10.5	5	21	23
Teerenhovi (185)	48	41	21	13	16	29
Percentage leukemic transformation by FAB subtype						
Kerkhofs (75)	25	16	64	60	18	37
Sanz (140)	21	39	57	82	15	—
Tricot (531)	11	11	56	56	56	—
Varela (536)	15	12	41	75	33	29
Foucar (84)	15	0	32	50	27	27
Coiffer (60)	15	20	44[a]	44[a]	40	32
Mufti (91)	11	5	28	55	13	—
Teerenhovi (185)	14	17	38	75	28	26.5

FAB, French-American-British.
[a]Patients with refractory anemia with ringed sideroblasts and refractory anemia with excess of blasts in transformation were pooled in this study.

curves are shown in Figure 11-10. The variable results among studies can be accounted for in most cases by exclusion or inclusion of patients with t-MDS, by differences in median age, or by differences due to referral patterns. Variable methods for assignment of patients who seem to fall into two FAB subclasses may also account for some discrepancies; such patients should be assigned to the FAB class with the poorer prognosis, for example, RAEB instead of RARS or CMML, if greater than 5% marrow blasts are present (7,75). If this is done, RARS patients generally have a somewhat longer median survival than RA patients, followed by CMML, RAEB, and RAEB-t, in that order.

Because the range of survival times within each subtype of MDS, especially RA and RARS, may be variable, many investigators have sought additional parameters besides FAB subtype to improve the accuracy of predicting prognosis in patients. Circulating blasts, whether myeloid or erythroid, may be an ominous sign (60,83). Large numbers of circulating monocytes predict shorter survival in patients with CMML (156,535). Other studies found trilineage marrow dysplasia prognostically poor in all FAB subtypes (84,536). Increased erythroid activity, even if ineffective, is more favorable than a predominantly myeloid marrow (60,425,537,538). A high percentage of ringed sideroblasts is also a good sign and usually occurs in conjunction with a predominantly erythroid marrow (60,309,539). Paradoxically, a hypocellular marrow is either good or neutral prognostically (34,58,59,532,534).

Another predictive morphologic abnormality is the presence of ALIPs on bone marrow biopsy, which are clumps of myeloid blast cells or promyelocytes aberrantly localized at a distance from bony trabeculae (37). Median survival of patients with ALIPs is only 12 months, regardless of FAB subclass, and 50 months without ALIPs (69,298,531). ALIPs are most useful in identifying RA, RARS, or CMML patients with less favorable prognoses, because almost all patients with RAEB or RAEB-t have ALIPs (78,531,540). Although the presence of Auer rods dictates inclusion in the RAEB-t FAB category, these rods have not been clearly shown to herald a higher rate of transformation (53,84).

In vitro cell culture has also been a source of prognostically useful information. Severely curtailed CFU-GM growth from the bone marrow has been associated with shorter survival in

both primary and t-MDS (30,60,423). For unknown reasons, dependence of marrow cells on phytohemagglutinin for growth *in vitro* is associated with an increased risk for leukemia (541).

Clinical parameters have also been investigated for their prognostic significance in MDS, both as single variables and by multivariate analysis. As might be expected, most investigators have found pancytopenia (542), thrombocytopenia (60,83,185), neutropenia (60,531), and severe anemia or transfusion dependence (83,86,185,534) to independently predict shorter survival. Several years ago, Mufti and co-workers (91) combined degree of cytopenias and bone marrow blast percentages into the Bournemouth scoring system, shown in Table 11-12. The system is simple and prognostically useful and has been modified to better accommodate CMML (543), or subdivided based on bone marrow blast percentage for better accuracy (140) (Table 11-12). Survival curves generated by this scoring system compared with the FAB system in a large cohort of patients with MDS are shown in Figure 11-10.

Most studies have not found gender to be prognostically important, and the predictive value of patient age is limited. Younger patients (defined as from less than 40 years to less than 65 years old, according to the study) have been found by some studies to have longer survival rates (140,534) but by others to have a worse prognosis, especially due to leukemic transformation (185,266,531). These discrepancies may stem from the inclusion of younger patients with t-MDS in some cohorts because primary myelodysplasia in patients under 40 years of age is extremely rare. There is also a recent report clearly showing that the apparent incidence of MDS is increasing as physicians become more aware of the syndrome and screen their elderly patients (531a). This increased prevalence may affect the interpretation of previous studies relating age and prognosis.

The few published pediatric studies all define MDS or preleukemia only retrospectively after the onset of acute leukemia (95–98,279). Refractory cytopenias with dysplastic changes precede 5% to 17% of childhood AML cases (95,98,279). It is not clear how frequently children with clinical and morphologic characteristics of MDS fail to progress rapidly to AML because an indolent course in children has not been reported. Survivals are brief because resultant leukemias are often refractory to chemotherapy, and a high incidence of serious infections, especially in children

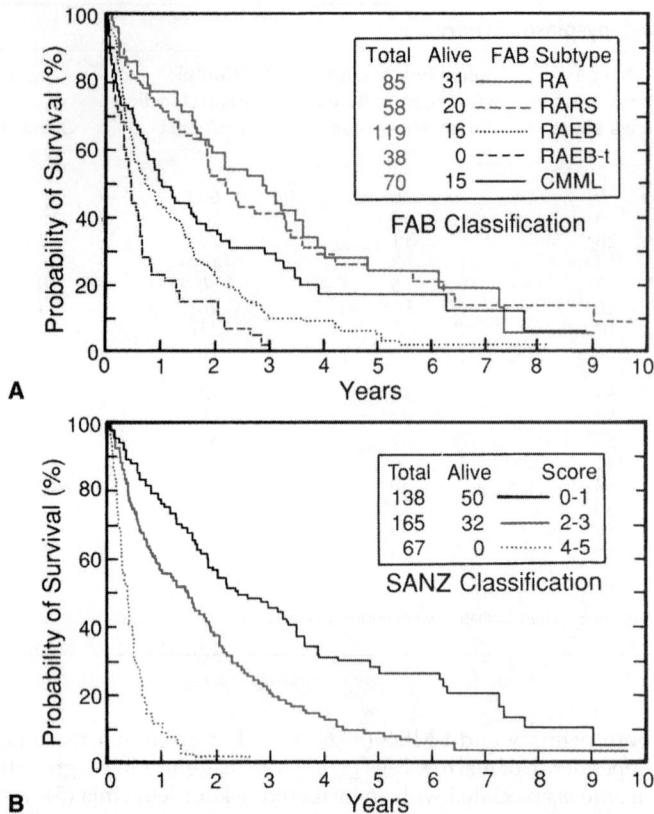

Figure 11-10. A: Survival according to French-American-British (FAB) subtype of 370 patients with myelodysplastic syndrome. The Kaplan-Meier product limit was used to estimate probability of survival. **B:** Survival according to the Sanz scoring system (Table 11-11) of the same 370 patients. CMML, chronic myelomonocytic leukemia; RA, refractory anemia; RAEB, refractory anemia with excess of blasts; RAEB-t, refractory anemia with excess of blasts in transformation; RARS, refractory anemia with ringed sideroblasts. (Adapted from Sanz GF, Sanz MA, Vallespi T, et al. Two regression models and a scoring system for predicting survival and planning treatment in myelodysplastic syndromes: a multivariate analysis of prognostic factors in 370 patients. *Blood* 1989;74:400.)

with monosomy 7, is seen (95,98,303,544–546). The incidence of monosomy 5 or 7 in childhood preleukemic disorders has suggested that a potent mutagen is involved in pathogenesis because the same cytogenetic changes are commonly found in t-MDS and in patients with significant chemical exposures (193).

Complex formulas have been devised for more precise prediction of prognosis based on clinical, morphologic, and bio-

TABLE 11-12. Prognostic Scoring Systems

Criteria	Points	Class	Points
Bournemouth score (reference 91)			
Bone marrow blast >5%	1	A	0–1
Platelets <100,000/μL	1	B	2–3
Hemoglobin <10 g/dL	1	C	4
Neutrophils <2500/μL	1	—	—
Sanz et al. modification (reference 140)			
Age older than 60 yr	1	A	0–1
Platelets			
<100,000/μL	1	B	2–3
<50,000/μL	2	C	4–5
Bone marrow blast			
5–10%	1	—	—
>10%	2	—	—

TABLE 11-13. International Prognostic Scoring System

Cytogenetic Variables		
Prognosis	Cytogenetic Finding	Score
Good	Normal karyotype; del(5q); del(20q); -Y	0
Intermediate	Any one or two other chromosome aberrations except those involving chromosome 7	0.5
Poor	Three or more chromosome changes, or any aberration involving chromosome 7	1

Noncytogenetic Finding	Value Range	Score
Number of cytopenias	0 or 1	0
	2 or 3	0.5
Percent of blasts in marrow	<5%	0
	5–10%	0.5
	11–20%	1.5
	21–30%	2

Data from Greenberg P, Cox C, LeBeau MM, et al. International scoring system for evaluating prognosis in myelodysplastic syndromes. *Blood* 1997;89(6):2079–2088.

logic variables found to be relevant by multivariate analysis (547–549). This approach may be useful for research purposes but is too complicated for general clinical usage and offers no significant advantage over the FAB classification tempered with clinical and cytogenetic data.

International Prognostic Scoring System

A new and simple method for prognostication has recently gained wide acceptance and has been cross-validated in several systems (277). The IPSS was designed in part to address the substantial overlap in survival curves associated with the FAB criteria (Fig. 11-10). The investigators focused on clinical criteria, including degree of pancytopenia, percent of blasts in the bone marrow, and developed a novel cytogenetic grading system (Table 11-13). They demonstrated that the patient population chosen for analysis, when stratified for risk by FAB criteria, had similar survival curves to those previously reported (550). However, when using risk stratification based on the low, intermediate-1, intermediate-2, and high-risk categories, there was well-delineated outcome between these groups (Fig. 11-11 and Table 11-14). These data have been validated in several different clinical contexts internationally (550–560) and are likely to be quite useful in risk stratification and assessment of novel therapeutic approaches to MDS.

Cytogenetic Abnormalities and Prognosis

Cytogenetic studies have provided a major source of prognostic information. It was previously noted that the occurrence of single nonspecified karyotypic abnormalities is not consistently a poor prognostic sign (69,260,264,266,561), whereas the presence of complex karyotypic changes, that is, multiple chromosomal abnormalities within one clone or coexisting multiple abnormal clones, accurately predicts a shorter survival (130,258,260,264,266,269,296). An exception is monosomy 7, which has a prognosis as poor as complex abnormalities (260,264,266,561). An isolated 5q- abnormality has a more favorable prognosis than any other single karyotype in MDS, including a normal karyotype (130).

Figure 11-12 shows survival curves based on the cytogenetic subgroupings of the IPSS system (550). In this system, normal karyotype, or isolated del(5q), del(20q), or –Y all carry a favor-

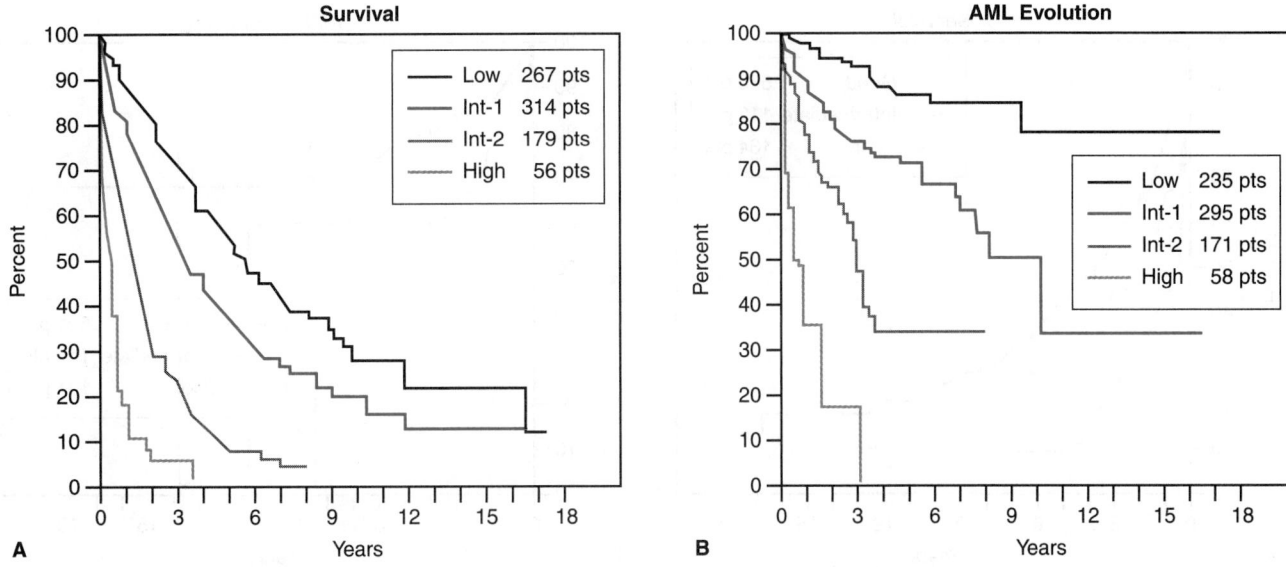

Figure 11-11. Survival by International Prognostic Scoring System for patients under and over the age of 60 years. AML, acute myelogenous leukemia. [From Greenberg P, Cox C, LeBeau MM, et al. International scoring system for evaluating prognosis in myelodysplastic syndromes. *Blood* 1997;89(6):2079–2088, with permission.]

able prognosis. Intermediate prognosis is assigned to patients with any one or two other chromosome aberrations except those involving chromosome 7. Poor prognosis is reserved for those patients with complex (more than three) rearrangements, or any aberration involving chromosome 7 (Table 11-13). Based on this scoring system, cytogenetics has a strong correlation with outcome in Kaplan-Meier survival curves (Figs. 11-11 and 11-12).

Other observations that may have relevance to prognosis include the observations that coexistence of cells with both normal and abnormal karyotypes in the bone marrow is less ominous than complete replacement by karyotypically abnormal cells (75). Sequential determinations may allow assessment of disease extent and pace (267,301). Cellular DNA content, as measured by flow cytometry, is also prognostically useful; hypodiploidy is associated with shorter survival (309).

Complex karyotypic changes are associated not only with lower survival rate but also with a higher rate of transformation to leukemia (258,262). Many case reports, as well as several larger studies, suggest that acquisition of a new cytogenetic abnormality coincides with transformation to acute leukemia (178,295,297,298,301,303,562,563). On the other hand, in many cases, acute leukemia has developed without a detectable new karyotypic change, and in other cases, a new karyotypic change was not accompanied by transformation or any other significant clinical event (297,298).

Prognosis of Therapy-Related Myelodysplastic Syndromes

t-MDS almost uniformly has an extremely poor prognosis, with median survival of only 3 to 8 months (189,191,201,202,564–566). The rate of leukemic transformation is higher than in primary MDS (50% to 87%), but length of survival in patients with t-MDS is similar with or without progression to AML (30,201,202,258). The percentage of myeloblasts at diagnosis, the presence of ringed sideroblasts, and other morphologic criteria seem to have little prognostic meaning in patients with t-MDS; thus, the FAB system has no real usefulness for these patients. Complex chromosomal abnormalities are associated with particularly short survival, but patients with t-MDS and isolated monosomy 7 have relatively good prognoses. This is especially true after leukemic transformation and may result from better responsiveness to chemotherapy (193,201).

Leukemic Transformation

The IPSS scoring system provides useful information about the likelihood of leukemia transformation, although it should be reiterated that many patients die of complications related to cytopenias before progression to frank AML (Table 11-14). Most acute leukemias supervening in patients with MDS are mye-

TABLE 11-14. International Prognostic Scoring System Risk Stratification

Risk Category	Overall International Prognostic Scoring System Score	Median Survival (yr)	Time to Acute Myeloid Leukemia (yr)[a]
Low	0	5.7	9.4
Intermediate-1	0.5–1.0	3.5	3.3
Intermediate-2	1.5–2.0	1.2	1.1
High	>2.5	0.4	0.2

[a]Time for 25% of patients to undergo evolution to acute myeloid leukemia.
Data from Greenberg P, Cox C, LeBeau MM, et al. International scoring system for evaluating prognosis in myelodysplastic syndromes. *Blood* 1997;89(6):2079–2088.

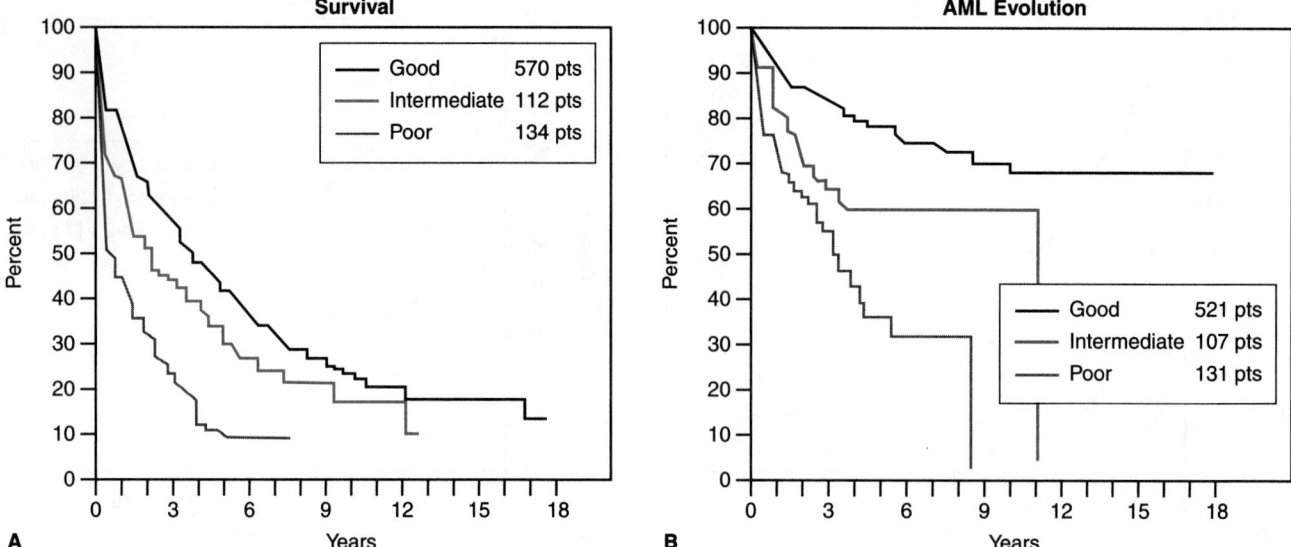

Figure 11-12. Cytogenic risk groups. Correlation of survival **(A)** and freedom from acute myelogenous leukemia (AML) evolution **(B)** of myelodysplastic syndrome related to risk-based categorical cytogenetic subgroups: Good, Intermediate, and Poor. Good, normal, del(5q) only, del(20q) only, −Y only; Intermediate, all other abnormalities; Poor, complex (i.e., >3 anomalies) or chromosome 7 abnormalities. (Kaplan-Meier curves). [From Greenberg P, Cox C, LeBeau MM, et al. International scoring system for evaluating prognosis in myelodysplastic syndromes. *Blood* 1997;89(6):2079–2088, with permisison.]

loid. Relative incidences of FAB leukemia subtypes M1 to M7 are not appreciably different from *de novo* AML, with the possible exception that a preponderance of CMML patients transform to M5 leukemia (76,84,85,536). As mentioned in previous sections, coexisting populations of both myeloid and lymphoid blasts (253,567–569), blast populations exhibiting lineage infidelity (55,252), and pure lymphoid leukemias (249,250) have been observed occasionally.

TREATMENT

At least three difficulties are inherent in designing and implementing treatment strategies for patients with MDS. First, our current lack of basic understanding of the pathogenesis of these syndromes makes the tailoring of specific therapeutic approaches and the prediction of which patients might benefit limited to a very small group of patients. Second, the heterogeneity of the patient population with respect to manifestations and prognosis means that interpretation of clinical trials is difficult and that results may vary radically depending on types of patients enrolled. This circumstance is likely to be improved with the implementation of the IPSS system, but better classification schemes based on molecular correlates are likely to be useful as well. In addition, inclusion of patients with t-MDS has complicated the interpretation of some clinical trials. In addition, most studies have been small, uncontrolled, and short term. Third, the advanced age of most patients with MDS means that unrelated comorbid conditions are common, complicating survival predictions and often precluding aggressive, potentially toxic therapies.

Another problem in design and interpretation of results from clinical trials has been variability in response criteria. Some trials have overestimated the value of some therapies, using marginal improvements in hematologic indices as evidence of response. There has also been wide variability in response criteria between clinical trials, adding to the difficulty in comparing efficacy of various regimens. Recent efforts

have focused on development of standardized response criteria for MDSs that include criteria for altering disease natural history, cytogenetic responses, quality of life responses, and improvement in hematologic indices (570). For example, it has been suggested that a major erythroid response should be characterized by a greater than 2-g/dL increase in hemoglobin for patients with a pretreatment hemoglobin of 11 g/dL, or, for RBC transfusion dependent patients, conversion to transfusion independence. A major platelet response was defined as an absolute increase of 30,000/mm³ for patients with a pretreatment platelet count less than 100,000/mm³, or, for platelet transfusion–dependent patients, stabilization of platelet counts and transfusion independence. Finally, for a major neutrophil response, there should be at least a 100% increase if the absolute neutrophilic count is less than 1500/mm³ before therapy, or an absolute increase of more than 500/mm³, whichever is greater. Although definitions of response criteria are also evolving (571), it is clear that uniform criteria are essential for evaluation and comparison of clinical trials, especially in the context of the heterogeneity of MDS.

The results of most clinical trials performed thus far are not encouraging. During the past decade, several interventions initially generated excitement but were later shown to have unacceptable side effects or no survival benefit, delay of leukemic transformation, or improvement in cytopenias (572–574). Allogeneic bone marrow transplantation for selected candidates remains the only known potential cure for MDS, but application is often limited due to the age of the patient (575–577).

Supportive Care

GENERAL MEASURES

Careful supportive care of patients with MDS may allow maintenance of a normal lifestyle and prevention of necessary morbidity and mortality. Medications that further suppress or damage bone marrow should be avoided, as should excessive amounts of alcohol. Because of neutrophil dysfunction in MDS, patients need counseling on the importance of obtaining prompt medical evaluation of any symptoms or signs of infection, even if they are not actually neutropenic. Aggressive parenteral antibiotic treatment of documented serious infections or neutropenic fevers is essential, as for any immunocompromised patient. The decision to discontinue antibiotic or antifungal agents is more difficult in patients with MDS than in patients who are neutropenic from chemotherapy, because bone marrow recovery is unlikely. In most patients, platelets should be transfused only when bleeding becomes a clinical problem or in preparation for surgical procedures.

CHELATION THERAPY

Because most patients with MDS become dependent on RBC transfusions, complications of iron overload are a significant cause of mortality and morbidity (578,579). Even untransfused or minimally transfused patients can sustain clinically significant organ damage, because ineffective erythropoiesis stimulates hyperabsorption of iron (144,145,148). Elderly patients with underlying cardiac, hepatic, or pancreatic dysfunction may be especially sensitive to further iron-induced organ damage.

The assessment of total body iron stores is not simple in patients with MDS. Serum iron, percentage of iron-binding capacity saturation, and even ferritin values become elevated early in the course of the disease and fluctuate widely, depending on intercurrent illnesses or status of erythropoiesis (580). Liver biopsy is the best diagnostic test, but an invasive procedure in patients with MDS with thrombocytopenia or platelet dysfunction is impractical and inadvisable. An accurate noninvasive magnetic interference technique for quantitation of liver iron has been developed that is gaining acceptance as a measure of iron burden (581). The number of units of packed RBCs given is an important determinant of iron stores, but excessive iron absorption also increases the total body iron burden and is harder to quantify.

Daily subcutaneous administration of deferoxamine, 1.5 to 2.0 g, effectively prevents progressive iron overload in transfusion-dependent patients. Chelation therapy is most effective when used for preventing iron overload than for reversing organ dysfunction such as in diabetes mellitus or cardiac disease after damage is clinically evident. Prophylactic chelation therapy is of little value for a patient with a poor prognosis in whom the total transfusion burden is unlikely to reach the level of 100 units of packed RBCs regularly associated with clinical hemochromatosis. Early chelation therapy is most appropriate in patients with RARS. Removal of iron by chelation or phlebotomy can improve erythropoiesis and help to correct anemia in patients with hereditary sideroblastic anemia and possibly those with primary myelodysplasia. Most often, patients with RARS are severely anemic or transfusion dependent before the diagnosis is unequivocally established, rendering phlebotomy impractical. Subcutaneous deferoxamine should be initiated early, because RARS patients are likely to survive long enough to develop complications of iron overload, which are preventable with regular chelation. Patients with RA, CMML, and RAEB may be observed on transfusion with periodic monitoring for endocrine or cardiac dysfunction. If no significant clinical worsening of complications occurs after 12 to 18 months of transfusion (50 to 75 units), chelation should be instituted.

Marrow Stimulation and Immune Suppression

HEMATINICS

Some physicians have advocated initially treating all patients with MDS with varying combinations of vitamin B_{12}, folate, pyridoxine, riboflavin, and vitamin C (145). Now that assays for B_{12} and folate are routinely available, this approach can no longer be justified and is not beneficial. A trial of pharmacologic doses of pyridoxine alone may be considered. Before the realization that ringed sideroblasts accompany several different types of anemia (Table 11-8), all patients with ringed sideroblasts received pyridoxine. Some responded at least partially and became transfusion independent (486,487,494,496,511,512). No evidence has been found that such patients had pyridoxine deficiency, and pharmacologic doses of 100 mg/day were required for a response.

Most, if not all, pyridoxine-responsive patients probably had hereditary or drug-induced sideroblastic anemia. Pharmacologic doses of pyridoxine might overcome a functional or absolute deficiency of ALA-S and improve erythropoiesis. Hereditary sideroblastic anemia is the only disorder with evidence for ALA-S deficiency. In recent trials in patients with RARS or RA, after careful exclusion of those with hereditary sideroblastic anemia, pyridoxine had no effect (145,506). Occasionally, the diagnosis of hereditary sideroblastic anemia is difficult to exclude. Because pyridoxine is a safe drug, a 3-month trial of 100 mg/day orally is warranted in suspected MDS if the patient has isolated anemia and ringed sideroblasts on bone marrow examination.

Heme arginate has been used in 26 patients with MDS (582). The hemoglobin concentrations of six patients increased significantly, accompanied by a reduction in ringed sideroblast count in the bone marrow. All responders initially had low levels of marrow ferrochelatase activity; heme arginate may allow bypass of this step in heme synthesis. Even though deficiency of this mitochondrial enzyme is unlikely to be the primary cause of the anemia in patients with MDS, secondary ferrochelatase deficiency from mitochondrial iron deposition and damage may contribute to the degree of anemia. Larger cohorts, especially of RARS patients, should be studied using this compound.

ANDROGENS

Androgen treatment has been investigated in several large trials. In an uncontrolled initial study, Najean and Pecking (583) treated 90 RAEB or RAEB-t patients with different androgen compounds. Less than 10% showed an increase in hemoglobin concentration or platelet count, and none had significant improvement in neutrophil counts. Side effects were common, including jaundice, muscle cramping, and virilization of female patients. The rate of transformation to leukemia in this androgen-treated cohort was higher than in historical controls. The same investigators then conducted a randomized trial comparing supportive care to androgen therapy, methenolone 2.5 mg/kg/day, or ara-C (cytosine arabinoside), 20 mg/m^2/12 hours subcutaneously (538). Neither modality affected survival or progression to leukemia. Several smaller studies have also reached similar conclusions (584–586); no evidence suggests that these drugs should be used in most patients with MDS.

Some data suggest that patients with MDS who have hypocellular bone marrows may benefit from androgen therapy. Testosterone enanthate, 7 to 10 mg/week intramuscularly, was given to 92 patients with either aplastic anemia or MDS (59). Some patients with MDS responded with clinically significant improvement in peripheral blood counts. Almost all of these responders initially had a hypocellular bone marrow. Those who responded survived longer than nonresponders, but there was no untreated control group. A 3-month trial of androgen therapy could be considered for patients with a hypocellular marrow and no other therapeutic options.

CORTICOSTEROIDS

In most patients with MDS, corticosteroids should be avoided because they are ineffective as well as toxic to already immunocompromised patients (20,587). Bagby and co-workers (587) found that prednisone improved the peripheral counts of a few patients with MDS and that response could be predicted by the *in vitro* enhancement of bone marrow CFU-GM by cortisol. These responders did not live demonstrably longer and suffered appreciable toxicity. The potential to improve peripheral blood counts was small and was outweighed by the toxicity of the treatment and the impracticability of performing bone marrow cultures on all patients to identify rare potential responders.

Conventional Chemotherapy

The attainment of complete and often sustained hematologic remissions in most patients with AML given standard antileukemic chemotherapy has prompted clinical trials of this approach in MDS. Several problems with high-dose chemotherapy in these patients could be predicted from the outset. They are on average older and thus less able to tolerate full-scale chemotherapy than patients with *de novo* AML. The bone marrow may not recover after chemotherapy, because patients with MDS have trilineage marrow replacement with abnormal clonal precursors. No functional repopulating hematopoietic stem cells may remain after chemotherapy-induced aplasia. Finally, it is hard to decide when to initiate chemotherapy, because the clinical course in individual patients varies so widely.

An early retrospective study included 45 patients with RAEB, RAEB-t, or CMML treated with one of several antileukemic chemotherapy regimens (588). Forty-five percent of the patients with RAEB or RAEB-t, and 64% of the patients with CMML achieved complete remission, but these remissions were brief (median of 8.4 and 6.2 months, respectively). Toxicity and treatment-related mortality rates did not differ from those of patients with *de novo* AML who were treated during the same period on the same regimens. This cohort of patients with MDS was relatively young (median age of 52 years).

A similar retrospective review of 20 patients with MDS of a more typical median age (69 years) treated with a variety of antileukemic regimens showed a complete remission rate of only 20%. Responding patients were, on average, younger than the rest of the cohort (589). Nonresponders had a median survival of only 1 month; this was shorter than the survival of five untreated patients from the same cohort and suggested increased mortality from chemotherapy. A more recent study of 29 patients with RAEB or RAEB-t, CMML, or AML evolving from MDS showed a higher complete remission rate (48%), but this was significantly less than the 73% complete remission rate that the same investigators found in treating *de novo* AML with the same regimen (590). However, 35% of the patients died during induction. No difference in complete remission rate or survival time after chemotherapy was found between patients treated in the MDS phase and those who had transformed to AML.

The ability to achieve complete remission in patients with MDS after transformation (t-MDS) to AML supports delaying the use of aggressive chemotherapy until transformation has occurred. Remission rates are not as high as in *de novo* AML, their duration is shorter, and toxicity is greater, but 22% to 50% of patients obtain complete remission (588,591–594). Standard regimens of ara-C plus daunorubicin or single agent high-dose ara-C, 3 g/m²/12 hours for 12 doses, have been successfully used. For patients younger than 50 years with RAEB, RAEB-t, or life-threatening cytopenias, some researchers have advocated treating with chemotherapy at presentation instead of waiting for progression to AML (592,595–598). No data from controlled trials support this approach.

In t-MDS, no formal studies of chemotherapy before acute transformation have been published, perhaps because the time until transformation or death from other complications is so brief. Patients with t-MDS treated with standard antileukemic chemotherapy after transformation attained a 41% to 45% complete remission rate, but remissions are short, and no evidence of an increase in survival duration has been found (201,202,596).

It should be noted that in one large cooperative group trial, patients treated with intensive AML treatment protocols but were later classified as having FAB, RAEB, or RAEB-t did as well as their counterparts with AML (599). However, these observations appear not to be readily generalizable to the general MDS population.

Differentiation Therapy

During the 1980s, much attention focused on the treatment of patients with MDS with agents that could, at least theoretically, induce the differentiation of abnormal hematopoietic progenitors (572,600). This approach seemed promising for several reasons (601). First, maturation of immature progenitors might increase the number of the functional hematopoietic cells and decrease complications such as infection, bleeding, and iron overload. Second, immature cells might be pushed out of the mitotic compartment into a nonmitotic compartment, from which they might be less likely to overrun remaining normal marrow elements. Finally, toxicity to normal marrow precursors and other rapidly dividing cells might be less from differentiating agents than from cytoreductive regimens. Unfortunately, these agents have not yet fulfilled the promise that they showed *in vitro* and in early clinical trials; in some instances, their mechanisms of action have been more cytostatic than differentiating.

The initial stimulus to investigation of differentiation induction was the observation that cell lines derived from leukemic mice became more mature by morphologic and functional criteria when exposed to several compounds *in vitro* (572,600,602,603). Lotem (603) and Sachs (600) discovered that only certain leukemic cell lines retain the ability to differentiate, suggesting more than one mechanism for maturation arrest. Clinical interest was generated by demonstration that ara-C, retinoic acid, vitamin D, interferon, dactinomycin, methotrexate, hypoxanthine, 5-azacytidine, and other compounds all induced differentiation of human cells (572,604–606). *In vitro* maturation of cells from patients with AML or MDS were less striking than that seen in cell lines, and varied from patient to patient (607–609). Striking synergism with combinations of different agents, such as retinoic acid and ara-C, has been demonstrated both in cell lines and in primary cells from patients with MDS or AML (610,611). The mechanism of induction by these compounds is not fully understood and probably varies among inducers. Concentrations of these compounds high enough to produce differentiation also generally inhibit proliferation. No one yet knows whether growth inhibition is a necessary side effect or a consequence of maturation (600,606).

Several of these above-mentioned agents—alone and in combination—have been tested in clinical trials. Although the clinical trials were based on the hypothesis that these agents would have differentiating ability *in vivo*, their mechanism of action might involve differential killing of dysplastic cells and hematopoietic repopulation by normal or less severely affected subclones.

Low-Dose Cytosine Arabinoside

Ara-C is the arabinoside analog of deoxycytidine. In its phosphorylated form, ara-C is incorporated into DNA, acting as a chain synthesis terminator. At doses of 100 to 200 mg/m²/day, in combination with daunorubicin, it is part of the standard regimen for remission induction of *de novo* AML. Low-dose ara-C, 10 to 20 mg/m^2/day by continuous intravenous infusion, or every 12 hours by subcutaneous injection, produces plasma levels high enough to induce differentiation of human promyelocytic (HL-60) cells *in vitro* without irreversible cytostasis. These concentrations are also high enough to inhibit DNA synthesis (572,606,612–614). There were initial reports of complete responses in three patients with AML using this low-dose regimen (615).

Interpretation of clinical trials with low-dose Ara-C is made difficult by their small size, intracohort and intercohort heterogeneity, inclusion of patients with frank acute leukemia, lack of untreated controls in all studies but one, differing dose schedules and treatment durations, and differing definitions of response. Najean and Pecking (538) carried out the only controlled trial. They compared supportive care with androgen or low-dose ara-C treatment and found no survival advantage for either therapy. Ara-C was given for only 2 days each month.

More encouraging results were obtained by Griffin and coworkers (616,617). Eleven of 16 patients had significant improvement in blood counts of one or more lineage, and some became transfusion independent for 2 to 14 months. Other investigators have generally not reported such a high response or complete remission rate. Even among responders, duration of improvement in counts or bone marrow remission has generally been only 2 to 3 months. In some patients, several courses of ara-C were required before a response occurred (616,618,619). Significant toxicity was often observed. Even at these low dosages, patients became extremely pancytopenic and required more RBC and platelet transfusions (614,619–623). Marrow recovery back to pre–ara-C counts did not occur in some cases for up to 1 month after treatment (616,623). Therapy-related deaths have been reported frequently (619,622,623).

Some investigators have argued that the mechanism of *in vivo* response to these dosages of ara-C was mainly differentiation, without significant cytoreduction (614,615,619). The detection of mature granulocytes with Auer rods in several patients after ara-C treatment and persistent abnormal cytogenetics in patients with complete hematologic remissions support this hypothesis (614,616). Even in AML before treatment, circulating mature granulocytes that originate from the abnormal clone have been detected (241). Many investigators have instead argued that the major mechanism of action of low-dose ara-C must be cytoreductive, with preferential killing or inhibition of the most severely dysregulated immature populations, allowing less severely affected progenitors to restore hematopoiesis (572,612,624). This hypothesis is supported by the documentation in many clinical trials of significant marrow aplasia in patients after ara-C treatment before hematopoietic recovery (616,620–622,625). In two patients with complete hematologic remissions after ara-C therapy, X-chromosome RFLP analysis showed that polyclonal hematopoiesis was restored.

The relatively low response rates, short response durations, and high toxicity and mortality rates associated with low-dose ara-C treatment have not encouraged more general application of these regimens (572,624). In an attempt to decrease toxicity, a few patients have been treated with very-low-dose ara-C, 6 mg/m^2/day for 21 days (626). Marrow suppression was not as severe as at the higher doses, and six of eight patients showed improvement in their counts; three had complete normalization. One study of more than 100 patients found that an adverse outcome after treatment with ara-C could be related to advanced age, low platelet count, the presence of the pseudo-Pelger in leukocytes, and multiple chromosomal abnormalities (627). The authors proposed that these parameters be used to

develop a predictive model for ara-C therapy. Another small study used low-dose oral 6-thioguanine, but only 4 of 18 patients showed any improvement (628). These studies have been presented to emphasize the major difficulties in evaluating new therapies. Although this approach showed some promise, a randomized trial was completed, showing no improvement in survival compared with supportive care (629).

Retinoids

Unlike ara-C, the retinoid class of vitamin A analogs are generally not cytostatic at concentrations sufficient to induce differentiation of HL-60 cells, although their mechanism of action is not completely understood (604). They are known to regulate the expression of several protooncogenes *in vitro*. When given to animals before mutagen exposure, they decrease the risk of subsequent development of neoplasms. Retinoids may also increase the sensitivity of hematopoietic precursors to stimulation by growth factors (634).

In a phase I study of 13-*cis*-retinoic acid, 15 of 45 courses of 25 to 125 mg/m^2/day orally were accompanied by some improvement in counts, generally in granulocytes (630). Similar results were reported in other smaller cohorts (631,632). Hepatotoxicity was dose limiting, and other side effects included cheilosis, hyperkeratosis, stomatitis, and increased serum lipid levels. In another uncontrolled trial, 22% of patients showed appreciable toxicity, including worsening thrombocytopenia (633).

Two randomized placebo-controlled trials have been published, with conflicting results. In one study, 70 patients with RA or RARS received 13-*cis*-retinoic acid, 20 mg/m^2/day, or placebo. Overall survival in the entire cohort was worse than in historical controls, but the 1-year survival rate in RA patients given the drug was 77% compared with 36% in the placebo group, which was statistically significant (634). Because no significant difference in blood counts or rate of transformation to acute leukemia was found between the two groups, the survival advantage remains unexplained. Sequential bone marrow examinations were not performed. In a second randomized, controlled trial, 68 patients with MDS of all subtypes received 13-*cis*-retinoic acid, 100 mg/m^2/day, or placebo for 6 months (635). Cytopenias were not significantly improved, and the overall course did not improve in the *cis*-retinoic acid–treated group. More than 90% sustained appreciable dermatologic toxicity. The reasons for the discrepancy in results between these two trials are unclear (636). On balance, the lack of documented hematologic improvement in the patients in the first study and their unusually short overall survival generates skepticism about a beneficial effect of retinoids.

Vitamin D

1,25-Dihydroxyvitamin D$_3$ effectively differentiates HL-60 cells *in vitro* at concentrations of 5 × 10^{-9} mol/L, and AML blasts at 10^{-6} to 10^{-7} mol/L^2. A clinical trial used 2 µg/day orally in 18 patients with MDS (2). Minimal transient increases in platelet and white blood cell counts were seen in 8 of 18 patients, but nine developed clinically significant hypercalcemia. Serum levels of only 2 × 10^{-10} mol/L were achieved, and higher doses were not practical because of hypercalcemia. Seven of 18 patients developed acute leukemia during treatment.

Interferon

Interferon-α also induces differentiation of leukemic cells *in vitro* and has been given to a small number of patients with MDS in uncontrolled studies. Apart from inducing differentiation, it may stimulate NK cell activity, which was found lacking in patients with MDS. Remarkable sustained responses even after discontinuation of therapy have been reported in two patients (637,638). Trisomy 8, detectable in most of the marrow metaphases in one patient before treatment, disappeared after interferon-α was given. Only one-eighth of patients demonstrated a response in the only clinical trial yet published, which was uncontrolled (638). Toxicity was minimal.

The possibility that combinations of interferon, vitamin D, retinoic acid, and ara-C could provide *in vivo* synergy is being investigated. All four given simultaneously are not well tolerated, but the first three given without ara-C produced a 44% response rate in one uncontrolled study (639).

5-Azacytidine

5-Azacytidine interferes with methylation and may partially correct deregulated gene expression in MDS, such as the p15 INK locus described above (397). Several studies have demonstrated significant response rates, and a recent randomized study by the Cancer and Leukemia Group B demonstrated an improved median time to progression to AML and a longer overall median survival when compared with best supportive care (640,641).

Amifostine

Amifostine is a phosphorylated organic thiol that may protect the hematopoietic stem cell from metabolic stress and promote progenitor growth, though the precise mode of action is not fully understood. There have been conflicting data from small, uncontrolled trials thus far, and it is likely that additional study will be needed to define a role for amifostine in MDS (642–645).

Hematopoietic Growth Factors

The potent abilities of recently isolated growth factors to support and stimulate hematopoiesis both *in vitro* and in experimental animals has focused scientific, economic, and clinical attention on their possible usefulness in treating hematologic disease (646–648). The human genes for at least 15 of these factors have been cloned during the past 5 years (417,646). Recombinant DNA technology allows production of pharmacologic quantities of the proteins in bacteria, yeast, or cultured mammalian cell systems. The lack of normal glycosylation of these recombinant human proteins might affect activity or immunogenicity, although neither has been a problem in clinical trials. Four factors are undergoing active clinical investigation in patients with MDS, and several more are certain to be released for initial studies soon.

A deficiency in production of any particular growth factor has not been shown in MDS, despite the mapping of several growth factor genes to the area deleted from the 5q chromosome. As noted, higher concentrations of these factors may be necessary to stimulate colony formation from MDS marrow than from normal bone marrow (443,444). Several possible growth factor effects might result in clinical improvement. These include differentiation of abnormal precursors, stimulation of residual normal hematopoietic elements, and enhancement of the function of mature cells. Conversely, adverse effects can also be imagined, such as stimulation of blast cell proliferation without differentiation. At least in culture, hematopoietic growth factors enhance the growth of both leukemic cell lines and primary blasts (649–651). In the future, combination therapy with two or more growth factors may prove desirable because synergy has already been demonstrated (652–655). An

agent acting early in hematopoietic development, such as IL-3, might be more effective in conjunction with a late-acting agent such as EPO.

Granulocyte-Macrophage Colony-Stimulating Factor

More patients with MDS have received GM-CSF than any other growth factor. Vadhan-Raj and co-workers (656) published a phase I/II trial using 30 to 500 μg/m^2/day by continuous intravenous infusion for 14 days to eight patients. All had a 5- to 70-fold increase in total leukocyte count, due mainly to increases in granulocytes and eosinophils. Three patients also had an increase in their reticulocyte or platelet counts. The percentage of myeloblasts in the bone marrow decreased in some patients, although small numbers of circulating blasts appeared during extreme leukocytosis. Toxicity was minimal, consisting mainly of nonspecific bone pain and fatigue.

Several small, uncontrolled studies have been subsequently published using 7- to 21-day courses of GM-CSF at equivalent doses. An increase in white blood cells occurred in nearly all patients (657,658). Consistent beneficial effects on platelet count, RBC count, and transfusion requirement have not been observed. Investigators have reported clinically significant decreases in platelet count in some patients receiving GM-CSF, necessitating discontinuation of therapy in several patients (659). The same study reported similar improvements in neutrophil count using up to 20 times lower doses of GM-CSF, with milder nonhematologic toxicity. One patient with t-MDS experienced a trilineage remission after two courses of GM-CSF, with disappearance of a documented cytogenetic abnormality (660). Relapse occurred after 1 year. The pathophysiology of this unusual response may have involved terminal differentiation of an abnormal clone precluding further proliferation.

In one study, 5 of 11 treated patients progressed to acute leukemia while on GM-CSF or within 4 weeks of completing a GM-CSF course (658). All had bone marrow myeloblast percentages of more than 15% before beginning therapy. It is unclear whether GM-CSF actually accelerated the progression to leukemia or whether the timing of transformation was coincidental.

Most patients do respond to GM-CSF with an increase in their neutrophil count, but the impact of this numeric change on ability to fight infection and on longer-term morbidity and mortality, both from infection and from leukemic progression is unclear. A multicenter, randomized, controlled trial has been carried out, with only preliminary results available (661). Median neutrophil counts were significantly increased in the treatment arm, but no effect on anemia, transfusion requirements, or platelet counts was seen. Patients on the GM-CSF arm experienced significantly fewer infections during the 3-month treatment period. There was no higher rate of leukemic transformation in the patients given GM-CSF, but follow-up has been brief.

Granulocyte Colony-Stimulating Factor

Response rates and patterns in small, uncontrolled trials of G-CSF have been similar to GM-CSF: More than 80% of patients significantly increase their neutrophil counts, but only rare responses in erythroid or platelet lineages have been seen (662–664). G-CSF, 0.1 to 5.0 μg/kg/day, has been used for up to 3 months. The first two trials did not report progression to acute leukemia while on therapy (662,663), but longer follow-up of subsequent patients did reveal progression to AML in several patients with marrow blast percentages of over 10% before therapy (664). Those patients with abnormal cytogenetics before therapy experienced no change in the percentage of abnormal metaphases detected in bone marrow while on therapy. One large randomized trial of G-CSF was conducted in MDS. The results have only been reported in abstract form, but did not show any survival benefit even though the majority of patients had a meaningful neutrophil response (665). G-CSF, as noted below, however, may potentiate the effects of EPO in MDS. Because of the clear evidence for neutrophil response in the majority of patients, G-CSF is most frequently used in the setting of febrile neutropenia in the MDS patient.

Interleukin-3

Only a limited number of patients in MDS have received IL-3 (666); there is no evidence that IL-3 offers any clinical advantages over GM-CSF or G-CSF. Most patients responded with increases in neutrophil count but to a less pronounced degree than with G-CSF or GM-CSF. Despite increases in reticulocyte counts, only one patient had decreased transfusion requirements. Patients did not show significant responses in the platelet lineage, a particularly disappointing outcome because IL-3 stimulates all lineages *in vitro* and has increased platelet and reticulocyte counts in primates as well as in humans with normal marrow function (652,654,667–668a).

Erythropoietin

EPO can improve the hematocrit and decrease transfusion requirements in as many as 25% of patients (669). The best predictors of response include low serum EPO levels (<200 mU/mL), low risk MDS, and minimal transfusion requirements. The current National Comprehensive Cancer Network (NCCN) guidelines recommend EPO therapy for patients with RA and serum EPO less than 500 mU/mL at a dose of 150 to 300 U/kg/day for 2 to 3 months (670). The overall response rate from compilation of data from multiple trials is approximately 20% and is best predicted by low (<200) serum EPO levels in the setting of anemia. It should also be noted that iron therapy will potentiate the therapeutic benefit of EPO in MDS, even if the patient is not iron deficient. However, iron therapy should not be used in the iron-overloaded MDS patient.

Erythropoietin Plus Granulocyte Colony-Stimulating Factor

There is now ample evidence that the combination of EPO and G-CSF results in improved erythroid responses in MDS patients. The NCCN currently recommends use of this combination for patients with RARS. EPO is given at the same dose as above, in conjunction with G-CSF 0.3 to 3.0 µg/kg/day for 3 months, based on data that indicates synergy between EPO and G-CSF (577,671–673). However, most of the phase II literature supports a broader application for the combination therapy (671,674–679). The overall response rate in one large phase II trial was approximately 38% (676). As noted above, iron therapy should accompany the combination of EPO and G-CSF except in those patients who are iron overloaded at the time of initiation of cytokine therapy. A randomized trial demonstrated little or no synergy between EPO and GM-CSF (680).

Thrombopoietin and Interleukin-11

Although there are little data on the value of thrombopoietin or IL-11 in stimulating platelet production in MDS, the available evidence indicates that neither IL-11 nor thrombopoietin has any significant benefit in the context of AML and is not likely to be therapeutically useful in MDS (681).

Immunosuppressive Therapy

As noted above, several clinical observations have suggested an overlap between aplastic anemia and MDS. These include progression to MDS or AML in some aplastic anemia patients, the presence of abnormal cytogenetic clones in some patients with aplastic anemia, and hematologic responses in some MDS patients treated with immunosuppressive therapy such as ATG and cyclosporin A (677,682–684). Twenty-five transfusion-dependent MDS patients with less than 20% blasts were treated in a phase II study with ATG (233). Eleven patients (44%) responded and became transfusion dependent, with more frequent responses in RA versus RAEB patients. ATG was well-tolerated, with mild serum sickness observed in all patients. Similar results have been observed in smaller studies, some of which also incorporated the use of cyclosporin A (228,231,234). Other studies using only cyclosporin in patients with hypoplastic MDS have also reported responses (235,236,685). It has been suggested that responses may be more frequent in patients who retain some degree of polyclonal hematopoiesis (230), and that response to immunosuppression may be due to ATG-mediated reversal of lymphocyte-mediated inhibition of CFU-GM (232). Immunosuppressive therapy may thus be a useful approach in some MDS patients. Additional studies will be necessary to determine the mechanism of action, and predictors of response to immunosuppressive therapy. For example, it is not clear whether hypoplastic MDSs (that might formally have been diagnosed as aplastic anemia) are more likely to respond than normal or hypercellular MDS. Thus, treatment should be undertaken in the context of a clinical trial.

Other Agents

Other agents that may have promise but still require further study include histone deacetylase inhibitors such as phenylbutyrate and others (686,687); UCN-01, a protein kinase C inhibitor; farnesyl transferase inhibitors FTI of RAS; and anti-angiogenesis agents (686). A 30% response rate has recently been reported in abstract form for the FTI R115777 (tipifarmib, Zarnestra) in small numbers of MDS patients, although responses did not correlate with activating mutations in RAS, or even with inhibition of farnesyl transferase activity, suggesting that there may be other targets for this drug. FLT3 inhibitors are also being investigated in clinical trials using several different small molecule inhibitors (336). Other promising agents include topoisomerase I inhibitors, such as topotecan (686,688), and antibody-mediated approaches using anti-CD33 humanized antibody conjugated to a novel toxin calicheamicin (gemtuzumab ozogamicin, Mylotarg) (689). Further clinical trials are necessary to assess the utility of these approaches alone and in combination.

Bone Marrow Transplantation

Bone marrow transplantation offers the only real opportunity for cure of MDS, and significant strides have been made in the past several years. These include extensive investigation of the role of autologous HSCT, allogeneic HSCT from sibling and alternative donors, and nonmyeloablative HSCT, which has lower acute transplant-related morbidity and mortality than conventional transplant (556,690–701).

Over the past two decades, more than 700 cases of allogeneic bone marrow transplant have been reported, with lead patients that have been disease-free for more than 16 years (697). The overall survival in combined studies has been approximately 46%. However, RA patients transplanted with fully matched related donors have as high as 75% long-term disease-free survival. Factors associated with increased risk of relapse include increased blast percentage and poor-risk karyotype (697). Factors associated with increased risk of nonrelapse mortality include longer disease duration, advanced patient age, t-MDS, and use of mismatched or unrelated donors. In addition, although numbers are small, favorable results have been seen in patients in the 55- to 66-year-old age group (702). Fifty patients in this age group had an overall 3-year disease-free survival of 53%. As in younger patients, relapse-free survival was decreased in patients with high-risk IPSS score or poor-risk cytogenetics. There is higher morbidity and mortality among patients receiving mismatched or unrelated donor transplant, although initial results in this context have been encouraging (699). For patients with advanced disease defined as greater than 5% blasts, 3-year survival is approximately 25% to 30% (556). Finally, use of nonmyeloablative bone marrow transplantation is being actively investigated in several centers (693,695). It is too early to assess the value of this approach in MDS, but the lower acute toxicities related to transplantation may be useful in older patients with MDS.

Collectively, these data suggest that younger patients with suitable sibling or alternative donors and an IPSS intermediate or high-risk score should be considered for HSCT. The use of induction chemotherapy before HSCT is controversial, but is probably most appropriate in the context of high blast count. With new WHO criteria for AML of greater than 20% marrow blasts, this problem may be obviated to a certain extent in that patients who formerly would have been diagnosed as RAEB-t are now more likely to receive induction chemotherapy as therapy of AML.

Because of substantial transplant-related morbidity and mortality related to allogeneic, mismatched, or unrelated donor transplantation, it has been suggested that consolidation of conventional chemotherapy with autologous HSCT may be a viable therapeutic option (691,693,694,696). One recent trial prospectively treated patients who developed AML after antecedent MDS with induction chemotherapy followed by alloHSCT for those with histocompatible sibling donors, and autologous HSCT for the remainder. The remission induction rate was 54%, and the 4-year disease-free survival was comparable between the two groups at 31% and 27%, respectively (703). It is not yet clear whether similar data would be obtained in MDS patients treated with a similar regimen, or whether autologous HSCT offers any advantage over conventional induction chemotherapy. These questions are currently being addressed in European Organization for Research and Treatment of Cancer cooperative trials.

Recommendations for Treatment

There are few therapies that have been proven effective for treatment of MDS. Supportive care remains a mainstay of treatment, and many MDS patients may enjoy a reasonable quality of life with attentive care. A trial of EPO should be considered for patients with symptomatic anemia and EPO levels lower than 500 mU/mL. For some patients with RA or RARS, response rates may be improved with addition of G-CSF and oral iron supplementation as long as the patient is not iron overloaded. Although use of G-CSF does not seem to accelerate progression to AML, G-CSF should be reserved in general for evidence of infection in the setting of neutropenia. Monitoring, and in some cases prophylaxis, may help prevent infectious complications of MDS; and iron overload should be treated with chelation therapy in appropriate MDS patients. It is possi-

ble that further improvements in treatment will ensue from progress in our understanding of molecular disease pathogenesis. For example, farnesyl transferase inhibitors may be useful in patients with activating mutations in RAS; specific tyrosine kinase inhibitors such as STI571 (imatinib mesylate; Gleevec) may be useful in treatment of CMML patients with activating mutations in PDGFβR; FLT3 inhibitors may have activity in treatment of MDS associated with FLT3 activating mutation; and all-*trans*-retinoic acid is likely to be useful in t-MDS patients with t(15;17). Histone deacetylase inhibitors have potential to reverse the block in differentiation that is induced by products of specific translocations such as the AML1/EVI1 fusion, and a number of both empiric and molecularly targeted therapies are being explored in clinical trials. Thus, there is continued hope for improvement in therapy and outcome of these complex and heterogeneous syndromes.

With the possible exception of 5-azacytidine treatment, which has demonstrated efficacy in a phase III randomized trial, all patients should be treated in the context of well-designed clinical trials that incorporate known risk factors according to the IPSS and account for the particularly poor prognosis of t-MDS. Immunosuppressive therapy may be an option for patients for whom HSCT is not an option.

HSCT offers the only real hope for cure of MDS at present. In general, younger patients with IPSS intermediate or high-risk MDS and a suitable related or unrelated donor, should be considered for allogeneic HSCT. Autologous HSCT is being investigated in clinical trials and may be a suitable alternative for patients without a suitable donor, especially with progression to advanced MDS or AML. Further guidance for the practitioner may be gleaned from review of the NCCN guidelines for therapy of MDS.

It is hoped that further progress and improvement in our understanding of the molecular pathogenesis of MDS over the next several years will lead to further progress in therapy.

REFERENCES

1. Yoshida Y. Biology of myelodysplastic syndromes. *Int J Cell Clon* 1987;5:356.
2. Koeffler HP. Myelodysplastic syndromes (preleukemia). *Semin Hematol* 1986;23:284.
3. Hoelzer D. Cytobiology and clinical findings of myelodysplastic syndromes. *Recent Results Cancer Res* 1988;106:172.
4. Geary CG. Clinical annotation: the diagnosis of preleukaemia. *Br J Haematol* 1983;55:1.
5. Mufti GJ, Galton DAG. Myelodysplastic syndromes: natural history and features of prognostic importance. *Clin Haematol* 1986;15:953.
6. Koeffler HP. Preleukaemia. *Clin Haematol* 1986;15:829.
7. Bennett JM. Classification of the myelodysplastic syndromes. *Clin Haematol* 1986;15:909.
8. Beris P. Primary clonal myelodysplastic syndromes. *Semin Hematol* 1989;26:216.
9. Jacobs A, Clark RE. Pathogenesis and clinical variations in the myelodysplastic syndromes. *Clin Haematol* 1986;15:925.
10. Bagby G. *The preleukemic syndrome.* Boca Raton: CRC Press, 1985.
11. Galton DAG. The myelodysplastic syndromes. *Scand J Haematol* 1986;36(Suppl 45):11.
12. Rhoads CP, Barker WH. Refractory anemia. *JAMA* 1938;110:794.
13. Bjorkman SE. Chronic refractory anemia with sideroblastic bone marrow: a study of four cases. *Blood* 1956;11:250.
14. Vilter RW, Jarrold T, Will JJ, et al. Refractory anemia with hyperplastic bone marrow. *J Haematol* 1960;15:1.
15. Hamilton-Paterson JL. Preleukaemic anaemia. *Acta Haematol* 1949;2:302.
16. Rheingold JJ, Kaufman R, Adelson E, Lear A. Smoldering acute leukemia. *N Engl J Med* 1963;268:812.
17. Meacham GC, Weisberger AS. Early atypical manifestations of leukemia. *Ann Intern Med* 1954;41:780.
18. Block M, Jacobson LO, Bethard WF. Preleukemic acute human leukemia. *JAMA* 1953;152:1018.
19. Boggs DR, Wintrobe MM, Cartwright GE. The acute leukemias. *Medicine* 1962;41:163.
20. Linman JW, Bagby GC. The preleukemic syndromes (hemopoietic dysplasia). *Cancer* 1978;42:854.

21. Hayhoe FGJ, Quaglino D. Refractory sideroblastic anaemia and erythraemic myelosis: possible relationship and cytochemical observations. *Br J Haematol* 1960;6:381.
22. Dameshek W. Sideroblastic anemia: is this a malignancy? *Br J Haematol* 1965;2:52.
23. Dreyfus B, Rochant H, Salmon C, et al. Anémies réfractaires états préleucemiques et anomalies enzymatiques multiples. *C R Acad Sci* 1968;266:1627.
24. Dreyfus B, Rochant H, Sultan C, et al. Les anémies réfractaires avec execs de myeloblastes dans la moelle. Étude de onze observations. *Presse Med* 1970; 78:359.
25. Saarni M, Linman J. Preleukemia: hematologic syndrome preceding acute leukemia. *Am J Med* 1973;55:38.
26. Bennett JM, Catovsky D, Daniel MT, et al. Proposals for the classification of the acute leukemias. *Br J Haematol* 1976;33:451.
27. Bennett JM, Catovsky D, Daniel MT, et al. Proposals for the classification of the myelodysplastic syndromes. *Br J Haematol* 1982;51:189.
28. Pedersen-Bjergaard J, Larsen SO. Incidence of acute nonlymphocytic leukemia, preleukemia, and acute myeloproliferative syndrome up to 10 years after treatment of Hodgkin's disease. *N Engl J Med* 1982;307:965.
29. Foucar K, McKenna RW, Bloomfield CD, et al. Therapy-related leukemia: a panmyelosis. *Cancer* 1979;43:1285.
30. Mortensen BT, Pedersen-Bjergaard J, Pedersen NT, et al. Predictive value of bone marrow cultures in 48 patients with acute myeloblastic leukaemia or myelodysplasia both secondary to treatment of other malignant diseases. *Scand J Haematol* 1985;35:423.
31. Bennett JM. World Health Organization classification of the acute leukemias and myelodysplastic syndrome. *Int J Hematol* 2000;72(2):131–133.
32. Wolf BC, Neiman RS. The bone marrow in myeloproliferative and dysmyelopoietic syndromes. *Hematol Oncol Clin North Am* 1988;2:669.
33. Krause JR. An appraisal of the value of the bone marrow biopsy in the assessment of proliferative lesions of the bone marrow. *Histopathology* 1983;7: 627.
34. Frisch B, Bartl R. Bone marrow histology in myelodysplastic syndromes. *Scand J Haematol* 1986;36(Suppl 45):21.
35. Georgii A, Vykoupil KF, Buhr T. Preleukemia: bone marrow histopathology in myelodysplasia and preleukemic syndrome. *Recent Results Cancer Res* 1988;106:159.
36. Jacot-Des-Combes E, Beris P, Kapanci Y. Plastic embedded bone marrow biopsy in the evaluation of myelodysplastic syndromes. *Pathol Res Pract* 1985;180:280.
37. Tricot G, DeWolfe-Peeters C, Hendrick B, Verwilghen RL. Bone marrow histology in myelodysplastic syndromes. *Br J Haematol* 1984;57:423.
38. Fohlmeister I, Fischer R, Schaefer H-E. Preleukemic myelodysplastic syndromes (MDS): pathogenetical considerations based on retrospective clinicomorphological sequential studies. *Anticancer Res* 1985;5:179.
39. Mitrou PS, Fischer M, Hubner K. Proliferation of ineffective erythropoiesis with nuclear abnormalities and megaloblastoid appearance in preleukaemia. *Acta Haematol* 1975;54:271.
40. Bethlenfalvey NC, Phaure TAJ, Phyliky RL, Bowman RP. Nuclear bridging of erythroblasts in acquired dyserythropoiesis: an early and transient preleukemic marker. *Am J Hematol* 1986;21:315.
41. Juneja SK, Imbert M, Sigaux F, et al. Prevalence and distribution of ringed sideroblasts in primary myelodysplastic syndromes. *J Clin Pathol* 83;36:566.
42. Bottomley SS. Sideroblastic anaemia. *Clin Haematol* 1982;11:389.
43. Hast R. Sideroblasts in myelodysplasia: their nature and clinical significance. *Scand J Haematol* 1986;45:53.
44. Caroli J, Bernard J, Bessis M, et al. Hémochromatose avec anémie hypochrome et absence d'hémoglobine anormale. *Presse Med* 1957;65:1991.
45. Goodman JR, Hall SG. Accumulation of iron in mitochondria of erythroblasts. *Br J Haematol* 1967;13:335.
46. Smith WB, Ablin A, Goodman JR, Brecher G. Atypical megakaryocytes in preleukemic phase of acute myeloid leukemia. *Blood* 1973;42:535.
47. Queisser W, Queisser U, Ansmann M, et al. Megakaryocyte polyploidization in acute leukemia and preleukemia. *Br J Haematol* 1974;28:261.
48. Thiede T, Enquist L, Billstrom R. Application of megakaryocytic morphology in diagnosing 5q-syndrome. *Eur J Haematol* 1988;41:434.
49. Thiele J, Krech R, Wienhold S, et al. The use of the anti-factor VIII method on trephine biopsies of the bone marrow for the identification of immature and atypical megakaryocytes in myeloproliferative diseases and allied disorders: a morphometric study. *Virchows Arch* 1987;54:89.
50. Hokland P, Kerndrup G, Griffin JD, Ellegaard J. Analysis of leukocyte differentiation antigens in blood and bone marrow from preleukemia (refractory anemia) patients using monoclonal antibodies. *Blood* 1986;67:898.
51. Scott CS, Cahill A, Bynoe AG, et al. EsteRASe cytochemistry in primary myelodysplastic syndromes and megaloblastic anaemias: demonstration of abnormal staining patterns associated with dysmyelopoiesis. *Br J Haematol* 1983;55:411.
52. Harris NL, Jaffe ES, Diebold J, et al. The World Health Organization classification of neoplastic diseases of the hematopoietic and lymphoid tissues. Report of the Clinical Advisory Committee meeting, Airlie House, Virginia, November, 1997. *Ann Oncol* 1999;10(12):1419–1432.
53. Seigneurin D, Audhuy B. Auer rods in refractory anemia with excess of blasts: presence and significance. *Am J Clin Pathol* 1983;80:359.
54. Kass L, Elias JM. Cytochemistry and immunocytochemistry in bone marrow examination: contemporary techniques for the diagnosis of acute leukemia and myelodysplastic syndromes. *Hematol Oncol Clin North Am* 1988;2:537.
55. San Miguel JF, Gonzalez M, Canizo MC, et al. The nature of blast cells in myelodysplastic syndromes evolving to acute leukaemia. *Blut* 1986;52:357.
56. Woessner S, Lafuente R, Florensa L, et al. Acquired refractory anaemia with excess of blasts of promegakaryoblastic type. *Blut* 1986;53:293.
57. Nand S, Godwin JE. Hypoplastic myelodysplastic syndrome. *Cancer* 1988; 62:958.
58. Yoshida Y, Oguma S, Uchino H, Maekawa T. Refractory myelodysplastic anaemias with hypocellular bone marrow. *J Clin Pathol* 1988;41:763.
59. Riccardi A, Giordano M, Girino M, et al. Refractory cytopenias: clinical course according to bone marrow cytology and cellularity. *Blut* 1987;54:153.
60. Coiffier B, Adeleine P, Viala JJ, et al. Dysmyelopoietic syndromes: a search for prognostic factors in 193 patients. *Cancer* 1983;52:83.
61. Sultan C, Sigaux F, Imbert M, Reyes F. Acute myelodysplasia with myelofibrosis: a report of eight cases. *Br J Haematol* 1981;49:11.
62. Pagliuca A, Layton DM, Manohara A, et al. Myelofibrosis in primary myelodysplastic syndromes: a clinico-morphological study of 10 cases. *Br J Haematol* 1989;71:499.
63. Bested AC, Cheng G, Pinkerton PH, et al. Idiopathic acquired sideroblastic anaemia transforming to acute myelosclerosis. *J Clin Pathol* 1984;37:1032.
64. Assoian RK, Grotendorst GR, Miller DM, Sporn MB. Cellular transformation by coordinated action of three peptide growth factors from human platelets. *Nature* 1984;309:804.
65. Gersuk GM, Carmel R, Pattengale PK. Platelet-derived growth factor concentrations in platelet-poor plasma and urine from patients with myeloproliferative disorders. *Blood* 1989;74:2330.
66. Gordon MY. Extracellular matrix of the marrow microenvironment. *Br J Haematol* 1988;70:1.
67. Gordon MY, Riley GP, Watt SM, Greaves MF. Compartmentalization of a haematopoietic growth factor (GM-CSF) by glycosaminoglycans in the bone marrow microenvironment. *Nature* 1987;326:403.
68. Islam A, Catovsky D, Goldman JM, Galton DAG. Studies on cellular interactions between stromal and hematopoietic stem cells in normal and leukemic bone marrows. *Bibl Haematol* 1984;50:17.
69. Tricot G, De Wolf-Peeter C, Vlietinck R, Verwilghen RL. Bone marrow histology in myelodysplastic syndromes. *Br J Haematol* 1984;58:217.
70. Greenberg P, Bagby G. Biologic rather than morphologic markers in myelodysplastic syndromes. *Br J Haematol* 1983;52:532.
71. Bagby GC Jr. The concept of preleukemia: clinical and laboratory studies. *CRC Crit Rev Oncol Hematol* 1980;4:203.
72. Spitzer TR, Goldsmith GH Jr. Myelodysplastic syndromes: is another classification necessary? *Br J Haematol* 1982;52:343.
73. Greenberg PL. The smoldering myeloid leukemic states: clinical and biologic features. *Blood* 1983;61:1035.
74. Ibbot JW, Whitelaw DM, Thomas JW. The significant percentage of blast cells in the bone marrow in the diagnosis of acute leukemia. *Can Med Assoc J* 1960;82:358.
75. Kerkhofs H, Hermans J, Haak HL, Leeksma CHW. Utility of the FAB classification for myelodysplastic syndromes: investigation of prognostic factors in 237 cases. *Br J Haematol* 1987;65:73.
76. Vallespi T, Torrabadella M, Julia A, et al. Myelodysplastic syndromes: a study of 101 cases according to the FAB classification. *Br J Haematol* 1985;61:83.
77. Bennett JM, Catovsky D, Daniel MT, et al. Proposed revised criteria for the classification of acute myeloid leukemia. *Ann Intern Med* 1985;103:620.
78. Kerndrup G, Bendix-Hansen K, Pedersen B. The prognostic significance of cytological, histological and cytogenetic findings in refractory anaemia (RA) and RA with sideroblasts. *Blut* 1987;54:231.
79. Cazzola M, Bergamaschi G, Huebers HA, Finch CA. Pathophysiological classification of acquired bone marrow failure based on quantitative assessment of erythroid function. *Eur J Haematol* 1987;38:426.
80. Kushner JP, Lee GR, Wintrobe MM, Cartwright GE. Idiopathic refractory sideroblastic anemia: clinical and laboratory investigation of 17 patients and review of the literature. *Medicine* 1971;50:139.
81. Bennett JM, Berger R, Brunning RD, et al. Recommendations for a morphologic, immunologic, and cytogenetic (MIC) working classification of the primary and therapy-related myelodysplastic disorders. *Cancer Genet Cytogenet* 1988;32:1.
82. Khaleeli M, Keane WM, Lee GR. Sideroblastic anemia in multiple myeloma: a preleukemic change. *Blood* 1973;41:17.
83. Garcia S, Sanz MA, Amigo V, et al. Prognostic factors in chronic myelodysplastic syndromes: a multivariate analysis in 107 cases. *Am J Hematol* 1988;27:163.
83a. Ballen KK, Gilliland DG, Kalish LA, et al. Bone marrow dysplasia in patients with newly diagnosed acute myelogenous leukemia does not correlate with history of myelodysplasia or with remission rate and survival. *Cancer* 1994;73:314.
84. Foucar K, Langdon RM II, Armitage JO, et al. Myelodysplastic syndromes: a clinical and pathologic analysis of 109 cases. *Cancer* 1985;56:553.
85. Weisdorf DJ, Oken MM, Johnson GJ, Rydell RE. Chronic myelodysplastic syndrome: short survival with or without evolution to acute leukaemia. *Br J Haematol* 1983;55:691.
86. van der Weide M, Sizoo W, Nauta JJP, et al. Myelodysplastic syndromes: analysis of clinical and prognostic features in 96 patients. *Eur J Haematol* 1988;41:115.
87. Schmalzl F, Lechleitner M. Disappearance of a sideroblastic cell clone during the chronic phase of a preleukemic myelodysplastic syndrome. *Br J Haematol* 1986;64:410.
88. Bursztyn B, Douer D, Ramot B. Chronic myelomonocytic leukemia following refractory anemia with sideroblasts: report of two cases. *Eur J Haematol* 1987;38:197.

89. Fenaux P, Estienne MH, Lepelley P, et al. Refractory anaemia according to the FAB classification: a report on 69 cases. *Eur J Haematol* 1988;40:318.
90. Weisdorf DJ, Oken MM, Johnson GJ, Rydell RE. Auer rod positive dysmyelopoietic syndrome. *Am J Hematol* 1981;11:397.
91. Mufti GJ, Stevens JR, Oscier DG, et al. Myelodysplastic syndromes: a scoring system with prognostic significance. *Br J Haematol* 1985;59:425.
92. Novitzky N. Myelodysplastic syndromes in children. A critical review of the clinical manifestations and management. *Am J Hematol* 2000;63(4):212–222.
93. Van Dijk JM, Sonnenblick M, Kornberg A, Rosin AJ. Preleukemic syndrome in elderly patients—report of 11 cases. *Israel J Med Sci* 1985;21:292.
94. Gardner FH. Refractory anemia in the elderly. *Adv Intern Med* 1987;32:155.
95. Wegelius R. Preleukaemic states in children. *Scand J Haematol* 1986;36(Suppl 45):133.
96. Blank J, Lange B. Preleukemia in children. *J Pediatr* 1981;98:565.
97. Saarinen UM, Wegelius R. Preleukemic syndrome in children: report of four cases and review of literature. *Am J Pediatr Hematol Oncol Clin North Am* 1984;6:137.
98. Blank J, Lange B. Preleukemia in children. *J Pediatr* 1981;98:565.
99. Niebrugge DJ. Preleukemia in children. *J Pediatr* 1981;100:507.
100. Paul B, Reid MM, Davison EV, et al. Familial myelodysplasia: progressive disease associated with emergence of monosomy 7. *Br J Haematol* 1987;65:321.
101. Li FP, Marchetto DJ, Vawter GF. Acute leukemia and preleukemia in eight males in a family: an X-linked disorder? *Am J Hematol* 1979;6:61.
102. Palmer CG, Heerema NA, Greist A, et al. Cytogenetic findings in siblings with a myelodysplastic syndrome. *Cancer Genet Cytogenet* 1987;27:241.
103. Shannon KM, Turhan AG, Chang SSY, et al. Familial bone marrow monosomy 7: evidence that the predisposing locus is not on the long arm of chromosome 7. *J Clin Invest* 1989;84:984.
104. Kamiyama R, Ishikawa Y, Hatakeyama S, et al. Clinicopathological study of hematological disorders after ThorotRASt administration in Japan. *Blut* 1988;56:153.
105. Yoosufani Z, Slavin JD, Hellman RM, et al. Preleukemia following large dose radioiodide therapy for metastatic thyroid carcinoma. *J Nuclear Med* 1987;28:1348.
106. Kamada N, Uchino H. Preleukemic states in atomic bomb survivors in Japan. *Blood Cells* 1976;2:57.
107. Farrow A, Jacobs A, West RR. Myelodysplasia, chemical exposure, and other environmental factors. *Leukemia* 1989;3:33.
108. Van Den Berghe H, Louwagie A, Broeckaert-Van Orshoven A, et al. Chromosome analysis in two unusual malignant blood disorders presumably induced by benzene. *Blood* 1979;53:558.
109. de Planque MM, Kluin-Nelemans HC, van Krieken HJM, et al. Evolution of acquired severe aplastic anemia to myelodysplasia and subsequent leukemia in adults. *Br J Haematol* 1988;70:55.
110. Tichelli A, Gratwohl A, Wursch A, et al. Late haematological complications in severe aplastic anaemia. *Br J Haematol* 1988;69:413.
111. Orlandi E, Alessandrino EP, Caldera D, Bernasconi C. Adult leukemia developing after aplastic anemia: report of 8 cases. *Acta Haematol* 1988;79:174.
112. Orlandi E, Alessandrino EP, Caldera D, Bernasconi C. Adult leukemia developing after aplastic anemia: report of 8 cases. *Acta Haematol* 1988;79:174.
113. Fohlmeister I, Fischer R, Modder B, et al. Aplastic anaemia and the hypocellular myelodysplastic syndrome: histomorphological, diagnostic, and prognostic features. *J Clin Pathol* 1985;38:1218.
114. Young NS. The problem of clonality in aplastic anemia: Dr Dameshek's riddle, restated. *Blood* 1992;79:1385.
115. Ng J-P, Pati A, Strevens MJ, Swart S. Myelodysplastic relapse of de novo acute myeloid leukaemia with trilineage myelodysplasia. *Br J Haematol* 1988;69:578.
116. Brito-Babapulle F, Catovsky D, Galton DAG. Myelodysplastic relapse of de novo acute myeloid leukaemia with trilineage myelodysplasia: a previously unrecognized correlation. *Br J Haematol* 1988;68:411.
117. Copplestone JA, Mufti GJ, Hamblin TJ, Oscier DG. Immunological abnormalities in myelodysplastic syndromes. *Br J Haematol* 1986;63:149.
118. Tranchida L, Palutke M, Poulik MD, Prasad AS. Primary acquired sideroblastic anemia preceding monoclonal gammopathy and malignant lymphoma. *Am J Med* 1973;55:559.
119. Greenberg BR, Miller C, Cardiff RD, et al. Concurrent development of preleukaemic, lymphoproliferative and plasma cell disorders. *Br J Haematol* 1983;53:125.
120. Takagi S, Kitagawa S, Takeda A, et al. Natural killer-interferon system in patients with preleukaemic states. *Br J Haematol* 1984;58:71.
121. Kerndrup G, Meyer K, Ellegaard J, Hokland P. Natural killer (NK)-cell activity and antibody-dependent cellular cytotoxicity (ADCC) in primary preleukemic syndrome. *Leuk Res* 1984;8:239.
122. Zanger B, Dorsey HN. Fever: a manifestation of preleukemia. *JAMA* 1976;236:1266.
123. Soppi E, Nousiainen T, Seppa A, Lahtinen R. Acute febrile neutrophilic dermatosis (Sweet's syndrome) in association with myelodysplastic syndromes: a report of three cases and a review of the literature. *Br J Haematol* 1989;73:43.
124. Tikjob G, Kassis V, Thomsen HK, Jensen G. Acute febrile neutrophilic dermatosis and abnormal bone marrow chromosomes as a marker for preleukemia. *Acta Derm Venereol* 1985;65:177.
125. Vilter RW, Wiltse D. Preleukemia and urticaria pigmentosa followed by acute myelomonoblastic leukemia. *Arch Intern Med* 1985;145:349.
126. Sadick N, Edlin D, Myskowski PL, et al. Granulocytic sarcoma: a new finding in the setting of preleukemia. *Arch Dermatol* 1984;120:1341.
127. Stoll DB, Blum S, Pasquale D, Murphy S. Thrombocytopenia with decreased megakaryocytes. *Ann Intern Med* 1981;94:170.
128. Gardner FH, Bessman JD. Thrombocytopenia due to defective platelet production. *Clin Haematol* 1983;12:23.
129. Najean Y, Lecompte T. Chronic pure thrombocytopenia in elderly patients. An aspect of the myelodysplastic syndrome. *Cancer* 1989;64:2506.
130. Dewald GW, Davis MP, Pierre RV, et al. Clinical characteristics and prognosis of 50 patients with a myeloproliferative syndrome and deletion of part of the long arm of chromosome 5. *Blood* 1985;66:189.
131. Juneja SK, Imbert M, Jouault H, et al. Haematological features of primary myelodysplastic syndromes (PMDS) at initial presentation: a study of 118 cases. *J Clin Pathol* 1983;36:1129.
132. Tulliez M, Testa U, Rochant H, et al. Reticulocytosis, hypochromia, and microcytosis: an unusual presentation of the preleukemic syndrome. *Blood* 1982;59:293.
133. White JM, Hoffbrand AV. Haem deficiency and chain synthesis. *Nature* 1974;248:88.
134. Maldonado J. Platelet granulopathy. *Mayo Clin Proc* 1976;51:452.
135. Pintado T, Maldonado J. Ultrastructure of platelet aggregation in refractory anemia and myelomonocytic leukemia. *Mayo Clin Proc* 1976;51:443.
136. Weil SC, Rose VL. A variant myelodysplastic syndrome with multilineage pelgeroid chromatin. *Am J Clin Pathol* 1986;85:176.
137. Felman P, Bryon P, Gentilhomme O, et al. The syndrome of abnormal chromatin clumping in leucocytes: a myelodysplastic disorder with proliferative features? *Br J Haematol* 1988;70:49.
138. Varma N, Dash S, Marwaha N, Varma S. A case of myelodysplastic syndrome with abnormal chromatin clumping in leucocytes. *Br J Haematol* 1989; 73:135.
139. Rassam SMB, Roderick P, Al-Hakim I, Hoffbrand AV. A myelokathexis-like variant of myelodysplasia. *Eur J Haematol* 1989;42:99.
140. Sanz GF, Sanz MA, Vallespi T, et al. Two regression models and a scoring system for predicting survival and planning treatment in myelodysplastic syndromes: a multivariate analysis of prognostic factors in 370 patients. *Blood* 1989;74:395.
141. Zittoun R. Subacute and chronic myelomonocytic leukaemia: a distinct haematological entity. *Br J Haematol* 1976;32:1.
142. Solal-Celigny P, Desaint B, Herrera A, et al. Chronic myelomonocytic leukemia according to FAB classification: analysis of 35 cases. *Blood* 1984;63:634.
143. Youman JD, Saarni M, Linman JW. Diagnostic value of muraminidase (lysozyme) in acute leukemia and preleukemia. *Mayo Clin Proc* 1970;45:219.
144. Weintraub LR, Conrad ME, Crosby WH. Regulation of intestinal absorption of iron by the rate of cytopoiesis. *Br J Haematol* 1965;11:432.
145. Beris P, Graf J, Miescher PA. Primary acquired sideroblastic and primary acquired refractory anemia. *Semin Hematol* 1983;20:101.
146. Cartwright GE, Edwards CQ, Skolnick MH, Amos DB. Association of HLA-linked hemochromatosis with idiopathic refractory sideroblastic anemia. *J Clin Invest* 1980;65:989.
147. Simon M, Beaumont C, Briere J, et al. Is the HLA-linked haemochromatosis allele implicated in idiopathic refractory sideroblastic anaemia? *Br J Haematol* 1985;60:75.
148. Peto TEA, Pippard MJ, Weatherall DJ. Iron overload in mild sideroblastic anaemias. *Lancet* 1983;1:375.
149. Simon M. Secondary iron overload and the haemochromatosis allele. *Br J Haematol* 1985;60:1.
150. Sinn CM, Dick FW. Monocytic leukemia. *Am J Med* 1956;20:588.
151. Pretlow TG. Chronic monocytic dyscrasia culminating in acute leukemia. *Am J Med* 1968;49:130.
152. Saarni MI, Linman JW. Myelomonocytic leukemia: disorderly proliferation of all marrow cells. *Cancer* 1971;27:1221.
153. Miescher PA, Farquet JJ. Chronic myelomonocytic leukemia in adults. *Semin Hematol* 1974;11:129.
154. Geary CG, Catovsky D, Wiltshaw E, et al. Chronic myelomonocytic leukemia. *Br J Haematol* 1975;30:289.
155. Skinnider LF, Card RT, Padmanabh S. Chronic myelomonocytic leukemia: an ultrastructural study by transmission and scanning electron microscopy. *Am J Clin Pathol* 1977;67:339.
156. Ribera J-M, Cervantes F, Rozman C. A multivariate analysis of prognostic factors in chronic myelomonocytic leukaemia according to the FAB criteria. *Br J Haematol* 1987;65:307.
157. Golub TR, Barker GF, Lovett M, Gilliland DG. Fusion of PDGF receptor beta to a novel ets-like gene, tel, in chronic myelomonocytic leukemia with t(5;12) chromosomal translocation. *Cell* 1994;77:307–316.
158. Golub TR, Goga A, Barker G, et al. Oligomerization of the ABL tyrosine kinase by the ETS protein TEL in human leukemia. *Mol Cell Biol* 1996;16:4107–4116.
159. Papadopoulos P, Ridge SA, Boucher CA, et al. The novel activation of ABL by fusion to an ets-related gene, TEL. *Cancer Res* 1995;55:34–38.
160. Ross TS, Bernard OA, Berger R, Gilliland DG. Fusion of Huntingtin interacting protein 1 to PDGFβR in chronic myelomonocytic leukemia with t(5;7)(q33;q11.2). *Blood* 1998;91:4419–4426.
161. Ross TS, Gilliland DG. Transforming properties of the Huntingtin interacting protein 1/ platelet-derived growth factor beta receptor fusion protein. *J Biol Chem* 1999;274(32):22328–22336.
162. Schwaller J, Anastasiadou E, Cain D, et al. H4(D10S170), a gene frequently rearranged in papillary thyroid carcinoma, is fused to the platelet-derived growth factor receptor beta gene in atypical chronic myeloid leukemia with t(5;10)(q33;q22). *Blood* 2001;97(12):3910–3918.
163. Schwaller J, Frantsve J, Tomasson M, et al. Transformation of hematopoietic cell lines to growth-factor independence and induction of a fatal myeloid

and lymphoproliferative disease in mice by retrovirally transduced TEL/JAK2 fusion gene. *EMBO J* 1998;17:5321–5333.

164. Magnusson MK, Meade KE, Brown KE, et al. Rabaptin-5 is a novel fusion partner to platelet-derived growth factor beta receptor in chronic myelomonocytic leukemia. *Blood* 2001;98(8):2518–2525.

165. Lacronique V, Boureux A, Valle VD, et al. A TEL-JAK2 fusion protein with constitutive kinase activity in human leukemia. *Science* 1997;278(5341):1309–1312.

166. Peeters P, Raynaud SD, Cools J, et al. Fusion of TEL, the ETS-variant gene 6 (ETV6), to the receptor-associated kinase JAK2 as a result of t(9;12) in a lymphoid and t(9;15;12) in a myeloid leukemia. *Blood* 1997;90:2535–2540.

167. Tomasson MH, Williams IR, Hasserjian R, et al. TEL/PDGFβR induces hematologic malignancy in mice that responds to the tyrosine kinase inhibitor CGP57148. *Blood* 1999;93:1707–1714.

168. Druker BJ, Talpaz M, Resta DJ, et al. Efficacy and safety of a specific inhibitor of the BCR-ABL tyrosine kinase in chronic myeloid leukemia. *N Engl J Med* 2001;344(14):1031–1037.

169. Magnusson MK, Meade KE, Nakamura R, et al. Activity of STI571 in chronic myelomonocytic leukemia with a platelet-derived growth factor β-receptor fusion oncogene. *Blood* 2002:(in press).

170. Apperly JF, Schultheis B, Steer J, Dimitrijevic S, et al. Chronic myeloproliferative diseases with t(5;12) and a PDGFβR fusion gene: complete cytogenetic remissions on STI571 (Abstract). *Blood* 2001;98:726a.

171. Van den Berghe H, Cassiman J-J, Fryns J-P. Distinct haematological disorder with deletion of long arm of No. 5 chromosome. *Nature* 1974;251:437.

172. Sokal G, Michaux JL, Van Den Berghe H, et al. A new hematologic syndrome with a distinct karyotype: the 5q- chromosome. *Blood* 1975;46:519.

173. Nimer SD, Golde DW. The 5q- abnormality. *Blood* 1987;70:1705.

174. Bunn HF. 5q- and disordered haematopoiesis. *Clin Haematol* 1986;15:1023.

175. Van Den Berghe H. The 5q- syndrome. *Scand J Haematol* 1986;45:78.

176. Tinegate H, Gaunt L, Hamilton PJ. The 5q-syndrome: an underdiagnosed form of macrocytic anaemia. *Br J Haematol* 1983;54:103.

177. Mahmood T, Robinson WA, Hamstra RD, Wallner SF. Macrocytic anemia, thrombocytosis and nonlobulated megakaryocytes. *Am J Med* 1979;66:946.

177a. Boultwood J, Fidler C, Lewis S, et al. Allelicloss of IRF1 in myelodysplasia and acute myeloid leukemia: retention of IRF1 on the 5q- chromosome in some patients with the 5q- syndrome. *Blood* 1993;82:2611.

178. Donti E, Tabilio A, Donti GV, et al. 5q- syndrome terminating in acute myeloid leukemia: karyotype evolution and immunologic characterization of blast cells. *Cancer Genet Cytogenet* 1988;32:205.

179. Jume'an HG, Libnoch JA. 5q- myelodysplasia terminating in acute leukemia. *Ann Intern Med* 1979;91:748.

180. Brusamolino E, Orlandi E, Morra E, et al. Hematologic and clinical features of patients with chromosome 5 monosomy or deletion (5q). *Med Pediatr Oncol* 1988;16:88.

181. Dowton SB, Beardsley D, Jamison D, et al. Studies of a familial platelet disorder. *Blood* 1985;65:557–563.

182. Ho CY, Otterud B, Legare RD, et al. Linkage of a familial platelet disorder with a propensity to develop myeloid malignancies to human chromosome 21q22.1-22.2. *Blood* 1996;87:5218–5224.

183. Song W-J, Sullivan MG, Legare RD, et al. Haploinsufficiency of CBFA2 (AML1) causes familial thrombocytopenia with propensity to develop acute myelogenous leukemia (FPD/AML). *Nat Genet* 1999;23:166–175.

184. Boice JD, Greene MH, Killen JY, et al. Leukemia and preleukemia after adjuvant treatment of gastrointestinal cancer with semustine (methyl-CCNU). *N Engl J Med* 1983;309:1079.

185. Teerenhovi L, Lintula R. Natural course of myelodysplastic syndromes—Helsinki experience. *Scand J Haematol* 1986;36(Suppl 45):102.

186. Calabresi P. Leukemia after cytotoxic chemotherapy—a pyrrhic victory? *N Engl J Med* 1983;309:1118.

187. Canellos G. Therapy-related leukemia: a necessary complication of successful systemic chemotherapy? *J Clin Oncol* 1984;2:1077.

188. Coltman CA, Dahlberg S. Treatment-related leukemia. *N Engl J Med* 1990;322:52.

189. De Gramont A, Louvet C, Krulik M, et al. Preleukemic changes in cases of nonlymphocytic leukemia secondary to cytotoxic therapy. *Cancer* 1986;58: 630.

190. Pedersen-Bjergaard J, Ersboll J, Sorensen HM, et al. Risk of acute nonlymphocytic leukemia and preleukemia in patients treated with cyclophosphamide for non-Hodgkin's lymphomas. *Ann Intern Med* 1985;103:195.

191. Bennett JM, Moloney WC, Greene MH, Boice JD. Acute myeloid leukemia and other myelopathic disorders following treatment with alkylating agents. *Hematol Pathol* 1987;1:99.

192. Pedersen-Bjergaard J, Osterlind K, Hansen M, et al. Acute nonlymphocytic leukemia, preleukemia, and solid tumors following intensive chemotherapy of small cell carcinoma of the lung. *Blood* 1985;66:1393.

193. LeBeau MM, Albain KS, Larson RA, et al. Clinical and cytogenetic correlations in 63 patients with therapy-related myelodysplastic syndromes and acute nonlymphocytic leukemia: further evidence for characteristic abnormalities of chromosomes No. 5 and 7. *J Clin Oncol* 1986;4:325.

194. Kaldor JM, Day NE, Pettersson F, et al. Leukemia following chemotherapy for ovarian cancer. *N Engl J Med* 1990;322:1.

195. Kaldor JM, Day NE, Clarke EA, et al. Leukemia following Hodgkin's disease. *N Engl J Med* 1990;322:7.

196. Giles FJ, Koeffler HP. Secondary myelodysplastic syndromes and leukemias. *Curr Opin Hematol* 1994;1(4):256–260.

197. Park DJ, Koeffler HP. Therapy-related myelodysplastic syndromes. *Semin Hematol* 1996;33(3):256–273.

198. La Starza R, Sambani C, Crescenzi B, et al. AML1/MTG16 fusion gene from a t(16;21)(q24;q22) translocation in treatment-induced leukemia after breast cancer. *Haematologica* 2001;86(2):212–213.

199. Tulliez M, Ricard MF, Jan F, Sultan C. Preleukaemic abnormal myelopoiesis induced by chlorambucil: a case study. *Scand J Haematol* 1974;13:179.

200. Pedersen-Bjergaard J, Larsen SO, Struck J, et al. Risk of therapy-related leukaemia and preleukaemia after Hodgkin's disease: relation to age, cumulative dose of alkylating agents, and time from chemotherapy. *Lancet* 1987;2:83.

201. Pedersen-Bjergaard J, Philip P, Pedersen NT, et al. Acute nonlymphocytic leukemia, preleukemia, and acute myeloproliferative syndrome secondary to treatment of other malignant diseases. *Cancer* 1984;54:452.

202. Michels SD, McKenna RW, Arthur DC, Brunning RD. Therapy-related acute myeloid leukemia and myelodysplastic syndrome: a clinical and morphologic study of 65 cases. *Blood* 1985;65:1364.

203. Rowley JD, Golomb HM, Vardiman JW. Nonrandom chromosome abnormalities in acute leukemia and dysmyelopoietic syndromes in patients with previously treated malignant disease. *Blood* 1981;58:759.

204. Zarrabi MH, Rosner F, Grunwald HW. Second neoplasms in acute lymphoblastic leukemia. *Cancer* 1983;52:1712.

205. Rustin GJS, Rustin F, Dent J, et al. No increase in second tumors after cytotoxic therapy for gestational trophoblastic tumors. *N Engl J Med* 1983;308:473.

206. International Agency for Research on Cancer Overall evaluation of carcinogenicity: an update of IARC monographs volumes 1–42(Suppl 7). Lyons, France: International Agency for Research on Cancer, 1987.

207. Andersen MK, Christiansen DH, Jensen BA, et al. Therapy-related acute lymphoblastic leukaemia with MLL rearrangements following DNA topoisomerase II inhibitors, an increasing problem: report on two new cases and review of the literature since 1992. *Br J Haematol* 2001;114(3):539–543.

208. Yagita M, Ieki Y, Onishi R, et al. Therapy-related leukemia and myelodysplasia following oral administration of etoposide for recurrent breast cancer. *Int J Oncol* 1998;13(1):91–96.

209. Pui CH, Ribeiro RC, Hancock ML, et al. Acute myeloid leukemia in children treated with epipodophyllotoxins for acute lymphoblastic leukemia. *N Engl J Med* 1991;325(24):1682–1687.

210. Krishnan A, Bhatia S, Slovak ML, et al. Predictors of therapy-related leukemia and myelodysplasia following autologous transplantation for lymphoma: an assessment of risk factors. *Blood* 2000;95(5):1588–1593.

211. Stone R. Myelodysplastic syndrome after autologous transplantation for lymphoma: the price of progress. *Blood* 1994;83:3437–3440.

212. Andre M, Henry-Amar M, Blaise D, et al. Treatment-related deaths and second cancer risk after autologous stem-cell transplantation for Hodgkin's disease. *Blood* 1998;92(6):1933–1940.

213. Bhatia S, Ramsay NK, Steinbuch M, et al. Malignant neoplasms following bone marrow transplantation. *Blood* 1996;87(9):3633–3639.

214. Darrington DL, Vose JM, Anderson JR, et al. Incidence and characterization of secondary myelodysplastic syndrome and acute myelogenous leukemia following high-dose chemoradiotherapy and autologous stem-cell transplantation for lymphoid malignancies. *J Clin Oncol* 1994;12(12):2527–2534.

215. Friedberg JW, Neuberg D, Stone RM, et al. Outcome in patients with myelodysplastic syndrome after autologous bone marrow transplantation for non-Hodgkin's lymphoma. *J Clin Oncol* 1999;17(10):3128–3135.

216. Harrison CN, Gregory W, Hudson GV, et al. High-dose BEAM chemotherapy with autologous haemopoietic stem cell transplantation for Hodgkin's disease is unlikely to be associated with a major increased risk of secondary MDS/AML. *Br J Cancer* 1999;81(3):476–483.

217. Miller JS, Arthur DC, Litz CE, et al. Myelodysplastic syndrome after autologous bone marrow transplantation: an additional late complication of curative cancer therapy. *Blood* 1994;83(12):3780–3786.

218. Milligan DW, Ruiz De Elvira MC, Kolb HJ, et al. Secondary leukaemia and myelodysplasia after autografting for lymphoma: results from the EBMT. EBMT Lymphoma and Late Effects Working Parties. European Group for Blood and Marrow Transplantation. *Br J Haematol* 1999;106(4):1020–1026.

219. Pedersen-Bjergaard J, Pedersen M, Myhre J, Geisler C. High risk of therapy-related leukemia after BEAM chemotherapy and autologous stem cell transplantation for previously treated lymphomas is mainly related to primary chemotherapy and not to the BEAM-transplantation procedure. *Leukemia* 1997;11(10):1654–1660.

220. Milligan DW. Secondary leukaemia and myelodysplasia after autografting for lymphoma: is the transplant to blame? *Leuk Lymphoma* 2000;39(3-4):223-8.

221. Pedersen-Bjergaard J, Andersen MK, Christiansen DH. Therapy-related acute myeloid leukemia and myelodysplasia after high-dose chemotherapy and autologous stem cell transplantation. *Blood* 2000;95(11):3273–3279.

222. Abruzzese E, Radford JE, Miller JS, et al. Detection of abnormal pretransplant clones in progenitor cells of patients who developed myelodysplasia after autologous transplantation. *Blood* 1999;94(5):1814–1819.

223. Traweek S, Slovak M, Nademanee A, et al. Myelodysplasia occurring after autologous bone marrow transplantation (ABMT) for Hodgkin's disease and non-Hodgkin's lymphoma. *Blood* 1993;82:455a (abstr).

224. Traweek ST, Slovak ML, Nademanee AP, Brynes RK, Niland JC, Forman SJ. Clonal karyotypic hematopoietic cell abnormalities occuring after autologous bone marrow transplantation for Hodgkin's disease and non-Hodgkin's lymphoma. *Blood* 1994;84:957–963.

225. Mach-Pascual S, Legare RD, Lu D, et al. Predictive value of clonality assays in patients with non-Hodgkin's lymphoma undergoing autologous bone marrow transplant: a single institution study. *Blood* 1998;91 (12):4496–4503.

226. Ingram L, Mott MG, Mann JR, et al. Second malignancies in children treated for non-Hodgkin's lymphoma and T-cell leukaemia with the UKCCSG regimens. *Br J Haematol* 1987;55:463.

227. Kurtzman GJ, Ozawa K, Cohen B, et al. Chronic bone marrow failure due to persistant B19 parvovirus infection. *N Engl J Med* 1987;317:287.

228. Geary CG, Harrison CJ, Philpott NJ, et al. Abnormal cytogenetic clones in patients with aplastic anaemia: response to immunosuppressive therapy. *Br J Haematol* 1999;104(2):271–274.

229. Howe RB, Bloomfield CD, McKenna RW. Hypocellular acute leukemia. *Am J Med* 1982;72:391.

230. Aivado M, Rong A, Stadler M, et al. Favourable response to antithymocyte or antilymphocyte globulin in low-risk myelodysplastic syndrome patients with a 'non-clonal' pattern of X-chromosome inactivation in bone marrow cells. *Eur J Haematol* 2002;68(4):210–216.

231. Asano Y, Maeda M, Uchida N, et al. Immunosuppressive therapy for patients with refractory anemia. *Ann Hematol* 2001;80(11):634–638.

232. Molldrem JJ, Jiang YZ, Stetler-Stevenson M, et al. Haematological response of patients with myelodysplastic syndrome to antithymocyte globulin is associated with a loss of lymphocyte-mediated inhibition of CFU-GM and alterations in T-cell receptor Vbeta profiles. *Br J Haematol* 1998;102(5):1314–1322.

233. Molldrem JJ, Caples M, Mavroudis D, et al. Antithymocyte globulin for patients with myelodysplastic syndrome. *Br J Haematol* 1997;99(3):699–705.

234. Biesma DH, van den Tweel JG, Verdonck LF. Immunosuppressive therapy for hypoplastic myelodysplastic syndrome. *Cancer* 1997;79(8):1548–1551.

235. Shimamoto T, Iguchi T, Ando K, et al. Successful treatment with cyclosporin A for myelodysplastic syndrome with erythroid hypoplasia associated with T-cell receptor gene rearrangements. *Br J Haematol* 2001;114(2):358–361.

236. Jonasova A, Neuwirtova R, Cermak J, et al. Cyclosporin A therapy in hypoplastic MDS patients and certain refractory anaemias without hypoplastic bone marrow. *Br J Haematol* 1998;100(2):304–309.

237. Raskind WH, Fialkow PJ. The use of cell markers in the study of human hematopoietic neoplasia. *Adv Cancer Res* 1987;49:127.

238. Prchal JT, Throckmorton DW, Carroll AJ, et al. A common progenitor for human myeloid and lymphoid cells. *Nature* 1978;274:590.

239. Raskind WH, Tirumali N, Jacobson R, et al. Evidence for a multistep pathogenesis of a myelodysplastic syndrome. *Blood* 1984;63:1318.

240. Abkowitz JL, Fialkow PJ, Niebrugge DJ, et al. Pancytopenia as a clonal disorder of a multipotent hematopoietic stem cell. *J Clin Invest* 1984;73:258.

241. Fearon ER, Burke PJ, Schiffer CA, et al. Differentiation of leukemia cells to polymorphonuclear leukocytes in patients with acute nonlymphocytic leukemia. *N Engl J Med* 1986;315:15.

242. Vogelstein B, Fearon ER, Hamilton SR, Feinberg AP. The use of restriction fragment length polymorphisms to determine the clonal origin of human tumors. *Science* 1985;227:642.

243. Fearon ER, Hamilton SR, Vogelstein B. Clonal analysis of human colorectal tumors. *Science* 1987;238:193.

244. Janssen JWG, Buschle M, Layton M, et al. Clonal analysis of myelodysplastic syndromes: evidence of multipotent stem cell origin. *Blood* 1989;73:248.

245. Phelan JT, 2nd, Prchal JT. Clonality studies in cancer based on X chromosome inactivation phenomenon. *Methods Mol Med* 2002;68:251–270.

246. Grier HE, Weinstein HJ, Revesz T, et al. Cytogenetic evidence for involvement of erythroid progenitors in a child with therapy linked myelodysplasia. *Br J Haematol* 1986;64:513.

247. Amenomori T, Tomonaga M, Jinnai I, et al. Cytogenetic and cytochemical studies on progenitor cells of primary acquired sideroblastic anemia (PASA): involvement of multipotential myeloid stem cells in PASA clone and mosaicism with normal clone. *Blood* 1987;70:1367.

248. Lawrence HJ, Broudy VC, Magenis RE, et al. Cytogenetic evidence for involvement of B lymphocytes in acquired sideroblastic anemia. *Blood* 1987;70:1003.

248a. Kroef MJ, Fibbe WE, Mout R. Myeloid but not lymphoid cells carry the 5q deletion: polymerase chain reaction analysis of loss of heterozygosity using mini-repeat sequence on highly purified cell fractions. *Blood* 1994;81:1849.

249. Inoshita T. Acute lymphoblastic leukemia following myelodysplastic syndrome. *Am J Clin Pathol* 1985;84:233.

250. Barton JC, Conrad ME, Parmley RT. Acute lymphoblastic leukemia in idiopathic refractory sideroblastic anemia: evidence for a common lymphoid and myeloid progenitor cell. *Am J Hematol* 1980;9:109.

251. Ariel I, Weiler-Ravell D, Stalnikowicz R. Preleukemia in acute lymphoblastic leukemia. *Acta Haematol* 1981;66:50.

252. Brusamolino E, Isernia P, Alessandrino EP, et al. Terminal deoxynucleotidyl transferase-positive acute leukemias evolving from a myelodysplastic syndrome. *Am J Hematol* 1985;20:187.

253. Eridani S, Chan LC, Halil O, Pearson TC. Acute biphenotypic leukaemia (myeloid and null-ALL type) supervening in a myelodysplastic syndrome. *Br J Haematol* 1985;61:525.

254. Heim S, Mitelman F. Chromosome abnormalities in the myelodysplastic syndromes. *Clin Haematol* 1986;15:1003.

255. Michels VV, Hoagland HC. Chromosome abnormalities in preleukemic or myelodysplastic syndromes. *Mayo Clin Proc* 1985;60:555.

256. Nowell PC. Cytogenetics of preleukemia. *Cancer Genet Cytogenet* 1982;5:265.

256a. Ohyashiki K, Sasao I, Ohyashiki JH, et al. Cytogenetic and clinical findings of myelodysplastic syndromes with a poor prognosis: an experience with 97 cases. *Cancer* 1992;70:94.

257. Billstrom R, Nilsson PG, Mitelman F. Cytogenetic analysis in 941 consecutive patients with haematologic disorders. *Scand J Haematol* 1986;37:29.

258. Anderson RL, Bagby GC. The prognostic value of chromosome studies in patients with the preleukemic syndrome (hemopoietic dysplasia). *Leuk Res* 1982;6:175.

259. Gold EJ, Conjalka M, Pelus LM, et al. Marrow cytogenetic and cell-culture analyses of the myelodysplastic syndromes: insights to pathophysiology and prognosis. *J Clin Oncol* 1983;1:627.

260. Nowell P, Besa EC, Stelmach T, Finan JB. Chromosome studies in preleukemic states. *Cancer* 1986;58:2571.

261. Lawler SD, Swansbury GJ. Cytogenetic studies in primary and secondary preleukaemic states. *Haematologica (Pavia)* 1987;72:49.

262. Jacobs RH, Cornbleet MA, Vardiman JW, et al. Prognostic implications of morphology and karyotype in primary myelodysplastic syndromes. *Blood* 1986;67:1765.

263. Ayraud N, Donzeau M, Raynaud S, Lambert J-C. Cytogenetic study of 88 cases of refractory anemia. *Cancer Genet Cytogenet* 1983;8:243.

264. Billstrom R, Thiede T, Hansen S, et al. Bone marrow karyotype and prognosis in primary myelodysplastic syndromes. *Eur J Haematol* 1988;41:341.

265. Estey EH, Keating MJ, Dixon DO, et al. Karyotype is prognostically more important than the FAB system's distinction between myelodysplastic syndrome and acute myelogenous leukemia. *Hematol Pathol* 1987;1:203.

266. Musilova J, Michalova K. Chromosome study of 85 patients with myelodysplastic syndrome. *Cancer Genet Cytogenet* 1988;33:39.

267. Horiike S, Taniwaki M, Misawa S, Abe T. Chromosome abnormalities and karyotypic evolution in 83 patients with myelodysplastic syndrome and predictive value for prognosis. *Cancer* 1988;62:1129.

268. Knapp RH, Dewald GW, Pierre RV. Cytogenetic studies in 174 consecutive patients with preleukemic or myelodysplastic syndromes. *Mayo Clin Proc* 1985;60:507.

269. Yunis JJ, Rydell RE, Oken MM, et al. Refined chromosome analysis as an independent prognostic indicator in de novo myelodysplastic syndromes. *Blood* 1986;67:1721.

270. Yunis JJ. Should refined chromosomal analysis be used routinely in acute leukemias and myelodysplastic syndrome? *N Engl J Med* 1986;315:322.

271. Mrozek K, Heinonen K, Bloomfield CD. Acute myeloid leukemia and myelodysplastic syndromes: clinical implications of cytogenetic abnormalities. *Adv Oncol* 2001;16(4):10–16.

272. Mecucci C. Molecular features of primary MDS with cytogenetic changes. *Leuk Res* 1998;22(4):293–302.

273. Sawyers CL. Molecular abnormalities in myeloid leukemias and myelodysplastic syndromes. *Leuk Res* 1998;22(12):1113–1122.

274. Willman CL. Molecular genetic features of myelodysplastic syndromes (MDS). *Leukemia* 1998;12(Suppl 1):S2–S6.

275. Mecucci C, La Starza R. Cytogenetics of myelodysplastic syndromes. *Forum (Genova)* 1999;9(1):4–13.

276. Olney HJ, Le Beau MM. The cytogenetics of myelodysplastic syndromes. *Best Pract Res Clin Haematol* 2001;14(3):479–495.

277. Greenberg P, Cox C, LeBeau MM, et al. International scoring system for evaluating prognosis in myelodysplastic syndromes. *Blood* 1997;89(6):2079–2088.

278. Heaney ML, Golde DW. Myelodysplasia. *N Engl J Med* 1999;340(21):1649–1660.

279. Nowell P, Wilmoth D, Lange B. Cytogenetics of childhood preleukemia. *Cancer Genet Cytogenet* 1983;6:261.

280. Nowell PC, Besa EC. Prognostic significance of single chromosomal abnormalities in preleukemic states. *Cancer Genet Cytogenet* 1989;42:1.

281. Carbonell F, Heimpel H, Kubanek B, Fliedner TM. Growth and cytogenetic characteristics of bone marrow colonies from patients with 5q-syndrome. *Blood* 1985;66:463.

282. Gyger M, Perreault C, Pichette R, et al. Interstitial deletion of the long arm of chromosome 5 (5q-) in leukemia and other hematological disorders: clinical and biological relevance of variable breakpoint patterns. *Leuk Res* 1986;10:9.

283. Mitelman F, Manolova Y, Manolov G, et al. High resolution analysis of the 5q- marker chromosome in refractory anemia. *Hereditas* 1986;105:49.

284. Wisniewski LP, Hirschorn K. Acquired partial deletion of the long arm of chromosome 5 in hematologic disorders. *Am J Hematol* 1983;15:295.

285. Haas OA, Bettelheim P, Schmidmeier W, et al. 5q- chromosome in acute leukemia with lymphoid morphology and expression of myeloid membrane determinants. *Blood* 1985;65:1342.

286. Swolin B, Weinfeld A, Ridell B, et al. On the 5q- deletion: clinical and cytogenetic observations in ten patients and review of the literature. *Blood* 1981;58:986.

287. Kerkhofs H, Hagemeijer A, Leeksma HW, et al. The 5q- chromosome abnormality in haematological disorders: a collaborative study of 34 cases from the Netherlands. *Br J Haematol* 1982;52:365.

288. Mitelman F. *Catalog of chromosome aberrations in cancer*, 3rd. New York: Alan R Liss, 1988.

289. Lavezzi AM, Maiolo AT, Chiorboli O, Mozzana R. The bone marrow karyotype in seventeen cases of refractory anemia with excess of blasts (RAEB). *Ann Genet* 1983;26:220.

290. Gyger M, Forest L, Vuong TE, et al. Therapy-induced preleukaemia in patients treated for Hodgkin's lymphoma: clinical and therapeutic relevance of sequential chromosome banding studies. *Br J Haematol* 1984;58:61.

291. Pedersen-Bjergaard J, Philip P. Cytogenetic characteristics of therapy-related acute nonlymphocytic leukaemia, preleukaemia and acute myeloproliferative syndrome: correlation with clinical data for 61 consecutive cases. *Br J Haematol* 1987;66:199.

292. Levin M, Le Coniat M, Bernheim A, Berger R. Complex chromosomal abnormalities in acute nonlymphocytic leukemia. *Cancer Genet Cytogenet* 1986;22:113.

293. Wilmoth D, Feder M, Finan J, Nowell P. Preleukemia and leukemia with 12p- and 19q+ chromosome alterations following Alkeran therapy. *Cancer Genet Cytogenet* 1985;15:95.

294. Kledsen N, Philip P, Pedersen-Bjergaard J. Translocations and deletions with breakpoint on 21q are nonrandomly associated with treatment-related acute nonlymphocytic leukemia and preleukemia. *Cancer Genet Cytogenet* 1987;29:43.

295. Tomonaga M, Tomonaga Y, Kusano M, Ichimaru M. Sequential karyotypic evolutions and bone marrow aplasia preceding acute myelomonocytic transformation from myelodysplastic syndrome. *Br J Haematol* 1984;58:53.

296. Yunis JJ, Lobell M, Arnesen MA, et al. Refined chromosome study helps define prognostic subgroups in most patients with primary myelodysplastic syndrome and acute myelogenous leukaemia. *Br J Haematol* 1988;68:189.

297. Pierre RV. Cytogenetic studies in preleukemia: studies before and after transition to acute leukemia in 17 subjects. *Blood Cells* 1975;1:163.

298. Tricot G, Boogaerts MA, De Wolf-Peeters C, et al. The myelodysplastic syndromes: different evolution patterns based on sequential morphological and cytogenetic investigations. *Br J Haematol* 1985;59:659.

299. Struli RA, Testa JR, Vardiman JW, et al. Dysmyelopoietic syndrome: sequential clinical and cytogenetic studies. *Blood* 1980;55:636.

300. Donti E, Tabilio A, Venti Donti G, et al. 5q- syndrome terminating in acute myeloid leukemia: karyotype evolution and immunologic characterization of blast cells. *Cancer Genet Cytogenet* 1988;32:205.

301. Benitez J, Carbonell F, Sanchez Fayos J, Heimpel H. Karyotypic evolution in patients with myelodysplastic syndromes. *Cancer Genet Cytogenet* 1985;16:157.

302. Ringressi A, Mecucci C, Grossi A, et al. 6p+ and 9q- in two chromosomally distinct clones occurring in a case of myelodysplastic syndrome evolving to acute nonlymphocytic leukemia. *Cancer Genet Cytogenet* 1988;35:213.

303. Miller BA, Weinstein HJ, Nell M, et al. Sequential development of distinct clonal chromosome abnormalities in a patient with preleukaemia. *Br J Haematol* 1985;59:411.

304. Smadja N, Krulik M, De Gramont A, et al. Acquired idiopathic sideroblastic anemia and terminal deletion of chromosome 11. *Cancer Genet Cytogenet* 1985;16:275.

305. Heim S, Mitelman F. Cytogenetically unrelated clones in hematological neoplasms. *Leukemia* 1989;3:6.

306. Knuutila S, Vuopio P, Borgstrom GH, De La Chapelle A. Higher frequency of 5q-clone in bone marrow mitoses after culture than by a direct method. *Scand J Haematol* 1980;25:358.

307. Wang WC, Dow LW, Presbury GJ, et al. Serial cell culture and cytogenetic studies of marrow cells from a patient with monosomy 7 syndrome. *Am J Pediatr Hematol Oncol* 1985;7:321.

308. Okuda T, Yokota S, Maekawa T, et al. Heterogeneous colony forming ability in vitro of the abnormal clone-derived granulocyte-macrophage precursors in myelodysplastic syndromes. *Leuk Res* 1988;12:687.

309. Clark R, Peters S, Hoy T, et al. Prognostic importance of hypodiploid hemopoietic precursors in myelodysplastic syndromes. *N Engl J Med* 1986; 314:1472.

310. Auffermann W, Fohlmeister I, Bocking A. Diagnostic and prognostic value of DNA image cytometry in myelodysplasia. *J Clin Pathol* 1988;41:604.

311. Thein SL, Oscier DG, Jeffreys AJ, et al. Detection of chromosomal 7 loss in myelodysplasia using an extremely polymorphic DNA probe. *Br J Cancer* 1988;57:131.

312. Kere J, Ruutu T, De La Chapelle A. Monosomy 7 in granulocytes and monocytes in myelodysplastic syndrome. *N Engl J Med* 1987;316:499.

313. Kere J. Chromosome 7 long arm deletion breakpoints in preleukemia: mapping by pulsed field gel electrophoresis. *Nucl Acid Res* 1989;17:1511.

314. Kelly L, Clark J, Gilliland DG. Comprehensive genotypic analysis of leukemia: clinical and therapeutic implications. *Curr Opin Oncol* 2002;14(1):10–18.

315. Barbacid M. RAS genes. *Annu Rev Biochem* 1987;56:779.

316. Tabin CJ, Bradley SM, Bargmann CI, et al. Mechanism of activation of a human oncogene. *Nature* 1982;300:143.

317. Bos JL. The RAS gene family and human carcinogenesis. *Mutat Res* 1988; 195:255.

318. Lyons J, Janssen JWG, Bartram C, et al. Mutation of Ki-RAS and N-RAS oncogenes in myelodysplastic syndromes. *Blood* 1988;71:1707.

319. Bar-Eli M, Ahuja H, Gonzalez-Cadavid N, et al. Analysis of N-RAS exon-1 mutations in myelodysplastic syndromes by polymeRASe chain reaction and direct sequencing. *Blood* 1989;73:281.

319a. Paquette RL, Landaw EM, Pierre RV, et al. N-RAS mutations are associated with poor prognosis and increased risk of leukemia in myelodysplastic syndrome. *Blood* 1993;82:590.

320. Padua RA, Carter G, Hughes D, et al. RAS mutations in myelodysplasia detected by amplification, oligonucleotide hybridization, and transformation. *Leukemia* 1988;2:503.

321. Toksoz T, Farr CJ, Marshall CJ. RAS genes and acute myeloid leukaemia. *Br J Haematol* 1989;71:1.

322. Bartram CR. Mutations in RAS genes in myelocytic leukemias and myelodysplastic syndromes. *Blood Cells* 1988;14:533.

323. Janssen JWG, Steenvoorden AGM, Lyons J, et al. RAS gene mutations in acute and chronic myelocytic leukemia, chronic myeloproliferative disorders, and myelodysplastic syndromes. *Proc Natl Acad Sci U S A* 1987;84:9228.

324. Hirai H, Koyabashi Y, Mano H, et al. A point mutation at codon 13 of the N-RAS oncogene in myelodysplastic syndrome. *Nature* 1987;327:430.

325. Liu E, Hjelle B, Morgan R, et al. Mutations of the Kirsten-RAS protooncogene in human preleukemia. *Nature* 1987;330:186.

326. Yunis JJ, Boot AJ, Mayer MG, Bos JL. Mechanisms of RAS mutation in myelodysplastic syndrome. *Oncogene* 1989;4:609.

327. Guerrero I, Calzada P, Mayer A, Pellicer A. A molecular approach to leukemogenesis: mouse lymphomas contain an activated c-RAS oncogene. *Proc Natl Acad Sci U S A* 1984;81:202.

328. Pedersen-Bjergaard J, Janssen JWG, Lyons J, et al. Point mutations of the RAS protooncogenes and chromosome aberrations in acute nonlymphocytic leukemia and preleukemia related to therapy with alkylating agents. *Cancer Res* 1988;48:1812.

329. Hirai H, Okada M, Mizoguchi H, et al. Relationship between an activated N-RAS oncogene and chromosomal abnormality during leukemic progression from myelodysplastic syndrome. *Blood* 1988;71:256.

330. Nakao M, Yokota S, Iwai T, et al. Internal tandem duplication of the flt3 gene found in acute myeloid leukemia. *Leukemia* 1996;10(12):1911–1918.

331. Kiyoi H, Naoe T, Nakano Y, et al. Prognostic implication of FLT3 and N-RAS gene mutations in acute myeloid leukemia. *Blood* 1999;93(9):3074–3080.

332. Hayakawa F, Towatari M, Kiyoi H, et al. Tandem-duplicated Flt3 constitutively activates STAT5 and MAP kinase and introduces autonomous cell growth in IL-3-dependent cell lines. *Oncogene* 2000;19(5):624–631.

333. Yamamoto Y, Kiyoi H, Nakano Y, et al. Activating mutation of D835 within the activation loop of FLT3 in human hematologic malignancies. *Blood* 2001;97(8):2434–2439.

334. Kelly LM, Liu Q, Kutok JL, et al. FLT3 internal tandem duplication mutations associated with human acute myeloid leukemias induce myeloproliferative disease in a murine bone marrow transplant model. *Blood* 2002;99(1):310–318.

335. Pedersen-Bjergaard J, Andersen MK, Christiansen DH, Nerlov C. Genetic pathways in therapy-related myelodysplasia and acute myeloid leukemia. *Blood* 2002;99(6):1909–1912.

336. Sawyers CL. Finding the next Gleevec: FLT3 targeted kinase inhibitor therapy for acute myeloid leukemia. *Cancer Cell* 2002;1:413–415.

337. Levis M, Allebach J, Tse KF, et al. A FLT3-targeted tyrosine kinase inhibitor is cytotoxic to leukemia cells in vitro and in vivo. *Blood* 2002;99(11):3885–3891.

338. Kelly LM, Yu J-C, Boulton CL, et al. CT53518, a novel selective FLT3 antagonist for the treatment of acute myelogenous leukemia. *Cancer Cell* 2002;1:421–432.

339. Weisberg E, Boulton CL, Kelly LM, et al. Inhibition of mutant FLT3 receptors in leukemia cells by the small molecule tyrosine kinase inhibitor PKC412. *Cancer Cell* 2002;1:433–443.

340. Speck NA, Gilliland DG. Core-binding factors in haematopoiesis and leukemia. *Nat Rev Cancer* 2002;2:502–513.

341. Castilla LH, Garrett L, Adya N, Orlic D, Dutra A, Anderson S, et al. The fusion gene Cbfβ blocks myeloid differentiation and predisposes mice to acute myelomonocytic leukemia. *Nat Genet* 1999;23:144–146.

342. Higuchi M, O'Brien D, Kumaravelu P, et al. Expression of a conditional AML1-ETO oncogene bypasses embryonic lethality and establishes a murine model of human t(8;21) acute myeloid leukemia. *Cancer Cell* 2002;1:63–74.

343. Fenaux P. Chromosome and molecular abnormalities in myelodysplastic syndromes. *Int J Hematol* 2001;73(4):429–437.

344. Nucifora G. The EVI1 gene in myeloid leukemia. *Leukemia* 1997;11(12):2022–2031.

345. Peeters P, Wlodarska I, Baens M, et al. Fusion of ETV6 to MDS1/EVI1 as a result of t(3;12)(q26;p13) in myeloproliferative disorders. *Cancer Res* 1997;57(4):564–569.

346. Russell M, List A, Greenberg P, et al. Expression of EVI1 in myelodysplastic syndromes and other hematologic malignancies without 3q26 translocations. *Blood* 1994;84:1243–1248.

347. Cuenco GM, Nucifora G, Ren R. Human AML1/MDS1/EVI1 fusion protein induces an acute myelogenous leukemia (AML) in mice: a model for human AML. *Proc Natl Acad Sci U S A* 2000;97:1760–1765.

348. Osato M, Asou N, Abdalla E, et al. Biallelic and heterozygous point mutations in the runt domain of the AML1/PEBP2alphaB gene associated with myeloblastic leukemias. *Blood* 1999;93(6):1817–1824.

349. Rowley JD, Reshmi S, Sobulo O, et al. All patients with the t(11;16)(q23;p13.3) that involves MLL and CBP have treatment-related hematologic disorders. *Blood* 1997;90:535–539.

350. Lavau C, Du C, Thirman M, Zeleznik-Le N. Chromatin-related properties of CBP fused to MLL generate a myelodysplastic-like syndrome that evolves into myeloid leukemia. *EMBO J* 2000;19(17):4655–4664.

351. Luo RT, Lavau C, Du C, et al. The elongation domain of ELL is dispensable but its ELL-associated factor 1 interaction domain is essential for MLL-ELL-induced leukemogenesis. *Mol Cell Biol* 2001;21(16):5678–5687.

352. Lavau C, Luo RT, Du C, Thirman MJ. Retrovirus-mediated gene transfer of MLL-ELL transforms primary myeloid progenitors and causes acute myeloid leukemias in mice. *Proc Natl Acad Sci U S A* 2000;97(20):10984–10989.

353. Slany RK, Lavau C, Cleary ML. The oncogenic capacity of HRX-ENL requires the transcriptional transactivation activity of ENL and the DNA binding motifs of HRX. *Mol Cell Biol* 1998;18(1):122–129.

354. Corral J, Lavenir I, Impey H, et al. An Mll-AF9 fusion gene made by homologous recombination causes acute leukemia in chimeric mice: a method to create fusion oncogenes. *Cell* 1996;14:853–861.

355. Dobson CL, Warren AJ, Pannell R, et al. The mll-AF9 gene fusion in mice controls myeloproliferation and specifies acute myeloid leukaemogenesis. *EMBO J* 1999;18(13):3564–3574.

356. Pollock JL, Westervelt P, Walter MJ, et al. Mouse models of acute promyelocytic leukemia. *Curr Opin Hematol* 2001;8(4):206–211.

357. He LZ, Tribioli C, Rivi R, et al. Acute leukemia with promyelocytic features in PML/RARalpha transgenic mice. *Proc Natl Acad Sci U S A* 1997;94:5302–5307.

358. Kelly LM, Kutok JL, Williams IR, et al. PML/RARalpha and FLT3-ITD induce an APL-like disease in a mouse model. *Proc Natl Acad Sci U S A* 2002;99(12):8283–8288.

359. Le Beau MM, Chandrasekharappa SC, Lemons RS, et al. Molecular and cytogenetic analysis of chromosome 5 abnormalities in myeloid disorders: chromosomal localization and physical mapping of IL-4 and IL-5. In: *Cancer cells 7/molecular diagnostics of human cancer.* Cold Spring Harbor, New York: Cold Spring Harbor Laboratory, 1989:53.

360. Huebner K, Isobe M, Croce CM, et al. The human gene encoding GM-CSF is at 5q21–q32, the chromosome region deleted in the 5q- anomaly. *Science* 1985;230:1282.

361. Sherr CJ, Rettenmier CW, Sacca R, et al. The c-fms proto-oncogene product is related to the receptor for the mononuclear phagocyte growth factor, CSF-1. *Cell* 1985;41:665.

362. Nienhuis AW, Bunn HF, Turner PH, et al. Expression of the human c-fms proto-oncogene in hematopoietic cells and its deletion in the 5q- syndrome. *Cell* 1985;42:421.

363. Pettenati MJ, Le Beau MM, Lemons RS, et al. Assignment of CSF-1 to 5q33.1: evidence for clustering of genes regulating hematopoiesis and for their involvement in the deletion of the long arm of chromosome 5 in myeloid disorders. *Proc Natl Acad Sci U S A* 1987;84:2970.

364. Le Beau MM, Epstein ND, O'Brien SJ, et al. The interleukin 3 gene is located on human chromosome 5 and is deleted in myeloid leukemias with a deletion of 5q. *Proc Natl Acad Sci U S A* 1987;84:5913.

365. Yamg YC, Kovacic S, Kriz R, et al. The human genes for GM-CSF and IL-3 are closely linked in tandem on chromosome 5. *Blood* 1988;71:958.

366. Sutherland GR, Baker E, Callen DF, et al. Interleukin-5 is at 5q31 and is deleted in the 5q- syndrome. *Blood* 1988;71:1150.

367. Le Beau MM, Lemons RS, Espinosa R III, et al. Interleukin-4 and interleukin-5 map to human chromosome 5 in a region encoding growth factors and receptors and are deleted in myeloid leukemias with a del(5q). *Blood* 1989;73:647.

368. van Leeuwen BH, Martinson ME, Webb GC, Young IG. Molecular organization of the cytokine gene cluster, involving the human IL-3, IL-4, IL-5, and GM-CSF genes, on human chromosome 5. *Blood* 1989;73:1142.

369. Yarden Y, Escobedo A, Kuang WJ, et al. Structure of the receptor for platelet-derived growth factor helps define a family of closely related growth factor receptors. *Nature* 1986;323:226.

370. Roberts WM, Loo AT, Roussel MF, Sherr CJ. Tandem linkage of human CSF-1 receptor (c-fms) and PDGF receptor genes. *Cell* 1988;55:655.

371. Kolbilka BK, Cison RAF, Frielle T, et al. cDNA for the human beta2-adrenergic receptor: a protein with multiple membrane-spanning domains and encoded by a gene whose chromosomal localization is shared with that of the receptor for platelet-derived growth factor. *Proc Natl Acad Sci U S A* 1987;84:46.

372. Jaye M, Howk R, Burgess W, et al. Human endothelial cell growth factor: cloning, nucleotide sequence and chromosomal localization. *Science* 1986;233:541.

373. Francke U, Foellmer BE. The glucocorticoid receptor gene is in 5q31–q32. *Genomics* 1989;4:610.

374. Goyert SM, Ferrero E, Rettig WJ, et al. The CD14 monocyte differentiation antigen maps to a region encoding growth factors and receptors. *Science* 1988;243:497.

375. Sukhatme VP, Cao X, Chang LC, et al. A zinc finger-encoding gene coregulated with c-fos during growth and differentiation and after cellular depolarization. *Cell* 1988;53:37.

376. Jaju RJ, Boultwood J, Oliver FJ, et al. Molecular cytogenetic delineation of the critical deleted region in the 5q- syndrome. *Genes Chromosomes Cancer* 1998; 22(3):251–256.

377. Boultwood J, Strickson AJ, Jabs EW, et al. Physical mapping of the human ATX1 homologue (HAH1) to the critical region of the 5q- syndrome within 5q32, and immediately adjacent to the SPARC gene. *Hum Genet* 2000;106(1): 127–129.

378. Westbrook CA, Hsu WT, Chyna B, et al. Cytogenetic and molecular diagnosis of chromosome 5 deletions in myelodysplasia. *Br J Haematol* 2000;110(4): 847–855.

379. Hu Z, Gomes I, Horrigan SK, et al. A novel nuclear protein, 5qNCA (LOC51780) is a candidate for the myeloid leukemia tumor suppressor gene on chromosome 5 band q31. *Oncogene* 2001;20(47):6946–6954.

380. Lai F, Godley LA, Joslin J, et al. Transcript map and comparative analysis of the 1.5-Mb commonly deleted segment of human 5q31 in malignant myeloid diseases with a del(5q). *Genomics* 2001;71(2):235–245.

381. Lai F, Godley LA, Fernald AA, et al. cDNA cloning and genomic structure of three genes localized to human chromosome band 5q31 encoding potential nuclear proteins. *Genomics* 2000;70(1):123–130.

382. Xie H, Hu Z, Chyna B, Horrigan SK, Westbrook CA. Human mortalin (HSPA9): a candidate for the myeloid leukemia tumor suppressor gene on 5q31. *Leukemia* 2000;14(12):2128–2134.

383. Westbrook CA, Hsu WT, Chyna B, et al. Cytogenetic and molecular diagnosis of chromosome 5 deletions in myelodysplasia. *Br J Haematol* 2000;110(4):847–855.

384. Horrigan SK, Arbieva ZH, Xie HY, et al. Delineation of a minimal interval and identification of 9 candidates for a tumor suppressor gene in malignant myeloid disorders on 5q31. *Blood* 2000;95(7):2372–2377.

385. Westbrook CA, Le Beau MM, Neuman WL, et al. Physical and genetic map of 5q31: use of fluorescence in situ hybridization data to identify errors in the CEPH database. Centre d'Etude de Polymorphisme Humain. *Cytogenet Cell Genet* 1994;67(2):86–93.

386. Le Beau MM, Espinosa R, Neuman WL, et al. Cytogenetic and molecular delineation of the smallest commonly deleted region of chromosome 5 in malignant myeloid diseases. *Proc Natl Acad Sci U S A* 1993;90(12):5484–5488.

387. Boultwood J, Fidler C, Strickson AJ, et al. Narrowing and genomic annotation of the commonly deleted region of the 5q- syndrome. *Blood* 2002;99(12):4638–4641.

388. Castro PD, Liang JC, Nagarajan L. Deletions of chromosome 5q13.3 and 17p loci cooperate in myeloid neoplasms. *Blood* 2000;95(6):2138–2143.

389. Castro PD, Fairman J, Nagarajan L. The unexplored 5q13 locus: a role in hematopoietic malignancies. *Leuk Lymphoma* 1998;30(5–6):443–448.

390. Bench AJ, Nacheva EP, Hood TL, et al. Chromosome 20 deletions in myeloid malignancies: reduction of the common deleted region, generation of a PAC/BAC contig and identification of candidate genes. UK Cancer Cytogenetics Group (UKCCG). *Oncogene* 2000;19(34):3902–3913.

391. Bench AJ, Aldred MA, Humphray SJ, et al. A detailed physical and transcriptional map of the region of chromosome 20 that is deleted in myeloproliferative disorders and refinement of the common deleted region. *Genomics* 1998;49(3):351–362.

392. Asimakopoulos FA, Green AR. Deletions of chromosome 20q and the pathogenesis of myeloproliferative disorders. *Br J Haematol* 1996;95(2):219–226.

393. Wang PW, Eisenbart JD, Espinosa R, et al. Refinement of the smallest commonly deleted segment of chromosome 20 in malignant myeloid diseases and development of a PAC-based physical and transcription map. *Genomics* 2000;67(1):28–39.

394. Wang PW, Iannantuoni K, Davis EM, et al. Refinement of the commonly deleted segment in myeloid leukemias with a del(20q). *Genes Chromosomes Cancer* 1998;21(2):75–81.

395. Kratz CP, Emerling BM, Donovan S, et al. Candidate gene isolation and comparative analysis of a commonly deleted segment of 7q22 implicated in myeloid malignancies. *Genomics* 2001;77(3):171–180.

396. Le Beau MM, Espinosa R, Davis EM, et al. Cytogenetic and molecular delineation of a region of chromosome 7 commonly deleted in malignant myeloid diseases. *Blood* 1996;88(6):1930–1935.

397. Quesnel B, Fenaux P. P15INK4b gene methylation and myelodysplastic syndromes. *Leuk Lymphoma* 1999;35(5–6):437–443.

398. Merlat A, Lai JL, Sterkers Y, et al. Therapy-related myelodysplastic syndrome and acute myeloid leukemia with 17p deletion. A report on 25 cases. *Leukemia* 1999;13(2):250–257.

399. Soenen V, Preudhomme C, Roumier C, et al. Myelodysplasia during the course of myeloma. Restriction of 17p deletion and p53 overexpression to myeloid cells. *Leukemia* 1998;12(2):238–241.

400. Soenen V, Preudhomme C, Roumier C, et al. 17p Deletion in acute myeloid leukemia and myelodysplastic syndrome. Analysis of breakpoints and deleted segments by fluorescence in situ. *Blood* 1998;91(3):1008–1015.

401. Preudhomme C, Fenaux P. The clinical significance of mutations of the P53 tumour suppressor gene in haematological malignancies. *Br J Haematol* 1997;98(3):502–511.

402. Rimsza LM, Kopecky KJ, Ruschulte J, et al. Microsatellite instability is not a defining genetic feature of acute myeloid leukemogenesis in adults: results of a retrospective study of 132 patients and review of the literature. *Leukemia* 2000;14(6):1044–1051.

403. Greenberg PL. Apoptosis and its role in the myelodysplastic syndromes: implications for disease natural history and treatment. *Leuk Res* 1998;22(12):1123–1136.

404. Shetty V, Hussaini S, Alvi S, et al. Excessive apoptosis, increased phagocytosis, nuclear inclusion bodies and cylindrical confronting cisternae in bone marrow biopsies of myelodysplastic syndrome patients. *Br J Haematol* 2002;116(4):817–825.

405. Mundle SD, Shetty VT, Raza A. Caspases and apoptosis in myelodysplastic syndromes. *Exp Hematol* 2000;28(12):1310–1312.

406. Arlett CF. Human DNA repair defects. *J Inherit Metab Dis* 1986;9:69.

407. Chaganti RSK, Schonberg S, German J. A manyfold increase in sister chromatid exchanges in Bloom's syndrome lymphocytes. *Proc Natl Acad Sci U S A* 1974;71:4508.

408. Schimke RT, Sherwood SW, Hill AB, Johnston RN. Overreplication and recombination of DNA in higher eukaryotes: potential consequences and biological implications. *Proc Natl Acad Sci U S A* 1986;83:2157.

409. Murthy PB, Kamada N, Kuramoto A. Increased sister chromatid exchange frequency in bone marrow cells of myelodysplastic syndromes. *Cancer Genet Cytogenet* 1985;15:151.

410. de Vinuesa ML, Larripa I, de Pargament MM, de Salum SB. Heterochromatic variants and their association with neoplasias. II preleukemic states. *Cancer Genet Cytogenet* 1985;14:31.

411. Murthy PB, Kamada N, Kuramoto A. Defective ultraviolet-induced DNA repair in bone marrow cells and peripheral lymphocytes of patients with refractory anemia with excess of blasts. *Jpn J Clin Oncol* 1984;14:87.

412. Temin HM. Evolution of cancer genes as a mutation-driven process. *Cancer Res* 1988;48:1697.

413. Knuutila S, Teerenhovi L, Borgstrom GH. Chromosome instability is associated with hypodiploid clones in myelodysplastic syndromes. *Hereditas* 1984;101:19.

414. Dash A, Gilliland DG. Molecular genetics of acute myeloid leukaemia. *Best Pract Res Clin Haematol* 2001;14(1):49–64.

415. Gilliland DG. Hematologic malignancies. *Curr Opin Hematol* 2001;8(4):189–191.

416. Gilliland DG, Tallman MS. Focus on acute leukemias. *Cancer Cell* 2002;1:417–420.

417. Metcalf D. *The hematopoeitic colony stimulating factors.* Amsterdam: Elsevier, 1984.

418. Milner GR, Testa NG, Geary CG, et al. Bone marrow culture studies in refractory cytopenia and "smouldering leukaemia." *Br J Haematol* 1977;35:251.

419. Mizoguchi H, Kubota K, Suda T, et al. Erythroid and granulocyte/macrophage progenitor cells in primary acquired sideroblastic anemia. *Intl J Cell Clon* 1983;1:15.

420. Baines P, Masters GS, Lush C, Jacobs A. Enrichment of haemopoietic progenitor cells from the marrow of patients with myelodysplasia. *Br J Haematol* 1988;68:159.

421. Geissler K, Hinterberger W, Jager U, et al. Deficiency of pluripotent hemopoietic progenitor cells in myelodysplastic syndromes. *Blut* 1988;57:45.

422. Tennant G, Jacobs A, Bailey-Wood R. Peripheral blood granulocyte-macrophage progenitors in patients with the myelodysplastic syndromes. *Exp Hematol* 1986;14:1063.

423. Greenberg PL, Mara B. The preleukemic syndrome: correlation of in vitro parameters of granulopoiesis with clinical features. *Am J Med* 1979;66:951.

424. Lidbeck J. In vitro colony and cluster growth in haemopoietic dysplasia (the preleukaemic syndrome). *Scand J Haematol* 1980;25:113.

425. Rosenthal DS, Moloney WC. Refractory dysmyelopoietic anemia and acute leukemia. *Blood* 1984;63:314.

426. Elstner E, Schulze E, Ihle R, et al. Proliferation and maturation of hemopoietic cells from patients with preleukemia and aplastic anemia in agar and diffusion chamber cultures. *Haematol Blood Transfus* 1983;28:358.

427. Zwierzina H, Sepp N, Ringler E, Schmalzl F. Delayed maturation of skin window macrophages in myelodysplastic syndromes. *Leuk Res* 1989;13:433.

428. May SJ, Smith SA, Jacobs A, et al. The myelodysplastic syndrome: analysis of laboratory characteristics in relation to the FAB classification. *Br J Haematol* 1985;59:311.

429. Senn JS, Messne HA, Pinkerton PH, et al. Peripheral blood blast cell progenitors in human preleukemia. *Blood* 1979;54:106.

430. Greenberg P. Clinical relevance of in vitro study of granulocytopoiesis. *Scand J Haematol* 1980;25:369.

431. Greenberg PL, Nichols WC, Schrier SL. Granulopoiesis in acute myeloid leukemia and preleukemia. *N Engl J Med* 1971;284:1225.

432. Everson MP, Brown CB, Lilly MB. Interleukin-6 and granulocyte-macrophage colony-stimulating factor are candidate growth factors for chronic myelomonocytic leukemia cells. *Blood* 1989;74:1472.

433. Geissler K, Hinterberger W, Bettelheim P, et al. Colony growth characteristics in chronic myelomonocytic leukemia. *Leuk Res* 1988;12:373.

434. Juvonen E, Partanen S, Knuutila S, Ruutu T. Megakaryocyte colony formation by bone marrow progenitors in myelodysplastic syndromes. *Br J Haematol* 1986;63:331.

435. Koeffler HP, Cline MJ, Golde DW. Erythropoiesis in preleukemia. *Blood* 1978;51:1013.

436. Geissler D, Zwierzina H, Pechlaner C, et al. Abnormal megakaryopoiesis in patients with myelodysplastic syndromes: analysis of cellular and humoral defects. *Br J Haematol* 1989;73:29.

437. Juvonen E, Partanen S, Knuutila S, Ruutu T. Colony formation by megakaryocyte progenitors in myelodysplastic syndromes. *Eur J Haematol* 1989;42:389.

438. Carbonell F, Heimpel H, Kubanek B, Fleidner TM. Growth and cytogenetic characteristics of bone marrow colonies from patients with 5q- syndrome. *Blood* 1985;66:463.

439. Koeffler HP, Golde DW. Cellular maturation in human preleukemia. *Blood* 1978;52:355.

440. Queisser U, Olischlager A, Queisser W, Heimpel H. Cell proliferation in the "preleukaemic" phase of acute leukaemia. *Acta Haematol* 1972;47:21.

441. Dormer P, Ucci G, Hershko C, Wilmanns W. Cell kinetics in leukemia and preleukemia. *Haematol Blood Transfus* 1987;30:3.

442. Montecucco C, Riccardi A, Traversi E, et al. Proliferative activity of bone marrow cells in primary dysmyelopoietic (preleukemic) syndromes. *Cancer* 1983;52:1190.

443. Stella CC, Cazzola M, Bergamaschi G, et al. Growth of human hematopoietic colonies from patients with myelodysplastic syndromes in response to recombinant human granulocyte-macrophage colony-stimulating factor. *Leukemia* 1989;3:363.

444. Mayani H, Baines P, Bowen DT, Jacobs A. In vitro growth of myeloid and erythroid progenitor cells form myelodysplastic patients in response to recombinant human granulocyte-macrophage colony-stimulating factor. *Leukemia* 1989;3:29.

445. Merchav S, Nagler A, Fleischer-Kurtz G, Tatarsky I. Regulatory abnormalities in the marrow of patients with myelodysplastic syndromes. *Br J Haematol* 1989;73:158.

446. Merchav S, Nagler A, Sahar E, Tatarsky I. Production of human pluripotent progenitor cell colony stimulating activity (CFU-GEMM-CSA) in patients with myelodysplastic syndromes. *Leuk Res* 1987;11:273.

447. Francis GE, Miller EJ, Wonke B, et al. Use of bone-marrow culture in prediction of acute leukaemic transformation in preleukaemia. *Lancet* 1983;1409.

448. Morris TCM, McNeill TA, Bridges JM. Inhibition of normal in vitro colony forming cells by cells from leukaemic patients. *Br J Cancer* 1975;31:641.

449. Quesenberry PJ, Rappeport JM, Fountebuoni A, et al. Inhibition of normal murine hematopoiesis by leukemic cells. *N Engl J Med* 1978;299:71.

450. Geissler D, Thaler J, Konwalinka G, Peschel C. Progressive preleukemia presenting amegakaryocytic thrombocytopenic purpura: association of the 5q-syndrome with a decreased megakaryocytic colony formation and a defective production of Meg-CSF. *Leuk Res* 1987;11:731.

451. Putintseva E, Garcia-Triana E. Thrombopoietic inhibitory activity in serum of patients with refractory anaemia. *Br J Haematol* 1987;265.

452. Kerndrup G, Hokland P. Natural-killer cell-mediated inhibition of bone marrow colony formation (CFU-GM) in refractory anemia (preleukemia): evidence for patient-specific cell populations. *Br J Haematol* 1988;69:457.

453. Jacobs A, Janowska-Wieczorek A, Caro J, et al. Circulating erythropoietin in patients with myelodysplastic syndromes. *Br J Haematol* 1989;73:36.

454. Wallner SF, Kurnick JE, Vautrin RM, et al. Levels of erythropoietin in patients with the anemias of chronic diseases and liver failure. *Am J Hematol* 1977;3:37.

455. Sherwood JB, Goldwasser E, Chilcote R, et al. Sickle cell anemia patients have low erythropoietin levels for their degree of anemia. *Blood* 1986;67:46.

456. de Klerk G, Rosengarten PCJ, Vet RJWM, Goudsmit R. Serum erythropoietin (ESF) titers in anemia. *Blood* 1981;58:1164.

457. Ward HP, Kurnick JE, Pisarczyk MJ. Serum level of erythropoietin in anemias associated with chronic infection, malignancy, and primary hematopoietic disease. *J Clin Invest* 1971;50:332.

458. Lutton JD, Ibraham NG, Hoffman R, et al. Sideroblastic anemia: differences in bone marrow erythroid colony (CFUE) growth responses to erythropoietin in plasma clot and methylcellulose cultures. *Am J Hematol* 1984;16:219.

459. Sporn MB, Roberts AB. Autocrine growth factors and cancer. *Nature* 1985;313:745.

460. Browder TM, Dunbar CE, Nienhuis AW. Private and public autocrine loops in neoplastic cells. *Cancer Cells* 1989;1:9.

461. Young DC, Griffin JD. Autocrine secretion of GM-CSF in acute myeloblastic leukemia. *Blood* 1986;68:1178.

462. Griffin JD, Young DC. The role of colony stimulating factors in leukaemogenesis. *Clin Haematol* 1986;15:995.

463. Russell NH, Reilly AG. Role of autocrine growth factors in the leukemic transformation of the myelodysplastic syndromes. *Leukemia* 1989;3:83.

464. Chang JM, Metcalf D, Lang RA, et al. Nonneoplastic hematopoietic myeloproliferative syndrome induced by dysregulated multi-CSF (IL-3) expression. *Blood* 1989;73:1487.

465. Wong PMC, Chung SW, Dunbar CE, et al. Retrovirus-mediated transfer and expression of the interleukin-3 gene in mouse hematopoietic cells result in a myeloproliferative disorder. *Mol Cell Biol* 1989;9:798.

466. Johnson GR, Gonda TJ, Metcalf D, et al. A lethal myeloproliferative syndrome in mice transplanted with bone marrow cells infected with a retrovirus expressing granulocyte-macrophage colony stimulating factor. *EMBO J* 1989;8:441.

467. Valentine WN, Konrad PN, Paglia DE. Dyserythropoiesis, refractory anemia, and "preleukemia": metabolic features of the erythrocytes. *Blood* 1973;41:857.

468. Boivin P, Galand C, Hakim J, Kahn A. Acquired erythroenzymopathies in blood disorders: study of 200 cases. *Br J Haematol* 1975;31:531.

469. Dreyfus B, Sultan C, Rochant H, et al. Anomalies of blood group antigens and erythrocyte enzymes in two types of chronic refractory anemia. *Br J Haematol* 1969;16:303.

470. Nano R, Invernizzi R, Rezzani R, Gerzeli G. Qualitative 2nd quantitative study of dihydrofolate reductase in myelodysplastic syndromes. *Acta Haematol* 1988;79:198.

471. Kanno H, Fujii H, Tani K, et al. Elevated erythrocyte adenosine deaminase activity in a patient with primary acquired sideroblastic anemia. *Am J Hematol* 1988;27:216.

472. van der Weyden MB, Harrison C, Hallam L, et al. Elevated red cell adenosine deaminase and haemolysis in a patient with a myelodysplastic syndrome. *Br J Haematol* 1989;73:129.

473. Helmstadter V, Arnold H, Blume KG, et al. Acquired pyruvate kinase deficiency with hemolysis in preleukemia. *Acta Haematol* 1977;57:339.

474. Kornberg A, Goldfarb A. Preleukemia manifested by hemolytic anemia with pyruvate-kinase deficiency. *Arch Intern Med* 1986;146:785.

475. Salmon C. Blood group changes in preleukemic states. *Blood Cell* 1976;2:211.

476. Yoshida A, Kumazaki T, Dave V, Dzik WH. Suppressed expression of blood group B antigen and blood group galactosyltransferase in a preleukemic subject. *Blood* 1985;66:990.

477. Rochant H, Dreyfus B, Bouguerra M, Tont-Hat H. Refractory anemias, preleukemic conditions, and fetal erythropoiesis. *Blood* 1972;39:721.

478. Abbondanzo SL, Anagnou NP, Sacher RA. Myelodysplastic syndrome with acquired hemoglobin H disease: evolution through megakaryoblastic transformation into myelofibrosis. *Am J Clin Pathol* 1988;89:401.

479. Peters RE, May A, Jacobs A. Globin chain synthesis ratios in sideroblastic anaemia. *Br J Haematol* 1983;53:201.

480. Anagnou NP, Ley TJ, Chesbro B, et al. Acquired alpha-thalassemia in preleukemia is due to decreased expression of all four alpha-globin genes. *Proc Natl Acad Sci U S A* 1983;80:6051.

481. Jacobs A. Primary acquired sideroblastic anemia. *Br J Haematol* 1986;64:415.

482. Pasanen A, Tenhunen R. Heme synthesis in sideroblastic anaemias. *Scand J Haematol* 1986;45:60.

483. Hast R, Reizenstein P. Sideroblastic anemia and development of leukemia. *Blut* 1981;42:223.

484. Bottomley SS. Porphyrin and iron metabolism in sideroblastic anemia. *Semin Hematol* 1977;14:169.

485. Verwilghen R, Reybrouck G, Callens L, Cosemans J. Antituberculous drugs and sideroblastic anaemia. *Br J Haematol* 1965;II:92.

486. Horrigan DL, Harris JW. Pyridoxine-responsive anemia: analysis of 62 cases. *Adv Intern Med* 1989;12:103.

487. Raab SO, Haut A, Cartwright GE, Wintrobe MM. Pyridoxine-responsive anemia. *Blood* 1961;18:285.

488. Ibraham NG, Lutton JD, Hoffman R, Levere RD. Regulation of heme metabolism in normal and sideroblastic bone marrow cells in culture. *J Lab Clin Med* 1985;105:593.

489. Konopka L, Hoffbrand AV. Haem synthesis in sideroblastic anaemia. *Br J Haematol* 1979;42:73.

490. Bottomley SS, Tan aka M, Self J. Delta-aminolevulinic acid synthetase activity in normal human bone marrow and in patients with idiopathic sideroblastic anemia. *Enzyme* 1973;16:138.

491. Aoki Y, Urata G, Takaku F. Delta-aminolevulinic acid synthetase activity in erythroblasts of patients with primary sideroblastic anemia. *Acta Haematol Jpn* 1973;36:74.

492. Bottomley SS, Healy HM, May BK. 5-Aminolevulinic acid synthetase in sideroblastic anemia revisited. *Blood* 1989;74:103a.

493. Aoki Y, Muranaka S, Nakabayashi K, Ueda Y. Delta-aminolevulinic acid synthetase in erythroblasts of patients with pyridoxine-responsive anemia. *J Clin Invest* 1979;64:1196.

494. Meier PJ, Fehr J, Meyer UA. Pyridoxine-responsive primary acquired sideroblastic anaemia. *Scand J Haematol* 1982;29:421.

495. Sutherland GR, Baker E, Callen DF, et al. 5-Aminolevulinate synthetase is at 3p21 and thus not the primary defect in X-linked sideroblastic anemia. *Am J Hum Genet* 1988;43:331.

496. Elves MW, Bourne MS, Israels MCG. Pyridoxine-responsive anaemia determined by an X-linked gene. *J Med Genet* 1966;3:1.

497. Jamel BCJ, Schretlen EDA. Sideroblastic anaemia: a review of seven paediatric cases. *Eur J Pediatr* 1982;138:130.

498. Pasanen AVO, Eklof M, Tenhunen R. Coproporphyrinogen oxidase activity and porphyrin concentrations in peripheral red blood cells in hereditary sideroblastic anaemia. *Scand J Haematol* 1985;34:235.

499. Prasad AS, Tranchida L, Konno ET, et al. Hereditary sideroblastic anemia and glucose-6-phosphate dehydrogenase deficiency in a Negro family. *J Clin Invest* 1968;47:1415.

500. Pagon RA, Bird TD, Detter JC, Pierce I. Hereditary sideroblastic anaemia and ataxia: an X linked recessive disorder. *J Med Genet* 1985;22:267.

501. Partanen S, Pasanen A, Juvonen E, et al. Erythroid colony formation and effect of hemin in vitro in hereditary sideroblastic anemias. *Exp Hematol* 1988;16:313.

502. Cox TC, Bottomley SS, Wiley JS, et al. X-linked pyridoxine-responsive sideroblastic anemia due to a Thr388-to-Ser substitution in erythroid 5-aminolevulinate synthase. *N Engl J Med* 1994;330(10):675–679.

503. Romslo I, Brun A, Sandberg S, et al. Sideroblastic anemia with markedly increased free erythrocyte protoprophyrin without dermal photosensitivity. *Blood* 1982;59:628.

504. Rothstein G, Lee GR, Cartwright GE. Sideroblastic anemia with dermal photosensitivity and greatly increased erythrocyte protoporphyrin. *N Engl J Med* 1969;280:587.

505. May A, De Souza P, Barnes K, et al. Erythroblast iron metabolism in sideroblastic marrows. *Br J Haematol* 1982;52:611.

506. Solomon LR, Hillman RS. Vitamin B6 metabolism in idiopathic sideroblastic anaemia and related disorders. *Br J Haematol* 1979;42:239.

507. Bottomley SS, Tanaka M, Everett MA. Diminished erythroid ferrochelatase activity in protoporphyria. *J Lab Clin Med* 1975;86:126.

508. Bottomley SS, Moore MZ. Acquired erythropoietic protoporphyria and sideroblastic anemia. *Clin Res* 1989;38a.

509. Grasso JA, Myers TJ, Hines JD, Sullivan AL. Energy-dispersive x-ray analysis of the mitochondria of sideroblastic anaemia. *Br J Haematol* 1980; 46:57.

510. Kushner JP, Steinmuller DP, Lee GR. Inhibition of uroporphyrinogen decarboxylase activity by iron. *Clin Res* 1973;21:266.

511. Hines JD. Effect of pyridoxine plus chronic phlebotomy on the function and morphology of bone marrow and liver in pyridoxine-responsive sideroblastic anemia. *Semin Hematol* 1976;13:133.

512. Weintraub LR, Conrad ME, Crosby WH. Iron-loading anemia: treatment with repeated phlebotomies and pyridoxine. *N Engl J Med* 1966;275:169.

513. Jensen PD, Jensen IM, Ellegaard J. Desferrioxamine treatment reduces blood transfusion requirements in patients with myelodysplastic syndrome. *Br J Haematol* 1992;80:121.

514. Aoki Y. Multiple enzymatic defects in mitochondria in hematological cells of patients with primary sideroblastic anemia. *J Clin Invest* 1980;66:43.

515. Rasi V, Lintula R. Platelet function in the myelodysplastic syndromes. *Scand J Haematol* 1986;36(Suppl 45):71.

516. Rao AK, Walsh PN. Acquired qualitative platelet disorders. *Clin Haematol* 1983;12:201.

517. Clark RE, Hoy TE, Jacobs A. Granulocyte and monocyte surface membrane markers in the myelodysplastic syndromes. *J Clin Pathol* 1985;38:301.

518. Boogaerts MA, Nelissen V, Roelant C, Goossens W. Blood neutrophil function in primary myelodysplastic syndromes. *Br J Haematol* 1983;55:217.

519. Cech P, Markert M, Perrin LH. Partial myeloperoxidase deficiency in preleukemia. *Blut* 1983;47:21.

520. Lehrer RI, Goldberg LS, Apple MA, Rosenthal NP. Refractory megaloblastic anemia with myeloperoxidase-deficient neutrophils. *Ann Intern Med* 1972; 76:447.

521. Breton-Gorius J, Houssay D, Dreyfus B. Partial myeloperoxidase deficiency in a case of preleukemia. *Br J Haematol* 1975;30:273.

522. Breton-Gorius J, Houssay D, Vilde JL, Dreyfus B. Partial myeloperoxidase deficiency in a case of preleukemia: defects of degranulation and abnormal bactericidal activity of blood neutrophils. *Br J Haematol* 1975;30:279.

523. Kletter Y, Nagler A. Function of peripheral blood and bone-marrow monocytes in preleukemic patients: normal phagocytosis and intracellular killing of Candida albicans. *Acta Haematol* 1984;72:379.

524. Bynoe AG, Scott CS, Ford P, Roberts BE. Decreased T helper cells in the myelodysplastic syndromes. *Br J Haematol* 1983;54:97.

525. Knox SJ, Greenberg BR, Anderson RW, Rosenblatt LS. Studies of T-lymphocytes in preleukemic disorders and acute nonlymphocytic leukemia: in vitro radiosensitivity, mitogenic responsiveness, colony formation, and enumeration of lymphocytic subpopulations. *Blood* 1983;61:449.

526. Colombat PH, Renoux M, Lamagnere JP, Renoux G. Immunologic indices in myelodysplastic syndromes. *Cancer* 1988;61:1075.

527. Janowska-Wieczorek A, Jakobisiak M, Dobaczewska H. Decreased antibody-dependent cellular cytotoxicity in preleukemic syndromes. *Acta Haematol* 1983;69:132.

528. Mufti GJ, Figes A, Hamblin TJ, et al. Immunological abnormalities in myelodysplastic syndromes. I. Serum immunoglobulins and autoantibodies. *Br J Haematol* 1986;63:143.

529. Anderson RW, Volsky DJ, Greenberg B, et al. Lymphocyte abnormalities in preleukemia. I. Decreased NK activity, anomalous immunoregulatory cell subsets and deficient EBV receptors. *Leuk Res* 1983;7:389.

530. Oblakowski P. Natural killer activity in preleukemic states. *Haematol Blood Transfus* 1987;31:132.

531. Tricot G, Vlietinck R, Boogaerts MA, et al. Prognostic factors in the myelodysplastic syndromes: importance of initial data on peripheral blood counts, bone marrow cytology, trephine biopsy and chromosomal analysis. *Br J Haematol* 1985;60:19.

531a. Aul C, Gattermann N, Schneider W. Age-related incidence and other epidemiologic aspects of myelodysplastic syndromes. *J Haematol* 1992;82:358.

532. Barlogie B, Johnston DA, Keating M, et al. Evolution of oligoleukemia. *Cancer* 1984;53:2115.

533. Heimpel H, Drings P, Mitrou P, Queiber W. Verlauf und prognostische kriterien bei patienten mit "praleukamie." *Klin Wochenschr* 1979;57:21.

534. Riccardi A, Giordano M, Giordano P, et al. Prognostic parameters in myelodysplastic syndromes: a multiple regression analysis. *Eur J Haematol* 1988;40: 158.

535. Jaworkowsky LI, Solovey DY, Rhausova LY, Udris OY. Monocytosis as a sign of subsequent leukemia in patients with cytopenias (preleukemia). *Folia Haematol Leipzig* 1983;110:395.

536. Varela BL, Chuang C, Woll JE, Bennett JM. Modifications in the classification of primary myelodysplastic syndromes: the addition of a scoring system. *Hematol Oncol* 1985;3:55.

537. Cazzola M, Barosi G, Gobbi PG, et al. Natural history of idiopathic refractory sideroblastic anemia. *Blood* 1988;71:305.

538. Najean Y, Pecking A. Refractory anemia with excess of blast cells: prognostic factors and effect of treatment with androgens or cytosine arabinoside. *Cancer* 1979;44:1976.

539. Vandermolen L, Rice L, Rose MA, Lynch EC. Ringed sideroblasts in primary myelodysplasia. *Arch Intern Med* 1988;148:653.

540. Kerndrup G, Pedersen B, Ellegaard J, Hokland P. Prognostic significance of some clinical, morphological and cytogenetic findings in refractory anaemia (RA) and RA with sideroblasts. *Blut* 1986;52:35.

541. Schipperus MR, Hagemeijer A, Ploemacher RE, et al. In myelodysplastic syndromes progression to leukemia is directly related to PHA dependency for colony formation and independent of in vitro maturation capacity. *Leukemia* 1988;2:433.

542. Greenberg PL, Mara B. The preleukemic syndrome: correlation of in vitro parameters of granulopoiesis with clinical features. *Am J Med* 1979;66:951.

543. Worsley A, Oscier DG, Stevens J, et al. Prognostic features of chronic myelomonocytic leukaemia: a modified Bournemouth score gives the best prediction of survival. *Br J Haematol* 1988;68:17.

544. Smith WB, Ablin A, Goodman JR, Brecher G. Atypical megakaryocytes in preleukemic phase of acute myeloid leukemia. *Blood* 1973;42:535.

545. Weiss K, Stass S, Williams D, et al. Childhood monosomy 7 syndrome: clinical and in vitro studies. *Leukemia* 1987;1:97.

546. Sieff CA, Chessells JM, Harvey BA, et al. Monosomy 7 in childhood: a preleukemic state. *Br J Haematol* 1981;49:129.

547. Oguma S, Yoshida Y, Uchino H, Maekawa T. Factors influencing leukemic transformation in refractory anemias with excess of blasts, with ringed sideroblasts, and without ringed sideroblasts. *Cancer Res* 1986;46:3698.

548. Oguma S, Yoshida Y, Uchino H, Maekawa T. Factors influencing nonleukemic death in refractory anemia, refractory anemia with ringed sideroblasts, and refractory anemia with excess blasts. *Cancer Res* 1987;47:3599.

549. Jaworkowsky LI, Solovey DY, Rhausova LY, et al. A simple mathematical method revealing the early stage of acute leukemia in patients with cytopenias. *Folia Haematol Leipzig* 1984;111:701.

550. Greenberg PL. Risk factors and their relationship to prognosis in myelodysplastic syndromes. *Leuk Res* 1998;22(Suppl 1):S3–S6.

551. Belli C, Acevedo S, Bengio R, et al. Detection of risk groups in myelodysplastic syndromes. A multicenter study. *Haematologica* 2002;87(1):9–16.

552. Kita-Sasai Y, Horiike S, Misawa S, et al. International prognostic scoring system and TP53 mutations are independent prognostic indicators for patients with myelodysplastic syndrome. *Br J Haematol* 2001;115(2):309–312.

553. Nosslinger T, Reisner R, Koller E, et al. Myelodysplastic syndromes, from French-American-British to World Health Organization: comparison of classifications on 431 unselected patients from a single institution. *Blood* 2001; 98(10):2935–2941.

554. Mirza I, Garzon R, Burns J, et al. Myelodysplastic syndromes: a community hospital-based study of prognostic factors and International Prognostic Scoring System. *Conn Med* 2001;65(8):455–463.

555. Sperr WR, Wimazal F, Kundi M, et al. Survival analysis and AML development in patients with de novo myelodysplastic syndromes: comparison of six different prognostic scoring systems. *Ann Hematol* 2001;80(5):272–277.

556. Deeg HJ, Appelbaum FR. Hematopoietic stem cell transplantation in patients with myelodysplastic syndrome. *Leuk Res* 2000;24(8):653–663.

557. Maes B, Meeus P, Michaux L, et al. Application of the International Prognostic Scoring System for myelodysplastic syndromes. *Ann Oncol* 1999;10(7):825–829.

558. Pfeilstocker M, Reisner R, Nosslinger T, et al. Cross-validation of prognostic scores in myelodysplastic syndromes on 386 patients from a single institution confirms importance of cytogenetics. *Br J Haematol* 1999;106(2):455–463.

559. Appelbaum FR, Anderson J. Allogeneic bone marrow transplantation for myelodysplastic syndrome: outcomes analysis according to IPSS score. *Leukemia* 1998;12(Suppl 1):S25–S29.

560. Sanz GF, Sanz MA, Greenberg PL. Prognostic factors and scoring systems in myelodysplastic syndromes. *Haematologica* 1998;83(4):358–368.

561. Nowell PC, Besa EC. Prognostic significance of single chromosomal abnormalities in preleukemic states. *Cancer Genet Cytogenet* 1989;42:1.

562. Berghe HVD, David G, Michaux JL, et al. 5q- acute myelogenous leukemia. *Blood* 1976;48:624.

563. Michiels JJ, Mallios-Zorbala H, Prins MEF, Hahlen K. Simple monosomy 7 and myelodysplastic syndrome in thirteen patients without previous cytostatic treatment. *Br J Haematol* 1986;64:425.

564. Larson RA. Treatment of acute myeloid leukemia with antecedent myelodysplastic syndrome. *Leukemia* 1996;10(Suppl 1):S23–S25.

565. Estey EH. Prognosis and therapy of secondary myelodysplastic syndromes. *Haematologica* 1998;83(6):543–549.

566. Dann EJ, Rowe JM. Biology and therapy of secondary leukaemias. *Best Pract Res Clin Haematol* 2001;14(1):119–137.

567. Camba LL, Joyner MV. Refractory anaemia terminating in a combined lymphoproliferative and myeloproliferative disorder. *J Clin Pathol* 1985;38:297.

568. Hehlmann R, Zonnchen B, Thiel E, Walther B. Idiopathic refractory sideroachrestic anemia (IRSA) progressing to acute mixed lymphoblastic-myelomonoblastic leukemia. *Blut* 1983;46:11.

569. Bonati A, Delia D, Starcich R. Progression of a myelodysplastic syndrome to pre-B acute lymphoblastic leukaemia with unusual phenotype. *Br J Haematol* 1986;64:487.

570. Cheson BD, Bennett JM, Kantarjian H, et al. Report of an international working group to standardize response criteria for myelodysplastic syndromes. *Blood* 2000;96(12):3671–3674.

571. Cheson BD, Bennett JM, Kantarjian H, et al. Myelodysplastic syndromes standardized response criteria: further definition. *Blood* 2001;98(6):1985.

572. Spriggs DR, Stone RM, Kufe DW. The treatment of myelodysplastic syndromes. *Clin Haematol* 1986;15:1081.

573. Larson RA. Management of myelodysplastic syndromes. *Ann Intern Med* 1985;103:136.

574. Treatment for pre-leukaemia? *Lancet* 1984;1:943.

575. Legare RD, Gilliland DG. Myelodysplastic syndrome. *Curr Opin Hematol* 1995;2(4):283–292.

576. Koeffler HP. Myelodysplastic syndromes. *Semin Hematol* 1996;33(2):87–94.

577. Cazzola M. Alternatives to conventional or myeloablative chemotherapy in myelodysplastic syndrome. *Int J Hematol* 2000;72(2):134–138.

578. Schafer AI, Cheron RG, Dluhy R, et al. Clinical consequences of acquired transfusional iron overload in adults. *N Engl J Med* 1981;304:319.

579. Pippard MJ, Callender ST. Clinical annotation: the management of iron chelation therapy. *Br J Haematol* 1983;54:503.

580. Ley TJ, Griffith P, Nienhuis AW. Transfusion haemosiderosis and chelation therapy. *Clin Haematol* 1982;11:437.

581. Brittenham GM, Zanzucchi PE, Farrell DE, et al. Non-invasive in vivo measurement of human iron overload by magnetic susceptibility studies. *Trans Assoc Am Phys* 1980;43:156.

582. Volin L, Tuutu T, Knuutila S, Tenhunen R. Heme arginate treatment for myelodysplastic syndromes. *Leuk Res* 1988;12:423.

583. Najean Y, Pecking A. Refractory anaemia with excess of myeloblasts in the bone marrow: a clinical trial of androgens in 90 patients. *Br J Haematol* 1977;37:25.

584. Doll DC, Ringenberg QS, Yarbro JW. Danazol therapy in acquired idiopathic sideroblastic anemia. *Acta Haematol* 1987;77:170.

585. Aviles A, Rubio E. Danazol in idiopathic sideroblastic anemia. *Acta Haematol* 1988;79:229.

586. Hupperets P, De Witte T, Haanen CA. Retrospective study of the effect of anabolic steroids on the dyshaematopoietic syndrome (preleukaemic syndrome). *Neth J Med* 1983;26:181.

587. Bagby GC, Gabourel JD, Linman JW. Gluticocorticoid therapy in the preleukemic syndrome (hemopoietic dysplasia). *Ann Intern Med* 1980;92:55.

588. Mertelsmann R, Thaler HT, To L, et al. Morphological classification, response to therapy, and survival in 263 adult patients with acute nonlymphoblastic leukemia. *Blood* 1980;56:773.

589. Armitage JO, Dick FR, Needleman SW, Burns CP. Effect of chemotherapy for the dysmyelopoietic syndrome. *Cancer Treat Rep* 1981;65:601.

590. Fenaux P, Lai JL, Jouet JP, et al. Aggressive chemotherapy in adult primary myelodysplastic syndromes. *Blut* 1988;57:297.

591. Murray C, Cooper B, Kitchens LW Jr. Remission of acute myelogenous leukemia in elderly patients with prior refractory dysmyelopoietic anemia. *Cancer* 1983;52:967.

592. Tricot G, Boogaerts MA. The role of aggressive chemotherapy in the treatment of the myelodysplastic syndromes. *Br J Haematol* 1986;63:477.

593. Preisler HD, Raza A, Barcos M, et al. High-dose cytosine arabinoside in the treatment of preleukemic disorders: a Leukemia Intergroup study. *Am J Hematol* 1986;23:131.

594. Martiat P, Ferrant A, Michaux JL, Sokal G. Intensive chemotherapy for acute non-lymphoblastic leukemia after primary myelodysplastic syndrome. *Hematol Oncol* 1988;6:299.

595. Tricot G, Boogaerts MA, Verwilghen RL. Treatment of patients with myelodysplastic syndromes: a review. *Scand J Haematol* 1986;36(Suppl 45):121.

596. Gyger M, Perreault C, Carnot J, et al. Treatment of therapy-induced preleukemic syndrome. *Blut* 1984;48:117.

597. Aul C, Schneider W. The role of low-dose cytosine arabinoside and aggressive chemotherapy in advanced myelodysplastic syndromes. *Cancer* 1989;64:1812.

598. Richard C, Iriondo A, Garijo J, et al. Therapy of advanced myelodysplastic syndrome with aggressive chemotherapy. *Oncology* 1989;46:6.

599. Bernstein SH, Brunetto VL, Davey FR, et al. Acute myeloid leukemia-type chemotherapy for newly diagnosed patients without antecedent cytopenias having myelodysplastic syndrome as defined by French-American-British criteria: a Cancer and Leukemia Group B Study. *J Clin Oncol* 1996;14(9):2486–2494.

600. Sachs L. Control of normal cell differentiation and the phenotypic reversion of malignancy in myeloid leukaemia. *Nature* 1978;274:535.

601. Morosetti R, Koeffler HP. Differentiation therapy in myelodysplastic syndromes. *Semin Hematol* 1996;33(3):236–245.

602. Friend C, Scher W, Holland J, Sato T. Hemoglobin synthesis in murine virus-induced leukemic cells in vitro: stimulation of erythroid differentiation by dimethyl sulfoxide. *Proc Natl Acad Sci U S A* 1971;68:378.

603. Lotem J, Sachs L. Different blocks in the differentiation of myeloid leukemic cells. *Proc Natl Acad Sci U S A* 1974;71:3507.

604. Sporn MB, Roberts AB. Role of retinoids in differentiation and carcinogenesis. *Cancer Res* 1983;43:3034.

605. Koeffler HP, Hirji K, Itri L, et al. 1,25-Dihydroxyvitamin D3: in vivo and in vitro effects on human preleukemic and leukemic cells. *Cancer Treat Rep* 1985;69:1399.

606. Griffin J, Munroe D, Major P, Kufe D. Induction of differentiation of human myeloid leukemia cells by inhibitors of DNA synthesis. *Exp Hematol* 1982;10:774.

607. Honma Y, Fujita Y, Kasukabe T, et al. Induction of differentiation of human acute non-lymphocytic leukemia cells in primary culture by inducers of differentiation of human myeloid leukemia line HL-60. *Eur J Cancer Clin Oncol* 1983;19:251.

608. Breitman TR, Collins SJ, Keene BR. Terminal differentiation of human promyelocytic leukemic cells in primary culture in response to retinoic acid. *Blood* 1981;57:1000.

609. Swanson G, Picozzi V, Morgan R, et al. Responses of hemopoietic precursors to 13-cis retinoic acid and 1,25-dihydroxyvitamin D3 in the myelodysplastic syndromes. *Blood* 1986;67:1154.

610. Gullberg U, Nilsson E, Einhorn S, Olsson I. Combinations of interferon-gamma and retinoic acid or 1-alpha, 25-dihydroxycholecalciferol induce differentiation of the human monoblast leukemia cell line U-937. *Exp Hematol* 1985;13:675.

611. Francis GE, Guimaraes JETE, Berney JJ, Wing MA. Synergistic interaction between differentiation inducers and DNA synthesis inhibitors: a new approach to differentiation induction in myelodysplasia and acute myeloid leukaemia. *Leuk Res* 1985;9:573.

612. Kufe DW, Griffin JD, Spriggs DR. Cellular and clinical pharmacology of low-dose Ara-C. *Semin Oncol* 1985;12:200.

613. Kreis W, Chaudhri F, Chan K, et al. Pharmacokinetics of low-dose 1-beta-D-arabinofuranosylcytosine given by continuous intravenous infusion over twenty-one-days. *Cancer Res* 1985;45:6498.

614. Ishikura H, Sawada H, Okazaki T, et al. The effect of low dose ara-C in acute nonlymphoblastic leukemias and atypical leukaemia. *Br J Haematol* 1984;58:9.

615. Housset M, Daniel MT, Degos L. Small doses of ARA-C in the treatment of acute myeloid leukemia: differentiation of myeloid leukemia cells? *Br J Haematol* 1982;51:125.

616. Wisch JS, Griffin JD, Kufe DW. Response of preleukemic syndromes to continuous infusion of low-dose cytarabine. *N Engl J Med* 1983;309:1599.

617. Griffin JD, Spriggs DR, Wisch JS. Treatment of preleukemic syndromes with continuous intravenous infusion of low dose cytosine arabinoside. *J Clin Oncol* 1985;3:982.

618. Izumi Y, Sawada H, Okazaki T, et al. Favourable remission rate by repeating low dose ARA-C treatment in ANNL and RAEB. *Br J Haematol* 1985;61:187.

619. Castaigne S, Daniel MT, Tilly H, et al. Does treatment with ARA-C in low dosage cause differentiation of leukemic cells? *Blood* 1983;62:85.

620. Jehn U, DeBock R, Haanen C. Clinical trial of low-dose ara-C in the treatment of acute leukemia and myelodysplasia. *Blut* 1984;48:255.

621. Winter JN, Variakojis D, Gaynor ER, et al. Low-dose cytosine arabinoside (ara-C) therapy in the myelodysplastic syndromes and acute leukemia. *Cancer* 1985;56:443.

622. Tricot G, de Bock R, Dekker AW, et al. Low dose cytosine arabinoside (Ara C) in myelodysplastic syndromes. *Br J Haematol* 1984;58:231.

623. Alessandrino EP, Orlandi E, Brusamolino E, et al. Low-dose arabinosyl cytosine in acute leukemia after a myelodysplastic syndrome and in elderly leukemia. *Am J Hematol* 1985;20:191.

624. Desforges JF. Cytarabine: low-dose, high-dose, no dose? *N Engl J Med* 1983;309:1637.

625. Baccarani M, Zaccaria A, Bandini G, et al. Low dose arabinosyl cytosine for treatment of myelodysplastic syndromes and subacute myeloid leukemia. *Leuk Res* 1983;7:539.

626. Worsley A, Mufti GJ, Copplestone JA, et al. Very-low-dose cytarabine for myelodysplastic syndromes and acute myeloid leukaemia in the elderly. *Lancet* 1986;1:966.

627. Hwellstrom-Lindber E, Robert KH, Gahrton G, et al. A predictive model for the clinical response to low dose ara-C: a study of 102 patients with myelodysplastic syndrome or acute leukemia. *Br J Haematol* 1992;81:503.

628. Spitzer TR, Lazarus HM, Crum ED, Weisman R. Treatment of myelodysplastic syndromes with low-dose oral 6-thioguanine. *Med Pediatr Oncol* 1988;16:17.

629. Cheson BD. Standard and low-dose chemotherapy for the treatment of myelodysplastic syndromes. *Leuk Res* 1998;22(Suppl 1):S17-21.

630. Gold EJ, Mertelsmann RH, Itri LM, et al. Phase I clinical trial of 13-cis-retinoic acid in myelodysplastic syndromes. *Cancer Treat Rep* 1983;67:981.

631. Kerndrup G, Bendix-Hansen K, Pedersen B, et al. Primary myelodysplastic syndrome: treatment of 6 patients with 13-cis-retinoic acid. *Scand J Haematol* 1986;45:128.

632. Leoni F, Ciolli S, Longo G, et al. 13-cis-retinoic acid treatment in patients with myelodysplastic syndrome. *Acta Haematol* 1988;80:8.

633. Greenberg BR, Durie BGM, Barnett TC, Meyskens FL Jr. Phase I-II study of 13-cis-retinoic acid in myelodysplastic syndrome. *Cancer Treat Rep* 1985;69:1369.

634. Clark RE, Lush CJ, Jacobs A, Smith SA. Effect of 13-cis-retinoic acid on survival of patients with myelodysplastic syndrome. *Lancet* 1987;1:763.

635. Koeffler HP, Heitjan D, Mertelsmann R, et al. Randomized study of 13-cis retinoic acid v placebo in the myelodysplastic disorders. *Blood* 1988;71:703.

636. Jacobs A, Clark RE. 13-cis-retinoic acid v placebo in myelodysplasia. *Br J Haematol* 1988.

637. Blok WL, Lowenberg B, Sizoo W. Disappearance of trisomy 8 after alpha-2 interferon in a patient with myelodysplastic syndrome. *N Engl J Med* 1988;318:787.

638. Galvani DW, Nethersell ABW, Cawley JC. Alpha-interferon in myelodysplasia: clinical observations and effects on NK cells. *Leuk Res* 1988;12:257.

639. Hellstrom E, Robert K-H, Gahrton G, et al. Therapeutic effects of low-dose cytosine arabinoside, alpha-interferon, 1-alpha-hydroxyvitamin D3 and retinoic acid in acute leukemia and myelodysplastic syndromes. *Eur J Haematol* 1988;40:449.

640. Kornblith AB, Herndon JE, Silverman LR, et al. Impact of azacytidine on the quality of life of patients with myelodysplastic syndrome treated in a randomized phase III trial: a Cancer and Leukemia Group B study. *J Clin Oncol* 2002;20(10):2441–2452.

641. Silverman LR, Demakos EP, Peterson BL, et al. Randomized controlled trial of azacitidine in patients with the myelodysplastic syndrome: a study of the cancer and leukemia group B. *J Clin Oncol* 2002;20(10):2429–2440.

642. Bowen DT, Denzlinger C, Brugger W, et al. Poor response rate to a continuous schedule of Amifostine therapy for 'low/intermediate risk' myelodysplastic patients. *Br J Haematol* 1998;103(3):785–787.

643. List AF, Heaton R, Glinsmann-Gibson B, Capizzi RL. Amifostine protects primitive hematopoietic progenitors against chemotherapy cytotoxicity. *Semin Oncol* 1996;23(4 Suppl 8):58–63.

644. List AF, Brasfield F, Heaton R, et al. Stimulation of hematopoiesis by amifostine in patients with myelodysplastic syndrome. *Blood* 1997;90(9):3364–3369.

645. List AF. Use of amifostine in hematologic malignancies, myelodysplastic syndrome, and acute leukemia. *Semin Oncol* 1999;26(2 Suppl 7):61–65.

646. Groopman JE, Molina J, Scadden DT. Hematopoietic growth factors: biology and clinical applications. *N Engl J Med* 1989;321:1449.

647. Clark SC, Kamen R. The human hematopoietic colony-stimulating factors. *Science* 1987;236:1229.

648. Nienhuis A. Hematopoietic growth factors: biologic complexity and clinical promise. *N Engl J Med* 1988;318:916.

649. Delwel R, Salem M, Pellens C, et al. Growth regulation of human acute myeloid leukemia: effects of five recombinant hematopoietic factors in a serum-free culture system. *Blood* 1988;72:1944.

650. Vellenga E, Ostapovicz D, O'Rourke B, Griffin JD. Effects of recombinant IL-3, GM-CSF and G-CSF on proliferation of leukemic clonogenic cells in short-term and long-term cultures. *Leukemia* 1987;1:584.

651. Vellenga E, Young DC, Wagner K, et al. The effects of GM-CSF and G-CSF in promoting growth of clonogenic cells in acute myeloblastic leukemia. *Blood* 1987;69:1771.

652. Bruno E, Miller ME, Hoffman R. Interacting cytokines regulate in vitro human megakaryocytopoiesis. *Blood* 1989;73:671.

653. Ikebuchi K, Wong GG, Clark SC, et al. Interleukin 6 enhancement of interleukin 3-dependent proliferation of multipotential hemopoietic progenitors. *Proc Natl Acad Sci U S A* 1987;84:9035.

654. Donahue RE, Seehra J, Metzger M, et al. Human IL-3 and GM-CSF act synergistically in stimulating hematopoiesis in primates. *Science* 1988;241:1820.

655. Broxmeyer HE, Williams DE, Hangoc G, et al. Synergistic myelopoietic actions in vivo after administration to mice of combinations of purified natural murine colony-stimulating factor 1, recombinant murine interleukin 3, and recombinant murine granulocyte/macrophage colony-stimulating factor. *Proc Natl Acad Sci U S A* 1987;84:3871.

656. Vadhan-Raj S, Keating M, LeMaistre A, et al. Effects of recombinant human granulocyte-macrophage colony-stimulating factor in patients with myelodysplastic syndromes. *N Engl J Med* 1987;317:1546.

657. Antin JH, Smith BR, Holmes W, Rosenthal DS. Phase I/II study of recombinant human granulocyte-macrophage colony-stimulating factor in aplastic anemia and myelodysplastic syndrome. *Blood* 1988;72:705.

658. Ganser A, Volkers B, Greher J, et al. Recombinant human granulocyte-macrophage colony-stimulating factor in patients with myelodysplastic syndromes: a phase I/II trial. *Blood* 1989;73:31.

659. Estey EH, Kurzrock R, Talpaz M, et al. Effects of low doses of recombinant human granulocyte-macrophage colony stimulating factor (GM-CSF) in patients with myelodysplastic syndromes. *Br J Haematol* 1991;77:291.

660. Vadhan-Raj S, Broxmeyer HE, Spitzer G, et al. Stimulation of nonclonal hematopoiesis and suppression of the neoplastic clone after treatment with recombinant human granulocyte-macrophage colony-stimulating factor in a patient with therapy-related myelodysplastic syndrome. *Blood* 1989;74:1491.

661. Schuster MW, Larson RA, Thompson JA, et al. Granulocyte-macrophage colony-stimulating factor (GM-CSF) for myelodysplastic syndrome (MDS): results of a multi-center randomized controlled trial. *Blood* 1990;76:318a.

662. Negrin RS, Haeuber DH, Nagler A, et al. Treatment of myelodysplastic syndromes with recombinant human granulocyte colony-stimulating factor. *Ann Intern Med* 1989;110:976.

663. Kobayashi Y, Okabe T, Ozawa K, et al. Treatment of myelodysplastic syndromes with recombinant human granulocyte colony-stimulating factor: a preliminary report. *Am J Med* 1989;86:178.

664. Negrin RS, Haeuber DH, Nagler A, et al. Maintenance therapy of patients with myelodysplastic syndromes using recombinant human granulocyte colony-stimulating factor. *Blood* 1990;76:36.

665. Greenberg PL, Taylor K, Larson RA, et al. Phase III randomized multicenter trial of G-CSF vs observation for myelodysplastic syndromes. *Blood* 1993;82:196a.

666. Ganser A, Seipelt G, Lindemann A, et al. Effects of recombinant human interleukin-3 in patients with myelodysplastic syndromes. *Blood* 1990;76:455.

667. Ganser A, Bartram CR, Ottman OG, et al. Stimulation of non-clonal hematopoiesis in patients with hematological disorders by recombinant human GM-CSF or interleukin-3. *Blood* 1990;76:1449.

668. Sonoda Y, Yang Y, Wong GG, et al. Analysis in serum-free culture of the targets of recombinant human hemopoietic growth factors: interleukin 3 and granulocyte/macrophage-colony-stimulating factor are specific for early developmental stages. *Proc Natl Acad Sci U S A* 1988;85:4360.

668a. Nand S, Sosman J, Godwin JE, et al. A phase I/II study of sequential interleukin 3 and granulocyte-macrophage colony-stimulating factor in myelodysplastic syndromes. *Blood* 1994;83:357.

669. Rose EH, Abels RI, Nelson RA, McCullough DM, Lessin L. The use of r-HuEpo in the treatment of anaemia related to myelodysplasia (MDS). *Br J Haematol* 1995;89(4):831–837.

670. Greenberg PL, Bishop M, Deeg J, et al. NCCN practice guidelines for the myelodysplastic syndromes. *Oncology* 1998;12:53–80.

671. Miller K. Erythropoietin, with and without granulocyte-colony stimulating factor (G-CSF), in the treatment of myelodysplastic syndrome (MDS) patients. *Leuk Res* 1998;22(Suppl 1):S13–S16.

672. Ganser A. Hematopoietic growth factors in the treatment of the myelodysplastic syndromes. *Curr Opin Hematol* 1995;2(3):204–209.

673. Seipelt G, Ottmann OG, Hoelzer D. Cytokine therapy for myelodysplastic syndrome. *Curr Opin Hematol* 2000;7(3):156–160.

674. Mantovani L, Lentini G, Hentschel B, et al. Treatment of anaemia in myelodysplastic syndromes with prolonged administration of recombinant human granulocyte colony-stimulating factor and erythropoietin. *Br J Haematol* 2000;109(2):367–375.

675. Remacha AF, Arrizabalaga B, Villegas A, et al. Erythropoietin plus granulocyte colony-stimulating factor in the treatment of myelodysplastic syndromes. Identification of a subgroup of responders. The Spanish Erythropathology Group. *Haematologica* 1999;84(12):1058–1064.

676. Hellstrom-Lindberg E, Ahlgren T, Beguin Y, et al. Treatment of anemia in myelodysplastic syndromes with granulocyte colony-stimulating factor plus erythropoietin: results from a randomized phase II study and long-term follow-up of 71 patients. *Blood* 1998;92(1):68–75.

677. Negrin RS, Stein R, Doherty K, et al. Maintenance treatment of the anemia of myelodysplastic syndromes with recombinant human granulocyte colony-stimulating factor and erythropoietin: evidence for in vivo synergy. *Blood* 1996;87(10):4076–4081.

678. Hellstrom-Lindberg E, Birgegard G, Carlsson M, et al. A combination of granulocyte colony-stimulating factor and erythropoietin may synergistically improve the anaemia in patients with myelodysplastic syndromes. *Leuk Lymphoma* 1993;11(3–4):221–228.

679. Negrin RS, Stein R, Vardiman J, et al. Treatment of the anemia of myelodysplastic syndromes using recombinant human granulocyte colony-stimulating factor in combination with erythropoietin. *Blood* 1993;82(3):737–743.

680. Thompson JA, Gilliland DG, Prchal JT, et al. Effect of recombinant human erythropoietin combined with granulocyte/macrophage colony-stimulating factor in the treatment of patients with myelodysplastic syndrome. GM/EPO MDS Study Group. *Blood* 2000;95(4):1175–1179.

681. Kaushansky K. Use of thrombopoietic growth factors in acute leukemia. *Leukemia* 2000;14(3):505–508.

682. Rosenfeld C, List A. A hypothesis for the pathogenesis of myelodysplastic syndromes: implications for new therapies. *Leukemia* 2000;14(1):2–8.

683. Dansey R. Myelodysplasia. *Curr Opin Oncol* 2000;12(1):13–21.

684. Barrett J, Saunthararajah Y, Molldrem J. Myelodysplastic syndrome and aplastic anemia: distinct entities or diseases linked by a common pathophysiology? *Semin Hematol* 2000;37(1):15–29.

685. Itoh M, Yago K, Shimada H, Tohyama K. Reversible acceleration of disease progression following cyclosporin A treatment in a patient with myelodysplastic syndrome. *Int J Hematol* 2002;75(3):302–304.

686. Cheson BD, Zwiebel JA, Dancey J, Murgo A. Novel therapeutic agents for the treatment of myelodysplastic syndromes. *Semin Oncol* 2000;27(5):560–577.

687. Minucci S, Nervi C, Lo Coco F, Pelicci PG. Histone deacetylases: a common molecular target for differentiation treatment of acute myeloid leukemias? *Oncogene* 2001;20(24):3110–3115.

688. Kouides PA, Bennett JM. Advances in the therapy of the myelodysplastic syndromes. *Cancer Treat Res* 1999;99:335–362.

689. Matthews DC. Immunotherapy in acute myelogenous leukemia and myelodysplastic syndrome. *Leukemia* 1998;12(Suppl 1):S33–S36.

690. Forman SJ. Myelodysplastic syndrome. *Curr Opin Hematol* 1996;3(4):297–302.

691. Oosterveld M, de Witte T. Intensive treatment strategies in patients with high-risk myelodysplastic syndrome and secondary acute myeloid leukemia. *Blood Rev* 2000;14(4):182–189.

692. Anderson JE, Appelbaum FR. Myelodysplasia and myeloproliferative disorders. *Curr Opin Hematol* 1997;4(4):261–267.

693. Deeg HJ, Appelbaum FR. Hemopoietic stem cell transplantation for myelodysplastic syndrome. *Curr Opin Oncol* 2000;12(2):116–120.

694. Boogaerts MA. Stem cell transplantation and intensified cytotoxic treatment for myelodysplasia. *Curr Opin Hematol* 1998;5(6):465-471.

695. Margolis J, Borrello I, Flinn IW. New approaches to treating malignances with stem cell transplantation. *Semin Oncol* 2000;27(5):524–530.

696. De Witte T. Stem cell transplantation for patients with myelodysplastic syndrome and secondary leukemias. *Int J Hematol* 2000;72(2):151–156.

697. Anderson JE. Bone marrow transplantation for myelodysplasia. *Blood Rev* 2000;14(2):63–77.

698. Anderson JE, Appelbaum FR, Fisher LD, et al. Allogeneic bone marrow transplantation for 93 patients with myelodysplastic syndrome. *Blood* 1993;82(2):677–681.

699. Anderson JE, Anasetti C, Appelbaum FR, Schoch G, Gooley TA, Hansen JA, et al. Unrelated donor marrow transplantation for myelodysplasia (MDS) and MDS-related acute myeloid leukaemia. *Br J Haematol* 1996;93(1):59–67.

700. Anderson JE, Appelbaum FR, Schoch G, et al. Allogeneic marrow transplantation for myelodysplastic syndrome with advanced disease morphology: a phase II study of busulfan, cyclophosphamide, and total-body irradiation and analysis of prognostic factors. *J Clin Oncol* 1996;14(1):220–226.

701. Anderson JE, Appelbaum FR, Schoch G, et al. Allogeneic marrow transplantation for refractory anemia: a comparison of two preparative regimens and analysis of prognostic factors. *Blood* 1996;87(1):51–58.

702. Deeg HJ, Shulman HM, Anderson JE, et al. Allogeneic and syngeneic marrow transplantation for myelodysplastic syndrome in patients 55 to 66 years of age. *Blood* 2000;95(4):1188–1194.

703. de Witte T, Suciu S, Verhoef G, et al. Intensive chemotherapy followed by allogeneic or autologous stem cell transplantation for patients with myelodysplastic syndromes (MDSs) and acute myeloid leukemia following MDS. *Blood* 2001;98(8):2326–2331.

704. van der Weide M, Sizoo W, Krefft J, Langenhuijsen MMAC. Myelodysplastic syndromes: analysis of morphological features related to the FAB-classification. *Eur J Haematol* 1988;41:58.

705. Weatherall DJ, Pembrey ME, Hall EG, et al. Familial sideroblastic anaemia: problem of Xg and X chromosome inactivation. *Lancet* 1970;2:744.

706. Hast R, Miale T, Westin J, et al. Hereditary ring sideroblastic anaemia and Christmas disease in a Swedish family. *Scand J Haematol* 1983;30:444.

707. van Waveren Hogervorst GD, van Roermund HPC, Snijders PJ. Hereditary sideroblastic anaemia and autosomal inheritance of erythrocyte dimorphism in a Dutch family. *Eur J Haematol* 1987;38:405.

708. Claustres M, Vannereau H, Bellet J, et al. A paediatric case of sideroblastic anaemia: ultrastructural studies of erythroblasts cultured from marrow BFU-E in a methylcellulose micromethod. *Eur J Pediatr* 1986;145:422.

709. Patterson WP, Winkelmann M, Perry MC. Zinc-induced copper deficiency: megamineral sideroblastic anemia. *Ann Intern Med* 1985;103:385.

CHAPTER 12

Myeloproliferative Disorders

Jerry L. Spivak

The chronic myeloproliferative disorders—polycythemia vera, idiopathic myelofibrosis, essential thrombocytosis, and chronic myelogenous leukemia (CML)—have been traditionally classified together (1) because they share a clonal origin in a multipotent hematopoietin progenitor cell, overproduction of one or more of the formed elements of the blood in the absence of a physiologic stimulus, and extramedullary hematopoiesis. Of the four disorders, only CML has a defined molecular defect, the 9-22 translocation, a unique cytogenetic abnormality (2), and, as a consequence, the constitutively active chimeric tyrosine kinase bcr-abl, that is necessary for disease activity (3). CML also differs from the other chronic myeloproliferative disorders because it has a shorter clinical course and, inevitably, terminates in acute leukemia or refractory bone marrow failure, whereas the others may not. Although it was once thought that polycythemia vera, idiopathic myelofibrosis, essential thrombocytosis, and CML were interrelated, we now understand that this contention was due to phenotypic mimicry, and that each disorder is not only a separate entity, but evolution into CML is not a clinical feature of any of the other three disorders (4), which are the subject of this chapter and, appropriately, considered separately from CML.

The major impediment to understanding the chronic myeloproliferative disorders is their low incidence, which has denied most physicians the opportunity to become familiar with them, promoted reliance on clinical anecdote, hindered basic research into molecular mechanisms, and prevented the development of evidence-based therapy.

POLYCYTHEMIA VERA

Polycythemia vera is the most common of the chronic myeloproliferative disorders and is characterized by the overproduction of morphologically normal red cells, white cells, and platelets and extramedullary hematopoiesis, most prominently in the spleen, to the exclusion of normal (polyclonal) hematopoiesis. Although first described in 1892 by the French physician Vaquez (5), widespread attention to the disorder did not occur until Osler's seminal publication in 1903 (6), and it is ironic that ten decades later little has changed with respect to the diagnostic criteria for the disease, and we are not closer to understanding its molecular basis.

Epidemiology

The incidence of polycythemia vera is approximately 2/100,000 (7), although estimates from 1/100,000 (8) to greater than 18/100,000 (7,9) have been made depending on the population studied and its age. Rare in children (10), polycythemia vera spares no age group among adults, although its peak frequency occurs in the fifth and sixth decades (8,9). There is a slight male predominance at 1.3:1, which is not seen for secondary forms of erythrocytosis. Polycythemia vera occurs in all ethnic groups but is less common in African-Americans and Asians than in Caucasians (11), and there appears to be a predilection for Ashkenazi Jews (12). Familial occurrence has been documented but is uncommon (13–18).

Pathogenesis

Hematopoiesis is the orderly, continuous process by which primitive, uncommitted hematopoietic progenitor cells give rise to the mature blood cells that transport oxygen, defend against microbial invasion, and promote hemostasis. Hematopoiesis is clonal (Fig. 12-1) and, normally, polyclonal with more than one pluripotent hematopoietic stem cell giving rise to the cells responsible for populating the bone marrow and the peripheral blood. In polycythemia vera, as well as the other chronic myeloproliferative disorders, hematopoiesis is monoclonal with a single pluripotent hematopoietic stem cell that gives rise to the cells populating the peripheral blood (Table 12-1). This observation, originally established using informative female patients with polycythemia vera who were heterozygous for the expression of glucose-6-phosphate dehydrogenase (G6PD) isoenzymes (19), has been confirmed using other X chromosome–linked DNA polymorphisms (20). A characteristic feature of hematopoiesis in polycythemia vera, as well as the other chronic myeloproliferative disorders, is clonal dominance, whereby the contribution of normal (polyclonal) pluripotent hematopoietic stem cells to hematopoiesis is suppressed over time until only the progeny of the abnormal clone are present in the peripheral blood (19), although normal hematopoietic progenitor cells persist in the bone marrow (21). The mechanism for this is unknown but could be due to the production of inhibitory factors by the malignant clone (22) or a differential sensitivity of the clonal hematopoietic progenitor cells to hematopoietic growth factors such as insulin-like growth factor (IGF)-1 (23). Because it involves a multipotent hematopoietic progenitor cell, the hallmark of polycythemia vera is multilineage hematopoietic cell hyperplasia. Erythrocytosis, however, is its most important clinical manifestation—the basis for its most common clinical complications and the essential requirement for its diagnosis (24). Thus, with respect to its pathogenesis, most investigations of polycythemia vera have focused on erythropoiesis.

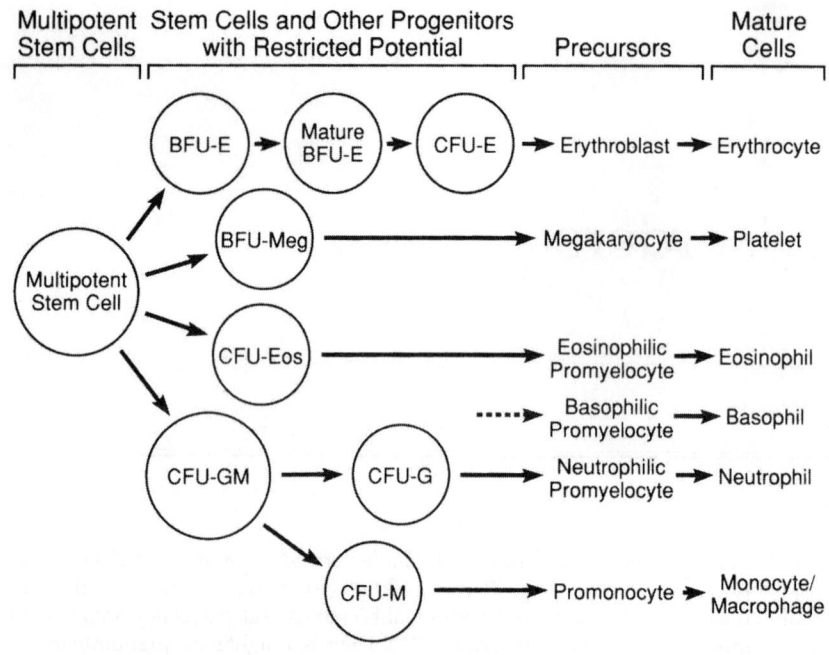

Figure 12-1. Current model of the cellular compartments in hematopoiesis. BFU-E, burst-forming unit erythrocyte; BFU-Meg, burst-forming unit megakaryocyte; CFU-E, colony-forming unit erythrocyte; CFU-Eos, colony-forming unit eosinophil; CFU-M, colony-forming unit megakaryocyte; CFU-G, colony-forming unit granulocyte; CFU-GM colony-forming unit granulocyte-macrophage. (After Stamatoyannopoulos G, Nienhuis AW. Hemoglobin switching. In: Stamatoyannopoulos G, Nienhuis AW, Leder P, et al., eds. *The molecular basis of blood diseases.* Philadelphia: WB Saunders, 1987:85.)

Red cell lifespan is not prolonged in polycythemia vera (25), nor is the erythroid progenitor cell pool expanded at the expense of the myeloid progenitor cell pool (26). Within the physiologic range of the erythropoietin dose-response curve, polycythemia vera erythroid progenitor cells respond like normal erythroid progenitor cells (27). At the same time, neither hyperoxia (28) nor renal failure (29) suppresses erythropoiesis *in vivo* in polycythemia vera patients, serum erythropoietin levels are lower than in any other disease (Fig. 12-2), and *in vitro*, polycythemia vera erythroid progenitor cells appear to be hypersensitive to erythropoietin or capable of proliferation in its absence (27,30). Indeed, this unusual behavior has been used as a diagnostic test to establish the presence of the disorder when, in fact, it is an *in vitro* artifact. In serum-free cultures, polycythemia vera erythroid progenitor cells are not more sensitive to erythropoietin than normal erythroid progenitor cells but, rather, are more sensitive to IGF-1 (23). Furthermore, the ability to proliferate *in vitro* in the absence of erythropoietin does not define the limits of the abnormal clone because not all polycythemia vera erythroid progenitor cells display this behavior (31). Primitive polycythemia vera erythroid progenitor cells exhibiting either erythropoietin independence or dependence could give rise to both erythropoietin-independent or -dependent progeny (31) and this characteristic remained fixed when these progenitor cells were analyzed in long-term *in vitro* cultures. It is also important to note that the *in vitro* proliferation of polycythemia vera erythroid progenitor cells in the absence of erythropoietin was not robust (31), which may be due to the tendency of these cells to differentiate faster *in vitro* in the absence of erythropoietin (32). This could provide these progenitor cells an advantage in the low erythropoietin milieu that characterizes polycythemia vera. The growth factor hypersensitivity of polycythemia vera erythroid progenitor cells is not limited to IGF-1 but extends to interleukin (IL)-3, granulocyte-macrophage colony-stimulating factor (GM-CSF) (33), and stem cell factor (SCF) (34).

The *in vitro* hypersensitivity of polycythemia vera erythroid progenitor cells to multiple hematopoietic growth factors has led

---

TABLE 12-1. Relative Amounts of Glucose-6-Phosphate Dehydrogenase Isoenzymes in Various Mesenchymal Tissues in Two Patients with Polycythemia Vera

Tissue	%A:%B	
	Case 1	Case 2
Skin	55:45	55:45
Lymphocytes	85:15[a]	55:45
Erythrocytes	100:0	100:0
Granulocytes	100:0	100:0
Platelets	100:0	100:0

[a]Contaminated with erythrocytes.
From Adamson JW, Fialkow PJ, Murphy S, et al. Polycythemia vera: stem-cell and probable clonal origin of the disease. *N Engl J Med* 1976;295:913–916.

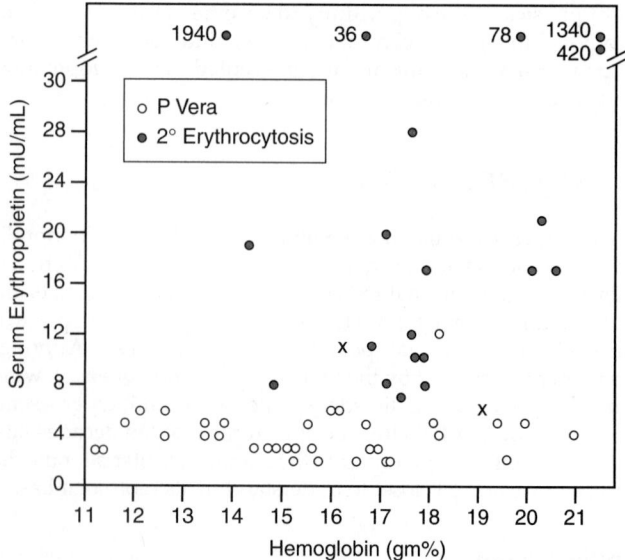

Figure 12-2. Serum immunoreactive erythropoietin in patients with polycythemia vera (○), pseudoerythrocytosis (X), and various forms of secondary erythrocytosis (●). The range of normal is 4–26 mU/mL.

to an examination of hematopoietic growth factor receptor function in these cells. This approach was also supported by the observations that mutations within the ligand-binding domain of the erythropoietin receptor led to its constitutive activation, whereas truncation of its cytoplasmic domain caused erythropoietin hypersensitivity (35). Importantly, a form of familial erythrocytosis is characterized by deletion of 41 to 90 amino acids in the terminal portion of the erythropoietin receptor cytoplasmic domain (36). Interestingly, this type of C-terminal truncation, which involves a region rich in tyrosines, was initially thought to release the receptor from the negative regulatory effect of the tyrosine phosphatase SHP-1. However, it has subsequently been demonstrated that erythropoietin receptors with this type of truncation are actually hyposensitive to erythropoietin and hypersensitive to IGF-1 (37). Studies of erythropoietin receptor expression and ligand binding by polycythemia vera erythroid progenitor cells were also not different from normal (38), nor have amplification, rearrangements, or functional mutations of the erythropoietin receptor been identified in polycythemia vera patients (39). Importantly, forced expression of a normal erythropoietin receptor in primitive hematopoietic progenitor cells neither led to autonomous proliferation nor stimulated trilineage hematopoietic cell hyperplasia (40), which are essential features of polycythemia vera; although expression of a constitutively active erythropoietin receptor caused both erythrocytosis and thrombocytosis, myeloid hyperplasia was not induced (41). Finally, no difference in the behavior of the receptors for IL-3 or SCF has been observed in polycythemia vera erythroid progenitor cells as compared to normal (42,43).

Although the erythropoietin receptor cannot be implicated in the pathogenesis of polycythemia vera, two candidate receptors that can are the IGF-1 receptor and the thrombopoietin receptor Mpl. Polycythemia vera erythroid progenitor cells were hypersensitive to IGF-1 (23), whereas the IGF-1 receptors of polycythemia vera peripheral blood mononuclear cells were constitutively tyrosine phosphorylated and more sensitive to IGF-1 than normal peripheral blood mononuclear cells (44). The serum concentration of IGF-1 binding protein 1 was also increased in polycythemia vera patients, and this protein could stimulate erythroid burst proliferation *in vitro* (45). IGF-1 is an antiapoptotic factor, and this could explain the ability of erythroid progenitor cells to survive in the absence of erythropoietin.

Mpl is a candidate receptor in the pathogenesis of polycythemia vera for several reasons. It is expressed in pluripotent hematopoietic stem cells (46) as well as megakaryocytes, platelets (47), and erythroid progenitor cells (48), and its cognate ligand thrombopoietin enhanced the survival of these cells (49). Thrombopoietin can also act synergistically with IL-3 and SCF to promote the proliferation of pluripotent hematopoietic stem cells (50) and the production of myeloid cells (51). Exposure to excessive concentrations of thrombopoietin in mice caused granulocytosis, thrombocytosis, osteomyelofibrosis, and extramedullary hematopoiesis (52,53), whereas ectopic Mpl expression caused fatal erythroblastosis (54). Importantly, the retroviral myeloproliferative leukemia virus (MPLV), which encodes a truncated Mpl gene fused with a viral envelope protein gene (55), induced a syndrome in mice mimicking polycythemia vera (56), whereas hematopoietic progenitor cells infected with MPLV were growth factor independent *in vitro* and capable of terminal differentiation in the absence of growth factors (55). Finally, recent studies have demonstrated that Mpl expression in polycythemia vera megakaryocytes and platelets was defective due to impaired posttranslational glycosylation that became more severe with disease duration and extent (57,58). However, the molecular basis for these latter observations and their role in the pathogenesis of polycythemia vera remains to be determined.

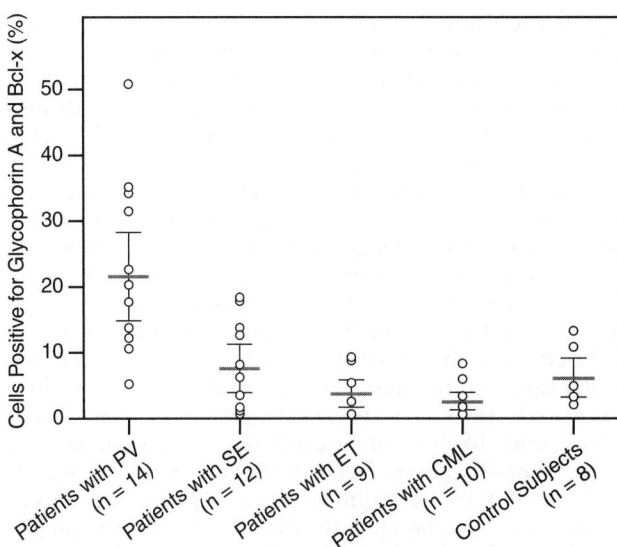

Figure 12-3. Mean (± standard deviation) percentage of glycophorin A–positive cells expressing Bcl-x in bone marrow of patients with polycythemia vera (PV), secondary erythrocytosis (SE), essential thrombocythemia (ET), or chronic myeloid leukemia (CML) and control subjects. The results were obtained by flow cytometry. (Modified from Silva M, Richard C, Benito A, et al. Expression of Bcl-x in erythroid precursors from patients with polycythemia vera. *N Engl J Med* 1998;338:564–571.)

Although a number of nonrandom cytogenetic defects principally involving chromosomes 1, 8, 9, 13, or 20 have been documented in polycythemia vera, these were present in less than 20% of patients at the time of diagnosis (59) and were not specific for polycythemia vera, and extensive analysis of the deleted portions of the long arm of chromosome 20 has failed, to date, to identify the loss of a specific tumor suppressor gene (60). In addition, expression of a cytogenetic abnormality was not always consistent within the malignant clone (61), suggesting that such abnormalities were secondary events. No abnormalities of p53 or the RAS gene family (62) have been observed in polycythemia vera, and, although calcitonin gene hypermethylation has been observed, this has not been a consistent observation, particularly early in the disease (63). Analysis of the gene for SHP-1, a negative regulatory tyrosine phosphatase, has also failed to define any abnormalities (64).

Perhaps the most important advance to date with respect to the molecular mechanisms involved in the pathogenesis of polycythemia vera has been the observation that erythroid progenitor cells in this disorder overexpress Bcl-xl, an antiapoptotic member of the Bcl-2 family (65) (Fig. 12-3). Under normal circumstances, early erythroid progenitor cells are largely dormant and require erythropoietin as a mitogen for entry into the cell cycle (66); late erythroid progenitor cells [colony-forming unit erythrocytes (CFU-E)] are, largely, cycling and require erythropoietin for their survival (67). Deprivation of erythropoietin caused cycling erythroid progenitor cells to arrest in G_0/G_1 (68), down-regulated Bcl-2 and Bcl-xl, and activated programmed cell death (69). Overexpression of either Bcl-2 or Bcl-xl permitted erythroid progenitor cells to maintain their viability and differentiate in the absence of erythropoietin (69). Similar behavior has been observed with multipotent hematopoietic progenitor cells overexpressing Bcl-2 (70). *In vitro* in the absence of serum, these cells arrested in a G_0/G_1 state and spontaneously differentiated in a stochastic fashion into erythroid, myeloid, or megakaryocytic lineages (70), mimicking the behavior of polycythemia vera cells.

A significant feature of Bcl-2 overexpression was prolongation of the G_1 phase of the cell cycle (70). Importantly, in this regard, the duration of G_1 in erythroid progenitor cells appears to be erythropoietin dependent; low concentrations of erythropoietin were associated with G_1 prolongation and initiation of differentiation, whereas higher concentrations caused G_1 shortening and cell proliferation (71). Therefore, Bcl-xl overexpression could explain the observed *in vitro* behavior of polycythemia vera erythroid progenitor cells, which not only differentiate faster than their normal counterparts but also survive longer in the absence of erythropoietin. It could explain their growth advantage *in vivo* where erythropoietin production is suppressed because both situations promote G_1 arrest and terminal differentiation. Because there is no difference in the cell cycle behavior of normal and polycythemia vera erythroid progenitor cells nor in the proportion of cells in cycle, the excess of erythroid cells that defines this disorder is more likely a consequence of cell accumulation than rapid cell proliferation. This contention is consistent with the incremental nature of erythrocytosis in polycythemia vera, because only a fraction (5% to 25%) of the erythroid progenitor cell population exhibited erythropoietin independence, and expression of this behavior appeared to be random (31). The molecular basis for Bcl-xl overexpression in polycythemia vera is unknown, but could be linked to IGF-1 hypersensitivity (23). Whether resistance to apoptosis is a feature of myelopoiesis or thrombopoiesis in this disease remains to be determined.

Clinical Manifestations

SYMPTOMS

With few exceptions, the presenting clinical manifestations of polycythemia vera, although they largely reflect the elevated red cell mass, are nonspecific and nondiagnostic (Table 12-2). Generalized weakness and fatigue are the most common symptoms, followed closely by headache, dizziness, vertigo, hemorrhage, dyspnea, abdominal pain, and scotomata or blurred vision (72). Pruritus, usually aquagenic, is a distinctive feature of polycythemia vera, occurring in approximately 30% of patients; extremity pain or paresthesias, usually due to erythromelalgia or circulatory stasis, and joint complaints, due to hyperuricemia, are other symptoms directly related to the disease, but, when they occur alone, their diagnostic significance is frequently overlooked. A history of thrombosis is not uncommon and may extend back as far as 5 years before diagnosis (73). Less common symptoms are weight loss, dyspepsia, and chest pain. If iron deficiency due to gastrointestinal blood loss is present, patients may experience pica, the abnormal gustatory craving for substances such as ice (pagophagia) or particular foods (74), but patients usually do not mention such behavior unless asked.

TABLE 12-2. Presenting Symptoms in Polycythemia Vera

	Percentage (%)	Range
Weakness or fatigue	51	31–66
Headache	50	31–90
Dizziness or vertigo	48	28–70
Bleeding or bruising	34	30–40
Dyspnea	31	17–40
Abdominal pain	30	23–50
Visual symptoms	29	7–37
Paresthesias or extremity pain	27	13–60
Pruritus	27	10–50
Thrombosis	26	17–45
Dyspepsia	13	8–19

TABLE 12-3. Laboratory Abnormalities in Polycythemia Vera

	Percentage (%)	Range
Erythrocytosis	91	88–99
Leukocytosis	67	43–84
Thrombocytosis	52	40–63
Reticulocytosis	35	6–54
Elevated leukocyte alkaline phosphatase	81	63–100

SIGNS

Because of its insidious nature, polycythemia vera is frequently recognized incidentally in the course of routine examination or diagnostic evaluation for an unrelated condition. Arterial or venous thrombosis may be the presenting manifestation of the disease; no area of the vasculature is spared, but the cerebral and abdominal vasculature is particularly at risk (75,76). Indeed, polycythemia vera is the most common cause of hepatic vein thrombosis in the western hemisphere (77). This may be the first manifestation of the illness and a catastrophic one to which younger patients, particularly women, are prone (78). Plethora of the skin and mucous membranes, conjunctival and retinal venous engorgement, acne rosacea, and systolic and diastolic hypertension are other manifestations of the elevated red cell mass. Easy bruising, epistaxis, gingival bleeding, or upper gastrointestinal hemorrhage are not infrequent, and, as a consequence of chronic blood loss, patients may initially present with iron deficiency anemia in the setting of splenomegaly. The hemorrhagic tendency may be a consequence of vascular damage due to circulatory stasis, severe thrombocytosis with consumption of large-molecular-weight von Willebrand's factor (vWF) multimers (79), or peptic ulceration or gastritis due to excess histamine or cytokine release by basophils and other leukocytes (80). Gouty arthritis or renal stone formation can also be early manifestations of the illness (81).

The most common physical abnormality is splenomegaly, which is present in approximately 70% of patients at the time of diagnosis and is usually modest in extent. Hepatomegaly is found in approximately 30% of patients (72) but not in the absence of splenomegaly. Lymphadenopathy is not a feature of polycythemia vera. It is noteworthy that splenomegaly is most frequent in young individuals, particularly women (82), in whom hepatic vein thrombosis may be the presenting manifestation (7).

LABORATORY ABNORMALITIES

An absolute erythrocytosis is the hallmark of polycythemia vera and is present in virtually every patient at diagnosis (Table 12-3); exceptions are usually the consequence of bleeding leading to iron deficiency anemia, but, occasionally, patients present initially with isolated leukocytosis (83) or thrombocytosis (84). Although trilineage hematopoietic cell hyperplasia is the defining characteristic of polycythemia vera, an increase in red cells, white cells, and platelets is seen at first presentation in only 40% of patients (9,85) (Table 12-4), whereas isolated erythrocytosis and combinations of erythrocytosis and leukocytosis or thrombocytosis are encountered at lesser frequencies. The reticulocyte count is mildly elevated in more than 50% of patients, and the leukocyte alkaline phosphatase is elevated in 70% (86). The MCV can be normal or low, but the combination of microcytic erythrocytosis associated with polycythemia vera or erythropoietin-driven erythrocytosis will not be confused with the microcytic erythrocytosis due to the thalassemia trait if one remembers that, in the latter, the red cell distribution width is normal, whereas in the former disorders, it is elevated (87). This

TABLE 12-4. Presenting Blood Counts in Polycythemia Vera

Normal WBC and Platelets (%)	Elevated WBC and Platelets (%)	Elevated WBC (%)	Elevated Platelets (%)
17[a]	38	29	16
18[b]	40	31	11
12[c]	43	15	26

WBC, white blood cell.

[a]From Berglund S, Zettervall O. Incidence of polycythemia vera in a defined population. *Eur J Haematol* 1992;48:20–26.
[b]From Szur L, Lewis SM, Goolden AWG. Polycythemia vera and its treatment with radioactive phosphorus. *QJM* 1959;397–424.
[c]Author's data.

is because iron deficiency causes anisocytosis as well as microcytosis, but the thalassemia trait usually does not.

The leukocyte count is usually between 10,000 and 20,000/mm³ at the time of diagnosis and rarely greater than 30,000/mm³ initially (72,85). Mature neutrophils predominate; myelocytes are present in low numbers in 20% to 40% of patients, but blast cells and nucleated red cells are uncommon unless the disorder presents with myelofibrosis (88), in which case there is a leukoerythroblastic blood picture replete with teardrop-shaped red cells. However, perhaps the most striking feature of the blood smear in newly diagnosed polycythemia vera is red cell crowding. Although not specific for this cause of erythrocytosis, the sea of red cells, edge to edge, is sufficiently striking on a well-made blood smear to demand a red cell mass determination.

Other laboratory abnormalities in polycythemia vera include elevation of the serum vitamin B_{12} level to greater than 900 pg/mL and an elevated saturated B_{12}-binding capacity (>2000 pg/mL) (86), primarily due to an elevation of TC III (89). Elevation of serum histamine also occurs, but its clinical significance is unclear because similar elevations occur in CML patients who do not have pruritus (80). Hyperuricemia occurs in approximately 30% of patients (72), but it is generally more marked later in the illness with the development of extramedullary hematopoiesis than in its beginning (81). Arterial oxygen saturation is greater than 92% in virtually all patients (90), but a few patients with coexisting emphysema have been described (91). The serum erythropoietin level is characteristically more depressed in this illness than in any other, but a low to normal serum erythropoietin level can be seen with other forms of erythrocytosis, including those due to hypoxia (92) (Fig. 12.2 and Fig. 12-4). Due to the expansion of hematopoiesis, the basal metabolic rate can be elevated in these patients (72).

The bone marrow in untreated polycythemia vera is typically hypercellular (>80% as compared with 60% normally) with a reduction in fat cells, an increase in erythroid precursors, and an increase in megakaryocyte number and size (93,94). Bone marrow–stainable iron is typically decreased or absent. However, in 10% to 20% of patients, bone marrow cellularity was normal at the time of diagnosis, and these patients did not differ clinically from those with a hypercellular bone marrow (88,93). A small proportion of patients with polycythemia vera present with a bone marrow histology that is compatible with idiopathic myelofibrosis (88,95). In the Polycythemia Vera Study Group (PVSG) analysis, a substantial increase in bone marrow reticulin was present in 11% of patients at the time of diagnosis (93), but this had no prognostic significance. It should be emphasized, however, that an increase in reticulin is not synonymous with myelofibrosis, which requires collagen deposition and disruption of marrow architecture (95). In polycythemia vera, the increase in reticulin usually is proportional

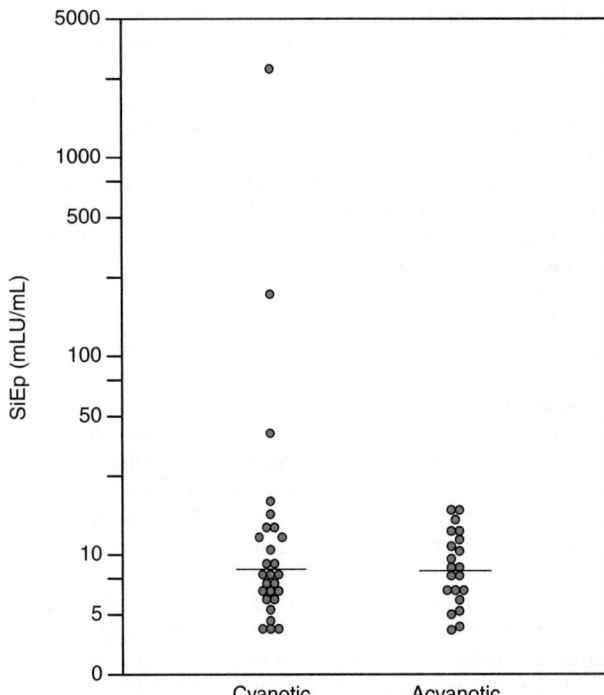

Figure 12-4. Serum immunoreactive erythropoietin (SiEp) levels in 27 cyanotic and 21 acyanotic children with congenital heart disease. Horizontal lines depict the geometric mean values for the two groups (the two highest values in the cyanotic group were omitted in the statistical evaluation). (Modified from Haga P, Cotes PM, Till JA, et al. Serum immunoreactive erythropoietin in children with cyanotic and acyanotic congenital heart disease. *Blood* 1987;70:822–826.)

to the degree of bone marrow cellularity. Because marrow cellularity correlates with the hematocrit and with splenomegaly (95), it is clear that an increase in reticulin per se is not necessarily associated with impaired bone marrow function, contrary to some contentions (96).

COAGULATION ABNORMALITIES

Polycythemia vera shares abnormalities of platelet structure and function with its companion myeloproliferative disorders. None is specific for a particular myeloproliferative disorder, and most correlate poorly with the propensity to hemorrhage and thrombosis that is characteristic of these disorders. The most common abnormality was defective platelet aggregation in response to adenosine diphosphate (ADP), epinephrine or collagen, alone or in combination (97). The bleeding time was prolonged in approximately 20% of patients without correlation with platelet aggregation defects or the platelet count (97). Platelet hyperfunction was observed in the form of spontaneous platelet aggregation (98), increased *in vivo* thromboxane biosynthesis (99), increased expression of platelet activation markers such as P-selectin, thrombospondin, and glycoprotein (GP) IV (100), and increased fibrinogen turnover (101); expression of platelet GPs Ib, IIb, and IIIa, however, was reduced (100), but there was an increased affinity of platelets for fibrinogen (102). Evidence of storage pool defects was reflected morphologically by a reduction in platelet-dense bodies and alpha granules as well as reduced intraplatelet levels of β-thromboglobulin, platelet factor 4 (PF4), platelet-derived growth factor (PDGF), fibrinogen, vWF, ADP, and 5-hydroxytyramine (103–107). Uptake and storage of the latter were also impaired (103). Loss of prostaglandin D_2 (PGD_2) receptors (108) and impaired lipoxygenase activity (109) are other platelet abnormalities, the etiology of which is unknown. Evidence for increased platelet turnover was observed in some studies (110) but not in others (111), and the ability of monocytes to increase tissue factor production on exposure to endotoxin *in vitro* was also increased (112). Given the morphologic abnormalities observed in myeloproliferative disorder megakaryocytes such as reduced alpha granule content, a disordered canalicular system, dilatation of the dense tubular system, and increased endoplasmic reticulum (113), it is likely that some of the platelet defects observed are intrinsic to the disorder. Other abnormalities, however, such as decreased platelet alpha granule content, may be exacerbated by extrinsic factors because improvement—although not complete correction—was observed after phlebotomy (104,114). Whether this was due to reduced interaction of the platelets with the vessel wall with the reduction in red cell mass (115) is unknown.

Although high-molecular-weight vWF multimers can be reduced with extremely high platelet counts, leading to impaired ristocetin cofactor activity (79), and homocysteine elevations (116), possibly due to folic acid deficiency, have been observed, there is no consistent evidence of underlying defects of coagulation proteins (117).

However, it must be remembered that when erythrocytosis is uncorrected, coagulation tests can be prolonged simply because the ratio of anticoagulant to plasma in polycythemic blood is greater than when the red cell mass is normal. As a consequence, because many patients with polycythemia vera are undertreated with respect to phlebotomy, if they are given coumadin therapy, such patients will also be undertreated with respect to their anticoagulation therapy because of artificial prolongation of the prothrombin time.

CYTOGENETICS

Nonrandom chromosome abnormalities are present in up to 17% of untreated patients at the time of diagnosis (59,118) and appear in more than 50% of patients sometime during the course of the disease. The most frequently observed cytogenetic abnormalities were trisomy 8, trisomy 9, trisomy 1q, and trisomy 9p, 12q⁻, 13q⁻ and 12p⁻; balanced translocations [t(1:3), t(1;5) and t(6:12)] have also been documented. A correlation does not exist between the presence of a cytogenetic abnormality at diagnosis and evolution to acute leukemia, nor is the development of a cytogenetic abnormality necessarily predictive for the development of acute leukemia (59,119). However, the presence of 5q– in association with other cytogenetic abnormalities appeared to be a marker for acute transformation (119,120). The 13q– abnormality was associated with evolution to myelofibrosis in some series (59). Cytogenetic abnormalities were present in 45% of patients who developed myelofibrosis in one series as compared to 30% of patients who did not develop complications (59). Therapy with alkylating agents, hydroxyurea, or phosphorus 32 (^{32}P) was associated with an increased rate of cytogenetic conversion (118,120). Compared to patients not exposed to chemotherapy, the frequency of cytogenetic abnormalities was increased threefold, as was the frequency of complex cytogenetic abnormalities (118,120). Clonal evolution, clonal expansion, and clonal reversion have been observed, and some clones harbored more than one abnormality, such as trisomy 8 and 9 or trisomy 9p and 1q (121,122). The high frequency of 20q–, which is due to an interstitial deletion (123), is of interest, but this abnormality is not specific for polycythemia vera (124), nor has the loss of a specific suppressor gene been identified. However, it has been associated with erythroid and megakaryocytic dysplasia (124), suggesting that when expressed in polycythemia vera, it reflects the nature of the involved progenitor cell. The cytogenetic abnormalities associated with the acute leukemic transformation of polycythemia vera are typical of

those seen in either *de novo* acute leukemia or therapy-related acute leukemia (120,125).

Differential Diagnosis

The diagnosis of polycythemia vera is straightforward when there is an excess of red cells, white cells, and platelets in the absence of a definable cause. However, in more than one-half of patients, trilineage hematopoietic cell hyperplasia is not present at the time of diagnosis. Because there are no distinguishing morphologic abnormalities of the blood cells in polycythemia vera nor a clinically applicable clonal marker, recognizing the disorder is difficult when its presenting manifestations are isolated erythrocytosis (9,85), isolated thrombocytosis (less common) (84), or isolated leukocytosis (rare) (83). Osler was the first to realize the need for a set of diagnostic criteria to distinguish the newly recognized entity, polycythemia vera, from the then-known causes of erythrocytosis (6) (Table 12-5). In 1966, the PVSG proposed an expanded set of diagnostic criteria, enlarging the Oslerian version by including abnormalities of the leukocytes and platelets as well as several biochemical measurements, with the intent of improving diagnostic accuracy in distinguishing polycythemia vera from the many other causes of erythrocytosis (Table 12-5) and creating unanimity among physicians with respect to this disease entity (24). The PVSG diagnostic criteria are as remarkable for what they do not include as for what they do. First, there is no stipulation that clonality be established even though polycythemia vera is a clonal disorder. This stipulation is absent because we still lack a clinically applicable clonal marker, but its absence cannot be ignored when the use of leukemogenic therapeutic agents is being considered. Second, there is no requirement for a bone marrow examination. However, virtually every patient evaluated for polycythemia vera undergoes this procedure. Given that bone marrow morphology and cellularity are normal in a substantial proportion of patients at the time of diagnosis (88,93), that even if they are abnormal, the abnormalities are not diagnostic, and that cytogenetic abnormalities are also infrequent initially and without prognostic significance (59), a bone marrow examination need not be part of the diagnostic evaluation. Examination of the bone marrow is only useful when some other diagnosis such as idiopathic myelofibrosis or CML is a consideration.

An erythropoietin assay was also not stipulated in the PVSG diagnostic criteria because no clinically reliable assay was available when the criteria were devised. Although we now have a sensitive and specific erythropoietin assay based on recombinant reagents, it is less useful than originally hoped. This is because of the physiology of erythropoietin production. Erythropoietin production is controlled at the level of gene transcription. Normally, there is constitutive production of erythropoietin

---

TABLE 12-5. Diagnosis of Polycythemia Vera

1903	1971 (PVSG Criteria)
Erythrocytosis	Elevated red cell mass
Chronic cyanosis	Normal arterial O₂ saturation
Splenomegaly	Splenomegaly
	Plus any two below if no splenomegaly
	Leukocytosis >12,000/μL
	Thrombocytosis >400,000/μL
	Elevated leukocyte alkaline phosphatase >100
	Elevated B$_{12}$ >900 pg/mL, or UB$_{12}$BC >2200 pg/mL

From Osler W. Chronic cyanosis, with polycythemia and enlarged spleen: a new clinical entity. *Am J Med Sci* 1903;126:176–201; and Wasserman L. The management of polycythemia vera. *Br J Haematol* 1971;21:371–376.

in an amount sufficient to maintain the red cell mass at a constant level that is consistent with the tissue oxygen needs of the individual. With tissue hypoxia, additional renal interstitial cells are recruited to produce erythropoietin (126), and the half-life of erythropoietin mRNA is also increased (127), thereby increasing the erythroid progenitor cell pool. When the red cell mass is sufficiently expanded, tissue hypoxia is corrected, and erythropoietin production is down-regulated at the level of transcription. At the same time with the expansion of the erythroid progenitor cell pool, there is increased catabolism of erythropoietin by these cells (128). In polycythemia vera, erythropoietin production is suppressed more than in any other condition because the expanded red cell mass ensures a high degree of tissue oxygenation, whereas the expanded erythroid progenitor cell pool ensures increased catabolism of erythropoietin. However, with hypoxic erythrocytosis, unless the hypoxia is severe, a similar compensation occurs, and the serum erythropoietin level is maintained in the normal range (92) (Fig. 12-4). Furthermore, as an additional brake on erythropoiesis, an increase in blood viscosity, for unknown reasons, results in a reduction in erythropoietin production (129). As a consequence, the serum erythropoietin level is often not a useful guide to the presence of tissue hypoxia and has no diagnostic value in the evaluation of isolated erythrocytosis unless it is elevated.

Erythropoietin-independent colony formation is another hallmark of the autonomous erythropoiesis associated with polycythemia vera (23,30,31) and has been used diagnostically (130,131). This assay is not widely available, is unstandardized, and is positive in idiopathic myelofibrosis (132), essential thrombocytosis (133), and, occasionally, the nonclonal form of erythrocytosis (134). As a consequence, it cannot be recommended as a routine diagnostic test.

The most important criterion that the PVSG diagnostic criteria do stipulate is an increased red cell mass. Although this criterion does not distinguish polycythemia vera from other disorders causing erythrocytosis, it distinguishes an absolute erythrocytosis from a spurious or relative erythrocytosis due to plasma volume contraction. Unfortunately, because measurement of the red cell mass (and plasma volume) requires the use of radioisotopes and is subject to imprecision based on body habitus, it has fallen into disuse in favor of predictive formulas and clinical maxims. However, it cannot be emphasized too strongly with respect to the latter that even with a hematocrit as high as 60%, there is no assurance that true erythrocytosis is present. Indeed, attempts to divine the red cell mass from the hematocrit are as futile as predicting total body sodium on the basis of the serum sodium concentration. With respect to predictive formulas, they are based on the assumption that the red cell mass and plasma volume have a constant relationship that holds time in disease as well as health. This is simply erroneous. Under normal circumstances, the distribution of red cells and plasma within the circulatory system is not uniform (135). As demonstrated by independent determination of the red cell mass and plasma volume, the ratio of red cells to plasma is higher in the peripheral vessels (venous or arterial) than in the body as a whole (i.e., the whole body hematocrit (derived from measurements of the red cell mass and plasma volume) divided by the peripheral hematocrit [derived by centrifugation of venous (or arterial) blood]) averages 0.92 (136). This is due to the slower flow of peripherally displaced plasma as compared with axially located red cells (137). With disease, independent changes occur in the plasma volume and red cell mass as well as in their distribution that are neither evident by a hematocrit determination nor predictable by the disease process. This situation is particularly confounded by splenomegaly, which leads not only to red cell sequestration but also to plasma volume

expansion (138–141). Tissue hypoxia, or any form of erythropoietin-driven erythrocytosis, has the opposite effect on the plasma volume; as the red cell mass increases, there is usually a concomitant reduction in plasma volume, the extent of which varies. This is as true in patients treated with androgens (142) or recombinant erythropoietin (143) as it is for high-altitude hypoxia (144), cyanotic congenital heart disease (145), and chronic carbon monoxide poisoning due to tobacco abuse (146). However, in polycythemia vera, in which erythropoiesis is autonomous and erythropoietin production is suppressed, the plasma volume either stays the same or increases as the red cell mass increases (147). Indeed, the plasma volume may expand to the point of masking the increase in red cell mass; this can occur even in the absence of splenomegaly (148). In this regard, it should also be evident that measuring only the plasma volume, which is technically easier, and calculating the red cell mass by extrapolation (or vice versa) are unacceptable practices (149) because of the lack of dependency of these two variables (136,140). Thus, measuring both the red cell mass and plasma volume to establish the presence of an absolute erythrocytosis is unchallengable not only from a physiologic perspective but also as a standard of care—although the issue is often ignored due to ignorance or economic concerns. As a corollary, it is possible that plasma volume expansion can mask an elevated red cell mass, so if polycythemia vera is suspected, a red cell mass and plasma volume determination are mandatory (148). Indeed, it is safe to state, based on PVSG data, that a normal hematocrit in an untreated patient with polycythemia vera should never be considered normal (Fig. 12-5).

Red cell mass and plasma volume determinations are conducted using the technique of isotope dilution (150). With this technique, an aliquot of the patient's red cells is labeled with chromium 51 and reinfused. Serial blood samples are taken over a time that is sufficient for adequate equilibration, which, if there is substantial splenomegaly, can be as long as 90 minutes. Simultaneous measurement of the plasma volume is performed using iodine 125–labeled albumin. Based on the dilution factor between the counts/unit volume injected and the counts/unit volume observed at equilibrium, the red cell mass and plasma volume can be calculated. Inaccuracies inherent in red cell mass and plasma volume determinations are

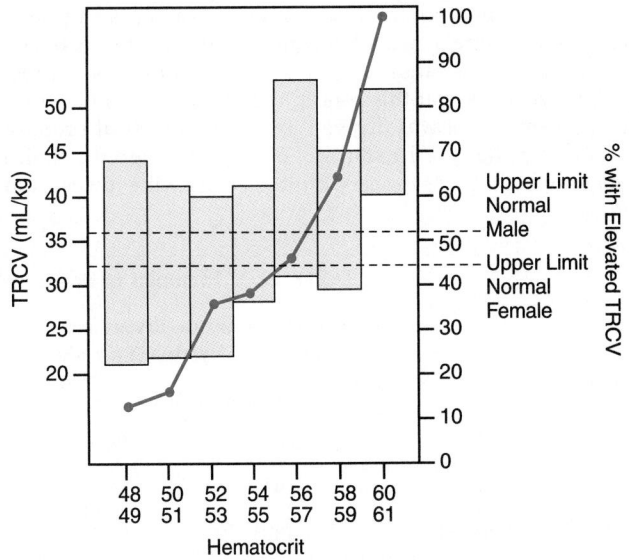

Figure 12-5. The range of observed total red cell volume (TRCV) as a function of hematocrit. (Modified from Berlin NI. Diagnosis and classification of the polycythemias. *Semin Hematol* 1975;12:339–351.)

TABLE 12-6. Recommendations for the Calculation of Standards for the Red Cell Mass (RCM) and Plasma Volume (PV)[a,b]

Males
  Mean normal RCM (mL): $(1486 \times S) - 825$
  Mean normal PV (mL): $1578 \times S$
Females
  Mean normal RCM (mL): $(1.06 \times age) + (822 \times S)$
  Mean normal PV (mL): $1395 \times S$

S, surface area.
[a]$S = w^{0.425} \times h^{0.725} \times 0.007148$; w, weight in kg; h, height in cm; S in M².
[b]Age is in years.
From Pearson TC, Botterill CA, Glass UH, et al. Interpretation of measured red cell mass and plasma volume in males with elevated venous PCV values. *Scand J Haematol* 1984;33:68–74.

largely due to body habitus effects. For example, adipose tissue is relatively avascular. Consequently, the expression of red cell mass and plasma volume measurements as a function of body weight (i.e., mL/kg) understate these measurements (151). However, correction formulas have been established that account for this problem (Tables 12-6 and 12-7). With the currently accepted confidence limits, the false-positive rate is approximately 1% (151).

Once the presence of an elevated red cell mass is established, its cause needs to be determined (Table 12-8). Exclusion of hypoxic causes requires direct measurement of arterial oxygen saturation. Arterial oxygen saturation can be misleading if the cause of the erythrocytosis is a high-affinity hemoglobin, in which case a hemoglobin P_{50} measurement is required. A serum erythropoietin level is only helpful if it is elevated. Hepatic and renal scans and a urinalysis complete the evaluation. Patients with acquired isolated erythrocytosis for which no etiology is apparent can be observed while being treated with phlebotomy for signs of evolution into polycythemia vera or for the emergence of another underlying cause.

Clinical Course

According to the current concept of the natural history of polycythemia vera, the disease evolves progressively through a series of phases beginning with an asymptomatic phase and proceeding through erythrocytotic, compensated or inactive, and spent or postpolycythemic myeloid metaplasia phases before terminating in acute leukemia, if the patient does not die first from another cause (152). What is generally not appreciated, however, is that this conception of the natural history of polycythemia vera was derived from a hypothetical proposal that rapidly attained the status of dogma, although the clinical data on which it was based would not satisfy the lowest stan-

dards of evidence-based medicine (153). Although it is well established that polycythemia vera has an asymptomatic phase, and that myeloid metaplasia, myelofibrosis, anemia, and acute leukemia can complicate the disorder, what has never been established is whether myeloid metaplasia and myelofibrosis have an adverse effect on bone marrow function or disease prognosis and whether acute leukemia is an inevitable complication of polycythemia vera.

There are many reasons for this situation—not the least of which is the low incidence of the disease as well as its chronic nature, which precludes most physicians from seeing more than a few of these patients or even following them for a time sufficient to encompass the full scope of the disease. The most important reason, however, has been failure to consider the effect of radiation or chemotherapy on bone marrow function. Indeed, the basis for the currently held concept of the natural history of polycythemia vera (152) is a publication from 1938 describing 13 polycythemia patients from a series of 75 who were thought to be representative of the various hematologic manifestations of the disease (153). Two of these patients were anemic and were considered to have spent phase of the disease, a concept that was first proposed in 1923 by Minot and Buckman on the basis of three patients from a series of 15 (42). What has not been appreciated is that all five of these patients had been treated with radiation. This same criticism also applies to the first reported case of polycythemia vera complicated by osteomyelosclerosis (154).

Only rarely, however, have polycythemia vera patients been followed long enough without exposure to therapeutic interventions that alter bone marrow function for any meaningful appreciation of the natural history of the disorder to be obtained. When this has been done, a different picture of the disease emerges (155,156). Furthermore, it is not widely appreciated that the disease may have different manifestations depending on the age at onset (78) and the patient's gender (82). Adding to the confusion has been the uncritical acceptance of terms such as *spent phase* and *postpolycythemic myeloid metaplasia*, as well as the assumption that the various chronic myeloproliferative diseases including CML are interrelated (1) when there is no evidence substantiating this claim (4).

Although the development of anemia due to marrow exhaustion has been considered to be an inevitable event in the natural history of polycythemia vera and possibly a forerunner of leukemia (152), in a large series of patients managed without irradiation, anemia was most often due to chemotherapy, hemorrhage, a deficiency of iron, folic acid, or vitamin B_{12}, or another disease—but not to intrinsic marrow failure (155). The importance of iron deficiency was not recognized in early descriptions of the disease, and the extent to which plasma volume expansion associated with splenomegaly could mask an

TABLE 12-7. Examples of Red Cell Mass and Plasma Volume Determinations

	(A) Pulmonary Atrial/Ventricular Shunt with Hypoxia (S = 1.85)		(B) Androgen Therapy (S = 2.15)		(C) Polycythemia Vera (S = 1.64)	
	50-yr-old man (Hct = 58.4%)		52-yr-old Man (Hct = 56.4%)		68-yr-old Woman (Hct = 47%)	
	Expected[a]	Observed	Expected[a]	Observed	Expected[a]	Observed
Red cell mass (mL)	1924	3982	2370	2661	1420	2217
Plasma volume (mL)	2919	2499	3393	1824	1288	2500
Total blood volume (mL)	4843	6481	5763	4485	3708	4717

Hct, hematocrit.
[a]The expected values were derived from the formulas in Table 12-6.

TABLE 12-8. Causes of Erythrocytosis

Relative erythrocytosis
    Hemoconcentration secondary to dehydration, androgens, or
      tobacco abuse
Absolute erythrocytosis
    Hypoxia
    Carbon monoxide intoxication
    High-affinity hemoglobin
    High altitude
    Pulmonary disease
    Right to left shunts
    Sleep apnea syndrome
    Neurologic disease
Renal disease
    Hydronephrosis
    Cysts
    Renal artery stenosis
    Focal sclerosing glomerulonephritis
    Renal transplantation
Tumors
    Hypernephroma
    Hepatoma
    Cerebellar hemangioblastoma
    Uterine fibronyoma
    Adrenal tumors
    Meningioma
    Pheochromocytoma
Androgen therapy
Erythropoietin abuse
Bartter syndrome
Familial with normal hemoglobin function
Polycythemia vera

increase in red cell mass was also not appreciated. Importantly, ferrokinetic studies have not indicated any diminution in marrow erythroid activity in many patients with advanced disease (157,158), and, in some patients, the so-called spent phase was reversed with chemotherapy, suggesting that it did not represent terminal marrow failure (159). It thus appears that the development of anemia in polycythemia vera is not necessarily a harbinger of marrow failure or impending leukemia in the absence of irradiation or chemotherapy.

The term *spent phase* has also been used to describe a phase of polycythemia vera with splenomegaly and erythrocytosis in the absence of myeloid metaplasia and myelofibrosis, in which the extent of the erythrocytosis was masked by plasma volume expansion (160). Others have described such patients as being in the "normal" (152) or "stationary" (161) phase of the disease. All of these designations are clinically inaccurate because bone marrow erythroid activity was clearly neither spent nor static. *Postpolycythemic myeloid metaplasia* is another designation that only adds confusion to the understanding of the natural history of polycythemia vera without conveying any useful information (162). The term is imprecise because it implies a state beyond polycythemia vera or a conversion to another disorder when, in fact, myeloid metaplasia is an integral feature of polycythemia vera, and there is no evidence that myeloid metaplasia, per se, influences bone marrow function in this disorder (88,95,157–159,163). Postpolycythemic myeloid metaplasia has also been considered synonymous with the spent phase of polycythemia vera (162). However, most of the patients so described were treated with radiation or chemotherapy, making it difficult to distinguish the effects of exogenous toxins from endogenous marrow behavior.

It should not be surprising that similar confusion surrounds the significance of myelofibrosis in polycythemia vera. This is because the mechanisms for marrow fibrosis are poorly understood, the means for quantitating myelofibrosis are imprecise, and the criteria for its recognition are variable (95,164). It has

also been assumed that polycythemia vera and idiopathic myelofibrosis are related diseases (1), but this has never been unequivocally established. Using an increase in marrow reticulin as the definition for myelofibrosis, this process has a frequency of 3% (155) to 19% (96) in polycythemia vera patients. Importantly, myelofibrosis was present at the time of diagnosis in 11% of patients in one prospective study—a finding that appeared to have no prognostic significance (93). This is, of course, in contrast to CML, in which the development of the myelofibrosis is generally associated with disease acceleration (165). It also appears that there is a higher incidence of myelofibrosis in polycythemia vera patients exposed to either radiation or chemotherapy (166–168) as opposed to those treated with phlebotomy alone, although there is not absolute agreement on this point (96). However, an increase in marrow reticulin is not synonymous with bone marrow failure in polycythemia vera (84), and there are no data to support the contention that the myelofibrosis is a progressive process or commonly contributory to bone marrow failure (88,95).

The relationship between polycythemia vera and acute leukemia has been a subject of contention since Osler's seminal paper, and it has been widely assumed that the development of leukemia was an inevitable event in the natural history of polycythemia vera (152,169). Initially, this was because of the failure to distinguish the leukemoid reaction of polycythemia vera from that of CML (169) and, subsequently, because of the failure to appreciate the leukemogenic effects of radiation and chemotherapy in polycythemia vera (170,171). Ironically, because external radiation or ^{32}P diminished myeloid metaplasia and corrected leukocytosis, these forms of therapy were considered not only to be efficacious against chronic leukemia but also to prolong survival (170). As a consequence, the development of acute leukemia was considered an expected outcome associated with prolonged survival. This contention was challenged first by the 1964 landmark study by Modan and Lilienfeld that demonstrated unequivocally that the leukemogenic effects of radiation or ^{32}P were not a consequence of prolonged survival (168). Subsequently, a prospective multicenter trial conducted by the PVSG confirmed the retrospective observations of Modan and Lilienfeld with regard to ^{32}P, demonstrated the leukemogenic effect of alkylating agents in this disorder, and showed that survival was not diminished in patients treated with phlebotomy alone (172). Subsequent studies have confirmed these observations with respect to the leukemogenic effect of ^{32}P (173) and have extended them to include hydroxyurea (174) and pipobroman (175). The combination of hydroxyurea with ^{32}P or an alkylating agent was also found to be deleterious (176,177).

The development of therapy-related secondary acute leukemia is, of course, not unique to polycythemia vera, nor is there any quantitative or qualitative difference between it and other neoplasms treated with the same agents (178) with respect to alkylating agent or radiation exposure, latency, type of leukemia (177,179–181), cytogenetic abnormalities (120,125), or response to antileukemic therapy (122,182,183). As a corollary, therapy-induced acute leukemia has also been observed in patients with secondary erythrocytosis who were mistakenly treated with chemotherapy or radiation (168). Although data have been presented indicating that myeloid metaplasia and myelofibrosis were predisposing factors for treatment-associated acute leukemia in polycythemia vera (93,162), the number of patients studied was small, and the observations were not confirmed in other studies (181). The development of treatment-related acute leukemia in patients with secondary erythrocytosis also speaks against an obligatory role for myeloid metaplasia or myelofibrosis in this process (168).

Polycythemia vera patients also appear to be at risk of sponta-neously developing acute leukemia. The exact frequency of this is unclear because there has been only one prospective study (172). In a review of 83 reported cases of polycythemia vera com-plicated by acute leukemia up to 1950, Schwartz and Ehrlich accepted only one as valid (184). In the same year, Dameshek reported that one of his 50 patients and one of 100 patients at the Mayo Clinic treated by phlebotomy had developed acute leuke-mia spontaneously (161). Since then, there have been 12 pub-lished case reports and an additional 13 patients identified by a questionnaire (179), whereas in three retrospective studies com-prising 371 patients treated with phlebotomy alone and repre-senting 23 to 28 years of observation, two cases of acute leukemia were observed (155,166,168). The demographic characteristics of the group of patients are of interest because they were predomi-nately men (90%) with a mean age of 60.5 years, in contrast to those polycythemia vera patients developing secondary acute leukemia, of whom 54% were men with a mean age of 52.5 years (179). The interval between the onset of the polycythemia vera and the onset of acute leukemia was 4 to 8 years (range, 1 to 13 years), indicating that the leukemia was not a consequence of prolonged survival, myeloid metaplasia, myelofibrosis, or the "spent phase" of polycythemia vera. It is also of interest in this regard that three of the ten patients developing spontaneous acute leukemia, for which information was available, had under-gone splenectomy 2 to 8 years before the onset of the leukemia.

The mechanisms involved in the development of spontaneous acute leukemia in polycythemia vera are unknown; however, given the increasing incidence of acute leukemia with age in gen-eral (185), the mean age of onset of polycythemia vera (8,9), and the restoration of the polycythemic state with successful antileu-kemic therapy (122,182), the possibility of coincidental occur-rence cannot be excluded. At the same time, given the evidence for clonal evolution and succession in polycythemia vera (59), the possibility of leukemia arising from the malignant clone is also likely. The potential role of splenectomy is intriguing because of its implication by some in the development of spontaneous acute leukemia in idiopathic myelofibrosis (186), Hodgkin's disease (187), and aplastic anemia (188). Because of the difference in

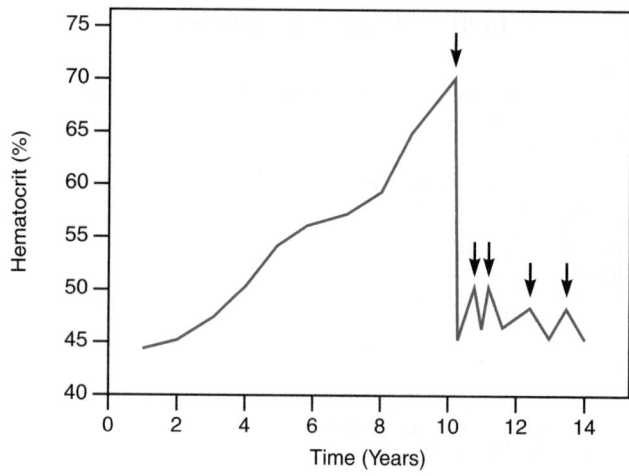

Figure 12-7. The natural history of untreated polycythemia vera. Arrows indicate phlebotomy therapy. (Adapted from Conley CL. Polycythemia vera diagnosis and treatment. *Hosp Pract* 1987;22:181–210.)

demographics between those polycythemia vera patients who develop spontaneous acute leukemia and those who develop treatment-related acute leukemia, the possibility exists that the development of spontaneous acute leukemia in polycythemia vera patients is similar to the development of Richter's syndrome in chronic lymphocytic leukemia (189). Regardless of the mecha-

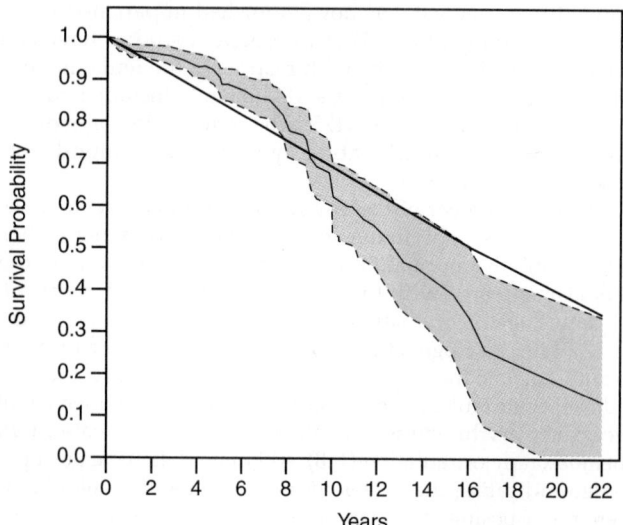

Figure 12-6. Polycythemia vera. Actuarial survival (*thin line*) and 95% con-fidence limits (*shadowed area*) of 454 patients are compared with the sur-vival of age-matched and sex-matched population (*thick line*). (Modified from Rozman C, Giralt M, Feliu E, et al. Life expectancy of patients with chronic nonleukemic myeloproliferative disorders. *Cancer* 1991;67:2658–2663.)

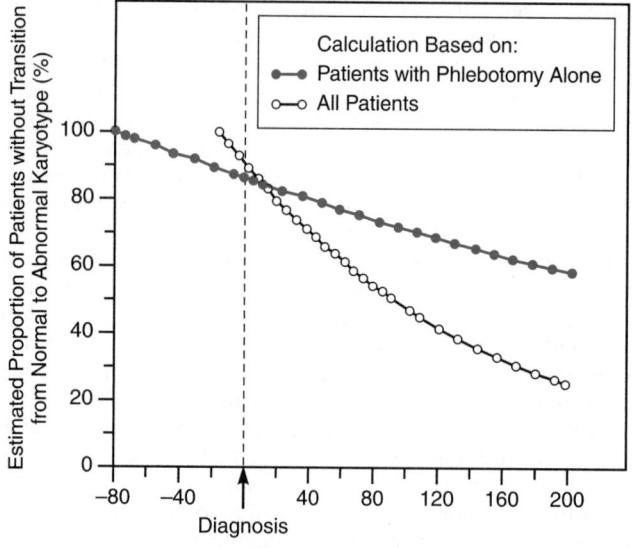

Figure 12-8. An estimation of the decline in the proportion of patients with a normal karyotype in relation to the time of the polycythemia vera (PV) diagnosis. The right part of the curves (the time *after* diagnosis) was calcu-lated from the data available in the cytogenetic studies during the follow-up period. The left part of the curves (the time *before* diagnosis) is a hypotheti-cal estimation based on two assumptions: The rate of the development of chromosome abnormalities was constant, and it was the same both before and after the PV diagnosis. Each dot in the curves is an estimation of the proportion of patients who, at that time, still had a normal karyotype. One curve uses data from all patients (-○-), the other curve uses data from patients treated with phlebotomy alone (-●-). The model suggests that the risk of transition from a normal to an abnormal karyotype first started some-time between 17 and 80 months before the diagnosis. These figures may also be considered an indication of the length of the preclinical phase of the disorder. (Modified from Swolin B, Weinfeld A, Westin J. A prospective long-term cytogenetic study in polycythemia vera in relation to treatment and clinical course. *Blood* 1988;72:386–395.)

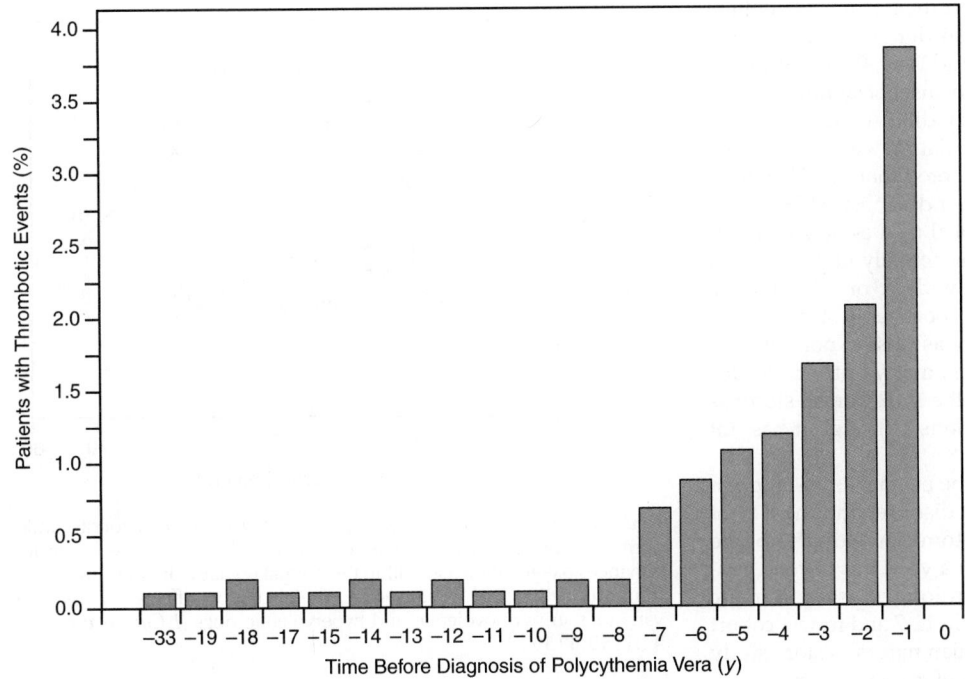

Figure 12-9. Thrombotic events in the years before the diagnosis of polycythemia vera. The y-axis represents the percentage of patients who had at least one thrombotic event each year before the diagnosis of polycythemia vera. (Modified from Polycythemia vera: the natural history of 1213 patients followed for 20 years. Gruppo Italiano Studio Policitemia. *Ann Intern Med* 1995;123:656–664.)

nisms involved, the development of acute leukemia in polycythemia vera is not common and certainly not inevitable in the absence of exposure to leukemogenic drugs.

Lack of a definitive diagnostic test, the uncommon nature of the disorder, its chronic course, the protean nature of its compli-

cations, reliance on anecdotal case reports with respect to its natural history, and lack of consensus concerning therapy as well as the widespread employment of leukemogenic agents in its treatment have made it difficult to reach a definitive conclusion about the prognosis of polycythemia vera. Substantial longevity

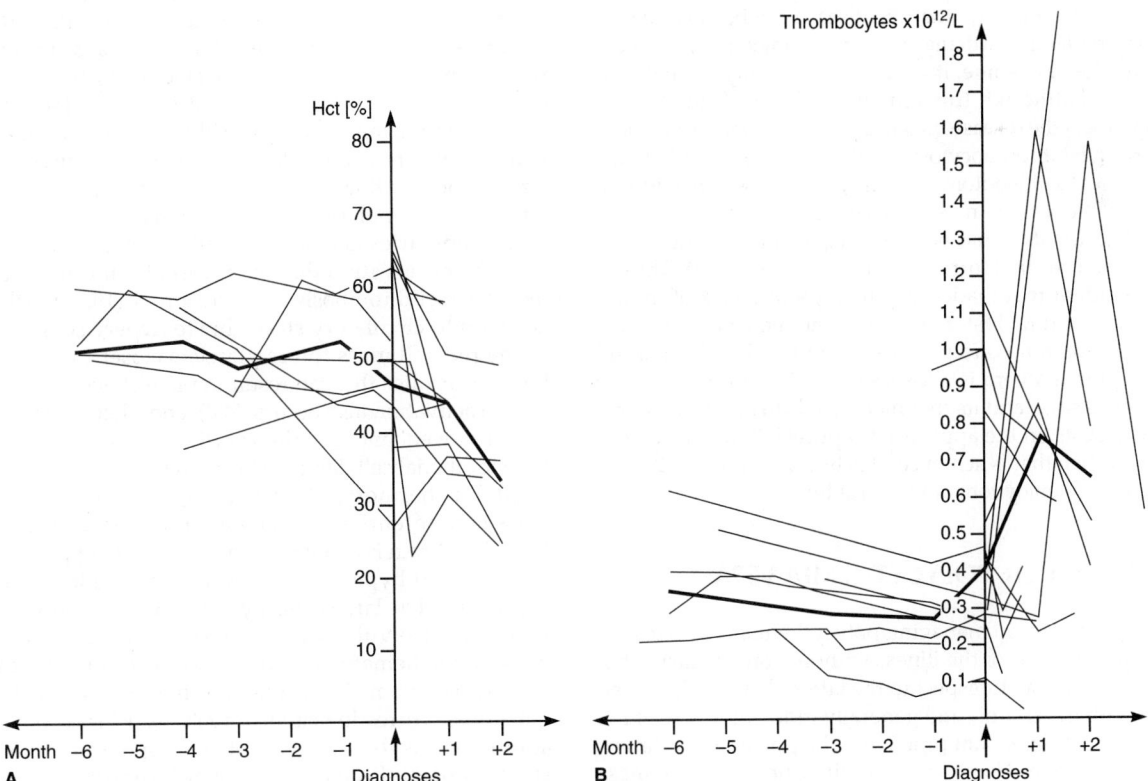

Figure 12-10. A: Hematocrit (Hct) values during the 6-month period before the thrombotic complication. Thick line, median values. **B:** Thrombocytic counts during the 6-month period before the thrombotic complication. Thick line, median values. (Modified from Anger BR, Seifried E, Scheppach J, et al. Budd-Chiari syndrome and thrombosis of other abdominal vessels in the chronic myeloproliferative diseases. *Klin Wochenschr* 1989;67:818–825.)

was a constant theme of the early literature at a time when there was no consistent treatment of the disorder (190). However, a retrospective Danish study in 1962 found that 50% of untreated patients died within 18 months after the onset of symptoms, and 50% of patients treated by phlebotomy died within 3.5 years, whereas 50% of patients treated by irradiation were alive at 12.5 years (166). Subsequent to this, it was noted that the lifespan of patients was proportional to their age at diagnosis (179), while the only prospective multicenter clinical trial established that patients treated with phlebotomy alone actually had a survival that equaled their counterparts treated with ^{32}P or chlorambucil (172). Furthermore, a recent Spanish report suggested that the lifespan of polycythemia vera patients was close to normal (156) (Fig. 12-6). Despite these observations, many authorities, for unknown reasons, continue to rely on the 1962 Danish study as a basis for therapeutic recommendations although it has not been corroborated by subsequent data.

Major issues in this regard include the erroneous assumption that polycythemia vera is a monolithic disorder and the lack of understanding of the role of phlebotomy. Although no one would withhold therapy in polycythemia vera, it is beyond contention that the disease can have a prolonged asymptomatic phase, as illustrated anecdotally in Figure 12-7 and from a cohort study in Figure 12-8 (59). Indeed, an Italian natural history study also documented a significant incidence of thrombosis more than 5 years before the diagnosis of polycythemia vera (Fig. 12-9) (73), whereas in another study, 11 of 13 patients with an intraabdominal venous thrombosis had an elevated hematocrit for 6 or more months before the thrombotic episode (Fig. 12-10) (191). With regard to the latter, it appears that hepatic vein thrombosis does not initiate in a major vessel but rather starts in small vessels and is gradually progressive (192). Furthermore, the assumption that disease behavior is similar in all patients with polycythemia is simply erroneous. It is clear that the disease can be very aggressive in some patients, particularly young women (78), and very indolent in others. In some, it is possible that only the red cells may be clonal, although this remains to be confirmed (193), whereas in others the disease masquerades as idiopathic myelofibrosis or essential thrombocytosis until it is recognized (84,192).

With respect to phlebotomy therapy, as discussed below, failure to reduce the red cell mass to a safe level in women as well as men and keep it there has been the major cause for the dismal results reported for this form of therapy (166,172,173). Thus, it should be evident that inadequate therapy and lack of understanding of the natural history of polycythemia vera have had a greater impact on our concept of its prognosis than the disease itself. Polycythemia vera is a disease of cell accumulation, the rate of which is slow, and its treatment needs to be based on this premise as well as on the appropriate appreciation of its pathophysiology. When that is achieved, it is likely that polycythemia vera patients will enjoy long and useful lives.

MANAGEMENT OF POLYCYTHEMIA VERA

The primary objective in managing polycythemia vera is to prevent the complications of the illness without compromising the patient's longevity; with respect to the latter, therapy should be consonant with the chronic and generally indolent nature of the disease. The most significant problem is the potential for thrombosis or hemorrhage. These are primarily due to red cell mass elevation and hyperviscosity. From the perspective of pathophysiology, elevation of the red cell mass in polycythemia vera is a gradual process (Figs. 12-7 and 12-8) that, in contrast to the red cell mass elevation–associated hypoxic or erythropoietin-driven erythrocytosis, is generally associated with an increase

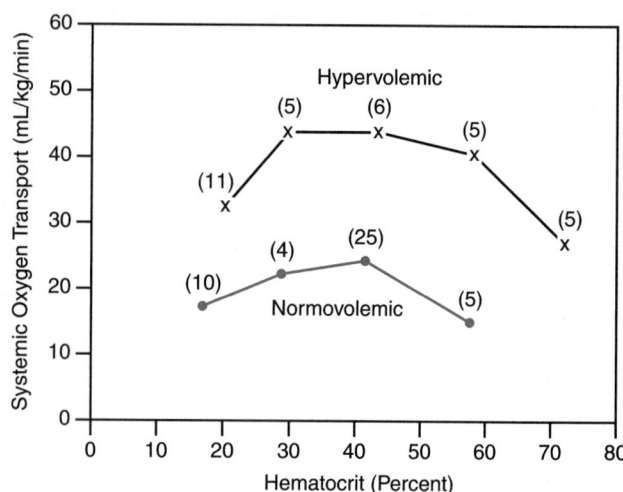

Figure 12-11. Systemic oxygen transport at varying hematocrits under normovolemic and hypervolemic conditions. Plasma volume expansion enhances oxygen transport within the normal hematocrit range. (Modified from Murray JF, Gold P, Johnson BL. The circulatory effects of hematocrit variations in normovolemic and hypervolemic dogs. *J Clin Invest* 1963; 42:1150–1159.)

in the plasma volume (148,194,195). Thus, as both the red cell mass and plasma volume increase, the total blood volume expands, particularly when there is splenomegaly (140,141). This results in an increase in cardiac output, vasodilation, and a reduction in peripheral vascular resistance (196) (Fig. 12-11). The spleen also serves as a reservoir for the expanded blood volume (141,197). Of course, as the hematocrit rises, blood viscosity increases (198). Initially, this is partially offset by the expanded plasma volume, increased cardiac output, and reduced peripheral vascular resistance (196), but eventually viscosity effects predominate (Fig. 12-12). The relationship of viscosity to the hematocrit is logarithmic, and small increments in hematocrit can produce large increments in viscosity, particularly at the low flow rates that might occur in the venous circulation (198). Capillary microscopy suggests that stasis is greatest in the capillaries and small venules (199), which is consistent with the observation that microvascular thrombosis preceded major vessel thrombosis in this disorder (192). Furthermore, in addition to circulatory stasis due to hyperviscosity, expansion of the red cell mass forces platelets closer to vessel walls. At high shear rates this can result in platelet activation (115). Leukocyte activation also occurs (200), and platelet-leukocyte interactions are enhanced at the vessel wall (201), as is the potential for endothelial cell damage due to hypoxia and abluminal stress (202). Furthermore, no scavenging by the increased red cell mass can potentiate platelet aggregation and hypertension (203). The brain is at a particular risk due to hyperoxic vasoconstriction and hyperviscosity caused by the increased red cell mass (204). The large capacity and low flow abdominal venous system is also vulnerable to stasis caused by hyperviscosity. Because the hematocrit is the major determinant of blood viscosity, phlebotomy is the most effective and the most immediate remedy for correcting circulatory stasis. What is not commonly appreciated is that the physiologic response to phlebotomy is an increase in plasma volume, which contributes to the reduction in blood viscosity (205). This is true even with pseudo-erythrocytosis due to plasma volume reduction (206). By contrast, reduction of the hematocrit by an agent such as ^{32}P neither increases the plasma volume nor lowers peripheral vascular resistance (Table 12-9) (205). The contention that iron-deficient

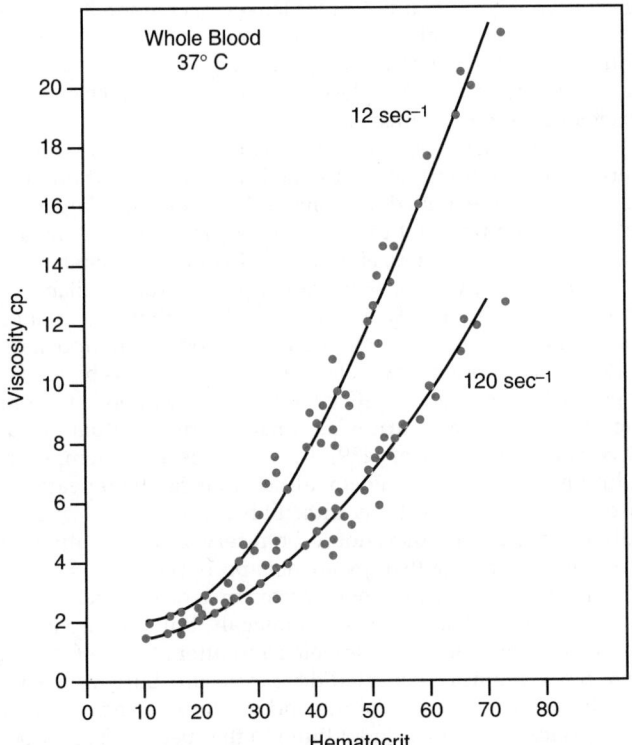

Figure 12-12. Comparison of viscosity-hematocrit relationships at two different shear rates. (Modified from Wells RE, Merrill EW. Influence of flow properties of blood upon viscosity hematocrit relationship. *J Clin Invest* 1962;41:1591–1598.)

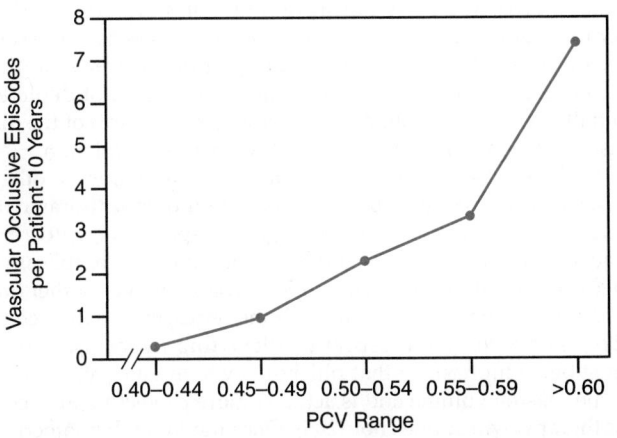

Figure 12-13. Relation of polycythemia vera (PCV) range to number of vascular occlusive episodes/10 patient years in patients with primary proliferative polycythemia. (Modified from Pearson TC, Weatherly-Mein G. Vascular occlusive episodes and venous haematocrit in primary proliferative polycythaemia. *Lancet* 1978;2:1219–1221.)

red cells increase blood viscosity due to their rigidity is erroneous (207,208); iron deficiency in the absence of anemia is not harmful in adults (209). Phlebotomy therapy is only ineffective when it is incomplete.

Phlebotomy is thus useful in two ways: mechanically, to alleviate hyperviscosity by reducing the total red cell mass, and biochemically, to induce a state of iron deficiency that prevents the rapid reaccumulation of red cells while assuring that those that accumulate are small and contribute little to the red cell mass. Concerns that phlebotomy therapy creates a hypercoagulable state, stimulates erythropoiesis, exacerbates thrombocytosis, causes crippling iron-deficiency, and promotes hyperviscosity through the production of iron-deficient red cells merely reflect a total misunderstanding of the pathophysiology of both polycythemia vera and iron deficiency. First, by lowering blood viscosity, phlebotomy actually corrects a hypercoagulable state and, at the same time, appears to reduce the tendency to hemorrhage, which is also a constant threat in polycythemia vera patients (104,114,210). Second, hematopoiesis is autonomous in

polycythemia vera and, thus, cannot be stimulated endogenously by phlebotomy (211,212). Third, in adults, in the absence of anemia, iron deficiency is not a liability except for the development of pica (74,209). Fourth, iron-deficient red cells are not significantly more rigid than normal red cells (213), and their small size not only compensates for their increased numbers but also reduces platelet-red cell interactions (214). Finally, reducing the red cell mass increases cerebral blood flow (215), in part by increasing the plasma volume (216).

Unsuccessful phlebotomy therapy in polycythemia vera has simply been due to insufficient reduction of the red cell mass to fully alleviate hyperviscosity. The principal reason for this was lack of recognition that, in polycythemia vera, the hematocrit or hemoglobin level does not reflect the true extent of elevation of the red cell mass (148). For example, at a hematocrit of 50%, which is within the range of normal for men, 20% of men with polycythemia vera have an elevated red cell mass (Fig. 12-5) (86). Of course, at this hematocrit, 100% of women have an elevated red cell mass. Initially, however, a hematocrit of 50% was the therapeutic target in the PVSG prospective multicenter trial (24). Although this target was later reduced to 45% (217) based on actual data (218), it was still too high for women, and it is not surprising that the incidence of thrombosis ranged from 20% to 30% in all three treatment arms of the PVSG trial (172). Thus, it is not unexpected that the PVSG was left with the therapeutic conundrum that the patients treated with phlebotomy alone had an unacceptable rate of serious early thrombotic events, whereas those treated with chemotherapy had an unacceptable later incidence of leukemia (217).

Unsuccessful intensive chemotherapy to reduce the incidence of thrombotic events in the Italian natural history study can probably be attributed to the same problem (Fig. 12-9) (73). Simply stated, to eliminate the issue of thrombosis in polycythemia vera, the hematocrit must be kept below 42% in women and 45% in men (Fig. 12-13) (218). It is important to emphasize that this is not a one-time goal (82). Once the red cell mass is reduced, periodic phlebotomies are required to keep it reduced: first, by physical removal of blood; second, by inducing a continual state of iron deficiency. Claims that the red cell mass cannot be controlled by phlebotomy merely reflect confusion about the amount of blood that needs to be removed initially and the role of iron available for red cell regeneration. Polycythemia vera patients absorb iron maximally (219), and, once their iron stores

---

TABLE 12-9. Effect of Phosphorus 32 or Phlebotomy on Systemic Vascular Resistance (SVR) and Hematocrit (Hct)

Phosphorus 32	Phlebotomy
SVR before: 1421	SVR before: 1504
SVR after: 1990	SVR after: 1464
Hct before: 64	Hct before: 63
Hct after: 44	Hct after: 47

From Segel N, Bishop JM. Circulatory studies in polycythemia vera at rest and during exercise. *Clin Sci* 1967;32:527–549.

are depleted, at an iron absorption rate of 3 mg/day, it takes approximately 3 months for an iron-depleted patient to produce a unit of blood. A rate of blood production greater than this merely means that the patient's iron stores were not depleted initially as opposed to having a more aggressive form of the disease, particularly because this is a disease of accumulation.

Initially, based on the red cell mass determination, in otherwise healthy patients, 500 mL of blood should be withdrawn on a daily basis until the appropriate gender-specific hematocrit is reached. For patients with cardiac disease or other complicating medical conditions, removal of 250 mL daily or every other day with replacement of the fluid volume removed is satisfactory (220). However, with respect to alleviating hyperviscosity, it must be reemphasized that phlebotomy stimulates an increase in the plasma volume and is actually more protective than chemotherapy, which does not (205). Once the target hematocrit is achieved, monthly blood counts are sufficient for monitoring the need for phlebotomy; once a state of iron deficiency is achieved, phlebotomy is generally only required at 3-month intervals.

An important feature of phlebotomy therapy is that its effects are immediate. Headache and generalized malaise or fatigue are alleviated, spleen size is reduced, and, in some patients, pruritus is controlled. Patients are protected from thrombosis, and their risk of surgical morbidity is reduced (221). Repeated phlebotomies do impose an inconvenience, and erythrocytapheresis has been proposed as a means to restore the red cell mass to normal with a single procedure (222). However, erythrocytapheresis does not eliminate the need for periodic phlebotomies to maintain the red cell mass at a normal level, and the appropriate clinical trials to demonstrate that it represents no greater or lesser risk than multiple phlebotomies have not been conducted.

The increase in cell turnover in polycythemia vera can lead to hyperuricemia, uric acid stones, and secondary gout (81,155). Minor degrees of hyperuremia in an asymptomatic patient require no treatment. However, a uric acid greater than 10 mg%, a history of gout or renal stones, and the use of chemotherapy to reduce cell number or spleen size are indications to inhibit uric acid metabolism with allopurinol. In the absence of tophaceous gout, there is no need to pretreat patients with colchicine.

There appears to be an increased incidence of acid-peptic disease in polycythemia vera that may be independent of *Helicobacter* infection (155). Whether this reflects circulatory stasis due to hyperviscosity, an increase in histamine production, the use of salicylates, or a combination of these is unclear, but symptoms are usually easily alleviated with an H_2 blocker.

Aquagenic pruritus is the most intolerable symptom of polycythemia vera and often the one most difficult to alleviate. The etiology is unknown, and evidence for (223) and against (224) mast cell involvement has been obtained. The itching, stinging, and burning sensations that are associated with exposure to water—or that even occur spontaneously—can be unbearable for patients, interfering with their daily activities and degrading their quality of life. As mentioned, minor degrees of pruritus can be alleviated with phlebotomy. Antihistamines or ataractics are often effective, although it is impossible to predict which of the many varieties will be useful *a priori*, but a long-acting formulation is usually the most effective. Psoralen and ultraviolet A light therapy should be used if simpler remedies are not sufficient, but this has its own toxicities, such as skin burns and hyperpigmentation, and is not always effective (225). Interferon-α has been effective when other treatments have not been successful, but its success rate is still only 60% (226). Reduction of the leukocyte count with hydroxyurea is highly

effective, but because this agent is leukemogenic and its effect is transient, its use should be reserved for cases of intractable pruritus. Danazol has been effective in some patients (227), but androgens can reduce the plasma volume (142), which could be deleterious in these patients.

Extramedullary hematopoiesis complicates polycythemia vera most commonly with splenic involvement, although no organ is immune to its development. Mild splenic enlargement needs no attention, but progressive splenomegaly can lead to early satiety, weight loss, abdominal discomfort, splenic infarction, and portal hypertension. Four approaches are available for control of splenomegaly: irradiation, chemotherapy, splenectomy, and interferon-α. Splenic irradiation is a temporizing solution that is not always effective and can depress bone marrow function because the effective dose of radiation is not predictable (228). Bone marrow suppression in this situation can have fatal consequences (229). Irradiation is also a temporary solution to a chronic problem, although it can be repeated. It also may make splenectomy difficult because of the creation of adhesions (229). Its use should be reserved for situations in which other forms of therapy are not appropriate.

Chemotherapy with either hydroxyurea or busulfan can be used to control distressing splenomegaly, but both are leukemogenic agents, and, like splenic irradiation, their effects are temporary, requiring repeated drug exposure. Surgery has the disadvantages of the morbidity and mortality associated with any surgical procedure, in addition to the specific risks associated with removal of a massive spleen. The most important of these are hemorrhage and thrombosis. The risk of either is increased if the red cell mass is elevated (221), and the risk of hemorrhage may also be increased if there is extreme thrombocytosis (230). One risk factor for thrombosis is the size of the splenic vein remnant, a factor that is not amenable to surgical control by virtue of the local anatomy. Another may be enhanced platelet function post splenectomy (231). Splenic, portal, or mesenteric vein thrombosis occurs in approximately 6% of polycythemia vera patients post splenectomy and has no correlation with the degree of thrombocytosis (232). The complication usually occurs within 4 weeks of surgery (232,233) and may be difficult to detect by ultrasound during the immediate postoperative period (234). Thus, it may be prudent to institute prophylactic anticoagulation postoperatively and maintain it for 6 weeks. Before splenectomy, the patient should be evaluated for portal hypertension, as splenectomy alone does not alleviate this if varices are present. Importantly, both the mechanical effects of the splenomegaly and the caloric demands of a massively enlarged spleen frequently create an unfavorable metabolic environment. The patient's nutritional status should, therefore, be evaluated preoperatively, and, if necessary, parenteral hyperalimentation should be instituted to correct cachexia before surgery to avoid postoperative complications. Pneumococcal vaccine should also be administered before splenectomy.

Postoperatively, leukocytosis and thrombocytosis can be expected, and these are frequently out of proportion to what is normally observed in the postsplenectomy state in the absence of a myeloproliferative disorder (235). Indeed, it almost appears as though the spleen has had an inhibitory influence on hematopoiesis, rather than having acted merely as a site of sequestration. Asymptomatic leukocytosis or thrombocytosis requires no therapy other than correction of hyperuricemia with allopurinol. A less common but more difficult issue is the development of progressive hepatomegaly due to extramedullary hematopoiesis. Hepatic failure in this situation is more common in idiopathic myelofibrosis, and, usually, the problem is self limited or can be alleviated by chemotherapy. The use of 2-CDA has been advocated to avoid the use of hydroxyurea or busulfan but has the risk of severe neutropenia (236).

Hydroxyurea, alkylating agents, and irradiation are associated with an increased risk of acute leukemia in polycythemia vera patients without significantly altering the natural history of the disorder. The introduction of interferon-α, a biologic response modifier that suppresses hematopoietic progenitor cell proliferation (237) for the control of the complications of polycythemia vera, was a major therapeutic advance (238). Although not without significant toxicity (239–241), inconvenience, and expense, this biologic modulator does not introduce the risk of acute leukemia, addresses a broad spectrum of problems, and has a reasonable therapeutic to toxic ratio. In a review of published reports that involved 279 patients, 82% required fewer phlebotomies, and 50% required none; pruritus was alleviated in 81%, and splenomegaly was alleviated in 77% (242). In a few patients, cytogenetic abnormalities regressed partially or completely with interferon therapy (243–246). Induction doses ranged from 3 to 30 million units/week, and the time to response varied with the specific disease manifestation, requiring much longer for the reduction in organomegaly, for example, than for the alleviation of pruritus. Interferon-α appeared effective whether given early in the disease or at an advanced stage. However, toxicity led to discontinuation of the drug in 21%, mostly in the first year (242). Current data, unfortunately, do not answer the question of whether interferon-α therapy can permanently eradicate the malignant clone because a widely applicable clonal marker is lacking or whether it can improve survival. The substantial longevity of patients with polycythemia vera with the prudent use of phlebotomy therapy and avoidance of DNA-damaging agents makes the latter a difficult question to answer. Marrow fibrosis does not appear to be appreciably affected (247). The varying response rate and the difference in the required dose of interferon-α suggest that there are either patient-specific or disease-specific variables that need to be identified to optimize the use of this agent. Until more data are available, it seems most appropriate to use interferon-α to control complications such as intractable pruritus, symptomatic organomegaly, and excessive leukocytosis or thrombocytosis—the management of which would otherwise require mutagenic drugs. Interferon-α should not be considered a surrogate for phlebotomy to control the red cell mass. The biggest issue with respect to the use of interferon-α is patient compliance. This can be improved by starting at a very low dose, 500,000 units three times a week, and advancing the dose gradually. In some patients, the addition of an antidepressant may improve tolerance to the drug (248).

Thrombocytosis causes otherwise astute clinicians to suspend disbelief more often than any other condition does. From the time that an elevated platelet count was first observed in polycythemia vera, physicians have assumed that thrombocytosis must contribute to the thrombotic complications associated with this disorder (153), when, in fact, there is no proof that this is the case. Indeed, there is substantial proof to the contrary (249,250). Thrombocytosis, particularly when the platelet count is greater than 1.5 million/mm^3, is associated with hemorrhage due to a reduction in high-molecular-weight von Willebrand's multimers (79). Thrombocytosis is also associated with two other distressing problems: migrainelike syndromes (251) and erythromelalgia (252). The migrainelike syndromes include headache, dizziness, and ocular symptoms such as scintillating scotomata and transient blindness (amaurosis fugax). These conditions are reversible by lowering the platelet count or inactivating the platelets with salicylates (251). *Erythromelalgia* is a syndrome characterized by burning and pain in the fingers and toes and, rarely, on the torso, and it is associated with warmth

and erythremia. Occasionally, digital ulcers develop, and, in some patients, there may be extreme pain without physical signs. Erythromelalgia can be the presenting manifestation of polycythemia vera, primarily in the lower extremities, and its presentation can be asymmetric and may only involve a few digits (252). The pulse is preserved in the affected appendage, but acrocyanosis, skin necrosis, and digital ulcers can develop. The underlying lesions are arteriolar with vessel wall thickening, endothelial cell damage, and platelet thrombi (251). Symptoms can be evanescent or persistent (see Figs. 12-27, 12-28).

In most patients, erythromelalgia responds to salicylates. It is also responsive to platelet count reduction without the need to reduce the platelet count to normal; when aspirin is not effective or when it is contraindicated due to gastrointestinal bleeding, it is necessary to reduce the platelet as an alternate means of alleviating the problem. Anagrelide, an oral imidazoquinazolin derivative, has been successfully used for this purpose (253). Anagrelide, which is discussed in more detail in the section Essential Thrombocytosis, has significant cardiac, neurologic, and gastrointestinal side effects. They include postural hypotension, fluid retention, palpitations, tachycardia, headache, nausea, vomiting, abdominal pain, and diarrhea. It can also cause anemia and thrombocytopenia but does not appear to influence platelet function in the doses used therapeutically. It is contraindicated in patients with cardiac disease. Anagrelide should be initiated slowly at a dose of 0.5 mg twice daily p.o., and the dose should be advanced according to tolerance and the platelet count. Usually, 2.0 to 3.0 mg/ day in divided doses is sufficient to lower the platelet count over 2 to 4 weeks, and a lower dose may be sufficient once the platelet count is reduced. When the drug is stopped, the platelet count increases over 4 days.

Thrombocytosis can also be controlled by interferon-α if anagrelide is not effective. Again, the dose should be titrated to obtain the required effect, and a lesser dose may be effective for maintenance if the initial requirement was not substantial. Given the toxicities associated with interferon-α, it should not be used to lower the platelet count in an asymptomatic patient. If neither anagrelide nor interferon-α is effective in relieving salicylate-insensitive erythromelalgia or neurologic symptoms, hydroxyurea can be used—but only intermittently. Busulfan has also been used; however, considering the substantial toxicities of this drug (not the least of which is bone marrow failure), daily low-dose oral Cytoxan appears to be a better choice, although experience with this agent in polycythemia vera is limited.

Pregnancy

Given the average age of onset of polycythemia vera, pregnancy is not a common occurrence in this patient population. Yet there remains a small segment of patients for whom it is a significant issue. In contrast to essential thrombocytosis, the published experience with pregnant polycythemia vera patients is limited (254). Erythrocytosis is the most significant clinical issue, particularly because it may be masked by the physiologic hydremia of pregnancy. Considering the experience in polycythemia vera patients in general, it would be prudent to consider a normal hematocrit, including that expected for the particular pregnancy stage, as indicative of an elevated red cell mass and an indication for phlebotomy. Stated differently, the hematocrit in a pregnant polycythemia vera patient should never exceed 36%. This approach should also reduce the potential for hypertension and hemorrhage before or after delivery. Iron supplementation is contraindicated, but folic acid supplementation is mandatory.

In polycythemia vera, as well as essential thrombocytosis, it is of interest that the platelet count can fall spontaneously during pregnancy. Asymptomatic thrombocytosis requires no therapy, whereas aspirin can be used for erythromelalgia or headache. Leukocytosis is usually mild and also requires no therapy. Splenomegaly may need to be corrected in anticipation of conception or during the pregnancy. Interferon-α is the agent of choice because it poses no risk to the fetus. Anagrelide, chemotherapeutic agents, and irradiation have no role in the management of the pregnant polycythemia vera patient. Managed appropriately with regard to control of the red cell mass, these patients can safely carry to term.

IDIOPATHIC MYELOFIBROSIS

Idiopathic myelofibrosis is a clonal disorder of unknown etiology that involves a multipotent hematopoietic progenitor cell and results in abnormalities of red cell, white cell, and platelet production in association with extramedullary hematopoiesis and bone marrow fibrosis. Idiopathic myelofibrosis is the least common of the chronic myeloproliferative disorders, but was the first to have been recognized by Heuck in 1897. It also has the distinction of having the largest number of names (255). Currently, the most commonly used are *idiopathic myelofibrosis*; *myelofibrosis with myeloid metaplasia; agnogenic myeloid metaplasia; primary myelofibrosis*; and *primary osteomyelofibrosis*. The multiplicity of names reflects a lack of understanding of not only the disorder's etiology but also the nonspecific nature of its dominant clinical manifestations.

Epidemiology

The incidence of idiopathic myelofibrosis, based on a national tumor registry in the United Kingdom, was 0.7/100,000 person years (185), and it was 1.4/100,000 person years in a smaller U.S. survey (256). In the former study but not the latter, there was male predominance; overall, in most published series, there is no gender bias—in contrast to polycythemia vera, with its male predominance and essential thrombocytosis, which is more common in women. The median age of 61 years (range, 15 to 94 years) at diagnosis is similar to its companion myeloproliferative disorders, as is the increase in frequency of the disorder with increasing age. Although irradiation, either iatrogenic (^{32}P, x-ray, thorium dioxide) (168,257) or accidental (258), and exposure to chemicals such as toluene and benzene (259,260) have been associated with marrow fibrosis, no consistent environment risk factors have been identified for idiopathic myelofibrosis, and familial transmission is rare (18).

Pathogenesis

The clonal nature of idiopathic myelofibrosis and its origin in a multipotent hematopoietic stem cell have been established by G6PD isoenzyme analysis (261) and restriction fragment length polymorphism analysis using X chromosome–linked gene inactivation patterns in informative women patients who were heterozygous for the genes of interest (262,263); cytogenetic analysis of hematopoietic progenitor cells cultured *in vitro* (264); and expression of N-RAS mutations (265). In the initial studies, expression of a single G6PD isoenzyme in red cells, white cells, and platelets (261), a single restriction fragment length polymorphism in isolated granulocytes (262,263), or expression of a specific cytogenetic marker in the erythroid, myeloid, and megakaryocyte cells harvested from *in vitro* cultures of peripheral blood nonnuclear cells (264), indicated that idiopathic myelofibrosis involved a multipotent hematopoietic progenitor cell. However, a subsequent study also based on restriction

fragment length polymorphism analysis, suggested that in some patients, circulating granulocytes were actually polyclonal (266). The potential for the disease to arise in a pluripotent stem cell was confirmed in a single patient in whom an N-RAS mutation was present in granulocytes, monocytes, B cells, and T cells (265). In contrast to CML, polyclonal granulocytes have also been observed in polycythemia vera and essential thrombocytosis, as well as in idiopathic myelofibrosis (266). Whether the clinical course of the disease differs according to its origin in a pluripotent hematopoietic stem cell or a multipotent stem cell or as a polyclonal phenomenon is unknown. Like the other chronic myeloproliferative disorders, mutations of p53, Ras, or Rb are uncommon unless there is transformation to acute leukemia (62); although multiple cytogenetic abnormalities have been identified in patients with idiopathic myelofibrosis, none is specific for the disorder, and in approximately 70% of patients, a cytogenetic abnormality is not present at the time of diagnosis (267).

In keeping with a clonal origin in a multipotent hematopoietic progenitor cell in most patients, both quantitative and qualitative abnormalities of circulating hematopoietic progenitor cells have been identified in idiopathic myelofibrosis. The number of circulating hematopoietic progenitor cells is markedly increased in idiopathic myelofibrosis, and this increase includes pluripotent (CD34$^+$) stem cells as well as multilineage [colony-forming unit granulocyte-erythroid-macrophage-megakaryocyte (CFU-GEMM)] and restricted lineage precursors [burst-forming unit erythroid, colony-forming unit granulocyte-monocyte, and colony-forming unit megakaryocyte (CFU-MK)], with CFU-MK being increased the most (132,268–272). In one study, the increase in the number of circulating hematopoietic progenitor cells was more marked with idiopathic myelofibrosis than when myelofibrosis was secondary to other types of hematologic malignancies (273). Whereas endogenous colony formation was observed for CFU-E, burst-forming unit erythroid, and CFU-MK in two studies (268,270), endogenous erythroid colony formation in another study was not seen in idiopathic myelofibrosis, in contrast to polycythemia vera (274). Importantly, splenectomy was associated with a reduction in circulating GFU-GEMM, burst-forming unit erythroid, and CFU-MK, in contrast to colony-forming unit granulocyte-monocyte (275), but this effect may be temporary in some patients (276).

The mechanisms involved in the preferential increase in circulating megakaryocyte progenitor cells in idiopathic myelofibrosis has been the subject of much investigation because of the potential relationship between megakaryocyte hyperplasia and marrow fibrosis. Although spontaneous *in vitro* colony formation in idiopathic myelofibrosis as well as essential thrombocytosis has been observed by some investigators (269), others have noted a requirement for accessory cells (277) and, in particular, those cells that release IL-3 (278); researchers have also noted a requirement for a functional thrombopoietin receptor (279). In one study, CD34$^+$ cells gave rise to spontaneous megakaryocyte colonies (269), but, in another, they did not (278). The hypersensitivity of idiopathic myelofibrosis CFU-MK to IL-3 is similar to that observed for these progenitor cells in polycythemia vera. In polycythemia vera, spontaneous erythroid colony formation in the absence of erythropoietin appears to be due to overexpression of the antiapoptotic protein Bcl-xl (65), possibly due to IGF-1 hypersensitivity (23), but the mechanisms involved in spontaneous megakaryocyte colony formation in idiopathic myelofibrosis are undefined. Although megakaryocytes constitutively produce and secrete IL-1α, IL-3, IL-6, and GM-CSF (280,281), spontaneous megakaryocyte colony formation was not abolished by antibodies against IL-3, IL-6, or GM-CSF (282). With respect to spontaneous megakaryocyte colony formation *in*

TABLE 12-10. Common Causes of Extramedullary Hematopoiesis and Leukoerythroblastosis

Carcinoma metastatic to the marrow (prostate, breast, lung, stomach)
Lymphoma involving the marrow
Idiopathic myelofibrosis
Polycythemia vera
Chronic myelogenous leukemia
Myelodysplasia
Hepatitis
Hemolytic anemia

vitro in idiopathic myelofibrosis, it is important to emphasize that the bulk of the megakaryocyte progenitors, as well as the other hematopoietic progenitor cells, require hematopoietic growth factors to proliferate (269), and, in idiopathic myelofibrosis, there is an increase in the serum level of β-thromboglobulin, PF4, PDGF (283), colony-stimulating factor-1 (284), IL-6, thrombopoietin (285), and, occasionally, erythropoietin (286). The serum levels of transforming growth factor (TGF)-β_1 and basic fibroblast growth factor (bFGF) are also increased (287). Whereas PF4 (288) and TGF-β (289) inhibit megakaryocyte production, bFGF promotes it (290). However, CD34$^+$ cells in idiopathic myelofibrosis have a reduced expression of the type II receptor for TGF-β_1 and an increase in expression of bFGF receptors (types I and II) and of bFGF itself (291). This would provide these cells with either a proliferative or survival advantage in comparison to normal (polyclonal) hematopoietic progenitor cells in a milieu in which there is overproduction of negative regulatory proteins such as TGF-β_1 and PF4.

Myeloid metaplasia due to extramedullary hematopoiesis is a hallmark of idiopathic myelofibrosis but is not specific for it because extramedullary hematopiesis can be observed in a variety of conditions (Table 12-10). The clinical manifestations of extramedullary hematopoiesis include circulating nucleated red cells, myelocytes, promyelocytes, and blast cells as well as teardrop-shaped erythrocytes, splenomegaly, and, occasionally, hepatomegaly. In some instances, such as thalassemia or other types of chronic anemia associated with ineffective erythropoiesis, extramedullary hematopoiesis appears to recapitulate embryonic erythropoiesis by its appearance in the spleen and liver, but there are no tissue boundaries to its expression. In idiopathic myelofibrosis and polycythemia vera, however, extramedullary hematopoiesis is not a recapitulation of ontogeny in the sense that hematopoiesis is initiated in the spleen, liver, and other sites to compensate for bone marrow failure due to myelofibrosis. Indeed, there is no correlation between extramedullary hematopoiesis in the spleen and marrow cellularity or marrow fibrosis (95,292). Rather, in this situation, extramedullary hematopoiesis reflects the reappearance of intravascular hematopoiesis in the marrow sinusoids with dissemination of hematopoietic progenitor cells into the circulation where they are filtered out by the spleen and liver (293).

Support for this contention comes from both histologic and cell kinetic studies. Extramedullary hematopoiesis in the fetal spleen is at best marginal with the presence of late erythroblasts but few early erythroblasts or myeloid precursors and no megakaryocytes (294). Hematopoiesis is absent in the normal adult spleen, whereas in the chronic myeloproliferative disorders, both early and late erythroid and myeloid cells as well as megakaryocytes are present (294). In idiopathic myelofibrosis and polycythemia vera of long duration, extramedullary hematopoiesis in the spleen was associated with intravascular hematopoiesis in marrow sinusoids, some of which were extremely dilated. This led to the proposal that the spleen and other organs acted as reservoirs for immature hematopoietic cells, filtering them from the circulation rather than serving as sites of autonomous production (293). Furthermore, when extramedullary hematopoiesis was associated with carcinoma metastatic to the marrow, intravascular hematopoiesis was also identified in distended marrow sinusoids (295). Thus, extramedullary hematopoiesis appears to be a consequence of the marrow stromal changes associated with myelofibrosis (296). Because angiogenesis with neovascularization is intense in idiopathic myelofibrosis (297) and, embryologically, both vascular endothelial cells and definite pluripotent hematopoietic stem cells arise from a common progenitor in the aorta-gonadal-mesonephric region (298), it is possible these processes are involved in the development of extramedullary hematopoiesis in idiopathic myelofibrosis. It is only in this sense that hematopoiesis in the chronic myeloproliferative disorders can be seen as a recapitulation of ontogeny. Because hematopoiesis is clonal and autonomous in these disorders, it can never be viewed as reacting in a compensatory manner.

Progenitor cell kinetic studies are also in keeping with the concept that the spleen acts as a hematopoietic cell reservoir because, in contrast to the peripheral blood, the spleen in idiopathic myelofibrosis is largely the site of stromal and committed hematopoietic progenitor cells incapable of long-term *in vitro* culture–repopulating ability, whereas circulating hematopoietic progenitor cells in this disorder are capable of long-term *in vitro* repopulation without forming an adherent layer (299). However, after splenic irradiation (300), there was a reduction in the number of hematopoietic progenitor cells in the circulation, suggesting that the spleen does act as a site for these cells to replicate.

Myelofibrosis is another hallmark of idiopathic myelofibrosis, and, as with extramedullary hematopoiesis, the diagnosis of idiopathic myelofibrosis cannot be made in its absence. At the same time, marrow fibrosis is not specific to idiopathic myelofibrosis but occurs in association with a variety of benign and malignant disorders (Table 12-11). It should not be surprising, therefore, that marrow fibroblasts in idiopathic myelofibrosis are polyclonal and not part of the malignant clone as demonstrated by G6PD isoenzyme expression (261) and cytogenetic studies (301,302). As a consequence, marrow fibrosis is a reversible phenomenon with suppression or eradication of the malignant clone by chemotherapy (303) or bone marrow transplantation (304), and, rarely, the clone is suppressed or

TABLE 12-11. Causes of Myelofibrosis

Malignant
    Acute leukemia (lymphocytic, myelogenous, and megakaryocytic)
    Chronic myelogenous leukemia
    Hairy cell leukemia
    Hodgkin's disease
    Idiopathic myelofibrosis
    Lymphoma
    Multiple myeloma
    Myelodysplasia
    Metastatic carcinoma
    Polycythemia vera
    Systemic mastocytosis
Nonmalignant
    Human immunodeficiency virus infection
    Hyperparathyroidism
    Renal osteodystrophy
    Systemic lupus erythematosus
    Tuberculosis
    Vitamin D deficiency
    Thorium dioxide exposure
    Gray platelet syndrome

eradicated spontaneously (305). The mechanisms responsible for marrow fibrosis and neoangiogenesis are not completely understood, but recent histologic and biochemical studies have provided insight to the nature of this process, particularly with respect to the role of the megakaryocyte.

Normally, in adults, hematopoiesis is extravascular and within the marrow cavity, hematopoietic progenitor cells and their maturing progeny are enmeshed in a highly specialized environment consisting of accessory cells such as fibroblasts, adipocytes, macrophages, reticulum cells, and endothelial cells and an extracellular matrix composed of collagens (types 1, 3, and 4); laminin; adhesive proteins such as fibronectin, vitronectin, and hemonectin; proteoglycans and glycosaminoglycans such as chondroitin and heparan sulphates; and hyaluronic acid, a nonsulfated glycosaminoglycan (306). These cells and the various protein and nonprotein components of the extracellular matrix including collagen are involved in the provision of soluble and membrane-bound growth factors and selective sites of attachment for these growth factors and the hematopoietic cells that require them, in addition to providing a supporting framework. With respect to physical support, collagen types 1 and 3 form a delicate, branched, and discontinuous supporting network among hematopoietic progenitor cells and their progeny and periosteal, endosteal, and trabecular bone (307). Type 3 collagen is also associated with sinus and capillary adventitia, whereas type 4 collagen, laminin, and fibronectin are localized in a continuous fashion along the basement membranes of blood vessels and in a discontinuous fashion along marrow sinusoids (308). With increasing cellularity, there is an increase in this collagenous network, which retains its characteristically delicate strands (164). With the development of myelofibrosis, there are not only changes in the characteristics of the collagenous network but also simultaneous changes in matrix proteins and accessory cells.

The histologic hallmark of myelofibrosis is an increase in the quantity of collagen fibers and a change in their physical characteristics with an increase in the number of fibers, an increase in their thickness, and a change from a discrete linear or branched network to connected wavy fibers that are refractile when viewed by polarized light (95). Under normal and pathologic circumstances, this collagenous network is argyrophilic, staining black when exposed to silver but not staining with the trichrome stains classically used to identify collagenous deposits, whereas the latter are also not argyrophilic. As a consequence, the silver-stained marrow fibers have been considered to be an immature form of collagen designated as *reticulin*. However, by electron microscopy, these so-called reticulin fibers have the typical striated structure of true collagen (309), and the argyrophilia of the reticulin fibers is actually not an intrinsic property, but a consequence of the deposition of matrix substances such as hyaluronic acid on them (309,310). Thus, the differences in staining between collagen and reticulin reflect the abundance of the collagen relative to other constituents of the extracellular matrix such as fibronectin, hyaluronic acid, and other glycosaminoglycans. Supporting this contention is the observation that the increase in marrow reticulin is paralleled by an increase in the major collagen constituent hydroxyproline (311). Furthermore, with time, there is an increase in the content of highly cross-linked collagen and a decrease in the concentration of glycosaminoglycans (311). Advanced stages of myelofibrosis are also accompanied by an increase in fibroblasts, lymphocytes, and plasma cells and a reduction in hematopoietic cells, with the exception of megakaryocytes (255). In some patients, there is also an increase in trabecular bone leading to osteosclerosis, but, in contrast to the process associated with metabolic bone disease, there is little increase in osteoblastic or

osteoclastic activity, and the neoossification can be considered to be largely a consequence of the chemical deposition of mineral (255). With this exception, there are no histologic differences between the myelofibrotic processes associated with the various disorders listed in Table 12-11, although their etiologies vary.

Myelofibrosis is, however, not merely the sum of the synthesis and deposition of types 1 and 3 collagen in the marrow matrix by stromal cells accompanied by an increase in the deposition of type 4 collagen, laminin, and fibronectin in sinus basement membranes, which become continuous with resultant sinusoidal dilatation and obliteration and capillary neovascularization (255,297). Endothelial cells, which synthesize laminin and type 4 collagen as well as fibronectin, are also involved in the process of myelofibrosis (312,313), as are megakaryocytes, which also synthesize fibronectin (314). Neoangiogenesis in idiopathic myelofibrosis appears to correlate more with marrow cellularity and megakaryocyte hyperplasia than with the degree of reticulin deposition, suggesting that these are actually parallel processes (315). Importantly, the extent of neoangiogenesis may correlate with prognosis, while the degree of myelofibrosis does not (315,316). With increased marrow vascularity, there is an increase in skeletal blood flow (317). In contrast to multiple myeloma in which the 13q deletion was associated with bone marrow neovascularization (318), no correlation between this cytogenetic abnormality and increased marrow angiogenesis was observed for idiopathic myelofibrosis (315). Furthermore, when the Masson trichrome technique was used for staining collagen, there was no correlation between bone marrow fiber content in idiopathic myelofibrosis and splenomegaly or disease duration, but there was a correlation with the leukocyte count (319).

The central role of the megakaryocyte in the pathogenesis of idiopathic myelofibrosis is suggested by the following observations. First, in idiopathic myelofibrosis, marrow megakaryocytes are closely associated anatomically with fibroblasts and collagen deposits. Second, it has been observed that megakaryocytes, particularly young ones, secrete both TGF-β (320) and PDGF, and this process could be up-regulated by IL-3 (321), a growth factor to which myeloproliferative hematopoietic progenitor cells are usually hypersensitive. Third, acute megakaryocyte leukemia is associated with intense myelofibrosis (322), and, in this disorder, there is up-regulation of both PDGF and TGF-β gene expression in the neoplastic cells (323,324) in conjunction with elevated plasma levels of both cytokines, as well as biochemical evidence of active matrix protein synthesis (325). Importantly, TGF-β appears to be secreted in an active rather than a latent state by leukemic megakaryoblasts (323), and biochemical and morphologic evidence of inappropriate megakaryocyte cytokine secretion was also provided by the elevated plasma level of another alpha granule constituent, β-thromboglobulin, and a deficiency of alpha granules in the neoplastic cells (326). Fourth, in the gray platelet syndrome, a hereditary disorder of unknown etiology, there is a deficiency of megakaryocyte and platelet alpha granules associated with nonprogressive myelofibrosis and splenomegaly (327). Because patients with the gray platelet syndrome have elevated blood levels of platelet alpha granule proteins, it has been assumed that the premature local release of these proteins from dysfunctional alpha granules in the marrow was responsible for the myelofibrosis (328). Fifth, in addition to PDGF, endothelial growth factor, and TGF-β, megakaryocytes synthesize other proteins involved in tissue repair and angiogenesis. These include growth factors such as bFGF (329) and vascular endothelial growth factor (330); calmodulin, a fibroblast mitogen (331); matrix proteins such as fibronectin (314) and thrombospondin (332); and protease inhibitors such as PF4 (333); plasminogen activator inhibitor-1 (334); and the tissue inhibitors of matrix metalloproteinases (TIMP 1 and 2) (335). Sixth, in idiopathic myelofibrosis megakaryocytes, PDGF and TGF-β expression is increased in contrast to endothelial growth factor, another alpha granule constituent (336–338); in other studies, there was a reduction in PDGF, PF4, and β-thromboglobulin content (255), with increased plasma levels of these mitogens (255,339), as well as increased urinary excretion of bFGF, calmodulin (340), and PF4 (341). As in the case of acute megakaryocytic leukemia (323), plasma TGF-β in idiopathic myelofibrosis was largely in the active form (287). Seventh, perhaps the most important evidence that megakaryocytes are involved in pathologic marrow fibrogenesis derives from studies using the principal regulator of megakaryocytopoiesis, thrombopoietin. Chronic overexposure to thrombopoietin in rodents either endogenously by gene transfer (342) or exogenously by direct infection (343) with a thrombopoietin-producing retrovirus resulted in thrombocytosis, anemia, leukocytosis, myeloid hyperplasia, extramedullary hematopoiesis in the spleen, liver, and lymph nodes, myelofibrosis, and osteosclerosis, which are features identical to those of idiopathic myelofibrosis (255). Interestingly, in one study, thrombopoietin-overexpressing mice that developed extramedullary hematopoiesis and osteomyelofibrosis had a normal survival in comparison to control mice (344); however, in another study in which extremely high plasma levels of thrombopoietin were achieved, fatal severe pancytopenia developed and leukemic transformation occurred in some mice (53). Cessation of exogenous or endogenous thrombopoietin overexposure was sufficient to reverse the osteomyelofibrosis and extramedullary hematopoiesis and to correct the hematologic abnormalities (343,344). Importantly, in some (343,344) but not all studies (53), plasma and marrow levels of TGF-β$_1$ and PDGF were elevated in the animals exposed to very high plasma levels of thrombopoietin, but the plasma and marrow TGF-β$_1$ was in an inactive form, and direct incubation of megakaryocytes with thrombopoietin did not result in TGF-β release, whereas megakaryocyte and platelet alpha granule content was increased rather than decreased, suggesting that this model did not faithfully recapitulate the clinical situation.

Histologic studies of the marrow of mice exposed to high thrombopoietin levels revealed megakaryocyte fragmentation, suggesting an alternate mechanism for TGF-β release (343,345). Examination of the bone marrow of thrombopoietin-overexpressing mice by immunohistochemistry revealed no differences in the alpha granule protein content with respect to TGF-β or the cellular localization of these granules as compared to control animals; however, there was an increase in cytoplasmic vacuoles, ruptured alpha granules, and a dystrophic demarcation membrane system in the megakaryocytes of the thrombopoietin-overexpressing mice, as well as increased reticulin deposition adjacent to the affected megakaryocytes (345). Furthermore, increased expression of P-selectin, an alpha granule constituent and neutrophil receptor, was observed with localization in the cytoplasmic vacuoles and the demarcation membrane system of these megakaryocytes. Importantly, emperipolesis, the usually random passage of cells through other cells (346), was increased in the megakaryocytes of the thrombopoietin-overexpressing mice, and the cell types involved were limited to neutrophils and eosinophils (345). Although emperipolesis is generally considered to be a benign phenomenon, there was a correlation between its extent and the severity of the myelofibrosis, as well as evidence of neutrophil damage and apoptosis with liberation of myeloperoxidase-positive lytic granules into the megakaryocyte cytoplasm (345). Given the up-regulation of P-selectin in the megakaryocyte demarcation membrane system, it was likely that neutrophils penetrating this system, presumably due to the release of chemotactic factors such as TGF-β and PDGF by the

megakaryocytes, were trapped by binding to P-selectin and activated to release their lytic granules.

The relevance of this model system to the pathophysiology of idiopathic myelofibrosis was confirmed by the observation that there is almost a fivefold increase in megakaryocyte emperipolesis by neutrophils in patients with idiopathic myelofibrosis, with a similar increase in megakaryocyte P-selectin expression, neutrophil activation, release of lytic granules, and apoptosis (345). However, this is unlikely to be the only process involved and could even be an end-stage process because thrombopoietin levels are elevated in polycythemia vera (57) and essential thrombocytosis patients (347) who do not have myelofibrosis.

Initially, PDGF was considered the important cytokine in the process of marrow fibrogenesis (348), but it is more likely that TGF-β$_1$ is the most relevant cytokine in this regard. TGF-β is a ubiquitous protein consisting of at least four isoforms of essentially identical behavior of which TGF-β$_1$ is the most important with respect to tissue fibrogenesis (349). TGF-β is widely expressed in epithelial, mesenchymal, and hematopoietic cells, and it is a component of the extracellular matrix (350). Generally secreted in an inactive or latent form due to noncovalent binding to a dimeric peptide, TGF-β$_1$ is activated by the extracellular matrix protein thrombospondin (351), which supports the clinical relevance of increased circulating inactive TGF-β$_1$. Once activated, TGF-β$_1$ is chemotactic for neutrophils, monocytes, T lymphocytes, and fibroblasts, which it also activates (349). Activated monocytes produce bFGF, tumor necrosis factor-α, and IL-1, whereas fibroblasts and other types of cells synthesize collagen. TGF-β$_1$ also enhances its own production (349). IL-1 not only stimulates TGF-β production (352) but also is itself a fibroblast mitogen. TGF-β$_1$ stimulates the synthesis of collagen and fibronectin by fibroblasts. However, these effects of TGF-β$_1$, as well as its effects on fibroblast proliferation, are concentration dependent, with inhibition dominating at high TGF-β$_1$ levels (353). For example, a low concentration TGF-β$_1$ enhances erythroid progenitor cell differentiation (354), but at a high level, by inducing tumor necrosis factor-α production, it inhibits erythropoietin production and erythropoiesis (355) and also down-regulates PDGF production (356). TGF-β also stimulates thrombopoietin production by marrow stromal cells (289).

With respect to its influence on the extracellular matrix, TGF-β$_1$ induces collagen, fibronectin, and proteoglycan synthesis, increases the production of protease inhibitors, decreases the production of collagen proteases, and up-regulates the expression of integrin receptors for collagen and fibronectin (349,357). Many of TGF-β$_1$ effects are mediated through connective tissue growth factor, a 38-kd GP expressed in a variety of cells including fibroblasts and endothelial cells, that potentiates the activity of bFGF and stimulates fibroblast adhesion, as well as the synthesis of collagen types 1 and 4 and fibronectin (358). Although PDGF undoubtedly has a role in the processes of myelofibrosis and neoangiogenesis with respect to being chemotactic for and activating neutrophils, monocytes, and fibroblasts and acting as a competence factor for fibroblast and smooth muscle cell proliferation (356,359,360), its role remains to be defined because PDGF also enhances collagenase synthesis and is rapidly neutralized by α$_2$ macroglobulin (361) in addition to having its receptor expression down-regulated by TGF-β$_1$ (356). Furthermore, overexpression of PDGF in mice, although inducing a fatal myeloproliferative syndrome characterized by anemia, leukocytosis, and extramedullary hematopoiesis, did not cause myelofibrosis (362), and plasma PDGF levels are as high in essential thrombocytosis as they are in idiopathic myelofibrosis (363).

Given the prominence histologically of megakaryocytes in myelofibrotic bone marrow and the nature of their alpha granule protein constituents, it is easy to overlook the role of other hematopoietic cells in the pathogenesis of myelofibrosis. Yet there is compelling evidence for their participation over and above the role of neutrophils in megakaryocyte emperipolesis and destruction. For example, not all studies have demonstrated an increase in plasma TGF-β_1 levels in the experimental myelofibrosis model of thrombopoietin overproduction (53), and whereas elevated levels of platelet PDGF, TGF-β_1, and bFGF have been observed in idiopathic myelofibrosis patients (255,287,329,336), because megakaryocyte bFGF lacks a secretory leader sequence, elevated plasma and urine bFGF in these patients must come from another source (340). Peripheral blood mononuclear cells and, in particular, monocytes are likely candidates because they synthesize PDGF, TGF-β_1, and bFGF. In idiopathic myelofibrosis, the plasma level of the major monocyte growth factor, colony-stimulating factor-1, is also elevated, in contrast to the other chronic myeloproliferative disorders (284); the mechanism for this is unknown. Nonlymphoid peripheral blood mononuclear cells that are isolated from patients with polycythemia vera, idiopathic myelofibrosis, or essential thrombocytosis also overexpress PDGF and other growth and transforming factors (22). Circulating idiopathic myelofibrosis monocytes are activated and produce greater than normal quantities of IL-1α, IL-1β, and TGF-β_1 in its active form (352,364), but they require adhesion that is mediated through CD44 for the secretion of these cytokines (364,365); adhesion also induces bFGF expression by idiopathic myelofibrosis monocytes, but, in contrast to TGF-β_1, an increase in serum bFGF levels was not a constant finding in patients with this disorder (287). As a corollary, serum bFGF levels were also elevated in some patients with polycythemia vera and essential thrombocytosis in the absence of myelofibrosis (287,366), suggesting that an increase in the circulating level of this cytokine is neither necessary nor sufficient for the induction of marrow fibrosis. On the other hand, immunohistochemical studies of TGF-β_1 in myelofibrotic states associated with a variety of hematologic neoplasms demonstrated the presence of TGF-β_1 in myeloid cells as well as in the extracellular matrix, supporting the contention that monocytes, myeloid cells, and megakaryocytes are involved in the pathogenesis of idiopathic myelofibrosis (287,367).

Perhaps the most compelling evidence for a role of monocytes in the pathogenesis of myelofibrosis comes from studies of thrombopoietin overexpression in immunodeficient mice. In severe combined immunodeficiency (SCID) mice, thrombopoietin overexpression that was induced by infection with an adenovirus vector containing the cDNA for thrombopoietin led to fibrosis in bone marrow and spleen and extramedullary hematopoiesis (368,369). However, when nonobese diabetic-SCID mice were infected with the same adenovirus vector, the expected increase in megakaryocytes and platelets was not accompanied by myelofibrosis and extramedullary hematopoiesis (369). Because nonobese diabetic-SCID monocytes, in contrast to those of SCID mice, are functionally deficient, it appears that an increase in megakaryocytes alone is insufficient to cause myelofibrosis, and that normally functioning monocytes are also necessary for this process.

Clinical Features

SYMPTOMS
Table 12-12 lists the most common presenting symptoms in patients with idiopathic myelofibrosis compiled from clinical reviews published over the past five decades (370,371). Clearly, nothing is diagnostic about these symptoms, but the usually indolent nature of the disorder is emphasized by the substantial proportion of patients who were asymptomatic at the time of diagnosis. This notion is reinforced by the observation that,

TABLE 12-12. Presenting Symptoms in Idiopathic Myelofibrosis

	Percentage (%)	Range
Fatigue	64	16–77
Weight loss	32	7–50
Abdominal pain	23	4–48
Dyspnea	22	9–48
None	21	3–38
Bleeding	14	5–21
Night sweats	13	6–21
Bone pain	11	4–20
Gout or renal stones	8	4–17
Fever	7	2–30
Diarrhea	4	3–5

although splenomegaly was present in virtually every patient at the time of diagnosis (often to a significant degree), symptoms that were referable to the spleen or a consequence of its enlargement were present in less than 25% of patients. Furthermore, in many patients, symptoms had been present for as long as 10 years before medical attention was sought (372), although more often the duration of symptoms before diagnosis was measured in months. Fatigue or weakness, often associated with dyspnea, was the most common symptom, followed by weight loss, which was usually due to early satiety, anorexia, hypermetabolism, or a combination of these; gout, renal stones, bleeding or purpura, bone pain, erythromelalgia, and constitutional symptoms such as fever and night sweats were less common presenting manifestations, and, considering the generally indolent nature of idiopathic myelofibrosis, it should not be surprising that constitutional symptoms such as fever and night sweats in the absence of infection correlated with a more aggressive phase of the disease (371,373–375). Hearing loss, probably due to otosclerosis, was observed in a few studies and may have been overlooked in others (255,371). In general, with disease progression, the proportion of patients experiencing the symptoms listed increased (255).

PHYSICAL ABNORMALITIES
Table 12-13 lists the physical abnormalities observed at the time of diagnosis of idiopathic myelofibrosis (370). As with the presenting symptoms, none of the physical findings is specific for idiopathic myelofibrosis; one finding, congestive heart failure, presumably reflects the age or composition of the particular patient populations surveyed because cardiac function is not directly impaired in this disease. Palpable splenomegaly is the rule in idiopathic myelofibrosis, and in its absence, the diagnosis cannot be made. Although hematologic abnormalities and marrow fibrosis can precede the development of splenomegaly in idiopathic myelofibrosis, there is no way of predicting that in an individual patient and in the absence of splenomegaly, the diagnosis cannot be established. In this regard, surrogate techniques such as ultrasound or scanning have been used to detect splenomegaly. How-

TABLE 12-13. Physical Abnormalities in Idiopathic Myelofibrosis

	Percentage (%)	Range
Splenomegaly	98	89–100
Hepatomegaly	63	33–86
Purpura	16	3–26
Congestive heart failure	16	6–27
Lymphadenopathy	9	1–29
Arthritis	4	1–13

ever, this approach cannot be recommended because no established standards exist for this purpose using an appropriate control population. An early study also suggested a correlation between the extent of splenomegaly and disease duration (255), but this has not been confirmed (371). The rate of splenic enlargement is variable and ranges from modest to very rapid. When splenomegaly is prominent, careful consideration should be given to the possibility of portal hypertension and variceal formation (376,377). Ascites may also develop in this situation, but consideration should also be given to the possibility of primary implants of extramedullary hematopoiesis as its cause. Extramedullary hematopoiesis can also present as intraabdominal masses, and, in women, it can be confused with an ovarian tumor or cyst.

Splenomegaly in idiopathic myelofibrosis is the consequence of trilineage extramedullary hematopoiesis in the splenic sinuses and red pulp with preservation of the white pulp and its follicles—in contrast to chronic myelogenous leukemia (255). Fibrosis also occurs in the spleen and occasionally the liver but to a much lesser degree than in the marrow. There is also no correlation between splenic hematopoiesis and bone marrow cellularity, fibrosis, or disease duration (255,292), but the largest spleens are usually associated with the most cellular marrows (292).

Hepatomegaly, usually of a modest degree, is never present in the absence of splenomegaly and is always of a lesser extent than the splenic enlargement. Liver architecture is preserved in idiopathic myelofibrosis with extramedullary hematopoiesis. Most hematopoietic activity is concentrated in the hepatic sinusoids with lesser infiltration in the portal triads; little fibrosis occurs as a consequence of myeloid metaplasia (255,376,378). Lymphadenopathy is uncommon, particularly if localized to a particular region, and never substantial. Gouty arthritis or renal stone formation due to uric acid overproduction is also present in a small proportion of patients at the time of diagnosis. In contrast to the extramedullary hematopoiesis that is responsible for the enlargement of the liver and spleen, extramedullary hematopoiesis at other sites is uncommon at presentation, and its development is most likely a reflection of disease acceleration or transformation (93). Table 12-14 lists the various sites at which extramedullary hematopoiesis has been identified. Occasionally, this process can become tumorlike with extensive fibrous change, particularly in the retroperitoneum, mesentery, and pleura (372,379,380).

LABORATORY ABNORMALITIES

The range of blood abnormalities present at the time of diagnosis of idiopathic myelofibrosis is listed in Table 12-15. Anemia is the most common abnormality, and in the presence of splenomegaly, a normal hemoglobin or hematocrit should suggest the possibility of

TABLE 12-14. Sites of Extramedullary Hematopoiesis in Idiopathic Myelofibrosis[a]

Spleen
Liver
Lymph nodes
Kidneys and ureters
Retroperitoneum
Peritoneum and mesentery
Lungs and pleura
Adrenals
Skin
Heart
Dura mater
Breasts
Ovaries

[a]In order of frequency.

TABLE 12-15. Blood Abnormalities in Idiopathic Myelofibrosis

	Percentage (%)
Hemoglobin (g%)	
<10	57
>10	43
Reticulocyte count (%)	
<2	34
3–10	60
>10	6
White cell count (mm^3)	
<4000	15
4000–10,000	37
>10,000	48
Platelet count (mm^3)	
<150,000	27
150,000–400,000	42
>400,000	31
Circulating blast cells (%)	
<2	64
≥2	36

polycythemia vera, a disorder that can present with myelofibrosis but requires a red cell mass determination for diagnosis. Indeed, most published series of patients with idiopathic myelofibrosis contain a small number of patients with polycythemia vera (372,381), but this was not always appreciated by the authors (158,382). In general, the anemia of idiopathic myelofibrosis is normochromic and normocytic, and its etiology is multifactorial. With substantial splenomegaly, there is hemodilution and splenic red cell sequestration (383). Consistently, red cell survival studies have demonstrated a mild shortening of red cell lifespan, but one that should be within the range of compensation for a normal bone marrow (384,385). However, despite an increase in blood production in the majority of patients as indicated by the reticulocyte count (255,386), such compensation is not achieved. The process leading to reduced red cell survival is extrinsic to the idiopathic myelofibrosis red cell (386), and only rarely is there immune hemolysis mediated by red cell autoantibodies (387). Increased red cell turnover can lead to an increased demand for folic acid and megaloblastic maturation with the resultant development of anemia if the supply of this vitamin is deficient (388). Bleeding due to thrombocytopenia or esophageal varices secondary to portal hypertension can lead to iron deficiency. When constitutional symptoms are present, the underlying but unexplained inflammatory process associated with idiopathic myelofibrosis, often accompanied by immune complexes (389,390), also suppresses erythropoiesis and erythropoietin production. In some patients, borderline to low vitamin B_6 levels have been observed, and, with supplemental pyridoxine, anemia was corrected in a few, although no evidence of sideroblastic changes was observed (391).

Extramedullary hematopoiesis is generally ineffective with respect to maintaining the red cell mass but may prove to be a sink for diverting iron from reaching the bone marrow (392). Although myelofibrosis per se can alter marrow histology and is associated with axial and extramedullary marrow expansion, there is no evidence that the latter occurs as compensation for the former (292) or that myelofibrosis per se affects erythropoiesis (157,158). Rather, it is more likely that the primary defect resides within the abnormal hematopoietic progenitor cells and may also in part be a consequence of their dominant negative effect on normal hematopoietic progenitors, a process that could be mediated by inflammatory cytokines such as TGF-β_1 and tumor necrosis factor-α. The reversal of hematopoietic failure with clonal evolution in a few patients (305,393) supports this contention, as does the presence of active and effective erythropoiesis in polycythemia vera patients who have myelofibrosis

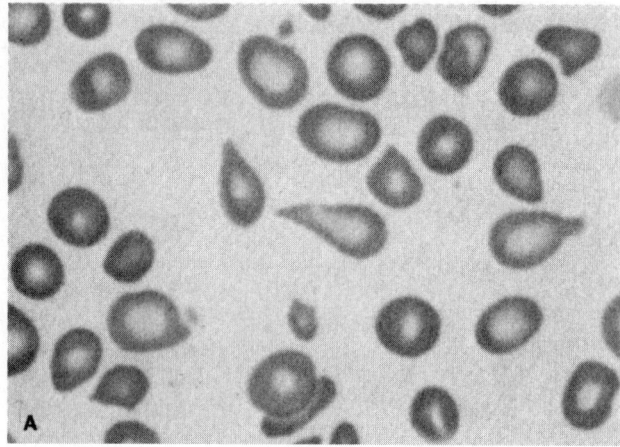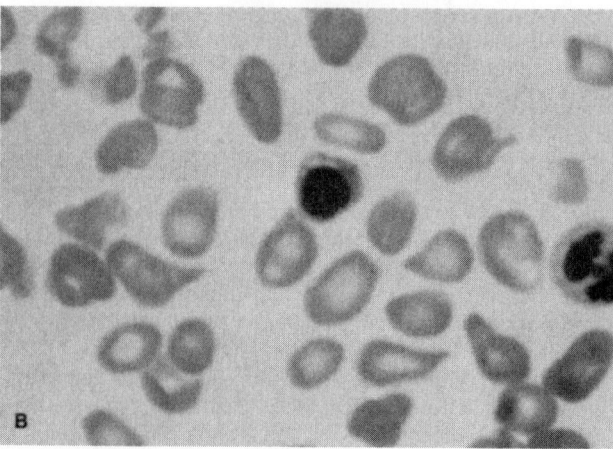

Figure 12-14. Teardrop-shaped red blood cells (RBCs), poikilocytes (**A** and **B**), and a nucleated RBC (**B**) from the blood of a patient with myofibrosis (Wright's stain, ×1000). (See Color Figure 12-14.)

(88,157). Although a paroxysmal nocturnal hemoglobinuria–like defect has been observed in association with myelofibrosis (394,395), there is no evidence that this process is involved in the anemia of idiopathic myelofibrosis.

Although hemolysis or deficiency of folic acid or iron can impart specific morphologic changes on the red cell in idiopathic myelofibrosis, the most distinctive abnormality is the teardrop-shaped red cell or dacrocyte (Fig. 12-14). The generation of these distinctive cells appears to require the presence of both an intact spleen and extramedullary hematopoiesis (396,397). As a consequence, in the absence of teardrop-shaped red cells, the diagnosis of idiopathic myelofibrosis is tenuous, although the presence of such cells is, of course, not specific for the disease. Nucleated erythrocytes are also a feature of extramedullary hematopoiesis in idiopathic myelofibrosis. They are present in virtually every patient, but their number can vary from 1/100 to greater than 20/100 leukocytes. Nucleated red cells and circulating immature leukocytes constitute the characteristic leukoerythroblastic blood picture associated with extramedullary hematopoiesis. Leuko-erythroblastosis, although an integral feature of idiopathic myelofibrosis, is, of course, not specific for it and can be seen in polycythemia vera and CML as well as a variety of benign and malignant conditions (Table 12-11) (398).

Leukocytosis is the rule in idiopathic myelofibrosis, but the count rarely exceeds 50,000 mm³, and in contrast to CML, the disorder that it mimics most closely, the leukocyte count is usually less than 25,000/mm³. In the majority of patients, there is a left shift in the neutrophil series, with promyelocytes, myelocytes, and metamyelocytes present. Blast cells are present in approximately 30% to 40% of patients without relationship to the total leukocyte count (255), but the number of blast cells is usually low. Occasionally, basophils or eosinophils are slightly increased, and in some patients, there is a reduction in lymphocytes and, in particular, natural killer (NK) cells and NK cell activity (399–401).

The leukocyte alkaline phosphatase score is usually normal or elevated but can be low as in CML (255,371,402,403). Thrombocytopenia and thrombocytosis appear to occur with equal frequency, and large bizarre platelets and megakaryocyte nuclei are not uncommon on the peripheral blood smear. Platelet dysfunction with prolongation of the bleeding time and impaired aggregation similar to that observed in polycythemia vera and essential thrombocytosis are also features of idiopathic myelofibrosis and can be even more severe than in the other myeloproliferative disorders (136). The most common biochemical abnormalities in idiopathic myelofibrosis are hyperuricemia, with higher values in men in whom gout was also more frequent (255), and abnormalities in liver function tests. Elevation of liver alkaline phosphatase is present in approximately 50% of patients and presumably reflects liver sinusoidal involvement with extramedullary hematopoiesis (255,378). After splenectomy, there is a substantial increase in the alkaline phosphatase level. Elevations of the bilirubin, lactic dehydrogenase, and transaminases also occur, but these cannot always be assumed to be due to myeloid metaplasia because folic acid deficiency, hemolysis, and hepatitis are more likely causes.

BONE MARROW ABNORMALITIES

In most patients with idiopathic myelofibrosis, bone marrow is inaspirable due to the presence of myelofibrosis (Fig. 12-15). Even when aspirable, the specimens are generally dilute and consist of disorganized clumps of cells without the characteristic marrow spicules. Failure to obtain an adequate bone marrow aspirate requires a bone marrow biopsy to distinguish marrow hypoplasia or aplasia from myelofibrosis or some other intramedullary process. Three characteristic histologic patterns have been described in idiopathic myelofibrosis (255). The first is bone marrow hypercellularity with trilineage hematopoietic hyperplasia. Megakaryocyte hyperplasia with clustering of these cells is particularly striking, and megakaryocyte morphology is dysplastic with nuclear cytoplastic asynchrony, bizarre nuclear shapes with hyper- and hypolobulation, and a reticulated chromatin pattern. Sinusoidal dilatation is prominent with intravascular hematopoiesis and increased marrow capillaries; the increase in reticulin deposition is mild to moderate. A second pattern is marrow hypocellularity with persistence of megakaryocytes, plasma cells, lymphocytes, and occasional islands of erythroid or myeloid cells and an increase in the collagenous matrix. The third pattern is that of osteosclerosis with an increase in trabecular bone collagen and osteoid seams with marrow hypoplasia and persistence of sinusoidal hematopoiesis (Fig. 12-16).

Although correlations between marrow megakaryocyte number and the extent of marrow fibrosis (255), between circulating granulocyte count and marrow collagen deposition (316), between myelofibrosis and osteosclerosis (404), and between osteosclerosis and spleen size (255) have been observed, there is no uniformity with respect to the expression of the three marrow morphologic patterns described above because each can be seen in the same biopsy specimen (292,386,405); thus, these patterns cannot be relied on to stage the disorder. Indeed, there has been an ongoing debate as to whether marrow fibrosis is progressive in idiopathic myelofibrosis, and the weight of the evidence supports the contention that it is not (316,372,406); suggestions to the contrary may reflect sampling error (407).

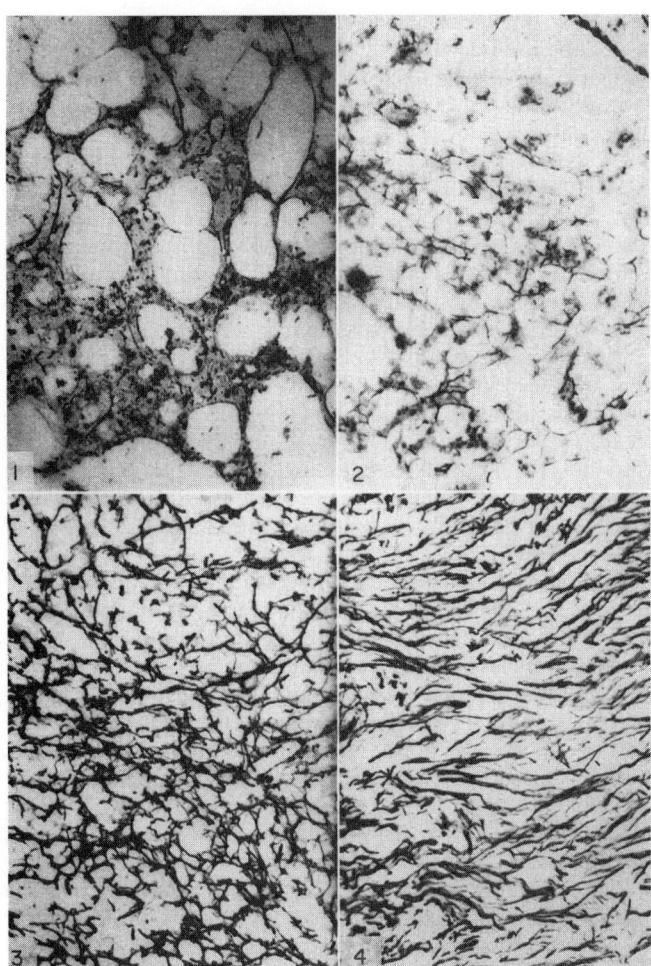

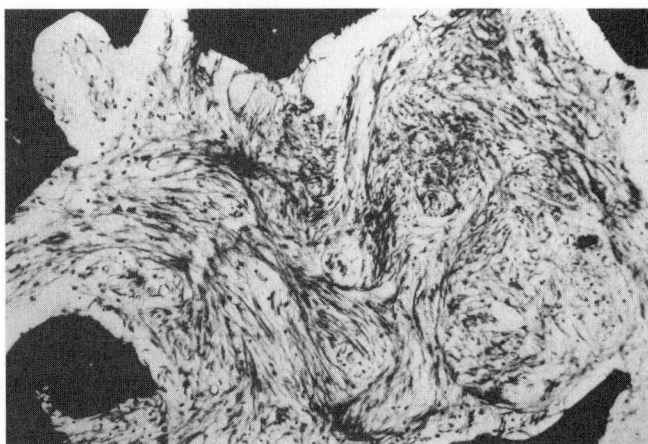

Figure 12-16. Idiopathic myelofibrosis, stage 4. Extensive fibrosis with collagen fibers and dilated, probably newly formed, sinusoids and local presence of fat cells. Irregular widened bone trabeculae (Sirius red, ×40). (Modified from Buyssens N, Bourgeois NH. Chronic myelolytic leukemia versus idiopathic myelofibrosis: a diagnostic problem in bone marrow biopsies. *Cancer* 1977;40:1548–1561.)

ganization of the open canalicular system, hypertrophy of the dense tubular system, and reduction in both alpha and dense granules (410). The same reduction in platelet GPs and increase in activation markers has been observed (100), as well as a reduction in platelet PGD_2 receptors (411), vWF, fibrinogen, ADP, 5-hydroxy-tryptamine, PF4, PDGF, and β-thromboglobulin (103,106,107); defective aggregation has been observed in response to one or more of the following: ADP, epinephrine, or collagen (412), and, as in the other chronic myeloproliferative disorders, platelet lipoxy-

Figure 12-15. Reticulin patterns. **1:** Grade +; transmitted light, from a normal marrow (×420). **2:** Grade ++; transmitted light (×420). **3:** Grade +++; transmitted light (×420). **4:** Grade ++++; transmitted light (×420). (Modified from Roberts BE, Miles DW, Woods CG. Polycythaemia vera and myelosclerosis: a bone marrow study. *Br J Haematol* 1969;16:75–85.)

RADIOLOGIC ABNORMALITIES

Osteosclerosis was detected radiologically in 20% to 50% of idiopathic myelofibrosis patients. The most common radiographic change was an increase in medullary density producing a "ground glass" appearance that was most evident in the humerus and femur. Rib involvement gives a "jail bars" appearance across the chest. In the vertebral bodies, bony sclerosis adjacent to the endplates gives a "rugger jersey" effect (Fig. 12-17) (408). The sclerosis usually involves more than one bone with the ribs, with the proximal femur and humerus and vertebrae most commonly involved, but the process may be generalized, and the skull is not immune to this complication (408). Osteosclerosis evident on x-ray suggests that at least 40% of the marrow cavity is involved; myelofibrosis per se is not radiologically detectable. Osteosclerosis appears to be related to the degree of myelofibrosis and spleen size but not to disease duration, age, or gender, and there is no correlation with prognosis (408).

COAGULATION ABNORMALITIES

The incidence of thrombosis and hemorrhage is much lower in idiopathic myelofibrosis than in the other chronic myeloproliferative disorders, but qualitative abnormalities of platelet function actually may be more severe in idiopathic myelofibrosis (Fig. 12-18) (409). Morphologically, idiopathic myelofibrosis platelets share the same abnormalities with respect to increased size, disor-

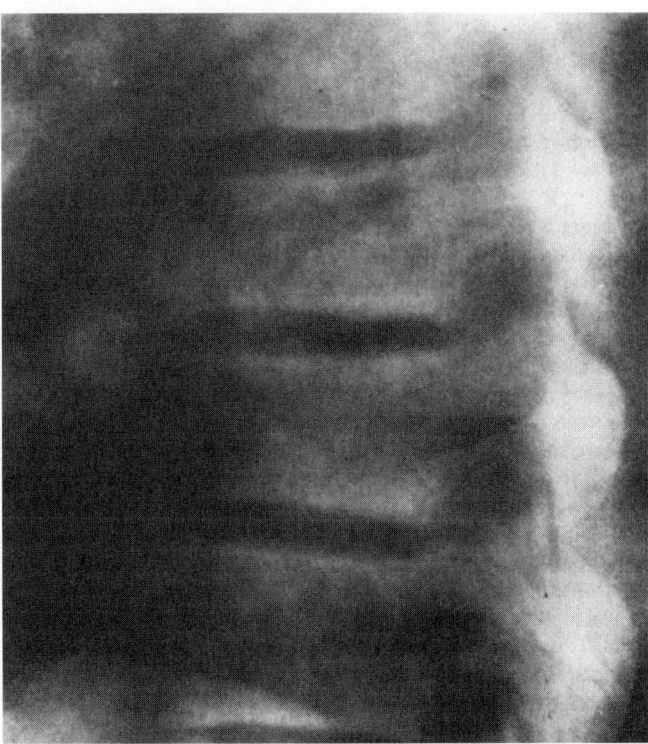

Figure 12-17. Osteosclerosis of the vertebral bodies with increased bone density adjacent to the vertebral endplates. [Modified from Ward HP, Block MH. The natural history of agnogenic myeloid metaplasia (AMM) and a critical evaluation of its relationship with the myeloproliferative syndrome. *Medicine* 1971;50:357–420.]

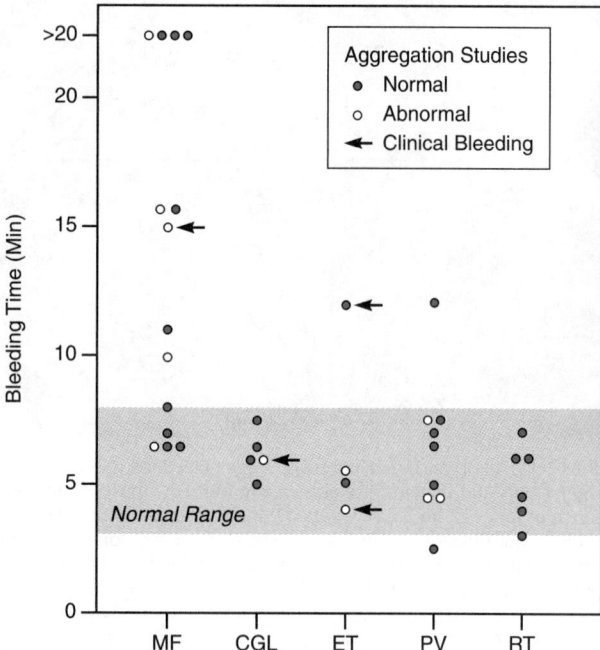

Figure 12-18. Template bleeding time in myeloproliferative disorders. Subclassifications are myelofibrosis (MF); chronic granulocytic leukemia (CGL); essential thrombocythemia (ET); polycythemia vera (PV); and reactive thrombocytosis (RT). Bleeding time was usually elevated in MF but rarely elevated in other diseases. Open circles, patients in whom one or more aggregation abnormalities were demonstrated; closed circles, patients with normal findings from aggregation studies; arrows, patients with clinical bleeding; horizontal lines, normal range. (Modified from Murphy S, Davis JL, Walsh PN, et al. Template bleeding time and clinical hemorrhage in myeloproliferative disease. *Arch Intern Med* 1978;138: 1251–1253.)

genase activity can be reduced (413). Platelet hyperfunction also was observed with spontaneous platelet aggregation (412). Circulating levels of PF4 and β-thromboglobulin are also elevated (104). This might be a reflection of megakaryocyte damage in the marrow or platelet injury in circulation (345,414). As a corollary, the bleeding time was more often prolonged in idiopathic myelofibrosis patients (409), and bleeding has been a more common complication than thrombosis (415).

CYTOGENETIC ABNORMALITIES

Cytogenetic abnormalities are present in approximately 30% of patients with idiopathic myelofibrosis at the time of diagnosis (416–419), which is a frequency higher than that in polycythemia vera or essential thrombocytosis patients and, therefore, more useful with respect to diagnosis and prognosis. As in polycythemia vera and essential thrombocytosis, none of the cytogenetic abnormalities is specific for idiopathic myelofibrosis. The most common abnormalities are del 20q, del 13q, trisomy 8, trisomy 9, trisomy 21, del 5, del 5q, del 7, del 7q, and partial trisomy 1q (253,254,306,323). More complex chromosomal abnormalities have also been documented. There are few data from serial studies, but in several patients with clinical deterioration, additional cytogenetic abnormalities were identified suggesting clonal instability or evolution (416). Although RB-1 is located on 13q, there is no evidence that it is lost as a consequence of the interstitial deletion on the long arm of chromosome 13 (420). However, it is of interest that del 13q is also seen in polycythemia vera in conjunction with the development of myelofibrosis (59) and in multiple myeloma in which it is associated with increased bone marrow angiogenesis (318). In idiopathic myelofibrosis, in contrast to polycythemia vera or essential thrombocytosis, expression of an abnormal karyotype was an adverse prognostic sign (416,417), making cytogenetic evaluation useful in this disorder prognostically as well as diagnostically.

IMMUNOLOGIC ABNORMALITIES

Immune dysfunction is a curious and unexplained feature in some patients with idiopathic myelofibrosis. The dysfunctional immunologic state is manifested by circulating immune complexes, cryoglobulins, antinuclear and anti–smooth muscle antibodies, rheumatoid factor, hypocomplementemia due to reduced C3, Coombs' test positivity, polyclonal hypergammaglobulinemia, decreased levels of B_{1H} and C3 inactivator, and a reduction in NK cell numbers and activity (389–401). The immune complexes were composed of IgG and, occasionally, IgA (421). In one study, the immune complexes contained C3 and fibronectin in addition to IgG, and plasma fibronectin was reduced (422). The frequency of immune complexes varied from 25% to 80% of patients (389,422,423) and was associated with symptomatic disease (423), advanced myelofibrosis (389), and an increased incidence of infection (390). It is also of interest that polycythemia vera patients with myelofibrosis but not those without myelofibrosis also had evidence of immunologic dysfunction with immune complex formation and anti–smooth muscle and antinuclear antibodies (389). The mechanisms for these abnormalities are unknown, but it is of note that myelofibrosis can complicate systemic lupus erythematosus (424). Most of the patients were women, and the lupus could antedate or occur simultaneously with the myelofibrosis; hypocomplementemia and a positive Coombs' test were common. In contrast to idiopathic myelofibrosis, arthritis was also common. Whereas the mechanisms for the autoimmune abnormalities in idiopathic myelofibrosis are unknown, rheumatic-type symptoms or vasculitis have also been observed in patients with myelodysplasia (425), suggesting that such manifestations in idiopathic myelofibrosis constitute a paraneoplastic process (426). Furthermore, PDGF can depress NK cell function and number (400), and circulating immune complexes could activate platelets to release PDGF and other cytokines by interacting with platelet Fc receptors. Finally, soluble IL-2 receptors are increased in the plasma of idiopathic myelofibrosis patients, and this was associated with more aggressive disease (427); the mechanisms involved are unknown.

Differential Diagnosis of Idiopathic Myelofibrosis

Idiopathic myelofibrosis is classically defined as a clinical syndrome characterized by bone marrow fibrosis and extramedullary hematopoiesis as manifested by splenomegaly and a leukoerythroblastic blood picture. However, as indicated in Table 12-10, many other disorders share the same clinical manifestations, but their etiology and management differ from that of idiopathic myelofibrosis, for which there is no currently applicable diagnostic test. To address this clinical problem, diagnostic criteria for idiopathic myelofibrosis have been proposed (428). These are listed in Table 12-16. These criteria are, of course, incomplete because they include no stipulation for clonality; although specifically demanding the exclusion of CML, they fail to exclude an equally important companion myeloproliferative disorder: polycythemia vera. Thrombocytosis also occurs in idiopathic myelofibrosis, but myelofibrosis is not a feature of essential thrombocytosis. Currently, there is no solution for the diagnostic dilemma involving idiopathic myelofibrosis other than to attempt to exclude in a methodic but parsimonious manner all those disorders that mimic it. It also needs to be

TABLE 12-16. Diagnostic Criteria for Idiopathic Myelofibrosis[a]

Necessary criteria
    Diffuse bone marrow fibrosis
    Absence of the Philadelphia chromosome or BCR-ABL rearrangement
       in peripheral blood cells
Optional criteria
    Splenomegaly of any grade
    Anisopoikilocytosis with teardrop erythrocytes
    Presence of circulating immature myeloid cells
    Presence of circulating erythroblasts
    Presence of clusters of megakaryocytes and anomalous megakaryo-
       cytes in bone marrow biopsy sections
    Myeloid metaplasia

[a]Diagnosis of idiopathic myelofibrosis is acceptable if the following combinations are present: the two necessary criteria plus any other two optional criteria when splenomegaly is present, or the two necessary criteria plus any four optional criteria when splenomegaly is absent.
From Barosi G, Ambrosetti A, Finelli C, et al. The Italian Consensus Conference on Diagnostic Criteria for Myelofibrosis with Myeloid Metaplasia. *Br J Haematol* 1999;104:730–737.

stated that attempts to diagnose idiopathic myelofibrosis in the absence of marrow fibrosis are illogical. Although the characteristics of this phase of idiopathic myelofibrosis have been identified, such identification was only validated retrospectively (429), an approach that has no clinical relevance and, if used prospectively, can only lead to the misdiagnosis and mismanagement of illnesses that mimic idiopathic myelofibrosis.

CHRONIC MYELOGENOUS LEUKEMIA

This disorder is the one most likely to be confused phenotypically with idiopathic myelofibrosis, because it can present with granulocyte and megakaryocyte hyperplasia, splenomegaly, anemia, a leukoerythroblastic blood picture, and myelofibrosis (430–432). Although uncommon, osteosclerosis can occur as well, and the histologic picture may be similar to advanced idiopathic myelofibrosis with dilated sinusoids and neoangiogenesis (432,433). Although the leukocyte alkaline phosphatase is typically low in CML, it can increase with the development of myelofibrosis (430). Furthermore, in idiopathic myelofibrosis, the leukocyte alkaline phosphatase can be normal, low, or high, making this test unhelpful for diagnostic purposes (255,402,403). Megakaryocyte morphology can he helpful because CML megakaryocytes are usually small and hypolobulated. The leukocyte count is usually much higher in CML, hepatomegaly is uncommon, and there is rarely lymphadenopathy during the chronic phase (403). Of course, the most important difference diagnostically is the expression of the chimeric tyrosine kinase, bcr-abl, in CML due to the t(9-21) translocation, which can easily be identified by fluorescence *in situ* hybridization analysis.

POLYCYTHEMIA VERA

This disorder, which can present with myelofibrosis, splenomegaly, and a leukoerythroblastic blood picture, is frequently overlooked because the increase in plasma volume associated with splenomegaly masks the elevated red cell mass (148). Indeed, the many patients with idiopathic myelofibrosis reported to convert to polycythemia vera are really patients with polycythemia vera with myelofibrosis in whom the red mass elevation only became apparent after splenic irradiation (228) or splenectomy (192,434). Polycythemia that presents with myelofibrosis will not be confused with idiopathic myelofibrosis if a red cell mass and plasma volume determination are performed in any patient with splenomegaly and myelofibrosis who has a normal or elevated hemoglobin level.

ACUTE MYELOFIBROSIS

Acute myelofibrosis, like idiopathic myelofibrosis, has a medley of names including *malignant myelosclerosis, acute megakaryocytic myelofibrosis, acute myelosclerosis,* and *acute megakaryocytic leukemia* (435,436). The syndrome is a rapidly progressive disorder with constitutional symptoms, pancytopenia, and myelofibrosis in the absence of splenomegaly and with minimal abnormalities in red cell morphology. Generally, the bone marrow is hypercellular with an increase in blast cells and dysplastic megakaryocytes. Circulating blast cells may be absent from the circulation or few in number, but the leukoerythroblastic blood picture of idiopathic myelofibrosis including teardrop-shaped red cells can be seen, although not usually to the extent characteristic of idiopathic myelofibrosis (436–438). Although it is clear that in many instances the syndrome of acute myelofibrosis is due to megakaryocytic leukemia (436,439), it can also be due to a stem cell leukemia (438) and either acute lymphocytic or myeloblastic leukemia (440). Furthermore, a similar clinic presentation can occur in therapy-related acute leukemia (441) or myelodysplasia (442). Although some authors consider acute myelofibrosis to be part of the spectrum of idiopathic myelofibrosis (443), its clinical course and features are distinctly different. Regardless of etiology, the important issue is to determine if the myelofibrotic process is a consequence of acute leukemia—a task that can be accomplished by cytogenetic analysis of peripheral blood cells or cells obtained from the marrow biopsy core, and immunohistochemical staining of the biopsy specimen for CD34+ cells.

MYELODYSPLASIA

Myelofibrosis complicates myelodysplasia with a frequency of 8% to 43% depending on the composition of the particular series (444–446), because it is a more common complication of chronic myelomonocytic leukemia than the other categories of myelodysplasia (444). Cytogenetic abnormalities are more frequent in myelodysplasia associated with myelofibrosis than its absence and are often multiple or complex (446). Myelofibrosis is more often a presenting manifestation or early complication of the myelodysplasia than a late complication and is associated with a poorer prognosis (446). Morphologically, trilineage dysplasia with an increase in megakaryocytes and, occasionally, ringed sideroblasts are present; cellularity can be normal, increased, or decreased, and a leukoerythroblastic blood picture with teardrop-shaped red cells can be present (447). The degree of fibrosis is not diagnostic. Splenomegaly is usually modest but with thrombocytosis can make the distinction between myelodysplasia and idiopathic myelofibrosis difficult. Cytogenetic abnormalities are also not distinctive unless −5 or −7 is present. Once again, severe depression of the white cell and platelet counts, as well as an increase in CD34+ cells in the marrow, favors myelodysplasia.

LYMPHOMAS

In one early series of patients with idiopathic myelofibrosis, retrospective analysis revealed patients with hairy cell leukemia misdiagnosed as idiopathic myelofibrosis (371). In an era when hairy cell leukemia was not well recognized nor its association with myelofibrosis widely appreciated, it is easy to understand how indolent pancytopenia with substantial splenomegaly and myelofibrosis due to hairy cell leukemia could be mistaken for idiopathic myelofibrosis. This is unlikely to be a diagnostic issue today, and this is also true for other lymphomas involving the bone marrow as well multiple myeloma, which can be associated with myelofibrosis (448).

METASTATIC CARCINOMA

Carcinoma metastatic to the bone marrow can stimulate fibrogenesis and extramedullary hematopoiesis producing the typical leukoerythroblastic blood picture, although not to the extent found in idiopathic myelofibrosis (449). Often, there is dense fibrosis with sparse tumor cells, and this with biopsy crush artifact can cause the tumor cells to be overlooked. Touch preparations and immunohistochemical staining for tumor-specific antigens are helpful in establishing the presence of marrow tumor.

SYSTEMIC MASTOCYTOSIS

Systemic mastocytosis can cause myelofibrosis, splenomegaly, and osteosclerotic as well as osteolytic bone lesions, and, in the absence of the characteristic maculopapular rash of urticaria pigmentosa, it can be confused with idiopathic myelofibrosis. The diagnostic difficulty is compounded when the marrow exhibits granulocytic hyperplasia (450). Anemia, leukocytosis, thrombocytopenia, and constitutional symptoms are other diagnostic confounders (451). Furthermore, in some patients, systemic mastocytosis is associated with a hematologic disorder such as myelodysplasia, polycythemia vera, idiopathic myelofibrosis, or essential thrombocytosis (452,453). Importantly, when there is an associated hematologic disorder, the frequency of urticaria pigmentosa is reduced (452). The diagnosis then rests on demonstrating mast cell infiltrates in the marrow or in other extracutaneous tissue and the presence of mast cell mediators such as histamine and PGD_2 and their metabolites in the blood and urine, although these are not specific for the disorder (451). The association of systemic mast cell disease with a hematologic disorder has adverse prognostic significance (452). Because systemic mastocytosis is responsive to interferon-α (454) while idiopathic myelofibrosis may not be (455), it is important to consider it the differential diagnosis of idiopathic myelofibrosis.

OTHER CAUSES OF MYELOFIBROSIS

Myelofibrosis can complicate a number of nonmalignant disorders, which are listed in Table 12-11. However, the clinical presentation and histopathology are usually indicative of the underlying disorder.

Clinical Course and Prognosis

The natural history of idiopathic myelofibrosis is, in general, characterized by progressive extramedullary hematopoiesis and bone marrow failure leading to splenic and hepatic enlargement, portal hypertension, splenic infarction, cachexia, hyperuricemia, anemia, thrombocytopenia, infection, heart failure, hemorrhage, thrombosis, and transformation to acute leukemia. Infection was a common complication and cause of death, with the lungs being the site most often involved in early studies (255,370,372,418). Hemorrhage, either superficial or originating in the gastrointestinal tract, occurred in approximately 30% of patients, whereas thrombotic events (which generally involved the spleen, heart, lungs or peripheral veins, and, uncommonly, the mesenteric vessels) occurred in 11% of patients (370). Hyperuricemia was very common, but gout (13%) and renal stones (7.5%) were not (255,370,371). Portal hypertension with esophageal varies and ascites occurs in approximately 10% of patients, probably from a combination of increased portal blood flow due to splenomegaly as well as sinusoidal obstruction due to extramedullary hematopoiesis (255,370). Heart failure, as a secondary complication, occurred in 23% of patients (370,418), and, in one series, hepatic failure due to extensive myeloid metaplasia was the

cause of death in 10% of patients even in the absence of splenectomy (373).

Acute leukemia, usually myelogenous, monocytic, or megakaryoblastic, occurs in approximately 14% of patients (range, 2% to 27%) (370) with idiopathic myelofibrosis with an actuarial frequency of 21% at 8 years—a frequency much higher than in polycythemia vera or essential thrombocytosis (456). Furthermore, in contrast to the latter disorders, acute leukemia is more often spontaneous in idiopathic myelofibrosis, can occur early in the course of illness, and is neither age nor gender restricted as in polycythemia (457). Risk factors for leukemia transformation, in addition to exposure to alkylating agents or irradiation, include an abnormal karyotype and a white count greater than $30,000/mm^3$ (82,405). N RAS mutations have also been observed with leukemic transformation (62).

Splenectomy has been a controversial procedure in patients with idiopathic myelofibrosis. It has been claimed by some observers to be a precipitating event for leukemic transformation (186), but this has been denied by others (381,458). Exuberant extramedullary hematopoiesis can precede leukemic transformation and could be the causal link between splenectomy and acute leukemia (379,459). The leukemia can either be abrupt or insidious in onset (456), appearing first in an extramedullary site (460). Interestingly, spontaneous regression of myelofibrosis has also been followed by acute leukemia (305,393).

Extramedullary hematopoiesis involving organs other than the spleen, liver, and lymph nodes is an uncommon but serious complication of idiopathic myelofibrosis. Virtually no organ is spared (379), and serious consequences can occur when enclosed structures such as the brain or spinal cord are involved (461,462). Mesenteric and intestinal myeloid metaplasia can cause bowel obstruction or diarrhea; retroperitoneal involvement can lead to ureteral obstruction; and peritoneal and pleural involvement causes ascites and effusions, whereas pulmonary parenchymal or intravascular hematopoiesis can cause pulmonary artery occlusion and infarction (379,463). The development of predominantly fibrous tumors with few hematopoietic elements is an uncommon but interesting feature of idiopathic myelofibrosis. These have been found in the mesentery, pleura, lungs, peritoneum, and retroperitoneum (372,379,380). Exuberant hepatic extramedullary hematopoiesis leading to hepatocellular failure has also been observed, usually post splenectomy (373,458,464,465). Once again, this is less likely a reaction to the absence of the spleen than it is a part of a generalized phenomenon that led to the splenectomy (186,379). This contention is supported by the observation that the development of portal hypertension was associated with increased (>2%) circulating blasts, leukocytosis (>30,000 mm³), hepatomegaly, and splenomegaly (316). Aggressive extramedullary hematopoiesis must, therefore, be considered as a sign of disease acceleration.

The median reported survival of patients with idiopathic myelofibrosis has been considered to be 3.3 to 5.7 years (140,255,372)—a duration not different than that for CML before the introduction of interferon-α and distinctly inferior to polycythemia vera and essential thrombocytosis for which survival approximates normal (156). However, it has long been recognized that the tempo of disease progression in idiopathic myelofibrosis can be extremely variable, with some patients experiencing a very short course and others enjoying substantial longevity (255,373,466). Therefore, a number of studies have addressed the prognostic value of the various manifestations of the disease at presentation (316,370,371,373–375,416,418,467,468). Given the heterogeneity of the patient populations examined, there has been remarkable agreement

TABLE 12-17. Two Scoring Systems for Predicting Survival in Idiopathic Myelofibrosis

(1) Prognostic factors
   Hemoglobin <10 g%
   White blood cell <4000 or >30,000/mm³

Number of Prognostic Factors	Risk Group	Median Survival (mo)
0	Low	93
1–2	High	17

(2) Prognostic factors
   Hemoglobin <10 g%
   Constitutional symptoms
   Blast cells ≥1%

Number of Prognostic Factors	Risk Group	Median Survival (mo)
0–1	Low	99
2–3	High	21

From Dupriez B, Morel P, Demory JL, et al. Prognostic factors in agnogenic myeloid metaplasia: a report on 195 cases with a new scoring system. *Blood* 1996;88:1013–1018; and Cervantes F, Barosi G, Demory JL, et al. Myelofibrosis with myeloid metaplasia in young individuals: disease characteristics, prognostic factors and identification of risk groups. *Br J Haematol* 1998;102:684–690.

on the clinical factors with adverse prognostic implications in idiopathic myelofibrosis. They include a short interval between the onset of symptoms and diagnosis; constitutional symptoms such as fevers, night sweats, and weight loss; anemia (hemoglobin <10 g%); greater than 1% circulating blasts cells; a white cell count less than 4000/mm³ or greater than 30,000/mm³; age greater than 64 years; thrombocytopenia; hepatomegaly; and an abnormal karyotype. Factors that did not appear to have prognostic significance were marrow cellularity, degree of fibrosis (reticulin or collagen), osteosclerosis, thrombocytosis, splenomegaly, and gender.

Based on this type of analysis and mathematic modeling, a number of prognostic scoring systems have devised to identify high-risk and low-risk patients at the time of diagnosis; two of them, chosen for their clinical applicability, are listed in Table 12-17 (316,373), and the corresponding survival curves are illustrated in Figure 12-19. Both scoring systems have been validated in individuals younger than 55 years of age (418,467). Cytogenetic analysis was not an option in these scoring systems owing to lack of sufficient data. However, cytogenetic analysis is extremely relevant to prognosis, particularly with respect to bone marrow failure and acute leukemia (416,417) and in patients younger than 68 years of age and anemic patients regardless of age (417). Recently, neoangiogenesis has also been suggested as a prognostic factor in idiopathic myelofibrosis (315). Bone marrow microvessel density was most marked in idiopathic myelofibrosis as compared with polycythemia vera or essential thrombocytosis and also the most closely correlated with marrow hypercellularity, age, and circulating blast cells. However, it was not predictive of survival from the time of first recognition (315).

Measurements of the serum level collagen metabolites such as the aminoterminal peptide of procollagen III and the 7S domain of type 4 collagen, as well as the connective tissue constituents, hyaluronan, fibronectin, and laminin P1, have also been employed as a means of assessing marrow fibrogenic activity in idiopathic myelofibrosis. Elevation of serum procol-

lagen III peptide was observed in some patients with idiopathic myelofibrosis, CML, and polycythemia vera, with the highest levels occurring in idiopathic myelofibrosis, including those patients with osteosclerosis, and CML (469). The serum 7S domain of type 4 collagen was increased in all of the above groups except in the osteosclerosis patients (469). Serum levels of both collagen fragments were highest with moderately advanced grades of fibrosis, and they correlated well with each other, with the leukocyte count, and with the serum alkaline phosphatase. It was thus initially proposed that serum procollagen peptide III was a quantitative marker for myelofibrosis (469,470). However, this contention was untenable because the highest serum procollagen peptide III levels were found in patients with constitutional symptoms, and the levels correlated well with the serum ferritin, megakaryocyte number, and leukocytosis but less well with the extent of marrow fibrosis (471,472). Indeed, serial measurements suggested that the procollagen III peptide was a marker of the disease acceleration or transformation rather than collagen deposition (471). As a corollary, the peptide level fell with a response to chemotherapy. Serum hyaluronan (473) and laminin P1 (474) paralleled the procollagen III peptide level, and for laminin P1 as well as fibronectin (475), substantial splenomegaly was associated with a reduction in their serum concentration. To date, correlation of the serum levels of these substances with any of the prognosis scoring systems has not been performed.

Management

Currently, there is no potentially curative therapy for idiopathic myelofibrosis other than allogeneic bone marrow transplantation and none known to prolong survival. Therefore, the first obligation in the management of a patient with idiopathic myelofibrosis is to ensure that all treatable disorders causing marrow fibrosis have been excluded (Table 12-11). Next, the patient should be staged using a scoring system for risk stratification, like those described in Table 12-17, with cytogenetic analysis, which can be performed using peripheral blood. With respect to survival, those patients younger than 55 years who are in a high-risk category with a potentially short median survival when treated with conventional therapy should be considered for allogeneic bone marrow transplantation if an HLA-matched, related donor is available. In a recent multicenter study of 55 idiopathic myelofibrosis patients younger than age 55 years, most of whom were at high risk, allogeneic bone marrow transplantation was associated with a probable overall 5-year survival of 47% (54% if a matched, related donor was used) (476). The overall year transplantation-related mortality was 27% (22% with a matched, related donor). Severe acute graft-versus-host disease occurred in 33% and correlated with the development of extensive chronic graft-versus-host disease. Pretransplant splenectomy, absence of osteomyelosclerosis or severe anemia, and a high number of nucleated cells infused were the factors associated with a shorter time to neutrophil and platelet recovery. By multivariate analysis, osteomyelosclerosis and a hemoglobin level of ≤10 g% or more, particularly in association with a large transfusion pretransplant requirement, were independent predictors for decreased survival. Treatment failure was associated with recipient age, a cytogenetic abnormality, and absence of grade II-IV acute graft-versus-host disease, the latter suggesting graft-versus-disease effect.

Unfortunately, enthusiasm for allogeneic bone marrow transplantation needs to be tempered by its lesser impact on survival in intermediate- and high-risk patients. In one study, 24% of patients at least 45 years of age were in a high-risk category (418), which correlates with recent data that an age of at

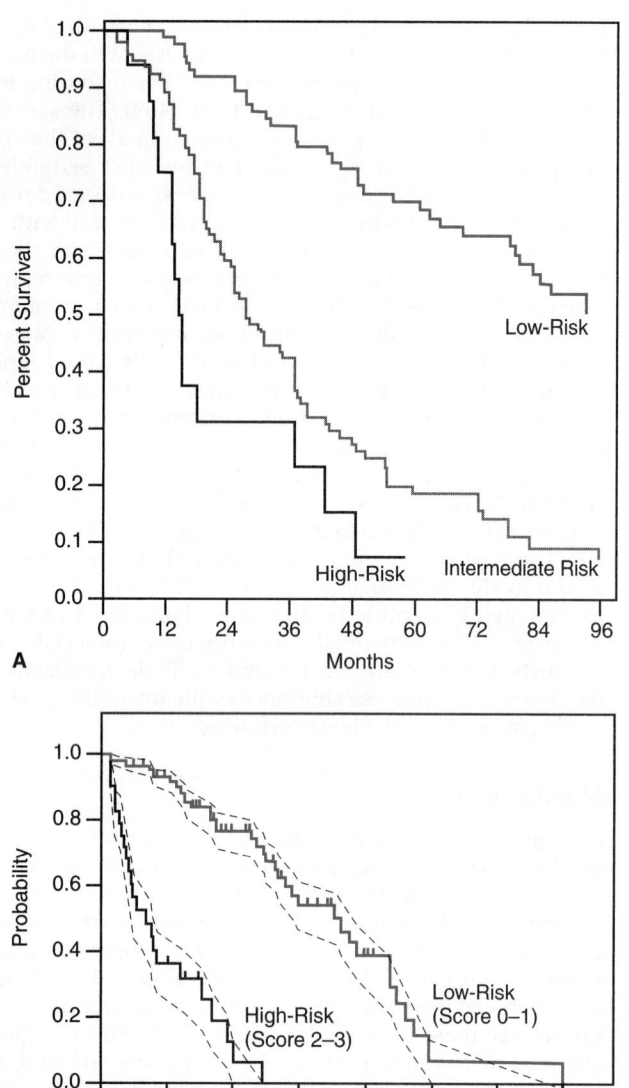

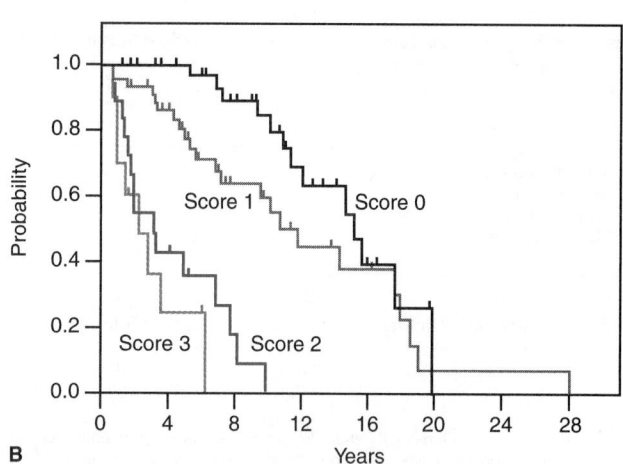

Figure 12-19. A: Survival of 195 patients according to high, intermediate, and low risk. **B:** Actuarial survival curves of the patients according to the number of bad prognostic factors at diagnosis [score 0, number (n) = 44; score 1, n = 4; score 2, n = 18; score 3, n = 10]. (Modified from Dupriez B, Morel P, Demory JL, et al. Prognostic factors in agnogenic myeloid metaplasia: a report on 195 cases with a new scoring system. *Blood* 1996;88:1013–1018.) **C:** Actuarial survival curves of low-risk (n = 88) and high-risk (n = 28) young patients with myelofibrosis with myeloid metaplasia. The dotted lines indicate the standard error of the probability of survival. (Modified from Cervantes F, Barosi G, Demory JL, et al. Myelofibrosis with myeloid metaplasia in young individuals: disease characteristics, prognostic factors and identification of risk groups. *Br J Haematol* 1998;102: 684–690.)

least 45 years had an adverse impact on survival after bone marrow transplantation, further narrowing the window of opportunity (477). Although more experience needs to be obtained and other forms of transplantation such as autologous stem cell transplantation need to be evaluated, allogeneic bone marrow transplantation using a matched, related donor should be considered as an early option for intermediate- and high-risk patients who are younger than 45 years of age; for low-risk patients, this approach should reserved for the acquisition of adverse risk factors such as increasing anemia, leukocytosis, thrombocytopenia, a cytogenetic abnormality, or constitutional symptoms in the absence of an identifiable cause. With increased experience, the mortality and morbidity of HLA-matched unrelated donor transplants are vastly improved, and nonmyeloablative transplants (minitransplants) are under study for this and other conditions.

The major problems imposed by idiopathic myelofibrosis are bone marrow failure and progressive organomegaly due to extramedullary hematopoiesis. Anemia is the most common consequence associated with bone marrow failure and the most important with respect to impact on survival (Table 12-17; Fig. 12-19). As mentioned previously, the anemia of idio-

pathic myelofibrosis is multifarious, having various contributions by hemodilution, iron, folic acid (388) or vitamin B_6 deficiency (391), blood loss due to gastrointestinal hemorrhage, hemolysis that is usually not autoimmune, suppression of erythropoietin production (286), and loss of effective marrow volume. Red cell aplasia has been considered to be a complication of idiopathic myelofibrosis, but review of these cases indicates that they represent either *de novo* or treatment-related myelodysplasia or acute myelofibrosis (478,479). Because there is evidence that correction of anemia is associated with improved survival (480), it is important to identify correctable causes of anemia. In the era before recombinant erythropoietin was available, androgens were a popular remedy (480,481). However, it is difficult to condone their use today because of the risks of liver damage, fluid retention, and heart failure and because often their effect is more apparent than real, which is due in part to a reduction in plasma volume (142). Furthermore, the response rate to androgen therapy was not only low (<30%), but survival was also not influenced in one study as compared with transfusions (481). Whether the impeded androgen Danazol will be more effective than other formulations remains to be determined (482,483).

The serum erythropoietin level in idiopathic myelofibrosis appears to be appropriately elevated to the degree of anemia in most patients (286), but this observation may be misleading because the observed increase in circulating erythropoietin was obviously not sufficient to correct the anemia—a situation common to the anemia of chronic disease (484). Thus, with symptomatic anemia in the absence of a correctable cause and when the serum erythropoietin level is less than 200 mU/mL, a trial of recombinant human erythropoietin at 40,000 U s.c. weekly is appropriate, although many patients do not respond (485,486). A caveat here is the tendency for stimulation of extramedullary hematopoiesis by recombinant erythropoietin with organ enlargement, particularly of the spleen but the liver may also enlarge. Thus, recombinant erythropoietin therapy should be carefully monitored using the minimal effective dose.

Many patients with idiopathic myelofibrosis have constitutional symptoms, which are in some instances associated with evidence of autoimmune phenomena. Anecdotal experience in patients with idiopathic myelofibrosis and myelofibrosis associated with myelodysplasia suggests that corticosteroid therapy might be effective in the correction of anemia (487,488). Although no controlled studies have been performed, a trial of pulse dexamethasone, 10 mg q.i.d. for 4 days seems reasonable when constitutional symptoms or evidence of autoimmune phenomena are present, particularly in association with symptomatic anemia.

Progressive organomegaly, particularly splenomegaly, is the second major management challenge in idiopathic myelofibrosis, giving rise to mechanical problems such as early satiety, diarrhea, abdominal distention, and discomfort; sequestration of platelets and white cells; local circulatory insufficiency leading to splenic infarction; diversion of nutritional and energy resources leading to cachexia; and increased splenic blood flow, which leads to portal hypertension, esophageal varies, and ascites. In the setting of myelofibrosis, it is often difficult to determine the contribution of splenomegaly to anemia, leukopenia, or thrombocytopenia. With respect to anemia, ferrokinetic studies have not been revealing with regard to bone marrow function owing to the confounding presence of extramedullary hematopoiesis (392), and splenectomy was associated with an improvement in the hemoglobin level or a reduction in transfusion requirements in only 30% of patients (371,458). If hypersplenism is considered a possibility, this should be confirmed by red cell survival and splenic sequestration studies with the caveat that if bone marrow function is also impaired, removal of the spleen may not lead to resolution of low blood counts.

Progressive splenomegaly needs to be addressed aggressively because it can lead to portal hypertension and cachexia and may be a manifestation of disease acceleration. The latter cause of splenomegaly may be the reason for the apparent associations of splenectomy with transformation to acute leukemia (186,459) and progressive hepatomegaly (464,465). Splenomegaly can often be controlled by oral chemotherapy using either an alkylating agent, such as busulfan, or hydroxyurea. Busulfan or thioguanine therapy has been demonstrated to relieve constitutional symptoms, reverse myelofibrosis, reduce splenomegaly and hepatomegaly, and, occasionally, increase the hemoglobin level (489,490). It is of interest that the reduction in marrow fibrosis observed with busulfan was not accompanied by a change in marrow megakaryocyte number (303). Suppression of the neutrophil and platelet count can occur, and the presence of leukopenia or thrombocytopenia can limit the use of this agent. Hydroxyurea is also effective in reducing organomegaly but can also cause significant bone marrow suppression. Both alkylating agents and hydroxyurea are leukemogenic; therefore, their use should be judicious. They also have significant other side effects as well.

Interferon-α therapy is an alternative approach to suppressing extramedullary hematopoiesis and controlling disease progression in idiopathic myelofibrosis because it impairs the proliferation of both hematopoietic and fibroblast progenitor cells (272,491). However, its side effects limit its usefulness, particularly in older patients, whereas its myelosuppressive effects can also be limiting when there is significant initial leukopenia or thrombocytopenia. Anecdotally, interferon-α has been used successfully to reduce splenomegaly (492), alleviate bony pain, and ameliorate anemia (493), but the response was not uniform (455,493,494), and it was inferior to that observed in polycythemia vera and essential thrombocytosis (495). Unfortunately, as with the types of conventional therapy used in the management of idiopathic myelofibrosis, no controlled prospective studies have been caused in patients stratified by risk group (Table 12-17). Overall, in 120 patients treated to date with doses of interferon ranging from 1 to 5 million units/day, a response rate of approximately 50% was observed for reduction in spleen size, leukocytosis, and thrombocytosis (496). Anemia was less likely to be alleviated and myelofibrosis only occasionally (493). In older patients, it is important to start at a very low dose with gradual increments as tolerated and to allow sufficient time for a response to occur.

The roles of splenectomy and splenic irradiation in the management of splenomegaly in idiopathic myelofibrosis have been the subject of much debate. Historically, splenectomy has been associated with a high morbidity (45%) and mortality rate (13%) with postoperative hemorrhage, mesenteric vein thrombosis, infection, exuberant leukocytosis and thrombocytosis, and leukemic transformation being the major problems encountered. Splenectomy has not been demonstrated to improve survival, and it continues in more recent studies to have substantial perioperative morbidity and mortality. In one study, splenectomy was shown to effectively alleviate the mechanical distress imposed by splenomegaly, provide relief from constitutional symptoms in 67% of patients, correct portal hypertension due to increased blood flow in 50%, and alleviate anemia in more than 20% of patients. Thrombocytopenia, however, was not appreciably improved (458). Postoperative complications (bleeding in 15%, infection in 9%, and thrombosis in 7%) occurred in 31% of patients—a frequency lower than in previous series. The mortality rate of 9% was also lower but still substantial with deaths due to hemorrhage, infection, or thrombosis. Thrombocytosis, which occurred in 22% of patients, was correlated with postoperative thrombosis and a hypo- or normocellular marrow was also associated with a lower postoperative survival. Marrow cellularity, collagen fibrosis, and cytogenetic abnormalities did not correlate with the effect of splenectomy on anemia (458). Postsplenectomy hepatomegaly occurred in 16% of patients, was not predictable, and did not have an impact on survival. Postsplenectomy hepatomegaly was also associated with an increase in serum alkaline phosphatase and gamma glutamyl transferase levels. Chemotherapy may be needed to control hepatic extramedullary hematopoiesis post splenomegaly. Hydroxyurea, busulfan, and even 2-CDA (236) have been used for this purpose, although the risk of severe myelosuppression must be considered, particularly with the latter agent.

The frequency of leukemic transformation post splenectomy in one series was 16%, but survival in these patients was not different from postsplenectomy patients who did not develop acute leukemia (458). This is in contrast to another report in which the frequency of leukemic transformation post splenectomy was twice that of nonsplenectomized patients (186). In this latter study, splenectomized patients were younger and had lower leukocyte counts and higher numbers of circulating blasts than their nonsplenectomized counterparts; most importantly, 72% had received chemotherapy as compared to 56% of the nonsplenectomized patients. The criteria for leukemic transformation were also less stringent than in other studies. Postsplenectomy blast transformation was also associated with a much lower median survival: 52 months versus 114 months. Although it is of interest that splenectomy is associated with an increased risk of leukemia in Hodgkin's disease (187) and aplastic anemia (188), suggesting an immunologic mechanism, it is more likely that in idiopathic myelofibrosis, the association is the result of disease acceleration causing splenomegaly, rather than splenectomy causing disease acceleration. It is also likely that chemotherapy pre splenectomy may provoke the leukemic transformation.

When splenectomy is considered, it is imperative that the patient has optimal nutritional status. This may entail parenteral hyperalimentation before surgery to prevent the postoperative morbidity and mortality related to a cachectic state. Furthermore, the surgeon should be familiar with the removal of a massive spleen because the presence of multiple adhesions, hypertrophied vessels, splenic varices, and the hemorrhagic diathesis associated with idiopathic myelofibrosis represent substantial challenges. Usually, the splenic vein remnant is not resectable, and it provides a potential site for postoperative thrombosis. Splenic, portal, and mesenteric vein thrombosis post splenectomy do not correlate with the platelet count (232) and may occur without symptoms (233). Ultrasound or radiologic imaging is recommended after splenectomy in patients with idiopathic myelofibrosis to monitor the development of intraabdominal venous thrombosis (233,234). Importantly, the risk of intraabdominal venous thrombosis is not limited to the immediate postoperative period (232). Whether prophylactic anticoagulation post splenectomy would be beneficial is unknown, but it seems reasonable because platelet aggregation is enhanced post splenectomy (231).

Splenic irradiation is another effective means of temporarily reducing spleen size and alleviating spleen-related pain. Splenomegaly was reduced in 95% of patients with a 50% or greater reduction in spleen size, and subjective relief of pain was reduced in approximately 90% of patients. Weight loss was also stabilized or reversed, and neither the efficiency nor the duration of response was reduced after multiple courses of irradiation (229,497). The response can be dramatic, but the median duration is usually 6 months. Complete hematologic remission has been obtained, but this was usually in patients with myelofibrosis complicating polycythemia vera in which, unlike idiopathic myelofibrosis, bone marrow failure is not an issue if the patient has not had prior chemotherapy exposure (228). Blood count suppression is the major toxicity of splenic irradiation. Myelosuppression occurred in 44% of patients in one series and contributed to a 50% mortality rate. Myelosuppression is probably due to either collateral marrow irradiation or damage to circulating hematopoietic progenitor cells in the spleen (300). Because irradiation can also mobilize hematopoietic progenitor cells (300), it may play a role in potentiating its own toxicity. Prior splenic irradiation can also complicate subsequent splenectomy (229).

Pretreatment factors such as blood counts, prior therapy, or disease duration were not predictive of radiation cytotoxicity, nor was monitoring of blood counts or the radiation dose useful

in this regard (229). Because intermittent therapy was as effective as daily fractionated therapy (498), using a conservative approach and adjusting the irradiation dose based on changes in spleen size is the safest policy. Irradiation is also useful for controlling localized extramedullary hematopoiesis and for the occasional patient with painful periostitis (499) and painful hepatomegaly (500).

The frequency of acute leukemia as the terminal event in idiopathic myelofibrosis varies in reported series from 5% to 27% with an actuarial probability of 8% at 5 years and 20% at 10 years (456). The onset can be acute or insidious, manifested mainly by exuberant and inappropriate extramedullary hematopoiesis. Invariably, the disorder is resistant to conventional chemotherapy, and the terminal course is rapid.

Recently, there has been substantial interest in the use of agents such as thalidomide, which inhibit fibrogenesis or angiogenesis, in the management of idiopathic myelofibrosis (501). At this juncture, the use of such agents is experimental and based on the assumptions that myelofibrosis and neoangiogenesis are either causal or pejorative in this disease. However, neither assumption has been proved.

ESSENTIAL THROMBOCYTOSIS

Essential thrombocytosis (other designations include *essential thrombocythemia, idiopathic thrombocytosis, primary thrombocytosis,* and *hemorrhagic thrombocythemia*) is a clonal disorder of unknown etiology (502,503) that involves a multipotent hematopoietic progenitor cell causing overproduction of platelets in the absence of a definable stimulus. Essential thrombocytosis is the least defined of the chronic myeloproliferative disorders because it lacks a clinically applicable clonal marker and the physiology of thrombopoiesis is not completely understood. As a consequence, because thrombocytosis is a feature of many benign and malignant disorders that do not involve the bone marrow (Table 12-18) and also a presenting manifestation of polycythemia vera, idiopathic myelofibrosis, CML, myelodysplasia, or systemic mastocytosis (453), the diagnosis of essential thrombocytosis has been customarily one of exclusion, although diagnostic criteria for it have been proposed (Table 12-19) (504). However, just as the assumption that the absence of evidence is proof of its absence is fallacious, the assumption that all patients identified by exclusion

TABLE 12-18. Causes of Thrombocytosis

Tissue inflammation
    Collagen vascular disease
    Inflammatory bowel disease
Malignancy
Infection
Myeloproliferative disorders
    Polycythemia vera
    Idiopathic myelofibrosis
    Essential thrombocytosis
    Chronic myelogenous leukemia
Myelodysplastic disorders
    5q– syndrome
    Idiopathic refractory sideroblastic anemia
Postsplenectomy or hyposplenism
Hemorrhage
Renal disease
Iron deficiency anemia
Surgery
Rebound
    Correction of vitamin B_{12} or folate deficiency, post ethanol abuse
Hemolysis

TABLE 12-19. Diagnostic Criteria for Essential Thrombocytosis

PVSG criteria
    Platelet count >600,000/mm³
    Hemoglobin <13 g% or normal red cell mass for gender
    Presence of marrow-stainable iron or failure of hemoglobin to increase >1 g% after 1-mo trial of iron therapy
    Megakaryocyte hyperplasia
    Absence of significant myelofibrosis
    Absence of the Philadelphia chromosome
    No more than two of the following:
        Mild myelofibrosis (<¹/₃ of biopsy area)
        Splenomegaly
        Leukoerythroblastic reaction
        Absence of a cause for reactive thrombocytosis
Rotterdam criteria of the Thrombocythemia Study Group
    Diagnostic
        Platelet count >400,000/mm³
        A_1: No known cause of thrombocytosis
        A_2: Increase and clustering of enlarged mature megakaryocytes with hyperploid nuclei in a bone marrow biopsy
    Confirmative
        B_1: Normal or elevated leukocyte alkaline phosphatase score, normal ESR, and no fever or infection
        B_2: Normal or increased cellularity of the bone marrow with or without the presence of reticulin fibers in biopsy material
        B_3: Splenomegaly on palpation, isotope or ultrasound scan, or computed tomogram
        B_4: Spontaneous erythroid colony formation (EEC) and/or spontaneous megakaryocyte colony formation
    Exclusion criteria: proposed by the PVSG
        I: Philadelphia chromosome or other chromosome abnormality
        II: Collagen fibrosis of the bone marrow in biopsy sections
        III: Osteosclerosis of the bone marrow in biopsy sections
        IV: Myelodysplastic features

From Michiels JJ, Juvonen E. Proposal for revised diagnostic criteria of essential thrombocythemia and polycythemia vera by the Thrombocythemia Vera Study Group. *Semin Thromb Hemost* 1997;23:339–347.

---

as having essential thrombocytosis actually have that particular illness is equally fallacious. Precedent for this contention is found in the variety of disorders discovered to date that cause isolated erythrocytosis in the absence of hypoxia (36), and this is probably no less true for essential thrombocytosis because even less is known about the regulation of platelet production.

The association of thrombocytosis with bone marrow disorders was first recognized by Di Guglielmo in 1920 (505). The term *hemorrhagic thrombocythemia* was first used by Reid in 1940 (506), who was the first to suggest that hemorrhagic thrombocythemia constituted a distinct clinical syndrome; in 1951, Dameshek included the disorder in the constellation of the chronic myeloproliferative diseases (1). It was Dameshek's hypothesis that polycythemia vera, idiopathic myelofibrosis, essential thrombocytosis, and CML each represented a different manifestation of the same disorder involving a multipotent hematopoietic stem cell, and as a corollary, transitions between them were to be expected. Although Dameshek's proposal was useful in codifying the chronic myeloproliferative disorders, he was misled with respect to transitions among them because of phenotypic mimicry. Only with respect to thrombocytosis is there any link between the chronic myeloproliferative disorders, and that is because thrombocytosis can be the sole presenting manifestation of each, even though their pathogenesis differs. Indeed, in a 1955 review of the published reports to date of hemorrhagic thrombocythemia (507), McCabe and co-workers raised substantial questions about the validity of considering hemorrhagic thrombocythemia as a unique clinical entity. However, it was not until 1960 that two major reviews (508,509) swayed clinicians to the consensus that "hemorrhagic thrombocythe-

mia" was a distinct disorder. It is, therefore, ironic that many of the patients in these two reviews actually had polycythemia vera rather than essential thrombocytosis. It is further ironic that although hemorrhagic complications were the major clinical manifestations observed in the reported patients, current publications stress the thrombotic complications of essential thrombocytosis. In denying that hemorrhage could be a significant feature of polycythemia vera or that microvascular occlusive events could occur in essential thrombocytosis, and in failing to consider the presence of masked erythrocytosis (148), these early reports, while raising clinical awareness and building clinical consensus, only served to confuse the situation. Indeed, although current clinical evidence supports the contention that essential thrombocytosis constitutes a distinct chronic myeloproliferative disorder, it needs to be continually reemphasized that not every patient with an elevated platelet count of unknown etiology necessarily has essential thrombocytosis. Consequently, although the term *thrombocythemia* was proposed to distinguish this disorder from the many known secondary causes of thrombocytosis, much as the term *erythremia* was once used to distinguish polycythemia vera from nonclonal forms of erythrocytosis, it seems more appropriate to use the designation *essential thrombocytosis* rather than *thrombocythemia* given the continued element of clinical uncertainty. Such a designation emphasizes that until a clinically applicable clonal marker becomes available, the diagnostic evaluation must be thorough and therapy must be judicious to avoid exposing patients with an unrecognized but benign cause for thrombocytosis to mutagenic agents or mistreating patients with other clonal disorders complicated by thrombocytosis.

Epidemiology

The epidemiology of essential thrombocytosis is not well defined because there is not a definitive test to distinguish clonal thrombocytosis from the many nonclonal causes (Table 12-18) and, for many years, enumeration of platelets for clinical purposes was not routine. Furthermore, because most patients with the disorder are asymptomatic and symptomatic patients are more likely to be referred to academic medical centers, ascertainment bias has been an inevitable feature of most clinical reports. Finally, several different sets of diagnostic criteria for essential thrombocytosis have been proposed (Table 12-19), and the particular diagnostic criteria chosen, especially the platelet count threshold, also influence case ascertainment.

In the era before platelet counts were performed routinely, review of 14,000 blood smears for an increase in platelet number over 10 months at a major academic medical center yielded 82 patients (0.6%) in whom a subsequent platelet count was greater than 400,000/mm³ (510). Of these 82 patients, only four (5%) had a chronic myeloproliferative disorder. With the advent of routine platelet counts, the incidence of thrombocytosis, defined as a platelet count greater than 500,000/mm³, increased, but the proportion due to myeloproliferative disorders remained essentially unchanged at approximately 3% to 6%/year (511–513). If, however, only platelet counts greater than 1 million/mm³, the so-called platelet millionaires (235), were considered, the proportion due to myeloproliferative disorders increased to 13.5% (514); when a bone marrow examination was also part of the evaluation, the proportion was 56% (515). With respect to the individual myeloproliferative disorders, among a total of 263 reported patients, 34% had essential thrombocytosis, 26% had polycythemia vera, 23% had CML, 8% had idiopathic myelofi-

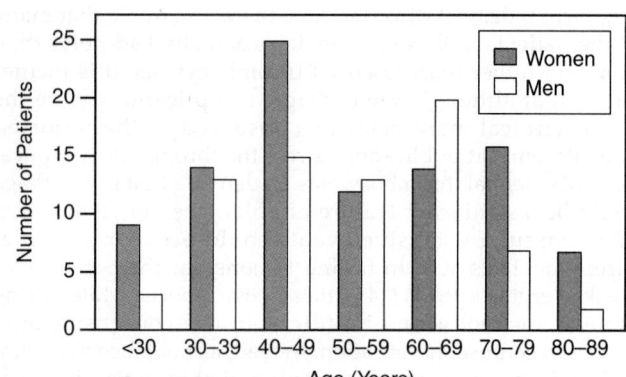

Figure 12-20. Age and sex distribution of essential thrombocythemia patients at diagnosis. (Modified from Jantunen R, Juvonen E, Ikkala E, et al. Essential thrombocythemia at diagnosis: causes of diagnostic evaluation and presence of positive diagnostic findings. *Ann Hematol* 1998; 77:101–106.)

brosis, and 9% had an unclassifiable myeloproliferative disorder. Taken together, chronic myeloproliferative disorders constitute less than 10% of patients identified as having thrombocytosis in an unselected patient population, but the proportion doubles when the platelet count is greater than 1 million/mm^3, and approximately a third of these patients have essential thrombocytosis.

Given the same caveats for population-based studies, the overall age- and gender-adjusted incidence rate/100,000 person years for essential thrombocytosis was 0.8 for the United Kingdom, with a female predominance (185). In a smaller U.S.-based population, the incidence rate was 2.53, again with female predominance (256), whereas in a single county in Denmark, the incidence rate was 0.59, with a 3.2-fold increase in incidence over the 21-year interval of observation and a female to male ratio of 2.6:1.0 (516). The overall female to male ratio, based on ten published reports totaling 956 patients, was approximately 1.5:1.0 (517–524). The mean age of onset for essential thrombocytosis was 51 years, with a range of 6 to 90 years. Interestingly, the incidence of essential thrombocytosis appears to be biphasic in women, with an initial peak at age 50 and a second peak at age 70, whereas in men there is a steady increase with age (Fig. 12-20) (523). This may reflect the frequency with which health care, particularly in the reproductive age range, is sought because women were more likely to be asymptomatic at diagnosis than men (523). Familial transmission is uncommon (18,525–531) and must be distinguished from benign hereditary thrombocytosis (532,533) and the initial manifestations of polycythemia vera (84) or myelofibrosis.

Pathogenesis

The megakaryocyte is the least common of the hematopoietic progenitor cells and the only one whose maturation is characterized by endomitosis. Until the discovery and cloning of its essential growth factor, thrombopoietin (534), and the thrombopoietin receptor, Mpl (535), the physiology of megakaryocytopoiesis was not well defined, and, as a consequence, the pathophysiology of disorders characterized by excessive platelet production was also poorly understood. Now, however, as is the case with erythrocytosis, it has been possible to define thrombocytosis into primary and secondary forms. As with erythrocytosis, however, the boundary between the two in a given patient is not always distinct.

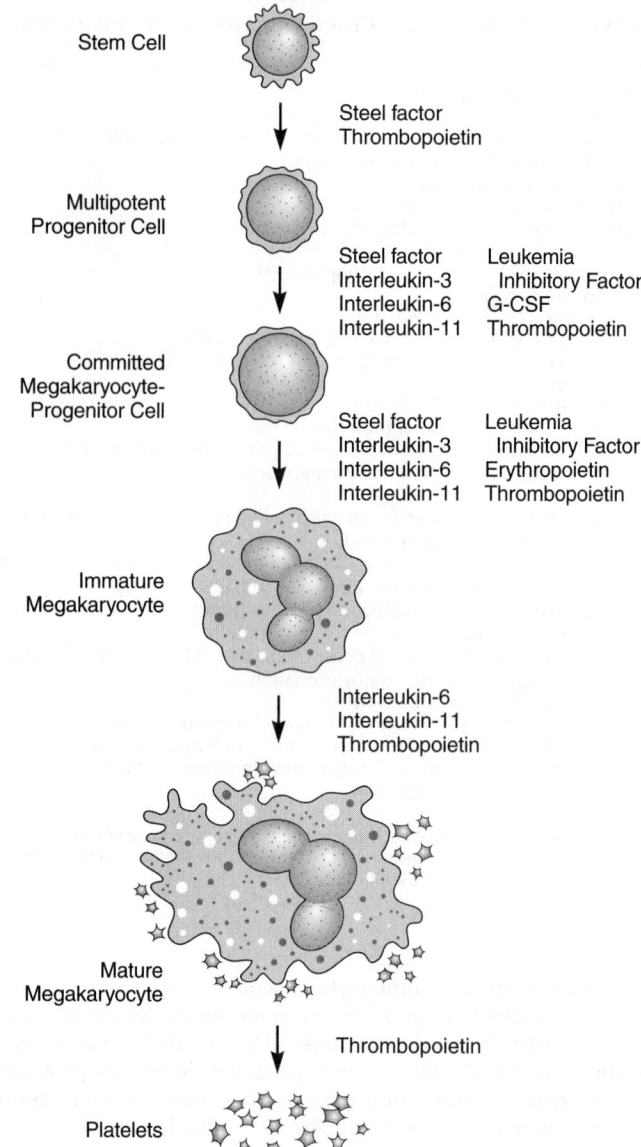

Figure 12-21. A scheme of megakaryocytopoiesis. G-CSF, granulocyte colony-stimulating factor. (Modified from Kaushansky K. Thrombopoietin. *N Engl J Med* 1998;339:746–754.)

Megakaryocytopoiesis is a complex process that, like erythropoiesis, involves the cooperative behavior of a number of hematopoietic growth factors in addition to thrombopoietin. Indeed, like erythropoiesis in which the initial stages can proceed in the absence of erythropoietin or its receptor (536), megakaryocytopoiesis can also proceed in the absence of thrombopoietin or its receptor (537). Knockout mice lacking either produce approximately 15% of the platelets found in normal animals, and these platelets were morphologically and functionally normal (538). The mechanism for this lies in the redundancy of hematopoiesis, in which multiple growth factors have overlapping functions. For example, in mice lacking erythropoietin receptors, erythropoiesis, at least *in vitro*, can be rescued by thrombopoietin (539). Figure 12-21 illustrates a current scheme of megakaryocytopoiesis, in which a variety of hematopoietic growth factors act in concert to promote the proliferation and differentiation of megakaryocyte progenitor cells to mature megakaryocytes capable of releasing functional platelets (540,551). Although only the committed megakaryocyte progenitor cell is illustrated, it is

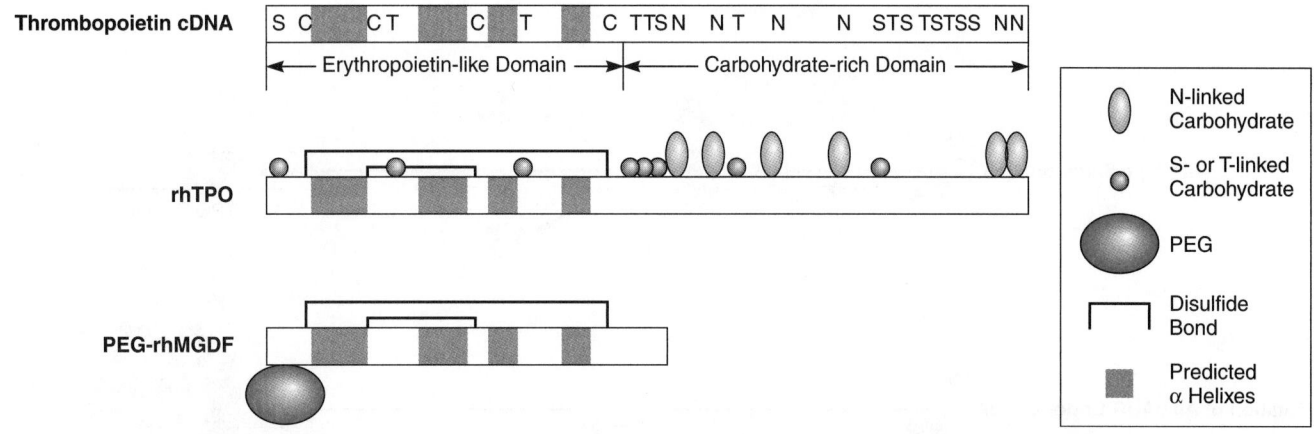

Thrombopoietin cDNA S C CT C T C TTSN NT N   N STS TSTSS NN

Erythropoietin-like Domain ——— Carbohydrate-rich Domain ———

rhTPO

PEG-rhMGDF

N-linked Carbohydrate

S- or T-linked Carbohydrate

PEG

Disulfide Bond

Predicted α Helixes

Figure 12-22. The structure of the thrombopoietin gene and its clinical derivatives. A model of the thrombopoietin polypeptide (*top*) can be derived from analysis of its complementary DNA (cDNA) structure. Amino acids responsible for important properties of the molecule are highlighted and include serine (S), cysteine (C), threonine (T), and asparagine (N) residues. Several of the disulfide bonds and the sites at which modifications of N-, T-, or S-linked carbohydrates occur in the recombinant protein produced in mammalian cells [recombinant human thrombopoietin (rhTPO)] have been identified (*middle*). The site of truncation and the addition of polyethylene glycol (PEG) are shown (*bottom*) for PEG-conjugated recombinant human megakaryocyte growth and development factor (PEG-rhMGDF). This form of thrombopoietin is produced in *Escherichia coli* and is devoid of carbohydrate. (Modified from Kaushansky K. Thrombopoietin. *N Engl J Med* 1998;339:746–754.)

important to remember that hematopoiesis is a stochastic or random process in which a multipotent hematopoietic progenitor cell has multiple lineage-specific commitment options. Such commitment decisions, although not entirely understood, are directed in part by local microenvironmental factors such as the presence of specific growth factors and in part by the expression within the progenitor cell of the appropriate receptors and transcription factors, for example, Mpl and NF-E2 for megakaryocytes (541). In this regard, it is also important to emphasize that thrombopoietin, although initially operationally defined as a megakaryocyte-specific growth factor, in contrast to the erythroid-specific growth factor erythropoietin, has a much broader progenitor cell target population. The thrombopoietin receptor is expressed in primitive CD34+ cells (46), and knockout mice lacking this receptor have reduced numbers of hematopoietic progenitor cells (542). As a corollary, thrombopoietin can enhance erythropoiesis and myelopoiesis (50) and act as a survival factor for not only megakaryocytes (543) but also erythroid progenitor cells (49) and pluripotent (CD34+) hematopoietic stem cells (544). This behavior is not unique for thrombopoietin because granulocyte colony-stimulating factor, a supposedly granulocyte-specific growth factor, also has activity at the pluripotent stem cell level (545) and at the level of the early committed erythroid progenitor cell (546). Thrombopoietin's interaction with erythroid progenitor cells may also have implications with respect to the pathophysiology of the chronic myeloproliferative disorders because there exist not only bipotent erythroid and megakaryocytic progenitor cells (547) but also erythroid progenitor cells expressing megakaryocyte markers such as CD41 and Mpl that are sensitive to thrombopoietin (48). Polycythemia vera can present with erythrocytosis and thrombocytosis, whereas erythropoietin-independent erythroid colonies are frequently observed in essential thrombocytosis (548), suggesting the specific involvement in these disorders of the class of erythroid progenitor cells expressing megakaryocytic markers.

Within the context of megakaryocyte physiology, thrombopoietin is essential for the proliferation and maturation of megakaryocyte progenitor cells (549) but is not required for their terminal differentiation (550). This behavior is similar to

that of erythropoietin, which is not required for terminal maturation of erythroid cells (69). Thrombopoietin is an 80- to 90-kd GP (Fig. 12-22) produced primarily in the liver and kidneys but also in the bone marrow, spleen, and lung. Like other members of the hematopoietic growth factor family, thrombopoietin has a four alpha-helical bundle structure, but it differs from the other family members not only with respect to its large size but also because, in addition to the four helix bundle structure represented in its *N*-terminal 153 amino acids, it also contains a 182–amino acid *C*-terminal domain that is heavily N and O glycosylated (551). The *N*-terminal thrombopoietin domain has 23% homology with erythropoietin and represents the biologically relevant portion of the ligand. The *C*-terminal domain is required for secretion of the protein and for its survival in the circulation (552). Like erythropoietin, which is also synthesized in the liver and kidneys, thrombopoietin synthesis is constitutive, as befits a hematopoietic growth factor with such important biologic functions. However, in contrast to erythropoietin whose synthesis is regulated at the level of gene transcription by changes in tissue oxygenation, thrombopoietin gene expression appears to be fixed, at least in the liver and spleen, and its plasma level is largely determined by its catabolism in megakaryocytes and platelets (553). Thus, in bone marrow failure states when megakaryocytes and platelet number are reduced, the circulating thrombopoietin level was high and declined with bone marrow recovery (554). Thrombocytopenia due to increased platelet destruction with active marrow thrombopoiesis was associated with a low thrombopoietin level, reflecting an increase in megakaryocyte mass (554). With liver disease, plasma thrombopoietin is also low (555).

Tight regulation of the thrombopoietin gene was confirmed by the discovery of several families in which family members had thrombocytosis and elevated thrombopoietin levels as an autosomal dominant trait. In each family, there was either a single base deletion (532) or mutation (533) in the 5' untranslated region (UTR) of the thrombopoietin gene. In both instances, either by activating a splice donor site (533) or causing a frameshift in the 5' UTR (532), the efficiency of thrombopoietin mRNA

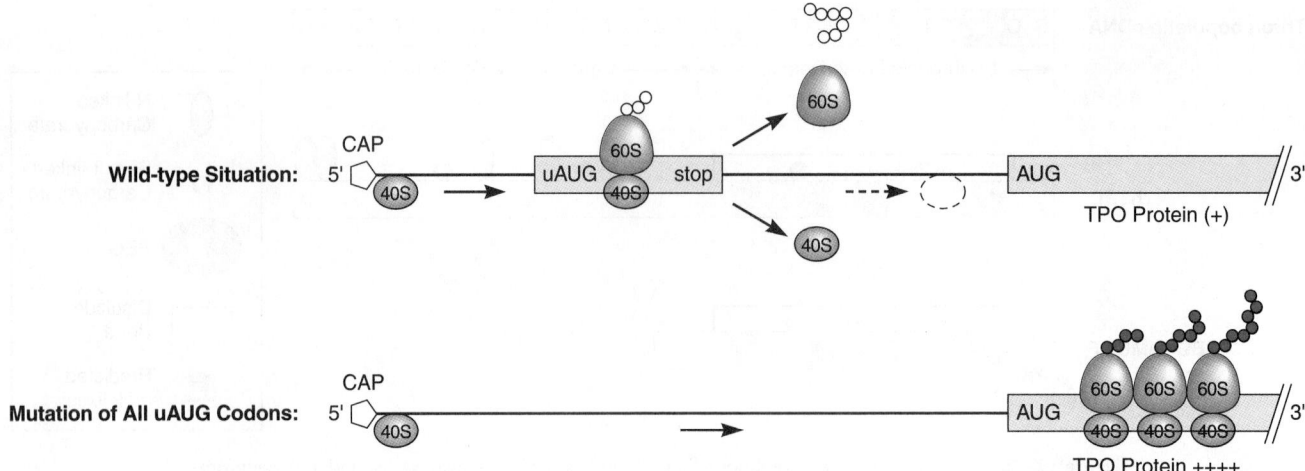

Figure 12-23. Effect of upstream ORFs on thrombopoietin (TPO) messenger RNA (mRNA) translation. Simplified drawing (*top*) of TPO mRNA with only one uORF in the 5' untranslated region (UTR) followed by the TPO-coding region (*open boxes*). According to the ribosomal scanning model, the 40S ribosomal subunit binds the cap structure at the 5' end of the mRNA and scans the mRNA until it encounters the first AUG, where a functional ribosome is assembled. The ribosome initiates translation and synthesizes a short peptide unit until a stop codon is reached. Here, the ribosome dissociates from the mRNA. This prevents the ribosome from reaching the physiologic TPO start codon. However, a minor proportion of 40S subunits may remain associated with the mRNA and continue scanning for a downstream AUG. TPO 5' UTR (*bottom*) with point mutation in all uAUG codons allows the 40S subunit to reach the physiologic start site more efficiently and initiate translation of the TPO protein. (Modified from Ghilardi N, Wiestner A, Skoda RC. Thrombopoietin production is inhibited by a translational mechanism. *Blood* 1998;92:4023–4030.)

translation was improved. Analysis of the thrombopoietin 5' UTR revealed the presence of eight AUG codons, only one of which represented the physiologic initiation site (Fig. 12-23). Experimental removal of certain of the redundant AUG codons resulted in enhanced thrombopoietin mRNA translation (556), explaining the effect of the genetic defects on thrombopoietin production (557) as well as the mechanism for its tight regulation. An additional regulatory mechanism may also be provided by differential splicing (558). This could allow an increase in thrombopoietin mRNA translation without an increase in thrombopoietin gene transcription. Other mechanisms such as activation of gene transcription could be operative in different organs because bone marrow stromal cell thrombopoietin mRNA synthesis and marrow thrombopoietin levels increased in patients with thrombocytopenia (559), but the contribution of bone marrow thrombopoietin production to thrombopoiesis has not yet been established.

A number of studies have evaluated blood thrombopoietin levels in the chronic myeloproliferative disorders and reactive thrombocytosis with conflicting results, which may reflect, in part, the sensitivity and specificity of the various assays used and, in part, the wide range of normal for circulating thrombopoietin levels. In polycythemia vera, idiopathic myelofibrosis, and essential thrombocytosis, circulating thrombopoietin levels were either normal or inappropriately elevated with respect to the platelet count in most studies (57,285,560–569). The thrombopoietin level in reactive thrombocytosis was also frequently elevated (570), preventing a distinction between the benign and malignant causes of thrombocytosis on this basis. There was also no evidence of the activating splice mutation in the thrombopoietin gene in patients with nonfamilial thrombocytosis (571). Finally, although the IL-6 level is elevated in idiopathic myelofibrosis (285) and IL-1, IL-4, and IL-6 levels are elevated in reactive thrombocytosis (570,572,573), none of these was elevated in essential thrombocytosis, indicating that essen-

tial thrombocytosis is not a cytokine-driven illness. At the same time, in contrast to polycythemia vera in which the plasma erythropoietin level is usually lower than normal, given the normal to elevated levels of thrombopoietin in essential thrombocytosis, it is clear that production of this hormone is not suppressed in this disorder.

Thrombopoietin interacts with its target cells through the thrombopoietin receptor Mpl. This receptor is a member of the hematopoietic growth factor receptor superfamily, sharing with them four positionally conserved cysteine residues in the extracellular domain cytokine receptor binding module as well as a WSWS motif and no tyrosine kinase domain in its cytoplasmic segment (534). Like several other family members, Mpl also has a reduplicated cytokine receptor binding module in its extracellular domain, but only the distal cytokine receptor binding module is required for ligand binding (574). Mpl, however, is unique among the hematopoietic growth factors because it is a protooncogene, deriving its name from the MPLV, a murine retrovirus in which a truncated form of the protein, v-Mpl, acts as an oncogene (55). Mice infected with MPLV develop a syndrome similar to polycythemia vera (56), and infected hematopoietic cells exhibit growth factor independence (55). Given this background, there has been substantial interest in Mpl expression in essential thrombocytosis. To date, no mutation of the Mpl gene has been identified in essential thrombocytosis (269). Some patients, however, similar to their polycythemia vera and idiopathic myelofibrosis counterparts, have impaired expression of platelet Mpl (575), but to date no clinical features have been identified that distinguish these patients from those in whom Mpl expression is normal (565).

Hematopoietic growth factor independence is a hallmark of hematopoietic progenitor cells in polycythemia vera and idiopathic myelofibrosis, and essential thrombocytosis is no exception to this rule. Not only was there an increase in circulating megakaryocyte progenitor cells in this disorder (576), as in polycythemia vera (577) and idiopathic myelofibrosis (132,270), but these progenitors were also capable of *in vitro* colony formation in the absence of added growth factors, in contrast to progenitor cells from normal individuals or patients with reactive thrombocytosis (269,576–582). It is important to emphasize in this regard that first, not all patients with essential thrombocytosis, as identified clinically, exhibited spontaneous megakaryocyte colony formation *in vitro*, particularly from peripheral blood progenitor cells (576,578–581). Second, as is the case in polycythemia vera (31), not all of the colonies were spontaneous (578,579,582). Third, these colony-forming cells were still growth factor responsive (582). Fourth, the thrombopoietin receptor appeared to be essential for spontaneous colony formation (279), and, finally, accessory cells appeared to be necessary for *in vitro* colony formation (277). Like polycythemia vera hematopoietic progenitor cells, those of essential thrombocytosis were hypersensitive to IL-3 (278) as well as thrombopoietin (583), and their thrombopoietin hypersensitivity, like erythropoietin hypersensitivity in polycythemia vera (23), has been considered a defining feature of the disease (583). At the same time, evidence has been presented that antisense oligonucleotides to IL-3, IL-6, GM-CSF (282), or a soluble thrombopoietin receptor (269) do not inhibit spontaneous megakaryocyte colony formation, suggesting an endogenous source of growth factors in this disorder. This is compatible with the observation that megakaryocytes synthesize many cytokines and growth factors (280,281), and that thrombopoietin is also capable of stimulating the production of some of these in its target cells (289,584).

Endogenous erythroid colony formation is another feature of essential thrombocytosis (548,584,585), but also one that is not present in every patient (586,587). Erythropoietin-independent colony formation was highly correlated with increased progenitor cell cycling and granulocyte monoclonality (584). However, monoclonality could be present without abnormal progenitor cell growth, whereas erythropoietin-independent colony formation was observed in patients with polyclonal granulocytes (238). Furthermore, one study suggests that some patients with spontaneous colony formation may actually have polycythemia vera (586).

Additional megakaryocyte abnormalities in essential thrombocytosis include a shift to the right with an increase in the number of mature marrow megakaryocytes compared to patients with CML (587,588), with ploidys as high as 512N (589). However, a high ploidy is not specific to essential thrombocytosis and can also be seen in polycythemia vera and reactive thrombocytosis, although an extreme increase in ploidy is not seen in these latter disorders (587,588). Megakaryocyte progenitors in essential thrombocytosis, like those in idiopathic myelofibrosis, are also insensitive to TGF-β_1 (337), giving them an apparent proliferative advantage over their normal counterparts.

In summary, megakaryocyte progenitor cells in essential thrombocytosis share a number of features with the other chronic myeloproliferative disorders. These include expansion of the progenitor cell pool; hypersensitivity to hematopoietic growth factors, in particular thrombopoietin and IL-3, or growth factor independence; hyposensitivity to inhibitory cytokines such as TGF-β_1; and hypermaturation. Autonomous erythroid colony formation is also in keeping with the concept that essential thrombocytosis is a clonal disorder involving red cells, white cells, and platelets (502,503). However, whether the same mechanisms are involved as in polycythemia vera—namely, resistance to apoptosis in the absence of growth factors, and why only megakaryocyte hyperplasia occurs as opposed to the trilineage hyperplasia characteristic

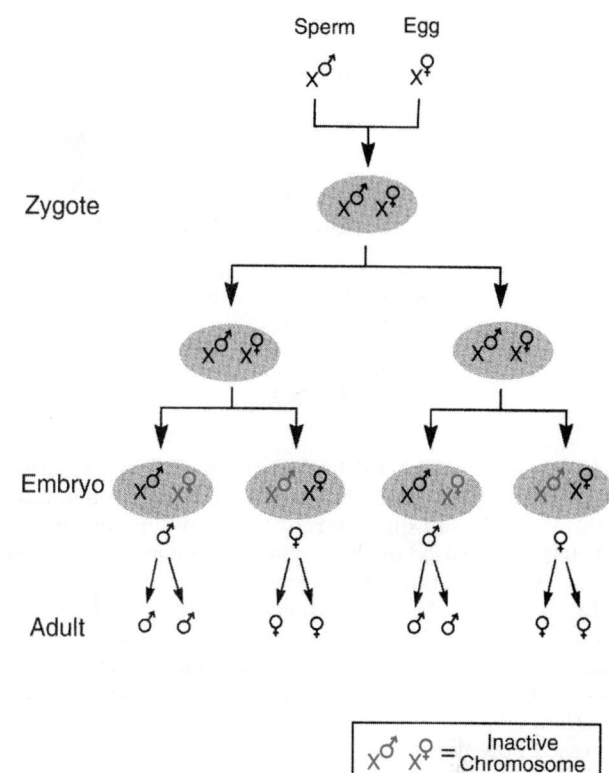

Figure 12-24. Diagrammatic representation of X chromosome inactivation. See text for explanation. (After Fialkow PJ. Clonal and stem cell origin of blood cell neoplasms. *Contemp Hematol Oncol* 1980;1:1.)

of polycythemia vera and idiopathic myelofibrosis because essential thrombocytosis involves also a pluripotent stem cell—remains to be determined.

Clonality

Involvement of a pluripotent or multipotent hematopoietic progenitor cell is a feature shared by all the chronic myeloproliferative disorders, and this clonal origin distinguishes them from the many nonclonal disorders that mimic them clinically. However, absent a cytogenetic abnormality, which is usually the situation in the chronic myeloproliferative disorders, particularly essential thrombocytosis (519,521–523), there is no clinically applicable diagnostic marker for use diagnostically. In informative women, however, clonality can be established using X chromosome–linked polymorphisms. This approach is based on the physiologic, random, and irreversible inactivation in females of one X chromosome in each somatic cell during a specific time interval in embryogenesis with transmission of the chromosome inactivation pattern to subsequent cellular progeny (Fig. 12-24). Because X chromosome inactivation is random as well as stable, active and inactive X chromosomes should normally be present in a 1:1 ratio in a given cell population. Dominant expression of only one allele of an X chromosome–linked gene in a given cell type is either the consequence of the clonal expansion of a single progenitor cell of that population or constitutive or acquired skewing favoring one allele. Excess acquired skewing does occur in hematopoietic cells, particularly myeloid cells, and is an age-related phenomenon that is observed in 38% of women older than age 60 (590–592); the exact age at which it starts to increase is unknown. Constitutive T-cell skewing also occurs but at a lower (9%) frequency (590).

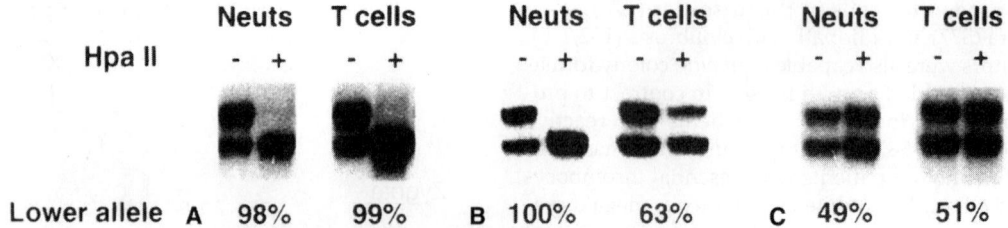

Figure 12-25. Representative HUMARA (human androgen receptor) analyses of DNA from neutrophils and T cells of essential thrombocytosis patients in each of the results groups. **A:** XCIPs skewed in both samples; **(B)** neutrophil XCIP skewed, T cell balanced; **(C)** both XCIPs balanced. (Modified from Harrison CN, Gale RE, MacHin SJ, et al. A large proportion of patients with a diagnosis of essential thrombocythemia do not have a clonal disorder and may be at lower risk of thrombotic complications. *Blood* 1999;93:417–424.)

X chromosome inactivation analysis can be performed using protein-, DNA-, or RNA-based methods. Protein-based methods are based on differential isoenzyme expression (502,503); DNA-based methods analyze gene methylation patterns on X chromosome genes known to be polymorphic (593). Of these genes, the human androgen receptor (HUMARA) has a highly polymorphic CAG repeat for which up to 80% of women are heterozygous, as well as a stable methylation pattern, making this a highly informative gene for clonality analysis (592–595). RNA-based methods currently rely on expressed polymorphisms in the G-GPD, P55, and IDS genes (596), which, when used together, are informative in more than 70% of women (597). This approach also is useful in analyzing the clonality of platelets that lack a nucleus. There is a high correlation between DNA- and RNA-based assays, as well as between marrow and peripheral blood samples (598). The accepted standard for a nonrandom or skewed X chromosome inactivation pattern is an allele expression ratio of at least 3:1 for the particular gene analyzed (Fig. 12-25). All methods, of course, rely on clonal dominance of the affected cells over their normal counterparts. In one study of essential thrombocytosis, a nonrandom or skewed pattern of X chromosome inactivation compatible with the clonal derivation of hematopoietic cells was present in 69% of patients using HUMARA, in contrast to 22% of age-matched controls (595). In another study, 74% of essential thrombocytosis patients had clonal hematopoiesis by HUMARA and 68% by RNA-based assays (597). In this study, T cells as well as neutrophils and platelets were monoclonal in four patients, and the platelets alone were monoclonal in three patients. T-cell monoclonality has also been observed in other essential thrombocytosis patients (20,84), suggesting that, like idiopathic myelofibrosis (265), the disease can arise in a pluripotent stem cell. In one study, no clinical differences were apparent between the clonal and nonclonal patient groups (597), whereas in another, clonal patients had a higher incidence of thrombosis (598). The significance of these latter observations was limited because of the small number of patients involved.

In conclusion, clonality analysis in essential thrombocytosis is limited diagnostically because it is restricted to women and, even then, only to those who are heterozygous for the analyzable genes. The problems of age-related and constitutional skewing of X chromosome inactivation in myeloid cells and T cells also make interpretation of the results difficult. The data to date, however, serve to emphasize that essential thrombocytosis, like idiopathic erythrocytosis, most likely represents a mixture of disorders, some clonal and some not, of differing etiologies that are not definable by current clinical testing. Therapy, therefore, should always be congruent with this reality.

Clinical Manifestations

SYMPTOMS

More than 50% (range, 36% to 84%) of reported patients with essential thrombocytosis were asymptomatic at the time of diagnosis (517–519,521–523) (Table 12-20). This was more true for women than men and did not vary with age. The most common presenting manifestations were due to microvascular events (26%) such as headache, visual disturbances, dizziness, or erythromelalgia. Arterial thrombotic events—cerebral, cardiac, or peripheral—were the initial manifestation in 18%, and venous thrombosis—cerebral, abdominal, or peripheral—was the initial manifestation in 6%. Hemorrhage, usually superficial or gastrointestinal or surgically involved and generally mild, was the initial manifestation in 14%. Bleeding symptoms were more common when the platelet count was greater than $1 \times 10^6/mm^3$ (517,519,521), and thrombotic complications were greater when the platelet count was less than this (521,523,524).

SIGNS

The physical signs of essential thrombocytosis are few. Splenomegaly is seen in less than 30% of patients (range, 16% to 43%), and when palpable, the spleen was usually not enlarged more than 4 cm below the left coastal margin (517–519,521–523). Hepatomegaly is even less frequent, being palpable in less than 10% of patients and never without splenomegaly. Even when ultrasound or radiologic imaging was used, the frequency of splenic or hepatic enlargement was not substantial, although this approach has no clinical merit diagnostically. Substantial splenomegaly, hepatomegaly, or lymphadenopathy should lead to the consideration of other causes for the thrombocytosis (Table 12-18).

LABORATORY FINDINGS

The hematologic abnormalities typical of essential thrombocytosis are shown in Table 12-21. In most patients, thrombocytosis is

---

TABLE 12-20. Presenting Manifestations of Essential Thrombocytosis and Major Vessel Thrombosis

	Percentage (%)	Range
Essential thrombocytosis		
Any symptoms	45	16–70
Splenomegaly	21	16–44
Hepatomegaly	7	4–9
Hemorrhage	11	0–38
Major vessel thrombosis		
Arterial	20	4–29
Venous	7	2–20
Microvascular occlusion	29	8–40
Cytogenetic abnormalities	6	0–25

TABLE 12-21. Hematologic Abnormalities in Essential Thrombocytosis

	Incidence (%)	Range
Hemoglobin (g%)		
<12	14	9–24
12–16	74	64–91
>16	7	0–22
Leukocyte count (×10³/mm³)		
<10	44	15–68
10–20	45	35–66
>20	11	5–25
Platelet count (×10⁶/mm³)		
<1.0	41	10–62
1.0–2.0	50	28–77
>2.0	9	7–13

the only abnormality, but a minor degree of anemia or leukocytosis is not unusual. The platelet count is usually higher in essential thrombocytosis than in secondary or reactive thrombocytosis, but there are numerous exceptions to this observation (514) so that it is not useful diagnostically and certainly does not permit distinction of essential thrombocytosis from the other chronic myeloproliferative disorders or myelodysplasia. Differences in mean platelet volume and distribution width also show overlap (599,600). Marked anemia, leukocytosis, or a leukoerythroblastic reaction should lead to the consideration of another myeloproliferative disorder as should elevation of the hematocrit. Finally, it is important to remember that thrombocytosis can cause artifactual hyperkalemia and, possibly, hypercalcemia due to the release of these substances from the excessive number of platelets present when blood clots to yield serum (601).

Bone marrow aspiration is often frustrated by obstruction of the aspiration needle with masses of platelets, but, except for an increase in the proportion of megakaryocytes and their hypermature appearance, marrow morphology is normal. Bone marrow cellularity and architecture are also usually normal when assessed by bone marrow biopsy, but the number of megakaryocytes is usually increased with nuclear hyperlobulation and clustering. An increase in mononuclear megakaryocytes should lead to the consideration of CML or a myelodysplastic disorder like the 5q- syndrome. There is considerable indecision in the literature as to the amount of reticulin fibrosis that occurs in essential thrombocytosis, a situation made more difficult by the fact that an inaspirable marrow in this disorder may be an artifact of platelet plugging. Reticulin may be increased (519,521), but if there is significant fibrosis as identified by either silver or trichrome stains, a diagnosis other than essential thrombocytosis should be considered. Iron deficiency is observed not infre-

quently in patients considered to have essential thrombocytosis given the percentage of women with this disorder. This demands an explanation because iron deficiency can cause thrombocytosis (602), as can many illnesses such as gastrointestinal cancers and polycythemia vera. Serum vitamin B_{12} and uric acid levels can be increased (519). The leukocyte alkaline phosphatase score is usually normal (603,604).

COAGULATION STUDIES

Global abnormalities of platelet structure and function are characteristic of the chronic myeloproliferative disorders (Table 12-22; Fig. 12-26) and consistent with the propensity to hemorrhage and thrombosis, both microvascular and macrovascular, that are also characteristic of these disorders. Although such abnormalities are less marked in CML and possibly more severe in idiopathic myelofibrosis (136), none of the structural or functional platelet abnormalities described to date is either specific or diagnostic for any of these disorders. Mean platelet volume is increased in these disorders when compared to normal individuals and patients with reactive or secondary thrombocytosis because of the pres-

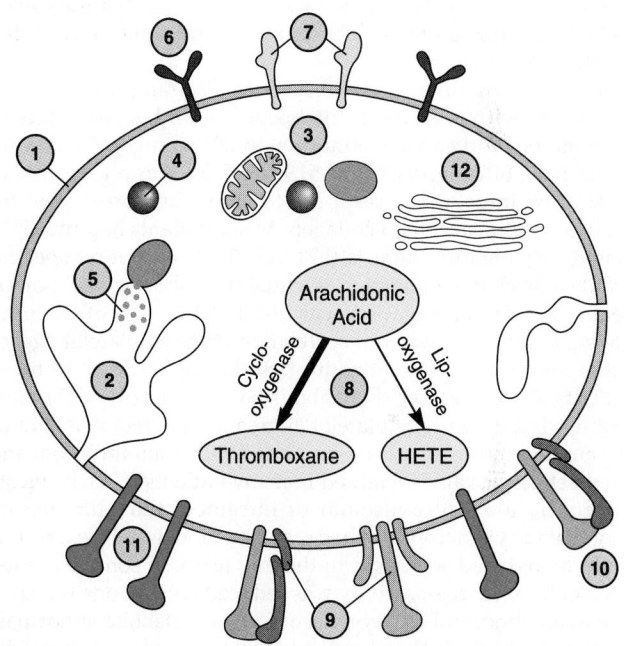

Figure 12-26. Characteristic abnormalities of platelets in chronic myeloproliferative disorders. *1*, Increased platelet volume heterogeneity, megathrombocytes with loss of discoid shape; *2*, increase of membranous structures, dilation, and disorganization of the open canalicular system; *3*, reduced concentration of platelet granules and mitochondria, low platelet buoyant density; *4*, storage pool defect of dense granules, impaired uptake and storage of serotonin; *5*, elevated plasma levels of platelet-specific proteins (β-thromboglobulin, platelet factor 4, platelet-derived growth factor); *6*, decreased concentration of α_1-adrenoreceptors in the platelet membrane, impaired platelet aggregation with adrenaline and other agonists in platelet-rich plasma *in vitro*; *7*, decreased concentration of prostaglandin D_2 receptors in the platelet membrane, resistance of the platelets to inhibitory prostaglandins; *8*, increased platelet thromboxane generation, impaired production of lipoxygenase products; *9*, decreased concentrations of platelet membrane glycoproteins IIIa and Ib, abnormally low sialation of platelet glycoproteins; *10*, heterogeneous affinity and decreased concentration of fibrinogen binding sites, expression of activation-dependent receptor-induced binding sites without exogenous stimulation of platelets; *11*, increased expression of glycoprotein IV on the platelet surface; *12*, impaired calcium mobilization on platelet stimulation, defective transduction mechanisms. (Modified from Wehmeier A, Sudhoff T, Meierkord F. Relation of platelet abnormalities to thrombosis and hemorrhage in chronic myeloproliferative disorders. *Semin Thromb Hemost* 1997;23:391–402.)

TABLE 12-22. Platelet Function Abnormalities in Essential Thrombocytosis

	Percentage (%)	Range
None	23	0–57
Defective aggregation[a]		
Epinephrine	72	8–100
Adenosine diphosphate	32	16–100
Collagen	22	0–39
Ristocetin	42	30–36
Arachidonic acid	10	0–31
Spontaneous aggregation	15	0–40
Prolonged bleeding time	19	0–26

[a]Multiple defects can be present simultaneously.

ence of giant platelets. The platelet distribution width is also increased but, again, is not diagnostic for a particular myeloproliferative disorder (599,600). Morphologically, a reduction in platelet-dense bodies and alpha granules is seen (605), which is compatible with the observed low levels of ADP, β-thromboglobulin, PDGF, and PF4 that are also characteristic of myeloproliferative disorder platelets (103,105,283). Disorganization of the microtubular system, hypertrophy of the dense tubular and open canalicular systems, increased endoplasmic reticulum and ribosomes intent and persistence of the Golgi apparatus are other morphologic abnormalities (605).

Changes in plasma membrane proteins include a reduction in GpIb, GpIIb/IIIa (CD41) (606), as well as in their sialation (607); a reduction in PGD_2 (411) and α-adrenergic receptor expression (608); and an increase in GPIV (CD36) (609). Impaired expression of the platelet thrombopoietin receptor Mpl is also present in some patients (575). In unstimulated essential thrombocytosis platelets, there was also increased expression of activation markers such as P-selectin and thrombospondin (100,610,611), the latter of which was also proteolytically cleaved (612). Intraplatelet concentrations of ADP, β-thromboglobulin, 5-hydroxytryptamine, PF4, vWF, fibrinogen, and PDGF were reduced (103,106,283), whereas the CD36 concentration was increased (609). Intracellular platelet Ca^{2+} homeostasis is abnormal, but the significance of this is unknown (613).

The bleeding time was increased in 16% (range, 0% to 26%) of patients with essential thrombocytosis, and in vitro platelet aggregation studies were abnormal in 80% (range, 0% to 90%) at the time of diagnosis (517,519,521,522). Aggregation was most often impaired in response to epinephrine followed by ADP, ristocetin, and then collagen. Many patients had multiple platelet aggregation defects (521,523,614–616), but no specific profile was characteristic for essential thrombocytosis. Spontaneous platelet aggregation was observed in 18% of patients (range, 0% to 50%) without correlation with the platelet aggregation defects or platelet count (98,106,519,521,522). In most patients, arachidonic acid metabolism was intact (519,617), suggesting that the in vitro platelet aggregation defect was due to impaired stimulus-response coupling (618). Total thromboxane B_2 excretion was also increased in many patients (619), suggesting continuous intravascular or intramedullary platelet or megakaryocyte activation because thromboxane B_2 excretion could be reduced with aspirin therapy (619). In some patients, platelet lipoxygenase activity was reduced (109) in one instance due to an abnormal lipoxygenase (620), a metabolic abnormality congruent with the observed increase in thromboxane B_2 synthesis. The latter was also marked in older patients and those with platelets counts greater than 1 million/mm^3 (619). There was also increased catabolism of fibrinogen and prothrombin (101). Finally, thrombopoietin, which usually augments platelet responses to ADP, epinephrine, and collagen, was less effective in patients with a myeloproliferative disorder (621), particularly if the plasma thrombopoietin level was already elevated (622).

In most patients with essential thrombocytosis, the prothrombin and partial thromboplastin time are normal (519,522), and abnormalities of protein C or S have been negligible (117,623,624). Although mild elevations of homocysteine have been observed, they did not correlate with a thrombotic tendency (116). A role for increased release of plasminogen activator inhibitor-1 has been proposed (625) and refuted (626), and there has been no evidence of endothelial cell hyperactivity (202,626). More important functionally is the reduction in the plasma concentration of high-molecular-weight vWF multimers together with decreased platelet ristocetin cofactor activity and an increase in vWF

multimer catabolism that correlated with the platelet count (79,627–631).

A paradox with respect to bleeding and thrombosis in the chronic myeloproliferative disorders is the lack of correlation between the various observed platelet structural and functional abnormalities and these two processes. This lack of correlation may be more apparent than real. First, in patients with polycythemia, it is the red cell mass that dictates the development of large vessel thrombosis, a fact frequently overlooked because of the assumption that a normal hematocrit in a polycythemia vera patient is automatically associated with a normal red cell mass. This assumption is simply erroneous and accounts for the observation of thrombosis occurring in such patients, despite antiplatelet therapy (250). Second is the misdiagnosis of essential thrombocytosis, when the patient really has polycythemia vera, which is basically an extension of the erroneous behavior described above. Third, many patients with so-called essential thrombocytosis came to medical attention because of a thrombotic episode, which is immediately attributed to the elevated platelet count when, in fact, no prospective study has ever proved this type of association. Considering the large number of causes for a hypercoagulable state, some of which also cause thrombocytosis, it is important to be cautious in assigning blame to the platelet count. Fourth, most platelet function studies in essential thrombocytosis have been performed with platelet-rich plasma. In some instances, adjustment of the platelet count prevented spontaneous platelet aggregation (412,519). Fifth, whole blood aggregometry, which avoids platelet manipulation and more closely reflects the in vivo situation, may be a more useful method to identify at-risk patients. In one study using whole blood aggregometry, patients could be segregated into hypersensitive, hypoactive, mixed activity, or normal with respect to platelet function (98). Hyperactivity was most common when there was a history of previous thrombosis; normal or hypoactive platelets were not associated with thrombosis (98). Sixth, there does appear to be a correlation between the plasma concentration of high-molecular-weight vWF multimers, excessive bleeding, and excessive prolongation of the bleeding time by aspirin (630). Finally, aspirin may also have a differential effect on platelet lipoxygenase activity in essential thrombocytosis platelets and, by impairing the activity of this enzyme, potentiate its cyclooxygenase inhibitory activity and the risk of bleeding (632).

A final issue, with respect to the thrombotic tendency in essential thrombocytosis, is the potential to confuse the manifestations of the peculiar syndrome of erythromelalgia with the propensity for major vessel thrombosis. Erythromelalgia is characterized by burning pain, erythema, and increased temperature primarily in the feet but also in the hands; aggravated by dependency, exercise, or heat; and relieved by cooling or elevation of the affected appendage (633) (Fig. 12-27). Erythromelalgia can manifest as an idiopathic disorder in children or adults or as a consequence of another disorder. Although a variety of diseases have been associated with erythromelalgia, the most common are the myeloproliferative disorders, and among these, the incidence is highest in polycythemia vera and essential thrombocytosis (252,633,634). Erythromelalgia can be the presenting manifestation of these disorders, and pain can predominate with only minimal erythema. Asymmetric involvement of the extremities is not uncommon, and the process can lead to acrocyanosis and cutaneous ulceration or necrosis of the affected digits despite normal peripheral pulses. Tissue involvement is primarily arteriolar with endothelial cell swelling, fibromuscular intimal proliferation, and thrombotic occlusion (633,635) (Fig. 12-28).

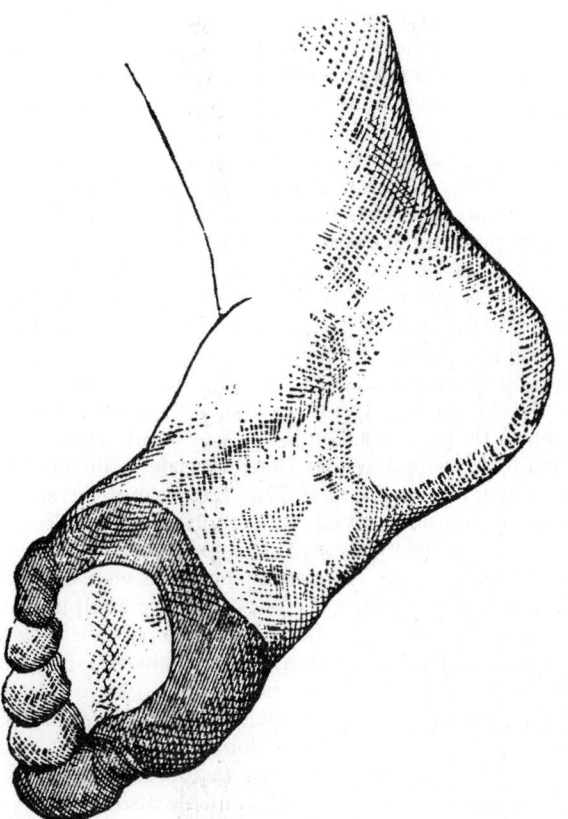

Figure 12-27. Area of pain in the foot. (From *Am J Med Sci* 1878;76:2.)

A single dose of aspirin relieves erythromelalgia due to a myeloproliferative disorder, and the response is so predictable that it is essentially diagnostic of this disease complex (633). The response to aspirin, as well as the histology of the arteriolar lesions, suggests that intravascular platelet activation and endothelial cell damage are the cause of erythromelalgia (636), a concept that is supported by the observation that urinary excretion of the arachidonic acid metabolite thromboxane B_2 increased before the onset of symptoms due to erythromelalgia (637). Platelet survival is also shortened with erythromelalgia and restored with aspirin therapy (638). Finally, a reduction in the platelet count can relieve erythromelalgia.

Patients with thrombocytosis due to a chronic myeloproliferative disorder are also subject to neurologic disturbances such as migraine, scintillating scotomata, dizziness, and transient ischemic attacks that are usually brief in duration and are undoubtedly the central nervous system's equivalent of erythromelalgia because they are also relieved by aspirin therapy or a reduction in the platelet count (639,640).

CYTOGENETIC ABNORMALITIES

In contrast to the other chronic myeloproliferative disorders, cytogenetic abnormalities in untreated patients with essential thrombocytosis are uncommon, usually occurring in no more than 25% of patients, and none is pathognomonic for the disorder or has any prognostic significance (519,521–523). The cytogenetic abnormalities encountered include trisomy 1q (641), t(x;5) (q13;q33) (642), t(13;14)(q32;q37) (643), 21q⁻ (644), –21 (522), 1q⁻, and 20q⁻; trisomy 3 (519); and trisomy 8, 9, and 21 (521,522). Of greater diagnostic and prognostic importance, however, is the clinical overlap between CML and essential thrombocytosis. This usually occurs in women, and conventional cytogenetics as well as the leukocyte alkaline phosphatase score can be normal (603,604,645,646), but megakaryocyte morphology and an increase in basophils usually suggest the diagnosis, which can be confirmed by bcr-abl fluorescence *in situ* hybridization. Molecular studies indicate that the molecular rearrangements are identical to those formed in classic CML (647,648). In keeping with this, the clinical course of Philadelphia chromosome (Ph¹)–positive essential thrombocytosis, although often longer than classic CML, is shorter than that for Ph¹-negative essential thrombocytosis and more likely to terminate in acute leukemia (604,649). The frequency with which bcr-abl–positive essential thrombocytosis occurs is a matter of debate (650,651), but testing for its presence is mandatory in the evaluation of every patient with unexplained thrombocytosis because of the therapeutic implications. In keeping with the low incidence of cytogenetic abnormalities in essential thrombocytosis, abnormalities of p53 and Ras are also uncommon (652).

Differential Diagnosis

Similar to the other chronic myeloproliferative disorders, the diagnosis of essential thrombocytosis is made by excluding the many nonclonal and malignant disorders that mimic it clinically, including the other chronic myeloproliferative disorders (Table 12-18). From a statistical perspective, it needs to be emphasized that chronic myeloproliferative disorders constitute only a small fraction of all the disorders associated with thrombocytosis. Furthermore, the proposed diagnostic criteria for essential thrombocytosis are more ambiguous than definitive (504) (Table 12-19), and even when the diagnosis appears certain, there are no clinical means for distinguishing those patients with essential thrombo-

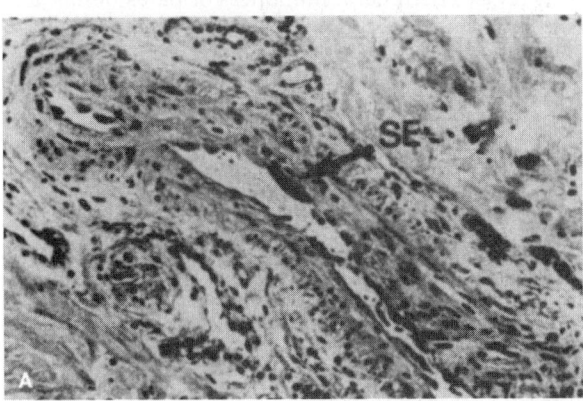
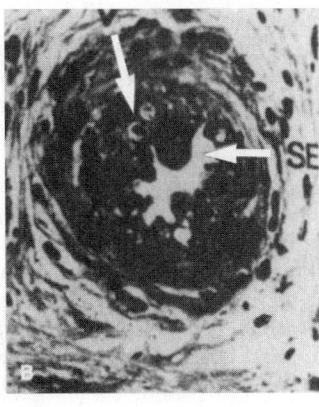

Figure 12-28. Arterioles with swollen endothelial cells (SE) and cell proliferation of the inner part of the media with associated degenerative vascular cytoplasmic swelling (V) (hematoxylin-azophyloxine; **A**, ×120; **B**, ×300). (After Michiels JJ, Ten Kate FWJ, Vuzevski VD, et al. Histopathology of erythromelalgia in thrombocythaemia. *Histopathology* 1984;8:669.)

cytosis associated with clonal hematopoiesis from those with polyclonal hematopoiesis. Although it is true that platelet counts tend to be higher in essential thrombocytosis and its myeloproliferative disease counterparts than in reactive or secondary thrombocytosis, there is still significant overlap between the two, particularly when the platelet count threshold is reduced to $600,000/mm^3$ or less. A normal erythrocyte sedimentation rate is usual in essential thrombocytosis but can also occur in secondary thrombocytosis and in polycythemia vera presenting as thrombocytosis. The leukocyte alkaline phosphatase score can be low in essential thrombocytosis and normal in CML presenting as essential thrombocytosis (604). Platelet aggregation abnormalities are uncommon but not absent in reactive thrombocytosis (615) and can also be absent in essential thrombocytosis (608). The bone marrow aspirate and biopsy can be helpful in the diagnostic process to the extent that disorders associated with the trilineage dysplasia, such as myelodysplasia or granulocytic hyperplasia, and small hypolobular or mononuclear megakaryocytes, such as CML, or disorders associated with marrow fibrosis, such as idiopathic myelofibrosis and systemic mastocytosis (453), can be distinguished from essential thrombocytosis. The extent of megakaryocyte hyperplasia and clustering is also useful for distinguishing essential thrombocytosis, polycythemia vera, or idiopathic myelofibrosis from reactive or secondary thrombocytosis (653), but this is not absolute. The bone marrow aspirate is also useful as a source of cells for cytogenetic analysis to exclude the presence of CML. However, if such a study is negative, a search for bcr-abl by fluorescence *in situ* hybridization is mandatory to identify the small fraction of patients, usually women, in whom CML presents as Ph^1 chromosome–negative but bcr-abl–positive. Such patients can have a more abbreviated clinical course than patients with essential thrombocytosis, just as thrombocytosis occurring in the setting of classic CML is associated with disease acceleration (654). The 5q– syndrome may also not always be easily distinguishable from essential thrombocytosis clinically (655).

Absence of bone marrow iron is not uncommon in essential thrombocytosis given the high proportion of women in the reproductive age range who develop this disorder and also the technical difficulties associated with histochemical evaluation of bone marrow iron. This is an important issue because iron deficiency causes thrombocytosis and because polycythemia vera, in which iron deficiency is common, can also masquerade as essential thrombocytosis, and its treatment differs from the latter. Therefore, not only is a trial of iron therapy mandatory if iron stores are absent, but also a red cell mass and plasma volume determination should always be considered in any nonanemic woman discovered to have a high platelet count.

Clinical Course

Based on the current clinical literature, it is difficult to reach unequivocal conclusions about the natural history of essential thrombocytosis. This is due to many factors, including differences in the composition of the study populations with respect to age, duration of observation, proportion of symptomatic patients, presence of underlying cardiovascular risk factors, the diagnostic criteria used for essential thrombocytosis—in particular, the platelet count threshold, the extent of the diagnostic evaluation, especially with respect to excluding polycythemia vera or other reasons for hypercoagulability, lack of a means for distinguishing clonal thrombocytosis from nonclonal forms, the retrospective nature of most reports, the differences in treatment protocols and intention to treat, the definition of significant complications and the choice of control groups or the lack of them. Additionally, the

assumption that essential thrombocytosis actually defines a single entity may well be erroneous. Indeed, the emergence of polycythemia vera or idiopathic myelofibrosis in patients presenting with thrombocytosis alone can take as long as 4 years (84).

In some studies, case ascertainment bias was probably responsible for a high rate of complications (656), whereas in others, reportorial bias was responsible (657). Indeed, although there are substantial data supporting the contention that treatment reduces the complication rate in essential thrombocytosis, there are no data proving that any therapy prolongs survival in this disorder. This is largely due to the fact that the survival of essential thrombocytosis patients can approach normal (156,517,524). It is clear from virtually every study that the platelet count per se was not a prognostic factor, and although there is not complete agreement, platelet counts greater than 1.5 million mm^3 were associated with an increased rate of hemorrhage (517,519,521). Furthermore, even chemotherapy could not prevent thrombotic complications (657), whereas antiplatelet therapy was associated with an increased risk of bleeding (249). Platelet function tests were also not reliable in predicting either the occurrence of complications or their type (521,658), nor was older age or gender necessarily associated with a higher complication rate (522–524,658,659) as claimed (660). The most significant predictor of a future thrombotic event was a prior one (517,518,657,660,661). Other significant risk factors included tobacco abuse (659), underlying cardiovascular disease or risk factors for same (518), and the presence of another hypercoagulable disorder such as the antiphospholipid syndrome (662). Failure to exclude polycythemia vera, in which thrombocytosis can be a presenting manifestation, is another reason for the development of thrombotic complications, particularly intraabdominal venous thrombosis. Indeed, in one study of hepatic vein thrombosis, most patients had a high hematocrit before this catastrophic event and a high platelet count afterward (191).

Although chronic myeloproliferative disorders are most common in individuals older than 50 years of age, younger individuals are not immune to these disorders, and the natural history of essential thrombocytosis in young patients has been the subject of several studies. Reportorial bias is evident in some of these (663,664), which essentially provide numerators without an appropriate denominator. In others, the clinical course has been benign (661,665,666), including a controlled, prospective study (520), which indicated that the incidence of thrombosis is not increased in this age group.

The most common problem confronting essential thrombocytosis patients in the absence of cardiovascular risk factors is the microvascular syndrome characterized by headache, often migrainous in nature, scintillating scotomata, unstable gait, transient ischemic attacks, blurred vision, transient blindness (amaurosis fugax), peripheral numbness or paresthesias, and erythromelalgia causing digital ischemia, necrosis, and ulceration. Overall, from a prognostic prospective, the incidence of complications in previously asymptomatic patients has been estimated at 5% to 8% per year, with thrombotic events occurring more frequently than hemorrhagic ones and microvascular events being the most common (663). Myocardial infarction and cerebrovascular infarction are the most serious reported arterial thrombotic events associated with essential thrombocytosis, whereas cerebral venous and intraabdominal venous thrombosis are the most serious venous occlusive events. The latter, however, are uncommon and most likely to occur in the younger patients (191), whereas the former in some series were clearly correlated with cardiovascular risk factors (518,659). Although not emphasized, there was a significant incidence of sudden death in several series (517,524), the epidemiology of which has not been defined but should be. It must be remembered, however, that ascertainment bias has a major confounding role in these statistics. For example, in one study, more than 50% of asymptomatic patients did not develop a complication, whereas in one of the few truly prospective studies, the rate of arterial or venous thrombosis of essential thrombosis patients younger than 60 years of age was not different from the control group (520). Furthermore, when the mortality rate of essential thrombocytosis patients was evaluated (excluding treatment-related deaths due to leukemia and those unrelated to the disease itself), it ranged from 0% to 14% (517–519,521,522,524), most of which was accounted for by patients 70 years of age or older.

Acute Leukemia

Spontaneous acute leukemia is an uncommon event in essential thrombocytosis in the absence of chemotherapy or irradiation. In 896 patients from seven different series, 19 cases of acute leukemia were observed (517–519,521,522,524,661), all of which developed in patients receiving irradiation, an alkylating agent, or hydroxyurea. Of 28 additional reported cases, only three of the patients who developed acute leukemia had not been exposed to irradiation or chemotherapy (667–671). Transformation appeared to occur independently of cytogenetic abnormalities (672), and mutations of p53 or Ras were rare during the chronic phase of the illness (652). Although megakaryocytic leukemia was observed, all other French-American-British types of acute nonlymphocytic leukemia were also observed (671), and lymphoblastic transformation has also been described (673). As mentioned previously, thrombocytosis is not only an adverse prognostic event in CML (654), it may also be the sole presenting manifestation of the disorder in a small number of patients (604,645). The average age of patients developing acute leukemia after treatment with either chemotherapy or irradiation was 60 years (range, 43 to 77 years), and while the numbers are very small, patients developing acute leukemia spontaneously were all older than 65 years. The mean time to transformation was approximately 6 years, but shorter and much longer durations have also been recorded. Acute leukemia has been associated with busulfan, melphalan, pipobroman, hydroxyurea, and ^{32}P therapy (670,671). Although hydroxyurea had been considered safe to use in essential thrombocytosis, its use was recently linked to the development of a specific cytogenetic abnormality, 17p, together with mutation of p53 and distinctive neutrophil morphologic abnormalities (674). As in the case of polycythemia vera, exposure to hydroxyurea with another chemotherapeutic agent or ^{32}P increases the risk of leukemic transformation in essential thrombocytosis (675).

Pregnancy

Essential thrombocytosis is most common in women, many of whom are in the reproductive age range. Periparturient thrombocytopenia, usually of a modest extent, is common in pregnancy, and a spontaneous reduction in platelet count (676–678) as well as an increased sensitivity to interferon-α have been observed during pregnancy in essential thrombocytosis patients (676) as well as suppression of the abnormal clone with reexpression postpartum (679,680). Anecdotal reports of fetal wastage in essential thrombocytosis patients must be balanced by the experience in larger studies. There has been a consensus that first trimester abortions were increased, but, otherwise, obstetric complications were uncommon (661,681,682). There was not a correlation between the preconception platelet count, preconception complications, or treatment and the pregnancy outcome, nor did pregnancy adversely affect the course of the essential thrombocytosis (681). In one study, therapy, including plateletpheresis, had no effect on the outcome (681), whereas in another, low-dose aspirin followed by low-molecular-weight heparin at term was associated with a more favorable outcome, but the number of patients studied was small (682). Interferon-α has also been used successfully to reduce the platelet count without adverse effects on the fetus (683). It is important to remember that recurrent abortion can be caused by other disorders such as the antiphospholipid syndrome (684) and not to assume that the platelet count is the problem in the pregnant patient with essential thrombocytosis. For example, in one such report, it is more probable that one of the patients had unrecognized polycythemia vera than essential thrombocytosis (685).

Management of Essential Thrombocytosis

It is unlikely that any other laboratory abnormality causes otherwise astute clinicians to suspend disbelief more often than thrombocytosis, and this abandonment of clinical perspective or judgment is reflected in the lack of consensus with respect to the platelet count threshold for the diagnosis of essential thrombocytosis, the indications for therapeutic intervention, and the most appropriate type of therapy. As emphasized above, given the inadequacy of current diagnostic procedures, it cannot be assumed that what is currently classified as essential thrombocytosis represents a single entity. In this regard, there appears to be no difference in the clinical features of clonal and polyclonal essential thrombocytosis. Whether their prognosis or their susceptibility to the mutagenic effects of chemotherapeutic agents differ remains unknown. Although autonomous in vitro erythroid and megakaryocyte colony formation and abnormalities of platelet function are features of essential thrombocytosis, they are neither diagnostically specific nor always present. Bone marrow abnormalities (i.e., change in megakaryocyte number and morphology) are also not diagnostically specific. Both hemorrhage and thrombosis occur in patients with reactive or secondary thrombocytosis, and, while their incidence is less (514), in an individual patient, this type of behavior is also not useful diagnostically. Abnormalities in platelet function tests are a feature of essential thrombocytosis, but they are also neither sensitive nor specific. Furthermore, rarely in any series of patients with essential thrombocytosis has there been an adequate investigation of other possible causes for hypercoagulability, including the antiphospholipid syndrome and oral contraceptive use by women. In addition, given the unfounded intuition that a high platelet count predisposes to thrombosis, there is a large collection of anecdotal reports of vascular catastrophes in patients with thrombocytosis that comprises a numerator without any meaningful denominator. However, in most large series of patients, the actual number of significant major vessel thromboses was low and unrelated to the height of the platelet count or even to platelet function tests. Whether the reticulated platelet count as a measure of increased platelet turnover (686) and, therefore, thrombotic activity will prove useful prognostically remains to be substantiated (687). Also, as emphasized above, thrombocytosis is often the presenting manifestation of polycythemia vera, and, in the absence of red cell mass and plasma volume determinations, the latter disorder can be missed, particularly in women, if the hematocrit is not markedly increased (148). Furthermore, not enough emphasis has been given to the potential importance of cardiovascular risk factors in patients with essential thrombocytosis, the frequency of which varied from 12% to 75% in six large series (517,518,523,659,660,688).

When this has not been considered important, it was because the frequency in the particular series was low in both patient and control groups. It is generally conceded that bleeding does not pose a major hazard except when the platelet count is greater than 1.5 million/mm^3 or when excessive concentrations of aspirin are used (689). Most studies also support the contention that risk of major vessel thrombosis is low in individuals younger than 60 years of age in the absence of cardiovascular risk factors or a prior thrombotic event. Furthermore, the most common thrombotic events are microvascular and usually evanescent, although their clinical manifestations may be worrisome (663). There is also no consensus as to what level the platelet count should be reduced in essential thrombocytosis—an issue confounded by the fact that if the disorder is clonal, the platelets will be abnormal no matter what the height of the platelet count is.

Given these issues and problems, the principal rule of treatment in essential thrombocytosis is "first do no harm." A high platelet count in the absence of symptoms for which no underlying cause is apparent requires no therapy, and age is not a criterion because published evidence for this is not convincing with respect to survival (657), while the evidence for the induction of leukemia with the use of alkylating agents, hydroxyurea, or ^{32}P is very convincing (670,671,674). The concept that it is acceptable to expose individuals older than the age of 60 years to such drugs with the attendant risk of acute leukemia because their life expectancy is already reduced is simply unacceptable.

Patients with significant cardiovascular risk factors and those presenting with hemorrhage or thrombosis are candidates for treatment with the acknowledgment that such therapy may reduce hemorrhage or thrombosis, but its impact on survival has yet to be substantiated. When hemorrhage is the issue, causes other than the platelet count such as drugs, liver disease, vitamin K deficiency and other coagulation abnormalities, and anatomic lesions need to be addressed first. If no other cause is present and renal function is normal, epsilon aminocaproic acid (Amicar) reliably corrects the problem when given as a 5-g loading dose i.v. or p.o. followed by 2 g every 4 hours with a maximum frequency of 2 g every 2 hours. Long-term use of epsilon aminocaproic acid can cause reversible muscle damage with weakness and myoglobinuria (690). Epsilon aminocaproic acid should be avoided when there is evidence of microvascular thrombosis. A reduction in platelet number may also be helpful if the count is greater than 1.5 million/mm^3, as this may be associated with a reduction in high-molecular-weight vWF multimers and reduced ristocetin cofactor activity (627,629). Plateletpheresis has been used for this purpose and improved platelet function (691–694). However, the beneficial effect of this approach is transient and, therefore, not efficacious unless combined with suppression of platelet production as discussed below.

Microvascular thrombosis, either in the central nervous system or peripherally, is the most common problem in patients with essential thrombocytosis and, in most patients, can be managed with low-dose aspirin therapy (100 to 300 mg p.o. q.d.). In fact, relief of symptoms with aspirin is virtually diagnostic for this process. There is a risk of bleeding, especially if a large dose of aspirin is used and when the platelet count is very high (630). Some essential thrombocytosis patients are very sensitive to aspirin, which may be a consequence of platelet function abnormalities such as lipoxygenase deficiency (632,695). In some patients, a cyclooxygenase-1 inhibitor may be as effective as aspirin but with the disadvantage (or advantage) that its antiplatelet effects are transient. Some investigators have advocated the chronic administration of low-dose aspirin in patients with essential thrombocytosis as a means of reducing the incidence of thrombotic events (696), but this is not always successful (657).

Major vessel thrombosis is the most serious consequence of essential thrombocytosis, but the assumption that such thromboses were due to the platelet count alone is never warranted. Immediate therapy should be no different from that for such a thrombotic event when the platelet count is normal. An exception might be myocardial ischemia or infarction with isolated single vessel stenosis when rapid lowering of the platelet count by plateletpheresis might be considered, although there is no proof of the efficacy of this approach. In one such patient, abciximab was used (697). In addition to anticoagulation for the appropriate period of time, chronic aspirin therapy may be beneficial in some patients (640).

Reducing the platelet count has also been widely used to alleviate the thrombotic proclivity of thrombocytosis even though there is no correlation between the height of the platelet count and the incidence of thrombosis or long-term survival. The fastest method is plateletpheresis—the effect of which is transient and rarely necessary. After plateletpheresis, platelet function has been observed to improve, presumably through the selective removal of larger platelets (694). Given the temporary nature of plateletpheresis, consideration should be given to some other method for controlling platelet number in combination with the procedure. The two safest for this purpose are anagrelide and agent interferon-α.

Anagrelide, an oral imidazoquinazolin derivative originally studied for its ability to impair platelet aggregation through its phosphodiesterase inhibitory activity, was observed to cause thrombocytopenia in humans at concentrations far less than those required to inhibit platelet function (253). The mechanisms by which thrombocytopenia is induced appear to involve postmitotic inhibition of megakaryocyte maturation with a reduction in ploidy, maturation stage, and cell diameter without an appreciable effect on cell proliferation except at very high concentrations (698,699). Because the effect of anagrelide on megakaryocyte size requires exposure to these cells at an earlier time during their development than its effects on ploidy or maturation stage (698), it appears that more than one mechanism is involved in its effect on thrombopoiesis. The drug does not alter platelet survival, and while it can increase platelet volume, this effect is not marked, and it has no significant *in vivo* influence on the abnormal platelet function observed in essential thrombocytopenia (699,700). It also does not influence marrow fibrosis (701).

Extensive clinical experience has indicated that anagrelide in doses of 0.5 to 1.0 mg four times daily can reduce the platelet count by 50% in more than 90% of patients (range, 60% to 93%) within 2 to 4 weeks, with most patients requiring approximately 2.5 mg (702). The response is usually sustained with continuous treatment; drug resistance has not developed, and, for maintenance, a lower dose may be effective. With cessation of therapy, the platelet count increases in less than a week. There appears to be no difference on response to anagrelide among the various chronic myeloproliferative disorders. In this regard, it is worth emphasizing that no controlled study has been performed to demonstrate that reduction of the platelet count with anagrelide is associated with a reduction in the thrombotic or hemorrhagic consequences of essential thrombocytosis or improved survival.

Anagrelide does not alter bone marrow cellularity, and the leukocyte count usually remains unchanged, but it has reduced the hematocrit in up to 36% of patients (702) and can induce significant thrombocytopenia. As a consequence of its vasodilatory and inotropic effects, it can also cause significant cardiovascular toxicity, including postural hypotension, particularly if 5 mg or more is taken as a single dose (702). Fluid retention, edema, and frank congestive heart failure have also been observed as well as palpitations, new onset angina or exacerbations of the same, tachycardia, and supraventricular arrhythmias. Unfortunately, anagrelide causes some of the same symptoms (i.e., headache and dizziness) that it was expected to relieve; gastrointestinal toxicity can be substantial, including nausea, vomiting, pain, bloating, and diarrhea, in part due to its lactose content. Pancreatitis has also been documented as well as skin rashes and interstitial pneumonitis. Overall, in the largest clinical trial, the drug was discontinued in 16% of patients because of toxicity (702).

Given the risk of leukemia associated with platelet count reduction by chemotherapy in a disease in which longevity is the rule and in which no study has demonstrated improved survival with chemotherapy, anagrelide offers a reasonable treatment option. Its drawbacks include its substantial toxicities, the need for continuous therapy, and the lack of proof of its impact on survival. Because no controlled studies have been performed, its use must by definition be empiric. Given that the major vascular problems in patients with essential thrombocytosis are microvascular and usually amenable to aspirin therapy, anagrelide appears to be most suitable for situations when aspirin is not effective or when the platelet count is greater than 1.5 million/mm^3 and the risk of hemorrhage can be potentiated by aspirin. Its use is proscribed when there is cardiovascular disease and during pregnancy, and there is no indication for its use in asymptomatic thrombocytosis. Because of its cardiovascular and gastrointestinal toxicity, the drug should be introduced slowly in 0.5-mg doses twice daily and escalated slowly to achieve the desired effect. Acetaminophen (Tylenol) and lactase preparations may be helpful, but patient education and a deliberate approach are even more important. If the desired effect is achieved, then dose reduction should be evaluated for maintenance. Because the platelet count declines spontaneously in some patients with essential thrombocytosis, it is appropriate to revisit the need for anagrelide periodically.

Interferon-α has proved to be an effective agent in reducing the platelet count in all of the myeloproliferative diseases as well as suppressing the malignant clone in CML and reducing organomegaly due to extramedullary hematopoiesis (238,703). Its effectiveness in suppressing the clonal population in the other myeloproliferative disorders is mixed, and, as a corollary, its effect in most patients was not sustained (704) and platelet function was not restored to normal (705), although there was a reduction in the surface expression of GPIV and thrombospondin but without a change in thrombospondin size (706). Interferon-α has the drawback of requiring administration by injection, and in some patients, daily administration is required. Its toxic profile is also substantial. Hematologic side effects include profound lowering of the leukocyte and platelet counts. Its nonhematologic side effects, in addition to the initial flulike symptoms and persistent fatigue, are numerous and often debilitating. The most serious of these are neurologic toxicity with memory loss, depression, and peripheral neuropathy, cardiac toxicity with arrhythmias and congestive heart failure, hair loss, nephrotoxicity, and suppression of thyroid function (239–241). While interferon-α is safe for use during pregnancy, it is most toxic in patients older than 60 years of age who are likely to need it most. In essential thrombocytosis, it is thought to act by impairing megakaryocyte progenitor cell proliferation (707), though, of course, it has a global inhibitory effect on all hematopoietic progenitor cells (237,272) including those of the neoplastic clone (708). The clinical experience to date in essential

thrombocytosis indicates a response rate for platelet count reduction of 69% to 100% if doses of 1 to 9 million units of interferon-α are administered subcutaneously on a daily basis, with the desired effect being achieved within 2 months and often sooner (709,710). Reduction in spleen size can take longer. Once the desired platelet count reduction has been achieved, the interferon dose should be titrated down to the minimally effective one (711). Induction and maintenance doses vary for individual patients. In general, those requiring the least amount of interferon for maintenance are the most likely to achieve a sustained, unmaintained remission (711). Otherwise, once the drug is stopped, the platelet count rises rapidly.

Interferon-α was a welcome addition to the agents useful for platelet count reduction. It has the advantage of not causing genetic damage in hematopoietic progenitor cells or to the fetus. Its toxicity profile, however, can be daunting, particularly in the elderly. Therefore, its use needs to be judicious. Interferon, like anagrelide, may be contraindicated in patients with heart failure or underlying neurologic disorders. It should also never be used to lower the platelet count in an asymptomatic patient because no controlled trial has demonstrated its efficacy in prolonging survival or preventing thrombosis or hemorrhage. It would appear to be most useful in patients with very high platelet counts who have failed an anagrelide trial and who are at risk of bleeding with the use of aspirin and, if necessary, during pregnancy. Interferon-α is always preferable to chemotherapy. However, to achieve patient compliance, it needs to be introduced slowly at doses less than 1 million U and given less often than daily in older individuals and combined with Tylenol for the inevitable headache, myalgias, and fever. Dose escalation should be gradual in response to patient tolerance, proceeding to the level required for an effect. Certainly, there is no rationale in using interferon-α to obtain a rapid response. Once the desired effect is achieved, dose reduction should be initiated to the minimal amount required. Surveillance for toxicity is mandatory, and periodic assessment for a durable remission is appropriate. Addition of an antidepressant may also improve patient tolerance and compliance (248).

Despite the leukemogenic risk (674,712), there is a place for chemotherapy in the management of essential thrombocytosis. Hydroxyurea can be useful in patients in whom anagrelide or interferon-α is ineffective or intolerable but only as intermittent therapy. There is no excuse for chronic maintenance therapy, as there is no evidence that platelet count reduction improves survival or prevents thrombosis, and there is substantial evidence that hydroxyurea is leukemogenic (674). Although busulfan is the alkylating agent most often used, it is possible that intermittent daily oral Cytoxan might be just as effective but with fewer long-term side effects.

REFERENCES

1. Damesek W. Some speculations on the myeloproliferative syndromes. *Blood* 1951;6:372–375.
2. Nowell PC, Hungerford DA. A minute chromosome in chronic granulocytic leukemia. *Science* 1960;132:1499–1504.
3. Daley GQ, Van Etten RA, Baltimore D. Induction of chronic myelogenous leukemia in mice by the P210bcr/abl gene of the Philadelphia chromosome. *Science* 1990;247:824–830.
4. Glasser RM, Walker RI. Transitions among the myeloproliferative disorders. *Ann Intern Med* 1969;71:285–307.
5. Vaquez H. Sur une forme speciale de cyanose s'accompagnant d'hyperglobulie excessive et peristante. *C R Soc Biol (Paris)* 1892;44:384–388.
6. Osler W. Chronic cyanosis, with polycythemia and enlarged spleen: a new clinical entity. *Am J Med Sci* 1903;126:176–201.

7. Ania BJ, Suman VJ, Sobell JL, et al. Trends in the incidence of polycythemia vera among Olmsted County, Minnesota residents, 1935–1989. *Am J Hematol* 1994;47:89–93.

8. Prochazka AV, Markowe HL. The epidemiology of polycythaemia rubra vera in England and Wales 1968–1982. *Br J Cancer* 1986;53:59–64.

9. Berglund S, Zettervall O. Incidence of polycythemia vera in a defined population. *Eur J Haematol* 1992;48:20–26.

10. Danish EH, Rasch CA, Harris JW. Polycythemia vera in childhood: case report and review of the literature. *Am J Hematol* 1980;9:421–428.

11. Damon A, Holub DA. Host factors in polycythemia vera. *Ann Intern Med* 1958;49:43.

12. Modan B, Kallner H, Zemer D, et al. A note on the increased risk of polycythemia vera in Jews. *Blood* 1971;37:172–176.

13. Brubaker LH, Wasserman LR, Goldberg JD, et al. Increased prevalence of polycythemia vera in parents of patients on polycythemia vera study group protocols. *Am J Hematol* 1984;16:367–373.

14. Ratnoff WD, Gress RE. The familial occurrence of polycythemia vera: report of a father and son, with consideration of the possible etiologic role of exposure to organic solvents, including tetrachloroethylene. *Blood* 1980;56:233–236.

15. Manoharan A, Garson OM. Familial polycythaemia vera: a study of 3 sisters. *Scand J Haemat* 1976;17:10–16.

16. Miller RL, Purvis JD III, Weick JK. Familial polycythemia vera. *Cleve Clin J Med* 1989;56:813–818.

17. Friedland ML, Wittels EG, Robinson RJ. Polycythemia vera in identical twins. *Am J Hematol* 1981;10:101–103.

18. Perez-Encinas M, Bello JL, Perez-Crespo S, et al. Familial myeloproliferative syndrome. *Am J Hematol* 1994;46:225–229.

19. Adamson JW, Fialkow PJ, Murphy S, et al. Polycythemia vera: stem-cell and probable clonal origin of the disease. *N Engl J Med* 1976;295:913–916.

20. Tsukamoto N, Morita K, Maehara T, et al. Clonality in chronic myeloproliferative disorders defined by X-chromosome linked probes: demonstration of heterogeneity in lineage involvement. *Br J Haematol* 1994;86:253–258.

21. Adamson JW, Singer JW, Catalano P, et al. Polycythemia vera. Further in vitro studies of hematopoietic regulation. *J Clin Invest* 1980;66:1363–1368.

22. Eid J, Ebert RF, Gesell MS, et al. Intracellular growth factors in polycythemia vera and other myeloproliferative disorders. *Proc Natl Acad Sci U S A* 1987;84: 532–536.

23. Correa PN, Eskinazi D, Axelrad AA. Circulating erythroid progenitors in polycythemia vera are hypersensitive to insulin-like growth factor-1 in vitro: studies in an improved serum-free medium. *Blood* 1994;83:99–112.

24. Wasserman L. The management of polycythemia vera. *Br J Haematol* 1971;21: 371–376.

25. London IM, Shemin D, West R, et al. Heme synthesis and red blood cell dynamics in normal humans and in subjects with polycythemia vera, sickle-cell anemia, and pernicious anemia. *J Biol Chem* 1949;179:463–484.

26. Eaves AC, Henkelman DH, Eaves CJ. Abnormal erythropoiesis in the myeloproliferative disorders: an analysis of underlying cellular and humoral mechanisms. *Exp Hematol* 1980;8[Suppl 8]:235–247.

27. Eaves CJ, Eaves AC. Erythropoietin (Ep) dose-response curves for three classes of erythroid progenitors in normal human marrow and in patients with polycythemia vera. *Blood* 1978;52:1196–1210.

28. Lawrence JH, Elmlinger PJ, Fulton G. Oxygen and the control of red cell production in primary and secondary polycythemia: effects on iron turnover pattern with Fe[59] as a tracer. *Cardiologia* 1952;21:346.

29. Spivak JL, Cooke CR. Polycythemia vera in an anephric man. *Am J Med Sci* 1976;272:339–344.

30. Prchal JF, Axelrad AA. Letter: Bone-marrow responses in polycythemia vera. *N Engl J Med* 1974;290:1382.

31. Cashman J, Henkelman D, Humphries K, et al. Individual BFU-E in polycythemia vera produce both erythropoietin dependent and independent progeny. *Blood* 1983;61:876–884.

32. Papayannopoulou T, Buckley J, Nakamoto B, et al. Hb F production of endogenous colonies of polycythemia vera. *Blood* 1979;53:446–454.

33. de Wolf JT, Beentjes JA, Esselink MT, et al. In polycythemia vera human interleukin 3 and granulocyte-macrophage colony-stimulating factor enhance erythroid colony growth in the absence of erythropoietin. *Exp Hematol* 1989;17:981–983.

34. Dai CH, Krantz SB, Green WF, et al. Polycythaemia vera. III. Burst-forming units-erythroid (BFU-E) response to stem cell factor and c-kit receptor expression. *Br J Haematol* 1994;86:12–21.

35. Yoshimura A, Longmore G, Lodish HF. Point mutation in the exoplasmic domain of the erythropoietin receptor resulting in hormone-independent activation and tumorigenicity. *Nature* 1990;348:647–649.

36. Gregg XT, Prchal JT. Erythropoietin receptor mutations and human disease. *Semin Hematol* 1997;34:70–76.

37. Damen JE, Krosl J, Morrison D, et al. The hyperresponsiveness of cells expressing truncated erythropoietin receptors is contingent on insulin-like growth factor-1 in fetal calf serum. *Blood* 1998;92:425–433.

38. Broudy VC, Kin N, Papayannopoulou T. Erythropoietin receptors in polycythemia vera. *Exp Hematol* 1990;18:576.

39. Hess G, Rose P, Gamm H, et al. Molecular analysis of the erythropoietin receptor system in patients with polycythaemia vera. *Br J Haematol* 1994; 88:794–802.

40. Lu L, Ge Y, Li ZH, et al. Retroviral transfer of the recombinant human erythropoietin receptor gene into single hematopoietic stem/progenitor cells from human cord blood increases the number of erythropoietin-dependent erythroid colonies. *Blood* 1996;87:525–534.

41. Longmore GD, Pharr P, Neumann D, et al. Both megakaryocytopoiesis and erythropoiesis are induced in mice infected with a retrovirus expressing an oncogenic erythropoietin receptor. *Blood* 1993;82:2386–2395.

42. Minot G, Buckman TE. The development of anemia; the relation to leukemia; consideration of the basal metabolism, blood formation and destruction and fragility of the red cells. *Am J Med Sci* 1923;166:469–488.

43. Harrop G. Polycythemia. *Medicine* 1928;7:291–344.

44. Mirza AM, Correa PN, Axelrad AA. Increased basal and induced tyrosine phosphorylation of the insulin-like growth factor I receptor beta subunit in circulating mononuclear cells of patients with polycythemia vera. *Blood* 1995;86:877–882.

45. Mirza AM, Ezzat S, Axelrad AA. Insulin-like growth factor binding protein-1 is elevated in patients with polycythemia vera and stimulates erythroid burst formation in vitro. *Blood* 1997;89:1862–1869.

46. Solar GP, Kerr WG, Zeigler FC, et al. Role of c-mpl in early hematopoiesis. *Blood* 1998;92:4–10.

47. Debili N, Wendling F, Cosman D, et al. The Mpl receptor is expressed in the megakaryocytic lineage from late progenitors to platelets. *Blood* 1995;85:391–401.

48. Papayannopoulou T, Brice M, Farrer D, et al. Insights into the cellular mechanisms of erythropoietin-thrombopoietin synergy. *Exp Hematol* 1996;24:660–669.

49. Ratajczak MZ, Ratajczak J, Marlicz W, et al. Recombinant human thrombopoietin (TPO) stimulates erythropoiesis by inhibiting erythroid progenitor cell apoptosis. *Br J Haematol* 1997;98:8–17.

50. Young JC, Bruno E, Luens KM, et al. Thrombopoietin stimulates megakaryocytopoiesis, myelopoiesis, and expansion of CD34+ progenitor cells from single CD34+Thy-1+Lin- primitive progenitor cells. *Blood* 1996;88:1619–1631.

51. Sawai Y, Koike K, Ito S, et al. Neutrophilic cell production by combination of stem cell factor and thrombopoietin from CD34(+) cord blood cells in long-term serum-deprived liquid culture. *Blood* 1999;93:509–518.

52. Ulich TR, del Castillo J, Senaldi G, et al. Systemic hematologic effects of PEG-rHuMGDF-induced megakaryocyte hyperplasia in mice. *Blood* 1996;87:5006–5015.

53. Villeval JL, Cohen-Solal K, Tulliez M, et al. High thrombopoietin production by hematopoietic cells induces a fatal myeloproliferative syndrome in mice. *Blood* 1997;90:4369–4383.

54. Cocault L, Bouscary D, Le Bousse KC, et al. Ectopic expression of murine TPO receptor (c-mpl) in mice is pathogenic and induces erythroblastic proliferation. *Blood* 1996;88:1656–1665.

55. Souyri M, Vigon I, Penciolelli JF, et al. A putative truncated cytokine receptor gene transduced by the myeloproliferative leukemia virus immortalizes hematopoietic progenitors. *Cell* 1990;63:1137–1147.

56. Wendling F, Varlet P, Charon M, et al. MPLV: a retrovirus complex inducing an acute myeloproliferative leukemic disorder in adult mice. *Virology* 1986; 149:242–246.

57. Moliterno AR, Hankins WD, Spivak JL. Impaired expression of the thrombopoietin receptor by platelets from patients with polycythemia vera. *N Engl J Med* 1998;338:572–580.

58. Moliterno AR, Spivak JL. Posttranslational processing of the thrombopoietin receptor is impaired in polycythemia vera. *Blood* 1999;94:2555–2561.

59. Swolin B, Weinfeld A, Westin J. A prospective long-term cytogenetic study in polycythemia vera in relation to treatment and clinical course. *Blood* 1988; 72:386–395.

60. Bench AJ, Nacheva EP, Hood TL, et al. Chromosome 20 deletions in myeloid malignancies: reduction of the common deleted region, generation of a PAC/BAC contig and identification of candidate genes. UK Cancer Cytogenetics Group (UKCCG). *Oncogene* 2000;19:3902–3913.

61. Kanfer E, Price CM, Colman SM, et al. Erythropoietin-independent colony growth in polycythaemia vera is not restricted to progenitor cells with trisomy of chromosome 8. *Br J Haematol* 1992;82:773–774.

62. Gaidano G, Guerrasio A, Serra A, et al. Mutations in the P53 and RAS family genes are associated with tumor progression of BCR/ABL negative chronic myeloproliferative disorders. *Leukemia* 1993;7:946–953.

63. Ihalainen J, Juvonen E, Savolainen ER, et al. Calcitonin gene methylation in chronic myeloproliferative disorders. *Leukemia* 1994;8:230–235.

64. Asimakopoulos FA, Hinshelwood S, Gilbert JG, et al. The gene encoding hematopoietic cell phosphatase (SHP-1) is structurally and transcriptionally intact in polycythemia vera. *Oncogene* 1997;14:1215–1222.

65. Silva M, Richard C, Benito A, et al. Expression of Bcl-x in erythroid precursors from patients with polycythemia vera. *N Engl J Med* 1998;338:564–571.

66. Spivak JL, Pham T, Isaacs M, et al. Erythropoietin is both a mitogen and a survival factor. *Blood* 1991;77:1228–1233.

67. Koury MJ, Bondurant MC. Erythropoietin retards DNA breakdown and prevents programmed death in erythroid progenitor cells. *Science* 1990;248:378–381.

68. Spivak JL, Ferris DK, Fisher J, et al. Cell cycle-specific behavior of erythropoietin. *Exp Hematol* 1996;24:141–150.

69. Silva M, Grillot D, Benito A, et al. Erythropoietin can promote erythroid progenitor survival by repressing apoptosis through Bcl-XL and Bcl-2. *Blood* 1996;88:1576–1582.

70. Fairbairn LJ, Cowling GJ, Reipert BM, et al. Suppression of apoptosis allows differentiation and development of a multipotent hemopoietic cell line in the absence of added growth factors. *Cell* 1993;74:823–832.

71. Carroll M, Zhu Y, D'Andrea AD. Erythropoietin-induced cellular differentiation requires prolongation of the G1 phase of the cell cycle. *Proc Natl Acad Sci U S A* 1995;92:2869–2873.
72. Calbresi P, Meyer OO. Polycythemia vera I. Clinical and laboratory manifestations. *Ann Intern Med* 1958;50:1182–1216.
73. Polycythemia vera: the natural history of 1213 patients followed for 20 years. Gruppo Italiano Studio Policitemia. *Ann Intern Med* 1995;123:656–664.
74. Moore DF, Sears DA. Pica, iron deficiency, and the medical history. *Am J Med* 1994;97:390–393.
75. Anger B, Haug U, Seidler R, et al. Polycythemia vera. A clinical study of 141 patients. *Blut* 1989;59:493–500.
76. Barabas AP, Offen DN, Meinhard EA. The arterial complications of polycythaemia vera. *Br J Surgery* 1973;50:183–187.
77. Parker RG. Occlusion of the hepatic veins in man. *Medicine* 1959;38:369–402.
78. Najean Y, Mugnier P, Dresch C, et al. Polycythaemia vera in young people: an analysis of 58 cases diagnosed before 40 years. *Br J Haematol* 1987;67:285–291.
79. Budde U, Scharf RE, Franke P, et al. Elevated platelet count as a cause of abnormal von Willebrand factor multimer distribution in plasma. *Blood* 1993;82:1749–1757.
80. Westin J, Granerus G, Weinfeld A, et al. Histamine metabolism in polycythaemia vera. *Scand J Haematol* 1975;15:45–57.
81. Fan Yu T, Weissmann B, Sharney L, et al. On the biosynthesis of uric acid from glycine-n in primary and secondary polcythemia. *Am J Med* 1956;901–917.
82. Videbaek A. Polycythemia vera. Course and prognosis. *Acta Med Scand* 1950;138:179–187.
83. Taylor KM, Shetta M, Talpaz M, et al. Myeloproliferative disorders: usefulness of X-linked probes in diagnosis. *Leukemia* 1989;3:419–422.
84. Janssen JW, Anger BR, Drexler HG, et al. Essential thrombocythemia in two sisters originating from different stem cell levels. *Blood* 1990;75:1633–1636.
85. Szur L, Lewis SM, Goolden AWG. Polycythemia vera and its treatment with radioactive phosphorus. *QJM* 1959;397–424.
86. Berlin NI. Diagnosis and classification of the polycythemias. *Semin Hematol* 1975;12:339–351.
87. Bessman DJ. Microcytic polycythemia: frequency of nonthalassemic causes. *JAMA* 1977;238:2391–2392.
88. Ikkala E, Rapola J, Kotilainen M. Polycythaemia vera and myelofibrosis. *Scand J Haematol* 1967;4:453–464.
89. Zittoun J, Zittoun R, Marquet J, et al. The three transcobalamins in myeloproliferative disorders and acute leukaemia. *Br J Haematol* 1975;31:287–298.
90. Bader R, Bader M, Duberstein JL. Polycythemia vera and arterial oxygen saturation. *Am J Med* 1963;34:435–439.
91. Lertzman M, Frome BM, Israels LG, et al. Hypoxia in polycythemia vera. *Ann Intern Med* 1963;60:409–417.
92. Haga P, Cotes PM, Till JA, et al. Serum immunoreactive erythropoietin in children with cyanotic and acyanotic congenital heart disease. *Blood* 1987;70:822–826.
93. Ellis JT, Peterson P, Geller SA, et al. Studies of the bone marrow in polycythemia vera and the evolution of myelofibrosis and second hematologic malignancies. *Semin Hematol* 1986;23:144–155.
94. Lundin PM, Ridell B, Weinfeld A. The significance of bone marrow morphology for the diagnosis of polycythaemia vera. *Scand J Haematol* 1972;9:271–282.
95. Roberts BE, Miles DW, Woods CG. Polycythaemia vera and myelosclerosis: a bone marrow study. *Br J Haematol* 1969;16:75–85.
96. Najean Y, Dresch C, Rain JD. The very-long-term course of polycythaemia: a complement to the previously published data of the Polycythaemia Vera Study Group. *Br J Haematol* 1994;86:233–235.
97. Berger S, Aledort LM, Gilbert HS, et al. Abnormalities of platelet function in patients with polycythemia vera. *Cancer Res* 1973;33:2683–2687.
98. Manoharan A, Gemmell R, Brighton T, et al. Thrombosis and bleeding in myeloproliferative disorders: identification of at-risk patients with whole blood platelet aggregation studies. *Br J Haematol* 1999;105:618–625.
99. Landolfi R, Ciabattoni G, Patrignani P, et al. Increased thromboxane biosynthesis in patients with polycythemia vera: evidence for aspirin-suppressible platelet activation in vivo. *Blood* 1992;80:1965–1971.
100. Jensen MK, de Nully BP, Lund BV, et al. Increased platelet activation and abnormal membrane glycoprotein content and redistribution in myeloproliferative disorders. *Br J Haematol* 2000;110:116–124.
101. Martinez J, Shapiro SS, Holburn RR. Metabolism of human prothrombin and fibrinogen in patients with thrombocytosis secondary to myeloproliferative states. *Blood* 1973;42:35–46.
102. Landolfi R, De Cristofaro R, Castagnola M, et al. Increased platelet-fibrinogen affinity in patients with myeloproliferative disorders. *Blood* 1988;71:978–982.
103. Pareti FI, Gugliotta L, Mannucci L, et al. Biochemical and metabolic aspects of platelet dysfunction in chronic myeloproliferative disorders. *Thromb Haemost* 1982;47:84–89.
104. Wehmeier A, Fricke S, Scharf RE, et al. A prospective study of haemostatic parameters in relation to the clinical course of myeloproliferative disorders. *Eur J Haematol* 1990;45:191–197.
105. Malpass TW, Savage B, Hanson SR, et al. Correlation between prolonged bleeding time and depletion of platelet dense granule ADP in patients with myelodysplastic and myeloproliferative disorders. *J Lab Clin Med* 1984;103:894–904.
106. Meschengieser S, Blanco A, Woods A, et al. Intraplatelet levels of vWF: Ag and fibrinogen in myeloproliferative disorders. *Thromb Res* 1987;48:311–319.
107. Baglin TP, Price SM, Boughton BJ. A reversible defect of platelet PDGF content in myeloproliferative disorders. *Br J Haematol* 1988;69:483–486.
108. Cooper B, Ahern D. Characterization of the platelet prostaglandin D2 receptor. Loss of prostaglandin D2 receptors in platelets of patients with myeloproliferative disorders. *J Clin Invest* 1979;64:586–590.
109. Schafer AI. Deficiency of platelet lipoxygenase activity in myeloproliferative disorders. *N Engl J Med* 1982;306:381–386.
110. Brodsky I, Kahn SB, Ross EM, et al. Platelet and fibrinogen kinetics in the chronic myeloproliferative disorders. *Cancer* 1972;30:1444–1450.
111. Harker LA, Finch CA. Thrombokinetics in man. *J Clin Invest* 1969;48:963–974.
112. Kornberg A, Rahimi-Levene N, Yona R, et al. Enhanced generation of monocyte tissue factor and increased plasma prothrombin fragment1+2 levels in patients with polycythemia vera: mechanism of activation of blood coagulation. *Am J Hematol* 1997;56:5–11.
113. Maldonado JE, Pintado T, Pierre RV. Dysplastic platelets and circulating megakaryocytes in chronic myeloproliferative diseases. I. The platelets: ultrastructure and peroxidase reaction. *Blood* 1974;43:797–809.
114. Boughton BJ. Chronic myeloproliferative disorders: improved platelet aggregation following venesection. *Br J Haematol* 1978;39:589–598.
115. Kroll MH, Hellums JD, McIntire LV, et al. Platelets and shear stress. *Blood* 1996;88:1525–1541.
116. Gisslinger H, Rodeghiero F, Ruggeri M, et al. Homocysteine levels in polycythaemia vera and essential thrombocythaemia. *Br J Haematol* 1999;105:551–555.
117. Bucalossi A, Marotta G, Bigazzi C, et al. Reduction of antithrombin III, protein C, and protein S levels and activated protein C resistance in polycythemia vera and essential thrombocythemia patients with thrombosis. *Am J Hematol* 1996;52:14–20.
118. Diez-Martin JL, Graham DL, Petitt RM, et al. Chromosome studies in 104 patients with polycythemia vera. *Mayo Clin Proc* 1991;66:287–299.
119. Testa JR, Kanofsky JR, Rowley JD, et al. Karyotypic patterns and their clinical significance in polycythemia vera. *Am J Hematol* 1981;11:29–45.
120. Rege-Cambrin G, Mecucci C, Tricot G, et al. A chromosomal profile of polycythemia vera. *Cancer Genet Cytogenet* 1987;25:233–245.
121. Iland HJ, Laszlo J, Case DC Jr, et al. Differentiation between essential thrombocythemia and polycythemia vera with marked thrombocytosis. *Am J Hematol* 1987;25:191–201.
122. Hazani A, Tatarsky I, Barzilai D. Prolonged remission of leukemia associated with polycythemia vera. *Cancer* 1977;40:1297–1299.
123. Asimakopoulos FA, Gilbert JG, Aldred MA, et al. Interstitial deletion constitutes the major mechanism for loss of heterozygosity on chromosome 20q in polycythemia vera. *Blood* 1996;88:2690–2698.
124. Kurtin PJ, Dewald GW, Shields DJ, et al. Hematologic disorders associated with deletions of chromosome 20q: a clinicopathologic study of 107 patients. *Am J Clin Pathol* 1996;106:680–688.
125. Berger R, Bernheim A, Flandrin G, et al. Cytogenetic studies on acute nonlymphocytic leukemias following polycythemia vera. *Cancer Genet Cytogenet* 1984;11:441–451.
126. Koury ST, Koury MJ, Bondurant MC, et al. Quantitation of erythropoietin-producing cells in kidneys of mice by in situ hybridization: correlation with hematocrit, renal erythropoietin mRNA, and serum erythropoietin concentration. *Blood* 1989;74:645–651.
127. Goldberg MA, Gaut CC, Bunn HF. Erythropoietin mRNA levels are governed by both the rate of gene transcription and posttranscriptional events. *Blood* 1991;77:271–277.
128. Cazzola M, Guarnone R, Cerani P, et al. Red blood cell precursor mass as an independent determinant of serum erythropoietin level. *Blood* 1998;91:2139–2145.
129. Singh A, Eckardt KU, Zimmermann A, et al. Increased plasma viscosity as a reason for inappropriate erythropoietin formation. *J Clin Invest* 1993;91:251–256.
130. Lemoine F, Najman A, Baillou C, et al. A prospective study of the value of bone marrow erythroid progenitor cultures in polycythemia. *Blood* 1986;68:996–1002.
131. Dudley JM, Westwood N, Leonard S, et al. Primary polycythaemia: positive diagnosis using the differential response of primitive and mature erythroid progenitors to erythropoietin, interleukin 3 and alpha-interferon. *Br J Haematol* 1990;75:188–194.
132. Colovic MD, Wiernik PH, Jankovic GM, et al. Circulating haemopoietic progenitor cells in primary and secondary myelofibrosis: relation to collagen and reticulin fibrosis. *Eur J Haematol* 1999;62:155–159.
133. Eridani S, Dudley JM, Sawyer BM, et al. Erythropoietic colonies in a serum-free system: results in primary proliferative polycythaemia and thrombocythaemia. *Br J Haematol* 1987;67:387–391.
134. Dainiak N, Hoffman R, Lebowitz AI, et al. Erythropoietin-dependent primary pure erythrocytosis. *Blood* 1979;53:1076–1084.
135. Smith HP, Arnold HR, Whipple GH. Comparative values of Welcker, carbon monoxide and dye methods for blood volume determinations. Accurate estimation of absolute blood volume. *Am J Physiol* 1921;56:336–360.
136. Berson SA, Yalow RS. The use of K^{42} or P^{32} labeled erythrocytes and I131 tagged human serum albumin in simultaneous blood volume determinations. *J Clin Invest* 1952;31:572–580.
137. Fahraeus R, Lindqvist T. The viscosity of the blood in narrow capillary tubes. *Am J Physiol* 1931;96:562–568.

138. Hess CH, Ayers CR, Sandusky WR, et al. Mechanism of dilutional anemia in massive splenomegaly. *Blood* 1976;47:629–644.
139. Campbell A, Emery EW, Godlee JN, et al. Diagnosis and treatment of primary polycythaemia. *Lancet* 1970;1:1074–1077.
140. Zhang B, Lewis SM. The splenomegaly of myeloproliferative disorders: effects on blood volume and red blood count. *Eur J Haematol* 1989;42:250–253.
141. Rothschild MA, Bauman A, Yalow RS, et al. Effect of splenomegaly on blood. *J Appl Physiol* 1954;6:701–706.
142. Besa EC, Gorshein D, Gardner FH. Androgens and human blood volume changes. Comparison in normal and various anemic states. *Arch Intern Med* 1974;133:418–425.
143. Lim VS, DeGowin RL, Zavala D, et al. Recombinant human erythropoietin treatment in pre-dialysis patients. A double-blind placebo-controlled trial. *Ann Intern Med* 1989;110:108–114.
144. Sanchez C, Merino C, Figallo M. Simultaneous measurement of plasma volume and cell mass in polycythemia of high altitude. *J Appl Physiol* 1970;28:775–778.
145. Rosenthal A, Button LN, Nathan DG, et al. Blood volume changes in cyanotic congenital heart disease. *Am J Cardiol* 1971;27:162–167.
146. Smith JR, Landaw SA. Smokers' polycythemia. *N Engl J Med* 1978;298:972–973.
147. Cobb LA, Kramer RJ, Finch CA. Circulatory effects of chronic hypervolemia in polycythemia vera. *J Clin Invest* 1960;39:1722–1728.
148. Lamy T, Devillers A, Bernard M, et al. Inapparent polycythemia vera: an unrecognized diagnosis. *Am J Med* 1997;102:14–20.
149. Strumia MM, Strumia PV, Dugan A. Significance of measurement of plasma volume and of indirect estimation of red cell volume. *Transfusion* 1968;8:197–209.
150. Recommended methods for measurement of red-cell and plasma volume: International Committee for Standardization in Haematology. *J Nucl Med* 1980;21:793–800.
151. Pearson TC, Botterill CA, Glass UH, et al. Interpretation of measured red cell mass and plasma volume in males with elevated venous PCV values. *Scand J Haematol* 1984;33:68–74.
152. Wasserman LR. Polycythemia vera—its course and treatment relation to myeloid metaplasia and leukemia. *Bull N Y Acad Med* 1954;30:343–375.
153. Rosenthal N, Bassen F. Course of polycythemia. *Arch Intern Med* 1938;62:903–917.
154. Hirsch EF. Case Reports, laboratory methods and technical notes. *Arch Path* 1935;19:91–97.
155. Perkins J, Israels MCG, Wilkinson JF. Polycythemia vera: clinical studies on a series of 127 patients managed without radiation therapy. *QJM* 1964;33:499–518.
156. Rozman C, Giralt M, Feliu E, et al. Life expectancy of patients with chronic nonleukemic myeloproliferative disorders. *Cancer* 1991;67:2658–2663.
157. Pollycove M, Winchell HS, Lawrence JH. Classification and evolution of patterns of erythropoiesis in polycythemia vera as studied by iron kinetics. *Blood* 1966;28:807–829.
158. Barosi G, Cazzola M, Frassoni F, et al. Erythropoiesis in myelofibrosis with myeloid metaplasia: recognition of different classes of patients by erythrokinetics. *Br J Haematol* 1981;48:263–272.
159. Pettit JE, Lewis SM, Nicholas AW. Transitional myeloproliferative disorder. *Br J Haematol* 1979;43:167–184.
160. Najean Y, Arrago JP, Rain JD, et al. The "spent" phase of polycythaemia vera: hypersplenism in the absence of myelofibrosis. *Br J Haematol* 1984;56:163–170.
161. Damesek W. Physiopathology and course of polycythemia vera as related to therapy. *JAMA* 1950;142:790–797.
162. Silverstein MN. Postpolycythemia myeloid metaplasia. *Arch Intern Med* 1974;134:113–117.
163. Kurnick JE, Mahmood T, Napoli N, et al. Extension of myeloid tissue into the lower extremities in polycythemia. *Am J Clin Pathol* 1980;74:427–431.
164. Burston J, Pinniger JL. The reticulin content of bone marrow in haematological disorders. *Br J Haematol* 1963;9:172–184.
165. Dekmezian R, Kantarjian HM, Keating MJ, et al. The relevance of reticulin stain-measured fibrosis at diagnosis in chronic myelogenous leukemia. *Cancer* 1987;59:1739–1743.
166. Chevitz E, Torben T. Complications and causes of death in polycythemia vera. *Acta Med Scand* 1962;172:513–523.
167. Leonard BJ, Israels MCG, Wilkinson JF. Myelosclerosis: a clinicopathological study. *QJM* 1957;26:131–149.
168. Modan B, Lilienfeld AM. Polycythemia vera and leukemia—the role of radiation treatment. *Medicine* 1965;44:305–339.
169. Lawrence JH, Berlin NI, Huff RL. The nature and treatment of polycythemia. *Medicine* 1953;32:323–388.
170. Osgood EE. Polycythemia vera: age relationships and survival. *Blood* 1965;26:243–256.
171. Lawrence JH, Winchell HS, Donald WG. Leukemia in polycythemia vera: relationship to splenic myeloid metaplasia and therapeutic radiation dose. *Ann Intern Med* 1969;70:763–771.
172. Berk PD, Goldberg JD, Silverstein MN, et al. Increased incidence of acute leukemia in polycythemia vera associated with chlorambucil therapy. *N Engl J Med* 1981;304:441–447.
173. Najean Y, Rain J. The very long-term evolution of polycythemia vera: an analysis of 318 patients initially treated by phlebotomy or ^{32}P between 1969 and 1981. *Semin Hematol* 1997;34:6–16.
174. Weinfeld A, Swolin B, Westin J. Acute leukaemia after hydroxyurea therapy in polycythaemia vera and allied disorders: prospective study of efficacy and leukaemogenicity with therapeutic implications. *Eur J Haematol* 1994;52:134–139.
175. Brusamolino E, Salvaneschi L, Canevari A, et al. Efficacy trial of pipobroman in polycythemia vera and incidence of acute leukemia. *J Clin Oncol* 1984;2:558–561.
176. Najean Y, Rain J. Treatment of polycythemia vera: use of ^{32}P alone or in combination with maintenace therapy using hydroxyurea in 461 patients greater than 65 years of age. *Blood* 1997;89:2319–2327.
177. Nand S, Messmore H, Fisher SG, et al. Leukemic transformation in polycythemia vera: analysis of risk factors. *Am J Hematol* 1990;34:32–36.
178. Leone G, Mele L, Pulsoni A, et al. The incidence of secondary leukemias. *Haematologica* 1999;84:937–945.
179. Landaw S. Acute leukemia in polycythemia vera. *Semin Hematol* 1976;13:33–48.
180. Landaw SA. Acute leukemia in polycythemia vera. *Semin Hematol* 1986;23:156–165.
181. Najean Y, Deschamps A, Dresch C, et al. Acute leukemia and myelodysplasia in polycythemia vera. A clinical study with long-term follow-up. *Cancer* 1988;61:89–95.
182. Neu LT, Shuman MA, Brown EB. Polycythemia vera and acute leukemia. *Ann Intern Med* 1975;83:672–673.
183. Lundberg WB, Farber LR, Cadman EC, et al. Spontaneous acute leukemia in polycythemia vera. *Ann Intern Med* 1976;84:294–295.
184. Schwartz SO, Ehrlich L. The relationship of polycythemia vera to leukemia; a critical review. *Acta Med Scand* 1950;4:129–147.
185. McNally RJ, Rowland D, Roman E. Age and sex distributions of hematological malignancies in the U.K. *Hematol Oncol* 1997;15:173–189.
186. Barosi G, Ambrosetti A, Centra A, et al. Splenectomy and risk of blast transformation in myelofibrosis with myeloid metaplasia. Italian Cooperative Study Group on Myeloid with Myeloid Metaplasia. *Blood* 1998;91:3630–3636.
187. Tura S, Fiacchini M, Zinzani PL, et al. Splenectomy and the increasing risk of secondary acute leukemia in Hodgkin's disease. *J Clin Oncol* 1993;11:925–930.
188. Socie G, Henry-Amar M, Bacigalupo A, et al. Malignant tumors occurring after treatment of aplastic anemia. European Bone Marrow Transplantation-Severe Aplastic Anaemia Working Party. *N Engl J Med* 1993;329:1152–1157.
189. McDonnell JM, Beschorner WE, Staal SP, et al. Richter's syndrome with two different B-cell clones. *Cancer* 1986;58:2031–2037.
190. Tinney WS, Hall BE, Giffin HZ. The prognosis of polycythemia vera. *Proc Staff Meet Mayo Clin* 1945;227–230.
191. Anger BR, Seifried E, Scheppach J, et al. Budd-Chiari syndrome and thrombosis of other abdominal vessels in the chronic myeloproliferative diseases. *Klin Wochenschr* 1989;67:818–825.
192. Wanless IR, Wong F, Blendis LM, et al. Hepatic and portal vein thrombosis in cirrhosis: possible role in development of parenchymal extinction and portal hypertension. *Hepatology* 1995;21:1238–1247.
193. Gilliland DG, Blanchard KL, Levy J, et al. Clonality in myeloproliferative disorders: analysis by means of the polymerase chain reaction. *Proc Natl Acad Sci U S A* 1991;88:6848–6852.
194. Hume R, Goldberg A. Actual and predicted-normal red-cell and plasma volumes in primary and secondary polycythemia. *Clin Sci* 1964;26:499–508.
195. Verel D. Blood volume changes in cyanotic congenital heart disease and polycythemia rubra vera. *Circulation* 1961;23:749–753.
196. Murray JF, Gold P, Johnson BL. The circulatory effects of hematocrit variations in normovolemic and hypervolemic dogs. *J Clin Invest* 1963;42:1150–1159.
197. Fudenberg H, Baldini M, Mahoney J, et al. The body hematocrit/venous hematocrit ratio and the "splenic reservoir." *Blood* 1960;71–82.
198. Wells RE, Merrill EW. Influence of flow properties of blood upon viscosity hematocrit relationship. *J Clin Invest* 1962;41:1591–1598.
199. Brown G, Giffin HZ. Studies of capillaries and blood volume in polycythemia vera. *Am J Med Sci* 1923;166:489–502.
200. Falanga A, Marchetti M, Evangelista V, et al. Polymorphonuclear leukocyte activation and hemostasis in patients with essential thrombocythemia and polycythemia vera. *Blood* 2000;96:4261–4266.
201. Kaplar M, Kappelmayer J, Kiss A, et al. Increased leukocyte-platelet adhesion in chronic myeloproliferative disorders with high platelet counts. *Platelets* 2000;11:183–184.
202. Friedenberg WR, Roberts RC, David DE. Relationship of thrombohemorrhagic complications to endothelial cell function in patients with chronic myeloproliferative disorders. *Am J Hematol* 1992;40:283–289.
203. Houston DS, Robinson P, Gerrard JM. Inhibition of intravascular platelet aggregation by endothelium-derived relaxing factor: reversal by red blood cells. *Blood* 1990;76:953–958.
204. Fiermonte G, Aloe Spiriti MA, Latagliata R, et al. Polycythaemia vera and cerebral blood flow: a preliminary study with transcranial Doppler. *J Intern Med* 1993;234:599–602.
205. Segel N, Bishop JM. Circulatory studies in polycythemia vera at rest and during exercise. *Clin Sci* 1967;32:527–549.
206. Humphrey PR, Michael J, Pearson TC. Red cell mass, plasma volume and blood volume before and after venesection in relative polycythaemia. *Br J Haematol* 1980;46:435–438.
207. Pearson TC, Grimes AJ, Slater NG, et al. Viscosity and iron deficiency in treated polycythaemia. *Br J Haematol* 1981;49:123–127.
208. Birgegard G, Carlsson M, Sandhagen B, et al. Does iron deficiency in treated polycythemia vera affect whole blood viscosity? *Acta Med Scand* 1984;216:165–169.

209. Rector WG, Fortuin NJ, Conley CL. Non-hematologic effects of chronic iron deficiency. A study of patients with polycythemia vera treated solely with venesections. *Medicine* 1982;61:382–389.
210. Challoner T, Briggs C, Rampling MW, et al. A study of the haematological and haemorheological consequences of venesection. *Br J Haematol* 1986;62:671–678.
211. Stephens DJ, Kaltreider N. The therapeutic use of venesection in polycythemia. *Ann Intern Med* 1933;10:1565–1581.
212. Kutti J, Weinfeld A. Platelet survival in active polycythaemia vera with reference to the haematocrit level. An experimental study before and after phlebotomy. *Scand J Haematol* 1971;8:405–414.
213. Tillmann W, Schroter W. Deformability of erythrocytes in iron deficiency anemia. *Blut* 1980;40:179–186.
214. Aarts PA, Bolhuis PA, Sakariassen KS, et al. Red blood cell size is important for adherence of blood platelets to artery subendothelium. *Blood* 1983;62:214–217.
215. Thomas DJ, du Boulay GH, Marshall J, et al. Cerebral blood-flow in polycythaemia. *Lancet* 1977;2:161–163.
216. Humphrey PR, Michael J, Pearson TC. Management of relative polycythaemia: studies of cerebral blood flow and viscosity. *Br J Haematol* 1980;46:427–433.
217. Berk PD, Goldberg JD, Donovan PB, et al. Therapeutic recommendations in polycythemia vera based on Polycythemia Vera Study Group protocols. *Semin Hematol* 1986;23:132–143.
218. Pearson TC, Weatherly-Mein G. Vascular occlusive episodes and venous haematocrit in primary proliferative polycythaemia. *Lancet* 1978;2:1219–1221.
219. Finch S, Haskins D, Finch CA. Iron metabolism hematopoiesis following phlebotomy iron as a limiting factor. *J Clin Invest* 1950;1078–1086.
220. Kiraly JF, Feldmann JE, Wheby MS. Hazards of phlebotomy in polycythemic patients with cardiovascular disease. *JAMA* 1976;236:2080–2081.
221. Wasserman LR, Gilbert HS. Surgical bleeding in polycythemia vera. *Ann N Y Acad Sci* 1964;115:122–138.
222. Kaboth U, Rumpf KW, Lipp T, et al. Treatment of polycythemia vera by isovolemic large-volume erythrocytapheresis. *Klin Wochenschr* 1990;68:18–25.
223. Jackson N, Burt D, Crocker J, et al. Skin mast cells in polycythaemia vera: relationship to the pathogenesis and treatment of pruritus. *Br J Dermatol* 1987;116:21–29.
224. Buchanan JG, Ameratunga RV, Hawkins RC. Polycythemia vera and water-induced pruritus: evidence against mast cell involvement. *Pathology* 1994;26:43–45.
225. Morison WL, Nesbitt JA. Oral psoralen photochemotherapy (PUVA) for pruritus associated with polycythemia vera and myelofibrosis. *Am J Hematol* 1993;42:409–410.
226. Finelli C, Gugliotta L, Gamberi B, et al. Relief of intractable pruritus in polycythemia vera with recombinant interferon alfa. *Am J Hematol* 1993;43:316–318.
227. Kolodny L. Danazole is safe and effective in relieving refractory pruritus in patients with myeloproliferative disorders and other diseases. *Am J Hematol* 1996;51:112–116.
228. Parmentier C, Charbord P, Tibi M, et al. Splenic irradiation in myelofibrosis clinical findings and ferrokinetics. *Int J Radiat Oncol Biol Phys* 1977;2:1075–1081.
229. Elliott MA, Chen MG, Silverstein MN, et al. Splenic irradiation for symptomatic splenomegaly associated with myelofibrosis with myeloid metaplasia. *Br J Haematol* 1998;103:505–511.
230. Brenner B, Nagler A, Tatarsky I, et al. Splenectomy in agnogenic myeloid metaplasia and postpolycythemic myeloid metaplasia. A study of 34 cases. *Arch Intern Med* 1988;148:2501–2505.
231. Aviram M, Carter A, Tatarsky I, et al. Increased platelet aggregation following splenectomy in patients with myeloproliferative disease. *Isr J Med Sci* 1985;21:415–417.
232. Broe PJ, Conley CL, Cameron JL. Thrombosis of the portal vein following splenectomy for myeloid metaplasia. *Surg Gynecol Obstet* 1981;152:488–492.
233. Petit P, Bret PM, Atri M, et al. Splenic vein thrombosis after splenectomy: frequency and role of imaging. *Radiology* 1994;190:65–68.
234. Chaffanjon PC, Brichon PY, Ranchoup Y, et al. Portal vein thrombosis following splenectomy for hematologic disease: prospective study with Doppler color flow imaging. *World J Surg* 1998;22:1082–1086.
235. Schilling RF. Platelet millionaires. *Lancet* 1980;2:372–373.
236. Tefferi A, Silverstein MN, Li CY. 2-Chlorodeoxyadenosine treatment after splenectomy in patients who have myelofibrosis with myeloid metaplasia. *Br J Haematol* 1997;99:352–357.
237. Castello G, Lerza R, Cerutti A, et al. The in vitro and in vivo effect of recombinant interferon alpha-2a on circulating haemopoietic progenitors in polycythemia vera. *Br J Haematol* 1994;87:621–623.
238. Silver RT. Interferon alfa: effects of long-term treatment for polycythemia vera. *Semin Hematol* 1997;34:40–50.
239. Silver RT, Woolf SH, Hehlmann R, et al. An evidence-based analysis of the effect of busulfan, hydroxyurea, interferon, and allogeneic bone marrow transplantation in treating the chronic phase of chronic myeloid leukemia: developed for the American Society of Hematology. *Blood* 1999;94:1517–1536.
240. Sacchi S, Kantarjian H, O'Brien S, et al. Immune-mediated and unusual complications during interferon alfa therapy in chronic myelogenous leukemia. *J Clin Oncol* 1995;13:2401–2407.
241. Kurschel E, Metz-Kurschel U, Niederle N, et al. Investigations on the subclinical and clinical nephrotoxicity of interferon alpha-2B in patients with myeloproliferative syndromes. *Ren Fail* 1991;13:87–93.
242. Lengfelder E, Berger U, Hehlmann R. Interferon alpha in the treatment of polycythemia vera. *Ann Hematol* 2000;79:103–109.
243. Messora C, Bensi L, Vecchi A, et al. Cytogenetic conversion in case of polycythaemia vera treated with interferon-alpha. *Br J Haematol* 1994;86:402–404.
244. Massaro P, Foa P, Pomati M, et al. Polycythemia vera treated with recombinant interferon-alpha 2a: evidence of a selective effect on the malignant clone. *Am J Hematol* 1997;56:126–128.
245. Sacchi S, Leoni P, Liberati M, et al. A prospective comparison between treatment with phlebotomy alone and with interferon-alpha in patients with polycythemia vera. *Ann Hematol* 1994;68:247–250.
246. Hino M, Futami E, Okuno S, et al. Possible selective effects of interferon alpha-2b on a malignant clone in a case of polycythemia vera. *Ann Hematol* 1993;66:161–162.
247. Kreft A, Nolde C, Busche G, et al. Polycythaemia vera: bone marrow histopathology under treatment with interferon, hydroxyurea and busulphan. *Eur J Haematol* 2000;64:32–41.
248. Valentine AD, Meyers CA, Kling MA, et al. Mood and cognitive side effects of interferon-alpha therapy. *Semin Oncol* 1998;1:39–47.
249. Kessler CM, Klein HG, Havlik RJ. Uncontrolled thrombocytosis in chronic myeloproliferative disorders. *Br J Haematol* 1982;50:157–167.
250. Tartaglia AP, Goldberg JD, Berk PD, et al. Adverse effects of antiaggregating platelet therapy in the treatment of polycythemia vera. *Semin Hematol* 1986;23:172–176.
251. Michiels JJ. Erythromelalgia and vascular complications in polycythemia vera. *Semin Thromb Hemost* 1997;23:441–454.
252. Kurzrock R, Cohen PR. Erythromelalgia and myeloproliferative disorders. *Arch Intern Med* 1989;149:105–109.
253. Spencer CM, Brogden RN. Anagrelide. A review of its pharmacodynamic and pharmacokinetic properties, and therapeutic potential in the treatment of thrombocythaemia. *Drugs* 1994;47:809–822.
254. Ferguson JE, Ueland K, Aronson WJ. Polycythemia rubra vera and pregnancy. *Obstet Gynecol* 1983;62:16s–20s.
255. Ward HP, Block MH. The natural history of agnogenic myeloid metaplasia (AMM) and a critical evaluation of its relationship with the myeloproliferative syndrome. *Medicine* 1971;50:357–420.
256. Mesa RA, Silverstein MN, Jacobsen SJ, et al. Population-based incidence and survival figures in essential thrombocythemia and agnogenic myeloid metaplasia: an Olmsted County Study, 1976–1995. *Am J Hematol* 1999;61: 10–15.
257. Da Silva HJ, Da Motta C, Tavares MH. Thorium dioxide effects in man. Epidemiological, clinical, and pathological studies (experience in Portugal). *Environ Res* 1974;8:131–159.
258. Anderson R, Hoshino T, Tsutomu Y. Myelofibrosis with myeloid metaplasia in survivors of the atomic bomb in Hiroshima. *Ann Intern Med* 1964;60:1–18.
259. Hu H. Benzene-associated myelofibrosis. *Ann Intern Med* 1987;106:171–172.
260. Bosch X, Campistol JM, Montoliu J, et al. Toluene-associated myelofibrosis. *Blut* 1989;58:219–220.
261. Jacobson RJ, Salo A, Fialkow PJ. Agnogenic myeloid metaplasia: a clonal proliferation of hematopoietic stem cells with secondary myelofibrosis. *Blood* 1978;51:189–194.
262. Kreipe H, Jaquet K, Felgner J, et al. Clonal granulocytes and bone marrow cells in the cellular phase of agnogenic myeloid metaplasia. *Blood* 1991;78:1814–1817.
263. Anger B, Janssen JW, Schrezenmeier H, et al. Clonal analysis of chronic myeloproliferative disorders using X-linked DNA polymorphisms. *Leukemia* 1990;4:258–261.
264. Sato Y, Suda T, Suda J, et al. Multilineage expression of haemopoietic precursors with an abnormal clone in idiopathic myelofibrosis. *Br J Haematol* 1986;64:657–667.
265. Buschle M, Janssen JW, Drexler H, et al. Evidence for pluripotent stem cell origin of idiopathic myelofibrosis: clonal analysis of a case characterized by a N-ras gene mutation. *Leukemia* 1988;2:658–660.
266. Ferraris AM, Mangerini R, Racchi O, et al. Heterogeneity of clonal development in chronic myeloproliferative disorders. *Am J Hematol* 1999;60:158–160.
267. Reilly JT, Wilson G, Barnett D, et al. Karyotypic and ras gene mutational analysis in idiopathic myelofibrosis. *Br J Haematol* 1994;88:575–581.
268. Partanen S, Ruutu T, Vuopio P. Circulating haematopoietic progenitors in myelofibrosis. *Scand J Haematol* 1982;29:325–330.
269. Taksin AL, Couedic JP, Dusanter-Fourt I, et al. Autonomous megakaryocyte growth in essential thrombocythemia and idiopathic myelofibrosis is not related to a c-mpl mutation or to an autocrine stimulation by Mpl-L. *Blood* 1999;93:125–139.
270. Han ZC, Briere J, Nedellec G, et al. Characteristics of circulating megakaryocyte progenitors (CFU-MK) in patients with primary myelofibrosis. *Eur J Haematol* 1988;40:130–135.
271. Chikkappa G, Carsten AL, Chanana AD, et al. Increased granulocytic, erythrocytic, and megakaryocytic progenitors in myelofibrosis with myeloid metaplasia. *Am J Hematol* 1978;4:121–131.
272. Carlo-Stella C, Cazzola M, Gasner A, et al. Effects of recombinant alpha and gamma interferons on the in vitro growth of circulating hematopoietic progenitor cells (CFU-GEMM, CFU-Mk, BFU-E, and CFU-GM) from patients with myelofibrosis with myeloid metaplasia. *Blood* 1987;70:1014–1019.
273. Wang JC, Cheung CP, Ahmed F, et al. Circulating granulocyte and macrophage progenitor cells in primary and secondary myelofibrosis. *Br J Haematol* 1983;54:301–307.
274. Kornberg A, Fibach E, Treves A, et al. Circulating erythroid progenitors in patients with "spent" polycythaemia vera and myelofibrosis with myeloid metaplasia. *Br J Haematol* 1982;52:573–578.
275. Hibbin JA, Njoku OS, Matutes E, et al. Myeloid progenitor cells in the circulation of patients with myelofibrosis and other myeloproliferative disorders. *Br J Haematol* 1984;57:495–503.

276. Partanen S, Ruutu T, Juvonen E, et al. Effect of splenectomy on circulating haematopoietic progenitors in myelofibrosis. *Scand J Haematol* 1986;37:87–90.

277. Battegay EJ, Thomssen C, Nissen C, et al. Endogenous megakaryocyte colonies from peripheral blood in precursor cell cultures of patients with myeloproliferative disorders. *Eur J Haematol* 1989;42:321–326.

278. Kobayashi S, Teramura M, Hoshino S, et al. Circulating megakaryocyte progenitors in myeloproliferative disorders are hypersensitive to interleukin-3. *Br J Haematol* 1993;83:539–544.

279. Li Y, Hetet G, Kiladjian JJ, et al. Proto-oncogene c-mpl is involved in spontaneous megakaryocytopoiesis in myeloproliferative disorders. *Br J Haematol* 1996;92:60–66.

280. Wickenhauser C, Lorenzen J, Thiele J, et al. Secretion of cytokines (interleukins-1 alpha, -3, and -6 and granulocyte-macrophage colony-stimulating factor) by normal human bone marrow megakaryocytes. *Blood* 1995;85:685–691.

281. Jiang S, Levine JD, Fu Y, et al. Cytokine production by primary bone marrow megakaryocytes. *Blood* 1994;84:4151–4156.

282. Li Y, Hetet G, Maurer AM, et al. Spontaneous megakaryocyte colony formation in myeloproliferative disorders is not neutralizable by antibodies against IL3, IL6 and GM-CSF. *Br J Haematol* 1994;87:471–476.

283. Rueda F, Pinol G, Marti F, et al. Abnormal levels of platelet-specific proteins and mitogenic activity in myeloproliferative disease. *Acta Haematol* 1991;85:12–15.

284. Gilbert HS, Praloran V, Stanley ER. Increased circulating CSF-1 (M-CSF) in myeloproliferative disease: association with myeloid metaplasia and peripheral bone marrow extension. *Blood* 1989;74:1231–1234.

285. Wang JC, Chen C, Lou LH, et al. Blood thrombopoietin, IL-6 and IL-11 levels in patients with agnogenic myeloid metaplasia. *Leukemia* 1997;11:1827–1832.

286. Barosi G, Liberato LN, Guarnone R. Serum erythropoietin in patients with myelofibrosis with myeloid metaplasia. *Br J Haematol* 1993;83:365–369.

287. Rameshwar P, Chang VT, Thacker UF, et al. Systemic transforming growth factor-beta in patients with bone marrow fibrosis—pathophysiological implications. *Am J Hematol* 1998;59:133–142.

288. Han ZC, Sensebe L, Abgrall JF, et al. Platelet factor 4 inhibits human megakaryocytopoiesis in vitro. *Blood* 1990;75:1234–1239.

289. Sakamaki S, Hirayama Y, Matsunaga T, et al. Transforming growth factor-beta1 (TGF-beta1) induces thrombopoietin from bone marrow stromal cells, which stimulates the expression of TGF-beta receptor on megakaryocytes and, in turn, renders them susceptible to supression by TGF-beta itself with high specificity. *Blood* 1999;94:1961–1970.

290. Avraham H, Banu N, Scadden DT, et al. Modulation of megakaryocytopoiesis by human basic fibroblast growth factor. *Blood* 1994;83:2126–2132.

291. Le Bousse-Kerdiles MC, Chevillard S, Charpentier A, et al. Differential expression of transforming growth factor-beta, basic fibroblast growth factor, and their receptors in CD34+ hematopoietic progenitor cells from patients with myelofibrosis and myeloid metaplasia. *Blood* 1996;88:4534–4546.

292. Wolf BC, Neiman RS. Myelofibrosis with myeloid metaplasia: pathophysiologic implications of the correlation between bone marrow changes and progression of splenomegaly. *Blood* 1985;65:803–809.

293. Wolf BC, Banks PM, Mann RB, et al. Splenic hematopoiesis in polycythemia vera. A morphologic and immunohistologic study. *Am J Clin Pathol* 1988;89:69–75.

294. Wilkins BS, Green A, Wild AE, et al. Extramedullary haemopoiesis in fetal and adult human spleen: a quantitative immunohistological study. *Histopathology* 1994;24:241–247.

295. O'Keane JC, Wolf BC, Neiman RS. The pathogenesis of splenic extramedullary hematopoiesis in metastatic carcinoma. *Cancer* 1989;63:1539–1543.

296. Rubins JM. The role of myelofibrosis in malignant leukoerythroblastosis. *Cancer* 1983;51:308–311.

297. Thiele J, Rompcik V, Wagner S, et al. Vascular architecture and collagen type IV in primary myelofibrosis and polycythaemia vera: an immunomorphometric study on trephine biopsies of the bone marrow. *Br J Haematol* 1992;80:227–234.

298. de Bruijn MF, Speck NA, Peeters MC, et al. Definitive hematopoietic stem cells first develop within the major arterial regions of the mouse embryo. *EMBO J* 2000;19:2465–2474.

299. Douay L, Laporte JP, Lefrancois G, et al. Blood and spleen haematopoiesis in patients with myelofibrosis. *Leuk Res* 1987;11:725–730.

300. Koeffler HP, Cline MJ, Golde DW. Splenic irradiation in myelofibrosis: effect on circulating myeloid progenitor cells. *Br J Haematol* 1979;43:69–77.

301. Wang JC, Lang HD, Lichter S, et al. Cytogenetic studies of bone marrow fibroblasts cultured from patients with myelofibrosis and myeloid metaplasia. *Br J Haematol* 1992;80:184–188.

302. Greenberg BR, Woo L, Veomett IC, et al. Cytogenetics of bone marrow fibroblastic cells in idiopathic chronic myelofibrosis. *Br J Haematol* 1987;66:487–490.

303. Manoharan A, Pitney WR. Chemotherapy resolves symptoms and reverses marrow fibrosis in myelofibrosis. *Scand J Haematol* 1984;33:453–459.

304. Anderson JE, Sale G, Appelbaum FR, et al. Allogeneic marrow transplantation for primary myelofibrosis and myelofibrosis secondary to polycythaemia vera or essential thrombocytosis. *Br J Haematol* 1997;98:1010–1016.

305. Ragni MV, Shreiner DP. Spontaneous "remission" of agnogenic myeloid metaplasia and termination in acute myeloid leukemia. *Arch Intern Med* 1981;141:1481–1484.

306. Gordon MY. Extracellular matrix of the marrow microenvironment. *Br J Haematol* 1988;70:1–4.

307. Bentley SA, Alabaster O, Foidart JM. Collagen heterogeneity in normal human bone marrow. *Br J Haematol* 1981;48:287–291.

308. Apaja-Sarkkinen M, Autio-Harmainen H, Alavaikko M, et al. Immunohistochemical study of basement membrane proteins and type III procollagen in myelofibrosis. *Br J Haematol* 1986;63:571–580.

309. Irving EA, Tomlin SG. Collagen, reticulum and their argyrophilic properties. *Proc R Soc Lond B Biol Sci* 1953;142:113–126.

310. Puchtler H, Waldrop FW. Silver impregnation methods for reticulum fibers and reticulin: a re-investigation of their origins and specificity. *Histochemistry* 1978;57:177–187.

311. Charron D, Robert L, Couty MC, et al. Biochemical and histological analysis of bone marrow collagen in myelofibrosis. *Br J Haematol* 1979;41:151–161.

312. Reilly JT, Nash JR, Mackie MJ, et al. Endothelial cell proliferation in myelofibrosis. *Br J Haematol* 1985;60:625–630.

313. Reilly JT, Nash JR, Mackie MJ, et al. Immuno-enzymatic detection of fibronectin in normal and pathological haematopoietic tissue. *Br J Haematol* 1985;59:497–504.

314. Schick PK, Wojenski CM, Bennett VD, et al. The synthesis and localization of alternatively spliced fibronectin EIIIB in resting and thrombin-treated megakaryocytes. *Blood* 1996;87:1817–1823.

315. Mesa RA, Hanson CA, Rajkumar SV, et al. Evaluation and clinical correlations of bone marrow angiogenesis in myelofibrosis with myeloid metaplasia. *Blood* 2000;96:3374–3380.

316. Dupriez B, Morel P, Demory JL, et al. Prognostic factors in agnogenic myeloid metaplasia: a report on 195 cases with a new scoring system. *Blood* 1996;88:1013–1018.

317. Van Dyke D, Parker H, Anger HO, et al. Markedly increased bone blood flow in myelofibrosis. *J Nucl Med* 1971;12:506–512.

318. Schreiber S, Ackermann J, Obermair A, et al. Multiple myeloma with deletion of chromosome 13q is characterized by increased bone marrow neovascularization. *Br J Haematol* 2000;110:605–609.

319. Bentley SA, Herman CJ. Bone marrow fibre production in myelofibrosis: a quantitative study. *Br J Haematol* 1979;42:51–59.

320. Fava RA, Casey TT, Wilcox J, et al. Synthesis of transforming growth factor-beta 1 by megakaryocytes and its localization to megakaryocyte and platelet alpha-granules. *Blood* 1990;76:1946–1955.

321. Wickenhauser C, Hillienhof A, Jungheim K, et al. Detection and quantification of transforming growth factor beta (TGF-beta) and platelet-derived growth factor (PDGF) release by normal human megakaryocytes. *Leukemia* 1995;9:310–315.

322. den Ottolander GJ, te VJ, Brederoo P, et al. Megakaryoblastic leukaemia (acute myelofibrosis): a report of three cases. *Br J Haematol* 1979;42:9–20.

323. Terui T, Niitsu Y, Mahara K, et al. The production of transforming growth factor-beta in acute megakaryoblastic leukemia and its possible implications in myelofibrosis. *Blood* 1990;75:1540–1548.

324. Marcus RE, Hibbin JA, Matutes E, et al. Megakaryoblastic transformation of myelofibrosis with expression of the c-sis oncogene. *Scand J Haematol* 1986;36:186–193.

325. Reilly JT, Barnett D, Dolan G, et al. Characterization of an acute micromegakaryocytic leukaemia: evidence for the pathogenesis of myelofibrosis. *Br J Haematol* 1993;83:58–62.

326. Breton-Gorius J, Bizet M, Reyes F, et al. Myelofibrosis and acute megakaryoblastic leukemia in a child: topographic relationship between fibroblasts and megakaryocytes with an alpha-granule defect. *Leuk Res* 1982;6:97–110.

327. Jantunen E, Hanninen A, Naukkarinen A, et al. Gray platelet syndrome with splenomegaly and signs of extramedullary hematopoiesis: a case report with review of the literature. *Am J Hematol* 1994;46:218–224.

328. Caen JP, Deschamps JF, Bodevin E, et al. Megakaryocytes and myelofibrosis in gray platelet syndrome. *Nouv Rev Fr Hematol* 1987;29:109–114.

329. Martyre MC, Le Bousse-Kerdiles MC, Romquin N, et al. Elevated levels of basic fibroblast growth factor in megakaryocytes and platelets from patients with idiopathic myelofibrosis. *Br J Haematol* 1997;97:441–448.

330. Mohle R, Green D, Moore MA, et al. Constitutive production and thrombin-induced release of vascular endothelial growth factor by human megakaryocytes and platelets. *Proc Natl Acad Sci U S A* 1997;94:663–668.

331. Eastham JM, Reilly JT, Mac NS. Raised urinary calmodulin levels in idiopathic myelofibrosis: possible implications for the aetiology of fibrosis. *Br J Haematol* 1994;86:668–670.

332. Long MW, Dixit VM. Thrombospondin functions as a cytoadhesion molecule for human hematopoietic progenitor cells. *Blood* 1990;75:2311–2318.

333. Hiti-Harper J, Wohl H, Harper E. Platelet factor 4: an inhibitor of collagenase. *Science* 1978;199:991–992.

334. Madoiwa S, Komatsu N, Mimuro J, et al. Developmental expression of plasminogen activator inhibitor-1 associated with thrombopoietin-dependent megakaryocytic differentiation. *Blood* 1991;94:475–482.

335. Murate T, Yamashita K, Isogai C, et al. The production of tissue inhibitors of metalloproteinases (TIMPs) in megakaryopoiesis: possible role of platelet- and megakaryocyte-derived TIMPs in bone marrow fibrosis. *Br J Haematol* 1997;99:181–189.

336. Martyre MC, Magdelenat H, Bryckaert MC, et al. Increased intraplatelet levels of platelet-derived growth factor and transforming growth factor-beta in patients with myelofibrosis with myeloid metaplasia. *Br J Haematol* 1991;77:80–86.

337. Zauli G, Visani G, Catani L, et al. Reduced responsiveness of bone marrow megakaryocyte progenitors to platelet-derived transforming growth factor beta 1, produced in normal amount, in patients with essential thrombocythaemia. *Br J Haematol* 1993;83:14–20.

338. Katoh O, Kimura A, Itoh T, et al. Platelet derived growth factor messenger RNA is increased in bone marrow megakaryocytes in patients with myeloproliferative disorders. *Am J Hematol* 1990;35:145–150.

339. Bernabel P, Arcangeli A, Casini M, et al. Platelet-derived growth factor(s) mitogenic activity in patients with myeloproliferative disease. *Br J Haematol* 1986;63:353–357.

340. Dalley A, Smith JM, Reilly JT, et al. Investigation of calmodulin and basic fibroblast growth factor (bFGF) in idiopathic myelofibrosis: evidence for a role of extracellular calmodulin in fibroblast proliferation. *Br J Haematol* 1996;93:856–862.

341. Burstein SA, Malpass TW, Yee E, et al. Platelet factor-4 excretion in myeloproliferative disease: implications for the aetiology of myelofibrosis. *Br J Haematol* 1984;57:383–392.

342. Yan XQ, Lacey D, Fletcher F, et al. Chronic exposure to retroviral vector encoded MGDF (mpl-ligand) induces lineage-specific growth and differentiation of megakaryocytes in mice. *Blood* 1995;86:4025–4033.

343. Yanagida M, Ide Y, Imai A, et al. The role of transforming growth factor-beta in PEG-rHuMGDF-induced reversible myelofibrosis in rats. *Br J Haematol* 1997;99:739–745.

344. Yan XQ, Lacey D, Hill D, et al. A model of myelofibrosis and osteosclerosis in mice induced by overexpressing thrombopoietin (mpl ligand): reversal of disease by bone marrow transplantation. *Blood* 1996;88:402–409.

345. Schmitt A, Jouault H, Guichard J, et al. Pathologic interaction between megakaryocytes and polymorphonuclear leukocytes in myelofibrosis. *Blood* 2000;96:1342–1347.

346. Cashell AW, Buss DH. The frequency and significance of megakaryocytic emperipolesis in myeloproliferative and reactive states. *Ann Hematol* 1992;64: 273–276.

347. Griesshammer M, Hornkohl A, Nichol JL, et al. High levels of thrombopoietin in sera of patients with essential thrombocythemia: cause or consequence of abnormal platelet production? *Ann Hematol* 1998;77:211–215.

348. Castro-Malaspina H, Moore MA. Pathophysiological mechanisms operating in the development of myelofibrosis: role of megakaryocytes. *Nouv Rev Fr Hematol* 1982;24:221–226.

349. Border WA, Noble NA. Transforming growth factor beta in tissue fibrosis. *N Engl J Med* 1994;331:1286–1292.

350. Thompson NL, Flanders KC, Smith JM, et al. Expression of transforming growth factor-beta 1 in specific cells and tissues of adult and neonatal mice. *J Cell Biol* 1989;108:661–669.

351. Crawford SE, Stellmach V, Murphy-Ullrich JE, et al. Thrombospondin-1 is a major activator of TGF-beta1 in vivo. *Cell* 1998;93:1159–1170.

352. Rameshwar P, Narayanan R, Qian J, et al. NF-kappa B as a central mediator in the induction of TGF-beta in monocytes from patients with idiopathic myelofibrosis: an inflammatory response beyond the realm of homeostasis. *J Immunol* 2000;165:2271–2277.

353. Kimura A, Katoh O, Hyodo H, et al. Transforming growth factor-beta regulates growth as well as collagen and fibronectin synthesis of human marrow fibroblasts. *Br J Haematol* 1989;72:486–491.

354. Krystal G, Lam V, Dragowska W, et al. Transforming growth factor beta 1 is an inducer of erythroid differentiation. *J Exp Med* 1994;180:851–860.

355. Chuncharunee S, Carter CD, Studtmann KE, et al. Chronic administration of transforming growth factor-beta suppresses erythropoietin-dependent erythropoiesis and induces tumour necrosis factor in vivo. *Br J Haematol* 1993;84:374–380.

356. Battegay EJ, Raines EW, Seifert RA, et al. TGF-beta induces bimodal proliferation of connective tissue cells via complex control of an autocrine PDGF loop. *Cell* 1990;63:515–524.

357. Czaja MJ, Weiner FR, Flanders KC, et al. In vitro and in vivo association of transforming growth factor-beta 1 with hepatic fibrosis. *J Cell Biol* 1989;108: 2477–2482.

358. EL-Din E, Moussad A, Brigstock D. Connective tissue growth factor: what's in a name? *Mol Genet Metab* 2000;71:276–292.

359. Deuel TF, Huang JS. Platelet-derived growth factor. Structure, function, and roles in normal and transformed cells. *J Clin Invest* 1984;74:669–676.

360. Battegay EJ, Rupp J, Iruela-Arispe L, et al. PDGF-BB modulates endothelial proliferation and angiogenesis in vitro via PDGF beta-receptors. *J Cell Biol* 1994;125:917–928.

361. Raines EW, Bowen-Pope DF, Ross R. Plasma binding proteins for platelet-derived growth factor that inhibit its binding to cell-surface receptors. *Proc Natl Acad Sci U S A* 1984;81:3424–3428.

362. Yan XQ, Brady G, Iscove NN. Overexpression of PDGF-B in murine hematopoietic cells induces a lethal myeloproliferative syndrome in vivo. *Oncogene* 1994;9:163–173.

363. Gersuk GM, Carmel R, Pattengale PK. Platelet-derived growth factor concentrations in platelet-poor plasma and urine from patients with myeloproliferative disorders. *Blood* 1989;74:2330–2334.

364. Rameshwar P, Denny TN, Stein D, et al. Monocyte adhesion in patients with bone marrow fibrosis is required for the production of fibrogenic cytokines. Potential role for interleukin-1 and TGF-beta. *J Immunol* 1994;153:2819–2830.

365. Rameshwar P, Chang VT, Gascon P. Implication of CD44 in adhesion-mediated overproduction of TGF-beta and IL-1 in monocytes from patients with bone marrow fibrosis. *Br J Haematol* 1996;93:22–29.

366. Wehmeier A, Sudhoff T. Elevated plasma levels of basic fibroblast growth factor in patients with essential thrombocythaemia and polycythaemia vera [letter; comment]. *Br J Haematol* 1997;98:1050–1051.

367. Johnston JB, Dalal BI, Israels SJ, et al. Deposition of transforming growth factor-beta in the marrow in myelofibrosis, and the intracellular localization and secretion of TGF-beta by leukemic cells. *Am J Clin Pathol* 1995;103:574–582.

368. Abina MA, Tulliez M, Lacout C, et al. Major effects of TPO delivered by a single injection of a recombinant adenovirus on prevention of septicemia and anemia associated with myelosuppression in mice: risk of sustained expression inducing myelofibrosis due to immunosuppression. *Gene Ther* 1998;5:497–506.

369. Frey BM, Rafii S, Teterson M, et al. Adenovector-mediated expression of human thrombopoietin cDNA in immune-compromised mice: insights into the pathophysiology of osteomyelofibrosis. *J Immunol* 1998;160:691–699.

370. Hasselbalch H. Idiopathic myelofibrosis. *Dan Med Bull* 1993;40:39–55.

371. Varki A, Lottenberg R, Griffith R, et al. The syndrome of idiopathic myelofibrosis. A clinicopathologic review with emphasis on the prognostic variables predicting survival. *Medicine* 1983;62:353–371.

372. Pitcock JA, Reinhard EH, Justus BW, et al. A clinical and pathological study of seventy cases of myelofibrosis. *Ann Intern Med* 1962;57:73–84.

373. Cervantes F, Pereira A, Esteve J, et al. Identification of "short-lived" and "long-lived" patients at presentation of idiopathic myelofibrosis. *Br J Haematol* 1997;97:635–640.

374. Rupoli S, Da Lio L, Sisti S, et al. Primary myelofibrosis: a detailed statistical analysis of the clinicopathological variables influencing survival. *Ann Hematol* 1994;68:205–212.

375. Visani G, Finelli C, Castelli U, et al. Myelofibrosis with myeloid metaplasia: clinical and haematological parameters predicting survival in a series of 133 patients. *Br J Haematol* 1990;75:4–9.

376. Ligumski M, Polliack A, Benbassat J. Nature and incidence of liver involvement in agnogenic myeloid metaplasia. *Scand J Haematol* 1978;21:81–93.

377. Silverstein MN, Wollaeger EE, Baggenstoss AH. Gastrointestinal and abdominal manifestations of agnogenic myeloid metaplasia. *Arch Intern Med* 1973;131:532–537.

378. Pereira A, Bruguera M, Cervantes F, et al. Liver involvement at diagnosis of primary myelofibrosis: a clinicopathological study of twenty-two cases. *Eur J Haematol* 1988;40:355–361.

379. Glew RH, Haese WH, McIntyre PA. Myeloid metaplasia with myelofibrosis. The clinical spectrum of extramedullary hematopoiesis and tumor formation. *Johns Hopkins Med J* 1973;132:253–270.

380. Beckman EN, Oehrle JS. Fibrous hematopoietic tumors arising in agnogenic myeloid metaplasia. *Hum Pathol* 1982;13:804–810.

381. Bouroncle B, Doan CA. Myelofibrosis clinical, hematologic and pathologic study of 110 patients. *Am J Med Sci* 1962;243:697–715.

382. Najean Y, Cacchione R, Castro-Malaspina H, et al. Erythrokinetic studies in myelofibrosis: their significance for prognosis. *Br J Haematol* 1978;40:205–217.

383. Bowdler AJ. Blood volume studies in patients with splenomegaly. *Transfusion* 1970;10:171–181.

384. Szur L, Smith M. Red-cell production and destruction in myelosclerosis. *Br J Haematol* 1961;7:147–168.

385. Milner GR, Geary CG, Wadsworth LD, et al. Erythrokinetic studies as a guide to the value of splenectomy in primary myeloid metaplasia. *Br J Haematol* 1973;25:467–484.

386. Korst D, Clatanoff DV, Schilling RF. On myelofibrosis. *Arch Intern Med* 1955; 169–183.

387. Khumbandoda M, Horowitz HI, Eyster ME. Coombs' positive hemolytic anemia in myelofibrosis with myeloid metaplasia. *Am J Med Sci* 1969;258:89–93.

388. Hoffbrand AV, Chanarin I, Kremenchuzky S, et al. Megaloblastic anaemia in myelosclerosis. *Q J Med* 1968;37:493–514.

389. Rondeau E, Solal-Celigny P, Dhermy D, et al. Immune disorders in agnogenic myeloid metaplasia: relations to myelofibrosis. *Br J Haematol* 1983;53: 467–475.

390. Gordon BR, Coleman M, Kohen P, et al. Immunologic abnormalities in myelofibrosis with activation of the complement system. *Blood* 1981;58:904–910.

391. Rojer RA, Mulder NH, Nieweg HO. Response to pyridoxine hydrochloride in refractory anemia due to myelofibrosis. *Am J Med* 1978;65:655–660.

392. Ferrant A, Rodhain J, Cauwe F, et al. Assessment of bone marrow and splenic erythropoiesis in myelofibrosis. *Scand J Haematol* 1982;29:373–380.

393. Pamphilon DH, Creamer P, Keeling DH, et al. Restoration of active haemopoiesis in a patient with myelofibrosis and subsequent termination in acute myeloblastic leukaemia: case report and review of the literature. *Eur J Haematol* 1987;38:279–283.

394. Lewis SM, Pettit JE, Tattersall MH, et al. Myelosclerosis and paroxysmal nocturnal haemoglobinuria. *Scand J Haematol* 1971;8:451–460.

395. Kuo C, van Voolen GA, Morrison AN. Primary and secondary myelofibrosis: its relationship to "PNH-like defect." *Blood* 1972;40:875–880.

396. DiBella NJ, Silverstein MN, Hoagland HC. Effect of splenectomy on teardrop-shaped erythrocytes in agnogenic myeloid metaplasia. *Arch Intern Med* 1977;137:380–381.

397. Farolino DL, Rustagi PK, Currie MS, et al. Teardrop-shaped red cells in autoimmune hemolytic anemia. *Am J Hematol* 1986;21:415–418.

398. Weick JK, Hagedorn AB, Linman JW. Leukoerythroblastosis. Diagnostic and prognostic significance. *Mayo Clin Proc* 1974;49:110–113.

399. Cervantes F, Hernandez-Boluda JC, Villamor N, et al. Assessment of peripheral blood lymphocyte subsets in idiopathic myelofibrosis. *Eur J Haematol* 2000;65:104–108.

400. Gersuk GM, Carmel R, Pattamakom S, et al. Quantitative and functional studies of impaired natural killer (NK) cells in patients with myelofibrosis, essential thrombocythemia, and polycythemia vera. I. A potential role for platelet-derived growth factor in defective NK cytotoxicity. *Nat Immun* 1993;12:136–151.

401. Froom P, Aghai E, Kinarty A, et al. Decreased natural killer (NK) activity in patients with myeloproliferative disorders. *Cancer* 1989;64:1038–1040.
402. Mitus W, Bergna L, Mednicoff I, et al. Alkaline phosphatase of mature neutrophils in chronic forms of the myeloproliferative syndrome. *Am J Clin Pathol* 1958;30:285–294.
403. Rosenthal DS, Moloney WC. Myeloid metaplasia: a study of 98 cases. *Postgrad Med* 1969;45:136–142.
404. Borgstrom GH, Knuutila S, Ruutu T, et al. Abnormalities of chromosome 13 in myelofibrosis. *Scand J Haematol* 1984;33:15–21.
405. Pereira A, Cervantes F, Brugues R, et al. Bone marrow histopathology in primary myelofibrosis: clinical and haematologic correlations and prognostic evaluation. *Eur J Haematol* 1990;44:95–99.
406. Hasselbalch H, Lisse I. A sequential histological study of bone marrow fibrosis in idiopathic myelofibrosis. *Eur J Haematol* 1991;46:285–289.
407. Lohmann TP, Beckman EN. Progressive myelofibrosis in agnogenic myeloid metaplasia. *Arch Pathol Lab Med* 1983;107:593–594.
408. Pettigrew JD, Ward HP. Correlation of radiologic, histologic, and clinical findings in agnogenic myeloid metaplasia. *Radiology* 1969;93:541–548.
409. Murphy S, Davis JL, Walsh PN, et al. Template bleeding time and clinical hemorrhage in myeloproliferative disease. *Arch Intern Med* 1978;138:1251–1253.
410. Raman BK, Van Slyck EJ, Riddle J, et al. Platelet function and structure in myeloproliferative disease, myelodysplastic syndrome, and secondary thrombocytosis. *Am J Clin Pathol* 1989;91:647–655.
411. Cooper B, Schafer AI, Puchalsky D, et al. Platelet resistance to prostaglandin D2 in patients with myeloproliferative disorders. *Blood* 1978;52:618–626.
412. Balduini CL, Bertolino G, Noris P, et al. Platelet aggregation in platelet-rich plasma and whole blood in 120 patients with myeloproliferative disorders. *Am J Clin Pathol* 1991;95:82–86.
413. Okuma M, Uchino H. Altered arachidonate metabolism by platelets in patients with myeloproliferative disorders. *Blood* 1979;54:1258–1271.
414. Boughton BJ, Corbett WE, Ginsburg AD. Myeloproliferative disorders: a paradox of in-vivo and in-vitro platelet function. *J Clin Pathol* 1977;30:228–234.
415. Wehmeier A, Daum I, Jamin H, et al. Incidence and clinical risk factors for bleeding and thrombotic complications in myeloproliferative disorders. A retrospective analysis of 260 patients. *Ann Hematol* 1991;63:101–106.
416. Demory JL, Dupriez B, Fenaux P, et al. Cytogenetic studies and their prognostic significance in agnogenic myeloid metaplasia: a report on 47 cases. *Blood* 1988;72:855–859.
417. Reilly JT, Snowden JA, Spearing RL, et al. Cytogenetic abnormalities and their prognostic significance in idiopathic myelofibrosis: a study of 106 cases. *Br J Haematol* 1997;98:96–102.
418. Cervantes F, Barosi G, Demory JL, et al. Myelofibrosis with myeloid metaplasia in young individuals: disease characteristics, prognostic factors and identification of risk groups. *Br J Haematol* 1998;102:684–690.
419. Mertens F, Johansson B, Heim S, et al. Karyotypic patterns in chronic myeloproliferative disorders: report on 74 cases and review of the literature. *Leukemia* 1991;5:214–220.
420. Pastore C, Nomdedeu J, Volpe G, et al. Genetic analysis of chromosome 13 deletions in BCR/ABL negative chronic myeloproliferative disorders. *Genes Chromosomes Cancer* 1995;14:106–111.
421. Cappio FC, Vigliani R, Novarino A, et al. Idiopathic myelofibrosis: a possible role for immune-complexes in the pathogenesis of bone marrow fibrosis. *Br J Haematol* 1981;49:17–21.
422. Baglin TP, Simpson AW, Price SM, et al. Composition of immune complexes and their relation to plasma fibronectin in chronic myeloproliferative disorders. *J Clin Pathol* 1987;40:1468–1471.
423. Hasselbalch H, Nielsen H, Berild D, et al. Circulating immune complexes in myelofibrosis. *Scand J Haematol* 1985;34:177–180.
424. Paquette RL, Meshkinpour A, Rosen PJ. Autoimmune myelofibrosis. A steroid-responsive cause of bone marrow fibrosis associated with systemic lupus erythematosus. *Medicine* 1994;73:145–152.
425. Pirayesh A, Verbunt RJ, Kluin PM, et al. Myelodysplastic syndrome with vasculitic manifestations. *J Intern Med* 1997;242:425–431.
426. Longley S, Caldwell JR, Panush RS. Paraneoplastic vasculitis. Unique syndrome of cutaneous angiitis and arthritis associated with myeloproliferative disorders. *Am J Med* 1986;80:1027–1030.
427. Wang JC, Wang A. Plasma soluble interleukin-2 receptor in patients with primary myelofibrosis. *Br J Haematol* 1994;86:380–382.
428. Barosi G, Ambrosetti A, Finelli C, et al. The Italian Consensus Conference on Diagnostic Criteria for Myelofibrosis with Myeloid Metaplasia. *Br J Haematol* 1999;104:730–737.
429. Thiele J, Kvasnicka HM, Boeltken B, et al. Initial (prefibrotic) stages of idiopathic (primary) myelofibrosis (IMF)—a clinicopathological study. *Leukemia* 1999;13:1741–1748.
430. Gralnick HR, Harbor J, Vogel C. Myelofibrosis in chronic granulocytic leukemia. *Blood* 1971;37:152–162.
431. Clough V, Geary CG, Hashmi K, et al. Myelofibrosis in chronic granulocytic leukaemia. *Br J Haematol* 1979;42:515–526.
432. Lazzarino M, Morra E, Castello A, et al. Myelofibrosis in chronic granulocytic leukaemia: clinicopathologic correlations and prognostic significance. *Br J Haematol* 1986;64:227–240.
433. Buyssens N, Bourgeois NH. Chronic myelolytic leukemia versus idiopathic myelofibrosis: a diagnostic problem in bone marrow biopsies. *Cancer* 1977;40:1548–1561.
434. Barosi G, Baraldi A, Cazzola M, et al. Polycythaemia following splenectomy in myelofibrosis with myeloid metaplasia. A reorganization of erythropoiesis. *Scand J Haematol* 1984;32:12–18.
435. Bearman RM, Pangalis GA, Rappaport H. Acute ("malignant") myelosclerosis. *Cancer* 1979;43:279–293.
436. Truong LD, Saleem A, Schwartz MR. Acute myelofibrosis. A report of four cases and review of the literature. *Medicine* 1984;63:182–187.
437. Lubin J, Rozen S, Rywlin M. Malignant myelosclerosis. *Arch Intern Med* 1976;136:141–145.
438. Schreeder MT, Prchal JT, Parmley RT, et al. An acute myeloproliferative disorder characterized by myelofibrosis and blast cells that express phenotypic properties associated with multiple hematopoietic lineages. *Am J Clin Pathol* 1985;83:114–121.
439. Cervantes F, Pereira A, Esteve J, et al. The changing profile of idiopathic myelofibrosis: a comparison of the presenting features of patients diagnosed in two different decades. *Eur J Haematol* 1998;60:101–105.
440. Manoharan A, Horsley R, Pitney WR. The reticulin content of bone marrow in acute leukaemia in adults. *Br J Haematol* 1979;43:185–190.
441. Tabilio A, Herrera A, D'Agay MF, et al. Therapy-related leukemia associated with myelofibrosis. Blast cell characterization in six cases. *Cancer* 1984;54:1382–1391.
442. Sultan C, Sigaux F, Imbert M, et al. Acute myelodysplasia with myelofibrosis: a report of eight cases. *Br J Haematol* 1981;49:11–16.
443. Hasselbalch H. Idiopathic myelofibrosis: a clinical study of 80 patients. *Am J Hematol* 1990;34:291–300.
444. Rios A, Canizo MC, Sanz MA, et al. Bone marrow biopsy in myelodysplastic syndromes: morphological characteristics and contribution to the study of prognostic factors. *Br J Haematol* 1990;75:26–33.
445. Maschek H, Georgii A, Kaloutsi V, et al. Myelofibrosis in primary myelodysplastic syndromes: a retrospective study of 352 patients. *Eur J Haematol* 1992;48:208–214.
446. Ohyashiki K, Sasao I, Ohyashiki JH, et al. Clinical and cytogenetic characteristics of myelodysplastic syndromes developing myelofibrosis. *Cancer* 1991;68:178–183.
447. Pagliuca A, Layton DM, Manoharan A, et al. Myelofibrosis in primary myelodysplastic syndromes: a clinico-morphological study of 10 cases. *Br J Haematol* 1989;71:499–504.
448. Krzyzaniak RL, Buss DH, Cooper MR, et al. Marrow fibrosis and multiple myeloma. *Am J Clin Pathol* 1988;89:63–68.
449. Spector JI, Levine PH. Case report. Carcinomatous bone marrow invasion simulating acute myelofibrosis. *Am J Med Sci* 1973;266:144–148.
450. Webb TA, Li CY, Yam LT. Systemic mast cell disease: a clinical and hematopathologic study of 26 cases. *Cancer* 1982;49:927–938.
451. Travis WD, Li CY, Bergstralh EJ, et al. Systemic mast cell disease. Analysis of 58 cases and literature review. *Medicine* 1988;67:345–368.
452. Travis WD, Li CY, Yam LT, et al. Significance of systemic mast cell disease with associated hematologic disorders. *Cancer* 1988;62:965–972.
453. Le Tourneau A, Gaulard P, D'Agay MF, et al. Primary thrombocythaemia associated with systemic mastocytosis: a report of five cases. *Br J Haematol* 1991;79:84–89.
454. Kluin-Nelemans HC, Jansen JH, Breukelman H, et al. Response to interferon alfa-2b in a patient with systemic mastocytosis. *N Engl J Med* 1992;326:619–623.
455. List AF, Doll DC. Alpha-interferon in the treatment of idiopathic myelofibrosis. *Br J Haematol* 1992;80:566–567.
456. Cervantes F, Tassies D, Salgado C, et al. Acute transformation in nonleukemic chronic myeloproliferative disorders: actuarial probability and main characteristics in a series of 218 patients. *Acta Haematol* 1991;85:124–127.
457. Silverstein MN, Brown AL, Linman J. Idiopathic myeloid metaplasia: its evolution into acute leukemia. *Arch Intern Med* 1973;132:709–712.
458. Tefferi A, Mesa RA, Nagorney DM, et al. Splenectomy in myelofibrosis with myeloid metaplasia: a single-institution experience with 223 patients. *Blood* 2000;95:2226–2233.
459. Porcu P, Neiman RS, Orazi A. Splenectomy in agnogenic myeloid metaplasia. *Blood* 1999;93:2132–2134.
460. Barnes HM, Prchal JT, Scott CW. Extramedullary blast transformation in the central nervous system in idiopathic myelofibrosis. *Am J Hematol* 1981;11:305–308.
461. Ligumski M, Polliack A, Benbassat J. Myeloid metaplasia of the central nervous system in patients with myelofibrosis and agnogenic myeloid metaplasia. Report of 3 cases and review of the literature. *Am J Med Sci* 1978;275:99–103.
462. Price F, Bell H. Spinal cord compression due to extramedullary hematopoiesis. Successful treatment in a patient with long-standing myelofibrosis. *JAMA* 1985;253:2876–2877.
463. Garcia-Manero G, Schuster SJ, Patrick H, et al. Pulmonary hypertension in patients with myelofibrosis secondary to myeloproliferative diseases. *Am J Hematol* 1999;60:130–135.
464. Towell BL, Levine SP. Massive hepatomegaly following splenectomy for myeloid metaplasia. Case report and review of the literature. *Am J Med* 1987;82:371–375.
465. Lopez-Guillermo A, Cervantes F, Bruguera M, et al. Liver dysfunction following splenectomy in idiopathic myelofibrosis: a study of 10 patients. *Acta Haematol* 1991;85:184–188.
466. Linman J, Bethell F. Agnogenic myeloid metaplasia. *Am J Med* 1957;22:107–122.

467. Morel P, Demory JL, Dupriez B. Relevance of prognostic features in myeloid metaplasia to selection of patients for bone marrow transplantation *Blood* 1997;89:2219–2220.

468. Kvasnicka HM, Thiele J, Werden C, et al. Prognostic factors in idiopathic (primary) osteomyelofibrosis. *Cancer* 1997;80:708–719.

469. Hasselbalch H, Junker P, Lisse I, et al. Serum markers for type IV collagen and type III procollagen in the myelofibrosis-osteomyelosclerosis syndrome and other chronic myeloproliferative disorders. *Am J Hematol* 1986;23:101–111.

470. Hochweiss S, Fruchtman S, Hahn EG, et al. Increased serum procollagen III aminoterminal peptide in myelofibrosis. *Am J Hematol* 1983;15:343–351.

471. Hasselbalch H, Junker P, Horslev-Petersen K, et al. Procollagen type III aminoterminal peptide in serum in idiopathic myelofibrosis and allied conditions: relation to disease activity and effect of chemotherapy. *Am J Hematol* 1990;33:18–26.

472. Barosi G, Costa A, Liberato LN, et al. Serum procollagen-III-peptide level correlates with disease activity in myelofibrosis with myeloid metaplasia. *Br J Haematol* 1989;72:16–20.

473. Hasselbalch H, Junker P, Lisse I, et al. Circulating hyaluronan in the myelofibrosis/osteomyelosclerosis syndrome and other myeloproliferative disorders. *Am J Hematol* 1991;36:1–8.

474. Hasselbalch H, Junker P. Serum laminin P1 in idiopathic myelofibrosis and related diseases. *Leuk Res* 1994;18:623–628.

475. Norfolk DR, Bowen M, Roberts BE, et al. Plasma fibronectin in myeloproliferative disorders and chronic granulocytic leukaemia. *Br J Haematol* 1983;55:319–324.

476. Guardiola P, Anderson JE, Bandini G, et al. Allogeneic stem cell transplantation for agnogenic myeloid metaplasia: a European Group for Blood and Marrow Transplantation, Societe Francaise de Greffe de Moelle, Gruppo Italiano per il Trapianto del Midollo Osseo, and Fred Hutchinson Cancer Research Center Collaborative Study. *Blood* 1999;93:2831–2838.

477. Guardiola P, Anderson JE, Gluckman E. Myelofibrosis with myeloid metaplasia. *N Engl J Med* 2000;343:659–660.

478. Bentley SA, Murray KH, Lewis SM, et al. Erythroid hypoplasia in myelofibrosis: a feature associated with blastic transformation. *Br J Haematol* 1977; 36:41–47.

479. Barosi G, Baraldi A, Cazzola M, et al. Red cell aplasia in myelofibrosis with myeloid metaplasia. A distinct functional and clinical entity. *Cancer* 1983; 52:1290–1296.

480. Besa EC, Nowell PC, Geller NL, et al. Analysis of the androgen response of 23 patients with agnogenic myeloid metaplasia: the value of chromosomal studies in predicting response and survival. *Cancer* 1982;49:308–313.

481. Brubaker LH, Briere J, Laszlo J, et al. Treatment of anemia in myeloproliferative disorders: a randomized study of fluoxymesterone v transfusions only. *Arch Intern Med* 1982;142:1533–1537.

482. Levy V, Bourgarit A, Delmer A, et al. Treatment of agnogenic myeloid metaplasia with danazol: a report of four cases. *Am J Hematol* 1996;53:239–241.

483. Cervantes F, Hernandez-Boluda JC, Alvarez A, et al. Danazol treatment of idiopathic myelofibrosis with severe anemia. *Haematologica* 2000;85:595–599.

484. Spivak JL. The blood in systemic disorders. *Lancet* 2000;355:1707–1712.

485. Tefferi A, Silverstein MN. Recombinant human erythropoietin therapy in patients with myelofibrosis with myeloid metaplasia. *Br J Haematol* 1994;86:893.

486. Mohr B, Herrmann R, Huhn D. Recombinant human erythropoietin in patients with myelodysplastic syndrome and myelofibrosis. *Acta Haematol* 1993;90:65–70.

487. Jack FR, Smith SR, Saunders PW. Idiopathic myelofibrosis: anaemia may respond to low-dose dexamethasone. *Br J Haematol* 1994;87:877–878.

488. Watts EJ, Majer RV, Green PJ, et al. Hyperfibrotic myelodysplasia: a report of three cases showing haematological remission following treatment with prednisolone. *Br J Haematol* 1991;78:120–122.

489. Manoharan A, Chen CF, Wilson LS, et al. Ultrasonic characterization of splenic tissue in myelofibrosis: further evidence for reversal of fibrosis with chemotherapy. *Eur J Haematol* 1988;40:149–154.

490. Chang JC, Gross HM. Remission of chronic idiopathic myelofibrosis to busulfan treatment. *Am J Med Sci* 1988;295:472–476.

491. Wang JC, Lang HD, Liao P, et al. Recombinant alpha-interferon inhibits colony formation of bone marrow fibroblast progenitor cells (CFU-F). *Am J Hematol* 1992;40:81–85.

492. Parmeggiani L, Ferrant A, Rodhain J, et al. Alpha interferon in the treatment of symptomatic myelofibrosis with myeloid metaplasia. *Eur J Haematol* 1987; 39:228–232.

493. Dalla KP, Zeigler ZR, Shadduck RK. alpha-Interferon in myelofibrosis: a case report. *Br J Haematol* 1994;86:654–656.

494. McCarthy D, Clark J, Giles F. The treatment of myelofibrosis with alfa-interferon. *Br J Haematol* 1991;78:590–591.

495. Gilbert HS. Long term treatment of myeloproliferative disease with interferon-alpha-2b: feasibility and efficacy. *Cancer* 1998;83:1205–1213.

496. Barosi G. Myelofibrosis with myeloid metaplasia: diagnostic definition and prognostic classification for clinical studies and treatment guidelines. *J Clin Oncol* 1999;17:2954–2970.

497. Greenberger JS, Chaffey JT, Rosenthal DS, et al. Irradiation for control of hypersplenism and painful splenomegaly in myeloid metaplasia. *Int J Radiat Oncol Biol Phys* 1977;2:1083–1090.

498. Wagner H Jr, McKeough PG, Desforges J, et al. Splenic irradiation in the treatment of patients with chronic myelogenous leukemia or myelofibrosis with myeloid metaplasia. Results of daily and intermittent fractionation with and without concomitant hydroxyurea. *Cancer* 1986;58:1204–1207.

499. Mason BA, Kressel BR, Cashdollar MR, et al. Periostitis associated with myelofibrosis. *Cancer* 1979;43:1568–1571.

500. Tefferi A, Jimenez T, Gray LA, et al. Radiation therapy for symptomatic hepatomegaly in myelofibrosis with myeloid metaplasia. *Eur J Haematol* 2001;66:37–42.

501. Talks KL, Harris AL. Current status of antiangiogenic factors. *Br J Haematol* 2000;109:477–489.

502. Fialkow PJ, Faguet GB, Jacobson RJ, et al. Evidence that essential thrombocythemia is a clonal disorder with origin in a multipotent stem cell. *Blood* 1981;58:916–919.

503. Gaetani GF, Ferraris AM, Galiano S, et al. Primary thrombocythemia: clonal origin of platelets, erythrocytes, and granulocytes in a GdB/Gd Mediterranean subject. *Blood* 1982;59:76–79.

504. Michiels JJ, Juvonen E. Proposal for revised diagnostic criteria of essential thrombocythemia and polycythemia vera by the Thrombocythemia Vera Study Group. *Semin Thromb Hemost* 1997;23:339–347.

505. Di Guglielmo G. Entroleucemia e Piastrinemia. *Folia Med* 1920;1:36.

506. Reid J. Hemorrhagic thrombocythemia. *Lancet* 1940;2:584–587.

507. McCabe W, Bird R, McLaughlin R. Is primary hemorrhagic thrombocythemia a clinical myth? *Ann Intern Med* 1955;43:182–190.

508. Gunz F. Hemorrhagic thrombocythemia: a critical review. *Blood* 1960;15:706–722.

509. Ozer F, Truax W, Miesch D, et al. Primary hemorrhagic thrombocythemia. *Am J Med* 1960;28:807–823.

510. Levin J, Conley CL. Thrombocytosis associated with malignant disease. *Arch Intern Med* 1964;114:497–500.

511. Santhosh-Kumar CR, Yohannan MD, Higgy KE, et al. Thrombocytosis in adults: analysis of 777 patients. *J Intern Med* 1991;229:493–495.

512. Griesshammer M, Bangerter M, Sauer T, et al. Aetiology and clinical significance of thrombocytosis: analysis of 732 patients with an elevated platelet count. *J Intern Med* 1999;245:295–300.

513. Davis WM, Ross AO. Thrombocytosis and thrombocythemia: the laboratory and clinical significance of an elevated platelet count. *Am J Clin Pathol* 1973; 59:243–247.

514. Buss DH, Cashell AW, O'Connor ML, et al. Occurrence, etiology, and clinical significance of extreme thrombocytosis: a study of 280 cases. *Am J Med* 1994; 96:247–253.

515. Buss DH, Stuart JJ, Lipscomb GE. The incidence of thrombotic and hemorrhagic disorders in association with extreme thrombocytosis: an analysis of 129 cases. *Am J Hematol* 1985;20:365–372.

516. Jensen MK, de Nully BP, Nielsen OJ, et al. Incidence, clinical features and outcome of essential thrombocythaemia in a well defined geographical area. *Eur J Haematol* 2000;65:132–139.

517. Lengfelder E, Hochhaus A, Kronawitter U, et al. Should a platelet limit of $600 \times 10(9)/l$ be used as a diagnostic criterion in essential thrombocythaemia? An analysis of the natural course including early stages. *Br J Haematol* 1998;100:15–23.

518. Besses C, Cervantes F, Pereira A, et al. Major vascular complications in essential thrombocythemia: a study of the predictive factors in a series of 148 patients. *Leukemia* 1999;13:150–154.

519. Bellucci S, Janvier M, Tobelem G, et al. Essential thrombocythemias. Clinical evolutionary and biological data. *Cancer* 1986;58:2440–2447.

520. Ruggeri M, Finazzi G, Tosetto A, et al. No treatment for low-risk thrombocythaemia: results from a prospective study. *Br J Haematol* 1998;103:772–777.

521. Fenaux P, Simon M, Caulier MT, et al. Clinical course of essential thrombocythemia in 147 cases. *Cancer* 1990;66:549–556.

522. Colombi M, Radaelli F, Zocchi L, et al. Thrombotic and hemorrhagic complications in essential thrombocythemia. A retrospective study of 103 patients. *Cancer* 1991;67:2926–2930.

523. Jantunen R, Juvonen E, Ikkala E, et al. Essential thrombocythemia at diagnosis: causes of diagnostic evaluation and presence of positive diagnostic findings. *Ann Hematol* 1998;77:101–106.

524. Bazzan M, Tamponi G, Schinco P, et al. Thrombosis-free survival and life expectancy in 187 consecutive patients with essential thrombocythemia. *Ann Hematol* 1999;78:539–543.

525. Slee PH, van Everdingen JJ, Geraedts JP, et al. Familial myeloproliferative disease. Hematological and cytogenetic studies. *Acta Med Scand* 1981;210:321–327.

526. Fickers M, Speck B. Thrombocythaemia. Familial occurrence and transition into blastic crisis. *Acta Haematol* 1974;51:257–265.

527. Williams EC, Shahidi NT. Benign familial thrombocytosis. *Am J Hematol* 1991; 37:124–125.

528. Schlemper RJ, van der Maas AP, Eikenboom JC. Familial essential thrombocythemia: clinical characteristics of 11 cases in one family. *Ann Hematol* 1994;68: 153–158.

529. Eyster ME, Saletan SL, Rabellino EM, et al. Familial essential thrombocythemia. *Am J Med* 1986;80:497–502.

530. Cohen N, Almoznino-Sarafian D, Weissgarten J, et al. Benign familial microcytic thrombocytosis with autosomal dominant transmission. *Clin Genet* 1997;52:47–50.

531. Randi ML, Fabris F, Vio C, et al. Familial thrombocythemia and/or thrombocytosis—apparently a rare disorder. *Acta Haematol* 1987;78:63.

532. Kondo T, Okabe M, Sanada M, et al. Familial essential thrombocythemia associated with one-base deletion in the 5'-untranslated region of the thrombopoietin gene. *Blood* 1998;92:1091–1096.

533. Wiestner A, Schlemper RJ, van der Maas AP, et al. An activating splice donor mutation in the thrombopoietin gene causes hereditary thrombocythaemia. *Nat Genet* 1998;18:49–52.

534. Lok S, Kaushansky K, Holly RD, et al. Cloning and expression of murine thrombopoietin cDNA and stimulation of platelet production in vivo. *Nature* 1994;369:565–568.

535. Vigon I, Mornon JP, Cocault L, et al. Molecular cloning and characterization of MPL, the human homolog of the v-mpl oncogene: identification of a member of the hematopoietic growth factor receptor superfamily. *Proc Natl Acad Sci U S A* 1992;89:5640–5644.

536. Wu H, Liu X, Jaenisch R, et al. Generation of committed erythroid BFU-E and CFU-E progenitors does not require erythropoietin or the erythropoietin receptor. *Cell* 1995;83:59–67.

537. Gurney AL, Carver-Moore K, de Sauvage FJ, et al. Thrombocytopenia in c-mpl-deficient mice. *Science* 1994;265:1445–1447.

538. Bunting S, Widmer R, Lipari T, et al. Normal platelets and megakaryocytes are produced in vivo in the absence of thrombopoietin. *Blood* 1997;90:3423–3429.

539. Kieran MW, Perkins AC, Orkin SH, et al. Thrombopoietin rescues in vitro erythroid colony formation from mouse embryos lacking the erythropoietin receptor. *Proc Natl Acad Sci U S A* 1996;93:9126–9131.

540. Kaushansky K. Thrombopoietin: the primary regulator of platelet production. *Blood* 1995;86:419–431.

541. Shivdasani RA, Rosenblatt MF, Zucker-Franklin D, et al. Transcription factor NF-E2 is required for platelet formation independent of the actions of thrombopoietin/MGDF in megakaryocyte development. *Cell* 1995;81:695–704.

542. Carver-Moore K, Broxmeyer HE, Luoh SM, et al. Low levels of erythroid and myeloid progenitors in thrombopoietin- and c-mpl-deficient mice. *Blood* 1996;88:803–808.

543. Zauli G, Vitale M, Falcieri E, et al. In vitro senescence and apoptotic cell death of human megakaryocytes. *Blood* 1997;90:2234–2243.

544. Borge OJ, Ramsfjell V, Cui L, et al. Ability of early acting cytokines to directly promote survival and suppress apoptosis of human primitive CD34+. *Blood* 1997;90:2282–2292.

545. Spivak JL, Hogans BB, Stuart RK. Tumor-promoting phorbol esters support the in vitro proliferation of murine pluripotent hematopoietic stem cells. *J Clin Invest* 1989;83:100–107.

546. Miles SA, Mitsuyasu RT, Moreno J, et al. Combined therapy with recombinant granulocyte colony-stimulating factor and erythropoietin decreases hematologic toxicity from zidovudine. *Blood* 1991;77:2109–2117.

547. Debili N, Coulombel L, Croisille L, et al. Characterization of a bipotent erythro-megakaryocytic progenitor in human bone marrow. *Blood* 1996;88: 1284–1296.

548. Eridani S, Batten E, Sawyer B. Erythropoietic activity in primary proliferative polycythaemia. *Br J Haematol* 1983;55:557–558.

549. Debili N, Wendling F, Katz A, et al. The Mpl-ligand or thrombopoietin or megakaryocyte growth and differentiative factor has both direct proliferative and differentiative activities on human megakaryocyte progenitors. *Blood* 1995;86:2516–2525.

550. de Sauvage FJ, Carver-Moore K, Luoh SM, et al. Physiological regulation of early and late stages of megakaryocytopoiesis by thrombopoietin. *J Exp Med* 1996;183:651–656.

551. Kaushansky K. Thrombopoietin. *N Engl J Med* 1998;339:746–754.

552. Linden HM, Kaushansky K. The glycan domain of thrombopoietin enhances its secretion. *Biochemistry* 2000;39:3044–3051.

553. Stoffel R, Wiestner A, Skoda RC. Thrombopoietin in thrombocytopenic mice: evidence against regulation at the mRNA level and for a direct regulatory role of platelets. *Blood* 1996;87:567–573.

554. Emmons RV, Reid DM, Cohen RL, et al. Human thrombopoietin levels are high when thrombocytopenia is due to megakaryocyte deficiency and low when due to increased platelet destruction. *Blood* 1996;87:4068–4071.

555. Goulis J, Chau TN, Jordan S, et al. Thrombopoietin concentrations are low in patients with cirrhosis and thrombocytopenia and are restored after orthotopic liver transplantation. *Gut* 1999;44:754–758.

556. Ghilardi N, Wiestner A, Skoda RC. Thrombopoietin production is inhibited by a translational mechanism. *Blood* 1998;92:4023–4030.

557. Ghilardi N, Skoda RC. A single-base deletion in the thrombopoietin (TPO) gene causes familial essential thrombocythemia through a mechanism of more efficient translation of TPO mRNA. *Blood* 1999;94:1480–1482.

558. Wu X, Nakayama M, Adamson JW. Identification of five new isoforms of murine thrombopoietin mRNA. *Biochem Biophys Res Commun* 2000;276:137–143.

559. Hirayama Y, Sakamaki S, Matsunaga T, et al. Concentration of thrombopoietin in bone marrow in normal subjects and in patients with idiopathic thrombocytopenic purpura, aplastic anemia, and essential thrombocythaemia correlate with its mRNA expression of bone marrow stromal cells. *Blood* 1998;92:46–52.

560. Griesshammer M, Kubanek B, Beneke H, et al. Serum erythropoietin and thrombopoietin levels in patients with essential thrombocythaemia. *Leuk Lymphoma* 2000;36:533–538.

561. Tomita N, Motomura S, Sakai R, et al. Strong inverse correlation between serum TPO level and platelet count in essential thrombocythaemia. *Am J Hematol* 2000;63:131–135.

562. Tahara T, Usuki K, Sato H, et al. A sensitive sandwich ELISA for measuring thrombopoietin in human serum: serum thrombopoietin levels in healthy volunteers and in patients with haemopoietic disorders. *Br J Haematol* 1996;93:783–788.

563. Espanol I, Hernandez A, Cortes M, et al. Patients with thrombocytosis have normal or slightly elevated thrombopoietin levels. *Haematologica* 1999;84: 312–316.

564. Wang JC, Chen C, Novetsky AD, et al. Blood thrombopoietin levels in clonal thrombocytosis and reactive thrombocytosis. *Am J Med* 1998;104:451–455.

565. Harrison CN, Gale RE, Pezella F, et al. Platelet c-mpl expression is dysregulated in patients with essential thrombocythaemia but this is not of diagnostic value. *Br J Haematol* 1999;107:139–147.

566. Pitcher L, Taylor K, Nichol J, et al. Thrombopoietin measurement in thrombocytosis: dysregulation and lack of feedback inhibition in essential thrombocythaemia. *Br J Haematol* 1997;99:929–932.

567. Usuki K, Tahara T, Iki S, et al. Serum thrombopoietin level in various hematological diseases. *Stem Cells* 1996;14:558–565.

568. Hou M, Carneskog J, Mellqvist UH, et al. Impact of endogenous thrombopoietin levels on the differential diagnosis of essential thrombocythaemia and reactive thrombocytosis. *Eur J Haematol* 1998;61:119–122.

569. Cerutti A, Custodi P, Duranti M, et al. Thrombopoietin levels in patients with primary and reactive thrombocytosis. *Br J Haematol* 1997;99:281–284.

570. Uppenkamp M, Makarova E, Petrasch S, et al. Thrombopoietin serum concentration in patients with reactive and myeloproliferative thrombocytosis. *Ann Hematol* 1998;77:217–223.

571. Harrison CN, Gale RE, Wiestner AC, et al. The activating splice mutation in intron 3 of the thrombopoietin gene is not found in patients with non-familial essential thrombocythaemia. *Br J Haematol* 1998;102:1341–1343.

572. Haznedaroglu IC, Ertenli I, Ozcebe OI, et al. Megakaryocyte-related interleukins in reactive thrombocytosis versus autonomous thrombocythemia. *Acta Haematol* 1996;95:107–111.

573. Tefferi A, Ho TC, Ahmann GJ, et al. Plasma interleukin-6 and C-reactive protein levels in reactive versus clonal thrombocytosis. *Am J Med* 1994;97:374–378.

574. Sabath DF, Kaushansky K, Broudy VC. Deletion of the extracellular membrane-distal cytokine receptor homology module of Mpl results in constitutive cell growth and loss of thrombopoietin binding. *Blood* 1999;94:365–367.

575. Horikawa Y, Matsumura I, Hashimoto K, et al. Markedly reduced expression of platelet c-mpl receptor in essential thrombocythemia. *Blood* 1997;90:4031–4038.

576. Mazur EM, Cohen JL, Bogart L. Growth characteristics of circulating hematopoietic progenitor cells from patients with essential thrombocythemia. *Blood* 1988;71:1544–1550.

577. Rolovic Z, Basara N, Gotic M, et al. The determination of spontaneous megakaryocyte colony formation is an unequivocal test for discrimination between essential thrombocythaemia and reactive thrombocytosis. *Br J Haematol* 1995;90:326–331.

578. Florensa L, Besses C, Woessner S, et al. Endogenous megakaryocyte and erythroid colony formation from blood in essential thrombocythaemia. *Leukemia* 1995;9:271–273.

579. Juvonen E, Ikkala E, Oksanen K, et al. Megakaryocyte and erythroid colony formation in essential thrombocythaemia and reactive thrombocytosis: diagnostic value and correlation to complications. *Br J Haematol* 1993;83:192–197.

580. Kimura H, Ishibashi T, Sato T, et al. Megakaryocytic colony formation (CFU-Meg) in essential thrombocythemia: quantitative and qualitative abnormalities of bone marrow CFU-Meg. *Am J Hematol* 1987;24:23–30.

581. Abgrall JF, Berthou C, Cauvin JM, et al. Spontaneous in vitro megakaryocyte colony formation in primary thrombocytemia: relation to platelet factor 4 plasma level and beta-thromboglobulin/platelet factor 4 ratio. *Acta Haematol* 1992;87:118–121.

582. Komatsu N, Suda T, Sakata Y, et al. Megakaryocytopoiesis in vitro of patients with essential thrombocythaemia: effect of plasma and serum on megakaryocytic colony formation. *Br J Haematol* 1986;64:241–252.

583. Axelrad AA, Eskinazi D, Correa PN, et al. Hypersensitivity of circulating progenitor cells to megakaryocyte growth and development factor (PEG-rHu MGDF) in essential thrombocythemia. *Blood* 2000;96:3310–3321.

584. Ozaki S, Kosaka M, Ozaki K, et al. Thrombopoietin-responsive essential thrombocythaemia with myelofibrosis. *Br J Haematol* 1997;97:449–452.

585. Turhan AG, Cashman JD, Eaves CJ, et al. Variable expression of features of normal and neoplastic stem cells in patients with thrombocytosis. *Br J Haematol* 1992;82:50–57.

586. Ciaudo M, Hadjez JM, Teyssandier I, et al. Prognostic and diagnostic value of endogenous erythroid colony formation in essential thrombocythemia. *Hematol Cell Ther* 1998;40:171–174.

587. Shih LY, Lee CT. Identification of masked polycythemia vera from patients with idiopathic marked thrombocytosis by endogenous erythroid colony assay. *Blood* 1994;83:744–748.

588. Jacobsson S, Carneskog J, Ridell B, et al. Flow cytometric analysis of megakaryocyte ploidy in chronic myeloproliferative disorders and reactive thrombocytosis. *Eur J Haematol* 1996;56:287–292.

589. Tomer A, Friese P, Conklin R, et al. Flow cytometric analysis of megakaryocytes from patients with abnormal platelet counts. *Blood* 1989;74:594–601.

590. Gale RE, Fielding AK, Harrison CN, et al. Acquired skewing of X-chromosome inactivation patterns in myeloid cells of the elderly suggests stochastic clonal loss with age. *Br J Haematol* 1997;98:512–519.

591. Busque L, Mio R, Mattioli J, et al. Nonrandom X-inactivation patterns in normal females: lyonization ratios vary with age. *Blood* 1996;88:59–65.

592. Mitterbauer G, Winkler K, Gisslinger H, et al. Clonality analysis using X-chromosome inactivation at the human androgen receptor gene (Humara). Evaluation of large cohorts of patients with chronic myeloproliferative diseases, secondary neutrophilia, and reactive thrombocytosis. *Am J Clin Pathol* 1999;112:93–100.

593. Gale RE, Wainscoat JS. Clonal analysis using X-linked DNA polymorphisms. *Br J Haematol* 1993;85:2–8.

594. Allen RC, Zoghbi HY, Moseley AB, et al. Methylation of HpaII and HhaI sites near the polymorphic CAG repeat in the human androgen-receptor gene correlates with X chromosome inactivation. *Am J Hum Genet* 1992;51:1229–1239.

595. el Kassar N, Hetet G, Li Y, et al. Clonal analysis of haemopoietic cells in essential thrombocythaemia. *Br J Haematol* 1995;90:131–137.

596. Prchal JT, Guan YL. A novel clonality assay based on transcriptional analysis of the active X chromosome. *Stem Cells* 1993;11[Suppl 1]:62–65.

597. el Kassar N, Hetet G, Briere J, et al. Clonality analysis of hematopoiesis in essential thrombocythemia: advantages of studying T lymphocytes and platelets. *Blood* 1997;89:128–134.

598. Harrison CN, Gale RE, MacHin SJ, et al. A large proportion of patients with a diagnosis of essential thrombocythemia do not have a clonal disorder and may be at lower risk of thrombotic complications. *Blood* 1999;93:417–424.

599. Osselaer JC, Jamart J, Scheiff JM. Platelet distribution width for differential diagnosis of thrombocytosis. *Clin Chem* 1997;43:1072–1076.

600. Van der LJ, dem Borne AK. Platelet volume analysis for differential diagnosis of thrombocytosis. *J Clin Pathol* 1986;39:129–133.

601. Howard MR, Ashwell S, Bond LR, et al. Artefactual serum hyperkalaemia and hypercalcaemia in essential thrombocythaemia. *J Clin Pathol* 2000;53:105–109.

602. Schloesser L, Kipp MA, Wenzel F. Thrombocytosis in iron-deficiency anemia. *J Lab Clin Med* 1965;66:107–114.

603. Blickstein D, Aviram A, Luboshitz J, et al. BCR-ABL transcripts in bone marrow aspirates of Philadelphia-negative essential thrombocytopenia patients: clinical presentation. *Blood* 1997;90:2768–2771.

604. Stoll DB, Peterson P, Exten R, et al. Clinical presentation and natural history of patients with essential thrombocythemia and the Philadelphia chromosome. *Am J Hematol* 1988;27:77–83.

605. Barnhart MI, Kim TH, Evatt BL, et al. Essential thrombocythemia in a child: platelet ultrastructure and function. *Am J Hematol* 1980;8:87–107.

606. Mazzucato M, De Marco L, De Angelis V, et al. Platelet membrane abnormalities in myeloproliferative disorders: decrease in glycoproteins Ib and IIb/IIIa complex is associated with deficient receptor function. *Br J Haematol* 1989;73:369–374.

607. Clezardin P, McGregor JL, Dechavanne M, et al. Platelet membrane glycoprotein abnormalities in patients with myeloproliferative disorders and secondary thrombocytosis. *Br J Haematol* 1985;60:331–344.

608. Kaywin P, McDonough M, Insel PA, et al. Platelet function in essential thrombocythemia. Decreased epinephrine responsiveness associated with a deficiency of platelet alpha-adrenergic receptors. *N Engl J Med* 1978;299:505–509.

609. Thibert V, Bellucci S, Cristofari M, et al. Increased platelet CD36 constitutes a common marker in myeloproliferative disorders. *Br J Haematol* 1995;91:618–624.

610. Griesshammer M, Beneke H, Nussbaumer B, et al. Increased platelet surface expression of P-selectin and thrombospondin as markers of platelet activation in essential thrombocythaemia. *Thromb Res* 1999;96:191–196.

611. Wehmeier A, Tschope D, Esser J, et al. Circulating activated platelets in myeloproliferative disorders. *Thromb Res* 1991;61:271–278.

612. Booth WJ, Berndt MC, Castaldi PA. An altered platelet granule glycoprotein in patients with essential thrombocythemia. *J Clin Invest* 1984;73:291–297.

613. Fujimoto T, Fujimura K, Kuramoto A. Abnormal Ca2+ homeostasis in platelets of patients with myeloproliferative disorders: low levels of Ca2+ influx and efflux across the plasma membrane and increased Ca2+ accumulation into the dense tubular system. *Thromb Res* 1989;53:99–108.

614. Zahavi J, Zahavi M, Firsteter E, et al. An abnormal pattern of multiple platelet function abnormalities and increased thromboxane generation in patients with primary thrombocytosis and thrombotic complications. *Eur J Haematol* 1991;47:326–332.

615. Ginsburg AD. Platelet function in patients with high platelet counts. *Ann Intern Med* 1975;82:506–511.

616. Baker RI, Manoharan A. Platelet function in myeloproliferative disorders: characterization and sequential studies show multiple platelet abnormalities, and change with time. *Eur J Haematol* 1988;40:267–272.

617. Mayordomo O, Carcamo C, Vecino AM, et al. Arachidonic acid metabolism in platelets of patients with essential thrombocythaemia. *Thromb Res* 1995;78:315–321.

618. Castaldi PA, Berndt MC, Booth W, et al. Evidence for a platelet membrane defect in the myeloproliferative syndromes. *Thromb Res* 1982;27:601–609.

619. Rocca B, Ciabattoni G, Tartaglione R, et al. Increased thromboxane biosynthesis in essential thrombocythemia. *Thromb Haemost* 1995;74:1225–1230.

620. Tomo K, Takayama H, Kaneko Y, et al. Qualitative platelet 12-lipoxygenase abnormality in a patient with essential thrombocythemia. *Thromb Haemost* 1997;77:294–297.

621. Oda A, Miyakawa Y, Druker BJ, et al. Thrombopoietin primes human platelet aggregation induced by shear stress and by multiple agonists. *Blood* 1996;87:4664–4670.

622. Usuki K, Iki S, Endo M, et al. Influence of thrombopoietin on platelet activation in myeloproliferative disorders. *Br J Haematol* 1997;97:530–537.

623. Conlan MG, Haire WD. Low protein S in essential thrombocythemia with thrombosis. *Am J Hematol* 1989;32:88–93.

624. Wieczorek I, MacGregor IR, Ludlam CA. Low proteins C and S and activation of fibrinolysis in treated essential thrombocythemia. *Am J Hematol* 1995;49:277–281.

625. Posan E, Ujj G, Kiss A, et al. Reduced in vitro clot lysis and release of more active platelet PAI-1 in polycythemia vera and essential thrombocythemia. *Thromb Res* 1998;90:51–56.

626. Bellucci S, Ignatova E, Jaillet N, et al. Platelet hyperactivation in patients with essential thrombocythemia is not associated with vascular endothelial cell damage as judged by the level of plasma thrombomodulin, protein S, PAI-1, t-PA and vWF. *Thromb Haemost* 1993;70:736–742.

627. Budde U, Dent JA, Berkowitz SD, et al. Subunit composition of plasma von Willebrand factor in patients with the myeloproliferative syndrome. *Blood* 1986;68:1213–1217.

628. Raman BK, Sawdyk M, Saeed SM. Essential thrombocythemia with acquired von Willebrand's disease. *Am J Clin Pathol* 1987;88:102–106.

629. van Genderen PJ, Budde U, Michiels JJ, et al. The reduction of large von Willebrand factor multimers in plasma in essential thrombocythaemia is related to the platelet count. *Br J Haematol* 1996;93:962–965.

630. van Genderen PJ, van Vliet HH, Prins FJ, et al. Excessive prolongation of the bleeding time by aspirin in essential thrombocythemia is related to a decrease of large von Willebrand factor multimers in plasma. *Ann Hematol* 1997;75:215–220.

631. van Genderen PJ, Prins FJ, Lucas IS, et al. Decreased half-life time of plasma von Willebrand factor collagen binding activity in essential thrombocythaemia: normalization after cytoreduction of the increased platelet count. *Br J Haematol* 1997;99:832–836.

632. Cortelazzo S, Marchetti M, Orlando E, et al. Aspirin increases the bleeding side effects in essential thrombocythemia independent of the cyclooxygenase pathway: role of the lipoxygenase pathway. *Am J Hematol* 1998;57:277–282.

633. Michiels JJ, Abels J, Steketee J, et al. Erythromelalgia caused by platelet-mediated arteriolar inflammation and thrombosis in thrombocythemia. *Ann Intern Med* 1985;102:466–471.

634. Kalgaard OM, Seem E, Kvernebo K. Erythromelalgia: a clinical study of 87 cases. *J Intern Med* 1997;242:191–197.

635. Michiels JJ, ten Kate FW, Vuzevski VD, et al. Histopathology of erythromelalgia in thrombocythaemia. *Histopathology* 1984;8:669–678.

636. van Genderen PJ, Lucas IS, van Strik R, et al. Erythromelalgia in essential thrombocythaemia is characterized by platelet activation and endothelial cell damage but not by thrombin generation. *Thromb Haemost* 1996;76:333–338.

637. van Genderen PJ, Prins FJ, Michiels JJ, et al. Thromboxane-dependent platelet activation in vivo precedes arterial thrombosis in thrombocythaemia: a rationale for the use of low-dose aspirin as an antithrombotic agent. *Br J Haematol* 1999;104:438–441.

638. van Genderen PJ, Michiels JJ, van Strik R, et al. Platelet consumption in thrombocythemia complicated by erythromelalgia: reversal by aspirin. *Thromb Haemost* 1995;73:210–214.

639. Michiels JJ, Koudstaal PJ, Mulder AH, et al. Transient neurologic and ocular manifestations in primary thrombocythemia. *Neurology* 1993;43:1107–1110.

640. Koudstaal PJ, Koudstaal A. Neurologic and visual symptoms in essential thrombocythemia: efficacy of low-dose aspirin. *Semin Thromb Hemost* 1997;23:365–370.

641. Richard C, Conde E, Garijo J, et al. Trisomy 1q in a case of essential thrombocythemia with long survival. *Cancer Genet Cytogenet* 1987;25:185–186.

642. Munro LR, Stevenson DA, Culligan DJ. Translocation (X;5)(q13;q33) in essential thrombocythemia. *Cancer Genet Cytogenet* 1999;114:78–79.

643. Mitev L, Georgiev G, Petrov A, et al. Unusual chromosome aberration, t(13;14)(q32;q32.3), in a case of essential thrombocythemia with extreme thrombocytosis. *Cancer Genet Cytogenet* 1996;91:68–70.

644. Zaccaria A, Tura S. A chromosomal abnormality in primary thrombocythemia. *N Engl J Med* 1978;298:1422–1423.

645. Morris CM, Fitzgerald PH, Hollings PE, et al. Essential thrombocythaemia and the Philadelphia chromosome. *Br J Haematol* 1988;70:13–19.

646. LeBrun DP, Pinkerton PH, Sheridan BL, et al. Essential thrombocythemia with the Philadelphia chromosome and BCR-ABL gene rearrangement. An entity distinct from chronic myeloid leukemia and Philadelphia chromosome-negative essential thrombocythemia. *Cancer Genet Cytogenet* 1991;54:21–25.

647. Martiat P, Ifrah N, Rassool F, et al. Molecular analysis of Philadelphia positive essential thrombocythemia. *Leukemia* 1989;3:563–565.

648. Emilia G, Luppi M, Ferrari MG, et al. Chronic myeloid leukemia with thrombocythemic onset may be associated with different BCR/ABL variant transcripts. *Cancer Genet Cytogenet* 1998;101:75–77.

649. Michiels JJ, Prins ME, Hagemeijer A, et al. Philadelphia chromosome-positive thrombocythemia and megakaryoblast leukemia. *Am J Clin Pathol* 1987;88:645–652.

650. Marasca R, Luppi M, Zucchini P, et al. Might essential thrombocythemia carry Ph anomaly? *Blood* 1998;91:3084–3085.

651. Sole F, Florensa L, Espinet B, et al. Absence of bcr/abl rearrangement in 41 patients with essential thrombocythemia. *Haematologica* 2000;85:214–215.

652. Neri A, Fracchiolla NS, Radaelli F, et al. p53 tumour suppressor gene and RAS oncogenes: molecular analysis in the chronic and leukaemic phases of essential thrombocythaemia. *Br J Haematol* 1996;93:670–673.

653. Thiele J, Kvasnicka HM, Fischer R. Histochemistry and morphometry on bone marrow biopsies in chronic myeloproliferative disorders—aids to diagnosis and classification. *Ann Hematol* 1999;78:495–506.

654. Mason JE, DeVita VT, Canellos GP. Thrombocytosis in chronic granulocytic leukemia: incidence and clinical significance. *Blood* 1974;44:483–487.

655. Takahashi H, Furukawa T, Hashimoto S, et al. 5q- syndrome presenting chronic myeloproliferative disorders-like manifestation: a case report. *Am J Hematol* 2000;64:120–123.

656. Lahuerta-Palacios JJ, Bornstein R, Fernandez-Debora FJ, et al. Controlled and uncontrolled thrombocytosis. Its clinical role in essential thrombocythemia. *Cancer* 1988;61:1207–1212.

657. Cortelazzo S, Finazzi G, Ruggeri M, et al. Hydroxyurea for patients with essential thrombocythemia and a high risk of thrombosis. *N Engl J Med* 1995; 332:1132–1136.

658. Randi ML, Casonato A, Fabris F, et al. The significance of thrombocytosis in old age. *Acta Haematol* 1987;78:41–44.

659. Watson KV, Key N. Vascular complications of essential thrombocythaemia: a link to cardiovascular risk factors. *Br J Haematol* 1993;83:198–203.

660. Cortelazzo S, Viero P, Finazzi G, et al. Incidence and risk factors for thrombotic complications in a historical cohort of 100 patients with essential thrombocythemia. *J Clin Oncol* 1990;8:556–562.

661. Tefferi A, Fonseca R, Pereira DL, et al. A long-term retrospective study of young women with essential thrombocythemia. *Mayo Clin Proc* 2001;76:22–28.

662. Harrison CN, MacHin SJ. Antiphospholipid antibodies and essential thrombocythemia. *Am J Med* 1997;102:317–318.

663. Griesshammer M, Bangerter M, van Vliet HH, et al. Aspirin in essential thrombocythemia: status quo and quo vadis. *Semin Thromb Hemost* 1997;23:371–377.

664. Millard FE, Hunter CS, Anderson M, et al. Clinical manifestations of essential thrombocythemia in young adults. *Am J Hematol* 1990;33:27–31.

665. McIntyre KJ, Hoagland HC, Silverstein MN, et al. Essential thrombocythemia in young adults. *Mayo Clin Proc* 1991;66:149–154.

666. Randi ML, Rossi C, Fabris F, et al. Essential thrombocythemia in young adults: major thrombotic complications and complications during pregnancy—a follow-up study in 68 patients. *Clin Appl Thromb Hemost* 2000;6:31–35.

667. Geller SA, Shapiro E. Acute leukemia as a natural sequel to primary thrombocythemia. *Am J Clin Pathol* 1982;77:353–356.

668. Colovic MD, Jankovic GM, Suvajdzic ND, et al. Acute myeloid leukaemia evolving from haemorrhagic essential thrombocythaemia. *Eur J Haematol* 1998;61:280–281.

669. Andersson PO, Ridell B, Wadenvik H, et al. Leukemic transformation of essential thrombocythemia without previous cytoreductive treatment. *Ann Hematol* 2000;79:40–42.

670. Sedlacek SM, Curtis JL, Weintraub J, et al. Essential thrombocythemia and leukemic transformation. *Medicine* 1986;65:353–364.

671. Shibata K, Shimamoto Y, Suga K, et al. Essential thrombocythemia terminating in acute leukemia with minimal myeloid differentiation—a brief review of recent literature. *Acta Haematol* 1994;91:84–88.

672. Sessarego M, Defferrari R, Dejana AM, et al. Cytogenetic analysis in essential thrombocythemia at diagnosis and at transformation. A 12-year study. *Cancer Genet Cytogenet* 1989;43:57–65.

673. Murphy PT, Sivakumaran M, van Rhee F, et al. Acute lymphoblastic transformation of essential thrombocythaemia. *Br J Haematol* 1995;89:921–922.

674. Sterkers Y, Preudhomme C, Lai JL, et al. Acute myeloid leukemia and myelodysplastic syndromes following essential thrombocythemia treated with hydroxyurea: high proportion of cases with 17p deletion. *Blood* 1998;91:616–622.

675. Randi ML, Fabris F, Girolami A. Leukemia and myelodysplasia effect of multiple cytotoxic therapy in essential thrombocythemia. *Leuk Lymphoma* 2000; 37:379–385.

676. Shpilberg O, Shimon I, Sofer O, et al. Transient normal platelet counts and decreased requirement for interferon during pregnancy in essential thrombocythaemia. *Br J Haematol* 1996;92:491–493.

677. Chow EY, Haley LP, Vickars LM. Essential thrombocythemia in pregnancy: platelet count and pregnancy outcome. *Am J Hematol* 1992;41:249–251.

678. Jones EC, Mosesson MW, Thomason JL, et al. Essential thrombocythemia in pregnancy. *Obstet Gynecol* 1988;71:501–503.

679. Turhan AG, Humphries RK, Cashman JD, et al. Transient suppression of clonal hemopoiesis associated with pregnancy in a patient with a myeloproliferative disorder. *J Clin Invest* 1988;81:1999–2003.

680. Samuelsson J, Swolin B. Spontaneous remission during two pregnancies in a patient with essential thrombocythaemia. *Leuk Lymphoma* 1997;25:597–600.

681. Beressi AH, Tefferi A, Silverstein MN, et al. Outcome analysis of 34 pregnancies in women with essential thrombocythemia. *Arch Intern Med* 1995;155: 1217–1222.

682. Bangerter M, Guthner C, Beneke H, et al. Pregnancy in essential thrombocythaemia: treatment and outcome of 17 pregnancies. *Eur J Haematol* 2000; 65:165–169.

683. Schmidt HH, Neumeister P, Kainer F, et al. Treatment of essential thrombocythemia during pregnancy: antiabortive effect of interferon-alpha? *Ann Hematol* 1998;77:291–292.

684. Randi ML, Rossi C, Fabris F, et al. Essential thrombocythemia in young adults: treatment and outcome of 16 pregnancies. *J Intern Med* 1999;246:517–518.

685. Falconer J, Pineo G, Blahey W, et al. Essential thrombocythemia associated with recurrent abortions and fetal growth retardation. *Am J Hematol* 1987;25:345–347.

686. Ault KA, Rinder HM, Mitchell J, et al. The significance of platelets with increased RNA content (reticulated platelets). A measure of the rate of thrombopoiesis. *Am J Clin Pathol* 1992;98:637–646.

687. Rinder HM, Schuster JE, Rinder CS, et al. Correlation of thrombosis with increased platelet turnover in thrombocytosis. *Blood* 1998;91:1288–1294.

688. Randi ML, Fabris F, Cella G, et al. Cerebral vascular accidents in young patients with essential thrombocythemia: relation with other known cardiovascular risk factors. *Angiology* 1998;49:477–481.

689. van Genderen PJ, Mulder PG, Waleboer M, et al. Prevention and treatment of thrombotic complications in essential thrombocythaemia: efficacy and safety of aspirin. *Br J Haematol* 1997;97:179–184.

690. Brodkin HM. Myoglobinuria following epsilon-aminocaproic acid (EACA) therapy. Case report. *J Neurosurg* 1980;53:690–692.

691. Panlilio AL, Reiss RF. Therapeutic plateletpheresis in thrombocythemia. *Transfusion* 1979;19:147–152.

692. Goldfinger D, Thompson R, Lowe C, et al. Long-term plateletpheresis in the management of primary thrombocytosis. *Transfusion* 1979;19:336–338.

693. Baron BW, Mick R, Baron JM. Combined plateletpheresis and cytotoxic chemotherapy for symptomatic thrombocytosis in myeloproliferative disorders. *Cancer* 1993;72:1209–1218.

694. Orlin JB, Berkman EM. Improvement of platelet function following plateletpheresis in patients with myeloproliferative diseases. *Transfusion* 1980;20: 540–545.

695. Barbui T, Buelli M, Cortelazzo S, et al. Aspirin and risk of bleeding in patients with thrombocythemia. *Am J Med* 1987;83:265–268.

696. Randi ML, Rossi C, Fabris F, et al. Aspirin seems as effective as myelosuppressive agents in the prevention of rethrombosis in essential thrombocythemia. *Clin Appl Thromb Hemost* 1999;5:131–135.

697. Michaels AD, Whisenant B, MacGregor JS. Multivessel coronary thrombosis treated with abciximab (ReoPro) in a patient with essential thrombocythemia. *Clin Cardiol* 1998;21:134–138.

698. Mazur EM, Rosmarin AG, Sohl PA, et al. Analysis of the mechanism of anagrelide-induced thrombocytopenia in humans. *Blood* 1992;79:1931–1937.

699. Solberg LA, Tefferi A, Oles KJ, et al. The effects of anagrelide on human megakaryocytopoiesis. *Br J Haematol* 1997;99:174–180.

700. Bellucci S, Legrand C, Boval B, et al. Studies of platelet volume, chemistry and function in patients with essential thrombocythaemia treated with Anagrelide. *Br J Haematol* 1999;104:886–892.

701. Yoon SY, Li CY, Mesa RA, et al. Bone marrow effects of anagrelide therapy in patients with myelofibrosis with myeloid metaplasia. *Br J Haematol* 1999;106: 682–688.

702. Anagrelide, a therapy for thrombocythemic states: experience in 577 patients. Anagrelide Study Group. *Am J Med* 1992;92:69–76.

703. Talpaz M, Kurzrock R, Kantarjian H, et al. Recombinant interferon-alpha therapy of Philadelphia chromosome-negative myeloproliferative disorders with thrombocytosis. *Am J Med* 1989;86:554–558.

704. Bentley M, Taylor K, Grigg A, et al. Long-term interferon-alpha 2A does not induce sustained hematologic remission in younger patients with essential thrombocythemia. *Leuk Lymphoma* 1999;36:123–128.

705. Catani L, Gugliotta L, Cascione ML, et al. Platelet function and interferon alpha-2a treatment in essential thrombocythaemia. *Eur J Haematol* 1991;46:158–162.

706. Legrand C, Bellucci S, Disdier M, et al. Platelet thrombospondin and glycoprotein IV abnormalities in patients with essential thrombocythemia: effect of alpha-interferon treatment. *Am J Hematol* 1991;38:307–313.

707. Gugliotta L, Bagnara GP, Catani L, et al. In vivo and in vitro inhibitory effect of alpha-interferon on megakaryocyte colony growth in essential thrombocythaemia. *Br J Haematol* 1989;71:177–181.

708. Petrini M, Simi P, Saglio G. Cytogenetic remission induced by interferon-alpha in a myeloproliferative disorder with trisomy 8. *Br J Haematol* 1996; 92:941–943.

709. Sacchi S, Tabilio A, Leoni P, et al. Interferon alpha-2b in the long-term treatment of essential thrombocythemia. *Ann Hematol* 1991;63:206–209.

710. Sacchi S, Gugliotta L, Papineschi F, et al. Alfa-interferon in the treatment of essential thrombocythemia: clinical results and evaluation of its biological effects on the hematopoietic neoplastic clone. Italian Cooperative Group on ET. *Leukemia* 1998;12:289–294.

711. Sacchi S, Tabilio A, Leoni P, et al. Sustained complete hematological remission in essential thrombocythemia after discontinuation of long-term alpha-IFN treatment. *Ann Hematol* 1993;66:245–246.

712. Finazzi G, Ruggeri M, Rodeghiero F, et al. Second malignancies in patients with essential thrombocythaemia treated with busulphan and hydroxyurea: long-term follow-up of a randomized clinical trial. *Br J Haematol* 2000;110: 577–583.

713. Wehmeier A, Sudhoff T, Meierkord F. Relation of platelet abnormalities to thrombosis and hemorrhage in chronic myeloproliferative disorders. *Semin Thromb Hemost* 1997;23:391–402.

CHAPTER 13

Chronic Myelogenous Leukemia

Guillermo Garcia-Manero, Moshe Talpaz, Stefan Faderl, and Hagop M. Kantarjian

INTRODUCTION

Chronic myelogenous (myeloid, myelocytic, granulocytic) leukemia (CML) is a clonal myeloproliferative disorder of a pluripotent hematopoietic stem cell. It is characterized by leukocytosis with or without thrombocytosis and splenomegaly. The malignant clone carries a chromosomal translocation involving chromosomes 9 and 22, t(9;22)(q34;q11), known as the *Philadelphia* (Ph) *chromosome*, which produces the fusion of the *BCR-ABL* gene. The protein generated by this chimeric aberrant gene has increased tyrosine kinase activity and induces phosphorylation of multiple downstream protein targets that alter the signal transduction characteristics of the CML cell.

The natural history of CML is divided into three phases: chronic, accelerated, and blastic. The initial chronic phase usually lasts for 3 to 5 years with hydroxyurea and 6 to 7 years with interferon (IFN)-α regimens. Most patients (85% to 90%) present in chronic phase. Patients usually show accelerated phase features before blastic transformation. Although the accelerated phase criteria vary, patients often exhibit increased blasts and basophils, additional chromosomal abnormalities, and thrombocytopenia with or without anemia and leukocytosis. Accelerated phase CML lasts less than 1.5 years. Approximately 10% to 20% of patients die in this phase from complications of myelofibrosis and marrow failure—an event more often associated with busulfan therapy.

Therapy for CML is evolving rapidly with improvements in allogeneic stem cell transplantation (SCT), IFN-based combinations, and the discovery of new BCR-ABL tyrosine kinase inhibitors such as the signal transduction inhibitor imatinib mesylate. Patients in chronic phase can be treated with several options depending on their age, availability of matched donors, performance, and socioeconomic status. Standard options include the use of hydroxyurea for tumor debulking between more definitive therapies or in combination, IFN-α and cytosine arabinoside (ara-C) combinations, and allogeneic SCT. There is a debate as to which patients should be transplanted in early chronic phase—a situation frequently reassessed as results of imatinib mesylate therapy mature. Patients in blastic phase are treated according to their immunophenotype with acute lymphocytic leukemia (ALL)–type programs if lymphoid and with high-dose ara-C–containing programs or investigational therapies if myeloid. However, results are poor, and prognosis of patients in this terminal phase is dismal.

The increasing knowledge of the molecular biology, signal transduction, and antigenic characteristics of CML is promoting the development of new targeted therapies for this disease, such as imatinib mesylate, an inhibitor of BCR-ABL protein. Dissect-ing the relative biologic significance of the downstream events of the BCR-ABL cascade may produce other specific anti-CML therapies.

MOLECULAR BIOLOGY OF CHRONIC MYELOGENOUS LEUKEMIA

Philadelphia Chromosome and the *BCR-ABL* Gene

CML is defined by the presence of the Ph chromosome, the *BCR-ABL* gene, or both. Among patients with a morphologic picture of CML, 90% show the Ph abnormality (Ph-positive CML) (1). The remaining 10% (Ph-negative CML) are a heterogeneous group with some atypical features (older age, dysplastic changes, monocytosis) and include some cases of proliferative myelodysplastic syndrome and chronic myelomonocytic leukemia. However, a subset of Ph-negative CML shows the *BCR-ABL* gene (2): These Ph-negative, *BCR-ABL*–positive cases have clinicopathologic features and prognoses identical to Ph-positive CML and respond similarly to therapy (3–7). The Ph chromosome is also present in 5% of pediatric ALL, in 15% to 30% of adult ALL, and in 1% to 2% of AML (1).

Nowell first described the Ph abnormality in 1960 as a shortened chromosome 22 (8), which lacks approximately half of the distal segment of its long arm. It was initially abbreviated as Ph^1 because it was thought that other abnormalities would be soon described and termed Ph^n; this was later changed to Ph (9). In 1973, using chromosome banding techniques, Rowley described the Ph abnormality as a balanced translocation between chromosomes 9 and 22 and located the precise positions of the chromosomal breaks at t(9;22)(q34;q11) (10,11). The Ph abnormality was identified in myeloid (including monocytes, basophils, and eosinophils), erythroid, megakaryocytic, and lymphoid precursor cells (B-lymphoid was frequent; T-lymphoid was rare) (12–16) but not in bone marrow fibroblasts (17,18). This indicated that CML originates in a pluripotent hematopoietic stem cell. At presentation, most patients are 100% Ph-positive, but few show a mixture of Ph-positive and normal cells. These patients with chimeric marrow findings were suggested to have a better prognosis (19,20). Variant chromosomal abnormalities have been described in CML, including simple and complex Ph translocations, as well as "masked" Ph translocations (between chromosome 9 and chromosomes other than 22), depending on the number and particular chromosomes involved.

In 1983, C-ABL was found to be involved in t(9;22) (21), and a year later a chromosomal breakpoint area on 22q11, now known as the breakpoint cluster region (BCR), was also implicated (22). C-ABL has 11 exons and expands over 230 kilobases (kb). It is located on chromosome 9q34 and encodes a 140-kilodalton (kd) protein, p140, with weak tyrosine kinase activity (23). Of importance, C-ABL has to alternate exon 1 sequences that are differentially transcribed from two different promoters. These exons are designated 1a and 1b and their respective promoters, Pa and Pb (24,25). Exon 1b is located at the 5' end of the gene and is 150 to 200 kb upstream of exon 1a. The first common exon of C-ABL is exon 2. The proximal promoter (Pa) and the distal promoter (Pb) are separated by 175 kb. They direct the synthesis of two different mRNA species of 6 and 7 kb, respectively. In approximately 90% of Ph chromosome translocations, the Pa is nested within the BCR-ABL transcriptional unit (26). In most cases of CML, the translocation breakpoint occurs between exons 1b and 1a, and therefore the Ph chromosome contains the entire coding sequence of C-ABL (exons 2 to 11) and an intact exon 1a and its promoter. This genomic DNA fragment, the 3' end of C-ABL, is transposed into the major breakpoint cluster region of BCR (M-BCR). This region is located between exons 12 and 16 (also known as b1 to b5) of BCR on chromosome 22 and extends over 5.8 kb (22). Generally, the breakpoints in BCR are located between introns b2 and b3 or b3 and b4. As a consequence, a BCR-ABL fusion gene is generated that can have either b2a2 or b3a2 junction (denoting the exons in BCR and ABL that are involved). This hybrid gene is transcribed into an 8.5-kb mRNA (27–29), which is translated into a hybrid protein, p210$^{BCR-ABL}$ (30). Patients with b3a2 tend to have higher platelet counts (31,32), but their clinicopathologic features, response to therapy, and prognosis are similar to those with b2a2 disease prognosis. Five percent of patients express both b2a2 and b3a2 due to alternative splicing mechanisms.

The BCR gene contains a second breakpoint cluster region, the minor breakpoint cluster region or m-BCR (33,34), located 5' of M-BCR and involved in 50% to 80% of Ph-positive ALL cases (33) and in rare cases of CML. The m-BCR breakpoint is within a long intron separating alternative exon e2' from exon 2. Secondary splicing of alternative exons e1' and e2' generates an e1a2 junction between BCR and ABL. e1 refers to the 3' distal exon of BCR present at the junction, and a2 refers to the proximal 5' exon transposed from C-ABL. Because of the proximal location of m-BCR, the BCR-ABL fusion gene generated is smaller and encodes a fusion protein of 190 kd, p190$^{BCR-ABL}$ (35). p190$^{BCR-ABL}$ has been associated with monocytosis (36). A third breakpoint cluster region, μ-BCR, located at the 3' end of M-BCR has recently been described. It is located between exons e19 and e20, creating an e19a2 junction (37). The fusion protein generated has a molecular weight of 230 kd and is known as p230$^{BCR-ABL}$. p230$^{BCR-ABL}$ has been described in cases of chronic neutrophilic leukemia, a rare disorder marked by sustained mature neutrophilic expansion, a more indolent behavior than classic CML, less tendency to transform (38), and thrombocytosis (39,40). In two-thirds of patients with CML, the cells also carry an ABL-BCR translocation (8,10) of no known pathophysiologic role (41). Figure 13-1 represents the cytogenetic and molecular aberrations of the Ph chromosome.

Signal Transduction Cascades Generated by BCR-ABL

The protein product of BCR-ABL, p210, has increased constitutive tyrosine kinase activity (27,42,43). p210$^{BCR-ABL}$ is the cellular homolog of p160$^{GAG/V-ABL}$, the product of v-abl. This viral protein has the capacity to transform NIH 3T3 cells (44) and lymphoid cells (45) and to relieve growth factor dependency of hematopoietic cell lines (46). In 1988, Daley et al. (47) demonstrated the transforming capacity of p210$^{BCR-ABL}$ and established a causal association between Ph/BCR-ABL abnormalities and CML disease. In their experiments, they infected an interleukin-3 (IL-3)–dependent murine bone marrow–derived cell

line, Ba/F3, with a retroviral vector encoding BCR-ABL. On infection, Ba/F3 became IL-3 independent and acquired malignant potential. The C-ABL sequences that are deleted both in p210 and p160 share homology with several nonreceptor tyrosine kinases including SRC (48). Deletion of these sequences activates the transforming capacity of C-ABL. The transforming activity of BCR-ABL is also regulated by the first exon of BCR (49). This first exon of BCR binds to the SRC homology (SH) 2 domain of ABL. This binding is essential for the transforming capacity of BCR-ABL (50). The three different BCR-ABL oncoproteins (p190, p210, and p230) are constitutively active tyrosine kinases. They exert their leukemogenic effect via autophosphorylation and phosphorylation of downstream effectors, including RAS, RAF, ERK, JNK, MYC, JAK/STAT, PI-3kinase–AKT, and NF-κB pathways (12,40). Multiple substrates are involved in these reactions, such as CRKL, p62Dok, paxillin, CBL, RIN, SHC, and GRB2 (1,12). GRB2 is fundamental in linking p210$^{BCR-ABL}$ to RAS (51). GRB2 is a 26-kd protein composed of one SH2 domain and two SH3 domains (52). It couples receptor tyrosine kinases to SOS, a RAS activator (53,54). GRB2 performs its docking function by binding with its SH2 domain to phosphorylated tyrosine kinases and with its SH3 domains to SOS. GRB2 binds to BCR-ABL via its SH2 domain. GRB2 cannot bind to either BCR or ABL alone. It specifically binds to amino acid residue Y177F in the first exon of BCR (55). This interaction, as expected, is essential for RAS signaling. Mutation of Y177F inhibits the transforming capacity of BCR-ABL, implicating the Ras pathway at the core of the transforming signals generated by BCR-ABL. The N-terminus of ABL contains an SH2 domain, an SH3 domain, a catalytic domain, and a myristoylation sequence that allows the binding of BCR-ABL to plasma membrane proteins. The C-terminus contains a DNA-binding domain, nuclear localization signals, and an actin-binding site (1). BCR potentiates the leukemogenic potential of ABL: The N-terminal segment of BCR, with a coiled-coil motif, increases tyrosine kinase activity and potentiates ABL's binding to F-actin (56). BCR also interferes with the SH3 domain of ABL. As the SH3 domain has a negative regulatory effect on the tyrosine kinase activity of ABL, this interference constitutively activates the phosphotyrosine kinase activity of ABL. The different domains found in the different BCR-ABL oncoproteins may have important clinicobiologic implications, as each one of these proteins has been related to a different phenotype of leukemia (40). p190 contains a dimerization, binding, and SH2 and serine/threonine kinase domains. In addition, p210 also contains a Pleckstrin homology domain and a Dbl-like domain, whereas p230 contains a calcium-phospholipid binding and the partial sequence of GAP^{rac} (40). The interpretation of these data is difficult, as there is no universal specificity between the BCR-ABL oncoprotein and the phenotype of the disease (i.e., not all patients with Ph-positive ALL carry p190), and animal and cellular models may differ in their phenotypic characteristics (12). BCR-ABL also activates ubiquitin-dependent degradation of targeted proteins (57). BCR-ABL may also induce the proteasomal degradation of cyclin-dependent kinase inhibitors, such as p27 (58), and thus promotes cell cycle progression. BCR-ABL also has been reported to have antiapoptotic activity (59). Expression of BCR-ABL protects growth factor–dependent cells from apoptotic death after cytokine withdrawal (60) and up-regulates Bcl-2 and Bcl-X$_L$ (61). Although data are conflicting, in vitro BCR-ABL may mediate cell adhesion to extracellular matrix proteins by regulating integrin function (62). CML cells show decreased expression of cytoadhesion molecules such as lymphocyte function–associated antigen 3 (63), which is restored with IFN-α exposure (63). Other integrins, such as α4, α5, and β1 chains, may pathologically be also involved in CML (64,65). Figure 13-2

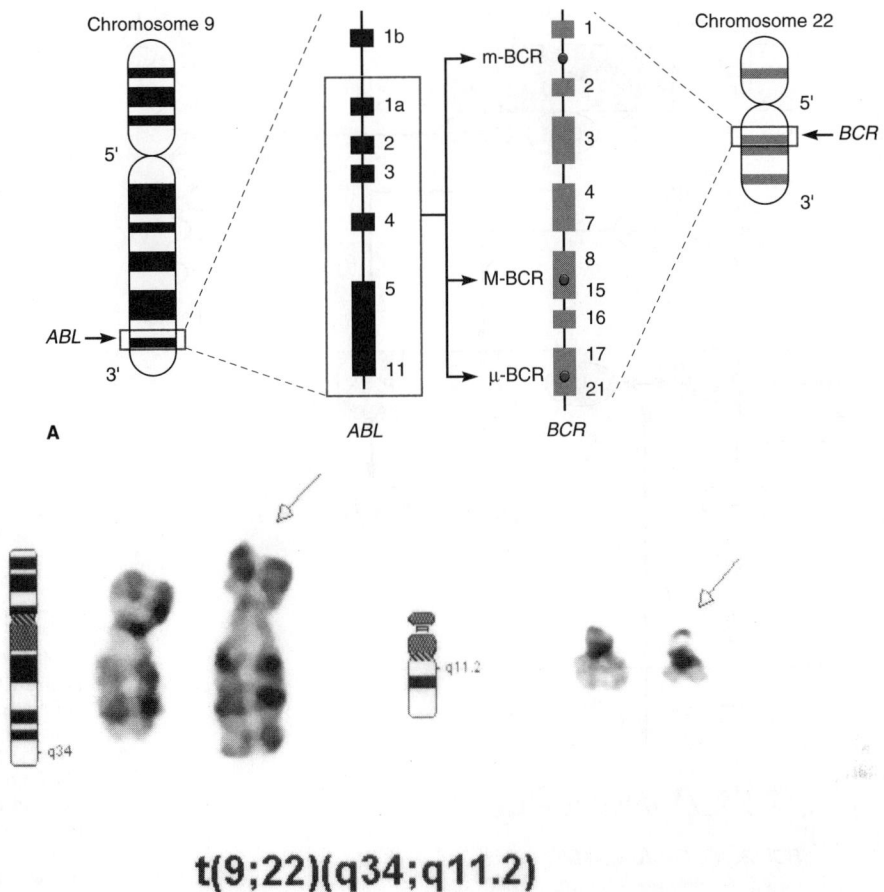

Figure 13-1. A: Schematic representation of the Philadelphia chromosome. The breakpoint in chromosome 9 generally occurs between exons 1b and 1a of *C-ABL*. This genomic DNA fragment (exons 1a to 11, inside the box) fuses with breakpoint areas on chromosome 22. Three known breakpoints exist on 22q11. *M-BCR*, located between exons 12 and 16, is the most common translocation site and generates p210$^{BCR-ABL}$. m-BCR, located between exons 1 and 2, is involved in p190$^{BCR-ABL}$. μ-BCR, located between exons 19 and 20, is involved in p230$^{BCR-ABL}$. **B:** Karyotype representing the Philadelphia chromosome, t(9;22)(q34;q11.2). Arrows indicate chromosomal changes.

summarizes the signal transduction cascade generated by BCR-ABL.

Molecular Events in Transformed Chronic Myelogenous Leukemia

New chromosomal alterations often herald the transition to CML transformation, suggesting that molecular events other than BCR-ABL may play a critical role in transformation. The dissection of key molecular events leading to transformation is important for understanding CML biology and for development of new therapeutic strategies.

Additional nonrandom cytogenetic abnormalities are found in 50% to 80% of patients in blastic phase (1,66). These include the presence of a double Ph, trisomy 8, isochromosome 17 or other chromosome 17 abnormalities, additional chromosomes 19 and 21, monosomies of chromosome 7, and t(3;21)(q26;q22) (67). Isochromosome 17 is associated with myeloid blastic phase. Molecular abnormalities include clonal immunoglobulin and T-cell receptor rearrangements in patients with lymphoid transformation (68,69), mutations in the *RAS* oncogene (70), and abnormalities in *p53*, *RB1*, and, rarely, in *C-MYC*, *p16^{INK4}*, and *AML-EVI-1*. Most such abnormalities have a cytogenetic counterpart (1) and are associated with particular phenotypic characteristics: *p53* abnormalities are frequently associated with myeloid blastic phase and, at times, linked to isochromosome 17, whereas *rb1* abnormalities are usually found in lymphoid blastic phase (1). Mutations in *p53* have

been found in transformed phases but not in chronic phase CML (71–73), suggesting that functional loss of *p53* may be involved in disease evolution. Recently, a transgenic mouse CML model has been generated in which a hematopoietic mouse promoter has been cloned and coupled to *BCR-ABL* (74). Although founder mice developed an ALL-like picture (75), transgenic offspring developed a clinical picture similar to CML. Crossmating of these transgenic mice with *p53* heterozygous mice generated compound transgenic-heterozygous mice that developed a blastic phase CML-like T-cell phenotype (74). Other experiments using *in vitro* transfection of bone marrow cells with p210$^{BCR-ABL}$ in a *p53*-deficient background have also shown blastic-like features (76).

Animal Models of Chronic Myelogenous Leukemia Disease

Several animal models have been developed to study CML. The aims of these studies were to re-create biologically significant models that can be used to analyze the molecular mechanisms of disease evolution and to evaluate preclinically the efficacy of new drugs. Models included the use of syngeneic (77) and immunodeficient mice (78) engrafted with *BCR-ABL*–transformed or –positive cell lines. Another approach is the generation of transgenic mice. Some of these models resemble ALL with a lymphoid immunophenotype (79). The use of newer promoters such as Tec is allowing the generation of transgenic mice models resembling human CML-like disease (75). Another model is

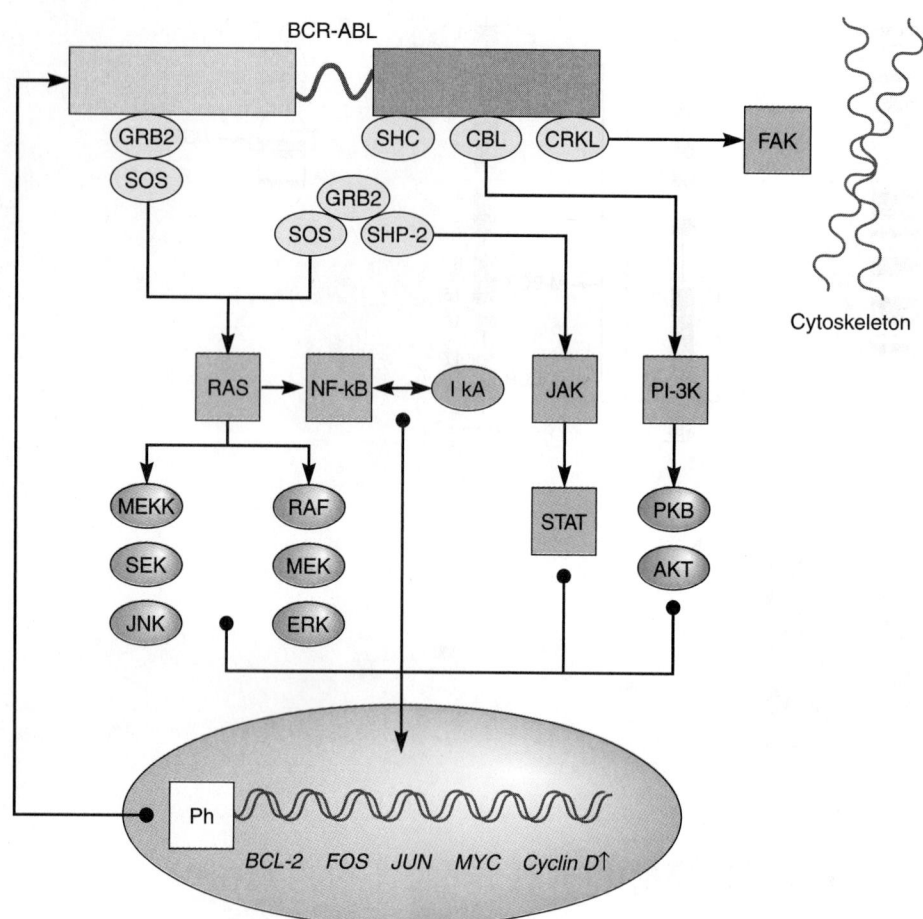

BCR-ABL

Cytoskeleton

Figure 13-2. Signal transduction cascades generated by BCR-ABL. The BCR-ABL proteins are constitutively active tyrosine kinases. Multiple downstream effectors are phosphorylated, including RAS, NF-κB, PI-3K, and FAK. These, in turn, phosphorylate other downstream proteins such as MEKK, RAF, ERK, STAT, and AKT that eventually interact with several transcription factors and nuclear proteins (BCL-2, FOS, JUN, MYC), leading to gene activation.

known as the transduction-transplantation system: Murine bone marrow cells are transduced with *BCR-ABL* retroviruses and are subsequently infused into secondary irradiated syngeneic mice. Approximately 25% of the transplanted animals develop a CML-like myeloproliferative syndrome, and the rest develop other hematologic malignancies such as ALL, erythroleukemia, and macrophage tumors (80,81). Recent technical advances of this model have allowed the induction of transplantable CML-like disease in 100% of recipients (82,83).

EPIDEMIOLOGY AND ETIOLOGY

Approximately 5000 to 7000 patients are diagnosed with CML every year in the United States. The annual incidence is 1 to 2 cases per 100,000 individuals. CML accounts for approximately 15% of all leukemias and 7% to 20% of adult leukemias. The incidence has not changed over the last fifty years (30,65,84–86). CML affects male individuals more often than female individuals (ratio of 1.3 to 2.2:1) (30,65,87). The median age at presentation is 45 to 55 years (30,65). The incidence increases with age; 30% of patients are older than 60 years in some studies (30,85), although this figure was 12% in studies of investigational agents in study groups referred to tertiary centers (65,88). This could be due to earlier detection by routine peripheral blood analysis, better exclusion of other myeloproliferative syndromes by cytogenetic and molecular analysis, or selection or referral patterns for investigational strategies (65). In the recent studies with imatinib mesylate, the median age of the study group was 57 years (89,90). Although the disease can be observed in all age groups, it comprises less than 5% of pediatric leukemias. There are no familial, ethnic, or social associations.

What promotes the development of CML is unknown. Leukemogenesis, like all neoplastic processes, is a multistep phenomenon divided into initiation, promotion, and progression phases. The initiation phase involves acquisition of a genetic defect that confers the cell survival advantage. What triggers the generation of the initiation step is unknown. In experiments in which leukemic cell lines were exposed to γ-irradiation (91), fusion genes characteristic of leukemia were induced, although these defects were also detected at a low level in untreated cells. There is no evidence supporting hereditary genetic factors: BCR-ABL is only found in hematopoietic cells, and there is no increased incidence in monozygotic twins or in relatives of patients with CML (92). The incidence of CML is higher in survivors of the atomic bomb or nuclear exposures, as well as following ionizing radiation (93,94). No chemical or infectious exposures have been linked to CML (65). Assuming that the generation of *BCR-ABL* is the key molecular event leading to CML, what induces this molecular rearrangement is still unknown. Using molecular techniques that amplify detection of *BCR-ABL* in $1/10^8$ cells, transcripts were detected in marrow cells of 25% to 30% of healthy volunteers (95,96). This raises several questions: (a) the dormancy of CML or other cancers or their clonal burnout in many cases; (b) the role of the host immune system in controlling cancerous events; and (c) the definition of cure (functional, molecular) in the presence of minimal residual disease.

CLINICAL FEATURES

CML follows a biphasic or triphasic course. The initial chronic phase is followed by an intermediate accelerated phase that

TABLE 13-1. Chronologic Evolution of Clinical Presentation of Patients with Ph-Positive Chronic Phase Chronic Myelogenous Leukemia (M. D. Anderson Cancer Center Experience)

Characteristic	Category	Percentage with Characteristic			
		Before 1980 (n = 334)	1981–1990 (n = 494)	1991–Present (n = 797)	p Value
Age (yr)	≥60	18	12	17	.016
Asymptomatic at diagnosis	Yes	16	46	40	.0001
Splenomegaly	Yes	65	55	45	.0001
Hepatomegaly	Yes	35	27	9	.0001
Hemoglobin (g/dL)	<10	26	23	15	.0001
White blood cell count (×10^9/L)	>99	62	55	49	.001
Platelet count (×10^9/L)	>700	21	19	13	.002
Peripheral blasts	Yes	69	53	47	.0001
Peripheral basophils (%)	>6	13	13	13	Not significant
Marrow blasts (%)	>4	10	7	5	.018
Marrow basophils (%)	>3	36	32	25	.001

eventually terminally transforms into the blastic phase. At diagnosis, more than 90% of patients are in chronic phase; approximately 80% first evolve into the accelerated phase before developing the blastic phase (65). Presenting features are changing in time due to earlier diagnosis—a result of routine physical examinations and blood testing. For example, the incidence of asymptomatic presentation in chronic phase has increased from 15% to approximately 40% to 50%. Features of increased tumor burden or aggressive disease (splenomegaly, basophilia, high-risk presentation) are also decreasing (Table 13-1) (88). Symptoms at presentation are often due to anemia or splenomegaly and include fatigue and left upper abdominal pain or mass (97). Less common presentations relate to a hypermetabolic state with fever, anorexia, weight loss, or gout or to consequences of platelet dysfunction such as hemorrhage, ecchymosis, hematomas, or thromboembolic events. Retinal hemorrhages are not uncommon (98). Findings of hyperleukocytosis and hyperviscosity include priapism reported in 1% of patients (99), tinnitus, stupor, and cerebrovascular accidents. On physical examination, palpable splenomegaly is present in 50% to 80% and hepatomegaly in 10%

to 20%. Manifestations of extramedullary hematopoiesis such as subcutaneous lesions or lymphadenopathy are rare and identify a subgroup with poor prognosis (88,100). Presenting features of CML are summarized in Table 13-1.

Cardinal features of accelerated phase are evidence of progressive maturation arrest with increased blasts and basophils, resistance to therapy, increased constitutional symptoms, progressive splenomegaly, cytogenetic clonal evolution, appearance of extramedullary disease, leukocytosis, and thrombocytosis or thrombocytopenia (65,101). Approximately 10% to 20% of patients die in accelerated phase (101), which usually lasts for 1.0 to 1.5 years (88). Table 13-2 summarizes accelerated and blastic phase criteria.

Patients who develop blastic phase are often symptomatic with weight loss, fever, night sweats, and bone pains, as well as infections and bleeding. Extramedullary hematopoiesis is also frequent, involving lymph nodes, skin, subcutaneous tissues, bone, and the central nervous system (30% of lymphoid blastic phase) (65). Fifty percent of the patients have myeloid, 25% have lymphoid, and 25% have undifferentiated or other rare blastic phenotypes (megakaryocytic, erythroid, basophilic) (65,102). Lymphoid blastic phase is more frequent in younger patients (40% if age is <40 years). Chemotherapy response rates (60% vs. 20%) are better with lymphoid compared with myeloid blastic phase (median survival, 9 months vs. 3 months), as are median survivals (9 to 12 months vs. 2 to 3 months).

TABLE 13-2. Features and Definitions of Accelerated and Blastic Phase Chronic Myelogenous Leukemia (CML)

Blastic phase CML
  30% or more marrow or peripheral blasts
  Extramedullary hematopoiesis with immature blasts
Accelerated phase CML
  Multivariate analysis–derived criteria
    Peripheral blasts 15% or more
    Peripheral blasts + promyelocytes 30% or more
    Peripheral basophils 20% or more
    Platelets <100 × 10^9/L unrelated to therapy
    Cytogenetic clonal evolution
  Criteria commonly used in clinical practice
    Marrow or peripheral blasts 10% or more
    Marrow or peripheral basophils and eosinophils 20% or more
    Frequent Pelger-Huët–like neutrophils nucleated red cells or megakaryocytic nuclear fragments
    Increased marrow reticulin or collagen fibrosis
    Leukocytosis (>50 × 10^9/L), anemia (hematocrit <25%), thrombocytopenia (<100 × 10^9/L) not responsive to antileukemic therapy
    Marked thrombocytosis (>1000 × 10^9/L)
    Progressive splenomegaly unresponsive to therapy
    Unexplained fever or bone pain
    Requirement of increased doses of medication

Adapted from Faderl S, Talpaz M, Estrov Z, et al. The biology of chronic myeloid leukemia. *N Engl J Med* 1999;341(3):164–172; and Kantarjian HM, Deisseroth A, Kurzrock R, et al. Chronic myelogenous leukemia: a concise update. *Blood* 1993;82(3):691–703.

LABORATORY CHARACTERISTICS

The most common feature in chronic phase is leukocytosis; 50% to 70% present with white blood cell (WBC) counts greater than 100×10^9/L (39). Cyclic variations in the WBC counts have been described in 10% to 20% of patients (97), attesting that CML, unlike other cancers, may remain under some regulatory control process. This may explain its response to immune approaches such as donor lymphocyte infusions (DLIs). These cyclic patterns are difficult to control with hydroxyurea. Thrombocytosis is observed in 30% to 50% of patients, occasionally at levels higher than 1000×10^6/L. Platelet aggregation abnormalities are frequent (65). Anemia (hemoglobin <10 g/dL) is observed in 20%. WBC differential shows myeloid cells in all stages of maturation. Basophils and eosinophils may be increased (101,103) (Fig. 13-3). The leukocyte alkaline phosphatase score is low, which may differentiate CML from other myeloproliferative disorders (104). The bone marrow is hypercellular with an elevated myeloid to erythroid ratio of 10:1 to 30:1 (105) (Fig. 13-3). Megakaryocytes are also increased, and Gaucher-like cells and sea-blue histiocytes

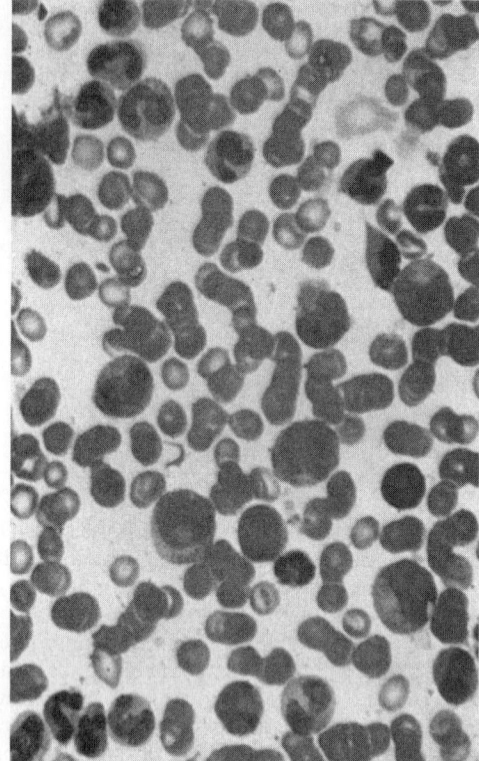 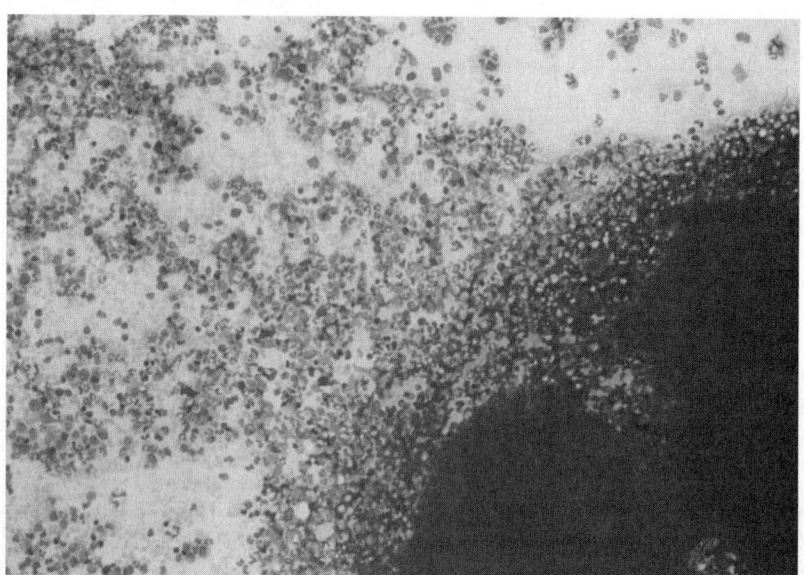

Figure 13-3. Photomicrographs of a blood peripheral smear **(A)** and bone marrow aspiration **(B)** from a patient with chronic myelogenous leukemia. The peripheral blood smear reveals the presence of multiple mature and immature myeloid forms and an increased number of eosinophils and basophils. Bone marrow is hypercellular, with excess myeloid precursors, megakaryocytes, and mild fibrosis.

are observed in 10% of cases. Grades 3 to 4 reticulin stain–measured myelofibrosis is found in 40% of cases (106) and may be associated with worse prognosis. Giemsa stain–measured fibrosis is rare and, when present, suggests transformation.

Different accelerated phase criteria are shown in Table 13-2. Increased number of blasts (15% or more), blasts and promyelocytes (30% or more), and basophils (20% or more) in the blood or marrow; thrombocytopenia unrelated to therapy; and cytogenetic clonal evolution have been defined by multivariate analysis to predict for a survival of 1.5 years or less. Criteria commonly used based on current practices to define accelerated phase include blasts (10% or more), blasts and promyelocytes (20% or more), myelofibrosis, and nucleated red cells (101).

The *blastic phase* is defined by the presence of 30% or more blasts or extramedullary blastic infiltrates. *Lymphoid blastic origin* is defined by a negative peroxidase stain, positive terminal deoxynucleotidyl transferase, and the expression of pre–B-cell markers, including CD19, CD20, and the common acute lymphoid leukemia antigen, CD10. Most such patients (80%) also express myeloid markers.

PROGNOSTIC FACTORS AND RISK GROUPS

The clinical course of CML patients is heterogeneous. With hydroxyurea or busulfan therapy, the median survival is 3.0 to 4.2 years (107), and the risk of death is 10% to 12% in the first 2 years and 15% to 25% subsequently (108).

Consistent pretreatment-poor prognostic factors for survival include the presence of splenomegaly, hepatomegaly, older age, leukocytosis, increased blast or basophil counts, thrombocytosis or thrombocytopenia, and cytogenetic clonal evolution.

Several multivariate-derived prognostic models and staging systems have been proposed (Table 13-3). These models are

helpful in defining individual prognosis, assigning patients to different strategies based on risk, evaluating the effects of newer therapies, and comparing the relative benefits of existing therapies (IFN-α, allogeneic SCT) within risk groups (108–114). The percentage of patients in good, intermediate, and poor risk categories has varied in different study groups. The median survival ranges were 50 to 60 months, 36 to 40 months, and 24 to 30 months, respectively, with chemotherapy. With IFN-α, the median survivals were 102 months, 80 to 95 months, and 45 to 60 months, respectively (115) (Table 13-3). A prognostic score has been developed by the European Collaborative CML Prognostic Factors Project Group (114) and recently updated (116). This

---

TABLE 13-3. Chronic Myelogenous Leukemia Characteristics Associated with Worse Prognosis

Older age (continuous variable, worse older than 60 yr)
Splenomegaly (continuous variable, worse greater than 10 cm)
Increased percentage of peripheral blasts (continuous variable, 3 or more in blood or 5 or more in marrow)
Thrombocytosis (worse over 700×10^9/L)
Increased percentage of basophil count (7 or more in blood, 3 or more in marrow)
Additional chromosomal abnormalities

Risk Group Distributions, Cytogenetic Responses, and Median Survivals		
Risk Group	**% Major Cytogenetic Response**	**Median Survival (mo)**
Good	46–52	102–204
Intermediate	32–38	82–95
Poor	14–26	47–62

score considers age, spleen size, and blast, eosinophil, basophil, and platelet counts as variables. Using this model, Hasford et al. have evaluated 1400 patients with CML treated with IFN-α. Forty-two percent of the patients were low risk, 45% were intermediate risk, and 13% were high risk. The 10-year survival rates were 42%, 18%, and 5%, respectively.

Response to IFN-α is a very powerful treatment-associated prognostic factor. Long-term survival rates in patients achieving a complete cytogenetic response are in excess of 80% (117–119). In the study by Hasford et al. (116), the 10-year survival rate of low-risk patients achieving complete or major cytogenetic responses in the first 21 months of therapy was 74% (116).

Several molecular markers have been investigated for their prognostic significance. The breakpoint location within M-BCR (3' vs. 5') and the corresponding messages (b3a2 vs. b2a2) were not prognostic for response or survival (120–122). However, large deletions at the t(9;22) breakpoint have been observed in a subgroup of patients (30%) and were associated with poor prognosis (123). Methylation of the Pa promoter of C-ABL has been associated with late chronic phase and with transformation but not with differences in response to IFN-α or with survival in early chronic phase (124,125). Telomere length, a marker of cell senescence, has also been associated with disease progression. Telomeres were shorter (a) in patients with CML compared with normal individuals, (b) in Ph-positive CML compared with Ph-negative CML (126), and (c) in transformation compared with chronic phase (126). Telomere shortening in chronic phase has been associated with faster progression to accelerated phase (127) and with increased risk of blastic transformation within 2 years (126). Expression of proteins of the interferon regulatory family—in particular, interferon regulatory factor 4—has been shown to be down-regulated in T cells from patients with CML and to predict for response to interferon treatment (128).

DIAGNOSTIC EVALUATION

Diagnosis is often suspected because of persistent unexplained leukocytosis, splenomegaly, or both. Workup includes a complete blood, differential, and platelet count to evaluate blastosis, basophilia, thrombocytosis, and thrombocytopenia and a marrow aspiration and biopsy to quantify the percentage of blasts and basophils and degree of fibrosis for cytogenetic analysis. Cytogenetic studies document the t(9;22)(q34;q11) or its variants in 90% of cases. Cytogenetic clonal evolution, a marker of disease progression, is found in 5% to 10% of patients at diagnosis. Ten percent of patients have morphologic features of CML but do not show Ph by cytogenetic studies; one-third of them are BCR-ABL–positive by molecular studies. Patients with true Ph-negative, BCR-ABL–negative CML have an intermediate prognosis between Ph-positive CML and chronic myelomonocytic leukemia with a median survival of 2.5 years (3,129). Genomic polymerase chain reaction (PCR) and Southern blot can detect the exact breakpoint. Reverse transcriptase PCR and Northern blot detect BCR-ABL transcripts, and antibodies against BCR or ABL detect the BCR-ABL protein. Occasionally, patients have p190 Ph-positive CML detectable by PCR but not by Southern blot analysis. Another rare entity, p230 CML, may manifest as Ph-positive, BCR-ABL–negative CML. Special attention to the PCR studies (specific primers) and protein analysis diagnoses p230 CML.

Monitoring Response to Therapy and Minimal Residual Disease

Several techniques can detect the Ph chromosome or its products at the DNA, RNA, or protein levels. Cytogenetic analysis remains the gold standard for the diagnosis of CML. The major advantage of conventional cytogenetics is the detection of other cytogenetic abnormalities, a marker of disease acceleration. Conventional cytogenetic analysis is limited by the number of metaphases analyzed (20 to 25 with a good harvest), is time consuming (12-hour technical work), and has a sensitivity of 1% to 5% (130). Cytogenetic analysis has a limited role in studying minimal residual disease, which is better evaluated with other techniques. Fluorescence *in situ* hybridization (FISH) is typically performed by cohybridization of a BCR, and ABL probes to denatured metaphase chromosomes or interphase nuclei. Applications of FISH, such as hypermetaphase FISH (H-FISH) and interphase FISH (I-FISH), have been developed. FISH techniques allow rapid evaluation ($1/2$ hour technical work) of several hundred cells (100 to 1000). H-FISH may detect persistent disease in patients in complete cytogenetic response and gives a precise measure of response (standard error of a measurement is <2%). A patient categorized to have 50% Ph-positive cells by routine cytogenetic analysis (10 of 20 metaphases) may have a response rate range of 35% to 65% (standard error ± 15%); by H-FISH, the measurement range is only 48% to 52% (131). The technique has a false positivity of less than 1% but requires bone marrow sampling. I-FISH allows the analysis of nondividing cells and does not depend on the cycling status of the cells (although this may not have relevance). Quantification of I-FISH is limited by the high rate of false-positives and -negatives (132) but can be performed on peripheral blood. Double-probe FISH (D-FISH) is a highly sensitive FISH procedure that uses two different probes, one for BCR and the other for ABL. This reduces the false-positive rates seen with I-FISH. D-FISH can be used to evaluate both blood and bone marrow (133). Table 13-4 summarizes the characteristics and uses of each technique.

Several molecular techniques can be used to detect the BCR-ABL gene. With Southern blot (134), restriction enzyme–digested genomic DNA is probed with a molecular probe encompassing the area of interest. The technique is limited by the amount of DNA required, the need to perform restriction enzyme digestion, and, in most laboratories, the use of radioactive reagents. False-positives and -negatives with Southern blot are rare but can occur due to changes in the size of the rearranged band. Southern blot measures the level of BCR-ABL positivity; results usually correspond with cytogenetic results. Southern blot has a low sensitivity and cannot be used to assess minimal residual disease (134). Its best use is in patients who are Ph-negative. It cannot be used to detect p190 or p230. BCR-ABL protein detection and quantification can be performed by Western blot analysis (135) through probing protein lysates, either from blood or bone marrow with an antibody against ABL, thus allowing the detection of the three BCR-ABL protein isoforms, although detection of p230[bcr-abl] is usually limited by its low expression level.

Other molecular techniques use PCR to detect BCR-ABL. PCR is the most sensitive technique: One Ph-positive cell can be detected in a background of 10^4 to 10^8 normal cells (136). PCR techniques are important to assess minimal residual disease in CML. Most studies have used PCR and a more sensitive variant known as *nested PCR*. Original studies involved patients postallogeneic SCT (137). In an analysis of 346 patients postallogeneic SCT, nested PCR positivity at 6 and 12 months posttransplantation significantly correlated with relapse (138). Not all studies were able to reproduce the prognostic significance of BCR-ABL positivity (139). Newer PCR techniques, including quantitative and real-time PCR, may allow rapid quantification of tumor burden (134). A recent report suggests that patients expressing p190[BCR-ABL] postallogeneic SCT have a higher relapse rate (140).

TABLE 13-4. Monitoring Chronic Myelogenous Leukemia Course and Detection of Minimal Residual Disease

Parameter	CG	I-FISH	D-FISH	H-FISH	Quantitative Polymerase Chain Reaction
N° cells analyzed	20–25	100–200	100–200	100–1000	>10,000
Technical time (hr)	12	<1	<1	<1	2–6
Current application	Frequent	Frequent	Rare	Rare	Rare
Detection of other chromosomal abnormalities	Yes	No	No	No	No
False-positive if true cytogenetic CR	NA	10%	1–5%	1%	NA
Precision of response estimation	±15%	±4%	±4%	±2%	NA
Overestimates response if 1005 Ph-positive	No	Yes	Yes	No	NA
Sample source	Marrow	Blood or marrow	Blood or marrow	Marrow	Blood or marrow
Best use	At diagnosis and every year	During therapy until Ph <10%	During therapy until Ph <10%	During therapy until Ph <10%	When Ph = 0%

CG, cytogenetics; CR, complete remission; D-FISH, double-probe fluorescent *in situ* hybridization; H-FISH, hypermetaphase fluorescent *in situ* hybridization; I-FISH, interphase fluorescent *in situ* hybridization; NA, not available; N°, number.

The molecular analysis of minimal residual disease in patients with CML treated with IFN-α is more complex. A competitive PCR (141) exploits a two-step reverse-transcriptase PCR procedure and the use of ABL amplification as an internal control. Patients with CML on IFN-α therapy who have a *BCR-ABL/ABL* ratio of 0.04% corresponded to those patients that had achieved complete cytogenetic responses, whereas patients who had partial, minor, or no cytogenetic responses had ratios of 7%, 21%, and 58%, respectively. A recent update of this analysis showed that a ratio level of 0.045% predicted for long-term event-free survival in patients in complete cytogenetic remission after IFN-α therapy (134,142). Table 13-5 summarizes the available tests to evaluate CML.

TABLE 13-5. Practical Guidelines to Diagnose and Monitor Chronic Myelogenous Leukemia (CML)

Test	Guidelines
Routine cytogenetic analysis	At diagnosis and every year
I-FISH	Pretreatment to have baseline percent of Ph-positive cells, then every 2–3 mo until Ph <10%.
D-FISH	As for I-FISH. Reliability for lack of false positivity when Ph 5–10% under investigation.
H-FISH	As for I-FISH. No false-positives; can be used when Ph <10%.
Southern blot	At diagnosis, particularly if patient has morphologic CML but is Ph-negative by routine cytogenetics; does not detect p190 or p230.
PCR quantification	Monitor minimal residual disease status in patients who are 0% Ph-positive; critical *BCR-ABL* to *ABL* ratio of 0.045 may be used for treatment decisions.[a]
Detection of p190 disease	Specific PCR primers.
Detection of p230 disease	Specific PCR primers.

D-FISH, double-probe fluorescence *in situ* hybridization; H-FISH, hypermetaphase fluorescence *in situ* hybridization; I-FISH, interphase fluorescent *in situ* hybridization; PCR, polymerase chain reaction.
[a] Data from Hochhaus A, Reiter A, Saussele S, et al. Molecular heterogeneity in complete cytogenetic responders after interferon-alpha therapy for chronic myelogenous leukemia: low levels of minimal residual disease are associated with continuing remission. *Blood* 2000;95:62–66.

TREATMENT OF CHRONIC MYELOGENOUS LEUKEMIA

Treatment of CML depends on the phase of disease, patient age, and risk group. With hydroxyurea and busulfan, the standard of care before the 1980s, the median survival was 3 years; fewer than 20% of patients survived more than 5 years. With modern approaches, the median survival is 5 to 7 years and 9 years in good-risk patients. The survival rates at 10 years are 30% to 50% (143).

Historic Perspective, Busulfan, and Hydroxyurea

Arsenicals, such as Fowler's solution, were used in CML therapy in the nineteenth century. Radiation therapy became the standard of care in the 1920s until the discovery of the efficacy of busulfan in the 1950s. Busulfan, an oral alkylating agent (144), provided long-term effective hematologic control but was associated with pulmonary toxicity, organ fibrosis, Addison's-like disease, and delayed and prolonged myelosuppression. Marrow terminal fibrosis (burn-out marrow) was not uncommon with this therapy, occurring in 20% to 30% of patients as a terminal phase. Introduced in the early 1970s, hydroxyurea, a cell cycle–specific inhibitor of DNA synthesis, gradually replaced busulfan as the treatment of choice for CML (145). Both agents can induce hematologic response rates of 50% to 80%, but cytogenetic responses are rare, and neither drug changes significantly the natural history of the disease (88). Hydroxyurea provides tighter control of the counts, whereas busulfan has to be discontinued when the WBC count reaches $20 \times 10^9/L$ because of potential delayed prolonged myelosuppression. Therefore, achievement of complete hematologic response (CHR) is better with hydroxyurea, explaining perhaps its better results compared with busulfan. Busulfan is usually given at 2 to 8 mg orally daily until the WBC count is reduced to $20 \times 10^9/L$; it is then discontinued and the patient observed until the WBC count rises above 40 to $50 \times 10^9/L$, at which time a subsequent course is instituted. Busulfan should not be used except in rare instances. Patients allergic to or intolerant of hydroxyurea may be controlled with 6-mercaptopurine or 6-thioguanine rather than busulfan. Hydroxyurea is usually given at an appropriate dose to keep the WBC count between 2 and $5 \times 10^9/L$. For patients presenting with a WBC above $100 \times 10^9/L$, hydroxyurea may be started at 5 to 8 g daily and the dose reduced by 50% for each 50% reduction of counts. A general

TABLE 13-6. Results of Allogeneic Stem Cell Transplantation in First Chronic Phase Chronic Myelogenous Leukemia (CML)

Reference	No. of Patients	Category	Percentage Survival/Disease-Free Survival (yr)	Percentage Mortality (yr)
German CML group (214)	137	Related	63/NS (3)	23 TRM (1)
	99	MUD	NS/NS	28 TRM (1)
	389	Interferon-α	78/NS (3)	NA
NMDP (180)	914	MUD	NS/43 (3)	<35 yr: 37% (5)
				>35 yr: 53% (5)
Morton (166)	184	MUD	45/NS (5)	55 (5)
Snyder (267)	94	Related	73/64 (5)	27 (5)
Clift (153)	142	Related	80/69 (3)	20 (3)
Clift (268)	116	Related	60–66/58–66 (4)	40–42 (4)
Biggs (269)	62	Related	58 (3)	22 TRM (1)
van Rhee (156)	373	Related	64/59 (1)	36 TRM (1)
Bortin (270)	1426	Related	NS/45 (5)	NS
Goldman (149)	450	Related	NS/45–61 (3)	33–55 (3)
Gratwohl (151)	947	Related	47/34 (8)	42 TRM (5)

MUD, matched-unrelated donor; NA, not available; NS, not significant; related, HLA-related donor; TRM, transplant-related mortality.

schedule would be 4 g daily for a WBC count of 60 to $100 \times 10^9/$L; 3 g daily for a WBC count of 40 to $60 \times 10^9/L$; 2 g daily for a WBC count of 20 to $40 \times 10^9/L$; 1 g daily for a WBC count of 10 to $20 \times 10^9/L$; and 0.5 to 1.0 g daily for a WBC count less than 10 $\times 10^9/L$. Hydroxyurea is an excellent initial tumor debulking agent and can be used later in combination with or in between more definitive therapies. In one randomized study comparing hydroxyurea and busulfan (146), the median survival (58 months vs. 45 months, $p = .008$) and median duration of chronic phase (47 months vs. 37 months) were superior with hydroxyurea. A metaanalysis of five other trials supported the benefit of hydroxyurea over busulfan (147). The outcome of allogeneic SCT is worse in patients previously exposed to busulfan (148,149).

Allogeneic Stem Cell Transplantation

Allogeneic SCT is an effective and curative form of therapy in chronic phase CML. Allogeneic SCT can prolong survival and cure a subgroup of selected patients with suitable donors. Projected actuarial 3- to 5-year survival rates range from 40% to 80%. Transplant-related mortality (TRM) ranges from 15% to 68%, depending on patient age, whether the donor is related or unrelated, the degree of matching (molecular), cytomegalovirus (CMV) status, patient and donor gender, and, perhaps, the antifungal prophylaxis, preparative regimen, and institutional expertise (Table 13-6). Most recent studies report 3- to 5-year survival rates of 50% to 60% with relapse rates less than 20%. The risk of relapse plateaus at 5 to 7 years posttransplantation (150). The two most significant factors influencing transplantation outcome negatively are older age and advanced phase of disease. Patients younger than 30 years have an excellent outcome, with disease-free survival rates of 60% to 70%, TRM rates of less than 10%, and relapse rates of 20%. Beyond age 30, the outcome worsens gradually as the TRM increases. Results from large series report 5-year survival rates of 30% in patients older than 50 years. Results of the European Bone Marrow Transplantation Registry (EBMTR) observed a TRM of 47% and a 5-year disease-free survival (DFS) of 25% in patients older than 45 years (151). Recent studies have reported better results. For example, some centers report 2-year estimated survival rates of 80% in carefully selected patients older than 50 years (152). Patients transplanted in chronic phase CML have an estimated DFS of 40% to 60%, compared with 15% when transplanted in blastic phase (88,149). Patients whose only criteria for acceleration is clonal evolution have a favorable prognosis when trans-

planted, with a DFS of 60% (153). Based on these data, most transplant centers recommend transplantation in early chronic phase (154). However, several recent updates show little difference in long-term outcome among patients transplanted in the first 12 months after diagnosis, compared with those transplanted during the first 24 months (155,156).

Other factors that influence transplant outcome include choice of pretransplant chemotherapy, preparative regimens, graft-versus-host disease (GVHD) prophylaxis, CMV status, and molecular matching in the setting of unrelated donor transplant. Patients treated with hydroxyurea pretransplant have a higher 3-year leukemia-free survival than those treated with busulfan (61% vs. 45%, $p = .0003$) (149). The use of IFN-α before transplantation did not negatively influence the outcome of matched related allogeneic SCT in seven of eight series (157–165) or the outcome of unrelated allogeneic SCT in 3 of 4 studies (158,159,162,164–166), provided that it was discontinued for at least 3 months before transplant in one study (164). The Seattle experience with unrelated transplant indicated a higher incidence of GVHD and mortality in patients treated with IFN-α for longer than 6 months before unrelated transplant. A recent analysis of the International Bone Marrow Transplant Registry (IBMTR) experience analyzed 740 patients who underwent unrelated transplant, 65% of whom were exposed to IFN-α before SCT. By multivariate analysis, IFN-α had no effect on survival, DFS, TRM, engraftment, or chronic GVHD. This was regardless of whether IFN-α was for less or more than 6 months, or whether it was discontinued within or longer than 3 months before transplant (167). Thus, literature evidence does not support an adverse effect of IFN-α before allogeneic SCT, whether in the setting of related or unrelated donor transplant.

Toxicity from preparative regimens is observed in 100% of patients. Severe oral mucositis occurs in 50% of patients (168,169). Preparative regimens of busulfan with cyclophosphamide or cyclophosphamide with total body irradiation (TBI) are commonly used, but the former has better toxicity profiles. Recent reports suggest that outcome is superior for cyclophosphamide-TBI in patients with acute myelogenous leukemia (AML) in first complete remission (170) and that the incidence of venoocclusive disease of the liver is less frequent (171). An update of 4 randomized trials comparing both combinations (172) has shown that death rates and late pulmonary toxicities are similar for the TBI-containing programs compared with the busulfan, but that patients treated with TBI had a higher incidence of cataract formation and avascular necrosis. Intravenous busulfan may be safer than oral busulfan because of better control of its pharmacokinetics (173,174). The incidence of severe acute and extensive chronic GVHD (most associated with mortality and morbidity) varies with patient age, degree of donor matching, preparative regimens, and GVHD prophylaxis. Overall, acute GVHD occurs in 8% to 63% of patients and is the cause of death in 13% (149). Chronic GVHD occurs in 75% of patients, and its associated mortality is 10%. Methotrexate, cyclosporine, and prednisone combinations are commonly used to prevent GVHD and are superior to single agents (175). Another strategy used to minimize GVHD includes the use of T-cell–depleted grafts, which improve TRM and transplant tolerance but increase rates of relapse and secondary lymphoproliferative disorders (176,177). The increased relapse associated with T-cell–depleted grafts demonstrates the graft-versus-leukemia effect in CML. This is further confirmed by the activity of DLIs as a salvage therapy in patients who relapse posttransplant, with response rates of 60% to 80% and 3-year DFS rates of 40% to 85% (178).

Another important problem associated with allogeneic SCT is the development of secondary malignancies posttransplantation (179). In a report from the National Marrow Donor Program (180), 41 patients (2.8%) who had received unrelated donor SCT had developed a second malignancy, 30 of which were B-cell lymphoproliferative disorders. These occurred at a median of 3 months posttransplant and were observed more frequently in patients treated with TBI or receiving a T-cell–depleted graft. Mortality with lymphoproliferative disorders was 80% (24 of 30).

The most common causes of mortality posttransplant are acute GVHD (2% to 13%) (150); chronic GVHD (8% to 10%) (150); interstitial pneumonitis (4% to 32%); opportunistic infections (3% to 24%); venoocclusive disease (1% to 4%); and resistant relapse (5% to 10%). Long-term posttransplant sequelae also include infertility and cataracts (150).

SALVAGE TREATMENT POSTTRANSPLANTATION

Patients who relapse postallogeneic SCT do not have a very adverse outcome as previously thought. In fact, the survival rates postallogeneic SCT are different from DFS rates because of effective salvage therapies including DLI. This led investigators to propose alternate measures of outcome, including overall DFS postallogeneic SCT plus salvage therapies (181). In such a review of the experience, the initial DFS rate was 36%, the overall DFS rate was 49%, and the overall survival rate was 61% (181). Salvage strategies postallogeneic SCT relapse include DLI, which is currently the most successful approach but is associated with recurrence of GVHD, myelosuppression, and procedure-related mortality. Incremental DLI dosing may alleviate some of these problems. Other strategies include IFN-α with or without ara-C, second transplant if the time to relapse is longer than 1 to 2 years, and the use of imatinib mesylate. Although experience with the latter agent is minimal, it may soon be quite effective alone or in combination with IFN-α, ara-C, or low-dose DLI.

Relapses posttransplant can be classified as hematologic, cytogenetic, or molecular. In a retrospective analysis of the EBMTR (182), 42% of evaluable patients relapsed cytogenetically, 27% relapsed hematologically in chronic phase, and 31% relapsed in accelerated or blastic phase. Sixty-four percent of cytogenetic relapses progressed to hematologic relapse after a median of 8 months. The actuarial 5-year survival rate was 34%. IFN-α, DLI, and second allogeneic SCT were successful in inducing second cytogenetic remissions in these patients. Salvage allogeneic SCT has been performed in relapsed transplanted patients with a reported DFS of 30% (183). Outcome of patients receiving a second transplant is better for those with a long first remission (184).

MATCHED UNRELATED DONOR TRANSPLANT

One limitation of allogeneic SCT is the availability of related donors. HLA-compatible unrelated donors can now be found in 50% of patients who lack a related donor. Median time from donor search to transplant is 3 to 6 months. The use of unrelated donors is associated with a higher morbidity and mortality (185,186). More than 50% of mortality associated with unrelated allogeneic SCT is secondary to acute and chronic GVHD. The National Marrow Donor Program has recently updated its results of unrelated allogeneic SCT in CML (180). Of more than 7000 searches, 23% were successful, translating into 1423 unrelated transplants. Early and late graft failure occurred in 17% of cases, grades III to IV acute GVHD in 33%, and extensive chronic GVHD in 60%. Relapse rate at 3 years was 6%, and DFS was 43%. The best results with unrelated allogeneic SCT were noted in patients younger than 30 years with transplant in early chronic phase, with CMV seronegative status, and with non-T-cell–depleted grafts (185). CMV seropositivity has been reported to be the most important factor influencing survival and TRM in unrelated SCT (187). Molecular matching is a major and underestimated factor, which influences outcome significantly: Matching at the HLA-DRB1 locus is the most significant factor influencing overall survival, DFS, and TRM. TRM in HLA-DRB1 mismatches was 80%. Patients matched at HLA-DRB1 transplanted in first chronic phase, and those receiving non-T-cell–depleted grafts had a 2-year survival of 51%, a TRM of 47%, and a relapse rate of 2% (188). Table 13-6 summarizes allogeneic SCT results.

NONMYELOABLATIVE PREPARATIVE REGIMENS

In an attempt to expand the indications of allogeneic SCT to older patients, investigators have resorted to nonablative regimens, currently referred to as "transplant-lite," "mini-SCT," or "nonablative" regimens. The rationale behind these approaches is that nonablative regimens result in less host antigenic exposure and, thus, fewer GVHD complications. Eradication of tumor does not rely on the ablation of the preparative regimen but rather on the graft-versus-leukemia effect produced by the expansion of the engrafted donor lymphocytes. Several preparative regimens have been proposed, which rely on immunosuppressive therapy to allow for donor cell engraftment (fludarabine, low-dose TBI, others). Early results of nonablative regimens in patients not eligible for standard transplant (older age, organ dysfunctions, others) are showing acceptable degrees of engraftment, less GVHD and mortality, and feasibility in older groups (age 60 years or older) but also more persistence or recurrence of disease, which may be handled with incremental DLI or other salvage approaches (i.e., imatinib mesylate). A recent report of the EBMTR has shown a 1-year survival of 65% and a TRM of 35% in 46 patients treated with nonablative allogeneic SCT in first chronic phase (189).

Principles of New Therapies in Chronic Myelogenous Leukemia

Investigational strategies in CML targeted suppression of Ph-positive CML cells (115) or the molecular consequences of the BCR-ABL abnormality or associated molecular events. Evidence to support these investigations was (a) the pathophysiologic association of BCR-ABL to development of CML, as demonstrated by the recapitulation of human CML-like disease following transfection of Ph-associated BCR-ABL molecular abnormalities in animal models (47,81); (b) the reduction of CML burden in preclinical models through suppression of BCR-ABL; and (c) the association between the achievement of minimal residual disease (complete hematologic response, cytogenetic response) and improved survival in CML (118,119,190–192) (Table 13-7).

TABLE 13-7. Minimal Residual Burden and Survival with Interferon-α Therapy

| Reference | Survival Advantage with Achievement of | |
	Complete Hematologic Response	Cytogenetic Response
MDACC (118)	Yes	Yes
Ozer (271)	Not done	No
Mahon (272)	Yes	Yes
ICSG-CML (119)	Yes	Yes
Hehlmann (190)	Yes	Trend
Allan (191)	Yes	Yes
Ohnishi (197)	Not done	Trend
Guilhot (117)	Yes	Yes

Interferon-α

Interferons are naturally occurring proteins produced by eukaryotic cells in response to multiple stimuli. Based on their structural and functional characteristics, they are divided into IFN-α, -β, and -γ. IFN-α is the most commonly used interferon in hematologic malignancies. IFN-γ has minimal activity in CML. Their mechanisms of action are not well defined but may include antiproliferative effects, regulation of cell adhesion, immunomodulation, and antiangiogenesis.

Single-agent IFN-α therapy has been used in different schedules. The M. D. Anderson Cancer Center (MDACC) studies advocated IFN-α at 5 MU/m^2 daily or the maximally tolerated dose. Most other cooperative groups have used lower dose schedules of 3 to 5 MU daily or three times weekly. Two ongoing studies are comparing lower versus higher dose schedules of IFN-α. Although there may be a dose response association, toxicity is also worse with higher doses, particularly in older patients. The differences in hematologic and cytogenetic response rates may be due to differences in the study group characteristics, risk groups, physician practices, patient enthusi-

asm and compliance, and dose schedule used. The median survivals with IFN-α therapy have ranged from 56 to 89 months. The initial IFN-α studies at MDACC showed CHR rates of 80%, cytogenetic response rates (Ph-positive cell reduction to ≤90%) of 58% [major 38% (Ph-positive, <35%), complete 26% (Ph-positive, 0%)], and a median survival of 89 months. Among good-risk patients (50% of total), the major cytogenetic response rate was 50% and the median survival was 102 months (115). Achieving a major cytogenetic response was associated with a greater than 80% 8- to 10-year survival rate (118,193). Most patients in long-term complete cytogenetic remission (Ph-positive, 0%) continued to have detectable *BCR-ABL* transcripts (194). Other large-scale studies with IFN-α have reported CHR rates of 50% to 80% and cytogenetic response rates of 20% to 50%. Achieving a complete hematologic or cytogenetic response with IFN-α is an independent favorable prognostic factor for survival (Table 13-7). The response rates and duration of survival with single-agent IFN-α are shown in Table 13-8.

Several randomized studies have compared IFN-α to conventional therapy with hydroxyurea or busulfan. In most studies, IFN-α was associated with significantly higher response rates and longer survival. A metaanalysis confirmed the benefit of IFN-α survival by risk group (147). These studies are summarized in Table 13-8. IFN-α toxicity is well described. Management of IFN-α side effects has been reviewed (195). The only absolute contraindication to its use is history of major depression. Overall, 16% to 25% of patients do not tolerate IFN-α administration, and 50% require dose reductions (115,119,196). Early side effects include fever, chills, headache, postnasal drip, and anorexia. These symptoms are usually not dose limiting and abate once tachyphylaxis develops after the first 1 or 2 weeks of therapy. Chronic side effects include fatigue, depression, insomnia, weight loss, reduced libido, and impotence (117,119,190,191,197). Some of these symptoms can be managed by administering IFN-α at bedtime, premedicating with acetaminophen, gradually escalating the dose of IFN-α at the initiation of therapy, and reducing the WBC count to the 10 to 20 ×

TABLE 13-8. Results of Interferon (IFN)-α in Early Chronic Phase Chronic Myelogenous Leukemia (CML)

| Reference | Treatment | No. | Complete Hematologic Response | Cytogenetic Response | | | Median Survival (mo) |
				Any	Major	Complete	
Single-agent IFN-α							
MDACC (118)	IFN	274	80	56	38	26	89
Mahon (272)	IFN	52	81	—	44	38	—
Alimena (273)	IFN	65	46	55	12	—	—
Ozer (271)	IFN	107	59	—	29	13	66
Randomized Studies							
ICSG-CML (119)	IFN	218	62	55	19.0	8.0	72
	Chemotherapy	104	53	34	1.0	0.0	52
Hehlmann (190)	IFN	133	31	18	10.0	7.0	66
	BUS	186	23	4	1.0	0.0	45
	HU	194	39	5	1.5	1.0	56
Allan (191)	IFN	293	68	22	11.0	6.0	61
	Chemotherapy	294	—	—	—	—	41
Ohnishi (197)	IFN	80	39	44	7.5	9.0	65+
	BUS	79	54	29	2.5	2.5	50
Cumulative Data on IFN-α from Nine Studies							
	IFN	1632	60	—	22	14	57[a]

BUS, busulfan; HU, hydroxyurea.
[a]Data taken from reference 147.

10^9/L level with hydroxyurea before starting IFN-α (88). Neurotoxicity is observed more commonly in patients older than 60 years or in patients with psychiatric problems (198). Neuropsychiatric side effects include lack of concentration, depression, psychosis, and dysautonomia. Autoimmune phenomena have been described in less than 5% of patients, including hemolytic anemia, thrombocytopenia, Raynaud's phenomenon, collagen vascular disorders, hypothyroidism, and nephrotic syndrome. Discontinuation of therapy is mandated in patients who develop cardiac arrhythmias, congestive heart failure, severe autoimmune phenomena, severe neurotoxicity, refractory depression, and pulmonary complications (199).

IFN-α can induce abortions in monkeys (200). Although its teratogenic potential has not been demonstrated, its use should be avoided during pregnancy because of its antiproliferative and antiangiogenic effects. Pregnant patients with CML are usually treated with leukopheresis during the first trimester of pregnancy and with hydroxyurea during the last 6 months.

Interferon-α and Low-dose Cytosine Arabinoside in Chronic Phase Chronic Myelogenous Leukemia

The rationale for combining IFN-α and low-dose ara-C includes (a) the selective *in vitro* suppression of CML cells versus normal with ara-C (201); (b) cytogenetic responses obtained with single-agent ara-C in 7 of 9 patients (202,203); and (c) the pilot studies of IFN-α plus ara-C in late chronic phase CML, which established the safety and efficacy of the combination (204). Several single-arm trials of IFN-α plus ara-C have been conducted (205,206) in early chronic phase, as well as randomized studies of IFN-α plus ara-C versus IFN-α. Two schedules of ara-C were used: (a) ara-C subcutaneously (s.c.), 10 to 20 mg/m² daily for 7 to 21 days every 4 to 6 weeks, and (b) ara-C, 10 mg s.c. daily. Daily low-dose ara-C combinations with IFN-α may be more effective and easier to manage than intermittent higher dose schedules given for 7 to 10 days every month. With IFN-α, 5 MU/m² daily, and ara-C, 10 mg s.c. daily, CHR was achieved in 92% of patients, and a cytogenetic response was achieved in 74%: major in 50% and complete in 31% (Table 13-9). The median IFN-α dose was 3.7 MU/m² daily, and the median ara-C dose was 7.5 mg daily. The CHR rate was higher with IFN-α and daily ara-C, compared with IFN-α and intermittent ara-C or IFN-α alone (92% vs. 84% vs. 80%, p = .01), as were the rates of cytogenetic response (74% vs. 73% vs. 58%, p = .003) and major cytogenetic response (50% vs. 38% vs. 38%, p = .06). The median time to achievement of major cytogenetic response was also significantly shorter (7 months vs. 10 months vs. 12 months, p <.01). Results of other combination schedules of IFN-α and low-dose ara-C were also reported by others (206–208) (Table 13-9). In most studies, there was a trend for higher response rates with the combination compared with IFN-α alone.

Two randomized trials comparing IFN-α plus ara-C with IFN-α have so far been reported. In a French multicenter trial in CML, Guilhot et al. randomized patients to IFN-α alone, 5 MU/m² daily (n = 361), or IFN-α plus low-dose ara-C, 20 mg/m² daily for 10 days every month (n = 360) (117). IFN-α plus ara-C was associated with a significantly higher CHR rate at 6 months (66% vs. 55%, p <.01); a higher cytogenetic response rate at 12 months, overall (61% vs. 50%) and major (38% vs. 26%, p <.01); and significantly better survival (5-year rate 70% vs. 60%, p = .02). A landmark analysis at 2 years showed an association of cytogenetic response with survival: The 7-year survival rate was 85% with complete or partial cytogenetic response, 62% with minor cytogenetic response, and 25% for others. Cytogenetic response, whether obtained with IFN-α alone or with IFN-α plus ara-C, translated into significant survival prolongation.

The Italian Cooperative Study Group on CML also randomized patients to similar schedules of IFN-α plus ara-C versus IFN-α. Among 540 evaluable patients, 275 received IFN-α and ara-C, and 265 received IFN-α alone. So far, the combination of IFN-α plus ara-C has demonstrated superior response rates to IFN-α alone (209). The 6-month CHR rates were 87% versus 80%; the cytogenetic response rates were 48% versus 44%; the major cytogenetic response rates were 28% versus 19%, p = .01; and the complete cytogenetic response rates were 14% versus 7%, respectively. The survival rates appear to be similar, but longer follow-up and more mature analysis are needed before a final assessment of the benefit of adding ara-C can be made. In both the French and Italian studies, ara-C was given for only 12 and 8 months, respectively. Daily ara-C schedules may reduce toxicities (mucositis, diarrhea), provide fewer interruptions of treatment because of myelosuppression, and allow more extended treatment durations with ara-C.

A novel oral prodrug analog of ara-C, YNK01, has been developed. In combination with IFN-α, this agent has shown activity in advanced CML (210) and in newly diagnosed patients

TABLE 13-9. Combination Interferon (IFN)-α and Cytosine Arabinoside (ara-C)

Reference	No. of Patients	Complete Hematologic Response	Cytogenetic Response (%)	
			Major	Complete
Single-arm studies				
MDACC (204)				
Daily ara-C	134	94	50	31
Intermittent ara-C	54	84	38	20
Arthur (207)	30	93	53	30
Thaler (206)	84	54	25	18
Silver (274)	88	72	51	15
Randomized Studies				
Guilhot (117)				
IFN + ara-C	360	66	38	15
IFN	361	55	26	9
ICSG-CML (209)				
IFN + ara-C	275	87	28	14
IFN	265	80	19	7

TREATMENT ALGORITHMS OF PATIENTS WITH EARLY CHRONIC PHASE CML

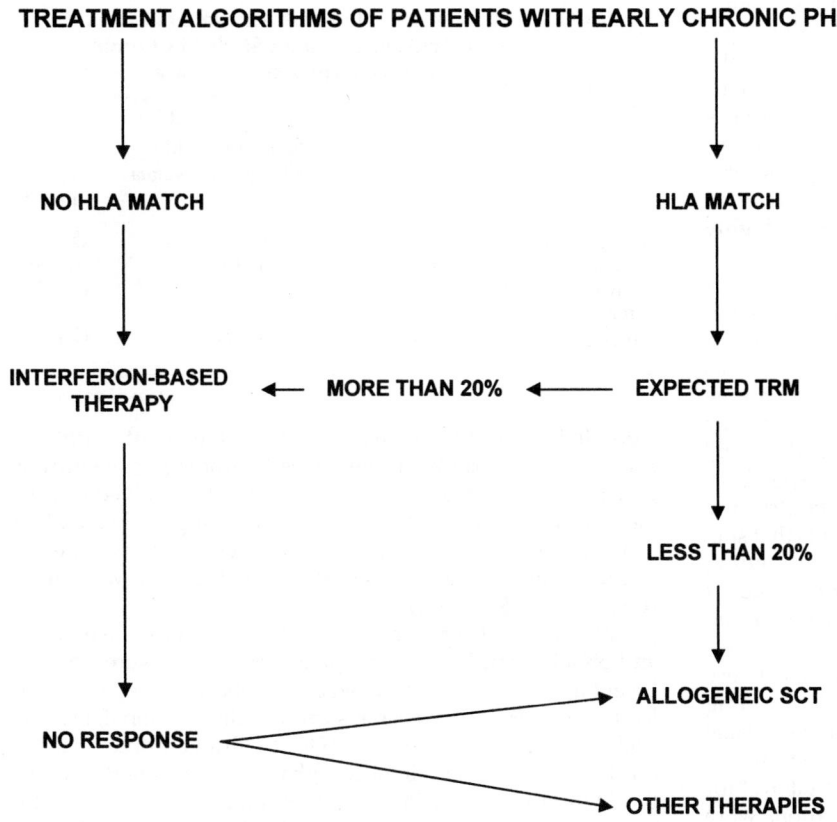

Figure 13-4. Treatment algorithm for patients with early chronic phase chronic myelogenous leukemia (CML). Current treatment choices include allogeneic stem cell transplantation (SCT) and interferon (IFN)-α–based therapies. The proposed algorithm is based on the excessive early mortality associated with allogeneic SCT and the lack of evidence supporting a deleterious effect of IFN-α on transplant outcome (see text for details). For those patients without an (HLA)–matched donor or for those with an expected transplant-related mortality (TRM) of more than 20%, IFN-α therapy is recommended. Patients who do not experience a cytogenetic response by 12 months are then offered allogeneic SCT if an HLA-matched donor is available or other therapies. Patients with an expected TRM of less than 20%, who are usually younger patients, should be offered allogeneic SCT if a donor is available.

(211). An oral ara-C–like formulation with equivalent efficacy will have a significant impact on patients' quality of life and will facilitate combinations with other active drugs.

Choice of Initial Therapy for Patients with Chronic Phase Chronic Myelogenous Leukemia

Until data from imatinib mesylate trials mature, patients with newly diagnosed chronic phase CML are generally offered therapy either with IFN-α or allogeneic SCT. The choice of therapy may be based on (a) the benefit to risk ratio of SCT versus IFN-α (early transplant mortality, long-term cure with SCT, survival with IFN-α), (b) patient risk group, and (c) patient preference. Although there is no universally accepted standard of care (150), treatment algorithms are based on the following principles: (a) postponing allogeneic SCT for up to 24 months (155,156) and pretransplantation use of IFN-α do not influence transplant outcome adversely (157,160,164); (b) the 1-year transplant-related mortality is age related and may define what is a reasonably acceptable risk of transplant in exchange for long-term outcome; and (c) median survival with IFN-α–based regimens is 6 to 7 years, whereas for good-risk patients it is 9 years, and for those patients who achieve a major or complete cytogenetic response, the 10-year survival is 70% to 90%. Thus, for patients with a 1-year TRM of less than 20%, up-front allogeneic SCT is reasonable; for those with an expected 1-year TRM of more than 20%, initial treatment with IFN-α is reasonable (Fig. 13-4).

Several studies have retrospectively (193,212,213) and prospectively (214) compared allogeneic SCT with IFN-α. In the Italian study (193), allogeneic SCT provided a survival advantage in patients younger than 32 years and those with high-risk CML. However, no survival advantage was demonstrated at 10 years among older patients and those with low-risk CML, who constituted 52% of the total population. A second study (212) compared the survival of 548 recipients of HLA-matched identical sibling transplants, reported to the IBMTR, with patients treated with IFN-α (n = 75) or hydroxyurea (n = 121) in a German CML study group trial (190,212). The 7-year probability of survival for low-risk patients was 58% with transplant and 49% for IFN-α or hydroxyurea, this difference being not statistically significant. Among intermediate- and high-risk patients, outcome was significantly better with allogeneic SCT after 4.7 years (58% vs. 21%). In a recent report from the French CML Intergroup and the IBMTR (213) comparing matched related allogeneic SCT (n = 373) with combination IFN-α and ara-C (n = 186), the predicted probabilities of survival at 6 years were 73% for patients transplanted in the first 6 months after diagnosis and 56% for those transplanted in months 6 to 12, compared with 77% for low–Sokal risk IFN-treated patients, 67% for intermediate-risk, and 35% for high-risk patients. No significant differences were detected at 6 years overall. However, low-risk patients had a better outcome with IFN therapy, and high-risk patients had a better outcome with SCT (213). German investigators, using a genetic randomization approach, have compared the outcome of allogeneic SCT versus IFN-α (214). Of 901 patients, 524 were genetically randomized: 165 (18% of total) for SCT and 389 for IFN-α therapy. During the first 4 years of observation, survival was better with IFN-α ($p = .014$), but the survival curves were expected to cross at 5 years. Although the authors suggest that SCT outcome will be more favorable with longer follow-up among intermediate-high risk patients, this is not observed for low-risk patients, although they speculate it may occur with much longer follow-up.

Imatinib Mesylate

Imatinib mesylate is one of the most important conceptual and therapeutic advances in CML and may serve as a paradigm for the development of similar small targeted molecules in other malignancies. The encouraging results with the maturing experience of imatinib mesylate may soon change the therapeutic algorithm regarding the indications and timing of allogeneic SCT and the value of IFN-α therapy in CML. The experience with imatinib mesylate provides an example of how understanding the disease's biology and pathophysiology can produce successful molecular-targeted approaches. CML is an ideal disease, because the molecular target is unique, highly expressed in most patients, and disease specific.

Several naturally occurring compounds manifest inhibitory activity against protein tyrosine kinases, including the isoflavinoid genistein, herbimycin A (an antibiotic), the flavinoid quercetin, and erbstatin (215,216). Synthetic compounds known as *tyrphostins* were rationally designed to compete with adenosine triphosphate or substrate for the binding site in the catalytic center of the kinase (217), including AG1112 and AG957 (218,219). These were the first compounds to display specificity for tyrosine kinases (220). Determination of the crystal structure of several protein kinases led to designing compounds that specifically interfered with the adenosine triphosphate–binding site or the enzyme active sites. One such class of compounds is the 2-phenylaminopyrimidine derivatives to which imatinib mesylate belongs.

Imatinib mesylate inhibits the ABL tyrosine kinases at very low concentrations [1 to 10 micromolar (μmol/L)], including p210$^{BCR-ABL}$, p190$^{BCR-ABL}$, V-ABL, and C-ABL. Imatinib mesylate inhibits equally effectively c-kit and platelet-derived growth factor receptor tyrosine kinases (221,223). This is of interest for several reasons: (a) The submicromolar concentrations were easily achievable in clinical trials, and once the imatinib mesylate dose reached 300 mg orally daily, serum levels of at least 1 μmol/L were achieved, and patients in chronic phase had a CHR greater than 90% and cytogenetic response rates of 30% to 50%; (b) imatinib mesylate may demonstrate significant activity in Ph-positive ALL and, in combination with chemotherapy, may improve its prognosis; and (c) imatinib mesylate therapeutic activity may extend beyond Ph-positive to c-kit and platelet-derived growth factor receptor–positive disorders including gastrointestinal sarcomatous tumors, AML, myeloproliferative disorders, prostate cancer, brain tumors, sarcomas, and others. Preclinical studies have confirmed the selective inhibitory effects of imatinib mesylate against p210$^{BCR-ABL}$ and p190$^{BCR-ABL}$ leukemias (222–224) with minimal inhibition of normal hematopoiesis. Inhibitory activity resulted in apoptosis. Anti–BCR-ABL efficacy was also demonstrated in syngeneic or nude mice injected with *BCR-ABL*–expressing cells and treated with imatinib mesylate (223,225). Animal toxicology studies with oral imatinib mesylate demonstrated its oral bioavailability and showed hepatic toxicity at the highest dose of 100 mg/kg. Other toxicities were vomiting, diarrhea, and myelosuppression (anemia, neutropenia).

Imatinib mesylate has undergone relatively rapid evaluations in phase I and phase II pivotal trials for the purpose of approval by the U.S. Food and Drug Administration (FDA). These studies involved patients in all CML phases. The results of the phase I study in patients in chronic phase CML and a parallel study in blastic phase and Ph-positive ALL have been reported (226,227). The dose of imatinib mesylate was escalated from 25 to 1000 mg orally daily. Common but rarely serious side effects included nausea and vomiting, diarrhea, skin rash, muscle cramps, bone or joint aches, myelosuppression, and weight gain. Less common side effects occurring at higher doses were fluid retention, periorbital and peripheral edema, fever, occasional liver dysfunction, and rarely decreased skin pigmentation. No maximum tolerated dose or dose-limiting toxicities

TABLE 13-10. Results of Imatinib Mesylate in Chronic Myelogenous Leukemia: Phase I Study in Chronic Myelogenous Leukemia Blastic Phase

	Myeloid (%)	Lymphoid and Ph-positive Acute Lymphocytic Leukemia (%)	Total (%)
Number treated	38	20	58
Complete response	4 (11)	4 (20)	8 (14)
Marrow complete remission	8 (21)	7 (35)	15 (26)
Partial response	9 (24)	3 (15)	12 (21)

were defined, but toxicities were more significant at doses of 600 mg or more daily. In the phase I chronic phase study, 83 patients were treated. Among 54 patients who received imatinib mesylate at doses of 300 mg or more, the complete hematologic response rate was 98%, and the cytogenetic response rate 31% (complete in 13%). In CML blastic phase, the marrow complete remission (CR) rate (marrow blasts <5% with or without peripheral count recovery) was 32% in myeloid blastic phase and 55% in lymphoid blastic phase; responses were transient except in a few cases of myeloid blastic phase (Table 13-10). This led to the three Novartis-sponsored multiinstitutional, multinational, and pivotal studies in IFN-α failure chronic phase, in accelerated phase, and in blastic phase, which were the basis of the FDA approval of imatinib mesylate for the treatment of CML. A phase II study in patients in chronic phase CML and IFN-α failure (89) accrued 532 patients: 30% had hematologic resistance, 34% had cytogenetic resistance, and 36% had severe IFN-α toxicities. The median time from diagnosis was 32 months, and the median duration of IFN-α therapy was 14 months. The dose of imatinib mesylate was 400 mg orally daily. Major cytogenetic responses were observed in 60% of patients, which were complete in 41%. The estimated 18-month event-free survival rate was 89%, and the survival rate was 95%. By multivariate analysis, absence of blasts in the peripheral blood, a hemoglobin level of more than 12 g/dL, less than 5% blasts in the bone marrow, and a time from diagnosis of CML to start of treatment of less than 1 year independently predicted a high rate of major cytogenetic response (89).

The phase II study of imatinib mesylate in accelerated phase accrued 235 patients (228). Doses were 400 mg daily (62 patients) or 600 mg daily (119 patients). Overall, 34% of patients achieved CHR, with an overall response rate of 82% (Table 13-11). Major cytogenetic responses were observed in 24% of patients, including 17% complete. Estimated 12-month progression-free and overall survival rates were 59% and 74%, respectively.

TABLE 13-11. Responses in Chronic Phase Chronic Myelogenous Leukemia

Category (No.)	Complete (%)	Partial (%)	Major (%)
IFN-α hematologic resistance (157)	28 (18)	26 (17)	54 (34)
IFN-α cytogenetic resistance (183)	53 (29)	36 (20)	89 (49)
IFN intolerant (192)	69 (36)	38 (20)	107 (56)
Total (532)	150 (28)	100 (19)	250 (47)

IFN, interferon.

In the phase II study in blastic phase (229), the imatinib mesylate daily doses were 400 mg (37 patients) or 600 mg (225 patients). Sixty patients were evaluable at 4 weeks and 34 patients at 8 weeks. In previously untreated patients, the overall response rate was 48% (15 of 31 patients) at 4 weeks and 47% (5 of 17 patients) at 8 weeks. In previously treated patients, the response rates were 38% (11 of 29 patients) and 33% (5 of 15 patients) at 4 and 8 weeks, respectively.

A randomized study of imatinib mesylate versus IFN-α and ara-C in newly diagnosed patients in chronic phase CML has completed accrual. The study has accrued 1032 patients over 6 months. The preliminary results demonstrate the superiority of imatinib mesylate in relation to higher major and complete cytogenetic responses, time to progression, and lower toxicity [American Society of Clinical Oncology (ASCO), 2002]. Ongoing studies at MDACC include the use of imatinib mesylate at a dose of 400 mg or 800 mg orally daily in newly diagnosed patients in chronic phase, with the provision for adding IFN-α and ara-C at 1 year if no cytogenetic response has been achieved. The preliminary findings with the 400 mg daily schedule showed that after only 6 months of therapy, the complete cytogenetic response rate was 52% and the major cytogenetic response rate was 80%. Combination studies using idarubicin, ara-C, and imatinib mesylate for patients in myeloid blastic phase and imatinib mesylate plus the hyper-CVAD (hyper–cyclophosphamide, vincristine, Adriamycin, and dexamethasone) chemotherapy program (230) for patients in lymphoid blastic phase are ongoing. Future studies include the use of high doses of imatinib mesylate (800 mg daily), imatinib mesylate plus IFN-α or ara-C in newly diagnosed patients, and combinations of imatinib mesylate with decitabine in advanced CML phases.

Homoharringtonine

Homoharringtonine (HHT) is a semisynthetic plant alkaloid studied initially in China. Phase I and II studies in the United States confirmed its activity in AML and myelodysplastic syndrome, but the HHT doses used, 5 to 9 mg/m^2 daily for 5 to 7 days, were associated with severe cardiovascular and hypotensive toxicities. A lower-dose, longer exposure schedule of HHT (2.5 mg/m^2 by continuous infusion daily for 14 to 21 days) reduced significantly the cardiovascular toxicity. HHT alone (2.5 mg/m^2 daily × 14 days for induction, then × 7 days every month for maintenance) (231) and HHT plus ara-C (HHT, 2.5 mg/m^2 daily × 5, and ara-C, 15 mg/m^2 daily × 5, every month) were investigated in late chronic phase CML. Among 173 patients treated with HHT alone or with ara-C, the CHR (approximately 65%) and cytogenetic response rates (approximately 30%) were similar, but survival was significantly longer with HHT plus ara-C (38% vs. 58%, p = .02) after accounting for risk groups and by multivariate analysis (232). HHT was also investigated in early chronic phase CML alone and in combinations, with favorable results (233). HHT may be a valuable addition to our future front-line therapies, which could include IFN-α, ara-C, imatinib mesylate, and others. Current investigations include combinations of HHT, IFN-α, and ara-C; subcutaneous routes of HHT delivery; and possible future combination of HHT and imatinib mesylate. Several new semisynthetic HHTs have been developed with more potent cytotoxic activity and ability to overcome P-glycoprotein efflux (234,235).

5-Aza-2'-deoxycytidine (Decitabine)

Aberrant methylation of promoter-associated CpG islands is a well-established oncogenic mechanism. Multiple genes are known to be abnormally methylated in leukemias and myelodysplastic syndromes (236). In CML, disease progression is associated with hypermethylation of the Pa promoter region within BCR-ABL (124,125). 5-Azacytidine and decitabine are cytidine analogs capable of inducing hypomethylation through inhibition of DNA methyltransferase enzyme. Decitabine, 50 to 100 mg/m^2 over 6 hours every 12 hours for 10 doses (500 to 1000 mg/m^2/course), produced response rates of 28% in blastic phase and 50% to 60% in accelerated phase disease (237). Compared with intensive chemotherapy as initial therapy for CML blastic phase, decitabine was associated with significantly better survival among patients 50 years or older (p <.01). By multivariate analysis, decitabine therapy remained an independent favorable prognostic factor for survival (p = .047). Lower dose schedules of decitabine (e.g., 5 to 10 mg/m^2 daily for 10 to 20 days) to target hypomethylation as the molecular endpoint are of interest and may provide a less myelosuppressive and perhaps equally effective regimen. Decitabine combinations with IFN-α or imatinib mesylate are under discussion.

Polyethylene Glycol Interferon

Polyethylene glycol (PEG) IFN (PEG-IFN) is a modified IFN-α molecule covalently linked to PEG, which has a longer half-life and is administered once weekly. In a phase I study (238), 27 patients with CML in chronic phase were treated with escalating doses of the PEG-IFN (PEG-Intron), 0.75 to 9.00 µg/kg weekly. The dose chosen for phase II studies of PEG-Intron was 6 µg/kg weekly (presumably equivalent to regular IFN-α 180 MU weekly = 15 MU/m^2 daily). Dose-limiting toxicities were neurotoxicity, thrombocytopenia, fatigue, and liver function abnormalities, similar to IFN-α but occurring at higher doses than with IFN-α. All 6 patients intolerant of IFN-α were able to receive PEG-Intron; 9 of 27 patients improved their responses, including three complete and three partial cytogenetic responses. Thus, PEG-Intron was easier to deliver (once weekly), was less toxic, and may be more effective than IFN-α. Current studies are investigating the two different formulations of PEG-IFN, PEG-Intron and Pegasus (PEG-Roferon), alone and in combination with ara-C in early chronic phase CML. In a phase II study completed at the MDACC (239), 76 patients in early chronic phase have received PEG-IFN, 6 µg/kg s.c. weekly (24 patients) or 4.5 µg/kg s.c. weekly (52 patients), and ara-C, 10 mg s.c. daily. The dose of the PEG-IFN was decreased because of unexpected chronic toxicities. The median follow-up time is 60 weeks. Fifty-nine (78%) patients achieved CHR; 45 (59%) had cytogenetic responses, complete (Ph, 0%) in 16 (21%). Seventy-five patients were alive at the follow-up time, the 2-year survival rate being 98%. Grades 3 to 4 nonhematologic toxicity was 61%: mainly neurologic side effects, fatigue, and aches. The median PEG-IFN dose delivered was 3.25 µg/kg. Thus, we propose, based on the phase II experience, to continue PEG-IFN at significantly lower doses than previously anticipated (e.g., 1 to 2 µg/kg weekly). Pegasus (PEG-IFN α-2a) is a different formulation with a larger molecular weight; it may offer less CNS penetration but more hepatic uptake. Combinations of these agents with an oral ara-C prodrug (YNK01) and imatinib mesylate are of interest. PEG-IFN preparations may replace IFN-α in the future if the favorable efficacy to toxicity profile is confirmed with longer follow-up.

Farnesyl Transferase Inhibitors

Activation of the Ras signal transduction pathway is a central event in BCR-ABL–induced malignant transformation (1). Several new agents, known as *farnesyl transferase inhibitors* (FTIs), have been developed that inhibit the enzyme farnesyl protein transferase, disrupt Ras prenylation, alter proper subcellular localization, and result in inhibition of Ras-dependent cellular transformation (240). FTIs have been shown to be active in murine animal models (241,242). R115777 is an FTI with activity in acute myeloid leukemia and blastic phase of CML (243). A study using R115777 at a dose of 600 mg orally taken twice a day for 28 days every 6 weeks in patients with CML has been conducted at the MDACC (244). Twenty-one patients with CML (10 in chronic phase, five in accelerated phase, and six in blastic phase) have been treated: All had failed at least one prior treatment; 16 (76%) had received prior IFN-α; and 15 (71%) had received imatinib mesylate. Six patients in chronic phase responded with complete (n = 5) or partial (n = 1) hematologic response; three of them achieved a minor cytogenetic response. One patient in accelerated phase CML had a complete hematologic response and minor cytogenetic response; none of the six patients in blastic phase CML responded. The preliminary results suggests that R115777 may be active in chronic phase CML. Further studies with FTIs alone and in combinations are ongoing.

Antisense Oligonucleotides

Antisense oligonucleotides are short DNA sequences that bind to targeted RNA sequences and block the translation of the message encoded by the RNA. This technology has been studied in CML using oligonucleotides against different molecules including BCR-ABL, RAS, PI-3-kinase, C-MYB, and C-MYC. A strategy using ex vivo cell purging with an antisense against BCR-ABL has shown preclinical activity (245).

Immunotherapy

Immunotherapy approaches have been used to treat patients with CML, frequently in the context of minimal residual disease posttransplant. One patient in accelerated phase CML postallogeneic SCT achieved complete remission following therapy with in vitro selected expanded leukemia reactive cytotoxic T-lymphocytes (246). Vaccination of patients with CML with BCR-ABL fusion peptides has been reported to be safe and to elicit specific immune responses (247). Autoantibodies against BCR-ABL have been demonstrated in patients with CML (248), suggesting that immunotherapy programs may need to circumvent humoral tolerance. Other discussed strategies include the use of T-cell–depleted allogeneic SCT to reduce transplant toxicity, followed by T-cell reinfusions at incremental doses to eradicate minimal residual disease (249).

Initial studies at the MDACC had shown that the addition of granulocyte-macrophage colony-stimulating factor (GM-CSF) to IFN-α–sensitive patients (those with a complete hematologic response but who had failed to achieve or who had lost a major cytogenetic response) induced significant cytogenetic responses in 29% of patients (250). Smith et al. recently reported (251) that the combination of GM-CSF and IFN-α induced rapid cytogenetic responses in patients with CML. The rationale for this approach was that both GM-CSF and IFN-α induced cell differentiation of CML progenitors in vitro. GM-CSF also induced increased expression of HLA-DR, facilitating recognition of CML cells by killer lymphocytes. In this study (251), patients were first started on IFN-α alone until hematologic remission was achieved and then given GM-CSF for 6 months, the dose adjusted to keep the WBC count at or below 10×10^9. The actuarial probability of achieving a major cytogenetic response was 74% in the 38 patients so far evaluated. All five patients who completed the treatment achieved major cytogenetic responses, three of them at the molecular level.

Intensive Chemotherapy and Autologous Stem Cell Transplantation

Several acute leukemia-like programs have been investigated in CML with modest results (252,253). Intensive chemotherapy regimens induced transient cytogenetic responses in 40% to 70% of patients and survival prolongation in poor-risk patients (254). Other strategies have combined intensive chemotherapy and IFN-α. Three cycles of intensive chemotherapy followed by IFN-α maintenance did not improve outcome (255). Addition of periodic cyclic (every 6 months) intensive chemotherapy in patients who had not achieved a favorable cytogenetic response to IFN-α after 6 or 12 months of therapy resulted in a projected 10-year survival of 50% compared with 35% for other IFN-α combinations. In another study, 213 evaluable patients were initially treated with IFN-α and hydroxyurea for 6 months and subsequently received 1 to 3 cycles of intensive chemotherapy, depending on their cytogenetic response. Patients who had a donor received allogeneic SCT, whereas patients who became Ph-negative received autologous SCT. After 6 months of IFN-α and hydroxyurea, 4% of patients achieved a complete cytogenetic response. After 2 cycles of systemic chemotherapy the percentage of complete cytogenetic responses was 28%. Among 39 patients who ultimately underwent autologous SCT, 24 have relapsed cytogenetically and 12 remain Ph-negative (256).

Autologous SCT has been investigated in CML in an attempt to maximize the intensity of chemotherapy. A major problem of autologous SCT is the reinfusion of Ph-positive cells and subsequent relapse (257). In vitro and in vivo purging approaches included incubation with IFN-α and -γ, positive and negative stem cell selection, long-term in vitro cultures, incubation with anti–C-MYB antisense, immunomodulation (linomide) (258), and priming patients with intensive chemotherapy and growth factor mobilization followed by peripheral stem cell collection (259). The latter approach, pioneered by Carella et al., showed promising results (259,260). However, most studies analyzing different priming programs have shown little added advantage of the autologous SCT approach (261,262). The value of autologous SCT is now being addressed in a multiinstitutional, multinational randomized trial.

Therapy for Accelerated and Blastic Phase Chronic Myelogenous Leukemia

Except for patients in accelerated phase CML based only on clonal evolution (153,263), results of current therapies in patients with transformed CML are suboptimal (264). Treatment approaches include hydroxyurea, other intensive chemotherapy regimens that provide short-term disease control, palliative splenectomy in cases of massive painful splenomegaly, combination IFN-α and ara-C (204), or investigational strategies including decitabine, imatinib mesylate, or others. Of all these strategies, imatinib mesylate appears the most promising, yielding overall hematologic response rates of 90% and cytogenetic response rates of approximately 40%. Allogeneic SCT in accelerated phase offers a potential for cure of 20% to 50%, depending on the definition of accelerated phase, and is the treatment of choice. Treatment for patients in blastic phase CML depends on the leukemia immunophenotype. IFN has no role in blastic phase CML (264). Patients with lymphoid phenotype have a complete remission rate of 60%, and 30% achieve cytogenetic responses. Remission duration is 9 to 12 months. Chemotherapy programs in this setting are modeled after ALL-like programs such as the hyperCVAD (265). Response rates in myeloid blastic phase are only

20% to 30% and are short-lived; cytogenetic responses are rare. High-dose ara-C regimens are often used but are of limited benefit. Experimental approaches are indicated in this setting, and ones with activity in myeloid blastic phase CML include imatinib mesylate, which provides transient disease control in 30% to 40% of patients (90); decitabine, which induces responses in 25% to 30% (237); and others (troxacitabine, tiazofurin).

PHILADELPHIA CHROMOSOME–NEGATIVE CHRONIC MYELOGENOUS LEUKEMIA

Approximately 5% to 10% of patients with clinical and laboratory features of CML do not show the Ph abnormality (3,65). One-third are BCR-ABL–positive by molecular studies (2,266). Ph-negative, BCR-ABL–positive patients have clinicopathologic features and prognosis identical to Ph-positive CML, respond similarly to therapy, and should be treated as Ph-positive cases (3–7). Characteristics of patients with true Ph-negative, BCR-ABL–negative CML include older age, thrombocytopenia, monocytosis, and lesser degree of leukocytosis and basophilia (65). Median survival is significantly shorter than Ph-positive CML (25 months vs. 70 months) (65). Of interest, only 50% of patients transform into a blastic phase; the others develop progressive hyperleukocytosis, organomegaly, extramedullary disease, and marrow failure (129).

The other subsets of Ph-negative myeloproliferative disorders include a wide variety of conditions, including chronic myelomonocytic leukemia and proliferative myelodysplastic syndrome. Allogeneic SCT is potentially curative in these subgroups and should be considered when possible. Other approaches include palliation with hydroxyurea, splenectomy, topotecan plus ara-C combinations, and novel investigations (oral topotecan, 9NC, farnesyl transferase inhibitors, others).

SUMMARY

The prognosis of patients with CML has improved dramatically over the last decade. Milestones of therapeutic advances have included (a) allogeneic SCT (curative but with high morbidity and mortality risks); (b) IFN-α therapy, the first biologic therapy to durably suppress the Ph abnormality; (c) DLI, the first example of highly successful cancer immunotherapy (molecular complete remissions in 70% of patients with active CML who relapse postallogeneic SCT); and (d) the recent BCR-ABL tyrosine kinase inhibitors, an example of a highly successful molecularly targeted therapy.

The gradual unraveling of the molecular pathogenesis of CML over 40 years—from the first description of the Ph abnormality to the subsequent definition of the precise cytogenetic translocation and, later, the BCR-ABL–associated molecular events—has finally resulted in a rationally designed molecular targeted approach: the BCR-ABL signal transduction inhibitor imatinib mesylate. Other such targeted approaches are likely to be soon developed, which will hopefully further improve our treatment results and prognosis in CML. Other promising approaches include IFN-α combinations, new PEG-IFN preparations, new chemotherapy agents (HHT, decitabine), immunomodulatory strategies (DLI), vaccines, and nonablative SCT modifications. Today, the outlook of a patient diagnosed with CML is much more hopeful than it was 30 years ago, when such a diagnosis implied a short survival and an invariable fatal outcome.

REFERENCES

1. Faderl S, Talpaz M, Estrov Z, et al. The biology of chronic myeloid leukemia. N Engl J Med 1999;341(3):164–172.
2. Wiedemann LM, Karhi KK, Shivji MK, et al. The correlation of breakpoint cluster region rearrangement and p210 phl/abl expression with morphological analysis of Ph-negative chronic myeloid leukemia and other myeloproliferative diseases. Blood 1988;71(2):349–355.
3. Kantarjian HM, Kurzrock R, Talpaz M. Philadelphia chromosome-negative chronic myelogenous leukemia and chronic myelomonocytic leukemia. Hematol Oncol Clin North Am 1990;4(2):389–404.
4. Ezdinli EZ, Sokal JE, Crosswhite L, et al. Philadelphia-chromosome-positive and -negative chronic myelocytic leukemia. Ann Intern Med 1970;72(2):175–182.
5. Canellos GP, Whang-Peng J, DeVita VT. Chronic granulocytic leukemia without the Philadelphia chromosome. Am J Clin Pathol 1976;65(4):467–470.
6. Pugh WC, Pearson M, Vardiman JW, et al. Philadelphia chromosome-negative chronic myelogenous leukaemia: a morphological reassessment. Br J Haematol 1985;60(3):457–467.
7. Kantarjian HM, Keating MJ, Walters RS, et al. Clinical and prognostic features of Philadelphia chromosome-negative chronic myelogenous leukemia. Cancer 1986;58(9):2023–2030.
8. Nowell PC HD. A minute chromosome in human chronic granulocytic leukemia. Science 1960;132:1497.
9. Sandberg AA, Hecht BK, Hecht F. Nomenclature: the Philadelphia chromosome or Ph without superscript. Cancer Genet Cytogenet 1985;14(1–2):1.
10. Rowley JD. Letter: a new consistent chromosomal abnormality in chronic myelogenous leukaemia identified by quinacrine fluorescence and Giemsa staining. Nature 1973;243(5405):290–293.
11. Whang-Peng J, Lee EC, Knutsen TA. Genesis of the Ph chromosome. J Natl Cancer Inst 1974;52(4):1035–1036.
12. Sawyers CL. Chronic myeloid leukemia [see comments]. N Engl J Med 1999; 340(17):1330–1340.
13. Martin PJ, Najfeld V, Hansen JA, et al. Involvement of the B-lymphoid system in chronic myelogenous leukaemia. Nature 1980;287(5777):49–50.
14. Bernheim A, Berger R, Preud'homme JL, et al. Philadelphia chromosome positive blood B lymphocytes in chronic myelocytic leukemia. Leuk Res 1981;5(4–5):331–339.
15. Hernandez P, Carnot J, Cruz C. Chronic myeloid leukaemia blast crisis with T-cell features. Br J Haematol 1982;51(1):175–177.
16. Griffin JD, Tantravahi R, Canellos GP, et al. T-cell surface antigens in a patient with blast crisis of chronic myeloid leukemia. Blood 1983;61(4):640–644.
17. Maniatis AK, Amsel S, Mitus WJ, et al. Chromosome pattern of bone marrow fibroblasts in patients with chronic granulocytic leukaemia. Nature 1969;222(200):1278–1279.
18. Greenberg BR, Wilson FD, Woo L, et al. Cytogentics of fibroblastic colonies in Ph1-positive chronic myelogenous leukemia. Blood 1978;51(6):1039–1044.
19. Sokal JE. Significance of Ph1-negative marrow cells in Ph1-positive chronic granulocytic leukemia. Blood 1980;56(6):1072–1076.
20. Golde DW, Bersch NL, Sparkes RS. Chromosomal mosaicism associated with prolonged remission in chronic myelogenous leukemia. Cancer 1976; 37(4):1849–1852.
21. Heisterkamp N, Stephenson JR, Groffen J, et al. Localization of the c-abl oncogene adjacent to a translocation break point in chronic myelocytic leukaemia. Nature 1983;306(5940):239–242.
22. Groffen J, Stephenson JR, Heisterkamp N, et al. Philadelphia chromosomal breakpoints are clustered within a limited region, bcr, on chromosome 22. Cell 1984;36(1):93–99.
23. Heisterkamp N, Groffen J, Stephenson JR. The human v-abl cellular homologue. J Mol Appl Genet 1983;2(1):57–68.
24. Shtivelman E, Lifshitz B, Gale RP, et al. Alternative splicing of RNAs transcribed from the human abl gene and from the bcr-abl fused gene. Cell 1986;47(2):277–284.
25. Ben-Neriah Y, Bernards A, Paskind M, et al. Alternative 5' exons in c-abl mRNA. Cell 1986;44(4):577–586.
26. Jiang XY, Trujillo JM, Dao D, et al. Studies of BCR and ABL gene rearrangements in chronic myelogenous leukemia patients by conventional and pulsed-field gel electrophoresis using gel inserts. Cancer Genet Cytogenet 1989;42(2):287–294.
27. Gale RP, Canaani E. An 8-kilobase abl RNA transcript in chronic myelogenous leukemia. Proc Natl Acad Sci U S A 1984;81(18):5648–5652.
28. Shtivelman E, Gale RP, Dreazen O, et al. bcr-abl RNA in patients with chronic myelogenous leukemia. Blood 1987;69(3):971–973.
29. Collins SJ, Groudine MT. Chronic myelogenous leukemia: amplification of a rearranged c-abl oncogene in both chronic phase and blast crisis. Blood 1987;69(3):893–898.
30. Faderl S, Kantarjian HM, Talpaz M. Chronic myelogenous leukemia: update on biology and treatment. Oncology (Huntingt) 1999;13(2):169–180.
31. Melo JV. The molecular biology of chronic myeloid leukaemia. Leukemia 1996;10(5):751–756.
32. Shepherd P, Suffolk R, Halsey J, et al. Analysis of molecular breakpoint and m-RNA transcripts in a prospective randomized trial of interferon in chronic myeloid leukaemia: no correlation with clinical features, cytogenetic response, duration of chronic phase, or survival. Br J Haematol 1995;89(3):546–554.
33. Hermans A, Heisterkamp N, von Linden M, et al. Unique fusion of bcr and c-abl genes in Philadelphia chromosome positive acute lymphoblastic leukemia. Cell 1987;51(1):33–40.

34. Goldman JM, Grosveld G, Baltimore D, et al. Chronic myelogenous leukemia—the unfolding saga. *Leukemia* 1990;4(3):163–167.

35. Kurzrock R, Shtalrid M, Romero P, et al. A novel c-abl protein product in Philadelphia-positive acute lymphoblastic leukaemia. *Nature* 1987;325(6105):631–635.

36. Melo JV, Myint H, Galton DA, et al. P190BCR-ABL chronic myeloid leukaemia: the missing link with chronic myelomonocytic leukaemia? *Leukemia* 1994;8(1):208–211.

37. Saglio G, Guerrasio A, Rosso C, et al. New type of Bcr/Abl junction in Philadelphia chromosome-positive chronic myelogenous leukemia. *Blood* 1990;76(9):1819–1824.

38. Pane F, Frigeri F, Sindona M, et al. Neutrophilic-chronic myeloid leukemia: a distinct disease with a specific molecular marker (BCR/ABL with C3/A2 junction). *Blood* 1996;88(7):2410–2414.

39. Faderl S, Talpaz M, Estrov Z, et al. Chronic myelogenous leukemia: biology and therapy. *Ann Intern Med* 1999;131(3):207–219.

40. Quackenbush RC, Reuther GW, Miller JP, et al. Analysis of the biologic properties of p230 Bcr-Abl reveals unique and overlapping properties with the oncogenic p185 and p210 Bcr-Abl tyrosine kinases. *Blood* 2000;95(9):2913–2921.

41. Melo JV, Hochhaus A, Yan XH, et al. Lack of correlation between ABL-BCR expression and response to interferon-alpha in chronic myeloid leukaemia. *Br J Haematol* 1996;92(3):684–686.

42. Konopka JB, Watanabe SM, Witte ON. An alteration of the human c-abl protein in K562 leukemia cells unmasks associated tyrosine kinase activity. *Cell* 1984;37(3):1035–1042.

43. Heisterkamp N, Stam K, Groffen J, et al. Structural organization of the bcr gene and its role in the Ph' translocation. *Nature* 1985;315(6022):758–761.

44. Scher CD, Siegler R. Direct transformation of 3T3 cells by Abelson murine leukaemia virus. *Nature* 1975;253(5494):729–731.

45. Rosenberg N, Baltimore D, Scher CD. In vitro transformation of lymphoid cells by Abelson murine leukemia virus. *Proc Natl Acad Sci U S A* 1975;72(5):1932–1936.

46. Cook WD, Fazekas de St. Groth B, Miller JF, et al. Abelson virus transformation of an interleukin 2-dependent antigen-specific T-cell line. *Mol Cell Biol* 1987;7(7):2631–2635.

47. Daley GQ, Baltimore D. Transformation of an interleukin 3-dependent hematopoietic cell line by the chronic myelogenous leukemia-specific P210bcr/abl protein. *Proc Natl Acad Sci U S A* 1988;85(23):9312–9316.

48. Stahl ML, Ferenz CR, Kelleher KL, et al. Sequence similarity of phospholipase C with the non-catalytic region of src. *Nature* 1988;332(6161):269–272.

49. Muller AJ, Young JC, Pendergast AM, et al. BCR first exon sequences specifically activate the BCR/ABL tyrosine kinase oncogene of Philadelphia chromosome-positive human leukemias. *Mol Cell Biol* 1991;11(4):1785–1792.

50. Pendergast AM, Muller AJ, Havlik MH, et al. BCR sequences essential for transformation by the BCR-ABL oncogene bind to the ABL SH2 regulatory domain in a non-phosphotyrosine-dependent manner. *Cell* 1991;66(1):161–171.

51. Sawyers CL, McLaughlin J, Witte ON. Genetic requirement for Ras in the transformation of fibroblasts and hematopoietic cells by the Bcr-Abl oncogene. *J Exp Med* 1995;181(1):307–313.

52. Lowenstein EJ, Daly RJ, Batzer AG, et al. The SH2 and SH3 domain-containing protein GRB2 links receptor tyrosine kinases to ras signaling. *Cell* 1992;70(3):431–442.

53. Hunter T. Protein kinases and phosphatases: the yin and yang of protein phosphorylation and signaling. *Cell* 1995;80(2):225–236.

54. Hunter T. Cooperation between oncogenes. *Cell* 1991;64(2):249–270.

55. Pendergast AM, Quilliam LA, Cripe LD, et al. BCR-ABL-induced oncogenesis is mediated by direct interaction with the SH2 domain of the GRB-2 adaptor protein. *Cell* 1993;75(1):175–185.

56. McWhirter JR, Galasso DL, Wang JY. A coiled-coil oligomerization domain of Bcr is essential for the transforming function of Bcr-Abl oncoproteins. *Mol Cell Biol* 1993;13(12):7587–7595.

57. Dai Z, Quackenbush RC, Courtney KD, et al. Oncogenic Abl and Src tyrosine kinases elicit the ubiquitin-dependent degradation of target proteins through a Ras-independent pathway. *Genes Dev* 1998;12(10):1415–1424.

58. Jonuleit T, van Der Kuip H, Miething C, et al. Bcr-Abl kinase down-regulates cyclin-dependent kinase inhibitor p27 in human and murine cell lines. *Blood* 2000;96(5):1933–1939.

59. Evans CA, Owen-Lynch PJ, Whetton AD, et al. Activation of the Abelson tyrosine kinase activity is associated with suppression of apoptosis in hemopoietic cells. *Cancer Res* 1993;53(8):1735–1738.

60. Bedi A, Zehnbauer BA, Barber JP, et al. Inhibition of apoptosis by BCR-ABL in chronic myeloid leukemia. *Blood* 1994;83(8):2038–2044.

61. Sanchez-Garcia I, Grutz G. Tumorigenic activity of the BCR-ABL oncogenes is mediated by BCL2. *Proc Natl Acad Sci U S A* 1995;92(12):5287–5291.

62. Bazzoni G, Carlesso N, Griffin JD, et al. Bcr/Abl expression stimulates integrin function in hematopoietic cell lines. *J Clin Invest* 1996;98(2):521–528.

63. Upadhyaya G, Guba SC, Sih SA, et al. Interferon-alpha restores the deficient expression of the cytoadhesion molecule lymphocyte function antigen-3 by chronic myelogenous leukemia progenitor cells. *J Clin Invest* 1991;88(6):2131–2136.

64. Bhatia R, Wayner EA, McGlave PB, et al. Interferon-alpha restores normal adhesion of chronic myelogenous leukemia hematopoietic progenitors to bone marrow stroma by correcting impaired beta 1 integrin receptor function. *J Clin Invest* 1994;94(1):384–391.

65. Cortes JE, Talpaz M, Kantarjian H. Chronic myelogenous leukemia: a review. *Am J Med* 1996;100(5):555–570.

66. Alimena G, Dallapiccola B, Gastaldi R, et al. Chromosomal, morphological and clinical correlations in blastic crisis of chronic myeloid leukaemia: a study of 69 cases. *Scand J Haematol* 1982;28(2):103–117.

67. Mitelman F. The cytogenetic scenario of chronic myeloid leukemia. *Leuk Lymphoma* 1993;11[Suppl 1]:11–15.

68. Bakhshi A, Minowada J, Arnold A, et al. Lymphoid blast crises of chronic myelogenous leukemia represent stages in the development of B-cell precursors. *N Engl J Med* 1983;309(14):826–831.

69. Chan LC, Furley AJ, Ford AM, et al. Clonal rearrangement and expression of the T cell receptor beta gene and involvement of the breakpoint cluster region in blast crisis of CGL. *Blood* 1986;67(2):533–536.

70. Liu E, Hjelle B, Bishop JM. Transforming genes in chronic myelogenous leukemia. *Proc Natl Acad Sci U S A* 1988;85(6):1952–1956.

71. Ahuja H, Bar-Eli M, Advani SH, et al. Alterations in the p53 gene and the clonal evolution of the blast crisis of chronic myelocytic leukemia. *Proc Natl Acad Sci U S A* 1989;86(17):6783–6787.

72. Kelman Z, Prokocimer M, Peller S, et al. Rearrangements in the p53 gene in Philadelphia chromosome positive chronic myelogenous leukemia. *Blood* 1989;74(7):2318–2324.

73. Feinstein E, Cimino G, Gale RP, et al. p53 in chronic myelogenous leukemia in acute phase. *Proc Natl Acad Sci U S A* 1991;88(14):6293–6297.

74. Honda H, Ushijima T, Wakazono K, et al. Acquired loss of p53 induces blastic transformation in p210(bcr/abl)-expressing hematopoietic cells: a transgenic study for blast crisis of human CML. *Blood* 2000;95(4):1144–1150.

75. Honda H, Oda H, Suzuki T, et al. Development of acute lymphoblastic leukemia and myeloproliferative disorder in transgenic mice expressing p210bcr/abl: a novel transgenic model for human Ph1-positive leukemias. *Blood* 1998;91(6):2067–2075.

76. Skorski T, Nieborowska-Skorska M, Wlodarski P, et al. Blastic transformation of p53-deficient bone marrow cells by p210bcr/abl tyrosine kinase. *Proc Natl Acad Sci U S A* 1996;93(23):13137–13142.

77. Ilaria RL Jr, Van Etten RA. The SH2 domain of P210BCR/ABL is not required for the transformation of hematopoietic factor-dependent cells. *Blood* 1995;86(10):3897–3904.

78. Sawyers CL, Gishizky ML, Quan S, et al. Propagation of human blastic myeloid leukemias in the SCID mouse. *Blood* 1992;79(8):2089–2098.

79. Heisterkamp N, Jenster G, ten Hoeve J, et al. Acute leukaemia in bcr/abl transgenic mice. *Nature* 1990;344(6263):251–253.

80. Daley GQ, Van Etten RA, Baltimore D. Induction of chronic myelogenous leukemia in mice by the P210bcr/abl gene of the Philadelphia chromosome. *Science* 1990;247(4944):824–830.

81. Kelliher MA, McLaughlin J, Witte ON, et al. Induction of a chronic myelogenous leukemia-like syndrome in mice with v-abl and BCR/ABL. *Proc Natl Acad Sci U S A* 1990;87(17):6649–6653.

82. Pear WS, Miller JP, Xu L, et al. Efficient and rapid induction of a chronic myelogenous leukemia-like myeloproliferative disease in mice receiving P210 bcr/abl-transduced bone marrow. *Blood* 1998;92(10):3780–3792.

83. Zhang X, Ren R. Bcr-Abl efficiently induces a myeloproliferative disease and production of excess interleukin-3 and granulocyte-macrophage colony-stimulating factor in mice: a novel model for chronic myelogenous leukemia. *Blood* 1998;92(10):3829–3840.

84. Call TG, Noel P, Habermann TM, et al. Incidence of leukemia in Olmsted County, Minnesota, 1975 through 1989. *Mayo Clin Proc* 1994;69(4):315–322.

85. Kinlen LJ. Leukaemia. *Cancer Surv* 1994;20:475–491.

86. Morrison VA. Chronic leukemias. *CA Cancer J Clin* 1994;44(6):353–377.

87. Brincker H. Population-based age- and sex-specific incidence rates in the 4 main types of leukaemia. *Scand J Haematol* 1982;29(3):241–249.

88. Kantarjian HM, Deisseroth A, Kurzrock R, et al. Chronic myelogenous leukemia: a concise update. *Blood* 1993;82(3):691–703.

89. Kantarjian H, Sawyers C, Hochhaus A, et al. Hematologic and cytogenetic responses to imatinib mesylate in chronic myelogenous leukemia. *N Engl J Med* 2002;346(9):645–652.

90. Talpaz MSC, Kantarjian HM, Resta D, et al. Activity of an ABL specific tyrosine kinase inhibitor in patients with BCR-ABL positive acute leukemias, including chronic myelogenous leukemia in blast crisis. *Proc Am Soc Clin Oncol* 2000;19:4a.

91. Deininger MW, Bose S, Gora-Tybor J, et al. Selective induction of leukemia-associated fusion genes by high-dose ionizing radiation. *Cancer Res* 1998;58(3):421–425.

92. Hasle H, Olsen JH. Cancer in relatives of children with myelodysplastic syndrome, acute and chronic myeloid leukaemia. *Br J Haematol* 1997;97(1):127–131.

93. Tanaka K, Takechi M, Hong J, et al. 9;22 translocation and bcr rearrangements in chronic myelocytic leukemia patients among atomic bomb survivors. *J Radiat Res (Tokyo)* 1989;30(4):352–358.

94. Corso A, Lazzarino M, Morra E, et al. Chronic myelogenous leukemia and exposure to ionizing radiation—a retrospective study of 443 patients. *Ann Hematol* 1995;70(2):79–82.

95. Bose S, Deininger M, Gora-Tybor J, et al. The presence of typical and atypical BCR-ABL fusion genes in leukocytes of normal individuals: biologic significance and implications for the assessment of minimal residual disease. *Blood* 1998;92(9):3362–3367.

96. Biernaux C, Loos M, Sels A, et al. Detection of major bcr-abl gene expression at a very low level in blood cells of some healthy individuals. *Blood* 1995;86(8):3118–3122.

97. Spiers AS. The clinical features of chronic granulocytic leukaemia. *Clin Haematol* 1977;6(1):77–95.

98. Mehta AB, Goldman JM, Kohner E. Hyperleucocytic retinopathy in chronic granulocytic leukaemia: the role of intensive leucapheresis. *Br J Haematol* 1984;56(4):661–667.

99. Suri R, Goldman JM, Catovsky D, et al. Priapism complicating chronic granulocytic leukemia. *Am J Hematol* 1980;9(3):295–299.

100. Savage DG, Szydlo RM, Goldman JM. Clinical features at diagnosis in 430 patients with chronic myeloid leukaemia seen at a referral centre over a 16-year period. *Br J Haematol* 1997;96(1):111–116.

101. Kantarjian HM, Dixon D, Keating MJ, et al. Characteristics of accelerated disease in chronic myelogenous leukemia. *Cancer* 1988;61(7):1441–1446.

102. Derderian PM, Kantarjian HM, Talpaz M, et al. Chronic myelogenous leukemia in the lymphoid blastic phase: characteristics, treatment response, and prognosis. *Am J Med* 1993;94(1):69–74.

103. Dowding C, Th'ng KH, Goldman JM, et al. Increased T-lymphocyte numbers in chronic granulocytic leukemia before treatment. *Exp Hematol* 1984;12(10):811–815.

104. Rosner F, Schreiber ZR, Parise F. Leukocyte alkaline phosphatase. Fluctuations with disease status in chronic granulocytic leukemia. *Arch Intern Med* 1972;130(6):892–894.

105. Knox WF, Bhavnani M, Davson J, et al. Histological classification of chronic granulocytic leukaemia. *Clin Lab Haematol* 1984;6(2):171–175.

106. Dekmezian R, Kantarjian HM, Keating MJ, et al. The relevance of reticulin stain-measured fibrosis at diagnosis in chronic myelogenous leukemia. *Cancer* 1987;59(10):1739–1743.

107. Bolin RW, Robinson WA, Sutherland J, et al. Busulfan versus hydroxyurea in long-term therapy of chronic myelogenous leukemia. *Cancer* 1982;50(9):1683–1686.

108. Sokal JE, Cox EB, Baccarani M, et al. Prognostic discrimination in "good-risk" chronic granulocytic leukemia. *Blood* 1984;63(4):789–799.

109. Kantarjian HM, Keating MJ, Smith TL, et al. Proposal for a simple synthesis prognostic staging system in chronic myelogenous leukemia. *Am J Med* 1990;88(1):1–8.

110. Sokal JE, Baccarani M, Tura S, et al. Prognostic discrimination among younger patients with chronic granulocytic leukemia: relevance to bone marrow transplantation. *Blood* 1985;66(6):1352–1357.

111. Tura S, Baccarani M, Corbelli G. Staging of chronic myeloid leukaemia. *Br J Haematol* 1981;47(1):105–119.

112. Cervantes F, Rozman C. A multivariate analysis of prognostic factors in chronic myeloid leukemia. *Blood* 1982;60(6):1298–1304.

113. Oguma S, Takatsuki K, Uchino H, et al. Factors influencing survival in Philadelphia chromosome positive chronic myelocytic leukemia. *Cancer* 1982;50(12):2928–2934.

114. Hasford J, Pfirrmann M, Hehlmann R, et al. A new prognostic score for survival of patients with chronic myeloid leukemia treated with interferon alfa. Writing Committee for the Collaborative CML Prognostic Factors Project Group. *J Natl Cancer Inst* 1998;90(11):850–858.

115. Kantarjian HM, O'Brien S, Anderlini P, et al. Treatment of myelogenous leukemia: current status and investigational options. *Blood* 1996;87(8):3069–3081.

116. Hasford J. Prognosis of patients with CML: updated results of the collaborative CML prognostic factors project. *Blood* 2000;96:546a.

117. Guilhot F, Chastang C, Michallet M, et al. Interferon alfa-2b combined with cytarabine versus interferon alone in chronic myelogenous leukemia. French Chronic Myeloid Leukemia Study Group. *N Engl J Med* 1997;337(4):223–229.

118. Kantarjian HM, Smith TL, O'Brien S, et al. Prolonged survival in chronic myelogenous leukemia after cytogenetic response to interferon-alpha therapy. The Leukemia Service. *Ann Intern Med* 1995;122(4):254–261.

119. Interferon alfa-2a as compared with conventional chemotherapy for the treatment of chronic myeloid leukemia. The Italian Cooperative Study Group on Chronic Myeloid Leukemia. *N Engl J Med* 1994;330(12):820–825.

120. Mills KI, Benn P, Birnie GD. Does the breakpoint within the major breakpoint cluster region (M-bcr) influence the duration of the chronic phase in chronic myeloid leukemia? An analytical comparison of current literature. *Blood* 1991;78(5):1155–1161.

121. Verschraegen CF, Kantarjian HM, Hirsch-Ginsberg C, et al. The breakpoint cluster region site in patients with Philadelphia chromosome-positive chronic myelogenous leukemia. Clinical, laboratory, and prognostic correlations. *Cancer* 1995;76(6):992–997.

122. Kurzrock R, Gutterman JU, Talpaz M. The molecular genetics of Philadelphia chromosome-positive leukemias. *N Engl J Med* 1988;319(15):990–998.

123. Sinclair PB, Nacheva EP, Leversha M, et al. Large deletions at the t(9;22) breakpoint are common and may identify a poor-prognosis subgroup of patients with chronic myeloid leukemia. *Blood* 2000;95(3):738–743.

124. Ben-Yehuda D, Krichevsky S, Rachmilewitz EA, et al. Molecular follow-up of disease progression and interferon therapy in chronic myelocytic leukemia. *Blood* 1997;90(12):4918–4923.

125. Issa JP, Kantarjian H, Mohan A, et al. Methylation of the ABL1 promoter in chronic myelogenous leukemia: lack of prognostic significance. *Blood* 1999;93(6):2075–2080.

126. Brummendorf TH, Holyoake TL, Rufer N, et al. Prognostic implications of differences in telomere length between normal and malignant cells from patients with chronic myeloid leukemia measured by flow cytometry. *Blood* 2000;95(6):1883–1890.

127. Boultwood J, Peniket A, Watkins F, et al. Telomere length shortening in chronic myelogenous leukemia is associated with reduced time to accelerated phase. *Blood* 2000;96(1):358–361.

128. Schmidt M, Hochhaus A, Konig-Merediz SA, et al. Expression of interferon regulatory factor 4 in chronic myeloid leukemia: correlation with response to interferon alfa therapy. *J Clin Oncol* 2000;18(19):3331–3338.

129. Kurzrock R, Kantarjian HM, Shtalrid M, et al. Philadelphia chromosome-negative chronic myelogenous leukemia without breakpoint cluster region rearrangement: a chronic myeloid leukemia with a distinct clinical course. *Blood* 1990;75(2):445–452.

130. Faderl S, Estrov Z. The clinical significance of detection of residual disease in childhood ALL. *Crit Rev Oncol Hematol* 1998;28(1):31–55.

131. Seong DC, Kantarjian HM, Ro JY, et al. Hypermetaphase fluorescence in situ hybridization for quantitative monitoring of Philadelphia chromosome-positive cells in patients with chronic myelogenous leukemia during treatment. *Blood* 1995;86(6):2343–2349.

132. Seong DC, Song MY, Henske EP, et al. Analysis of interphase cells for the Philadelphia translocation using painting probe made by inter-Alu-polymerase chain reaction from a radiation hybrid. *Blood* 1994;83(8):2268–2273.

133. Buno I, Wyatt WA, Zinsmeister AR, et al. A special fluorescent in situ hybridization technique to study peripheral blood and assess the effectiveness of interferon therapy in chronic myeloid leukemia. *Blood* 1998;92(7):2315–2321.

134. Hochhaus A, Weisser A, La Rosee P, et al. Detection and quantification of residual disease in chronic myelogenous leukemia. *Leukemia* 2000;14(6):998–1005.

135. Guo JQ, Lian J, Glassman A, et al. Comparison of bcr-abl protein expression and Philadelphia chromosome analyses in chronic myelogenous leukemia patients. *Am J Clin Pathol* 1996;106(4):442–448.

136. Sklar J. Polymerase chain reaction: the molecular microscope of residual disease [editorial, comment]. *J Clin Oncol* 1991;9(9):1521–1524.

137. Roth MS, Antin JH, Ash R, et al. Prognostic significance of Philadelphia chromosome-positive cells detected by the polymerase chain reaction after allogeneic bone marrow transplant for chronic myelogenous leukemia. *Blood* 1992;79(1):276–282.

138. Radich JP, Gehly G, Gooley T, et al. Polymerase chain reaction detection of the BCR-ABL fusion transcript after allogeneic marrow transplantation for chronic myeloid leukemia: results and implications in 346 patients. *Blood* 1995;85(9):2632–2638.

139. Faderl S, Talpaz M, Kantarjian HM, et al. Should polymerase chain reaction analysis to detect minimal residual disease in patients with chronic myelogenous leukemia be used in clinical decision making? *Blood* 1999;93(9):2755–2759.

140. Serrano J, Roman J, Sanchez J, et al. Molecular analysis of lineage-specific chimerism and minimal residual disease by RT-PCR of p210(BCR-ABL) and p190(BCR-ABL) after allogeneic bone marrow transplantation for chronic myeloid leukemia: increasing mixed myeloid chimerism and p190(BCR-ABL) detection precede cytogenetic relapse. *Blood* 2000;95(8):2659–2665.

141. Hochhaus A, Lin F, Reiter A, et al. Quantification of residual disease in chronic myelogenous leukemia patients on interferon-alpha therapy by competitive polymerase chain reaction. *Blood* 1996;87(4):1549–1555.

142. Hochhaus A, Reiter A, Saussele S, et al. Molecular heterogeneity in complete cytogenetic responders after interferon-alpha therapy for chronic myelogenous leukemia: low levels of minimal residual disease are associated with continuing remission. *Blood* 2000;95:62–66.

143. Kantarjian HM, Giles FJ, O'Brien SM, et al. Clinical course and therapy of chronic myelogenous leukemia with interferon-alpha and chemotherapy. *Hematol Oncol Clin North Am* 1998;12(1):31–80.

144. Galton DA. Some problems in the management of leukaemia and lymphoma. *Proc R Soc Med* 1966;59(12):1268–1272.

145. Kennedy BJ. Hydroxyurea therapy in chronic myelogenous leukemia. *Cancer* 1972;29(4):1052–1056.

146. Hehlmann R, Heimpel H, Hasford J, et al. Randomized comparison of busulfan and hydroxyurea in chronic myelogenous leukemia: prolongation of survival by hydroxyurea. The German CML Study Group. *Blood* 1993;82(2):398–407.

147. Interferon alfa versus chemotherapy for chronic myeloid leukemia: a meta-analysis of seven randomized trials: Chronic Myeloid Leukemia Trialists' Collaborative Group. *J Natl Cancer Inst* 1997;89(21):1616–1620.

148. Brodsky I, Biggs JC, Szer J, et al. Treatment of chronic myelogenous leukemia with allogeneic bone marrow transplantation after preparation with busulfan and cyclophosphamide (BuCy2): an update. *Semin Oncol* 1993;20[4 Suppl 4]:27–31, quiz 32.

149. Goldman JM, Szydlo R, Horowitz MM, et al. Choice of pretransplant treatment and timing of transplants for chronic myelogenous leukemia in chronic phase. *Blood* 1993;82(7):2235–2238.

150. Silver RT, Woolf SH, Hehlmann R, et al. An evidence-based analysis of the effect of busulfan, hydroxyurea, interferon, and allogeneic bone marrow transplantation in treating the chronic phase of chronic myeloid leukemia: developed for the American Society of Hematology. *Blood* 1999;94(5):1517–1536.

151. Gratwohl A, Hermans J, Niederwieser D, et al. Bone marrow transplantation for chronic myeloid leukemia: long-term results. Chronic Leukemia Working Party of the European Group for Bone Marrow Transplantation. *Bone Marrow Transplant* 1993;12(5):509–516.

152. Clift R, Appelbaum F, Thomas E. Treatment of chronic myeloid leukemia by marrow transplantation. *Blood* 1993;82:1954–1956.

153. Clift RA, Buckner CD, Thomas ED, et al. Marrow transplantation for patients in accelerated phase of chronic myeloid leukemia. *Blood* 1994;84(12):4368–4373.

154. Lee SJ, Anasetti C, Horowitz MM, et al. Initial therapy for chronic myelogenous leukemia: playing the odds. *J Clin Oncol* 1998;16(9):2897–2903.

155. Clift RA, Anasetti C. Allografting for chronic myeloid leukaemia. *Baillieres Clin Haematol* 1997;10(2):319–336.

156. van Rhee F, Szydlo RM, Hermans J, et al. Long-term results after allogeneic bone marrow transplantation for chronic myelogenous leukemia in chronic phase: a report from the Chronic Leukemia Working Party of the European Group for Blood and Marrow Transplantation. *Bone Marrow Transplant* 1997;20(7):553–560.

157. Giralt SA, Kantarjian HM, Talpaz M, et al. Effect of prior interferon alfa therapy on the outcome of allogeneic bone marrow transplantation for chronic myelogenous leukemia. *J Clin Oncol* 1993;11(6):1055–1061.

158. Beelen DW, Graeven U, Elmaagacli AH, et al. Prolonged administration of interferon-alpha in patients with chronic-phase Philadelphia chromosome-positive chronic myelogenous leukemia before allogeneic bone marrow transplantation may adversely affect transplant outcome. *Blood* 1995;85(10):2981–2990.

159. Sheperd P, Richards S, Allan N. Survival after allogeneic bone marrow transplantation in patients randomized into a trial of IFN alpha versus chemotherapy: no significant adverse effect of prolonged IFN alpha administration. *Blood* 1995;86[Suppl 1]:94a.

160. Tomas JF, Lopez-Lorenzo JL, Requena MJ, et al. Absence of influence of prior treatment with interferon on the outcome of allogeneic bone marrow transplantation for chronic myeloid leukemia. *Bone Marrow Transplant* 1998;22(1):47–51.

161. Beelen DW, Elmaagacli AH, Schaefer UW. The adverse influence of pretransplant interferon-alpha (IFN-alpha) on transplant outcome after marrow transplantation for chronic phase chronic myelogenous leukemia increases with the duration of IFN-alpha exposure. *Blood* 1999;93(5):1779–1810.

162. Pigneaux A, Tanguy M, Michallet M. Prior treatment with alpha interferon does not adversely affect the outcome of allogeneic transplantation for CML. *Blood* 1998;92[Suppl 1]:495a.

163. Zuffa E, Bandini G, Bonini A, et al. Prior treatment with alpha-interferon does not adversely affect the outcome of allogeneic BMT in chronic phase chronic myeloid leukemia. *Haematologica* 1998;83(3):231–236.

164. Hehlmann R, Hochhaus A, Kolb HJ, et al. Interferon-alpha before allogeneic bone marrow transplantation in chronic myelogenous leukemia does not affect outcome adversely, provided it is discontinued at least 90 days before the procedure. *Blood* 1999;94(11):3668–3677.

165. Kantarjian HM, Giles FJ, O'Brien S, et al. Therapeutic choices in younger patients with chronic myelogenous leukemia. *Cancer* 2000;89(8):1647–1658.

166. Morton AJ, Gooley T, Hansen JA, et al. Association between pretransplant interferon-alpha and outcome after unrelated donor marrow transplantation for chronic myelogenous leukemia in chronic phase. *Blood* 1998;92(2):394–401.

167. Lee S, Klein J, Anasetti C, et al. Effect of interferon-alpha (IFN) on outcome of unrelated donor (URD) bone marrow transplantation (BMT). *Blood* 2000;96:841a.

168. Nevill TJ, Barnett MJ, Klingemann HG, et al. Regimen-related toxicity of a busulfan-cyclophosphamide conditioning regimen in 70 patients undergoing allogeneic bone marrow transplantation. *J Clin Oncol* 1991;9(7):1224–1232.

169. Storb R, Deeg HJ, Pepe M, et al. Methotrexate and cyclosporine versus cyclosporine alone for prophylaxis of graft-versus-host disease in patients given HLA-identical marrow grafts for leukemia: long-term follow-up of a controlled trial. *Blood* 1989;73(6):1729–1734.

170. Blaise D, Maraninchi M, Michallet J, et al. Ten year follow-up of a national randomized trial comparing CYTBI vs BUSCY as conditioning regimen for patients administered HLa-identical marrow grafts for CR1 AML. *Blood* 2000;96:480a.

171. Litzow MR, Bolwell BJ, Camitta BM, et al. Comparison of allogeneic bone marrow transplantation (BMT) with cyclophosphamide-total body irradiation (CyTBI) versus busulfan-cyclophosphamide (BuCy) conditioning regimens for acute myelogenous leukemia (AML) in first remission (CR1). *Blood* 2000;96:480a.

172. Socié G, Clift RA, Blaise D, et al. Busulfan (BU)-cyclophosphamide (CY) versus CY-total body irradiation as conditioning regimen before bone marrow transplantation (BMT) for acute myelogenous leukemia (AML) or chronic myelogenous leukemia (CML): long-term follow-up of 4 randomized trials. *Blood* 2000;96:557a.

173. Bhagwatwar HP, Phadungpojna S, Chow DS, et al. Formulation and stability of busulfan for intravenous administration in high-dose chemotherapy. *Cancer Chemother Pharmacol* 1996;37(5):401–408.

174. Clift RA, Buckner CD, Thomas ED, et al. Marrow transplantation for chronic myeloid leukemia: a randomized study comparing cyclophosphamide and total body irradiation with busulfan and cyclophosphamide. *Blood* 1994;84(6):2036–2043.

175. Chao NJ, Schmidt GM, Niland JC, et al. Cyclosporine, methotrexate, and prednisone compared with cyclosporine and prednisone for prophylaxis of acute graft-versus-host disease. *N Engl J Med* 1993;329(17):1225–1230.

176. Horowitz MM, Gale RP, Sondel PM, et al. Graft-versus-leukemia reactions after bone marrow transplantation. *Blood* 1990;75(3):555–562.

177. Goldman JM, Gale RP, Horowitz MM, et al. Bone marrow transplantation for chronic myelogenous leukemia in chronic phase. Increased risk for relapse associated with T-cell depletion. *Ann Intern Med* 1988;108(6):806–814.

178. Giralt SA, Kolb HJ. Donor lymphocyte infusions. *Curr Opin Oncol* 1996;8(2):96–102.

179. Curtis RE, Rowlings PA, Deeg HJ, et al. Solid cancers after bone marrow transplantation. *N Engl J Med* 1997;336(13):897–904.

180. McGlave PB, Shu XO, Wen W, et al. Unrelated donor marrow transplantation for chronic myelogenous leukemia: 9 years' experience of the national marrow donor program. *Blood* 2000;95(7):2219–2225.

181. Craddock C, Szydlo RM, Klein JP, et al. Estimating leukemia-free survival after allografting for chronic myeloid leukemia: a new method that takes into account patients who relapse and are restored to complete remission. *Blood* 2000;96(1):86–90.

182. Guglielmi C, Arcese W, Hermans J, et al. Risk assessment in patients with Ph+ chronic myelogenous leukemia at first relapse after allogeneic stem cell transplant: an EBMT retrospective analysis. The Chronic Leukemia Working Party of the European Group for Blood and Marrow Transplantation. *Blood* 2000;95(11):3328–3334.

183. Arcese W, Goldman JM, D'Arcangelo E, et al. Outcome for patients who relapse after allogeneic bone marrow transplantation for chronic myeloid leukemia. Chronic Leukemia Working Party. European Bone Marrow Transplantation Group. *Blood* 1993;82(10):3211–3219.

184. Mrsic M, Horowitz MM, Atkinson K, et al. Second HLA-identical sibling transplants for leukemia recurrence. *Bone Marrow Transplant* 1992;9(4):269–275.

185. Hansen JA, Gooley TA, Martin PJ, et al. Bone marrow transplants from unrelated donors for patients with chronic myeloid leukemia. *N Engl J Med* 1998;338(14):962–968.

186. McGlave P, Bartsch G, Anasetti C, et al. Unrelated donor marrow transplantation therapy for chronic myelogenous leukemia: initial experience of the National Marrow Donor Program. *Blood* 1993;81(2):543–550.

187. Kroeger N, Zabelina T, Krueger W, et al. CMV-seropositivity of the patient with or without reactivation is the most important prognostic factor for survival and TRM in stem cell transplantation from unrelated donors using pretransplant in-vivo T-cell depletion with ATG. *Blood* 2000;96:417a.

188. Devergie A, Apperley JF, Labopin M, et al. European results of matched unrelated donor bone marrow transplantation for chronic myeloid leukemia. Impact of HLA class II matching. Chronic Leukemia Working Party of the European Group for Blood and Marrow Transplantation. *Bone Marrow Transplant* 1997;20(1):11–19.

189. Lalancette M, Rezvani K, Szydlo R, et al. Favorable outcome of non-myeloablative stem cell transplant (NMSCT) for chronic myeloid leukemia (CML) in first chronic phase: a retrospective study of the European Group for Blood and Marrow Transplantation (EBMT). *Blood* 2000;96:545a.

190. Hehlmann R, Heimpel H, Hasford J, et al. Randomized comparison of interferon-alpha with busulfan and hydroxyurea in chronic myelogenous leukemia. The German CML Study Group. *Blood* 1994;84(12):4064–4077.

191. Allan NC, Richards SM, Shepherd PC. UK Medical Research Council randomised, multicentre trial of interferon-alpha n1 for chronic myeloid leukemia: improved survival irrespective of cytogenetic response. The UK Medical Research Council's Working Parties for Therapeutic Trials in Adult Leukaemia. *Lancet* 1995;345(8962):1392–1397.

192. Long-term follow-up of the Italian trial of interferon-alpha versus conventional chemotherapy in chronic myeloid leukemia. The Italian Cooperative Study Group on Chronic Myeloid Leukemia. *Blood* 1998;92(5):1541–1548.

193. Monitoring treatment and survival in chronic myeloid leukemia. Italian Cooperative Study Group on Chronic Myeloid Leukemia and Italian Group for Bone Marrow Transplantation. *J Clin Oncol* 1999;17(6):1858–1868.

194. Kurzrock R, Estrov Z, Kantarjian H, et al. Conversion of interferon-induced, long-term cytogenetic remissions in chronic myelogenous leukemia to polymerase chain reaction negativity. *J Clin Oncol* 1998;16(4):1526–1531.

195. O'Brien S, Kantarjian H, Talpaz M. Practical guidelines for the management of chronic myelogenous leukemia with interferon alpha. *Leuk Lymphoma* 1996;23(3–4):247–252.

196. Quesada JR, Talpaz M, Rios A, et al. Clinical toxicity of interferons in cancer patients: a review. *J Clin Oncol* 1986;4(2):234–243.

197. Ohnishi K, Ohno R, Tomonaga M, et al. A randomized trial comparing interferon-alpha with busulfan for newly diagnosed chronic myelogenous leukemia in chronic phase. *Blood* 1995;86(3):906–916.

198. Trask PC, Esper P, Riba M, et al. Psychiatric side effects of interferon therapy: prevalence, proposed mechanisms, and future directions. *J Clin Oncol* 2000;18(11):2316–2326.

199. Sacchi S, Kantarjian H, O'Brien S, et al. Immune-mediated and unusual complications during interferon alfa therapy in chronic myelogenous leukemia. *J Clin Oncol* 1995;13(9):2401–2407.

200. Vassiliadis S, Athanassakis I. Type II interferon may be a potential hazardous therapeutic agent during pregnancy [letter]. *Br J Haematol* 1992;82(4):782–783.

201. Sokal JE, Leong SS, Gomez GA. Preferential inhibition by cytarabine of CFU-GM from patients with chronic granulocytic leukemia. *Cancer* 1987;59(1):197–202.

202. Robertson MJ, Tantravahi R, Griffin JD, et al. Hematologic remission and cytogenetic improvement after treatment of stable-phase chronic myelogenous leukemia with continuous infusion of low-dose cytarabine. *Am J Hematol* 1993;43(2):95–102.

203. Sokal J BS. Low-dose cytosine arabinoside by subcutaneous infusion in early and advanced chronic granulocytic leukemia. *Blood* 1986;68:233a.

204. Kantarjian HM, Keating MJ, Estey EH, et al. Treatment of advanced stages of Philadelphia chromosome-positive chronic myelogenous leukemia with interferon-alpha and low-dose cytarabine. *J Clin Oncol* 1992;10(5):772–778.

205. Kantarjian HM, O'Brien S, Smith TL, et al. Treatment of Philadelphia chromosome-positive early chronic phase chronic myelogenous leukemia with daily doses of interferon alpha and low-dose cytarabine. *J Clin Oncol* 1999;17(1):284–292.

206. Thaler J, Hilbe W, Apfelbeck U, et al. Interferon-alpha-2C and LD ara-C for the treatment of patients with CML: results of the Austrian multi-center phase II study. *Leuk Res* 1997;21(1):75–80.

207. Arthur CK MD. Combined interferon alpha-2a and cytosine arabinoside as first-line treatment for chronic myeloid leukemia. *Acta Haematol* 1993; 89[Suppl 1]:15–21.

208. Silver RST, Peterson B, et al. Combined a-interpheron and low-dose cytosine arabinoside for Ph+ chronic phase myeloid leukemia. *Blood* 1996;88:638a.

209. Rosti GBF, De Vivo, et al. Cytarabine increases karyotypic response in IFNα treated chronic myeloid leukemia patients: results of a national prospective randomized trial of the Italian Cooperative Study Group on CML. *Blood* 1999;94:600a.

210. Kuhr T, Eisterer W, Apfelbeck U, et al. Treatment of patients with advanced chronic myelogenous leukemia with interferon-alpha-2b and continuous oral cytarabine ocfosfate (YNK01): a pilot study. *Leuk Res* 2000;24(7):583–587.

211. Mollee P, Taylor K, Arthur C, et al. A phase II study of interferon alpha (IFN) and intermittent oral cytarabine (YNK01) in the treatment of newly diagnosed chronic myeloid leukemia (CML). *Blood* 2000;96:545a.

212. Gale RP, Hehlmann R, Zhang MJ, et al. Survival with bone marrow transplantation versus hydroxyurea or interferon for chronic myelogenous leukemia. The German CML Study Group. *Blood* 1998;91(5):1810–1819.

213. Guilhot F, Sobocinski K, Guilhot J, et al. Comparison of HLA-identical sibling bone marrow transplants (BMT) versus interferon plus cytarabine (IFN/Ara-C) for chronic myelogenous leukemia (CML) in chronic phase (CP). *Blood* 2000;96:545a.

214. Hehlmann R, Berger U, Hochhaus A, et al. Randomized comparison of allogeneic bone marrow transplantation and IFN based drug treatment in CML. *Proc ASCO* 1999;19:10.

215. Carlo-Stella C, Dotti G, Mangoni L, et al. Selection of myeloid progenitors lacking BCR/ABL mRNA in chronic myelogenous leukemia patients after in vitro treatment with the tyrosine kinase inhibitor genistein. *Blood* 1996;88(8):3091–3100.

216. Okabe M, Uehara Y, Miyagishima T, et al. Effect of herbimycin A, an antagonist of tyrosine kinase, on bcr/abl oncoprotein-associated cell proliferations: abrogative effect on the transformation of murine hematopoietic cells by transfection of a retroviral vector expressing oncoprotein P210bcr/abl and preferential inhibition on Ph1-positive leukemia cell growth. *Blood* 1992;80(5):1330–1338.

217. Levitzki A, Gazit A. Tyrosine kinase inhibition: an approach to drug development. *Science* 1995;267(5205):1782–1788.

218. Anafi M, Gazit A, Zehavi A, et al. Tyrphostin-induced inhibition of p210bcr-abl tyrosine kinase activity induces K562 to differentiate. *Blood* 1993;82(12):3524–3529.

219. Bhatia R, Munthe HA, Verfaillie CM. Tyrphostin AG957, a tyrosine kinase inhibitor with anti-BCR/ABL tyrosine kinase activity restores beta1 integrin-mediated adhesion and inhibitory signaling in chronic myelogenous leukemia hematopoietic progenitors. *Leukemia* 1998;12(11):1708–1717.

220. Yaish P, Gazit A, Gilon C, et al. Blocking of EGF-dependent cell proliferation by EGF receptor kinase inhibitors. *Science* 1988;242(4880):933–935.

221. Carroll M, Ohno-Jones S, Tamura S, et al. CGP 57148, a tyrosine kinase inhibitor, inhibits the growth of cells expressing BCR-ABL, TEL-ABL, and TEL-PDGFR fusion proteins. *Blood* 1997;90(12):4947–4952.

222. Druker BJ, Tamura S, Buchdunger E, et al. Effects of a selective inhibitor of the Abl tyrosine kinase on the growth of Bcr-Abl positive cells. *Nat Med* 1996;2(5):561–566.

223. Beran M, Cao X, Estrov Z, et al. Selective inhibition of cell proliferation and BCR-ABL phosphorylation in acute lymphoblastic leukemia cells expressing Mr 190,000 BCR-ABL protein by a tyrosine kinase inhibitor (CGP-57148). *Clin Cancer Res* 1998;4(7):1661–1672.

224. Deininger MW, Vieira S, Mendiola R, et al. BCR-ABL tyrosine kinase activity regulates the expression of multiple genes implicated in the pathogenesis of chronic myeloid leukemia. *Cancer Res* 2000;60(7):2049–2055.

225. le Coutre P, Mologni L, Cleris L, et al. In vivo eradication of human BCR/ABL-positive leukemia cells with an ABL kinase inhibitor. *J Natl Cancer Inst* 1999;91(2):163–168.

226. Druker BJ, Talpaz M, Resta DJ, et al. Efficacy and safety of a specific inhibitor of the BCR-ABL tyrosine kinase in chronic myeloid leukemia. *N Engl J Med* 2001;344(14):1031–1037.

227. Druker BJ, Sawyers CL, Kantarjian H, et al. Activity of a specific inhibitor of the BCR-ABL tyrosine kinase in the blast crisis of chronic myeloid leukemia and acute lymphoblastic leukemia with the Philadelphia chromosome. *N Engl J Med* 2001;344(14):1038–1042.

228. Talpaz M, Silver R, Druker B, et al. Glivec (imatinib mesylate) induces durable hematologic and cytogenetic responses in patients with accelerated phase chronic myelogenous leukemia: results of a phase II study. *Blood* 2002;(in press).

229. Sawyers C, Hochhaus A, Feldman E, et al. A phase II study to determine the safety and anti-leukemic effects of STI571 in patients with Philadelphia chromosome positive chronic myelogenous leukemia in myeloid blast crisis. *Blood* 2000;96:503a.

230. Garcia-Manero G, Kantarjian HM. The hyper-CVAD regimen in adult acute lymphocytic leukemia. *Hematol Oncol Clin North Am* 2000;14(6):1381–1396.

231. O'Brien S, Kantarjian H, Keating M, et al. Homoharringtonine therapy induces responses in patients with chronic myelogenous leukemia in late chronic phase. *Blood* 1995;86(9):3322–3326.

232. Kantarjian HM, Talpaz M, Smith TL, et al. Homoharringtonine and low-dose cytarabine in the management of late chronic-phase chronic myelogenous leukemia. *J Clin Oncol* 2000;18(20):3513–3521.

233. O'Brien S, Kantarjian H, Koller C, et al. Sequential homoharringtonine and interferon-alpha in the treatment of early chronic phase chronic myelogenous leukemia. *Blood* 1999;93(12):4149–4153.

234. Robin J-P, Radosevic N, Pasco S, et al. A new series of homoharringtonine (HHT) analogs exhibiting a potent antileukemic activity in vitro. *Blood* 2000;96:306a.

235. Radosevic N, Pasco S, Drouyé F, et al. OP5215, a new semisynthetic homoharringtonine derivative, is highly cytotoxic on multidrug-resistant cell lines. *Blood* 2000;96(306a).

236. Issa JP, Baylin SB, Herman JG. DNA methylation changes in hematologic malignancies: biologic and clinical implications. *Leukemia* 1997;11[Suppl]1: S7–S11.

237. Kantarjian HM, O'Brien SM, Keating M, et al. Results of decitabine therapy in the accelerated and blastic phases of chronic myelogenous leukemia. *Leukemia* 1997;11(10):1617–1620.

238. Talpaz M, O'Brien S, Rose E, et al. Phase 1 study of polyethylene glycol formulation of interferon alpha-2B (Schering 54031) in Philadelphia chromosome-positive chronic myelogenous leukemia. *Blood* 2001;98(6):1708–1713.

239. Garcia-Manero G, Talpaz M, Giles F, et al. Treatment of Philadelphia chromosome positive chronic phase chronic myelogenous leukemia (Ph+ CML) with pegylated interferon alpha 2B (Peg-IFN/SCH54031) and low dose cytosine arabinoside. *Blood* 2001;98:258b.

240. Reuter CW, Morgan MA, Bergmann L. Targeting the Ras signaling pathway: a rational, mechanism-based treatment for hematologic malignancies? *Blood* 2000;96(5):1655–1669.

241. Reichert A, Heisterkamp N, Daley GQ, et al. Treatment of Bcr/Abl-positive acute lymphoblastic leukemia in P190 transgenic mice with the farnesyl transferase inhibitor SCH66336. *Blood* 2001;97(5):1399–1403.

242. Peters DG, Hoover RR, Gerlach MJ, et al. Activity of the farnesyl protein transferase inhibitor SCH66336 against BCR/ABL-induced murine leukemia and primary cells from patients with chronic myeloid leukemia. *Blood* 2001;97(5):1404–1412.

243. Karp JE, Lancet JE, Kaufmann SH, et al. Clinical and biologic activity of the farnesyltransferase inhibitor R115777 in adults with refractory and relapsed acute leukemias: a phase 1 clinical-laboratory correlative trial. *Blood* 2001; 97(11):3361–3369.

244. Thomas D, Cortes J, O'Brien S, et al. R115777, a farnesyl transferase inhibitor (FTI), has significant anti-leukemia activity in patients with chronic myelogenous leukemia (CML). *Blood* 2001;98:727a.

245. Skorski T, Nieborowska-Skorska M, Wlodarski P, et al. Antisense oligodeoxynucleotide combination therapy of primary chronic myelogenous leukemia blast crisis in SCID mice. *Blood* 1996;88(3):1005–1012.

246. Falkenburg JH, Wafelman AR, Joosten P, et al. Complete remission of accelerated phase chronic myeloid leukemia by treatment with leukemia-reactive cytotoxic T lymphocytes. *Blood* 1999;94(4):1201–1208.

247. Pinilla-Ibarz J, Cathcart K, Korontsvit T, et al. Vaccination of patients with chronic myelogenous leukemia with bcr-abl oncogene breakpoint fusion peptides generates specific immune responses. *Blood* 2000;95(5):1781–1787.

248. Talpaz M, Qiu X, Cheng K, et al. Autoantibodies to Abl and Bcr proteins. *Leukemia* 2000;14(9):1661–1666.

249. Choudhury A, Gajewski JL, Liang JC, et al. Use of leukemic dendritic cells for the generation of antileukemic cellular cytotoxicity against Philadelphia chromosome-positive chronic myelogenous leukemia. *Blood* 1997;89(4):1133–1142.

250. Cortes J, Kantarjian H, O'Brien S, et al. GM-CSF can improve the cytogenetic response obtained with interferon-alpha therapy in patients with chronic myelogenous leukemia. *Leukemia* 1998;12(6):860–864.

251. Smith D, Matsui W, Miller C, et al. GM-CSF and interferon (INF) rapidly induce cytogenetic remissions in chronic myeloid leukemia (CML). *Blood* 2000;96:544a.

252. Cunningham I, Gee T, Dowling M, et al. Results of treatment of Ph'+ chronic myelogenous leukemia with an intensive treatment regimen (L-5 protocol). *Blood* 1979;53(3):375–395.

253. Kantarjian HM, Vellekoop L, McCredie KB, et al. Intensive combination chemotherapy (ROAP 10) and splenectomy in the management of chronic myelogenous leukemia. *J Clin Oncol* 1985;3(2):192–200.

254. Kantarjian HM, Smith TL, McCredie KB, et al. Chronic myelogenous leukemia: a multivariate analysis of the associations of patient characteristics and therapy with survival. *Blood* 1985;66(6):1326–1335.

255. Kantarjian HM, Talpaz M, Keating MJ, et al. Intensive chemotherapy induction followed by interferon-alpha maintenance in patients with Philadelphia chromosome-positive chronic myelogenous leukemia. *Cancer* 1991;68(6): 1201–1207.

256. Simonsson B, Oberg G, Linder O, et al. Intensive treatment in order to minimize the Ph-positive clone in CML. *J Mol Med* 1997;75(7):B223.

257. Deisseroth AB, Zu Z, Claxton D, et al. Genetic marking shows that Ph+ cells present in autologous transplants of chronic myelogenous leukemia (CML) contribute to relapse after autologous bone marrow in CML. *Blood* 1994;83(10):3068–3076.

258. Rowe J, Ryan D, Dipersio J, et al. Autografting in chronic myelogenous leukemia followed by immunotherapy. *Stem Cells* 1993;11[Suppl]3:34–42.

259. Carella AM, Podesta M, Frassoni F, et al. Selective overshoot of Ph-negative blood hemopoietic cells after intensive idarubicin-containing regimen and their repopulating capacity after reinfusion. *Stem Cells* 1993;11[Suppl]3:67–72.

260. Carella AM, Lerma E, Corsetti MT, et al. Autografting with Philadelphia chromosome-negative mobilized hematopoietic progenitor cells in chronic myelogenous leukemia. *Blood* 1999;93(5):1534–1539.

261. Khouri IF, Kantarjian HM, Talpaz M, et al. Results with high-dose chemotherapy and unpurged autologous stem cell transplantation in 73 patients

with chronic myelogenous leukemia: the MD Anderson experience. *Bone Marrow Transplant* 1996;17(5):775–779.

262. Verfaillie CM, Bhatia R, Steinbuch M, et al. Comparative analysis of autografting in chronic myelogenous leukemia: effects of priming regimen and marrow or blood origin of stem cells. *Blood* 1998;92(5):1820–1831.

263. Cortes J, Talpaz M, O'Brien S, et al. Suppression of cytogenetic clonal evolution with interferon alfa therapy in patients with Philadelphia chromosome-positive chronic myelogenous leukemia. *J Clin Oncol* 1998;16(10): 3279–3285.

264. Kantarjian HM, Keating MJ, Talpaz M, et al. Chronic myelogenous leukemia in blast crisis. Analysis of 242 patients. *Am J Med* 1987;83(3):445–454.

265. Kantarjian HM, O'Brien S, Smith TL, et al. Results of treatment with hyper-CVAD, a dose-intensive regimen, in adult acute lymphocytic leukemia. *J Clin Oncol* 2000;18(3):547–561.

266. Dobrovic A, Morley AA, Seshadri R, et al. Molecular diagnosis of Philadelphia negative CML using the polymerase chain reaction and DNA analysis: clinical features and course of M-bcr negative and M-bcr positive CML. *Leukemia* 1991;5(3):187–190.

267. Snyder DS, Negrin RS, O'Donnell MR, et al. Fractionated total-body irradiation and high-dose etoposide as a preparatory regimen for bone marrow transplantation for 94 patients with chronic myelogenous leukemia in chronic phase. *Blood* 1994;84(5):1672–1679.

268. Clift RA, Buckner CD, Appelbaum FR, et al. Allogeneic marrow transplantation in patients with chronic myeloid leukemia in the chronic phase: a randomized trial of two irradiation regimens. *Blood* 1991;77(8):1660–1665.

269. Biggs JC, Szer J, Crilley P, et al. Treatment of chronic myeloid leukemia with allogeneic bone marrow transplantation after preparation with BuCy2. *Blood* 1992;80(5):1352–1357.

270. Bortin MM, Horowitz MM, Rowlings PA, et al. 1993 progress report from the International Bone Marrow Transplant Registry. Advisory Committee of the International Bone Marrow Transplant Registry. *Bone Marrow Transplant* 1993;12(2):97–104.

271. Ozer H, George SL, Schiffer CA, et al. Prolonged subcutaneous administration of recombinant alpha 2b interferon in patients with previously untreated Philadelphia chromosome-positive chronic-phase chronic myelogenous leukemia: effect on remission duration and survival: Cancer and Leukemia Group B study 8583. *Blood* 1993;82(10):2975–2984.

272. Mahon F, Faberes C, Boiron J, et al. High response rate using recombinant alpha interpheron in patients with newly diagnosed chronic myeloid leukemia—analysis of predictive factors. *Blood* 1996;88:638a.

273. Alimena G, Morra E, Lazzarino M, et al. Interferon alpha-2b as therapy for Ph'-positive chronic myelogenous leukemia: a study of 82 patients treated with intermittent or daily administration. *Blood* 1988;72(2):642–647.

274. Silver R, Szatrowski T, Peterson B, et al. Combined interferon and low-dose cytosine arabinoside for Ph+ chronic phase myeloid leukemia. *Blood* 1996; 88:638a.

PART 4

White Blood Cells

Neutrophils and Monocytes: Normal Physiology and Disorders of Neutrophil and Monocyte Production

David C. Dale and W. Conrad Liles

This chapter describes the normal production of neutrophils and monocytes and nonmalignant conditions causing reduced or increased production of these cells. Subsequent chapters describe disorders affecting the function of neutrophils and monocytes and the involvement of phagocytes in immunologic processes.

NEUTROPHIL LIFE CYCLE

Neutrophils play a critical role in host defense against microbial invasion and are important mediators of inflammatory responses. Approximately 1×10^9 neutrophils/kg are produced in the bone marrow daily (1,2). Production and deployment of mature neutrophils involves an orderly series of morphologic and functional changes coincident with changes in gene expression. The production of these cells and their state of activation are tightly regulated to maintain a supply for host defenses while avoiding self-injury.

General Features of Neutrophil Development

Two distinctive morphologic processes characterize the formation of mature neutrophils from their precursors (3,4). First, neutrophil precursors acquire cytoplasmic granules (primary, secondary, and tertiary granules) and vesicles, which are critical for the function of these cells (Fig. 14-1). Second, the nuclei of the immature cells become progressively smaller, more dense, more lobulated, and less functionally active.

The earliest morphologically identifiable neutrophil precursors are *myeloblasts*, large (15 to 20 μm) round cells with large nuclei and scant cytoplasm. Their nuclei contain fine chromatin and several nucleoli, and their cytoplasm is lightly basophilic and generally without granules. Myeloblasts mature into promyelocytes, which are characterized by the presence of abundant primary granules, also referred to as *azurophilic* or *nonspecific* granules (Fig. 14-2). Granule formation occurs in the Golgi apparatus, which appears as a clear zone in the cytoplasm when the cells are examined by light microscopy. The nuclear chromatin of the promyelocyte often shows some condensation or clumping.

Promyelocytes evolve into myelocytes, which are the most differentiated myeloid cells capable of undergoing mitosis. These cells are considerably smaller than promyelocytes and have distinct clumping of nuclear chromatin. The nuclei of myelocytes are usually eccentrically placed, and myelocytes have no visible nucleoli. At this developmental stage, primary and secondary granule formation continues in the Golgi appa-

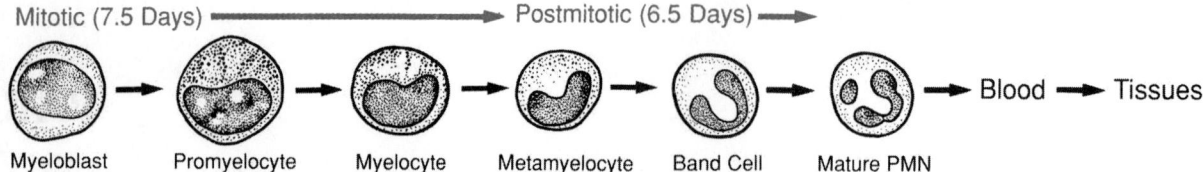

Figure 14-1. Development of the neutrophil. (Adapted from Bainton DF, Ullyot JL, Farquhar MG. The development of neutrophilic polymorphonuclear leukocytes in human bone marrow. *J Exp Med* 1971;134:907.)

ratus. Myeloblasts, promyelocytes, and myelocytes constitute the proliferative myeloid compartment and normally account for 20% to 30% of the myeloid cell population (2).

Myelocytes develop into metamyelocytes, the first cells of the neutrophil lineage that cannot divide; thus, by definition, metamyelocytes do not incorporate tritiated thymidine (^{3}H-TdR). The predominant feature at this transition is the condensation of nuclear chromatin with shrinkage toward a C-shaped or horseshoe-shaped nucleus. Although metamyelocytes have tertiary granules and vesicles, secondary granules predominate. In Giemsa- or Wright-stained preparations, the cytoplasm shifts from a blue hue in promyelocytes and myelocytes to a faint pink in cells of the metamyelocyte stage and beyond.

As the chromatin further condenses, but before the nucleus is distinctly segmented, the cells are called *bands* or *band neutrophils*. The usual definition of a mature marrow neutrophil is a leukocyte with a faintly staining pinkish cytoplasm and a segmented nucleus, usually with two or more nuclear lobes separated by narrow filaments. Mature neutrophils have a relatively limited capacity for protein synthesis and have no endoplasmic reticulum or Golgi apparatus (Fig. 14-3). During development, the cells shrink, and the mature neutrophil in the marrow has a diameter approximately two-thirds that of the promyelocyte. Postmitotic cells (i.e., metamyelocytes, bands, and mature neutrophils) constitute approximately two-thirds of the cells of the neutrophil series in the marrow. Normally, more than one-half of the cells in a marrow differential count are neutrophils and their precursors (2).

Formation of Neutrophil Granules

The formation and storage of proteins in the primary, secondary, and tertiary granules are important features of neutrophil development (5). All granule proteins are synthesized with the same general features. Translation of the specific gene leads to protein synthesis within the endoplasmic reticulum. Packaging of the

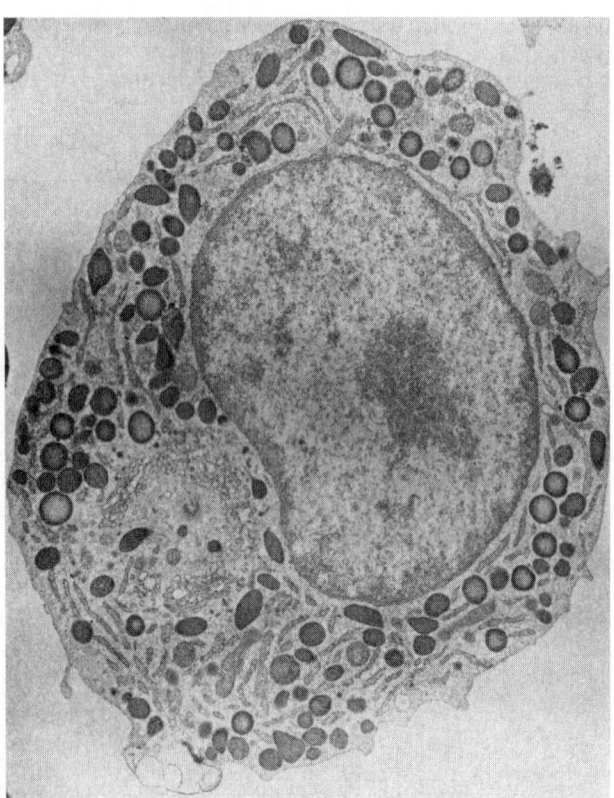

Figure 14-2. Promyelocyte stained for peroxidase. A prominent Golgi apparatus and spherical and elliptoid azurophilic granules can be seen. (Adapted from Bainton DF, Ullyot JL, Farquhar MG. The development of neutrophilic polymorphonuclear leukocytes in human bone marrow: origin and content of azurophil and specific granules. *J Exp Med* 1971;134:907; copyright 1971 Rockefeller University Press.)

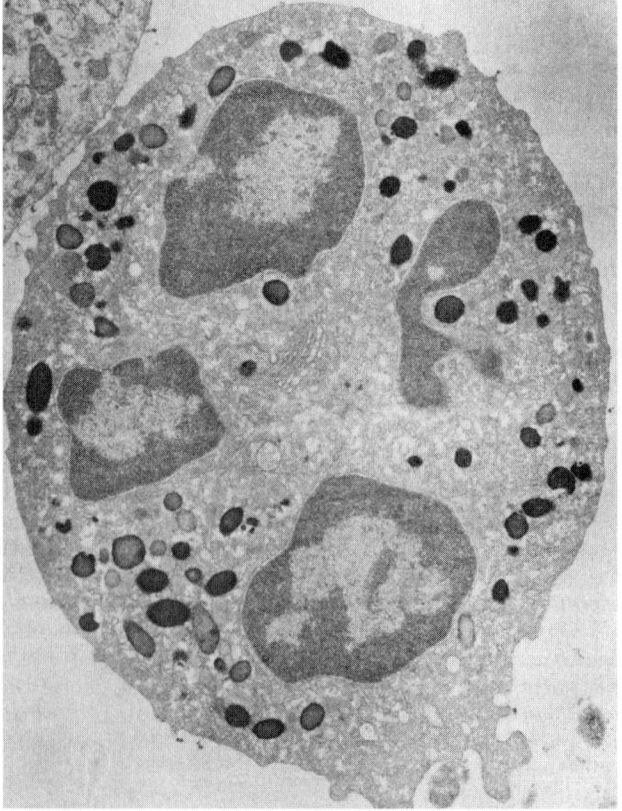

Figure 14-3. Normal blood neutrophil as seen under the electron microscope. (Adapted from Bainton DF, Ullyot JL, Farquhar MG. The development of neutrophilic polymorphonuclear leukocytes in human bone marrow: origin and content of azurophil and specific granules. *J Exp Med* 1971;134:907; copyright 1971 Rockefeller University Press.)

proteins in the Golgi apparatus and storage in granules characteristic for each stage in development follow. The process occurs in a rigidly maintained sequence (6,7). Cells at the beginning of the transition from myeloblasts to promyelocytes produce primary granule enzymes, such as myeloperoxidase, neutrophil elastase, and the defensins. Synthesis of these enzymes then ceases as the cell switches to production of secondary granule proteins (e.g., collagenase, lysozyme, and lactoferrin) at the myelocyte stage in development (8–11). Formation of the tertiary granules, also called *gelatinase granules*, follows. Secretory vesicles, which are formed last in the developmental process, contain neutrophil (leukocyte) alkaline phosphatase (12,13).

There are several important differences between primary and secondary granules. The primary granules are formed from the inner, convex surface of the Golgi apparatus, whereas the secondary granules form from the outer, convex surface (14–16). The sequence of fusion of the granules within phagocytic vacuoles may be related to these different properties. In Giemsa-stained smears, primary granules appear deep bluish-purple in color, whereas the secondary granules appear faintly pink, owing to differences in protein content between the two granule types. The secondary granules are also more abundant, outnumbering primary granules approximately tenfold. Finally, primary granules are more dense than secondary granules. This difference in density facilitates separation of the granule types for biochemical studies.

Recent studies have characterized the synthesis of granule proteins and defined steps in this process that may be altered in diseases affecting neutrophil development (6–9). In general, these proteins are synthesized as proenzymes and glycosylated while in the Golgi apparatus. Enzymatic activity is inhibited by peptide extensions at both the amino and carboxyl ends. These terminal sequences may be either removed at the time of granule incorporation, resulting in the storage of fully active enzyme, or retained, permitting storage of inactive enzyme. Myeloperoxidase, cathepsin G, neutrophil elastase, and the defensins are stored in their active forms (7,17–19), while secondary granule proteins (e.g., lactoferrin and gelatinase) are stored as glycosylated proteins that are activated after release from secondary granules (6).

Functional Development

During development, neutrophils acquire many cytoplasmic and surface features to facilitate trafficking from marrow to tissue sites and to enhance microbicidal activity. For example, bone marrow neutrophils accumulate a large quantity of cytoplasmic glycogen for the burst of metabolic activity that occurs later when engaged in phagocytic and bactericidal functions (Chapter 16). Neutrophils develop an elaborate cytoskeletal machinery to enable efficient migration from the blood to tissue sites of inflammation (Chapter 16). Neutrophils synthesize a multicomponent enzyme, nicotinamide adenine dinucleotide phosphate (NADPH) oxidase, that plays a critical role in their bactericidal activity (Chapter 16). Glycogen accumulation, cytoskeletal formation, and the synthesis of the cytoplasmic components of NADPH oxidase all occur relatively late in neutrophil development within the bone marrow, after formation of most of the granule proteins.

The surface of the neutrophil is highly specialized to assist in its physiologic functions. As demonstrated by scanning electron microscopy, the surface of mature neutrophils contains ruffles and deep folds that spread behind the cell as it moves through the environment (15,16). Earlier in development, the surface is smoother and apparently not specialized for phagocytosis of particulate matter. Cells of the mitotic precursor pool in the

marrow have numerous growth factor receptors on their surface, such as the receptors for kit-ligand (also called *stem cell factor*), flt-3 ligand, interleukin 3 (IL-3), granulocyte colony-stimulating factor (G-CSF), and granulocyte-macrophage colony-stimulating factor (GM-CSF). Most of these growth factor receptors are lost as the cells proceed down their developmental pathway (20–23). Mature neutrophils, however, retain functionally active receptors for G-CSF and GM-CSF that serve to enhance the metabolic burst of the mature neutrophil when it engages in phagocytosis (a phenomenon known as *priming*), illustrating how the function of receptors can adapt as the cells mature (24).

The antigens on the surface of leukocytes are designated by the cluster differentiation (CD) system (Table 14-1). Many of these antigens are useful markers of specific stages of cell development. Others serve as cell-surface receptors for physiologically important ligands. For example, CD34, a marker expressed on early precursor cells, is widely used for selecting and counting hematopoietic stem cells capable of repopulating the marrow following hematopoietic transplantation. By contrast, the CD11/18 family of surface antigens, also know as the β_2 integrins, is expressed late in development (25–27). The three members of the β_2-integrin family (CD11a/CD18, CD11b/CD18, CD11c/CD18) have distinctive functions and are composed of variable α-subunits and a common β-subunit. CD11b/CD18 is the C3bi receptor, a critical surface protein for neutrophil adherence and migration (28). CD11a/CD18 and CD11c/18 are also involved in cell adhesion (Chapter 16) (29).

Functional development is virtually completed by the time the neutrophil leaves the marrow and enters the blood. Adherence proteins expressed on hematopoietic cells and matrix proteins, produced by fibroblasts and stromal cells, normally retain developing cells within the marrow until fully mature. Mobilization of both immature and mature myeloid elements from marrow to blood is presumed to involve changes in adherence proteins or receptors to which adherence proteins bind (30). Undifferentiated neutrophil precursors (i.e., CD34+ cells) express several adhesion molecules, including the fibronectin receptors [i.e., very late activation antigen 4 (VLA-4) (CD49d/CD2), VLA-5 (CD49e/CD29)], and platelet/endothelial cell adhesion molecule-1 (CD31)]. Expression of all these proteins decreases as cells differentiate via the myeloid pathway (31–34). CD44 and CD62L (L-selectin) are both expressed on CD34+ cells and mature neutrophils but are down-regulated during the intermediate stages of development. By contrast, CD67, another adhesion molecule, is maximally expressed during the intermediate stages of cell development. The factors governing the sequential expression and disappearance of these adhesions and the molecular mechanisms governing cell release from marrow to blood are not yet fully understood.

Chemotaxis, the active and directed migration of cells, depends on the functional integrity of cytoskeletal elements and stimuli from environmental chemotactic factors (35,36). These factors act through specific cell surface receptors. Primitive myeloid cells lack these capacities, because of the lack of chemotactic receptors and the required cytoskeletal elements, which are both late features of myeloid development (37). Responsiveness to chemotactic factors becomes detectable at the metamyelocyte stage in development (37). There are several well-characterized chemoattractants, including N-formylated peptides, the activated fifth component of complement (C5a), leukotriene B$_4$, platelet-activating factor, the CXC chemokines, IL-8, GROα, neutrophil-activating protein-2, and the C-C chemokines, macrophage inhibitor protein 1α (MIP-1α) and MIP-1β (Table 14-1). Chemoattractants can be exogenous (e.g., microbial) or endogenous (e.g., derived from monocytes, plate-

TABLE 14-1. Expression of Cluster Differentiation Antigens on Human Neutrophils and Monocytes

Surface Antigen	Distribution	Ligand(s)	Function(s)
CD9 (motility related protein 1)	Leukocytes	Associates with CD63, CD81, CD82	Modulation of cell adhesion/migration and myeloid development
CD10 (common acute lympho-blastic leukemia antigen, enkephalinase)	Neutrophils	Unknown	Unknown
CD11a (lymphocyte function antigen-1α, α_L integrin)	Leukocytes	CD54, CD102, CD50	Cell adhesion, co-stimulation
CD11b (CR3, Mac-1, α_M integrin)	Neutrophils, monocytes	iC3b, fibrinogen, CD23	Cell adhesion, phagocytosis
CD11c (CR4, α_X integrin)	Neutrophils, monocytes	iC3b, fibrinogen, CD23	Cell adhesion, phagocytosis
CDw12	Neutrophils, monocytes	Unknown	Unknown
CD13 (aminopeptidase N)	Neutrophils, monocytes	Unknown	Cleavage of peptides bound to MHC-II
CD14	Monocytes, neutrophils (weak)	LPS	Docking receptor for LPS
CD15 (LewisX)	Neutrophils, monocytes	Selectins	Cell adhesion
CD15s (sialyl LewisX)	Neutrophils, monocytes	CD62E	Cell adhesion
CD16a (FcγRIIIa, LEU-11)	Neutrophils, monocytes	IgG	Low-affinity receptor for IgG, antibody-dependent cellular cytotoxicity, cytokine production
CD16b (FcγRIIIb)	Neutrophils	IgG	Low-affinity receptor for IgG
CDw17 (lactosylceramide)	Neutrophils, monocytes	Unknown	Unknown
CD18 (β_2 integrin common subunit)	Leukocytes	Ligands for CD11a, CD11b, CD11c	Associates with CD11a–c; cell adhesion and migration
CD23 (FcϵRII, B6, LEU-20, BLAST-2)	Monocytes	IgE, CD21, CD11b, CD11c	Regulates cytokine release from mono-cytes
CD24 (BA-1, HAS)	Neutrophils	CD62P (P-selectin)	Unknown
CD25 (IL-2Rα, TAC)	Monocytes	IL-2	Low-affinity IL-2R α chain
CD29 (β_1 integrin common subunit)	Leukocytes	Ligands for CD49a–f	Associates with CD49a–f; cell adhesion
CD31 (PECAM-1)	Neutrophils, monocytes	CD31, $\alpha_v\beta_3$ integrin	Cell adhesion
CD32 (FcγRII)	Monocytes, macrophages	IgG	Low-affinity receptor for IgG; mediates endocytosis, cytotoxicity, immuno-modulation
CD33	Neutrophils, monocytes, macro-phages	Unknown	Unknown
CD35 (CR1, C3bR, C4bR)	Neutrophils, monocytes	C3b, C4b, iC3b, C3dg, iC3, iC4	Binding of C4b/C3b-coated particles; removal and processing of immune complexes
CD36 (GPIIIb, GPIV)	Mature monocytes, macrophages	Oxidized LDL, long-chain fatty acids, collagen, thrombospondin	Scavenger receptor for oxidized LDL; cell adhesion
CD39	Monocytes	Unknown	Unknown
CD40	Macrophages	CD154	Cell activation; inhibition of apoptosis
CD43 (leukosialin, sialophorin)	Leukocytes (except B cells)	CD54	Cell adhesion
CD44 (H-CAM, Hermes, Pgp-1)	Leukocytes	MIP-1β, hyaluronan, osteopontin, ankyrin	Cell adhesion, signaling, activation
CD44R (CD44v)	Monocytes, other activated leuko-cytes	MIP-1β, hyaluronan, bFGF, osteopontin, ankyrin	Possible role in cell migration through extracellular matrix
CD45 (leukocyte common antigen, T200, B220)	Leukocytes	CD2, CD3, CD4, galectin-1	Signal transduction
CD48 (BLAST-1)	Leukocytes, except neutrophils	CD2	Cell adhesion
CD49a (VLA-1, α_1 integrin)	Monocytes	Laminin, collagen I, collagen IV	Associates with CD29; cell adhesion
CD49d (VLA-4, α_4 integrin)	Monocytes	CD106, MAdCAM-1, fibronectin, invasin, thrombospondin	Associates with CD29; cell adhesion
CD49e (VLA-5, α_5 integrin, FNRα)	Monocytes	Fibronectin	Associates with CD29; cell adhesion, migration, and matrix assembly
CD49f (VLA-6, α_6 integrin)	Monocytes	Laminin	Associates with CD29; cell adhesion, spreading, and migration
CD50 (ICAM-3)	Leukocytes	CD11a/CD18	Cell adhesion, co-stimulation
CD51 (α_v integrin, VNR-α)	Monocytes	Vitronectin, fibrinogen, vWF, throm-bospondin, fibronectin, collagen	Associates with CD61; cell adhesion
CD52 (CAMPATH-1)	Monocytes	Unknown	Unknown
CD54 (ICAM-1)	Monocytes	CD11a/CD18, CD11b/CD18, rhi-novirus	Cell adhesion; receptor for rhinovirus
CD55 (decay accelerating factor)	Leukocytes	C3b/C3bBb convertase, C4b/C4b2a convertase, CD97, echo-virus, coxsackie B virus	Complement regulation; receptor for echovirus and coxsackie B virus
CD61 (β_3 integrin, GPIIb/IIIa)	Monocytes	Vitronectin, fibrinogen, vWF, thrombospondin, fibronectin, collagen	Associates with CD51; cell adhesion
CD62L (L-selectin, LAM-1, LECAM-1, LEU-8)	Neutrophils	GlyCAM-1, MAdCAM-1, CD34	Leukocyte rolling on activated endothe-lial cells
CD63 (LIMP, LAMP-3, NGA)	Monocytes, degranulated neutrophils	Unknown	Unknown
CD64 (FcγRI)	Neutrophils, monocytes	IgG	Binding of IgG

CD65 (ceramide dodecasaccharide)	Neutrophils, monocytes	Unknown	Unknown
CD66	Neutrophils	CD62, CD66	Cell adhesion and signaling
CD69 (AIM, MLR3, EA-1)	Monocytes	Unknown	Monocyte activation and signal transduction
CD74 (invariant chain)	Monocytes	Unknown	Intracellular sorting of MHC-II molecules
CDw78	Macrophages	Unknown	Unknown
CD82	Activated leukocytes	MHC-I, MHC-II, β_1 integrins, CD4, CD8	Signal transduction
CD84	Monocytes	Unknown	Unknown
CD87 (UPAR)	Neutrophils, monocytes	u-PA, vitronectin	Cell migration
CD88 (C5aR)	Neutrophils, monocytes	C5a, anaphylatoxin	Granulocyte activation, signal transduction
CD89 (FcαR)	Myeloid cells	IgA	Phagocytosis, degranulation, respiratory burst, microbicidal activity
CD91 (α_2-M-R, LDL-R)	Monocytes	α_2-microglobulin, plasminogen activator complex	Endocytosis of α_2-microglobulin, plasminogen activator complexes, chylomicrons, and lipoprotein lipase
CDw92	Neutrophils, monocytes	Unknown	Unknown
CD93	Neutrophils, monocytes	Unknown	Unknown
CD95 (Fas, APO-1)	Leukocytes	Fas ligand (CD95L)	Apoptosis; cell activation in certain circumstances
CD97 (BL-KDD/F12)	Neutrophils, monocytes	Unknown	Unknown
CD98 (4F2)	Leukocytes	Unknown	Integrin-associated protein that regulates expression of the high-affinity forms of integrins; regulation of cell activation
CD101	Neutrophils, monocytes	Unknown	Unknown
CD102 (ICAM-2)	Monocytes	CD11a/CD18	Cell adhesion; co-stimulation
CD104 (β4 integrin)	Monocytes	Laminin-1, -4, -5	Cell adhesion and migration
CD105 (endoglin)	Activated monocytes	Unknown	Modulation of cell responses to transforming growth factor-β1
CD106 (VCAM-1, INCAM-1)	Monocytes	CD49d/CD29 (VLA-4, $\alpha_4\beta_1$), $\alpha_4\beta_7$	Cell adhesion and activation
CD107a (LAMP-1)	Activated neutrophils	Unknown	Unknown
CD107b (LAMP-2)	Activated neutrophils	Unknown	Unknown
CD114 (G-CSFR)	Myeloid cells	G-CSF	Regulation of granulocyte proliferation and differentiation
CD115 (M-CSFR, CSF-1R)	Monocytes, macrophages	M-CSF	Differentiation, survival, and proliferation of monocytes and macrophages
CD116 (GM-CSFR-α)	Myeloid cells	GM-CSF	Differentiation, survival, and proliferation of myeloid cells
CDw119 (IFNγR-α)	Leukocytes	IFNγ	Associates with IFNγRII (β chain) to form the IFNγ receptor
CD120a (TNFR type 1)	Neutrophils, activated monocytes	TNF	Induction of inflammatory mediators; up-regulation of adhesion molecules
CD120b (TNFR type 2)	Neutrophils, monocytes	TNF	Induction of inflammatory mediators; up-regulation of adhesion molecules
CD121a (IL-1R type 1)	Leukocytes	IL-1α, IL-1β, IL-1Ra	Functional receptor for IL-1
CDw121b (IL-1R type 2)	Monocytes	IL-1α, IL-1β, IL-1Ra	Decoy receptor for IL-1
CD122 (IL-2R-β)	Monocytes	IL-2, IL-15	Associates with CD25 and CD132 to form the high-affinity receptor for IL-2
CDw123 (IL-3R-α)	Myeloid cells	IL-3	Low-affinity receptor for IL-3; associates with CDw131 to form high-affinity IL-3R
CD126 (IL-6R)	Monocytes	IL-6	Associates with CD130 to form IL-6R; inflammation
CDw128 (IL-8R types A and B, CXCR1, CXCR2)	Neutrophils, monocytes	—	Chemotaxis and cell activation
CD130	Leukocytes	IL-6, IL-11, oncostatin M, LIF, CNF, cardiotropin-1	Signal transduction component of the IL-6, IL-11, oncostatin M, LIF, CNF, and cardiotropin-1 receptors
CDw131	Myeloid cells	IL-3, IL-5, GM-CSF	Signal transduction component (common β chain subunit) of the IL-3, IL-5, and GM-CSF receptors
CD132	Neutrophils, monocytes	IL-2, IL-4, IL-7, IL-9, IL-15	Signal transduction component (common γ chain subunit) of the IL-2, IL-4, IL-7, IL-9, and IL-15 receptors
CDw137 (4-1BB)	Monocytes	4-1BB	Cell stimulation
CD139	Neutrophils, monocytes	Unknown	Unknown
CD140b (PDGFRb)	Neutrophils, monocytes	PDGF-β	Signal transduction, cell proliferation, cell migration

(continued)

TABLE 14-1. (continued)

Surface Antigen	Distribution	Ligand(s)	Function(s)
CD141 (thrombomodulin)	Neutrophils, monocytes	Thrombin	Cofactor for thrombin-mediated activation of protein C and anticoagulation
CD142 (tissue factor)	Activated monocytes	Factor VIIa, factor Xa/TFPI	Forms an enzyme when associated with factor VIIa involved in initiation of coagulation cascade
CD143 (ACE, peptidyl dipeptidase A)	Leukocytes	Angiotensin I, bradykinin, substance P	Metabolism of angiotensin and bradykinin
CD147 (neurothelin, basigin, EMMPRIN, M6)	Leukocytes	Unknown	Unknown
CD148 (HPTP-eta)	Leukocytes	Unknown	Tyrosine phosphatase
CDw149	Neutrophils, monocytes	Unknown	Unknown
CD154 (CD40L)	Monocytes	CD40	Monocyte activation
CD155 (poliovirus receptor)	Monocytes	Poliovirus	Poliovirus receptor
CD156 (ADAM-8)	Neutrophils, monocytes	Unknown	Unknown
CD157 (Mo5, BST-1)	Myeloid cells	Nicotinamide adenine dinucleotide, cyclic ADP-ribose	ADP-ribosyl cyclase
CD162 (PSGL-1)	Neutrophils, monocytes	CD62P, CD62E	Rolling of leukocytes over endothelial cells, platelets, and other leukocytes
CD163 (M130)	Activated monocytes, macrophages	Unknown	Unknown
CD164	Monocytes	Unknown	Cell adhesion
CD165 (AD2)	Monocytes	Unknown	Cell adhesion
CD166 (ALCAM, CD6L)	Activated leukocytes	CD6, CD166	Cell adhesion

ACE, angiotensin converting enzyme; ADAM, a disintegrin and metalloproteinase; ADCC, antibody-dependent cellular cytotoxicity; ADP, adenosine diphosphate; AIM, activation inducer molecule; ALCAM, activated leukocyte cell adhesion molecule; bFGF, basic fibroblast growth factor; BST, bone marrow stroma cell antigen; CALLA, common acute lymphoblastic leukemia antigen; CNF, ciliary neurotropic factor; CSF-1, colony-stimulating factor-1; CXCR, CXC chemokine receptor; EMMPRIN, extracellular matrix metalloproteinase inducer; G-CSF, granulocyte colony-stimulating factor; GlyCAM, glycosylation-dependent cell adhesion molecule; GM-CSF, granulocyte-macrophage colony-stimulating factor; H-CAM, homing-associated cell adhesion molecule; HPTP-eta, human protein tyrosine phosphatase eta; ICAM, intracellular adhesion molecule; IFN-γ, interferon-γ; IgA, immunoglobulin A; IgE, immunoglobulin E; IgG, immunoglobulin G; IL, interleukin; INCAM, inducible cell adhesion molecule; LAM, leukocyte adhesion molecule; LAMP, lysosome-associated membrane protein; LDL, low-density lipoprotein; LECAM, lectin cell adhesion molecule; LEU, leucine; LIF, leukemia inhibitory factor; LIMP, lysosomal integral membrane protein; LPS, lipopolysaccharide; MAdCAM, mucosal addressin cell adhesion molecule; M-CSF, macrophage colony-stimulating factor; MHC-I, major histocompatibility complex class I; MHC-II, major histocompatibility complex class II; MIP-1β, macrophage inflammatory protein-1β; NGA, neuroglandular antigen; PDGF, platelet-derived growth factor; PECAM, platelet/endothelial cell adhesion molecule; PSGL, P-selectin glycoprotein ligand; TNF, tumor necrosis factor; u-PA, urokinase plasminogen activator; VCAM, vascular cell adhesion molecule; VLA, very late activation antigen; vWF, von Willebrand's factor.

lets, and endothelial cells). Although tumor necrosis factor-alpha (TNF-α) and IL-1 are not direct chemoattractants, both induce production of chemoattractants from many types of cells at an inflammatory focus (36). For each attractant, there is a corresponding receptor on the neutrophil.

Phagocytosis of bacteria and other particles is facilitated by immunoglobulin G (IgG) and complement (e.g., CR3) receptors on neutrophils (Chapter 16). Two IgG Fc receptors are normally expressed, namely, FcγRIII (CD16) and FcγRII (CD32). A third receptor [i.e., FcγRI (CD64)] is induced during inflammation by proinflammatory cytokines (38). CD16 and CD32, as well as CR3, are expressed at the metamyelocyte stage in neutrophil development. Inducible CD64 can also be detected at this stage in development (39,40).

Gene Expression with Myeloid Differentiation

The differentiation of hematopoietic stem cells to form neutrophils and monocytes is quite complex and is not yet completely understood. Major advances, however, followed the discovery of the hematopoietic growth factors, particularly G-CSF and GM-CSF. These factors not only stimulate cell division but also affect the synthesis of many cytoplasmic components of these cells. For example, G-CSF treatment increases expression of primary granule proteins, such as the enzyme myeloblastin. Expression of the G-CSF receptor on the cell is necessary for this response (41). The discovery of transcription factors, such as PU.1, Sp-1, C/EBPα, and Oct-1, with specific effects on myeloid differentiation was a second major advance in understanding this process (42,43). For

example, the promoter for the myeloblastin gene has binding sites for PU.1, C/EBP, and cMyb, but the response to the growth factor G-CSF is associated mainly with PU.1 (41). Genes associated with cell proliferation, such as junB and DNA topoisomerase II, are also responsive to G-CSF (44,45).

Recent research suggests that PU.1 may serve as a major regulator of differentiation and commitment to the myeloid pathway. PU.1 is a member of the Ets family of transcription factors and a product of the Spi-1 oncogene (43). The PU.1 protein contains 272 amino acids and binds to a specific DNA winged helix-turn-motif (46). It is expressed in myeloid and B cells, including human CD34+ cells, and specifically up-regulated in myeloid differentiation. PU.1 can interact directly with other promoters such as GATA-1, a promoter of erythroid differentiation, to block its effect and, thereby, direct cells toward the myeloid pathway (47,48). Within the myeloid pathway, PU.1 induces expression of the receptor for macrophage colony-stimulating factor (M-CSF), whereas C/EBPα up-regulates expression of the G-CSF receptor and is necessary for neutrophil formation (49). Thus, the relative expression levels and interactions between growth factors and transcription factors are currently presumed to govern the final properties as well as the number of phagocytes produced.

REGULATION OF PHAGOCYTE PRODUCTION (MYELOPOIESIS)

All the cellular elements of blood are derived from pluripotent stem cells in the bone marrow. There is a hierarchy of

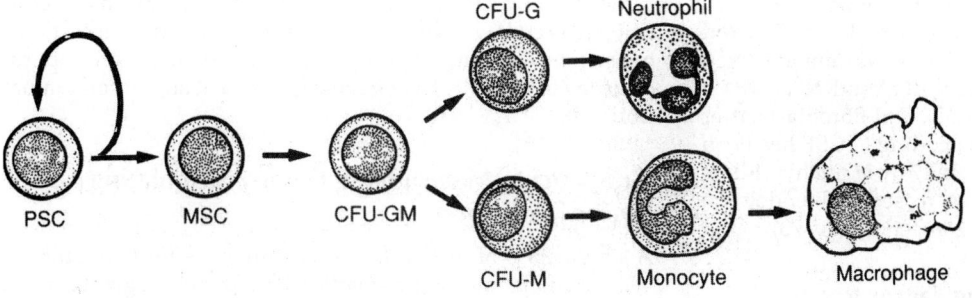

Figure 14-4. Stem cell development of neutrophils and macrophages. CFU-G, colony-forming unit, granulocyte; CFU-GM, colony-forming unit, granulocyte-macrophage; CFU-M, colony-forming unit, monocyte; MSC, myeloid stem cell; PSC, totipotent hematopoietic stem cell.

stem cells, the earliest of which have the capacity to give rise to cells of myeloid, erythroid, lymphoid, and megakaryocyte lineages (50,51). Stem cells are not morphologically recognizable but possess the capacity for extensive self-replication. The earliest stem cells give rise to more restricted stem cells, with the ultimate appearance of committed progenitors, which can proliferate and mature along only a single pathway (Fig. 14-4).

Differentiation in the stem cell compartment is manifested by expression of cellular receptors for various growth factors that allow progenitor cells to respond to hormonal signals in the environment, regulating the body's requirements for blood cell production. For example, expression of erythropoietin receptors is a characteristic of cells committed to erythroid differentiation, whereas expression of G-CSF and GM-CSF receptors is associated with neutrophil and monocyte development (52,53).

A variety of *in vivo* and *in vitro* models have been used to study multipotent stem cells. The first assay used to identify stem cells was based on their ability to form hematopoietic colonies in the spleens of lethally irradiated mice. This assay, developed by Till and McCulloch, defined the colony-forming unit, spleen (CFU-S), which is capable of forming erythroid, granulocytic, megakaryocytic, and mixed colonies in the spleen (54). Since then, a number of investigations have shown that the CFU-S has limited self-renewal properties and, thus, does not represent the true pluripotent hematopoietic stem cell (55).

The initial development of semisolid culture techniques provided a system that could be used to study the clonal proliferation of hematopoietic progenitors (56,57). In this system, colonies of maturing myeloid cells develop from progenitors in response to the presence of colony-stimulating factors (CSFs) (Fig. 14-5). In humans, a primitive myeloid progenitor cell, the *CFU-blast*, can be identified in *in vitro* culture assays and is characterized by high *in vitro* self-renewal capability and complete myeloid potential. However, these cells probably do not represent true hematopoietic stem cells (58). Stem cells can be puri-

fied from mouse bone marrow with properties characteristic of pluripotent hematopoietic stem cells. These stem cells, isolated with monoclonal antibodies, are weakly *Thy-1*–positive, lineage marker-negative, and *Sca-1*–positive and can completely reconstitute hematopoiesis in lethally irradiated mice (59). Similar populations with long-term proliferative capacity can also be identified in humans (60).

Studies in humans and mice (thymidine suicide, 5-fluorouracil resistance of CFU-S) demonstrate that most stem cells are not actively cycling but are resting in the nonproliferating state of the cell cycle (G_0) (60,61). Various hormonal signals have been identified that can act to stimulate movement of cells from phase G_0 to G_1, including kit ligand (stem cell factor), IL-3, and G-CSF (62). Proliferation of primitive hematopoietic progenitors in culture is factor-dependent, and IL-3, kit ligand, and flt-3 ligand are the most effective factors in supporting proliferation of multipotent progenitors (63–67).

Growth Factors

In vitro clonogenic culture systems have been used to identify and isolate factors regulating hematopoietic cell proliferation and maturation. Characterization of these factors in mice led to the description of four distinct CSFs, named according to the type of colonies resulting from the addition of the factor to murine bone marrow cultures. These factors are known as *G-CSF*, *GM-CSF*, *M-CSF* (also referred to as *CSF-1*) and *IL-3* (or *multi-CSF*).

Granulocyte Colony-Stimulating Factor

G-CSF is a species-nonspecific growth factor with activity on both human and murine cells (68). Human and mouse G-CSFs are approximately 75% homologous. Human G-CSF is an 18- to 22-kd glycoprotein originally purified from the CHO-2 squamous lung carcinoma cell line, the 5637 human bladder carci-

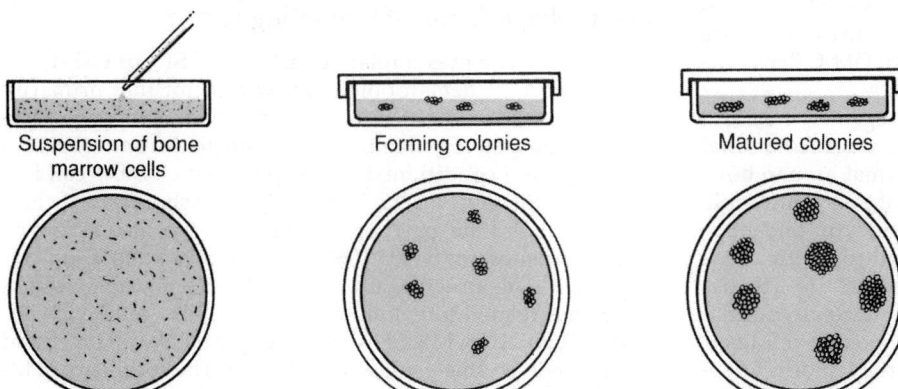

Suspension of bone marrow cells

Forming colonies

Matured colonies

Figure 14-5. Colony assay for colony-forming unit, granulocyte-macrophage.

noma cell line, and human placenta–conditioned medium (69). Complementary DNA (cDNA) clones were isolated (70), and the nonglycosylated bacteria-derived G-CSF was initially used in clinical trials (71). G-CSF messenger RNA (mRNA) can be detected in monocytes, endothelial cells, and fibroblasts after cytokine stimulation, and the gene encoding G-CSF has been localized to the long arm of chromosome 17 by *in situ* hybridization (69). G-CSF levels are markedly increased with endotoxin exposure and with naturally occurring infections (70–73).

Granulocyte Colony-Stimulating Factor Receptor

G-CSF acts via its specific high-affinity cell-surface receptor expressed on myeloid cells (74). Approximately 560 receptors (K_d of 250 pmol) have been demonstrated on human neutrophils using a modified human G-CSF ligand (75). Chemical cross-linking of ligand to its receptor results in a complex of 170 kd, indicating that the G-CSF receptor is a 150-kd molecule. Studies using radiolabeled mouse G-CSF have demonstrated G-CSF receptor expression in mouse and human bone marrow, human neutrophils, and a variety of murine myelomonocytic cell lines (76). G-CSF receptors have also been identified on blood monocytes and myeloid leukemia cells (77,78).

On binding to myeloid cells, G-CSF forms a tetrameric complex consisting of two G-CSF and two G-CSF receptor molecules (79). Signal translation occurs via sulfhydryl groups on the internal domain of the receptor which interact with Janus kinase (JAK)-2 (80). In mice, targeted disruption ("knock-out") of the gene for G-CSF or its receptor results in severe chronic neutropenia, probably due to decreased mobilization of neutrophils from the marrow to the blood (81). However, experimental infections in these animals increases blood neutrophils, similar to normal animals, suggesting redundancy in the pathways for mobilizing cells from the marrow to the blood (82). In humans, G-CSF receptor expression on neutrophils but not on monocytes is decreased by *in vivo* or *in vitro* exposure to endotoxin (83).

Granulocyte-Macrophage Colony-Stimulating Factor

Human GM-CSF is a 19-kd to 32-kd glycoprotein initially purified from a human T-lymphoblastic cell line infected with human T-cell leukemia virus type II (84). Isolation of GM-CSF cDNA permitted generation of large amounts of recombinant GM-CSF protein for characterization of its *in vitro* and *in vivo* activities (85,86). Cellular sources of GM-CSF are limited; GM-CSF is made by activated but not resting T-lymphocytes, and by all T-cell lines infected by human T-cell leukemia virus II (84). GM-CSF is also produced by monocytes, fibroblasts, endothelial cells, and keratinocytes stimulated by cytokines such as IL-1, TNF, or other cellular activators (87,88). Although low-level constitutive transcription of the GM-CSF gene can be demonstrated under certain *in vitro* conditions, there appears to be little constitutive production of GM-CSF by normal human cells.

GM-CSF has activity on bone marrow progenitor cells and mature myeloid effector cells, enhancing their functional activities (89). Addition of GM-CSF to normal human bone marrow in gel culture results in formation of pure neutrophil, pure eosinophil, mixed neutrophil–monocyte, and pure monocyte colonies. In the presence of erythropoietin, GM-CSF can support the growth of erythroid bursts. GM-CSF has weak stimulatory activity on megakaryocyte colony formation and stimulates colony formation of leukemia cell lines, such as KG-1 and HL-60. GM-CSF has a variety of direct (primary) and indirect effects on mature neutrophils, eosinophils, and monocytes, enhancing their functions and stimulating

cytokine production (90,91). Serum concentrations of GM-CSF are very low or undetectable even with severe infections, consistent with the hypothesis that GM-CSF acts in a paracrine fashion locally in bone marrow and at sites of inflammation (73).

Granulocyte-Macrophage Colony-Stimulating Factor Receptor

A single class of high-affinity binding sites for GM-CSF has been demonstrated on human bone marrow progenitors and mature neutrophils, eosinophils, and monocytes (92,93). The GM-CSF receptor shares a common β-subunit with the receptors for IL-3 and IL-5, which is essential for signaling (93). Binding of GM-CSF to its receptor induces phosphorylation of the receptor β-chain and activates JAK-2 and signal transducers and activators of transcription (STAT)-5 (94–97). Increased proliferation and survival of hematopoietic cells follows activation of these intracellular proteins (96,97). GM-CSF receptors have been identified on many nonhematopoietic cells, and various tumor cell lines can respond to GM-CSF.

Interleukin-3

Murine IL-3 was the first of the hematopoietic growth factors to be molecularly cloned (98). After isolation of a gibbon ape IL-3 cDNA, the human gene for IL-3 was identified and cloned (99). IL-3 is produced primarily by activated T lymphocytes, natural killer cells, and mast cells (100). The genes encoding both IL-3 and GM-CSF are located in close proximity on the long arm of chromosome 5, separated by only 9 kB. The structure of the genes for IL-3 and GM-CSF is similar, suggesting evolution from a common ancestral gene. IL-3 (or multi-CSF) acts at an earlier level of stem cell development than GM-CSF. Studies in human culture systems show that IL-3 can influence replication of both CFU-blasts and primitive uncommitted progenitors, as well as stimulate growth of committed progenitor cells. IL-3 is more effective than human GM-CSF in supporting proliferation of multipotential progenitors. IL-3 does not direct movement of stem cells from phase G_0 to G_1 but synergizes with IL-1, G-CSF, and IL-6 to stimulate formation of early progenitor cell–derived colonies. Addition of IL-3 to normal human bone marrow results in formation of colonies containing mast cells, neutrophils, monocytes, erythroblasts, eosinophils, and megakaryocytes.

The receptor for IL-3 is expressed on early hematopoietic precursors and mature leukocytes, but not on neutrophils (101). It shares a common β-subunit with both GM-CSF and IL-5 and signals via the same pathways (102).

Macrophage Colony-Stimulating Factor

Macrophage colony-stimulating factor (M-CSF), or CSF-1, is a lineage-specific hematopoietic growth factor that primarily influences cells committed to the monocyte-macrophage pathway. Human M-CSF was originally purified from urine and from medium conditioned by the pancreatic cancer cell line (103,104). The M-CSF gene is located on the short arm of chromosome 1, and the gene for its receptor, *c-fms*, is on the long arm of chromosome 5 (105,106). M-CSF is a 70-kd to 90-kd glycoprotein. The structure of M-CSF places it in the family of hormones related to insulin and relaxin. Also unlike G-CSF, GM-CSF, and IL-3, M-CSF is produced by many cell types and is readily detectable in plasma and urine. The specificity of M-CSF is determined by its receptors, which are expressed on monocytes, macrophages, and their precursors (107,108).

Interleukin-1 and Interleukin-6

Several other factors have demonstrated important effects on the growth and function of myeloid progenitor cells. IL-6 is a 26-kd glycoprotein produced by IL-1 or TNF-α stimulated fibroblasts, activated T lymphocytes, and monocytes (109,110). IL-6 has a wide range of biologic activities and is known also as hepatocyte-stimulating factor, hybridoma growth factor, B-cell stimulatory factor 2, and interferon-β_2 (IFN-β_2). Some effects attributed to IL-1, may be the result of IL-1–induced expression of IL-6. IL-6 appears to serve as a competence factor for proliferation of progenitor cells, which also requires the presence of IL-3. In *in vitro* culture systems, IL-6 may synergize with IL-3 and other growth factors (111). IL-6 may also exert important effects on hematopoiesis through its influence on expression of transcription factors (112,113).

IL-1 appears to play an important role in host defense because of its central involvement in inflammatory and immune responses. Both IL-1α and IL-1β function as endogenous pyrogens and activate a wide range of cells, including B and T lymphocytes, fibroblasts, endothelial cells, and osteoclasts. When exposed to IL-1, these target cells demonstrate enhanced functional activity and secrete a variety of cytokines, including IL-2, IFN-γ, GM-CSF, G-CSF, IL-3, and IL-6. IL-1, therefore, has numerous indirect effects on hematopoiesis, rendering it somewhat difficult to determine its direct effect on hematopoietic cell growth (114). The toxicities of IL-1 have limited its potential clinical applications (115).

Inhibitors of Hematopoiesis

A variety of inhibitors of hematopoiesis resulting in neutropenia have been identified (principally using *in vitro* culture techniques) in aplastic anemia, myelodysplasia, and T-cell disorders, such as T-γ disease (116–119). Cytokines from T cells are probably the principle extracellular factors involved in these processes. Identified inhibitory factors include IFN-α, IFN-β, IFN-γ, TNF-α, MIP-1α, prostaglandins E_1 and E_2, and transforming growth factor–β (120–126). Lactoferrin, a constituent of the secondary granules of neutrophils, was proposed as a specific inhibitor of neutrophil production (127), but this hypothesis is controversial (128). Recent studies have indicated that accelerated apoptosis of neutrophil precursors is probably the cellular mechanism responsible for neutropenia in myelodysplasia (129,130), myelokathexis, and cyclic and congenital neutropenia (131). The molecular mechanisms for suppression of cell production in these conditions may involve, in part, Fas-Fas ligand interactions (127), dysregulation of Bcl-x expression (132), and genetic mutations of neutrophil elastase, an enzyme of the primary granules of neutrophils (133).

KINETICS OF NEUTROPHIL PRODUCTION

Bone Marrow

Kinetic studies of neutrophil production are largely based on *in vivo* and *in vitro* labeling studies using radioisotopes. These studies indicate that approximately five cell divisions occur between the myeloblast and myelocyte stages (117,134). In the bone marrow, myelocytes probably undergo three cycles of cell division; thus, the major expansion of the neutrophil pool probably occurs at the myelocyte stage. Myeloblasts, promyelocytes, and myelocytes constitute the mitotic pool, whose size is estimated at 2×10^9 cells/kg (Fig. 14-6) (2). The postmitotic pool (metamyelocytes, bands, and segmented neutrophils) constitutes a maturation-storage compartment of approximately 6.5 to 8.0×10^9 cells/kg (2). Radionuclide studies suggest that cells spend approximately 135 hours in transit from myeloblast to myelocyte, with 14 hours at the myeloblast stage, 19 hours as a promyelocyte, and 102 hours as a myelocyte. The transit time from myelocyte to mature blood neutrophil has been estimated at 131 to 158 hours. Data from one study indicate that the neutrophil spends approximately 30 hours as a metamyelocyte, 50 hours as a band neutrophil, and 72 hours as a segmented neutrophil. Thus, approximately 11 or 12 days are required normally for the mature neutrophil to form from the precursor to the myeloblast (117).

Thymidine incorporation studies show an orderly progression from metamyelocytes to neutrophils, which then exit the storage compartment of bone marrow to the bloodstream. Labeled metamyelocytes can be identified by autoradiography approximately 3 hours after injection of ^{3}H-TdR. Labeled neutrophils appear in the blood 4 to 7 days after administration of ^{3}H-TdR; thus, the transition time from myelocyte to circulating neutrophil is approximately 5 to 7 days (2). In the presence of active infection, the myelocyte-neutrophil transit time may be reduced to only 48 hours. At any given time, the reserve of mature neutrophils in the bone marrow greatly exceeds the number of neutrophils circulating in the blood. Under stress conditions, the number of myeloid progenitors increases, and maturation times are shortened; however, release of functionally mature neutrophils from the storage compartment is the mechanism used initially in the response to the need for additional circulating neutrophils (1).

Blood

Once the neutrophil leaves the bone marrow storage compartment and enters the blood, no significant reentry into the marrow occurs (117–122,134). The total blood neutrophil pool consists of

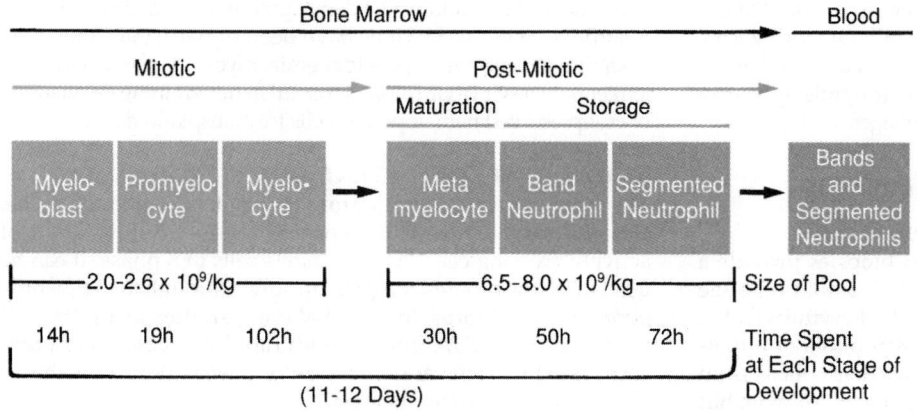

Figure 14-6. Neutrophil kinetics.

TABLE 14-2. Absolute Blood Phagocyte Concentrations

Population	Concentration [cells/µL; 95% range (mean)]			
	Band Forms	Segmented Forms	Band and Segmented Forms	Monocytes
American adults[a]				
White subjects	200–2150 (600)	1500–6050 (3000)	—	220–950 (460)
Black subjects	60–1650 (300)	1100–6700 (2700)	—	210–1050 (470)
European adults[b]				
White subjects	—	—	3487–9206	221–843
American infants and children[c]				
Birth	—	—	6000–26,000 (11,000)	400–3100 (1050)
7 d	—	—	1500–10,000 (5500)	300–2700 (1100)
4 yr	—	—	1500–8500 (3800)	0–800 (450)
10 yr	—	—	1800–8000 (4400)	0–800 (350)

[a]Orfanakis NG, Ostlund RE, Bishop CR, Athens JW. Normal blood leukocyte concentration values. *Am J Clin Pathol* 1970;53:647.
[b]England JM, Bain BJ. Total and differential leukocyte count. *Br J Haematol* 1976;33:1.
[c]Altman PL, Katz DD. Human health and disease. In: *FASEB biology handbooks II*. Washington, DC: FASEB, 1977:161.

cells that circulate freely in vascular spaces [referred to as the *circulating neutrophil pool* (CNP)] and neutrophils that adhere to the endothelium of capillaries and postcapillary venules [referred to as the *marginated blood pool* (MBP)] (118). Marginated neutrophils are particularly common in the lung, liver, and spleen. When labeled neutrophils are injected into normal subjects, approximately 50% remain in the CNP, while the other 50% enter the MBP, suggesting that these pools are roughly of equal size (estimated at 31×10^7 cells/kg; Table 14-2) (119).

Many factors affect the size of the CNP and MBP. Stress, exercise, and epinephrine injection redistribute neutrophils from the MBP to the CNP (120–125). The effects of stress and exercise are probably mediated in part by changes in circulating levels of epinephrine and glucocorticoids. Glucocorticoids increase the total blood neutrophil pool, as well as the proportion of neutrophils in the CNP (125). The increase in blood neutrophils is the result of an increased efflux of neutrophils from marrow storage and a decreased rate of loss of neutrophils from the circulation. Whereas neutrophils normally leave the circulation with a mean disappearance time of 6 to 8 hours, the half-life of circulating neutrophils increases to 10 hours in the presence of glucocorticoids. The disappearance time of neutrophils from the circulation should not be confused with the granulocyte life span, because the granulocyte spends most of its life in the bone marrow and at tissue sites.

Neutrophils that have migrated into tissue do not return to the bloodstream. Although they appear to leave the bone marrow in a first-in, first-out manner (126), movement of neutrophils from the circulation into tissue is random. Thus, neutrophils newly released from the bone marrow are as likely to leave the blood as neutrophils that have been circulating for several hours. In contrast, senescent neutrophils may be removed from the circulation by the mononuclear phagocyte (MNP) network with a different set of kinetics. The fate of neutrophils in tissue is largely unknown, although senescent, apoptotic neutrophils appear to be readily phagocytized by resident macrophages.

Evaluation of Neutrophil Production

BONE MARROW ASPIRATION AND BIOPSY
Expertly read bone marrow aspirates and biopsies provide a rough estimate of leukocyte production. By combining bone marrow biopsy cellularity data with the myeloid-erythroid ratio, one can determine whether granulocytic hypoplasia or hyperplasia is present and distinguish granulocytic hypoplasia from erythroid hyperplasia. Bone marrow examination, however, has

several limitations. For example, a bone marrow specimen showing diminished neutrophil development beyond the myelocyte stage may be due to a defect in cellular maturation as occurs in myelodysplasia or rapid mobilization of cells from marrow as may occur with septic shock. The proliferative activity of this is difficult to judge from the proportions of cells or the frequency of mitoses, especially when there is only one marrow sample. Marrow differential counting requires careful attention to the details of cell morphology. Despite these limitations, when absolute neutrophil count and marrow cellularity (ascertained from a bone marrow biopsy) are used together, they provide a practical and useful guide in most clinical settings. For example, an absolute neutrophil count of less than 1.0×10^9/L in the presence of a hypocellular marrow invariably reflects impaired production of neutrophils. Similarly, a reduced blood neutrophil count associated with a hypercellular marrow and an increased proportion of early precursors suggests ineffective production.

IN VITRO BONE MARROW CULTURE
The colony-forming unit, granulocyte-macrophage (CFU-GM), which is usually regarded as the committed progenitor of neutrophils and macrophages, gives rise to colonies of neutrophils, monocytes, and macrophages in semisolid culture (53). The maximal number of colonies formed in agar from marrow aspirates is reflective of the number of CFU-GM existing *in vivo*, or the relative concentration of CFU-GM among all nucleated marrow cells. It does not provide information about the total number of these progenitors in the bone marrow. Although circulating CFU-GM can be quantified in peripheral blood, this determination may be more reflective of the distribution of CFU-GM than of its production in the bone marrow. *In vitro* culture techniques permit assessment of abnormalities of granulocytic development in various hematologic disorders. These techniques have been of particular interest in assessing patients with aplastic anemia, myelodysplasia, and acute leukemia. The CFU-GM assay is useful in determining the viability of cryopreserved hematopoietic cells for transplantation.

³H-THYMIDINE LABELING AND DNA MEASUREMENT
The proliferation of bone marrow progenitors is reflected by the amount or rate of ³H-TdR incorporation into cellular DNA of actively growing cells. ³H-TdR labels cells in S phase. It can be used to follow progression of neutrophils through the sequential bone marrow compartments. Labeling studies using ³H-TdR allow selective DNA labeling with rapid degradation of unincorporated material and emission of a weak β-particle that is ideal for radioautography (117).

MITOTIC INDEX

Cell division can be assessed directly by measuring the mitotic index (MI). The *MI* is the ratio of cells in mitosis to the total number of cells in the population. MI and ³H-TdR–labeling studies were useful to establish the rates of cell turnover in hematologic malignancies, especially in diseases associated with uniform cell populations, such as multiple myeloma and chronic myelogenous leukemia (CML). These techniques are rarely used presently.

DIISOPROPYL FLUOROPHOSPHATE AND CHROMIUM-51 LABELING

Diisopropyl fluorophosphate (DFP) containing radioactive phosphate (^{32}P) was introduced as a granulocyte marker in the late 1950s (126). This radiolabeled compound binds to mature granulocytes, monocytes, and erythrocytes; thus, cell populations must be carefully separated for kinetic studies. Kinetic studies of intravenously administered ^{32}P-DFP have been used to measure marrow transit times, neutrophil reserves, and marrow myelocyte turnover rates under steady-state and non–steady-state conditions. This radiopharmaceutical is no longer available for clinical or research studies. ³H-TdR–labeled DFP has been employed in some more recent studies (135).

GALLIUM-67, TECHNETIUM-99M, AND INDIUM-111 LABELING

The fate of neutrophils leaving the blood and entering tissues can be traced by radiolabeling the cells with a γ-particle–emitting isotope (136–141). This technique is most useful for evaluation of patients with infections and inflammatory diseases that have eluded diagnosis using other studies or modalities. The isotopes used for this purpose are gallium-67 (^{67}Ga), technetium-99m (^{99m}Tc), and indium-111 (^{111}In) (138–140). Because of nonspecific accumulation of ^{67}Ga in the liver and gut and binding of ^{67}Ga to serum proteins and tumors, ^{67}Ga has not proved reliable as a leukocyte label. ^{99m}Tc has a shorter half-life and has been used widely, although it also accumulates in the liver (138). ^{111}In-labeled leukocytes have demonstrated the greatest *in vivo* and *in vitro* stability, and labeled cells retain most functional activities. Unlike the β-emitters ^{32}P and ^{3}H, ^{111}In emits two γ-photons that can be detected externally with commercially available radioactivity detectors. Using an ^{111}In-oxine complex and separated leukocytes, approximately 75% to 90% of the label appears in the neutrophils. ^{111}In-tropolone complexes have also been used to facilitate labeling. ^{111}In-labeled leukocytes and whole-body scanning with a γ-counter may be used to identify or localize inflammatory or infectious processes that cannot be identified using other diagnostic studies. Recently, the specificity of neutrophil scanning has increased with the use of ^{99m}Tc-labeled antineutrophil antibodies (141).

Using ^{111}In labeling, the estimated half-life of neutrophils in circulating blood has been calculated at 4 to 5 hours, which is somewhat shorter than that measured by other techniques. A drawback to the use of ^{111}In as a label for neutrophils is that the half-life of this isotope (2.8 days) is relatively long compared with the clearance time for neutrophils (6 to 7 hours). Thus, radioactive neutrophils taken up by the mononuclear phagocytic system can deliver significant radiation to the liver, spleen, and bone marrow.

NEUTROPENIA

Definition

The mean blood neutrophil count normally is approximately 3.6 $\times 10^9$/L, including segmented forms and bands (Table 14-2). The normal range is rather broad, ranging from approximately 2.0 to 8.0 $\times 10^9$/L. In persons of African origin and some other populations (142,143), counts as low as 1.0 $\times 10^9$/L should be regarded as normal. The level of the neutrophil count normally varies considerably with physical and emotional states, as well as with the time of day. Neutropenia is usually described as "mild" (1.0 to 1.5 $\times 10^9$/L), "moderate" (0.5 to 1.0 $\times 10^9$/L), or "severe" (less than 0.5 $\times 10^9$/L). *Agranulocytosis*, a term often used synonymously with severe neutropenia, implies an absence of circulating neutrophils.

Neutrophils serve primarily to prevent and contain bacterial and fungal infections. Patients with severe neutropenia frequently develop fevers and infections of the oropharynx, sinuses, ears, lungs, and skin. With protracted severe neutropenia, bacterial invasion from the gastrointestinal tract frequently occurs. The pattern of infection, infecting organisms, prognosis, and clinical outcome depend on many factors in addition to the level of the neutrophil count. For serious infections in neutropenic patients, recovery from neutropenia is the most important determinant of clinical outcome.

Causes

Neutropenia can be divided on a kinetic basis into disorders secondary to abnormalities of production, distribution, or rapid use or turnover of cells in the peripheral blood. Because disorders of production are far more common than those in other categories, it is usually more helpful to categorize neutropenia on an etiologic basis. This approach divides neutropenia into primary forms caused by intrinsic disorders of the hematopoietic system and secondary forms caused by extrinsic factors, including drugs, radiation, autoimmune disorders, and infections (Table 14-3).

TABLE 14-3. Neutropenia

Primary hematologic disorders
Congenital
    Severe congenital neutropenia (Kostmann's syndrome)
    Cyclic neutropenia
    Myelokathexis
    Shwachman-Diamond syndrome
    Neutropenia with congenital immunodeficiency diseases
    Cartilage-hair hypoplasia syndrome
    Diamond-Blackfan syndrome
    Griscelli syndrome
    Chédiak-Higashi syndrome
    Barth syndrome
Acquired
    Acute myelogenous leukemia
    Myelodysplastic syndromes
    Chronic lymphocytic leukemia
    Hodgkin's disease
    Lymphoma
    Aplastic anemia
    Chronic idiopathic neutropenia
Secondary disorders
Immune neutropenias
    Alloimmune neutropenia
    Isoimmune neutropenia
    Autoimmune neutropenia
Neutropenia with autoimmune diseases
    Systemic lupus erythematosus
    Rheumatoid arthritis
    Felty's syndrome
    Sjögren's syndrome
Neutropenia with large granular lymphocytes
Neutropenia with splenomegaly
Neutropenia with infectious diseases
    Sepsis
    Viral—mononucleosis, parvovirus, human immunodeficiency virus
Drugs
    Dose and exposure related
    Idiosyncratic

Neutropenia as a Feature of Primary Hematologic Diseases

CONGENITAL DISORDERS

Severe congenital neutropenia, often referred to as *Kostmann's syndrome*, was first described in northern Sweden as an autosomal-recessive disorder affecting neutrophil production (144). More recently, many sporadic cases and cases with probable autosomal-dominant inheritance have been reported (145,146). Severe congenital neutropenia is usually recognized in a newborn with fever and evidence of serious bacterial infections. The absolute neutrophil count at diagnosis is often less than 0.2 to $10 \times 10^9/L$. Blood monocytes are often three to five times the normal. Platelets are generally moderately increased, and mild anemia is usually present as a consequence of attributable acute and chronic inflammation. The spleen is often modestly enlarged. Marrow studies characteristically reveal the presence of myeloblasts and promyelocytes with a markedly reduced proportion of myelocytes, metamyelocyte, band, and neutrophils. Marrow eosinophils are often increased in number, but other lineages are normal or near normal. There are no distinctive features of the cells; the percentage of myeloblasts is usually not increased and Auer rods are not present, but the granule development may appear mildly dysmorphic or normal. In a newborn, the differential diagnosis usually includes acute leukemia and alloimmune, isoimmune, and autoimmune neutropenia.

The histologic pattern in the marrow has long been described as "maturation arrest." Recent studies have demonstrated that this abnormality is due to accelerated apoptosis of developing neutrophil precursors and is attributable to mutation of the primary granule enzyme, neutrophil elastase (133). Development of neutrophil precursors appears to proceed to the myeloblast-promyelocyte stage, at which point the cells are damaged by the mutant enzyme and fail to complete the maturation process in sufficient quantities to achieve a normal blood neutrophil count (147). Monocytes are presumably increased because this lineage produces very limited amounts of the mutant neutrophil elastase and is, thus, spared from accelerated apoptosis. Current studies indicate that more than 90% of cases of severe congenital neutropenia may be attributed to this molecular mechanism (133).

Treatment of severe congenital neutropenia with G-CSF is usually effective in amelioration of neutropenia, with subsequent reduction in the occurrence of fevers and infections (146,148). More than 90% of patients respond to treatment with daily G-CSF (usually 5 to 10 µg/kg/day), titrated to achieve a neutrophil count at the lower limit of normal. Management also requires careful attention to oral hygiene. Splenic enlargement may occur but is infrequently of clinical significance. Patients who fail to respond to G-CSF therapy should be considered for hematopoietic stem cell transplantation.

Evolution of severe congenital neutropenia to myelodysplasia and acute myelogenous leukemia (AML) occurs with and without treatment with G-CSF (149). Presently, it is unclear if G-CSF treatment increases this risk. Because the first sign of evolution may be development of anemia or thrombocytopenia, monitoring with regular blood counts and periodic bone marrow examinations are advised. Dysplasia can also be recognized by appearance of abnormal clones marked by monosomy 7 or other chromosomal changes (149). Mutations in the receptor for G-CSF are also an early feature of this evolutionary process (150). These mutations may increase the survival of abnormal precursors, thereby accelerating leukemic evolution. Hematopoietic stem cell transplantation after ablative chemotherapy currently appears to be the best therapeutic option for patients with evidence of leukemic evolution (146).

CYCLIC NEUTROPENIA

Cyclic neutropenia occurs sporadically or as an autosomal-dominant disorder (151,152). Characteristically, peripheral blood neutrophil counts oscillate between approximately $0.1 \times 10^9/L$ and $1.5 \times 10^9/L$ every 21 days. Neutropenic periods typically last for 3 to 6 days and are accompanied by malaise, anorexia, fever, lymphadenopathy, and ulcerations of the mucous membranes both in the mouth and along the gastrointestinal tract. During neutropenic periods, patients are at risk for the development of bacteremias, usually with *Clostridium* species. Other deep tissue infections may occur, but inflammatory symptoms and signs generally resolve as the blood neutrophil count increases. Careful serial blood counts also show oscillations of blood monocytes, platelets, and reticulocytes. Cyclic neutropenia also occurs as an acquired disorder in association with clonal proliferation of large granular lymphocytes (153).

Recent genetic and molecular studies in families with autosomal-dominant cyclic neutropenia indicate that cyclic neutropenia is associated with mutations of the gene for neutrophil elastase, the same gene that is abnormal in patients with congenital neutropenia (154). In cyclic neutropenia, mutations appear to affect the enzyme active site. At the cellular level, neutropenia appears to be caused by accelerated apoptosis of developing neutrophils (155). Mathematical modeling studies indicate that oscillations of peripheral counts are a natural consequence of the apoptotic process involving early precursor cells (152).

The clinical diagnosis of cyclic neutropenia can only be made by serial differential leukocyte counts, performed at least two to three times/week for a minimum of 6 weeks. In families with autosomal-dominant cyclic neutropenia, there are substantial variations in both the amplitude of oscillations and the severity of clinical symptoms among affected family members (156).

Treatment of cyclic neutropenia with G-CSF is very effective (148). It reduces inflammatory symptoms and the occurrence of infections and shortens the duration of neutropenic periods and the overall cycle length (157). Other hematopoietic growth factors, androgens, and corticosteroids have not proved effective for therapy.

MYELOKATHEXIS

Myelokathexis is a rare cause of severe neutropenia and occurs sporadically or as an autosomal-dominant disorder (158). Characteristically, the total leukocyte count is very low, often less than $1.0 \times 10^9/L$, with a blood neutrophil count of less than $0.5 \times 10^9/L$. Marrow and blood neutrophils characteristically have very pyknotic nuclei; granulocyte hyperplasia is present in the bone marrow. Occasionally, marrow macrophages ladened with debris of senescent neutrophils can be seen. This disorder was recently attributed to accelerated apoptosis of marrow neutrophils, which was associated with abnormally decreased expression of the antiapoptotic protein, Bcl-x (159). G-CSF treatment can increase blood neutrophil counts in this disorder and is often helpful for patients with recurrent infections. However, G-CSF administration is often not necessary for patients with myelokathexis. Morphologic changes of myelokathexis can be observed in acute leukemia, but the congenital disorder is not currently classified as a preleukemic disorder.

SHWACHMAN-DIAMOND SYNDROME

Shwachman-Diamond syndrome is an autosomal-recessive disorder characterized by exocrine pancreatic dysfunction, bony metaphysical dysostosis, and varying degrees of neutropenia, anemia, and thrombocytopenia (160). Myelodysplasia and acute myeloid leukemia eventually develop in up to one-third of patients (161). Neutropenia may not be severe at birth, and the frequency of infectious complications varies considerably among patients. When neutropenia or pancytopenia is present, the marrow is usually hypocellular. Recent studies indicate that marrow CD34+ cells are reduced and have markedly impaired capacity for proliferation *in vitro* (162). Furthermore, the capacity of marrow stromal cells from patients with Shwachman-Diamond syndrome to support proliferation of normal hematopoietic precursor cells is impaired. Also, marrow stromal cells have an impaired capacity to support proliferation of normal hematopoietic precursor cells, suggesting both an intrinsic abnormality and an abnormality of the marrow microenvironment. The molecular mechanism responsible for the pathophysiology of Shwachman-Diamond syndrome is not yet known. The neutropenia of Shwachman-Diamond syndrome usually responds to treatment with G-CSF. At present, it is unclear whether G-CSF therapy alters the risk for evolution to leukemia.

CONGENITAL IMMUNODEFICIENCY DISEASES

Congenital immunodeficiency diseases are primary disorders of B-cell and T-cell development. Neutropenia contributes to the susceptibility to infection in some, but not all, of these conditions. In X-linked agammaglobulinemia, severe neutropenia is present in approximately one-fourth of patients in the common variable form of immunodeficiency (163). Neutropenia occurs in association with anemia and thrombocytopenia. In X-linked hyperimmunoglobulin M syndrome, approximately 50% of patients are neutropenic (164). In congenital severe combined immunodeficiency, neutropenia may occur but is not a consistent feature of this disorder. Neutropenia occurs as a prominent feature of reticular dysgenesis (165), but is rare in adenosine deaminase deficiency and Omenn's syndrome. Case reports suggest that G-CSF is an effective therapy for most patients with congenital immunodeficiency disorders complicated by neutropenia.

CARTILAGE-HAIR HYPOPLASIA SYNDROME

Cartilage-hair hypoplasia syndrome is a rare autosomal-recessive disorder, characterized by short limb dwarfism, hyperextensible digits, fine hair, neutropenia, and recurrent infections. The degree of neutropenia and pattern of infectious complications vary considerably (166). A disorder of lymphocyte proliferation in this syndrome appears to predispose patients to viral infections (167).

DIAMOND-BLACKFAN SYNDROME

Neutropenia is a rare complication of Diamond-Blackfan syndrome associated with congenital hypoplastic anemia and anomalies of the head and upper limbs.

GRISCELLI SYNDROME

Griscelli syndrome is a rare autosomal-recessive disorder which maps to chromosome 15q21 (168,169). Neutropenia occurs in association with pancytopenia, immunodeficiency, and hypopigmentation due to abnormal melanin formation. Hematocytophagia and myelodysplasia are complications, along with uncontrolled accumulations of lymphocytes and macrophages in many tissues. Hematopoietic stem cell transplantation is a potential therapy.

CHÉDIAK-HIGASHI SYNDROME

Chédiak-Higashi syndrome is a rare autosomal-recessive disorder characterized by partial albinism and giant granules in developing neutrophils, monocytes, and lymphocytes associated with neutropenia and recurrent infections (170). The neutropenia is usually mild, and the susceptibility to infection is largely attributable to abnormalities in the microbicidal activity of neutrophils and monocytes.

BARTH SYNDROME

Barth syndrome is an X-linked disorder characterized by cardioskeletal myopathy, abnormal mitochondria, and neutropenia (171). Mutational analysis has identified a locus at Xq28 in a gene encoding tafazzin, a protein which is essential for the structural integrity of mitochondria, which are present in neutrophil precursors in the bone marrow (172,173). There are also membrane-bound vacuoles in neutrophil precursors. The neutropenia is generally mild, and infectious complications are infrequent.

WISKOTT-ALDRICH SYNDROME

X-linked severe congenital neutropenia occurs due to mutations in the gene for the Wiskott-Aldrich protein. The affected family had neutropenia and monocytopenia, but they had normal platelet counts (174).

GLYCOGEN STORAGE DISEASE

Glycogen storage disease is an autosomal-recessive disease characterized by hypoglycemia, splenomegaly, and seizures due to mutations of the gene for glucose 6-phosphate translocase (175). Neutropenia is a feature of glycogen storage disease type 1b, but not other forms (176). In contrast to some other forms of neutropenia, the marrow is often hypercellular with an ample supply of neutrophils. The blood neutrophils have reduced oxidative (respiratory) burst activity and defective chemotaxis. The exact mechanism causing neutropenia is not known. Treatment with G-CSF can correct the neutropenia and improve the associated symptoms of inflammatory bowel disease. However, because extended G-CSF therapy can result in further hepatosplenomegaly, doses of G-CSF need to be titrated carefully.

Acquired Disorders

ACUTE MYELOGENOUS LEUKEMIA

Fever, fatigue, and severe neutropenia are common features of patients presenting with AML (177). The majority of patients at presentation have an absolute peripheral neutrophil count less than 1.0×10^9/L. One carefully performed study documented cytochemical abnormalities in the blood neutrophils from 34 of 35 patients (178) and an associated reduction in the functional activities of these abnormal cells (179) (Chapter 15). Although acute leukemia itself may be a cause of fever, febrile neutropenic patients with leukemia should generally receive empiric broad spectrum antibiotic therapy because of the potential for severe infectious sequelae in these patients (180).

MYELODYSPLASTIC SYNDROMES

Mild to moderate neutropenia is present at diagnosis in approximately one-third of patients with myelodysplasia (Chapter 11). The pattern of progression and the severity of the neutropenia vary markedly, even within a group of patients with the same disease classification. As in AML, functions of the circulating neutrophils are often defective, and the clinical complications are more severe than might be predicted solely from peripheral blood counts. As part of supportive therapy, colony-stimulating factors, usually G-CSF, are often administered to transiently increase blood neutrophil counts and aid in management of infections (181,182). Currently, there is insufficient evidence to support long-term CSF therapy for myelodysplastic syndromes (Chapter 11).

CHRONIC LEUKEMIA, LYMPHOMA, AND HODGKIN'S DISEASE

Neutropenia is rarely a feature at diagnosis in patients with chronic lymphocytic leukemia, Hodgkin's disease, non-Hodgkin's lymphoma, or CML. However, neutropenia is a common consequence of therapy. Autoimmune neutropenia develops rarely in the course of chronic lymphocytic leukemia and Hodgkin's disease, as part of the propensity for development of autoimmune complications in these diseases (183–185).

APLASTIC ANEMIA

Typically, all blood cells are reduced in patients with aplastic anemia. Neutropenia and monocytopenia are severe, with the consequent risk of severe infections. The incapacity of the marrow to generate new precursors often results in a fall, rather than a rise, in blood neutrophil counts during infections. When this development occurs, the prognosis is often extremely poor (Chapter 9).

NEUTROPENIA IN PREMATURE INFANTS

Epidemiologic studies show that approximately 50% of neonates with a birth weight less than 2 kg have neutrophil counts less than 1.5×10^9/L at birth (186–189). In some newborns, neutropenia is much more severe, with an accompanying threat of serious gram-negative infections. The precise mechanism responsible for neonatal neutropenia is unknown but presumably involves some aspect of the regulation of neutrophil proliferation that is not fully mature at birth. Some investigations have suggested an association with maternal hypertension (187). Differential diagnosis includes severe congenital neutropenia, cyclic neutropenia, allo- and isoimmune neutropenia, and sepsis. Longitudinal studies indicate that blood neutrophil levels gradually normalize.

CHRONIC IDIOPATHIC NEUTROPENIA

Chronic neutropenia, without other hematologic or systemic abnormalities, is occasionally found in both children and adults (190–193). Longitudinal data indicate that chronic idiopathic neutropenia is usually a benign condition that does not evolve to aplastic anemia, myelodysplasia, or leukemia. Bone marrow examinations are either normal or show reductions in the proportion of postmitotic cells (i.e., metamyelocytes, bands, and mature neutrophils), and chromosomal studies are characteristically normal. Experimental evidence indicates that marrow precursors, as measured by colony-forming unit studies, are normal, and that the syndrome is due to ineffective neutrophil production, with loss of cells in the late stages of development. There is overlap of the syndrome of chronic idiopathic neutropenia with autoimmune neutropenia, principally because reliable tests for antineutrophil antibodies are not widely available. The neutropenia for some patients with chronic idiopathic neutropenia is severe, with recurrent fevers and infectious complications. For these patients, long-term treatment with G-CSF (usually in doses of 1 to 2 μg/kg/day or every other day) is quite effective in increasing neutrophil counts and reducing infection-related morbidity (148). The prognosis for resolution of chronic benign idiopathic neutropenia is more favorable in children than in adults. In one series, neutropenia resolved in 23 of 37 children with a median duration of 19 months (193). Remissions in adults are quite uncommon (192).

SECONDARY FORMS OF NEUTROPENIA

Immune Neutropenias

There are numerous potential mechanisms for antibodies or cells of the immune system to cause neutropenia, ranging from damage to early cells, such as in aplastic anemia and pure white cell aplasia, to damage of mature neutrophils, such as in isoimmune neonatal neutropenia. In recent years, substantial progress has occurred in methods for detection of antibodies to neutrophil-specific antigens, particularly the antigens of the CD11/CD18 complex. Methods employing a panel of paraformaldehyde- or glutaraldehyde-preserved cells and fluorescence-activated cell sorting are now widely available and much more reproducible and reliable than older methods. Testing for cell-mediated immune injury to neutrophil precursors (e.g., studies coincubating marrow cells and a patient's serum), however, remains a research methodology.

ALLOIMMUNE AND ISOIMMUNE NEONATAL NEUTROPENIA

Alloimmune neonatal neutropenia occurs when a neonate's mother produces antibodies which cross the placenta and react with the infant's neutrophils (194). In isoimmune neutropenia, the antigen responsible for stimulation of antibody production is a paternal isotype of CD16 (FcγRIII, originally described as NA1 and NA2) that is different from the isotype of the mother (195,196). In mothers with autoimmune neutropenia, IgG antibodies transferred transplacentally cause alloimmune neutropenia in the infant. Bacterial infections may complicate this form of neutropenia, but spontaneous remission is expected. Short-term treatment of severely neutropenic neonates with G-CSF is probably effective in raising neutrophil counts and reducing susceptibility to infections, but clinical data on the benefits of treatment versus observation alone is limited.

AUTOIMMUNE NEUTROPENIA

Selective neutropenia unaccompanied by other hematologic abnormalities is often presumed to be caused by autoimmune destruction of developing neutrophils. This diagnosis is confirmed by marrow examinations usually showing minimal abnormalities and the finding of antineutrophil antibodies in the serum (197–199). There are now several tests used to detect antineutrophil antibodies. Neutrophil agglutination and binding of staphylococcal protein A to immunoglobulins on the surface of the neutrophils are older and less reliable tests than immunofluorescence testing by fluorescence-activated cell sorting with a standard panel of paraformaldehyde-fixed cells bearing the well-characterized neutrophil antigens: NA-1, NA-2, NB-1, NC-1, and 9a. Because affected patients usually have an insufficient supply of cells for these assays, indirect methods are commonly employed.

Because the neutropenia is not severe and infectious complications occur infrequently, treatment for autoimmune neutropenia is often not necessary in either children or adults. During infection, these patients may also develop a neutrophilic leukocytosis. In patients with severe neutropenia, recurrent fevers, and infections, treatment with G-CSF may be helpful.

NEUTROPENIA ASSOCIATED WITH AUTOIMMUNE DISEASES

Systemic Lupus Erythematosus

Leukopenia (neutropenia, monocytopenia, lymphocytopenia), anemia, and thrombocytopenia occur in greater than one-half of patients with systemic lupus erythematosus (SLE) (200). Both increased amounts of IgG and immune complexes are often present on the surface of neutrophils, suggesting the possibility that accelerated neutrophil turnover may contribute to neutropenia in affected patients (200,201). Usually, the marrow cellularity and the maturation of cells of the neutrophilic series are normal, and infections attributable to neutropenia are uncommon. Both G-CSF and GM-CSF, in conjunction with immunosuppressive therapies for patients with severe disease, have been used to treat SLE-related neutropenia (202).

Rheumatoid Arthritis, Felty's Syndrome, and Sjögren's Syndrome

Leukopenia and neutropenia are less common in rheumatoid arthritis and Sjögren's syndrome than in SLE. Patients with severely deforming rheumatoid arthritis, splenomegaly, and elevated rheumatoid factor titers may have associated severe neutropenia, a condition referred to as *Felty's syndrome* (203). Marrow findings vary from very severe depletion of cells of the neutrophil lineage to minimal abnormalities. In general, patients with more severe marrow findings have a more clinical course. Mechanisms responsible for neutropenia probably include suppression of early cell proliferation, splenic trapping, and antibody-mediated accelerated turnover of developing neutrophils. The clinical course varies remarkably. Some patients with extremely low neutrophil counts have long periods without infectious complications and require no therapy for neutropenia, whereas others have major problems. Treatment alternatives include weekly methotrexate, G-CSF, GM-CSF, or splenectomy (204). It is probably best to initiate therapy with a trial of methotrexate, followed by G-CSF, then splenectomy, if necessary. Corticosteroid therapy may elevate neutrophil counts but is associated with serious complications. Other immunosuppressive drugs are used for refractory patients. In Sjögren's syndrome, mild to moderate leukopenia, which is rarely associated with infectious complications, occurs in one-third of patients (205).

Neutropenia with Large Granular Lymphocyte Syndrome

A subset of patients with Felty's syndrome and a diverse group of other patients will develop severe neutropenia associated with increased numbers of circulating large granular lymphocytes, which are usually phenotyped as natural killer cells (206). Focal collections of these cells are often present in the marrow. Neutropenia may result from expression of high levels of Fas ligand, triggering accelerated apoptosis of neutrophils and their precursors (207). The clinical course of patients varies considerably, as does the response to therapy.

Other Causes of Neutropenia

Neutropenia occurs in a wide variety of disorders associated with splenomegaly, including sarcoidosis, malaria, kala-azar, and tuberculosis. Presumably, the mechanism causing neutropenia in these diseases is splenic trapping of cells. Neutropenia is also a feature of vitamin B_{12} and folate deficiency (Chapter 46).

Neutropenia with Infectious Diseases

Most bacterial infections cause neutrophilia. Exceptions include typhoid fever and severe gram-negative bacteremias (208). With viral infections, mild neutropenia may occur, particularly in infectious mononucleosis, infectious hepatitis, parvovirus B-19 (209), and human immunodeficiency virus (HIV) infections (210). Multiple mechanisms are involved, including enhanced adherence of neutrophils to activated or infected endothelial cells (increased margination), effects of cytokines generated in the marrow and periphery [which may impair neutrophil production (e.g., IFN-γ)], and effects of the virus on hematopoietic stem cells (decreased supply of

precursors). With some viral infections, such as infectious mononucleosis, infectious hepatitis, and particularly HIV infection, the neutropenia may be protracted and associated with pancytopenia. With the advent of highly active antiretroviral therapy for HIV infection, the problem of neutropenia has diminished remarkably.

Drug-Induced Neutropenia

Drug-related neutropenia is probably the most common cause of isolated neutropenia (211–213). Cytotoxic drugs predictably cause neutropenia, as does extensive bone marrow irradiation. Table 14-4 lists the different classes of drugs associated with idiosyncratic drug-induced neutropenia.

Aminopyrine, which was introduced as an analgesic in the 1920s, was probably the first drug to be convincingly associated with neutropenia. Administration often resulted in a total absence of granulocytes (agranulocytosis). Chloramphenicol, introduced in 1948, can cause a dose-related suppression of

TABLE 14-4. Drugs Associated with Neutropenia or Agranulocytosis

Analgesics	Methylthiouracil
Aminopyrine	Potassium perchlorate
Dipyrone	Propylthiouracil
Antibiotics	Cardiovascular agents
Cephalosporins	Captopril
Chloramphenicol	Diazoxide
Clindamycin	Hydralazine
Doxycycline	Methyldopa
Flucytosine	Pindolol
Gentamicin	Procainamide
Griseofulvin	Propanolol
Isoniazid	Quinidine
Lincomycin	Diuretics
Metronidazole	Acetazolamide
Nitrofurantoin	Bumetanide
Penicillins	Chlorothiazide
Rifampin	Hydrochlorothiazide
Streptomycin	Hydrochlorthalidone
Sulfonamides	Methazolamide
Vancomycin	Spironolactone
Anticonvulsants	Hypoglycemic agents
Carbamazepine	Chlorpropamide
Ethosuximide	Tolbutamide
Mephenytoin	Phenothiazines
Phenytoin	Chlorpromazine
Primidone	Methylpromazine
Trimethadione	Prochlorperazine
Antihistamines	Promazine
Brompheniramine	Thioridazine
Cimetidine	Trifluoperazine
Pyribenzamine	Trimeprazine
Ranitidine	Sedatives and neuropharmacologic
Thenalidine	agents
Antiinflammatory agents	Chlordiazepoxide
Fenoprofen	Clozapine
Gold salts	Desipramine
Ibuprofen	Diazepam
Indomethacin	Imipramine
Phenylbutazone	Meprobamate
Antimalarials	Metoclopramide
Amodiaquine	Miscellaneous
Dapsone	Allopurinol
Hydroxychloroquine	Colchicine
Pyrimethamine	Ethanol
Quinine	Levamisole
Antithyroid drugs	Levodopa
Carbimazole	D-Penicillamine
Methimazole	

Adapted from Vincent PC. Drug-induced aplastic anemia and agranulocytosis. *Drugs* 1986;31:52.

hematopoiesis and an idiosyncratic aplastic anemia with severe neutropenia that is often irreversible.

The phenothiazines are an important cause of drug-induced neutropenia, with an incidence of agranulocytosis of approximately 0.1%. Agranulocytosis due to phenothiazines occurs concomitantly with treatment, usually after a 10- to 20-g cumulative dose (20 to 40 days of therapy). Clozapine, a dibenzodiazepine antipsychotic drug that is now widely used for the treatment of schizophrenia refractory to phenothiazines, has an approximate 1% incidence of agranulocytosis usually occurring within the first 6 months of treatment (214). Olanzapine is similarly toxic (215).

The penicillins and cephalosporins are remarkably nontoxic agents but are a common cause of drug-induced neutropenia because of the frequency of their use. Nafcillin, oxacillin, cephalothin, and methicillin have been most frequently reported to cause neutropenia in high doses, but probably all β-lactam antibiotics can cause neutropenia. Most patients who develop neutropenia have been given a prolonged course (more than 10 days) of high-dose therapy.

Captopril has been associated with several cases of neutropenia or aplastic anemia. Certain patients are at high risk for developing captopril-induced neutropenia, particularly those with renal insufficiency who have delayed clearance of the drug.

Several mechanisms are probably involved in drug-induced neutropenia (213–215). Drugs such as the antithyroid agents phenothiazines and cloazepine are probably directly toxic to marrow precursors and are nonselective in their effects. Aminopyrine, the sulfonamides, penicillins, and cephalosporins probably cause neutropenia by immune-mediated mechanisms. Large studies suggest that women are more susceptible than men, the elderly more than the young, and agranulocytosis occurs more often in patients who are taking multiple drugs and who are more severely ill.

Patients developing severe neutropenia attributable to a medication should have the potentially offending drug stopped immediately. For most medications, there is a satisfactory substitute. Unless essential, the patient should not be reexposed to this agent. Patients beginning medications known to cause neutropenia should be so advised and arrangement made for monitoring blood counts, usually at weekly intervals for several weeks and then at increasing intervals. These patients should also be cautioned to contact their physician if they develop unexplained fever, chills, sore throat, or malaise within the first weeks to months after starting treatment. With the reversible drug-induced neutropenias, the leukocyte count usually begins to recover within 1 week of drug discontinuance, and long-term sequelae are uncommon. Patients with profound neutropenia usually require hospitalization for observation and treatment.

General Approach to the Neutropenic Patient

Evaluation of a patient with neutropenia begins with a careful history to determine the duration of neutropenia, associated illnesses, exposure to drugs and potential toxins, and whether there is a family history of neutropenia. Physical examination should include careful attention to the oropharynx, lymph nodes, spleen, and perirectal area. A bone marrow aspirate and biopsy should be performed to assess cellularity and myeloid maturation and to rule out neoplastic disorders and infiltrative diseases. Neutropenia associated with granulocytic hyperplasia and normal maturation in the bone marrow suggests increased destruction of neutrophils, either in the marrow itself (ineffective granulopoiesis) or in the circulation. A decreased myeloid-erythroid ratio associated with a normal or hypocellular marrow and peripheral neutropenia implies that marrow neutrophil production is decreased. Testing for the presence of antibodies associated with autoimmune diseases and antineutrophil antibodies is often helpful in evaluating patients with chronic neutropenia.

The most important concern with regard to management of neutropenia is the prevention and control of infection. Generally, infections tend to be more common and more severe when the absolute neutrophil count falls below 0.5×10^9/L. Most patients with severe neutropenia associated with fever should be hospitalized, and antibiotics should be administered after cultures are obtained. The most likely sources of infection are the lungs, skin, and venous catheters. The infecting organisms are usually endogenous. Systemic administration of prophylactic antibiotics to neutropenic patients without fever has not been proved useful. Neutrophil transfusion therapy can correct neutropenia, but the clinical benefits and risks of this therapy are not yet established.

Clinical Use of Colony-Stimulating Factors

The CSFs stimulate production of neutrophils and monocytes and enhance their functional activities. These agents are now widely used to reduce the duration and severity of neutropenia after chemotherapy or radiation therapy, to permit harvesting of peripheral blood hematopoietic stem cells for transplantation, to facilitate the recovery of allogeneic and autologous transplants, and to treat severe chronic neutropenia. Numerous other clinical applications are under investigation (Table 14-1).

GRANULOCYTE COLONY-STIMULATING FACTOR

In normal human subjects, administration of G-CSF causes a dose-dependent increase in the blood neutrophil counts and a marked increase in neutrophil production by the bone marrow. This occurs by a combination of changes: increased cell division, shortening of the time between generations, and acceleration of transit through the postmitotic compartment in the marrow with early entry of developing neutrophils into the blood (216,217). Neutrophils from subjects given G-CSF have enhanced metabolic responses to a variety of agonists. For some (but not all) microorganisms, G-CSF induces enhanced microbicidal activity (218,219). G-CSF and the corticosteroid, dexamethasone, have been shown to exert additive effects in the induction of neutrophilia, thereby facilitating collection of large numbers of neutrophils for neutrophil (granulocyte) transfusion therapy (220).

G-CSF is widely used to accelerate neutrophil recovery after chemotherapy. In one pivotal study, G-CSF was administered to patients receiving combination chemotherapy for small cell lung cancer (221). Although the depth of the neutrophil nadir was not altered, G-CSF treatment shortened the duration of severe neutropenia and reduced febrile episodes during the recovery period. Other studies using G-CSF to abrogate chemotherapy-induced neutropenia confirmed these results, generally using a dose of 5 µg/kg administered subcutaneously on a daily basis until neutrophils returned to normal levels (222). Bone pain and headache were the most frequent adverse effect in all of these trials.

G-CSF is also widely used to aid in collection of peripheral blood hematopoietic stem progenitor cells for autologous and allogeneic transplantation and to stimulate the recovery of blood counts after infusion of these cells (Chapter 61).

A randomized clinical trial established the benefits of long-term G-CSF treatment for congenital, cyclic, and idiopathic neutropenia (148). Treatment increased blood neutrophil counts to normal levels in more than 90% of patients. The occurrence of fever, oropharyngeal inflammation, and infection-related events was decreased for all patient groups.

G-CSF has also been used on a chronic basis for therapy of neutropenia in patients with HIV infection, myelodysplasia, hairy cell leukemia, and a variety of autoimmune diseases. In the majority of these patients, increases in blood neutrophil counts occur within a few days and are sustained as long as therapy is continued. Specific clinical benefits of G-CSF for these patients (e.g., reducing the frequency of febrile episodes) have not been established by randomized trials.

GRANULOCYTE-MACROPHAGE COLONY-STIMULATING FACTOR

GM-CSF was first administered to patients with neutropenia due to HIV infection (222). Dose-dependent increases in circulating neutrophils, eosinophils, and monocytes occurred. Side effects included low-grade fever, myalgia, headache, facial flushing, or faint macular skin rash. Subsequent studies in normal human subjects established that GM-CSF increases marrow myeloid cell proliferation and blood neutrophil counts, but the increase in neutrophil production and counts is less than for G-CSF (223).

GM-CSF is used to facilitate the collection of hematopoietic progenitor cells and to accelerate hematopoietic recovery after bone marrow or peripheral progenitor cell transplantation (Chapter 61). After chemotherapy, GM-CSF will hasten the recovery of blood neutrophil counts and has been demonstrated to reduce the occurrence of infections in older patients treated for AML (224). Studies of GM-CSF in myelodysplastic syndromes and aplastic anemia have also demonstrated the capacity of GM-CSF to raise leukocyte counts with primary bone marrow disorders.

NEUTROPHILIA

Neutrophilia is arbitrarily defined as an absolute blood neutrophil count greater than $7.5 \times 10^9/L$ in adults (225). Most commonly, neutrophilia results from increased production or release of cells from the bone marrow, although it may also result from a shift of blood neutrophils from the marginated to circulating pools. This change in distribution of neutrophils is sometimes referred to as *pseudoneutrophilia*. Acute neutrophilia can occur in response to severe pain, exercise, extremes of heat and cold, epileptic seizures, or emotional stress. This neutrophilia results from adrenergic stimulation, which increases the neutrophil count up to twofold within a few minutes.

Glucocorticosteroids can cause acute neutrophilia by releasing neutrophils from the marrow and diminishing the rate of egress of neutrophils from the circulation (226). Neutrophilia occurs in Cushing's syndrome and with therapeutic use of glucocorticosteroids. A single dose of hydrocortisone (200 mg) or prednisone (40 mg) elevates the neutrophil count by an average of 4000/μL within 5 to 6 hours, and counts remain elevated if treatment continues.

The most common reason for neutrophilia in the clinical setting is inflammatory disease due to microbial infection or to ischemic, autoimmune, or traumatic injury causing tissue necrosis. Multiple mechanisms may contribute to the neutrophilia, including release of microbial and host tissue constituents that cause neutrophil mobilization from the bone marrow, adrenergic stimulation, increased corticosteroid release, and enhanced elaboration of cytokines that promote myelopoiesis. When the combination of factors is intense, very high neutrophil counts can be encountered as well as immature myeloid forms in the blood. This picture is designated a *leukemoid reaction*.

Lithium can produce a neutrophilia in patients with psychiatric disorders (227) and can ameliorate neutrophilia in some patients (228). Lithium acts by stimulating leukocyte production rather than altering the distribution, function, or lifespan of neutrophils. Lithium may cause neutrophilia through enhanced production of CSF, direct stimulation of hematopoietic stem cells, or potentiation of the *in vitro* effects of CSF on myeloid colony formation (229). Lithium has neurologic and endocrinologic toxicities and is not currently recommended to treat neutropenia.

Lung cancer, gastric cancer, and renal carcinoma have all been associated with elevated leukocyte counts. Production of CSF has been postulated as the mechanism for the sustained neutrophilia associated with certain tumors. A variety of hereditary conditions associated with neutrophilia have been reported (230), as has neutrophilia after splenectomy.

The major distinction to be made in an elevated leukocyte count consisting of predominantly mature blood neutrophils is whether the patient has a leukemoid reaction, CML, or another myeloproliferative disorder. Absence of eosinophilia, thrombocytosis, nucleated red blood cells, splenomegaly, and a normal bone marrow cell karyotype favor the diagnosis of leukemoid reaction. The leukocyte alkaline phosphatase score should be normal or elevated in a leukemoid reaction and markedly decreased in CML (Chapter 13). Chromosomal analysis for the Philadelphia chromosome or molecular studies to detect the *bcr/abl* rearrangement are useful in the diagnosis of CML (Chapter 13).

LIFE CYCLE OF MONONUCLEAR PHAGOCYTES

Morphologic Development

Both monocytes and neutrophils are derived from a common progenitor cell, the CFU-GM. Monoblasts develop from monocyte-committed progenitor cells derived from the CFU-GM. Monoblasts mature into promonocytes, which are the first morphologically identifiable cells in the monocyte-macrophage lineage (Fig. 14-7). In general, the decision to differentiate toward monocytes or granulocytes is thought to occur at the level of the CFU-GM. However, differentiation studies with both HL-60 and KG-1 myeloid leukemia cell lines suggest that morphologically identifiable myeloid cells (promyelocytes and myeloblasts, respectively) retain the capacity to differentiate along the monocyte-macrophage pathway.

By light microscopy, monoblasts appear identical to myeloblasts. Both are approximately 15 μm in diameter and have a clear, deep-blue cytoplasm when stained with Giemsa. The nucleus in both cell types is large, indented, and eccentrically placed, with prominent nucleoli. The promonocyte is larger than the monoblast (up to 18 μm in diameter) and contains a few peroxidase-positive primary granules in a basophilic cytoplasm. The promonocyte nucleus is usually irregularly shaped and indented, containing minimally condensed chromatin and one nucleolus. The monocyte is the largest cell circulating in the peripheral blood (12 to 20 μm in diameter) and has a characteristically folded ("kidney bean–shaped") nucleus that is eccentrically placed. Both peroxidase-positive and peroxidase-negative granules, as well as many vacuoles, are characteristically present in the abundant gray-blue cytoplasm.

Electron microscopy demonstrates a progression of ultrastructural features associated with maturation from the monoblast to the monocyte stage (231,232). The promonocyte has a well-developed endoplasmic reticulum and an active Golgi apparatus synthesizing peroxidase and other granule components. Promonocytes contain unique bundles of cytoplasmic filaments, which distinguish them from promyelocytes. Peripheral blood monocytes exhibit surface features consistent with their phagocytic and motile capabilities. Viewed under the scanning electron microscope, the monocyte surface is exten-

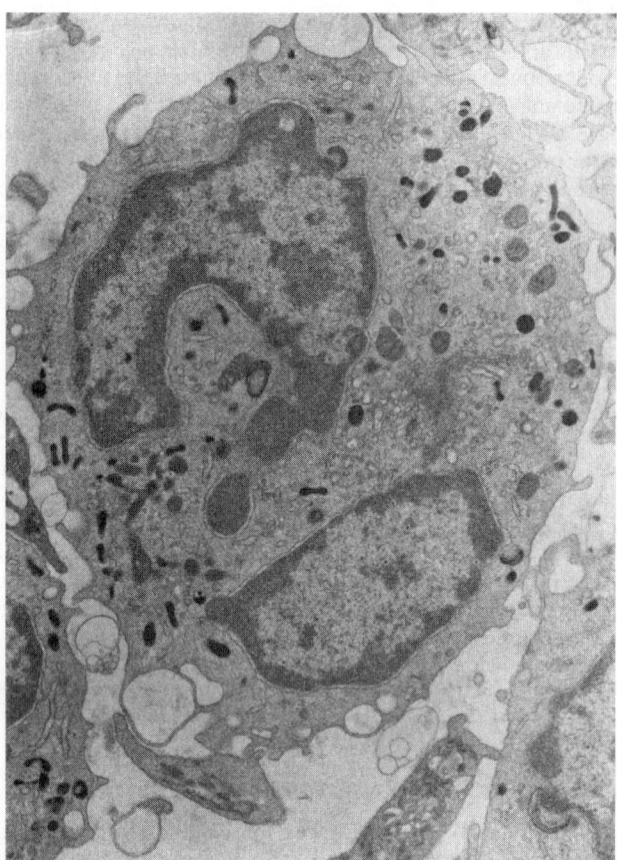

Figure 14-7. Development of mononuclear phagocytes. (Adapted from Cline MJ, Golde DW. A review and reevaluation of the histiocytic disorders. *Am J Med* 1973;55:49.)

sively ruffled, with fingerlike microvilli that extend in a polar fashion during cell movement. The monocyte cytoplasm has many microtubules, filament bundles, mitochondria, and an active Golgi apparatus (Fig. 14-8).

The macrophage is a large cell (15 to 80 μm in diameter), oval in shape and containing an eccentric nucleus (233). Its cell membrane is highly ruffled with frequent pseudopodia (arm-like projections). The cytoplasm is clear and often contains ingested particulate matter. The macrophage characteristically contains an extensive endoplasmic reticulum, a prominent Golgi complex, and peroxidase-negative granules. During transformation from the monocyte to the macrophage stage, the cell enlarges five- to tenfold, develops vacuoles, begins to spread over surfaces, and loses its peroxidase-positive granules. The nuclear chromatin becomes clumped, and the potential for more active oxidative metabolism is evidenced by an increase in number and activity of mitochondria and more active glycolysis. Activated macrophages are larger than rest-

ing cells and have a greater number of cytoplasmic granules, enhanced ability to phagocytize particles, and increased metabolism of glucose through the hexose monophosphate shunt.

Functional Maturation

As MNPs mature from bone marrow precursors to tissue macrophages, they acquire increasing capacity for the phagocytosis of microorganisms. Although the promonocyte has few receptors for the Fc portion of IgG and has limited phagocytic capability, mature monocytes express greater numbers of Fc and complement receptors and contain a greater amount of lysozyme. Both promonocytes and monocytes adhere to glass.

Two functionally distinct populations of granules can be detected in bone marrow promonocytes and blood monocytes. Monocytes contain a number of hydrolytic enzymes also found in neutrophils, including lysozyme, peroxidase, acid phosphatase, β-glucuronidase, sulfatase, N-acetylglucosaminidase, cathepsins, lipases, elastases, collagenases, plasminogen activator, and nucleases (233). Monocytes cannot hydrolyze naphthol AS-D chloroacetate, but they hydrolyze esters such as β-naphthyl butyrate and β-naphthyl acetate, which are nonspecific esterase markers for MNPs (234,235). Monocyte esterase is inhibited by sodium fluoride (236).

Two major subsets of monocytes have been identified, based on functional and morphologic criteria (237–239). One subset has receptors for the chemoattractant, f-MLP, and receptors for C5a. These monocyte subsets can also be separated by size and density. The slightly larger cells have more intense peroxidase activity and strongly express M1 antigen. The monocyte subset with low peroxidase activity lacks both M1 antigen and a receptor for pokeweed mitogen. The subsets are apparently not a reflection of age of the monocyte.

As described in Chapter 16, monocytes and macrophages play a vital role in multiple host functions, including initiation and regulation of the immune response, phagocytosis and killing of microorganisms, phagocytosis and degradation of aging cells and cellular debris, secretion of various biologically active substances, and antitumor effects. Monocytes and macrophages are considered "professional" phagocytes. Their ability to phagocytose organisms can be enhanced by a variety of means, including coating of these organisms by complement or immunoglobulin and activation of the macrophage by exposure to bacterial products, adherence to glass, or exposure to various cytokines. Denatured proteins, antigen complexes, activating clotting factors, and aging red blood cells are all cleared by macrophages. MNPs are also important in the removal of blood cells coated by antibodies. Thus, in autoimmune hemolytic anemias, thrombocytopenia, or neutropenia, the macrophage plays an important role in reducing the number of circulating cells, a process that may occur by means of the macrophage C3b and IgG-1 and IgG-3 Fc receptors.

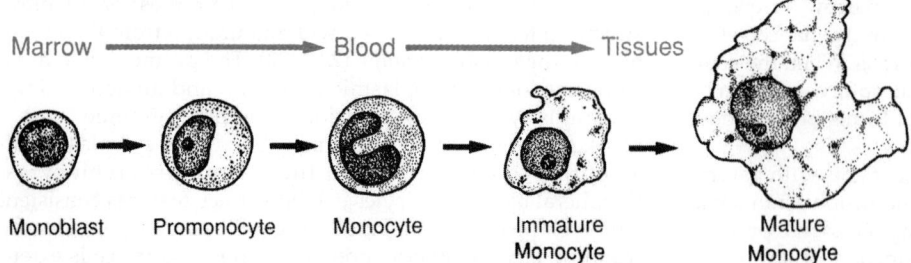

Marrow → Blood → Tissues

Monoblast   Promonocyte   Monocyte   Immature Monocyte   Mature Monocyte

Figure 14-8. Mature monocyte. A nucleolus is clearly visible; the abundance of cytoplasmic organelles (Golgi apparatus, rough endoplasmic reticulum, mitochondria) reflects the functional capabilities of the monocyte. (Adapted from Morris RB, Nichols BA, Bainton DF. Ultrastructure and peroxidase cytochemistry of normal human leukocytes at birth. *Dev Biol* 1975;44:233.)

Monocytes and macrophages express a large number of surface proteins, classified as CD molecules, which play important functional roles in the regulation of MNP biology (Table 14-1). Among these CD molecules are important receptors for immunoglobulin binding (e.g., Fc receptors), cell adhesion (e.g., integrins and selectins), phagocytosis (e.g., scavenger receptor, CD36, and the phosphatidylserine receptor), chemotaxis (e.g., chemokine receptors), and pathogen recognition (e.g., Toll-like receptors and CD14) (240–259). Expression of specific receptors on macrophages also confers the ability to respond to C5a, N-formylated bacterial peptides, and hydroxylated derivatives of arachidonic acid. Activated macrophages release a large variety of cytokines and other mediators (Chapter 16) that can serve as either autocrine factors or paracrine factors to activate other MNPs, neutrophils (e.g., TNF, GM-CSF, neutrophil-activating factor) and mesenchymal cells (e.g., IL-1, TNF, platelet-derived growth factor). The major cytokines produced by monocytes and macrophages and their respective cell targets and biologic effects are outlined in Table 14-5. One important proinflammatory cytokine is IL-8, an 8- to 10-kd peptide (260), also known as *monocyte-derived neutrophil chemotactic factor* or *neutrophil-activating factor*, produced by human monocytes stimulated by lipopolysaccharide, phytohemagglutinin or Con A (261), lectin-stimulated lymphocytes (262,263), and stimulated fibroblasts and endothelial cells. IL-8 serves as a chemotactic factor for neutrophils and can enhance many of their functional activities. IL-8 induces neutrophil shape change, respiratory burst, and the exocytosis of specific and azurophilic neutrophil granules (264,265). IL-8 is partially homologous to β-thromboglobulin and platelet-activating factor-4 (266).

The human immune system has been traditionally divided into innate immunity and adaptive (acquired) immunity. MNPs play critical effector and regulatory roles in both arms of the immune response (267–269). The immediate, innate immune response, which represents the first line of defense against invading microbial pathogens, is mediated largely by neutrophils and monocyte-derived macrophages. Recent evidence indicates that the Toll-like receptor family of pattern-recognition receptors plays a fundamental role in detection and recognition of a wide range of pathogens by monocytes and macrophages (257,270–273). At least nine distinct human Toll-like receptors have been identified by DNA sequencing, and specific members of the family recognize lipopolysaccharide, bacterial lipoproteins, bacterial peptidoglycan, lipoteichoic acid, zymosan (yeast cell wall), mycobacteria-derived lipoarabinomannan, and bacterial DNA (274–284). The human Toll-like receptors are differentially expressed among leukocytes, and it appears that specific family members can interact and cooperate to mediate proinflammatory signaling (285–287). Upon activation, the Toll-like receptors signal via a pathway involving the adaptor protein MyD88 to activate NF-κB and stimulate cytokine production by the host cell (288–293).

Macrophages and T lymphocytes interact extensively to provide cellular immune function during adaptive (acquired) immunity (294–296). Macrophages present antigen to T cells in the setting of class II major histocompatibility complex compatibility (297), and macrophage products such as IL-1 are involved in activating T cells to perform effector functions. Activated T cells can release substances, including IFN-γ, GM-CSF, and IL-3, which can enhance various macrophage functions.

Circulating monocytes can also give rise to dendritic cells, which are distinctive, potent antigen-presenting cells (298–303). TNF-α, CD40L, GM-CSF, and IL-4 are important stimuli for the development of dendritic cells from monocytes (298,304–308). In contrast to macrophages, mature dendritic cells are nonadherent, CD83+, CD40+, and CD14−. Dendritic cells also express high levels of MHC class II antigen and low levels of Fc receptors (298,309).

Mononuclear Phagocyte Kinetics

It is difficult to measure precisely the behavior of monoblasts because they lack distinctive features separating them from myeloblasts. The mature monocyte is derived from its earliest morphologically identifiable precursor after at least three divisions. The generation time for promonocytes from earlier progenitors is approximately 30 to 48 hours in humans, and tritiated thymidine-labeling studies suggest that approximately 80% of promonocytes are in S phase (310). The time required for a promonocyte to undergo division is approximately 19.5 hours. After completing their last division, most monocytes leave the bone marrow space within 24 hours. Promonocytes constitute approximately 3% of bone marrow cells, and blood monocytes represent 3% to 11% of circulating leukocytes. The total number of monocytes in the bone marrow is estimated to be approximately 7.3×10^9 cells (310). Unlike neutrophils, no significant storage pool of monocytes exists in the bone marrow (311). The presence of an MBP of peripheral monocytes in humans has been suggested (312) but not definitively shown (310,313). Circulating monocytes leave the blood randomly; that is, their exit from the blood is independent of their time of entry into the blood from bone marrow. Tritiated thymidine-labeled monocytes are cleared from the circulation with a half-life of approximately 71 hours (range of 36 to 104 hours), although estimates of the monocyte half-life in blood have varied widely depending on the methods used (310,314). Once monocytes leave the blood, they do not reenter the circulation.

Blood monocytes can enter tissue, where they may participate in inflammatory reactions or die by unknown means. The monocytes can also provide a renewal source for tissue macrophages and dendritic cells. Studies in animal and human bone marrow transplantation indicate that the resident tissue macrophages ultimately are derived from bone marrow precursors. Thus, pulmonary alveolar macrophages, Kupffer's cells, and dermal Langerhans' cells become of donor type after successful bone marrow engraftment (315,316). It has been estimated that by day 100 posttransplantation, all recipient alveolar macrophages are replaced by cells of donor type (317). Peritoneal and pleural macrophages, osteoclasts (318), and microglial cells of the brain are also resident macrophages derived from bone marrow precursors. Consequently, osteopetrosis, a disease caused by a deficiency in osteoclast activity, can be successfully treated by bone marrow transplantation (319).

Although tissue macrophage populations are derived from bone marrow, they are not dependent on an influx of marrow-derived cells to maintain their numbers (320,321). Tissue macrophages have proliferative capability and can sustain their populations by replication *in situ*. The precise relation between local macrophage replication and mononuclear cell influx from the bone marrow in the maintenance of resident macrophage populations is uncertain. In general, tissue macrophages have a low ³H-TdR–labeling index (313), suggesting that a small proportion of the cells are in active cell cycle. Studies using fluorescent dyes for *in situ* labeling of resident peritoneal macrophages and recruited macrophages have demonstrated no replacement of resident macrophages by recruited blood monocytes in the steady state over a 7-week period (322). Macrophages in inflammatory tissue exudates, however, are largely derived from circulating blood monocytes (311).

Gene Expression

Protooncogenes are thought to play a critical role in the process of cellular growth and differentiation. Whereas tissue plasminogen activator (TPA)-induced differentiation of HL-60 cells toward

TABLE 14-5. Cytokines Produced by Monocytes and Macrophages

Cytokine	Receptor	Cell Target	Biologic Activity
G-CSF	G-CSFR; gp130	Myeloid cells	Stimulation of myelopoiesis; enhancement of neutrophil survival and function
GM-CSF	GM-CSFR	Monocytes, macrophages, neutrophils, eosinophils, fibroblasts	Regulation of myelopoiesis; up-regulation of macrophage bactericidal and tumoricidal activity; mediator of dendritic cell maturation and function; stimulation of NK cell function
GROα/MGSA	CXCR2	Neutrophils, epithelial cells, endothelial cells	Chemoattractant for and activator of neutrophils; suppression of hematopoiesis; angiogenic activity
GROβ/MIP-2α	CXCR2	Neutrophils, endothelial cells	Chemoattractant for neutrophils; activator of neutrophils; angiogenic activity
IFNα	Type I IFN receptor	All cells	Antiviral and antitumor activity; stimulation of T cell, macrophage, and NK cell activity; up-regulation of MHC class I antigen expression
IFNβ	Type I IFN receptor	All cells	Antiviral and antitumor activity; stimulation of T cell, macrophage, and NK cell activity; up-regulation of MHC class I antigen expression
IL-1α/β	Type I IL-1R, type II IL-1R	All cells	Inflammation; up-regulation of adhesion molecule expression; endogenous pyrogen; neutrophil and macrophage emigration; up-regulation of hepatic acute phase protein production
IL-6	IL-6R, gp 130	Monocytes, macrophages, T cells, B cells, hepatocytes, epithelial cells	Induction of acute phase protein production; T- and B-cell growth and differentiation; osteoclast growth and differentiation
IL-8	CXCR1, CXCR2	Neutrophils, monocytes, macrophages, T cells, endothelial cells, basophils	Chemoattractant for neutrophils, monocytes, and T cells; stimulation of neutrophil adherence to endothelium; stimulation of histamine release from basophils; angiogenesis; suppression of hepatic precursor proliferation
IL-10	IL-10R	Monocytes, macrophages, T cells, B cells, NK cells, mast cells	Inhibition of macrophage proinflammatory cytokine production; inhibition of T_H1 cell differentiation and NK cell function; down-regulation of CD80 (B7-1) and CD86 (B7-2) expression; stimulation of mast cell proliferation and function; B-cell activation and differentiation
IL-12	IL-12R	T cells, NK cells	T_H1 induction; stimulation of proinflammatory cytokine expression in PBMC; lymphokine-activated killer cell formation
IL-15	IL-15Rα, IL-2Rβ	T cells	T-cell activation and proliferation; angiogenesis
IFNγ-inducible protein–10	CXCR3	Activated T cells, tumor infiltrating lymphocytes	Chemoattractant (IFNγ-inducible protein) for T cells; suppression of hematopoietic precursor proliferation
MCP-1	CCR2	Monocytes, macrophages, memory T cells, NK cells, basophils	Chemoattractant for monocytes, activated memory T cells, and NK cells; stimulation of granule release from CD8+ T cells and NK cells; potent stimulus for histamine release from basophils; inhibition of hematopoiesis; regulation of monocyte protease production
MCP-2	CCR1, CCR2	Monocytes, macrophages, T cells, eosinophils, basophils, NK cells	Chemoattractant for monocytes, T cells, and eosinophils; activation of eosinophils and basophils; regulation of monocyte protease production
MCP-3	CCR1, CCR2	Monocytes, macrophages, T cells, eosinophils, basophils, NK cells, dendritic cells	Chemoattractant for monocytes, T cells, dendritic cells, and eosinophils; activation of eosinophils and basophils; regulation of monocyte protease production
M-CSF	M-CSFR (FMS protooncogene)	Monocytes, macrophages	Regulation of monocyte/macrophage production and function
MDC	CCR4	Activated T cells	Chemoattractant for activated T cells
MIG	CXCR3	Activated T cells, tumor-infiltrating lymphocytes	Chemoattractant for T cells; suppression of hematopoiesis
MIP-1α	CCR1, CCR5	Monocytes, macrophages, T cells, eosinophils, basophils, NK cells, dendritic cells	Chemoattractant for monocytes, T cells, dendritic cells, and NK cells; weak chemoattractant for eosinophils and basophils; activation of NK cell function; suppression of hematopoiesis
MIP-1β	CCR5	Monocytes, macrophages, T cells, NK cells, dendritic cells	Chemoattractant for monocytes, T cells, and NK cells; activation of NK cell function
OSM	OSMR, gp130	Neurons, hepatocytes, monocytes, macrophages, adipocytes, alveolar epithelial cells, embryonic stem cells, endothelial cells, fibroblasts, melanocytes, myeloma cells	Hepatic acute phase protein induction; stimulation of macrophage differentiation and growth of myeloma cells and hematopoietic progenitors; thrombopoiesis
RANTES	CCR1, CCR2, CCR5	Monocytes, macrophages, T cells, eosinophils, basophils, NK cells, dendritic cells	Chemoattractant for
TGFβ	Type I, type II, TGFβ receptor	Most cell types	Down-regulation of T cell, macrophage, and granulocyte responses; stimulation of matrix protein synthesis and angiogenesis
TNF-α	TNF-RI, TNF-RII	All cells except erythrocytes	Endogenous mediator of fever, anorexia/cachexia, shock, and capillary leak syndrome; proinflammatory cytokine induction; stimulation of acute phase protein synthesis; enhancement of leukocyte toxicity and NK cell function

CCR, CC-type chemokine receptor; CXCR, CXC-type chemokine receptor; G-CSF, granulocyte colony-stimulating factor; GM-CSF, granulocyte-macrophage colony-stimulating factor; IFN, interferon; Ig, immunoglobulin; IL, interleukin; LIF, leukemia inhibitory factor; NK, natural killer; MCP, monocyte chemotactic protein; M-CSF, macrophage colony-stimulating factor; MDC, macrophage-derived chemokine; MHC, major histocompatibility complex; MIG, monteine induced by IFNγ; IP-10, IFNγ-inducible protein-10; MIP, macrophage inflammatory protein; NK, natural killer; OSM, oncostatin M; PBMC, peripheral blood mononuclear cells; RANTES, regulated on activation, normally T cell expressed and secreted; SCF, stem cell factor; TGF, transforming growth factor; TNF, tumor necrosis factor.

macrophages results in decreased expression of c-*myc* (323) and c-*myb* (324), increased amounts of c-*fos* and c-*fms* accumulate in hematopoietic cells as monocytic maturation proceeds. Expression of these oncogenes may be directly related to the differentiation process (325–327). Rapid induction of c-*fos* is seen in TPA-induced monocytic differentiation of the HL-60 and U937 cell lines (328), and high levels of c-*fos* have also been detected in primary cultures of peritoneal macrophages (329). Low basal levels of c-*fos* transcripts are seen in pure myeloid subtypes of AML, whereas high constitutive c-*fos* expression has been detected in the M4 and M5 monocytic subtypes of AML (330). The levels of c-*fos* RNA correlate with expression of CD14 (Mo-2) and expression of sodium fluoride-inhibitable β-naphthyl acetate esterase. Nonetheless, studies examining differentiation of HL-60 variants by vitamin D_3 or TPA have demonstrated that c-*fos* expression is not essential for monocyte differentiation (331).

HL-60 cells can be differentiated toward monocytes by incubation with phorbol diesters (332,333) or 1,25 dihydroxyvitamin D_3 (334,335) or stimulated lymphocyte-conditioned medium (PHA-LCM). These agents can have differential effects on gene expression. For example, PHA-LCM [which contains IFN-γ (336) and other lymphokines] induces expression of Mo-1 and Mo-2 surface antigens, whereas phorbol diesters, such as phorbol myristate acetate (PMA), induce only Mo-1 expression (337). Morphologic differentiation of HL-60 cells toward monocytes by vitamin D derivatives is accompanied by increases in secreted lysozyme, nonspecific acid esterase activity, nitroblue tetrazolium (NBT) reduction, phagocytic activity, f-MLP receptor, and Mac-120 surface antigen expression (338). In contrast, PMA-treated HL-60 cells demonstrate only weak NBT reduction (339), and although they show a marked increase in OKM-1 positivity, they do not express the monocyte-specific marker, 61D3. Deprivation of a single essential amino acid also results in differentiation of HL-60 cells toward monocytes (340), defined by CD11 (OKM-1) or CD14 (Leu M3) antigen expression.

TNF-α can also induce differentiation of myeloid leukemia cells toward monocyte-like cells (341). Treatment of HL-60 cells with TNF-α had no effect on cell growth or thymidine incorporation but did enhance the nonspecific esterase activity and increase superoxide production, NBT reduction, and acid phosphatase content of the cells. TNF-α synergized with both IFN-γ and 1,25 dihydroxyvitamin D_3 in its effects on the functional activity of these cells and on the expression of monocyte antigens such as CD14 (Leu M3) and CD11 (OKM-1) (342).

HL-60 cells differentiated toward monocytes still display granulocyte-specific markers (343); thus, they are not fully suitable for studying monocyte differentiation processes. IFN-γ treatment increases antibody-dependent cell-mediated cytotoxicity and surface antigen expression on HL-60 cells (336). IFN-γ also induces an increase in Fc receptor expression on both HL-60 and U937 cells (344), which may not be linked to monocytoid differentiation. Additional polypeptide factors capable of inducing monocyte differentiation of HL-60 cells have been characterized and are referred to as *differentiation-inducing factors* (DIFs, also referred to as *leukemia inhibitory factors*). DIFs were originally described as products of mitogen-stimulated human mononuclear cells (345) but are also produced by T cells (346) and T-cell and monocytic cell lines, such as HUT-102 (347) and THP-1 (348), respectively. The DIFs represent a family of polypeptides, originally described as a murine factor (D factor) capable of inducing differentiation of murine myeloid leukemia M1 cells. Human macrophage DIF is equivalent to murine leukemia inhibitory factor (348). Although DIFs have potent differentiation-inducing effects on HL-60 cells, many have little or no effect on U937 cells.

Differentiation of the U937 cell line into monocyte- or macrophage-like cells occurs in response to phorbol diesters, retinoic acid (349), vitamin D_3 (350), IFN-γ (351,352), TNF-α, GM-CSF (353), G-CSF (354), and a 45- to 55-kd, heat-stable T-cell lymphokine distinct from IFN-γ or GM-CSF (355). U937 cells cannot be induced to differentiate toward granulocytic lineages; thus, they have been useful in studying monocyte and macrophage development. Undifferentiated U937 cells do not express the c-*fms* gene (which encodes the M-CSF receptor) and therefore do not respond to M-CSF. Exposure of U937 cells to GM-CSF results in induction of c-*fms* expression, allowing the cells to respond to M-CSF and also leads to expression of C3bi receptors, prominent nonspecific esterase activity, and development of a respiratory (oxidative) burst, as measured by NBT reduction. GM-CSF also induces Mo-1 expression and stimulates TNF-α production, which may have additional effects on monocytes. M-CSF can increase CD14 (My4 antigen) expression on peripheral blood monocytes (354).

Expression of c-*mos* RNA has been observed in U937 cells as they differentiate into macrophages in response to TPA or macrophage differentiation-inducing factor. Inducible expression of the v-*mos* gene in U937 cells results in their differentiation into macrophages (356). Cell growth was inhibited in proportion to the amount of *mos* mRNA produced, and cells expressing *mos* became adherent and developed the ability to reduce NBT and generate superoxide anions. These cells also became phagocytic and increased their expression of IgG Fc receptors and the Mac-1 surface antigen. Continuous synthesis of *mos* was required for maintenance of the differentiated phenotype, and the quantity of macrophage-associated characteristics corresponded well with the amount of *mos* RNA present. Although *mos* expression by itself does not appear to be sufficient to trigger the differentiation process, expression of *mos* is closely related to activation of a variety of genes involved in macrophage differentiation.

Regulation of Mononuclear Phagocyte Production

Monocytes and macrophages elaborate a variety of factors that stimulate or inhibit MNP proliferation, including GM-CSF, M-CSF, IL-1, TNF, and IFN (357,358). Peripheral blood monocytes stimulated by IFN-γ, PMA, GM-CSF, or TNF (359) produce M-CSF, and mouse peritoneal macrophages produce GM-CSF after cycloheximide treatment or stimulation by adherence or endotoxin (125,205,206). Production of M-CSF and GM-CSF by MNPs is potentially important in stimulating monocyte production by an autocrine mechanism. Clearance of M-CSF by macrophages has also been implicated in controlling the rate of macrophage production (360).

Although active in generating murine macrophage colonies, human M-CSF by itself has relatively weak ability to stimulate human macrophage colony formation. However, in combination with IL-1184 or suboptimal concentrations of GM-CSF (163), M-CSF is a potent stimulator of macrophage proliferation. M-CSF is present in serum (158) and urine, and *in vivo* administration of M-CSF results in increased numbers of promonocytes and monocytes. M-CSF appears to be important in the day-to-day regulation of monocyte numbers.

GM-CSF can directly stimulate macrophage colony formation at low concentrations and can prime marrow precursor cells to respond to M-CSF. GM-CSF is produced by stromal cells, such as fibroblasts and endothelial cells, after stimulation by monocyte-derived IL-1 or TNF-α (126–128), and may also play an important role in controlling macrophage production, particularly during inflammation. Because GM-CSF can stimulate production of TNF by MNPs, several positive feedback loops may exist (361). The role of the T lymphocyte and its secretory products in the day-to-day control of monocyte proliferation is unknown. Activated T cells produce IL-3 and GM-

CSF, suggesting a role for these mediators in stimulating macrophage production and function during immune responses. IL-3 stimulates macrophage colony formation and may act to sensitize macrophage progenitors to more lineage-restricted growth factors, such as GM-CSF and M-CSF (362).

A variety of factors have been suggested to function as possible negative regulators of MNP proliferation. Of these, prostaglandin E, lactoferrin, and TNF have all been shown to have inhibitory effects on formation of phagocytic cells *in vitro* (363,364). By contrast, TNF-α reportedly supports the viability of skin macrophages (Langerhans' cells) in culture but does not affect the maturation of monocytes (365). Because prostaglandin E is produced by macrophages, it may serve in negative-feedback regulation (366). Lactoferrin, which is produced by neutrophils, suppresses CSF production by MNPs (190,367). Tumor growth factor-β (TGF-β), which is secreted by activated macrophages (368), can inhibit proliferation of macrophages in response to M-CSF (369).

Monocytosis

In the normal adult, between 1% and 9% of the circulating leukocytes are monocytes. Absolute monocyte counts range from 300 to 700 cells/μL. Monocyte counts of more than 800 cells/μL represent monocytosis in adults (370). Monocytosis is normal during the first few weeks of life (Table 14-2) (371), and children tend to have higher monocyte counts than adults. Increases in monocyte numbers frequently accompany neutrophilia. Because the monocyte plays an important role in immunologic reactions and the host response to neoplasia, a variety of inflammatory, neoplastic, and immune conditions can be associated with monocytosis (372). Tuberculosis is associated with a brisk monocytosis (373), as are chronic infections such as subacute bacterial endocarditis (374) and secondary syphilis (375). Monocytosis is also seen in response to malignancies (376), especially lymphomas and Hodgkin's disease (377,378), and can accompany lipid storage or connective tissue diseases, such as rheumatoid arthritis, systemic lupus erythematosus, sarcoidosis, and polyarteritis nodosum. Modest monocytosis is seen in preleukemic conditions (379). A variety of malignant monocyte disorders have been identified, including acute monocytic leukemia and acute or chronic myelomonocytic leukemia (380–383).

Monocytosis may also occur after recovery from chemotherapy or drug-induced agranulocytosis or as a compensatory event in association with neutropenic disorders such as cyclic neutropenia. This stem cell disorder is marked by striking periodicity of neutrophil production, often reciprocal to the periodicity affecting monocytes; monocyte numbers change reciprocally to neutrophil numbers and may reach peaks of over 5000 cells/μL.

Monocytopenia

Monocytopenia is observed in patients receiving chronic corticosteroid therapy, even when prednisone is administered on an alternate-day basis (384,385). Monocytopenia can also occur in conjunction with neutropenia in diseases such as hairy cell leukemia (386,387), aplastic anemia (388), acquired immunodeficiency syndrome, and infiltrative diseases of the bone marrow.

REFERENCES

1. Boggs DR. The kinetics of neutrophilic leukocytes in health and in disease. *Semin Hematol* 1967;4:359.
2. Dancey JT, Deubelbeiss KA, Harker LA, et al. Neutrophil kinetics in man. *J Clin Invest* 1976;58:705.
3. Bainton DF, Ullyot JL, Farquhar MG. The development of neutrophilic polymorphonuclear leukocytes in human bone marrow. *J Exp Med* 1971;134:907.
4. Bainton DF. Neutrophilic leukocyte granules: from structure to function. *Adv Exp Med Biol* 1993;336:17.
5. Borregaard N. Development of neutrophil granule diversity. *Ann N Y Acad Sci* 1997;832:62.
6. Gullberg U, Andersson E, Garwicz D, et al. Biosynthesis, processing and sorting of neutrophil proteins: insight into neutrophil granule development. *Eur J Haematol* 1997;58:137.
7. Gullberg U, Bengtsson N, Bulow E, et al. Processing and targeting of granule proteins in human neutrophils. *J Immunol Methods* 1999;232:201.
8. Borregaard N, Lollike K, Kjeldsen L, et al. Human neutrophil granules and secretory vesicles. *Eur J Haematol* 1993;51:187.
9. Borregaard N. Current concepts about neutrophil granule physiology. *Curr Opin Hematol* 1996;3:11.
10. Saito N, Takemori N, Hirai K, et al. Ultrastructural localization of lactoferrin in the granules other than typical secondary granules of human neutrophils. *Hum Cell* 1993;6:42.
11. Nauseef WM. Neutrophil granules: heterogeneity of their contents reflects targeting by timing. *J Leukoc Biol* 1999;66:867.
12. Rustin GJ, Wilson PD, Peters TJ. Studies on the subcellular localization of human neutrophil alkaline phosphatase. *J Cell Sci* 1979;36:401.
13. Borregaard N, Kjeldsen L, Sengelov H, et al. Changes in subcellular localization and surface expression of L-selectin, alkaline phosphatase, and Mac-1 in human neutrophils during stimulation with inflammatory mediators. *J Leukoc Biol* 1994;56:80.
14. Bainton DF, Farquhar MG. Origin of granules in polymorphonuclear leukocytes. Two types derived from opposite faces of the Golgi complex in developing granulocytes. *J Cell Biol* 1966;28:277.
15. Scott RE, Horn RG. Ultrastructural aspects of neutrophil granulocyte development in humans. *Lab Invest* 1970;23:202.
16. Bainton DF, Ullyot JL, Farquhar MG. The development of neutrophilic polymorphonuclear leukocytes in human bone marrow. *J Exp Med* 1971;134:907.
17. Martin E, Ganz T, Lehrer RI. Defensins and other endogenous peptide antibiotics of vertebrates. *J Leukoc Biol* 1995;58:128.
18. Levy O. Antibiotic proteins of polymorphonuclear leukocytes. *Eur J Haematol* 1996;56:263.
19. Ganz T, Lehrer RI. Antimicrobial peptides of leukocytes. *Curr Opin Hematol* 1997;4:53.
20. Ebihara Y, Xu MJ, Manabe A, et al. Exclusive expression of G-CSF receptor on myeloid progenitors in bone marrow CD34+ cells. *Br J Haematol* 2000;109:153.
21. Lund-Johansen F, Houck JD, Hoffman R, et al. Primitive human hematopoietic progenitor cells express receptors for granulocyte-macrophage colony-stimulating factor. *Exp Hematol* 1999;27:762.
22. Xiao M, Oppenlander BK, Plunkett JM, et al. Expression of Flt3 and c-kit during growth and maturation of human CD34+CD38- cells. *Exp Hematol* 1999;27:916.
23. De Bruyn C, Delforge A, Lagneaux L, et al. Characterization of CD34+ subsets derived from bone marrow, umbilical cord blood and mobilized peripheral blood after stem cell factor and interleukin 3 stimulation. *Bone Marrow Transplant* 2000;25:377.
24. Pitrak DL. Effects of granulocyte colony-stimulating factor and granulocyte-macrophage colony-stimulating factor on the bactericidal functions of neutrophils. *Curr Opin Hematol* 1997;4:183.
25. Rosmarin AG, Weil SC, Rosner GL, et al. Differential expression of CD11b/CD18 (Mo1) and myeloperoxidase genes during myeloid differentiation. *Blood* 1989;73:131.
26. Hickstein DD, Back AL, Collins SJ. Regulation of expression of the CD11b and CD18 subunits of the neutrophil adherence receptor during human myeloid differentiation. *J Biol Chem* 1989;264:21812.
27. Kansas GS, Muirhead MJ, Dailey MO. Expression of the CD11/CD18, leukocyte adhesion molecule 1, and CD44 adhesion molecules during normal myeloid and erythroid differentiation in humans. *Blood* 1990;76:2483.
28. Carlos TM, Harlan JM. Leukocyte-endothelial adhesion molecules. *Blood* 1994;84:2068.
29. Dransfield I. Granulocyte adhesion molecules—structure/function relations. *Semin Cell Biol* 1995;6:337.
30. Kronenwett R, Martin S, Haas R. The role of cytokines and adhesion molecules for mobilization of peripheral blood stem cells. *Stem Cells* 2000;18:320.
31. Yamaguchi M, Ikebuchi K, Hirayama F, et al. Different adhesive characteristics and VLA-4 expression of CD34(+) progenitors in G0/G1 versus S+G2/M phases of the cell cycle. *Blood* 1998;92:842.
32. Kovach NL, Lin N, Yednock T, et al. Stem cell factor modulates avidity of alpha 4 beta 1 and alpha 5 beta 1 integrins expressed on hematopoietic cell lines. *Blood* 1995;85:159.
33. Le Marer N, Skacel PO. Up-regulation of alpha2,6 sialylation during myeloid maturation: a potential role in myeloid cell release from the bone marrow. *J Cell Physiol* 1999;179:315.
34. Lund-Johansen F, Terstappen LW. Differential surface expression of cell adhesion molecules during granulocyte maturation. *J Leukoc Biol* 1993;54:47.
35. Bokoch GM. Chemoattractant signaling and leukocyte activation. *Blood* 1995;86:1649.
36. Wagner JG, Roth RA. Neutrophil migration mechanisms, with an emphasis on the pulmonary vasculature. *Pharmacol Rev* 2000;52:349.
37. Fontana JA, Wright DG, Schiffman E, et al. Development of chemotactic responsiveness in myeloid precursor cells: studies with a human leukemia cell line. *Proc Natl Acad Sci U S A* 1980;77:3644.

38. Takano K, Kaganoi J, Yamamoto K, et al. Rapid and prominent up-regulation of high-affinity receptor for immunoglobulin G (Fc gamma RI) by cross-linking of beta 2 integrins on polymorphonuclear leukocytes. *Int J Hematol* 2000; 72:48.

39. Fleit HB, Writhe SD, Durie CJ, et al. Ontogeny of Fc receptors and complement receptor (CR3) during human myeloid differentiation. *J Clin Invest* 1984;73:516.

40. Rosenberg JS, Melnicoff MJ, Wilding P. Fc receptors for IgG on human neutrophils: analysis of structure and function by using monoclonal antibody probes. *Clin Chem* 1985;31:1444.

41. Lutz PG, Moog-Lutz C, Coumau-Gatbois E, et al. Myeloblastin is a granulocyte colony-stimulating factor-responsive gene conferring factor-independent growth to hematopoietic cells. *Proc Natl Acad Sci U S A* 2000;97:1601.

42. Ward AC, Loeb DM, Soede-Bobok AA, et al. Regulation of granulopoiesis by transcription factors and cytokine signals. *Leukemia* 2000;14:973.

43. Tenen DG, Hromas R, Licht JD, et al. Transcription factors, normal myeloid development, and leukemia. *Blood* 1997;90:489.

44. Adachi K, Saito H. Induction of junB expression, but not c-jun, by granulocyte colony-stimulating factor or macrophage colony-stimulating factor in the proliferative response of human myeloid leukemia cells. *J Clin Invest* 1992;89:1657.

45. Towatari M, Ito Y, Morishita Y, et al. Enhanced expression of DNA topoisomerase II by recombinant human granulocyte colony-stimulating factor in human leukemia cells. *Cancer Res* 1990;50:7198.

46. Zeng W, Remold-O'Donnell E. Human monocyte/neutrophil elastase inhibitor (MNEI) is regulated by PU.1/Spi-1, Sp1, and NF-kappaB. *J Cell Biochem* 2000;78:519.

47. Zhang P, Zhang X, Iwama A, et al. PU.1 inhibits GATA-1 function and erythroid differentiation by blocking GATA-1 DNA binding. *Blood* 2000;96:2641.

48. Nerlov C, Querfurth E, Kulessa H, et al. GATA-1 interacts with the myeloid PU.1 transcription factor and represses PU.1-dependent transcription. *Blood* 2000;95:2543.

49. Behre G, Zhang P, Zhang DE, et al. Analysis of the modulation of transcriptional activity in myelopoiesis and leukemogenesis. *Methods* 1999;17:231.

50. Ogawa M. Differentiation and proliferation of hematopoietic stem cells. *Blood* 1993;81:2844.

51. Sieff CA. Hematopoietic cell proliferation and differentiation. *Curr Opin Hematol* 1994;1:310.

52. Migliaccio AR, Vannucchi AM, Migliaccio G. Molecular control of erythroid differentiation. *Int J Hematol* 1996;64:1.

53. Metcalf D. Cellular hematopoiesis in the twentieth century. *Semin Hematol* 1999;36:5.

54. Till JE, McCulloch EA. A direct measurement of the radiation sensitivity of normal mouse bone marrow cells. *Radiat Res* 1961;14:213.

55. Schofield R. The relationship between spleen colony-forming cells and the haematopoietic stem cell. *Blood Cells* 1978;4:7.

56. Bradley TR, Metcalf D. The growth of mouse bone marrow cells in vitro. *Aust J Exp Biol Med Sci* 1966;44:287.

57. Pluznik DH, Sachs L. The cloning of normal "mast" cells in tissue culture. *J Cell Physiol* 1965;66:319.

58. Nakahata T, Ogawa M. Identification in culture of a class of hematopoietic colony-forming units with extensive capability to self-renew and generate multipotential colonies. *Proc Natl Acad Sci U S A* 1982;79:3843.

59. Zhao Y, Lin Y, Zhan Y, et al. Murine hematopoietic stem cell characterization and its regulation in BM transplantation. *Blood* 2000;96:3016.

60. Vassort F, Winterholer M, Frindel E, et al. Kinetic parameters of bone marrow stem cells using in vivo suicide by tritiated thymidine or by hydroxyurea. *Blood* 1973;41:789.

61. Hodgson GS, Bradley TR. Properties of haematopoietic stem cells surviving 5-fluorouracil treatment: evidence for a pre-CFU-S cell? *Nature* 1979;281:381.

62. Glimm H, Oh IH, Eaves CJ. Human hematopoietic stem cells stimulated to proliferate in vitro lose engraftment potential during their S/G(2)/M transit and do not reenter G(0). *Blood* 2000;96:4185.

63. Duarte RF, Frank DA. SCF and G-CSF lead to the synergistic induction of proliferation and gene expression through complementary signaling pathways. *Blood* 2000;96:3422.

64. Holm M, Thomsen M, Hoyer M, et al. Dynamic cell cycle kinetics of normal CD34+ cells and CD38+/− subsets of haemopoietic progenitor cells in G-CSF-mobilized peripheral blood. *Br J Haematol* 1999;105:1002.

65. Gilmore GL, DePasquale DK, Lister J, et al. Ex vivo expansion of human umbilical cord blood and peripheral blood CD34(+) hematopoietic stem cells. *Exp Hematol* 2000;28:1297.

66. Won JH, Cho SD, Park SK, et al. Thrombopoietin is synergistic with other cytokines for expansion of cord blood progenitor cells. *J Hematother Stem Cell Res* 2000;9:465.

67. Bryder D, Jacobsen SE. Interleukin-3 supports expansion of long-term multilineage repopulating activity after multiple stem cell divisions in vitro. *Blood* 2000;96:1748.

68. Nicola NA, Begley CG, Metcalf D. Identification of the human analogue of a regulator that induces differentiation in murine leukaemic cells. *Nature* 1985;314:625.

69. Welte K, Platzer E, Lu L, et al. Purification and biochemical characterization of human pluripotent hematopoietic colony-stimulating factor. *Proc Natl Acad Sci U S A* 1985;82:1526.

70. Nagata S, Tsuchiya M, Asano S, et al. Molecular cloning and expression of cDNA for human granulocyte colony-stimulating factor. *Nature* 1986;319:415.

71. Souza LM, Boone TC, Gabrilove J, et al. Recombinant human granulocyte colony-stimulating factor: effects on normal and leukemic myeloid cells. *Science* 1986;232:61.

72. Simmers RN, Webber LM, Shannon MR, et al. Localization of the G-CSF gene on chromosome 17 proximal to the breakpoint in the t(15;17) in acute promyelocytic leukemia. *Blood* 1987;70:330.

73. Presneill JJ, Waring PM, Layton JE, et al. Plasma granulocyte colony-stimulating factor and granulocyte-macrophage colony-stimulating factor levels in critical illness including sepsis and septic shock: relation to disease severity, multiple organ dysfunction, and mortality. *Crit Care Med* 2000;28:2344.

74. Uzumaki H, Okabe T, Sasaki N, et al. Characterization of receptor for granulocyte colony-stimulating factor on human circulating neutrophils. *Biochem Biophys Res Commun* 1988;156:1026.

75. Nicola NA, Metcalf D. Binding of ^{125}I-labeled granulocyte colony-stimulating factor to normal murine hemopoietic cells. *J Cell Physiol* 1985;124:313.

76. Ebihara Y, Xu MJ, Manabe A, et al. Exclusive expression of G-CSF receptor on myeloid progenitors in bone marrow CD34+ cells. *Br J Haematol* 2000;109:153.

77. Boneberg EM, Hareng L, Gantner F, et al. Human monocytes express functional receptors for granulocyte colony-stimulating factor that mediate suppression of monokines and interferon-gamma. *Blood* 2000;95:270.

78. Kawada H, Sasao T, Yonekura S, et al. Clinical significance of granulocyte colony-stimulating factor (G-CSF) receptor expression in acute myeloid leukemia. *Leuk Res* 1998;22:31.

79. Layton JE, Shimamoto G, Osslund T, et al. Interaction of granulocyte colony-stimulating factor (G-CSF) with its receptor. Evidence that Glu19 of G-CSF interacts with Arg288 of the receptor. *J Biol Chem* 1999;274:17445.

80. Ward AC, Oomen SP, Smith L, et al. The SH2 domain-containing protein tyrosine phosphatase SHP-1 is induced by granulocyte colony-stimulating factor (G-CSF) and modulates signaling from the G-CSF receptor. *Leukemia* 2000;14:1284.

81. Semerad CL, Poursine-Laurent J, Liu F, et al. A role for G-CSF receptor signaling in the regulation of hematopoietic cell function but not lineage commitment or differentiation. *Immunity* 1999;11:153.

82. Basu S, Hodgson G, Zhang HH, et al. "Emergency" granulopoiesis in G-CSF-deficient mice in response to Candida albicans infection. *Blood* 2000;95:3725.

83. Dekkers PE, Juffermans NP, Hove T, et al. Granulocyte colony-stimulating factor receptors on granulocytes are down-regulated after endotoxin administration to healthy humans. *J Infect Dis* 2000;181:2067.

84. Gasson JC, Weisbart RH, Kaufman SE, et al. Purified human GM-colony-stimulating factor: direct action on neutrophils. *Science* 1984;226:1339.

85. Kaushansky K, O'Hara PJ, Berkner K, et al. Genomic cloning, characterization and multilineage growth-promoting activity of human granulocyte-macrophage colony-stimulating factor. *Proc Natl Acad Sci U S A* 1986;83:3101.

86. Chan JY, Slamon DJ, Nimer SD, et al. Regulation of expression of human granulocyte-macrophage colony-stimulating factor (GM-CSF). *Proc Natl Acad Sci U S A* 1986;83:8669.

87. Kupper TS, Dower S, Birchall N, et al. Interleukin-1 binds to specific receptors on keratinocytes and induces granulocyte/macrophage colony stimulating factor (GM-CSF) mRNA and protein: a potential autocrine role for IL-1 in epidermis. *J Clin Invest* 1988;82:1787.

88. Metcalf D, Begley CG, Johnson GR, et al. Biologic properties in vitro of a recombinant human granulocyte-macrophage colony-stimulating factor. *Blood* 1986;67:37.

89. Gasson JD. Molecular physiology of granulocyte-macrophage colony-stimulating factor. *J Am Soc Hematol* 1995;77:1131.

90. Rapoport AP, Abboud CN, DiPersio JF. Granulocyte-macrophage colony-stimulating factor (GM-CSF) and granulocyte colony-stimulating factor (G-CSF): receptor biology, signal transduction, and neutrophil activation. *Blood Rev* 1992;6:43.

91. You A, Kitagawa S, Ohsaka A, et al. Stimulation and priming of human neutrophils by granulocyte colony-stimulating factor and granulocyte-macrophage colony-stimulating factor: qualitative and quantitative differences. *Biochem Biophys Res Commun* 1990;171:491.

92. Woodcock JM, Bagley CJ, Lopez AF. The functional basis of granulocyte-macrophage colony stimulating factor, interleukin-3 and interleukin-5 receptor activation, basic and clinical implications. *Int J Biochem Cell Biol* 1999;31:1017.

93. Militi S, Riccioni R, Parolini I, et al. Expression of interleukin 3 and granulocyte-macrophage colony-stimulating factor receptor common chain betac, betaIT in normal haematopoiesis: lineage specificity and proliferation-independent induction. *Br J Haematol* 2000;111:441.

94. D'Andrea RJ, Gonda TJ. A model for assembly and activation of the GM-CSF, IL-3 and IL-5 receptors: insights from activated mutants of the common beta subunit. *Exp Hematol* 2000;28:231.

95. Okuda K, Smith L, Griffin JD, et al. Signaling functions of the tyrosine residues in the betac chain of the granulocyte-macrophage colony-stimulating factor receptor. *Blood* 1997;90:4759.

96. Al-Shami A, Mahanna W, Naccache PH. Granulocyte-macrophage colony-stimulating factor-activated signaling pathways in human neutrophils. Selective activation of Jak2, Stat3, and Stat5b. *J Biol Chem* 1998;273:1058.

97. Al-Shami A, Naccache PH. Granulocyte-macrophage colony-stimulating factor-activated signaling pathways in human neutrophils. Involvement of Jak2 in the stimulation of phosphatidylinositol 3-kinase. *J Biol Chem* 1999;274:5333.

98. Fung MC, Hapel AJ, Ymer S, et al. Molecular cloning of cDNA for murine interleukin-3. *Nature* 1984;307:233.

99. Yang YC, Ciarletta AB, Temple PA, et al. Identification by expression cloning of a novel hematopoietic growth factor related to murine IL-3. *Cell* 1986;47:3.

100. Mangi MH, Newland AC. Interleukin-3 in hematology and oncology: current state of knowledge and future directions. *Cytokines Cell Mol Ther* 1999;5:87.

101. Reddy EP, Korapati A, Chaturvedi P, et al. IL-3 signaling and the role of Src kinases, JAKs and STATs: a covert liaison unveiled. *Oncogene* 2000;19:2532.

102. Guthridge MA, Stomski FC, Barry EF, et al. Site-specific serine phosphorylation of the IL-3 receptor is required for hemopoietic cell survival. *Mol Cell* 2000;6:99.

103. Stanley ER, Hansen G, Woodcock J, et al. Colony stimulating factor and the regulation of granulopoiesis and macrophage production. *Fed Proc* 1975;34:2272.

104. Wu M, Cini JK, Yunis AA. Purification of a colony stimulating factor from cultured pancreatic cells. *J Biol Chem* 1979;254:6226.

105. Wong GG, Temple PA, Leary AC, et al. Human CSF-1: molecular cloning and expression of a 4 kb cDNA encoding the hematopoietin and determination of the complete amino acid sequence of the human urinary protein. *Science* 1987;235:1504.

106. Yasukawa K, Hirano T, Watanabe Y, et al. Structure and expression of human B cell stimulatory factor-2 (BSF-2/IL-6) gene. *EMBO J* 1987;6:2939.

107. Hamilton JA. CSF-1 signal transduction. *J Leukoc Biol* 1997;62:145.

108. Bourette RP, Rohrschneider LR. Early events in M-CSF receptor signaling. *Growth Factors* 2000;17:155.

109. Nienhuis AW, Bunn HF, Turner PH, et al. Expression of the human c-*fms* proto-oncogene in hematopoietic cells and its deletion in the 5q-syndrome. *Cell* 1985;42:421.

110. Zilberstein A, Ruggieri R, Korn JH, et al. Structure and expression of cDNA and genes for human interferon-beta-2, a distinct species inducible by growth-stimulatory cytokines. *EMBO J* 1986;5:2529.

111. Hoang T, Goncalves HO, Wong GG, et al. Interleukin-6 enhances growth factor-dependent proliferation of the blast cells of acute myeloblastic leukemia. *Blood* 1988;72:823.

112. Akira S. IL-6 regulated transcription factors. *Int J Biochem Cell Biol* 1997;12:1401.

113. Venden Berghe W, Vermeulen L, De Wilde G, et al. Signal transduction by tumor necrosis factor and gene regulation of the inflammatory cytokine interleukin-6. *Biochem Pharmacol* 2000;60:1185.

114. Hannen M, Banning U, Bonig H, et al. Cytokine-mediated regulation of granulocyte colony-stimulating factor production. *Scand J Immunol* 1999;50:461.

115. Veltri S, Smith JW 2nd. Interleukin 1 trials in cancer patients: a review of the toxicity, antitumor and hematopoietic effects. *Stem Cells* 1996;14:164.

116. Warner HR, Athens JW. An analysis of granulocyte kinetics in blood and bone marrow. *Ann N Y Acad Sci* 1964;113:523.

117. Cronkite EP, Vincent PC. Granulocytopoiesis. *Ser Haematol II* 1969;4:3.

118. Athens JW, Haab OP, Raab SO, et al. Leukokinetic studies. IV. The total blood, circulating and marginal granulocyte pools and the granulocyte turnover rate in normal subjects. *J Clin Invest* 1961;40:989.

119. Athens JW, Raab SO, Haab OP, et al. Leukokinetic studies. III. The distribution of granulocytes in the blood of normal subjects. *J Clin Invest* 1961;40:159.

120. Cartwright GE, Athens JW, Wintrobe MM. The kinetics of granulopoiesis in normal man. *Blood* 1964;24:780.

121. Cronkite EP, Fliedner TM. Granulocytopoiesis. *N Engl J Med* 1964;270:1403.

122. Fliedner TM, Cronkite EP, Robertson JS. Granulocytopoiesis. 1. Senescence and random loss of neutrophilic granulocytes in human beings. *Blood* 1964;24:402.

123. Boggs DR, Athens JW, Cartwright GE, et al. "Masked" granulocytosis. *Proc Soc Exp Biol Med* 1965;118:753.

124. Walker RI, Herion JC, Herring WB, et al. Leukocyte kinetics in hematologic disorders studied by DNA-phosphorus labeling. *Blood* 1964;23:795.

125. Bishop CR, Athens JW, Boggs DR, et al. Leukokinetic studies. XIII. A non-steady-state kinetic evaluation of the mechanism of cortisone-induced granulocytosis. *J Clin Invest* 1968;47:249.

126. Maloney M, Patt HM. Granulocyte transit from bone marrow to blood. *Blood* 1968;31:195.

127. Liu JH, Wei S, Lamy T, et al. Chronic neutropenia mediated by fas ligand. *Blood* 2000;95:3219.

128. Aprikyan AA, Liles WC, Park JR, et al. Myelokathexis, a congenital disorder of severe neutropenia characterized by accelerated apoptosis and defective expression of bcl-x in neutrophil precursors. *Blood* 2000;95:320.

129. Dale DC, Person RE, Bolyard AA, et al. Mutations in the gene encoding neutrophil elastase in congenital and cyclic neutropenia. *Blood* 2000;96:2317.

130. Shetty V, Hussaini S, Broady-Robinson L, et al. Intramedullary apoptosis of hematopoietic cells in myelodysplastic syndrome patients can be massive: apoptotic cells recovered from high-density fraction of bone marrow aspirates. *Blood* 2000;96:1388.

131. Aprikyan AA, Liles WC, Dale DC. Emerging role of apoptosis in the pathogenesis of severe neutropenia. *Curr Opin Hematol* 2000;7:131.

132. Aprikyan AA, Liles WC, Park JR, et al. Myelokathexis, a congenital disorder of severe neutropenia characterized by accelerated apoptosis and defective expression of bcl-x in neutrophil precursors. *Blood* 2000;95:320.

133. Dale DC, Person RE, Bolyard AA, et al. Mutations in the gene encoding neutrophil elastase in congenital and cyclic neutropenia. *Blood* 2000;96:2317.

134. Warner HR, Athens JW. An analysis of granulocyte kinetics in blood and bone marrow. *Ann N Y Acad Sci* 1964;113:523.

135. Price TH. Comparison of 3H-diisopropyl fluorophosphate and 32P-diisopropyl fluorophosphate for neutrophil kinetic studies. *Acta Haematol* 1982;67:175.

136. Thakur ML, Seifert CL, Madsen MT, et al. Neutrophil labeling: problems and pitfalls. *Semin Nucl Med* 1984;14:107.

137. Weiner RE, Thakur ML. Imaging infection/inflammations. Pathophysiologic basis and radiopharmaceuticals. *Q J Nucl Med* 1999;43:2.

138. Schauwecker DS, Park HM, Mock BH, et al. Evaluation of complicating osteomyelitis with Tc-99m MDP, In-111 granulocytes, and Ga-67 citrate. *J Nucl Med* 1984;25:849.

139. Harwood SJ, Camblin JG, Hakki S, et al. Use of technetium antigranulocyte monoclonal antibody Fab' fragments for the detection of osteomyelitis. *Cell Biophys* 1994;24–25:99.

140. Thakur ML, Marcus CS, Henneman P, et al. Imaging inflammatory diseases with neutrophil-specific technetium-99m-labeled monoclonal antibody anti-SSEA-1. *J Nucl Med* 1996;37:1789.

141. Kipper SL, Rypins EB, Evans DG, et al. Neutrophil-specific 99mTc-labeled anti-CD15 monoclonal antibody imaging for diagnosis of equivocal appendicitis. *J Nucl Med* 2000;41:449.

142. Sahr F, Hazra PK, Grillo TA. White blood cell count in healthy Sierra Leoneans. *West Afr J Med* 1995;14:105.

143. Weingarten MA, Pottick-Schwartz EA, Brauner A. The epidemiology of benign leukopenia in Yemenite Jews. *Isr J Med Sci* 1993;29:297.

144. Kostmann R. Infantile genetic agranulocytosis. *Acta Paediatr* 1956;45:1.

145. Briars GL, Parry HF, Ansari BM. Dominantly inherited severe congenital neutropenia. *J Infect* 1996;33:132.

146. Zeidler C, Boxer L, Dale DC, et al. Management of Kostmann syndrome in the G-CSF era. *Br J Haematol* 2000;109:490.

147. Dale DC, Liles WC, Garwicz D, et al. Clinical implications of mutations of neutrophil elastase in congenital and cyclic neutropenia. *J Pediatr Hematol Oncol* 2001;23:208.

148. Dale DC, Bonilla MA, Davis MW, et al. A randomized controlled phase III trial of recombinant human granulocyte colony-stimulating factor (filgrastim) for treatment of severe chronic neutropenia. *Blood* 1993;81:2496.

149. Freedman MH, Bonilla MA, Fier C, et al. Myelodysplasia syndrome and acute myeloid leukemia in patients with congenital neutropenia receiving G-CSF therapy. *Blood* 2000;96:429.

150. Ward AC, van Aesch YM, Schelen AM, et al. Defective internalization and sustained activation of truncated granulocyte colony-stimulating factor receptor found in severe congenital neutropenia/acute myeloid leukemia. *Blood* 1999;93:447.

151. Dale DC, Hammond WP 4th. Cyclic neutropenia: a clinical review. *Blood Rev* 1988;3:178.

152. Haurie C, Dale DC, Mackey MC. Cyclical neutropenia and other periodic hematological disorders: a review of mechanisms and mathematical models. *Blood* 1998;92:2629.

153. Loughran TP Jr, Hammond WP 4th. Adult-onset cyclic neutropenia is a benign neoplasm associated with clonal proliferation of large granular lymphocytes. *J Exp Med* 1986;164:2089.

154. Horwitz M, Benson KF, Person RE, et al. Mutations in ELA2, encoding neutrophil elastase, define a 21-day biological clock in cyclic haematopoiesis. *Nat Genet* 1999;23:433.

155. Aprikyan AA, Liles WC, Rodger E, et al. Impaired survival of bone marrow hematopoietic progenitor cells in cyclic neutropenia. *Blood* 2001;97:147.

156. Palmer SE, Stephens K, Dale DC. Genetics, phenotype, and natural history of autosomal dominant cyclic hematopoiesis. *Am J Med Genet* 1996;66:413.

157. Hammond WP 4th, Price TH, Souza LM, et al. Treatment of cyclic neutropenia with granulocyte colony-stimulating factor. *N Engl J Med* 1989;320:1306.

158. Zuelzer WW. Myelokathexis: a new form of chronic granulocytopenia. *N Engl J Med* 1964;270:699.

159. Aprikyan AA, Liles WC, Park JR, et al. Myelokathexis, a congenital disorder of severe neutropenia characterized by accelerated apoptosis and defective expression of bcl-x in neutrophil precursors. *Blood* 2000;95:320.

160. Schwachman H, Diamond LK, Oski FA, et al. The syndrome of pancreatic insufficiency and bone marrow dysfunction. *J Pediatr* 1964;65:645.

161. Smith OP, Hann IM, Chessells JM, et al. Haematological abnormalities in Schwachman-Diamond syndrome. *Br J Haematol* 1996;94:279.

162. Dror Y, Freedman MH. Schwachman-Diamond syndrome: an inherited preleukemic bone marrow failure disorder with aberrant hematopoietic progenitors and faulty marrow microenvironment. *Blood* 1999;9:3048.

163. Levy J, Espanol-Boren T, Thomas C, et al. Clinical spectrum of X-linked hyper-IgM syndrome. *J Pediatr* 1997;131:47.

164. Farrar JE, Rohrer J, Conley ME. Neutropenia in X-linked agammaglobulinemia. *Clin Immunol Immunopathol* 1996;81:271.

165. Bujan W, Ferster A, Sariban E, et al. Effect of recombinant human granulocyte colony-stimulating factor in reticular dysgenesis. *Blood* 1993;82:1684.

166. Lux SE, Johnston RB, August CS, et al. Chronic neutropenia and abnormal cellular immunity in cartilage-hair hypoplasia. *N Engl J Med* 1970;282:231.

167. Makitie O, Kaitila I, Savilahti E. Deficiency of humoral immunity in cartilage-hair hypoplasia. *J Pediatr* 2000;137:487.

168. Mancini AJ, Chan LS, Paller AS. Partial albinism with immunodeficiency: Griscelli syndrome: report of a case and review of the literature. *J Am Acad Dermatol* 1998;38:295.

169. Menasche G, Pastural E, Feldmann J, et al. Mutations in RAB27A cause Griscelli syndrome associated with haemophagocytic syndrome. *Nat Genet* 2000;25:173.

170. Introne W, Boissy RE, Gahl WA. Clinical, molecular, and cell biological aspects of Chediak-Higashi syndrome. *Mol Genet Metab* 1999;68:283.

171. Barth PG, Scholte HR, Berden JA, et al. An X-linked mitochondrial disease affecting cardiac muscle, skeletal muscle and neutrophil leukocytes. *J Neurol Sci* 1983;62:327.

172. Barth PG, Wanders RJ, Vreken P, et al. X-linked cardioskeletal myopathy and neutropenia (Barth syndrome). *J Inherit Metab Dis* 1999;22:555.

173. Cantlay AM, Shokrollahi K, Allen JT, et al. Genetic analysis of the G4.5 gene in families with suspected Barth syndrome. *J Pediatr* 1999;135:311.

174. Devriendt K, Kim AS, Mathijs G, et al. Constitutively activating mutation in WASP causes X-linked severe congenital neutropenia. *Nat Genet* 2001;27:313.

175. Veiga-da-Cunha M, Gerin I, Chen YT, et al. The putative glucose 6-phosphate translocase gene is mutated in essentially all cases of glycogen storage disease type I non-a. *Eur J Hum Genet* 1999;7:717.

176. Visser G, Rake JP, Fernandes J, et al. Neutropenia, neutrophil dysfunction, and inflammatory bowel disease in glycogen storage disease type I: results of the European Study on Glycogen Storage Disease type I. *J Pediatr* 2000;173:187.

177. Bodey GP, Rodriguez V, Chang HY, et al. Fever and infection in leukemic patients: a study of 494 consecutive patients. *Cancer* 1978;41:1610.

178. Suda T, Onai T, Maekawa T. Studies on abnormal polymorphonuclear neutrophils in acute myelogenous leukemia: clinical significance and changes after chemotherapy. *Am J Hematol* 1983;15:45.

179. Powell BL, Olbrantz P, Bicket D, et al. Altered oxidative product formation in neutrophils of patients recovering from therapy for acute leukemia. *Blood* 1986;67:1624.

180. Fanci R, Paci C, Martinez RL, et al. Management of fever in neutropenic patients with acute leukemia: current role of ceftazidime plus amikacin as empiric therapy. *J Chemother* 2000;12:232.

181. Thompson JA, Gilliland DG, Prchal JT, et al. Effect of recombinant human erythropoietin combined with granulocyte/macrophage colony-stimulating factor in the treatment of patients with myelodysplastic syndrome. GM/EPO MDS Study Group. *Blood* 2000;95:1175.

182. Seipelt G, Ottmann OG, Hoelzer D. Cytokine therapy for myelodysplastic syndrome. *Curr Opin Hematol* 2000;7:156.

183. Keating MJ. Chronic lymphocytic leukemia. *Semin Oncol* 1999;26:107.

184. Stern SC, Shan S, Costello C. Probable autoimmune neutropenia induced by fludarabine treatment for chronic lymphocytic leukaemia. *Br J Haematol* 1999;106:836.

185. Heyman MR, Walsh TJ. Autoimmune neutropenia and Hodgkin's disease. *Cancer* 1987;59:1903.

186. Omar S, Salhadar A, Wooliever DE, et al. Late-onset neutropenia in very low birth weight infants. *Pediatrics* 2000;106:E55.

187. Gray PH, Rodwell RL. Neonatal neutropenia associated with maternal hypertension poses a risk for nosocomial infection. *Eur J Pediatr* 1999;158:71.

188. Ferreira PJ, Bunch TJ, Albertine KH, et al. Circulating neutrophil concentration and respiratory distress in premature infants. *J Pediatr* 2000;136:466.

189. Juul SE, Calhoun DA, Christensen RD. "Idiopathic neutropenia" in very low birthweight infants. *Acta Paediatr* 1998;87:963.

190. Zuelzer WW, Bajoghli M, Evans RM. Chronic granulocytopenia in childhood. *Blood* 1964;23:359.

191. Pincus SH, Boxer LA, Stossel TP. Chronic neutropenia in childhood. *Am J Med* 1976;61:849.

192. Dale DC, Guerry D, Wewerka JR, et al. Chronic neutropenia. *Medicine* 1979;58:128.

193. Jonsson OG, Buchanan GR. Chronic neutropenia during childhood. A 13-year experience in a single institution. *Am J Dis Child* 1991;145:232.

194. Boxer LA, Yokoyama M, Lalezari P. Isoimmune neonatal neutropenia. *J Pediatr* 1972;80:783.

195. Satoh T, Kobayashi M, Kaneda M, et al. Genotypical classification of neutrophil Fc gamma receptor III by polymerase chain reaction-single-strand conformation polymorphism. *Blood* 1994;83:3312.

196. Bux J, Jung KD, Kauth T, et al. Serological and clinical aspects of granulocyte antibodies leading to alloimmune neonatal neutropenia. *Transfus Med* 1992;2:143.

197. Boxer LA, Greenberg MS, Boxer GJ, et al. Autoimmune neutropenia. *N Engl J Med* 1975;293:748.

198. Shastri KA, Logue GL. Autoimmune neutropenia. *Blood* 1993;81:1984.

199. Bux J, Behrens G, Jaeger G, et al. Diagnosis and clinical course of autoimmune neutropenia in infancy: analysis of 240 cases. *Blood* 1998;91:181.

200. Kurien BT, Newland J, Paczkowski C, et al. Association of neutropenia in systemic lupus erythematosus (SLE) with anti-Ro and binding of an immunologically cross-reactive neutrophil membrane antigen. *Clin Exp Immunol* 2000;120:209.

201. Hayashi S, Kiyokawa T, Aochi H, et al. Characterization of elevated neutrophil-associated IgG in various autoimmune disorders: not anti-neutrophil autoantibodies, but possibly immune complexes, bind to neutrophils. *Autoimmunity* 1997;26:195.

202. Hellmich B, Schnadel A, Gross WL. Treatment of severe neutropenia due to Felty's syndrome or systemic lupus erythematosus with granulocyte colony-stimulating factor. *Semin Arthritis Rheum* 1999;29:82.

203. Campion G, Maddison PJ, Goulding N, et al. The Felty syndrome: a case-matched study of clinical manifestations and outcome, serologic features, and immunogenetic associations. *Medicine (Baltimore)* 1990;69:69.

204. Rashba EJ, Rowe JM, Packman CH. Treatment of the neutropenia of Felty syndrome. *Blood Rev* 1996;10:177.

205. Ramakrishna R, Chaudhuri K, Sturgess A, et al. Haematological manifestations of primary Sjogren's syndrome: a clinicopathological study. *QJM* 1992;83:547.

206. Lamy T, Loughran TP Jr. Current concepts: large granular lymphocyte leukemia. *Blood Rev* 1999;13:230.

207. Liu JH, Wei S, Lamy T, et al. Chronic neutropenia mediated by fas ligand. *Blood* 2000;95:3219.

208. Mammen EF. The haematological manifestations of sepsis. *J Antimicrob Chemother* 1998;41[Suppl A]:17.

209. Brown KE, Young NS. Parvovirus B19 in human disease. *Annu Rev Med* 1997;48:59.

210. Kuritzkes DR. Neutropenia, neutrophil dysfunction, and bacterial infection in patients with human immunodeficiency virus disease: the role of granulocyte colony-stimulating factor. *Clin Infect Dis* 2000;30:256.

211. Van der Klauw MM, Wilson JH, Stricker BH. Drug-associated agranulocytosis: 20 years of reporting in the Netherlands (1974-1994). *Am J Hematol* 1998;57:206.

212. Kaufman DW, Kelly JP, Jurgelon JM et al. Drugs in the aetiology of agranulocytosis and aplastic anaemia. *Eur J Haematol* 1996;60[Suppl]:23.

213. Palmblad J. Drug-induced neutropenias: now and then. *Arch Intern Med* 1999;159:2745.

214. Tschen AC, Rieder MJ, Oyewumi LK, et al. The cytotoxicity of clozapine metabolites: implications for predicting clozapine-induced agranulocytosis. *Clin Pharmacol Ther* 1999;65:526.

215. Benedetti F, Cavallaro R, Smeraldi E. Olanzapine-induced neutropenia after clozapine-induced neutropenia. *Lancet* 1999;354:567.

216. Chatta GS, Price TH, Allen RC, et al. The effects of in vivo recombinant methionyl human granulocyte colony stimulating factor (rhG-CSF) on the neutrophil response and peripheral blood colony-forming cells in healthy young and elderly volunteers. *Blood* 1994;84:2923.

217. Price TH, Chatta GS, Dale DC. The effect of recombinant granulocyte colony-stimulating factor on neutrophil kinetics in normal young and elderly humans. *Blood* 1996;88:335.

218. Liles WC, Huang JE, van Burik JH, et al. Granulocyte colony-stimulating factor (G-CSF) administered in vivo augments neutrophil-mediated activity against opportunistic fungal pathogens. *J Infect Dis* 1997;175:1012.

219. Root RK, Dale DC. Granulocyte colony-stimulating factor and granulocyte-macrophage colony-stimulating factor: comparisons and potential for use in the treatment of infections in non-neutropenic patients. *J Infect Dis* 1999;179:S352.

220. Liles WC, Huang JE, Llewellyn C, et al. A comparative trial of granulocyte colony-stimulating factor (G-CSF) and dexamethasone alone and in combination for the mobilization of neutrophils in the peripheral blood of normal human volunteers. *Transfusion* 1997;37:182.

221. Crawford J, Ozer H, Stoller R, et al. Reduction by granulocyte colony-stimulating factor of fever and neutropenia induced by chemotherapy in patients with small-cell lung cancer. *N Engl J Med* 1991;325:164.

222. Groopman JE, Mitsuyasu RT, DeLeo MJ, et al. Effect of recombinant human granulocyte-macrophage colony-stimulating factor on myelopoiesis in the acquired immunodeficiency syndrome. *N Engl J Med* 1987;317:593.

223. Dale DC, Liles WC, Llewellyn C, et al. The effects of granulocyte macrophage colony-stimulating factor (GM-CSF) on neutrophil kinetics and function in normal human volunteers. *Am J Hematol* 1998;57:7.

224. Heil G, Hoelzer D, Sanz MA, et al. A randomized, double-blind, placebo-controlled, phase III study of filgrastim in remission induction and consolidation therapy for adults with de novo acute myeloid leukemia. *Blood* 1997;90:4710.

225. Bishop CR, Rothstein G, Ashenbrucker HE, et al. Leukokinetic studies. XIV. Blood neutrophil kinetics in chronic, steady-state neutropenia. *J Clin Invest* 1971;50:1678.

226. Dale DC, Fauci AS, Guerry D, et al. Comparison of agents producing a neutrophilic leukocytosis in man: hydrocortisone, prednisone, endotoxin and etiocholanolone. *J Clin Invest* 1975;56:808.

227. O'Connell RA. Leukocytosis during lithium carbonate treatment. *Int J Pharmacopsychiatric* 1970;4:30.

228. Stein RS, Beaman C, Ali MY, et al. Lithium carbonate attenuation of chemotherapy-induced neutropenia. *N Engl J Med* 1977;297:430.

229. Barr RD, Koekebakker M, Brown EA, et al. Putative role for lithium in human hematopoiesis. *J Lab Clin Med* 1987;109:159.

230. Herring WB, Smith LG, Walker RI, et al. Hereditary neutrophilia. *Am J Med* 1974;56:729.

231. Nichols BA, Bainton DF, Farquhar MG. Differentiation of monocytes: origin, nature, and fate of their azurophilic granules. *J Cell Biol* 1971;50:498.

232. Nichols BA, Bainton DF. Differentiation of human monocytes in bone marrow and blood: sequential formation of two granule populations. *Lab Invest* 1973;29:27.

233. Nathan CF, Murray HW, Cohn ZA. The macrophage as an effector cell. *N Engl J Med* 1980;303:622.

234. Bozdech MJ, Bainton DF. Identification of alpha-naphthyl butyrate esterase as a plasma membrane ectoenzyme of monocytes and as a discrete intracellular membrane-bound organelle in lymphocytes. *J Exp Med* 1981;153:182.

235. Braunsteiner H, Schmalzl F. Cytochemistry of monocytes and macrophages. In: Van Furth F, ed. *Mononuclear phagocytes*. Oxford: Blackwell, 1970:62.

236. Li CY, Lam KW, Yam LT. Esterases in human leukocytes. *J Histochem Cytochem* 1973;21:1.

237. Akiyama Y, Miller PJ, Thurman GB, et al. Characterization of a human blood monocyte subset with low peroxidase activity. *J Clin Invest* 1983;71:1093.

238. Figdor CG, Bont WS, Touw I, et al. Isolation of functionally different human monocytes by counterflow centrifugation elutriation. *Blood* 1982;60:46.

239. Norris DA, Morris RM, Sanderson RJ, et al. Isolation of functional subsets of human peripheral blood monocytes. *J Immunol* 1979;123:166.

240. Daeron M. Fc receptor biology. *Annu Rev Immunol* 1997;15:203.

241. Ravetch JV. Fc receptors. *Curr Opin Immunol* 1997;9:121.

242. De Villiers W, Fraser IP, Hughes DA, et al. M-CSF selectively enhances macrophage scavenger receptor expression and function. *J Exp Med* 1994; 180:705.

243. Ren Y, Silverstein RL, Allen J, et al. CD36 gene transfer confers capacity for phagocytosis of cells undergoing apoptosis. *J Exp Med* 1995;181:1857.

244. Pearson AM. Scavenger receptors in innate immunity. *Curr Opin Immunol* 1996;8:20.

245. Platt N, Suzuki H, Kurihara Y, et al. Role for the class A macrophage scavenger receptor in the phagocytosis of apoptotic thymocytes. *Proc Natl Acad Sci U S A* 1996;93:12456.

246. Haworth R, Platt N, Keshav S, et al. The macrophage scavenger receptor type A (SR-A) is expressed by activated macrophages and protects the host against lethal endotoxic shock. *J Exp Med* 1997;186:1431.

247. Suzuki H, Kurihara Y, Takeya M, et al. A role for macrophage scavenger receptors in atherosclerosis and susceptibility to infection. *Nature* 1997;386: 292.

248. Trinchieri G. Cytokines acting on or secreted by mononuclear phagocytes during intracellular infection (IL-10, IL-12, IFN-gamma). *Curr Opin Immunol* 1997;9:17.

249. Fraser IP, Koziel H, Ezekowitz RA. The serum mannose-binding protein and the macrophage mannose receptor are pattern recognition molecules that link innate and adaptive immunity. *Semin Immunol* 1998;10:363.

250. Thomas CA, Li Y, Kodama T, et al. Protection from lethal gram-positive infection by macrophage scavenger receptor-dependent phagocytosis. *J Exp Med* 2000;191:147.

251. Fadok VA, Bratton DL, Rose DM, et al. A receptor for phosphatidylserine-specific clearance of apoptotic cells. *Nature* 2000;405:85.

252. Fadok VA, deCathelineau A, Daleke DL, et al. Loss of phospholipid asymmetry and surface exposure of phosphatidylserine is required for phagocytosis of apoptotic cells by macrophages and fibroblasts. *J Biol Chem* 2001; 276:1071.

253. Premack BA, Schall TJ. Chemokine receptors: gateways to inflammation and infection. *Nat Med* 1996;2:1174.

254. Rollins B. Chemokines. *Blood* 1997;90:909.

255. Luster AD. Chemokines—chemotactic cytokines that mediate inflammation. *N Engl J Med* 1998;338:436.

256. Epstein J, Eichbaum Q, Sheriff S, et al. The collectins in innate immunity. *Curr Opin Immunol* 1996;8:29.

257. Aderem A, Ulevitch RJ. Toll-like receptors in the induction of the innate immune response. *Nature* 2000;406:782.

258. Wright SD, Tobias PS, Ulevitch RJ, et al. Lipopolysaccharide (LPS) binding protein opsonizes LPS-bearing particles for recognition by a novel receptor on macrophages. *J Exp Med* 1989;170:1231.

259. Wright SD, Ramos RA, Tobias PS, et al. CD14, a receptor for complexes of lipopolysaccharide (LPS) and LPS binding protein. *Science* 1990; 249:1431.

260. Lindley I, Aschauer H, Seifert JM, et al. Synthesis and expression in *Escherichia coli* of the gene encoding monocyte-derived neutrophil-activating factor: biological equivalence between natural and recombinant neutrophil-activating factor. *Proc Natl Acad Sci U S A* 1988;85:9199.

261. Yoshimura T, Matsushima K, Tanaka S, et al. Purification of a human monocyte-derived neutrophil chemotactic factor that has peptide sequence similarity to other host defense cytokines. *Proc Natl Acad Sci U S A* 1987;84:9233.

262. Gregory H, Young J, Schroder JM, et al. Structure determination of a human lymphocyte derived neutrophil activating peptide (LYNAP). *Biochem Biophys Res Commun* 1988;151:883.

263. Van Damme J, van Beeumen J, Opdenakker G, et al. A novel, NH₂-terminal sequence-characterized human monokine possessing neutrophil chemotactic, skin-reactive, and granulocytosis-promoting activity. *J Exp Med* 1988;167: 1364.

264. Peveri P, Walz A, Dewald B, et al. A novel neutrophil-activating factor produced by human mononuclear phagocytes. *J Exp Med* 1988;167:1547.

265. Thelen M, Peveri P, Kernen P, et al. Mechanism of neutrophil activation by NAF, a novel monocyte-derived peptide agonist. *FASEB J* 1988;2:2702.

266. Schmid J, Weissmann C. Induction of mRNA for a serine protease and a β-thromboglobulin-like protein in mitogen-stimulated human leukocytes. *J Immunol* 1987;139:250.

267. Gordon S. Development and distribution of mononuclear phagocytes: relevance to inflammation. In: *Inflammation: basic principles and clinical correlates*, 3rd ed. Gallin JI, Snyderman R, eds. Philadelphia: Lippincott Williams & Wilkins, 1999:35–48.

268. Medzhitov R, Janeway CA Jr. Innate immunity: impact on the adaptive immune response. *Curr Opin Immunol* 1997;9:4.

269. Medzhitov R, Janeway C Jr. Innate immunity. *N Engl J Med* 2000;343:338.

270. Medzhitov R, Preston-Hurlburt P, Janeway CA Jr. A human homologue of the Drosophila Toll protein signals activation of adaptive immunity. *Nature* 1997;388:394.

271. Rock FL, Hardiman G, Timans JC, et al. A family of human receptors structurally related to Drosophila Toll. *Proc Natl Acad Sci U S A* 1998;95:588.

272. Brightbill HD, et al. Host defense mechanisms triggered by microbial lipoproteins through toll-like receptors. *Science* 1999;285:732.

273. Anderson KV. Toll signaling pathways in the innate immune response. *Curr Opin Immunol* 2000;12:13.

274. Hemmi H, Takeuchi O, Kawai T, et al. A Toll-like receptor recognizes bacterial DNA. *Nature* 2000;408:740.

275. Hoshino K, Takeuchi O, Kawai T, et al. Toll-like receptor 4 (TLR4)-deficient mice are hyporesponsive to lipopolysaccharide: evidence for TLR4 as the LPS gene product. *J Immunol* 1999;162:3749.

276. Kirschning CJ, Wesche H, Merrill AT, et al. Human toll-like receptor 2 confers responsiveness to bacterial lipopolysaccharide. *J Exp Med* 1998;188: 2091.

277. Lien E, Sellati TJ, Yoshimura A, et al. Toll-like receptor 2 functions as a pattern recognition receptor for diverse bacterial products. *J Biol Chem* 1999; 274: 33419.

278. Lien E, Means TK, Heine H, et al. Toll-like receptor 4 imparts ligand-specific recognition of bacterial lipopolysaccharide. *J Clin Invest* 2000;105:497.

279. Poltorak A, He X, Smirnova I, et al. Defective LPS signaling in C3H/HeJ and C57BL/10ScCr mice: mutations in Tlr4 gene. *Science* 1998;282:2085.

280. Quershi ST, Lariviere L, Leveque G, et al. Endotoxin-tolerant mice have mutations in Toll-like receptor 4. *J Exp Med* 1999;189:615.

281. Takeuchi O, Hoshino K, Kawai T, et al. Differential roles of TLR2 and TLR4 in recognition of gram-negative and gram-positive bacterial cell wall components. *Immunity* 1999;11:443.

282. Takeuchi O, Hoshino K, Akira S. TLR2-deficient and MyD88-deficient mice are highly susceptible to *Staphylococcus aureus* infection. *J Immunol* 2000;165: 5392.

283. Underhill DM, Ozinsky A, Hajjar AM, et al. The Toll-like receptor 2 is recruited to macrophage phagosomes and discriminates between pathogens. *Nature* 1999;401:811.

284. Yang RB, Mark MR, Gray A, et al. Toll-like receptor-2 mediates lipopolysaccharide-induced cellular signalling. *Nature* 1998;395:284.

285. Muzio M, Bosisio D, Polentarutti N, et al. Differential expression and regulation of Toll-like receptors (TLR) in human leukocytes: selective expression of TLR3 in dendritic cells. *J Immunol* 2000;164:5998.

286. Ozinsky A, Underhill DM, Fontenot JD, et al. The repertoire for pattern recognition of pathogens by the innate immune system is defined by cooperation between Toll-like receptors. *Proc Natl Acad Sci U S A* 2000;97:13766.

287. Hajjar AM, O'Mahony DS, Ozinsky A, et al. Functional interactions between Toll-like receptor (TLR) 2 and TLR1 or TLR6 in response to phenol-soluble modulin. *J Immunol* 2001;166:15.

288. Kawai T, Adachi O, Ogawa T, et al. Unresponsiveness of MyD88-deficient mice to endotoxin. *Immunity* 1999;11:115.

289. Medzhitov R, Preston-Hurlburt P, Kopp E, et al. MyD88 is an adaptor protein in the hToll/IL-1 receptor family signaling pathways. *Mol Cell* 1998;2:253.

290. Muzio M, Natoli G, Saccani S, et al. The human toll signaling pathway: divergence of nuclear factor kappaB and JNK/SAPK activation upstream of tumor necrosis factor receptor-associated factor 6 (TRAF6). *J Exp Med* 1998;187:2097.

291. Takeuchi O, Kauffman A, Grote K, et al. Preferentially the R-stereoisomer of the mycoplasma lipopeptide macrophage-activating lipopeptide-2 activates immune cells through a Toll-like receptor 2- and MyD88-dependent signaling pathway. *J Immunol* 2000;164:554.

292. Wesche H, Henzel WJ, Shillinglaw W, et al. MyD88: an adapter that recruits IRAK to the IL-1 receptor complex. *Immunity* 1997;7:837.

293. Yang RB, Mark MR, Gurney AL, et al. Signaling events induced by lipopolysaccharide-activated toll-like receptor 2. *J Immunol* 1999;163:639.

294. Rosenthal AS. Regulation of the immune response: role of the macrophage. *N Engl J Med* 1980;303:1153.

295. Unanue ER. Cooperation between mononuclear phagocytes and lymphocytes in immunity. *N Engl J Med* 1980;303:977.

296. Unanue ER. The regulation of lymphocyte functions by the macrophage. *Immunol Rev* 1978;40:227.

297. Nossal GVJ. The basic components of the immune system. *N Engl J Med* 1987;316:1320.

298. Steinman RM, Bhardwaj N. Dendritic cells. In: *Inflammation: basic principles and clinical correlates*, 3rd ed. Gallin JI, Snyderman R, eds. Philadelphia: Lippincott Williams & Wilkins, 1999:49–59.

299. Cella M, Sallusto F, Lanzavecchia A. Origin, maturation and antigen presenting function of dendritic cells. *Curr Opin Immunol* 1997;9:10.

300. Palucka KA, Tacquet N, Sanchez-Chapuis F, et al. Dendritic cells as the terminal stage of monocyte differentiation. *J Immunol* 1998;160:4587.

301. Romani N, Gruner S, Brang D, et al. Proliferating dendritic cell progenitors in human blood. *J Exp Med* 1994;180:83.

302. Szabolcs P, Avigan D, Gezelter S, et al. Dendritic cells and macrophages can mature independently from a human bone marrow-derived, post-CFU intermediate. *Blood* 1996;87:4520.

303. Zhou LJ, Tedder TF. CD14+ blood monocytes can differentiate into functionally mature CD83+ dendritic cells. *Proc Natl Acad Sci U S A* 1996;93:2588.

304. Bender A, Sapp M, Schuler G, et al. Improved methods for the generation of dendritic cells from nonproliferating progenitors in human blood. *J Immunol Methods* 1996;196:121.

305. Caux C, Vanbervliet B, Massacrier C, et al. CD34⁺ hematopoietic progenitors from human blood differentiate along two independent dendritic cell pathways in response to GM-CSF and TNF-alpha. *J Exp Med* 1996;184:695.

306. Reddy A, Sapp M, Feldman M, et al. A monocyte conditioned medium is more effective than defined cytokines in mediating the terminal maturation of human dendritic cells. *Blood* 1997;90:3640.

307. Young JW, Szabolcs P, Moore MAC. Identification of dendritic cell colony-forming units among normal CD34⁺ hematopoietic progenitors that are expanded by c-kit ligand and yield pure dendritic cell colonies in the pres-

ence of granulocyte/macrophage colony-stimulating factor and tumor necrosis factor alpha. *J Exp Med* 1995;182:1111.

308. Young JW. Dendritic cells: expansion and differentiation with hematopoietic growth factors. *Curr Opin Hematol* 1999;6:135.

309. Hashimoto SI, Suzuki T, Nagai S, et al. Identification of genes specifically expressed in human activated and mature dendritic cells through serial analysis of gene expression. *Blood* 2000;96:2206.

310. Van Furth R, Baeburn JA, van Zwet TL. Characteristics of human mononuclear phagocytes. *Blood* 1979;54:485.

311. Van Furth R, Diesselhoff-den Dulk MC, Mattie H. Quantitative study on the production and kinetics of mononuclear phagocytes during an acute inflammatory reaction. *J Exp Med* 1973;138:1314.

312. Van Furth R, Sluiter W. Distribution of blood monocytes between a marginating and a circulating pool. *J Exp Med* 1986;163:474.

313. Van Furth R, Cohn ZA. The origin and kinetics of mononuclear phagocytes. *J Exp Med* 1968;128:415.

314. Whitelaw DM. Observations on human monocyte kinetics after pulse labeling. *Cell Tissue Kinet* 1972;5:311.

315. Gale RP, Sparkes RS, Golde DW. Bone marrow origin of hepatic macrophages (Kupffer cells) in humans. *Science* 1978;201:937.

316. Katz SI, Tamaki K, Sachs DH. Epidermal Langerhans cells are derived from cells originating in bone marrow. *Nature* 1979;282:324.

317. Thomas ED, Ramberg RE, Sale GE, et al. Direct evidence for a bone marrow origin of the alveolar macrophage in man. *Science* 1976;192:1016.

318. Ash P, Loutit JF, Townsend KMS. Osteoclasts derived from haemopoietic stem cells. *Nature* 1980;283:669.

319. Coccia PF, Krivit W, Cervenka J, et al. Successful bone-marrow transplantation for infantile malignant osteopaetrosis. *N Engl J Med* 1980;302:701.

320. Golde DW, Byers LA, Finley TN. Proliferative capacity of human alveolar macrophage. *Nature* 1974;247:373.

321. Golde DW, Finley TN, Cline MJ. The pulmonary macrophage in acute leukemia. *N Engl J Med* 1974;290:875.

322. Melnicoff MJ, Horan PK, Breslin EW, et al. Maintenance of peritoneal macrophages in the steady state. *J Leukoc Biol* 1988;44:367.

323. Reitsma PH, Rothberg PG, Astrin SM, et al. Regulation of *myc* gene expression in HL-60 leukaemia cells by a vitamin D metabolite. *Nature* 1983;306:492.

324. Westin EH, Gallo RC, Arya SK, et al. Differential expression of the *amv* gene in human hematopoietic cells. *Proc Natl Acad Sci U S A* 1982;79:2194.

325. Gonda TJ, Metcalf D. Expression of *myb*, *myc* and *fos* proto-oncogenes during differentiation of murine myeloid leukaemias. *Nature* 1984;310:249.

326. Muller R, Curran T, Muller D, et al. Induction of c-*fos* during myelomonocytic differentiation and macrophage proliferation. *Nature* 1985;314:546.

327. Sariban E, Mitchell T, Kufe D. Expression of the c-*fms* proto-oncogene during human monocyte differentiation. *Nature* 1985;316:64.

328. Mitchell RL, Zokas L, Schreiber RD, et al. Rapid induction of expression of proto-oncogene *fos* during human monocytic differentiation. *Cell* 1985;40:209.

329. Muller R, Muller D, Guilbert L. Differential expression of c-*fos* in hematopoietic cells: correlation with differentiation of monomyelocytic cells in vitro. *EMBO J* 1984;3:1887.

330. Pinto A, Colletta G, Vecchio LD, et al. c-*fos* Oncogene expression in human hematopoietic malignancies is restricted to acute leukemias with monocytic phenotype and to subsets of B cell leukemias. *Blood* 1987;70:1450.

331. Mitchell RL, Henning-Chubb C, Huberman E, et al. C-*fos* expression is neither sufficient nor obligatory for differentiation of monomyelocytes to macrophages. *Cell* 1986;45:497.

332. Cooper RA, Braunwald AD, Kuo AL. Phorbol ester induction of leukemic cell differentiation is a membrane-mediated process. *Proc Natl Acad Sci U S A* 1982;79:2865.

333. Koeffler HP, Bar-Eli M, Territo MC. Phorbol ester effect on differentiation of human myeloid leukemia cell lines blocked at different stages of maturation. *Cancer Res* 1981;41:919.

334. Bar-Shavit Z, Teitelbaum SL, Reitsma P, et al. Induction of monocytic differentiation and bone resorption by 1,25-dihydroxyvitamin D₃. *Proc Natl Acad Sci U S A* 1983;80:5907.

335. McCarthy DM, San Miguel JF, Freake HC, et al. 1,25-Dihydroxyvitamin D₃ inhibits proliferation of human promyelocytic leukaemia (HL60) cells and induces monocyte-macrophage differentiation in HL60 and normal human bone marrow cells. *Leuk Res* 1983;7:51.

336. Ball ED, Guyre PM, Shen L, et al. Gamma interferon induces monocytoid differentiation in the HL-60 cell line. *J Clin Invest* 1983;73:1072.

337. Todd RF III, Griffin JD, Ritz J, et al. Expression of normal monocyte-macrophage differentiation antigens on HL60 promyelocytes undergoing differentiation induced by leukocyte-conditioned medium or phorbol diester. *Leuk Res* 1981;5:491.

338. Mangelsdorf DJ, Koeffler HP, Donaldson CA, et al. 1,25-Dihydroxy-vitamin D3-induced differentiation in a human promyelocytic leukemia cell line (HL-60): receptor-mediated maturation to macrophage-like cells. *J Cell Biol* 1984;98:391.

339. Newburger PE, Baker RD, Hansen SL, et al. Functionally deficient differentiation of HL-60 promyelocytic leukemia cells induced by phorbol myristate acetate. *Cancer Res* 1981;41:1861.

340. Nichols KE, Weinberg JB. Essential amino acid deprivation induces monocyte differentiation of the human HL-60 myeloid leukemia cell line. *Blood* 1989;73:1298.

341. Takeda K, Iwamoto S, Sugimoto H, et al. Identity of differentiation inducing factor and tumour necrosis factor. *Nature* 1986;323:338.

342. Weinberg JB, Larrick JW. Receptor-mediated monocytoid differentiation of human promyelocytic cells by tumor necrosis factor: synergistic actions with interferon-γ and 1,25-dihyroxyvitamin D3. *Blood* 1987;70:994.

343. Ferrero D, Pessano S, Pagliardi GL, et al. Induction of differentiation of human myeloid leukemias: surface changes probed with monoclonal antibodies. *Blood* 1983;61:171.

344. Guyre PM, Morganelli PM, Miller R. Recombinant immune interferon increases immunoglobulin G Fc receptors on cultured human mononuclear phagocytes. *J Clin Invest* 1983;72:393.

345. Olsson I, Olofsson T, Mauritzon N. Characterization of mononuclear blood cell-derived differentiation inducing factors for the human promyelocytic leukemia cell line HL-60. *J Natl Cancer Inst* 1981;67:1225.

346. Leung K, Chiao JW. Human leukemia cell maturation induced by a T-cell lymphokine isolated from medium conditioned by normal lymphocytes. *Proc Natl Acad Sci U S A* 1985;82:1209.

347. Olsson IL, Sarngadharan MG, Breitman TR, et al. Isolation and characterization of a T lymphocyte-derived differentiation inducing factor for the myeloid leukemic cell line HL-60. *Blood* 1984;63:510.

348. Abe T, Murakami M, Sato T, et al. Macrophage differentiation inducing factor from human monocytic cells is equivalent to murine leukemia inhibitory factor. *J Biol Chem* 1989;246:8941.

349. Olsson I, Breitman TR. Induction of differentiation of the human histiocytic lymphoma cell line, U-937, by retinoic acid and cyclic AMP-inducing agents. *Cancer Res* 1982;42:3924.

350. Dodd RC, Cohen MS, Newman SL, et al. Vitamin D metabolites change the phenotype of monoblastic U937 cells. *Proc Natl Acad Sci U S A* 1983;80:7538.

351. Hattori T, Pack M, Bougnoux P, et al. Interferon-induced differentiation of U937 cells. Comparison with other agents that promote differentiation of human myeloid or monocytelike cell lines. *J Clin Invest* 1983;72:237.

352. Ralph P, Harris PE, Punjabi CJ, et al. Lymphokine inducing "terminal differentiation" of the human monoblast leukemia line U937: a role for gamma interferon. *Blood* 1983;62:1169.

353. Zuckerman SH, Surprenant YM, Tang J. Synergistic effect of granulocyte-macrophage colony-stimulating factor and 1,25-dihydroxyvitamin D3 on the differentiation of the human monocytic cell line U937. *Blood* 1988;71:619.

354. Geissler K, Harrington M, Srivastava C, et al. Effects of recombinant human colony stimulating factors (CSF) (granulocyte-macrophage CSF, granulocyte CSF, and CSF-1) on human monocyte/macrophage differentiation. *J Immunol* 1989;143:140.

355. Clement LT, Roberts RL, Martin AM. Characterization of a monocyte differentiation factor distinct from gamma-interferon, tumor necrosis factor, or G,M-colony-stimulating factor that regulates the growth and function capabilities of the U937 monocytic cell line. *J Leukoc Biol* 1988;44:101.

356. Kurata N, Akiyama H, Taniyama T, et al. Dose-dependent regulation of macrophage differentiation by mos mRNA in a human monocytic cell line. *EMBO J* 1989;8:457.

357. Stanley ER, Heard PM. Factors regulating macrophage production and growth. *J Biol Chem* 1977;252:4305.

358. Nathan CF. Secretory products of macrophages. *J Clin Invest* 1987;79:319.

359. Oster W, Lindemann A, Horn S, et al. Tumor necrosis factor (TNF)-alpha but not TNF-beta induces secretion of colony-stimulating factor for macrophages (CSF-1) by human monocytes. *Blood* 1987;70:1700.

360. Bartocci A, Mastrogiannis DS, Migliorati G, et al. Macrophages specifically regulate the concentration of their own growth factor in the circulation. *Proc Natl Acad Sci U S A* 1987;84:6179.

361. Cannistra SA, Rambaldi A, Spriggs DR, et al. Human granulocyte-macrophage colony-stimulating factor induces expression of the tumor necrosis factor gene by the U937 cell line and by normal human monocytes. *J Clin Invest* 1987;79:1720.

362. Zhou YQ, Stanley ER, Clark SC, et al. Interleukin-3 and interleukin-1 alpha allow earlier bone marrow progenitors to respond to human colony-stimulating factor-1. *Blood* 1988;72:1870.

363. Kurland JI, Broxmeyer HE, Pelus LM, et al. Role for monocyte-macrophage-derived colony-stimulating factor and prostaglandin E in the positive and negative feedback control of myeloid stem cell proliferation. *Blood* 1978;52:388.

364. Kurland JI, Bockman RS, Broxmeyer HE, et al. Limitation of excessive myelopoiesis by the intrinsic modulation of macrophage-derived prostaglandin E. *Science* 1978;199:552.

365. Koch F, Heufler C, Kämpgen E, et al. Tumor necrosis factor α maintains the viability of murine epidermal Langerhans cells in culture, but in contrast to granulocyte/macrophage colony-stimulating factor, without inducing their functional maturation. *J Exp Med* 1990;171:159.

366. Williams N, Jackson H. Limitation of macrophage production in long term marrow cultures containing prostaglandin E. *J Cell Physiol* 1980;103:239.

367. Pelus LM, Broxmeyer HE, Kurland JI, et al. Regulation of macrophage and granulocyte proliferation: specificities of prostaglandin E and lactoferrin. *J Exp Med* 1979;150:277.

368. Assoian RK, Fleurdelys BE, Stevenson HC, et al. Expression and secretion of type β transforming growth factor by activated human macrophages. *Proc Natl Acad Sci U S A* 1987;84:6020.

369. Strassmann G, Cole MD, Newman W. Regulation of colony-stimulating factor 1-dependent macrophage precursor proliferation by type b transforming growth factor. *J Immunol* 1988;140:2645.

370. Munan L, Kelly A. Age-dependent changes in blood monocyte populations in man. *Clin Exp Immunol* 1979;35:161.

371. Kato K. Leukocytes in infancy and childhood. *J Pediatr* 1935;7:7.

372. Maldonado JE, Hanlon DG. Monocytosis: a current appraisal. *Mayo Clin Proc* 1965;40:248.

373. Flinn JW. A study of differential blood count in one thousand cases of active pulmonary tuberculosis. *Ann Intern Med* 1929;2:622.

374. Daland GA, Gottlieb L, Wallerstein RO, et al. Hematologic observations in bacterial endocarditis: especially the prevalence of histiocytes and the elevation and variation of the white cell count in blood from the ear lobe. *J Lab Clin Med* 1956;48:827.

375. Rosahn PD, Pearce L. The blood cytology in untreated and treated syphilis. *Am J Med Sci* 1934;187:88.

376. Barrett O Jr. Monocytosis in malignant disease. *Ann Intern Med* 1970;73:991.

377. Levinson B, Walter BA, Wintrobe MM, et al. A clinical study in Hodgkin's disease. *Arch Intern Med* 1957;99:519.

378. Ultman JE. Clinical features and diagnosis of Hodgkin's disease. *Cancer* 1966;19:297.

379. Saarni MI, Liman JW. Preleukemia: the hematologic syndrome preceding acute leukemia. *Am J Med* 1973;55:38.

380. Bearman RM, Kjeldsberg CR, Pangalis GA, et al. Chronic monocytic leukemia in adults. *Cancer* 1981;48:2239.

381. Brynes RK, Golomb HM, Desser RK, et al. Acute monocytic leukemia. *Am J Clin Pathol* 1976;65:471.

382. Geary CG, Catovsky D, Wiltshaw E, et al. Chronic myelomonocytic leukemia. *Br J Haematol* 1975;30:289.

383. Saarni MI, Liman JW. Myelomonocytic leukemia. *Cancer* 1971;27:1221.

384. Dale DC, Fauci AS, Wolff SM. Alternate-day prednisone: leukocyte kinetics and susceptibility to infections. *N Engl J Med* 1974;291:1154.

385. Thompson J, van Furth R. The effect of glucocorticosteroids on the proliferation and kinetics of promonocytes and monocytes of the bone marrow. *J Exp Med* 1973;137:10.

386. Seshardi RS, Brown EJ, Zipursky A. Leukemic reticuloendotheliosis: a failure of monocyte production. *N Engl J Med* 1976;295:181.

387. Turner A, Kjeldsberg CR. Hairy cell leukemia. *Medicine* 1978;57:477.

388. Twomey JJ, Douglass CC, Sharkey O Jr. The monocytopenia of aplastic anemia. *Blood* 1973;41:187.

CHAPTER 15

Acute Myelogenous Leukemia

D. Gary Gilliland and Martin S. Tallman

Acute myelogenous leukemia (AML) is a disorder caused by the malignant transformation of a bone marrow hematopoietic stem cell. This transformed stem cell has an increased rate of self-renewal and is inevitably associated with aberrant or absent differentiation, leading to an accumulation of cells in the marrow with phenotypic features of immature phagocytes, conventionally designated *myeloid cells*. This usurpation of normal bone marrow by leukemic cells ultimately suppresses normal hematopoiesis and produces the clinical signs and symptoms of bone marrow failure. During the past decade, the application of new techniques in molecular biology, cytogenetics, and immunology to the study of AML has greatly improved our understanding of this disease. Furthermore, important advances in the treatment of AML with chemotherapy or bone marrow transplantation have improved the prognosis for most patients with this disease. However, the majority of adults who develop AML still die from their disease or therapy. There is thus a compelling need to develop more efficacious and less toxic treatments for AML.

Although Virchow (1) recognized leukemia ("white blood") as a clinical entity in 1845, it is likely that most or all of Virchow's cases represented chronic lymphocytic or myeloid leukemias. Leukemia with an acute course was not reported until 1857 by Friedreich (2). Such cases were considered to be lymphocytic in origin until Naegeli (3) described the myeloblast in 1900 as a precursor of blood neutrophilic granulocytes. It then became evident that many cases of leukemia, both acute and chronic, originated from marrow myeloid cells, and were thus *myeloid*. Subtypes of AML were recognized as early as 1913 with the report of a possible case of acute monocytic leukemia (4). Later, subsets of monocytic leukemia were described, including myelomonocytic (Naegeli's type) and pure monocytic (Schilling's type) leukemia (5). In 1946, DiGuglielmo reported an acute disorder that involved primarily the erythroid series (6). Morphologic subtypes continue to be defined, including acute promyelocytic leukemia (APL) in 1957 (7), acute megakaryoblastic leukemia in 1963 (8), and the microgranular variant of APL in 1980 (9–11). Organization of the various subtypes of AML into a widely accepted classification system has been accomplished in the past by the French/American/British (FAB) (12–15) cooperative group, and this has greatly facilitated studies of prognostic features and interpretation of clinical trials in AML (15).

EPIDEMIOLOGY

AML accounts for 15% to 20% of the acute leukemias in children and 80% of the acute leukemias in adults. The overall annual incidence of AML in the United States is approximately 2.3 per 100,000 people (16). The estimated number of new cases of AML in the United States in 2001 is 10,000 (17). The age-specific incidence of AML increases from fewer than 1 per 100,000 people under age 30 years to approximately 15 per 100,000 people over age 80 years. The median age of patients with AML is approximately 63 years. However, a recent study suggested that the incidence of APL is constant with respect to age, suggesting a single genetic event to initiate the disease (18). In contrast to acute lymphoblastic leukemia (ALL), there is no peak age incidence of AML in childhood (19). Both ALL and AML are slightly more common in males than females, and the reported incidence is similar in patients of different races. Geographic variations in both incidence and subtypes of leukemia have been observed in children (20). In Japan and several African countries, in contrast to the United States and Europe, the incidence of childhood AML is greater than childhood ALL. In Turkey, the M4 subtype of AML (discussed in the section M4: Myelomonocytic Leukemia) has often been associated with orbital chloromas and accounts for approximately 35% of all cases of childhood leukemia (21). In a recent comparison of biologic characteristics of *de novo* AML in Australia and Japan, cases of M2 were more common in Japan than Australia, whereas M4 was more common in Australia (22). Among cases of M2, leukemic cells from patients in Japan had a higher incidence of t(8;21) than in Australia (33.1% vs. 15.3%, $p < .05$). The t(15;17), inv/del(16), 11q23, and 5/7/8 abnormalities were similar in the two countries. In Japan, cases of M4/M5 more frequently expressed CD13, and HLA-DR was expressed in M3 cases more in Australia than Japan.

ETIOLOGY

Although the cause of AML in humans is unknown, several predisposing factors as well as inciting agents are well established. Risk factors such as exposure to high-dose radiation, occupational exposure to benzene, and previous chemotherapy for other cancers or benign conditions have been well established. These factors have historically accounted for only a fraction of AML cases in adults and children. However, the incidence of therapy-related myelodysplastic syndrome (MDS) and AML has increased in recent years due in part to increased intensity of therapy for other cancers and improved long-term survival in these patients, allowing the development of AML as a late complication of therapy.

Radiation

Ionizing radiation is the most conclusively identified leukemogenic factor in humans (23). Physicians and scientists exposed to excessive amounts of radiation during the early years of research on medical application of x-rays (24), patients given low-dose radiation for rheumatoid spondylitis (25), and atomic bomb survivors in Hiroshima and Nagasaki have all been found to have an increased incidence of leukemia (26). Children and adults exposed to radiation from the atomic bombs in Japan had a 20-fold increased incidence of both AML and chronic myeloid leukemia (CML) that peaked 5 to 9 years after the explosion, and 20 years later, the incidence of acute leukemia remained elevated (27).

Considerable controversy still surrounds whether the developing fetus is unusually susceptible to radiation-induced carcinogenesis (23). Studies of atomic bomb survivors have not confirmed an increased risk for leukemia after low-dose intrauterine or preconception irradiation (28). There are also conflicting reports about whether prenatal exposure to diagnostic x-rays is associated with an increased risk of leukemia and other childhood cancers (29). An increased risk of leukemia has also been reported to be associated with nuclear power reactors (30) and with occupational or residential exposure to electromagnetic radiation. These reports are controversial and inconclusive (31,32).

Chemical Agents

Both chemotherapy and occupational chemical exposure are associated with an increased risk for AML (33,34). High-dose occupational benzene exposure increases the risk of AML, with bone marrow hypoplasia or pancytopenia often preceding the diagnosis of leukemia. Less convincing reports have implicated chloramphenicol (35) and phenylbutazone (36) as leukemogenic agents. The use of alkylating agents such as nitrogen mustard, chlorambucil, and melphalan for both neoplastic and benign conditions has resulted in an increased risk for developing AML or MDS (discussed in Chapter 12) (37–39). In many cases, these secondary leukemias have developed in the absence of radiation therapy or a predisposing immunodeficiency. From 2% to 10% of patients treated with a regimen of mechlorethamine, Oncovin (vincristine), procarbazine, and prednisone chemotherapy for Hodgkin's disease developed AML within 2 to 12 years after completing chemotherapy, with the peak incidence at 6 years. In several of these Hodgkin's disease studies, splenectomy was an additional risk factor for developing AML (38). Until recently, patients given nonalkylating cytotoxic agents as cancer chemotherapy had not been reported to develop AML as a second neoplasm. Recent reports of children treated for ALL (40) and adults treated for small cell lung cancer (41) suggested that the epipodophyllotoxins (VM 26 or VP 16) may also be leukemogenic.

Viruses

Retroviruses are clearly capable of inducing acute leukemia in mice, domestic cats, cattle, chickens, and gibbon apes (42,43). With one exception, attempts to identify leukemogenic viruses in humans have been inconclusive. It was only recently demonstrated that any human leukemia was caused by a virus. Clusters of adult T-cell leukemia in Japan and in islands of the Caribbean were independently found to be due to the retrovirus human T-cell leukemia virus type 1 (44,45).

Recent studies have focused on investigating the role of dominant and recessive cellular oncogenes in the pathogenesis of AML rather than continuing the search for leukemogenic viruses in humans. These investigations aim to establish causal relations between altered gene expression and leukemic hematopoiesis.

Oncogenes and Human Leukemogenesis

Many genes involved in the regulation of cell growth and development have been found in mutated forms in retroviruses capable of transforming animal cells (46). The normal cellular versions of these genes, protooncogenes, are typically involved in stimulating cell proliferation in normal cells and include growth factors, growth factor receptors, and signal-transducing molecules (47–49) (discussed in Chapter 6). In addition to growth-stimulating oncogenes, a growing number of human tumors have been found to have deletions of tumor-suppressor genes such as the retinoblastoma gene or p53 (50,51). Such genes are believed to regulate cell growth normally at specific checkpoints in the cell cycle. A third class of oncogene is typified by bcl-2, which encodes a protein that decreases programmed cell death, or apoptosis.

Retroviruses that contain mutated versions of growth-stimulating genes such as tyrosine kinases have been shown to transform hematopoietic cells effectively in several nonhuman animals (52,53). For example, retroviruses with activated versions of src, abl, fgr, and yes readily cause leukemias or other tumors in animals. Except for abl, activating mutations in tyrosine kinase protooncogenes are uncommon in human leukemias. In CML, the activation of abl tyrosine kinase activity by the bcr/abl rearrangement has been well described (54,55). However, as described in more detail below, recent evidence indicates that activating mutations in certain hematopoietic kinases such as FLT3 may play an important role in the pathogenesis of AML.

Mutations in members of the ras family in human AML and MDS have been reported in as many as 25% to 44% of patients (56–58), although analysis by direct DNA sequence analysis indicates that the overall frequency is closer to 20% (59). The human genome has three ras genes, N-ras at chromosome 1p11-13, H-ras at 11p14.1, and K-ras at 12p12.1 (60,61). The three protooncogenes encode proteins of 21-kd molecular mass, which are similar structurally and functionally. The ras proteins are guanosine triphosphate (GTP)-binding proteins, have GTPase activity, and have some homology with the γ-subunit of G proteins involved in transmembrane cellular signal transduction (60,61). Unlike the classic G proteins, however, human ras proteins are not thought to modulate the activity of adenyl cyclase. It is likely, however, that members of this family transduce some type of signal from membrane receptors. For example, some receptors of the hematopoietic growth factor receptor family are known to activate p21 ras in normal cells (62). The ras proteins are activated when GTP is bound and inactivated after hydrolysis of the GTP to guanosine diphosphate and Pi (63). Point mutations that reduce the GTPase activity lead to transformation, presumably by producing a prolonged active state of ras. Mutations in ras genes have been found to occur primarily in codons 12, 13, 59, and 61 (60,61). These codons all encode for regions of ras that are directly involved in guanosine diphosphate–GTP binding (64). Animal model studies suggest that activation of a ras gene is by itself insufficient to cause tumor development. Complementing mutations in other protooncogenes are likely required in most tumors. Point mutations have been detected in each of the three ras genes in AML but are most common in N-ras (56–58). Mutations in ras do not clearly correlate with morphology (65), but recent studies indicate that ras mutations confer a poor prognosis (66,67). When relapse samples have been compared with initial diagnostic samples, occasional ras mutations are no longer detected (68), an observation suggesting that ras mutations may be acquired in a subclone of a leukemia and thus may be more important for progression than for initiation of the clone. As discussed in more detail below, the possibility to pharmacologically inhibit *ras* function with farnesyl transferase inhibitors forms the basis for a new strategy of treatment for AML (69).

Overall, although many oncogenes can be identified that cause leukemias in lower animals, only a small number have been shown to be leukemogenic in humans. In contrast, the cloning of genes at the breakpoints of chromosomal translocations has been used to identify several novel genes that are likely involved in causing human myeloid leukemias. These include the *PML-RAR-α* fusion gene produced as a result of the t(15;17)(q22;q12-21) translocation in APL (70–72); the *AML1/ETO* fusion gene produced by the t(8;21) translocation (73–77); the *CBFβ/SMMHC* fusion produced by the inv(16) (78); the *MLL/AF4* fusion gene produced by the t(4;11) translocation (79–83); and the *DEK/CAN* fusion gene produced as a result of the t(6;9)(p23,q24) translocation (84). The role of these fusion proteins in pathogenesis of leukemia is discussed in more detail later in this chapter.

The deletion or mutation of tumor-suppressor genes may also play an important role in human myeloid leukemias. Mutations in the retinoblastoma gene and decreased expression of the Rb protein have been described in some cases (85). Similarly, mutations in the p53 gene have been observed in AML and the blast crisis phase of CML (86).

Host Susceptibility

Clinical observations have identified unusual susceptibility to AML in monozygotic twins (89) and people with certain heritable disorders and genetic syndromes. Hereditary conditions associated with chromosomal instability and a predisposition to AML include Bloom's syndrome and Fanconi's anemia (90). Congenital bone marrow failure syndromes such as Diamond-Blackfan anemia (91) (discussed in Chapter 10) and Kostmann's syndrome (92) (discussed in Chapter 17) also predispose patients to an increased risk for AML.

Children with Down's syndrome have a tenfold to 20-fold increased risk of leukemia during the first decade of life (93). The types of leukemia follow the usual distribution of acute leukemia in the United States and Europe (ALL/AML ratio is 4:1) in childhood, except during the neonatal period. Neonates with Down's syndrome are more likely to develop AML or MDS than ALL. However, these data may be biased by inclusion of neonates with trisomy 21 and a disorder called *transient myeloproliferative syndrome* (TMS) (94). TMS is invariably diagnosed during the first month of life and is clinically and hematologically indistinguishable from congenital AML (95). In contrast to congenital AML, however, spontaneous regression with normalization of blood counts occurs in most of these infants within weeks to months without specific antileukemia therapy. The blasts associated with this unique syndrome have been shown to have cell-surface antigens that are characteristic of megakaryoblasts (96,97), and data from several cases show that this proliferation is clonal (97). TMS has also been observed in newborns without the clinical features of Down's syndrome but with a mosaic karyotype and trisomy 21 (98,99). Approximately 20% to 30% of infants with TMS eventually develop AML, often type M7 (100,101).

BIOLOGY

Hematopoietic Stem Cells

AML cells are derived from immature hematopoietic cells and retain many biologic features of their cell of origin. Understanding the nature of the cellular defects in AML requires an appreciation of normal hematopoiesis, particularly the regulation of granulocyte and monocyte production. Briefly, mature granulocytes, monocytes, and their immediate precursors (myeloid cells) are derived from a small population of pluripotent stem cells that have extensive capacity to self-renew and to differentiate (102–107). These stem cells reside in and interact with a complex microenvironment composed of endothelial cells, fibroblasts, adipocytes, macrophages, and T lymphocytes, the bone marrow "stroma." Evidence for the existence of self-renewing stem cells first came from the work of Till and McCulloch (102) and Becher et al. (105), who noted 40 years ago that injection of syngeneic marrow into lethally irradiated mice resulted in the formation of macroscopic colonies of hematopoietic cells in the spleen. The colonies were shown to be the product of single cells, termed *colony-forming unit-spleen* (CFU-S), through the use of marker chromosomes (105). Self-renewal of CFU-S was demonstrated by showing that colonies could be excised, homogenized, and reinjected into new irradiated recipients, resulting in the growth of new CFU-S colonies. At approximately the same time, Pluznick and Sachs (103), Pike and Robinson (104), Bradley and Metcalf (106), and others initiated efforts to define *in vitro* culture conditions that would support growth of hematopoietic precursor cells. In semisolid media, marrow cells exhibited little spontaneous proliferation, but colonies of single or multiple lineages were readily produced when colony-stimulating factors (CSFs) were added (initially in the form of media conditioned by exposure to spleen cells, mononuclear blood cells, or certain tumor cell lines) (108–110). The *in vitro* assays continue to be refined but have made it possible to identify a hierarchy of hematopoietic progenitor cells and determine their individual growth factor requirements. The most primitive and most recently identified clonogenic cell, termed the *CFU-blast cell* by Suda et al. (110), gives rise to a small colony composed of blasts with a high secondary plating efficiency. The CFU-blast cell also has some degree of self-renewal. Evidence from murine marrow transplantation studies suggests that blast colony cells are close to true hematopoietic (transplantable) stem cells. The recent efforts of Spangrude et al. (111) to purify murine hematopoietic stem cells are likely to clarify the relation of CFU-S and CFU-blast to true stem cells.

Several other distinct stages of progenitor cells have been identified that fall between stem cells and mature myeloid elements. The colony-forming unit-granulocyte, erythrocyte, monocyte, megakaryocyte (CFU-GEMM) is a cell that is multipotent by virtue of its ability to give rise to multiple cell lineages (granulocyte, erythrocyte, monocyte, and megakaryocyte) but has a limited capacity for self-renewal (112). Of particular interest for the study of AML is the existence of several different levels of progenitor cells committed to granulocyte and monocyte differentiation that produce colonies containing only neutrophils, both neutrophils and monocytes, only monocytes, or only eosinophils. These cells, termed *CFU-G, CFU-GM, CFU-M,* or *CFU-Eo,* respectively, have no self-renewal potential, and a high fraction are actively cycling (113,114). Similarly, clonogenic cells committed to erythroid differentiation can be assayed as burst-forming units (BFU-E) or the more mature CFU-E (115).

Colony-Stimulating Factors

The factors that regulate the growth of normal stem cells are also important in the growth of AML cells (116). The conditioned media that were originally used to support the growth of clonogenic cells have been shown to contain several specific factors, including interleukin (IL)-3, granulocyte-macrophage colony-stimulating factor (GM-CSF), granulocyte colony-stimulating factor (G-CSF), or macrophage colony-stimulating factor (M-CSF or CSF-1) (117–122). There is clear evidence that these factors act directly on some progenitor cells to stimulate production of neutrophils or monocytes, and there is evidence to suggest that they are active *in vivo* as well (123–130). The complementary DNAs for all CSF genes have been cloned and recombinant human and murine factors produced (117–122). The availability of pure CSFs has allowed precise characterization of their functions and specificity. The cellular and molecular characteristics of IL-3, GM-CSF, G-CSF, and M-CSF are summarized in Table 15-1.

In Vitro Growth of Acute Myelogenous Leukemia Cells

Many advances in our understanding of AML cell biology are a result of studies of the proliferation of leukemic cells in tissue culture (117). AML cells from the blood or marrow of more than 90% of cases grow in semisolid media or liquid suspension culture for periods of 7 days to 6 months or more. The assay of leukemic clonogenic cells (CFU-AML) has been particularly informative (117). Only a small subset of cells (typically 0.1% to 1%) proliferate in agar or methylcellulose to form a colony of leukemic blasts (129). The remaining cells are either nonproliferative or can undergo only one to four cell divisions. The CFU-AMLs have several properties of leukemic stem cells, including self-renewal capacity (130,131) and the ability to produce daughter cells that have undergone partial differentiation as assessed by analysis of cell-surface antigens (131). Thus, studies of CFU-AML suggest that production of leukemic leukocytes is similar in some respects to normal myelopoiesis. Small numbers of highly proliferative, self-renewing, leukemic stem cells produce large numbers of partially differentiated but nonfunctional leukemic cells, which fill the marrow and physically suppress normal hematopoiesis. The self-renewal capacity of CFU-AML is limited in culture, and permanent cell lines are only rarely obtained (132). This finding suggests that leukemic stem cells may exist that are even earlier than CFU-AML and that have not been successfully cultured.

The gross appearance of AML colonies in semisolid media is different from that of normal CFU-GM–derived colonies. The leukemic colonies are smaller and tend not to display the heterogeneity of normal granulocyte and monocyte colonies (117). Typical AML colony morphology can be seen in preleukemic disorders that may herald the onset of acute leukemia (133,134). In remission, colony morphology usually returns to a normal pattern. The degree of CFU-AML self-renewal has also been investigated as a prognostic factor in AML. Higher secondary plating efficiency (higher self-renewal) has been associated with a significantly worse treatment outcome (135). The secondary plating efficiency assay is technically difficult and is not recommended for routine analysis. The sensitivity of CFU-AML to cytotoxic drugs can be readily assessed, and in general, there is a positive correlation between *in vitro* sensitivity and patient response to induction therapy (117). However, considerable overlap exists between sensitive and resistant cases, and the technique has not found widespread acceptance.

Cell Cycle Analysis and Kinetic Properties of Acute Myelogenous Leukemia Cells

Extensive studies of cell cycle kinetics have been conducted in AML in an effort to understand better the clinical heterogeneity of these patients. Initial studies by Clarkson et al. (136), Killmann (137), and Mauer et al. (138) estimated the fraction of cells in S phase by infusing pulses of ^{3}H-thymidine into patients with advanced disease. The labeling indexes were surprisingly low (5% to 7%). More sophisticated studies in which bromodeoxyuridine was infused, followed by detection of labeled cells in marrow biopsy specimens by immunofluorescence, gave a slightly higher value (mean, 17%), but this value was still lower than the estimates of 35% to 55% labeling index of myeloblasts in normal bone marrow (139,140). These results suggest that most leukemic cells are not proliferating and thus do not incorporate nucleic acids into DNA. These *in vivo* results are consistent with *in vitro* studies of clonogenic AML cells that indicate that only a small fraction of leukemic cells have extensive proliferative capacity and that most leukemic cells rapidly become quiescent (115).

Limited studies of cell cycle parameters have also been undertaken on clonogenic cells using the technique of "thymidine suicide" or some variation thereof. Marrow or blood cells are briefly (30 to 60 minutes) exposed to high-specific-activity ^{3}H-thymidine. Cells in S phase incorporate a lethal dose of tritium, and the subsequent loss of clonogenic cells (compared with unexposed cells) represents the fraction in S. Such studies have shown that clonogenic cells have a high S phase fraction (30% to 50%). Recent studies suggest that this fraction can be further increased both *in vitro* and *in vivo* by exposure of leukemic cells to GM-CSF or other growth factors. This observation

---

TABLE 15-1. Biologic Characteristics of Human Colony-Stimulating Factors (CSFs) Affecting Acute Myelogenous Leukemia (AML) Cell Growth

Factor	Alternate Name	Major Target Cells	Protein Size (kd)	Chromosome	Effect on AML[a]
Interleukin-3	Multi-CSF	CFU-GEMM, CFU-GM, BFU-E, CFU-meg, CFU-Eo, monocyte	20–26 (133 amino acids)	5q23-31	++++
GM-CSF	CSF-α, pluripoietin-α	CFU-GEMM, CFU-GM, BFU-E, CFU-meg, CFU-Eo, granulocyte, monocyte	14–30 (127 amino acids)	5q23-31	++++
G-CSF	CSF-β, pluripoietin	CFU-G, neutrophil	18–22 (177 amino acids)	17q11.2-q21	+++
M-CSF	CSF-1	CFU-M, monocyte	Dimer 40–44 × 2 or 18–26 × 2 (3 different complementary DNAs; 3 different 1 proteins; 2 different secreted M-CSFs)	5q33.1	+

BFU, burst-forming unit; CFU, colony-forming unit; E, erythroid; Eo, eosinophil; G, granulocyte; GEMM, granulocyte, erythrocyte, monocyte, megakaryocyte; GM, granulocyte-macrophage; M, macrophage; meg, megakaryocyte.
[a]Growth of AML cells in reponse to the cited cytokines is graded from "+," indicating modest effect, to "++++," indicating marked proliferative effect.

has led to the suggestion that it may be possible to augment the effectiveness of S phase–specific chemotherapy drugs, such as cytarabine, by combining such drugs with GM-CSF (141).

Leukemic cell cycle time has been measured by exposing cells to two separate pulses of labeling agents, such as an *in vivo* pulse of bromodeoxyuridine followed by an *in vitro* pulse of ^{3}H-thymidine (139,140). Cell cycle times have been extremely variable, ranging from approximately 24 hours to more than 10 days. Such studies are complicated by the heterogeneity of proliferative potential of leukemic cells in each patient. The cell cycle time of clonogenic cells is considerably shorter, with estimates of 9 to 22 hours.

The clinical utility of measuring cell cycle parameters in AML has not been determined. Limited studies have suggested that patients with either very low or very high labeling indexes may have a poorer prognosis. In general, however, technical difficulties with the assays and leukemic cell heterogeneity have limited the clinical usefulness of these studies.

Growth Factors for Acute Myelogenous Leukemia Cells in Tissue Culture

In 20% to 25% of cases, leukemic cells proliferate spontaneously *in vitro* in fetal calf serum-containing media (142,143). Such spontaneous proliferation is not observed with normal marrow cells or cells from myelodysplastic patients. In most AML cases, however, proliferation of leukemic cells requires the addition of specific growth factors. With few exceptions, the same factors that support the growth of normal myeloid cells also support the growth of AML cells, including GM-CSF, IL-3, G-CSF, M-CSF, and IL-1 (142–145). The most effective factors to promote growth of AML cells in both semisolid media and in liquid suspension culture are GM-CSF and IL-3 (Table 15-1). Combinations of CSFs, such as GM-CSF and G-CSF, are more active than single factors (142). There is no evidence from tissue culture studies that any of these CSFs enhance differentiation of AML cells. In limited clinical trials in myelodysplasia and AML, GM-CSF, G-CSF, and IL-3 were shown to accelerate leukemic cell proliferation in some cases (146–152). This finding suggests both that these CSFs are important growth factors *in vivo* and that supply of CSF may be a limiting factor in the rate of leukemic cell proliferation in patients. However, most patients with MDS receiving CSFs do not progress to AML. Preliminary studies suggest that patients with more advanced disease (refractory anemia with excess blasts in transformation) are more likely to convert to AML with CSF stimulation. The rate of transformation may be particularly low with G-CSF.

The response of AML cells *in vitro* and *in vivo* to CSFs suggests that a supply of these factors may be critical for progression of AML in patients (153). Indirect evidence supports this concept in murine leukemias (154). Several cloned hematopoietic cell lines such as FDC-P1 have been developed that are immortal but remain dependent on GM-CSF or IL-3 for growth (154). Such cell lines are not leukemic in syngeneic animals despite an extremely high rate of self-renewal. When FDC-P1 cells are made to secrete GM-CSF or IL-3 after retroviral insertion of a CSF complementary DNA, these cells rapidly become factor-independent and fully leukemogenic (155). The autocrine production of CSFs has also been demonstrated in spontaneous and virus-induced murine leukemias (156,157). In some examples, virus insertion has been shown to occur adjacent to or within a CSF gene (158). Human leukemias are usually not factor-independent, however, and only approximately one-fifth of cases proliferate spontaneously in culture (143,144). Some of these spontaneously proliferating cases produce a CSF in culture, usually GM-CSF, IL-1, or G-CSF (159–162). Evidence that

CSFs are being produced *in vivo* is lacking, although cases have been reported in which serum G-CSF levels have been elevated (163). Thus, it is possible that autocrine and paracrine stimulation of AML cells occurs in some cases. However, excess growth factor supply by itself would not be leukemogenic. The primary transforming event must cause an increase in the rate of self-renewal and a decrease in differentiation. Nonetheless, autonomous proliferation in culture indicates a poor prognosis (164).

Leukemic Cell Lines

Extensive studies on the growth properties and differentiation of several myeloid leukemia cell lines have been conducted (132). The most useful cell lines have included the promyelocytic line HL-60 (165), the Philadelphia chromosome erythroleukemic cell line K562 (166), and the monocytic lines U937 (167) and THP-1 (168). These cell lines have some common features, including that they are all factor-independent for growth and that they can be induced to undergo some degree of differentiation in response to agents such as phorbol ester, tumor necrosis factor, retinoic acid, or 1,25-dihydroxyvitamin D_3 (132). HL-60 has been particularly valuable because of the large variety of effective differentiating agents and the finding that it can differentiate to either macrophages or to a neutrophil-like cell in response to different inducing agents (169). Differentiation of all the cell lines is associated with cessation or diminishment of proliferation. Studies with HL-60 in particular have been used to identify agents for clinical trials of differentiation therapy. Unfortunately, preliminary clinical studies of such inducers, including interferon-γ, tumor necrosis factor, 13-*cis*-retinoic acid, hexamethylene bisacetamide, and low-dose cytarabine, have produced only modest evidence of either significant *in vivo* differentiation of AML cells or significant clinical benefit (170). However, all-*trans*-retinoic acid (ATRA) is an effective differentiating agent for patients with APL with a t(15;17) chromosomal translocation, as discussed in more detail below (171–173).

Although the leukemic cell lines are valuable models of primary AML, there are a number of fundamental biologic differences between the cell lines listed previously and primary AML cells. First, primary AML cells are almost always dependent on CSFs for *in vitro* growth, whereas all the commonly used cell lines are factor-independent. Also, primary AML cells have a limited lifespan in tissue culture, possibly indicating that they require a stromal cell microenvironment for optimal growth and self-renewal. Improvements in long-term culture of AML cells would solve many of these problems. Finally, many of the cell lines have evolved in culture, acquiring (or losing) new characteristics, including karyotypic changes.

Clonality

In contrast to normal blood cells, myeloid leukemic cells are monoclonal, derived from a single stem cell that has become neoplastic (174). Evidence for the monoclonal nature of AML comes from three lines of evidence. First, studies of female patients heterozygous for isoenzymes of the X-linked gene encoding glucose-6-phosphate dehydrogenase (G6PD) indicate that, whereas normal cells in heterozygous people are always polyclonal (have approximately equal amounts of G6PD isoenzymes A and B), AML cells express only a single isoenzyme and are therefore derived from a single cell (175). Second, cytogenetic analysis of AML cells frequently shows specific chromosomal markers that are present in all metaphases (176–180). Finally, restriction fragment length polymorphism (RFLP) studies of X-chromosomal genes, such as phosphoglycerol kinase, have confirmed the clonality of AML and further indicated that remission cells in occasional patients with AML may also be clonal (181,182). Although the significance of clonal remissions is not clear, one explanation is that AML in some patients arises in the setting of a clonal blood disorder, such as a myelodysplastic or myeloproliferative syndrome. Successful therapy of the acute leukemia leads to reemergence of the underlying preleukemic disorder. These data also support the hypothesis that more than one mutation may be necessary for the development of the AML phenotype.

Cell of Origin

Karyotype, G6PD isoenzyme, and RFLP analyses have been used to investigate clonality of individual lineages in AML to determine at what point in the hierarchy of hematopoietic stem cells the leukemic cells arise (183,184). Similar studies have suggested that in contrast to CML, in which the cell of origin is always a pluripotent stem cell (185), AML may have as many as two-thirds of cases arise at levels more mature than the pluripotent stem cell. Specifically, the erythroid and megakaryocytic lineages are involved in approximately one-third of *de novo* cases of AML, whereas in two-thirds, only the granulocytic and monocytic lineage is clonal (175,176). Additional evidence comes from immunophenotype analysis of leukemic clonogenic cells using monoclonal antibodies that identify restricted stages of differentiation of myeloid cells (186–201). Approximately one-third of cases are found to be related to multipotent progenitor cells and two-thirds to committed progenitor cells, such as the CFU-GM. Morphologic abnormalities of erythroid or megakaryocytic cells are observed in up to half of cases. Limited data suggest that patients with AML arising in a multipotent stem cell tend to be older, have secondary (therapy-related) leukemia, or have had MDS. These data suggest that AML may arise at any point within the proliferating compartment of the bone marrow, from the pluripotent stem cell to the promyelocyte. This wide variability of the cell of origin of AML is likely to account for some of the striking morphologic, molecular, and heterogeneous clinical manifestations and behavior of AML.

Clonal Remissions

Studies using RFLP and G6PD techniques have documented clonal hematopoiesis in 1% to as many as 26% of patients with AML in complete remission (CR) (181–185). Discrepancies in these incidence figures of clonal remission can be partly explained by extreme lyonization of polyclonal cells (184). The significance of this observation has not been determined. It is possible that such patients have an unrecognized underlying clonal stem cell disorder and that, after successful elimination of a frankly leukemic subclone with chemotherapy, morphologically normal but clonal hematopoiesis continues. Alternatively, CR induction in these cases may have altered the biologic behavior of AML by selecting out a subclone of leukemic stem cells that can differentiate nearly normally. Long-term follow-up of additional cases is warranted.

CLASSIFICATIONS

French/American/British Classification System

Although all cases of AML share many common biologic features, such as cell of origin, clonality, growth factor requirement, and aberrant differentiation, the morphology is strikingly heterogeneous. The most widely accepted classification scheme, the FAB system, divides AML cases into seven major groups (M1

through M7) and several subgroups (12–15) (Fig. 15-1 and Table 15-2). The FAB classification depends on identifying the lineage of the major population of blasts (myeloblast, monoblast, erythroblast, or megakaryoblast) and the degree of differentiation present. Cytochemical identification of myeloperoxidase, specific esterase, nonspecific esterase enzymes, and staining for Sudan black and periodic acid-Schiff (PAS) are used to confirm or extend interpretation of Romanowsky-stained specimens (13,15).

Of the specimens, 5% to 20% are difficult to classify by the FAB system, and this problem seems to be particularly common in leukemias arising in the setting of preleukemic disorders. Satisfactory classification systems for hybrid or biphenotypic leukemias, hypoplastic leukemias, basophilic leukemias, and primitive erythroblast leukemias have not been devised. Nonetheless, the FAB system is invaluable in providing common ground for comparing patients in different studies and for providing useful prognostic information.

M1: Myeloblastic Leukemia without Maturation

In this category, marrow cells show minimal evidence of granulocytic maturation, with 3% or more of the blasts being myeloperoxidase-positive or Sudan black–positive and a varying proportion of the cells expressing a few needle-shaped azurophilic granules (Auer rods), or both. More than 90% of nonerythroid cells are blasts, and the remaining cells are monocytes or maturing granulocytes. Two types of M1 blasts have been defined. Type I blasts are primitive cells that lack granules and usually contain one or more nucleoli. Type II blasts are slightly larger, have a lower nucleus to cytoplasm ratio, and contain one to six azurophilic granules. Unlike in promyelocytes, the nucleus of the type II blast is central, the nuclear chromatin is uncondensed, and the Golgi zone is not prominent.

M2: Myeloblastic Leukemia with Maturation

In M2, the sum of type I and II blasts is 30% to 89% of nonerythroid cells, and there is evidence of maturation to the stage of promyelocyte or beyond. Monocytic precursor cells account for less than 20%. Nucleoli, azurophilic granules, and Auer rods are common. Myeloblasts with bilobed or reniform nuclei can be distinguished from monocytes by the fine chromatin pattern of the blast.

M3: Hypergranular Promyelocytic Leukemia

Most M3 cells are heavily granulated promyelocytes. The nuclei may be reniform, and the cytoplasmic granules may be coalescent. Auer rods are common, and bundles of Auer rods called *Faggot cells* may be seen and are pathognomonic for this subtype (Fig. 15-2).

M3 Variant: Microgranular Promyelocytic Leukemia

The promyelocytes contain large numbers of tiny granules that may be difficult to distinguish by light microscopy (9,10). The cytoplasm is usually strikingly myeloperoxidase-positive, however, and the combination of agranular cytoplasm and strong myeloperoxidase staining should suggest this variant. The nuclei may be reniform, and the diagnosis of M4 is initially made in some cases. The diagnosis can be confirmed by cytogenetics, which reveals t(15:17) translocation, or molecular studies, which reveal the PML-RAR-α fusion transcript. Electron microscopy shows multiple dark primary granules and Auer rods.

M4: Myelomonocytic Leukemia

More than 20% but less than 80% of the M4 nonerythroid cells are of the monocytic lineage, often *promonocytes*. More than 30% of all nonerythroid cells must be blasts. In addition, the blood monocyte concentration should exceed $5 \times 10^9/L$ or the serum (or urine) lysozyme should exceed three times normal. In some cases, the marrow picture may be more consistent with M2, but if there is blood monocytosis or elevated lysozyme, the diagnosis is M4. Esterase stains can be particularly useful to distinguish promonocytes from promyelocytes (Table 15-2).

M5: Monocytic Leukemia

Two forms are recognized: M5a, in which more than 80% of marrow nonerythroid cells are monoblasts, and M5b, in which less than 80% of nonerythroid cells are monoblasts but more than 80% are monoblasts, promonocytes, and monocytes.

M6: Erythroleukemia

Over 30% of nonerythroid cells are type I or II blasts in M6, but half or more of marrow cells are erythroblasts. Cases in which more than half of marrow cells are erythroblasts but less than

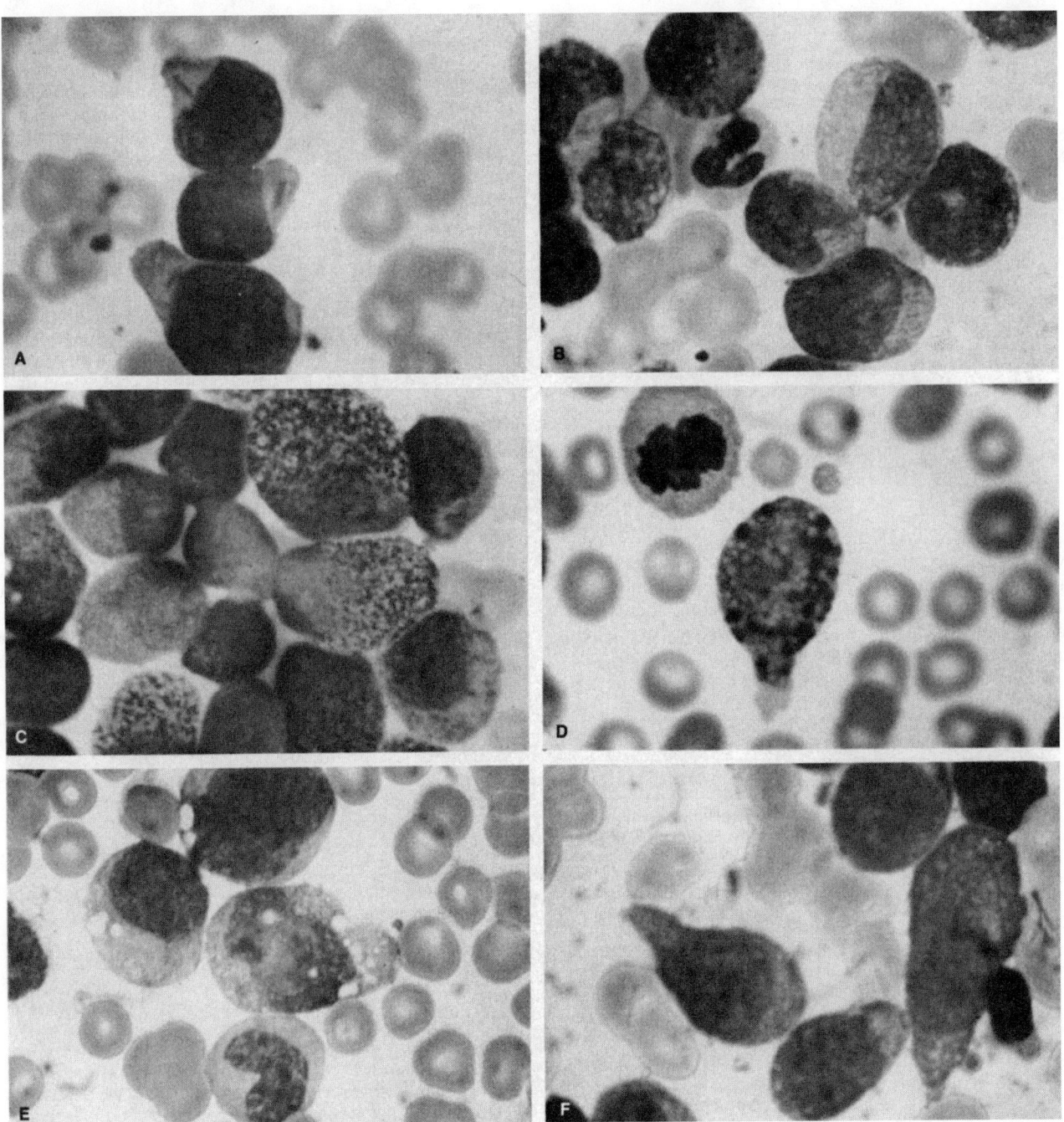

Figure 15-1. Morphologic appearance of bone marrow in Wright-Giemsa–stained films for each French/American/British type of acute myelogenous leukemia. **A:** M1: myeloblastic without maturation; the blasts contain Auer rods. **B:** M2: myeloblastic with maturation. **C:** M3: hypergranular promyelocytic. **D:** M4: myelomonocytic. **E:** M4Eo: myelomonocytic with abnormal eosinophilic and basophilic granules. **F:** M5: monocytic. (*continued*)

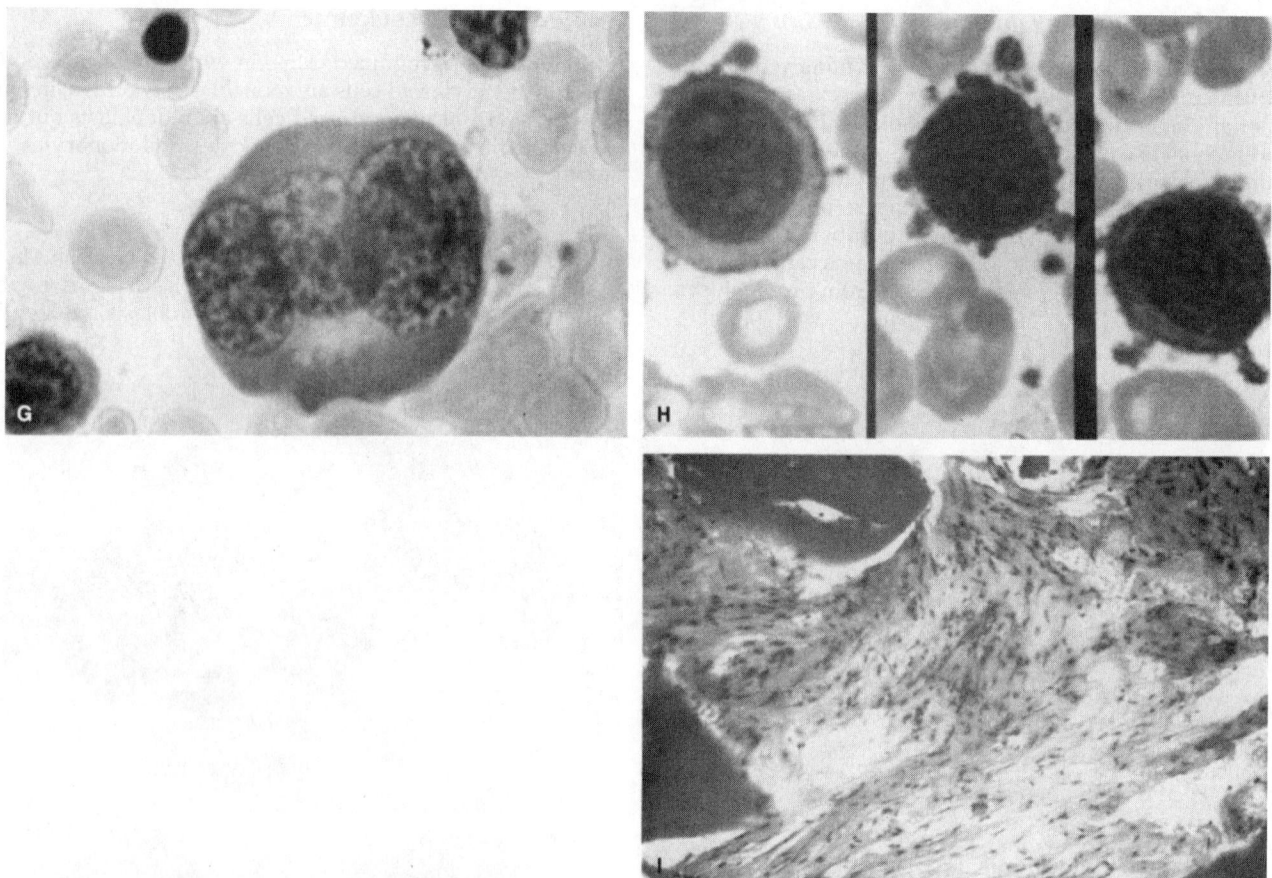

Figure 15-1. (*continued*) **G:** M6: erythroleukemic. **H:** M7: megakaryoblastic. **I:** M7: myelofibrotic. (See Color Fig. 15-1.) (Courtesy of Pearl Leavitt and Dr. Arthur Skarin, Dana-Farber Cancer Institute, Boston.)

30% of nonerythroid cells are myeloblasts fall into the category of MDS (refractory anemia with excess blasts in transformation). In rare cases, there is a monomorphic population of erythroblasts without a significant myeloblast component. These cases are not classifiable within the FAB system but are being recognized more frequently with immunophenotype analysis.

M7: Megakaryoblastic Leukemia

In M7, the blast cells are typically polymorphic with round nuclei and finely reticulated nuclear chromatin. Cytoplasmic blebs may be seen, as may bare nuclei surrounded by clusters of platelets. Megakaryocytic fragments may be seen in the blood

TABLE 15-2. French/American/British (FAB) Classification of Acute Myelogenous Leukemia

FAB Subtype	Morphologic and Cytochemical Characteristics	Frequency, %
M0	Large, agranular myeloblasts, sometimes resembling lymphoblasts of FAB subtype L2. Stain negative for myeloperoxidase and Sudan black. Express CD13 or CD33 antigens on cell surface.	2–3
M1	Acute myeloblastic leukemia without maturation to at least promyelocyte stage: large, poorly differentiated myeloblasts represent 90% or more of the nonerythroid cells. At least 3% of the myeloblasts stain positive for myeloperoxidase.	20
M2	Acute myeloblastic leukemia with maturation: between 30% and 89% of the nonerythroid cells are myeloblasts having abundant cytoplasm with moderate to many granules. Auer rods are often visible. Myeloblasts are myeloperoxidase-positive.	25–30
M3	Leukemia cells usually contain heavy azurophilic granulation. Nuclear size varies greatly. Nuclei are often bilobed or kidney-shaped. Some cells contain bundles of Auer rods (Faggot cells). Leukemia cells strongly positive for myeloperoxidase. Microgranular variant. Usually HLA-DR–negative.	8–15
M4	Myeloblasts, promyelocytes, myelocytes, and other granulocytic precursors account for more than 30% of the nonerythroid cells but do not exceed 80%. Monocytic cells account for up to 20% of the nonerythroid cells. Nonspecific esterase and chloroacetate esterase cytochemical reactions are positive. Auer rods may be present.	20–25
M4Eo	Myelomonoblasts with cytochemically and morphologically abnormal eosinophils.	5
M5	Monoblasts, promonocytes, or monocytes account for 80% or more of the nonerythroid cells. In M5a, 80% or more of all the monocytic cells are monoblasts negative for myeloperoxidase and usually positive for nonspecific esterase. In the well-differentiated subtype M5b, <80% are monoblasts. Nonspecific esterase positivity is lost with NaF.	10
M6	>50% of the nucleated marrow cells are erythroid. Erythroblasts usually strongly periodic acid-Schiff–positive. Myeloblasts represent 30% or more of the nonerythroid cells.	5
M7	Large and small megakaryoblasts with high nuclear to cytoplasm ratio. Cytoplasm is pale and agranular. Standard cytochemical stains not definitive. Platelet peroxidase and platelet-specific antibodies often positive. Factor VIII may be positive.	1–2

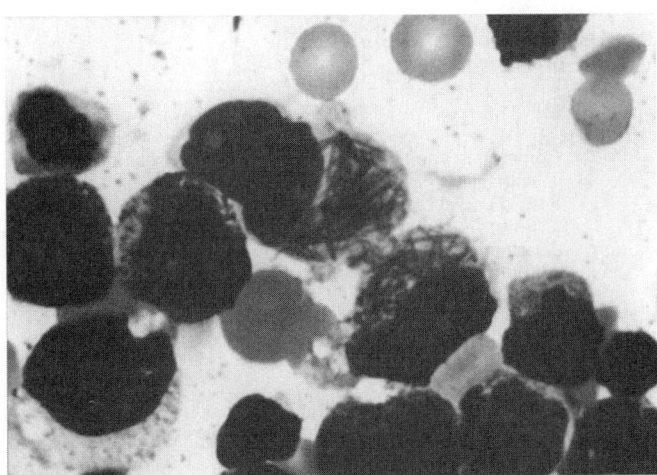

Figure 15-2. Faggot cell containing numerous Auer rods in the bone marrow aspirate from a patient with acute promyelocytic leukemia (French/American/British M3). (See Color Fig. 15-2.) (Courtesy of Dr. Martin Tallman, Northwestern University Medical School, Chicago.)

film. The blasts are peroxidase-negative and Sudan black–negative but may stain for fluoride-inhibitable nonspecific esterase activity. The PAS and acid phosphatase reactions are frequently positive. Bone marrow fibrosis is a frequent accompaniment of the M7 subtype. The diagnosis should be confirmed with ultrastructural histochemistry, demonstrating platelet peroxidase activity exclusively on the nuclear membrane and the endoplasmic reticulum. Immunophenotype analysis is also useful to confirm the diagnosis of M7. The blasts typically express platelet glycoproteins IIb/IIIa or Ib. Factor VIII antibodies may also react with cells.

World Health Organization Classification

A new proposed World Health Organization classification takes into account cytogenetics and molecular genetics (202) (Table 15-3). Patients are classified into those with well recognized and characterized clonal cytogenetic abnormalities, those with mul-

---

TABLE 15-3. Proposed World Health Organization Classification of Myeloid Neoplasms: Acute Myelogenous Leukemias (AMLs)

1. AMLs with recurrent cytogenetic translocations
    AML with t(8;21)(q22;q22), AML1 (CBF-α)/ETO
    Acute promyelocytic leukemias [AML with t(15;17)(q22;q11) and variants, PML/RAR-α]
    AML with abnormal bone marrow eosinophils inv(16)(p13q22) or t(16;16)(p13;q11), CBFβ/MYH11X
    AML with 11q23 (MLL) abnormalities
2. AML with multilineage dysplasia
    With previous myelodysplastic syndrome
    Without previous myelodysplastic syndrome
3. AML and myelodysplastic syndromes, therapy-related
    Alkylating agent-related
    Epipodophyllotoxin-related (some may be lymphoid)
    Other types
4. AML not otherwise categorized
    AML minimally differentiated
    AML with maturation
    AML without maturation
    Acute monocytic leukemia
    Acute erythroid leukemia
    Acute panmyelosis with myelofibrosis
5. Acute biphenotypic leukemias

---

tilineage dysplasia, those with therapy-related AMLs (divided into AMLs that are alkylating agent-induced and those that are epipodophyllotoxin-related because they define very different clinical syndromes, as discussed later), those not easily classifiable, and those with biphenotypic leukemias.

Myelodysplastic Syndrome–Related versus *De Novo* Acute Myelogenous Leukemia Classification

An alternative classification has been proposed by Head (203) that divides AMLs into two categories: those MDS-related with characteristic clonal cytogenetic changes, including -5 and -7, associated with an antecedent MDS, multistep evolution, and poor response to chemotherapy; and those occurring in younger patients with an antecedent MDS, often associated with favorable karyotypes (discussed later) and a good response to chemotherapy (Table 15-4).

Separation of Acute Myelogenous Leukemia from Acute Lymphoblastic Leukemia

Distinguishing AML from ALL is essential for treatment planning and is relatively simple in 80% to 90% of cases. The presence of Auer rods or myeloperoxidase-positive primary granules is pathognomonic of AML. AML cells tend to be larger and are more heterogeneous in size and nuclear morphology than ALL cells. Useful cytochemical stains include myeloperoxidase, Sudan black B, naphthol-ASD chloroacetate esterase, and lysozyme. The PAS stain is negative in M1, M2, and M3 but may be positive in M4, M5 (punctate staining), and M6. The PAS stain may be particularly useful in M6, in which blocks of PAS-positive material are identified in the abnormal erythroid cells of this disease. Terminal deoxynucleotidyl transferase is more commonly expressed by ALL cells than AML cells, but it is not lineage-specific and is consistent with lymphoid differentiation only if other lymphoid-specific markers are present (186–188). Up to 25% of patients with AML have cells that express terminal deoxynucleotidyl transferase; when this expression is associated with the expression of CD7, these patients tend to have a lower CR rate and shorter overall survival (OS) compared to patients with AML with cells lacking expression of either marker or expressing only one of the two (188).

In the 10% to 20% of cases in which morphology and cytochemistry are inconclusive or insufficient to distinguish AML and ALL, immunophenotype analysis provides the diagnosis in virtually all cases (189). A large number of monoclonal antibodies have been generated that recognize antigens expressed on the surface of AML but not ALL cells (190,191). All the antibodies studied also react with subsets of normal hematopoietic cells, indicating that leukemia-specific antigens in human myeloid leukemias are rare or nonexistent. These antibodies have been grouped into clusters of differentiation (CDs) by International Workshops on Leukocyte Differentiation Antigens, and antibodies of several clusters have been shown in extensive studies to be useful in distinguishing myeloid from lymphoid leukemias (189–194) (Table 15-5). Using a combination of antibodies specifically recognizing B-cell, T-cell, and myeloid antigens, it is possible to distinguish AML from ALL in 95% to 99% of cases. Many of the most useful myeloid antigens are expressed by normal cells at specific stages of differentiation, and some investigators have attempted to correlate surface phenotype of AML cells with a normal cell counterpart (194). There appears to be only a limited utility to this type of approach. Cells from AML patients with immature morphology (M1) tend to have an immature phenotype, whereas cells from patients with M3 or M5 tend to express an immunophenotype typical of the normal promyelocyte or promonocyte (195–198). Also, limited informa-

TABLE 15-4. Characterization of Myelodysplastic Syndrome (MDS)-Acute Myelogenous Leukemia (AML) versus True *De Novo* AML

Feature	MDS-Related AML	True *De Novo* AML
Incidence	Common in elderly; exponential increase with age	Common in younger patients; approximately flat incidence with age
Cytogenetics	-5, 5q-, -7, 7q-, +8, 20q-, +9, 11q-, 12p-, -18, +19, +21, 3q21-26 abnormalities, t(1;7), t(2;11)	t(15;17), t(9;11), t(8;21), inv(16), t(16;16), t(8;16), t(11;17), t(6;9)
Previous MDS	Frequent documented MDS; sequential multistep evolution	Absent
Morphologic dysplasia	Frequent multilineage myelodysplastic features	Absent
Hematopoiesis	Clonal at presentation and remission	Nonclonal
Treatment response	Poor response to chemotherapy: resistant disease, early relapse, impaired marrow reserve, frequent MDR1 expression at presentation	Good response to appropriate chemotherapy, infrequent MDR1 expression at presentation
Remissions	May revert to MDS or pre-MDS	True with chemotherapy
Cell of origin	Multipotential myeloid stem cell	Lineage-restricted stem cell
Iatrogenic model	AML postalkylating agent chemotherapy	AML postepipodophyllotoxins or complex combination therapy

tion may be available from surface antigen phenotype (195,197,198). Some studies have indicated that expression of CD13, CD14, or CD34 may be associated with a lower than average rate of CR (195,198–200). Overall, however, the primary value of surface antigen analysis in most cases of AML is in distinguishing AML and ALL.

Hybrid or Biphenotypic Leukemia

Approximately 5% of cases of acute leukemia have morphologic, cytochemical, immunophenotypic, or genetic evidence of more than one hematopoietic lineage (204–210). This promiscuity may be due to the simultaneous presence of two distinct leukemic populations (bilineage or biclonal) or, more commonly, to the presence of features of more than one lineage in the same cells (hybrid or biphenotypic). This phenomenon has been best studied with immunophenotype analysis, and cases in which there is coexpression of myeloid–T-cell, myeloid–B-cell, and T-cell–B-cell phenotypes are commonly reported (205–211). The pathogenesis of these mixed leukemias has been the subject of much speculation, but it remains poorly understood (205–213). One popular school of thought is that leukemic cells represent frozen stages of differentiation and that a biphenotypic leukemia represents a clonal expansion of a normal cell that expresses features of more than one lineage. It has been difficult to identify such cells in normal marrow, however, and it is more likely that the molecular events that determine the orderly commitment to one or another lineage in normal hematopoiesis are disrupted in AML. Lineage switching can also be observed in a small fraction of cases (212). A typical example would be a patient with features of a T-cell phenotype at diagnosis but with a mixed T-cell–myeloid or pure myeloid phenotype at relapse. Hybrid leukemias may be more common in patients with antecedent myelodysplastic disorders; secondary leukemias; translocations involving chromosome 11q23, particularly t(4;11); the Philadelphia chromosome; or age younger than 6 months (206–214). A better understanding of the

TABLE 15-5. Immunophenotype Analysis of Acute Myelogenous Leukemia

CD	Antibodies	M1/M2	M3	M4/M5	M6	M7	B-ALL	T-ALL
Myeloid lineage								
CD11b	Anti-Mo1	–	+	++	–	–	–	–
CD13	Anti-MY7	+	+	++	+	+	–	–
CD14	Anti-Mo2, MY4	–	–	++	–	–	–	–
CD15	Anti-MY1	+	++	++	–	–	–	–
CD33	Anti-MY9	++	++	++	++	++	–	–
CD34	Anti-MY10	++	+	+	+	+	+	+
T Lineage								
CD2	Anti-T11	–	–	–	–	–	–	++
CD3	Anti-T3	–	–	–	–	–	–	+
CD5	Anti-T1	–	–	–	–	–	–	++
CD7	3A1	+	+	+	+	+	+	++
B Lineage								
CD10	Anti-CALLA	–	–	–	–	–	+	–
CD19	Anti-B4	–	–	–	–	–	+	–
CD20	Anti-B1	–	–	–	–	–	+	–
Erythroid lineage								
	Antiglycophorin A	–	–	–	++	–	–	–
Megakaryocyte lineage								
CD41	Anti-gpIIb/IIIa	–	–	–	–	++	–	–
CD42	Anti-gpIb	–	–	–	–	++	–	–

B-ALL, B-lineage acute lymphoblastic leukemia; CALLA, common acute lymphoblastic leukemia antigen; gp, glycoprotein; T-ALL, T-lineage acute lymphoblastic leukemia; ++, expressed by over 20% of blasts in 20% to 50% of cases; +, expressed by over 20% of blasts in 5% to 20% of cases; –, expressed by less than 5% of cases.

molecular control of lineage commitment is likely to be required before the precise mechanisms responsible for biphenotypic leukemias are identified.

It is controversial whether patients with hybrid leukemias have a poorer prognosis than patients with classic AML or ALL. Recent pediatric data suggest that the expression of lymphoid-associated cell-surface antigens on leukemic cells from children with AML lacks prognostic significance (208,209). The significance of hybrid acute leukemia in adults may depend on whether the cells are primarily myeloid (AML with lymphoid markers) or lymphoid (ALL with myeloid markers). In a prospective Cancer and Leukemia Group B (CALGB) study of adults with ALL, 31% of patients coexpressed lymphoid and myeloid surface antigens (215). These hybrid cases had a statistically significant lower CR rate than nonhybrid cases (30% vs. 73%, p <.01) when treated with an aggressive ALL regimen. In contrast, patients whose disease is primarily myeloid but who coexpress lymphoid markers may have a favorable prognosis (216).

M0: Undifferentiated Myeloid Leukemia

M0 is defined as cases of AML lacking morphologic or cytochemical analyses (217–220). Evidence of myeloid differentiation can be obtained from immunophenotype analysis with expression of CD13, CD33, or other surface markers (221–226) or with demonstration of peroxidase-positive granules by electron microscopy (224). If platelet peroxidase is positive by electron microscopy, the case should be considered M7.

CYTOGENETIC ABNORMALITIES

Chromosomal analysis has proved to be a valuable aspect of diagnostic, prognostic, and biologic studies of AML (176–179)

(discussed in Chapter 5). Nonrandom chromosomal abnormalities have been detected in 50% to 90% of cases of AML using high-resolution banding techniques (227–232). These abnormalities include balanced reciprocal translocations, such as t(8;21) or t(15;17); internal deletions of single chromosomes, such as 5q- or 7q-; gain or loss of whole chromosomes, such as +8 or -7; or chromosome inversions, such as inv(3) or inv(16). Complex chromosomal defects are observed in approximately 15% of *de novo* cases (i.e., without a preceding myelodysplastic disorder) and constitute a clinical group of patients with particularly poor prognoses. Common cytogenetic abnormalities observed in AML are annotated in Table 15-6 in relation to FAB subtype and discussed in more detail below (176–179,227–233).

Cloning of chromosomal translocation breakpoints has provided important insights into pathophysiology of AML. Several themes have emerged from the analysis of the more than 300 recurring chromosomal translocations associated with human leukemias, of which approximately 100 have been cloned (233,234). First, different chromosomal abnormalities have been associated with the same FAB subtype of AML, indicating that although chromosomal translocations may involve different genes in disparate parts of the human genome, they presumably target similar signal transduction or transcriptional pathways in leukemic cells. Second, most chromosomal translocations in AML target transcription factors that are required for normal hematopoietic development. As detailed below, examples include core binding factor (CBF), the retinoic acid receptor-α (RAR-α) gene, and HOX gene family members. Third, a physiologic consequence of many translocations is disruption of normal hematopoietic development. Fourth, gene rearrangements induced by chromosomal translocation appear in general to be necessary but not sufficient to cause AML.

TABLE 15-6. Selected Recurring Structural Rearrangements in Malignant Myeloid Diseases

Disease	Chromosome Abnormality	Involved Genes
AML		
AML-M2	t(8;21)(q22;q22)	ETO-AML1
APL-M3, M3V	t(15;17)(q22;q21)	PML-RAR-α
Atypical APL	t(11;17)(q23;q21)	PLZF-RAR-α
AMMoL-M4E0	inv(16)(p13q22) or	MYH11-CBFβ
	t(16;16)(p13;q22)	MYH11-CBFβ
AMMoL-M4/AmoL-M5	t(6;11)(q27;q23)	AF6-MLL
	t(9;11)(p22;q23)	AF9-MLL
	t(4;11)(q21;q23)	AF4-MLL
AMegL-M7	t(1;22)(p13;q13)	MAL-OTT/RBM15-MLK1
AML	t(3;3)(q21;q26)	RPN1-EVI1
	or inv(3)(q21;q26)	
	t(3;5)(q21;q26)	
	t(3;5)(q25;q34)	MLF1-NPM1
	t(6;9)(p23;q34)	DEK-CAN (NUP214)
	t(7;11)(p15;p15)	HOXA9-NUP98
	t(8;16)(q34;p13)	MOZ-CBP
	t(9;12)(q34;p13)	TEL-ABL
	t(12;22)(p13;q13)	TEL-NM1
	t(16;21)(p11;q22)	TLS(FUS)-ERG
	-5 or del(5q)	
	-7 or del(7q)	
	del(20q)	
	del(12p)	?TEL,?p27^{KIP1}
Therapy-related AML	-7 or del(7q)	
	and/or	
	-5 or del(5q)	
	t(11q23)	MLL
	t(3;21)(q26;q22)	EAP/MDS1/EVI1-AML1

AML, acute myeloid leukemia; APL, acute promyelocytic leukemia.

Translocations Involving the Retinoic Acid Receptor-α Gene

For example, the translocation t(15;17))(q22;q11-12) associated with M3 has been extensively studied. Several groups showed that the RAR-α gene on chromosome 17, which plays an important role in hematopoietic differentiation, was rearranged in patients with APL with a t(15;17)(q22;q12-21) translocation (70–72). The RAR-α gene is fused with a gene on chromosome 15 that encodes a putative zinc finger transcription factor, PML, named for its involvement in promyelocytic leukemia (236–238). Two reciprocal types of fusion RNA species are produced: RAR-α-PML and PML-RAR-α. The PML-RAR-α species contains the zinc finger of PML fused to the DNA-binding and protein-binding domains of RAR-α. The aberrant PML-RAR-α fusion protein functions as a dominant inhibitory oncogene for RAR-α interacting proteins, including RXR-α (238). In addition, the PML-RAR-α fusion interferes with the function of the native PML protein, which is thought to function as a tumor-suppressor gene based on analysis of mice that are deficient in PML (239–241). Collectively, the dominant interfering activities of the PML-RAR-α fusion protein result in a block in differentiation at the promyelocyte stage of development. The clinical response of these patients to ATRA, as discussed in more detail below, is explained by the ability of this retinoid to bind to the PML-RAR-α fusion protein and reverse repression of target genes required for normal hematopoietic development (171,173,242–246). It has recently been appreciated that the ability of the PML-RAR-α fusion protein to repress transcription is due in part to the aberrant recruitment of the nuclear corepressor complex, including histone deacetylase (247–249). This observation, in turn, has suggested that pharmacologic agents that inhibit histone deacetylases may be useful in therapy of APL (250–252).

Murine models have provided clear evidence for the role of the PML-RAR-α fusion protein in APL. Expression of the PML-RAR-α fusion protein from the cathepsin G promoter, which is expressed in promyelocytes during hematopoietic development, results in an acute leukemia syndrome with features of APL in humans (253,254). The murine model also demonstrates sensitivity to ATRA and has allowed testing of various agents that may have therapeutic activity in humans, such as arsenic trioxide (255–257). The murine model has also allowed analysis of the role of the reciprocal RAR-α-PML fusion protein in disease pathogenesis. Coexpression of both the PML-RAR-α and the RAR-α-PML fusion from the cathepsin G promoter increases the penetrance of the disease in the murine model, suggesting that the reciprocal fusion protein may facilitate the acquisition of second mutations required for the acute leukemia phenotype (258). Data from the murine model also provide convincing evidence that the t(15;17) is not sufficient for the leukemia phenotype in the transgenic model. In transgenic models, there is not complete penetrance of disease, and there is a long latency of at least 3 months before leukemia develops. As discussed in more detail below, activating mutations of the hematopoietic tyrosine kinase FLT3 occur in up to 40% of APL and may be one example of second mutations in APL.

Translocations Involving Core Binding Factor

Core binding factor is another example of an important hematopoietic transcription factor that is targeted by chromosomal translocations in AML, including the t(8;21) and inv(16) translocations. In general, patients with translocations involving CBF have a good clinical outcome, especially when treated with regimens containing high-dose cytosine arabinoside (259,260). CBF is composed of an AML1 (RUNX1, CBFA2) subunit that contacts DNA,

and its heterodimeric partner CBFβ that does not contact DNA but facilitates transactivation of CBF target genes (261–263). CBF targets include cytokines and cytokine receptors important for normal hematopoietic development. Perhaps the most convincing evidence of the importance of CBF in hematopoiesis is that knockout mice that are deficient for both alleles of either AML1 or CBFβ have a complete lack of definitive hematopoiesis (264–266).

Thus, a mutation or gene rearrangement that resulted in loss of function of either AML1 or CBFβ would be predicted to impair hematopoietic differentiation. Several chromosomal translocations target CBF and result in loss of function through dominant negative activity. The translocation t(8;21)(q22;q22) is the most frequently occurring translocation in de novo AML, found in 18% of M2 cases. The t(8;21) produces a fusion protein involving the AML1 gene on chromosome 21 and the ETO gene on chromosome 8 (73–77). The inv(16)(p12;q22) and t(16;16)(p13;q22), associated with the unique syndrome of M4 with abnormal eosinophils (M4Eo) (267–269), targets CBFβ and results in expression of the CBFβ/SMMHC fusion gene (78,270). Both the AML1/ETO and the CBFβ/SMMHC fusions are dominant negative inhibitors of CBF and impair differentiation (271,272). For example, expression of either the AML1/ETO or CBFβ/SMMHC fusion genes from their endogenous promoter mice completely inhibits the function of the residual AML1 or CBFβ alleles, resulting in a lack of definitive hematopoiesis (273–275). Repression of CBF target genes by the AML1/ETO or CBFβ/SMMHC fusions, as for the PML/RAR-α fusion, is mediated by recruitment of the nuclear corepressor complex (276–278). Thus, it has been suggested that histone deacetylase, a component of the corepressor complex, may also be a therapeutic target for leukemias associated with CBF loss of function (13,14).

There is convincing evidence, as there is for PML/RAR-α fusion protein, that expression of AML1/ETO and CBFβ/SMMHC is necessary but not sufficient to cause AML. For example, murine models of leukemia have been developed that allow for expression of each of these fusion proteins in adult hematopoietic cells. Expression of AML1/ETO or CBFβ/SMMHC alone is not sufficient to cause AML. Chemical mutagens such as ethylnitrosourea must be used in these systems to induce second mutations and subsequent AML (276,279,280).

Translocations Involving HOX Family Members

Members of the extended family of HOX transcription factors play an important role in hematopoietic development (281) and are also involved in translocations associated with AML. Examples include the NUP98/HOXA9 and NUP98/HOXD13 fusions, associated with t(7;11) and t(2;11), respectively (282–284). HOX family members are directly involved in leukemia-associated translocations, and proteins thought to be upstream regulators of HOX gene expression are also found in translocations. These include CDX2, an upstream regulator of HOX gene expression in colonic epithelial cells, which is involved in a TEL/CDX2 fusion associated with t(12;13) (285,286), and a diverse group of translocations involving the MLL gene product, also thought to be an upstream regulator of HOX gene expression (287–290).

HOX gene expression is tightly regulated during hematopoietic development. HOXA9, for example, is expressed in early hematopoietic progenitor cells but is down-regulated during hematopoietic differentiation and is undetectable in terminally differentiated cells. Thus, unregulated overexpression of the HOXA9 moiety from the constitutively active NUP98 promoter may result in aberrant differentiation. Experimental support for this hypothesis includes the observation that the NUP98/HOXA9 fusion protein can transform 3T3 fibroblasts, an activity that requires the HOXA9 DNA binding domain (291). The NUP98 moiety may also provide more than just an active promoter. First, there is now a spectrum of fusion proteins that involve components of the nuclear pore. These include NUP98 and NUP214 fused to a diverse group of partners: NUP98 to HOX family members HOXA9 and HOXD13, and NUP214 to the DDX10, PMX1, and DEK genes (292–295).

It is plausible that these fusions also result in aberrant nuclear pore function in leukemic cells. In addition, the NUP98 moiety itself has been reported to have transactivating function in the context of the NUP98/HOXA9 fusion in that deletion of FG repeat elements within NUP98 impairs transactivation by NUP98/HOXA9 (291). Furthermore, this domain has been shown to interact with transcriptional coactivator CBP/p300 (291). Together, these data indicate that the NUP98/HOXA9 fusion transforms hematopoietic progenitors in part through dysregulated overexpression, and through transactivation mediated through the NUP98 transactivation domain that recruits CBP. Recent evidence indicates, however, that like the other gene rearrangements involving hematopoietic transcription factors, expression of NUP98/HOXA9 alone is not sufficient to cause leukemia. In murine bone marrow transplant models, NUP98/HOXA9 induces AML only after markedly prolonged latencies, indicative of a requirement for second mutation (291).

Translocations Involving the MLL (ALL1, HRX, HTRX) Gene

MLL (for mixed lineage leukemia 1) is also known as ALL1 (acute lymphoblastic leukemia 1), as well as HRX and Htrx, based on homology to the *Drosophila* developmental gene trithorax. It is located at human chromosome band 11q23 and is involved in more than 40 different chromosomal translocations with a remarkably diverse group of fusion partners (234,296). The majority of patients with 11q23 abnormalities have M5 or M4 leukemias, and a smaller fraction have M2 leukemias (230). Therapy-related MDS/AML often has abnormalities in 11q23, especially in patients with previous therapy with topoisomerase inhibitors such as epipodophyllotoxins. In fact, the t(11;16)(q23;p13.3) translocation resulting in a MLL-CBP fusion is associated exclusively with previous therapy (297). The consequence of 11q23 translocations is expression of a fusion gene containing amino terminal MLL sequences fused to a wide variety of fusion partners. Although the function of most of the fusion partners is poorly understood, specific fusions may correspond to a specific phenotype. For example, the MLL-AF4 fusion associated with t(4;11) is frequently observed in infant leukemias and is associated with an ALL phenotype in more than 90% of cases, whereas the MLL-AF9 fusion associated with the t(9;11) is almost exclusively associated with AML (298,299). In addition, the MLL fusion genes may carry specific prognostic information. For example, a study conducted by the CALGB suggested that patients with t(9;11)(p22;q23) have a better outcome than patients with other translocations involving 11q23 (300) (Fig. 15-3).

The *MLL* gene encodes a large, ubiquitously expressed protein. Based on homology with the *Drosophila* protein trithorax, it was thought that MLL might be required for maintenance of *HOX* gene activity. In support of this hypothesis, mice that lack *Mll* express HoxA7 but are not able to maintain expression (287,289). Mice that have homozygous deficiency for *Mll* have an embryonic lethal phenotype at day postconception 10.5. Even heterozygous animals have development anomalies in the axial skeleton and hematopoietic defects including anemia (287,289). Thus, as for other genes targeted by chromosomal translocations, *MLL* is important for normal hematopoietic development.

The function of the *MLL* fusion genes in leukemia is not well understood, but cell culture and murine models have provided some insights into transforming activity of the fusion proteins. The MLL protein of the fusion protein retains the amino termi-

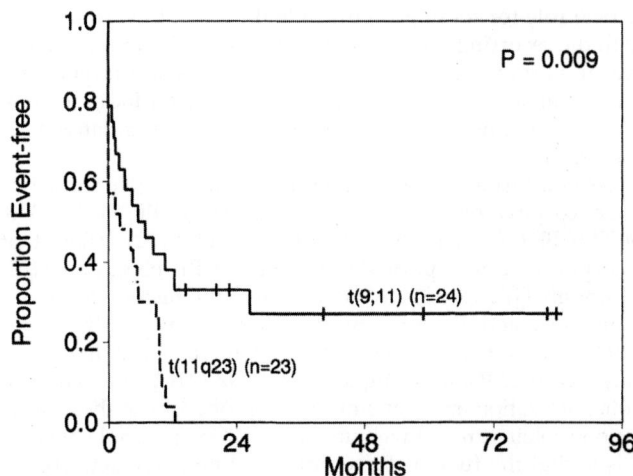

Figure 15-3. Probability of overall survival for patients with t(9;11) compared with those with t(11q23). [From Mrozek K, Heinonen K, Lawrence D, et al. Adult patients with de novo acute myeloid leukemia and t(9;11)(p22;q23) have a superior outcome to patients with other translocations involving band 11q23: a Cancer and Leukemia Group B study. *Blood* 1997;90:4532–4538.]

nal AT hooks that facilitate binding to DNA as well as a methyltransferase domain. With exception of CBP/p300, the function of the broad spectrum of divergent fusion partners is poorly understood. In fact, the remarkable divergence of partners has suggested that alteration in the MLL gene itself is a critical required event for transformation. In support of a central role of *MLL* rearrangement in AML, it has recently been reported that internal tandem duplications of MLL are associated with AML, in particular AML associated with +11 (301).

MLL fusion genes have transforming properties both in serial replating assays in retrovirally transduced hematopoietic progenitors (296) and in murine models of disease (302–304). Although various MLL fusions have similar transforming properties *in vitro*, there are distinctive differences in disease penetrance and latency in the murine models depending on the fusion partner. Thus, the MLL gene rearrangement may be critical for transformation, whereas the fusion partners confer properties related to differences in disease phenotype. The long latency of disease in murine knock-in and bone marrow transplant models of leukemia supports the hypothesis that MLL fusions, like the PML/RAR-α and CBF-related fusion proteins, require second mutations to cause leukemia (302–304).

The t(4;11)(q21;q23) may also be observed in AML, particularly in infants and children (214,305–307). This translocation was originally described in association with ALL, but later studies documented the myeloid or hybrid nature of blasts in some of the patients (308). New insights into pathogenesis of infant acute leukemia associated with the t(4;11) MLL-AF4 fusion have been gained from analysis of global patterns of gene expression (290). These analyses indicate that infant leukemia with the MLL-AF4 fusion represents a distinct subclass of leukemia that can be readily delineated from AML or ALL by gene expression profiles. These data, and the target genes that are overexpressed in infant leukemia with the MLL-AF4 fusion such as FLT3 (290), suggest novel approaches to therapy of this subtype of leukemia.

Transcriptional Regulatory Proteins Involved in Chromosomal Translocations

The recruitment of transcriptional coactivators and corepressors by transcription factors involved in leukemia suggests a critical role for these proteins in leukemogenesis. In keeping with the recurring theme that the diverse and numerous chromosomal translocations in leukemia may share targets and functional activity, there are chromosomal translocations that involve proteins that modulate and facilitate regulated gene expression.

Several fusions associated with leukemia involve transcriptional coactivators. These include the MLL/CBP, MLL/p300, MOZ/CBP (297,309,310), and MOZ/TIF2 (311,312) fusions that incorporate transcriptional coactivators CBP, p300, and TIF2. Although TIF2 itself is not known to have histone acetylase transferase activity, a hallmark of the coactivators CBP and p300, it has a well characterized CBP interaction domain that may recruit CBP into a complex with MOZ/TIF2. The transcriptional activation and transformation properties of these large fusion proteins are not well understood. One plausible hypothesis is that the fusions have dominant negative activity for CBP/p300, or that the translocation leads to simple loss of function of CBP expressed from one allele. In support of this hypothesis, loss of a single allele of CBP/p300 in the human Rubenstein-Taybi syndrome increases predisposition to malignancies, including colon cancer.

Deletions and Numeric Abnormalities of Chromosomes

Deletions of all or part of chromosomes 5 and 7 and trisomy 8 are generally not associated with a specific FAB subtype of AML (313–315). They are considerably more frequent in older patients, whereas the frequency of the specific translocations and inversions decreases with age (316). In addition, older adults have high expression of the multidrug resistance glycoprotein MDR1 (71%), which is associated with a lower CR rate than nonexpression of MDR1 (316). These same abnormalities (+8, -7, -5/5q-) are more common in patients with an antecedent MDS (178,179), therapy-related AML, and suspected exposure to environmental mutagens (317). In contrast, specific translocations are relatively less common in these patient groups. An exception is AML that develops in patients who have received high doses of epipodophyllotoxins (VP 16 or VM 26) for treatment of a previous malignancy (282,283). Translocations involving 11q23 are commonly observed in this setting (318,319). Trisomy 8 is the most frequent numeric cytogenetic abnormality in AML (320). The outcome of patients with trisomy 8 appears to depend on the prognosis of associated cytogenetic abnormalities (320).

The frequent involvement of chromosome 5q is of interest because the genes encoding several hematopoietic growth factors and their receptors are located in this arm, including GM-CSF (5q23-31), IL-3 (5q23-31), and IL-4 (5q23-31) (321). The M-CSF receptor, c-*fms*, and the PDGFβR are also on this chromosome, at 5q33. The genes for GM-CSF and IL-3 and for c-*fms* and the PDGFβR are structurally similar and appear to have arisen from gene duplication events (243,322). In some 5q- chromosome defects, one or more of these genes may be deleted (321). There has been an intensive effort to identify putative tumor-suppressor genes in several critically deleted regions of chromosome 5q, as well as 7q and 20q (323–330). In addition, genomic-wide loss of heterozygosity screens have identified a spectrum of other deletions associated with AML (331).

Thus far, however, no gene has been identified that meets the criteria for a classic tumor suppressor in which one allele is deleted and the other allele contains loss of function mutations in the 5q, 7q, or 20q deleted regions in MDS or AML. There are several possible explanations for the difficulty in identification of classic tumor suppressors, despite availability of complete genomic sequence and detailed annotations of expressed sequences in these regions. The residual allele may be affected by mutations that interfere with expression, such as promoter or aberrant methylation or both, but do not affect coding sequence. These types of mutations are more difficult to detect. Alternatively, it is possible that haploinsufficiency for one or more genes in the critically deleted loci is responsible for the MDS/AML phenotype. Haploinsufficiency for the transcription factor AML1 has been reported in a familial leukemia syndrome and has been increasingly identified as the genetic basis for human inherited diseases (332,333).

Point Mutations in Acute Myelogenous Leukemia

RAS

There is an extensive literature that documents the presence of activating mutations in RAS associated with AML and MDS, typically at codons 12; 13 or 61, or N- and K-RAS (Fig. 15-4). The reported incidence varies widely between studies, from 25% to 44% [reviewed in (1)]. One carefully conducted cooperative group trial reported an 18% incidence of N-RAS or K-RAS mutations and indicated that RAS mutations conferred a poor prognosis (2). There has been considerable effort to develop small molecule inhibitors of RAS activation, with a focus on farnesyl transferase and geranylgeranylation inhibitors that preclude appropriate targeting of activated RAS to the plasma membrane (334,335). This remains an attractive approach to target activating mutations in RAS specifically. Although prenyl transferases inhibitors appear to have activity in AML, it is not clear that activity correlates with activating mutations in RAS

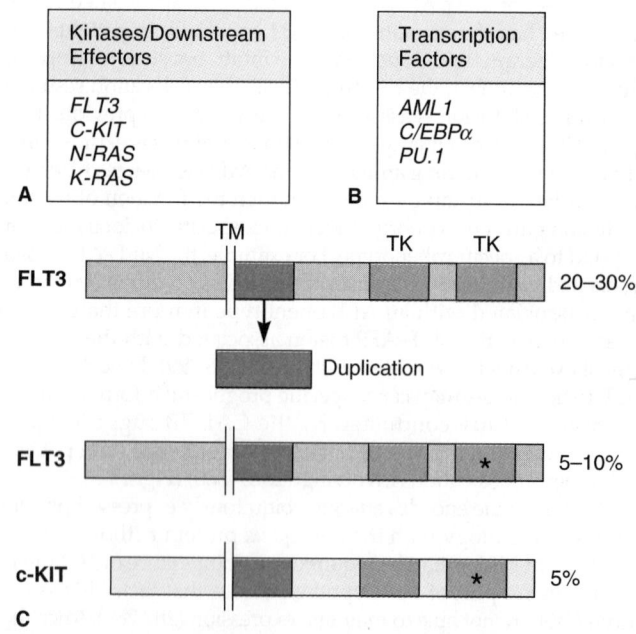

Figure 15-4. Point mutations in leukemia. Point mutations have been discovered in a spectrum of genes. These include the following. **A:** Mutations in the RAS family members and the hematopoietic receptor tyrosine kinases FLT3 and c-KIT confer proliferative and survival signals to cells. **B:** Loss-of-function point mutations in AML1, C/EPBα, and PU.1 are likely to impair hematopoietic differentiation. **C:** Activating mutations in FLT3 and c-KIT. Of AML, 20% to 25% have juxtamembrane repeats of amino acids ranging from 3 to 42 amino acids in length that activate the FLT3 kinase. So-called activating loop mutations occur in FLT3 and in c-KIT in approximately 5% and 10% of AML, respectively. TK, tyrosine kinase domain; TM, transmembrane domain.

(336). There are several possible interpretations of these observations, including the possibility that RAS is activated by mechanisms other than intrinsic point mutations, or that other proteins that are targets of prenylation are important in leukemia pathogenesis.

FLT3 AND C-KIT

However, perhaps the most exciting recent development in pathogenesis of acute myeloid leukemias over the past several years has been identification and characterization of activating mutations in hematopoietic tyrosine kinases. There is substantial evidence that chromosomal translocations that activate tyrosine kinases can contribute to the pathogenesis of chronic myeloid leukemia syndromes. The most common of these is the BCR/ABL gene rearrangement, but other examples include the TEL/ABL, TEL/PDGFβR, TEL/JAK2, H4/PDGFβR, and HIP1/PDG-FβR and rapabtin/PDGFβR fusion proteins (337–345). However, these fusion genes are only rarely encountered in acute myeloid leukemias. Approximately 1% to 2% of cases of de novo AML have the BCR/ABL gene rearrangement (346–348). In addition, there are very rare cases of disease progression from CML to AML associated with acquisition of second mutations such as the NUP98/HOXA9, AML1/ETO, or AML1/EVI1 rearrangement noted. However, until recently, there had been no direct evidence for involvement of activated tyrosine kinases in the vast majority of cases of AML by cytogenetic, fluorescence in situ hybridization, or spectral karyotype analysis. However, point mutations and unusual juxtamembrane repeat mutations that activate FLT3 and c-KIT have been identified in a significant proportion of AML cases. These findings may have important therapeutic implications with the recent demonstration of the efficacy of molecular targeting of the ABL kinase in BCR/ABL-positive CML and CML blast crisis with STI571 (349–352).

Activating mutations in FLT3 have been reported in approximately 30% to 35% of cases of AML. In 20% to 25% of cases, there are tandem internal duplications of the juxtamembrane domain (353) that are now known to result in constitutive activation of FLT3. In an additional 5% to 10% of cases, there are so-called activating loop mutations that occur at position D835 in the tyrosine kinase (354,355). Several large studies have confirmed the frequency of these mutations in both adult and pediatric AML populations and indicated that mutations in FLT3 appear to confer a poor prognosis (356–358). In addition, it has been observed that FLT3 mutations may occur in conjunction with known gene rearrangements such as AML1/ETO, PML/RAR-α, CBFβ/SMMHC, or MLL. Analogous activating loop mutations at position D816 have also been reported in c-KIT in approximately 5% of cases of AML. These data suggest that constitutive activation of tyrosine kinases may play an important role in the pathogenesis of acute leukemia as well as in CML. Based on these data, it is plausible that additional mutations that activate hematopoietic tyrosine kinases may be discovered.

AML1

AML1 (also known as RUNX1 or CBFA2) is a frequent target of translocations in human leukemias. In addition, it has recently been determined that loss of function mutations in AML1 are responsible for the inherited leukemia syndrome familial platelet disorder with propensity to develop acute myelogenous leukemia (332). In addition, approximately 3% to 5% of sporadic cases of AML harbor loss of function mutations in AML1 (359,360), with a higher frequency in M0 AML (25%) and in AML or MDS with trisomy 21. It is not known whether loss of function mutations in AML1 confer the favorable prognosis associated with translocations involving the AML1 gene.

C/EBPα

C/EBPα is a hematopoietic transcription factor required for normal myeloid lineage development. Because many translocations associated with acute myeloid leukemia phenotypes result in loss of function of hematopoietic transcription factors, it has been hypothesized that C/EBPα may also be a target of loss of function mutations in human leukemia. Evidence to support this hypothesis has recently been reported. Point mutations that result in expression of a mutant C/EBPα protein that has dominant negative activity for wild-type C/EBPα (361) have been reported in a fraction of M2 AML cases. Thus, these mutations would be predicted to impair hematopoietic differentiation.

Cooperating Oncogenes in Acute Myelogenous Leukemia

There are several lines of evidence that demonstrate that more than one mutation is necessary for the pathogenesis of AML. First, there is evidence for acquisition of additional cytogenetic abnormalities with disease progression from CML to AML (i.e., CML blast crisis). Published examples of progression in BCR/ABL-positive CML include acquisition of t(3;21) AML1/EVI1 or t(7;11) NUP98/HOXA9 gene rearrangements. Progression of CMML to AML in a patient with the TEL/PDGFβR gene rearrangement was associated with acquisition of a t(8;21) AML1/ETO gene rearrangement (337). Second, expression of the AML1/ETO or CBFβMYH11 fusion proteins in murine models is not sufficient to cause AML (279,280). Chemical mutagens must be used in these contexts to generate second mutations that cause the AML phenotype. Third, recent evidence indicates that, in some cases, the TEL/AML1 gene rearrangement may be acquired in utero, but ALL does not develop until years later, indicating a requirement for a second mutation (362–364). Fourth, transgenic mice that express the PML/RAR-α fusion protein develop AML only after a long latency of 3 to 6 months, with incomplete penetrance, indicating a need for a second mutation.

What is the nature of the cooperating mutations? The cases of disease progressions from CML to AML suggest the hypothesis that constitutively activated tyrosine kinases or RAS cooperates with mutations in hematopoietic transcription factors to cause the AML phenotype (Fig. 15-5B). In this model, the constitutively activated tyrosine kinase or RAS confers a proliferative or survival advantage, or both, to cells, but does not affect differentiation. The second mutation, such as AML1/ETO or PML/RAR-α serves primarily to impair hematopoietic differentiation. In support of this hypothesis, expression of BCR/ABL (365) or TEL/PDGFβR (366), as well as activated N-RAS (367), causes a myeloproliferative syndrome but does not cause acute leukemia in murine bone marrow transplantation models. In addition, as noted, genotypic analysis of some patients has shown concurrence of activating mutations in tyrosine kinases such as FLT3 or c-KIT and loss of function mutations in, for example, the AML1 gene. This two-hit hypothesis can be tested in animal models and may have important therapeutic implications. For example, it may be possible to improve AML outcome by incorporating specific tyrosine kinase inhibitors into therapeutic regimens. Proof of principle for this approach has been demonstrated in treatment of CML blast crisis with the ABL-specific inhibitor STI571.

In summary, specific karyotypic abnormalities are common in AML and may be associated with specific clinical syndromes, such as the association of t(15;17) with promyelocytic leukemia and inv(16) with eosinophilia and M4 AML. Cytogenetics abnormalities can be divided into those associated with favorable prognosis [t(8;21), t(16;16) and inv(16), t(15;17)]; those with an intermediate prognosis (normal karyotype, trisomy 8); and

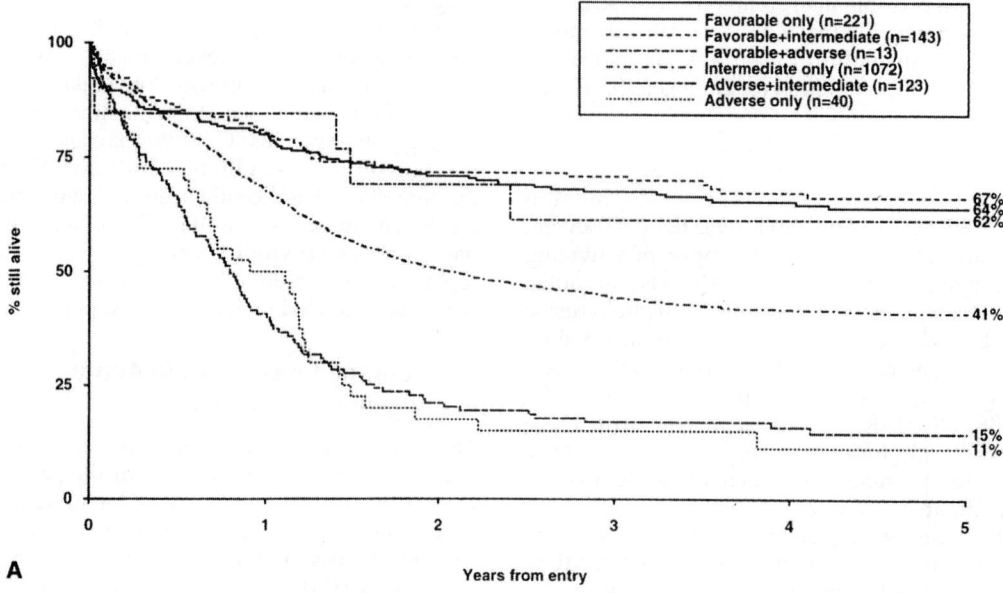

A

Years from entry

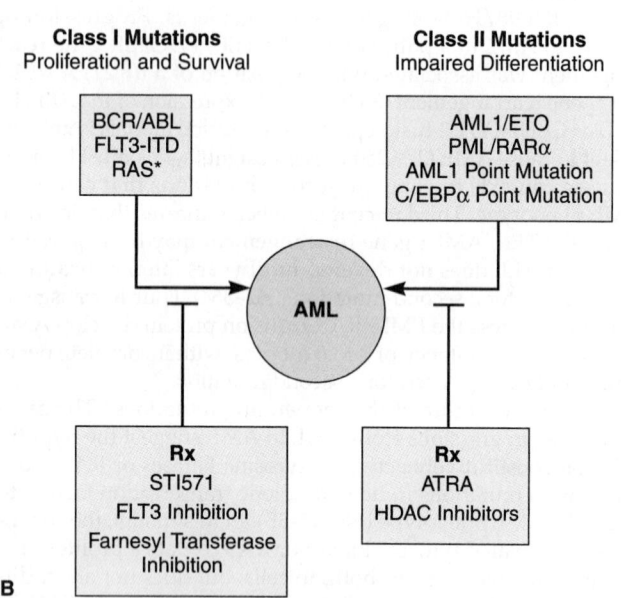

Class I Mutations
Proliferation and Survival

Class II Mutations
Impaired Differentiation

B

Figure 15-5. A: Influence of additional cytogenetic abnormalities on overall survival in acute myelogenous leukemia. (From Grimwade D, Walker H, Oliver F, et al. The importance of diagnostic cytogenetics on outcome in AML: analysis of 1,612 patients entered into the MRC AML 10 trial. The Medical Research Council Adult and Children's Leukaemia Working Parties. *Blood* 1998;92:2322–2333, with permission.) **B:** Model for cooperation between gene rearrangements and mutations that confer a proliferative advantage, a survival advantage, or both to leukemia cells, and those that impair hematopoietic differentiation. Class 1 mutations, exemplified by activating mutations in tyrosine kinases such as BCR/ABL or FLT3, or their downstream effectors such as RAS, result in enhanced proliferative and survival advantage for cells. These mutations can be targeted by specific inhibitors of ABL, such as STI571, or specific FLT3 inhibitors, whereas RAS may be targeted with prenyltransferase inhibitors. Class II mutations are loss of function mutations in hematopoietic receptor tyrosine kinases, as exemplified by the AML1/ETO or PML/RAR-α gene rearrangements, or point mutations in AML1 and C/EBPα. Treatment that targets this class of mutations can include agents that specifically induce differentiation and apoptosis of leukemic cells, as demonstrated by the use of all-*trans*-retinoic acid (ATRA) in PML/RAR-α–positive acute promyelocytic leukemia, and potentially by histone deacetylase inhibitors.

those with an unfavorable prognosis (-5, -7, -5q, 7q-, most 11q23, complex karyotypes) (368,369) (Fig. 15-5A). Identification and characterization of the other new genes involved in AML represents a major challenge for the next decades of research in AML. It is likely that the specific translocations activate or otherwise dysregulate genes controlling proliferation and differentiation of myeloid cells, contributing to leukemogenesis. New therapeutic interventions such as ATRA or histone deacetylase inhibitors may relieve impaired differentiation in hematopoietic cells mediated by fusion genes involving hematopoietic transcription factors. In addition, it is plausible that small molecule inhibitors that target activated tyrosine kinases such as FLT3 may prove to be useful additions to the armamentarium of AML drugs.

CLINICAL PRESENTATION

The symptoms of AML may be as nonspecific as weight loss, fatigue, and weakness but more commonly include pallor, fever, and bleeding (370). These symptoms are usually due to

anemia, neutropenia, and thrombocytopenia, which are secondary to decreased normal myelopoiesis from leukemic replacement of the bone marrow. Patients rarely have symptoms for more than 6 months before diagnosis and often for only 1 to several months. AML rarely presents as an incidental finding on a routine blood count in an asymptomatic patient.

Approximately one-third of patients have petechiae, bruising, oral bleeding, or epistaxis. Patients with APL often have more extensive and life-threatening bleeding because of disseminated intravascular coagulation (DIC) and fibrinolysis (Fig. 15-6). Another one-third of patients present with fever and a serious bacterial infection. Common sites of infection include the respiratory tract, gums, teeth, sinuses, urinary tract, perirectal area, and skin. Approximately 5% of patients present with signs and symptoms that reflect pulmonary or intracerebral leukostasis (371,372). These may include tachypnea, rales, stupor, coma, or stroke.

The most common sites of clinically overt extramedullary leukemic infiltration include superficial lymph nodes, liver, spleen, gingiva, central nervous system (CNS), and skin. Bulky lymphadenopathy and mediastinal involvement are rare in

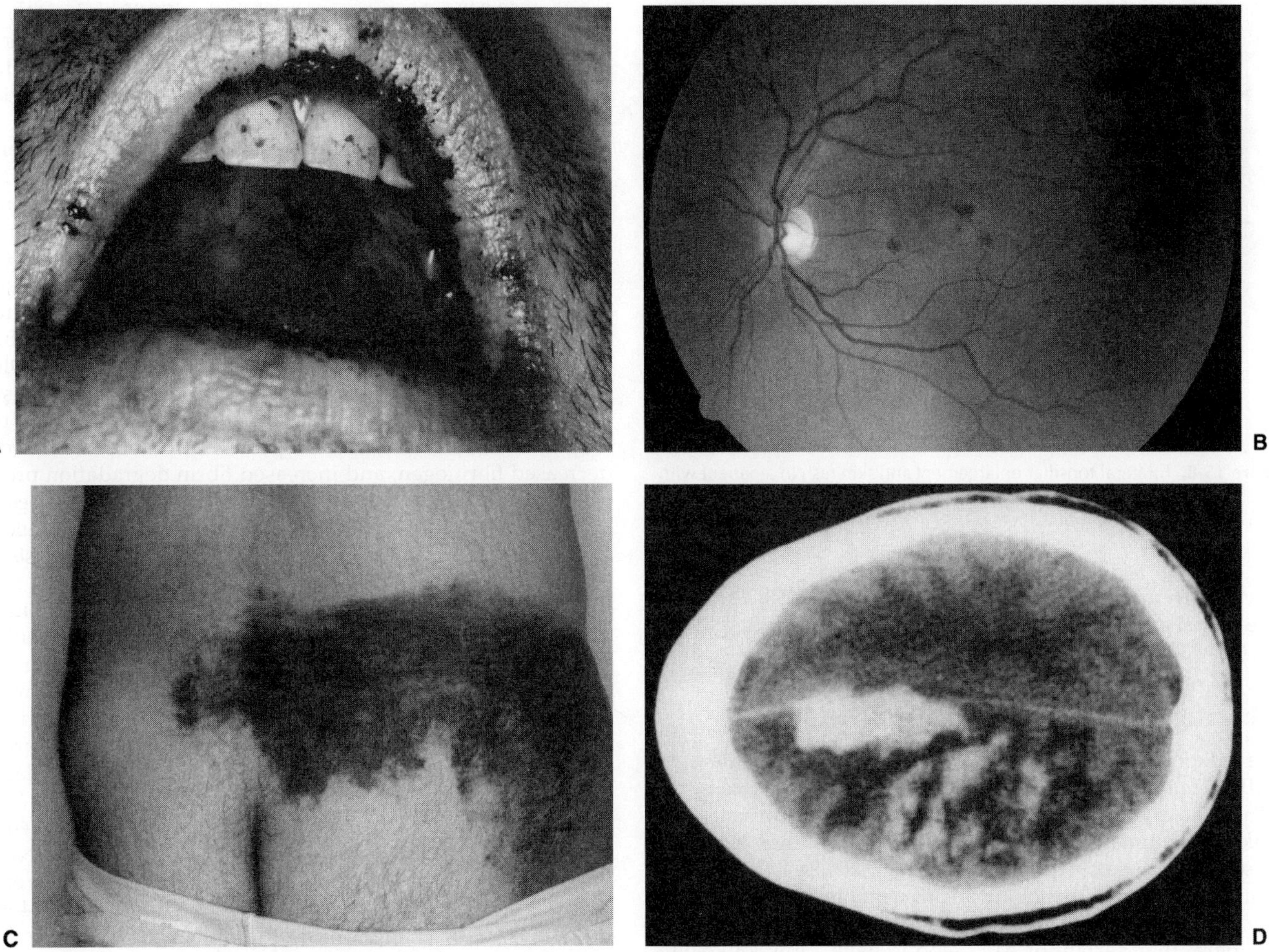

Figure 15-6. Various hemorrhagic complications at presentation in patients with acute promyelocytic leukemia, including **(A)** oral mucosal bleeding, **(B)** retinal hemorrhages, **(C)** extensive subcutaneous bleeding, and **(D)** intracerebral hemorrhage. (See Color Fig. 15-6A–C.)

patients with AML. Leukemic infiltrates in the adenoids, tonsils, or paratracheal area may result in airway obstruction. Splenomegaly is found in approximately 25% of patients. Bone pain or tenderness and joint pain or swelling may be initial presenting complaints, but these symptoms are more commonly associated with ALL.

Gingival hypertrophy, signs of meningeal leukemia, and leukemia cutis (Fig. 15-7) are much more commonly associated with the monocytic or myelomonocytic subtypes (M4, M5) of AML (373–376). Interestingly, most neonates with AML have the M5 subtype and present with skin infiltrates that often appear as slate-blue, subcutaneous nodules (377). Skin infiltration in acute monocytic leukemia may be associated with the expression of T-cell antigens (378) (Fig. 15-8).

Approximately 2% of patients with AML present with signs and symptoms related to discrete tumors. These tumors are composed of immature myeloid cells and are referred to as *myeloblastomas, chloromas,* or *granulocytic sarcomas* (379–381). Myeloblastomas may be the initial clinical manifestation of AML or may herald bone marrow and blood involvement by weeks to months (381–383). They may be found in virtually any location but especially the orbit, paranasal sinuses, brain, spinal cord, bone, breast, skin, and subcutaneous tissues. These tumors were originally called *chloromas* because of their greenish color secondary to a high myeloperoxidase content. In the past, these tumors were often misdiagnosed as diffuse lymphomas or anaplastic

carcinomas. Histochemical and immunoperoxidase studies are helpful in establishing the correct diagnosis. There appears to be an association between the FAB M2 subtype with t(8;21) and extramedullary disease (384–386) (Fig. 15-9). This association

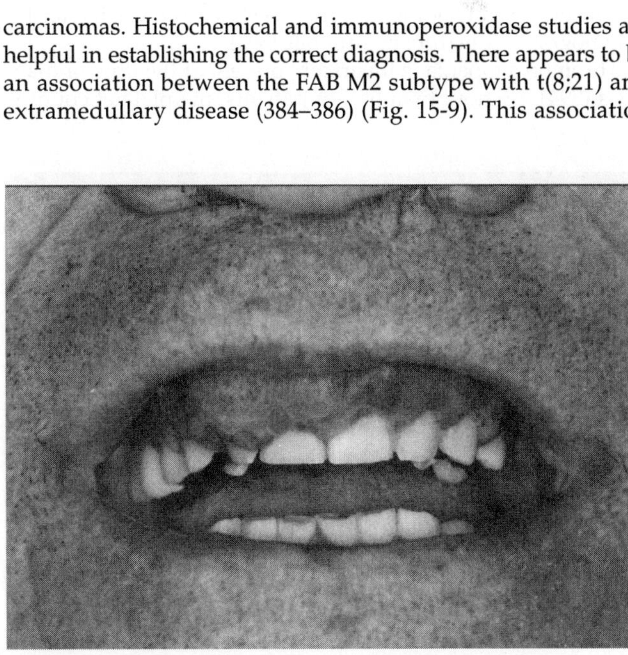

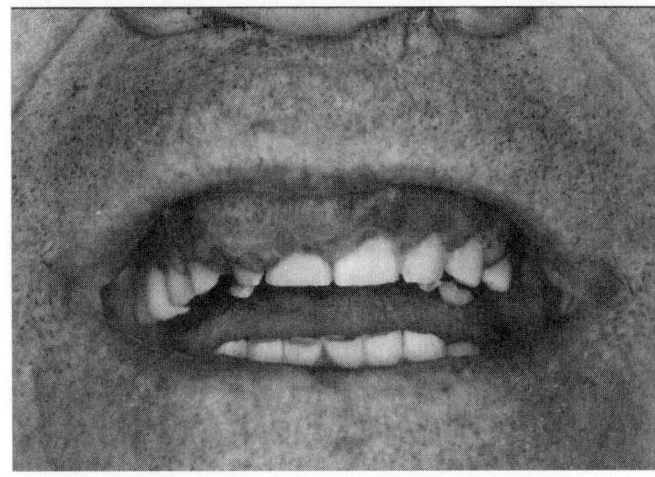

Figure 15-7. Gingival hypertrophy in a patient with French/American/British M5. (See Color Fig. 15-7.) (Courtesy of Dr. Martin Tallman, Northwestern University Medical School, Chicago.)

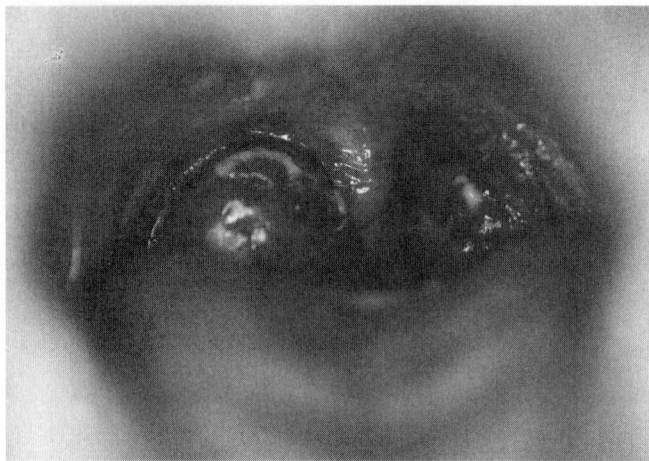

Figure 15-8. Bilateral tonsillar enlargement and skin rash in a patient with M5a. (See Color Fig. 15-8.) (Courtesy of Dr. Martin Tallman, Northwestern University Medical School, Chicago.)

may be attributable in part to the expression of CD56, a cell surface neural adhesion molecule responsible for trafficking of the cell (387,388).

Laboratory Findings at Diagnosis

The leukocyte counts at the time of diagnosis in patients with AML can vary from 100 cells/µL to more than 1,000,000 cells/µL (176,389). Approximately 15% to 20% of patients present with leukocyte counts greater than 100,000/µL, but most patients present with leukocyte counts less than 50,000/µL. The highest counts have been observed in patients with the M4 and M5 subtypes of AML (390,391), whereas patients with M3, except the microgranular variant of APL, tend to have a low leukocyte count at diagnosis (392). The differential leukocyte count reveals less than 1000 neutrophils/µL and a variable percentage of blasts in most patients. In approximately 10% of patients, no peripheral blasts are detectable. Other leukocyte abnormalities may be present, including Pelger-Huët (discussed in Chapter 19) or hypogranular mature neutrophils (393).

Thrombocytopenia is invariably present at the time of diagnosis (394). In more than half of patients, the platelet count is

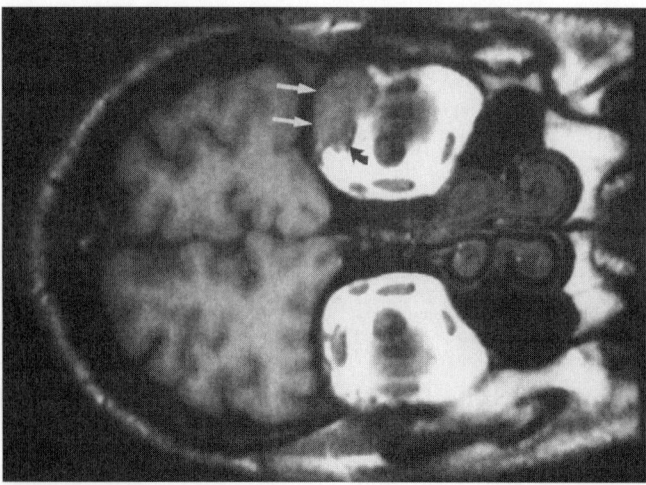

Figure 15-9. Chloroma (*arrows*) in a patient with M2 t(8;21) otherwise in complete remission. (Courtesy of Dr. Martin Tallman, Northwestern University Medical School, Chicago.)

less than 50,000/µL, and counts of less than 20,000/µL are common. Giant platelets and poorly granulated platelets with functional abnormalities can occur (395). Thrombocytopenia is due to decreased platelet production, reduced megakaryocytes accompanying leukemic infiltration of the bone marrow, or DIC. Hypersplenism as a cause of thrombocytopenia is uncommon in patients with acute leukemia.

Almost all patients have a normocytic, normochromic anemia (hematocrit, 25% to 35%) with occasional nucleated red blood cells (RBCs) and teardrop forms seen on peripheral blood smear (176,307). The anemia is secondary to either decreased RBC production or blood loss (396). The rare hemolytic anemia associated with AML is usually not immune-mediated but rather a microangiopathic hemolytic anemia secondary to DIC. The serum uric acid and lactate dehydrogenase (LDH) are usually modestly elevated (307). Laboratory evidence of DIC (prolonged prothrombin time and partial thromboplastin time, decreased fibrinogen, and increased fibrin degradation products) is commonly associated with the M3 and M5 subtypes of AML (397–401). In patients with the M3 subtype, the coagulopathy is a complex process and includes primary fibrinolysis in addition to DIC (400,401).

The typical bone marrow findings include a hypercellular biopsy sample and an aspirate showing more than half leukemic cells (more than 30% are required by FAB criteria for the diagnosis of AML) (307,370). The bone marrow biopsy may be hypocellular, especially in elderly men and in patients with an antecedent hematologic disorder (i.e., paroxysmal nocturnal hemoglobinuria, Fanconi's anemia, or MDS) or therapy-related AML (402,403). Patients with AML rarely have fewer than 30% bone marrow blasts but more than 30% peripheral blasts (404). Patients with AML, especially those with M6 or M7 or a preceding MDS, may show morphologic abnormalities in the erythroid, granulocytic, and megakaryocytic lineages (405,406). These dysplastic changes of multiple lineages are consistent with a malignant transformation of a primitive multipotential progenitor or stem cell.

Differential Diagnosis

Most cases of AML can be readily diagnosed after an examination of the peripheral blood and bone marrow aspirate and biopsy. As discussed, AML in infants with Down's syndrome needs to be differentiated from the transient myeloproliferative syndrome (96). In some situations, it may be difficult to distinguish MDS from AML (407), such as in the setting of a hypoplastic marrow with occasional blasts or M2 AML with marked myeloid differentiation and a low percentage of typical blasts (384).

In a small percentage of patients, other diagnoses must be entertained and systematically excluded. For example, bacterial sepsis may cause either a leukemoid reaction or profound neutropenia (408,409). In this circumstance, the bone marrow aspirate may be confusing. There may be an apparent maturation arrest at the promyelocytic stage of myeloid maturation. This morphologic picture has been confused with APL. With resolution of the sepsis, normal myeloid maturation ensues. Patients with acute infectious mononucleosis may have signs and symptoms similar to those seen in patients with AML. On rare occasions, the atypical lymphocytes have a bizarre mononuclear appearance that may mimic monoblasts, but normal findings on bone marrow examination exclude AML. Acute monocytic leukemia may occasionally be difficult to distinguish from malignant lymphoma because of the clinical presentation of adenopathy, mass lesions, or both, and because of the cytologic appearance of the cells (410–412). Acute monocytic leukemia can also present with myelofibrosis or rash (413,414).

Patterns of Spread

CENTRAL NERVOUS SYSTEM

CNS involvement in patients with AML can be due to meningeal infiltration (415–417), epidural or brain parenchymal myeloblastomas (418), or leukostasis (419–421). Meningeal leukemia is much more common in ALL than in AML. Approximately 5% to 20% of patients with AML either present with (usually with no symptoms) or develop meningeal leukemia during the course of their disease (415–417). It has been postulated that leukemic cells reach the meninges by either hematogenous spread or by direct extension from cranial bone marrow (421). Hematogenous spread may occur as a result of direct perivascular invasion or deposition from petechial hemorrhages in the pia-arachnoid. Alterations in adhesion molecules may be responsible for many of the manifestations of hyperleukocytosis (422). Adhesion molecules such as ICAM-1 and P-selectins play a role in neutrophil-induced lung injury in the setting of sepsis (423,424). Up-regulation of CD54, CD62E, CD62P, and CD106 on the endothelial cells in patients with AML and leukostasis has been observed (425). The most common signs and symptoms of meningeal leukemia reflect increased intracranial pressure and include nausea, vomiting, lethargy, headache, and papilledema. Other signs and symptoms may include meningism, cranial nerve palsy, root pain, and paresthesia. Symptomatic meningeal leukemia is usually not observed at initial diagnosis. Plasma levels of E-selectin, VCAM-1, and ICAM-1 have been found to be elevated significantly in patients with acute leukemia compared to healthy controls, with the highest levels in acute myelomonocytic leukemia, perhaps contributing to the migration of blasts to extramedullary sites (426).

Clinical or laboratory features at diagnosis that have been strongly associated with the development of CNS leukemia include the M4 and M5 subtypes (415,416), high leukocyte counts (371), elevated levels of lysozyme (427), chromosome abnormality inv(16) (270), high serum LDH levels, and extramedullary involvement at other sites. High blood lysozyme and LDH levels and extramedullary leukemia are associated with M4 and M5 AML, probably accounting for their association with meningeal leukemia. The diagnosis of meningeal leukemia is made by examining a cytocentrifuged preparation of cerebrospinal fluid (428). There is usually an increased number of cells in the CSF, with blast cells present. The cytocentrifuge technique is important because this method may reveal blasts despite a normal routine cell count. The spinal fluid is examined only when blasts are cleared from the blood in the absence of neurologic symptoms. On occasion, patients may have clinical evidence of CNS leukemia (i.e., cranial nerve palsy) with negative CSF cytology. In this situation, appropriate CNS therapy should be instituted.

Central nervous system disease in patients with AML may also be secondary to intracranial or epidural myeloblastomas (418). These solid tumors of myeloblasts are believed to arise from hematopoietic tissue and traverse the haversian canals to reach the subperiosteum and dura, and eventually penetrate to the subarachnoid and Virchow-Robin spaces.

Patients with cerebral leukostasis may also develop intraparenchymal brain lesions (419). These nodular leukemic lesions result from blasts invading and penetrating vessel walls.

INTEGUMENTARY

Leukemia cutis has been reported to occur in 2% to 13% of cases of AML (429–434). Skin involvement is associated with M5 AML (especially in neonates) and with extramedullary infiltration at other sites (Fig. 15-8). Such infiltration usually results in small (2-mm to 5-mm) raised pink or salmon-colored nodules or bluish-gray, firm, rubbery nodules (414). The skin lesions are painless and are most common on the extremities or trunk but may involve the face, scalp, and other areas. These lesions may be difficult to distinguish from infection, hemorrhage, or neutrophilic dermatosis (434). Biopsy specimens show dense infiltration of the dermis with or without subcutaneous infiltration by myeloblasts or monoblasts, often with eosinophilic myelocytes. Leukemia cutis may antedate bone marrow involvement or may be a harbinger of imminent marrow relapse. Leukemia cutis can also be associated with vasculitis with vessel involvement ranging from mild microvascular injury to necrotizing arteritis (433).

CARDIAC

Cardiovascular abnormalities due to leukemic infiltration are rarely clinically significant (435,436). Leukemic infiltration of the pericardium, conduction system, and endocardium have been associated with arrhythmia, heart failure, and death.

RESPIRATORY

Leukemic infiltration or myeloblastomas may lead to laryngeal obstruction, pulmonary parenchymal infiltrates, alveolar septal infiltration, or pleural seeding (437–439). Pulmonary leukostasis can also lead to respiratory distress with abnormal radiologic findings (440,441). Pneumonia remains the most common pulmonary lesion associated with AML.

GASTROINTESTINAL

Functional disturbances of the gastrointestinal tract secondary to leukemic infiltration are uncommon. Gingival hypertrophy secondary to leukemic infiltration is commonly associated with AML, especially with acute myelomonocytic and monocytic leukemia (442) (Fig. 15-7). It is not unusual for the dentist to raise the first suspicion of leukemia after seeing the patient with gingival disease. Esophagitis, enterocolitis, and proctitis usually result from chemotherapy-induced mucosal changes and infection during periods of neutropenia (443). Leukemic infiltration of the gastrointestinal tract rarely causes significant bleeding, perforation, or other symptoms (i.e., obstruction).

GENITOURINARY

The kidneys may be diffusely enlarged secondary to leukemic infiltration in a small proportion of cases, but functional abnormalities are extremely unusual (444). Rare cases of bladder neck, prostatic, or testicular involvement with AML have been described (445). Testicular leukemia has been observed in several young boys with M4 or M5 AML (410,446,447).

OSTEOARTICULAR

Osteoarticular symptoms other than bone pain are infrequent in patients with AML (307). Migratory polyarthritis or arthralgia is more common in children with ALL, but these conditions have been observed in patients with AML (448). The most common radiologic findings of bone seen in children with leukemia are osteoporosis and submetaphyseal lucent lines (growth arrest lines), whereas thinning of the cortex of the long bones is seen in adults (449). Periosteal elevation or osteolytic lesions are uncommon. Myeloblastomas of bone may give the radiologic appearance of an expanding geographic lesion with well-defined but irregular nonsclerotic margins.

OCULAR

Approximately 40% to 50% of patients with AML have ocular manifestations of leukemia at diagnosis (450–452). Leukemic infiltration of the optic nerve, choroid, and retina is rare, but secondary ophthalmic manifestations, including intraretinal

TABLE 15-7. Patient Characteristics Related to Complete Remission Rate

Characteristic	Favorable Value
Cytogenetics	t(8;21) or inv(16)
Secondary acute myelogenous leukemia	Not present
Age	<60 yr
Leukocyte count	<100,000/µL
French/American/British subtype	M1, M2, M4, M5
Auer rods	Present
Albumin	>3.5 g/dL
Creatinine	<1.1 mg/dL
Leukemia blast self-renewal	Low
Fibrinogen	>250 mg%

hemorrhage, cotton-wool spots, white-centered retinal hemorrhages, central vein obstruction, and vitreous hemorrhage, are more commonly observed. Controversy exists concerning the relation between fundus findings in leukemic retinopathy and hematologic parameters, such as platelet count, hematocrit, and leukocyte count (452). In all studies, patients with retinopathy had significantly lower platelet counts than those without retinopathy. Some studies have found a relation between retinopathy and low hematocrit.

Leukemic infiltration of the eye requires prompt recognition to save vision. Local irradiation combined with intrathecal chemotherapy is recommended in such cases. Leukemic ocular infiltrates are often associated with other evidence of CNS leukemia but may represent the first detectable site of relapse. Anterior chamber involvement is rare but has been reported as the site of first or subsequent relapse in both ALL and AML (453). The conjunctiva may also be the site of relapse (454).

PROGNOSTIC FACTORS

Achieving remission is the prime determinant of survival in patients with AML. The likelihood of achieving remission is age-dependent (Table 15-7), but it is also related to other clinical and laboratory variables (455–463). Factors that have been consistently associated with lower remission rates include age greater than 60 years, poor-risk (unfavorable) chromosomal abnormalities (-5/5q- or -7/7q-), poor performance status, therapy-related AML, and AML that develops secondary to MDS. In many studies, additional adverse prognostic variables have included leukocyte count higher than 100,000/µL, M6 or

M7 AML, low fibrinogen, elevated creatinine, low serum albumin, absence of Auer rods, blasts with low S phase, and a high leukemic blast self-renewal rate (405,463–467).

Failure to achieve remission may result from early death secondary to infection, hemorrhage, leukostasis, or therapy-resistant leukemia. Several of the prognostic variables mentioned, including poor performance status, leukocyte count higher than 100,000/µL, and low albumin, identify patients who are not likely to survive induction because of complications of leukemia and its treatment. On the other hand, the lower remission rates associated with low labeling index (S phase), unfavorable cytogenetics, and therapy-related AML or AML that develops secondary to MDS are chiefly due to resistant leukemia (i.e., persistence of bone marrow blasts after one or two cycles of induction chemotherapy). In addition to having more resistant leukemia, patients with secondary AML or previous MDS have a slow recovery of blood counts after induction chemotherapy, placing them at increased risk for fungal infections and other complications associated with prolonged pancytopenia. The adverse influence of older age on the remission rate is due to a greater risk of early death from toxicity but also to disease-related factors, including a higher incidence of previous MDS and unfavorable cytogenetics (468).

The absence of Auer rods has been shown in some studies to be associated with a low remission rate (463,469). In a recent pediatric AML report (470), the absence of Auer rods in the M1 group was correlated with both a low CR rate and a short duration of remission. The biologic significance of this association is unknown, but Auer rod–negative M1 AML may represent a less differentiated subtype of AML that is relatively chemotherapy resistant.

Prediction of durations of remission in patients with AML based on various clinical, laboratory, or therapy-related factors has been difficult and not consistent from one study to another. For example, there is not a clear relation between age at diagnosis and duration of remission (457,468,471). The Eastern Cooperative Oncology Group has recently analyzed the outcome of 1882 patients treated in clinical trials for newly diagnosed patients conducted between 1974 and 1996, with management including an anthracycline and cytarabine for induction and increasingly intensive postremission therapy (472) (Fig. 15-10). The shortest remissions were observed in patients older than 55 years. Such older adults had a 5-year OS of 7.6%, compared to patients younger than 55 years, who had a 5-year survival of 24% (472). A previous MDS and therapy-related AML are unfavorable factors for both induction response and CR duration (461,462). In several

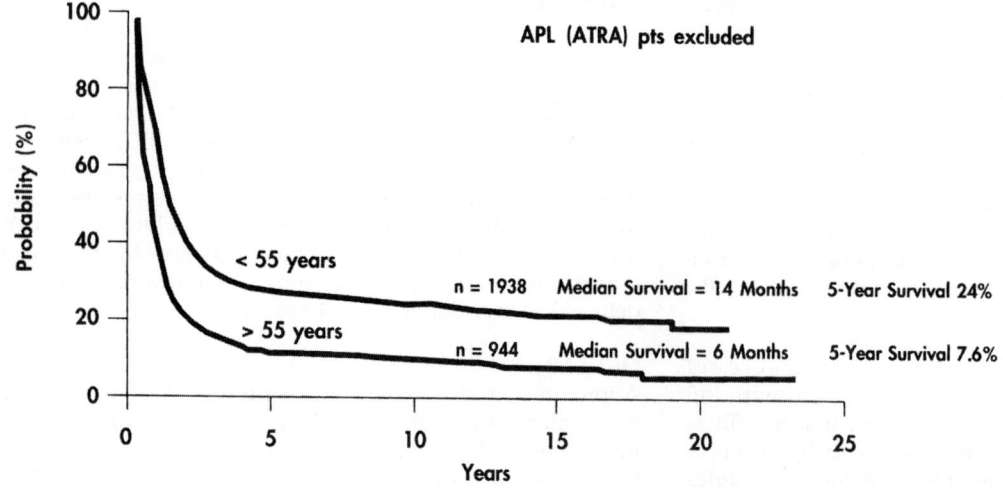

Figure 15-10. Kaplan-Meier analysis of overall survival for adults with acute myeloid leukemia who were treated on Eastern Cooperative Oncology Group protocols between 1974 and 1996. Outcome by age group is statistically significant (p <.001). APL, acute promyelocytic leukemia; ATRA, all-*trans*-retinoic acid. (From Rowe JM. Treatment of acute myelogenous leukemia in older adults. *Leukemia* 2000;14: 480–487, with permission.)

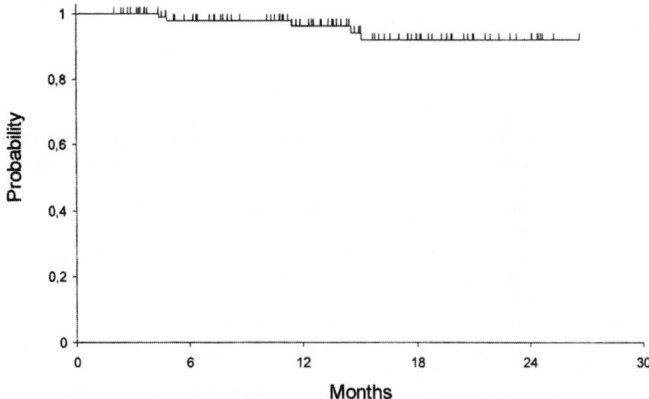

Figure 15-11. Disease-free survival of acute promyelocytic leukemia patient treated with all-*trans*-retinoic acid plus idarubicin, anthracycline-based consolidation, and all-*trans*-retinoic acid + 6-MP + methotrexate maintenance. (From Sanz MA, Martin G, Rayon C, et al. A modified AIDA protocol with anthracycline-based consolidation results in high antileukemic efficacy and reduced toxicity in newly diagnosed PML/RARalpha-positive acute promyelocytic leukemia. PETHEMA group. *Blood* 1999;94:3015–3021, with permission.)

studies, patients (especially children) with M4 and M5 AML and leukocyte counts higher than 30,000/µL have had statistically significant shorter durations of remission compared with those with other FAB subtypes or lower leukocyte counts (405,473). Other studies have not confirmed these findings. Because many prognostic factors are treatment-dependent, more effective or different therapies will likely influence what emerge as important prognostic variables. It is possible, for example, that the adverse impact of M4 and M5 AML is lost with protocols that include an epipodophyllotoxin (446,474).

The cytogenetic findings that predict a low remission rate (-5/5q- and -7/7q-) also associate with short durations of response (457). It appears that patients with inv/del(16)(q22) and t(8;21) have high CR rates and relatively favorable durations of remission (475–477). In several adult studies, patients with rearrangements of band 16q22 also have among the longest remissions (369). It has been recognized for many years that patients with M3 AML can have long remissions if they survive the hemorrhagic complications of remission-induction therapy (478,479). Patients with M3 AML now have the highest cure rates with the introduction of ATRA (478) (Fig. 15-11). In a recently reported pediatric AML trial, children with structural abnormalities involving 11q23 were infants (median age, 6 months) with M4 or M5 AML, hyperleukocytosis, and frequent coagulation abnormalities (480). These infants relapsed early during postremission therapy. This result contrasted with that for children with M5 AML and t(9;11), who had favorable durations of remission, similar to adults with t(9;11) AML (Fig. 15-3).

The Berlin-Frankfurt-Münster Study Group has identified low-risk and high-risk groups of children with AML (470). The low-risk group accounted for 37% of the patients who achieved remission and included those with M1 and Auer rods, M2 with leukocyte counts lower than 20,000/µL, M3, and M4 with eosinophilia. The 6-year relapse-free survival was 91% for the low-risk children and 42% for those in the high-risk category.

THERAPY

The goal of therapy is to reduce and eventually eradicate the leukemic cell population while restoring normal hematopoiesis (allowing return of normal bone marrow function). This goal presupposes that both normal and leukemic cells coexist at diagnosis and that effective therapy will sufficiently reduce the leukemic cell burden to allow regrowth of normal myeloid progenitors. The available data (cytogenetics, G6PD isoenzyme studies, RFLP analyses) suggest that nonneoplastic cells repopulate the marrow after chemotherapy-induced remissions in most patients with AML. If untreated, AML progresses rapidly in most patients, but it may remain indolent or smolder for many weeks in a small percentage of patients (481).

Before the late 1940s, there was no treatment available that could reduce the leukemic cell mass and induce a return of normal marrow function. There were rare reports of spontaneous remissions after viral or bacterial infections or transfusions (482–484). Irradiation with x-rays or γ emissions was successful in reducing high peripheral blast counts or extramedullary organ infiltration, but CR was not achieved (485,486). It was not until the clinical trials of Farber et al. (487) with the folic acid antagonist aminopterin that systemic chemotherapy became the mainstay of therapy for the acute leukemias (Table 15-8). Since 1955, there has been a formal anticancer drug development program supported with public funds at the National Cancer Institute (488). The private sector is also active in drug development. During the period from 1970 to 1985, the National Cancer Institute introduced 83 drugs into clinical trial. Many of these agents, including amsacrine, 5-azacytidine, doxorubicin, etoposide, mitoxantrone, and homoharringtonine, have been shown to be active in AML. During the 1960s, the anthracyclines (doxorubicin, daunorubicin) and cytarabine (cytosine arabinoside), the two most active agents in the treatment of AML, entered clinical trial (489,490). New drug development has had a major impact on therapeutic outcome, but improvements in supportive care made it safe and feasible to treat patients with myelosuppressive therapies. In addition, carefully designed clinical trials in single institutions and through the cooperative group mechanism, and increasing numbers of physicians trained in the complex medical treatment of patients with leukemia, also contributed to increased survival rates.

Until the 1970s, there were few long-term (more than 5 years) survivors of AML. The first chemotherapy regimens that resulted in long-term disease-free survival (DFS) usually included cytarabine and often involved the administration of prolonged courses of maintenance chemotherapy (cytarabine and thioguanine) or rotating combinations of drugs with or without concomitant immunotherapy (491–494). The average remission durations ranged from 6 to 15 months, with approximately 10% to 15% of complete responders remaining in continuous remission for 5 or more years. Actuarial life-table analyses indicated a decreasing hazard of relapse after 3 to 4 years of remission, suggesting that a small proportion of these patients were cured of their AML.

Supportive Care

With the exception of APL, the treatment of AML is rarely an emergent situation, but rather is subacute. The initial hours of treatment are directed toward stabilizing the patient with respect to metabolic parameters, bleeding, fever and infection, and other life-threatening problems, such as a high peripheral blast count or extramedullary leukemic spread (e.g., CNS, epidural chloromas). An indwelling central venous catheter (e.g., Hickman or Broviac) should be placed by a surgeon early in the treatment course unless the patient has APL, in which case the placement of a central catheter should be delayed until any coagulopathy has resolved (495,496) (Table 15-9). This access facilitates administration of chemotherapy, antibiotics, and blood components and also permits repetitive sampling of blood for diagnostic purposes.

TABLE 15-8. Supportive Care in the Treatment of Acute Myelogenous Leukemia

Clinical Problem	Treatment	Comment
Vascular access	Semipermanent central venous catheter	Delay placement in APL until coagulopathy resolves.
Disseminated intravascular coagulation/fibrinolysis	Replacement of factors with FFP and fibrinogen with cryoprecipitate; exclude sepsis	Most common in APL. All-*trans*-retinoic acid in APL corrects coagulopathy. If factor replacement not successful, consider low-dose heparin, especially if evidence of end organ thrombosis.
Anemia	Packed red blood cell transfusion	No clear role for erythropoietin. If increment less than expected, think of alloimmunization.
Thrombocytopenia	Platelet transfusions	Single donor or random donor pooled units. Prophylactic transfusions indicated for level <10,000/μL. If inadequate increment, consider sepsis, DIC, alloimmunization.
Transfusion-refractory thrombocytopenia	Transfusions	HLA-compatible units or crossmatch compatible units
	Other	Consider amino caproic acid if no evidence of DIC and bleeding is significant and platelet count <10,000/μL.
Fever and neutropenia	Empiric broad-spectrum antibiotics	Broad-spectrum antibacterial agents initiated at time of fever. Choice dictated by local microbiology. May require empiric antifungal therapy if prolonged (>3 days) or recurrent fever.
Neutropenia	Protective isolation	May reduce prevalence of disseminated aspergillosis.
	Hematopoietic colony-stimulating factors: G-CSF or GM-CSF	Use reduces median duration of neutropenia. Inconsistent effect on morbidity or hospital stay; no clear impact on survival.
	Prophylactic antibiotics	Does not substantially reduce significant morbidity or mortality. Concern is emergence of resistance.
Tumor lysis syndrome	Preventive measures	Allopurinol and saline hydration to maintain adequate urinary output. Careful attention to serum electrolytes.
Hyperleukocytosis	Therapeutic cytapheresis	Indicated if signs of microvascular compromise or if blasts >50,000/μL.

APL, acute promyelocytic leukemia; DIC, disseminated intravascular coagulation; FFP, fresh frozen plasma; G-CSF, granulocyte colony-stimulating factor; GM-CSF, granulocyte-macrophage colony-stimulating factor.

RBC transfusions should be given to a patient with a modest degree of anemia (hemoglobin, 7 to 8 g/dL) who is about to begin remission-induction therapy. During this phase of therapy, there is an expected 3- to 4-week period of complete bone marrow suppression with profound thrombocytopenia and mucosal (skin, mouth, gastrointestinal tract) injury from chemotherapy. In this situation, maintaining a relatively high hemoglobin level provides some reserve in the case of a major bleeding episode. The blood component of choice is packed RBCs (497). A partial exchange transfusion is sometimes preferred in the severely anemic patient (especially a young infant) with congestive heart failure (498). Many blood banks are beginning to advocate the use of leukocyte-poor or fresh frozen packed RBCs (499,500). Their use minimizes exposure to leukocyte antigens and thus reduces the likelihood of allergic and febrile transfusion reactions. These red cell products have not been known to transmit cytomegalovirus. Several studies also suggest that leukocyte-poor blood products decrease the risk of alloimmunization (501). A continuing controversy surrounds the issue of whether to irradiate blood products to avoid the potentially fatal syndrome of transfusion-associated graft-versus-host disease (GVHD) (502). Although the incidence of transfusion-associated GVHD is exceedingly rare in patients with AML, many investigators recommend irradiation of blood products because it is safe and effective in preventing this disease.

Hemorrhage in the patient with AML is usually secondary to thrombocytopenia. Thrombocytopenia in this setting is nearly always due to decreased production of platelets caused by reduced numbers of megakaryocytes accompanying leukemia cell infiltration of the bone marrow. It may also result from mechanical platelet injury, as seen in patients with M3 AML and DIC (300,301). Bleeding in APL may also arise from a fibrinolytic disorder (397,398,400,401,503). Severe hemorrhage is uncommon until the platelet count falls below 20,000/μL (504). Intensive platelet support is required in a patient with AML who has severe thrombocytopenia and is bleeding. Controversies surrounding the use of single-donor or leukocyte-poor platelet units are discussed elsewhere. Prophylactic platelet transfusions have histori-

TABLE 15-9. Remission-Induction Results in Untreated Patients with Acute Myelogenous Leukemia

Regimen	Percentage Achieving Complete Remission			References
	Children	Age <60 Years	Age >60 Years	
7-and-3 (cytarabine and daunorubicin)	79	70	31	578,580,583
7-and-3 (cytarabine and doxorubicin)	73	58	34	582
Daunorubicin, thioguanine, and cytarabine	82	70	51	574
Cytarabine and mitoxantrone	—	80	46	585
High-dose cytarabine	—	67[a]	—	473

[a]Mean age, 54 ± 17.5 yr. Data not shown for younger than or older than 60 years of age.

cally been recommended by many physicians for patients with AML whose platelet counts are less than 20,000/μL, because these patients have no marrow compensation for bleeding and are believed to be at risk for diffuse mucosal ulceration and bleeding from the toxicity of chemotherapy. The risk of fatal intracranial hemorrhage can theoretically also be reduced if the platelet count is maintained above 5000/μL. These recommendations notwithstanding, there are no controlled studies to support the efficacy of prophylactic platelet transfusions in the nonbleeding thrombocytopenic patient with AML (505,506). However, recent studies show that the threshold for platelet transfusion can be safely lowered to 10,000/μL (507,508). Recent studies evaluating thrombopoietic agents have not shown significant benefit (509).

Disseminated intravascular coagulation and fibrinolysis are seen primarily in patients with septicemia and with M3 (acute promyelocytic leukemia) and M5 (monocytic) AML (510–516). In acute monocytic leukemia, a heparin-like anticoagulant has been described (511). The primary therapy for DIC is treatment of the leukemia (effective cytoreductive chemotherapy) or complicating infectious disease. Platelet and fresh frozen plasma transfusions should be given to patients with DIC. The use of heparin remains controversial in patients with APL but has been all but abandoned with the introduction of ATRA (400,401). In several retrospective studies, the use of heparin (low-dose, 10 to 20 IU/kg/hour, or standard-dose) has been shown to reduce the likelihood of fatal hemorrhagic complications during remission-induction therapy (514,515). This potential benefit of heparin for patients with M3 AML has never been prospectively evaluated in a controlled study (516). Furthermore, ATRA induces rapid correction of the coagulopathy at a median of approximately 4 days (243–246). Therefore, heparin is no longer administered unless there is evidence of end organ damage attributable to thrombolic events.

Most patients with AML are febrile (over 38.5°C) at the time of diagnosis or become febrile within several days after initiation of cytotoxic therapy. Although some of these patients may have fever because of their leukemia, it is probable that most have an overt or occult infection (517). These patients should be rapidly evaluated and given empiric broad-spectrum antibiotic therapy, even if the site of infection is not defined. The use of empiric antibiotics for the febrile, neutropenic (>500 neutrophils/μL) patient has markedly reduced morbidity and mortality rates (518,519).

Most microbiologically documented infections at diagnosis or early during the course of remission induction in patients with AML are caused by endogenous microflora, and some of the responsible pathogens are nosocomially acquired shortly after admission to the hospital (520). The neutropenic AML patient with skin disrupted by chemotherapy or by intravenous catheters is especially susceptible to infection. The patient with AML may first come to medical attention because of an infection (respiratory, dental, sinus, perirectal, urinary tract, or skin) that never fully responds to antibiotic therapy (520). Most pathogens associated with fevers in newly diagnosed patients with AML are bacterial. The antibiotic regimen must cover a broad spectrum to encompass both Gram-positive and enteric Gram-negative bacteria (521).

With the increased use of indwelling venous access devices (Broviac catheters, port-a-caths), catheter-associated bacteremia has become more frequent, and most of these infections are caused by Gram-positive organisms (coagulase-negative staphylococci or hemolytic streptococci) (522). Bacterial pathogens usually predominate as the cause of localized pulmonary infiltrates within the first 2 weeks of induction.

If a period of neutropenia persists to the second to fourth week of induction, patients are more prone to develop a fungal infection, usually *Candida albicans* or *Aspergillus* species (519). It is therefore appropriate to institute empiric antifungal treatment for the patient with AML who is febrile for more than 3 days while on antibiotics or who develops a new pulmonary infiltrate (523,524). Studies have shown that liposomal formulations of amphotericin B are as effective and less toxic than conventional amphotericin B in the setting of persistent fever and neutropenia (524). Bronchoalveolar lavage or open-lung biopsy may also be indicated to establish the diagnosis. Localized pneumonia caused by *Legionella* species must also be considered in the differential diagnosis (525). It is uncommon for a patient with AML to develop *Pneumocystis carinii* infection, herpes simplex virus, or cytomegalovirus pneumonitis during remission induction.

The most common lesions of the oral cavity during remission induction are superficial infections due to *C. albicans* (526). This infection is easily controlled by nystatin suspension 1 million IU four times a day or clotrimazole troches 10 mg four times a day. Herpes simplex is the most common viral pathogen isolated from mucosal lesions (527), and intravenous acyclovir 250 mg/m^2 every 8 hours for 7 to 14 days is the preferred treatment (528). Both *C. albicans* and herpes simplex may cause clinically significant esophagitis (529). Chemotherapeutic agents (especially doxorubicin in combination with cytarabine) are frequently responsible for oral mucositis and esophagitis during remission induction.

The most serious intraabdominal complication observed during remission induction is typhlitis, also called *necrotizing enterocolitis* (530–533), an inflammatory cellulitis that involves the distal ileum, cecum, ascending colon, and appendix and occurs in the setting of neutropenia and cytotoxic drug–related mucosal injury. Several of the chemotherapeutic agents commonly associated with typhlitis include daunorubicin, doxorubicin, cytarabine, and methotrexate. Typhlitis is characterized by fever, right lower quadrant abdominal pain, and diarrhea. Gram-negative bacillary and, occasionally, anaerobic organisms are responsible for the bacteremia in this setting. Abdominal radiography may show a lack of gas in the right lower quadrant and minimal distention of the small bowel. An abdominal ultrasound examination may show thickness and edema of the wall of the cecum (534). The management of typhlitis includes cessation of oral feeding, parenteral nutrition, and administration of broad-spectrum antibiotics. Exploratory laparotomy is reserved for the rare occurrence of perforation, uncontrollable lower gastrointestinal hemorrhage, or abdominal wall fasciitis (530,531). Supportive care guidelines in the treatment of AML are provided in Table 15-8.

Metabolic Complications

Metabolic complications of AML may result from both spontaneous and treatment-induced leukemic cell lysis (370). Tumor lysis can lead to hyperuricemia, hyperkalemia, and hyperphosphatemia with concomitant hypocalcemia and hyperphosphaturia (535–537). The increase in uric acid is caused by catabolism of purines and may result in precipitation of uric acid in the renal collecting system with subsequent renal failure (538). Uric acid nephropathy is avoided by prompt attention to intravenous hydration, alkalinization of the urine, and administration of allopurinol, although patients with a massive leukemia burden and a concentrated, acidic urine remain at risk for this complication. Potassium release by leukemic cells during clotting of blood samples may lead to a spurious reporting of hyperkalemia (536).

Hypercalcemia has been observed on rare occasions in patients with AML (539–541). The pathogenesis is probably multifactorial, but cases with increased ectopic parathormone-like activity in the plasma have been described (542). Severe hypernatremia as a consequence of diabetes insipidus can be an initial manifestation (542), and marked hyponatremia associated with

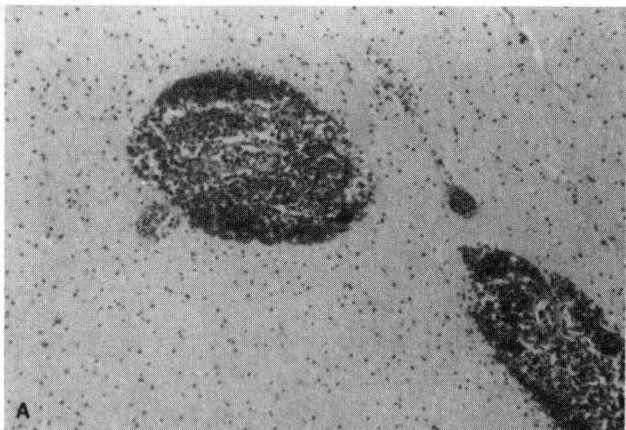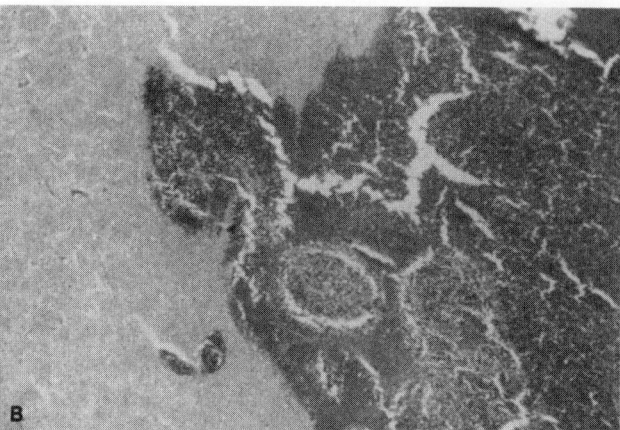

Figure 15-12. Central nervous system leukostasis in a patient with acute myelogenous leukemia. **A:** Plugging of vessels by myeloblasts. **B:** Hemorrhage and infarction.

inappropriate antidiuretic hormone secretion has also occurred at presentation (536). The presence of monosomy 7 may be associated with diabetes insipidus (543). Spurious hypoglycemia and hyperkalemia may occur (544,545). Spurious hypoxia from the effects of a high blast count also can occur (546). Patients with very high serum lysozyme levels (370), as in M4 or M5 AML, may develop hypokalemia secondary to renal tubular injury from high levels of urinary lysozyme (427).

Leukostasis

Extreme leukocytosis is often associated with early morbidity and mortality among patients with AML (370,547–551). Histopathologic studies have revealed leukocyte thrombi and aggregates in the vasculature of AML patients with leukocyte counts greater than 150,000/μL, but especially in those with counts over 300,000/μL (550,552). This phenomenon of leukostasis (white thrombi) affects blood flow in the lung, brain, and other organs and eventually leads to infarction and hemorrhage (Fig. 15-12). The blasts can also compete for oxygen in the microcirculation and invade and damage vessel walls.

Leukostasis can occur in any organ, but the brain and lung appear to be the major target organs. The most common manifestations of leukostasis include stupor, coma, retinal engorgement, acute respiratory distress, and priapism. Chest radiographs may show diffuse pulmonary infiltrates, vascular engorgement, cardiomegaly, and pleural effusions. The immediate goal of therapy is to lower rapidly the peripheral blast count in an attempt to prevent infarction and hemorrhage. This goal may be achieved by the use of a rapidly acting chemotherapeutic agent, such as hydroxyurea 3 g/m²/day orally for 2 days (553), sometimes in conjunction with leukapheresis once daily. Leukapheresis is recommended for the patient who already has clinical signs and symptoms of leukostasis (554). However, leukapheresis has been reported to be ineffective and detrimental in patients with APL who present with a high white blood count (555). Potentially fatal hemorrhage may be initiated or exacerbated, presumably due to lysis of the leukemic promyelocytes during the procedure. In the newly diagnosed patient with AML and a leukocyte count greater than 150,000/μL, it is critical to initiate promptly remission-induction chemotherapy along with intravenous hydration and allopurinol.

Remission Induction

The first step required to provide a significant prolongation of survival for patients with AML is to induce CR (489). For treatment purposes, CR has been defined as the reduction of leukemic blasts to less than 5% in the bone marrow and restoration of normal marrow function without evidence of extramedullary leukemia (556). Peripheral blood counts should approach normal values and any organomegaly, lymphadenopathy, or other extramedullary evidence of leukemic infiltration should resolve. The patient should also have returned to a normal performance status.

It has been estimated that the leukemic cell burden is reduced by at least 2 to 3 logs (10^9 to 10^{12} cells) during the remission-induction period (557). Additional therapy therefore is required to eradicate the residual leukemic cell mass. Therapy administered to patients after the induction of CR has been referred to as either *consolidation*, *intensification* (both imply intensive chemotherapy rendering the bone marrow temporarily hypoplastic or aplastic associated with blood product support), or *maintenance treatment* (implies less intensive, usually outpatient chemotherapy often not requiring blood product support).

The remission-induction phase of therapy for patients with AML is more toxic than ALL induction because of several factors, including the toxicities of the active drugs in AML and greater impairment of normal marrow reserve in the AML patient.

The induction of CR is successful in 70% to 80% of children and adults who are younger than 60 years with AML (558,559). Lower remission rates are seen in older adults and in patients with therapy-related AML or certain cytogenetic findings (456–458,461,462). The cause of the lower remission rates in older adults may be attributable to the inability of the older patient to tolerate intensive chemotherapy, reluctance to administer intensive chemotherapy in this setting, and more resistant leukemia cells (560).

A bone marrow aspirate and biopsy specimen should be assessed within 10 to 14 days after initiation of the first cycle of induction chemotherapy. A period of profound marrow hypoplasia and pancytopenia usually precedes a remission marrow. Patients with M3 AML or those receiving low-dose cytarabine (20 mg/m² for 10 to 20 days) may achieve CR after only modest decreases in bone marrow cellularity or, in fact, no period of aplasia (561,562). Posttreatment marrow biopsy specimens in M3 AML are often cellular and contain residual dysplastic promyelocytes. Follow-up marrow aspirates in the absence of additional chemotherapy usually show CR. If it is difficult to distinguish leukemic blasts or promyelocytes from a recovering myeloid picture, a bone marrow sample should be obtained again in several days. If the repeat marrow in patients with AML other than M3 shows persistence of blasts, a second

TABLE 15-10. Acute Myelogenous Leukemia Remission-Induction Regimens

Drug	Dosage (mg/m²)	Route	Course 1 (day)	Course 2 (day)
Daunorubicin	45	i.v.	1, 2, 3	1, 2
Cytarabine (7-and-3)	100–200	Continuous i.v. infusion	1–7	1–5
Daunorubicin	60	i.v.	1, 2, 3	1, 2
Cytarabine	100	i.v. q12h	1–7	1–5
Thioguanine	100	p.o. q12h	1–7	1–5
Mitoxantrone	12	i.v.	1, 2, 3	1, 2
Cytarabine	100	Continuous i.v. infusion	1–7	1–5
Cytarabine	3000	i.v. q12h	1, 2	8, 9
L-Asparaginase	6000 U/m²	i.m.	[a]	[a]

[a]L-Asparaginase is administered at hour 42.

induction cycle should commence. Approximately two-thirds of patients who achieve CR do so after one cycle of induction, and the remainder of patients destined to respond do so after a second cycle.

Current induction protocols (Tables 15-9 and 15-10) for patients with AML usually involve drug regimens with two or more agents, including anthracycline and cytarabine. Cytarabine was introduced into clinical trial in the 1960s and remains the single most effective drug in the treatment of AML (489). The original studies with cytarabine were patterned after preclinical trials in mice bearing the L1210 leukemia, which illustrated significant schedule dependency (563). This finding provided the basis for prolonged exposure (5 to 10 days) to cytarabine at the commonly used dosages of 100 to 200 mg/m²/day (564). It was subsequently shown by CALGB that the combination of cytarabine and thioguanine was superior to single-agent cytarabine for inducing CR (565).

After daunorubicin and doxorubicin were shown to be useful in the treatment of AML (490,566), induction regimens added daunorubicin to cytarabine and thioguanine (DAT) and showed that the three-drug regimen was superior to the two-drug regimen (567). At approximately the same time, other investigators demonstrated the efficacy of 3 days of daunorubicin combined with a 7-day continuous infusion of cytarabine (7-and-3 regimen) (568). The 7-and-3 combination has been compared with DAT in several randomized clinical trials and was found to be of equal efficacy (569). Subsequent studies have attempted to define the optimal dose and schedule of cap C as well as the choice of anthracycline (daunorubicin or doxorubicin). Results of several randomized clinical trials have shown a slight advantage for continuous infusion versus twice-daily intravenous bolus cytarabine and a statistically significant advantage for a 7-and-3 versus a 5-and-2 schedule (570). CALGB could not demonstrate a further advantage for a more prolonged course of cytarabine (10-and-3) (569).

Several cooperative group studies have shown that daunorubicin is preferable to doxorubicin when three daily equally myelosuppressive doses of either anthracycline are combined with a 7-day infusion of cytarabine (571). There has been less oral mucositis and gastrointestinal toxicity (necrotizing enterocolitis) with daunorubicin compared with doxorubicin, especially in patients older than 60 years and in infants. The increased toxicity associated with doxorubicin led to more deaths during induction and a lower overall CR rate. Data from the Children's Cancer Study Group (CCSG) were similar to the adult experience but also showed greater toxicity of the 7-and-3 regimen in infants when doses were calculated by milligram per square meter rather than by milligram per kilogram (572). It has been recommended that children younger than 1 year or smaller than 0.6 m² should have doses of chemotherapy calculated on a milligram-per-kilogram

basis. The best dose of anthracycline in younger adults has never been evaluated in a prospective randomized trial. The optimal dose of daunorubicin with respect to response in induction in adults is approximately 280 mg/m² (573).

Several newer chemotherapeutic agents, including mitoxantrone and idarubicin, have been combined with cytarabine and compared with daunorubicin and cytarabine for remission-induction efficacy as well as toxicity (574–577). These new combinations have resulted in higher CR rates in younger adults and may have other advantages. For example, a significantly higher percentage of patients achieved CR after a single induction course of mitoxantrone and cytarabine compared with daunorubicin and cytarabine in one randomized trial (578). This result may indicate a greater antileukemic efficacy of mitoxantrone compared with daunorubicin at doses that produced comparable toxicity. Because the median time to CR was shorter in patients treated with mitoxantrone compared with daunorubicin (35 vs. 43 days), less supportive care was required during induction. In the randomized trials of idarubicin compared to daunorubicin, the dose of idarubicin was 12 to 13 mg/m²/day for 3 days and daunorubicin 45 mg/m²/day for 3 days. It may be possible that a higher dose of daunorubicin (60 to 70 mg/m² or higher) confers the same potential benefits as idarubicin.

The epipodophyllotoxins (VP 16 or VM 26) have been increasingly used in AML protocols (579,580). They are particularly active single agents in patients with M4 and M5 AML. The addition of etoposide (VP 16) to daunorubicin and cytarabine during induction, however, did not improve the induction response in an adult AML randomized study (580,581).

In an attempt to increase the CR rate or achieve greater leukemic cell kill early during induction, several groups have intensified therapy by using high-dose cytarabine alone or in combination with either daunorubicin, amsacrine, or L-asparaginase (582–584). There are sufficient clinical pharmacologic and biochemical data to suggest that intermittent infusions of high-dose cytarabine, 1 to 3 g/m² given as a 1-hour to 3-hour infusion every 12 hours for 8 to 12 doses, may be more optimal than standard dosing (488). Clinical responses to high-dose cytarabine have been observed in patients with AML who were refractory to standard doses (583,584). Early data from these high-dose cytarabine studies show CR rates comparable to those achieved after standard-dose cytarabine (584,585). Serious nonhematologic toxicity of high-dose cytarabine has been limited to cerebellar dysfunction (586,587). Most studies indicate that age older than 50 years is the major risk factor for cerebellar toxicity.

Other novel approaches to increase leukemia cell kill during the induction phase have been based on leukemia cell kinetics and biochemistry. Researchers at Johns Hopkins Medical Center designed a study for adults with AML based on both a rodent model of AML (588) and principles developed in the laboratory (589). In this model, initial reduction of leukemia with intensive chemotherapy results in predictable leukemic regrowth that is stimulated by host-derived humoral stimulatory activities. A second cycle of chemotherapy is timed to coincide with this increase in DNA synthesis in the blast population. This approach has been termed *timed sequential chemotherapy*. The original study that tested this concept achieved only a modest remission rate but long, unmaintained durations of remission in a small fraction of patients (590). In a follow-up study, patients who entered CR received a second course of timed sequential chemotherapy. There was an impressive long-term leukemia-free survival for the patients who were able to receive the second cycle (591). It is not known whether this timed sequential therapy is more effective than conventionally timed high-dose intensive therapies for adults with AML, although in children, this strategy has proven beneficial (592). Several recent studies testing high-dose cytarabine given during induction have suggested that the initial CR rate is higher than with a standard induction regimen (593,594); however, two randomized cooperative group trials did not confirm any improvement in CR rate (595,596). The German AML Cooperative Group conducted a randomized trial of high-dose cytarabine in induction and showed an improved CR rate and better event-free survival and OS in high-risk patients identified by more than 40% residual blasts on day 16 bone marrow, unfavorable karyotype, and high LDH level (597).

Other experimental remission-induction approaches have included the use of colony-stimulating or hematopoietic growth factors (G-CSF or GM-CSF) to recruit leukemic cells into cycle to enhance their susceptibility to certain cell cycle-specific drugs (141). Hematopoietic growth factors have also been used in combination with standard chemotherapy in an attempt to shorten the period of chemotherapy-induced pancytopenia, especially in the higher-risk elderly population (598–608). In the aggregate experience, several trials showed an improvement in CR rate, but only one study showed an improvement in survival, and the shortening of the period of neutropenia varied from 2 to 7 days (Table 15-11).

Postremission Therapy

Most patients with AML who enter CR still have occult residual leukemia. Regrowth of these leukemic cells leads to relapse in most patients. Consequently, several postremission strategies have emerged to prevent relapse. These include consolidation chemotherapy maintenance or marrow ablation followed by either allogeneic or autologous bone marrow transplantation. *Consolidation* generally refers to repetitive course of the induction regimen or higher doses of chemotherapy (with or without different drugs) than used during induction (609). Consolidation courses result in severe myelosuppression. Maintenance chemotherapy includes weekly or monthly cycles of therapy for several months or years and is less myelosuppressive.

Because the type of induction regimen (e.g., single-agent versus intensive combination chemotherapy) impacts the subsequent duration of remission, postremission therapies must be evaluated in the context of the induction therapy (590,610). The more intensive induction programs have been associated with longer durations of unmaintained remission because of a presumed greater leukemia cell kill during the first several weeks of treatment.

By the early 1970s, it was clear that patients induced into remission with one or more courses of remission-induction therapy were almost certain to relapse within a few months if they received no further treatment. However, there were no successfully conducted randomized trials that objectively assessed the merits of maintenance therapy only after remission was achieved. Moreover, the results of one nonrandomized study suggested that no further therapy after initial remission provided a median duration of remission comparable to the results of maintenance therapy (590). Therefore, the Eastern Cooperative Oncology Group (ECOG) (611) in 1984 began a randomized study comparing no postremission therapy to prolonged maintenance therapy. Induction therapy consisted of one or two courses of daunorubicin, cytarabine, and thioguanine (5 days). The maintenance therapy consisted of thioguanine 40 mg/m^2 orally every 12 hours for 4 days of the week followed by cytarabine 60 mg/m^2 on the fifth day of the week subcutaneously (total duration of 2 years). Patients receiving no postremission therapy experienced significantly shorter remission durations compared with patients receiving maintenance. Each of the 26 patients in the group who were administered no postremission therapy relapsed (median remission duration of 4 months). In contrast, 16% of the patients who received maintenance therapy remained disease-free, with a median duration of remission of 8 months. Because of these results, the trial was terminated early. CALGB (570,571) studied the optimal duration of maintenance treatment in patients with AML. Maintenance consisted of 8 to 36 months of rotating pairs of drug combinations. These studies did not show a benefit for prolonged maintenance therapy.

TABLE 15-11. Randomized Trials of Growth Factor after Induction Therapy in Acute Myelogenous Leukemia

Author	Patients (n)	Growth Factor	Start Day	Marrow Aplasia	CR (%) Growth Factor	vs.	CR (%) Control	Median Days ANC to 1000/µL
Rowe	117	GM-CSF	11	Yes	60/44			12/18
Dombret	173	G-CSF	8	No	70/47[a]			21/27[a]
Heil	521	G-CSF	8	No	69/68			20/25
Godwin	234	G-CSF	11	Yes	42/49			3–4 d
Stone	379	GM-CSF	8	No	52/54			15/17
Zittoun	53	GM-CSF	8	No	48/77[a]			Not different
Löwenberg	316	GM-CSF	1–8	No	63/61			26/31[a]
Link	187	G-CSF	9	No	60/43[a]			12/18[a]
Goldstone	800	G-CSF	8	No	72/75			15/20
Witz	209	GM-CSF	1	No	63/61			22/26[a]

ANC, absolute neutrophil count; CR, complete remission; G-CSF, granulocyte colony-stimulating factor; GM-CSF, granulocyte-macrophage colony-stimulating factor.
[a]$p \leq .05$.
Adapted from Rowe JM, Liesveld JL. Hematopoietic growth factors in acute leukemia. *Leukemia* 1997;11:328–341.

**TABLE 15-12. Comparison of Treatment Results in Clinical Trials
for Pediatric Acute Myelogenous Leukemia**

Trial (Reference)	Patients (n)	Complete Remission (%)	Actuarial DFS (%)	% Actuarial EFS (yr)
BFM-78 (597)	151	80	47	38 (6)
BFM-83 (597)	182	80	61	49 (4)
DFCI-VAPA (585)	125	72	45	31 (5)
POG-8498 (II) (588)	145	85	41	38 (2)
St. Jude (ANLL-83) (584)	68	85	—	33 (2)
LAM-8204 (582)	133	80	41	33 (3)

DFS, disease-free survival (measured from the time of complete remission; failure is defined as relapse or death in remission from any cause); EFS, event-free survival (measured from the time of initial therapy; failure is defined as induction failure for any reason or termination of remission).

In the early 1980s, the contribution of maintenance therapy after one or more courses of consolidation was also prospectively evaluated. In a Swiss study (612), patients were randomized to receive maintenance therapy or no therapy after one to three cycles of consolidation therapy. There was no improvement in duration of CR (median, 18 months) in the maintenance therapy group. Patients who relapsed before randomization were excluded from the analysis, leading to longer remission durations than those reported in other studies. In contrast, Buchner et al. (613,614) gave only one course of consolidation before randomizing patients to maintenance or no further therapy. In the patients receiving maintenance, the median duration of remission was 15 months and the probability of remission after 7 years was 22%, versus 7 months and 6%, respectively, for the observation arm. The monthly maintenance courses in this study were more myelosuppressive than several of the previously described maintenance regimens. This study has been criticized because the median duration of remission in the no maintenance arm was inferior to that reported for several uncontrolled trials of consolidation therapy alone.

The ECOG (615) and the British Medical Research Council (MRC) (616) both prospectively assessed the contribution of consolidation therapy in adults who were receiving maintenance chemotherapy. In these two large clinical trials, there was no statistically significant benefit for consolidation as defined by either two or six cycles of additional DAT induction courses. The median durations of remission ranged from 8 to 15 months, with less than 30% of complete responders still in remission after 2 years.

Data from these well-conducted randomized trials indicate that consolidation of remission (repetition of the induction regimen) for one or more courses offers a similar outcome compared with less intensive maintenance therapy continued for months or years. There was also evidence that increasing the intensity of consolidation increased the median duration of remission, but most patients still relapsed.

In one of the earlier studies to use the concept of intensification, both children and young adults (under 50 years of age) with AML were treated with 16 months of sequentially administered combinations of active, non–cross-resistant drugs (617). Cytarabine was given at two times the induction dose. In adults, the relapse-free survival was comparable to that found in studies using short-course consolidation therapy, but the results in children were more impressive. Their 5-year probability of relapse-free survival was 45%, with an event-free survival of 31%. The German BFM Study Group (470) also completed several studies for childhood AML that included prolonged induction and consolidation over 8 weeks followed by 2 years of maintenance treatment. This approach has been promising for children with AML.

Results of selected chemotherapy protocols for AML in children are summarized in Table 15-12 (617–620).

Subsequent clinical trials have intensified therapy with high-dose cytarabine 1 to 3 g/m^2 alone or combined with an anthracycline, amsacrine, or L-asparaginase (621–623). Cytarabine has been the prototype drug for dose intensification. It is the single most active agent in AML, and laboratory and clinical studies have indicated that at least a log increase in its dose can overcome certain patterns of resistance and lead to CR in patients with AML who were previously refractory to conventional cytarabine treatment. Intensification therapy has been given for one to three courses. Death secondary to drug toxicity or infection occurred in 5% to 17% of patients. The prolonged periods of pancytopenia have necessitated long hospitalizations. These studies have been uncontrolled and biased with a young patient population, but nevertheless have produced encouraging results. In a CALGB randomized trial, 596 patients in CR were randomized to receive four courses of cytarabine at one of three doses: 100 $mg/m^2/day$ by intravenous infusion for 5 days; 400 $mg/m^2/day$ by intravenous infusion for 5 days; or 3 $g/m^2/day$ twice daily on days 1, 3, and 5. High rates of CNS toxicity were observed in patients older than 60 years randomized to the high-dose regimen. Among patients younger than 60 years, the DFS rate was 21% in the 100-mg arm, 25% in the 400-mg arm, and 39% in the 3-g arm (Fig. 15-13). The high cytarabine dose and schedule used in this trial have become widely adopted; however, it is important to recognize that patients were scheduled to receive four monthly cycles of cytarabine 100 mg/m^2 every 12 hours for 5 days by subcutaneous infusion and daunorubicin 45 mg/m^2 intravenous infusion on day 1 ($p = .004$) (624,625) (Fig. 15-14). The Finnish Leukemia Study Group randomized younger patients in CR after two courses of induction to either four courses of additional consolidation after two courses of high-dose cytarabine or observation (626) (Fig. 15-15). No benefit was observed for patients randomized to the longer consolidation arm, suggesting that early intensive consolidation is more important than the number of cycles. In the interim, a reasonable option is to treat patients younger than 60 years who have a good performance status with two to four cycles of a postremission high-dose cytarabine–containing regimen.

TREATMENT OF OLDER ADULTS

Treatment of older patients with AML requires special considerations because of both patient-related and leukemia-related factors (468). Older adult patients often have a poor performance status and therefore do not tolerate intensive chemotherapy.

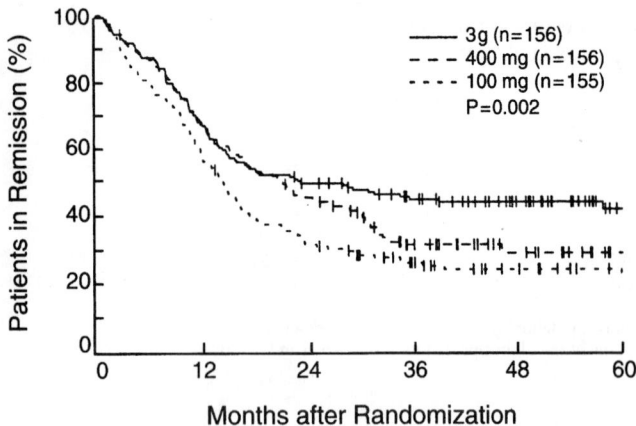

Figure 15-13. Disease-free survival of adults younger than 60 years with *de novo* acute myelogenous leukemia treated with three different doses of cytarabine. (From Mayer RJ, Davis RB, Schiffer CA, et al. Intensive postremission chemotherapy in adults with acute myeloid leukemia. Cancer and Leukemia Group B. *N Engl J Med* 1994;331:896–903, with permission.)

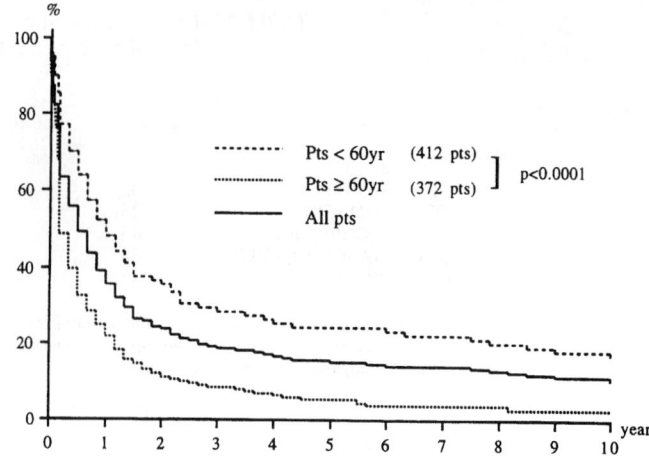

Figure 15-15. Overall survival according to age for 784 consecutive newly diagnosed acute myeloid leukemia patients treated between 1980 and 1995. (From Baudard M, Beauchamp-Nicoud A, Delmer A, et al. Has the prognosis of adult patients with acute myeloid leukemia improved over years? A single institution experience of 784 consecutive patients over a 16-year period. *Leukemia* 1999;13:1481–1490, with permission.)

Therapy is frequently complicated by concomitant organ system (especially cardiovascular, pulmonary, and renal) disease. As mentioned earlier, AML in older patients is also associated with poor prognostic characteristics (317).

Because of these factors, elderly patients have a greater risk of early death from drug toxicity or infection. They also have more resistant leukemia than do younger patients. Therefore, the CR rates for patients older than 60 years have ranged between 40% and 50%, well below those observed in younger patients.

Although a large proportion of patients with AML are over 65 years of age, few studies have specifically addressed optimal therapy for this age group. Some investigators have questioned whether older patients with AML should be treated at all. A study conducted by the Dutch-Belgian Hematology-Oncology Cooperative Group (HOVON) compared immediate standard induction chemotherapy versus supportive care with or with-

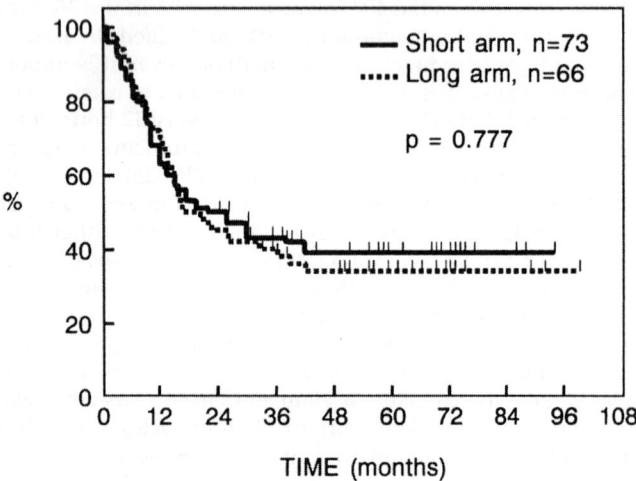

Figure 15-14. Projected relapse-free survival of 139 patients with acute myeloid leukemia in complete remission randomized to either two courses of high-dose cytarabine consolidation or the same two courses followed by four additional courses of intensive chemotherapy (the last including high-dose cytarabine). (From Elonen E, Almqvist A, Hanninen A, et al. Comparison between four and eight cycles of intensive chemotherapy in adult acute myeloid leukemia: a randomized trial of the Finnish Leukemia Group. *Leukemia* 1998;12:1041–1048, with permission.)

out mild cytotoxic therapy (given only for relief of progressive symptoms related to an increased leukemic cell burden) (627). This study showed that a strategy based on supportive care yielded only extremely poor results. Complete remission was not achieved in the supportive care group, compared with a 58% CR rate in the chemotherapy-treated group. There was also a significantly longer survival for the latter group (median survival, 21 vs. 11 weeks).

Another approach used for older patients and others in poor-risk categories has been treatment with low-dose cytarabine (628,629). Low-dose cytarabine has been used on the assumption that it is less toxic than conventional-dose cytarabine. There is also *in vitro* but not *in vivo* evidence that low-dose cytarabine induces differentiation of leukemic blasts (630). In a recently reported randomized trial comparing low-dose cytarabine (20 mg/m^2 for 21 days) with an intensive chemotherapy regimen (rubidazone 100 mg/m^2 for 4 days and cytarabine 200 mg/m^2 for 7 days) in patients over 65 years of age with *de novo* AML, there were a higher number of cases of CR with intensive chemotherapy, but with low-dose cytarabine there was a lower early death rate, resulting in similar OSs (628). The ECOG randomized older patients with AML to either full-dose induction with DAT or attenuated-schedule (reduced-dose) DAT and found no difference in the CR rate (28%) or survival (631). Prognostic factors important in predicting response and outcome in older adults include age greater than 67 years and CD7 expression, and abnormal karyotype and CD14 expression, respectively (632). High CR rates (55%) can be achieved in older adults with mitoxantrone plus etoposide without cytarabine (633). In a single-institution experience of 784 patients with newly diagnosed AML, there has been little, if any, improvement in the outcome of treatment of older (≥60 years) adults (634) (Fig. 15-15).

Central Nervous System Prophylaxis

In contrast to studies in ALL (635,636), early treatment or prophylaxis of the CNS with intrathecal chemotherapy (methotrexate or cytarabine) alone or combined with cranial irradiation has not been shown to prolong DFS in children or adults with AML. However, most pediatric AML studies include some form of CNS prophylaxis (375,470,473,474). This practice evolved because childhood AML studies that did not include CNS prophylaxis reported as many as 20% of children having isolated CNS relapse during their first hematologic remission. CNS prophylaxis included intrathecal chemotherapy (methotrexate or cytarabine) alone or intrathecal methotrexate combined with cranial irradiation. These treatments have resulted in little additional acute toxicity and a low incidence of CNS relapse. Most adult therapy studies do not use CNS prophylaxis but rely on systematically administered chemotherapy (cytarabine) to eradicate occult meningeal leukemia. Ultimately, 5% to 10% of adults manifest meningeal involvement, usually in the setting of bone marrow relapse. Patients with high peripheral blast counts at diagnosis and M4 or M5 AML have the highest incidence of CNS leukemia (405,637). The recommended therapy for CNS relapse includes four to six doses of intrathecal chemotherapy (methotrexate or cytarabine) and an intensified regimen of systemic reinduction. This is sometimes followed by cranial spinal irradiation or bone marrow transplantation.

Chloromas

Because most patients with isolated chloromas eventually manifest bone marrow involvement, immediate systemic AML treatment has been recommended for these patients (381,382). There is, however, little data to indicate that this approach has been successful. In most patients with AML and a chloroma, it has not been necessary to administer local radiation therapy in addition to chemotherapy to achieve local control. However, in an emergency situation (i.e., acute spinal cord compression secondary to an epidural myeloblastoma), several days of local irradiation 175 to 250 cGy/day may be indicated.

Hematopoietic Stem Cell Transplantation

Marrow ablative doses of chemotherapy with or without total body irradiation (TBI) followed by bone marrow (stem cell) transplantation from an HLA-matched sibling donor have been increasingly applied to young adults and children with AML in first remission (638,639). Only a small proportion of patients with AML are considered for an allogeneic bone marrow transplantation because of age restrictions (<50 years) and the lack of a histocompatible donor. The initial transplantation studies for AML involved patients with advanced refractory leukemia who had failed to respond or relapsed after multiple courses of chemotherapy (640). Even in this setting, 10% to 15% of patients with AML became long-term disease-free survivors. Beginning in the mid-1970s, allogeneic marrow transplantation for young patients with AML in first remission was investigated (641–643). It was hoped that an allogeneic transplantation early in the course of the disease would be associated with less infectious morbidity and mortality and a lower leukemic relapse rate (Fig. 15-16). Several conclusions became apparent from these early uncontrolled studies. The actuarial relapse rates (15% to 25%) were lower for patients who underwent transplantation in first remission compared with second or subsequent remissions, and the relapse rates were also lower than those achieved after consolidation or maintenance chemotherapy. Outcome was also related to recipient age in most studies, with 50% to 70% relapse-free survival in patients younger than 30 years and 30% to 50% relapse-free survival in patients between 30 and 50 years of age.

These studies were criticized because of the bias in timing and selection of patients referred for marrow transplantation. The median age of the patients who underwent transplantation was less than 35 years. The average time between documenting CR and referral to a transplantation center was

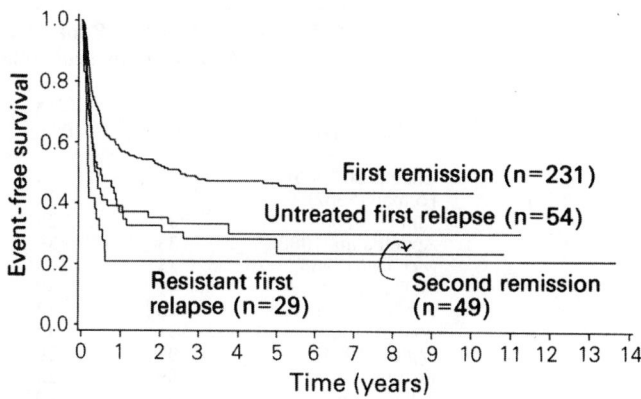

Figure 15-16. Outcome after HLA-matched sibling allogeneic bone marrow transplantation for acute myelogenous leukemia in first complete remission and other phases of the disease. (From Clift RA, Buckner CD, Thomas ED, et al. The treatment of acute nonlymphoblastic leukemia by allogeneic marrow transplantation. *Bone Marrow Transplant* 1987;2:243, with permission.)

several months (range, 1 month to 1 year); therefore, patients who had more resistant or aggressive AML would most likely have relapsed before undergoing transplantation. Because of these controversies, several prospective studies in adults and children with AML were initiated to compare the outcomes of allogeneic bone marrow transplantation and chemotherapy (644–646).

Several of these studies have reported a statistically significant leukemia-free survival advantage for the transplant recipients compared with those receiving chemotherapy. These studies have also been criticized for lack of intensity in the chemotherapy regimens, the unusually high percentage of patients with histocompatible donors, and the young patient population.

Based on the cumulative published experience, it appears that patients younger than 30 years with AML in first remission are the most likely to benefit from allogeneic marrow transplantation (638,647). Because of the higher mortality associated with bone marrow transplantation in the group 30 to 50 years old, there is less of a survival advantage for those receiving transplants compared with chemotherapy. However, not all studies have reported an adverse effect of increasing age on outcome after allogeneic transplantation (643). The preliminary data from intensive chemotherapy protocols are comparable to results achieved after allogeneic bone marrow transplantation, especially in the group 30 to 50 years old (591,621,624,625). During the last decade, several prospective and randomized studies were performed (639,643–658) (Table 15-13).

Stimulated by the promising results of allogeneic marrow transplantation, an increasing number of patients with AML have been treated with cytoreductive therapy followed by autologous marrow rescue (659–674). The advantages of autologous marrow transplantation or rescue include the elimination of problems associated with GVHD and the expansion of patient eligibility. Disadvantages include possible leukemic contamination of infused marrow and the loss of the graft-versus-leukemia effect. The early experience with autologous marrow transplantation included several uncontrolled clinical trials in adults with AML (659–661). Transplantation preparation regimens included chemotherapy and TBI or high-dose chemotherapy alone. Purged (pharmacologic or monoclonal antibody-treated) and unpurged autologous marrow were used in these studies. The actuarial relapse rates were approximately 50%, with 30% to 65% of patients remaining in remission 2 to 4 years after transplantation, and the outcome appeared to be related to the timing of the transplantation. For

TABLE 15-13. Allogeneic Bone Marrow (Stem Cell) Transplantation for Acute Myelogenous Leukemia in First Complete Remission

Author (Year)	Patients (n)	TRM (%)	RR (%)	% Disease-Free Survival (yr)	% Overall Survival (yr)
Champlin (1985)	23	43	40	60[d] (4)	40
Forman (1987)	69[e]	30	16	51 (4)	NA
Clift (1987)	231	25	25	46 (5)	48 (5)
Appelbaum (1988)	33	36	15	48 (5)	48 (5)
McGlave (1988)	73	7	9	62 (7)	NA
Geller[f] (1989)	49	49	8	45 (3)	46
Schiller (1992)	28	32	32	48 (5)	45 (5)
Young[c] (1992)	31	42	13	45 (3)	45 (3)
Fagioli (1994)	91	26	29	NA	53 (5)
Keating (1996)	169	22	23	60 (3)	NA
Labar (1996)	46	18	12	71 (7)	NA
Mehta (1996)	85	33[b]	25[b]	48 (10)	NA
Reiffers (1996)	36	12	24	67 (3)	65 (3)
Ferrant[a] (1997)	346	NA	22	57 (3)	59 (3)
Soiffer[c] (1997)	14	16	25	63 (4)	71 (4)

NA, not available; RR, relapse rate; TRM, toxicity-related mortality.
[a]Results for standard-risk patients.
[b]At 10 years; only two relapses beyond 2 years.
[c]T-cell depletion.
[d]Freedom from relapse.
[e]Includes 20 patients age 1–19 years.
[f]Includes 27 patients who received low-dose cyclophosphamide ± methylprednisone or intramuscular cyclosporine as graft-versus-host disease prophylaxis.

patients who underwent transplantation within 3 months of achieving remission, there was only a 30% DFS, compared with 50% to 60% for patients who underwent transplantation later in first remission (more than 9 months) (661). It was argued by many that the latter patients were already cured by the time they underwent transplantation. Whether marrow purging contributed to the success of these autologous transplants remains unknown, but a recent retrospective review suggests a benefit of purging for a subset of patients in first remission (661). Several prospective studies have recently been initiated to compare autologous bone marrow transplantation to either allogeneic bone marrow transplantation or chemotherapy. In a Dutch AML study, allogeneic bone marrow transplantation resulted in more rapid hematopoietic reconstitution, was followed by fewer relapses, and provided better survival than autologous bone marrow transplantation (660). A recently reported pediatric study showed comparable results (50% DFS) after autologous and allogeneic marrow transplantation (675). The results of autologous stem cell transplantation for patients with AML in first CR are detailed in Table 15-14 (659–674,676).

Autologous stem cell transplantation involves the administration of higher chemotherapy doses but is limited by the lack of graft-versus-leukemia effect associated with allogeneic transplantation. Furthermore, there is a theoretic risk of infusion of occult residual leukemic cells. Allogeneic transplantation provides the

TABLE 15-14. Autologous Bone Marrow (Stem Cell) Transplantation for Acute Myelogenous Leukemia in First Complete Remission

Author (Year)	Patients (n)	TRM (%)	RR (%)	% Disease-Free Survival (yr)	% Overall Survival (yr)
Gorin (1986)	60	NA	NA	67 (2)	45 (2)
Löwenberg (1990)	32	9	53	35 (3)	33 (3)
Gorin (1991)	671	NA	41	48 (7)	NA
Gulati (1992)	15	0	27	72 (4)	NA
Cassileth (1993)	39	6	33	54 (3)	NA
Linker (1993)	58	3	22	76 (3)	NA
Sanz (1993)	24	13	60	35 (2.5)	~53 (2.5)
Sierra (1993)	24	4	48	48 (3)	NA
Laporte (1994)	64	18	25	58 (8)	NA
Cahn (1995)	111	28	52	34 (4)	35 (4)
Cahn (1995)	786	14	50	43 (4)	48 (4)
Miggiano (1996)	51	0	24	71 (5)	77 (5)
Stein (1996)	60	8	44	49 (2)	NA
Schiller (1997)	59	33	54	42 (3)	47 (3)
Gondo (1997)	42	0	21	79 (3)	NA
Martin (1998)	35	0	47	52 (4)	52 (4)
Visani (1999)	44	NA	52	~45 (4)	NA

NA, not applicable; RR, relapse rate; TRM, toxicity-related mortality.

TABLE 15-15. Prospective Randomized Trials of Consolidation Chemotherapy versus Bone Marrow Transplantation (BMT) in Acute Myelogenous Leukemia

Author (Year)	Disease-Free/Overall Survival: 4-Year (%)		
	Consolidation Chemotherapy	Autologous BMT	Assigned Allogeneic BMT
Zittoun (1995)	30/46	48/56	55/59
Cassileth (1998)	34/52	34/43	43/46
Harousseau (1997)	43/59	48/52	49/55
Burnett (1998)	40/57[a]	54/45	—

[a]Seven years.

best antileukemic potential but is consistently associated with a higher risk of treatment-related mortality than the other two strategies. All of these studies *assign* younger patients with an HLA-matched donor to allogeneic transplantation and *randomize* other patients to either consolidation chemotherapy or autologous transplantation or between the latter two strategies (676–679) (Table 15-15). The earliest study carried out as a collaboration between the European Organization for Research and Treatment of Cancer and Gruppo Italiano Malattie Ematologiche Magligne dell'Adulto (GIMEMA) assigned 168 patients in first CR to allogeneic transplantation and randomized 126 patients to a second cycle of consolidation with cytarabine 2 g/m^2 every 12 hours days 1 to 4 plus daunorubicin 45 mg/m^2 days 5 to 7, and 128 patients to autologous transplantation with cyclophosphamide/TBI or busulfan/TBI (55% of patients) as the preparative regimen (677). Only 74% of patients randomized to autologous transplantation actually completed the treatment because of early relapse and toxicity. Nevertheless, the DFS at 4 years, by an intention-to-treat analysis, was approximately 50%. This outcome is not different from that achieved in patients undergoing allogeneic transplantation (cyclophosphamide/TBI in approximately 66% of patients as the preparative regimen and Bu/Cy in 34%) who had a DFS of 55% at 4 years. These results were significantly better than those observed among patients receiving consolidation (30%). However, the OS at 4 years for all three treatment groups was similar (59% allogeneic, 56% autologous, 46% consolidation). Whereas relapse was more frequent among patients randomized to autologous transplantation, treatment-related mortality was higher among those assigned allogeneic transplantation.

Despite a similar trial design, although the autologous transplants were carried out with purged bone marrow, different observations were made in the trial conducted by ECOG, the Southwest Oncology Group, and CALGB (680). The DFS associated with allogeneic transplantation was not significantly longer (43% at 4 years) than that associated with autologous transplantation (34%) or consolidation with high-dose cytarabine (34%). However, OS after high-dose cytarabine was longer than that after autologous or allogeneic transplantation. The discrepancy between DFS and OS likely relates to the opportunity to undergo transplantation at relapse among patients initially assigned consolidation chemotherapy.

In a study by Harousseau et al. (678), there was no difference in the 4-year DFS or OS between patients randomized to autologous transplantation and those randomized to consolidation. The trial conducted by the MRC was unique because it demonstrated that the addition of autologous transplantation after three cycles of consolidation (two similar to induction and one including cytarabine 1 g/m^2 every 12 hours for 3 days) reduced the risk of relapse, and a statistical effect was seen on OS (679).

The interpretations of these studies require caution. First, in all studies, a significant number of patients randomized to autol-

ogous transplantation do not receive the assigned treatment. Second, although allogeneic transplantation offers the potential for graft-versus-leukemia effect and is associated with the lowest risk of relapse, higher treatment-related mortality compared to that with autologous transplantation and consolidation chemotherapy diminishes the impact of the greater antileukemic potential; therefore, a benefit in OS is not observed. Third, the mortality rate associated with autologous transplantation has decreased to less than 3%, and that for allogeneic transplantation will likely continue to decrease as the techniques of transplantation improve, such as improvements in T-cell depletion techniques for allogeneic transplantation (658,681). Furthermore, recent studies suggest that the outcome for allogeneic transplantation in patients older than age 40 may not be worse than for younger patients (682). There are improvements in all three postremission strategies, so frequent reappraisal of the benefits and hazards of each approach is required.

In an effort to reduce the mortality and morbidity of allogeneic bone marrow transplantation, attempts have been made to modify or prevent GVHD through the *ex vivo* depletion of T lymphocytes (683) from donor marrow or the intensification of pharmacologic approaches (684). Although these methods have been successful in reducing the incidence and severity of GVHD, fewer cases of this disease in some studies have resulted in an increased probability of posttransplantation leukemic relapse (i.e., loss of graft-versus-leukemia effect). Because of the higher likelihood of relapse and an increased risk of graft failure, *ex vivo* T-cell depletion of donor marrow has not resulted in a survival advantage for patients with leukemia (685).

Refractory Acute Myelogenous Leukemia

Patients with refractory or resistant AML include those who survived the initial induction chemotherapy but failed to achieve CR and those who achieved a remission but eventually relapsed. Only a few studies provide therapeutic guidelines for these patients (686,687). The initial management choices include introducing previously effective drugs, using new classes of drugs, or proceeding directly to bone marrow transplantation. Bone marrow transplantation probably offers the greatest likelihood for a long-term second remission in this setting (639).

Patients treated with chemotherapy alone for refractory (induction failure) or relapsed AML have little possibility of long-term DFS (687). In most of the reported studies, there have been few relapsed patients with second remissions lasting longer than the initial remission. The likelihood of achieving a second CR is lowest in patients with primary refractory AML and in patients who had short initial remission durations (less than 6 months) (687,688). Patients in whom AML developed secondary to MDS or was therapy-induced were relatively resistant to primary therapy and particularly resistant to subsequent therapy. Results from the MRC support these generalizations. In the eighth MRC trial, 155 (29%) of 531 relapsed patients achieved a second CR (616). Age above 60 years in addition to short initial CR duration adversely influenced second CR rates in that study. The M. D. Anderson Cancer Center data are in accord with MRC results and also indicate longer second CR durations in the group of patients with longer first remissions (687,688).

A variety of different reinduction regimens were used in these patients. Is there a best second-line induction regimen, and in what circumstance should the initial induction regimen be used? Several factors, including duration of first CR and significant other medical problems such as cardiac dysfunction or liver disease, influence subsequent choice of therapy. For patients who have had long initial remissions (more than 12 months) and who have not had high cumulative doses of an anthracycline or cardiac toxicity, it is reasonable to reuse the original effective remission-induction regimen (689). For the remainder of patients, newer treatment approaches should be considered. It could also be argued that new drugs should be tested in a favorable group of relapsed patients, because the goal is to identify active agents that might eventually be used as initial therapy.

High-dose cytarabine has been extensively studied in patients with refractory AML (582–585). The mechanism of leukemia cell resistance to standard-dose cytarabine (100 to 200 mg/m^2/day for 5 to 7 days by intermittent or continuous parenteral administration) is not completely understood but may be overcome by using very high doses of cytarabine (2 to 3 g/m^2 every 12 hours for 8 to 12 doses). Although CR can be achieved in this setting, it is not clear that the high-dose cytarabine approach is of long-term value in such patients. Other active drugs include VP 16 (579), idarubicin (689), diaziquone (690), mitoxantrone, amsacrine (583), and azacytidine (691,692). Both the prednisone, vincristine, mercaptopurine, and methotrexate combination (693) and the regimen of methotrexate and L-asparaginase (694) have been effective in patients with either refractory or relapsed AML.

Allogeneic or autologous bone marrow transplantation appears to offer the possibility of long-term survival in 20% to 35% of patients with advanced AML (639,695–697). The best timing of an allogeneic transplantation (at initial relapse or in second remission) and the potential benefit of *in vitro* treatment (purging) of marrow for an autologous transplantation remain unanswered questions. The Seattle bone marrow transplantation group has reported that the results of allogeneic transplantation in early relapse were equivalent to those achieved in second remission (639). Because of these data, it may be prudent to follow the marrow status of patients closely to identify early relapse and to be able to refer such patients quickly for transplantation. This approach would especially apply to patients with an initial short remission because of their low likelihood of achieving a second remission.

Autologous bone marrow transplantation for patients who lack HLA-matched donors also appears promising (676,695). However, most of these transplantations have been performed in second remission, thereby selecting a group of patients with less resistant leukemia. In addition, the second remissions have been durable enough that patients could be referred to a transplantation center. Not unlike the situation in first remission, the role of marrow purging with drugs or antimyeloid monoclonal antibodies is unknown. Purging of marrow appears to delay engraftment and therefore should be prospectively studied before it is more widely applied (696). New transplantation strategies include matched unrelated donor transplantation

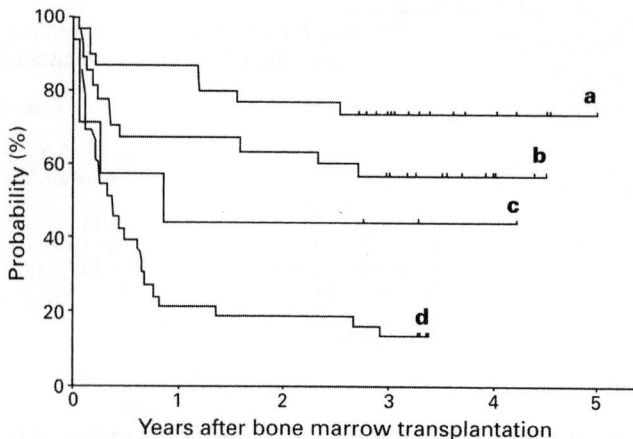

Figure 15-17. Probability of disease-free survival among patients with acute myelogenous leukemia transplanted in (a) first remission (*n* = 29), (b) second remission (*n* = 27), and (c) third or subsequent remission (*n* = 9), and (d) at the time of relapse of the disease (*n* = 33). [From Kodera Y, Morishima Y, Kato S, et al. Analysis of 500 bone marrow transplants from unrelated donors (UR-BMT) facilitated by the Japan marrow donor program: confirmation of UR-BMT as a standard therapy for patients with leukemia and aplastic anemia. *Bone Marrow Transplant* 1999;24:995–1003, with permission.]

(697–699) (Fig. 15-17) and both matched and unrelated umbilical cord stem cell transplantation (700–702) and the administration of large doses of T-cell–depleted stem cells with an intensive conditioning regimen and immunosuppression (703). Other novel approaches have included attempts at modulating multidrug resistance with cyclosporine (704); PSC-835 (705–707); topotecan, a topoisomerase I inhibitor, either alone (708) or in combination with other agents (709); the purine analog 2-chlorodeoxyadenosine either alone (710) or in combination therapy (711); and farnesyl-transferase inhibitors (69). Inhibitor of angiogenesis is also being investigated (712–714). Gemtuzumab ozogamicin (Mylotarg) is an immunoconjugate of an anti-CD33 antibody linked to a potent cytotoxic drug, calicheamicin (Fig. 15-18). This immunoconjugate induces remission in approximately 30% of patients in first relapse (715,716). Selected trials of various drugs for patients with relapse or refractory AML are presented in Table 15-16 (717–723). The outcome of high-dose cytarabine in patients with relapsed and refractory AML is shown in Figure 15-19 (723).

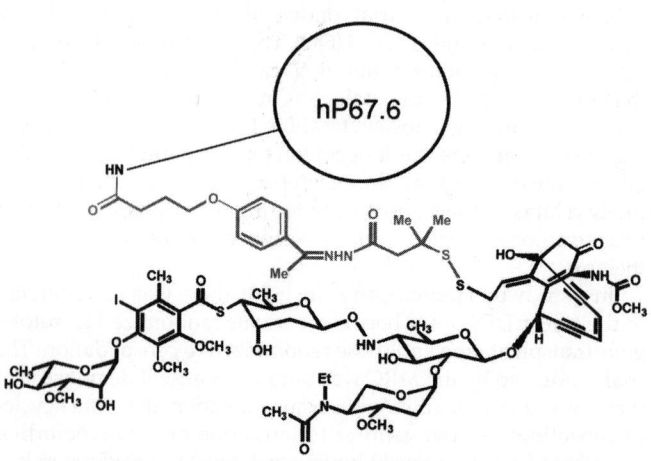

hP67.6 - humanized anti-CD33 antibody; **gray** - linker; **black** - calicheamicin

Figure 15-18. Chemical structure of Mylotarg.

TABLE 15-16. Therapy for Relapsed or Refractory Patients and Induction Failures: Studies with More Than 100 Patients

Author (Year)	Type of Therapy	n	Complete Remission (%)	Duration of Response (mo)	Survival (mo)
Keating (1985)	Various	243	33	6	4.5
Rees (1986)	DAT	531	29	NA	NA
Hiddemann (1990)	DAT	146	47	5	8
Davis (1993)	Various	162	30	7	4
Archimbaud (1995)	MEC	133	60	8	7
Greenberg (1999)	MEC ± PSC-833	113	21	6.4 (MEC)	NA
Thalhammer (1996)	Various	168	39	7.5	NA
Karanes (1999)	HiDAC ± Mitox	162	38	5.1	5.1
Sievers (2000)	Mylotarg	142	30	6.8	5.9
		142	17[a]	4.4	11

DAT, daunorubicin, cytarabine, thioguanine; HiDAC, high-dose cytarabine; MEC, mitoxantrone, etoposide, cytarabine; PSC-833, valspodar excluded.
[a]Complete response excluding platelets.

Biologic Response Modifiers

During the past 2 decades, there have been extensive attempts to use immunologic agents to treat AML. The early studies used adjuvant and nonspecific agents such as *Corynebacterium parvum* and bacillus Calmette-Guérin alone or in combination with chemotherapy to enhance antileukemic immunity (724,725). The administration of irradiated or chemically modified autologous or allogeneic leukemia cells was part of some of these protocols (726). These forms of immunotherapy failed to improve the long-term DFS of patients with AML. Interferon has also been used in the treatment of AML, but the data do not indicate that it is an active drug (727). Recent investigational efforts have focused on enhancing the activity of lymphokine-activated killer cells or natural killer cells using IL-2 in patients with AML in remission (728). Phase I and II studies using such approaches are under way.

Another experimental approach has been to use growth factors (i.e., G-CSF or GM-CSF) either to recruit malignant myeloblasts into cell cycle or to shorten the duration of neutropenia associated with chemotherapy protocols (142,597–608). As discussed earlier in the chapter, these growth factors may induce proliferation of myeloblasts and therefore have the potential to increase blast counts in these patients. Nevertheless, these innovative studies are proceeding with caution in relapsed or high-risk, newly diagnosed patients (>60 years of age) with AML. IL-2 has shown activity in patients with limited residual disease (729–732).

Differentiation Agents

Another potential approach to the treatment of AML is to induce maturation of leukemic blasts to terminal, nonproliferating cells. Many agents can induce myeloid leukemic cells to differentiate *in vitro*, including vitamin D analogs, phorbol esters, retinoid agents, and low doses of chemotherapy drugs (e.g., cytarabine). Retinoic acid has been studied in patients with AML and MDS and, with rare exceptions, has not resulted in CR. Several reports, however, indicate that ATRA rather than the commonly used *cis*-isomer is a very effective agent for inducing CR in patients with M3 AML (171–173). Clinical response to this agent is associated with leukemic cell differentiation and is linked to the expression of an aberrant RAR nuclear receptor. The proper role of ATRA in the treatment of patients with M3 AML has been established. Low-dose cytarabine has also been extensively studied and is active in approximately 20% of patients with AML, but it probably acts through cytotoxicity rather than differentiation (629).

Treatment of Acute Promyelocytic Leukemia

Acute promyelocytic leukemia is treated differently from all other subtypes of AML and has become the most curable subtype of AML in adults. Phase II trials have confirmed the effectiveness of the vitamin A derivative ATRA as differentiation therapy in patients with APL (171–173,242–246). Two prospective randomized trials have compared ATRA with or without chemotherapy to chemotherapy alone for induction (733,734). After CR, patients in both trials received two cycles of consolidation: 7+3, then intermediate-dose cytarabine plus daunorubicin in the APL91 trial; and 7+3, then HiDAC plus daunorubicin in the North American Intergroup trial (733). In the latter trial, patients in CR after two cycles of consolidation were randomized to either 1 year of daily maintenance ATRA or observation. In both trials, the CR rates in both arms were not statistically different. However, event-free survival, DFS, and OS were markedly improved with ATRA such that approximately 70% of patients remain disease-free at 4 years. This benefit was attributable to a decrease in the relapse rate with

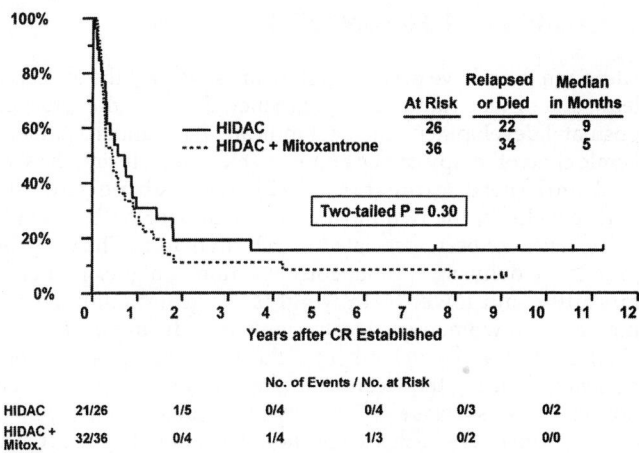

Figure 15-19. Relapse-free survival by induction therapy of patients with relapsed or refractory acute myelogenous leukemia treated with high-dose cytarabine (HIDAC) with or without the addition of mitoxantrone. Kaplan-Meier estimates of the distribution of relapse-free survival, measured for onset of complete remission (CR) until relapse or death from any case. [From Karanes C, Kopecky KJ, Head DR, et al. A phase III comparison of high-dose cytarabine (HIDAC) versus HIDAC plus mitoxantrone in the treatment of first relapsed or refractory acute myeloid leukemia Southwest Oncology Group study. *Leuk Res* 1999;23:787–794, with permission.]

ATRA. In the North American Intergroup trial, patients induced with standard induction chemotherapy and maintained with ATRA had an outcome identical to those patients who received ATRA during induction. The most serious and life-threatening complication of differentiation therapy with ATRA is the retinoic acid syndrome, a cardiorespiratory distress syndrome manifested by interstitial pulmonary infiltrates, pleural or pericardial effusions, hypoxemia, and episodic hypotension with otherwise unexplained weight gain (735,736). The syndrome may be related to the rapid development of hyperleukocytosis, which can be observed with ATRA induction. The syndrome usually resolves quickly if corticosteroids (dexamethasone 10 mg b.i.d. for at least 3 days) are administered at the earliest sign or symptom. The APL93 trial showed that administering concurrent ATRA plus chemotherapy reduces the relapse rate compared to sequential ATRA for induction followed by chemotherapy (734). This was observed even among patients presenting with a relatively low white blood count. Therefore, the standard induction strategy for APL now includes ATRA plus chemotherapy for all patients. The MRC randomized patients to either a short course of ATRA (5 days) in an effort to reduce the coagulopathy but avoid the retinoic acid syndrome with chemotherapy, or concomitant ATRA plus chemotherapy initial CR, and found that the latter strategy was associated with an improved outcome (737). Although the best chemotherapy regimen to include in induction is not established, anthracycline alone during induction is sufficient. The best consolidation regimen has not been established; however, it appears that all patients should receive at least two cycles of consolidation with either anthracycline plus cytarabine, as in the APL91 trial; anthracycline plus cytarabine followed by HiDAC, as in the North American Intergroup Trial; or intermediate-dose cytarabine plus idarubicin, then mitoxantrone plus etoposide plus cytarabine plus 6-thioguanine, as in the GIMEMA trial. Anthracyclines alone as consolidation may well be sufficient. The precise role of maintenance therapy with ATRA continues to evolve. The North American Intergroup Trial and the APL93 trial both suggest a beneficial role. Arsenic trioxide is an extremely effective therapy for patients with relapsed or refractory APL, even with previous ATRA exposure, including a CR rate of approximately 80% (738–741).

TREATMENT OF PREGNANT PATIENTS

Although there have been no systematic studies of the effects of leukemia or its treatment on pregnancy, delivery, the fetus, or postnatal development, the data indicate that standard antileukemic chemotherapy can be administered safely during the second and third trimesters (742). Cytarabine and the anthracyclines, the two most active drugs for patients with AML, have not been associated with birth defects. The risks for premature delivery, spontaneous abortion, a higher perinatal mortality, and lower birth weights for gestational age are increased in women treated for leukemia during pregnancy (743). Growth and development of the newborn exposed to chemotherapy during the second and third trimesters appear to be normal. Issues such as elective delivery before term and vaginal delivery versus cesarean section should be individualized. Only one reasonably well-documented case of maternal–fetal transmission of AML has been reported (744). In a report of 7 cases and a review of the literature, Reynoso et al. (745) presented 50 live births among 58 cases of leukemia during pregnancy, of whom 28 were born premature and 4 had low birth weight for gestational age. Thirty-three percent of the newborns exposed to chemotherapy during the third trimester had cytopenias at birth. A single newborn had congenital malformations.

TABLE 15-17. Escalating Intensity of Postremission Therapy in Patients Younger Than 55 Years in Five Eastern Cooperative Oncology Group Trials

Postremission Therapy	% 5-year DFS (95% CI)	% 5-year OS (95% CI)
Observation	0 (0,0)	10 (0,23)
Maintenance	13 (7,19)	19 (12,26)
Maintenance and intermediate-dose consolidation × 2	24 (14,33)	33 (22,43)
Intensive consolidation × 1	24 (14,34)	29 (18,39)
Autologous BMT	55 (40,70)	53 (38,69)
Allogeneic BMT	40 (22,58)	45 (27,63)

BMT, bone marrow transplantation; CI, confidence interval; DFS, disease-free survival; OS, overall survival.
From Bennett JM, Young ML, Andersen JW, et al. Long-term survival in acute myeloid leukemia: the Eastern Cooperative Oncology Group experience. *Cancer* 1997;80 [Suppl 11]:2205–2209, with permission.

LONG-TERM SURVIVAL

During the past 20 years, the long-term prognosis for patients with AML has improved considerably. The CCSG reported an increase in 4-year survival probabilities from 19% to 36% for 1000 children with AML who were treated on CCSG protocols between 1972 and 1983 (746). The risk of death or relapse in each year of follow-up decreased progressively from a high of 43% in the first year to 8% by the fourth year and remained close to 5% for the next 5 years. The German BFM Study Group treated more than 300 children with AML between 1978 and 1986 with intensive induction and consolidation chemotherapy followed by 2 years of maintenance and demonstrated an improvement in event-free survival from 38% to 49% (470).

The OS for adults with AML treated according to ECOG protocols between 1974 and 1996 increased from approximately 10% to approximately 30% to 40% (Table 15-17) (747). Age older than 60 years was an adverse prognostic factor for relapse-free survival in the CALGB trials as well as in other studies of older adults with AML. In the early CALGB studies (studies 7421, 7521, and 7721), the relapse curves did not plateau until the eighth year of remission (748). The detection of

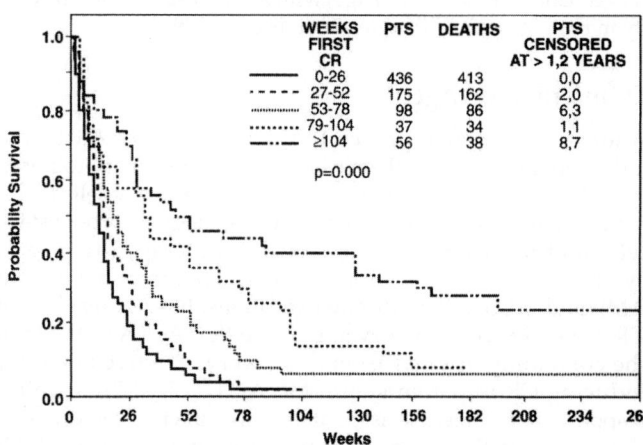

Figure 15-20. Probability of survival for 806 patients (PTS) with relapsed or refractory acute myelogenous leukemia treated generally with high-dose cytarabine-containing regimens at the M.D. Anderson Cancer Center. CR, complete remission. (From Estey E. Treatment of refractory AML. *Leukemia* 1996;10:932, with permission.)

minimal residual disease by immunophenotyping is now possible and may be useful in predicting relapse (749,750).

As previously discussed, survival after a relapse of AML is very poor. The M. D. Anderson Cancer Center reviewed their treatment experience for adults with AML in first relapse (686,687). Thirty-three percent of patients obtained a second CR. The median survival after relapse was only 18 weeks. The OS at 5 years from relapse was 5%, and the 5-year survival probability for the CR patients was 16%. Estey (751) has shown that among the most important prognostic factors predicting outcome in relapsed and refractory AML is the duration of first CR (751) (Fig. 15-20).

LATE EFFECTS OF ACUTE MYELOGENOUS LEUKEMIA AND ITS TREATMENT

Relatively little is known about the late effects of therapy in long-term survivors of AML. This lack of knowledge is not surprising, because most patients with AML have not remained in remission for 5 or more years. The biologic and psychologic late effects of surviving childhood ALL and its treatment have been well studied in the recent past (discussed in Chapter 27). Somatic complications have included inhibition of linear growth, sterility, CNS and cardiac dysfunction, hepatic and renal toxicities, and second malignancies. The psychologic problems have included learning disabilities, academic failure, behavioral and other adjustment problems, and depression. There are no studies reporting late neuropsychologic effects or brain abnormalities after treatment for AML, probably reflecting the minimal use of CNS therapy (cranial irradiation or intrathecal chemotherapy).

Infertility in leukemia survivors is a major concern. Results from a large retrospective cohort study of fertility in survivors of cancer during childhood and adolescence demonstrated that previous therapy with alkylating agents reduced fertility by approximately 60% in men, and there was no apparent effect among women (752). Previous therapy with nonalkylating agents resulted in no apparent decrease in fertility in either sex. Further screening for gonadal toxicity caused by anthracyclines and cytarabine is necessary to assess reproductive function and pregnancy outcome in treated patients.

Second malignant tumors have rarely been reported in survivors of AML, not surprisingly, because there have been few long-term survivors and because a limited number of patients have been treated with alkylating agents or irradiation (except in bone marrow transplantation studies).

Because the percentage of long-term survivors with AML is steadily increasing (747), studies should be initiated to examine the late sequelae of AML and its treatment as well as issues such as libido, sexual function, marital patterns, and overall psychologic adjustment. Among 215 cured patients (in first or second CR for at least 3 years), 163 (76%) were found on long-term follow-up to be alive in CR (753). Seventy-four percent of the patients who were working full-time and who were under age 50 at treatment were working at follow-up (754).

REFERENCES

1. Virchow R. Weisses Blut and Milztumoren. *Med Z* 1847;16:19.
2. Freidreich N. Ein neuer Fall von Leukamie. *Arch Pathol Anat* 1857;12:37.
3. Naegeli O. Ueber rotes Knochenmark und myeloblasten. *Dtsch Med Wochenschr* 1900;26:287.
4. Reschad H, Schilling-Torgau V. Ueber eine neue Leukamie durch echte uebergangsformen (Splenocytenleukemie) und ihre Bedeutung fur die Selbstandigkeit dieser Zellen. *Munchen Med Wochenschr* 1913;60:1981.
5. Watkins CH, Hall BE. Monocytic leukemia of the Naegeli and Schilling types. *Am J Clin Pathol* 1940;10:387.
6. DiGuglielmo G. Les maladies erythremisques. *Rev Hematol* 1946;1:355.
7. Hillstad LK. Acute promyelocytic leukemia. *Acta Med Scand* 1957;159:189.
8. Lewis SM, Szur L. Malignant myelosclerosis. *BMJ* 1963;2:472.
9. Golomb HM, Rowley JD, Vardiman J, et al. "Microgranular" acute promyelocytic leukemia: a distinct clinical, ultrastructural, and cytogenetic entity. *Blood* 1980;55:253.
10. McKenna RW, Parkin J, Bloomfield CD, et al. Acute promyelocytic leukaemia: a study of 39 cases with identification of a hyperbasophilic microgranular variant. *Br J Haematol* 1982;50:201–214.
11. Rovelli A, Biondi A, Cantu Rajnoldi A, et al. Microgranular variant of acute promyelocytic leukemia in children. *J Clin Oncol* 1992;10:1413–1418.
12. Bennett JM, Catovsky D, Daniel MT, et al. Proposals for the classification of the acute leukemias. *Br J Haematol* 1976;33:451.
13. Bennett JM, Catovsky D, Daniel MT, et al. Proposed revised criteria for the classification of acute myeloid leukemia. *Ann Intern Med* 1985;103:626.
14. Bennett JM, Catovsky D, Daniel MT, et al. Criteria for the diagnosis of acute leukemia of megakaryocytic lineage (M7). *Ann Intern Med* 1985;103:460.
15. Stanley M, McKenna RW, Ellinger G, et al. Classification of 358 cases of acute myeloid leukemia by FAB criteria: analysis of clinical and morphologic features. In: Bloomfield CD, ed. *Chronic and acute leukemias in adults*. Boston: Martinus Niijhoff, 1985:147–174.
16. Cutler SJ, Young JL, eds. *Third national cancer: incidence data*. National Cancer Institute Monograph No. 41. Washington, DC: US Government Printing Office, 1975.
17. Greenlee RT, Hill-Harmon MB, Murray T, et al. Cancer statistics, 2001. *CA Cancer J Clin* 2001;51:15.
18. Vickers M, Jackson G, Taylor P. The incidence of acute promyelocytic leukemia appears constant over most of a human lifespan, implying only one rate limiting mutation. *Leukemia* 2000;14:722.
19. Young JL, Ries LG, Silverberg E, et al. Cancer incidence, survival, and mortality for children younger than age 15 years. *Cancer* 1986;58:598.
20. Linet MS. The leukemias: epidemiologic aspects. In: Lilienfeld AM, ed. *Monographs in epidemiology and biostatistics*. New York: Oxford University Press, 1985:1.
21. Cavdar AO, Arcasoy A, Babacan E, et al. Ocular granulocytic sarcoma (chloroma) with acute myelomonocytic leukemia in Turkish children. *Cancer* 1978;41:1606.
22. Nakase K, Bradstock K, Sartor M, et al. Geographic heterogeneity of cellular characteristics of acute myeloid leukemia: a comparative study of Australian and Japanese adult cases. *Leukemia* 2000;14:163.
23. Committee on the Biological Effects of Ionizing Radiations, National Research Council. Health effects of exposure to low levels of ionizing radiation (BEIRV). Washington, DC: National Academy Press, 1990.
24. Matanoski GM, Seltser R, Sartwell PE. The current mortality rates of radiologists and other physician specialists: specific causes of death. *Am J Epidemiol* 1975;101:199.
25. Court-Brown WM, Doll R. Mortality from cancer and other causes after radiotherapy for ankylosing spondylitis. *BMJ* 1965;2:1327.
26. Ichimaru M, Ishimaru T, Belsky JL. Incidence of leukemia in atomic bomb survivors belonging to a fixed cohort in Hiroshima and Nagasaki, 1950–1971: radiation dose, years after exposure, age at exposure, and type of leukemia. *J Radiat Res* 1978;19:262.
27. Shimizu Y, Schull WJ, Kato H. Cancer risk among atomic bomb survivors: the RERF Life Span Study. *JAMA* 1990;264:601.
28. Stewart A, Webb J, Hewitt D. A survey of children malignancies. *BMJ* 1958;1:1495.
29. Graham S, Levin M, Lilienfeld A, et al. Preconception, intra-uterine, and postnatal irradiation as related to leukemia. *Natl Cancer Inst Monogr* 1966;19: 347.
30. Gilbert ES, Marks S. An analysis of the mortality of workers in a nuclear facility. *Radiat Res* 1979;79:122.
31. Savitz DA, Calle E. Leukemia and occupational exposure to electromagnetic fields: review of epidemiologic surveys. *J Occup Med* 1987;29:47.
32. Severson RK, Stevens RG, Kaune WT, et al. Acute non-lymphocytic leukemia and residential exposure to power frequency magnetic fields. *Am J Epidemiol* 1988;128:10.
33. Adamson RH, Seiber SM. Chemically induced leukemia in humans. *Environ Health Perspect* 1981;39:93.
34. Austin A, Delzell E, Cole P. Benzene and leukemia: a review of the literature and risk assessment. *Am J Epidemiol* 1988;127:419.
35. Cohen HJ, Huang ATF. A marker chromosome abnormality: occurrence in chloramphenicol-associated acute leukemia. *Arch Intern Med* 1973;132:440.
36. Friedman GD. Phenylbutazone, musculoskeletal disease, and leukemia. *J Chronic Dis* 1982;35:233.
37. Tucker MA, Meadows AT, Boice JD, et al. Leukemia after therapy with alkylating agents for childhood cancer. *J Natl Cancer Inst* 1977;78:459.
38. Kaldor JM, Day NE, Clarke EA, et al. Leukemia following Hodgkin's disease. *N Engl J Med* 1990;322:7.
39. Kaldor JM, Day NE, Pettersson F, et al. Leukemia following chemotherapy for ovarian cancer. *N Engl J Med* 1990;322:1–6.
40. Pui CH, Behm FG, Raimondi SC, et al. Secondary acute myeloid leukemia in children treated for acute lymphoid leukemia. *N Engl J Med* 1989;321:136.
41. Ratain MJ, Kaminer LS, Bitran JD, et al. Acute nonlymphocytic leukemia following etoposide and cisplatin combination chemotherapy for advance non-small-cell carcinoma of the lung. *Blood* 1987;70:1412.

42. Gallo C, Wong-Staal F. Retroviruses and etiologic agents of some animal and human leukemias and lymphoma and as tools for elucidating the molecular mechanism of leukemogenesis. *Blood* 1982;60:545.

43. Deinhardt F, Wolfe LG, Theilen GH, et al. ST-feline fibrosarcoma virus: induction of tumors in marmoset monkeys. *Science* 1970;167:881.

44. Poiesz BJ, Ruscetti FW, Gazdar AF, et al. Detection and isolation of type C retrovirus particles from fresh and cultured lymphocytes of a patient with cutaneous T-cell lymphoma. *Proc Natl Acad Sci U S A* 1980;77:7415.

45. Wong Staal F, Gallo RC. Human T-lymphotropic retroviruses. *Nature* 1985; 317:395.

46. Bishop JM. Viral oncogenes. *Cell* 1985;42:23.

47. Varmus HE. The molecular genetics of cellular oncogenes. *Annu Rev Genet* 1984;18:553.

48. Weinberg RA. The action of oncogenes in the cytoplasm and nucleus. *Science* 1985;230:770.

49. Bishop JM. The molecular genetics of cancer. *Science* 1987;235:305.

50. Friend SH, Horowitz JM, Gerber MR, et al. Deletions of a DNA sequence in retinoblastomas and mesenchymal tumors: organization of the sequence and its encoded protein. *Proc Natl Acad Sci U S A* 1987;84:9059.

51. Finlay CA, Hinds PW, Levine AJ. The p53 proto-oncogene can act as a suppressor of transformation. *Cell* 1989;57:1083.

52. Blasi E, Mathieson BJ, Varesio L, et al. Selective immortalization of murine macrophages from fresh bone marrow by a raf/myc recombinant murine retroviruses. *Nature* 1985;18:667.

53. Graf T, von Kirchbach A, Beug H. Characterization of the hematopoietic target cells of AEV, MC29, and AMV avian leukemia viruses. *Exp Cell Res* 1981;131:331.

54. Bartram CR, de Klein A, Hagemeijer A, et al. Translocation of the c-abl oncogene correlates with the presence of a Philadelphia chromosome myelocytic leukemia. *Nature* 1983;306:239.

55. Heisterkamp N, Stephenson JR, Groffen J, et al. Localization of the c-abl oncogene adjacent to a translocation break point in chronic myelocytic leukemia. *Nature* 1983;306:277.

56. Bos JL, Toksoz D, Marchall CJ, et al. Amino-acid substitutions at codon 13 of the N-ras oncogene in human acute myeloid leukemia. *Nature* 1985; 315:726.

57. Needleman SW, Kraus MH, Srivastava SK, et al. High frequency of N-ras activation in acute myelogenous leukemia. *Blood* 1986;67:753.

58. Farr CJ, Saiki RK, Erlich HA, et al. Analysis of RAS gene mutations in acute myeloid leukemia by polymerase chain reaction and oligonucleotide probes. *Proc Natl Acad Sci U S A* 1988;85:1629.

59. Beaupre DM, Kurzrock R. RAS and leukemia: from basic mechanisms to gene-directed therapy. *J Clin Oncol* 1999;17:1071–1079.

60. Barbicid M. Ras genes. *Annu Rev Biochem* 1987;56:779.

61. Varmus HE. The molecular genetics of cellular oncogenes. *Annu Rev Genet* 1984;18:553.

62. Satoh T, Nakafuku M, Miyajima A, et al. Involvement of rasp21 protein in signal transduction pathways from interleukin 2, interleukin 3, and granulocyte/macrophage colony-stimulating factor, but not from interleukin 4. *Proc Natl Acad Sci U S A* 1991;88:3314.

63. Lochrie MA, Simon MI. G. protein multiplicity in eukaryotic signal transduction systems. *Biochemistry* 1988;27:4957.

64. DeVos AM, Tong L, Milburn MV, et al. Three dimensional structure of an oncogene protein: catalytic domain of human c-H-vas p21. *Science* 1988;239:888.

65. Bos JL, Verlaan-de Vries M, van der Eb AJ, et al. Mutations in N-ras predominate in acute myeloid leukemia. *Blood* 1987;69:1237.

66. Neubauer A, Greenberg P, Negrin R, et al. Mutations in the ras proto-oncogenes in patients with myelodysplastic syndromes. *Leukemia* 1994;8:638–641.

67. Neubauer A, Dodge RK, George SL, et al. Prognostic importance of mutations in the ras proto-oncogenes in de novo acute myeloid leukemia. *Blood* 1994;83:1603–1611.

68. Senn HP, Jiricny J, Fopp M, et al. Relapse cell population differ from acute onset clone as shown by absence of the initially activated N-ras oncogene in a patient with acute myelomonocytic leukemia. *Blood* 1988;72:931.

69. Karp J, Lancet JE, Kaufmann SH, et al. Clinical and biologic activity of the farnesyltransferase inhibitor R115777 in adults with refractory and relapsed acute leukemias: a phase 1 clinical-laboratory correlative trial. *Blood* 2001;97:3361–3369.

70. Borrow J, Goddard AD, Sheer D, et al. Molecular analysis of acute promyelocytic leukemia breakpoint cluster region on chromosome 17. *Science* 1990; 240:1577.

71. Alcalay M, Zangrilli D, Pandolfi PP, et al. Translocation breakpoint of acute promyelocytic leukemia lies within the retinoic acid receptor alpha locus. *Proc Natl Acad Sci U S A* 1991;88:1977.

72. de The H, Chomienne C, Lanotte M, et al. The t(15;17) translocation of acute promyelocytic leukaemia fuses the retinoic acid receptor gene to a novel transcribed locus. *Nature* 1990;347:558.

73. Miyoshi H, Shimizu K, Kozu T, et al. The t (8;21) breakpoints on chromosome 21 in acute myeloid leukemia clustered within a limited region of a novel gene AMLI. *Proc Natl Acad Sci U S A* 1991;88:10431.

74. Gao J, Erickson P, Gardiner K, et al. Isolation of a yeast artificial chromosome spanning the 8;21 translocation breakpoint, t(8;21)(q22.3) in acute myelogenous leukemia. *Proc Natl Acad Sci U S A* 1991;88:4882.

75. Erickson P, Gao J, Chang K-S, et al. Identification of breakpoints in t(8;21) AML and isolation of a fusion transcript with similarity to *Drosophila* segmentation gene runt. *Blood* 1992;80:1825.

76. Nucifora G, Larson RA, Rowley JD. Persistence of the 8;21 translocation in patients with acute myeloid leukemia type M2 in long-term remission. *Blood* 1993;82:712.

77. Kozu T, Miyoshi H, Shimizu K, et al. Junctions of the AML 1/MTG8(ETO) fusion are constant in t(8;21) acute myeloid leukemia detected by reverse transcription polymerase chain reaction. *Blood* 1993;82:1270.

78. Liu P, Tarle SA, Hajra A, et al. Fusion between transcription factor CBF beta/PEBA2 beta and a myosin heavy chain in acute myeloid leukemia. *Science* 1993;261:1041.

79. Domer PH, Fakharzadeh SS, Chen CS, et al. Acute mixed-lineage leukemia t(4;11)(q21;q23) generates an MLL-AF4 fusion product. *Proc Natl Acad Sci U S A* 1993;90:7884.

80. Thirman MJ, Gill HJ, Burnett RC, et al. Rearrangement of the MLL gene in acute lymphoblastic and acute myeloid leukemias with 11q23 chromosomal translocations. *N Engl J Med* 1993;329:909.

81. Kobayashi H, Espinosa R III, Thirman MJ, et al. Heterogeneity of breakpoints of 11q23 rearrangements in hematologic malignancies identified with fluorescence in situ hybridization. *Blood* 1993;82:547.

82. McCabe NR, Burnett RC, Gill HJ, et al. Cloning of cDNAs of the MLL gene that detect DNA rearrangements and altered RNA transcripts in human leukemic cells with 11q23 translocations. *Proc Natl Acad Sci U S A* 1992;89: 11794.

83. Zieman-van der Poel S, McCabe NR, Gill HJ, et al. Identification of a gene, MLL, that spans the breakpoint in 11q.23 translocations associated with human leukemias. *Proc Natl Acad Sci U S A* 1991;88:10735.

84. von Lindern M, Poutska AM, Lehrach H, et al. The (6;9) chromosome translocation, associated with a specific subtype of acute nonlymphocytic leukemia, leads to aberrant transcription of a target gene on 9q34. *Mol Cell Biol* 1990;10:4016.

85. Ahuja HG, Jat PS, Foti A, et al. Abnormalities of the retinoblastoma gene in the pathogenesis of acute leukemia. *Blood* 1991;78:3259.

86. Ahuja HG, Bar-Eli M, Advani SH, et al. Alterations in the p53 gene and the clonal evolution of the blast crisis of chronic myeloid leukemia. *Proc Natl Acad Sci U S A* 1989;86:6783.

87. Reference deleted.

88. Reference deleted.

89. Linet MS. The leukemias: epidemiologic aspects. In: Lilienfeld AM, ed. *Monographs in epidemiology and biostatistics.* New York: Oxford University Press, 1985:1.

90. Mulvihill JJ. Congenital and genetic diseases. In: Fraumeni JF, ed. *Persons at high risk of cancer.* San Diego: Academic Press, 1975:3.

91. Garriga S, Crosby WH. The incidence of leukemia in families of patients with hypoplasia of the marrow. *Blood* 1959;14:1008.

92. Rosen RB, Kang S-JA. Congenital agranulocytosis terminating in acute myelomonocytic leukemia. *J Pediatr* 1979;94:406.

93. Rosner F, Lee SL. Down's syndrome and acute leukemia: myeloblastic or lymphoblastic? *Am J Med* 1972;53:203.

94. Weinstein HJ. Congenital leukemia and the neonatal myeloproliferative disorders associated with Down's syndrome. *Clin Hematol* 1978;7:147.

95. Hayashi Y, Eguchi M, Sugita K, et al. Cytogenetic findings and clinical features in acute leukemia and transient myeloproliferative disorder in Down's syndrome. *Blood* 1988;72:15.

96. Eguchi M, Sakakibara H, Suda J, et al. Ultrastructural and ultracytochemical differences between transient myeloproliferative disorder and megakaryoblastic leukemia in Down's syndrome. *Br J Haematol* 1989;73:315.

97. Kurahashi H, Hara J, Yumura-Yagi K, et al. Monoclonal nature of transient abnormal myelopoiesis in Down's syndrome. *Blood* 1991;77:1161.

98. Seibel NL, Sommer A, Miser J. Transient neonatal leukemoid reactions in mosaic trisomy 21. *J Pediatr* 1984;104:251.

99. Brodeur GM, Dahl GV, Williams DL, et al. Transient leukemoid reaction and trisomy 21 mosaicism in a phenotypically normal newborn. *Blood* 1980;55: 691.

100. Zipursky A, Peeters M, Poon A. Megakaryoblastic leukemia and Down's syndrome: a review. *Proc Clin Biol Res* 1987;246:33.

101. Homans A, Verissimo AM, Vlacha V. Transient abnormal myelopoiesis of infancy associated with trisomy 21. *Am J Pediatr Hematol Oncol* 1993;15: 392.

102. Till JE, McCulloch EA. A direct measurement of the radiation sensitivity of normal mouse bone marrow cells. *Radiat Res* 1961;14:213

103. Pluznik DH, Sachs L. The cloning of normal "mast" cells in tissue culture. *J Cell Physiol* 1965;66:319.

104. Pike BL, Robinson WA. Human bone marrow colony growth in agar-gel. *J Cell Physiol* 1970;76:77.

105. Becher AJ, McCulloch EA, Till JE. Cytological demonstration of the clonal nature of spleen colonies derived from transplanted mouse marrow cells. *Nature* 1963;197:452.

106. Bradley TR, Metcalf D. The growth of mouse bone marrow cells in vitro. *Aust J Exp Biol Med Sci* 1966;44:287.

107. Chervenick PA, Boggs DR. Bone marrow colonies: stimulation in vitro by supernatant from incubated human blood cells. *Science* 1970;69:691.

108. Sheridan JW, Stanley ER. Tissue sources of bone marrow colony stimulating factor. *J Cell Physiol* 1971;78:451.

109. Golde DW, Clive MJ. Identification of the colony-stimulating cell in human peripheral blood. *J Clin Invest* 1972;51:2981.

110. Suda J, Suda T, Ogawa M. Analysis of differentiation of mouse hemopoietic stem cells in culture by sequential replating of paired progenitors. *Blood* 1984;64:393.

111. Spangrude GJ, Heimfeld S, Weissman IL. Purification and characterization of mouse hematopoietic stem cells. *Science* 1988;241:58.

112. Fauser AA, Messner HA. Identification of megakaryocytes, macrophages and eosinophils in colonies of human bone marrow containing neutrophilic granulocytes and erythroblasts. *Blood* 1979;53:1023.

113. Till JE, McCulloch EA. Hematopoietic stem cell differentiation. *Biochem Biophys Acta* 1980;605:431.

114. Ogawa M, Porter PN, Nakahata T. Renewal and commitment to differentiation of hemopoietic stem cells. *Blood* 1983;61:823.

115. Stephenson JR, Axelrod AA, McLeod DL, et al. Induction of colonies of hemoglobin synthesizing cells by erythropoietin in vitro. *Proc Natl Acad Sci U S A* 1971;68:1542.

116. Griffin JD, Lowenberg B. Clonogenic cells in acute myeloblastic leukemia. *Blood* 1986;68:1185.

117. Metcalf D. The granulocyte-macrophage colony stimulating factors. *Science* 1985;229:16.

118. Dinarello CA, Mier JW. Lymphokines. *N Engl J Med* 1987;317:940.

119. Nienhuis AW. Hematopoietic growth factors: biological complexity and clinical promise. *N Engl J Med* 1988;318:916.

120. Clark SC, Kamen R. The human hematopoietic colony-stimulating factors. *Science* 1987;236:1229.

121. Metcalf D. The molecular biology and functions of the granulocyte colony-stimulating factors. *Blood* 1986;67:257.

122. Sieff CA. Hematopoietic growth factors. *J Clin Invest* 1987;79:1549.

123. Bronchud MH, Scarffe JH, Thatcher N, et al. Phase I/II study of recombinant human granulocyte colony-stimulating factor in patients receiving intensive chemotherapy for small cell lung cancer. *Br J Cancer* 1987;56:809.

124. Gabrilove JL, Jakubowski A, Scher H, et al. Effect of granulocyte colony-stimulating factor on neutropenia and associated morbidity due to chemotherapy for transitional–cell carcinoma of the urothelium. *N Engl J Med* 1988; 318:1414.

125. Antman KS, Griffin JD, Elias A, et al. Effect of recombinant human granulocyte-macrophage colony-stimulating factor on chemotherapy-induced myelosuppression. *N Engl J Med* 1988;319:593.

126. Ganser A, Volkers B, Ottmann OG, et al. Recombinant human granulocyte-macrophage colony-stimulating factor in patients with myelodysplastic syndromes: a phase I/II trial. *Blood* 1989;73:31.

127. Leischke GJ, Maher D, Cebon J, et al. Effects of bacterially synthesized recombinant human granulocyte-macrophage colony stimulating factor in patients with advanced malignancy. *Ann Intern Med* 1989;110:357.

128. Moore MAS, Williams N, Metcalf D. In vitro colony formation by normal and leukemic human hematopoietic cells: characterization of the colony forming cells. *J Natl Cancer Inst* 1973;50:603.

129. Minden MD, Till JE, McCulloch EA. Proliferative state of blast cells progenitors in acute myeloblastic leukemia (AML). *Blood* 1978;52:592.

130. Wouters R, Lowenberg B. On the maturation order of AML cells: a destruction on the basis of self renewal properties and immunologic phenotypes. *Blood* 1984;63:684.

131. Griffin JD, Larcom P, Schlossman SF. Use of surface markers to identify a subset of acute myelomonocytic leukemia cells with progenitor cells properties. *Blood* 1983;62:1300.

132. Koeffler HP, Golde DW. Human myeloid leukemia cell lines: a review. *Blood* 1980;56:344.

133. Greenberg PL. The smouldering myeloid leukemic states: clinical and biologic features. *Blood* 1983;61:1035.

134. Verma DS, Spitzer G, Dicke KA, et al. In vitro agar culture patterns in preleukemia and their clinical significance. *Leuk Res* 1979;3:41.

135. McCulloch EA, Curtis JE, Messner HA, et al. The contribution of blast cell properties to outcome variation in acute myeloblastic leukemia. *Blood* 1982;59:601.

136. Clarkson B, Fried J, Strife A, et al. Studies of cellular proliferation in human leukemia, III: behavior of leukemic cell in three adults with acute leukemia given continuous infusions of 3H-thymidine for 8 or 10 days. *Cancer* 1970;25:1237.

137. Killmann SA. Proliferative activity of blast cells in leukemia and myelopoiesis: morphological differences between proliferating and non-proliferating blast cells. *Acta Med Scand* 1965;178:263.

138. Mauer AM, Saunders EF, Lampkine BC. Possible significance of nonproliferating leukemia cells. *Natl Cancer Inst Monogr* 1969;30:63.

139. Raza A, Maheshwari Y, Ucar K, et al. Proliferative characteristics of acute nonlymphocytic leukemia in vivo. *Acta Haematol (Basel)* 1987;77:140.

140. Raza A, Maheshwari Y, Yasin Z, et al. A new method for studying cell cycle characteristics in ANLL using double-labeling with BrdU and 3 HHTdr. *Leuk Res* 1987;11:1079.

141. Cannistra SA, Groshek P, Griffin JD. Granulocyte-macrophage colony-stimulating factor enhances the cytotoxic effects of cytosine arabinoside in acute myeloblastic leukemia and in the myeloid blast crisis phase of chronic myeloid leukemia. *Leukemia* 1989;3:328.

142. Vellenga E, Young DC, Wagner K, et al. The effects of GM-CSF and G-CSF in promoting growth of clonogenic cells in acute myeloblastic leukemia. *Blood* 1987;69:1771.

143. Vellenga E, Ostapovicz D, O'Rourke B, et al. Effects of recombinant IL-3, GM-CSF and G-CSF on proliferation of leukemic clonogenic cells in short-term and long-term cultures. *Leukemia* 1987;1:584.

144. Hoang T, Nara N, Wong G, et al. Effects of recombinant GM-CSF on the blast cells of acute myeloblastic leukemia. *Blood* 1986;68:313.

145. Hoang T, Haman A, Goncalves O, et al. Interleukin 1 enhances growth factor-dependent proliferation of the clonogenic cells in acute myeloblastic leukemia and of normal human hemopoietic precursors. *J Exp Med* 1988;168:463.

146. Vadhan-Raj S, Keating M, LeMaistre A, et al. Effects of recombinant human granulocyte-macrophage colony-stimulating factor in patients with myelodysplastic syndromes. *N Engl J Med* 1987;317:1545.

147. Ganser A, Volkers B, Greher J, et al. Recombinant human granulocyte-macrophage colony-stimulating factor in patients with myelodysplastic syndromes: a phase I/II trial. *Blood* 1988;73:31.

148. Kobayashi Y, Okabe T, Ozawa K, et al. Treatment of myelodysplastic syndromes with recombinant human granulocyte colony-stimulating factor: a preliminary report. *Am J Med* 1989;86:178.

149. Negrin RS, Haeuber DH, Nagler AN, et al. Treatment of myelodysplastic syndromes with recombinant human granulocyte colony-stimulating factor: a phase I-II trial. *Ann Intern Med* 1989;110:976.

150. Herrmann F, Lindermann A, Klein H, et al. Effect of recombinant human granulocyte-macrophage colony-stimulating factor in patients with myelodysplastic syndrome with excess of blasts. *Leukemia* 1989;3:335.

151. Ganser A, Seipelt G, Lundermann A, et al. Effects of recombinant human interleukin 3 in patients with myelodysplastic syndromes. *Blood* 1990;76:455.

152. Cannistra SA, DiCarlo J, Groshek P, et al. Simultaneous administration of granulocyte-macrophage colony stimulating factor and cytosine arabinoside for the treatment of relapsed acute myeloid leukemia. *Leukemia* 1991;5:230.

153. Dexter TM, Garland J, Scott D, et al. Growth factor-dependent hemopoietic precursor cell lines. *J Exp Med* 1980;152:1036.

154. Lang RA, Metcalf D, Gough NM, et al. Expression of a hemopoietic growth factor cDNA in a factor-dependent cell line results in autonomous growth and tumorigenicity. *Cell* 1985;43:531.

155. Adkins B, Leutz A, Graf T. Autocrine growth factor induced by svc-related oncogenes in transformed chicken myeloid cells. *Cell* 1984;39:439.

156. Baumbach WR, Stanley ER, Cole MD. Induction of clonal monocyte-macrophage tumors in vivo by mouse c-myc retrovirus: rearrangement of the CSF-1 gene as a secondary transforming event. *Mol Cell Biol* 1987;7:664.

157. Ymer S, Tucker WQJ, Sanderson CJ, et al. Constitutive synthesis of interleukin 3 by leukemia cell line WEHI-3B is due to retroviral insertion near the gene. *Nature* 1985;317:255.

158. Young DC, Griffin JD. Autocrine secretion of GM-CSF in acute myeloblastic leukemia. *Blood* 1986;68:1178.

159. Young DC, Wagner K, Griffin JD. Constitutive expression of the granulocyte-macrophage colony-stimulating factor gene in acute myelocytic leukemia. *J Clin Invest* 1987;79:100.

160. Kaufman DC, Baer MR, Gao XZ, et al. Enhanced expression of the granulocyte-macrophage colony-stimulating factor gene in acute myelocytic leukemia cells following in vitro blast cell enrichment. *Blood* 1988;1329:1332.

161. Oster W, Lindemann A, Ganser A, et al. Constitutive expression of hematopoietic growth factors in acute myeloblastic leukemia cells. *Behring Inst Mitt* 1987;83:68.

162. Griffin JD, Rambaldi A, Vellenga E, et al. Secretion of interleukin 1 by acute myeloblastic leukemia cells in vitro induces endothelial cells to secrete colony-stimulating factors. *Blood* 1987;70:1218.

163. Watari K, Asano S, Shirafuji N, et al. Serum granulocyte colony stimulating factor levels in healthy volunteers and patients with various disorders as estimated by enzyme immunoassay. *Blood* 1989;73:117.

164. Löwenberg B, van Putten WL, Touw IP, et al. Autonomous proliferation of leukemic cells in vitro as a determinant of prognosis in adult acute myeloid leukemia. *N Engl J Med* 1993;328:614.

165. Collins SJ, Gallo RC, Gallagher RE. Continuous growth and differentiation of human myeloid leukemic cells in suspension culture. *Nature* 1977;270:347.

166. Lozzio CB, Lozzio BB. Human chronic myelogenous leukemia cell line with positive Philadelphia chromosome. *Blood* 1975;45:321.

167. Sundstrom C, Nilsson K. Establishment and characterization of a human histocytic lymphoma cell line (U-937). *Int J Cancer* 1976;17:565.

168. Tsuchiya S, Yamabe M, Yamaguchi Y, et al. Establishment and characterization of a human acute monocytic leukemic cell line (THP-1). *Int J Cancer* 1980;26:171.

169. Collins SJ. The HL-60 promyelocytic leukemia cell line: proliferation, differentiation, and cellular oncogene expression. *Blood* 1987;70:1233.

170. Hoffman SJ, Robinson WA. Use of differentiation-inducing agents in the myelodysplastic syndrome and acute non-lymphocytic leukemia. *Am J Hematol* 1988;28:124.

171. Huang ME, Ye YC, Chen SR, et al. Use of all-trans retinoic acid in the treatment of acute promyelocytic leukemia. *Blood* 1988;72:567.

172. Wang ZY, Sun GL, Lu JX, et al. Treatment of acute promyelocytic leukemia with all-trans retinoic acid in China. *Nouv Rev Fr Hematol* 1990;32:34.

173. Castaigne S, Chomienne C, Daniel MT, et al. All-trans retinoic acid as a differentiation therapy for acute promyelocytic leukemia, I: clinical results. *Blood* 1990;76:1704.

174. Fialkow PJ, Singer JW, Adamson JW, et al. Acute nonlymphocytic leukemia: heterogeneity of stem cell origin. *Blood* 1981;57:1068.

175. Fialkow PJ, Singer JW, Raskind WH, et al. Clonal development, stem cell differentiation, and clinical remissions in a acute nonlymphocytic leukemia. *N Engl J Med* 1987;317:468.

176. Rowley JD. Recurring chromosome abnormalities in leukemia and lymphoma. *Semin Hematol* 1990;27:122.

177. Rowley JD, LeBeau MM. Cytogenetic and molecular analysis of therapy-related leukemia. *Ann N Y Acad Sci* 1989;567:130.

178. Yunis JJ, Brunning RD. Prognostic significance of chromosomal abnormalities in acute leukaemias and myelodysplastic syndromes. *Clin Haematol* 1986;15:597.
179. Bloomfield CD, de la Chapelle A. Chromosome abnormalities in acute non-lymphocytic leukemia: clinical and biological significance. *Semin Oncol* 1987;14:372.
180. Fearon ER, Burke PJ, Schiffer CA, et al. Differentiation of leukemia cells to polymorphonuclear leukocytes in patients with acute nonlymphocytic leukemia. *N Engl J Med* 1986;315:15.
181. Jacobsen RJ, Temple MJ, Singer JW, et al. A clonal complete remission in a patient with acute nonlymphocytic leukemia originating in a multi-potent stem cell. *N Engl J Med* 1984;310:1513.
182. LoCoco F, Pelicci PG, D'Adamo F, et al. Polyclonal hematopoietic reconstitution in leukemia patients at remission after suppression of specific gene rearrangements. *Blood* 1993;82:606.
183. Busque L, Gilliland DG. Clonal evolution in acute myeloid leukemia. *Blood* 1993;82:337.
184. Fialkow PJ, Gartler SM, Yoshida A. Clonal origin of chronic myelocytic leukemia in man. *Proc Natl Acad Sci U S A* 1967;58:1468.
185. Sabbath KD, Ball ED, Larcom P, et al. Heterogeneity of clonogenic cells in AML. *J Clin Invest* 1985;75:746.
186. Lee EJ, Yang J, Leavitt RD, et al. The significance of CD34 and TdT determinations in patients with untreated de novo acute myeloid leukemia. *Leukemia* 1992;6:1203–1209.
187. Huh YO, Smith TL, Collins P, et al. Terminal deoxynucleotidyl transferase expression in acute myelogenous leukemia and myelodysplasia as determined by flow cytometry. *Leuk Lymphoma* 2000;37:319–331.
188. Venditti A, Del Poeta G, Buccisano F, et al. Prognostic relevance of the expression of Tdt and CD7 in 335 cases of acute myeloid leukemia. *Leukemia* 1998;12:1056–1063.
189. Chan LC, Pegram SM, Greaves MF. Contribution of immunophenotype to the classification and differential diagnosis of acute leukemia. *Lancet* 1985;1:475.
190. Freedman AS, Nadler LM. Cell surface markers in hematologic malignancies. *Semin Oncol* 1987;14:193.
191. Drexter HG, Minowada J. The use of monoclonal antibodies for the identification and classification of acute myeloid leukemias. *Leuk Res* 1986;10:279.
192. Foon KA, Todd RF. Immunologic classification of leukemia and lymphoma. *Blood* 1986;68:1.
193. McMichael AJ, ed. *Leucocyte typing, III: white cell differentiation antigens.* Oxford, UK: Oxford University Press, 1987.
194. Griffin JD, Ritz J, Nadler LM, et al. Expression of myeloid differentiation antigens on normal and malignant myeloid cells. *J Clin Invest* 1981;68:932.
195. Griffin JD, Davis R, Nelson DA, et al. Use of surface marker analysis to predict outcome of adult acute myeloblastic leukemia. *Blood* 1986;68:1232.
196. Drexter HG. Classification of acute myeloid leukemias: a comparison of FAB and immunophenotyping. *Leukemia* 1987;1:697.
197. Campos L, Guyotat D, Archimbaud E, et al. Surface marker expression in adult acute myeloid leukemia: correlations with initial characteristics, morphology and response to therapy. *Br J Haematol* 1989;72:161.
198. Schwarzinger I, Valent P, Koller U, et al. Prognostic significance of surface marker expression on blasts of patients with de novo acute myeloblastic leukemia. *J Clin Oncol* 1990;8:423.
199. Borowitz MJ, Gockerman JP, Moore JP, et al. Clinicopathologic and cytogenetic features of CD34 (My10)-positive acute nonlymphocytic leukemia. *Am J Clin Pathol* 1989;91:265.
200. Solary E, Casasnovas RO, Campos L, et al. Surface markers in adult acute myeloblastic leukemia: correlation of CD19+, CD34+ and CD14+/DR- phenotypes with shorter survival. Groupe d'Etude Immunologique des Leucemies (GEIL). *Leukemia* 1992;6:393–399.
201. Bradstock K, Matthews J, Benson E, et al. Prognostic value of immunophenotyping in acute myeloid leukemia. Australian Leukaemia Study Group. *Blood* 1994;84:1220–1225.
202. Harris NL, Jaffe ES, Diebold J, et al. World Health Organization classification of neoplastic diseases of the hematopoietic and lymphoid tissues: report of the Clinical Advisory Committee Meeting—Airlie House, Virginia, November, 1997. *J Clin Oncol* 1999;17:3835–3849.
203. Head DR. Revised classification of acute myeloid leukemia. *Leukemia* 1996; 10:1826.
204. Greaves MF, Chan LC, Furley AJW, et al. Lineage promiscuity in hemopoietic differentiation and leukemia. *Blood* 1986;67:1.
205. Paietta F, Bettleheim P, Schwarzmeier JD, et al. Distinct lymphoblastic and myeloblastic populations in TdT positive acute myeloblastic leukemia: evidence by double fluorescence staining. *Leuk Res* 1983;7:301.
206. Cross AH, Goorha RM, Nuss R, et al. Acute myeloid leukemia with T-lymphoid features: a distinct biological and clinical entity. *Blood* 1988;72:579.
207. Hurwitz C, Raimondi S, Head D, et al. Distinctive immunophenotypic features of t(8;21) (q22;q22) acute myeloblastic leukemia in children. *Blood* 1992;80:3182.
208. Pui CH, Raimondi SC, Head D, et al. Characterization of childhood acute leukemia with multiple myeloid and lymphoid markers at diagnosis and relapse. *Blood* 1991;78:1327.
209. Smith FO, Lampkin BC, Versteeg C, et al. Expression of lymphoid-associated cell surface antigens by childhood acute myeloid leukemia cells lacks prognostic significance. *Blood* 1992;79:2415.
210. Jensen AW, Hokland M, Jorgensen H, et al. Solitary expression of CD7 among T-cell antigens in acute myeloid leukemia: identification of a group of

211. patients with similar T cell receptor beta and delta rearrangements and course of disease suggestive of poor prognosis. *Blood* 1991;78:1292.
211. Drexler HG, Thiel E, Ludwig W-D. Acute myeloid leukemia expressing lymphoid-associated antigens: diagnostic incidence and prognostic significance. *Leukemia* 1993;7:489.
212. Smith LJ, Curtis JE, Messner HA, et al. Lineage infidelity in acute leukemia. *Blood* 1983;61:1138.
213. Hershfield MS, Kurtzberg J, Harden E, et al. Conversion of a stem cell leukemia from a T- lymphoid to a myeloid phenotype induced by the adenosine deaminase inhibitor 2'-deoxycoformycin. *Proc Natl Acad Sci U S A* 1984;81:253.
214. Pui CH, Frankel LS, Carroll AJ, et al. Clinical characteristics and treatment outcome of childhood acute lymphoblastic leukemia with the t(4;11)(q21;q23): a collaborative study of 40 cases. *Blood* 1991;77:440.
215. Sobol RE, Mick R, Royston I, et al. Clinical importance of myeloid antigen expression in adult acute lymphoblastic leukemia. *N Engl J Med* 1987;316:1111.
216. Ball ED, Davis RB, Griffin JD, et al. Prognostic value of lymphocyte surface markers in acute myeloid leukemia. *Blood* 1991;77:2242.
217. Lee EJ, Pollak A, Leavitt RD, et al. Minimally differentiated acute nonlymphocytic leukemia: a distinct entity. *Blood* 1987;70:1400.
218. Cohen PL, Hoyer JD, Kurtin PJ, et al. Acute myeloid leukemia with minimal differentiation: a multiple parameter study. *Am J Clin Pathol* 1998;109:32–38.
219. Venditti A, Del Poeta G, Buccisano F, et al. Minimally differentiated acute myeloid leukemia (AML-M0): comparison of 25 cases with other French-American-British subtypes. *Blood* 1997;89:621–629.
220. Cuneo A, Ferrant A, Michaux JL, et al. Cytogenetic profile of minimally differentiated (FAB M0) acute myeloid leukemia: correlation with clinicobiologic findings. *Blood* 1995;85:3688–3694.
221. Raghavachar A, Bartram CR, Ganser A, et al. Acute undifferentiated leukemia: implications for cellular origin and clonality suggested by analysis of surface markers and immunoglobulin gene rearrangement. *Blood* 1986;68:658.
222. Pombo de Oliveira MS, Matutes E, Rani S, et al. Early expression of MCS2 (CD13) in the cytoplasm of blast cells from acute myeloid leukemia. *Acta Haematol (Basel)* 1988;80:61.
223. Parreira A, Pombo de Oliveira MS, Matutes E, et al. Terminal deoxynucleotidyl transferase positive acute myeloid leukemia: an association with immature myeloblastic leukaemia. *Br J Haematol* 1988;69:219.
224. Vainchenker W, Villeval JL, Tabilio A, et al. Immunophenotype of leukemic blasts with small peroxidase-positive granules detected by electron microscopy. *Leukemia* 1988;2:274.
225. Lo Coco F, De Rossi G, Pasqualetti D, et al. CD7 positive acute myeloid leukaemia: a subtype associated with cell immaturity. *Br J Haematol* 1989;73:480.
226. Matutes E, Pombo de Oliveira M, Foroni L, et al. The role of ultrastructural cytochemistry and monoclonal antibodies in clarifying the nature of undifferentiated cells in acute leukaemia. *Br J Haematol* 1988;69:205.
227. Larson RA, LeBeau MM, Vardiman JW, et al. The predictive value of initial cytogenetic studies in 148 adults with acute nonlymphocytic leukemia: a 12 year study (1970–1982). *Cancer Genet Cytogenet* 1983;10:219.
228. Berger R, Bernheim A, Flandrin G, et al. Valeur pronostique de anomalies chromosomiques dans les leucemies aigues non lymphoblastiques. *Nouv Rev Fr Hematol* 1983;25:87.
229. Keating MJ, Cork A, Broach Y, et al. Toward a clinically relevant cytogenetic classification of acute myelogenous leukemia. *Leuk Res* 1987;11:119.
230. The Fourth International Workshop on Chromosomes in Leukemia. A prospective study of acute nonlymphocytic leukemia. *Cancer Genet Cytogenet* 1984;11:249.
231. Yunis JJ, Brunning RD, Howe RB, et al. High-resolution chromosomes as an independent prognostic indicator in adult acute nonlymphocytic leukemia. *N Engl J Med* 1984;311:812.
232. Arthur DC, Berger R, Golcomb HM, et al. The clinical significance of karyotype in acute myelogenous leukemia. *Cancer Genet Cytogenet* 1989;40:203.
233. Rowely JD. The role of chromosome translocations in leukemogenesis. *Semin Hematol* 1999;36:59–72.
234. Rowley JD. Molecular genetics in acute leukemia. *Leukemia* 2000;14:513–517.
235. Reference deleted.
236. Goddard AD, Borrow J, Freemont PS, et al. Characterization of a zinc finger gene disrupted by the t(15;17) in acute promyelocytic leukemia. *Science* 1991; 4:1371.
237. Kakizuka A, Miller WH, Umesono K, et al. Chromosomal translocation t(15;17) in human acute promyelocytic leukemia fuses RARα with a novel putative transcription factor, PML. *Cell* 1991;66:663.
238. de The H, Lavau C, Marchio A, et al. The PML-RAR alpha fusion mRNA generated by the t(15;17) translocation in acute promyelocytic leukemia encodes a functionally altered RAR. *Cell* 1991;66:675.
239. Wang ZG, Delva L, Gaboli M, et al. Role of PML in cell growth and the retinoic acid pathway. *Science* 1998;279:1547–1551.
240. Wang ZG, Ruggero D, Ronchetti S, et al. PML is essential for multiple apoptotic pathways. *Nat Genet* 1998;20:266–272.
241. Salomoni P, Pandolfi PP. The role of PML in tumor suppression. *Cell* 2002;108:165–170.
242. Fenaux P, Castaigne S, Dombret H, et al. All-trans retinoic acid followed by intensive chemotherapy gives a high complete remission rate and may prolong remissions in newly diagnosed acute promyelocytic leukemia: a pilot study on 26 cases. *Blood* 1992;80:2176–2181.

243. Warrell RP Jr, Maslak P, Eardley A, et al. Treatment of acute promyelocytic leukemia with all-trans retinoic acid: an update of the New York experience. *Leukemia* 1994;8:929–933.

244. Kanamaru A, Takemoto Y, Tanimoto M, et al. All-trans retinoic acid for the treatment of newly diagnosed acute promyelocytic leukemia. Japan Adult Leukemia Study Group. *Blood* 1995;85:1202–1206.

245. Mandelli F, Diverio D, Avvisati G, et al. Molecular remission in PML/RAR alpha-positive acute promyelocytic leukemia by combined all-trans retinoic acid and idarubicin (AIDA) therapy. Gruppo Italiano-Malattie Ematologiche Maligne dell'Adulto and Associazione Italiana di Ematologia ed Oncologia Pediatrica Cooperative Groups. *Blood* 1997;90:1014–1021.

246. Lengfelder E, Reichert A, Schoch C, et al. Double induction strategy including high dose cytarabine in combination with all-trans retinoic acid: effects in patients with newly diagnosed acute promyelocytic leukemia. German AML Cooperative Group. *Leukemia* 2000;14:1362–1370.

247. Grignani F, De Matteis S, Nervi C, et al. Fusion proteins of the retinoic acid receptor-alpha recruit histone deacetylase in promyelocytic leukaemia. *Nature* 1998;391:815–818.

248. He LZ, Guidez F, Triboli C, et al. Distinct interactions of PML-RARalpha and PLZF-RARalpha with co-repressors determine differential responses to RA in APL. *Nat Genet* 1998;18:126–135.

249. Lin RJ, Nagy L, Inoue S, et al. Role of the histone deacetylase complex in acute promyelocytic leukaemia. *Nature* 1998;391:811–814.

250. He LZ, Tolentino T, Grayson P, et al. Histone deacetylase inhibitors induce remission in transgenic models of therapy-resistant acute promyelocytic leukemia. *J Clin Invest* 2001;108:1321–1330.

251. Pandolfi PP. Histone deacetylases and transcriptional therapy with their inhibitors. *Cancer Chemother Pharmacol* 2001;48:S17–S19.

252. Pandolfi PP. Transcription therapy for cancer. *Oncogene* 2001;20:3116–3127.

253. Grisolano JL, Wesselschmidt RL, Pelicci PG, et al. Altered myeloid development and acute leukemia in transgenic mice expressing PML-RAR alpha under control of cathepsin G regulatory sequences. *Blood* 1997;89:376–387.

254. He LZ, Triboli C, Rivi R, et al. Acute leukemia with promyelocytic features in PML/RARalpha transgenic mice. *Proc Natl Acad Sci U S A* 1997;94:5302–5307.

255. Tallman MS. Arsenic trioxide: its role in acute promyelocytic leukemia and potential in other hematologic malignancies. *Blood Rev* 2001;15:133–142.

256. Tallman MS, Nabhan C, Feusner JH, et al. Acute promyelocytic leukemia: evolving therapeutic strategies. *Blood* 2002;99:759–767.

257. Hong SH, Yang Z, Privalsky ML. Arsenic trioxide is a potent inhibitor of the interaction of SMRT corepressor with its transcription factor partners, including the PML-retinoic acid receptor alpha oncoprotein found in human acute promyelocytic leukemia. *Mol Cell Biol* 2001;21:7172–7182.

258. Zimonjic DB, Pollock JL, Westervelt P, et al. Acquired, nonrandom chromosomal abnormalities associated with the development of acute promyelocytic leukemia in transgenic mice. *Proc Natl Acad Sci U S A* 2000;97:13306–13311.

259. Bloomfield CD, Shuma C, Regal L, et al. Long-term survival of patients with acute myeloid leukemia: a third follow-up of the Fourth International Workshop on Chromosomes in Leukemia. *Cancer* 1997;80:2191–2198.

260. Bloomfield CD, Herzig GP, Peterson BA, et al. Long-term survival of patients with acute myeloid leukemia: updated results from two trials evaluating postinduction chemotherapy. *Cancer* 1997;80:2186–2190.

261. Speck NA, Stacy T, Wang Q, et al. Core-binding factor: a central player in hematopoiesis and leukemia. *Cancer Res* 1999;59:1789s–1793s.

262. Downing JR. AML1/CBFbeta transcription complex: its role in normal hematopoiesis and leukemia. *Leukemia* 2001;15:664–665.

263. Downing JR. The AML1-ETO chimaeric transcription factor in acute myeloid leukaemia: biology and clinical significance. *Br J Haematol* 1999;106:296–308.

264. Wang Q, Stacy T, Miller JD, et al. The CBFbeta subunit is essential for CBFalpha2 (AML1) function in vivo. *Cell* 1996;87:697–708.

265. Wang Q, Stacy T, Binder M, et al. Disruption of the Cbfa2 gene causes necrosis and hemorrhaging in the central nervous system and blocks definitive hematopoiesis. *Proc Natl Acad Sci U S A* 1996;93:3444–3449.

266. Okuda T, van Deursen J, Hiebert SW, et al. AML1, the target of multiple chromosomal translocations in human leukemia, is essential for normal fetal liver hematopoiesis. *Cell* 1996;84:321–330.

267. Arthur DC, Bloomfield CD. Partial deletion of the long arm of chromosome 16 and bone marrow eosinophilia in acute nonlymphocytic leukemia: a new association. *Blood* 1983;61:994.

268. LeBeau MM, Larson RA, Bitter MA, et al. Association of an inversion of chromosome 16 with abnormal marrow eosinophils in acute myelomonocytic leukemia. *N Engl J Med* 1983;309:630.

269. Marlton P, Keating M, Kantarjian H, et al. Cytogenetic and clinical correlates in AML patients with abnormalities of chromosome 16. *Leukemia* 1995;9:965–971.

270. LeBeau MM, Diaz MO, Karin M, et al. Metallothionein gene cluster is split by chromosome 16 rearrangements in myelomonocytic leukaemia. *Nature* 1985;313:709.

271. Frank R, Zhang J, Uchida H, et al. The AML1/ETO fusion protein blocks transactivation of the GM-CSF promoter by AML1B. *Oncogene* 1995;11:2667–2674.

272. Meyers S, Lenny N, Hiebert SW. The t(8;21) fusion protein interferes with AML-1B-dependent transcriptional activation. *Mol Cell Biol* 1995;15:1974–1982.

273. Castilla LH, Wijmenga C, Wang Q, et al. Failure of embryonic hematopoiesis and lethal hemorrhages in mouse embryos heterozygous for a knocked-in leukemia gene CBFB-MYH11. *Cell* 1996;87:687–696.

274. Yergeau DA, Hetherington CJ, Wang Q, et al. Embryonic lethality and impairment of haematopoiesis in mice heterozygous for an AML1-ETO fusion gene. *Nat Genet* 1997;15:303–306.

275. Okuda T, Cai Z, Yang S, et al. Expression of a knocked-in AML1-ETO leukemia gene inhibits the establishment of normal definitive hematopoiesis and directly generates dysplastic hematopoietic progenitors. *Blood* 1998;91:3134–3143.

276. Lutterbach B, Westendorf JJ, Linggi B, et al. ETO, a target of t(8;21) in acute leukemia, interacts with the N-CoR and mSin3 corepressors. *Mol Cell Biol* 1998;18:7176–7184.

277. Amann JM, Nip J, Strom DK, et al. ETO, a target of t(8;21) in acute leukemia, makes distinct contacts with multiple histone deacetylases and binds mSin3A through its oligomerization domain. *Mol Cell Biol* 2001;21:6470–6483.

278. Lutterbach B, Westendorf JJ, Linggi B, et al. A mechanism of repression by acute myeloid leukemia-1, the target of multiple chromosomal translocations in acute leukemia. *J Biol Chem* 2000;275:651–656.

279. Castilla LH, Garrett L, Adya N, et al. The fusion gene Cbfβ blocks myeloid differentiation and predisposes mice to acute myelomonocytic leukemia. *Nat Genet* 1999;23:144–146.

280. Higuchi M, O'Brien D, Kumaravelu P, et al. Expression of a conditional AML1-ETO oncogene bypasses embryonic lethality and establishes a murine model of human t(8;21) acute myeloid leukemia. *Cancer Cell* 2002;1:63–74.

281. Thorsteinsdottir U, Sauvageau G, Humphries RK. Hox homeobox genes as regulators of normal and leukemic hematopoiesis. *Hematol Oncol Clin North Am* 1997;11:1221–1237.

282. Borrow J, Shearman AM, Stanton JR, et al. The t(7;11)(p15;p15) translocation in acute myeloid leukaemia fuses the genes for nucleoporin NUP98 and class I homeoprotein HOXA9. *Nat Genet* 1996;12:159–167.

283. Raza-Egilmez SZ, Jani-Sait SN, Grossi M, et al. NUP98-HOXD13 gene fusion in therapy-related acute myelogenous leukemia. *Cancer Res* 1998;58:4269–4273.

284. Nakamura T, Largaespada DA, Lee MP, et al. Fusion of the nucleoporin gene NUP98 to HOXA9 by the chromosome translocation t(7;11)(p15;p15) in human myeloid leukaemia. *Nat Genet* 1996;12:154–158.

285. Chase A, Reiter A, Burci L, et al. Fusion of ETV6 to the caudal-related homeobox gene CDX2 in acute myeloid leukemia with the t(12;13)(p13;q12). *Blood* 1999;93:1025–1031.

286. Downing JR, Look AT. MLL fusion genes in the 11q23 acute leukemias. *Cancer Treat Res* 1996;84:73–92.

287. Yu BD, Hess JL, Horning SE, et al. Altered Hox expression and segmental identity in Mll-mutant mice. *Nature* 1995;378:505–508.

288. Hanson RD, Hess JL, Yu BD, et al. Mammalian trithorax and polycomb-group homologues are antagonistic regulators of homeotic development. *Proc Natl Acad Sci U S A* 1999;96:14372–14377.

289. Yu BD, Hanson RD, Hess JL, et al. MLL, a mammalian trithorax-group gene, functions as a transcriptional maintenance factor in morphogenesis. *Proc Natl Acad Sci U S A* 1998;95:10632–10636.

290. Armstrong SA, Staunton JE, Silverman LB, et al. MLL translocations specify a distinct gene expression profile that distinguishes a unique leukemia. *Nat Genet* 2002;30:41–47.

291. Kasper LH, Brindle PK, Schnabel CA, et al. CREB binding protein interacts with nucleoporin-specific FG repeats that activate transcription and mediate NUP98-HOXA9 oncogenicity. *Mol Cell Biol* 1999;19:764–776.

292. Nakamura T, Yamazaki Y, Hatano Y, et al. NUP98 is fused to PMX1 homeobox gene in human acute myelogenous leukemia with chromosome translocation t(1;11)(q23;p15). *Blood* 1999;94:741–747.

293. Raza-Egilmez SZ, Jani-Sait SN, Grossi M, et al. NUP98-HOXD13 gene fusion in therapy-related acute myelogenous leukemia. *Cancer Res* 1998;58:4269–4273.

294. Arai Y, Hosoda F, Kobayashi H, et al. The inv(11)(p15q22) chromosome translocation of de novo and therapy-related myeloid malignancies results in fusion of the nucleoporin gene, NUP98, with the putative RNA helicase gene, DDX10. *Blood* 1997;89:3936–3944.

295. von Lindern M, Fornerod M, van Baal S, et al. The translocation (6;9), associated with a specific subtype of acute myeloid leukemia, results in the fusion of two genes, dek and can, and the expression of a chimeric, leukemia-specific dek-can mRNA. *Mol Cell Biol* 1992;12:1687–1697.

296. Ayton PM, Cleary ML. Molecular mechanisms of leukemogenesis mediated by MLL fusion proteins. *Oncogene* 2001;20:5695–5707.

297. Rowley JD, Reshmi S, Sobulo O, et al. All patients with the t(11;16)(q23;p13.3) that involves MLL and CBP have treatment-related hematologic disorders. *Blood* 1997;90:535–539.

298. Bain BJ, Moorman AV, Johansson B, et al. Myelodysplastic syndromes associated with 11q23 abnormalities. European 11q23 Workshop Participants. *Leukemia* 1998;12:834–839.

299. Secker-Walker LM, Moorman AV, Bain BJ, et al. Secondary acute leukemia and myelodysplastic syndrome with 11q23 abnormalities. EU Concerted Action 11q23 Workshop. *Leukemia* 1998;12:840–844.

300. Mrozek K, Heinonen K, Lawrence D, et al. Adult patients with de novo acute myeloid leukemia and t(9;11)(p22;q23) have a superior outcome to patients with other translocations involving band 11q23: a Cancer and Leukemia Group B study. *Blood* 1997;90:4532–4538.

301. Whitman SP, Strout MP, Marcucci G, et al. The partial nontandem duplication of the MLL (ALL1) gene is a novel rearrangement that generates three distinct fusion transcripts in B-cell acute lymphoblastic leukemia. *Cancer Res* 2001;61:59–63.

302. Corral J, Lavenir I, Impey H, et al. An Mll-AF9 fusion gene made by homologous recombination causes acute leukemia in chimeric mice: a method to create fusion oncogenes. *Cell* 1996;14:853–861.

303. Dobson CL, Warren AJ, Pannell R, et al. The mll-AF9 gene fusion in mice controls myeloproliferation and specifies acute myeloid leukaemogenesis. *EMBO J* 1999;18:3564–3574.

304. Lavau C, Du C, Thirman M, et al. Chromatin-related properties of CBP fused to MLL generate a myelodysplastic-like syndrome that evolves into myeloid leukemia. *EMBO J* 2000;19:4655–4664.

305. Arthur DC, Bloomfield CD, Lindquist LL, et al. Translocation 4:11 in acute lymphoblastic leukemia: clinical characteristics and prognostic significance. *Blood* 1982;59:96.

306. Nagasaka M, Maeda S, Maeda H, et al. Four cases of t(4;11) acute leukemia and its myelomonocytic nature in infants. *Blood* 1983;61:1174.

307. Boggs DR, Wintrobe MM, Cartwright GE. The acute leukemias: analysis of 322 cases and review of the literature. *Medicine* 1987;41:163.

308. Choi S-I, Simone JV. Acute non-lymphoblastic leukemia in 171 children. *Med Pediatr Oncol* 1976;2:119.

309. Giles RH, Dauwerse JG, Higgins C, et al. Detection of CBP rearrangements in acute myelogenous leukemia with t(8;16). *Leukemia* 1997;11:2087–2096.

310. Taki T, Sako M, Tsuchida M, et al. The t(11;16)(q23;p13.3) translocation in myelodysplastic syndrome fuses the MLL gene to the CBP gene. *Blood* 1997;89:3945–3949.

311. Carapeti M, Aguiar RCT, Goldman JM, et al. A novel fusion between MOZ and the nuclear receptor coactivator TIF2 in acute myeloid leukemia. *Blood* 1998;91:3127–3133.

312. Liang J, Prouty L, Williams BJ, et al. Acute mixed lineage leukemia with an inv(8)(p11q13) resulting in fusion of the genes for MOZ and TIF2. *Blood* 1998;92:2118–2122.

313. Le Beau MM, Albain KS, Larson RA, et al. Clinical and cytogenetic correlation in 63 patients with therapy-related myelodysplastic syndromes and acute non-lymphocytic leukemia: further evidence for characteristic abnormalities of chromosomes no. 5 and 7. *J Clin Oncol* 1986;4:325.

314. Rowley JD. Recurring chromosome abnormalities in leukemia and lymphoma. *Semin Hematol* 1990;27:122–136.

315. Levine EG, Bloomfield CD. Secondary myelodysplastic syndromes and leukemias. *Clin Haematol* 1986;15:1037.

316. Leith CP, Kopecky KJ, Godwin J, et al. Acute myeloid leukemia in the elderly: assessment of multidrug resistance (MDR1) and cytogenetics distinguishes biologic subtypes with remarkably distinct responses to standard chemotherapy: a Southwest Oncology Group study. *Blood* 1997;89:3323–3329.

317. Pedersen-Bjergaard J, Philip P, Larsen SO, et al. Therapy-related myelodysplastic and acute myeloid leukemia: cytogenetic characteristics of 115 consecutive cases and risks in seven cohorts of patients treated intensively for malignant diseases in the Copenhagen series. *Leukemia* 1993;7:1975–1986.

318. Rubnitz JE, Behm FG, Downing JR. 11q23 rearrangements in acute leukemia. *Leukemia* 1996;10:74–82.

319. Archimbaud E, Charrin C, Magaud JP, et al. Clinical and biological characteristics of adult de novo and secondary acute myeloid leukemia with balanced 11q23 chromosomal anomaly or MLL gene rearrangement compared to cases with unbalanced 11q23 anomaly: confirmation of the existence of different entities with 11q23 breakpoint. *Leukemia* 1998;12:25–33.

320. Schoch C, Haase D, Fonatasch C, et al. The significance of trisomy 8 in de novo acute myeloid leukemia: the accompanying chromosome aberrations determine the prognosis. *Br J Haematol* 1997;99:605–611.

321. Nimer SD, Golde DW. The 5q- abnormality. *Blood* 1987;70:1705.

322. Roberts WM, Look AT, Roussel MF, et al. Tandem linkage of human CSF-1 receptor (c-fms) and PDGF receptor genes. *Cell* 1988;55:655.

323. Olney HJ, Le Beau MM. The cytogenetics of myelodysplastic syndromes. *Best Pract Res Clin Haematol* 2001;14:479–495.

324. Lai F, Godley LA, Joslin J, et al. Transcript map and comparative analysis of the 1.5-Mb commonly deleted segment of human 5q31 in malignant myeloid diseases with a del(5q). *Genomics* 2001;71:235–245.

325. Asimakopoulos FA, Gilbert JG, Aldred MA, et al. Interstitial deletion constitutes the major mechanism for loss of heterozygosity on chromosome 20q in polycythemia vera. *Blood* 1996;88:2690–2698.

326. Asimakopoulos FA, Green AR. Deletions of chromosome 20q and the pathogenesis of myeloproliferative disorders. *Br J Haematol* 1996;95:219–226.

327. Jaju RJ, Boultwood J, Oliver FJ, et al. Molecular cytogenetic delineation of the critical deleted region in the 5q- syndrome. *Genes Chromosomes Cancer* 1998; 22:251–256.

328. Ning Y, Liang JC, Nagarajan L, et al. Characterization of 5q deletions by subtelomeric probes and spectral karyotyping. *Cancer Genet Cytogenet* 1998; 103:170–172.

329. Kratz CP, Emerling BM, Donovan S, et al. Candidate gene isolation and comparative analysis of a commonly deleted segment of 7q22 implicated in myeloid malignancies. *Genomics* 2001;77:171–180.

330. Westbrook CA, Hsu WT, Chyna B, et al. Cytogenetic and molecular diagnosis of chromosome 5 deletions in myelodysplasia. *Br J Haematol* 2000;110:847–855.

331. Sweetser DA, Chen CS, Blomberg AA, et al. Loss of heterozygosity in childhood de novo acute myelogenous leukemia. *Blood* 2001;98:1188–1194.

332. Song W-J, Sullivan MG, Legare RD, et al. Haploinsufficiency of *CBFA2 (AML1)* causes familial thrombocytopenia with propensity to develop acute myelogenous leukemia (FPD/AML). *Nat Genet* 1999;23:166–175.

333. Seidman JG, Seidman C. Transcription factor haploinsufficiency: when half a loaf is not enough. *J Clin Invest* 2002;109:451–455.

334. Karp JE. Farnesyl protein transferase inhibitors as targeted therapies for hematologic malignancies. *Semin Hematol* 2001;38:16–23.

335. Peters DG, Hoover RR, Gerlach MJ, et al. Activity of the farnesyl protein transferase inhibitor SCH66336 against BCR/ABL-induced murine leukemia and primary cells from patients with chronic myeloid leukemia. *Blood* 2001;97:1404–1412.

336. Sebti S, Hamilton AD. Inhibitors of prenyl transferases. *Curr Opin Oncol* 1997;9:557–561.

337. Golub TR, Barker GF, Lovett M, et al. Fusion of PDGF receptor beta to a novel ets-like gene, tel, in chronic myelomonocytic leukemia with t(5;12) chromosomal translocation. *Cell* 1994;77:307–316.

338. Golub TR, Goga A, Barker G, et al. Oligomerization of the ABL tyrosine kinase by the ETS protein TEL in human leukemia. *Mol Cell Biol* 1996;16:4107–4116.

339. Ross TS, Bernard OA, Berger R, et al. Fusion of Huntingtin interacting protein 1 to PDGFβR in chronic myelomonocytic leukemia with t(5;7)(q33;q11.2). *Blood* 1998;91:4419–4426.

340. Schwaller J, Frantsve J, Tomasson M, et al. Transformation of hematopoietic cell lines to growth-factor independence and induction of a fatal myeloid and lymphoproliferative disease in mice by retrovirally transduced TEL/JAK2 fusion gene. *EMBO J* 1998;17:5321–5333.

341. Schwaller J, Anastasiadou E, Cain D, et al. H4(D10S170), a gene frequently rearranged in papillary thyroid carcinoma, is fused to the platelet-derived growth factor receptor beta gene in atypical chronic myeloid leukemia with t(5;10)(q33;q22). *Blood* 2001;97:3910–3918.

342. Lacronique V, Boureux A, Valle VD, et al. A TEL-JAK2 fusion protein with constitutive kinase activity in human leukemia. *Science* 1997;278:1309–1312.

343. Peeters P, Raynaud SD, Cools J, et al. Fusion of TEL, the ETS-variant gene 6 (ETV6), to the receptor-associated kinase JAK2 as a result of t(9;12) in a lymphoid and t(9;15;12) in a myeloid leukemia. *Blood* 1997;90:2535–2540.

344. Papadopoulos P, Ridge SA, Boucher CA, et al. The novel activation of ABL by fusion to an ets-related gene, TEL. *Cancer Res* 1995;55:34–38.

345. Magnusson MK, Meade KE, Brown KE, et al. Rabaptin-5 is a novel fusion partner to platelet-derived growth factor beta receptor in chronic myelomonocytic leukemia. *Blood* 2001;98:2518–2525.

346. Kurzrock R, Shtalrid M, Talpaz M, et al. Expression of c-abl in Philadelphia-positive acute myelogenous leukemia. *Blood* 1987;70:1584.

347. Kurzrock R, Gutterman JU, Talpaz M. The molecular genetics of Philadelphia-positive leukemias. *N Engl J Med* 1988;319:990.

348. Oshimura M, Freeman AI, Sandberg AA. Chromosomes and causation of human cancer and leukemia (ALL). *Cancer* 1977;40:1161.

349. Druker BJ, Sawyers CL, Kantarjian H, et al. Activity of a specific inhibitor of the BCR-ABL tyrosine kinase in the blast crisis of chronic myeloid leukemia and acute lymphoblastic leukemia with the Philadelphia chromosome. *N Engl J Med* 2001;344:1038–1042.

350. Druker BJ, Talpaz M, Resta DJ, et al. Efficacy and safety of a specific inhibitor of the BCR-ABL tyrosine kinase in chronic myeloid leukemia. *N Engl J Med* 2001;344:1031–1037.

351. Sawyers CL. Molecular studies in chronic myeloid leukemia patients treated with tyrosine kinase inhibitors. *Semin Hematol* 2001;38:15–21.

352. Appelbaum FR. Perspectives on the future of chronic myeloid leukemia treatment. *Semin Hematol* 2001;38:35–42.

353. Kiyoi H, Towatari M, Yokota S, et al. Internal tandem duplication of the FLT3 gene is a novel modality of elongation mutation which causes constitutive activation of the product. *Leukemia* 1998;12:1333–1337.

354. Yamamoto Y, Kiyoi H, Nakano Y, et al. Activating mutation of D835 within the activation loop of FLT3 in human hematologic malignancies. *Blood* 2001;97:2434–2439.

355. Griffin JD. Point mutations in the FLT3 gene in AML. *Blood* 2001;97:2193A–2193.

356. Meshinchi S, Woods WG, Stirewalt DL, et al. Prevalence and prognostic significance of Flt3 internal tandem duplication in pediatric acute myeloid leukemia. *Blood* 2001;97:89–94.

357. Abu-Duhier F, Goodeve A, Wilson G, et al. FLT3 internal tandem duplication mutations in adult acute myeloid leukaemia define a high-risk group. *Br J Haematol* 2000;111:190–195.

358. Kiyoi H, Naoe T, Nakano Y, et al. Prognostic implication of FLT3 and N-RAS gene mutations in acute myeloid leukemia. *Blood* 1999;93:3074–3080.

359. Osato M, Asou N, Abdalla E, et al. Biallelic and heterozygous point mutations in the runt domain of the AML1/PEBP2alphaB gene associated with myeloblastic leukemias. *Blood* 1999;93:1817–1824.

360. Michaud J, Wu F, Osato M, et al. In vitro analyses of known and novel RUNX1/AML1 mutations in dominant familial platelet disorder with predisposition to acute myelogenous leukemia: implications for mechanisms of pathogenesis. *Blood* 2002;99:1364–1372.

361. Pabst T, Mueller BU, Zhang P, et al. Dominant-negative mutations of CEBPA, encoding CCAAT/enhancer binding protein-alpha (C/EBPalpha), in acute myeloid leukemia. *Nat Genet* 2001;27:263–270.

362. Ford AM, Bennett CA, Price CM, et al. Fetal origins of the TEL-AML1 fusion gene in identical twins with leukemia. *Proc Natl Acad Sci U S A* 1998;95:4584–4588.

363. Wiemels JL, Cazzaniga G, Daniotti M, et al. Prenatal origin of acute lymphoblastic leukaemia in children. *Lancet* 1999;354:1499–1503.

364. Wiemels JL, Ford AM, Van Wering ER, et al. Protracted and variable latency of acute lymphoblastic leukemia after TEL-AML1 gene fusion in utero. *Blood* 1999;94:1057–1062.

365. Daley GQ, Van Etten RA, Baltimore D. Induction of chronic myelogenous leukemia in mice by the P210*bcr/abl* gene of the Philadelphia chromosome. *Science* 1990;247:824–830.

366. Tomasson MH, Sternberg DW, Williams IR, et al. Fatal myeloproliferation, induced in mice by TEL/PDGFβR expression, depends on PDGFβR tyrosines 579/581. *J Clin Invest* 2000;105:423–432.

367. MacKenzie KL, Dolnikov A, Millington M, et al. Mutant N-ras induces myeloproliferative disorders and apoptosis in bone marrow repopulated mice. *Blood* 1999;93:2043–2056.

368. Dastugue N, Payen C, Lafage-Pochitaloff M, et al. Prognostic significance of karyotype in de novo adult acute myeloid leukemia. The BGMT Group. *Leukemia* 1995;9:1491–1498.

369. Grimwade D, Walker H, Oliver F, et al. The importance of diagnostic cytogenetics on outcome in AML: analysis of 1,612 patients entered into the MRC AML 10 trial. The Medical Research Council Adult and Children's Leukaemia Working Parties. *Blood* 1998;92:2322–2333.

370. Burns P, Armitage JO, Frey AL, et al. Analysis of presenting features of adult leukemia. *Cancer* 1981;47:2460.

371. Ventura GJ, Hestar JP, Smith TL, et al. Acute myeloblastic leukemia with hyperleukocytosis: risk factors for early mortality in induction. *Am J Hematol* 1988;27:34.

372. Creutzig U, Ritter J, Budde M, et al. Early deaths due to hemorrhage and leukostasis in childhood acute myelogenous leukemia. *Cancer* 1987;60:3071.

373. Stanley M, McKenna RW, Ellinger G, et al. Classification of 358 cases of acute myeloid leukemia by FAB criteria: analysis of clinical and morphologic features. In: Bloomfield CD, ed. *Chronic and acute leukemia in adults.* Hingham, MA: Marinus Nijhoff, 1985:155.

374. Straus DJ, Mertelsmann R, Koziner B, et al. The acute monocytic leukemias: multidisciplinary studies in 45 patients. *Medicine* 1980;59:409.

375. Pui CH, Dahl GV, Kalwinksy DK, et al. Central nervous system leukemia in children with nonlymphoblastic leukemia. *Blood* 1982;66:1062.

376. Fung H, Shepherd J, Naiman SC, et al. Acute monocytic leukemia: a single institution experience. *Leuk Lymphoma* 1995;19:259–265.

377. Pui CH, Kalwinsky D, Schell MJ, et al. Acute nonlymphoblastic leukemia in infants. *J Clin Oncol* 1988;6:1008.

378. Schwonzen M, Kuehn N, Vetten B, et al. Phenotype of acute myelomonocytic (AMMoL) and monocytic leukemia (AmoL): association of T-cell related antigens and skin infiltration in AmoL. *Leuk Res* 1989;13:893–898.

379. Muss H, Moloney W. Chloroma and other myeloblastic tumors. *Blood* 1973; 42:721.

380. Neiman RS, Barcos M, Berard C, et al. Granulocytic sarcoma: a clinicopathologic study of 61 biopsied cases. *Cancer* 1981;48:1426.

381. Eshghabadi M, Shojania AM, Carr I. Isolated granulocytic sarcoma: report of a case and review of the literature. *J Clin Oncol* 1986;4:912.

382. Meiss JM, Butler JJ, Osborne BM, et al. Granulocytic sarcoma in nonleukemic patients. *Cancer* 1986;56:2697.

383. Byrd JC, Edenfield WJ, Shields DJ, et al. Extramedullary myeloid cell tumors in acute nonlymphocytic leukemia: a clinical review. *J Clin Oncol* 1995;13: 1800–1816.

384. Swirsky DM, Li YS, Matthews JG, et al. 8;21 translocation in acute granulocytic leukemia: cytological, cytochemical, and clinical features. *Br J Haematol* 1984;56:199.

385. Tallman MS, Hakimian D, Shaw JM, et al. Granulocytic sarcoma is associated with the 8;21 translocation in acute myeloid leukemia. *J Clin Oncol* 1993;11:690–697.

386. Byrd JC, Weiss RB. Recurrent granulocytic sarcoma: an unusual variation of acute myelogenous leukemia associated with 8;21 chromosomal translocation and blast expression of the neural cell adhesion molecule. *Cancer* 1994;73:2107–2112.

387. Hurwitz CA, Raimondi SC, Head DR, et al. Distinctive immunphenotypic features of t(8;21)(q22;q22) acute myeloblastic leukemia in children. *Blood* 1992;80:3182.

388. Byrd JC, Weiss RB, Arthur DC, et al. Extramedullary leukemia adversely affects hematologic complete remission rate and overall survival in patients with t(8;21)(q22;q22): results from Cancer and Leukemia Group B 8461. *J Clin Oncol* 1997;15:406.

389. Rowe JM. Clinical and laboratory feature of the myeloid and lymphoid leukemias. *Am J Med Technol* 1983;49:103.

390. Kaneko Y, Maseki N, Takasakin, et al. Clinical and hematologic characteristics in acute leukemia with 11q23 translocations. *Blood* 1986;67:484.

391. Creutzig U, Ritter J, Budde M, et al. Early deaths due to hemorrhage and leukostasis in childhood acute myelogenous leukemia: associations with hyperleukocytosis and acute monocytic leukemia. *Cancer* 1987;60:3071–3079.

392. McKenna RW, Parkin J, Bloomfield C, et al. Acute promyelocytic leukemia: a study of 39 cases with identification of a hyperbasophilic microgranular variant. *Br J Haematol* 1982;50:201.

393. Suda T, Onai T, Maekawa T. Studies on abnormal polymorphonuclear neutrophils in acute myelogenous leukemia. *Am J Hematol* 1983;15:45.

394. Cowan DH. Thrombokinetics in acute non-lymphocytic leukemia. *J Lab Clin Med* 1973;82:911.

395. Woodcock BE, Cooper PC, Brown PR, et al. The platelet defect in acute myeloid leukemia. *J Clin Pathol* 1984;37:1339.

396. Gavosto F, Gabritti V, Masera P, et al. The problem of anaemia in the acute leukemias. *Eur J Cancer Clin Oncol* 1970;6:33.

397. Bauer KA, Rosenberg RD. Thrombin generation in acute promyelocytic leukemia. *Blood* 1984;64:791.

398. Kantarjian HM, Keating MJ, Walters RS. Acute promyelocytic leukemia. *Am J Med* 1986;80:789.

399. McKenna RW, Bloomfield CD, Dick F, et al. Acute monoblastic leukemia: diagnosis and treatment of ten cases. *Blood* 1975;46:481.

400. Tallman MS, Kwaan HC. Reassessing the hemostatic disorder associated with acute promyelocytic leukemia. *Blood* 1992;79:542–546.

401. Barbui T, Finazzi G, Falanga A. The impact of all-trans retinoic acid on the coagulopathy of acute promyelocytic leukemia. *Blood* 1998;91:3093.

402. Needleman SW, Burns CP, Dick FR, et al. Hypoplastic acute leukemia. *Cancer* 1981;48:1410.

403. Howe RB, Bloomfield CD, McKenna RW. Hypocellular acute leukemia. *Am J Med* 1982;72:391.

404. Carson JD, Trujillo JM, Estey EH, et al. Peripheral acute leukemia: high pest count. *Blood* 1989;74:1758.

405. Peterson BA, Levine EG. Uncommon subtypes of acute non-lymphocytic leukemia: clinical features and management of FAB M5, M6, and M7. *Semin Oncol* 1987;14:425.

406. Babapulle FB, Catovsky D, Galton DAG. Clinical and laboratory features of de novo acute myeloid leukaemia with trilineage myelodysplasia. *Br J Haematol* 1987;66:445.

407. Fohlmeister F, Fischer R, Modder B, et al. Aplastic anemia and the hypocellular myelodysplastic syndrome. *J Clin Pathol* 1985;38:1218.

408. Lanham GR, Dahl GV, Billings FT, et al. Pseudomonas aeruginosa infection with marrow suppression simulating acute promyelocytic leukemia. *Am J Med* 1983;14:147.

409. Sanal SM, Campbell EW, Bowdler AJ, et al. Pseudoleukemia. *Postgrad Med* 1983;65:143.

410. Peterson LA, Dehner LP, Brunning RD. Extramedullary masses as presenting features of acute monoblastic leukemia. *Am J Clin Pathol* 1981;75:140–148.

411. Bain B, Manoharan A, Lampert I, et al. Lymphoma-like presentation of acute monocytic leukaemia. *J Clin Pathol* 1983;36:559–565.

412. Schwarzmeier JD, Bettelheim P, Radaszkiewicz T, et al. Acute leukemia with mediastinal mass, lymphadenopathy, and monocytic precursor cells. *Am J Hematol* 1986;22:313–321.

413. Janin A, Nelken B, Dufour S, et al. Acute monoblastic leukemia with osteosclerosis and extensive myelofibrosis. *Am J Pediatr Hematol Oncol* 1988;10: 319–322.

414. Gottesfeld E, Silverman RA, Coccia PF, et al. Transient blueberry muffin appearance of a newborn with congenital monoblastic leukemia. *J Am Acad Dermatol* 1989;21:347–351.

415. Peterson BA, Brunning RD, Bloomfield CD, et al. Central nervous system involvement in acute nonlymphocytic leukemia: a prospective study of adults in remission. *Am J Med* 1987;83:464.

416. Pui CA, Dahl GV, Kalwinnsky DK, et al. Central nervous system leukemia in children with acute nonlymphoblastic leukemia. *Blood* 1985;66:1062.

417. Meyer RJ, Ferreira P, Cuttner J, et al. Central nervous system involvement at presentation in acute granulocytic leukemia: a prospective cytocentrifuge study. *Am J Med* 1980;68:691.

418. Takave Y, Culbert S, Baram T, et al. Therapeutic modalities for central nervous system involvement by granulocytic sarcoma (chloroma) in children with acute nonlymphocytic leukemia. *J Neurooncol* 1987;4:371.

419. Fritz RD, Forkner CD Jr, Freireich EJ. The association of fatal intracranial hemorrhage and "blastic crisis" in patients with acute leukemia. *N Engl J Med* 1959;261:59.

420. Porcu P, Cripe LD, Ng EW, et al. Hyperleukocytic leukemias and leukostasis: a review of pathophysiology, clinical presentation and management. *Leuk Lymphoma* 2000;39:1–18.

421. Price RA, Johnson WW. The central nervous system in childhood leukemia, I: the arachnoid. *Cancer* 1973;31:520.

422. Opdenakker G, Fibbe WE, Van Dammer J. The molecular basis of leukocytosis. *Immunol Today* 1998;12:182–189.

423. Doerschuck CM, Quinlan WM, Doyle NA, et al. The role of p-selection and ILAM-1 in acute lung injury as determined using anti-adhesion molecule antibodies and mutant mice. *J Immunol* 1996;157:4609–4614.

424. Kumasaka T, Quinlan WM, Doyle NA, et al. Role of the intercellular adhesion molecule-1(ICAM-1) in endotoxin-induced pneumonia evaluated using ICAM-1 antisense oligonucleotides, anti-ICAM-1 monoclonal antibodies, and ICAM-1 mutant mice. *J Clin Invest* 1996;97:2362–2369.

425. Stucki A, Cordey AS, Monai N, et al. Activation of vascular endothelial cells by leukemic blasts: a mechanism of leukostasis. *Blood* 1995;86:4359.

426. Sudhoff T, Wehmeier A, Kliche KO, et al. Levels of circulating endothelial adhesion molecules (sE-selectin) and sVCAM-1 in adult patients with acute leukemia. *Leukemia* 1996;10:682.

427. Wiernik PH, Serpick AA. Clinical significance of serum and urinary muramidase activity in leukemia and other hematologic malignancies. *Am J Med* 1969;46:330.

428. Woodruff KH. Cerebrospinal fluid cytomorphology using cytocentrifugation. *Am J Clin Pathol* 1973;60:621.

429. Beuchner SA, Li C-Y, Su WPD. Leukemia cutis. *Am J Dermatol* 1985;7:109.

430. Long JC, Mihm MC. Multiple granulocytic sarcomas of the skin: report of six cases of myelogenous leukemia with initial manifestation in the skin. *Cancer* 1977;39:2004.

431. Baer MR, Barcos M, Farrell H, et al. Acute myelogenous leukemia with leukemia cutis: eighteen cases seen between 1969 and 1986. *Cancer* 1989;63:2192–2220.

432. Longacre TA, Smoller BR. Leukemia cutis. *Am J Clin Pathol* 1993;100:276–284.

433. Jones D, Dorfman DM, Barnhill RL, et al. Leukemia vasculitis: a feature of leukemia cutis in some patients. *Am J Clin Pathol* 1997;107:637–642.

434. Cooper PH, Innes DJ, Greer KE. Acute febrile neutrophilic dermatosis (Sweet's syndrome) and myeloproliferative disorders. *Cancer* 1983;51:1518.

435. Roberts WC, Bodey GD, Wertlake PT. The heart in acute leukemia: a study of 420 autopsy cases. *Am J Cardiol* 1968;21:338.

436. Wiernik PH, Sutherland JC, Stechmiller BK, et al. Clinically significant cardiac infiltration in acute leukemia, lymphocytic lymphoma, and plasma cell myeloma. *Med Pediatr Oncol* 1976;2:75.

437. Ti M, Villafuerte R, Chase PH, et al. Acute leukemia presenting as laryngeal obstruction. *Cancer* 1974;34:427.

438. Wu KK, Burns CP. Leukemic pleural infiltrates during bone marrow remission of acute myelocytic leukemia. *Cancer* 1974;33:1179.

439. Armstrong P, Dyer R, Alford BA, et al. Leukemic pulmonary infiltrates: rapid development mimicking pulmonary edema. *AJR Am J Roentgenol* 1980;135:373.

440. Nagler A, Brenner B, Zuckerman E, et al. Acute respiratory failure in hyperleukocytic acute myeloid leukemia. *Am J Hematol* 1988;27:65.

441. Lester TJ, Johnson JW, Cuttner J. Pulmonary leukostasis as the single worst prognostic factor in patients with acute myelocytic leukemia and hyperleukocytosis. *Ann Intern Med* 1985;79:43.

442. Duffy JH, Driscoll EJ. Oral manifestations of leukemia. *Oral Surg* 1958;11:484.

443. Hunter TB, Bjelland JC. Gastrointestinal complications of leukemia and its treatment. *AJR Am J Roentgenol* 1984;142:513.

444. Norris NH, Weiner J. The renal lesions in leukemia. *Am J Med Sci* 1961;241:512.

445. Frame R, Head D, Lee R, et al. Granulocytic sarcoma of the prostate: two cases causing urinary obstruction. *Cancer* 1987;59:142.

446. Odom LF, Gordon EM. Acute monoblastic leukemia in infancy and early childhood: successful treatment with an epipodophyllotoxin. *Blood* 1984;64:875.

447. Roberts JP, Atwell JD. Testicular enlargement as a presenting feature of monocytic leukemia in an infant. *J Pediatr Surg* 1989;24:1306–1307.

448. Spilberg I, Meyer GJ. The arthritis of leukemia. *Arthritis Rheum* 1972;15:630.

449. Parker BR, Marglin S, Castellino RA, et al. Skeletal manifestations of leukemia, Hodgkin's disease, and non-Hodgkin lymphoma. *Semin Roentgenol* 1980;4:302.

450. Karesh JW, Goldman EJ, Reck K, et al. A prospective ophthalmic evaluation of patients with acute myeloid leukemia: correlation of ocular and hematologic findings. *J Clin Oncol* 1989;7:1528.

451. Guyer DR, Schachat AP, Vitale S, et al. Leukemic retinopathy: relationship between fundus lesions and hematologic parameters at diagnosis. *Ophthalmology* 1989;96:860.

452. Rowan PJ, Sloan JB. Iris and anterior chamber involvement in leukemia. *Ann Ophthalmol* 1976;8:1081.

453. Hertler AA, Rosenwasser GO, Gluck WL. Isolated anterior chamber relapse in acute monoblastic leukemia. *Am J Hematol* 1986;23:401–403.

454. Font RL, Mackay B, Tang R. Acute monocytic leukemia recurring as bilateral perilimbal infiltrates. *Ophthalmology* 1985;92:1681–1685.

455. Estey E, Smith TL, Keating MJ, et al. Prediction of survival during induction therapy in patients with newly diagnosed acute myeloblastic leukemia. *Leukemia* 1989;3:257.

456. Keating MJ, Smith TL, Kantarjian H, et al. Cytogenetic pattern in acute myelogenous leukemia: a major reproducible determinant of outcome. *Leukemia* 1988;2:403.

457. Schiffer CA, Lee EJ, Tomiyasu T, et al. Prognostic impact of cytogenetic abnormalities in patients with de novo acute non-lymphocytic leukemia. *Blood* 1989;73:63.

458. Billstrom R, Nilsson PG, Mitelman F. Chromosomes, Auer rods, and prognosis in acute myeloid leukemia. *Eur J Haematol* 1988;40:273.

459. Swirsky DM, de Bastos M, Parish SE, et al. Features affecting outcome during remission induction of myeloid leukemia in 619 adult patients. *Br J Haematol* 1986;64:435.

460. Cheson BD. The myelodysplastic syndromes: current approaches to therapy. *Ann Intern Med* 1990;112:932.

461. Hoyle CF, de Bastos M, Wheatley K, et al. AML associated with previous cytotoxic therapy, MDS, or myeloproliferative disorders: results from the MRC's 9th AML trial. *Br J Haematol* 1989;72:45.

462. Gajewski JL, Ho WG, Nimer SD, et al. Efficacy of intensive chemotherapy for acute myelogenous leukemia associated with a preleukemic syndrome. *J Clin Oncol* 1989;7:1637.

463. Mertelsmann R, Thaler HT, To L, et al. Morphological classification, response to therapy, and survival in 263 adult patients with acute non-lymphoblastic leukemia. *Blood* 1980;56:773.

464. Report of the Medical Research Council's Working Party on Leukemia in Adults: the relationship between morphology and other features of acute myeloid leukemia, and their prognostic significance. *Br J Haematol* 1975;31:165.

465. Preisler HD, Azarnia N, Raza A, et al. Relationship between the percent of marrow cells in S phase and the outcome of remission-induction therapy of acute myelogenous leukemia. *Br J Haematol* 1984;56:399.

466. Curtis JE, Messner HA, Mindin MD, et al. High-dose cytosine arabinoside in the treatment of acute myelogenous leukemia: contributions to the outcome of clinical and laboratory attributes. *J Clin Oncol* 1987;5:532.

467. Frei E, Yankee R, Krishan A. Cytokinetic evaluation of the effectiveness of remission induction treatment in patients with acute leukemia. *Adv Biosci* 1975;14:15.

468. Champlin RE, Gajewski JL, Golde DW. Treatment of acute myelogenous leukemia in the elderly. *Semin Oncol* 1989;16:51.

469. Keating MJ, Smith TL, Gehan EL, et al. A prognostic factor analysis for use in the development of predictive models for response in adult leukemia. *Cancer* 1982;50:457.

470. Creutzig U, Ritter J, Schellong G, for the AML-BFM Study Group. Identification of two risk groups in childhood acute myelogenous leukemia after therapy intensification in study AML-BFM-83 as compared with study AML-BFM-78. *Blood* 1990;75:1932.

471. Champlin R, Gajewski J, Nimer S, et al. Postremission chemotherapy for adults with acute myelogenous leukemia: improved survival with high-dose cytarabine and daunorubicin consolidation treatment. *J Clin Oncol* 1990;8:1199.

472. Rowe JM. Treatment of acute myelogenous leukemia in older adults. *Leukemia* 2000;14:480–487.

473. Grier HE, Gelber RD, Camitta BM, et al. Prognostic factors in childhood acute myelogenous leukemia. *J Clin Oncol* 1987;5:1026.

474. Dahl GV, Kalwinsky DK, Mirro J Jr, et al. Allogeneic bone marrow transplantation in a program of intensive sequential chemotherapy for children and young adults with acute non-lymphocytic leukemia in first remission. *J Clin Oncol* 1990;8:295.

475. Byrd JL, Weiss RB, Arthur DC, et al. Extramedullary leukemia adversely affects hematologic complete remission rate and overall survival in patients with t(8;21)(q22;q22): results from Cancer and Leukemia Group B 8461. *J Clin Oncol* 1997;15:466–475.

476. Rege K, Swansbury GJ, Aitra AA, et al. Disease features in acute myeloid leukemia with t(8;21) (q22;q22): influence of age, secondary karyotype abnormalities, CD19 status, and extramedullary leukemia on survival. *Leuk Lymphoma* 2000;40:67–77.

477. Byrd JC, Dodge RK, Carroll A, et al. Patients with t(8;21)(q22;q22) and acute myeloid leukemia have superior failure-free and overall survival when repetitive cycles of high-dose cytarabine are administered. *J Clin Oncol* 1999;17:3767–3775.

478. Cunningham I, Gee TS, Reich LM, et al. Acute promyelocytic leukemia: treatment results during a decade at Memorial Hospital. *Blood* 1989;13:1116.

479. Sanz MA, Martin G, Rayon C, et al. A modified AIDA protocol with anthracycline-based consolidation results in high antileukemic efficacy and reduced toxicity in newly diagnosed PML/RARalpha-positive acute promyelocytic leukemia. PETHEMA group. *Blood* 1999;94:3015–3021.

480. Kalwinsky DK, Raimondi SC, Schell MT, et al. Prognostic importance of cytogenetic subgroups in de novo pediatric acute non-lymphocytic leukemia. *J Clin Oncol* 1990;8:75.

481. Barlogie B, Johnston DA, Keating M, et al. Evolution of oligoleukemia. *Cancer* 1984;53:2115.

482. Ifrah N, James J-M, Viguie J-PM, et al. Spontaneous remission in adult acute leukemia. *Cancer* 1985;56:1187.

483. Robert EE. Spontaneous complete remission in acute promyelocytic leukemia. *N Y State J Med* 1985;86:622.

484. Wetherly-Mein G, Cottom DG. Fresh blood transfusion in leukemia. *Br J Haematol* 1956;2:25.

485. Ridings GR. Radiotherapy in the leukemias. *Radiol Clin North Am* 1968;6:83.

486. Thomas E, Epstein RB, Eschbach JW, et al. Treatment of leukemia by extracorporeal irradiation. *N Engl J Med* 1965;273:6.

487. Farber S, Diamond LK, Mercer RD, et al. Temporary remissions in acute leukemia in children produced by folic acid antagonist 4-aminopteroyl-glutamic acid (aminopterin). *N Engl J Med* 1948;238:787.

488. Marsoni S, Hoth D, Simon R, et al. Clinical drug development: an analysis of phase II trials, 1970–1985. *Cancer Treat Rep* 1987;71:71.

489. Ellison RR, Holland JF, Weil M, et al. Arabinoside cytosine, a useful agent in the treatment of acute leukemia in adults. *Blood* 1986;4:507.

490. Weil M, Glidewell OJ, Jacquillant CL, et al. Daunorubicin in the treatment of acute granulocytic leukemia. *Cancer Res* 1973;33:921.

491. Lewis JP. Clinical trials of adult acute non-lymphocytic leukemia: evidence of progress. *Cancer Treat Rev* 1985;12:133.

492. Clarkson BD, Gee T, Mertelsmann R, et al. Current status of treatment of acute leukemia in adults: an overview of the Memorial experience and review of the literature. *Crit Rev Oncol Hematol* 1986;4:221.

493. Peterson BA, Bloomfield CD. Long-term disease-free survival in acute non-lymphocytic leukemia. *Blood* 1981;6:1144.

494. Baehner RL, Kennedy MD, Sather H, et al. Characteristics of children with acute non-lymphocytic leukemia in long-term continuous remission: a report for the Children's Cancer Study Group. *Med Pediatr Oncol* 1981;9:393.

495. Wade JC, Newman KA, Schimpff SC, et al. Two methods for improved venous access in acute leukemia patients. *JAMA* 1981;246:140.

496. Mirro J, Bhaskar NR, Stokes DC, et al. A prospective study of Hickman/Broviac catheters and implantable ports in pediatric oncology patients. *J Clin Oncol* 1989;7:214.

497. Allegretta GJ, Weisman SJ, Altman AJ. Hematologic and infectious complications of cancer and cancer treatment. *Pediatr Clin North Am* 1985;32:613.

498. Neiburg PI, Stockman JA III. Rapid correction of anemia with partial exchange transfusion. *Am J Dis Child* 1977;131:60.

499. Hughes ASB, Brozovic B. Leucocyte depleted blood: an appraisal of available techniques. *Br J Haematol* 1982;50:381.

500. Chaplin H Jr. The proper use of previously frozen red blood cells for transfusion. *Blood* 1982;59:1118.

501. Schiffer CA, Wade JC. Supportive care: issues in the use of blood products and treatment of infection. *Semin Oncol* 1987;14:454.

502. Anderson K, Weinstein HJ. Transfusion associated graft-versus-host disease. *N Engl J Med* 1990;323:315.

503. Avvisati G, Wouter Ten Cate J, Buller HR, et al. Tranexamic acid for control of haemorrhage in acute promyelocytic leukemia. *Lancet* 1989;1:122.

504. Gaydos AL, Freireich EJ, Mantel N. The quantitative relation between platelet count and hemorrhage in patients with acute leukemia. *N Engl J Med* 1962;266:905.

505. Feusner J. The use of platelet transfusion. *Am J Pediatr Hematol Oncol* 1984;6:255.

506. Aderka D, Praff G, Santo M, et al. Bleeding due to thrombocytopenia in acute leukemias and reevaluation of the prophylactic platelet transfusion policy. *Am J Med Sci* 1986;291:147.

507. Rebulla P, Finazzi G, Marangoni F, et al. The threshold for prophylactic platelet transfusions in adults with acute myeloid leukemia. Gruppo Italiano Malattie Ematologiche Maligne dell'Adulto. *N Engl J Med* 1997;337:1870–1875.

508. Heckman KD, Weiner GJ, Davis CS, et al. Randomized study of prophylactic platelet transfusion threshold during induction therapy for adult acute leukemia: 10,000/microL versus 20,000/microL. *J Clin Oncol* 1997;15:1143–1149.

509. Schiffer CA, Miller K, Larsen RA, et al. A double-blind, placebo-controlled trial of pegylated recombinant human megakaryocyte growth and development factor as an adjunct to induction and consolidation therapy for patients with acute myeloid leukemia. *Blood* 2000;95:2530–2535.

510. Ribeiro R, Pui CH. The clinical and biologic correlates of coagulopathy in children with acute leukemia. *J Clin Oncol* 1986;4:1212.

511. Fenaux P, Vanhaesbroucke C, Estienne MH, et al. Acute monocytic leukemia in adults: treatment and prognosis in 99 cases. *Br J Haematol* 1990;75:41.

512. Mangal AK, Grossman L, Vickars L. Disseminated intravascular coagulation in acute monoblastic leukemia: response to heparin therapy. *Can Med Assoc J* 1984;130:731–733.

513. Bussel JB, Steinherz PG, Miller DR, et al. A heparin-like anticoagulant in an 8-month-old boy with acute monoblastic leukemia. *Am J Hematol* 1984;16:83–90.

514. Gralnick HR, Bagley J, Abrell E. Heparin treatment for the hemorrhagic diathesis of acute promyelocytic leukemia. *Br J Haematol* 1990;75:41.

515. Hayle CF, Swirsky DM, Freedman L, et al. Beneficial effects of heparin in the management of patients with APL. *Br J Haematol* 1988;68:283.

516. Goldberg MA, Ginsburg D, Mayer RJ, et al. Is heparin administration necessary during induction chemotherapy for patients with acute promyelocytic leukemia? *Blood* 1987;69:187.

517. Pizzo PA, Robichaud KJ, Wesley R, et al. Fever in the pediatric and young adult patient with cancer: a prospective study of 1001 episodes. *Medicine* 1982;61:153.

518. Schimpff SC. Overview of empiric antibiotic therapy for the febrile neutropenic patient. *Rev Infect Dis* 1985;7:S734.

519. Pizzo PA, Robichaud KJ, Gill FA, et al. Empiric antibiotic and antifungal therapy for cancer patients with prolonged fever and granulocytopenia. *Am J Med* 1982;72:101.

520. Sickles EA, Greene WH, Wiernik PH. Clinical presentation in granulocytopenic patients. *Arch Intern Med* 1975;135:715.

521. Hughes WT, Bodey G, Feld G, et al. Guidelines for the use of antimicrobial agents in neutropenic patients with unexplained fever. *J Infect Dis* 1990;161: 381.

522. Hiemenz J, Skelton J, Pizzo PA. Perspective on the management of catheter related infections in cancer patients. *Pediatr Infect Dis J* 1986;5:6.

523. Prentice HG, Hann IM, Herbrecht R, et al. A randomized comparison of liposomal versus conventional amphotericin B for the treatment of pyrexia of unknown origin in neutropenia patients. *Br J Haematol* 1997;98:711.

524. Kelsey SM, Goldman JM, McCann S, et al. Liposomal amphotericin (AmBisome) in the prophylaxis of fungal infections in neutropenic patients: a randomized, double-blind, placebo-controlled study. *Bone Marrow Transplant* 1999;23:163.

525. Kirby BD, Synder KM, Meyer RD, et al. Legionnaire's disease: report of sixty-five nosocomially acquired cases and review of the literature. *Medicine* 1980; 59:188.

526. Kostiala I, Kostiala AAI, Kahanpaa A, et al. Acute fungal stomatitis in patients with hematologic malignancies: quantity and species of fungi. *J Infect Dis* 1982;146:101.

527. Lam MT, Pazin GJ, Armstrong JA, et al. Herpes simplex infection in acute myelogenous leukemia and other hematologic malignancies: a prospective study. *Cancer* 1981;48:2169.

528. Meyers JD, Wade JC, Mitchell CD, et al. Multicenter collaborative trial of intravenous acyclovir for treatment of mucocutaneous herpes simplex infection in the immunocompromised host. *Am J Med* 1982;73:229.

529. Buss DH, Scharyj M. Herpes virus infection of the esophagus and other visceral organs in adults: incidence and clinical significance. *Am J Med* 1979; 66:457.

530. Skibber JM, Matler GJ, Lotze MT, et al. Right lower quadrant complications in young patients with leukemia: a surgical prospective. *Ann Surg* 1987; 206:711.

531. Shamberger RC, Weinstein HJ, Delorey MJ, et al. The medical and surgical management of typhlitis in children with acute non-lymphocytic (myelogenous) leukemia. *Cancer* 1986;57:603.

532. Moir CR, Scudamore CH, Benny WB. Typhlitis: selective surgical management. *Am J Surg* 1986;151:563.

533. Katz JA, Wagner MK, Gresik MV, et al. Typhlitis: an 18-year experience and postmortem review. *Cancer* 1990;65:1041–1047.

534. Alexander JE, Williamson SL, Seibert JJ, et al. The ultrasonographic diagnosis of typhlitis (neutropenic colitis). *Pediatr Radiol* 1988;18:200.

535. O'Regan S, Carson S, Chesney RW, et al. Electrolyte and acid base disturbances in the management of leukemia. *Blood* 1977;49:345.

536. Mir WA, Delamore IW. Metabolic disorders in acute myeloid leukemia. *Br J Haematol* 1978;40:79.

537. Zusman J, Brow DM, Nesbit ME. Hyperphosphatemia, hyperphosphaturia, and hypocalcemia in acute lymphoblastic leukemia. *N Engl J Med* 1973;289: 1335.

538. Kjellstrand CM, Campbell DC, Von Hartitzsch B, et al. Hyperuricemic acute renal failure. *Arch Intern Med* 1974;133:349.

539. Palva IP, Salokannel SJ. Hypercalcemia in acute leukemia. *Blut* 1972;24:209.

540. Gewirtz AM, Stewart AF, Vignery A, et al. Hypercalcemia complicating acute myelogenous leukemia: a syndrome of multiple aetiologies. *Br J Haematol* 1983;54:133.

541. Zidar BL, Shadduck RK, Winkelstein A, et al. Acute myeloblastic leukemia and hypercalcemia. *N Engl J Med* 1976;295:692.

542. Bergman GE, Balvarte HJ, Naiman JL. Diabetes insipidus as a presenting manifestation of acute myelogenous leukemia. *J Pediatr* 1976;88:355.

543. de la Chapelle A, Lahtinen R. Monosomy 7 predisposes to diabetes insipidus in leukaemia and myelodysplastic syndrome. *Eur J Haematol* 1987;39:404–411.

544. Salomon J. Spurious hypoglycemia and hyperkalemia in myelomonocytic leukemia. *Am J Med Sci* 1974;267:359.

545. Bellvue R, Dosik H, Speigel G, et al. Pseudohyperkalemia and extreme leukocytosis. *J Lab Clin Med* 1975;85:660.

546. Fox MJ, Brody JS, Weintraub LR, et al. Leukocyte larceny: a cause of spurious hypoxia. *Am J Med* 1979;67:742.

547. Dutcher J, Schiffer CA, Wiernik PH. Hyperleukocytosis in adult acute nonlymphocytic leukemia: impact on remission rate, duration and survival. *J Clin Oncol* 1987;5:1364.

548. Dearth J, Salter M, Wilson E, et al. Early death in acute leukemia in children. *Med Pediatr Oncol* 1983;11:225.

549. Wald BR, Heisel MA, Ortega JA. Frequency of early death in children with acute leukemia presenting with hyperleukocytosis. *Cancer* 1982;50:150.

550. Freireich EJ, Thomas LB, Frei E III, et al. A distinctive type of intracerebral hemorrhage associated with "blastic crisis" in patients with leukemia. *Cancer* 1960;13:146.

551. Bunin NJ, Pui CH. Differing complications in hyperleukocytosis in children with acute lymphoblastic leukemia or acute nonlymphoblastic leukemias. *J Clin Oncol* 1985;3:1590.

552. McKee LC, Collins RD. Intravascular leukocyte thrombi and aggregates as a cause of morbidity and mortality in leukemia. *Medicine* 1974;53:463.

553. Grund FM, Armitage JU, Burns CP. Hydroxyurea in the prevention of the effects of leukostasis in acute leukemia. *Arch Intern Med* 1977;137:1246.

554. Cuttner J, Holland JF, Norton L, et al. Therapeutic leukapheresis for hyperleukocytosis in acute myelocytic leukemia. *Med Pediatr Oncol* 1983;11:76.

555. Vahdat L, Maslak P, Miller WH Jr, et al. Early mortality and the retinoic acid syndrome in acute promyelocytic leukemia: impact of leukocytosis, low-dose chemotherapy, PMN/RAR-alpha isoform, and CD13 expression in patients treated with all-trans retinoic acid. *Blood* 1994;84:3843–3849.

556. Cheson BD, Cassileth PA, Head DR, et al. Report of the National Cancer Institute-Sponsored Workshop on definition of diagnosis and response in acute myeloid leukemia. *J Clin Oncol* 1990;8:813.

557. Frei E III, Freireich EJ. Progress and perspectives in the chemotherapy of acute leukemias. *Adv Chemother* 1965;2:269.

558. Champlin RE, Gale RP. Acute myelogenous leukemia. *Blood* 1987;69:1551.

559. Mayer RJ. Current chemotherapeutic treatment approaches to the management of previously untreated adults with de novo acute myelogenous leukemia. *Semin Oncol* 1987;14:384.

560. Leith C, Chen I-M, Kopecky KJ, et al. Correlation of multidrug resistance (MDR1) protein expression with functional dye/drug efflux in acute myeloid leukemia by multiparameter flow cytometry: identification of discordant MDR-/efflux+ and MDR1+/efflux- cases. *Blood* 1995;86:2329–2342.

561. Worsely A, Mufti GJ, Copplestone JA, et al. Very-low-dose cytarabine for myelodysplastic syndromes and acute myeloid leukemia in the elderly. *Lancet* 1986;1:966.

562. Stone RM, Maguire M, Goldberg MA, et al. Complete remission in acute promyelocytic leukemia despite persistence of abnormal marrow promyelocytes during induction therapy: experience in 34 patients. *Blood* 1988;71:690.

563. Skipper HE, Schabel FM, Wilcox WS. Experimental evaluation of potential anti-cancer agents, XXI: scheduling of arabinosylcytosine to take advantage of its S phase specificity against leukemic cells. *Cancer Chemother Rep* 1967; 51:125.

564. Southwest Oncology Group. Cytarabine for acute leukemia in adults: effect of schedule on therapeutic response. *Arch Intern Med* 1974;133:251.

565. Carey RW, Ribas-Mundo M, Ellison RR, et al. Comparative study of cytosine arabinoside therapy alone and combined with thioguanine, mercaptopurine, or daunorubicin in acute myelocytic leukemia. *Cancer* 1975;36:1560.

566. Wilson HE, Bodey GP, Moon TE, et al. Adriamycin therapy in previously treated adult acute leukemia. *Cancer Treat Rep* 1977;61:905.

567. Gale RP, Cline MS. High remission-induction rate in acute myeloid leukemia. *Lancet* 1977;1:497.

568. Yates JW, Wallace JH, Ellison RR, et al. Cytosine arabinoside (NSC-63878) and daunorubicin (NSC-83142) therapy in acute non-lymphocytic leukemia (part I). *Cancer Chemother Rep* 1973;57:485.

569. Preisler H, Davis RB, Krishner J, et al. Comparison of three induction regimens and two postinduction strategies for the treatment of acute non-lymphocytic leukemia: a Cancer and Leukemia Group B study. *Blood* 1987;69: 1441.

570. Rai KR, Holland JF, Glidewell OJ, et al. Treatment of acute myelocytic leukemia: a study by Cancer and Leukemia Group B. *Blood* 1981;58:1203.

571. Yates J, Glidewell OJ, Wiernik P, et al. Cytosine arabinoside with daunorubicin or Adriamycin for therapy of acute myelocytic leukemia: a CALGB study. *Blood* 1982;60:454.

572. Buckley JD, Lampkin BC, Nesbit ME, et al. Remission induction in children with acute non-lymphocytic leukemia using cytosine arabinoside and doxorubicin or daunorubicin: a report from the Children's Cancer Study Group. *Med Pediatr Oncol* 1989;17:382.

573. Usui N, Dobashi N, Kobayashi T, et al. Role of daunorubicin in the induction therapy for adult acute myeloid leukemia. *J Clin Oncol* 1998;16:2086–2092.

574. Vogler WR, Velex-Garcia E, Omura G, et al. A phase III trial comparing daunorubicin and idarubicin in combination with cytosine arabinoside as induction therapy for acute myelogenous leukemia. *Blood* 1987;70:240.

575. Berman E, Heller G, Santorsa J, et al. Results of a randomized trial comparing idarubicin and cytosine arabinoside with daunorubicin and cytosine arabinoside in adult patients with newly diagnosed acute myelogenous leukemia. *Blood* 1991;77:1666–1674.

576. Wiernik PH, Banks PLC, Case DC, et al. Cytarabine plus idarubicin or daunorubicin as induction and consolidation therapy for previously untreated adult patients with acute myeloid leukemia. *Blood* 1992;79:313–319.

577. Mandelli F, Petti MC, Ardia A, et al. A randomised clinical trial comparing idarubicin and cytarabine to daunorubicin and cytarabine in the treatment of acute non-lymphoid leukaemia: a multicentric study from the Italian Cooperative Group GIMEMA. *Eur J Cancer* 1991;27:750–755.

578. Arlin Z, Case DC, Moore J, et al. Randomized multi-center trial of cytosine arabinoside with mitoxantrone or daunorubicin in previously untreated adult patients with acute nonlymphocytic leukemia (ANLL). *Leukemia* 1990;4:177.

579. Mathe G, Schwarzenberg L, Pouillart P, et al. Two epipodophyllotoxin derivatives, VM 26 and VP 16213, in the treatment of leukemias, hematosarcomas, and lymphomas. *Cancer* 1974;34:985.

580. Bishop JF, Lowenthal RM, Joshua D, et al. Etoposide in acute non-lymphocytic leukemia. *Blood* 1990;75:21.

581. Hann IM, Stevens RF, Goldstone AH, et al. Randomized comparison of DAT versus ADE as induction chemotherapy in children and younger adults with acute myeloid leukemia: results of the Medical Research Council's 10th AML trial (MRC AML10). Adult and Childhood Leukaemia Working Parties of the Medical Research Council. *Blood* 1997;89:2311–2318.

582. Herzig RH, Lazarus HM, Wolff SM, et al. High-dose cytosine arabinoside therapy with and without anthracycline antibiotics for remission reinduction of acute non-lymphoblastic leukemia. *J Clin Oncol* 1985;3:992.

583. Arlin ZA, Ahmed T, Mittelman A, et al. A new regimen of amsacrine with high dose cytarabine is safe and effective therapy for acute leukemia. *J Clin Oncol* 1987;5:371.

584. Capizzi RL, Davis R, Powell B, et al. Synergy between high-dose cytarabine and asparaginase in the treatment of adults with refractory and relapsed acute myelogenous leukemia: a Cancer and Leukemia Group B study. *J Clin Oncol* 1988;6:499.

585. Rudnick S, Cadman EC, Capizzi RL, et al. High dose cytosine arabinoside in refractory acute leukemia. *Cancer* 1979;44:1189.

586. Capizzi RL, Yang JL, Rathmell JP, et al. Dose-related pharmacologic effects of high dose ara-C. *Semin Oncol* 1985;12:65.

587. Herzig RH, Hines JD, Herzig GP, et al. Cerebellar toxicity with high dose cytosine arabinoside. *J Clin Oncol* 1987;5:927.

588. Martens ACM, Van Bekkum DW, Hagenbeek A. The BN acute myelocytic leukemia (BNML): a rat model for studying human acute myelocytic leukemia. *Leukemia* 1990;4:244.

589. Karp JE, Donehower RC, Dole GB, et al. Correlation of drug perturbed marrow cell growth kinetics and intracellular 1-B-D-arabino furanosylcytosine metabolism with clinical response in adult acute myelogenous leukemia. *Blood* 1987;69:1134.

590. Vaughn WP, Karp JE, Burke PJ. Long chemotherapy-free remissions after single cycle timed sequential chemotherapy for acute myelocytic leukemia. *Cancer* 1980;45:859.

591. Burke PJ, Karp JE, Geller RB, et al. Cures of leukemia with aggressive postremission treatment: an update of timed sequential therapy (Ac-D-Ac). *Leukemia* 1989;3:692.

592. Woods WG, Kobrinsky N, Buckley JD, et al. Timed-sequential induction therapy improves postremission outcome in acute myeloid leukemia: a report from the Children's Cancer Group. *Blood* 1996;87:4979–4989.

593. Mitus AJ, Miller KB, Schenkien DP, et al. Improved survival for patients with an acute myelogenous leukemia. *J Clin Oncol* 1995;13:560–569.

594. Stein AS, O'Donnell MR, Slovak ML, et al. High-dose cytosine arabinoside and daunorubicin induction therapy for adult patients with de novo nonM3 acute myelogenous leukemia: impact of cytogenetics on achieving a complete remission. *Leukemia* 2000;14:1191–1196.

595. Cassileth PA, Lee SJ, Miller KB, et al. Feasibility study of adding high-dose cytarabine (HDAC) in induction (IND) and in consolidation (cons) before autologous stem cell transplant (ASCT) in adult acute myeloid leukemia. *Blood* 1998;92:4559(abst).

596. Petersdorf S, Rankin C, Terebolo H, et al. A phase III study of standard-dose daunorubicin and cytosine arabinoside (Ara-C) with high-dose Ara-C induction followed by sequential high-dose Ara-C consolidation for adults with previously untreated acute myelogenous leukemia: a Southwest Oncology Group Study (SWOG 9500). *Proc Am Soc Clin Oncol* 1998;17:55(abst).

597. Buchner T, Hiddemann W, Worman B, et al. Double induction strategy for acute myeloid leukemia: the effect of high-dose cytarabine with mitoxantrone instead of standard-dose cytarabine with daunorubicin and 6-thioguanine: a randomized trial by the German AML Cooperative Group. *Blood* 1996;93:4116–4124.

598. Estey EH, Dixon D, Kantarjian HM, et al. Treatment of poor-prognosis, newly diagnosed acute myeloid leukemia with ara-C and recombinant human granulocyte-macrophage colony-stimulating factor. *Blood* 1990;75:1766.

599. Rowe JM, Andersen J, Mazza JJ, et al. A randomized placebo-controlled study of granulocyte-macrophage colony stimulating factor in adult patients (>55-70 years of age) with acute myelogenous leukemia (AML): a study of the Eastern Cooperative Oncology Group (E1490). *Blood* 1995;86:457–462.

600. Dombret H, Chastang C, Fenaux P, et al. A controlled study of recombinant human granulocyte colony-stimulating factor in elderly patents after treatment for acute myelogenous leukemia. *N Engl J Med* 1995;332:1678–1683.

601. Heil G, Hoelzer D, Sanz MA, et al. A randomized, double-blind placebo-controlled, phase III study of filgrastim in remission induction and consolidation therapy for adults with de novo acute myeloid leukemia. *Blood* 1997;90:4710–4718.

602. Godwin JR, Kopecky KJ, Head DR, et al. A double-blind placebo-controlled trial of granulocyte colony-stimulating factor in elderly patients with previously untreated acute myeloid leukemia: a Southwest Oncology Group study (903). *Blood* 1998;91:3607–3615.

603. Stone RM, Berg DT, George SL, et al., for Cancer and Leukemia Group B. Granulocyte-macrophage colony-stimulating factor after initial chemotherapy for elderly patients with primary acute myelogenous leukemia. *N Engl J Med* 1995;332:1671–1677.

604. Zittoun R, Suciu S, Mandelli F, et al. Granulocyte-macrophage colony-stimulating factor associated with induction treatment of acute myelogenous leukemia: a randomized trial by the European Organization for Research and Treatment of Cancer and Leukemia Cooperative Groups. *J Clin Oncol* 1996;14:2150–2159.

605. Löwenberg B, Suciu S, Archimbaud E, et al. Use of recombinant GM-CSF during and after remission induction chemotherapy in patients aged 61 years and older with acute myeloid leukemia: final report of AML-11, a phase III randomized study of the Leukemia Cooperative Group of the European Organization for the Research and Treatment of Cancer and the Dutch-Belgium Hemato-Oncology Cooperative Group. *Blood* 1997;90:2952–2961.

606. Link H, Wandt H, Schonrock-Nabulski P, et al. G-CSF (lenograstim) after chemotherapy for acute myeloid leukemia: a placebo controlled trial. *Blood* 1996;88:2654(abst).

607. Goldstone AH, Burnett AK, Milligan DW, et al. Lack of benefit of G-CSF on complete remission and possible increased relapsed risk in AML: an MRC study of 800 patients. *Blood* 1997;90:2595(abst).

608. Witz F, Harousseau JL, Sadoun A, et al. GM-CSF during and after remission induction treatment for elderly patients with acute myeloid leukemia (AML). *Hematol Blood Trans* 1997;40:852–856.

609. Bloomfield CD. Postremission therapy in acute myeloid leukemia. *J Clin Oncol* 1985;3:1570.

610. Wiernik PH, Serpick AA. A randomized trial of daunorubicin and a combination of prednisone, vincristine, 6-mercaptopurine, and methotrexate in adult non-lymphocytic leukemia. *Cancer Res* 1972;32:2032.

611. Cassileth P, Harrighton DP, Hines JD, et al. Maintenance chemotherapy prolongs initial complete remission duration in adult acute non-lymphocytic leukemia. *J Clin Oncol* 1988;6:583.

612. Sauter C, Berchtold W, Foop M, et al. Acute myelogenous leukemia: maintenance chemotherapy after early consolidation does not prolong survival. *Lancet* 1984;1:379.

613. Buchner T, Urbanitz D, Hiddeman W, et al. Intensified induction and consolidation with or without maintenance chemotherapy for acute myeloid leukemia (AML): two multicenter studies of the German AML Cooperative Group. *J Clin Oncol* 1985;3:1583.

614. Buchner T, Hiddeman W, Nowrousian M, et al. Long-term effect on monthly myelosuppressive maintenance chemotherapy in acute myeloid leukemia (AML): a randomized study by the AMLCG. *Proc Am Soc Clin Oncol* 1990;9:202.

615. Cassileth PA, Begg CB, Bennett JM, et al. A randomized study of the efficacy of consolidation therapy in adult acute non-lymphocytic leukemia. *Blood* 1984;63:843.

616. Rees JKH, Gray RG, Swirsky D, et al. Principal results of the Medical Research Council's 8th acute myeloid leukaemia trial. *Lancet* 1986;2:1236.

617. Weinstein HJ, Mayer RJ, Rosenthal DS, et al. Chemotherapy for acute myelogenous leukemia in children and adults: VAPA update. *Blood* 1983;62:315.

618. Kalwinksy D, Mirro J, Schell M, et al. Early intensification of chemotherapy for childhood acute nonlymphoblastic leukemia: improved remission induction with a five drug regimen including etoposide. *J Clin Oncol* 1988;6:1134.

619. Amadori S, Ceci A, Correlli A, et al. Treatment of acute myelogenous leukemia in children: results of the Italian Cooperative study AISOP/LAM8204. *J Clin Oncol* 1987;5:1356.

620. Steuber CP, Culbert SJ, Ravindranath Y, et al. Therapy of childhood acute nonlymphocytic leukemia: the Pediatric Oncology Group experience (1977–1988). In: Buechner T, Schellong G, Hiddeman W, eds. *Haematology and blood transfusion acute leukemias II.* New York: Springer-Verlag, 1990;33:198.

621. Wolff SW, Herzig RN, Fay JW, et al. High-dose cytarabine and daunorubicin as consolidation therapy for acute myeloid leukemia in first remission: long-term follow-up and results. *J Clin Oncol* 1989;7:1260.

622. Cassileth PA, Begg CB, Silber R, et al. Prolonged unmaintained remission after intensive consolidation therapy in adult acute nonlymphocytic leukemia. *Cancer Treat Rep* 1987;71:137.

623. Rohatiner AZS, Gregory WM, Bassan R, et al. Short-term therapy for acute myelogenous leukemia. *J Clin Oncol* 1988;6:218.

624. Stone R, Mayer R. Treatment of the newly diagnosed adult with de novo acute myeloid leukemia. *Hematol Oncol Clin North Am* 1993;7:47.

625. Mayer RJ, Davis RB, Schiffer CA, et al. Intensive postremission chemotherapy in adults with acute myeloid leukemia. Cancer and Leukemia Group B. *N Engl J Med* 1994;331:896–903.

626. Elonen E, Almqvist A, Hanninen A, et al. Comparison between four and eight cycles of intensive chemotherapy in adult acute myeloid leukemia: a randomized trial of the Finnish Leukemia Group. *Leukemia* 1998;12:1041–1048.

627. Lowenberg B, Zittoun R, Kerkhofs H, et al. On the value of intensive remission-induction chemotherapy in elderly patients of 65+ years with acute myeloid leukemia: a randomized phase III study of the European organization for research and treatment of Cancer Leukemia Group. *J Clin Oncol* 1989;7:1268.

628. Tilly H, Castaigne S, Bordessoule D, et al. Low-dose cytarabine versus intensive chemotherapy in the treatment of acute nonlymphocytic leukemia in the elderly. *J Clin Oncol* 1990;8:272.

629. Cheson BD, Jasperse DM, Simon R, et al. A critical appraisal of low-dose cytosine arabinoside in patients with acute non-lymphocytic leukemia and myelodysplastic syndromes. *J Clin Oncol* 1986;4:1857.

630. Sachs L. The differentiation of myeloid leukemia cells: new possibilities for therapy. *Br J Haematol* 1978;40:509.

631. Kahn SB, Begg CB, Mazza JJ, et al. Full dose versus attenuated dose daunorubicin, cytosine arabinoside, and 6-thioguanine in the treatment of acute nonlymphocytic leukemia in the elderly. *J Clin Oncol* 1984;2:865–870.

632. Stasi R, Venditti A, Del Poeta G, et al. Intensive treatment of patients age 60 years and older with de novo acute myeloid leukemia: analysis of prognostic factors. *Cancer* 1996;77:2476–2488.

633. Bow EJ, Sutherland JA, Kilpatrick MG, et al. Therapy of untreated acute myeloid leukemia in the elderly: remission-induction using a non-cytarabine-containing regimen of mitoxantrone plus etoposide. *J Clin Oncol* 1996;14:1345–1352.

634. Baudard M, Beauchamp-Nicoud A, Delmer A, et al. Has the prognosis of adult patients with acute myeloid leukemia improved over years? A single institution experience of 784 consecutive patients over a 16-year period. *Leukemia* 1999;13:1481–1490.

635. Aur RJA, Simone JV, Husto HO, et al. Central nervous system therapy and combination chemotherapy of childhood lymphocytic leukemia. *Blood* 1971;37:272.

636. Nesbit ME, Sather HN, Robison LL, et al. Presymptomatic central nervous system therapy in previously untreated childhood acute lymphoblastic leukemia: comparison of 1800 rad and 2400 rad: a report for the Children's Cancer Study Group. *Lancet* 1981;1:461.

637. Cassileth PA, Sylvester LS, Bennett JM, et al. High peripheral blast count in adult acute myelogenous leukemia is a primary risk factor for CNS leukemia. *J Clin Oncol* 1988;6:495.

638. Santos GW. Marrow transplantation in acute nonlymphocytic leukemia. *Blood* 1989;74:901.

639. Clift RA, Buckner CD, Thomas ED, et al. The treatment of acute nonlymphoblastic leukemia by allogeneic marrow transplantation. *Bone Marrow Transplant* 1987;2:243.

640. Thomas ED, Buckner CD, Banaji M, et al. One hundred patients with acute leukemia treated by chemotherapy, total body irradiation, and allogeneic marrow transplantation. *Blood* 1977;49:511.

641. Thomas ED, Buckner CD, Clift RA, et al. Marrow transplantation for acute non-lymphoblastic leukemia in first remission. *N Engl J Med* 1979;301:597.

642. Dinsmore R, Kirkpatrick D, Flomenberg N, et al. Allogeneic bone marrow transplantation for patients with acute nonlymphocytic leukemia. *Blood* 1984;63:649.

643. McGlave PB, Haake RJ, Bostrom BC, et al. Allogeneic bone marrow transplantation for acute nonlymphocytic leukemia in first remission. *Blood* 1988;72:1512–1517.

644. Champlin RE, Ho WG, Gale RP, et al. Treatment of acute myelogenous leukemia: a prospective controlled trial of bone marrow transplantation versus consolidation chemotherapy. *Ann Intern Med* 1985;102:285–291.

645. Appelbaum FR, Fisher LD, Thomas ED. Chemotherapy or marrow transplantation for adults with acute non-lymphocytic leukemia: a five year follow-up. *Blood* 1988;72:179.

646. Nesbit M, Buckley J, Feig S, et al. Chemotherapy for induction of remission of childhood acute myeloid leukemia followed by marrow transplantation or multiagent chemotherapy: a report from the Children's Cancer Group. *J Clin Oncol* 1994;12:127.

647. Hurd DD. Allogeneic and autologous bone marrow transplantation (BMT) for acute nonlymphocytic leukemia. *Semin Oncol* 1987;14:407.

648. Forman SJ, Krance RA, O'Donnell MR, et al. Bone marrow transplantation for acute nonlymphoblastic leukemia during first complete remission: an analysis of prognostic factors. *Transplantation* 1987;43:650–653.

649. Geller RB, Saral R, Piantadosi S, et al. Allogeneic bone marrow transplantation after high-dose busulfan and cyclophosphamide in patients with acute nonlymphocytic leukemia. *Blood* 1989;73:2209–2218.

650. Schiller GJ, Nimer SD, Territo MC, et al. Bone marrow transplantation versus high-dose cytarabine-based consolidation chemotherapy for acute myelogenous leukemia in first remission. *J Clin Oncol* 1992;10:41–46.

651. Young JW, Papdopoulos EB, Cunningham I, et al. T-cell-depleted allogeneic bone marrow transplantation in adults with acute nonlymphocytic leukemia in first remission. *Blood* 1992;79:3380–3387.

652. Fagioli F, Bacigalupo A, Frassoni F, et al. Allogeneic bone marrow transplantation for acute myeloid leukemia in first complete remission: the effect of FAB classification and GVHD prophylaxis. *Bone Marrow Transplant* 1994;13:247–252.

653. Keating S, Suciu S, de Witte T, et al. Prognostic factors of patients with acute myeloid leukemia (AML) allografted in first complete remission: an analysis of the EORTC-GIMEMA AML 8A trial. The European Organization for Research and Treatment of Cancer (EORTC) and the Gruppo Italiano Malattie Ematologiche Maligne dell' Adulto (GIMEMA) Leukemia Cooperative Groups. *Bone Marrow Transplant* 1996;17:993–1001.

654. Labar B, Masszi T, Morabito F, et al. Allogeneic bone marrow transplantation for acute leukemia—IGCI experience. *Bone Marrow Transplant* 1996;17:1009–1012.

655. Mehta J, Powles R, Treleaven J, et al. Long-term follow-up of patients undergoing allogeneic bone marrow transplantation for acute myeloid leukemia in first complete remission after cyclophosphamide-total body irradiation and cyclosporine. *Bone Marrow Transplant* 1996;18:741–746.

656. Reiffers J, Stoppa AM, Attal M, et al. Allogeneic vs autologous stem cell transplantation in patients with acute myeloid leukemia in first remission: the BGMT 87 study. *Leukemia* 1996;10:1874–1882.

657. Ferrant A, Labopin M, Frassoni F, et al. Karyotype in acute myeloblastic leukemia: prognostic significance for bone marrow transplantation in first remission: a European Group for Blood and Marrow Transplantation study. Acute Leukemia Working Party of the European Group for Blood and Marrow Transplantation (EBMT). *Blood* 1997;90:2931–2938.

658. Soiffer RJ, Fairclough D, Robertson M, et al. CD6-depleted allogeneic bone marrow transplantation for acute leukemia in first complete remission. *Blood* 1997;89:3039–3047.

659. Gorin NC, Herve P, Aegerter P, et al. Autologous bone marrow transplantation for acute leukemia in remission. *Br J Haematol* 1986;64:385.

660. Lowenberg B, Verdonck LG, Dekker AW, et al. Autologous bone marrow transplantation in acute myeloid leukemia in first remission: results of a Dutch prospective study. *J Clin Oncol* 1990;8:287.

661. Gorin NC, Aegerter P, Auvert B, et al. Autologous bone marrow transplantation for acute myelocytic leukemia in first remission: a European survey of the role of marrow purging. *Blood* 1990;75:1606.

662. Gulati S, Acaba L, Yahalom J, et al. Autologous bone marrow transplantation for acute myelogenous leukemia using 4-hydroperoxycyclophosphamide and VP-16 purged bone marrow. *Bone Marrow Transplant* 1992;10:129–134.

663. Cassileth PA, Andersen JW, Lazarus HM, et al. Autologous bone marrow transplant in acute myeloid leukemia in first remission. *J Clin Oncol* 1993; 11:314–319.

664. Linker CA, Ries CA, Damon LE, et al. Autologous bone marrow transplantation for acute myeloid leukemia using busulfan plus etoposide as a preparative regimen. *Blood* 1993;81:311–318.

665. Sanz M, de la Rubia J, Guillermo F, et al. Busulfan plus cyclophosphamide followed by autologous blood stem-cell transplantation for patients with acute myeloblastic leukemia in first complete remission: a report from a single institution. *J Clin Oncol* 1993;11:1661–1667.

666. Sierra J, Grañena A, Garcia J, et al. Autologous bone marrow transplantation for acute leukemia: results and prognostic factors in 90 consecutive patients. *Bone Marrow Transplant* 1993;12:517–523.

667. Laporte JP, Douay L, Lopez M, et al. One hundred twenty-five adult patients with primary acute leukemia autografted with marrow purged by mafosfamide: a 10-year single institution experience. *Blood* 1994;84:3810–3818.

668. Cahn JY, Labopin M, Mandelli F, et al. Autologous bone marrow transplantation for first remission acute myeloblastic leukemia in patients older than 50 years: a retrospective analysis of the European Bone Marrow Transplant Group. *Blood* 1995;85:575–579.

669. Miggiano MC, Gherlinzoni F, Rosti G, et al. Autologous bone marrow transplantation in late first complete remission improves outcome in acute myelogenous leukemia. *Leukemia* 1996;10:402–409.

670. Stein AS, O'Donnell MR, Chai A, et al. In vivo purging with high-dose cytarabine followed by high-dose chemoradiotherapy and reinfusion of unpurged bone marrow for adult acute myelogenous leukemia in first complete remission. *J Clin Oncol* 1996;14:2206–2216.

671. Schiller J, Lee M, Miller T, et al. Transplantation of autologous peripheral blood progenitor cells procured after high-dose cytarabine-based consolidation chemotherapy for adults with acute myelogenous leukemia in first remission. *Leukemia* 1997;11:1533–1539.

672. Gondo H, Harada M, Miyamoto T, et al. Autologous peripheral blood stem cell transplantation for acute myeloid leukemia. *Bone Marrow Transplant* 1997;20:821–826.

673. Martin C, Torres A, Leon A, et al. Autologous peripheral blood stem cell transplantation (PBSCT) mobilized with G-CSF in AML in first complete remission: role of intensification therapy in outcome. *Bone Marrow Transplant* 1998;21:375–382.

674. Visani G, Lemoli R, Tosi P, et al. Use of peripheral blood stem cells for autologous transplantation in acute myeloid leukemia patients allows faster engraftment and equivalent disease-free survival compared with bone marrow cells. *Bone Marrow Transplant* 1999;24:467–472.

675. Woods W, Kobrinsky N, Neudorf S, et al. Intensively timed induction therapy followed by autologous or allogeneic bone marrow transplantation for children with acute myeloid leukemia or myelodysplastic syndrome: a Children's Cancer Group pilot study. *J Clin Oncol* 1993;11:1448.

676. Gorin NC. Autologous stem cell transplantation in acute myeloid leukemia. *Blood* 1998;92:1073–1090.

677. Zittoun RA, Mandelli F, Willemze R, et al. Autologous or allogeneic bone marrow transplantation compared with intensive chemotherapy in acute myelogenous leukemia. European Organization for Research and Treatment of Cancer (EORTC) and the Gruppo Italiano Malattie Ematologiche Maligne dell'Adulto (GIMEMA) Leukemia Cooperative Groups. *N Engl J Med* 1995;332:217–223.

678. Harousseau JL, Cahn JY, Pignon B, et al. Comparison of autologous bone marrow transplantation and intensive chemotherapy as postremission therapy in adult acute myeloid leukemia. The Groupe Ouest Est Leucemies Aigues Myeloblastiques (GOELAM). *Blood* 1997;90:2978–2986.

679. Burnett AK, Goldstone AH, Stevens RMF, et al. Randomized comparison of addition of autologous bone marrow transplantation to intensive chemotherapy for acute myeloid leukemia in first remission: results of MRC AML 10 trial. *Lancet* 1998;351:700–708.

680. Cassileth PA, Harrington DP, Appelbaum FR, et al. Chemotherapy compared with autologous or allogeneic bone marrow transplantation in the management of acute myeloid leukemia in first remission. *N Engl J Med* 1998;339:1649–1656.

681. Papdopoulos EB, Carabasi MH, Castro-Malaspina H, et al. T-cell-depleted allogeneic bone marrow transplantation as postremission therapy for acute myelogenous leukemia: freedom from relapse in the absence of graft-versus-host disease. *Blood* 1998;91:1083–1090.

682. Cahn JY, Labopin M, Schattenberg A, et al. Allogeneic bone marrow transplantation for acute leukemia in patients over the age of 40 years. Acute Leukemia Working Party of the European Group for Bone Marrow Transplantation (EBMT). *Leukemia* 1997;11:416–419.

683. Gale RP. T cells, bone marrow transplantation, and immunotherapy. *Ann Intern Med* 1987;106:257.

684. Storb R, Deeg HJ, Whitehead J, et al. Methotrexate and cyclosporine compared with cyclosporine alone for prophylaxis of acute graft-versus-host disease after marrow transplantation for leukemia. *N Engl J Med* 1986;314:729.

685. Mitsuyasu R, Champlin RE, Gale RP, et al. Depletion of T lymphocytes from donor bone marrow for prevention of graft-versus-host disease following bone marrow transplantation. *Ann Intern Med* 1986;105:20.

686. Grever MR. Treatment of patients with acute nonlymphocytic leukemia not in remission. *Semin Oncol* 1987;14:416.

687. Keating MJ, Kantarjian H, Smith TL, et al. Response to salvage therapy and survival after relapse in acute myelogenous leukemia. *J Clin Oncol* 1989;7:1071.

688. Kantarjian HM, Keating MJ, Walters RS, et al. The characteristics and outcome of patients with late relapse acute myelogenous leukemia. *J Clin Oncol* 1988;6:232.

689. Carella AM, Santini G, Martinengo M, et al. 4-Demethoxy daunorubicin (idarubicin) in refractory or relapsed acute leukemia: a pilot study. *Cancer* 1985;55:1452.

690. Lee EJ, Van Echo DA, Egorin MJ, et al. Diaziquone given as a continuous infusion is an active agent for relapsed adult acute nonlymphocytic leukemia. *Blood* 1986;67:182.

691. Glover AB, Leyland-Jones BR, Chun HG, et al. Azacitidine: 10 years later. *Cancer Treat Rep* 1987;71:737.

692. Kalwinsky DK, Dahl GV, Mirro J, et al. Induction failures in childhood acute nonlymphocytic leukemia: etoposide/5-azacytidine for cases refractory to daunorubicin/cytarabine. *Med Pediatr Oncol* 1986;14:245.

693. Leone G, Pagano L, Marra R, et al. Combination of 6-mercaptopurine, vincristine, methotrexate, and prednisone in resistant or relapsed acute nonlymphoid leukemia. *Cancer Treat Rep* 1987;71:751.

694. Amadori S, Tribalto M, Pastore S, et al. Sequential combination of methotrexate (mtx) and L-asparaginase (asp) in advanced acute nonlymphocytic leukemia (ANLL). *Am Assoc Cancer Res* 1980;21:131(abst).

695. Korbling M, Hunstein W, Fliedner TM, et al. Disease-free survival after autologous bone marrow transplantation in patients with acute myelogenous leukemia. *Blood* 1989;74:1898.

696. Ball ED, Mills LE, Cornwell III GG, et al. Autologous bone marrow transplantation for acute myeloid leukemia using monoclonal antibody-purged bone marrow. *Blood* 1990;75:1199.

697. Schiller G, Feig SA, Territo M, et al. Treatment of advanced acute leukaemia with allogeneic bone marrow transplantation from unrelated donors. *Br J Haematol* 1994;88:72–78.

698. Chown SR, Marks DI, Cornish JM, et al. Unrelated donor bone marrow transplantation in children and young adults with acute myeloid leukemia in remission. *Br J Haematol* 1997;99:36.

699. Kodera Y, Morishima Y, Kato S, et al. Analysis of 500 bone marrow transplants from unrelated donors (UR-BMT) facilitated by the Japan Marrow Donor Program: confirmation of UR-BMT as a standard therapy for patients with leukemia and aplastic anemia. *Bone Marrow Transplant* 1999;24:995.

700. Kurtzberg J, Laughlin M, Graham ML, et al. Placental blood as a source of hematopoietic stem cells for transplantation into unrelated recipients. *N Engl J Med* 1996;335:157–166.

701. Gluckman E, Rocha V, Boyer-Chammard A, et al. Outcome of cord-blood transplantation from related and unrelated donors. Eurocord Transplant Group and the European Blood and Marrow Transplantation Group. *N Engl J Med* 1997;337:373–381.

702. Laughlin MJ, Barker J, Bambach B, et al. Hematopoietic engraftment and survival in adult recipients of umbilical-cord blood from unrelated donors. *N Engl J Med* 2001;344:1815–1822.

703. Aversa F, Tabilio A, Velardi A, et al. Treatment of high-risk acute leukemia with T-cell-depleted stem cells from related donors with one fully mismatched HLA haplotype. *N Engl J Med* 1998;339:1186–1193.

704. Tallman MS, Lee S, Sikic BJ, et al. Mitoxantrone, etoposide, and cytarabine plus cyclosporine for patients with relapsed or refractory acute myeloid leukemia. *Cancer* 1999;85:358–367.

705. Advani R, Saba HI, Tallman M, et al. Treatment of refractory and relapsed acute myeloid leukemia with combination chemotherapy plus the multidrug resistance modulator PSC-833 (Valspodar). *Blood* 1999;93:787–795.

706. Lee EJ, George SL, Caligiuri M, et al. Parallel phase I studies of daunorubicin given with cytarabine and etoposide with or without the multidrug resistance modulator PSC-833 in previously untreated patients 60 years of age or older with acute myeloid leukemia: results of Cancer and Leukemia Group B study 9420. *J Clin Oncol* 1999;17:2831–2839.

707. Visani G, Milligan D, Leoni F, et al. Combined action of PSC-833 (Valspodar), a novel MDR reversing agent, with mitoxantrone, etoposide and cytarabine in poor-prognosis acute myeloid leukemia. *Leukemia* 2001;15:764–771.

708. Kantarjian HM, Beran M, Ellis A, et al. Phase I study of topotecan, a new topoisomerase I inhibitor, in patients with refractory or relapsed acute leukemia. *Blood* 1993;81:1146–1151.

709. Cortes J, Estey E, Beran M, et al. Cyclophosphamide, ara-C and topotecan (CAT) for patients with refractory or relapsed acute leukemia. *Leuk Lymphoma* 2000;36:479–484.

710. Gordon MS, Young ML, Tallman MS, et al. Phase II trial of 2-chlorodeoxyadenosine in patients with relapsed/refractory acute myeloid leukemia: a study of the Eastern Cooperative Oncology Group (ECOG), E5995. *Leuk Res* 2000;24:871–875.

711. Robak T, Wrzesien-Kus A, Lech-Maranda E, et al. Combination regimen of cladribine (2-chlorodeoxyadenosine), cytarabine and G-CSF (CLAG) as induction therapy for patients with relapsed or refractory acute myeloid leukemia. *Leuk Lymphoma* 2000;39:121–129.

712. Aguayo A, Kantarjian H, Manshouri T, et al. Angiogenesis in acute and chronic leukemias and myelodysplastic syndromes. *Blood* 2000;96:2240–2245.

713. Padro T, Ruiz S, Bieker R, et al. Increased angiogenesis in the bone marrow of patients with acute myeloid leukemia. *Blood* 2000;95:2637–2644.

714. Kini AR, Peterson LC, Tallman MS, et al. Angiogenesis in acute promyelocytic leukemia: induction by vascular endothelial growth factor and inhibition by all-trans retinoic acid. *Blood* 2001;97:3919–3924.

715. Sievers EL, Appelbaum FR, Spielberger RT, et al. Selective ablation of acute myeloid leukemia using antibody-targeted chemotherapy: a phase I study of an anti-CD33 calicheamicin immunoconjugate. *Blood* 1999;93:3678–3684.

716. Sievers EL, Larson RA, Stadtmauer EA, et al. Efficacy and safety of gemtuzumab ozogamicin in patients with CD33-positive acute myeloid leukemia in first relapse. *J Clin Oncol* 2001;19:3244–3254.

717. Keating MJ, Estey E, Plunkett W, et al. Evolution of clinical studies with high-dose cytosine arabinoside, etoposide, cytarabine (PSC-MEC) vital signs show a temperature of MEC: randomized phase IV trial (E2995). *Blood* 1999;94:383a (abst).

718. Hiddemann W, Martin WR, Saverland CM, et al. Definition of refractoriness against conventional chemotherapy in acute myeloid leukemia: a proposal based on the results of retreatment by thioguanine, cytosine arabinoside, and daunorubicin (TAD 9) in 150 patients with relapse after standardized first line therapy. *Leukemia* 1990;4:184–188.

719. Davis CL, Rohatiner AZ, Lim J, et al. The management of recurrent acute myelogenous leukemia at a single centre over a fifteen-year period. *Br J Haematol* 1993;83:404–411.

720. Archimbaud E, Thomas X, Leblond V, et al. Timed sequential chemotherapy for previously treated patients with acute myeloid leukemia: long-term follow-up of the etoposide, mitoxantrone, and cytarabine-86 trial. *J Clin Oncol* 1995;13:11–18.

721. Advani R, Saba HI, Tallman MS, et al. Treatment of refractory and relapsed acute myelogenous leukemia with combination chemotherapy plus the multi drug resistance modulator PSC 833 (Valdospar). *Blood* 1999;93:787–795.

722. Thalhammer F, Geissler K, Jager U, et al. Duration of second complete remission in patients with acute myeloid leukemia treated with chemotherapy: a retrospective single-center study. *Ann Hematol* 1996;72:216–222.

723. Karanes C, Kopecky KJ, Head DR, et al. A phase III comparison of high-dose ARA-C (HIDAC) versus HIDAC plus mitoxantrone in the treatment of first relapsed or refractory acute myeloid leukemia Southwest Oncology Group study. *Leuk Res* 1999;23:787–794.

724. Baehner RL, Bernstein ID, Sather H, et al. Improved remission induction rate with D-ZAPO but unimproved remission duration with addition of immunotherapy to chemotherapy in previously untreated children with ANLL. *Med Pediatr Oncol* 1979;7:127.

725. Lister TA, Whitehouse JMA, Oliver RTD, et al. Chemotherapy and immunotherapy for acute myelogenous leukemia. *Cancer* 1980;46:2142.

726. Holland JF, Bekesi JG, Cuttner J, et al. Chemoimmunotherapy in acute myelocytic leukemia. *Isr J Med Sci* 1977;13:694.

727. Mirro J, Dow LW, Kalwinsky DK, et al. Phase I–II study of continuous-infusion high-dose human lymphoblastoid interferon and in vitro sensitivity of leukemic progenitors in nonlymphocytic leukemia. *Cancer Treat Rep* 1986;70:363.

728. Adler A, Albo V, Blatt J, et al. Interleukin-2 induction of lymphokine-activated killer (CAk) activity in the peripheral blood and bone marrow of acute leukemia patients, II: feasibility of LAK generation in children with active disease and in remission. *Blood* 1989;74:1690.

729. Maraninchi D, Blaise D, Viens P, et al. High-dose recombinant interleukin-2 and acute myeloid leukemias in relapse. *Blood* 1991;78:2182–2187.

730. Foa R. Does interleukin-2 have a role in the management of acute leukemia? *J Clin Oncol* 1993;11:1817–1825.

731. Meloni G, Foa R, Vignetti M, et al. Interleukin-2 may induce prolonged remissions in advanced acute myelogenous leukemia. *Blood* 1994;84:2158–2163.

732. Meloni G, Vignetti M, Andrizzi C, et al. Interleukin-2 for the treatment of advanced acute myelogenous leukemia patients with limited disease: updated experience with 20 cases. *Leuk Lymphoma* 1996;21:429–435.

733. Tallman MS, Andersen JW, Schiffer CA, et al. All-trans-retinoic acid in acute promyelocytic leukemia. *N Engl J Med* 1997;337:1021–1028.

734. Fenaux P, Chastang C, Chevret P, et al. A randomized comparison of all trans-retinoic acid (ATRA) followed by chemotherapy and ATRA plus chemotherapy and the role of maintenance therapy in newly diagnosed acute promyelocytic leukemia. The European APL Group. *Blood* 1999;94:1192–1200.

735. De Botton S, Dombret H, Sanz M, et al. Incidence, clinical features, and outcome of all trans-retinoic acid syndrome in 413 cases of newly diagnosed acute promyelocytic leukemia. The European APL Group. *Blood* 1998;92:2712–2718.

736. Tallman MS, Andersen JW, Schiffer CA, et al. Clinical description of 44 patients with acute promyelocytic leukemia who developed the retinoic acid syndrome. *Blood* 2000;95:90–95.

737. Burnett AK, Grimwade D, Soloman E, et al. Presenting white blood cell count and kinetics of molecular remission predict prognosis in acute promyelocytic leukemia treated with all-trans retinoic acid: result of the Randomized MRC Trial. *Blood* 1999;93:4131–4143.

738. Chen GQ, Zhu J, Shi XG, et al. In vitro studies on cellular and molecular mechanisms of arsenic trioxide (As2O3) in the treatment of acute promyelocytic leukemia: As2O3 induces NB4 cell apoptosis with downregulation of Bcl-2 expression and modulation of PML-RAR alpha/PML proteins. *Blood* 1996;88:1052–1061.

739. Chen GQ, Shi XG, Tang W, et al. Use of arsenic trioxide (As2O3) in the treatment of acute promyelocytic leukemia (APL), I: As2O3 exerts dose-dependent dual effects on APL cells. *Blood* 1997;89:3345–3353.

740. Soignet SL, Maslak P, Wang Z-G, et al. Complete remission after treatment of acute promyelocytic leukemia with arsenic trioxide. *N Engl J Med* 1998;339:1341–1348.

741. Niu C, Yan H, Yu T, et al. Studies on treatment of acute promyelocytic leukemia with arsenic trioxide: remission induction follow-up, and molecular monitoring in 11 newly diagnosed and 47 relapsed acute promyelocytic leukemia patients. *Blood* 1999;94:3315.

742. Doll DC, Ringenberg QS, Yarbro JW. Antineoplastic agents and pregnancy. *Semin Oncol* 1989;16:337.

743. Caligiuri MA, Mayer RJ. Pregnancy and leukemia. *Semin Oncol* 1989;16:388.

744. Osada S, Horibe K, Oiwak K, et al. A case of infantile acute monocytic leukemia caused by vertical transmission of the mother's leukemia cells. *Cancer* 1990;65:1146.

745. Reynoso EE, Shepherd FA, Messner HA, et al. Acute leukemia during pregnancy: the Toronto Leukemia Study Group experience with long-term follow-up of children exposed in utero to chemotherapeutic agents. *J Clin Oncol* 1987;5:1098–1106.

746. Buckley JD, Chard RL, Baehner RL, et al. Improvement in outcome for children with acute nonlymphocytic leukemia. *Cancer* 1989;63:1457.

747. Bennett JM, Young ML, Andersen JW, et al. Long-term survival in acute myeloid leukemia: the Eastern Cooperative Oncology Group experience. *Cancer* 1997;80[Suppl 11]:2205–2209.

748. Preisler HD, Anderson K, Rai K, et al. The frequency of long-term remission in patients with acute myelogenous leukemia treated with conventional maintenance chemotherapy: a study of 760 patients with a minimal follow-up time of 6 years. *Br J Haematol* 1989;71:189.

749. Campana D, Coustan-Smith E, Janossy G. The immunologic detection of minimal residual disease in acute leukemia. *Blood* 1990;76:163.

750. San Miguel JF, Martinez A, Macedo A, et al. Immunophenotyping investigation of minimal residual disease is a useful approach for predicting relapse in acute myeloid leukemia patients. *Blood* 1997;90:2465.

751. Estey E. Treatment of refractory AML. *Leukemia* 1996;10:932.

752. Byrne J, Mulvihill JJ, Myers MH, et al. Effects of treatment on fertility in long-term survivors of childhood or adolescent cancer. *N Engl J Med* 1987;317:135.

753. de Lima M, Strom SS, Keating M, et al. Implications of potential cure in acute myelogenous leukemia: development of subsequent cancer and return to work. *Blood* 1997;90:4719.

754. Rowe JM, Liesveld JL. Hematopoietic growth factors in acute leukemia. *Leukemia* 1997;11:328–341.

CHAPTER 16

Structure, Function, and Functional Disorders of the Phagocyte System

Thomas P. Stossel and Bernard M. Babior

The phagocyte system consists of bone marrow–derived cells with the common feature of efficient engulfment of particulate material. The development of these cells from the pluripotent and committed stem cells, covered in detail in Chapter 7, leads to the differentiation and deployment of two major phagocyte classes: the neutrophilic polymorphonuclear leukocytes (PMNs) and the mononuclear phagocytes (MNPs). The MNPs consist of two morphologically distinct cell types: the blood monocytes and the tissue macrophages into which they develop. Eosinophilic PMNs (eosinophils) qualify as phagocytes, but because they seem to have functions distinct from those of neutrophilic PMNs, they are usually separated conceptually from the phagocyte system (see Chapter 14). Chapter 13 covers the acute myelogenous leukemias, neoplastic diseases of the cell lineage normally committed to development of the phagocyte system. Malignancies of mature-appearing MNP, the histiocytoses, are discussed in Chapter 28, which also mentions enzyme deficiencies of MNP leading to so-called storage disorders. Phagocytes, especially MNPs, participate in immune responses engineered primarily by cells of the lymphoid system, and Chapter 15 provides information on this important function. This chapter describes structural and functional properties of mature PMNs and MNPs, focusing on the role of these cells in host defense against microbial infection and in certain types of inflammation.

Although many have attributed the discovery of phagocytosis to the Russian comparative zoologist Elie Metchnikoff, it was a German clergyman and amateur naturalist named Johann Goeze (1731 to 1793) who, in 1777, published the first account of protists ingesting other protists (Fig. 16-1). In the following year, a German nobleman, Wilhelm F. von Gleichen-Russworm (1717 to 1783) described his experiments feeding carmine particles to lower eukaryotes. The emigration of leukocytes from blood into tissues was observed by Waller and by Addison in the early part of the 19th century, and Schultze first described phagocytosis by human leukocytes in 1865. Metchnikoff, however, deserves (and received) much credit for recognizing, beginning in 1888, the significance of this system of cells in physiology and pathology. Metchnikoff consolidated his theory that phagocytes mediate host defense and cause inflammation by a series of brilliant experiments using comparative pathology. By showing that animals without circulatory systems exhibited collections of phagocytes at sites of inflammation, Metchnikoff overcame the objection by his critics, who espoused the earlier views of Virchow and Cohnheim that vascular permeability was the cause, not the effect, of phagocyte emigration (1). The discovery of serum opsonins by Wright and Douglas, and their identification as antibody and complement by Ward and Enders and others in the early 20th century, provided an important step in ascertaining how phagocytes act specifically against pathogens and pointed to a source other than the phagocytes for that specificity.

The modern era of phagocytosis research began in the 1950s and 1960s with a number of important advances. One was recognition by Robert McKannes and his colleagues of macrophage activation in the containment of facultative intracellular parasites. Another was the cultivation and extensive characterization of MNPs by Zanvil Cohn and co-workers at Rockefeller University. Still another was the beginning use of phagocytes as subjects of biochemical research by Manfred Karnovsky at Harvard, who was interested in the metabolic basis of ingestion. These investigations and others by Filipo Rossi in Trieste led to new insights into the molecular mechanisms of microbicidal and inflammatory activities of phagocytes, especially the importance of oxygen metabolites. The elucidation of the antimicrobial myeloperoxidase (MPO) and hydrogen peroxide system by Seymour Klebanoff had a major influence in the development of this field. James Hirsch, Cohn, and later, Marco Baggiolini at Rockefeller, Dorothy Bainton and Marilyn Farquhar at the University of California, and John Spitznagel in Chapel Hill contributed landmark investigations on the composition and microbicidal function of phagocyte subcellular organelles. Peter Elsbach at New York University and, later, Bengt Samuelsson at the Karolinska Institute made phagocyte lipids important focuses of research. The introduction by Stephen Boyden in 1963 of a simple method for measuring leukocyte locomotion *in vitro* was the impetus for studies by Elmer Becker and Peter Ward at Walter Reed Army Institute for Medical Research and ultimately led to the discovery of a large number of humoral factors, *chemoattractants*, that controlled the direction of migration of leukocytes. Nobuyuki Senda in Osaka, Japan, pioneered studies on the role of contractile proteins in phagocyte motility. Also of great importance was the recognition that a qualitative disorder of phagocytes, *chronic granulomatous disease (CGD)*, first described by Robert Good and colleagues at the University of Minnesota, led to susceptibility to infection. This group and others later documented that this

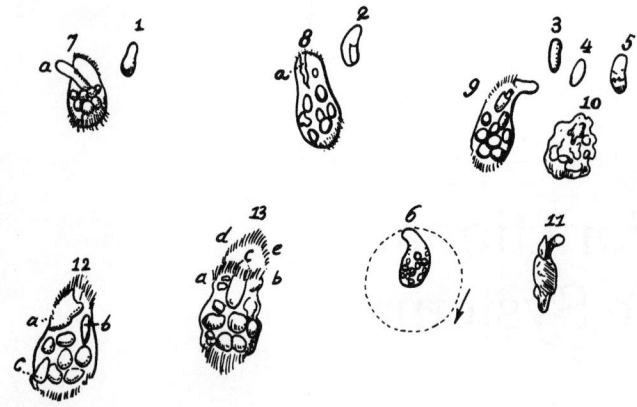

Figure 16-1. Original description of phagocytosis: reproduction by Joy Marlowe of drawings by Johann Goeze (1) showing small protists, which Goeze called *small oval animals*, ingested by larger ones, which he called *Haarwanzen* ("hairbugs").

disease resulted from a disorder of phagocyte bactericidal deficiency related to faulty oxygen metabolism.

GENERAL FUNCTIONS AND CLASSIFICATION OF PHAGOCYTES

The most clearly defined function of the phagocyte system is as a scavenger of senescent or damaged cells and macromolecules and as a powerful defense mechanism against infection by microorganisms. To the extent that these cells must use biochemical activities that are cytolytic or destructive of macromolecules in their degrading and defensive roles, they have the capacity to damage host tissue. When this destruction occurs, either as a by-product of the combat between phagocytes and invading microorganisms or as a direct attack on the host in autoimmune disorders, the phagocytes contribute importantly to inflammation and host cell destruction. The target range of phagocytes is relatively nonspecific, and the cells depend heavily on the lymphoid system for directions (see Chapter 18).

Phagocytes also elaborate an enormous variety of compounds (Table 16-1), some of which participate in the local regulation of cell growth and development, in immune responses, in blood coagulation, and even in atherogenesis and carcinogenesis.

Because PMNs and MNPs arise from a common committed stem cell, it is not surprising that they share many characteristics. Indeed, their functional similarities outweigh their differences sufficiently that it is reasonable to economize by summarizing much of their physiology together. Nevertheless, PMNs and MNPs have important differences. In addition to indicating these variations throughout the chapter, we highlight major differences here.

Mobility

Both PMNs and MNPs arise from the bone marrow and circulate. In their life cycles, both exhibit invasive properties when they enter the blood from the marrow sinuses and leave it to penetrate body tissues by active motility. In this motile activity, PMNs are more active than monocytes; indeed, PMNs are among the most motile eukaryotic cells in the human body. As monocytes become macrophages, they lose most of their capacity to move translationally (i.e., mobility), although they remain actively *motile* in terms of surface ruffling, spreading, and phagocytosis.

TABLE 16-1. Substances Secreted by Mononuclear Phagocytes

Cytokines	Aryl sulfatase A, B
Thymosin B_4	Iduronate sulfatase
Interferon-γ	Heparan-N-sulfatase
IL-6	N-acetylgalactosamine-6-
TGF-α, -β	sulfate sulfatase
Fibroblast growth factor	N-acetylglucosamine sulfatase
Erythropoietin	β-Glucuronidase
IL-1α, β	Lipoprotein lipase
Tumor necrosis factor-α, -β	β-Glucosidase
Platelet-derived growth factor	β-Galactosidase
IL-8	α-Mannosidase
IL-1	α-L-Fucosidase
Bombesin	α-Iduronidase
Granulocyte-macrophage CSF	α-Neuraminidase
Granulocyte CSF	Aspartylglycosaminidase
Macrophage CSF	N-acetyl-β-glucosaminidase
IL-1 inhibitor	N-acetyl-β-galactosaminidase
IL-12	Oxidants
IL-18	Superoxide
Chemokines	Hydroxyl radical
Complement system proteins	Hydrogen peroxide
C1, C4, C2, C3, C5	Hypohalous acids
Factors B, D, H	Nitric oxide
Properdin	Coagulation system proteins
C3b inactivator	Factors V, VII, IX, X, XIII
Binding proteins	Tissue factor
Transcobalamin II	Plasminogen activator
Haptoglobin	Urokinase
Transferrin	Thrombospondin
$α_1$-Antiprotease	Lipid metabolites
$α_2$-Macroglobulin	Prostaglandin E_2, $F_{2α'}$ I
$α_1$-Antichymotrypsin	Thromboxane A_2
Gelsolin	Leukotriene B, C, D, E
Apolipoprotein E	Malonyldialdehyde
Enzymes	Mono-, diHETE
Lysozyme	Platelet-activating factor
Arginase	Other metabolites, peptides, and
Angiotensin-converting enzyme	proteins
Acid lipase	Glutathione
Acid phosphatase	Purines
Acid RNAase	Pyrimidines
Acid DNAase	Biopterin
α-Naphthylesterase	Serum amyloid A, P
Leucine-2-naphthylaminidase	Fibronectin
Acid deramidase	Defensins
Sphingomyelinase	Cathelicidin
Phospholipase A_2	1,25-hydroxyvitamin D_3
Elastase	Renin
Collagenase	Chondroitin sulfate proteogly-
Acid sulfatase	can

CSF, colony-stimulating factor; IL, interleukin; HETE, hydroxyeicosatetraenoic acid; TNF, tumor growth factor.

Life Cycle

The growth and development of phagocytes are described in detail in Chapter 14. Although neither mature PMNs nor MNPs are able to self-replicate, they differ in the degree to which they are end cells. A relatively brief lifetime (days at most) is characteristic of PMNs, whereas MNPs persist for months as macrophages in the tissues. Nearly all the biosynthetic activity of PMNs takes place during their period of maturation in the bone marrow, whereas MNPs retain the ability to make an amazing variety of products throughout their lifetime. Both PMNs and MNPs are relegated to function in their final resting place in the tissue, in contrast to free-living phagocytic cells such as amebae, which they resemble in many other ways and which have the ability to crawl about and ingest particulate matter wherever they please. This apparent lack of economy in the failure to recycle phagocytic cells, which requires the human organism to generate billions of PMNs daily, seems wasteful at face value.

Functional Versatility

In keeping with their short lifespan and limited biosynthetic capacity, PMNs have a narrower spectrum of functional roles than do MNPs, although recent studies suggest that they are less biosynthetically impaired than previously recognized (2). PMNs are of prime importance in the defense against many species of bacteria, and their rapid concentration in huge numbers at the site of attack by such organisms in the form of pus explains why these microbes are called *pyogenic*. PMNs also collect in necrotic tissues, where they participate in the digestion of macromolecules. In these activities, PMNs depend on immunoproteins, immunoglobulin M (IgM), IgG, and complement protein fragments to recognize where to mobilize (see later discussion). MNPs also participate in the defense against pyogenic infection and in the digestion of denatured macromolecules, and they become increasingly prominent when such processes become chronic. Unlike PMNs, however, MNPs, in the form of tissue macrophages, have the major share of the task of clearance of senescent cells and macromolecules under normal circumstances (3). Moreover, MNPs play an important role in the containment and eradication of so-called facultative intracellular parasites and interact in the exercise of this function with T lymphocytes (see Chapter 18). In light of the numerous digestive enzymes, binding proteins, and cytokines produced by MNPs (Table 16-1), these remarkable cells undoubtedly have many functions that are yet to be defined.

Why More Than One Kind of Phagocyte?

Relatively little comparative hematology has used modern tools of cell biology, so we can only speculate about reasons for different characteristics of phagocytes in various species. Some of the mysteries include the absence of MPO in chicken phagocytes, the abundant neutral protease content of human PMNs but not of PMNs from other species, the lack of N-formyloligopeptide (FMLP) chemotactic factor receptors in bovine phagocytes, and the residence of MNPs in the lumen of pulmonary blood vessels of horse, sheep, pig, dogs, and cats, but not rabbits or humans (4). Most curious of all is that only mammals have clearly defined populations of PMNs and MNPs. Lower organisms have phagocytes with characteristics resembling PMNs, but the phagocytes are more nearly akin to MNPs, and only mammals form true pus. It may be that the need for this particularly aggressive phagocyte evolved from the high risk of tissue infection associated with mammalian parturition.

PHAGOCYTIC FUNCTION—GENERAL OVERVIEW

The many functional activities of phagocytes share certain common features. Most phagocyte functions are not constitutive, but rather become manifest when soluble or particulate molecules in the environment of the cell perturb externally disposed plasma membrane receptors on the phagocyte (Table 16-2). We allude to the acute initiation of such functions as phagocyte excitation to distinguish it from the phenomena to be defined below and known, respectively, as stimulation and activation of MNPs.

PMNs, monocytes, and macrophages can ingest a wide variety of pathogenic microorganisms, but many of these, known as *facultative intracellular parasites*, are not contained or killed after ingestion. Examples of such microorganisms include *Listeria monocytogenes*, *Salmonella* spp, mycobacteria causing tuberculosis and leprosy, certain fungi such as *Candida albicans*, and metazoan parasites like *Toxoplasma gondii* and *Leishmania donovanii*. Macrophages that have interacted with T lymphocytes from

TABLE 16-2. Phagocyte Chemotactic, Adhesion, and Phagocytic Receptors

Receptor	Ligands
Chemoattractants	
C5a	C5a
Formyl-peptide	FMLP
Platelet-activating factor	PAF
CXCR1	IL8
CXCR2	IL8, Gros, NAP, ENA, GCP
CX3CR1	Fractaline
CCR1	RANTES, MIPs, HCC, MCP
CCR2	MIPs
CCR5	RANTES, MIPs
L-selectins	sLe^x on GlyCAM, CD34, MadCAM-1
Integrins	
αvβ3	Many extracellular matrix components
αLβ2	ICAM-1–3
αMβ2	C3bi, fibrinogen, factor X, ICAM-1, platelet Gp1b
αxβ2	C3bi, fibrinogen
αdβ2	ICAM-3
α1β1	Collagen, laminin
α2β1	Collagen, laminin
α4β1	Fibronectin, VCAM-1
α5β1	Fibronectin
α6β1	Laminin
α9β1	?
Scavenger receptors	
SR-A I and II (macrophages)	Oxidized LDL, HDL, apoptotic cells
CD36 (monocytes)	
Complement receptor 1 (CR1)	C3b
Mannose receptor (MNP)	Oligosaccharides on diverse microorganisms
Immunoglobulin receptors	
FcRI (macrophages, inducible in monocytes)	IgG monomers, soluble immune complexes
FcRII (PMN, MNP)	IgG aggregates, particulate immune complexes
FcRIIIA (MNP)	IgG aggregates, particulate immune complexes
FcRIIIB (PMN)	

FcR, Fc receptor; FMLP, N-formyloligopeptide; HDL, high-density lipoprotein; ICAM-1, intercellular adhesion molecule-1; Ig, immunoglobulin; LDL, low-density lipoprotein; MCC, monocyte chemoattractant protein; MIP, macrophage inflammatory protein; MNP, mononuclear phagocyte; PAF, platelet-activating factor; PMN, polymorphonuclear leukocyte; vascular cell adhesion molecule-1 (VCAM-1).

immunocompetent subjects previously exposed to these microorganisms acquire the ability to deal with them. This acquisition of defensive function is part of a cellular program known as *MNP activation* (Table 16-3). Activated MNPs also demonstrate enhanced cytotoxicity against mammalian cells, especially neoplastic cells, a phenomenon of great interest regarding immunity against malignant tumors. MNP activation is to be distinguished from the phenomenon known as *MNP stimulation*, the panel of alterations that takes place when MNPs ingest digestible material (Table 16-3). A classic experimental technique for preparing stimulated MNPs is to harvest them from the peritoneal cavities of mice 12 hours after intraperitoneal injection of thioglycolate broth.

T cells activate MNPs by secretion of interferon-γ (IFN-γ), which interacts with receptors on the MNP surface. One of the most important consequences of IFN-γ action on MNPs is stimulation of synthesis of components of the respiratory burst superoxide-producing nicotinamide adenine dinucleotide phosphate (NADPH) oxidase, described in more detail later. Although monocytes respond acutely to stimuli with a respiratory burst, unactivated monocyte-derived macrophages do not, unless activated by IFN-γ. Another antimicrobial effector system

TABLE 16-3. Characteristics of Activated and Stimulated Mononuclear Phagocytes

Activated
- Increased killing of facultative parasites
- Increased superoxide anion production
- Increased plasminogen-activator secretion
- Increased tissue transglutaminase activity
- Increased neopterin secretion
- Increased expression of IgA receptors, class II HLA antigens, FcRI receptors
- Decreased endocytosis of mannose glycoconjugates
- Synthesis of macrophage-inflammatory proteins
- Increased metabolism of vitamin D_3
- Increased TGF-β synthesis
- Increased TNF and IL-1 secretion, PAF-related proteins
- Increased α_1-proteinase–inhibitor secretion
- Increased nitrate and nitrite secretion
- Decreased transferrin receptor expression
- Decreased CD4 expression
- Increased C2 and factor B synthesis
- Increased expression of Mo-3 antigen

Stimulated
- Increased CR1- and CR3-mediated phagocytosis
- Increased acid hydrolase content
- Increased elastase and collagenase secretion
- Decreased icosanoid synthesis
- Decreased PAF accumulation
- Decreased 5' nucleotide activity
- Increased apoprotein E secretion
- Increased synthesis of complement factor proteins
- Increased glutathione release
- Increased expression of heat-shock proteins

Ig, immunoglobulin; IL, interleukin; PAF, platelet-activating factor; TGF, tumor growth factor; TNF, tumor necrosis factor.

of MNPs induced by activation is a biopterin-linked metabolic pathway that catalyzes the oxidation of arginine to citrulline, concomitant with the elaboration of cytotoxic nitrogen dioxide. T cells elaborate other mediators, such as tumor necrosis factor (TNF), macrophage colony-stimulating factor (M-CSF), and interleukin-2 (IL-2), which may contribute to macrophage activation. Because activated MNPs have increased expression of TNF, this may explain, in part, enhanced MNP cytotoxicity against tumor cells. Other alterations in MNPs associated with activation are listed in Table 16-3. Presumably, the activation process is a mechanism for limiting autotoxicity of MNPs and eliciting the numerous cytotoxic products of MNPs only in the face of microbial challenge. The activation of MNPs can be

inhibited by glucocorticosteroids. The cytokines, tumor growth factor-β, and IL-4 also deactivate MNPs.

The number of agonists that affect phagocytes and membrane receptors that these agents bind is large and represents many inflammatory systems (Table 16-2). Receptor-ligand complexes initiate the various responses of phagocytes, which include adhesion, locomotion, phagocytosis, pinocytosis (fluid endocytosis), and the secretion of many substances, either by exocytosis of preformed constituents or by the biosynthesis of molecules in the membrane, such as oxygen reduction products (known as "the respiratory burst") or metabolites of arachidonic acid. In addition, MNPs have a metabolic function in the organism, which is to process important constituents such as heme and iron (5) and to degrade circulating proteins when they have fulfilled their lifespan. The numerous molecules that affect phagocytes appear to work through molecular events in the plasma membrane and subjacent cytoplasm, known collectively as *transmembrane signaling*, and phagocytes are a particularly active area of research in this realm. The diverse agonists affecting phagocytes appear to use common signals in eliciting varied responses.

SPECIFIC FEATURES OF PHAGOCYTE FUNCTIONS

General Features of Receptor-Ligand Interactions on Phagocytes

Consistent with the importance of phagocyte emigration in host defense is the existence of multiple molecules that have the capacity to influence the movement of phagocytes throughout their life cycle, so as to guide them from bone marrow to appropriate tissue sites. Most of the agents listed in Table 16-1 are chemotactic factors, that is, molecules that, when originating from a source in a gradient, focus the direction of phagocytes up the concentration gradient. Most chemotactic factors attract both PMNs and MNPs, although some appear to be specific for MNPs or PMNs. A few other factors are *chemokinetic agents*, molecules that increase the speed at which phagocytes move, and yet others, fragments of C3, are *mobilizing compounds*, substances that cause phagocytes to leave the bone marrow to enter the circulation. There are also inhibitors of phagocyte mobility.

Table 16-4 shows that chemoattractants arise from microorganisms and degraded and denatured tissue components, as well as many sources that are likely to be involved in defense and inflammatory functions of the host. These include products

TABLE 16-4. Molecules That Attract Phagocytes (Chemoattractants)

Source	Molecules
Complement system (plasma and mononuclear phagocyte)	C5a, C5a-des-arg plus vitamin D–binding protein
Membrane phospholipids	Leukotriene B_4, lipoxin A and B, acetylglycerophosphatidylcholine (platelet-activating factor), diacylglycerol, lysophosphatidylcholine
Coagulation system (plasma and platelets)	Thrombin,[a] fibrinopeptides A and Bb1-42, platelet factor 4, platelet-derived growth factor, urokinase, heparin cofactor II–reaction products, interleukin-8–like peptide derived from platelet factor 4 by monocyte proteinases
Mononuclear phagocytes, tumor cells, endothelial cells, lymphocytes, epithelial cells	Interleukin-8 (monocyte-derived chemotactic factor),[b] tumor necrosis factor, oxidized low-density lipoprotein, chemokines
Neutrophils	Defensins[a]
Denatured proteins	Maleyl albumin, casein, collagen fragments, elastase–α_1-proteinase inhibitor complex
Bacteria, mitochondria	N-formyloligopeptides
Metabolites, alkaloids	Adenosine, nicotine

[a]Reportedly chemotactic only for monocytes.
[b]Only for neutrophils.

of the complement system, the coagulation system, and the lipoxygenase pathway of arachidonic acid metabolism. Of special note is the central role of MNPs in generating chemotactic molecules, either by producing them in response to stimulation or by processing plasma protein. This involvement of MNPs is teleologically reasonable in view of the wide distribution of these cells in a sentry network poised for first exposure to pathogens. An important chemotactic product of MNP is a class of small polypeptides known as *chemokines* (6). The signature of this large chemokine family is a pair of cysteines, and depending on the positioning of these residues, the chemokines sort into four classes (7).

The agents described in Table 16-4 bind specific and distinct receptors on phagocytes. The receptors for C5a, FMLP, platelet-activating factor (PAF), leukotriene B_4 (LTB_4), and the chemokines are seven-membrane spanning–proteins (8–12). The dissociation constant for agonist binding of these receptors agrees reasonably with the median effective dose for potency in assays of chemotaxis. The physiology of ligand-receptor interaction, however, is more complex than can be ascertained by equilibrium binding studies, as the on and off rates of the ligands appear to be important and because enzymatic hydrolysis of ligands, as well as internalization of receptor-ligand complexes by receptor-mediated endocytosis and changes in ligand avidity due to phosphorylation, occur under physiologic conditions. Collectively, these effects have been grouped under the term *desensitization* (13).

The concentration of agonist, the affinity of the receptor for the agonist, and the association and dissociation rates between receptor and ligand all influence subsequent events. These factors determine the extent to which the receptor exists in a state that leads to the generation of signals. Agonists, receptors, and signals interact in remarkably complex patterns. In some cases, a single agonist may act through a single receptor to elicit multiple responses, although the number of receptors occupied may determine which response predominates. For example, low concentrations (approximately 10 nmol) of the agonists C5a, FMLP, PAF, and chemokine chemotactic factors have chemotactic activities, whereas higher concentrations (100 to 1000 nmol/L) elicit secretion and the respiratory burst of phagocytes. In other instances, agonists elicit more limited effects (14).

An additional element of complexity is the phenomenon known as priming. Phagocytes may respond to agonists only if some predisposing event has occurred, presumably one that altered the intracellular set of signals or the responsiveness of intracellular signal targets. For example, PMNs carefully prepared using endotoxin-free solutions do not release superoxide in response to chemotactic peptides, but will do so if first allowed to spread on protein-coated glass or if exposed to lipopolysaccharide (LPS) endotoxin. Other agents that prime phagocytes for these responses are tetradecanoyl phorbol myristate acetate (usually abbreviated TPA or PMA), purine and pyrimidine nucleotides, serine proteinases, granulocyte-macrophage CSF (GM-CSF), cytochalasins, and substance P. Spreading of cells on a surface can also have a priming effect. The responses induced by agonists with or without priming usually occur rapidly (within seconds) and are of short duration (minutes) (15).

Phagocyte Adhesion Molecules

The L-selectins are constitutively expressed on all phagocytes and bind fucosyl groups expressed on the surface of the partner cell that the selectin-bearing cell ligates, and these are part of O-linked, mucin-like molecules that represent the blood group sialy-Le^x (16).

The integrins represent a superfamily of heterodimeric molecules that includes the fibronectin receptor, platelet glycoprotein IIb/IIIa, and receptors first identified on activated lymphocytes, called *very late antigens* (VLA) (17). The VLA integrins are expressed on MNP but not PMN. They bind to extracellular matrix components such as collagen, laminin, and vitronectin. Common to the integrin family is an amino acid sequence, arg-gly-asp-ser, in the externally disposed domain of the larger (α) subunit. The predominant phagocyte integrin family is designated β_2-integrin; its members include $\alpha L\beta 2$ (LFA-1), $\alpha M\beta 2$ (Mac-1, Mo-1), $\alpha x\beta 2$ (p150,95), and $\alpha d\beta 2$. The α chain of the two transmembrane polypeptide subunits that characterize β_2-integrins determines the specific identity of these receptors, as they all express an identical β chain. The various members of the β_2-integrin family may interact cooperatively with each other and with other adhesion molecules to mediate adhesion under different circumstances (18).

The β_2-integrins are synthesized by PMNs and MNPs during maturation in the bone marrow. Circulating phagocytes express β_2-integrins on their surfaces but also have a pool of these receptors within the cell. Exposure of phagocytes to a variety of agents, including chemotactic peptides, TPA, LPS-binding protein complexes, and fibronectin, increases not only the number of β_2-integrin molecules on the cell surface, but also their functional avidity for ligands (19). This up-regulation of phagocyte adhesion receptors on circulating phagocytes is demonstrable in humans after exposure of their circulation to foreign surfaces such as hemodialysis coils or extracorporeal cardiopulmonary assist devices. There is evidence that these maneuvers activate the alternative pathway of complement, which generates the chemotactic polypeptide C5a, which in turn up-regulates the β_2-integrins.

The events leading to integrin activation are complex and involve signaling traffic that moves both directions across the plasma membrane. The integrins require extracellular divalent cations for stability and function. Ligation of integrins perturbs the orientation of the two subunits such that the cytoplasmic domains, too, change configuration and can engage complexes of intracellular signaling molecules described later, mostly via the β subunit ("outside-in signaling"). Conversely, engagement of intracellular cascades can change the extracellular structure of the integrins such that their avidity for ligands increases ("inside-out signaling"). The molecules associating with the cytoplasmic domains of integrins include phospholipases, phosphoinositide kinases, tyrosine kinases of the *Src* oncogene family, enzymes participating in serine-threonine kinase phosphorylating cascades, such as focal adhesion kinase, protein kinase C, the MAP/ERK system, and so-called adaptor proteins, including integrin-associated protein and others, some of which harbor src-homology domains (Grb, Crk, IRS-1, and SHC). Many of these same players are involved in signaling via immunoglobulin (Fc) receptors on phagocytic cells. Part of the effect of outside-in signaling is to cause reorganization of the submembrane actin cytoskeleton; in reverse, inside-out signaling is, to some degree, a result of cytoskeletal rearrangements brought about by other receptor-mediated pathways that then impact on the integrins. The activation processes can either release integrins from the cytoskeleton to change their avidity for ligands or promote their attachment to the cytoskeleton to create transmembrane adhesive complexes (20).

Phagocytes express receptors for the Fc domain of immunoglobulins (FcRs). PMNs have polymorphic low-affinity FcRs, FcRII and FcRIII, that bind Fc domains expressed in immune complexes. The FcRIII exist as transmembrane or as peptidoglycan-linked proteins. The PMN FcRIIA and FcRIIB isoforms are targets of iso- and autoantibodies in immune neutropenia syndromes. Macrophages have isoforms of these receptors and, in addition, express a high-affinity receptor for monomeric IgG (FcRI) after stimulation by IFN-γ. Signaling after FcR ligation involves recruitment of transmembrane proteins originally identified in T-cell receptor complexes (21). These cofactors either activate (ITAMs) or desensitize (ITIMs) FcR-mediated responses. ITAM activation is required for signaling from monomeric IgG ligation of FcRI and results from phosphorylation reactions mediated by *Syk*, a tyrosine kinase of the *Src* family that causes dimerization of ITAM subunits. The activation of ITAM and subsequent events resemble the signaling reactions induced by integrins. The downstream consequences of this activation include increases in cytosolic calcium, induction of phosphorylation cascades, synthesis of phosphoinositides, and activation of Rho guanosine triphosphatases (GTPases). ITIM activation occurs when membrane protein phosphatases, such as SHC, dephosphorylate the ITIM subunit, and the ITIM inactivates ITAM by dimerizing with it, thereby removing the activating ITAM homodimer from play.

A receptor for mannose oligosaccharides mediates the binding of phagocytes to numerous microorganisms and, in some cases, the phagocytosis of these targets (22). A nonintegrin complement receptor binds C3b and catalyzes the proteolysis of the ligand.

Transmembrane Signaling in Phagocytes

GUANOSINE TRIPHOSPHATASES

GTPases, G proteins named because of their GTP-binding properties, provide an amplification step between receptor occupancy and signal transduction. G proteins amplify signal production because they cycle on and off activated receptors (Fig. 16-2).

The amplifying role of G proteins helps to explain why chemotactic oligopeptides can cause structural changes in PMNs when as few as 1% of the receptors for that peptide are ligated. One major class of G proteins consists of three polypeptide subunits of approximately 40 kd, designated α, β, and γ. The α subunit is generally the module that interacts with targets such as the signal-transducing enzyme adenylate cyclase or phospholipases A_2 (PLA$_2$) or C, although the other subunits can sometimes serve that purpose. The way in which G proteins amplify signaling is that the trimeric complex binds to the cytoplasmic domain of transmembrane receptors activated by bound ligands. This binding causes the exchange of guanosine diphosphate (GDP) bound to the α subunit for GTP, and the α subunit complex dissociates from the β and γ subunits. The free α subunit activates or inhibits its target, dependent on the particular

G protein; stimulatory G proteins are designated G_s, inhibitory G_i. Hydrolysis of the bound GTP to GDP and Pi restores the α subunit to a conformation in which it binds β and γ partners (23). The reformation of the trimeric complex terminates signal transduction and restores the G protein to a form ready for further messages from receptors. Thus, a single ligated receptor can excite multiple cycles of G-protein activation of target enzymes. Nonhydrolyzable GTP analogs lock G-α subunits in a conformation that prohibits reassociation, and signal generation is inhibited. The active form of the receptor associates with G protein and may be bound to the submembrane cytoskeleton (24). Studies with mutant C5a receptors suggest that ligand binding by the receptor alters the orientation of two of the seven helical membrane-spanning domains to accommodate triggering of G proteins (25).

A second major class of G proteins known as *Rho family proteins* are approximately 20 kd in mass and are homologous to the oncogene product H$_{ras}$. Of the Rho proteins, specific family members named *Rac* (especially Rac2 in myeloid cells), *Rho, Arf*, and *Cdc42* have well-defined roles in signaling by phagocytes, leading to motility and to the synthesis of microbicidal and inflammatory reactive oxygen metabolites. Rho GTPases work as single subunits together with several types of regulatory proteins. When ligated to GTP, these Rho GTPases interact with effector targets. One of the Rho regulators, GTPase activating protein, catalyzes the hydrolysis of GTP to GDP, thereby inactivating the effector-stimulating function of the GTPase. Another factor, the guanine-nucleotide exchange factor, promotes the exchange of bound GDP for ambient GTP, recycling an inactive Rho to its active state. A third control factor, guanine nucleotide dissociation inhibitor, inhibits guanine nucleotide exchange, thereby locking the GTPase in an inactive form. This constellation of control factors permits small GTPases to serve a wide variety of signaling functions (26). Rac2 in PMN is important for signaling to actin rearrangements required for locomotion and for activation of antimicrobial oxidase activity. The importance of Rac2 for these functions is manifest in knock-out mice that fail to express Rac2. These mice have impaired PMN migration, actin assembly, and oxidase activity to some, but not all, stimuli (27).

One experimentally useful property of some G proteins is that they are targets of an adenosine diphosphate (ADP) ribosylation reaction catalyzed by bacterial toxins. Depending on the toxin and the G protein, the consequence of ADP ribosylation varies. *Vibrio cholera* toxin, for example, causes the permanent activation of the G-α protein, which stimulates adenylate cyclase, causing the accumulation of large quantities of intracellular cyclic adenosine monophosphate in the poisoned target cell. Conversely, *Bordetella pertussis* toxin inactivates G-α proteins that transduce activation signals for several phagocyte functions mediated by calcium transients and phosphoinositide turnover (discussed later). *Clostridium botulinum* exoenzyme 3 and *Clostridium difficile* toxin, respectively, ADP ribosylate and glycosylate Rho proteins and inactivate them.

CALCIUM TRANSIENTS AND PHOSPHOINOSITIDE METABOLISM

One of the responses of phagocytes to binding of an agonist is a transient rise in cytosolic calcium (Fig. 16-3) (28). Mammalian phagocytes live in an environment that contains millimolar ionized calcium concentrations. This calcium can slowly leak down a concentration gradient across lipid bilayers from the outside of the cell or from internalized membrane vesicles within. The resting cell, however, keeps its cytosolic calcium in the nanomolar range. The cell actively extrudes calcium against a 1000-fold concentration gradient with an adenosine triphosphate (ATP)–

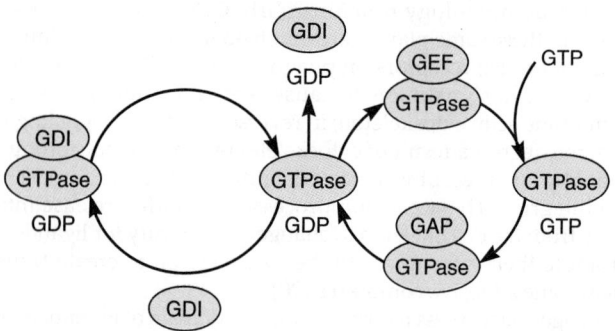

Figure 16-2. Role of heterotrimeric guanosine triphosphate (GTP)–binding proteins in phagocyte signal–response coupling. Regulation of small monomeric GTP-binding proteins is similar. Not shown is that additional cofactors, GTPase activating proteins (GAPs), stimulate GTP hydrolysis; others, GTP-dissociation inhibitors (GDIs), inhibit GTP/GDP exchange.

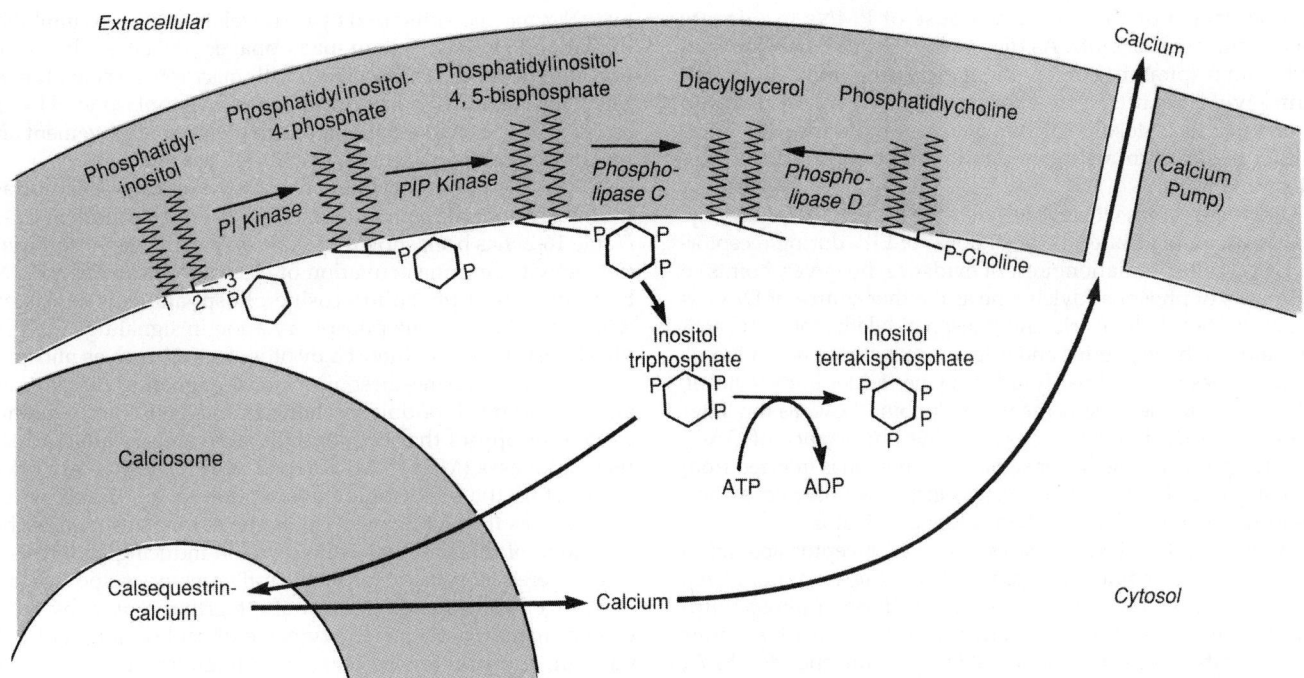

Figure 16-3. Signal transduction pathways in phagocytes showing the interrelation between membrane phospholipid metabolism and the regulation of cytosolic calcium concentrations. ADP, adenosine diphosphate; ATP, adenosine triphosphate; PI, phosphatidylinositol; PIP, phosphatidylinositol-4-phosphate.

driven plasma membrane pump. Should the calcium concentration rise into the micromolar range, calcium can bind to a number of calcium-binding proteins that, in turn, activate signaling reactions. One well-known, high-affinity, calcium-binding protein is calmodulin. The calcium-calmodulin complex is involved in triggering some responses, but it also promotes the removal of calcium by activating the membrane extrusion pump. The cell also sequesters calcium in internal compartments. Mitochondria represent a low-affinity reservoir for calcium, but other vesicular structures analogous to the sarcoplasmic reticulum or striated muscle cells take up calcium with high avidity. In phagocytes, such vesicles have been shown to contain a protein immunoreactive with calsequestrin, the low-affinity, high-capacity, calcium-binding protein of striated muscle, and these vesicles have been named calciosomes (29).

Stimulation of many cell receptors, including chemoattractant receptors of phagocytes, leads to activation of G proteins that increase the activity of cytoplasmic phospholipase C enzymes, which eventually leads to rises in cytosolic calcium. These enzymes catalyze the hydrolysis of the phosphodiester bond between the glycerol backbone and the head group of membrane phospholipids, generating water-soluble base phosphates and diacylglycerols (DAG), the latter of which remain in the membrane bilayer (30). Phospholipase C appears to be specific for particular phospholipids, but the most important for signal transduction hydrolyze the phosphoinositide phosphatidylinositol-4,5-bisphosphate (PIP$_2$) and phosphatidylcholine. The number and position of phosphates on the inositol ring of phosphoinositides influences the expression, metabolism, and signaling activities of these lipids. D3 phosphoinositides have a phosphate atom in the 3-position of the inositol ring, and D4 phophoinositides have phosphate in the 4-position. D3 phosphoinositide levels increase in chemoattractant-stimulated PMN, and forced elevation of PMN phosphatidylinositol-3,4,5-triphosphate stimulates migration of the cells (31). Mouse PMN lacking an enzyme that synthesizes D3 phosphoinosi-

tides, phosphoinositide 3-kinase γ, have impaired chemotactic responsiveness (32,33).

The breakdown of the D4 phosphoinositides and their subsequent resynthesis by different kinases are important in signaling (34). PIP$_2$ breakdown, for example, leads to the accumulation of inositol-4,5-triphosphate, which has the important property of releasing calcium from the high-affinity intracellular vesicles. This mechanism is the basis for rises in cytosolic calcium accompanying cell stimulation, even when calcium is removed from the extracellular medium. When extracellular calcium is present, however, receptor perturbation also opens a channel in the membrane that permits calcium to pour down its concentration gradient. One effect of cytoplasmic calcium is that it increases the patency of this calcium leak (35). The efficiency, therefore, of this pathway in increasing cytosolic calcium allows much lower agonist concentrations to elicit responses in the presence than in the absence of extracellular calcium.

Just as the cell performs ATP-consuming work to keep cytosolic calcium at low levels, so does it dispose of DAG and regenerate the phospholipids hydrolyzed during the first phase of the cellular response to agonist. Separate ATP-dependent kinases phosphorylate phosphatidylinositol to phosphatidylinositol-4-phosphate (PIP), PIP$_2$, and PIP$_3$, respectively, and some of the phosphatidylinositol and PIP kinases respond to unique receptor-activated G proteins (36).

Calcium is a pleiotropic signal that can theoretically influence metabolic, motile, and membrane reactions. It activates enzymes of phospholipid metabolism and of glycogenolysis, and it regulates some proteins important for cell motility, as described later. Certain phagocyte functions, however, do not absolutely require a sustained or possibly even an acute rise in cytosolic calcium (37). Exposure of PMNs to chemotactic peptides induces an abrupt increase in cytosolic calcium, after which the calcium level falls to baseline, yet PMN locomotion continues. Lowering of the cytosolic calcium of PMNs and macrophages to nanomolar levels does not impair the extent of phagocytosis nor the initial response of PMNs to migrate toward chemoattractants. As discussed later, PMNs express an exuberant respiratory burst without increasing intracellular calcium levels. Secretion by exocytosis, however, appears to require that the cytosolic calcium increase, and raising the intracellular free calcium with ionophoric compounds induces exocytosis in PMNs.

Diradylglycerols, where *radyl* refers to acyl, alkyl, or alk-1'-enyl groups, accumulate after the breakdown of PIP_2 during receptor-mediated cell stimulation. Recent evidence, however, points to hydrolysis of phosphatidylcholine as another source of DAG as well as of phosphatidic acid and phosphatidylethanol. DAG activates a phosphatidylserine and calcium-activating protein kinase (protein kinase C). Ordinarily, this enzyme resides in the cytosol, but it moves to the plasma membrane to bind DAG as the latter accumulates during cell excitation. The importance of DAG-activated protein kinase C for signal transduction is inferred from the ability of PMA to stimulate many functions of phagocytes and to substitute for DAG as a protein kinase C activator.

In addition to phospholipases C and D, receptor activation activates another phospholipid hydrolyzing enzyme, PLA_2. PLA_2 cleaves the fatty acid in the sn-2 position of phospholipids, yielding free fatty acids and lysophosphatides; other enzymes catalyze the reacylation of the lysophosphatides. PLA_2 is activated by receptor-mediated perturbation of phagocytes and by increasing the cytosolic calcium of the cell with appropriate ionophores.

Lysophosphatidic acid and a related compound, sphingosine 1-phosphate, bind to specific receptors on target cells related to inflammatory responses (38,39). Also of great importance is the free fatty acid product of the PLA_2 reaction. Polyphosphoinositides are preferred substrates for PLA_2, and the sn-2 fatty acid of these phospholipids is arachidonate. Arachidonic acid can have two messenger functions. In one function, the fatty acid is the substrate of the enzyme 5' lipoxygenase, which catalyzes the first of a series of reactions in phagocytes, leading to the biosynthesis of the bioactive metabolites, the leukotrienes. Leukotrienes, the synthetic pathways for which are described later, either directly or after subsequent metabolism by neighboring cells act as potent mediators of inflammation. Because phagocytes have leukotriene receptors, this pathway can be seen as autostimulatory (40). In another function, arachidonic acid has been shown to participate as one cofactor in activation of the respiratory burst oxidase of phagocytes.

Stimulated phagocytes also release free arachidonic acid, which can activate cellular responses, but lipid-binding proteins such as albumin can modulate this activity, and its physiologic importance is unclear. When PLA_2 attacks the membrane phospholipid alkylacylphosphatidylcholine, the resulting reactions (described later) lead to the synthesis of acetyl glyceryl phosphatidylcholine, also known as PAF or PAF acether. PAF is a potent bioactive compound that, like the leukotrienes, can act on phagocyte receptors (Table 16-2). Other bioactive products of arachidonate metabolism are leukotriene-related molecules, the lipoxins (41).

OTHER SIGNALS

As is seen with mitogen-stimulated cultured cells, phagocytes respond to some agonists with proton extrusion, resulting in a temporary rise in intracellular pH, presumably mediated by an Na^+-H^+ antiporter (42). In contrast to excitable cells such as nerve and muscle, phagocytes appear functionally impervious to broad variations in their intracellular monovalent ion composition and engage in acute responses to agonists, with either Na^+ or K^+ as the dominant extracellular cation. On the other hand, more delayed effects of stimuli, such as the activation of MNPs

by IFN-γ, may be influenced by monovalent cations, as inhibition of Na^+ and H^+ exchange in macrophages prevented the induction of gene products associated with macrophage activation by this lymphokine. In addition, changes in cytoplasmic pH were associated with marked alterations in membrane movement and the distribution of lysosomes in cultured macrophages.

Reversible phosphorylation of tyrosine residues is important for transmembrane signaling. The leukocyte glycoprotein CD45 (Table 16-2) has been shown to express tyrosine dephosphorylation activity, and the activation of electropermeabilized PMNs by inhibitors of phosphotyrosine phosphatases is consistent with a role for tyrosine phosphorylation in signaling (43). This phosphorylation is influenced by other factors, such as phosphatidic acid (44). Serine-threonine kinase–signaling cascades are also important. Lipopolysaccharides and TNF family ligands engage receptors that sequentially activate so-called stress-related kinases (MEKK, MKK3, p38 MAPK), ultimately phosphorylating the pleiotropic transcription factor NF-κB, which translocates to the nucleus (15). Some evidence suggests that activation of this pathway is involved in inducing apoptosis in PMN, thereby serving to terminate inflammatory responses (45). TNF, together with engagement of integrin receptors by extracellular matrix, activates the tyrosine phosphorylation of Pyk, paxillin, and PI-3 kinase (46). Immunoglobulin receptor and formyl peptide receptor engagement also activate serine-threonine and tyrosine kinase phosphorylation (47,48).

Another interesting cell modification associated with phagocyte excitation is the acylation of certain intracellular polypeptides, which causes a fatty acid to be added covalently to proteins, possibly enhancing their association with hydrophobic lipid membranes. In fact, one protein that becomes acylated in stimulated phagocytes acquires a membrane localization in association with myristoylation and is also a target for phosphorylation by protein kinase C (49).

Irreversible proteolysis of intracellular proteins has also been proposed as a mechanism for cellular excitation. Cell excitation activates a calcium-dependent proteinase (calpain) that degrades a number of proteins, including protein kinase C, rendering it constitutively active rather than capable of being regulated by its usual cofactors.

CYTOSKELETON

Cytoskeletal polymers determine shape and movement of nonmuscle cells, and because of their active motility, the cytoskeletal structure and function of phagocytes have been actively studied. The shape of phagocytes is determined by a cortical layer of cytoplasm that contains predominantly the nonmuscle-cell isoform of the protein actin (designated β-actin) in nearly millimolar concentrations. Actin subunits polymerize reversibly into linear and three-dimensional polymers, and the balance between these states accounts for changes in cell-surface configuration associated with phagocyte movements. A number of actin-binding proteins control the interconversion between the states of actin, and these proteins are in turn regulated by the signal molecules, calcium, polyphosphoinositides, Rho GTPases, and phosphorylation reactions discussed previously (Table 16-5). Actin-binding toxins directly inhibit actin assembly and agonist-elicited phagocyte movements. Other toxins operate indirectly by inactivating Rho GTPases. Actin assembles by a nucleation condensation mechanism in which spontaneous nucleation *in vitro* is highly unfavorable. Elongation is more efficient than nucleation and is proportional to the monomer concentration, although the rate of growth is asymmetric on an actin polymer. Actin filaments to which myosin head fragments are bound look like strings adorned with arrowheads, and such decoration of actin filaments defines a

TABLE 16-5. Actin-Binding Proteins Involved in Phagocyte Responses

Protein	Function	Regulators
Profilin, thymosin	Sequester monomeric actin	—
Actin-related protein 2/3	Branching nucleation	WASP, Cdc42, PIP_2
Gelsolin, CapG	Sever and cap actin filaments	Calcium, PIP_2
CapZ, adducin	Cap actin filament barbed ends	PIP_2
Tropomyosin	Stabilize actin filaments	—
Filamin A	Stabilize actin filaments in orthogonal arrays; link actin filaments to membranes	—
Alpha actinin, fimbrin	Stabilize actin filament bundles	Calcium, phosphorylation
Ezrin-radixin-moesin proteins	Link actin filaments to membranes	PIP_2, phosphorylation

PIP_2, phosphoinositide phosphatidylinositol-4,5-bisphosphate; WASP, Wiskott-Aldrich syndrome protein.

"barbed" and "pointed" polarity. The growth of actin is 15 to 20 times faster at the barbed ends than at the pointed ends of actin filaments. Each actin monomer contains an ATP prosthetic group, which hydrolyzes to ADP and Pi during assembly. When ADP monomers dissociate from filaments, ambient ATP rapidly exchanges with the ADP to yield ATP monomers. At steady state, therefore, actin exists in an ATP-consuming dynamic equilibrium, and a lower-than-micromolar concentration of monomeric actin coexists with actin filaments *in vitro*. By contrast, nearly half the millimolar actin in resting phagocytes is unpolymerized, indicating that control of the competence of actin monomers to assemble in filaments is fundamental to the control of actin assembly in phagocytic cells.

An abundant actin subunit–binding protein, β-thymosin, helps to keep much cellular actin unpolymerized by stoichiometric formation of an equimolar complex in which the actin is sequestered, unable to nucleate (50). Free barbed ends of actin filaments can compete with thymosin for actin monomers, and so it is a combination of thymosin and proteins that "cap" the barbed ends of actin filaments that can maintain a large pool of monomeric actin. Uncapping of these filaments provides a place and time for actin filament elongation. The assembly of actin in the cell takes place when and where polyphosphoinositides accumulate in the membrane and interact with barbed-end capping proteins, releasing them from filaments (Fig. 16-4) (51). Nucleation at the barbed ends of actin filaments can be amplified by a group of seven proteins, the actin-related protein 2/3 (Arp2/3) complex (52). Arp2/3 is proposed to simulate the pointed end of an actin filament offset from the barbed end of a filament so that elongation can occur in two directions separated by precisely 70° (53). Although phosphoinositides can release capping proteins directly, they also participate in the activation of Arp2/3 by stimulating the Wiskott-Aldrich syndrome protein (WASP) to increase the ability of Arp2/3 to accelerate branched actin nucleation. This action of WASP also follows its binding to the Rho GTPase Cdc42 (54), and all of these maneuvers work by unfolding WASP from an autoinhibited conformation (55). Engagement of FMLP receptors activates Cdc42, and activated Cdc42 in turn activates WASP as well as Rac. Because Rac stimulates phosphoinositide 4 phosphate-5 kinase, this pathway powerfully leads to actin polymerization by barbed-end uncapping and by branching amplification (56).

Additional proteins serve to stabilize the elongating actin filaments by organizing them into three-dimensional architectures, such as bundles and gels, and by linking the filaments to plasma membrane receptors. Some actin filament cross-linking proteins promote the formation of actin bundles (α-actinin, L-plastin), and others stabilize three-dimensional orthogonal gels (filamins). Filamins are also implicated, along with talin, fimbrin, and vinculin, in the linkage of actin filaments to leukocyte integrins (57,58). Proteins of the ezrin-radixin-moesin family

bind actin filaments to nonintegrin membrane structures, such as hyaluronate receptors (CD44) or integrin counter receptors (59). Contraction of actin filaments by myosin filaments can occur when the regulatory subunits of the myosin molecules are in a phosphorylated state. Calcium and MAP kinase (60) promote such phosphorylation by activating a specific myosin light chain kinase (61). Phosphorylation also occurs when Rho in the GTP-bound state activates Rho kinase, which inactivates a myosin light chain phosphatase by phosphorylating it (62).

Remodeling of actin networks occurs by forced depolymerization of actin filaments. This process occurs constitutively due to the action of actin-depolymerizing factor, also called *cofilin*, which weakly severs actin filaments by preferentially attacking subunits containing ADP and also by accelerating the rate of monomer loss from pointed filament ends. A serine phosphorylation reaction catalyzed by LIM kinase inactivates actin-depolymerizing factor/cofilin (63,64), and the protein phosphatases PP1 and PP2 are involved in activating it (65). Rapid breakdown of actin networks is the purview of proteins of the gelsolin family. In the presence of micromolar calcium ions, gelsolin severs the noncovalent bonds holding actin filaments together at random locations and then caps the barbed ends of the severed filaments (66). Actin subunits released by depolymerization are in the ADP form and are bound by thymosin. When circumstances promote elongation of filaments, a protein called *profilin* catalyzes exchange of ATP for ADP on the actin monomers, and this reaction accelerates elongation (67).

Microtubules are hollow fibers composed of helical assemblies of tubulin heterodimers, and their outer surfaces are coated with a large number of proteins known as *microtubule-associated proteins*. In interphase cells, as in phagocytes, microtubules originate in a perinuclear structure, the centriole, and radiate outward to enter the actin-rich cell periphery (68). Intermediate filaments, polymers of the protein vimentin, maintain a perinuclear distribution in phagocytic cells. Phosphorylation reactions regulate the reversible assembly of vimentin, but relatively little is known about this regulation in phagocytes. Alterations in intermediate filament structure accompany induced secretion in PMN (69).

SPECIFIC PHAGOCYTE ACTIVITIES

Circulation of Phagocytes

Translational movement becomes manifest at the band state of PMN development. Some fraction of PMNs and monocytes move out of the bone marrow. This form of motility involves active crawling. The cell extends one or more organelle-excluding pseudopodia in the direction of locomotion, and these attach to the surface (Fig. 16-5A). The cell body is drawn forward toward the pseudopodia, which extend outward again. In addition to actual

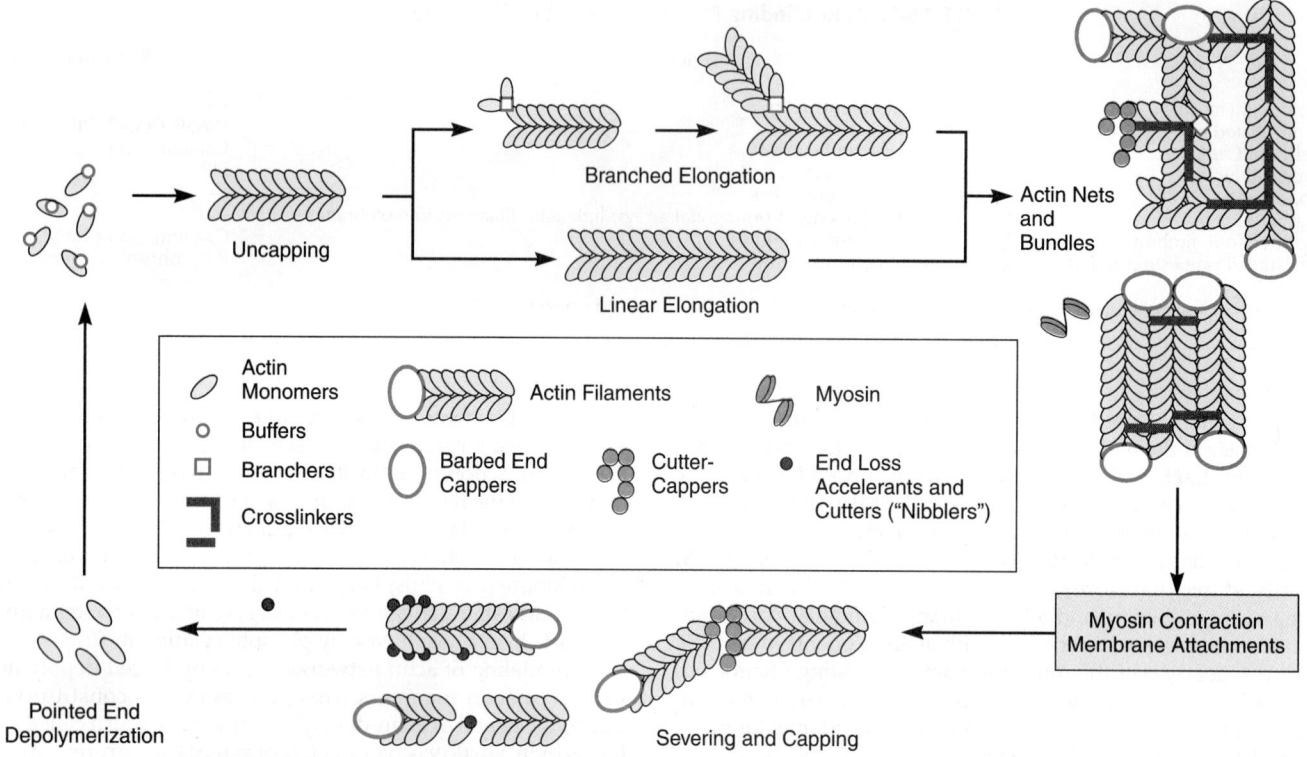

Figure 16-4. Postulated mechanism for regulation of actin assembly coordinated with signal–response coupling in phagocytes. The major actin subunit buffering protein is β-thymosin (not shown). IP$_3$, inositol triphosphate; ABP, actin-binding protein.

movement, the phagocytes cause the lining cells of the bone marrow to separate and to be sufficiently pliable so they can negotiate the marrow–blood barrier and enter the peripheral circulation.

Once in the peripheral blood, the asymmetry of the extruded phagocytes dissipates, and the cells appear round as they roll along the walls of blood vessels in the so-called marginal blood pool. An undetermined number of PMNs become senescent and undergo the sequence of events known as *programmed cell death* or *apoptosis*. In experimental conditions, PMN apoptosis includes degradation of nuclear DNA, membrane blebbing, and loss of the asymmetric distribution of membrane phospholipids characteristic of living cells (70). In particular, phosphatidylserine, normally located on the inner leaflet of the plasma membrane, becomes externally disposed and recognizable by scavenger receptors on fixed MNPs. Presumably, many circulating PMNs are cleared by this mechanism (71).

However, under normal circumstances, some PMNs attach to the endothelium with sufficient avidity to resist being moved by the flow of blood, and they leave the circulation by the process known as *diapedesis*. Diapedesis ordinarily takes place in capillary beds exposed to microbes, such as the skin, the oral cavity and the large intestine, and it occurs in a markedly augmented manner when infection or inflammation becomes established. At this point, the cells again acquire the elongated configuration of motility and extend pseudopodia in the direction of movement. Insofar as phagocytes move several millimeters into the tissues, the daily net movement of billions of these cells in an adult amounts to a distance greater than the circumference of the earth.

Phagocyte-Initial Vessel Wall Interactions

The interaction between circulating PMNs and the endothelium is a tightly orchestrated process. Most of these interactions occur in postcapillary venules, and a few generalities are invokable, although the specific details vary depending on the vascular bed. When inflammatory mediators, including cytokines, chemokines, and mechanical disruption, cause up-regulation of E- and P-selectin, these receptors bind to L-selectin molecules, which cluster constitutively on microvilli extended by the circulating PMNs. Pushed along by the circulatory flow, the PMNs roll like gears on a ratchet of microvilli. The relative slowing of movement along the vessel incurred by the rolling increases the exposure of the PMNs to secreted and membrane-bound molecules expressed by the inflamed endothelium. This process eventuates in the up-regulation and increased avidity of PMN integrins, and the interaction between PMNs and endothelial selectins positions the PMNs near the borders of endothelial cells (72). An additional factor involved in phagocyte-vessel interaction is the ability of agonists to distort phagocyte shape and stiffen them (responses related to intracellular actin assembly), and there is evidence that these mechanical changes in phagocytes can cause their retention in pulmonary capillaries, independent of changes in cell-surface adhesiveness related to β$_2$-integrins (73). A cooperative interaction facilitates the interaction between PMNs, monocytes, and endothelial cells as the phagocytes emigrate into the tissues (74). Part of this process involves secretion of chemokines by the phagocytes, leading to induction of increased free calcium levels in the endothelial cells, which promotes contractility. It also inactivates adhesion molecules, the platelet-endothelial cell adhesion molecule-1 and junctional adhesion molecule, that maintain intercellular endothelial junctions. The net effect is to open conduits that the phagocytes navigate (75,76). Once in the extravascular space, complex interactions of extracellular matrix, chemoattractants, and other factors program the retention of specific phagocytes in particular types of inflammatory lesions (77).

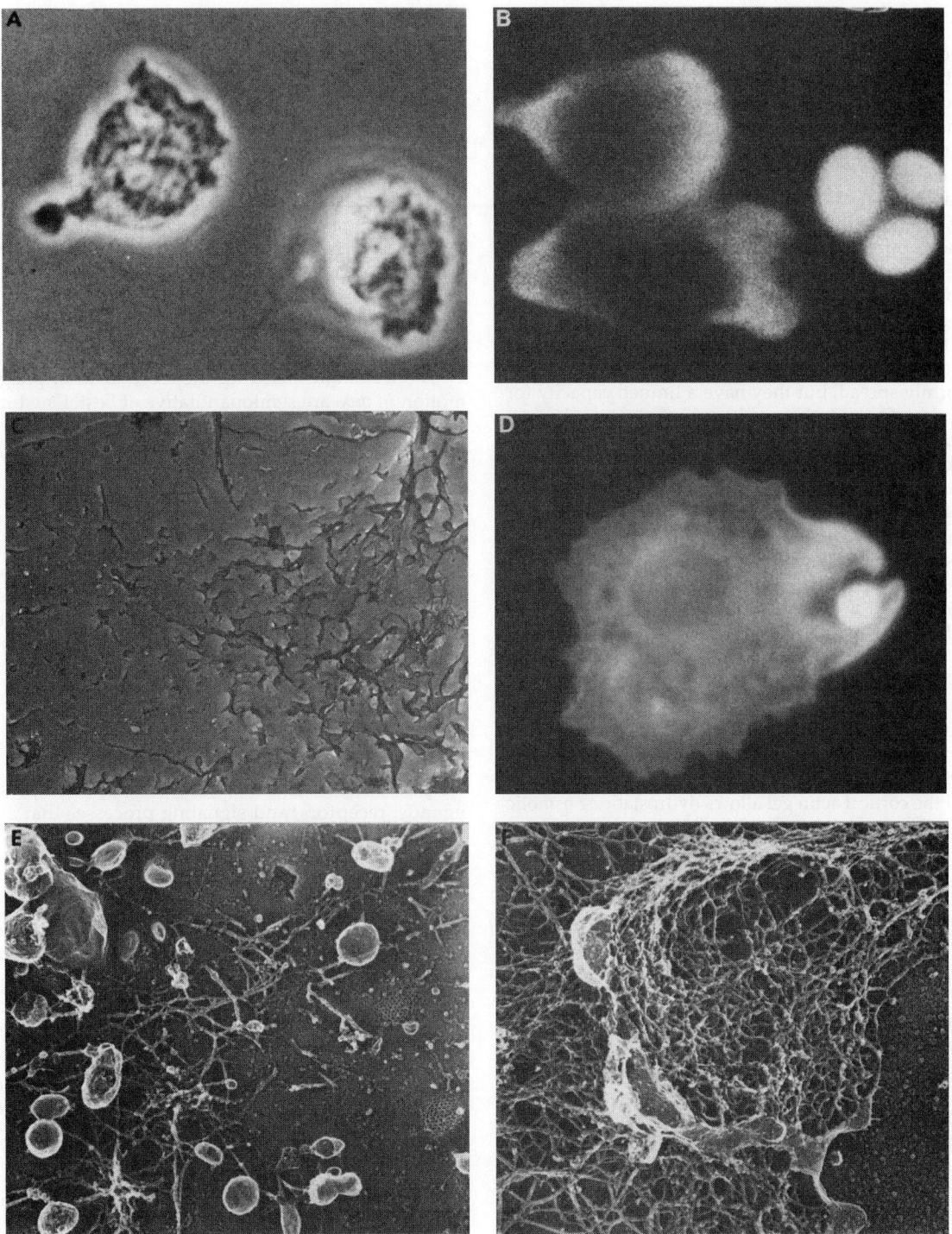

Figure 16-5. Morphology of neutrophils and mononuclear phagocytes. **A:** Phase contrast photomicrograph of a neutrophil in the characteristic pose of locomotion. Note the asymmetric shape, anterior pseudopod, and posterior knoblike tail. **B:** Immunofluorescence photomicrograph showing rhodamine staining of myosin in the pseudopodia of a neutrophil undergoing chemotaxis toward a fluorescein-stained yeast particle. **C:** Scanning electron photomicrograph of the surface of a monocyte or macrophage revealing pleats and ruffles extended from the surface. **D:** Immunofluorescence photomicrograph of a macrophage stained with rhodamine for actin-binding protein showing pseudopodia engulfing a fluorescein-stained yeast particle. **E:** Cytoplasmic membrane surface of an adherent macrophage revealed by tearing of part of the membrane, rapid freezing, and metal casting. Actin filaments and basketlike clathrin-coating of endocytic vesicles are visible. **F:** The cortical orthogonal actin network of a macrophage shown in a detergent-permeabilized cell that was then rapidly frozen and metal-shadowed. (Courtesy of John Hartwig, PhD, Division of Experimental Medicine, Brigham and Women's Hospital, Boston.)

Cellular Responses to Chemotactic Factors

When chemotactic factors engage phagocytes that are in a rounded state, they first "cringe" by wrinkling their surface, and then they begin to spread uniformly on the substrate. PMNs and monocytes soon acquire the characteristic polarity of locomotion in which pseudopodia extend in a preferred direction, even when the chemotactic factor is not present in a gradient. If such a gradient exists, PMNs move toward it, not in a straight line, but with frequent deviations from the gradient source; as they approach higher concentrations of the factor, however, their turn angles decrease. If the chemoattractant is removed and replaced by a new supply, but from the opposite side, PMNs may round up and extend a pseudopod in the direction of the new gradient, but they prefer to retain their original polarity and make a U-turn. Macrophages tend to remain uniformly spread, but they have a limited capacity for slow locomotion. Despite the wealth of information known about the reception of chemotactic molecules, the signaling cascades this reception generates, and the cellular responsiveness to those cascades (78), a detailed explanation of the way in which phagocytes orient and move directionally is still a subject requiring wholesale speculation (79,80).

Organelle-excluding pseudopodia can be dissociated from the cell by heat treatment, and these structures exhibit rudimentary locomotion, suggesting that all the sensory and motor components reside in the cortical regions of the cell. The mechanisms underlying the cell-surface shape changes involve focal increases in the turgor of the peripheral cytoplasm, and evidence indicates that the assembly of actin, by mechanisms discussed previously, is responsible for these increases. It is unclear whether actin assembly mechanically pushes against the membrane to effect propulsion of pseudopodia (81) or whether a weakening of the cortical actin gel allows hydrostatic or osmotic forces to push the membrane outwards (82). Both mechanisms may occur at times.

The sequence of events in translational locomotion appears to be that pseudopodia extend in the direction of movement, they attach to the substrate, and then the cell body is pulled forward. If attachment fails, then the pseudopod may be retracted. These findings suggest that a contractile mechanism based on myosins within the cytoplasm is operative.

The translational movement of PMNs requires that they adhere to the substrate in vitro or to the fibers of connective tissue in vivo. The advancing pseudopod attaches to surfaces, and the cell body drags along behind. The adherent regions must then become unattached for the cell to move, and the mechanism of letting go is unknown. Proteases may digest adhesion proteins, or else some more complex process may cause them to lose their avidity for their ligands. In some instances, parts of the cell fail to disengage, and long processes are drawn out; these may either break off or tether the cell, preventing its forward progress. Although β_2-integrin–dependent adhesion is extremely important for normal locomotion in vitro and in vivo, PMNs can undergo rudimentary locomotion in the absence of integrin-based adhesion by using a set of writhing movements (83) that have been called "chimneying."

Measurement of Phagocyte Locomotion

Of many methods applicable to the study of leukocyte movement in vitro, the simplest is to observe cells directly under the phase-contrast microscope. One way to do this is to allow blood taken by finger prick to clot on a slide in a humidified Petri dish, wash off the clot with 10% autologous plasma in buffered salt solution, place a coverslip over it, and then look for characteristic polarized shapes and movements of the PMNs and monocytes, preferably at 37°C. This method detects gross defects in leukocyte adhesion and motility in that cells appear rounded, fail to attach to the surface, and do not move translationally. For more sophisticated laboratory assessment of leukocyte locomotion, a system in which a cell monolayer is separated by a slit from the source of a chemotactic factor allows quantitation of the fraction of cells that polarize in the direction of the gradient. A two-compartment chamber in which cells crawl through porous filters toward the source of a chemotactic gradient has been used extensively in chemotaxis studies. Another technique is to inject leukocytes under one part of an agarose sheet and a chemotactic factor under another part and to stain the sheet after a suitable time and observe the extent to which the front of leukocytes has moved away from the site of injection.

The techniques used for the assessment of phagocyte locomotion in vivo are semiquantitative at best. One time-honored method is to abrade the skin of a subject and apply a coverslip or sponge, sometimes impregnated with a chemotactic agent, and to assess by microscopy the number of cells in the inflammatory exudate. A more complex variation is to use a subcutaneous chamber and count the cells in the accumulated fluid. Some advocate the counting of leukocytes in isotonic salt solution mouthwashes as an index of phagocyte exudation. With all these approaches, it must be remembered that the supply of phagocytes in the circulation ultimately determines the number of cells available to the tissues, so that the measurement of locomotion in vivo in leukopenic patients yields abnormal results.

PHAGOCYTOSIS

Despite many mechanistic similarities, phagocytosis involves ligands, receptors, and signaling processes that are different from chemotaxis.

Opsonins and Opsonin Receptors

Opsonins are molecules that coat particulate objects and promote their phagocytosis. Particle-bound opsonins interact with specific cell-surface receptors. When this interaction only promotes strong attachment of the particle to the phagocyte, requiring additional interactions for engulfment, the opsonin is "incomplete." If the encounter leads directly to internalization, the opsonin is "complete." The Fcγ receptors of phagocytes are complete. They induce phagocytosis when they ligate the Fc domains of immunoglobulins bound to particles. The mannose receptor that binds to mannose residues on the surface of microorganisms such as yeasts is also a complete opsonin.

The CR3 receptor has broad specificity, including, in addition to the iC3b fragment of C3, fibrinogen, certain microbial coat components, and intercellular adhesion molecule-1 (ICAM-1), which is found on the surface of a variety of human cells, including endothelial cells. Other phagocyte receptors mediate the phagocytosis of cells undergoing apoptosis. These include the β_1-, β_3-, and β_5-integrins that bind thrombospondin, which in turn binds to a thrombospondin receptor on target cells. Phosphatidylserine exposed on apoptotic cells binds C3bi, which in turn binds β_2-integrin. β_2-integrin also ligates a receptor called B2, a phosphatidylinositol-linked protein on target cells. Apoptotic cells bind C1q, and the complex binds to the C1q receptor on phagocytic cells. A recently defined class of receptors designated SRs binds CD36 and oxidized low-density lipoprotein (LDL) on target cells, and CD14 on the phagocyte also recognizes ICAM-3 on apoptotic cells. Lectin-sugar interactions are also important (3). Phagocytes also recognize phosphatidylserine, which transfers from its normal location at the inner membrane leaflet to the outer in cells undergoing apoptosis (84). Receptors for fibronectin, LPS-binding protein, and mannose-binding protein are incomplete and mediate only attachment of phagocytes to their homologous ligand-coated surfaces or particles.

The C3 fragment receptors, CR1 and CR3, may be complete or incomplete depending on the state of the phagocyte. CR1 (C3b) receptors primarily mediate attachment, but they may signal ingestion in PMNs if the cells are previously exposed to TPA or to fibronectin. Resting mouse macrophages attach only to C3b-coated erythrocytes, but they ingest them if previously stimulated by exposure to denatured proteins. The reason for these effects is unknown. Some of the treatments that render CR1 and CR3 molecules competent to signal ingestion switch them from being dispersed in the plasma membrane to being aggregated in concert with phosphorylation of their cytoplasmic domains. Incomplete opsonin-receptor complexes may act cooperatively to permit small numbers of complete complexes to trigger ingestion (19).

Engulfment

The phagocytic response to certain particles, such as iC3b-coated objects, is localized to the region of receptor-ligand interaction such that particles are engulfed by the progressive extension of pseudopodia around recognition molecules on the particle surface, a phenomenon known as "zippering." The mechanism of pseudopod extension that leads to the enclosure of objects within phagocytic vacuoles is similar to that encountered in locomotion, in that actin assembly and complex remodeling occurs in the submembrane zone of particle contact, although the signals used to elicit this actin assembly may be different in phagocytosis (85). A further complication is that the signals and the mechanical events involved in different phases of phagosome formation vary. Fc-mediated phagocytosis characteristically involves active extension of large lamellae, whereas ingested C3 fragment–opsonized particles and microorganisms entering cells by interactions with integrins appear to sink into an invagination on the phagocyte surface. The GTPases Rac and Cdc42 are implicated in Fc-mediated phagocytosis. On the other hand, the GTPase Rho appears important for C3-mediated phagocytosis, which is calcium-independent in PMNs (86–88). Mechanisms also are cell-type specific; PMNs, but not MNPs, require gelsolin for uptake of Fc-coated particles (89), and murine MNPs can ingest Fc-coated erythrocytes without increasing intracellular calcium levels (90). PI-3 kinases and myosin-based actin contractions seem to be important for the closure of phagosomes at the end of engulfment of antibody-opsonized erythrocytes (91,92). The Arp2/3 complex also has a role in the actin assembly associated with phagocytosis (93), as do many other actin-binding proteins that mediate the polymerization, depolymerization, and cross-linking of actin (94).

At the pit of forming phagocytic vacuoles in PMNs, cytoplasmic granules fuse with the plasma membrane and secrete their contents onto the engulfed particle, and the phagocytic vesicle becomes a phagolysosome, the inside of which contains the secretory products of the granules and the membrane of which acquires proteins previously embedded in the granule membrane. The secretion of large granules, which can be seen with the light microscope, is known as *degranulation.* The vesicle contents are discharged into phagocytic vacuoles. As a result, this cellular compartment comes to contain a vast number of macromolecules derived from the plasma membrane from fusing granules, as well as cytosolic components that regulate this process (95). Some of this material leaks out of incompletely closed vacuoles into the extracellular medium. Direct fusion of granules with the plasma membrane can also occur, resulting in exocytosis.

Phagosome-lysosome fusion is a key part of the digestive process discussed later and is representative of a general class of membrane fusion events in phagocytes and other cells. During all forms of phagocyte cellular and subcellular movement, large amounts of membrane traffic to and from the cell surface and between cell compartments. Indeed, some of this membrane cycling must contribute to the surface-to-volume changes that have to accommodate the cell-shape changes associated with motility and endocytosis in general (96,97). Chemotactic factor-receptor complexes are internalized in less than 0.1-μm diameter structures known as *coated pits.* The "coats" of these vesicles were first recognized as electron-dense particles lining their cytoplasmic surfaces and are basketlike networks composed mainly of a complex of proteins collectively called *clathrin.* MNPs also endocytose IgG-containing immune complexes in coated pits, and a specific determinant in the cytoplasmic domain of the transmembrane tail of FcRII mediates this process. Macrophages internalize and return to the surface their entire plasma membrane every 20 minutes in the form of such vesicles, called *endosomes,* some coated and some not. The membrane cycling process in which membrane is shuttled among intracellular compartments, especially the Golgi cisternae, is somewhat vectorial, in that it concentrates near areas of cell interaction with surfaces or with phagocytic particles.

Advances in understanding of the mechanisms of membrane cycling and of the membrane fusion events associated with it have occurred in recent years. Membrane-to-membrane recognition and fusion involve specific macromolecular components. Vesicle membrane fusion proteins called v-SNAREs bind to and activate homologous target membrane SNAREs (t-SNAREs); the interaction brings lipid bilayers into close apposition, allowing additional energy-dependent steps to bring about fusion (98). Whereas certain pairs of these fusion proteins mediate polarized redistribution of intracellular vesicles, others target membrane to sites where additional membrane is required to provide membrane area during phagocytic particle engulfment and extension of surface protrusions involved in locomotion (99). One of the factors imparting specificity to targeting of membranes between cell compartments is small GTPases of the Rab family. Certain microorganisms secrete molecules that interact with these messengers, thereby redirecting the trafficking of internalized microbes to avoid antimicrobial mechanisms (100). The distribution of intracellular organelles involved in endocytosis and exocytosis also involves, in part, the function of microtubules. One species of microtubule-associated proteins, known as *dyneins* and *kinesins,* may attach large intracellular secretory granules (described later) and, using ATP as an energy source, motor the granules outward (kinesin) and inward (dynein). Localized disaggregation of the submembrane actin networks permits the granules to approach the plasmalemma for fusion. The fusion of coated vesicles involves ATP-dependent removal of clathrin from the endosome surface, and the pH of the vesicle as well as a protein called *dynamin* regulate the uncoating process. Approximation of granules to the membrane before fusion may also be facilitated by a family of calcium- and phospholipid-binding proteins. Phagocytes have at least two of these, lipocortin (annexin III) and synexin (101,102). The actin cytoskeleton has both positive and negative roles in membrane fusion. It serves as a barrier to keep fusogenic organelles away from the plasma membrane, but in as-yet-undefined ways it also facilitates the fusion events. Actin filaments can provide tracks for the movement of granules, and there is evidence that actin polymerization induced by phagosomes facilitates phagosome-endosome fusion (103).

Measurement of Phagocytosis and Secretion

Few situations arise in which evaluation of patients requires measurement of these parameters, because all clinical disorders associated with cell-based abnormalities of phagocytosis or exocytosis have even more profound impairments of adhesion and locomotion. For laboratory assessment of phagocytosis and exocytosis, a variety of methods are available. The simplest involve morphologic observation of ingestion by phagocytes by light microscopy. More sophisticated assays measure the uptake of radioactively or otherwise-labeled particles by the cells. Detection of granule contents, usually hydrolytic enzymes, in the extracellular medium is a simple method of measuring phagocyte exocytosis.

DISORDERS OF PHAGOCYTE MOTILITY AND INGESTION

Deficiencies in the synthesis of the immunoproteins IgM, IgG, or C3 lead to the impairment of opsonic function. Microorganisms are not rendered recognizable to phagocytic cells, and affected patients suffer from recurrent or severe infections, usually caused by encapsulated bacteria. From the pattern of infections, one can infer that the role of these immunoproteins in phagocytosis is primarily to promote clearance of certain pathogenic bacteria by MNPs and is less directed toward defending the tissue-environmental interfaces. This latter task appears to be the responsibility of the moving phagocytes, the PMNs, and the monocytes, as neutropenia and monocytopenia predispose to bacterial infections affecting the skin, lungs, and gastrointestinal tract.

Leukocyte Adhesion Deficiency

In 1978, a boy was encountered who suffered from recurrent tissue bacterial infections. The patient had a neutrophilic leukocytosis, but the blood neutrophils did not enter infected sites and were deficient in migration assays *in vitro*. The locomotion defect was localized to an inability of the cells to adhere to surfaces. A surface glycoprotein of normal PMNs was missing from the PMNs of this patient, and the PMNs of the boy's parents had this glycoprotein in reduced amounts compared with amounts in normal adults, indicating autosomal-recessive inheritance. This case was the first example of what has become established as a rare but conceptually important genetic disease affecting phagocytes and termed *leukocyte adhesion deficiency* (LAD). LAD type I is a family of related diseases affecting β_2-integrins. All cases of the disease arise from defects affecting β-chain synthesis or its primary amino acid sequence, but the dimeric complex is either totally or partially missing, suggesting that both components must be present for normal deployment to the cell surface. For this reason, affected patients underexpress all members of the adhesion molecule family, although the degree of reduced expression varies depending on the underlying biosynthetic defect.

The clinical manifestations of LAD type I (Table 16-6) are similar to those seen in neutropenic patients, but LAD patients have normal to elevated peripheral blood phagocyte counts. The major functional defect appears to be that mobile phagocytes simply do not enter the tissues to control microorganisms, and the bone marrow attempts to compensate by increasing phagocyte production. These facts tend to minimize the importance of

TABLE 16-6. Phagocyte Adhesion Molecule Deficiency

Clinical Features	Laboratory Features
Autosomal-recessive inheritance	Neutrophilic and monocytic leukocytosis
Delayed separation of umbilical stump	Variably impaired adhesion, locomotion, spreading, phagocytosis by neutrophils and monocytes
Variable incidence of pyogenic infections; periodontal disease	Decreased expression of β_2-integrins or L-selectins

some of the other phagocyte adhesion molecules that have been identified by their activities *in vitro*. The lung is an exception to this rule, implying that a different adhesion and recognition system mediates transit of phagocytes into that organ, but their phagocyte function may be impaired even if they access the lung. LAD phagocytes are also variably defective in phagocytosis of a variety of particles, not just iC3b-opsonized ones, indicating that adhesion required for phagocytosis is a cooperative phenomenon. The clinical severity of LAD correlates well with the extent of expression of β_2-integrin on the phagocyte surface. Patients with mildly reduced β_2-integrin expression may only have neutrophilia, gingivitis, and moderate infections, whereas patients with severely deficient phagocytes have life-threatening infections, especially necrotizing enterocolitis, and have died from such infections (104,105).

A second type of LAD, LAD type II, has been described in patients with a generalized impairment of a fucosyltransferase activity that completes the terminal structure of fucose-bearing cell-surface receptors, including L-selectin and E-selectin molecules on PMNs and endothelial cell surfaces, respectively. Affected patients have documentable deficiencies of PMN rolling behavior on endothelial surfaces and suffer from recurrent pyogenic infections (106). Treatment of cultured cells from these patients and of the patients themselves with five oral doses of 400 mg/kg of fucose daily restores selectin expression to near-normal levels and reduces high circulating PMN counts ordinarily found in these patients (107).

Mutant Rac

A single patient has been described who had recurrent pyogenic infections and PMN dysfunction cured by bone marrow transplantation. The patient was found to have a spontaneous point mutation in the coding sequence at the heart of the catalytic GTPase site of Rac2. The evidence to date indicates that this mutant Rac2 acts as a dominant-negative inhibitor of wild-type Rac in the patient's cells, inhibiting responses leading to migration, actin assembly, and oxidase activity, much like the Rac2 knock-out mice (108,109).

Leukocyte Actin Dysfunction

A male infant was described who suffered from severe tissue infections and did not mobilize PMNs to make pus. Like LAD patients, this patient had a peripheral blood neutrophilia. The infant's PMNs were quantitatively defective in adhesion and locomotion and less so in phagocytosis. A severe deficiency in the extent of actin assembly was detected in PMN extracts of the patient, and a partial deficiency was identified in both intact PMNs and extracts of the PMNs of the patient's parents and siblings. The patient's father's PMNs expressed β_2-integrin receptors at approximately half of normal levels. The basis of the actin polymerization deficiency is not known, and because most

LAD patients polymerize actin normally in response to various stimuli, the relation of this disorder to LAD is unclear. Two additional families with patients and relatives demonstrating this constellation of findings have been identified, and all of their PMNs have been shown to contain supranormal quantities of LSP-1, an actin-binding protein, possibly because of abnormal processing of this protein. Overexpression of LSP-1 confers a phenotype resembling cells from the affected patients (110,111).

Another form of phagocyte dysfunction associated with the actin system was reported from Japan. The affected patient had severe, recurrent infections and died in infancy. The patient's PMNs had gross defects in locomotion, phagocytosis, and metabolic responses. The only biochemical abnormality detected in a survey of the patient's PMNs and in cultured lymphoid cells revealed a population of β actin molecules with a point mutation near the N-terminus, where actin interacts with numerous actin-binding proteins. Presumably this actin functioned in a dominant-negative manner to inhibit actin-based reactions associated with normal PMN function (112).

Other Disorders

The complexity of phagocyte locomotion causes considerable variation in the results of assays measuring it, and as a result, the literature contains numerous reports correlating phagocyte (especially PMN) chemotaxis deficiency with various diseases for which a clear-cut linkage is unclear. Examples include reduced in vitro PMN motility associated with neutropenia (lazy leukocyte syndrome), with periodontal disease, with the hyper IgE syndrome, and with a variety of systemic disorders, including bacterial sepsis, burns, malnutrition, rheumatoid arthritis, systemic lupus erythematosus, multiple myeloma, and hepatic cirrhosis. The neutrophils of newborns also have functional abnormalities detectable in in vitro assays. It is possible that these findings reflect the stress of childbirth and infusion of substances released from the destruction of the placenta and umbilical cord. As-yet-unspecified microtubule abnormalities have been invoked to explain abnormal locomotion and chemotactic behavior of PMNs from patients with primary ciliary dyskinesia, a rare autosomal-recessive disorder characterized by bronchopulmonary infections, situs inversus, and infertility, ascribable to impaired ciliary motion (113). Phagocytes of patients with Wiskott-Aldrich syndrome (described in Chapter 22) lack the myeloid cell-specific form of WASP. Although these patients have immunodeficiency, they do not suffer from infections characteristic of PMN disorders. Actin polymerization responses to formyl peptides are normal in these patients' PMNs (114), although morphologic abnormalities of adhesion foci are detectable in MNPs (115), possibly contributing to disordered antigen responsiveness. PMN from patients with glycogen storage disease type Ib have neutropenia and documented PMN migration abnormalities. Recently, the neutropenia has been shown to respond to therapy with G-CSF (116).

PHAGOCYTE GRANULES

Neutrophil Granules

Neutrophil granules fall into two general categories: secretory granules, whose contents are mostly secreted into the external medium, and lysosome-like granules, whose contents are mostly used within the neutrophil. The secretory granules include the specific granules (also called *secondary granules*) and the gelatinase granules, which may actually be a subset of the

specific granules. Neutrophils also contain a set of very small secretory vesicles. There is only one type of lysosome-like granule—the primary or azurophil granule.

AZUROPHIL GRANULES

The azurophil granules are the blue-staining granules seen in neutrophils as they appear in blood films treated with Wright's stain. These granules, generally approximately 0.5 μm in diameter, are first detected in the promyelocyte, where, on staining with Wright-Giemsa, they are recognized as purple granules that are dark in hue compared with their appearance in more mature stages of the neutrophil. Their biosynthesis ceases at the myelocyte stage (117), by which time they have taken on their final staining characteristics.

The contents of the azurophil granules are used almost exclusively for the disposal of ingested microorganisms. Accordingly, these granules almost invariably deliver their contents into phagocytic vesicles, with little discharge outside the cell except for release from disintegrating neutrophils or leakage as the granules expel their contents prematurely into developing vesicles still in communication with the exterior. Some of the azurophil granule components, however, are highly corrosive, and the portion of these that manage to escape from the neutrophils is responsible for much of the damage sustained by tissues in the neighborhood of an inflammatory reaction (118). In functional terms, the azurophil granules contain two groups of constituents: microbicidal agents, which kill ingested microorganisms, and hydrolytic enzymes, which dispose of the remains. They also contain proteoglycans, which curb the activity of the hydrolases before their release from the granules.

Microbicidal Agents. Five kinds of microbicidal agents are known to occur in the azurophil granules. All are cationic at physiologic pH, so they all adhere firmly to the negatively charged surfaces of their targets. One of these microbicidal agents, MPO, is involved in the oxygen-dependent microbicidal mechanisms that account for much of the killing power of neutrophils. These are discussed in detail in Microbicidal Oxidant Production and the Respiratory Burst. The rest are able to destroy bacteria under anaerobic conditions.

Oxygen-Independent Microbicidal Agents
Defensins. The defensins are a group of three small peptides with potent lethal activity against a wide variety of microorganisms, including bacteria, viruses, and fungi (119). Identical except for their N-terminal amino acids, the three peptides are all rigid, bicyclic structures with positively charged amino acids at one end and hydrophobic amino acids at the other (Fig. 16-6), a distribution that gives them the properties of cationic detergents. In the neutrophil, the defensins occur at high concentrations, constituting over 5% of the total protein of the cell. They are not uniformly distributed among the azurophil granules, however, but are found only in a morphologically distinct subset (Fig. 16-7).

The defensins appear to kill bacteria by destroying the barrier function of their membranes. Defensins only affect bacteria that are engaged in energy production; bacteria maintained in a nutrient-free environment are resistant to their action (120). One of the principal uses of metabolic energy in a microorganism is for the maintenance of the transmembrane potential. It may be that, as with mellitin, one of the active principles of bee venom, the membrane-permeabilizing activity of the defensins is only expressed in the presence of a transmembrane potential of a certain magnitude. Some microorganisms manage to synthesize specific gene products under direction of a transcriptional regulatory protein known as *PhoP*, which renders them resistant to the microbicidal action of defensins.

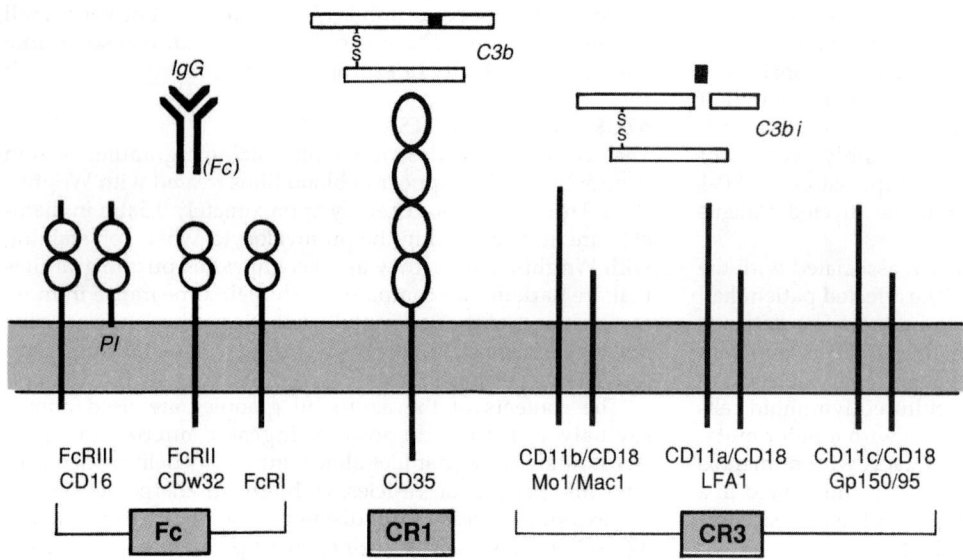

Figure 16-6. Schematic summary of the major opsonins and their receptors on phagocytic cells. FcR, Fc receptor; Ig, immunoglobulin; PI, phosphatidylinositol.

BACTERICIDAL PERMEABILITY-INCREASING PROTEIN. Bactericidal permeability-increasing protein (BPI) is a 60-kd cationic protein of known sequence (121). Its crystal structure discloses a symmetric molecule with a highly cationic N-terminal half able to neutralize endotoxin and a C-terminal half that can opsonize gram-negative bacteria. Like the defensins, BPI kills by causing the membranes of its targets to become leaky. Whereas the target range of the defensins is broad, BPI is only active against gram-negative bacteria. In a process antagonized by Ca^{2+} and Mg^{2+}, it binds to the outer walls of these bacteria (i.e., their LPS) (122), then works its way through these walls to disorganize their cell membranes. Within minutes of exposure to BPI, the membrane barrier becomes sufficiently dysfunctional to allow actinomycin C to leak in, but macromolecule synthesis remains intact for some hours. The membrane leak, however, destroys the microorganism as a colony-forming unit.

LYSOZYME. The interior of a bacterium is hypertonic with respect to its environment, and as a result, the microorganism tends to take in water from surrounding fluids. Rupture of the organism through the unopposed influx of water is prevented, however, by peptidoglycan, a huge polymer of N-acetylglucosamine and muramic acid extensively cross-linked by short peptides, that lies between the cell wall and the plasma membrane. The densely woven peptidoglycan forms a strong, nonexpandable net that envelops the microorganism and protects it from the hypotonic medium in which it lives.

Lysozyme, a 14-kd enzyme found in both the azurophil and specific granules (123), destroys peptidoglycan by hydrolyzing the glycosidic bonds in the glucosamine-muramic acid polymers. It operates most effectively at pH 4 to 5, the typical pH in the interior of the phagosome (124). With the lysis of the peptidoglycan, the force opposing the osmotic gradient between the microorganism and its environment is lost. Water then moves freely into the bacterium, causing it to swell and burst.

The peptidoglycans of most bacteria contain substituents that render them resistant to the action of lysozyme. Their resistance to lysozyme is broken down, however, by exposure to oxidants of the kind generated by stimulated neutrophils. In these cases, lysozyme appears to serve an auxiliary role, acting in concert with the oxidants to destroy the targets. In a few microorganisms, however, the peptidoglycan is readily hydrolyzed by lysozyme. Toward these, the enzyme alone is a potent microbicidal agent.

SERPROCIDINS. The serprocidins (125) are large, microbicidal proteins in the azurophil granules, weighing 25 to 37 kd. They include four species: three neutral proteases—elastase, cathepsin G, and proteinase 3—and a structurally related protein without catalytic activity known as *azurocidin/CAP37*. All are microbicidal, probably killing as membrane-active agents as well as by virtue of their proteolytic action (except for azurocidin/CAP37). They have a very broad spectrum of activity, killing gram-positive and gram-negative bacteria, fungi such as *C. albicans*, and protozoa.

The proteolytic activities of the neutral proteases are maximum at pH values close to neutrality, a pH optimum that distinguishes them from the other azurophil granule hydrolases, most of which show optimal activity at pH near 4 or 5. As mentioned previously, these proteases act as microbicidal agents. Their pH optimum suggests that they act during the earliest stages of phagocytosis, before the phagosomes have become acidified.

It is evident that these proteases, as enzymes of broad specificity active at physiologic pH, have the potential to inflict considerable damage when they are released from the neutrophil

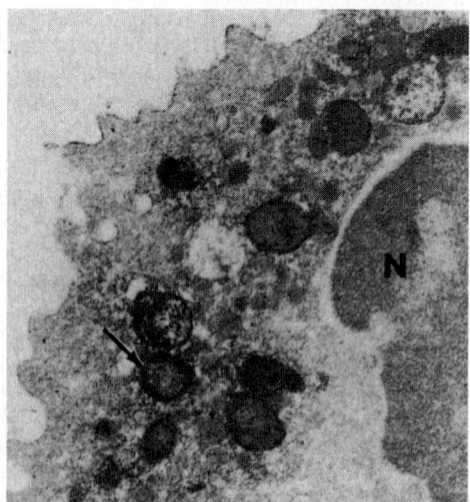

Figure 16-7. Morphologic characteristics of defensin-containing azurophil granules. In this section of a neutrophil stained for peroxidase and viewed by electron microscopy, azurophil granules appear black because of their myeloperoxidase content. Defensin-containing granules are stained only at the periphery because myeloperoxidase is excluded from their centers, possibly by crystals of defensin (*arrow*). N, nucleus.

into surrounding tissues. Normally, tissue destruction by the liberated neutral proteases is controlled through rapid inactivation by a group of antiproteinases (α_1-antiproteinase, β_2-macroglobulin, and so forth) that are found at high concentrations in plasma and extracellular fluids (126). When the antiproteinases fail, however, the destructive potential of these enzymes is realized. This is best seen in the emphysema of α_1-antiproteinase deficiency, which has been attributed to the unopposed action of neutrophil elastase and proteinase 3 on pulmonary tissues. Destruction of the lung by tobacco smoke may be another example of the effects of neutral proteases (127); lung tissue, in this case, is destroyed by a smoldering inflammatory reaction featuring an abundance of both neutrophils, which bring their neutral proteases to the inflamed site, and oxidants (from tobacco smoke and stimulated phagocytes), which inactivate α_1-antiproteinase by oxidizing a critical methionine residue. Further investigation probably will show that these neutral proteases mediate tissue destruction at other sites of inflammation. Neutral PMN proteinase has been identified as one antigen reactive with autoantibodies found in the plasma of patients with Wegener's granulomatosis (128,129).

ACID HYDROLASES. The azurophil granules are the lysosomes of the neutrophils and, as such, contain a wide variety of hydrolytic enzymes that are maximally active at the relatively low pH of a fully acidified phagocytic vesicle (124). These enzymes are probably not involved in microbial killing, but rather are responsible for breaking down the macromolecules of the ingested targets to their low-molecular-weight constituents. Included among the acid hydrolases of the azurophil granules are proteases (e.g., cathepsin D, an aspartate protease active at pH 4.0 to 5.0), glycosidases (e.g., lysozyme), lipid-hydrolyzing enzymes (130), and RNase (131). Neutrophils have surprisingly little ability to degrade DNA (132). A partial listing of acid hydrolases is given in Table 16-7.

TABLE 16-7. Contents of Human Neutrophil Secretory Granules

Primary (azurophilic) granules
    Acid phosphatase
    N-acetyl-β-glucosaminidase
    α-Mannosidase
    β-Glucuronidase
    Cathepsins B, D, and G
    Elastase
    Proteinase 3
    Azurocidin
    Azurophil granule protein 7
    Bacterial permeability inducer
    Lysozyme
    Defensins
    (Myelo)peroxidase
Secondary (specific) granules
    Vitamin B_{12}–binding protein
    N-formyloligopeptide receptors
    Laminin receptors
    Lactoferrin
    Collagenase
    Lysozyme
    NADPH oxidase (cytochrome *b*)
    β_2-Microglobulin
    Gelatinase
    CD11b/CD18 (CR3 receptors)
    Vitronectin receptors
Tertiary (microvesicular) granules
    Class 1
        Gelatinase
        CD11b/CD18
        Plasminogen activator
    Class 2
        Alkaline phosphatase
        Tetranectin

Oxygen-Dependent Microbicidal Agent

MYELOPEROXIDASE. MPO plays an important role in the oxygen-dependent microbicidal mechanisms that account for much of the killing power of neutrophils. It is composed of two 60-kd peptides and two 12-kd peptides, the larger of which is glycosylated, and it carries two iron-containing porphyrin molecules as prosthetic groups (133). An abundant protein, MPO constitutes over 5% of the dry weight of the neutrophil, and through the color of its prosthetic groups [green instead of red because of a domed configuration of the heme on the MPO molecule (17)], endows the cell with its characteristic greenish hue. The sequence of the enzyme has been determined by cloning its gene, which is located on chromosome 17 and encodes both subunits of the enzyme as a single long polypeptide (134). MPO is synthesized as a 92-kd glycosylated precursor (pro-MPO), then undergoes limited deglycosylation followed by proteolysis to release a short glycopeptide and cut the remaining fragment into the 60-kd and 12-kd peptides. Dimerization and delivery to the azurophil granule complete the formation of the enzyme.

MPO catalyzes the oxidation of Cl^- by the H_2O_2 generated by neutrophils when they are exposed to a target microorganism (135). This oxidation produces hypochlorous acid, a powerful microbicidal oxidant:

$$Cl^- + H_2O_2 \overset{MPO}{\rightarrow} HOCl + OH^-$$

The microbicidal role of MPO is aided by a high isoelectric point that confers a positive charge on the enzyme at physiologic pH, allowing it to bind directly to the negatively charged surface of an ingested microorganism. From this location, it can deliver its lethal products to the target with maximal efficiency. MPO can also catalyze the oxidation of Br^- and I^- to the corresponding hypohalous acids, but Cl^- is its physiologic substrate. Like many lysosomal enzymes, it operates best at pH 4 to 5.

Like antibodies against neutral PMN proteinase, circulating antibodies against MPO may be associated with collagen vascular disease (135).

Proteoglycans. Proteoglycans, or mucopolysaccharides, are molecules composed of a serine- and glycine-rich polypeptide extensively substituted with highly anionic polysaccharide chains rich in uronic acids and sulfate groups. In neutrophils and their precursors, the azurophil granules (but not the specific granules) contain substantial concentrations of proteoglycans, principally chondroitin sulfate. The rich purple color of the azurophil granules in the promyelocytes is due to their proteoglycan content, and the loss of color as the cells mature is thought to result from the masking of the proteoglycan sulfate groups as the granules mature (136).

In proteoglycan-containing granules, not only in phagocytes but also in mast cells and natural killer cells, hydrolases and other positively charged proteins are held as complexes in a dense network of anionic polysaccharide chains. Although the hydrolases are active when complexed to proteoglycan, their access to substrates is greatly restricted; the attachment of the enzymes to the proteoglycan matrix prevents them from diffusing to potential substrates, whereas substrate molecules more than a few kilodaltons are screened away from the active sites of the complexed enzymes by the close mesh of the polysaccharide network. Autolysis of the granules is therefore prevented by the proteoglycan, which appears to be largely responsible for maintaining the structural integrity of granules despite their content of potentially destructive hydrolytic enzymes.

SPECIFIC GRANULES

The specific granules (137) are smaller than the azurophil granules (average size approximately 0.2 µm) and appear pink on Wright-stained blood films. They are first seen in the myelocytes, but unlike the azurophil granules, whose production ceases at the myelocyte stage, their numbers continue to increase throughout most of the later stages of neutrophil maturation (117). By the time the cell is mature, it contains approximately two specific granules for every azurophil granule.

The specific granules resemble the azurophil granules in delivering their contents into phagocytic vesicles. Unlike the azurophil granules, however, the specific granules also secrete their contents deliberately into the extracellular medium (138). Secretion occurs in response to many agents, including such physiologic stimuli as the anaphylatoxin C5a, liberated during complement activation; N-formylated peptides, released from bacteria and from the mitochondria of damaged cells; and lipid mediators, such as LTB_4 and PAF (139). Secretion takes place by the fusion of the specific granule with the plasma membrane, a process that transfers the granule membrane, with its complement of proteins, to the plasma membrane. Accordingly, secretion releases proteins into the extracellular medium and transfers other proteins to the outer layer of the neutrophil.

Among the specific granule membrane components relocated in this way are the formyl-peptide receptor, the CD11/ CD18 family of adhesion glycoproteins (discussed previously), and cytochrome b_{558}, a heme protein that participates in microbicidal oxidant production, as explained later.

The contents of the specific granule include lysozyme, also found in the azurophil granules; certain ligand-binding proteins; cathelicidin; and a few proteases with highly restricted substrate specificities. Lysosomal hydrolases are absent from this granule.

Ligand-Binding Proteins.
The specific granules contain two ligand-binding proteins: apolactoferrin and cobalamin-binding protein. One binds iron tightly, and the other takes up cobalamin and related corrinoids.

Apolactoferrin.
Apolactoferrin is the iron-binding protein of the specific granules (140). Each molecule of apolactoferrin contains two sites that bind ferric (Fe^{3+}) iron with very high affinity (K_a 10^{22} mol^{-1}). When one or both of these sites is occupied, the protein is called *lactoferrin*.

Some have proposed that the iron bound to the protein in its lactoferrin form catalyzes the production of the very reactive hydroxyl radical (OH•) from the oxidants generated by stimulated neutrophils (the so-called Haber-Weiss reaction, discussed later). It is more likely, however, that lactoferrin-bound iron is unable to participate in the Haber-Weiss reaction. Apolactoferrin may therefore play a protective role at sites of inflammation, controlling nonspecific oxidant damage by sequestering loose iron and suppressing its reactivity (141). The protein may also potentiate microbial killing by preventing the ingested bacteria from obtaining the iron they require metabolically. In addition, it can kill bacteria directly, presumably through an effect on their membranes. Finally, lactoferrin appears to exert some control over granulopoiesis by inhibiting GM-CSF secretion by MNPs.

Cobalamin-Binding Protein.
The corrinoids are a family of compounds that all contain a *corrin ring*, a partly reduced tetrapyrrole with a cobalt at its center. Biologic systems contain many kinds of corrinoids, some direct products of biosynthesis and others arising through chemical modification of the biosynthetically produced compounds. Only one group of corrinoids, however, is active in humans; these are the *cobalamins*. Humans assimilate other classes of corrinoids, acquiring them in part from bacteria (142). These nonphysiologic corrinoids must be disposed of to prevent them from interfering with the function of the cobalamins in the tissues.

The specific granules contain a cobalamin-binding glycoprotein, sometimes called *transcobalamin III*, that is closely related to transcobalamin I, the principal cobalamin-binding protein of plasma. The specific granule cobalamin binder takes up a wide variety of corrinoids with high affinity (143). It is thought that this protein aids in the elimination of nonphysiologic corrinoids by binding them where they are released and transporting them to the liver, which excretes them in bile.

Cathelicidins.
Cathelicidins (144) are a heterogeneous group of antimicrobial polypeptides that are released by proteolysis from the C-terminal ends of inactive precursors. The precursors have a highly conserved proregion, but the structures of the cathelicidins themselves are very diverse. They are found in many species. The human cathelicidin, variably called *hCAP-18*, *FALL-39*, or *LL-37* and located in the neutrophil specific granule, has a molecular weight of approximately 45 kd. It has chemoattractant properties as well as antimicrobial activity against a broad spectrum of microorganisms. It is liberated from its precursor by elastase. Because specific granules are secretory, the cathelicidin is released into the external environment, where it can presumably act against extracellular microorganisms.

Protegrin, a cathelicidin from pigs, only weighs 2 kd and has structural features resembling defensins.

Collagenase and Gelatinase.
As its name implies, collagenase catalyzes the hydrolysis of native collagen. Like other collagenases, the specific granule collagenase splits the collagen molecule asymmetrically into two fragments by hydrolyzing a specific peptide bond; further degradation of the incised collagen molecule is accomplished by other proteases (145). It is likely that collagenase serves as a demolition unit, helping to clear away debris at damaged and inflamed sites preparatory to reconstruction.

Collagenase is a metalloproteinase, bearing a Ca^{2+} ion at its active site. It exists in the specific granules as a proenzyme but is converted to the active enzyme by exposure to the microbicidal oxidants manufactured by stimulated neutrophils, or by treatment with elastase (146). Like other components of the specific granules, the enzyme is secreted when the neutrophils are exposed to activators of degranulation.

Gelatinase is also found in the specific granules, but is discussed in the section Gelatinase (Tertiary) Granules in connection with the gelatinase granules.

C5-Activating Protease.
Contained within the specific granules and released into the extracellular medium when neutrophils are stimulated is a protease that splits the circulating complement component C5 into C5a and C5b (146). The C5a liberated through the action of this enzyme is both a chemotactic factor that calls more neutrophils to its site of production and (at higher concentrations) a stimulating agent that induces the newly arrived neutrophils to release their specific granule contents, including the C5-activating protease. The release of the C5a-activating enzyme therefore introduces a positive feedback loop that amplifies the inflammatory reaction, drawing progressively increasing numbers of neutrophils into the inflamed site.

GELATINASE (TERTIARY) GRANULES
Gelatinase granules (147) are a third set of granules found in the neutrophil. Smaller than the specific granules, they are characterized by the ease with which they degranulate, liberating their contents in response to stimuli too weak to cause the generalized release of the specific granule contents. As suggested by their name, they contain a great deal of gelatinase—a quantity amounting to half the gelatinase in the granulocyte—the remainder being located in the specific granules. They also con-

tain other components, including acetyltransferase and β_2-microglobulin (148). Their membranes contain the adhesion protein CD11b/CD18 and cytochrome b_{558}, a component of the neutrophil NADPH oxidase (29).

Gelatinase. Gelatinase resembles collagenase in many ways. Like collagenase, it is a metalloenzyme with Ca^{2+} at its active site. It exists in the granule as a proenzyme that is activated by an oxidative mechanism as well as by elastase (29). Its classic substrate is denatured collagen, but it also digests type IV and type V collagens (29). Gelatinase, like collagenase, probably serves as a demolition enzyme. By digesting the type IV collagen in the basement membrane beneath the endothelial cell layer, gelatinase may also participate in the egress of neutrophils from the vascular tree (148).

SECRETORY VESICLES
Secretory vesicles (149) are very small vesicles contained within the neutrophil. They are the most rapidly mobilized of the granules (although they are not strictly granules). Produced by endocytosis, their contents consist of plasma proteins such as albumin. Their critical components are their membranes, which are loaded with important proteins such as alkaline phosphatase, the oxidase component cytochrome b_{558}, the adhesion protein complex CD11b/CD18, the endotoxin receptor CD14, the formylated peptide receptor, the vacuolar H^+-ATPase, and the complement antagonist DAF. Mobilization of the secretory granules causes all these membrane proteins to be exposed on the surface of the neutrophil.

Granules of Mononuclear Phagocytes

Unlike neutrophils, MNPs contain only one type of granule. Sometimes, a distinction is made between an early MPO-containing granule that occurs in monocytes and the later MPO-free granule that is found in macrophages. Apart from their differences in peroxidase content, however, the two kinds of granules are similar in composition and function and therefore are considered to represent a single granule type. Although this granule has not been as well characterized as those of the neutrophil, studies have shown that it closely resembles the neutrophil azurophil granule. Like the latter, the granule of the MNP contains a large number of acid hydrolases, giving it the character of a lysosome (150). In addition, it contains several other constituents found in azurophil granules, including several microbicidal proteins: the defensins, lysozyme, and (at certain stages) MPO (150). Because of their content of microbicidal proteins, these granules, like the azurophil granules of the neutrophil, are able to participate in the killing of ingested microorganisms. In addition, the acid hydrolases in these granules are responsible for the degradation of materials ingested by the cell, which, in the case of MNPs, include invading microorganisms and superannuated cells [e.g., red blood cells (RBCs) at the end of their lifespans and assorted debris that accumulates at sites of injury]. The various lipid storage diseases (e.g., Gaucher's disease, Niemann-Pick disease) are caused by deficiencies of one or another of these lysosomal acid hydrolases (see Chapter 30).

During their lifetimes, which may last months, MNPs can undergo many changes in morphology and function in response to exogenous influences (e.g., LPS, IFN-γ) as they transform from circulating monocytes to tissue macrophages (151) (Table 16-2). Included among these changes are major alterations affecting their granules. Granule numbers increase continuously as the monocyte, maturing under the influence of cytokines and tissue location, enlarges to a macrophage (first resting, then activated), then with continued stimulation to an epithelioid cell, and finally to a giant cell, the latter arising through the fusion of epithelioid cells that have been subjected to prolonged stimula-

tion by cytokines (Fig. 16-8). The composition of the granules also changes; for example, levels of defensins and acid hydrolases increase, whereas MPO, abundant in monocyte granules, declines greatly as the cell transforms into a macrophage. These changes and others that occur as MNPs come under the influence of their local environment may enable them to accomplish their tasks of demolition and destruction in an optimal fashion, regardless of the circumstances or the targets.

Macrophages are highly secretory cells, releasing a large number of substances into their environment when appropriately stimulated (151) (Table 16-1). Among these substances are the acid hydrolases, which, unlike most of these secreted materials (discussed later), are not synthesized *de novo* in response to the stimulus but exist as preformed proteins in the macrophage granules. Release of these lysosomal hydrolases takes place in part through leakage due to premature fusion of the granules with partly formed phagocytic vesicles and in part through deliberate exocytosis of the granule contents. The liberated hydrolases, which include cathepsins, glycosidases, aryl sulfatases, and other catabolic enzymes, participate in the tissue repair process at inflammatory sites and also alter the nature of the inflammatory reaction by destroying protein mediators such as C5a and immunoglobulins.

DISEASES AFFECTING PHAGOCYTE GRANULES

Chédiak-Higashi Syndrome
Chédiak-Higashi syndrome (152,153) is an inherited disorder of granule morphogenesis affecting tissues throughout the body. Its most prominent and dangerous clinical manifestations are a greatly increased susceptibility to bacterial infections resulting from serious abnormalities in the function of affected phagocytes and a lymphoma-like illness that eventually kills most patients who survive the bacterial infections.

PATHOGENESIS
The pathogenetic basis for Chédiak-Higashi syndrome is readily apparent on inspecting affected cells under the microscope. Phagocytes, instead of containing granules that are relatively regular in size and shape, contain a highly inhomogeneous population of granules, some normal but many huge and misshapen. These grossly distorted granules are also seen in other cells, including melanocytes, platelets, lymphocytes, and cells of the nervous system, all of which contribute to the clinical manifestations of the disease. In neutrophils, the defective organelles contain constituents from both the azurophil and specific granules, some in decreased amounts, whereas some components (e.g., cathepsin G and elastase) are absent altogether. The abnormal granules are seen in mature cells, in myeloid precursors, and in colonies derived from affected marrow stem cells.

These abnormal granules cause disturbances in the function of various types of blood cells in Chédiak-Higashi patients. In neutrophils, both phagocytosis and O_2^- production are normal, but bacterial killing is impaired, degranulation is delayed and incomplete, and chemotaxis is defective, perhaps because the enlarged granules pass only with difficulty through the narrow spaces of the tissues. Defects in degranulation and chemotaxis may be partly attributable to disruption in the function of the microtubules, which show abnormalities in polymerization and in interaction with the granule membranes. A high proportion of the cells are destroyed in the marrow (ineffective granulopoiesis), leading to a mild to moderate neutropenia and the excretion of abnormally large amounts of lysozyme (muramidase) in the urine. In the platelets, storage pools of ADP and serotonin are decreased, possibly because of a deficiency in dense granule pre-

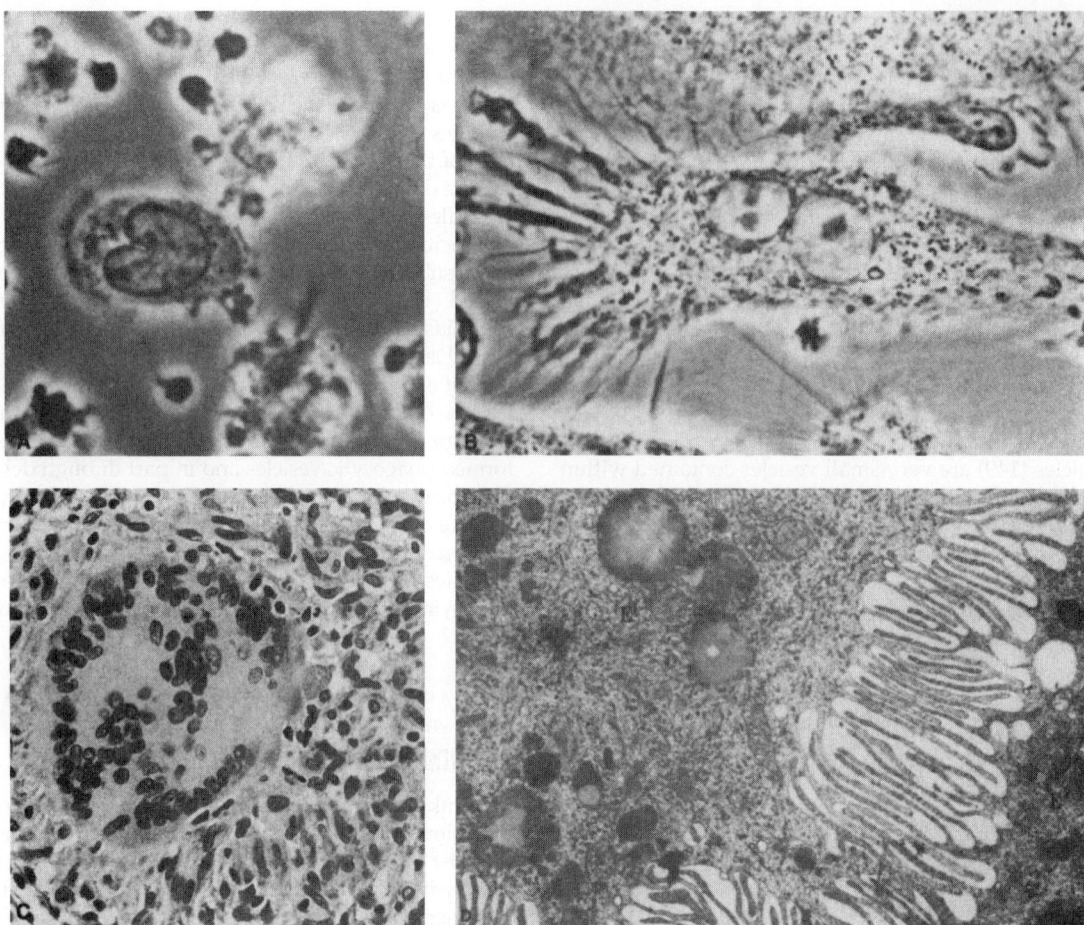

Figure 16-8. Stages in the transformation of a monocyte to a giant cell at an inflammatory site. **A:** Monocyte. **B:** Macrophage. This cell is much larger and more granular than the monocyte. Its membrane is thrown into irregular folds and projections, through which it adheres to nearby cells and substratum. **C:** Granuloma, showing a large giant cell surrounded by tightly packed epithelioid cells. **D:** The junction between two epithelioid cells, showing that they are tightly joined through a complex system of interdigitating membrane folds. E^1, first epithelioid cell; E^2, second epithelioid cell.

cursors in the megakaryocytes. Lymphocytes show an impairment of both antibody-dependent (ADCC) and natural killer cell–mediated cytotoxicity, demonstrating in particular a problem in handling Epstein-Barr virus infections (154).

Studies with myeloid precursors have suggested that the giant granules of Chédiak-Higashi syndrome arise through the progressive coalescence of smaller granules as the defective cells mature. The molecular lesion underlying this abnormality in granule morphogenesis is a mutation in a gene known as *LYST* (for lysosomal trafficking regulator). LYST, which is located on chromosome 1q43, encodes a 429-kd polypeptide that resembles a yeast protein involved in vacuolar sorting (38). A variety of different mutations affecting LYST have been described in patients with Chédiak-Higashi syndrome (155).

CLINICAL FEATURES

Chédiak-Higashi is a rare disorder inherited as an autosomal-recessive trait. In the past, patients with Chédiak-Higashi syndrome have typically died of bacterial infections in their first or second decade. The prevention of infections by prophylactic antibiotics and other measures have recently altered this pattern, and patients are living longer. Of those who survive the infections, however, most succumb to the *accelerated phase*, a progressive lymphoproliferative syndrome that leads inevitably to death through pancytopenia.

Infections begin in early infancy. They are serious and recurrent, typically involving the skin and subcutaneous tissues (abscess and pyoderma) and the upper and lower respiratory tracts (sinusitis, otitis media, pneumonia). Severe gum disease with bone atrophy and loss of teeth is also seen in Chédiak-Higashi syndrome, as it is in several other disorders of neutrophil function. *Staphylococcus aureus* is the most frequent pathogen, but infections by other bacteria (e.g., *Streptococcus pneumoniae*, *Streptococcus pyogenes*) are also seen, as well as infections by *Aspergillus* and *Candida* spp. The infections tend to be protracted, responding only slowly to antibiotic treatment.

Other signs of the disease also appear in infancy. Diffuse hypopigmentation (partial albinism) is evident at birth, with pale skin and eyegrounds and a silvery sheen to the hair. These pigmentary abnormalities are manifestations of the granular abnormalities that occur in Chédiak-Higashi melanocytes. Neurologic signs, which are manifestations of abnormalities affecting the neurons, glia, and Schwann's cells, may include peripheral neuropathy, ataxia, weakness, and seizures (155).

Total leukocyte counts of Chédiak-Higashi patients are low (1000 to 3000/μL), and urine muramidase (lysozyme) levels are high, both reflecting intramedullary destruction of granulocytes. The bleeding time is prolonged and platelet aggregation is abnormal as a result of the storage pool defect in Chédiak-Higashi platelets, resulting in a mild to moderate bleeding dia-

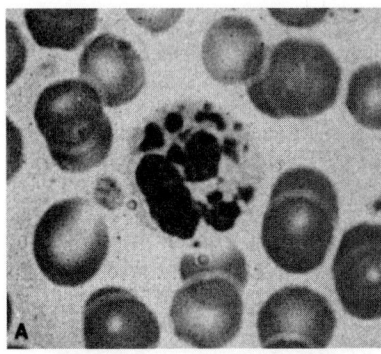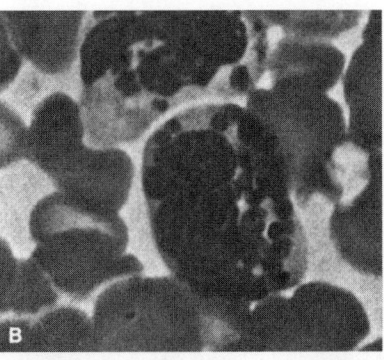

Figure 16-9. Neutrophils in Chédiak-Higashi syndrome. **A:** Peripheral blood. **B:** Bone marrow. The large, malformed granules that are pathognomonic of Chédiak-Higashi syndrome are readily identified. In the bone marrow, precursors as well as mature cells contain the defective granules, which are found in all leukocyte lines.

thesis in Chédiak-Higashi patients. The diagnosis is made by examination of the blood film, which shows the pathognomonic giant granules in most members of the leukocyte series, including neutrophils, eosinophils, monocytes, and occasional granular lymphocytes (Fig. 16-9). The giant granules are also seen in hematopoietic precursors in the marrow.

In most Chédiak-Higashi patients who survive for a sufficiently long time, the disease enters an accelerated phase. This is a lymphoma-like illness characterized by an uncontrolled and ultimately fatal proliferation of normal-appearing lymphocytes and histiocytes (Fig. 16-10) (156). Affected patients begin to develop recurrent fevers, rash, and prostration, perhaps due to the release of lymphokines from the proliferating cells, and infections increase in frequency. The neutrophil counts begin to decline from their already diminished levels, and anemia and (less often) thrombocytopenia appear. The liver, spleen, and lymph nodes enlarge as they become infiltrated with the proliferating cells, which also fill the marrow, accounting for the progressively worsening pancytopenia. Death from the complications of pancytopenia is inevitable after a relentless downhill course of a few months to 2 years.

TREATMENT

The treatment of Chédiak-Higashi syndrome amounts to the prevention and treatment of the infectious complications. Patients should be placed on prophylactic antibiotic therapy: trimethoprim, 160 mg/day, plus sulfamethoxazole, 800 mg/day (the combination is available as Septra, Bactrim, or generic equivalents, and all are sold as elixirs for children, in whom the dose is 5 mL/10 kg); or for patients with allergy to sulfonamides, dicloxacillin, 500 mg (250 mg in children) twice daily.

Infections that develop should be treated vigorously with high doses of appropriate antibiotics and surgical drainage as necessary. High-dose ascorbic acid, 200 mg/day, has been reported to improve neutrophil function and ameliorate the clinical manifestations in some patients.

As to the accelerated phase, steroids, vincristine, and antithymocyte globulin have been used for treatment, but with only modest success. Marrow transplantation, however, is curative (157). Only small numbers of donor leukocytes are needed to prevent the development of the accelerated phase. Failure of engraftment, however, leads to death in the accelerated phase.

Specific Granule Deficiency

INHERITED

Inherited specific granule deficiency is a condition whose most characteristic feature is the absence of specific granules from affected neutrophils (158). In these cells, specific granules cannot be detected by either light or electron microscopy (Fig. 16-11). Cells from one patient contained small, flat vesicles that were tentatively identified as empty specific granules. Moreover, many individual specific granule components are missing from these cells. Cobalamin-binding protein and lactoferrin are absent, as is gelatinase, ordinarily found in both specific granules and the readily discharged gelatinase granules. Lactoferrin mRNA is greatly diminished in marrow cells from patients deficient in specific granules. In addition, unlike normal neutrophils, specific granule–deficient cells fail to deliver additional CD11/CD18, formyl peptide receptors, and cytochrome b_{558} [part of the superoxide (O_2^-)-forming apparatus, discussed later] to the plasma membrane in response to stimuli, suggesting that

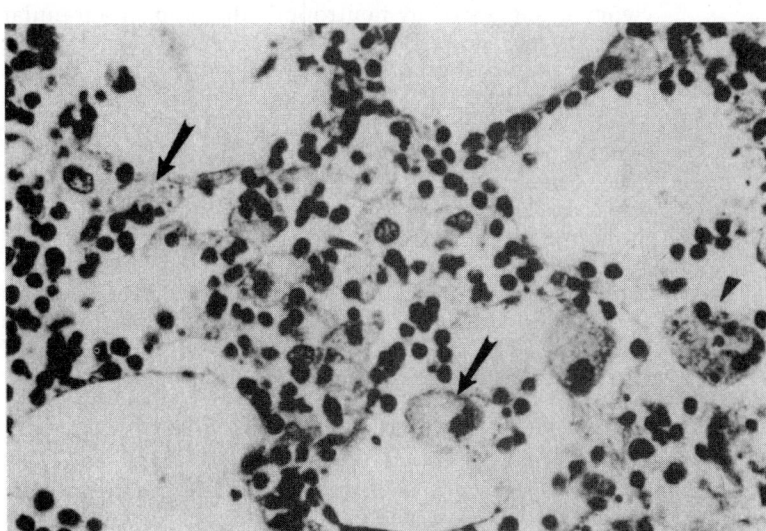

Figure 16-10. The accelerated phase of Chédiak-Higashi syndrome. The involved bone marrow infiltrated with large, benign-appearing mononuclear cells (*arrows*). This marrow also shows hematophagocytosis (*arrowhead*), another typical feature of the accelerated phase of Chédiak-Higashi syndrome.

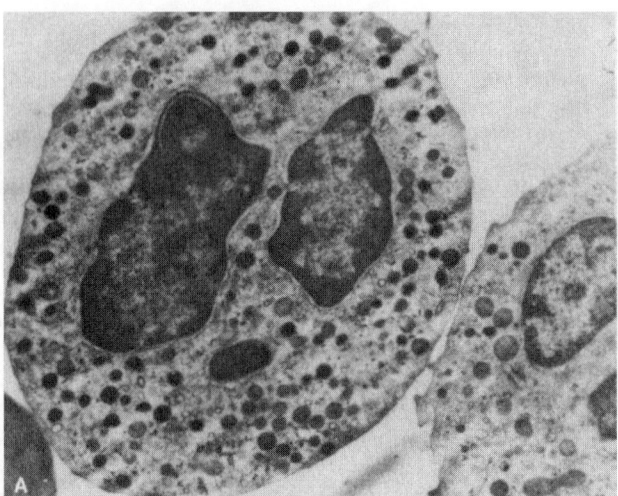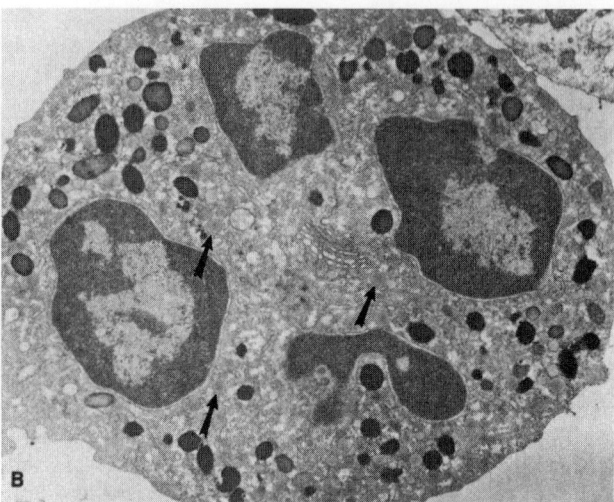

Figure 16-11. Electron micrographs of neutrophils from a patient with specific granule deficiency (**A**) and a normal patient (**B**). Darkly stained azurophil granules are present in both neutrophil profiles, but smaller, lighter-staining specific granules (*arrows*) are seen only in the normal cell.

pools of these components normally found in the specific granule membranes are also missing from these cells.

The term *specific granule deficiency* is somewhat of a misnomer, because several other structures are also involved. In the azurophil granules, complex carbohydrates stain abnormally, and the defensins, a group of potent antimicrobial peptides restricted to the azurophil granules, are completely absent, although MPO appears to be normal. Nuclei are abnormal in shape, frequently bilobed (pseudo–Pelger-Huët), with redundant membranes (Fig. 16-12). Finally, leukocyte alkaline phosphatase activity is absent from the plasma membrane. These findings suggest that inherited specific granule deficiency actually represents a general defect in membrane biosynthesis that affects all the membranes of the neutrophil.

The biochemical deficiencies in inherited specific granule deficiency result in characteristic abnormalities in neutrophil function. Chemotaxis is abnormal (158), possibly because of defects in neutrophil adherence and chemotactic sensing due to the failure of the defective neutrophils to up-regulate CD11/CD18 adherence proteins and chemotactic receptors on activation. In contrast, no consistent abnormality in O_2^- production has been demonstrated, and MPO levels are normal. Bacterial

killing (*S. aureus, Escherichia coli*), however, is depressed in specific granule–deficient neutrophils despite the presence of normal oxidative killing mechanisms, probably because of the lack of defensins in these cells.

Inherited specific granule deficiency is rare, having been reported in only five patients to date. Genetic transmission appears to occur by an autosomal-recessive mechanism. A clue as to the gene that might be defective in specific granule deficiency was provided by the finding that specific granule proteins were missing in a knock-out mouse lacking the CCAAT/enhancer binding protein epsilon (C/EBPε) (159). Pursuing this lead, the C/EBPε-containing region of the genome of a patient with specific granule deficiency was sequenced and was found to contain a deletion in exon 2. Therefore, in this patient, and perhaps in others, specific granule deficiency is caused by an abnormality in C/EBPε.

As with other inherited disorders of neutrophils, patients with specific granule deficiency show a marked susceptibility to recurrent bacterial infections involving the skin, subcutaneous tissues, and upper and lower respiratory tracts. *S. aureus* is the most common infecting organism, but enterobacterial and candidal infections have also been seen. In the appropriate clinical setting, the diagnosis of inherited specific granule deficiency is suggested by neutrophils that appear agranular under the microscope (Wright's stain normally reveals specific but not azurophil granules), with bilobed nuclei. The cells stain normally for MPO, but leukocyte alkaline phosphatase is usually low. If necessary, the diagnosis of specific granule deficiency can be established definitively either by demonstrating that the neutrophils are deficient in a specific granule component (lactoferrin or cobalamin-binding protein) or by showing through electron microscopy that the specific granules are missing from the neutrophils. Management involves vigorous antibiotic treatment of infections, with drainage of abscesses as necessary. Prophylactic antibiotics may be useful in this condition, as they are in other abnormalities of neutrophil function. With proper treatment, the prognosis of inherited specific granule deficiency is good.

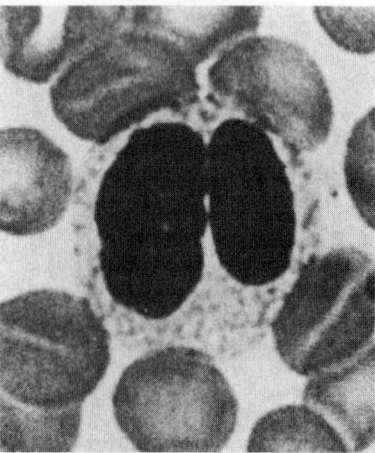

Figure 16-12. A specific granule–deficient neutrophil, showing its abnormal nucleus. The nucleus is much larger than normal, bilobed, and highly atypical in appearance.

ACQUIRED

Acquired specific granule deficiency has been reported in neonates (158) and in burned patients (160). In the latter group, the deficiency may reflect the presence in the circulation of neutrophils that have undergone partial degranulation in response to the thermal injury. Neutrophils from both groups show decreased chemotaxis. Acquired specific granule deficiency is also seen in patients with certain stem cell disorders. This is discussed later.

GRANULE-INDEPENDENT SECRETION

In addition to secreting substances produced at an earlier time and stored in secretory granules until needed, phagocytes are also able to secrete freshly synthesized materials. These materials include a large number of proteins, an array of lipid mediators, and a group of low-molecular-weight oxygen- and nitrogen-containing compounds, some of which are used as microbicidal agents. Some of these materials exert their effects only in the immediate vicinity of the secreting cell, whereas others are distributed throughout the tissues by the circulation and operate far from their site of production.

Proteins

Newly synthesized proteins are secreted by both neutrophils and MNPs, usually in response to stimulation by an external agent. MNPs secrete a remarkable number of peptides with diverse functions, most related to aspects of host defense and inflammation (Table 16-1). Neutrophils are generally thought to have little capacity for protein synthesis, but recent work has shown that these cells too are able to manufacture and secrete certain proteins when the need arises.

MONONUCLEAR PHAGOCYTES

Cytokines. Cytokines are intercellular messengers that coordinate the host response to infection or injury. They are released in small amounts by cells that participate in this response (e.g., inflammatory cells, endothelial cells, fibroblasts), then they bind to specific receptors on target cells (often including the secreting cells themselves) and instruct these cells to alter their growth and function. At last count, the cytokines numbered over three dozen, each produced by many types of cells and each binding to many kinds of targets. Moreover, many different cytokines are generated by each type of producer cell, whereas each target cell responds to many different cytokines, each of which affects the target's response to all the others. It is clear that the cytokines, with their array of producer and target cells, form a regulatory network of fantastic intricacy and complexity.

A large number of the cytokines are produced by MNPs. As a rule, these cells generate the cytokines only after stimulation, either by direct interaction with a T cell during antigen presentation (discussed later) or by exposure to cytokines secreted by other cells (e.g., the T-lymphocyte product IFN-γ, usually in the presence of LPS). The cytokines known to be produced by MNPs are listed in Table 16-1. A few deserve special mention.

Interleukin-1 and Tumor Necrosis Factor. IL-1 and TNF, both 17 kd, are regarded as the major proinflammatory peptides released by MNPs. IL-1, originally known as *leukocyte pyrogen*, consists of two 17-kd peptides, designated IL-1α and IL-1β, with considerable sequence homology and similar actions (161,162). TNF was initially recognized for two of its activities: its ability to cause certain malignancies to undergo hemorrhagic necrosis and its role in the pathogenesis of wasting in trypanosome-infected mice.

TABLE 16-8. Some Actions of Interleukin-1 and Tumor Necrosis Factor

IL-1
  Central nervous system
    Pyrogenic
    Induces slow-wave sleep
    Suppresses appetite
  Liver: acute-phase response
  Fat and muscle: induces catabolic state
  Endothelial cells: induces procoagulant state (tissue factor, plasminogen-activator inhibitor)
  Lymphocytes: activates IL-2 production and expression of IL-2 receptors
  Endocrine system: stresses hormone response (secretion of endorphins, corticotropin-releasing factor, ACTH, somatostatin)
Tumor necrosis factor
  Central nervous system
    Pyrogenic
    Suppresses appetite
  Liver: acute-phase response
  Fat: induces catabolic state[a]
  Bone and cartilage: promotes resorption[a]
  Endothelial cells
    Stimulates IL-1 production
    Induces procoagulant state[a]
  Increases surface adhesion proteins (integrins)[a]
  Phagocytes: causes general increase in PMN and monocyte and macrophage activity (adhesion, phagocytosis, respiratory burst)
  Bone marrow: a cause of the anemia of chronic disease (suppresses erythropoiesis, shortens red blood cell lifespan)
  Miscellaneous
    Kills tumor cells with fragmentation of DNA (apoptosis)
    Causes hypotension and capillary leak (responsible for many of the manifestations of endotoxin shock)[a]
    No effect on lymphocytes

ACTH, adrenocorticotropic hormone; IL, interleukin; PMN, polymorphonuclear leukocyte.
[a]Potentiated by IL-1.

Both IL-1 and TNF are produced by MNPs in response to stimulation by endotoxin or IFN-γ (163). In combination, endotoxin and IFN-γ act synergistically to amplify cytokine production. Corticosteroids antagonize the effects of endotoxin and IFN-γ on MNPs, suppressing the production of both cytokines. IL-1 production is also stimulated by phagocytosis, leukotrienes, C5a, and GM-CSF, whereas TNF production is stimulated by the combination of GM-CSF and IL-3, but not by either agent acting individually. Finally, IL-1 and TNF each stimulate the production of the other.

Extensive studies of both IL-1 and TNF have shown them to have similar effects on a wide variety of cells and tissues. A partial list of these effects is given in Table 16-8. It is evident from this list that the actions of these two cytokines are responsible for many of the systemic manifestations of inflammation. In particular, TNF appears to be largely responsible for septic shock, the systemic catastrophe that accompanies massive endotoxemia.

Colony-Stimulating Factors. The CSFs are a group of peptide hormones that are necessary for the production of neutrophils and MNPs. These factors include IL-3 and GM-CSF, which stimulate the growth and differentiation of early hematopoietic precursors, and G-CSF and M-CSF, which act on hematopoietic precursors that are already committed to the phagocyte lineage, directing them to differentiate into neutrophils and monocytes, respectively. Of these four CSFs, all but IL-3 are made by MNPs (164). For the production of G-CSF and GM-CSF, the MNPs must be stimulated by other cytokines (IL-3, IFN-γ) or by endotoxin; M-CSF, however, is made by unstimulated MNPs, although its production is increased when the cells are exposed to cytokines (e.g., IL-3).

In addition to influencing cell proliferation and differentiation, the CSFs exert many effects on the function and behavior of mature phagocytes. These effects are discussed elsewhere in the chapter.

Tissue Factor. MNPs make a number of procoagulant proteins. Of these, the most important is tissue factor (165). Unlike the other proteins discussed in this section, tissue factor is not a secreted protein but rather is associated with the cell surface, where its active site faces the exterior. Here, tissue factor accelerates clotting by binding factor VII to its active site to form a tissue factor–factor VII complex that is much more effective than free factor VII as an activator of factor X.

Tissue factor is found in both monocytes and macrophages. On the surface of unstimulated MNPs, it is detectable in only small amounts, but its surface expression increases sharply over a few hours when the phagocytes are activated by exposure to IFN-γ plus LPS, to TNF (166), or to 12-hydroxyeicosatetraenoic acid (12-HETE), which is released by activated platelets (167). Much of the coagulation that occurs in regions of inflammation may be due to the increased surface tissue factor activity of MNPs activated by cytokines released into the inflamed tissues. The hypercoagulable state seen in patients with inflammatory diseases may be attributable in part to the same cause.

Complement Components. MNPs are important sources of early complement components. Components C2 through C5 are manufactured by MNPs, as are the specific alternative pathway components factor B, factor D, and properdin. Factors H and I, which together greatly accelerate the destruction of component C3b, are also produced by MNPs. The production of some of these factors is augmented by exposure of the cells to endotoxin. IFN-γ also augments the secretion of complement components by MNPs (168).

Proteases and Protease Antagonists. MNPs synthesize a variety of proteases and antiproteases that participate in the demolition necessary for tissue repair at inflammatory sites. These include elastase and collagenase, which degrade connective tissue, and tissue plasminogen activator (169), which binds to the fibrin in a thrombus and there initiates lysis of the thrombus by activating the fibrin-splitting enzyme plasmin. Antagonists of these proteases are also manufactured by MNPs. Among these antagonists are α_1-antiproteinase and β_2-macroglobulin, which inactivate serine proteases such as phagocyte elastase; a collagenase inhibitor; and inhibitors of fibrinolysis, including plasminogen-activator inhibitor and α_2-antiplasmin. α_2-Antiplasmin is a powerful, specific, and rapidly acting inactivator of circulating plasmin that has relatively little effect on fibrin-bound plasmin (170). Deficiency of plasminogen-activator inhibitor leads to a hypercoagulable state, whereas α_2-Antiplasmin deficiency results in a severe bleeding disorder in which all the usual coagulation screening tests are normal.

Lysozyme. Lysozyme, whose properties were discussed previously, is secreted continuously by MNPs. Its rate of secretion remains invariant regardless of whether the phagocytes have been exposed to cytokines, LPS, or other modifying influences. Lysozyme is able to destroy bacteria, sometimes as a single agent but more often in concert with antimicrobial oxidants of phagocytic origin. The steady release of lysozyme into the tissues thus provides extracellular fluids with a certain degree of intrinsic antimicrobial activity.

NEUTROPHILS

Neutrophils also secrete newly synthesized proteins into the surrounding medium, but to a much smaller extent than MNPs. In response to stimuli present at an inflamed site, neutrophils manufacture and secrete cytokines that further influence the nature of the inflammatory and repair processes occurring at that site. Activated neutrophils also secrete fibronectin (171). Further investigations have revealed other proteins that are secreted by neutrophils under appropriate circumstances (172).

Lipid Agonists. Phagocytes secrete lipid agonists that can exert powerful effects on surrounding cells. These lipid agonists include leukotrienes, prostaglandins, thromboxanes, and PAF. All are derived from arachidonic acid except PAF, which is generated from a phospholipid.

Leukotrienes. Leukotrienes are the principal arachidonate-derived inflammatory mediators manufactured by phagocytes (173). Their production begins with the phospholipase A_2–catalyzed release of arachidonic acid from a phospholipid (a phosphatidylcholine or phosphatidylinositol) in response to a stimulus that raises the intracellular concentration of Ca^{2+}, a cofactor for the phospholipase. Commitment to the leukotriene pathway occurs with the 5-lipoxygenase–catalyzed conversion of the arachidonate to leukotriene A_4 (LTA_4), an oxidation in which the double bonds of the arachidonate are shifted and a 5,6-epoxide group is introduced into the molecule (Fig. 16-13). Activation of the 5-lipoxygenase is associated with its translocation from the cytosol to the plasma membrane and requires a cofactor protein of 18 kd (174). The unstable LTA_4 is then rapidly converted into the inflammatory mediators: LTB_4, an agent with powerful pleiotropic effects on the phagocytes; and the cysteine-containing leukotrienes LTC_4, LTD_4, and LTE_4, which permeate small blood vessels and cause protracted spasms of the bronchi, arterioles, and intestine through their agonist effect on smooth muscle, but do little to phagocytes. LTB_4 is produced through the action of an epoxide hydrolase (175), which opens the epoxide ring and places a hydroxyl group at the 12 position of the molecule, whereas LTC_4 is generated by the alkylation of LTA_4 at its epoxide group by glutathione, and LTD_4 and LTE_4 are produced by the successive removal of glutamic acid and glycine from the glutathione of LTC_4. Cytochrome P-450$_{LTB}$ of neutrophils oxidizes 12-HETE to 12,20-diHETE and then further to the inactive 12-HETE-1,20-dioic acid. Conversely, the phagocyte product 5-HETE is converted by platelets to 5,12-diHETE. Pulmonary epithelial cells release arachidonic acid, which is converted by alveolar macrophages to LTB_4 (176), whereas neutrophils feed LTA_4 to pulmonary tissues, which convert it to LTB_4, 20-OH LTB_4, and the cysteine leukotrienes LTC_4, LTD_4, and LTE_4. It is likely that increasing numbers of these transcellular interactions will be recognized as more is learned about these lipid mediators.

Other Arachidonate-Derived Agonists. Other arachidonate-derived agonists manufactured by phagocytes include prostaglandins, which increase intracellular cyclic adenosine monophosphate levels in many tissues by activating membrane adenylate cyclase, and thromboxanes, which act on platelets to promote thromboxane A_2 (TxA_2) or inhibit prostacyclin aggregation (177). Prostaglandin E_2 (PGE_2) is released in large amounts by macrophages in response to many kinds of stimuli:

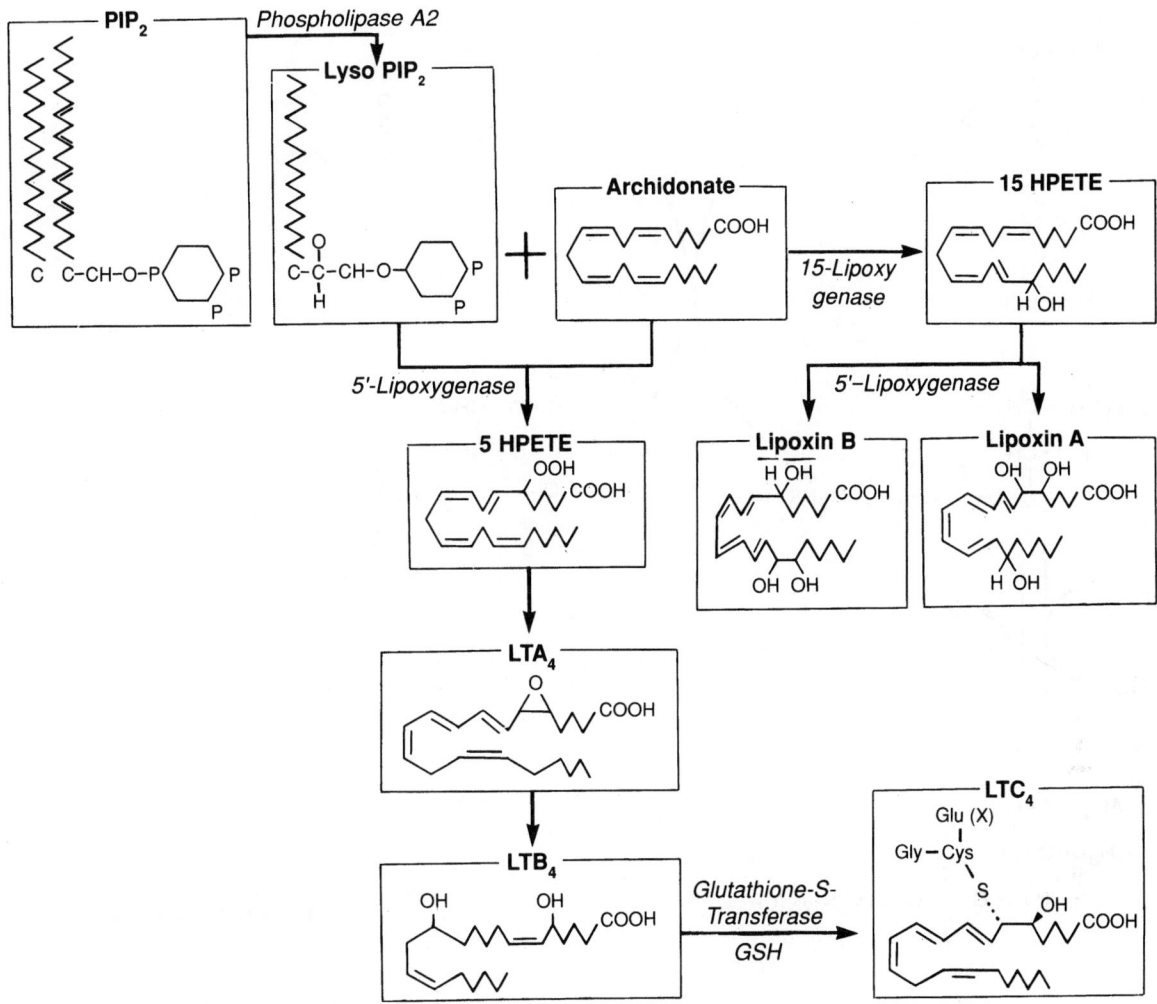

Figure 16-13. Biosynthesis of the leukotrienes. GSH, reduced glutathione; HPETE, hydroperoxyeicosatet-raenoic acid; LTA$_4$, leukotriene A$_4$; LTB$_4$, leukotriene B$_4$; LTC$_4$, leukotriene C$_4$; PIP$_2$, phosphoinositide phosphatidylinositol-4,5-bisphosphate.

- Opsonized zymosan
- Unopsonized zymosan (through the α-glucan receptor)
- Endotoxin (LPS)
- IL-1
- C3b
- Late complement components
- PAF
- Immune complexes

The production of PGE$_2$ is suppressed, however, by exposure of the macrophage to IFN-γ, perhaps a result of the maturation of the macrophage into an epithelioid-like cell under the influence of the cytokine. Most of the agents that elicit PGE$_2$ formation also stimulate macrophages to produce TxA$_2$ (detected as its footprint, TxB$_2$) (178). TxA$_2$ is also manufactured by neutrophils; its production in these cells does not require the activity of the O$_2^-$-forming respiratory burst oxidase. Prostacyclin (detected as 6-ketoPGF$_1$α) is also formed by macrophages under certain circumstances (179).

Platelet-Activating Factor. Another lipid mediator of inflammation is PAF. An exceedingly powerful inflammatory agonist, PAF exerts major effects on a variety of cells and tissues. Its potency is such that, when given intravenously to baboons in

submilligram quantities, it is able to cause an immediate and highly lethal anaphylactic reaction (180).

PAF is 1-O-alkyl-2-acetylglycero-3-phosphocholine, a phospholipid that bears a structural resemblance to the common phospholipid phosphatidylcholine. It is manufactured by both neutrophils and MNPs. In the principal route of PAF synthesis, lyso-PAF is formed by the release of arachidonate from 1-O-alkyl-2-arachidonylphosphatidylcholine, an abundant membrane lipid. The lyso-PAF is then acylated with acetyl coenzyme A to yield the final product (Fig. 16-14). The release of arachidonic acid from the alkylacylphospholipid is accomplished by means of a Ca^{2+}-activated cytosolic phospholipase A$_2$ (181), whereas the subsequent acetylation is catalyzed by a highly specific membrane-associated acetyltransferase (182).

The newly synthesized PAF is initially found in the membrane of the cell that produced it. There, it is rapidly inactivated by removal of the acetate group and reacylation with long-chain fatty acids to regenerate alkylacylphosphatidylcholine, the starting material from which PAF was originally formed. The fraction of PAF that is not inactivated is released over minutes into the extracellular medium, where it can act on other cells.

PAF is not manufactured by resting phagocytes (183) but only by phagocytes that have been suitably stimulated. A vari-

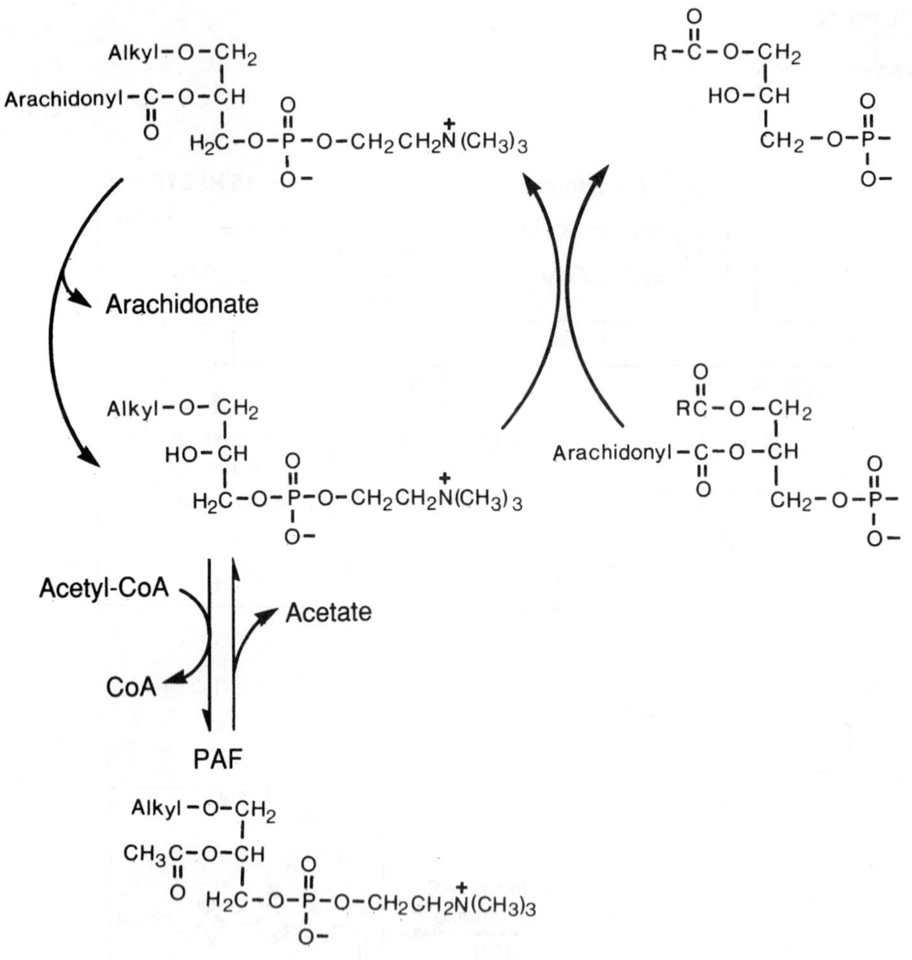

Figure 16-14. Biosynthesis of platelet-activating factor (PAF). CoA, coenzyme A.

ety of agents induce PAF production by neutrophils, including opsonized zymosan, 5-HETE, LTB_4, FMLP, C5a, TNF, and PAF. PAF production elicited by formylpeptides and C5a is greatly increased by prior exposure of the cells to GM-CSF. Agents that stimulate PAF production by MNPs include opsonized zymosan and TNF. PAF production in stimulated phagocytes appears to result from a rapid increase in acetyltransferase activity (184), combined with a decrease in the activity of acetylhydrolase, the enzyme that converts PAF to lyso-PAF. Synthesis of PAF declines greatly as monocytes mature into macrophages, a feature ascribed to an increase in acetylhydrolase that occurs during the monocyte-to-macrophage transition (184). As with leukotrienes, the biosynthesis of PAF is suppressed in subjects on diets containing large amounts of eicosapentaenoic acid. PAF has significant effects on phagocytes, binding to specific receptors to stimulate many functions directly and priming the cells for augmented responses to other stimuli (185). The ability of PAF to stimulate its own synthesis lends a self-reinforcing character to inflammatory processes in which this mediator is released.

MICROBICIDAL OXIDANT PRODUCTION AND THE RESPIRATORY BURST

When exposed to appropriate stimuli, most phagocytes change their pattern of oxygen metabolism, increasing their oxygen uptake sharply and at the same time releasing large amounts of superoxide (O_2^-) and hydrogen peroxide (H_2O_2)

into their environment. This change in oxygen metabolism, which usually lasts from a few seconds to 10 to 15 minutes, is known as the *respiratory burst*. Its purpose is the production of microbicidal oxidants by the partial reduction of oxygen. Mature PMNs and blood monocytes constitutively express the components required to engage in the respiratory burst in response to excitation of appropriate receptors. As monocytes mature into macrophages *in vitro*, they lose the capacity to have a respiratory burst unless exposed to the cytokine IFN-γ, although Kupffer's cells do not develop a respiratory burst ability even after cultivation with IFN-γ (186). Considerable evidence indicates that the phenomenon of macrophage activation, in which these cells acquire the ability to contain or kill a variety of facultative intracellular parasites, depends on this development of a respiratory burst in response to IFN-γ.

Oxidase activity begins to decline, however, even with continued exposure to the activating agent, until, by 1 week, the cells are no longer able to express a respiratory burst. In other respects, however, the macrophages are, at this point, highly activated and well on their way to the epithelioid state. Macrophages are thus only transiently capable of expressing a respiratory burst, with oxidase activity appearing and disappearing during the first week of activation.

Respiratory Burst Oxidase

The key reaction of the respiratory burst is the one-electron reduction of oxygen to O_2^- at the expense of NADPH (187):

$$2O_2 + NADPH \rightarrow 2\,O_2^- + NADPH^+ + H^+$$

The O_2^- produced in this reaction serves as the precursor of a group of powerful microbicidal oxidants that are deployed by the phagocyte as microbicidal agents, whereas the $NADP^+$ is reconverted to NADPH by glucose-6-phosphate dehydrogenase (G6PD) and 6-phosphogluconate dehydrogenase, the first two enzymes of the hexosemonophosphate shunt.

The reduction of oxygen to O_2^- is catalyzed by a membrane-bound enzyme known as the *NADPH oxidase*. This enzyme is dormant in resting cells but acquires catalytic activity when the cells are exposed to certain activating agents. A wide variety of agents are able to activate the oxidase, including particulate (e.g., opsonized bacteria) and soluble stimuli [e.g., C5a or the formylated peptide intermediates of bacterial protein synthesis (188)]. With agents whose association with the phagocyte can be reversed (e.g., F^-, or N-formylpeptides), oxidase activation may also be reversed, the enzyme returning to the dormant state on removal of the activating agent. With other activators, especially particulate agents, activation is irreversible; oxidase activated by these agents continues to manufacture O_2^- until the enzyme is eventually destroyed by its own products.

The activation of the oxidase involves an assembly of components (189). The electron transporting oxidase is cytochrome b_{558}, a membrane-associated heterodimer containing a 91-kd and a 22-kd polypeptide. The 91-kd polypeptide binds heme and flavin adenine dinucleotide. Its activity requires its binding to a number of molecules that become membrane-attached after activation. These molecules include two cytosolic proteins, p47^{PHOX} and p67^{PHOX}, and two small GTPases, Rac 2 (cytosolic) and Rap 1A (membrane-bound). During activation, Rap 1A exchanges a bound GDP for GTP, and Rac 2 dissociates from an inhibitor guanine nucleotide dissociation inhibitor and also exchanges bound GDP for GTP. Posttranslationally added isoprenyl groups are involved in the membrane binding of the two GTPases. In cells containing a competent oxidase, O_2^- production is stimulated by a broad range of agents. Those that evoke the largest O_2^- responses are particulate stimuli such as opsonized bacteria and opsonized yeast cell walls. Soluble stimuli such as immune complexes, C5a, N-formylated peptides, and LTB$_4$ also elicit O_2^- production, but generally for a much shorter period of time than the particulate stimuli. Neutrophils incubated with a substimulatory concentration of a soluble stimulus, however, produce much more O_2^- than usual when previously primed (i.e., previously exposed to a subactivating concentration of a soluble stimulus).

REACTIVE OXIDANTS

The O_2^- produced in the respiratory burst has little antimicrobial activity of its own, although it can break down iron-sulfur clusters (190). Rather, it is the precursor of a complex battery of reactive oxidants that together represent the real microbicidal oxidizing power of the phagocyte. These reactive oxidants fall into three groups: the oxidized halogens, the oxidizing radicals, and singlet oxygen.

The production of all three groups of microbicidal oxidants begins with the dismutation of O_2^- to oxygen and H_2O_2:

$$2O_2^- \rightarrow O_2 + H_2O_2$$

Oxidized halogen production is then initiated by the H_2O_2-mediated oxidation of Cl^- to hypochlorite (OCl^-), a reaction catalyzed by MPO (described previously) (191):

$$H_2O_2 + Cl^- \overset{MPO}{\rightarrow} OCl^- + H_2O$$

OCl^- itself is a powerful microbicidal agent. It also reacts with the many amines that occur in biologic systems, producing a vast number of chloramines:

$$OCL^- + R\text{-}NH_2 \rightarrow R\text{-}NHCl + OH^-$$

$$OCl^- + R\text{-}NHCl \rightarrow R\text{-}NCl_2 + OH^-$$

Some of these chloramines, especially those that are lipid-soluble (e.g., NH_2Cl), are even more toxic than OCl^-; others such as taurine chloramine are stable and may furnish protection for the phagocyte against the potentially lethal products of its own metabolism. The reactive oxidized halogens then kill by inactivating proteins and other susceptible molecules in the target through oxidation and halogenation. Iron-sulfur proteins are particularly liable to inactivation by oxidized halogens (192).

The production of oxidizing radicals is generally ascribed to the Haber-Weiss reaction, in which a metal ion (iron or copper) catalyzes the oxidation of O_2^- by H_2O_2, yielding oxygen and hydroxyl radical ($OH\bullet$). For example:

$$O_2^- + Fe^{3+} \rightarrow O_2 + Fe^{2+}$$

$$\underline{H_2O_2 + Fe^{2+} \rightarrow OH\bullet + Fe^{3+} + OH^-}$$

$$O_2^- + H_2O_2 \rightarrow OH\bullet + O_2 + OH^-$$

Other oxidizing radicals are manufactured by phagocytes, but radicals other than $OH\bullet$ have not been specifically identified as yet, nor have their routes of production been elucidated. The oxidizing radicals provide a backup system to the oxidized halogens, killing less rapidly but just as efficiently as the oxidized halogens. One particularly important target of hydroxyl radicals is the bases comprising DNA. Phagocyte-induced DNA damage may account in part for the association between chronic inflammation and malignancy (193).

Singlet oxygen is a form of oxygen in which its valence electrons, instead of being unpaired with parallel spins (its lowest energy state), are paired, with antiparallel spins. It is a very short-lived but highly reactive species, reacting particularly with double bonds. It is produced by the reaction of hydrogen peroxide with hypohalous acids:

$$H_2O_2 + HOCl \rightarrow singlet\ O_2 + H_2O + HCl$$

OXIDASES OF NITROGEN

It has recently become evident that reactive nitrogen compounds are important oxidants in biologic systems. These originate from nitric oxide (NO), which is produced in phagocytes by inducible NO synthase, a 130-kd enzyme that contains heme, flavin adenine dinucleotide, flavin mononucleotide, tetrahydrobiopterin, and a tightly bound molecule of calmodulin (194). The source of the NO is arginine, which is converted in an NADPH- and oxygen-dependent reaction to NO and citrulline:

$$Arginine + NADPH + O_2 \rightarrow NO + Citrulline$$

In this reaction, one of the guanidine nitrogens of arginine is converted to the nitrogen of NO. NO is generated by activated (i.e., IFN-γ–treated) MNPs, and in much smaller quantities by neutrophils (195). The production of NO by neutrophils is stimulated by several inflammatory mediators, including LTB$_4$, formylated peptides, and PAF (196).

Once formed, the NO can exert its direct biologic effects. The principal known biologic effect of NO is its well-established ability to activate guanylate cyclase (197). Its action as a vasodilator appears to be mediated through this effect. Alternatively, it can be oxidized further to NO_2^- and NO_3^-

(82). NO_2^- is potentially dangerous, because at low pH it can add to amino nitrogens to form carcinogenic nitrosamines (198); the extent to which nitrosamines formed in this way are responsible for endogenous carcinogenesis is not known. NO_3^- is excreted in the urine, and its excretion increases greatly in infection, perhaps a result of an increase in the rate of production of NO and its derivatives by macrophages activated by the cytokines (especially IFN-γ) released during infection.

A very important reaction of NO is its reaction with O_2^- (199). This extremely rapid reaction leads to the formation of peroxynitrite, which in turn is transformed to a nitrating agent of unknown character. This nitrating agent is able to convert protein-bound tyrosine to nitrotyrosine, with deleterious effects on the function of the affected protein. Better-defined nitrating agents are produced in an MPO-dependent process by the reaction of NO_2^- with HOCl, which gives rise to the nitrating agents NO_2Cl and NO_2 (200).

Antioxidant Defenses

Like other cells, phagocytes are equipped with systems that destroy the highly reactive oxidants that arise in the course of the cells' activity. These include enzymes and low-molecular-weight antioxidants.

ANTIOXIDANT ENZYMES
Phagocytes contain antioxidant enzymes that can destroy O_2^- and H_2O_2, the two compounds that together represent the ultimate source of all the microbicidal oxidants deployed in the respiratory burst.

Superoxide Dismutase. Superoxide dismutase (190) catalyzes a reaction in which one molecule of O_2^- is reduced by another, converting the two O_2^- molecules into H_2O_2 and oxygen, respectively:

$$2O_2^- + 2H^+ \rightarrow O_2 + H_2O_2$$

This enzyme is present in virtually all prokaryotic and eukaryotic cells, where it protects them from the deleterious effects of O_2^-. Its importance in antioxidant defense has been best shown in *E. coli* dismutase-less mutants, which grow poorly in the presence of oxygen and are highly susceptible to further mutation. Phagocytes, like most mammalian cells, contain two forms of the dismutase: a copper- and zinc-containing enzyme that is found in the cytosol and a manganese-containing enzyme located in the mitochondria. These enzymes protect the cells from the O_2^- routinely generated in the course of mitochondrial oxygen metabolism and from the O_2^- that leaks back into the cytoplasm during the respiratory burst. Not surprisingly, the phagosomes containing the target organisms are free of phagocyte superoxide dismutase.

Glutathione Peroxidase–Glutathione Reductase System
In this system, glutathione and the enzymes glutathione peroxidase and glutathione reductase catalyze the reduction of H_2O_2 to H_2O using NADPH as electron donor. The first step in this system is the reduction of H_2O_2 to H_2O by glutathione, a reaction catalyzed by glutathione peroxidase, a selenium-containing enzyme:

$$2GSH + H_2O_2 \xrightarrow{\text{GSH peroxidase}} GSSG + H_2O$$

where *GSH* is reduced glutathione and *GSSG* is oxidized glutathione.

In the second step, the oxidized glutathione is converted back to the reduced form by NADPH in a reaction catalyzed by glutathione peroxidase:

$$GSSG + NADPH + H^+ \xrightarrow{\text{GSH reductase}} 2GSH + NADP^+$$

Because glutathione peroxidase has a high turnover number, the glutathione peroxidase–glutathione reductase system is an efficient scavenger of H_2O_2, eliminating it even when it is present at low concentrations. Lipid hydroperoxides, readily formed in biologic systems by the autooxidation of polyunsaturated fatty acids, are detoxified by phospholipid hydroperoxide glutathione peroxidase, another selenium-containing enzyme (201):

$$2GSH + ROOH \xrightarrow{\text{GSH peroxidase}} GSSG + ROH + H_2O$$

Catalase. Catalase is a large, heme-containing protein that catalyzes the conversion of H_2O_2 to oxygen and water:

$$2H_2O_2 \rightarrow O_2 + 2H_2O$$

The enzyme is found in the cytoplasm of phagocytes and other cells. It has a high turnover number, but under the usual assay conditions, it also shows a high K_m (i.e., a low affinity) fluxes that result in high steady-state concentrations of H_2O_2. Catalase, however, possesses a tightly bound NADPH that prevents inactivation of the enzyme by H_2O_2 (202). It is therefore likely that, under physiologic conditions, catalase is able to deal effectively with H_2O_2 even at the relatively low concentrations that are likely to prevail in tissues.

A few families have been reported whose tissues contain very low levels of catalase. Members of these families show little pathology except for oral ulcerations (203). The lack of unusual susceptibility to bacterial infections in patients with acatalasemia indicates that the glutathione peroxidase–glutathione reductase system alone is sufficient to protect the phagocytes from the peroxide stress to which they are normally exposed.

Low-Molecular-Weight Antioxidants. The major low-molecular-weight oxidants found in the neutrophil are ascorbic acid, taurine, and α-tocopherol. In the form of dehydroascorbate, ascorbic acid is actively transported into the cytosol of the phagocyte, where it is found in high concentrations. It is highly effective as an antioxidant and is probably the principal scavenger of reactive radicals in the phagocyte cytosol. Taurine (204), also present in phagocytes in high concentrations, reacts readily with OCl^- to form the relatively stable taurine chloramine ($=O_3S-CH_2CH_2-NHCl$), protecting the phagocyte from the harmful effects of OCl^- and at the same time providing a relatively long-lived source of oxidized halogen.

α-Tocopherol (vitamin E) is a lipid-soluble antioxidant that is found in the organelles and plasma membranes of the phagocytes (205). It reacts rapidly with oxidizing radicals and, like ascorbate, serves as a primary radical scavenger, but in lipid rather than aqueous environments. In neonates and infants, α-tocopherol deficiency causes a hemolytic anemia that appears to arise because of oxidant damage to the red-cell membrane.

METHODS FOR MEASURING COMPONENTS OF PHAGOCYTIC OXYGEN METABOLISM
MPO activity of phagocytes is easily determined histochemically on air-dried blood smears. In the clinical laboratory, an historic test for O_2^- is a histochemical application of nitroblue tetrazolium (NBT) reduction. It has been used as a diagnostic test for CGD. A preferred test, however, is a fluorescence-activated cell sorter (FACS) test using dihydrorhodamine 123 as the fluorescent dye.

DISORDERS OF THE OXYGEN-DEPENDENT MICROBICIDAL SYSTEM

Myeloperoxidase Deficiency

MPO deficiency (19,90) is the most common inherited disorder of phagocytes. Its estimated prevalence is approximately 1 in 2000, but only a small number of MPO-deficient patients are clinically ill from the disease (206).

PATHOGENESIS

Inherited MPO deficiency has been shown to be caused by any of several mutations affecting the MPO gene. A common mutation is R569W (207). In this mutation, the genetic defect results in a posttranslational processing abnormality, because apopro-MPO is detected in the phagocytes but heme insertion, which generates pro-MPO, does not take place. In five unrelated patients, pro-MPO was detected in the phagocytes but MPO was not. Restriction maps of the MPO genes from these patients gave three different fragment patterns (208). Cells from a sixth patient contained neither MPO, pro-MPO, nor processed MPO mRNA, although unprocessed message was detected. These findings suggest the existence of at least five different kinds of genetic lesions in patients with MPO deficiency.

The deficiency of the enzyme can be partial or complete; the aggregate ratio of partial to complete deficiency in two recent series was approximately 3:1 (206). In terms of neutrophil function, MPO-deficient cells show normal phagocytosis, but the respiratory burst is significantly altered. O_2^- and H_2O_2 production are increased in amount and duration probably because the usual MPO-mediated inactivation of the respiratory burst oxidase is retarded, but OCl^- production is low to nil depending on the level of residual MPO. Killing of bacteria (*S. aureus, E. coli*) by MPO-deficient phagocytes, although significantly delayed, reaches normal values by 1 hour (207). On the other hand, certain fungi that are readily killed by normal neutrophils, such as the hyphal stages of *C. albicans* and *Aspergillus fumigatus,* are highly resistant to killing by MPO-deficient cells (209,210).

MPO deficiency can also be an acquired condition. It is a frequent accompaniment of myeloproliferative disorders (discussed later). In newborns, neutrophil MPO levels are normal at birth, fall by 75% after 1 to 2 days, then return to normal levels at 1 week (211).

CLINICAL FEATURES

Most patients with MPO deficiency suffer no ill effects from their condition. This fact attests to the redundancy of the microbicidal mechanisms of phagocytes, which include oxidizing radicals and several microbicidal proteins in addition to the MPO-dependent microbicidal agents. In those rare patients in whom MPO deficiency results in clinical disease, the most frequent manifestation has been disseminated candidiasis, usually in patients who also have diabetes mellitus (212). A few other patients have been described in whom MPO deficiency has been associated with recurrent bacterial infections, most frequently skin infections, sometimes combined with *Candida* infections of the perianal region (213). It is not known why this small minority of MPO-deficient patients is so susceptible to infections, although mixed defects in phagocyte function have been postulated.

DIAGNOSIS

The diagnosis is made by demonstrating that peroxidase in the neutrophils and monocytes is deficient or absent. This can be accomplished by a spectrophotometric assay or by staining a blood film for MPO; the latter is probably better because eosino-phil peroxidase, a distinct enzyme that is unaltered in MPO deficiency (212), can be a source of confusion in a spectrophotometric assay but does not affect an assay in which the peroxidase-positive cells are individually identified.

TREATMENT

Because MPO deficiency is a silent abnormality in most patients, treatment is usually not necessary. In those few patients with recurrent infections, management is based on the usual measures of vigorous antibiotic therapy and drainage of abscesses as indicated. If recurrent bacterial infections are a problem, prophylactic antibiotics may be tried, but these are of no value for the prevention of fungal infections. In patients with diabetes mellitus, control of blood glucose levels should be optimized.

Chronic Granulomatous Disease

CGD (214) is an inherited disorder in which phagocytes are unable to express a respiratory burst. As a result, all oxygen-dependent microbial killing is ablated, and patients suffer recurrent infections that eventually lead to chronic organ pathology and an early death.

PATHOGENESIS

CGD results when the respiratory burst oxidase or its activating apparatus is defective. Four types of CGD have been described, each caused by an abnormality affecting one of the four oxidase polypeptides identified to date. The most common type of CGD, accounting for approximately three-fourths of reported cases, is due to an abnormality involving the 91-kd subunit of the cytochrome. Phagocytes from most patients with this type lack cytochrome b_{558}. The gene encoding the 91-kd subunit is on the X chromosome, so transmission of this type of the disease is X-linked. A few patients have been described in whom the primary lesion affects the 67-kd cytosolic polypeptide or the 22-kd subunit of the cytochrome. These rare types of CGD are transmitted according to an autosomal-recessive pattern. A variety of genetic lesions are responsible for the defects in the 91-, 67-, and 22-kd genes, including deletions, missense and nonsense mutations, frameshifts, splice mutations, and mutations involving the regulatory regions. The remaining patients, amounting to approximately one-fifth of the total, lack the 47-kd protein. In these patients, the disease is inherited as an autosomal-recessive trait. This form is almost always due to a rearrangement involving the 47-kd gene and its pseudogene that results in the deletion of a GT pair from the second exon of the 47-kd gene. The various types can be classified by spectroscopy, which reveals whether or not cytochrome b_{558} is present, and immunoblotting, which shows the presence or absence of the individual subunits.

Cytochrome b_{558} is absent from neutrophils lacking the 22-kd subunit. In each of the cytochrome b_{558}–deficient types of CGD, both cytochrome subunits are missing, possibly because in the absence of one subunit the other is unstable and is destroyed by intracellular proteases. The various types of CGD are summarized in Table 16-9.

In the X chromosome, the gene encoding the 91-kd subunit is located on the short arm at Xp21.1. Nearby are other genes that, when defective, result in clinical abnormalities, and several patients have been reported with multiple diseases caused by an abnormality that simultaneously affects two or more of these genes. The most common inherited disorder associated with CGD is the McLeod phenotype, a condition that results from a deficiency of the K_x antigen, a precursor of the Kell blood group antigen family (215). K_x, encoded by a gene that is closely linked to the 91-kd gene on the X-chromosome, is normally found on

TABLE 16-9. Types of Chronic Granulomatous Disease

Mode of Inheritance	Status of Cytochrome b_{558}	Deficient Components[a]	Abnormal Gene
X-linked	Absent	p22 and gp91	gp91
X-linked	Present	gp91 (his → pro)	gp91 (missense)
Autosomal recessive	Absent	p22 and gp91	p22
Autosomal recessive	Present	p47	p47
Autosomal recessive	Present	p67	p67

[a]Cytochrome b_{558} is a membrane-associated component made up of gp91 and p22, whereas p47 and p67 are found in the cytosol; p47 is phosphorylated during oxidase activation.

the surfaces of RBCs and phagocytes but is missing from one or both in most patients with X-linked CGD. Its absence from the RBCs results in a mild hemolytic anemia. Inherited disorders less frequently combined with CGD include retinitis pigmentosa and Duchenne's muscular dystrophy. Combinations of X-linked CGD, the McLeod phenotype, and retinitis pigmentosa, with or without Duchenne's muscular dystrophy, have been reported in patients with small deletions involving the Xp21 locus (216).

The motor functions of CGD neutrophils (chemotaxis, phagocytosis, and degranulation) are normal. Respiratory burst activity, however, is grossly deficient, whether determined as O_2^- production, H_2O_2 production, or oxygen uptake, and whether measured in neutrophils, monocytes, or eosinophils. Because they are unable to produce microbicidal oxidants, neutrophils from patients with CGD have great difficulty killing most species of bacteria, including *S. aureus* and *Enterobacteriaceae* spp. Fungal killing is also defective. CGD neutrophils, however, have no problem with catalaseless organisms such as *S. pneumoniae* and *S. pyogenes*, in part perhaps because these bacteria excrete H_2O_2 into the surrounding medium, thereby providing the defective neutrophils with the OCl⁻ precursor they cannot produce.

CLINICAL FEATURES

Recurrent infection beginning in infancy is the major clinical manifestation of CGD (217), although in mild cases, the presentation may be delayed until adolescence or even adulthood (218,219). Infections usually take the form of abscesses involving deep subcutaneous tissues, lymph nodes, or liver or serious respiratory tract infections involving the sinuses or lungs. They are long-lasting and respond only sluggishly to antibiotic therapy. Because these repeated infections lead to chronic activation of the immune system, most patients with CGD also manifest generalized lymphadenopathy, sometimes prominent, as well as enlarged livers and spleens.

The organism found most frequently in these infections is *S. aureus*, but infections due to certain fungi, especially *Aspergillus*, are very common. By far, the most common cause of pneumonia in CGD is *Aspergillus* spp. Infections with unusual microorganisms, however, are also to be expected. In particular, *Burkholderia cepacia* infections, rare under other circumstances, are frequent causes of death in CGD, perhaps because this species may be unusually resistant to the anaerobic mechanisms that represent the residual microbicidal capacity of CGD phagocytes. *A. nidulans* is particularly virulent in patients with CGD, but rarely infects normal patients. Mycobacterial infections also occur at a greater-than-normal frequency, and death at an early age from miliary tuberculosis has been described. On the other hand, infections with streptococci (including pneumococci) are

not a problem, a clinical reflection of the ability of CGD cells to kill bacteria of this genus.

In addition to abscesses and other acute infections, patients with CGD also develop chronic inflammatory processes, probably the result of granulomatous reactions and fibrosis in the neighborhood of imperfectly suppressed infections. These inflammatory processes may lead to masses and strictures affecting a variety of hollow organs, including the stomach, intestine, ureter, and bladder (Fig. 16-15). Recurrent vomiting may suggest gastric obstruction, whereas a patient with obstruction of the urogenital tract may present with symptoms of chronic cystitis or pyelonephritis. Intractable chronic pulmonary inflammation, through bronchiectasis and emphysema, leads to the eventual destruction of the lung. With the recent practice of treating these patients with prophylactic antibiotics, these chronic processes have become more common. In addition, *Aspergillus* spp. pneumonia has become a frequent cause of death in these patients as their incidence of acute bacterial infections has declined.

DIAGNOSIS

The diagnosis of CGD is usually made by FACS using dihydrorhodamine 123, a nonfluorescent dye that is oxidized to the fluorescent rhodamine 123 by cells expressing a respiratory burst. Because they make little or no oxidants, CGD cells produce little to no fluorescence from dihydrorhodamine 123. The diagnosis may also be made by means of the NBT test (220), in which neutrophils are incubated with an activating agent in the presence of NBT, a yellow, water-soluble dye. The O_2^- liberated from the activated neutrophils reduces the dye to an insoluble, dark blue formazan that is deposited on the activated cells as a granular precipitate, easily seen under the microscope (Fig. 16-16A). Because they are unable to manufacture O_2^-, neutrophils from patients with CGD form no formazan precipitate when activated in the presence of NBT (Fig. 16-16B). Appropriate radiologic examinations are used to identify the abscesses and obstructive complications that occur frequently in patients with CGD.

Female carriers of the X-linked type of CGD can be identified by either FACS or the NBT test. Because of random X-chromosome inactivation, the gene encoding the normal 91-kd subunit is expressed in approximately half of the neutrophils of such a carrier, whereas the gene encoding the defective subunit is expressed in the remainder of the cells. Therefore, the dihydrorhodamine test and the NBT test show two populations of neutrophils in a carrier of X-linked CGD: a normal population that reduces oxidized dihydrorhodamine or reduces NBT, and an abnormal population that does not (the NBT test is shown in Fig. 16-16C).

Prenatal diagnosis can be made by performing an NBT test on blood obtained at fetoscopy (221). It is necessary to wait until the 18th week of pregnancy to obtain fetal blood by this procedure, which carries a small but distinct risk of fetal loss. A pair of single nucleotide polymorphisms (222), a restriction fragment length polymorphism, or a polymorphic repeat within the 91-kd gene (223) allows prenatal diagnosis to be made by restriction mapping of fetal DNA obtained by the much less hazardous procedure of amniocentesis.

A second condition in which the respiratory burst may be impaired enough to affect microbial killing is severe G6PD deficiency. A few patients with G6PD deficiency have displayed a CGD-like picture, presenting with recurrent bacterial infections and a greatly diminished respiratory burst (224). It is likely that, in the neutrophils of these patients, G6PD levels were so low that NADPH production was severely curtailed, leading to a failure of O_2^- generation because of a deficiency of reducing agent. The clue that the disease responsible for the recurrent infections in this group of patients was something other than CGD was the simultaneous existence in each of the patients of a

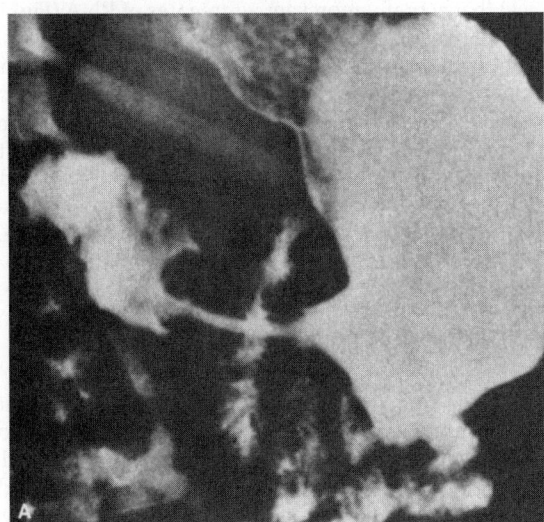
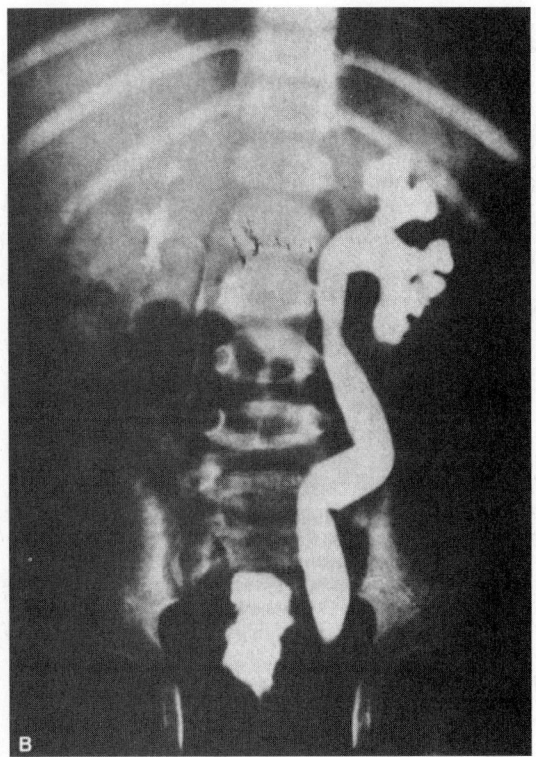

Figure 16-15. Some complications of chronic granulomatous disease (CGD). **A:** Gastric antral lesion. Characteristic roentgenographic appearance of the gastric antral lesion in a 4-year-old boy with X-linked CGD who presented with persistent vomiting. A concentric prepyloric narrowing was associated with delayed gastric emptying. Biopsy of the lesion revealed granulomatous inflammation. Cultures for bacteria and fungi were negative. The patient was managed conservatively with small frequent feedings. The lesion spontaneously improved over 1 year. **B:** Obstructive uropathy. Intravenous pyelogram of a boy with X-linked CGD demonstrating hydronephrosis and hydroureter on the left side. The obstruction was due to compression by a large inflammatory mass in the pelvis between the rectum and the bladder.

hemolytic anemia, a feature that is typical of G6PD deficiency but not of CGD. The diagnosis is easily made by measuring red-cell G6PD levels.

Recently, a third condition in which the respiratory burst is defective has been described (109). Neutrophils from the affected patient showed a complex mixture of defects involving migration, phagocytosis, and degranulation, as well as the respiratory burst defect. The molecular abnormality was a dominant negative mutation of Rac2 that interfered with the normal function of Rac2 in the activation of the respiratory burst.

TREATMENT

As with other disorders of phagocyte function, the treatment of CGD mainly involves the prevention and treatment of the infections that complicate the disorder. Prophylactic antibiotics have been shown to reduce inpatient days and prolong life expectancy in patients with CGD (225) and are used routinely in this and other disorders of phagocyte function. The usual program is similar to that used for Chédiak-Higashi syndrome: trimethoprim, 160 mg/day, plus sulfamethoxazole, 800 mg/day, with a reduced dose for children; or, for patients allergic to sulfonamides or trimethoprim, dicloxacillin, 500 mg (250 mg for children) twice daily. Itroconazole as prophylactic against fungal infections is currently under study in the United States and has been used with success in England. When infections occur, vigorous therapy must be applied using large doses of appropriate antibiotics. Surgery may be required to drain collections. Although relief of obstructions may require surgery, such obstructions may gradually resolve under long-term antibiotic therapy to treat the underlying infection, plus or minus steroids;

the choice between medical and surgical therapy for such a complication can be difficult. Granulocyte transfusions have been used as adjunct therapy, but with equivocal results (226). Bone marrow transplantation has cured some patients with CGD, but some patients have died as a result of the procedure (227).

A multicenter, placebo-controlled, clinical trial of 128 patients with X-linked or autosomal CGD led to the conclusion that recombinant IFN-γ, 50 μg/m² subcutaneously three times per week, was well tolerated and reduced the number of serious infections by approximately half. Despite the clinical benefits, none of the IFN-treated patients' phagocytes showed any improvement in respiratory activity (228). Newer modes of antimicrobial prophylaxis may reduce the need for IFN-γ in CGD patients.

Miscellaneous Granulocyte Abnormalities

MORPHOLOGIC VARIANTS

Inherited. There are a few inherited conditions in which normally functioning neutrophils show well-defined morphologic abnormalities.

Pelger-Huët Anomaly. The Pelger-Huët anomaly is an inherited trait in which the nuclei in most neutrophils of heterozygotes are hyposegmented, having only one or two lobes instead of the usual three to five (229). In Pelger-Huët homozygotes, neutrophil nuclei are uniformly unsegmented (230) (Fig. 16-17A). The incidence of this trait has been estimated at 1 in 5000. Pelger-Huët neutrophils are normal in size and show fully

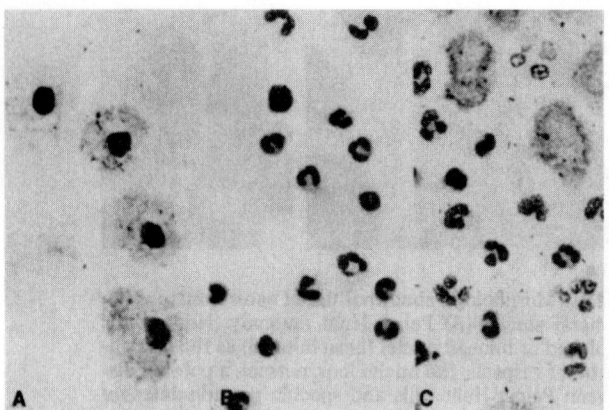

Figure 16-16. Nitroblue tetrazolium (NBT) test for the diagnosis of chronic granulomatous disease (CGD). A drop of blood is placed on an endotoxin-coated coverslip and incubated to allow the granulocytes and monocytes to adhere to the glass surface. The coverslip is then incubated with a solution of serum and NBT dye, then washed, fixed, counterstained, and mounted. **A:** Normal control. All the neutrophils are NBT-positive, appearing as large, exploded cells with cytoplasm stained blue by reduced NBT. **B:** Patient with CGD. All the neutrophils are NBT-negative. They retain their typical morphologic appearance and show no blue (reduced) dye. **C:** Carrier of CGD. Two populations of cells coexist, one NBT-positive and the other NBT-negative.

condensed chromatin, features that serve to distinguish them from normal neutrophil precursors such as myelocytes and metamyelocytes. The function of Pelger-Huët neutrophils is entirely normal, and the trait is of no clinical significance.

An acquired Pelger-Huët anomaly, usually termed *pseudo–Pelger-Huët*, has been reported in a remarkably large number of conditions. Most frequently seen in disorders of myeloid stem

cells (231), it has also been described *inter alia* in infections such as tuberculosis, mycoplasma pneumonia, allergic reactions, and lymphoid malignancies.

May-Hegglin Anomaly. The May-Hegglin anomaly is a rare but dominantly inherited trait affecting neutrophils and platelets. On a Wright-stained blood film, most of the neutrophils are seen to contain small homogeneous blue inclusions (Döhle bodies) that actually represent aggregates of RNA (Fig. 16-17B). The platelets are abnormally large (as large as in Bernard-Soulier syndrome) and hypogranular, the platelet counts are low, and platelet survival is shortened by approximately half (232). In approximately half of cases, the May-Hegglin anomaly is associated with a bleeding disorder, usually mild (epistaxis, bruising) (116) but sometimes more serious. The bleeding time is prolonged to a value consistent with the reduced platelet count, but platelet function studies have been variable. The May-Hegglin anomaly has also been reported in a few patients with hereditary nephritis (Alport's syndrome) (233); the term *Fechtner's syndrome* has been used to refer to this combination of Alport's nephritis and May-Hegglin anomaly.

Alder-Reilly Anomaly. Alder-Reilly bodies are deeply basophilic granules that are sometimes seen in neutrophils from patients with disorders of mucopolysaccharide degradation (e.g., Hunter's, Hurler's, and Maroteaux-Lamy syndromes; Fig. 16-17C). These granules may also be present in lymphocytes and monocytes. Although often absent from circulating leukocytes, Alder-Reilly bodies can usually be found in the marrow, where they appear as darkly staining granules in mononuclear cells (Buhot cells). Alder-Reilly bodies appear to be lysosomes that stain abnormally due to their content of incompletely degraded mucopolysaccharides.

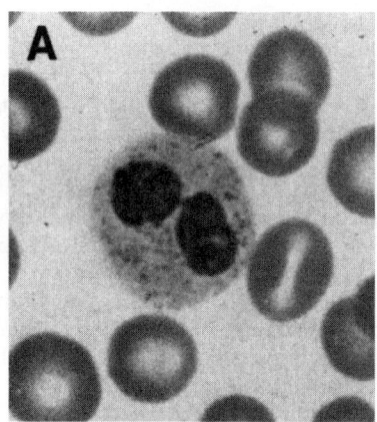
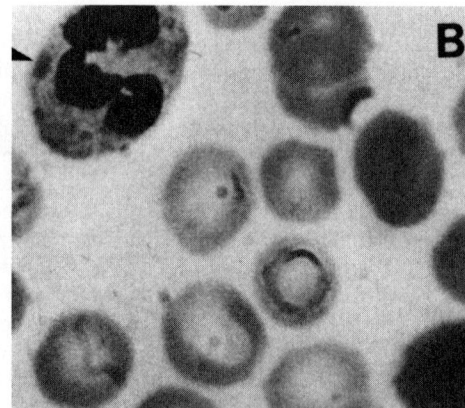
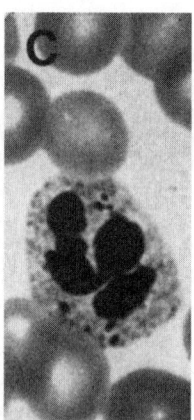
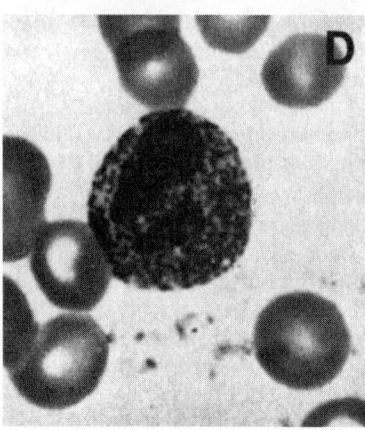

Figure 16-17. Morphologic abnormalities of neutrophils as seen on the peripheral smear. **A:** Pelger-Huët anomaly. Neutrophils contain monolobed or bilobed nuclei (here bilobed) as the sole abnormality. In other respects, the nuclei look normal, a point of distinction between Pelger-Huët cells and specific granule–deficient neutrophils. **B:** May-Hegglin anomaly. Masses of pale blue–staining RNA, known as *Döhle bodies,* are present in the neutrophil cytoplasm (*arrow*). A giant platelet, as large as an RBC, is seen in the lower right corner of this figure. **C:** Alder-Reilly anomaly. Darkly stained granules are seen in most of the leukocytes (neutrophils, monocytes, and lymphocytes). These granules appear to be lysosomes that stain abnormally because of their content of incompletely degraded mucopolysaccharides. **D:** Toxic granulation. The neutrophil contains a multitude of darkly stained granules (the toxic granules). These are azurophil granules whose mucopolysaccharides have not matured. Döhle bodies and vacuoles may accompany the toxic granulation.

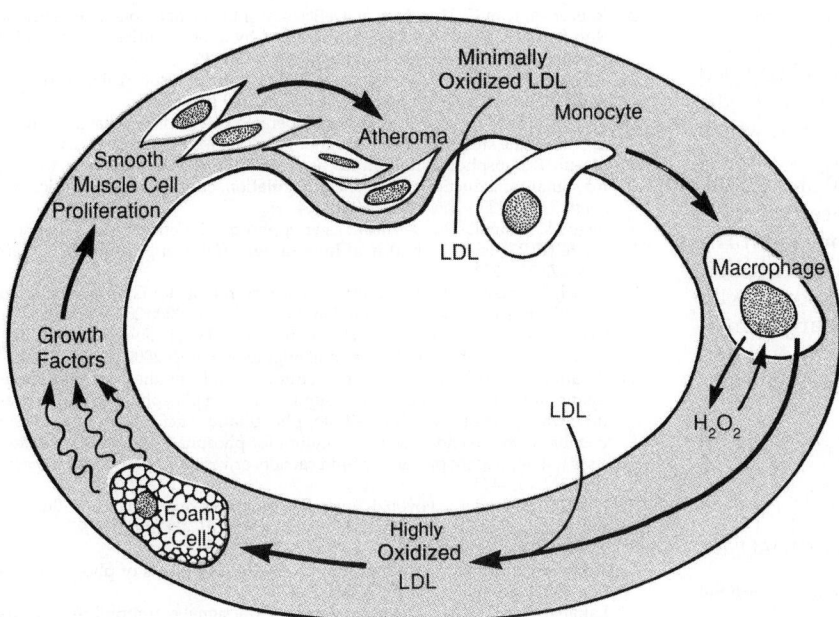

Figure 16-18. Role of mononuclear phagocytes in the pathogenesis of atherosclerosis. LDL, low-density lipoprotein.

Toxic Phagocytes. Circulating neutrophils from patients with a variety of inflammatory conditions can show characteristic morphologic changes (Fig. 16-17D). These include cytoplasmic vacuoles, Döhle bodies, and toxic granules. Döhle bodies appear as greenish inclusions on Wright-stained smears, and electron micrographs reveal them to be aggregates of rough endoplasmic reticulum (234). Toxic granules are azurophilic granules that do not appear stained in normal neutrophils. Because of a degree of immaturity of neutrophils produced in response to inflammatory demands, however, the mucopolysaccharide content of the toxic neutrophils is increased, causing them to appear as dark dots in the cytoplasm (235). They do not take on the deep violet hue of azurophilic granules seen in the normal promyelocyte.

The toxic changes seen in neutrophils are nonspecific in that they are often associated with, but do not necessarily reflect, the presence of bacterial infections. From a functional standpoint, toxic neutrophils appear "primed" and excited. They have abnormally high resting rates of oxygen consumption, reactive oxygen metabolite release, and surface expression of Fc and complement receptors. They also may have reduced contents of granule enzymes. These changes presumably represent exposure of the neutrophils to bacteria or to microbial products such as endotoxin. Toxic neutrophils appear to characterize neutrophils that are in a state of heightened responsiveness to an infection, but whether neutrophils in such a condition in the circulation can get to the source of infection is unclear.

In patients with rheumatoid arthritis, neutrophils may contain amorphous eosinophilic material, presumably representing ingested rheumatoid factor immune complexes. Such neutrophils, as well as those from patients with systemic lupus erythematosus, another immune complex disorder, reportedly have reduced antimicrobial functional activity. Whether these abnormalities are of clinical importance is not clear.

Monocytes from patients with infections or with other inflammatory conditions may also appear abnormal. They tend to resemble macrophages on Wright-stained smears in that they are larger than monocytes; they have a rounder, more eccentric nucleus with more condensed chromatin than monocyte nuclei; and, rather than the characteristic gray hue of the monocyte cytoplasm, they have a bluish tinge with prominent azurophilic cytoplasmic granules.

Myelodysplasia and Myeloproliferative Disorders. Neutrophils and neutrophil precursors derived from abnormal stem cells frequently show morphologic abnormalities. These may include pseudo–Pelger-Huët changes in the nucleus (236), an agranular appearance due to loss of the specific granules (120), and loss of stainable MPO on the blood film. These abnormalities may be seen in any stem cell disorder: aplastic anemia, myeloid metaplasia, and acute and chronic myelogenous leukemia. They are perhaps most characteristic of myelodysplasia, in which their presence indicates clinically significant involvement of the myeloid series, a finding that places the disorder into the *excess blasts* or the *chronic myelomonocytic leukemia* category. PMNs from patients with chronic myelogenous leukemia have, in addition to low or absent alkaline phosphatase activity (see Chapter 13), moderately reduced locomotion, phagocytosis, and oxidant release in response to excitation (237). These functional abnormalities detectable *in vitro* do not appear to predispose patients with this disease to pyogenic infection so long as they have normal or high peripheral blood neutrophil counts.

PHAGOCYTES IN ATHEROSCLEROSIS

Atherosclerosis is a highly complex process in which monocytes play a key role (Fig. 16-18) (238). It begins with the diffusion of LDL through the endothelium and into the subendothelial matrix. There, the LDL is slightly modified by oxidation, acylation, or other processes, giving rise to what is known as "minimally oxidized" LDL. This minimally oxidized LDL stimulates the endothelium to manufacture molecules that attract monocytes: adhesion molecules such as E-selectin and P-selectin; integrin counterligands such as vascular cell adhesion molecule-1 (VCAM-1), which binds tightly to the MNP integrin VLA-4; and the monocyte chemotactic factor MCP-1. The growth factor M-CSF is also produced. The net effect of these adhesion molecules and cytokines is to draw the monocytes into the subendothelial matrix and stimulate their conversion into macrophages. Meanwhile the LDL is undergoing further modification—oxidation by MPO and other changes catalyzed by sphingomyelinase and phospholipase—converting it into "highly oxidized" LDL that is taken up by macrophages to form foam cells. The fatty streak that is often seen subjacent to the endothelium of large blood vessels is a subendothelial collection of foam cells. Uptake of the highly oxidized

LDL is mediated by the scavenger receptors on the macrophages: SR-A and CD36. The lipid-stuffed foam cells die, releasing their contents, which aggregate to form debris-filled necrotic masses surmounted by a fibrous cap produced via the extracellular matrix secreted by smooth muscle cells, which migrate into the lesion—the atherosclerotic plaque. Foam cells also continue to migrate into these plaques. CD40 and CD40L are important for the production of these advanced, fibrotic, debris-laden lesions. (CD40 is expressed on macrophages.) The rupture of a plaque exposes macrophage tissue factor, which is at least in part responsible for the thrombosis that occurs with that event. Atherosclerotic plaques that are particularly vulnerable to rupture have thin, fibrous caps attenuated by enzymes of macrophage origin—collagenases, gelatinases, cathepsins, stromelysins—and many inflammatory cells.

REFERENCES

1. Stossel T. In: Gordon S, ed. *Phagocytosis: the host.* Stamford, CT: JAI Press, 1999:3–18.
2. Newburger P, Subrahmanyam Y, Weissman S. Global analysis of neutrophil gene expression. *Curr Opin Hematol* 2000;7:6–20.
3. Savill J, Fadok V. Corpse clearance defines the meaning of death. *Nature* 2000;407:784–788.
4. Miyamoto K, Schultz E, Heath T, et al. Pulmonary intravascular macrophages and hemodynamic effects of liposomes in sheep. *J Appl Physiol* 1988; 64:1143–1152.
5. Kristiansen M, Graversen JH, Jacobsen C, et al. Identification of the haemoglobin scavenger receptor. *Nature* 2001;409:198–201.
6. Rossi D, Zlotnik A. The biology of chemokines and their receptors. *Annu Rev Immunol* 2000;18:217–242.
7. Baggiolini M. Chemokines and leukocyte traffic. *Nature* 1998;392:565–658.
8. Gerard C, Gerard N. C5A anaphylatoxin and its seven transmembrane-segment receptor. *Annu Rev Immunol* 1994;12:775–808.
9. Murdoch C, Finn A. Chemokine receptors and their role in inflammation and infectious diseases. *Blood* 2000;95:3032–3043.
10. Geva A, Lassere T, Lichtarge O, et al. Genetic mapping of the human C5a receptor. Identification of transmembrane amino acids critical for receptor function. *J Biol Chem* 2000;275:35993–35401.
11. Serhan C, Prescott S. The scent of a phagocyte: advances on leukotriene B4 receptors. *J Exp Med* 2000;192:F5–F8.
12. Mills J, Miettinen H, Cummings D, et al. Characterization of the binding site on the formyl peptide receptor using three receptor mutants and analogs of Met-Leu-Phe and Met-Met-Trp-Leu-Leu. *J Biol Chem* 2000;275:39012–39017.
13. Maestes D, Potter R, Prossnitz E. Differential phosphorylation paradigms dictate desensitization and internalization of the N-formyl peptide receptor. *J Biol Chem* 1999;274:29791–29795.
14. Haribabu B, Zhelev D, Pridgen B, et al. Chemoattractant receptors activate distinct pathways for chemotaxis and secretion. Role of G-protein usage. *J Biol Chem* 1999;274;37087–37092.
15. Nick JA, Avdi NJ, Young SK, et al. Selective activation and functional significance of p38α mitogen-activated protein kinase in lipopolysaccharide-stimulated neutrophils. *J Clin Invest* 1999;103:851–858.
16. Somers W, Tang J, Shaw G, et al. Insights into the molecular basis of leukocyte tethering and rolling revealed by structures of P- and E-selectin bound to SLex and PSGL-1. *Cell* 2000;03:467–479.
17. Blystone S, Brown E. In: Gordon S, ed. *Phagocytosis: the host.* Stamford, CT: JAI Press, 1999:103–147.
18. Forlow SB, White EJ, Barlow SC, et al. Severe inflammatory defect and reduced viability in CD18 and E-selectin double-mutant mice. *J Clin Invest* 2000;106:1457–1466.
19. Williams M, Solomkin J. Integrin-mediated signaling in human neutrophil functioning. *J Leukoc Biol* 1999;65:725–736.
20. Jones S, Knaus U, Bokoch G, et al. Two signaling mechanisms for activation of αMβ2 avidity in polymorphonuclear neutrophils. *J Biol Chem* 1998;273: 10556–10566.
21. Sánchez-Mejorada G, Rosales C. Signal transduction by immunoglobulin Fc receptors. *J Leukoc Biol* 1998;63:521–533.
22. Fraser I, Ezekowitz R. In: Gordon S, ed. *Phagocytosis: the host.* Stamford, CT: JAI Press, 1999.
23. Hamm H. The many faces of G protein signaling. *J Biol Chem* 1998;273:669–672.
24. Miettinen H, Gripentrog J, Mason M, et al. Identification of putative sites of interaction between the human formyl peptide receptor and G protein. *J Biol Chem* 1999;274:27934–27942.
25. Gerber B, Meng E, Dötsch V, et al. An activation switch in the ligand binding pocket of the C5a receptor. *J Biol Chem* 2001;276:3394–3400.
26. Bokoch G. Chemoattractant signaling and leukocyte activation. *Blood* 1995; 86:1649–1660.
27. Roberts A, Kim C, Zhen L, et al. Deficiency of the hematopoietic cell-specific Rho family GTPase Rac2 is characterized by abnormalities in neutrophil function and host defense. *Immunity* 1999;10:183–196.
28. Alteraifi A, Zhelev D. Transient increase of free cytosolic calcium during neutrophil motility responses. *J Cell Sci* 1997;110:1967–1977.
29. Favre C, Nüsse O, Lew D. Store-operated Ca2+ influx: what is the message from the stores to the membrane? *J Lab Clin Med* 1996;128:19–26.
30. Martin T. Phosphoinositide lipids as signaling molecules: common themes for signal transduction, cytoskeletal regulation, and membrane trafficking. *Annu Rev Cell Dev Biol* 1998;14:231–264.
31. Niggli V. A membrane-permeant ester of phosphatidylinositol 3,4,5-trisphosphate (PIP3) is an activator of human neutrophil migration. *FEBS Lett* 2000;473:217–221.
32. Hirsch E, Katanaev VI, Garlanda C, et al. Central role for G protein-coupled phosphoinositide 3-kinase γ in inflammation. *Science* 2000;287:1049–1053.
33. Sasaki T, Irie-Sasaki J, Jones RG, et al. Function of PI3Kγ in thymocyte development, T cell activation, and neutrophil migration. *Science* 2000;287:1040–1046.
34. Whatmore J, Wiedemann C, Somerharju P, et al. Resynthesis of phosphatidylinositol in permeabilized neutrophils following phospholipase Cβ activation: transport of the intermediate, phosphatidic acid, from the plasma membrane to the endoplasmic reticulum for phosphatidylinositol resynthesis is not dependent on soluble lipid carriers or vesicular transport. *Biochem J* 1999;341:435–444.
35. Nüsse O, Serrander L, Foyouzi-Youssefi R, et al. Store-operated Ca2+ influx and stimulation of exocytosis in HL-60 granulocytes. *J Biol Chem* 1997;272:28360–28367.
36. Toker A, Cantley L. Signaling through the lipid products of phosphoinositide-3-OH kinase. *Nature* 1997;387:673–676.
37. Laffafian I, Hallett M. Does cytosolic free Ca2+ signal neutrophil chemotaxis in response to formylated chemotactic peptide? *J Cell Sci* 1995;108:3199–3205.
38. Gaits F, Fourcade O, Le Balle F, et al. Lysophosphatidic acid as a phospholipid mediator: pathways of synthesis. *FEBS Lett* 1997;410:54–58.
39. Moolenaar W. Bioactive lysophospholipids and their G protein-coupled receptors. *Exp Cell Res* 1999;253:230–238.
40. Scott K, Bryant K, Bidgood M. Functional coupling and differential regulation of the phospholipase A2-cyclooxygenase pathways in inflammation. *J Leukoc Biol* 1999;66:535–541.
41. Rådmark O. The molecular biology and regulation of 5-lipoxygenase. *Am J Respir Crit Care Med* 2000;161:S11–S15.
42. Chow C, Demaurex N, Grinstein S. Ion transport and the function of phagocytic cells. *Curr Opin Hematol* 1995;1:89–95.
43. Berton G. Tyrosine kinases in neutrophils. *Curr Opin Hematol* 1999;6:51–58.
44. Sergeant S, Waite K, Heravi J, et al. Phosphatidic acid regulates tyrosine phosphorylating activity in human neutrophils. Enhancement of Fgr activity. *J Biol Chem* 2001;276:4737–4746.
45. Avdi N, Nick JA, Whitlock BB, et al. Tumor necrosis factor-α activation of the c-Jun N-terminal kinase pathway in human neutrophils. Integrin involvement in a pathway leading from cytoplasmic tyrosine kinases to apoptosis. *J Biol Chem* 2001;276:2189–2190.
46. Fuortes M, Melchior M, Han H, et al. Role of the tyrosine kinase pyk2 in the integrin-dependent activation of human neutrophils by TNF. *J Clin Invest* 1999;104:327–335.
47. Brumell J, Chan CK, Butler J, et al. Regulation of Src homology 2-containing tyrosine phosphatase 1 during activation of human neutrophils. Role of protein kinase C. *J Biol Chem* 1997;272:875–882.
48. Rane M, Arthur J, Prossnitz E, et al. Activation of mitogen-activated protein kinases by formyl peptide receptors is regulated by the cytoplasmic tail. *J Biol Chem* 1998;273:20916–20923.
49. Laux T, Fukami K, Telen M, et al. GAP43, MARCKS, and CAP23 modulate PI(4,5)P2 at plasmalemmal rafts, and regulate cell cortex actin dynamics through a common mechanism. *J Cell Biol* 2000;149:1455–1471.
50. Cassimeris L, Safer D, Nachmias V, et al. Thymosin β4 sequesters the majority of G-actin in resting human polymorphonuclear leukocytes. *J Cell Biol* 1992;119:1261–1270.
51. Botelho R, Teruel M, Dierckman R, et al. Localized biphasic changes in phosphatidylinositol-4,5-bisphosphate at sites of phagocytosis. *J Cell Biol* 2000;151:1353–1367.
52. Higgs H, Pollard T. Regulation of actin polymerization by Arp2/3 complex and WASp/SCAR proteins. *J Biol Chem* 1999;274:32531–32534.
53. Pantaloni D, Boujemaa R, Didry D, et al. The Arp2/3 complex branches filament barbed ends: functional antagonism with capping proteins. *Nat Cell Biol* 2000;2:385–391.
54. Zigmond S, Joyce M, Yang C, et al. Mechanism of Cdc42-induced actin polymerization in neutrophil extracts. *J Cell Biol* 1998;142:1001–1012.
55. Wear M, Schafer D, Cooper J. Actin dynamics: assembly and disassembly of actin networks. *Curr Biol* 2000;10:R891–R895.
56. Glogauer M, Hartwig J, Stossel T. Two pathways through Cdc42 couple the N-formyl receptor to actin nucleation in permeabilized human neutrophils. *J Cell Biol* 2000;150:785–796.
57. Jones S, Wang J, Turck C, et al. A role for the actin-bundling protein L-plastin in the regulation of leukocyte integrin function. *Proc Natl Acad Sci U S A* 1998;95:9331–9336.
58. Calderwood D, Shattil S, Ginsberg M. Integrins and actin filaments: reciprocal regulation of cell adhesion and signaling. *J Biol Chem* 2000;275:22607–22610.
59. Tsukita S, Tsukita S. Cortical actin organization: lessons from ERM (ezrin/radixin/moesin) proteins. *J Biol Chem* 1999;274:34507–34510.

60. Mansfield P, Shayman J, Boxer L. Regulation of polymorphonuclear leukocyte phagocytosis by myosin light chain kinase after activation of mitogen-activated protein kinase. *Blood* 2000;95:2407–2412.

61. Eddy R, Pierini L, Matsumura F, et al. Ca2+-dependent myosin II activation is required for uropod retraction during neutrophil migration. *J Cell Sci* 2000;113:1287–1298.

62. Kaibuchi K, Kuroda S, Amano M. Regulation of the cytoskeleton and cell adhesion by the Rho family GTPases in mammalian cells. *Annu Rev Biochem* 1999;68:459–486.

63. Heyworth P, Robinson J, Ding J, et al. Cofilin undergoes rapid dephosphorylation in stimulated neutrophils and translocates to ruffled membranes enriched in products of the NADPH oxidase complex. Evidence for a novel cycle of phosphorylation and dephosphorylation. *Histochem Cell Biol* 1997;108:221–233.

64. Bamburg J. Proteins of the ADF/cofilin family: essential regulators of actin dynamics. *Annu Rev Cell Dev Biol* 1999;15:185–230.

65. Ambach A, Konstandin S, Wesselborg S, et al. The serine phosphatases PP1 and PP2A associate with and activate the actin binding protein cofilin in human T lymphocytes. *Eur J Immunol* 2000;12:3422–3431.

66. Sun H, Yamamoto M, Mejillano M, et al. Gelsolin, a multifunctional actin regulatory protein. *J Biol Chem* 1999;274:33179–33182.

67. Carlier M-F. Control of actin dynamics. *Curr Opin Cell Biol* 1998;10:45–51.

68. Rosania G, Swanson J. Microtubules can modulate pseudopod activity from a distance inside macrophages. *Cell Motil Cytoskeleton* 1996;34:230–245.

69. Pryzwanski K, Merricks E. Chemotactic peptide-induced changes of intermediate filament organization in neutrophils during granule secretion: role of cyclic guanosine monophosphate. *Mol Biol Cell* 1998;9:2933–2947.

70. Suzuki K, Hasegawa T, Sakamoto C, et al. Cleavage of mitogen-activated protein kinases in human neutrophils undergoing apoptosis: role in decreased responsiveness to inflammatory cytokines. *J Immunol* 2001;166:1185–1192.

71. Knepper-Nicolai B, Savill J, Brown S. Constitutive apoptosis in human neutrophils requires synergy between calpains and the proteasome downstream of caspases. *J Biol Chem* 1998;273:30530–30536.

72. Burns A, Bowden RA, Abe Y, et al. P-selectin mediates neutrophil adhesion to endothelial cell borders. *J Leukoc Biol* 1999;65:299–306.

73. Doherty D, Downey G, Schwab B, et al. Lipopolysaccharide-induced monocyte retention in the lung. Role of monocyte stiffness, actin assembly, and CD18-dependent adherence. *J Immunol* 1994;153:241–255.

74. Johnson-Léger C, Aurrand-Lions M, Imhof B. The parting of the endothelium: miracle, or simply a junctional affair? *J Cell Sci* 2000;113:921–933.

75. Hixenbaugh E, Goeckeler A, Papaiya N, et al. Stimulated neutrophils induce myosin light chain phosphorylation and isometric tension in endothelial cells. *Am J Physiol* 1997;273:H981–H988.

76. Hu W-H, Chen H-I, Huang J-P, et al. Endothelial [Ca2+]i signaling during transmigration of polymorphonuclear leukocytes. *Blood* 2000;96:3816–3822.

77. Loike J, Cao L, Budhu S, et al. Differential regulation of β1 integrins by chemoattractants regulates neutrophil migration through fibrin. *J Cell Biol* 1999;144:1047–1056.

78. Vanhaesenbroeck B, Jones GE, Allen WE, et al. Distinct PI(3)Ks mediate mitogenic signalling and cell migration in macrophages. *Nat Cell Biol* 2000;1:69–71.

79. Sánchez-Madrid F, del Pozo M. Leukocyte polarization in cell migration and immune interactions. *EMBO J* 1999;18:501–511.

80. Rickert P, Weiner O, Wang F, et al. Leukocytes navigate by compass: roles of PI3Kγ and its lipid products. *Trends Cell Biol* 2000;10:466–473.

81. Weiner O, Servant G, Welch M, et al. Spatial control of actin polymerization during neutrophil chemotaxis. *Nat Cell Biol* 1999;1:75–81.

82. Keller H, Babie H. Protrusive activity quantitatively determines the rate and direction of cell locomotion. *Cell Motil Cytoskeleton* 1996;33:241–251.

83. Malawista S, de Boisfleury Chevance A, Boxer L. Random locomotion and chemotaxis of human blood polymorphonuclear leukocytes from a patient with leukocyte adhesion deficiency-1: normal displacement in close quarters via chimneying. *Cell Motil Cytoskeleton* 2000;46:183–189.

84. Fadok V, de Cathelineau A, Daleke D, et al. Loss of phospholipid asymmetry and surface exposure of phosphatidylserine is required for phagocytosis of apoptotic cells by macrophages and fibroblasts. *J Biol Chem* 2001;276:1071–1077.

85. Aderem A, Underhill D. Mechanisms of phagocytosis in macrophages. *Annu Rev Immunol* 1999;17:593–623.

86. Lew PD, Andersson T, Hed J, et al. Ca2+-dependent and Ca2+-independent phagocytosis in human neutrophils. *Nature* 1985;315:509–511.

87. Caron E, Hall A. Identification of two distinct mechanisms of phagocytosis controlled by different Rho GTPases. *Science* 1998;282:1717–1721.

88. Chimini G, Chavrier P. Function of Rho family proteins in actin dynamics during phagocytosis and engulfment. *Nat Cell Biol* 2000;2:E191–E196.

89. Serrander L, Skarman P, Rasmussen B, et al. Selective inhibition of IgG-mediated phagocytosis in gelsolin-deficient murine neutrophils. *J Immunol* 2000;165:2451–2457.

90. DiVirgilio F, Meyer BC, Greenberg S, et al. Fc receptor-mediated phagocytosis occurs in macrophages at exceedingly low cytosolic Ca2+ levels. *J Cell Biol* 1988;106:657–666.

91. Araki N, Johnson M, Swanson J. A role for phosphoinositide 3-kinase in the completion of macropinocytosis and phagocytosis by macrophages. *J Cell Biol* 1996;135:1249–1260.

92. Swanson J, Johnson M, Beningo K, et al. A contractile activity that closes phagosomes in macrophages. *J Cell Sci* 1999;112:307–316.

93. May R, Caron E, Hall A, et al. Involvement of the Arp2/3 complex in phagocytosis mediated by FcγR or CR3. *Nat Cell Biol* 2000;2:246–248.

94. Stossel T. In: Gallin J, Snyderman R, eds. *Inflammation. Basic principles and clinical correlates.* Philadelphia: Lippincott, Williams & Wilkins, 1999:661–680.

95. Garin J, Diez R, Kieffer S, et al. The phagosome proteome: insight into phagosomal functions. *J Cell Biol* 2001;152:165–180.

96. Bretscher M, Aguado-Velasco C. Membrane traffic during cell locomotion. *Curr Opin Cell Biol* 1998;10:537–541.

97. Mellman I. *Quo vadis*: polarized membrane recycling in motility and phagocytosis. *J Cell Biol* 2000;149:529–530.

98. McNew J, Weber T, Parlati F, et al. Close is not enough: SNARE-dependent membrane fusion requires an active mechanism that transduces force to membrane anchors. *J Cell Biol* 2000;150:105–117.

99. Bajno L, Peng X-R, Schreiber A, et al. Focal exocytosis of VAMP3-containing vesicles at sites of phagosome formation. *J Cell Biol* 2000;149:697–705.

100. Alvarez-Dominguez C, Mayorga L, Stahl P. In: Gordon S, ed. *Phagocytosis: the host.* Stamford, CT: JAI Press, 1999:285–297.

101. Pittis M, Garcia R. Annexins VII and XI are present in a human macrophage-like cell line. Differential translocation on FcR-mediated phagocytosis. *J Leukoc Biol* 1999;66:845–850.

102. Ayala-Sanmartin J, Gouache P, Henry J. N-terminal domain of annexin 2 regulates Ca(2+)-dependent aggregation by the core domain: a site directed mutagenesis study. *Biochemistry* 2000;39:15190–15198.

103. Jahrhaus A, Egeberg M, Hinner B, et al. ATP-dependent membrane assembly of F-actin facilitates membrane fusion. *Mol Biol Cell* 2001;12:155–170.

104. Holland S, Gallin J. Evaluation of the patient with recurrent bacterial infections. *Annu Rev Med* 1998;49:185–199.

105. Lekstrom-Himes J, Gallin J. Immunodeficiency diseases caused by defects in phagocytes. *N Engl J Med* 2000;343:1703–1714.

106. Becker D, Lowe J. Leukocyte adhesion deficiency type II. *Biochim Biophys Acta* 1999;1455:193–204.

107. Lühn K, Marquardt T, Harms E, et al. Discontinuation of fucose therapy in LADII causes rapid loss of selectin ligands and rise of leukocyte counts. *Blood* 2001;97:330–332.

108. Ambruso D, Knall C, Abell AN, et al. Human neutrophil immunodeficiency syndrome is associated with an inhibitory Rac2 mutation. *Proc Natl Acad Sci U S A* 2000;97:4654–4659.

109. Williams D, Tao W, Yang F, et al. Dominant negative mutation of the hematopoietic-specific Rho GTPase, Rac2, is associated with a human phagocyte immunodeficiency. *Blood* 2000;96:1646–1654.

110. Li Y, Zhang Q, Aaron R. LSP1 modulates the locomotion of monocyte-differentiated U937 cells. *Blood* 2000;96:1100–1105.

111. Zhang Q, Li Y, Howard T. Human lymphocyte-specific protein 1, the protein overexpressed in neutrophil actin dysfunction with 47-kDa and 89-kDa protein abnormalities (NAD 47/89), has multiple F-actin binding domains. *J Immunol* 2000;165:2052–2058.

112. Nunoi H, Yamazaki T, Tsuchiya H, et al. A heterozygous mutation of β-actin associated with neutrophil dysfunction and recurrent infection. *Proc Natl Acad Sci U S A* 1999;96:8693–8698.

113. Meeks M, Bush A. Primary ciliary dyskinesia. *Pediatr Pulmonol* 2000;29:307–316.

114. Rengan R, Ochs HD, Sweet LI, et al. Actin cytoskeletal function is spared, but apoptosis is increased in WAS patient hematopoietic cells. *Blood* 2000;95:1283–1292.

115. Linder S, Nelson D, Weiss M, et al. Wiskott-Aldrich syndrome protein regulates podosomes in primary human macrophages. *Proc Natl Acad Sci U S A* 1999;96:9648–9653.

116. Calderwood S, Kilpatrick L, Douglas SD, et al. Recombinant human granulocyte colony-stimulating factor therapy for patients with neutropenia and/or neutrophil dysfunction secondary to glycogen storage disease. *Blood* 2001;97:376–382.

117. Bainton DF, Ullyot JL, Farquhar MG. The development of neutrophilic polymorphonuclear leukocytes in human bone marrow. *J Exp Med* 1971;2673:907–934.

118. Henson PM, Johnston RB Jr. Tissue injury in inflammation: oxidants, proteinases, and cationic proteins. *J Clin Invest* 1987;79:669–674.

119. Lehrer R, Ganz T, Selsted M. Defensins: endogenous antibiotic peptides of animal cells. *Cell* 1991;64:229–230.

120. Lichtenstein AK, Ganz T, Nguyen TM, et al. Mechanism of target cytolysis by peptide defensins: target cell metabolic activities, possibly involving endocytosis, are crucial for expression of cytotoxicity. *J Immunol* 1988;140:2686–2694.

121. Gray PW, Flaggs G, Leong SR, et al. Cloning of the cDNA of a human neutrophil bactericidal protein. *J Biol Chem* 1989;264:9505–9509.

122. Weiss J, Hutzler M, Kao L. Environmental modulation of lipopolysaccharide chain length alters the sensitivity of *Escherichia coli* to the neutrophil bactericidal/permeability-increasing protein. *Infect Immun* 1986;51:594–599.

123. Jensen MS, Bainton DF. Temporal changes in pH within the phagocytic vacuole of the polymorphonuclear neutrophilic leukocyte. *J Cell Biol* 1973;56:379–388.

124. Salton MRJ. The properties of lysozyme and its action on microorganisms. *Bact Rev* 1957;21:82–99.

125. Levy O. Antimicrobial proteins and peptides of blood: templates for novel antimicrobial agents. *Blood* 2000;96:2664–2672.

126. Travis J, Salvesen GS. Human plasma proteinase inhibitors. *Annu Rev Biochem* 1983;52:655–709.

127. Janoff A, Carp H, Laurent P, et al. The role of oxidative processes in emphysema. *Am Rev Respir Dis* 1983;127:S31–S38.

128. Wilde CG, Snable JL, Griffeth JE, et al. Characterization of two azurophil granule proteases with active-site homology to neutrophil elastase. *J Biol Chem* 1990;265:2038–2041.

129. Gross WL, Schmitt WH, Csernok E. ANCA and associated diseases: immunodiagnostic and pathogenetic aspects. *Clin Exp Immunol* 1993;91:1–12.

130. Hack NJ, Smith GP, Peters TJ. Subcellular localization and properties of lipase activities in human polymorphonuclear leukocytes. *Biochim Biophys Acta* 1985;833:406–411.

131. Sznajd J, Naskalski JW. Ribonuclease from human granulocytes. *Biochim Biophys Acta* 1973;302:282–292.

132. Fox HB, DeTogni P, McMahon G, et al. Fate of the DNA in plasmid-containing E coli minicells ingested by human neutrophils. *Blood* 1987;69:1394–1400.

133. Fenna R, Zeng J, Davey C. Structure of the green heme in myeloperoxidase. *Arch Biochem Biophys* 1995;316:653–656.

134. Nauseef WM, Cogley M, McCormick S. Effect of the R569W missense mutation on the biosynthesis of myeloperoxidase. *J Biol Chem* 1996;271:9546–9549.

135. Winterbourn CC, Vissers MC, Kettle AJ. Myeloperoxidase. *Curr Opin Hematol* 2000;7:53–58.

136. Parmley RT, Hurst RE, Takagi M, et al. Glycosaminoglycans in human neutrophils and leukemic myeloblasts: ultrastructural, cytochemical, immunologic, and biochemical characterization. *Blood* 1983;61:257–266.

137. Gallin JI. Neutrophil specific granule deficiency. *Annu Rev Med* 1985;36:263–274.

138. Wright DG, Gallin JI. Secretory responses of human neutrophils: exocytosis of specific (secondary) granules by human neutrophils during adherence in vivo and during exudation in vivo. *J Immunol* 1979;123:285–294.

139. Takasaki J, Kawauchi Y, Masuho Y. Synergistic effect of type II phospholipase A2 and platelet-activating factor on Mac-1 surface expression and exocytosis of gelatinase granules in human neutrophils: evidence for the 5-lipoxygenase-dependent mechanism. *J Immunol* 1998;160:5066–5072.

140. Anderson BF, Baker HM, Dodson EJ, et al. Structure of human lactoferrin at 32-A resolution. *Proc Natl Acad Sci U S A* 1987;84:1969–1773.

141. Weinberg ED. Iron withholding: a defense against infection and neoplasia. *Physiol Rev* 1984;64:65–102.

142. Murphy MF, Sourial NA, Burman JF, et al. Megaloblastic anaemia due to vitamin B12 deficiency caused by small intestinal bacterial overgrowth: possible role of vitamin B12 analogues. *Br J Haematol* 1986;62:7–12.

143. Burger RL, Mehlman CS, Allen RH. Human plasma R-type vitamin B_{12}-binding proteins. I. Isolation and characterization of transcobalamin I: transcobalamin III and the normal granulocyte vitamin B_{12}-binding protein. *J Biol Chem* 1975;250:7700–7706.

144. Weiss SJ, Peppin GJ. Collagenolytic metalloenzymes of the human neutrophil: characteristics, regulation and potential function in vivo. *Biochem Pharmacol* 1986;35:3189–3197.

145. Borregaard N, Cowland JB. Granules of the human neutrophilic polymorphonuclear leukocyte. *Blood* 1997;89:3503–3521.

146. Wright DG, Gallin JI. A functional differentiation of human neutrophil granules: generation of C5a by a specific (secondary) granule product and inactivation of C5a by azurophil (primary) granule products. *J Immunol* 1977;119:1068–1076.

147. Dewald B, Bretz U, Baggiolini M. Release of gelatinase from a novel secretory compartment of human neutrophils. *J Clin Invest* 1982;70:518–525.

148. Baggiolini M, Schnyder J, Bretz U, et al. Cellular mechanisms of proteinase release from inflammatory cells and the degradation of extracellular proteins. *Ciba Found Symp* 1979;75:105–121.

149. Johnston RB. Monocytes and macrophages. *N Engl J Med* 1988;318:747–752.

150. Johnson J, Mei B, Cohn ZA. The separation, long-term cultivation and maturation of the human monocyte. *J Exp Med* 1977;146:1613–1630.

151. Nathan CF. Secretory products of macrophages. *J Clin Invest* 1987;79:319–326.

152. Introne W, Boissy RE, Gahl WA. Clinical, molecular, and cell biological aspects of Chediak-Higashi syndrome. *Mol Genet Metab* 1999;68:283–303.

153. Rubin CM, Burke BA, McKenna RW, et al. The accelerated phase of Chediak-Higashi syndrome: an expression of the virus-associated hemophagocytic syndrome. *Cancer* 1985;56:524–530.

154. Mechanisms of disease. *N Engl J Med* 2000;343:1101.

155. Certain S, Barrat F, Pastural E, et al. Protein truncation test of LYST reveals heterogenous mutations in patients with Chediak-Higashi syndrome. *Blood* 2000;95:979–983.

156. Pettit RE, Berdal KG. Chediak-Higashi syndrome: neurologic appearance. *Arch Neurol* 1984;41:1001–1005.

157. Haddad E, Le Deist F, Blanche S, et al. Treatment of Chediak-Higashi syndrome by allogenic bone marrow transplantation: report of 10 cases. *Blood* 1995;85:3328–3333.

158. Gallin JI, Fletcher MP, Seligmann BE, et al. Human neutrophil-specific granule deficiency: a model to assess the role of neutrophil-specific granules in the evolution of the inflammatory response. *Blood* 1982;59:1317–1329.

159. Lekstrom-Himes JA, Dorman SE, Kopar P, et al. Neutrophil-specific granule deficiency results from a novel mutation with loss of function of the transcription factor CCAAT/enhancer binding protein epsilon. *J Exp Med* 1999;189:1847–1852.

160. Davis JM, Dineen J, Gallin JI. Neutrophil degranulation and abnormal chemotaxis after thermal injury. *J Immunol* 1980;124:1467–1471.

161. Dinarello CA. Biology of interleukin I. *FASEB J* 1988;2:198–215.

162. Beutler B, Cerami A. Tumor necrosis, cachexia, shock, and inflammation: a common mediator. *Annu Rev Biochem* 1988;57:505–518.

163. Beutler B, Cerami A. The history, properties, and biological effects of cachectin. *Biochemistry* 1988;27:7575–7582.

164. Clark SC, Kamen R. The human hematopoietic colony-stimulating factors. *Science* 1987;236:1229–1237.

165. Schwartz BS, Levy A, Fair DS, et al. Murine lymphoid procoagulant activity induced by bacterial lipopolysaccharide and immune complexes in a monocyte prothrombinase. *J Exp Med* 1982;155:1464–1479.

166. Conkling PR, Chua CC. Clinical trials with human tumor necrosis factor: in vivo and in vitro effects on human mononuclear phagocyte function. *Cancer Res* 1988;48:5604–5609.

167. Lorenzet R, Niemetz J, Marcus AJ, et al. Enhancement of mononuclear procoagulant activity by platelet 12-hydroxyeicosatetraenoic acid. *J Clin Invest* 1986;78:418–423.

168. Hamilton AO, Jones L, Morrison L, et al. Modulation of monocyte complement synthesis by interferons. *Biochem J* 1987;242:809–815.

169. Vassalli J, Dayer J, Wohlwend A, et al. Concomitant secretion of prourokinase and of plasminogen activator-specific inhibitor by cultured human monocytes-macrophages. *J Exp Med* 1985;159:1653–1668.

170. Aoki N, Harpel PC. Inhibitors of the fibrinolytic enzyme system. *Semin Thromb Hemost* 1984;10:24–41.

171. LaFleur M, Beaulieu AD, Kreis C, et al. Fibronectin gene expression in polymorphonuclear leukocytes: accumulation of mRNA in inflammatory cells. *J Biol Chem* 1987;262:2111–2115.

172. Newburger PE, Subrahmanyam YV, Weissman SM. Global analysis of neutrophil gene expression. *Curr Opin Hematol* 2000;7:16–20.

173. Samuelsson B, Dahlen S-E, Lindgren J-A, et al. Leukotrienes and lipoxins: structures, biosynthesis and biological effects. *Science* 1987;237:1171–1176.

174. Miller DK, Gillard JW, Vickers PJ, et al. Identification and isolation of a membrane protein necessary for leukotriene production. *Nature* 1990;343:278–281.

175. Rådmark O, Shimizu T, Jornvall H, et al. Leukotriene A4 hydrolase in human leukocytes: purification and properties. *J Biol Chem* 1984;259:12339–12345.

176. Chauncey JB, Simon RH, Peters-Golden M. Rat alveolar macrophages synthesize leukotriene B4 and 12-hydroxyeicosatetraenoic acid from alveolar epithelial cell–derived arachidonic acid. *Am Rev Respir Dis* 1988;138:928–935.

177. Samuelsson B, Goldyne M, Granstrom E, et al. Prostaglandins and thromboxanes. *Annu Rev Biochem* 1978;47:997–1029.

178. Browning JL, Ribolini A. Interferon blocks interleukin 1-inducted prostaglandin release from human peripheral monocytes. *J Immunol* 1987;138:2857–2863.

179. Lim LK, Hunt NH, Eichner RD, et al. Cyclic AMP and the regulation of prostaglandin production by macrophages. *Biochem Biophys Res Commun* 1983;114:248–254.

180. McManus LM, Pinckard N, Fitzpatrick FA, et al. Acetyl glyceryl ether phosphorylcholine: intravascular alterations following intravenous infusion into the baboon. *Lab Invest* 1981;45:303–307.

181. Alonso F, Henson PM, Leslie CC. A cytosolic phospholipase in human neutrophils that hydrolyzes arachidonoyl-containing phosphatidylcholine. *Biochim Biophys Acta* 1986;878:273–280.

182. Mollinedo F, Gomez-Cambronero J, Cano E, et al. Intracellular localization of platelet-activating factor synthesis in human neutrophils. *Biochem Biophys Res Commun* 1988;154:1232–1239.

183. Roubin R, Dulioust A, Haye-Legrand I, et al. Biosynthesis of paf-acether. VIII. Impairment of paf-acether production in activated macrophages does not depend upon acetyltransferase activity. *J Immunol* 1986;136:1796–1802.

184. Elstad MR, Stafforini DM, McIntyre TM, et al. Platelet-activating factor acetylhydrolase increases during macrophage differentiation: a novel mechanism that regulates accumulation of platelet-activating factor. *J Biol Chem* 1989;264:8467–8470.

185. Dewald B, Baggiolini M. Platelet-activating factor as a stimulus of exocytosis in human neutrophils. *Biochim Biophys Acta* 1986;888:42–48.

186. Nathan CF, Tsunawaki S. Secretion of toxic oxygen products by macrophages: regulatory cytokines and their effects on the oxidase. *Ciba Found Symp* 1986;118:211–230.

187. Babior BM. The respiratory burst oxidase. *Trends Biochem Sci* 1987;12:241–243.

188. Wymann MP, von Tscharner V, Deranleau DA, et al. The onset of the respiratory burst in human neutrophils: real-time studies of H2O2 formation reveal a rapid agonist-induced transduction process. *J Biol Chem* 1987;262:12048–12053.

189. Babior BM. NADPH oxidase: an update. *Blood* 1999;93:1464–1476.

190. Fridovich I. Superoxide radical and superoxide dismutases. *Annu Rev Biochem* 1995;64:97–112.

191. Klebanoff SJ. Oxygen-dependent cytotoxic mechanisms of phagocytes. *Adv Host Defense Mech* 1982;1:111.

192. Rosen H, Rakita RM, Waltersdorph AM, et al. Myeloperoxidase-mediated damage to the succinate oxidase system of *Escherichia coli*: evidence for selective inactivation of the dehydrogenase component. *J Biol Chem* 1987;242:15004–15010.

193. Weitzman SA, Weitberg AB, Clark EP, et al. Phagocytes as carcinogens: malignant transformation produced by human neutrophils. *Science* 1985;227:1231–1233.

194. Griffith OW, Stuehr DJ. Nitric oxide synthases: properties and catalytic mechanism. *Annu Rev Physiol* 1995;57:707–736.

195. Wright CD, Mulsch A, Busse R, et al. Generation of nitric oxide by human neutrophils. *Biochem Biophys Res Commun* 1989;160:813–819.

196. Schmidt HH, Seifert R, Bohme E. Formation and release of nitric oxide from human neutrophils and HL-60 cells induced by a chemotactic peptide, platelet activating factor and leukotriene B4. *FEBS Lett* 1989;44:357–360.

197. Arnold WP, Mittal CK, Katsuki S, et al. Nitric oxide activates guanylate cyclase and increases guanosine 3':5'-cyclic monophosphate levels in various tissue preparations. *Proc Natl Acad Sci U S A* 1977;74:3203–3207.

198. Iyengar R, Stuehr DJ, Marletta MA. Macrophage synthesis of nitrite, nitrate, and N-nitrosamines: precursors and role of the respiratory burst. *Proc Natl Acad Sci U S A* 1987;84:6369–6373.

199. Beckman JS, Koppenol WH. Nitric oxide, superoxide, and peroxynitrite: the good, the bad, and the ugly. *Am J Physiol Cell Physiol* 1996;271:C1424–C1437.

200. Eiserich JP, Hristova M, Cross CE, et al. Formation of nitric oxide-derived inflammatory oxidants by myeloperoxidase in neutrophils. *Nature* 1998;39:393–397.

201. Brigelius-Flohe R. Tissue-specific functions of individual glutathione peroxidases. *Free Radic Biol Med* 1999;27:951–965.

202. Gaetani GF, Galiano S, Canepa L, et al. Catalase and glutathione peroxidase are equally active in detoxification of hydrogen peroxide in human erythrocytes. *Blood* 1989;73:334–339.

203. Aebi H, Suter H. Acatalasemia. *Adv Hum Genet* 1971;2:143–199.

204. Weiss SJ, Klein R, Slivka A, et al. Chlorination of taurine by human neutrophils. *J Clin Invest* 1982;70:598–607.

205. Baehner RL, Boxer LA. Role of membrane vitamin E and cytoplasmic glutathione in the regulation of phagocytic functions of neutrophils and monocytes. *Am J Pediatr Hematol Oncol* 1979;1:71–76.

206. Parry MF, Root RK, Metcalf JA, et al. Myeloperoxidase deficiency: prevalence and clinical significance. *Ann Intern Med* 1981;95:283–301.

207. Nauseef WM. Insights into myeloperoxidase biosynthesis from its inherited deficiency. *J Mol Med* 1998;76:661–668.

208. Nauseef WM. Aberrant restriction endonuclease digests of DNA from subjects with hereditary myeloperoxidase deficiency. *Blood* 1989;73:290–295.

209. Lehrer RI, Hanifin J, Cline MJ. Defective bactericidal activity in myeloperoxidase-deficient human neutrophils. *Nature* 1969;223:78–79.

210. Diamond RD, Clark RA, Haudenschild CC. Damage to *Candida albicans* hyphae and pseudohyphae by the myeloperoxidase system and oxidative products of neutrophil metabolism in vitro. *J Clin Invest* 1980;66:908–917.

211. Rider ED, Christensen RD, Hall DC, et al. Myeloperoxidase deficiency in neutrophils of neonates. *J Pediatr* 1988;112:648–651.

212. Salmon SE, Cline MJ, Schultz J, et al. Myeloperoxidase deficiency: immunological study of a genetic leukocyte defect. *N Engl J Med* 1970;282:250–253.

213. Stendahl O, Lindgren S. Function of granulocytes with deficient myeloperoxidase-mediated iodination in a patient with generalized pustular psoriasis. *Scand J Haematol* 1976;16:144–153.

214. Johnston RB Jr. Clinical aspects of chronic granulomatous disease. *Curr Opin Hematol* 2001;8:17–22.

215. Marsh WL. Chronic granulomatous disease, the McLeod syndrome, and the Kell blood groups. *Birth Defects* 1978;14:9–25.

216. deSaint-Basile G, Bohler MC, Fischer A, et al. Xp21 DNA microdeletion in a patient with chronic granulomatous disease, retinitis pigmentosa, and McLeod phenotype. *Hum Genet* 1988;80:85–90.

217. Johnston RB, Newman SL. Chronic granulomatous disease. *Pediatr Clin North Am* 1977;24:365–376.

218. Dilworth JA, Mandell GL. Adults with chronic granulomatous disease of childhood. *Am J Med* 1977;63:233–266.

219. Perry HB, Boulanger M, Pennoyer D. Chronic granulomatous disease in an adult with recurrent abscesses. *Arch Surg* 1980;115:200–202.

220. MacPherson BR. The clinical laboratory diagnosis of chronic granulomatous disease in childhood. *CRC Crit Rev Clin Lab Sci* 1977;8:81–103.

221. Alter BP. Advances in the prenatal diagnosis of hematologic diseases. *Blood* 1984;64:329–340.

222. Hossle JP, de Boer M, Seger RA, et al. Identification of allele-specific p22-phox mutations in a compound heterozygous patient with chronic granulomatous disease by mismatch PCR and restriction enzyme analysis. *Hum Genet* 1994;93:437–442.

223. Gorlin JB. Identification of (CA/GT) in polymorphisms within the X-linked chronic granulomatous disease (X-CGD) gene: utility for prenatal diagnosis. *J Pediatr Hematol Oncol* 1998;20:112–119.

224. Cooper MR, DeChatelet LR, McCall CE, et al. Complete deficiency of leukocyte glucose-6-phosphate dehydrogenase with defective bactericidal activity. *J Clin Invest* 1972;51:769–778.

225. Gonzalez LA, Hill HR. Advantages and disadvantages of antimicrobial prophylaxis in chronic granulomatous disease in childhood. *Pediatr Infect Dis J* 1988;7:83–85.

226. Fanconi S, Seger J, Gmur J, et al. Surgery and granulocyte transfusions for life-threatening infections in chronic granulomatous disease. *Helv Paediatr Acta* 1985;40:277–284.

227. Horwitz ME, Barret J, Brown MR, et al. Treatment of chronic granulomatous disease with nonmyeloablative conditioning and a T-cell-depleted hematopoietic allograft. *N Engl J Med* 2001;344:881–888.

228. Group TICGDS. A controlled trial of interferon gamma to prevent infection in chronic granulomatous disease. *N Engl J Med* 1991;324:509–516.

229. Aznar J, Vaya A. Homozygous form of the Pelger-Huet leukocyte anomaly in man. *Acta Haematol* 1981;66:59–62.

230. Dorr AD, Moloney WC. Acquired pseudo-Pelger anomaly of granulocytic leukocytes. *N Engl J Med* 1959;261:742–748.

231. Heyns ADP, Badenhorst PN, Wessels P, et al. Kinetics, in vitro redistribution and sites of sequestration of indium-111–labeled platelets in giant platelet syndromes. *Br J Haematol* 1985;60:323–330.

232. Coller BS, Zarrabi MH. Platelet membrane studies in the May-Hegglin anomaly. *Blood* 1981;58:279–284.

233. Brivet F, Girot R, Barbanel C, et al. Hereditary nephritis associated with May-Hegglin anomaly. *Nephron* 1981;29:59–62.

234. Peterson LC, Rao KV, Crosson JT, et al. Fechtner syndrome: a variant of Alport's syndrome with leukocyte inclusions and macrothrombocytopenia. *Blood* 1985;65:397–406.

235. Schofield KP, Stone PCW, Beddall AC, et al. Quantitative cytochemistry of the toxic granulation blood neutrophil. *Br J Haematol* 1983;53:15–22.

236. Kuriyama K, Tomonaga M, Matsuo T, et al. Diagnostic significance of detecting pseudo-Pelger-Huet anomalies and micro-megakaryocytes in myelodysplastic syndrome. *Br J Haematol* 1986;63:665–669.

237. Olofsson T, Odeberg H, Olsson I. Granulocyte function in chronic granulocytic leukemia. II. Bactericidal capacity, phagocytic rate, oxygen consumption and granule protein composition in isolated granulocytes. *Blood* 1976;48:581–593.

238. Lusis AJ. Atherosclerosis. *Nature* 2000;407:233–241.

CHAPTER 17

Eosinophils, Basophils, and Mast Cells

Peter F. Weller, Mindy Tsai, and Stephen J. Galli

EOSINOPHILS

Eosinophils, a distinct class of bone marrow–derived granulocytes, normally circulate in low numbers in the blood. Increased blood or tissue eosinophilia typically accompanies allergic diseases and helminth parasite infections and may occur with other disorders. Traditionally, roles for eosinophils as terminally differentiated, end-stage leukocytes have been sought to define the acute "effector" mechanisms by which eosinophils participate in the immunopathogenesis of allergic diseases and parasite host defense. In addition, eosinophils have further functional roles in varied responses not conventionally associated with eosinophilia, including wound healing (1,2), fibrosis (3), and graft rejection (4). Eosinophils express receptors for diverse cytokines and other immunologic mediators and notably contain multiple preformed cytokines stored within cytoplasmic granules. Eosinophils can engage in cognate cell–cell interactions with other cells, including lymphocytes (5,6). Thus, as recently reviewed (7–10), eosinophils can be both end-stage effector cells and participants in physiologic and pathologic responses not necessarily accompanied by prominent eosinophilia.

Eosinophil Development and Tissue Distribution

Eosinophils develop from interleukin (IL)-5 responsive CD34+ bone marrow progenitor cells. Granulocyte-macrophage colony-stimulating factor (GM-CSF) and IL-3 can stimulate development of eosinophils as well as other lineages, but IL-5 specifically promotes development and differentiation of eosinophils (and basophils). Although IL-5 may be produced by various cells, including mast cells and eosinophils, IL-5 is a prototypical cytokine product of CD4+ Th2 cells. IL-5 produced by this T-cell subset accounts for the eosinophilia seen with the Th2-mediated immune responses characteristic of allergic diseases and helminth infections. GM-CSF, IL-3, and IL-5 receptors are composed of cytokine-specific, low-affinity α chains, which combine with a common β chain to constitute high affinity αβ receptors. Mice with genetic deletions of IL-5, the IL-5 receptor α chain, or the common receptor β chain do not develop eosinophilia in response to allergic or helminthic challenges but still exhibit basal eosinophilia, indicating that other, currently unknown, mediators also contribute to eosinophilopoiesis.

Eosinophil maturation in the marrow develops over approximately a week to generate a pool of mature yet marrow-retained eosinophils. IL-5, alone and in concert with the chemokine

eotaxin, can release this marrow pool of mature eosinophils to rapidly increase blood eosinophilia (11). Eosinophils circulate in the blood with a half-life of 8 to 18 hours and normally leave the circulation to localize in tissues, especially those with mucosal interfaces with the external environment, including the respiratory and gastrointestinal tracts. Mechanisms governing eosinophil tropism for mucosal tissues are not known, although eotaxin is involved in the homing of eosinophils to the gastrointestinal, but not respiratory, tract (12). Eosinophils are tissue-dwelling cells; and for every eosinophil present in the circulation, 300 to 500 eosinophils are estimated to be in tissues. Eosinophils live longer than neutrophils and persist in tissues for days, if not several weeks.

The tissue accumulation of eosinophils, especially at specific sites of inflammation, is dependent on multiple adherence molecules expressed on eosinophils that regulate their egress from the marrow, circulation through the bloodstream, and subsequent entry into tissues. As with other leukocytes, eosinophil recruitment into tissue sites uses combinatorial interactions involving specific adhesion molecules (via their expression and altered affinity states) that mediate cellular interactions with the vascular endothelium and the actions of chemoattractant molecules (13,14). Eosinophils express several adhesion molecules broadly shared with other leukocytes that mediate their initial rolling and subsequent adherence to endothelial cells (13). Eosinophils express P-selectin glycoprotein ligand-1. Unlike neutrophils, but similar to lymphocytes, eosinophils express two α4 integrins, α4β1 and α4β7, that bind to vascular cell adhesion molecule-1 (VCAM-1). Both IL-4 and IL-13 enhance expression of VCAM-1 and P-selectin on human endothelial cells and thereby may contribute to preferential eosinophil localization in specific sites of inflammation (13,15).

Eosinophil recruitment into tissues is also governed by receptor-mediated chemoattractants that promote the directed migration of eosinophils and may enhance their adhesion and migration through the vascular endothelium. Many compounds have been identified as eosinophil chemoattractants (16), including immune mediators, such as platelet-activating factor (PAF) and the complement anaphylatoxins (C5a and C3a), certain cytokines, and several chemokines, most notably the eotaxins. None of these is specific solely for eosinophils, but eotaxin, eotaxin-2, and eotaxin-3 exhibit the most restricted specificity for eosinophils (17). The eotaxins signal through CCR3 receptors expressed on eosinophils as well as basophils, some Th2 cells and some mast cells. Prostaglandin (PG) D_2 attracts eosinophils via a novel recep-

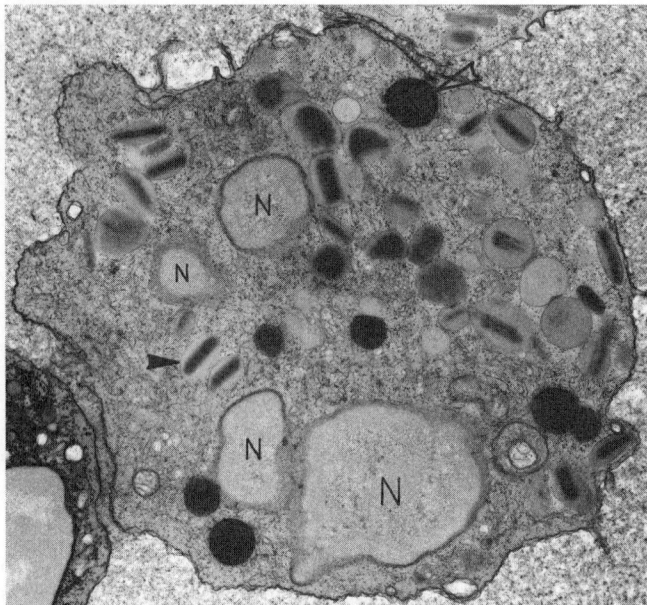

Figure 17-1. Mature peripheral blood eosinophil. Multiple nuclear lobes (N) are visible. The cytoplasm contains diffuse monoparticulate glycogen, a few vesicles, and mitochondria. Numerous specific granules (*closed arrowhead*) contain the distinctive electron-dense crystalline core. Lipid bodies (*open arrowhead*) are darkly stained with osmium. 18,500×. (Adapted from Dvorak AM, Weller PF. Ultrastructural analysis of human eosinophils. *Chem Immunol* 2000;76:1.)

tor, CRTH2, expressed on eosinophils, basophils, and Th2 cells (18). Thus, the recruitment of eosinophils to sites of immunologic reactions is governed by (1) the responsiveness of eosinophils to chemoattractants (chemokines, cytokines, and other mediators) that facilitate eosinophil emigration from the vasculature and elicit directed migration of eosinophils and (2) the expression and functional states of eosinophil adherence molecules and the differential expression of endothelial cell adherence ligands.

Eosinophil Morphology, Constituents, Products, and Mechanisms of Activation for Mediator Release

MORPHOLOGY

The distinguishing feature of eosinophils are their specific granules, which are morphologically unique because within each is located one or more crystalloid cores (Fig. 17-1) (19). Eosinophils at sites of inflammatory responses can exhibit morphologic changes within these granules, including loss of the matrix or core components from intact granules, due to extracellular release of granule components (19).

Lipid bodies, cytoplasmic structures that are distinct from granules, lack a delimiting membrane but contain an internal honeycomb-like membranous structure often obscured by an overlying lipid (19) (Fig. 17-1). Lipid bodies are found in other cells, especially in association with inflammation; but eosinophils typically contain more lipid bodies than neutrophils (20). Lipid body formation in eosinophils is rapidly inducible within minutes by signaling pathways that may be activated via PAF and CCR3 receptors (21–24). In eosinophils, key eicosanoid-forming enzymes, including cyclooxygenase, the 5- and 15-lipoxygenases and leukotriene C_4 synthase, are localized, in part, at lipid bodies (22,25).

CELL-SURFACE RECEPTORS AND PROTEINS

Eosinophils express receptors for a multitude of immunologic ligands (Table 17-1) (9). The immunoglobulin G (IgG) receptor on

TABLE 17-1. Eosinophil Plasma Membrane Proteins and Receptors

Immunoglobulin (Ig) receptors
IgA receptor: FcαR (CD89)
IgG receptors: FcγRII (CD32)
  FcγRIII (CD16) (on some activated eosinophils)
IgE receptors: FcεRI
  FcεRII (CD23)
  εBP (Mac-2)
Complement receptors and proteins
C3a receptor
C5a receptor (CD88)
CR1 (CD35): C3b, C1q, C4b, MBL
CR3 (Mac-1, CD11b/CD18): iC3b, ICAM-1
p150, 95 (CD11c/CD18): iC3b, ICAM-1
CD46
DAF (CD55)
CD59
Chemokine receptors
CCR-1: MIP-1α, MCP-3, RANTES
CCR-3: Eotaxins-1, -2, - 3; MCP-3; RANTES
CCR ?: MDC
CXCR4: SDF-1α
Other receptors
PAF receptor
PGE₂ receptor
LTB₄ receptor
Cysteinyl leukotriene receptors
PGD₂ receptor (CRTH2)
Histamine receptor(s)
β-adrenergic receptors
fMLP receptor
Cytokine receptors
IL-1
IL-2 (CD25/CD123/CD132)
IL-3 (CDw123/CDw131)
IL-4 (CD124/CD132)
IL-5 (CDw125/CDw131)
IL-12
IL-13
IL-16 (CD4)
GM-CSF (CD116/CDw131)
IFN-α
IFN-γ
TNF-α
SCF (c-*kit*)
Other immune receptors/ligands
HLA class I
HLA class II (inducible)
CD40
CD40L (CD154)
CD30L (CD153)
CD28
CD86 (B7-2)
Transmembrane 4 superfamily
CD9
CD37
CD53
CD63
CD81
Other
Fas (CD95)
CAMPATH-1 (CD52)
CD69 (on "activated" eosinophils)
CD63
CD137

CCR, C-C chemokine receptor; CD, clusters of differentiation; CR, complement receptor; CRTH2, chemoattractant receptor–homologous molecule expressed on Th2 cells; DAF, decay accelerating factor; fMLP, formylmethionylleucylphenylalanine; GM-CSF, granulocyte-macrophage colony-stimulating factor; ICAM, intercellular adhesion molecule; IFN, interferon; IL, interleukin; LTB, leukotriene B₄; MBL, mannan-binding lectin; MCP, macrophage chemotactic protein; MDC, macrophage-derived chemokine; MIP, macrophage inhibitory protein; PAF, platelet-activating factor; PG, prostaglandin; RANTES, regulated on activation normal T-cell expressed and secreted; SCF, stem cell factor; SDF-1α, stromal cell–derived factor-1α; TNF, tumor necrosis factor.

eosinophils is principally the low-affinity FcγRII (CD32). Human eosinophils do not usually express CD16, although expression of CD16 is elicitable with some stimuli (e.g., interferon-γ) and may be found on eosinophils from some eosinophilic patients. Human eosinophils have three receptors for IgE, including the high affinity IgE receptor FcεRI, found on basophils and mast cells (26). FcεRI α chain protein is detectable within eosinophils, although its surface expression can be low or undetectable (27). Whether engagement of eosinophil FcεRI elicits degranulation of eosinophils, as it does on basophils and mast cells, remains the subject of controversy. Eosinophils also express FcεRII, a low-affinity IgE receptor (CD23) (28), and a lectin-like protein, εBP/Mac-2, that binds IgE with low affinity (29). Eosinophil FcεRI (CD89) potently binds secretory IgA, and FcαRI engagement triggers eosinophil release of granule proteins (30).

Eosinophils have receptors for complement components, including C1q (CR1), C3b/C4b (CR1), iC3b (CR3), C3a, and C5a. Eosinophils express specific chemokine receptors, including CCR1 [for macrophage inhibitory protein–1α, macrophage chemotactic protein-3, and regulated upon activation normal T-cell expressed and secreted (RANTES)], CCR3 (for eotaxin, eotaxin-2, eotaxin-3, macrophage chemotactic protein-3, and RANTES), and CXCR4 (for stromal cell–derived factor-1α).

Monocyte-derived chemokine induces eosinophil chemotaxis via an undefined receptor (31). Eosinophils express receptors for GM-CSF, IL-3, and IL-5, which promote eosinophilopoiesis and stimulate the functioning of mature eosinophils. In addition, eosinophils have receptors for a broad range of other cytokines (Table 17-1), including IL-1α, IL-2, IL-4, IL-12, IL-13, interferons α and γ, tumor necrosis factor-α (TNF-α), stem cell factor (SCF) (c-kit), and IL-16 (which signals via CD4 on eosinophils). Thus, eosinophils are capable of responding to diverse cytokines, although the functional consequences of these eosinophil cytokine receptor-mediated responses are not yet well understood.

Of potential importance for cognate interactions between eosinophils and B and T lymphocytes, eosinophils express several relevant plasma membrane proteins. The expression of class II major histocompatibility complex (MHC) proteins, generally absent on blood eosinophils, can be induced *in vitro* and are found *in vivo* on eosinophils recruited into tissues sites of inflammation. Eosinophils also express CD40, CD154 (CD40 ligand), CD153 (CD30 ligand), CD28 (B7-2), and CD86.

Eosinophil lipid mediator receptors include those for PAF, leukotriene (LT) B$_4$, prostaglandin E$_2$ (PGE$_2$), and prostaglandin D$_2$ (PGD$_2$) (CRTH2) and both known cysteinyl leukotriene receptors (9,18,32,33). The functions of eosinophil cysteinyl leukotriene receptors have not been defined.

CONSTITUENTS OF EOSINOPHILS

Eosinophil-specific granules, stores of preformed proteins packaged for ready extracellular release, contain a range of proteins that include specific cationic proteins and diverse cytokines and chemokines.

Four cationic eosinophil granule proteins have been extensively studied, in part because of their abundance in granules and their ability to produce major effects pertinent to eosinophils' potential roles in host defense against helminth parasites and in contributing to tissue dysfunction and damage in eosinophil-related allergic and other diseases (34). Major basic protein (MBP) is a markedly cationic (pI ~11), 13.8- to 14.0-kD protein that is packaged in the core of specific granules. A homolog of MBP that is smaller (13.4 kD) and less basic (pI 8.7) has been identified recently (35). MBP lacks any enzymatic activity and likely exerts its varied effects based on its markedly cationic nature.

The other three cationic proteins, eosinophil peroxidase (EPO), eosinophil cationic protein (ECP) and eosinophil-derived neurotoxin (EDN), are localized in the granule matrix. EPO, distinct from the myeloperoxidase, uses hydrogen peroxide and halide ions, especially bromide and the pseudohalide, thiocyanate, in preference to chloride, to catalyze the formation of hypohalous acids. ECP (18 kD, pI 10.8) and EDN (18–19 kD, pI 8.9) share sequence homology with pancreatic ribonuclease (RNase) (36). EDN expresses 100-fold more RNase activity than does ECP (37), although their toxic effects on bacterial, parasitic, and mammalian target cells apparently are not due to their RNase catalytic activities. Eosinophil specific granules also contain enzymes similar to those in neutrophil granules, although the content of enzymes present within eosinophil granules has never been thoroughly studied. Eosinophils are a source of a 92-kD metalloproteinase, a gelatinase (38).

Eosinophils can elaborate diverse cytokines and chemokines (39). The potential activities of eosinophil-derived cytokines are protean. Eosinophil-derived cytokines include those with potential autocrine growth factor activities for eosinophils and those with potential roles in acute and chronic inflammatory responses. A notable feature of eosinophils as sources of cytokines is that eosinophils contain cytokine proteins stored within specific granules. Thus, in contrast to most lymphocytes that must be induced to synthesize *de novo* cytokines destined for release, eosinophils can immediately release preformed cytokine and chemokine proteins. This local and rapid release of eosinophil-derived cytokines in tissues can readily effect responses of varied adjoining cell types.

Eosinophils synthesize GM-CSF, IL-3, and IL-5. These growth factor cytokines act on mature eosinophils to promote their survival, antagonizing apoptosis, and enhance their effector responses. Other cytokines elaborated by human eosinophils that may have activities in acute and chronic inflammatory responses include IL-1α, IL-6, IL-8, TNF-α, macrophage inhibitory protein-1α, macrophage inhibition factor, nerve growth factor, and SCF. Human eosinophils can elaborate other various "growth" factors, including transforming growth factor (TGF)-α, TGF-β1, vascular endothelial growth factor, platelet-derived growth factor-β, and heparin-binding epidermal growth factor–like growth factor. These cytokines may have roles in contributing to epithelial hyperplasia and fibrosis, as well as other activities. In addition, eosinophils are sources of specific cytokines and chemokines capable of stimulating or inhibiting lymphocyte responses, including IL-2, IL-4, IL-9, IL-10, IL-12, IL-13, IL-16, RANTES, and TGF-β1.

PRODUCTS OF EOSINOPHILS

Eosinophils have the capacity to release a broad range of products (40), including oxidative products and newly formed lipid mediators as well as the preformed granule-derived cationic proteins and cytokines noted above. The release of granule proteins, including cytokines, does not occur via granule exocytosis, but rather by selective incorporation into small vesicles that traffic to the cell surface and release these granule contents (i.e., by a process of "piecemeal" degranulation based on vesicular transport) (19,41–43). How this process of vesicular transport is regulated to selectively mobilize specific granule-derived cytokines or cationic proteins is under study.

The oxidative products released by eosinophils include hydrogen peroxide, superoxide anion, hydroxyl radical, and singlet oxygen. In addition, eosinophil peroxidase, as noted above, may catalyze the formation of longer-lived hypohalous oxidants, including brominating oxidants (44).

Eosinophils, upon stimulation, form and release biologically active lipids. The oxidative metabolism of arachidonic acid by the 5-lipoxygenase pathway in eosinophils leads to the production of LTC_4, in contrast to neutrophils that form LTB_4 (40). Eosinophils also elaborate products from the 15-lipoxygenase pathway of arachidonic acid metabolism (40). Arachidonic acid metabolism via cyclooxygenase pathways in eosinophils forms predominantly PGE_2 and thromboxane B_2 (40). In addition to perinuclear membranes, sites of eicosanoid formation include lipid bodies in eosinophils; lipid body domains likely contribute to the augmented formation of lipoxygenase and cyclooxygenase products in primed eosinophils (22). Increased numbers of eosinophil lipid bodies correlate with increased capacities to release LTC_4 and PGE_2 (22). Moreover, lipid bodies in eosinophils are sites of specific LTC_4 formation in eotaxin and RANTES primed and stimulated cells (21). In addition to their roles as paracrine mediators, cysteinyl leukotrienes also have autocrine effects antagonizing eosinophil apoptosis (45).

Eosinophils are also a source PAF, a potent paracrine mediator with a wide range of biologic activities. PAF also functions in autocrine signaling in eosinophils, including pathways stimulated by IL-5 receptor and Fcγ receptor engagement (23).

Functions of Eosinophils

Eosinophils have functional roles in diseases characteristically marked by eosinophilia, including host defense against helminth infections and the immunopathogenesis of allergic and other eosinophilic diseases, as well as other immune or inflammatory responses not conventionally recognized to contain abundant eosinophils.

ROLES IN HOST DEFENSE
In contrast to unicellular protozoan parasites, multicellular helminth parasites characteristically stimulate Th2-mediated blood or tissue eosinophilia (46). In such infections, which are often associated with augmented IgE antibody formation, eosinophils can have roles in killing helminthic parasites, especially during their larval stages. Eosinophils adhere to the surface of parasite targets too large to be ingested by CR1 binding to C3b deposited on the worm's surface or by FcγR- or FcεR-mediated binding with antiparasite IgG or IgE, respectively. *In vitro*, deposition of eosinophil cationic granule contents onto the surface of the parasite follows, accompanied by a tighter binding of the eosinophil to the parasite. Cell products that can contribute to the death of the parasite include MBP, ECP, EDN, and EPO. Oxidative products, such as hydrogen peroxide, may also contribute to parasite cytotoxicity. While eosinophil killing of helminths is readily demonstrated *in vitro*, the interactions *in vivo* are likely very complex, as evidenced by difficulties demonstrating eosinophil killing of parasites in several models of helminth infection in mice deficient in eosinophils or overproducing eosinophils (47,48). Eosinophils likely have roles in killing infective larval stages, but not adults, of most helminth parasites (47); however, given that helminths persist in the face of eosinophilia even in naturally infected hosts, eosinophil helminthotoxicity does not totally protect hosts against these parasitic infections.

Eosinophils do not have major roles in host defense against bacteria and most other small microbial pathogens. With most bacterial and viral infections, eosinopenia, rather than eosinophilia, develops. One viral infection in which eosinophils may play a role is that due to respiratory syncytial virus. Respiratory syncytial virus infections elicit eosinophilia and associated bronchial hyperreactivity (49). The eosinophil granule proteins, EDN and ECP, based on their RNase activities, can exert antiviral activity for this single-stranded RNA virus (50).

ROLES IN DISEASE PATHOGENESIS
The capacities of eosinophils to release biologically active lipids as paracrine mediators of inflammation and to release their preformed cationic and cytokine granule constituents enable eosinophils to contribute to the immunopathogenesis of various diseases. Eosinophils are potential sources of two major types of mediator lipids, LTC_4 and PAF. LTC_4 and its derivative cysteinyl leukotrienes have bronchoconstrictor activity, constrict terminal arterioles, dilate venules, and stimulate airway mucous secretion. Oxidants released by eosinophils, including superoxide anion, hydroxyl radical, and singlet oxygen, and EPO-catalyzed hypothiocyanous acid and other hypohalous acids have the potential to damage host tissues (44).

Released eosinophil granule proteins are immunochemically detectable in fluids, including sputum, and in tissues, including the respiratory and gastrointestinal tracts, skin, and heart, in association with various eosinophil-related diseases (34). The eosinophil cationic proteins can damage various cell types (34). Release of mediators of inflammation from other cell types may also follow stimulation by eosinophil granule cationic proteins. For instance, MBP can activate basophils, mast cells, and neutrophils to release their inflammatory mediators (34). Thus, extracellular release of eosinophil granule proteins could contribute to local tissue damage by causing dysfunction and damage to adjacent cells.

OTHER EOSINOPHIL FUNCTIONS
Other functional roles for the eosinophil are likely, but as yet not fully delineated. In addition to the acute release of lipid, peptide, and cytokine mediators of inflammation, eosinophils likely contribute to chronic inflammation, including the development of fibrosis. Eosinophils are the major source of the fibrosis-promoting cytokine TGF-β1 in nodular sclerosing Hodgkin's disease and idiopathic pulmonary fibrosis (51). Additional roles of the eosinophil in modulating extracellular matrix deposition and remodeling are suggested by studies of normal wound healing. During dermal wound healing, eosinophils infiltrate into the wound sites and sequentially express TGF-α early and TGF-β1 later during wound healing (1).

Additional functions for the eosinophil are suggested by the findings that eosinophils may be induced to express class II MHC proteins and can function as antigen-presenting cells. Both murine and human eosinophils can function as class II MHC-restricted antigen-presenting cells in stimulating proliferation of T cells (52,53). *In vivo*, murine eosinophils can process exogenous antigens within the airways, traffic to regional lymph nodes, and function as antigen-specific antigen-presenting cells to stimulate responses of $CD4^+$ T cells (6). For potential interactions with lymphocytes, human eosinophils express relevant membrane proteins, including CD40, CD28, and CD86, and express receptors for varied cytokines, such as IL-2, as noted above.

Because eosinophils normally become resident in submucosal tissues, eosinophils likely have functional roles in ongoing homeostatic immune responses at these sites. Moreover, broader functional contributions are suggested by the multitude of cytokine receptors expressed on eosinophils and their potential to release a diversity of cytokines that are stored, preformed, in their granules. Interactions of eosinophils with other cells, including lymphocytes, are feasible. Thus, eosinophil functions will likely extend beyond their currently more defined roles as effector cells contributing to allergic inflammation.

TABLE 17-2. **Eosinophil-Associated Diseases and Disorders**

Allergic or atopic diseases
Allergic rhinitis, asthma, atopic dermatitis
Infectious diseases
Helminth parasites
Coccidioidomycosis
Immunologic reactions
Immunodeficiency diseases: Job's syndrome and Omenn's syndrome
Transplant rejections
Medication-related eosinophilias
Myeloproliferative and neoplastic disorders
Hypereosinophilic syndrome
Leukemia
Lymphoma- and tumor-associated
Mastocytosis
Pulmonary syndromes
Parasite-induced eosinophilic lung diseases:
  Löffler's syndrome: migratory infiltrates resolving over weeks; seen with transpulmonary migration of helminth parasites (especially *Ascaris*)
  Tropical pulmonary eosinophilia: miliary lesions and fibrosis seen with heightened immune response in lymphatic filariasis; increased IgE and antifilarial antibodies
Pulmonary parenchymal invasion: paragonimiasis
Heavy hematogenous seeding with helminths: trichinosis, schistosomiasis, larva migrans
Allergic bronchopulmonary aspergillosis
Chronic eosinophilic pneumonia: dense peripheral infiltrates; fever; progressive; blood eosinophilia may be absent; steroid responsive
Acute eosinophilic pneumonia: acute presentation diagnosed by bronchoalveolar lavage or biopsy
Churg-Strauss vasculitis: small and medium sized arteries; granulomas, necrosis; asthma often antecedent; extrapulmonary (e.g., neurologic, cutaneous, cardiac, or gastrointestinal involvement likely)
Drug- and toxin-induced eosinophilic lung diseases
Other: Hypereosinophilic syndrome, neoplasia, bronchocentric granulomatosis
Skin and subcutaneous diseases
Skin diseases: atopic dermatitis, blistering diseases, including bullous pemphigoid, urticarias, and drug reactions
Diseases of pregnancy: pruritic urticarial papules and plaques syndrome, herpes gestationis
Eosinophilic pustular folliculitis
Eosinophilic cellulitis (Well's syndrome)
Kimura's disease and angiolymphoid hyperplasia with eosinophilia
Shulman's syndrome (eosinophilic fasciitis)
Episodic angioedema with eosinophilia: recurrent periodic episodes with fever, angioedema, and secondary weight gain; may be longstanding without untoward cardiac dysfunction
Gastrointestinal disorders
Eosinophilic gastroenteritis: (a) blood eosinophilia, (b) eosinophil cell infiltrates, (c) edema of stomach or intestines, and (d) absence of extraintestinal involvement; may involve mucosa, muscularis or serosa
Inflammatory bowel disease: eosinophils in lesions; occasionally blood eosinophilia with ulcerative colitis
Rheumatologic diseases
Churg-Strauss vasculitis
Cutaneous necrotizing eosinophilic vasculitis
Endocrine
Hypoadrenalism: Addison's disease, adrenal hemorrhage, hypopituitarism
Other causes of eosinophilia
Atheromatous cholesterol embolization
Hereditary
Serosal surface irritation, including peritoneal dialysis and pleural eosinophilia

Adapted from Wilson ME, Weller PF. Approach to the patient with eosinophilia. In: Guerrant RL, Walker DH, Weller PF, eds. *Tropical infectious diseases: principles, pathogens and practice.* New York: Churchill Livingstone, 1999:1400.

Eosinophilic Syndromes

Various infectious, allergic, neoplastic, and other, often idiopathic, diseases can be associated with increased eosinophil numbers in the peripheral blood or tissues (Table 17-2). Eosino-phil numbers greater than 450/μL of blood define blood eosinophilia. Blood eosinophil numbers exhibit a mild diurnal variation, being higher in the early morning and falling as endogenous glucocorticosteroid levels increase. Blood eosinophil numbers can be decreased by stress and intercurrent bacterial and viral infections.

A propensity for endomyocardial damage is a recognized complication of varied diseases marked by sustained eosinophilia. This cardiac involvement can include early necrosis and subsequent formation of intraventricular thrombi and endomyocardial fibrosis with secondary mitral or tricuspid regurgitation. The damage to the heart occurs identically whether the eosinophilia is due to the idiopathic hypereosinophilic syndrome or other etiologies (54). Eosinophilic diseases associated at times with endomyocardial damage include eosinophilic leukemia, eosinophilia with carcinomas or Hodgkin's or non-Hodgkin's lymphomas, eosinophilia from GM-CSF or IL-2 administration or drug-reactions, and eosinophilia from helminth infections. While diverse eosinophilic diseases can cause identical forms of cardiac disease, most patients with eosinophilia develop no evidence of endomyocardial damage. Thus, the pathogenesis of eosinophil-mediated cardiac damage involves both heightened numbers of eosinophils and some activating events, as yet ill-defined, that promote eosinophil-mediated endomyocardial damage. Patients with sustained eosinophilia should be monitored by echocardiography for evidence of cardiac disease.

The idiopathic hypereosinophilic syndrome is not a single entity but rather a constellation of leukoproliferative disorders characterized by sustained overproduction of eosinophils (54,55). The three diagnostic criteria for this syndrome are (a) eosinophilia in excess of 1500/μL of blood persisting for longer than 6 months; (b) lack of an identifiable parasitic, allergic, or other etiology for eosinophilia and an absence of other, even idiopathic, eosinophilic syndromes clinically distinct from the hypereosinophilic syndrome; and (c) signs and symptoms of organ involvement (54). Not all patients with prolonged eosinophilia develop organ involvement, and many have benign courses. The clinical manifestations, severity, and therapeutic responsiveness vary for different patients with the hypereosinophilic syndrome. Because the above diagnostic criteria are sufficiently broad to include a diversity of eosinophilic disorders, the hypereosinophilic syndrome represents a collection of varied disorders. In some patients, the disorder has been correlated with either clonal expansions of CD4+, CD3−, CD8−, and Th2-like lymphocytes (56–58) or other aberrant T cells elaborating IL-5 (59). A case with eosinophilia associated with polyclonal expansion of activated CD3+ T cells expressing natural killer cell markers (CD16 and CD56) associated with IL-2 and IL-15 overproduction has been reported (60). In other eosinophilic patients, however, it appears that overproduction of IL-5 is not solely responsible for the eosinophilia (54). Clonal abnormalities in the eosinophil lineage have been reported in few patients (61–63). For many patients with the hypereosinophilic syndrome, the etiologies of the eosinophilia are not currently understood.

BASOPHILS AND MAST CELLS

Basophils, like eosinophils, are circulating granulocytes that can infiltrate tissues or appear in exudates during a variety of inflammatory or immunologic processes (Table 17-3). By contrast, morphologically identifiable mast cells do not normally circulate but reside in virtually all vascularized tissues. Despite significant differences in their natural history and distribution,

TABLE 17-3. Natural History and Major Mediators of Human Mast Cells and Basophils

	Basophils	Mast Cells
Natural history		
Origin of precursor cells	Marrow	Marrow
Site of maturation	Marrow	Connective tissue (a few in marrow)
Mature cells in circulation	Yes (usually <1% of blood leukocytes)	No
Mature cells recruited into tissues from circulation	Yes (during immunologic, inflammatory responses)	No
Mature cells normally residing in connective tissues	No (not detectable by microscopy)	Yes
Proliferative ability of morphologically mature cells	None reported	Yes (limited; under certain circumstances)
Life span	Days (like other granulocytes)	Weeks to months (according to studies in rodents)
Major growth factor	Interleukin-3 (IL-3)	Stem cell factor
Mediators		
Major mediators stored preformed in cytoplasmic granules	Histamine, chondroitin sulfates, neutral protease with bradykinin-generating activity, β-glucuronidase, elastase, cathepsin G–like enzyme, major basic protein, Charcot-Leyden crystal protein, peroxidase[a], carboxypeptidase A[b]	Histamine, heparin and/or chondroitin sulfates, neutral proteases (chymase and/or tryptase[b]), major basic protein, many acid hydrolases, cathepsin, carboxypeptidases, peroxidase
Major lipid mediators produced on appropriate activation	Leukotriene C_4	Prostaglandin D_2, leukotriene C_4, platelet-activating factor
Cytokines released on appropriate activation[c]	IL-4, IL-13	TNF-α, MIP-1α, VPF/VEGF, IL-3, IL-4, IL-5, IL-6, IL-8, IL-10, IL-11, IL-13, IL-16, GM-CSF, MCP-1 (Mouse and perhaps human mast cells produce many more.)

GM-CSF, granulocyte-macrophage colony-stimulating factor; MCP, macrophage chemotactic protein; MIP, macrophage inhibitory protein; TNF, tumor necrosis factor; VPF/VEGF, vascular permeability factor/vascular endothelial growth factor.
[a]The peroxidase of basophil granules may be similar or identical to eosinophil peroxidase. Adapted from Toba KK, Shibata T, Hashimoto A, et al. Novel technique for the direct flow cytofluorometric analysis of human basophils in unseparated blood and bone marrow, and the characterization of phenotype and peroxidase of human basophils. *Cytometry* 1999;35:249.
[b]Under certain conditions, tryptase+, chymase+, carboxypeptidase A+ and c-*kit*+ granulated cells that appear to be basophils by morphology and are reactive with an antibody against BSP-1 (which stains basophils but not mast cells) can be observed in the peripheral blood. Adapted from Li L, Li Y, Reddel SW, et al. Identification of basophilic cells that express mast cell granule proteases in the peripheral blood of asthma, allergy, and drug-reactive patients. *J Immunol* 1998;161:5079–5086.
[c]Several lines of evidence indicate that certain cytokines produced by mast cells, such as TNF-α and VPF/VEGF, are released in part from preformed stores, some of which may be physically associated with the cells' cytoplasmic granules.

both basophils and mast cells have prominent cytoplasmic granules with affinity for certain basic dyes. They store (or release on appropriate stimulation) a similar (not identical) pattern of biochemical mediators (Table 17-3), and they express cell-surface receptors (FcεRI) that bind the Fc portion of IgE class antibodies with high affinity (Table 17-4). Most important, they participate in mechanisms of host defense and in IgE-associated allergic disorders. To highlight their many similarities and also emphasize their differences, the features of basophils and mast cells are presented together.

Basophil and Mast Cell Development and Tissue Distribution

The derivation of basophils from precursors shared by other granulocytes and monocytes is suggested by cytogenetic evidence (64,65), analyses of cell-surface phenotype (66–70), and observations made *in vitro* in which colonies of bone marrow–derived cells that include basophils also usually contain eosinophils and other granulocytes (71,72). Studies of the production and circulation of human basophils suggest that the kinetics of basophil production and peripheral circulation are similar to those of eosinophils (73,74). Basophils and eosinophils also share certain biochemical constituents, exhibit some similarities in the regulation of their numbers in the circulation (see Basophilopenia and Basophilia), and often represent the two most prevalent lineages when human hematopoietic cells are cultured in suspension in the presence of IL-3 and IL-4 (68,75,76). In addition, a single family has been reported

with a hereditary syndrome in which crystalline inclusions appear in the cytoplasmic granules of eosinophils and basophils but not in neutrophils or mast cells (77). Taken together, these findings suggest that basophils and eosinophils may be more closely related to each other than to neutrophils or other differentiated products of the hematopoietic system, including mast cells.

The basophil is the least common of human blood granulocytes, with a normal mean incidence of less than 0.5% of total circulating leukocytes and about 0.3% of total nucleated bone marrow cells (78). The basophil's prominent, metachromatic cytoplasmic granules permit it to be identified easily in Wright-Giemsa–stained preparations of peripheral blood or bone marrow cells, but because of the cell's rarity, accurate estimates of basophil numbers require absolute counting methods (78,79). The absolute numbers of circulating basophils exhibit wide individual variation, with normal ranges in two studies of 20–45/μL and 10–80/μL (64,79). Unlike the eosinophil, the basophil ordinarily does not occur in peripheral tissues in significant numbers. Basophils can infiltrate sites of many immunologic or inflammatory processes (often in association with eosinophils) and are represented in the reactions to some tumors (80). In such cases, the basophils are readily distinguishable from mast cells residing in the same tissues (81).

In contrast to the basophil, mast cells do not normally circulate in mature form. Although a circulating lineage-committed precursor of the mast cell has not been identified in humans, studies in mice indicate that some mast cell precursors are bone

TABLE 17-4. Plasma Membrane Proteins of Human Mast Cells and Basophils

	Basophils	Mast Cells
Immunoglobulin receptors	FcεRI, FcγRII (CDw32)	FcεRI, FcγRI, FcγRII, FcγRIII (only mRNA)
Cytokine and growth factor receptors	IL-1RII (CD121b), IL-2Rα (CD25), IL-3R, IL-4R (CD124), IL-5R (CD125),and IL-8R (CD128) and GM-CSFR (CD116), IFN-α/βR (CD118), IFN-γR (CD119); c-*kit* (CD117) (some basophils express low numbers of c-*kit* receptors[a])	c-*kit* (CD117) [only mRNA: IL-3R, IL-4R, IL-5R, IL-6R]
Complement receptors and proteins	CR1 (CD35), CR3/C3biR (CD11b/18),CR4 (CD11c/18) C5aR (CD88), C3aR, MCP (CD46), DAF (CD55), MACIF (CD59)	C5aR(CD88), MCP(CD46), DAF(CD55), MACIF(CD59)
Chemokine receptors	CCR1, CCR2, CCR3, , CXCR1, CXCR2, CXCR4	CXCR-1, CXCR-2, CCR3
Other immune receptors/ligands	CD40L (CD154), CD40, CD4[b]	CD40L (CD154), HLA-DR, HLA-DQ
Other receptors	fMLPR, PAFR, histamine H$_2$ receptor, PGD$_2$ receptor	Histamine H$_2$ receptor, PGD$_2$ receptor, urokinase receptor (CD87)
Transmembrane 4 superfamily	CD37, CD53, CD63, CD81	CD53, CD63, CD81
Cell adhesion structures (underlined structures are apparently expressed on just one of the two cell types)	P24 (CD09), LFA-1β chain, PECAM (CD31), β1 integrins (CD29, CD49d, CD49e), ICAM-1 (CD54) (low level), ICAM-2 (CD102), ICAM-3 (CD50), β2 integrins (CD18, CD11a, CD11b, CD11c), VCAM-1 , LFA-1(CD11a/18), LFA-3 (CD58), Leukosialin (CD43), Pgp-1 (CD44)	P24(CD09), LFA-1β chain, β1 integrins (CD29, CD49d, CD49e), ICAM-1 (CD54) (low level), ICAM-2 (CD102), ICAM-3(CD50)(+), β3 integrins (CD61, CD51), LFA-3(CD58), Leukosialin (CD43), Pgp-1(CD44)
Others	LCA (CD45), ME491 (CD63), bsp-1, CD46, CD54, CD13, CD26	LCA (CD45), ME491 (CD63), CD46, CD54

CCR, C-C chemokine receptor; CD, clusters of differentiation; CR, complement receptor; DAF, decay accelerating factor; fMLPR, formylmethionylleucylphenylalanine receptor; GM-CSFR, granulocyte-macrophage colony-stimulating factor receptor; ICAM, intercellular adhesion molecule; IFN, interferon; IL, interleukin; LCA, leukocyte common antigen; LFA, lymphocyte function–associated antigen; MACIF, membrane attack complex inhibition factor; MCP, membrane co-factor protein; mRNA, messenger ribonucleic acid; PAFR, platelet-activating factor receptor; PECAM, platelet endothelium cellular adhesion molecule; PGD, prostaglandin D; SCF, stem cell factor; SDF-1α, stromal cell–derived factor-1α; TNF, tumor necrosis factor; VCAM, vascular adhesion molecule; VLA, very late antigen; VNR, vitronectin receptor.
Data regarding CD antigens are from analysis of blood basophils (references 67–70) and lung or uterine mast cells (references 67–69).
[a]See references 101 and 102.
[b]It appears that at least some peripheral blood basophils can express CD4 (reference 183).

marrow–derived cells lacking morphologically identifiable cytoplasmic granules (82,83), whereas an apparently lineage-committed mast cell precursor, the "promastocyte" identified in fetal mouse blood, does contain small numbers of cytoplasmic granules like those of mast cells (84). The hypothesis that basophils can represent circulating precursors of mast cells has not been formally excluded, but it seems unlikely for several reasons:

1. No evidence has been presented indicating that mature circulating basophils are capable either of division or of differentiation into mast cells.
2. The rare reports of patients with hereditary or acquired abnormalities affecting basophil numbers or morphology indicate that eosinophils but not mast cells may also be affected in these disorders (77,85,86).
3. Morphologically identifiable human tissue mast cells can exhibit mitotic activity, indicating that this lineage can replicate independently of a stage resembling the circulating basophil (87).
4. Studies of the differentiation potential of human hematopoietic cells *in vitro* indicate that peripheral blood basophils can not give rise to mast cells (88), whereas mast cells can be generated from circulating progenitors that are CD34+, c-*kit*+, Ly−, CD14−, CD17− (or from CD34+, CD38+, HLADR− progenitors in the cord blood) (89).

Mast cells occur throughout virtually all vascularized tissues, although their numbers in individual anatomic sites exhibit considerable variation (80,89–95). In humans and many other mammalian species, mast cells, like eosinophils, are particularly abundant near surfaces exposed to environmental antigens or parasites, such as the skin, gastrointestinal tract, and respiratory system. Mast cells also represent a numerically minor component of human bone marrow (0.02% or less of nucleated cells in sternal aspirates) (78). The anatomic distribution of mast cells within individual organs or tissues varies, although in most sites, mast cells occur in close association with blood vessels or nerves (90–95).

Under some circumstances, such as in association with certain inflammatory or immunologic reactions, mast cells can appear within the respiratory or gastrointestinal epithelium and in secretions at these sites (92). The numbers of mast cells at sites of chronic inflammation due to a variety of different causes can often be many times higher than in the corresponding normal tissues (see Secondary Changes in Mast Cell Numbers) (90–95). The extent to which such changes in mast cell number reflect proliferation of resident mast cell populations compared with recruitment and differentiation of mast cell precursors remains to be determined.

Variation in multiple morphologic, biochemical, or functional characteristics, including sensitivity to pharmacologic agents, has been identified in mast cells derived from different anatomic locations (and even among mast cells in the same tissue or organ) in humans and several other mammalian species (82,90–95). This phenomenon, called *mast cell heterogeneity*, suggests that mast cells of different phenotype may express different functions in health and disease. Mast cell phenotype may be regulated by multiple mechanisms influencing the maturation and differentiation or function of the cells (82,91–97).

In humans, IL-3 promotes basophil production and survival *in vitro* (66,72) and can induce basophilia *in vivo* (98). These findings suggest that IL-3 may contribute to the regulation of normal levels of blood basophils and raise the possibility that increased production of IL-3 by T cells may promote the baso-philia associated with certain immunologic responses. Findings in IL-3 −/− mice indicate that IL-3 is not necessary for the development of normal numbers of bone marrow or blood basophils but is very important for the bone marrow and blood basophilia associated with certain Th2 cell-associated immunologic responses (99,100). Basophils also express receptors for several cytokines besides IL-3 (Table 17-4), and some basophils express small numbers of c-*kit*, the receptor for SCF (101,102). IL-3 and some of these other cytokines can modulate basophil function, for example, by inducing mediator release directly or by augmenting the cell's ability to release mediators in response to challenge with IgE and specific antigen (66,103).

In vitro and *in vivo* studies in murine rodents, nonhuman primates, and humans indicate that many individual aspects of mast cell development are critically regulated by SCF (96,97,104,105). SCF is produced by many different cell types in membrane-associated and soluble forms, both of which are biologically active (96,104). In addition to promoting the migration, survival, proliferation, and maturation of cells in the mast cell lineage, SCF also can directly promote release of mast cell cytokines (106) or other mediators (101,107) and, at even lower concentrations, can augment mast cell mediator release in response to stimulation by IgE and antigen (101,108). Thus, SCF not only regulates the normal development of mast cells but also influences the functional repertoire of these cells. Recent reports indicate that human mast cells (109) and human eosinophils (110) represent potential sources of SCF.

Factors in addition to SCF may also contribute to mast cell development or survival in humans. Although the binding of FcεRI by IgE is thought to primarily regulate the effector function of mast cells, IgE can also promote mouse mast cell survival *in vitro* by suppressing apoptosis (111,112). Whether IgE has antiapoptotic effects on human basophils or mast cells remains to be determined, and, even in mice, the biologic significance of such findings is not yet clear.

Basophil and Mast Cell Morphology, Cellular Constituents, and Products

MORPHOLOGY

Morphologic distinctions between mature basophils and mast cells have been appreciated in all mammalian species that have been carefully studied (80,81). Typical human basophils and mast cells can be distinguished from each other in appropriately fixed and processed light microscopic sections, but the differences between the two cell types are particularly evident by transmission electron microscopy (81). Mature human basophils contain round cytoplasmic granules with electron-dense particles and, rarely, large crystals (Fig. 17-2) (81). As in other mature granulocytes, the nucleus typically is segmented and the chromatin is heavily condensed, the cytoplasm contains glycogen particles and aggregates, and the rough endoplasmic reticulum and Golgi apparatus are inconspicuous.

In vivo, human mast cells generally appear larger than basophils and contain a round-to-oval nucleus that typically is not segmented and generally occupies an eccentric location within the cell (Fig. 17-3) (80,81). Mature human mast cells have granules that are more numerous, smaller, and more variable in shape than those of basophils. The granule content also is much more heterogeneous than that of basophils and can appear as scrolls, particles, or crystals, either alone or in combination (80,81). Human basophil granules can also contain occasional multilamellar arrays and scroll-like structures (81). In contrast to the blunt surface projections of basophils, quiescent mast cells (those not participating in a degranulation event) are covered by uni-

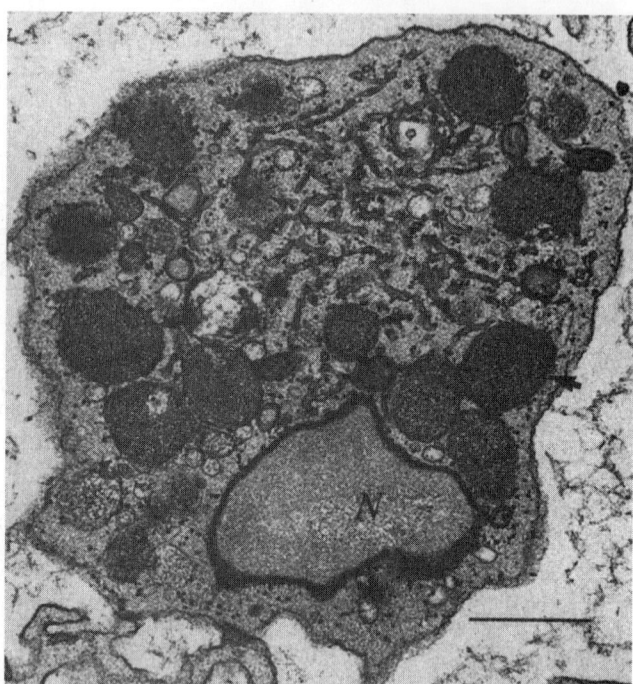

Figure 17-2. Transmission electron micrograph of a human basophil in a preparation of peripheral blood leukocytes obtained by separation over Ficoll-Hypaque density gradient. All cytoplasmic granules (some indicated by *solid arrows*) contain particulate electron-dense material. N, nucleus; bar = 1 μm. (From Dvorak AM, Newball HH, Dvorak HF, et al. Antigen-induced IgE-mediated degranulation of human basophils. *Lab Invest* 1980;43:126, with permission.)

formly distributed, thin surface processes. Mast cells also differ from basophils in having many more cytoplasmic filaments and in lacking cytoplasmic glycogen deposits (80,81). Human mast cells can also contain numerous cytoplasmic lipid bodies, structures uncommonly observed in basophils (80,81,113,114).

BASOPHIL AND MAST CELL CONSTITUENTS AND PRODUCTS

Basophils and mast cells contain or elaborate on appropriate stimulation, a diverse array of potent, biologically active mediators (Table 17-3) (115–117). Some of these are stored preformed in the cells' cytoplasmic granules (proteoglycans, proteases, histamine); others are synthesized on activation of the cell by IgE and antigen or other stimuli (products of arachidonic acid oxidation through the cyclooxygenase or lipoxygenase pathways, and, in some cells, PAF). Individually, these agents can have diverse effects in inflammation, immunity, and tissue remodeling and can influence the clotting, fibrinolytic, complement, and kinin systems (115–117).

Human mast cell populations contain variable mixtures of heparin and chondroitin sulfate proteoglycans (118,119). Although the sulfated glycosaminoglycans of normal human blood basophils have not been characterized, heparin has not been detected consistently in basophils of patients with myelogenous leukemia (118,119). Although the biologic functions of basophil and mast cell proteoglycans are not yet fully understood, in mice, heparin is required for normal packaging of certain neutral proteases in mast cell cytoplasmic granules (120,121).

Human basophils and mast cells synthesize histamine and store histamine in their cytoplasmic granules in ionic association with the granule proteoglycans (115,116). Basophils are the source of most, if not all, of the histamine present in normal

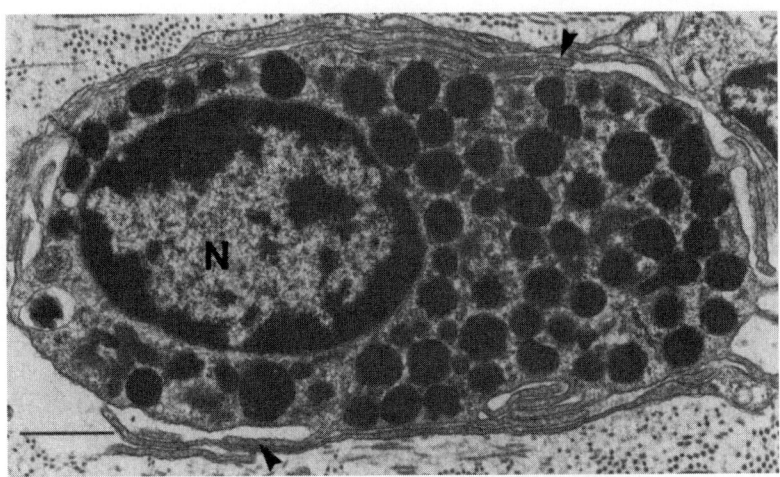

Figure 17-3. Transmission electron micrograph of a human mast cell from a breast fibroadenoma specimen. The nucleus (N) is monolobed; narrow surface folds (*arrowheads*) and numerous cytoplasmic granules are seen. Bar = 1 μm. (From Dvorak AM. Human mast cells. In: Beck F, Hild W, Kriz W, et al, eds. *Advances in anatomy embryology and cell biology*, Vol. 114. Berlin: Springer-Verlag, 1989;1, with permission.)

human blood (122). Studies in genetically mast cell–deficient and congenic normal mice indicate that mast cells represent the source of virtually all of the histamine stored in normal tissues, with the notable exceptions of the stomach and the central nervous system (123). Mouse and rat mast cells contain significant quantities of serotonin, but this amine has not been detected in populations of human mast cells or basophils.

Neutral proteases represent the major protein component of mast cell secretory granules. Human mast cell tryptase is a serine endopeptidase that exists in the granule in active form as a tetramer of 134 kD containing subunits of 31 to 35 kD, each of which contains an active site (124). The active tetrameric form of tryptase is stabilized by its association with heparin and perhaps other proteoglycans within the mast cell granule (124). Recent work indicates that there are multiple, closely related genes for human tryptase, which raises the possibility that the corresponding products may have some distinct functions (125). Mast cell chymase is also a serine protease that is stored in active form in the mast cell granule but as a monomer with a molecular weight of 30 kD (126,127). Chymase is present in relatively high levels of some mast cell populations, including those of the skin and gastrointestinal submucosal tissue [these mast cells have been designated MC_{TC} because of their content of tryptase and chymase (128)] but is present in low or undetectable levels in many of the mast cells in other anatomic sites such as the lung and gastrointestinal mucosa (128,129) [these mast cells have been designated MC_T (128)]. Mast cells that express chymase but little or no tryptase (MC_C) have also been reported (130).

A population of basophilic cells isolated from the blood of patients with allergic disorders closely resemble basophils by morphology, but these cells express tryptase, chymase, or carboxypeptidase A in their granules (102). In addition, it was recently reported that basophils isolated from some normal individuals express tryptase in an amount comparable to that found in mast cells (131). One interpretation of these findings is that basophils, like mast cells, can exhibit heterogeneity in multiple phenotypic characteristics, such as content of tryptase, chymase, and carboxypeptidase A, and extent of expression of the SCF receptor, c-*kit* (101,102).

The human mast cell cytoplasmic granule-associated carboxypeptidase can convert angiotensin I to des-leu$_{10}$ angiotensin I (132). Human basophils, like eosinophils, can form Charcot-Leyden crystals (133,134) and contain Charcot-Leyden crystal protein (lysophospholipase) in quantities similar to that of eosinophils (133).

In addition to the preformed, cytoplasmic granule-associated mediators, basophils and mast cells can release products of

arachidonic acid oxidation after appropriate stimulation (e.g., with IgE and specific antigen) (115,116). The specific products released by different populations of mast cells or by blood basophils vary considerably. For example, mast cells isolated from a variety of different human tissues release both LTC_4 and PGD_2, whereas peripheral blood basophils release LTC_4 but no detectable PGD_2 (115,116).

Platelet-activating factor [originally PAF, more recently designated PAF-acether or alkylglyceryletherphosphoryl-choline (AGEPC)] and its inactive derivative, lyso-PAF, appear in biologic fluids after antigen challenge in humans (135), but it is unclear whether human basophils or mast cells represent important potential sources of this mediator. Production of AGEPC by human basophils has not been demonstrated (136). Purified human lung mast cells can generate AGEPC on immunologic activation, but the compound apparently remains cell-associated (137).

Mast cells represent a potential source of many different cytokines and growth factors (117,138–140). For example, appropriately stimulated mouse or human mast cells can release the cytokine TNF-α (141–143), and both mouse and human mast cells and basophils can produce IL-4 (138,140,144–146). Work with mouse and human mast cells indicates that mast cells may also represent a potential source of many additional cytokines with effects in inflammation, immunity, hematopoiesis, tissue remodeling, and many other biologic processes (117,147). At least two of the mast cell–associated cytokines, TNF-α and vascular permeability factor/vascular endothelial growth factor (VPF/VEGF), can be released by mast cells from both preformed stores and, in even larger amounts, from a newly synthesized pool (141,143,148). Thus, TNF-α and VPF/VEGF represent mast cell–associated mediators that are preformed and newly synthesized. The spectrum of basophil-derived cytokines appears to be more limited than that of mast cells but includes IL-4 and IL-13 (144,146,149).

Basophil and Mast Cell Functions and Mechanisms of Activation for Mediator Release

The actual roles of basophils and mast cells in health and host defense have been remarkably difficult to ascertain. In part, this reflects the rarity of "experiments of nature" affecting these populations. Few patients lacking basophils have been reported, and these persons usually also have other abnormalities that might potentially affect immune or inflammatory responses (150,151). We are not aware of reports of humans with a profound mast cell deficiency.

In the absence of information derived from patients with isolated abnormalities of basophil or mast cell numbers or function, concepts of the roles of these cells in human health and disease have been developed based on more indirect lines of evidence, including animal experiments. This work indicates that the major roles of basophils and mast cells in host defense are in the orchestration of local immunologic and inflammatory reactions, especially those associated with parasitic infections, and that their major role in disease is to represent an important source of the mediators responsible for many reactions of immediate hypersensitivity and related IgE-associated disorders (94,115–117,147). In both of these contexts—host defense against parasites and IgE-associated disorders—the roles of basophils and mast cells are expressed primarily by the release to the exterior of preformed, granule-associated mediators, cytokines, or newly generated (lipid) mediators. Although the ability of basophils or mast cells to phagocytose bacteria and other particles has been reported (152), it is not yet clear whether this represents an important aspect of their contribution to host defense or pathology (152,153). On the other hand, studies in "mast cell knock-in mice" [i.e., genetically mast cell–deficient mice that have been selectively repaired of their mast cell deficiency (95,117)] have shown that mast cells can contribute significantly to "innate immunity" by promoting host defense against some bacterial infections (154,155). This role of the mast cell in "innate" or "natural" immunity appears to be due in part to complement-dependent activation of mast cells (156) and in part to TNF-α production by mast cells (154–157), although other mechanisms of mast cell activation [e.g., via fimbrial adhesions and CD48 (152) and via lipopolysaccharide (LPS) and Toll-like receptor 4 (158)], as well as other meditators, can contribute to the role of mast cells in innate immunity (152,153).

In vitro studies also indicate that basophils and mast cells can internalize and store in their granules certain products of other cell types, including eosinophil peroxidase (159,160). This mechanism may contribute to the limitation of the toxicity or other biologic activities of the internalized compounds or, alternatively, may place the expression of the compounds' biologic activity under the regulation of signals that elicit basophil or mast cell degranulation.

MECHANISMS OF ACTIVATION FOR MEDIATOR RELEASE

The dominant cellular event that underlies expression of basophil or mast cell function is the process of *degranulation*, a stereotyped constellation of stimulus-activated biochemical (161,162) and morphologic (81) events that result in the fusion of the cytoplasmic granule membranes with the plasma membrane (with external release of granule-associated mediators), associated with the generation and release of products of arachidonic acid oxidation (Fig. 17-4). Although a variety of stimuli can initiate basophil or mast cell degranulation, the best-studied pathway of stimulation is that transduced through FcεRI expressed on the basophil or mast cell surface (161,162). Human basophils generated *in vitro* can express approximately 2.7×10^5 FcεRI per cell, which bind monovalent IgE immunoglobulin with a K_A of approximately 2.8×10^9 mol/L (163). The FcεRI consists of one α chain, which binds the Fc portion of IgE, one β chain, which amplifies signaling via the receptor and promotes its expression on the cell surface, and two identical disulfide-linked γ chains, which transmit the signal into the cell (161,162). When adjacent FcεRIs are aggregated, either by bivalent or multivalent antigens interacting with receptor-bound IgE or by antibodies directed against receptor-bound IgE or the receptor itself, activation of the cells for release of stored and newly generated mediators is rapidly triggered (161,162). Notably, as plasma levels of IgE increase (as typically occurs in subjects with allergic diseases or parasite infections), levels of FcεRI expression on the surface of basophils and mast cells also

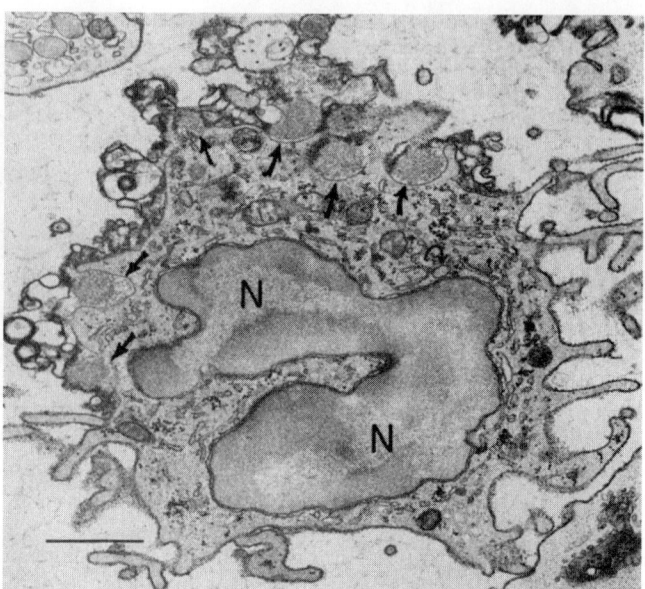

Figure 17-4. Transmission electron micrograph of a human basophil 2 minutes after exposure to antigen *in vitro*. The cell, undergoing immunoglobulin E– and antigen-dependent degranulation, exhibits extrusion of granules from six separate sites on plasma membrane (*arrows*). At this time, after cell stimulation, particle-filled granules retain shape and characteristic structure even after exposure to extracellular milieu. Electron-dense deposits of cationized ferritin coat the cell surface and enter cul-de-sacs that contain exteriorized granules. The cell exhibits no fully intracytoplasmic, typical basophilic granules, but one of the smaller kind of granules (*curved arrow*) can be observed in perinuclear region. N, nucleus; bar = 1 μm. (From Dvorak AM, Newball HH, Dvorak HF, et al. Antigen-induced IgE-mediated degranulation of human basophils. *Lab Invest* 1980;43:126, with permission.)

increase (117,147,164). Compared to cells with low "baseline" levels of FcεRI expression, such cells can bind more IgE, release mediators in response to lower concentrations of allergens, and produce significantly larger amounts of preformed and lipid mediators and cytokines (117,164). Thus, basophils and mast cells in subjects with higher levels of IgE are significantly enhanced in their ability to express IgE-dependent effector or immunoregulatory functions (117,147,164). Degranulation by the FcεRI is also associated with activation of membrane-associated serine proteases, phospholipase C, methyltransferase and adenylate cyclase, the stimulation of phosphatidylinositol turnover and generation of diacylglycerol, and activation of protein kinase C and phospholipase A_2 (161,162).

In addition to IgE and specific antigen, a variety of biologic substances, chemical agents, and physical stimuli can elicit release of basophil or mast cell mediators, including products of complement activation (C3a, C5a), products of bacteria and viruses (some of which appear to act directly and some by interacting with IgE bound to the cells' surface, thus functioning as "super antigens"), certain chemokines and cytokines, some neuropeptides, morphine and other narcotics, and hyperosmolar mannitol (115–117,153). However, the responsiveness of basophils and mast cells to individual examples of these stimuli varies, and significant differences have been reported in the responses of mast cells derived from different anatomic sites. Some of these agents, when administered systemically, can induce a clinical picture indistinguishable from IgE-dependent anaphylaxis (165). Others may release certain cytokines in preference to preformed mediators or proportionately more histamine than products of arachidonic acid oxidation (115–117,153). Mast cells and basophils may be able to release granule contents by a process of vesicle-mediated "piece-meal granulation," as well as by classical degranulation (80,81). The molecular regulation of this process remains to be determined.

BASOPHIL AND MAST CELL FUNCTIONS IN IGE-ASSOCIATED AND OTHER BIOLOGIC RESPONSES

The rapid release of mediators from IgE-primed basophils and mast cells activated by exposure to parasite-associated antigens is thought to contribute significantly to the local inflammation associated with IgE-dependent immune responses to parasites (115–117,153). When the same events are triggered by antigens that are intrinsically innocuous or of limited toxicity, such as pollen, food components, pharmacologic agents, or insect venom, the result is a disorder of immediate hypersensitivity (116,117). The latter can range in severity from the simply annoying (allergic rhinitis) to the catastrophic and life-threatening (systemic anaphylaxis) (165). In addition to such acute manifestations of IgE-dependent disorders, basophils and mast cells also contribute significantly to late-phase reactions, inflammatory reactions involving the skin, respiratory tract, or gastrointestinal tract, which follow by hours the exposure of sensitive subjects to specific antigen (117,166). It is widely believed that much of the morbidity associated with chronic allergic conditions, such as allergic asthma, reflects the actions of leukocytes recruited to sites of late-phase reactions and which persist at sites of chronic allergic inflammation (117,166).

Although there is much circumstantial evidence suggesting an important role for mast cells and basophils in IgE-associated immune responses to multicellular parasites, theories about the specific functions and potential importance of basophils and mast cells in this setting have far outdistanced hard evidence documenting the cells' actual contributions. This reflects, in large part, the difficulties of effectively manipulating these populations *in vivo* (117,147). The most compelling evidence supporting a role for basophils and mast cells in defense against parasites is found in immune responses to ectoparasites such as ticks. However, the relative importance of basophils or mast cells in orchestrating the effector limb of the immune response to ticks may vary according to species of host and species of tick (147,167–170).

Mast cell activation and infiltration of circulating basophils also can occur during a variety of T-cell–dependent immunologic responses that are not associated with IgE production in humans and experimental animals (117,171,172). However, in mice, examples of such responses generally can be expressed in the absence of mast cells, at least under certain conditions of testing, indicating that mast cells are not essential for the responses (117,171,172). On the other hand, under some conditions, mast cells appear to be required for the optimal expression of the responses. Thus, studies in mast cell knock-in mice indicate that mast cells can contribute to neutrophil recruitment at sites of cutaneous contact hypersensitivity reactions (173) and to airway hyperreactivity, airway inflammation and eosinophil recruitment, and airway epithelial cell proliferation at sites of allergen challenge in an asthma model (174). These studies and others indicate that mast cells may have a major "amplifying" function in regulating the extent of inflammation at sites of T-cell–dependent responses, particularly under conditions of antigen sensitization and challenge that might, in the absence of mast cells, be associated with relatively weak responses (117,175,176).

In addition to their participation in immune responses, basophils or mast cells have been implicated in a wide variety of biologic responses, including diverse acute inflammatory responses and examples of angiogenesis and wound healing, inflammatory bowel disease, scleroderma, and the reactions to certain neoplasms (80,81,117,171,177). The roles of basophils or mast cells in most of the responses mentioned are uncertain, but stud-

ies in mast cell knock-in mice indicate that mast cells can augment the intensity or rate of development of immunologically nonspecific acute inflammatory reactions and also may accelerate the development of blood vessels in association with certain experimental tumors (177–180).

Recently, several lines of evidence suggest that mast cells and basophils may play a role in human immunodeficiency virus (HIV) infections. HIV-1 gp120 can activate human basophils and lung mast cells *in vitro* by binding to the V_H3 region of IgE, and thereby induce the release of IL-4 and IL-13 from human basophils and histamine from both basophils and lung mast cells (181). Tat, the HIV-1 viral *trans*-activator protein, was shown to be a potent chemoattractant for basophils and mast cells by interacting with the chemokine receptor CCR3 (182). Li et al. detected the expression of CD4 and the HIV retrovirus co-receptors, CCR5 and CXCR4, on the surface of basophilic cells (with many features of basophils) isolated from the blood of allergic patients; moreover, HIV-1 viral protein can be detected in such cells in acquired immunodeficiency syndrome (AIDS) patients (183).

Basophilopenia and Basophilia

Except when numbers of basophils are extraordinarily elevated, such as in chronic myelogenous leukemia (CML) and other myeloproliferative disorders, accurate determination of blood basophil levels requires absolute methods of quantification (78,79). Because most laboratories do not routinely perform such determinations, information about conditions associated with elevation or diminution of numbers of basophils is more limited than it is for other granulocytes (Table 17-5). Basophilopenia has

---

TABLE 17-5. Disorders Associated with Alterations in Numbers of Blood Basophils

Decreased numbers (basophilopenia)
Hereditary absence of basophils (very rare)
Elevated levels of glucocorticoids
Hyperthyroidism or treatment with thyroid hormones
Ovulation
Hypersensitivity reactions
  Urticaria (acute)
  Anaphylaxis
  Drug-induced reactions
Leukocytosis (in association with diverse disorders) such as the following:
  Acute myocardial infarction
  Lobar pneumonia
  Bleeding peptic ulcer
Lipemia
Solid tumors (some patients)
Increased numbers (basophilia)
Allergy or inflammation
  Ulcerative colitis
  Drug, food, or inhalant hypersensitivity
  Erythroderma, urticaria (chronic)
  Juvenile rheumatoid arthritis
Endocrinopathy
  Diabetes mellitus
  Estrogen administration
  Hypothyroidism (myxedema)
Infection
  Chickenpox
  Influenza
  Smallpox
  Tuberculosis
Iron deficiency
Exposure to ionizing radiation
Neoplasia
  Leukemias associated with basophilia (see Table 17-6)
  Myeloproliferative diseases (especially chronic myelogenous leukemia; also polycythemia vera, idiopathic myelofibrosis, primary thrombocythemia)
  Carcinoma (certain examples)

been recorded immediately after anaphylaxis and in urticaria, especially when angioedema is present (184,185). These findings probably reflect, at least partly, a loss of metachromatic staining of degranulated basophils rather than an actual drop in basophil numbers (184). Diurnal variations in basophil levels, with lowest levels in the morning, have been reported in some persons (184,186) but not in others (184). Some authors have detected slight variations in adult basophil counts with age or sex, whereas this was not observed in other studies (184,187,188). Basophils have been reported to almost double within 24 hours of birth, to drop to values less than half of the adult levels by 1 week, then to increase nearly to adult levels by 6 weeks after birth (187). Most authors found blood basophil levels in children to be similar to those of adults (184,187).

Perhaps the most common clinical settings in which basophilopenia can be documented (often in association with a parallel eosinophilopenia) are during the reactive leukocytoses associated with disorders such as acute myocardial infarction, lobar pneumonia, and bleeding peptic ulcer (189,190). These findings may reflect effects of release of increased levels of corticosteroids during these conditions, because administration of adrenocorticotropic hormone or corticosteroids results in marked reductions in basophil and eosinophil counts (191–193). Basophils can be greatly diminished in thyrotoxicosis or after treatment with thyroid hormones and may be increased after ablation of thyroid function or in myxedema (188,190,194). Ovulation has been associated with a rapid and significant (up to 50%) drop in basophil levels; the mechanisms and significance of this phenomenon are not clear (195). Basophil degranulation can also be observed during lipemia (196). One study has reported that patients with solid malignant tumors exhibited a modest (approximately 30% to 40%) diminution of levels of blood histamine, basophils, and eosinophils compared with those of control groups (197).

Basophil levels are variably increased in patients with chronic myeloproliferative disorders, a finding that can be useful in distinguishing these conditions from leukemoid reactions in which absolute basophil levels generally are low (198). Basophils may be moderately elevated to 1000/μL or more in myeloid metaplasia and polycythemia vera (198) and can be strikingly elevated in CML, in which basophils often account for 2% to 20% of circulating leukocytes (Table 17-6) (198). Basophil counts exceeding 30% can occur intermittently during the course of CML, particularly late in the disease, often in association with its terminal phase (199). The basophils found in CML patients are best considered neoplastic cells, which in some patients have been reported to possess the Ph chromosome (65,200) (and presumably also the breakpoint cluster gene rearrangement on chromosome 22) and which can exhibit a variety of morphologic and histochemical alterations (201,202). At least some basophils from patients with CML can be triggered to degranulate in vitro (203).

Immature forms may circulate, particularly during the terminal basophil crisis, and some cases of apparently acute myelogenous leukemia with high levels of immature basophils have been reported (201,204).

Cells resembling normal basophils may rarely account for over 80% of circulating leukocytes even early in CML (205). Such cases sometimes have been designated *basophil leukemia*. Indeed, Ph chromosome–positive "acute basophilic leukemia" may be a presenting manifestation of CML (206). However, the basis for designating some cases as basophil leukemia, as opposed to examples of myelogenous leukemia with a pronounced associated basophilia, is not always clear. As a result, we prefer to refer to these conditions as *leukemias associated with basophilia* (Table 17-6). Occasional patients with CML with extremely high levels of circulating basophils may exhibit clinical effects (e.g., episodes of flushing, pruritus, and hypotension) attributable to the liberation of histamine and perhaps other basophil mediators (207,208). The treatment of patients with extremely high levels of circulating basophils is particularly problematic, because the cytolysis of these basophils during chemotherapy can result in shock as a result of the massive release of histamine and perhaps other basophil-associated mediators (207).

Basophilia has been reported in patients in the chronic phases of drug allergies (224,225), in subjects with ulcerative colitis (189) or myxedema (189,190,194) or in those recovering from acute illnesses (190), and in children with juvenile rheumatoid arthritis (226). Generally, the recorded elevations in basophil counts were modest and overlapped the normal range. A single report has been made of a patient with a leukemoid reaction in association with disseminated tuberculosis, whose basophil count was markedly elevated (11% to 56%) (227).

Alterations in Mast Cell Numbers and the Spectrum of Mast Cell Neoplasia

Although mast cells cannot be identified in the blood of healthy individuals by standard techniques, mast cells can be observed in the blood of monkeys that have been treated chronically with large amounts of SCF (96) and in the blood of some patients with systemic mastocytosis (228). Increases in tissue mast cells can reflect a combination of enhanced influx and retention of progenitors and proliferation of resident mast cells (82,96). Changes in tissue mast cell numbers can occur because of neoplasms affecting this cell type or can reflect "secondary" effects of diverse processes that result in an expansion or reduction of populations of nonneoplastic mast cells.

SECONDARY CHANGES IN MAST CELL NUMBERS
Although long-term treatment with glucocorticoids, particularly topical treatment of the skin, can result in diminished mast cell numbers (229,230), there has been no report of a clinical disorder whose primary feature is a reduction in levels of tissue mast cells. The numbers of one mast cell subpopulation, containing cytoplasmic granules with tryptase but with little or no chymase (i.e., MC_T), can be markedly reduced in the intestinal mucosa and submucosa of patients with either congenital combined immunodeficiency disease or AIDS (231). Two hypotheses have been proposed that may account for this local mast cell deficiency in AIDS patients. Irani et al. proposed that these subjects may have a deficit of CD4+ T-cell–derived mast cell growth factors (231). More recently, based on the demonstration that an "M-tropic" strain of HIV-1 can infect cells with many features of basophils that can be found in the peripheral blood of AIDS patients, it has been proposed that HIV-1 also may be able to infect mast cells, and thereby contribute to their elimination from the gut of AIDS patients (183).

TABLE 17-6. Leukemias Associated with Basophilia

Chronic myelogenous leukemia with exaggerated basophilia (references 200,207–210)
Acute basophilic transformation of chronic myelogenous leukemia (references 207 and 211)
Ph chromosome–positive "acute basophilic leukemia" (reference 206)
Acute myelogenous leukemia with t(6;9), t(3;6), or inv(16) and marrow basophilia (references 212–215)
Acute promyelocytic leukemia with basophilic maturation (references 216–218)
"Acute basophilic leukemia" (references 211 and 219–223)

Several disorders are associated with small to severalfold local increases in mast cell numbers, so-called reactive mastocytosis. Tissues at sites of recurrent IgE-associated allergic reactions (i.e., allergic rhinitis, asthma, and urticaria) often exhibit increases in mast cell numbers to levels up to approximately fourfold normal (232,233). Small increases in mast cell numbers have been observed at sites of pathology in rheumatoid arthritis, psoriatic arthritis, scleroderma, and systemic lupus erythematosus (234,235). Mast cells have been reported to be increased in osteoporosis (236), but it is unclear to what extent this may reflect a decrease in bone matrix or decreases in other cell types. Numbers of marrow mast cells can be increased in patients with chronic liver or renal diseases (237). Increases in mast cells have also been reported in infectious diseases, including tuberculosis, syphilis, and parasitic diseases, particularly at sites of infection with parasites such as *Strongyloides*, in which a greater than fourfold increase in mast cell numbers can occur (238). In such settings, mast cell numbers can return toward normal on resolution of the infection. Finally, mast cell numbers can be increased severalfold in lymph nodes draining areas of tumor growth (237,239) and in subjects with hematopoietic stem cell diseases or lymphoproliferative diseases, including Waldenström's macroglobulinemia, CLL, and lymphoma involving the bone marrow, as well as in association with CML (237,240–242).

DISORDERS OF MAST CELL HYPERPLASIA AND NEOPLASIA

"Mastocytosis" refers to a group of systemic disorders associated with significant increases in mast cell numbers in the skin and internal organs. In addition to such systemic disorders, apparently localized cutaneous aggregates of mast cells ranging from "mast cell nevuses" and "mastocytomas" in infants and children to multiple nodules in older children have also been reported (243,244). The solitary "mastocytomas" typically present before 6 months of age and usually involute spontaneously; in rare cases, they have been followed by urticaria pigmentosa (UP) (244). Because the pathogenesis of such lesions has not yet been elucidated, the remainder of this section focuses on mastocytosis.

Notably, the clinical patterns of disease in mastocytosis and the prognosis can vary significantly from patient to patient (see Therapy and Course and Prognosis). However, guidelines regarding prognosis and treatment have been incorporated into a consensus classification for mastocytosis (245) (Table 17-7). Category I ("indolent mastocytosis") comprises the great majority of subjects with mastocytosis; these patients can expect a normal life span. In category II disease, subjects have a prognosis determined by the associated hematologic disorder. Patients with category III disease ("aggressive mastocytosis") generally have a 3–5 year survival rate, and mastocytic leukemia (category IV disease, see Mast Cell Leukemia) typically is rapidly fatal.

TABLE 17-7. Mastocytosis Classification

Category I: Indolent mastocytosis [can occur as primarily cutaneous disease (e.g., urticaria pigmentosa) with involvement of both skin and other organs, or, more rarely, without skin involvement]
Category II: Mastocytosis with an associated hematologic disorder (usually a myeloproliferative or myelodysplastic disease)
Category III: Aggressive mastocytosis (also known as *lymphadenopathic mastocytosis with eosinophilia*)
Category IV: Mastocytic leukemia (also known as *mast cell leukemia*)

Modified from Metcalfe DD. Clinical advances in mastocytosis—conclusions. *J Invest Dermatol* 1991;96:64S.

Etiology and Pathogenesis. Several lines of evidence indicate that activating mutations in c-*kit*, which encodes the receptor for SCF, can be involved in the pathogenesis of mastocytosis. The most common mutation (Asp816Val), which results in ligand-independent activation of the c-*kit* receptor, was first identified in a cell line derived from a patient with mast cell leukemia (246). It was then detected in mononuclear cells in the peripheral blood of patients with mastocytosis and an associated hematologic disorder (247) as a somatic mutation in lesional tissue obtained from one patient with an aggressive form of mastocytosis and from a second patient with an indolent form of UP (248) and in the skin, but not the bone marrow and peripheral blood, of an 11-month-old child with mastocytosis (249).

These findings suggest that the mutation may occur initially in a mast cell progenitor and that, as the clone expands, it first becomes detectable in mastocytosis skin lesions. In patients with more severe disease, and thus with a larger clonal expansion, it can also be identified in circulating cells. The Asp816Val mutation or similar 816 activating mutations that result in the substitution of valine or tyrosine for aspartate are now believed to occur in virtually all adult patients with mastocytosis; the mutation can be readily identified in the UP skin lesions of such patients (250). Mutations at codon 816 (valine, tyrosine, or phenylalanine for aspartate) have also been identified in a small subset of pediatric patients, whereas other pediatric patients exhibit a dominant inactivating c-*kit* mutation, in which lysine is substituted for glutamic acid in position 839, the site of a potential salt bridge (250).

It is not yet clear to what extent the presence of various c-*kit* mutations or the anatomic distribution of the affected cells can be used to predict prognosis or disease severity. Moreover, some children with mastocytosis appear to lack any c-*kit* mutations (250). Perhaps additional "gain-of-function" mutations of c-*kit* in human subjects with mastocytosis remain to be characterized. In dogs, a species in which up to 20% of all neoplasms are mast cell tumors, 5 of 11 analyzed mast cell tumors exhibited tandem duplications involving exons 11 and 12 of c-*kit* (251). Analysis of a dog mastocytoma cell line indicates that such mutations, which affect the juxtamembrane portion of the cytoplasmic domain of the c-*kit* receptor, result in ligand-independent activation of the receptor (251). Gain-of-function mutations of c-*kit* have also been reported in gastrointestinal stromal tumors (252), in one pedigree as a germline mutation (253). However, in these subjects, it is not yet clear whether mast cell numbers are increased.

Clinical Features. The organs that are most frequently involved in systemic mastocytosis are the skin, lymph nodes, liver, spleen, bone marrow, and gastrointestinal tract. UP is the usual presenting lesion of cutaneous mast cell disease. UP lesions appear as small yellowish-tan to reddish-brown macules or slightly raised papules, which can exhibit Darier's sign (urticaria after mild friction of the skin) (228,254). The palms, soles, face, and scalp generally remain free of lesions. In many cases, UP can develop before the age of 2 years and can subside by puberty; however, in adults with UP, extracutaneous involvement by mastocytosis is common (228,254–256). Notably, some patients, particularly those with mastocytosis and an associated hematologic disorder, may entirely lack cutaneous lesions. In such cases, other organs must be biopsied to make the diagnosis (see below). Diffuse cutaneous mastocytosis is an unusual manifestation of mastocytosis (244,256). The skin appears yellowish-brown and is thickened. Young children with cutaneous disease may have bullous eruptions with hemorrhage (244). Some adult patients develop prominent vascularity in association with the skin lesions, a condition termed *telangiectasia macularis eruptiva perstans* (244).

Lymphadenopathy tends to be most prominent in patients with category II or III disease; in one series, peripheral lymphadenopathy occurred in 26% and central lymphadenopathy in 19% of patients at diagnosis (257). Mast cell infiltrates occur in the paracortex, follicles, medullary cords, and sinuses. Findings also can include prominent infiltrates of eosinophils (thus the alternative term for aggressive mastocytosis: *lymphadenopathic mastocytosis with eosinophilia*), blood vessel proliferation in association with mast cells in the paracortical areas, and extramedullary hematopoiesis.

Many patients exhibit involvement of the liver and often have some pathology associated with the mast cell infiltrates, but severe liver disease is uncommon (228). When severe liver disease occurs, it typically affects those with category II or III disease. In one series of 41 patients, 61% had some liver disease and elevated alkaline phosphatase, aminotransamidases, 5' nucleotidase, or gamma-glutamyltranspepidase was detected in the serum of approximately half of the patients (258). Hepatomegaly, prominent infiltration of the liver with mast cells, and hepatic fibrosis are positively correlated with elevated levels of alkaline phosphatase and were observed more frequently in patients with aggressive disease, and ascites or portal hypertension occurred in some of these individuals. Portal fibrosis was observed in 68% and was positively correlated with hepatic inflammation and mast cell infiltrates. Venopathy and associated venoocclusive disease were observed in four patients who had an associated hematologic disorder.

Approximately one-half of the patients with systemic disease have splenic involvement at diagnosis (257,259,260). Mast cells most commonly occurred in a paratrabecular distribution followed by perifollicular, follicular, and diffuse infiltrates. Trabecular and capsular fibrosis and eosinophilic infiltration were observed, and extramedullary hematopoiesis was present in the majority of biopsies. Splenomegaly of greater than 700 g generally occurred in patients within unfavorable categories of mastocytosis.

Focal mast cell lesions occur in the bone marrow of more than 90% of adults with mastocytosis (259,261–264), typically appearing as perivascular, paratrabecular, or intertrabecular foci of spindle-shaped mast cells in a fibrotic background (sometimes with associated eosinophils and lymphocytes). There may be an increase in staining for reticulin and collagen. In specimens that are extensively involved by mast cell lesions, the bony trabeculae may be moderately to markedly thickened. In hematoxylin and eosin (H&E) stained sections, the mast cells typically exhibit a spindle-shaped or oval nucleus, and fine eosinophilic granules are apparent in the cytoplasm at high power magnification; mast cells with bilobed nuclei also may be seen in these lesions, a finding associated with a poor prognosis (259). Wright-Giemsa and toluidine blue stains can be used, especially with nondecalcified, plastic-embedded specimens, for a more definitive visualization of mast cells. However, these stains are less effective on ethylenediaminetetraacetic acid-decalcified, paraffin-embedded material. Mast cells also stain positively for chloracetate esterase and aminocaproate esterase and, in suitably processed specimens, for mast cell tryptase by immunohistochemistry. Aspirate smears or clot sections alone cannot be used to diagnose mast cell disease in the bone marrow. Although increased numbers of mast cells may be present in bone marrow aspirate smears of patients with systemic mast cell diseases, similar findings have been reported in patients without mast cell disorders or when there is a reactive increase in marrow mast cells. Bone marrow involvement appears to be less common in children (264). Moreover, the focal lesions found in children were uniformly small and perivascular. The progression of bone marrow involvement in systemic mast cell disease is variable. While many adults with indolent disease appear to have stable or even decreasing marrow involvement over time (259), patients with more aggressive patterns of disease more commonly exhibit a progressive increase in focal mast cell lesions.

Clinical Presentation. All patients within a given category of mastocytosis generally exhibit similar clinical features, which largely reflect the local and systemic consequences of mediator release from tissue mast cells. There also may be effects due to the disruption of normal structures by local collections of mast cells.

At presentation, patients may complain of vague and nonspecific constitutional symptoms, such as fatigue, weakness, flushing, and musculoskeletal pain, and some experience fever or weight loss (228,258). A few may present with recurrent episodes of unexplained anaphylaxis (265). However, most patients with indolent mastocytosis and a hematologic disorder are usually diagnosed on the basis of bone marrow biopsy findings during the investigation of their hematologic disease (256,259). Those with aggressive disease often present with unexplained lymphadenopathy and splenomegaly or hepatomegaly. Patients often have gastrointestinal disease and associated symptoms, either at presentation or as the disease progresses (256,266). Findings include nausea, vomiting, abdominal pain, and diarrhea. Peptic ulcer disease, which may reflect (at least in part) the promotion of gastric acid secretion by elevated histamine levels, occurs in up to 50% of those with systemic disease (266). With progressive disease, patients may develop mild malabsorption (266). If systemic involvement is already advanced at the time of diagnosis, patients may also exhibit lymphadenopathy, hepatomegaly, and splenomegaly during the initial evaluation (228,256). Because osteoporosis may accompany systemic disease, rare patients present with pathologic fractures (267).

Laboratory Evaluation. If mastocytosis is suspected based on the history and physical examination, a routine workup in adults should consist of a gross and microscopic examination of the skin, a bone marrow biopsy and aspirate (228,245,256), and serum for alpha and beta tryptase levels (two forms of trypase, a protease that is produced abundantly by most, if not all, human mast cells, but which also may be found in at least some human basophils) (268). Additional studies may include a skeletal survey and bone scan, as indicated by the need to assess the extent of disease or to evaluate pain. A gastrointestinal evaluation, including radiographic studies of the upper gastrointestinal tract and small intestines, a computed tomography scan of the abdomen, and endoscopy, may also be indicated. The requirements for the diagnosis of mastocytosis remain the presence of substantial increases in mast cell numbers in one or more tissues. Slight increases (e.g., up to fourfold) in mast cell numbers in target tissues, such as the skin, gastrointestinal tract, or bone marrow, are not diagnostic because they may only reflect normal variation or inflammatory or reactive processes. In skin biopsies of sites that lack other causes of increased numbers of mast cells, such as chronic inflammatory processes, a tenfold increase in mast cells numbers is generally considered diagnostic of mastocytosis (233,244,256). Mast cell aggregates or the presence of confluent infiltrates of mast cells is required for the diagnosis of bone marrow involvement. In patients with advanced category II or III disease, mast cells may be detectable in the peripheral blood, and rare patients can progress to mast cell leukemia (256,259,269–272).

Although plasma or urinary histamine levels are frequently increased in systemic mastocytosis (273), the isolated findings of increased levels of histamine or histamine metabolites may reflect many other problems, including anaphylaxis. Similarly, serum beta tryptase may be elevated after anaphylaxis. Alpha tryptase is more specific for mastocytosis but may sometimes be normal, even in patients with a diagnostic bone marrow biopsy (268). Because no single laboratory test is diagnostic of mastocytosis, the demonstration of mast cell mediators in blood or urine should prompt further investigation for the presence of mastocytosis.

Differential Diagnosis. The differential diagnosis of systemic mastocytosis includes several disorders that may produce a similar clinical picture, such as allergic diseases, the hyper-IgE syndrome, hereditary or acquired angioneurotic edema, idiopathic flushing or anaphylaxis, carcinoid tumor, and idiopathic capillary leak syndrome. When episodic hypertension is a major finding, pheochromocytoma should be considered. Significant unexplained gastroduodenal ulcer disease requires that a Zollinger-Ellison/gastrinoma syndrome be ruled out. *Helicobacter pylori* infection should be considered in all patients with ulcer disease, even those diagnosed with mastocytosis.

Therapy. There currently is no cure for mastocytosis (274). There also is no evidence that symptomatic therapy significantly alters the course of the underlying disease (274). Management of mastocytosis includes instruction on the avoidance of factors that may trigger symptoms (presumably by the direct or indirect activation of mast cell mediator production); these can include temperature extremes, physical exertion, or, in some unusual cases, the ingestion of ethanol, nonsteroidal antiinflammatory drugs, or opiate analgesics (256,274). Anaphylaxis may sometimes follow insect stings even in the absence of evidence of allergic sensitivity. For these reasons, consideration should be given to providing epinephrine-filled syringes to all patients. Patients with mast cell disease and a history of anaphylaxis clearly should be advised to carry epinephrine-filled syringes and taught to self-medicate. Such patients may also benefit from the concurrent prophylactic use of H_1 and H_2 antihistamines. Because mastocytosis patients may experience severe reactions to iodinated contrast materials, consideration should be given to premedicating these patients with H_1 and H_2 antihistamines and prednisone. Nonsedative H_1 antihistamines decrease the irritability of the skin and pruritus (256,274–276). More potent H_1 blockers, such as hydroxyzine and doxepin (277), may be useful in more severe cases. Pruritus may also be relieved by approaches that maintain the hydration of the skin. H_2 antihistamines, including ranitidine and famotidine, are used to treat the gastritis and peptic ulcer disease associated with mastocytosis (256,274,278). H_2 antihistamines may be adjusted based on symptom control or to a particular level of gastric secretion. Proton pump inhibitors (omeprazole) are also useful in the management of gastric hypersecretion (256,274).

The oral administration of disodium cromoglycate has been reported to be useful in the treatment of gastrointestinal cramping and diarrhea (279,280) and in cutaneous mast cell disease in children and infants (281). Ketotifen, widely used outside of the United States, has been reported to be effective in the relief of pruritus and wheal formation in cutaneous mastocytosis (282) and even to improve osteoporosis (283); however, one pediatric study found ketotifen to be no more effective than hydroxyzine (284). In another study, azelastine offered only minimal benefit over chlorpheniramine (285). Diphosphonates have been reported to be useful in the treatment of the osteopenia associated with mastocytosis (286).

Cutaneous lesions have been treated with either corticosteroids (287) or 8-methoxypsoralen plus ultraviolet A (PUVA) (288,289) largely to reduce pruritus or for cosmetic improvement. There is no evidence that such approaches alter the progression of systemic disease, and relapses 3 to 6 months after cessation of PUVA therapy are common. Patients may also experience a decrease in the intensity of lesions after exposure to natural sunlight. Repeated or extensive application of corticosteroids may result in cutaneous atrophy or adrenocortical suppression (287).

Nonsteroidal antiinflammatory agents have been useful in some patients whose primary manifestations are recurrent episodes of flushing or syncope, or both (274). However, these agents may also exacerbate ulcer disease. Patients with a history of aspirin sensitivity should not be placed on this therapy, unless they first undergo desensitization.

In patients with advanced disease, systemic corticosteroids are used to decrease significant malabsorption and ascites (290). In adults, oral prednisone (40 to 60 mg/day) usually results in a decrease in symptoms over a 2- to 3-week period. After initial improvement, steroids usually may be tapered to an alternate-day regime. Unfortunately, the ascites frequently recur; such patients may benefit from a portacaval shunt (290).

Patients with mastocytosis and an associated hematologic disorder are managed as dictated by the specific hematologic abnormality. Interferon-α-2β may have contributed to a decrease in mast cell infiltration in one patient with mastocytosis and an associated hematologic disorder (291), but a subsequent study reported that interferon-α-2β was of no benefit in three patients (292), and there is a report of an anaphylactic-like syndrome after treatment with interferon-α (293).

A small number of patients with mastocytosis may have a syndrome resembling non-Hodgkin's lymphoma, an aggressive myeloproliferative disease or, rarely, an overt nonlymphocytic leukemia (294). Two patients have been reported with systemic mast cell disease associated with primary mediastinal germ cell tumor (295,296). In such patients, traditional chemotherapy directed toward the neoplastic process may be appropriate. Chemotherapy with cyclophosphamide, vincristine, and prednisone has been used in some mastocytosis patients whose clinical picture is that of a non-Hodgkin's lymphoma, although the response to chemotherapy was variable (294). Radiotherapy has been used in a limited number of patients to control local disease (297). One patient with a myelodysplastic syndrome of recent onset, a leukemic spread of immature mast cells, and hyperfibrinolysis, possibly related to mast cell–derived tissue plasminogen activator, responded well to remission-induction polychemotherapy followed by two cycles of consolidation with intermediate dose cytarabine (298).

Splenectomy has been performed on patients with severe aggressive mastocytosis in an attempt to improve their limiting cytopenias (299). Based on comparisons to historic controls, splenectomy increased survival by an average of 12 months. Patients who had undergone splenectomy also appeared to be better able to tolerate chemotherapy. Splenectomy appears to be of no value in the management of indolent mast cell disease (299).

Recent findings indicate that the 2-phenylaminopyrimidine derivative, STI 571, an inhibitor of the c-abl, bcr-abl, and platelet-derived growth factor receptor tyrosine kinases, also inhibits c-*kit* receptor tyrosine kinase activity (300). STI 571 is U.S. Food and Drug Administration–approved (as imatinib mesylate capsules, marketed by Novartis Pharmaceuticals Corporation as Gleevec) for the treatment of CML in blast crisis, accelerated phase, and chronic phase after failure of interferon-α treatment (301,302). Very early results indicate that STI 571 also may have benefit in patients with metastatic gastrointestinal stromal tumors (303), another neoplasm in which gain-of-function mutations of c-*kit* have a pathogenetic role (252,253). Unfortunately, *in vitro* studies indicate that the Asp816Val c-*kit* mutation, which is the most common c-*kit* mutation associated with sporadic adult mastocytosis, is resistant to STI571 (304).

Course and Prognosis. The prognosis of adults with mast cell disorders is related to the disease category. The great majority of patients who present with UP and have indolent (category I) disease have a chronic protracted course that responds to symptomatic medical management. A normal life span is the expectation, and few of these cases progress to more severe forms of the disease; some patients may even experience a diminution in the severity of skin lesions in later years (256,259,305). An elevated serum lactate dehydrogenase level, a late age of onset, and, in category II patients, the presence of a significant hematologic abnormality (e.g., a myeloproliferative or myelodysplastic disorder or, more rarely, overt leukemia) indicate a poor prognosis and shortened survival (259). Indeed, the prognosis for patients in category II ("mastocytosis with an associated hematologic disorder") depends on the course of the associated hematologic disorder (259). Patients with category III disease ("aggressive mastocytosis") have a guarded prognosis owing to complications arising from rapid and profound increases in mast cell numbers; these patients usually have a 3- to 5-year survival (259). Patients with mast cell leukemia (category IV disease) typically die within approximately 6 months of diagnosis (270).

Mast Cell Leukemia. This rapidly fatal disorder either develops in a small minority of patients with category II or III disease (269–272) or can represent the initial clinical presentation of the mast cell disorder (270,306,307). Patients may have fever, anorexia, weight loss, fatigue, severe abdominal cramping, nausea, vomiting, diarrhea, flushing, hypotension, pruritus, or bone pain. Peptic ulcer and gastrointestinal bleeding are frequent, as are hepatomegaly, splenomegaly, and lymph node enlargement. Anemia is a constant feature, and most subjects have thrombocytopenia (270,306,307). The total leukocyte count varies from 10,000 to 150,000/μL (10 to 150×10^9/L), with mast cells representing 10% to 90% of the leukocytes. Marrow biopsy invariably shows a striking increase in mast cells, sometimes up to 90% of marrow cells, although the leukemic mast cells are often hypogranular or agranular. Leukemic mast cells generally stain with Sudan black and Alcian blue and are positive for chloracetate esterase and acid phosphatase and are negative in the peroxidase and α-naphthylesterase reactions (270,306). Electron microscopy may show the characteristic scroll-like ultrastructural features of the mast cell granule (202).

Mast Cell Sarcoma. This exceedingly rare tumor is characterized by nodules at various cutaneous and mucosal sites and, eventually, by involvement of virtually all organs with extensive infiltrates of mast cells (237). Terminally, nearly all of the blood cells are immature mast cells with a monocytoid appearance.

ACKNOWLEDGMENTS

We thank the many colleagues who critically read sections of the chapter, and we thank Ann M. Dvorak for the electron micrographs. The following grants have supported our research: NIH CA72074, NIH R37AI23990, and NIH HL67674.

REFERENCES

1. Wong DTW, Donoff RB, Yang J, et al. Sequential expression of TGF-α and TGF-β_1 during cutaneous wound healing in the hamster. *Am J Pathol* 1993;143:130.
2. Blumenthal RD, Samoszuk M, Taylor AP, et al. Degranulating eosinophils in human endometriosis. *Am J Pathol* 2000;156:1581.
3. Gharaee-Kermani M, Phan SH. The role of eosinophils in pulmonary fibrosis (Review). *Int J Mol Med* 1998;1:43.
4. Goldman M, Le Moine A, Braun M, et al. A role for eosinophils in transplant rejection. *Trends Immunol* 2001;22:247.
5. Douglas IS, Leff AR, Sperling AI. CD4+ T cell and eosinophil adhesion is mediated by specific ICAM-3 ligation and results in eosinophil activation. *J Immunol* 2000;164:3385.
6. Shi H, Humbles A, Gerard C, et al. Lymph node trafficking and antigen presentation by endobronchial eosinophils. *J Clin Invest* 2000;105:945.
7. Rothenberg ME. Eosinophilia. *New Engl J Med* 1998;338:1592.
8. Weller PF. Human eosinophils. *J Allergy Clin Immunol* 1997;100:283.
9. Giembycz MA, Lindsay MA. Pharmacology of the eosinophil. *Pharmacol Rev* 1999;51:213.
10. Gleich GJ. Mechanisms of eosinophil-associated inflammation. *J Allergy Clin Immunol* 2000;105:651.
11. Palframan RT, Collins PD, Severs NJ, et al. Mechanisms of acute eosinophil mobilization from the bone marrow stimulated by interleukin 5: the role of specific adhesion molecules and phosphatidylinositol 3-kinase. *J Exp Med* 1998;188:1621.
12. Mishra A, Hogan SP, Lee JJ, et al. Fundamental signals that regulate eosinophil homing to the gastrointestinal tract. *J Clin Invest* 1999;103:1719.
13. Bochner BS, Schleimer RP. Mast cells, basophils, and eosinophils: distinct but overlapping pathways for recruitment. *Immunol Rev* 2001;179:5.
14. Wardlaw AJ. Molecular basis for selective eosinophil trafficking in asthma: a multistep paradigm. *J Allergy Clin Immunol* 1999;104:917.
15. Woltmann G, McNulty CA, Dewson G, et al. Interleukin-13 induces PSGL-1/P-selectin-dependent adhesion of eosinophils, but not neutrophils, to human umbilical vein endothelial cells under flow. *Blood* 2000;95:3146.
16. Resnick MB, Weller PF. Mechanisms of eosinophil recruitment. *Am J Respir Cell Mol Biol* 1993;8:349.
17. Bandeira-Melo C, Herbst A, Weller PF. Eotaxins. Contributing to the diversity of eosinophil recruitment and activation. *Am J Respir Cell Mol Biol* 2001;24:653.
18. Hirai H, Tanaka K, Yoshie O, et al. Prostaglandin D2 selectively induces chemotaxis in T helper type 2 cells, eosinophils, and basophils via seven-transmembrane receptor CRTH2. *J Exp Med* 2001;193:255.
19. Dvorak AM, Weller PF. Ultrastructural analysis of human eosinophils. *Chem Immunol* 2000;76:1.
20. Weller PF, Monahan-Earley RA, Dvorak HF, et al. Cytoplasmic lipid bodies of human eosinophils: subcellular isolation and analysis of arachidonate incorporation. *Am J Pathol* 1991;138:141.
21. Bandeira-Melo C, Phoofolo M, Weller PF. Extranuclear lipid bodies, elicited by CCR3-mediated signaling pathways, are the sites of chemokine-enhanced leukotriene C$_4$ production in eosinophils and basophils. *J Biol Chem* 2001;276:22779.
22. Bozza PT, Yu W, Penrose JF, et al. Eosinophil lipid bodies: specific, inducible intracellular sites for enhanced eicosanoid formation. *J Exp Med* 1997;186:909.
23. Bartemes KR, McKinney S, Gleich GJ, et al. Endogenous platelet-activating factor is critically involved in effector functions of eosinophils stimulated with IL-5 or IgG. *J Immunol* 1999;162:2982.
24. Bozza PT, Payne JL, Goulet JL, et al. Mechanisms of PAF-induced lipid body formation: a central role for 5-lipoxygenase in the compartmentalization of leukocyte lipids. *J Exp Med* 1996;183:1515.
25. Bozza PT, Yu W, Cassara J, et al. Pathways for eosinophil lipid body induction: differing signal transduction in cells from normal and hypereosinophilic subjects. *J Leukocyte Biol* 1998;64:563.
26. Gounni AS, Lamkhioued B, Ochiai K, et al. High-affinity IgE receptor on eosinophils is involved in defence against parasites. *Nature* 1994;367:183.
27. Seminario MC, Saini SS, MacGlashan DW, et al. Intracellular expression and release of Fc epsilon RI alpha by human eosinophils. *J Immunol* 1999;162:6893.
28. Abdelilah SG, Bouchaib L, Morita M, et al. Molecular characterization of the low-affinity IgE receptor FcϵRII/CD23 expressed by human eosinophils. *Int Immunol* 1998;10:395.
29. Truong MJ, Gruart V, Liu FT, et al. IgE-binding molecules (Mac-2/ϵBP) expressed by human eosinophils. Implication in IgE-dependent eosinophil cytotoxicity. *Eur J Immunol* 1993;23:3230.
30. Motegi Y, Kita H. Interaction with secretory component stimulates effector functions of human eosinophils, but not of neutrophils. *J Immunol* 1998;161:4340.
31. Bochner BS, Bickel CA, Taylor ML, et al. Macrophage-derived chemokine induces human eosinophil chemotaxis in a CC chemokine receptor 3- and CC chemokine receptor 4-independent manner. *J Allergy Clin Immunol* 1999;103:527.
32. Heise CE, O'Dowd BF, Fugueroa DJ, et al. Characterization of the human cysteinyl leukotriene 2 (CysLT$_2$) receptor. *J Biol Chem* 2000;275:30531.
33. Lynch KR, O'Neill GP, Liu Q, et al. Characterization of the human cysteinyl leukotriene CysLT1 receptor. *Nature* 1999;399:789.
34. Kita H, Adolphson CR, Gleich GJ. Biology of eosinophils. In: Adkinson NF Jr, Busse WW, Ellis EF, et al, eds. *Allergy: principles and practice*, 5th ed. St. Louis: Mosby, 1998:242.
35. Plager DA, Loegering DA, Weiler DA, et al. A novel and highly divergent homolog of human eosinophil granule major basic protein. *J Biol Chem* 1999;274:14464.
36. Gleich GJ, Loegering DA, Bell MP, et al. Biochemical and functional similarities between eosinophil-derived neurotoxin and eosinophil cationic protein: homology with ribonuclease. *Proc Natl Acad Sci U S A* 1986;83:3146.

37. Slifman NR, Loegering DA, McKean D, et al. Ribonuclease activity associated with human eosinophil-derived neurotoxin and eosinophil cationic protein. *J Immunol* 1986;137:2913.

38. Stahle-Backdahl M, Parks WC. 92-kd gelatinase is actively expressed by eosinophils and stored by neutrophils in squamous cell carcinoma. *Am J Pathol* 1993;142:995.

39. Lacy P, Moqbel R. Eosinophil cytokines. *Chem Immunol* 2000;76:134.

40. Weller PF. Lipid, peptide and cytokine mediators elaborated by eosinophils. In: Smith JH, Cook RM, eds. *Immunopharmacology of eosinophils: the handbook of immunopharmacology.* London: Academic Press, 1993:25.

41. Lacy P, Mahmudi-Azer S, Bablitz B, et al. Rapid mobilization of intracellularly stored RANTES in response to interferon-γ in human eosinophils. *Blood* 1999;94:23.

42. Bandeira-Melo C, Gillard G, Ghiran I, et al. EliCell: a solid-phase dual antibody capture and detection assay to detect cytokine release by eosinophils. *J Immunol Methods* 2000;244:105.

43. Bandeira-Melo C, Sugiyama K, Woods L, et al. Cutting edge: eotaxin elicits rapid, vesicular transport-mediated release of preformed IL-4 from human eosinophils. *J Immunol* 2001;166:4813.

44. Wu W, Samoszuk MK, Comhair SA, et al. Eosinophils generate brominating oxidants in allergen-induced asthma. *J Clin Invest* 2000;105:1455.

45. Lee E, Robertson T, Smith J, et al. Leukotriene receptor antagonists and synthesis inhibitors reverse survival in eosinophils of asthmatic individuals. *Am J Respir Crit Care Med* 2000;161:1881.

46. Wilson ME, Weller PF. Approach to the patient with eosinophilia. In: Guerrant RL, Walker DH, Weller PF, eds. *Tropical infectious diseases: principles, pathogens and practice.* New York: Churchill Livingstone, 1999:1400.

47. Meeusen ENT, Balic A. Do eosinophils have a role in the killing of helminth parasites? *Parasitol Today* 2000;16:95.

48. Behm CA, Ovington KS. The role of eosinophils in parasitic helminth infections: insights from genetically modified mice. *Parasitol Today* 2000;16:202.

49. Schwarze J, Hamelmann E, Bradley KL, et al. Respiratory syncytial virus infection results in airway hyperresponsiveness and enhanced airway sensitization to allergen. *J Clin Invest* 1997;100:226.

50. Domachowske JB, Dyer KD, Bonville CA, et al. Recombinant human eosinophil-derived neurotoxin/RNase 2 functions as an effective antiviral agent against respiratory syncytial virus. *J Infect Dis* 1998;177:1458.

51. Kadin M, Butmarc J, Elovic A, et al. Eosinophils are the major source of transforming growth factor-beta 1 in nodular sclerosing Hodgkin's disease. *Am J Pathol* 1993;142:11.

52. Weller PF, Rand TH, Barrett T, et al. Accessory cell function of human eosinophils: HLA-DR dependent, MHC-restricted antigen-presentation and interleukin-1α formation. *J Immunol* 1993;150:2554.

53. Del Pozo V, De Andrés B, Martín E, et al. Eosinophil as antigen-presenting cell: activation of T cell clones and T cell hybridoma by eosinophils after antigen processing. *Eur J Immunol* 1992;22:1919.

54. Weller PF, Bubley GJ. The idiopathic hypereosinophilic syndrome. *Blood* 1994;83:2759.

55. Fauci AS, Harley JB, Roberts WC, et al. NIH Conference. The idiopathic hypereosinophilic syndrome. Clinical, pathophysiologic, and therapeutic considerations. *Ann Intern Med* 1982;97:78.

56. Cogan E, Schandené L, Crusiaux A, et al. Clonal proliferation of type 2 helper T cells in a man with the hypereosinophilic syndrome. *New Engl J Med* 1994;330:535.

57. Brugnoni D, Airo P, Rossi G, et al. A case of hypereosinophilic syndrome is associated with the expansion of a CD3-CD4+ T-cell population able to secrete large amounts of interleukin-5. *Blood* 1996;87:1416.

58. Kitano K, Ichikawa N, Mahbub B, et al. Eosinophilia associated with proliferation of CD(3+)4-(8-) alpha beta+ T cells with chromosome 16 anomalies. *Br J Haematol* 1996;92:315.

59. Simon HU, Plotz SG, Dummer R, et al. Abnormal clones of T cells producing interleukin-5 in idiopathic eosinophilia. *N Engl J Med* 1999;341:1112.

60. Means-Marwell M, Burgess T, deKeraty D, et al. Eosinophilia with aberrant T cells and elevated serum levels of interleukin-2 and interleukin-15. *N Engl J Med* 2000;342:1568.

61. Malbrain ML, Van den Bergh H, Zachee P. Further evidence for the clonal nature of the idiopathic hypereosinophilic syndrome: complete haematological and cytogenetic remission induced by interferon-alpha in a case with a unique chromosomal abnormality. *Br J Haematol* 1996;92:176.

62. Luppi M, Marasca R, Morselli M, et al. Clonal nature of hypereosinophilic syndrome. *Blood* 1994;84:349.

63. Chang HW, Leong KH, Koh DR, et al. Clonality of isolated eosinophils in the hypereosinophilic syndrome. *Blood* 1999;93:1651.

64. Parwaresch MR. *The human blood basophil.* New York: Springer-Verlag, 1976.

65. Denegri JF, Naiman SC, Gillen J, et al. *In vitro* growth of basophils containing the Philadelphia chromosome in the acute phase of chronic myelogenous leukemia. *Br J Haematol* 1978;40:351.

66. Valent P, Bettelheim P. The human basophil. *Crit Rev Oncol Hematol* 1990;10:327.

67. Valent P. The phenotype of human eosinophils, basophils, and mast cells. *J Allergy Clin Immunol* 1994;94:1177.

68. Agis H, Fureder W, Bankl HC, et al. Comparative immunophenotypic analysis of human mast cells, blood basophils and monocytes. *Immunology* 1996;87:535.

69. Valent P. Immunophenotypic characterization of human basophils and mast cells. *Chem Immunol* 1995;61:34.

70. Toba KK, Shibata T, Hashimoto A, et al. Novel technique for the direct flow cytofluorometric analysis of human basophils in unseparated blood and bone marrow, and the characterization of phenotype and peroxidase of human basophils. *Cytometry* 1999;35:249.

71. Denburg JA, Tanno Y, Bienenstock J. Growth and differentiation of human basophils, eosinophils, and mast cells. In: Befus AD, Bienenstock J, Denburg JA, eds. *Mast cell differentiation and heterogeneity.* New York: Raven Press, 1986:71.

72. Ishizaka T, Dvorak AM, Conrad DH, et al. Morphological and immunological characterization of human basophils developed in cultures of cord blood mononuclear cells. *J Immunol* 1985;134:532.

73. Steinbach KH, Schick P, Trepel F, et al. Estimation of kinetic parameters of neutrophilic, eosinophilic, and basophilic granulocytes in human blood. *Blut* 1979;39:27.

74. Murakami I, Ogawa M, Amo H, et al. Studies on kinetics of human leukocytes *in vivo* with ³H-thymidine autoradiography. II. Eosinophils and basophils. *Acta Haematol* 1969;32:384.

75. Saito H, Hatake K, Dvorak AM, et al. Selective differentiation and proliferation of hematopoietic cells induced by recombinant human interleukins. *Proc Natl Acad Sci U S A* 1988;85:2288.

76. Ishizaka T, Saito H, Furitsu T, et al. Growth of human basophils and mast cells *in vitro*. In: Galli SJ, Austen KF, eds. *Mast cell and basophil differentiation and function in health and disease.* New York: Raven Press, 1989:39.

77. Tracey R, Smith H. An inherited anomaly of human eosinophils and basophils. *Blood Cells* 1978;4:291.

78. Juhlin L. Basophil leukocyte differential in blood and bone marrow. *Acta Haematol* 1963;29:89.

79. Gilbert HS, Ornstein L. Basophil counting with a new staining method using alcian blue. *Blood* 1975;46:279.

80. Dvorak AM. Human mast cells. In: Beck F, Hild W, Kriz W, et al, eds. *Advances in anatomy, embryology and cell biology,* Vol. 114. Berlin: Springer-Verlag, 1989:1.

81. Dvorak AM. *Blood cell biochemistry: basophil and mast cell degranulation and recovery,* Vol. 4. New York: Plenum Press, 1991.

82. Kitamura Y. Heterogeneity of mast cells and phenotypic changes between subpopulations. *Annu Rev Immunol* 1989;7:59.

83. Kitamura Y, Nakayama H, Fujita J. Mechanism of mast cell deficiency in mutant mice of W/Wᵛ and Sl/Slᵈ genotype. In: Galli SJ, Austen KF, eds. *Mast cell and basophil differentiation and function in health and disease.* New York: Raven Press, 1989:15.

84. Rodewald H-R, Dressing M, Dvorak AM, et al. Identification of a committed precursor for the mast cell lineage. *Science* 1996;87:326.

85. Mitchell EB, Platts-Mills TAE, Pereira RS, et al. Acquired basophil and eosinophil deficiency in a patient with hypogammaglobulinaemia associated with thymoma. *Clin Lab Haematol* 1983;5:253.

86. Juhlin L, Michäelsson G. A new syndrome characterized by absence of eosinophils and basophils. *Lancet* 1977;1:1233.

87. Dvorak AM, Mihm MC Jr, Dvorak HF. Morphology of delayed-type hypersensitivity reactions in man. II. Ultrastructural alterations affecting the microvasculature and the tissue mast cells. *Lab Invest* 1976;34:179.

88. Agis H, Willheim M, Sperr WR, et al. Monocytes do not make mast cells when cultured in the presence of SCF. Characterization of the circulating mast cell progenitor as a c-Kit+, CD34+, Ly–, CD14–, CD17–, colony-forming cell. *J Immunol* 1993;151:4221.

89. Kempuraj D, Saito H, Kaneko A, et al. Characterization of mast cell-committed progenitors present in human umbilical cord blood. *Blood* 1999;93:3338.

90. Selye H. *The mast cells.* Washington, DC: Butterworths, 1965.

91. Bienenstock J, Befus AD, Denburg JA. Mast cell heterogeneity: basic questions and clinical implications. In: Befus AD, Bienenstock J, Denburg JA, eds. *Mast cell differentiation and heterogeneity.* New York: Raven Press, 1986:391.

92. Enerbäck L, Pipkom U, Aldenborg F, et al. Mast cell heterogeneity in man: properties and function of human mucosal mast cells. In: Galli SJ, Austen KF, eds. *Mast cell and basophil differentiation and function in health and disease.* New York: Raven Press, 1989:27.

93. Bienenstock J, Blennerhassett M, Kakuta Y, et al. Evidence for central and peripheral nervous system interaction with mast cells. In: Galli SJ, Austen KF, eds. *Mast cell and basophil differentiation and function in health and disease.* New York: Raven Press, 1989:275.

94. Galli SJ. New insights into "the riddle of the mast cells": microenvironmental regulation of mast cell development and phenotypic heterogeneity. *Lab Invest* 1990;62:5.

95. Galli SJ. New concepts about the mast cell. *N Engl J Med* 1993;328:257.

96. Galli SJ, Zsebo KM, Geissler EN. The kit ligand, stem cell factor. *Adv Immunol* 1994;55:1.

97. Huang C, Sali A, Stevens RL. Regulation and function of mast cell proteases in inflammation. *J Clin Immunol* 1998;18:169.

98. Ganser A, Lindemann A, Seipelt G, et al. Effects of recombinant human interleukin-3 in patients with normal hemopoiesis and in patients with bone marrow failure. *Blood* 1990;76:666.

99. Lantz CS, Boesiger J, Song CH, et al. Role for interleukin-3 in mast cell and basophil development and immunity to parasites. *Nature* 1998;293:445.

100. Lantz CS, Song CH, Dranoff G, et al. Interleukin-3 (IL-3) is required for blood basophilia, but not for increased IL-4 production, in response to parasite infection in mice. *FASEB J* 1999;13:A325.

101. Columbo M, Horowitz EM, Botana LM, et al. The human recombinant *c-kit* receptor ligand, rhSCF, induces mediator release from human cutaneous

mast cells and enhances IgE-dependent mediator release from both skin mast cells and peripheral blood basophils. *J Immunol* 1992;149:599.

102. Li L, Li Y, Reddel SW, et al. Identification of basophilic cells that express mast cell granule proteases in the peripheral blood of asthma, allergy, and drug-reactive patients. *J Immunol* 1998;161:5079–5086.

103. Alam R, Welter JB, Forsythe PA, et al. Comparative effects of recombinant IL-1, -2, -3, -4, and -6, INF-γ, granulocyte-macrophage-colony-stimulating factor, tumor necrosis factor-α, and histamine-releasing factors on the secretion of histamine from basophils. *J Immunol* 1989;142:3431.

104. Broudy VC. Stem cell factor and hematopoiesis. *Blood* 1997;90:1345.

105. Costa JJ, Demetri, GD, Harrist TJ, et al. Recombinant human stem cell factor (kit ligand) promotes human mast cell and melanocyte hyperplasia and functional activation *in vivo*. *J Exp Med* 1996;183:2681.

106. Gargari E, Tsai M, Lantz CS, et al. Differential release of mast cell interleukin-6 via c-Kit. *Blood* 1997;89:2654.

107. Wershil BK, Tsai M, Geissler EN, et al. The rat *c-kit* ligand, stem cell factor, induces *c-kit* receptor-dependent mouse mast cell activation *in vivo*: evidence that signaling through the *c-kit* receptor can induce expression of cellular function. *J Exp Med* 1992;175:245.

108. Bischoff SC, Dahinden CA. *c-kit* Ligand: a unique potentiator of mediator release by human lung mast cells. *J Exp Med* 1992;175:237.

109. Patella V, Marino I, Arbustini E, et al. Stem cell factor in mast cells and increased mast cell density in idiopathic and ischemic cardiomyopathy. *Circulation* 1998;97:971.

110. Hartman M, Piliponsky AM, Temkin V, et al. Human peripheral blood eosinophils express stem cell factor. *Blood* 2001;97:1086.

111. Asai K, Kitaura J, Kawakami Y, et al. Regulation of mast cell survival by IgE. *Immunity* 2001;14:791.

112. Kalesnikoff J, Huber M, Lam V, et al. Monomeric IgE stimulates signaling pathways in mast cells that lead to cytokine production and cell survival. *Immunity* 2001;14:801.

113. Dvorak AM, Hammel I, Schulman ES, et al. Differences in the behavior of cytoplasmic granules and lipid bodies during human lung mast cell degranulation. *J Cell Biol* 1984;99:1678.

114. Hammel I, Dvorak AM, Peters SP, et al. Differences in the volume distributions of human lung mast cell granules and lipid bodies: evidence that the size of these organelles is regulated by distinct mechanisms. *J Cell Biol* 1985; 100:1488.

115. Schwartz LB, Huff TF. Biology of mast cells. In: Middleton E Jr, Reed CE, Ellis EF, et al, eds. *Allergy principles and practice*, 5th ed. St. Louis: Mosby, 1998:261.

116. Wedemeyer J, Galli SJ. Mast cells and basophils. In: Rich RR, Fleisher TA, Shearer WT, et al, eds. *Clinical immunology: principles and practice*, 2nd ed. London: Mosby, 2001:23.1.

117. Williams CMM, Galli SJ. The diverse potential effector and immunoregulatory roles of mast cells in allergic disease. *J Allergy Clin Immunol* 2000;105: 847.

118. Stevens RL, Fox CC, Lichtenstein LM, et al. Identification of chondroitin sulfate E proteoglycans and heparin proteoglycans in the secretory granules of human lung mast cells. *Proc Natl Acad Sci U S A* 1988;85:2284.

119. Thompson HL, Schulman ES, Metcalfe DD. Identification of chondroitin sulfate E in human lung mast cells. *J Immunol* 1988;140:2708.

120. Humphries DE, Wong GW, Friend DS, et al. Heparin is essential for the storage of specific granule proteases in mast cells. *Nature* 1999;400:769.

121. Forsberg E, Pejler G, Ringvall M, et al. Absence of heparin and altered mast cell mediator content in NDST-2 deficient mice. *Nature* 1999;400:773.

122. Porter JF, Mitchell RGL. Distribution of histamine in human blood. *Physiol Rev* 1972;52:361.

123. Yamatodani A, Maeyama K, Watanabe T, et al. Tissue distribution of histamine in a mutant mouse deficient in mast cells: clear evidence for the presence of non-mast cell histamine. *Biochem Pharmacol* 1982;31:305.

124. Schwartz LB, Bradford TM. Regulation of tryptase from human lung mast cells by heparin: stabilization of the active tetramer. *J Biol Chem* 1986;261: 7372.

125. Caughey GH. Mast cell chymases and tryptases: phylogeny, family relations and biogenesis. In: *Mast cell proteases in immunology and biology*. New York: Marcel Dekker, 1995:305.

126. Schechter NM, Franki JE, Geesin JC, et al. Human skin chymotryptic proteinase. I. Isolation and relation to cathepsin G and rat mast cell protease. *J Biol Chem* 1983;31:276.

127. Johnson LA, Moon KE, Eisenberg M. Purification to homogeneity of the human skin chymotryptic proteinase "chymase." *Anal Biochem* 1986;155:358.

128. Irani AA, Schechter NM, Craig SS, et al. Two human mast cell subsets with different neutral protease composition. *Proc Natl Acad Sci U S A* 1986;83:4464.

129. Craig SS, Schechter NM, Schwartz LB. Ultrastructural analysis of maturing human T and TC mast cells in situ. *Lab Invest*, 1989;60:147.

130. Weidner N, Austen KF. Heterogeneity of mast cells at multiple body sites. Fluorescent determination of avidin binding and immunofluorescent determination of chymase, tryptase, and carboxypeptidase content. *Pathol Res Pract* 1993;189:156.

131. Foster B, Schwartz DD, Metcalfe C, et al. Tryptase is expressed by human basophils independent of disease status. *J Allergy Clin Immunol* 2000;105:S89.

132. Goldstein SM, Kaempfer CE, Proud D, et al. Detection and partial characterization of a human mast cell carboxypeptidase. *J Immunol* 1987;139:2724.

133. Ackerman SJ, Weil GJ, Gleich GJ. Formation of Charcot-Leyden crystals by human basophils. *J Exp Med* 1982;155:1597.

134. Dvorak AM, Ackerman SJ. Ultrastructural localization of the Charcot-Leyden crystal protein (lysophospholipase) to granules and intragranular crystals in mature human basophils. *Lab Invest* 1989;60:557.

135. Hammarström S, Lindgren JA, Marcelo C, et al. Arachidonic acid transformations in normal and psoriatic skin. *J Invest Dermatol* 1979;73:180.

136. Betz SJ, Lotner GZ, Henson PM. Generation and release of platelet-activating factor (PAF) from enriched preparations of rabbit basophils; failure of human basophils to release PAF. *J Immunol* 1980;125:2749.

137. Schleimer RP, MacGlashan DW, Peters SP, et al. Characterization of inflammatory mediator release from purified human lung mast cells. *Am Rev Respir Dis* 1986;133:614.

138. Plaut M, Pierce JH, Watson CJ, et al. Mast cell lines produce lymphokines in response to cross-linkage of FcεRI or to calcium ionophores. *Nature* 1989;339:64.

139. Wodnar-Filipowicz A, Heusser CH, Moroni C. Production of the haemopoietic growth factors GM-CSF and interleukin-3 by mast cells in response to IgE receptor-mediated activation. *Nature* 1989;339:150.

140. Burd PR, Rogers HW, Gordon JR, et al. IL-3–dependent and –independent mast cells stimulated with IgE and antigen express multiple cytokines. *J Exp Med* 1989;170:245.

141. Gordon JR, Galli SJ. Mast cells as a source of both preformed and immunologically inducible TNF-α/cachectin. *Nature* 1990;346:274.

142. Walsh LJ, Trincheri G, Waldorf HA, et al. Human dermal mast cells contain and release tumor necrosis factor-α, which induces endothelial leukocyte adhesion molecule 1. *Proc Natl Acad Sci U S A* 1991;88:4220.

143. Gordon JR, Galli SJ. Release of both preformed and newly synthesized tumor necrosis factor α (TNF-α)/cachectin by mouse mast cells stimulated by the FcεRI: a mechanism for the sustained action of mast cell-derived TNF-α during IgE-independent biological responses. *J Exp Med* 1991;174:103.

144. Seder RA, Paul WE, Dvorak AM, et al. Mouse splenic and bone marrow cell populations that express high-infinity Fc receptors and produce interleukin 4 are highly enriched in basophils. *Proc Natl Acad Sci U S A* 1991;88:2835.

145. Bradding P, Feather IH, Howarth PH, et al. Interleukin 4 is localized to and released by human mast cells. *J Exp Med* 1992;176:1381.

146. Brunner T, Heusser CH, Dahinden CA. Human peripheral blood basophils primed by interleukin 3 (IL-3) produce IL-4 in response to immunoglobulin E receptor stimulation. *J Exp Med* 1993;177:605.

147. Wedemeyer J, Tsai M, Galli SJ. Roles of mast cells and basophils in innate and acquired immunity. *Curr Opin Immunol* 2000;12:624.

148. Boesiger J, Tsai M, Maurer M, et al. Mast cells can secrete VPF/VEGF and exhibit enhanced release after IgE-dependent upregulation of FcεRI expression. *J Exp Med* 1998;188:1135.

149. Li H, Sim TC, Alam R. IL-13 released by and localized in human basophils. *J Immunol* 1996;156:4833.

150. Mitchell EB, Platts-Mills TAE, Pereirà RS, et al. Acquired basophil and eosinophil deficiency in a patient with hypogammaglobulinaemia associated with thymoma. *Clin Lab Haematol* 1983;5:253.

151. Juhlin L, Michäelsson G. A new syndrome characterized by absence of eosinophils and basophils. *Lancet* 1977;1:1233.

152. Malaviya R, Abraham SN. Mast cell modulation of immune responses to bacteria. *Immunol Rev* 2001;179:16.

153. Galli SJ, Maurer M, Lantz CS. Mast cells as sentinels of innate immunity. *Curr Opin Immunol* 1999;11:53.

154. Echtenacher B, Mannel DN, Hultner L. Critical protective role of mast cells in a model of acute septic peritonitis. *Nature* 1996;381:75.

155. Malaviya R, Ikeda T, Ross E, et al. Mast cell modulation of neutrophil influx and bacterial clearance at sites of infection through TNF-alpha. *Nature* 1996;381:77.

156. Prodeus AP, Zhou X, Maurer M, et al. Impaired mast cell-dependent natural immunity in complement C3-deficient mice. *Nature* 1997;390:172.

157. Maurer M, Echtenacher B, Hültner L, et al. The c-kit ligand, stem cell factor, can enhance innate immunity through effects on mast cells. *J Exp Med* 1998;188:2343.

158. Supajatura V, Ushio H, Nakao A, et al. Protective roles of mast cells against enterobacterial infection are mediated by toll-like receptor 4. *J Immunol* 2001; 167:2250.

159. Dvorak AM, Klebanoff SJ, Henderson WR, et al. Vesicular uptake of eosinophil peroxidase by guinea pig basophils and by cloned mouse mast cells and granule-containing lymphoid cells. *Am J Pathol* 1985;118:425.

160. Dvorak AM, Ishizaka T, Galli SJ. Ultrastructure of human basophils developing *in vitro*. Evidence of acquisition of peroxidase by basophils and for different effects of human and murine growth factors on human basophil and eosinophil maturation. *Lab Invest* 1985;53:57.

161. Beavan MA, Metzger H. Signal transduction by Fc receptors: the FcεRI case. *Immunol Today* 1993;14:222.

162. Kinet J-P. The high affinity IgE receptor (FcεRI) from physiology to pathology. *Annu Rev Immunol* 1999;17:931.

163. Ogawa M, Nakahata T, Leary AG, et al. Suspension culture of human mast cells/basophils from umbilical cord blood mononuclear cells. *Proc Natl Acad Sci U S A* 1983;80:4494.

164. MacGlashan D Jr, Lavesn-Phillips S, Miura K. Perspectives on the regulation of secretion from human basophils and mast cells. In: Marone G, Lichtenstein LM, Galli SJ, eds. *Mast cells and basophils*. London: Academic Press, 2000:195.

165. Lieberman P. Anaphylaxis and anaphylactoid reactions. In: Middleton E Jr, Reed CE, Ellis EF, et al, eds. *Allergy principles and practice*, 5th ed. St. Louis: Mosby, 1998:1079.

166. Peters SP, Zangrilli JG, Fish JE. Late phase allergic reactions. In: Middleton E Jr, Reed CE, Ellis EF, et al, eds. *Allergy principles and practice*, 5th ed. St. Louis: Mosby, 1998:342.

167. Brown SJ, Galli SJ, Gleich GJ, et al. Ablation of immunity to *Amblyomma americanum* by anti-basophil serum: cooperation between basophils and eosinophils in expression of immunity to ectoparasites (ticks) in guinea pigs. *J Immunol* 1982;129:790.

168. Matsuda H, Watanabe N, Kiso Y, et al. Necessity of IgE antibodies and mast cells for manifestation of resistance against larval *Haemaphysalis longicornis* ticks in mice. *J Immunol* 1990;144:259.

169. Reed ND. Function and regulation of mast cells in parasite infections. In: Galli SJ, Austen KF, eds. *Mast cell and basophil differentiation and function in health and disease.* New York: Raven Press, 1989:205.

170. Steeves EB, Allen JR. Basophils in skin reactions of mast cell-deficient mice infected with Dermacentor variabilis. *Int J Parasitol* 1990;20:655.

171. Galli SJ, Dvorak AM, Dvorak HF. Basophils and mast cells: morphologic insights into their biology, secretory patterns and function. *Prog Allergy* 1984;34:1.

172. Galli SJ, Askenase PW. Cutaneous basophil hypersensitivity. In: Abramoff P, Phillips SM, Escobar MR, eds. *The reticuloendothelial system: a comprehensive treatise,* Vol. 9. New York: Plenum Press, 1986:321.

173. Biedermann T, Kneilling M, Mailhammer R, et al. Mast cells control neutrophil recruitment during T cell-mediated delayed-type hypersensitivity reactions through tumor necrosis factor and macrophage inflammatory protein 2. *J Exp Med* 2000;192:1441.

174. Williams CMM, Galli SJ. Mast cells can amplify airway reactivity and features of chronic inflammation in an asthma model in mice. *J Exp Med* 2000;192:455.

175. Kobayashi T, Miura T, Haba T, et al. An essential role of mast cells in the development of airway hyperresponsiveness in a murine asthma model. *J Immunol* 2000;164:3855.

176. Secor VH, Secor WE, Gutekunst CA, et al. Mast cells are essential for early onset and severe disease in a murine model of multiple sclerosis. *J Exp Med* 2000;191:813.

177. Crowle PK, Starkey JR. Mast cells and tumor-associated angiogenesis. In: Galli SJ, Austen KF, eds. *Mast cell and basophil differentiation and function in health and disease.* New York: Raven Press, 1989:307.

178. Wershil BK, Murakami T, Galli SJ. Mast cell-dependent amplification of an immunologically nonspecific inflammatory response: mast cells are required for the full expression of cutaneous acute inflammation induced by phorbol 12-myristate 13-acetate. *J Immunol* 1988;140:2356.

179. Yano H, Wershil BK, Arizono N, et al. Substance P-induced augmentation of cutaneous vascular permeability and granulocyte infiltration in mice is mast cell-dependent. *J Clin Invest* 1989;84:1276.

180. Qureshi R, Jakschik BA. The role of mast cells in thioglycollate-induced inflammation. *J Immunol* 1988;141:2090.

181. Patella V, Florio G, Petraroli A, et al. HIV-1 gp120 induces IL-4 and IL-13 release from human FcεRI+ cells through interaction with the VH3 region of IgE. *J Immunol* 2000;164:589.

182. dePaulis A, De Palma R, Di Gioia L, et al. Tat protein is an HIV-1-encoded β-chemokine homolog that promotes migration and up-regulates CCR3 expression on human FcεRI+ cells. *J Immunol* 2000;165:7171.

183. Li Y, Li L, Wadley R, et al. Mast cells/basophils in the peripheral blood of allergic individuals who are HIV-1 susceptible due to their surface expression of CD4 and the chemokine receptors CCR3, CCR5, and CXCR4. *Blood* 2001;97:3484–3490.

184. Rorsman II. Studies on basophil leukocytes with special reference to urticaria and anaphylaxis. *Acta Derm Venereol* 1962;42:1.

185. Shelley WB, Juhlin I. New test for detecting anaphylactic sensitivity: basophil reaction. *Nature* 1961;191:1056.

186. Osada Y. Diurnal rhythms of three numbers in circulating basophils and eosinophils in healthy adults. *Bull Inst Public Health* 1956;5:5.

187. Mitchell RG. Circulating basophilic leukocyte counts in the newborn. *Arch Dis Child* 1955;30:130.

188. Thonnard-Neumann E. Studies of basophils: variations with age and sex. *Acta Haematol* 1963;30:221.

189. Juhlin L. Basophil and eosinophil leukocytes in various internal disorders. *Acta Med Scand* 1963;174:249.

190. Mitchell RG. Basophilic leukocytes in children in health and disease. *Arch Dis Child* 1958;33:193.

191. Kelemen E, Bikich G. Insufficiency of acute response of basophil and eosinophil leukocytes and of blood histamine after the administration of ACTH and cortisone in untreated myelocytic leukemia. *Acta Haematol* 1956;15:202.

192. Boseila A-WA, Uhrbrand H. Basophil-eosinophil relationship in human blood. Studies on the effect of corticotrophin (ACTH). *Acta Endocrinol* 1958;28:49.

193. Juhlin L. The effect of corticotropin and corticosteroids on the basophil and eosinophil granulocytes. *Acta Haematol* 1963;29:157.

194. Inagaki S. The relationship between the level of circulating basophil leucocytes and thyroid function. *Acta Endocrinol* 1957;26:477.

195. Mettler L, Shirwani D. Direct basophil count for timing ovulation. *Fertil Steril* 1974;25:718.

196. Shelley WB, Juhlin L. Degranulation of the basophil of man induced by lipemia. *Am J Med Sci* 1961;242:211.

197. Galoppin L, Noirot C, Wastiaux JP, et al. Comparison between number of basophils, blood histamine, and histamine release in cancer and non cancer patients. *J Allergy Clin Immunol* 1989;84:501.

198. Fredericks RE, Moloney WC. The basophilic granulocyte. *Blood* 1959;14:571.

199. Doan CA, Reinhart HL. The basophil granulocyte, basophilicytosis and myeloid leukemia basophil and mixed granule types: an experimental, clinical and pathological study, with the report of a new syndrome. *Am J Clin Pathol* 1941;11:1.

200. Goh KO, Anderson FW. Cytogenetic studies in basophilic chronic myelocytic leukemia. *Arch Pathol Lab Med* 1979;103:288.

201. Dvorak AM, Monahan RA, Dickersin GR. Diagnostic electron microscopy. I. Hematology: differential diagnosis of acute lymphoblastic and acute myeloblastic leukemia—use of ultrastructural peroxidase cytochemistry and routine electron microscopic technology. In: Sommers SC, Rosen PP, eds. *Pathology annual,* Part I. New York: Appleton-Century-Crofts, 1981;16:101.

202. Galli SJ, Wedemeyer J, Zucker-Franklin D. Basophils. In: Zucker-Franklin D, Greaves MF, Grossi CE, Marmont AM, eds. *Atlas of blood cells function and pathology,* 3rd ed. Milan: Edi.Ermes s.r.l.-Milano, 2001; In press.

203. Lewis RA, Goetzl EJ, Wasserman SI, et al. The release of four mediators of immediate hypersensitivity from human leukemic basophils. *J Immunol* 1975;114:87.

204. Mitrakul C, Othaganonda BO, Manothal P, et al. Basophilic leukemia: report of a case. *Clin Pediatr* 1969;8:178.

205. Lennert K, Koster E, Martin H. Über die Mastzellen-leukaemie. *Acta Haematol* 1956;16:255.

206. Kue Y, Gus Y, Lu D, et al. A case of basophilic leukemia bearing simultaneous translocations t(8;21) and t(9;22). *Cancer Genet Cytogenet* 1991;51:215.

207. Youman JD, Taddeini L, Cooper T. Histamine excess, symptoms in basophilic chronic granulocytic leukemia. *Arch Intern Med* 1973;131:560.

208. Rosenthal S, Schwartz JH, Canellos GP. Basophilic chronic granulocytic leukaemia with hyperhistaminaemia. *Br J Haematol* 1977;36:367.

209. Valimaki M, Vuopio P, Salaspuro M. Plasma histamine and serum pepsinogen 1 concentration in chronic myelogenous leukaemia. *Acta Med Scand* 1985;217:89.

210. Anderson W, Helman CA, Hirschowitz BI. Basophilic leukemia and the hypersecretion of gastric acid and pepsin. *Gastroenterology* 1988;95:195.

211. Peterson LC, Parkin JL, Arthur DC, et al. Acute basophilic leukemia. *Am J Clin Pathol* 1991;96:160.

212. Pearson MG, Vardiman JW, LeBeau MM, et al. Increased numbers of marrow basophils may be associated with t(6;9) in ANLL. *Am J Haematol* 1985;18:393.

213. Horsman DE, Kalousek DK. Acute myelomonocytic leukemia (AML-M4) and translocation t(6;9)(p23;q34): two additional patients with prominent myelodysplasia. *Am J Hematol* 1987;26:77.

214. Hoyle CF, Sherrington P, Hayhoe FG. Translocation (3;6)(q21;p21) in acute myeloid leukemia with abnormal thrombopoiesis and basophilia. *Cancer Genet Cytogenet* 1988;30:261.

215. Matsura Y, Sato N, Kimura F, et al. An increase in basophils in a case of acute myelomonocytic leukaemia associated with marrow eosinophilia and inversion of chromosome 16. *Eur J Haematol* 1987;39:457.

216. Moir DJ, Pearson J, Buckle VJ. Acute promyelocytic transformation in a case of acute myelomonocytic leukemia. *Cancer Genet Cytogenet* 1984;12:359.

217. Umeda M, Nojima Z, Yamaguchi R, et al. Two cases of acute promyelocytic leukemia with marked basophilia—a variant type of APL with the capability of differentiating into basophils. *Rinsho Ketsueki* 1987;28:2004.

218. Gotoh H, Murakami S, Oku N, et al. Translocations t(15;17) and t(9;14)(q34;q22) in a case of acute promyelocytic leukemia with increased number of basophils. *Cancer Genet Cytogenet* 1988;36:103.

219. Cecio A, Dini E, Quattrin N. Preliminary observations with the electron microscope of two cases of acute basophilic leukemia. *Boll Soc Ital Biol Sper* 1970;46:459.

220. Lertprasertsuke N, Tsutsumi Y. An unusual form of chronic myeloproliferative disorder. *Acta Pathol Jpn* 1991;41:473.

221. Wick MR, Li CY, Pierre RV. Acute nonlymphocytic leukemia with basophilic differentiation. *Blood* 1982;60:38.

222. Dvorak AM, Dickersin GR, Connell A, et al. Degranulation mechanisms in human leukemic basophils. *Clin Immunol Immunopathol* 1976;5:235.

223. Quattrin N. Follow up of sixty-two cases of acute basophilic leukemia. *Biomedicine* 1978;28:72.

224. Shelley WB. The circulating basophil as an indicator of hypersensitivity in man. *Arch Dermatol* 1963;88:759.

225. Shelley WB, Parnes HM. The absolute basophil count. *JAMA* 1965;192:368.

226. Athreya BH, Moser G, Raghavan TES. Increased circulating basophils in juvenile rheumatoid arthritis: a preliminary report. *Am J Dis Child* 1975;129:935.

227. Paar JA, Scheinman MM, Weaver RA. Disseminated nonreactive tuberculosis with basophilia, leukemoid reaction and terminal pancytopenia. *N Engl J Med* 1966;274:335.

228. Travis WD, Li C-Y, Bergstralh EJ, et al. Systemic mast cell disease: analysis of 58 cases and literature review. *Medicine* 1988;67:345.

229. Lavker RM, Schechter NM. Cutaneous mast cell depletion results from topical steroid usage. *J Immunol* 1985;135:2368.

230. Finotto S, Mekori YA, Metcalfe DD. Glucocorticoids decrease tissue mast cell number by reducing the production of the c-Kit ligand, stem cell factor; by resident cells. *In vitro* and *in vivo* evidence in murine systems. *J Clin Invest* 1997;99:1721.

231. Irani AA, Craig SS, DeBlois G, et al. Deficiency of the tryptase-positive, chymase-negative mast cell type in gastrointestinal mucosa of patients with defective T lymphocyte function. *J Immunol* 1987;138:4381.

232. Irani AA, Garriga MM, Metcalfe DD, et al. Mast cells in cutaneous mastocytosis: accumulation of the MC_{tc} type. *Clin Exp Allergy* 1990;20:52.

233. Garriga MM, Friedman MM, Metcalfe DD. A survey of the number and distribution of mast cells in the skin of patients with mast cell disorders. *J Allergy Clin Immunol* 1988;82:425.

234. Malone DG, Irani AA, Schwartz LB, et al. Mast cell numbers and histamine levels in synovial fluids from patients with diverse arthritides. *Arthritis Rheum* 1986;29:956.

235. Malone DG, Wilder RL, Saavedra-Delgado AM, et al. Mast cell numbers in rheumatoid synovial tissues. *Arthritis Rheum* 1987;30:130.

236. Frame B, Nixon RK. Bone marrow mast cells in osteoporosis of aging. *N Engl J Med* 1968;279:626.

237. Lennert K, Parwaresch MR. Mast cells and mast cell neoplasia—a review. *Histopathology* 1979;3:349.

238. Barrett KE, Neva FA, Gam AA, et al. The immune response to nematode parasites: modulation of mast cell numbers and function during Strongyloides stercoralis infections in nonhuman primates. *Am J Trop Med Hyg* 1988;30:574.

239. Bowers HM, Mahapatro RC, Kennedy JW. Numbers of mast cells in the axillary lymph nodes of breast cancer patients. *Cancer* 1979;43:568.

240. Yoo D, Lessin LS, Jensen WN. Bone marrow mast cells in lymphoproliferative disorders. *Ann Intern Med* 1978;88:753.

241. Yoo D, Lessin LS. Bone marrow mast cell content in preleukemic syndrome. *Am J Med* 1982;73:539.

242. Fohlmeister I, Reber T, Fischer R. Bone marrow mast cell reaction in preleukemic myelodysplasia and in aplastic anemia. *Virchows Arch* 1985;405:503.

243. Fine JD. Mastocytosis (review). *Int Soc Trop Dermatol* 1980;19:117.

244. Soter NA. The skin in mastocytosis. *J Invest Dermatol* 1991;3:32S.

245. Metcalfe DD. Clinical advances in mastocytosis—conclusions. *J Invest Dermatol* 1991;96:64S.

246. Furitsu T, Tsujimura T, Tono T, et al. Identification of mutations in the coding sequences of the proto-oncogene c-kit in a human mast cell leukemia cell line causing ligand independent activation of c-kit product. *J Clin Invest* 1993;92:1736.

247. Nagata H, Worobec AS, Oh CK, et al. Identification of a point mutation in the catalytic domain of the proto-oncogene c-kit in the peripheral blood mononuclear cells of patients with mastocytosis. *Proc Natl Acad Sci U S A* 1995;92:10560.

248. Longley BJ, Tyrell L, Lu SZ, et al. Somatic c-kit activating mutation in urticaria pigmentosa and aggressive mastocytosis: establishment of clonality in a human mast cell neoplasm. *Nat Genet* 1996;12:312.

249. Nagata H, Okada T, Worobec AS, et al. c-Kit mutation in a population of patients with mastocytosis. *Int Arch Allergy Immunol* 1997;113:184.

250. Longley BJ, Metcalfe DD, Tharp M, et al. Activating and dominant inactivating c-Kit catalytic domain mutations in distinct clinical forms of human mastocytosis. *Proc Natl Acad Sci U S A* 1999;96:1609.

251. London CA, Galli SJ, Yuuki T, et al. Spontaneous canine in mast cell tumors express tandem duplications in the proto-oncogene c-kit. *Exp Hematol* 1999;27:689.

252. Hiroto S, Isozaki K, Moriyami Y, et al. Gain-of-function mutations of c-kit in human gastrointestinal stromal tumors. *Science* 1998;279:577.

253. Nishida T, Hirota S, Taniguchi M, et al. Familial gastrointestinal stromal tumors with germline mutation of the KIT gene. *Nat Genet* 1998;19:323.

254. Czarnetzki BM, Behrendt H. Urticaria pigmentosa: Clinical picture and response to oral disodium cromoglycate. *Br J Dermatol* 1981;105:563.

255. Tharp MD. The spectrum of mastocytosis. *Am J Med Sci* 1985;289:117.

256. Kirshenbaum AS, Metcalfe DD. The biology and therapy of mastocytosis. In: Galli SJ, Austen KF, eds. *Mast cell and basophil differentiation and function in health and disease.* New York: Raven, 1989:317.

257. Travis WD, Li C-Y. Pathology of the lymph node and spleen in systemic mast cell disease. *Mod Pathol* 1988;1:4.

258. Mican JM, DiBisceglie AM, Fong T-L, et al. Hepatic involvement in mastocytosis: clinicopathologic correlations in 41 cases. *Hepatology* 1995;22:1163.

259. Lawrence JB, Friedman GB, Travis WD, et al. Hematologic manifestations of systemic mast cell disease: a prospective study of laboratory and morphologic features and their relation to prognosis. *Am J Med* 1991;91:612.

260. Horny H-P, Ruck MT, Kaiserling E. Spleen findings in generalized mastocytosis. *Cancer* 1992;70:459.

261. Horny H-P, Parwaresch MR, Lennart K. Bone marrow findings in systemic mastocytosis. *Hum Pathol* 1985;16:808.

262. Ridell B, Olafsson JH, Roupe G, et al. The bone marrow findings in systemic mastocytosis. *Hum Pathol* 1985;16:808.

263. Parker RI. Hematologic aspects of mastocytosis I. Bone marrow pathology in adult and pediatric systemic mast cell disease. *J Invest Dermatol* 1991;96:47S.

264. Kettlehut BV, Parker RI, Travis WD, et al. Hematopathology of the bone marrow in pediatric cutaneous mastocytosis: a study of 17 patients. *Am J Clin Pathol* 1989;91:558.

265. Roberts LJ, Fields JP, Oats JA. Mastocytosis without urticaria pigmentosa: a frequently unrecognized cause of recurrent syncope. *Trans Assoc Am Physicians* 1982;95:36.

266. Cherner JA, Jensen RT, Dubois A, et al. Gastrointestinal dysfunction in systemic mastocytosis. *Gastroenterology* 1988;95:657.

267. Rafü M, Birooznia H, Colimbu C, et al. Pathologic fracture in systemic mastocytosis. *Clin Orthop* 1983;180:260.

268. Schwartz LB, Sakai K, Bradford TR, et al. The α form of human tryptase is the predominant type present in blood at baseline in normal subjects and is elevated in those with systemic mastocytosis. *J Clin Invest* 1995;96:2702.

269. Joachim G. Über mastzellenleukämie. *Dtsch Arch Klin Med* 1906;87:437.

270. Travis WD, Li C-Y, Hoaglan HC, et al. Mast cell leukemia: report of a case and review of the literature. *Mayo Clinic Proc* 1986;61:957.

271. Torrey E, Simpson K, Wilbur S, et al. Malignant mastocytosis with circulating mast cells. *Am J Med* 1990;34:283.

272. Lennert K, Koster E, Martin H. Über die Mastzellen-leukaemie. *Acta Haematol* 1956;16:255.

273. Friedman BS, Steinberg S, Meggs WJ, et al. Analysis of plasma histamine levels in patients with mast cell disorders. *Am J Med* 1989;87:649.

274. Metcalfe DD. The treatment of mastocytosis: an overview. *J Invest Dermatol* 1991;96:5S.

275. Frieri M, Alling DW, Metcalfe DD. Comparison of the therapeutic efficacy of cromolyn sodium with that of combined chlorpheniramine and cimetidine in systemic mastocytosis. *Am J Med* 1985;78:9.

276. Roberts LJ II, Marney SR Jr, Oates JA. Blockade of the flush associated with metastatic gastric carcinoid by combined histamine H_1 and H_2 receptor-antagonists. *N Engl J Med* 1979;300:236.

277. Sullivan TJ. Pharmacologic modulation of the whealing response to histamine in human skin: identification of doxepin as a potent in vivo inhibitor. *J Allergy Clin Immunol* 1982;69:260.

278. Hirschowitz BI, Broarke JF. Effect of cimetidine on gastric hypersecretion and diarrhea in systemic mastocytosis. *Ann Intern Med* 1979;90:769.

279. Soter NA, Austen KF, Wasserman ST. Oral disodium cromoglycate in the treatment of systemic mastocytosis. *N Engl J Med* 1979;310:465.

280. Frieri M, Alling DW, Metcalfe DD. Comparison of the therapeutic efficacy of cromolyn sodium with that of combined chlorpheniramine and cimetidine in systemic mastocytosis: results of double-blind clinical trial. *Am J Med* 1985;78:9.

281. Welch EA, Alper JC, Boggars H, et al. Treatment of bullous mastocytosis with disodium cromoglycolate. *J Am Acad Dermatol* 1983;9:349.

282. Czarnetzki BM. A double-blind cross-over study of the effect of ketotifen in urticaria pigmentosa. *Dermatologica* 1983;166:44.

283. Graves L III, Stechschulty DJ, Morris DC, et al. Inhibition of mediator release in systemic mastocytosis is associated with reversal of bone changes. *J Bone Miner Res* 1990;5:113.

284. Kettlehut BV, Berkebile C, Bradely D, et al. A double-blind placebo controlled trial of ketotifen versus hydroxyzine in the treatment of pediatric mastocytosis. *J Allergy Clin Immunol* 1989;83:866.

285. Friedman BS, Santiago ML, Berkebile C, et al. Comparison of azelastine and chlorpheniramine in the treatment of mastocytosis. *J Allergy Clin Immunol* 1993;92:520.

286. Cundy T, Beneton MNC, Darby AJ, et al. Osteopenia in systemic mastocytosis: natural history and responses to treatment with inhibitors of bone resorption. *Bone* 1987;8:149.

287. Barton J, Lauker RM, Schecter NM, et al. Treatment of urticaria pigmentosa with corticosteroids. *Arch Dermatol* 1985;121:1516.

288. Czarnetzki PM, Rosenbach T, Kolde G, et al. Phototherapy of urticaria pigmentosa: clinical response and changes of cutaneous reactivity, histamine and chemotactic leukotrienes. *Arch Dermatol* 1985;227:105.

289. Kolde G, Frosch PJ, Czarnetzki BM. Responses of cutaneous mast cells to PUVA in patients with urticaria pigmentosa: histomorphometric, ultrastructural and biochemical investigations. *J Invest Dermatol* 1984;83:175.

290. Reisberg IR, Oyakawa S. Mastocytosis with malabsorption, myelofibrosis, and massive ascites. *Am J Gastroenterol* 1987;82:54.

291. Klunin-Nelemans HC, Jansen JH, Breukelman H, et al. Response to interferon alfa-2β in a patient with systemic mastocytosis. *N Engl J Med* 1992;326:619.

292. Worobec AS, Kirshenbaum AS, Schwartz L. Treatment of three patients with systemic mastocytosis with interferon alpha-2β. *Leuk Lymphoma* 1995;18:179.

293. Pardini S, Bosincu L, Bonfigli S, et al. Anaphylactic-like syndrome in systemic mastocytosis treated with alpha-2-interferon. *Acta Haematol* 1991;85:220.

294. Hutchinson RM. Mastocytosis and co-existent non-Hodgkin's lymphoma and myeloproliferative disorders. *Leuk Lymphoma* 1992;7:29.

295. Chariot P, Monnet I, LeLong F, et al. Systemic mast cell disease associated with primary mediastinal germ cell tumor. *Am J Med* 1991;90:381.

296. Chariot P, Monnet I, Guarland P, et al. Systemic mastocytosis following mediastinal germ cell tumor: an association confirmed. *Hum Pathol* 1993;24:111.

297. Johnstone PA, Mican JM, Metcalfe DD, et al. Radiotherapy of refractory bone pain due to systemic mast cell disease. *Am J Clin Oncol* 1994;17:328.

298. Wimazal F, Sperr WR, Horny HP, et al. Hyperfibrinolysis in a case of myelodysplastic syndrome with leukemic spread of mast cells. *Am J Hematol* 1999;61:66.

299. Friedman B, Darling G, Norton J, et al. Splenectomy in the management of systemic mast cell disease. *Surgery* 1990;107:94.

300. Heinrich MC, Griffith DJ, Druker BJ, et al. Inhibition of c-kit receptor tyrosine kinase activity by STI 571, a selective tyrosine kinase inhibitor. *Blood* 2000;96:925.

301. Druker BJ, Talpaz M, Resta DJ, et al. Efficacy and safety of a specific inhibitor of the BCR-ABL tyrosine kinase in chronic myeloid leukemia. *N Engl J Med* 2001;344:1031.

302. Schwetz BA. New treatment for chronic myelogenous leukemia. *JAMA* 2001;286:35.

303. Berman R, O'Leary TJ. Gastrointestinal stromal tumor workshop. *Hum Pathol* 2001;32:578.

304. Ma Y, Zeng S, Metcalfe DD, et al. The c-KIT mutation causing human mastocytosis is resistant to STI571 and other KIT kinase inhibitors; kinases with enzymatic site mutations show different inhibitor sensitivity profiles with wild-type kinases and those with regulatory-type mutations. *Blood* 2002;99:741.

305. Horan RF, Austen KF. Systemic mastocytosis: a retrospective view of a decade's clinical experience at the Brigham and Women's Hospital. *J Invest Dermatol* 1991;96:55.

306. Coser P, Quaglino D, DePasquale A, et al. Cytobiological and clinical aspects of tissue mast cell leukemia. *Br J Haematol* 1980;45:5.

307. Dalton R, Chan L, Batten E, et al. Mast cell leukemia: evidence for bone marrow origin of the pathological clone. *Br J Haematol* 1984;64:397.

CHAPTER 18

Cellular and Molecular Biology of Lymphoid Cells

Maria Paola Martelli and Barbara E. Bierer

The mammalian immune response has evolved to protect the species from foreign agents that are potentially harmful to the body. Protection involves not only the defense of the species from invasion of microorganisms (e.g., viruses, bacteria, or parasites) but also from spontaneous but dangerous changes, such as mutation and malignant degeneration. Immunity is conferred by two distinct but overlapping networks of defending cells and structures, one provided by innate (or "natural") immunity and the other by acquired (or adaptive) immunity (Table 18-1). Innate immunity depends on the defenses with which an individual is born: effective barriers against invasion (skin, mucosal tissues), secreted products (serum proteins, soluble mediators such as cytokines and chemokines) and cellular elements [e.g., granulocytes, monocytes, and natural killer (NK) cells], among others. Each component, although nonspecific, cooperates to provide an immediate and rapid defense against any number of foreign or toxic invaders.

The adaptive immune response has evolved more recently in evolutionary times and, unlike innate immunity, has only been identified in vertebrate species. The distinctive characteristics of the adaptive immune response are the ability to distinguish self from nonself; the ability to generate a specific response to a specific foreign intruder; and the ability, on second and subsequent exposure to a foreign element, to respond with a more vigorous and rapid reaction. This latter property of immunologic memory, by which the response on reexposure is increased, is termed an *anamnestic response*. The cells that are responsible for adaptive immunity are principally T and B lymphocytes, distinguished not by morphology but by their genetic program and expression of specific T-cell and immunoglobulin receptors, respectively, on their cell surface. These specific receptors each bind to and recognize one specific foreign peptide or molecule, termed an *antigen*. Each T cell bears, on its surface, many copies of only one given T-cell receptor (TcR) and each B cell expresses and secretes an immunoglobulin molecule of only one specificity; antigen specificity is the hallmark of the adaptive immune response. The ability to recognize and respond to literally millions of foreign proteins derives from the great diversity of differentiated cells; the anamnestic response is mediated by the clonal proliferation and functional capacity of the responders.

The adaptive immune response is further subdivided into two general categories, one termed *humoral immunity* and one termed *cell-mediated* (or *cellular*) *immunity*. B cells mediate humoral immunity: B cells produce and secrete specific immunoglobulin or antibody molecules that bind to foreign molecules, coating their surfaces and targeting them for destruction

or lysis. Because antibodies are secreted into the plasma, humoral immunity can be transferred to another member of the species in serum. T cells, responsible for cell-mediated immunity, express antigen-specific TcRs; T cells develop in the thymus, where they acquire their unique specificity for antigen. In the periphery, T cells further differentiate into multiple different T-cell subpopulations with different functions, including cytotoxicity and the secretion of soluble factors termed *cytokines*. A multiplicity of cytokines have now been identified, including 25 interleukin (IL) molecules and more than 40 chemokines, their functions, including growth promotion, differentiation, chemotaxis, and cell stimulation, are diverse (1). In the absence of T-cell cytokine production, B cells fail to differentiate and secrete antibody; T-cell help, and therefore cellular immunity, is required for humoral responses. In the absence of lymphocyte (T- and B-) cell development and appropriate function, immunodeficiency results. Furthermore, in the absence of appropriate control and regulation of development and function, autoimmunity may result.

Our understanding of the complexities of the immune response increased greatly in the 1980s and 1990s. Initially, the generation of monoclonal antibodies—antibodies with a singular and unique specificity derived from a single clone of cells—allowed the identification, characterization, and genetic cloning of molecules and discrete subsets of cells. For clarity, a nomenclature for cloned cell-surface molecules has been developed; each molecule is assigned to a cluster of differentiation (CD) that is uniquely numbered. The list of CD designations is continuously updated, annotated, and available at http://www.ncbi.nlm.nih.gov/prow/. The vast majority of CD molecules are cell-surface proteins involved in adhesion or signaling, but the nomenclature has now been generally adopted and is no longer restricted to human leukocyte cells. In concert with the identification and characterization of molecules involved in the immunity, molecular genetic and biochemical techniques, coupled with the development of animal models, have contributed to an explosion of information regarding the development, regulation, and control of the immune response. This chapter reviews essential concepts of the molecular and cellular biology of lymphoid cells.

IMMUNE CELL DIFFERENTIATION

In the embryo, self-renewing hematopoietic stem cells, developing initially in the primitive yolk sac, migrate to fetal liver. In fetal liver and, after birth, in bone marrow, these pluripotential,

TABLE 18-1. Innate versus Adaptive Immunity

TABLE 18-1. Innate versus Adaptive Immunity

	Innate or Natural Immunity	Adaptive or Acquired Immunity
Specificity	Nonself	Random
Effector cell type	Phagocytic cells: granulocytes, monocytes, macrophages, natural killer cells, natural killer T cells, etc.	Lymphocytes: B and T cell
Cell-surface receptors	Germline	Antigen-specific, rearranged somatically
Distribution	Nonclonal: each cell can express one or more than one receptor, each with different specificities	Clonal: single receptor expressed by single lymphocyte
Response time	Rapid and immediate: neither proliferation nor expansion required for response	Slow: requires clonal proliferation for response

CD34+, hematopoietic stem cells give rise to the earliest myeloid and lymphoid progenitors (Fig. 18-1). Myeloid progenitors give rise to granulocytes, monocytes, and macrophages, NK cells, dendritic cells (DCs), and a variety of other differentiated cells (megakaryocytes, eosinophils, basophils) (2). B cells develop from lymphoid progenitors in the bone marrow and at sites at which the B cell encounters antigen (e.g., secondary lymphoid organs). T cells develop in the thymus and in a variety of extrathymic tissues (i.e., gut) from a lymphoid precursor (3,4); both B- and T-cell differentiation are discussed in detail below. With the fine analysis of mice rendered genetically deficient in single genes and the ability to mark lineage development, it is now appreciated that lineage commitment is not dictated at a single checkpoint nor is there a single precursor to product relationship (5,6). Lymphoid precursors have been shown to be capable, under certain circumstances, of B-cell differentiation in the thymus (7). Bipotent T cell/NK cells and T cell/DC primitive thymocytes have been identified by single-cell analysis (4,8,9). Circulating progenitor cells in the blood have been identified that retain osteogenic potential and that can differentiate to muscle. It is important to recognize that progenitors often maintain the ability to differentiate along different lineages, and only by the expression of lineage-specific genes is cell fate determined and (retrospectively) identified. Indeed, the potential ability of cells to reprogram is currently being exploited as an approach to regeneration (10).

INNATE OR NATURAL IMMUNITY

The innate or natural immune response provides the first defense against microbial invasion. In addition, cell-bound and soluble products of innate immunity stimulate and regulate B and T cells, components of the adaptive immune response. Reciprocally, antigen-specific B and T lymphocytes can regulate innate responses. The two arms of immune defense are intricately interconnected (Fig. 18-2).

In addition to physical (e.g., mucosal and epithelial) barriers to infection, the principal mediators of innate immunity include NK cells (discussed in the section Natural Killer Cells), polymorphonuclear leukocytes (neutrophils), monocytes and macrophages, and soluble proteins, such as complement, inflammatory mediators, chemokines, and cytokines. Neutrophils, like lymphocytes and other hematopoietic elements, circulate in the bloodstream and, by a process of binding to and detaching from endothelial molecules, roll along endothelial surfaces (Fig. 18-3) (11,12). Members of the selectin family of adhesion molecules mediate neutrophil adhesion; the selectins generally regulate initial adhesion and binding of hematopoietic cells (13). L-selectin (CD62L) expressed on leukocytes, P-selectin (CD62P) expressed on platelets, and E-selectin (CD62E) expressed on endothelial surfaces all bind to modified carbohydrate structures (14); the selectin-carbohydrate interaction mediates adhesion independent of antigen-specific binding. Although initial adhesion of neutrophils is mediated by selectins, neutrophil recognition of a chemokine gradient results in stable and tight adhesion, after which the cell may transmigrate through the endothelial barrier to the tissue. Tight adhesion is mediated by members of the integrin family of adhesion molecules. Members of the integrin family are heterodimeric molecules composed of variable α and one of a limited number of β subunits that, in aggregate, regulate cell-cell and cell-extracellular matrix adhesion (15–18). Recruited to sites of inflammation by soluble mediators, neutrophils mediate phagocytosis and bacterial killing via the nicotinamide adenine dinucleotide phosphate reduced form (NADPH) oxidase system. That mutation of any single member of the NADPH oxidase system ($p47^{phox}$, $p67^{phox}$, $p22^{phox}$, and $p91^{phox}$) results in chronic granulomatous disease (see Chapter 16) (19,20) demonstrates that each of these proteins is essential for an effective inflammatory response.

The efficiency of neutrophil killing of microorganisms is enhanced if the bacterium is first coated with antibody (the product of B cells and discussed further below) or complement. The complement system is composed of at least 20 different serum glycoproteins that are activated sequentially and cooperatively in a cascade to amplify the response. Complement activation results in opsonization, leukocyte chemotaxis and activation, and development of the membrane attack complex, resulting in killing of bacteria (21,22). Complement activation is initiated by either the classic or alternative pathway or, more recently appreciated, by the mannose-binding lectin pathway (23). Deficiencies of complement components both result in and are the result of a number of disorders, including membranoproliferative glomerulonephritis, systemic lupus erythematosus, and hereditary angioedema (21,22). In addition, complement activation provides a link to the adaptive immune response; complement products, for instance, bind to B lymphocytes and regulate B-cell responses (21,22).

Circulating monocytes and tissue macrophages function as accessory cells in the activation of both B and T cells. Monocytes and macrophages do not express antigen-specific receptors, but they are capable of processing foreign proteins for presentation to T cells. In addition, mononuclear cells differentiate to specialized antigen-presenting cells (APCs) termed *DCs*, of which many subsets and separable lineages have now been defined (24,25). Contrary to the early belief that innate immunity was nonspecific, it is now clear that innate immunity is tightly regulated and, in addition, has the capacity to distinguish pathogens from self. The ability to recognize pathogenic structures expressed by microorganisms is conferred by germline receptors, termed *pattern-recognition receptors*, that are expressed on a variety of immune cells, including monocytes, macrophages, and DCs. In mammals, the Toll-like receptors (TLRs) function as pattern-recognition receptors and recognize not only microbial products but also some endogenous ligands. Ten members of the TLR, each encoded in the germline and nonclonal, have been identified to date. The TLRs share significant homology in their cytoplasmic domain to the type I IL-1 receptor (26,27). TLR4 is the receptor for the gram-negative bacterial component

37. Krausa P, Bodmer JG, Browning M. Defining the common subtypes of HLA-A9, A10, A28 and A19 by use of ARMS/PCR. *Tissue Antigens* 1993;42:91–99.

38. Bunce M, Welsh KI. Rapid DNA typing for HLA-C using sequence-specific primers (PCR-SSP): identification of serological and nonserologically defined HLA-C alleles including several new alleles. *Tissue Antigens* 1994;43:7–17.

39. Sadler AM, Petronzelli F, Krausa P, et al. Low-resolution DNA typing for HLA-B using sequence-specific primers in allele or group specific ARMS/PCR. *Tissue Antigens* 1994;44:148–154.

40. Guttridge MG, Burr C, Klouda PT. Identification of HLA-B35, B53, B18, B5, B78 and B17 alleles by the polymerase chain reaction using sequence-specific primers (PCR-SSP). *Tissue Antigens* 1994;44:43–46.

41. Hein J, Bottcher K, Grundmann R, et al. Low resolution DNA typing of the HLA-B5 cross-reactive group by nested PCR-SSP. *Tissue Antigens* 1995;45:27–35.

42. Bugawan TL, Begovich AB, Erlich HA. Rapid HLA DPB typing using enzymatically amplified DNA and nonradioactive sequence-specific oligonucleotide probes. *Immunogenetics* 1990;32:231–241.

43. Petersdorf EW, Smith AG, Mickelson EM, et al. Ten HLA-DR4 alleles defined by sequence polymorphisms within the DRB1 first domain. *Immunogenetics* 1991;33:267–275.

44. Allen M, Liu L, Gyllensten U. A comprehensive polymerase chain reaction-oligonucleotide typing system for the HLA-class I A locus. *Hum Immunol* 1994;40:25–32.

45. Levine JE, Yang SY. SSOP typing of the Tenth International Histocompatibility Workshop reference cell lines for HLA-C alleles. *Tissue Antigens* 1994;44:174–183.

46. Scharf SJ, Griffith RL, Erlich HA. Rapid typing of DNA sequence polymorphism at the HLA-DRB1 locus using the polymerase chain reaction and nonradioactive oligonucleotide probes. *Hum Immunol* 1991;30:190–201.

47. Bugawan TL, Apple R, Erlich HA. A method for typing polymorphism at the HLA-A locus using PCR amplification and immobilized oligonucleotide probes. *Tissue Antigens* 1994;44:137–147.

48. Santamaria P, Lindstrom AL, Boyce-Jacino MT, et al. HLA class I sequence-based typing. *Hum Immunol* 1993;37:39–50.

49. Versluis LF, Rozemuller E, Tonks S, et al. High-resolution HLA-DPB typing based upon computerized analysis of data obtained by fluorescent sequencing of the amplified polymorphic exon 2. *Hum Immunol* 1993;38:277–283.

50. Petersdorf EW, Hansen JA. A comprehensive approach for typing the alleles of the HLA-B locus by automated sequencing. *Tissue Antigens* 1995;46:73–85.

51. Marcadet A, O'Connell P, Cohen D. Standardized southern blot workshop technique. In: Dupont B, ed. *Immunobiology of HLA*, Vol. 1. New York: Springer-Verlag, 1989:553–560.

52. Clay TM, Bidwell JL, Howard MR, et al. PCR-fingerprinting for selection of HLA matched unrelated marrow donors. Collaborating centres in the IMUST Study. *Lancet* 1991;337:1049–1052.

53. Tong JR, Hammad A, Rudert WA, et al. Heteroduplexes for HLA-DQB1 identity of family members and kidney donor-recipient pairs. *Transplantation* 1994;57:741–745.

54. Orita M, Suzuki Y, Sekiya T, et al. Rapid and sensitive detection of point mutations and DNA polymorphisms using polymerase chain reaction. *Genomics* 1989;5:874–879.

55. Blasczyk R, Hahn U, Wehling J, et al. Complete amplification followed by direct sequencing or single-strand conformation polymorphism analysis. *Tissue Antigens* 1995;46:86–95.

56. Arguelo JR, Little A-M, Bohan E, et al. High resolution HLA class I typing by reference strand mediated conformation analysis (RSCA). *Tissue Antigens* 1998;52:57–66.

57. Arguello R, Avakian H, Goldman JM, et al. A novel method for simultaneous high resolution identification of HLA-A, HLA-B and HLA-Cw alleles. *Proc Natl Acad Sci U S A* 1996;93:10961–10965.

58. Madrigal JA, Arguello R, Gallardo D, et al. High resolution HLA class I and II typing for unrelated bone marrow donors. *Eur J Immunogenet* 1997;24:70(abst).

59. Maskos U, Southern EM. Oligonucleotide hybridizations on glass supports: a novel linker for oligonucleotide synthesis and hybridization properties of oligonucleotides synthesized in situ. *Nucleic Acids Res* 1992;20:1679–1684.

60. Blanchard AP, Kaiser RJ, Hood LE. High-density oligonucleotide arrays. *Biosens Bioelectron* 1996;11:687–690.

61. Lilly F, Boyse EA, Old LJ. Genetic basis of susceptibility to viral leukaemogenesis. *Lancet* 1964;ii:1207–1209.

62. Amiel JL. Study of the leucocyte phenotypes in Hodgkin's disease. In: Curtoni ES, Mattiuz PL, Tosi RM, eds. *Histocompatibility testing 1967*. Copenhagen: Munksgaard, 1967:115–133.

63. Schlosstein L, Terasaki PI, Bluestone R, et al. High association of an HL-A antigen, W27, with ankylosing spondylitis. *N Engl J Med* 1973;288:704–706.

64. Brewerton DA, Caffrey M, Hart FD, et al. Ankylosing spondylitis and HL-A27. *Lancet* 1973;1:904–907.

65. Tiwari JL, Terasaki PI, eds. *HLA and disease associations*. New York: Springer-Verlag, 1985.

66. Caillat-Zucman S, Djilali-Saiah I, Timsit J, et al. Insulin dependent diabetes mellitus (IDDM): 12th International Histocompatibility Workshop study. In: Charron D, ed. *HLA: genetic diversity of HLA—functional and medical implication*, Vol. 1. Sevres: EDK, 1997:389–398.

67. Thorsby E. Invited anniversary review: HLA associated diseases. *Hum Immunol* 1997;53:1–11.

68. Yankee RA, Grumet FC, Rogentine GN. Platelet transfusion. The selection of compatible platelet donors for refractory patients by lymphocyte HL-A typing. *N Engl J Med* 1969;281:1208–1212.

69. Kunicki TJ. Human platelet antigens. In: Hoffman R, Benz EJ Jr, Shattil SJ, et al., eds. *Hematology: basic principles and practice*, 3rd ed. New York: Churchill Livingstone, 1998.

70. Friedman JM, Aster RH. Neonatal alloimmune thrombocytopenic purpura and congenital porencephaly in two siblings associated with a "new" maternal antiplatelet antibody. *Blood* 1985;65:1412–1415.

71. Noris P, Simsek S, de Bruijne-Admiraal LG, et al. Max (a), a new low-frequency platelet-specific antigen localized on glycoprotein IIb, is associated with neonatal alloimmune thrombocytopenia. *Blood* 1995;86:1019–1026.

72. Collaborative Transplant Study. http://www.ctstransplant.org.

73. Takemoto SK, Terasaki PI, Gjertson DW, et al. Twelve years' experience with national sharing of HLA-matched cadaveric kidneys for transplantation. *N Engl J Med* 2000;343:1078–1084.

74. Hansen JA, Petersdorf E, Martin PJ, et al. Hematopoietic stem cell transplants from unrelated donors. *Immunol Rev* 1997;157:141–151.

75. Beatty PG, Clift RA, Mickelson EM, et al. Marrow transplantation from related donors other than HLA-identical siblings. *N Engl J Med* 1985;313:765–771.

76. Anasetti C, Amos D, Beatty PG, et al. Effect of HLA compatibility on engraftment of bone marrow transplants in patients with leukemia or lymphoma. *N Engl J Med* 1989;320:197–204.

77. Anasetti C, Beatty PG, Storb R, et al. Effect of HLA incompatibility on graft-versus-host disease, relapse, and survival after marrow transplantation for patients with leukemia or lymphoma. *Hum Immunol* 1990;29:79–91.

78. Petersdorf EW, Longton GM, Anasetti C, et al. Association of HLA-C disparity with graft failure after marrow transplantation from unrelated donors. *Blood* 1997;89:1818–1823.

79. Erlich H. Principles and applications of the polymerase chain reaction. *Rev Immunogenet* 1999;1:127–134.

80. Anasetti C. Hematopoietic cell transplantation from HLA partially matched related donors. In: Thomas ED, Blume KG, Forman SJ, eds. *Hematopoietic cell transplantation*, 2nd ed. Boston: Blackwell Science, 1999:904–914.

81. National Marrow Donor Program (NMDP). http://www.marrow.org.

82. Bone Marrow Donors Worldwide. http://www.bmdw.org.

83. Petersdorf EW, Hansen JA, Martin PJ, et al. Sequence polymorphisms of major histocompatibility class I genes that define the HLA barrier in hematopoietic cell transplantation. *N Engl J Med*, submitted, 2001.

84. Petersdorf EW, Gooley TA, Anasetti C, et al. Optimizing outcome after unrelated marrow transplantation by comprehensive matching of HLA class I and II alleles in the donor and recipient. *Blood* 1998;92:3515–3520.

85. Sasazuki T, Juji T, Morishima Y, et al. Importance of HLA class I allele matching for clinical outcome after unrelated donor hematopoietic stem cell transplantation. *N Engl J Med* 1998;339:1177–1185.

86. Hansen JA, Yamamoto K, Petersdorf E, et al. The role of HLA matching in hematopoietic cell transplantation. *Rev Immunogenet* 1999;1:359–373.

CHAPTER 20

Reactive Lymphocyte Disorders and Lymphadenopathy

Kenneth B. Miller

Lymphadenopathy is a common presenting finding in a patient with benign and malignant disorders. This chapter reviews the history of the discovery of the lymphatic system and its function, the anatomy of lymphatic organs, and the causes and evaluation of lymphadenopathy.

HISTORY

The lymphatic system, from the Latin word *lympha* meaning clear spring water, was recognized in the seventeenth century as distinct from the arterial and venous systems. Jean Pecquet (1) noted in 1651 that the lymphatics, like the venous system, are composed of numerous small vessels that gradually combine to form larger and larger trunks, eventually emptying into the subclavian vein through the thoracic duct. William Hewson, one of the fathers of hematology, in his treatise on the lymphatic system, described its anatomy in detail, including the basic architecture of the lymph nodes and the dual circulation within them (2). Hewson noted prominent lymphadenopathy in some patients with syphilis, cancer, and abscesses, and he concluded that the primary function of the lymph nodes was to act as "absorbants" to drain adjacent areas of noxious agents (3). He also noticed that the lymph fluid contains colorless nucleated cells, which he speculated were formed in the lymph nodes and thymus. He postulated that the entire hematopoietic system is derived from these colorless lymphocytes, calling the lymph corpuscles "central particles." The lymphocytes, according to Hewson, form the central colorless area of the red blood cells (RBCs), hence the term *central*. Noting the enlarged thymus in children, he speculated on its biologic importance in the normal development of the lymphoid system. Hewson's career was tragically cut short when he died at the age of 35 from an infection sustained during a dissection.

By the late nineteenth century, the spleen and lymph nodes were known to be involved in different disorders such as tuberculosis, leukemia, and cancer. Virchow, a leading pathologist of the day, attempted to address the morphologic and biologic differences between lymphoid hyperplasia and neoplasia (4). Virchow studied the spleen and lymph nodes in patients with leukemia. He commented on the change in the normal architecture, using the word *neoplasia* to describe new growth and to distinguish these findings from hyperplasia. In 1875, Louis

Antoine Ranvier published the then-definitive text on the lymphatic system. His 1100-page volume, *Traité Technique d'Histologie*, described the structure and function of the lymph nodes and lymphatic vessels (5). Ranvier speculated that the lymphocytes were involved in healing and tissue repair, presumably because of their ability to migrate through blood vessel walls. He asserted that the lymphocyte is a carrier cell that supplies nutrients and essential metabolites to tissues with sudden or unusual metabolic requirements. Fleming, using new staining techniques developed by Ehrlich and newly improved microscopes, described the follicles in the spleen, lymph nodes, and tonsils. He called the central pale areas "germinal centers" because of their many dividing cells (6).

Ehrlich's method of staining thin, dried films of blood had a profound influence on all areas of hematology, including studies of the lymphatics. He was able to distinguish the lymphocyte from the leukocyte and proposed that the lymphocyte represented a separate cell lineage, originating in the lymph nodes and spleen, in contrast to the cellular elements formed in the bone marrow.

In the seventeenth century, Marcello Malphigi described the glandular appearance of the spleen and the densely packed cells now known as the *malpighian corpuscles* (7). In 1854, Theodore Billroth identified the unique vascular structures of the spleen (8). He described the splenic red pulp, now called the *cords of Billroth*, and the splenic sinuses, referred to as the *sinuses of Billroth*.

Throughout the centuries, the spleen was given many roles and names reflecting its pivotal anatomic position juxtaposed between the liver and the stomach but unknown functional importance.

The ancients considered the spleen to be part of the digestive system (9). Galen, a father of modern science, believed the spleen functioned to extract liquid from the stomach. He was perplexed by this role, referring to the spleen as a "plenum mysterii organon" (an organ filled with mystery) (10). Erasistratus, one of the first anatomists, saw the spleen as a counterbalance to the mighty liver, preserving the symmetry of the abdomen. Plato was also intrigued by the spleen and its proximity to the liver. He suggested that it served to keep the liver clean and healthy. Hippocrates believed that the spleen balanced the four essential humors of man: blood, phlegm, golden bile, and black bile. The liver was thought to be the source of the all-important golden bile, and the spleen was thought to be the source of black bile. The Greeks and Romans believed that the spleen affected athletic ability, and they consumed certain beverages before athletic competition, purportedly to shrink the spleen and enhance their performance.

The spleen, as a ductless gland occupying so much of the anterior abdomen, has fascinated physician and philosopher alike. The spleen was considered as both the center of violent ill tempers, as in "venting one's spleen," and as the origin of amusement and laughter. The Talmud describes the spleen as the source of both laughter and joy (11). *Melt* was another word for the spleen, reflecting its key anatomic position. This term was derived from the verb *to melt*, meaning to knock down by a blow to the side (12). In battle, a blow to the melt, or spleen, could be fatal. This anatomic weakness was well known in Southeast Asia, where massively swollen spleens were commonplace, presumably caused by malaria. A sharp blow to the left upper quadrant, rupturing the spleen, was a quick and effective tactic for assassins (13).

These observations on the origin and function of the lymphatic system by the founders of modern medicine and science have laid the foundation for the study of immunology and pathology.

LYMPHOID CELLS AND THE LYMPHATIC SYSTEM

Lymph Nodes

The lymphatic system consists of the peripheral lymph nodes, the spleen, Waldeyer's ring (including the oropharyngeal lymphoid tissues), and lymphoid aggregates in the lamina propria and submucosa of the respiratory and gastrointestinal tract, including Peyer's patches. These are referred to as the *secondary lymphoid tissues*, which are in contrast to the bone marrow and thymus that are the primary lymphoid tissues. Afferent and efferent vessels carry lymph into and out of the nodes. Normal lymph nodes vary in size from 2 to 20 mm, averaging 15 mm in

longitudinal diameter. Size and structure vary according to the node's location and the person's age. Lymph nodes draining areas of active antigenic stimulation, such as the neck, inguinal area, and abdomen, have proportionally larger and more numerous germinal centers, whereas mesenteric nodes have wider medullary sinuses and fewer germinal centers. Peripheral nodes are more common in younger persons and are absent in newborns (14).

Changes that occur in the different nodal compartments are helpful in differentiating a reactive node from one involved with a lymphoproliferative disorder (Fig. 20-1) (15). The lymph node has a limited repertoire of morphologic responses to the wide variety of specific and nonspecific stimuli that it receives (16). Histochemistry, immunochemistry, and molecular studies are helpful in evaluating the histologic changes observed in an enlarged lymph node.

Immunohistochemical markers, using monoclonal antibodies capable of recognizing differentiation antigens and surface markers on distinct populations of B, T, and natural killer (NK) cells and monocytes, have defined the distribution and compartmentalization of lymphocytes in normal lymph nodes. These antibodies form a cluster and, therefore, could be grouped together because they recognize the same cell-surface molecules. Thus a given molecule was assigned a "cluster of differentiation" (CD) number. The CD nomenclature has become the standard way of referring to these cell-surface molecules recognized by specific monoclonal antibodies. The use of immunophenotyping and flow cytometry has become an important part of the diagnosis and classification of lymphoid malignancies (17). In peripheral lymph nodes, T cells are usually restricted to the paracortical or interfollicular areas, whereas B cells are concentrated in the lymphoid follicles and medullary zones. Most cells in the follicle area, which includes the mantle zone and the germinal centers, are B lymphocytes that are positive for the pan-B-cell marker, CD20. The expression of surface immunoglobulins (Igs) is highly variable within these regions. The B cells in the mantle zone are positive for

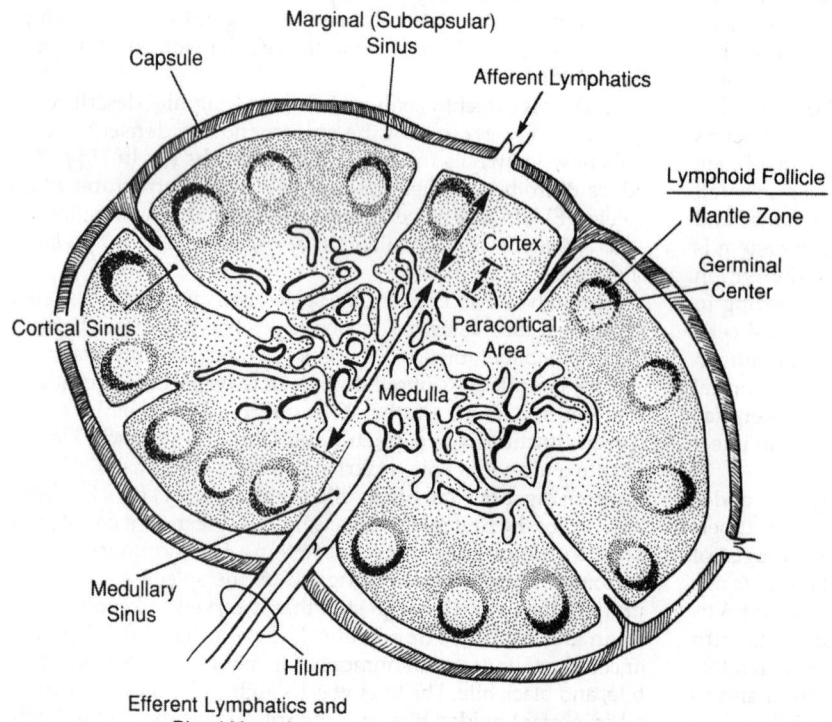

Figure 20-1. Schematic view of the organization of the human lymph node.

μ– and δ–heavy chains. The B-cell population of a normal lymph node is polyclonal and, therefore, contains roughly equal populations of cells that express either κ– or λ–light chains on their surfaces. The germinal centers are generated by activated B cells and are the part of the lymphoid follicle that reflects the events of antigenic stimulation and the normal steps of B-lymphocyte differentiation. There are two subsets of B cells recognized: B1 and B2. The B1 cells develop earliest during ontogeny and are self-renewing and long lived (18). A majority of B1 cells express CD5, an adhesion and signaling cell molecule. The majority of B cells in the lymph node are the B2 subtype and produce antibodies. The B2 cells develop later in ontogeny and lack the CD5 molecule. Naïve B2 cells, before they encounter antigens, coexpress IgM and IgD antibodies on their cell surface, but by the time they become memory cells, they switch to the expression of surface IgG, IgA, or IgE as their antigen receptors (19). B lymphocytes bearing the surface IgM and surface IgD are found throughout the normal node but are concentrated primarily in the mantle zone. In the germinal centers of lymph nodes and the spleen, B cells encounter antigens and undergo immunoglobulin class switching and begin to produce IgG, IgA, or IgE. Memory cells and plasma cell precursors are generated in the germinal centers, but the final differentiation of B2 cells into antigen-bearing plasma cells occurs outside the germinal centers but within the spleen and lymph nodes. More mature lymphocytes bearing surface IgG or surface IgA are rarely found in the normal lymph node.

T cells present in the normal lymph node stain with a number of monoclonal antibodies. T cells that mark with the pan-T-cell marker, CD2, are found diffusely throughout the paracortical and intrafollicular area of the normal lymph node. In the paracortical areas, CD4+ (helper and inducer T cells) and CD8+ (suppressor-cytotoxic cells) are normally present in a ratio of 2 to 3:1, a ratio similar to that found normally in the blood. The T cells in the germinal centers, although rare, are usually of the helper-inducer phenotype (CD4); the suppressor-cytotoxic T cell (CD8+) is virtually absent.

In response to an antigenic stimulus, the lymph node rapidly increases the proportion of CD4+ cells two- to threefold. An increase of the CD8+ population in a hyperplastic node is rare (20). In the germinal centers and mantle zones, T cells make up between 5% and 20% of the total cells (20). CD57, which includes cells of the NK phenotype, can also be found in the germinal centers. Moreover, many of these CD57+ cells are localized to the upper poles of the germinal centers and double-stain with CD4 (19).

The interdigitating reticulum dendritic cells are usually strongly positive for HLA-DR and are most numerous in the paracortical area and germinal centers (21). These interdigitating dendritic cells are a key cellular component of the immune response and, when activated, become antigen presenting to specific T cells (22).

Spleen

The distribution of lymphocytes in the spleen closely resembles that in the normal lymph node (22). The splenic follicles, like the lymph node follicles, contain mostly B cells that stain with the pan-B-cell marker, CD20. The B lymphocytes in the mantle zone also express surface Ig of the μ– and δ–heavy chains. Most of the lymphocytes in the periarteriolar sheaths are CD4+ T cells, and the ratio of CD4+ to CD8+ cells is approximately 3:1 (23). In the marginal zone, the T and B cells are mixed with occasional HLA-DR+ monocytes, reflecting the extensive blood supply to this area and the branching trabeculae. Within the splenic sinusoids and cords, T and B cells are randomly distributed. The red pulp contains few resident lymphocytes, most of which are cells that are CD8+, suppressor-cytotoxic T cells.

Lymphocytes are a heterogeneous collection of cells with different origins, functions, and lifespans. In the peripheral blood, lymphocytes make up 20% to 40% of total blood leukocytes. Most of the circulating lymphocytes are small (10 μm or less) and are referred to by their morphologic appearance (small, medium, large, or clefted); their functional characteristics (helper, suppressor, or NK); or their surface phenotype markers (e.g., CD4, CD8).

Viral infections are the most common causes of transient lymphocytosis. Varicella, mumps, cytomegalovirus (CMV), and Epstein-Barr virus (EBV) are associated with prominent lymphocytosis. Viral infections are characterized by the increased numbers of large, reactive, atypical-appearing lymphocytes. Lymphocytosis rarely occurs during most bacterial infections, with the exception of pertussis, in which the total white blood cell count may range between 20,000/μL and 50,000/μL with 60% or more lymphocytes. Patients with hyposplenism may have a persistently high lymphocyte count (24). In these reactive settings, a polyclonal increase in lymphocytes is found, which is in contrast to that found in patients with early chronic lymphocytic leukemia and other lymphoproliferative disorders in which there is an increase in a clonal populations of cells. Flow cytometry and molecular studies demonstrating immunoglobulin or T-cell receptor gene rearrangements have made it possible to distinguish a clonal lymphoproliferative disorder from reactive lymphocytosis (25–27). In most patients, persistent chronic lymphocytosis is associated with an underlying monoclonal malignant lymphoproliferative disorder (28).

The percentage of circulating lymphocytes in the peripheral blood varies according to the person's age (29). The lymphocyte concentration is high at birth and may rise to 22,000/μL in apparently healthy infants during the first year of life. Then, a gradual decline throughout childhood occurs, which stabilizes after age 7 years at approximately 4000/μL. The increased total lymphocyte count in infants reflects the high relative proportion of surface Ig–positive B cells with a relative decrease in circulating T cells. The percentage of T cells slowly increases after the second year of life to reach adult levels by the age of 7 years (29). In adults, the total number of T or B lymphocytes does not appear to change with age (30). However, the relative distribution of T lymphocytes in the peripheral blood does change with age. Activated (HLA-DR+) and memory (CD45RO+) T cells and CD3+ cells that express the NK marker CD56 are expanded in healthy elderly individuals (31). There are also changes in B-cell antigen expression, including the increased expression of CD20 (32). The lymphoid organs gradually decrease in size with advancing age, with a decrease in the number and size of germinal centers in lymph nodes and an increase in plasma cells.

CLINICAL EVALUATION OF LYMPHOID TISSUES

Lymphadenopathy is a common physical finding that affects patients of all ages and is associated with benign and malignant disorders. Benign, reactive disorders account for the majority of enlarged lymph nodes. Reactive hyperplasia and atypical lymphoid hyperplasia are nonmalignant proliferations of cells of one or more of the different anatomic and immunologic compartments of lymphoid tissue. Hyperplasia may involve the follicles (B-cell and plasma cell regions), the interfollicular or paracortical regions (T cells), or the sinuses of the lymph nodes (macrophages and histiocytes). The morphologic appearance of reactive lymph nodes varies with the patient's age, immunologic status, and the offending agent. The etiologic agent in

TABLE 20-1. Causes of Atypical, Reactive Lymphoid Hyperplasia

Infections
    Cat-scratch disease
    Epstein-Barr virus
    Cytomegalovirus disease
    Herpesvirus infection
    Human immunodeficiency virus
    Toxoplasmosis
    Syphilis
    Postvaccination
    Rubella
    Rickettsial infection
    Tularemia
    Lymphogranuloma venereum
    Yersinia infection
Drug-associated
    Dilantin
    Carbamazepine
    Gold derivative
    Phenylbutazone
Autoimmune
    Rheumatoid arthritis
    Systemic lupus erythematosus
    Still's disease
    Hyperthyroidism
    Sjögren's syndrome
    Autoimmune lymphoproliferative syndrome
Other
    Sarcoid
    Angioimmunoblastic lymphadenopathy
    Castleman's disease
    Kikuchi's disease
    Inflammatory pseudotumor of lymph nodes
    Reactive follicular hyperplasia (nonspecific)

most instances of reactive lymphoid hyperplasia is not known. The changes in reactive lymph nodes may be the result of an atypical response to a bacterial or viral infection (Table 20-1).

Palpable cervical nodes are common both in young children and adults. Soft, movable, and nontender cervical lymph nodes between 0.5 and 1.0 cm are frequently felt in the submandibular and posterior cervical regions in healthy children and adolescents (33). The evaluation of symptomatic or asymptomatic lymphadenopathy relies on the physical examination, a detailed medical history, and consideration of the anatomy and different functions of the lymphatic system. The evaluation should consider the dual function of lymphatic organs as both immunologic agents and mechanical filters that trap foreign antigens and malignant cells. In approaching a patient with lymphadenopathy, it is important to determine which nodes are likely to be associated with a benign, self-limited disorder and should be followed versus those lymph nodes that are pathologic and need to be biopsied. A range of variables, including the patient's age, node location and size, tenderness to palpation, and systemic symptoms, provides important clues to the cause of lymphadenopathy and the need for a biopsy (34).

Age is the most important factor in predicting the likelihood if the lymphadenopathy is due to a benign or malignant disorder (35). Children and adolescents commonly have palpable lymph nodes that reflect exposure to new antigens or recurrent viral infections (36). In adolescents, infections are the most common causes of lymphadenopathy. Infectious mononucleosis is a common cause of cervical lymphadenopathy and, although usually associated with an acute pharyngitis, may occur without apparent pharyngeal symptoms. Toxoplasmosis or CMV infections may mimic mononucleosis. The likelihood of finding a malignant process in a palpable peripheral lymph node increases with age. In patients younger than 20 years of age, 75% to 85% of all biopsy specimens of nodes are benign,

whereas less than 30% of the specimens in patients older than 60 years of age are benign (35).

The location, size, and duration of the lymphadenopathy are important variables when deciding if or when a biopsy is needed (37). For example, large bilateral hilar nodes without other detectable lymphadenopathy in a young asymptomatic black patient is suggestive of sarcoidosis (38). Hilar and anterior mediastinal adenopathy are common findings on chest x-rays. Neoplastic disorders associated with hilar adenopathy include bronchogenic carcinoma, metastatic breast and gastrointestinal cancers, and Hodgkin's or non-Hodgkin's lymphoma. Anterior mediastinal fullness on chest x-rays may represent a thymoma, teratoma, or other germ cell tumor, intrathoracic goiter, or Hodgkin's or non-Hodgkin's lymphoma. Generalized tender lymphadenopathy is consistent with a bacterial or viral infection (39). Supraclavicular and scalene lymphadenopathy is more suggestive of carcinoma, whereas a solitary axillary node suggests a diagnosis of lymphoma. Inguinal nodes are more often involved with a reactive process (Table 20-2).

Superficial lymphadenopathy in the head and neck most often results from an intercurrent or recovering acute bacterial or viral illness. Neoplasms or infectious processes originating in the lung or retroperitoneal area produce supraclavicular and scalene lymphadenopathy. Axillary lymphadenopathy occurs from changes in the upper extremities, including infections, trauma, or even insect bites to the extremities. Epitrochlear adenopathy historically has been associated with secondary syphi-

TABLE 20-2. Common Causes of Lymphadenopathy

Region	Etiology
Occipital lymph nodes	Scalp infections, insect bites (children), ringworm, very rarely lymphoma or metastatic tumors, cat-scratch disease
Posterior auricular	Rubella, oculoglandular syndromes
Anterior auricular	Infections of eyelids and conjunctiva, epidemic keratoconjunctivitis
Posterior and anterior cervical	Toxoplasmosis, adenovirus syndromes, infections of oral cavity and pharynx
Posterior cervical and submental	Scalp infections, dental infections, tuberculosis
Cervical (suppurative)	Tuberculosis
Supraclavicular (hard and fixed)	Metastases from intrathoracic or intraabdominal carcinoma, Hodgkin's disease
Axillary	Infection of upper extremities, cat-scratch disease, brucellosis, sporotrichosis, non-Hodgkin's lymphomas
Epitrochlear	
Unilateral	Infections of hands, Hodgkin's disease
Bilateral	Viral disease in children, sarcoidosis, tularemia
Inguinal	
Unilateral	Lymphogranuloma venereum, syphilis, chancroid; gonococcal, herpetic venereal infections; mycoplasma; urethritis, tularemia, plague, loiasis, onchocerciasis, lymphoma, metastatic pelvic carcinoma, gynecologic malignancies
Bilateral	
Pulmonary hilar	
Unilateral	Metastatic lung carcinoma
Bilateral	Sarcoidosis, tuberculosis, histoplasmosis, coccidioidomycosis
Mediastinal, symmetric	Hodgkin's disease, lymphoma
Intraabdominal and retroperitoneal	Lymphoma, metastatic carcinoma, tuberculosis in mesenteric lymph nodes
Regional involvement in systemic infections	Infectious mononucleosis, viral hepatitis, cytomegalovirus disease, rubella, influenza, leprosy, toxoplasmosis, acquired immunodeficiency syndrome
Generalized lymphadenopathy	Sarcoidosis, hyperthyroidism, systemic lupus erythematosus, lymphoma, syphilis

lis, leprosy, and rubella but is also associated with a number of systemic infections and non-Hodgkin's lymphoma but rarely with Hodgkin's lymphoma (40). Small, 0.5- to 1.0-cm, non-tender inguinal adenopathy is frequently noted in the region of the inguinal ligament and femoral triangle and usually reflects prior inflammation in the perirectal and vaginal areas or lower extremities. Small abrasions of the toes or infections in the nail beds can cause prominent reactive lymphadenopathy in the extremity involved. The node of Cloquet, a deep inguinal lymph node near the femoral canal, can be mistaken for a inguinal hernia when it is enlarged (41).

Enlarged nodes in the supraclavicular fossa are more likely to be involved with a malignant disorder. The Virchow's node, a pathologic enlarged anterior left supraclavicular node, is associated with diseases in the chest, gastrointestinal tract, or retroperitoneum (42).

The threshold size for defining an abnormal lymph node is controversial and depends, in part, on its location and the imaging technique used to define its size. Mediastinal nodes greater than 1.0 cm for the short axis in the transverse diameter on computed tomographic (CT) scans are pathologically enlarged (43). In the abdomen, the upper limits of normal adenopathy by location are retrocrural 6.0 mm, paracardiac 0.8 cm, and paraaortic 0.9 to 1.1 cm, whereas in all others, 1 cm is considered the upper limit of normal (44).

The texture of the node may provide clues to its cause. Bacterial infections are associated with warm, tender, or fluctuant adenopathy from the draining area, whereas lymphadenopathy that is firm, fixed, matted, and painless is suggestive of involvement with metastatic disease. However, the node consistency is the least helpful physical finding in distinguishing a benign from a malignant lesion (35).

Infections are common causes of localized or diffuse lymphadenopathy (39). Patients should be questioned about recent travel or exposure to infections. International travel has changed the distribution of many infections (45). A detailed sexual history is also needed on all patients with unexplained lymphadenopathy. Sexually transmitted diseases such as syphilis, chancroid, and herpes simplex can present with prominent lymphadenopathy (46,47). Diffuse lymphadenopathy may be one of the early signs of a human immunodeficiency virus (HIV) infection (48,49).

Reactive, hyperplastic lymphadenopathy has been associated with a number of drugs, including phenylbutazone, methyldopa, meprobamate, hydralazine, gold derivative, and the phenytoin derivatives (50–55). Dilantin can produce a clinical syndrome that is similar to Hodgkin's lymphoma, with the development of fever, eosinophilia, and diffuse or localized lymphadenopathy that develops within weeks to months after starting the drug (52,54).

Endocrine or autoimmune disorders can present with lymphadenopathy or splenomegaly. Patients with hyperthyroidism can present with findings suggestive of a lymphoproliferative disorder, including a history of weight loss, diffuse sweating, and generalized firm lymphadenopathy and splenomegaly. Autoimmune disorders such as systemic lupus erythematosus and Sjögren's syndrome may present with diffuse or localized lymphadenopathy (56–58).

When and whether to perform a biopsy on an enlarged lymph node depends on the patient's symptoms and the location of the adenopathy. A patient with symptoms of weight loss, night sweats, or gradually enlarging nontender, asymmetric lymphadenopathy without an obvious source of infection requires a lymph node biopsy. More difficult is the patient with an isolated, enlarged lymph node and a recent bacterial or viral infection. An enlarged lymph node that does not decrease in

size within 2 months after resolution of the infection should be biopsied.

The initial evaluation of a patient with lymphadenopathy should include a complete physical examination. The physician should carefully note the location, size, shape, and consistency of the enlarged lymph nodes. Whenever possible, the nodes should be measured in two dimensions. Close attention should be paid to the area draining the involved nodes. Isolated cervical lymphadenopathy requires a detailed head and neck examination, paying close attention to the tongue, gums, and hard and soft palates. For patients with a solitary submandibular or submental node, a thorough head and neck examination including indirect laryngoscopy is necessary before proceeding with a biopsy. In patients with a history of tobacco use, a careful oral examination is required.

Occipital lymphadenopathy may be caused by a lesion on the head and scalp. Small areas of eczema on the hairline can produce prominent cervical adenopathy. Reactive inguinal adenopathy is common in both children and adults and may be caused by infections in the inguinal, pelvic, and retroperitoneal areas.

Multiple studies have attempted to define algorithms for the evaluation of lymphadenopathy (33,34,59,60). A patient with a node larger than 2 cm, with an abnormal chest radiograph, and without fevers or chills is likely to require a biopsy for diagnosis. An enlarged scalene, supraclavicular, or solitary nontender axillary node is highly suggestive of a malignant or granulomatous disorder and should be biopsied.

The initial investigation should focus on likely causes of the lymphadenopathy. The location of the enlarged lymph node should direct the evaluation. Supraclavicular adenopathy of more than 1 cm is highly suggestive of intrathoracic or retroperitoneal disease, and a chest and abdominal radiograph or CT scan should be obtained. Patients with newly diagnosed asymptomatic generalized symmetric cervical lymphadenopathy and a negative chest radiograph can usually be followed before proceeding with a biopsy. If all evaluations are negative or nondiagnostic and the lymphadenopathy persists or increases for greater than 2 months, a biopsy should be obtained.

A sample of the lymph node for evaluation can be obtained by excisional biopsy, core-needle biopsy, or fine-needle biopsy. The procedure of choice, in part, depends on the location and clinical status of the patient. In a patient with a prior malignant disorder, a core- or fine-needle biopsy is usually sufficient to diagnose metastatic or recurrent disease. In patients suspected of an infectious etiology, a fine-needle biopsy with smears and cultures may be sufficient (61). A needle biopsy may be sufficient to establish a diagnosis in many patients with unexplained adenopathy (62–64). In patients without accessible peripheral adenopathy, the use of an imaging-guided core-needle biopsy is an alternative to excisional biopsy (65). Core-needle biopsies should have sufficient material for immunophenotyping and immunohistochemical studies (66). A fine-needle biopsy, however, may not provide sufficient material to diagnose and subclassify a Hodgkin's or non-Hodgkin's lymphoma. A needle biopsy may not allow for adequate immunophenotyping or studies of nodal architecture or mitotic activity. In addition, a needle sample may not obtain enough representative material from certain pleomorphic malignancies, such as Hodgkin's lymphoma, which may result in a misdiagnosis. If a high suspicion of an underlying malignant lymphoma exists and the patient has an accessible enlarged lymph node, it is best to proceed with a definitive excisional biopsy rather than a needle biopsy.

The diagnostic yield from the first node biopsy depends on the location of the node; inguinal nodes have the lowest yield, and supraclavicular and axillary nodes have the highest yield. In patients with a nondiagnostic or reactive node on the initial biopsy, approximately 20% have a specific diagnosis confirmed on a subsequent biopsy from a different nodal site (67). The use of immunophenotyping and molecular studies has increased the yield of lymph node biopsies (66). The diagnosis of lymphoma requires the close coordination of cytopathologists and hematopathologists. A cytologic diagnosis of lymphoma is not sufficient for planning therapy and assigning prognosis. If a core- or fine-needle biopsy is planned, sufficient material should be obtained for cytomorphology and immunophenotyping. A consultation with the evaluating pathologist before a planned surgical or needle biopsy helps in directing the diagnostic studies.

LYMPHADENOPATHY DUE TO INFECTIONS

Lymphadenopathy due to an infection may be either localized and draining an infected area or generalized from a systemic infection. The gross and microscopic changes in a lymph node depend on the nature of the infectious organism, the host's defense, and the antimicrobial therapy that the patient has received (39,67). A variety of bacterial, rickettsial, chlamydial, spirochetal, protozoal, and helminthic agents can cause localized and generalized lymphadenopathy (Table 20-2). Many common viral syndromes typically present with generalized prominent lymphadenopathy, including rubella, measles, HIV, infectious mononucleosis, and CMV infections.

Certain infections produce distinctive pathologic findings. Caseous necrosis results from infections with *Mycobacterium tuberculosis, Histoplasma capsulatum, Coccidioides immitis*, and the various atypical mycobacteria (61,68). Cat-scratch disease, tularemia, and lymphogranuloma venereum produce stellate abscesses surrounded by palisading epithelioid cells (69–73). Toxoplasmosis produces follicular hyperplasia with reactive germinal centers and clusters of epithelial cells in the paracortex and germinal centers (74). Acute lymphadenitis due to pyogenic bacteria produces tender, enlarged nodes, which are firm or fluctuant to palpation and usually at least 3 cm in diameter. Acute lymphadenitis, more common in children than adults, is usually due to *Staphylococcus aureus* or group A streptococci (75). The most common nodes of involvement, in descending order of rate of occurrence, are submandibular, anterior and posterior cervical, inguinal, and axillary. Cervical lymphadenopathy from these infections is usually unilateral and tender and is often associated with swelling of the face or neck, which is sometimes so pronounced as to interfere with the opening of the mouth.

Lymphadenopathy is caused by lymphatic drainage of the involved area. The iliac nodes, located along the external and common iliac arteries, receive lymphatic drainage from the lower abdominal wall and superficial and deep inguinal structures. Iliac and inguinal lymphadenopathy reflect infections of the lower extremities, lower abdominal wall, perineum, and pelvis. Patients may develop limping, back pain, or hip pain because the lymphadenopathy causes pain on extension of the thigh.

Scrofula, or tuberculous cervical lymphadenopathy, was frequently acquired from milk infected with bovine tuberculosis or was lymphohematogenically spread from an initial pulmonary focus. Most mycobacterial cervical lymphadenitis is now caused by atypical mycobacteria, such as *Mycobacterium scrofulaceum* or *Mycobacterium avium*-intracellulare rather than *M. tuberculosis* (76,77). An enlarging nontender cervical mass usually brings the patient to seek medical attention, and most patients have no additional clinical evidence of tuberculosis. Defining the species of mycobacteria is important. The atypical mycobacteria are frequently resistant to standard antituberculosis therapy.

The paratracheal and mediastinal nodes may be sites of tuberculosis adenitis. On biopsy, the caseous necrosis characteristic of tuberculosis is coagulative with total necrosis that leaves no cellular traces or nuclear debris. The diagnosis is confirmed by demonstrating the typical acid-fast bacilli on smears or sections of the node or by culturing the organism, which is more sensitive because the smear may be positive in less than one-third of patients with a positive culture (78).

Reactive lymphoid hyperplasia is seen in a number of infectious diseases. In most instances of reactive hyperplasia, the etiologic agent is not known; however, in some disorders the histologic findings are so characteristic that a specific diagnosis can be made on morphologic criteria alone. These disorders include cat-scratch disease, lymphogranuloma venereum, syphilis, toxoplasmosis, and a variety of viral illnesses. Cat-scratch disease is an indolent, self-limited illness, which is characterized by tender, regional lymphadenopathy. The etiologic agent is a pleomorphic gram-negative bacillus, *Rochalimaea henselae*, which is identified by the Warthin-Starry silver stain (79,80). Cultures of material aspirated from the node are usually nonrevealing, and the diagnosis is made on the basis of the appropriate exposure and the clinical picture. Patients are usually not ill, despite impressive regional nontender lymphadenopathy. Some patients may complain of a recent influenza-like illness with diffuse myalgia and low-grade fever (81). Over 90% of patients give a history of contact with a cat, and the mode of transmission is presumably from a scratch, bite, or lick. A primary lesion consisting of a small papule or vesicle usually develops at the site of the scratch 7 to 14 days after contact with the cat. The primary lesion may persist for 1 to 3 weeks, and it heals without scar formation. Regional lymphadenopathy develops within 2 weeks of the appearance of the skin papule. Any peripheral lymph node may be involved, but axillary, cervical, and occipital nodes, respectively, are most frequently involved. Epitrochlear adenopathy is rare, despite the frequent inoculation of the hands and forearms. The node biopsy reveals follicular hyperplasia with little distortion of the general nodal architecture. The germinal centers are enlarged, with a diffuse proliferation of immunoblasts, macrophages, and scattered plasma cells. Later in the disease, granuloma forms with central microabscesses. The use of serologic and skin tests to diagnose this disease is still controversial (81).

Bilateral inguinal adenopathy in a young, sexually active, otherwise healthy patient may be caused by one of several venereal diseases. The primary lesion of syphilis, the *chancre*, is usually accompanied by discrete, firm, painless enlarged inguinal nodes (60). The histologic findings in the lymph node include reactive hyperplasia and interfollicular plasmacytosis. Spirochetes are readily demonstrated by immunofluorescence studies. In secondary syphilis, the follicular hyperplasia is more pronounced, and large clusters of epithelioid histiocytes and sarcoidlike granulomas may be present. In late syphilis, the intrafollicular areas show vascular proliferation with prominent endothelial cells, plasma cells, and immunoblasts.

Lymphogranuloma venereum results in large, tender, discrete, and movable bilateral adenopathy. The inguinal nodes are most often involved, but both cervical and supraclavicular adenopathy can occur (84). There is prominent follicular hyperplasia with well-developed suppurative granulomas. Toxoplasmosis lymphadenopathy characteristically affects cervical lymph nodes. Histologically, there is striking follicular hyperplasia with tingible body macrophages and many mitotic figures (74).

Inguinal adenopathy can also be a manifestation of nonvenereal systemic infections. In bubonic plague, caused by *Yersinia pestis*, the inguinal nodes are frequently involved because the flea bite introducing the infection commonly occurs on the lower extremity (85,87). The buboes of the plague produce rapidly enlarging tender lymphadenopathy that quickly becomes suppurative and frequently drains spontaneously. Tularemia may mimic some of the features of the plague and produce regional suppurative adenopathy. In these infections, blood cultures are usually positive early in the disease. Helminthic infections such as loiasis and onchocerciasis can also produce impressive local, inguinal lymphadenopathy.

EPSTEIN-BARR VIRUS: INFECTIOUS MONONUCLEOSIS

Pathogenesis

Infectious mononucleosis is caused by EBV, a DNA virus and a member of the human herpesvirus group. EBV infections occur worldwide and usually result in subclinical early childhood infections (87). Over 90% of American adults have demonstrable antibodies to EBV (88). The illness generally develops before age 30 years; in underdeveloped countries, it usually occurs by age 10 years. In contrast, only 30% to 40% of American children are infected with EBV by age 10 years (90).

EBV receptors have been detected on human B lymphocytes, complement receptor-positive non-B and non-T lymphocytes, and nasopharyngeal epithelial cells (89,90). The EBV receptor is the receptor for the third complement component, the C3d receptor (also known as *CD21*) (91). The major histocompatibility complex serves as a cofactor for the infection of B cells (92). Infection with EBV usually occurs by contact with oral secretions. The virus replicates in the cells of the oropharynx. The B cells are infected by contact with these cells or directly by B cells in the oropharynx (90). The virus interacts with the B cell in a number of defined steps. First, it attaches to the receptor; then, it gains entry into the susceptible B lymphocyte. Epstein-Barr nuclear antigens (EBNAs) appear within cell nuclei within 6 hours of infection and before virus-directed protein synthesis is detectable (93). Each of the EBNA proteins coded for by the EBV plays a different role in the growth and transformation of B cells (87,94). The EBNA up-regulates the expression of EBV latent membrane proteins. The latent membrane proteins are important controls of latent viral infection and may play a role in enabling the EBV to evade the host immune response (87). During the initial phase of primary EBV infection, up to 18% of peripheral B lymphocytes express one or more EBNA proteins (95).

In the normal host, EBV infection results in the proliferation of transformed B cells, which are contained by a vigorous immune response involving both the T- and B-cell network. The humoral response to EBV infections is characterized by both non–EBV-specific (heterophil antibody and autoantibodies) and EBV-specific antibodies, directed against EBV viral capsid antigen (VCA), early antigen, and EBNA. Although the antibodies directed against viral structural proteins and EBNAs are important for the diagnosis of a recent EBV infection, the cellular immune response is more important for the control of EBV disease. In the primary infection, NK cells and CD4+ and CD8+ cytotoxic T cells control EBV-infected B cells (96). The cytotoxic T cells generated during an acute infection are EBV specific: EBV activates B cells, resulting in their polyclonal stimulation (Fig. 20-2). This response elicits a corresponding T-cell response (97). After convalescence, EBV persists in resting memory B cells for the life of the individual.

The serologic response includes production of neutralizing antibodies to glycoproteins on the cell membranes of EBV-infected cells. EBV infection also produces antibodies to a num-

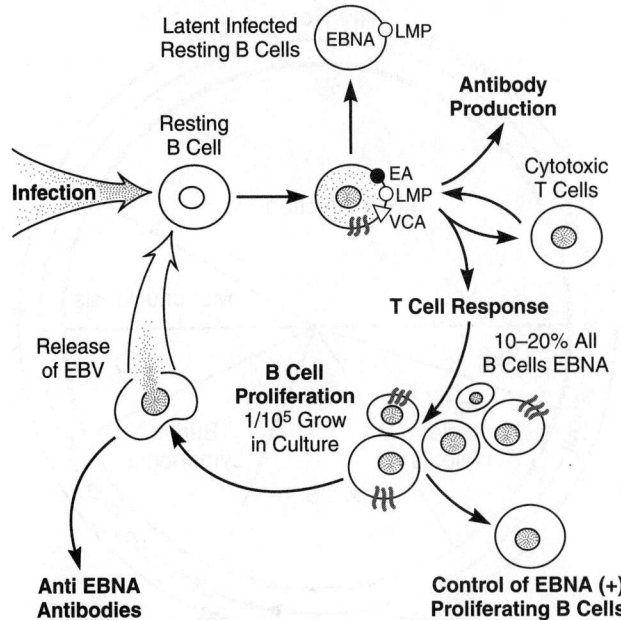

Figure 20-2. The cellular and humoral immune response in infectious mononucleosis. The Epstein-Barr virus (EBV) infects B cells and results in the synthesis of circulating antibodies directed against viral antigens as well as unrelated antigens. These later antigens are the heterophile antibodies. The responding T lymphocytes are cytotoxic to EBV-infected B cells and appear as atypical lymphocytes found in the peripheral blood. The T-cell response is important in the control of the EBV-infected B lymphocytes. Cytotoxic EBV-specific T cells lyse infected B cells. Latently infected B cells express latent membrane protein (LMP) and are long-lived infected cells. EA, early antigen; EBNA, Epstein-Barr nuclear antigen; VCA, viral capsid antigen.

ber of unrelated antigens found in sheep, horse, and beef RBCs (98). These heterophile antibodies, which are detected as sheep and horse RBC agglutinins and beef cell hemolysins, do not cross-react with specific antibodies against EBV antigens. They are IgM antibodies with no clear role in the pathogenesis of the infection, recovery, or control of the disease.

Clinical Features

Infection with EBV causes a broad spectrum of illness in humans (Fig. 20-3). EBV is associated with the development of African Burkitt lymphoma, nasopharyngeal carcinoma, and lymphoproliferative disease in immunosuppressed patients (Table 20-3) (99,100). The EBV genome has been demonstrated by DNA hybridization studies in biopsy specimens of African patients with Burkitt lymphoma and nasopharyngeal carcinoma. In addition, the virus can be recovered from biopsy specimens, and the EBNA is demonstrable in the nuclei of cells obtained from the involved nodes (101–103). The geographic restriction of Burkitt lymphoma in Africa suggests the role of associated genetic or environmental factors (malaria infection and possibly other viral infections) in the development of the disease (102). EBV does not appear to be associated with Burkitt lymphoma in Americans (103). In patients with Duncan syndrome, a rare familial X-linked recessive lymphoproliferative disorder, EBV infection is overwhelming and may result in agammaglobulinemia, B-cell lymphomas, or death during the acute phase (104,105). Primary EBV infection may also evolve into a fatal immunoblastic lymphoma (106,107). EBV is associated with lymphoproliferative disease in patients with congenital and acquired immunodeficiency (108–110). EBV-related lymphomas have been observed in patients

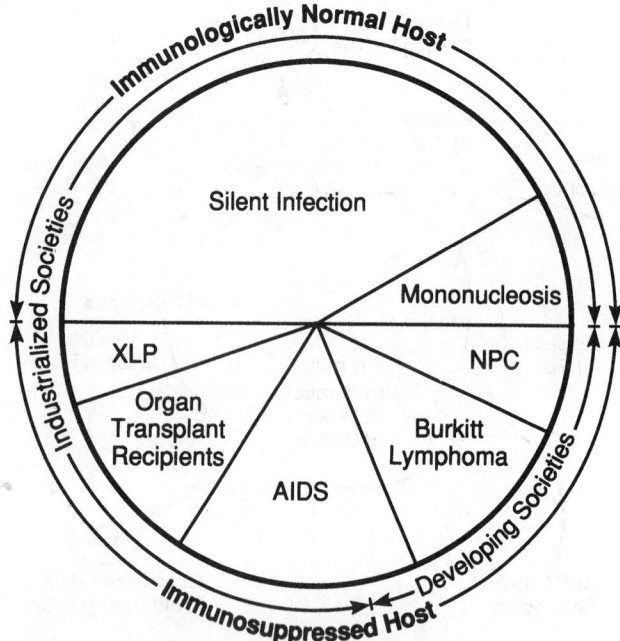

Figure 20-3. The spectrum of infections with Epstein-Barr virus. The immune status of the host determines the outcome of an Epstein-Barr virus infection. AIDS, acquired immunodeficiency syndrome; NPC, nasopharyngeal carcinoma; XLP, X-linked lymphoproliferative disorder.

after renal, cardiac, and bone marrow transplants. The lymph nodes from EBV lymphoproliferative disease show plasmacytic hyperplasia, B-cell hyperplasia, B-cell lymphoma, or immunoblastic lymphoma. The disorders may be monoclonal, oligoclonal, or polyclonal. The polyclonal lesions have the best prognosis (87). None of the lymphoproliferative diseases has the characteristic 8;14 translocation of Burkitt lymphoma. The diagnosis of EBV lymphoproliferative disease requires the demonstration of EBV DNA or RNA in tissue biopsy. Patients on prolonged immunosuppression, particularly with cyclosporine (Cyclosporin-A) after solid organ transplant, and recipients of a T-cell–depleted or HLA-mismatched bone marrow transplant are at risk for EBV-

---

TABLE 20-3. Epstein-Barr Virus (EBV)–Associated Disorders

Clinical syndromes
  Infectious mononucleosis
  Chronic active EBV infection
  Fatal EBV infection in X-linked lymphoproliferative disease
  Oral hairy leukoplakia in HIV infection
  Lymphoid interstitial pneumonitis
  Angioimmunoblastic lymphadenopathy[a]
Malignancies
  Nasopharyngeal carcinomas
  Burkitt lymphoma
  EBV-associated lymphoproliferative disease
  Hodgkin's lymphoma[a]
  Non-Hodgkin's lymphoma
  Leiomyosarcoma in HIV infection[a]
  Nasal T-cell/natural killer cell lymphoma[a]
  Lymphomatoid granulomatosis[a]
  Central nervous lymphoma in nonimmunosuppressed patients[a]
  Peripheral T-cell lymphomas[a]
  Gastric carcinoma[a]
  Smooth muscle tumors[a]

HIV, human immunodeficiency virus.
[a]EBV viral DNA or proteins have been found in these disorders, but etiologic role of EBV is unclear.

associated lymphoproliferative disease/lymphoma (110). EBV DNA has been detected in some patients with Hodgkin's lymphoma (111). In addition, seroepidemiologic studies have suggested a possible relationship between Hodgkin's lymphoma and EBV infection (112). These studies demonstrated that the titers to EBV antigens were elevated both at the time of diagnosis of Hodgkin's lymphoma and several years before the diagnosis. However, the etiologic relationship between the EBV virus and Hodgkin's lymphoma remains controversial. EBV infection may also have a role in other cancers. EBV DNA or proteins have been detected in nasal T-cell lymphoma/NK cell lymphoma, smooth muscle tumors, gastric carcinomas, and central nervous lymphomas in nonimmunocompromised patients (87,99,106,113).

The patient's age affects the clinical course of EBV infection. In children younger than 5 years of age, the primary EBV infection is usually asymptomatic or associated with mild, nonspecific symptoms such as a rash or mild pharyngitis. In most children, the disease is self-limited and lasts 2 or 3 weeks. Adolescents and adults usually develop acute infectious mononucleosis. The clinical manifestations of mononucleosis are summarized in Table 20-3. Malaise, fatigue, fever, headache, diffuse myalgias, a feeling of abdominal fullness, and anorexia are common symptoms during the acute illness (99). The most common complaint is the sudden onset of a severe sore throat with accompanying dysphagia. The pharynx is typically erythematous with a thick white exudate and develops during the first week and lasts for 7 to 10 days. Palatal petechiae are also common but are not diagnostic of infectious mononucleosis and can be seen in other viral illnesses. Tonsillar enlargement is prominent and, in some patients, may become severe enough to interfere with deglutition or cause respiratory obstruction (114).

Fever is present early in the course in over 90% of patients with infectious mononucleosis. Cervical lymphadenopathy, present in 80% to 90% of patients, is symmetric and most frequently involves the posterior and anterior cervical chain. Moderate splenomegaly occurs in most cases and is most prominent 10 to 14 days after the pharyngitis. Hepatomegaly is noted in 10% to 20% of cases, and jaundice is noted in 5% to 10%, which usually peaks in the second week of the illness. Mild to moderate hepatic dysfunction is common, but occasionally patients develop marked hyperbilirubinemia (115). Liver biopsies have revealed infiltration of the sinusoids with atypical lymphocytes. A macular papular rash is noted in approximately 5% of all infected patients. A pruritic macular papular rash, however, develops in 90% to 100% of patients who take ampicillin during the acute illness (116).

The complications of infectious mononucleosis are outlined in Table 20-4. Hemolytic anemia and thrombocytopenia are the most common hematologic complications and occur in 0.5% to 5.0% of patients. Hemolytic anemia, usually mild, occurs in approximately 3% of cases (117,118). In 70% of cases, the Coombs' test is positive, but a severe hemolytic anemia is rare (119). Seventy percent to 90% of patients develop a cold agglutinin, usually IgM and rarely of the IgG class, that is specific for the RBC antigen i (small i) (120). The development of hemolysis from the cold agglutinin is related to the thermal amplitude of the antibody or other associated antibodies (118). Thrombocytopenia is a frequent complication, more common in children than adults, but is rarely sufficient to produce bleeding (121,122). Usually occurring during the first 2 weeks of the illness, thrombocytopenia may be related to the development of antiplatelet antibodies. Mild neutropenia is frequently found during the first weeks of infection (123). Antineutrophil antibodies are common manifestations of the polyclonal B-cell activation induced by EBV.

Aplastic anemia can occur in association with EBV infections, possibly caused by the direct viral infection of bone mar-

TABLE 20-4. Complications of Infectious Mononucleosis

Hematologic (0.5%–5.0%)
  Autoimmune hemolytic anemia
  Thrombocytopenia
  Neutropenia
  Aplastic anemia
  Splenic rupture (<1%)
Cardiac (1%–6%)
  Pericarditis
  Myocarditis
  Bradycardia
  Electrocardiogram abnormalities
Nervous system (0.5%–2.0%)
  Encephalitis
  Meningitis
  Guillain-Barré syndrome
  Optic neuritis
  Cranial nerve palsies
  Myelitis—psychiatric disorders
Pulmonary (1%–5%)
  Cough
  Interstitial infiltrate
  Adult respiratory distress syndrome
  Pleural effusions

row progenitor cells or the effect of circulating T cells that suppress hematopoietic progenitor cells (124,125). DNA hybridization studies have revealed EBV DNA and proteins in the bone marrow of patients with aplastic anemia who have no recent history of infectious mononucleosis (124).

Rapid enlargement of the spleen that may occur during the course of infectious mononucleosis leaves it vulnerable to rupture. This rare but potentially fatal complication generally occurs during the second and third weeks of the illness. Splenic rupture may occur spontaneously or with minimal trauma to the left upper quadrant (126). Abdominal pain is infrequent in patients with infectious mononucleosis. Therefore, the presence of abdominal or left shoulder pain may signal a potential splenic rupture. The onset of such pain may be insidious or abrupt and signs of peritoneal irritation, such as rebound tenderness or shifting dullness from intraabdominal bleeding, may dominate the clinical picture. Laboratory findings include the sudden onset of anemia without evidence of hemolysis, which is frequently associated with neutrophilia (125). Neutrophilia is infrequent in uncomplicated mononucleosis, and its presence may be an early signal of impending splenic rupture. The abdominal CT scan is the study of choice to confirm a suspected ruptured spleen (126). The treatment of a ruptured spleen is the surgical removal of the spleen. Patients should be warned of the potential for this complication and instructed to avoid strenuous exercise for at least 1 month and contact sports for at least 3 months after onset of the illness (127).

Neurologic complications of infectious mononucleosis occur in less than 1% of all patients but may be the first or only manifestation of the illness (128). The clinical picture may be atypical with minimal lymphadenopathy, a negative Monospot test, and rare circulating atypical lymphocytes (129,130). Encephalitis is the most common neurologic complication (130). Aseptic meningitis from EBV infection may be acute in onset and rapidly progressive. Spinal fluid analysis reveals a mononuclear pleocytosis with a normal to mildly elevated protein and a normal glucose. The cerebrospinal fluid may have low titers of EBV VCA (130). Other neurologic complications include Guillain-Barré syndrome (130), optic neuritis (131), cranial nerve palsies, and transverse myelitis (131).

Hepatic involvement is usually manifest as a self-limited elevation of hepatocellular enzymes in most patients (132). Rare

cases of severe, fatal hepatitis have occurred during the course of infectious mononucleosis (133). Cardiac involvement is rare and represents as nonspecific anterior chest pain, arrhythmias, electrocardiogram abnormalities, pericarditis, and myocarditis (134).

Laboratory Features

The laboratory abnormalities in infectious mononucleosis occur in response to virally infected B cells, polyclonal B-cell proliferation, and specific antibodies to EBV. The infection produces a prominent lymphocytosis with circulating atypical lymphocytes. The atypical lymphocytes are activated T cells and have round or irregular nuclei with prominent clumped chromatin. The cytoplasm is intensely basophilic with numerous vacuoles. The atypical cells may be confused with lymphoblasts. The monocyte counts may rise transiently, but the term *mononucleosis* refers to the rise in the number of lymphocytes, not monocytes. These cytologic alterations are not pathognomonic of infectious mononucleosis and are noted in a number of viral illnesses, including CMV infections, acute hepatitis A and B, and varicella.

The heterophile antibody, a sheep erythrocyte agglutinin, is present in the sera at some time during the course of infectious mononucleosis in 90% of patients. The presence of this antibody is not specific for infectious mononucleosis. In patients with infectious mononucleosis, the heterophile antibodies are absorbed by bovine red cells and not by other antigens such as those found in guinea pig kidneys (Table 20-5). This provides the basis for the sensitive Monospot test. Test serum is mixed with a suspension of finely ground guinea pig kidney on one part of the slide and a suspension of bovine erythrocyte stroma on the other. Horse erythrocytes, more sensitive than the originally described sheep RBCs, are added to each spot and mixed. The sera from a patient with infectious mononucleosis agglutinates with the horse erythrocytes in the serum absorbed with guinea pig kidney but not in the serum absorbed with bovine erythrocyte stroma.

Newer Monospot tests use a suspension of latex particles that are coated with highly purified bovine RBC membranes. The RBC membrane antigens are highly specific for infectious mononucleosis heterophile antibodies and differential absorption is, therefore, not necessary. A positive test in either serum or plasma result is agglutination of the latex suspension (135).

False-negative tests occur mainly in young children who produce limited amounts of the IgM heterophile antibody. In these patients, the diagnosis requires the assay of specific antibodies to the EBV. False-positive Monospot tests have been noted rarely in patients with lymphomas and non-EBV–related acute hepatitis (135).

Several virus-specific antibodies produced by the host in response to EBV infection appear at different times during the

TABLE 20-5. Heterophile Antibodies

Source of Serum	Unabsorbed[a]	After Absorption[a] Beef Red Blood Cells	Guinea Pig Kidney
Infectious mononucleosis[b]	++++	0	+++
Serum sickness	+++	0	0
Normal serum (Forssman)	+	+	0

+, 1–25%; +++, 50–75%; ++++, 75–100%.
[a]Sheep RBC agglutination.
[b]Sixty percent positive during first 2 weeks of Epstein-Barr virus infection; 80% to 90% positive by 1 month; usually negative after 3 to 6 months.

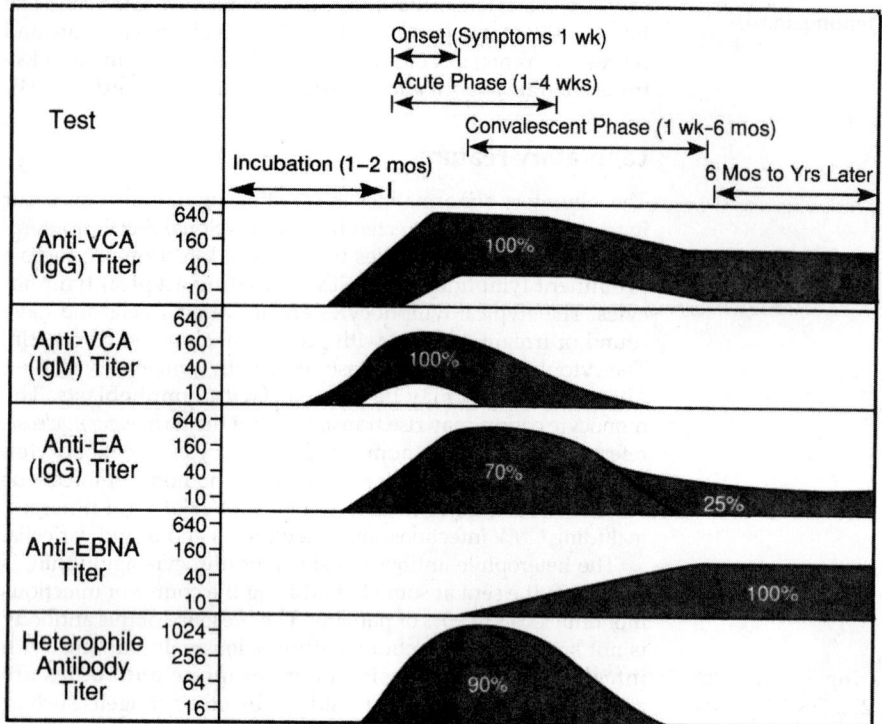

Figure 20-4. Antibody response to Epstein-Barr virus (EBV) infection. Antibodies to the viral capsid antigen (VCA) are measured by immunofluorescence and rise early in the course of the illness. Immunoglobulin (Ig) G antibodies to the VCA are present in 100% of patients exposed to EBV. The highest titers are found at the onset of clinical illness. The IgG VCA antibody is present for life after an EBV infection. The IgM anti-VCA antibodies are sensitive and specific for a recent EBV infection. They are found in almost all individuals and occur at the onset of infection. Titers usually fall within 4 weeks after the onset of infection, and most individuals have negative titers at 4 months. The presence of anti-VCA IgM titer is virtually diagnostic in an acute EBV infection. Anti–early antigen (anti-EA) antibodies persist for 3 to 6 months and correlate in part with the severity of the disease. Anti–Epstein-Barr nuclear antigen (anti-EBNA) is found in all patients, appearing late in the course of clinical infection. The peak titer occurs 2 to 4 weeks after the onset of clinical symptoms. EBNA persists for years and may be helpful in the diagnosis of heterophile-negative cases. (Adapted from Henle W, Henle GE, Horwitz CA. Epstein-Barr virus-specific diagnostic tests in infectious mononucleosis. *Hum Pathol* 1974;5:551.)

course of the illness (Fig. 20-4). Because over 90% of cases are heterophile positive and have a positive Monospot test, determination of these antibodies is rarely necessary for diagnosis. In the atypical or heterophile-negative case, however, determination of EBV-specific antibodies is necessary for the diagnosis of infectious mononucleosis (136). Antibodies to VCA occur early in the course of infectious mononucleosis in all patients. Those who are acutely ill already have IgG antibodies to VCA when they present for evaluation. The IgG anti-VCA persists for life and, therefore, is not helpful in establishing a diagnosis of an acute or ongoing infection. The IgM anti-VCA antibody is highly sensitive and specific for a recent EBV infection. The IgM anti-VCA falls rapidly after the first 4 to 8 weeks.

Serum antibodies to specific early antigens are demonstrable in the first month of infection. The early antigen antibodies persist for only a few years. Specific antibodies to EBNA develop after the acute phase of the illness, usually after 4 weeks, and persist for life. A recent primary EBV infection is indicated by the presence of VCA-specific IgM antibodies, high titers of VCA-specific IgG antibodies (>1:320), detection of anti–early antigen antibodies, and the absence of anti-EBNA by the immunofluorescent antibody test. The presence of anti-EBNA antibodies should not be used to make a diagnosis of chronic EBV infection because normal individuals may have high titers for years after an uncomplicated infection.

EBV may be cultured from oropharyngeal washings or cultured peripheral blood B lymphocytes in most patients with infectious mononucleosis (137). Many normal persons without an acute infection may also shed the virus, and therefore, culturing the virus is of questionable clinical use.

In most cases, the diagnosis of infectious mononucleosis is clear from the clinical manifestations, appropriate setting, circulating atypical lymphocytes, and positive heterophile Monospot test. The diagnosis becomes difficult when clinical manifestations are atypical, blunted, or severe and when they occur in heterophile-negative infections. CMV infection is the most common cause of heterophile-negative infectious mononucleosis. CMV can produce an illness that is similar clinically

to EBV infection. CMV infection, however, usually presents with less pharyngitis and lymphadenopathy and rarely induces anti–i-specific cryoglobulins (138). Toxoplasmosis may also mimic many of the features of infectious mononucleosis. In addition, many other viral illnesses may present with features of infectious mononucleosis, including hepatitis A and B, coxsackievirus, and HIV infections.

Treatment

Infection with EBV causes a variety of clinical manifestations that are partly dependent on the immune response elicited in the infected host. Most patients who develop infectious mononucleosis require no specific therapy, and the symptoms resolve spontaneously over a 2- to 3-week period. The sore throat is usually maximal for 3 to 5 days early in the course, and then it gradually resolves within 1 week to 10 days and responds to supportive therapy and mild analgesics. The patient should avoid all sports or strenuous activity because of the risk of splenic rupture. Some patients may experience severe tonsillar enlargement, which can result in airway obstruction.

Corticosteroids are effective for the treatment of impending airway obstruction (139). Prednisone or an equivalent steroid preparation, 40 to 80 mg/day in divided doses tapering over 7 to 10 days, can have a dramatic effect on tonsillar enlargement and pharyngitis. Corticosteroids do not appear to change the pattern of the lymphocyte response during the early phase of the illness or to alter the serologic response to EBV (140). Corticosteroids are generally only administered to patients who have had one of the complications associated with an acute EBV infection such as severe thrombocytopenia, hemolytic anemia, neurologic complications, myocarditis, and pericarditis (141).

Treatment with acyclovir does not affect the clinical course, duration of symptoms, or laboratory parameters but may decrease oropharyngeal viral shedding early in the course in patients with infectious mononucleosis (142,143). Antibiotics have no effect on the course of EBV infection. Approximately 20% of patients during an acute infection have a concurrent β-hemolytic streptococcal pharyngitis and should, therefore, receive appropriate antibiotics. Almost all patients develop a rash if ampicillin is administered, but other penicillins or erythromycin can be safely administered.

The treatment of EBV-associated disorders remains controversial. The aggressive and potentially fatal infectious mononucleosis that occurs in patients with the X-linked lymphoproliferative syndrome generally does not respond to acyclovir (144). The EBV-associated lymphoproliferative disease in immunocompromised hosts may respond to a reduction in the dose of immunosuppressive medication. Some patients have had a complete resolution of lesions after the reduction of their immunosuppressive drugs (145,146). Surgical removal or irradiation of localized lymphoproliferative lesions, especially in the gastrointestinal tract, has been effective in selected patients (87). The use of acyclovir, although widely administered, is generally not effective. Monoclonal antibody therapy has been used with encouraging results. The use of rituximab, a monoclonal antibody directed against the CD20 B-cell antigen, has resulted in complete and durable remissions in some patients (106,147). EBV-specific cytotoxic T cells have been administered to selected patients with posttransplant lymphoproliferative disease with encouraging results (148). In high-risk patients for EBV infection after a T-cell–depleted bone marrow transplant, EBV-specific cytotoxic T cells have been used to prevent EBV-associated lymphoproliferative disease (149).

The chronic mononucleosis syndrome is a poorly defined clinical entity. The disorder is linked to EBV because its symptoms are similar to the prodrome of infectious mononucleosis. It is marked by prolonged fever and malaise in young and middle-aged adults (150,151). Other prominent symptoms are difficulty in concentrating, arthralgias, myalgias, recurrent sore throat, and fluctuating lymphadenopathy. At this point, no one etiologic agent has been identified for the chronic mononucleosis syndrome. Possible infectious agents are CMV, HIV, influenza A, coxsackievirus, and *Borrelia burgdorferi*. Many studies of chronic mononucleosis and chronic fatigue syndrome are frustrated by a lack of objective findings. At this time, it is unlikely that EBV infection is the source of this disorder in most patients (151).

CYTOMEGALOVIRUS

Pathogenesis and Clinical Features

CMV is a member of the herpes group and produces a clinical syndrome similar to EBV. CMV presents many unique problems for immunocompromised hosts, including bone marrow and organ transplant patients, immature neonates, and persons with acquired immunodeficiency syndrome.

The epidemiology of CMV infections is like that of other herpesviruses. The infection is widespread and usually inapparent. In the United States, approximately 40% of adults have antibodies to CMV. In underdeveloped countries, the percent of individuals exposed to CMV is significantly higher than in the United States and Europe (152). In third world countries, 30% to 50% of children acquire the infection in the perinatal period.

CMV can be transmitted through the contaminated uterine cervix during birth as well as through human milk (153). Transmission is also common from exposure in nurseries and day care centers (154). Infected children generally carry the virus for long periods in the respiratory tract and urine (155). Another significant source of CMV transmission is through blood products. The risk of infection is proportional to the number of units received, with estimates varying from 1% to 12% per unit (156–158). The overall risk of acquiring a CMV infection is two sero-

conversions per 100 units of RBCs transfused (158). The risk of CMV transmission is decreased by using cryopreserved blood, leukocyte-poor blood, or blood from seronegative donors (158). Many blood products are now being tested for CMV, and CMV-negative blood products are available for selected patients. Special care must be taken when blood products are used with seronegative neonates because they are at high risk for primary fatal CMV infection.

CMV is also transmitted sexually. The incidence of asymptomatic CMV virus in the cervix ranges from 1% to 35% in different populations (159). CMV has also been found in high titers in the semen of both heterosexual and homosexual men (160). Liver, heart, and bone marrow transplant patients are at high risk for severe, fatal CMV infection (161). The clinical manifestations of the reactivation of CMV infections include CMV hepatitis, pneumonitis, and colitis (161,162). Congenital CMV infections can produce jaundice, hepatosplenomegaly, multiple system organ failures, macrocephaly, chorioretinitis, and cerebral calcification (163).

CMV infection in most adults presents with fever, malaise, and splenomegaly. CMV infection may be more prolonged than an EBV infection, with fevers persisting for 1 to 2 months.

CMV also has many of the laboratory features of EBV infections. Lymphocytosis is prominent, with an elevated total lymphocyte count and many circulating atypical lymphocytes. Immunologic abnormalities are uncommon in CMV-associated infections. Hepatitis is more common in patients with CMV. As with other herpesviruses, CMV can be cultured from urine, semen, white blood cells, and other infected tissues, but this does not necessarily reflect an acute infection. The antibodies to the different CMV antigens are less well defined than are those to EBV.

Therapy

Most patients with CMV infection recover without therapy. Treating immunocompromised patients with CMV infections presents a number of special problems. Ganciclovir treatment for patients with CMV retinitis is encouraging, although responses with other serious CMV infections have been variable (164–166). Ganciclovir, either alone or in combination with high-dose intravenous immunoglobulin has been effective in selected immunosuppressed bone marrow transplant patients with CMV pneumonitis (167). The use of sensitive tests to detect the presence of CMV has made preemptive therapy possible in high-risk patients. The purpose of monitoring is to restrict the exposure of ganciclovir to patients at highest risk for developing CMV disease. The currently available CMV assays include shell vial culture, CMV antigenemia assay, polymerase chain reaction for CMV DNA, and detection of CMV RNA by nucleic acid sequence–based amplification (166,169,170).

The pathogenesis of CMV-associated disease in marrow and stem cell transplant recipients is defined by the exposure or reactivation of CMV, the presence of graft-versus-host disease, and the absence of T-cell immunity against CMV. The adoptive transfer of CMV-specific CD8+ cytotoxic T lymphocytes may protect high-risk patients from CMV disease (171–173).

ATYPICAL LYMPHOPROLIFERATIVE DISEASE

Atypical lymphoproliferative diseases are a heterogeneous group of disorders characterized by atypical lymph node hyperplasia. These disorders demonstrate an abnormal lymph node histologic pattern but do not meet the criteria for a malignancy. The etiology is not known and the clinical course is variable in these uncommon disorders. The atypical lymphoproliferative diseases include autoimmune lymphoproliferative syndrome, angioimmunoblastic lymphadenopathy with dysproteinemia, Castleman's disease, and Kikuchi's disease.

Autoimmune lymphoproliferative syndrome is a rare disorder characterized by generalized lymphadenopathy, hepatosplenomegaly, hypergammaglobulinemia, B-cell lymphocytosis, and autoimmune disorders (174,175). The autoimmune manifestations include Guillain-Barré syndrome, urticarial rash, glomerulonephritis, and immune thrombocytopenia. The majority of cases occur in young children under the age of 2 years. The enlarged lymph nodes generally reveal follicular hyperplasia and an expansion of double-negative T cells, CD4⁻, and CD8⁻ in the paracortical regions. There is also a diffuse infiltrate composed of plasma cells, small lymphocytes, and immunoblasts. The lymph node findings may resemble those of patients with a posttransplant lymphoproliferative disease (174). The disorder appears to be due to an impairment of apoptosis due to a inherited heterozygous mutation in the *fas* gene (174,176). The natural history is very variable with some patients progressing to T-cell rich, B-cell lymphomas or lymphocyte-predominant Hodgkin's lymphoma, whereas in others the disease has resolved spontaneously (177).

Angioimmunoblastic lymphadenopathy with dysproteinemia is an acute systemic illness characterized by generalized lymphadenopathy, hepatosplenomegaly, polyclonal hypergammaglobulinemia, skin rashes, and fevers (178). Many cases present with a polyclonal hypergammaglobulinemia and Coombs'-positive hemolytic anemia. The disease often begins after viral infection. Histologically, angioimmunoblastic lymphadenopathy with dysproteinemia is characterized by obliteration of the lymph node architecture; loss of germinal centers; marked proliferation of small, mature-appearing lymphocytes; plasma cells and immunoblasts (transformed lymphoid cells of medium and large sizes). Eosinophils are prominent, and there is an amorphous intercellular material that is PAS-positive and dispersed throughout the node. Many cases have clonal T-cell rearrangements and are variants of a peripheral T-cell lymphoma (180). A majority of patients die from infectious complications or progress to a T-cell lymphoma. The treatment remains controversial and disappointing for most patients (180,181).

Castleman's disease has many synonyms, including lymph nodal hamartoma, angiofollicular mediastinal lymph node hyperplasia, giant lymph node hyperplasia, and lymph node hyperplasia of Castleman (183). The clinical manifestations vary from a localized solitary mass to a systemic disorder with generalized adenopathy. Fevers, autoimmune phenomena, and recurring infections generally occur with the multicentric form. The course is very variable from an indolent disorder to one that is rapidly fatal. Patients can present with a solitary lesion consisting of a round mass, most frequently in the mediastinum ranging in size from 1.5 to 16.0 cm (184). The multicentric form presents with multiple areas of lymph node enlargement and prominent splenomegaly and hepatomegaly (185). A majority of the patients with the multicenter form are older men, with a median age of 57 years. Approximately one-third of patients develop a malignant lymphoma during the course of their disease. Patients are typically anemic with hypoalbuminemia and polyclonal hypergammaglobulinemia. Proteinuria and renal insufficiency are occasionally seen. Histologically, Castleman's disease is divided into the hyaline-vascular and plasma cell subtypes. A majority of the cases are of the hyaline-vascular type, which is characterized by abnormal nodal follicles and interfollicular vascularity. The follicles contain small blood vessels that have thickened, hyalinized walls giving rise to diffuse hyalin staining within the follicles. Other follicles are characterized by the concentric layering of cells around the germinal cen-

ter. The node has an "onion skin" pattern, which includes the shrunken germinal centers with concentrically arranged lymphocytes in the expanded surrounding mantle zone (184).

The vascularity is increased in the intrafollicular regions with plasma cells, immunoblasts, and eosinophils. The appearance of the hyaline-vascular germinal center is not specific for Castleman's disease and is seen in the lymph nodes of patients with acquired immunodeficiency syndrome and angioimmunoblastic lymphadenopathy (186,187). The rare plasma cell variant is characterized by a solid sheet of plasma cells in the intrafollicular area. The follicles are hyperplastic and with many mitotic figures and tingible body macrophages. The lymphocytes are generally polyclonal (188).

The etiology of Castleman's disease is unknown. In some cases, the cytokine interleukin-6 appears to be involved in the progression of Castleman's disease (189,190). Treatment with anti–interleukin-6 receptor antibody has been reported to ameliorate some of the systemic symptoms of the disease. The treatment is controversial. Patients with localized Castleman's disease can be treated with surgical removal of the solitary mass or local radiotherapy (193). In patients with multicenter disease, corticosteroids are sometimes successful in controlling symptoms. The use of combination chemotherapy regimens utilized for lymphoma is associated with an increased risk of infectious complications and a poor overall response.

Kikuchi-Fujimoto disease is a self-limited disorder characterized by prominent cervical adenopathy (194). The disorder generally affects young women who present with fevers and localized adenopathy. The etiology is unknown, and in most patients the symptoms and adenopathy resolve spontaneously within 4 months. Histologically, Kikuchi-Fujimoto disease can be confused with a malignant lymphoma. The lymph node demonstrates areas of necrosis without a neutrophilic infiltrate. The necrotic area contains karyorrhectic debris, which contains immunoblasts, histiocytes, and plasmacytoid monocytes. In some patients, the necrosis is absent, and therefore, differentiating this benign, self-limited disorder from a localized lymphoma can be difficult (195).

Inflammatory pseudotumor of lymph nodes is a rare benign disorder, which mimics many of the features of a malignant lymphoma (196). The disorder may be localized or involve multiple lymph nodes. Patients present with fevers, splenomegaly, and tender adenopathy. Histologically, there is a proliferation of spindle cells expanding the connective tissue framework of the lymph node associated with a plasma cell and a small lymphocyte infiltrate. There are variable numbers of macrophages, neutrophils, and eosinophils, and there is fibrosis. Immunoblasts and histiocytes may be noted in the lymphocyte infiltrate, and the finding in the lymph node can be confused with the pattern of Hodgkin's lymphoma.

REFERENCES

1. Joffey JM, Courtice FC. *Lymphocytes, lymph and the lymphomyeloid complex.* London: Academic Press, 1970:942.
2. Hewson W. Part the Third, containing a description of the red particles of the blood in the human subject and other animals, with an account of the structure and offices of the lymphatic gland, of the thymus gland, and of the spleen. In: Falconar M, ed. *Experimental inquiries.* London: T Longman, 1777:133.
3. Gulliver G, ed. *The works of William Hewson FRS.* London: Sydenham Society, 1848:360.
4. Virchow R. *Die Leukämie, in Gesammelte Abhandlungen zur wissenschaftlichen Medizin.* Frankfurt: Meidinger, 1956:190.
5. Ranvier LA. *Triate technique d'histologie.* Paris: Librairie F Savy, 1875.
6. Fleming W. *Studien über Regeneration der Gewebe. I. Die Zellvermebrung in den lymphdrusen und verwandten Organen, und ihr Einflus auf Deren Bau.* Bonn: Max Cohen & Sohn, 1885:66.
7. Malphighi M. Chapter IV. *De Viscerum structura exercitatio anatomica.* Bonn: De Liene, 1666:101.

8. Billroth T. Neue Beitragezur vergleichenden Histologie der Milz. *Arch Anat Physiol* 1857;24:88.

9. Gray H. *On the structure and use of the spleen.* London: John W Parker, 1854:380.

10. May MT. *Galen: on the usefulness of the parts of the body.* Ithaca, NY: Cornell University Press, 1968:232.

11. Rosner F. The spleen in the Talmud and other early Jewish writing. *Bull Hist Med* 1972;40:82.

12. Crosby WH. The spleen. In: Wintrube MM, ed. *Blood pure and eloquent.* New York: McGraw-Hill, 1980.

13. Muller J. Uber die Strucktur der eigenthumlichen Korperchen in der Milz einiger planzefresser: Saugetiere. *Arch Anat Physiol* 1834;1:80.

14. MacDonald RH, Moretta L. The definition of lymphocyte subpopulations: new approaches to an old problem. *Semin Oncol* 1984;21:223.

15. Lennert K, Stein HH. The germinal center: morphology, histochemistry, and immunohistology. In: Goos M, Christophe E, eds. *Lymphoproliferative diseases of the skin.* Berlin: Springer-Verlag, 1982:3.

16. Mann RB, Jaffe ES, Berard CW. Malignant lymphomas: a conceptual understanding of morphological diversity. *Am J Pathol* 1979;94:105.

17. Jennings CD, Foon KA. Recent advances in flow cytometry: application to the diagnosis of hematologic malignancy. *Blood* 1997;90:2863.

18. Mackay I, Rosen F. The immune system. *N Engl J Med* 2000;343:37.

19. Hsu S, Cossman J, Jaffe ES. Lymphocyte subsets in normal human lymphoid tissues. *Am J Clin Pathol* 1983;80:21.

20. Aisenberg AC. Current concepts in immunology: cell-surfaced markers in lymphoproliferative disease. *N Engl J Med* 1981;304:331.

21. Bell D, Young JW, Banchereau J. Dendritic cells. *Adv Immunol* 1999;72:255.

22. Butler JJ. Pathology of the spleen in benign and malignant conditions. *Histopathology* 1983;7:453.

23. Stein H, Gerdes J, Mason DY. The normal and malignant germinal centre. *Clin Haematol* 1982;11:531.

24. Wilkinson L, Tang A, Gjedrteda A. Marked lymphocytosis suggesting chronic lymphocytic leukemia in three patients with hyposplenism. *Am J Med* 1983;75:1053.

25. Bleesing JJ, Fleisher TA. Immunophenotyping. *Semin Hematol* 2001;38:100.

26. Crotty PL, Smith BR, Tallini G. Morphologic, immunophenotypic and molecular evaluation of bone marrow involvement in non-Hodgkin's lymphoma. *Diagn Mol Pathol* 1998;7:90.

27. Stetler-Stevenson M, Braylan RC. Flow cytometric analysis of lymphomas and lymphoproliferative disorders. *Semin Hematol* 2001;38:111.

28. Tefferi A, Phyliky R. Role of immunotyping in chronic lymphocytosis: review of the natural history of the condition in 145 adult patients. *Mayo Clin Proc* 1988;63:801.

29. Falcao RP. Human blood lymphocyte subpopulations from birth to eight years. *Clin Exp Immunol* 1980;39:203.

30. Weksler ME. Senescence of the immune system. *Med Clin North Am* 1983;67:263.

31. Ginaldi L, De Martinis M, Modesti M, et al. Immunophenotypical changes of T lymphocytes in the elderly. *Gerontology* 2000;46:242.

32. Ginaldi L, De Martinis M, Modesti M, et al. Changes in the expression of surface receptors on lymphocyte subsets in the elderly: quantitative flow cytometric analysis. *Am J Hematol* 2001;67:63.

33. Kelly CS, Kelly RE Jr. Lymphadenopathy in children. *Pediatr Clin North Am* 1998;45:875.

34. Vassilokopoulos TP, Pangalis GA. Application of a prediction rule to select which patients presenting with lymphadenopathy should undergo a lymph node biopsy. *Medicine* 2000;79:338.

35. Lee Y, Terry R, Lukes RJ. Lymph node biopsy for diagnosis: a statistical study. *J Surg Oncol* 1980;14:53.

36. Dajani AS, Garcia RE, Wolinski E. Etiology of cervical lymphadenitis in children. *N Engl J Med* 1963;268:1329.

37. Haberman J, Steensma DP. Lymphadenopathy. *Mayo Clin Proc* 2000;75:723.

38. Sap GB, Brooks JSJ, Schwartz J. When to perform biopsies of enlarged peripheral lymph nodes in young patients. *JAMA* 1984;252:1321.

39. Heitman B, Irizarry A. Infectious disease causes of lymphadenopathy: localized versus diffuse. *Lippincotts Prim Care Pract* 1999;3:19.

40. Selby CD, Marcus HS. Enlarged epitrochlear lymph nodes: an old physical sign revisited. *J R Coll Physicians Lond* 1992;26:159.

41. Connelly JH, Osborne BM, Butler JJ. Lymphoreticular disease masquerading as or associated with inguinal or femoral hernia. *Surg Gynecol Obstet* 1990;170:309.

42. Morgenstern L. The Virchow-Troisler node: a historical note. *Am J Surg* 1979;138:703.

43. Glazer GM, Gross BH, Quint LE, et al. Normal mediastinal lymph nodes: numbers and size according to American Thoracic Society mapping. *AJR Am J Roentgenol* 1985;144:261.

44. Dorfman RE, Alpern MD, Gross BH, et al. Upper abdominal lymph nodes: criteria for normal size determined with CT. *Radiology* 1991;180:319.

45. Raoult D, Fournier P, Fenollar F, et al. Rickettsia Africae, a tick-borne pathogen in travelers to sub-Saharan Africa. *N Engl J Med* 2001;344:1504.

46. Drusin LM, Singer C, Valtni AJ, et al. Infectious syphilis mimicking neoplastic disease. *Arch Intern Med* 1977;137:156.

47. Epstein JI, Ambinder RF, Kuhajda FP, et al. Localized herpes simplex lymphadenitis. *Am J Clin Pathol* 1986;86:444.

48. Metroka CE, Cunningham-Rundles S, Pollack MS, et al. Generalized lymphadenopathy in homosexual men. *Ann Intern Med* 1983;99:585.

49. Houn HY, Pappas AA, Walker EM Jr. Lymph node pathology of acquired immunodeficiency syndrome (AIDS). *Ann Clin Lab Sci* 1990;20:337.

50. Weisenburger DD. Immunoblastic lymphadenopathy associated with methyldopa therapy. *Cancer* 1978;42:2322.

51. Gams RA, Neal JA, Conrad FG. Hydantoin-induced pseudolymphoma. *Ann Intern Med* 1968;69:557.

52. Schlienger RG, Shear NH. Antiepileptic drug hypersensitivity syndrome. *Epilepsia* 1998;39[Suppl]:S3.

53. DeVriese AS, Philippe J, Van Renterghem DM, et al. Carbamazepine hypersensitivity syndrome: report of 4 cases and review of the literature. *Medicine* 1995;74:144.

54. Vittorio CC, Muglia JJ. Anticonvulsant hypersensitivity syndrome. *Arch Intern Med* 1995;155:2285.

55. Rothschild B, Marshall H. Lymphadenopathy and lymph node infarction in the course of gold therapy. *Am J Med* 1986;80:537.

56. Shapira Y, Weinberger A, Wysenbeek AJ. Lymphadenopathy in systemic lupus erythematosus: prevalence and relation to disease manifestations. *Clin Rheumatol* 1996;15:335.

57. Moutsopoulos HM, Chiesed TM, Mann DL, et al. Sjögren syndrome: current issues. *Ann Intern Med* 1980;92:212.

58. Kelly CA, Malcolm AJ, Griffiths I. Lymphadenopathy in rheumatic patients. *Ann Rheum Dis* 1987;46:224.

59. Greenfield S, Jordan C. The clinical investigation of lymphadenopathy in primary care practice. *JAMA* 1978;240:1388.

60. Knight PJ, Mulne AF, Vassy LE. When is lymph node biopsy indicated in children with enlarged peripheral nodes? *Pediatrics* 1982;69:391.

61. Prasoon D. Acid-fast bacilli in fine needle aspiration smears from tuberculous lymph nodes. Where to look for them. *Acta Cytol* 2000;44:297.

62. Saboorian MH, Ashfaq R. The use of needle aspiration biopsy in the evaluation of lymphadenopathy. *Semin Diagn Pathol* 2001;18:110.

63. Wiersema MJ, Vazques-Sequeriros E, Wiersema LM. Evaluation of mediastinal lymphadenopathy with endoscopic US-guided fine needle biopsy aspiration biopsy. *Radiology* 2001;219:252.

64. Ponder TB, Smith D, Ramzy I. Lymphadenopathy in children and adolescents: role of fine needle aspiration in management. *Cancer Detect Prev* 2000;24:228.

65. Pappa VI, Hussain HK, Reznek RH, et al. Role of image-guided biopsy in the management of patients with lymphoma. *J Clin Oncol* 1996;14:2427.

66. Knowles DM. Immunophenotypic and immunogenotypic approaches useful in distinguishing benign and malignant lymphoid proliferation. *Semin Oncol* 1993;20:583.

67. Swartz M. *Lymphadenitis and lymphangitis. V.* New York: McGraw-Hill, 1990:818.

68. Iles PB, Emerson PA. Tuberculous lymphadenitis. *BMJ* 1974;1:143.

69. Carithers HA. Cat-scratch disease: an overview based on a study of 1,200 patients. *Am J Dis Child* 1985;139:1124.

70. Stastny JF, Wakeley PE, Frable WJ. Cytologic features of necrotizing granulomatous inflammation consistent with cat-scratch disease. *Diagn Cytopathol* 1996;15:108.

71. Becker LE. Lymphogranuloma venereum. *Int J Dermatol* 1976;15:26.

72. Young LS, Bicknell DS, Archer BG, et al. Tularemia epidemic: Vermont 1968: forty-seven cases linked to contact with muskrats. *N Engl J Med* 1969;280:1253.

73. Jacobs RF, Condrey YM, Yamauchi T. Tularemia in adults and children: changing presentation. *Pediatrics* 1985;76:818.

74. Stansfield AG. The histological diagnosis of toxoplasmic lymphadenitis. *J Clin Pathol* 1961;14:565.

75. Scobie WG. Acute suppurative adenitis in children. *Scott Med J* 1969;14:352.

76. Lincoln EM, Gilbert LA. Disease in children due to mycobacteria other than Mycobacterium tuberculosis. *Am Rev Respir Dis* 1972;683:105.

77. Spark RP, Fried ML, Bean CK, et al. Nontuberculous mycobacterial adenitis of childhood: the ten-year experience at a community hospital. *Am J Dis Child* 1988;142:106.

78. Boyd JC, Marr JJ. Decreasing reliability of acid fast smear techniques for detection of tuberculosis. *Ann Intern Med* 1975;82:481.

79. Tappero JN, Mohle-Boetani J, Koehler JE, et al. The epidemiology of bacillary angiomatosis and bacillary peliosis. *JAMA* 1993;269:770.

80. Dolan MJ, Wong MT, Regnery RL, et al. Syndrome of *Rochalimaea henselae* adenitis suggesting cat scratch disease. *Ann Intern Med* 1993;118:331.

81. Conrad DA. Treatment of cat-scratch disease. *Curr Opin Pediatr* 2001;13:56.

82. Stastny JF, Wakely PE, Frable WJ. Cytologic features of necrotizing granulomatous inflammation consistent with cat-scratch disease. *Diagn Cytopathol* 1996;15:108.

83. Hartsock RJ, Halling IW, King FM. Luetic lymphadenitis: a clinical and histologic study of 20 cases. *Am J Clin Pathol* 1973;53:304.

84. Walzer PD, Armstrong D. Lymphogranuloma venereum presenting as superclavicular and inguinal lymphadenopathy. *Sex Transm Dis* 1977;4:12.

85. Crook LD, Tempest B. Plague: a clinical review of 27 cases. *Arch Intern Med* 1992;152:1253.

86. Shapira Y, Weinberger A, Wysenbeek AJ. Lymphadenopathy in systemic lupus erythematosus: prevalence and relation to disease manifestations. *Clin Rheumatol* 1996;15:3355.

87. Cohen JI. Epstein-Barr virus infection. *N Engl J Med* 2000;343:481.

88. Straus S, Cohen JI, Tosato G, et al. Epstein-Barr virus infections: biology, pathogenesis and management. *Ann Intern Med* 1993;118:45.

89. Sixbey JW, Davis DS, Young LS, et al. Human epithelial cell expression of an Epstein-Barr virus receptor. *J Gen Virol* 1987;68:805.

90. Niedobitek G, Agathanggelou A, Herbst H, et al. Epstein-Barr virus (EBV) infection in infectious mononucleosis: virus latency, replication and phenotype of EBV-infected cells. *J Pathol* 1997;182:151.

91. Fingeroth JD, Weiss JJ, Tedder TF, et al. Epstein-Barr virus receptor of human B lymphocytes is the C3d receptor CR2. *Proc Natl Acad Sci U S A* 1984;81:4510.

92. Li Q, Spriggs MK, Kovats S, et al. Epstein virus uses HLA class II as a cofactor for infection of B lymphocytes. *J Virol* 1997;71:4657.

93. Hennesy K, Kieff E. One of two Epstein-Barr virus nuclear antigens contains a glycine-alanine copolymer domain. *Proc Natl Acad Sci U S A* 1983;80:5665.

94. Thorley-Lawson DA, Mann KP. Early events in Epstein-Barr virus infection provide a model for B cell activation. *J Exp Med* 1985;162:45.

95. Robinson J, Smith RW, Niederman JC. Mitotic EBNA-positive lymphocytes in peripheral blood during infectious mononucleosis. *Nature* 1980;287:334.

96. Callan MFC, Tan L, Anneks N, et al. Direct visualization of antigen specific CD 8+ T cells during the primary immune response to Epstein-Barr virus in vivo. *J Exp Med* 1998;187:1395.

97. De Waele M, Theilemans C, VanCamp BKG. Characterization of immunoregulatory T cells in EBV-induced infectious mononucleosis by monoclonal antibodies. *N Engl J Med* 1981;304:460.

98. Paul JR, Bunnel WW. The presence of heterophile antibodies in infectious mononucleosis. *Am J Med Sci* 1932;183:90.

99. Strauss SE, Cohen JI, Tosato G, et al. Epstein-Barr virus infections: biology, pathogenesis, and management. *Ann Intern Med* 1993;118:45.

100. Zur Hausen H, Schulte-Holthausen H, Klein G, et al. EBV DNA in biopsies of Burkitt's tumors and anaplastic carcinomas of the nasopharynx. *Nature* 1970;228:1056.

101. deThe G, Geser A, Day NE, et al. Epidemiological evidence for causal relationship between Epstein-Barr virus and Burkitt's lymphoma from a Ugandan prospective study. *Nature* 1978;274:756.

102. Tao Q, Robertson KD, Manns A, et al. Epstein-Barr virus (EBV) in endemic Burkitt's lymphoma: molecular analysis of primary tumor tissue. *Blood* 1998;91:1373.

103. Pagano JS, Huang CH, Levine P. Absence of Epstein-Barr viral DNA in American Burkitt's lymphoma. *N Engl J Med* 1973;289:1395.

104. Sullivan JL, Byron KS, Brewster FE, et al. X-linked lymphoproliferative syndromes: natural history of the immunodeficiency. *J Clin Invest* 1983;71:1765.

105. Grierson H, Purtilo DT. Epstein-Barr virus infection in males with the X-linked lymphoproliferative syndrome. *Ann Intern Med* 1987;106:538.

106. Ambinder RF, Lemas MV, Moore S, et al. Epstein-Barr virus and lymphoma. *Cancer Treat Res* 1999;99:27.

107. Snydman DR, Rudders RA, Daoust P, et al. Infectious mononucleosis in an adult progressing to fatal immunoblastic lymphoma. *Ann Intern Med* 1982;96:737.

108. Hanto DW, Frizzera G, Gajl-Peczalska KJ, et al. Epstein-Barr virus induced B-cell lymphoma after renal transplantation: acyclovir therapy and transition from polyclonal to monoclonal B-cell proliferation. *N Engl J Med* 1982;306:913.

109. Hanto DW, Frizzera G, Gajl-Peczalska J, et al. The Epstein-Barr virus (EBV) in the pathogenesis of post-transplant lymphoma. *Transplant Proc* 1981;13:756.

110. Curtis RE, Travis LB, Rowlings PA, et al. Risk of lymphoproliferative disorders after bone marrow transplantation: a multi-institutional study. *Blood* 1999;94:2208.

111. Weiss LM, Movahed LA, Warnke RA, et al. Epstein-Barr viral denomes in Reed Sternberg cells of Hodgkin's disease. *N Engl J Med* 1989;320:502.

112. Glaser SL, Lin RJ, Stewart SL, et al. Epstein-Barr virus associated Hodgkin's disease: epidemiologic characteristics in international data. *Int J Cancer* 1997;70:375.

113. Baumforth KR, Young LS, Flavell KJ, et al. The Epstein-Barr virus and its association with human cancers. *Mol Pathol* 1999;52:307.

114. Catling SJ, Astbury AJ, Latif M. Airway obstruction in infectious mononucleosis. A case report. *Anaesthesia* 1984;39:699.

115. Kilpatrick ZM. Structural and functional abnormalities of the liver in infectious mononucleosis. *Arch Intern Med* 1966;117:47.

116. Pullen H, Wright N, Murdock J. Hypersensitivity reactions to antibacterial drugs in infectious mononucleosis. *Lancet* 1967;2:1176.

117. Troxel DB, Innella F, Cohen RJ. Infectious mononucleosis complicated by hemolytic anemia due to anti-i. *Am J Clin Pathol* 1966;46:625.

118. Horwitz CA, Moulds J, Henle W, et al. Cold agglutinins in infectious mononucleosis and heterophil-antibody-negative mononucleosis-like syndromes. *Blood* 1977;50:195.

119. Silber M, Richards JD, Jacobs P. Life threatening haemolytic anemia and infectious mononucleosis: a case report. *S Afr Med J* 1985;67:183.

120. Wilkinson LS, Petz LD, Garraty G. Reappraisal of the role of anti-i in haemolytic anemia in infectious mononucleosis. *Br J Haematol* 1973;25:715.

121. Clark BF, Davies SH. Severe thrombocytopenia in infectious mononucleosis. *Am J Med Sci* 1964;248:703.

122. Winiarski J. Antibodies to platelet membrane glycoprotein antigens in three cases of infectious mononucleosis-induced thrombocytopenic purpura. *Eur J Haematol* 1989;43:29.

123. Schooley RT, Densen P, Harmon D, et al. Antineutrophil antibodies in infectious mononucleosis. *Am J Med* 1984;76:85.

124. Baranski B, Armstrong G, Truman JT, et al. Epstein-Barr virus in the bone marrow of patients with aplastic anemia. *Ann Intern Med* 1988;109:695.

125. Frecentese DF, Cogbill TH. Spontaneous splenic rupture in infectious mononucleosis. *Am Surg* 1987;53:521.

126. Vezina WC, Nicholson RL, Cohen P, et al. Radionuclide diagnosis of splenic rupture in infectious mononucleosis. *Clin Nucl Med* 1984;9:341.

127. Haines JD Jr. When to resume sports after infectious mononucleosis: how soon is safe? *Postgrad Med* 1987;81:331.

128. Silverstein A, Steinberg S, Nathanson M. Nervous system involvement in infectious mononucleosis: the heralding and/or major manifestation. *Arch Neurol* 1972;26:353.

129. Grose C, Henle W, Henle G, et al. Primary Epstein-Barr virus infections in acute neurologic diseases. *N Engl J Med* 1975;292:392.

130. Silber MH. Acute transverse myelopathy in Epstein-Barr virus infection: case reports. *S Afr Med J* 1983;64:753.

131. Tanner OR. Ocular manifestations of infectious mononucleosis. *Arch Ophthalmol* 1954;51:229.

132. Finkel M, Parker GW, Fanselau HA. The hepatitis of infectious mononucleosis: experience with 235 cases. *Mil Med* 1964;129:533.

133. Markin RS, Linder J, Zuerlein K, et al. Hepatitis in fatal infectious mononucleosis. *Gastroenterology* 1987;93:1210.

134. Butler T, Pastore J, Simon G, et al. Infectious mononucleosis myocarditis. *J Infect* 1981;3:172.

135. Titton RC, Dias P, Ryan RW. Comparative evaluation of three commercial tests for detections of heterophile antibody in patients with infectious mononucleosis. *J Clin Microbiol* 1988;26:278.

136. Halpring J, Scott AL, Jacobson L, et al. Enzyme-linked immunosorbent assay of antibodies to Epstein-Barr virus nuclear and early antigens in patients with infectious mononucleosis and nasopharyngeal carcinoma. *Ann Intern Med* 1986;104:331.

137. Niederman JC, Miller G, Pearson HA, et al. Infectious mononucleosis: Epstein-Barr virus shedding in saliva and the oropharynx. *N Engl J Med* 1976;294:1355.

138. Betts RF. Syndrome of cytomegalovirus infection. *Adv Intern Med* 1980;26:447.

139. Synderman NL, Stool SE. Management of airway obstruction in children with infectious mononucleosis. *Otolaryngol Head Neck Surg* 1982;90:168.

140. Brandfonbrener A, Epstein A, Wu S, et al. Corticosteroid therapy in Epstein-Barr virus infection: effect on lymphocyte class, subset, and response to early antigen. *Arch Intern Med* 1986;146:337.

141. Andersson J, Ernberg I. Management of Epstein-Barr virus infections. *Am J Med* 1988;85:107.

142. Tynell E, Aurelius E, Brandell A, et al. Acyclovir and prednisolone treatment of acute mononucleosis: a multicenter, double-blind placebo-controlled study. *J Infect Dis* 1996;174:324.

143. Andersson J, Britton S, Ernberg I, et al. Effect of acyclovir on infectious mononucleosis: a double-blind, placebo-controlled study. *J Infect Dis* 1986;153:283.

144. Green M, Michaels MG, Webber SA, et al. The management of Epstein-Barr virus associated post-transplant lymphoproliferative disorders in pediatric solid organ transplant recipients. *Pediatr Transplant* 1999;3:271.

145. Craig FE, Gulley ML, Ganks PM. Posttransplantation lymphoproliferative disorders. *Am J Clin Pathol* 1993;99:265.

146. Ho M, Jaffe R, Miller G, et al. The frequency of Epstein-Barr virus infection and associated lymphoproliferative syndrome after transplantation and its manifestations in children. *Transplantation* 1988;45:719.

147. Kuehnle I, Huls MH, Lui A, et al. CD20 monoclonal antibody (rituximab) for therapy of Epstein-Barr virus lymphoma after hemopoietic stem-cell transplantation. *Blood* 2000;95:1502.

148. Rooney CM, Smith CA, Ng CY, et al. Infusion of cytotoxic T cells for the prevention and treatment of Epstein-Barr virus-induced lymphoma in allogeneic transplant recipients. *Blood* 1998;92:1549.

149. Lucas KG, Small TN, Heller G, et al. The development of cellular immunity to Epstein-Barr virus after allogeneic bone marrow transplantation. *Blood* 1996;87:2594.

150. Straus SE. The chronic mononucleosis syndrome. *J Infect Dis* 1988;157:405.

151. Schooley RT. Chronic fatigue syndrome: a manifestation of Epstein-Barr virus infection? *Curr Clin Top Infect Dis* 1988;9:126.

152. Krech U. Complement-fixing antibodies against cytomegalovirus in different parts of the world. *Bull World Health Organ* 1973;49:103.

153. Stagno S, Reynolds DW, Pass RF, et al. Breast milk and the risk of cytomegalovirus infection. *N Engl J Med* 1980;312:1073.

154. Pass RF, August AM, Dworsky M, et al. Cytomegalovirus infection in a day care center. *N Engl J Med* 1982;307:477.

155. Dworsky ME, Welder K, Cassaday G, et al. Occupational risk for primary cytomegalovirus infection among pediatric health care workers. *N Engl J Med* 1983;309:950.

156. Prince AM, Szmuness W, Millian SJ, et al. A serologic study of cytomegalovirus infections associated with blood transfusions. *N Engl J Med* 1971;284:1125.

157. Chou S, Kim DY, Normal DJ. Transmission of cytomegalovirus by pretransplant leukocyte transfusions in renal transplant candidates. *J Infect Dis* 1987;155:565.

158. Bowden RA, Slichter SJ, Sayers MH, et al. Use of leukocyte-depleted platelets and cytomegalovirus-seronegative red blood cells for prevention of primary cytomegalovirus infection after marrow transplant. *Blood* 1991;79:246.

159. Stagno S, Reynolds D, Tsiantos A, et al. Cervical cytomegalovirus excretion in pregnant and non-pregnant women: suppression in early gestation. *J Infect Dis* 1975;131:522.

160. Lang DJ, Kummer JF. Demonstration of cytomegalovirus in semen. *N Engl J Med* 1972;287:756.

161. Meyers JD, Flournoy N, Thomas ED. Risk factors for cytomegalovirus infection after human marrow transplantation. *J Infect Dis* 1986;153:478.

162. Verdonck LF, Dekker AW, Rozenberg-Arska M, et al. A risk-adapted approach with a short course of ganciclovir to prevent cytomegalovirus

(CMV) pneumonia in CMV-seropositive recipients of allogeneic bone marrow transplants. *Clin Infect Dis* 1997;24:901.

163. Trincado DE, Rawlinson WD. Congenital and perinatal infections with cytomegalovirus. *J Paediatr Child Health* 2001;37:187.

164. Winston DJ, Ho WG, Bartoni K, et al. Ganciclovir prophylaxis of cytomegalovirus infection and disease in allogeneic bone marrow transplant recipients: results of a placebo-controlled, double-blind trial. *Ann Intern Med* 1993;118:179.

165. Zaia JA, Schmidt GM, Chao NJ. Preemptive ganciclovir based solely on asymptomatic pulmonary cytomegalovirus infection in allogeneic bone marrow transplant recipients. *Biol Blood Marrow Transplant* 1995;1:88.

166. Einsele H, Ehninger G, Hebert H, et al. Polymerase chain reaction monitoring reduces the incidence of cytomegalovirus disease and the duration and side effects of antiviral therapy after bone marrow transplantation. *Blood* 1995;86:2815.

167. Emmanuel D, Cunningham I, Julie-Elysee K. Cytomegalovirus pneumonia after bone marrow transplantation successfully treated with the combination of ganciclovir and high dose intravenous globulin. *Ann Intern Med* 1988;109:777.

168. Boeckh M, Gooley TA, Myerson D. Cytomegalovirus pp65 antigenemia-guided early treatment with ganciclovir at engraftment after allogeneic marrow transplantation: a randomized double-blind study. *Blood* 1996;10:4063.

169. Hebart H, Gamer D, Loeffler J, et al. Evaluation of Murex CMV DNA hybrid capture assay for the detection and quantitation of cytomegalovirus infection in patients following allogeneic stem cell transplantation. *J Clin Microbiol* 1998;36:1333.

170. Retiere C, Prod'homme V, Imbert-Marcille BM, et al. Generation of cytomegalovirus specific human T-lymphocyte clones by using autologous B-lymphoblastoid cells with stable expression of pp65 of IE1 proteins: a tool to study the fine specificity of the antiviral response. *J Virol* 2000;74:3948.

171. Walter EA, Greenberg PD, Gilbert MJ, et al. Reconstitution of cellular immunity against cytomegalovirus in recipients of allogeneic bone marrow by transfer of T-cell clones from the donor. *N Engl J Med* 1995;334:601.

172. Greenberg PD, Reusser P, Goodrich JM, et al. Development of a treatment regimen for human cytomegalovirus (CMV) infection in bone marrow transplantation recipients by adoptive transfer of donor-derived CMV-specific T cell clones expanded in vitro. *Ann N Y Acad Sci* 1991;636:184.

173. Sneller MC, Wang J, Dale JK, et al. Clinical, immunologic, and genetic features of an autoimmune lymphoproliferative syndrome associated with abnormal lymphocyte apoptosis. *Blood* 1997;89:1341.

174. Lim MS, Straus SE, Dale JK, et al. Pathological findings in human autoimmune lymphoproliferative syndrome. *Am J Pathol* 1998;153:1541.

175. Avila NA, Dwyer AJ, Dale JK, et al. Autoimmune lymphoproliferative syndrome: a syndrome associated with inherited genetic defects that impair lymphocytic apoptosis—CT and US features. *Radiology* 1999;212:257.

176. Jackson CE, Puck JM. Autoimmune lymphoproliferative syndrome, a disorder of apoptosis. *Curr Opin Pediatr* 1999;11:521.

177. Stobel P, Nanan R, Gattenlohner S, et al. Reversible monoclonal lymphadenopathy in autoimmune lymphoproliferative syndrome with functional FAS(CD95/APO-1) deficiency. *Am J Surg Pathol* 1999;23:829.

178. Frizzera G, Moran EM, Rappaport H. Angio-immunoblastic lymphadenopathy: diagnosis and clinical course. *Am J Med* 1975;59:803.

179. Ree HJ, Kadin ME, Kikuchi M, et al. Angioimmunoblastic lymphoma (AILD-type T cell lymphoma) with hyperplastic germinal centers. *Am J Surg Pathol* 1998;22:643.

180. Harris NL, Jaffe ES, Diebold H, et al. World Health Organization classification of neoplastic diseases of the hematopoietic and lymphoid tissues: report of the clinical advisory committee meeting—Airlie House, Virginia, November 1997. *J Clin Oncol* 1999;147:3835.

181. Pautier P, Devidas A, Delmer A, et al. Angioimmunoblastic-like T cell non-Hodgkin's lymphoma: outcome after chemotherapy in 33 patients and review of the literature. *Leuk Lymphoma* 1999;32:545.

182. Sallah S, Webbie R, Depera P, et al. The role of 2-chlorodeoxyadenosine in the treatment of patients with refractory angioimmunoblastic lymphadenopathy with dysproteinemia. *Br J Haematol* 1999;104:163.

183. Peterson BA, Frizzera G. Multicentric Castleman's disease. *Semin Oncol* 1993;20:636.

184. Keller AR, Hocholzer L, Castleman B. Hyalin-vascular and plasma cell types of giant lymph node hyperplasia of mediastinum and other locations. *Cancer* 1972;29:670.

185. Gaba AR, Stein RS, Sweet DL, et al. Multicentric giant lymph node hyperplasia. *Am J Clin Pathol* 1978;68:86.

186. Sohn CC, Sheibani K, Winberg CD, et al. Monocytoid B lymphocytes: their relationship to the patterns of the acquired immunodeficiency syndrome (AIDS) and AIDS-related lymphadenopathy. *Hum Pathol* 1985;16:979.

187. Frizzera G. Castleman's disease and related disorders. *Semin Diagn Pathol* 1988;5:346.

188. Soulier J, Grollet L, Oksenhendler E, et al. Molecular analysis of clonality in Castleman's disease. *Blood* 1995;86:1131.

189. Brandt SJ, Bodine DM, Dunbar CE, et al. Dysregulated interleukin 6 expression produces a syndrome resembling Castleman's disease in mice. *J Clin Invest* 1990;86:592.

190. Leger-Ravet MB, Peuchmaur M, Devergne O, et al. Interleukin-6 gene expression in Castleman's disease. *Blood* 1991;78:2923.

191. Nishimoto N, Sasai M, Shima Y, et al. Improvement in Castleman's disease by humanized anti-interleukin-6 receptor antibody therapy. *Blood* 2000;95:56.

192. Beck JT, Hsu SM, Wijdenes J, et al. Brief report: alleviation of systemic manifestations of Castleman's disease by monoclonal anti-interleukin-6 antibody. *N Engl J Med* 1994;330:602.

193. Bowne WB, Lewis JJ, Filippa DA, et al. The management of unicentric and multicentric Castleman's disease: a report of 16 cases and a review of the literature. *Cancer* 1999;85:706.

194. Dorfamn RF, Berry GJ. Kikuchi's histiocytic necrotising lymphadenitis; an analysis of 108 cases with emphasis on differential diagnosis. *Semin Diagn Pathol* 1988;5:329.

195. Chamulak GA, Brynes RK, Nathwani BN. Kikuchi-Fujimoto disease mimicking malignant lymphoma. *Am J Surg Pathol* 1990;14:514.

196. New NE, Bishop PW, Stewart PW, et al. Inflammatory pseudotumor of lymph nodes. *J Clin Pathol* 1005;48:37.

197. Kemper CA, Davis RE, Deresinski SC, et al. Inflammatory pseudotumour of intra-abdominal lymph nodes manifesting as recurrent fever of unknown origin. *Am J Med* 1991;90:519.

CHAPTER 21

Disorders of the Spleen

Chad T. Jacobsen and Susan B. Shurin

Hippocrates' and Aristotle's writings describe the gross anatomy of the spleen, which was regarded in ancient times as an "organ of mystery" (*misterii organum plenum*), as described by Galen. The earliest function ascribed to the spleen was the extraction of "melancholic humours," so large spleens resulted in more systemic humor. (Pliny the Elder, in A.D. 150, said, "great laughers have great spleens.") By the seventeenth century, localization of unhappiness in the spleen connoted spite, which is an attribute that persists. Anatomists of the seventeenth century described the microscopic structure of the spleen for the first time. In 1777, William Hewson assigned the spleen to the lymphatic system, recognizing a hematopoietic function as well. Virchow identified the malpighian follicles as being composed of lymphocytes (1). The filtration function was described in 1885 by Ponfick, who recognized the role of the spleen in the destruction of blood cells. The spleen was considered a nonessential organ because patients survived splenectomy without apparent ill effects. The association of asplenia with increased susceptibility to infection was not clear until 1952 (2).

EMBRYOLOGY, ANATOMY, AND PHYSIOLOGY

A number of homeobox genes (i.e., genes that activate downstream target genes, which are often involved in embryologic development) (3) that are crucial for the development of the spleen in other species have been identified. Mice lacking the gene *Hox11* have no spleen but are otherwise normal (3). Mice lacking *Bapx1* (a homeobox-containing gene in the *Nk-2* family) do not produce splenic progenitor cells in the corresponding area of mesoderm early in development, nor do they produce *Hox11* (4). Absence of the *Nkx2-3* gene leads to asplenia in some mice and to disordered development of the white pulp of the spleen in the others (5). Finally, the *Xenopus* tadpole gene *Nkx2-5* appears to function locally in the determination of sidedness (i.e., the development of the spleen on the left side, not the right) in splenic development (6).

In humans, the spleen arises from the mesoderm, which is first evident at the fifth week of gestation (0.8- to 1.0-cm embryo) (7). Layers of the left dorsal mesogastrium condense, and blood vessels appear in the eighth to ninth week of development (7). Reticular cells and fibers form sheaths around arterioles as they develop. During the fourth month, lymphocytes appear; B cells [surface immunoglobulin (Ig)–bearing] and T cells (E-rosetting cells) are identifiable by the thirteenth week, with B cells predominating throughout gestation (7). Red and

white pulp can be identified by the sixth month, but germinal centers are not evident in fetal spleen (7). Primitive inactive follicles are present at birth, with IgM and small amounts of IgG synthesized in the last trimester (7). Macrophages in the cords of the spleen possess phagocytic activity by the end of the first trimester (12 weeks) (7).

Fetal studies on mammals other than humans demonstrate significant hematopoiesis (production of formed elements of blood) within the spleen. Human fetal spleen also has been regarded as a hematopoietic organ. The spleen certainly has the capacity to support hematopoiesis later in life in conditions of bone marrow dysfunction with extramedullary hematopoiesis (e.g., myelofibrosis) and hemolytic anemias (e.g., thalassemia). Hematopoietic precursors are seen in the spleen, peaking in the second trimester and tapering off during the last trimester (8). Immature erythroid and myeloid precursors circulate in large numbers during fetal life, and their presence in the spleen may indicate little more than the filtering function of the spleen. The least mature blast forms and those in the mitotic pool are present in small numbers (7). Because conditions of congenital asplenia are not associated with hematopoietic failure (8), it appears that splenic hematopoiesis is not essential for normal maturation of blood cell production.

The anatomy of the spleen is shown schematically in Figure 21-1. The spleen is covered with a fibrous capsule and coated by peritoneal mesothelium (8). The capsule contains blood vessels, lymphatics, and nerves but no muscular elements, and, therefore, it has none of the contractile ability of the spleens of many animal species. The splenic artery exits from the celiac axis, enters the capsule at the hilum of the spleen, and branches into trabecular arteries. The central arteries branch from the trabecular arteries and enter the white pulp. The white pulp is grossly visible as white nodules 0.1 to 0.2 cm in diameter. The central arteries branching from the trabecular arteries are surrounded by a cuff of T lymphocytes, plasma cells, and macrophages; this is called the *periarterial lymphoid sheath*. As the arteries branch further, the sheath diminishes but continues down to the level of the penicilliary arterioles. At arterial branch points, follicles of B lymphocytes appear as clusters along the periarterial lymphoid sheath (8). A reticulin network and supporting stromal cells with long cytoplasmic processes connect the parts of the white pulp. The appearance of the white pulp varies with age and antigenic stimulation. At the time of birth, the white pulp is fully developed. The size of the nodules of the white pulp increases in childhood, especially with immunization and infection, peaks at puberty, and begins to involute in adulthood.

White Pulp

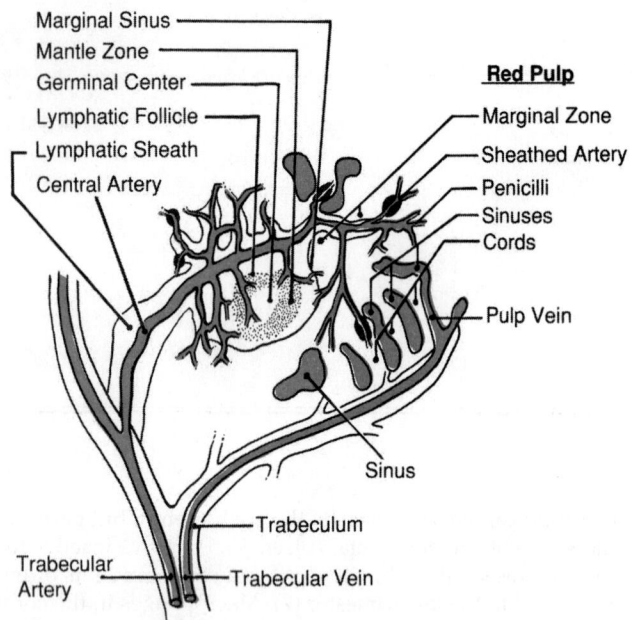

Figure 21-1. Schematic depiction of the spleen. (Bellanti JA. *Immunology, basic processes.* Philadelphia: WB Saunders, 1979.)

Uninfected adults who are immunologically normal usually have no evident germinal centers in contrast to children and adolescents (8). The secondary germinal center, or follicle, is surrounded by a mantle zone of B lymphocytes, which are, in turn, engulfed by the marginal zone where the white and red pulps meet (9). The marginal zone is part of the periarterial lymphoid sheath, so it consists mostly of T cells (10). Around the marginal zone is an area of perifollicular venous sinuses. Some of the central arteries end within the periarterial lymphoid sheaths, some arteries enter the marginal zones, and some branches exit from the marginal zones into the red pulp as penicilliary arteries. The marginal zone of the white pulp is the site of initial antigen trapping and processing (11).

The red pulp of the spleen consists of the vascular sinuses, the cords of Billroth, and the terminal branches of the penicilliary arteries. Vascular sinuses are lined with endothelial cells with long cytoplasmic processes, and a basement membrane beneath that has ring fibers at right angles to the endothelial cell processes. These ring fibers are attached to the macrophages' dendritic processes (12). The cytoplasmic processes are close together without tight junctions or interdigitations. Intact blood cells can be seen squeezing through the potential spaces between these cells and between the ring fibers. Outside the sinus walls are processes of the reticular cells of the cords of Billroth, which also surround the periarterial lymphoid sheath and the marginal zones of the follicles. These macrophages attach to the ring fibers surrounding the sinuses (12). The cords of Billroth are thus interspersed between the sinuses and receive the terminations of the arterial capillaries. The cords are not lined with endothelium, unlike the sinuses and pulp veins. Circulation of blood through red pulp that is entirely lined with endothelial cells is relatively rapid and is referred to as *closed circulation* (12,13). Circulation that goes directly into the cords is referred to as *open circulation*, is significantly slower, and encourages the cordal macrophages to remove cells that are damaged or aged in the hypoxic, hypoglycemic, and acidotic environment with stagnant flow (14).

SPLENIC FUNCTIONS

Fetal and Extramedullary Hematopoiesis

Many studies have reported that active hematopoiesis can be seen in the fetal spleen throughout the second trimester and, to a decreasing extent, in the third trimester (15,16). Erythroid and megakaryocytic elements predominate, but myeloid elements are also present. After the fifth month *in utero*, bone marrow is the major hematopoietic organ, and the presence of immature hematopoietic elements may represent pooling of fetal blood in the spleen, because hematopoietic elements circulate in considerable numbers in fetal blood (17,18). Because the cells are represented in the approximate proportion that they are present in peripheral blood, it has been argued that the fetal spleen is not a hematopoietic organ (19,20). Evidence that it can be a hematopoietic organ comes from both mice and humans. In lethally irradiated mice given compatible bone marrow infusion, the spleen is the initial site of hematopoietic colonies (21). Spleen cells reconstitute hematopoietic function in mice, but mononuclear cells from other lymphoid organs (nodes, thymus, and thoracic duct) do not (22).

Extramedullary hematopoiesis is a major cause of splenomegaly in human diseases affecting the bone marrow. It is most common in hemolytic anemias, either congenital (e.g., thalassemia) or acquired, but production of myeloid and megakaryocytic elements is seen as well in myelofibrosis with myeloid metaplasia. It appears that the stromal cells of the spleen are capable of supporting hematopoiesis, which suggests that they resemble those of the bone marrow and produce the c-kit ligand needed for growth of stem cells (23,24). Production of growth factors in the spleen is poorly defined, but the presence of appropriate cell types (lymphocytes, monocytes, fibroblasts, and stromal cells) and the occurrence of hematopoiesis in conditions of stress on the bone marrow make it clear that the spleen is capable of fulfilling this role. The normal bone marrow architecture seems to keep immature cells from circulating. The process of exiting from the marrow appears to require more active participation on the part of the cell than does exiting the spleen, and circulating nucleated erythroid elements and immature myeloid cells in addition to large platelets are characteristic of states in which splenic and other extramedullary sites of hematopoiesis are occurring. Reticulocytes mature in the spleen for 36 hours after leaving the bone marrow and then reenter the circulation (12) (Table 21-1).

Culling and Pitting of Erythrocytes

The adult spleen receives approximately 2 L/minute of blood, or 5% of the cardiac output (25), giving it an opportunity to view all circulating cells on a regular basis. The term *culling* is used to describe destruction of erythrocytes and may refer to either normal removal of aging erythrocytes or removal of damaged cells in pathologic conditions (26). Other formed elements—leukocytes and platelets—are also culled from the blood by the spleen, especially when they are damaged. The spleen is probably not the normal site of destruction of most leukocytes and platelets, which adhere to vessel walls and migrate into tissues where they die and are removed (27).

The removal of inclusions from within erythrocytes while releasing the cell back into the circulation is termed the *pitting function*. It is accomplished by passage of erythrocytes between or through the cordal macrophages, through the fenestrations of the basement membrane of the sinus, and then between the endothelial cells (Fig. 21-2). Cells that are poorly deformable are unable to enter the sinuses. The close apposition of the erythrocyte membrane with the macrophage membrane during this

TABLE 21-1. Splenic Functions

Clearance and filtration
  Clearance of blood cells, microorganisms, and other particles by macrophages. Optimal clearance with antibody or complement-coated particles.
  Culling and pitting of normal red blood cells; trapping of abnormal red blood cells by the reticular meshwork.
Immune function
  Marginal zone
    Promotes interaction of antigens with cells of monocytic and lymphocytic lines.
    Initiation of the immune response; processing of antigens.
  White pulp
    Periarteriolar lymphatic sheath (T cells): immune recognition.
    Lymphoid follicles (B cells): antibody production, immunoregulation.
  Red pulp: macrophages
    Antigen processing; antigen preservation.
    Phagocytosis.
Hematologic function
  Hematopoiesis perhaps *in utero* and during stem cell reconstitution, in severe hemolysis, and in myeloid metaplasia.
  Storage pool for erythrocytes, leukocytes, and platelets.
Hemostatic function
  Production of factor VIII and von Willebrand's factor by endothelial cells.

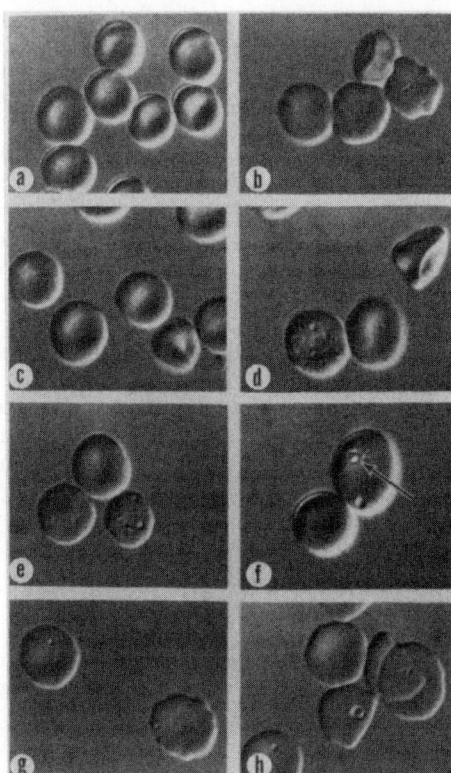

Figure 21-3. Pitted red blood cells **(a–h)**. Arrow points to a red blood cell pit **(f)**. (Holroyde CP, Oski RA, Gardner FH. The "pocked" erythrocyte: red cell surface alterations in reticuloendothelial immaturity of the neonate. *N Engl J Med* 1969;281:516.)

process enables the macrophage to identify aged or damaged membrane glycoproteins or the presence of antibody or complement and to phagocytize the cell. Cells that are poorly deformable (e.g., spherocytes) may lyse in the process of passage into the sinus. Particulate matter within the erythrocyte is concentrated in the last part of the cell to pass through the sinusoidal wall, where it is removed by macrophages (28). Among the particulate matter removed are Howell-Jolly bodies (remnants of nuclear material), Heinz bodies (denatured hemoglo-

bin, usually adherent to the membrane), Pappenheimer bodies (iron-containing granules), and intraerythrocytic parasites, such as malarial organisms. Fragmentation of erythrocytes, with return of the rest of the red blood cells (RBCs) to the circulating blood, is termed *erythroclasis* and occurs in autoimmune hemolysis, the thalassemias, and RBC membrane disorders. These damaged fragments may be less deformable and may be removed on a subsequent passage through the spleen.

"Polishing" of the erythrocyte membrane also takes place in the spleen, with removal of excess membrane and "pocks" or "pits." These internal vesicles appear as if they are on the surface of the RBC when using interference (Nomarski) optics (29,30) (Fig. 21-3). These pits are dramatically visible using scanning electron microscopy, but they are also visible when glutaraldehyde-fixed erythrocytes are examined under phase contrast microscopy. This simple examination is the easiest, cheapest, and least invasive approach to the identification of asplenia, and it is increasingly available in clinical laboratories. Less than 2% of the RBCs contain pits in individuals with normal splenic function (31). Nearly one-half the erythrocytes of asplenic individuals may demonstrate pits. There is an inverse relationship between the pit count and the degree of splenic dysfunction or the amount of remaining splenic tissue (32). Pits are removed with the protein-lipid components as the reticulocytes are polished by the spleen (33). Another morphologic change seen when the spleen is removed is an increased number of target cells and acanthocytes (34).

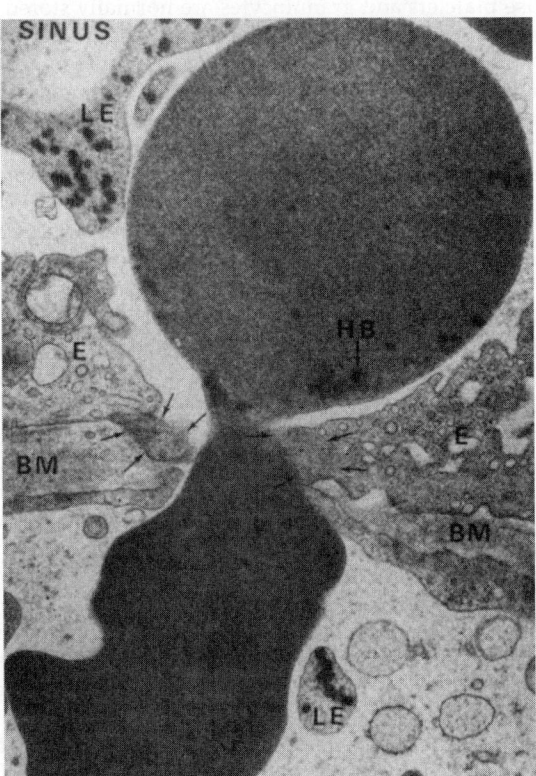

Figure 21-2. Heinz body (HB) being removed (culled) from an erythrocyte. BM, basement membrane; E, sinus endothelial cell; LE, hemolyzed erythrocyte fragments. (Chen LT, Weiss L. Role of the sinus wall in the passage of erythrocytes through the spleen. *Blood* 1973;41:529.)

Senescence of Blood Cells

The blood in the pulp cords is concentrated and viscous, with a higher hematocrit than the blood in the splenic artery or vein. The environment is acidotic. Precise measurements within the red pulp are difficult to obtain without contamination by blood flowing more rapidly through the spleen. Best estimates indicate that pH within the red pulp ranges between 6.8 and 7.2. The oxygen tension appears to go as low as 54 mm Hg, and the glucose concentration is approximately 60% of that within the venous blood (12,35). Normal erythrocytes tolerate such conditions, though glycolysis is probably impaired by acidosis and relative hypoglycemia. Normal reticulocytes are capable of oxidative phosphorylation and are imperiled by the hypoxic environment (36). The importance of energy generation is demonstrated by pyruvate kinase deficiency, in which adenosine triphosphate generation from glucose is impaired. The spleen appears to be especially hostile to reticulocytes in pyruvate kinase deficiency. Reticulocytes also have a less negative surface charge than mature erythrocytes and repel each other less (33). They also are larger than mature erythrocytes and have excess membrane. Remodeling of erythrocytes and their removal from the circulation as they age are splenic contributions to erythrocyte maturation.

Host Defense

The white pulp of the spleen is the largest collection of lymphoid tissue in the body. The spleen is able to recognize and process antigens, produce lymphokines, activate T lymphocytes, and generate activated B cells to produce antibodies. Other lymphoid organs recognize and process antigens that enter locally; the spleen recognizes antigens in the bloodstream and those administered systemically (12,37–40).

The marginal zone, with abundant blood supply and a large number of macrophages, appears to be most important in trapping and processing antigens (41). After initial localization in the marginal zones, antigens penetrate the germinal center. T lymphocytes predominate in the periarterial lymphoid sheaths, whereas B lymphocytes predominate in the germinal centers and mantle zones (42). The marginal zone lymphocytes appear to be particularly adept at recognizing carbohydrate antigens, whose processing is markedly different from that of protein antigens (43). Morphologic and metabolic (DNA synthesis) evidence of lymphocyte activation after administration of antigen occurs first in the periarterial lymphoid sheath and red pulp (T-cell areas) and is followed 3 to 4 days later by enlargement of the primary follicles and development of germinal centers (activation of B-lymphocyte areas) (44). These changes resolve over the month after the removal of the antigenic stimulus. With reexposure to antigen (anamnestic response), the same sequence of events is repeated but greatly sped up.

The key role of the spleen in defense against encapsulated organisms appears to derive from the marginal zone lymphocytes (particularly important in recognizing the carbohydrate antigens found in bacterial capsules) and from the great sensitivity of splenic macrophages to small amounts of opsonin on the surface of particles. The spleen is particularly capable of recognizing and processing particulate antigens that the host has not previously encountered (40,45). When an antigen is administered intravenously, an asplenic individual may fail to recognize it altogether (45,46). Hepatic recognition of antigens is less efficient because of more rapid transit of blood through the liver with less opportunity for macrophages to recognize and process the antigen.

The major impairment in antibody response after splenectomy is in IgM production (47). Antigen-specific IgM antibody may not be made at all in an asplenic individual, even if IgG is produced (46,47). The initial antibody response to an antigen is IgM, so the blunting of IgM production results in low levels of specific antibody early in an infectious process. Some splenecto-mized patients have low IgM levels (48), but in immunologically normal adults, the total antibody levels are normal. Specific IgM production may still be impaired, however (46).

Splenic macrophages phagocytize particles more effectively than hepatic macrophages when antibody is absent or present in low levels (32,49–52). The receptors on the surface of splenic macrophages for the constant region of the Ig molecule (Fc receptors) appear to bind to and recognize antibody more effectively than those in the liver (53). This may be largely a function of longer exposure of opsonized particles to macrophages in the splenic sinusoids compared with the liver. When particles are well opsonized, with abundant surface IgG or C3b, they are removed with equal efficiency by the liver and spleen (51,53).

Other Functions

RESERVOIR FUNCTION

The normal adult human spleen holds 20 to 40 mL of blood (54) and does not serve as a storage site for erythrocytes. Platelets and granulocytes are normally stored in the spleen, primarily in the red pulp. Up to one-third of the total platelet mass is available for release into the systemic blood supply when factors that affect adhesiveness are released (55). In some animals, the splenic capsule contains smooth muscle and is able to affect intravascular volume by relaxing and contracting, but this is not the case in humans.

In conditions associated with splenomegaly, the spleen does serve as a reservoir for all formed elements, including RBCs. Widening of the pulp cords creates an organ with greater volume, and secondary hypersplenism, or vascular pooling of cells within the cords and sinuses, occurs regardless of the underlying cause of the splenomegaly (56). Thus, hypersplenism is a pathologic extension of the spleen's normal reservoir function. Because platelets and granulocytes are normally stored in the spleen, granulocytosis and thrombocytosis occur immediately after splenectomy. The increase in granulocyte and platelet counts partially resolves in the first 2 weeks after surgery, but the white blood cell and platelet counts are usually chronically elevated relative to normal values. In children, this is rarely a cause of difficulty. In children with polycythemia, however, and in adults with myeloproliferative disease, the thrombocytosis may lead to vascular complications, and antiplatelet agents may be needed (34,57). Low-dose aspirin (81 mg/day) and dipyridamole are commonly used agents.

RESPONSE TO INFECTION AND PORTAL HYPERTENSION

The increase in spleen size with pathologic conditions is associated with different microscopic findings, depending on the process involved. With hemolysis or any destructive cytopenia, the major changes are in the red pulp and splenic sinusoids, with erythrophagocytosis or phagocytosis of leukocytes or platelets. The size of the spleen inversely correlates with the leukocyte and platelet counts (58) (Fig. 21-4). When the spleen is responding to infection, most of the increase in size is due to hyperplasia of the periarterial lymphoid tissue and germinal centers (59). Regardless of the cause of splenomegaly, the increase in blood flow to the spleen increases the portal venous pressure (60,61). Portal hypertension may be mild, but it may increase with time and with the degree of splenomegaly. The incidence and the severity of hypersplenism in patients with portal hypertension depend on the underlying pathology. Portal hypertension may decrease intravascular volume, with secondary renin and aldosterone secretion followed by an increase in plasma volume (62). These changes reverse after splenectomy when the portal hypertension is secondary to the splenomegaly.

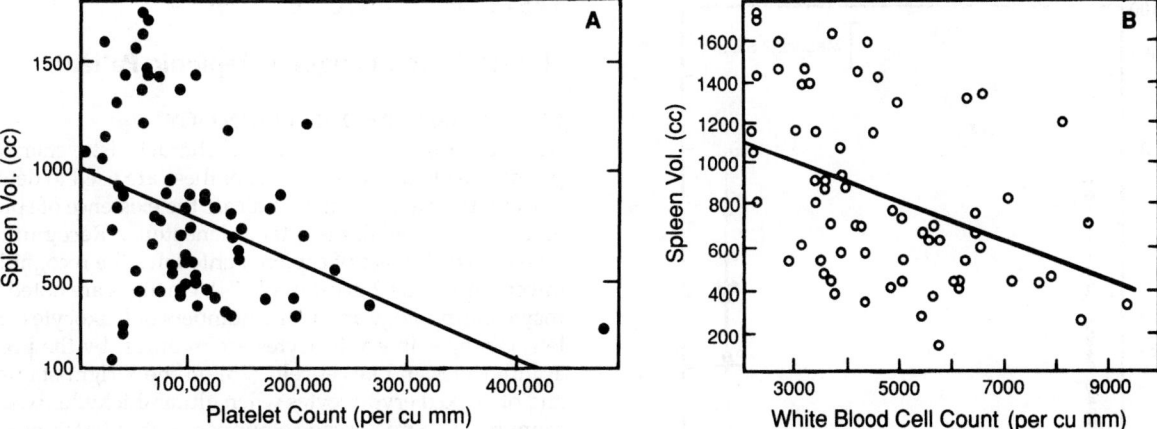

Figure 21-4. A,B: Correlation between spleen size and blood counts. Vol., volume. (El Khishen MA, Henderson JM, Millikan WJ, et al. Splenectomy is contraindicated for thrombocytopenia secondary to portal hypertension. *Surg Gynecol Obstet* 1985;160:233.)

ERYTHROKINETICS

As the graveyard of normal and damaged erythrocytes, the spleen is the site of degradation of the contents of erythrocytes. Hemoglobin is broken down to bilirubin, which is released into the plasma, further metabolized in the liver, and excreted in bile and urine. The other major breakdown products that are handled by the spleen are membrane lipids and iron. Normally, the lipids in the membrane are also fully degraded and released into the plasma. In the lipid-storage diseases, absence of various degradative enzymes leads to accumulation of these membrane-lipid products, with engorgement of the macrophages and splenic enlargement.

Iron is also stored in the macrophages as ferritin and hemosiderin (63). In conditions of iron overload associated with hemolysis (e.g., thalassemia major), splenic macrophages become engorged with iron. The bioavailability of iron stored in splenic macrophages is limited (64). That transfused erythrocytes are the source of the iron in secondary hemochromatosis is demonstrated by the fact that the spleen, unlike the liver, does not store iron in primary hemochromatosis. As long as the spleen is in place, other organs that are affected by severe hemosiderosis (endocrine organs and the heart) appear to be somewhat protected (65). In thalassemia, splenectomy for hypersplenism is usually performed late in the first decade or early in the second—about the time that iron overload is becoming clinically significant—and all subsequent iron absorption is directed to less expendable organs. In aplastic anemia and pure RBC aplasia in which iron is not reused, the presence of a normal spleen does not protect other organs from damage caused by iron (66).

DEVELOPMENTAL CHANGES IN SPLENIC FUNCTION

Neonates have Howell-Jolly bodies in their erythrocytes and an increased number of pocked erythrocytes, with a mean of 24% of erythrocytes pocked in the blood of term infants and 47% in preterm infants (30) (Fig. 21-5). Some of the findings may be because of the high rate of erythrocyte production in the third trimester and because neonatal erythrocytes develop more membrane vesicles when incubated *in vitro* than adult erythrocytes do (67). Nevertheless, the filtering function of the spleen is immature at birth (68).

Both the Howell-Jolly bodies and the pocked erythrocytes disappear during the first few weeks of life (Fig. 21-6), and their persistence beyond a month in a term neonate should raise the suspicion of congenital hyposplenia or asplenia (30). A consequence of normal maturation of splenic function is that neonates with isoimmune hemolytic disease who have well-compensated hemolysis without anemia at birth may accelerate the rate of erythrocyte destruction as the spleen matures. Consequently, anemia may develop at a time when erythropoiesis has temporarily ceased because of decreased endogenous erythropoiesis (69).

The relative impairment in the phagocytic function of the spleen of neonates may contribute to their immunoincompetence and susceptibility to infection, particularly with bacterial pathogens (68). Macrophage dysfunction is also manifested by impaired processing of carbohydrate antigens (46), which is a T-cell–independent function important in acquiring specific

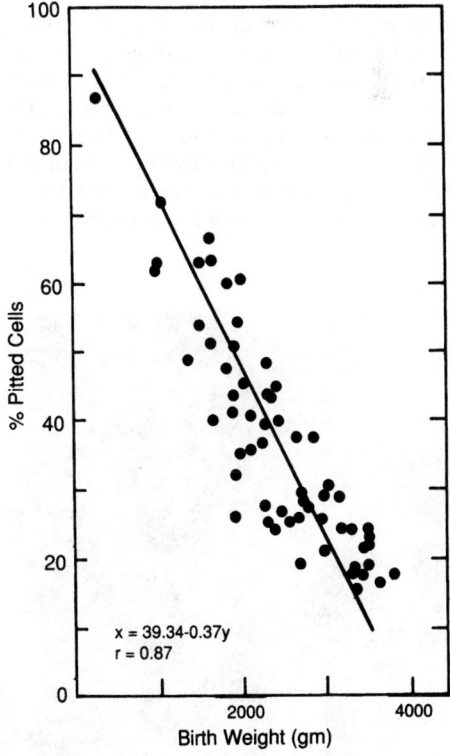

Figure 21-5. Graph of pit count versus birth weight. (Holroyde CP, Oski RA, Gardner FH. The "pocked" erythrocyte: red cell surface alterations in reticuloendothelial immaturity of the neonate. *N Engl J Med* 1969;281:516.)

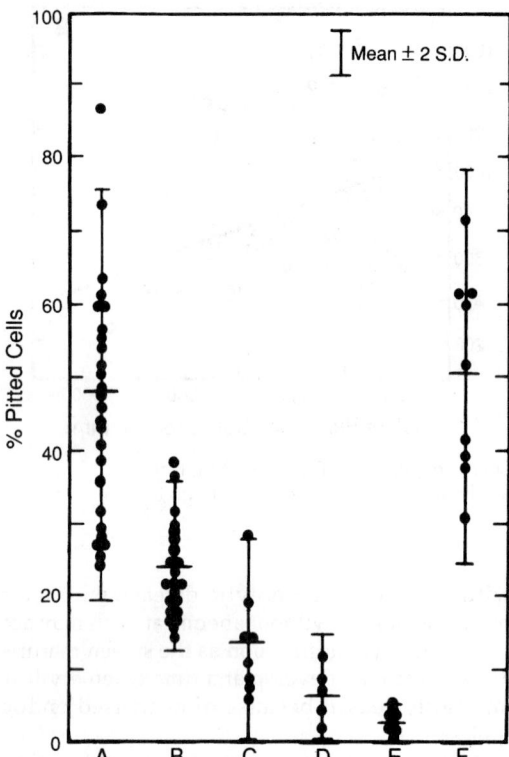

Figure 21-6. Disappearance of pitted cells relative to age. Premature infants in first 24 hours (A); term infants in first 24 hours (B); term infants at 1 month (C); term infants at 2 months (D); adults (E); splenectomized adults (F). (Holroyde CP, Oski RA, Gardner FH. The "pocked" erythrocyte: red cell surface alterations in reticuloendothelial immaturity of the neonate. *N Engl J Med* 1969;281:516.)

humoral immunity to many of the same particulate pathogens (encapsulated bacteria) phagocytosed by splenic macrophages (70,71). Maturation of splenic phagocytic function is complete in term neonates by 2 months of age and slightly later in premature infants, as assessed by pit counts (which may underestimate splenic function) (30,67). Development of the ability to process carbohydrate antigens occurs much later, progressing to adult norms by approximately 2 years of age (72).

TESTS OF SPLENIC FUNCTION

Hematologic Changes in Asplenic Patients

CELL NUMBERS AND MORPHOLOGY

Absence of the spleen results in characteristic changes in the peripheral blood picture. Some of these are used to detect asplenia, and their absence may indicate the existence of splenosis or accessory splenic tissue after splenectomy. Recognition of the hematologic impact of asplenia antedates the recognition of an infectious risk by 2 decades (73,74). Changes are noted in erythrocyte morphology and in the numbers of leukocytes and platelets. Changes in erythrocytes are manifest by the presence of acanthocytes and target cells (75) on the Wright-stained smear and of pocked erythrocytes when glutaraldehyde-fixed cells are examined in a microscope equipped with interference (Nomarski) optics (30). Because the spleen removes senescent erythrocytes, the survival of erythrocytes is lengthened in asplenic conditions, but only if the RBC survival was shorter than normal initially, as it is in many hemolytic anemias (76). More dramatic than the changes in erythrocyte shape are the inclusions that are normally pitted from erythrocytes by the spleen. These include Howell-Jolly bodies, Heinz bodies, and Pappenheimer bodies (77,78). Both leukocytes and platelets tend to pool in the spleen, and both are increased in number in asplenic patients compared with those with functional spleens (79). The increase in leukocyte count is primarily mature neutrophils (27,34). The increase in platelet count may be dramatic immediately after splenectomy, especially if there was a shortened platelet survival that was compensated before splenectomy (55,80,81).

HOWELL-JOLLY BODIES

The most characteristic finding on the asplenic blood smear is the presence of Howell-Jolly bodies, which are dense, dark purple to black spheroidal inclusions (0.5 to 1.5 μm) that represent retained (incompletely extruded) nuclear material (34) (Fig. 21-7). Howell-Jolly bodies are visible and striking on routine peripheral blood smears with standard stains and, thus, represent the simplest screening test for hyposplenism. Although Howell-Jolly bodies are fairly specific for hyposplenism, they are not seen unless splenic function is largely ablated (82) and may not be seen with lesser degrees of hyposplenism. Conversely, they may be seen with extensive hemolysis resulting in

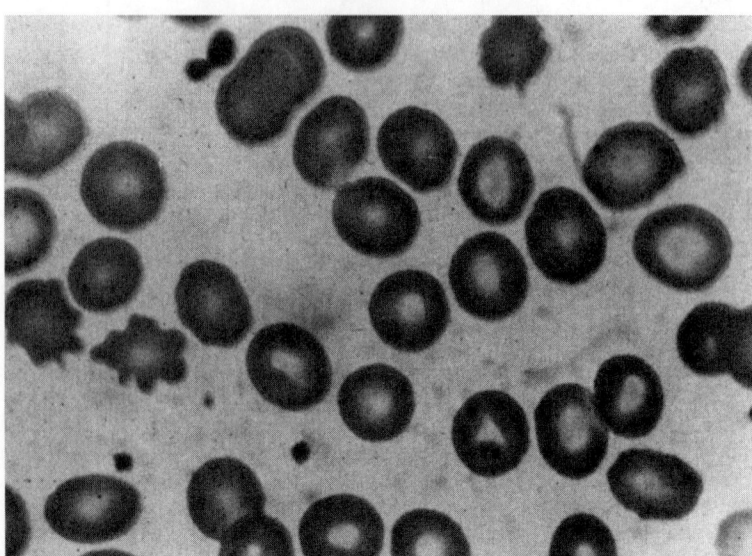

Figure 21-7. Postsplenectomy smear with acanthocytes and Howell-Jolly bodies.

an overload of splenic clearance of particles, indicating relative hyposplenia rather than anatomic or functional asplenia. The same is true for Pappenheimer bodies, which are siderotic granules that are normally removed by the spleen. Pappenheimer bodies tend to be particularly numerous in patients with hemolysis, especially after splenectomy (63).

PITTED ERYTHROCYTES

Erythrocytes fixed in 0.5% to 1.0% buffered glutaraldehyde may be examined under interference optics for pocks or pits on their surface (29,30) (Fig. 21-3). These pits are vesicles containing ferritin, hemoglobin, and remnants of mitochondria, which form spontaneously in erythrocytes (26,28). They form in mature RBCs and, thus, indicate ongoing membrane remodeling by the spleen (83). Normally, less than 2% of erythrocytes have surface pits (83). The number of cells that have pits is scored rather than the total number of pits. The number of pitted cells is inversely proportional to the degree of splenic function. The loss of splenic function with age in sickle cell disease has been examined using the pit count; this count reveals loss of splenic function earlier than radiologic methods (84,85). In part, this may reflect the short RBC survival in sickle cell disease and the reticulocytosis that results in a higher proportion of the cells having pits to begin with; the total splenic burden is proportionally greater than when RBC survival is normal (84).

Radionuclide Scans

In addition to assessing splenic size, a number of radionuclide scans provide information about splenic function. To assess the phagocytic function of the spleen, erythrocytes can be labeled with chromium 51, mercury 197, rubidium 81, or technetium 99m (^{99m}Tc) and deliberately damaged with heat, antibody, or chemicals *in vitro* before reinfusion into the patient (86). These manipulations ensure removal of the erythrocytes from the circulation by splenic macrophages, and the cytoplasmic radionuclide label permits external visualization (87). These techniques have been supplanted by use of sulfur colloidal suspensions of radionuclides (e.g., ^{99m}Tc) that are also sequestered in the spleen and are safer for patients. Other isotopes (e.g., gold 198 and indium 113m) have also been used (86), but they are not standard in most centers. A major use for these techniques is visualization of accessory or regenerated splenic tissue, particularly after splenectomy (88).

To evaluate the extent to which particles or cells are sequestered in the spleen, reinfusion of the patient's own indium 111–labeled erythrocytes or platelets can be used to determine survival time (89). Information is obtained about the *in vivo* survival of the cells and their relative extent of sequestration in liver and spleen. The half-life of platelet survival appears to predict response to splenectomy in immune thrombocytopenia (ITP) (90). The extent to which radioactivity accumulates in the spleen correlates poorly with the extent of prolongation of cell survival postsplenectomy in immunologically mediated processes. Because the liver is not a major site of cell destruction in many nonimmune cytopenias (e.g., RBC membrane disorders), the spleen-to-liver accumulation is more meaningful in predicting response to splenectomy in these disorders (90).

A third radionuclide imaging technique that may demonstrate splenic function is the use of iron 59 to identify hematopoietic tissue. If the spleen is a site of extramedullary hematopoiesis, iron 59 is concentrated in the spleen when ferrokinetic studies are performed. Often, these studies also demonstrate impaired hematopoiesis in the bone marrow.

Ultrasound

Ultrasound is a noninvasive, readily available procedure for evaluation of splenic anatomy. Splenic size and shape and several aspects of anatomy can be readily evaluated (91). Cysts and abscesses are particularly readily identified. The technique is not sufficiently sensitive to exclude the presence of accessory spleens, which are frequently too small to be accurately identified.

Computed Tomographic Scanning

Computed tomography (CT) is the most useful imaging modality for evaluation of splenic pathology because it elucidates both anatomy and certain aspects of function (92). The visceral surface of the spleen is adjacent to the stomach, left kidney, tail of the pancreas, and splenic flexure of the colon. Thus, contrast media in the stomach, small bowel, and colon by oral administration may help identify splenic tissue when there is an external indentation on these organs. Intravenous administration of contrast is usually necessary to detect splenic lesions that are the same density as normal splenic parenchyma. The contrast is given as a bolus, but it is important not to scan during the arterial phase of the contrast administration. Inhomogeneous enhancement is often seen if scans are obtained in the first minute after the bolus is given, probably because of variable rates of blood flow in the red pulp (93,94). Rapid scans may help distinguish accessory spleens from hilar lymph nodes (which do not enhance) (95), pancreatic tail masses, or vascular structures, however (93). Without contrast medium, the spleen is slightly less dense than liver. With contrast enhancement, it fills just after the aorta. The liver has a delayed peak of contrast enhancement because of the later arrival of blood from the portal veins. Abscesses show rim enhancement and show up well on CT (96).

The size of the spleen varies with the size of the patient and with age (97). Children have relatively more splenic tissue than adults. Normal splenic volume in an adult is less than 175 mL (98). With an electronic cursor, the volume of the spleen can be estimated by adding together areas of contiguous 1-cm slices on CT scans (99). Accessory spleens have the same attenuation values and contrast enhancement as normal spleen and are usually located in the gastrosplenic ligament near the hilum (92,95).

Diffuse splenomegaly without evident abscess formation is seen with many viral infections (including Epstein-Barr virus, human immunodeficiency virus, and cytomegalovirus); parasitic infections (malaria, schistosomiasis); and some bacterial infections, including subacute bacterial endocarditis (100). Most granulomatous diseases (including histoplasmosis and tuberculosis) cause diffuse splenomegaly acutely, followed by calcified granulomata in a normal-sized spleen, often noted incidentally (101). Fungal infections also show focal lesions (102). Leukemia, myeloproliferative disorders, Langerhans' cell histiocytosis, and benign hematologic disorders (including hemolysis of any cause) produce diffuse splenomegaly (103). The infarcted spleens of sickle cell disease are small and densely calcified (104). Other inflammatory diseases (systemic lupus erythematosus, sarcoid, and rheumatoid arthritis) and storage diseases (Gaucher's, Niemann-Pick) also show diffuse splenomegaly (105).

Congestive splenomegaly due to portal hypertension, splenic vein occlusion, or thrombosis is associated with a nodular liver, ascites, gastroesophageal varices, and collateral veins. A dynamic scan, with rapid injection of contrast, may demonstrate an occluded splenic vein (93).

Splenic trauma is extremely well visualized with CT (106). Both subcapsular or intrasplenic hematomas and splenic laceration can be clearly identified. Subcapsular hematomas have a collection of low-density fluid in a crescent shape with a flattening of the surface (106). Acutely (up to 4 hours), they are usually evident only with contrast enhancement, because the blood has the same density as the splenic tissue. As the hematoma organizes, it is evident without contrast administration and often keeps a crescent shape. This is then replaced with fluid of water density, which appears as a false cyst (i.e., without epithelial lining) just below the capsule. Lacerations are subtler. The splenic margins may be less clear, the parenchyma inhomogeneous, and lacerations may actually be evident. More commonly, a hematoma adjacent to the spleen or free blood or fluid in the left subphrenic space or in the peritoneal cavity is demonstrated on CT imaging. Contrast in the bowel is especially helpful to separate perisplenic blood or fluid from bowel.

Other focal abnormalities evident on CT scan include infarction, cysts, abscesses, and tumors. Infarction resulting from occlusion of a portion of the splenic artery is usually due to emboli (including tumor emboli) or to diseases of the arteries, such as atherosclerosis or polyarteritis (104). It usually appears as a low-density, peripheral, wedge-shaped lesion without contrast enhancement. The rim of the infarcted region does enhance (104).

Splenic cysts may be due to *Echinococcus granulosus* (92), or they may be nonparasitic. Splenic hydatid cysts appear as well-defined, low-density masses with multiple septae and a thick, enhancing cyst wall. The CT findings are characteristic; with a suggestive history, serology, and eosinophilia, the diagnosis can be made before any invasive procedures are undertaken, because rupture poses the risk of hemorrhage and dissemination of infection. Nonparasitic cysts may be lined with epithelium (true cyst) or unlined (false cyst). This differentiation cannot be made on CT scan images. They are frequently not loculated, are thin walled, and do not enhance with contrast. True cysts are developmental in origin. Unlined cysts represent previous splenic trauma with replacement of the hematoma by a cavity with serous fluid (107). Cystic hemangiomas of the spleen may be multiple and contain lymph (108). Their attenuation is higher than other cystic lesions. Pancreatic pseudocysts may occur in, or immediately adjacent or adherent to, the spleen, usually in the context of pancreatitis. The fluid is rich in amylase (107).

Splenic abscesses produce focal cystic abnormalities on CT scan. Bacterial endocarditis, intravenous drug abuse, alcoholism, trauma, diabetes, sickle cell disease, myeloproliferative disease, and immunosuppression all predispose to splenic abscess formation. Systemic signs and symptoms suggestive of infection are usually present but may be absent, particularly in immunosuppressed or partially treated patients. Splenomegaly is more common than tenderness (101,102). Blood cultures are frequently negative, necessitating percutaneous drainage or splenectomy (95).

Malignancies involving the spleen may be focal on CT scan. Involvement with Hodgkin's disease may be evident on CT scan if the granulomas exceed 1 cm in diameter. For staging, CT does not exclude splenic involvement. Non-Hodgkin's lymphoma more often diffusely involves the spleen but may be nodular. Splenic enlargement and involvement with lymphoma may be more common in patients with acquired immunodeficiency syndrome. Metastatic disease is seen in the spleen, usually in the context of widespread metastasis to other organs and rarely as the sole site of disease on CT scanning (109,110).

CT-guided aspiration of cysts, drainage of hematomas and abscesses, and biopsies of lesions permit both diagnostic and therapeutic intervention in instances in which anatomic lesions are demonstrated. The availability of thin needles permits safe puncture of the splenic capsule as long as vascular structures have been excluded and portal hypertension is not present.

Magnetic Resonance Imaging

Magnetic resonance imaging (MRI) of the spleen may give better resolution than CT scanning but rarely displays abnormalities not evident on CT scanning. MRI is more expensive than CT scanning. It also is more difficult to image upper-abdominal contents, because there is motion artifact accompanying respiration and it takes longer to obtain the images with MRI. MRI complements CT scanning in imaging the spleen primarily for identification of vascular lesions that otherwise would require angiography.

MRI appears to be uniquely suited for evaluation of the spleen for suspected fungal infection. Semelka et al. have recently reported that evaluation with MRI for acute fungal disease yields a sensitivity of 100% and a specificity of 97% (111). The lesions noted were typically less than 1 cm in diameter and were all well defined and of high signal intensity on T2-weighted images. Subacute and chronic lesions were also readily identifiable on MRI.

STRUCTURAL DEFECTS

Accessory Spleens

Accessory spleens are noted in approximately 30% of autopsies and may range from one to six in number (94). They are identical to normal spleens anatomically and functionally but are usually small. They may be located at the splenic hilum or in the lienorenal and gastrosplenic ligaments, the jejunal wall, and the tail of the pancreas, mesentery, and omentum. Their major importance is that they may hypertrophy after splenectomy for hematologic indications and may cause late (up to 25 years) relapse of a process for which splenectomy was performed (112,113).

Splenic-Gonadal Fusion

During embryonic development, the spleen is close to the mesonephros. Occasionally, fusion of the spleen with the left gonad is noted (114). Splenic-gonadal fusion occurs into the fifth to eighth week of intrauterine life before the descent of the gonad and involution of the mesonephros. The majority of cases reported in the literature occurred in males, and approximately 20% of cases were found at autopsy (115). In the discontinuous variant of this anomaly, there is no physical connection between the spleen and the accessory splenic tissue associated with the gonad. In the continuous variant, fibrous connective tissue and ectopic splenic tissue link the spleen and gonad. The most common presentation is scrotal mass, but patients may also present incidentally on evaluation of their cryptorchidism (116). Associated hernias can be found. Approximately one-third of the cases that have been described were associated with other congenital anomalies, with the majority of those anomalies involving limb defects (115). A significant number of the described cases of splenic-gonadal fusion limb defects were further associated with orofacial malformations, an association prompting some to recommend that babies born with oromandibular-limb hypogenesis also be evaluated for the presence of splenic-gonadal fusion (117).

Asplenia-Polysplenia Syndrome

More serious congenital anomalies occur in association with major cardiovascular malformations. Asplenia is associated with severe cyanotic congenital heart disease and bilateral right-sidedness; polysplenia is associated with bilateral left-sidedness (118). Asplenia is often accompanied by life-threatening cyanotic congenital heart lesions, including transposition of the great vessels, pulmonary artery atresia or stenosis, septal defects, anomalous venous drainage, and a single atrioventricular valve (119). Typically, both lungs have three lobes, the liver is central, and the stomach is on the right side (119). Although the cardiovascular lesions are often fatal in early infancy, increased survival with better surgical management has resulted in survival of sufficient numbers of patients to permit clear identification of greatly increased risk of bacterial sepsis with a high mortality (120). These patients have peripheral blood smears suggestive of asplenia. Imaging studies and autopsy demonstrate multiple small splenic nodules or no splenic tissue. In polysplenia, the splenic tissue is divided into two or more (up to nine described) masses (121). Dextrocardia, bilateral superior venae cavae, septal defects, and anomalous pulmonary venous return are associated lesions. Both lungs tend to have two lobes, the liver is midline, and bowel malrotation is common (122). These patients do not usually have evidence of hyposplenia on peripheral blood examination, and increased risk of infection has not been attributed to impaired splenic function.

Asplenia also may occur without heart disease, in which case it is less likely to be detected early in life than when it is associated with life-threatening lesions (123). When it occurs with situs inversus, it represents a milder and later-occurring variant of the developmental processes of the syndromes described above. Less often, asplenia occurs without any other anatomic defect. In at least one case, isolated asplenia appears to have led to the death of an otherwise healthy adult from pneumococcal septicemia (68). Some of these patients, like asplenic mice, may be found to have defects in the *Hox11* gene (124).

Both of these conditions have been associated with an increased incidence of intestinal rotation disorders, putting both of these patient populations at risk for volvulus (125,126).

Splenic Cysts

Splenic cysts may be (a) parasitic (*E. granulosus*), (b) true cysts with epithelial lining, or (c) false cysts without such linings (127).

Echinococcal (hydatid) cysts occur in patients with potential exposure, eosinophilia, and positive blood serology. The thick cyst wall is characteristic but not diagnostic, and there are usually multiple septate daughter cysts within the larger cyst, which are not seen with other types of cysts. *E. granulosus* is endemic to the Mediterranean area, South America, Australia, and Alaska. The reported prevalence of splenic involvement varies from 0.9% to 8.0%, and in some series, the spleen is the third most common location of hydatid disease involvement after the liver and the lungs (128,129). The fluid within the cyst is infected with organisms and is under pressure. The presence of daughter cysts and the serologic evidence of infection usually permit diagnosis of echinococcal cysts preoperatively. Total splenectomy is the treatment of choice and must be done with care to avoid spillage of the infectious contents within the abdomen, which may induce anaphylaxis. Surgery is easier if the cysts are drained and 1% formalin or 3% sodium chloride is used to kill the organisms. Mebendazole is used when spillage occurs or if cysts are present in other organs.

Nonparasitic true cysts (with an epithelial lining) develop as a consequence of several anomalies. The peritoneal mesothelium may infold after rupture of the splenic capsule, resulting in an intrasplenic cyst with mesothelial lining. Peritoneal mesothelial cells may be trapped in the sulci of the spleen, and these aggregates may form a cyst—also lined with mesothelium. Additionally, the lymphatics within the spleen may be dilated, creating lymphangiomata that are true cysts. Epidermoid and

dermoid cysts are most common in young patients. Cystic lymphangiomas and true mesothelial cysts are often identified in older patients (107,130,131). They tend to increase in size with time and present with pressure, rupture, or secondary infection (132). They are generally asymptomatic until enlarged. The treatment of choice is partial splenectomy, which can be performed by enucleating the cyst along a plane external to it and achieving hemostasis in the residual splenic tissue (133).

Non–epithelial-lined cysts, termed *false cysts* or *pseudocysts*, are generally posttraumatic in origin. Resolution of subcapsular or intraparenchymal hematomas results in a cavity with a thin, fibrous wall. The serous fluid replaces the earlier hematoma. The rim may be calcified. Pseudocysts do not tend to enlarge with time to the extent that true cysts do, because they lack an epithelial lining (134). When they need surgery, splenic conservation or CT-guided aspiration usually can be performed. It is likely that these cysts increase in frequency with the increasing use of splenic conservation for trauma and are more commonly diagnosed with more sensitive, noninvasive diagnostic techniques such as ultrasound and CT. With a previous history of trauma, their nature should be evident. Unless they pose a diagnostic dilemma or cause symptoms, no treatment is necessary (133).

Splenic cysts may become large and may hemorrhage or lead to splenic rupture. When this is the case, splenectomy may be necessary to prevent rupture. Increasingly, as a consequence of spleen preservation techniques developed for management of acute trauma, subtotal splenectomy with preservation of normal splenic tissue may be feasible and is desirable when possible (133).

Pancreatic pseudocysts may be adjacent to, or actually extend into, the spleen. These occasionally are loculated. Because pancreatic pseudocysts occur in the setting of acute or chronic pancreatitis, and the adjacent pancreas is inflamed, it is usually evident that this is the diagnosis. If questions remain, aspiration of the cyst yields fluid with a high amylase content (135), which confirms the diagnosis. Specific treatment is not needed for the splenic cyst when it represents a pancreatic pseudocyst.

SPLENIC TUMORS

Benign Tumors

Benign splenic hamartomas, cavernous hemangiomata, and adenomas are histologically similar to each other and to normal splenic tissue. These consist of large, thin-walled vascular spaces lined with endothelium and interspersed with normal pulp tissue (136). Multiple benign tumors have been described at autopsy in the spleen (137). These include dermoids, fibromata, leiomyomata, osteomata, chondromata, and lipomas. Because these rarely cause clinical problems, they do not require intervention.

Angiosarcoma

Splenic angiosarcoma is virtually the only primary malignant tumor seen in the spleen other than lymphoma. Angiosarcoma of the spleen has a high rate of metastasis (approximately 80%), and one-third of patients experience spontaneous splenic rupture. Concomitant malignancies (breast carcinoma, colon cancer, non-Hodgkin's lymphoma, and so forth) are noted in approximately 5% of cases (138). It has previously been reported that both hepatic and splenic angiosarcoma are associated with previous administration of the contrast medium Thorotrast (109). However, in a review of the medical literature in which 73 cases of primary splenic angiosarcoma were found, there was no documented association of the administration of

Thorotrast with the development of the splenic angiosarcoma (138). The dye has been replaced by other contrast media.

Lymphomas

Lymphomas are the most common malignant tumors involving the spleen (139). As detailed in the section on CT of the spleen, imaging is unreliable in determining splenic involvement with lymphoma. Hodgkin's disease frequently involves the spleen with macroscopically visible nodules that are 1 cm or less in diameter and thus tend not to be evident on CT scan. Additionally, granulomatous lesions that are not Hodgkin's disease (including tuberculosis, histoplasmosis, sarcoid, and lymphoid granulomatosis) may involve both the liver and spleen, so the presence of nodules in the spleen does not confirm Hodgkin's disease. The spleen may be involved without being enlarged, and it may be enlarged without being involved with Hodgkin's disease. The frequency of splenic involvement varies with the histologic subtype and is more common in mixed cellularity, nodular sclerosing, and lymphocyte depletion than in lymphocyte-predominant Hodgkin's disease. Staging laparotomy has been standardly performed because of the 25% discordance between clinical and pathologic staging, which is primarily due to findings in the spleen at splenectomy. However, because of the association of irradiation therapy with the development of second malignancies (140,141), other therapeutic modalities have begun to be adopted in the treatment of low-stage disease (141,142), including combination chemotherapy and lower dose irradiation or chemotherapy alone. Thus, with the advent of systemic therapy and the advances in imaging techniques, splenectomy in staging of Hodgkin's disease has become much less common (142).

Non-Hodgkin's lymphomas may be primary in the spleen. All histologies are seen in the spleen. Splenic involvement may be a manifestation of more widespread disease. In young patients, non-Hodgkin's lymphoma is virtually never truly a localized disease, and systemic therapy is needed regardless of histology or staging. In older patients, disease truly limited to the spleen, especially of low-grade histology, may be treated with splenectomy alone (143,144). Non-Hodgkin's lymphomas may cause either diffuse or nodular splenomegaly, depending on the histologic type. Splenic involvement is usually an indication of disseminated disease, although this is not always the case.

Splenomegaly is common in all the leukemias. The closest relation between disease activity and splenic function is seen in hairy cell leukemia (145). Splenomegaly is a constant in hairy cell leukemia, and splenectomy remains front-line therapy for this disease. The pancytopenia accompanying hairy cell leukemia usually improves if the marrow cellularity is less than 85%, and systemic therapy can often be delayed in these patients. Survival is unaffected, but clinical manifestations improve with splenectomy (146).

Metastatic Tumors

Metastatic lesions involving the spleen develop as a consequence of the filtering function of the spleen for bloodborne contaminants. Unlike the lung (another filter organ), the spleen is rarely an isolated site of metastatic disease. The incidence of splenic metastases has been reported to range from 0.3% to 7.3% (147). Splenic metastasis occurs in the setting of widespread metastatic disease in other organs. Metastatic breast carcinoma may cause splenomegaly, which develops largely in response to splenic infarction from tumor clumps in the splenic arterial supply, with infarction and reactive splenomegaly (148). Other metastatic tumors may also cause infarction. The tumors most likely to involve the spleen include melanoma, choriocarcinoma, seminoma, lung, pancreas, stomach, colon, breast, and neuroblastoma (110,149–151).

FUNCTIONAL HYPOSPLENIA

Functional hyposplenia refers primarily to the phagocytic function of the spleen. It is defined by lack of uptake of heat-damaged labeled erythrocytes, sulfur colloid, ^{99m}Tc, or other radionuclide imaging materials, and evidence of impaired remodeling of erythrocytes (increased numbers of pocked erythrocytes and Howell-Jolly bodies). In general, this appears to correlate well with macrophage processing of antigens, especially carbohydrate antigens and intravenously administered antigens such as sheep erythrocytes (82,152). Actual atrophy of the spleen is less common than evidence of hypofunction without any change in the size of the spleen. Atrophy is seen in Fanconi's anemia (153), after the administration of Thorotrast (154), after irradiation therapy (155,156), with infarction in sickle cell disease (85), and accompanying a number of inflammatory disorders (157–160) (Table 21-2).

Sickle Cell Disease

SPLENIC INFARCTION

The spleen is a particularly hostile environment for sickle cells, which respond poorly to hypoxia, acidosis, and hypoglycemia. Sickle hemoglobin crystallizes when deoxygenated, and the poorly deformable cells then adhere to and block the small blood vessels in which they are circulating. Infarction of multiple organs is a major manifestation of the disease. Because the environment of the spleen predisposes to sickling, damage to the splenic vasculature is one of the earliest permanent consequences of sickle cell disease. The other major organ affected by these events in early childhood is the renal medulla, and both the concentrating ability of the kidney and the phagocytic function of the spleen can be restored by transfusion in young children with sickle cell disease (younger than approximately 2 years) (161). With time, however, the damage becomes perma-

---

TABLE 21-2. Causes of Hyposplenism

Hematologic
  Sickle cell disease and variants
  Lymphoma (Hodgkin's, non-Hodgkin's)
  Fanconi's anemia
Immunologic
  Systemic lupus erythematosus
  Rheumatoid arthritis
  Thyroiditis
  Chronic active hepatitis
  Sjögren's syndrome
  Mixed connective tissue disease
  Ulcerative colitis
  Crohn's disease
  Celiac disease
  Tropical sprue
  Intestinal lymphangiectasia
  Chronic graft-versus-host disease
Anatomic
  Congenital absence or hypoplasia
  Sarcoidosis
  Amyloidosis
  Occlusion of splenic artery or vein
  Celiac artery thrombosis
  Irradiation
  Hemangiosarcoma

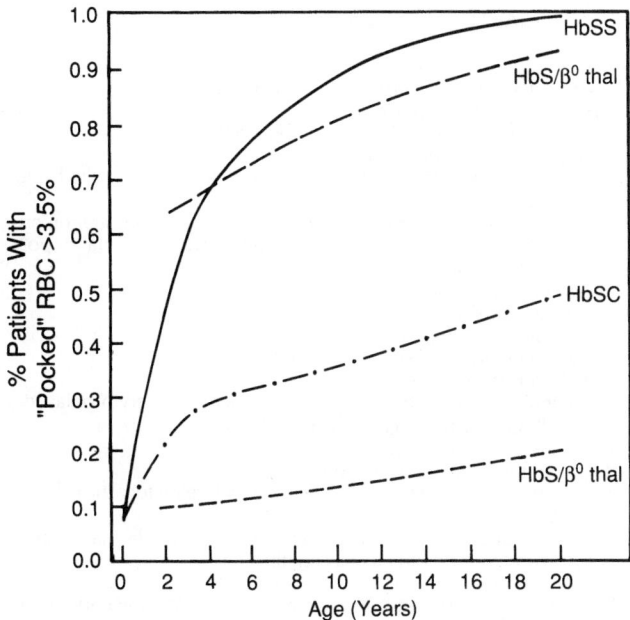

Figure 21-8. Development of asplenia in sickle syndrome. HbSS, hemoglobin SS disease; HbS/β⁰ thal, hemoglobin Sβ-thalassemia disease; HbSC, hemoglobin SC disease; RBC, red blood cell. (Pearson HA, Gallagher D, Chilcote R, et al. Developmental pattern of splenic dysfunction in sickle cell disorders. *Pediatrics* 1985;76:392.)

nent, and transfusion fails to restore the organs to health. By 6 to 8 years of age, the spleen is reduced to a fibrotic nubbin by repeated infarction, a process termed *autosplenectomy.*

The time course of splenic infarction and the development of hyposplenia in sickle cell disease are assessed with liver-spleen scans and by counting pocked erythrocytes (54). Because a count of greater than 2% pocked erythrocytes correlates well with failure to visualize the spleen by ^{99m}Tc scanning (85,161), this noninvasive and inexpensive test can be used to screen for hyposplenia. In homozygous sickle cell disease and Sβ⁰-thalassemia, hyposplenia is demonstrable in virtually all children by the time of their first birthday (85) (Fig. 21-8). In patients with hemoglobin S-C and Sβ⁺-thalassemia, hyposplenia develops considerably later. The best predictor of hyposplenia is the level of fetal hemoglobin (162,163). With more than 15% to 20% of fetal hemoglobin, splenic function is preserved. This is predicted from observations of sickle cell patients in the eastern province of Saudi Arabia who retain fetal hemoglobin levels of above 20% and do not infarct their spleens (164).

Patients with hemoglobin S-C and Sβ⁺-thalassemia often have persistent splenomegaly with evidence of impaired phagocytic function, despite the enlarged size (165). It is important that those caring for such patients recognize that they are, in fact, hyposplenic (163) and, therefore, susceptible to infection with encapsulated organisms, although the frequency of such events is less than for patients with SS- or Sβ⁰-thalassemia (161).

The poor function of the spleen in sickle cell disease is reversible with transfusion in young children (161). Neither the amount of blood needed to reverse the hypofunction nor the length of this reversibility is entirely clear. In general, sickling manifestations persist as long as hemoglobin S is the predominant hemoglobin; it is probable that transfusion to at least 50% of hemoglobin A is needed to significantly affect sickling in the spleen as well. By 6 years of age, transfusion fails to restore splenic function.

The splenic infarction that leads to hyposplenia occurs primarily in the sinusoids. In sickling disorders, most of the infarc-

tion occurs in the capillaries and venules (where hemoglobin S is deoxygenated and sickled) rather than in the arterioles (where oxyhemoglobin S is in solution within the erythrocyte).

SPLENIC SEQUESTRATION CRISIS

When sickling occurs in the venules and extends into the larger veins of the spleen, the immediate consequence is not infarction but obstruction of venous outflow. With unimpeded arterial blood supply and a distensible capsule, the spleen is capable of enlarging massively, and a significant portion of the systemic blood supply may pool within the spleen. This is termed a *splenic sequestration crisis* (166,167). Similar events may occur within the liver but are rarely life-threatening because the hepatic capsule is not as distensible. This is an event of early childhood, rarely occurring after 4 years of age, and it may be fatal as a result of acute hypovolemia and severe anemia, with impaired perfusion, shock, and acidosis (168). Because acute splenic sequestration tends to recur and may be fatal, splenectomy is frequently recommended after the first episode (168).

IMMUNOLOGIC-AUTOIMMUNE DISEASES

Hyposplenia occurs in a number of inflammatory and autoimmune disorders. In many instances, the function of the Fc receptors is impaired, with poor clearance of particles opsonized with IgG antibodies (169). This common theme is demonstrated in systemic lupus erythematosus (169), rheumatoid arthritis (170), sarcoidosis (160), systemic vasculitis (170), ulcerative colitis (82), amyloidosis (171), and celiac disease or sprue (172,173).

Hyposplenia is an occasional feature of a variety of other diseases, including dermatitis herpetiformis (174), sarcoidosis (160), systemic mastocytosis (157), thyrotoxicosis (159), Fanconi's anemia (153), splenic angiosarcoma (154), and graft-versus-host disease (158). In the late stages of acquired immunodeficiency syndrome, atrophy of lymphoid follicles and severe depletion of all T-cell–dependent areas are seen (175). Splenomegaly is common in acquired immunodeficiency syndrome (176). There is evidence that macrophage activation is impaired in the spleens of human immunodeficiency virus–infected individuals (143). In many of the conditions mentioned, immunosuppressive therapy is administered, and patients are immunologically compromised for a variety of primary and secondary reasons. The fact that specific antibody production may be impaired adds to the risk of Fc receptor dysfunction. From the standpoint of patient management, rapid intervention to detect and treat infection with encapsulated organisms and gram-negative organisms that afflict hyposplenic patients may be life-saving. Immunization is rarely effective because of the underlying immunosuppression, but antibiotic administration with amoxicillin or equivalent coverage is recommended for febrile patients. The need for hospitalization and parenteral administration of antibiotics depends on the severity of the underlying process and concurrent immunosuppression.

Iatrogenic Splenic Dysfunction

CORTICOSTEROIDS

Acquired splenic dysfunction accompanies several therapeutic maneuvers, especially treatment with systemic corticosteroids and irradiation therapy that affects the spleen. Corticosteroids decrease the affinity of the Fc receptors on splenic macrophages for the Fc fragment and may actually decrease the numbers of receptors on the macrophages themselves (177). In addition, the phagocytic function of neutrophils and monocytes is diminished by corticosteroid treatment because of diminished surface adherence. This is also usually the cause of the acute effect of corticosteroid therapy on many processes mediated by humoral antibodies. The steroid-induced increase in the platelet count in ITP or the rise in hemoglobin in autoimmune hemolysis is due to diminished splenic clearance of opsonized particles (177). The effect on hepatic macrophage function is much less marked than on splenic macrophages. Diminished antibody production is a later effect of steroid treatment but also affects the spleen, where antibody production takes place (178).

IMMUNOGLOBULIN G

Blockade of Fc receptors in the liver and spleen is thought to be a major mechanism of action of high-dose intravenously administered IgG given for immune cytopenias, especially ITP (179,180). This effect is transient and reversible within several weeks of administration, and therapy needs to be repeated to maintain Fc receptor blockade. The same mechanism is attributed to use of intravenous anti-D antibody in Rh-positive patients with ITP (181–183).

Samuelsson and his colleagues have recently proposed another mechanism of intravenously administered IgG in the treatment of ITP (184). Their research has shown that in the murine model of ITP, intravenously administered IgG acts by inducing the expression of FcγRIIB, an inhibitory receptor on the effector cells of the reticuloendothelial system. Engagement of the FcγRIIB receptor appears to counterbalance the activation responses triggered by FcγRIII binding in the reticuloendothelial system, thereby inhibiting the clearance of the opsonized platelets.

IRRADIATION THERAPY

Irradiation therapy to the spleen affects functions differently depending on the total dose administered. Lymphocytes are extremely sensitive to irradiation therapy, but the extent to which irradiation ablates lymphocyte function depends, in part, on the cell type and the extent to which the cell is activated. Less than 500 cGy ablates much B-cell function (185). Exposure to 3000 cGy eliminates over 95% of T-lymphocyte thymidine incorporation (185). Because blastogenesis and proliferation are an integral part of specific lymphocyte responses, low doses to areas that include the spleen impair lymphocyte function. These changes are transient because circulating blood lymphocytes originating in the bone marrow, thymus, and lymph nodes repopulate the spleen within a matter of weeks, and no pathologic changes are noted years after 600 to 800 cGy of irradiation exposure (186). In contrast, macrophages are much more tolerant of irradiation exposure than lymphocytes, and the phagocytic function of the spleen is rarely affected by doses below 2000 cGy. It is, however, ablated at high doses, and functional hyposplenia (i.e., phagocytic dysfunction) can be expected with the doses of irradiation (4000 cGy) given for Hodgkin's disease (155,156). Thus, a child receiving 1080 cGy to the left renal bed for a Wilms' tumor may lose some lymphocyte function but is not likely to have increased susceptibility to bacterial infection on the basis of poor clearance of particles by the spleen. The anatomic changes with higher-dose irradiation are similar to those seen with infarction of the spleen for any reason, and susceptibility to bacterial infection is well known (156).

SPLENECTOMY AND RELATED PROCEDURES

Indications

Some indications for splenectomy are listed in Table 21-3. None of these indications is absolute. In each instance, the relative risks and benefits must be weighed to make a rational decision.

TABLE 21-3. Indications for Splenectomy

Chronic hemolytic anemias
  Diseases that respond reliably to splenectomy
    Hereditary spherocytosis
    Hereditary elliptocytosis or pyropoikilocytosis
    Hereditary stomatocytosis[a]
    Thalassemia with increasing transfusion requirement due to hypersplenism
    Hemoglobin S syndromes with recurrent splenic sequestration crises
  Diseases that respond variably to splenectomy when a partial response would be clinically significant
    Autoimmune hemolytic anemia
    Glycolytic defects
    Unstable hemoglobinopathies
    Congenital erythropoietic porphyria
    Thalassemia intermedia
    Congenital dyserythropoietic anemia II (hereditary erythroblastic multinuclearity with a positive acid serum test)
Chronic thrombocytopenias
  Idiopathic thrombocytopenic purpura
  Human immunodeficiency virus infection with refractory thrombocytopenia
  Thrombotic thrombocytopenic purpura refractory to plasma therapy
  Wiskott-Aldrich syndrome (occasionally)
Chronic neutropenias
  Rheumatoid arthritis (Felty's syndrome) and recurrent infections (occasionally)
Primary splenic malignancies
  Splenic lymphoma
  Angiosarcoma
Severe hypersplenism (severe cytopenias) or other symptoms of marked splenomegaly (pressure symptoms, splenic infarction)
  Lymphoproliferative diseases
    Hairy cell leukemia (leukemic reticuloendotheliosis)
    Chronic lymphocytic leukemia
  Myeloproliferative diseases (without significant splenic hematopoiesis)
    Myeloid metaplasia
    Spent polycythemia vera (occasionally)
  Congestive splenomegaly
    Cirrhosis
    Portal, splenic, or hepatic vein thrombosis
  Storage diseases (e.g., Gaucher's disease refractory to enzyme replacement therapy)
  Renal disease on chronic hemodialysis (occasionally)
Surgical indications
  Staging for Hodgkin's disease (as indicated)
  Splenic cysts, including echinococcal cysts
  Ruptured spleen that cannot be repaired
  En bloc resection for certain carcinomas
  Splenorenal shunt
Diagnostic splenectomy

[a]Splenectomy is effective but is associated with an extremely high risk of thromboembolic disease (*Br J Haematol* 1996;93:303) and probably should only be used for life-threatening hemolysis.

In hemolytic disorders, splenectomy is indicated if the patient has significant compromise related to anemia (poor physical growth, inadequate stamina), requires repeated exposure to blood products, demonstrates impaired function and energy sufficient to interfere with normal activities, or requires medications that have significant side effects. These indications apply only if the disorder can be expected to improve or if the medication (such as corticosteroids) can be discontinued or decreased to significantly fewer toxic doses after splenectomy. Newer approaches to gallstones and better recognition that such stones are frequently silent and cause no symptoms make prevention of gallstones a poor sole indicator for splenectomy in hemolytic anemia. When splenectomy is needed, it is worthwhile to delay it as long as practically feasible. The lymphoid activity of the spleen matures most notably during the first 5 years of life. Therefore, by delaying splenectomy, one allows maturation of lymphoid immunity to a degree sufficient to minimize the risk of postsplenectomy septicemia and increases the probability of a good response to active immunization measures. This is particularly important when considering splenectomy in young children. Some would recommend delaying splenectomy until well into grade school because of the high numbers of febrile illnesses children develop on entering preschool and grade school. Each of these acute illnesses would necessitate a trip to either the child's physician or the emergency room in splenectomized children to rule out sepsis. However, delaying splenectomy should not be done at the expense of the patient's clinical status; the risks and benefits of each case must be carefully weighed in the decision on splenectomy.

Young children with sickle cell disease are susceptible to acute splenic sequestration crises in which the venous drainage of the spleen is occluded by sickled cells, and the arterial supply is patent. The result is rapid distention of the spleen with pooling of a substantial portion of the total blood volume. This complication is accompanied by a high mortality rate unless rapid intervention with either transfusion, splenectomy, or both occurs (167). Exchange transfusion is usually successful in reversing the venous occlusion, but the relapse rate is high, and acute splenic sequestration is usually considered an indication for splenectomy (167). Because this is a process primarily seen in very young children, chronic transfusion to delay splenectomy until the child is 2 years of age is commonly undertaken. This permits the lymphoid function of the spleen to mature, and it may lessen the risk of postsplenectomy sepsis. Prophylactic antibiotics are imperative in these children.

In ITP, the indication for splenectomy depends heavily on the age of the patient and whether the thrombocytopenia is acute or chronic. In children, most acute ITP resolves without requiring splenectomy or long-term steroid therapy. In adults and older children with chronic ITP, spontaneous resolution is uncommon, and splenectomy may be indicated early in the course of the illness. In both instances, it is important to use clinical rather than laboratory indications for splenectomy to prevent potentially hazardous surgery that results in patient improvement on paper but does not result in better function.

Splenectomy should be undertaken with extreme caution in patients with underlying immunologic impairment (e.g., Wiskott-Aldrich syndrome and acquired immunodeficiency syndrome) because the loss of lymphocyte and macrophage mass may further compromise an already tenuous balance between host and pathogens (187,188). With antibiotic prophylaxis, this may be manageable if the indications are strong. Autoantibodies may cause splenic destruction of platelets and worsen the primary thrombocytopenia in Wiskott-Aldrich syndrome. In these instances, the platelet count may improve with splenectomy.

Thrombotic thrombocytopenic purpura that is relapsing and recurrent has been successfully treated with splenectomy. The mechanism of benefit is unclear but appears to relate to abnormal platelet aggregation and von Willebrand multimers (189). In addition, it has been demonstrated that in many instances acute TTP is mediated by the production of autoantibodies to von Willebrand's factor–cleaving protease (190,191). Those individuals with recurrent TTP and who have identifiable antibodies to von Willebrand's factor–cleaving protease may benefit from the associated decreases in the number of B cells and circulating antibody associated with splenectomy.

Splenectomy is indicated in hypersplenism when hypersplenism is the principal cause of uncontrollable thrombocytopenia that is associated with significant bleeding, unremitting neutropenia associated with recurrent infections, or persistent anemia necessitating an increasing number of transfusions. Splenomegaly may cause substantial local symptoms (especially in portal hypertension and cirrhosis in which the spleen presses on the stomach), including impaired growth and nutri-

tion. Clinical problems, such as infection or bleeding, rather than laboratory abnormalities should be used in determining whether splenectomy is needed in portal hypertension.

The indications for splenectomy in Gaucher's disease have been somewhat modified due to the introduction of enzyme replacement therapy (ERT), because much of the hepatosplenomegaly and hematologic manifestations secondary to the disease are often ameliorated by ERT [usually within the first 6 months of therapy (192)]. It has been recommended that splenectomy be reserved for those patients who, despite ERT, suffer from severe cytopenias, persistent abdominal pain secondary to recurrent splenic infarction, growth retardation, or pressure effects secondary to splenomegaly (e.g., cardiopulmonary compromise, left-sided hydronephrosis, early satiety) (193,194). Because ERT may not lead to a complete correction of bony disease, and the spleen protects the bones against accumulation of material that causes thinning of the cortex, splenectomy may be followed by increased orthopedic problems and hepatomegaly (195). Timing of splenectomy should be carefully balanced so that the consequences of hypersplenism (which is not responsive to ERT) are sufficiently great enough to justify this additional risk. Specific benefits (improved blood counts or nutrition) should be anticipated from splenectomy, which, if necessary, should be delayed until after the teen years if possible.

In thalassemia and other disorders in which patients are transfusion dependent, the spleen may absorb a considerable amount of iron that is to be stored in other, less expendable organs such as the liver and heart. Again, documentation that the transfusion requirement is increased sufficiently to warrant this possible risk is imperative before splenectomy is performed.

Splenectomy is performed to ameliorate the pancytopenia of hairy cell leukemia. Some patients with enlarged spleens are not cytopenic, and some fail to respond to splenectomy, which should be done for clinical rather than laboratory indications (146). This remains a useful modality despite the availability of systemic therapies for this disease.

In addition to staging of Hodgkin's disease, splenectomy may be useful for treatment if the spleen is massively enlarged. Irradiating a large spleen subjects the stomach and the left kidney to doses of irradiation that are poorly tolerated by those organs—both acutely and in the long term. Thus, splenectomy with irradiation only to the splenic pedicle may be a less damaging approach to massive involvement of the spleen in Hodgkin's disease. The indications for staging laparotomy with splenectomy have changed during the past 20 years as therapies have changed. The late effects of 4000 cGy of total nodal irradiation are significant, and systemic chemotherapy is being used in a greater number of patients with lower-stage disease, particularly children (141).

Occasionally, it is necessary to do a splenectomy to make a diagnosis (196). Under no circumstances should a splenectomy be undertaken for diagnostic purposes without confirmation that the bone marrow is not fibrotic. Conditions associated with myelofibrosis may result in myeloid metaplasia, with hematopoiesis occurring in the spleen. This is perhaps one of the few true contraindications to splenectomy (197,198), because splenectomy performed under these circumstances leaves a patient without adequate resources for hematopoiesis, and it may be followed by aplasia. The risks of the splenectomy itself must be acceptable if the procedure is to be performed.

The risks of splenectomy should also be weighed carefully when considering it in the treatment of hereditary stomatocytosis. Although splenectomy is useful in decreasing the amount of hemolysis associated with hereditary stomatocytosis, there has been clear evidence of an increased incidence of thromboembolic disease in those patients who have undergone splenectomy for their disease (199,200). As such, splenectomy should probably be reserved for those with truly life-threatening situations.

Techniques of Splenectomy

PARTIAL SPLENECTOMY

Surgical procedures have become more sophisticated in recent years because of improvements in surgical techniques motivated by the observation that splenectomy leaves patients at risk for serious medical complications in later years. The intrasplenic surgical arterial anatomy is sufficiently defined (57) to permit subtotal splenectomy in instances in which total splenectomy is not desirable. Hemostatic techniques have been developed for partial excision, including mattress sutures, wedge resection with sutures, cyanoacrylate adhesives, and microfibrillar collagen omental packs (201). Hilar artery ligation minimizes blood loss. By approaching the spleen through the intersegmental planes, partial excision with lesser degrees of blood loss can be planned. These techniques are appropriate for elective partial resection [e.g., for removal of cysts (202) or tumors], for some studies on patients with Hodgkin's disease, and for splenic preservation after traumatic rupture (201,203–205).

Partial splenectomy leaves an obvious risk of regeneration of splenic tissue and is not generally indicated when the spleen is causing cell destruction. It is potentially desirable for the removal of cysts or other localized anatomic structures and for Hodgkin's disease staging. The lack of homogeneous involvement of the spleen in Hodgkin's disease has relegated this procedure to a minor or investigational role, as failure to identify disease of clinical significance is clearly possible with partial splenectomy. Partial splenectomy, splenic repair, and nonoperative management have become prominent in the management of splenic trauma and permit the salvage of more than half of ruptured spleens (201). Improvements in nonoperative diagnosis (CT scan and ultrasound) and a greater appreciation of the risks of postsplenectomy sepsis contribute substantially to the development of conservative management plans (205).

Partial splenectomy has also been advocated in the treatment of hereditary spherocytosis (HS). Partial splenectomy has been shown to decrease the rate of hemolysis in HS (206,207); however, in some patients, mild to moderate hemolysis did persist and was associated with secondary gallstone formation and aplastic crisis (207). This small risk may be deemed acceptable when considering using this procedure in young children with HS because of the protective immunologic effect afforded by leaving a portion of their spleen in place.

One should not be lulled into a false sense of security simply because some splenic tissue remains in place after a subtotal splenectomy. There has been a report of overwhelming sepsis that developed in a patient with $S\beta^0$-thalassemia who was treated with a subtotal splenectomy (208). It may be beneficial to assess splenic function after subtotal splenectomy and counsel and prophylax the patient accordingly.

TOTAL SPLENECTOMY

Massive splenomegaly presents some challenges to the surgeon, because the risk of intraoperative splenic rupture is significantly greater than when the spleen is moderately enlarged (209,210). A sufficiently large incision to permit full visualization and mobilization is imperative (211–213). A flank incision may permit identification of the vessels at the splenic hilum, through which the splenic artery may be ligated, but removal of a massively enlarged spleen is rarely possible through such an approach.

When splenectomy is performed for hematologic indications to reduce the rate of destruction of formed elements of the blood, a thorough search for accessory spleens must be performed. Because most accessory spleens are located at the splenic hilum, gastrosplenic ligament, and tail of the pancreas (113), most are readily identified at the time of splenectomy. They may be found at any place in the peritoneal cavity (214), however, and may later hypertrophy to resume destruction of formed elements. Thus, late relapse after splenectomy for ITP, autoimmune hemolytic anemia, hereditary spherocytosis, or pyruvate kinase deficiency should raise the question of whether an accessory spleen has hypertrophied and is causing destruction of cells.

Preliminary ligation of the splenic artery should be performed in the lesser sac before the spleen is mobilized to permit control of the major blood supply to the spleen. Accessory spleens should be sought at the beginning of the dissection and again after the spleen is mobilized. Many surgeons request preoperative ultrasonography so that they can identify accessory spleens, which they cannot detect through the laparoscope or may miss with an open procedure. The lateral peritoneal attachments must be incised, followed by the gastrosplenic and splenocolic ligaments. The lower pole of the spleen is raised by division of the gastroepiploic vessels and the upper by division of the short gastric vessels. This leaves the spleen attached at the hilum and the tail of the pancreas. Dissection of the splenic artery and vein must be done with special attention to protection of the tail of the pancreas, which may extend into the splenic hilum. The artery should be ligated before the vein so that blood is not sequestered in the spleen. An inflamed or massively enlarged spleen may be particularly difficult to free because of dense adhesions to the pancreas or diaphragm.

Surgical complications of splenectomy include splenic rupture with bleeding, postoperative atelectasis (especially in the lower lobes), pancreatitis, and subphrenic abscess (213,215). When splenectomy is performed for causes associated with serious systemic disease (especially portal hypertension), operative and postoperative complications, including bleeding, are more likely to develop. Postoperative splenic vein thrombosis with bleeding varices is an occasional complication (216). In patients without underlying disease, splenectomy is extremely well tolerated and has been performed without significant bleeding in many patients with thrombocytopenia (215).

LAPAROSCOPIC SPLENECTOMY

One of the more profound changes in the past 15 years in the surgical management of splenic disorders has been the introduction of laparoscopic splenectomy.

Difficulties in the adaptation of the laparoscopic approach to splenectomy have included concerns about exposure of the spleen in the left upper quadrant (especially in obese patients), acquiring the techniques necessary for achieving adequate control of the splenic blood supply, potential for injury to the pancreas due to its proximity to the splenic hilum, and risk of morbidity secondary to the complications commonly seen in patients undergoing splenectomy for hematologic disease (e.g., splenomegaly, hypervascularity from portal congestion, thrombocytopenia) (217).

Laparoscopic splenectomy for hematologic diseases has produced immediate response rates similar to open splenectomy, and the later relapse rates are similar as well (218). In addition, it has been reported that laparoscopic splenectomy is superior to open splenectomy in terms of degree of postoperative pain, amount of parenteral analgesic use, duration of ileus, length of hospital stay, duration of postoperative disability, and time to recovery of normal activity (217,219). In most cases, however, the operative time is greater for laparoscopic splenectomy than for open splenectomy; as such, the procedural cost is higher for laparoscopic splenectomy.

Indications for laparoscopic splenectomy mirror those for open splenectomy (217). Relative indications include massive splenomegaly, splenic artery aneurysm, portal hypertension, splenic abscesses, ascites, and traumatic splenic injuries (217). Uncorrectable coagulopathy and the presence of severe comorbid illness that makes the operative risk excessive should be considered absolute contraindications to laparoscopic splenectomy (217).

One of the surgical approaches used for laparoscopic splenectomy is the lateral technique (220). The patient is first placed in a right lateral decubitus position, and the surgeon stands at the patient's right side. The table is placed in the reverse Trendelenburg position to allow blood and irrigation to flow away from the surgical field. Three to four ports are then placed in the patient, with the optimal positions allowing the instruments to be 4 mm below the spleen but within reach of the diaphragm. The most lateral port should be approximately at the level of the eleventh rib, the medial site should be in proximity to the midline, and the middle port should be halfway between the others. The middle trocar is placed first with an open technique; the others are placed under direct visualization with a 30- or 45-degree laparoscope (220). A pneumoperitoneum is then created with carbon dioxide, and pressure is maintained at 13 to 15 mm Hg (221).

Before any surgical dissection, careful abdominal exploration should be done to evaluate for any accessory splenic tissue. Dissection is then begun by mobilizing the splenic flexure of the colon inferiorly (if needed). Proceeding in a caudal to cranial direction, the peritoneal attachments are divided close to the spleen. Dissection continues in a lateral to medial direction, with special care given when approaching the pancreas and splenic hilum. The inferior pole is mobilized, including the branch from the epiploic vessels, with use of either the harmonic scalpel or surgical clips (220).

Dissection continues up to the superior pole, with care taken to identify the greater curvature of the stomach and the short gastric vessels. The final division of the hilum can then be done with a vascular gastrointestinal anastomosis stapler (or a right-angled clamp may be used to individually dissect the hilar and short gastric vessels, which can then be clipped and divided) (220).

The spleen is then placed into an impermeable retrieval bag of an appropriate size. The bag is delivered through the middle port and excised in chunks with a ringed forceps (220). If it is desirable to remove an intact specimen for pathologic review, the inferior incision can be enlarged to allow for removal of the bag without tearing (221).

In recent years, the technique of laparoscopic splenectomy has been further adapted to allow surgeons to perform laparoscopic subtotal splenectomies (222). The advantages of laparoscopic subtotal splenectomy are the same as those for laparoscopic total splenectomies; in addition, laparoscopic subtotal splenectomy adds the advantage of leaving a portion of the spleen in place, thereby preserving some of the immunologic function of the spleen.

SPLENIC EMBOLIZATION

Splenic embolization is used to diminish splenic blood flow in patients with portal hypertension (223–226). This can be done in patients whose condition makes surgery risky. The procedure may raise the platelet count for a period of months (227,228). Because collateral blood vessels tend to develop readily, responses may not be sustained (229). Embolization appears to be of greatest use in patients whose surgical risks and anticipated survival times make a less invasive approach desirable (230–232).

SPLENIC AUTOTRANSPLANTATION

Autotransplantation, or the deliberate introduction of splenic tissue into the peritoneal cavity with the intention of inducing splenosis, can be performed in an attempt to minimize the risk of postsplenectomy septicemia in patients for whom residual splenic tissue is not a problem. This is done primarily during splenectomy for trauma or removal of cysts (233). Animal studies show improved clearance of bacterial inocula after autotransplantation (234,235). Animal studies also have shown improved humoral response to polysaccharide vaccine administration in autotransplanted subjects compared to subjects that have undergone total splenectomy (236). It is unclear if this benefit translates to improvement in host defenses in humans. Although autotransplantation may demonstrate some degree of restoration of a localized group of Fc receptor–bearing cells by radionuclide scan, the function of these cells does not appear to be characteristic of adequate restoration of splenic function (237). An additional apparent difficulty with autotransplantation is the restoration of the arterial blood supply to the splenic remnant (238). Random regeneration in the peritoneum appears not to restore the blood supply to the autotransplanted splenic tissue as growth of splenic tissue in the gastrosplenic ligament does.

SPLENOSIS

Splenosis is the regrowth of splenic tissue after splenic rupture (239). This may occur during the traumatic rupture that occasioned splenectomy (240) or after intraoperative rupture of the spleen. Splenosis may occur throughout the peritoneal cavity, on the pleural and pericardial surfaces, and in skin scars (239). Usually, these growths range from 1 to 7 cm in diameter (233). The splenic function of these regenerated remnants is sufficient to be visualized on radionuclide scans, and these remnants remodel erythrocyte membranes sufficiently to normalize the pit count in some patients (241). Because the risk of postsplenectomy septicemia is already low in patients who undergo splenectomy for trauma, it is difficult to assess whether patients with splenosis actually have a lower risk of such infections. The functional capacity of these splenotic nodules is real, however, and splenosis appears to be potentially beneficial for patients whose spleens were removed for nonhematologic indications. Animal studies of splenosis suggest that preservation of the arterial supply and of the architecture of splenic tissue is important for the splenic nodules to retain their protective filter function (10,238,242–244). Splenic implants without adequate blood supply may not be protective against pneumococcal septicemia even if the volume of tissue is considerable (204,233,245–247). The volume of splenic tissue appears to be regulated by humoral factors that are poorly defined (248). After splenectomy, the accessory spleens or implants hypertrophy in response to these factors.

SPLENIC IRRADIATION

There have been reports of small series of very poor surgical candidates who have undergone splenic irradiation for management of their underlying splenic disorder after failing pharmacologic management. Recently reported series include the use of splenic irradiation in the treatment of cytopenias, splenomegaly, or splenic pain in conditions such as myelofibrosis with myeloid metaplasia (249); hypersplenism due to congestive splenomegaly (250); HIV-associated ITP (251,252); and idiopathic myelofibrosis (253). Total doses of radiation administered have ranged from 500 to 9800 cGy (249–253), and reported side effects consisted primarily of cytopenias (249,253). Response rates have been variable and, in most cases, short lived. However, the responses have been significant enough to suggest that the use of splenic irradiation could be a viable method of palliative care for those patients who fail medical intervention and cannot tolerate surgical intervention.

**TABLE 21-4. Organisms Causing Severe
Infections in Asplenic Patients**

Bacteria
  Streptococcus pneumoniae
  Haemophilus influenzae types b and f
  Neisseria meningitidis
  Pseudomonas aeruginosa
  Escherichia coli
  Dysgenic fermenter 2
  Other encapsulated organisms
Protozoa
  Babesia species
  Plasmodium species

POSTSPLENECTOMY SEPSIS

Bacterial infection with septicemia rapidly progressing to circulatory collapse and death is a recognized syndrome after splenectomy (254–256). Abrupt onset, rapid development of shock, and frequent accompaniment of meningitis are characteristic of overwhelming postsplenectomy sepsis (257). Its occurrence is more frequent in younger patients (258) and during the first few years after splenectomy, but it may occur in older patients and years after splenectomy (259–261). Patients generally run high fevers and may appear well at the time of initial evaluation (254). Once cardiovascular decompensation occurs, the process is frequently fatal regardless of therapy. Adrenal hemorrhage (Waterhouse-Friderichsen syndrome) can accompany cardiovascular collapse with the septicemia (262). Encapsulated organisms that evade normal clearance mechanisms and intraerythrocyte parasites are the greatest threats to these patients.

Streptococcus pneumoniae is the most common cause of septicemia in asplenic children and adults, accounting for 60% of cases (263,264) (Table 21-4). *Neisseria meningitidis* and *Haemophilus influenzae* type b account for another 25%, with the remainder caused by *Escherichia coli*, *Streptococcus* spp, *Staphylococcus aureus*, *Klebsiella* spp, *Salmonella* spp, anaerobic oral organisms such as the DF-2 group, and *Pseudomonas aeruginosa* (265–272). Severe infections with *Brucella* spp and *Pasteurella tularensis* are also described after splenectomy. Fatal malaria (273) and severe babesiosis (274) are other potential infectious complications of asplenia.

Bacteria proliferate in the bloodstream when they are not cleared by the splenic macrophages. Studies in animals demonstrate the intravascular growth of bacteria in the absence of the spleen (27). The ability of hepatic, pulmonary, and bone marrow macrophages to compensate for the absence of the spleen is especially compromised in the absence of specific antibody to the encapsulated organisms (53). Splenic macrophages ingest particles with far fewer antibody and complement molecules on their surfaces than hepatic macrophages do, and the contact between particles and the phagocytes is much closer in the spleen than in the liver (275). Deposition of complement via the alternative pathway is insufficient in the absence of type-specific antibody to opsonize bacteria for the liver (53,275). In the presence of type-specific antibody, the liver is able to recognize encapsulated organisms, and complement is activated by means of the classic pathway (276). The role of antibody is important in the prevention of postsplenectomy sepsis and contributes to the greater susceptibility of younger (preimmune) children to the development of this complication (Fig. 21-9). Because young children do not respond well to carbohydrate antigens (277,278), immunization with purified polysaccharide vaccines is frequently not protective for the group at highest risk (53,279). However, the introduction of protein-conjugated polysaccharide vaccines (e.g., the heptavalent conjugate pneumococcal vaccine), which have been shown to be effective in young children (280), may further aid in the prevention of postsplenectomy sepsis.

The incidence of overwhelming postsplenectomy septicemia is affected by not only the age and immune status of the patient but also his or her underlying disease. Whereas children who undergo splenectomy as a result of trauma have a 58 times greater risk of death from sepsis than healthy children, those who undergo splenectomy for thalassemia have a 1000 times greater risk (257). The patients at lowest risk have no associated underlying immunologic deficits (e.g., ITP and congenital hemolytic anemias). Those at highest risk have associated reticuloendothelial blockade, especially associated with iron overload (thalassemia), or lymphoid immunodeficiency [including Hodgkin's disease, other lymphomas, and congenital or acquired immunodeficiency (e.g., Wiskott-Aldrich syndrome)] (281). Additionally, patients with nonsurgical asplenia induced by irradiation or splenic infarction (156), as in sickle cell disease (32), share the high risk of sepsis accompanying asplenia. Complicating factors may be genetic differences in antibody production in response to carbohydrate antigens, which appear to develop later or to a lesser extent in African

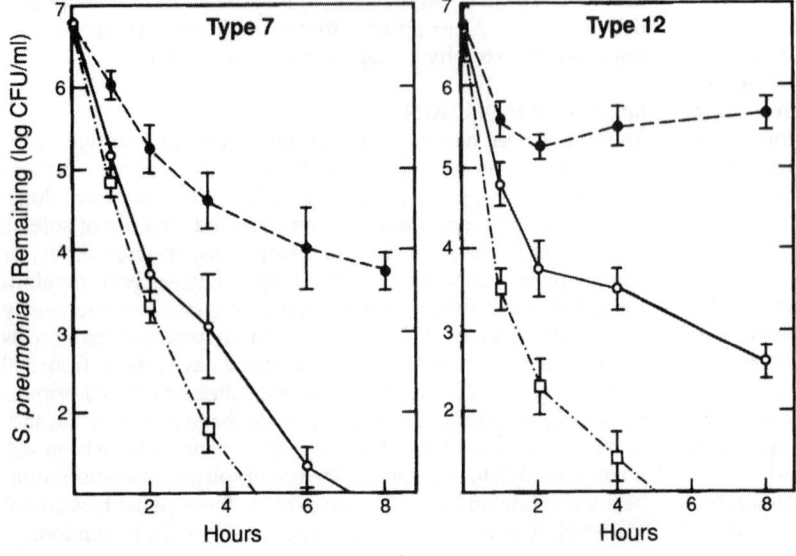

Figure 21-9. Clearance of pneumococci from the blood of guinea pigs. Immunization corrects the clearance defect for both types of pneumococci. *Squares*, splenectomized guinea pig immunized to the specific pneumococcal serotype indicated; *open circles*, intact, unimmunized guinea pig; *filled circles*, splenectomized, unimmunized guinea pig. (Brown EJ, Hosea SW, Frank MM. The role of the spleen in experimental pneumococcal bacteremia. *J Clin Invest* 1981;67:975.)

TABLE 21-5. Immunization Recommendations for Patients at High Risk for Pneumococcal Invasive Infection[a]

Age	Number of Previous Doses	Recommendations
<24 mo	None	PCV7 as recommended for infants and toddlers
24–59 mo	4 doses PCV7	1 dose of 23-PS at 24 mo, at least 6–8 wk after last dose of PCV7
24–59 mo	1–3 doses PCV7	1 dose of PCV7; 1 dose of 23-PS 6–8 wk after last dose of PCV7; 1 dose 23-PS 3–5 yr after last dose of 23-PS
24–59 mo	1 dose 23-PS	2 doses PCV7 6–8 wk apart beginning 6–8 wk after last dose of 23-PS; 1 dose 23-PS 3–5 yr after last dose of 23-PS
24–59 mo	None	2 doses PCV7 6–8 wk apart; 1 dose 23-PS 6–8 wk after the last dose of PCV7; 1 dose of 23-PS 3–5 yr after last dose of 23-PS
6–13 yr	None	1 dose of PCV7; 1 dose of 23-PS 6–8 wk after PCV7; repeat 23-PS 3–5 yr after first dose OR 1 dose 23-PS; repeat 23-PS 3–5 yr after the first dose
>13 yr	None	1 dose of 23-PS; repeat 3–5 yr after the first dose

PCV7, heptavalent pneumococcal conjugate vaccine; 23-PS, 23-valent pneumococcal capsular polysaccharide vaccine.
[a]Patients undergoing elective splenectomy or who are to receive immunocompromising therapy should receive either the 23-PS or PCV7 immunization at least 2 wk before surgery/treatment.
Adapted from American Academy of Pediatrics. Committee on Infectious Diseases. Policy statement: recommendations for the prevention of pneumococcal infections, including the use of pneumococcal conjugate vaccine (Prevnar), pneumococcal polysaccharide vaccine, and antibiotic prophylaxis. *Pediatrics* 2000:106:362–366.

Americans and Native Americans, and coexisting Ig subtype deficiency, such as IgG2 (277,278).

Gorse (282) combined several series of reports and estimated the incidence of postsplenectomy septicemia in various conditions. The number of fatalities ranged from 33% to 71% in those who developed septicemia (282). These data are imperfect because the studies were all retrospective, and most reflected splenectomies that occurred before the era of antibiotic prophylaxis and pneumococcal vaccination.

The risk of infection appears to be greatest in the first 2 years after splenectomy (269) but may occur years later (259,270,271). Infants and children appear to be at greater risk (255–258). In Singer's review (257), serious bacterial infection occurred in 21.0% of children who underwent splenectomy for HS before 1 year of age but in only 3.5% of children who underwent splenectomy later in life (Fig. 21-9). Chaikof (260), in a retrospective review done 10 to 20 years after surgery, found an incidence of overwhelming postsplenectomy septicemia of 3.77% in children who underwent splenectomy before 16 years of age and 0.34% in patients who underwent splenectomy as adults. Again, these data reflect many cases of splenectomy done very early in life and during a time when few patients received postsplenectomy immunization or antibiotic prophylaxis.

Other data suggest that, in fact, the true rate of overwhelming postsplenectomy infection (OPSI) is actually lower than that cited in the previous paragraphs. This view is supported by the report by Schwartz and his colleagues that showed a rate of fulminant sepsis in splenectomized individuals of 0.18/100 person-years and a mortality rate from fulminant sepsis of only 0.9/1000 person-years (283). In addition, in a review of fatal fulminant postsplenectomy sepsis in patients with HS, Schilling found that the rate of fatal infection was only 0.73/1000 person-years (284). Of note, none of those who died was receiving prophylactic penicillin, and none had been immunized against pneumococcus (284).

The previous data that describe the risk of overwhelming sepsis after splenectomy certainly are concerning to all who care for patients with hyposplenia/asplenia. Because of these data, the medical community has been alerted to these risks and has responded to them appropriately by immunizing and providing antibiotic prophylaxis for these patients. As such, the risk for OPSI has diminished notably over the past couple of decades. This is best demonstrated in the review by Konradsen and colleagues in which they reported on all cases of invasive pneumococcal infection in splenectomized patients from Denmark for the time before pneumococcal vaccination and penicil-

lin prophylaxis were initiated (1969 to 1978) and after these precautions were put in place (1979 to 1987) (285). Konradsen found that the incidence of culture-proven postsplenectomy pneumococcal infections decreased from 3.9% in the former group to 0.0% in the latter group (285).

Prevention of the devastating consequences of OPSI in hyposplenia/asplenia depends primarily on having the patient, family, and medical staff recognize the risk, undertake preventive measures, and treat with antibiotics at the first sign of a possible infection. All patients who are at risk of having or developing splenic hypofunction because of an underlying disease should have their splenic function assessed. When indicated, they should be immunized and receive prophylactic antibiotics (286). Early recognition of splenic hypofunction is most important in children with sickle cell syndromes and cardiac lesions associated with asplenia or polysplenia. Vaccination against *S. pneumoniae, H. influenzae* type b, and *N. meningitidis* is extremely important in the prevention of invasive bacterial infection.

In August of 2000, the American Academy of Pediatrics released a policy statement on the prevention of pneumococcal disease in children (287). Patients at high risk were defined as those with sickle cell anemia, other types of functional or anatomic asplenia, human immunodeficiency virus infection, or primary immunodeficiency and children who are receiving immunosuppressive therapy (287). It is recommended that those children receive the heptavalent pneumococcal conjugate vaccine if younger than 6 years of age or the 23-valent pneumococcal capsular polysaccharide vaccine if older than 6 years of age (see Table 21-5 for complete details). It is recommended that the polyvalent polysaccharide pneumococcal vaccine be repeated every 3 to 5 years thereafter. The statement also recommends administering antibiotic prophylaxis beginning before 2 months of age. This can be discontinued after the patient's fifth birthday if there has been no history of invasive pneumococcal disease and the patient has been on the prophylactic antibiotics for more than 2 years.

Patients scheduled for elective splenectomy should receive either the polyvalent polysaccharide pneumococcal vaccine or the heptavalent pneumococcal conjugate vaccine (depending on age), the trivalent meningococcal vaccine, and (if not previously given) the *H. influenzae* type b vaccine at least 72 hours before splenectomy for greatest efficacy. This permits antigen processing and maximizes the immune response to the vaccine before splenectomy (286). Ideally, splenectomy should be delayed until a child is at least 5 years of age to permit lymphoid maturation and minimize the risks of postsplenectomy sepsis.

TABLE 21-6. Antibiotic Doses for Prophylaxis for Patients with Asplenia/Hyposplenia

Age	Penicillin V	Amoxicillin	Erythromycin (EES)[a]
2 mo to 3 yr	125 mg p.o. b.i.d.	125 mg p.o. b.i.d.	125 mg p.o. q.i.d.
3 yr and older	250 mg p.o. b.i.d.	250 mg p.o. b.i.d.	250 mg p.o. q.i.d.

[a]To be used only for patients with a penicillin allergy.

Prophylactic antibiotics are of demonstrated benefit in the prevention of bacterial infections in patients with sickle cell syndromes (279). All children with sickle cell disease and Sβ^0-thalassemia should receive prophylactic antibiotics through 5 years of age. There is no clear benefit to continuing prophylactic antibiotics beyond 5 years of age in patients with sickle cell anemia who have not had a history of invasive pneumococcal disease (288). If compliance is poor, the risk of selecting resistant organisms by intermittent use of prophylactic antibiotics must be considered.

The use of prophylactic antibiotics in young children with congenital asplenia and those who have undergone splenectomy is also advised. There are no clear guidelines on how long to continue prophylaxis, but in the authors' opinion, young children should be continued on prophylactic antibiotics at least until 5 years of age or, at minimum, for 2 years after splenectomy.

The issue of antibiotic prophylaxis is even more unclear for adults who are noted to have hyposplenia or who received a splenectomy. Again, the authors would recommend placing these individuals on prophylactic antibiotics for at least 2 years after their diagnosis or splenectomy. In addition, some groups also recommend that patients with hyposplenia/asplenia keep a supply of antibiotics on hand and use them immediately for episodes of fever, malaise, and chills (289). Recommended dosages of prophylactic antibiotics can be found in Table 21-6. Table 21-7 gives further recommendations for the prevention of OPSI.

The single best protection against overwhelming postsplenectomy septicemia is a high index of suspicion and a rapid response to fever on the part of the patient, family, and medical staff. Antibiotics should be readily available, and patients with documented fever exceeding 38.5°C should be treated. It is possible to treat selected outpatients with oral or parenteral agents (290). It is important to keep in mind that patients may appear well minutes before developing circulatory collapse, and these patients must be considered at high risk regardless of how well they appear. The risk of infection with organisms other than those sensitive to penicillin, including gram-negative organisms, must be kept in mind (291). Choice of empiric antibiotics depends on local epidemiology. In areas where penicillin-

TABLE 21-7. Prevention of Postsplenectomy Septicemia

Avoid splenectomy when possible.
Delay splenectomy until patient is older than 5 yr.
Immunize before splenectomy with pneumococcal vaccine, polyvalent meningococcal vaccine, and conjugated haemophilus vaccine.
Daily prophylactic antibiotic administration (penicillin or amoxicillin by mouth or erythromycin for penicillin-allergic patients) for all patients at high risk of development of sepsis (i.e., younger patients, underlying disease).
Aggressive education of patient and family to ensure rapid medical attention.
Obtain MedicAlert or equivalent warning system.

TABLE 21-8. Emergency Management of Febrile Asplenic Patients

Temperature below 38.5°C
  Examine patient (vital signs, localizing findings, especially any indication of meningitis).
  Obtain blood culture and other cultures as indicated.
  Administer stat intravenous or intramuscular antibiotics (ceftriaxone, ampicillin, or equivalent coverage).
  Begin oral antibiotics to cover encapsulated organisms (choice depends on local epidemiology and whether the patient is receiving prophylactic antibiotics).
Temperature above 38.5°C
  Examine patient (vital signs, localizing findings, especially any indication of meningitis).
  Obtain blood cultures, complete blood cell count, and other cultures as indicated.
  Administer stat intravenous antibiotics (ceftriaxone, ampicillin, or equivalent coverage).
  Maintain intravenous hydration and observe patient for at least 6–12 hr in medical facility.
  Consider hospital admission, depending on local circumstances, ability to monitor patient, and proximity to medical facility. Discharge requires a responsible adult immediately available to bring patient back in event of change in clinical status.

resistant pneumococcus and ampicillin-resistant *Haemophilus* are uncommon, ampicillin may be sufficient, but a second- or third-generation cephalosporin is more commonly chosen. A well-educated patient and family are the best first-line defenses and prevent most fatal outcomes (292) (Table 21-8).

OTHER COMPLICATIONS OF SPLENECTOMY

Thrombosis is a known potential complication of splenectomy. Again, those with hereditary stomatocytosis are at an increased risk for thrombosis after splenectomy (199). Although the mechanism is not fully defined, some have postulated that the continued circulation of fragmented red blood cells—fragments that would be cleared by the intact spleen—is thrombogenic due to exposed phospholipids from the fragmented red blood cell membrane (199). In addition, one may see a marked increase in the platelet count after splenectomy for other conditions. This may be associated with a tendency to develop thrombosis in adults. Antiplatelet agents (aspirin and dipyridamole) may be used to reduce the risk of thrombosis (293). Even marked thrombocytosis rarely causes clinical problems in children, but thrombosis may occur in older patients with myeloproliferative disorders or coexisting arteriosclerosis.

Removal of the spleen also removes a major site of antibody production. Serum IgM and properdin levels are lower after splenectomy (48,276).

The risk of ischemic heart disease may also increase after splenectomy. In one study (294), death from ischemic heart disease was 1.86 times more frequent during a 28-year follow-up in splenectomized men than in men whose spleens were intact—a statistically significant difference. Chronically elevated platelet counts may contribute to this risk, as many of the lipids present in arteriosclerotic plaques originate in platelet membranes. Arteriosclerosis involves neutrophil activation as well; as such, the chronically higher neutrophil count in asplenic patients may also contribute to a higher incidence of cardiovascular disease.

SPLENOMEGALY

Spleens that are palpable more than 2 cm below the left costal margin are usually abnormal (248). Many enlarged spleens are

TABLE 21-9. Diseases Associated with Splenomegaly

Anatomic
  Cysts
  Hamartomas
  Pseudocysts
  Peliosis
  Systemic cystic angiomatosis
  Hemangiomas
Hyperplasia due to hematologic disorders
  Acute and chronic hemolysis
    HS, HE, SS, SC, S-thal, thalassemias, unstable hemoglobins, pyruvate kinase deficiency, autoimmune hemolytic anemia, isoimmune hemolysis, etc.
  Extramedullary hematopoiesis
    Severe hemolytic anemias, especially in fetus and neonates
    Myeloproliferative diseases: polycythemia vera, chronic myelogenous leukemia, thrombocythemia, myelofibrosis with myeloid metaplasia
    Osteopetrosis
Infections
  Bacterial
    Acute sepsis: *Salmonella* (typhoid fever), *Streptococcus pneumoniae, Haemophilus influenzae, Staphylococcus aureus,* etc.
    Chronic infections: subacute bacterial endocarditis, chronic meningococcemia, brucellosis, tularemia, etc.
    Local infections: splenic abscess, pyogenic liver abscess, cholangitis
  Viral
    Acute viral infections, especially in children
    Congenital: cytomegalovirus, herpes simplex, rubella
    Hepatitis A, B, and C, cytomegalovirus
    Epstein-Barr virus
    Psittacosis
    Viral hemophagocytic syndromes
    Human immunodeficiency virus
  Spirochetal
    Syphilis (especially congenital)
    Lyme disease
    Leptospirosis
  Rickettsial
    Rocky Mountain spotted fever
    Q fever
    Typhus
  Fungal or mycobacterial
    Disseminated tuberculosis
    Disseminated histoplasmosis
    South American blastomycosis

Parasitic
  Malaria
  Babesiosis
  Toxoplasmosis, especially congenital
  Visceral larval migrans (*Toxocara canis, Toxocara catis*)
  Leishmaniasis (kala-azar)
  Schistosomiasis
  Trypanosomiasis
  Fascioliasis
Immunologic, inflammatory
  Collagen vascular
    Systemic lupus erythematosus
    Rheumatoid arthritis (Felty's syndrome)
    Mixed connective tissue disease
    Systemic vasculitis
  Other
    Serum sickness
    Drug hypersensitivity, especially phenytoin
    Graft-versus-host disease
    Sjögren's syndrome
    Cryoglobulinemia
    Amyloidosis
    Inflammatory bowel disease
    Myasthenia gravis
    Sarcoidosis
    Large granular lymphocytosis and neutropenia
    Hyperimmune B-lymphocyte disorder
    Weber-Christian disease
    Familial Mediterranean fever
    Histiocytosis syndromes
    Systemic mastocytosis
Malignancies
  Primary: leukemia, lymphoma, angiosarcoma, etc.
  Metastatic disease
Storage diseases
  Gaucher's disease, Niemann-Pick disease, GM-1 gangliosidosis, etc.
  Glycogen storage disease type IV
  Tangier disease
  Wolman's disease
  Hyperchylomicronemia types I and V
  Mucopolysaccharidoses
Congestive disorders
  Congestive heart failure
  Intrahepatic cirrhosis
  Extrahepatic portal, splenic, hepatic vein obstruction (Budd-Chiari syndrome)
Idiopathic disorders

not palpable on physical examination, however, because of their relationship to other organs and the thoracic cage. No clear etiology is found for some spleens that are repeatedly found to be enlarged. Patients with low diaphragms often have palpable spleens. Approximately 3% of college freshmen (136) and 5% to 15% of younger children (295) have palpable spleens. A relaxed patient must be examined supine and in the right lateral decubitus position with the knees up to maximize the probability that a palpable spleen is appreciated by the examiner. In adults, the spleen ranges from 100 to 250 g, with an upper limit of 15 cm in length on ultrasound examination. The spleen is proportionally larger in normal children and adolescents and involutes with age so that a barely palpable spleen in an older person is far more likely to represent pathology than in a younger patient.

A variety of conditions can cause splenomegaly (Table 21-9). Chronic splenomegaly may be due to several types of processes, such as the "work hypertrophy" seen with acute and chronic infections and in hemolytic anemias; congestive enlargement due to heart failure, cirrhosis, or portal hypertension; infiltration with sarcoidosis, amyloidosis, or storage diseases such as Gaucher's; myeloproliferation as in chronic myelogenous leukemia and myeloid metaplasia; and neoplastic causes, as in lymphomas, hemangiomas, and cysts. Acute

enlargement of the spleen is usually due to trauma or to sequestration crises in sickle syndromes.

REFERENCES

1. Virchow R. Weisses Lut und Ilztumoren. *Med Zeit* 1846;15:157.
2. King H, Shumacher HB. Splenic studies. 1. Susceptibility to infection after splenectomy performed in infancy. *Ann Surg* 1952;136:239.
3. Dear TN, Colledge WH, Carlton MB, et al. The Hox11 gene is essential for cell survival during spleen development. *Development* 1995;121:2909.
4. Lettice LA, Purdie LA, Carlson GJ, et al. The mouse bagpipe gene controls development of axial skeleton, skull, and spleen. *Proc Natl Acad Sci U S A* 1999;96:9695.
5. Pabst O, Zweigerdt R, Arnold HH. Targeted disruption of the homeobox transcription factor Nkx2-3 in mice results in postnatal lethality and abnormal development of small intestine and spleen. *Development* 1999;126:2215.
6. Patterson KD, Drysdale TA, Krieg PA. Embryonic origins of spleen asymmetry. *Development* 2000;127:167.
7. Tischendorf F. On the evolution of the spleen. *Experientia* 1985;41:145.
8. Weiss L. The spleen. In: Weiss L, ed. *Histology, cell, and tissue biology.* Vol. 5. New York: Elsevier, 1983:236.
9. Eikelenboom P, Dijkstra CD, Boorsma DM, et al. Characterization of lymphoid and nonlymphoid cells in the white pulp of the spleen using immunohistoperoxidase techniques and enzyme histochemistry. *Experientia* 1985;41:209.
10. van Wyck DB, Witte MH, Witte CL. Compensatory spleen growth and protective function in rats. *Clin Sci (Lond)* 1986;71:573.

11. Kashimura M, Fujita T. A scanning electron microscope study of the human spleen: relationship between the microcirculation and function. *Scanning Microsc* 1987;1:841.
12. Groom AC. Microcirculation of the spleen: new concepts, new challenges. *Microvasc Res* 1987;34:269.
13. Weiss L. A scanning electron microscopic study of the spleen. *Blood* 1974;43:665.
14. Weiss L. The red pulp of the spleen: structural basis of blood flow. *Clin Haematol* 1983;12:375.
15. Theil GA, Downey H. The development of the mammalian spleen with special reference to its hematopoietic activity. *Am J Anat* 1921;28:279.
16. Freeman MH, Saunders EF. Hematopoiesis in the human spleen. *Am J Hematol* 1981;11:271.
17. Playfair JHL, Wolfendale MR, Kay HEM. The leukocytes of the peripheral blood in the human foetus. *Br J Haematol* 1963;9:336.
18. Linch DC, Knott RJ, Rodeck CH, et al. Studies of circulating hematopoietic progenitor cells in human fetal blood. *Blood* 1982;59:976.
19. Wolf BC, Luevano E, Neiman RS. Evidence to suggest that the human fetal spleen is not a hematopoietic organ. *Am J Clin Pathol* 1983;80:140.
20. Calhoun DA, Li Y, Braylan RC, et al. Assessment of the contribution of the spleen to granulocytopoiesis and erythropoiesis of the mid-gestation human fetus. *Early Hum Dev* 1996;46:217.
21. McCulloch AE, Till JE. The sensitivity of cells from normal mouse bone marrow to gamma radiation in vitro and in vivo. *Radiat Res* 1962;16:882.
22. Ford CE, Micklem HS. The thymus and lymph nodes in radiation chimaeras. *Lancet* 1963;1:359.
23. Copeland NG, Gilbert DJ, Cho BC. Mast cell growth factor maps near the steel locus on mouse chromosome 10 and is deleted in a number of steel alleles. *Cell* 1990;63:175.
24. Flanagan JG, Leder P. The kit ligand: a cell surface molecule altered in steel mutant fibroblasts. *Cell* 1990;63:185.
25. Bowdler AJ. Regional variations in the proportion of red cells in the blood in man. *Br J Haematol* 1969;16:557.
26. Weiss L, Javassoli M. Anatomical hazards to the passage of erythrocytes through the spleen. *Semin Hematol* 1970;7:372.
27. McBride JA, Dacie JV, Shapley R. The effect of splenectomy on the leucocyte count. *Br J Haematol* 1968;14:225.
28. Nathan DG. Rubbish in the red cell. *N Engl J Med* 1969;281:558.
29. Crosby WH. Splenic remodeling of red cell surfaces. *Blood* 1977;50:643.
30. Holroyde CP, Oski RA, Gardner FH. The "pocked" erythrocyte: red cell surface alterations in reticuloendothelial immaturity of the neonate. *N Engl J Med* 1969;281:516.
31. Corrigan JJ Jr, VanWyck DB, Crosby WH. Clinical disorders of splenic function: the spectrum from asplenism to hypersplenism. *Lymphology* 1983;16:101.
32. Buchanan GR, Holtkamp CA, Horton JA. Formation and disappearance of pocked erythrocytes: studies in human subjects and laboratory animals. *Am J Hematol* 1987;25:243.
33. Lux SE, John KM. Isolation and partial characterization of a high molecular weight red cell membrane protein complex which is normally removed by the spleen. *Blood* 1977;50:625.
34. Lipson RL, Bayrd ED, Watkins CH. The post-splenectomy blood picture. *Am J Clin Pathol* 1959;32:526.
35. Groom AC, Levesque MJ, Bruckschweiger D. Flow stasis, blood gases and glucose levels in the red pulp of the spleen. *Adv Exp Med Biol* 1977;94:567.
36. Song SH, Groom AC. Sequestration and possible maturation of reticulocytes in the normal spleen. *Can J Physiol Pharmacol* 1972;50:400.
37. Aguado MT, Mannik M. Clearance kinetics and organ uptake of complement-solubilized immune complexes in mice. *Immunology* 1987;60:255.
38. Amlot PL, Hayes AE. Impaired human antibody response to the thymus-independent antigen, DNP-Ficoll, after splenectomy: implications for post-splenectomy infections. *Lancet* 1985;1:1008.
39. Mitchell J, Abbot A. Antigens in immunity. XVI. A light and electron microscope study of antigen localization in the rat spleen. *Immunology* 1971;21:207.
40. Nossal GJV, Austin CM, Pye J, et al. Antigens in immunity. XII. Antigen trapping in the spleen. *Int Arch Allergy Appl Immunol* 1966;29:368.
41. Humphrey JH, Grennan D. Different macrophage populations distinguished by means of fluorescent polysaccharides: recognition and properties of marginal-zone macrophages. *Eur J Immunol* 1981;11:221.
42. Kumararatne DS, Bazin H, MacLennan ICM. Marginal zones: the major B cell compartment of rat spleens. *Eur J Immunol* 1981;11:858.
43. Hammarstrom L, Smith CIE. Development of anti-polysaccharide antibodies in asplenic children. *Clin Exp Immunol* 1986;66:457.
44. MacLennan ICM. The lymphocytes of splenic marginal zones: a distinct B cell lineage. *Immunol Today* 1981;3:305.
45. Brown JC, De Jesus DG, Holborow EJ, et al. Lymphocyte-mediated transport of aggregated gamma-globulin into germinal centre areas of normal mouse spleen. *Nature* 1973;228:367.
46. Sullivan JL, Schiffman G, Miser J, et al. Immune response after splenectomy. *Lancet* 1978;1:178.
47. Claret I, Morales L, Montaner A. Immunological studies in the post-splenectomy syndrome. *J Pediatr Surg* 1975;10:59.
48. Schumacher MJ. Serum immunoglobulin and transferrin levels after childhood splenectomy. *Arch Dis Child* 1970;45:114.
49. Jandl J, Greenberg MS, et al. Clinical determination of the sites of red cell destruction in the hemolytic anemias. *J Clin Invest* 1956;35:842.
50. Brown EJ, Hosea SW, Hammer CH, et al. A quantitative analysis of the interactions of antipneumococcal antibody and complement in experimental pneumococcal bacteremia. *J Clin Invest* 1982;69:85.
51. Brown EJ, Hosea SW, Frank MM. The role of antibody and complement in the reticuloendothelial clearance of pneumococci from the bloodstream. *Rev Infect Dis* 1983;5[Suppl]:8797.
52. Brown EJ, Hosea SW, Frank MM. The role of the spleen in experimental pneumococcal bacteremia. *J Clin Invest* 1981;67:975.
53. Hosea SW, Brown EJ, Hamburger MI, et al. Opsonic requirements for intravascular clearance after splenectomy. *N Engl J Med* 1981;304:245.
54. Davies BN, Withrington PG. The action of drugs on smooth muscle of the capsule and blood vessels of the spleen. *Pharmacol Rev* 1973;25:373.
55. Aster RH. Pooling of platelets in the spleen: role in the pathogenesis of "hypersplenic" thrombocytopenia. *J Clin Invest* 1966;45:645.
56. Jandl JH, Aster RH. Increased splenic pooling and the pathogenesis of hypersplenism. *Am J Med Sci* 1967;253:383.
57. Dawson AA, Bennett B, Jones PF, et al. Thrombotic risks of staging laparotomy with splenectomy in Hodgkin's disease. *Br J Surg* 1981;68:842.
58. el-Khishen MA, Henderson JM, Millikan WJ Jr, et al. Splenectomy is contraindicated for thrombocytopenia secondary to portal hypertension. *Surg Gynecol Obstet* 1985;160:233.
59. Jandl JH, Files NM, et al. Proliferative response of the spleen and liver to hemolysis. *J Exp Med* 1965;122:299.
60. Blendis LM, Banks DC, Ramboer C, et al. Spleen blood flow and splanchnic haemodynamics in blood dyscrasia and other splenomegalies. *Clin Sci* 1970;38:73.
61. Stathers GM, Ma MH, Blackburn CRB. Extra-hepatic portal hypertension: the clinical evaluation, investigation and results of treatment of 28 patients. *Aust Ann Med* 1968;17:12.
62. Hess CE, Ayers CR, Sandusky WR, et al. Mechanism of dilutional anemia in massive splenomegaly. *Blood* 1976;47:629.
63. Crosby WH. Siderocytes and the spleen. *Blood* 1956;12:165.
64. Barzanju J, Every JL. Changes in the spleen related to birth. *J Anat* 1979;129:819.
65. Blendis LM, Modell CB, Bowdler AJ, et al. Some effects of splenectomy in thalassemia major. *Br J Haematol* 1974;28:77.
66. Heaton LD, Crosby WH, et al. Splenectomy in the treatment of hypoplasia of the bone marrow: with a report of 12 cases. *Ann Surg* 1957;146:634.
67. Sills RH, Tamburlin JH, Barrios NJ, et al. Formation of intracellular vesicles in neonatal and adult erythrocytes: evidence against the concept of neonatal hyposplenism. *Pediatr Res* 1988;24:703.
68. Freeman RM, Johnston D, Mahoney MJ, et al. Development of splenic reticuloendothelial function in neonates. *J Pediatr* 1980;96:466.
69. Diamond LK. The concept of functional asplenia. *N Engl J Med* 1969;281:958.
70. Llende M, Santiago-Delpin EA, Lavergne J. Immunobiological consequences of splenectomy: a review. *J Surg Res* 1986;40:85.
71. Timens W, Poppema A. Impaired immune response to polysaccharides. *N Engl J Med* 1987;317:837.
72. Ozsoylu S, Hosain F, McIntyre PA. Functional development of phagocytic activity of the spleen. *J Pediatr* 1977;90:560.
73. Polhemus DW, Schaefer WB. Absent spleen syndrome: hematologic findings as an aid to diagnosis. *Pediatrics* 1959;24:254.
74. Krumbhaar EB. The changes produced in the blood by removal of the normal mammalian spleen. *Am J Med Sci* 1932;184:215.
75. Dean HW. Acanthocytes after splenectomy. *N Engl J Med* 1968;279:947.
76. Weiss L. The role of the spleen in the removal of normal aged red cells. *Am J Anat* 1962;111:175.
77. Douglas AS, Dacie JV. Incidence and significance of iron-containing granules in human erythrocytes and their precursors. *J Clin Pathol* 1953;6:307.
78. Acevedo G, Mauer AM. The capacity for removal of erythrocytes containing Heinz bodies in premature infants and patients following splenectomy. *J Pediatr* 1963;61.
79. Peters AM. Splenic blood flow and blood cell kinetics. *Clin Haematol* 1983;12:421.
80. Penny R, Rozenberg MC, Firkin BG. The splenic platelet pool. *Blood* 1966;27:1.
81. Libre EB, Cowan DH, Watkins SP Jr, et al. Relationship between spleen, platelets, and factor VIII levels. *Blood* 1968;31:358.
82. Robertson DAF, Bullen AW, Hall R, et al. Blood film appearances in the hyposplenism of coeliac disease. *Br J Clin Pract* 1983;37:19.
83. Holyroyde CP, Gardner FH. Acquisition of autophagic vacuoles by human erythrocytes: physiological role of the spleen. *Blood* 1970;36:566.
84. Pearson HA, Gallagher D, Chilcote R, et al. Developmental patterns of splenic dysfunction in sickle cell disorders. *Pediatrics* 1985;76:392.
85. Pearson HA. Developmental aspects of splenic function in sickle cell disease. *Blood* 1979;53:358.
86. Mettler FA. Essentials of nuclear medicine imaging. In: Stratton G, ed. *Essentials of Nuclear Medicine Imaging*, 2nd ed. Orlando: Grune & Stratton, 1986:223.
87. Armas RR, Thakur ML, Gottschalk A. A simplified method of selective spleen scintigraphy with Tc-99m-labeled erythrocytes: clinical applications. *J Nucl Med* 1980;21:413.
88. Nielsen JL, Ellegaard J, Marqversen J, et al. Detection of splenosis and ectopic spleens with 99mTc-labelled heat damaged autologous erythrocytes in 90 splenectomized patients. *Scand J Haematol* 1981;27:51.
89. Peters AM, Walport MJ, Bell RN, et al. Methods of measuring splenic blood flow and platelet transit time with "In-labelled" platelets. *J Nucl Med* 1984;25:86.

90. Siegel RS, Rae JL, Barth S, et al. Platelet survival and turnover: important factors in predicting response to splenectomy in immune thrombocytopenic purpura. *Am J Hematol* 1989;30:206.
91. Cooperberg PL. Ultrasonography of the spleen. In: Sarti DA, ed. *Diagnostic ultrasound: text and cases.* Chicago: Year Book, 1987:312.
92. Federle M, Moss AA. Computer tomography of the spleen. *Crit Rev Diagn Imaging* 1983;19:1.
93. Glazer GM, Axel L, Goldberg HI, et al. Dynamic CT of the normal spleen. *Am J Radiol* 1981;137:343.
94. Paterson A, Frush DP, Donnelly LF, et al. A pattern-oriented approach to splenic imaging in infants and children. *Radiographics* 1999;19:1465.
95. Beahrs JR, Stephens DH. Enlarged accessory spleens: CT appearance in postsplenectomy patients. *Am J Radiol* 1980;135:483.
96. Johnson FD, Raff MJ, Drasin GF, et al. Radiology in the diagnosis of splenic abscess. *Rev Infect Dis* 1985;7:10.
97. Heymsfield SB, Fulenwider T, Nordlinger B, et al. Accurate measurement of liver, kidney and spleen volume and mass by computerized axial tomography. *Ann Intern Med* 1979;90:185.
98. Henderson JM, Heymsfield SB, Horowitz J, et al. Measurement of liver and spleen volume by CT. Assessment of reproducibility and changes found following a selective distal splenorenal shunt. *Radiology* 1981;141:525.
99. Moss AA, Friedman MA, Brito AC. Determination of liver, kidney and spleen volumes by computed tomography: an experimental study in dogs. *J Comput Assist Tomogr* 1981;5:12.
100. Pierkarski J, Goldberg HI, Royal SA, et al. Difference between liver and spleen CT numbers in the normal adult: its usefulness in predicting the presence of diffuse liver disease. *Radiology* 1980;137:727.
101. Miller JH, Greenfield LD, Wald BR. Candidiasis of the liver and spleen in childhood. *Radiology* 1982;142:375.
102. Bartley DL, Hughes WT, Parvey LS, et al. Computed tomography of hepatic and splenic fungal abscesses in leukemic children. *Pediatr Infect Dis* 1982;1:317.
103. Ellert J, Kneel L. The role of computed tomography in the initial staging and subsequent management of the lymphomas. *J Comput Assist Tomogr* 1980;4:368.
104. Balcar I, Seltzer SE, Davis S, et al. CT patterns of splenic infarction: a clinical and experimental study. *Radiology* 1984;151:723.
105. Pierkarski J, Federle MP, Moss AA, et al. Computed tomography of the spleen. *Radiology* 1980;135:683.
106. Federle MP, Goldberg HI, Kaiser JA, et al. Evaluation of abdominal trauma by computed tomography. *Radiology* 1981;138:637.
107. Dachman AH, Ros PR, Murari PJ, et al. Nonparasitic splenic cysts: a report of 52 cases with radiologic-pathologic correlation. *AJR Am J Roentgenol* 1986;147:537.
108. Ros PR, Moser RP Jr, Dachman AH, et al. Hemangioma of the spleen: radiologic pathologic correlation in ten cases. *Radiology* 1987;162:73.
109. Levy DW, Rindsberg S, Friedman AC, et al. Thorotrast-induced hepatosplenic neoplasia: CT identification. *AJR Am J Roentgenol* 1986;146:997.
110. Berge T. Splenic metastases: frequencies and patterns. *Acta Pathol Microbiol Scand [A]* 1974;82:499.
111. Semelka RC, Kelekis NL, Sallah S, et al. Hepatosplenic fungal disease: diagnostic accuracy and spectrum of appearances on MR imaging. *AJR Am J Roentgenol* 1997;169:1311.
112. Bart JB, Appel MF. Recurrent hemolytic anemia secondary to accessory spleens. *South Med J* 1978;71:608.
113. Wallace D, Fromm D, Thomas D. Accessory splenectomy for idiopathic thrombocytopenic purpura. *Surgery* 1982;91:134.
114. Putschar WGJ, Manion WC. Splenic-gonadal fusion. *Am J Pathol* 1986;32:15.
115. Balaji KC, Caldamone AA, Rabinowitz R, et al. Splenogonadal fusion. *J Urol* 1996;156:854.
116. Cortes D, Thorup JM, Visfeldt J. The pathogenesis of cryptorchidism and splenogonadal fusion: a new hypothesis. *Br J Urol* 1996;77:285.
117. Bonneau D, Roume J, Gonzalez M, et al. Splenogonadal fusion limb defect syndrome: report of five new cases and review. *Am J Med Genet* 1999;86:347.
118. Moller JH, Nakib A, Anderson RC, et al. Congenital cardiac disease associated with polysplenia: a development complex of bilateral "leftsidedness." *Circulation* 1967;36:789.
119. Ivemark BI. Implications of agenesis of the spleen on the pathogenesis of cono-truncus anomalies in childhood: analysis of the heart malformations of the splenic agenesis syndrome with fourteen new cases. *Acta Paediatr* 1955;44[Suppl 104]:1.
120. Waldman JD, Rosenthal A, Smith AL, et al. Sepsis and congenital asplenia. *J Pediatr* 1977;90:555.
121. van Mierop LHS, Gessner IHS, Schiebler GL. Asplenia and polysplenia syndromes. *Birth Defects* 1972;8:36.
122. Freedom RM. The asplenia syndrome: a review of significant extracardiac structural abnormalities in twenty-nine necropsied patients. *J Pediatr* 1972;81:1130.
123. Pearson HA, Schiebler GL, Spencer RP. Functional hyposplenia in cyanotic congenital heart disease. *Pediatrics* 1971;48:277.
124. Roberts CWM, Shutter JR, Korsmeyer SJ. Hox 11 controls the genesis of the spleen. *Nature* 1994;368:747.
125. Ditchfield MR, Hutson JM. Intestinal rotational abnormalities in polysplenia and asplenia syndromes. *Pediatr Radiol* 1998;28:303.
126. Nakada K, Kawaguchi F, Munechika W, et al. Digestive tract disorders associated with asplenia/polysplenia syndrome. *J Pediatr Surg* 1997;32:91.
127. Burrig KF. Epithelial (true) splenic cysts: pathogenesis of the mesothelial and so-called epidermoid cyst of the spleen. *Am J Surg Pathol* 1988;12:275.
128. Pedrosa I, Saiz A, Arrazola J, et al. Hydatid disease: radiologic and pathologic features and complications. *Radiographics* 2000;20:795.
129. Safioleas M, Misiakos E, Manti C. Surgical treatment for splenic hydatidosis [see comments]. *World J Surg* 1997;21:374; discussion 378.
130. Browne MK. Epidermoid cyst of the spleen. *Br J Surg* 1963;50:838.
131. Sirinek KR, Evans WE. Nonparasitic splenic cysts: case report of epidermoid cyst with review of the literature. *Am J Surg* 1973;126:8.
132. Didlake RH, Miller RC. Epidermoid cyst of the spleen manifested as an abdominal abscess. *South Med J* 1986;79:635.
133. Morgenstern L, Shapiro SJ. Partial splenectomy for nonparasitic splenic cysts. *Am J Surg* 1980;139:278.
134. Martin JW. Congenital splenic cysts. *Am J Surg* 1958;96:302.
135. Ugochukwu AI, Irving M. Intraperitoneal low-pressure suction drainage following splenectomy. *Br J Surg* 1985;72:247.
136. Rappaport H. Tumors of the hematopoietic system. In: *Atlas of tumor pathology.* Fascicle 8, section 3, 1966:357.
137. Garvin DF, King FM. Cysts and nonlymphomatous tumors of the spleen. *Pathol Annu* 1981;16:61.
138. Hai SA, Genato R, Gressel I, et al. Primary splenic angiosarcoma: case report and literature review. *J Natl Med Assoc* 2000;92:143.
139. Mauch P, Larson D, Osteen R, et al. Prognostic factors for positive surgical staging in patients with Hodgkin's disease. *J Clin Oncol* 1989;8:257.
140. Clemons M, Loijens L, Goss P. Breast cancer risk following irradiation for Hodgkin's disease. *Cancer Treat Rev* 2000;26:291.
141. Eghbali H, Soubeyran P, Tchen N, et al. Current treatment of Hodgkin's disease. *Crit Rev Oncol Hematol* 2000;35:49.
142. Advani RH, Horning SJ. Treatment of early-stage Hodgkin's disease. *Semin Hematol* 1999;36:270.
143. Falk S, Stutte JH. Primary malignant lymphomas of the spleen. *Cancer* 1990;64:2612.
144. Kehoe J, Straus DJ. Primary malignant lymphomas of the spleen. Clinical features and outcome after splenectomy. *Cancer* 1988;62:1433.
145. Ratain MJ, Vardiman JW, Barker CM, et al. Prognostic variables in hairy cell leukemia after splenectomy as initial therapy. *Cancer* 1988;62:2420.
146. Golomb HM. The treatment of hairy cell leukemia. *Blood* 1987;69:979.
147. Lam KY, Tang V. Metastatic tumors to the spleen: a 25-year clinicopathologic study. *Arch Pathol Lab Med* 2000;124:526.
148. Klein B, Stein M, Kuten A, et al. Splenomegaly and solitary spleen metastasis in solid tumors. *Cancer* 1987;60:100.
149. Zamora JU, Halpern NB. Splenectomy for metastatic neoplasms. *South Med J* 1987;80:805.
150. Willey RF, Ridger A, Webb JN. Seminoma presenting as gross splenomegaly. *Scott Med J* 1982;27:254.
151. Carr AJ, Jacob G, Glanfield PA, et al. Male choriocarcinoma of the spleen: a case report. *Eur J Surg Oncol* 1987;13:75.
152. Spencer RP, et al. "Reversible" functional asplenia in combined immunodeficiency. *Int J Nucl Med Biol* 1978;5:125.
153. Garriga S, Crosby WH. The incidence of leukemia in families with hypoplasia of the marrow. *Blood* 1959;14:1008.
154. Bensinger TA, Keller AR, Merrell LF, et al. Thorotrast-induced reticuloendothelial blockade in man. *Am J Med* 1970;51:663.
155. Dailey MO, Coleman CN, Kaplan HS. Radiation-induced splenic atrophy in patients with Hodgkin's disease and non-Hodgkin's lymphoma. *N Engl J Med* 1980;302:215.
156. Coleman CN, McDougall IR, Dailey MO, et al. Functional hyposplenia after splenic irradiation for Hodgkin's disease. *Ann Intern Med* 1982;96:44.
157. Roth J, Brudler O, Henze E. Functional asplenia in malignant mastocytosis. *J Nucl Med* 1985;26:1149.
158. Al-Eid MA, Tutschka PJ, Wagner HN Jr, et al. Functional asplenia in patients with graft-versus-host disease. *J Nucl Med* 1983;24:1123.
159. Jellinek EH, Ball K. Hashimoto's disease, encephalopathy and splenic atrophy. *Lancet* 1976;1:1248.
160. Stone RW, McDaniel WR, Armstrong EM, et al. Acquired functional asplenia in sarcoidosis. *J Natl Med Assoc* 1985;77:930.
161. Pearson HA, Cornelius EA, Schwartz AD, et al. Transfusion reversible functional asplenia in young children with sickle cell anemia. *N Engl J Med* 1970;283:334.
162. Stevens MCG, Vaidya S, Serjeant GR. Fetal hemoglobin and clinical severity of homozygous sickle cell disease in early childhood. *J Pediatr* 1981;98:37.
163. Rogers DW, Serjeant BE, Serjeant GR. Early rise in "pitted" red cell count as a guide to susceptibility to infection in childhood sickle cell anaemia. *Arch Dis Child* 1982;57:338.
164. Al-Alwamy B, Wilson W, Pearson HA. Splenic function in sickle cell disease in the eastern province of Saudi Arabia. *J Pediatr* 1984;104:714.
165. Rogers DW, Vaidya S, Serjeant GR. Early splenomegaly in homozygous sickle cell disease: an indicator of susceptibility to infection. *Lancet* 1978;2:963.
166. Seeler RA, Shwaiki MZ. Acute splenic sequestration crises (ASSC) in young children with sickle cell anemia. *Clin Pediatr* 1972;11:701.
167. Emond AM, Collis R, Darvill D, et al. Acute splenic sequestration in homozygous sickle cell disease: natural history and management. *J Pediatr* 1985;107:201.
168. Topley DW, Rogers MC, Stevens C, et al. Acute splenic sequestration and hypersplenism in the first five years in homozygous sickle cell disease. *Arch Dis Child* 1981;56:765.

169. Frank MM, Hamburger MI, Lawley TJ, et al. Defective reticuloendothelial system Fc-receptor function in systemic lupus erythematosus. *N Engl J Med* 1979;300:518.

170. Frank MM, Lawley TJ, Hamburger MI, et al. Immunoglobulin G Fc-receptor-mediated clearance in autoimmune diseases. *Ann Intern Med* 1983;98:206.

171. Gertz MA, Kyle RA, Griepp RP. Hyposplenism in primary systemic amyloidosis. *Ann Intern Med* 1983;98:475.

172. Corazza GR, Lazzari R, Frisoni M, et al. Splenic function in childhood coeliac disease. *Gut* 1982;23:415.

173. Corazza GR, Frisoni M, Vaira D, et al. Effect of gluten-free diet on splenic hypofunction of adult coeliac disease. *Gut* 1983;24:228.

174. Corazza GR, Bullen AW, Hall R, et al. Simple method of assessing splenic function in coeliac disease. *Clin Sci (Lond)* 1981;60:109.

175. Bender BS, Quinn TC, Lawley TJ. Acquired immune deficiency syndrome (AIDS): a defect in Fc-receptor-specific clearance. *Clin Res* 1984;32:511a(abstr).

176. Falk S, Muller H, Stutte HJ. The spleen in acquired immunodeficiency syndrome (AIDS). *Pathol Res Pract* 1988;183:425.

177. Schreiber AD, Parsons J, McDermott P, et al. The effects of corticosteroids on the human monocyte IgG and complement receptors. *J Clin Invest* 1975;56:1189.

178. Rosse WF. Quantitative immunology of immune hemolytic anemia: II. the relationship of cell-bound antibody to hemolysis and the effect of treatment. *J Clin Invest* 1971;50:734.

179. Kelton JG. Platelet and red cell clearance is determined by the interaction of the IgG and complement on the surface of the cells and activity of the reticuloendothelial system. *Transfus Med Rev* 1987;1:75.

180. Kawada K, Terasaki PI. Evidence for immunosuppression by high-dose gammaglobulin. *Exp Hematol* 1987;15:133.

181. Petri IB, Lorincz A, Berek I. Detection of Fc-receptor blocking antibodies in anti-Rh (D) hyperimmune gammaglobulin. *Lancet* 1984;2:1478.

182. Bussel JB, Graziano JN, Kimberley RP, et al. Intravenous anti-D treatment of immune thrombocytopenic purpura: analysis of efficacy, toxicity and mechanism of effect. *Blood* 1991;77:1884.

183. Ware RE, Zimmerman SA. Anti-D: mechanisms of action. *Semin Hematol* 1998;35:14.

184. Samuelsson A, Towers TL, Ravetch JV. Anti-inflammatory activity of IVIG mediated through the inhibitory Fc receptor. *Science* 2001;291:484.

185. Paule B, Cosset HN, LeBourgeois JP. The possible role of radiotherapy in chronic lymphocytic leukaemia: a critical review. *Radiother Oncol* 1985;4:45.

186. Singh AK, Bates T, Wetherley-Mein G. A preliminary study of low-dose splenic irradiation for the treatment of chronic lymphocytic and prolymphocytic leukemias. *Scand J Haematol* 1986;37:50.

187. Barbui T, Cortelazzo S, Minetti B, et al. Does splenectomy enhance risk of AIDS in HIV-positive patients with chronic thrombocytopenia? *Lancet* 1987;2:342.

188. Lum LG, Tubergen DG, Corash L, et al. Splenectomy in the management of the thrombocytopenia of the Wiskott-Aldrich syndrome. *N Engl J Med* 1980;302:892.

189. Rowe JM, Francis CW, Cyran EM, et al. Thrombotic thrombocytopenic purpura: recovery after splenectomy associated with persistence of unusually large von Willebrand's factor multimers. *Am J Hematol* 1985;20:161.

190. Tsai HM, Chen E, Lian CY. Antibodies to von Willebrand factor-cleaving protease in acute thrombotic thrombocytopenic purpura. *N Engl J Med* 1998;339:1585.

191. Furlan M, Robles R, Solenthaler M, et al. Acquired deficiency of von Willebrand factor-cleaving protease in a patient with thrombotic thrombocytopenic purpura. *Blood* 1998;91:2839.

192. Beutler E. Enzyme replacement therapy for Gaucher's disease. *Baillieres Clin Haematol* 1997;10:751.

193. Cox TM, Schofield JP. Gaucher's disease: clinical features and natural history. *Baillieres Clin Haematol* 1997;10:657.

194. Mistry PK, Abrahamov A. A practical approach to diagnosis and management of Gaucher's disease. *Baillieres Clin Haematol* 1997;10:817.

195. Ashkenazi A, Zizov R, Mathoth Y. Effect of splenectomy on destructive bone changes in children with chronic (type I) Gaucher disease. *Eur J Pediatr* 1986;145:138.

196. Goonewardene A, Bourke JB, Ferguson R, et al. Splenectomy for undiagnosed splenomegaly. *Br J Surg* 1979;66:62.

197. Coon WW, Liepman MK. Splenectomy for agnogenic myeloid metaplasia. *Surg Gynecol Obstet* 1982;154:561.

198. Towell BL, Levine SP. Massive hepatomegaly following splenectomy for myeloid metaplasia. *Am J Med* 1987;82:371.

199. Stewart GW, Amess JAL, Eber SW, et al. Thrombo-embolic disease after splenectomy for hereditary stomatocytosis. *Br J Haematol* 1996;93:303.

200. Kemahli S, Canatan D, Cin S, et al. Post-splenectomy thrombosis and haemolytic anaemiaes. *Br J Haematol* 1997;97:505.

201. Sherman R. Management of trauma to the spleen. In: Shires GT, ed. *Advances in surgery*. Vol. 17. Chicago: Year Book, 1984.

202. Kamel R, Dunn MA. Segmental splenectomy in schistosomiasis. *Br J Surg* 1982;69:311.

203. Dixon JA, Miller F, McCloskey D, et al. Anatomy and techniques in segmental splenectomy. *Surg Gynecol Obstet* 1980;150:520.

204. Scher KS, Scott-Conner C, Jones CW, et al. Methods of splenic preservation and their effect on clearance of pneumococcal bacteremia. *Ann Surg* 1985;202:595.

205. Luna GK, Dellinger EP. Nonoperative observation treatment for splenic injuries: a safe therapeutic option? *Am J Surg* 1987;153:462.

206. Tchernia G, Gauthier F, Mielot F, et al. Effect of partial splenectomy in hereditary spherocytosis. *Blood* 1993;81:2014.

207. Bader-Meunier B, Gauthier F, Archambaud F, et al. Long-term evaluation of the beneficial effect of subtotal splenectomy for management of hereditary spherocytosis. *Blood* 2001;97:399.

208. Svarch E, Nordet I, Gonzalez A. Overwhelming septicaemia in a patient with sickle cell/beta(o) thalassemia and partial splenectomy. *Br J Haematol* 1999;104:930.

209. Wobbes T, Van der Sluis RF, Lubbers EJ. Removal of the massive spleen: a surgical risk? *Am J Surg* 1984;147:800.

210. Goldstone J. Splenectomy for massive splenomegaly. *Am J Surg* 1978;135:385.

211. Taylor MA, Kaplan HS, Nelson TS. Staging laparotomy with splenectomy for Hodgkin's disease: the Stanford experience. *World J Surg* 1985;9:449.

212. Williams SF, Golomb HM. Perspective on staging approaches in the malignant lymphomas. *Surg Gynecol Obstet* 1986;163:193.

213. Kiesewetter WB. Pediatric splenectomy: indications, technique, complications, and mortality. *Surg Clin North Am* 1975;55:449.

214. Appel MF, Bart JB. The surgical and hematologic significance of accessory spleens. *Surg Gynecol Obstet* 1976;143:191.

215. Ellison EC, Fabri PJ. Complications of splenectomy: etiology, prevention and management. *Surg Clin North Am* 1983;63:1313.

216. Roder OC. Splenic vein thrombosis with bleeding gastroesophageal varices: reports of two splenectomised cases and review of the literature. *Acta Chir Scand* 1984;150:265.

217. Glasgow RE, Mulvihill SJ. Laparoscopic splenectomy. *World J Surg* 1999;23:384.

218. Katkhouda N, Hurwitz MB, Rivera RT, et al. Laparoscopic splenectomy: outcome and efficacy in 103 consecutive patients. *Ann Surg* 1998;228:568.

219. Minkes RK, Lagzdins M, Langer JC. Laparoscopic versus open splenectomy in children. *J Pediatr Surg* 2000;35:699.

220. Walsh RM, Heniford BT. Role of laparoscopy for Hodgkin's and non-Hodgkin's lymphoma. *Semin Surg Oncol* 1999;16:284.

221. Katkhouda N, Mavor E. Minimal access surgery: laparoscopic splenectomy. *Surg Clin North Am* 2000;80:1285.

222. Sheshadri PA, Poulin EC, Mamazza J, et al. Technique for laparoscopic partial splenectomy. *Surg Laparosc Endosc Percutan Tech* 2000;10:106.

223. Jonasson O, Spigos DG, Mozes MF. Partial splenic embolisation: experience in 136 patients. *World J Surg* 1985;9:461.

224. Levy JM, Wasserman P, Pitha N. Presplenectomy transcatheter occlusion of the splenic artery. *Arch Surg* 1979;114:198.

225. Back LM, Bagwell CE, Greenbaum BH, et al. Hazards of splenic embolization. *Clin Pediatr* 1987;26:292.

226. Yoshioka H, Kuroda C, Hori S, et al. Splenic embolization for hypersplenism using steel coils. *AJR Am J Roentgenol* 1985;144:1269.

227. Maddison FE. Embolic therapy of hypersplenism. *Invest Radiol* 1973;8:280.

228. Chuang VP, Reuter SR. Experimental diminution of splenic function by selective embolization of the splenic artery. *Surg Gynecol Obstet* 1975;140:715.

229. Politis E, Spigos DG, Georgiopoulou P, et al. Partial splenic embolisation for hypersplenism of thalassaemia major: five year follow up. *BMJ* 1987;294:665.

230. Owman T, Lunderquist A, Alwmark A, et al. Embolization of the spleen for treatment of splenomegaly and hypersplenism in patients with portal hypertension. *Invest Radiol* 1979;14:457.

231. Mozes MF, Spigos DG, Pollack R, et al. Partial splenic embolization: an alternative to splenectomy—results of a prospective, randomized study. *Surgery* 1984;96:694.

232. Thanopoulos BD, Frimas CA. Partial splenic embolisation in the management of hypersplenism secondary to Gaucher disease. *J Pediatr* 1982;101:740.

233. Pabst R, Kamran D. Autotransplantation of splenic tissue. *J Pediatr Surg* 1986;21:120.

234. Dickerman JD, Horner SR, Coil JA, et al. The protective effect of intraperitoneal splenic autotransplants in mice exposed to an aerosolized suspension of type III Streptococcus pneumoniae. *Blood* 1979;54:354.

235. Patel J, Williams JS, Shmigel B, et al. Preservation of splenic function by autotransplantation of traumatized spleen in man. *Surgery* 1981;90:683.

236. Leemans R, Harms G, Rijkers GT, et al. Spleen autotransplantation provides restoration of functional splenic lymphoid compartments and improves the humoral immune response to pneumococcal polysaccharide vaccine [see comments]. *Clin Exp Immunol* 1999;117:596.

237. Leemans R, Beekhuis H, Timens W, et al. Fc-receptor function after human splenic autotransplantation. *Br J Surg* 1996;83:543.

238. Horton J, Ogden ME, Williams S, et al. The importance of splenic blood flow in clearing pneumococcal organisms. *Ann Surg* 1982;195:172.

239. Fleming CR, Dickson E, Harrison EG. Splenosis: autotransplantation of splenic tissue. *Am J Med* 1976;61:414.

240. Willis BK, Deitch EA, McDonald JC. The influence of trauma to the spleen on postoperative complications and mortality. *J Trauma* 1986;26:1073.

241. Pearson HA, Johnston D, Smith KA, et al. The born-again spleen: return of splenic function after splenectomy for trauma. *N Engl J Med* 1978;298:1389.

242. Traub A, Giebink GS, Smith C, et al. Splenic reticuloendothelial function after splenectomy, spleen repair and spleen autotransplantation. *N Engl J Med* 1987;317:559.

243. Steely WM, Satava RM, Harris RW, et al. Comparison of omental splenic autotransplant to partial splenectomy: protective effect against septic death. *Am Surg* 1987;53:702.

244. Livingston CD, Levine BA, Sirinek KR. Improved survival rate for intraperitoneal autotransplantation of the spleen after pneumococcal pneumonia. *Surg Gynecol Obstet* 1983;156:761.

245. Moore GE, Stevens RE, Moore EE, et al. Failure of splenic implants to protect against fatal postsplenectomy infection. *Am J Surg* 1983;146:413.
246. Sass W, Bergholz M, Kehl A, et al. Overwhelming infection after splenectomy in spite of some spleen remaining and splenosis: a case report. *Klin Wochenschr* 1983;61:1075.
247. Rice HM, James PD. Ectopic splenic tissue failed to prevent fatal pneumococcal septicemia after splenectomy for trauma. *Lancet* 1980;1:565.
248. Jacob HS, McDonald RA, Jandl JH. Regulation of spleen growth and sequestering function. *J Clin Invest* 1963;42:1476.
249. Elliott MA, Tefferi A. Splenic irradiation in myelofibrosis with myeloid metaplasia: a review. *Blood Rev* 1999;13:163.
250. Kenawi MM, el-Ghamrawi KA, Mohammad AA, et al. Splenic irradiation for the treatment of hypersplenism from congestive splenomegaly. *Br J Surg* 1997;84:860.
251. Blauth J, Fisher S, Henry D, et al. The role of splenic irradiation in treating HIV-associated immune thrombocytopenia. *Int J Radiat Oncol Biol Phys* 1999;45:457.
252. Soum F, Trille JA, Auvergnat JC, et al. Low-dose splenic irradiation in the treatment of immune thrombocytopenia in HIV-infected patients. *Int J Radiat Oncol Biol Phys* 1998;41:123.
253. Bouabdallah R, Coso D, Gonzague-Casabianca L, et al. Safety and efficacy of splenic irradiation in the treatment of patients with idiopathic myelofibrosis: a report on 15 patients. *Leuk Res* 2000;24:491.
254. Bisno AL, Freeman JC. The syndrome of asplenia, pneumococcal sepsis, and disseminated intravascular coagulation. *Ann Intern Med* 1970;72:389.
255. Heier HE. Splenectomy and serious infections. *Scand J Haematol* 1980;24:5.
256. Horan M, Colebatch FH. Relation between splenectomy and subsequent infection: a clinical study. *Arch Dis Child* 1962;37:398.
257. Singer DB. Postsplenectomy sepsis. *Perspect Pediatr Pathol* 1973;1:285.
258. Eraklis AJ, Kevy SV, Diamond LK, et al. Hazard of overwhelming infection after splenectomy in childhood. *N Engl J Med* 1967;276:1225.
259. Rosner F, Zarrabi MH. Late infections following splenectomy in Hodgkin's disease. *Cancer Invest* 1983;1:57.
260. Chaikof EL, McCabe CJ. Fatal overwhelming postsplenectomy infection. *Am J Surg* 1985;149:534.
261. O'Neal BJ, McDonald JC. The risk of sepsis in the asplenic adult. *Ann Surg* 1981;194:775.
262. Kingston ME, MacKenzie CR. The syndrome of pneumococcemia, disseminated intravascular coagulation and asplenia. *Can Med Assoc J* 1979;121:57.
263. Wara DW. Host defense against Streptococcus pneumoniae: the role of the spleen. *Rev Infect Dis* 1981;3:299.
264. Barrett-Connor E. Bacterial infection and sickle cell anemia: an analysis of 250 infections in 166 patients and a review of the literature. *Medicine* 1971;50:97.
265. Mower WR, Hawkins JA, Nelson EW. Postsplenectomy infection in patients with chronic leukemia. *Am J Surg* 1986;152:583.
266. Askergren J, Bjorkholm M. Postsplenectomy septicaemia in Hodgkin's disease and other disorders. *Acta Chir Scand* 1980;146:569.
267. Buchanan GR, Smith SJ, Holtkamp CE, et al. Bacterial infection and splenic reticuloendothelial function in children with hemoglobin SC disease. *Pediatrics* 1983;72:93.
268. Loggie BW, Hinchey J. Does splenectomy predispose to meningococcal sepsis? An experimental study and clinical review. *J Pediatr Surg* 1986;21:326.
269. Hitzig WH. Immunological and hematological consequences of deficient function of the spleen. *Prog Pediatr Surg* 1985;18:132.
270. Wahlby L, Domellof L. Splenectomy after blunt abdominal trauma: a retrospective study of 413 children. *Acta Chir Scand* 1981;147:131.
271. Zarrabi MH, Rosner F. Serious infections in adults following splenectomy for trauma. *Arch Intern Med* 1984;144:1421.
272. Hicklin H, Verghese A, Alvarez S. Dysgonic fermenter 2 septicemia. *Rev Infect Dis* 1987;9:884.
273. Israeli A, Shapiro M, Ephros MA. Plasmodium falciparum malaria in an asplenic man. *Trans R Soc Trop Med Hyg* 1987;81:233.
274. Rosner F, Zarrabi MH, Benach JL, et al. Babesiosis in splenectomized adults: review of 22 reported cases. *Am J Med* 1984;76:696.
275. Jandl JH, Jones AR, et al. The destruction of red cells by antibodies in man: I. observations on the sequestration and lysis of red cells altered by immune mechanisms. *J Clin Invest* 1957;36:1428.
276. Carlisle HN, Saslaw S. Properdin levels in splenectomized persons. *Proc Soc Exp Biol Med* 1959;102:150.
277. Petersen GM, Silimperi DR, Rotter JI, et al. Genetic factors in Haemophilus influenzae type b disease susceptibility and antibody acquisition. *J Pediatr* 1987;110:228.
278. Siber GR, Santosham M, Reid GR, et al. Impaired antibody response to Haemophilus influenzae type b polysaccharide and low IgG2 and IgG4 concentrations in Apache children. *N Engl J Med* 1990;323:1387.
279. Gaston MH, Verter JI, Woods G, et al. Prophylaxis with oral penicillin in children with sickle cell anemia: a randomized trial. *N Engl J Med* 1986;314:1593.
280. Overturf GD. Infections and immunizations of children with sickle cell disease. *Adv Pediatr Infect Dis* 1999;14:191.
281. Chilcote RR, Baehner RL, Hammond D, et al. Septicemia and meningitis in children splenectomized for Hodgkin's disease. *N Engl J Med* 1980;302:892.
282. Gorse GJ. The relationship of the spleen to infection. In: Bowlder AJ, ed. *The spleen: structure, function, and clinical significance.* New York: van Nostrand Reinhold, 1990:269.
283. Schwartz PE, Sterioff S, Mucha P, et al. Postsplenectomy sepsis and mortality in adults. *JAMA* 1982;248:2279.
284. Schilling RF. Estimating the risk for sepsis after splenectomy in hereditary spherocytosis. *Ann Intern Med* 1995;122:187.
285. Konradsen HB, Henrichsen J. Pneumococcal infections in splenectomized children are preventable. *Acta Paediatr Scand* 1991;80:423.
286. Goodman RA, Ahtone JL, Finton RJ. Prevention of fatal bacterial infection in patients with anatomic or functional asplenia. *Ann Intern Med* 1982;96:117.
287. American Academy of Pediatrics. Committee on Infectious Diseases. Policy statement: recommendations for the prevention of pneumococcal infections, including the use of pneumococcal conjugate vaccine (Prevnar), pneumococcal polysaccharide vaccine, and antibiotic prophylaxis. *Pediatrics* 2000;106:362.
288. Falletta JM, Woods GM, Verter JI, et al. Discontinuing penicillin prophylaxis in children with sickle cell anemia. Prophylactic Penicillin Study II. *J Pediatr* 1995;127:685.
289. Working Party of the British Committee for Standards in Haematology Clinical Haematology Task Force. Guidelines for the prevention and treatment of infection in patients with an absent or dysfunctional spleen. *BMJ* 1996;312:430.
290. Rogers ZR, Morrison RA, Vedro DA, et al. Outpatient management of febrile illness in infants and young children with sickle cell anemia. *J Pediatr* 1990;117:736.
291. Istre GR, Tarpay M, Anderson M, et al. Invasive disease due to Streptococcus pneumoniae in an area with a high rate of relative penicillin resistance. *J Infect Dis* 1987;156:732.
292. Zarrabi MH, Rosner F. Rarity of failure of penicillin prophylaxis to prevent postsplenectomy sepsis. *Arch Intern Med* 1986;146:1207.
293. Pedersen AK, FitzGerald GA. Dose-related kinetics of aspirin: presystemic acetylation of platelet cyclooxygenase. *N Engl J Med* 1984;311:1206.
294. Robinette CD, Fraumeni JF Jr. Splenectomy and subsequent mortality in veterans of the 1939-45 war. *Lancet* 1977;2:127.
295. DeLand FH. Normal spleen size. *Radiology* 1970;97:589.

CHAPTER 22

Primary Immunodeficiency Diseases and Immunoproteins

Francisco A. Bonilla and Raif S. Geha

The immune system is a complex web of interacting cells and factors that provides protection against infection and malignancy, and orchestrates inflammatory processes such as wound healing. The system is composed of elements that are specific in their interactions with various immune challenges, as well as other components that become nonspecifically engaged during these reactions. The specificity of immunity resides in antibodies and T-cell antigen receptors. Thus, defects in T lymphocytes, which mediate cellular immunity and provide help to B cells, or defects in B lymphocytes, which make antibodies, result in deficiencies of specific immune responses. Repeated microbial infections of varying severity, increased rates of malignancy, and autoimmune disease are the consequences of these defects (1).

The complement system contributes to immune protection via innate mechanisms of activation that operate against a broad range of microbes. It also partakes of specific immunity via antibody-dependent mechanisms of activation. Defects in components of the complement system are also associated with susceptibility to various infections, as well as immune dysregulation manifested by autoimmune disease. Figure 22-1 shows the relative frequencies of various categories of primary immunodeficiency in a cohort of 91 patients identified through retrospective review in a single center (2).

We begin this chapter with an overview of combined immune deficiencies, involving cellular and humoral arms of specific immunity. We also briefly discuss definitive modes of therapy, bone marrow transplantation, and gene therapy. We then present the physiology of immunoglobulins, as well as immune deficiencies arising from lesions principally affecting specific humoral immunity. We conclude with the physiology of the complement system and diseases resulting from aberrant function of its components.

SEVERE COMBINED IMMUNODEFICIENCY

The term *severe combined immunodeficiency* (SCID) describes a clinical phenotype that is genetically determined, but has many different genetic bases. The X-linked form of the disease is distinct from autosomal-recessive forms, and the latter may result from deficiencies in a variety of molecules important in immune system function. SCID is characterized by a profound absence of T lymphocytes, with the resultant absence of cell-mediated immunity and help for specific antibody production; it is invariably fatal to affected infants (1).

Infants with SCID develop severe, recurrent, and persistent infections, usually by 3 months of age. The most common are moniliasis of the mouth and skin, protracted diarrhea, and severe pertussis-like cough owing to interstitial pneumonia. The latter is most frequently caused by *Pneumocystis carinii* and, inadequately treated, is the most frequent cause of death. In European countries where universal bacille Calmette-Guérin (BCG) vaccination is practiced, progressive infection with BCG is fatal to infants with SCID. In earlier times, when smallpox vaccination was universally applied, infants with SCID died of progressive vaccinia. Infection with varicella, herpes, and adenoviruses also are frequent causes of death.

Because these infants are immunologically incompetent, they are also extremely susceptible to the development of graft-versus-host disease (GVHD) when they are transfused with immunologically competent cells. Blood transfusions are the most frequent sources of such cells (i.e., lymphocytes) and, therefore, blood must be irradiated to inactivate lymphocytes before administration to infants with SCID.

Infants with SCID have no cell-mediated immunity. Thus, they are unable to reject tissue grafts (e.g., of skin). The blood mononuclear cells are unresponsive to nonspecific mitogens, such as phytohemagglutinin, and to specific antigens, such as tetanus or diphtheria toxoids. Although their mononuclear cells are capable of stimulating allogeneic cells *in vitro*, their own lymphocytes do not respond to such a stimulus. Infants with SCID are often profoundly lymphopenic. When CD3+ T cells are encountered in the circulation, they usually are of maternal origin (3,4). When a weak response is found *in vitro* to any stimulus, one must be certain that the cells responding are not maternal. In infants with SCID, the histology of the thymus gland is markedly abnormal. Paucicellular remnants of thymus are usually found in the neck; the organ almost always fails to become lymphoid and to descend into the anterior mediastinum. The thymus cannot be seen in a chest radiograph of a SCID patient, and this may aid in diagnosis.

In the following sections we discuss clinical and laboratory characteristics of several of the forms of SCID whose molecular bases have been determined.

X-Linked Severe Combined Immunodeficiency (Common γ-Chain Deficiency)

X-linked SCID (XSCID) accounts for one-half of cases of SCID in males (5). These patients have the general SCID phenotype as described previously. T cells are absent, and B cells are present

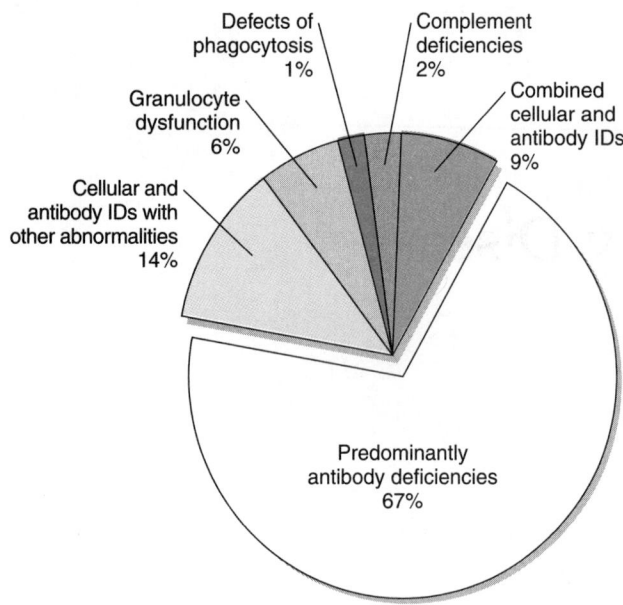

Figure 22-1. Relative incidence of different primary immunodeficiency disorders (IDs) diagnosed in patients seen during an 8-year period in a pediatric tertiary hospital. (From Javier FC III, Moore CM, Sorensen RU. Distribution of primary immunodeficiency diseases diagnosed in a pediatric tertiary hospital. *Ann Allergy Asthma Immunol* 2000;84:25–30, with permission.)

in normal or increased numbers. For this reason, this phenotype is often referred to as T^-B^+ *SCID*. Despite the presence of B cells, agammaglobulinemia is the rule. This results mainly from the absence of T-cell help for antibody production. B cells are not completely normal, however, and their function can only be complemented partially by normal T cells (6).

XSCID is caused by mutations in a gene encoding a signal-transducing component of five different cytokine receptor complexes (7,8). The common γ-chain, or $γ_c$, is a component of the receptors for interleukin (IL)-2, -4, -7, -9, -15, and -21 (9–11a). Thus, a single gene defect disrupts several signaling pathways essential for normal immune function.

T cells in female XSCID carriers show a highly skewed pattern of lyonization, that is, nonrandom X-chromosome inactivation. This may be studied using DNA probes specific for highly polymorphic repetitive sequence regions which may be associated with specific genetic loci such as monoamine oxidase A (12), coagulation factor IX (13), or the androgen receptor (14). Female XSCID carriers express a single allele at the polymorphic locus being studied in more than 95% of T lymphocytes. This represents the preferential survival of T cells retaining the functional gene on the active X chromosome. The expression of alleles in other tissues is less unbalanced. Approximately 50% of patients have a mother who is a carrier (13). This may be helpful in early evaluation and is critical for genetic counseling. Similar analyses are useful with other X-linked immunodeficiency disorders, such as Wiskott-Aldrich syndrome (WAS) and X-linked agammaglobulinemia (XLA) (see below).

Large numbers of mutations in X-linked SCID have been cataloged (15,16). Databases of these mutations can be accessed via the World Wide Web (Table 22-1). There is heterogeneity in the phenotype depending on the specific mutation, and poorly understood interacting polymorphisms of other genes. Some cases of combined immunodeficiency with normal T-cell number and partial function are caused by $γ_c$ mutations (17,18). Cases of XSCID with absence of B cells have also been described (19). Expansion of T cells bearing the γδ form of the T-cell antigen receptor (TCR) has been described in a few patients with

TABLE 22-1. Databases of Mutations in Human Primary Immunodeficiencies Accessible via the World Wide Web

Gene	URL
IL-2RG ($γ_c$)	http://www.nhgri.nih.gov/DIR/GMBB/SCID/IL2RGbase.html
ATM	http://www.vmresearch.org/atm.htm
	http://www.med.jhu.edu/ataxia/mutate.htm
CD154/CD40L	http://www.expasy.ch/cd40lbase/
NBS	http://www.vmresearch.org/nbs.htm
Many genes	http://www.uta.fi/imt/bioinfo/mutdat-bas.html#idmdb

ATM, ataxia-telangiectasia mutated; IL-2RG, interleukin-2 receptor γ chain (common γ chain); NBS, Nijmegen breakage syndrome.

mutations of $γ_c$ (20), suggesting that this type of T cell is somewhat less dependent on $γ_c$ for development and function.

XSCID has been cured by bone marrow transplantation (BMT) and gene therapy (see Therapy of Severe Combined Immunodeficiency). Gene therapy is completely curative, as may be BMT. Because $γ_c$ mutations affect both B- and T-cell function, however, many patients are left with residual defects of humoral immunity after BMT, because B cells may remain of host origin (see Bone Marrow Transplantation).

Autosomal-Recessive Forms of Severe Combined Immunodeficiency

JAK3 DEFICIENCY
A form of SCID phenotypically very similar to XSCID is associated with defects of the tyrosine kinase Jak3 (21,22). The similarity with XSCID is easily understood, because Jak3 is a critical signal-transducing molecule associated with the $γ_c$ chain. Oligoclonal and poorly functional T cells may develop in some of these patients (23). This diagnosis should be sought in T^-B^+ SCID females and in males having normal $γ_c$. Jak3 deficiency is also curable by BMT. Persistence of autologous B cells with aberrant function may still permit reconstitution of complete humoral immunity after BMT (24).

INTERLEUKIN-7 RECEPTOR α-CHAIN DEFICIENCY
IL-7 receptor α-chain deficiency has been described in a very small number of patients (25,26). The disease is also phenotypically similar to XSCID and is curable by BMT.

AUTOSOMAL-RECESSIVE SEVERE COMBINED IMMUNODEFICIENCY OWING TO DEFECTS IN PURINE NUCLEOTIDE METABOLISM: DEFECTS OF ADENOSINE DEAMINASE AND PURINE NUCLEOSIDE PHOSPHORYLASE
Adenosine deaminase (ADA) deficiency accounts for approximately 20% of SCID and 50% of SCID with autosomal-recessive inheritance (27). Purine nucleoside phosphorylase (PNP) deficiency is quite rare (30+ cases reported) (28). ADA catalyzes the deamination of adenosine and deoxyadenosine to inosine and deoxyinosine. In the absence of ADA, adenosine and deoxyadenosine accumulate within cells and are converted to adenosine triphosphate (ATP) and deoxyadenosine triphosphate (dATP). The latter is particularly toxic to ribonucleotide reductase, an enzyme required for DNA synthesis. In addition, high amounts of adenosine inside cells inhibit the enzyme S-adenosyl homocysteine hydrolase, which is required for the methylation of DNA. There is approximately 13 times more ADA in thymocytes than in other cells. Furthermore, these biochemical consequences of ADA deficiency are especially noxious to lymphoid cells because they are relatively lacking in ribonucleotide reductase activity, which would prevent accumulation of deoxyadenosine monophos-

phate and, thus, dATP (29). PNP catalyzes the dephosphorylation of guanosine and inosine as well as of deoxyguanosine and deoxyinosine. Analogous to ADA deficiency, PNP deficiency leads to accumulation of guanosine triphosphate and deoxyguanosine triphosphate. The latter has the same effects as dATP in inhibiting ribonucleotide reductase.

Approximately 85% of ADA-deficient patients have an SCID phenotype with markedly reduced numbers of both T and B cells (i.e., T⁻B⁻ SCID), and hypo- or agammaglobulinemia. Ten percent to 15% of patients may have a delayed or late onset form, which may present in late infancy or early childhood (29). These patients have variable numbers of lymphocytes and some humoral immunity, which may subsequently wane. The severity of the phenotype correlates with the amount of residual ADA activity. Variability of the expression of this defect is associated with mutant ADA molecules possessing as little as 5% to 28% of normal activity (30). Some patients bearing ADA mutations have been diagnosed as adults (31). Several mutations have been observed in this gene that do not have clinical consequences, but result in an absence of ADA from red blood cells (RBCs); apparently, there is enough residual ADA activity in the lymphocytes to prevent the untoward biochemical consequences that result in SCID (29).

PNP deficiency is a somewhat selective defect in cellular immunity, with extreme susceptibility to viral and fungal infections. These patients have decreased circulating T cells, with normal numbers of B cells and serum immunoglobulin levels. With time, humoral immunity usually deteriorates (28).

ADA and PNP activities are readily measurable in RBC and white blood cell lysates. In symptomatic patients, activity is usually 1% or less compared to normals. Serum and urine levels of uric acid are decreased in PNP deficiency because this enzyme is required for production of hypoxanthine, a urate precursor. This is not the case in ADA deficiency.

ADA and PNP deficiency have been cured by BMT. Alternative therapies have also been successful for ADA deficiency. RBCs contain high levels of ADA, and transfusions can ameliorate the enzyme defect (32). Such treatment is effective in approximately 50% of patients, mainly those with some residual immune function. Another therapy that avoids the long-term risks of blood transfusion is infusion of polyethylene glycol–conjugated bovine ADA (33). ADA deficiency was the first disease for which a cure was attempted through gene therapy (see Gene Therapy). A patient with an apparent spontaneous reversion of an ADA mutation also has been described (34).

DEFECTS IN RECOMBINASE-ACTIVATING GENES 1 AND 2 (RAG1, RAG2)
SCID with absence of T cells and B cells (T⁻B⁻ SCID), or alymphocytosis, has historically been referred to as *Swiss-type agammaglobulinemia*, or *autosomal-recessive SCID*, even though it is not the only form of SCID with autosomal-recessive inheritance. Approximately 50% of alymphocytic patients without defects of ADA or PNP have a defect in either of recombinase-activating genes 1 or 2 (*RAG1* or *RAG2*) (35). These genes are required for the somatic assembly of mature immunoglobulin and T-cell receptor genes from the gene segments in their germline configurations (see section Immunoglobulins). B- and T-cell precursors are arrested at an early stage of development. This form of SCID is often called *B⁻ SCID* to distinguish it from forms in which B cells are usually present, such as XSCID and Jak3 deficiency.

Omenn's syndrome is a variant of autosomal-recessive SCID, with a distinct phenotype characterized by a presentation similar to acute GVHD (36). Symptoms are as for SCID in general, with a prominent erythroderma with exfoliation and exudation. Hepatosplenomegaly, anemia, hypogammaglobulinemia with elevated immunoglobulin (Ig) E, decreased peripheral blood B cells, along with infiltration of the skin, intestinal mucosa, liver,

and spleen with histiocytes and an oligoclonal population of T cells are characteristic. Poorly functional oligoclonal immature CD4⁺CD8⁺ T cells are found in the circulation, whereas the thymus, spleen, and other peripheral lymphoid tissues are generally devoid of normal lymphocytes.

Omenn's syndrome results from RAG1 or -2 defects that allow partial function of these proteins (37,38). All Omenn's syndrome patients studied and reported to date have had mutations in one of these two genes. The highly restricted nature of the T-cell repertoire in these patients has been demonstrated at the genetic level (39,40). T⁻B⁻ SCID owing to defects of RAG1 or -2 has been cured by BMT.

SEVERE COMBINED IMMUNODEFICIENCY OWING TO DEFECTS IN MAJOR HISTOCOMPATIBILITY COMPLEX CLASS II MOLECULES: BARE LYMPHOCYTE SYNDROME
The products of the major histocompatibility complex (MHC) class II genes play critical roles in the development and activation of CD4⁺ T cells, and in the interaction of B cells and other antigen-presenting cells with T cells (41). An intricate complex of several DNA-binding proteins and regulatory components controls the transcription of these genes. Deficiencies of several of these proteins have been identified in patients with a distinctive form of SCID. Their leukocytes lack surface MHC class II molecules, and this heterogeneous group of diseases bears the eponym *bare lymphocyte syndrome* (42). Approximately 50 such patients have been reported to date. Most of the patients cluster in northern Africa, and occur in kindreds with consanguinity. Five complementation groups (A–E) have been defined; each apparently corresponds to mutations of one component within the group of factors regulating MHC class II gene expression. Mutations in *CIITA* (class II *trans*-activator) correspond to group A, mutations in *RFX-B* (the B subunit of the regulatory factor X complex) to group B (43), mutations in *RFX5* (another subunit of RFX) to group C (44), and *RFXAP* to group D (45). The genetic basis for group E has not yet been identified.

These patients usually present within the first weeks of life; the phenotype is that of classic SCID (41,42). BMT is the only mode of successful therapy. Lymphocyte numbers are normal; no form of MHC class II is expressed. Levels of MHC class I expression are frequently depressed, but never to the same degree as class II. Peripheral CD4⁺ T cells are greatly diminished, whereas CD8⁺ T cells may be increased. Patients show cutaneous anergy, and most have agammaglobulinemia. A few patients have appreciable serum immunoglobulin, but they do not make specific antibody. *In vitro* alloreactivity may be seen, possibly driven by differences in MHC class I. The phenotype is somewhat distinct from classic SCID in the lack of disseminated disease after BCG vaccination, or GVHD after transfusion of blood products containing viable lymphocytes.

DEFECTS OF TRANSPORTERS OF ANTIGENIC PEPTIDES 1 AND 2: MAJOR HISTOCOMPATIBILITY COMPLEX CLASS I DEFICIENCY
Although not associated with a classic SCID phenotype, we discuss MHC class I deficiency here because it is often considered as a subtype within the eponym *bare lymphocyte syndrome*. MHC class I molecules are necessary for the development, activation, and target recognition of CD8⁺ T cells (46). The molecule transporters of antigenic peptide-1 and -2 (TAP-1 and TAP-2), as their names imply, are critical for the transfer of antigenic peptides from the cytosol into the endoplasmic reticulum, where MHC class I molecules are being synthesized (47). If TAP-1 or -2 is absent or nonfunctional, MHC class I molecules are not loaded with peptides, and they cannot be stably expressed on the cell surface.

A few patients with defects of these molecules have been described. Children with TAP-2 defects exhibit mainly infections that are associated with antibody deficiency, that is, recurrent bacterial sinopulmonary infections (48,49). The phenotype of circulating lymphocytes may be normal; one patient had an abnormal $CD4^+CD8^+$ (double positive) population. The percentage of T cells bearing the $\gamma\delta$ form of the TCR, which normally constitute only 1% to 5% of the total, may be increased. The basis for this is not entirely clear, because specific antibody production was preserved. A patient with TAP-1 mutations and MHC class I deficiency with a similar phenotype was recently reported (50).

DEFECT OF THE ζ-ASSOCIATED PROTEIN OF 70 KD

Defects in the ζ-associated protein of 70-kd tyrosine kinase, a critical intermediary in T-cell receptor signaling, result in a form of SCID characterized by lack of peripheral $CD8^+$ T cells, with high numbers of nonfunctional $CD4^+$ T cells in the periphery (51–53).

Other Forms of Combined Immunodeficiency

The distinction between SCID and CID may be occasionally somewhat arbitrary, and is based on the degree of the susceptibility to infections. Severe and moderate combined immunodeficiencies have been associated with a wide variety of phenotypes. In some cases, the gene defect is known; in many cases, it is not. Some known defects in molecules important in T-cell activation have been reported in a few patients associated with manifestations of SCID or CID. These include mutations of the protein tyrosine phosphatase CD45 (54), and mutations in the CD3 complex γ (55) and ε (56,57) chains. The Griscelli syndrome is a form of SCID associated with pigmentary dilution (partial albinism) (58–60). Two genes have been implicated in this disorder: *myosin Va*, important for melanosome trafficking, and *RAB27A*, a guanosine triphosphatase–binding protein required for cytotoxic granule exocytosis.

A rapidly fatal form of SCID owing to the absence of T and B lymphocytes, as well as myeloid cells, is called *reticular dysgenesis* (61–64). The molecular defect is unknown. Other reported SCID/CID phenotypes with unknown defects include patients with failure to produce IL-1 (65) or IL-2 (66,67), or inability to produce multiple cytokines owing to failure in the assembly of the transcription factor nuclear factor of activated T cells (68). For additional examples of CID associated with various genetic syndromes, see Rosen and colleagues (1).

Therapy of Severe Combined Immunodeficiency

BONE MARROW TRANSPLANTATION

A variety of techniques of BMT have been applied for the cure of various forms of SCID. Sources of stem cells include HLA antigen–identical siblings, haploidentical parents, HLA-matched unrelated donors, and partially matched umbilical cord blood (69–75). Bone marrow has most often been used as a source of stem cells, and various means have been applied to deplete mature T cells to reduce the risk of GVHD. The type of conditioning required depends mainly on the type of SCID and the source of stem cells. Similar considerations guide the need for posttransplantation prophylactic immunosuppression to prevent GVHD. In some cases, stem cells have been infused *in utero*, to take advantage of the relative immunologic immaturity of the fetus, with a lower risk of graft rejection (76,77). This must be balanced against the risk of fetal loss as a result of intrauterine manipulations. Worldwide experience with BMT for SCID is now well in excess of 500 patients.

Although the thymus is often rudimentary in SCID patients, it appears to function normally in T-cell development after BMT (78). A state of cellular chimerism is frequent after BMT for SCID. RBCs usually remain of host origin (79). Myeloid chimerism is variable (74,80). B-cell chimerism is common, and depends on the type of SCID and the particular techniques applied for BMT (80). Although many patients with SCID achieve complete reconstitution of B- and T-cell function, many remain with defects of humoral immunity requiring long-term replacement with intravenous immunoglobulin (IVIG).

Infection is the most common complication of BMT for SCID, and it is also the most frequent cause of death in these patients. Additional complications may include lymphoproliferative disease, most often associated with Epstein-Barr virus (EBV) (81). Also, the fragile regulation of immune function during reconstitution may result in autoimmune processes such as anemia (82) and thrombocytopenia (83).

GENE THERAPY

Gene therapy technology is another method having the potential for the complete cure of genetically determined immune deficiency, apart from BMT. A variety of viruses have been altered by molecular biologic techniques to carry functional human genes into infected cells. This therapy has been undertaken for the treatment of a few immunodeficiency diseases.

The first applications of gene therapy for the treatment of immunodeficiency were attempts to correct ADA deficiency (84). Two patients who were already undergoing treatment with bovine ADA (see Autosomal-Recessive Severe Combined Immunodeficiency Owing to Defects in Purine Nucleotide Metabolism: Defects of Adenosine Deaminase and Purine Nucleoside Phosphorylase) received infusions of their own peripheral blood T cells which had been transduced with ADA complementary DNA. In one patient, T-cell–ADA levels increased; peripheral T-cell numbers became normal; *in vitro* mitogen activation and cytotoxicity, as well as cutaneous delayed hypersensitivity were restored; and isohemagglutinins were produced. The second patient also showed clinical improvement, although ADA levels never rose significantly, and the T-cell number declined after an initial rise. Bovine ADA treatment was continued, although reduced, after transduced T-cell infusion. This may have blunted a survival advantage of transduced cells. ADA-deficient newborns have also received infusions of transduced umbilical cord blood hematopoietic stem cells (85). These patients have also improved, although the frequency of transduced T cells in the circulation was low, and some had reduction in immune function with reduction or withdrawal of bovine ADA treatment.

The most dramatic success of gene therapy in the treatment of SCID to date has been for XSCID (γ_c deficiency) by the *ex vivo* introduction of a retroviral vector bearing a functional γ_c gene *IL2RG* into the stem cells of two patients (86). Ten months after infusion of these transduced cells, reconstitution of immune function appeared to be complete. Various vectors carrying functional genes have been used to reconstitute lymphocyte function *in vitro* from patients with MHC class II deficiency (CIITA gene) (87), Jak3 deficiency (88), and ζ-associated protein of 70-kd deficiency (89), although no patients treated with cells transduced with these genes have yet been reported.

COMBINED IMMUNODEFICIENCIES

Wiskott-Aldrich Syndrome

WAS is a rare, X-linked immunodeficiency (1). Affected males have thrombocytopenia, eczema, and recurrent sinopulmonary bacterial infections. Petechiae and bloody diarrhea are frequent, and may be part of the clinical presentation. Autoimmune disorders such as vasculitis and glomerulonephritis have also been observed in WAS.

The number of platelets in the blood of WAS-affected children is markedly decreased, and the platelets are abnormally small (effective average diameter 1.82 + 0.1 mm, compared with the normal diameter of 2.23 + 0.1 mm). The platelets are also often coated with IgG. The size of the platelets has been noted to increase after splenectomy, and the amount of surface IgG decreases to normal (90). Immune thrombocytopenia may sometimes be confused with WAS; however, the other clinical manifestations usually clarify the differential diagnosis. Approximately 20% of WAS patients also develop an immune thrombocytopenia, so the disorders may coexist (91).

Cell-mediated immunity progressively declines with age, but the number and phenotype of the blood lymphocytes are often normal. T cells from WAS patients may have diminished proliferation to mitogens, particularly to anti-CD3 antibodies (92). Antigen-specific proliferation is usually diminished, and cutaneous anergy to recall antigens is also common. Serum immunoglobulins are abnormal; concentrations of IgA and IgE are elevated and the concentration of IgM is decreased, whereas IgG is normal. Affected males do not respond to polysaccharide antigens, whereas the response to protein antigens is normal or nearly so. Like the platelets, the blood lymphocytes are also small, and their size increases after splenectomy. By scanning electron microscopy, these blood elements have a characteristic reduction of surface membrane ruffling, and this has proved useful in the perinatal and prenatal diagnosis of WAS (93) (Fig. 22-2).

The gene that is affected in WAS has been identified, and the protein it encodes is the WAS protein, or WASP (94–96). WASP is expressed in CD34+ hematopoietic precursor cells, and in all derived lineages, including dendritic cells (97). Patients with X-linked thrombocytopenia (XLT) also harbor WASP mutations, showing the phenotypic variability that may result from lesions in this gene. One female patient with classic WAS has been reported (98). She expressed the defect as a result of extreme nonrandom lyonization of the chromosome carrying the functional WASP gene in all of her tissues. Otherwise, normal female carriers of WAS generally show nonrandom X inactivation in leukocytes, and this may aid in diagnosis.

WASP mutations do not show clear correlations with phenotype either in WAS or XLT (95,99,100). Many WASP mutations, regardless of the severity of the clinical phenotype, lead to absence of the protein, which may be established by Western blotting leukocyte lysates with specific antiserum. A database of WASP mutations may be found on the World Wide Web (Table 22-1).

Recent studies have defined WASP as an important intermediate in controlling the reorganization of the cytoskeleton that occurs in leukocytes during development and activation via various surface receptors (101). CD34+ precursors from WAS patients show reduced development along megakaryocyte, erythroid, and myeloid lineages (102). This was not seen in cells from patients with XLT. Megakaryocytes from patients with either diagnosis showed reduced generation of proplatelets after stimulation with thrombopoietin. Platelets from WAS patients express high levels of surface phosphatidylserine, a signal for macrophage clearance (103). Spleens from these patients show high levels of platelet phagocytosis by macrophages. Although biochemical and cytoskeletal abnormalities have been observed in WAS platelets, no clear defects in structure or in function (aggregation) have been demonstrated (101,104).

Studies in WASP-deficient mice have demonstrated impaired intrathymic T-cell development, as well as diminished concentrations of intracellular calcium, proliferation, and IL-2 production after T-cell stimulation via the TCR (105). Actin polymerization in T cells after activation was markedly reduced. WASP has been shown to associate with the Bruton's tyrosine kinase (btk) and is phosphorylated after Ig receptor cross-linking in B-cell lines from WAS patients (106). However, studies in WASP-deficient mice have not shown reduction in B-cell stimulation by Ig cross-linking (107). IgG-mediated phagocytosis by monocytes, macrophages, and neutrophils is impaired in WAS patients (105,108). WAS macrophages also show reduced che-

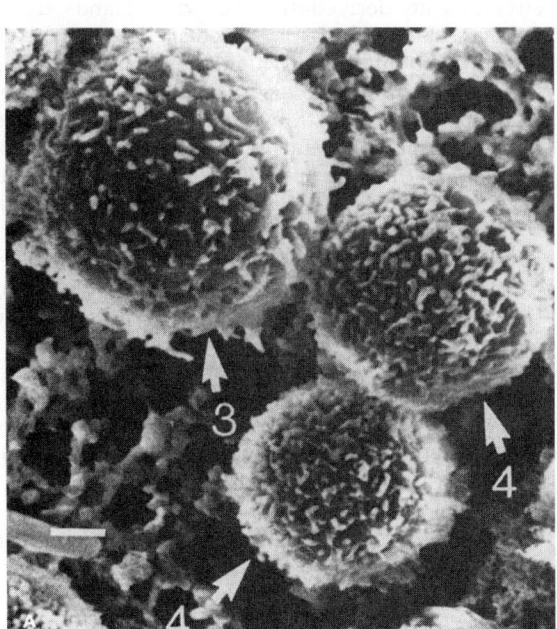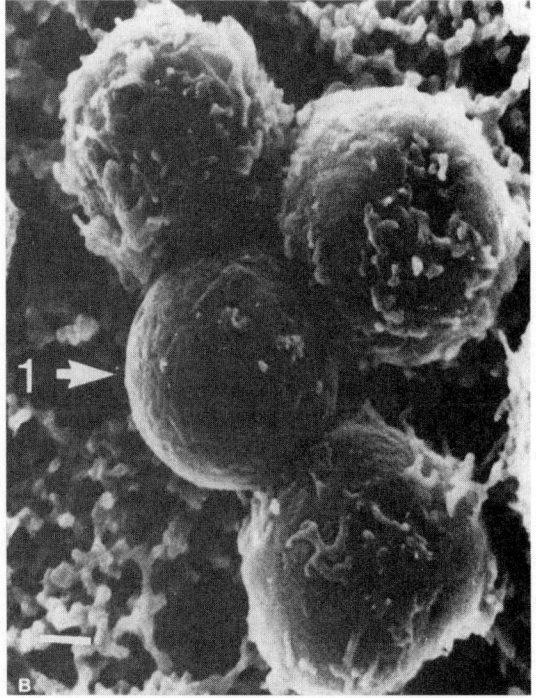

Figure 22-2. Scanning electron micrographs of lymphocytes from a normal subject **(A)** and from a patient with Wiskott-Aldrich syndrome **(B)**. Note the baldness of the affected cells. (From Kenney D, Cairns L, Remold-O'Donnell E, et al. Morphological abnormalities in the lymphocytes of patients with Wiskott-Aldrich syndrome. *Blood* 1986;68:1329, with permission.)

motaxis (109). Dendritic cells from WAS patients show abnormal mobility and polarization during antigen presentation (110).

Median survival in WAS may be increased from 5 years to 25 years by splenectomy (91,111). IVIG and antibiotic prophylaxis are also very useful therapies, although replacement therapy with IVIG does not usually lead to significant increases in platelet counts in thrombocytopenic WAS patients (112). In general, BMT with a matched sibling donor is highly successful and is considered the treatment of choice for WAS. HLA-matched unrelated donors are also good sources of stem cells. To date, the results of partially matched or haploidentical BMT have been disappointing, predominantly owing to a high rate of graft rejection (91,113). Retrovirus-mediated introduction of a functional WAS gene has corrected cytoskeletal (114) and surface glycoprotein (115) abnormalities in cells from WAS patients *in vitro*.

Ataxia-Telangiectasia

Ataxia-telangiectasia (A-T) is inherited as an autosomal-recessive characteristic. Affected children may exhibit ataxia from the time they begin to walk, which often is delayed beyond the first year (116). Beginning in approximately the fifth or sixth year of life, fine telangiectasias develop in the conjunctivae, on the ear lobes, and on other exposed parts of the body, often in skin creases. Most patients develop persistent sinopulmonary infections. The diagnosis can be established early by detecting the characteristic elevation of serum α-fetoprotein seen in approximately 95% of patients.

Populations of peripheral T and B cells are most often normal. Interestingly, T cells bearing the γδ form of the T-cell receptor may constitute up to 50% or more of the total number in patients with A-T (117). These cells normally comprise only 1% to 5% of peripheral T cells in normal individuals. Decrease or absence of cutaneous delayed hypersensitivity responses, as well as diminished T-cell mitogen and antigen responses *in vitro*, are common. Approximately 80% of patients are deficient in IgA. Some of these patients have a concomitant deficiency of IgG2 and IgG4, and susceptibility to recurrent bacterial sinopulmonary infections is most frequently encountered in these patients. Hypergammaglobulinemia occurs in approximately 40% of A-T patients. It is usually of the IgM isotype, although elevated levels of IgG and IgA have also been observed (118). Approximately one-fifth of these are oligo- or monoclonal. Patients with A-T develop malignancies, principally of the lymphoreticular organs, usually by the end of the second decade of life. Additional manifestations such as oral motor problems with drooling, dysphagia, and aspiration are also common (119).

The diagnosis may be missed early in life because the characteristic telangiectasias do not appear until approximately 3 to 5 years of age. Many of these children are misdiagnosed as having cerebral palsy and other neurological disorders (120). This delay in diagnosis may lead to missed opportunities for therapy such as IVIG replacement, and for genetic counseling. Elevated serum α-fetoprotein distinguishes A-T from other conditions, and some advocate routine screening of α-fetoprotein in children with persistent ataxia (120).

Patients with A-T are susceptible to the effects of ionizing radiation. Cultured cells, such as fibroblasts, exhibit many chromosomal breaks after such exposure. Fibroblasts from A-T patients exhibit radioresistant DNA synthesis: That is, the cells fail to detect radiation-induced damage to their DNA, and do not normally shut down the cell cycle under these circumstances. Lymphocytes frequently exhibit breaks at the loci of the rearranging T-cell receptor and immunoglobulin genes.

The gene mutated in A-T has been identified, and is designated *ATM* (A-T mutated) (121). A portion of the ATM protein has structural similarity to phosphatidyl inositol 3' kinase.

Other regions contain leucine zipper motifs. ATM has additional regions of homology with highly conserved proteins from yeast and humans, which regulate telomere structure and detection of DNA damage and its repair. In response to ionizing radiation, the ATM protein phosphorylates the tumor-suppressor gene p53 and breast cancer gene 1, important in the development of a variety of cancers (122,123).

Most A-T patients are compound heterozygotes, and there is a high proportion of unique mutations (124–127). Most mutations (>80%) are truncating, leading to lack of expression of ATM. Some missense mutations have been associated with milder phenotypes, such as absence of immune deficiency (128) or telangiectasia (125). Approximately 1.4% of whites in the United States are heterozygous carriers of A-T (129). Some early investigations suggested that there was a substantially increased risk of cancer in these carriers, particularly of breast cancer in women (130). Recent studies do not agree, however, and there is not yet a consensus regarding this issue (131–133).

The treatment of A-T is generally preventive and supportive. Modalities include IVIG replacement and prophylactic antibiotics. Therapy of lymphoma in A-T with chemotherapy has had disappointing results (134). In 21 patients treated with standard chemotherapy, complete remission was induced in 76%, but relapses and other complications led to median survival of only 9 months. A functional ATM gene introduced into A-T T cells with a viral vector has resulted in normal responses to ionizing radiation *in vitro* (135).

The Nijmegen breakage syndrome is a disorder of chromosome fragility with autosomal-recessive inheritance. The phenotype is similar to A-T with growth retardation, microcephaly, immune deficiency, radiation sensitivity, and a high rate of lymphoma (136). The affected gene maps to chromosome 8q21, and was recently cloned and called *NBS1* (137). NBS1 is another substrate of ATM in the cellular response to ionizing radiation (138,139).

DiGeorge Anomaly

The thymus gland is derived early in embryogenesis from the third and fourth pharyngeal arches. From these same embryonic structures are derived the parathyroid glands, the cardiac outflow vessels, and the hyomandibular elements of the face. By the sixth week of human gestation, the thymus becomes lymphoid owing to an immigration of lymphoid stem cells from the yolk sac and subsequently from the fetal liver. Neural crest cells also make up important elements of the mature thymus. By 20 weeks of gestation, fully competent T lymphocytes begin to emigrate from the thymus to populate the secondary lymphoid organs.

The DiGeorge anomaly (DGA) and related conditions, such as the velocardiofacial syndrome, result from faulty development of the organs derived from the third and fourth pharyngeal arches (140–142). This may lead to neonatal hypocalcemia and tetany as a result of hypoplasia of the parathyroid glands, and an absence or severe hypoplasia of the thymus. Affected infants may have poor cell-mediated immunity and a decrease in the number of circulating T cells. They also have anomalies of the great vessels and a variety of cardiac defects, tetralogy of Fallot being the most common. A facies characterized by low-set ears, shortened philtrum of the upper lip, and an increased interocular space is common. Death is most often a result of the cardiac abnormalities.

So-called partial and complete forms of DGA have been distinguished (141–144). This distinction reflects the amount of thymus that develops. In complete DGA, the thymus is absent, and no mature T cells develop, although oligoclonal populations of nonfunctional T cells are occasionally encountered (145). In partial DGA, some thymus develops. It is often ectopic, found within the structures of the neck. A very small thymus, weighing as little as a few grams, may be able to support protective T-cell function, although the number of peripheral T cells may be reduced. Despite this, the recurrent infections characteristic of partial DGA are those associated more commonly with antibody defects (146). Total IgG is usually normal; mild hypogammaglobulinemia may be seen. A 13% prevalence of IgA deficiency (IgAD) has been noted in patients with DGA (147). Humoral responses to immunization as well as natural infection are usually robust in patients with partial DGA, despite variable reductions in peripheral blood T cells (145,148). Immune function often improves with time in partial DGA (149). Complete DGA is universally fatal without immune reconstitution (see the following paragraphs). Partial forms outnumber complete forms by approximately 10 to 1.

DGA most often (>90%) results from chromosomal abnormalities at position 22q11. Most patients have a large 2–3 megabase deletion in this region (150). These may be detected easily by fluorescent *in situ* hybridization with 22q11 specific probes. There appear to be five distinct subregions important for the development of DGA (151). A variety of candidate genes from the DGA critical region have been identified, but none has yet been demonstrated to play a definitive role in the DGA phenotype (152–157). The gene encoding the transcription factor TBX-1 has recently emerged as an important element in the phenotype of DGA. Mice that are heterozygous for targeted disruption of this gene recapitulate the cardiac defects of DGA, although thymus development appears to be normal (157a).

As in many other immune deficiencies, the phenotype is variable, even with the same chromosomal deletion (158). The phenotype of DGA is a spectrum with other disorders resulting from 22q11 deletions such as velocardiofacial syndrome, which has features of DGA without hypocalcemia or immune dysfunction. Clinical immune deficiency was found in approximately 6% of one large (n = 130) cohort of patients with demonstrable 22q11 deletion (159). However, another study found abnormal cellular and humoral immunity in 77% of individuals with 22q11 deletion, although the frequency of clinical symptoms was not stated (150).

DGA has also been associated with chromosomal deletions and rearrangements of chromosome 10p (160). There do not appear to be any clinical or immunological differences between patients who have chromosome 22q11 deletions detectable by fluorescent *in situ* hybridization versus those who do not (146).

Most patients with partial DGA do very well with preventive and supportive therapy with antibiotics and IVIG replacement, when necessary. Complete DGA may be quite difficult to treat. Transplantation of neonatal thymus tissue has been successful in the reconstitution of immune function in complete DGA. However, survival is achieved in only approximately one-third of these cases (161,162). The thymus need not be completely matched for functional T cells to develop. All of the determinants of successful thymic transplantation are not known.

Bone marrow transplantation has also been successful in DGA (163–165). Because all of the donors were HLA-identical siblings and the marrow was not T-cell depleted, some have speculated that these patients were reconstituted by mature T cells in the graft. In fact, partial reconstitution of T-cell number and function with good antibody function has been achieved in a patient with complete DGA by infusion of purified mature peripheral T cells from an HLA-identical sibling (166).

X-Linked Hyperimmunoglobulin M Syndrome (or CD154 Deficiency)

CD154, also known as *CD40 ligand*, is principally a marker of activated T cells, although it may be found on other leukocytes (167). It is a member of the tumor necrosis factor (TNF) family of cytokines. Its only ligand is CD40, expressed mainly by B cells and antigen-presenting cells, although it may be found on other types of cells. CD40 is a member of the TNF receptor family of cytokines and plays a critical role in T-cell interactions with antigen-presenting cells during antigen-specific priming. It is also critical for the process of Ig class-switching, the change in B-cell production of IgM to the synthesis of other isotypes such as IgG, A, and E. X-linked hyper-IgM syndrome is caused by mutations in the gene encoding CD154 (168–172).

The median age at presentation is 8 months (173). The major clinical manifestations include recurrent viral and bacterial infections, as well as opportunistic infections such as *P. carinii* pneumonia. Also found frequently are chronic diarrhea owing to cryptosporidium, neutropenia, anemia owing to parvovirus, stomatitis, sclerosing cholangitis, and inflammatory arthritis.

The disorder derives its name from its most characteristic immunological abnormalities: low levels of IgG with normal or elevated levels of IgM (173,174). This phenotype results from an inability of T cells to provide the signals necessary for B cells to switch Ig isotype during an antibody response. Specific antibody production is relatively poor, and generally only of the IgM class. The susceptibility to viral and other opportunistic infections results from disruption of T-cell interactions with antigen-presenting cells in the process of antigen priming. Lymphocyte subset analysis is usually normal. T-cell proliferation with mitogens *in vitro* is normal; response to a specific antigen is frequently reduced.

Treatment of X-linked hyper-IgM syndrome is usually supportive with IVIG infusions, and trimethoprim/sulfamethoxazole or other prophylaxis for *P. carinii* pneumonia (173,174). Neutropenia may be treated with granulocyte colony–stimulating factor, although response is variable. Several patients have been successfully treated with BMT.

Defects of the Interleukin-12–Interferon-γ Axis

Patients with defects of the IL-12–interferon (IFN)-γ axis have highly selective susceptibility to organisms that replicate within phagocytic cells. They were identified initially in a cohort of infants and young children suffering disseminated infection after BCG vaccination (175). Other mycobacterial and salmonella infections are also often seen (176). These situations are not infrequently encountered in SCID, however, these infants had none of the laboratory immunological features of SCID; lymphocyte numbers and *in vitro* function were normal. Some of these patients harbor mutations in the α-chain of the IFN-γ receptor (IFNGR1) (175,176). Additional patients with defects of the β-chain (IFNGR2) have also been described (177,178).

IL-12 is produced by macrophages and monocytes and is the principal stimulus for production of IFN-γ by natural killer (NK) cells. IFN-γ then stimulates mononuclear cells to increase function as antigen-presenting cells and activate intracellular cytotoxic mechanisms. Additional patients exhibiting the previously mentioned clinical phenotype bear mutations in the genes encoding the IL-12 p40 subunit (179) or the β1-chain of the IL-12 receptor (180).

X-Linked Lymphoproliferative Disease

The most dramatic presentation of X-linked lymphoproliferative disease is that of a boy with fulminant and fatal infectious mononucleosis with hemophagocytosis owing to infection with EBV (181). Mortality is greater than 90%. Most children are healthy before the fatal infection, although a few have recurrent viral or bacterial infections. Some may also exhibit alterations in the composition of Ig classes and subclasses (e.g., increased IgA or IgM, decreased IgG1 and/or IgG3). Less-distinct presentations of this disorder include lymphoid necrosis with dysgammaglobulinemia, malignant lymphoma, aplastic anemia, and pulmonary lymphomatoid granulomatosis with vasculitis. More than one of these may occur in a single patient.

The signaling lymphocyte activation molecule is a lymphocyte homotypic adhesion molecule important in activation. The gene responsible for X-linked lymphoproliferative disease encodes a cytoplasmic adaptor protein known as the signaling lymphocyte activation molecule–associated protein (182–184). This molecule links the signaling lymphocyte activation molecule to downstream signaling pathways. The mechanism of the exquisite susceptibility to EBV is not yet understood. Acute mononucleosis in some patients has been successfully treated with antiinflammatory and chemotherapeutic regimens (181). BMT can be curative (185).

Chronic Mucocutaneous Candidiasis

Chronic mucocutaneous candidiasis is a heterogeneous group of disorders characterized principally by recurrent and severe infections of the skin, nails, and mucous membranes with *Candida albicans* (186). A predisposition to infection with a variety of microbes is also seen. Additional manifestations include asplenia or hyposplenism, and higher rates of malignancy (particularly thymoma). Most patients have impairment of *in vitro* and *in vivo* (delayed hypersensitivity) responses to *Candida* antigens. Ig levels, lymphocyte numbers, and function with respect to non-*Candida* antigens are normal. Some patients presenting early with more severe disease may exhibit somewhat more global impairment of cellular immunity, alterations in Ig classes and subclasses, and specific antibody production have also been noted.

Some patients with chronic mucocutaneous candidiasis exhibit autoimmune endocrinopathy. Different organs may be affected, such as thyroid, parathyroid, adrenal, or ovary. Autoimmune hepatitis may also occur. This form of the disease has been called *autoimmune polyendocrinopathy–Candidiasis–ectodermal dystrophy* or *autoimmune polyglandular syndrome type 1* (187). A gene defect has been identified in this group of patients; the gene is called *autoimmune regulator* (188–191). The encoded protein has structural features of transcription regulators, and is expressed in primary (thymic medulla) and secondary lymphoid organs. A few patients have been treated successfully with BMT or infusions of lymphocytes from donors with anti-*Candida* immunity (192,193).

Hyperimmunoglobulin E Syndrome

The classic clinical features of hyper-IgE syndrome are recurrent bacterial infections, mainly skin and sinopulmonary abscesses, chronic dermatitis resembling eczema, and elevated serum IgE (194). Mucocutaneous candidiasis may be seen in newborns. The infections are generally not life-threatening and respond to standard antimicrobial regimens. Some patients have been diagnosed in adulthood (195). The most frequent pathogenic organisms are *Staphylococcus aureus* and *Aspergillus*. Neutrophils often display impaired chemotaxis, and they do not migrate properly to sites of infection, thus inflammation is reduced and abscesses are "cold." For this reason, some classify this disease with the neutrophil disorders. Serum IgE levels range from 3000 IU/mL to more than 50,000 IU/mL. Levels may fall later in life (194). Associated nonimmunologic findings are asymmetric and coarse facial features, delay of shedding of primary teeth, bone fragility and frequent fractures, hyperextensible joints, scoliosis, and keratoconjunctivitis with corneal ulceration.

Characteristic clinical features may suggest the diagnosis. The great majority of patients exhibit elevated IgE, together with positive immediate cutaneous hypersensitivity (skin-prick test) with *S. aureus*, and serum antibodies binding staphylococci and staphylococcal toxins. All of these may be seen in some patients with atopic dermatitis, however, a disease that shares many features with hyper-IgE syndrome. Gene mutations have not been described in these patients.

Antibiotic prophylaxis and aggressive antimicrobial treatment of established infections are the mainstays of management. Experimental alternatives for which insufficient clinical data exist include IFN-γ, IFN-α, and intravenous gamma globulin (196–198).

IMMUNOGLOBULINS

Igs are a heterogeneous group of proteins found in the blood plasma and body fluids; they are secreted solely by lymphocytes of the B-cell lineage. Ig molecules also occupy the surfaces of B lymphocytes, where they are known as the *B-cell receptor*, or the *Ig receptor*. Ig proteins are all related in structure and function as antibodies, that is, they recognize and bind specifically to antigen. These proteins are generally referred to as *immunoglobulins* when their specificity is not of concern. The term *antibody* is more appropriate when one is considering only Igs that bind to a specific antigen(s). Ig is the major effector of specific humoral immunity. They function in concert with Ig Fc receptors on leukocytes and other cells, as well as with the complement system (see Immunoglobulin Fc Receptors) to exert their effector functions.

Structure

All Ig molecules consist of a pair of identical polypeptide chains linked by disulfide bonds and electrostatic forces. The prototype molecule consists of a pair of identical heavy chains that determine the Ig class, found in combination with a pair of identical light chains (Fig. 22-3). Each Ig-synthesizing cell secretes only one type of heavy and light chain. Each Ig mole-

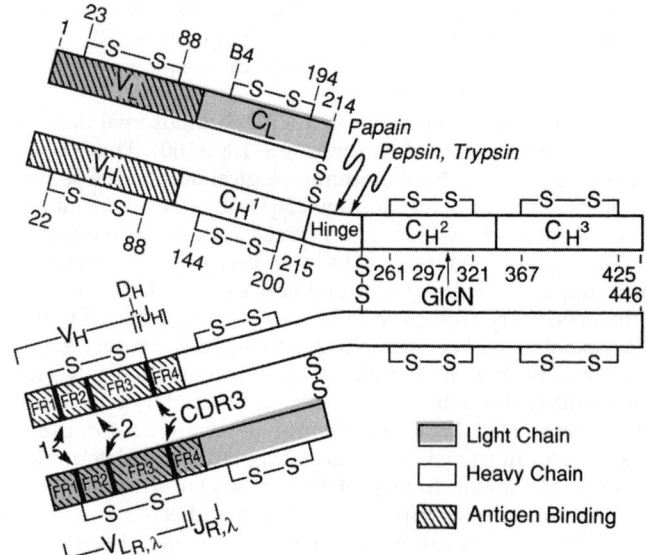

Figure 22-3. Schematic depiction of a prototypic immunoglobulin molecule (monomer). The identical light (L) and heavy (H) chains are shown linked by interchain disulfide bonds. The unique amino acid sequences of the complementarity-determining regions (CDRs) and the framework regions (FRs) of the antibody-binding site of the H and L chains are illustrated in one of two identical halves of the molecule. N-linked oligosaccharide sites are located on each H chain within the C_H2 domain (GlcN). Cleavage sites for proteases (papain, pepsin, trypsin) are indicated. Papain digestion of an Ig molecule yields two types of fragments: two Fab (antigen-binding) pieces each consisting of the amino terminal half of a heavy chain with a light chain; and the Fc (crystallizable) piece, consisting of the two carboxy-terminal halves of the heavy chains that remain joined at the hinge region. After pepsin digestion of Ig, the two Fab fragments remain joined by one or more disulfide links, forming a bivalent fragment called $F(ab)_2$' ("f-a-b-prime-two").

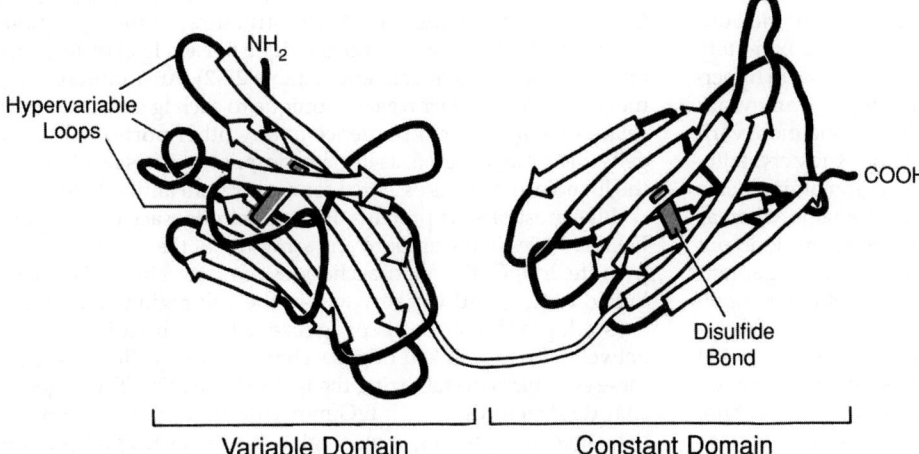

Figure 22-4. Tertiary structure of an immunoglobulin light chain. The characteristic immunoglobulin fold is seen in the V_L and C_L domains as two β-pleated sheets connected by an intrachain disulfide bond. In the V_L, the hypervariable amino acid regions (CDR1 to CDR3) are seen as loops independent of the fold that, together with the V_H complementarity-determining regions, determine the three-dimensional structure of the antibody-binding site. (COOH, carboxyl group; NH_2, amino group.) (From Schiffer M, Girling RL, Ely KR, Edmunson AB. Structure of the lambda-type Bence Jones protein at 3.5Å resolution. *Biochemistry* 1970;12:4620, with permission.)

cule (monomer) has two antigen-combining sites, which are contained within the Fab fragment (Fig. 22-3) and involve regions on the heavy and light chains. Sequences in the Fc region of the heavy chain mediate Ig effector functions.

Amino acid sequence analysis reveals that the heavy and light chains are composed of a series of distinct repeating homology units termed the *Ig domains* (199,200). These domains consist of regions of 100 to 120 amino acids containing an intrachain disulfide bond. X-ray crystallography indicates that each Ig domain consists of two β sheets of three or four antiparallel strands that contain five to ten amino acids each (Fig. 22-4). The domain structures are stabilized by the interior hydrophobic region between each sheet and by the intrachain disulfide bond. The Ig domains function as independent structural determinants that permit a variety of interactions through the accessible surfaces of the Ig molecule. Interactions between domains occur on the faces of the β sheets, whereas interactions with other molecules (e.g., antigens, complement) occur on contact residues near the ends of the domains. X-ray crystallography of an entire Ig molecule reveals that each pair of homologous domains compacts together to form a globular unit (201,202) (Fig. 22-5). In this model, molecular flexibility is provided by the sequences in the interdomain regions.

A considerable number of cell-surface and secreted molecules are constructed from similar Ig-like domains. Collectively, these proteins are members of the Ig superfamily, which includes a variety of receptors and adhesion molecules within the immune system, such as the T-cell receptor CD3 complex, histocompatibility molecules, adhesion molecules, Ig Fc receptors, and cytokine receptors (203). These molecules are found in tissues of other organ systems as well, such as the nervous system (e.g., neural cell adhesion molecule, myelin-associated glycoprotein, and contactin). In each case, the known functions of these molecules involve cell-surface interactions and triggering of signaling mechanisms within. The Ig domain functions as a protein framework for displaying determinants that permit molecular recognition of other molecules and transduction of biologic effects, usually via association with other molecules as part of a complex.

Systematic analysis of the amino acid sequences of light and heavy chains reveals an enormous diversity of sequences in the N-terminal half of each chain. This region on each chain is termed the *variable region* (V_L and V_H), and the antigen-binding sites are determined by the amino acid sequences of these regions (Fig. 22-3). The V_L and V_H region sequence variations are concentrated in three regions, termed the *hypervariable* or *complementarity-determining regions* (CDR1, CDR2, and CDR3) (204) (Fig. 22-6). The remainder of the V region is more con-

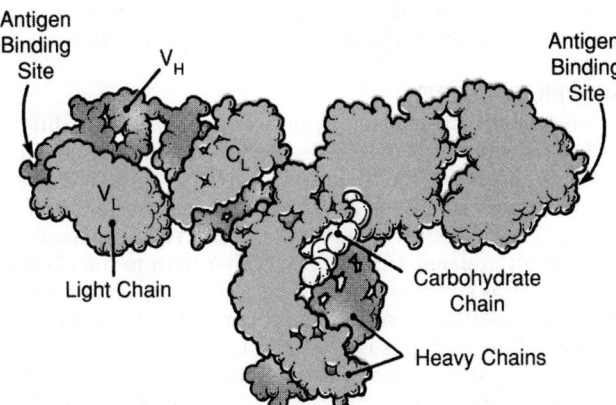

Figure 22-5. The quaternary structure of an immunoglobulin G molecule. The interactions among H- and L-chain components are displayed at the level of individual amino acids. A stabilizing carbohydrate structure on C_H2 is shown as occurring between each C_H2 chain. (From Silverton EW, Navia MA, Davis DR. The dimensional structure of an intact human Ig. *Proc Natl Acad Sci U S A* 1977;74:5140, with permission.)

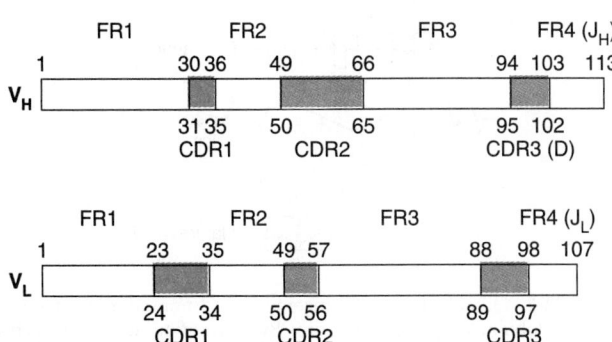

Figure 22-6. Immunoglobulin V regions are subdivided into four framework regions (FR) with three complementarity-determining regions (CDR) between them. A V_H gene encodes through the end of FR3. CDR3 is encoded by a D gene (see text and Figs. 22-7 and 22-8), and FR4 by a J_H gene. V_L genes encode almost to the end of CDR3; the remainder and FR4 are encoded by a J_L gene. The numbering scheme shown here are from Kabat and colleagues (583). (Reprinted from Bona CA, Bonilla FA. *Textbook of immunology,* 2nd ed. Amsterdam: Harwood Academic Publishers GmbH, 1996:72; with permission from Gordon and Breach Publishers.)

served throughout all light and heavy chains and is termed the *framework region*, which consists of four clusters of framework segments (FR1 through FR4; Fig. 22-6). In all, approximately one-third of the amino acid sequences in the V region are hypervariable, the remaining two-thirds consisting of framework regions. The heavy-chain CDR3 is slightly longer and more variable in amino acid sequence than in light chains. X-ray crystallographic studies reveal that the framework-region amino acids are organized as the β strands of the V region domains, whereas the amino acids constituting the hypervariable regions loop out of the domain structure (205) (Fig. 22-4). This arrangement allows considerable variability in the sequence of the complementarity-determining regions without disturbing the framework of the Ig V domains. The constraints on amino acids necessary to stabilize the hydrophobic β-sheet interior provide the stringent requirements that produce sequence conservation. The antibody-binding site is thus viewed as an exposed surface formed from the six complementarity-determining regions and built on the framework region scaffold.

The Ig molecule is encoded in a series of three unlinked gene families in the human genome: the κ and λ light-chain genes (on chromosomes 2p12 and 22q12, respectively), and the heavy-chain genes (chromosome 14q32). A complete mature light-chain gene is assembled in a process of somatic rearrangement from three segments (206) (Fig. 22-7). The amino-terminal half of each light chain is encoded by a series of germline V_κ or V_λ genes, together with a J_κ or J_λ (J = joining) gene. The carboxy-terminal half of each light chain is encoded by germline C_κ or C_λ (C = constant) genes, which determine the light-chain class.

Mature heavy-chain genes are assembled from four gene segments: V_H, D (diversity), J_H, and a C_H gene (206) (Fig. 22-8). Ig heavy chains are divided into five principal classes: IgM, IgD, IgG, IgA, and IgE. IgG is further divided into four subclasses, IgG1, IgG2, IgG3, and IgG4; IgA is subdivided into IgA1 and IgA2. Each distinct class and subclass of Ig corresponds to a distinct C_H gene. The heavy-chain locus also contains a few pseudogenes, which do not encode functional proteins. The order of the C_H genes on chromosome 14q32 is C_μ, C_δ, $C_{\gamma3}$, $C_{\gamma1}$, ψ_ϵ, $C_{\alpha1}$, ψ_γ, $C_{\gamma2}$, $C_{\gamma4}$, C_ϵ, $C_{\alpha2}$ (ψ = pseudogene). The structures of the C_H regions determine the biologic functions unique to each Ig class (e.g., cell binding, complement activation; Table 22-2). An additional segment, termed the *hinge region*, is unique to each Ig class and is not related by amino acid sequence to any other portion of the Ig genes. The hinge region, as its name implies, confers flexibility on the Ig molecule and is essential for multivalent antibody binding.

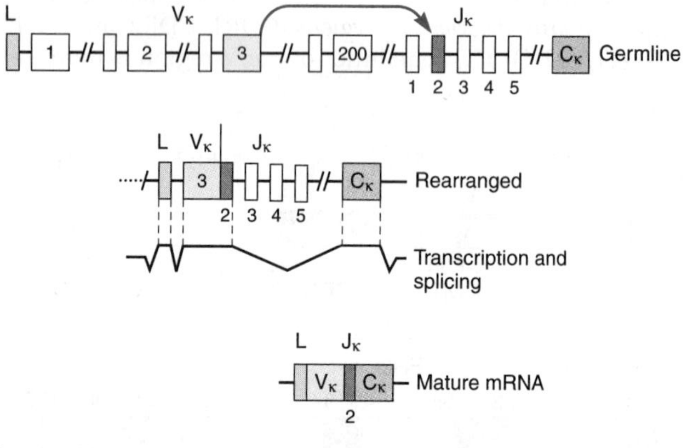

Like most plasma proteins, Ig contains oligosaccharides. Each Ig class varies in the amount and structure of the attached carbohydrate. In IgG, the oligosaccharides are found in the Fc region linked to C_H2, and variably within the Fab region (207). X-ray crystallographic analysis of IgG reveals a direct interaction between the C_H2-linked oligosaccharides, suggesting a role for these structures in stabilizing the Ig molecule (208). The oligosaccharide structures of each IgG molecule show a large degree of heterogeneity, resulting in many glycoforms of each polypeptide. This heterogeneity is found in each molecule and is not the result of polyclonality, because similar results are seen in myeloma- and hybridoma (monoclonal)-derived Ig (209). The occurrence of oligosaccharides in the Fab region further increases the diversity of antibodies and has been implicated in IgG aggregation and cryoprecipitation (210,211). IgG oligosaccharides have also been implicated in complement binding and activation, and in Fc-receptor binding and immune clearance (212).

Genetic and biochemical features of different Ig classes are summarized in Table 22-3. Biologic functions of the various classes and subclasses are summarized in Table 22-2.

Diversity

Ig diversity is entirely genetically determined. The nomenclature of this diversity is based on differences in structure identified by specific antiglobulin antibodies before the genetic basis of this diversity was understood. Diversity in the C region is limited and results in the Ig heavy- and light-chain classes (isotypes) and the genetic polymorphisms of these classes (allotypes). Diversity in the V regions is much greater and forms the basis of antigen recognition by antibodies, as well as the antigenic determinants of the Ig V regions themselves (idiotypes). The tremendous diversity of the Ig V regions is created during the process of gene rearrangement described previously. Diversity arises from multiple gene segments with differing structures, their assembly in various distinct combinations, the imprecise joining of the gene segment ends, template-independent insertion of nucleotides, the accumulation of point mutations during B-cell activation, and gene conversion events [reviewed by Oettinger (213)].

ISOTYPIC DIVERSITY

Ig determinants recognized by antisera prepared in a different (iso) species are termed *isotypes*. Each C region gene encodes a specific Ig isotype (see the previous paragraph). The heavy-chain isotypes define the Ig classes and the subclasses of IgG and IgA (Table 22-3). The isotype differences in subclasses are antigenically related more to each other than to the class isotypes, and it is speculated that subclasses represent a relatively late evolutionary diversification in mammals (214). Diversity of the light-chain isotypes is confined to the λ-chain in humans (215). Four distinct λ isotypes have been characterized, each corresponding to a distinct functional C_λ gene (Fig. 22-9).

Because the isotypes each represent distinct gene products, every individual has the capacity to produce each isotypic variant. In addition to determining the unique functions of each antibody class or subclass, isotypes may play a role in immune regulation. Isotypic determinants on membrane-bound antibody molecules may interact directly with T lymphocytes and, thus, regulate anti-

Figure 22-7. Organization, rearrangement, and transcription of human immunoglobulin κ–light-chain genes. By convention, diagrams such as this are drawn with left to right corresponding to the direction of messenger RNA (mRNA) transcription, 5' to 3'. This corresponds to the direction of protein synthesis, beginning with the amino terminus and ending with the carboxyl terminus. In the germline configuration, a few hundred V_κ genes are arrayed 5' to the five J_κ genes and the single C_κ gene. A single DNA rearrangement event joins one V_κ gene to one J_κ gene. After transcription, introns are spliced out yielding mature mRNA encoding a κ–light chain. (Reprinted from Bona CA, Bonilla FA. *Textbook of immunology*, 2nd ed. Amsterdam: Harwood Academic Publishers GmbH, 1996:63; with permission from Gordon and Breach Publishers.)

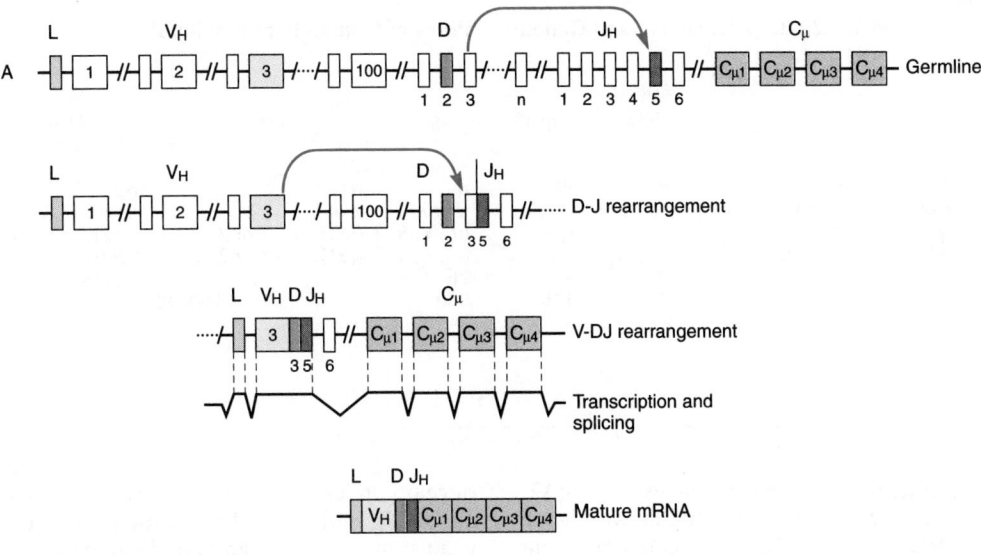

Figure 22-8. Organization, rearrangement, and transcription of human immunoglobulin (Ig) heavy-chain genes. **A:** The heavy-chain locus contains approximately 100 variable region (V$_H$) genes (many are nonfunctional pseudogenes), approximately 20 to 30 diversity (D) genes, and nine joining (J$_H$) region genes. Only six J$_H$ genes are functional; three are pseudogenes (not shown). Also shown here is C$_\mu$, the most 5' constant region gene. Some human D genes are interspersed with the 3' V$_H$ genes. The first DNA rearrangement step joins D to J$_H$; the second brings V$_H$ to DJ$_H$. As with light chains, introns are spliced out of primary transcripts to give mature heavy-chain messenger RNA (mRNA). **B:** There are 11 constant region genes, each encoding one of the Ig isotypes: μ (IgM), δ (IgD), γ3 (IgG3), γ1 (IgG1), ψ$_\varepsilon$ (epsilon pseudogene), α1 (IgA1), ψ$_\gamma$ (pseudo-gamma), γ2 (IgG2), γ4 (IgG4), ε (IgE), and α2 (IgA2). The relative positions of the VDJ regions and the enhancer region (E) are shown (not to scale). (Reprinted from Bona CA, Bonilla FA. *Textbook of immunology,* 2nd ed. Amsterdam: Harwood Academic Publishers GmbH, 1996:64; with permission from Gordon and Breach Publishers.)

body responses during antigenic challenge (216). Consistent with this possibility, isotype-restricted antibody expression has been observed in humans in response to specific bacterial and viral infections (217). Antiisotypic antibodies (C-region autoantibodies) are found in low abundance in the sera of most normal people and in increased amounts in patients with certain autoimmune disorders.

ALLOTYPIC DIVERSITY

Genetically determined allelic differences in antibody structure are termed allotypes. These determinants are recognized by antisera prepared from different individuals of the same species (allo) in which they occur. These represent allelic variants or polymorphisms within a given class or subclass. Antibody allotypes represent individual genetic alternatives, and thus occur only in certain members in a given population. Rheumatoid factors are IgM (sometimes IgG) antiallotype antibodies (218). Owing to the relative lack of specificity of most rheumatoid factors, allotypes are now generally characterized using the sera of multiply transfused patients. The detection system involves inhibition of red cell agglutination, and the antiallotypic IgG antibodies found in the transfusion sera are termed serum normal agglutinins. In addition, because allotypes represent inherited differences in Ig amino acid sequence, these differences can be identified directly by DNA analysis using specific probes (219).

TABLE 22-2. Biologic Properties of Human Immunoglobulins

Biologic Properties	IgG				IgM	IgA		IgE	IgD
	IgG1	IgG2	IgG3	IgG4		IgA1	IgA2		
Primary antibody response		−			+	−		−	−
Secondary antibody response		++			−		+	+	−
Complement activation									
Classic pathway	+	+	+	−	+		−	−	−
Alternative pathway	−	−	−	−	−		±	±	±
Transplacental transport	+	+	+	+	−		−	−	−
Opsonization	+	+	+	+	++		−	−	−
Reaginic activity	−	−	−	−	−		−	++	−

−, negative; +, positive; ±, varibale; Ig, immunoglobulin.

TABLE 22-3. Biochemical and Genetic Features of Human Immunoglobulins

Biochemical Properties	IgG				IgM	IgA		IgE	IgD
	IgG1	IgG2	IgG3	IgG4		IgA1	IgA2		
Structure									
Heavy chain	$\gamma1$	$\gamma2$	$\gamma3$	$\gamma4$	μ	$\alpha1$	$\alpha2$	ϵ	δ
Light chain	κ or λ	κ or λ	κ or λ	κ or λ	κ or λ	κ or λ	κ or λ	κ or λ	κ or λ
Molecular formula	$(\gamma1)_2, \kappa_2$; $(\gamma1)_2, \lambda_2$	$(\gamma2)_2, \kappa_2$; $(\gamma2)_2, \lambda_2$	$(\gamma3)_2, \kappa_2$; $(\gamma3)_2, \lambda_2$	$(\gamma4)_2, \kappa_2$; $(\gamma4)_2, \lambda_2$	$(\mu_2, \kappa_2)5$; $(\mu_2, \lambda_2)5$	$([\alpha1]_2, \kappa_2)$ 1 or 2; $([\alpha1]_2, \lambda_2)$ 1 or 2	$([\alpha2]_2, \kappa_2)$ 1 or 2; $([\alpha2]_2, \lambda_2)$ 1 or 2	ϵ_2, κ_2; ϵ_2, λ_2	δ_2, κ_2; δ_2, λ_2
Interchain S–S bonds	4	6	14	4	26	4	3 (or 4)	4	3
Molecular mass (kd)	146	146	155 165	146	900	160–385		190	180
Number of heavy chain domains	3	3	3	3	4	3	3	4	3

Ig, immunoglobulin.

Allotypes have been defined for IgG subclasses 1–4, IgA2, and κ–light chains. An allotype designation is built from a letter denoting the antibody class (G, A, or K), a number denoting the subclass, and the letter m followed by a number in parentheses, e.g., Km(1), G1m(2), G3m(10), A2m(1). There are three allotypes of κ-chains, two of IgA2, and 20 among the various subclasses of IgG (most for IgG3).

The biologic correlates of allotypic diversity are unclear. There are no well-defined associations between immunological disorders and allotypic haplotypes. In some cases, specific Gm alleles are associated with a twofold variation in the serum level of specific IgG subclasses, but the significance of this variation appears minimal for host defense (220). The antibody response to certain polysaccharide antigens may also be related to allotypic diversity. In one study, the response to *Haemophilus influenzae* vaccination was tenfold greater in children lacking the Km(1) allotype (221). The anti-Gm antibodies seen after exogenous gamma globulin administration or exposure of pregnant women to paternally derived Gm allotypes have not been associated with alterations in the pattern of IgG synthesis (222,223).

IDIOTYPIC DIVERSITY

Antigenic differences among all antibodies are due to differences in the amino acid sequences found in the V regions of the Ig molecule. The V-region sequence determines the unique specificity of each antibody molecule, and the unique structure created by this sequence is termed an idiotype. The determinants of idiotypes may be recognized by antisera from the same individual in which they occur. The individual antigenic components that determine a given idiotype are called idiotopes. Although some idiotopes can be localized to light- or heavy-chain V regions, most require an intact region of both chains for antigenic recognition (224).

All idiotypes are capable of eliciting an antibody response in an appropriate host, and these elicited antibodies are termed *antiidotypic*. Antiidotypic antibodies arise during the normal course of many immune responses (225). Antiidotypic antibodies that develop under these circumstances are autoantibodies directed against Ig molecules. These autoantibodies are directed only against the V regions and are distinct from rheumatoid factors directed against C-region allotypes. Antiidotypic antibodies themselves also have unique idiotopes, possibly resulting in multiple additional generations of antiidotypic responses. The recurrent nature of the antiidotypic response prompted Jerne to propose a fundamental role for these antibodies in a network of immune regulation linking antibodies and lymphocytes in the modulation of the immune response (226). The role of such idiotypic networks in the regulation of immune responses has been the focus of much controversy. Many studies in mice have shown that it is possible to alter the character of immune responses by exogenously administered antiidotype antibody (227). More recently, attention has focused on the potential role of idiotype-determined interactions in the pathophysiology of autoimmune disease (228,229), and in the therapeutic effects of IVIG for the treatment of autoimmune disease (230). Furthermore, antibody idiotopes may have structural similarity to protein structures on microbes or cancer cells (they function directly as tumor-associated antigens on Ig-bearing B-cell malignancies). Thus, they have been used with some success as antimicrobial and anticancer vaccines (231,232).

Immunoglobulin Function and Properties of Immunoglobulin Classes

The dual function of all antibody molecules is to recognize antigen and to communicate with host effector systems (humoral and cellular). Although the V-region structural diversity determines the antigenic specificity of each antibody molecule, it is the C-region diversity that determines the range of biologic functions of these molecules. Indeed, the evolution of C-region diversity has resulted in an expanded range of functions for each antibody molecule. These functions are different but overlapping for each Ig class (Table 22-2).

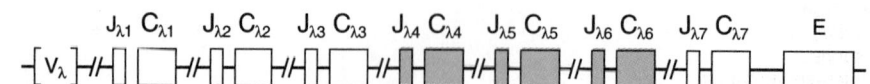

Figure 22-9. Organization of human immunoglobulin λ–light-chain genes. V_λ genes are located 5' to seven J_λ and seven C_λ genes. In contrast to heavy-chain and κ–light-chain loci, each J_λ gene is associated with one C_λ gene. As with κ–light chains, a single DNA rearrangement event joins a V_λ gene to J_λ. Again, introns are spliced out to yield mature messenger RNA. The fourth, fifth, and sixth J_λ –C_λ units are pseudogenes and are not expressed. The box labeled E shows the location of the λ enhancer region. (Reprinted from Bona CA, Bonilla FA. *Textbook of immunology*, 2nd ed. Amsterdam: Harwood Academic Publishers GmbH, 1996:65; with permission from Gordon and Breach Publishers.)

IMMUNOGLOBULIN G

IgG is the most abundant Ig class in human serum, accounting for more than 75% of all the antibody activity found in this compartment. This protein circulates as a 155-kd monomer in the plasma; normally, approximately 45% of the total body IgG is in the extravascular compartment. Patients deficient in Ig production best illustrate the essential nature of Ig in host defense. They suffer recurrent infections, and eventually succumb if not treated with exogenous Ig (see Antibody Deficiency Diseases). IgG is the sole isotype transported in any significant amount across the placenta, providing the human newborn with adequate passive immunity for the first 3 to 4 months of life (233). The human fetus is able to mount an effective humoral response *in utero*, and IgG synthesis has been detected in the human conceptus by eleven weeks of gestation, but under normal conditions, fetal IgG synthesis contributes little to total IgG in the newborn (234).

IgG mediates host defense in several ways. IgG can bind directly to a variety of toxins, resulting in their neutralization in the plasma. After antigen binding, IgG may activate the complement system. This activation is the result of direct protein interaction with the initial components of the complement pathway and is determined by unique sequences in the heavy-chain C region of this isotype and IgM. The activation of complement results in mononuclear phagocyte uptake of antigen-antibody complexes and the enzymatic production of anaphylatoxins, which promote inflammatory cell chemotaxis, migration, phagocytosis, and target cell lysis (see C3 and C5). In addition, IgG can interact directly with receptors on the surface of cells by means of determinants in the Fc region (see Immunoglobulin Fc Receptors). The presence of these receptors on mononuclear phagocytes and neutrophils promotes immune complex uptake and phagocytosis of particulate antigens. These interactions also mediate a variety of other cell functions essential to host survival during inflammation and tissue injury. Finally, the presence of IgG on defined target cell antigens such as tumors or allogeneic transplant tissue mediates the processes of antibody-dependent cellular cytotoxicity whereby lymphocyte cell populations are directed to lyse cells recognized as foreign.

As mentioned previously, differences in IgG-effector protein interactions and IgG–cell-surface binding account for the biologic differences seen among the IgG subclasses 1–4 (235,236) (Tables 22-1 to 22-3). The importance of IgG isotype differences in biologic function is further highlighted by the predominance of certain isotypes such as IgG1 in immune complex–mediated disorders (237). Patients have been described with isolated IgG subclass deficiency in association with increased susceptibility to infection (see Immunoglobulin G Subclass Deficiency). Although some of these patients have deficient antibody responses and additional immunological deficits, a specific role for IgG isotypes in the regulation of the humoral immune response remains unclear.

IMMUNOGLOBULIN M

IgM monomers have four C_H domains, and circulate in the serum as a pentamer of disulfide-linked Ig molecules joined by a single cross-linking peptide, the J chain (238,239) (Fig. 22-10). Under normal circumstances, the size of this pentameric structure (over 900 kd) limits the distribution of IgM to the vascular compartment. In contrast to IgG, the affinity of monomeric IgM is low. This is balanced, however, by high IgM antibody avidity owing to the multivalent structure of the molecule. In addition, this multivalent structure provides flexibility to the IgM antibody molecule that is important in mediating the specific biologic functions of this isotype.

IgM antibodies are the first isotype to appear in the plasma after antigenic stimulation. These antibodies usually appear within 3 to 5 days, are transient in nature, and are not associated with the development of immunological memory. For this reason, the presence of specific IgM antibodies can be indicative of recent antigenic exposure. Active synthesis of IgM has been detected in the human conceptus as early as 10.5 weeks of gestation (240). Because this isotype is not transported across the placenta, the presence of specific IgM antibodies in the human fetus or newborn can be used as prima facie evidence of intrauterine infection. Certain polysaccharide antigens result in an antibody response that is predominantly IgM. An example is the naturally occurring isohemagglutinins, which are IgM antibodies to erythrocyte blood group antigens. Allotype-specific autoantibodies, such as rheumatoid factors, are also predominantly IgM.

IgM antibodies mediate host defense in several important ways. The IgM molecule is more efficient in activating the classic complement cascade than any other Ig isotype, and many of the biologic effects of IgM are mediated by means of complement activation. The pentameric structure confers multivalency to the IgM molecule, and the molecular structure appears to afford a range of motion (flexibility) that permits conformational changes to accommodate this multivalent ligand binding. The localization of IgM antibodies in the serum, combined with efficient complement activation, results in a prominent role for this isotype in serum particle clearance by macrophages. Thus, IgM functions as a first line of specific immunological defense in the serum.

IgM is the first isotype expressed during human B lymphoid ontogeny, and under these circumstances, the molecule is found as a monomer on the B-lymphocyte cell surface (241). IgM monomers can sometimes be detected free in the plasma, generally in association with immunodeficiency or autoimmune disorders. These IgM monomers have been found to have antibody activity, and in certain cases, this involves the common blood-group isoantigens (242). Defects in IgM polymerization or J-chain production can also result in IgM monomer formation. The J chain, a 137–amino acid polypeptide, is synthesized only in Ig-producing cells, and preferentially in those cells secreting polymeric Ig (IgM or IgA) (238,239). Note that this J chain is completely distinct from the J region or segment of the heavy- and light-chain V regions. The amino acid sequence of the J chain is not homologous to the Ig domains.

IMMUNOGLOBULIN A

IgA is by far the most abundant Ig isotype found in humans (243). In the serum, IgA exists as a monomer (160 kd), accounting for approximately 10% of the total amount of Ig in this compartment. IgA is also abundant in all external secretions. This secretory IgA (S-IgA) exists as a dimer (500 kd) attached to the same J-chain peptide in pentameric IgM. S-IgA is not derived from the serum, but rather is produced by plasma cells localized in and around mucosal tissues. S-IgA is generally found in secretions attached to an additional protein termed the *secretory component*. The secretory component is synthesized by epithelial cells of mucosal tissues and hepatocytes and is derived from proteolytic cleavage of the receptor used to facilitate the secretion of polymeric IgA (receptor-mediated transcytosis) into body fluids and bile (see Polyimmunoglobulin Receptor). Although difficult to quantify, the amount of S-IgA produced each day exceeds all other Ig isotypes combined. Two IgA subclasses (isotypes) have been identified (designated IgA1 and IgA2; see previous and Tables 22-1 to 22-3). Differences in the amino acid sequence of the hinge region of IgA2 (found preferentially in secretions) confer partial resistance to bacterial proteases (243).

Despite the presence of IgA antibodies in the plasma, the primary role of IgA in host defense appears to be localized to mucosal surfaces (244). After antigenic stimulation, lymphoid tissues associated with specific organs, such as the lung and gastrointes-

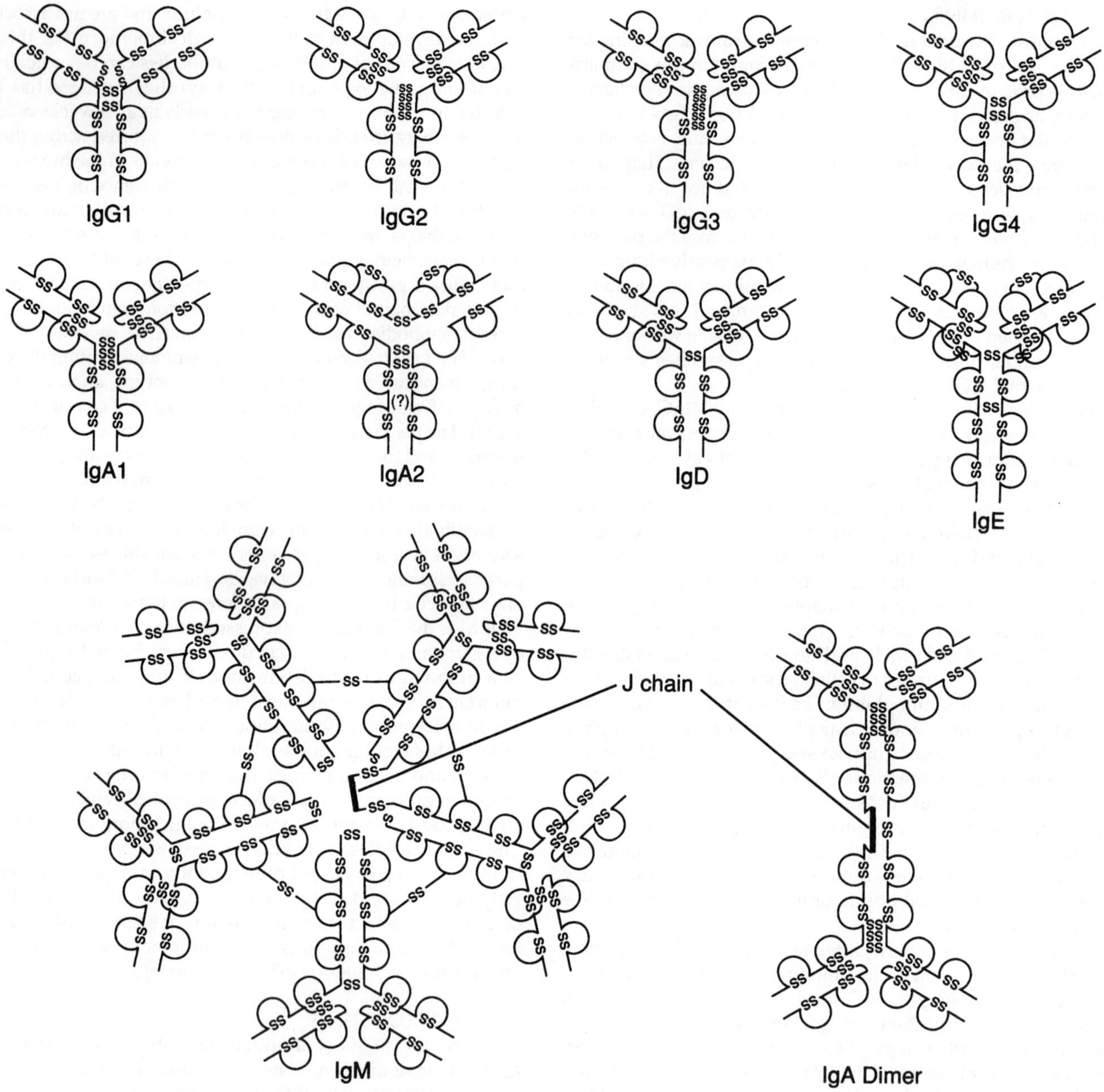

Figure 22-10. Structural characteristics of individual immunoglobulin (Ig) isotypes. Dimeric structure of serum IgA and pentameric structure of Ig M are illustrated linked by unique J-chain component. Variations in isotype structure are noted among isotype subclasses and each isotype in terms of both disulfide bond structure and number of domains. (From Gally J. Structure of Ig. In: Sela M, ed. *The antigens.* New York: Academic Press, 1973, with permission.)

tinal tract, mediate the local synthesis and secretion of specific polymeric IgA antibodies. In addition, homing of locally sensitized cells to distant tissue sites results in an elaborate system of mucosal defense in which specific IgA antibodies are present at all potential portals of entry. IgA antibodies do not activate the classic complement pathway and are not particularly effective in promoting phagocytosis. The overall importance of IgA in host defense is not known. Many individuals may have very low or absent serum IgA and suffer no apparent increase in susceptibility to infection or other apparent immune abnormality (see Immunoglobulin A Deficiency).

IMMUNOGLOBULIN E

The concentration of IgE in normal plasma is below the limits of conventional immunochemical detection, normally accounting for less than 0.01% of the Ig concentration in serum. IgE circulates in the plasma in monomeric form (190 kd). This isotype lacks a hinge region and contains four C-region heavy-chain domains. IgE is synthesized in most lymphoid tissues in the body but probably in greatest abundance in the lung and gastrointestinal tract. Unlike IgA, this isotype is not secreted at mucosal surfaces, and appears in increased concentrations in certain body fluids only during inflammatory exudation. Two forms of secreted IgE (εS1, εS2) are produced via alternative messenger RNA (mRNA) splicing of the Cε4 exon. The εS2 form is produced only in very small amounts, and is less active in IgE receptor binding in comparison to εS1 (245). The biologic implications of the two IgE isoforms are not known.

The primary biologic function of IgE appears to be the mediation of immediate hypersensitivity reactions (246). Antigen-specific IgE interacts with tissue mast cells by means of a receptor specific for the IgE Fc region (see Immunoglobulin E Fc Receptors). On antigenic stimulation, Fc-bound IgE mediates mast cell degranulation, with resultant bronchoconstriction, vasodilation, tissue edema, and urticaria. Although these responses may be beneficial in some way to the host, the presence of IgE-mediated allergic reactions are at best a nuisance and at times life-threatening. The presence of elevated serum IgE in patients with certain parasitic infections suggests that this isotype may play a role in host defense, and that encounter with parasites may be the evolutionary driving force for the persistence of an otherwise disadvantageous Ig (247). IgE can mediate cytotoxicity by eosinophils bearing IgE Fc receptors (see Immunoglobulin E Fc Receptors). IgE antibodies cannot activate complement.

IMMUNOGLOBULIN D

IgD is found in small quantities in human plasma and appears to have no direct role as a soluble antibody molecule. IgD antibody does not activate the complement cascade and does not interact directly with effector cells. The membrane-bound form of IgD is widely distributed on mature B cells, and appears to have some functional differences in signaling in comparison to membrane IgM (248).

Immunoglobulin Metabolism

The concentration of Ig in the plasma can be qualitatively assessed by serum protein electrophoresis. For example, in most cases of hypogammaglobulinemia, the gamma globulin fraction is reduced or absent, whereas the other separated protein fractions appear normal (Fig. 22-11). Serum protein electrophoresis is also useful in differentiating cases of secondary Ig deficiency (e.g., generalized protein loss) because, in these cases, the level of other protein fractions also is decreased. Finally, in cases of monoclonal and oligoclonal gammopathies, when the total concentration of Ig may be normal or even elevated, the monoclonal nature of the Ig can be appreciated on serum electrophoresis as a well-focused band (or series of bands) distinct from the normal diffuse pattern (Fig. 22-12). Quantitative Ig determination should always accompany serum protein electrophoresis. Enzyme-linked immunoassays using antisera specific to a given Ig isotype are sensitive and specific and can be readily adapted to the clinical laboratory. Ig subclasses and genetic variants can be similarly quantified providing the appropriate specific antisera are available. A caveat in all methods for quantifying Ig is that each antiserum and each Ig standard used is heterogeneous. Thus, variation in sample measurements between and even within laboratories can result. Fortunately, the normal biologic variation in Ig metabolism is much broader than the usual degree of uncertainty in these determinations, so that these measurements are still useful in the clinical setting.

Several important limitations in the interpretation of serum Ig measurements should be noted. First, all values must be interpreted in light of the changes that occur during development and aging. Although the variations in Ig levels are considerable under such circumstances, these have been carefully defined, and reference values allow adequate interpretation (Table 22-4). Second, the assessment of Ig levels provides no information regarding antibody activity. Such information is important because some patients with normal Ig levels have marked deficiency in specific antibody production after antigen exposure. The diagnostic approach in such cases is a part of the overall evaluation of immunologic competence (see Antibody Deficiency Diseases). Finally, the static measurement of Ig concentration in the plasma provides no

information about Ig flux, synthesis rates, body fluid distribution, or catabolism.

Most of the data concerning Ig metabolism have been obtained using passively administered (intravenous) radioiodinated purified proteins. These studies have revealed that each Ig isotype has a characteristic synthesis, transport, distribution, and catabolism (249) (Table 22-4). It is apparent from these data that differences in the rates of catabolism are as important as changes in the rates of synthesis in determining serum Ig concentration for each isotype. For some, including IgM and IgA, the fractional catabolic rate remains constant over a wide range of plasma concentrations, implying that short-term changes in the rate of synthesis have little or no effect on plasma concentration. On the other hand, the mean half-life of IgG is inversely proportional to the plasma IgG concentration (250). A decrease in the IgG synthetic rate resulting in a decrease in serum IgG thus results in an increase in the IgG half-life. This serves to diminish the impact of decreased IgG synthesis on the plasma IgG concentration. Thus, although the mean half-life of IgG is 23 days (longer than any other serum protein), in patients with agammaglobulinemia, this value may be prolonged to 30 days (251). The plasma levels of other Ig isotypes do not affect the half-life of IgG.

The transfer of Ig to the fetus takes place directly through the placenta and indirectly through the amniotic fluid (252,253). All Ig isotypes are exchanged from mother to fetus and from fetus to mother by both of these routes, albeit in small amounts. However, the placental transfer of IgG from mother to fetus in the later portion of gestation is much more efficient than is the transfer of any other isotype. Indeed, this process is so efficient that by term, the human infant is born with an IgG concentration equal to or greater than that of the mother. The kinetics of IgG transport across the placenta has been carefully studied and is consistent with both passive and active transport mechanisms. IgG is transported across the placenta by the so-called neonatal Fc receptor, or FcRn (254) (see Neonatal Immunoglobulin G Fc Receptor). Because the transport process begins at approximately 20 weeks of gestation, premature infants are born with lower IgG levels, but it is unclear if this contributes to the increased susceptibility to infection seen in these patients.

Immunoglobulin Fc Receptors

The highly conserved molecular framework of the Ig Fc region mediates the biologic effects of antibody molecules. The mechanisms determining these biologic effects involve interaction of this Fc domain with either fluid-phase or cell-surface-bound Fc receptor (FcR) molecules.

As the general designation indicates, these receptors specifically bind the Fc region of the Ig molecule, and are found on a variety of cells that participate in the immune response (239). FcRs mediate phagocytosis of antigen-antibody complexes, acquisition of passive immunity during development, stimulation of mediator release during inflammation, Ig clearance and catabolism, and antibody-dependent cell-mediated cytotoxicity. In addition, these receptors influence B-cell proliferation and thereby influence the synthesis and secretion of Ig. Most FcRs are members of the Ig superfamily (see Structure, under Immunoglobulins) differing in ligand affinity and primary structure. The diversity of the cytoplasmic regions of each receptor determines the unique signals transmitted and the distinct cellular functions.

IMMUNOGLOBULIN G FC RECEPTORS (FCγ RECEPTORS I, II, AND III)

Three classes of FcγR are recognized, each of which is encoded by genes located on chromosome 1 (239,255). Several of these

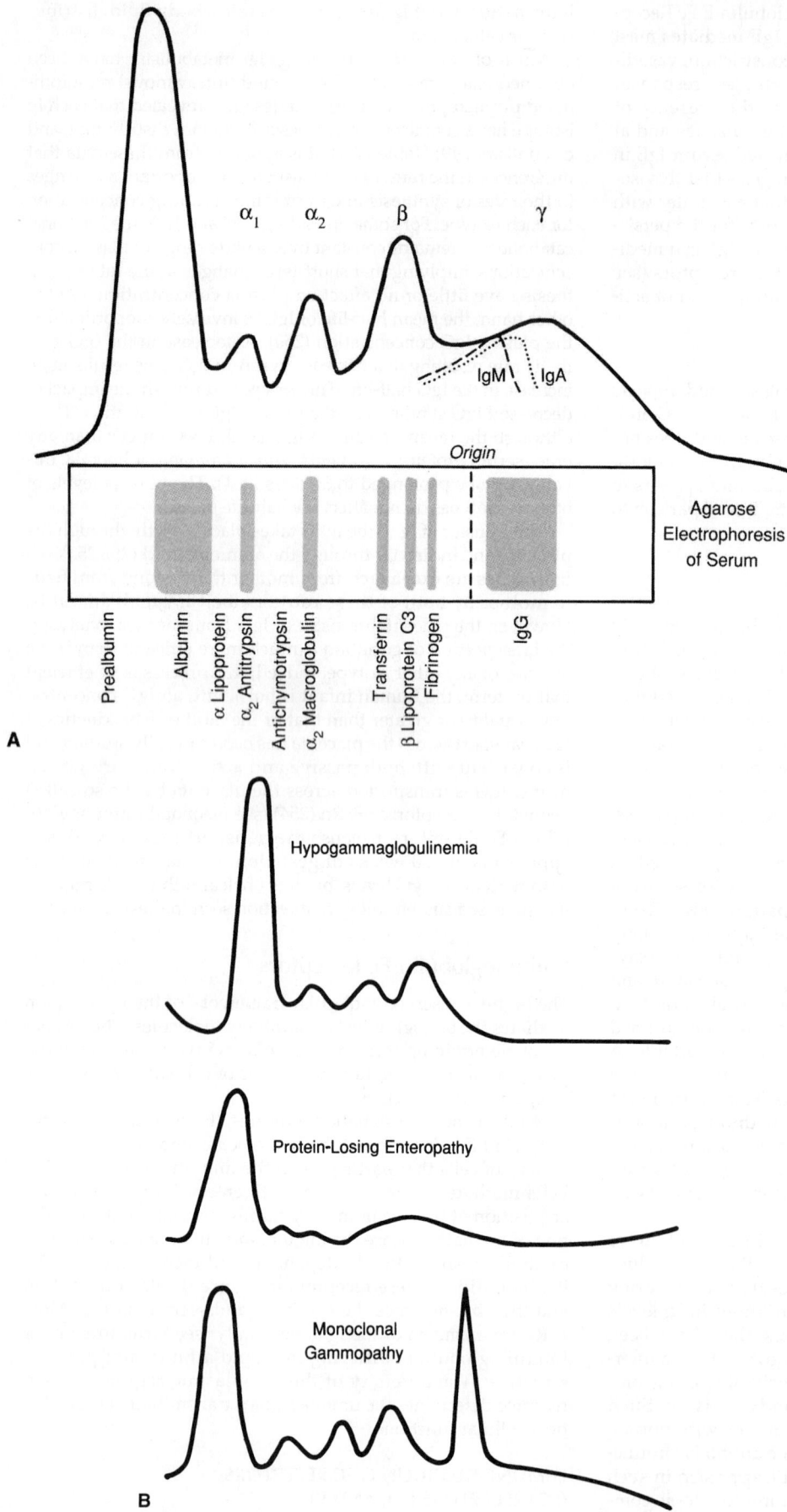

Figure 22-11. A: Agarose gel electrophoresis of serum with notation of major protein components and the fractions (α_1, α_2, β, γ) obtained by densitometry. The immunoglobulins (IgM and IgA) are contained within the β fractions as well as the predominant γ (IgG) fraction. **B:** Illustrative patterns of serum protein electrophoresis in various disorders of Ig metabolism. There is a selective loss of fraction in hypogammaglobulinemia as opposed by the general decrease in all fractions in protein-losing enteropathy. A single homogeneous spike is illustrated in monoclonal gammopathy.

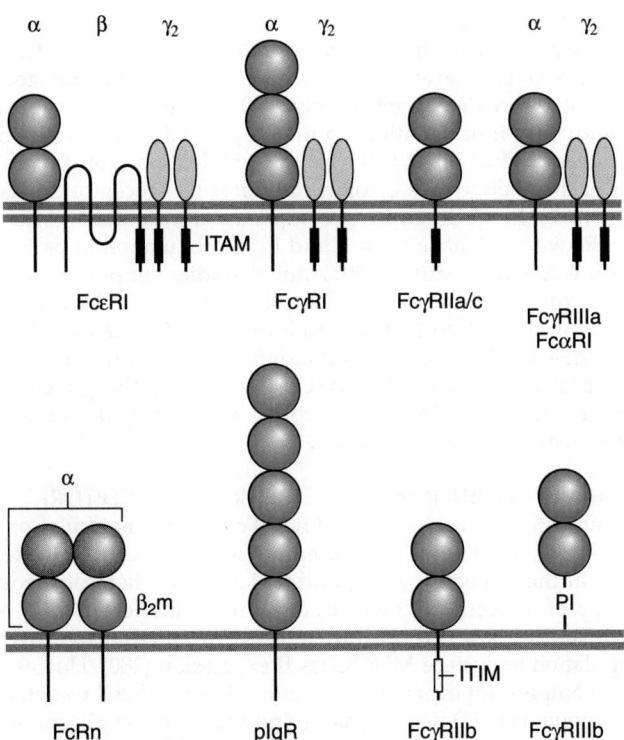

Figure 22-12. Structures of immunoglobulin (Ig) Fc receptors. Ig homology domains are depicted as spheres. The immunoreceptor tyrosine-based activation motifs (ITAM; see text) are filled boxes; the immunoreceptor tyrosine-based inhibitory motif (ITIM) is an open box. β_2m, β_2-microglobulin; PI, phosphatidylinositol linkage. See text for a description of each receptor.

activation signals after IgG binding (256). IgG subclasses differ in their affinity for various FcγRs: FcγRI has highest affinity for IgG1 and IgG3, followed by IgG4; affinity for IgG2 is relatively low. FcγRI is expressed on macrophages, monocytes, neutrophils, and mast cells (257); IFN-γ stimulates increased surface expression on all of these cells. FcγRI binds to the C_H2 domain of IgG, and has roles in antibody-dependent cytotoxicity by macrophages and monocytes, endocytosis, and phagocytosis. FcγRI cross-linking also stimulates release of inflammatory cytokines and intracellular superoxide production, and induces the transcription factor nuclear factor κB.

There are three different genes encoding FcγRI α-chains, designated FcγRI A, B, and C. Only the form encoded by FcγRIA appears to be expressed on cell surfaces. Four individuals in a single family have been found to lack expression of FcγRI owing to a mutation in FcγRIA that affects mRNA stability (258). These individuals are healthy, indicating that there is redundancy for FcγRI functions in immunity.

FcγRII (CD32) is a low-affinity receptor which binds primarily aggregated IgG molecules (239,255). Affinity is highest for IgG1 and 3, low for IgG2 and 4. FcγRII molecules are monomeric transmembrane chains with two extracellular Ig homology domains (Fig. 22-12). These chains bear their own cytoplasmic signaling motifs, and do not rely on associations with other molecules within the membrane to initiate signal transduction. There are three different forms of FcγRII, encoded by distinct genes A, B, and C. FcγRIIA and C are activating receptors; they carry ITAMs in their cytoplasmic domains. FcγRIIA and C are expressed mainly on myeloid cells, dendritic cells, and megakaryocytes and platelets. FcγRIIA is also found on lymphocytes. These receptors have roles in phagocytosis, and also stimulate the respiratory burst and mediator release. Two alleles of FcγRIIA have been found. They are designated high-responder and low-responder based on the ability of monocytes to provide costimulation for T cells on activation with antibodies binding the TCR. These alloforms also show differences in phagocytosis (259,260).

At least two soluble forms of FcγRIIA have been identified. One is generated by alternative mRNA splicing, another by cleavage of the extracellular portion of the molecule (261). The biologic role of these molecules is not well understood. They are capable of blocking interaction of IgG with cellular FcγR (262), and may play a role in suppressing B-cell activation and Ig secre-

exist as complexes with other molecules that modulate intracellular signaling after ligand binding (Fig. 22-12). FcγRI (also called CD64) is the only IgG FcR that has high affinity for monomeric IgG. It is a heterotrimeric complex of an α-chain that contains three Ig homology domains, together with a dimer of γ-chains (Fig. 22-12). These gamma chains participate in signaling of several different FcRs, and are often called FcRγ. These molecules have motifs in their cytoplasmic domains called *immunoreceptor tyrosine-based activation motifs* (ITAMs) critical for

TABLE 22-4. Metabolic Parameters of Human Immunoglobulins

	IgG				IgM	IgA			IgE	IgD
	IgG1	IgG2	IgG3	IgG4		IgA1	IgA2			
Serum concentration (mg/dL)										
Adult										
Range (total)		600–1500			75–150		200–300		0.02–0.06	0.01–3.00
Mean (total)		1200			97		250		0.04	2.2
Mean (subclasses)	840	240	80	40	—	220	30		—	—
Fetus (6 mo, mean)		300			20	ND			0.003	0.05
Newborn		1200 (all maternal)			30	ND			0.003	0.1
6-Month-old		400			40	25			0.006	0.1
1-Yr-old		800			60	60			0.01	0.3
Fraction of total serum Ig (%)		75–80			10	10–15			<0.01	<1
Fraction of total serum IgG (%)	70	18	8	4	—	—			—	—
Intravascular fraction (%)		45			80	42			50	75
Half-life (d)		23			5.1	5.8			2.5	2.6
	23	23	9	23						

Ig, immunoglobulin; ND, not determined.

tion (261). Elevated levels of FcγRIIA have been found in patients with stage C of B-cell chronic lymphocytic leukemia (262). FcγRIIA polymorphisms also appear to correlate with susceptibility to infection in patients with properdin deficiency (263).

FcγRIIB exists in two forms (FcγRIIB1 and 2) derived from different mRNA splicing from a single transcript (239,255). This receptor has general structural features similar to FcγRIIA and C, however, FcγRIIB does not have ITAMs in the cytoplasmic domain; instead, FcγRIIB has a distinct tyrosine-based inhibitory motif (264). The immunoreceptor tyrosine-based inhibitory motif recruits signaling molecules which act to down-regulate positive signals derived from other receptors. FcγRIIB1 is expressed primarily by lymphocytes, FcγRIIB2 by myeloid cells. Although these are not activating receptors, they still play a role in endocytosis and phagocytosis. FcγRIIB has been shown to down-regulate signaling by the B-cell receptor (265), and by the high-affinity receptor for IgE (266).

FcγRIII (CD16) is another low-affinity receptor for aggregated IgG molecules with subclass specificity similar to FcγRII (239,255). There are two forms, FcγRIIIA and B, encoded by distinct genes. FcγRIIIA is an activating receptor. The α-chain, with two Ig homology domains, associates with a dimer of FcRγ (see previous and Fig. 22-12). FcγRIIIB is unique among this group of receptors. Its truncated α-chain does not cross the membrane, but is anchored to phosphatidylinositol. FcγRIIIA is expressed on macrophages, monocytes, NK cells, pre-B cells, and T cells with the γδ form of the antigen receptor. FcγRIIIA is the only type of FcγR expressed on NK cells where it mediates antibody-dependent cytotoxicity. On other cells, FcγRIIIA participates in endocytosis and phagocytosis and promotes inflammation. Expression of FcγRIIIB is restricted to neutrophils. Two alleles are known, NA-1 and NA-2, distinguished by reactivity with antineutrophil antibodies from patients with autoimmune neutropenia. Some studies have shown differences in phagocytosis mediated by these alloforms (267), whereas others have not (260).

Soluble forms of FcγRIII also exist. Biologic functions for these molecules also are obscure. One study suggested that they could activate dendritic cells for antigen presentation and production of cytokines such as IL-12 (268). They may also play a role in inhibition of B-cell activity (261). Soluble FcγRIIIA is derived from NK cells by proteolytic cleavage at the membrane (269). Soluble FcγRIIIB is also generated by cleavage. Measurement of soluble FcγRIII in serum has been used as an indicator of inflammatory disease. For example, it has been found in relatively high amounts in gut lavage fluid from patients with inflammatory bowel disease (270), and serum levels correlate with clinical condition in sepsis (271). Low levels appear to correlate with susceptibility to infection in patients with chronic idiopathic neutropenia; low levels have also been observed in association with acute myelogenous leukemia (272).

Genetic defects involving FcγRIIIB have a prevalence of approximately 1.2/1000 in one survey in France (273). Women with absence of CD16 may have a greater rate of sensitization to CD16 present on cells from fetuses and resulting alloimmune neonatal neutropenia. In one study of 21 individuals with mutations of FcγRIIIB, 67% were healthy, 14% had incidental infections, 19% had recurrent or serious infections, and two patients had autoimmune thyroiditis (274).

IMMUNOGLOBULIN A FC RECEPTORS
(FCα RECEPTOR I, CD89)

FcαRI, or CD89, is structurally similar to many other Ig FcR. It is a heterotrimeric complex consisting of a ligand-binding α-chain, together with a dimer of FcRγ (Fig. 22-12) (275). Alternative mRNA splicing yields α-chains of differing structures with unknown functional correlates (276). FcαRI is expressed on monocytes, macrophages, neutrophils, and eosinophils. CD89 appears to function as an opsonic receptor, permitting phagocytosis of IgA-coated targets by myeloid cells. It also has a role in attenuating inflammation. In monocytes, CD89 cross-linking reduces production of TNF and IL-6, while it promotes synthesis of the endogenous cytokine inhibitor IL-1 receptor antagonist (277). Large amounts of complexes of the soluble form of FcαRI with IgA have been found in the circulation in patients with IgA nephropathy (278). Animal studies support a pathogenic role for these complexes, although the mechanisms of aberrant regulation that lead to formation of these complexes and disease remain to be elucidated. A novel IgA-binding receptor distinct from FcαRI/CD89 and the poly-Ig receptor (see Polyimmunoglobulin Receptor) has recently been identified on intestinal epithelial cells (279).

IMMUNOGLOBULIN M FC RECEPTORS (FCμ RECEPTOR)

Several studies have identified IgM Fc-binding molecules on a variety of cell types. These receptors remain poorly characterized at the molecular level, and this may be a heterogeneous group of molecules. The FcμR of natural killer cells has been reported to have an inhibitory function, mediating down-regulation of surface MHC class II expression (280). However, this complex appears to contain either FcRγ or T-cell receptor ζ components (281). Cross-linking induces tyrosine phosphorylation of Src and Syk family kinases, usually associated with activating stimuli. B cells express a receptor for IgM Fc joined to the membrane by a glycosyl phosphatidylinositol linkage (282). It is expressed mainly on B cells after activation. T cells appear to express a FcμR that is biochemically distinct (283). It is found mainly on resting T cells, and expression is reduced after activation.

IMMUNOGLOBULIN E FC RECEPTORS
(FCε RECEPTORS I AND II)

FcεRI is a high-affinity receptor for IgE. It is a tetrameric complex consisting of a ligand-binding α chain containing two Ig homology domains (Fig. 22-12), a signal-amplifying β-chain, and a signal-transducing γ-chain, the same FcRγ found in FcγRI and FcγRIIIA (284). The receptor is expressed as the full complex on mast cells and basophils, and may be expressed without the β-chain on monocytes, dendritic cells, and eosinophils. FcεRI is constitutively occupied by IgE on mast cells and basophils. Allergen cross-linking of specific receptor-bound IgE causes degranulation (release of preformed inflammatory mediators such as histamine and tryptase) and synthesis of additional mediators (arachidonate metabolites, cytokines). FcεRI cross-linking leads to increased receptor expression (285). FcεRI on antigen-presenting cells may mediate uptake of allergen-IgE complexes, enhancing presentation of allergens to T cells (286,287). FcεRI also mediates an IgE-dependent cellular cytotoxicity executed by eosinophils against eukaryotic parasites (247,288).

FcεRII (CD23) is a low-affinity receptor for IgE. It is a member of the family of proteins bearing C-type lectin domains, and is expressed as a homotrimer (289). It is found on monocytes, macrophages, dendritic cells, eosinophils, platelets, and B and T lymphocytes. Two forms are produced by alternative transcription; FcεRIIa is expressed only by B cells, whereas FcεRIIb is found on B cells, as well as other cell types. Biologic differences between these two types of receptors have not been described. FcεRII may also participate in IgE-dependent cellular cytotoxicity against parasites (290). By binding to FcεRII, IgE immune complexes increase its cell-surface expression (291) while they down-regulate IgE production (292). IgE-allergen complexes may also enhance antigen presentation via uptake by CD23 (293). Soluble forms of FcεRII (sCD23) are produced by cleavage of the extracellular portion. This molecule is capable of enhancing IgE production *in vitro*; its *in vivo* function is unknown (294).

IMMUNOGLOBULIN D FC RECEPTORS (FCδ RECEPTOR)

FcδR have been identified only on a subset of T cells (295–298). The function of this molecule remains unclear, and its structure is not known. In humans, the receptor behaves as a lectin, binding to oligosaccharides found on IgD, as well as IgA1. In comparison to T cells lacking FcδR, T cells induced to express FcδR generate more effective B-cell help for antibody production (298). This activity is reduced by addition of soluble IgD. The ability to respond to influenza vaccine has been correlated with the ability of T cells to up-regulate FcδR expression *in vitro* (295,296).

POLYIMMUNOGLOBULIN RECEPTOR

The polyimmunoglobulin receptor (pIgR) is expressed only on epithelial cells and appears to transport IgA and IgM across the epithelial cell surface (299). The pIgR consists of five Ig homology domains (Fig. 22-12). Polymeric IgA (or IgM) binds to the pIgR on the basolateral surfaces of mucosal epithelial cells via the J chain. Pinocytosis creates vesicles that are then transported across the cytoplasm to the apical surface of the cell. The pIgR undergoes proteolytic cleavage, and a fragment known as *secretory component* remains attached to the IgA or IgM molecule. In the case of IgA, the pIgR binds specifically to the C_H3 domain (300). Approximately 4 g of IgA is secreted in this way every day. Secretory IgA and IgM are critical for the protection of the mucosal surfaces of the intestines and airways. These antibodies may neutralize microbes and provide a first line of defense against pathogens that invade via these routes.

NEONATAL IMMUNOGLOBULIN G FC RECEPTOR

FcRn is expressed on human placental syncytiotrophoblast, capillary endothelial cells, and intestinal epithelium, and in other tissues such as liver, mammary gland, and kidney (254,301). FcRn has two apparent principal roles in IgG trafficking: It is responsible for most, if not all, of the transplacental transfer of IgG during the third trimester of gestation; it also protects IgG from degradation in endothelial cells after it is taken up by pinocytosis. The latter is responsible for the unique characteristics of the regulation of serum IgG levels (see Immunoglobulin Metabolism). Endothelial cells pinocytose serum proteins, including IgG. The IgG bound to FcRn is protected from degradation within the endothelial cell, and returns to the circulation. As the concentration of serum IgG rises, FcRn becomes saturated, and a greater fraction of IgG is available for degradation (i.e., the fractional catabolic rate increases). FcRn also mediates bidirectional transport of IgG across intestinal epithelium (302). The role of this transport process in intestinal immune surveillance is not clear.

The FcRn α-chain has homology to the α-chains of MHC class I molecules, and FcRn also functions in association with β_2 microglobulin (Fig. 22-12). The gene encoding the FcRn α-chain is located on chromosome 19, not in the MHC complex (chromosome 6) (303). Analysis of the crystal structure of FcRn has revealed differences in its interactions with different IgG subclasses and allotypes, but these do not appear to correlate clearly with differences in serum half-life (304).

IMMUNOGLOBULIN-BINDING FACTORS

A variety of Ig-binding activities have been described in various tissues, secretions, and culture supernatants. Few have

been characterized at the molecular level. One molecule now known as *Ig-binding factor* (IgBF) was identified initially by its interaction with a monoclonal antibody specific for FcγRIII. A recent analysis of protein structure suggests that IgBF itself may be a heterogeneous family of proteins (305). At least one IgBF may be what has been previously called *β-microseminoprotein*. This has been found in semen and prostate cells, and is a useful clinical marker of prostate cancer (306,307). IgBF has also been found in cervical and vaginal fluid (308). Extracellular enzymes in cervical secretions activate IgBF by cleaving inactive homodimers to yield the active monomers. IgBF has been found coating sperm cells (309); it may serve to mask alloantigens from immune surveillance in the female reproductive tract, or to block opsonization by antisperm antibodies (308). IgBF is also found in the healthy lower respiratory tract. Its concentration in bronchoalveolar secretions is higher in various inflammatory lung conditions and in smokers (310,311).

ANTIBODY DEFICIENCY DISEASES

A variety of primary immunodeficiencies have as their principal manifestation the impairment of humoral immunity, with general preservation of cellular immunity. Defects in this group of diseases may impair B-cell development, may affect specific antibody production, or the synthesis only of specific Ig classes or subclasses.

X-Linked Agammaglobulinemia

XLA was described in 1952 and was the first well-defined immunodeficiency disease (312). Affected males are well during the first 9 to 12 months of life owing to passive protection provided by transplacentally acquired IgG (313). Subsequently, these boys develop recurrent pyogenic infections of the upper and lower respiratory tract, middle ear, and the skin. They are generally free of urinary tract infections and diarrhea, and recover from the ordinary viral infections of childhood in the usual manner, although they may be prone in such situations to secondary pyogenic infections. The most common pathogenic bacteria in affected males are *Haemophilus influenzae*, pneumococci, streptococci, and staphylococci, and, to a lesser extent, *Pseudomonas* spp. These infections can generally be prevented by treatment with IVIG. Vaccine-associated paralytic poliomyelitis may be a complication of XLA.

Additional manifestations include arthritis, which may be owing to infection with mycoplasma or ureaplasma organisms (314). A syndrome much resembling dermatomyositis occurs in some patients. This is owing to infection of the central nervous system with echoviruses, which can be readily recovered from cerebrospinal fluid (315). These infections may be controlled with IVIG; however, high doses are required, and fatality or some degree of neurological impairment is common in this situation. It is important to test the various IVIG products and lots for the best titer against the relevant echovirus in each patient. Another rare finding in XLA (as well as in common variable immunodeficiency, or CVID) is the occurrence of sarcoidlike granulomas in the skin and viscera; the cause of this is unknown. Patients with all forms of agammaglobulinemia are extremely susceptible to infection with *Giardia lamblia*, which causes diarrhea, steatorrhea, and weight loss. Opportunistic infections such as *P. carinii* pneumonia are rare in XLA, but they have been described in a few cases (316).

The only striking and consistent finding on physical examination of boys with XLA is the virtual absence of tonsillar tissue, which is composed mostly of B lymphocytes. Their blood contains

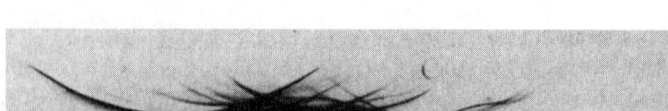

Figure 22-13. Immunoelectrophoresis of the serum of an agammaglobulinemic person (*top*) and a normal subject (*bottom*). The anode is to the left. The pattern was developed with horse antihuman serum. The precipitin bands for immunoglobulins G, A, and M are missing from the agammaglobulinemic serum.

no B lymphocytes, nor do their lymph nodes; as a consequence, there is little architectural organization and an absence of follicular structures. Plasma cells cannot be found in the lymphoid tissue or in the bone marrow. The bone marrow contains normal numbers of pre-B cells. The serum contains little IgG (approximately 10% of normal) and no IgA, IgM, IgD, and IgE (Fig. 22-13). In many patients with XLA, a few "leaky" B cells may develop (317). These B cells may be capable of normal or almost normal function, and some low specific antibody responses may even be demonstrated *in vivo*. T-cell number and function is normal in XLA. Normal delayed-type hypersensitivity can be elicited with the usual skin test antigens. Skin grafts are rejected in the usual manner.

XLA is caused by mutations in a protein tyrosine kinase that is now known as btk (318,319). Btk is expressed during all stages of B-cell development, as well as in monocytes, macrophages, mast cells, and erythroid cells. A tremendous variety of btk gene defects have been described in various patients with XLA. Databases of btk mutations are accessible via the World Wide Web (Table 22-1).

The identification of btk led to the discovery that the spectrum of phenotypes associated with this gene defect ranged from the severity of classic XLA, to a clinically silent mutation. The identification of atypical clinical phenotypes associated with btk mutations has led to reassignment of some diagnoses. For example, some patients initially thought to have CVID (see Common Variable Immunodeficiency) have been found to harbor mutations in btk (320). There are no distinct genotype-phenotype correlations in XLA: Even siblings harboring the same mutation may have distinct phenotypes (321–324). Btk protein is frequently undetectable even in patients with mild phenotypes (322); some of these may even be diagnosed in adulthood (325). These observations suggest that there is some redundancy in btk function that is polymorphic.

Btk has roles in signaling via the B-cell receptor, as well as FcεRI (326). In B-cell receptor signaling, btk is required for production of inositol triphosphate, a key intermediate in the release of intracellular calcium stores essential for B-cell activation (327). Btk also has a role in platelet activation by the gpVI collagen receptor (328). Collagen induction of protein tyrosine phosphorylation, calcium mobilization, and dense granule secretion were all reduced in XLA platelets. Responses to thrombin were preserved.

A recent retrospective study of IVIG therapy in 31 patients with XLA has shown a reduction in the incidence of bacterial infections from 0.40 to 0.06 per patient per year (329). Viral infections still developed, including enteroviral meningoencephalitis, which caused the only death in the study (median period of observation 10 years). IVIG was given at a dose of 250 mg/kg every 3 weeks, and trough serum IgG concentrations ranged from 500 to 1140 mg/dL (median, 700 mg/dL). Because T-cell function is completely normal in XLA, killed viral vaccines may be of benefit, because they may stimulate protective or partially protective cellular immunity (330).

Autosomal-Recessive Agammaglobulinemia

Several female patients with agammaglobulinemia and lack of mature B cells, as well as men with a similar phenotype lack-

ing btk mutations have been identified. Several molecular defects have been defined in this group of patients with agammaglobulinemia with autosomal-recessive inheritance. Mutations involving the Ig μ–heavy-chain locus prevent formation of the IgM heavy chain, required for formation of the Ig receptors on pre-B cells and mature B cells (331). Defects of the λ5 (surrogate light chain) gene prevent formation of the pre-B cell Ig receptor required for B-cell development (332). Igα (CD79a) is required for signal transduction via the pre-B cell and mature B-cell Ig receptors. Lesions in this gene prevent Ig receptor signaling and B-cell development (333). Most recently, defects in the signal transduction adapter B-cell linker protein have been found in some of these patients (334,335). This molecule is also required for normal signaling in B cells. All of these mutations arrest B-cell development at early stages in the bone marrow.

Common Variable Immunodeficiency

CVID may be acquired at any time in life, and affects men and women equally. There are two peaks in the age of onset, one in the first decade, and the other in the third or fourth (336–338). There is no clear inheritance pattern for the acquisition of CVID, and the cause of the disease is unknown, although it may follow an infection with EBV (339), or solid organ transplantation (340), in rare instances. The diagnosis rests on the demonstration of hypogammaglobulinemia and impairment of specific antibody production (1,341).

Patients with CVID are susceptible to recurrent pyogenic infections, as are males with XLA, and any survey of a population with chronic obstructive pulmonary disease reveals some patients with undiagnosed CVID. Additional manifestations include chronic enteroviral infections, including meningoencephalitis; arthropathy, which may be owing to mycoplasma or ureaplasma; and symptoms suggestive of asthma and allergic rhinitis, although no allergen-specific IgE is found (336,338). These patients are prone to developing a variety of autoimmune pathologies such as inflammatory bowel disease, cytopenias, and pernicious anemia and becoming vitamin B12–dependent. This complication should always be suspected when a serious infection does not respond to antibiotic therapy in a patient with CVID who is receiving adequate γ-globulin replacement.

Many patients may develop a benign lymphoproliferative disorder with splenomegaly and giant lymphoid hyperplasia of the intestine. There is an increased rate of lymphoma as well; the relative risk has been estimated between 30- and greater than 400-fold in comparison to the general population (336,338,342). Noncaseating granulomatous disease resembling sarcoid may be encountered in the skin or viscera. It often responds well to steroid therapy (343,344). There also appears to be an increased incidence of gastrointestinal malignancy in patients with CVID. Diarrhea and steatorrhea are common and often due to infestation with *G. lamblia*.

Reduced levels of IgG are universal, by definition. Reduction of IgA is seen in the majority of patients, as well. IgM may be normal or reduced. Ig levels most often are static, or fall with time. In rare cases, they may rise (345,346). Other immunological manifestations of CVID are heterogeneous. B cells may be reduced or normal. In most patients, they produce antibody normally when stimulated *in vitro* (347). However, a subgroup of patients have normal numbers of peripheral blood B cells that do not secrete antibody *in vitro* (348). These cells fail to up-regulate CD86 (B7-2, important for interactions with T cells) after stimulation via the B-cell receptor and CD40. Others have demonstrated impairment of Ig gene somatic mutation in B cells in CVID (349).

Reductions of CD4+ T-cell numbers have been reported in some cases of CVID, and some have demonstrated impairment of cytokine production (IL-2, IL-4, IL-5, and IFN-γ) (350–352) or expression of CD154 (353) after T-cell stimulation *in vitro*. A few studies have shown an approximately sixfold reduction in the frequency of peripheral antigen-specific CD4+ T cells in CVID patients (354,355). Lymphopenia in CVID patients has been associated with increases in CD95 (Fas) expression and spontaneous apoptosis (356).

There is significant immunological heterogeneity among CVID patients (357). No single gene defect has yet been described in any patient with CVID. Most cases appear to be sporadic. Homozygosity at HLA class II loci, particularly HLA DQ, has been found in greater frequency among CVID patients in comparison to controls (358). Some studies also suggest associations with IgAD and extended MHC haplotypes (359).

CVID should be treated with regular administration of IVIG (336,338). The occurrence of anaphylactic reactions in IgA-deficient CVID patients after infusion of blood products containing IgA has been associated with anti-IgA antibodies (360,361), but these correlations are not supported in all studies (362). Therapeutic and prophylactic antibiotic therapy is also frequently required in CVID. Alternative therapies have also been attempted. A double-blind placebo-controlled crossover study of IL-2 therapy in ten CVID patients has been reported (363). The group that received IL-2 first, followed by placebo, had a significant drop in the rate of infections in the placebo phase of the study. The authors speculated that specific antibody responses occurred during the IL-2 phase, and the protection was manifested during the placebo phase. Alternatively, the sustained administration of IL-2 followed by its withdrawal may have led to a restoration of a normal cytokine balance.

Immunoglobulin A Deficiency

Approximately 1 in 700 American caucasions is IgA-deficient; thus, IgAD is the most common immunodeficiency in this group (364). On the other hand, IgAD is encountered much more rarely in other ethnic groups, such as the Japanese (365). There are usually no apparent clinical consequences of note in the majority of patients with low IgA, but some have a predisposition to bacterial respiratory tract infections. Extended (20-year) follow-up of apparently healthy blood donors with IgAD found higher relative rates of respiratory tract infection and autoimmune disease (366). Infections are seen more consistently when IgAD occurs together with IgG subclass deficiency (IgGSD), usually IgG2 and/or IgG4 (see Immunoglobulin G Subclass Deficiency), or when antigen responses, such as to pneumococcal polysaccharide, are impaired (367,368). IgGSD occurs in approximately one-third of IgAD patients (367).

In a survey of patients with rheumatoid arthritis, it was found that IgAD was more frequent than in the normal control population. This is true of many autoimmune diseases, which also occur with greater frequency in IgA-deficient persons (369). Circulating autoantibodies against a variety of antigens

(e.g., cardiolipin, Sm, collagen) are found more frequently even in healthy people with low IgA (370). Syndromes otherwise associated with atopy also occur in IgAD (371), and these patients also encounter an increased rate of the forms of malignancy associated with CVID (372). Clearly, there are many parallels between the clinical manifestations of CVID and IgAD. Some cases of IgAD have even evolved over time into CVID (345,373). As with CVID, rare cases of IgAD may improve with time (345).

Many IgAD patients have normal numbers of circulating B cells bearing surface α-chains, but they appear to be blocked in their development (374). One study has demonstrated low expression of Cα mRNA after class switching to the IgA locus in B cells from IgA-deficient patients (375). Usually, serum levels of IgA1 and IgA2 subclasses are affected equally. Results of studies of *in vitro* IgA production by B cells from IgAD patients have been mixed (376–379). Defects in class switching to IgA, or in the development of cells after switching to IgA, have been reported (380,381). The cytokine transforming growth factor-β (TGF-β) is important for IgA class switching in humans. One study found reduced levels of TGF-β in serum from IgAD patients (382), whereas another reported normal TGF-β mRNA in IgAD (381). Mice with targeted disruption of the TGF-β1 gene have reduced serum IgA (383).

Anaphylactoid reactions in IgAD patients with anti-IgA antibodies have been reported after administration of IgA-containing blood products (360). However, one recent study found anti-IgA antibodies in 76% of IgA-deficient blood donors, but only in 18% of IgAD samples being analyzed for possible anaphylactic transfusion reactions (362). The expected frequency of IgAD with anti-IgA was calculated to be much greater than the rate of anaphylactic transfusion reactions. These authors suggest that anti-IgA is not pathologic in these instances.

The inheritance of IgA deficiency is variable, and genetic studies have not identified clear molecular associations. IgA gene deletions are found in a tiny fraction of individuals, often associated with other gene deletions (see Immunoglobulin G Subclass Deficiency). An IgAD susceptibility locus (called by some *IGAD1*) appears to lie within the telomeric part of the MHC class II region, or the centromeric part of the class III region (384). IgAD has been associated with the northern European haplotype HLA-A1, -B8, -DR3 (385–387). This haplotype is also associated with CVID (359,387). A case of phenytoin-induced IgAD has been reported (388). The serum IgA rose again after the drug was discontinued.

Treatment of IgA deficiency generally focuses on the management of complications as they arise. IVIG may be useful in some patients, particularly when IgAD is associated with IgGSD (see the next section).

Immunoglobulin G Subclass Deficiency

Each of the four subclasses of IgG is found within a characteristic range of serum concentrations (Table 22-4). Thus, IgG subclass deficiency is the relative reduction of one or more IgG subclasses, most often in the context of a normal total concentration of serum IgG. Molecular defects in the vast majority of patients have not been described. Most individuals are asymptomatic. Some may present with recurrent sinopulmonary infections caused by common respiratory bacterial pathogens (389), as well as recurrent diarrhea, often of infectious origin; inhalant and food allergies; autoimmune disease; and seizure disorders (390). There is great overlap in clinical features even when different subclasses are affected.

A variety of distinct patterns of subclass deficiency have been reported. IgG1 deficiency may occur alone, with elevated

IgG2, and with low IgG3 (391,392). Low levels of IgG2 are detected most commonly in pediatric patients; most of these are male. It is frequently associated with deficiency of IgG4 and/or IgA (367,393–396). Deficiency of IgG3 alone is found more commonly in adult females (394,397,398). Finally, low levels of IgG4 may occur alone (399,400).

Most individuals with IgG subclass deficiency are asymptomatic, and frequent infections and impaired antibody responses may occur in people with normal IgG subclasses. Thus, the clinical significance of low IgG subclass concentrations in patients with recurrent infections is controversial. Some suggest that assessing the response to antigen challenge is the most important element in evaluation of these patients. Indeed, a clinical entity has been distinguished from IgG subclass deficiency by the association of impairment in antibody responses to vaccines and/or natural infectious challenge, with normal levels of Ig and IgG subclasses (389,401–403). This entity has been called *specific* or *functional* antibody deficiency. However, several studies have shown an increased proportion of subclass-deficient individuals among patients with recurrent infections (394–396,404–406). Not all of these patients have demonstrably impaired vaccine responses.

In children, therapy of these disorders consists mainly of antibiotic treatment and prophylaxis of bacterial infections, as well as therapy of any associated disorders such as environmental allergies and asthma. In the more severe cases that do not respond well to preventive antibiotic treatment, a period of IVIG replacement therapy is warranted. The natural history of these syndromes is often slow spontaneous resolution. Most patients have a greatly reduced frequency of infections by late childhood. When recurrent infections have their onset in adulthood, the clinical course most often resembles CVID. These patients frequently respond to IVIG. However, therapy may have to be lifelong, as infections may recur when IVIG therapy is discontinued.

There is only one case report of clinically significant IgG2 deficiency with mutations identified in the IgG2 genes (407). These brothers were both homozygous for an insertion mutation that resulted in the loss of the transmembrane and cytoplasmic domains, prohibiting formation of a functional surface IgG2 molecule. Interestingly, large deletions of Ig C region genes are found commonly (up to 10%) in the general population; six multigene deletion haplotypes have been identified (408). In one analysis of 16 individuals from consanguineous kindreds with homozygous or compound heterozygous deletions, only one had recurrent infections, although all completely lacked one or more IgG subclasses and/or IgA1. Healthy individuals with homozygous deletions of IgA1, IgG2, IgG4, and IgE have also been described (409). Among 33 patients with CVID studied, only two were heterozygous for Ig C region gene deletions (410).

Transient Hypogammaglobulinemia of Infancy

Transient hypogammaglobulinemia of infancy (THI) is defined as a serum IgG concentration below normal in an infant or young child that spontaneously resolves by approximately three to four years of age (411). The disorder is most frequently sporadic, but may be familial. No molecular defects have been described. A delay in the development of T-cell help for antibody production may occur in some individuals (412). There are no abnormalities of lymphocyte subsets, or *in vivo* or *in vitro* measures of cellular immunity. B-cell numbers are normal.

Many infants with low IgG levels are healthy. Between 6 and 12 months of age, some begin to have the typical recurrent respiratory tract infections associated with hypogammaglobulin-

emia. One 10-year prospective analysis of 35 patients who presented with hypogammaglobulinemia under the age of 4 years (one-third with associated impairment in specific antibody production) showed three patterns over time (413). In group 1, comprised of 29 patients (83%), IgG and IgG subclass levels and antibody responses all became normal and infections ceased; in group 2 (three patients, or 9%) IgG levels remained low, and antibody production was poor; in the remaining three patients (group 3), IgG levels became normal, but antibody production remained poor. Group 1 would be classified as THI; and group 3 as specific antibody deficiency. Group 2 consists of uncharacterized persistent hypogammaglobulinemia: This could include atypical XLA, CVID, HIGM, or undefined conditions. Invasive infections and low tetanus antibody level at presentation were the most significant predictors of persistent immune abnormalities.

In THI, specific antibody production is often normal at presentation. In most children, antibody response is robust before their serum antibody levels enter the normal range (414); however, this is not true in all cases (415). Before its resolution, THI is a diagnosis of exclusion. Thus, these patients deserve close attention to look for the appearance of other symptoms or signs of other distinct forms of hypogammaglobulinemia.

Antibiotic prophylaxis is almost always adequate to prevent infections in THI. A poor response to antibiotics may warrant a period of IVIG replacement. If such therapy is required, infusions should be stopped after 6 to 12 months, and antibody production reevaluated. Children who have a slow rise in antibody production, invasive infections, or who fail to respond to IVIG therapy must be thoroughly re-evaluated with respect to immune function.

COMPLEMENT SYSTEM

The complement system consists of approximately 30 plasma and cell membrane proteins. The system is divided into the classic and alternative pathways, which have distinct modes of activation and interactions with innate and specific immune effector mechanisms. However, both pathways are activated more or less together in many situations. The physiologic roles of the complement system have perhaps been most clearly indicated by the clinical consequences of genetic defects in this system (Table 22-5). Through their role as major opsonic factors for phagocytosis, complement proteins protect the host from a variety of bacterial infections. In addition, via mechanisms that are not yet well understood, complement is required for the formation of immunological memory, and for the establishment and/or maintenance of B-cell tolerance. Autoimmune disease often results from a failure of complement function.

TABLE 22-5. Clinical Conditions Associated with Complement Deficiencies

Component(s)	Syndrome(s)
C1, C2, C3, C4, factor I	Recurrent bacterial infections, mainly of the respiratory tract
C5, C6, C7, C8, C9, factor H	Recurrent meningococcal meningitis
C1, C2, C4, C5, properdin	Autoimmune disease, including discoid or systemic lupus, vasculitis, other
Factor H	Familial relapsing hemolytic uremic syndrome
C1 inhibitor	Hereditary angioedema

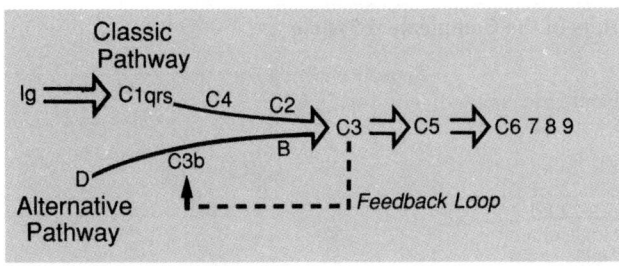
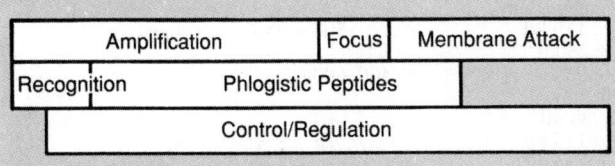

Figure 22-14. Classic and alternative complement activation pathways leading to assembly of the membrane attack complex. Ig, immunoglobulin.

The interaction of antigens with antibodies of several Ig classes and subclasses initiates binding and activation of the classic complement pathway. Specificity of the classic pathway reaction is imposed by antibody. In a few instances, such as viral agents (416), C-reactive protein (417), and mitochondrial membranes (418), activation of the classic pathway can proceed in the absence of antibody. The recently described lectin pathway is another mode of classic pathway activation that bypasses C1 and antibody (see Lectin Complement Pathway).

Activation of the alternative complement pathway involves antibody-independent recognition of structures, such as repeating polysaccharides and endotoxin of bacteria, and extracellular matrix components which are either highly represented among pathogenic microorganisms, or signal tissue injury. This activation, therefore, involves relatively nonspecific binding. Localization of the alternative pathway reaction is accomplished by propagation of the cascade under conditions when inactivation of the effector proteins is limited. Amplification is an important feature of classic and alternative pathways because deposition of one or few initiating complexes can yield enzymatic cleavage of thousands of later components in the cascade. In the course of complement activation, numerous biologically active complement-derived polypeptides are released in the fluid phase. The effects of these may be exerted at great distance and, in most instances, through interaction with specific cell-surface receptors. Modulation of the complement cascade is accomplished by fluid-phase and membrane proteins (inhibitors/cofactors) as well as intrinsic decay or instability of several of the complement components or fragments. Figure 22-14 diagrams the complement pathways.

The soluble complement proteins are designated numerically (e.g., C1 through C9) or by uppercase letters (e.g., factor B, factor D); their cleavage products by lowercase letters (e.g., C2a, C3b); and the polypeptide subunits of the multichain proteins by lowercase Greek letters (e.g., C4α, β, γ). Table 22-6 outlines several physicochemical properties of the complement proteins and their approximate serum concentrations. In the following paragraphs we consider each complement component and its role in the system separately, along with the clinical conditions associated with genetic defects of that component. Table 22-5 contains a summary of the clinical consequences of complement component deficiencies.

Early Components of the Classic Complement Pathway

C1

The C1 complement component is a Ca^{2+}-dependent metalloprotein complex of a collagen-like recognition molecule C1q and dimers of the serine proteases C1r and C1s (419). C1q is composed of six globular domains connected by triple helical regions to a central fibril (420) (Fig. 22-15). The globular heads interact with the C_H2 domain of IgG (421) and C_H3 or C_H4 of IgM (422). Binding to Ig distorts C1q, and activates C1r, which cleaves and activates the C1s serine protease (423). C1q is present in normal human serum mostly in the complex $C1qr_2s_2$, but up to 20% to 30% may be found as free C1q and $C1r_2s_2$. Binding of C1q to Ig increases the affinity of C1r2s2 for C1q by an order of magnitude. On cell surfaces, a single IgM or an IgG doublet (30 to 50 nm or less from each other) in complex with antigen is capable of binding a single C1 molecule and initiating the classic pathway complement cascade. C1 may also bind effectively to certain structures independently of Ig, such as β amyloid (424), bacterial cell walls (425), or C-reactive protein (417). C1 is synthesized in epithelial cells, mononuclear phagocytes, and fibroblasts and hepatocytes.

Defects in any component of the C1qrs complex causes loss of C1 function. Clinical manifestations include susceptibility to recurrent infections, and a systemic lupus-like syndrome. There are three C1q genes (A, B, C); mutations in C1qB and C1qC have been described (426,427). Mutations in C1r (428), and C1s (429,430) have also been reported. C1q-deficient mice generated by targeted gene disruption are prone to autoimmune disease and glomerulonephritis (431).

C4

C4, the natural substrate of the C1s enzyme, is a disulfide-linked heterotrimer consisting of α-, β-, and γ-chains generated by posttranslational cleavage of a single polypeptide precursor (419). Cleavage of an amino-terminal fragment of C4 (C4a) from the α chain exposes the binding site for the C4b fragment to Ig, antigen, or cell surfaces. Two isoforms of C4, products of the separate genes C4A and C4B, are found in human serum. The previously identified red cell antigens Rodgers and Chido are, in fact, cleavage fragments of C4A and C4B proteins, respectively (432). The two forms differ by only four residues, but these differences account for a profound difference in affinity for hydroxyl (C4B) or amino group (C4A) acceptor sites. Both forms of C4b serve as binding sites for the cleavage product of C2 activation (C2a), thus generating the classic pathway C3 convertase enzyme. The C4a fragment is an anaphylatoxin, and has distinct biologic effects mediated by a specific receptor (see Receptors for the Anaphylatoxins: C5aR(CD88), C3aR, C4aR).

The C4 genes are located in the class III region of the MHC complex on chromosome 6. Null alleles are found at these loci quite frequently; 35% of individuals have one of either C4AQ0 or C4BQ0. Approximately 10% have two null alleles, and 1% have three (433). Complete C4 deficiency (four null alleles) is quite rare. Partial C4 deficiency usually does not lead to symptoms. However, MHC haplotypes containing C4 null alleles are found with relatively greater frequency in patients with systemic lupus (434), CVID, and IgAD (359). Complete C4 deficiency is associated with severe glomerulonephritis with a systemic lupus-like syndrome, and susceptibility to bacterial infections.

C2

C2 is a single-chain glycoprotein that binds to C4b in the presence of Mg^{2+} and is cleaved into an amino-terminal polypeptide (C2b), and a carboxy-terminal fragment (C2a), which contains

TABLE 22-6. Proteins, Regulators, and Receptors of the Complement System

	Molecular Mass (kd)	Subunit Structure	Serum Concentration (μg/mL)
Complement protein			
C1q	410	6A: 24 kd 6B: 23 kd 6C: 22 kd	70
C1r	95	Single chain	35
C1s	87	Single chain	35
C2	110	Single chain	25
Factor B	93	Single chain	200
Factor D	24	Single chain	1
C3	185	α: 110 kd β: 75 kd	1500
C4	200	α: 93 kd β: 78 kd γ: 33 kd	400–600
C5	190	α: 115 kd β: 75 kd	75
C6	115	Single chain	75
C7	115	Single chain	65
C8	163	α: 64 kd β: 64 kd γ: 22 kd	55
C9	71	Single chain	60
C1 inhibitor	104 (34% CHO)	Single chain	150
Properdin	~224	6: 56,000	25
C4bp	500	7: 70,000 (6α: 70,000) (1β: 45,000)	~150
Factor I	88	46,000 39,000	35
Factor H	155	Single chain	500
S protein	~80	Single chain	500
Membrane receptors and regulators			
Decay-accelerating factor	70	Single chain	—
Membrane cofactor protein	58–63	Single chain	—
Homologous restriction factor	20	Single chain	—
CR1	A: 190[a] B: 220 C: 160 D: 250	Single chain	—
CR2	140	Single chain	—
CR3	260	α: 165,000 β: 95,000	—
C5aR	~45	Single chain	—
C1qR	~70	Not determined	—

CHO, carbohydrate; CR, complement receptor.
[a]Allotypes.

the active site (419). C4b and C2a deposit on a cell membrane as a complex (C4b2a), which has C3-cleaving activity. Thus, it is often called a *C3 convertase*. The C4b2a complex is unstable. First-order decay is an intrinsic control mechanism in the classic pathway, but decay is accelerated by cell-surface control proteins, described in the following paragraphs. On the cell membrane, a single C1 molecule can generate a cluster of C4b2a molecules that function to generate membrane lesions at or near the recognition site. C2 is synthesized in the liver, mononuclear phagocytes, fibroblasts, and perhaps in other cells. There are three C2 isoforms, one large and two smaller. The largest form is glycosylated and secreted in approximately 60 minutes, but the other two forms remain cell-associated. The function of these cell-associated C2 proteins has not been determined.

The C2 gene is also within the MHC class III region on chromosome 6p. A null C2 allele (C2Q0) is found in approximately 1.0% to 1.5% of caucasians, thus, approximately 1:10,000 individuals is homozygous and completely C2-deficient (435). Other genetic

defects leading to C2 deficiency have been described. Type I deficiency results from inability to synthesize C2; in type II deficiency the protein is not secreted (436–439). Approximately one-half of individuals lacking C2 are asymptomatic. Possible clinical manifestations include vasculitides such as discoid or systemic lupus, Henoch-Schönlein purpura, polymyositis, and recurrent pyogenic infections (440). Some of these patients have been treated successfully with infusions of fresh-frozen plasma (441).

The relatively high frequencies of C2 and C4 null alleles lead to combined heterozygous partial deficiencies of both in approximately 1:1000 caucasians. Approximately one-third of these patients exhibits systemic lupus erythematosus (SLE) and other autoimmune diseases (442).

Lectin Complement Pathway

Mannose-binding lectin (MBL) is a member of the collectin family of proteins (443,444). MBL is synthesized in the liver, and is

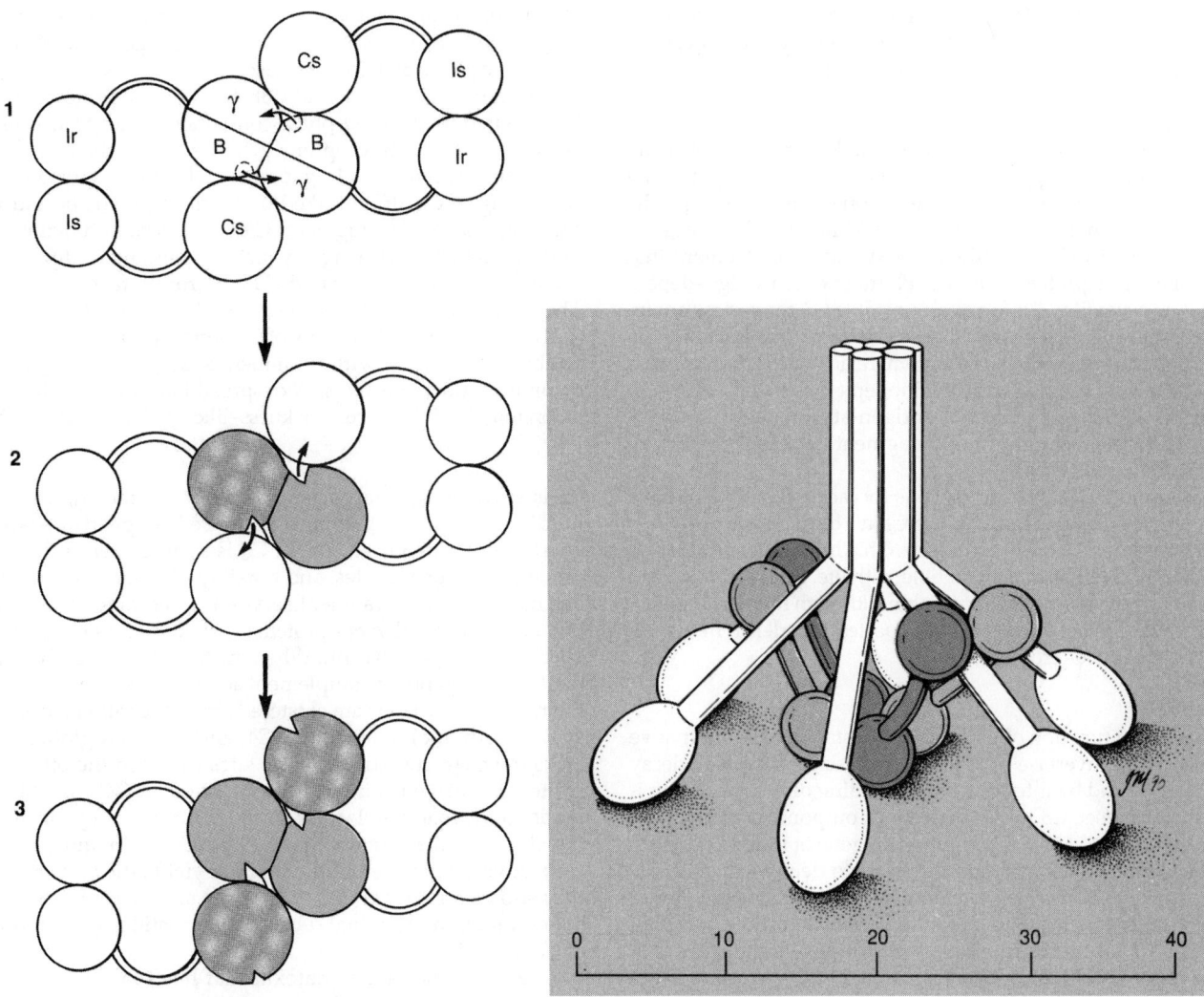

Figure 22-15. A: Schematic representation of the C1r–C1s catalytic subunit of the first component of complement. The diagram shows the autoactivation of C1r (1), C1s activation by C1r (2), leading to full activation of C1s–C1r–C1r–C1s macromolecular complex (3). Dotted circles represent active sites in zymogen form; nicks represent true active sites; and curved arrows represent proteolytic cleavage sites. Cs, catalytic domain of C1s; Ir and Is, interaction domains of C1r and C1s. (From Arlaud GJ, et al. Molecular characterization of the catalytic domains of human complement serine protease C1r. *Biochemistry* 1986;25:5177, with permission.) **B:** Model of C1r–C1s with C1q: C1q is white and C1r2–C1s2 is dark. The ruler is in nanometers. (From Colomb MG, Arlaud GJ, Viliers CL. Activation of C1. *Trans R Soc Biol Lond* 1984;306:283, with permission.)

an acute phase reactant; it interacts with mannose-containing oligosaccharides that may be found on viruses, bacteria, fungi, and parasites. Two serine proteases associated with MBL (MBL-associated proteases 1 and 2) are similar to C1r and C1s, and are activated when MBL binds to a saccharide ligand (445,446). C2 and C4 are substrates for these proteases, and complement activation proceeds via the classic pathway.

Mutations and polymorphisms within the promoter region and first exon of the MBL gene have been associated with an increased risk of bacterial infection, although low levels of MBL and similar polymorphisms may also be found in healthy people (447). One study found an association with MBL deficiency and IgG subclass deficiency, indicating that other characteristics of an individual's immune system influence the expression of a particular MBL genotype (448). MBL polymorphism has been studied in a great variety of clinical settings. MBL genotype has been reported to affect the progression of chronic hepatitis B infection (449), the susceptibility to SLE (450) and to infections in patients

with SLE (451), and the severity of lung disease and survival in cystic fibrosis (452). MBL genotypes have also been correlated with an early age of onset of CVID (453), as well as recurrent spontaneous abortion. An actual pathophysiologic role played by MBL in any of these situations has not been defined.

Early Components of the Alternative Complement Pathway

FACTOR D

Factor D is a serine protease present in serum at extremely low concentrations, apparently in its active form (419). The enzyme can circulate in plasma as an active enzyme because it is not susceptible to inactivation by the serine proteinase inhibitor family of proteins. Factor D cleaves factor B when it is bound to C3b, yielding fragments Ba and Bb. Factor D is synthesized in mononuclear phagocytes, adipocytes, and peripheral nerves (perhaps Schwann cells). Three patients with factor D defects have been described. Their clinical presentations were recurrent neisserial infections (454), recurrent respiratory tract infections (455), and neonatal pneumococcal sepsis (456).

FACTOR B

Factor B is the structural and functional alternative pathway homolog of the C2 protein of the classic pathway (419). The gene for factor B is near the C2 gene on chromosome 6p. The factor B protein is activated by factor D-mediated cleavage of the zymogen to yield Bb, the carboxy-terminal fragment that bears the serine protease site. The Bb fragment in a Mg^{2+}-dependent complex with C3b forms an unstable C3 convertase analogous to the classic pathway C4b2a complex. In addition to its role in alternative pathway complement activation, factor B also has a role in activation of plasminogen (457) and as a growth factor for clonal expansion of antigen-stimulated B lymphocytes (458). Interestingly, the Ba fragment appears to inhibit B-cell proliferation (459).

Several individuals heterozygous for factor B mutations have been identified (460). However, there have been no reported cases of homozygous factor B deficiency: This has led to speculation that this condition is not compatible with life. Mice with targeted disruption of factor B genes are viable, although homozygous factor B$^{-/-}$ mice are not born with the expected Mendelian frequency from heterozygous crosses (461,462).

PROPERDIN

The principal function of properdin is to stabilize the alternative pathway C3 convertase (C3bBb) by decreasing the rate of decay dissociation and by interfering with binding of the cofactor protein factor H (see C3 under Terminal Components of Complement Activation) (419). The properdin gene is located on the X chromosome. A lack of properdin leads to decreased efficiency of alternative pathway complement activation. Reported clinical manifestations include susceptibility to meningococcal infection and discoid lupus erythematosus (463,464). Simultaneous lack of properdin and C2 has been associated with recurrent pneumococcal bacteremia (465).

Terminal Components of Complement Activation

C3

The classic and alternative pathways converge on C3 (Fig. 22-14). The C3 protein is a disulfide-linked heterodimer of α- and β-chains produced by cleavage of a single precursor protein (419). It is the most abundant of the complement proteins in serum (100 to 150 mg/dL) and is synthesized principally by the liver. Genetically determined polymorphic variants of C3 have been identified, each with approximately the same activity. Cleavage of the C3 α chain liberates the C3a fragment, a potent anaphylatoxin that elicits histamine release, smooth muscle contraction, and liberation of arachidonate metabolites (466). These effects are mediated by specific receptors for C3a [see Receptors for the Anaphylatoxins: C5aR (CD88), C3aR, C4aR].

Covalent binding of C3b to a carboxyl- or amino-acceptor site is accomplished by its labile thioester. Deposition of C3 on a cell is relatively inefficient (less than 5% to 10% is bound under optimal conditions), so that much of the metastable C3b reacts with water and cannot bind to target cell or immune complex. Nevertheless, C3b, whether surface-bound or hydrolyzed, can bind the C4b2a complex, C5, factors B and H, properdin, and the C3b receptor, complement receptor 1 (CR1).

Binding and activation of factor B to C3b generates the alternative pathway amplification loop, which is controlled by decay of the enzyme C3bBb complex and cleavage of C3b (419). Addition of a second C3b to the C3bBb complex generates

(C3b)$_2$Bb, the alternative pathway C5 convertase. Binding of C3b to the C4b2a complex on a cell surface generates C4b2a3b, the classic pathway C5 convertase.

Proteolytic inactivation of C3b by a control protein, factor I, is facilitated by the fluid-phase component factor H, and on cell surfaces by the C3b receptor, CR1. The C3b α-chain is cleaved by factor I at two sites to generate C3bi (often written iC3b), consisting of disulfide-linked α-chain fragments bound to β-chain, and a smaller fragment (C3f) of uncertain function. C3bi undergoes further cleavage by factor I, yielding C3dg, which is further degraded to C3g and C3d, a growth factor for B cells. The remainder of the molecule is the C3c fragment.

The clinical manifestations of C3 deficiency resemble those of antibody deficiency, with prominent susceptibility to pyogenic respiratory tract infections. Widespread immune complex deposition may lead to a serum sickness–like syndrome (467–472).

C5

C5 is encoded by a large gene on chromosome 9q; it is a heterodimer of α- and β-chains, produced by posttranslational cleavage of a precursor (419). C5 is synthesized in the liver, mononuclear phagocytes, and possibly in other cells. On cleavage of C5, the C5b fragment serves as a nidus for assembly of the terminal complement proteins, also known as the *membrane attack complex* (MAC) (419). When the target of antibody-dependent or -independent complement activation is on a cell surface, the membrane lesions are clustered about the initial recognition site. C5 is homologous to C3, C4, and α$_2$-macroglobulin, but lacks the characteristic thioester sites found in the other three proteins. Native C5 interacts with sites on C4b or C3b, and binds to the macromolecular complex C5-cleaving enzymes of the classic and alternative pathways: C4b2a3b and (C3b)$_2$Bb, respectively. Cleavage of the α-chain yields the C5a fragment that shows structural and functional similarity to the corresponding amino-terminal α-chain polypeptides (C3a and C4a) of C3 and C4.

C5a is another anaphylatoxin that has spasmogenic activity, induces chemotaxis, increases adherence and noncytotoxic release of intracellular enzymes, and induces an oxidative burst and arachidonate metabolism in granulocytes (473). Carboxy-peptidase-N in plasma cleaves the carboxy-terminal arginine in C5a (or C3a or C4a) to generate C5a-des-Arg with modification of several of these biologic activities. C5a-des-Arg is approximately 100 times less potent as a chemotactic factor than C5a. C5a and C5a-des-Arg have an amplifying effect on antibody responses and T-cell proliferation. C3a has similar, but less potent, effects.

C5b, the remaining portion of the C5 molecule, remains bound to the convertase, where it expresses a binding site for C6 and the assembly of the proteins of the MAC. This C5b6 complex is unstable and decays with a relatively short half-life. C5b6 can remain bound or transfer to other cells generating sites for the phenomenon of reactive lysis and diffusion of the effects of complement activation, but its short half-life limits this phenomenon unless the complex is stabilized by addition of C7 and C8.

Genetic defects of C5 have been associated with recurrent neisserial infections and rheumatic disease (474,475).

C6 AND C7

The single-chain glycoproteins C6 and C7 are considered together because of similarities in the functions of these two proteins in the MAC. The amino-terminal two-thirds of C7 is approximately 30% homologous with C8α and C8β chains and C9. Several other proteins show sequence homology with a cysteine-rich region of the C7 molecule: These include the low-density lipoprotein receptor, thrombospondin, factors IX and X of the coagulation system, and many other proteins. Functional and structural data support the concept that binding of C7 to C5b6 generates an amphiphilic complex from the hydrophilic precursors (C5b6 and C7) that permits insertion of the complex into a lipid bilayer and generation of a discrete membrane lesion.

Recurrent neisserial infections and autoimmune disease have been noted in patients with defects of C6 (476), C7 (477), and both together (478).

C8

The penultimate component in the complement cascade leading to cytolysis, C8 is a complex of three polypeptides: disulfide-linked α- and γ-chains, and a non–covalently associated β-chain (419). The polypeptides are translated from three separate mRNA species derived from three genes: two (α and β) on chromosome 1p, and γ on 9q (479,480). As indicated previously, C8β and C8α chains show sequence homology with other MAC and functionally unrelated membrane plasma proteins. C8 binds the 5b67 complex; its α-γ subunit inserts into the membrane and forms a lesion with an effective pore size of about 10 to 30 nm. Thus, slow lysis of a cell can occur in the absence of C9. Defects in C8 genes may result in susceptibility to neisserial infections (481).

C9

In plasma, C9 is a soluble glycoprotein with amino-terminal hydrophilic and carboxy-terminal relatively hydrophobic domains (419). When C9 interacts with a single C5b678 complex, it expresses amphiphilic properties, inserts in the membrane, and polymerizes with 10 to 15 additional C9 molecules to generate an effective lesion of approximately 100 nm (482). These pores result in disruption of osmotic integrity of the cell, loss of small intracellular molecular species, and then loss and degradation of macromolecules. Complement-dependent hemolysis is efficient, but lysis of nucleated cells is less so because the latter are capable of repairing these membrane lesions. Perforin, a protein produced by cytolytic T lymphocytes and natural killer cells, is a 70-kd channel-forming protein that bears striking functional and structural homology with C9 (483). That is, the mechanisms of fluid-phase and cell-mediated cytolysis seem to be rather similar. Most patients with C9 deficiency are healthy; a few are susceptible to recurrent infections with *Neisseria* (484).

Complement Regulatory Proteins

The complement cascade is modulated to some extent by (a) the intrinsic decay of multimolecular enzyme complexes (e.g., C4b2a, C3bBb, C4b2a3b, C3b$_2$3b); (b) labile reactive sites with microsecond half-lives (e.g., the thioester of C3); and (c) dissociation of incompletely assembled MAC from cell surfaces. Nevertheless, the absence of regulatory proteins of the system results in uncontrolled wasteful activation and consumption of complement (see the following section). Many of the regulatory proteins are products of extended gene families, including some with no apparent functional relation to the complement system.

SOLUBLE COMPLEMENT REGULATORS

Factor I. Factor I is a disulfide-linked, heterodimeric glycoprotein synthesized in the liver and in extrahepatic tissues as a single-chain precursor (419). It is also sometimes called *C3b inactivator*, or *C3b-INA*. Factor I, like factor D, circulates in plasma as an active serine protease. The active serine esterase site is on the light chain, a polypeptide with extensive primary sequence homology to tissue plasminogen activator. The heavy chain shows homology with low-density lipoprotein and epidermal growth factor receptors, as well as the terminal complement components C8 and C9. Factor I displays exquisite substrate specificity for C3b and C4b. The cleavage of these substrates is facilitated in fluid phase by factor H and C4-binding protein (C4bp) and on cell surfaces by the complement C3b/C4b receptor, CR1. As indicated previously, cleavage of C3b and C4b renders these proteins hemolytically inactive, but at least for C3b, several new biologic activities are generated by factor I–mediated cleavage.

The absence of factor I leads to increased consumption of C3 (and factor B), owing to the inability to control constitutive low-level activity of the alternative pathway of activation (485). These patients have manifestations of C3 deficiency, such as recurrent infections (486,487). Immune complex disease such as glomerulonephritis has also been reported (488,489). The gene-encoding factor I is located on chromosome 4; mutations have been characterized only in a few patients (490,491).

Factor H. The complement-regulatory glycoprotein factor H is synthesized in the liver, macrophages, fibroblasts, and possibly platelets (in which it is found in the α granules) (419). The liver is also the site of synthesis of a truncated form of factor H, but its function and fate are unknown (492). Recent studies have identified multiple factor H–related proteins in serum, some of which are derived from distinct genes, but the function of these proteins in complement regulation is unknown (493). The gene for factor H is on chromosome 1, within the regulators of complement activation (RCA) gene complex. Other molecules encoded by genes within this complex include membrane cofactor protein, decay-accelerating factor (DAF), CR1 (CD35), and complement receptor 2 (CD21) (494).

The primary structure of factor H shows homology to several other proteins displaying a characteristic 60-residue cysteine-rich repeating unit (493). Based on physicochemical properties, amino acid composition, and electron microscopic data, the protein is thought to have an unusual higher-order structure and elongated shape. Factor H binds to C3b, thereby leading to dissociation and decay of the alternative pathway C3 convertase (C3bBb) and the C5 convertase, (C3b)$_2$Bb (419). This interaction facilitates cleavage of C3b by factor I.

As with deficiency of factor I, a low level or lack of factor H leads to reductions of C3 and factor B. Clinical associations with factor H mutations include recurrent infections with *Neisseria meningitidis* (495), membranoproliferative glomerulonephritis (496), and sporadic and familial relapsing hemolytic uremic syndrome (497–499).

C4-Binding Protein. C4bp is the classic pathway functional homolog of the alternative pathway regulator factor H (500). C4bp is a disulfide-linked multimer of several α- and β-chains; each of these chains is built up of several repeating structural units. Various isoforms of C4bp may be generated, having different ratios of α:β-chains (501). The amounts of the different isoforms vary among individuals and appear to be genetically regulated. In plasma, C4bp is free or noncovalently complexed with protein S, a cofactor in protein C degradation of clotting factors Va and VIIIa (502). Multiple sites facilitate association of the binding protein with C4b, leading to dissociation of the C4b2a complex and consequent inhibition of C3 degradation. In addition, C4bp acts as a cofactor to enhance generation of the products of factor I cleavage and dissociation of C4b to C4c and C4d fragments.

Vitronectin/S-protein. Vitronectin, or S-protein, binds to C5b and C8 and functions as an inhibitor of the MAC (503) and in the heparin-accelerated inactivation of thrombin by antithrombin III (504). This protein must be distinguished from the vitamin K–dependent protein S, another cofactor in the clotting system alluded to previously. Several distinct structural domains of vitronectin mediate its multiple functional activities. A sequence characteristic of integrins facilitates cell-surface binding and enhancement of Fc-mediated phagocytosis. NK cells express an integrin ($\alpha_v\beta_3$) receptor for vitronectin (505). Signals via this receptor synergize with cross-linking FcγRIII, or IL-2 to promote cellular proliferation, and production of IFN-γ and TNF. Vitronectin also binds to insulin-like growth factor II; the biologic importance of this interaction remains to be clarified.

Clusterin. Clusterin is another inhibitor of the MAC that prevents membrane deposition of the C5b67 complex (506). It is a heterodimer of α- and β-chains, and is found in association with inactive MAC complexes in a variety of complement-dependent pathological processes, such as glomerulonephritis. Depletion of clusterin exacerbates complement-mediated tissue injury. It is also found in high amounts in semen, and may play a role in protecting sperm from destruction by complement in the female reproductive tract.

C1 Esterase Inhibitor and Hereditary Angioedema. C1 esterase inhibitor (C1-INH) is a highly glycosylated plasma protein member of the serine protease inhibitor family. It is the only known inhibitor of the C1r and C1s enzymes, but it also forms 1:1 stoichiometric complexes with factors XII and XI of the coagulation cascade, kallikrein, and plasmin (507). C1-INH is synthesized in the liver, and by mononuclear phagocytes, fibroblasts, and perhaps megakaryocytes. The importance of C1-INH as a regulator of complement activation is evidenced by the profound life-threatening symptoms associated with genetically determined and acquired deficiencies of the protein.

Genetic defects of C1-INH lead to a clinical syndrome known as *hereditary angioedema* (HAE) with autosomal-dominant inheritance (507,508). Up to 25% of patients may express new mutations (509). The principal manifestations of this disorder are recurrent bouts of acute subepithelial edema most often affecting the extremities, genitalia, intestinal mucosa, and the pharyngeal mucosa (507). Physical trauma may precipitate an attack at the site of injury. Edema of the extremities is painless; swelling of intestinal mucosa frequently leads to painful obstruction and vomiting; swelling of the pharynx may be fatal owing to airway obstruction. Symptoms typically develop to their maximum over approximately 12 hours, and wane slowly over 1 to 2 days. Episodes may occur in childhood, but typically become more frequent during puberty.

Approximately 85% of affected patients have HAE type I, a result of abnormally low levels of C1-INH. The remainder has HAE type II, with normal serum levels of a nonfunctional protein (510). Absence of functional C1-INH leads to increased activity of C1r, C1s, and kallikrein. As a consequence, levels of the substrates C2, C4, and bradykinin are reduced, and this may aid in diagnosis. Activation of the coagulation cascade also accompanies acute attacks (511). The clinical symptoms of HAE result from the vasoactive properties of the peptides released from these proteins (512,513).

HAE is transmitted with autosomal-dominant inheritance, that is, the presence of a mutant gene somehow prevents the expression of the functional gene. This appears to arise via inhibition of transcription, but the mechanism is unknown (514). A wide variety of genetic lesions have been identified in patients with HAE (515–520). The C1-INH gene is located on chromosome 11 (521).

Medications commonly used to treat anaphylactic angioedema (e.g., epinephrine, H1 receptor antagonists, corticosteroids) are not generally useful in HAE owing to its distinct pathophysiology. Fresh-frozen plasma contains C1-INH, but it also contains C2, C4, and bradykinin, and may exacerbate an attack. Supportive care depends on the site(s) of swelling. Airway protection (which may include intubation or tracheotomy) is critical for pharyngeal involvement; analgesia is indicated for painful abdominal attacks. Purified human C1-INH for intravenous administration has been used successfully to arrest attacks of HAE (522–524). This product is not licensed for general use in the United States. In addition to replacement therapy for HAE, purified C1-INH may be useful in limiting the complement activation associated with sepsis, cytokine-induced vascular leak syndrome, acute myocardial infarction, or other diseases (525,526). Impeded androgens, such as danazol and stanozolol, are useful as chronic prophylaxis for reducing the frequency of attacks (527). These hormones act to increase the expression of the normal C1-INH gene.

Recurrent angioedema with decreased levels of C1-INH may also be an acquired disorder (528–530). Acquired angioedema type I results from abnormally low levels of C1-INH, and is seen in association with lymphoma and lymphoproliferative disorders. The mechanism of the reduction in C1-INH is unknown. Acquired angioedema type II is caused by autoantibodies against C1-INH. These may arise sporadically, but have also been associated with lymphoproliferation. Two groups have reported a clinical syndrome indistinguishable from HAE in which C1 inhibitor level and function, as well as C4 levels are normal (525,526). Some have been shown to have normal C1-INH gene sequences. The molecular basis of this disorder is unknown.

MEMBRANE-ASSOCIATED COMPLEMENT REGULATORS

Membrane Cofactor Protein (CD46). The membrane cofactor protein (MCP) is one of the several fluid-phase and membrane proteins that inhibit the C3 convertases by facilitating factor I-mediated cleavage of C3b/C4b deposited on cell membranes (531). MCP does not promote dissociation and decay of convertase complexes. MCP is encoded by a gene on chromosome 1q within the RCA complex. More than eight different isoforms are generated by differential mRNA processing. MCP is an integral membrane protein; it is expressed on all nucleated cells. It is found in a complex with β_1 integrins and tetraspan molecules (532). MCP/CD46 is a receptor for a variety of pathogens including measles virus (531), the M protein of group A streptococci (533), and pili of *Neisseria* (534). Elevated levels of soluble forms of CD46 have been described in the blood of patients with SLE (535) and in the urine of patients with a variety of glomerular diseases (536).

Decay-Accelerating Factor (CD55). DAF, another member of the supergene family exhibiting characteristic highly repetitive homology units, is encoded by a gene on chromosome 1p within the RCA complex (537,538). It is a 70-kd polypeptide anchored to membranes of erythrocytes, leukocytes (T and B lymphocytes, monocytes, neutrophils), platelets, and vascular endothelium by means of a glycolipid. DAF and proteins such as acetylcholinesterase, 5-nucleotidase, and many others are released from cell surfaces by a phosphatidylinositol-specific phospholipase C. A secreted form of DAF may also be generated by alternative mRNA splicing. DAF promotes dissociation of the C3 convertases C4b2a and C3bBb and the C5 convertases C4b2a3b and $(C3b)_2Bb$, but it does not serve as cofactor for factor I cleavage of C3b/C4b. DAF bears the determinants of the Cromer group of blood antigens (539). DAF is also a receptor for *Coxsackie* and echoviruses (540).

Homologous Restriction Factor (CD59). Homologous restriction factor (HRF, CD59) is a glycophospholipid-anchored membrane protein that restricts lysis of platelets, leukocytes, and erythrocytes by disrupting the MAC (541,542). The CD59 glycolipid anchor permits lateral mobility in the lipid bilayer, facilitating blocking of the randomly distributed MAC on a cell surface by a minimal number of HRF molecules per cell. Only approximately 9000 HRF molecules per erythrocyte are required for effective blockade of lysis.

Paroxysmal Nocturnal Hemoglobinuria. Approximately 200 patients with paroxysmal nocturnal hemoglobinuria (PNH) have been described. This disorder is a fascinating example of an acquired genetic disease (543–546). The phosphatidylinositol glycan class A (PIG-A) gene lies on the X chromosome; its product is required for the first step of glycophosphoinositol biosynthesis. A hemopoietic stem cell acquires a mutation in a PIG-A gene. This prevents the coupling of more than 20 different proteins that depend on this type of linkage for cell-surface expression. These include DAF/CD55 and HRF/CD46. RBCs that develop from these stem cells are more sensitive to complement lysis. Thus, affected individuals have nocturnal episodes of RBC lysis after or during certain situations, such as surgery, infection, or trauma.

By an unknown mechanism, the PIG-A mutation must yield an advantage in proliferation and/or survival for the stem cell. This supposition is supported by one case report in which a ten-year-old girl with PNH received an infusion of HLA-identical marrow without a conditioning regimen (547). Hemolysis ceased initially owing to engraftment of normal donor stem cells. However, a mutant host clone persisted, and over a 17-month period expanded until, again, a majority of cells were PIG-A deficient, and hemolysis recurred. Interestingly, populations of PIG-A mutant cells may be found in some normal individuals (548), suggesting that the survival advantage accruing to stem cells which mutate PIG-A is variable. Also, there appears to be a threshold level of PIG-A mutant RBCs below which clinical symptoms and signs are not evident. PNH may be treated with corticosteroids, but not all patients respond. Successful use of danazol has also been reported in PNH (549).

Complement Receptors

COMPLEMENT RECEPTOR 1 (CD35)

CR1/CD35 binds the C3b and C4b complement fragments, as well as C1q (550,551). CR1 is a single-chain integral membrane glycoprotein found on erythrocytes, lymphocytes, monocytes, granulocytes, glomerular podocytes, and dendritic cells; it carries the determinants of the Knops blood group antigens (552). CR1 is detected early in B-cell development and is present on circulating B cells, but expression is down-regulated just before plasma cell differentiation (553). CR1, like many other products of the RCA, displays a repeating structural motif of approximately 60 residues. Multiples of these short consensus repeats are found within larger homologous repeating units. These structural features are thought to be important in the interaction with C3 and C4 cleavage products. A substantial intracellular pool of CR1 is translocated to the cell surfaces of polymorphonuclear leukocytes after exposure to several stimuli, including C5a, fMet-Leu-Phe (554), TNF, and viral agents such as herpes simplex (555). This phenomenon is potentially important in the pathogenesis of several disorders characterized by neutropenia and sequestration.

CR1/CD35 is encoded by a single-copy gene on chromosome 1q32 within the RCA complex, but four codominantly expressed allelic size variants have been recognized (556). These allelic variants arise from intragenic duplications within the C3b-binding portion of CRI, thus varying the number of C3b-binding sites from one to four among each variant. Another variant resulting in decreased CR1 expression may be a disease susceptibility marker for SLE (557). The finding of reduced CR1 on cells of patients with SLE also results from nongenetic factors, hence, the meaning of relative CR1 deficiency in this disorder remains uncertain.

CR1 exhibits saturable, relatively high-affinity binding of multimeric C3b or C4b (550). The cleavage products, C3bi and C4bi also bind to CR1, but with lower affinity. CR1 is also a complement-regulatory protein that mediates decay and dissociation of classic and alternative complement activation pathways, and is a cofactor for factor I-mediated cleavage of C3b on leukocytes. In addition, CR1 on erythrocyte membranes plays an important role as a carrier for complement-fixing immune complexes that are cycled to fixed mononuclear phagocytes for removal (558). This mechanism reduces the concentration of free soluble immune complexes in plasma. CD35 cross-linking on B cells enhances the expression of molecules important in their interactions with T cells, B7-1 (CD80), and B7-2 (CD86) (559).

COMPLEMENT RECEPTOR 2 (CD21)

Complement receptor 2 (CR2) has a more limited cellular distribution than the other complement receptors; it is found primarily on B lymphocytes and follicular dendritic cells (560). The CR2 binds C3 fragments C3dg and C3bi, and it is the cellular receptor for EBV. The mature form of CR2/CD21 is a 145-kd glycoprotein encoded by a gene within the RCA complex on chromosome 1q32. It also displays the 60- to 75-residue repeating structure, a typical transmembrane region, and a 34-amino acid cytoplasmic tail.

CD21 is part of a complex with molecules of CD19, CD81, and Leu-13 (561). This signaling complex reduces the threshold for B-cell activation via the Ig receptor, and enhances the humoral immune response (560,562). This signaling has important roles in B-cell activation and in the formation of the B-cell repertoire (i.e., the induction and maintenance of tolerance). C3d-containing immune complexes may enhance the antigen uptake and antigen-presenting functions of B cells, and they may also serve as bridges between dendritic cells and B cells in germinal centers. The link between early complement component deficiencies and autoimmune diseases (see Early Components of the Classic Complement Pathway) may result from diminished signaling via CR2/CD21.

COMPLEMENT RECEPTORS 3 AND 4

Complement receptors 3 (CR3) and 4 (CR4) are members of the β_2 integrin family (563,564). CR3 is also known as *CD11c/CD18, Mac-1*, or $\alpha_M\beta_2$ *integrin*. Synonyms for CR4 are *p150/95, CD11c/ CD18*, and $\alpha_X\beta_2$ *integrin*. The other member of this family is leukocyte function-associated antigen 1 (LFA-1, CD11a/CD18, $\alpha_L\beta_2$ integrin). CR3 and CR4 are distributed on mononuclear phagocytes, polymorphonuclear leukocytes, NK cells, and a subset of lymphocytes. In the presence of calcium, they bind to the C3 cleavage product C3bi with high affinity. These receptors also bind to yeast cell wall constituents and can, by this means, facilitate ingestion of unopsonized particles. Other functions of CR3 and CR4 include binding to endothelium and phagocytosis.

Intercellular adhesion molecule 1 (CD54) is another ligand for CR3. CR3 is the predominant integrin found on mononuclear cells and polymorphonuclear leukocytes and plays a key role in host defense during the initial stages of leukocyte extravasation and phagocytosis. CR3 and CR4 may serve as signal-transducing adapter molecules for some glycosylphosphatidylinositol-anchored proteins on the cell membrane, such as the receptor for lipopolysaccharide binding protein, CD14 (565–567).

Genetic defects of the β_2 integrin CD18 prevent expression of any of the members of this family and lead to severe neutrophil and mononuclear cell functional defects (568). The disease is known as *leukocyte adhesion deficiency*. Leukocytes are trapped within the circulation, and cannot extravasate into areas of inflammation and infection.

RECEPTORS FOR THE ANAPHYLATOXINS: C5AR (CD88), C3AR, C4AR

As mentioned previously, the C3a, C4a, and C5a complement fragments are grouped together with the designation *anaphylatoxins* (473,569). The term derives from the biologic effects exerted by these substances on various tissues, which are analogous to processes occurring during anaphylactic reactions, and which share some mediators, such as histamine. The relative potencies of the anaphylatoxins are C5a > C3a > C4a. Biologic activities include airway smooth muscle contraction, mast cell histamine release, increased vascular permeability and relaxation of vascular smooth muscle, degranulation of neutrophils, activation of the respiratory burst, and alterations in adhesion molecule expression. The actions of each of the anaphylatoxins are similar, but there may be some distinctions that remain to be clarified. For example, C5a is the most potent chemotactic factor for granulocytes. Anaphylatoxins are inactivated by carboxypeptidase-N-dependent cleavage of the C-terminal arginine residue, yielding C5a-des-Arg, C3a-des-Arg, and C4a-des-Arg. These molecules have severely reduced affinity for the respective receptors, although they may retain some biologic activity (570,571).

The C5a and C3a receptors have been cloned; they are both members of the rhodopsin family of receptors. The ligand-binding chain has seven transmembrane regions, and is linked to G proteins that mediate signal transduction. The C5a receptor has been identified on granulocytes and mononuclear cells. Some have reported C5aR expression on a variety of other cell types such as hepatocytes, lung bronchial and alveolar epithelium, lung vascular smooth muscle and endothelial cells, heart, kidney, intestine (572), and renal proximal tubule (573). Others suggest that expression in some of these tissues (e.g., liver) is limited to mononuclear-derived cells (574). The distribution of the C3a receptor may not be as widespread as that of C5a, but this requires further study. C5aR and C3aR have been identified on neurons and glial cells as well (575,576). The C4a receptor has not yet been cloned, although there is evidence that C4a signals through a distinct receptor (577).

C1Q (COLLECTIN) RECEPTOR

A variety of biologic activities have been attributed to C1q binding to cell-surface proteins. These include stimulation of phagocytosis and the respiratory burst, microbial killing, and chemotaxis by granulocytes and mononuclear cells. Additional activities include increasing Ig production by B cells; expression of adhesion molecules on platelets, and stimulation of fibroblast cell division and migration (578). A cellular receptor for C1q (C1qRp) also interacts with other members of the collectin family, such as MBL (see Lectin Complement Pathway) (579). C1qRp is expressed on leukocytes, including platelets, and endothelial cells. C1qRp enhances phagocytosis (hence, the "p" in its name) mediated by FcγR and CR1 (580). C1qRp is also able to inhibit complement activation by sequestering C1q and inhibiting its association with C1r and C1s (581). Zinc-dependent interactions between C1qRp and high-molecular-weight kininogen and coagulation factor XII have also been described (582). As mentioned previously, CR1/CD35 also binds to C1q and mediates some of its biologic effects. A third receptor, called $C1qR_{O2}^-$, is thought to mediate the up-regulation of the respiratory burst that follows C1q binding to granulocytes.

REFERENCES

1. Rosen FS, Wedgwood RJP, Eibl M, et al. Primary immunodeficiency diseases. Report of a WHO scientific group. *Clin Exp Immunol* 1997;109[Suppl 1]:1–28.
2. Javier FC III, Moore CM, Sorensen RU. Distribution of primary immunodeficiency diseases diagnosed in a pediatric tertiary hospital. *Ann Allergy Asthma Immunol* 2000;84:25–30.
3. Plebani A, Stringa M, Prigione I, et al. Engrafted maternal T cells in human severe combined immunodeficiency: evidence for a TH2 phenotype and a potential role of apoptosis on the restriction of T-cell receptor variable beta repertoire. *J Allergy Clin Immunol* 1998;101:131–134.
4. Sottini A, Quiros-Roldan E, Notarangelo LD, et al. Engrafted maternal T cells in a severe combined immunodeficiency patient express T-cell receptor variable beta segments characterized by a restricted V-D-J junctional diversity. *Blood* 1995;85:2105–2113.
5. Conley MA, Buckley RH, Hong R, et al. X-linked severe combined immunodeficiency. Diagnosis in males with sporadic severe combined immunodeficiency and clarification of clinical findings. *J Clin Invest* 1990;85:1548–1554.
6. White H, Thrasher A, Veys P, et al. Intrinsic defects of B cell function in X-linked severe combined immunodeficiency. *Eur J Immunol* 2000;30:732–737.
7. Noguchi M, Yi H, Rosenblatt HM, et al. Interleukin-2 receptor gamma chain mutation results in X-linked severe combined immunodeficiency in humans. *Cell* 1993;73:147–157.
8. Voss SD, Hong R, Sondel PM. Severe combined immunodeficiency, interleukin-2 (IL-2), and the IL-2 receptor: experiments of nature continue to point the way. *Blood* 1994;83:626–635.
9. Leonard WJ, Noguchi M, Russsell SM, et al. The molecular basis of X-linked severe combined immunodeficiency: the role of the interleukin-2 receptor gamma chain as a common gamma chain, gammac. *Immunol Rev* 1994;138:61–86.
10. Kimura Y, Takeshita T, Kondo M, et al. Sharing of the IL-2 receptor gamma chain with the functional IL-9 receptor complex. *Int Immunol* 1995;7:115–120.
11. Grabstein KH, Eisenman J, Shanebeck K, et al. Cloning of a T cell growth factor that interacts with the beta chain of the interleukin-2 receptor. *Science* 1994;264:965.
11a. Asao H, Okuyama C, Kumaki S, et al. Cutting edge: the common gamma-chain is an indispensable subunit of the IL-21 receptor complex. *J Immunol* 2001;167:1–5.
12. Hendriks RW, Chen ZY, Hinds H, et al. Carrier detection in X-linked immunodeficiencies. I. A PCR-based X chromosome inactivation assay at the MAOA locus. *Immunodeficiency* 1993;4:209–211.
13. Puck JM, Nussbaum RL, Conley ME. Carrier detection in X-linked severe combined immunodeficiency based on patterns of X chromosome inactivation. *J Clin Invest* 1987;79:1395–1400.
14. Allen RC, Zoghbi HY, Moseley AB, et al. Methylation of HpaII and HhaI sites near the polymorphic CAG repeat in the human androgen-receptor gene correlates with X chromosome inactivation. *Am J Hum Genet* 1992;51:1229–1239.
15. Niemela JE, Puck JM, Fischer RE, et al. Efficient detection of thirty-seven new IL2RG mutations in human X-linked severe combined immunodeficiency. *Clin Immunol* 2000;95:33–38.
16. Puck JM, Pepper AE, Henthorn PS, et al. Mutation analysis of IL2RG in human X-linked severe combined immunodeficiency. *Blood* 1997;89:1968–1977.
17. Mella P, Imberti L, Brugnoni D, et al. Development of autologous T lymphocytes in two males with X-linked severe combined immune deficiency: molecular and cellular characterization. *Clin Immunol* 2000;95:39–50.
18. Sharfe N, Shahar M, Roifman CM. An interleukin-2 receptor gamma chain mutation with normal thymus morphology. *J Clin Invest* 1997;100:3036–3043.
19. Jones AM, Clark PA, Katz F, et al. B-cell-negative severe combined immunodeficiency associated with a common gamma chain mutation. *Hum Genet* 1997;99:677–680.
20. Jung EY, Heike T, Katamura K, et al. X-linked severe combined immunodeficiency with gamma delta T cells. *Acta Paediatr Jpn* 1997;39:442–447.
21. Candotti F, Oakes SA, Johnston JA, et al. Structural and functional basis for JAK3-deficient severe combined immunodeficiency. *Blood* 1997;90:3996–4003.
22. Russell SM, Tayebi N, Nakajima H, et al. Mutation of Jak3 in a patient with SCID: essential role of Jak3 in lymphoid development. *Science* 1995;270:797–800.
23. Brugnoni D, Notarangelo LD, Sottini A, et al. Development of autologous, oligoclonal, poorly functioning T lymphocytes in a patient with autosomal recessive severe combined immunodeficiency caused by defects of the Jak3 tyrosine kinase. *Blood* 1998;91:949–955.
24. Bozzi F, Lefranc G, Villa A, et al. Molecular and biochemical characterization of JAK3 deficiency in a patient with severe combined immunodeficiency over 20 years after bone marrow transplantation: implications for treatment. *Br J Haematol* 1998;102:1363–1366.
25. Puel A, Ziegler SF, Buckley RH, et al. Defective IL7R expression in T(-)B(+)NK(+) severe combined immunodeficiency. *Nat Genet* 1998;20:394–397.
26. Puel A, Leonard WJ. Mutations in the gene for the IL-7 receptor result in T(-)B(+)NK(+) severe combined immunodeficiency disease. *Curr Opin Immunol* 2000;12:468–473.
27. Aldrich MB, Blackburn MR, Kellems RE. The importance of adenosine deaminase for lymphocyte development and function. *Biochem Biophys Res Commun* 2000;272:311–315.

28. Markert ML. Purine nucleoside phosphorylase deficiency. *Immunodefic Rev* 1991;3:45–81.
29. Hirschhorn R. Adenosine deaminase deficiency. *Immunodefic Rev* 1990;2:175–198.
30. Arredondo-Vega FX, Santisteban I, Daniels S, et al. Adenosine deaminase deficiency: genotype-phenotype correlations based on expressed activity of 29 mutant alleles. *Am J Hum Genet* 1998;63:1049–1059.
31. Ozsahin H, Arredondo-Vega FX, Santisteban I, et al. Adenosine deaminase deficiency in adults. *Blood* 1997;89:2849–2855.
32. Polmar SH. Red cell therapy: its clinical and immunological efficacy in ADA deficiency. In: Pollara B, Meuwisen HJ, Pickering RJ, eds. *Inborn errors of specific immunity*. New York: Academic Press, 1979:343–348.
33. Hershfield MS. PEG-ADA: an alternative to haploidentical bone marrow transplantation and an adjunct to gene therapy for adenosine deaminase deficiency. *Hum Mutat* 1995;5:107–112.
34. Hirschhorn R, Yang DR, Puck JM, et al. Spontaneous in vivo reversion to normal of an inherited mutation in a patient with adenosine deaminase deficiency. *Nat Genet* 1996;13:290–295.
35. Schwarz K, Gauss GH, Ludwig L, et al. RAG mutations in human B cell-negative SCID. *Science* 1996;274:97–99.
36. Businco L, DiFazio A, Ziruolo MG, et al. Clinical and immunological findings in Omenn's syndrome: a form of severe combined immunodeficiency with phenotypically normal T cells, elevated IgE, and eosinophilia. *Clin Immunol Immunopath* 1987;44:123–133.
37. Villa A, Santagata S, Bozzi F, et al. Partial V(D)J recombination activity leads to Omenn syndrome. *Cell* 1998;93:885–896.
38. Wada T, Takei K, Kudo M, et al. Characterization of immune function and analysis of RAG gene mutations in Omenn syndrome and related disorders. *Clin Exp Immunol* 2000;119:148–155.
39. Mathioudakis G, Good RA, Chernajovsky Y, et al. Selective gamma-chain T-cell receptor gene rearrangements in a patient with Omenn's syndrome: absence of V-II subgroup (V gamma 9) transcripts. *Clin Diagn Lab Immunol* 1996;3:616–619.
40. Rieux-Laucat F, Bahadoran P, Brousse N, et al. Highly restricted human T cell repertoire in peripheral blood and tissue-infiltrating lymphocytes in Omenn's syndrome. *J Clin Invest* 1998;102:312–321.
41. Mach B, Steimle V, Martinez-Soria E, et al. Regulation of MHC class II genes: lessons from a disease. *Annu Rev Immunol* 1996;14:301–331.
42. Klein C, Lisowska-Grospierre B, LeDeist F, et al. Major histocompatibility complex class II deficiency: clinical manifestations, immunologic features, and outcome. *J Pediatr* 1993;123:921–928.
43. Nagarajan UM, Louis-Plence P, DeSandro A, et al. RFX-B is the gene responsible for the most common cause of the bare lymphocyte syndrome, an MHC class II immunodeficiency. *Immunity* 1999;10:153–162.
44. Villard J, Reith W, Barras E, et al. Analysis of mutations and chromosomal localisation of the gene encoding RFX5, a novel transcription factor affected in major histocompatibility complex class II deficiency. *Hum Mutat* 1997;10:430–435.
45. Durand B, Sperisen P, Emery P, et al. RFXAP, a novel subunit of the RFX DNA binding complex is mutated in MHC class II deficiency. *Embo J* 1997;16:1045–1055.
46. York IA, Rock KL. Antigen processing and presentation by the class I major histocompatibility complex. *Annu Rev Immunol* 1996;14:369–396.
47. Pamer E, Cresswell P. Mechanisms of MHC class I–restricted antigen processing. *Annu Rev Immunol* 1998;16:323–358.
48. de la Salle H, Hanau D, Fricker D, et al. Homozygous human TAP peptide transporter mutation in HLA class I deficiency. *Science* 1994;265:237–240.
49. Donato L, de la Salle H, Hanau D, et al. Association of HLA class I antigen deficiency related to a TAP2 gene mutation with familial bronchiectasis. *J Pediatr* 1995;127:895–900.
50. Furukawa H, Murata S, Yabe T, et al. Splice acceptor site mutation of the transporter associated with antigen processing-1 gene in human bare lymphocyte syndrome. *J Clin Invest* 1999;103:755–758.
51. Elder ME. ZAP-70 and defects of T-cell receptor signaling. *Semin Hematol* 1998;35:310–320.
52. Gelfand EW, Weinberg K, Mazer BD, et al. Absence of ZAP-70 prevents signaling through the antigen receptor on peripheral blood T cells but not on thymocytes. *J Exp Med* 1995;182:1057–1065.
53. Arpaia E, Shahar M, Dadi H, et al. Defective T cell receptor signaling and CD8+ thymic selection in humans lacking Zap-70 kinase. *Cell* 1994;76:947–958.
54. Kung C, Pingel JT, Heikinheimo M, et al. Mutations in the tyrosine phosphatase CD45 gene in a child with severe combined immunodeficiency disease. *Nat Med* 2000;6:343–345.
55. Arnaiz-Villena A, Timon M, Corell A, et al. Primary immunodeficiency caused by mutations in the gene encoding the CD3-gamma subunit of the T-lymphocyte receptor. *N Engl J Med* 1992;327:529–533.
56. Thoenes G, Le Deist F, Fischer A, et al. Immunodeficiency associated with defective expression of the T-cell receptor-CD3 complex. *N Engl J Med* 1990;322:1399.
57. Thoenes G, Soudais C, le Deist F, et al. Structural analysis of low TCR-CD3 complex expression in T cells of an immunodeficient patient. *J Biol Chem* 1992;267:487–493.
58. Menasche G, Pastural E, Feldmann J, et al. Mutations in RAB27A cause Griscelli syndrome associated with haemophagocytic syndrome. *Nat Genet* 2000;25:173–176.
59. Tezcan I, Sanal O, Ersoy F, et al. Successful bone marrow transplantation in a case of Griscelli disease which presented in accelerated phase with neurological involvement. *Bone Marrow Transplant* 1999;24:931–933.
60. Mancini AJ, Chan LS, Paller AS. Partial albinism with immunodeficiency: Griscelli syndrome: report of a case and review of the literature. *J Am Acad Dermatol* 1998;38:295–300.
61. Roper MA, Parmely RT, Crist WM, et al. Severe congenital leukopenia (reticular dysgenesis): Immunologic and morphologic characterization of leukocytes. *Am J Dis Child* 1985;139:832.
62. De Santes KB, Lai SS, Cowan MJ. Haploidentical bone marrow transplants for two patients with reticular dysgenesis. *Bone Marrow Transplant* 1996;17:1171–1173.
63. De La Calle-Martin O, Badell I, Garcia A, et al. B cells and monocytes are not developmentally affected in a case of reticular dysgenesis. *Clin Exp Immunol* 1997;110:392–396.
64. Emile JF, Geissmann F, Martin OC, et al. Langerhans cell deficiency in reticular dysgenesis. *Blood* 2000;96:58–62.
65. Sahdev I, O'Reilly R, Hoffman MK. Correlation between interleukin-1 production and engraftment of bone marrow stem cells in patients with lethal immunodeficiencies. *Blood* 1989;73:11712–11719.
66. Disanto JP, Keever CA, Small TN, et al. Absence of interleukin 2 production in a severe combined immunodeficiency disease syndrome with T cells. *J Exp Med* 1990;171:1697–1704.
67. Weinberg K, Parkman R. Severe combined immunodeficiency due to a specific defect in the production of interleukin-2. *N Engl J Med* 1990;322:1718–1723.
68. Castigli E, Geha RS, Chatila T. Severe combined immunodeficiency with selective T-cell cytokine genes. *Pediatr Res* 1993;33:S20–S22.
69. Buckley RH, Schiff SE, Schiff RI, et al. Hematopoietic stem-cell transplantation for the treatment of severe combined immunodeficiency. *N Engl J Med* 1999;340:508–516.
70. Dalal I, Reid B, Doyle J, et al. Matched unrelated bone marrow transplantation for combined immunodeficiency. *Bone Marrow Transplant* 2000;25:613–621.
71. Knutsen AP, Wall DA. Kinetics of T-cell development of umbilical cord blood transplantation in severe T-cell immunodeficiency disorders. *J Allergy Clin Immunol* 1999;103:823–832.
72. Toren A, Nagler A, Amariglio N, et al. Successful human umbilical cord blood stem cell transplantation without conditioning in severe combined immune deficiency. *Bone Marrow Transplant* 1999;23:405–408.
73. Bertrand Y, Landais P, Friedrich W, et al. Influence of severe combined immunodeficiency phenotype on the outcome of HLA non-identical, T-cell-depleted bone marrow transplantation: a retrospective European survey from the European group for bone marrow transplantation and the European society for immunodeficiency. *J Pediatr* 1999;134:740–748.
74. Haddad E, Landais P, Friedrich W, et al. Long-term immune reconstitution and outcome after HLA-nonidentical T-cell-depleted bone marrow transplantation for severe combined immunodeficiency: a European retrospective study of 116 patients. *Blood* 1998;91:3646–3653.
75. Fischer A. Thirty years of bone marrow transplantation for severe combined immunodeficiency. *N Engl J Med* 1999;340:559–561.
76. Touraine JL. In utero transplantation of fetal liver stem cells into human fetuses. *J Hematother* 1996;5:195–199.
77. Wengler GS, Lanfranchi A, Frusca T, et al. In-utero transplantation of parental CD34 haematopoietic progenitor cells in a patient with X-linked severe combined immunodeficiency (SCIDXI). *Lancet* 1996;348:1484–1487.
78. Patel DD, Gooding ME, Parrott RE, et al. Thymic function after hematopoietic stem-cell transplantation for the treatment of severe combined immunodeficiency. *N Engl J Med* 2000;342:1325–1332.
79. Brady KA, Cowan MJ, Leavitt AD. Circulating red cells usually remain of host origin after bone marrow transplantation for severe combined immunodeficiency. *Transfusion* 1996;36:314–317.
80. Haddad E, Le Deist F, Aucouturier P, et al. Long-term chimerism and B-cell function after bone marrow transplantation in patients with severe combined immunodeficiency with B cells: A single-center study of 22 patients. *Blood* 1999;94:2923–2930.
81. O'Reilly RJ, Small TN, Papadopoulos E, et al. Biology and adoptive cell therapy of Epstein-Barr virus-associated lymphoproliferative disorders in recipients of marrow allografts. *Immunol Rev* 1997;157:195–216.
82. Horn B, Viele M, Mentzer W, et al. Autoimmune hemolytic anemia in patients with SCID after T cell-depleted BM and PBSC transplantation. *Bone Marrow Transplant* 1999;24:1009–1013.
83. Ting SS, Ziegler JB, Vowels MR. Acquired autoimmune thrombocytopenia post-bone marrow transplantation for severe combined immunodeficiency. *Bone Marrow Transplant* 1998;21:841–843.
84. Blaese RM, Culver KW, Miller D, et al. T lymphocyte-directed gene therapy for ADA-SCID: initial trial results after 4 years. *Science* 1995;270:475–480.
85. Kohn DB, Parkman R. Gene therapy for newborns. *FASEB J* 1997;11:635–639.
86. Cavazzana-Calvo M, Hacein-Bey S, de Saint Basile G, et al. Gene therapy of human severe combined immunodeficiency (SCID)-X1 disease. *Science* 2000;288:669–672.
87. Bradley MB, Fernandez JM, Ungers G, et al. Correction of defective expression in MHC class II deficiency (bare lymphocyte syndrome) cells by retroviral transduction of CIITA. *J Immunol* 1997;159:1086–1095.
88. Candotti F, Oakes SA, Johnston JA, et al. In vitro correction of JAK3-deficient severe combined immunodeficiency by retroviral-mediated gene transduction. *J Exp Med* 1996;183:2687–2692.
89. Taylor N, Bacon KB, Smith S, et al. Reconstitution of T cell receptor signaling in ZAP-70-deficient cells by retroviral transduction of the ZAP-70 gene. *J Exp Med* 1996;184:2031–2036.

90. Lum LG, Tubergen DG, Corash L, et al. Splenectomy in the management of the thrombocytopenia of the Wiskott- Aldrich syndrome. *N Engl J Med* 1980; 302:892–896.

91. Mullen CA, Anderson KD, Blaese RM. Splenectomy and/or bone marrow transplantation in the management of the Wiskott-Aldrich syndrome: long-term follow-up of 62 cases. *Blood* 1993;82:2961–2966.

92. Molina IJ, Sancho J, Terhorst C, et al. T cells of patients with the Wiskott-Aldrich syndrome have a restricted defect in proliferative responses. *J Immunol* 1993;151:4383.

93. Kenney D, Cairns L, Remold-O'Donnell E, et al. Morphological abnormalities in the lymphocytes of patients with the Wiskott-Aldrich syndrome. *Blood* 1986;68:1329–1332.

94. Derry JM, Kerns JA, Weinberg KI, et al. WASP gene mutations in Wiskott-Aldrich syndrome and X-linked thrombocytopenia. *Hum Mol Genet* 1995; 4:1127–1135.

95. Kolluri R, Shehabeldin A, Peacocke M, et al. Identification of WASP mutations in patients with Wiskott-Aldrich syndrome and isolated thrombocytopenia reveals allelic heterogeneity at the WAS locus. *Hum Mol Genet* 1995;4: 1119–1126.

96. Villa A, Notarangelo L, Macchi P, et al. X-linked thrombocytopenia and Wiskott-Aldrich syndrome are allelic diseases with mutations in the WASP gene. *Nat Genet* 1995;9:414–417.

97. Parolini O, Berardelli S, Riedl E, et al. Expression of Wiskott-Aldrich syndrome protein (WASP) gene during hematopoietic differentiation. *Blood* 1997;90:70–75.

98. Parolini O, Ressmann G, Haas OA, et al. X-linked Wiskott-Aldrich syndrome in a girl. *N Engl J Med* 1998;338:291–295.

99. Schindelhauer D, Weiss M, Hellebrand H, et al. Wiskott-Aldrich syndrome: no strict genotype-phenotype correlations but clustering of missense mutations in the amino-terminal part of the WASP gene product. *Hum Genet* 1996;98:68–76.

100. Schwarz K. WASPbase: a database of WAS- and XLT-causing mutations. *Immunol Today* 1996;17:496–502.

101. Snapper SB, Rosen FS. The Wiskott-Aldrich syndrome protein (WASP): roles in signaling and cytoskeletal organization. *Annu Rev Immunol* 1999;17:905–929.

102. Kajiwara M, Nonoyama S, Eguchi M, et al. WASP is involved in proliferation and differentiation of human haemopoietic progenitors in vitro. *Br J Haematol* 1999;107:254–262.

103. Shcherbina A, Rosen FS, Remold-O'Donnell E. Pathological events in platelets of Wiskott-Aldrich syndrome patients. *Br J Haematol* 1999;106:875–883.

104. Gross BS, Wilde JI, Quek L, et al. Regulation and function of WASp in platelets by the collagen receptor, glycoprotein VI. *Blood* 1999;94:4166–4176.

105. Zhang J, Shehabeldin A, da Cruz LA, et al. Antigen receptor-induced activation and cytoskeletal rearrangement are impaired in Wiskott-Aldrich syndrome protein-deficient lymphocytes. *J Exp Med* 1999;190:1329–1342.

106. Baba Y, Nonoyama S, Matsushita M, et al. Involvement of Wiskott-Aldrich syndrome protein in B-cell cytoplasmic tyrosine kinase pathway. *Blood* 1999;93:2003–2012.

107. Snapper SB, Rosen FS, Mizoguchi E, et al. Wiskott-Aldrich syndrome protein-deficient mice reveal a role for WASP in T but not B cell activation. *Immunity* 1998;9:81–91.

108. Lorenzi R, Brickell PM, Katz DR, et al. Wiskott-Aldrich syndrome protein is necessary for efficient IgG-mediated phagocytosis. *Blood* 2000;95:2943–2946.

109. Zicha D, Allen WE, Brickell PM, et al. Chemotaxis of macrophages is abolished in the Wiskott-Aldrich syndrome. *Br J Haematol* 1998;101:659–665.

110. Binks M, Jones GE, Brickell PM, et al. Intrinsic dendritic cell abnormalities in Wiskott-Aldrich syndrome. *Eur J Immunol* 1998;28:3259–3267.

111. Litzman J, Jones A, Hann I, et al. Intravenous immunoglobulin, splenectomy, and antibiotic prophylaxis in Wiskott-Aldrich syndrome. *Arch Dis Child* 1996;75:436–439.

112. Mathew P, Conley ME. Effect of intravenous gammaglobulin (IVIG) on the platelet count in patients with Wiskott-Aldrich syndrome. *Pediatr Allergy Immunol* 1995;6:91–94.

113. Ozsahin H, Le Deist F, Benkerrou M, et al. Bone marrow transplantation in 26 patients with Wiskott-Aldrich syndrome from a single center. *J Pediatr* 1996;129:238–244.

114. Candotti F, Facchetti F, Blanzuoli L, et al. Retrovirus-mediated WASP gene transfer corrects defective actin polymerization in B cell lines from Wiskott-Aldrich syndrome patients carrying 'null' mutations. *Gene Ther* 1999;6:1170–1174.

115. Huang MM, Tsuboi S, Wong A, et al. Expression of human Wiskott-Aldrich syndrome protein in patients' cells leads to partial correction of a phenotypic abnormality of cell surface glycoproteins. *Gene Ther* 2000;7:314–320.

116. Gatti A, Swift M. *Ataxia-telangiectasia: genetics, neuropathology, and immunology of a degenerative disease of childhood.* New York: Alan R. Liss, Inc., 1985.

117. Carbonari M, Cherchi M, Paganelli R, et al. Relative increase of T cells expressing the gamma/delta rather than the alpha/beta receptor in ataxia-telangiectasia. *N Engl J Med* 1990;322:73–76.

118. Sadighi Akha AA, Humphrey RL, Winkelstein JA, et al. Oligo-/monoclonal gammopathy and hypergammaglobulinemia in ataxia-telangiectasia. A study of 90 patients. *Medicine (Baltimore)* 1999;78:370–381.

119. Lefton-Greif MA, Crawford TO, Winkelstein JA, et al. Oropharyngeal dysphagia and aspiration in patients with ataxia-telangiectasia. *J Pediatr* 2000; 136:225–231.

120. Cabana MD, Crawford TO, Winkelstein JA, et al. Consequences of the delayed diagnosis of ataxia-telangiectasia. *Pediatrics* 1998;102:98–100.

121. Savitsky K, Bar-Shira A, Gilad S, et al. A single ataxia telangiectasia gene with a product similar to PI-3 kinase. *Science* 1995;268:1749–1753.

122. Gatei M, Scott SP, Filippovitch I, et al. Role for ATM in DNA damage-induced phosphorylation of BRCA1. *Cancer Res* 2000;60:3299–3304.

123. Lavin MF, Khanna KK. ATM: the protein encoded by the gene mutated in the radiosensitive syndrome ataxia-telangiectasia. *Int J Radiat Biol* 1999;75:1201–1214.

124. Concannon P, Gatti RA. Diversity of ATM gene mutations detected in patients with ataxia-telangiectasia. *Hum Mutat* 1997;10:100–107.

125. Gilad S, Chessa L, Khosravi R, et al. Genotype-phenotype relationships in ataxia-telangiectasia and variants. *Am J Hum Genet* 1998;62:551–561.

126. Li A, Swift M. Mutations at the ataxia-telangiectasia locus and clinical phenotypes of A-T patients. *Am J Med Genet* 2000;92:170–177.

127. Wright J, Teraoka S, Onengut S, et al. A high frequency of distinct ATM gene mutations in ataxia-telangiectasia. *Am J Hum Genet* 1996;59:839–846.

128. Toyoshima M, Hara T, Zhang H, et al. Ataxia-telangiectasia without immunodeficiency: novel point mutations within and adjacent to the phosphatidylinositol 3-kinase-like domain. *Am J Med Genet* 1998;75:141–144.

129. Swift M, Morrell D, Cromartie E, et al. The incidence and gene frequency of ataxia telangiectasia in the United States. *Am J Hum Genet* 1986;39:573–583.

130. Swift M, Reitnauer PJ, Morrell D, et al. Breast and other cancers in families with ataxia-telangiectasia. *N Engl J Med* 1987;316:1289–1294.

131. Angele S, Hall J. The ATM gene and breast cancer: is it really a risk factor? *Mutat Res* 2000;462:167–178.

132. Broeks A, Urbanus JH, Floore AN, et al. ATM-heterozygous germline mutations contribute to breast cancer-susceptibility. *Am J Hum Genet* 2000;66:494–500.

133. FitzGerald MG, Bean JM, Hegde SR, et al. Heterozygous ATM mutations do not contribute to early onset of breast cancer. *Nat Genet* 1997;15:307–310.

134. Sandoval C, Swift M. Treatment of lymphoid malignancies in patients with ataxia-telangiectasia. *Med Pediatr Oncol* 1998;31:491–497.

135. Ziv Y, Bar-Shira A, Pecker I, et al. Recombinant ATM protein complements the cellular A-T phenotype. *Oncogene* 1997;15:159–167.

136. van der Burgt I, Chrzanowska KH, Smeets D, et al. Nijmegen breakage syndrome. *J Med Genet* 1996;33:153–156.

137. Matsuura S, Tauchi H, Nakamura A, et al. Positional cloning of the gene for Nijmegen breakage syndrome. *Nat Genet* 1998;19:179–181.

138. Wu X, Ranganathan V, Weisman DS, et al. ATM phosphorylation of Nijmegen breakage syndrome protein is required in a DNA damage response. *Nature* 2000;405:477–482.

139. Zhao S, Weng YC, Yuan SS, et al. Functional link between ataxia-telangiectasia and Nijmegen breakage syndrome gene products. *Nature* 2000;405:473–477.

140. Conley MA, Beckwith JB, Mancer JFK, et al. The spectrum of the DiGeorge syndrome. *J Pediatr* 1979;94:883–890.

141. Muller W, Peter HH, Wilken M, et al. The DiGeorge syndrome. I. Clinical evaluation and course of partial and complete forms of the syndrome. *Eur J Pediatr* 1988;147:496–502.

142. Muller W, Peter HH, Kallfelz HC, et al. The DiGeorge syndrome. II. Immunologic findings in partial and complete forms of the disorder. *Eur J Pediatr* 1989;149:96–103.

143. Bastian J, Law S, Vogler L, et al. Prediction of persistent immunodeficiency in the DiGeorge anomaly. *J Pediatr* 1989;115:391–396.

144. Markert ML, Hummell DS, Rosenblatt HM, et al. Complete DiGeorge syndrome: persistence of profound immunodeficiency. *J Pediatr* 1998;132:15–21.

145. Collard HR, Boeck A, McLaughlin TM, et al. Possible extrathymic development of nonfunctional T cells in a patient with complete DiGeorge syndrome. *Clin Immunol* 1999;91:156–162.

146. Kornfeld SJ, Zeffren B, Christodoulou CS, et al. DiGeorge anomaly: a comparative study of the clinical and immunologic characteristics of patients positive and negative by fluorescence in situ hybridization. *J Allergy Clin Immunol* 2000;105:983–987.

147. Smith CA, Driscoll DA, Emanuel BS, et al. Increased prevalence of immunoglobulin A deficiency in patients with the chromosome 22q11.2 deletion syndrome (DiGeorge syndrome/velocardiofacial syndrome). *Clin Diagn Lab Immunol* 1998;5:415–417.

148. Junker AK, Driscoll DA. Humoral immunity in DiGeorge syndrome. *J Pediatr* 1995;127:231–237.

149. Sullivan KE, McDonald-McGinn D, Driscoll DA, et al. Longitudinal analysis of lymphocyte function and numbers in the first year of life in chromosome 22q11.2 deletion syndrome (DiGeorge syndrome/velocardiofacial syndrome). *Clin Diagn Lab Immunol* 1999;6:906–911.

150. McDonald-McGinn DM, Kirschner R, Goldmuntz E, et al. The Philadelphia story: the 22q11.2 deletion: report on 250 patients. *Genet Couns* 1999;10:11–24.

151. Amati F, Conti E, Novelli A, et al. Atypical deletions suggest five 22q11.2 critical regions related to the DiGeorge/velo-cardio-facial syndrome. *Eur J Hum Genet* 1999;7:903–909.

152. Pizzuti A, Novelli G, Ratti A, et al. UFD1L, a developmentally expressed ubiquitination gene, is deleted in CATCH 22 syndrome. *Hum Mol Genet* 1997;6:259–265.

153. Yamagishi H, Garg V, Matsuoka R, et al. A molecular pathway revealing a genetic basis for human cardiac and craniofacial defects. *Science* 1999;283: 1158–1161.

154. Chieffo C, Garvey N, Gong W, et al. Isolation and characterization of a gene from the DiGeorge chromosomal region homologous to the mouse Tbx1 gene. *Genomics* 1997;43:267–277.

155. Kurahashi H, Akagi K, Inazawa J, et al. Isolation and characterization of a novel gene deleted in DiGeorge syndrome. *Hum Mol Genet* 1995;4:541–549.

156. Lindsay EA, Harvey EL, Scambler PJ, et al. ES2, a gene deleted in DiGeorge syndrome, encodes a nuclear protein and is expressed during early mouse development, where it shares an expression domain with a Goosecoid-like gene. *Hum Mol Genet* 1998;7:629–635.

157. Wilming LG, Snoeren CA, van Rijswijk A, et al. The murine homologue of HIRA, a DiGeorge syndrome candidate gene, is expressed in embryonic structures affected in human CATCH22 patients. *Hum Mol Genet* 1997;6:247–258.

157a. Lindsay EA, Vitelli F, Su H, et al. Tbx1 haploinsufficiency in the DiGeorge syndrome region causes aortic arch defects in mice. *Nature* 2001;410:97–101.

158. Kasprzak L, Der Kaloustian VM, Elliott AM, et al. Deletion of 22q11 in two brothers with different phenotype. *Am J Med Genet* 1998;75:288–291.

159. Vantrappen G, Devriendt K, Swillen A, et al. Presenting symptoms and clinical features in 130 patients with the velo-cardio-facial syndrome. The Leuven experience. *Genet Couns* 1999;10:3–9.

160. Van Esch H, Groenen P, Daw S, et al. Partial DiGeorge syndrome in two patients with a 10p rearrangement. *Clin Genet* 1999;55:269–276.

161. Hong R. Disorders of the T cell system. In: Stiehm ER, ed. *Immunologic disorders in infants and children*, 4th ed. Philadelphia: WB Saunders, 1996:339–408.

162. Markert ML, Boeck A, Hale LP, et al. Transplantation of thymus tissue in complete DiGeorge syndrome. *N Engl J Med* 1999;341:1180–1189.

163. Borzy MS, Ridgway D, Noya FJ, et al. Successful bone marrow transplantation with split lymphoid chimerism in DiGeorge syndrome. *J Clin Immunol* 1989;9:386–392.

164. Goldsobel AB, Haas A, Stiehm ER. Bone marrow transplantation in DiGeorge syndrome. *J Pediatr* 1987;111:40–44.

165. Matsumoto T, Amamoto N, Kondoh T, et al. Complete-type DiGeorge syndrome treated by bone marrow transplantation. *Bone Marrow Transplant* 1998;22:927–930.

166. Bowers DC, Lederman HM, Sicherer SH, et al. Immune constitution of complete DiGeorge anomaly by transplantation of unmobilised blood mononuclear cells. *Lancet* 1998;352:1983–1984.

167. van Kooten C, Banchereau J. CD40-CD40 ligand. *J Leukoc Biol* 2000;67:2–17.

168. Aruffo A, Farrington M, Hollenbaugh D, et al. The CD40 ligand, gp39, is defective in activated T cells from patients with X-linked hyper-IgM syndrome. *Cell* 1993;72:291–300.

169. Allen RC, Armitage RJ, Conley ME, et al. CD40 ligand gene defects responsible for X-linked hyper-IgM syndrome. *Science* 1993;259:990–993.

170. DiSanto JP, Bonnefoy JY, Gauchat JF, et al. CD40 ligand mutations in x-linked immunodeficiency with hyper-IgM. *Nature* 1993;361:541–543.

171. Fuleihan R, Ramesh N, Loh R, et al. Defective expression of the CD40 ligand in X chromosome-linked immunoglobulin deficiency with normal or elevated IgM. *Proc Natl Acad Sci U S A* 1993;90:2170–2173.

172. Korthauer U, Graf D, Mages HW, et al. Defective expression of T-cell CD40 ligand causes X-linked immunodeficiency with hyper-IgM. *Nature* 1993;361:539–541.

173. Bonilla FA, Geha RS. CD154 deficiency and related syndromes. *Immunol Allergy Clin North Am* 2001;21:65–89.

174. Levy J, Espanol-Boren T, Thomas C, et al. Clinical spectrum of X-linked hyper-IgM syndrome. *J Pediatr* 1997;131:47–54.

175. Jouanguy E, Altaire F, Lamhamedi S, et al. Interferon-γ-receptor deficiency in an infant with fatal bacille Calmette-Guerin infection. *N Engl J Med* 1996; 335:1956–1961.

176. Newport MJ, Huxley CM, Huston S, et al. A mutation in the interferon-γ-receptor gene and susceptibility to mycobacterial infection. *N Engl J Med* 1996;335:1941–1949.

177. Doffinger R, Jouanguy E, Dupuis S, et al. Partial interferon-gamma receptor signaling chain deficiency in a patient with bacille Calmette-Guerin and Mycobacterium abscessus infection. *J Infect Dis* 2000;181:379–384.

178. Dorman SE, Holland SM. Mutation in the signal-transducing chain of the interferon-gamma receptor and susceptibility to mycobacterial infection. *J Clin Invest* 1998;101:2364–2369.

179. Altare F, Lammas D, Revy P, et al. Inherited interleukin 12 deficiency in a child with bacille Calmette-Guerin and *Salmonella enteritidis* disseminated infection. *J Clin Invest* 1998;102:2035–2040.

180. de Jong R, Altare F, Haagen IA, et al. Severe mycobacterial and Salmonella infections in interleukin-12 receptor-deficient patients. *Science* 1998;280:1435–1438.

181. Seemayer TA, Gross TG, Egeler M, et al. X-linked lymphoproliferative disease: twenty-five years after the discovery. *Pediatr Res* 1995;38:471–478.

182. Sayos J, Wu C, Morra M, et al. The X-linked lymphoproliferative-disease gene product SAP regulates signals induced through the co-receptor SLAM. *Nature* 1998;395:462–469.

183. Howie D, Sayos J, Terhorst C, et al. The gene defective in X-linked lymphoproliferative disease controls T cell dependent immune surveillance against Epstein-Barr virus. *Curr Opin Immunol* 2000;12:474–478.

184. Coffey AJ, Brooksbank RA, Brandau O, et al. Host response to EBV infection in X-linked lymphoproliferative disease results from mutations in an SH2-domain encoding gene. *Nat Genet* 1998;20:129–135.

185. Vowels MR, Tang RL, Berdoukas V, et al. Brief report: correction of X-linked lymphoproliferative disease by transplantation of cord-blood stem cells. *N Engl J Med* 1993;329:1623–1625.

186. Kirkpatrick CH. Chronic mucocutaneous candidiasis. *J Am Acad Dermatol* 1994;31:S14–S17.

187. Obermayer-Straub P, Manns MP. Autoimmune polyglandular syndromes. *Baillieres Clin Gastroenterol* 1998;12:293–315.

188. Aaltonen J, Bjorses P. Cloning of the APECED gene provides new insight into human autoimmunity. *Ann Med* 1999;31:111–116.

189. Bjorses P, Aaltonen J, Horelli-Kuitunen N, et al. Gene defect behind APECED: a new clue to autoimmunity. *Hum Mol Genet* 1998;7:1547–1553.

190. Heino M, Peterson P, Kudoh J, et al. Autoimmune regulator is expressed in the cells regulating immune tolerance in thymus medulla. *Biochem Biophys Res Commun* 1999;257:821–825.

191. Heino M, Scott HS, Chen Q, et al. Mutation analyses of North American APS-1 patients. *Hum Mutat* 1999;13:69–74.

192. Hoh MC, Lin HP, Chan LL, et al. Successful allogeneic bone marrow transplantation in severe chronic mucocutaneous candidiasis syndrome. *Bone Marrow Transplant* 1996;18:797–800.

193. Kirkpatrick CH, Rich RR, Graw RG, Jr., et al. Treatment of chronic mucocutaneous moniliasis by immunologic reconstitution. *Clin Exp Immunol* 1971; 9:733–748.

194. Grimbacher B, Holland SM, Gallin JI, et al. Hyper-IgE syndrome with recurrent infections—an autosomal dominant multisystem disorder. *N Engl J Med* 1999;340:692–702.

195. Desai K, Huston DP, Harriman GR. Previously undiagnosed hyper-IgE syndrome in an adult with multiple systemic fungal infections. *J Allergy Clin Immunol* 1996;98:1123–1124.

196. King CL, Gallin JI, Malech HL, et al. Regulation of immunoglobulin production in hyperimmunoglobulin E recurrent-infection syndrome by interferon gamma. *Proc Natl Acad Sci U S A* 1989;86:10085–10089.

197. Pung YH, Vetro SW, Bellanti JA. Use of interferons in atopic (IgE-mediated) diseases. *Ann Allergy* 1993;71:234–238.

198. Kimata H. High-dose intravenous gamma-globulin treatment for hyperimmunoglobulinemia E syndrome. *J Allergy Clin Immunol* 1995;95:771–774.

199. Amzel LM, Poljak RJ. Three-dimensional structure of immunoglobulins. *Annu Rev Biochem* 1979;48:961–997.

200. Schiffer M, Girling RL, Ely KR, et al. Structure of a lambda-type Bence-Jones protein at 3.5-A resolution. *Biochemistry* 1973;12:4620–4631.

201. Silverton EW, Navia MA, Davies DR. Three-dimensional structure of an intact human immunoglobulin. *Proc Natl Acad Sci U S A* 1977;74:5140–5144.

202. Alzari PM, Lascombe MB, Poljak RJ. Three-dimensional structure of antibodies. *Annu Rev Immunol* 1988;6:555–580.

203. Williams AF, Barclay AN. The immunoglobulin superfamily—domains for cell surface recognition. *Annu Rev Immunol* 1988;6:381–405.

204. Wu TT, Kabat EA. An analysis of the sequences of the variable regions of Bence Jones proteins and myeloma light chains and their implications for antibody complementarity. *J Exp Med* 1970;132:211–250.

205. Edmundson AB, Ely KR, Abola EE, et al. Conformational isomerism, rotational allomerism, and divergent evolution in immunoglobulin light chains. *Fed Proc* 1976;35:2119–2123.

206. Schatz DG, Oettinger MA, Schlissel MS. V(D)J recombination: molecular biology and regulation. *Annu Rev Immunol* 1992;10:359–383.

207. Rademacher TW, Homans SW, Parekh RB, et al. Immunoglobulin G as a glycoprotein. *Biochem Soc Symp* 1986;51:131–148.

208. Sutton BJ, Phillips DC. The three-dimensional structure of the carbohydrate within the Fc fragment of immunoglobulin G. *Biochem Soc Trans* 1983;11 Pt 2:130–132.

209. Burton DR. Immunoglobulin G: functional sites. *Mol Immunol* 1985;22:161–206.

210. Middaugh CR, Litman GW. Atypical glycosylation of an IgG monoclonal cryoimmunoglobulin. *J Biol Chem* 1987;262:3671–3673.

211. Rademacher TW, Parekh RB, Dwek RA. Glycobiology. *Annu Rev Biochem* 1988;57:785–838.

212. Lund J, Takahashi N, Pound JD, et al. Multiple interactions of IgG with its core oligosaccharide can modulate recognition by complement and human Fc gamma receptor I and influence the synthesis of its oligosaccharide chains. *J Immunol* 1996;157:4963–4969.

213. Oettinger MA. V(D)J recombination: on the cutting edge. *Curr Opin Cell Biol* 1999;11:325–329.

214. Takahashi N, Ueda S, Obata M, et al. Structure of human immunoglobulin gamma genes: implications for evolution of a gene family. *Cell* 1982;29:671–679.

215. Vasicek TJ, Leder P. Structure and expression of the human immunoglobulin lambda genes. *J Exp Med* 1990;172:609–620.

216. del Guercio P. Regulatory structures on the V and C regions of immunoglobulin molecules. *Immunol Today* 1987;8:304–308.

217. Ferrante A, Beard LJ, Feldman RG. IgG subclass distribution of antibodies to bacterial and viral antigens. *Pediatr Infect Dis J* 1990;9:S16–S24.

218. Sutton B, Corper A, Bonagura V, et al. The structure and origin of rheumatoid factors. *Immunol Today* 2000;21:177–183.

219. Grubb R. Advances in human immunoglobulin allotypes. *Exp Clin Immunogenet* 1995;12:191–197.

220. Yount WJ, Kunkel HG, Litwin SD. Studies of the Vi (gamma-2c) subgroup of gamma-globulin. A relationship between concentration and genetic type among normal individuals. *J Exp Med* 1967;125:177–190.

221. Granoff DM, Pandey JP, Boies E, et al. Response to immunization with Haemophilus influenzae type b polysaccharide-pertussis vaccine and risk of Haemophilus meningitis in children with the Km(1) immunoglobulin allotype. *J Clin Invest* 1984;74:1708–1714.

222. Allen JC, Kunkel HG. Antibodies against gamma-globulin after repeated blood transfusions in man. *J Clin Invest* 1966;45:29–39.

223. Fudenberg HH, Fudenberg BR. Antibody to hereditary human gamma-globulin (GM) factor resulting from maternal-fetal incompatibility. *Science* 1964;145:170.

224. Poskitt DC, Jean-Francois MJ, Turnbull S, et al. The nature of immunoglobulin idiotypes and idiotype-anti-idiotype interactions in immunological networks. *Immunol Cell Biol* 1991;69:61–70.

225. Geha RS. Presence of auto-anti-idiotypic antibody during the normal human immune response to tetanus toxoid antigen. *J Immunol* 1982;129:139–144.

226. Jerne NK. Towards a network theory of the immune system. *Ann Immunol (Paris)* 1974;125C:373–389.

227. Takemori T, Rajewsky K. Mechanism of neonatally induced idiotype suppression and its relevance for the acquisition of self-tolerance. *Immunol Rev* 1984;79:103–117.

228. Zouali M, Isenberg DA, Morrow WJ. Idiotype manipulation for autoimmune diseases: where are we going? *Autoimmunity* 1996;24:55–63.

229. Mackworth-Young CG, Madaio MP. Anti-DNA idiotype network: therapeutic considerations. *Lupus* 1992;1:339–340.

230. DeKeyser F, DeKeyser H, Kazatchkine MD, et al. Pooled human immunoglobulins contain anti-idiotypes with reactivity against the SLE-associated 4B4 cross-reactive idiotype. *Clin Exp Rheumatol* 1996;14:587–591.

231. Bhattachary-Chatterjee M, Nath Baral R, Chatterjee SK, et al. Counterpoint. Cancer vaccines: single-epitope anti-idiotype vaccine versus multiple-epitope antigen vaccine. *Cancer Immunol Immunother* 2000;49:133–141.

232. Hefty PS, Kennedy RC. Immunoglobulin variable regions as idiotype vaccines. *Infect Dis Clin North Am* 1999;13:27–37,vi.

233. Story CM, Mikulska JE, Simister NE. A major histocompatibility complex class I-like Fc receptor cloned from human placenta: possible role in transfer of immunoglobulin G from mother to fetus. *J Exp Med* 1994;180:2377–2381.

234. Gitlin D, Biasucci A. Development of gamma G, gamma A, gamma M, beta IC-beta IA, C 1 esterase inhibitor, ceruloplasmin, transferrin, hemopexin, haptoglobin, fibrinogen, plasminogen, alpha 1-antitrypsin, orosomucoid, beta-lipoprotein, alpha 2-macroglobulin, and prealbumin in the human conceptus. *J Clin Invest* 1969;48:1433–1446.

235. Garred P, Michaelsen TE, Aase A. The IgG subclass pattern of complement activation depends on epitope density and antibody and complement concentration. *Scand J Immunol* 1989;30:379–382.

236. Jefferis R, Pound J, Lund J, et al. Effector mechanisms activated by human IgG subclass antibodies: clinical and molecular aspects. Review article. *Ann Biol Clin* 1994;52:57–65.

237. Bielory L, Kemeny DM, Richards D, et al. IgG subclass antibody production in human serum sickness. *J Allergy Clin Immunol* 1990;85:573–577.

238. Sorensen V, Rasmussen IB, Sundvold V, et al. Structural requirements for incorporation of J chain into human IgM and IgA. *Int Immunol* 2000;12:19–27.

239. Daeron M. Fc receptor biology. *Annu Rev Immunol* 1997;15:203–234.

240. Rosen FS, Janeway CA. Immunologic competence of the newborn infant. *Pediatrics* 1964;33:159.

241. Burrows PD, Cooper MD. B cell development and differentiation. *Curr Opin Immunol* 1997;9:239–244.

242. Metzger H. Structure and function of gamma M macroglobulins. *Adv Immunol* 1970;12:57–116.

243. Hexham JM, Carayannopoulos L, Capra JD. Structure and function in IgA. *Chem Immunol* 1997;65:73–87.

244. Lamm ME, Nedrud JG, Kaetzel CS, et al. IgA and mucosal defense. *Apmis* 1995;103:241–246.

245. Lorenzi R, Jouvin MH, Burrone OR. Functional Fc epsilonRI engagement by a second secretory IgE isoform detected in humans. *Eur J Immunol* 1999;29:936–945.

246. Maggi E, Macchia D, Parronchi P, et al. The IgE response in atopy and infections. *Clin Exp Allergy* 1991;21[Suppl 1]:72–78.

247. McSharry C, Xia Y, Holland CV, et al. Natural immunity to Ascaris lumbricoides associated with immunoglobulin E antibody to ABA-1 allergen and inflammation indicators in children. *Infect Immun* 1999;67:484–489.

248. Kim KM, Reth M. The B cell antigen receptor of class IgD induces a stronger and more prolonged protein tyrosine phosphorylation than that of class IgM. *J Exp Med* 1995;181:1005–1014.

249. Waldmann TA. Methods for the study of the metabolism of immunoglobulins. *Methods Enzymol* 1985;116:201–210.

250. Masson PL. Elimination of infectious antigens and increase of IgG catabolism as possible modes of action of IVIg. *J Autoimmun* 1993;6:683–689.

251. Fischer SH, Ochs HD, Wedgwood RJ, et al. Survival of antigen-specific antibody following administration of intravenous immunoglobulin in patients with primary immunodeficiency diseases. *Monogr Allergy* 1988;23:225–235.

252. Gitlin D, Kumate J, Morales C. Metabolism and maternofetal transfer of human growth hormone in the pregnant woman at term. *J Clin Endocrinol Metab* 1965;25:1599–1608.

253. Gitlin D, Kumate J, Morales C, et al. The turnover of amniotic fluid protein in the human conceptus. *Am J Obstet Gynecol* 1972;113:632–645.

254. Ghetie V, Ward ES. Multiple roles for the major histocompatibility complex class I-related receptor FcRn. *Annu Rev Immunol* 2000;18:739–766.

255. Gessner JE, Heiken H, Tamm A, et al. The IgG Fc receptor family. *Ann Hematol* 1998;76:231–248.

256. Isakov N. Immunoreceptor tyrosine-based activation motif (ITAM), a unique module linking antigen and Fc receptors to their signaling cascades. *J Leukoc Biol* 1997;61:6–16.

257. Okayama Y, Kirshenbaum AS, Metcalfe DD. Expression of a functional high-affinity IgG receptor, Fc gamma RI, on human mast cells: Up-regulation by IFN-gamma. *J Immunol* 2000;164:4332–4339.

258. van de Winkel JG, de Wit TP, Ernst LK, et al. Molecular basis for a familial defect in phagocyte expression of IgG receptor I (CD64). *J Immunol* 1995;154:2896–2903.

259. Bredius RG, de Vries CE, Troelstra A, et al. Phagocytosis of *Staphylococcus aureus* and *Haemophilus influenzae* type B opsonized with polyclonal human

IgG1 and IgG2 antibodies. Functional hFc gamma RIIa polymorphism to IgG2. *J Immunol* 1993;151:1463–1472.

260. Salmon JE, Edberg JC, Brogle NL, et al. Allelic polymorphisms of human Fc gamma receptor IIA and Fc gamma receptor IIIB. Independent mechanisms for differences in human phagocyte function. *J Clin Invest* 1992;89:1274–1281.

261. Fridman WH, Teillaud JL, Bouchard C, et al. Soluble Fc gamma receptors. *J Leukoc Biol* 1993;54:504–512.

262. Astier A, Merle-Beral H, de la Salle H, et al. Soluble Fcgamma receptor, Fc gammaRIIa2, is present in two forms in human serum and is increased in patients: with stage C chronic lymphocytic leukemia. *Leuk Lymphoma* 1997;26:317–326.

263. Fijen CA, Bredius RG, Kuijper EJ, et al. The role of Fcgamma receptor polymorphisms and C3 in the immune defence against *Neisseria meningitidis* in complement-deficient individuals. *Clin Exp Immunol* 2000;120:338–345.

264. Daeron M, Latour S, Malbec O, et al. The same tyrosine-based inhibition motif, in the intracytoplasmic domain of Fc gamma RIIB, regulates negatively BCR-, TCR-, and FcR-dependent cell activation. *Immunity* 1995;3:635–646.

265. Koncz G, Pecht I, Gergely J, et al. Fcgamma receptor-mediated inhibition of human B cell activation: the role of SHP-2 phosphatase. *Eur J Immunol* 1999;29:1980–1989.

266. Kepley CL, Cambier JC, Morel PA, et al. Negative regulation of FcepsilonRI signaling by FcgammaRII costimulation in human blood basophils. *J Allergy Clin Immunol* 2000;106:337–348.

267. Bredius RG, Fijen CA, De Haas M, et al. Role of neutrophil Fc gamma RIIa (CD32) and Fc gamma RIIIb (CD16) polymorphic forms in phagocytosis of human IgG1- and IgG3-opsonized bacteria and erythrocytes. *Immunology* 1994;83:624–630.

268. de la Salle H, Galon J, Bausinger H, et al. Soluble CD16/Fc gamma RIII induces maturation of dendritic cells and production of several cytokines including IL-12. *Adv Exp Med Biol* 1997;417:345–352.

269. de Haas M, Kleijer M, Minchinton RM, et al. Soluble Fc gamma RIIIa is present in plasma and is derived from natural killer cells. *J Immunol* 1994;152:900–907.

270. Hommes DW, Meenan J, de Haas M, et al. Soluble Fc gamma receptor III (CD 16) and eicosanoid concentrations in gut lavage fluid from patients with inflammatory bowel disease: reflection of mucosal inflammation. *Gut* 1996;38:564–567.

271. Muller Kobold AC, Zijlstra JG, Koene HR, et al. Levels of soluble Fc gammaRIII correlate with disease severity in sepsis. *Clin Exp Immunol* 1998;114:220–227.

272. Fleit HB, Kobasiuk CD. Soluble Fc gamma RIII is present in lower concentrations in the serum of patients with acute myelogenous leukemia (AML): a retrospective study. *Leukemia* 1993;7:1250–1252.

273. Fromont P, Bettaieb A, Skouri H, et al. Frequency of the polymorphonuclear neutrophil Fc gamma receptor III deficiency in the French population and its involvement in the development of neonatal alloimmune neutropenia. *Blood* 1992;79:2131–2134.

274. de Haas M, Kleijer M, van Zwieten R, et al. Neutrophil Fc gamma RIIIb deficiency, nature, and clinical consequences: a study of 21 individuals from 14 families. *Blood* 1995;86:2403–2413.

275. Saito K, Suzuki K, Matsuda H, et al. Physical association of Fc receptor gamma chain homodimer with IgA receptor. *J Allergy Clin Immunol* 1995;96:1152–1160.

276. Pleass RJ, Andrews PD, Kerr MA, et al. Alternative splicing of the human IgA Fc receptor CD89 in neutrophils and eosinophils. *Biochem J* 1996;318:771–777.

277. Wolf HM, Hauber I, Gulle H, et al. Anti-inflammatory properties of human serum IgA: induction of IL-1 receptor antagonist and Fc alpha R (CD89)-mediated down-regulation of tumour necrosis factor-alpha (TNF-alpha) and IL-6 in human monocytes. *Clin Exp Immunol* 1996;105:537–543.

278. Launay P, Grossetete B, Arcos-Fajardo M, et al. Fcalpha receptor (CD89) mediates the development of immunoglobulin A (IgA) nephropathy (Berger's disease). Evidence for pathogenic soluble receptor-Iga complexes in patients and CD89 transgenic mice. *J Exp Med* 2000;191:1999–2009.

279. Kitamura T, Garofalo RP, Kamijo A, et al. Human intestinal epithelial cells express a novel receptor for IgA. *J Immunol* 2000;164:5029–5034.

280. Pricop L, Rabinowich H, Morel PA, et al. Characterization of the Fc mu receptor on human natural killer cells. Interaction with its physiologic ligand, human normal IgM, specificity of binding, and functional effects. *J Immunol* 1993;151:3018–3029.

281. Rabinowich H, Manciulea M, Metes D, et al. Physical and functional association of Fc mu receptor on human natural killer cells with the zeta- and Fc epsilon RI gamma-chains and with src family protein tyrosine kinases. *J Immunol* 1996;157:1485–1491.

282. Ohno T, Kubagawa H, Sanders SK, et al. Biochemical nature of an Fc mu receptor on human B-lineage cells. *J Exp Med* 1990;172:1165–1175.

283. Nakamura T, Kubagawa H, Ohno T, et al. Characterization of an IgM Fc-binding receptor on human T cells. *J Immunol* 1993;151:6933–6941.

284. Kinet JP. The high-affinity IgE receptor (Fc epsilon RI): from physiology to pathology. *Annu Rev Immunol* 1999;17:931–972.

285. Yamaguchi M, Sayama K, Yano K, et al. IgE enhances Fc epsilon receptor I expression and IgE-dependent release of histamine and lipid mediators from human umbilical cord blood-derived mast cells: synergistic effect of IL-4 and IgE on human mast cell Fc epsilon receptor I expression and mediator release. *J Immunol* 1999;162:5455–5465.

286. Maurer D, Fiebiger E, Reininger B, et al. Fc epsilon receptor I on dendritic cells delivers IgE-bound multivalent antigens into a cathepsin S-dependent pathway of MHC class II presentation. *J Immunol* 1998;161:2731–2739.

287. Maurer D, Ebner C, Reininger B, et al. Mechanisms of Fc epsilon RI-IgE-facilitated allergen presentation by dendritic cells. *Adv Exp Med Biol* 1997;417:175–178.

288. Gounni AS, Lamkhioued B, Delaporte E, et al. The high-affinity IgE receptor on eosinophils: from allergy to parasites or from parasites to allergy? *J Allergy Clin Immunol* 1994;94:1214–1216.

289. Conrad DH. Fc epsilon RII/CD23: the low affinity receptor for IgE. *Annu Rev Immunol* 1990;8:623–645.

290. Capron M, Grangette C, Torpier G, et al. The second receptor for IgE in eosinophil effector function. *Chem Immunol* 1989;47:128–178.

291. Kisselgof AB, Oettgen HC. The expression of murine B cell CD23, in vivo, is regulated by its ligand, IgE. *Int Immunol* 1998;10:1377–1384.

292. Sherr E, Macy E, Kimata H, et al. Binding the low affinity Fc epsilon R on B cells suppresses ongoing human IgE synthesis. *J Immunol* 1989;142:481–489.

293. Mudde GC, Bheekha R, Bruijnzeel-Koomen CA. Consequences of IgE/CD23-mediated antigen presentation in allergy. *Immunol Today* 1995;16:380–383.

294. Pene J, Chretien I, Rousset F, et al. Modulation of IL-4-induced human IgE production in vitro by IFN-gamma and IL-5: the role of soluble CD23 (s-CD23). *J Cell Biochem* 1989;39:253–264.

295. Swenson CD, Cherniack EP, Russo C, et al. IgD-receptor up-regulation on human peripheral blood T cells in response to IgD in vitro or antigen in vivo correlates with the antibody response to influenza vaccination. *Eur J Immunol* 1996;26:340–344.

296. Swenson CD, Thorbecke GJ. The effect of aging on IgD receptor expression by T cells and its functional implications. *Immunol Rev* 1997;160:145–157.

297. Swenson CD, Patel T, Parekh RB, et al. Human T cell IgD receptors react with O-glycans on both human IgD and IgA1. *Eur J Immunol* 1998;28:2366–2372.

298. Yang YJ, Coico RF. In vitro enhancement of antibody responses by T delta cells expressing IgD receptors. *Cell Immunol* 1996;168:107–116.

299. Norderhaug IN, Johansen FE, Schjerven H, et al. Regulation of the formation and external transport of secretory immunoglobulins. *Crit Rev Immunol* 1999;19:481–508.

300. Hexham JM, White KD, Carayannopoulos LN, et al. A human immunoglobulin (Ig)A calpha3 domain motif directs polymeric Ig receptor-mediated secretion. *J Exp Med* 1999;189:747–752.

301. Haymann JP, Levraud JP, Bouet S, et al. Characterization and localization of the neonatal Fc receptor in adult human kidney. *J Am Soc Nephrol* 2000;11:632–639.

302. Dickinson BL, Badizadegan K, Wu Z, et al. Bidirectional FcRn-dependent IgG transport in a polarized human intestinal epithelial cell line. *J Clin Invest* 1999;104:903–911.

303. Mikulska JE, Pablo L, Canel J, et al. Cloning and analysis of the gene encoding the human neonatal Fc receptor. *Eur J Immunogenet* 2000;27:231–240.

304. West AP Jr, Bjorkman PJ. Crystal structure and immunoglobulin G binding properties of the human major histocompatibility complex-related Fc receptor(,). *Biochemistry* 2000;39:9698–9708.

305. Kamada M, Mori H, Maeda N, et al. beta-Microseminoprotein/prostatic secretory protein is a member of immunoglobulin binding factor family. *Biochim Biophys Acta* 1998;1388:101–110.

306. Maegawa M, Kamada M, Maeda N, et al. Colocalization of immunoglobulin binding factor and prostate specific antigen in human prostate gland. *Arch Androl* 1996;37:149–154.

307. Maeda N, Kamada M, Daitoh T, et al. Immunoglobulin binding factor: a new tumor marker for prostatic tumors. *Prostate* 1994;24:125–130.

308. Mori H, Kamada M, Maegawa M, et al. Enzymatic activation of immunoglobulin binding factor in female reproductive tract. *Biochem Biophys Res Commun* 1998;246:409–413.

309. Hirano M, Kamada M, Maeda N, et al. Presence of immunoglobulin binding factor on human sperm surface as sperm coating antigen. *Arch Androl* 1996;37:163–170.

310. Ogushi F, Sone S, Tani K, et al. Identification and localization of immunoglobulin binding factor in bronchoalveolar lavage fluid from healthy smokers. *Am J Respir Crit Care Med* 1995;152:2133–2137.

311. Ichikawa W, Ogushi F, Tani K, et al. Characterization of immunoglobulin binding factor in sputum from patients with chronic airway diseases. *Respirology* 1999;4:375–381.

312. Bruton OC. Agammaglobulinemia. *Pediatrics* 1952;9:722.

313. Ochs HD, Smith CI. X-linked agammaglobulinemia. A clinical and molecular analysis. *Medicine (Baltimore)* 1996;75:287–299.

314. Furr PM, Taylor-Robinson D, Webster AD. Mycoplasmas and ureaplasmas in patients with hypogammaglobulinaemia and their role in arthritis: microbiological observations over twenty years. *Ann Rheum Dis* 1994;53:183–187.

315. Wilfert CM, Buckley RH, Mohanakumar T, et al. Persistent and fatal central-nervous-system ECHOvirus infections in patients with agammaglobulinemia. *N Engl J Med* 1977;296:1485–1489.

316. Alibrahim A, Lepore M, Lierl M, et al. Pneumocystis carinii pneumonia in an infant with X-linked agammaglobulinemia. *J Allergy Clin Immunol* 1998;101:552–553.

317. Nonoyama S, Tsukada S, Yamadori T, et al. Functional analysis of peripheral blood B cells in patients with X-linked agammaglobulinemia. *J Immunol* 1998;161:3925–3929.

318. Tsukada S, Saffran DC, Rawlings DJ, et al. Deficient expression of a B cell cytoplasmic tyrosine kinase in human X-linked agammaglobulinemia. *Cell* 1993;72:279.

319. Vetrie D, Vorechovsky I, Sideras P, et al. The gene involved in X-linked agammaglobulinemia is a member of the *src* family of protein-tyrosine kinases. *Nature* 1993;361:226.

320. Kanegane H, Tsukada S, Iwata T, et al. Detection of Bruton's tyrosine kinase mutations in hypogammaglobulinaemic males registered as common variable immunodeficiency (CVID) in the Japanese Immunodeficiency Registry. *Clin Exp Immunol* 2000;120:512–517.

321. Bykowsky MJ, Haire RN, Ohta Y, et al. Discordant phenotype in siblings with X-linked agammaglobulinemia. *Am J Hum Genet* 1996;58:477–483.

322. Gaspar HB, Lester T, Levinsky RJ, et al. Bruton's tyrosine kinase expression and activity in X-linked agammaglobulinaemia (XLA): the use of protein analysis as a diagnostic indicator of XLA. *Clin Exp Immunol* 1998;111:334–338.

323. Holinski-Feder E, Weiss M, Brandau O, et al. Mutation screening of the BTK gene in 56 families with X-linked agammaglobulinemia (XLA): 47 unique mutations without correlation to clinical course. *Pediatrics* 1998;101:276–284.

324. Kornfeld SJ, Haire RN, Strong SJ, et al. Extreme variation in X-linked agammaglobulinemia phenotype in a three-generation family. *J Allergy Clin Immunol* 1997;100:702–706.

325. Hashimoto S, Miyawaki T, Futatani T, et al. Atypical X-linked agammaglobulinemia diagnosed in three adults. *Intern Med* 1999;38:722–725.

326. Kawakami Y, Kitaura J, Hata D, et al. Functions of Bruton's tyrosine kinase in mast and B cells. *J Leukoc Biol* 1999;65:286–290.

327. Rawlings DJ. Bruton's tyrosine kinase controls a sustained calcium signal essential for B lineage development and function. *Clin Immunol* 1999;91:243–253.

328. Quek LS, Bolen J, Watson SP. A role for Bruton's tyrosine kinase (Btk) in platelet activation by collagen. *Curr Biol* 1998;8:1137–1140.

329. Quartier P, Debre M, De Blic J, et al. Early and prolonged intravenous immunoglobulin replacement therapy in childhood agammaglobulinemia: a retrospective survey of 31 patients. *J Pediatr* 1999;134:589–596.

330. Plebani A, Fischer MB, Meini A, et al. T cell activity and cytokine production in X-linked agammaglobulinemia: implications for vaccination strategies. *Int Arch Allergy Immunol* 1997;114:90–93.

331. Yel L, Minegishi Y, Coustan-Smith E, et al. Mutations in the mu heavy-chain gene in patients with agammaglobulinemia. *N Engl J Med* 1996;335:1486–1493.

332. Minegishi Y, Coustan-Smith E, Wang YH, et al. Mutations in the human lambda5/14.1 gene result in B cell deficiency and agammaglobulinemia. *J Exp Med* 1998;187:71–77.

333. Minegishi Y, Coustan-Smith E, Rapalus L, et al. Mutations in Igalpha (CD79a) result in a complete block in B-cell development. *J Clin Invest* 1999;104:1115–1121.

334. Minegishi Y, Rohrer J, Coustan-Smith E, et al. An essential role for BLNK in human B cell development. *Science* 1999;286:1954–1957.

335. Pappu R, Cheng AM, Li B, et al. Requirement for B cell linker protein (BLNK) in B cell development. *Science* 1999;286:1949–1954.

336. Cunningham-Rundles C. Clinical and immunologic analyses of 103 patients with common variable immunodeficiency. *J Clin Immunol* 1989;9:22–33.

337. Spickett GP, Webster ADB, Farrant J. Cellular abnormalities in common variable immunodeficiency. In: Rosen FS, Seligmann M, eds. *Immunodeficiencies*. Amsterdam: Harwood Academic Publishers GmbH, 1993:111–126.

338. Cunningham-Rundles C, Bodian C. Common variable immunodeficiency: clinical and immunological features of 248 patients. *Clin Immunol* 1999;92:34–48.

339. Zuccaro G, Della Bella S, Polizzi B, et al. Common variable immunodeficiency following Epstein-Barr virus infection. *J Clin Lab Immunol* 1997;49:41–45.

340. Miller BW, Brennan DC, Korenblat PE, et al. Common variable immunodeficiency in a renal transplant patient with severe recurrent bacterial infection: a case report and review of the literature. *Am J Kidney Dis* 1995;25:947–951.

341. Conley ME, Notarangelo LD, Etzioni A. Diagnostic criteria for primary immunodeficiencies. Representing PAGID (Pan-American Group for Immunodeficiency) and ESID (European Society for Immunodeficiencies). *Clin Immunol* 1999;93:190–197.

342. Cunningham-Rundles C, Lieberman P, Hellman G, et al. Non-Hodgkin lymphoma in common variable immunodeficiency. *Am J Hematol* 1991;37:69–74.

343. Fasano MB, Sullivan KE, Sarpong SB, et al. Sarcoidosis and common variable immunodeficiency. Report of 8 cases and review of the literature. *Medicine (Baltimore)* 1996;75:251–261.

344. Sutor G, Fabel H. Sarcoidosis and common variable immunodeficiency. A case of a malignant course of sarcoidosis in conjunction with severe impairment of the cellular and humoral immune system. *Respiration* 2000;67:204–208.

345. Johnson ML, Keeton LG, Zhu ZB, et al. Age-related changes in serum immunoglobulins in patients with familial IgA deficiency and common variable immunodeficiency (CVID). *Clin Exp Immunol* 1997;108:477–483.

346. Seligmann M, Aucouturier P, Danon F, et al. Changes in serum immunoglobulin patterns in adults with common variable immunodeficiency. *Clin Exp Immunol* 1991;84:23–27.

347. Nonoyama S, Farrington M, Ishida H, et al. Activated B cells from patients with common variable immunodeficiency proliferate and synthesize immunoglobulin. *J Clin Invest* 1993;92:1282–1287.

348. Denz A, Eibel H, Illges H, et al. Impaired up-regulation of CD86 in B cells of "type A" common variable immunodeficiency patients. *Eur J Immunol* 2000;30:1069–1077.

349. Levy Y, Gupta N, Le Deist F, et al. Defect in IgV gene somatic hypermutation in common variable immuno-deficiency syndrome. *Proc Natl Acad Sci U S A* 1998;95:13135–13140.

350. Sneller MC, Strober W. Abnormalities of lymphokine gene expression in patients with common variable immunodeficiency. *J Immunol* 1990;144:3762–3769.

351. Fischer MB, Hauber I, Vogel E, et al. Defective interleukin-2 and interferon-γ gene expression in response to antigen in a subgroup of patients with common variable immunodeficiency. *J Allergy Clin Immunol* 1993;92:340–352.

352. Eisenstein EM, Jaffe JS, Strober W. Reduced interleukin-2 (IL-2) production in common variable immunodeficiency is due to a primary abnormality of CD4+ T cell differentiation. *J Clin Immunol* 1993;13:247–258.

353. Farrington M, Grosmaire LS, Nonoyama S, et al. CD40 ligand expression is defective in a subset of patients with common variable immunodeficiency. *Proc Natl Acad Sci U S A* 1994;91:1099–1103.

354. Funauchi M, Farrant J, Moreno C, et al. Defects in antigen-driven lymphocyte responses in common variable immunodeficiency (CVID) are due to a reduction in the number of antigen-specific CD4+ T cells. *Clin Exp Immunol* 1995;101:82–88.

355. Kondratenko I, Amlot PL, Webster AD, et al. Lack of specific antibody response in common variable immunodeficiency (CVID) associated with failure in production of antigen-specific memory T cells. MRC Immunodeficiency Group. *Clin Exp Immunol* 1997;108:9–13.

356. Iglesias J, Matamoros N, Raga S, et al. CD95 expression and function on lymphocyte subpopulations in common variable immunodeficiency (CVID); related to increased apoptosis. *Clin Exp Immunol* 1999;117:138–146.

357. Spickett GP, Farrant J, North ME, et al. Common variable immunodeficiency: how many diseases? *Immunol Today* 1997;18:325–328.

358. De La Concha EG, Fernandez-Arquero M, Martinez A, et al. HLA class II homozygosity confers susceptibility to common variable immunodeficiency (CVID). *Clin Exp Immunol* 1999;116:516–520.

359. Schaffer FM, Palermos J, Zhu ZB, et al. Individuals with IgA deficiency and common variable immunodeficiency share polymorphisms of major histocompatibility complex class III genes. *Proc Natl Acad Sci U S A* 1989;86:8015–8019.

360. Burks AW, Sampson HA, Buckley RH. Anaphylactic reactions after gamma globulin administration in patients with hypogammaglobulinemia. *N Engl J Med* 1986;314:560.

361. Cunningham-Rundles C, Zhou Z, Mankarious S, et al. Long-term use of IgA-depleted intravenous immunoglobulin in immunodeficient subjects with anti-IgA antibodies. *J Clin Immunol* 1993;13:272–278.

362. Sandler SG, Mallory D, Malamut D, et al. IgA anaphylactic transfusion reactions. *Transfus Med Rev* 1995;9:1–8.

363. Rump JA, Jahreis A, Schlesier M, et al. A double-blind, placebo-controlled, crossover therapy study with natural human IL-2 (nhuIL-2) in combination with regular intravenous gammaglobulin (IVIG) infusions in 10 patients with common variable immunodeficiency (CVID). *Clin Exp Immunol* 1997;110:167–173.

364. Ropars C, Muller A, Paint N, et al. Large scale detection of IgA deficient blood donors. *J Immunol Methods* 1982;54:183.

365. Kanoh T, Mizumoto T, Yasuda N, et al. Selective IgA deficiency in Japanese blood donors: frequency and statistical analysis. *Vox Sang* 1986;50:81.

366. Koskinen S, Tolo H, Hirvonen M, et al. Long-term follow-up of anti-IgA antibodies in healthy IgA-deficient adults. *J Clin Immunol* 1995;15:194–198.

367. Sandler SG, Trimble J, Mallory DM. Coexistent IgG2 and IgA deficiencies in blood donors. *Transfusion* 1996;36:256–258.

368. French MA, Denis KA, Dawkins R, et al. Severity of infections in IgA deficiency: correlation with decreased serum antibodies to pneumococcal polysaccharides and decreased serum IgG2 and/or IgG4. *Clin Exp Immunol* 1995;100:47–53.

369. Amman AJ, Hong R. Selective IgA deficiency: presentation of 30 cases and a review of the literature. *Medicine* 1971;50:223.

370. Barka N, Shen GQ, Shoenfeld Y, et al. Multireactive pattern of serum autoantibodies in asymptomatic individuals with immunoglobulin A deficiency. *Clin Diagn Lab Immunol* 1995;2:469–472.

371. Plebani A, Monafo V, Ugazio AG, et al. Comparison of the frequency of atopic diseases in children with severe and partial IgA deficiency. *Int Arch Allergy Appl Immunol* 1987;82:485.

372. Kersey JH, Shapiro RS, Filipovich AH. Relationship of immune deficiency to lymphoid malignancy. *Pediatr Infect Dis J* 1988;7:S10.

373. Espanol T, Catala M, Hernandez M, et al. Development of a common variable immunodeficiency in IgA-deficient patients. *Clin Immunol Immunopathol* 1996;80:333–335.

374. Conley ME, Cooper MD. Immature IgA B cells in IgA deficient patients. *N Engl J Med* 1986;305:495.

375. Wang Z, Yunis D, Irigoyen M, et al. Discordance between IgA switching at the DNA level and IgA expression at the mRNA level in IgA-deficient patients. *Clin Immunol* 1999;91:263–270.

376. King MA, Wells JV, Nelson DS. IgA synthesis by peripheral blood mononuclear cells from normal and selectively IgA deficient subjects. *Clin Exp Immunol* 1979;38:306.

377. Schwartz SA. Heavy-chain-specific suppression of immunoglobulin synthesis and secretion by lymphocytes from patients with selective IgA deficiency. *J Immunol* 1980;124:2034.

378. Inoue T, Okubo H, Kudo J, et al. Selective IgA deficiency: analysis of Ig production in vitro. *J Clin Immunol* 1984;4:235.

379. Friman V, Hanson LA, Bridon JM, et al. IL-10-driven immunoglobulin production by B lymphocytes from IgA-deficient individuals correlates to infection proneness. *Clin Exp Immunol* 1996;104:432–438.

380. Islam KB, Baskin B, Nilsson L, et al. Molecular analysis of IgA deficiency—evidence for impaired switching to IgA. *J Immunol* 1994;152:1442.

381. van Vlasselaer P, Punnonen J, de Vries JE. Transforming growth factor-beta directs IgA class-switching in human cells. *J Immunol* 1992;152:2062.

382. Muller F, Aukrust P, Nilssen DE, et al. Reduced serum level of transforming growth factor-beta in patients with IgA deficiency. *Clin Immunol Immunopathol* 1995;76:203–208.

383. van Ginkel FW, Wahl SM, Kearney JF, et al. Partial IgA-deficiency with increased Th2-type cytokines in TGF-beta 1 knockout mice. *J Immunol* 1999;163:1951–1957.

384. Vorechovsky I, Cullen M, Carrington M, et al. Fine mapping of IGAD1 in IgA deficiency and common variable immunodeficiency: identification and characterization of haplotypes shared by affected members of 101 multiple-case families. *J Immunol* 2000;164:4408–4416.

385. Cucca F, Zhu ZB, Khanna A, et al. Evaluation of IgA deficiency in Sardinians indicates a susceptibility gene is encoded within the HLA class III region. *Clin Exp Immunol* 1998;111:76–80.

386. Hammarstrom L, Axelsson U, Bjorkander U, et al. HLA antigens in selective IgA deficiency. *Tissue Antigens* 1984;24:35.

387. Schroeder HW Jr, Zhu ZB, March RE, et al. Susceptibility locus for IgA deficiency and common variable immunodeficiency in the HLA-DR3, -B8, -A1 haplotypes. *Mol Med* 1998;4:72–86.

388. Braconier JH. Reversible total IgA deficiency associated with phenytoin treatment. *Scand J Infect Dis* 1999;31:515–516.

389. Umetsu DT, Ambrosino DM, Quinti I, et al. Recurrent sinopulmonary infection and impaired antibody response to bacterial capsular polysaccharide antigen in children with selective IgG-subclass deficiency. *N Engl J Med* 1985;313:1247.

390. Morgan G, Levinsky RJ. Clinical significance of IgG subclass deficiency. *Arch Dis Child* 1988;63:771–773.

391. Lacombe C, Aucouturier P, Preud'homme JL. Selective IgG1 deficiency. *Clin Immunol Immunopathol* 1997;84:194–201.

392. Van Kessel DA, Horikx PE, Van Houte AJ, et al. Clinical and immunological evaluation of patients with mild IgG1 deficiency. *Clin Exp Immunol* 1999;118:102–107.

393. Ainsworth SB, Baraitser M, Mueller RF, et al. Selective IgG2 subclass deficiency—a marker for the syndrome of pre/postnatal growth retardation, developmental delay, hypotrophy of distal extremities, dental anomalies and eczema. *Clin Dysmorphol* 1997;6:139–146.

394. De Gracia J, Rodrigo MJ, Morell F, et al. IgG subclass deficiencies associated with bronchiectasis. *Am J Respir Crit Care Med* 1996;153:650–655.

395. Masin JS, Hostoffer RW, Arnold JE. Otitis media following tympanostomy tube placement in children with IgG2 deficiency. *Laryngoscope* 1995;105:1188–1190.

396. Ojuawo A, Milla PJ, Lindley KJ. Serum immunoglobulin and immunoglobulin G subclasses in children with allergic colitis. *West Afr J Med* 1998;17:206–209.

397. Barlan IB, Geha RS, Schneider LC. Therapy for patients with recurrent infections and low serum IgG3 levels. *J Allergy Clin Immunol* 1993;92:353–355.

398. Coskun Y, Bayraktaroglu Z. Immunoglobulin isotypes and IgG subclasses in recurrent infections. *Turk J Pediatr* 1997;39:347–352.

399. Schur PH, Borel H, Gelfand EW, et al. Selective gamma-G globulin deficiencies in patients with recurrent pyogenic infections. *N Engl J Med* 1970;283:631.

400. Schur PH. IgG human subclasses—a review. *Ann Allergy* 1987;58:89.

401. Antall PM, Meyerson H, Kaplan D, et al. Selective antipolysaccharide antibody deficiency associated with peripheral blood CD5+ B-cell predominance. *J Allergy Clin Immunol* 1999;103:637–641.

402. Epstein MM, Gruskay F. Selective deficiency in pneumococcal antibody response in children with recurrent infections. *Ann Allergy Asthma Immunol* 1995;75:125–131.

403. Ambrosino DM, Umetsu DT, Siber GR, et al. Selective defect in the antibody response to Haemophilus influenzae type b in children with recurrent infections and normal serum IgG subclass levels. *J Allergy Clin Immunol* 1988;81:1175.

404. Guneser S, Antmen B, Altintas D, et al. The frequency of IgG subclass deficiency in children with recurrent respiratory infections. *Turk J Pediatr* 1996;38:161–168.

405. Karaman O, Uguz A, Uzuner N. IgG subclasses in wheezing infants. *Indian J Pediatr* 1999;66:345–349.

406. May A, Zielen S, von Ilberg C, et al. Immunoglobulin deficiency and determination of pneumococcal antibody titers in patients with therapy-refractory recurrent rhinosinusitis. *Eur Arch Otorhinolaryngol* 1999;256:445–449.

407. Tashita H, Fukao T, Kaneko H, et al. Molecular basis of selective IgG2 deficiency. The mutated membrane-bound form of gamma2 heavy chain caused complete IGG2 deficiency in two Japanese siblings. *J Clin Invest* 1998;101:677–681.

408. Lefranc MP, Hammarstrom L, Smith CI, et al. Gene deletions in the human immunoglobulin heavy chain constant region locus: molecular and immunological analysis. *Immunodef Rev* 1991;2:265–281.

409. Plebani A, Ugazio AG, Meini A, et al. Extensive deletion of immunoglobulin heavy chain constant region genes in the absence of recurrent infections: when is IgG subclass deficiency clinically relevant? *Clin Immunol Immunopathol* 1993;68:46–50.

410. Olsson PG, Hofker MH, Walter MA, et al. Ig H chain variable and C region genes in common variable immunodeficiency. Characteristics of two new deletion haplotypes. *J Immunol* 1991;147:2540–2546.

411. Tiller TLJ, Buckley RH. Transient hypogammaglobulinemia of infancy: review of the literature, clinical and immunologic features of 11 new cases, and long-term follow-up. *J Pediatr* 1978;92:347.

412. Siegal RL, Issekutz T, Schwaber J, et al. Deficiency of helper T cells in transient hypogammaglobulinemia of infancy. *N Engl J Med* 1981;305:1307–1313.

413. Dalal I, Reid B, Nisbet-Brown E, et al. The outcome of patients with hypogammaglobulinemia in infancy and early childhood. *J Pediatr* 1998;133:144–146.

414. McGeady SJ. Transient hypogammaglobulinemia of infancy: need to reconsider name and definition. *J Pediatr* 1987;110:47–50.

415. Cano F, Mayo DR, Ballow M. Absent specific viral antibodies in patients with transient hypogammaglobulinemia of infancy. *J Allergy Clin Immunol* 1990;85:510–513.

416. Bartholomew RM, Esser AF. Mechanism of antibody-independent activation of the first component of complement (Cl) on retrovirus membranes. *Biochemistry* 1980;19:2847–2853.

417. Richards RL, Gewurz H, Siegel J, et al. Interactions of C-reactive protein and complement with liposomes. II. Influence of membrane composition. *J Immunol* 1979;122:1185–1189.

418. Storrs SB, Kolb WP, Olson MS. C1q binding and C1 activation by various isolated cellular membranes. *J Immunol* 1983;131:416–422.

419. Whaley K, Schwaeble W. Complement and complement deficiencies. *Semin Liver Dis* 1997;17:297–310.

420. Reid KB, Porter RR. The proteolytic activation systems of complement. *Annu Rev Biochem* 1981;50:433–464.

421. Burton DR, Boyd J, Brampton AD, et al. The Clq receptor site on immunoglobulin G. *Nature* 1980;288:338–344.

422. Hurst MM, Volanakis JE, Hester RB, et al. The structural basis for binding of complement by immunoglobulin M. *J Exp Med* 1974;140:1117–1121.

423. Dobo J, Gal P, Szilagyi K, et al. One active C1r subunit is sufficient for the activity of the complement C1 complex: stabilization of C1r in the zymogen form by point mutations. *J Immunol* 1999;162:1108–1112.

424. Jiang H, Burdick D, Glabe CG, et al. beta-Amyloid activates complement by binding to a specific region of the collagen-like domain of the C1q A chain. *J Immunol* 1994;152:5050–5059.

425. Clas F, Euteneuer B, Stemmer F, et al. Interaction of fluid phase C1/C1q and macrophage membrane-associated C1q with gram-negative bacteria. *Behring Inst Mitt* 1989;236–254.

426. Hannema AJ, Kluin-Nelemans JC, Hack CE, et al. SLE-like syndromes and functional deficiency of C1q in members of a large family. *Clin Exp Immunol* 1984;55:106–114.

427. Leyva-Cobian F, Moneo I, Mampaso R, et al. Familial C1q deficiency associated with renal and cutaneous disease. *Clin Exp Immunol* 1981;44:173–180.

428. Loos M, Heinz H. Component deficiencies. I. The first component: C1q, C1r, C1s. *Prog Allergy* 1986;39:212–231.

429. Endo Y, Kanno K, Takahashi M, et al. Molecular basis of human complement C1s deficiency. *J Immunol* 1999;162:2180–2183.

430. Inoue N, Saito T, Masuda R, et al. Selective complement C1s deficiency caused by homozygous four-base deletion in the C1s gene. *Hum Genet* 1998;103:415–418.

431. Botto M. C1q knock-out mice for the study of complement deficiency in autoimmune disease. *Exp Clin Immunogenet* 1998;15:231–234.

432. O'Neill GJ, Yang SY, Tegoli J, et al. Chido and Rodgers blood groups are distinct antigenic components of human complement C4. *Nature* 1978;273:668–670.

433. Hauptmann G, Tappeiner G, Schifferli JA. Inherited deficiency of the fourth component of human complement. *Immunodef Rev* 1988;1(1):3–22.

434. Fielder AHL, Walport MJ, Batchelor HR, et al. Family study of the major histocompatibility complex in patients with systemic lupus erythematosus: importance of null alleles of C4A and C4B in determining disease susceptibility. *BMJ* 1983;286:425–428.

435. Awdeh ZL, Raum DD, Glass D, et al. Complement human histocompatibility antigen haplotypes in C2 deficiency. *J Clin Invest* 1981;67:581–583.

436. Wang X, Circolo A, Lokki ML, et al. Molecular heterogeneity in deficiency of complement protein C2 type I. *Immunology* 1998;93:184–191.

437. Wetsel RA, Kulics J, Lokki ML, et al. Type II human complement C2 deficiency. Allele-specific amino acid substitutions (Ser189 → Phe; Gly444 → Arg) cause impaired C2 secretion. *J Biol Chem* 1996;271:5824–5831.

438. Zhu ZB, Atkinson TP, Volanakis JE. A novel type II complement C2 deficiency allele in an African-American family. *J Immunol* 1998;161:578–584.

439. Johnson CA, Densen P, Hurford RK Jr, et al. Type I human complement C2 deficiency. A 28-base pair deletion causes skipping of exon 6 during RNA splicing. *J Biol Chem* 1991;268:2268.

440. Perlmutter DH, Colten HR. Molecular basis of complement deficiencies. *Immunodef Rev* 1989;1:105–134.

441. Hudson-Peacock MJ, Joseph SA, Cox J, et al. Systemic lupus erythematosus complicating complement type 2 deficiency: successful treatment with fresh frozen plasma. *Br J Dermatol* 1997;136:388–392.

442. Hartmann D, Fremeaux-Bacchi V, Weiss L, et al. Combined heterozygous deficiency of the classical complement pathway proteins C2 and C4. *J Clin Immunol* 1997;17:176–184.

443. Turner MW. Mannose-binding lectin (MBL) in health and disease. *Immunobiology* 1998;199:327–339.

444. Fraser IP, Koziel H, Ezekowitz RA. The serum mannose-binding protein and the macrophage mannose receptor are pattern recognition molecules that link innate and adaptive immunity. *Semin Immunol* 1998;10:363–372.

445. Vorup-Jensen T, Petersen SV, Hansen AG, et al. Distinct pathways of mannan-binding lectin (MBL)- and C1-complex autoactivation revealed by reconstitution of MBL with recombinant MBL-associated serine protease-2. *J Immunol* 2000;165:2093–2100.

446. Matsushita M, Thiel S, Jensenius JC, et al. Proteolytic activities of two types of mannose-binding lectin-associated serine protease. *J Immunol* 2000;165:2637–2642.

447. Babovic-Vuksanovic D, Snow K, Ten RM. Mannose-binding lectin (MBL) deficiency. Variant alleles in a midwestern population of the United States. *Ann Allergy Asthma Immunol* 1999;82:134–138,141; quiz 142–143.

448. Aittoniemi J, Baer M, Soppi E, et al. Mannan binding lectin deficiency and concomitant immunodefects. *Arch Dis Child* 1998;78:245–248.

449. Yuen MF, Lau CS, Lau YL, et al. Mannose binding lectin gene mutations are associated with progression of liver disease in chronic hepatitis B infection. *Hepatology* 1999;29:1248–1251.

450. Ip WK, Chan SY, Lau CS, et al. Association of systemic lupus erythematosus with promoter polymorphisms of the mannose-binding lectin gene. *Arthritis Rheum* 1998;41:1663–1668.

451. Garred P, Madsen HO, Halberg P, et al. Mannose-binding lectin polymorphisms and susceptibility to infection in systemic lupus erythematosus. *Arthritis Rheum* 1999;42:2145–2152.

452. Garred P, Pressler T, Madsen HO, et al. Association of mannose-binding lectin gene heterogeneity with severity of lung disease and survival in cystic fibrosis. *J Clin Invest* 1999;104:431–437.

453. Mullighan CG, Marshall SE, Welsh KI. Mannose binding lectin polymorphisms are associated with early age of disease onset and autoimmunity in common variable immunodeficiency. *Scand J Immunol* 2000;51:111–122.

454. Hiemstra PS, Langeler E, Compier N, et al. Complete and partial deficiencies of complement factor D in a Dutch family. *J Clin Invest* 1989;84:1957–1961.

455. Kluin-Nelemans HC, van VelzenBlad H, van Helden HP, et al. Functional deficiency of complement factor D in a monzygous twin. *Clin Exp Immunol* 1984;58:724–730.

456. Weiss SJ, Ahmed AE, Bonagura VR. Complement factor D deficiency in an infant first seen with pneumococcal neonatal sepsis. *J Allergy Clin Immunol* 1998;102:1043–1044.

457. Sundsmo JS, Wood LM. Activated factor B (Bb) of the alternative pathway of complement activation cleaves and activates plasminogen. *J Immunol* 1981;127:877–880.

458. Peters MG, Ambrus JL Jr, Fauci AS, et al. The Bb fragment of complement factor B acts as a B cell growth factor. *J Exp Med* 1988;168:1225–1235.

459. Ambrus JL Jr, Peters MG, Fauci AS, et al. The Ba fragment of complement factor B inhibits human B lymphocyte proliferation. *J Immunol* 1990;144:1549–1553.

460. Tokunaga K, Omoto K, Yukiyama Y, et al. Further study on a BF silent allele. *Hum Genet* 1984;67:449–451.

461. Matsumoto M, Fukuda W, Circolo A, et al. Abrogation of the alternative complement pathway by targeted deletion of murine factor B. *Proc Natl Acad Sci U S A* 1997;94:8720–8725.

462. Pekna M, Hietala MA, Landin A, et al. Mice deficient for the complement factor B develop and reproduce normally. *Scand J Immunol* 1998;47:375–380.

463. Sjoholm AG, Kuijper EJ, Tijssen CC, et al. Dysfunctional properdin in a Dutch family with meningococcal disease. *N Engl J Med* 1988;319:33–37.

464. Holme ER, Veitch J, Johnston A, et al. Familial properdin deficiency associated with chronic discoid lupus erythematosus. *Clin Exp Immunol* 1989;76:76–81.

465. Gelfand EW, Rao CP, Minta JO, et al. Inherited deficiency of properdin and C2 in a patient with recurrent bacteremia. *Am J Med* 1987;82:671–675.

466. Hugli TE. Structure and function of C3a anaphylatoxin. *Curr Top Microbiol Immunol* 1990;153:181–208.

467. Winkelstein JA, Colten HR. Genetically determined disorders of the complement system. In: Scriver CR, Beaudet AL, Sly WS, et al., eds. *The metabolic basis of inherited diease,* 6th ed. St. Louis: McGraw-Hill, 1989:2711–2737.

468. Botto M, Fong KY, So AK, et al. Molecular basis of hereditary C3 deficiency. *J Clin Invest* 1990;86:1158–1163.

469. Botto M, Fong KY, So AK, et al. Homozygous hereditary C3 deficiency due to a partial gene deletion. *Proc Natl Acad Sci U S A* 1992;89:4957–4961.

470. Katz Y, Singer L, Wetsel RA, et al. Inherited complement C3 deficiency: a defect in C3 secretion. *Eur J Immunol* 1994;24:1517–1522.

471. Katz Y, Wetsel RA, Schlesinger M, et al. Compound heterozygous complement C3 deficiency. *Immunology* 1995;84:5–7.

472. Singer L, Van Hee ML, Lokki ML, et al. Inherited complement C3 deficiency: reduced C3 mRNA and protein levels in a Laotian kindred. *Clin Immunol Immunopathol* 1996;81:244–252.

473. Wetsel RA. Structure, function and cellular expression of complement anaphylatoxin receptors. *Curr Opin Immunol* 1995;7:48–53.

474. Sanal O, Loos M, Ersoy F, et al. Complement component deficiencies and infection: C5, C8 and C3 deficiencies in three families. *Eur J Pediatrics* 1992;151:676–679.

475. Asghar SS, Venneker GT, van Meegen M, et al. Hereditary deficiency of C5 in association with discoid lupus erythematosus. *J Am Acad Dermatol* 1991;24:376–378.

476. Lim D, Gewurz A, Lint TF, et al. Absence of the sixth component of complement in a patient with repeated episodes of meningocal meningitis. *J Pediatrics* 1976;89:42.

477. Boyer JT, Gall EP, Norman ME, et al. Hereditary deficiency of the seventh component of complement. *J Clin Invest* 1975;56:905.

478. Morgan BP, Vora JP, Bennett JA, et al. A case of hereditary combined deficiency of complement components C6 and C7 in man. *Clin Exp Immunol* 1989;83:43–47.

479. Rao AG, Howard OMZ, Ng SC, et al. Complementary DNA and derived amino acid sequence of the alpha subunit of human complement protein C8. Evidence for the existence of a separate alpha subunit messenger RNA. *Biochemistry* 1987;26:1556–1564.

480. Howard OMZ, Rao AG, Sodetz JM. Complementary DNA and derived amino acid sequence of the beta subunit of human complement protein C8: identification of a close structural and ancestral relationship to the alpha subunit and C9. *Biochemistry* 1987;26:3565–3570.

481. Tedesco F. Component deficiencies 8: the eighth component. *Prog Allergy* 1986;39:295–306.

482. Acosta JA, Benzaquen LR, Goldstein DJ, et al. The transient pore formed by homologous terminal complement complexes functions as a bidirectional route for the transport of autocrine and paracrine signals across human cell membranes. *Mol Med* 1996;2:755–765.

483. Stepp SE, Mathew PA, Bennett M, et al. Perforin: more than just an effector molecule. *Immunol Today* 2000;21:254–256.

484. Ross SD, Densen P. Complement deficiency states and infection: epidemiology, pathogenesis and consequences of neisserial and other infections in an immune deficiency. *Medicine* 1984;63:243–273.

485. Abramson N, Alper CA, Lachmann PJ, et al. Deficiency of C3 inactivator in man. *J Immunol* 1971;107:19–27.

486. Teisner B, Brandslund I, Folkerson J, et al. Factor I deficiency and C3 nephritic factor: immunochemical findings and association with *Neisseria meningitidis* infection in two patients. *Scand J Immunol* 1984;20:291.

487. Naked GM, Florido MP, Ferreira de Paula P, et al. Deficiency of human complement factor I associated with lowered factor H. *Clin Immunol* 2000;96:162–167.

488. Sadallah S, Gudat F, Laissue JA, et al. Glomerulonephritis in a patient with complement factor I deficiency. *Am J Kidney Dis* 1999;33:1153–1157.

489. Solal-Celigny P, Laviolette M, Hebert J, et al. C3b inactivator deficiency with immune complex manifestations. *Clin Exp Immunol* 1982;47:197.

490. Vyse TJ, Morley BJ, Bartok I, et al. The molecular basis of hereditary complement factor I deficiency. *J Clin Invest* 1996;97:925–933.

491. Morley BJ, Bartok I, Spath PJ, et al. Molecular basis of hereditary factor I deficiency. *Mol Immunol* 1998;35:344.

492. Schwaeble W, Zwirner J, Schulz TF, et al. Human complement factor H: expression of an additional truncated gene product of 43 kDa in human liver. *Eur J Immunol* 1987;17:1485–1489.

493. Zipfel PF, Jokiranta TS, Hellwage J, et al. The factor H protein family. *Immunopharmacology* 1999;42:53–60.

494. Rodriguez de Cordoba S, Diaz-Guillen MA, Heine-Suner D. An integrated map of the human regulator of complement activation (RCA) gene cluster on 1q32. *Mol Immunol* 1999;36:803–808.

495. Nielsen HE, Christensen KC, Koch C, et al. Hereditary, complete deficiency of complement factor H associated with recurrent meningococcal disease. *Scand J Immunol* 1989;30:711–718.

496. Levy M, Halbwachs-Mecarelli L, Gubler M-C, et al. H deficiency in two brothers with atypical dense intramembranous deposit disease. *Kidney Int* 1986;30:949–956.

497. Rougier N, Kazatchkine MD, Rougier JP, et al. Human complement factor H deficiency associated with hemolytic uremic syndrome. *J Am Soc Nephrol* 1998;9:2318–2326.

498. Warwicker P, Donne RL, Goodship JA, et al. Familial relapsing haemolytic uraemic syndrome and complement factor H deficiency. *Nephrol Dial Transplant* 1999;14:1229–1233.

499. Warwicker P, Goodship TH, Donne RL, et al. Genetic studies into inherited and sporadic hemolytic uremic syndrome. *Kidney Int* 1998;53:836–844.

500. Kristensen T, D'Eustachio P, Ogata RT, et al. The superfamily of C3b/C4b-binding proteins. *Fed Proc* 1987;46:2463–2469.

501. Sanchez-Corral P, Criado Garcia O, Rodriguez de Cordoba S. Isoforms of human C4b-binding protein. I. Molecular basis for the C4BP isoform pattern and its variations in human plasma. *J Immunol* 1995;155:4030–4036.

502. Suzuki K, Nishioka J. Binding site for vitamin K-dependent protein S on complement C4b-binding protein. *J Biol Chem* 1988;263:17034–17039.

503. Su HR. S-protein/vitronectin interaction with the C5b and the C8 of the complement membrane attack complex. *Int Arch Allergy Immunol* 1996;110:314–317.

504. Essex DW, Miller A, Swiatkowska M, et al. Protein disulfide isomerase catalyzes the formation of disulfide-linked complexes of vitronectin with thrombin-antithrombin. *Biochemistry* 1999;38:10398–10405.

505. Rabinowich H, Lin WC, Amoscato A, et al. Expression of vitronectin receptor on human NK cells and its role in protein phosphorylation, cytokine production, and cell proliferation. *J Immunol* 1995;154:1124–1135.

506. Jenne DE, Tschopp J. Clusterin: the intriguing guises of a widely expressed glycoprotein. *Trends Biochem Sci* 1992;17:154–159.

507. Davis AE 3rd. C1 inhibitor and hereditary angioneurotic edema. *Annu Rev Immunol* 1988;6:595–628.

508. Cicardi M, Bergamaschini L, Cugno M, et al. Pathogenetic and clinical aspects of C1 inhibitor deficiency. *Immunobiology* 1998;199:366–376.

509. Tosi M. Molecular genetics of C1 inhibitor. *Immunobiology* 1998;199:358–365.

510. Rosen FS, Alper CA, Pensky J, et al. Genetically determined heterogeneity of the C1 esterase inhibitor in patients with hereditary angioneurotic edema. *J Clin Invest* 1971;50:2143–2149.

511. Cugno M, Cicardi M, Bottasso B, et al. Activation of the coagulation cascade in C1-inhibitor deficiencies. *Blood* 1997;89:3213–3218.

512. Strang CJ, Cholin S, Spragg J, et al. Angioneurotic edema induced by a peptide derived from complement component C2. *J Exp Med* 1988;168:1685–1698.

513. Shoemaker LR, Schurman SJ, Donaldson VH, et al. Hereditary angioneurotic oedema: characterization of plasma kinin and vascular permeability-enhancing activities. *Clin Exp Immunol* 1994;95:22–28.

514. Kramer J, Rosen FS, Colten HR, et al. Transinhibition of C1 inhibitor synthesis in hereditary angioneurotic edema. *J Clin Invest* 1993;91:1258–1262.

515. Aulak KS, Cicardi M, Harrison RA. Identification of a new P1 residue mutation (444 Arg-Ser) in a dysfunctional C1 inhibitor protein contained in a type II hereditary angioedema plasma. *FEBS Lett* 1990;266:13–16.

516. Frangi D, Cicardi M, Sica A, et al. Nonsense mutations affect C1 inhibitor mRNA levels in patients with type I hereditary angioneurotic edema. *J Clin Invest* 1991;88:755–759.

517. Levy NJ, Ramesh N, Cicardi M, et al. Type II hereditary angioneurotic edema that may result from a single nucleotide change in the codon for alanine 436 in the C1 inhibitor gene. *Proc Natl Acad Sci U S A* 1990;87:265–268.

518. Parad RB, Kramer J, Strunk RC, et al. Dysfunctional C1 inhibitor Ta: deletion of Lys-251 results in acquisition of an N-glycosylation site. *Proc Natl Acad Sci U S A* 1990;87:6786–6790.

519. Skriver K, Wikoff WR, Patston PA, et al. Substrate properties of C1 inhibitor Ma (alanine 434-glutamic acid). General and structural evidence suggesting that the P12-region contains critical determinants of serine protease inhibitor/substrate status. *J Biol Chem* 1991;266:9216–9221.

520. Stoppa-Lyonnet D, Carter PE, Meo T, et al. Clusters of intragenic Alu repeats predispose the human C1 inhibitor locus to deleterious rearrangements. *Proc Natl Acad Sci U S A* 1990;87:1551–1555.

521. Davis AE, Whitehead AS, Harrison RA, et al. Human C1 inhibitor: Characteristics of cDNA clones and localization of the gene to chromosome 11. *Proc Natl Acad Sci U S A* 1986;83:3161–3165.

522. Agostoni A, Cicardi M, Cugno M, et al. Clinical problems in the C1-inhibitor deficient patient. *Behr Inst Mitt* 1993;93:306–312.

523. Waytes AT, Rosen FS, Frank MM. Treatment of hereditary angioedema with a vapor-heated C1 inhibitor concentrate. *N Engl J Med* 1996;334:1630–1634.

524. Kunschak M, Engl W, Maritsch F, et al. A randomized, controlled trial to study the efficacy and safety of C1 inhibitor concentrate in treating hereditary angioedema. *Transfusion* 1998;38:540–549.

525. Binkley KE, Davis A III. Clinical, biochemical, and genetic characterization of a novel estrogen-dependent inherited form of angioedema. *J Allergy Clin Immunol* 2000;106:546–550.

526. Bork K, Barnstedt SE, Koch P, et al. Hereditary angioedema with normal C1-inhibitor activity in women. *Lancet* 2000;356:213–217.

527. Cicardi M, Castelli R, Zingale LC, et al. Side effects of long-term prophylaxis with attenuated androgens in hereditary angioedema: comparison of treated and untreated patients. *J Allergy Clin Immunol* 1997;99:194–196.

528. Valsecchi R, Reseghetti A, Pansera B, et al. Autoimmune C1 inhibitor deficiency and angioedema. *Dermatology* 1997;195:169–172.

529. Heymann WR. Acquired angioedema. *J Am Acad Dermatol* 1997;36:611–615.

530. Chevailler A, Arlaud G, Ponard D, et al. C-1-inhibitor binding monoclonal immunoglobulins in three patients with acquired angioneurotic edema. *J Allergy Clin Immunol* 1996;97:998–1008.

531. Seya T, Hirano A, Matsumoto M, et al. Human membrane cofactor protein (MCP, CD46): multiple isoforms and functions. *Int J Biochem Cell Biol* 1999;31:1255–1260.

532. Lozahic S, Christiansen D, Manie S, et al. CD46 (membrane cofactor protein) associates with multiple beta1 integrins and tetraspans. *Eur J Immunol* 2000;30:900–907.

533. Okada N, Liszewski MK, Atkinson JP, et al. Membrane cofactor protein (CD46) is a keratinocyte receptor for the M protein of the group A streptococcus. *Proc Natl Acad Sci U S A* 1995;92:2489–2493.

534. Kallstrom H, Liszewski MK, Atkinson JP, et al. Membrane cofactor protein (MCP or CD46) is a cellular pilus receptor for pathogenic Neisseria. *Mol Microbiol* 1997;25:639–647.

535. Kawano M, Seya T, Koni I, et al. Elevated serum levels of soluble membrane cofactor protein (CD46, MCP) in patients with systemic lupus erythematosus (SLE). *Clin Exp Immunol* 1999;116:542–546.

536. Shoji T, Nakanishi I, Kunitou K, et al. Urine levels of CD46 (membrane cofactor protein) are increased in patients with glomerular diseases. *Clin Immunol* 2000;95:163–169.

537. Nicholson-Weller A, Wang CE. Structure and function of decay accelerating factor CD55. *J Lab Clin Med* 1994;123:485–491.

538. Nicholson-Weller A. Decay accelerating factor (CD55). *Curr Top Microbiol Immunol* 1992;178:7–30.

539. Telen MJ, Rao N, Udani M, et al. Molecular mapping of the Cromer blood group Cra and Tca epitopes of decay accelerating factor: toward the use of recombinant antigens in immunohematology. *Blood* 1994;84:3205–3211.

540. Spiller OB, Goodfellow IG, Evans DJ, et al. Echoviruses and coxsackie B viruses that use human decay-accelerating factor (DAF) as a receptor do not bind the rodent analogues of DAF. *J Infect Dis* 2000;181:340–343.

541. Zalman LS. Homologous restriction factor. *Curr Top Microbiol Immunol* 1992;178:87–99.

542. Zalman LS, Muller-Eberhard H. Homologous restriction factor: effect on complement C8 and C9 uptake and lysis. *Mol Immunol* 1994;31:301–305.

543. Boccuni P, Del Vecchio L, Di Noto R, et al. Glycosyl phosphatidylinositol

(GPI)-anchored molecules and the pathogenesis of paroxysmal nocturnal hemoglobinuria. *Crit Rev Oncol Hematol* 2000;33:25–43.

544. Chrobak L. Paroxysmal nocturnal hemoglobinuria (membrane defect, pathogenesis, aplastic anemia, diagnosis). *Acta Medica* 2000;43:3–8.

545. Nishimura J, Murakami Y, Kinoshita T. Paroxysmal nocturnal hemoglobinuria: an acquired genetic disease. *Am J Hematol* 1999;62:175–182.

546. Tomita M. Biochemical background of paroxysmal nocturnal hemoglobinuria. *Biochim Biophys Acta* 1999;1455:269–286.

547. Endo M, Beatty PG, Vreeke TM, et al. Syngeneic bone marrow transplantation without conditioning in a patient with paroxysmal nocturnal hemoglobinuria: in vivo evidence that the mutant stem cells have a survival advantage. *Blood* 1996;88:742–750.

548. Araten DJ, Nafa K, Pakdeesuwan K, et al. Clonal populations of hematopoietic cells with paroxysmal nocturnal hemoglobinuria genotype and phenotype are present in normal individuals. *Proc Natl Acad Sci U S A* 1999;96:5209–5214.

549. Harrington WJ Sr, Kolodny L, Horstman LL, et al. Danazol for paroxysmal nocturnal hemoglobinuria. *Am J Hematol* 1997;54:149–154.

550. Krych M, Molina H, Atkinson JP. CD35: complement receptor type 1. *J Biol Regul Homeost Agents* 1999;13:229–233.

551. Klickstein LB, Barbashov SF, Liu T, et al. Complement receptor type 1 (CR1, CD35) is a receptor for C1q. *Immunity* 1997;7:345–355.

552. Petty AC, Green CA, Poole J, et al. Analysis of Knops blood group antigens on CR1 (CD35) by the MAIEA test and by immunoblotting. *Transfus Med* 1997;7:55–62.

553. Carroll M. Role of complement receptors CD21/CD35 in B lymphocyte activation and survival. *Curr Top Microbiol Immunol* 1999;246:63–68.

554. Fearon DT, Collins LA. Increased expression of C3b receptors on polymorphonuclear leukocytes induced by chemotactic factors and by purification procedures. *J Immunol* 1983;130:370–375.

555. Kubota Y, Gaither TA, Cason J, et al. Characterization of the C3 receptor induced by herpes simplex virus type 1 infection of human epidermal, endothelial, and A431 cells. *J Immunol* 1987;138:1137–1142.

556. Wong WW, Farrell SA. Proposed structure of the F' allotype of human CR1. Loss of a C3b binding site may be associated with altered function. *J Immunol* 1991;146:656–662.

557. Dykman TR, Hatch JA, Atkinson JP. Polymorphism of the human C3b/C4b receptor. Identification of a third allele and analysis of receptor phenotypes in families and patients with systemic lupus erythematosus. *J Exp Med* 1984;159:691–703.

558. Ross GD, Medof ME. Membrane complement receptors specific for bound fragments of C3. *Adv Immunol* 1985;37:217–267.

559. Kozono Y, Abe R, Kozono H, et al. Cross-linking CD21/CD35 or CD19 increases both B7-1 and B7-2 expression on murine splenic B cells. *J Immunol* 1998;160:1565–1572.

560. Fearon DT, Carroll MC. Regulation of B lymphocyte responses to foreign and self-antigens by the CD19/CD21 complex. *Annu Rev Immunol* 2000;18:393–422.

561. Tedder TF, Zhou LJ, Engel P. The CD19/CD21 signal transduction complex of B lymphocytes. *Immunol Today* 1994;15:437–442.

562. Carroll MC. The role of complement in B cell activation and tolerance. *Adv Immunol* 2000;74:61–88.

563. Ehlers MR. CR3: a general purpose adhesion-recognition receptor essential for innate immunity. *Microbes Infect* 2000;2:289–294.

564. Cabanas C, Sanchez-Madrid F. CD11c (leukocyte integrin CR4 alpha subunit). *J Biol Regul Homeost Agents* 1999;13:134–136.

565. Stockinger H. Interaction of GPI-anchored cell surface proteins and complement receptor type 3. *Exp Clin Immunogenet* 1997;14:5–10.

566. Todd RF III, Petty HR. Beta 2 (CD11/CD18) integrins can serve as signaling partners for other leukocyte receptors. *J Lab Clin Med* 1997;129:492–498.

567. Medvedev AE, Flo T, Ingalls RR, et al. Involvement of CD14 and complement receptors CR3 and CR4 in nuclear factor-kappaB activation and TNF production induced by lipopolysaccharide and group B streptococcal cell walls. *J Immunol* 1998;160:4535–4542.

568. Anderson DC, Springer TA. Leukocyte adhesion deficiency: an inherited defect in the Mac-1, LFA-1, and p150,95 glycoproteins. *Annu Rev Med* 1987;38:175–194.

569. Ember JA, Hugli TE. Complement factors and their receptors. *Immunopharmacology* 1997;38:3–15.

570. Crass T, Bautsch W, Cain SA, et al. Receptor activation by human C5a des Arg74 but not intact C5a is dependent on an interaction between Glu199 of the receptor and Lys68 of the ligand. *Biochemistry* 1999;38:9712–9717.

571. Wilken HC, Gotze O, Werfel T, et al. C3a(desArg) does not bind to and signal through the human C3a receptor. *Immunol Lett* 1999;67:141–145.

572. Wetsel RA. Expression of the complement C5a anaphylatoxin receptor (C5aR) on non-myeloid cells. *Immunol Lett* 1995;44:183–187.

573. Zahedi R, Braun M, Wetsel RA, et al. The C5a receptor is expressed by human renal proximal tubular epithelial cells. *Clin Exp Immunol* 2000;121:226–233.

574. Zwirner J, Fayyazi A, Gotze O. Expression of the anaphylatoxin C5a receptor in non-myeloid cells. *Mol Immunol* 1999;36:877–884.

575. Davoust N, Jones J, Stahel PF, et al. Receptor for the C3a anaphylatoxin is expressed by neurons and glial cells. *Glia* 1999;26:201–211.

576. Gasque P, Singhrao SK, Neal JW, et al. Expression of the receptor for complement C5a (CD88) is up-regulated on reactive astrocytes, microglia, and endothelial cells in the inflamed human central nervous system. *Am J Pathol* 1997;150:31–41.

577. Ames RS, Tornetta MA, Foley JJ, et al. Evidence that the receptor for C4a is distinct from the C3a receptor. *Immunopharmacology* 1997;38:87–92.

578. Eggleton P, Reid KB, Tenner AJ. C1q—how many functions? How many receptors? *Trends Cell Biol* 1998;8:428–431.

579. Malhotra R. Collectin receptor (C1q receptor): structure and function. *Behring Inst Mitt* 1993;254–261.

580. Nepomuceno RR, Tenner AJ. C1qRP, the C1q receptor that enhances phagocytosis, is detected specifically in human cells of myeloid lineage, endothelial cells, and platelets. *J Immunol* 1998;160:1929–1935.

581. van den Berg RH, Faber-Krol M, van Es LA, et al. Regulation of the function of the first component of complement by human C1q receptor. *Eur J Immunol* 1995;25:2206–2210.

582. Joseph K, Ghebrehiwet B, Peerschke EI, et al. Identification of the zinc-dependent endothelial cell binding protein for high molecular weight kininogen and factor XII: identity with the receptor that binds to the globular "heads" of C1q (gC1q-R). *Proc Natl Acad Sci U S A* 1996;93:8552–8557.

583. Kabat EA, Wu TT, Perry HM, et al. *Sequences of proteins of immunological interest*, 5th ed. U.S. Department of Health and Human Services, Public Health Service, National Institutes of Health, NIH Publication No. 91-3242, 1991.

CHAPTER 23

Acquired Immunodeficiency Syndrome

David T. Scadden

The number of individuals infected with the human immunodeficiency virus type 1 (HIV-1) worldwide is currently estimated at 36 million with 11 people infected every minute, eight of those in sub-Saharan Africa. The impact of the acquired immunodeficiency syndrome (AIDS) caused by this virus is enormous from virtually every perspective, entering even the geopolitical discourse as a major destabilizing force in world affairs. The advent of potent new therapies over the last half-decade has dramatically changed the course of the illness for many of those fortunate enough to have access to such medications. What was once a certain, inexorable decline to death has been transformed to a chronic illness for many in North America, Western Europe, and Australia. However, cost, limited duration of activity, and toxicity have made even this revolutionary advance less than a total success. New drugs, immunologic manipulation, and the development of vaccines are critically needed to help those infected and protect those at risk. For those without access to intensive antiretroviral therapy, the hematologic and oncologic complications are myriad and frequent; for those responding to anti-HIV therapy, the spectrum of disease is narrower, less frequent, and yet, complex. The focus of this chapter is to provide a detailed review of the broad range of abnormalities seen, including information as to how the perspective on these issues has changed for those receiving highly active antiretroviral therapy (HAART).

GENERAL

The development of antiretroviral agents of multiple classes has led to a complex array of treatment options available to patients newly infected with HIV-1. Critical in assessing patients on presentation is assessing their anti-HIV serologic status, their plasma HIV RNA level, and their CD4+ lymphocyte count. These simple parameters can be used to roughly gauge the severity of immunosuppression and prognosis. Importantly, for individuals presenting with a viral syndrome and detectable HIV RNA levels, but who are seronegative for HIV, the possibility of an acute HIV infection syndrome should be considered. The significance of this finding is that these patients have the potential to gain immunologic control of their virus if antiretroviral treatment is rapidly begun. In the acute phase of infection, CD4+ T–helper cell function specific for HIV is robustly activated, but also in danger of consumption by uncontrolled viral replication. Should antiretroviral therapy abort virus destruction of this population, control of virus without anti-HIV medi-

cation has been documented in over half the patients (1). For patients in whom seroconversion has already occurred, a series of guidelines have been proposed for initiation of combination drug therapy. In general, therapy should always be multiagent to avoid emergence of viral drug resistance.

The introduction of antiretroviral therapy can be guided by the underlying level of immune suppression induced by the virus. In any individual with symptomatic HIV infection, including the list of AIDS-defining concurrent conditions (Table 23-1), antiretroviral therapy should initiated. For those who are asymptomatic with CD4+ T-cell counts of <200 cells/mm^3, initiation of treatment is also generally recommended because of the risk of complications due to advanced immunodeficiency. Most practitioners also advocate adding medications if the CD4+ cell count is between 200 and 350 cells/mm^3, although the balance between potential toxicities or future development of resistance and clinical benefit is more tenuous. This choice needs to be made in frank discussion with the patient about the complexities of an antiretroviral regimen and possible complications. When the CD4+ cell count exceeds 350 cells/mm^3, there is active controversy, and no clear guidelines have been established.

The agents that comprise the current armamentarium against HIV include three distinct classes of drugs. These are (a) the nucleoside analogs, (b) nonnucleoside reverse transcriptase inhibitors, and (c) protease inhibitors (Table 23-2). The nucleoside analogs function to interrupt reverse transcription of the virus genome through high affinity for the viral polymerase [reverse transcriptase (RT)] relative to cellular polymerases. These drugs have variable toxicity, including peripheral neuropathy and mitochondrial toxicity. Zidovudine (ZDV) or azidothymidine (AZT) is unique among them in its propensity to induce myelosuppression, an issue discussed later in Anemia. Nonnucleoside RT inhibitors are associated with a rapid development of viral resistance if used as monotherapy and have effects on the p450 system of drug metabolism, variably affecting this drug clearance system in an agent-specific manner. Inhibitors of the HIV protease necessary for virus assembly have been highly successful in suppressing viremia when used in combination. These agents also may affect p450-mediated drug metabolism and often have associated gastrointestinal (GI) symptoms. Recommendations for combining agents of different classes are outlined in Table 23-3.

Problematic for each of the agents is the cross-resistance of viruses to several compounds of the same drug class. To assess resistance, genotyping and/or phenotyping of a virus is an often-used means of evaluating patients with suboptimal

TABLE 23-1. Concurrent Clinical Categories

Category A	Category B	Category C
Asymptomatic HIV infection Persistent generalized lymphadenopathy Acute (primary) HIV infection with accompanying illness or history of acute HIV infection	Bacillary angiomatosis Candidiasis, oropharyngeal (thrush) Candidiasis, vulvovaginal; persistent, frequent, or poorly responsive to therapy Cervical dysplasia (moderate or severe)/cervical carcinoma *in situ* Constitutional symptoms, such as fever (38.5°C) or diarrhea lasting greater than 1 mo Hairy leukoplakia, oral Herpes zoster (shingles), involving at least two distinct episodes or more than one dermatome Idiopathic thrombocytopenic purpura Listeriosis Pelvic inflammatory disease, particularly if complicated by tuboovarian abscess Peripheral neuropathy	Candidiasis of bronchi, trachea, or lungs Candidiasis, esophageal Cervical cancer, invasive[a] Coccidioidomycosis, disseminated or extrapulmonary Cryptococcosis, extrapulmonary Cryptosporidiosis, chronic intestinal (greater than 1 month's duration) Cytomegalovirus disease (other than liver, spleen, or nodes) Cytomegalovirus retinitis (with loss of vision) Encephalopathy, HIV related Herpes simplex: chronic ulcer(s) (greater than 1 month's duration); or bronchitis, pneumonitis, or esophagitis Histoplasmosis, disseminated or extrapulmonary Isosporiasis, chronic intestinal (greater than 1 month's duration) Kaposi's sarcoma Lymphoma, Burkitt (or equivalent term) Lymphoma, immunoblastic (or equivalent term) Lymphoma, primary, of brain *Mycobacterium avium* complex or *M. kansasii*, disseminated or extrapulmonary *M. tuberculosis*, any site (pulmonary[a] or extrapulmonary) Mycobacterium, other species or unidentified species, disseminated or extrapulmonary *Pneumocystis carinii* pneumonia Pneumonia, recurrent[a] Progressive multifocal leukoencephalopathy Salmonella septicemia, recurrent Toxoplasmosis of brain Wasting syndrome due to HIV

HIV, human immunodeficiency virus.
[a]Added in the 1993 expansion of the AIDS surveillance case definition.

responses to therapy or those who have re-emergence of a virus after a period of retroviral control. The use of these assays in altering clinical outcomes is still to be demonstrated, and no commonly adopted guidelines for use have been established.

The ability of anti-HIV agents to impair virus replication should not be equated with reconstitution of immunologic competence. In patients who present with an opportunistic infection or who have CD4+ cell counts below 200 cells/mm³, prophylaxis against infections is generally initiated. The risk of opportunistic infection is reflected in the CD4+ cell count with

Pneumocystis carinii infection risk documented below 200 cells/mm³; the risk of atypical mycobacterium or cytomegalovirus (CMV) disease is generally only below 50 cells/mm³. Recommendations for prophylactic therapy of these and other disorders have been established (2). If and when patients have a sustained improvement in their CD4+ cell counts, it appears that prophylactic measures for at least *P. carinii* pneumonia (PCP) can be discontinued without undue risk (3,4).

Although the vast majority of patients receiving combination antiretroviral therapy will have a virologic and immunologic response, breakthrough of virus resistant to therapy is common. In patients who either present with severe immunodeficiency or who have progressive attrition of immune function with antiviral failure, a spectrum of opportunistic disease may emerge. The formal definition of AIDS is based on the presence of such opportunistic disease. The full classification system may be obtained via the following Internet site: www.cdc.gov/mmwr.

HEMATOLOGIC ASPECTS

General Features

A signature laboratory abnormality of HIV-1 infection is declining blood cell counts, a finding that first indicated the primary pathophysiologic process of this infection in the early 1980s. This is most prominent in the CD4+ T-lymphocyte population, but cytopenias of diverse cell types are seen. HIV induces broad, if not equally distributed, abnormalities in the innate and adaptive immune response and blood cells, generally. It has been reported that, during the course of unchecked HIV disease, anemia occurs in 60%, thrombocytopenia in 40%, and neutropenia in 50% of infected individuals (5–8). Cytopenia tends to develop coincident with progressive deterioration of the immune system

TABLE 23-2. Nomenclature of Antiretroviral Medications

	Abbreviated Chemical Name	Generic Name	Trade Name
Nucleoside reverse transcriptase inhibitors	ABC	Abacavir	Ziagen
	ddI	Didanosine	Videx
	3TC	Lamivudine	Epivir
	d4T	Stavudine	Zerit
	ddC	Zalcitabine	Hivid
	AZT or ZDV	Zidovudine	Retrovir
	AZT/3TC (ZDV/3TC)	Zidovudine/lamivudine	Combivir
Nonnucleoside reverse transcriptase inhibitors		Delavirdine	Rescriptor
		Efavirenz	Sustiva
		Nevirapine	Viracept
Protease inhibitors		Amprenavir	Agenerase
		Indinavir	Crixivan
		Nelfinavir	Viracept
		Ritonavir	Norvir
		Saquinavir (soft gel capsules)	Fortovase
		Saquinavir (hard capsules)	Invirase

TABLE 23-3. Advantages and Disadvantages of Possible Initial Antiretroviral Regimens

Regimen	Advantages	Disadvantages
Recommended regimens		
Protease inhibitor + NRTIs	Clinical data	Complexity and high pill burden
	Longest experience for viral suppression	Compromises future protease inhibitor regimens
		Long-term toxicity
NNRTI + 2NRTIs	Defers protease inhibitor	Limited long-term data
	Low pill burden	Compromises future NNRTI regimens
2 Protease inhibitors + 2 NRTIs	High potency	High pill burden with some regimens
	Convenient dosing	Long-term toxicities unknown
Regimens under evaluation		
3 NRTIs	Defers protease inhibitor and NNRTI	Lower potency than 2-NRTI and protease inhibitor regimen in patients with high balance viral loads
		Limited long-term data
		Compromises future NRTI regimens
Protease inhibitor + NNRTI + NRTI	High potency	Complexity
		Compromises future regimens
		Multiple-drug toxicity

NNRTI, nonnucleoside reverse transcriptase inhibitor; NRTI, nucleoside reverse transcriptase inhibitor.
Adapted from Carpenter CC, Cooper DA, Fischl MA, et al. Antiretroviral therapy in adults: updated recommendations of the IAS-USA Panel. *JAMA* 2000;283:381–390.

of these patients, occurring less frequently in earlier stages of HIV-related illness. Thrombocytopenia is the exception to this generalization, as it may be the presenting manifestation of HIV infection. Potential mechanisms for thrombocytopenia in this setting and its management are discussed in the next section.

The cytopenias seen in advanced HIV infection may be the result of multiple interacting factors (9). In addition to possible direct and indirect roles for the virus, complicating opportunistic infections, neoplasms, and myelotoxic antiretroviral, antimicrobial, and antitumor therapies are frequently important. The differential diagnosis of low blood counts in HIV-infected patients is broad. The diagnostic approach to a patient with low blood counts who is known to be HIV infected differs from that in uninfected persons, primarily in its emphasis on a careful evaluation for infectious causes and attention to the possible myelotoxic effect of intercurrent therapy.

Evaluation of the Patient with Cytopenia

Standard laboratory approaches to cytopenias should be undertaken, but blood cultures for fungi and mycobacteria, evaluation of CMV antigenemia, and active parvovirus infection should be added to these. When proceeding with bone marrow sampling, cultures for fungi and mycobacteria and stains for their presence histologically are essential. *Mycobacterium avium*-intracellulare, *Mycobacterium tuberculosis*, *Cryptococcus neoformans*, *Histoplasma capsulatum*, *P. carinii*, and *Ehrlichia* are associated with hematologic abnormalities and may be found on examination of the bone marrow (10–15). Parvovirus infection is associated with giant pronormoblasts on histologic study and may cause profound anemia, or rarely, pancytopenia in patients with AIDS. CMV does not induce specific morphologic changes of the bone marrow, but it does alter hematopoiesis and may be identified by circulating antigenemia. In addition, bone marrow involvement by non-Hodgkin's lymphoma (NHL) may be the presenting site for that diagnosis, as marrow infiltration is common in HIV-infected patients with this neoplasm. Kaposi's sarcoma, the other major neoplastic complication of HIV infection, has only rarely been reported in the bone marrow (16).

Guidelines for proceeding with bone marrow aspirate and biopsy in an HIV-infected patient with low blood counts have not been well defined but may include the following: (a) cytopenia out of proportion to the stage of HIV-related illness, (b) rapidly developing cytopenia (other than anemia due to blood loss),

(c) severe systemic symptoms such as fever with an otherwise-negative evaluation, and (d) use of aspirate and biopsy as a staging modality in patients with a known malignancy. Although the use of bone marrow evaluation appears to be only equally sensitive to routine blood culture for the diagnosis of mycobacterial or fungal disease, the rapidity with which a histologic diagnosis can be made is often advantageous in AIDS patients with progressive systemic symptoms (17).

Even in the absence of the identifiable pathogenetic processes above, morphologic abnormalities are present in the bone marrow in most patients (Table 23-4). However, there is no pathognomonic appearance to an HIV-positive bone marrow sample; the abnormalities are nonspecific (Fig. 23-1). Cellularity tends to be increased or normal, with only 1 in 20 marrow specimens appearing hypocellular (7,18–20). The myeloid/erythroid ratio ranges from 2:1 to 5:1 (7,21). Abnormalities in cell maturation are common, with megaloblastic changes, ringed sideroblasts, and other dysplastic features identified (22–25). All cell types may be affected and typically show high nuclear/cytoplasmic ratios and aberrant nuclear contours. Morphologic abnormalities tend to increase with advanced immunosuppression, as patients with isolated thrombocytopenia occurring relatively early in HIV-1 disease often have increased megakaryocytes but otherwise-unremarkable bone marrow histology. Increased plasma cells, lymphoid aggregates, increased eosinophils, and a focal or diffuse increase in reticulin are also frequently seen. There may be granuloma-like collections of cells and a general increase in marrow histiocytes. Large, foamy histiocytes (pseudo–Gaucher cells) have been associated with infiltration of the marrow with *M.*

TABLE 23-4. Bone Marrow Morphology

Normal or increased cellularity
Mild dysplasia
Lymphoid aggregates
Increased reticulin
Increased plasma cells and eosinophils

From Spivak JL, Bender BS, Quinn TC. Hematologic abnormalities in the acquired immune deficiency syndrome. *Am J Med* 1984;77:224–228; Castella A, Croxson TS, Mildvan D, et al. The bone marrow in AIDS. A histologic, hematologic, and microbiologic study. *Am J Clin Pathol* 1985;84:425–432; and Karcher DS, Frost AR. The bone marrow in human immunodeficiency virus (HIV)-related disease: morphology and clinical correlation. *Am J Clin Pathol* 1991;95:63–71.

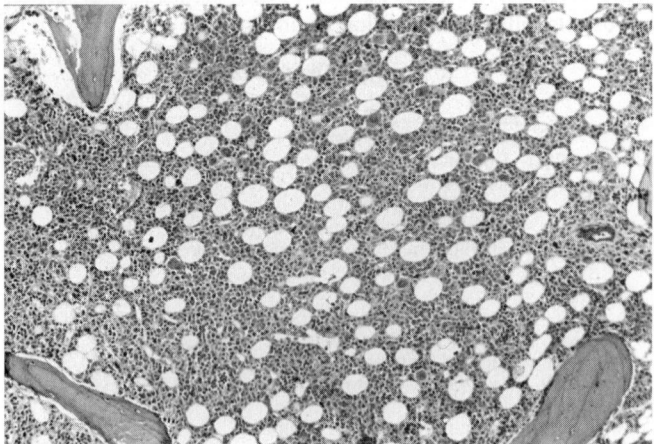

Figure 23-1. Bone marrow biopsy characteristic of patients with human immunodeficiency virus (HIV)–related pancytopenia. Despite low blood counts, the bone marrow often has normal to increased cellularity in the setting of advanced HIV disease. Cellular elements exhibit mild dysplastic morphology.

avium-intracellulare (10). The presence of lymphoid aggregates is common (reported in up to 50% of patients) and is nonspecific (7,18–21). The presence of paratrabecular lymphoid aggregates has been associated with lymphoma. Because the NHL that occurs in AIDS is often extranodal and involves the bone marrow in approximately 25% of patients, this finding should raise the suspicion of a lymphomatous process.

Hematopoietic Abnormalities in Human Immunodeficiency Virus Disease

The dysregulation of blood cell production in advanced HIV disease remains poorly understood, but specific hematopoietic cell types and events have now been evaluated in depth. Due to the broad diversity of cell types affected and the apparent inadequate compensatory response in cell production, the hematopoietic stem cell has often been regarded as a potential basis for altered blood cell production in AIDS. Contributing factors affecting stem cell function may be broadly viewed as due to either direct virus infection or indirect effects via perturbation of the cellular or cytokine milieu of the bone marrow microenvironment.

Stem cells have been reported to bear the surface receptor molecules necessary for HIV infection. They have been characterized to express CD4 and the chemokine receptors CXCR-4 and CCR-5 (26–30), yet, despite the presence of these structures, the stem cell is highly resistant to HIV infection (30–32). *In vitro, in vivo,* and animal models all point to the stem cell as a sanctuary cell not susceptible to direct infection. However, the lack of infection is not synonymous with lack of adverse effects of HIV due to direct interactions with the virus. The virus envelope glycoprotein, gp120, is capable of interacting with CXCR-4 and inducing intracellular signaling events as manifested by calcium flux, kinase activation, and functional changes such as chemotaxis of some cell types (33,34). Whether it may directly induce altered function of stem cells that express CXCR-4 is not clear, but there are data that suggest that apoptosis may be induced (35).

Evaluating more mature progenitor cells using colony-forming assays has yielded variable results, but most suggest a modest decrease in the colony-forming capacity of blood cell progenitors of multiple lineages (36–46). One study indicated a specific defect in the megakaryocytic colony-forming cells among patients with thrombocytopenia (47). Similar to data for the stem cell, however, evidence points away from direct infection of progenitors by HIV

as a major contributing factor (40,44–46,48). If HIV infection of progenitor cells occurs, it does so infrequently. In contrast, more differentiated cells of monocytic or megakaryocytic lineage appear to be readily infectible (47,49–51). Therefore, susceptibility to HIV infection is differentiation-stage dependent, with relative resistance seen with progressively more primitive cells.

Although direct HIV infection appears not to play a major role, *in vivo* evidence points to stem cell dysfunction as a result of the presence of HIV. Using immunodeficient mice engrafted with human hematopoietic tissue, reduced CD34+ cells and/or decreased colony-forming capacity has been shown to occur after HIV infection (52,53). The loss of cell number is more difficult to assess in humans, but clinical studies evaluating circulating pools of CD34+ cells after cytokine mobilization have supported the conclusions of the animal models. The concentration of CD34+ cells in the blood after granulocyte colony-stimulating factor (G-CSF) mobilization was reduced progressively in conjunction with lower CD4+ cell counts (54). With more advanced HIV disease, the mobilizable pool of stem cells appears to be diminished. Importantly, this study demonstrated that, despite lower concentrations of CD34+ cells, the stem cell numbers that could be harvested from patients with CD4 counts below 200 cells/mm^3 was within acceptable range for purposes of transplantation (54).

Participation of Hematopoiesis in Immune Decline and Regeneration

A causal relationship between lower CD4+ cells and CD34+ cell function has not been rigorously defined, but several lines of evidence provide supportive evidence. The first is the sequential analysis of stem cell and lymphocyte numbers in a mouse model engrafted with human cells. After HIV infection in that model, a decline in primitive cell numbers and function preceded the decline in thymocytes in a manner consistent with the kinetics expected if primitive cell dysfunction failed to replete thymocyte loss (53). The second is based on changes seen with antiretroviral therapy. Abnormal T-lymphocyte production from hematopoietic progenitors *ex vivo* has been correlated with the severity of immune suppression and reversed when patients were treated with antiretroviral therapy (55). T-lymphopoietic capacity was quantitatively affected by HIV. Similarly, other studies have noted that suppression of HIV replication is associated with an improvement in CD34+ cells, myeloid colony-forming capacity, and CD4+ T cells (56,57). Measuring T-cell kinetics directly has indicated that the observed increase in CD4+ cells is due less to improved T-cell survival than to increased rates of production (58). The increased production of lymphocytes appears to be biphasic, with the initial increase in CD4+ cells due to expansion of existing mature memory cells. However, *de novo* generation of T cells provides a later and sustained contribution of new T cells to the immune repertoire (59–61). Immunophenotypic markers for naïve cells and a method based on detecting the excised region of the T-cell receptor during T-cell ontogeny has permitted direct quantitation of T-lymphocyte production and indicated that hematopoiesis provides the driving force of immune reconstitution after antiretroviral treatment. The improvement in T-cell generation may reflect improved primitive cell number and function, but is also dependent on the health of the tissue microenvironments in which the differentiation of primitive cells occurs.

Thymic Function in Human Immunodeficiency Virus Disease

Disruption of thymic architecture has been well described with HIV infection with prominent infection and depletion of intrathymic progenitor cells (CD3–, CD4+, CD8–) (62), depletion of double positive (CD4+, CD8+) and, to a lesser extent, single positive CD4+ cells (63). In addition, thymic epithelial cells important in thymocyte differentiation and selection processes have been noted to be infected and disorganized (64,65). The issue of thymic integrity has taken on greater significance lately with the development of assays quantitating lymphocytes emigrating from the thymus, which have indicated that the thymus is active far longer in the human than previously thought (66,67). With the availability of HAART, the potential for restoring immunity by improved thymic function has been an area of great interest. Animal models have documented an improvement in T-cell generation from precursor populations, both endogenous and exogenous to the thymus, accompanying control of HIV viremia (60,68). In humans, radiographically detectable thymus is present in many HIV-infected patients (69), and it appears to increase in volume after initiation of active antiretroviral therapy (70). Indeed, thymic volume correlated with the basal level of CD4+ cells and the extent to which they rebounded after antiretroviral therapy. The ability of new T-cell generation to contribute to improved immunologic function is highly dependent on the successful control of viremia (71). Abnormalities of the tissues required for T lymphopoiesis appear to be reversible, although highly sensitive to HIV replication.

Bone Marrow Microenvironment in Human Immunodeficiency Virus Disease

The microenvironment of the bone marrow has several cellular constituents that are ready targets of HIV (lymphocytes and monocytes) and some that are less readily infectible (fibroblasts and endothelial cells) (72–74). Infection of these accessory cells of the bone marrow stroma may result in an altered milieu in which hematopoietic cells mature (74). Testing such a hypothesis has been done in two ways: long-term bone marrow culture techniques and measurement of cytokines released by individual accessory cell types. There are data suggesting that infection of bone marrow stroma alters the *in vitro* support of long-term bone marrow culture (75,76). Evidence for an altered production of cytokines in the presence of HIV or HIV products is more controversial. Ambiguity remains as to whether HIV directly induces cytokine alterations or whether they may be induced secondarily as the result of coincident effects on other aspects of immune function or intercurrent infections (77–81). However, patients with HIV disease have been demonstrated to have abnormally elevated levels of certain cytokines, such as tumor necrosis factor-α (TNF-α), interleukin-6 (IL-6), transforming growth factor-β (TGF-β), and interferon-α (82–85). Among these, TNF-α, TGF-β, and interferon-α are all known to have suppressive effects on hematopoiesis. It has also been observed that serum erythropoietin levels are abnormally depressed in patients with AIDS (86,87). The relative depression of erythropoietin to the extent of anemia mimics that of the anemia of chronic disease, although a direct effect of HIV on erythropoietin production has been reported (88). Exogenous erythropoietin administration may effectively overcome suppressed red cell production (see Anemia).

More difficult to evaluate is the role of immune phenomena on the bone marrow or mature blood cells in AIDS. It has been reported that the immunoglobulin fraction of the sera of AIDS patients or of an 84-kd glycoprotein derived from mononuclear cells of patients with AIDS are capable of inhibiting *in vitro* colony formation (36,37). Also, T-cell depletion has been reported to enhance colony growth of AIDS patients' bone marrow (39). Others have found that the changes in subsets of T cells are more closely linked to effects on colony formation and have proposed a causative role (46). The complex interactions of T

cells with other bone marrow elements are difficult to dissect experimentally, and our present understanding of the interplay between HIV, T cells, and hematopoiesis remains quite limited. What is clear, however, is that enhanced immune function with antiretroviral therapy results in improved bone marrow function (57,70,89,90).

Thrombocytopenia

Thrombocytopenia may occur as either an isolated hematologic abnormality at any stage of HIV disease or with other cytopenias in patients with advanced immunodeficiency. In one study evaluating the epidemiology of thrombocytopenia in HIV-seropositive patients, the incidence of a platelet count below 150,000/μL was 11%, below 100,000/μL was 4.2%, and below 50,000/μL was 1.5% (25). All risk groups for HIV disease may develop thrombocytopenia, but the incidence may be slightly higher among whites and lower in patients whose risk factor for HIV infection was heterosexual contact (25).

Because thrombocytopenia may be the clinical finding that first brings an HIV-infected person to medical attention, HIV infection should be considered in patients presenting with low platelet counts. Participation in high-risk behaviors should be specifically addressed when obtaining a history from a patient with unexplained thrombocytopenia. Those patients with isolated thrombocytopenia who are found to be HIV-seropositive and have no other HIV-related diseases apparently have the same risk over time for the development of AIDS as asymptomatic HIV-seropositive persons (91). The presence of thrombocytopenia does not define advanced HIV disease by Centers for Disease Control and Prevention criteria.

Thrombocytopenia in HIV infection may have multiple causes, including immune-mediated destruction, impaired hematopoiesis, or, rarely, syndromes resembling hemolytic uremic syndrome or thrombotic thrombocytopenia purpura (91). Isolated thrombocytopenia is generally associated with a clinical picture resembling that of classic autoimmune thrombocytopenic purpura (AITP). Affected patients have a normal to increased number of megakaryocytes in the bone marrow and elevated levels of platelet-bound immunoglobulin. The platelet-bound protein has been identified in homosexual men as immune complexes (92). The platelet-adherent immune complexes have been shown to include anti-HIV antibodies and antibodies directed against them (antiidiotype antibodies) (93,94). Cross-reactivity between anti-HIV antibodies and platelet antigen has been reported (94,95). Definitive evidence associating antibody with HIV-associated thrombocytopenia has arisen in studies in which antibody to platelet antigen GPIIIa has been found and correlated with platelet destruction (96–98). However, platelet clearance was shown to be mitigated by antiidiotype antibody directed against the anti-GPIIIa antibody. Therefore, the degree of thrombocytopenia appears to be based on the balance between antibody and antiidiotypic antibody (98). An additional contributing factor modulating the extent of thrombocytopenia may be altered reticuloendothelial cell function documented in HIV infection (99–101). Some patients with cell-associated antibodies may maintain higher cell counts because of impairment of the Fc receptor–mediated clearance of these cells.

Thrombocytopenic HIV-positive patients have been shown to have abnormalities in platelet production as well as decreased platelet survival times. *In vivo* measurements of platelet survival have indicated that the lifespan of autologous-labeled platelets is approximately one-third of that of controls (97). However, marrow platelet production also appears to be impaired (97,102). Megakaryocyte mass in the marrow is actually increased, but the ability of cells to generate platelets and

TABLE 23-5. Therapy for Idiopathic Thrombocytopenic Purpura–Like Syndrome

AZT associated with 50,000 or twofold increase in platelets by 8 weeks (112,113)
Response to AZT is dose related (353); at least 600 mg/d recommended to start
ddI associated with a small increase in platelets (354); overall other antivirals not as effective as AZT
Anti-RhD for Rh+ patients (124) or IVIG (355) for Rh– patients with severe thrombocytopenia
Corticosteroids (short term) (356)
Danazol (357)
Dapsone (130)
Interferon-α (358)
Splenectomy (359)
Splenic irradiation (360)

AZT, azidothymidine; ddI, didanosine.

the ability of CD34+ cells to generate megakaryocytes appears to be reduced (51,97,103). Megakaryocytes appear to be susceptible to HIV-1 infection, possibly resulting in diminished platelet formation (47). This phenomenon may be particularly associated with specific quasispecies of HIV-1 particularly effective at suppressing platelet production (104).

The complications from thrombocytopenia in HIV-infected patients are similar to those in uninfected persons with AITP. Fortunately, severe thrombocytopenia is uncommon in these patients, and major bleeding complications are rare. More significant problems may occur with HIV-infected hemophiliacs who develop complicating thrombocytopenia. The mechanism for thrombocytopenia in these patients appears to be similar to that seen in other subgroups of HIV-positive patients (105). Complications from thrombocytopenia may be severe in this population; therefore, maintenance of a more conservative threshold for initiation of therapy is recommended, although no specific thresholds have been established (106).

Therapeutically, an important distinction in approaching HIV-thrombocytopenic patients as opposed to seronegative patients with AITP is the improvement in platelet numbers documented with ZDV or AZT therapy (Table 23-5) (107–112). Approximately half of HIV-positive patients have been reported to increase their platelet counts (a threefold mean increase) within 12 weeks of initiating AZT therapy (112,113). For HIV-positive patients who do not respond to AZT and who have symptomatic thrombocytopenia, the range of therapeutic modalities used in AITP, such as corticosteroids (114–116), splenectomy (117–120), γ-globulin (121–123), anti-RhD (124,125), danazol (126), vincristine (127), interferon-α (128,129), and dapsone (130), has been reported to increase platelet numbers in some patients. The general approach we use when treating patients with HIV-associated thrombocytopenia is to treat those in immediate need with either anti-RhD or gammaglobulin. Patients not on ZDV or AZT should have this medication incorporated into their antiretroviral regime. Pulse corticosteroids may be added; however, one caveat when treating this already immunocompromised population is the theoretical risk of long-term use of immunosuppressive corticosteroids. Other than possible exacerbation of Kaposi's sarcoma (131), adverse effects have not been seen with short-term use of corticosteroids, but long-term consequences have not been defined. Further, when the use of an immunosuppressive agent or splenectomy is contemplated, excluding an infectious cause for the thrombocytopenia, such as mycobacteria, takes on even greater importance. Appropriate treatment of the infection may correct the thrombocytopenia, and immunosuppressive therapy and

splenectomy are clearly undesirable in the setting of disseminated mycobacterial disease. In the absence of a durable response to ZDV and pulse steroids, dapsone or danazol may be useful before considering splenectomy. The use of growth factors in HIV-associated thrombocytopenia has not yet been systematically evaluated.

A number of cases of thrombotic thrombocytopenic purpura (TTP) and hemolytic uremic syndrome (HUS) have been reported in patients with AIDS (132–137). No definitive epidemiologic studies have been done; however, clinical experience suggests that there is an increased frequency of this disorder in HIV-infected individuals and that it generally occurs in patients with advanced immunosuppression. The recent association of antibodies to von Willebrand's factor protease with TTP (138) appears to hold in patients with TTP in the setting of HIV disease and may be partly attributable to the abnormal antibody production accompanying HIV infection (see Gammopathy and Coagulopathy). TTP/HUS has also been seen with enterohemorrhagic *Escherichia coli* infection (*E. coli* O15:H7), and assessment of the stool for this organism should be performed. The use of plasma exchange for TTP/HUS has been effective in patients with HIV disease, and the guidelines for therapy of patients outside the context of HIV disease should be applied to the HIV-infected population. Steroid use is controversial in this disorder, and particular caution should be used in the HIV-infected individual in whom the immunosuppression accompanying steroid use may have more substantial ramifications.

Anemia

Anemia is the most common hematologic abnormality seen in HIV-infected patients. It occurs coincidentally with the development of advanced stages of immunosuppression. Typically, the anemia is normochromic and normocytic, with a depressed reticulocyte index and iron studies that are either normal or consistent with that of chronic disease. Antiglobulin tests have been reported to be positive in up to 85% of AIDS patients and 44% of asymptomatic homosexual men (139,140). The antibodies are occasionally of anti-i or other specificity, but nonspecific binding of antiphospholipid antibodies or immune complexes to erythrocytes is more common. As with platelets, the presence of red blood cell (RBC)–associated antibody does not correlate well with anemia, and hemolysis is rare (141).

The predominant mechanism resulting in anemia in HIV disease is inadequate erythropoiesis. A range of potential factors contribute to this problem and should be considered in the differential diagnosis. In addition to the complex changes in the bone marrow discussed earlier, toxic, infectious, endocrine, or nutritional abnormalities may play contributing roles.

Many patients with HIV disease experience GI disorders that may affect the hematopoietic system. Chronic blood loss from Kaposi's sarcoma, lymphoma, or infections of the gut may result in depletion of iron stores. A range of infectious intestinal insults or HIV itself may alter nutrient absorption and result in other deficiencies, particularly in the context of poor food intake that often occurs in persons with AIDS. Measurements of iron, folate, and B_{12} are important to exclude these treatable causes of anemia.

A caveat to the interpretation of an abnormal serum B_{12} level in patients with AIDS has been raised (142,143). Rather than a physiologic deficiency of B_{12}, transcobalamin transport has been shown to be affected, and supplemental B_{12} has had disappointing effects on anemia. Nevertheless, malabsorption of B_{12} is also prominent among patients with diarrhea and AIDS, mandating that appropriate diagnostic measures be undertaken to exclude a physiologically significant B_{12} deficiency.

Serum erythropoietin levels have been reported to be disproportionately low for the degree of anemia in AIDS patients compared with a control group (86). These alterations have been noted despite the absence of evidence for renal dysfunction, and the cause is not clear. One *in vitro* model system for this phenomenon suggested that it may be due to a direct action of HIV on the posttranslational events important in erythropoietin production (144). In addition, parvovirus infection has been documented as a cause of RBC aplasia in patients with AIDS and may be diagnosed by bone marrow examination or appropriate serologic tests. γ-Globulin has been reported to reverse this unusual cause of severe anemia (145).

Drug-induced anemia is particularly common in HIV-infected patients. AZT (ZDV), which remains among the antiretroviral drugs most commonly used, frequently causes anemia (108,146). The degree to which AZT affects the bone marrow is clearly dose related and varies widely, with the most severely immunocompromised tolerating the drug least well. At currently recommended doses, AZT is associated with the development of anemia (hemoglobin levels below 8 g/dL) in 29% of AIDS patients (compared with 34% to 39% using the previously recommended AZT dose of 1200 to 1500 mg/day). The anemia associated with AZT is usually macrocytic, although some patients have normal mean corpuscular volumes. The normocytic anemia of AZT is often more severe and refractory to erythropoietin therapy. Rarely, AZT may induce a profound depression of erythropoiesis resembling pure red cell aplasia (147). Whereas anemia associated with AZT generally responds to the withdrawal of AZT, this latter group may have a persistent defect in RBC production.

The changes AZT induces in blood cell formation are probably due to its effects on DNA synthesis. AZT is a thymidine analog that functions both to competitively inhibit thymidine kinase and to induce DNA-chain termination when incorporated into nascent DNA. The kinetics of its incorporation into DNA by the viral RT are one or two orders of magnitude above its incorporation by cellular DNA polymerases (148). However, inhibition of cellular proliferation occurs, and it occurs preferentially in erythroid cells compared with granulocytic cells (149,150). Anemia or other cytopenias do not appear to be toxicities common to all nucleoside analogs, as dideoxycytidine and didanosine (ddI) do not induce bone marrow depression. Stavudine (2',3'-didehydro-3'-deoxythymidine) has been noted to increase mean corpuscular volume, but it is not associated with anemia (151).

Recombinant erythropoietin has been shown to decrease the transfusion requirement and increase hemoglobin and hematocrit in anemic AIDS patients, even if their anemia was precipitated by AZT (152,153). Thus, erythropoietin may be an alternative to AZT dose reduction in some patients and an important adjunctive measure in the case of HIV-infected patients requiring frequent RBC transfusion. The benefits of exogenous erythropoietin are apparently limited to those in whom the pretreatment serum erythropoietin level is below 500 mU/mL (153).

Neutropenia

Neutropenia in association with decreases in other cell counts is seen with progressive deterioration of the immune system in HIV-infected patients. As with other cytopenias, neutropenia may be caused by a combination of decreased production and increased clearance of these cells. Antibody bound to granulocyte cell surfaces has been detected in approximately one-third of HIV-infected persons (140,154). The presence of neutrophil-associated antibodies in these studies again did not directly correlate with the presence of decreased neutrophil cell counts. The abnormalities in bone marrow function described in Hematopoietic Abnormalities in Human Immunodeficiency Virus Disease are likely to be major contributors to the neutropenia observed in HIV disease.

It is perhaps these underlying abnormalities in hematopoiesis that account for the particular sensitivity to the myelotoxic effects of drug therapies observed in patients with AIDS. Neutropenia accompanies the use of many common therapies in AIDS and often limits their use. Although ddI and ddC are not implicated in myelosuppression, AZT is commonly dose limited by neutropenia or anemia (108,146). In addition, therapy with trimethoprim-sulfamethoxazole for PCP, pyrimethamine-sulfadiazine for central nervous system (CNS) toxoplasmosis, ganciclovir (dihydroxyproproxymethylguanine) for CMV retinitis, and acyclovir for disseminated herpes simplex or herpes zoster may be complicated by dose-limiting neutropenia. Ganciclovir is particularly toxic for neutrophils, and isolated severe neutropenia is common when using this medication. Antitumor therapy is also often frustrated by neutropenia. Myelosuppression is therefore a fundamental problem in the treatment of both the underlying HIV infection and its complicating infectious or neoplastic diseases. This problem is mitigated by the availability of less-myelotoxic antiretroviral therapies and the use of hematopoietic growth factors.

In addition to low cell numbers, abnormalities in neutrophil function have been documented (155). Phagocytic and intracellular killing of microbes may be impaired in HIV disease. The extent to which these abnormalities contribute to the susceptibility of the patients to infection is not clear. A subset of AIDS patients seems particularly susceptible to recurrent infections with encapsulated bacteria, but no correlation with neutrophil dysfunction has been documented.

Hematopoietic Growth Factors

Because of the sensitivity of the bone marrow in HIV-infected persons to the toxic effects of therapy or coincident illness, hematopoietic growth factors have been used in the care of these patients. Erythropoietin (152,156), GM-CSF (157,158), G-CSF (156), and IL-3 (159) have been tested in patients with AIDS. Erythropoietin has been evaluated in four randomized, placebo-controlled trials and one expanded-access trial of patients experiencing anemia while receiving AZT (152,153). Analysis of the experience in the randomized trials indicated that benefit was significant only if the pretreatment serum erythropoietin level was below 500 mU/mL. (The previously stated depression of serum erythropoietin levels in AIDS patients who were anemic before AZT therapy does not hold when AZT therapy is introduced; in that setting, serum erythropoietin levels rise markedly.) Before considering erythropoietin therapy, a serum erythropoietin level should be obtained, as little benefit can be expected if the level is above 500 mU/mL. Approximately two-thirds of anemic AIDS patients receiving AZT fall into the group with erythropoietin levels below 500 mU/mL. In the subset of patients with hematocrits below 30% and erythropoietin levels below 500 mU/mL, recombinant human erythropoietin at a dose of 4000 U/day, 6 days a week, has been shown to improve the hematocrit and reduce transfusion requirements. Analysis of erythropoietin use in an inner-city population with HIV disease indicated an independent beneficial effect of erythropoietin on more than just anemia or symptoms. A benefit on survival was also noted, although other factors not measured cannot be excluded (160). In addition, patient perception of well-being and energy have also been noted to improve on erythropoietin therapy (161).

GM-CSF and G-CSF have been evaluated in neutropenic AIDS patients and are capable of improving neutrophil counts at relatively low doses. This ability to mitigate myelosuppression is apparent even in the presence of myelotoxic agents such as AZT, interferon-α, or ganciclovir (158,162–167). The hematologic effects have been sustained, despite chronic use of the growth factors, without evidence for tachyphylaxis or antibody formation (159). One note of concern was the development of thrombocytopenia in five of 17 patients treated with GM-CSF while receiving AZT (162). Although effects on hematologic parameters have been well documented, other clinical outcomes have been less well studied. Randomized trials have been completed in AIDS patients with CMV retinitis who were receiving ganciclovir (165) and in AIDS patients with lymphoma who were receiving cyclophosphamide, hydroxydaunorubicin, Oncovin, prednisone (CHOP) (166). The subjects were randomly assigned to receive GM-CSF or to a control group. The data in the CMV trial indicated reduced days with absolute neutrophil count below 750 cells/μL, but did not demonstrate a statistically significant benefit in either drug delivery or preservation of vision with GM-CSF. In the lymphoma trial, GM-CSF did result in improvements in days of fever and neutropenia, in days of hospitalization, and in drug delivery. A phase III study assessing the overall impact on GM-CSF in patients with HIV disease (but without neutropenia) has indicated that this cytokine may have additional effects on host defense besides raising the neutrophil count. CD4 cell counts and overall infection rates were modestly, but statistically significantly, improved in patients who received GM-CSF rather than placebo (168). Similarly, G-CSF has been assessed compared with control, and bacterial infections and days of hospitalization, among other parameters, were significantly reduced (169). Another study found that G-CSF increased CD4+, CD8+, and NK cells (170). However, for each of these parameters, the changes noted have been relatively minor when compared with the cost, and these agents at this time remain supportive care adjuncts for patients with profound neutropenia.

The side-effect profile of recombinant growth factors in HIV-infected individuals is similar to that of other patient groups. Several issues about growth factor use in HIV disease distinguish it from other clinical situations, however. Specifically, the growth factors may interact with the virus or with the other drugs that are frequently in concurrent use. In vitro data conflict but suggest that certain growth factors—most notably GM-CSF, IL-3, and M-CSF—are capable of enhancing HIV replication (171–175). The clinical data regarding this issue also conflict, with some studies suggesting that GM-CSF increases virologic parameters and others reporting no such changes (164–166). In the absence of more definitive data, caution suggests that GM-CSF should be used in conjunction with antiretroviral therapy. Within that context, GM-CSF has not affected HIV viral load any differently than placebo (168). Neither G-CSF nor erythropoietin were thought to have any effect on HIV-1 replication; however, the use of G-CSF to mobilize progenitor cells has been associated with increases in circulating HIV RNA levels. These increases were transient and occurred in patients not receiving antiretroviral therapy (176).

GAMMOPATHY AND COAGULOPATHY

The spectrum of immunohematologic abnormalities induced by HIV-1 is extremely broad and includes a variety of abnormalities in B-cell function, such as antibody production and proliferation. Elevation of immunoglobulin levels is a virtually uniform laboratory abnormality seen in HIV-1–seropositive people regardless of the stage of HIV disease. Generally, the immunoglobulins are polyclonal, but the incidence of oligoclonal or monoclonal increases has been reported to be as high as 9%

(177–183), and some of the clones appear to be specifically reactive to HIV-1 (184). These elevations are generally not accompanied by a decrease in other immunoglobulins and only rarely result in hyperviscosity (185). The abnormalities associated with the dysregulated immunoglobulins are the increased cell-associated immunoglobulin noted earlier and the formation of antibodies affecting coagulation.

Antiphospholipid antibodies have been reported in 20% to 70% of HIV-seropositive individuals (186–189). They generally are associated with laboratory findings of a lupus anticoagulant—namely, a prolonged activated partial thromboplastin time not corrected by normal plasma, often an increased prothrombin time, and an abnormal Russell viper venom time. The antibodies mediating these abnormalities are often IgM (186) and are common in symptomatic and asymptomatic patients alike, with a reported incidence in asymptomatic patients as high as 43% (190,191).

A subset of patients with antiphospholipid antibodies has anticardiolipid antibodies, which may or may not be associated with lupus anticoagulant characteristics. These appear to be unrelated in frequency to the clinical status of the patient and do not correlate with the risk of progression to AIDS or with thrombocytopenia (189,190). Indeed, some studies have documented a high incidence of anticardiolipin antibodies in patients at risk of, but negative for, HIV (190). There does not appear to be an associated increase in the false-positive rate of the Venereal Disease Research Laboratory test (186). Slight elevations (1:20 and, rarely, 1:160) of antinuclear antibodies have been reported in 13% of symptomatic HIV-positive patients. The correlation of these with anticardiolipin antibodies has not been defined in HIV disease.

Strong clinical associations with these laboratory abnormalities are not apparent. Thrombosis and embolism have been reported (187), but there does not appear to be an unusual predisposition to these events. Similarly, abnormal bleeding is uncommon, although one case in a patient with a decreased factor VII level has been reported (192), and qualitative platelet function abnormalities were documented (186). The most problem-filled scenario is that of patients with inherited coagulation disorders in whom the antibodies may distort the laboratory parameters used to measure replacement therapy.

The mechanisms underlying the abnormal development of antibodies in HIV disease remains obscure. Associations with opportunistic infections have been noted, but the incidence of the antibodies in asymptomatic individuals suggests otherwise (193). Rather, there appears to be a poorly understood dysregulation of the interactions between T cells and B cells that normally govern the modulation of B-cell proliferation and the antibodies their progeny produce. Introduction of antiretroviral therapy may mitigate the B-cell dysregulation, reduce gamma globulin production, and be expected to reduce pathogenic antibody levels.

In addition to abnormal antibody production, B-lymphoid proliferation commonly accompanies HIV disease and can result in lymph node enlargement and possibly contribute to lymphoid transformation.

LYMPHADENOPATHY

Depletion of the CD4–T lymphocyte, the primary target of HIV, is accompanied by altered function of other elements of the immune system. B-cell growth and immunoglobulin production are markedly abnormal, which may result in the hypergammaglobulinemia and lymphadenopathy that are common features of HIV infection.

Lymphadenopathy occurs in most patients infected with HIV at some time during the course of their illness. The possible causes of this abnormality are multiple, including HIV infection and a host of secondary infections such as Epstein-Barr virus (EBV), CMV, *M. avium*-intracellulare, *M. tuberculosis, C. neoformans, H. capsulatum,* and syphilis. In addition, lymphoma and Kaposi's sarcoma occur dramatically more frequently in HIV-infected persons and may result in marked lymph node enlargement.

The mechanism by which HIV affects B-cell function has not been well defined, but dysregulation of activation is apparent (194,195). Early in HIV infection, IgG and IgA antibody production is nonspecifically elevated (IgM synthesis may be decreased) and antigen-specific B-cell clonal proliferation occurs (196). Lymphadenopathy is clinically apparent during this phase of HIV infection and may persist for months to years. The presence of lymphadenopathy in two or more noninguinal lymph node sites of at least 3 months' duration without other secondary causes of adenopathy has been defined by the Centers for Disease Control and Prevention as persistent generalized lymphadenopathy. This phase of HIV infection has not been associated with a high incidence of opportunistic infection and is apparently not a harbinger of the imminent onset of an AIDS-defining illness (197–199).

Differentiating between HIV-related and secondary causes of lymph node enlargement is complex and may require lymph node biopsy. Reports have indicated that otherwise clinically indistinguishable patients undergoing lymph node biopsy may reveal a secondary cause of lymphadenopathy in approximately 15% of patients (200). The incidence of secondary conditions that result in a different treatment plan based on this diagnostic procedure is considerably lower. The site of lymph node enlargement is of little help in selecting patients for biopsy, as virtually any site (including the spleen) may be abnormal without a specific secondary cause. Cervical, axillary, and inguinal lymph nodes enlarge at some time in almost all persistent generalized lymphadenopathy and most HIV-infected patients. Guidelines for deciding which patients should undergo lymph node biopsy, modified from those proposed by Abrams (201), are the following:

- Disproportionate localized lymph node enlargement
- Rapidly evolving lymphadenopathy
- Marked constitutional symptoms with negative cultures including bone marrow
- Bulky mediastinal or abdominal adenopathy or a splenic mass

Patients with persistent generalized lymphadenopathy have nonspecific histologic features on lymph node biopsy. These hyperplastic nodes have several atypical features (202–206). Prominent follicular hyperplasia with disruption of the follicular structure or dendritic network, attenuation of mantle zones, multinucleated cells, and monocytoid cells are commonly noted. In addition, alterations in CD4 and CD8 lymphocyte populations within nodal zones are documented and reflect the decline in CD4 and increase in CD8-bearing lymphocytes seen in the circulation (207). With progression of the stage of HIV infection, lymphadenopathy tends to resolve, with involution of follicles, hyperplasia of paracortical histiocytes and blood vessels, and depletion of lymphocytes (208). Lymph nodes in AIDS frequently reveal absent or markedly atrophic follicles, a fibrotic capsule, and prominent sinus histiocytosis (209). Clinically, lymphadenopathy becomes less prominent with progression to AIDS unless involved with a previously noted secondary cause of lymph node enlargement.

Abundant HIV is found within the lymph nodes throughout the course of HIV disease (210,211). Early in infection, follicular dendritic cells are coated with viral particles and probably serve as a reservoir for infecting T cells that traffic through the lymph node follicle. An intercellular adhesion molecule-3 receptor on dendritic cells, DC-SIGN, binds to the HIV envelope and promotes efficient infection of CD4+ T cells (212). As the disease progresses, dendritic cells are lost and plasma virus levels increase while HIV in lymph node T cells can still be detected. With effective control of viral replication, alterations in the follicular dendritic cell network can be reversed and lymph node architecture improved (213).

NON-HODGKIN'S LYMPHOMA

Lymphoproliferation may occur when select subcomponents of the immune system are dysfunctional, whether from HIV infection, from immunosuppressive drugs as used after organ transplant, or from the genetic immunodeficiency states such as Wiskott-Aldrich syndrome and ataxia telangiectasia (214) (Table 23-6). Against these backgrounds, B-cell proliferation and malignant transformation to NHL occur with increased frequency. Levine and colleagues (209) have estimated that the rate of conversion from persistent generalized lymphadenopathy to lymphoma is approximately 3% per person per year, placing the relative risk of lymphoma in patients with persistent generalized lymphadenopathy at 850 times the expected rate for non–HIV-infected persons of comparable age. Other studies have estimated the risk of lymphoma in advanced HIV disease as 3% to 12% at 24 months (215,216). The contribution of

TABLE 23-6. Relative Risk (RR) of Lymphoma Associated with Selected Conditions That Entail Altered Immunity[a]

Magnitude of Relative Risk of Lymphoma		
High (RR >15)	Intermediate (RR >2)	Low (RR ≤ 2)
Multiple transplants	Sibling transplant	Splenectomy
Cadaver transplant	Mild sicca syndrome	Sarcoidosis
Severe sicca syndrome	Nontropical sprue	Hyperimmunization
Wiskott-Aldrich syndrome	Crohn's disease	Asthma
Ataxia-telangiectasia	Short-term HIV infection	Hansen's disease
Long-term HIV infection	Rheumatoid arthritis	Cytotoxic drug therapy
		Systemic lupus

HIV, human immunodeficiency virus.
[a]Risk of lymphoma in patients with the condition relative to a risk of 1.0 to comparable individuals without the condition.
Hoover RN. Lymphoma risks in populations with altered immunity: a search for mechanism. *Cancer Res* 1992;52:5477S.

AIDS-related lymphoma (ARL) NHL in the United States has been estimated at 8% to 27% (217).

Pathophysiology

The one clear feature of the pathophysiology of AIDS lymphoma is that HIV is not directly involved. There is no HIV in B-cell lymphoma cells; rather, the virus plays an indirect role, providing the immunodeficiency in which B-cell malignancy may occur. These tumors appear to be opportunistic neoplasms in a fashion similar to the multiple infectious agents these patients acquire. NHL in an HIV-positive person is now considered an AIDS-defining illness.

Unlike other immunodeficiency states, the presence of EBV in ARLs is consistently present in only a select subset, and its pathophysiologic role is less clear (217–221). Among the ARL settings, it is only those primary CNS lymphomas that demonstrate EBV in virtually all tumors and express EBV-encoded proteins in a pattern similar to that seen in lymphoproliferative disease posttransplantation (222,223). The EBV latent gene expression pattern is type III with expression of LMP1,2 and EBNA 1-6 (223).

Systemic lymphomas can be identified as EBV positive in 33% to 67% (224–226), and the pattern of EBV latent gene expression is more variable. There is also a small subset of systemic lymphomas, primary effusion lymphomas (PELs), which are consistently associated with another gamma herpesvirus, Kaposi's sarcoma herpesvirus (KSHV). PEL is a unique clinico-pathologic entity and is generally a manifestation of advanced AIDS. Cells from these tumors uniformly have KSHV DNA within them and are often coinfected with EBV (227,228).

Genetic mutations in AIDS lymphomas vary based on the histologic subtype. Among large cell lymphomas, Bcl-6 rearrangement, c-myc rearrangement, and p53 mutations occur in approximately 33%, 40%, and 25%, respectively (229). The small cell lymphomas are somewhat distinct in that c-myc rearrangements are common, but not Bcl-6 and rarely p53 mutations (230–233). There is no clear link between EBV and any specific genetic mutations other than those noted for the histologic subtype (230–233). The rearrangements of c-myc seen in AIDS lymphomas juxtapose c-myc with the immunoglobulin gene–heavy chain switch region (219,232,234–236), suggesting that the rearrangement occurs at the time of class switching in B-cell ontogeny. This occurs after that of VDJ rearrangement of the immunoglobulin locus and indicates that the cell of origin is likely to be postgerminal center or relatively late in B-cell ontogeny.

Genetic variation within the host has been reported to affect the relative risk of AIDS lymphoma. Those individuals with variant regulatory regions in the chemokine gene encoding stroma-derived growth factor-1 have an excess risk of developing the Burkitt lymphoma (BL) subtype of ARL (237). The basis for this altered susceptibility to lymphoid malignancy is not clear, but stroma-derived growth factor-1 was first identified by its ability to induce B-cell proliferation, suggesting that B-cell growth kinetics may be affected by the genetic alteration observed.

Immunocompetence also plays a critical role in lymphoma development. Those patients with advanced HIV disease are at increased risk of both primary CNS lymphoma and the more rare, KSHV-associated PEL. Systemic lymphoma generally is increased with progressive immune suppression, but is not as markedly associated with end-stage immunodeficiency. In treatment trials, the mean entry CD4+ cell count has ranged between 50 and 189 cells/mm², whereas the mean CD4+ cell count for those with primary CNS lymphoma is generally less than 50 cells/mm² (222). Within the systemic lymphomas, those with a BL or Burkitt-like lymphoma (BLL) histology tend to

have a higher CD4+ cell count than those with large cell lymphomas. The systemic lymphomas can occur at any point in HIV disease and may be the presenting evidence of underlying HIV infection.

The introduction of potent antiretroviral therapy has affected the incidence and type of AIDS lymphomas. As might be anticipated, those patients responding to antiretroviral therapy are less prone to develop the lymphoproliferative syndrome associated with poor control of EBV, specifically primary CNS lymphoma. Once commonplace in any center caring for patients with HIV disease, this entity is now rarely encountered and is generally found only among those who have either failed or not undertaken HAART. Although the number of systemic lymphomas is said to be relatively constant despite the introduction of HAART (238,239), there are emerging data that suggest a modest but real decrease in this tumor type as well (240–244).

Pathology

The pathology of ARLs is generally that of B-cell tumors, with rare T-cell tumors of various types identified. The T-cell tumors range from large granular lymphocyte disease, to large cell or anaplastic T-cell lymphoma, to Sézary's syndrome, to angiocentric T-cell proliferation (245–253). Within the T-cell malignancies noted, a subset has been identified in which HIV inserted into the host genome upstream of the c-fes protooncogene, suggesting a possible insertional mutagenesis mechanism in some of these tumors (254).

The B-cell tumor types seen (Fig. 23-2) can be broadly categorized as large cell, immunoblastic, and small cell. Among the small, noncleaved cell tumors are the BL and BLL subtypes. The BLL subtype more closely resembles the large cell phenotype. Characteristics that distinguish BLL from BL include a higher frequency of EBV, CD39, CD70, and CD11a among BLL tumors. Whereas BL is often found in a patient population with higher CD4 counts, the BLL patients have been noted to have lower counts similar to the large cell subsets (255,256).

Apart from the unusual case of low-grade lymphoma that may be associated with a less-aggressive clinical cause and perhaps a different pathogenesis, the histologic classification of HIV-associated NHL has not been consistently correlated with prognosis. Conflicting data have been presented and require further compilation of patient information to be clarified

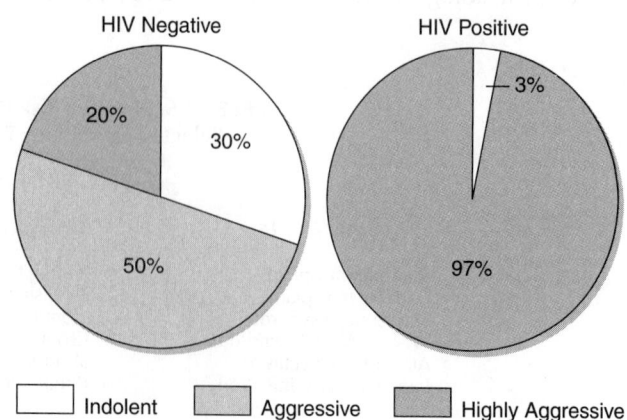

Figure 23-2. Comparison of the relative abundance of distinct histologic subgroups among patients with non-Hodgkin's lymphoma **(left)** versus acquired immunodeficiency syndrome–related non-Hodgkin's lymphoma **(right)**. HIV, human immunodeficiency virus.

TABLE 23-7. Location and Stage of Non-Hodgkin's Lymphoma in AIDS Patients

Study	Patients	Extranodal Sites				Stage	
		GI	Liver	CNS	Marrow	I or II	III or IV
Levine et al.	27	6	1	8	5	7	20
Kalter et al.	14	2	2	8	4	1	13
Gill et al.	22	5	5	3	7	1	21
Knowles et al.	89	14	14	19	19	27	57
Ziegler et al.	90	8	8	38	30	38	52
Bermudez et al.	31	6	6	8	10	1	30
Lowenthal et al.	43	11	6	11	13	9	26
Kaplan et al.	84	7	22	10	26	14	69
Kaplan et al.	30	?	?	?	7	12	14
Levine et al.	42	5	11	6	6	11	24
Remick et al.	18	5	?	?	?	5	13
Raphael et al.	113	18	3	22	17	—	—
Total	603	124 (21%)	78 (13%)	133 (23%)	138 (23%)	126 (27%)	339 (73%)

AIDS, acquired immunodeficiency syndrome; CNS, central nervous system; GI, gastrointestinal.

(222,231,257,258). In general, NHL in this setting is highly aggressive with histologic subsets not clearly identifying those with worse prognosis.

Clinical Presentation and Evaluation

ARLs can be generally broken down into two major groups: primary CNS lymphoma (PCNS) and systemic lymphoma. Within the systemic lymphomas there are several subgroups, including PEL and plasmablastic lymphoma, each of which is a rare occurrence. The relative frequency of PCNS versus systemic lymphoma in AIDS is changing with the use of potent antiretroviral therapy. Before the availability of HAART, PCNS accounted for approximately 15% of the AIDS lymphomas, a fraction that has dramatically declined in the era of HAART.

Systemic ARLs may present with a wide range of symptoms due to the propensity for extranodal disease (166,231,258–273). Sites of involvement in HIV, as in other settings of immunocompromised-associated NHL, are often outside the confines of the lymphatic system with a particular predilection for the GI tract, bone marrow, CNS, liver, and soft tissues (Table 23-7). Two thirds of all patients in one large series were diagnosed with NHL based on biopsies of nonnodal anatomic sites (266). The site of extranodal disease may correlate with histologic type, as in one series in which approximately 40% of patients with small, noncleaved cells had bone marrow involvement. This is a less common event in patients with an immunoblastic histology and rare in patients with a diffuse large cell histology (266). In contrast, GI involvement is noted more frequently with immunoblastic (48%) and diffuse, large, noncleaved cells (36%) than with small, noncleaved cells (8%). GI involvement may occur anywhere from esophagus to anus with an unusual predilection for anal or rectal involvement in homosexual males (274). The presentation of ARL does not appear to be appreciably affected by HAART, although one study has suggested a decline in the BL and BLL subset (238,275).

The incidence of CNS involvement in patients with systemic lymphoma has been estimated to be as high as 20% (264); thus, all HIV-positive patients presenting with systemic NHL should undergo careful assessment of the CNS. This generally includes an imaging technique [computed tomographic scan or magnetic resonance imaging (MRI)] and cerebrospinal fluid sampling; however, involvement is generally due to meningeal rather than parenchymal disease. CNS relapse has often occurred even in individuals with a negative evaluation at the time of presentation. Retrospective analysis of those patients in whom CNS involvement has occurred indicates that the presence of EBV in the tumor specimen is associated with CNS relapse (276). Patients whose tumor was EBV negative have a low frequency of CNS relapses and may therefore be considered at low risk, an issue with implications for prophylactic therapy discussed later.

At presentation, most HIV-infected patients with NHL have advanced-stage lymphoma. Systemic "B" symptoms (fever, weight loss, anorexia, malaise) are particularly common, although secondary infectious causes must be vigorously excluded. Staging the extent of tumor involvement should follow guidelines that are followed for NHL in other settings, with particular attention to the CNS, GI tract, and bone marrow.

Prognosis in patients with ARL has generally been poor, but with the advent of HAART, the improved prognosis from HIV-1 itself, as well as the improved tolerance of chemotherapy, long-term results are beginning to be more encouraging. Factors that have been indicative of higher risk have been variably reported based on the specific clinical trial. The largest experience to date is from the trial comparing methotrexate, bleomycin, doxorubicin (Adriamycin), cyclophosphamide, vincristine (Oncovin), dexamethasone (m-BACOD) with modified m-BACOD in 192 patients. Independent negative prognostic indicators on multivariant analysis were CD4 count less than 100 cells/mm^3, age greater than 35 years, intravenous drug user status, and stage III/IV disease (277). When one or none of these factors was present, the overall survival was 46 weeks, when two factors were present, 44 weeks, and when 3 or 4 factors were present, 18 weeks.

The International Prognostic Index (278), useful in other lymphoma groups, is likely to be useful in ARL, but experience with it has been limited to date. In one small study of 46 patients, it was found to be predictive of poor outcome (279). Although not formally assessed in the context of the International Prognostic Index, other studies have identified elevated lactate dehydrogenase (280) or age greater than 40 years as independent risk factors. Other factors that have been identified as indicative of worse outcome in some but not all reports include prior AIDS-defining illness, poor Karnofsky performance status, small cell histology, and bone marrow involvement (222,268,281–283). Polyclonality of the tumor in the absence of EBV and a CD4 count of greater than 300 cells/mm^3 were noted as positive prognostic indicators by Kaplan and colleagues (282).

Primary effusion lymphoma has a very distinct clinical presentation. These tumors are generally in liquid phase with mass lesions only very rarely noted (284–286). Body cavity involvement is the manner in which they present, with large anaplastic or immunoblastic-appearing cells seen on cytology. Immunophenotypic analysis often reveals surface CD45 (common leukocyte antigen), but staining for B- (CD20 or CD19) or T-cell (CD3) specific markers is absent. Characterization of these cells as of B-cell origin has depended on Southern blotting of the immunoglobulin locus to demonstrate rearrangement of the VDJ regions. Uniform among these tumors is the presence of the KSHV genome. EBV-encoded RNA may also be detected in the majority of tumors, but not with the consistency of KSHV.

Plasmablastic lymphomas of the jaw and oral cavity have also been described as a clinicopathologic subset of AIDS lymphomas (287,288). This tumor type typically presents with involvement restricted to the oral cavity, although involvement of additional sites may occur with late disease. Morphologically, these cells appear as cohesive sheets of monomorphic plasmablasts and they do not stain for CD45 or B- or T-cell markers. Discriminating them from nonhematologic malignancies can therefore be problematic. The cells typically do express CD138/syndecan-1, stain for VS38c, and have rearranged Ig loci. They are generally EBV positive by EBV-encoded RNA analysis.

PCNS lymphoma may provide particular diagnostic challenges given the range of other opportunistic diseases seen in the severely immunocompromised patients who are at greatest risk for this disease. In particular, PCNS lymphoma may be difficult to differentiate from progressive multifocal leukoencephalopathy or infection with *Toxoplasma gondii* or *M. tuberculosis*. Radiographically, progressive multifocal leukoencephalopathy may be distinguished by its lack of enhancement with gadolinium on nuclear MRI. Lymphomatous lesions may be isodense or hypodense and contrast enhancing on computed tomographic scans and enhancing on MRI scans, but so may toxoplasmal abscess (265). Other features may help discriminate among these diagnoses, such as the number of lesions (usually single in lymphoma, multiple in toxoplasmosis) and their location (lymphoma tends to be paraventricular and lymphoma may cross the midline, where toxoplasma does not), but there is no definitive radiographic appearance. Positron emission tomography and single photon emission computed tomography scanning have been useful in identifying CNS lymphomas and may provide important additional information. Nonradiographic information can be critical in assessing the relative risk of toxoplasma abscess versus lymphoma. Use of anti-PCP prophylaxis is common in the patients at highest risk for PCNS lymphoma. The most commonly used prophylactic agent, trimethoprim-sulfamethoxazole, is also excellent prophylaxis for toxoplasma. If a patient has been taking this medication and he or she does not have toxoplasma antibodies in his or her serum, the pathologic basis for a mass lesion has a likelihood of being lymphoma estimated at 74% (289). Evaluation of the cerebrospinal fluid for EBV by polymerase chain reaction also adds critical information to the evaluation of such patients. A positive EBV–polymerase chain reaction result in the context of a brain mass in patients with HIV disease has been reported to have a specificity for lymphoma of 100% in one study (290). However, the sensitivity of this test is less than perfect, calculated at 80% in the same report. If the above information is not definitive, and a patient is unwilling or unable to undergo biopsy, an empiric trial of antitoxoplasma therapy with sulfadiazine or clindamycin with pyrimethamine may be tried. This intervention generally halts the progression of toxoplasma abscess by 5 days and results in clinical or radiographic improvement by 14 days (291). When these milestones are not met, the likelihood of toxoplasmosis is low.

Therapy

Treatment of patients with HIV-associated NHL is complicated by the limited tolerance for chemotherapy in this patient popu-

lation as well as the aggressive biology of the malignancy. Bone marrow suppression and opportunistic infection commonly limit treatment, impeding optimal delivery of antitumor therapy. These complications occur more commonly with more advanced HIV disease and have been substantially mitigated by effective antiretroviral therapy. Patients on HAART who have control of HIV and restoration of CD4 counts tolerate antitumor therapy well, with the caveat of potential drug–drug interactions. Thus, selecting a treatment for patients with NHL should include consideration of the status of the HIV disease, including the treatment in place for the underlying HIV infection.

The treatment approaches for patients with advanced HIV disease or a failure to respond to HAART may be guided by studies conducted before the availability of potent anti-HIV medications. One regimen developed to accommodate the poor tolerance of chemotherapy in such patients was the modified m-BACOD protocol (264). This essentially half-dose regimen was compared with full-dose m-BACOD in a multicenter, phase III, randomized trial and found to be highly comparable in terms of tumor response and survival (283). There was no statistically significant difference in complete remission rate (50% vs. 46%), relapse after complete remission (19% vs. 23%), time to progression (22 weeks vs. 28 weeks), overall median survival (31 weeks vs. 34 weeks), death from AIDS (20 patients vs. 12 patients) or death from lymphoma (24 patients vs. 36 patients). There was, however, a difference in grade 4 neutropenia that occurred with greater frequency in patients receiving the standard dose regimen, despite the fact that all such patients received GM-CSF. Although these results are encouraging, subsequent studies have raised concern that the tumor response rates are inferior with low-dose regimens (270,292). Therefore, these approaches are generally reserved only for those patients in whom advanced AIDS precludes full-dose chemotherapy.

For those patients with either early HIV disease or with antiretroviral control of HIV-1, standard dose therapies with curative intent are appropriate (Table 23-8). Response rates to regimens such as CHOP have been generally well tolerated with response rates only slightly lower than those of the uninfected population (266–268,293–295).

More intensive regimens have also been tested, including the LNH84 regimen developed by the French-Italian Cooperative Group. In 140 patients, a complete remission rate of 65% with a relapse rate of 24% was observed (296). In a follow-up study, patients with CD4 counts greater than 100 cells/mm^3, no prior AIDS-defining illnesses, and good performance status were treated with either CHOP chemotherapy or ACVB (doxorubicin 75 mg/m^2 day 1, cyclophosphamide 1.2 g/m^2 day 1, vindesine 2 mg/m^2 day 1, bleomycin 10 mg days 1 to 5, prednisolone 60 mg days 1 to 5) with G-CSF support. Superior response rates in the ACVB arm were seen, balanced by a higher rate of toxicity (295).

Modifications in dose delivery with continuous infusion regimens have been tested with encouraging early results. Continuously infused cyclophosphamide 800 mg/m^2, doxorubicin 50 mg/m^2, and etoposide 240 mg/m^2, all per day for 4 days plus the antiretroviral ddI, achieved a complete response rate of 58% with a median response duration exceeding 18 months in a phase II trial (297). A follow-up multicenter study documented a complete remission rate of 46% with median survival of 8.2 months, although it should be noted that this was in an extremely immunocompromised population with median CD4 count of only 78 cells/µL (298). An alternative approach has been developed by the U.S. National Cancer Institute (NCI) using dose-adjusted etoposide, prednisone, Oncovin, cyclophosphamide, and hydroxydaunorubicin (299,300). The early results using this regimen are extremely encouraging, and multicenter evaluation is anticipated (301).

TABLE 23-8. Commonly Used Therapy Regimens for AIDS-Related Lymphoma

Regimen	Standard	Modified
CHOP		
Cyclophosphamide	750 mg/m², IVPB, day 1	375 mg/m², day 1
Doxorubicin	50 mg/m², IVPB day 1	25 mg/m², day 1
Vincristine	1.4 mg/m² (not to exceed 2 mg), IVPB, day 1	1.4 mg/m² (maximum 2 mg), day 1
Prednisone (each cycle q 21–28 d)	100 mg, PO, days 1–5	50–100 mg PO, days 1–5
Continuous infusion regimens		
CDE		
Cyclophosphamide	187.5 mg/m², CI, days 1–4	
Doxorubicin	12.5 mg/m², CI, days 1–4	
Etoposide	60 mg/m², CI, days 1–4	
Dose-adjusted EPOCH		
Etoposide	200 mg/m², days 1–4	
Vincristine	1.6 mg/m², days 1–4	
Doxorubicin	40 mg/m², days 1–4	
Cyclophosphamide	187 mg/m² (CD4 <100 µL), day 5	
	375 mg/m² (CD4 ≥100 µL), day 5	
Prednisone	60 mg/m², days 1–5	
G-CSF	5 µg/kg, day 6 (to ANC >5000/µL)	
Oral regimen		
CCNU	100 mg/m², PO, day1 (cycles 1, 3, 5)	
Etoposide	200 mg/m², PO, days 1–3	
Cyclophosphamide	100 mg/m², PO, days 22–31	
Procarbazine (each cycle q 42 d)	100 mg/m², PO, days 22–31	
ACVB dose-intensive chemotherapy regimen		
Induction[a]		
Adriamycin	75 mg/m², day 1	
Cyclophosphamide	1200 mg/m², day 1	
Vindesine	2 mg/m², days 1, 5	
Bleomycin	10 mg, days 1, 5	
Prednisolone	60 mg/m², days 1–5	
Consolidation		
Methotrexate (IV)	3 g/m², days 1, 5	
Folinic acid rescue (PO)	25 mg × 4, days 1–3, 15–17	
Ifosfamide (IV)	1.5 g/m², days 29, 33	
VP-16 (IV)	300 mg/m², days 29, 33	
L-Asparaginase (IM)	50,000 U/m², days 57, 64	
Ara-C (SC)	50 mg/m² q12h x 8, days 78, 92	
CNS prophylaxis		
Methotrexate (IT)	12 mg, days 1, 8, 15, 29	
CNS treatment		
Methotrexate (IT)	12 mg 2 × wk for 5 wk	
Radiation therapy	3000–3600 cGy	

AIDS, acquired immunodeficiency syndrome; Ara-C, cytarabine; CCNU, chloroethylcyclohexylnitrosourea (lomustine); CI, continuous infusion; VP-16, etoposide.
[a]Every 2 weeks for three cycles.

Enhancement of standard cytotoxic agents with monoclonal antibody therapy is currently being evaluated by the AIDS Malignancy Consortium sponsored by the NCI. This phase III trial compares CHOP alone with CHOP plus rituximab for previously untreated patients with systemic AIDS lymphoma.

Dose intensification with stem cell rescue is currently being tested in patients with ARL. Scattered reports have indicated reasonable tolerance and no difficulty with engraftment (302,303). These trials represent a potential opportunity to also test the ability of gene-modified cells to preferentially rebuild the immune system in HIV-infected individuals. Such gene therapy studies are under way. Allogeneic transplant is only beginning to be tested after early experience was tainted by substantial toxicity (292,304–311). Such approaches can only be recommended in the context of clinical trials at this time.

An unresolved issue in the care of patients with ARL is the extent to which therapy for HIV should be pursued during the time of cytotoxic chemotherapy. Two distinct approaches have been tested to date. The AIDS Malignancy Consortium has assessed the combination of stavudine (2',3'-didehydro-3'-deoxythymidine), lamivudine, and indinavir in combination with either modified or full-dose CHOP. The results indicate that no untoward or unexpected toxicity occurred. The pharma-

cokinetic profile of doxorubicin or indinavir was unaltered, whereas the clearance for cyclophosphamide was diminished by approximately 50% (312). Taking the position that pharmacodynamic interactions may have unpredicted untoward events, the NCI has studied EPOCH in the context of antiviral therapy interruption for the duration of cytotoxic chemotherapy. Preliminary results from this study indicate that the HIV viral load increase noted when antiretrovirals were stopped reverted to baseline on reintroduction of the drugs after lymphoma therapy completion. In addition, the change in CD4+ cell counts did not appear to be any greater than in other contexts. Therefore, physician and patient need to weigh relative tolerance of each type of medication and the possibility for side effects that could not be anticipated from new drugs or combinations of drugs and structure a specific plan.

In general, the approach to patients with HIV-related lymphomas requires consideration of three additional issues compared with the non-HIV–infected population. The first is that prophylaxis for P. carinii should be considered for all patients. The second is that myelotoxicity may be considerable in this patient population due to hematopoietic dysfunction, and growth factor is generally required. The third is that the potential for CNS involvement (266) has led some to advocate prophylactic intrathecal therapy for all. This issue remains highly controversial and the value of such an intervention has not been systematically studied. The risk factors of CNS involvement in other hematologic malignancies such as bone marrow, paranasal sinus, or testicular involvement should be considered in making this decision. Further, a recent study by Cingolani has assessed risk factors for CNS relapse and identified EBV in the primary tumor as highly associated with risk (p = .003) (276). Other identified risk factors were extranodal disease at presentation and extranodal relapse. These data suggest that CNS prophylaxis should be targeted to those with EBV in the tumor tissue, particularly emphasizing those with extranodal disease at presentation (313).

Treatment of PCNS lymphoma must be balanced with the severity of the underlying HIV disease. Radiation therapy is generally the approach used and may achieve responses in 60% to 79% of patients, but durable remissions are uncommon (265,314,315). Steroid therapy is often given in conjunction with radiation and is generally not associated with increased short-term morbidity in this patient population. However, it is important to proceed with tapering as rapidly as tolerated to prevent worsening the severe immune dysfunction of this patient group. High-dose methotrexate has been proposed as an alternative to radiation therapy and demonstrated to be active in this population with a tolerable side-effect profile (316). Combination cytotoxic chemotherapy and radiation therapy, however, cannot be recommended due to the severity of side effects generally observed. Due to the virtually uniform presence of EBV in tumor cells, antiherpesvirus or immune-modulating therapies have been tested in preliminary fashion. Ganciclovir in combination with ZDV (or AZT) and IL-2 was noted to have antitumor activity (317) and will be tested in larger clinical trials. Other EBV-directed genetic (318) or chemical (319) manipulations have also been proposed and await clinical assessment.

Due to the contribution of immune dysfunction to the development of this tumor type, it may be hypothesized that immune recovery with HAART may positively affect the outcome of disease. Although this has not been rigorously shown, there are reports of disease control on HAART (320) that suggest that adding HAART to the treatment program of individuals with AIDS-related PCNS lymphoma is appropriate.

HODGKIN'S DISEASE

The incidence of Hodgkin's disease (HD) has been estimated to be increased 2.5-fold to 8.5-fold above that of the uninfected population (321–327), with certain geographic populations reporting an increase of up to 18.3-fold (325). The risk of HD appears to be uniformly increased across the risk groups for HIV infection and independent of age or gender (328). The clinical features of the disease in HIV-positive persons are substantially different from those in uninfected counterparts, with a higher incidence of advanced-stage disease, "B" symptoms, and extranodal disease (329–332). Stage III or IV disease was reported in 91% of HIV-infected patients compared with 46% in individuals without HIV (333). Bone marrow may be involved in up to 50% of patients (334–336) in addition to involvement of less-common extranodal sites such as the tongue, rectum, skin, and lung (332). Staging procedures should follow guidelines in the HIV-uninfected population, but with particular care to assess for coincident infectious causes of "B" symptoms.

Pathologic features of HD are also different in the HIV-infected individual, with mixed-cellularity histology more commonly noted (281,329–331). EBV is also much more frequently detected in the tumor specimens. EBV has been estimated to be present in 80% to 100% of Hodgkin's tumors from individuals with HIV infection (337–339) and typically expressing LMP-1, but not EBNA2 (339). The transcription factor Bcl-6 expressed in germinal-center B cells is present on Reed-Sternberg cells from both HIV-1 infected and uninfected individuals. However, syndecan-1 (a proteoglycan associated with the postgerminal center) is restricted to the HIV-1 positive population (340,341), suggesting that the postgerminal-center B cell may be the cell of origin in HIV-1-related HD. In contrast, the germinal-center cell is considered to be the source of Reed-Sternberg cells in the HIV-negative patients with HD.

Therapy

Treatment guidelines for HD outside the context of HIV infection should generally be applied to the infected individual as well. The limited published experience with chemotherapy regimens for HD in HIV-positive patients suggests that response rates may be lower, possibly due to enhanced toxicity from therapy (281,342–344). However, these studies were generally conducted before the era of HAART, and patients with effective control of HIV often tolerate regimens such as ABVD or epirubicin, bleomycin, and vinblastine quite well (345). There is also a record of reasonable tolerance and activity of the Stanford V regimen in AIDS-related HD (346). Cure of HD is certainly possible in the setting of HIV disease and should be the goal of therapy except in the case of concurrent severe AIDS. In patients failing antiretroviral therapy with advanced AIDS and HD, a palliative approach may be warranted. Outside of this context, aggressive therapy is appropriate, and patients failing first-line therapy are now participating in clinical trials using autologous or allogeneic bone marrow transplantation.

In addition to cytotoxic therapy, consideration should be given to prophylaxis for opportunistic infection. In particular, medication to prevent *P. carinii* is commonly used in conjunction with HD therapy. Growth factor support for myelotoxicity is often effective in this population, and guidelines for their use in other contexts should be followed.

CASTLEMAN'S DISEASE

Multicentric Castleman's disease or angiofollicular lymph node hyperplasia has been reported in patients with advanced HIV disease (347). This process often presents with fever, peripheral adenopathy, weight loss, hepatosplenomegaly, pulmonary symptoms and anemia, or pancytopenia. Both the hyalin-vascular and plasma cell subtypes of Castleman's disease have been reported in AIDS, although the plasma cell subtype is more common. KSHV is found in the involved nodes, and there is a high prevalence of coincident or subsequent Kaposi's sarcoma (284,347–349). This lymphoproliferative process is regarded as a KSHV-related neoplasm that is aggressive with poor outcome, although responses to chemotherapy have been reported (347). No specific regimen can be regarded as standard, although reports of success using interferon-α (350), simple agent vinblastine (347), or HAART (351) have emerged.

REFERENCES

1. Rosenberg ES, Altfeld M, Poon SH, et al. Immune control of HIV-1 after early treatment of acute infection. *Nature* 2000;407:523–526.
2. Centers for Disease Control. 1992. Guidelines for prophylaxis against Pneumocystis carinii pneumonia for persons infected with human immunodeficiency virus. *MMWR Recommendations and Reports* 2001;41(No. RR-4):1–11.
3. Ledergerber B, Mocroft A, Reiss P, et al. Discontinuation of secondary prophylaxis against Pneumocystis carinii pneumonia in patients with HIV

infection who have a response to antiretroviral therapy. Eight European Study Groups. *N Engl J Med* 2001;344:168–174.

4. Lopez Bernaldo de Quiros JC, Miro JM, Pena JM, et al. A randomized trial of the discontinuation of primary and secondary prophylaxis against Pneumocystis carinii pneumonia after highly active antiretroviral therapy in patients with HIV infection. Grupo de Estudio del SIDA 04/98. *N Engl J Med* 2001; 344:159–167.

5. Spivak JL, Selonick SE, Quinn TC. Acquired immune deficiency syndrome and pancytopenia. *JAMA* 1983;250:3084–3087.

6. Spivak JL, Bender BS, Quinn TC. Hematologic abnormalities in the acquired immune deficiency syndrome. *Am J Med* 1984;77:224–228.

7. Zon LI, Arkin C, Groopman JE. Haematologic manifestations of the human immunodeficiency virus (HIV). *Br J Haematol* 1987;66:251–256.

8. Treacy M, Lai L, Costello C, et al. Peripheral blood and bone marrow abnormalities in patients with HIV related disease. *Br J Haematol* 1987;65:289–294.

9. Scadden DT, Zon LI, Groopman JE. Pathophysiology and management of HIV-associated hematologic disorders. *Blood* 1989;74:1455–1463.

10. Solis OG, Belmonte AH, Ramaswamy G, et al. Pseudogaucher cells in Mycobacterium avium intracellulare infections in acquired immune deficiency syndrome (AIDS). *Am J Clin Pathol* 1986;85:233–235.

11. Kovacs JA, Kovacs AA, Polis M, et al. Cryptococcosis in the acquired immunodeficiency syndrome. *Ann Intern Med* 1985;103:533–538.

12. Mandell W, Goldberg DM, Neu HC. Histoplasmosis in patients with the acquired immune deficiency syndrome. *Am J Med* 1986;81:974–978.

13. Rossi JF, Dubois A, Bengler C, et al. Pneumocystis carinii in bone marrow. *Ann Intern Med* 1985;102:868.

14. Raviglione MC, Garner GR, Mullen MP. Pneumocystis carinii in bone marrow. *Ann Intern Med* 1988;109:253.

15. Pearce CJ, Conrad ME, Nolan PE, et al. Ehrlichiosis: a cause of bone marrow hypoplasia in humans. *Am J Hematol* 1988;28:53–55.

16. Little BJ, Spivak JL, Quinn TC, et al. Kaposi's sarcoma with bone marrow involvement: occurrence in a patient with the acquired immunodeficiency syndrome. *Am J Med Sci* 1986;292:44–46.

17. Northfelt DW, Mayer A, Kaplan LD, et al. The usefulness of diagnostic bone marrow examination in patients with human immunodeficiency virus (HIV) infection. *J Acquir Immune Defic Syndr* 1991;4:659–666.

18. Mir N, Costello C, Luckit J, et al. HIV-disease and bone marrow changes: a study of 60 cases. *Eur J Haematol* 1989;42:339–343.

19. Osborne BM, Guarda LA, Butler JJ. Bone marrow biopsies in patients with the acquired immunodeficiency syndrome. *Hum Pathol* 1984;15:1048–1053.

20. Castella A, Croxson TS, Mildvan D, et al. The bone marrow in AIDS. A histologic, hematologic, and microbiologic study. *Am J Clin Pathol* 1985;84:425–432.

21. Perkocha LA, Rodgers GM. Hematologic aspects of human immunodeficiency virus infection: laboratory and clinical considerations. *Am J Hematol* 1988;29:94–105.

22. Franco CM, Hendrix LE, Lokey JL. Bone marrow abnormalities in the acquired immunodeficiency syndrome. *Ann Intern Med* 1984;101:275–276.

23. Geller SA, Muller R, Greenberg ML, et al. Acquired immunodeficiency syndrome. Distinctive features of bone marrow biopsies. *Arch Pathol Lab Med* 1985;109:138–141.

24. Hromas RA, Murray JL. Bone marrow in the acquired immunodeficiency syndrome. *Ann Intern Med* 1984;101:877.

25. Schneider DR, Picker LJ. Myelodysplasia in the acquired immune deficiency syndrome. *Am J Clin Pathol* 1985;84:144–152.

26. Aiuti A, Turchetto L, Cota M, et al. Human CD34(+) cells express CXCR4 and its ligand stromal cell-derived factor-1. Implications for infection by T-cell tropic human immunodeficiency virus. *Blood* 1999;94:62–73.

27. Lee B, Ratajczak J, Doms RW, et al. Coreceptor/chemokine receptor expression on human hematopoietic cells: biological implications for human immunodeficiency virus-type 1 infection. *Blood* 1999;93:1145–1156.

28. Viardot A, Kronenwett R, Deichmann M, et al. The human immunodeficiency virus (HIV)-type 1 coreceptor CXCR-4 (fusin) is preferentially expressed on the more immature CD34+ hematopoietic stem cells. *Ann Hematol* 1998;77:193–197.

29. Ruiz ME, Cicala C, Arthos J, et al. Peripheral blood-derived CD34+ progenitor cells: CXC chemokine receptor 4 and CC chemokine receptor 5 expression and infection by HIV. *J Immunol* 1998;161:4169–4176.

30. Shen H, Cheng T, Preffer FI, et al. Intrinsic human immunodeficiency virus type 1 resistance of hematopoietic stem cells despite coreceptor expression. *J Virol* 1999;73:728–737.

31. Weichold FF, Zella D, Barabitskaja O, et al. Neither human immunodeficiency virus-1 (HIV-1) nor HIV-2 infects most-primitive human hematopoietic stem cells as assessed in long-term bone marrow cultures. *Blood* 1998;91:907–915.

32. Koka PS, Jamieson BD, Brooks DG, et al. Human immunodeficiency virus type 1-induced hematopoietic inhibition is independent of productive infection of progenitor cells in vivo. *J Virol* 1999;73:9089–9097.

33. Iyengar S, Schwartz DH, Hildreth JE. T cell-tropic HIV gp120 mediates CD4 and CD8 cell chemotaxis through CXCR4 independent of CD4: implications for HIV pathogenesis. *J Immunol* 1999;162:6263–6267.

34. Misse D, Cerutti M, Noraz N, et al. A CD4-independent interaction of human immunodeficiency virus-1 gp 120 with CXCR4 induces their cointernalization, cell signaling, and T-cell chemotaxis. *Blood* 1999;93:2454–2462.

35. Zauli G, Furlini M, Vitale MC, et al. A subset of human CD34+ hematopoietic progenitors express low levels of CD4, the high-affinity receptor for human immunodeficiency virus-type 1. *Blood* 1994;84:1896–1905.

36. Donahue RE, Johnson MM, Zon LI, et al. Suppression of in vitro haematopoiesis following human immunodeficiency virus infection. *Nature* 1987;326:200–203.

37. Leiderman IZ, Greenberg ML, Adelsberg BR, et al. A glycoprotein inhibitor of in vitro granulopoiesis associated with AIDS. *Blood* 1987;70:1267–1272.

38. Sloand EM, Klein HG, Banks SM, et al. Epidemiology of thrombocytopenia in HIV infection. *Eur J Haematol* 1992;48:168–172.

39. Stella CC, Ganser A, Hoelzer D. Defective in vitro growth of the hemopoietic progenitor cells in the acquired immunodeficiency syndrome. *J Clin Invest* 1987;80:286–293.

40. Molina JM, Scadden DT, Sakaguchi M, et al. Lack of evidence for infection of or effect on growth of hematopoietic progenitor cells after in vivo or in vitro exposure to human immunodeficiency virus. *Blood* 1990;76:2476–2482.

41. von Laer D, Hufert FT, Fenner TE, et al. CD34+ hematopoietic progenitor cells are not a major reservoir of the human immunodeficiency virus. *Blood* 1990;76:1281–1286.

42. Davis BR, Schwartz DH, Marx JC, et al. Absent or rare human immunodeficiency virus infection of bone marrow stem/progenitor cells in vivo. *J Virol* 1991;65:1985–1990.

43. Steinberg HN, Crumpacker CS, Chatis PA. In vitro suppression of normal human bone marrow progenitor cells by human immunodeficiency virus. *J Virol* 1991;65:1765–1769.

44. Zauli G, Vitale M, Re MC, et al. In vitro exposure to human immunodeficiency virus type 1 induces apoptotic cell death of the factor-dependent TF-1 hematopoietic cell line. *Blood* 1994;83:167–175.

45. Zauli G, Re MC, Visani G, et al. Evidence for a human immunodeficiency virus type 1-mediated suppression of uninfected hematopoietic (CD34+) cells in AIDS patients. *J Infect Dis* 1992;166:710–716.

46. Ganser A, Ottmann OG, von Briesen H, et al. Changes in the haematopoietic progenitor cell compartment in the acquired immunodeficiency syndrome. *Res Virol* 1990;141:185–193.

47. Zauli G, Re MC, Gugliotta L, et al. Lack of compensatory megakaryocytopoiesis in HIV-1-seropositive thrombocytopenic individuals compared with immune thrombocytopenic purpura patients. *AIDS* 1991;5:1345–1350.

48. Folks TM, Kessler SW, Orenstein JM. Infection and replication of HIV-1 in purified progenitor cells of normal human bone marrow. *Science* 1988;242:919–922.

49. Kitano K, Abboud CN, Ryan DH. Macrophage-active colony-stimulating factors enhance human immunodeficiency virus type 1 infection in bone marrow stem cells. *Blood* 1991;77:1699–1705.

50. Schuitemaker H, Kootstra NA, Koppelman MH, et al. Proliferation-dependent HIV-1 infection of monocytes occurs during differentiation into macrophages. *J Clin Invest* 1992;89:1154–1160.

51. Louache F, Bettaieb A, Henri A, et al. Infection of megakaryocytes by human immunodeficiency virus in seropositive patients with immune thrombocytopenic purpura. *Blood* 1991;78:1697–1705.

52. Koka PS, Fraser JK, Bryson Y, et al. Human immunodeficiency virus inhibits multilineage hematopoiesis in vivo. *J Virol* 1998;72:5121–5127.

53. Jenkins M, Hanley MB, Moreno MB, et al. Human immunodeficiency virus-1 infection interrupts thymopoiesis and multilineage hematopoiesis in vivo. *Blood* 1998;91:2672–2678.

54. Mladenovic J, Sevin A, Chiu S, et al. Decreased mobilization of CD34+ cells in advanced HIV-1 disease: results of a multicenter prospective study. *Blood* 1998;92:2808.

55. Clark DR, Repping S, Pakker NG, et al. T-cell progenitor function during progressive human immunodeficiency virus-1 infection and after antiretroviral therapy. *Blood* 2000;96:242–249.

56. Adams GB, Pym AS, Poznansky MC, et al. The in vivo effects of combination antiretroviral drug therapy on peripheral blood CD34+ cell colony-forming units from HIV type 1-infected patients. *AIDS Res Hum Retroviruses* 1999;15:551–559.

57. Huang SS, Barbour JD, Deeks SG, et al. Reversal of human immunodeficiency virus type 1-associated hematosuppression by effective antiretroviral therapy. *Clin Infect Dis* 2000;30:504–510.

58. Hellerstein M, Hanley MB, Cesar D, et al. Directly measured kinetics of circulating T lymphocytes in normal and HIV-1-infected humans [see comments]. *Nat Med* 1999;5:83–89.

59. Douek DC, McFarland RD, Keiser PH, et al. Changes in thymic function with age and during the treatment of HIV infection [see comments]. *Nature* 1998;396:690–695.

60. Zhang ZQ, Notermans DW, Sedgewick G, et al. Kinetics of CD4+ T cell repopulation of lymphoid tissues after treatment of HIV-1 infection. *Proc Natl Acad Sci U S A* 1998;95:1154–1159.

61. Autran BG, Carcelain TS, Li C, et al. Positive effects of combined antiretroviral therapy on CD4+ T cell homeostasis and function in advanced HIV disease. *Science* 1997;277:112–116.

62. Su L, Kaneshima M, Bonyhadi S, et al. HIV-1 induced thymocyte depletion is associated with indirect cytopathicity and infection of progenitor cells in vivo. *Immunity* 1995;2:25–36.

63. Autran B, Guiet P, Raphael M, et al. Thymocyte and thymic microenvironment alterations during a systemic HIV infection in a severe combined immunodeficient mouse model. *AIDS* 1996;10:717–727.

64. Gaulton GN, Scobie JV, Rosenzweig M. HIV-1 and the thymus [Editorial]. *AIDS* 1997;11:403–414.

65. Stanley SK, McCune JM, Kaneshima H, et al. Human immunodeficiency virus infection of the human thymus and disruption of the thymic microenvironment in the SCID-hu mouse. *J Exp Med* 1993;178:1151–1163.

66. Jamieson BD, Douek DC, Killian S, et al. Generation of functional thymocytes in the human adult. *Immunity* 1999;10:569–575.
67. Poulin JF, Viswanathan MN, Harris JM, et al. Direct evidence for thymic function in adult humans. *J Exp Med* 1999;190:479–486.
68. Amado RG, Jamieson BD, Cortado R, et al. Reconstitution of human thymic implants is limited by human immunodeficiency virus breakthrough during antiretroviral therapy. *J Virol* 1999;73:6361–6369.
69. McCune JM, Loftus R, Schmidt DK, et al. High prevalence of thymic tissue in adults with human immunodeficiency virus-1 infection [see comments]. *J Clin Invest* 1998;101:2301–2308.
70. Smith KY, Valdez H, Landay A, et al. Thymic size and lymphocyte restoration in patients with human immunodeficiency virus infection after 48 weeks of zidovudine, lamivudine, and ritonavir therapy. *J Infect Dis* 2000;181:141–147.
71. Douek DC, Koup RA, McFarland RD, et al. Effect of HIV on thymic function before and after antiretroviral therapy in children. *J Infect Dis* 2000;181:1479–1482.
72. Scadden DT, Zeira M, Woon A, et al. Human immunodeficiency virus infection of human bone marrow stromal fibroblasts. *Blood* 1990;76:317–322.
73. Steffan AM, Lafon ME, Gendrault JL, et al. Primary cultures of endothelial cells from the human liver sinusoid are permissive for human immunodeficiency virus type 1. *Proc Natl Acad Sci U S A* 1992;89:1582–1586.
74. Moses AV, Williams ML, Heneveld J, et al. Human immunodeficiency virus infection of bone marrow endothelium reduces induction of stromal hematopoietic growth factors. *Blood* 1996;87:919–925.
75. Bahner I, Kearns K, Coutinho S, et al. Infection of human marrow immunodeficiency virus-1 (HIV-1) is both required and sufficient for HIV-1-inducted hematopoietic suppression in vitro: demonstration by gene modification of primary human stroma. *Blood* 1997;90:1787–1798.
76. Calenda V, Chermann JC. Severe in vitro inhibition of erythropoiesis and transient stimulation of granulopoiesis after bone-marrow infection with eight different HIV-2 isolates. *AIDS* 1992;6:943–948.
77. Wahl LM, Corcoran ML, Pyle SW, et al. Human immunodeficiency virus glycoprotein (gp120) induction of monocyte arachidonic acid metabolites and interleukin 1. *Proc Natl Acad Sci U S A* 1989;86:621–625.
78. Merrill JE, Koyanagi Y, Chen IS. Interleukin-1 and tumor necrosis factor alpha can be induced from mononuclear phagocytes by human immunodeficiency virus type 1 binding to the CD4 receptor. *J Virol* 1989;63:4404–4408.
79. Molina JM, Scadden DT, Amirault C, et al. Human immunodeficiency virus does not induce interleukin-1, interleukin-6, or tumor necrosis factor in mononuclear cells. *J Virol* 1990;64:2901–2906.
80. Zauli G, Davis BR, Re MC, et al. tat protein stimulates production of transforming growth factor-beta 1 by marrow macrophages: a potential mechanism for human immunodeficiency virus-1-induced hematopoietic suppression. *Blood* 1992;80:3036–3043.
81. Molina JM, Scadden DT, Byrn R, et al. Production of tumor necrosis factor alpha and interleukin 1 beta by monocytic cells infected with human immunodeficiency virus. *J Clin Invest* 1989;84:733–737.
82. Lahdevirta J, Maury CP, Teppo AM, et al. Elevated levels of circulating cachectin/tumor necrosis factor in patients with acquired immunodeficiency syndrome. *Am J Med* 1988;85:289–291.
83. Reddy MM, Sorrell SJ, Lange M, et al. Tumor necrosis factor and HIV P24 antigen levels in serum of HIV-infected populations. *J Acquir Immune Defic Syndr* 1988;1:436–440.
84. Breen EC, Rezai AR, Nakajima K, et al. Infection with HIV is associated with elevated IL-6 levels and production. *J Immunol* 1990;144:480–484.
85. Kekow J, Wachsman W, McCutchan JA, et al. Transforming growth factor-beta and suppression of humoral immune responses in HIV infection. *J Clin Invest* 1991;87:1010–1016.
86. Spivak JL, Barnes DC, Fuchs E, et al. Serum immunoreactive erythropoietin in HIV-infected patients. *JAMA* 1989;261:3104–3107.
87. Rarick MU, Loureiro C, Groshen S, et al. Serum erythropoietin titers in patients with human immunodeficiency virus (HIV) infection and anemia. *J Acquir Immune Defic Syndr* 1991;4:593–597.
88. Wang Z, Goldberg MA, Scadden DT. HIV-1 suppresses erythropoietin production in vitro. *Exp Hematol* 1993;21:683–688.
89. Isgro A, Mezzaroma I, Aiuti A, et al. Recovery of hematopoietic activity in bone marrow from human immunodeficiency virus type 1-infected patients during highly active antiretroviral therapy. *AIDS Res Hum Retroviruses* 2000;16:1471–1479.
90. Sloand EM, Maciejewski J, Kumar P, et al. Protease inhibitors stimulate hematopoiesis and decrease apoptosis and ICE expression in CD34(+) cells. *Blood* 2000;96:2735–2739.
91. Holzman RS, Walsh CM, Karpatkin S. Risk for the acquired immunodeficiency syndrome among thrombocytopenic and nonthrombocytopenic homosexual men seropositive for the human immunodeficiency virus. *Ann Intern Med* 1987;106:383–386.
92. Walsh CM, Nardi MA, Karpatkin S. On the mechanism of thrombocytopenic purpura in sexually active homosexual men. *N Engl J Med* 1984;311:635–639.
93. Yu JR, Lennette ET, Karpatkin S. Anti-F(ab')2 antibodies in thrombocytopenic patients at risk for acquired immunodeficiency syndrome. *J Clin Invest* 1986;77:1756–1761.
94. Hohmann AW, Booth K, Peters V, et al. Common epitope on HIV p24 and human platelets. *Lancet* 1993;342:1274–1275.
95. Bettaieb A, Fromont P, Louache F, et al. Presence of cross-reactive antibody between human immunodeficiency virus (HIV) and platelet glycoproteins in HIV-related immune thrombocytopenic purpura. *Blood* 1992;80:162–169.
96. Nardi MA, Liu LX, Karpatkin S. GPIIIa-(49-66) is a major pathophysiologically relevant antigenic determinant for anti-platelet GPIIIa of HIV-1-related immunologic thrombocytopenia. *Proc Natl Acad Sci U S A* 1997;94:7589–7594.
97. Cole JL, Marzec UM, Gunthel CJ, et al. Ineffective platelet production in thrombocytopenic human immunodeficiency virus-infected patients. *Blood* 1998;91:3239–3246.
98. Nardi M, Karpatkin S. Antiidiotype antibody against platelet anti-GPIIIa contributes to the regulation of thrombocytopenia in HIV-1-ITP patients. *J Exp Med* 2000;191:2093–2100.
99. Bender BS, Frank MM, Lawley TJ, et al. Defective reticuloendothelial system Fc-receptor function in patients with acquired immunodeficiency syndrome. *J Infect Dis* 1985;152:409–412.
100. Bender BS, Quinn TC, Spivak JL. Homosexual men with thrombocytopenia have impaired reticuloendothelial system Fc receptor-specific clearance. *Blood* 1987;70:392–395.
101. Kelton JG, Carter CJ, Rodger C, et al. The relationship among platelet-associated IgG, platelet lifespan, and reticuloendothelial cell function. *Blood* 1984;63:1434–1438.
102. Ballem PJ, Belzberg A, Devine DV, et al. Kinetic studies of the mechanism of thrombocytopenia in patients with human immunodeficiency virus infection [see comments]. *N Engl J Med* 1992;327:1779–1784.
103. Zauli G, Catani L, Gibellini D, et al. Impaired survival of bone marrow GPIIb/IIIa+ megakaryocytic cells as an additional pathogenetic mechanism of HIV-1-related thrombocytopenia. *Br J Haematol* 1996;92:711–717.
104. Voulgaropoulou F, Tan B, Soares M, et al. Distinct human immunodeficiency virus strains in the bone marrow are associated with the development of thrombocytopenia. *J Virol* 1999;73:3497–3504.
105. Karpatkin S, Nardi MA. Immunologic thrombocytopenic purpura in human immunodeficiency virus—seropositive patients with hemophilia. Comparison with patients with classic autoimmune thrombocytopenic purpura, homosexuals with thrombocytopenia, and narcotic addicts with thrombocytopenia. *J Lab Clin Med* 1988;111:441–448.
106. Ragni M, Bontempo F, Myers D, et al. Hemorrhagic sequelae of immune thrombocytopenic purpura (ITP) in HIV infected hemophiliacs. *Blood* 1989;90:127a(abstr).
107. Schmitt FA, Bigley JW, McKinnis R, et al. Neuropsychological outcome of zidovudine (AZT) treatment of patients with AIDS and AIDS-related complex. *N Engl J Med* 1988;319:1573–1578.
108. Richman DD, Fischl MA, Grieco MH, et al. The toxicity of azidothymidine (AZT) in the treatment of patients with AIDS and AIDS-related complex. A double-blind, placebo-controlled trial. *N Engl J Med* 1987;317:192–197.
109. Pottage JC, Benson CA, Spear JB, et al. Treatment of human immunodeficiency virus-related thrombocytopenia with zidovudine. *JAMA* 1988;260:3045–3048.
110. Gottlieb MS, Wolfe PR, Chafey S. Response of AIDS-related thrombocytopenia to intravenous and oral azidothymidine (3'-azido-3'-deoxythymidine). *AIDS Res Hum Retroviruses* 1987;3:109–114.
111. Fischl MA, Parker CB, Pettinelli C, et al. A randomized controlled trial of a reduced daily dose of zidovudine in patients with the acquired immunodeficiency syndrome. The AIDS Clinical Trials Group. *N Engl J Med* 1990;323:1009–1014.
112. Oksenhendler E, Bierling P, Ferchal F, et al. Zidovudine for thrombocytopenic purpura related to human immunodeficiency virus (HIV) infection. *Ann Intern Med* 1989;110:365–368.
113. The Swiss Group for Clinical Studies on the Acquired Immunodeficiency Syndrome (AIDS). Zidovudine for the treatment of thrombocytopenia associated with human immunodeficiency virus (HIV). A prospective study. *Ann Intern Med* 1988;109:718–721.
114. Immune thrombocytopenia in homosexual men. *Ann Intern Med* 1986;104:583–584.
115. Ratner L. Human immunodeficiency virus-associated autoimmune thrombocytopenic purpura: a review. *Am J Med* 1989;86:194–198.
116. Walsh C, Krigel R, Lennette E, et al. Thrombocytopenia in homosexual patients. Prognosis, response to therapy, and prevalence of antibody to the retrovirus associated with the acquired immunodeficiency syndrome. *Ann Intern Med* 1985;103:542–545.
117. Goldsweig HG, Grossman R, William D. Thrombocytopenia in homosexual men. *Am J Hematol* 1986;21:243–247.
118. Costello C, Treacy M, Lai L. Treatment of immune thrombocytopenic purpura in homosexual men. *Scand J Haematol* 1986;36:507–510.
119. Schneider PA, Abrams DI, Rayner AA, et al. Immunodeficiency-associated thrombocytopenic purpura (IDTP). Response to splenectomy. *Arch Surg* 1987;122:1175–1178.
120. Barbui T, Cortelazzo S, Minetti B, et al. Does splenectomy enhance risk of AIDS in HIV-positive patients with chronic thrombocytopenia? *Lancet* 1987;2:342–343.
121. Beard J, Savidge GF. High-dose intravenous immunoglobulin and splenectomy for the treatment of HIV-related immune thrombocytopenia in patients with severe haemophilia. *Br J Haematol* 1988;68:303–306.
122. Pollak AN, Janinis J, Green D. Successful intravenous immune globulin therapy for human immunodeficiency virus-associated thrombocytopenia. *Arch Intern Med* 1988;148:695–697.
123. Tertian G, Boue F, Lebras P, et al. Thrombocytopenia in ARC: management with high dose IV IgG. *Vox Sang* 1987;52:170.
124. Oksenhendler E, Bierling P, Brossard Y, et al. Anti-RH immunoglobulin therapy for human immunodeficiency virus-related immune thrombocytopenic purpura. *Blood* 1988;71:1499–1502.
125. Biniek R, Malessa R, Brockmeyer NH, et al. Anti-Rh(D) immunoglobulin for AIDS-related thrombocytopenia. *Lancet* 1986;2:627.

126. Fischl MA, Ahn YS, Klimas N, et al. Use of Danazol in autoimmune thrombocytopenia purpura associated with the acquired immunodeficiency syndrome. *Blood* 1984;64:236a(abstr).

127. Mintzer DM, Real FX, Jovino L, et al. Treatment of Kaposi's sarcoma and thrombocytopenia with vincristine in patients with the acquired immunodeficiency syndrome. *Ann Intern Med* 1985;102:200–202.

128. Ellis ME, Neal KR, Leen CL, et al. Alfa-2a recombinant interferon in HIV associated thrombocytopenia. *Br Med J (Clin Res Ed)* 1987;295:1519.

129. Lever AM, Brook MG, Yap I, et al. Treatment of thrombocytopenia with alfa interferon. *Br Med J (Clin Res Ed)* 1987;295:1519–1520.

130. Durand JM, Lefevre P, Hovette P, et al. Dapsone for thrombocytopenic purpura related to human immunodeficiency virus infection. *Am J Med* 1991;90:675–677.

131. Gill PS, Loureiro C, Bernstein-Singer M, et al. Clinical effect of glucocorticoids on Kaposi sarcoma related to the acquired immunodeficiency syndrome (AIDS). *Ann Intern Med* 1989;110:937–940.

132. Boccia RV, Gelmann EP, Baker CC, et al. A hemolytic-uremic syndrome with the acquired immunodeficiency syndrome. *Ann Intern Med* 1984;101:716–717.

133. Jokela J, Flynn T, Henry K. Thrombotic thrombocytopenic purpura in a human immunodeficiency virus (HIV)-seropositive homosexual man. *Am J Hematol* 1987;25:341–343.

134. Sutor GC, Schmidt RE, Albrecht H. Thrombotic microangiopathies and HIV infection: report of two typical cases, features of HUS and TTP, and review of the literature. *Infection* 1999;27:12–15.

135. Avery RA, Denunzio TM, Craig DB. Thrombotic thrombocytopenic purpura associated with HIV and visceral Kaposi's sarcoma treated with plasmapheresis and chemotherapy. *Am J Hematol* 1998;58:148–149.

136. Yospur LS, Sun NC, Figueroa P, et al. Concurrent thrombotic thrombocytopenic purpura and immune thrombocytopenic purpura in an HIV-positive patient: case report and review of the literature. *Am J Hematol* 1996;51:73–78.

137. Nosari AM, Landonio G, Caggese L, et al. Thrombotic thrombocytopenic purpura associated with HIV infection: report of two cases. *Haematologica* 1994;79:280–282.

138. Tsai HM, Lian EC. Antibodies to von Willebrand factor-cleaving protease in acute thrombotic thrombocytopenic purpura. *N Engl J Med* 1998;339:1585–1594.

139. Toy PT, Reid ME, Burns M. Positive direct antiglobulin test associated with hyperglobulinemia in acquired immunodeficiency syndrome (AIDS). *Am J Hematol* 1985;19:145–150.

140. McGinniss MH, Macher AM, Rook AH, et al. Red cell autoantibodies in patients with acquired immune deficiency syndrome. *Transfusion* 1986;26:405–409.

141. Simpson MB, Delong N. Autoimmune hemolytic anemia in a patient with acquired immunodeficiency syndrome. *Blood* 1987;705:127.

142. Burkes RL, Cohen H, Kramer M, et al. Low serum cobalamin levels occur frequently in the acquired immune deficiency syndrome and related disorders. *Eur J Haematol* 1987;38:141–147.

143. Remacha AF, Cadafalch J. Cobalamin deficiency in patients infected with the human immunodeficiency virus. *Semin Hematol* 1999;36:75–87.

144. Wang Z, Goldberg MA, Scadden DT. HIV-1 suppresses erythropoietin production in vitro. *Exp Hematol* 1993;21:683–688.

145. Frickhofen N, Abkowitz J, King L, et al. Red cell aplasia due to persistent B19 parvovirus infections in HIV-infected patients and its treatment with immunoglobulin. *Blood* 1989;74:44a(abstr).

146. Walker RE, Parker RI, Kovacs JA, et al. Anemia and erythropoiesis in patients with the acquired immunodeficiency syndrome (AIDS) and Kaposi sarcoma treated with zidovudine. *Ann Intern Med* 1988;108:372–376.

147. Forester G. Profound cytopenia secondary to azidothymidine. *N Engl J Med* 1987;317:772.

148. Palefsky JM. Anal human papillomavirus infection and anal cancer in HIV-positive individuals: an emerging problem. *AIDS* 1994;8:283–295.

149. Scadden DT, Wang A, Zsebo KM, et al. In vitro effects of stem-cell factor or interleukin-3 on myelosuppression associated with AIDS. *AIDS* 1994;8:193–196.

150. Dainiak N, Worthington M, Riordan MA, et al. 3'-Azido-3'-deoxythymidine (AZT) inhibits proliferation in vitro of human haematopoietic progenitor cells. *Br J Haematol* 1988;69:299–304.

151. Geene D, Sudre P, Anwar D, et al. Causes of macrocytosis in HIV-infected patients not treated with zidovudine. Swiss HIV Cohort Study. *J Infect* 2000;40:160–163.

152. Henry DH, Beall GN, Benson CA. Recombinant human erythropoietin in the treatment of anemia associated with human immunodeficiency virus (HIV) infection and zidovudine therapy: overview of four clinical trials. *Ann Intern Med* 1992;117:739–748.

153. Phair JP, Abels RI, McNeill MV, et al. Recombinant human erythropoietin treatment: investigational new drug protocol for the anemia of the acquired immunodeficiency syndrome. *Arch Intern Med* 1993;153:2669–2675.

154. Murphy MF, Metcalfe P, Walters AH. Incidence and mechanism of neutropenia and thrombocytopenia in patients with human immunodeficiency virus infection. *Br J Haematol* 1987;66:337–340.

155. Baldwin GC, Gasson JC, Quan SG. Granulocyte macrophage colony-stimulating factor enhances neutrophil function in acquired immunodeficiency syndrome patients. *Proc Natl Acad Sci U S A* 1988;85:2763–2766.

156. Miles SA, Mitsuyasu RT, Moreno M. Combined therapy with recombinant granulocyte-colony-stimulating factor and erythropoietin decreases the hematologic toxicity from zidovudine. *Blood* 1991;77:2109–2117.

157. Groopman JE, Mitsuyasu RT, DeLeo MJ, et al. Effect of recombinant human granulocyte-macrophage colony stimulating factor on myelopoiesis in the acquired immunodeficiency syndrome. *N Engl J Med* 1987;317:593–598.

158. Krown SE, Paredes J, Bundow D, et al. Interferon-alpha, zidovudine, and granulocyte-macrophage colony-stimulating factor: a phase I AIDS Clinical Trials Group study in patients with Kaposi's sarcoma associated with AIDS. *J Clin Oncol* 1992;10:1344–1351.

159. Scadden DT, Levine JD, Hammer S, et al. Recombinant human interleukin-3 for cytopenia in AIDS. *Blood* 1992;80:515a(abstr).

160. Moore RD, Keruly JC, Chaisson RE. Anemia and survival in HIV infection. *J Acquir Immune Defic Syndr Hum Retrovirol* 1998;19:29–33.

161. Revicki DA, Brown RE, Henry DH, et al. Recombinant human erythropoietin and health-related quality of life of AIDS patients with anemia. *J Acquir Immune Defic Syndr* 1994;7:474–484.

162. Levine JD, Allan JD, Tessitore JH. Recombinant human granulocyte-macrophage colony-stimulating factor ameliorates zidovudine-induced neutropenia in patients with acquired immunodeficiency syndrome (AIDS)/AIDS-related complex. *Blood* 1991;78:3148–3154.

163. Scadden DT, Bering HA, Levine JD, et al. Granulocyte-macrophage colony-stimulating factor mitigates the neutropenia of combined interferon alfa and zidovudine treatment of acquired immune deficiency syndrome-associated Kaposi's sarcoma [published erratum appears in *J Clin Oncol* 1992;10(2):346.] [see comments]. *J Clin Oncol* 1991;9:802–808.

164. Pluda JM, Yarchoan R, Smith PD, et al. Subcutaneous recombinant granulocyte-macrophage colony-stimulating factor used as a single agent and in an alternating regimen with azidothymidine in leukopenic patients with severe human immunodeficiency virus infection [see comments]. *Blood* 1990;76:463–472.

165. Hardy WD. Combined ganciclovir and recombinant human granulocyte-macrophage colony-stimulating factor in the treatment of cytomegalovirus retinitis in AIDS patients. *J Acquir Immune Defic Syndr* 1991;4[Suppl]:S22.

166. Kaplan LD, Kahn JO, Crowe S, et al. Clinical and virologic effects of recombinant human granulocyte-macrophage colony-stimulating factor in patients receiving chemotherapy for human immunodeficiency virus-associated non-Hodgkin's lymphoma: results of a randomized trial. *J Clin Oncol* 1991;9:929–940.

167. Davey RT Jr, Davey VJ, Metcalf JA, et al. A phase I/II trial of zidovudine, interferon-alpha, and granulocyte- macrophage colony-stimulating factor in the treatment of human immunodeficiency virus type 1 infection. *J Infect Dis* 1991;164:43–52.

168. Angel JB, High K, Rhame F, et al. Phase III study of granulocyte-macrophage colony-stimulating factor in advanced HIV disease: effect on infections, CD4 cell counts and HIV suppression. Leukine/HIV Study Group. *AIDS* 2000;14:387–395.

169. Kuritzkes DR, Parenti D, Ward DJ, et al. Filgrastim prevents severe neutropenia and reduces infective morbidity in patients with advanced HIV infection: results of a randomized, multicenter, controlled trial. G-CSF 930101 Study Group. *AIDS* 1998;12:65–74.

170. Aladdin H, Ullum H, Dam Nielsen S, et al. Granulocyte colony-stimulating factor increases CD4+ T cell counts of human immunodeficiency virus-infected patients receiving stable, highly active antiretroviral therapy: results from a randomized, placebo-controlled trial. *J Infect Dis* 2000;181:1148–1152.

171. Hammer SM, Gillis JM, Groopman JE, et al. In vitro modification of human immunodeficiency virus infection by granulocyte-macrophage colony-stimulating factor and gamma interferon. *Proc Natl Acad Sci U S A* 1986;83:8734–8738.

172. Koyanagi Y, O'Brien WA, Zhao JQ, et al. Cytokines alter production of HIV-1 from primary mononuclear phagocytes. *Science* 1988;241:1673–1675.

173. Perno CF, Cooney DA, Gao WY, et al. Effects of bone marrow stimulatory cytokines on human immunodeficiency virus replication and the antiviral activity of dideoxynucleosides in cultures of monocyte/macrophages. *Blood* 1992;80:995–1003.

174. Perno CF, Yarchoan R, Cooney DA, et al. Replication of human immunodeficiency virus in monocytes. Granulocyte/macrophage colony-stimulating factor (GM-CSF) potentiates viral production yet enhances the antiviral effect mediated by 3'-azido-2'3'-dideoxythymidine (AZT) and other dideoxynucleoside congeners of thymidine. *J Exp Med* 1989;169:933–951.

175. Schuitemaker H, Kootstra NA, van Oers MH, et al. Induction of monocyte proliferation and HIV expression by IL-3 does not interfere with anti-viral activity of zidovudine. *Blood* 1990;76:1490–1493.

176. Campbell TB, Sevin A, Coombs RW, et al. Changes in human immunodeficiency virus type 1 virus load during mobilization and harvesting of hemopoietic progenitor cells. Adult AIDS Clinical Trials Group 285 Study Team. *Blood* 2000;95:48–55.

177. Turbat-Herrera EA, Hancock C, Cabello-Inchausti B, et al. Plasma cell hyperplasia and monoclonal paraproteinemia in human immunodeficiency virus-infected patients. *Arch Pathol Lab Med* 1993;117:497–501.

178. Sala PG, Mazzolini S, Tonutti E, et al. Monoclonal immunoglobulins in HTLV III-positive sera [Letter]. *Clin Chem* 1986;32:574.

179. Papadopoulos NM, Lane HC, Costello R, et al. Oligoclonal immunoglobulins in patients with the acquired immunodeficiency syndrome. *Clin Immunol Immunopathol* 1985;35:43–46.

180. Crapper RM, Deam DR, Mackay IR. Paraproteinemias in homosexual men with HIV infection. Lack of association with abnormal clinical or immunologic findings. *Am J Clin Pathol* 1987;88:348–351.

181. Lefrere JJ, Fine JM, Lambin P, et al. Monoclonal gammopathies in asymptomatic HIV-seropositive patients. *Clin Chem* 1987;33:1697–1698.

182. Kouns DM, Marty AM, Sharpe RW. Oligoclonal bands in serum protein electrophoretograms of individuals with human immunodeficiency virus antibodies. *JAMA* 1986;256:2343.

183. Heriot K, Hallquist AE, Tomar RH. Paraproteinemia in patients with acquired immunodeficiency syndrome (AIDS) or lymphadenopathy syndrome (LAS). *Clin Chem* 1985;31:1224–1226.

184. Ng VL, Hwang KM, Reyes GR, et al. High titer anti-HIV antibody reactivity associated with a paraprotein spike in a homosexual male with AIDS related complex. *Blood* 1988;71:1397–1401.

185. Martin CM, Matlow AG, Chew E, et al. Hyperviscosity syndrome in a patient with acquired immunodeficiency syndrome. *Arch Intern Med* 1989;149:1435–1436.

186. Cohen AJ, Philips TM, Kessler CM. Circulating coagulation inhibitors in the acquired immunodeficiency syndrome. *Ann Intern Med* 1986;104:175–180.

187. Bloom EJ, Abrams DI, Rodgers G. Lupus anticoagulant in the acquired immunodeficiency syndrome. *JAMA* 1986;256:491–493.

188. Canoso RT, Zon LI, Groopman JE. Anticardiolipin antibodies associated with HTLV-III infection. *Br J Haematol* 1987;65:495–498.

189. Intrator L, Oksenhendler E, Desforges L, et al. Anticardiolipin antibodies in HIV infected patients with or without immune thrombocytopenic purpura. *Br J Haematol* 1988;68:269–270.

190. Panzer S, Stain C, Hartl H, et al. Anticardiolipin antibodies are elevated in HIV-1 infected haemophiliacs but do not predict for disease progression. *Thromb Haemost* 1989;61:81–85.

191. LeFrere JJ, Gozin D, Modai J, et al. Circulating anticoagulant in the acquired immunodeficiency syndrome. *Ann Intern Med* 1987;107:429–430.

192. Ndimbie OK, Raman BK, Saeed SM. Lupus anticoagulant associated with specific inhibition of factor VII in a patient with AIDS. *Am J Clin Pathol* 1989;91:491–493.

193. Di Prima MA, Sorice M, Vullo V, et al. Anticardiolipin antibody in the acquired immunodeficiency syndrome: a marker of Pneumocystis carinii infection? *J Infect* 1989;18:100–101.

194. Lane HC, Masur H, Edgar LC, et al. Abnormalities of B-cell activation and immunoregulation in patients with the acquired immunodeficiency syndrome. *N Engl J Med* 1983;309:453–458.

195. Yarchoan R, Redfield RR, Broder S. Mechanisms of B cell activation in patients with acquired immunodeficiency syndrome and related disorders. Contribution of antibody-producing B cells, of Epstein-Barr virus-infected B cells, and of immunoglobulin production induced by human T cell lymphotropic virus, type III/lymphadenopathy-associated virus. *J Clin Invest* 1986;78:439–447.

196. Wigzell H. Immunopathogenesis of HIV infection. *J Acquir Immune Defic Syndr* 1988;1:559–565.

197. Mathur-Wagh U, Enlow RW, Spigland I, et al. Longitudinal study of persistent generalised lymphadenopathy in homosexual men: relation to acquired immunodeficiency syndrome. *Lancet* 1984;1:1033–1038.

198. Fishbein DB, Kaplan JE, Spira TJ, et al. Unexplained lymphadenopathy in homosexual men. A longitudinal study. *JAMA* 1985;254:930–935.

199. Abrams DI, Lewis BJ, Beckstead JH, et al. Persistent diffuse lymphadenopathy in homosexual men: endpoint or prodrome? *Ann Intern Med* 1984;100:801–808.

200. Levine AM, Meyer PR, Gill PS, et al. Results of initial lymph node biopsy in homosexual men with generalized lymphadenopathy. *J Clin Oncol* 1986;4:165–169.

201. Abrams DI. AIDS-related lymphadenopathy: the role of biopsy. *J Clin Oncol* 1986;4:126–127.

202. Brynes RK, Chan WC, Spira TJ, et al. Value of lymph node biopsy in unexplained lymphadenopathy in homosexual men. *JAMA* 1983;250:1313–1317.

203. Burns BF, Wood GS, Dorfman RF. The varied histopathology of lymphadenopathy in the homosexual male. *Am J Surg Pathol* 1985;9:287–297.

204. Fernandez R, Mouradian J, Metroka C, et al. The prognostic value of histopathology in persistent generalized lymphadenopathy in homosexual men. *N Engl J Med* 1983;309:185–186.

205. Ewing EP, Chandler FW, Spira TJ, et al. Primary lymph node pathology in AIDS and AIDS-related lymphadenopathy. *Arch Pathol Lab Med* 1985;109:977–981.

206. Ioachim HL, Lerner CW, Tapper ML. The lymphoid lesions associated with the acquired immunodeficiency syndrome. *Am J Surg Pathol* 1983;7:543–553.

207. Wood GS, Garcia CF, Dorfman RF, et al. The immunohistology of follicle lysis in lymph node biopsies from homosexual men. *Blood* 1985;66:1092–1097.

208. O'Hara CT. The lymphoid and hematopoietic systems. In: Oh CJ, Harawi SJ, eds. *Pathology and pathophysiology of AIDS and HIV-related diseases.* London: Chapman & Hall, 1989:135.

209. Levine AM, Gill PS, Krailo M, et al. Natural history of persistent, generalized lymphadenopathy (PGL) in gay men: risk of lymphoma and factors associated with development of lymphoma. *Blood* 1986;68:5477(abstr).

210. Schnittman SM, Psallidopoulos MC, Lane HC, et al. The reservoir for HIV-1 in human peripheral blood is a T cell that maintains expression of CD4. *Science* 1989;245:305–308.

211. Psallidopoulos MC, Schnittman SM, Thompson LM, et al. Integrated proviral human immunodeficiency virus type 1 is present in CD4+ peripheral blood lymphocytes in healthy seropositive individuals. *J Virol* 1989;63:4626–4631.

212. Geijtenbeek TB, Torensma R, van Vliet SJ, et al. Identification of DC-SIGN, a novel dendritic cell-specific ICAM-3 receptor that supports primary immune responses. *Cell* 2000;100:575–585.

213. Zhang ZQ, Schuler T, Cavert W, et al. Reversibility of the pathological changes in the follicular dendritic cell network with treatment of HIV-1 infection. *Proc Natl Acad Sci U S A* 1999;96:5169–5172.

214. Hoover RN. Lymphoma risks in populations with altered immunity—a search for mechanism. *Cancer Res* 1992;52[19 Suppl]:5477S–5478S.

215. Pluda JM, Yarchoan R, Jaffe ES, et al. Development of non-Hodgkin lymphoma in a cohort of patients with severe human immunodeficiency virus (HIV) infection on long-term antiretroviral therapy. *Ann Intern Med* 1990;113:276–282.

216. Moore RD, Kessler H, Richman DD, et al. Non-Hodgkin's lymphoma in patients with advanced HIV infection treated with zidovudine. *JAMA* 1991;265:2208–2211.

217. Gail MH, Pluda JM, Rabkin CS, et al. Projections of the incidence of non-Hodgkin's lymphoma related to acquired immunodeficiency syndrome. *J Natl Cancer Inst* 1991;83:695–701.

218. Birx DL, Redfield RR, Tosato G. Defective regulation of Epstein-Barr virus infection in patients with acquired immunodeficiency syndrome (AIDS) or AIDS-related disorders. *N Engl J Med* 1986;314:874–879.

219. Petersen JM, Tubbs RR, Savage RA, et al. Small noncleaved B cell Burkitt-like lymphoma with chromosome t(8;14) translocation and Epstein-Barr virus nuclear-associated antigen in a homosexual man with acquired immune deficiency syndrome. *Am J Med* 1985;78:141–148.

220. Subar M, Neri A, Inghirami G, et al. Frequent c-myc oncogene activation and infrequent presence of Epstein-Barr virus genome in AIDS-associated lymphoma. *Blood* 1988;72:667–671.

221. Shibata D, Weiss LM, Nathwani BN, et al. Epstein-Barr virus in benign lymph node biopsies from individuals infected with the human immunodeficiency virus is associated with concurrent or subsequent development of non-Hodgkin's lymphoma. *Blood* 1991;77:1527–1533.

222. Levine AM, Sullivan-Halley J, Pike MC, et al. Human immunodeficiency virus-related lymphoma. Prognostic factors predictive of survival [see comments]. *Cancer* 1991;68:2466–2472.

223. Knowles DM. Immunodeficiency-associated lymphoproliferative disorders. *Mod Pathol* 1999;12:200–217.

224. Levine A, Shibata D, Weiss L. Molecular characteristics of intermediate/high (I/H) grade lymphomas (NHL) arising in HIV-positive vs. HIV-negative PTS: preliminary data from a population (POP) based study in the county of Los Angeles. *Blood* 1992;80:1028.

225. Hamilton-Dutoit SJ, Pallesen G, Franzmann MB, et al. AIDS-related lymphoma. Histopathology, immunophenotype, and association with Epstein-Barr virus as demonstrated by in situ nucleic acid hybridization. *Am J Pathol* 1991;138:149–163.

226. Hamilton-Dutoit SJ, Pallesen G, Karkov J, et al. Identification of EBV-DNA in tumour cells of AIDS-related lymphomas by in-situ hybridisation [Letter]. *Lancet* 1989;1:554–562.

227. Knowles DM. Etiology and pathogenesis of AIDS-related non-Hodgkin's lymphoma. *Hematol Oncol Clin North Am* 1996;10:1081–1109.

228. Knowles DM. Molecular pathology of acquired immunodeficiency syndrome-related non-Hodgkin's lymphoma. *Semin Diagn Pathol* 1977;14:67–82.

229. Gaidano G, Lo Coco F, Ye BH, et al. Rearrangements of the BCL-6 gene in acquired immunodeficiency syndrome-associated non-Hodgkin's lymphoma: association with diffuse large-cell subtype. *Blood* 1994;84:397–402.

230. Shiramizu B, Herndier B, Meeker T, et al. Molecular and immunophenotypic characterization of AIDS-associated, Epstein-Barr virus-negative, polyclonal lymphoma. *J Clin Oncol* 1992;10:383–389.

231. Levine AM. Acquired immunodeficiency syndrome-related lymphoma. *Blood* 1992;80:8–20.

232. Pelicci PG, Knowles DM, Arlin ZA, et al. Multiple monoclonal B cell expansions and c-myc oncogene rearrangements in acquired immune deficiency syndrome-related lymphoproliferative disorders. Implications for lymphomagenesis. *J Exp Med* 1986;164:2049–2060.

233. Ballerini P, Gaidano G, Gong JZ, et al. Multiple genetic lesions in acquired immunodeficiency syndrome-related non-Hodgkin's lymphoma. *Blood* 1993;81:166–176.

234. Chaganti RS, Jhanwar SC, Koziner B, et al. Specific translocations characterize Burkitt's-like lymphoma of homosexual men with the acquired immunodeficiency syndrome. *Blood* 1983;61:1265–1268.

235. Haluska FG, Russo G, Kant J, et al. Molecular resemblance of an AIDS-associated lymphoma and endemic Burkitt lymphomas: implications for their pathogenesis. *Proc Natl Acad Sci U S A* 1989;86:8907–8911.

236. Neri A, Barriga F, Knowles DM, et al. Different regions of the immunoglobulin heavy-chain locus are involved in chromosomal translocations in distinct pathogenetic forms of Burkitt lymphoma. *Proc Natl Acad Sci U S A* 1988;85:2748–2752.

237. Rabkin CS, Yang Q, Goedert JJ, et al. Chemokine and chemokine receptor gene variants and risk of non-Hodgkin's lymphoma in human immunodeficiency virus-1-infected individuals. *Blood* 1999;93:1838–1842.

238. Matthews GV, Bower M, Mandalia S, et al. Changes in acquired immunodeficiency syndrome-related lymphoma since the introduction of highly active antiretroviral therapy. *Blood* 2000;96:2730–2734.

239. Mocroft A, Katlama C, Johnson AM, et al. AIDS across Europe, 1994–98: the EuroSIDA study. *Lancet* 2000;356:291–296.

240. Jacobson LP, Yamashita TE, Detels R, et al. Impact of potent antiretroviral therapy on the incidence of Kaposi's sarcoma and non-Hodgkin's lymphomas among HIV-1-infected individuals. Multicenter AIDS Cohort Study. *J Acquir Immune Defic Syndr* 1999;21[Suppl 1]:S34–S41.

241. Rabkin CS, Testa MA, Huang J, et al. Kaposi's sarcoma and non-Hodgkin's lymphoma incidence trends in AIDS Clinical Trial Group study participants. *J Acquir Immune Defic Syndr* 1999;21[Suppl 1]:S31–S33.

242. Buchbinder SP, Holmberg SD, Scheer S, et al. Combination antiretroviral therapy and incidence of AIDS-related malignancies. *J Acquir Immune Defic Syndr* 1999;21[Suppl 1]:S23–26.

243. Grulich AE. AIDS-associated non-Hodgkin's lymphoma in the era of highly active antiretroviral therapy. *J Acquir Immune Defic Syndr* 1999;21[Suppl 1]:S27–S30.

244. Sparano JA, Anand K, Desai J, et al. Effect of highly active antiretroviral therapy on the incidence of HIV-associated malignancies at an urban medical center. *J Acquir Immune Defic Syndr* 1999;21[Suppl 1]:S18–S22.

245. Presant CA, Gala K, Wiseman C, et al. Human immunodeficiency virus-associated T-cell lymphoblastic lymphoma in AIDS. *Cancer* 1987;60:1459–1461.
246. Ruff P, Bagg A, Papadopoulos K. Precursor T-cell lymphoma associated with human immunodeficiency virus type 1 (HIV-1) infection. First reported case. *Cancer* 1989;64:39–42.
247. Tirelli U, Serraino D, Carbone A. Hodgkin disease and HIV [Letter; Comment]. *Ann Intern Med* 1993;118:313; discussion 313–314.
248. Shibata D, Brynes RK, Rabinowitz A, et al. Human T-cell lymphotropic virus type I (HTLV-I)-associated adult T-cell leukemia-lymphoma in a patient infected with human immunodeficiency virus type 1 (HIV-1). *Ann Intern Med* 1989;111:871–875.
249. Sternlieb J, Mintzer D, Kwa D, et al. Peripheral T-cell lymphoma in a patient with the acquired immunodeficiency syndrome. *Am J Med* 1988;85:445.
250. Gonzalez-Clemente JM, Ribera JM, Campo E, et al. Ki-1+ anaplastic large-cell lymphoma of T-cell origin in an HIV-infected patient. *AIDS* 1991;5:751–755.
251. Ciobanu N, Andreeff M, Safai B, et al. Lymphoblastic neoplasia in a homosexual patient with Kaposi's sarcoma. *Ann Intern Med* 1983;98:151–155.
252. Gold JE, Ghali V, Gold S, et al. Angiocentric immunoproliferative lesion/T-cell non-Hodgkin's lymphoma and the acquired immune deficiency syndrome: a case report and review of the literature. *Cancer* 1990;66:2407–2413.
253. Karp JE, Broder S. The pathogenesis of AIDS lymphomas: a foundation for addressing the challenges of therapy and prevention. *Leuk Lymphoma* 1992; 8:167–188.
254. Shiramizu B, Herndier BG, McGrath MS. Identification of a common clonal human immunodeficiency virus integration site in human immunodeficiency virus-associated lymphomas. *Cancer Res* 1994;54:2069–2072.
255. Davi F, Delecluse HJ, Guiet P, et al. Burkitt-like lymphoma in AIDS patients: characterization within a series of 103 human immunodeficiency virus-associated non-Hodgkin's lymphomas. Burkitt's Lymphoma Study Group. *J Clin Oncol* 1998;16:3788–3795.
256. Gaidano G, Pastore C, Gloghini A, et al. Genetic heterogeneity of AIDS-related small non-cleaved cell lymphoma. *Br J Haematol* 1997;98:726–732.
257. Kalter SP, Riggs SA, Cabanillas F, et al. Aggressive non-Hodgkin's lymphomas in immunocompromised homosexual males. *Blood* 1985;66:655–659.
258. Knowles DM, Chamulak GA, Subar M. Lymphoid neoplasia associated with the acquired immunodeficiency syndrome (AIDS): The New York University Medical Center experience with 105 patients. *Ann Intern Med* 1988;108:744–753.
259. Kalter SP, Riggs SA, Cabanillas F. Aggressive non-Hodgkin's lymphoma in immunocompromised homosexual males. *Blood* 1985;665–659.
260. Ioachim HL, Dorsett B, Cronin W, et al. Acquired immunodeficiency syndrome-associated lymphomas: clinical, pathologic, immunologic, and viral characteristics of 111 cases. *Hum Pathol* 1991;22:659–673.
261. Ziegler JL, Beckstead JA, Volberding PA, et al. Non-Hodgkin's lymphoma in 90 homosexual men. Relation to generalized lymphadenopathy and the acquired immunodeficiency syndrome. *N Engl J Med* 1984;311:565–570.
262. Lowenthal DA, Straus DJ, Campbell SW, et al. AIDS-related lymphoid neoplasia. The Memorial Hospital experience. *Cancer* 1988;61:2325–2337.
263. The Non-Hodgkin's Lymphoma Pathologic Classification Project. National Cancer Institute sponsored study of classifications of non-Hodgkin's lymphomas: summary and description of a working formulation for clinical usage. *Cancer* 1982;49:2112–2135.
264. Levine AM, Wernz JC, Kaplan L. Low-dose chemotherapy with central nervous system prophylaxis and zidovudine maintenance in AIDS-related lymphoma. *JAMA* 1991;266:84–88.
265. Gill PS, Levine AM, Meyer PR, et al. Primary central nervous system lymphoma in homosexual men. Clinical, immunologic, and pathologic features. *Am J Med* 1985;78:742–748.
266. Gill PS, Levine AM, Krailo M. AIDS-related malignant lymphoma: results of prospective treatment trials. *J Clin Oncol* 1987;5:1322–1328.
267. Bermudez MA, Grant KM, Rodvien R, et al. Non-Hodgkin's lymphoma in a population with or at risk for acquired immunodeficiency syndrome: indications for intensive chemotherapy. *Am J Med* 1989;86:71–76.
268. Kaplan LD, Abrams DI, Feigal E. AIDS-associated non-Hodgkin's lymphoma in San Francisco. *JAMA* 1989;261:719–724.
269. Kaplan MH, Susin M, Pahwa SG, et al. Neoplastic complications of HTLV-III infection. Lymphomas and solid tumors. *Am J Med* 1987;82:389–396.
270. Remick SC, McSharry JJ, Wolf BC. Novel oral combination chemotherapy in the treatment of intermediate-grade and high-grade AIDS-related non-Hodgkin's lymphoma. *J Clin Oncol* 1993;11:1691–1702.
271. Freter CE. Acquired immunodeficiency syndrome-associated lymphomas. *J Natl Cancer Inst Monogr* 1990;10:45–54.
272. von Gunten CF, Von Roenn JH. Clinical aspects of human immunodeficiency virus-related lymphoma. *Curr Opin Oncol* 1992;4:894–899.
273. Raphael M, Gentilhomme O, Tulliez M, et al. Histopathologic features of high-grade non-Hodgkin's lymphomas in acquired immunodeficiency syndrome. The French Study Group of Pathology for Human Immunodeficiency Virus-Associated Tumors. *Arch Pathol Lab Med* 1991;115:15–20.
274. Burkes RL, Meyer PR, Gill PS, et al. Rectal lymphoma in homosexual men. *Arch Intern Med* 1986;146:913–915.
275. Levine AM, Seneviratne L, Espina BM, et al. Evolving characteristics of AIDS-related lymphoma. *Blood* 2000;96:4084–4090.
276. Cingolani A, Gastaldi R, Fassone L, et al. Epstein-Barr virus infection is predictive of CNS involvement in systemic AIDS-related non-Hodgkin's lymphomas [In Process Citation]. *J Clin Oncol* 2000;18:3325–3330.
277. Straus DJ, Huang J, Testa MA, et al. Prognostic factors in the treatment of human immunodeficiency virus-associated non-Hodgkin's lymphoma: analysis of AIDS Clinical Trials Group protocol 142—low-dose versus standard-dose m-BACOD plus granulocyte-macrophage colony-stimulating factor. National Institute of Allergy and Infectious Diseases. *J Clin Oncol* 1998;16:3601–3606.
278. Shipp MA, Harrington DP, Klatt MM, et al. Identification of major prognostic subgroups of patients with large-cell lymphoma treated with m-BACOD or M-BACOD. *Ann Intern Med* 1986;104:757–765.
279. Navarro JT, Ribera JM, Oriol A, et al. International prognostic index is the best prognostic factor for survival in patients with AIDS-related non-Hodgkin's lymphoma treated with CHOP. A multivariate study of 46 patients. *Haematologica* 1998;83:508–513.
280. Vaccher E, Tirelli U, Spina M, et al. Age and serum lactate dehydrogenase level are independent prognostic factors in human immunodeficiency virus-related non-Hodgkin's lymphomas: a single-institute study of 96 patients. *J Clin Oncol* 1996;14:2217–2223.
281. Tirelli U, Errante D, Dolcetti R, et al. Hodgkin's disease and human immunodeficiency virus infection: clinicopathologic and virologic features of 114 patients from the Italian Cooperative Group on AIDS and Tumors. *J Clin Oncol* 1995;13:1758–1767.
282. Kaplan LD, Shiramizu B, Herndier B, et al. Influence of molecular characteristics on clinical outcome in human immunodeficiency virus-associated non-Hodgkin's lymphoma: identification of a subgroup with favorable clinical outcome. *Blood* 1995;85:1727–1735.
283. Kaplan LD, Straus DJ, Testa MA, et al. Low-dose compared with standard-dose m-BACOD chemotherapy for non-Hodgkin's lymphoma associated with human immunodeficiency virus infection. *N Engl J Med* 1997;336:1641–1648.
284. Cesarman E, Chang Y, Moore PS, et al. Kaposi's sarcoma-associated herpesvirus-like DNA sequences in AIDS-related body-cavity-based lymphomas [see comments]. *N Engl J Med* 1995;332:1186–1191.
285. Nador RG, Cesarman E, Chadburn A, et al. Primary effusion lymphoma: a distinct clinicopathologic entity associated with the Kaposi's sarcoma-associated herpes virus. *Blood* 1996;88:645–656.
286. Karcher DS, Alkan S. Human herpesvirus-8-associated body cavity-based lymphoma in human immunodeficiency virus-infected patients: a unique B-cell neoplasm. *Hum Pathol* 1997;28:801–808.
287. Delecluse HJ, Anagnostopoulos I, Dallenbach F, et al. Plasmablastic lymphomas of the oral cavity: a new entity associated with the human immunodeficiency virus infection. *Blood* 1997;89:1413–1420.
288. Carbone A, Gaidano G, Gloghini A, et al. AIDS-related plasmablastic lymphomas of the oral cavity and jaws: a diagnostic dilemma. *Ann Otol Rhinol Laryngol* 1999;108:95–99.
289. Antinori A, Ammassari A, De Luca A, et al. Diagnosis of AIDS-related focal brain lesions: a decision-making analysis based on clinical and neuroradiologic characteristics combined with polymerase chain reaction assays in CSF. *Neurology* 1997;48:687–694.
290. Cingolani A, De Luca A, Larocca LM, et al. Minimally invasive diagnosis of acquired immunodeficiency syndrome-related primary central nervous system lymphoma [see comments]. *J Natl Cancer Inst* 1998;90:364–369.
291. Luft BJ, Hafner R, Korzun AH, et al. Toxoplasmic encephalitis in patients with the acquired immunodeficiency syndrome. Members of the ACTG 077p/ANRS 009 Study Team. *N Engl J Med* 1993;329:995–1000.
292. Contu L, LaNasa G, Arras M, et al. Allogeneic bone marrow transplantation combined with multiple anti-HIV-1 treatment in a case of AIDS. *Bone Marrow Transplant* 1993;12:669–671.
293. Aviles A, Nambo MJ, Halabe J. Treatment of acquired immunodeficiency syndrome-related lymphoma with a standard chemotherapy regimen. *Ann Hematol* 1999;78:9–12.
294. Kaplan LD, Straus DJ, Testa MA, et al. Low-dose compared with standard-dose m-BACOD chemotherapy for non-Hodgkin's lymphoma associated with human immunodeficiency virus infection. National Institute of Allergy and Infectious Diseases AIDS Clinical Trials Group. *N Engl J Med* 1997;336: 1641–1648.
295. Gisselbrecht C, Gabarre J, Spina G, et al. Therapy of HIV related non-Hodgkin's lymphoma: an European multicentric randomized study in patients stratified according to their prognostic factors. *Proc ASCO* 1999;18:55(abstr).
296. Gisselbrecht C, Oksenhendler E, Tirelli U. Human immunodeficiency virus-related lymphoma: treatment with intensive combination chemotherapy. *Am J Med* 1993;95:188–196.
297. Sparano JA, Wiernik PH, Hu X, et al. Pilot trial of infusional cyclophosphamide, doxorubicin, and etoposide plus didanosine and filgrastim in patients with human immunodeficiency virus-associated non-Hodgkin's lymphoma. *J Clin Oncol* 1996;14:3026–3035.
298. Sparano JA, Lee S, Chen M, et al. Phase II trial of infusional cyclophosphamide, doxorubicin, and etoposide (CDE) in HIV-associated non-Hodgkin's lymphoma: an Eastern Cooperative Oncology Group Trial. *Proc Am Soc Clin Oncol* 1999;18:12a(abstr 41).
299. Wilson WH, Bryant G, Bates S, et al. EPOCH chemotherapy: toxicity and efficacy in relapsed and refractory non-Hodgkin's lymphoma. *J Clin Oncol* 1993; 11:1573–1582.
300. Gutierrez M, Chabner BA, Pearson D, et al. Role of a doxorubicin-containing regimen in relapsed and resistant lymphomas: an 8-year follow-up study of EPOCH. *J Clin Oncol* 2000;18:3633–3642.
301. Little R, Pearson D, Steinberg S, et al. Dose-adjusted EPOCH chemotherapy (CT) in previously untreated HIV-associated non-Hodgkin's lymphoma (HIV-NHL), Atlanta, GA, 1999.
302. Gabarre J, Leblond V, Sutton L, et al. Autologous bone marrow transplantation in relapsed HIV-related non-Hodgkin's lymphoma. *Bone Marrow Transplant* 1996;18:1195–1197.

303. Zaia J, et al. One year results after autologous stem cell transplantation using retrovirus-transduced peripheral blood progenitor cells in HIV-infected subjects. *Blood* 1998;92:665a(abstr).
304. Holland HK, Saral R, Rossi JJ, et al. Allogeneic bone marrow transplantation, zidovudine, and human immunodeficiency virus type 1 (HIV-1) infection. Studies in a patient with non-Hodgkin lymphoma. *Ann Intern Med* 1989;111:973–981.
305. Cooper MH, Maraninchi D, Gastaut JA, et al. HIV infection in autologous and allogeneic bone marrow transplant patients: a retrospective analysis of the Marseille bone marrow transplant population. *J Acquir Immune Defic Syndr* 1993;6:277–284.
306. Vilmer E, Rhodes-Feuillette A, Rabian C, et al. Clinical and immunological restoration in patients with AIDS after marrow transplantation, using lymphocyte transfusions from the marrow donor. *Transplantation* 1987;44:25–29.
307. Hassett JM, Zaroulis CG, Greenberg ML, et al. Bone marrow transplantation in AIDS [Letter]. *N Engl J Med* 1983;309:665.
308. Bowden RA, Coombs RW, Nikora BH, et al. Progression of human immunodeficiency virus type-1 infection after allogeneic marrow transplantation. *Am J Med* 1990;88:49N–52N.
309. Bardini G, Re MC, Rosti G, et al. HIV infection and bone-marrow transplantation [Letter; Comment]. *Lancet* 1991;337:1163–1164.
310. Giri N, Vowels MR, Ziegler JB. Failure of allogeneic bone marrow transplantation to benefit HIV infection. *J Paediatr Child Health* 1992;28:331–333.
311. Torlontano G, DiBartolomeo P, DiGirolamo G, et al. AIDS-related complex treated by antiviral drugs and allogeneic bone marrow transplantation following conditioning protocol with busulphas, cyclophosphamide and cyclosporin. *Haematologica* 1992;77:287–290.
312. Straus D, Redden D, Hamzeh F, et al. Excessive toxicity is not seen with low-dose chemotherapy for HIV-associated non-Hodgkin lymphoma (HIV-NHL) in combination with highly active antiretroviral therapy (HAART). *Blood* 1998;92:624a(abstr).
313. Scadden DT. Epstein-Barr virus, the CNS, and AIDS-related lymphomas: as close as flame to smoke. *J Clin Oncol* 2000;18:3323–3324.
314. Epstein L, DiCarlo F, Joshi V, et al. Primary lymphoma of the CNS in children with AIDS. *Pediatrics* 1988;82:355–363.
315. Baumgartner JE, Rachlin JR, Beckstead JH, et al. Primary central nervous system lymphomas: natural history and response to radiation therapy in 55 patients with acquired immunodeficiency syndrome. *J Neurosurg* 1990;73:206–211.
316. Jacomet C, Girard PM, Lebrette MG, et al. Intravenous methotrexate for primary central nervous system non-Hodgkin's lymphoma in AIDS [see comments]. *AIDS* 1997;11:1725–1730.
317. Raez L, Cabral L, Cai JP, et al. Treatment of AIDS-related primary central nervous system lymphoma with zidovudine, ganciclovir, and interleukin 2. *AIDS Res Hum Retroviruses* 1999;15:713–719.
318. Franken M, Estabrooks A, Cavacini L, et al. Epstein-Barr virus-driven gene therapy for EBV-related lymphomas. *Nat Med* 1996;2:1379–1382.
319. Robertson KD, Hayward SD, Ling PD, et al. Transcriptional activation of the Epstein-Barr virus latency C promoter after 5-azacytidine treatment: evidence that demethylation at a single CpG site is crucial. *Mol Cell Biol* 1995;15:6150–6159.
320. McGowan JP, Shah S. Long-term remission of AIDS-related primary central nervous system lymphoma associated with highly active antiretroviral therapy [Letter]. *AIDS* 1998;12:952–954.
321. Hessol NA, Katz MH, Liu JY, et al. Increased incidence of Hodgkin disease in homosexual men with HIV infection [see comments]. *Ann Intern Med* 1992;117:309–311.
322. Koblin BA, Hessol NA, Zauber AG, et al. Increased incidence of cancer among homosexual men, New York City and San Francisco, 1978–1990. *Am J Epidemiol* 1996;144:916–923.
323. Reynolds P, Saunders LD, Layefsky ME, et al. The spectrum of acquired immunodeficiency syndrome (AIDS)-associated malignancies in San Francisco, 1980–1987. *Am J Epidemiol* 1993;137:19–30.
324. Lyter DW, Bryant J, Thackeray R, et al. Incidence of human immunodeficiency virus-related and nonrelated malignancies in a large cohort of homosexual men. *J Clin Oncol* 1995;13:2540–2546.
325. Grulich A, Wan X, Law M, et al. Rates of non-AIDS defining cancers in people with AIDS. *J AIDS Hum Retrovirol* 1997;14:A18.
326. Serraino D, Pezzotti P, Dorrucci M, et al. Cancer incidence in a cohort of human immunodeficiency virus seroconverters. HIV Italian Seroconversion Study Group [see comments]. *Cancer* 1997;79:1004–1008.
327. Goedert JJ, Cote TR, Virgo P, et al. Spectrum of AIDS-associated malignant disorders [see comments]. *Lancet* 1998;351:1833–1839.
328. Franceschi S, Dal Maso L, Arniani S, et al. Risk of cancer other than Kaposi's sarcoma and non-Hodgkin's lymphoma in persons with AIDS in Italy. Cancer and AIDS Registry Linkage Study. *Br J Cancer* 1998;78:966–970.
329. Scheib RG, Siegel RS. Atypical Hodgkin's disease and the acquired immunodeficiency syndrome. *Ann Intern Med* 1985;102:554.
330. Schoeppel SL, Hoppe RT, Dorfman RF, et al. Hodgkin's disease in homosexual men with generalized lymphadenopathy. *Ann Intern Med* 1985;102:68–70.
331. Robert NJ, Schneiderman H. Hodgkin's disease and the acquired immunodeficiency syndrome. *Ann Intern Med* 1984;101:142–143.
332. Levine AM. Hodgkin's disease in the setting of human immunodeficiency virus infection. *J Natl Cancer Inst Monogr* 1998;23:37–42.
333. Kieff E. Current perspectives on the molecular pathogenesis of virus-induced cancers in human immunodeficiency virus infection and acquired immunodeficiency syndrome. *J Natl Cancer Inst Monogr* 1998;23:7–14.
334. Andrieu JM, Roithmann S, Tourani JM, et al. Hodgkin's disease during HIV1 infection: the French registry experience. French Registry of HIV-associated Tumors. *Ann Oncol* 1993;4:635–641.
335. Monfardini S, Tirelli U, Vaccher E, et al. Hodgkin's disease in 63 intravenous drug users infected with human immunodeficiency virus. Gruppo Italiano Cooperativo AIDS & Tumori (GICAT). *Ann Oncol* 1991;2[Suppl 2]:201–205.
336. Serrano M, Bellas C, Campo E, et al. Hodgkin's disease in patients with antibodies to human immunodeficiency virus. A study of 22 patients. *Cancer* 1990;65:2248–2254.
337. Carbone A, Weiss LM, Gloghini A, et al. Hodgkin's disease: old and recent clinical concepts. *Ann Otol Rhinol Laryngol* 1996;105:751–758.
338. Carbone A, Dolcetti R, Gloghini A, et al. Immunophenotypic and molecular analyses of acquired immune deficiency syndrome-related and Epstein-Barr virus-associated lymphomas: a comparative study. *Hum Pathol* 1996;27:133–146.
339. Spina M, Sandri S, Tirelli U. Hodgkin's disease in HIV-infected individuals [In Process Citation]. *Curr Opin Oncol* 1999;11:522–526.
340. Carbone A, Gloghini A, Larocca LM, et al. Human immunodeficiency virus-associated Hodgkin's disease derives from post-germinal center B cells. *Blood* 1999;93:2319–2326.
341. Carbone A, Gloghini A, Gaidano G, et al. Expression status of BCL-6 and syndecan-1 identifies distinct histogenetic subtypes of Hodgkin's disease. *Blood* 1998;92:2220–2228.
342. Levine AM, Li P, Cheung T, et al. Chemotherapy consisting of doxorubicin, bleomycin, vinblastine, and dacarbazine with granulocyte-colony-stimulating factor in HIV-infected patients with newly diagnosed Hodgkin's disease: a prospective, multi-institutional AIDS clinical trials group study (ACTG 149). *J Acquir Immune Defic Syndr* 2000;24:444–450.
343. Levy R, Colonna P, Tourani JM, et al. Human immunodeficiency virus associated Hodgkin's disease: report of 45 cases from the French Registry of HIV-Associated Tumors. *Leuk Lymphoma* 1995;16:451–456.
344. Rubio R. Hodgkin's disease associated with human immunodeficiency virus infection. A clinical study of 46 cases. Cooperative Study Group of Malignancies Associated with HIV Infection of Madrid. *Cancer* 1994;73:2400–2407.
345. Errante D, Gabarre J, Ridolfo AL, et al. Hodgkin's disease in 35 patients with HIV infection: an experience with epirubicin, bleomycin, vinblastine and prednisone chemotherapy in combination with antiretroviral therapy and primary use of G-CSF. *Ann Oncol* 1999;10:189–195.
346. Spina M, Gabarre J, Fasan M, et al. Stanford V regimen and concomitant highly active antiretroviral therapy is feasible and active in patients with Hodgkin's disease and HIV infection. *AIDS* 2000;14:1457–1458.
347. Oksenhendler E, Duarte M, Soulier J, et al. Multicentric Castleman's disease in HIV infection: a clinical and pathological study of 20 patients. *AIDS* 1996;10:61–67.
348. Herndier BG, Shiramizu BT, Jewett NE, et al. Acquired immunodeficiency syndrome-associated T-cell lymphoma: evidence for human immunodeficiency virus type 1-associated T-cell transformation. *Blood* 1992;79:1768–1774.
349. Soulier J, Grollet L, Oksenhendler E, et al. Kaposi's sarcoma-associated herpes virus-like DNA sequences in multicentric Castleman's disease [see comments]. *Blood* 1995;86:1276–1280.
350. Kumari P, Schechter GP, Saini N, et al. Successful treatment of human immunodeficiency virus-related Castleman's disease with interferon-alpha. *Clin Infect Dis* 2000;31:602–604.
351. Lanzafame M, Carretta G, Trevenzoli M, et al. Successful treatment of Castleman's disease with HAART in two HIV-infected patients. *J Infect* 2000;40:90–91.
352. Karcher DS, Frost AR. The bone marrow in human immunodeficiency virus (HIV)-related disease: morphology and clinical correlation. *Am J Clin Pathol* 1991;95:63–71.
353. Landonio G, Cinque P, Nosari A, et al. Comparison of two dose regimens of zidovudine in an open, randomized, multicentre study for severe HIV-related thrombocytopenia. *AIDS* 1993;7:209–212.
354. Schacter LP, Rozencweig M, Beltangady M, et al. Effects of therapy with didanosine on hematologic parameters in patients with advanced human immunodeficiency virus disease. *Blood* 1992;80:2969–2976.
355. Bussel JB, Pham LC, Aledort L, et al. Maintenance treatment of adults with chronic refractory immune thrombocytopenic purpura using repeated intravenous infusions of gammaglobulin [see comments]. *Blood* 1988;72:121–127.
356. Abrams DI, Kiprov DD, Goedert JJ, et al. Antibodies to human T-lymphotropic virus type III and development of the acquired immunodeficiency syndrome in homosexual men presenting with immune thrombocytopenia. *Ann Intern Med* 1986;104:47–50.
357. Oksenhendler E, Bierling P, Farcet JP, et al. Response to therapy in 37 patients with HIV-related thrombocytopenic purpura. *Br J Haematol* 1987;66:491–495.
358. Marroni M, Gresele P, Landonio G, et al. Interferon-alpha is effective in the treatment of HIV-1-related, severe, zidovudine-resistant thrombocytopenia. A prospective, placebo-controlled, double-blind trial. *Ann Intern Med* 1994;121:423–429.
359. Lord RV, Coleman MJ, Milliken ST. Splenectomy for HIV-related immune thrombocytopenia: comparison with results of splenectomy for non-HIV immune thrombocytopenic purpura. *Arch Surg* 1998;133:205–210.
360. Needleman SW, Sorace J, Poussin-Rosillo H. Low-dose splenic irradiation in the treatment of autoimmune thrombocytopenia in HIV-infected patients. *Ann Intern Med* 1992;116:310–311.

CHAPTER 24

Biology and Classification of Lymphoid Neoplasms

Nancy Lee Harris and Judith A. Ferry

PRINCIPLES OF LYMPHOMA CLASSIFICATION

From the 1980s through the early 1990s, two lymphoma classifications were used in different parts of the world—the Kiel Classification in Europe and the Working Formulation (WF) in the United States (Tables 24-1 and 24-2) (1,2). This lack of consensus on lymphoma classification and terminology caused problems for pathologists and clinicians and caused difficulty in interpreting published studies. In the United States, reliance of oncologists on the WF clinical groups led to the impression that specific disease entities were irrelevant, and only the WF clinical 0 "grades" were important in determining therapy. In addition, in the 1980s and 1990s, many new disease entities were described that were not included in either classification, leading to confusion among pathologists and oncologists about which were "real" diseases, that they should be recognizing in daily practice. Finally, the introduction of the new techniques of immunophenotyping and molecular genetic analysis led to confusion about what, if anything, should be the modern "gold standard" for defining disease entities.

Revised European-American Classification of Lymphoid Neoplasms and the World Health Organization Classification of Neoplasms of the Hematopoietic and Lymphoid Tissues

The International Lymphoma Study Group (ILSG)—consisting of 19 hematopathologists from the United States, Europe, and Asia—adopted a new approach to lymphoma classification in 1994 (Table 24-3). The ILSG developed a consensus on a list of diseases that could be recognized (using a combination of available morphologic, immunologic, and genetic information) and that appeared to be distinct clinical entities. All available information—morphology, immunophenotype, genetic features, and clinical features—is used to define a disease entity. The relative importance of each of these features varies among diseases. Morphology is always important, and some diseases are primarily defined by morphology [e.g., follicular lymphoma (FL), angioimmunoblastic T-cell lymphoma, nodular sclerosis Hodgkin's disease] with immunophenotype as backup in difficult cases. Some diseases have a virtually specific immunophenotype [e.g., mantle cell lymphoma (MCL), small lymphocytic lymphoma (SLL), anaplastic large-cell lymphoma (ALCL)] such

that one would hesitate to make the diagnosis in the absence of the immunophenotype. In some lymphomas, a specific genetic abnormality is an important defining criterion [e.g., t(11;14) in MCL; t(8;14) in Burkitt lymphoma (BL); t(14;18) in FL], whereas others lack specific genetic abnormalities [e.g., mucosa-associated lymphoid tissue (MALT) lymphoma and diffuse large B-cell lymphoma (DLBCL)]. Still others require knowledge of clinical features as well (e.g., nodal versus extranodal presentation in marginal zone B-cell lymphomas and peripheral T-cell lymphomas, and mediastinal location in mediastinal large B-cell lymphoma).

The emphasis on defining "real" disease entities, using all available information, represented a new paradigm in lymphoma classification. The consensus approach represented a second major departure from previous classifications, most of which represented the work of one or a few individuals. The ILSG recognized that the complexity of the field now makes it impossible for a single person or small group to be completely authoritative and also that broad agreement is necessary if the result is to be used by multiple pathologists, even if it requires compromise.

The ILSG consensus list was published in 1994 (3). Because it represented a revision of current or prior European and American lymphoma classifications, it was called the *Revised European-American Classification of Lymphoid Neoplasms* (REAL) (Tables 24-4 and 24-5). Although its initial publication incited considerable controversy, experience over the ensuing years showed that it can be used by most pathologists, and that the entities it describes have distinctive clinical features, making it a useful and practical classification, despite its apparent complexity (4–6).

In 1995, members of the European and American Hematopathology societies began collaborating on a new World Health Organization (WHO) classification of hematologic malignancies. This uses an updated version of the REAL classification for lymphomas and expands the principles of the REAL classification to the classification of myeloid and histiocytic neoplasms. The project also included a Clinical Advisory Committee of international expert hematologists and oncologists (7–9). Proponents of current classifications (i.e., WF, Kiel, REAL, and French/American/British) are in agreement that the final WHO consensus will replace existing classifications. Thus, it represents the first true international consensus on the classification of hematologic malignancies.

TABLE 24-1. Kiel Classification (1974, 1988)

B-Cell	T-Cell
Low-grade malignancy	
Lymphocytic	Lymphocytic
CLL	CLL
Hairy cell leukemia	Small cerebriform cell
Lymphoplasmacytoid/cytic	Lymphoepithelioid (Lennert's)
(immunocytoma)	
Plasmacytic (plasmacytoma)	Angioimmunoblastic
Centroblastic/centrocytic	T zone
Centrocytic	Pleomorphic, small cell (HTLVI±)
High-grade malignancy	
Centroblastic	Pleomorphic, medium and large cell
	(HTLVI±)
Immunoblastic	Immunoblastic (HTLVI±)
Lymphoblastic	Lymphoblastic
Burkitt lymphoma	
Anaplastic large cell (Ki-1+)	Anaplastic large cell (Ki-1+)

CLL, chronic lymphocytic leukemia; HTLV, human T-cell lymphotrophic virus.
Gerard-Marchant R, Hamlin I, Lennert K, et al. Classification of non-Hodgkin's lymphomas. *Lancet* 1974;2:406–408; and Stansfeld A, Diebold J, Kapanci Y, et al. Updated Kiel classification for lymphomas. *Lancet* 1988;1:292–293.

CATEGORIES OF LYMPHOID NEOPLASMS

The REAL and WHO classifications recognize three major categories of lymphoid malignancies that can be defined based on a combination of morphology and cell lineage: B-cell neoplasms, T/natural killer (NK) cell neoplasms, and Hodgkin's disease (HD)/Hodgkin's lymphoma (HL). Both lymphomas and lymphoid leukemias are included in this classification, because both solid and circulating phases are present in many lymphoid neoplasms, and distinction between them is artificial. Thus, B-cell chronic lymphocytic leukemia (B-CLL) and B-cell SLL are simply different manifestations of the same neoplasm, as are lymphoblastic lymphomas and acute lymphoid leukemias, and BL and Burkitt cell leukemia. In addition, HD and plasma cell myeloma are now recognized as lymphoid neoplasms of B lineage and therefore belong in a compilation of lymphoid neoplasms.

TABLE 24-2. Working Formulation for Clinical Usage (1982)

Low grade
Malignant lymphoma, small lymphocytic
  Consistent with chronic lymphocytic leukemia
  Plasmacytoid
Malignant lymphoma, follicular, predominantly small cleaved cell
Malignant lymphoma, follicular, mixed small cleaved and large cell
Intermediate grade
Malignant lymphoma, follicular, predominantly large cell
Malignant lymphoma, diffuse, small cleaved cell
Malignant lymphoma, diffuse, mixed small and large cell
Malignant lymphoma, diffuse, large cell
  Cleaved cell
  Noncleaved cell
High grade
Malignant lymphoma, large cell, immunoblastic
  Plasmacytoid
  Clear cell
  Polymorphous
Malignant lymphoma, lymphoblastic
  Convoluted
  Nonconvoluted
Malignant lymphoma, small noncleaved cell
  Burkitt lymphoma
  Non-Burkitt lymphoma

Non-Hodgkin's lymphoma pathologic classification project. National Cancer Institute sponsored study of classifications of non-Hodgkin's lymphomas: summary and description of a Working Formulation for clinical usage. *Cancer* 1982;49:2112–2135.

TABLE 24-3. Revised European-American Classification of Lymphoid Neoplasms/World Health Organization Classification of Lymphoid Neoplasms (1994, 1999–2001)[a]

B-cell neoplasms
Precursor B-cell neoplasm
  Precursor B-lymphoblastic leukemia/lymphoma (precursor B-cell acute lymphoblastic leukemia)
Mature (peripheral) B-cell neoplasms[a]
  Chronic lymphocytic leukemia/ B-cell small lymphocytic lymphoma
  B-cell prolymphocytic leukemia
  Lymphoplasmacytic lymphoma
  Splenic marginal zone B-cell lymphoma (splenic lymphoma with villous lymphocytes)
  Hairy cell leukemia
  Plasma cell myeloma/plasmacytoma
  Extranodal marginal zone B-cell lymphoma (mucosa-associated lymphoid tissue lymphoma)
  Nodal marginal zone B-cell lymphoma
  Follicular lymphoma
  Mantle cell lymphoma
  Diffuse large B-cell lymphomas
  Burkitt lymphoma/leukemia
T- and NK-cell neoplasms
Precursor T-cell neoplasm
  Precursor T-lymphoblastic leukemia/lymphoma (precursor T-cell acute lymphoblastic leukemia)
  Blastic NK-cell lymphoma[b]
Mature (peripheral) T-cell neoplasms
  T-cell prolymphocytic leukemia
  T-cell large granular lymphocytic leukemia
  Aggressive NK-cell leukemia
  Adult T-cell lymphoma/leukemia (human T-cell lymphotrophic virus 1+)
  Extranodal NK/T-cell lymphoma, nasal type
  Enteropathy-type T-cell lymphoma
  Hepatosplenic T-cell lymphoma
  Subcutaneous panniculitis-like T-cell lymphoma
  Mycosis fungoides/Sézary's syndrome
  Primary cutaneous anaplastic large cell lymphoma
  Peripheral T-cell lymphoma, not otherwise specified
  Angioimmunoblastic T-cell lymphoma
  Primary systemic anaplastic large cell lymphoma
Hodgkin's lymphoma (Hodgkin's disease)
Nodular lymphocyte predominant Hodgkin's lymphoma
Classic Hodgkin's lymphoma
  Nodular sclerosis Hodgkin's lymphoma (grades 1 and 2)
  Lymphocyte-rich classic Hodgkin's lymphoma
  Mixed cellularity Hodgkin's lymphoma
  Lymphocyte-depleted Hodgkin's lymphoma

NK, natural killer.
[a]B- and T/NK-cell neoplasms are grouped according to major clinical presentations (predominantly disseminated and leukemic, primary extranodal, and predominantly nodal).
[b]Neoplasm of uncertain lineage and stage of differentiation.

GRADING AND PROGNOSTIC GROUPS

The final WHO classification of lymphoid neoplasms includes over 30 distinct entities. These diseases are in most cases unrelated to one another [i.e., we can no longer talk about "lymphoma" or "non-Hodgkin's lymphoma" (NHL) as a single disease with a range of histologic grade and clinical aggressiveness]. One of the corollaries of defining distinct lymphoma entities is that it is neither possible nor helpful to sort them precisely according to histologic grade or clinical aggressiveness. For example, although it is true that many lymphomas composed of relatively small cells with a low proliferation fraction have a generally indolent course, at least one of them (MCL) is rather aggressive. In addition, each has a distinctive set of presenting features and, often, different treatments [e.g., hairy cell leukemia (HCL) versus B-CLL versus MALT lymphoma]. Several of the lymphomas that we can now recognize have within themselves a range of histologic grade (number of large cells or proliferation fraction) and clinical aggressiveness (e.g., FL, MCL, and probably MALT lymphoma). Thus, histo-

TABLE 24-4. Comparison of the Revised European-American Classification of Lymphoid (REAL) Neoplasms/World Health Organization (WHO) Classification with the Working Formulation

REAL/WHO Classification	Working Formulation
Precursor B-lymphoblastic lymphoma/leukemia	Lymphoblastic
Chronic lymphocytic leukemia/B-cell small lymphocytic lymphoma	Small lymphocytic, consistent with chronic lymphocytic leukemia Small lymphocytic, plasmacytoid
Lymphoplasmacytic lymphoma	Small lymphocytic, plasmacytoid Diffuse, mixed small and large cell
Splenic marginal zone B-cell lymphoma	Small lymphocytic Diffuse small cleaved cell
Hairy cell leukemia	—
Plasmacytoma/myeloma	Extramedullary plasmacytoma
Extranodal marginal zone B-cell lymphoma (mucosa-associated lymphoid tissue lymphoma)	Small lymphocytic Diffuse, small cleaved cell Diffuse, mixed small and large cell
Follicular lymphoma	
Grade 1	Follicular, predominantly small cleaved cell
Grade 2	Follicular, mixed small and large cell
Grade 3	Follicular, large cell
Follicle center lymphoma, diffuse	
Grade 1	Diffuse, small cleaved cell
Grade 2	Diffuse, mixed small and large cell
Nodal marginal zone B-cell lymphoma	Small lymphocytic Diffuse, small cleaved cell Diffuse, mixed small and large cell
Mantle cell lymphoma	Small lymphocytic Diffuse, small cleaved cell Follicular, small cleaved cell Diffuse, mixed small and large cell Diffuse, large cleaved cell
Diffuse large B-cell lymphoma	Diffuse, large cell Large cell immunoblastic Diffuse, mixed small and large cell
Burkitt lymphoma	Small noncleaved cell, Burkitt and non-Burkitt lymphoma
Precursor T-lymphoblastic lymphoma/leukemia	Lymphoblastic
T-cell prolymphocytic leukemia	Small lymphocytic Diffuse small cleaved cell
T-cell large granular lymphocytic leukemia	Small lymphocytic Diffuse, small cleaved cell
Adult T-cell lymphoma/leukemia	Diffuse, small cleaved cell Diffuse, mixed small and large cell Diffuse, large cell Large cell immunoblastic
Extranodal natural killer/T-cell lymphoma, nasal-type	Diffuse, small cleaved cell Diffuse, mixed small and large cell Diffuse, large cell Large cell immunoblastic
Enteropathy-type T-cell lymphoma	Diffuse, small cleaved cell Diffuse, mixed small and large cell Diffuse, large cell Large cell immunoblastic
Hepatosplenic T-cell lymphoma	—
Subcutaneous panniculitis-like T-cell lymphoma	Diffuse, mixed small and large cell Diffuse, large cell Large cell immunoblastic
Mycosis fungoides/Sézary's syndrome	Mycosis fungoides
Angioimmunoblastic T-cell lymphoma	Diffuse, mixed small and large cell Diffuse, large cell Large cell immunoblastic
Peripheral T-cell lymphomas, unspecified	Diffuse, small cleaved cell Diffuse, mixed small and large cell Diffuse, large cell Large cell immunoblastic
Anaplastic large cell lymphoma	Large cell immunoblastic

TABLE 24-5. Comparison of Revised European-American Classification of Lymphoid (REAL) Neoplasms/World Health Organization (WHO) Classification with the Rye Classification of Hodgkin's Lymphoma (HL)

REAL/WHO Classification	Rye Classification
Nodular lymphocyte predominant HL	Lymphocyte predominance, nodular (most cases)
Classic HL	
Nodular sclerosis HL	Nodular sclerosis
Mixed cellularity HL	Mixed cellularity (most cases)
Lymphocyte-rich classic HL	Lymphocyte predominance, nodular (most)
	Lymphocyte predominance, diffuse (some)
Lymphocyte depleted HL	Lymphocyte depletion
Unclassifiable classic HL	Mixed cellularity (some cases)

TABLE 24-6. Reproducibility of Lymphoma Diagnosis

Reproducibility	Contribution of Immunophenotype (%)
Reproducibility >85% (86% to 96%)	
B-cell chronic lymphocytic leukemia/small lymphocytic lymphoma	3
Mantle cell lymphoma	10
Follicular lymphoma	0
Marginal zone/mucosa-associated lymphoid tissue	2
Diffuse large B-cell lymphoma	15
T-Lymphoblastic lymphoma	40
Anaplastic large-cell lymphoma	39
Peripheral T-cell lymphoma, unspecified	41
Mycosis fungoides	—
Reproducibility 80%	
Angioimmunoblastic T-cell lymphoma	—
Extranodal natural killer/T-cell lymphoma	—
Reproducibility <50%	
Burkitt-like lymphoma	6
Lymphoplasmacytic lymphoma	—

A clinical evaluation of the International Lymphoma Study Group classification of non-Hodgkin's lymphoma. *Blood* 1997;89:3909–3918; and Armitage JO, Weisenburger DD. New approach to classifying non-Hodgkin's lymphomas: clinical features of the major histologic subtypes. *J Clin Oncol* 1998;16:2780–2795.

logic grade should be applied within a disease entity, not across the whole range of lymphoid neoplasms. Although several recent publications suggested clinical groupings of the entities in the REAL classification (10,11), the Clinical Advisory Committee for the WHO classification agreed that such groupings were neither necessary nor desirable for clinical practice. Both pathologists and oncologists must "get to know" each disease entity and its spectrum of morphology and clinical behavior. In practice, treatment of a specific patient is determined not by which broad "prognostic group" the lymphoma falls into but by the specific histologic type of lymphoma, with the addition of grade within the tumor type, if applicable, and clinical features such as stage, age, performance status, and the International Prognostic Index (IPI) (12).

Because of the impracticality of arranging the list of B- and T/NK-cell lymphoid neoplasms according to prognostic groups, the final WHO classification lists them first according to differentiation stage and secondarily according to predominant clinical presentation. Two major differentiation stages are recognized: precursor neoplasms (corresponding to the earliest stages of differentiation) and peripheral or mature neoplasms (corresponding to more differentiated stages). Three broad categories of clinical presentation are recognized: predominantly disseminated diseases that often involve bone marrow and may be leukemic, primary extranodal lymphomas, and predominantly nodal diseases that are often disseminated and may also involve extranodal sites (8). This approach is intended for convenience and ease of learning only, by placing diseases that are likely to resemble one another both clinically and histologically in proximity to one another in the list and in a text. It also has some biologic relevance, because there appear to be important biologic differences between primary nodal and primary extranodal lymphomas, particularly in the T/NK-cell diseases. However, any principle of sorting these neoplasms is artificial, and the lists can be regrouped in different ways for different purposes.

Clinical Relevance of the Revised European-American Classification of Lymphoid Neoplasms and World Health Organization Classification

An initial criticism of the REAL classification was that it had not been tested in a clinical study (13), although it only included diseases that had been previously published and for which the clinical features were known (14). To address this issue, an international group of oncologists and pathologists devised a clinical study of the classification, in which five expert pathologists reviewed over 1300 cases of NHL at centers around the

world (6,15). The aims of the study were (a) to see whether the classification could be used in practice, (b) to test its interobserver reproducibility, (c) to determine the need for immunophenotyping in diagnosis, (d) to determine whether the categories of disease identified in the classification were clinically distinctive either at presentation or in outcome, and (e) to determine the relative frequency of these diseases in the populations studied.

REPRODUCIBILITY

This study convincingly demonstrated that the classification could be used by expert hematopathologists: Over 95% of the cases with adequate material could be classified into one or another of the categories. The interobserver reproducibility was substantially better than that for other classifications and was better than 85% for most diseases (Table 24-6). Immunophenotyping had been done in all cases as a requirement for entry into the study to confirm the diagnosis of lymphoma and to identify lineage (B, T, NK). Immunophenotyping was helpful in improving interobserver reproducibility in some diseases, such as MCL and DLBCL, where it improved accuracy by 10% to 15% and was essential for all types of T-cell lymphoma, improving reproducibility from approximately 50% to over 90%. It was not required for many diseases, such as FL, B-cell SLL, and MALT lymphoma (6).

FREQUENCY OF LYMPHOID NEOPLASMS

The relative frequency of the different B and T/NK-cell lymphomas in the study population was similar to previous patterns reported in the literature (Tables 24-7 and 24-8). The most common lymphoma was DLBCL, followed by FL; together, these comprised 50% of the lymphomas in the study. New entities not specifically recognized in the WF accounted for 27% of the cases: MALT lymphoma, 8%; mantle cell, 7%; peripheral T-cell, 6%; nodal marginal zone, 2%; mediastinal large B-cell, 2%; anaplastic large T/null cell, 2%. These results are reassuring, confirming that the majority of the cases that will be encountered by oncologists and pathologists will be only a few subtypes with which they are already familiar. However, they also underscore the need for recognizing the more recently described entities,

TABLE 24-7. Frequency and Presenting Features of Common B- and T-Cell Neoplasms in the Revised European-American Classification of Lymphoid Neoplasms Classification

Neoplasm	Frequency[a]	Age	Male	Stage				B Symptoms	Any Extranodal Site (Including Bone Marrow)	Bone Marrow	Gastrointestinal Tract	International Prognostic Index		
				I	II	III	IV					0/1	2/3	4/5
Large B-cell	31	64	55	25	29	13	33	33	71	16	18	35	46	9
Mediastinal	2	37	34	10	56	3	31	38	56	3	0	52	37	11
Follicular	22	59	42	18	15	16	51	28	64	42	4	45	48	7
Chronic lymphocytic leukemia/small lymphocytic lymphoma	6	65	53	4	5	8	83	33	80	72	3	23	64	13
Mucosa-associated lymphoid tissue	8	60	48	39	28	2	31	19	98	14	50	44	48	8
Mantle cell	6	63	74	13	7	9	71	28	81	51	9	23	54	23
Peripheral T-cell	7	61	55	8	12	15	65	50	82	36	15	17	52	31
Anaplastic large cell lymphoma	2	34	69	19	32	10	39	53	59	13	9	61	18	21

[a]All numbers are percentages of cases in the international study.

Armitage JO, Weisenburger DD. New approach to classifying non-Hodgkin's lymphomas: clinical features of the major histologic subtypes. *J Clin Oncol* 1998;16:2780–2795.

TABLE 24-8. Lymphomas Presenting in Selected Extranodal Sites

Site	Lymphoma	Percent of Cases[a]
Stomach	Diffuse large B-cell lymphoma	55
	MALT lymphoma	40
	Burkitt lymphoma	3
	Mantle cell lymphoma	<1
	Follicular lymphoma	<1
Intestine	Diffuse large B-cell lymphoma	55
	MALT lymphoma	20
	Burkitt lymphoma	5
	Peripheral T-cell lymphomas	15
Bone	Diffuse large B-cell lymphoma (often multilobated)	>90
Central nervous system and eye	Diffuse large B-cell lymphoma	>90
Ocular adnexae	MALT lymphoma	40
	Follicular lymphoma	40
	Diffuse large B-cell lymphoma	20
Skin	Mycosis fungoides	45
	CD30+ cutaneous lymphoproliferative disorders (lymphomatoid papulosis, primary cutaneous anaplastic large cell lymphoma)	25
	Peripheral T-cell lymphomas, CD30-	10
	Follicle center lymphoma and diffuse large B-cell lymphoma	15
	MALT lymphoma	5

MALT, mucosa-associated lymphoid tissue.
[a]Data on gastrointestinal lymphomas from Radaszkiewicz T, Dragosics B, Bauer P. Gastrointestinal malignant lymphomas of the mucosa-associated lymphoid tissue: factors relevant to prognosis. *Gastroenterology* 1992;102:1628–1638; data on bone lymphomas from Pettit C, Zukerberg L, Gray M, et al. Primary lymphoma of bone: a B cell tumor with a high frequency of multilobated cells. *Am J Surg Pathol* 1990;14:329–334; data on central nervous system from Bashir R, Freedman A, Harris N, et al. Immunophenotypic profile of CNS lymphoma: a review of 18 cases. *J Neurooncol* 1989;7:249–254; data on ocular adnexal lymphomas from Ferry J, White W, Grove A, Harris N. Malignant lymphoma of ocular adnexa: a spectrum of B-cell neoplasia including low grade B-cell lymphoma of MALT type. *Lab Invest* 1992;66:77A; data on cutaneous lymphomas from Willemze R, Beljaards R, Meijer C, Rijlaarsdam J. Classification of primary cutaneous lymphomas. *Dermatology* 1994;189(suppl 2):8–15.

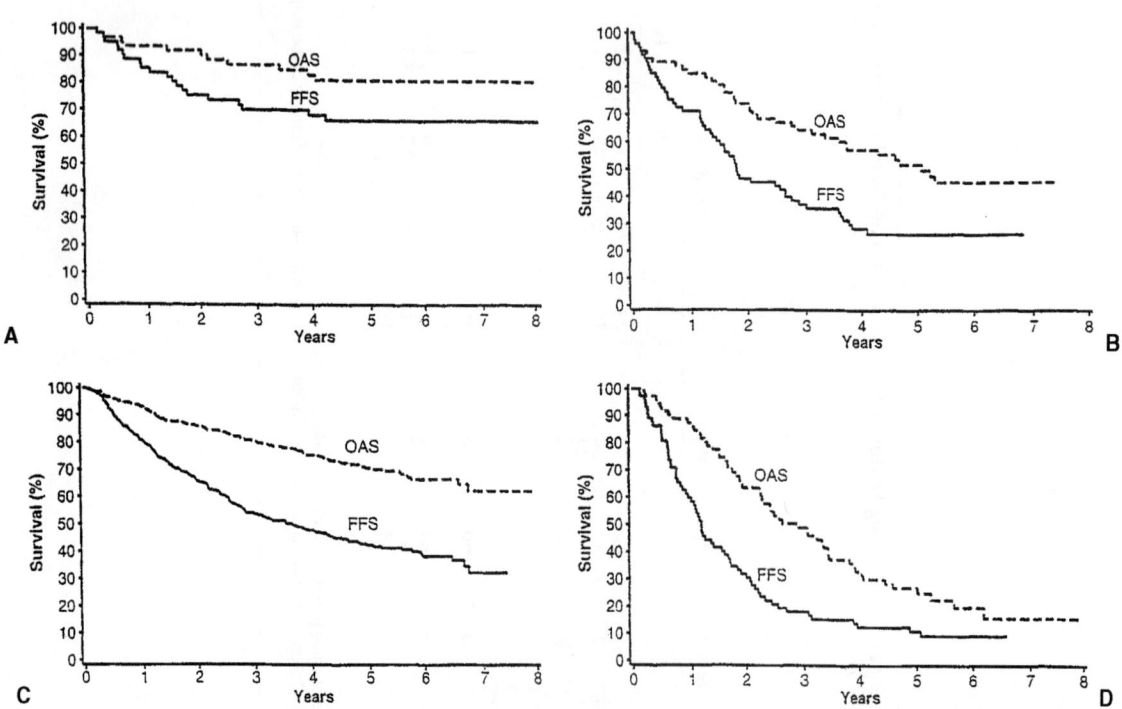

Figure 24-1. Overall survival of patients with lymphomas that would have been classified as "low grade" in the Working Formulation. **A:** Marginal zone lymphoma of mucosa-associated lymphoid tissue type has a good overall survival with a plateau in the curve suggesting the possibility of cure. **B,C:** Small lymphocytic lymphoma and follicular lymphoma have an intermediate prognosis typical of indolent lymphomas. **D:** Mantle cell lymphoma is shown to be a more aggressive disease with a median survival of 3 years. FFS, failure-free survival; OAS, overall actuarial survival. (From Armitage JO, Weisenburger DD. New approach to classifying non-Hodgkin's lymphomas: clinical features of the major histologic subtypes. *J Clin Oncol* 1998;16:2780–2795, with permission.)

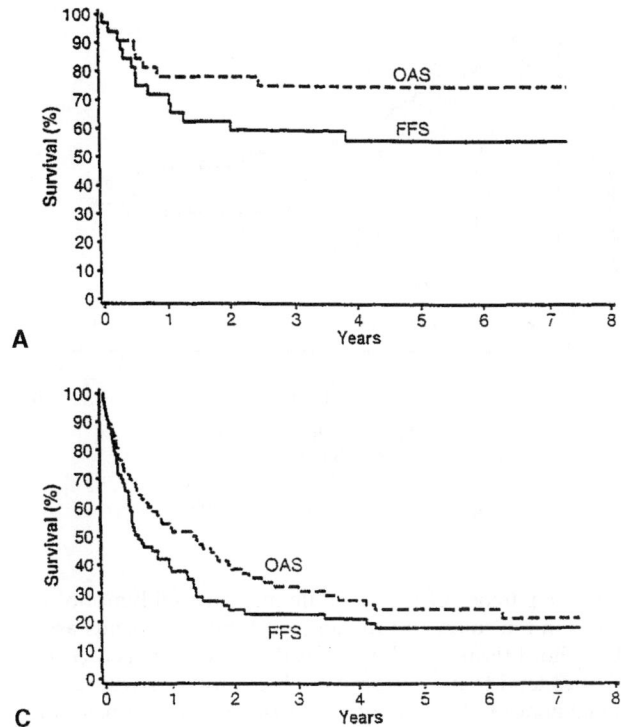

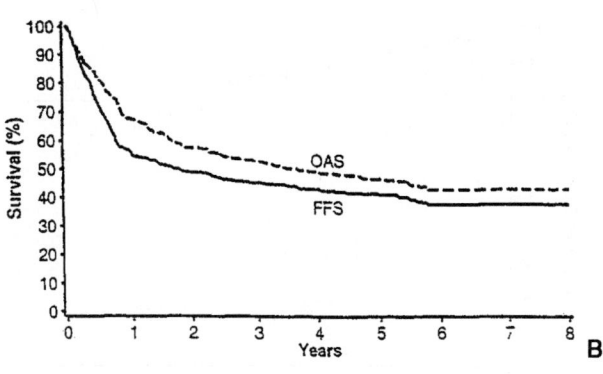

Figure 24-2. Overall survival of patients with lymphomas that would have been classified as "intermediate/high grade" in the Working Formulation. **A:** Anaplastic large-cell lymphoma has an excellent prognosis; **(B)** diffuse large B-cell lymphoma has a long-term survival of approximately 50%; and **(C)** peripheral T-cell lymphoma, unspecified, has an extremely poor prognosis, with median survival of one year. FFS, failure-free survival; OAS, overall actuarial survival. (From Armitage JO, Weisenburger DD. New approach to classifying non-Hodgkin's lymphomas: clinical features of the major histologic subtypes. *J Clin Oncol* 1998;16:2780–2795, with permission.)

which, although less common, have important clinical differences. The study also found differences in geographic distribution of the lymphoma types, with FL being more common in North America and western Europe, T-cell lymphomas more common in Hong Kong, and both mediastinal large B-cell lymphoma and MCL more common in Ticino (the Italian-speaking canton), Switzerland (16).

CLINICAL FEATURES OF LYMPHOID NEOPLASMS IN REVISED EUROPEAN-AMERICAN CLASSIFICATION OF LYMPHOID NEOPLASMS

The different entities recognized by the classification had significantly different clinical presentations and survivals. For example, diffuse aggressive lymphomas, which would be lumped as intermediate to high grade in the WF, include DLBCL, mediastinal large B-cell lymphoma, peripheral T-cell lymphoma, and anaplastic large T/null-cell lymphoma. The clinical features at presentation were strikingly different, with a younger age group for mediastinal large B-cell lymphoma and anaplastic large T-cell lymphoma, and striking differences in male to female ratios, suggesting that these are distinctive biologic entities (Table 24-7). When overall survivals were analyzed, entities that would have been lumped together as "low grade" or "intermediate to high grade" in the WF showed marked differences in survival, again confirming that they need to be recognized and treated as distinct entities (Figs. 24-1 and 24-2).

A critical finding in this study was that pathologic classification is not the only predictor of clinical outcome. Patients with any of these diseases could be stratified into better and worse prognostic groups according to the IPI (12). For example, although patients with FL typically have IPI scores of 1 to 3, those patients with scores of 4 or 5 had a predicted median overall survival of only 18 months (Fig. 24-3). Thus, to plan treatment for an individual patient, the oncologist must know not only the diagnosis but also the clinical prognostic factors that will influence that patient's course.

BIOLOGIC BASIS FOR CLASSIFICATION OF LYMPHOID NEOPLASMS

Although the normal counterpart of the neoplastic cell is not known for all types of lymphoid neoplasms, it can be postulated for many of them. Understanding the normal counterpart of neoplastic cells can provide a useful framework for understanding the morphology, immunophenotype, and to some extent, the clinical behavior of the neoplasms (Fig. 24-4).

Anatomy and Morphology of Normal Lymphoid Tissues

Lymphoid tissues can be divided into two major categories: (a) the central or primary lymphoid tissues, which harbor lymphoid precursor cells and provide for their maturation to a stage at which they are capable of performing their function in response to antigen; and (b) the peripheral or secondary lymphoid tissue, in which antigen-specific reactions occur.

PRIMARY (CENTRAL) LYMPHOID TISSUES

Bone Marrow (Bursa-Equivalent). Many of the early experiments that elucidated the basic biology of the lymphoid system used chickens and other avian species as experimental animals; in avian species, an organ known as the *bursa of Fabricius*, located in the region of the cloaca, proved to be the source of cells capable of producing antibody. Thus, these cells were termed *B cells*, for bursa-derived cells. In mammals, the bursa does not exist, and experiments have shown that the precursors of antibody-producing cells come from the bone marrow. The bone marrow is also the source of other hematopoietic cells, including T cells (so named because their crucial maturation steps cannot occur in the absence of the thymus).

Thymus. The thymus, located in the anterior mediastinum, is the site at which immature T-cell precursors (prethymocytes)

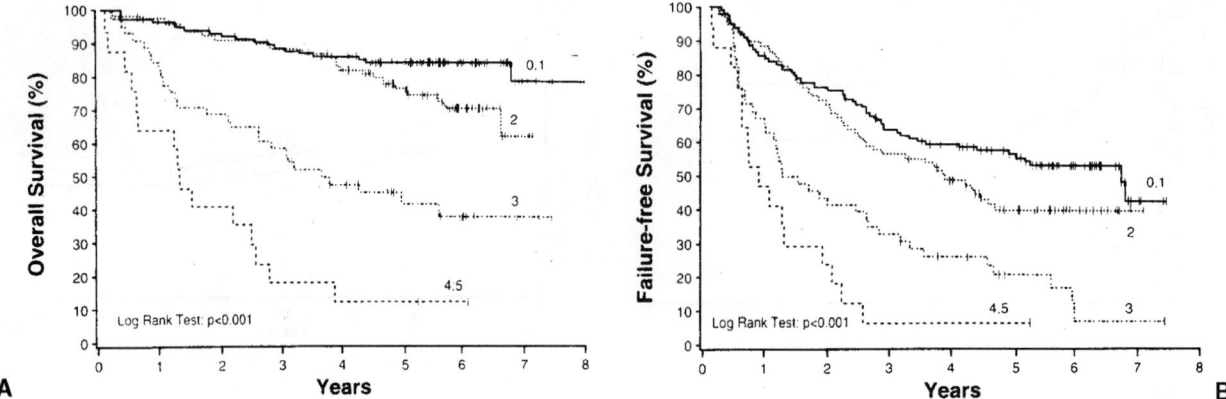

Figure 24-3. Overall **(A)** and failure-free **(B)** survival of follicular lymphoma, stratified by the International Prognostic Index. There are marked differences in outcome for patients with different International Prognostic Index scores, with the poorest group having a very poor prognosis. (From A clinical evaluation of the International Lymphoma Study Group classification of non-Hodgkin's lymphoma. *Blood* 1997;89:3909–3918, with permission.)

that migrate from the bone marrow undergo maturation and selection to become mature, naive T cells, which are capable of responding to antigen. The thymus is divided into a cortex and a medulla, each of which is characterized by specialized epithelium and accessory cells, which provide the milieu for T-cell maturation.

SECONDARY (PERIPHERAL) LYMPHOID TISSUES

Lymph Nodes. Lymph nodes are located at sites throughout the body, strategically placed to process antigens present in lymph drained from most organs via the afferent lymphatics. Lymph nodes have a capsule, a cortex, a medulla, and sinuses (subcapsular, cortical, and medullary) (Fig. 24-5). The sinuses contain macrophages that take up and process antigen, which may then be presented to lymphocytes. The cortex is divided into follicular and diffuse (paracortical) regions, and the medulla into medullary cords and sinuses. The paracortex contains high endothelial venules (HEV) (through which both T and B lymphocytes enter the node) and specialized antigen-presenting cells (APCs), the interdigitating dendritic cells, which may be related to the cutaneous Langerhans' cell, and which present antigen to T cells. Both T cell and early B cell reactions to antigen occur in the paracortex, while the germinal center (GC) reaction occurs in the follicular cortex. The follicular cortex also contains a specific type of accessory cell, the follicular dendritic cell (FDC); adhesion to the FDC-antigen complex is important in the differentiation of B cells in response to antigen. Plasma cells and effector T cells generated by immune reactions accumulate in the medullary cords and exit via the medullary sinuses.

Spleen. The spleen, located in the left upper abdomen, has two major compartments: the red pulp, which functions as a filter for particulate antigens and for the formed elements of the blood, and the white pulp, which is virtually identical in its compartments to the lymphoid tissue of the lymph node. Follicles and GCs are found in the malpighian corpuscles, whereas T cells and interdigitating dendritic cells are found in the adjacent periarteriolar lymphoid sheath. Plasma cells accumulate in the red pulp.

Mucosa-Associated Lymphoid Tissue. Specialized lymphoid tissue is found in association with certain epithelia, in particular the naso- and oropharynx (Waldeyer's ring: adenoids, tonsils), the gastrointestinal tract (gut-associated lymphoid tissue:

Peyer's patches of the distal ileum, mucosal lymphoid aggregates in the colon and rectum), and lung (bronchus-associated lymphoid tissue). Collectively, this is known as *MALT*. These tissues tend to have prominent B-cell follicles with broad marginal zones but also may have discrete T-cell zones, similar to the paracortex of lymph nodes. MALT is thought to function in responding to intraluminal antigens and the generation of mucosal immunity. Lymphoid cells that respond to antigen in the MALT acquire homing properties that enable them to return to these tissues (17,18).

B- and T-Cell Differentiation

In both the T- and B-cell systems, there are two major phases of differentiation: antigen-independent and antigen-dependent (Fig. 24-4). Antigen-independent differentiation occurs in the primary lymphoid organs [e.g., bursa-equivalent (bone marrow) and thymus] without exposure to antigen and produces a pool of lymphocytes that are capable of responding to antigen (naive or virgin T and B cells). The early stages are stem cells and lymphoblasts (also known as *precursor T and B cells*) that are self-renewing, whereas the later stages are resting cells with a finite lifespan ranging from weeks to years. On exposure to antigen, the naive lymphocyte undergoes "blast transformation," and becomes a large, proliferating cell that gives rise to progeny capable of direct activity against the inciting antigen, the antigen-specific effector cells. The earlier stages of antigen-dependent differentiation are proliferating cells, whereas the fully differentiated effector cells are less mitotically active. Thus, neoplasms that correspond to proliferating stages of either antigen-independent or antigen-dependent differentiation are likely to be aggressive, whereas those that correspond to naive or mature effector stages are likely to be indolent. Neoplasms corresponding to precursor cells tend to be more common in children (lymphoblastic lymphoma or leukemia), whereas those corresponding to mature effector cells tend to be seen more often in adults [(lymphoplasmacytic lymphoma (LPL), mycosis fungoides)].

B-CELL DIFFERENTIATION

Antigen-Independent B-Cell Differentiation

Precursor B cells. B-cell differentiation involves rearrangements of the genes involved in immunoglobulin (Ig) production (19,20). The genes that encode the constant and variable regions

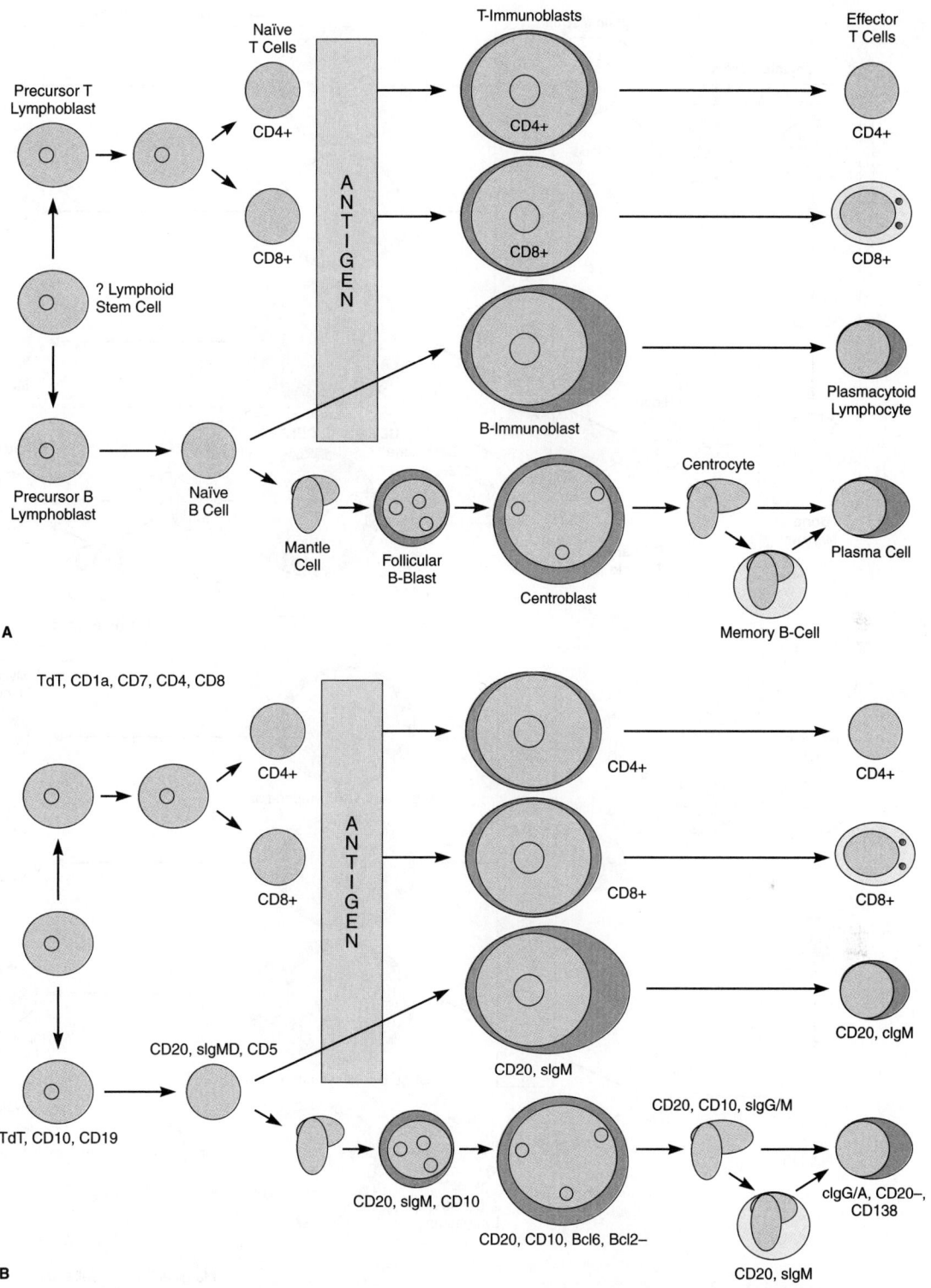

Figure 24-4. Hypothetical scheme of lymphocyte differentiation. **A:** In antigen-independent differentiation, precursor T and B cells mature to naive T and B cells. On exposure to antigen, they undergo blast transformation, proliferate, and mature into antigen-specific effector cells: helper and suppressor/cytotoxic T cells and plasma cells. **B:** Antigen expression distinguishes T cells from B cells and also changes during differentiation so that the differentiation stage of a normal or neoplastic cell can be inferred from the immunophenotype. Precursor T and B cells express the nuclear antigen terminal deoxynucleotidyl transferase (TdT). Immature T cells express CD1a and both CD4 and CD8; mature T cells lose TdT and express either CD4 or CD8. Immature B cells express CD10 and CD19, but not CD20; mature naive B cells express CD20, immunoglobulin M (IgM), and immunoglobulin D (IgD), and often CD5. Germinal center B cells down-regulate bcl-2, express CD10, and may switch their immunoglobulin heavy chain to immunoglobulin G (IgG) or IgA. Plasma cells lack surface Ig and CD20 and have cytoplasmic IgG or IgA. (*continued*)

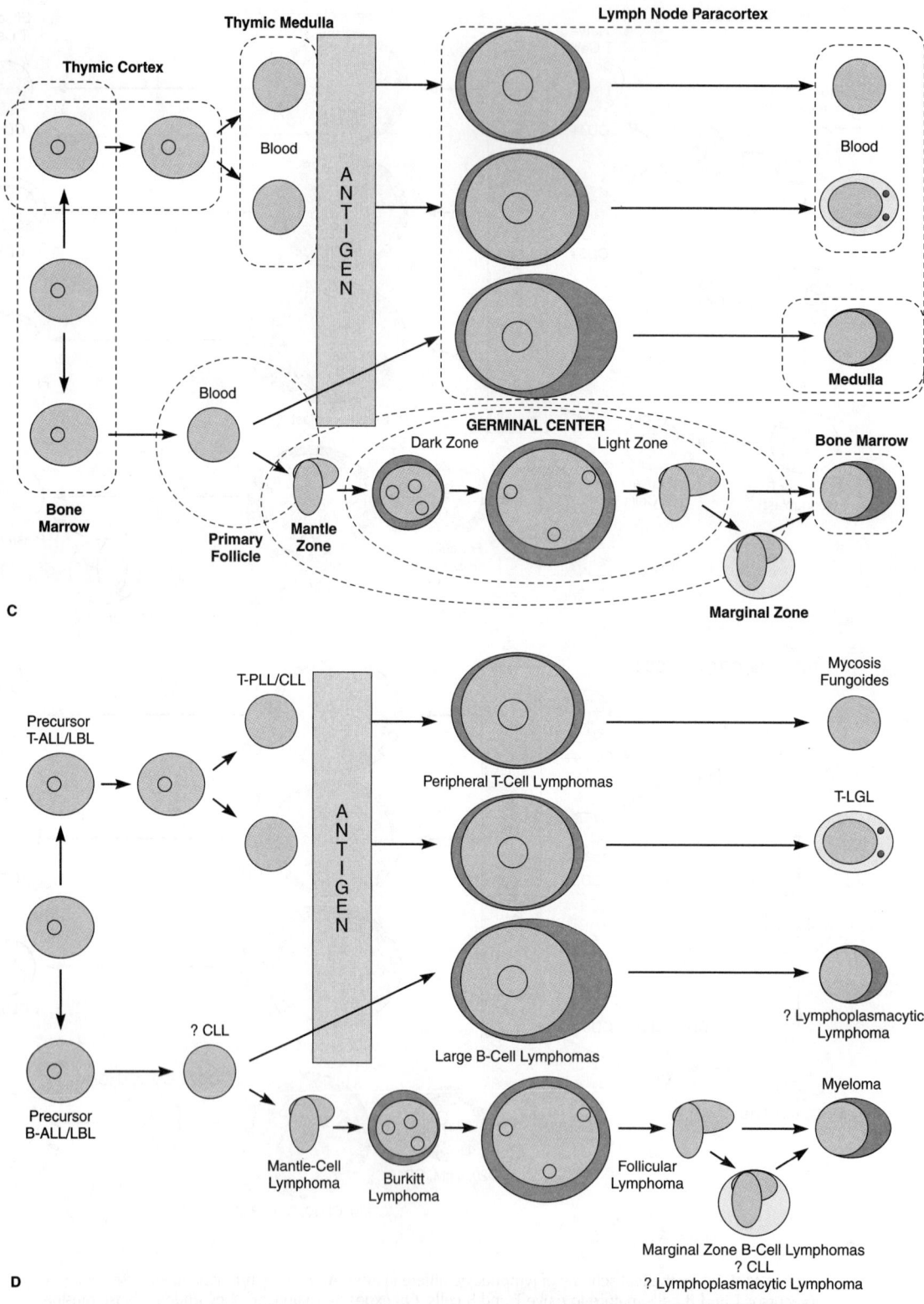

Figure 24-4. (*continued*) C: Lymphoid cell differentiation occurs in distinct anatomic sites and tissue compartments. **D:** Many lymphoid neoplasms have morphologic, immunophenotypic, and genetic similarities to normal stages of B- and T-cell differentiation. ALL, acute lymphoblastic leukemia; CLL, chronic lymphocytic leukemia; LBL, lymphoblastic lymphoma; LGL, large granular lymphocyte; PLL, prolymphocytic leukemia.

of the Ig heavy- and light-chain molecules are located far apart on the chromosomes in germline cells. To produce RNA for an Ig protein, many thousands of base pairs of DNA must be deleted from the genome to bring the different portions of the Ig gene together (Fig. 24-6). The earliest B cells have rearranged Ig heavy-

chain genes but lack surface Ig (SIg); the B cells at this stage are called *precursor B cells* (Fig. 24-4B) (20). At the next stage, the cells make cytoplasmic μ heavy chain, but no light chain, and do not express SIg. Both types of cells are lymphoblasts with dispersed chromatin and small nucleoli. They contain the intranuclear

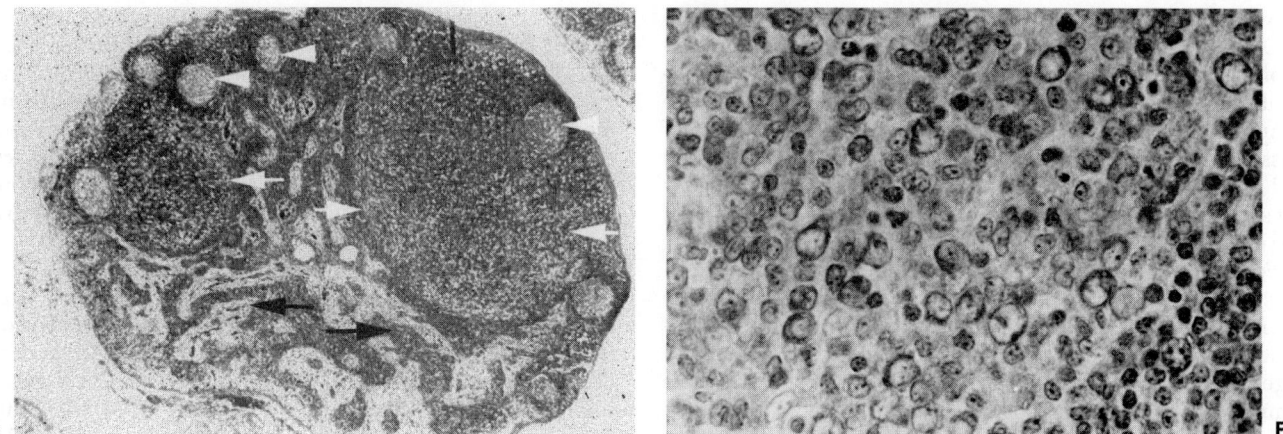

Figure 24-5. Normal lymph node. **A:** Low magnification showing architectural features: cortex with reactive follicles containing germinal centers (GCs) (*arrowheads*), expanded paracortical T-cell zones (*short arrows*), and medullary cords and sinuses (*long arrows*). **B:** High magnification of a GC, showing centroblasts (large cells with oval, vesicular nuclei, peripheral nucleoli, and basophilic cytoplasm) and centrocytes (smaller cells with irregular nuclei, inconspicuous nucleoli, and scant cytoplasm) (Giemsa stain). (From Harris NL, Ferry JA. Follicular lymphoma. In: Knowles DM, ed. *Neoplastic hematopathology*. Philadelphia: Lippincott Williams & Wilkins, 2001, with permission.)

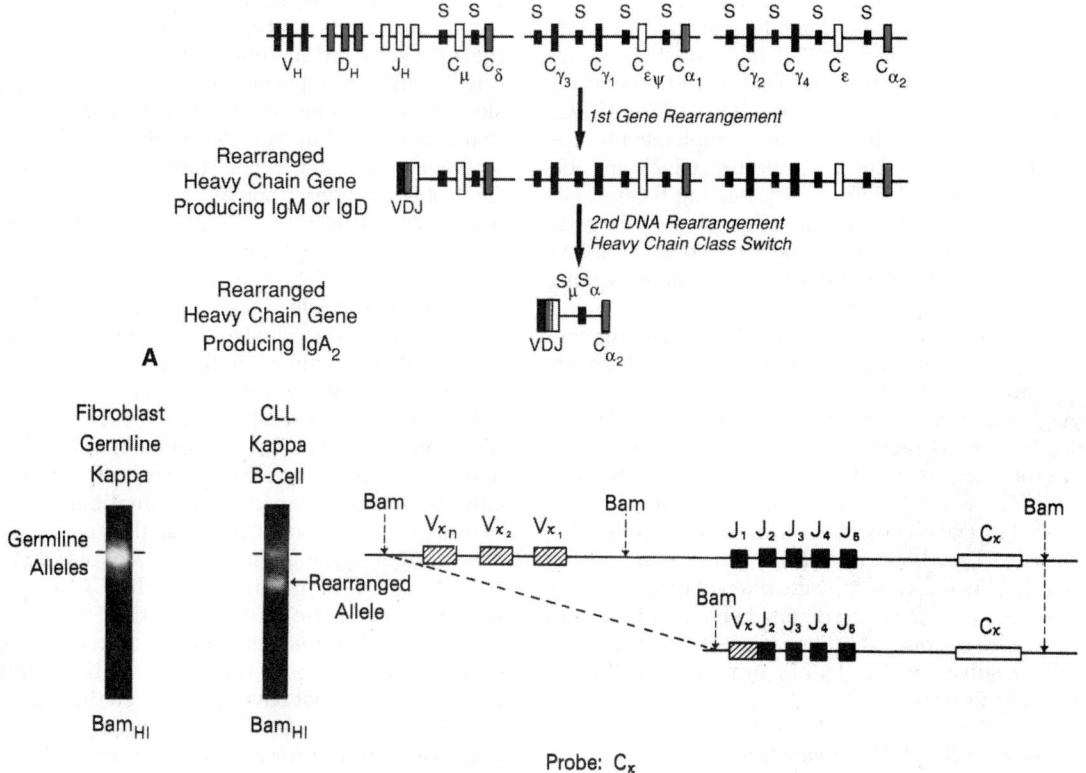

Figure 24-6. Immunoglobulin (Ig) gene rearrangement. **A:** Schematic representation of human germline heavy-chain gene locus on chromosome 14q32. The first DNA rearrangement assembles the variable (V), diversity (D), and joining (J) segments to complete the variable portion of the molecule, which now lies adjacent to the C_μ and C_δ genes. The cell can now produce IgM and IgD. In class switching, a second rearrangement occurs between the homologous heavy-chain class switch sites flanking each constant (C) region, moving a distal C region next to the assembled VDJ. In the example shown, the cell would now produce IgA. **B:** Rearrangement of a human kappa gene (right) and its detection by Southern blot (left). The upper diagram shows a germline gene with a 12-kb fragment delimited by 2 BamHI restriction cleavage sites, detected by a C_κ probe in the blot at left. In the lower diagram, the rearrangement placing the V_κ gene next to the J_2 gene has eliminated one of the BamHI restriction sites, resulting in a smaller fragment containing the C_κ region; this rearranged allele migrates differently on the Southern blot. CLL, chronic lymphocytic leukemia.

enzyme terminal deoxynucleotidyl transferase (TdT) and express CD34 (a glycoprotein present on immature cells of both lymphoid and myeloid lineage), HLA-DR [class II major histocompatibility complex (MHC) antigens], and the common acute lymphoblastic leukemia antigen (CD10) (21–24). Expression of class II MHC antigens persists throughout the life of the B cell and is important in interactions with T cells. Pan-B-cell antigens are sequentially expressed on precursor B cells: CD19, CD79a, and cytoplasmic CD22, followed by surface CD20 and CD45.

Fetal early B-cell development occurs in the liver, bone marrow, and spleen, whereas in adults it is restricted to the bone marrow (Fig. 24-4C). Cells with the morphologic and immunologic features of precursor B cells can be found in normal and regenerating bone marrow, where they correspond to the lymphocyte-like cells known as *hematogones* (25,26). Neoplasms of precursor B cells usually involve bone marrow and peripheral blood and are known as *common* or *precursor B acute lymphoblastic leukemia*; rarely, they present as solid tumors [precursor B lymphoblastic lymphoma (LBL)] (Fig. 24-4D).

Naive B Cells. The end stage of antigen-independent B-cell differentiation is the mature, naive (virgin) B cell, which expresses both complete surface IgM and IgD, lacks TdT and common acute lymphoblastic leukemia antigen and is capable of responding to antigen. Naive B cells have rearranged but unmutated Ig genes (27). Each individual B cell is committed to a single light chain, either kappa or lambda, and all of its progeny will express the same light chain (28). In contrast to precursor B cells, naive B cells lack CD10 and CD34. In addition to SIg, naive B cells express pan-B-cell antigens (CD19, CD20, CD22, CD40, and CD79a), HLA class II molecules, complement receptors (CD21 and CD35), CD44, Leu-8 (L-selectin), CD23, and the pan-T-cell antigen, CD5 (29) (Fig. 24-4B). Resting B cells also produce the bcl-2 protein, which promotes survival in the resting state (30). CD5-positive B cells produce Ig that often has broad specificity (cross-reactive idiotypes) and reactivity with self antigens (autoantibodies) (29).

Naive B cells are small resting lymphocytes. In fetal tissues, they are the predominant lymphoid cell in the spleen; in adults, they circulate in the blood and also comprise a minor fraction of the B cells in primary lymphoid follicles and follicle mantle zones (so-called recirculating B cells) (29,31) (Fig. 24-4C). Studies of single cells picked from the mantle zones of reactive follicles show that they are clonally diverse and contain unmutated Ig genes, consistent with naive B cells (32). Tumors of these cells are usually clinically indolent and histologically low grade. In addition, they are often widespread and leukemic, consistent with the recirculating behavior of the normal naive B cell. Two neoplasms appear to correspond to CD5-positive B cells: a subset of B-cell CLL, and mantle cell lymphoma (33–35) (Fig. 24-4D).

Antigen-Dependent B-Cell Differentiation

Immunoblastic and Plasma Cell Reaction. On encountering antigen, the naive B cell transforms into a proliferating cell, which ultimately matures into an antibody-secreting plasma cell. In T-cell–independent reactions and in the early primary immune response, naive B cells transform into IgM+ blast cells (B-blasts or immunoblasts) in the T-cell zones, proliferate, and differentiate into IgM-secreting plasma cells, producing the IgM antibody of the primary immune response (28,36,37) (Fig. 24-4A). Surface IgD is lost during blast transformation, as are some other antigens, such as CD21 and CD22. Other antigens associated with activation are up-regulated. With maturation to plasma cells, most surface antigens are lost, including pan-B-

cell antigens, HLA-DR, and the leukocyte common antigen, CD45 (38), and secretory cytoplasmic IgM accumulates (Fig. 24-4B). The immunoblastic reaction occurs in the lymph node paracortex, and IgM-producing plasma cells accumulate in the medullary cords (Fig. 24-4C). The corresponding neoplasm to the IgM-producing plasma cell may be lymphoplasmacytic lymphoma (immunocytoma), or Waldenström's macroglobulinemia (Fig. 24-4D), although at least some cases appear to correspond to post-GC cells.

GC Reaction. Later in the primary immune response (within 3 to 7 days of antigen challenge in experimental animals) and in secondary responses, the T-cell–dependent GC reaction occurs. Each GC is formed from between three and ten naive B cells and ultimately contains approximately 10,000 to 15,000 B cells; thus, more than ten generations are required to form a GC (32,37). Proliferating IgM-positive B-blasts formed from naive B cells that have encountered antigen in the T-cell zone (paracortex) migrate into the center of the primary follicle and fill the FDC meshwork, forming a GC (37,39) (Fig. 24-4A). These B-blasts differentiate into Ig-negative centroblasts (large noncleaved follicular center cells), which appear at approximately 4 days and accumulate at one pole of the GC, forming the "dark zone." *Centroblasts* are large, proliferating cells with vesicular nuclei; one to three prominent, peripheral nucleoli; and a narrow rim of basophilic cytoplasm. They lack SIg (37,40,41) and also switch off the gene that encodes the bcl-2 protein; thus, they and their progeny are susceptible to death through apoptosis (30) (Fig. 24-4B). An important event in GC development is expression of bcl-6 protein, a nuclear zinc-finger transcription factor that is expressed by both centroblasts and centrocytes but not by naive or memory B cells, mantle cells, or plasma cells (42,43). Centroblasts undergo somatic mutation of the Ig variable (Ig V) region, which alters the affinity for antigen of the antibody that will be produced by the cell (44,45).

Centroblasts mature to nonproliferating medium-sized cells with irregular nuclei, inconspicuous nucleoli, and scant cytoplasm, called *centrocytes* (small or large cleaved follicular center cells), which accumulate in the opposite pole of the GC, known as the "light zone," which also contains a high concentration of FDCs. Centrocytes reexpress SIg, which has the same variable diversity joining (VDJ) rearrangement as the parent naive B cell and the centroblast of the dark zone but has an altered antibody combining site because of the somatic mutations in the Ig V region (32). This somatic mutation thus results in marked diversity of antibody combining sites in a population of cells derived from only a few precursors. In the GC, the bcl-6 gene also undergoes somatic mutation of the 5' noncoding promoter region at a lower frequency than is seen in the Ig genes (46–48). Thus, both the Ig gene mutation and bcl-6 mutation serve as markers of cells that have experienced the GC.

Centrocytes whose Ig gene mutations have resulted in decreased affinity for antigen rapidly die by apoptosis (programmed cell death); the prominent "starry sky" pattern of phagocytic macrophages seen in GCs at this stage is a result of the apoptosis of centrocytes. In contrast, centrocytes whose Ig gene mutations have resulted in increased affinity are able to bind to antigen trapped in antigen–antibody complexes by the complement receptors on the processes of FDCs. The centrocytes present the antigen to T cells in the light zone of the GC. The activated T cells express CD40 ligand (CD40L), which engages CD40 on the B cell. Both ligation of the antigen receptor by antigen and ligation of CD40 on the surface of GC B cells "rescues" them from apoptosis (28,39–41,49). Interaction with surface molecules expressed by FDCs, such as CD23, directs differentiation of the centrocytes into plasma cells and stimulates class switching from IgM to IgG or IgA production (39,50), whereas interaction with T cells via CD40-CD40L appears to be important in the generation of memory B cells (37,39). In addition, both antigen-receptor ligation and CD40 ligation switch off bcl-6 messenger RNA production and bcl-6 protein expression (51). Through the mechanisms of Ig V region mutation and class switching, the GC reaction gives rise to the better-fitting IgG or IgA antibody of the late primary or secondary immune response (32,52).

FLs are tumors of GC B cells, in which centrocytes fail to undergo apoptosis because they have a chromosomal rearrangement, t(14;18), that prevents the normal switching off of the anti-apoptosis gene, bcl-2 (30,53). Most large B-cell lymphomas are composed of cells that at least in part resemble centroblasts and have mutated Ig V region genes and are therefore thought to derive from the GC stage of differentiation. Finally, it is thought that BL corresponds to the early SIgM+ B blast found in the early GC reaction in experimental animals (54) (Fig. 24-4D).

Marginal Zone and Monocytoid B Cells. When the GC polarizes into a dark and a light zone, the mantle zone becomes better defined and eccentric, with the broader portion surrounding the light zone. Antigen-specific B cells generated in the GC reaction leave the follicle and reappear in the outer mantle zone, to form a "marginal zone"; these are particularly prominent in mesenteric lymph nodes, Peyer's patches, and the spleen (40,55–58). Marginal zone B cells have slightly irregular nuclei, resembling those of centrocytes, but with more abundant, pale cytoplasm. The term centrocyte-like has been applied to similar neoplastic cells (59). Marginal zone B cells from spleen and Peyer's patches have mutated V region genes, consistent with post-GC cells (60–62). On rechallenge with antigen, splenic marginal zone B cells rapidly give rise to antigen-specific plasma cells, consistent with memory B cells (37). Memory B cells are also detectable in the peripheral blood, where they may be IgM+ and even CD5+ (63,64).

Monocytoid B lymphocytes are cells that resemble marginal zone B cells but with even more nuclear indentation and abundant cytoplasm. These are found in clusters adjacent to subcapsular and cortical sinuses of some reactive lymph nodes (65). In contrast to marginal zone B cells, monocytoid B cells in reactive lymph nodes have either unmutated Ig V region genes or show only a small number of randomly distributed mutations that do not suggest selection by antigen (62,66). Nodal and splenic tumors resembling normal marginal zone and monocytoid B cells have been described (67–70), but analysis of Ig V region genes from the tumors suggest that most of these have mutations consistent with GC exposure and antigen selection (71,72). Thus, the relationship of normal to neoplastic monocytoid B cells is not clear.

Bone Marrow Plasma Cells. IgG- and IgA-producing plasma cells accumulate in the lymph node medulla, but it appears that the immediate precursor of the bone marrow plasma cell leaves the node and migrates to the bone marrow. Plasma cells lose SIg, pan-B-cell antigens, HLA-DR, CD40, and CD45, and cytoplasmic IgG or IgA accumulates. Plasma cells also express CD38 and CD138; the latter may be important in adhesion to bone marrow stroma. They have rearranged and mutated Ig genes but do not have the ongoing mutations seen in follicle center cells. Tumors of these marrow-homing plasma cells correspond to plasmacytoma and multiple myeloma.

Mucosa-Associated Lymphoid Tissue. A subset of B cells, including all the differentiation stages listed above, are programmed for gut-associated rather than nodal lymphoid tissue. In these tissues (Waldeyer's ring, Peyer's patches, and mesen-

teric nodes), similar responses occur to antigen, but both the intermediate and end-stage B cells that originate in the gut or mesenteric lymph nodes preferentially return there, rather than to peripheral lymph nodes or bone marrow. Thus, the plasma cells generated in gut-associated lymphoid tissue home preferentially to the lamina propria, rather than to the bone marrow (17,18). MALT is characterized by reactive follicles with GCs and prominent marginal zones, as well as numerous plasma cells in the lamina propria. Marginal zone B cells in normal MALT typically infiltrate the overlying epithelium, forming a lymphoepithelium. Many extranodal low-grade B-cell lymphomas are thought to arise from MALT (59). Because most MALT lymphomas contain prominent marginal zone type B cells, in addition to small B lymphocytes and plasma cells, and because similar lymphomas occur in non-MALT sites, the term extranodal marginal zone lymphoma (MZL) of MALT type has been proposed for these tumors (3). MALT-type lymphomas have somatically mutated V-region genes, consistent with an antigen-selected post-GC B-cell stage (73).

T-CELL DIFFERENTIATION

Antigen-Independent T-Cell Differentiation

Cortical Thymocytes. The earliest antigen-independent stages of T-cell differentiation occur in the bone marrow; later stages occur in the thymic cortex. The exact site at which precursor cells become committed to the T lineage is not known, because the thymus contains cells that can differentiate into either T cells or NK cells, but not B cells (reviewed in 74) (Fig. 24-4A). Cortical thymocytes are lymphoblasts, which contain the intranuclear enzyme TdT, like B lymphoblasts. Within the thymus they sequentially acquire CD1a, CD2, CD5, and cytoplasmic CD3, and first the CD4 "helper" and then the CD8 "suppressor" antigen ("double positive"). A process of antigen-receptor gene rearrangement analogous to that seen in B cells also occurs during T-cell differentiation (74) (Fig. 24-7). Rearrangement of the T-cell receptor genes begins with the γ and Δ chains, followed by the β- and then the α-chain genes; these proteins are then expressed on the cell surface. Surface CD3 expression appears at the same time as expression of the T-cell antigen receptor β chain, with which it is closely associated and participates in signal transduction. Cortical thymocytes, like GC B cells, lack the antiapoptosis protein, bcl-2 (30), and are thus susceptible to apoptosis (Fig. 24-4B).

In addition to providing a pool of mature T cells through proliferation of precursor cells, the thymus plays a major role in the selection of T cells so that the resulting pool of mature T cells recognize self MHC molecules and do not react to "self" antigens. Both positive and negative selection occur in the thymus at the double positive (CD4+CD8+) stage. Thymocytes that have antiself specificity bind strongly via their T-cell receptor (TCR) complex to self antigens presented by the MHC on thymic dendritic cells and die by apoptosis. Those that lack antiself reactivity but bind strongly to MCH molecules undergo positive selection on thymic epithelial cells; they then express increased levels of surface CD3, lose CD1 and either CD4 or CD8, and express bcl-2, to become mature, naive T cells (74). The tumor that corresponds to the stages of T-cell differentiation in the thymic cortex is precursor T lymphoblastic lymphoma and leukemia; the variety of immunophenotypes and antigen receptor gene rearrangements found in precursor T-cell neoplasia correspond to the variety of stages of intrathymic T-cell differentiation.

Naive T Cells. Mature, naive (virgin) T cells have the morphologic appearance of small lymphocytes, have a low proliferation fraction, lack TdT and CD1, and express either (but not

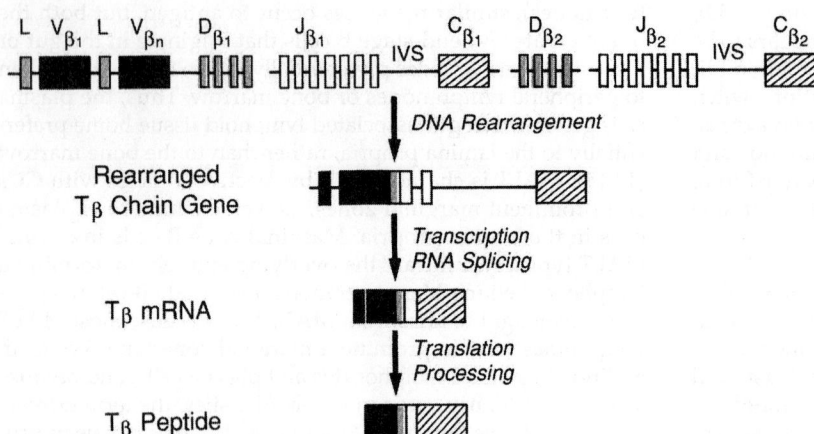

Figure 24-7. Schematic depiction of the beta chain gene of the T-cell receptor. Two constant regions ($C\beta_1$ and $C\beta_2$) each have their own joining and diversity segments and share a common pool of variable ($V\beta$) segments. The rearrangement associates one $V\beta$, one diversity ($D\beta$), and one joining ($J\beta$) gene with a $V\beta$ segment to form a rearranged gene. Transcriptional RNA splicing, translation, and processing generates the final beta chain.

both) CD4 or CD8, as well as surface CD3 and CD5 (75), and bcl-2 (30,76). These cells are found in the thymic medulla, in the circulation, and in the paracortex of lymph nodes (Fig. 24-4C). Some cases of T-cell prolymphocytic leukemia (PLL) and peripheral T-cell lymphoma may correspond to naive T cells (Fig. 24-4D).

Antigen-Dependent T-Cell Differentiation. In contrast to B cells, which can recognize unprocessed antigen free in the tissues, T cells can only recognize antigen after it has been processed by phagocytes and presented on the surface of APC in the "pocket" of the MHC molecule (reviewed in 77). On the T cell, the CD4 or CD8 molecules bind to MHC class II or class I molecules, respectively, on the APC. The T cell is then activated via CD40-CD40L and binding of CD28 and CTLA4 on the T cell to B7-1 and B7-2 (CD80/86) on the APC (78,79).

T-Immunoblasts. On encountering antigen, mature T cells transform into *immunoblasts*, which are large cells with prominent nucleoli and basophilic cytoplasm, which may be indistinguishable from B immunoblasts. T immunoblasts, in contrast to T lymphoblasts (thymocytes), are TdT and CD1a negative, strongly express pan-T-cell antigens, and continue to express either CD4 or CD8, not both. Antigen-dependent T-cell reactions occur in the paracortex of lymph nodes and the periarteriolar lymphoid sheath of the spleen, as well as at extranodal sites of immunologic reactions. Many peripheral T-cell lymphomas appear to correspond to proliferating peripheral T cells.

Effector T Cells. From the T-immunoblastic reaction come antigen-specific effector T cells of either CD4 or CD8 type, as well as memory T cells. Effector T cells of the CD4 type typically act as helper cells, and those of the CD8 type act as suppressor cells *in vitro*, but both types can be cytotoxic (80). CD4 cells are cytotoxic to cells that display antigen complexed with MHC class II antigen, whereas CD8 cells are cytotoxic to cells that display it complexed with MHC class I antigen. Cytotoxic T cells contain cytoplasmic granule–associated proteins that attack target cells (TIA-1, perforin, granzyme B), and which can be used to identify cytotoxic cells in tissue sections. In addition to cytotoxicity, effector T cells produce a variety of cytokines that affect the function of B cells and APCs, which modulate the immune response. Fully differentiated T effector cells are small lymphocytes, morphologically similar to other nonproliferating lymphocytes of either T or B type. In addition to differences in subset antigen (CD4 versus CD8 or double negative) expression, peripheral T cells may differ in their T-cell receptor expression ($\gamma\delta$ versus $\alpha\beta$). The majority of T cells in the circulation and

in most lymphoid tissues are $\alpha\beta^+$; $\gamma\delta$ T cells are more numerous in mucosae and in the spleen (81).

Some cases of peripheral T-cell lymphomas are thought to correspond to effector T cells. For example, mycosis fungoides corresponds to a mature, effector CD4$^+$ cell; hepatosplenic T-cell lymphoma to $\gamma\delta$ T cells that reside in the spleen; T-cell large granular lymphocyte (LGL) leukemia to a mature effector CD8$^+$ cell; and many extranodal T-cell lymphomas to cytotoxic T cells. However, the relationship between neoplastic and normal T cells is not nearly as well understood as in the B-cell system (Fig. 24-4C). The systemic symptoms such as fever, skin rashes, and hemophagocytic syndromes associated with some peripheral T-cell lymphomas may be a consequence of cytokine production by the neoplastic T cells.

NATURAL KILLER CELLS

A third line of lymphoid cells, called *NK cells* because they can kill certain targets without sensitization and without MHC restriction, appears to derive from a common progenitor with T cells (reviewed in 74). NK cells recognize self class I MHC molecules on the surfaces of cells and kill cells that lack these antigens. Immature NK cells have cytoplasmic CD3, but these cells do not rearrange their T-cell receptor genes or express T-cell receptors or surface CD3. They are characterized by certain NK-cell–associated antigens (CD16, CD56, and CD57) that can also be expressed on some T cells and also express some T-cell–associated antigens (CD2 and CD8). NK cells appear in the peripheral blood as a small proportion of circulating lymphocytes; they are usually slightly larger than most normal T and B cells, with abundant pale cytoplasm containing azurophilic granules, so-called LGLs. Extranodal T/NK cell lymphoma and some types of LGL leukemia appear to correspond to immature and mature NK cells, respectively.

Immunophenotyping of Lymphoid Cells

Individual B and T lymphoid cells as well as accessory cells of the mononuclear phagocyte system can be recognized in cell suspensions or tissue sections by the presence of surface or cytoplasmic molecules (antigens) that can be detected using antibodies labeled with either fluorescence or enzymatic (immunohistochemical) methods. A series of international workshops have developed a standardized nomenclature for many of the antigens detected by more than one monoclonal antibody (82) (Table 24-9). Immunophenotyping with monoclonal antibodies can be done using viable cell suspensions, frozen tissue sections, or paraffin-embedded tissue sections. For cells in body fluids, particularly the peripheral blood and bone

TABLE 24-9. Cluster Designations of Antigens Useful in the Classification of Lymphoid Neoplasms

Cluster Designations	Normal Cells	Neoplasms
1a	Cortical thymocytes (strong), Langerhans' cells	Precursor T lymphoblastic lymphoma/leukemia; Langerhans' cell neoplasms
2	T cells, NK cells	T-cell neoplasms
3	T cells, immature NK cells (cytoplasm)	T-cell neoplasms, some NK-cell neoplasms
4	T subset (MHC Class II restricted), monocytes	Some T-cell neoplasms
5	T cells, naive B cells	T-cell neoplasms, B-CLL, mantle cell lymphoma
7	T cells, NK cells	T-cell neoplasms, NK-cell neoplasms
8	T subset (MHC Class I restricted), NK subset, splenic sinus lining cells	Some T-cell neoplasms, some NK-cell neoplasms
10	Precursor B cells, GC B cells, granulocytes, fibroblasts, kidney epithelium	Precursor B lymphoblastic lymphoma/leukemia, Burkitt lymphoma, follicular lymphoma, diffuse large B-cell lymphoma (25%)
11c	Monocytes, granulocytes, activated CD8$^+$ T cells, NK cells, B-cell subset	B-CLL (some cases); hairy cell leukemia
15	Granulocytes, monocytes	Reed-Sternberg cells of classic HL
16	NK cells, granulocytes, macrophages	NK-cell neoplasms, some T-cell neoplasms
19	B cells, including precursor B	B-cell neoplasms
20	Mature B cells (not plasma cells), T-cell subset	Mature B-cell neoplasms, lymphocyte predominance HL, some classic HL
21	Mature B-cell subset, FDC	Mature B-cell neoplasms, FDCs in some lymphomas and FDC neoplasms
22	B cells (cytoplasm); B-cell subset (surface)	B-cell neoplasms
23	IgE Fc receptor: activated B cells, monocytes, FDC	B-CLL/ small lymphocytic lymphoma, FDCs in some lymphomas
25	Il2 receptor: activated T cells, activated B cells, activated monocytes	Hairy cell leukemia, Reed-Sternberg cells, ALCL, some T-cell neoplasms
30	Activated T cells, B cells, NK-cells, monocytes	Reed-Sternberg cells in classic HL, ALCL, some diffuse large B-cell lymphomas
43	T cells, B subset, NK cells, monocytes, plasma cells and myeloid cells	T-cell neoplasms, some B-cell neoplasms, myeloid neoplasms
45	Leukocyte common antigen, all leukocytes except plasma cells	Lymphoid and myeloid neoplasms
45RA	B-cells, naive T cells, NK cells	B-cell neoplasms, some T-cell neoplasms
45RO	T-cells (most), granulocytes, monocytes	T-cell neoplasms
56	Neural cell adhesion molecule: NK cells, activated T cells	NK cell neoplasms, some T-cell neoplasms
68	Monocytes, macrophages, activated T cells	Myeloid and histiocytic neoplasms, some T-cell neoplasms
57	T cell and NK cell subset, neural tissue	NK-cell neoplasms, some T-cell neoplasms
79a	B cells, including precursor B and plasma cells	B-cell neoplasms, rare T-lymphoblastic neoplasms, lymphocyte predominant HL, rare classic HL
95	Fas (apoptosis receptor): activated T cells, B cells	Some B- and T-cell neoplasms, HL
99	Cortical thymocytes	Precursor B- and T-cell neoplasms, Ewing's sarcoma
103	Mucosal intraepithelial lymphocytes	Hairy cell leukemia; enteropathy-type T-cell lymphoma
138	Syndecan 1(stromal binding): plasma cells	Plasma cell neoplasms, plasmablastic lymphomas

ALCL, anaplastic large-cell lymphoma; CLL, chronic lymphocytic leukemia; FDC, follicular dendritic cell; HL, Hodgkin's lymphoma; MHC, major histocompatibility complex; NK, natural killer.

marrow, flow cytometry with fluorescent-labeled antibodies is the method of choice; this method can also be applied to fine-needle aspiration biopsy specimens and to cell suspensions prepared from fresh tissue specimens, but sampling problems can occur due to selective loss of fragile neoplastic cells. Acetone-fixed frozen sections are the most reliable method for the pathologist to assess the phenotype of lymphoid cells in tissue sections. However, in recent years, the technology for detecting lymphocyte-associated antigens in paraffin-embedded tissue has greatly improved, so that most clinically necessary immunophenotyping can be accomplished using only routinely processed tissue. Nonetheless, it is still advisable to prepare fresh frozen tissue on all cases of suspected lymphoma, in case a diagnosis cannot be made with certainty on paraffin tissue section analysis, and also for possible molecular genetic analysis.

Chromosomal Translocations and Oncogene Rearrangements

In addition to rearrangements of antigen-receptor genes, hematologic malignancies frequently have specific chromosomal trans-

locations (Table 24-10) (83,84). Cellular oncogenes (genes that can cause malignant transformation when transfected in activated or altered form into cultured normal cells) and tumor-suppressor genes have been identified in association with some of the more common chromosome translocations that characterize lymphoid malignancies (85,86). The most common translocations involved in lymphoid neoplasms place a gene that is normally silent in resting cells under the influence of a promotor associated with either an Ig or T-cell receptor gene, resulting in activation of the gene and giving the cell either a growth or survival advantage. Examples include the t(8;14)(q24;q32) in BL (Fig. 24-8), which places the cMYC gene under the Ig heavy-chain promotor (83) (Fig. 24-8); the t(14;18)(q32;q32) of FL (Fig. 24-9), which places the BCL2 gene on chromosome 18 under the Ig promotor (86,87); and the t(11;14)(q13;q32) in MCL, which places the cyclin D1 gene (associated with the BCL1 breakpoint) on chromosome 11 under the Ig promotor (88). These translocations can be detected using DNA probes that hybridize to the breakpoint regions on the chromosomes carrying the Ig gene and containing the oncogene.

In some lymphoid neoplasms, a chromosomal translocation results in a fusion of two genes, resulting in an abnormal protein,

TABLE 24-10. Genetic Abnormalities in Lymphoid Neoplasms

Genetic Abnormality	Genes	Lymphoid Neoplasms	Detection
Translocations involving Ig genes (activation by Ig promotor)			
t(8;14)(q23;q32)	c-MYC/IgH	Burkitt lymphoma (30% to 100%);	CG, Southern blot, FISH (c-MYC)
t(2;8)(p12;q23)	c-MYC/Igκ	large B-cell lymphoma (approxi-	
t(8;22)(q23;q11)	c-MYC/Igλ	mately 10%)	
t(11;14)(q13;32)	BCL1(CCND1)/IgH	Mantle cell lymphoma; plasma cell	CG, PCR, FISH
		myeloma[a]	
t(14;18)(q32;q21)	BCL2/IgH	Follicular lymphoma (90%); large B-	CG, Southern blot, PCR, FISH
		cell lymphoma (20%)	
t(14;19)(q32;q13)	BCL3/IgH	CLL/B-SLL	CG
t(3;14)(q27;q32) and t(V;3q27)[b]	BCL6/IgH	Large B-cell lymphoma (30%); follicu-	CG, Southern blot, FISH
	Variable/BCL6	lar lymphoma (15%)	
t(1;14)(p22;q32)	BCL10/IgH	MALT lymphoma; large B-cell lym-	CG
		phoma	
t(9;14)(p13;q32)	PAX5(BSAP)/IgH	Lymphoplasmacytic lymphoma	CG
		(approximately 50%); plasma cell	
		myeloma (rare)	
t(4;14)(p16;q32)	MMSET(FGFR)/IgH	Plasma cell myeloma	Southern blot, FISH
t(6;14)(p25;q32)	IRF4(MUM1)/IgH		Southern blot, FISH
t(14;16)(q32;q23)	IgH/c-MAF		Southern blot, FISH
t(1;14)(q21;q32)	NUM2/IgH		CG, FISH
Translocations involving the TCR genes (activation by TCR promotors)			
t(1;14)(p32;q11)[c,e]	TAL1/TCRβ	Precursor T lymphoblastic lymphoma/	CG
		leukemia	
t(8;14)(q24;q11)	c-MYC/TCRβ		CG, FISH (c-MYC)
t(11;14)(p15;q11)[d]	RBTN1(TTG2)/TCRβ		CG
t(10;14)(q24;q11)	HOX11/TCRβ		CG
inv(14)(q11;q32)	TCRα/unknown	T-PLL (70%)	CG
t(14;14)(q11;q32)		T-PLL (10%)	CG
Translocations producing fusion genes/proteins (activation or inactivation)			
t(9;22)(q34;q11)	BCR/ABL	Precursor B lymphoblastic lym-	CG, FISH
		phoma/leukemia	
t(V)(11q23)	MLL		CG, PCR
t(12;21)(p12;q22)	TEL/AML1		CG, FISH
t(1;19)(q23;p13)	PBX/E2A		CG
t(11;18)(q21;q21)	API2/MLT	MALT lymphoma	CG, RT-PCR, FISH
t(2;5)(p23;q35)	NPM/ALK	Anaplastic large cell lymphoma	CG, RT-PCR, FISH (ALK)
Chromosomal additions and deletions			
i(7q)(q10)	Unknown	Hepatosplenic T-cell lymphoma	CG
+3	Unknown	MALT lymphoma; large B-cell lym-	CG, FISH
		phoma	
6q23-26	Unknown	B-cell lymphomas (10% to 40%)	CG
+8	Unknown	Peripheral T-cell lymphoma	CG, FISH
+3 +5 +X	Unknown	Angioimmunoblastic T-cell lym-	
		phoma	
+12	Unknown	CLL/B-SLL (30%)	CG, FISH
13q deletions	Unknown	CLL/B-SLL (25%)	CG, FISH
−13, 13q14 deletions	Unknown	Plasma cell myeloma	CG, FISH

CG, cytogenetics; CLL, chronic lymphocytic leukemia; FISH, fluorescence *in situ* hybridization; Ig, immunoglobulin; MALT, mucosa-associated lymphoid tissue; PCR, polymerase chain reaction; PLL, prolymphocytic leukemia; SLL, small lymphocytic lymphoma; TCR, T-cell receptor.
[a]In myeloma, translocation is into switch region of IgH; in mantle cell, into joining region.
[b]Promotors other than IgH activate BCL6.
[c]May involve 7q34 (TCRγ) instead of 14q11.
[d]May involve RBTN2 at 11p13.
[e]Deletions in the 5' regulatory region of TAL1 may also be seen.

which may be either abnormally activated or inactivated. Examples include the t(2;5)(p23;q35) found in ALCL, which produces a hybrid nucleophosmin–anaplastic lymphoma kinase (ALK) protein (89), and the t(11;18)(q21;q21) in MALT lymphoma, which produces an API2-MLT fusion protein (90).

Using a technique for amplifying unique DNA segments [polymerase chain reaction (PCR)], rare cells carrying a given translocation can be detected by using probes that span the breakpoint (91), or using a reverse transcriptase technique to detect RNA produced by an altered or fused gene (92) (Fig. 24-9). The PCR technique can be used to detect minimal residual dis-

ease in patients whose tumors carry a specific translocation (93,94). Numeric abnormalities of chromosomes are also found in lymphoid malignancies; both these and some of the translocations can be detected by fluorescence *in situ* hybridization, using probes to specific chromosomes or segments (95–97).

To the extent to which specific histologic subtypes or prognostic groups of lymphomas are associated with specific gene rearrangements, detection of these rearrangements is useful in the characterization of lymphomas (Table 24-10). In addition, this technique can be used to detect disseminated or recurrent lymphoma on very small biopsy specimens or in the blood.

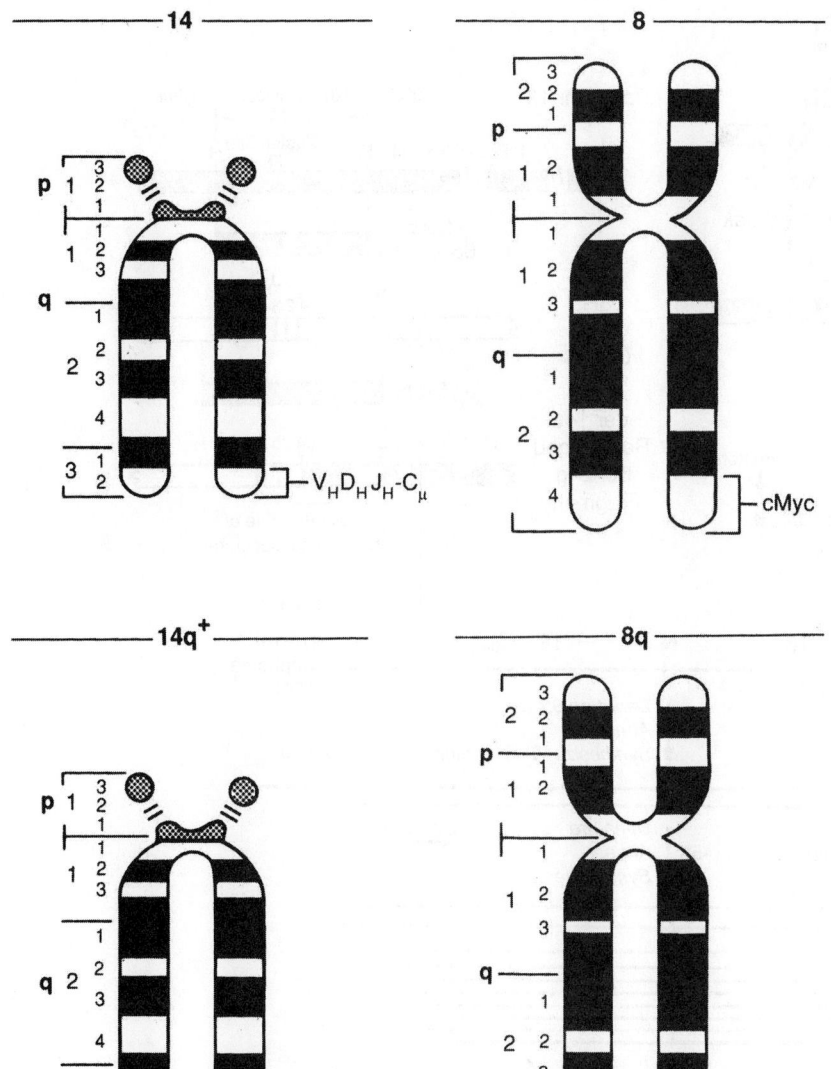

Figure 24-8. Schematic karyotype of Burkitt lymphoma translocation t(8;14)(q24;q32). The translocation introduces the c-Myc gene from chromosome 8 into the $V_H D_H J_H$ locus on chromosome 14, and a portion of the V_H gene on chromosome 14 is moved to the end of chromosome 8. The normal chromosome 14 retains a productively rearranged $V_H D_H J_H$ responsible for immunoglobulin M production. The normal chromosome 8 retains a germline copy of the c-Myc oncogene.

Finally, studies of the function of the translocated oncogenes are providing clues to the mechanisms of oncogenesis.

Use of Immunophenotyping and Genetic Studies in the Diagnosis of Lymphoid Neoplasms

Each of the lymphoid neoplasms has a characteristic morphology, which may be sufficient in a given case to permit diagnosis and classification on morphologic grounds alone, if well-prepared sections are available. Thus, many cases of lymphoma can be diagnosed and classified with reasonable certainty on the basis of routine histologic sections alone. However, there are many pitfalls in the histologic diagnosis of malignant lymphoma, and immunophenotyping or genetic studies can be useful in resolving major differential diagnostic problems. The major immunophenotypic and genetic features of the more common B- and T-cell neoplasms are listed in Tables 24-11 and 24-12.

Problems that can be resolved by these techniques include the following: (a) reactive versus neoplastic lymphoid infiltrates, (b) lymphoid versus nonlymphoid malignancies, and (c) subclassification of lymphoma. In a given case, if the morphology is typical of a given entity but the immunophenotypic or genetic features are unusual, the histologic sections should be reexamined; however, the case may still be accepted as an example of the entity suggested by morphologic features. If the morphology is atypical but the immunophenotype and genetic features are classic for a given entity, these features may override morphology in classification. If both the morphology and the immunophenotype are atypical, then the case is best regarded as unclassifiable or borderline.

LYMPHOID NEOPLASMS IN THE REVISED EUROPEAN-AMERICAN CLASSIFICATION OF LYMPHOID NEOPLASMS AND THE WORLD HEALTH ORGANIZATION CLASSIFICATION

Precursor (Lymphoblastic) Neoplasms

PRECURSOR B-CELL LYMPHOBLASTIC LEUKEMIA AND LYMPHOMA

Clinical Features. Precursor B-cell acute lymphoblastic leukemia (ALL) and precursor LBL occurs most frequently in

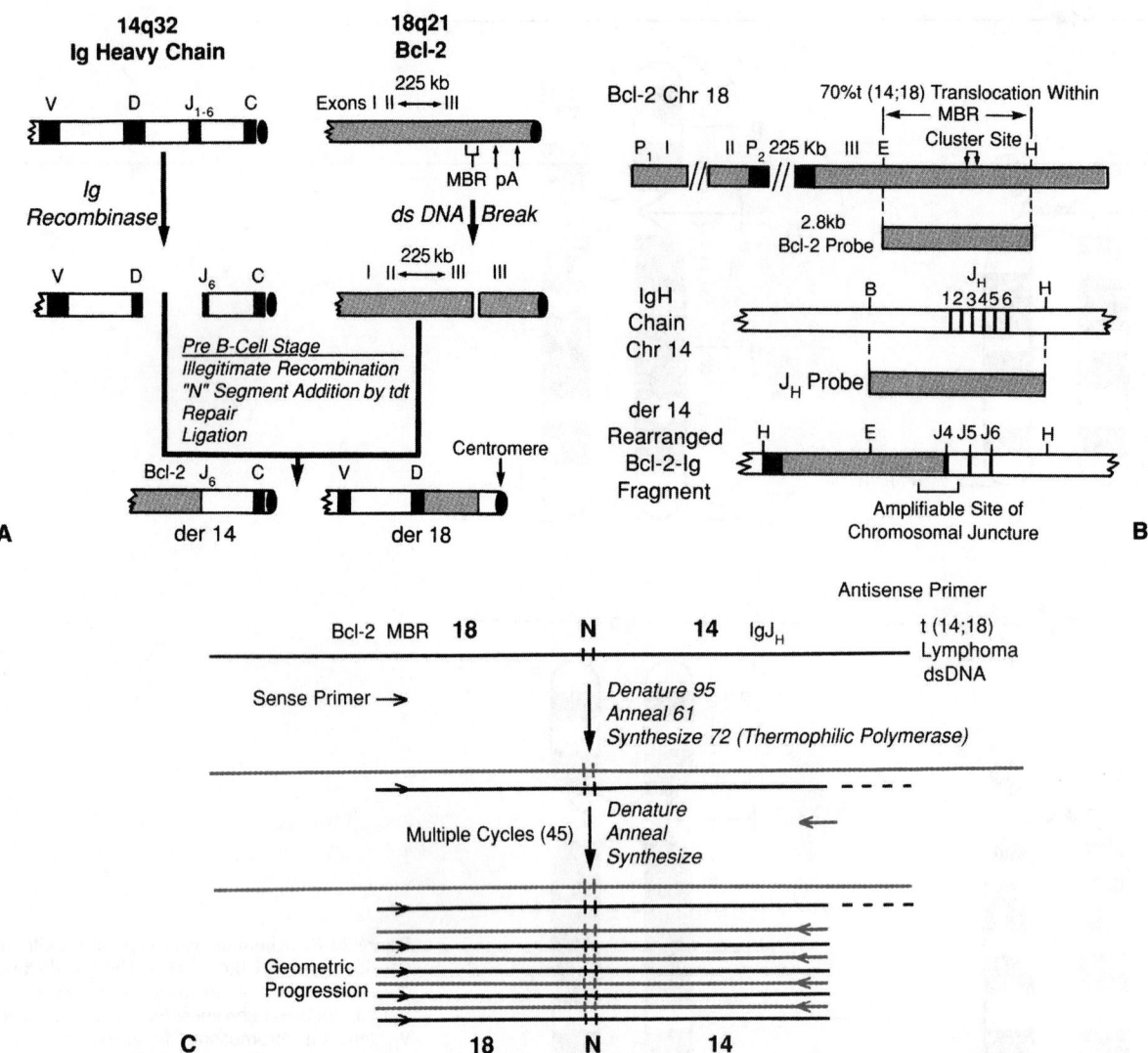

Figure 24-9. Mechanism and detection of the t(14;18) recombination. **A:** The derivative chromosome 14 demonstrates a breakpoint at a J segment, while the derivative chromosome 18 contains a breakpoint involving a D segment of the immunoglobulin (Ig) gene. This suggests that the translocation occurs in a precursor B cell when Ig recombinase has cleaved at a D and J segment; these ends, instead of joining to form a functional Ig molecule, recombine with a break at 18q21 within the major breakpoint region (MBR) of *BCL-2* exon III. **B:** Schematic representation of a molecular marker for the t(14;18) interchromosomal breakpoint. The der (14) chromosome possesses an altered size HKNDIII (H) DNA fragment that will hybridize to both a chromosome 18 *BCL-2* probe and a chromosome 14 J_H probe. **C:** Schematic representation of polymerase chain reaction amplification of the t(14;18) breakpoint. A sense oligonucleotide primer 5' to the BCL-2 MBR is used together with an antisense primer complementary to the JH region on chromosome 14. Successive cycles of denaturation, primer annealing, and synthesis with polymerase results in the specific amplification of a fragment containing both chromosome 18 and chromosome 14 information. dsDNA, double-stranded DNA; IgJ, immunoglobulin J; TdT, terminal deoxynucleotidyl transferase.

childhood, with a second peak in the elderly. Patients typically have involvement of bone marrow and peripheral blood. Occasionally patients present with isolated tumors of lymph nodes, skin, or bone (precursor B LBL); many of these eventually develop bone marrow involvement (98–101). The outcome is less favorable in infants less than 1 year of age and in adults. In addition to cytogenetic features, risk groups are based on age, leukocyte count, sex, and response to therapy. In infants, many cases have translocations involving the mixed lineage leukemia gene at 11q23, which is associated with a poor prognosis at any age (102); older children more often have hyperdiploidy or t(12;21), which confers a better prognosis (85% to 90% long-term survival) (103). Adult pre-

cursor B ALL is more often associated with the poor-prognosis t(9;22) or t(v11q23), and the survival is much poorer than that for childhood cases (104,105). Myeloid antigen expression does not seem to be an independent prognostic factor in ALL (106,107).

Morphology. On smears, lymphoblasts vary from small cells with scant cytoplasm, condensed nuclear chromatin, and indistinct nucleoli to larger cells with a moderate amount of cytoplasm, dispersed chromatin, and multiple nucleoli. Azurophilic granules may be present. In tissue sections, the cells are small to medium sized, with scant cytoplasm, round, oval, or convoluted nuclei, with fine chromatin and indistinct

TABLE 24-11. Immunophenotypic and Genetic Features of Common B-Cell Neoplasms

Neoplasm	Surface Ig; Intracytoplasmic Ig	CD5	CD10	CD23	CD43	CD103	Cyclin D1	Genetic Abnormality	Ig Genes[a]
B-cell small lymphocytic lymphoma/ chronic lymphocytic leukemia	+; –/+	+	–	+	+	–	–	Trisomy 12; 13q	R, U (50%); M (50%)
Lymphoplasmacytic lymphoma	+; +	–	–	–	+/–	–	–	t(9;14); del 6(q23)	R,M
Hairy cell leukemia	+; –	–	–	–	+	+	+/–	none known	R,M
Splenic marginal zone lymphoma	+; –/+	–	–	–	–	+/–	–	none known	R,M
Follicular lymphoma	+; –	–	+/–	–/+	–	–	–	t(14;18); bcl-2	R,M,O
Mantle cell lymphoma	+; –	+	–	–	+	–	+	t(11;14); bcl-1	R,U
Mucosa-associated lymphoid tissue lymphoma	+; +/–	–	–	–/+	–/+	–	–	t(11;18); trisomy 3; AP12/MLT1	R,M,O
Diffuse large B-cell lymphoma	+/–; –/+	–	–/+	NA	–/+	NA	–	t(14;18), t(8;14), 3q; bcl-2, myc, bcl-6	R,M
Burkitt lymphoma	+; –	–	+	–	–	NA	–	t(8;14), t(2;8), t(8;22); c-myc; Epstein-Barr virus –/+	R,M

+, greater than 90% positive; +/–, greater than 50% positive; –/+ less than 50% positive; –, less than 10% positive; Ig, immunoglobulin; M, mutated; NA, not available; O, ongoing mutations; R, rearranged; U, unmutated.
[a]Mutations in the Ig gene variable region indicate exposure to antigen.

TABLE 24-12. Immunophenotypic and Genetic Features of Common T-Cell Neoplasms

Neoplasm	CD3 S;C	CD5	CD7	CD4	CD8	CD30	T-Cell Receptor	NK CD16, CD56	Cytotox Granule	Epstein-Barr Virus	Genetic Abnormality	T-Receptor Genes
T-cell prolymphocytic leukemia	+	–	+	+/–	–/+	–	αβ	–	–	–	Inv 14; trisomy 8q	R
T-cell large granular lymphocyte	+	–	+	–	+	–	αβ	+, –	+	–	None known	R
NK-large granular lymphocyte	–	–	+	–	+/–	–	–	–,+	+	+	None known	G
Extranodal NK/T-cell lymphoma	–;+	–	+	–	–	–	–	NA, +	+	+	None known	G
Hepatosplenic T-cell lymphoma	+	–	+	–	–	–	γδ>αβ	+, –/+	+	–	Iso 7q	R
Enteropathy-type T-cell lymphoma	+	+	+	–	+/–	+/–	αβ>γδ	–	+	–	None known	R
Mycosis fungoides	+	+	–/+	+	–	–	αβ	–	–	–	None known	R
Cutaneous ALCL	+	+/–	+/–	+/–	–	++	αβ	–	–/+	–	None known	R
Subcutaneous panniculitis-like T-cell	+	+	+/–	–	+	–/+	αβ>γδ	+/–	+	–	None known	R
Peripheral T-cell lymphoma NOS	+/–	+/–	+/–	+/–	–/+	–/+	αβ>γδ	–/+	–/+	–/+	Inv 14; complex	R
Angioimmunoblastic	+	+	+/–	+/–	–/+	–	αβ	–	NA	+/–	+3, +5, +X	R
Primary systemic ALCL	+/–	+/–	NA	+/–	–/+	++	αβ	–	+	–	t(2;5); NPM/ ALK	R

+, greater than 90% positive; +/–, greater than 50% positive; –/+, less than 50% positive; –, less than 10% positive; ALCL, anaplastic large-cell lymphoma; C, cytoplasmic; G, gamma; NA, not available; NK, natural killer; NOS, not otherwise specified; R, rearranged; S, surface.

or small nucleoli. The pattern in lymph nodes is infiltrative rather than destructive, with partial preservation of the subcapsular sinus and GCs. The bone marrow shows varying degrees of involvement in most cases, and the peripheral blood is typically involved. Extramedullary presentations may be misdiagnosed as other types of small round-cell neoplasms (98–101).

Immunophenotype and Genetic Features. Precursor B lymphoblasts express nuclear TdT and variably express CD19, CD22, CD20, and CD79a, as well as CD45 and CD10. The constellation of antigens defines stages of differentiation, ranging from early precursor (membrane CD19 and CD79a and cytoplasmic CD22), to "common" ALL (CD10+) to late pre–B ALL (CD20+, cytoplasmic μ–heavy chain). CD34 is expressed on 40% of the cases, and coexpression of myeloid antigens is seen in up to 30%, most commonly CD13 (14%) or CD33 (16%) (104,107). Expression of CD13 and CD33 is associated with rearrangement of ETV6 [t(12;21)(p12;q22),ETV6-CBFA2/TEL-AML1], whereas expression of CD68, CD15, and CD33 is seen in cases with 11q23/MLL abnormalities (107).

Rearrangement of antigen receptor genes is variable in lymphoblastic neoplasms and may not be lineage-specific; thus, precursor B-cell neoplasms may have either or both Ig heavy-chain and T-cell receptor γ- or β- chain gene rearrangements or may show no rearrangements (108–110). Ig V region genes are unmutated.

Chromosomal abnormalities are common in precursor B lymphoblastic neoplasms and are related to prognosis. They are typically divided into 3 categories: hyperdiploidy greater than 50 chromosomes, hyperdiploidy less than 50 chromosomes, and pseudodiploidy and translocations. The frequency of these abnormalities varies between children and adults, and some are associated with characteristic immunophenotypes or clinical behavior. Hyperdiploidy with 51 to 65 chromosomes (DNA index 1.16 to 1.6) is seen in up to 50% of cases of childhood precursor B ALL and is associated with a good prognosis; it is less common in adult ALL.

Translocations involving four recurrent sites are seen in precursor B ALL:

t(9;22)(a34;q11) BCR/ABL: poor prognosis; 25% of adults
t(v;11q23); MLL rearranged: poor prognosis; infants less than 1 year of age and adults (102)
t(12;21)(p12;q22) TEL/AML1: good prognosis; children (103)
t(1;19)(q23;p13) PBX/E2A: poor prognosis; 25% of children

The t(9;22) and t(v;11q23) are often associated with an early pre-B immunophenotype and a poor prognosis (102,104), whereas the t(1;19) is often associated with a late pre-B immunophenotype (cytoplasmic μ+).

Postulated Normal Counterpart. Precursor B-cell neoplasms are thought to correspond to precursor B lymphoblasts at varying stages of differentiation.

PRECURSOR T-CELL LYMPHOBLASTIC LYMPHOMA AND LEUKEMIA

Clinical Features. Precursor T-cell neoplasia occurs most frequently in late childhood, adolescence, and young adulthood, with a male predominance; it comprises 15% of childhood and 25% of adult ALL (105). The prognosis is typically worse than that for precursor B-cell neoplasms and is not affected by immunophenotype or genetic abnormalities. Patients typically present with a very high leukocyte count and often a mediastinal mass. Clinically, a case is defined as *lymphoma* if there is a mediastinal or other mass and less than 25% blasts in the bone marrow and as *leukemia* if there are greater than 25% bone marrow blasts, with or without a mass. In children, treatment is generally more aggressive than that for precursor B ALL and is typically the same for lymphomatous and leukemic presentations (111).

Morphology. The morphologic features of precursor T lymphoblasts are identical to those of precursor B lymphoblasts (see Morphology under Precursor B-Lymphoblastic Leukemia and Lymphoma).

Immunophenotype and Genetic Features. The lymphoblasts express TdT and variably express CD2, CD7, CD3, CD5, CD1a, CD4, and CD8. Only surface CD3 is considered lineage-specific. The constellation of antigens defines stages of differentiation, ranging from early or pro-T (CD2, CD7, and cytoplasmic CD3), to "common" thymocyte (CD1a, sCD3, CD4, and CD8), to late thymocyte (CD4 or CD8). Although there is some correlation with presentation and differentiation stage [cases with bone marrow and blood presentation may show earlier differentiation stage than cases with thymic presentation (112,113)], there is overlap (114).

Rearrangement of antigen-receptor genes is variable in lymphoblastic neoplasms and may not be lineage-specific; thus, precursor T-cell neoplasms may have either or both TCR β- or γ- chain gene rearrangements and Ig heavy-chain gene rearrangements (115). Chromosomal translocations involving the TCR α and Δ loci at chromosome 14q11 and β and γ loci at 7q34 are present in approximately one-third of the cases (104,111); the partner genes are variable and include the transcription factors c-MYC (8q24), TAL1/SCL (1p32), RBTN1 (11p35), RBTN2 (11913), HOX11 (10q24), and the cytoplasmic tyrosine kinase LCK (1p34). In an additional 25%, the TAL1 locus at 1p32 has deletions in the 5' regulatory region (116).

Postulated Normal Counterpart. Precursor T-cell neoplasms are thought to correspond to precursor T lymphoblasts at varying stages of differentiation.

Mature (Peripheral) B-Cell Neoplasms

CHRONIC LYMPHOCYTIC LEUKEMIA AND SMALL LYMPHOCYTIC LYMPHOMA

Clinical Features. Cell CLL comprises 90% of chronic lymphoid leukemias in the United States and Europe; nonleukemic B SLL accounts for less than 5% of NHLs. In the International non-Hodgkin's Lymphoma Classification Project, 6.7% of 1378 cases were diagnosed as B CLL/SLL. The median age was 65 years, and 83% had stage IV disease (73% with bone marrow involvement). Generalized lymphadenopathy, hepatosplenomegaly, and extranodal infiltrates may occur. Sixty-four percent had an IPI score of 2 to 3. The 5-year overall actuarial survival (OAS) was 51%, with a failure-free survival of 25%; for those patients with an IPI of 0 to 1, the OAS was 76%, whereas for those with an IPI of 4 to 5, it was only 38%. Thus, the extent of the disease at the time of the diagnosis is the best predictor of survival; however, chromosomal abnormalities, morphology, and immunophenotype may also have prognostic importance (117). Occasional patients (<10%) present with aleukemic nodal involvement, but most will ultimately be found to have or develop marrow and blood infiltration. *B-cell SLL* is defined as a tissue infiltrate with the morphology and immunophenotype of CLL but without overt leukemia, or in which the status of the blood and bone marrow are not known.

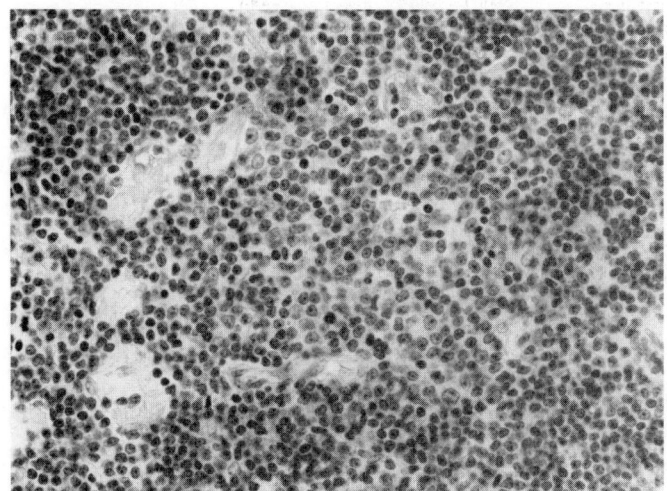

Figure 24-10. B-cell small lymphocytic lymphoma/chronic lymphocytic leukemia. There is a diffuse infiltrate of lymphocytes with an ill-defined pseudofollicle containing small lymphocytes, prolymphocytes, and paraimmunoblasts. (From Harris NL, Ferry JA. Classification of non-Hodgkin's lymphomas. In: Knowles DM, ed. *Neoplastic hematopathology.* Philadelphia: Lippincott Williams & Wilkins, 2001, with permission.)

Morphology. The lymph node infiltrate of CLL/SLL is composed predominantly of small lymphocytes with condensed chromatin, round nuclei, and occasionally a small nucleolus (118,119). Larger lymphoid cells (prolymphocytes and paraimmunoblasts) with more prominent nucleoli and dispersed chromatin are always present, usually clustered in pseudofollicles (Fig. 24-10). In some cases, the cells show moderate nuclear irregularity, which can lead to a differential diagnosis of MCL (120,121). Occasional cases show plasmacytoid differentiation. In the bone marrow and peripheral blood, the cells resemble normal lymphocytes but may have slightly more dispersed chromatin or small nucleoli. Most cases have less than 5% prolymphocytes (larger cells with prominent nucleoli); the designation CLL-PL is used for cases with increased prolymphocytes (5% to 55%), which may have a worse prognosis.

Immunophenotype and Genetic Features. The tumor cells of CLL have faint surface IgM and most coexpress IgD. Cytoplasmic Ig is detectable in approximately 5% of the cases. B-cell–associated antigens (CD19, CD20, CD79a) are positive, but CD20 may be very weak; tumor cells characteristically express both CD5 and CD23 (33). CD23 is useful in distinguishing B CLL/SLL from MCL and should be evaluated in every case, if possible (33); however, CD23 may be expressed in MCL and absent in CLL, so that analysis of cyclin D1 should be done whenever possible in this differential diagnosis. Expression of CD38 is seen in approximately 50% of the cases and may be associated with a worse prognosis (122,123).

Ig heavy- and light-chain genes are rearranged. Most cases in early studies did not show somatic mutation of their Ig V regions, suggesting that they corresponded to a naive B cell (124). However, recent studies have found up to 60% of the cases to have Ig V region mutations, consistent with exposure to the GC. Cases with mutations are reported to be associated with a better prognosis than cases without mutations (122,123).

Approximately 50% of cases have abnormal karyotypes (125). Trisomy 12 is reported in one-third of the cases with cytogenetic abnormalities (126) and correlates with atypical histology and an aggressive clinical course (121,127,128). Abnormalities of 13q are reported in up to 25% of the cases and are associated with long survival. t(11;14)(q13;q32) and bcl-1 gene rearrangement have

been reported (83,85), but many of these cases may be examples of leukemic MCL. Abnormalities of 11q23 are found in a small subset of cases and are associated with lymphadenopathy and an aggressive course (129,130).

Postulated Normal Counterpart. Many cases of CLL are thought to correspond to the recirculating CD5⁺ CD23⁺ naive B cells (29), which are found in the peripheral blood, primary follicle, and follicle mantle zone (28,31). It has been suggested that they are an anergic, self-reactive CD5⁺ B-cell subset (131,132). Cases that show V region mutations may correspond to a subset of peripheral blood CD5⁺ IgM⁺ B cells that appear to be memory B cells (133).

B-CELL PROLYMPHOCYTIC LEUKEMIA

Clinical Features. B-cell prolymphocytic leukemia is an extremely rare disease, comprising less than 1% of B-cell leukemias. If cases of MCL and atypical CLL and CLL/PLL are excluded, it may be vanishingly rare. The patients who have been reported typically present with very high white blood cell counts (>100 × 10⁹) and splenomegaly, with anemia and thrombocytopenia in 50%. The response to chemotherapy is poor. Responses have been reported to CHOP (cytoxan, adriamycin, vincristine, and prednisone), fludarabine, and 2-chlorodeoxyadenosine, and splenic irradiation or splenectomy. Patients usually live less than 3 years (134).

Morphology. *Prolymphocytes* are medium-sized cells, approximately twice the size of a small lymphocyte, with a round nucleus, moderately condensed chromatin, and a single, prominent nucleolus. These cells comprise by definition over 55% and typically over 90% of the neoplastic cells. The bone marrow is infiltrated in an interstitial pattern by similar cells. The spleen shows extensive white and red pulp infiltration by prolymphocytes. Involved lymph nodes may show vague nodularity, but pseudofollicles are absent (134–137). Distinction from leukemic MCL may be difficult.

Immunophenotype and Genetic Features. The cells express bright surface IgM and IgD and bright CD20 as well as other B-cell antigens (CD22, FMC7) and typically lack CD5 and CD23 (although up to one-third of cases may express CD5).

Translocations involving 14q32 are reported in two-thirds of the cases; the most common of these is the t(11;14)(q13;q32), which is characteristic of MCL. It has not been excluded that these cases are in fact examples of leukemic MCL. Trisomy 12 and complex karyotypes are also reported (138,139).

Postulated Normal Counterpart. B-cell prolymphocytic leukemia is thought to correspond to mature B cells at unknown differentiation stage.

LYMPHOPLASMACYTIC LYMPHOMA (WITH OR WITHOUT WALDENSTRÖM'S MACROGLOBULINEMIA)

Clinical Features. LPL comprised only 1.2% (16/1378) of the cases in the REAL classification clinical study (6). Similar to B-CLL/SLL, the median age was 63 years, and 53% were male; most (73%) had bone marrow involvement. Sixty-nine percent had an IPI of 2/3. Lymph node and splenic involvement is common. A monoclonal serum paraprotein of IgM type, with or without hyperviscosity syndrome (Waldenström's macroglobulinemia), is present in most patients (140); as with B-CLL, the paraprotein may have autoantibody or cryoglobulin activity. Cases with mixed cryoglobulinemia may be related to hepatitis C virus infection (141,142), and treatment with interferon to reduce viral load has been associated with regression of the lymphoma (143). Thus, some cases of LPL may be antigen-driven, similar to MALT-type lymphomas. Although extranodal infiltrates may occur in patients with LPL, localized extranodal lymphomas with plasmacytic differentiation are likely to be examples of MALT lymphoma.

The clinical course of LPL is indolent; in some European series it has been reported to be more aggressive than typical B-CLL (144,145), but in the REAL clinical study, 5-year OAS (58%) and failure-free survival (25%) were identical to that of CLL/SLL (6).

Morphology. The tumor consists of a diffuse proliferation of small lymphocytes, plasmacytoid lymphocytes, and plasma cells, with variable numbers of immunoblasts. By definition, features of other lymphomas—particularly MZLs and SLL—that may have plasmacytoid differentiation are absent. In the spleen, both red and white pulp may be infiltrated, but red pulp involvement is more prominent. The bone marrow infiltrate may be either diffuse or nodular and is often interstitial and rather subtle. Peripheral blood involvement is usually less prominent than in CLL, and the cells often have a plasmacytoid appearance.

Immunophenotype and Genetic Features. The cells have surface and cytoplasmic (some cells) Ig, usually of IgM type, usually lack IgD, and strongly express B-cell-associated antigens (CD19, CD20, CD22, CD79a). The cells are CD5⁻, CD10⁻, CD23⁻, and CD43±; CD25 or CD11c may be faintly positive in some cases (33,146–148). Lack of CD5 and CD23, strong SIg and CD20, and the presence of cytoplasmic Ig are useful in distinction from B-CLL.

Ig heavy- and light-chain genes are rearranged, and V-region genes show somatic mutations, suggesting that these cells arise from a population of B cells that have undergone antigen-driven selection (124,149–151). Translocation t(9;14)(p13;q32) and rearrangement of the PAX-5 gene is reported in up to 50% of the cases. PAX-5 encodes a protein, B-cell–specific activator protein, which is important in early B-cell development. Expression of B-cell–specific activator protein is restricted to B cells and appears to be independent of the translocation (152).

Postulated Normal Counterpart. LPL is thought to correspond to peripheral B lymphocytes stimulated to differentiate to plasma cells, possibly corresponding to the primary immune response to antigens, or to post-GC cells that have undergone somatic mutation but not heavy-chain class switch.

SPLENIC MARGINAL ZONE LYMPHOMA AND VILLOUS LYMPHOCYTES (SPLENIC LYMPHOMA WITH VILLOUS LYMPHOCYTES)

Clinical Features. Splenic MZL (SMZL) accounts for only 1% to 2% of chronic lymphoid leukemias found on bone marrow examination but up to 25% of low-grade B-cell neoplasms in splenectomy specimens (153–156). It may comprise the majority of chronic B-cell leukemias and low-grade splenic lymphomas that do not fit the defining criteria of B-cell CLL, LPL, MCL, FL, or HCL. Patients typically present with splenomegaly and lymphocytosis, usually without peripheral lymphadenopathy, and may have circulating neoplastic cells with short cytoplasmic villi, and a small M-component (69). Extranodal sites are not typically involved, and despite the "marginal zone" name, this disease appears to be completely distinct from extranodal MZL of MALT type. The course is extremely indolent, although the tumor may be surprisingly resistant to chemotherapy that would ordinarily be effective for CLL. Splenectomy may be followed by prolonged remission.

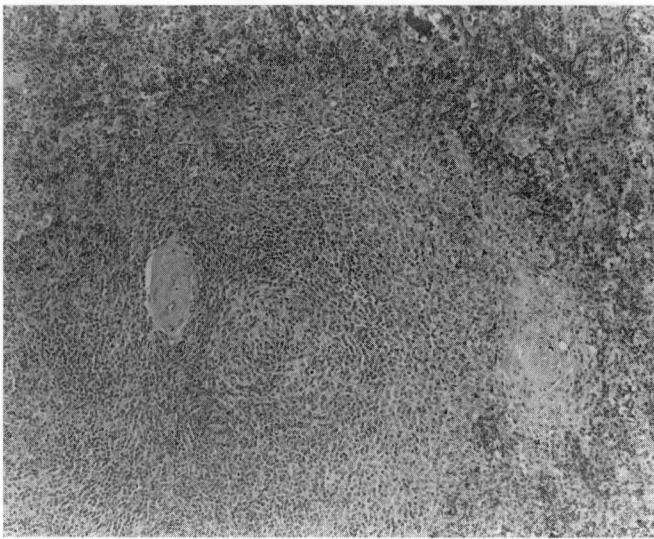

Figure 24-11. Splenic marginal zone B-cell lymphoma. There is expansion of the white pulp by an infiltrate of small lymphoid cells with scant cytoplasm, surrounded by a rim of small cells with slightly more abundant cytoplasm. The remnant of a reactive follicle is found in the center of the white pulp. (From Harris NL, Ferry JA. Classification of non-Hodgkin's lymphomas. In: Knowles DM, ed. *Neoplastic hematopathology*. Philadelphia: Lippincott Williams & Wilkins, 2001, with permission.)

Morphology. In the spleen, the neoplastic cells of SMZL/splenic lymphoma with villous lymphocytes (SLVL) occupy both the mantle and marginal zones of the splenic white pulp, usually with a central residual GC, which may be either atrophic or hyperplastic (153,154,157) (Fig. 24-11). The cells in the mantle zone are small, with slight nuclear irregularity and scant cytoplasm, while those in the marginal zone have more dispersed chromatin and abundant, pale cytoplasm, resembling marginal zone cells, and are admixed with centroblasts and immunoblasts. The red pulp is also involved, with both a diffuse and micronodular pattern and sinus infiltration. Epithelioid histiocytes may be present singly or in clusters and, particularly in the bone marrow, may give rise to the differential diagnosis of an infectious process. Splenic hilar lymph nodes are often involved; the neoplastic cells form vague nodules, often without a central GC, and a marginal zone pattern may or may not be present (158). The marrow usually contains discrete lymphoid aggregates, without a marginal zone pattern, with or without diffuse lymphoid infiltration, and often with intrasinusoidal neoplastic cells. When tumor cells are present in the peripheral blood, they often have abundant cytoplasm with small surface "villous" projections (i.e., SLVL), or may appear plasmacytoid.

Immunophenotype and Genetic Features. The tumor cells are IgM⁺, IgD⁺, CD5⁻, CD10⁻, CD43⁻, CD23⁻; express B-cell antigens (CD19, CD20, CD22) and bcl-2; and lack CD11c and CD25 (153,159). In the majority of cases, lack of CD5 will serve to distinguish this disorder from B-CLL, and lack of CD103 and CD25 are useful in distinguishing it from HCL. The cells are cyclin D1 negative by immunoperoxidase staining (160).

Analysis of the Ig V region genes indicates a high degree of somatic mutation, consistent with a post-GC stage of B-cell development (161). More recently, ongoing mutations of V region genes, similar to GC cells, have been reported (71). BCL-2 is germline. Early reports that t(11;14)(q13;132), BCL-1 rearrangement, and cyclin D1 overexpression were common are now thought to have reflected inclusion of cases of leukemic MCL (162,163). Deletions at 7q31–7q32 are found in some cases.

Trisomy 3, found in nodal and extranodal MZL, is detected in only a small number of cases (164,165), and the t(11;18)(q21;q21) has not been reported.

Postulated Normal Counterpart. SMZL and SLVL are thought to correspond to post-GCs, memory B cells of splenic type.

HAIRY CELL LEUKEMIA

Clinical Features. HCL is a rare disease; patients are adults with splenomegaly and pancytopenia and may have few circulating neoplastic cells. Monocytopenia is usually present. There is increased susceptibility to opportunistic infections. Prolonged remissions may follow splenectomy. HCL does not respond well to conventional lymphoma chemotherapy, but interferon, deoxycoformycin, or 2-chlorodeoxyadenosine can induce long-term remissions (166,167).

Morphology. Hairy cells are small lymphoid cells with an oval or bean-shaped nucleus, chromatin slightly less clumped than that of a normal lymphocyte, and abundant, pale cytoplasm with "hairy" projections on smear preparations. The bone marrow is always involved by a diffuse, interstitial infiltrate characterized by widely spaced, small nuclei, in contrast to the closely packed nuclei of most other low-grade lymphoid neoplasms involving the bone marrow. Lymphoid aggregates are not seen. Reticulin is increased, often resulting in a "dry tap." The diagnosis is best made on bone marrow biopsy. In the spleen, HCL involves the red pulp; the white pulp is usually atrophic.

Immunophenotype and Genetic Features. The tumor cells are SIg$^+$ (M$^+$/$^-$D, G, or A), and express B-cell–associated antigens (CD19, CD20, CD22, CD79a). They are typically CD5$^-$, CD10$^-$, and CD23$^-$, and express CD11c (strong), CD25 (strong) (168), FMC7, and CD103 (169–172). They may express nuclear cyclin D1, but do not have the t(11;14) associated with MCL. Tartrate-resistant acid phosphatase is present in most cases but is neither necessary nor specific for the diagnosis. No one marker is specific for distinguishing HCL from other B-cell leukemias, because CD22, CD11c, CD25, FMC7, and even tartrate-resistant acid phosphatase can be present in disorders other than HCL. Strong expression of these markers in association with CD103, together with the characteristic morphologic features, is most useful. In tissue sections, the monoclonal antibody DBA.44 gives strong staining of hairy cells, but other lymphomas may also express this antigen, as well as normal B cells (173,174). Ig heavy- and light-chain genes are rearranged (175). Ig variable region genes are mutated, consistent with a post-GC cell (151). No specific cytogenetic abnormality is described.

Postulated Normal Counterpart. HCL is thought to correspond to peripheral B cells of unknown post-GC stage.

PLASMA CELL MYELOMA

Clinical Features. Plasma cell myeloma is a disease of older adults, with a median survival of 3 years. Patients typically present with osteolytic lesions and a serum monoclonal Ig. The prognosis depends on the clinical stage of the disease at diagnosis. The 10% of patients with plasmablastic or other atypical morphologies have a worse prognosis.

Morphology. The bone marrow contains greater than 10% plasma cells (usually >30%), which are distributed in clusters and sheets in biopsy specimens, in contrast to the perivascular location of normal plasma cells. The neoplastic cells may resemble normal plasma cells or may have more dispersed chromatin, nucleoli, and decreased nuclear to cytoplasmic ratio, consistent with plasmablasts. Rare cases have multinucleated, polylobated, or pleomorphic cells (176).

Immunophenotype and Genetic Features. The plasma cells contain monotypic Ig, of IgG, IgA, or less often, IgD or IgE type; 10% have light chains only. They typically lack CD20, variably express CD45, and express CD38 and CD138 (syndecan-1). Ig heavy- and light-chain genes are rearranged and show variable region mutations consistent with post-GC cells (151). Cytogenetic abnormalities are common and are typically complex. The most common translocations involve the Ig heavy-chain locus at 14q32 with a variety of partners. Some cases have t(11;14)(q12;q32) and cyclin D1 rearrangement and overexpression (177,178). Rare cases have the t(9;14)(p13q32) associated with lymphoplasmacytic lymphoma, involving rearrangement of the PAX-5 gene (179).

Postulated Normal Counterpart. Plasma cell myeloma is thought to correspond to bone marrow plasma cells.

EXTRANODAL MARGINAL ZONE B-CELL LYMPHOMA OF MUCOSA-ASSOCIATED LYMPHOID TISSUE TYPE

Clinical Features. Extranodal marginal zone B-cell (MALT) lymphoma comprised 8% of the lymphomas in the recent study of the REAL classification (15). Fifty percent involve the gastrointestinal tract, and they comprise almost 50% of all gastric lymphomas (180). They also represent 40% to 60% of lymphomas in other glandular epithelial tissues, such as the ocular adnexae, thyroid, lung, breast, and salivary gland (181–185); skin or soft tissue may also be the primary site. Patients are usually older adults, although there is a broad age range, and cases have been reported in children. A slight female predominance has been reported in some series (33). The majority of patients present with localized (stage I or II) extranodal disease. The bone marrow is involved in 15% to 30%. Many patients have a history of autoimmune disease, such as Sjögren's syndrome or Hashimoto's thyroiditis, or of *Helicobacter gastritis* in the case of gastric MALT lymphoma. "Acquired MALT" secondary to autoimmune disease or infection in these sites is thought to be the substrate for lymphoma development (186).

Antibiotic therapy directed at *Helicobacter pylori* in gastric MALT lymphoma results in regression of most early lesions (187,188). Cases of gastric MALT lymphoma with the t(11;18)(q21;q21) have a lower frequency of response to antibiotic therapy (189). The long-term prognosis of patients treated with antibiotics is not known, and these patients require long and careful follow-up by an oncologist. For this reason, patients with gastric biopsies showing atypical lymphoid infiltrates associated with *H. pylori* should not be treated empirically with antibiotics until a diagnosis of lymphoma is either made or excluded.

The disease known as *Mediterranean abdominal lymphoma, alpha heavy chain disease,* and *immunoproliferative small intestinal disease,* which occurs in young adults in Eastern Mediterranean countries, is another example of a MALT-type lymphoma that may respond to antibiotic therapy in its early stages (186). Localized MALT lymphomas of the stomach that do not respond to antibiotics, and those occurring in other sites may be cured with local treatment, typically radiation (184,190–192). Dissemination or recurrence may occur; these are often in other localized extranodal sites, with long disease-free intervals (185,193,194).

Morphology. Extranodal marginal zone B-cell (MALT) lymphoma reproduces the morphologic features of normal MALT

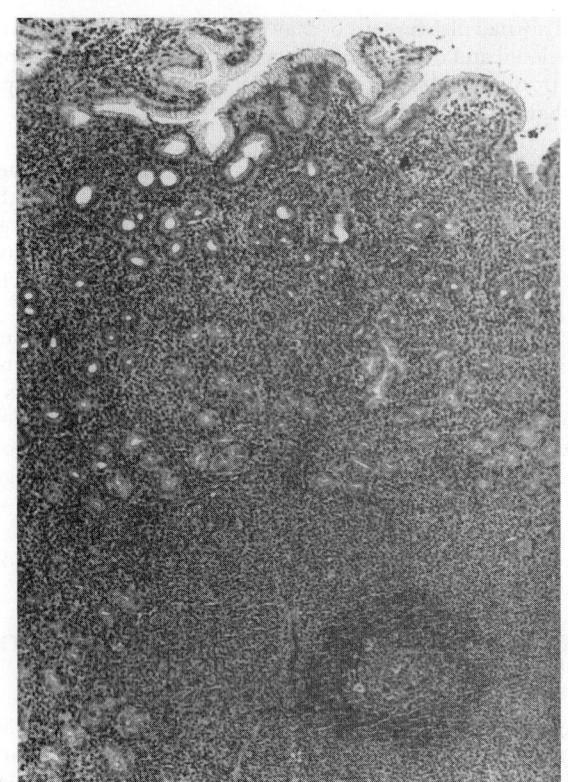
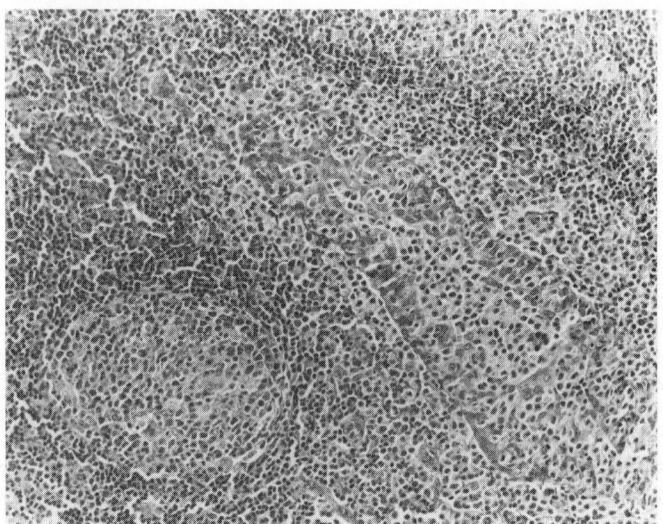

Figure 24-12. Extranodal marginal zone cell lymphoma (mucosa-associated lymphoid tissue lymphoma). **A:** Gastric lymphoma, showing infiltration of the lamina propria by small lymphocytes, marginal zone cells with epithelial infiltration (lymphoepithelial lesions), and plasma cells. **B:** Parotid lymphoma, showing a reactive follicle adjacent to a lymphoepithelial lesion, which consists of a dilated duct infiltrated and surrounded by neoplastic marginal zone/monocytoid B cells. (From Harris NL, Ferry JA. Classification of non-Hodgkin's lymphomas. In: Knowles DM, ed. *Neoplastic hematopathology.* Philadelphia: Lippincott Williams & Wilkins, 2001, with permission.)

(Fig. 24-12A), with a polymorphous infiltrate of small lymphocytes, marginal zone (centrocyte-like) B cells, monocytoid B cells, and plasma cells, as well as rare centroblast- or immunoblast-like cells. Reactive follicles are usually present, with the neoplastic cells occupying the marginal zone or the interfollicular region; occasional follicles may be "colonized" by marginal zone or monocytoid cells. In epithelial tissues, neoplastic cells typically infiltrate the epithelium, forming so-called lymphoepithelial lesions (59) (Fig. 24-12B). Blast cells are typically present, but are by definition in the minority in MALT lymphoma. Clusters or sheets of blasts sufficiently large to warrant a diagnosis of large cell lymphoma are associated with a worse prognosis. In these cases, a separate diagnosis of DLBCL should be made. The term *high-grade MALT lymphoma* should be avoided for large B-cell lymphomas in MALT sites, because it may lead to inappropriate treatment with antibiotics instead of aggressive antilymphoma therapy (8).

Immunophenotype and Genetic Features. The tumor cells express SIg (M>G>A), lack IgD, and 40% have monotypic cytoplasmic Ig, indicating plasmacytoid differentiation. They express B-cell–associated antigens (CD19, CD20, CD22, CD79a) and are usually negative for CD5 and CD10. Immunophenotyping studies are useful in confirming malignancy (light-chain restriction) and in excluding B-CLL (CD5+), mantle cell (CD5+), and follicle center (CD10+ CD43−, CD11c−, usually CIg−) lymphomas (33,157).

Ig genes are rearranged, and the V region has a high degree of somatic mutation as well as intraclonal diversity consistent with a GC or post-GC stage of B-cell development (73,195,196). Ig heavy-chain V regions are those often found in autoantibodies,

consistent with studies showing that the antibodies produced by the tumor cells have specificity against self antigens (73). The Bcl-1 and bcl-2 genes are germline (197); trisomy 3 (60%) and t(11;18)(q21;q21) (25% to 40%) are the most common reported cytogenetic abnormalities (164,198,199). Interestingly, neither of these abnormalities is common in primary large-cell lymphomas of the gastrointestinal tract (199,200). Recently, analysis of the t(11;18) breakpoint has shown fusion of the apoptosis-inhibitor gene API2 to a novel gene at 18q21, named *MLT*, in cases of MALT lymphoma (90). A gene involved in a breakpoint in MALT lymphomas with t(1;14) has recently been cloned; named *BCL-10*, it is an apoptosis-promoting gene, which, in mutated form, may cause cellular transformation (201).

Postulated Normal Counterpart. Extranodal marginal zone B-cell (MALT) is throught to correspond to post-GC B memory cells with capacity to differentiate into marginal zone, monocytoid, and plasma cells.

NODAL MARGINAL ZONE B-CELL LYMPHOMA
Clinical Features. By definition, nodal MZL involves lymph nodes and not extranodal sites or spleen. This diagnosis should not be made in a patient with known risk factors for MALT lymphoma, such as Sjögren's syndrome or Hashimoto's thyroiditis, or in a patient with a known extranodal MALT lymphoma—in these cases, MZL in a lymph node represents dissemination of extranodal MALT lymphoma. Primary nodal MZL is a rare disorder, comprising 1% of the cases in the international study of the REAL classification (6). Patients present with isolated or generalized nodal disease; bone marrow was involved in 30%;

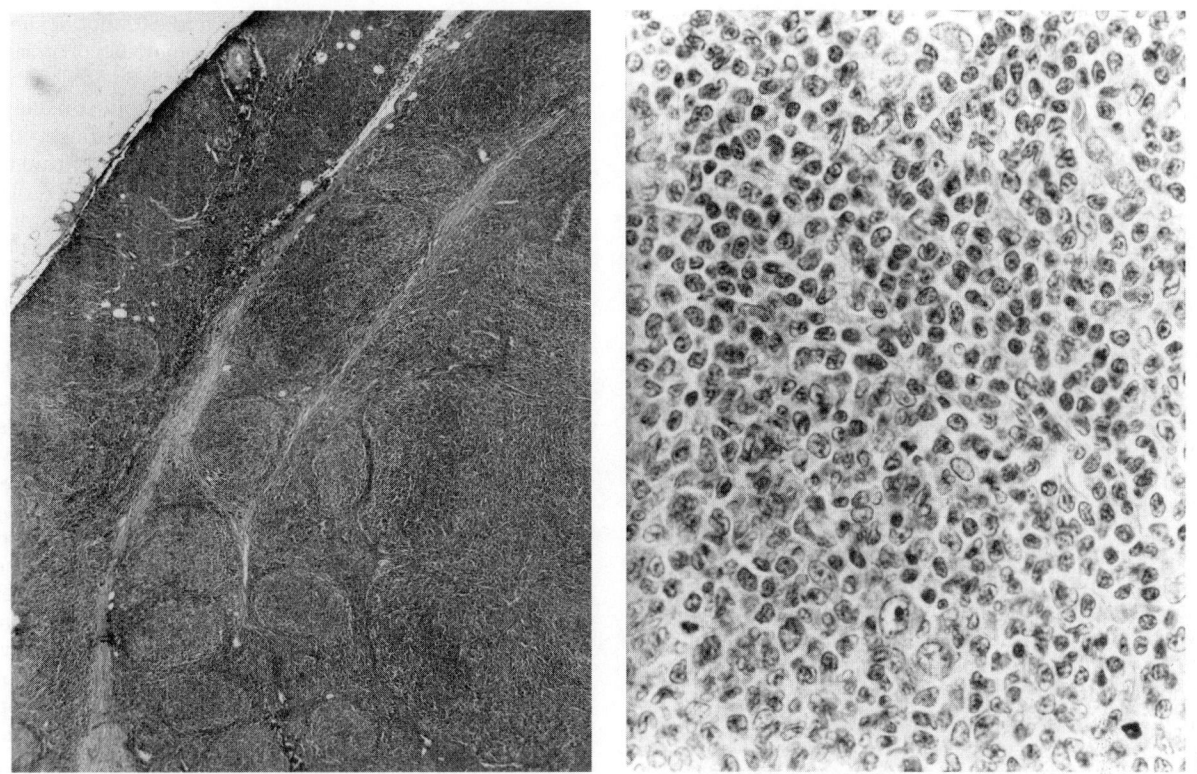

Figure 24-13. Follicular lymphoma. **A:** Low magnification showing multiple poorly circumscribed, crowded follicles extending beyond the lymph node capsule into perinodal fat. **B:** High magnification, showing a majority of centrocytes (cleaved cells) and a minority of centroblasts (large noncleaved cells). (From Harris NL, Ferry JA. Follicular lymphoma. In: Knowles DM, ed. *Neoplastic hematopathology.* Philadelphia: Lippincott Williams & Wilkins, 2001, with permission.)

rarely, peripheral blood may be involved (15,70,202). In one series of cases of nodal MZL that were morphologically similar to nodes involved by MALT lymphoma, 44% of those with follow-up developed an extranodal MALT lymphoma (70). The survival of primary nodal MZL appears to be similar to those of FL or SLL (15).

Morphology. Two morphologic types have been described: cases that resemble MALT lymphoma and cases that more closely resemble SMZL (70). Those that resemble MALT lymphoma show aggregates of monocytoid B cells in a parafollicular, perivascular, and perisinusoidal distribution, with preserved GCs and mantle zones. Those that resemble SMZL have infiltrates of marginal zone cells surrounding reactive follicles with GCs but with attenuated mantle zones.

Immunophenotype and Genetic Features. The cases that resembled SMZL express IgD and lack CD5, CD23, and cyclin D1. Those that resemble MALT lymphoma are IgD⁻ and have an immunophenotype identical to that of extranodal marginal zone B-cell lymphoma (MALT) (70).

Postulated Normal Counterpart. Nodal MZL is thought to correspond to nodal monocytoid or marginal zone B cells.

FOLLICULAR LYMPHOMA
Clinical Features. FL is the second most common lymphoma in the United States and western Europe, comprising 20% of all NHLs and up to 70% of low-grade lymphomas reported in American and European clinical trials (6,203). Thus, our understanding of the clinical features and response to treatment of low-grade lymphoma is essentially that of FL. FL affects pre-

dominantly older adults, with a median age of 59 years and a slight female predominance (1,6,15). Most patients have widespread disease at diagnosis, predominantly lymph nodes, but also spleen, bone marrow, and occasionally peripheral blood or extranodal sites. Despite the advanced stage, the clinical course is generally indolent, with median survivals in excess of 8 years; however, the disease is not usually curable with available treatment. The prognosis is related to the number of large cells (centroblasts), with grade 1 and grade 2 cases having a median survival of 7 to 8 years, which is unaffected by aggressive therapy, and grade 3 cases having a shorter median survival, which is significantly improved by treatment with anthracycline-containing regimens (204,205). In the recent international study of the REAL classification, the few patients (7%) with IPI scores of 4/5 have a much worse prognosis, with a median survival of only 1 year (6).

Morphology. The tumor is composed of a mixture of centrocytes (cleaved follicle center cells) and centroblasts (large noncleaved follicle center cells) and by definition has at least a partially follicular pattern (Fig. 24-13). Rare lymphomas with a follicular growth pattern consist almost entirely of centroblasts. The proportion of centroblasts varies from case to case, and the clinical aggressiveness of the tumor increases with increasing numbers of centroblasts. Numerous criteria have been proposed for grading FL, but reproducibility is poor. The WHO Classification uses the cell-counting method of Mann and Berard (Table 24-13) (8,206), which has been shown to have better reproducibility and predictive value than other schemes (207). The bone marrow is frequently involved by lymphoid aggregates that are typically paratrabecular. Splenic involvement is typically predominantly white pulp.

TABLE 24-13. Follicular Lymphoma: Grading and Variants

Grades
  Grade 1: 0–5 centroblasts/hpf
  Grade 2: 6–15 centroblasts/hpf
  Grade 3: >15 centroblasts/hpf
    3a: >15 centroblasts, but centrocytes are still present
    3b: Centroblasts form solid sheets with no residual centrocytes
Variants
  Cutaneous follicle center lymphoma
  Diffuse follicle center lymphoma
    Grade 1: 0–5 centroblasts/hpf
    Grade 2: 6–15 centroblasts/hpf

hpf, high-power field.

In addition to typical FL, two variants are recognized whose relationship to FL remains controversial: cutaneous follicle center lymphoma and diffuse follicle center lymphoma.

Immunophenotype and Genetic Features. The tumor cells of FL are usually SIg⁺ (IgM>IgG>IgA). The tumor cells express pan-B-cell–associated antigens. Approximately 60% are CD10⁺, and they are CD5⁻, CD23⁻/⁺, and CD43⁻ (most cases). Tightly organized meshworks of FDCs are present in follicular areas (146,208). Most cases are bcl-2⁺, and nuclear bcl-6 is expressed by at least some of the neoplastic cells (43,209). The Ki-67⁺ fraction is lower than that of reactive follicles. Ig heavy- and light-chain genes are rearranged, with extensive and ongoing somatic mutations, similar to normal GC cells (210,211). t(14;18)(q32;q21) and *BCL*-2 gene rearrangement are present in the majority of the cases. Abnormalities of 3q27 or *BCL6* rearrangement are found in approximately 15% of FLs, whereas 5' mutations of the *BCL6* gene are found in approximately 40% (46).

Postulated Normal Counterpart. FL is thought to correspond to GC B cells, both centrocytes and centroblasts.

MANTLE CELL LYMPHOMA

Clinical Features. MCL comprises 5% to 7% of adult NHLs in the United States and Europe (6,15,119,212). The median age is 63 years, and there is a marked male predominance (75%) (6). The majority (70%) of patients are in stage IV at diagnosis; sites involved include lymph nodes, spleen, Waldeyer's ring, bone marrow (>60%), blood (up to 50%), and extranodal sites, especially the gastrointestinal tract (lymphomatous polyposis) (213). The median overall survival in most series is 3 years, with no plateau in the curve, and failure-free survival is approximately 1 year. The blastoid variant is reported in some studies to be more aggressive (6,33,212,214–216). Some reports indicate a better prognosis for cases with a mantle zone pattern (217). Therapy with anthracycline-containing regimens does not improve the outcome, and initial results with high-dose therapy and marrow transplantation have been disappointing (218–221). Fludarabine is reported to be less effective in MCL than in CLL and FL (222).

Morphology. MCL may have a diffuse, nodular, mantle zone, or mixed pattern in lymph nodes. Most cases are composed of monomorphous small to medium-sized lymphoid cells, with slightly irregular or "cleaved," nuclei (Fig. 24-14); however, the morphology in different cases can range from lymphocyte-like to large cleaved or lymphoblast-like (33,119,223–225). Neoplastic centroblasts and immunoblasts are not seen, nor are pseudofollicles. Despite the small size and bland appearance of the cells, there is often more mitotic activity than in other small-cell lymphomas. Bone marrow involvement is typically nodular and may be paratrabecular, and the splenic white pulp may be involved. Gastrointestinal involvement may mimic MALT lymphoma; lymphoepithelial lesions are less common, but immunophenotyping may be required. On smears the cells may resemble small lymphocytes or prolymphocytes.

Immunophenotype and Genetic Features. The tumor cells express strong SIgM and IgD, which is often of λ light chain type, and strongly express B-cell–associated antigens; most coexpress CD5, similar to B-CLL/SLL, and are usually but not always CD23⁻ (216,226,227). A prominent, irregular meshwork of FDCs is found even in diffuse cases (33,146,208). Nuclear cyclin D1 protein is present in all cases and is the "gold standard" for the diagnosis (177,228).

Ig heavy- and light-chain genes are rearranged and lack somatic mutations in most cases, indicating a preGC stage of differentiation (35). A t(11;14)(q13;q32) in the majority of the cases results in rearrangement of the *BCL1* locus and overexpression the cyclin D1 gene, which encodes a cell cycle–associated protein that is not normally expressed in lymphoid

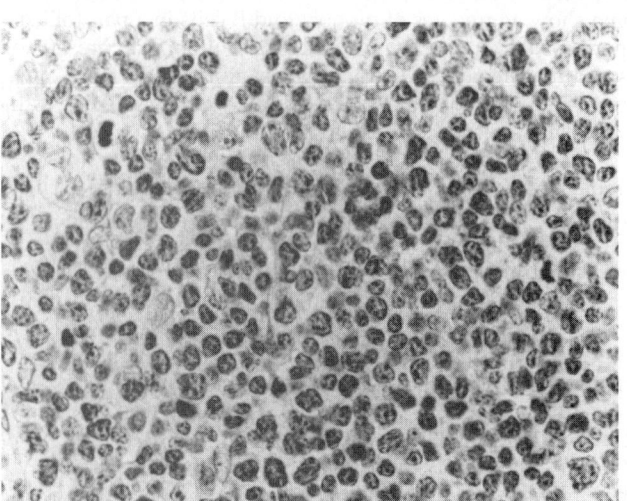

Figure 24-14. Mantle cell lymphoma, showing **(A)** a vaguely nodular pattern and **(B)** a monomorphous population of cells with irregular nuclei. (From Harris NL, Ferry JA. Classification of non-Hodgkin's lymphomas. In: Knowles DM, ed. *Neoplastic hematopathology*. Philadelphia: Lippincott Williams & Wilkins, 2001, with permission.)

cells (88,228–231). Overexpression of this protein may explain the high proliferation fraction and aggressive clinical course of this histologically low-grade lymphoma. The translocation can be detected by fluorescence *in situ* hybridization on touch preps, bone marrow or blood smears, or nuclei extracted from paraffin sections. There are often abnormalities in expression of other genes associated with the cell cycle, including mutations of the CDK inhibitors, p16 and p17, in blastoid variants and decreased expression of p27, another CDK inhibitor, in the majority of the cases (232). Cases of the blastoid variant have a high incidence of tetraploidy and p53 gene mutations (233–235).

Postulated Normal Counterpart. MCL is thought to correspond to naive B cells of follicle mantle or GC origin.

LARGE B-CELL LYMPHOMA

Clinical Features. DLBCL was the most common lymphoma in the international study of the REAL classification, comprising 31% of the cases. It may occur in both children and adults, but the median age is 64 years. Patients typically present with a rapidly enlarging, symptomatic mass, with "B" symptoms in one third of the cases (6,15). Approximately 50% have localized (stage I or II) disease; bone marrow involvement is seen in only 15% (15). Up to 40% of DLBCLs are extranodal; common sites include the gastrointestinal tract, bone, and central nervous system (CNS). The prognosis was highly associated with the IPI score (15) but not with histologic subclassification according to either the WF or the Kiel Classification. Large B-cell lymphoma is likely a heterogeneous category, but criteria for defining distinct subentities are in general lacking. Several clinically and morphologically distinct subtypes can be recognized at present, which are described below and summarized in Table 24-14. Large B-cell lymphoma may also occur as a high-grade transformation of several low-grade B-cell lymphomas (e.g., CLL, lymphoplasmacytic lymphoma, FL, MALT lymphoma, SMZL).

DLBCL is usually treated with combination chemotherapy containing anthracyclines (236); early-stage cases may be treated with shorter courses of chemotherapy followed by involved-field radiation therapy. DLBCLs of certain extranodal sites, such as the CNS, may be clinically distinctive and may have specific treatment protocols.

Morphology. DLBCL are a heterogeneous group of neoplasms. They are typically composed of large cells (three times the size of normal lymphocytes) that resemble centroblasts or immunoblasts, most often with a mixture of the two (Fig. 24-15). Several morphologic variants can be recognized, but their clinical significance is debated. The centroblastic type (80% of the cases) is composed of cells resembling centroblasts, with one to three peripheral nucleoli and a narrow rim of basophilic cytoplasm, often with a variable admixture of immunoblasts. Some cases have multilobated centroblasts. The immunoblastic type (10% of the cases) has more than 90% immunoblasts with a prominent central nucleolus and abundant, basophilic cytoplasm, often with plasmacytoid differentiation. These cases are more common in immunosuppressed patients. In nonimmunosuppressed patients, they have been reported in some studies to have a worse prognosis, whereas others have failed to confirm this (15,237). In the anaplastic type, the cells are morphologically similar to those of T/null ALCL, with pleomorphic nuclei, abundant cytoplasm and sinusoidal growth pattern, and CD30 expression. Although these have been called *B-ALCL*, they do not have the same distinctive clinical or genetic features of T/null ALCL and are considered a morphologic variant of large B-cell lymphoma. Two other distinctive morphologic and immu-

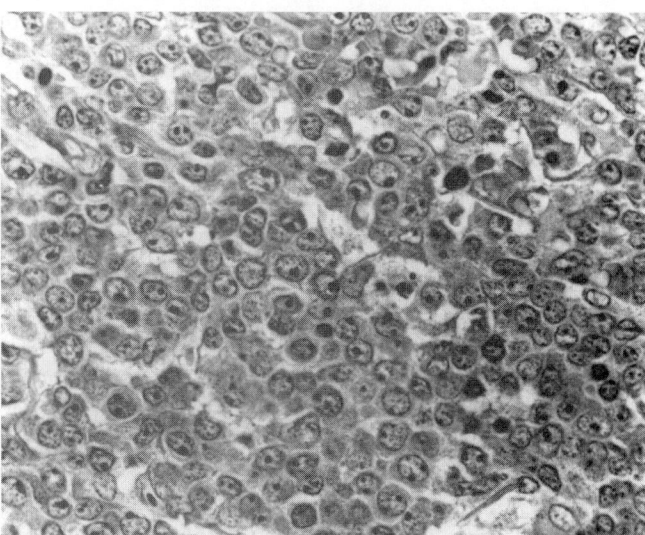

Figure 24-15. Diffuse large B-cell lymphoma. The most common type shows a mixture of cells resembling centroblasts (one to three peripheral nucleoli) and cells resembling immunoblasts (single central nucleolus). (From Harris NL, Ferry JA. Classification of non-Hodgkin's lymphomas. In: Knowles DM, ed. *Neoplastic hematopathology.* Philadelphia: Lippincott Williams & Wilkins, 2001, with permission.)

nophenotypic variants of DLBCL are the plasmablastic type and a rare variant expressing the full-length ALK protein.

Bone marrow involvement in DLBCL may take two forms. In approximately 10% of the cases, there is large-cell lymphoma in the marrow. However, a slightly higher proportion may show so-called discordant marrow involvement—aggregates of small atypical lymphoid cells consistent with involvement by low-grade lymphoma, particularly FL. Several studies have shown that discordant marrow involvement is not associated with a worse prognosis than cases without marrow involvement (238).

Immunophenotype and Genetic Features. DLBCLs express one or more B-cell–associated antigens (CD19, CD20, CD22, CD79a), as well as CD45, and often SIg. They may coexpress CD5 or CD10 (146,239). Twenty-five percent to 80% in various studies express bcl-2 protein, and this may be associated with a worse prognosis (240–244). Approximately 70% express bcl-6 protein, consistent with a GC origin (243,244), independent of bcl-6 gene rearrangement. Ig genes are rearranged, and most have somatic mutations in the variable region genes (64,245). The *BCL2* gene is rearranged in 15% to 30%; it is associated with disseminated nodal disease but not with either a worse prognosis or with bcl-2 protein expression (240). The *c-MYC* gene is rearranged in 5% to 15% (84,246), and the *BCL6* gene is rearranged in 20% to 40% of cases (246,247) and shows mutations in the 5' noncoding region in 70% (248,249). Both the 5' noncoding mutations of the bcl-6 gene (46,48) and the Ig V region gene mutations are found in normal GC cells (32); their presence in large B-cell lymphoma is consistent with a GC or post-GC stage of differentiation.

Postulated Normal Counterpart. Large B-cell lymphoma is thought to correspond to proliferating peripheral B cells: centroblasts or immunoblasts in most cases.

LARGE B-CELL LYMPHOMA SUBTYPES

As mentioned above, DLBCL is believed to be a heterogeneous category, which we currently lack the tools to dissect into clinically relevant diseases. However, several distinctive subtypes of DLBCL have been recognized; these are summarized in Table 24-14 and discussed briefly below.

Primary Mediastinal (Thymic) Large B-Cell Lymphoma. Primary mediastinal large B-cell lymphoma is a distinct clinico-pathologic entity, requiring knowledge of morphology, immunophenotype, and presenting site for the diagnosis (6). It comprised 7% of DLBCLs (2.4% of all NHLs) in the international REAL classification study (6,15). There is a female predominance and a median age in the fourth decade; patients present with a locally invasive anterior mediastinal mass originating in the thymus, with frequent airway compromise and superior vena cava syndrome (250). Relapses tend to be extranodal, including liver, gastrointestinal tract, kidneys, ovaries, and CNS. Although early studies suggested an unusually aggressive, incurable tumor, others have reported cure rates similar to those for other large-cell lymphomas with aggressive therapy, usually combining chemotherapy with mediastinal irradiation (250,251).

Primary mediastinal large B-cell lymphoma usually involves the thymus (252,253). The tumor cells may have pale or "clear" cytoplasm but otherwise resemble other large B-cell lymphomas. Many cases have fine, compartmentalizing sclerosis. The tumor cells are often Ig⁻ but express B-cell–associated antigens (CD19, CD20, CD22, CD79a) and CD45 (253). Most cases are bcl6⁺, and approximately 25% are CD10⁺ (254). Ig heavy- and light-chain genes are rearranged; the bcl-2 gene is usually germline (253,255,256). Bcl-6 gene rearrangements are uncommon (257). Amplification of the *REL* oncogene has been described in some cases (258).

Intravascular Large B-Cell Lymphoma. Rare cases of large-cell lymphoma, usually of B-cell type, present with a disseminated intravascular proliferation of large lymphoid cells involving small blood vessels without an obvious extravascular tumor mass or leukemia (259). This tumor has also been variously known as *intravascular lymphomatosis, angiotropic lymphoma,* and *malignant angioendotheliomatosis.* The neoplastic lymphoid cells are mainly lodged in the lumina of small vessels in many organs. The tumor cells may resemble centroblasts or immunoblasts and express B-cell–associated antigens. Malignant cells are rarely seen in cerebrospinal fluid, blood, or bone marrow. The organs most commonly involved are the CNS, kidneys, lungs, and skin, but virtually any site may be involved. Patients present with a variety of symptoms related to organ dysfunction secondary to vascular occlusion. Because of this, the diagnosis is difficult, and many reported cases were diagnosed at autopsy. If a timely diagnosis is made and combination chemotherapy instituted, many patients achieve complete remission, and long-term survival appears to be possible (260).

TABLE 24-14. Diffuse Large B-Cell Lymphoma, Variants and Subtypes

Diffuse large B-cell lymphoma, morphologic variants:
    Centroblastic
    Immunoblastic
    Anaplastic large B-cell
    Plasmablastic
    Anaplastic lymphoma kinase–positive
Diffuse large B-cell lymphoma, subtypes:
    Mediastinal (thymic) large B-cell lymphoma
    Intravascular large B-cell lymphoma
    T-cell/histiocyte-rich large B-cell lymphoma
    Lymphomatoid granulomatosis–type large B-cell lymphoma
    Primary effusion lymphoma

T-Cell–Rich/Histiocyte-Rich Large B-Cell Lymphoma. Some cases of large B-cell lymphoma have a prominent background of reactive T cells and, often, histiocytes—so-called T-cell–rich/histiocyte-rich large B-cell lymphoma (T/HRLBCL). The tumors may resemble HD of either lymphocyte predominance or mixed cellularity (MC) type (261,262). However, in contrast to either lymphocyte predominance or MC HD, patients with T/HRLBCL typically present with disseminated disease involving lymph nodes, liver, spleen, and bone marrow. They may respond to aggressive therapy for large-cell lymphoma but have a poor overall survival. The relationship of this disease to lymphocyte-predominance and/or classic HD remains to be elucidated.

Large B-Cell Lymphoma, Lymphomatoid Granulomatosis Type. Recently, the entity described as lymphomatoid granulomatosis has been shown in most cases to be an Epstein-Barr virus (EBV)⁺ large B-cell lymphoma with a T-cell–rich background (263–266). Patients typically present with extranodal disease, most commonly involving lung, CNS, or kidneys. Evidence of past or present immunosuppression may be found. The infiltrates show extensive necrosis, often with only a few atypical large B cells in a background of small T lymphocytes; the infiltrate may be both angiocentric and angioinvasive. Although the infiltrates may resemble those of nasal-type NK/T-cell lymphoma, there is no biologic and little clinical overlap, because the latter is an NK/T-cell neoplasm that involves the upper airway and midfacial region, skin, and sometimes the gastrointestinal tract, but only rarely the lung or CNS. Lymphomatoid granulomatosis is graded according to the number of large B cells. The lower-grade cases are not typically treated as lymphoma; grade 3 cases fulfill the criteria for large B-cell lymphoma in a T-cell–rich background and may be clinically aggressive (267).

Primary Effusion Lymphoma. This recently recognized disease occurs most often in immunosuppressed patients, either with human immunodeficiency virus (HIV) or in the posttransplant setting, but occasional cases in nonimmunosuppressed patients have been reported. Patients present with effusions in serous cavities—pleura, pericardium, or peritoneum. Occasionally, infiltration of other tissues may be seen (268). The clinical course is usually very aggressive. The tumor cells are large, often pleomorphic cells resembling either bizarre plasma cells or the cells of ALCL. They often lack B-cell associated antigens, such as CD20, and are bcl6⁻ but may be CD79a⁺ and CD45⁺, sometimes contain cytoplasmic Ig, and often express CD30 and the plasma cell–associated antigen CD138 (269). Ig genes are clonally rearranged. They typically contain both EBV and the recently described Kaposi's sarcoma herpes virus (human herpes virus 8) (270).

BURKITT LYMPHOMA

Clinical Features. There are three distinct forms of BL: endemic, sporadic, and immunodeficiency-associated (271). Although they are histologically identical and have similar clinical behavior, there are differences in epidemiology, clinical presentation, and genetic features between the three forms. Endemic and sporadic BLs are both most common in children, but the median age is younger in endemic patients, and the disease is found primarily in Africa. Sporadic BL comprises 30% of pediatric lymphomas in the United States but less than 1% of adult NHLs. Immunodeficiency-associated BL is seen most often in HIV-positive patients and occasionally in iatrogenically immunosuppressed patients. It typically occurs in patients with a relatively high CD4 count and no opportunistic infections.

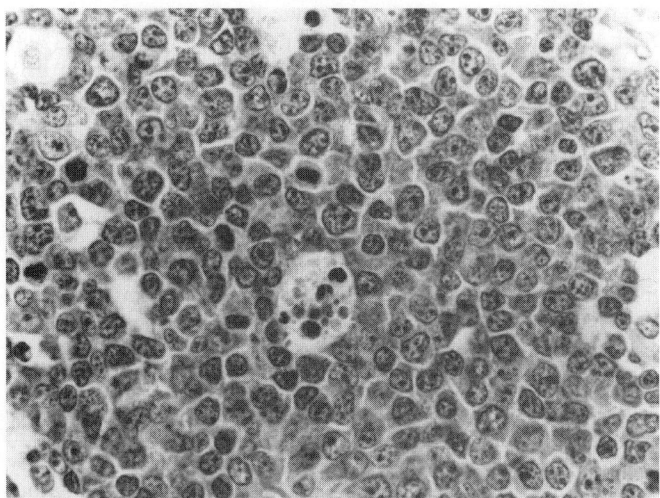

Figure 24-16. Burkitt lymphoma, endemic type, in an African child: the tumor is composed of medium-sized, relatively monomorphous cells with a high mitotic rate. Tingible body macrophages are present. (From Harris NL, Ferry JA. Classification of non-Hodgkin's lymphomas. In: Knowles DM, ed. *Neoplastic hematopathology*. Philadelphia: Lippincott Williams & Wilkins, 2001, with permission.)

In all groups, the majority of patients are male (3:1 to 4:1). Patients typically present with rapidly growing tumor masses and often have a very high serum lactate dehydrogenase. In endemic cases, the jaws and other facial bones are often involved, as well as the mesentery and gonads. In sporadic cases, the majority present with abdominal tumors, most often in the distal ileum, cecum, or mesentery; ovaries, kidneys, or breasts may be involved (272). Immunodeficiency-related cases more often involve lymph nodes, and both these and sporadic cases may present as acute leukemia (Burkitt cell leukemia). BL is highly aggressive but potentially curable with very aggressive therapy (272).

Morphology. BL cells are monomorphic, medium-sized cells with round nuclei, multiple nucleoli, and basophilic cytoplasm (Fig. 24-16). There is a very high rate of proliferation, with virtually every cell being in cycle; a "starry-sky" pattern is imparted by macrophages that have ingested apoptotic tumor cells. Although most cases present no problem in diagnosis, some cases may have larger cells or an admixture of immunoblast-like cells, and there is morphologic overlap with large B-cell lymphoma. These borderline cases are often called *non-Burkitt* (273) or *Burkitt-like* (3). In children and HIV-positive patients, these borderline cases often have a c-MYC translocation and behave similarly to typical BL, whereas in adults, cases classified as non-Burkitt or Burkitt-like lymphomas often have BCL-2 gene rearrangement and may represent variants of DLBCL (274). In the international study of the REAL classification (6), Burkitt-like lymphoma was a nonreproducible category, in which the pathologists agreed on the diagnosis only 50% of the time; disagreements were equally split between large B-cell and BL.

These borderline cases present a clinical problem, because treatment for BL is often more aggressive than that for large B-cell lymphoma. Patients with BL may not do well if treated as large-cell lymphoma, and patients with large B-cell lymphoma may have significant treatment-related morbidity if treated as BL (275). Unfortunately, there are no good data to indicate how to draw the line between large-cell lymphoma and BL so that morphologically borderline cases will be assigned to the correct category. The WHO Clinical Advisory Committee concluded that *Burkitt-like lymphoma* should be defined as a tumor that should be treated "like Burkitt lymphoma (8)."

The defining biologic feature of BL is believed to be *c-MYC* deregulation; this causes the tumor cells to remain constantly in cycle and presumably drives its clinical behavior. Unfortunately, detection of this translocation is not possible in most clinical specimens. The best surrogate for c-MYC deregulation is proliferation fraction: In a tumor with c-MYC deregulation, 100% of viable cells should express Ki-67. Thus, the WHO committees concluded that a diagnosis of Burkitt-like lymphoma should only be made in a tumor with morphologic features intermediate between BL and DLBCL, in which the Ki-67 fraction of viable cells is at least 99%. This tumor is considered a variant of BL in the WHO classification (8).

Immunophenotype and Genetic Features. BL cells express surface IgM and B-cell–associated antigens (CD19, CD20, CD22, CD79a), as well as CD10; they lack CD5, bcl-2, and CD23 (276). They show nuclear staining for BCL-6 protein, which is independent of bcl-6 gene rearrangement (277). Ig heavy- and light-chain genes are rearranged, and most studies of the variable region genes show somatic mutations and intraclonal heterogeneity, consistent with a GC cell (54,278–280). Most cases have a translocation of *c-MYC* from chromosome 8q to either the Ig heavy-chain region on chromosome 14q [t(8;14)(q24;q32)] or light-chain loci on 2q [t(2;8)] or 22q [t(8;22)]. In endemic cases, the breakpoint on chromosome 14 involves the heavy-chain joining region, whereas in nonendemic cases, the translocation involves the heavy-chain switch region (281,282). Mutations in the 5' noncoding region of the Bcl-6 gene, similar to those seen in large B-cell lymphoma, have been reported in 25% to 50% of the cases (283). Virtually all endemic cases contain EBV genomes, as do 25% to 40% of sporadic and immunodeficiency-associated cases (284).

Postulated Normal Counterpart. BL is thought to correspond to peripheral B cells of unknown stage, possibly the B blast of the early GC reaction.

Mature T-Cell and Natural Killer Cell Neoplasms

T-CELL PROLYMPHOCYTIC LEUKEMIA

Clinical Features. T-cell PLL (T-PLL) comprises 1% of cases classified morphologically as CLL but the majority of cases classified as PLL. Patients typically have a high white blood cell count (>100,000) and splenomegaly. Bone marrow, liver, and lymph nodes may be involved, as well as skin and mucosal sites. It is an aggressive disease, with most patients dying within 1 year, and is not usually curable with available therapy (285).

Morphology. The leukemic T-cells usually are slightly larger than normal lymphocytes and have prominent nucleoli, some nuclear irregularity, and moderately abundant nongranular cytoplasm. Some cases have smaller cells with inconspicuous nucleoli or cerebriform nuclei (285–287). This range of morphology has led to some cases being classified as T-CLL and others as T-PLL. However, all have the same genetic abnormalities and aggressive clinical course, so that the WHO classification defines all as T-PLL. Lymph node involvement is often paracortical, with sparing of follicles, and pseudofollicles are absent. HEV may be prominent and often contain atypical lymphoid cells (288). Splenic red pulp and hepatic sinusoids may be infiltrated. Bone marrow involvement is diffuse.

Immunophenotype and Genetic Features. The tumor cells express CD2, CD3, CD5, and CD7, as well as the TCR αβ chain, and usually lack CD25; most cases are CD4+ (65%), but some are

CD4$^+$8$^+$ (21%), and rare cases are CD4$^-$8$^+$ (285,287,289). T-cell receptor genes are clonally rearranged; inv 14 (q11;q32) is found in 80%; in 10% there is a reciprocal translocation t(14;14)(q11;q32). In 70% of cases there is also trisomy 8q, often as a consequence of iso (8q). Deletions or translocations of chromosome 11 are seen in 50% of cases.

Postulated Normal Counterpart. T-PLL is thought to correspond to circulating peripheral T cells.

T-CELL LARGE GRANULAR LYMPHOCYTE LEUKEMIA

Clinical Features. LGL leukemia is a rare disorder that presents in adulthood with mild to moderate stable lymphocytosis (5000 to 20,000/mm^3), neutropenia and anemia, and mild to moderate splenomegaly without significant lymphadenopathy or hepatomegaly. The course is usually indolent, with morbidity related to cytopenias rather than tumor burden—often, recurrent bacterial infections. Cyclosporine has been reported to ameliorate the neutropenia (290). Indolent cases may undergo histologic progression to a higher-grade neoplasm as a late event (291). Recently, aggressive T-cell LGLs have been reported in immunosuppressed patients (292,293).

Morphologic Features. Peripheral blood cells have round or oval nuclei with moderately condensed chromatin and rare nucleoli, eccentrically placed in abundant pale blue cytoplasm with azurophilic granules. This disorder corresponds to cases described as T8 lymphocytosis with neutropenia, CD8 or Tγ lymphoproliferative disease, and CD8$^+$ T-CLL (291). Bone marrow infiltration is usually sparse, with mild to moderate lymphocytosis as well as focal aggregates sometimes resembling B-cell lymphoma. There may be a myeloid maturation arrest or erythroid hypoplasia. The spleen is involved with an infiltrate in the red pulp cords and sinuses. Hepatic sinuses may be infiltrated (294).

Immunophenotype and Genetic Features. T-cell LGL cells (291) express CD2, CD3, and usually CD8, as well as the NK cell–associated antigens CD16 and CD57 (Leu-7), but not CD56, and TCR αβ. The TCR genes are clonally rearranged.

Postulated Normal Counterpart. T-cell LGL is thought to correspond to peripheral CD8$^+$ T lymphocytes with suppressor but no NK function.

AGGRESSIVE NATURAL KILLER CELL LEUKEMIA

Clinical Features. Aggressive NK cell leukemia is an uncommon disease that has been reported most often in Asia. Patients are usually adolescents or young adults who present with fever, hepatosplenomegaly, lymphadenopathy, and leukemia (295,296). The disease is usually rapidly fatal. Rare cases of nasal-type T/NK-cell lymphoma have progressed to aggressive NK-cell leukemia, and some believe it may be a leukemic manifestation of this disorder (297).

Morphology. Circulating leukemic cells are slightly larger than normal LGL cells and may have irregular, hyperchromatic nuclei and distinct nucleoli. The cytoplasm is abundant and contains azurophilic granules. The marrow is often involved, with a diffuse interstitial pattern. Lymph nodes and spleen show a diffuse infiltrate similar to that seen in acute leukemias. The cells often appear more primitive in tissue infiltrates than in the blood.

Immunophenotype and Genetic Features. The cells are CD2$^+$ CD56$^+$ and surface CD3$^-$. CD11b may be positive. CD16 is variable, and CD57 is usually negative. Rare cases of aggressive LGL leukemia with CD3 expression have been reported (298). The TCR genes are typically germline. Most contain EBV genomes, which are clonal.

Postulated Normal Counterpart. Aggressive NK cell leukemia is thought to correspond to immature NK cells.

ADULT T-CELL LYMPHOMA AND LEUKEMIA

Clinical Features. Most cases of adult T-cell lymphoma and leukemia occur in Japan or in the Caribbean, but sporadic cases are found elsewhere in the world (299–304). Patients are adults with antibodies to human T-cell lymphotrophic virus (HTLV) 1. Clinical variants include acute, lymphomatous, chronic, and smoldering types. The acute type is most common and presents with circulating neoplastic cells, skin rash, lymphadenopathy, hepatosplenomegaly, and hypercalcemia. The lymphomatous type has lymphadenopathy without blood involvement. The chronic type has skin lesions and blood involvement with absolute lymphocytosis, but no hypercalcemia. The smoldering type has normal blood lymphocyte counts with less than or equal to 5% circulating neoplastic cells (305). Progression from chronic or smoldering to acute types occurs in up to 25% of the cases. This is an aggressive disease with poor survival with currently available therapies and a median survival of less than 3 years.

Morphology. In lymph nodes, the infiltrates are diffuse with architectural effacement. Neoplastic cells are usually medium- to large-sized with nuclear pleomorphism (302). RS-like cells and giant cells with convoluted or cerebriform nuclei may be present (306). Rare cases may be composed of small atypical lymphocytes, or may resemble anaplastic large-cell lymphoma (307). Cells with hyperlobated nuclei (flower cells) are common in the peripheral blood in leukemic cases. Bone marrow infiltrates are usually patchy.

Immunophenotype and Genetic Features. Tumor cells express T-cell–associated antigens (CD2, CD3, CD5), but usually lack CD7. Most cases are CD4$^+$, CD8$^-$. Rare cases are CD4$^-$,CD8$^+$ or CD8$^+$, and CD4$^+$. CD25 is expressed in a majority of the cases. Anaplastic large-cell types react with CD30, but are ALK (p80) negative. Clonally integrated HTLV-1 genes are found in all cases (308). The TCR genes are clonally rearranged.

Possible Normal Counterpart. Adult T-cell lymphoma and leukemia are thought to correspond to peripheral CD4$^+$ T cells in various stages of transformation.

EXTRANODAL NATURAL KILLER/T-CELL LYMPHOMA, NASAL-TYPE (FORMERLY ANGIOCENTRIC LYMPHOMA)

Clinical Features. Nasal-type NK/T-cell lymphoma is a rare disorder in the United States and Europe but is more common in Asia and in native populations in Peru. It may affect children or adults. Extranodal sites are invariably involved, including nose, palate, upper airway, gastrointestinal tract, and skin (309–313). The clinical course is typically aggressive, with relapses in other extranodal sites, including gastrointestinal tract or testis (311,314,315). Hemophagocytic syndromes may occur. Some cases of the aggressive variant of NK-cell leukemia and lymphoma may be related to this disorder (297).

Morphologic Features. Extranodal NK/T-cell lymphoma is typically characterized by a polymorphous infiltrate composed of a mixture of normal-appearing small lymphocytes and atypical lymphoid cells of varying size (309,313), along with plasma

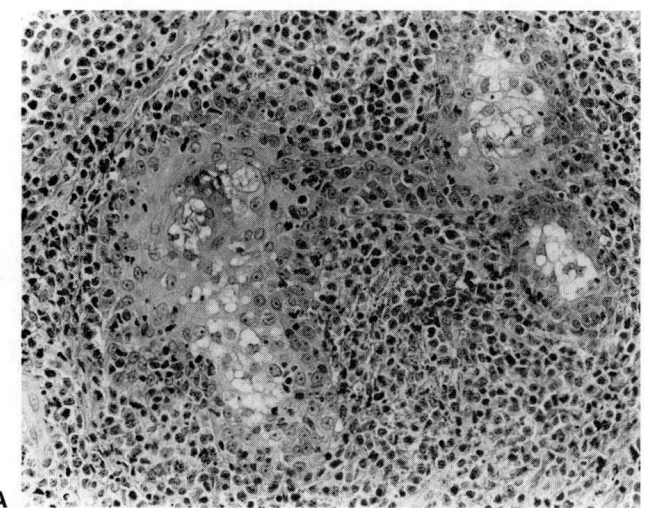
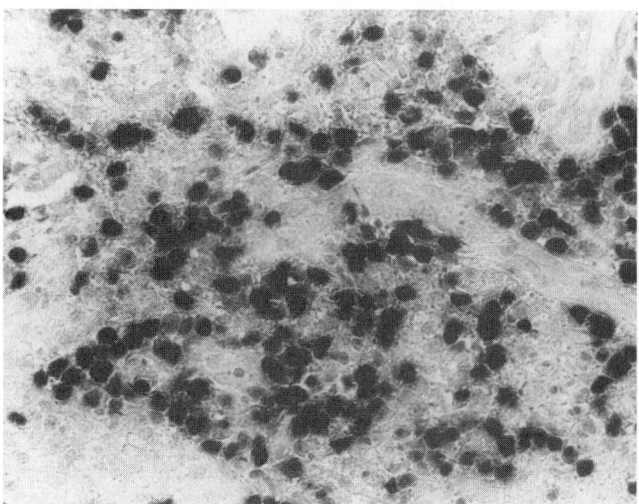

Figure 24-17. Nasal natural killer/T-cell lymphoma. **A:** There is an infiltrate of medium-sized pleomorphic cells associated with squamous metaplasia of epithelial structures. **B:** *In situ* hybridization shows that neoplastic cells are uniformly positive for Epstein-Barr virus latency-associated RNA. (From Harris NL, Ferry JA. Classification of non-Hodgkin's lymphomas. In: Knowles DM, ed. *Neoplastic hematopathology*. Philadelphia: Lippincott Williams & Wilkins, 2001, with permission.)

cells and occasionally eosinophils and histiocytes (Fig. 24-17). A characteristic feature is invasion of vascular walls and occlusion of lumina by lymphoid cells with varying degrees of cytologic atypia; however, this is not seen in all the cases. There is usually prominent ischemic necrosis of both tumor cells and normal tissue. The term *angiocentric lymphoma* has proven confusing, because angiocentricity is not evident in all cases. Because the most characteristic presentation is midfacial, and the cells have both T and NK-cell features, the term *extranodal NK/T-cell lymphoma, nasal-type* has been proposed (316).

Immunophenotype and Genetic Features. The atypical cells in most cases are CD2+ CD56+, surface CD3−, and cytoplasmic CD3+ (Leu 4− but positive with the polyclonal anti-CD3, which detects the epsilon chain of CD3). They are typically CD4−CD8− but may express CD4 or CD7 (309,311,317). Most cases express cytotoxic granule proteins such as granzyme B and TIA-1 (318).

The TCR and Ig genes are usually germline; EBV genomes are usually present, and are detectable in the majority of the cells in most cases by *in situ* hybridization for EBV-encoded RNA (311,319) (Fig. 24-17).

Postulated Normal Counterpart. Nasal-type NK/T-cell lymphoma is thought to correspond to immature NK cells.

ENTEROPATHY TYPE T-CELL LYMPHOMA

Clinical Features. This disorder was originally termed *malignant histiocytosis of the intestine* but has since been conclusively shown to be a T-cell lymphoma (320). The disease occurs in adults, who typically have a rather brief history of gluten-sensitive enteropathy. It may also occur as the initial event in a patient found to have villous atrophy in the resected intestine. Some patients without evidence of enteropathy have either or both antigliadin antibodies or the typical HLA type (DQA1*0501, DQB1*0201) of patients with celiac disease (321). It is uncommon in most areas of the United States and Europe but is seen with increased frequency in areas in which gluten-sensitive enteropathy is common, such as Ireland and Wales. Treatment of celiac disease with a gluten-free diet effectively prevents the development of lymphoma, so that patients diag-

nosed with celiac disease early in life usually do not develop lymphoma, and patients with lymphoma rarely have a long history of celiac disease (322,323).

Patients present with abdominal pain, often associated with jejunal perforation; stomach or colon is affected less often (324), and other viscera, skin, or soft tissues may be involved (325,326). The course is aggressive, and death usually occurs from multifocal intestinal perforation due to refractory malignant ulcers.

Morphology. On gross examination, circumferentially oriented jejunal ulcers are present, often multiple and with perforation. A mass may or may not be present. The tumors contain a variable admixture of small, medium and mixed, large, or anaplastic tumor cells, often with a high content of intraepithelial T cells in adjacent mucosa. The adjacent mucosa may or may not show villous atrophy (327); this varies depending on the segment analyzed, because in sprue, villous atrophy is most prominent in the proximal small intestine and may be absent in distal jejunum or ileum. Early lesions may show mucosal ulceration with only scattered atypical cells and numerous reactive histiocytes, without formation of large masses (328); these lesions are nonetheless clonal. Intraepithelial lymphocytes in apparently nonneoplastic mucosa may also be clonal (329). Clonal TCR gene rearrangements have been found in cases of celiac disease unresponsive to a gluten-free diet, suggesting that these cases may represent early T-cell lymphomas (330). The tumor may involve liver, spleen, lymph nodes, and other viscera such as the gallbladder.

Immunophenotype and Genetic Features. The tumor cells express pan-T antigens (CD3+ CD7+), usually CD8+ CD4−, and express the mucosal lymphoid antigen CD103 (331). CD30 may be positive in some cells. Expression of cytotoxic T-cell–associated proteins (Granzyme B, TIA-1, perforin) is seen in many of the cases (332,333). The TCRβ gene is clonally rearranged (320); no specific cytogenetic abnormality has been described.

Postulated Normal Counterpart. Enteropathy type T-cell lymphoma is thought to correspond to intestinal intraepithelial cytotoxic T cells in various stages of transformation.

HEPATOSPLENIC T-CELL LYMPHOMA

Clinical Features. Hepatosplenic T-cell lymphoma is a rare neoplasm, but because it has only recently been characterized, its frequency is not known. Patients are predominantly adolescent and young adult males, who present with marked hepatosplenomegaly; although circulating neoplastic cells are not usually prominent, subtle bone marrow involvement may be present (334,335). Several cases have been reported in immunosuppressed, solid-organ allograft recipients (336,337). Despite the relatively bland appearance of the cells, this is an aggressive tumor; although there is often an initial response to chemotherapy, relapse and death are common (338). The cells in most cases express the γδ T-cell receptor, but rare cases are αβ. Neoplasms of γδ T cells may occur in other sites, particularly mucosal or cutaneous locations; these appear to behave similarly to primary extranodal αβ T-cell or NK-cell neoplasms of the same sites and do not disseminate to spleen and liver (339,340). Thus, the site of presentation appears to be an important defining criterion for this disease.

Morphology. Hepatosplenic T-cell lymphoma produces a sinusoidal infiltrate in liver and spleen, as well as bone marrow, of medium-sized lymphoid cells with round nuclei, moderately condensed chromatin, and moderately abundant, pale cytoplasm (341). Mitotic activity is generally low (338). The white pulp is atrophic. Erythrophagocytosis may be prominent in splenic and bone marrow sinuses.

Immunophenotype and Genetic Features. The tumor cells are CD2+ and CD3+, CD5−, CD4−, CD8−, CD16+, and CD56±, and most cases lack the αβ T-cell receptor protein, expressing instead the γδ complex. Cytotoxic granule protein TIA-1 is typically expressed, but Granzyme-B and perforin are absent, indicating a nonactivated cytotoxic T-cell phenotype (342–344). The TCRγ and TCRδ genes are rearranged; the TCRβ gene may be rearranged or germline. The tumor cells are EBV negative. Isochromosome 7q and trisomy 8 have been reported in many cases (337,345,346).

Postulated Normal Counterpart. Hepatosplenic T-cell lymphoma is thought to correspond to T cells of splenic type, usually γδ but occasionally αβ.

SUBCUTANEOUS PANNICULITIS-LIKE T-CELL LYMPHOMA

Clinical Features. Patients with subcutaneous panniculitis-like T-cell lymphoma present with one or more subcutaneous nodules, which may resolve spontaneously and are often misdiagnosed as panniculitis. Hemophagocytic syndrome is common. The disease may present in an indolent fashion but typically becomes aggressive; patients may respond to aggressive therapy, and cure appears to be possible (347,348).

Morphologic Features. There is a variable mixture of small, medium, and large atypical cells in the subcutis, often containing irregular, hyperchromatic nuclei and pale cytoplasm (Fig. 24-18). Reactive histiocytes with phagocytized nuclear debris or lipid are numerous. Granulomas may be present. Individual adipocytes are rimmed by neoplastic cells (347,348).

Immunophenotype and Genetic Features. Most cases express pan-T antigens and usually CD8 (although they may be CD4+), cytotoxic granule proteins TIA-1 and perforin, and in most cases, the αβ T-cell receptor (349). Occasional cases derive from γδ T cells (348). T-cell receptor γ genes are rearranged; usually β- but occasionally δ-chain genes are rearranged (348). No specific cytogenetic abnormalities have been described.

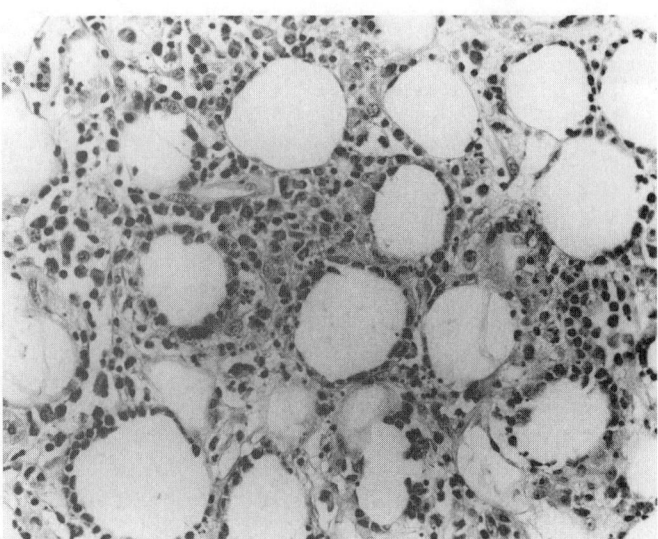

Figure 24-18. Subcutaneous panniculitis-like T-cell lymphoma. The subcutaneous tissue contains a dense interstitial infiltrate of atypical lymphoid cells, with rimming of individual fat cells by the lymphoid cells. (From Harris NL, Ferry JA. Classification of non-Hodgkin's lymphomas. In: Knowles DM, ed. *Neoplastic hematopathology.* Philadelphia: Lippincott Williams & Wilkins, 2001, with permission.)

Postulated Normal Counterpart. Subcutaneous panniculitis-like T-cell lymphoma is thought to correspond to mature cytotoxic T cells.

MYCOSIS FUNGOIDES

Clinical Features. Patients are almost exclusively adults, with single or multiple cutaneous lesions (350). The disease has an indolent course with progression from patches to plaques and eventually tumors. Peripheral blood involvement is absent or subtle, and lymphadenopathy is a late occurrence. Long-term remissions can be obtained in the early stages. Prognosis in advanced stages is less favorable. As a terminal event, transformation to a large T-cell lymphoma or ALCL may occur.

Morphology. Skin lesions show epidermotropic infiltrates consisting of small or medium-sized cells with irregular (cerebriform) nuclei. A minority of larger cells with similar nuclei may be present but are never prominent. Pautrier microabscesses, consisting of groups of cerebriform cells in the epidermis, are highly characteristic but not seen in all cases. Epidermal involvement with single cell exocytosis is more common. The dermal infiltrates may be patchy, bandlike, or diffuse depending on the stage of the disease. Involved lymph nodes may have the appearance of dermatopathic lymphadenitis or may show paracortical infiltrates of atypical cells similar to those seen in the skin, with architectural effacement.

Immunophenotype and Genetic Features. Tumor cells are CD2+, CD3+, TCR β+, CD5+, and CD7±. Most cases are CD4+. The expression of CD8 is less frequent. Aberrant T-cell phenotypes are frequent in tumor stages (351). The TCR genes are clonally rearranged (352). Consistent cytogenetic abnormalities have not been identified.

Possible Normal Counterpart. Mycosis fungoides is thought to correspond to peripheral, epidermotropic T-cells.

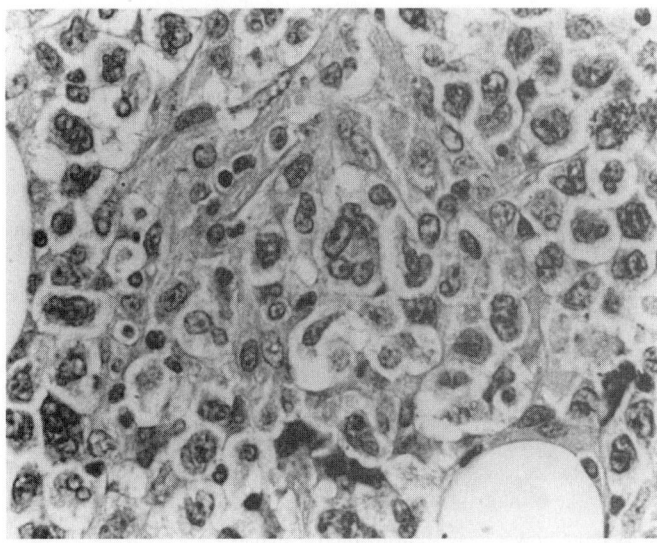

Figure 24-19. Primary cutaneous anaplastic large-cell lymphoma, showing large cells with abundant cytoplasm, large, often indented or horseshoe-shaped nuclei with conspicuous nucleoli, and scattered multinucleated cells. (From Harris NL, Ferry JA. Classification of non-Hodgkin's lymphomas. In: Knowles DM, ed. *Neoplastic hematopathology*. Philadelphia: Lippincott Williams & Wilkins, 2001, with permission.)

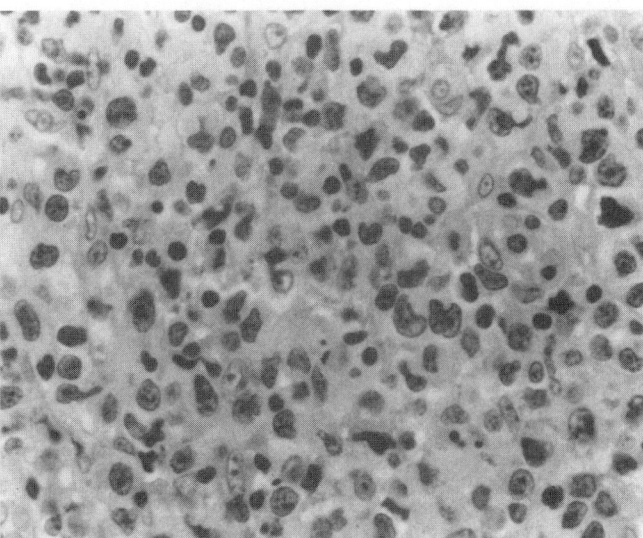

Figure 24-20. Peripheral T-cell lymphoma, not otherwise specified, composed predominantly of medium-sized and large cells with pleomorphic, irregular nuclei. (From Harris NL, Ferry JA. Classification of non-Hodgkin's lymphomas. In: Knowles DM, ed. *Neoplastic hematopathology*. Philadelphia: Lippincott Williams & Wilkins, 2001, with permission.)

PRIMARY CUTANEOUS ANAPLASTIC LARGE-CELL LYMPHOMA

Clinical Features. Primary cutaneous ALCL affects predominantly older adults and is rare in children. Most cases show limited disease with solitary or localized skin tumors or nodules; by definition, extracutaneous involvement is absent. The prognosis is favorable, with long-term remissions or even spontaneous regressions. Systemic disease develops occasionally, late in the course. This disorder appears to represent one end of a biologic spectrum that includes lymphomatoid papulosis at the clinically benign end: so-called cutaneous CD30+ lymphoproliferative disease (353,354).

Histology. The cytologic features are similar to those of systemic ALCL (Fig. 24-19). Infiltrates are diffuse and involve both the upper and deep dermis and the subcutaneous tissue. Most cases are nonepidermotropic.

Immunophenotype and Genetic Features. The neoplastic cells express T-cell antigens and CD30 and are usually CD4+. Unlike systemic ALCL, most cutaneous cases are negative for ALK and epithelial membrane antigen (355,356). One-half of the lesions are positive for the cutaneous lymphocyte antigen recognized by HECA 452 (353). The TCR genes are clonally rearranged. The t(2;5) is typically absent, and its presence should raise the concern that the tumor is a cutaneous manifestation of systemic ALCL (357).

PERIPHERAL T-CELL LYMPHOMA, UNSPECIFIED

Clinical Features. Mature T-cell lymphomas have variable morphologic features but consistent immunophenotypic, genetic, or clinical correlations have not been found. The term *peripheral T-cell lymphoma, unspecified* has been proposed for these cases. This category includes heterogeneous diseases that require further definition. Peripheral T-cell lymphomas comprised only 6% of lymphomas in the international study of the REAL classification (6,15), reflecting their rarity in American

and European populations. The median age was in the seventh decade, and 65% of the patients had stage IV disease. Blood eosinophilia, pruritus, and hemophagocytic syndromes may occur (358); lymph nodes, skin, liver, spleen, and other viscera may be involved (327,347). The clinical course is aggressive, and relapses are more common than in large B-cell lymphoma (6,359–362). In the international REAL classification study, this group had one of the lowest overall and failure-free survival rates (6,15).

Morphologic Features. Peripheral T-cell lymphomas typically contain a mixture of small and large atypical cells (288,363) and are classified as diffuse small cleaved, mixed, large cell, and immunoblastic in the WF (Fig. 24-20) (15,364). Admixed eosinophils or epithelioid histiocytes may be numerous (365); the term *lymphoepithelioid cell (Lennert's) lymphoma* has been used for cases rich in epithelioid cells (365). Because of their relative rarity and heterogeneity, it has been impossible to arrive at a generally useful classification (288,359,366–368). For the time being, these tumors are simply designated "peripheral T-cell lymphomas, unspecified."

Immunophenotype and Genetic Features. T-cell–associated antigens are variably expressed (CD3$^{-/+}$, CD2$^{-/+}$, CD5$^{-/+}$, CD7$^{-/+}$), CD4 is more often expressed than CD8, and tumors may be CD4$^-$CD8$^-$. B-cell–associated antigens are lacking (363,369). The TCR genes are usually but not always rearranged; Ig genes are germline (370,371). No specific cytogenetic or oncogene abnormality has been reported, although complex karyotypes are common in cases with larger cells.

Postulated Normal Counterpart. Unspecified peripheral T-cell lymphoma is thought to correspond to peripheral T cells in various stages of transformation.

ANGIOIMMUNOBLASTIC T-CELL LYMPHOMA

Clinical Features. Angioimmunoblastic T-cell lymphoma is one of the more common peripheral T-cell lymphomas encoun-

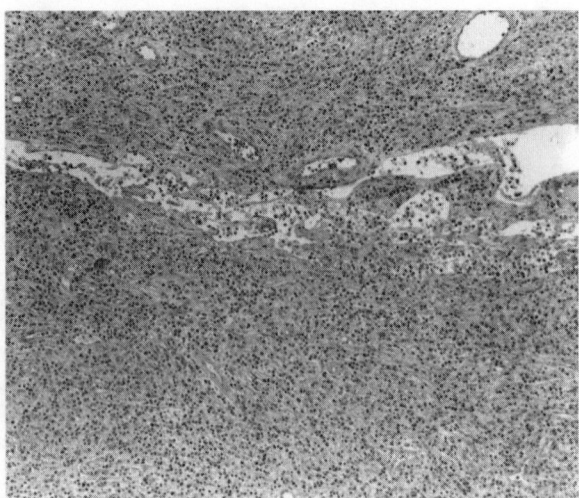
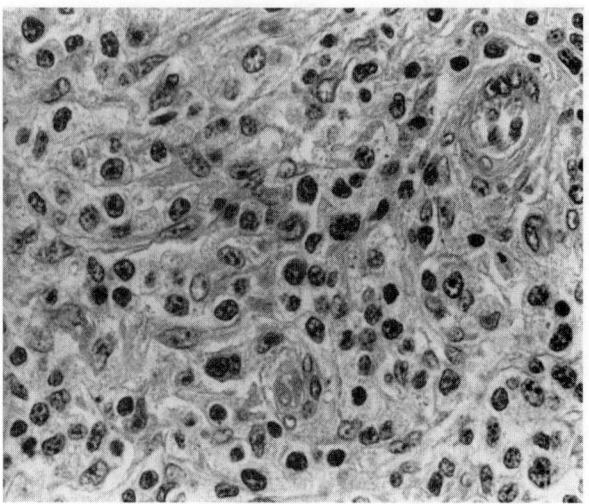

Figure 24-21. Angioimmunoblastic T-cell lymphoma. **A:** Medium-power view showing diffuse architectural effacement with widely patent subcapsular sinus and extension of the infiltrate beyond the nodal capsule. **B:** The infiltrate contains medium-sized cells with clear cytoplasm and increased numbers of blood vessels. (From Harris NL, Ferry JA. Classification of non-Hodgkin's lymphomas. In: Knowles DM, ed. *Neoplastic hematopathology*. Philadelphia: Lippincott Williams & Wilkins, 2001, with permission.)

tered in western countries. In the Kiel Registry, it accounted for 20% of all T-cell lymphomas and approximately 4% of all lymphomas (367). Angioimmunoblastic T-cell lymphoma is clinically distinctive: Patients typically have generalized lymphadenopathy, fever, weight loss, skin rash, and polyclonal hypergammaglobulinemia (372) and are susceptible to infections. The course is moderately aggressive, with occasional spontaneous remissions, and is not reliably predicted by the histologic appearance. Approximately 30% of the patients may have initial remission on steroids alone, but most require some form of chemotherapy. Median survivals range from 15 to 24 months, and its curability has not been well established. Some patients develop a secondary EBV+ large B-cell lymphoma.

Morphology. The nodal architecture is effaced; peripheral sinuses are typically open and even dilated, but the abnormal infiltrate often extends beyond the capsule into the perinodal fat (Fig. 24-21). There are prominent arborizing HEVs, many of which show thickened or hyalinized PAS+ walls. Clusters of epithelioid histiocytes and numerous eosinophils and plasma cells may be present. Expanded aggregates of FDCs, visible on immunostained sections, surround the proliferating blood vessels and may have the appearance of "burnt-out" GCs. The lymphoid cells are a mixture of small lymphocytes, immunoblasts, plasma cells, and medium-sized cells with round nuclei and clear cytoplasm. B-immunoblasts may be numerous.

Immunophenotype and Genetic Features. Tumor cells express T-cell–associated antigens and usually CD4, but many CD8+ cells are often present; expanded FDC clusters (CD21+) are present around proliferated venules (373). The latter feature is useful in distinguishing this disorder from other T-cell lymphomas (367). Polyclonal plasma cells and B-immunoblasts may be numerous. The TCR genes are rearranged in 75%, IgH in 10%, corresponding to expanded B-cell clones (373,374). EBV genomes are detected in many cases and may be present in either T or B cells (375,376); trisomy 3 or 5 may occur (377).

Postulated Normal Counterpart. Angioimmunoblastic T-cell lymphoma is thought to correspond to peripheral T cells of unknown subset in various stages of transformation.

ANAPLASTIC LARGE-CELL LYMPHOMA

Clinical Features. ALCL represents approximately 2% of all lymphomas but approximately 10% of childhood lymphomas and 50% of large cell pediatric lymphomas (4,6,15,367,378,379). Primary systemic ALCL may involve lymph nodes or extranodal sites, including the skin, but is not localized to the skin. Tumors that present with systemic disease (with or without skin involvement) have a bimodal age distribution in children and adults and are associated with the t(2;5)(p23;q35), particularly in children, in up to 80% of the cases. Patients may present with isolated lymphadenopathy or as extranodal disease in any site, including gastrointestinal tract and bone (378). Anaplastic large-cell lymphoma in children is characterized by frequent high stage but a good response to therapy with overall excellent survival (378–380). In adults, the tumor is aggressive but potentially curable, similar to other aggressive lymphomas (381). Cases with the t(2;5) have a significantly better prognosis than cases lacking the t(2;5) (382).

Morphologic Features. The tumor is usually composed of large blastic cells with round or pleomorphic (often horseshoe-shaped or multiple) nuclei with multiple or single prominent nucleoli with abundant cytoplasm, which gives the cells an epithelial or histiocyte-like appearance (Fig. 24-19). The so-called hallmark cell has an eccentric nucleus and a prominent, eosinophilic Golgi region (383). The tumor cells grow in a cohesive pattern and often preferentially involve the lymph node sinuses or paracortex (384) (Fig. 24-22). In some cases, the tumor cells may have a more monomorphous appearance, with round to oval nuclei and no RS–like cells; these cases have in common with the more anaplastic cases a low nuclear-cytoplasmic ratio, with dense, abundant cytoplasm and a cohesive, often sinusoidal growth pattern (385). Lymphohistiocytic and small-cell variants have been described, again, more commonly in children (386,387). Study of cytogenetic and molecular genetic abnormalities as well as clinical features suggest that these cases belong to the same disease entity as the more anaplastic cases (383,388).

A variant of ALCL resembling HL of nodular sclerosis (NS) type has been described (389,390), originally called *ALCL Hodgkin's-related*, and included as a provisional entity under the

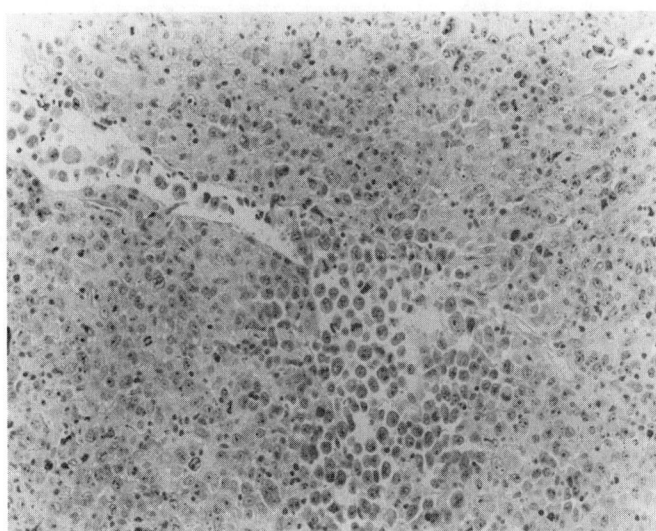

Figure 24-22. Anaplastic large-cell lymphoma involving lymph node, showing invasion of sinuses. (From Harris NL, Ferry JA. Classification of non-Hodgkin's lymphomas. In: Knowles DM, ed. *Neoplastic hematopathology.* Philadelphia: Lippincott Williams & Wilkins, 2001, with permission.)

name *ALCL Hodgkin's-like* (ALCL-HL), in the REAL classification (3). This subtype was defined as having architectural features of HD (nodularity and sclerosis) but cytologic features of ALCL (sheets of neoplastic cells and sinusoidal infiltration). Many reported patients were young adults with mediastinal masses, and the outcome was said to be intermediate between that of typical ALCL and NSHL. Several recent studies suggest that these are not true borderline cases. First, most cases of ALCL-HL lack the t(2;5) or ALK protein (356,391). Second, most cases of HD are now thought to be B-cell derived, based on single-cell studies showing Ig gene rearrangement (392–396), whereas ALCL is predominantly a T-cell disease; thus, there should be no true biologic borderline. Finally, a recent randomized study showed that patients with ALCL-HL responded equally well to the ABVD regimen for HD as to a MACOP-B regimen for aggressive NHL (397), suggesting a closer relationship to HD than to typical ALCL. The current consensus is that the majority of these cases can be resolved as either HD (CD15+, CD30+, T-cell antigen−, ALK−) or ALCL (CD15−, CD30+, T-cell antigen±, ALK±) by a combination of morphology and immunophenotype. Thus, this category has been eliminated from the WHO classification (8).

Immunophenotype and Genetic Features. The tumor cells are CD30+ and usually express CD25 and epithelial membrane antigen; they are typically CD45+ and CD15−; approximately 60% express one or more T-cell–associated antigens (CD3, CD43, or CD45RO). Recent studies have shown cytotoxic granule proteins in many of the cases (398,399). The ALK protein can be detected in 40% to 60% of the cases using the ALK1 monoclonal antibody, showing both nuclear and cytoplasmic staining in cases with the t(2;5), because nucleophosmin is a nuclear protein. ALK+ cases are more common in children and have a better prognosis than ALK− cases (356,382,391).

The majority of the cases have TCR genes rearranged; 20% to 30% have no rearrangement of TCR or Ig genes. Between 20% and 50% of primary systemic ALCL have a t(2;5)(p23;q35) (380,400), which results in a fusion of the nucleophosmin gene on chromosome 5 to a novel tyrosine kinase gene on chromosome 2, called *ALK*. The specificity of this translocation for ALCL has been debated, in part because of differing criteria for the diagnosis of ALCL. Using the reverse transcriptase PCR or an antibody

to the fusion protein, the fusion gene product can be detected in approximately 50% of ALCL of T and null type; however, it is also detected in some T-cell lymphomas without obvious anaplastic morphology (89,380,382). Based on illustrations published in some of these articles, the so-called nonanaplastic cases appear to represent examples of the monomorphic, small-cell or histiocyte-rich variants (380). Rare cases of B-cell lymphoma with the t(2;5) have been reported (379,382). Finally, variant translocations have been described, which also result in overexpression of ALK protein but without the nuclear localization (401).

Based on current information, t(2;5) and ALK expression are not considered defining features of ALCL; however, the positive cases appear clinically relatively homogeneous: young patients with a relatively good prognosis. Thus, ALK staining or t(2;5) should be assessed in all cases.

HODGKIN'S LYMPHOMAS (HODGKIN'S DISEASE)

HL differs from most other malignant tumors in its unique cellular composition: a minority of neoplastic cells (RS cells and their variants) in an inflammatory background. The clinical features and responses to treatment of HL differ dramatically from those of most so-called NHLs, suggesting that a specific immunologic reaction is important not only in the definition but also in the clinical behavior of this disease. Between 1980 and 2000, immunophenotypic and genetic studies showed that virtually all cases of HL derive from monoclonal B lymphocytes (392–394,402–409); thus the term *lymphoma* seems appropriate, rather than *disease*. In the same time period, two major types of HL were defined, based on morphology, immunophenotype, and clinical features: classic HL [NSHL, mixed cellularity HL (MCHL), and lymphocyte depletion HL (LDHL)] and nodular lymphocyte predominant HL (NLPHL) (410). Thus, it is appropriate to speak of *HLs* (plural) rather than *HL* (singular). Although we now know that the neoplastic cells in most cases of HL are monoclonal B cells, their distinctive pathologic and clinical features still warrant placing them together in a separate category from other lymphoid neoplasms (410). Thus, the HLs are defined *as lymphomas containing one of the characteristic types of RS cells in a background of nonneoplastic cells;* cases are subclassified according to the morphology and immunophenotype of the RS cells and the composition of the cellular background.

Nodular Lymphocyte Predominant Hodgkin's Lymphoma

CLINICAL FEATURES

NLPHL accounts for approximately 5% of the cases of HL in most series (411). The median age is in the mid-30s, but cases may be seen both in children and the elderly. The male to female ratio is 3 to 1 or greater. NLPHL usually involves peripheral lymph nodes, with sparing of the mediastinum. Approximately 80% of the patients in most series are stage I or II at the time of the diagnosis, but rare patients may present with stage III or IV disease, with a concomitantly worse prognosis (412). Over 90% of the patients have a complete response to therapy, and 90% are alive at ten years. Relapses occur as frequently as in classic HL, and both late and multiple relapses are more common than in other types of HL; however, these are usually isolated nodal recurrences and are not associated with poor survival (413–416). The cause of death is often NHL, other cancers, or complications of treatment rather than HL (412,414,415,417).

Patients with NLPHL have a slightly higher risk of development of NHL than patients with other types of HL (418). The

A
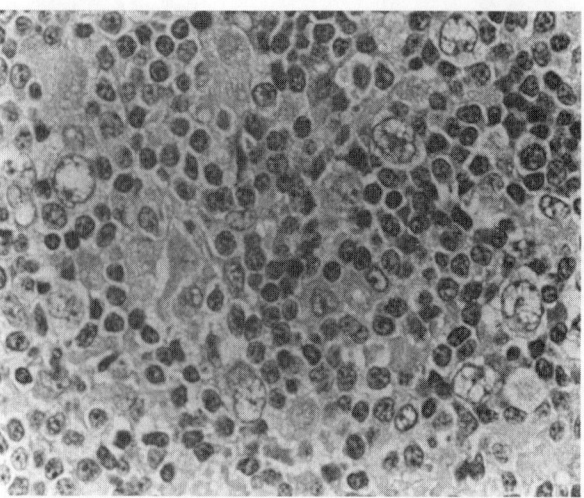
B

Figure 24-23. Nodular lymphocyte predominant Hodgkin's lymphoma. **A:** Nodular lymphocyte predominant Hodgkin's lymphoma, showing large nodules effacing the nodal architecture. **B:** Nodular lymphocyte predominant Hodgkin's lymphoma, high magnification, showing a background of small lymphocytes and numerous large mononuclear and multilobated "popcorn" cells.

frequency ranges from 2.0% to 6.5% (414,415,417–419). Transformation to large B-cell lymphoma is most common. In addition to the cases that progress to DLBCL, NLPHL may be composite with DLBCL in the same lymph node, either at the time of diagnosis or relapse (420). The frequency of this phenomenon is not known, but it appears to be rare in that most large series of NLPHL do not report any composite cases; a recent report of 66 cases, however, included one composite (414). In the reported cases, the prognosis of these patients appears to be significantly better than that for usual DLBCL, and patients who respond to treatment may later relapse with only NLPHL (420).

MORPHOLOGIC FEATURES
NLPHL by definition has at least a partially nodular growth pattern (Fig. 24-23A); diffuse areas are present in a minority of the cases, and it is controversial whether purely diffuse cases exist (411). The RS cell variants have vesicular, polylobated nuclei and distinct but small (usually peripheral) nucleoli (Fig. 24-23B). These have been called *lymphocytic and histiocytic* (L and H) cells in the Lukes and Butler classification or *popcorn* cells because of the resemblance of their nuclei to an exploded kernel of corn (421,422). In occasional cases, the RS cells may resemble classic or lacunar types; in such cases, immunophenotyping is helpful in establishing the diagnosis. The background is predominantly lymphocytes; clusters of epithelioid histiocytes may be numerous; plasma cells, eosinophils, and neutrophils are rarely seen and, if present, are not numerous (423). Occasional sclerosis may cause some cases to resemble NSHL.

PROGRESSIVE TRANSFORMATION OF GCs
A distinctive type of follicular lymphoid hyperplasia, known as *progressive transformation of GCs* (PTGC), is seen focally in approximately 20% of lymph nodes involved by NLPHL and may be seen in the absence of HL in other lymph nodes in the same patient (424,425). PTGC are enlarged follicles that contain numerous small B cells of mantle zone type and may resemble the nodules of NLPHL. PTGC are usually seen as single or only a few enlarged follicles in a setting of nonspecific reactive follicular lymphoid hyperplasia; however, on occasion, they may be numerous and associated with prominent lymph node enlargement, particularly in adolescents and young adults (426). In several studies of *de novo* PTGC in children, there appears to be a small but increased risk of subsequent development of NLPHL; this progression is rare and

may occur only after many years (419,427–429). Nonetheless, young patients with lymphadenopathy and florid PTGC should be followed closely for development of NLPHL.

IMMUNOPHENOTYPE AND GENETIC FEATURES
The tumor cells are CD45+ and express B-cell–associated antigens (CD19, CD20, CD22, and CD79a), but they lack CD15 and CD30. They also express the nuclear protein encoded by the bcl-6 gene, which is associated with normal GC B-cell development (430). The background lymphocytes in the nodules are a mixture of polyclonal B cells with a mantle zone phenotype (IgM and IgD+), and numerous T cells, many of which are CD57+, similar to the T cells in normal and progressively transformed GCs (431). T cells typically surround the neoplastic B cells, forming rings (432,433). A prominent concentric meshwork of FDC is present within the nodules (434).

Analysis of single cells from frozen sections shows clonally rearranged Ig heavy chain genes (82,84) with ongoing somatic mutation of the Ig gene variable regions, indicating a GC stage of differentiation (393,408,435). In contrast to classic HL, the Ig genes appear to be potentially functional, and light-chain messenger RNA can be detected in the cytoplasm of the RS cells in many cases.

Approximately 40% of the cases of NLPHL show abnormal metaphases, most with numeric abnormalities, including aneuploidy and hyperdiploidy (436,437). Molecular genetic analysis has not revealed abnormalities of the oncogenes typically involved in hematologic malignancies.

Classic Hodgkin's Lymphoma

Classic HL is defined by the presence of classic, diagnostic RS cells with the immunophenotype of classic HL (CD15+, CD30+, T- and B-cell–associated antigens usually negative). Classic HL includes NSHL, MCHL, and LDHL, as well as the new category of lymphocyte-rich classic HL (LRCHL).

CLINICAL FEATURES
NSHL is the most common subtype of HL in developed countries (60% to 80% in most series). It is most common in adolescents and young adults, but can occur at any age; females equal or exceed males. The mediastinum and other supradiaphragmatic sites are commonly involved. MCHL comprises 15% to

30% of HL cases in most series; it may be seen at any age and lacks the early adult peak of NSHL. Involvement of the mediastinum is less common than in NSHL, and abdominal lymph node and splenic involvement are more common. LDHL is the least common variant of HL, comprising less than 1% of the cases in recent reports. It is most common in older people, in HIV-positive individuals (438,439), and in nonindustrialized countries. LDHL frequently presents with abdominal lymphadenopathy, spleen, liver, and bone marrow involvement, without peripheral lymphadenopathy (439). The stage is usually advanced at diagnosis; however, response to treatment is reported not to differ from that of other subtypes (440).

LRCHL comprised 6% (116 cases) of 1959 cases of HL in a recent study, similar in frequency to NLPHL (411,441). The clinical features at presentation seem to be intermediate between those of NLPHL and classic HL. Similar to NLPHL, patients had early stage disease and lacked bulky disease or "B" symptoms; like both NLPHL and MCHL and in contrast to NLPHL, they lacked mediastinal disease and had a predominance of males, and like MCHL, they had an older median age than either NLPHL or NSHL. In one series, the overall survival of both LPHL and LRCHL were excellent, but not significantly different from other types of HL. However, cases of NLPHL had an increased frequency of multiple relapses and better survival after relapse compared to LRCHL, NSHL, and MCHL (412,442). In another study, the overall survival of LRCHL was significantly worse than that of NLPHL (411,441). These data do not clearly define LRCHL as a distinct entity but are consistent with either an early phase of MCHL or a novel subtype.

MORPHOLOGIC FEATURES
Classic HL is subclassified according to the cellular composition of the background infiltrate (Fig. 24-24A–D). NSHL has at least a partially nodular pattern, with fibrous bands separating the nodules. The characteristic cell is the lacunar type RS cell, with multilobated nucleolus, small nucleoli, and abundant, pale cytoplasm that retracts in formalin-fixed sections, producing an empty space, or *lacuna*. Diagnostic RS cells are also present but may be rare. In MCHL, the infiltrate is usually diffuse or at most vaguely nodular, without band-forming sclerosis, although fine interstitial fibrosis may be present. RS cells of the classic, diagnostic type and mononuclear variants are present. Diagnostic RS cells are large cells with bilobed, double, or multiple nuclei, with a large, eosinophilic, inclusion-like nucleolus in at least two lobes or nuclei. The infiltrate in both NS and MCHL typically contains lymphocytes, epithelioid histiocytes, eosinophils, and plasma cells (422). The infiltrate in LDHL is diffuse and often appears hypocellular owing to the presence of diffuse fibrosis and necrosis; there are large numbers of classic RS cells and bizarre "sarcomatous" variants, with a paucity of other inflammatory cells. Confluent sheets of RS cells and variants may occur and rarely predominate ("reticular" variant or "Hodgkin sarcoma") (422,439). Prior to the availability of immunophenotyping studies, many cases diagnosed as LDHL were, in reality, cases of large B-cell lymphoma or T-cell lymphomas, often of the ALCL type (440,443,444).

Some cases of HL with RS cells of classic type, both by morphology and immunophenotype, may have a background infiltrate that consists predominantly of lymphocytes, with rare or no eosinophils. The term *LRCHL* is used for these cases. The pattern may be diffuse or nodular, resembling NLPHL (445,446). Two studies of cases originally classified as LPHL revealed that only one-half were confirmed as NLPHL, whereas approximately one-fourth were lymphocyte-rich classic HL (411,446). Thus, cases of LRCHL may very closely resemble NLPHL and require immunophenotyping for differential diagnosis.

GRADING OF NODULAR SCLEROSIS HODGKIN'S LYMPHOMA
The British National Lymphoma Investigation developed a system for grading NSHL (grade 1 and grade 2) based on the number and atypia of the RS cells in the nodules (447–449). Approximately 80% of the cases in most series are grade 1, and 20% are grade 2. Recent results from American and European centers have had conflicting results, showing either no influence on outcome or a significantly worse outcome for NS2 patients (450–455). Grading is considered desirable for research purposes but optional for routine diagnosis.

IMMUNOPHENOTYPE AND GENETIC FEATURES
In 75% to 80% of the cases of classic HL, the tumor cells are CD15+ and CD30+. CD45 is typically absent. Expression of B-cell antigens occurs in 5% to 50%, usually only weakly and in a minority of the cells (405,441,456,457). Thus, expression of B-cell antigens does not exclude a diagnosis of HL if the morphologic features are typical. In contrast to NLPHL, the RS cells of many cases of classic HL lack the nuclear bcl-6 protein associated with follicle center B cells (430). In EBV+ cases, the tumor cells express EBV latent membrane protein but not EBV nuclear antigen.

One study found that cases that lacked CD15 but expressed CD30 had a significantly worse freedom from relapse and overall survival than CD15+ cases. Coexpression of CD20 with CD15 or CD30 had no impact on outcome, but cases that expressed CD20 alone had poor survival (441). This result raises the question whether the CD20 only cases may represent cases of T-cell–rich large B-cell lymphoma. The background lymphocytes in classic HL are predominantly CD4+ T cells, but in nodular areas of NS or LRCHL, the background lymphocytes are B cells, similar to LPHL, and follicular meshworks of FDC are seen with antibodies to CD21 or CD35.

IMMUNOGLOBULIN GENES
In classic HL, Ig and TCR genes are usually germline when studied by Southern blot, but rearrangements of Ig genes are reported in some cases, usually with faint bands (371,395,396). Using the more sensitive PCR technique on whole tissue sections to detect clonal VDJ rearrangements in cases of HL, several groups have documented Ig gene rearrangements 28% to 50% of cases of classic HL, and in 58% to 71% of cases with B-cell antigen expression (406,458). In some of the cases, there were somatic mutations in the VH segments, suggestive of a GC or post-GC stage of differentiation, while others lacked them, suggesting a pre-GC stage (406). Recently, several groups have used single cell assays of RS cells obtained by either micromanipulation of frozen sections or cell suspension, and subjecting them to PCR to detect VDJ rearrangements. These studies have convincingly shown that the vast majority of classic HL has shown clonal rearrangements of Ig genes (392–394).

Clonal cytogenetic abnormalities are found in the majority of the cases of classic HL; however, the abnormalities vary from case to case, and there is often intraclonal variability, indicating chromosome instability (459). Many cases show 14q abnormalities, similar to those found in B-cell lymphomas, but this only rarely involves a t(14;18). Using fluorescence *in situ* hybridization, with or without fluorescence immunophenotyping, two groups found that RS cells showed clonal numerical abnormalities in all cases of HL (407,460).

Bcl-2 rearrangement may be detected with the PCR in a variable proportion of the cases in some laboratories (461,462), but the rearrangement does not seem to be in the neoplastic cells (459). Although one group found the t(2;5) characteristic of anaplastic large T-cell lymphoma cases of HL (463), most other studies have found that it is not detectable in HL (464–467).

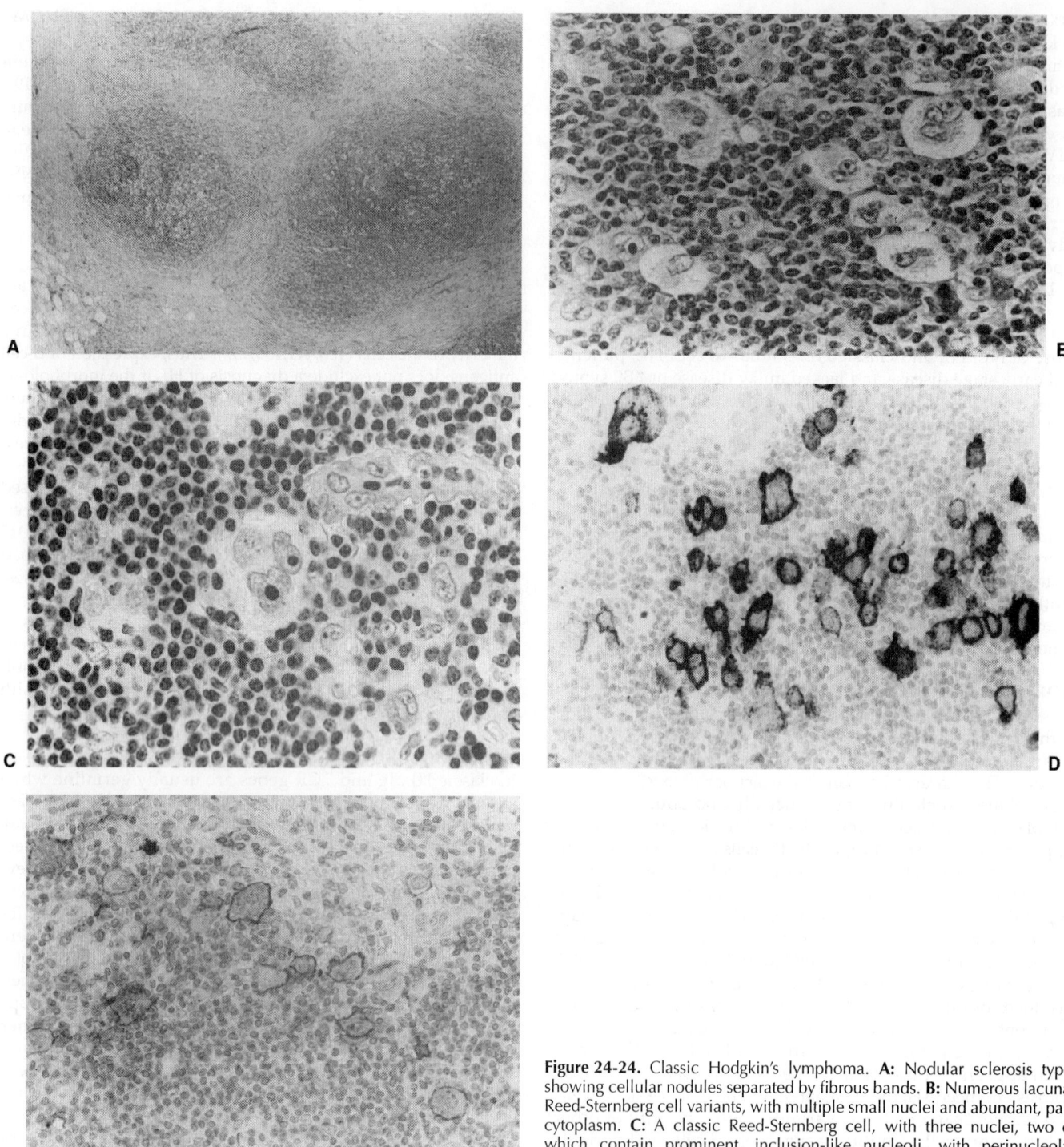

Figure 24-24. Classic Hodgkin's lymphoma. **A:** Nodular sclerosis type, showing cellular nodules separated by fibrous bands. **B:** Numerous lacunar Reed-Sternberg cell variants, with multiple small nuclei and abundant, pale cytoplasm. **C:** A classic Reed-Sternberg cell, with three nuclei, two of which contain prominent, inclusion-like nucleoli, with perinucleolar haloes and irregular nuclear membranes. **D:** Immunoperoxidase stain for CD15, showing membrane and focally paranuclear Golgi region staining. **E:** Immunoperoxidase stain for CD30, showing membrane staining.

SUMMARY AND CONCLUSIONS

Lymphoid neoplasms are a diverse group of tumors arising from cells of the immune system, and to various degrees, recapitulating stages of normal lymphocyte differentiation. A combination of morphologic, immunophenotypic, genetic, and clinical features defines each disease entity. The relative importance of these features varies from one entity to another, and there is no one "gold standard" at present. Although more than 30 distinct diseases can be recognized with current techniques, only approxi-

mately ten of them will be encountered in daily practice by most oncologists and pathologists. However, the less common entities must be recognized, and progress will be facilitated by defining homogeneous disease categories for clinical and basic research.

REFERENCES

1. Non-Hodgkin's lymphoma pathologic classification project. National Cancer Institute–sponsored study of classifications of non-Hodgkin's lympho-

mas: summary and description of a Working Formulation for clinical usage. *Cancer* 1982;49:2112–2135.

2. Gerard-Marchant R, Hamlin I, Lennert K, et al. Classification of non-Hodgkin's lymphomas. *Lancet* 1974;ii:406–408.

3. Harris NL, Jaffe ES, Stein H, et al. A revised European-American classification of lymphoid neoplasms: a proposal from the International Lymphoma Study Group. *Blood* 1994;84:1361–1392.

4. Weisenburger D. The International Lymphoma Study Group (ILSG) Classification of non-Hodgkin's lymphoma (NHL): pathology findings from a large multi-center study. *Mod Pathol* 1997;10:136A.

5. Weisenburger D. The International Lymphoma Study Group (ILSG) Classification of non-Hodgkin's lymphoma (NHL): clinical findings from a large multi-center study. *Mod Pathol* 1997;10:136A.

6. A clinical evaluation of the International Lymphoma Study Group classification of non-Hodgkin's lymphoma. *Blood* 1997;89:3909–3918.

7. Harris NL, Jaffe ES, Diebold J, et al. The World Health Organization Classification of Hematological Malignancies. Report of the Clinical Advisory Committee Meeting; Airlie House, Virginia, November, 1997. *Mod Pathol* 2000;13:193–207.

8. Harris NL, Jaffe ES, Diebold J, et al. The World Health Organization Classification of Hematological Malignancies. Report of the Clinical Advisory Committee Meeting; Airlie House, Virginia, November, 1997. *J Clin Oncol* 1999;17: 3835–3849.

9. Jaffe ES, Harris NL, Vardiman JW, Stein H. Pathology and genetics of tumours of the hematopoietic and lymphoid tissues. In: Kleihues P, Sobin L, eds. *World Health Organization classification of tumours*. Lyon: IARC Press, (in press).

10. Hiddemann W, Longo DL, Coiffier B, et al. Lymphoma classification: the gap between biology and clinical management is closing. *Blood* 1996;88:4085–4089.

11. Shipp M, Harris NL, Mauch P. Non-Hodgkin's lymphomas. In: DeVita V, Hellman S, Rosenberg S, eds. *Principles and practice of oncology*. Philadelphia: Lippincott, 1996.

12. A predictive model for aggressive non-Hodgkin's lymphoma. The International non-Hodgkin's Lymphoma Project. *N Engl J Med* 1993;329:987–994.

13. Rosenberg SA. Classification of lymphoid neoplasms. *Blood* 1994;84:1359–1360.

14. Harris NL, Jaffe ES, Stein H, et al. Lymphoma classification proposal: clarification. *Blood* 1995;85:857–860.

15. Armitage JO, Weisenburger DD. New approach to classifying non-Hodgkin's lymphomas: clinical features of the major histologic subtypes. *J Clin Oncol* 1998;16:2780–2795.

16. Anderson JR, Armitage JO, Weisenburger DD. Epidemiology of the non-Hodgkin's lymphomas: distributions of the major subtypes differ by geographic locations. Non-Hodgkin's Lymphoma Classification Project. *Ann Oncol* 1998;9:717–720.

17. Gowans J, Knight E. The route of recirculation of lymphocytes in the rat. *Proc R Soc (Lond) B Biol Sci* 1964;159:257.

18. Butcher E. Cellular and molecular mechanisms that direct leukocyte traffic. *Am J Pathol* 1990;136:3–12.

19. Arnold A, Cossman J, Bakhshi A, et al. Immunoglobulin gene rearrangements as unique clonal markers in human lymphoid neoplasms. *N Engl J Med* 1983;309:1594–1599.

20. Korsmeyer S, Hieter P, Ravetch J, et al. Developmental hierarchy of immunoglobulin gene rearrangements in leukemic pre-B cells. *Proc Natl Acad Sci U S A* 1981;78:7096–7100.

21. Pesando J, Ritz J, Lazarus H, et al. Leukemia-associated antigens in ALL. *Blood* 1979;54:1240–1248.

22. Janossy G, Bollum F, Bradstock K, Ashley J. Cellular phenotypes of normal and leukemic hematopoietic cells determined by selected antibody combinations. *Blood* 1980;56:430–441.

23. Shipp M, Richardson N, Sayre P, et al. Molecular cloning of the common acute lymphoblastic leukemia antigen (CALLA) identifies a type II integral membrane protein. *Proc Natl Acad Sci U S A* 1988;85:4819–4823.

24. Shipp M, Vuayaraghavan J, Schmidt E, et al. Common acute lymphoblastic leukemia antigen (CALLA) is active neutral endopeptidase 24.11 ("enkephalinase"): direct evidence by cDNA transfection analysis. *Proc Natl Acad Sci U S A* 1989;86:297–301.

25. Longacre T, Foucar K, Crago S, et al. Hematogones: a multiparameter analysis of bone marrow precursor cells. *Blood* 1989;73:543–552.

26. Loken M, Shah V, Dattilio K, Civin C. Flow cytometric analysis of human bone marrow. II. Normal B lymphocyte development. *Blood* 1987;70:1317–1324.

27. Klein U, Kuppers R, Rejewsky K. Human IgM+IgD+B cells, the major B cell subset in the peripheral blood, express Vh genes with no or little somatic mutation throughout life. *Eur J Immunol* 1993;23:3272.

28. MacLennan I, Liu Y, Oldfield S, et al. The evolution of B-cell clones. *Curr Top Microbiol Immunol* 1990;159:37–63.

29. Kipps T. The CD5 B cell. *Adv Immunol* 1989;47:117–185.

30. Hockenbery D, Zutter M, Hickey W, et al. BCL2 protein is topographically restricted in tissues characterized by apoptotic cell death. *Proc Natl Acad Sci U S A* 1991;88:6961–6965.

31. Inghirami G, Foitl D, Sabichi A, et al. Autoantibody-associated cross-reactive idiotype-bearing human B lymphocytes: distribution and characterization, including IgVH gene and CD5 antigen expression. *Blood* 1991;78:1503–1515.

32. Kuppers R, Zhao M, Hansmann M-L, Rajewsky K. Tracing B cell development in human germinal centres by molecular analysis of single cells picked from histological sections. *EMBO J* 1993;12:4955.

33. Zukerberg L, Medeiros L, Ferry J, Harris N. Diffuse low-grade B-cell lymphomas: four clinically distinct subtypes defined by a combination of morphologic and immunophenotypic features. *Am J Clin Pathol* 1993;100:373–385.

34. Kuppers R, Ganse A, Rajewsky K. B cells of chronic lymphatic leukemia express V genes in unmutated form. *Leuk Res* 1991;15:487.

35. Hummel M, Tamaru J, Kalvelage B, Stein H. Mantle cell (previously centrocytic) lymphomas express Vh genes with no or very little somatic mutations like the physiologic cells of the follicle mantle. *Blood* 1994;84:403–407.

36. Veldman J, Keuning F, Molenaar I. Site of initiation of the plasma cell reaction in the rabbit lymph node. *Virchows Arch B Cell Pathol* 1978;8:187–202.

37. Liu Y-J, Zhang J, Lane PJL, et al. Sites of specific B cell activation in primary and secondary responses to T cell-dependent and T cell-independent antigens. *Eur J Immunol* 1991;21:2951–2962.

38. Halper J, Fu S, Wang C, et al. Patterns of expression of IA-like antigens during the terminal stages of B cell development. *J Immunol* 1978;120:1480–1484.

39. MacLennan I. Germinal centers. *Annu Rev Immunol* 1994;12:117–139.

40. Liu Y-J, Oldfield S, MacLennan I. Memory B cells in T-cell dependent antibody responses colonise the splenic marginal zones. *Eur J Immunol* 1988;18:355–362.

41. Liu Y-J, Johnson G, Gordon J, MacLennan I. Germinal centres in T-cell-dependent antibody responses. *Immunol Today* 1992;13:1–39.

42. Cattoretti G, Chang CC, Cechova K, et al. BCL-6 protein is expressed in germinal-center B cells. *Blood* 1995;86:45–53.

43. Flenghi L, Bigerna B, Fizzotti M, et al. Monoclonal antibodies PG-B6a and PG-B6p recognize, respectively, a highly conserved and a formol-resistant epitope on the human BCL-6 protein amino-terminal region. *Am J Pathol* 1996;148:1543–1555.

44. French DL, Laskov R, Scharff MD. The role of somatic hypermutation in the generation of antibody diversity. *Science* 1989;244:1152.

45. Jacob J, Kelsoe G, Rajewsky K, Weiss U. Intraclonal generation of antibody mutants in germinal centres. *Nature* 1991;354:389.

46. Peng HZ, Du MQ, Koulis A, et al. Nonimmunoglobulin gene hypermutation in germinal center B cells. *Blood* 1999;93:2167–2172.

47. Pasqualucci L, Migliazza A, Fracchiolla N, et al. BCL-6 mutations in normal germinal center B cells: evidence of somatic hypermutation acting outside Ig loci. *Proc Natl Acad Sci U S A* 1998;95:11816–11821.

48. Shen HM, Peters A, Baron B, et al. Mutation of BCL-6 gene in normal B cells by the process of somatic hypermutation of Ig genes. *Science* 1998;280:1750–1752.

49. Liu Y-J, Joshua DE, Williams GT, et al. Mechanism of antigen-driven selection in germinal centres. *Nature* 1989;342:929–931.

50. Wabl M, Forni L, Loor F. Switch in immunoglobulin production observed in single clones of committed lymphocytes. *Science* 1978;199:1078–1079.

51. Allman D, Jain A, Dent A, et al. BCL-6 expression during B-cell activation. *Blood* 1996;87:5257–5268.

52. Berek C. The development of B cells and the B-cell repertoire in the microenvironment of the germinal centre. *Immunol Rev* 1992;126:5.

53. Pezzella F, Tse A, Cordell J, et al. Expression of the Bcl-2 oncogene protein is not specific for the 14-18 chromosomal translocation. *Am J Pathol* 1990;137:225–232.

54. Klein U, Klein G, Ehlin-Henriksson B, Rajewsky K, Kuppers R. Burkitt's lymphoma is a malignancy of mature B cells expressing somatically mutated V region genes. *Mol Med* 1995;1:495–505.

55. Van den Oord J, De Wolf-Peeters C, De Vos R, Desmet V. Immature sinus histiocytosis. Light- and electron-microscopic features, immunologic phenotype, and relationship with marginal zone lymphocytes. *Am J Pathol* 1985; 1985:266–277.

56. van Krieken J, von Schilling C, Kluin P, et al. Splenic marginal zone lymphocytes and related cells in the lymph node: a morphologic and immunohistochemical study. *Hum Pathol* 1989;20:320–325.

57. Smith-Ravin J, Spencer J, Beverley P, Isaacson P. Characterization of two monoclonal antibodies (UCL4D12 and UCL3D3) that discriminate between human mantle zone and marginal zone B cells. *Clin Exp Immunol* 1990; 82:181–187.

58. Spencer J, Finn T, Pulford K, et al. The human gut contains a novel population of B lymphocytes which resemble marginal zone cells. *Clin Exp Immunol* 1985;62:607–612.

59. Isaacson P, Spencer J. Malignant lymphoma of mucosa-associated lymphoid tissue. *Histopathol* 1987;11:445–462.

60. Dunn-Walters DK, Isaacson PG, Spencer J. Analysis of mutations in immunoglobulin heavy chain variable region genes of microdissected marginal zone (MGZ) B cells suggests that the MGZ of human spleen is a reservoir of memory B cells. *J Exp Med* 1995;182:559–566.

61. Dunn-Walters DK, Isaacson PG, Spencer J. Sequence analysis of rearranged IgVH genes from microdissected human Peyer's patch marginal zone B cells. *Immunology* 1996;88:618–624.

62. Tierens A, Delabie J, Michiels L, et al. Marginal-zone B cells in the human lymph node and spleen show somatic hypermutations and display clonal expansion. *Blood* 1999;93:226–234.

63. Klein U, Kuppers R, Rajewsky K. Evidence for a large compartment of IgM-expressing memory B cells in humans. *Blood* 1997;89:1288–1298.

64. Klein U, Goossens T, Fischer M, et al. Somatic hypermutation in normal and transformed human B cells. *Immunol Rev* 1998;162:261–280.

65. Cardoso de Almeida P, Harris N, Bhan A. Characterization of immature sinus histiocytes (monocytoid cells) in reactive lymph nodes by use of monoclonal antibodies. *Hum Pathol* 1984;15:330–335.

66. Stein K, Hummel M, Korbjuhn P, et al. Monocytoid B cells are distinct from splenic marginal zone cells and commonly derive from unmutated naive B cells and less frequently from postgerminal center B cells by polyclonal transformation. *Blood* 1999;94:2800–2808.

67. Nizze H, Cogliatti S, von Schilling C, et al. Monocytoid B-cell lymphoma: morphological variants and relationship to low-grade B-cell lymphoma of the mucosa-associated lymphoid tissue. *Histopathology* 1991;18:403–414.

68. Piris M, Rivas C, Morente M, et al. Monocytoid B-cell lymphoma, a tumour related to the marginal zone. *Histopathology* 1988;12:383–392.

69. Melo J, Hegde U, Parreira A, et al. Splenic B cell lymphoma with circulating villous lymphocytes: differential diagnosis of B cell leukaemias with large spleens. *J Clin Pathol* 1987;40:642–651.

70. Campo E, Miquel R, Krenacs L, et al. Primary nodal marginal zone lymphomas of splenic and MALT type. *Am J Surg Pathol* 1999;23:59–68.

71. Dunn-Walters DK, Boursier L, Spencer J, Isaacson PG. Analysis of immunoglobulin genes in splenic marginal zone lymphoma suggests ongoing mutation. *Hum Pathol* 1998;29:585–593.

72. Kuppers R, Hajadi M, Plank L, et al. Molecular Ig gene analysis reveals that monocytoid B cell lymphoma is a malignancy of mature B cells carrying somatically mutated V region genes and suggests that rearrangement of the kappa-deleting element (resulting in deletion of the Ig kappa enhancers) abolishes somatic hypermutation in the human. *Eur J Immunol* 1996;26:1794–1800.

73. Du M, Diss T, Xu C, et al. Somatic mutations and intraclonal variations in MALT lymphoma immunoglobulin genes. *Blood* 1995;86(Suppl):181a.

74. Spits H, Lanier L, Phillips J. Development of human T and natural killer cells. *Blood* 1995;85:2654–2670.

75. Bhan A, Reinherz E, Poppema S, et al. Location of T cell and major histocompatibility antigens in the human thymus. *J Exp Med* 1980;152:771–782.

76. Thomas M. The leukocyte common antigen family. *Ann Rev Immunol* 1989; 7:339–369.

77. Durie FH, Foy TM, Masters SR, et al. The role of CD40 in the regulation of humoral and cell-mediated immunity. *Immunol Today* 1994;15:406–410.

78. Engel P, Gribben J, Freeman G, et al. The B7-2 (B70) costimulatory molecule expressed by monocytes and activated B lymphocytes is the CD86 differentiation antigen. *Blood* 1994;84:1402–1407.

79. Gimmi C, Freeman J, Sugita K, et al. B7 provides a costimulatory signal which induces T cells to proliferate and secrete interleukin 2. *Proc Natl Acad Sci U S A* 1991;88:6575–6579.

80. Meurer S, Schlossman S, Reinherz E. Clonal analysis of human cytotoxic T lymphocytes: T4 and T8 effector T cells recognize products of different major histocompatibility regions. *Proc Natl Acad Sci U S A* 1982;79:4395–4399.

81. Inghirami G, Zhu B, Chess L, Knowles D. Flow cytometric and immunohistochemical characterization of the g/d T-lymphocyte population in normal human lymphoid tissue and peripheral blood. *Am J Pathol* 1990;136:357–367.

82. Knapp W, Dorken B, Rieber P, et al. *Leukocyte typing IV*. Oxford: Oxford University Press, 1989.

83. Croce C, Tsujimoto Y, Erikson J, Nowell P. Chromosome translocations and B cell neoplasia. *Lab Invest* 1984;51:258–267.

84. Yunis J, Mayer M, Arnesen M, et al. Bcl-2 and other genomic alterations in the prognosis of large-cell lymphoma. *N Engl J Med* 1989;320:1047–1054.

85. Tsujimoto Y, Yunis J, Onorato-Showe L, et al. Molecular cloning of the chromosomal breakpoint of B-cell lymphomas and leukemias with the t(11;14) chromosome translation. *Science* 1984;224:1406.

86. Tsujimoto T, Cossman J, Jaffe E, Croce C. Involvement of the bcl-2 gene in human follicular lymphoma. *Science* 1985;288:1440–1443.

87. McDonnell T, Deane N, Platt F, et al. Bcl-2-immunoglobulin transgenic mice demonstrate extended B cell survival and follicular lymphoproliferation. *Cell* 1989;57:79–88.

88. Rosenberg C, Wong E, Petty E, et al. Overexpression of PRAD1, a candidate BCL1 breakpoint region oncogene, in centrocytic lymphomas. *Proc Natl Acad Sci U S A* 1991;88:9638–9642.

89. Downing J, Shurtleff S, Zielenska M, et al. Molecular detection of the (2;5) translocation of non-Hodgkin's lymphoma by reverse transcriptase-polymerase chain reaction. *Blood* 1995;85:3416–3422.

90. Dierlamm J, Baens M, Wlodarska I, et al. The apoptosis inhibitor gene API2 and a novel 18q gene, MLT, are recurrently rearranged in the t(11;18)(q21;q21) associated with mucosa-associated lymphoid tissue lymphomas. *Blood* 1999;93:3601–3609.

91. Horsman DE, Gascoyne RD, Coupland RW, et al. Comparison of cytogenetic analysis, southern analysis, and polymerase chain reaction for the detection of t(14;18) in follicular lymphoma. *Am J Clin Pathol* 1995;103:472–478.

92. Wellmann A, Otsuki T, Vogelbruch M, et al. Analysis of the t(2;5)(p23;q35) translocation by reverse transcription-polymerase chain reaction in CD30+ anaplastic large-cell lymphomas, in other non-Hodgkin's lymphomas of T-cell phenotype, and in Hodgkin's disease. *Blood* 1995;86:2321–2378.

93. Lee M, Chang K, Cabanillas F, et al. Detection of minimal residual cells containing t(14;18) by DNA sequence amplification. *Science* 1987;237:175–178.

94. Ha CS, Cabanillas F, Lee MS, et al. Serial determination of the bcl-2 gene in the bone marrow and peripheral blood after central lymphatic irradiation for stages I-III follicular lymphoma: a preliminary report. *Clin Cancer Res* 1997;3:215–219.

95. Wotherspoon AC, Finn TM, Isaacson PG. Trisomy 3 in low-grade lymphomas of mucosa-associated lymphoid tissue. *Blood* 1995;85:2000–2004.

96. Matutes E, Oscier D, Garcia-Marco J, et al. Trisomy 12 defines a group of CLL with atypical morphology: correlation between cytogenetic, clinical and laboratory features in 544 patients. *Br J Haematol* 1996;92:382–388.

97. Siebert R, Matthiesen P, Harder S, et al. Application of interphase fluorescence in situ hybridization for the detection of the Burkitt translocation t(8;14)(q24;q32) in B-cell lymphomas. *Blood* 1998;91:984–990.

98. Ozdemirli M, Fanburg-smith J, Hartmann D-P, et al. Precursor B-lymphoblastic lymphoma presenting as a solitary bone tumor and mimicking Ewing's sarcoma. A report of four cases and review of the literature. *Am J Surg Pathol* 1998;22:795–804.

99. Nathwani BN, Diamond LW, Winberg CD, et al. Lymphoblastic lymphoma: a clinicopathologic study of 95 patients. *Cancer* 1981;48:2347–2357.

100. Sander C, Medeiros L, Abruzzo L, et al. Lymphoblastic lymphoma presenting in cutaneous sites: a clinicopathologic analysis of six cases. *J Am Acad Dermatol* 1991;25:1023–1031.

101. Soslow RA, Baergen RN, Warnke RA. B-lineage lymphoblastic lymphoma is a clinicopathologic entity distinct from other histologically similar aggressive lymphomas with blastic morphology. *Cancer* 1999;85:2648–2654.

102. Pui CH, Behm FG, Downing JR, et al. 11q23/MLL rearrangement confers a poor prognosis in infants with acute lymphoblastic leukemia. *J Clin Oncol* 1994;12:909–915.

103. Rubnitz JE, Downing JR. The role of TEL fusion genes in pediatric leukemias. *Leukemia* 1999;13:6–13.

104. Khalidi HS, Chang KL, Medeiros LJ, et al. Acute lymphoblastic leukemia. Survey of immunophenotype, French-American-British classification, frequency of myeloid antigen expression, and karyotypic abnormalities in 210 pediatric and adult cases. *Am J Clin Pathol* 1999;111:467–476.

105. Boucheix C, David B, Sebban C, et al. Immunophenotype of adult acute lymphoblastic leukemia, clinical parameters, and outcome: an analysis of a prospective trial including 562 tested patients (LALA87). French Group on Therapy for Adult Acute Lymphoblastic Leukemia. *Blood* 1994;84:1603–1612.

106. Uckun FM, Sather HN, Gaynon PS, et al. Clinical features and treatment outcome of children with myeloid antigen positive acute lymphoblastic leukemia: a report from the Children's Cancer Group. *Blood* 1997;90:28–35.

107. Pui CH, Rubnitz JE, Hancock ML, et al. Reappraisal of the clinical and biologic significance of myeloid-associated antigen expression in childhood acute lymphoblastic leukemia. *J Clin Oncol* 1998;16:3768–3773.

108. Kitchingman G, Robigatti U, Mauer A, et al. Rearrangement of immunoglobulin heavy chain genes in T cell acute lymphoblastic leukemia. *Blood* 1985; 65:725–729.

109. Tawa A, Hozumi N, Minden M, et al. Rearrangements of the T-cell receptor b chain gene in non-T-cell, non-B-cell acute lymphoblastic leukemia in childhood. *N Engl J Med* 1985;313:1033–1037.

110. Felix CA, Poplack DG, Reaman GH, et al. Characterization of immunoglobulin and T-cell receptor gene patterns in B-cell precursor acute lymphoblastic leukemia of childhood. *J Clin Oncol* 1990;8:431–442.

111. Uckun FM, Sensel MG, Sun L, et al. Biology and treatment of childhood T-lineage acute lymphoblastic leukemia. *Blood* 1998;91:735–746.

112. Bernard A, Boumsell L, Reinherz L, et al. Cell surface characterization of malignant T cells from lymphoblastic lymphoma using monoclonal antibodies: evidence for phenotypic differences between malignant T cells from patients with acute lymphoblastic leukemia and lymphoblastic lymphoma. *Blood* 1981;57:1105–1110.

113. Gouttefangeas C, Bensussan A, Boumsell L. Study of the CD3-associated T-cell receptors reveals further differences between T-cell acute lymphoblastic lymphoma and leukemia. *Blood* 1990;74:931–934.

114. Quintanilla L, Zukerberg LR, Harris NL. Pre-thymic adult lymphoblastic lymphoma. *Am J Surg Pathol* 1992;16:1075–1084.

115. Szczepanski T, Pongers-Willemse MJ, Langerak AW, et al. Ig heavy chain gene rearrangements in T-cell acute lymphoblastic leukemia exhibit predominant DH6-19 and DH7-27 gene usage, can result in complete V-D-J rearrangements, and are rare in T-cell receptor alpha beta lineage. *Blood* 1999; 93:4079–4085.

116. Begley CG, Green AR. The SCL gene: from case report to critical hematopoietic regulator. *Blood* 1999;93:2760–2770.

117. O'Brien A, del Giglio A, Keating M. Advances in the biology and treatment of B-cell chronic lymphocytic leukemia. *Blood* 1995;85:307–318.

118. Ben-Ezra J, Burke J, Swartz W, et al. Small lymphocytic lymphoma: a clinicopathologic analysis of 268 cases. *Blood* 1989;73:579–587.

119. Lennert K. *Malignant lymphomas other than Hodgkin's disease*. New York: Springer-Verlag, 1978.

120. Perry D, Bast M, Armitage J, Weisenburger D. Diffuse intermediate lymphocytic lymphoma: a clinicopathologic study and comparison with small lymphocytic lymphoma and diffuse small cleaved cell lymphoma. *Cancer* 1990; 66:1995–2000.

121. Bonato M, Pittaluga S, Tierens A, et al. Lymph node histology in typical and atypical chronic lymphocytic leukemia. *Am J Surg Pathol* 1998;22:49–56.

122. Oscier DG, Thompsett A, Zhu D, Stevenson FK. Differential rates of somatic hypermutation in V(H) genes among subsets of chronic lymphocytic leukemia defined by chromosomal abnormalities. *Blood* 1997;89:4153–4160.

123. Damle RN, Wasil T, Fais F, et al. Ig V gene mutation status and CD38 expression as novel prognostic indicators in chronic lymphocytic leukemia [see comments]. *Blood* 1999;94:1840–1847.

124. Aoki H, Takishita M, Kosaka M, Saito S. Frequent somatic mutations in D and/or Jh segments of Ig gene in Waldenstrom's macroglobulinemia and chronic lymphocytic leukemia (CLL) with Richter's syndrome but not in common CLL. *Blood* 1995;85:1913–1919.

125. Juliusson G, Oscier D, Fitchett M, et al. Prognostic subgroups in B-cell chronic lymphocytic leukemia defined by specific chromosomal abnormalities. *N Engl J Med* 1990;323:720–724.

126. Knuutila S, Elonen E, Teerenhovi L, et al. Trisomy 12 in B cells of patients with B-cell chronic lymphocytic leukemia. *N Engl J Med* 1986;314:865–869.

127. Oscier DG, Matutes E, Copplestone A, et al. Atypical lymphocyte morphology: an adverse prognostic factor for disease progression in stage A CLL independent of trisomy 12. *Br J Haematol* 1997;98:934–939.

128. Juliusson G, Merup M. Cytogenetics in chronic lymphocytic leukemia. *Semin Oncol* 1998;25:19–26.

129. Zhu Y, Monni O, El-Rifai W, et al. Discontinuous deletions at 11q23 in B cell chronic lymphocytic leukemia. *Leukemia* 1999;13:708–712.

130. Sembries S, Pahl H, Stilgenbauer S, et al. Reduced expression of adhesion molecules and cell signaling receptors by chronic lymphocytic leukemia cells with 11q deletion. *Blood* 1999;93:624–631.

131. Caligaris-Cappio F. B-chronic lymphocytic leukemia: a malignancy of anti-self B cells. *Blood* 1996;87:2615–2620.

132. Caligaris-Cappio F, Hamblin T. B-cell chronic lymphocytic leukemia: a bird of a different feather. *J Clin Oncol* 1999;17:399–408.

133. Klein U, Rajewsky K, Kuppers R. Human immunoglobulin (Ig)M+IgD+ peripheral blood B cells expressing the CD27 cell surface antigen carry somatically mutated variable region genes: CD27 as a general marker for somatically mutated (memory) B cells. *J Exp Med* 1998;188:1679–1689.

134. Melo J, Catovsky D, Galton D. The relationship between chronic lymphocytic leukaemia and prolymphocytic leukaemia. I. Clinical and laboratory features of 300 patients and characterization of an intermediate group. *Br J Haematol* 1985;63:377–387.

135. Bearman RM, Pangalis GA, Rappaport H. Prolymphocytic leukemia. Clinical, histopathological and cytochemical observations. *Cancer* 1978;42:2360–2372.

136. Galton D, Goldman J, Wiltshaw E, Catovsky D. Prolymphocytic leukaemia. *Br J Haematol* 1974;27:7–23.

137. Lampert I, Catovsky D, Marsh G, et al. The histopathology of prolymphocytic leukaemia with particular reference to the spleen: a comparison with chronic lymphocytic leukaemia. *Histopathology* 1980;4:3–19.

138. Lens D, Coignet LJ, Brito-Babapulle V, et al. B cell prolymphocytic leukaemia (B-PLL) with complex karyotype and concurrent abnormalities of the p53 and c-MYC gene. *Leukemia* 1999;13:873–876.

139. Sole F, Woessner S, Espinet B, et al. Cytogenetic abnormalities in three patients with B-cell prolymphocytic leukemia. *Cancer Genet Cytogenet* 1998; 103:43–45.

140. Dimopoulos MA, Alexanian R. Waldenstrom's macroglobulinemia. *Blood* 1994;83:1452–1459.

141. Agnello V, Chung RT, Kaplan LM. A role for hepatitis C virus infection in type II cryoglobulinemia [see comments]. *N Engl J Med* 1992;327:1490–1495.

142. Pozzato G, Mazzaro C, Crovatto M, et al. Low-grade malignant lymphoma, hepatitis C virus infection, and mixed cryoglobulinemia. *Blood* 1994;84:3047–3053.

143. Mazzaro C, Franzin F, Tulissi P, et al. Regression of monoclonal B-cell expansion in patients affected by mixed cryoglobulinemia responsive to alpha-interferon therapy. *Cancer* 1996;77:2604–2613.

144. Brittinger G, Bartels H, Common H, et al. Clinical and prognostic relevance of the Kiel classification of non-Hodgkin lymphomas: results of a prospective multicenter study by the Kiel lymphoma study group. *Hematol Oncol* 1984;2:269–306.

145. Engelhard M, Brittinger G, Heinz R, et al. Chronic lymphocytic leukemia (B-CLL) and immunocytoma (LP-IC): clinical and prognostic relevance of this distinction. *Leuk Lymphoma* 1991;Suppl:161–173.

146. Stein H, Lennert K, Feller A, Mason D. Immunohistological analysis of human lymphoma: correlation of histological and immunological categories. *Adv Cancer Res* 1984;42:67–147.

147. Harris N, Bhan A. B-cell neoplasms of the lymphocytic, lymphoplasmacytoid, and plasma cell types: immunohistologic analysis and clinical correlation. *Hum Pathol* 1985;16:829–837.

148. Lennert K, Tamm I, Wacker H-H. Histopathology and immunocytochemistry of lymph node biopsies in chronic lymphocytic leukemia and immunocytoma. *Leuk Lymphoma* 1991;Suppl:157–160.

149. Crouzier R, Martin T, Pasquali JL. Monoclonal IgM rheumatoid factor secreted by CD5-negative B cells during mixed cryoglobulinemia. Evidence for somatic mutations and intraclonal diversity of the expressed VH region gene. *J Immunol* 1995;154:413–421.

150. Sahota SS, Garand R, Bataille R, et al. VH gene analysis of clonally related IgM and IgG from human lymphoplasmacytoid B-cell tumors with chronic lymphocytic leukemia features and high serum monoclonal IgG. *Blood* 1998;91:238–243.

151. Wagner SD, Martinelli V, Luzzatto L. Similar patterns of Vk gene usage but different degrees of somatic mutation in hairy cell leukemia, prolymphocytic leukemia, Waldenstrom's macroglobulinemia, and myeloma. *Blood* 1994;83: 3647–3653.

152. Krenacs L, Himmelmann AW, Quintanilla-Martinez L, et al. Transcription factor B-cell-specific activator protein (BSAP) is differentially expressed in B cells and in subsets of B-cell lymphomas. *Blood* 1998;92:1308–1316.

153. Isaacson PG, Matutes E, Burke M, Catovsky D. The histopathology of splenic lymphoma with villous lymphocytes. *Blood* 1994;84:3828–3834.

154. Mollejo M, Menarguez J, Lloret E. Splenic marginal zone lymphoma: a distinctive type of low-grade B-cell lymphoma. A clinicopathologic study of 13 cases. *Am J Surg Pathol* 1995;19:1146–1157.

155. Pittaluga S, Verhoef G, Criel A, et al. "Small" B-cell non-Hodgkin's lymphomas with splenomegaly at presentation are either mantle cell lymphoma or marginal zone cell lymphoma. A study based on histology, cytology, immunohistochemistry, and cytogenetic analysis. *Am J Surg Pathol* 1996;20:211–223.

156. Arber DA, Rappaport H, Weiss LM. Non-Hodgkin's lymphoproliferative disorders involving the spleen. *Mod Pathol* 1997;10:18–32.

157. Schmid C, Kirkham N, Diss T, Isaacson P. Splenic marginal zone cell lymphoma. *Am J Surg Pathol* 1992;16:455–466.

158. Mollejo M, Lloret E, Menárguez J, et al. Lymph node involvement by splenic marginal zone lymphoma: morphological and immunohistochemical features. *Am J Surg Pathol* 1997;21:772–780.

159. Matutes E, Morilla R, Owusu-Ankomah K, et al. The immunophenotype of splenic lymphoma with villous lymphocytes and its relevance to the differential diagnosis with other B-cell disorders. *Blood* 1994;83:1558–1562.

160. Savilo E, Campo E, Mollejo M, et al. Absence of cyclin D1 protein expression in splenic marginal zone lymphoma. *Mod Pathol* 1998;11:601–606.

161. Zhu D, Oscier DG, Stevenson FK. Splenic lymphoma with villous lymphocytes involves B cells with extensively mutated Ig heavy chain variable region genes. *Blood* 1995;85:1603–1607.

162. Oscier DG, Matutes E, Gardiner A, et al. Cytogenetic studies in splenic lymphoma with villous lymphocytes. *Br J Haematol* 1993;85:487–491.

163. Jadayel D, Matutes E, Dyer MJS, et al. Splenic lymphoma with villous lymphocytes: analysis of bcl-1 rearrangements and expression of cyclin D1 gene. *Blood* 1994;83:3664–3671.

164. Finn T, Isaacson P, Wotherspoon A. Numerical abnormality of chromosomes 3, 7, 12, and 18 in low grade lymphomas of MALT-type and splenic marginal zone lymphomas detected by interphase cytogenetics on paraffin embedded tissue. *J Pathol* 1993;170:335A.

165. Brynes RK, Almaguer R, Leathery K, et al. Numerical cytogenetic abnormalities of chromosomes 3, 7, and 12 in marginal zone B-cell lymphomas. *Mod Pathol* 1996;9:995–1000.

166. Spiers A, Moore D, Cassileth P, et al. Remissions in hairy-cell leukemia with pentostatin (2'-deoxycoformycin). *N Engl J Med* 1987;316:825–830.

167. Piro L, Carrera C, Carson D, Beutler E. Lasting remissions in hairy cell leukemia induced by a single infusion of 2'-chlorodeoxyadenosine. *Cancer* 1990; 332:1117–1121.

168. Mason D, Cordell J, Tse A, et al. The IgM-associated protein mb-1 as a marker of normal and neoplastic B-cells. *J Immunol* 1991;147:2474–2482.

169. Moller P, Mielke B, Moldenhauer G. Monoclonal antibody HML-1, a marker for intraepithelial T cells and lymphomas derived thereof, also recognizes hairy cell leukemia and some B-cell lymphomas. *Am J Pathol* 1990;136:509–512.

170. Visser L, Shaw A, Slupsky J, et al. Monoclonal antibodies reactive with hairy cell leukemia. *Blood* 1989;74:320–325.

171. Moldenhauer G, Mielke B, Dorken B, et al. Identity of HML-1 antigen on intestinal intraepithelial T cells and of B-ly7 antigen on hairy cell leukaemia. *Scand J Immunol* 1990;32:77–82.

172. Flenghi L, Spinozzi F, Stein H, et al. LF61: a new monoclonal antibody directed against a trimeric molecule (150kD, 125kD, 105kD) associated with hairy cell leukaemia. *Br J Haematol* 1990;76:451–459.

173. Falini B, Pileri S, Flenghi L, et al. Selection of a panel of monoclonal antibodies for monitoring residual disease in peripheral blood and bone marrow of interferon-treated hairy cell leukemia patients. *Br J Haematol* 1990;76:460–468.

174. Hounieu H, Shashikant C, Saati T, et al. Hairy cell leukemia: diagnosis of bone marrow involvement in paraffin-embedded sections with monoclonal antibody DBA.44. *Am J Clin Pathol* 1992;28:26–33.

175. Korsmeyer S, Greene W, Cossman J. Rearrangement and expression of immunoglobulin genes and expression of Tac antigen in hairy cell leukemia. *Proc Natl Acad Sci U S A* 1983;80:4522–4528.

176. Zukerberg L, Ferry J, Conlon M, Harris N. Plasma cell myeloma with cleaved, multilobated, and monocytoid nuclei. *Am J Clin Pathol* 1990;93:657–661.

177. Zukerberg LR, Yang W-I, Arnold A, Harris NL. Cyclin D1 expression in non-Hodgkin's lymphomas: detection by immunohistochemistry. *Am J Clin Pathol* 1995;102:756–760.

178. Vasef MA, Medeiros LJ, Yospur LS, et al. Cyclin D1 protein in multiple myeloma and plasmacytoma: an immunohistochemical study using fixed, paraffin-embedded tissue sections. *Mod Pathol* 1997;10:927–932.

179. Sawyer J, Lukacs J, Munshi N, et al. Identification of new nonrandom translocation in multiple myeloma with multicolor spectral karyotyping. *Blood* 1998;92:4269–4278.

180. Radaszkiewicz T, Dragosics B, Bauer P. Gastrointestinal malignant lymphomas of the mucosa-associated lymphoid tissue: factors relevant to prognosis. *Gastroenterology* 1992;102:1628–1638.

181. Hyjek E, Isaacson P. Primary B cell lymphoma of the thyroid and its relationship to Hashimoto's thyroiditis. *Hum Pathol* 1988;19:1315–1326.

182. Hyjek E, Smith W, Isaacson P. Primary B cell lymphoma of salivary gland and its relationship to myoepithelial sialadenitis (MESA). *Hum Pathol* 1988;19:766–776.

183. Ferry J, White W, Grove A, Harris N. Malignant lymphoma of ocular adnexa: a spectrum of B-cell neoplasia including low grade B-cell lymphoma of MALT type. *Lab Invest* 1992;66:77A.

184. Cogliatti S, Schmid U, Schumacher U, et al. Primary B-cell gastric lymphoma: a clinicopathological study of 145 patients. *Gastroenterology* 1991;101:1159–1170.

185. Mattia A, Ferry J, Harris N. Breast lymphoma: a B-cell spectrum including the low grade B-cell lymphoma of mucosa associated lymphoid tissue. *Am J Surg Pathol* 1993;17:574–587.

186. Isaacson PG. Gastrointestinal lymphoma. *Hum Pathol* 1994;25:1020–1029.

187. Wotherspoon A, Doglioni C, Diss T, et al. Regression of primary low-grade B-cell gastric lymphoma of mucosa-associated lymphoid tissue type after eradication of Helicobacter pylori. *Lancet* 1993;342:575–577.

188. Pinotti G, Roggero E, Zucca E, et al. Primary low-grade gastric MALT lymphoma (Abstr). *Proc ASCO* 1995;14:393.

189. Liu H, Ruskon-Fourmestraux A, Lavergne-Slove A, et al. Resistance of t(11;18) positive gastric mucosa-associated lymphoid tissue lymphoma to Helicobacter pylori eradication therapy. *Lancet* 2001;357:39–40.

190. Li G, Hansmann M, Zwingers T, Lennert K. Primary lymphomas of the lung: morphological, immunohistochemical and clinical features. *Histopathology* 1990;16:519–531.
191. Fung CY, Grossbard ML, Linggood RM, et al. Mucosa-associated lymphoid tissue lymphoma of the stomach. Long term outcome after local treatment. *Cancer* 1999;85:9–17.
192. Fung C, Ferry J, Linggood R, et al. Extranodal marginal zone (MALT type) lymphoma of the ocular adnexae: a localized tumor with favorable outcome after radiation therapy. Proceedings of ASTRO 37th Annual Meeting. *Int J Radiat Oncol Phys* 1996;36:199.
193. Bailey EM, Ferry JA, Harris NL, et al. Marginal zone lymphoma (low-grade B-cell lymphoma of mucosa-associated lymphoid tissue type) of skin and subcutaneous tissue: a study of 15 patients [see comments]. *Am J Surg Pathol* 1996;20:1011–1023.
194. Zinzani PL, Magagnoli M, Ascani S, et al. Nongastrointestinal mucosa-associated lymphoid tissue (MALT) lymphomas: clinical and therapeutic features of 24 localized patients. *Ann Oncol* 1997;8:883–886.
195. Qin Y, Greiner A, Trunk MJF, et al. Somatic hypermutation in low-grade mucosa-associated lymphoid tissue-type B-cell lymphoma. *Blood* 1995;86:3528–3534.
196. Miklos J, Swerdlow S, Bahler D. Analysis of immunoglobulin VH genes used by low grade salivary gland lymphomas of the mucosa-associated lymphoid tissue (MALT) type. *Blood* 1995;86(Suppl):182a.
197. Pan L, Diss T, Cunningham D, Isaacson P. The bcl-2 gene in primary B-cell lymphomas of mucosa associated lymphoid tissue (MALT). *Am J Pathol* 1989;135:7–11.
198. Auer IA, Gascoyne RD, Connors JM, et al. t(11;18)(q21;q21) is the most common translocation in Malt lymphomas. *Ann Oncol* 1997;8:979–985.
199. Ott G, Katzenberger T, Greiner A, et al. The t(11;18)(q21;q21) chromosome translocation is a frequent and specific aberration in low-grade but not high-grade malignant non-Hodgkin's lymphomas of the mucosa-associated lymphoid tissue (MALT) type. *Cancer Res* 1997;57:3944–3948.
200. Barth TF, Dohner H, Werner CA, et al. Characteristic pattern of chromosomal gains and losses in primary large B-cell lymphomas of the gastrointestinal tract. *Blood* 1998;91:4321–4330.
201. Willis TG, Jadayel DM, Du MQ, et al. Bcl10 is involved in t(1;14)(p22;q32) of MALT B cell lymphoma and mutated in multiple tumor types [see comments]. *Cell* 1999;96:35–45.
202. Carbone A, Gloghini A, Pinto A, et al. Monocytoid B-cell lymphoma with bone marrow and peripheral blood involvement at presentation. *Am J Clin Pathol* 1989;92:228–236.
203. Glass A, Karnell L, Menck H. The National Cancer Data Base report on non-Hodgkin's lymphoma. *Cancer* 1997;80:2311–2320.
204. Bartlett NL, Rizeq M, Dorfman RF, et al. Follicular large-cell lymphoma: intermediate or low grade? *J Clin Oncol* 1994;12:1349–1357.
205. Kantarjian HM, McLaughlin P, Fuller LM, et al. Follicular large cell lymphoma: analysis and prognostic factors in 62 patients. *J Clin Oncol* 1984;2:811–819.
206. Mann R, Berard C. Criteria for the cytologic subclassification of follicular lymphomas: a proposed alternative method. *Hematol Oncol* 1982;1:187–192.
207. Weisenburger D, Anderson J, Armitage J, et al. Grading of follicular lymphoma: diagnostic accuracy, reproducibility, and clinical relevance. *Mod Pathol* 1998;11:142A.
208. Harris N, Nadler L, Bhan A. Immunohistologic characterization of two malignant lymphomas of germinal center type (centroblastic/centrocytic and centrocytic) with monoclonal antibodies: follicular and diffuse lymphomas of small cleaved cell types are related but distinct entities. *Am J Pathol* 1984;117:262–272.
209. Pittaluga S, Ayoubi TA, Wlodarska I, et al. BCL–6 expression in reactive lymphoid tissue and in B-cell non-Hodgkin's lymphomas. *J Pathol* 1996;179:145–150.
210. Cleary M, Mecker T, Levy S, et al. Clustering of extensive somatic mutations in the variable region of an immunoglobulin heavy chain gene from a human B cell lymphoma. *Cell* 1986;44:97–106.
211. Bahler D, Campbell M, Hart S, et al. Ig V(H) gene expression among human follicular lymphomas. *Blood* 1991;78:1561.
212. Fisher RI, Dahlberg S, Nathwani BN, et al. A clinical analysis of two indolent lymphoma entities: mantle cell lymphoma and marginal zone lymphoma (including the mucosa-associated lymphoid tissue and monocytoid B-cell subcategories): a Southwest Oncology Group study. *Blood* 1995;85:1075–1082.
213. Isaacson P, MacLennan K, Subbuswamy S. Multiple lymphomatous polyposis of the gastrointestinal tract. *Histopathology* 1984;8:641–656.
214. Meusers P, Engelhard M, Bartels H, et al. Multicentre randomized therapeutic trial for advanced centrocytic lymphoma: anthracycline does not improve the prognosis. *Hematol Oncol* 1989;7:365–380.
215. Berger F, Felman P, Sonet A, et al. Nonfollicular small B-cell lymphomas: a heterogeneous group of patients with distinct clinical features and outcome. *Blood* 1994;83:2829–2835.
216. Bosch F, Lopez-Guillermo A, Campo E, et al. Mantle cell lymphoma: presenting features, response to therapy, and prognostic factors. *Cancer* 1998;82:567–575.
217. Majlis A, Pugh WC, Rodriguez MA, et al. Mantle cell lymphoma: correlation of clinical outcome and biologic features with three histologic variants. *J Clin Oncol* 1997;15:1664–1671.
218. Stewart DA, Vose JM, Weisenburger DD, et al. The role of high-dose therapy and autologous hematopoietic stem cell transplantation for mantle cell lymphoma. *Ann Oncol* 1995;6:263–266.
219. Ketterer N, Salles G, Espinouse D, et al. Intensive therapy with peripheral stem cell transplantation in 16 patients with mantle cell lymphoma. *Ann Oncol* 1997;8:701–704.
220. Andersen NS, Donovan JW, Borus JS, et al. Failure of immunologic purging in mantle cell lymphoma assessed by polymerase chain reaction detection of minimal residual disease. *Blood* 1997;90:4212–4221.
221. Freedman AS, Neuberg D, Gribben JG, et al. High-dose chemoradiotherapy and anti-B-cell monoclonal antibody-purged autologous bone marrow transplantation in mantle-cell lymphoma: no evidence for long-term remission [see comments]. *J Clin Oncol* 1998;16:13–18.
222. Decaudin D, Bosq J, Tertian G, et al. Phase II trial of fludarabine monophosphate in patients with mantle-cell lymphomas. *J Clin Oncol* 1998;16:579–583.
223. Lardelli P, Bookman M, Sundeen J, et al. Lymphocytic lymphoma of intermediate differentiation. Morphologic and immunophenotypic spectrum and clinical correlations. *Am J Surg Pathol* 1990;14:752–763.
224. Ott M, Ott G, Kuse R, et al. The anaplastic variant of centrocytic lymphoma is marked by frequent rearrangements of the Bcl-1 gene and high proliferation indices. *Histopathol* 1994;24:329–334.
225. Banks P, Chan J, Cleary M, et al. Mantle cell lymphoma: a proposal for unification of morphologic, immunologic, and molecular data. *Am J Surg Pathol* 1992;16:637–640.
226. Dorfman DM, Pinkus GS. Distinction between small lymphocytic and mantle cell lymphoma by immunoreactivity for CD23. *Mod Pathol* 1994;7:326–331.
227. Kaptain S. CD5-negative mantle cell lymphoma. *Mod Pathol* 1998;11:133a.
228. Yang WI, Zukerberg LR, Motokura T, et al. Cyclin D1 (Bcl-1, PRAD1) protein expression in low-grade B-cell lymphomas and reactive hyperplasia. *Am J Pathol* 1994;145:86–96.
229. Vandenberghe E, De Wolf-Peeters C, Van den Oord J, et al. Translocation (11;14): a cytogenetic anomaly associated with B-cell lymphomas of non-follicle centre cell lineage. *J Pathol* 1991;163:13–18.
230. Swerdlow SH, Yang WI, Zukerberg LR, et al. Expression of cyclin D1 protein in centrocytic/mantle cell lymphomas with and without rearrangement of the BCL1/cyclin D1 gene. *Hum Pathol* 1995;26:999–1004.
231. de Boer CJ, Vaandrager JW, van Krieken JH, et al. Visualization of mono-allelic chromosomal aberrations 3' and 5' of the cyclin D1 gene in mantle cell lymphoma using DNA fiber fluorescence in situ hybridization. *Oncogene* 1997;15:1599–1603.
232. Quintanilla-Martinez L, Thieblemont C, Fend F, et al. Mantle cell lymphomas lack expresion of p27kip1, a cyclin-dependent kinase inhibitor. *Am J Pathol* 1998;153:175–182.
233. Greiner TC, Moynihan MJ, Chan WC, et al. p53 mutations in mantle cell lymphoma are associated with variant cytology and predict a poor prognosis. *Blood* 1996;87:4302–4310.
234. Ott G, Kalla J, Ott MM, et al. Blastoid variants of mantle cell lymphoma: frequent bcl-1 rearrangements at the major translocation cluster region and tetraploid chromosome clones. *Blood* 1997;89:1421–1429.
235. Dreyling MH, Bullinger L, Ott G, et al. Alterations of the cyclin D1/p16-pRB pathway in mantle cell lymphoma. *Cancer Res* 1997;57:4608–4614.
236. Fisher R, Gaynor E, Dahlberg S, et al. A phase III comparison of CHOP vs ProMACE-cytaBOM vs MACOP-B in patients with intermediate or high grade non-Hodgkin's lymphoma: results of SWOG-8576 (Inter group 0067), the national high priority lymphoma study. *N Engl J Med* 1993.
237. Engelhard M, Brittinger G, Huhn D, et al. Subclassification of diffuse large B-cell lymphomas according to the Kiel Classification: distinction of centro-blastic and immunoblastic lymphomas is a significant prognostic risk factor. *Blood* 1997;89:2291–2297.
238. Fisher D, Jacobson J, Ault K, Harris N. Diffuse large cell lymphoma with discordant bone marrow histology: clinical features and biologic implications. *Cancer* 1989;64:1879–1887.
239. Doggett R, Wood G, Horning S, et al. The immunologic characterization of 95 nodal and extranodal diffuse large cell lymphomas in 89 patients. *Am J Pathol* 1984;115:245–252.
240. Gascoyne RD, Adomat SA, Krajewski S, et al. Prognostic significance of Bcl-2 protein expression and Bcl-2 gene rearrangement in diffuse aggressive non-Hodgkin's lymphoma. *Blood* 1997;90:244–251.
241. Kramer MH, Hermans J, Parker J, et al. Clinical significance of bcl2 and p53 protein expression in diffuse large B-cell lymphoma: a population-based study. *J Clin Oncol* 1996;14:2131–2138.
242. Sanchez E, Chacon I, Plaza MM, et al. Clinical outcome in diffuse large B-cell lymphoma is dependent on the relationship between different cell-cycle regulator proteins. *J Clin Oncol* 1998;16:1931–1939.
243. Skinnider B, Horsman D, Dupuis B, Gascoyne R. Bcl-6 and Bcl-2 protein expression in diffuse large B-cell lymphoma and follicular lymphoma: correlation with 3q27 and 18q21 chromosomal abnormalities. *Hum Pathol* 1999;30:803–808.
244. de Leval L, Shipp M, Neuberger D, et al. Diffuse large B-cell lymphomas are tumors of germinal center origin. *Blood* (in press).
245. Kuppers R, Rajewsky K, Hansmann ML. Diffuse large cell lymphomas are derived from mature B cells carrying V region genes with a high load of somatic mutation and evidence of selection for antibody expression. *Eur J Immunol* 1997;27:1398–1405.
246. Kramer M, Hermans J, Wijburg E, et al. Clinical relevance of BCL2, BCL6 and MYC rearrangements in diffuse large B-cell lymphoma. *Blood* 1998;92:3152–3162.
247. Bastard C, Deweindt C, Kerckaert JP, et al. LAZ3 rearrangements in non-Hodgkin's lymphoma: correlation with histology, immunophenotype, karyotype, and clinical outcome in 217 patients. *Blood* 1994;83:2423–2427.

248. Migliazza A, Martinotti S, Chen W, et al. Frequent somatic hypermutation of the 5' noncoding region of the BCL6 gene in B cell lymphoma. *Proc Natl Acad Sci U S A* 1995;91:12520–12524.

249. Vitolo U, Gaidano G, Botto B, et al. Rearrangements of bcl-6, bcl-2, c-myc and 6q deletion in B-diffuse large-cell lymphoma: clinical relevance in 71 patients. *Ann Oncol* 1998;9:55–61.

250. Jacobson J, Aisenberg A, Lamarre L, et al. Mediastinal large cell lymphoma: an uncommon subset of adult lymphoma curable with combined modality therapy. *Cancer* 1988;62:1893–1898.

251. Lazzarino M, Orlandi E, Paulli M, et al. Treatment outcome and prognostic factors for primary mediastinal (thymic) B-cell lymphoma: a multicenter study of 106 patients. *J Clin Oncol* 1997;15:1646–1653.

252. Addis B, Isaacson P. Large cell lymphoma of the mediastinum: a B-cell tumor of probable thymic origin. *Histopathology* 1986;10:379–390.

253. Lamarre L, Jacobson JO, Aisenberg AC, Harris NL. Primary large cell lymphoma of the mediastinum. A histologic and immunophenotypic study of 29 cases. *Am J Surg Pathol* 1989;13:730–739.

254. de Leval L, Ferry J, Shipp M, Harris NL. Expression of bcl-6 in primary mediastinal diffuse large B-cell lymphoma: evidence for derivation from germinal center B cells? *Mod Pathol* 2000;13:146A.

255. Moller P, Moldenhauer G, Momburg F, et al. Mediastinal lymphoma of clear cell type is a tumor corresponding to terminal steps of B cell differentiation. *Blood* 1987;69:1087–1095.

256. Scarpa A, Bonetti F, Menestrina F. Mediastinal large cell lymphoma with sclerosis. Genotypic analysis establishes its B nature. *Virchows Arch* 1987;412:17–21.

257. Tsang P, Cesarman E, Chadburn A, et al. Molecular characterization of primary mediastinal B cell lymphoma. *Am J Pathol* 1996;148:2017–2025.

258. Joos S, Otano-Joos MI, Ziegler S, et al. Primary mediastinal (thymic) B-cell lymphoma is characterized by gains of chromosomal material including 9p and amplification of the REL gene. *Blood* 1996;87:1571–1578.

259. Ferry J, Harris N, Picker L, et al. Intravascular lymphomatosis (malignant angioendotheliomatosis): a B-cell neoplasm expressing surface homing receptors. *Mod Pathol* 1988;1:444–452.

260. DiGiuseppe J, Nelson W, Seifter E, et al. Intravascular lymphomatosis: a clinicopathologic study of 10 cases and assessment of response to chemotherapy. *J Clin Oncol* 1994;12:2573–2579.

261. Delabie J, Vandenberghe E, Kennes C, et al. Histiocyte-rich B-cell lymphoma. A distinct clinicopathologic entity possibly related to lymphocyte predominant Hodgkin's disease, paragranuloma subtype. *Am J Surg Pathol* 1992;16:37–48.

262. McBride JA, Rodriguez J, Luthra R, et al. T-cell-rich B large-cell lymphoma simulating lymphocyte-rich Hodgkin's disease [see comments]. *Am J Surg Pathol* 1996;20:193–201.

263. Guinee D, Kingma D, Fishback N, et al. Pulmonary lymphomatoid granulomatosis. Evidence for a proliferation of EBV infected B lymphocytes with a prominent T-cell component and vasculitis. *Am J Surg Pathol* 1994;18:753–764.

264. Haque AK, Myers JL, Hudnall SD, et al. Pulmonary lymphomatoid granulomatosis in acquired immunodeficiency syndrome: lesions with Epstein-Barr virus infection. *Mod Pathol* 1998;11:347–356.

265. Katzenstein A-L, Peiper S. Detection Epstein-Barr genomes in lymphomatoid granulomatosis: analysis of 29 cases by the polymerase chain reaction. *Mod Pathol* 1990;3:435.

266. Myers JL, Kurtin P, Katzenstein A, et al. Lymphomatoid granulomatosis. Evidence of immunophenotypic diversity and relationship to Epstein-Barr virus infection. *Am J Surg Pathol* 1995;19:1300–1312.

267. Wilson WH, Kingma DW, Raffeld M, et al. Association of lymphomatoid granulomatosis with Epstein-Barr viral infection of B lymphocytes and response to interferon-alpha 2b. *Blood* 1996;87:4531–4537.

268. Otsuki T, Kumar S, Ensoli B, et al. Detection of HHV-8/KSHV DNA sequences in AIDS-associated extranodal lymphoid malignancies. *Leukemia* 1996;10:1358–1362.

269. Carbone A, Gaidano G, Gloghini A, et al. Differential expression of BCL-6, CD138/syndecan-1, and Epstein-Barr virus-encoded latent membrane protein-1 identifies distinct histogenetic subsets of acquired immunodeficiency syndrome-related non-Hodgkin's lymphomas. *Blood* 1998;91:747–755.

270. Nador RG, Cesarman E, Chadburn A, et al. Primary effusion lymphoma: a distinct clinicopathologic entity associated with the Kaposi's sarcoma-associated herpes virus. *Blood* 1996;88:645–656.

271. Wright DH. What is Burkitt's lymphoma? [editorial]. *J Pathol* 1997;182:125–127.

272. Magrath I, Shiramizu B. Biology and treatment of small non-cleaved cell lymphoma. *Oncology* 1989;3:41–53.

273. Grogan T, Warnke R, Kaplan H. A comparative study of Burkitt's and non-Burkitt's "undifferentiated" malignant lymphoma: immunologic, cytochemical, ultrastructural, cytologic, histopathologic, clinical and cell culture features. *Cancer* 1982;49:1817–1828.

274. Yano T, van Krieken J, Magrath I, et al. Histogenetic correlations between subcategories of small noncleaved cell lymphomas. *Blood* 1992;79:1282–1290.

275. Sweetenham JW, Pearce R, Taghipour G, et al. Adult Burkitt's and Burkitt-like non-Hodgkin's lymphoma—outcome for patients treated with high-dose therapy and autologous stem-cell transplantation in first remission or at relapse: results from the European Group for Blood and Marrow Transplantation. *J Clin Oncol* 1996;14:2465–2472.

276. Garcia C, Weiss L, Warnke R. Small noncleaved cell lymphoma: an immunophenotypic study of 18 cases and comparison with large cell lymphoma. *Hum Pathol* 1986;17:454–461.

277. Falini B, Fizzotti M, Pileri S, et al. Bcl-6 protein expression in normal and neoplastic lymphoid tissues. *Ann Oncol* 1997;8(Suppl 2):101–104.

278. Carroll WL, Yu M, Link MP, Korsmeyer SJ. Absence of Ig V region gene somatic hypermutation in advanced Burkitt's lymphoma. *J Immunol* 1989;143:692.

279. Chapman C, Mockridge C, Rowe M, et al. Analysis of VH genes used by neoplastic B cells in endemic Burkitt's lymphoma shows somatic hypermutation and intraclonal heterogeneity. *Blood* 1995;85:2176–2181.

280. Chapman CJ, Zhou JX, Gregory C, et al. VH and VL gene analysis in sporadic Burkitt's lymphoma shows somatic hypermutation, intraclonal heterogeneity, and a role for antigen selection. *Blood* 1996;88:3562–3568.

281. Neri A, Barriga F, Knowles D, et al. Different regions of the immunoglobulin heavy-chain locus are involved in chromosomal translocations in distinct pathogenetic forms of Burkitt lymphoma. *Proc Natl Acad Sci U S A* 1988;85:2748–2752.

282. Pelicci P, Knowles D, Magrath I, Dalla-Favera R. Chromosomal breakpoints and structural alterations of the c-myc locus differ in endemic and sporadic forms of Burkitt lymphoma. *Proc Natl Acad Sci U S A* 1986;83:2984–2988.

283. Capello D, Carbone A, Pastore C, et al. Point mutations of the BCL-6 gene in Burkitt's lymphoma. *Br J Haematol* 1997;99:168–170.

284. Hamilton-Dutoit S, Pallesen G, Franzmann M, et al. AIDS-related lymphoma. Histopathology, immunophenotype, and association with Epstein-Barr virus as demonstrated by in situ nucleic acid hybridization. *Am J Pathol* 1991;138:149–163.

285. Matutes E, Brito-Babapulle V, Swansbury J, et al. Clinical and laboratory features of 78 cases of T-prolymphocytic leukemia. *Blood* 1991;78:3269–3274.

286. Brouet J, Sasportes M, Flandrin G, et al. Chronic lymphocytic leukemia of T cell origin. *Lancet* 1975;ii:890–893.

287. Bennett J, Catovsky D, Daniel M-T, et al. Proposals for the classification of chronic (mature) B and T lymphoid leukemias. *J Clin Pathol* 1989;42:567–584.

288. Suchi T, Lennert K, Tu L-Y. Histopathology and immunohistochemistry of peripheral T-cell lymphomas: a proposal for their classification. *J Clin Pathol* 1987;40:995–1015.

289. Knowles D. The human T-cell leukemias: clinical, cytomorphologic, immunophenotypic, and genotypic characteristics. *Hum Pathol* 1986;17:14–33.

290. Sood R, Stewart CC, Aplan PD, et al. Neutropenia associated with T-cell large granular lymphocyte leukemia: long-term response to cyclosporine therapy despite persistence of abnormal cells. *Blood* 1998;91:3372–3378.

291. Loughran T. Clonal diseases of large granular lymphocytes. *Blood* 1993;82:1–14.

292. Gentile TC, Hadlock KG, Uner AH, et al. Large granular lymphocyte leukaemia occurring after renal transplantation. *Br J Haematol* 1998;101:507–512.

293. Gelb AB, van de Rijn M, Regula DP Jr, et al. Epstein-Barr virus-associated natural killer-large granular lymphocyte leukemia. *Hum Pathol* 1994;25:953–960.

294. Agnarsson B, Loughran T, Starkebaum G, Kadin M. The pathology of large granular lymphocyte leukemia. *Hum Pathol* 1989;20:643–651.

295. Imamura N, Kusunoki Y, Kawa-Ha K, et al. Aggressive natural killer cell leukaemia/lymphoma: report of four cases and review of the literature. Possible existence of a new clinical entity originating from the third lineage of lymphoid cells. *Br J Haematol* 1990;76:49–59.

296. Kwong Y, Chan A, Liang R. Natural killer cell lymphoma/leukemia: pathology and treatment. *Hematol Oncol* 1997;15:71–79.

297. Soler J, Bordes R, Ortuni F, et al. Aggressive natural killer cell leukaemia/lymphoma in two patients with lethal midline granuloma. *Br J Haematol* 1994;86:659–662.

298. Gentile TC, Uner AH, Hutchison RE, et al. CD3+, CD56+ aggressive variant of large granular lymphocyte leukemia [see comments]. *Blood* 1994;84:2315–2321.

299. Uchiyama T, Yodoi J, Sagawa K, et al. Adult T-cell leukemia: clinical and hematologic features of 16 cases. *Blood* 1977;50:481–492.

300. Yamada Y. Phenotypic and functional analysis of leukemic cells from 16 patients with adult T cell leukemia/lymphoma. *Blood* 1983;61:192–199.

301. Chadburn A, Athan E, Wieczorek R, Knowles D. Detection and characterization of HTLV-I associated T neoplasms in an HTLV-I non-endemic region by polymerase chain reaction. *Blood* 1991;70:1500–1508.

302. Kikuchi M, Mitsui T, Takeshita M, et al. Virus associated adult T-cell leukemia (ATL) in Japan: clinical, histological and immunological studies. *Hematol Oncol* 1987;4:67.

303. Swerdlow S, Habeshaw J, Rohatiner A, et al. Caribbean T-cell lymphoma/leukemia. *Cancer* 1984;54:687–696.

304. Groopman J, Ferry J. Case record of the Massachusetts General Hospital: Case 36-1989. *N Engl J Med* 1989;321:663–675.

305. Abrams M, Sidawy M, Novich M. Smoldering HTLV-associated T-cell leukemia. *Arch Intern Med* 1985;145:2257–2258.

306. Duggan D, Ehrlich G, Davey F, et al. HTLV-I induced lymphoma mimicking Hodgkin's disease. Diagnosis by polymerase chain reaction amplification of specific HTLV-I sequences in tumor DNA. *Blood* 1988;71:1027–1032.

307. Jaffe E, Blattner W, Blayney D, et al. The pathologic spectrum of adult T-cell leukemia/lymphoma in the United States. *Am J Surg Pathol* 1984;8:263–275.

308. Poiesz B, Ruscetti F, Gazdar A. Detection and isolation of type C retrovirus particles from fresh and cultured lymphocytes of a patient with cutaneous T-cell lymphoma. *Proc Natl Acad Sci U S A* 1980;77:7415–7419.

309. Chan J, Ng C, Lau W, Ho S. Most nasal/nasopharyngeal lymphomas are peripheral T cell neoplasms. *Am J Surg Pathol* 1987;11:418–429.

310. Ho F, Srivastava G, Loke S, et al. Presence of Epstein-Barr virus DNA in nasal lymphomas of B and T cell type. *Hematol Oncol* 1990;8:271–281.

311. Ferry J, Sklar J, Zukerberg L, Harris N. Nasal lymphoma: a clinicopathologic study with immunophenotypic and genotypic analysis. *Am J Surg Pathol* 1991;15:268–279.

312. Lipford E, Margolich J, Longo D, et al. Angiocentric immunoproliferative lesions: a clinicopathologic spectrum of post-thymic T cell proliferations. *Blood* 1988;5:1674–1681.

313. Chan JKC, Sin VC, Wong KF, et al. Nonnasal lymphoma expressing the natural killer cell marker CD56: a clinicopathologic study of 49 cases of an uncommon aggressive neoplasm. *Blood* 1997;89:4501–4513.

314. Cuadra-Garcia I, Harris N, Proulx G, et al. Sinonasal lymphoma: an analysis of 57 cases. *Mod Pathol* 1999;12.

315. Cuadra-Garcia I, Proulx G, Wu C, et al. Sinonasal lymphoma: a clinicopathologic analysis of 58 cases. *Am J Surg Pathol* 1999;23(11):1356–1369.

316. Jaffe E, Chan J, Su I, et al. Report of the workshop on nasal and related extranodal angiocentric T/NK cell lymphomas: definitions, differential diagnosis, and epidemiology. *Am J Surg Pathol* 1996;20:103–111.

317. Ho F, Choy D, Loke S, et al. Polymorphic reticulosis and conventional lymphomas of the nose and upper aerodigestive tract—a clinicopathologic study of 70 cases, and immunophenotypic studies of 16 cases. *Hum Pathol* 1990; 21:1041–1050.

318. Elenitoba-Johnson KS, Zarate-Osorno A, Meneses A, et al. Cytotoxic granular protein expression, Epstein-Barr virus strain type, and latent membrane protein-1 oncogene deletions in nasal T-lymphocyte/natural killer cell lymphomas from Mexico [In Process Citation]. *Mod Pathol* 1998;11:754–761.

319. Chan JK, Yip TT, Tsang WY, et al. Detection of Epstein-Barr viral RNA in malignant lymphomas of the upper aerodigestive tract [published erratum appears in *Am J Surg Pathol* 1994 Dec;18(12):1274]. *Am J Surg Pathol* 1994;18:938–946.

320. Isaacson P, Spencer J, Connolly C, et al. Malignant histiocytosis of the intestine: a T-cell lymphoma. *Lancet* 1985;ii:688–691.

321. Howell WM, Leung ST, Jones DB, et al. HLA-DRB, -DQA, and -DQB polymorphism in celiac disease and enteropathy-associated T-cell lymphoma. Common features and additional risk factors for malignancy. *Hum Immunol* 1995;43:29–37.

322. Collin P, Reunala T, Pukkala E, et al. Coeliac disease—associated disorders and survival [see comments]. *Gut* 1994;35:1215–1218.

323. Egan LJ, Stevens FM, McCarthy CF. Celiac disease and T-cell lymphoma [letter; comment]. *N Engl J Med* 1996;335:1611–1612.

324. Case records of the Massachusetts General Hospital. Weekly clinicopathological exercises. Case 15-1996. A 79-year-old woman with anorexia, weight loss, and diarrhea after treatment for celiac disease [clinical conference] [see comments]. *N Engl J Med* 1996;334:1316–1322.

325. Mantovani G, Esu S, Astara G, et al. Primary T cell CD30-positive anaplastic large-cell lymphoma associated with adult-onset celiac disease and presenting with skin lesions. *Acta Haematol* 1995;94:48–51.

326. Shiboski CH, Greenspan D, Dodd CL, Daniels TE. Oral T-cell lymphoma associated with celiac sprue. A case report. *Oral Surg Oral Med Oral Pathol* 1993;76:54–58.

327. Chott A, Dragosics B, Radaszkiewicz T. Peripheral T-cell lymphomas of the intestine. *Am J Pathol* 1992;141:1361–1371.

328. Ashton-Key M, Diss TC, Pan L, et al. Molecular analysis of T-cell clonality in ulcerative jejunitis and enteropathy-associated T-cell lymphoma. *Am J Pathol* 1997;151:493–498.

329. Murray A, Cuevas EC, Jones DB, Wright DH. Study of the immunohistochemistry and T cell clonality of enteropathy-associated T cell lymphoma. *Am J Pathol* 1995;146:509–519.

330. Carbonnel F, Grollet-Bioul L, Brouet JC, et al. Are complicated forms of celiac disease cryptic T-cell lymphomas? *Blood* 1998;92:3879–3886.

331. Spencer J, Cerf-Bensussan N, Jarry A, et al. Enteropathy-associated T-cell lymphoma is recognized by a monoclonal antibody (HML-1) that defines a membrane molecule on human mucosal lymphocytes. *Am J Pathol* 1988; 132:1–5.

332. Daum S, Foss HD, Anagnostopoulos I, et al. Expression of cytotoxic molecules in intestinal T-cell lymphomas. The German Study Group on Intestinal Non-Hodgkin Lymphoma. *J Pathol* 1997;182:311–317.

333. de Bruin PC, Connolly CE, Oudejans JJ, et al. Enteropathy-associated T-cell lymphomas have a cytotoxic T-cell phenotype [published erratum appears in Histopathology 1997 Dec;31(6):578]. *Histopathology* 1997;31:313–317.

334. Wong KF, Chan JK, Matutes E. Hepatosplenic gamma delta T-cell lymphoma: a distinctive aggressive lymphoma type. *Am J Surg Pathol* 1995;19:718–726.

335. Cooke C, Greiner T, Raffeld M, et al. Gamma delta T-cell lymphoma: a distinct clinicopathologic entity. *Mod Pathol* 1994;7:106A.

336. Ross CW, Schnitzer B, Scheldon S, et al. Gamma/delta T-cell posttransplantation lymphoproliferative disorder primarily in the spleen. *Am J Clin Pathol* 1994;102:310–315.

337. François A, Lesesve J-F, Stamatoullas A, et al. Hepatosplenic gamma/delta T-cell lymphoma: a report of two cases in immunocompromised patients, associated with isochromosome 7q. *Am J Surg Pathol* 1997;21:781–790.

338. Farcet J, Gaulard P, Marolleau J, et al. Hepatosplenic T-cell lymphoma: sinusal/sinusoidal localization af malignant cells expressing the T-cell receptor gamma delta. *Blood* 1990;75:2213–2219.

339. Arnulf B, Copie-Bergman C, Delfau-Larue MH, et al. Nonhepatosplenic gammadelta T-cell lymphoma: a subset of cytotoxic lymphomas with mucosal or skin localization. *Blood* 1998;91:1723–1731.

340. Takimoto Y, Imanaka F, Sasaki N, et al. Gamma/delta T cell lymphoma presenting in the subcutaneous tissue and small intestine in a patient with capillary leak syndrome. *Int J Hematol* 1998;68:183–191.

341. Gaulard P, Bourquelot P, Kanavaros P, et al. Expression of the alpha/beta and gamma/delta T-cell receptors in 57 cases of peripheral T-cell lymphomas. Identification of a subset of gamma/delta T-cell lymphomas. *Am J Pathol* 1990;137:617–628.

342. Boulland ML, Kanavaros P, Wechsler J, et al. Cytotoxic protein expression in natural killer cell lymphomas and in alpha beta and gamma delta peripheral T-cell lymphomas. *J Pathol* 1997;183:432–439.

343. Salhany KE, Feldman M, Kahn MJ, et al. Hepatosplenic gammadelta T-cell lymphoma: ultrastructural, immunophenotypic, and functional evidence for cytotoxic T lymphocyte differentiation. *Hum Pathol* 1997;28:674–685.

344. Cooke CB, Krenacs L, Stetler-Stevenson M, et al. Hepatosplenic T-cell lymphoma: a distinct clinicopathologic entity of cytotoxic gamma delta T-cell origin [see comments]. *Blood* 1996;88:4265–4274.

345. Wang CC, Tien HF, Lin MT, et al. Consistent presence of isochromosome 7q in hepatosplenic T gamma/delta lymphoma: a new cytogenetic-clinicopathologic entity. *Genes Chromosomes Cancer* 1995;12:161–164.

346. Jonveaux P, Daniel MT, Martel V, et al. Isochromosome 7q and trisomy 8 are consistent primary, non-random chromosomal abnormalities associated with hepatosplenic T gamma/delta lymphoma. *Leukemia* 1996;10:1453–1455.

347. Gonzalez C, Medeiros L, Braziel R, Jaffe E. T-cell lymphoma involving subcutaneous tissue: a clinicopathologic entity commonly associated with hemophagocytic syndrome. *Am J Surg Pathol* 1991;15:17–27.

348. Salhany KE, Macon WR, Choi JK, et al. Subcutaneous panniculitis-like T-cell lymphoma: clinicopathologic, immunophenotypic, and genotypic analysis of alpha/beta and gamma/delta subtypes. *Am J Surg Pathol* 1998;22:881–893.

349. Kumar S, Krenacs L, Medeiros J, et al. Subcutaneous panniculitic T-cell lymphoma is a tumor of cytotoxic T lymphocytes. *Hum Pathol* 1998;29:397–403.

350. Lutzner M, Edelson R, Schein P, et al. Cutaneous T-cell lymphomas: the Sezary syndrome, mycosis fungoides, and related disorders. *Ann Intern Med* 1975;83:534–552.

351. Ralfkiaer E, Wantzin G, Mason D, et al. Phenotypic characterization of lymphocyte subsets in mycosis fungoides. *Am J Clin Pathol* 1985;84:610–619.

352. Aisenberg A, Krontiris T, Mak T, Wilkes B. The gene for the beta chain of the T-cell receptor is rearranged in mycosis fungoides and dermatopathic lymphadenopathy. *N Engl J Med* 1985;313:529–533.

353. de Bruin P, Beljaards R, van Heerde P, et al. Differences in clinical behaviour and immunophenotype between primary cutaneous and primary nodal anaplastic large cell lymphoma of T-cell or null cell phenotype. *Histopathology* 1993;23:127–135.

354. Kaudewitz P, Stein H, Dallenbach F, et al. Primary and secondary cutaneous Ki-1+ (CD30+) anaplastic large cell lymphomas: morphologic, immunohistologic, and clinical characteristics. *Am J Pathol* 1989;135:359–367.

355. Pittaluga S, Wiodarska I, Pulford K, et al. The monoclonal antibody ALK1 identifies a distinct morphological subtype of anaplastic large cell lymphoma associated with 2p23/ALK rearrangements. *Am J Pathol* 1997;151:343–351.

356. Pulford K, Lamant L, Morris S, et al. Detection of anaplastic lymphoma kinase (ALK) and nucleolar protein nucleophosmin (NPM)-ALD proteins in normal and neoplastic cells with the monoclonal antibody ALK1. *Blood* 1997;89:1394–1404.

357. Ott G, Katzenberger T, Siebert R, et al. Chromosomal abnormalities in nodal and extranodal CD30+ anaplastic large cell lymphomas: infrequent detection of the t(2;5) in extranodal lymphomas. *Genes Chromosomes Cancer* 1998;22:114–121.

358. Falini B, Pileri S, De Solas I, et al. Peripheral T-cell lymphoma associated with hemophagocytic syndrome. *Blood* 1990;75:434–444.

359. Weisenburger D, Linder J, Armitage J. Peripheral T cell lymphoma. A clinicopathologic study of 42 cases. *Hematol Oncol* 1987;5:175–187.

360. Armitage J, Greer J, Levine A, et al. Peripheral T-cell lymphoma. *Cancer* 1989;63:158–163.

361. Lippman S, Miller T, Spier C, et al. The prognostic significance of the immunotype in diffuse large-cell lymphoma: a comparative study of the T-cell and B-cell phenotype. *Blood* 1988;72:436–441.

362. Coiffier B, Brousse N, Peuchmaur M, et al. Peripheral T-cell lymphomas have a worse prognosis than B-cell lymphomas: a prospective study of 361 immunophenotyped patients treated with the LNH-84 regimen. *Ann Oncol* 1990;1:45–50.

363. Weiss L, Crabtree G, Rouse R, Warnke R. Morphologic and immunologic characterization of 50 peripheral T-cell lymphomas. *Am J Pathol* 1985;118:316–324.

364. Medeiros L, Lardelli P, Stetler-Stevenson M, et al. Genotypic analysis of diffuse, mixed cell lymphomas: comparison with morphologic and immunophenotypic findings. *Am J Clin Pathol* 1991;95:547.

365. Patsouris E, Noel H, Lennert K. Histological and immunohistological findings in lymphoepithelioid cell lymphoma (Lennert's lymphoma). *Am J Surg Pathol* 1988;12:341–350.

366. Chott A, Augustin I, Wra F, et al. Peripheral T-cell lymphomas: a clinicopathologic study of 75 cases. *Hum Pathol* 1990;21:1117–1125.

367. Lennert K, Feller A. *Histopathology of non-Hodgkin's lymphomas*. New York: Springer-Verlag, 1992.

368. Hastrup N, Hamilton-Dutoit S, Ralfkiaer E, Pallesen G. Peripheral T-cell lymphomas: an evaluation of reproducibility of the updated Kiel classification. *Histopathology* 1991;18:99–105.

369. Borowitz M, Reichert T, Brynes R, et al. The phenotypic diversity of peripheral T-cell lymphomas. The Southeastern Cancer Study Group experience. *Hum Pathol* 1986;17:567.

370. Weiss L, Trela M, Cleary M, et al. Frequent immunoglobulin and T cell receptor gene rearrangement in "histiocytic" neoplasms. *Am J Pathol* 1985;121:369–373.

371. Weiss L, Picker L, Grogan T, et al. Absence of clonal beta and gamma T-cell receptor gene rearrangements in a subset of peripheral T-cell lymphomas. *Am J Pathol* 1988;130:436–443.

372. Frizzera G, Moran E, Rappaport H. Angio-immunoblastic lymphadenopathy with dysproteinemia. *Lancet* 1974;i:1070–1073.

373. Feller A, Griesser H, Schilling C, et al. Clonal gene rearrangement patterns correlate with immunophenotype and clinical parameters in patients with angioimmunoblastic lymphadenopathy. *Am J Pathol* 1988;133:549–556.

374. Weiss L, Strickler J, Dorfman R, et al. Clonal T-cell populations in angioimmunoblastic lymphadenopathy and angioimmunoblastic lymphadenopathy-like lymphoma. *Am J Pathol* 1986;122:392–397.

375. Anagnostopoulos I, Hummel M, Finn T, et al. Heterogeneous Epstein-Barr virus infection patterns in peripheral T-cell lymphoma of angioimmunoblastic lymphadenopathy type. *Blood* 1992;80:1804–1812.

376. Weiss L, Jaffe E, Liu X, et al. Detection and localization of Epstein-Barr viral genomes in angioimmunoblastic lymphadenopathy and antiimmunoblastic lymphadenopathy-like lymphomas. *Blood* 1992;79:1789.

377. Schlegelberger B, Feller A, Godde W, Lennert K. Stepwise development of chromosomal abnormalities in angioimmunoblastic lymphadenopathy. *Cancer Genet Cytogenet* 1990;50:15.

378. Reiter A, Schrappe M, Tiemann M, et al. Successful treatment strategy for Ki-1 anaplastic large-cell lymphoma of childhood: a prospective analysis of 62 patients enrolled in three consecutive Berlin-Frankfurt-Munster group studies. *J Clin Oncol* 1994;12:899–908.

379. Sandlund J, Pui C-H, Santana V, et al. Clinical features and treatment outcome for children with CD30+ large-cell non-Hodgkin's lymphoma. *J Clin Oncol* 1994;12:895–898.

380. Weisenburger D, Gordon B, Vose J, et al. Occurrence of the t(2;5)(p23;q35) in non-Hodgkin's lymphoma. *Blood* 1996;87:3860–3868.

381. Greer J, Kinney M, Collins R, et al. Clinical features of 31 patients with Ki-1 anaplastic large-cell lymphoma. *J Clin Oncol* 1991;9:539–547.

382. Shiota M, Nakamura S, Ichinohasama R, et al. Anaplastic large cell lymphomas expressing the novel chimeric protein p80NPM/ALK: a distinct clinicopathologic entity. *Blood* 1995;86:1954–1960.

383. Benharroch D, Meguerian-Bedoyan Z, Lamant L, et al. ALK-positive lymphoma: a single disease with a broad spectrum of morphology. *Blood* 1998;91:2076–2084.

384. Stein H, Mason D, Gerdes J, et al. The expression of the Hodgkin's disease associated antigen Ki-1 in reactive and neoplastic lymphoid tissue: evidence that Reed-Sternberg cells and histiocytic malignancies are derived from activated lymphoid cells. *Blood* 1985;66:848–858.

385. Chan J, NG C, Hui P, et al. Anaplastic large cell Ki-1 lymphoma. Delineation of two morphological types. *Histopathology* 1989;15:11–34.

386. Pileri S, Falini B, Delsol G, et al. Lymphohistiocytic T-cell lymphoma (anaplastic large cell lymphoma CD30+/Ki1+) with a high content of reactive histiocytes. *Histopathology* 1990;16:383–391.

387. Kinney M, Collins R, Greer J, et al. A small-cell-predominant variant of primary Ki-1 (CD30)+ T-cell lymphoma. *Am J Surg Pathol* 1993;17:859–868.

388. Falini B, Bigerna B, Fizzotti M, et al. ALK expression defines a distinct group of T/null lymphomas ("ALK lymphomas") with a wide morphological spectrum. *Am J Pathol* 1998;153:875–886.

389. Pileri S, Bocchia M, Baroni C, et al. Anaplastic large cell lymphoma (CD30+/Ki-1+): results of a prospective clinicopathologic study of 69 cases. *Br J Haematol* 1994;86:513–523.

390. Zinzani P, Bendandi M, Martelli M, et al. Anaplastic large cell lymphoma (Ki-1/CD30+): clinical and prognostic evaluation of 90 adult patients. *J Clin Oncol* 1996;14:955.

391. Pittaluga S, Pulford K, Wlodarska I, et al. ALK-1 antibody staining pattern in anaplastic large cell lymphoma (ALCL) and ALCL-Hodgkin's like. *Mod Pathol* 1997;10:132A.

392. Kanzler H, Hansmann ML, Kapp U, et al. Hodgkin and Reed Sternberg cells in Hodgkin's disease represent the outgrowth of a dominant tumor clone derived from (crippled) germinal center B cells. *J Exp Med* 1996;184:1495–1505.

393. Kuppers R, Rajewsky K, Zhao M, et al. Hodgkin's disease: Hodgkin and Reed Sternberg cells picked from histological sections show clonal immunoglobulin gene rearrangements and appear to be derived from B cells at various stages of development. *Proc Nat Acad Sci U S A* 1994;91:1092–1096.

394. Hummel M, Ziemann K, Lammert H, et al. Hodgkin's disease with monoclonal and polyclonal populations of Reed-Sternberg cells. *N Engl J Med* 1995;333:901–906.

395. Sundeen J, Lipford E, Uppenkamp J, et al. Rearranged antigen receptor genes in Hodgkin's disease. *Blood* 1987;70:96–103.

396. Weiss L, Strickler J, Hu E, et al. Immunoglobulin gene rearrangements in tissues involved by Hodgkin's disease. *Hum Pathol* 1986;17:1006–1014.

397. Zinzani P, Martelli M, Magagnoli M, et al. Anaplastic large cell lymphoma, Hodgkin's-like: a randomized trial of ABVD versus MACOP-B with and without radiation therapy. *Blood* 1998;92:790–794.

398. Foss H, Anagnostopoulos I, Araujo I, et al. Anaplastic large-cell lymphomas of T-cell and null-cell phenotype express cytotoxic molecules. *Blood* 1996;88:4005–4011.

399. Krenacs L, Wellman A, Sorbara L, et al. Cytoxic cell antigen expression in anaplastic large cell lymphomas of T- and null-cell type and Hodgkin's disease: evidence for distinct cellular origin. *Blood* 1997;89:980–999.

400. Mason D, Bastard C, Rimokh R, et al. CD30-positive large cell lymphomas ("Ki-1 lymphoma") are associated with a chromosomal translocation involving 5q35. *Br J Haematol* 1990;74:161–168.

401. Wlodarska I, De Wolf-Peeters C, Falini B, et al. The cryptic inv(2)(p23q35) defines a new molecular genetic subtype of ALK-positive anaplastic large-cell lymphoma. *Blood* 1998;92:2688–2695.

402. Pinkus G, Said J. Hodgkin's disease, lymphocyte predominance type, nodular—a distinct entity? Unique staining profile of L&H variants of Reed-Sternberg cells defined by monoclonal antibodies to leukocyte common antigen, granulocyte specific antigen, and B-cell specific antigen. *Am J Pathol* 1985;116:1–6.

403. Pinkus G, Said J. Hodgkin's disease, lymphocyte predominance type, nodular—further evidence for a B cell derivation: L&H variants of Reed-Sternberg cells express L26, a pan B cell marker. *Am J Pathol* 1988;133:211–217.

404. Zukerberg L, Ferry J, Harris N. Expression of B lineage antigens by Reed-Sternberg cells in NS and MCHD. *Lab Invest* 1992;66:90A.

405. Schmid C, Pan L, Diss T, Isaacson P. Expression of B-cell antigens by Hodgkin's and Reed-Sternberg cells. *Am J Pathol* 1991;139:701–707.

406. Tamaru J, Hummel M, Zemlin M, et al. Hodgkin's disease with a B-cell phenotype often shows a VDJ rearrangement and somatic mutations in the VH genes. *Blood* 1994;84:708–715.

407. Inghirami G, Marci L, Rosati S, et al. The Reed-Sternberg cells of Hodgkin's disease are clonal. *Proc Natl Acad Sci U S A* 1994;91:9842–9846.

408. Marafioti T, Hummel. M, Anagnostopoulos I, et al. Origin of nodular lymphocyte-predominant Hodgkin's disease from a clonal expansion of highly mutated germinal-center B cells. *N Engl J Med* 1997;337:453–458.

409. Brauninger A, Kuppers R, Strickler JG, et al. Hodgkin and Reed-Sternberg cells in lymphocyte predominant Hodgkin disease represent clonal populations of germinal center-derived tumor B cells [published erratum appears in *Proc Natl Acad Sci U S A* 1997;94(25):14211]. *Proc Natl Acad Sci U S A* 1997;94:9337–9342.

410. Mason D, Banks P, Chan J, et al. Nodular lymphocyte predominance Hodgkin's disease: a distinct clinico-pathological entity. *Am J Surg Pathol* 1994;18:528–530.

411. von Wasielewski R, Werner M, Fischer R, et al. Lymphocyte-predominant Hodgkin's disease: an immunohistochemical analysis of 208 reviewed Hodgkin's disease cases from the German Hodgkin Study Group. *Am J Pathol* 1997;150:793–803.

412. Diehl V, Sextro M, Franklin J, et al. Clinical presentation, course, and prognostic factors in lymphocyte-predominant Hodgkin's disease and lymphocyte-rich classic Hodgkin's disease: report from the European Task Force on Lymphoma Project on Lymphocyte-Predominant Hodgkin's Disease [see comments]. *J Clin Oncol* 1999;17:776–783.

413. Regula D, Hoppe R, Weiss L. Nodular and diffuse types of lymphocyte predominance Hodgkin's disease. *N Engl J Med* 1988;318:214–219.

414. Orlandi E, Lazzarino M, Brusamolino E, et al. Nodular lymphocyte predominance Hodgkin's disease (NLPHD): clinical behavior and pattern of progression in 66 patients. Third International Symposium on Hodgkin's Lymphoma, Kolne, Germany, 1995.

415. Krayalcin G, Behm F, Geiser P, et al. Lymphocyte predominant Hodgkin disease: clinicopathologic features and results of treatment: the Pediatric Oncology Group experience. *Med Pediat Oncol* 1997;29:519–525.

416. Bodis S, Kraus MD, Pinkus G, et al. Clinical presentation and outcome in lymphocyte-predominant Hodgkin's disease. *J Clin Oncol* 1997;15:3060–3066.

417. Divine M, Brice P, Bastion Y, et al. Indolent, relapsing pattern in nodular lymphocyte predominance Hodgkin's disease (NLPHD): the GELA experience in a series of 70 patients. Third International Workshop on Hodgkin's Lymphoma, Kolne, Germany, 1995.

418. Bennett M, MacLennan K, Hudson G, Hudson B. Non-Hodgkin's lymphoma arising in patients treated for Hodgkin's disease in the BNLI: a 20-year experience. *Ann Oncol* 1991;2 Suppl 2:83–92.

419. Hansmann M, Stein H, Fellbaum C, et al. Nodular paragranuloma can transform into high-grade malignant lymphoma of B type. *Hum Pathol* 1989;20:1169–1175.

420. Sundeen J, Cossman J, Jaffe E. Lymphocyte predominant Hodgkin's disease, nodular subtype with coexistent "large cell lymphoma." Histological progression or composite malignancy? *Am J Surg Pathol* 1988;12:599–606.

421. Lukes RJ, Butler JJ. The pathology and nomenclature of Hodgkin's disease. *Cancer Res* 1966;26:1063–1081.

422. Lukes R, Butler J, Hicks E. Natural history of Hodgkin's disease as related to its pathological picture. *Cancer* 1966;19:317–344.

423. Burns B, Colby T, Dorfman R. Differential diagnostic features of nodular L&H Hodgkin's disease, including progressive transformation of germinal centers. *Am J Surg Pathol* 1984;8:253–261.

424. Poppema S, Kaiserling E, Lennert K. Nodular paragranuloma and progressively transformed germinal centers: ultrastructural and immunohistochemical findings. *Virchows Arch* 1979;31:211–225.

425. Poppema S, Kaiserling E, Lennert K. Hodgkin's disease with lymphocyte predominance, nodular type (nodular paragranuloma) and progressively transformed germinal centres: a cytohistological study. *Histopathology* 1979;3:295–308.

426. Ferry J, Zukerberg L, Harris N. Florid progressive transformation of germinal centers in young men without progression to nodular lymphocyte predominance Hodgkin's disease (NLPHD). *Am J Surg Pathol* 1992;16:252–258.

427. Hansmann M, Fellbaum C, Hui P, et al. Progressive transformation of germinal centers with and without association to Hodgkin's disease. *Am J Clin Pathol* 1990;93:219–226.

428. Osborne B, Butler J. Clinical implications of progressive transformation of germinal centers. *Am J Surg Pathol* 1984;8:725–733.

429. Osborne B, Butler J, Gresik M. Progressive transformation of germinal centers: comparison of 23 pediatric patients to the adult population. *Mod Pathol* 1993;5:135–140.
430. Falini B, Dalla Favara R, Pileri S, et al. BCL-6 gene rearrangement and expression in Hodgkin's disease. Third International Symposium on Hodgkin's Lymphoma, Kolne, Germany, 1995.
431. Timmens W, Visser L, Poppema S. Nodular lymphocyte predominance type of Hodgkin's disease is a germinal center lymphoma. *Lab Invest* 1986;54:457–461.
432. Poppema S. The nature of the lymphocytes surrounding Reed-Sternberg cells in nodular lymphocyte predominance and in other types of Hodgkin's disease. *Am J Pathol* 1989;135:351–357.
433. Kamel O, Gelb A, Shibuha R, et al. Leu-7 (CD57) reactivity distinguishes nodular lymphocyte predominance Hodgkin's disease from nodular sclerosing Hodgkin's disease, T-cell-rich B-cell lymphoma and follicular lymphoma. *Am J Pathol* 1993;142:541–546.
434. Hansmann M-L, Stein H, Dallenbach F, Feldbaum C. Diffuse lymphocyte predominant Hodgkin's disease (paragranuloma): a variant of the B cell-derived nodular type. *Am J Pathol* 1991;138:29–36.
435. Ohno T, Stribley JA, Wu G, et al. Clonality in nodular lymphocyte-predominant Hodgkin's disease [see comments]. *N Engl J Med* 1997;337:459–465.
436. Schouten HC, Sanger WG, Duggan M, et al. Chromosomal abnormalities in Hodgkin's disease. *Blood* 1989;73:2149–2154.
437. Tilly H, Bastard C, Delastre T, et al. Cytogenetic studies in untreated Hodgkin's disease. *Blood* 1991;77:1298–1304.
438. Pelstring R, Zellmer R, Sulak L, et al. Hodgkin's disease in association with human immunodeficiency virus infection. *Cancer* 1991;67:1865–1873.
439. Neiman R, Rosen P, Lukes R. Lymphocyte depletion Hodgkin's disease. A clinicopathological entity. *N Engl J Med* 1973;288:751–755.
440. Kant J, Hubbard S, Longo D, et al. The pathologic and clinical heterogeneity of lymphocyte-depleted Hodgkin's disease. *J Clin Oncol* 1986;4:284–294.
441. von Vasielewski R, Mengel M, Fischer R, et al. Classic Hodgkin's disease: clinical impact of the immunophenotype. *Am J Pathol* 1997;151:1123–1130.
442. Anagnostopoulos I, Hansmann ML, Franssila K, et al. European Task Force on Lymphoma project on lymphocyte predominance Hodgkin disease: histologic and immunohistologic analysis of submitted cases reveals 2 types of Hodgkin disease with a nodular growth pattern and abundant lymphocytes. *Blood* 2000;96:1889–1899.
443. Leoncini L, Del Vecchio M, Kraft R, et al. Hodgkin's disease and CD30-positive anaplastic large cell lymphomas: a continuous spectrum of malignant disorders. *Am J Pathol* 1990;137:1047–1057.
444. Stein H, Herbst H, Anagnostopoulos I, et al. The nature of Hodgkin and Reed-Sternberg cells, their association with EBV, and their relationship to anaplastic large-cell lymphoma. *Ann Oncol* 1991;2:33–38.
445. Ashton-Key M. Follicular Hodgkin's disease. *Am J Surg Pathol* 1995;19:1294–1299.
446. Diehl V, Stein H, Sextro M, et al. Lymphocyte predominant Hodgkin's disease: a European Task Force on Lymphoma project. *Blood* 1996;88:294a.
447. Bennett M, MacLennan K, Easterling M, et al. The prognostic significance of cellular subtypes in nodular sclerosing Hodgkin's disease: an analysis of 271 non-laparotomised cases (BNLI report no. 22). *Clin Radiol* 1983;34:497–501.
448. MacLennan K, Bennett M, Tu A, et al. Relationship of histopathologic features to survival and relapse in nodular sclerosing Hodgkin's disease. *Cancer* 1989;64:1686–1693.
449. Haybittle J, Easterling M, Bennett M, et al. Review of British National Lymphoma Investigation studies of Hodgkin's disease and development of prognostic index. *Lancet* 1985;1:967–972.
450. Wijlhuizen T, Vrints L, Jairam R, et al. Grades of nodular sclerosis (NSI-NSII)

in Hodgkin's disease: are they of independent prognostic value? *Cancer* 1989;63:1150–1153.
451. Ferry J, Linggood R, Convery K, et al. Hodgkin's disease, nodular sclerosis type: implications of histologic subclassification. *Cancer* 1993;71:457–463.
452. Hess J, Bodis S, Pinkus G, et al. Histopathologic grading of nodular sclerosis Hodgkin's disease. Lack of prognostic significance in 254 surgically staged patients. *Cancer* 1994;74:708–714.
453. Georgii A, Hasenclever D, Fischer R, et al. Histopathological grading of nodular sclerosis Hodgkin's reveals significant differences in survival and relapse rather under protocol therapy. Third International Symposium on Hodgkin's lymphoma, September, Kolne, Germany, 1995.
454. Michel G, Bouzourene H, Delacretaz F, et al. Histologic grade of nodular sclerosing Hodgkin's disease: is it a prognostic factor? Third International Symposium on Hodgkin's lymphoma, Kolne, Germany, 1995.
455. van Spronsen D, Vrints L, Erdkamp F, et al. Disappearance of prognostic value of subclassification of nodular sclerosing Hodgkin's disease in southeast Netherlands since 1972. Third International Symposium on Hodgkin's lymphoma, Kolne, Germany, 1995.
456. Falini B, Stein H, Pileri S, et al. Expression of T-cell antigens on Hodgkin's and Sternberg-Reed cells of Hodgkin's disease. A combined immunocytochemical and immunohistological study using monoclonal antibodies. *Histopathology* 1987;12:1229–1241.
457. Zukerberg L, Collins A, Ferry J, Harris N. Coexpression of CD15 and CD20 by Reed-Sternberg cells in Hodgkin's disease. *Am J Pathol* 1991;139: 475–483.
458. Orazi A, Jiang B, Lee C-H, et al. Correlation between presence of clonal rearrangements of immunoglobulin heavy chain genes and B-cell antigen expression in Hodgkin's disease. *Am J Clin Pathol* 1995;104:413–418.
459. Poppema S, Kaleta J, Hepperle B. Chromosomal abnormalities in patients with Hodgkin's disease: evidence for frequent involvement of the 14q chromosomal region but infrequent bcl-2 gene rearrangements in Reed-Sternberg cells. *J Natl Cancer Inst* 1992;84:1789–1793.
460. Weber-Mathisen K, Deerberg J, Poetsch M, et al. Numerical chromosome aberrations are present within the CD30+ Hodgkin and Reed Sternberg cells in 100% of analysed cases of Hodgkin's disease. *Blood* 1995;86:1464–1468.
461. Stetler-Stevenson M, Crush-Stanton S, Cossman J. Involvement of the bcl-2 gene in Hodgkin's disease. *J Natl Cancer Inst* 1990;82:855–858.
462. Athan E, Chadburn A, Knowles D. The bcl-2 gene translocation is undetectable in Hodgkin's disease by Southern blot hybridization and polymerase chain reaction. *Am J Pathol* 1992;141:193–201.
463. Orscheschek K, Merz H, Hell J, et al. Large cell anaplastic lymphoma-specific translocation (t[2;5][p23q35]) in Hodgkin's disease: indication of a common pathogenesis? *Lancet* 1995;345:87–90.
464. Elmberger P, Lozano M, Weisenburger D, et al. Transcripts of the npm-alk fusion gene in anaplastic large cell lymphoma, Hodgkin's disease, and reactive lymphoid lesions. *Blood* 1995;86:3517–3521.
465. Wellmann A, Otsuki T, Vogelbruch M, et al. Analysis of the t(2;5)(p23;q35) translocation by reverse transcription-polymerase chain reaction in CD30+ anaplastic large-cell lymphomas, in other non-Hodgkin's lymphomas of T-cell phenotype, and in Hodgkin's disease. *Blood* 1995;86: 2321–2328.
466. Sarris AH, Luthra R, Papadimitracopoulou V, et al. Long-range amplification of genomic DNA detects the t(2;5)(p23;q35) in anaplastic large-cell lymphoma, but not in other non-Hodgkin's lymphomas, Hodgkin's disease, or lymphomatoid papulosis. *Ann Oncol* 1997;8:59–63.
467. Trümper L, Daus H, Merz H, et al. NPM/ALK fusion mRNA expression in Hodgkin and Reed-Sternberg cells is rare but does occur: results from single-cell cDNA analysis. *Ann Oncol* 1997;8:83–87.

CHAPTER 25

Acute Lymphoblastic Leukemia

Lewis B. Silverman and Stephen E. Sallan

Acute leukemia refers to clonal malignant disorders of lymphoid or myeloid progenitor cells. In acute lymphoblastic leukemia (ALL), abnormalities of lymphoid cell differentiation, proliferation, or both, lead to excessive infiltration and accumulation of leukemic lymphoblasts in bone marrow and other organs. If untreated, the disease is rapidly fatal, with death usually caused by infection or bleeding. ALL accounts for approximately 80% of the childhood leukemias in the United States; the remaining 20% originate in cells of the myeloid lineage and collectively are called *acute myelogenous leukemia* (AML). This ratio is reversed in adults.

The development of effective therapy for children with ALL is one of the undisputed successes of modern clinical hematology-oncology. Fifty years ago, ALL was uniformly fatal, but currently, over three-fourths of children (Fig. 25-1) (1) and one-third of adults with ALL are cured. This extraordinary therapeutic progress resulted from a series of clinical trials that used combinations of antileukemia drugs, radiation, and supportive measures. More recently, advances in the understanding of leukemia cell biology and clinical risk factors have made it possible to recognize a spectrum of prognostically distinctive ALL subtypes. Current treatment regimens stratify therapy based on risk of relapse. For instance, patients with relatively favorable prognoses are treated on protocols that modify or eliminate certain intensive components of therapy with the goal of decreasing morbidity without compromising efficacy. Patients with relatively higher risk of relapse are more intensively treated to improve cure rates. This chapter reviews the epidemiology, classification, and clinical management of ALL, concentrating on the principles and strategies of therapy, with particular attention given to new findings in the biology of ALL and unresolved treatment controversies.

EPIDEMIOLOGY

Approximately 3000 cases of ALL are diagnosed in the United States each year (2). Nearly two-thirds of cases are diagnosed in children, constituting approximately 25% of all childhood cancers and 80% of childhood leukemias (3). Between 1975 and 1995, the annual incidence of ALL in the United States among children 19 years of age or younger was 29.2 cases/million (3). In adults, ALL represents approximately 1% to 2% of all cancers and 20% of all leukemias (2). The age-adjusted incidence of ALL in adults (over 15 years of age) is seven cases/million.

The peak incidence of ALL in the United States occurs in children between the ages of 2 and 4 years (3); a similar age distribution has been noted in Great Britain and Japan. T-cell ALL occurs more often in older children, whereas B-progenitor ALL usually develops in children younger than 7 years of age. No obvious peak incidence of ALL is observed during adulthood, although the incidence increases slightly after age 50 years (2).

ALL affects males more often than females in all age groups except infants, with a male:female ratio of 1.2:1.0 (3). Male predominance is even greater in adolescent patients and in those with T-cell immunophenotype (3,4). In the United States, white children have a higher incidence of ALL than do black children (incidence rates of 45.6 versus 27.8/million between 1985 and 1995) (3), an observation that lacks a clear explanation. Although the incidence of ALL for white children increased at an overall rate of approximately 1%/year between 1977 and 1995, there was no change in ALL incidence for black children during that time (3).

The frequency of ALL also varies by geography. The incidence of childhood ALL is lower in India, Turkey, and China than in the United States and other industrialized western nations (5). Cases of T-cell and mature B-cell ALL are more frequent than the progenitor B-cell subtype among African blacks and Arabs in the Gaza Strip (6,7). Reasons for this geographic variation are unclear, but may reflect underreporting of common ALL in developing countries or increased exposure to leukemogens in industrialized nations.

PREDISPOSING FACTORS

Certain genetic abnormalities, environmental exposures, viral infections, and immunodeficiency states have been linked to the development of ALL, although in the vast majority of cases, there is no identifiable risk factor.

Evidence of genetic factors includes the association of ALL with various chromosomal abnormalities, as well as the occurrence of familial leukemia. Siblings of pediatric leukemia patients are two to four times more likely to develop the disease than the general population (8). The concordance rate of acute leukemia in monozygotic twins is estimated to be as high as 25%, with highest risk of concordance during infancy and decreasing thereafter (9). By the age of 7 years, the risk of developing leukemia in monozygotic twins of pediatric leukemia patients no longer exceeds that of the general population. Concordant leukemia in monozygotic twins may reflect a common genetic determinant, shared intrauterine leukemogenic event, or placental spread of the disease from one twin to the other (10). The risk of vertical transmission of ALL appears low. Among 119 pregnant women with leukemia, including ALL, none had offspring with this disease (11).

Children with certain genetic disorders have an increased risk of developing ALL (9). Children with Down's syndrome (trisomy

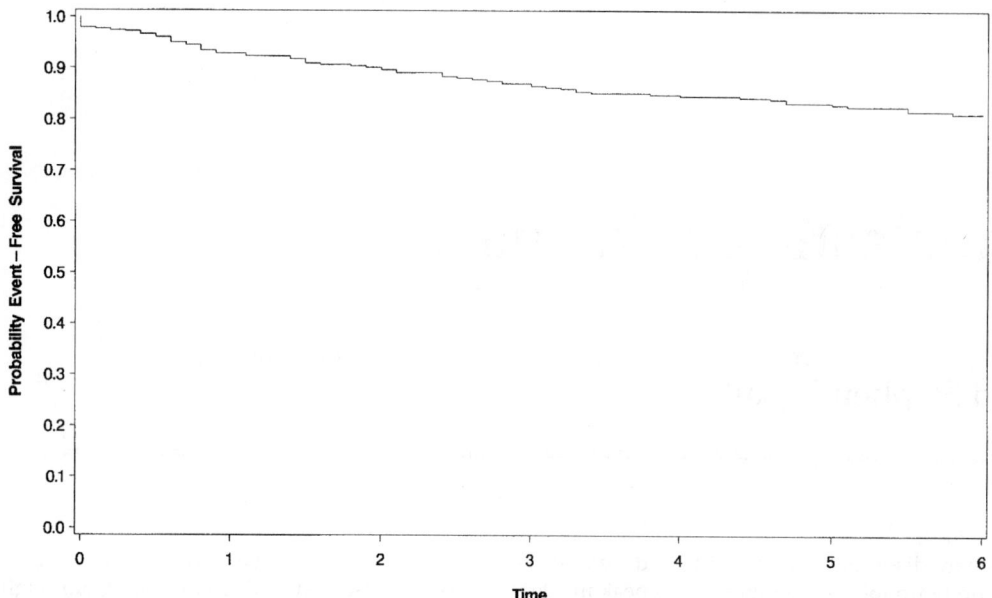

Figure 25-1. Event-free survival for 377 children (ages 1 to 18 years) treated on Dana-Farber Cancer Institute Acute Lymphoblastic Leukemia Consortium Protocol 91-01 between 1991 and 1995. The 5-year event-free survival rate (± standard error) was 83 + 2%.

21) have up to 15 times the risk of developing leukemia as nonaffected children, with ALL predominating in all but the neonatal age group (12). There is also an increased incidence of acute leukemia in Bloom's syndrome, a disorder associated with increased chromosomal fragility, although AML is more common than ALL in these patients (13). Patients with ataxia-telangiectasia have an increased risk of developing lymphoid malignancies, including T-cell ALL (14), although a clear link has not been established between ATM gene mutations and ALL in other children (15).

Certain environmental exposures, such as ionizing radiation, may predispose to ALL. Among Japanese within 1000 meters of the epicenters of atomic bomb blasts in Nagasaki and Hiroshima, the risk of ALL was 1 in 60 over 12 years, with ALL observed more frequently in children (9). Conversely, there was not any increased risk of leukemia in children exposed to these bomb blasts *in utero*. The excess risk, if any, of developing ALL from low-level diagnostic radiation, has not been clearly established (16,17). Similarly, there is conflicting and inconsistent data linking childhood ALL and residential exposure to electromagnetic fields from high-voltage power lines (16,17), although the preponderance of evidence does not support any association (18). Environmental carcinogens, such as hydrocarbons, have also been implicated in leukemogenesis, although such exposures are usually associated with AML and not ALL (19).

With the exception of Epstein-Barr virus and mature B-cell (Burkitt) leukemia, no virus or other infectious agent has been identified as an etiologic agent in childhood ALL. Retroviruses, such as human T-cell leukemia/lymphoma virus type 1, have a direct causative role in leukemogenesis in some adults, but they have not been convincingly linked to the childhood leukemias (20). Greaves has postulated that childhood ALL may result from a rare, abnormal response to common infections, perhaps due to host genetic susceptibility or delayed exposure in childhood to these infections (17). However, a large case-control analysis conducted by the Children's Cancer Group did not find any relationship between early childhood infections and risk of ALL, with the exception of an apparent protective effect of multiple ear infections in infancy (21).

CLASSIFICATION

ALL is a heterogeneous disorder which can be subclassified in terms of morphology, cytochemistry, and immunophenotype, as well as chromosomal and molecular genetic aberrations. Continued study of these subtypes may further improve classification systems, provide information of prognostic importance, and lead to an understanding of the mechanisms of leukemic transformation.

Morphology

Because leukemic lymphoblasts are morphologically indistinguishable from immature normal lymphoid cells, attempts to subclassify these cells on the basis of size, nuclear/cytoplasmic ratio, presence of cytoplasmic granules, or other features have been largely unsuccessful. A morphologic classification system devised by the French-American-British (FAB) Cooperative Working Group (Fig. 25-2) has gained wide acceptance (22). Approximately 90% of cases of childhood ALL are of the FAB L1 subtype, characterized by relatively small lymphoblasts with scanty cytoplasm and inconspicuous nucleoli. Cells in the L2 category, found in 5% to 15% of pediatric cases, are larger than those classified as L1, show marked variability in size, and have prominent nucleoli and more abundant cytoplasm. Only 1% to 2% of ALL cases in children have L3 lymphoblasts, which appear identical to Burkitt lymphoma cells. The distribution of FAB subtypes in adult ALL differs strikingly from that in children in that a much higher percentage of cases (60% to 70%) are classified as L2 (23). Other morphologic variants of ALL, including ALL with "hand-mirror" cells or granules, have been described but are of uncertain significance (24). Although L3 ALL is nearly always associated with mature B-cell immunophenotype, L1 and L2 lymphoblasts do not differ significantly in terms of cell-surface markers or genetic abnormalities (10). In some studies, L2 morphology has been associated with an inferior prognosis when compared with the L1 subtype, although this finding is controversial (25,26). Most investigators no longer consider the distinction between the L1 and L2 subtypes when risk-stratifying patients.

Cytochemistry

A variety of cytochemical stains can distinguish ALL from AML. In approximately 80% of cases of ALL, lymphoblasts react positively with periodic acid-Schiff, which stains cytoplasmic glycogen, whereas myeloid-specific stains, such as myeloperoxidase, specific and non-specific esterase, and Sudan black (a cytoplasmic lipid stain) are usually negative. Terminal deoxynucleotidyl transferase (TdT), an unusual enzyme that catalyzes the polymerization of

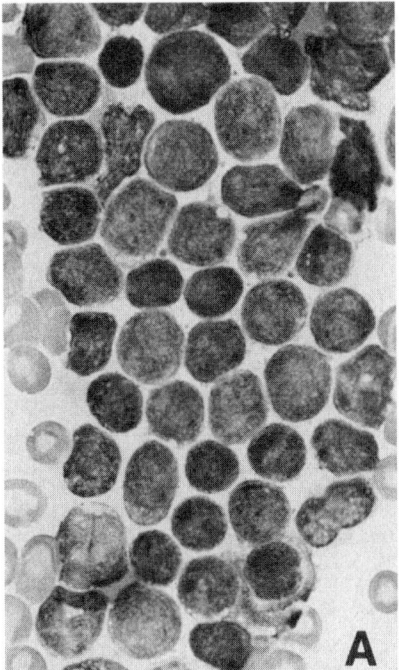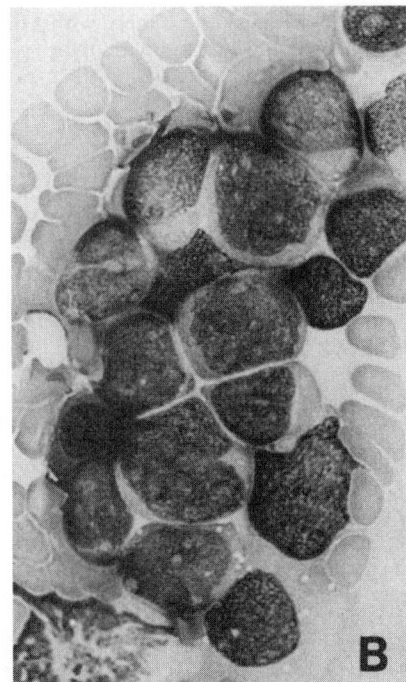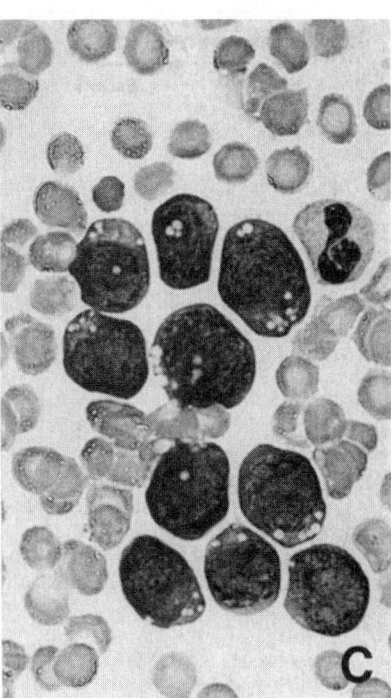

Figure 25-2. Morphologic appearance of leukemic lymphoblasts according to the French-American-British classification system. **A:** L1 blasts are small with scanty cytoplasm. **B:** L2 blasts are larger with increased amounts of cytoplasm, irregular nuclear membranes, and prominent nucleoli. **C:** L3 blasts have basophilic cytoplasm with vacuolization. (Adapted from Rivera G, Pui C-H. Acute lymphoblastic leukemia. In: Rudolph AM, ed. *Pediatrics.* Norwalk, CT: Appleton-Century-Crofts, 1987:1098.)

deoxynucleoside monophosphates into a single-strand DNA primer, can be demonstrated in the nuclei of both T- and B-cell lymphoblasts but is rarely present in cases of myeloid leukemia (27,28).

Cytochemical stains have also been studied for their ability to distinguish clinically relevant subsets of lymphoblasts. Although some strong correlations between blast cell–staining characteristics and subtype of ALL have been noted, the practical value of this type of information is limited. The acid phosphatase reaction, for example, can be used to distinguish cases of T-cell ALL from other immunologic subtypes; but it is not specific for the lymphoid lineage, nor does it identify all cases that express T-cell–specific antigens (29,30). TdT activity appears more relevant to identifying the maturational stage of a lymphoblast than to specifying its lineage and does not appear to have prognostic relevance.

Immunophenotype

Differences in surface membrane or cytoplasmic components of T and B lymphocytes (immunophenotype) can be used to identify and classify lymphoblasts as to cell of origin and stage of maturation (Fig. 25-1). Markers that are specific for or closely related to cell lineage or stage of differentiation have proved especially useful in this regard (4,31). Based on reactivity with a panel of lineage-associated antibodies, ALL has been subclassified into three broad categories: mature B-cell, B-progenitor, and T-cell. The immunophenotypic subsets are associated with distinctive clinical features, as shown in Table 25-1 (4,31).

MATURE B-CELL ACUTE LYMPHOBLASTIC LEUKEMIA
The mature B-cell phenotype accounts for 1% to 2% of cases of childhood ALL and up to 5% of adult ALL (31). It is characterized by surface immunoglobulin, most often immunoglobulin M, which is monoclonal for κ or λ light chain. The cells also express other B-cell antigens, including CD19, CD20, and HLA-DR. Morphologically, the blast cells tend to have FAB L3 features, with intensely

staining cytoplasmic basophilia similar to that of erythroblasts (Fig. 25-2). Nearly all of these cases have a translocation involving the c-*myc* oncogene on chromosome 8, most frequently also involving chromosome 14 [at the immunoglobulin–heavy chain (IgH) locus], but sometimes chromosomes 2 (the κ–light chain locus) or 22 (the λ–light chain locus) (32). Mature B-cell ALL is clinically indistinguishable from disseminated Burkitt lymphoma and is much more successfully treated with regimens used for that disease than with conventional childhood ALL therapy (33,34).

B-PROGENITOR ACUTE LYMPHOBLASTIC LEUKEMIA
Approximately 80% to 85% of children with ALL present with B-progenitor phenotype. These leukemia cells are characterized by reactivity with monoclonal antibodies specific for B-cell–associated antigens (e.g., CD9, CD19, and CD20) and are distinguished from mature B-cell ALL by the absence of surface immunoglobulin. The vast majority (80% to 90%) of B-progenitor ALL cells express CD10, also known as the *common ALL antigen* (35).

More than 90% of cases of B-progenitor ALL cases have evidence of immunoglobulin gene rearrangements, predominately involving the IgH gene (36). The pattern of immunoglobulin gene rearrangements in ALL cells may indicate the degree of differentiation of the precursor B-cell from which it derives, because normal B-cell maturation is characterized by sequential rearrangements of the IgH–, κ–, and then λ–light chain rearrangements (37). However, many B-progenitor ALL cells display an immunoglobulin gene rearrangement profile that is not consistent with any known stage of normal B-cell development, reflecting the disordered nature of the leukemic cell genome (38). Moreover, T-cell receptor gene rearrangements occur very frequently in B-progenitor ALL, and IgH gene rearrangements have been observed in T-cell ALL (36). Thus, the pattern of immunoglobulin and T-cell receptor gene rearrangements are insufficient to categorize the lineage or degree of differentiation of an individual patient's lymphoblasts.

TABLE 25-1. Initial Clinical and Laboratory Findings in Children with Acute Lymphoblastic Leukemia (ALL) According to Immunophenotype

Characteristic	Early Pre-B (cIg⁻) (%)	Pre-B (cIg⁺) (%)	T (%)	Mature B (%)	P Value for Statistical Comparison[a] Non-T, Non-B vs. T
Sex					
Male	521 (54)	144 (52)	131 (68)	6 (67)	.0001
Female	450 (46)	132 (48)	62 (32)	3 (33)	—
Race					
White	781 (80)	202 (73)	136 (70)	7 (78)	.0001
Black	89 (9)	36 (13)	36 (19)	1 (11)	—
Hispanic	69 (7)	30 (11)	9 (5)	1 (11)	—
Other	33 (4)	9 (3)	12 (6)	0 (0)	—
Age (yr)					
<1.5	60 (6)	25 (9)	5 (2)	3 (18)	.0001
1.5–7.0	654 (66)	175 (61)	98 (45)	8 (47)	—
7–10	130 (13)	43 (15)	56 (26)	2 (12)	—
≥10	149 (15)	42 (15)	57 (26)	4 (24)	—
Leukocyte count (×10⁸/L)					
<10	493 (50)	122 (43)	43 (20)	5 (31)	.0001
10–50	348 (35)	93 (33)	63 (29)	6 (38)	—
50–100	82 (8)	33 (12)	27 (13)	3 (19)	—
>100	71 (7)	37 (13)	83 (38)	2 (13)	—
Platelet count (×10⁹/L)					
<20	201 (21)	64 (23)	25 (13)	3 (38)	.0001
20–100	514 (53)	130 (47)	85 (44)	5 (62)	—
<100	252 (26)	80 (29)	84 (43)	0 (0)	—
Hemoglobin (g/dL)					
<7.5	482 (50)	120 (44)	50 (27)	4 (50)	.0001
7.5–10.0	311 (32)	76 (28)	42 (22)	1 (12)	—
>10	167 (17)	75 (28)	95 (51)	3 (38)	—
Hepatomegaly					
No	923 (93)	263 (92)	187 (87)	13 (81)	.001
Yes[b]	71 (7)	22 (8)	27 (13)	3 (19)	—
Splenomegaly					
No	905 (91)	254 (89)	170 (79)	14 (87)	.0001
Yes	86 (9)	31 (11)	44 (21)	2 (13)	—
Lymphadenopathy					
None	385 (39)	101 (35)	48 (22)	2 (12)	.0001
Minimal	392 (39)	114 (40)	59 (27)	10 (59)	—
Moderate	190 (19)	61 (21)	64 (30)	1 (6)	—
Marked	28 (3)	9 (3)	44 (20)	4 (24)	—
Mediastinal mass					
No	990 (95)	284 (99)	104 (48)	17 (100)	.0001
Yes	5 (5)	2 (1)	112 (52)	0 (0)	—
CNS disease					
No	954 (96)	272 (95)	205 (95)	14 (72)	—
Yes	41 (4)	13 (5)	11 (5)	3 (18)	—
Periodic acid-Schiff stain					
Positive (>50)	641 (65)	170 (60)	74 (35)	3 (19)	.0001
Negative	347 (35)	114 (40)	140 (65)	13 (81)	—
Glucocorticoid (receptors/cell)					
<2500	18 (5)	7 (7)	27 (25)	4 (31)	.0001
2500–6000	80 (20)	26 (25)	54 (49)	3 (23)	—
6000–10,000	102 (26)	27 (25)	16 (15)	2 (15)	—
10,000–20,000	159 (41)	35 (33)	11 (10)	4 (31)	—
>20,000	33 (8)	11 (10)	2 (2)	0 (0)	—
CD10 (common acute lymphoblastic leukemia antigen)					
Positive	895 (90)	260 (91)	65 (30)	8 (50)	.0001
Negative	98 (10)	25 (9)	150 (70)	8 (50)	—
HLA-DR					
Positive	974 (98)	277 (97)	36 (17)	15 (94)	.0001
Negative	19 (2)	8 (3)	180 (83)	1 (6)	—

cIg, cytoplasmic immunoglobulin; CNS, central nervous system.
[a]There were too few patients with B-cell ALL for statistical comparisons.
[b]Palpable to below umbilicus.
Pullen DJ, Boyett JM, Crist WM, et al. Pediatric Oncology Group utilization of immunologic markers in the designation of acute lymphocytic leukemia subgroups: influence on treatment response. *Ann N Y Acad Sci* 1984;428:26.

The presence of intracytoplasmic immunoglobulin along with various cell-surface markers have been used to distinguish different subsets of B-progenitor ALL based on their level of differentiation (Fig. 25-3). These subsets include pro-B ALL (3% to 4% of pediatric patients), early pre-B ALL (60% to 70% of pediatric patients), and pre-B ALL (20% to 30% of pediatric patients) (39).

Pro-B ALL, thought to be derived from a very immature B-cell precursor, is characterized by CD10⁻ immunophenotype and the absence of cytoplasmic immunoglobulin (cIg). It is most frequently observed in infants with ALL, especially those with abnormalities involving chromosome 11q23 (*MLL* gene locus) (40–42). Early pre-B ALL is thought to be derived from a more

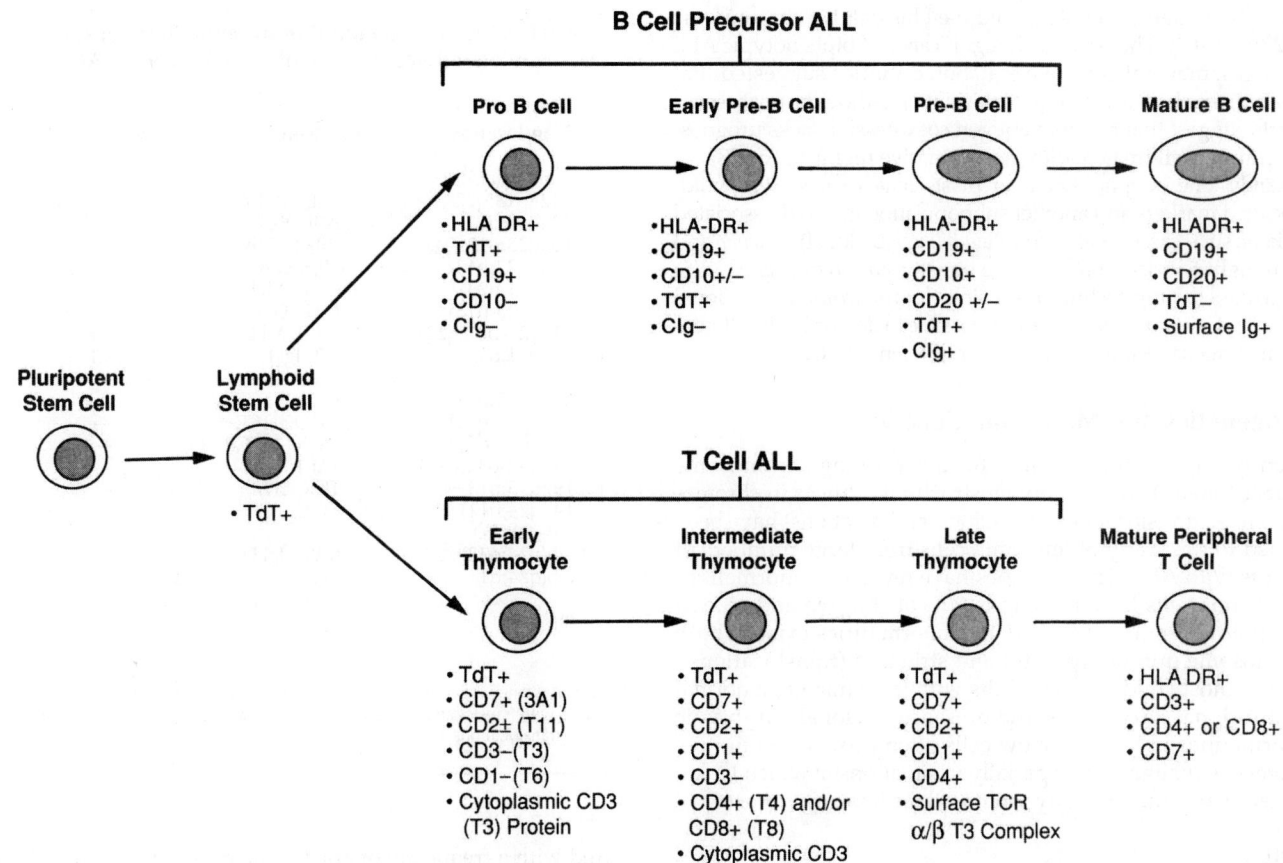

B Cell Precursor ALL

Pro B Cell
- HLA DR+
- TdT+
- CD19+
- CD10−
- CIg−

Early Pre-B Cell
- HLA-DR+
- CD19+
- CD10+/−
- TdT+
- CIg−

Pre-B Cell
- HLA-DR+
- CD19+
- CD10+
- CD20 +/−
- TdT+
- CIg+

Mature B Cell
- HLADR+
- CD19+
- CD20+
- TdT−
- Surface Ig+

Pluripotent Stem Cell

Lymphoid Stem Cell
- TdT+

T Cell ALL

Early Thymocyte
- TdT+
- CD7+ (3A1)
- CD2± (T11)
- CD3−(T3)
- CD1−(T6)
- Cytoplasmic CD3 (T3) Protein

Intermediate Thymocyte
- TdT+
- CD7+
- CD2+
- CD1+
- CD3−
- CD4+ (T4) and/or CD8+ (T8)
- Cytoplasmic CD3

Late Thymocyte
- TdT+
- CD7+
- CD2+
- CD1+
- CD4+
- Surface TCR α/β T3 Complex

Mature Peripheral T Cell
- HLA DR+
- CD3+
- CD4+ or CD8+
- CD7+

Figure 25-3. Model of lymphoid cell differentiation showing stages of cellular development based on terminal deoxynucleotidyl transferase (TdT) activity, cell-surface antigens, T-cell receptor (TCR) gene rearrangement, and the presence of immunoglobulin molecules. ALL, acute lymphoblastic leukemia; CD, cluster of differentiation group.

mature B-cell precursor than pro-B ALL. Early pre-B cells frequently express CD10, but still lack cIg. Pre-B cell ALL is characterized by the presence of cIg (43). It is thought to derive from an intermediate B-precursor cell, more mature than those lacking cIg (early pre-B cells) but not as mature as those with surface immunoglobulin (mature B cells). Like early pre-B cells, pre-B lymphoblasts typically express CD10 and HLA-DR. Approximately 25% of cases of pre-B (cIg+) ALL have the chromosomal translocation t(1;19)(q23;p13), which fuses the E2A gene on chromosome 19 with the PBX1 gene on chromosome 1 (44). This translocation is observed in only 1% of early pre-B ALL. Although initial studies suggested that patients with pre-B ALL (cIg+) had a worse outcome than those with early pre-B ALL (cIg−) (45), subsequent reports indicated that the adverse outcome of pre-B ALL was due to the subset with the t(1;19) translocation (46).

T-CELL ACUTE LYMPHOBLASTIC LEUKEMIA

Recognition of T-cell leukemia can be credited to Borella and Sen, who in 1973 reported on a boy with a very high initial leukocyte count and lymphoblasts that formed rosettes with sheep erythrocytes, a characteristic of T cells but not of B cells (47). Use of anti–T-cell heteroantisera with pan-T specificity and, more recently, monoclonal antibodies directed against epitopes of T-cell–associated antigens has improved the detection of leukemic T lymphoblasts (48). The frequency of T-cell ALL in large pediatric series ranges from 10% to 15% and in adults from 20% to 25% (39,49). In comparison with B-progenitor childhood ALL, T-cell ALL has a higher male predominance and is more frequently associated with older age at diagnosis, higher presenting leukocyte counts, and bulky extramedullary disease [including lymphadenopathy, hepatosple-

nomegaly, overt central nervous system (CNS) leukemia, and an anterior mediastinal thymic mass] (Table 25-1). Adults with T-cell ALL share this pattern of distinctive clinical features. Historically, patients with T-cell ALL had an inferior outcome compared to those with B-progenitor ALL, although this prognostic difference is not observed when more intensive regimens are used (50).

T-cell ALL can be subclassified by using monoclonal antibodies that recognize surface antigens expressed during discrete stages of normal T-cell development (51). In one such classification scheme, T-cell ALL has been subdivided into three categories, based on the maturational stage of its cell-surface antigen pattern (Fig. 25-3): early (stage I), intermediate (stage II), or late (stage III). Stage II cases occur most frequently (52). The clinical relevance, if any, of this subclassification scheme remains to be established (53); however, some investigators have reported that patients with more immature (stage I) T-cell ALL may have an inferior prognosis (52,54).

MIXED LINEAGE LEUKEMIAS

Mixed lineage (biphenotypic) leukemia refers to cases in which both lymphoid- and myeloid-associated surface antigens are expressed on the same cells. Mixed lineage leukemia may arise from a transformed pluripotent stem cell capable of differentiation in either the lymphoid or myeloid pathway, from aberrant gene expression in a committed precursor cell, or from transformation of a normal biphenotypic cell (55). The incidence of mixed lineage leukemia has been reported in up to 20% of cases of ALL (56,57). Biphenotypic ALL is associated with young age at diagnosis (less than 12 months) and also certain chromosomal abnormalities, such as rearrangements of chromosome 11q23 (frequently observed in infants with ALL) and the Philadelphia chromosome [t(9;22)] (58–60). The prognostic significance of biphenotypic ALL remains somewhat controversial. Some studies suggested that such patients had a worse prognosis (61), although most recent reports suggest that myeloid antigen coexpression lacks prognostic significance if treated with more intensive regimens (56,57).

Rarely, one subpopulation of blasts may express lymphoid-associated markers and another subpopulation myeloid-associated markers; such cases have been called *bilineal* (biclonal) *leukemia* and are thought to arise from separate transformation events. Studies with dual labeling techniques, using fluorochrome-monoclonal antibody conjugates, have made it possible to determine if differentiation antigens reside on the same or different blasts.

Cytogenetics and Molecular Genetics

Recently improved techniques for determining chromosome number (ploidy) and identifying structural changes in chromosomes (e.g., translocations, inversions, and deletions) have been applied to the study of leukemia cells from large numbers of patients with ALL. These studies have revealed abnormalities in leukemia cells from more than 90% of children and at least 65% of adults with ALL (62–64). Abnormalities exist in both chromosome number (ploidy) and structure (translocations). Because most children and adults with leukemia have normal constitutional karyotypes, the presence of clonal karyotypic abnormalities in bone marrow cells often provides definitive evidence of malignancy, especially in situations in which leukemic cells have only partially infiltrated the bone marrow (65).

PLOIDY

Ploidy can be determined by karyotypic analysis (counting modal number of chromosomes) or by measuring DNA content by flow cytometry (DNA index) (66). Most cases of childhood ALL are diploid, pseudodiploid, or hyperdiploid. Several investigators have demonstrated the prognostic significance of lymphoblast ploidy in both pediatric and adult ALL, with most favorable outcomes observed in cases of high hyperdiploidy (>50 chromosomes or DNA index ≥1.16) and least favorable in cases of hypodiploidy (<45 chromosomes) (64,66–71).

High hyperdiploidy is observed in approximately 30% of children with ALL (66,69). It occurs more frequently in CD10+, B-progenitor ALL than in mature B-cell, T-cell, or CD10- B-progenitor cases (72). It is also associated with low-risk features at diagnosis, including favorable age and low initial leukocyte count (66). The relatively favorable prognosis of high hyperdiploid ALL may be related to several features, including increased accumulation of intracellular methotrexate polyglutamates (73,74), increased sensitivity to antimetabolite agents (75), and a higher propensity to undergo apoptosis in comparison with other lymphoblasts (76). Among patients with hyperdiploid ALL, those with trisomies 10 and 17 appear to have more favorable prognoses, and those with trisomy 5 or any structural chromosomal abnormalities have relatively inferior outcomes (77,78). Regardless of ploidy, patients with B-progenitor ALL and trisomies of both chromosomes 4 and 10 have a very favorable prognosis (79).

STRUCTURAL CHROMOSOMAL ABNORMALITIES

Table 25-2 shows the distribution of chromosomal translocations, genes affected, and incidence of each genetic abnormality in childhood ALL and the association of these changes with immunophenotype. Most of the nonrandom structural chromosomal abnormalities found in children with ALL are also found in adults with this disease, although the frequency of specific abnormalities may differ considerably. For example, 15% to 30% of adults with ALL have the Philadelphia chromosome, as com-

TABLE 25-2. Nonrandom Chromosomal Translocations in Childhood Acute Lymphoblastic Leukemia (ALL)

Nonrandom Translocation	Involved Genes	Frequency (%)
B-progenitor ALL		
t(12;22)(p13;q22)	TEL, AML1	20–25
t(9;22)(q34;q11)	ABL, BCR	3–5
t(1;19)(q23;p13)	PBX1, E2A	5–6
t(17;19)(q22;p13)	HLF, E2A	<1
t(4;11)(q21;q23)	AF-4, MLL	2–3
t(11;19)(q23;p13)	MLL, ENL	<1
t(9;11)(p21-p22;q23)	AF-9, MLL	<1
t(5;14)(q31;q32)	IL3, IgH	<1
T-cell ALL		
t(11;14)(p15;q11)	LMO1, TCR	—
t(11;14)(p13;q11)	LMO2, TCR	—
t(10;14)(q24;q11)	HOX11, TCR	—
t(1;14)(p32-p34;q11)	TAL1, TCR	—
t(7;19)(q35;p13)	TCR, LYL1	—
t(8;14)(q24;q11)	MYC, TCR	—
Mature B-cell ALL		
t(8;14)(q24;q32)	MYC, IgH	2–3
t(8;22)(q24;q11)	MYC, IgLambda	<1
t(2;8)(p11-p12;q24)	IgKappa, MYC	<1

NOTE: Frequency estimates represent percentage of all newly diagnosed children with ALL with translocation based on karyotypic analysis. Frequency estimates for T-cell ALL translocations are not well characterized.

pared with a frequency of approximately 2% to 5% in pediatric patients (63,64,80,81).

Recurring chromosomal abnormalities have made it possible to pinpoint genetic lesions that appear to be involved in the molecular origin or progression of leukemia. For example, immunophenotype-specific translocations often have breakpoints that involve genes encoding immunoglobulin or T-cell receptor genes (Table 25-2). Also, several protooncogenes, including c-*myc* in Burkitt lymphoma and c-*abl* in ALL with the Philadelphia (Ph) chromosome [t(9;22)], have been linked to malignant transformation (65,82–86). Further identification and molecular characterization of such genes promise major advances in the understanding and treatment of ALL.

TEL/AML1 Gene Fusion. The *TEL/AML1* gene rearrangement, which fuses the *TEL* gene on chromosome 12p13 with the *AML1* gene on chromosome 21q22, is the most common structural abnormality yet identified in childhood ALL, occurring in approximately 20% to 25% of children with B-progenitor ALL (87–89). This translocation is much less frequently observed in adults (88,90). *TEL/AML1* fusions are cryptic by conventional cytogenetics but detectable using reverse transcriptase-polymerase chain reaction (PCR), Southern blot, and fluorescence *in situ* hybridization (91). They are frequently associated with deletion of the nontranslocated allele of *TEL* (92). They are also associated with favorable presenting features at diagnosis, including age and CD10+ B-progenitor phenotype (88,93). Based on retrospective data, several investigators have reported that the *TEL/AML1* fusion is associated with a very favorable outcome, with long-term event-free survival (EFS) rates exceeding 90% (88,93). However, there are conflicting data regarding the incidence of *TEL/AML1* fusion in patients at the time of relapse. Some investigators have reported a very low frequency at relapse (consistent with the hypothesis that *TEL/AML1* patients respond favorably to initial therapy) (94,95), whereas others have reported the frequency of *TEL/AML1* fusion at relapse is similar to that at initial diagnosis (suggesting that *TEL/AML1* fusion may not confer a reduced risk of relapse) (96,97). These discrepant results suggest that the prognosis of *TEL/AML1*-positive patients may, in part, be therapy-dependent. For example, *in vitro* drug sensitivity testing of *TEL/AML1*-positive lymphoblasts suggests a relative sensitivity to L-asparaginase (98), consistent with the finding that *TEL/AML1*-postive patients seemed to fare best with regimens that include intensive use of this agent (88,94). Results from prospective clinical studies will help to further clarify which therapies most effectively treat this patient subgroup.

Philadelphia Chromosome. The t(9;22)(q34;q11) translocation, originally identified in patients with chronic myelogenous leukemia, is found in approximately 2% to 5% of children and 15% to 30% of adults with ALL (63,64,99). Its frequency increases with age. The t(9;22) translocation involves the *ABL* gene on chromosome 9 and the *BCR* region on chromosome 22. In chronic myelogenous leukemia, the fusion transcript encodes a 210-kd hybrid protein (p210), whereas in ALL, a 185- to 190-kd hybrid protein (p190) is formed (83,84,100). Both fusion proteins exhibit tyrosine kinase activity (101). Philadelphia chromosome–positive ALL is associated with B-progenitor, CD10+ phenotype, and hyperleukocytosis (80,102). Both pediatric and adult patients with this translocation respond poorly to conventional chemotherapy, with high rates of induction failure and relapse (102). Long-term EFS estimates for these patients range from 0% to 25% (63,64,80,81,102), although some investigators have recently identified patient subsets who may respond better to intensive chemotherapy, such as those with low initial leukocyte counts or a favorable peripheral blood response to corticosteroids (103,104). Most patients with Philadelphia chromosome–positive ALL in first remission are treated with an allogeneic stem cell transplant, with estimated leukemia-free survival rates ranging between 30% and 40% (105–107). A report of 320 pediatric patients demonstrated that matched related donor transplant was associated with a lower risk of treatment failure compared with chemotherapy (102).

MLL Gene Rearrangements. Structural abnormalities of the *MLL* gene, located at chromosome 11q23, have been observed in approximately 80% of infants with ALL and between 5% and 10% of older children and adults (41,63,108). The most common *MLL* gene rearrangement is the t(4;11)(q21;q23), which fuses the *MLL* and *AF4* genes (109). Other common fusion partner genes are located on chromosomes 9 and 19. Molecular techniques, such as Southern blot analysis and reverse transcriptase PCR, more sensitively detect *MLL* rearrangements than do standard cytogenetics. *MLL* gene rearrangements are associated with a very young age at diagnosis (less than 6 months of age), very high presenting leukocyte counts, increased frequency of CNS leukemia at presentation, absence of CD10 expression, and presence of myeloid antigen coexpression (41,42,108,110). Infants with *MLL* gene expression have a dismal prognosis, with long-term EFS rates ranging from 10% to 30% (41,42,108). The prognosis of older patients with *MLL* gene rearrangements is more controversial, with some investigators suggesting that such patients may fare better than infants, especially older patients with *MLL* rearrangements that do not involve the AF4 gene (59,111). Others have reported that all patients with MLL gene rearrangements respond poorly to treatment, regardless of presenting age (110).

E2A/PBX1. The t(1;19)(q23;q11) translocation occurs in approximately 5% of childhood ALL and slightly less fre-

quently in adults (64,99). It is strongly associated with the pre-B (cIg+) subset of B-progenitor ALL and is present in 25% of cases with intracytoplasmic immunoglobulin (99). The translocation fuses the transcriptional activation domain of the *E2A* gene (on chromosome 19p) with the DNA binding domain of *PBX1* (on chromosome 1) (112–114). Initial studies suggested that the t(1;19) was associated with inferior outcomes (46), although recent studies suggest that with more intensive therapy, presence of the t(1;19) no longer has prognostic significance (115,116). Another fusion partner of the *E2A* gene, the *HLF* gene on chromosome 17(q21-q22), has been identified in childhood ALL (117,118). Because of its infrequent occurrence, distinct clinical features and prognostic significance of the t(17;19) have not been fully elucidated. Case reports suggest that this translocation is associated with disseminated intravascular coagulation at diagnosis in patients with B-progenitor immunophenotype (118).

Chromosome 9p Deletions. Deletions of chromosome 9p21-22 have been reported in up to 10% of cases of childhood ALL (119) and in a higher proportion of cases when molecular techniques are used in addition to karyotypic analysis (120–122). Chromosome 9p deletions appear to involve the interferon-α and β-1 genes (120), as well as the site of two cyclin D kinase inhibitors, p16 and p15 (121,122). 9p deletions are more frequently observed in patients who are older and have higher presenting white blood cell (WBC) counts and T-cell immunophenotype, but they are not restricted to this subset of patients (119).

T-Cell Receptor Gene Rearrangements. Several recurrent translocations have been described in T-cell ALL, many of which involve translocations of transcription factor genes to T-cell receptor loci located on chromosomes 7 or 14 (123,124). Involved transcription factors include *TAL1* (chromosome 1), *HOX 11* (chromosome 10), *LMO1/LMO2* (chromosome 11), and *LYL1* (chromosome 19). The *TAL1* gene on chromosome 1 is translocated to chromosome 14 in approximately 5% of childhood T-cell ALL (125). Using molecular techniques, partial *TAL1* deletions (which lead to an overexpression of the protein) have been identified in approximately 25% of T-cell cases (126–128). The t(10;14)(q24;q11), involving the *HOX 11* gene on chromosome 10, has been identified in approximately 5% of T-cell cases (124), as has the t(11;14), involving either the *LMO1* gene at chromosome 11p15 or the *LMO2* gene at 11p13 (123,129). A translocation involving the *myc* oncogene on chromosome 8q24 and the T-cell receptor locus on chromosome 14 has been described in patients with T-cell ALL and may be associated with a poor prognosis (130). This translocation is similar to that seen in mature B-cell ALL, in which *myc* is translocated to the immunoglobulin heavy chain gene on chromosome 14, resulting in overexpression of *myc*.

Immunoglobulin Gene Rearrangements. Nearly all adults and children with mature B-cell ALL have a pseudodiploid karyotype with a t(8;14)(q24;q23), involving the *myc* oncogene on chromosome 8 and the IgH gene on chromosome 14 (32,85). The t(8;14) translocation is the predominant translocation observed in Burkitt lymphoma, and patients with mature B-cell phenotype and the t(8;14) translocation are much more successfully treated on therapy used for Burkitt rather than standard ALL regimens (33,34). Alternative translocations observed less frequently in mature B-cell ALL and Burkitt lymphoma include t(2;8)(p11–13;q24) and t(8;22)(q24;q11), involving the *myc* gene on chromosome 8 and the light chain gene loci on chromosomes 2 or 22 (131,132). All of these translocations lead to overexpression of the *myc* oncogene.

The t(5;14)(q31;q32) has been described in B-precursor ALL, involving the interleukin-3 gene on chromosome 5 and the IgH gene on chromosome 14 (133). This translocation, resulting in an overexpression of interleukin-3, is characterized by hypereosinophilia at the time of diagnosis (133,134).

DIAGNOSIS

The diagnosis of ALL can be made in most patients by physical examination and assessment of the complete blood count and bone marrow specimen. The diagnosis cannot be made from examination of the peripheral blood smear alone. Lymphoblasts can be absent in a stained peripheral blood smear; also, some children have activated and atypical blood lymphocytes due to viral infections which can be confused with lymphoblasts even by experienced hematologists. Thus, it is essential to examine an adequate sample of well-stained bone marrow. In most cases, marrow is hypercellular with 60% to 100% blast cells, scattered normal myeloid or erythroid precursors, and few (if any) detectable megakaryocytes. By convention, at least 25% of the nucleated marrow cells must be blasts to establish the diagnosis of acute leukemia; if the FAB morphologic subtype is lymphoid and the myeloperoxidase stain is negative or the immunophenotype confirms a lymphoid rather than myeloid precursor, a diagnosis of ALL can be made. Packed red blood transfusion rarely alters bone marrow morphologic findings; hence, this supportive therapy can be given before marrow aspiration. Figure 25-4 illustrates the important steps in the initial evaluation of a patient with suspected ALL.

The frequencies of clinical and laboratory abnormalities commonly observed in children with ALL are shown in Table 25-1, according to immunophenotype. No indication has been found that these features differ substantially in adults. Patients with ALL present most frequently with signs and symptoms of leukemic cell infiltration of the marrow and other organs, including the failure of normal hematopoiesis. The differences noted among the immunophenotypic groups probably reflect basic biologic differences in these ALL subtypes. Peripheral blood counts and physical findings are almost always abnormal at the time of presentation, although the degree of abnormality varies widely. In rare cases, peripheral blood findings or physical examination may be normal.

Nearly all patients with acute leukemia have peripheral blood abnormalities at diagnosis. A normocytic anemia (usually with a low reticulocyte count) is present in the majority of patients, as is thrombocytopenia (platelet counts <100,000/ mm^3). Many patients present with severe neutropenia (<500 granulocytes/mm^3). Leukocyte counts are elevated above 50,000/mm^3 in approximately 20% of cases (135).

Fever at presentation may be due to infection (usually viral or bacterial) or to undetermined causes. Rarely, such fever reflects fungal or protozoan infections. Establishing a precise cause of fever is often difficult, but it should be attempted. Pallor, which is seen in most patients, is caused by low hemoglobin levels due to bone marrow infiltration by leukemic cells, leading to inadequate erythrocyte production. Malaise may be due to anemia, infection, or unknown causes. Bruising and petechiae are common and are usually secondary to thrombocytopenia resulting from replacement of normal marrow by lymphoblasts. Bleeding and hemorrhage is rarely observed. Disseminated intravascular coagulation is occasionally observed in patients with T-cell ALL as a result of thromboplastic substances released from T lymphoblasts (136). Bone

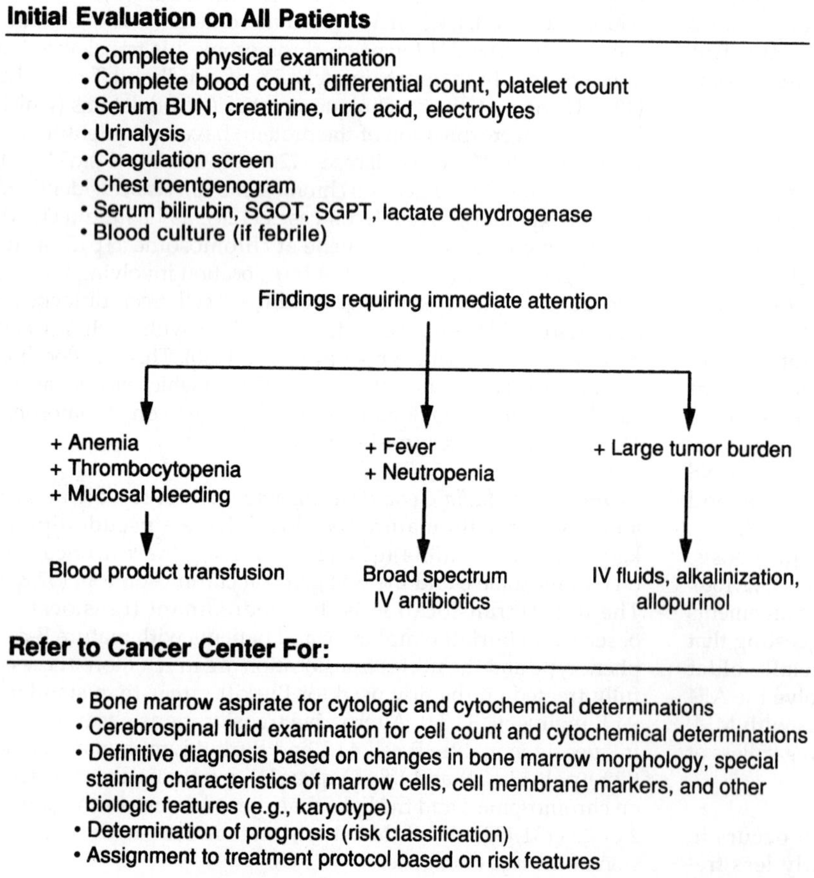

Initial Evaluation on All Patients

- Complete physical examination
- Complete blood count, differential count, platelet count
- Serum BUN, creatinine, uric acid, electrolytes
- Urinalysis
- Coagulation screen
- Chest roentgenogram
- Serum bilirubin, SGOT, SGPT, lactate dehydrogenase
- Blood culture (if febrile)

Findings requiring immediate attention

+ Anemia
+ Thrombocytopenia
+ Mucosal bleeding

+ Fever
+ Neutropenia

+ Large tumor burden

Blood product transfusion

Broad spectrum IV antibiotics

IV fluids, alkalinization, allopurinol

Refer to Cancer Center For:

- Bone marrow aspirate for cytologic and cytochemical determinations
- Cerebrospinal fluid examination for cell count and cytochemical determinations
- Definitive diagnosis based on changes in bone marrow morphology, special staining characteristics of marrow cells, cell membrane markers, and other biologic features (e.g., karyotype)
- Determination of prognosis (risk classification)
- Assignment to treatment protocol based on risk features

Figure 25-4. Flow diagram of the important steps in the initial evaluation and management of patients with newly diagnosed acute lymphoblastic leukemia. BUN, blood urea nitrogen; SGOT, serum glutamic-oxaloacetic transaminase; SGPT, serum glutamic-pyruvic transaminase.

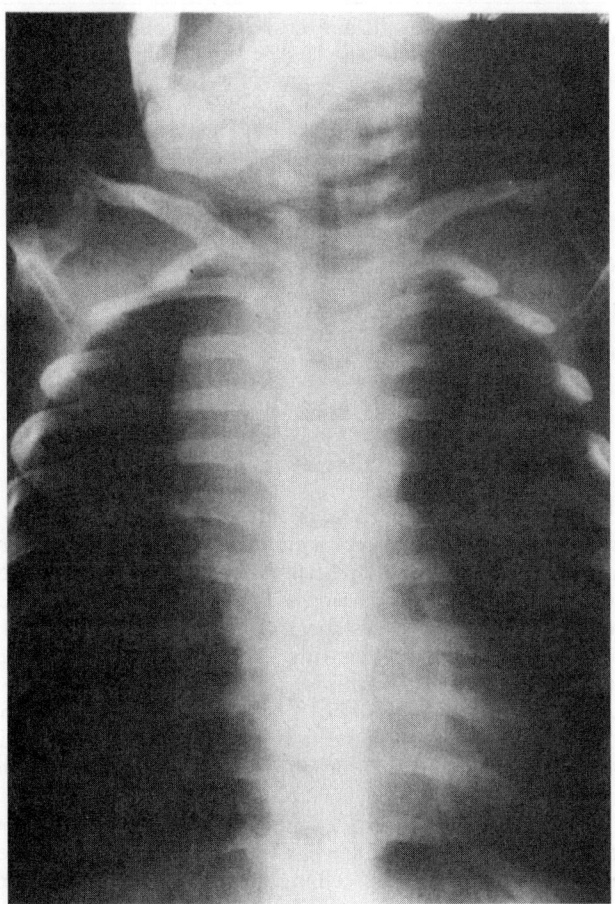

Figure 25-5. Chest roentgenogram showing an anterior mediastinal mass in a child with newly diagnosed acute lymphoblastic leukemia.

and joint pain are thought to reflect leukemia infiltration with secondary stretching of the periosteum or joint capsule, which contains sensory nerve endings. Children frequently present with limp or refusal to walk. Lymphadenopathy and hepatosplenomegaly, two frequently observed signs of ALL, often result from infiltration by leukemic cells. Signs and symptoms of CNS involvement are rarely observed at diagnosis. Respiratory distress and failure may result from an anterior mediastinal thymic mass, observed most frequently in T-cell ALL; thus, a chest roentgenogram should be performed in all patients at the time of diagnosis to exclude this potentially life-threatening condition (Fig. 25-5).

DIFFERENTIAL DIAGNOSIS

At the time of diagnosis, ALL may present with signs and symptoms of other malignant and nonmalignant conditions. The differential diagnosis of ALL includes other forms of leukemia, idiopathic thrombocytopenic purpura (ITP), aplastic anemia, juvenile rheumatoid arthritis, acute infectious mononucleosis, neutropenic conditions, metastatic solid tumors with marrow involvement, and advanced stage non-Hodgkin's lymphoma.

ITP can be distinguished from ALL with relative ease because isolated thrombocytopenia, often with large platelets seen on a blood smear, contrasts sharply with the more generalized blood cell abnormalities and small platelets typically observed in patients with ALL (137). Physical findings in ITP are usually limited to bruising or bleeding associated with thrombocytopenia. An occasional patient develops modest splenomegaly, probably caused by a recent viral infection. In most cases, the leukocyte level and differential count are unremarkable, and there is no anemia unless bleeding has been substantial or an unrelated anemia is present. If doubt exists, a bone marrow aspirate is diagnostic because the marrow elements appear normal or show increased megakaryocytes. Adults with ITP are more likely than children to have associated serious diseases, such as malignancy or collagen vascular disease.

Patients with aplastic anemia usually present with pancytopenia without blast cells in blood or bone marrow; blood cell precursors are either decreased or absent in a bone marrow biopsy specimen. Organs are not usually enlarged. Rarely, patients with ALL present with pancytopenia and have areas of bone marrow that are fibrotic and empty, impeding diagnosis. Repeated bone marrow aspirates or biopsies establish the correct diagnosis by demonstrating areas of marrow that are infiltrated with lymphoblasts.

Presenting symptoms shared by juvenile rheumatoid arthritis and ALL include lymphadenopathy, splenomegaly, pallor, fever, anemia, and joint pain. Some patients with positive antinuclear antibody tests have been later shown to have ALL (138). Bone marrow aspiration before beginning corticosteroid therapy for presumed juvenile rheumatoid arthritis should be performed to definitively rule out ALL.

Patients with acute infectious mononucleosis syndrome due to Epstein-Barr virus, cytomegalovirus, or *Toxoplasma* infection may have symptoms and signs similar to those seen in patients with ALL. Usually, the neutrophil and platelet counts remain normal in infectious mononucleosis, even when there is marked leukocytosis with atypical mononuclear cells (139). However, thrombocytopenia and anemia can be observed when there is marked splenomegaly. The diagnosis of infectious mononucleosis can usually be serologically confirmed. Bone marrow aspirate findings may be difficult to interpret in infectious mononucleosis because of atypical lymphocytosis. Rarely, patients with ALL may also have coexisting infectious mononucleosis.

Patients with congenital or acquired neutropenia or sepsis may present with neutropenia. No proliferation of lymphoid cells occurs, so confusion with ALL is unlikely in most cases. For the few patients with ALL who present with neutropenia as the primary abnormality, a bone marrow examination usually provides a definitive diagnosis.

ALL can usually be distinguished from other forms of leukemia based on morphology, histochemical stains, and immunophenotype, as discussed above. The morphology of lymphoblasts in ALL is generally sufficiently different from that of Sézary cells, plasma cells, or hairy cells to avoid confusion with these disorders. Occasionally, a case of ALL has relatively mature-appearing lymphoid cells, leading to some difficulty, on morphologic grounds alone, in distinguishing between this disease and chronic lymphocytic leukemia, which is characterized by relatively mature cells. The vastly different usual age at diagnosis (0 to 30 years for ALL and 30 or more years for chronic lymphocytic leukemia), presenting features, clinical courses, and complications of these two diseases make a distinction relatively easy.

Children with neuroblastoma frequently have malignant involvement of liver, lymph nodes, bone, or bone marrow; the marrow involvement may be extensive. Occasionally, neuroblasts are found on a peripheral blood smear, and their appearance may resemble that of lymphoblasts. A palpable or radiographically demonstrable abdominal nonhepatic mass is usually discernible, suggesting the true diagnosis. Neuroblasts tend to cluster and form pseudorosettes, in contrast to the diffuse involvement generally observed in ALL. The diagnosis can be confirmed by measurement of urinary catecholamines, radiologic examination, and biopsy of the mass. Other tumors (rhabdomyosarcoma, Ewing's sarcoma, or carcinomas) with extensive marrow involvement may also enter the differential diagnosis. If questions remain after bone marrow examination, including cytochemical, immunophenotypic, and cytogenetic evaluations, electron microscopy may disclose neurosecretory granules or other features helpful in specific diagnosis; use of monoclonal antibodies (conjugated to fluorochromes) to lineage-specific or lineage-associated cell-surface antigens may also be useful

There is some controversy regarding the distinction between ALL and advanced stage non-Hodgkin's lymphoma with bone marrow and blood involvement. The distinction between lymphoblastic lymphoma with marrow involvement and ALL with lymphomatous features has been arbitrarily defined, with many institutions using a cutoff of 25% or more blast cells in the bone marrow to define leukemia. The distinction may not be clinically important because advanced stage lymphoma and ALL of similar immunophenotype respond similarly to intensive ALL-type therapy (140,141).

CLINICAL OUTCOME AND PROGNOSTIC FACTORS

Tables 25-3 and 25-4 summarize EFS for children and overall survival (OS) rates for adults with ALL. In general, 70% to 80% of children and 30% to 50% of adults are cured of their disease. By comparing the presenting features of those patients who are cured with those who relapse, investigators have identified clinical and laboratory features that are prognostically significant. The ability to identify reliable prognostic factors has contributed importantly to explanations of disease outcome and to the design and evaluation of treatment protocols. An array of clinical and lymphoblast biologic features have been found to be prognostically significant, including age, presenting leukocyte count, immunophenotype, chromosomal abnormalities (ploidy, translocations), the presence of overt CNS leukemia at diagnosis, and the rapidity with which patients respond to initial induction chemotherapy (135). It is important to recognize that the impact of any prognostic factor depends on the efficacy of therapy—the single most clinicalinfluential predictor outcome.

TABLE 25-3. Results of Research Protocols for Acute Lymphoblastic Leukemia in Children

Study	No. of Children	5-Yr Event-Free Survival (%)	Reference
BFM-90 (1990–1995)	2178	78	148,149
CCG 1800–1900 series (1989–1995)	5121	75	244
DFCI 91-01 (1991–1995)	377	83	1,50
POG AlinC14 and 15 (1986–1994)	3828	71	239
SJCRH Total Therapy 13A (1991–1994)	165	77	182

TABLE 25-4. Results of Research Protocols for Acute Lymphoblastic Leukemia in Adults

Study	No. of Adults	Overall Survival (%)	Reference
MD Anderson (1992–1998)	204	39 at 5 yr	274
CALGB 8811 (1988–1991)	214	50 at 3 yr	143
HOVON (1988–1992)	130	22 at 5 yr	273
GIMEMA 0183 (1983–1987)	358	25 at 10 yr	272
GMALL 02/84 (1983–1987)	569	36 at 7 yr	271

Age

The age of patients with ALL significantly correlates with clinical outcome. In childhood ALL, infants and adolescents have a worse prognosis in comparison with patients in the intermediate age group (1). ALL in infancy (<1 year of age at diagnosis) is associated with high presenting leukocyte counts, increased frequency of CNS leukemia at presentation, and, as noted above, a very high frequency of *MLL* gene rearrangements (41,42,108,110). Infants, especially those with *MLL* gene rearrangements, have a dismal prognosis, with long-term EFS rates ranging from 10% to 30% (41,42,108).

Adolescents (ages 10 to 21 years) also have a relatively poor prognosis compared to other children with ALL. ALL in adolescence is associated with T-cell immunophenotype, higher presenting leukocyte levels, male predominance, and a lower incidence of the potentially favorable *TEL/AML1* gene rearrangement (88,142). Also, because of their unique stage of psychologic and physical development, adolescents often experience serious side effects and adjustment problems related to the diagnosis and treatment of ALL, both of which may impact their response to therapy (1).

The poor prognosis of ALL in adults in comparison to children is well known. Adults have a higher incidence of T-cell immunophenotype and of Philadelphia chromosome–positive ALL (2). In addition, adults experience more toxicity from intensive ALL regimens than do pediatric patients (49). Within the adult population, prognosis becomes worse with increasing age (143).

Leukocyte Count

In many series, the initial leukocyte count is a significant predictor of treatment outcome, with worsening outcomes as the leukocyte count increases (135). Since 1996, based on the recommendation of the Cancer Therapy Evaluation Program of the National Cancer Institute, many investigators consider a leukocyte count of $50 \times 10^9/L$ as the level separating patients with an unfavorable prognosis from those more likely to have a durable response (135). Within the context of intensive chemotherapy, some investigators have reported that presenting leukocyte count no longer has prognostic significance (1).

Immunophenotype

Historically, immunophenotype was an important predictor of outcome, with adverse prognoses observed in patients with mature B-cell and T-cell disease. With more intensive regimens, T-cell phenotype in childhood ALL no longer has prognostic significance, as such patients fare as well as those with B-progenitor disease (1). Interestingly, the T-cell phenotype in adults does not always connote a poor prognosis (144). As noted above, mature B-cell ALL is more effectively treated with the same therapy used for advanced stage Burkitt lymphoma.

Some investigators have reported prognostic differences within subsets of patients with B-progenitor ALL. Initial studies suggested that patients with pre-B ALL (cIg⁺) had a worse outcome than those with early pre-B ALL (cIg⁻) (45). Subsequent reports indicated that the adverse outcome of pre-B ALL was due to the subset with the t(1;19) translocation (46), and with greater treatment intensity, even patients with this cytogenetic abnormality may not have adverse prognosis (115,116). Preliminary findings suggested that children and adults with mixed lineage or bilineal leukemia fare less well than other patients with ALL (61); however, more recent reports indicate that myeloid antigen coexpression is not prognostically significant (56,57).

Chromosomal Abnormalities

As noted earlier, several recurrent chromosomal abnormalities are important predictors of outcome in childhood ALL. Favorable prognosis is associated with high hyperdiploidy (more than 50 chromosomes or DNA index ≥1.16) and trisomies of chromosome 4 and 10 (66,79,145). Many investigators have reported that patients with the cryptic t(12;21) translocation (*TEL/AML1* gene fusion) have a favorable prognosis, although this finding remains controversial (88,93–97). Adverse chromosomal abnormalities include hypodiploidy (<45 chromosomes) (67,70), rearrangements of the *MLL* gene (chromosome 11q23) (41,42,108,110), and the Philadelphia chromosome [t(9;22)] (63,64,80,81,102). The adverse prognostic significance of the t(1;19) translocation appears to be abrogated with more intensive therapy (115,116).

Early Response to Induction Chemotherapy

The rapidity with which a patient responds to initial induction chemotherapy is a significant predictor of long-term outcome (146). Patients who require two or more cycles of induction chemotherapy to achieve complete remission (CR) have a much worse prognosis than those who achieve CR within a month of diagnosis (147). The Berlin-Frankfurt-Munster (BFM) group treats patients with one week of corticosteroid monotherapy (and one dose of intrathecal methotrexate) before beginning multiagent induction chemotherapy and have reported that poor peripheral blood response at the end of that week (defined as an absolute blast count of 1000/mm³) is an independent predictor of adverse outcome (148,149). Others have reported that the rate of clearance of blasts from the peripheral blood after multiagent chemotherapy is also an independent predictor of relapse (150–152). Similarly, persistence of leukemia in bone marrow specimens obtained 7 or 14 days after beginning multiagent chemotherapy strongly correlates with poor outcome (146), although intensification of therapy can abrogate the adverse prognostic significance of slow early response (153).

Minimal Residual Disease

Many studies have focused on determining the prognostic significance of levels of minimal residual disease (MRD) at various time points in therapy. MRD evaluation involves identification of patient-specific leukemia clones at diagnosis (e.g., chromosomal translocations or patient-specific immunoglobulin or T-cell antigen receptor gene rearrangements) (154). Once patient-specific clones are identified, molecular techniques, such as the PCR, can be used to detect extremely small numbers of residual

leukemia cells in subsequent samples. Initial clinical studies using PCR technology yielded conflicting results. The majority of investigators reported that the presence of detectable residual disease late in treatment or at the completion of therapy was predictive of subsequent relapse (155–157), although some suggested that molecularly detectable leukemia could persist in off-therapy patients who remained in clinical remission (158,159). Additionally, the absence of detectable residual leukemia at the end of chemotherapy was insufficient to assure that a patient was cured (160).

More recently, many investigators have reported that MRD levels early in therapy may be significant predictors of outcome (161–164). In one study performed by the European Organization for Research and Treatment of Cancer group, patients in morphologic remission but with detectable MRD at the end of remission induction were at higher risk of subsequent relapse; increased levels of residual disease correlated with increased relapse rates (161). At all time points measured (during several phases of therapy), the risk of relapse was significantly higher in patients with detectable MRD, especially in those with the highest levels (161). Similar results have been obtained for patients treated on BFM and St. Jude Children's Research Hospital (SJCRH) protocols: High relapse rates were observed for patients with MRD at any time point but especially at the end of induction therapy and early on during postremission therapy (week 12 and week 14 of therapy, respectively) (162,164). On all of these studies, MRD levels were confirmed to be an independent risk factor for relapse by multivariate analyses. High MRD levels measured as early as day 15 of induction therapy have also been correlated with poor outcome (163).

Other Prognostic Factors

Sex, race, and patient-specific factors influencing drug metabolism may also be independent predictors of outcome. Some investigators have reported that males fare worse than female patients (165,166). This observation had been attributed, in part, to the risk of testicular relapse (165), although the higher relapse rate in males were observed even when testicular relapse rates were quite low (166). Race may also influence outcome, with lower EFS rates reported for black and Hispanic patients even after adjustment for differences in prognostically significant presenting features (167,168). The reasons why patients of different sex or race have varying responses to therapy on certain regimens have not been fully elucidated.

Recently, research has suggested that outcome may be affected by how rapidly and effectively an individual patient metabolizes certain chemotherapeutic agents. Polymorphisms within genes involved in chemotherapy drug metabolism have been associated with risk of relapse in childhood ALL. Favorable outcomes have been reported in patients with mutant thiopurine methyltransferase phenotypes (involved in the metabolism of thioguanines, such as 6-mercaptopurine) (169) and with certain polymorphisms of the glutathione S–transferase genes (encoding enzymes involved in the intracellular detoxification of various compounds) (170). In one study, concurrent therapy with long-term anticonvulsants was associated with inferior EFS, perhaps due to anticonvulsant-associated induction of drug-metabolizing enzymes (leading to increased clearance of antileukemia drugs, such as methotrexate) (171). In another randomized study, conventional dosing of methotrexate based on body surface area was compared to individualizing dosing based on pharmacokinetic measurements to adjust for patient-specific clearance of this agent. Individualized dosing was associated with an improvement in outcome in children with B-lineage ALL, suggesting that some relapses on the conventionally dosed arm may have been due to rapid drug clearance (172).

BACKGROUND FOR TREATMENT

Before 1947, when the first CR in childhood ALL was attained by Farber and co-workers (173), the median duration of survival from the time of diagnosis was 2 months (174). During the 1950s, drugs such as 6-mercaptopurine, methotrexate, and corticosteroids were found to be active in leukemia-bearing mice (175) and subsequently in human leukemias (176). The first controlled clinical trials were conducted by Frei and associates (177), who ushered in the era of single-agent (and soon thereafter combination-agent) antileukemic chemotherapy trials (178). Active drugs introduced in the 1960s and 1970s included the anthracyclines (doxorubicin and daunorubicin), asparaginase, and the epipodophyllotoxins (VP-16 and VM-26) (179–181).

Current regimens for the treatment of childhood ALL result in high proportions (>95%) of patients achieving CR and long-term EFS for 70% to 80% of patients (Table 25-3) (1,148,182). This is true despite the fact that, with few exceptions, the drugs used for the treatment of ALL today were all available by the late 1960s. Improvement in outcome over the last 30 to 40 years can be attributed the development of complex chemotherapeutic regimens designed to achieve clonal eradication, improvement in supportive care, the recognition of the CNS as a sanctuary site, and the application of risk-directed therapy.

Critical to the pioneering efforts of early clinical trials was an understanding of the principles of the first-order cytokinetic effect of chemotherapeutic agents and the need for clonal eradication. In the early 1960s, Skipper and associates initiated a series of studies that addressed the quantitative biology of leukemia in mice and its perturbation by chemotherapy (183). The first-order cytokinetic effect of chemotherapy on tumor (leukemia) cells means that for a given treatment there is a constant fractional reduction of leukemia cells that is independent of the total leukemia burden.

From Skipper and colleague's mouse leukemia models, it was shown that the time of death following treatment was a precise measure of the number of leukemia cells persisting at the end of treatment (183,184). They further demonstrated that having only one L1210 leukemic cell present was enough to cause the death of the animal. This observation led to the understanding of the need for clonal eradication. Moreover, their models provided important observations with respect to drug resistance, combination chemotherapy, and the cycling of chemotherapeutic agents. By the 1960s, effective systemic chemotherapy and the development of improved supportive care with blood products and antibiotics resulted in an increased percentage of CRs and an increase in the duration of remissions. The ability to support a patient through prolonged myelosuppression has permitted clinical investigations that have demonstrated the importance of using maximal tolerable doses of drugs (185,186).

In the 1960s, the incidence of CNS leukemia as an initial site of relapse became progressively more common (187,188), and the concept of the CNS as a "pharmacologic sanctuary" (i.e., an anatomic space that is poorly penetrated by systemically administered chemotherapeutic agents) emerged. Several avenues of approach to the problem of CNS leukemia and its treatment and prevention have been explored. These include intrathecal administration of drugs (189,190), craniospinal irradiation (191), cranial irradiation with intrathecal drugs (192), and high doses of systemically administered drugs that result in therapeutic concentrations in the cerebrospinal fluid (193,194).

The optimal delivery of CNS treatment remains controversial (see below).

Risk-Adapted Therapy

An important concept in the treatment of ALL in children is risk-directed therapy. Clinical trials conducted during the 1970s and early 1980s established groups of patients whose risk of subsequent relapse varied according to different characteristics. Current clinical trials use these outcome predictors to stratify therapy. For example, children with the least likelihood of relapse can be assessed to determine whether some of the more morbid components of therapy can be modified or eliminated. In contrast, individuals at a greater risk of relapse can be more intensively treated, and the potential higher risks of such intensified therapy can be limited to only these patients.

For many years, pediatric cooperative groups and institutions applied prognostic factors differently when defining risk categories. A more uniform approach to risk classification was proposed and agreed on at a National Cancer Institute sponsored workshop held in 1993 (135). For patients with B-precursor ALL, the "standard" risk category was defined as an age between 1 and 9 years and an initial leukocyte count lower than $50,000/mm^3$. Other presenting features used by some investigators to classify patients as "standard" risk included hyperdiploidy (DNA index >1.16) and trisomy of chromosomes 4 and 10. The remaining patients were considered to have "high" risk ALL. Other characteristics used by the various cooperative groups to classify patients as "high" risk include T-cell phenotype, certain cytogenetic translocations [e.g., t(9;22)], overt CNS leukemia at diagnosis, and slow early response to induction chemotherapy (135). Ultimately, treatment is the most important prognostic factor, and those factors which are used to risk-stratify patients on one regimen may be irrelevant for patients treated on a different regimen.

SUPPORTIVE CARE

Supportive care is an important determinant of outcome in children with acute leukemia. Before instituting chemotherapy, patients must be assessed and treated for any metabolic disturbances, hematologic abnormalities, and presumed or documented infections.

Rapid turnover of leukemia cells before and immediately following the initiation of chemotherapy leads to the release of intracellular contents, which can overwhelm the body's normal excretory mechanisms. The resultant metabolic disturbances include hyperkalemia, hyperuricemia, hyperphosphatemia, and hypocalcemia. Patients with high levels of uric acid are at risk for the development of acute renal failure secondary to uric acid deposition in the kidney (195). To ensure that uric acid remains in solution within the renal tubule for optimal excretion, intravenous hydration (usually with twice the maintenance volumes of fluids) and urinary alkalinization (pH 7 to 8), usually with bicarbonate-containing intravenous fluid, should be instituted immediately after diagnosis. In addition, administration of a xanthine oxidase inhibitor such as allopurinol should be started before institution of antileukemic drugs. Allopurinol prevents the formation of uric acid during cell lysis. For patients with WBC counts above $200,000/mm^3$, leukapheresis has been advocated to prevent hyperviscosity and lysis-related problems (196).

Thrombocytopenia, in association with neutropenia and anemia, is a common presenting feature of ALL (137); however, active bleeding is a relatively unusual feature at the time of diagnosis. Despite this fact, most investigators recommend prophylactic platelet transfusions for patients with thrombocytopenia, as opposed to transfusions only for active bleeding. Prophylactic transfusions have frequently been given when platelet counts fall below 15,000 to 20,000/mm³. A study of adults with AML demonstrated the safety of decreasing the prophylactic platelet transfusion threshold to a platelet count of 10,000/mm³ in clinically stable patients (197). Any active hemorrhage associated with a platelet count of less than 100,000/mm³ should be treated with platelet transfusions. Similarly, symptomatic anemia should be treated by transfusion of packed red blood cells. Most investigators recommend prophylactic transfusions for a hematocrit below 20 to 25 volume percent. Stabilization of these two hematologic parameters should take no longer than 12 to 24 hours and should therefore not delay the start of antileukemia therapy.

Patients should also be treated intensively for any documented or presumed infection before beginning chemotherapy (198). For a temperature above 38.5°C, broad-spectrum intravenous antibiotic coverage should be given after obtaining cultures but before laboratory confirmation of an infectious etiology. Chemotherapy should be started as soon as possible after diagnosis despite the need for antibiotics. Although newly diagnosed patients might not have severe neutropenia (granulocyte counts < 500/mm³), the usual state of marrow replacement with lymphoblasts and the anticipated marrow hypocellularity associated with antileukemia treatment make such antibiotic recommendations prudent. One series, which included pediatric patients already receiving chemotherapy, documented bacteremia in 21% of episodes of fever and neutropenia (199).

Various approaches have been used to prevent or reduce infections in patients once they have commenced with treatment. Prophylaxis with trimethoprim-sulfamethoxazole, usually from the time of CR, successfully prevents *Pneumocystis carinii* pneumonia (200). The optimal use of hematologic growth factors, such as granulocyte colony-stimulating factor (G-CSF), remains a matter of controversy. In prospective randomized studies, the use of G-CSF in children and adults receiving intensive therapy for ALL was associated with a shorter duration of neutropenia and a tighter adherence to the planned treatment schedule (201–204). However, although some investigators reported a significantly decreased incidence in severe infections in patients treated with G-CSF during ALL therapy (201,204), others have not confirmed this finding (202,203). Also, G-CSF treatment did not prolong survival or reduce the cost of supportive care for children with ALL (202).

PHASES OF THERAPY

In general, current treatment regimens for patients with newly diagnosed ALL include four phases—remission induction, intensification (or consolidation), continuation, and CNS treatment. The remission induction phase of therapy is designed to rapidly destroy measurable leukemic cells and minimize residual leukemia burden (i.e., the total number of leukemic cells in the body). The CNS treatment phase is used to address the issue of pharmacologic sanctuary sites (i.e., areas of the body, such as the brain and spinal cord, that are not well penetrated by conventional doses of most antileukemic drugs). The intensification (or consolidation) phase is designed to further reduce the total body leukemic cell burden and address issues of antileukemic drug resistance. Such treatment usually consists of higher doses of the same drugs used during induction, or of high doses of different drugs.

The continuation phase is designed to eradicate the residual leukemic cell burden. In the past, this part of treatment was referred to as *maintenance therapy*. However, because the current concept is to eradicate all remaining leukemia cells, as opposed to maintaining a low tumor burden, the newer terminology is preferred.

Remission Induction

As soon as the patient has been stabilized by the supportive measures discussed above, antileukemic chemotherapy is begun. The goal of induction therapy is to rapidly induce a CR. *Hematologic remission* is defined as attainment of a normocellular bone marrow with 5% or fewer blasts and peripheral blood without lymphoblasts and with a granulocyte count exceeding 500/mm³ and a platelet count exceeding 100,000/mm³. CR is defined as achievement of the above criteria plus the absence of any demonstrable signs and symptoms of leukemia. A CR must be induced before the next component of therapy is begun and is therefore essential in prolonging survival. The duration of most induction regimens is 3 to 4 weeks.

Using a two-drug regimen of weekly vincristine and daily prednisone, nearly 90% of children with ALL will achieve remission at the end of one month of therapy (205,206). With the addition of a third agent, such as asparaginase or an anthracycline, CRs can be induced in approximately 95% of children with ALL (207,208). In addition to improving remission rates, intensified three-drug induction regimens also prolong remission duration. The importance of induction intensity in determining OS was demonstrated in a study conducted at the Dana-Farber Cancer Institute (DFCI), in which children were randomly assigned to receive identical therapy except for induction drugs; one group received vincristine and prednisone and the other received those two drugs plus an anthracycline. Although the CR rates for both groups exceeded 90%, there was long-term benefit for the more intensively treated group (EFS for the two groups at 16 years were 37% and 63%, respectively) (208,209). In theory, the more intensive induction regimen may prevent the emergence of drug-resistant leukemic clones by an initial leukemic cell lysis of greater rapidity and magnitude (210).

Based on the hypothesis that early intensity may improve EFS, many groups have further intensified induction regimens. The benefit in terms of long-term survival of using four drugs during induction therapy (vincristine, prednisone, asparaginase, and an anthracycline) is widely accepted in higher risk patients (211) but less clear in lower risk patients (212). Other agents that have been added to induction regimens include alkylators (such as cyclophosphamide) (148,182), epipodophyllotoxins (teniposide, etoposide) (182), and antimetabolites (cytarabine, methotrexate) (50,148). Even with very intensive induction regimens, very few toxic deaths are reported (1,149).

Pharmacologic sanctuary sites, such as the CNS, should be treated during remission induction. Some commonly used systemic drugs such as glucocorticoids and asparaginase effectively treat CNS leukemic cells, but intrathecal agents such as cytarabine and methotrexate are also recommended. Intrathecal cytarabine has the advantage of having no additive myelosuppression because it is immediately inactivated by deaminases when it enters the blood.

Even after the induction of CR, leukemic cells remain in the marrow, undetected by light microscopy, and further therapy is necessary to achieve cure. Indirect evidence for this observation was derived from early clinical trials in which chemotherapy was stopped after induction of a clinical CR; all patients relapsed within 6 months (213). It is the remaining tumor burden that necessitates postinduction treatment. The use of PCR technology may aid in assessing whether the rate or degree of initial cell killing will be a predictive factor for long-term survival (see above).

Failure to achieve remission after 1 month of therapy (induction failure) is uncommon in children, occurring in fewer than 5% of patients (147). Successful treatment of refractory ALL has been reported with the use of drugs such as cytarabine, teniposide, daunomycin, and idarubicin (214–217). However, even after achieving remission, OS for patients with a history of initial induction failure is very poor (147), and these patients should be considered candidates for allogeneic stem cell transplant or other intensive therapies.

Treatment of the Central Nervous System

All current treatment regimens for ALL include therapy directed at treating CNS leukemia. In the 1960s, as systemic chemotherapy became more effective in prolonging the duration of hematologic remission in patients with ALL, investigators recognized that CNS recurrence represented a major cause of treatment failure. It was hypothesized that leukemic cells, even if subclinical, were present in the CNS in all patients, and that these cells were protected by the blood–brain barrier from systemically administered chemotherapy. The introduction of effective therapy for subclinical CNS leukemia in the 1970s was a pivotal step in boosting long-term disease-free survival rates in childhood ALL (218).

CNS-directed therapy is usually initiated during induction therapy, and definitive CNS treatment is usually begun immediately after induction of CR (to prevent seeding from the CNS to the periphery). This concept is based on data from the 1960s that demonstrated that most children who developed CNS leukemia did so during the first year of therapy. However, some clinical trials have delayed definitive CNS treatment for several months to permit more intensive systemic therapy (219,220). In these studies, there was no increase in CNS relapse, except in patients who had presented with leukemic blasts in their cerebrospinal fluid at diagnosis (221).

2400-CENTIGRAY CRANIAL RADIATION

Radiation therapy was the first modality successfully used to prevent CNS relapses. The use of radiation as CNS treatment was based on experiments demonstrating that L1210 murine leukemia could be cured by the addition of cranial radiation to systemic treatment with cyclophosphamide (222). In the 1960s and 1970s, studies performed at SJCRH documented the effectiveness of CNS radiation as preventive therapy (192). In one study, patients were randomized to receive either 2400-cGy craniospinal radiation or no radiation. The difference in CNS relapse rates was striking: Only two (4%) of 45 irradiated patients had their initial CRs ended by meningeal relapse, compared to 33 (67%) of 49 nonirradiated patients (205). The median time to CNS relapse was 8 months (range, 2 to 29 months). Moreover, 31 of the patients who received prophylactic radiation remained alive after 18 to 20 years, compared with only ten patients in the nonirradiated group. Subsequent studies demonstrated that 2400-cGy cranial radiation with intrathecal methotrexate was as effective in preventing CNS relapse as 2400-cGy craniospinal radiation without intrathecal chemotherapy (190,191). Because craniospinal radiation was associated with increased toxicity, including excessive myelosuppression and spinal growth retardation, radiation directed only to the cranium administered with intrathecal chemotherapy became the standard form of CNS treatment in the 1970s.

Although 2400-cGy cranial radiation (with intrathecal chemotherapy) effectively prevents CNS relapses in children with ALL, it is also associated with subsequent learning disabilities, growth and neuroendocrinologic abnormalities, and an increased risk of second malignant neoplasms (see Late Effects of Treatment). Thus, many investigators have studied alternative CNS treatments with the goal of minimizing CNS relapse rates with minimum morbidity. Alternative CNS treatment strategies include lower doses of cranial radiation, high-dose systemic chemotherapy (known to achieve therapeutic levels in cerebrospinal fluid), and intrathecal chemotherapy. Effective CNS treatment includes some or all of these therapies.

REDUCED DOSES OF CRANIAL RADIATION

Many pediatric protocols restrict the use of cranial radiation to higher risk patients, especially those with T-cell disease, high presenting leukocyte counts, or overt CNS leukemia at diagnosis (1,149,223,224). Cranial radiation is frequently administered at a dose of 1800 cGy, based on the finding that CNS and marrow relapse rates were not significantly different when the dose of cranial radiation was lowered from 2400 cGy to 1800 cGy on consecutive Children's Cancer Study Group trials (225). The BFM group has successfully used 1200-cGy radiation in the context of an intensive systemic regimen that included high-dose methotrexate (known to effectively penetrate the CNS) (148,226).

For those regimens that include cranial radiation, there is variability regarding the duration of intrathecal chemotherapy. It remains uncertain whether prolonged intermittent intrathecal chemotherapy is necessary in irradiated patients. However, trials with the lowest reported incidence of CNS relapse use this combination of cranial radiation and extended intrathecal chemotherapy (227).

HIGH-DOSE SYSTEMIC THERAPY

Systemic therapy plays an important role in the prevention of CNS leukemia. Penetration of the cerebrospinal fluid by drugs has been clearly demonstrated with the use of glucocorticoids (228) and high doses of methotrexate and cytarabine (193,194). It has also been shown that systemically administered asparaginase, whose efficacy is a function of asparagine depletion, effectively lowers cerebrospinal fluid asparagine levels and lowers the number of lymphoblasts in the cerebrospinal fluid of children with CNS disease (229).

INTRATHECAL CHEMOTHERAPY

Intrathecal chemotherapy, used in conjunction with intensive systemic therapy or cranial radiation, is an important component of CNS treatment. Many investigators have attempted to substitute cranial radiation with frequent dosing of intrathecal chemotherapy, especially in lower risk patients. In a study conducted by the Pediatric Oncology Group (POG), frequent doses of intrathecal chemotherapy (17 doses of intrathecal methotrexate, hydrocortisone, and cytarabine administered every 8 weeks) were administered instead of radiation to lower-risk patients with B-progenitor ALL, resulting in a 4.5% cumulative incidence of any CNS relapse (isolated or combined with another site) (230). Within the context of a randomized study, investigators from the Children's Cancer Group (CCG) demonstrated that administering intrathecal methotrexate throughout all phases of therapy was as effective in preventing CNS relapses in lower risk patients as 1800-cGy cranial radiation (with 6 months of intrathecal methotrexate), but only in the context of an intensified systemic regimen (231). When a less intensive systemic regimen was used (no delayed intensification), more CNS relapses were observed with intrathecal methotrexate than with cranial radiation (231). Similarly, in another study, excessive CNS relapses were observed in standard risk males when cranial radiation was eliminated without increasing the frequency of intrathecal chemotherapy or the intensity of systemic chemotherapy (232). Thus, those regimens that have successfully eliminated cranial radiation use extended or frequent dosing of intrathecal chemotherapy within the context of intensified systemic therapy, often including several doses of high-dose methotrexate (223,233,234).

The goal of eliminating cranial radiation in pediatric patients is to minimize long-term CNS sequelae (see Late Effects of Treatment). Although several studies have indicated that intrathecal chemotherapy and intensive systemic therapy can be as effective as cranial radiation in preventing CNS relapses, the relative late toxicities of these CNS treatment strategies remain unsettled. Moreover, higher rates of acute neurotoxicity, including seizures, have been observed with regimens that used high-dose methotrexate and intensive intrathecal chemotherapy (235). Thus, the optimal CNS treatment in childhood ALL remains uncertain.

Intensification Chemotherapy

Postinduction intensification or consolidation is a common component of most ALL treatment protocols. The goals of intensification therapy are to further reduce the disease burden and to adjust the intensity of treatment based on the risk of subsequent relapse (i.e., to formulate risk group–specific therapy). A wide variety of agents and schedules have been used during the intensification phase of treatment in pediatric trials. On some protocols, the intensification phase is administered immediately after achieving remission (early intensification), whereas on others it is given after a short period of less intensive therapy (delayed intensification).

Several childhood ALL protocols have used a phase of early intensification immediately after remission induction. For example, the DFCI ALL Consortium demonstrated that early intensification with weekly high-dose asparaginase for 20 to 30 weeks improved EFS for all patients (236) and that repeated doses of doxorubicin during this phase, in addition to asparaginase, favorably impacted the outcome of high-risk patients, including those with T-cell ALL (50,237,238). For patients with lower risk B-progenitor ALL, POG has successfully used an early intensification phase with repeated doses of intermediate-dose methotrexate (235,239,240) but has not observed any significant improvement in outcome for this patient subset with the addition of high-dose cytarabine, high-dose mercaptopurine, or high-dose asparaginase to this intensification regimen (235,239,240). Several other protocols also include a phase of early intensification with high-dose methotrexate immediately after remission induction for both high- and low-risk patients, often in place of cranial radiation, as described above (148,182,241,242).

Several groups have emphasized the use of a delayed intensification phase, an intensive cycle of chemotherapy administered weeks to months after achieving CR, often after a period of less intensive chemotherapy (interim maintenance). The BFM and CCG groups have demonstrated that patients with both low- and high-risk ALL benefit from such a strategy. On these protocols, the delayed intensification phase consists of an intensive reinduction cycle, including such agents as vincristine, corticosteroid, anthracycline, asparaginase, cyclophosphamide, cytarabine, and 6-thioguanine (148,211,212,243,244). By augmenting this regimen (including the use of two delayed intensification cycles instead of one), the CCG has improved outcome for high-risk patients who had responded slowly to initial induction therapy (153). The United Kingdom ALL

group reported that patients treated with both early and delayed intensification cycles (which included cytarabine, etoposide, 6-thioguanine, daunomycin, vincristine, and prednisone) had a superior outcome when compared with patients who received only one of these cycles (245) and that patients who received three cycles of intensification (separated by periods of less intensive therapy) fared better than those who received two (246).

Continuation Therapy

Nearly all current treatment regimens for ALL employ a phase of continuation therapy, in which patients are treated with less intensive chemotherapy to complete at least 2 years of therapy. Most continuation regimens consist of weekly low-dose methotrexate and daily oral 6-mercaptopurine. Some groups add regular pulses of vincristine and corticosteroid to this regimen (50,211,244), although the benefit of these pulses remains controversial (247,248).

The relative efficacy and toxicity of two corticosteroids used during continuation therapy, prednisone and dexamethasone, has been a major research focus for many investigators. Several reports have suggested that dexamethasone has more potent *in vitro* antileukemic activity, higher free plasma levels, and enhanced CSF penetration (228,249–251). The DFCI group and the Dutch Childhood Leukemia Study Group have both reported that the nonrandomized substitution of dexamethasone for prednisone may have favorably impacted EFS (1,234). The CCG reported the results of a randomized trial comparing the two agents in lower-risk patients, which indicated that dexamethasone was associated with a superior 5-year EFS (244). However, dexamethasone may also be associated with increased side effects, including higher rates of bony morbidity and infectious complications (252,253).

SJCRH protocols have included an intensified continuation therapy consisting of rotating pairs of non–cross-resistant drugs, including many agents not traditionally incorporated during the continuation phase, such as cyclophosphamide, epipodophyllotoxins, and cytarabine. This strategy has resulted in improved outcomes for higher-risk but not lower-risk patients (182,220).

Duration of Therapy

The optimal duration therapy remains unknown. Most investigators continue to treat patients for 2 to 3 years, based on results of older studies, in which patients received therapy that was less intensive than current regimens (254). Randomized studies conducted by CCG indicated that there was no significant difference in outcome when comparing 5 versus 3 years of therapy (255,256). In a randomized study of 2 versus 3 years of continuation therapy, the United Kingdom ALL group observed no significant survival advantage with longer therapy. In that study, patients receiving the shorter duration of therapy had a higher relapse rate, but this was counterbalanced by a higher remission death rate in those receiving 3 years of treatment (257). Some early studies suggested that the optimal duration of therapy may be different for boys and girls, with boys benefiting from a more prolonged continuation phase (258), although this finding may be less relevant with current, intensive regimens.

Even with intensive regimens, attempts to shorten therapy duration from 2 years have not been successful. The BFM group randomized patients to receive 18 or 24 months of treatment and observed a higher relapse rate with patients who received the shorter treatment (148,248). Similarly, high relapse rates were observed on a nonrandomized study conducted by the Tokyo Children's Cancer Study Group, in which patients received intensified therapy for only 12 months, suggesting that truncated therapy, even if intensive, is inadequate for most children with ALL (259). Ongoing studies of minimal residual disease (discussed above) may help to clarify the optimal therapy duration for patients in the era of intensive, multiagent chemotherapy.

Treatment of Special Patient Subsets

PHILADELPHIA CHROMOSOME–POSITIVE ACUTE LYMPHOBLASTIC LEUKEMIA

The Philadelphia chromosome t(9;22)(q34;q11) is detectable in approximately 5% of children and 20% of adults with ALL (63). Many investigators have reported that these patients have a dismal prognosis, with long-term EFS rates ranging from 0% to 25% (63,80,81). Although some preliminary studies suggested that patients with Philadelphia chromosome–positive ALL and low presenting leukocyte counts may be successfully treated with intensive chemotherapy (103), most investigators recommend allogeneic stem cell transplantation in first remission for all patients with this chromosomal translocation. One study reviewed the outcome of 267 children with Philadelphia chromosome–positive ALL treated by ten study groups between 1986 and 1996. Results suggested that transplantation in first remission from an HLA-matched related donor was superior to intensive chemotherapy alone for these patients (102). This finding confirmed the results of smaller series (105). Preliminary data suggests that unrelated donor stem cell transplantation in first remission may also effectively treat patients with Philadelphia chromosome–positive ALL (106,107). STI-571, a specific inhibitor of the BCR-ABL tyrosine kinase, is a promising new agent which may further improve the outcome of patients with Philadelphia chromosome–positive ALL. Pilot studies of STI-571 demonstrated its activity in patients with Philadelphia chromosome–positive ALL (260); further work is necessary to determine if and how it should be incorporated into the therapy of these patients.

INFANTS

Patients diagnosed with ALL during the first year of life also represent a special population because of their poor prognosis as well as their increased vulnerability to the toxic effects of therapy (261). Infants appear to have a biologically distinct form of ALL, characterized by a molecularly detectable rearrangement of the MLL gene on chromosome 11q23 (41,42,108,110). Their overall outcome is significantly worse than that for older children with ALL, with reported long-term EFS rates of less than 40% (262–264).

Some modest improvement in the therapy of infants with ALL has been reported. The DFCI group reported improved outcome for infants (50-month EFS of 54%) treated with a chemotherapy regimen that included early intensification with high-dose cytarabine, high-dose methotrexate, and delayed cranial radiation (delivered at age 12 months) (265). This finding was in accord with in vitro studies that demonstrated that lymphoblasts from infants were resistant to many agents, such as corticosteroids, anthracyclines, and L-asparaginase, but were more sensitive to cytarabine than cells from older children (266). The BFM group has reported that a favorable response to a prednisone prophase identified a subset of infants with a better prognosis (6-year EFS of 53%), independent of MLL gene status (267). Some investigators have treated patients diagnosed in infancy with allogeneic stem cell transplantation in first remission, especially those infants with detectable MLL gene rearrangements. However, there is little published data regarding the efficacy or toxicity of such an approach (268,269).

ADULT ACUTE LYMPHOBLASTIC LEUKEMIA

Adults with ALL have a poorer prognosis than pediatric patients, likely secondary to differences in underlying biology of their disease as well has higher rates of therapy-related morbidity. Currently, CR rates in adults range from 70% to 90%, and long-term OS is achieved by 20% to 50% of patients (Table 25-4) (270). Most adult protocols, similar to pediatric protocols, consist of four phases of therapy: remission induction, CNS-directed therapy, intensification, and continuation. Because of the relatively poor prognosis of adults, postremission therapy is frequently more intensive than on pediatric protocols, incorporating such agents as high-dose cytarabine, cyclophosphamide, epipodophyllotoxins, anthracyclines, and high-dose methotrexate (143,271–274).

Most adult studies routinely include cranial radiation, high-dose systemic therapy (methotrexate, cytarabine, dexamethasone), or extended intrathecal chemotherapy as CNS-directed therapy. However, fewer studies in adult patients than in children have addressed whether CNS prophylaxis is a necessary component of therapy. The Southwest Oncology Group randomized patients aged 15 years or greater to receive either CNS treatment (with 2400-cGy cranial radiation and intrathecal methotrexate) or no CNS-directed therapy, within the context of identical intensive multiagent systemic therapy. Irradiated patients had a much lower risk of CNS relapse, although overall remission duration and survival was not significantly different in the two arms (275).

There are conflicting data supporting the use of allogeneic stem cell transplantation in first remission in adult ALL. In general, results reported after allogeneic transplant have been superior to those reported with chemotherapy for adults with ALL, but direct comparisons have been difficult due to differences in patient selection criteria, variations in the interval from CR to transplant, and the paucity of randomized studies comparing the two modalities (276). In a comparative study using data from International Bone Marrow Transplant Registry and a German protocol, there was no significant difference in outcome between allogeneic stem cell transplantation and chemotherapy alone when results were adjusted according to prognostic factors and time to transplant (277). In that study, relapses were more frequent in the chemotherapy group, and remission deaths were higher in the transplanted patients (277). In a French study, allogeneic stem cell transplantation in first remission was found to be superior to either chemotherapy or autologous transplantation in high-risk patients, including those with Philadelphia chromosome–positive ALL, age greater than 35 years, high presenting leukocyte count, and initial induction failure (278). Based on these findings, stem cell transplantation in first remission is frequently recommended for high-risk, nonelderly adult patients, especially if they have a matched related donor.

LATE EFFECTS OF TREATMENT

The treatment of children with ALL has resulted in prolonged, EFS for 70% to 80% of patients (Table 25-3) (1,149,182,244). However, even for successfully treated children, long-term effects of the disease and its treatment often result in organ toxicity of varying but clinically significant magnitude. The consequences of treatment to the normal tissue are a function of the organ system involved and the type of therapy. The most common and often most problematic late effects involve the CNS (279), but other problems include cataracts (280), cardiac abnormalities (281), bony morbidity (252), short stature (282), obesity (283), abnormalities of gonadal function and reproduction (284,285), and second malignant neoplasms (286,287).

Low and low–average intelligence quotients have been frequent findings in survivors of ALL (288–291). More detailed neuropsychologic studies have demonstrated that learning disabilities are related to a slow speed of processing information, distractibility, and difficulty in dealing with complex or conceptually demanding material (292,293). The severity of neuropsychological sequelae varies, dependent on both treatment and patient characteristics. For example, younger children (<5 years of age) are more vulnerable than older children (288,289,291,294), and in some studies, girls are more vulnerable than boys (292,295,296).

Most long-term neuropsychologic effects have been attributed to cranial radiation (288–290,293). The most severely impaired long-term survivors are those who received cranial radiation doses (2400 to 2800 cGy) that are higher than doses used in current treatment regimens (1200 to 1800 cGy) (297,298). A recent study of long-term survivors treated on DFCI ALL protocols with 1800-cGy cranial radiation did not find any significant neuropsychologic impairments in patients who were 3 years of age or older at the time of diagnosis (294), suggesting that lower doses of cranial radiation may be associated with reduced risk of learning disabilities. Microcephaly has also been reported as a late effect of CNS treatment and was found to be dependent on the radiation dose (299).

The contribution of systemic and intrathecal chemotherapy to the development of neurocognitive toxicities has not been fully assessed. It has been demonstrated that systemic chemotherapy impacts the severity of radiation-associated neuropsychologic sequelae. In one study, the development of leukoencephalopathy was associated with escalating doses of systemic methotrexate in children who had received cranial radiation (300). In another series, intelligent quotient decline was associated with combined therapy of high-dose systemic methotrexate and 1800-cGy cranial radiation but not with either therapy alone (301). Moreover, there is evidence that cognitive deficits are present in long-term survivors treated without cranial radiation (302), and in one study, there were no significant difference in the severity and range of deficits between irradiated and nonirradiated patients (296).

Neuropathologic changes in the CNS have been identified in survivors of childhood ALL. Leukoencephalopathy, a relatively rare phenomenon, is characterized by multifocal demyelination visible on radiographic imaging (computed tomography or magnetic resonance imaging) (303). Patients may present with a wide range of neurologic and behavioral problems, including poor school performance, confusion, memory problems, personality changes, and, in its most severe form, even progressive dementia and coma (303). Risk factors for the development of leukoencephalopathy include large doses of cranial radiation (usually not observed in patients receiving 1800 cGy or less) or high cumulative doses of systemic and intrathecal methotrexate (303).

In some studies, survivors of ALL are shorter than expected for their age (282,304,305). The greatest impact on final height has been noted in patients treated with 2400-cGy cranial radiation, with less severe growth failure noted in patients whose CNS treatment included 1800 cGy or no cranial radiation (304,306). Young age and female sex are associated with greater growth failure (282,304). Short stature in survivors of childhood ALL is sometimes, but not always, associated with growth hormone deficiency (307–309), suggesting that growth hormone replacement may have a potential therapeutic role in some patients.

Bony morbidity, including osteopenia, fractures, and osteonecrosis, has been observed in up to 30% of children with ALL and is likely secondary to chronic exposure to corticosteroids while on therapy (252). Many investigators have demonstrated that children with ALL have reduced bone mineral density during and even many years after the completion of therapy (310–314), although the clinical relevance of this finding has not been clarified. *Osteonecrosis* (ON), also known as *avascular necrosis*, is a dis-

abling bony toxicity, frequently involving multiple joints. ON can lead to significant pain and loss of function, sometimes necessitating total joint replacement (315–317). The CCG and DFCI groups recently reported ON cumulative incidence rates of 9% and 7%, respectively, in survivors of childhood ALL, with the highest frequency observed in those diagnosed in adolescence (252,318).

Small, nonprogressive posterior subcapsular cataracts, which did not impair vision or require surgical treatment, were reported in over 50% of children treated for ALL (280). Although the cataracts were thought to be related to the administration of high cumulative doses of corticosteroids, these patients had also received cranial radiation (which included treatment of the posterior half of the globes and the optic nerves).

Echocardiographic abnormalities, particularly increased afterload and decreased contractility, are common late effects of anthracycline therapy (281,319). The mechanism of this toxicity is impairment of myocardial growth. The severity of cardiac dysfunction is correlated with higher cumulative doses of anthracycline and higher dose rates (281,319–321). Patients treated at a young age, females, and those with Down's syndrome appear to be more vulnerable to anthracycline-associated cardiac toxicity (320,321). Despite these echocardiographic abnormalities, congestive heart failure rarely occurs in long-term survivors who were treated with anthracycline (319,321), although longer follow-up is needed to fully assess the risk of late symptomatic cardiac disease.

Late-occurring hepatotoxicity is a relatively uncommon effect of ALL therapy (322,323). Elevations of transaminase levels are quite common while patients are receiving therapy but are not associated with chronic liver disease once therapy is completed (323).

Ovarian and testicular function are relatively unaffected on most current childhood ALL regimens (285,305,324) with the possible exception of programs that use alkylating agents (e.g., cyclophosphamide) (325,326), high doses of cytarabine (325), or prophylactic gonadal radiation (326). Thus, fertility is preserved in the vast majority of survivors of childhood ALL. In girls, puberty may occur early, and in both sexes, normal pubertal growth spurts may be blunted (285,305). Several normal children have been born of patients successfully treated for childhood ALL (327).

Second malignant neoplasms, including malignant gliomas (286,328–330), treatment-related AML (329,331,332), and carcinomas of the parotid and thyroid glands (286,329) have been reported in survivors of ALL. Risk factors for the development of secondary AML in survivors of childhood ALL include treatment with epipodophyllotoxins and alkylating agents (331–333). For example, the cumulative risk of secondary AML has been reported to be as high as 5% to 6% with epipodophyllotoxin-containing regimens (331,332) but is less than 1% with a regimen lacking both epipodophyllotoxins and alkylators (334,335). Secondary solid tumors have been observed in patients who received cranial or craniospinal radiation, especially those receiving higher doses (1800- to 2400-cGy cranial radiation) (286,330,336). In several large studies, the long-term cumulative incidences rates of secondary brain tumors in previously irradiated patients ranged from 1.0% to 1.6% (330,335,336).

TREATMENT OF RELAPSED ACUTE LYMPHOBLASTIC LEUKEMIA

Approximately 20% to 30% of children and 40% to 60% of adults with ALL who achieve remission after initial induction chemotherapy will subsequently relapse. Several factors have been identified that influence the outcome of patients with relapsed

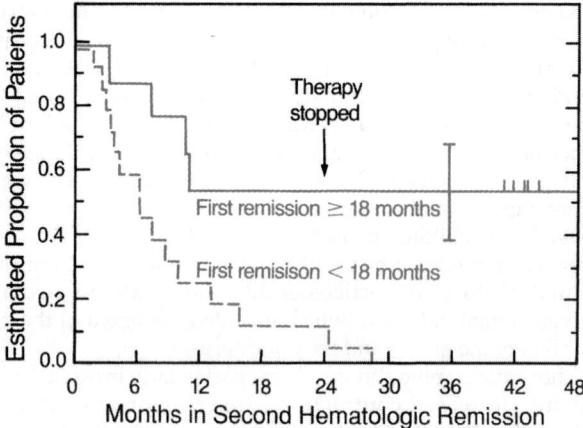

Figure 25-6. Influence of initial hematologic remission length on the outcome of secondary chemotherapy. Second remissions were significantly longer among patients with longer initial remissions ($p = .004$ by Cox life-table regression analysis). Tick marks represent patients still at risk; the bar at 36 months denotes the 95% confidence limit. (Adapted from Rivera GK, Buchanan G, Boyett JM, et al. Intensive retreatment of childhood acute lymphoblastic leukemia in first bone marrow relapse. *N Engl J Med* 1986;315:273.)

ALL, including duration of initial remission, site of relapse, immunophenotype, age, and presenting WBC count at relapse.

Many investigators have identified duration of initial remission as one of the most important prognostic factors, with significantly worse outcomes observed in patients who relapse early (defined as those occurring while on initial therapy or within 2 years of diagnosis) than in those with longer initial remissions (Fig. 25-6) (337–341). T-lineage immunophenotype and age greater than 10 years have also been associated with an adverse prognosis (338–340). Some authors have reported that patients with low presenting WBC counts at relapse have a superior prognosis (340), although most investigators have not confirmed this finding (337,338). The BFM group has reported that the absence of peripheral blasts at the time of a first late marrow relapse is associated with favorable outcome (342).

Site of relapse also has prognostic importance, with superior outcomes observed for patients experiencing isolated extramedullary relapses when compared with those with marrow relapses (339,343). Some authors have suggested that patients with combined marrow and extramedullary relapses have a better prognosis than those with isolated marrow relapses (339,344), although this finding may be confounded by the fact that the cohort with combined relapses had longer initial remissions (339). Among patients with isolated extramedullary relapses, those with testicular relapse appear to fare better than those with CNS relapse (339,345).

By using these prognostic factors, investigators have identified subsets of patients with a relatively favorable prognosis (e.g., patients experiencing a late extramedullary relapse) who may be able to maintain durable second remissions with less intensive therapies, such as conventional dose chemotherapy. Subsets of patients with a less favorable prognosis, such as those experiencing an early marrow relapse, are considered candidates for more intensive therapies, such as stem cell transplantation.

Marrow Relapse

Marrow relapse accounts for the majority of recurrences in childhood ALL. Induction of second CR can be expected in 70% to 90% of children with B-lineage ALL, but the percentage is lower in children with T-lineage ALL (337,346–350). After a sec-

ond CR has been attained, subsequent treatment may include conventional-dose chemotherapy or high-dose chemotherapy with stem cell transplantation.

Most trials of conventional dose chemotherapy have been unsuccessful at producing long-term survival in patients who have experienced a marrow relapse. In a review of 36 published reports of children with relapsed ALL, only 18% of 600 children treated with chemotherapy survived (351). In another large series, the 5-year probability of relapse was 80% for 540 children treated in second remission on POG chemotherapy protocols (352).

Most investigators have reported that the duration of initial remission significantly predicts outcome of children with relapsed ALL treated with chemotherapy in second remission (Fig. 25-6). In most reports, early relapse is associated with survival rates of less than 20% (337,338,346,349,352). The most successful chemotherapy trial results have been achieved with patients whose initial CRs exceeded 18 to 30 months. With intensive chemotherapy regimens, the probability of EFS for this subset of patients ranges from 30% to 40% (337,340,341,352,353). In a SJCRH pilot study, 34 children whose initial remissions exceeded 36 months were treated in second remission with intensified rotational combination chemotherapy and achieved a 5-year EFS of 65% (354). The BFM group has reported that the absence of peripheral blasts at the time of a first late marrow relapse is associated with a favorable response to chemotherapy, with such patients achieving a 10-year EFS of 64% (342).

Sibling-matched allogeneic stem cell transplantation for relapsed ALL has resulted in long-term survival in 25% to 60% of patients (352,353,355–360). Transplantation in second remission has generally been more favorable than in third or subsequent remission (356). In most published reports, the most common cause of failure after allogeneic stem cell transplantation is recurrence of leukemia (357–360). Therapy-related toxicity, including infections and severe graft-versus-host disease, is also a major cause of death, occurring in 15% to 30% of patients (352,353,358,359,361). In recent years, the incidence of treatment-related complications appears to be decreasing with improvements in supportive care (358). As has been demonstrated in chemotherapy trials for relapsed ALL, duration of initial remission is an important predictor of outcome after allogenic stem cell transplantation, with improved survival observed in patients with longer initial remissions (352,357).

Because there are no randomized trials comparing chemotherapy and allogeneic transplantation in relapsed ALL, published comparisons of the two modalities have generally been complicated by variability of patient selection and treatment. A retrospective, matched-pair analysis comparing sibling-matched allogeneic stem cell transplant with chemotherapy demonstrated that transplantation was associated with improved leukemia-free survival (5-year leukemia-free survival of 40% for transplanted patients versus 17% for chemotherapy-treated patients) (352). The superiority of outcome after transplantation was observed in patients with both short and long first remissions. Others have also observed that sibling-matched allogeneic stem cell transplantation conferred a survival advantage, especially in patients with short initial remissions (353,358,360).

Because over 80% of patients do not have histocompatible sibling donors, various methods have been developed to circumvent the lack of a matched related donor. Other potential stem cell sources for transplantation include matched unrelated donors and autologous marrow.

The efficacy of unrelated donor transplantation for patients with relapsed ALL is difficult to assess because of the small numbers of such patients reported in the literature. In most published series, which include patients treated after multiple

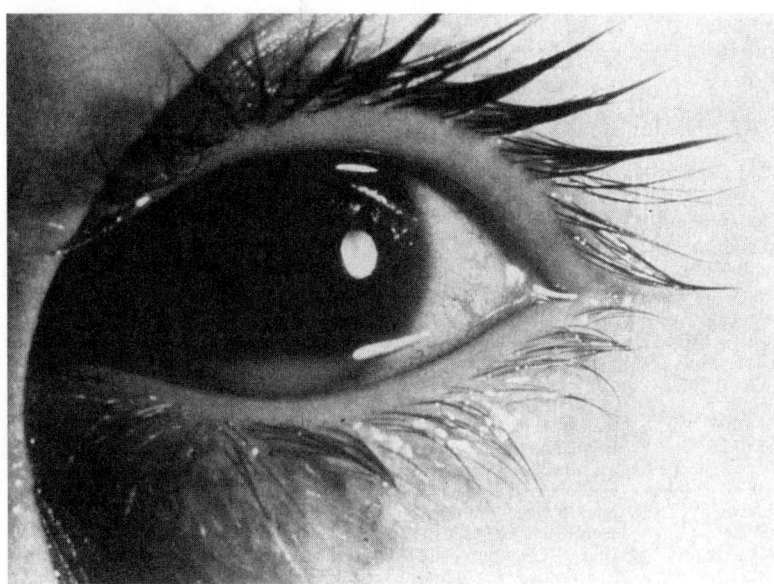

Figure 25-7. Hypopyon in the left eye of a child with acute lymphoblastic leukemia. Milky material can be seen at the base of the iris within the anterior chamber.

relapses, EFS ranges between 20% and 30% (362–365). The risk of treatment-related morbidity and mortality is substantial, often secondary to graft-versus-host disease. With improvements in supportive care and more accurate genomic typing of HLA class II antigens, treatment-related mortality with unrelated donor transplantation has been decreasing. In one nonrandomized study of pediatric patients in second CR, patients who received an unrelated SCT had equivalent EFS to those who received a matched sibling donor SCT (366).

Autologous transplantation is another option for patients in second or subsequent CR who do not have a matched related donor. Autologous transplantation is often performed in conjunction with *ex vivo* purging of residual leukemia in harvested marrow via immunologic or pharmacologic techniques (363,367–371). For patients with long initial remissions, results achieved after autologous transplantation are comparable to those observed after allogeneic transplantation, with EFS rates of 40% to 50% (361,368,370,372). Patients with short initial remissions fare less well (371,372). Relapse is the most common cause of treatment failure after autologous bone marrow transplantation, with a lower incidence of toxicity-related deaths than is observed after allogeneic transplantation (361). It is not clear that autologous transplantation offers any advantage over chemotherapy in the treatment of relapsed ALL (372).

Isolated Extramedullary Relapses

Isolated extramedullary relapses, occurring either in the CNS or testicle, are less frequent than marrow relapses in ALL. Isolated CNS relapse occurs in fewer than 10% of patients with ALL. Although CNS remission can be successfully induced in more than 90% of such patients with CNS-directed therapy, most patients treated without intensive systemic therapy will subsequently develop a bone marrow recurrence (373). Thus, in addition to CNS-directed therapy (usually radiation with intrathecal chemotherapy), patients with isolated CNS relapses are treated with either intensive chemotherapy or stem cell transplantation (374–377). Several reports have indicated that intensive chemotherapy regimens may provide adequate postremission therapy for patients with an isolated CNS relapse, with EFS rates of 45% to 70% (376–379). There is much less published data regarding outcome after stem cell transplantation in second remission for patients with an isolated CNS relapse.

As with marrow relapses, patients experiencing early isolated CNS relapses (within 24 months of initial diagnosis) have a much poorer prognosis than those whose relapses occur later (338,339,376,377). A patient's CNS prophylaxis at the time of initial diagnosis may also affect outcome after an isolated CNS relapse. Some studies have suggested that patients whose initial CNS prophylaxis included only intrathecal medications may have a somewhat better prognosis after an isolated CNS relapse than those whose initial CNS prophylaxis included cranial radiation (378,380).

Isolated testicular relapses rarely occur in the era of intensified chemotherapy regimens for patients with newly diagnosed ALL (50). For boys with isolated testicular relapses, systemic chemotherapy and testicular radiation have resulted in prolonged second remissions in greater than 80% of patients with late-occurring relapses (381,382). This approach has been less successful in patients whose testicular relapses occur during or soon after cessation of initial therapy, with long-term EFS ranging from 20% to 43% (381,383). Such patients could be considered candidates for stem cell transplantation, although data are insufficient to indicate whether this approach would be beneficial.

Other rare sites of extramedullary relapse include eyes (Fig. 25-7) and ovaries. Case reports have indicated successful treatment of such patients with local radiation and intensive systemic therapy (384,385).

FUTURE DIRECTIONS

Although risk-adapted therapy has resulted in marked improvement in the outcome of children with ALL over the last few decades, the results of recent studies suggest that we are reaching the limits of prognostic significance of currently applied clinical risk factors. The use of molecular techniques may identify biologically distinct leukemia subtypes, which may supplement or replace the epidemiologic factors currently used to determine risk-based therapy. Such research may also help identify molecular targets for therapy. STI-571, the selective inhibitor of the BCR-ABL encoded tyrosine kinase, may be the prototype of a new class of antileukemic agents that are more specific and less toxic than current chemotherapy (260). Other possible novel approaches to therapy include monoclonal antibodies linked to toxins (386,387), the stimulation of leukemia-specific immunity (388,389), and the use of antiangiogenesis factors (390). The development of patient-specific treatment regimens (based on *in vitro* cytotoxicity assays or individualized pharmacokinetic dosing of chemotherapeutic agents) is also promising new approaches to the improved treatment of this disease (172,391).

REFERENCES

1. Silverman LB, Gelber RD, Dalton VK, et al. Improved outcome for children with acute lymphoblastic leukemia: results of Dana-Farber Consortium Protocol 91-01. *Blood* 2001;97:1211.
2. Cortes JE, Kantarjian HM. Acute lymphoblastic leukemia. A comprehensive review with emphasis on biology and therapy. *Cancer* 1995;76:2393.
3. Ries LAG, Smith MA, Gurney JG, et al. Cancer Incidence and Survival among Children and Adolescents: United States SEER Program 1975–1995, vol. NIH Pub. No. 99-4649. Bethesda, MD, National Cancer Institute, SEER Program, 1999.
4. Pullen DJ, Boyett JM, Crist WM, et al. Pediatric oncology group utilization of immunologic markers in the designation of acute lymphocytic leukemia subgroups: influence on treatment response. *Ann N Y Acad Sci* 1984;428:26.
5. Pendergrass TW. Epidemiology of acute lymphoblastic leukemia. *Semin Oncol* 1985;12:80.
6. Miller RW. Ethnic differences in cancer occurrence: genetic and environmental influences with particular reference to neuroblastoma. In: Mulvhill JJ, Miller RW, Fraumeni JF Jr, eds. *Genetics of human cancer*. New York: Raven Press, 1977.
7. Greaves MF. Speculations on the cause of childhood acute lymphoblastic leukemia. *Leukemia* 1988;2:120.
8. Draper GJ, Heaf MM, Kinnier Wilson LM. Occurrence of childhood cancers among sibs and estimation of familial risks. *J Med Genet* 1977;14:81.
9. Miller RW. Persons with exceptionally high risk of leukemia. *Cancer Res* 1967;27:2420.
10. Pui CH. Childhood leukemias. *N Engl J Med* 1995;332:1618.
11. Harris LJ. Leukaemia and pregnancy. *Cancer Med Assoc J* 1953;68:234.
12. Miller R. Neoplasia and Down's syndrome. *Ann N Y Acad Sci* 1970;171:637.
13. Bloom D. The syndrome of congenital telangiectatic erythema and stunted growth. *J Pediatr* 1966;68:103.
14. Toledano SR, Lange BJ. Ataxia-telangiectasia and acute lymphoblastic leukemia. *Cancer* 1980;45:1675.
15. Takeuchi S, Koike M, Park S, et al. The ATM gene and susceptibility to childhood T-cell acute lymphoblastic leukaemia. *Br J Haematol* 1998;103:536.
16. Sandler DP. Recent studies in leukemia epidemiology. *Curr Opin Oncol* 1995;7:12.
17. Greaves MF. Aetiology of acute leukaemia. *Lancet* 1997;349:344.
18. Linet MS, Hatch EE, Kleinerman RA, et al. Residential exposure to magnetic fields and acute lymphoblastic leukemia in children. *N Engl J Med* 1997;337:1.
19. Rinsky RA, Smith AB, Hornung R, et al. Benzene and leukemia: an epidemiologic risk assessment. *N Engl J Med* 1987;316:1044.
20. Gallo RC. Human T-lymphotropic retroviruses. In: Gallo RC, Essex ME, Gross L, eds. *Human T-cell leukemia/lymphoma virus*. Cold Spring Harbor, N.Y.: Cold Spring Harbor Laboratory, 1984:1.
21. Neglia JP, Linet MS, Shu XO, et al. Patterns of infection and day care utilization and risk of childhood acute lymphoblastic leukaemia. *Br J Cancer* 2000;82:234.
22. Bennett JM, Catovsky D, Daniel MT, et al. Proposals for the classification of the acute leukaemias. French-American-British (FAB) co-operative group. *Br J Haematol* 1976;33:451.
23. Burns CP, Armitage JO, Frey AL, et al. Analysis of the presenting features of adult acute leukemia: the French-American-British classification. *Cancer* 1981;47:2460.
24. Miller DR, Steinherz PG, Feuer D, et al. Unfavorable prognostic significance of hand mirror cells in childhood acute lymphoblastic leukemia. A report from the Childrens Cancer Study Group. *Am J Dis Child* 1983;137:346.
25. van Eys J, Pullen J, Head D, et al. The French-American-British (FAB) classification of leukemia. The Pediatric Oncology Group experience with lymphocytic leukemia. *Cancer* 1986;57:1046.
26. Lilleyman JS, Hann IM, Stevens RF, et al. Cytomorphology of childhood lymphoblastic leukaemia: a prospective study of 2000 patients. United Kingdom Medical Research Council's Working Party on Childhood Leukaemia. *Br J Haematol* 1992;81:52.
27. McCaffrey R, Harrison TA, Parkman R, Baltimore D. Terminal deoxynucleotidyl transferase activity in human leukemic cells and in normal human thymocytes. *N Engl J Med* 1975;292:775.
28. Hutton JJ, Coleman MS. Terminal deoxynucleotidyl transferase measurements in the differential diagnosis of adult leukaemias. *Br J Haematol* 1976;34:447.
29. Shaw MT. The cytochemistry of acute leukemia: a diagnostic and prognostic evaluation. *Semin Oncol* 1976;3:219.
30. Head DR, Borowitz M, Cerezo L, et al. Acid phosphatase positivity in childhood acute lymphocytic leukemia. *Am J Clin Pathol* 1986;86:650.
31. Crist WM, Grossi CE, Pullen DJ, Cooper MD. Immunologic markers in childhood acute lymphocytic leukemia. *Semin Oncol* 1985;12:105.
32. Berger R, Bernheim A. Cytogenetic studies on Burkitt's lymphoma-leukemia. *Cancer Genet Cytogenet* 1982;7:231.
33. Murphy SB, Bowman WP, Abromowitch M, et al. Results of treatment of advanced-stage Burkitt's lymphoma and B cell (SIg+) acute lymphoblastic leukemia with high-dose fractionated cyclophosphamide and coordinated high-dose methotrexate and cytarabine. *J Clin Oncol* 1986;4:1732.
34. Patte C, Philip T, Rodary C, et al. High survival rate in advanced-stage B-cell lymphomas and leukemias without CNS involvement with a short intensive polychemotherapy: results from the French Pediatric Oncology Society of a randomized trial of 216 children. *J Clin Oncol* 1991;9:123.
35. Nadler LM, Korsmeyer SJ, Anderson KC, et al. B cell origin of non-T cell acute lymphoblastic leukemia. A model for discrete stages of neoplastic and normal pre-B cell differentiation. *J Clin Invest* 1984;74:332.
36. Felix CA, Poplack DG, Reaman GH, et al. Characterization of immunoglobulin and T-cell receptor gene patterns in B-cell precursor acute lymphoblastic leukemia of childhood. *J Clin Oncol* 1990;8:431.
37. Korsmeyer SJ, Hieter PA, Ravetch JV, et al. Developmental hierarchy of immunoglobulin gene rearrangements in human leukemic pre-B-cells. *Proc Natl Acad Sci U S A* 1981;78:7096.
38. Hurwitz CA, Loken MR, Graham ML, et al. Asynchronous antigen expression in B lineage acute lymphoblastic leukemia. *Blood* 1988;72:299.
39. Hann IM, Richards SM, Eden OB, Hill FG. Analysis of the immunophenotype of children treated on the Medical Research Council United Kingdom Acute Lymphoblastic Leukaemia Trial XI (MRC UKALLXI). Medical Research Council Childhood Leukaemia Working Party. *Leukemia* 1998;12:1249.
40. Stark B, Vogel R, Cohen IJ, et al. Biologic and cytogenetic characteristics of leukemia in infants. *Cancer* 1989;63:117.
41. Chen C-S, Sorensen PHB, Domer PH, et al. Molecular rearrangements on chromosome 11q23 predominate in infant acute lymphoblastic leukemia and are associated with specific biologic variables and poor outcome. *Blood* 1993;81:2386.
42. Pui CH, Behm FG, Downing JR, et al. 11q23/MLL rearrangement confers a poor prognosis in infants with acute lymphoblastic leukemia. *J Clin Oncol* 1994;12:909.
43. Vogler LB, Crist WM, Bockman DE, et al. Pre-B-cell leukemia. A new phenotype of childhood lymphoblastic leukemia. *N Engl J Med* 1978;298:872.
44. Carroll AJ, Crist WM, Parmley RT, et al. Pre-B cell leukemia associated with chromosome translocation 1;19. *Blood* 1984;63:721.
45. Crist W, Boyett J, Roper M, et al. Pre-B cell leukemia responds poorly to treatment: a pediatric oncology group study. *Blood* 1984;63:407.
46. Crist WM, Carroll AJ, Shuster JJ, et al. Poor prognosis of children with pre-B acute lymphoblastic leukemia is associated with the t(1;19)(q23;p13): a Pediatric Oncology Group study. *Blood* 1990;76:117.
47. Borella L, Sen L. T cell surface markers on lymphoblasts from acute lymphocytic leukemia. *J Immunol* 1973;111:1257.
48. Borowitz MJ, Dowell BL, Boyett JM, et al. Monoclonal antibody definition of T cell acute leukemia: a Pediatric Oncology Group study. *Blood* 1985;65:785.
49. Copelan EA, McGuire EA. The biology and treatment of acute lymphoblastic leukemia in adults. *Blood* 1995;85:1151.
50. Silverman LB, Declerck L, Gelber RD, et al. Results of Dana-Farber Cancer Institute Consortium protocols for children with newly diagnosed acute lymphoblastic leukemia (1981–1995). *Leukemia* 2000;14:2247.
51. Roper M, Crist WM, Metzgar R, et al. Monoclonal antibody characterization of surface antigens in childhood T- cell lymphoid malignancies. *Blood* 1983;61:830.
52. Uckun FM, Gaynon PS, Sensel MG, et al. Clinical features and treatment outcome of childhood T-lineage acute lymphoblastic leukemia according to the apparent maturational stage of T-lineage leukemic blasts: a Children's Cancer Group study. *J Clin Oncol* 1997;15:2214.
53. Crist WM, Shuster JJ, Falletta J, et al. Clinical features and outcome in childhood T-cell leukemia-lymphoma according to stage of thymocyte differentiation: a Pediatric Oncology Group Study. *Blood* 1988;72:1891.
54. Shuster JJ, Falletta JM, Pullen DJ, et al. Prognostic factors in childhood T-cell acute lymphoblastic leukemia: a Pediatric Oncology Group study. *Blood* 1990;75:166.
55. Uckun FM, Muraguchi A, Ledbetter JA, et al. Biphenotypic leukemic lymphocyte precursors in CD2+CD19+ acute lymphoblastic leukemia and their putative normal counterparts in human fetal hematopoietic tissues. *Blood* 1989;73:1000.
56. Pui CH, Behm FG, Singh B, et al. Myeloid-associated antigen expression lacks prognostic value in childhood acute lymphoblastic leukemia treated with intensive multiagent chemotherapy. *Blood* 1990;75:198.
57. Uckun FM, Sather HN, Gaynon PS, et al. Clinical features and treatment outcome of children with myeloid antigen positive acute lymphoblastic leukemia: a report from the Children's Cancer Group. *Blood* 1997;90:28.
58. Ludwig WD, Bartram CR, Harbott J, et al. Phenotypic and genotypic heterogeneity in infant acute leukemia. I. Acute lymphoblastic leukemia. *Leukemia* 1989;3:431.
59. Pui CH, Frankel LS, Carroll AJ, et al. Clinical characteristics and treatment outcome of childhood acute lymphoblastic leukemia with the t(4;11)(q21;q23): a collaborative study of 40 cases. *Blood* 1991;77:440.
60. Hirsch-Ginsberg C, Childs C, Chang KS, et al. Phenotypic and molecular heterogeneity in Philadelphia chromosome-positive acute leukemia. *Blood* 1988;71:186.
61. Wiersma SR, Ortega J, Sobel E, Weinberg KI. Clinical importance of myeloid-antigen expression in acute lymphoblastic leukemia of childhood. *N Engl J Med* 1991;324:800.
62. Williams DL, Raimondi S, Rivera G, et al. Presence of clonal chromosome abnormalities in virtually all cases of acute lymphoblastic leukemia. *N Engl J Med* 1985;313:640.

63. Bloomfield CD, Goldman AI, Alimena G, et al. Chromosomal abnormalities identify high-risk and low-risk patients with acute lymphoblastic leukemia. *Blood* 1986;67:415.

64. Secker-Walker LM, Prentice HG, Durrant J, et al. Cytogenetics adds independent prognostic information in adults with acute lymphoblastic leukaemia on MRC trial UKALL XA. MRC Adult Leukaemia Working Party. *Br J Haematol* 1997;96:601.

65. Look AT. The cytogenetics of childhood leukemia: clinical and biologic implications. *Pediatr Clin North Am* 1988;35:723.

66. Look AT, Roberson PK, Williams DL, et al. Prognostic importance of blast cell DNA content in childhood acute lymphoblastic leukemia. *Blood* 1985;65:1079.

67. Pui CH, Williams DL, Raimondi SC, et al. Hypodiploidy is associated with a poor prognosis in childhood acute lymphoblastic leukemia. *Blood* 1987;70:247.

68. Trueworthy R, Shuster J, Look T, et al. Ploidy of lymphoblasts is the strongest predictor of treatment outcome in B-progenitor cell acute lymphoblastic leukemia of childhood: a Pediatric Oncology Group study. *J Clin Oncol* 1992;10:606.

69. Chessells JM, Swansbury GJ, Reeves B, et al. Cytogenetics and prognosis in childhood lymphoblastic leukaemia: results of MRC UKALL X. Medical Research Council Working Party in Childhood Leukaemia. *Br J Haematol* 1997;99:93.

70. Heerema NA, Nachman JB, Sather HN, et al. Hypodiploidy with less than 45 chromosomes confers adverse risk in childhood acute lymphoblastic leukemia: a report from the children's cancer group. *Blood* 1999;94:4036.

71. Forestier E, Johansson B, Gustafsson G, et al. Prognostic impact of karyotypic findings in childhood acute lymphoblastic leukaemia: a Nordic series comparing two treatment periods. For the Nordic Society of Paediatric Haematology and Oncology (NOPHO) Leukaemia Cytogenetic Study Group. *Br J Haematol* 2000;110:147.

72. Pui CH, Williams DL, Roberson PK, et al. Correlation of karyotype and immunophenotype in childhood acute lymphoblastic leukemia. *J Clin Oncol* 1988;6:56.

73. Whitehead VM, Vuchich MJ, Lauer SJ, et al. Accumulation of high levels of methotrexate polyglutamates in lymphoblasts from children with hyperdiploid (greater than 50 chromosomes) B-lineage acute lymphoblastic leukemia: a Pediatric Oncology Group study. *Blood* 1992;80:1316.

74. Synold TW, Relling MV, Boyett JM, et al. Blast cell methotrexate-polyglutamate accumulation in vivo differs by lineage, ploidy, and methotrexate dose in acute lymphoblastic leukemia. *J Clin Invest* 1994;94:1996.

75. Kaspers GJ, Smets LA, Pieters R, et al. Favorable prognosis of hyperdiploid common acute lymphoblastic leukemia may be explained by sensitivity to antimetabolites and other drugs: results of an in vitro study. *Blood* 1995;85:751.

76. Ito C, Kumagai M, Manabe A, et al. Hyperdiploid acute lymphoblastic leukemia with 51 to 65 chromosomes: a distinct biological entity with a marked propensity to undergo apoptosis. *Blood* 1999;93:315.

77. Heerema NA, Sather HN, Sensel MG, et al. Prognostic impact of trisomies of chromosomes 10, 17, and 5 among children with acute lymphoblastic leukemia and high hyperdiploidy (>50 chromosomes). *J Clin Oncol* 2000;18:1876.

78. Pui CH, Raimondi SC, Dodge RK, et al. Prognostic importance of structural chromosomal abnormalities in children with hyperdiploid (greater than 50 chromosomes) acute lymphoblastic leukemia. *Blood* 1989;73:1963.

79. Harris MB, Shuster JJ, Carroll A, et al. Trisomy of leukemic cell chromosomes 4 and 10 identifies children with B-progenitor cell acute lymphoblastic leukemia with a very low risk of treatment failure: a Pediatric Oncology Group study. *Blood* 1992;79:3316.

80. Crist W, Carroll A, Shuster J, et al. Philadelphia chromosome positive childhood acute lymphoblastic leukemia: clinical and cytogenetic characteristics and treatment outcome. A Pediatric Oncology Group study. *Blood* 1990;76:489.

81. Fletcher JA, Lynch EA, Kimball VM, et al. Translocation (9;22) is associated with extremely poor prognosis in intensively treated children with acute lymphoblastic leukemia. *Blood* 1991;77:435.

82. Croce CM. Chromosome translocations and human cancer. *Cancer Res* 1986;46:6019.

83. Clark SS, McLaughlin J, Crist WM, et al. Unique forms of the abl tyrosine kinase distinguish Ph1-positive CML from Ph1-positive ALL. *Science* 1987;235:85.

84. Kurzrock R, Shtalrid M, Romero P, et al. A novel c-abl protein product in Philadelphia-positive acute lymphoblastic leukaemia. *Nature* 1987;325:631.

85. Dalla-Favera R, Bregni M, Erikson J, et al. Human c-myc onc gene is located on the region of chromosome 8 that is translocated in Burkitt lymphoma cells. *Proc Natl Acad Sci U S A* 1982;79:7824.

86. Lombardi L, Newcomb EW, Dalla-Favera R. Pathogenesis of Burkitt lymphoma: expression of an activated c-myc oncogene causes the tumorigenic conversion of EBV-infected human B lymphoblasts. *Cell* 1987;49:161.

87. Romana SP, Poirel H, Leconiat M, et al. High frequency of t(12;21) in childhood B-lineage acute lymphoblastic leukemia. *Blood* 1995;86:4263.

88. McLean TW, Ringold S, Neuberg D, et al. TEL/AML-1 dimerizes and is associated with a favorable outcome in childhood acute lymphoblastic leukemia. *Blood* 1996;88:4252.

89. Borkhardt A, Cazzaniga G, Viehmann S, et al. Incidence and clinical relevance of TEL/AML1 fusion genes in children with acute lymphoblastic leukemia enrolled in the German and Italian multicenter therapy trials. Associazione Italiana Ematologia Oncologia Pediatrica and the Berlin-Frankfurt-Munster Study Group. *Blood* 1997;90:571.

90. Aguiar RC, Sohal J, van Rhee F, et al. TEL-AML1 fusion in acute lymphoblastic leukaemia of adults. M.R.C. Adult Leukaemia Working Party. *Br J Haematol* 1996;95:673.

91. Golub TR, Barker GF, Bohlander SK, et al. Fusion of the TEL gene on 12p13 to the AML1 gene on 21q22 in acute lymphoblastic leukemia. *Proc Natl Acad Sci U S A* 1995;92:4917.

92. Raynaud S, Cave H, Baens M, et al. The 12;21 translocation involving TEL and deletion of the other TEL allele: two frequently associated alterations found in childhood acute lymphoblastic leukemia. *Blood* 1996;87:2891.

93. Rubnitz JE, Downing JR, Pui CH, et al. TEL gene rearrangement in acute lymphoblastic leukemia: a new genetic marker with prognostic significance. *J Clin Oncol* 1997;15:1150.

94. Loh ML, Silverman LB, Young ML, et al. Incidence of TEL/AML1 fusion in children with relapsed acute lymphoblastic leukemia. *Blood* 1998;92:4792.

95. Rubnitz JE, Behm FG, Wichlan D, et al. Low frequency of TEL-AML1 in relapsed acute lymphoblastic leukemia supports a favorable prognosis for this genetic subgroup. *Leukemia* 1999;13:19.

96. Harbott J, Viehmann S, Borkhardt A, et al. Incidence of TEL/AML1 fusion gene analyzed consecutively in children with acute lymphoblastic leukemia in relapse. *Blood* 1997;90:4933.

97. Seeger K, Adams HP, Buchwald D, et al. TEL-AML1 fusion transcript in relapsed childhood acute lymphoblastic leukemia. *Blood* 1998;91:1716.

98. Ramakers-van Woerden NL, Pieters R, Loonen AH, et al. TEL/AML1 gene fusion is related to in vitro drug sensitivity for L-asparaginase in childhood acute lymphoblastic leukemia. *Blood* 2000;96:1094.

99. Pui CH, Crist WM, Look AT. Biology and clinical significance of cytogenetic abnormalities in childhood acute lymphoblastic leukemia. *Blood* 1990;76:1449.

100. Chan LC, Karhi KK, Rayter SI, et al. A novel abl protein expressed in Philadelphia chromosome positive acute lymphoblastic leukaemia. *Nature* 1987;325:635.

101. Lugo TG, Pendergast AM, Muller AJ, Witte ON. Tyrosine kinase activity and transformation potency of bcr-abl oncogene products. *Science* 1990;247:1079.

102. Arico M, Valsecchi MG, Camitta B, et al. Outcome of treatment in children with Philadelphia chromosome-positive acute lymphoblastic leukemia. *N Engl J Med* 2000;342:998.

103. Ribeiro RC, Broniscer A, Rivera GK, et al Philadelphia chromosome-positive acute lymphoblastic leukemia in children: durable responses to chemotherapy associated with low initial white blood cell counts. *Leukemia* 1997;11:1493.

104. Schrappe M, Arico M, Harbott J, et al. Philadelphia chromosome-positive (Ph+) childhood acute lymphoblastic leukemia: good initial steroid response allows early prediction of a favorable treatment outcome. *Blood* 1998;92:2730.

105. Barrett AJ, Horowitz MM, Ash RC, et al. Bone marrow transplantation for Philadelphia chromosome-positive acute lymphoblastic leukemia. *Blood* 1992;79:3067.

106. Sierra J, Radich J, Hansen JA, et al. Marrow transplants from unrelated donors for treatment of Philadelphia chromosome-positive acute lymphoblastic leukemia. *Blood* 1997;90:1410.

107. Marks DI, Bird JM, Cornish JM, et al. Unrelated donor bone marrow transplantation for children and adolescents with Philadelphia-positive acute lymphoblastic leukemia. *J Clin Oncol* 1998;16:931.

108. Rubnitz JE, Link MP, Shuster JJ, et al. Frequency and prognostic significance of HRX rearrangements in infant acute lymphoblastic leukemia: a Pediatric Oncology Group Study. *Blood* 1994;84:570.

109. Gu Y, Nakamura T, Alder H, et al. The t(4;11) chromosome translocation of human acute leukemias fuses the ALL-1 gene, related to Drosophila trithorax, to the AF-4 gene. *Cell* 1992;71:701.

110. Behm FG, Raimondi SC, Frestedt JL, et al. Rearrangement of the MLL gene confers a poor prognosis in childhood acute lymphoblastic leukemia, regardless of presenting age. *Blood* 1996;87:2870.

111. Rubnitz JE, Camitta BM, Mahmoud H, et al. Childhood acute lymphoblastic leukemia with the MLL-ENL fusion and t(11;19)(q23;p13.3) translocation. *J Clin Oncol* 1999;17:191.

112. Mellentin JD, Nourse J, Hunger SP, et al. Molecular analysis of the t(1;19) breakpoint cluster region in pre-B cell acute lymphoblastic leukemias. *Genes Chromosomes Cancer* 1990;2:239.

113. Nourse J, Mellentin JD, Galili N, et al. Chromosomal translocation t(1;19) results in synthesis of a homeobox fusion mRNA that codes for a potential chimeric transcription factor. *Cell* 1990;60:535.

114. Kamps MP, Murre C, Sun XH, Baltimore D. A new homeobox gene contributes the DNA binding domain of the t(1;19) translocation protein in pre-B ALL. *Cell* 1990;60:547.

115. Raimondi SC, Behm FG, Roberson PK. Cytogenetics of pre-B-cell acute lymphoblastic leukemia with emphasis on prognostic implications of the t(1;19). *J Clin Oncol* 1990;8:1380.

116. Uckun FM, Sensel MG, Sather HN, et al. Clinical significance of translocation t(1;19) in childhood acute lymphoblastic leukemia in the context of contemporary therapies: a report from the Children's Cancer Group. *J Clin Oncol* 1998;16:527.

117. Raimondi SC, Privitera E, Williams DL, et al. New recurring chromosomal translocations in childhood acute lymphoblastic leukemia. *Blood* 1991;77:2016.

118. Hunger SP. Chromosomal translocations involving the E2A gene in acute lymphoblastic leukemia: clinical features and molecular pathogenesis. *Blood* 1996;87:1211.

119. Murphy SB, Raimondi SC, Rivera GK, et al. Nonrandom abnormalities of chromosome 9p in childhood acute lymphoblastic leukemia: association with high-risk clinical features. *Blood* 1989;74:409.

120. Diaz MO, Rubin CM, Harden A, et al. Deletions of interferon genes in acute lymphoblastic leukemia. *N Engl J Med* 1990;322:77.

121. Heyman M, Rasool O, Borgonovo Brandter L, et al. Prognostic importance of p15INK4B and p16INK4 gene inactivation in childhood acute lymphocytic leukemia. *J Clin Oncol* 1996;14:1512.

122. Kees UR, Burton PR, Lu C, Baker DL. Homozygous deletion of the p16/MTS1 gene in pediatric acute lymphoblastic leukemia is associated with unfavorable clinical outcome. *Blood* 1997;89:4161.

123. Heerema NA, Sather HN, Sensel MG, et al. Frequency and clinical significance of cytogenetic abnormalities in pediatric T-lineage acute lymphoblastic leukemia: a report from the Children's Cancer Group. *J Clin Oncol* 1998; 16:1270.

124. Schneider NR, Carroll AJ, Shuster JJ, et al. New recurring cytogenetic abnormalities and association of blast cell karyotypes with prognosis in childhood T-cell acute lymphoblastic leukemia: a pediatric oncology group report of 343 cases. *Blood* 2000;96:2543.

125. Carroll AJ, Crist WM, Link MP, et al. The t(1;14)(p34;q11) is nonrandom and restricted to T-cell acute lymphoblastic leukemia: a Pediatric Oncology Group study. *Blood* 1990;76:1220.

126. Brown L, Cheng JT, Chen Q, et al. Site-specific recombination of the tal-1 gene is a common occurrence in human T cell leukemia. *EMBO J* 1990;9:3343.

127. Aplan PD, Lombardi DP, Reaman GH, et al. Involvement of the putative hematopoietic transcription factor SCL in T-cell acute lymphoblastic leukemia. *Blood* 1992;79:1327.

128. Bash RO, Crist WM, Shuster JJ, et al. Clinical features and outcome of T-cell acute lymphoblastic leukemia in childhood with respect to alterations at the TAL1 locus: a Pediatric Oncology Group study. *Blood* 1993;81:2110.

129. Ribeiro RC, Raimondi SC, Behm FG, et al. Clinical and biologic features of childhood T-cell leukemia with the t(11;14). *Blood* 1991;78:466.

130. Lange BJ, Raimondi SC, Heerema N, et al. Pediatric leukemia/lymphoma with t(8;14)(q24;q11). *Leukemia* 1992;6:613.

131. Emanuel BS, Selden JR, Chaganti RS, et al. The 2p breakpoint of a 2;8 translocation in Burkitt lymphoma interrupts the V κ–locus. *Proc Natl Acad Sci U S A* 1984;81:2444.

132. Hollis GF, Mitchell KF, Battey J, et al. A variant translocation places the lambda immunoglobulin genes 3' to the c-myc oncogene in Burkitt's lymphoma. *Nature* 1984;307:752.

133. Grimaldi JC, Meeker TC. The t(5;14) chromosomal translocation in a case of acute lymphocytic leukemia joins the interleukin-3 gene to the immunoglobulin heavy chain gene. *Blood* 1989;73:2081.

134. Hogan TF, Koss W, Murgo AJ, et al. Acute lymphoblastic leukemia with chromosomal 5;14 translocation and hypereosinophilia: case report and literature review. *J Clin Oncol* 1987;5:382.

135. Smith M, Arthur D, Camitta B, et al. Uniform approach to risk classification and treatment assignment for children with acute lymphoblastic leukemia. *J Clin Oncol* 1996;14:18.

136. Ribeiro RC, Pui CH. The clinical and biological correlates of coagulopathy in children with acute leukemia. *J Clin Oncol* 1986;4:1212.

137. Dubansky AS, Boyett JM, Falletta J, et al. Isolated thrombocytopenia in children with acute lymphoblastic leukemia: a rare event in a Pediatric Oncology Group Study. *Pediatrics* 1989;84:1068.

138. Saulsbury FT, Sabio H, Conrad D, et al. Acute leukemia with features of systemic lupus erythematosus. *J Pediatr* 1984;105:57.

139. Sullivan JL. Epstein-Barr virus and lymphoproliferative disorders. *Semin Hematol* 1988;25:269.

140. Reiter A, Schrappe M, Ludwig WD, et al. Intensive ALL-type therapy without local radiotherapy provides a 90% event-free survival for children with T-cell lymphoblastic lymphoma: a BFM group report. *Blood* 2000;95:416.

141. Neth O, Seidemann K, Jansen P, et al. Precursor B-cell lymphoblastic lymphoma in childhood and adolescence: clinical features, treatment, and results in trials NHL-BFM 86 and 90. *Med Pediatr Oncol* 2000;35:20.

142. Crist W, Pullen J, Boyett J, et al. Acute lymphoid leukemia in adolescents: clinical and biologic features predict a poor prognosis—a Pediatric Oncology Group Study. *J Clin Oncol* 1988;6:34.

143. Larson RA, Dodge RK, Burns CP, et al. A five-drug remission induction regimen with intensive consolidation for adults with acute lymphoblastic leukemia: cancer and leukemia group B study 8811. *Blood* 1995;85:2025.

144. Czuczman MS, Dodge RK, Stewart CC, et al. Value of immunophenotype in intensively treated adult acute lymphoblastic leukemia: cancer and leukemia Group B study 8364. *Blood* 1999;93:3931.

145. Williams DL, Tsiatis A, Brodeur GM, et al. Prognostic importance of chromosome number in 136 untreated children with acute lymphoblastic leukemia. *Blood* 1982;60:864.

146. Gaynon PS, Desai AA, Bostrom BC, et al. Early response to therapy and outcome in childhood acute lymphoblastic leukemia: a review. *Cancer* 1997; 80:1717.

147. Silverman LB, Gelber RD, Young ML, et al. Induction failure in acute lymphoblastic leukemia of childhood. *Cancer* 1999;85:1395.

148. Schrappe M, Reiter A, Zimmermann M, et al. Long-term results of four consecutive trials in childhood ALL performed by the ALL-BFM study group from 1981 to 1995. Berlin-Frankfurt-Munster. *Leukemia* 2000;14:2205.

149. Schrappe M, Reiter A, Ludwig WD, et al. Improved outcome in childhood acute lymphoblastic leukemia despite reduced use of anthracyclines and cranial radiotherapy: results of trial ALL-BFM 90. German-Austrian-Swiss ALL-BFM Study Group. *Blood* 2000;95:3310.

150. Rautonen J, Hovi L, Siimes M. Slow disappearance of peripheral blast cells: an independent risk factor indicating poor prognosis in children with acute lymphoblastic leukemia. *Blood* 1988;71:989.

151. Gajjar A, Ribeiro R, Hancock ML, et al. Persistence of circulating blasts after 1 week of multiagent chemotherapy confers a poor prognosis in childhood acute lymphoblastic leukemia. *Blood* 1995;86:1292.

152. Griffin TC, Shuster JJ, Buchanan GR, et al. Slow disappearance of peripheral blood blasts is an adverse prognostic factor in childhood T cell acute lymphoblastic leukemia: a Pediatric Oncology Group study. *Leukemia* 2000; 14:792.

153. Nachman JB, Sather HN, Sensel MG, et al. Augmented post-induction therapy for children with high-risk acute lymphoblastic leukemia and a slow response to initial therapy. *N Engl J Med* 1998;338:1663.

154. Campana D, Pui C-H. Detection of minimal residual disease in acute leukemia: methodologic advances and clinical significance. *Blood* 1995;85:1416.

155. Dibenedetto SP, Nigro LL, Mayer SP, et al. Detectable molecular residual disease at the beginning of maintenance therapy indicates poor outcome in children with T-cell acute lymphoblastic leukemia. *Blood* 1997;90:1226.

156. Neale GA, Menarguez J, Kitchingman GR, et al. Detection of minimal residual disease in T-cell acute lymphoblastic leukemia using polymerase chain reaction predicts relapse. *Blood* 1991;78:739.

157. Cave H, Guidal C, Rohrlich P, et al. Prospective monitoring and quantitation of residual blasts in childhood acute lymphoblastic leukemia by polymerase chain reaction study of delta and gamma T-cell receptor genes. *Blood* 1994;83:1892.

158. Nizet Y, Van Daele S, Lewalle P, et al. Long-term follow-up of residual disease in acute lymphoblastic leukemia patients in complete remission using clonogenic IgH probes and the polymerase chain reaction. *Blood* 1993;82: 1618.

159. Roberts WM, Estrov Z, Ouspenskaia MV, et al. Measurement of residual leukemia during remission in childhood acute lymphoblastic leukemia. *N Engl J Med* 1997;336:317.

160. Ito Y, Wasserman R, Galili N, et al. Molecular residual disease status at the end of chemotherapy fails to predict subsequent relapse in children with B-lineage acute lymphoblastic leukemia. *J Clin Oncol* 1993;11:546.

161. Cave H, van der Werff ten Bosch J, Suciu S, et al. Clinical significance of minimal residual disease in childhood acute lymphoblastic leukemia. European Organization for Research and Treatment of Cancer—Childhood Leukemia Cooperative Group. *N Engl J Med* 1998;339:591.

162. van Dongen JJ, Seriu T, Panzer-Grumayer ER, et al. Prognostic value of minimal residual disease in acute lymphoblastic leukaemia in childhood. *Lancet* 1998;352:1731.

163. Panzer-Grumayer ER, Schneider M, Panzer S, et al. Rapid molecular response during early induction chemotherapy predicts a good outcome in childhood acute lymphoblastic leukemia. *Blood* 2000;95:790.

164. Coustan-Smith E, Sancho J, Hancock ML, et al. Clinical importance of minimal residual disease in childhood acute lymphoblastic leukemia. *Blood* 2000;96:2691.

165. Chessells JM, Richards SM, Bailey CC, et al. Gender and treatment outcome in childhood lymphoblastic leukaemia: report from the MRC UKALL trials. *Br J Haematol* 1995;89:364.

166. Shuster JJ, Wacker P, Pullen J, et al. Prognostic significance of sex in childhood B-precursor acute lymphoblastic leukemia: a Pediatric Oncology Group Study. *J Clin Oncol* 1998;16:2854.

167. Pui CH, Boyett JM, Hancock ML, et al. Outcome of treatment for childhood cancer in black as compared with white children. The St. Jude Children's Research Hospital experience, 1962 through 1992. *JAMA* 1995;273: 633.

168. Pollock BH, DeBaun MR, Camitta BM, et al. Racial differences in the survival of childhood B-precursor acute lymphoblastic leukemia: a Pediatric Oncology Group Study. *J Clin Oncol* 2000;18:813.

169. Relling MV, Hancock ML, Boyett JM, et al. Prognostic importance of 6-mercaptopurine dose intensity in acute lymphoblastic leukemia. *Blood* 1999; 93:2817.

170. Stanulla M, Schrappe M, Brechlin AM, et al. Polymorphisms within glutathione S-transferase genes (GSTM1, GSTT1, GSTP1) and risk of relapse in childhood B-cell precursor acute lymphoblastic leukemia: a case-control study. *Blood* 2000;95:1222.

171. Relling MV, Pui CH, Sandlund JT, et al. Adverse effect of anticonvulsants on efficacy of chemotherapy for acute lymphoblastic leukaemia. *Lancet* 2000; 356:285.

172. Evans WE, Relling MV, Rodman JH, et al. Conventional compared with individualized chemotherapy for childhood acute lymphoblastic leukemia. *N Engl J Med* 1998;338:499.

173. Farber S, Diamond LK, Mercer RD, et al. Temporary remissions in acute leukemia in children produced by folic acid antagonist, 4-aminopteroylglutamic acid (aminopterin). *N Engl J Med* 1948;238:787.

174. Frei E III. Acute leukemia in children. Model for the development of scientific methodology for clinical therapeutic research in cancer. *Cancer* 1984; 53:2013.

175. Elion G, Hitchings G. Metabolic basis for the actions of analogs of purines and pyrimidines. *Adv Chemother* 1965;2:91.

176. Burchenal JH, Murphy ML, Ellison RR, et al. Clinical evaluation of a new antimetabolite: 6-mercaptopurine in the treatment of leukemia and allied diseases. *Blood* 1953;8:965.

177. Frei E III, Holland JF, Schneiderman MA, et al. A comparative study of two regimens of combination chemotherapy in acute leukemia. *Blood* 1958;13:1126.

178. Freireich EJ, Frei E III. Recent advances in acute leukemia. *Prog Hematol* 1964;4:187.

179. Blum R, Carter S. Adriamycin. A new anticancer drug with significant clinical activity. *Ann Intern Med* 1974;80:249.
180. Tallal L, Tan C, Oettgen H, et al. *E. coli* L-asparaginase in the treatment of leukemia and solid tumors in 131 children. *Cancer* 1970;25:306.
181. Jaffe N, Traggis D, Das L, et al. Comparison of daily and twice-weekly schedule of L-asparaginase in childhood leukemia. *Pediatrics* 1972;49:590.
182. Pui CH, Boyett JM, Rivera GK, et al. Long-term results of Total Therapy studies 11, 12 and 13A for childhood acute lymphoblastic leukemia at St. Jude Children's Research Hospital. *Leukemia* 2000;14:2286.
183. Skipper HE, Schabel FM Jr, Wilcox WS. Experimental evaluation of potential anticancer agents: on the criteria and kinetics associated with "curability" of experimental leukemia. *Cancer Chemother Rep* 1964;35:1.
184. Frei E III, Freireich EJ. Progress and perspectives in the chemotherapy of acute leukemia. *Adv Chemother* 1965;2:269.
185. Pinkel D, Hernandez K, Borella L, et al. Drug dosage and remission duration in childhood lymphocytic leukemia. *Cancer* 1971;27:247.
186. Sallan SE, Gelber RD, Kimball V, et al. More is better! Update of Dana-Farber Cancer Institute/Children's Hospital childhood acute lymphoblastic leukemia trials. *Hamatol Bluttransfus* 1990;33:459.
187. Pinkel D. Five-year follow-up of "total therapy" of childhood lymphocytic leukemia. *JAMA* 1971;216:648.
188. Evans AE, Gilbert ES, Zandstra R. The increasing incidence of central nervous system leukemia in children. (Children's Cancer Study Group A). *Cancer* 1970;26:404.
189. Komp DM, Fernandez CH, Falletta JM, et al. CNS prophylaxis in acute lymphoblastic leukemia: comparison of two methods a Southwest Oncology Group study. *Cancer* 1982;50:1031.
190. Nesbit ME, Sather H, Robison LL, et al. Sanctuary therapy: a randomized trial of 724 children with previously untreated acute lymphoblastic leukemia: a report from Children's Cancer Study Group. *Cancer Res* 1982;42:674.
191. Aur RJ, Simone JV, Hustu HO, Verzosa MS. A comparative study of central nervous system irradiation and intensive chemotherapy early in remission of childhood acute lymphocytic leukemia. *Cancer* 1972;29:381.
192. Hustu HO, Aur RJ, Verzosa MS, et al. Prevention of central nervous system leukemia by irradiation. *Cancer* 1973;32:585.
193. Wang JJ, Freeman AI, Sinks LF. Treatment of acute lymphocytic leukemia by high-dose intravenous methotrexate. *Cancer Res* 1976;36:1441.
194. Frick J, Ritch PS, Hansen RM, Anderson T. Successful treatment of meningeal leukemia using systemic high-dose cytosine arabinoside. *J Clin Oncol* 1984;2:365.
195. Arrambide K, Toto RD. Tumor lysis syndrome. *Semin Nephrol* 1993;13:273.
196. Bunin NJ, Pui CH. Differing complications of hyperleukocytosis in children with acute lymphoblastic or acute nonlymphoblastic leukemia. *J Clin Oncol* 1985;3:1590.
197. Rebulla P, Finazzi G, Marangoni F, et al. The threshold for prophylactic platelet transfusions in adults with acute myeloid leukemia. *N Engl J Med* 1997;337:1870.
198. Pizzo PA. Management of fever in patients with cancer and treatment-induced neutropenia. *N Engl J Med* 1993;328:1323.
199. Rackoff WR, Gonin R, Robinson C, et al. Predicting the risk of bacteremia in children with fever and neutropenia. *J Clin Oncol* 1996;14:919.
200. Hughes WT, Rivera GK, Schell MJ, et al. Successful intermittent chemoprophylaxis for Pneumocystis carinii pneumonia. *N Engl J Med* 1987;316:1627.
201. Welte K, Reiter A, Mempel K, et al. A randomized phase-III study of the efficacy of granulocyte colony-stimulating factor in children with high-risk acute lymphoblastic leukemia. Berlin-Frankfurt-Munster Study Group. *Blood* 1996;87:3143.
202. Pui CH, Boyett JM, Hughes WT, et al. Human granulocyte colony-stimulating factor after induction chemotherapy in children with acute lymphoblastic leukemia. *N Engl J Med* 1997;336:1781.
203. Ottmann OG, Hoelzer D, Gracien E, et al. Concomitant granulocyte colony-stimulating factor and induction chemoradiotherapy in adult acute lymphoblastic leukemia: a randomized phase III trial. *Blood* 1995;86:444.
204. Geissler K, Koller E, Hubmann E, et al. Granulocyte colony-stimulating factor as an adjunct to induction chemotherapy for adult acute lymphoblastic leukemia—a randomized phase-III study. *Blood* 1997;90:590.
205. Simone J, Aur RJ, Hustu HO, Pinkel D. "Total therapy" studies of acute lymphocytic leukemia in children. Current results and prospects for cure. *Cancer* 1972;30:1488.
206. Holland JF, Glidewell O. Chemotherapy of acute lymphocytic leukemia of childhood. *Cancer* 1972;30:1480.
207. Ortega JA, Nesbit ME Jr, Donaldson MH, et al. L-Asparaginase, vincristine, and prednisone for induction of first remission in acute lymphocytic leukemia. *Cancer Res* 1977;37:535.
208. Sallan SE, Camitta BM, Cassady JR, et al. Intermittent combination chemotherapy with adriamycin for childhood acute lymphoblastic leukemia: clinical results. *Blood* 1978;51:425.
209. Hitchcock-Bryan S, Gelber R, Cassady JR, Sallan SE. The impact of induction anthracycline on long-term failure-free survival in childhood acute lymphoblastic leukemia. *Med Pediatr Oncol* 1986;14:211.
210. Goldie JH, Coldman AJ, Gudauskas GA. Rationale for the use of alternating non-cross-resistant chemotherapy. *Cancer Treat Rep* 1982;66:439.
211. Gaynon PS, Steinherz PG, Bleyer WA, et al. Improved therapy for children with acute lymphoblastic leukemia and unfavorable presenting features: a follow-up report of the Childrens Cancer Group Study CCG-106. *J Clin Oncol* 1993;11:2234.
212. Tubergen DG, Gilchrist GS, O'Brien RT, et al. Improved outcome with delayed intensification for children with acute lymphoblastic leukemia and intermediate presenting features: a Childrens Cancer Group phase III trial. *J Clin Oncol* 1993;11:527.
213. Freireich EJ, Gehan E, Frei E III, et al. The effect of 6-mercaptopurine on the duration of steroid-induced remissions in acute leukemia: a model for evaluation of other potentially useful therapy. *Blood* 1963;21:699.
214. Ochs J, Rivera GK, Pollock BH, et al. Teniposide (VM-26) and continuous infusion cytosine arabinoside for initial induction failure in childhood acute lymphoblastic leukemia. A Pediatric Oncology Group pilot study. *Cancer* 1990;66:1671.
215. Giona F, Testi AM, Annino L, et al. Treatment of primary refractory and relapsed acute lymphoblastic leukaemia in children and adults: the GIMEMA/AIEOP experience. Gruppo Italiano Malattie Ematologiche Maligne dell'Adulto. Associazione Italiana Ematologia ed Ocologia Pediatrica. *Br J Haematol* 1994;86:55.
216. Early AP, Preisler HD, Gottlieb AJ, Lanchant NA. Treatment of refractory adult acute lymphocytic leukaemia and acute undifferentiated leukaemia with an anthracycline antibiotic and cytosine arabinoside. *Br J Haematol* 1981;48:369.
217. Rivera G, Dahl GV, Bowman WP, et al. VM-26 and cytosine arabinoside combination chemotherapy for initial induction failures in childhood lymphocytic leukemia. *Cancer* 1980;46:1727.
218. Rivera GK, Pinkel D, Simone JV, et al. Treatment of acute lymphoblastic leukemia. 30 years' experience at St. Jude Children's Research Hospital. *N Engl J Med* 1993;329:1289.
219. Dahl GV, Rivera GK, Look AT, et al. Teniposide plus cytarabine improves outcome in childhood acute lymphoblastic leukemia presenting with a leukocyte count greater than or equal to 100×10^9/L. *J Clin Oncol* 1987;5:1015.
220. Rivera GK, Raimondi SC, Hancock ML, et al. Improved outcome in childhood acute lymphoblastic leukaemia with reinforced early treatment and rotational combination chemotherapy. *Lancet* 1991;337:61.
221. Mahmoud HH, Rivera GK, Hancock ML, et al. Low leukocyte counts with blast cells in cerebrospinal fluid of children with newly diagnosed acute lymphoblastic leukemia. *N Engl J Med* 1993;329:314.
222. Johnson R. An experimental therapeutic approach to L1210 leukemia in mice: combination chemotherapy and central nervous system irradiation. *J Natl Cancer Inst* 1964;32:133.
223. Pui CH, Mahmoud HH, Rivera GK, et al. Early intensification of intrathecal chemotherapy virtually eliminates central nervous system relapse in children with acute lymphoblastic leukemia. *Blood* 1998;92:411.
224. Conter V, Schrappe M, Arico M, et al. Role of cranial radiotherapy for childhood T-cell acute lymphoblastic leukemia with high WBC count and good response to prednisone. Associazione Italiana Ematologia Oncologia Pediatrica and the Berlin-Frankfurt-Munster groups. *J Clin Oncol* 1997;15:2786.
225. Nesbit ME Jr, Sather HN, Robison LL, et al. Presymptomatic central nervous system therapy in previously untreated childhood acute lymphoblastic leukaemia: comparison of 1800 rad and 2400 rad. A report for Children's Cancer Study Group. *Lancet* 1981;1:461.
226. Schrappe M, Reiter A, Henze G, et al. Prevention of CNS recurrence in childhood ALL: results with reduced radiotherapy combined with CNS-directed chemotherapy in four consecutive ALL-BFM trials. *Klin Padiatr* 1998;210:192.
227. Gelber RD, Sallan SE, Cohen HJ, et al. Central nervous system treatment in childhood acute lymphoblastic leukemia. Long-term follow-up of patients diagnosed between 1973 and 1985. *Cancer* 1993;72:261.
228. Balis FM, Lester CM, Chrousos GP, et al. Differences in cerebrospinal fluid penetration of corticosteroids: possible relationship to the prevention of meningeal leukemia. *J Clin Oncol* 1987;5:202.
229. Dibenedetto SP, Di Cataldo A, Ragusa R, et al. Levels of L-asparagine in CSF after intramuscular administration of asparaginase from Erwinia in children with acute lymphoblastic leukemia. *J Clin Oncol* 1995;13:339.
230. Pullen J, Boyett J, Shuster J, et al. Extended triple intrathecal chemotherapy trial for prevention of CNS relapse in good-risk and poor-risk patients with B-progenitor acute lymphoblastic leukemia: a Pediatric Oncology Group study. *J Clin Oncol* 1993;11:839.
231. Tubergen DG, Gilchrist GS, O'Brien RT, et al. Prevention of CNS disease in intermediate-risk acute lymphoblastic leukemia: comparison of cranial radiation and intrathecal methotrexate and the importance of systemic therapy: a Childrens Cancer Group report. *J Clin Oncol* 1993;11:520.
232. LeClerc JM, Billett AL, Gelber RD, et al. Treatment of childhood acute lymphoblastic leukemia: results of Dana-Farber ALL Consortium 87-01. *J Clin Oncol* 2002;20:237.
233. Conter V, Arico M, Valsecchi MG, et al. Extended intrathecal methotrexate may replace cranial irradiation for prevention of CNS relapse in children with intermediate-risk acute lymphoblastic leukemia treated with Berlin-Frankfurt-Munster-based intensive chemotherapy. The Associazione Italiana di Ematologia ed Oncologia Pediatrica. *J Clin Oncol* 1995;13:2497.
234. Veerman AJ, Hahlen K, Kamps WA, et al. High cure rate with a moderately intensive treatment regimen in non-high-risk childhood acute lymphoblastic leukemia. Results of protocol ALL VI from the Dutch Childhood Leukemia Study Group. *J Clin Oncol* 1996;14:911.
235. Mahoney DH Jr, Shuster JJ, Nitschke R, et al. Acute neurotoxicity in children with B-precursor acute lymphoid leukemia: an association with intermediate-dose intravenous methotrexate and intrathecal triple therapy—a Pediatric Oncology Group study. *J Clin Oncol* 1998;16:1712.

236. Sallan SE, Hitchcock-Bryan S, Gelber R, et al. Influence of intensive aspara-ginase in the treatment of childhood non-T-cell acute lymphoblastic leuke-mia. *Cancer Res* 1983;43:5601.
237. Clavell LA, Gelber RD, Cohen HJ, et al. Four-agent induction and intensive asparaginase therapy for treatment of childhood acute lymphoblastic leuke-mia. *N Engl J Med* 1986;315:657.
238. Schorin MA, Blattner S, Gelber RD, et al. Treatment of childhood acute lym-phoblastic leukemia: results of Dana-Farber Cancer Institute/Children's Hos-pital Acute Lymphoblastic Leukemia Consortium Protocol 85-01. *J Clin Oncol* 1994;12:740.
239. Maloney KW, Shuster JJ, Murphy S, et al. Long-term results of treatment studies for childhood acute lymphoblastic leukemia: Pediatric Oncology Group studies from 1986–1994. *Leukemia* 2000;14:2276.
240. Harris MB, Shuster JJ, Pullen DJ, et al. Consolidation therapy with antime-tabolite-based therapy in standard-risk acute lymphocytic leukemia of child-hood: a Pediatric Oncology Group Study. *J Clin Oncol* 1998;16:2840.
241. Kamps WA, Veerman AJ, van Wering ER, et al. Long-term follow-up of Dutch Childhood Leukemia Study Group (DCLSG) protocols for children with acute lymphoblastic leukemia, 1984–1991. *Leukemia* 2000;14:2240.
242. Gustafsson G, Schmiegelow K, Forestier E, et al. Improving outcome through two decades in childhood ALL in the Nordic countries: the impact of high-dose methotrexate in the reduction of CNS irradiation. Nordic Society of Pedi-atric Haematology and Oncology (NOPHO). *Leukemia* 2000;14:2267.
243. Reiter A, Schrappe M, Ludwig WD, et al. Chemotherapy in 998 unselected childhood acute lymphoblastic leukemia patients. Results and conclusions of the multicenter trial ALL-BFM 86. *Blood* 1994;84:3122.
244. Gaynon PS, Trigg ME, Heerema NA, et al. Children's Cancer Group trials in childhood acute lymphoblastic leukemia: 1983-1995. *Leukemia* 2000;14:2223.
245. Chessells JM, Bailey C, Richards SM. Intensification of treatment and sur-vival in all children with lymphoblastic leukaemia: results of UK Medical Research Council UKALL X. Medical Research Council Working Party on Childhood Leukaemia. *Lancet* 1995;345:143.
246. Eden OB, Harrison G, Richards S, et al. Long-term follow-up of the United Kingdom Medical Research Council protocols for childhood acute lympho-blastic leukaemia, 1980-1997. Medical Research Council Childhood Leu-kaemia Working Party. *Leukemia* 2000;14:2307.
247. Bleyer WA, Sather HN, Nickerson HJ, et al. Monthly pulses of vincristine and prednisone prevent bone marrow and testicular relapse in low-risk childhood acute lymphoblastic leukemia: a report of the CCG-161 study by the Childrens Cancer Study Group. *J Clin Oncol* 1991;9:1012.
248. Riehm H, Gadner H, Henze G, et al. Results and significance of six randomized trials in four consecutive ALL-BFM studies. *Hamatol Bluttransfus* 1990;33:439.
249. Jones B, Freeman AI, Shuster JJ, et al. Lower incidence of meningeal leuke-mia when prednisone is replaced by dexamethasone in the treatment of acute lymphocytic leukemia. *Med Pediatr Oncol* 1991;19:269.
250. Ito C, Evans WE, McNinch L, et al. Comparative cytotoxicity of dexametha-sone and prednisolone in childhood acute lymphoblastic leukemia. *J Clin Oncol* 1996;14:2370.
251. Kaspers GJ, Veerman AJ, Popp-Snijders C, et al. Comparison of the antileu-kemic activity in vitro of dexamethasone and prednisolone in childhood acute lymphoblastic leukemia. *Med Pediatr Oncol* 1996;27:114.
252. Strauss AJ, Su JT, Dalton VM, et al. Bony morbidity in children treated for acute lymphoblastic leukemia. *J Clin Oncol* 2001;19:3066.
253. Hurwitz CA, Silverman LB, Schorin MA, et al. Substituting dexamethasone for prednisone complicates remission induction in children with acute lym-phoblastic leukemia. *Cancer* 2000;88:1964.
254. Simone JV, Aur RJ, Hustu HO, et al. Three to ten years after cessation of ther-apy in children with leukemia. *Cancer* 1978;42:839.
255. Nesbit ME Jr, Sather HN, Robison LL, et al. Randomized study of 3 years versus 5 years of chemotherapy in childhood acute lymphoblastic leukemia. *J Clin Oncol* 1983;1:308.
256. Miller DR, Leikin SL, Albo VC, et al. Three versus five years of maintenance therapy are equivalent in childhood acute lymphoblastic leukemia: a report from the Childrens Cancer Study Group. *J Clin Oncol* 1989;7:316.
257. Eden OB, Lilleyman JS, Richards S, et al. Results of Medical Research Coun-cil Childhood Leukaemia Trial UKALL VIII (report to the Medical Research Council on behalf of the Working Party on Leukaemia in Childhood). *Br J Haematol* 1991;78:187.
258. Ravindranath Y, Soorya DT, Schultz GE, Lusher JM. Long-term survivors of acute lymphoblastic leukemia—risk of relapse after cessation of therapy. *Med Pediatr Oncol* 1981;9:209.
259. Toyoda Y, Manabe A, Tsuchida M, et al. Six months of maintenance chemo-therapy after intensified treatment for acute lymphoblastic leukemia of childhood. *J Clin Oncol* 2000;18:1508.
260. Druker BJ, Sawyers CL, Kantarjian H, et al. Activity of a specific inhibitor of the BCR-ABL tyrosine kinase in the blast crisis of chronic myeloid leukemia and acute lymphoblastic leukemia with the Philadelphia chromosome. *N Engl J Med* 2001;344:1038.
261. Biondi A, Cimino G, Pieters R, Pui CH. Biological and therapeutic aspects of infant leukemia. *Blood* 2000;96:24.
262. Chessells JM, Eden OB, Bailey CC, et al. Acute lymphoblastic leukaemia in infancy: experience in MRC UKALL trials. Report from the Medical Research Council Working Party on Childhood Leukaemia. *Leukemia* 1994;8:1275.
263. Frankel LS, Ochs J, Shuster JJ, et al. Therapeutic trial for infant acute lympho-blastic leukemia: the Pediatric Oncology Group experience (POG 8493). *J Pediatr Hematol Oncol* 1997;19:35.
264. Reaman GH, Sposto R, Sensel MG, et al. Treatment outcome and prognostic factors for infants with acute lymphoblastic leukemia treated on two consec-utive trials of the Children's Cancer Group. *J Clin Oncol* 1999;17:445.
265. Silverman LB, McLean TW, Gelber RD, et al. Intensified therapy for infants with acute lymphoblastic leukemia: results from the Dana-Farber Cancer Institute Consortium. *Cancer* 1997;80:2285.
266. Pieters R, den Boer ML, Durian M, et al. Relation between age, immunophe-notype and in vitro drug resistance in 395 children with acute lymphoblastic leukemia—implications for treatment of infants. *Leukemia* 1998;12:1344.
267. Dordelmann M, Reiter A, Borkhardt A, et al. Prednisone response is the strongest predictor of treatment outcome in infant acute lymphoblastic leu-kemia. *Blood* 1999;94:1209.
268. Pirich L, Haut P, Morgan E, et al. Total body irradiation, cyclophosphamide, and etoposide with stem cell transplant as treatment for infants with acute lymphocytic leukemia. *Med Pediatr Oncol* 1999;32:1.
269. Marco F, Bureo E, Ortega JJ, et al. High survival rate in infant acute leukemia treated with early high-dose chemotherapy and stem-cell support. Groupo Espanol de Trasplante de Medula Osea en Ninos. *J Clin Oncol* 2000;18:3256.
270. Verma A, Stock W. Management of adult acute lymphoblastic leukemia: moving toward a risk-adapted approach. *Curr Opin Oncol* 2001;13:14.
271. Hoelzer D, Thiel E, Ludwig WD, et al. Follow-up of the first two successive German multicentre trials for adult ALL (01/81 and 02/84). German Adult ALL Study Group. *Leukemia* 1993;7 Suppl 2:S130.
272. Mandelli F, Annino L, Rotoli B. The GIMEMA ALL 0183 trial: analysis of 10-year follow-up. GIMEMA Cooperative Group, Italy. *Br J Haematol* 1996;92:665.
273. Dekker AW, van't Veer MB, Sizoo W, et al. Intensive postremission chemother-apy without maintenance therapy in adults with acute lymphoblastic leuke-mia. Dutch Hemato-Oncology Research Group. *J Clin Oncol* 1997;15:476.
274. Kantarjian HM, O'Brien S, Smith TL, et al. Results of treatment with hyper-CVAD, a dose-intensive regimen, in adult acute lymphocytic leukemia. *J Clin Oncol* 2000;18:547.
275. Omura GA, Moffitt S, Vogler WR, Salter MM. Combination chemotherapy of adult acute lymphoblastic leukemia with randomized central nervous sys-tem prophylaxis. *Blood* 1980;55:199.
276. Finiewicz KJ, Larson RA. Dose-intensive therapy for adult acute lympho-blastic leukemia. *Semin Oncol* 1999;26:6.
277. Zhang MJ, Hoelzer D, Horowitz MM, et al. Long-term follow-up of adults with acute lymphoblastic leukemia in first remission treated with chemo-therapy or bone marrow transplantation. The Acute Lymphoblastic Leuke-mia Working Committee. *Ann Intern Med* 1995;123:428.
278. Sebban C, Lepage E, Vernant JP, et al. Allogeneic bone marrow transplanta-tion in adult acute lymphoblastic leukemia in first complete remission: a comparative study. French Group of Therapy of Adult Acute Lymphoblastic Leukemia. *J Clin Oncol* 1994;12:2580.
279. Roman DD, Sperduto PW. Neuropsychological effects of cranial radiation: current knowledge and future directions. *Int J Radiat Oncol Biol Phys* 1995;31:983.
280. Hoover DL, Smith LE, Turner SJ, et al. Ophthalmic evaluation of survivors of acute lymphoblastic leukemia. *Ophthalmology* 1988;95:151.
281. Lipshultz SE, Colan SD, Gelber RD, et al. Late cardiac effects of doxorubicin therapy for acute lymphoblastic leukemia in childhood. *N Engl J Med* 1991;324:808.
282. Schriock EA, Schell MJ, Carter M, et al. Abnormal growth patterns and adult short stature in 115 long-term survivors of childhood leukemia. *J Clin Oncol* 1991;9:400.
283. Van Dongen-Melman JE, Hokken-Koelega AC, Hahlen K, et al. Obesity after successful treatment of acute lymphoblastic leukemia in childhood. *Pediatr Res* 1995;38:86.
284. Chessells JM. Childhood acute lymphoblastic leukaemia: the late effects of treatment. *Br J Haematol* 1983;53:369.
285. Quigley C, Cowell C, Jimenez M, et al. Normal or early development of puberty despite gonadal damage in children treated for acute lymphoblastic leukemia. *N Engl J Med* 1989;321:143.
286. Neglia JP, Meadows AT, Robison LL, et al. Second neoplasms after acute lymphoblastic leukemia in childhood. *N Engl J Med* 1991;325:1330.
287. Dalton VMK, Gelber RD, Donnelly MJ, et al. Second malignant neoplasms in children treated for acute lymphoblastic leukemia. *Blood* 1997;90:559a.
288. Eiser C. Effects of chronic illness on intellectual development. A comparison of normal children with those treated for childhood leukaemia and solid tumours. *Arch Dis Child* 1980;55:766.
289. Meadows AT, Gordon J, Massari DJ, et al. Declines in IQ scores and cognitive dysfunctions in children with acute lymphocytic leukaemia treated with cra-nial irradiation. *Lancet* 1981;2:1015.
290. Rowland JH, Glidewell OJ, Sibley RF, et al. Effects of different forms of cen-tral nervous system prophylaxis on neuropsychologic function in childhood leukemia. *J Clin Oncol* 1984;2:1327.
291. Jankovic M, Brouwers P, Valsecchi MG, et al. Association of 1800 cGy cranial irradiation with intellectual function in children with acute lymphoblastic leukaemia. ISPACC. International Study Group on Psychosocial Aspects of Childhood Cancer. *Lancet* 1994;344:224.
292. Waber DP, Gioia G, Paccia J, et al. Sex differences in cognitive processing in children treated with CNS prophylaxis for acute lymphoblastic leukemia. *J Pediatr Psychol* 1990;15:105.
293. Butler RW, Hill JM, Steinherz PG, et al. Neuropsychologic effects of cranial irradiation, intrathecal methotrexate, and systemic methotrexate in child-hood cancer. *J Clin Oncol* 1994;12:2621.

294. Waber DP, Shapiro BL, Carpentieri SC, et al. Excellent therapeutic efficacy and minimal late neurotoxicity in children treated with 18 grays of cranial radiation therapy for high-risk acute lymphoblastic leukemia. *Cancer* 2001;92:15.

295. Waber DP, Tarbell NJ, Kahn CM, et al. The relationship of sex and treatment modality to neuropsychologic outcome in childhood acute lymphoblastic leukemia. *J Clin Oncol* 1992;10:810.

296. Mulhern RK, Fairclough D, Ochs J. A prospective comparison of neuropsychologic performance of children surviving leukemia who received 18-Gy, 24-Gy, or no cranial irradiation. *J Clin Oncol* 1991;9:1348.

297. Halberg FE, Kramer JH, Moore IM, et al. Prophylactic cranial irradiation dose effects on late cognitive function in children treated for acute lymphoblastic leukemia. *Int J Radiat Oncol Biol Phys* 1992;22:13.

298. Mulhern RK, Kovnar E, Langston J, et al. Long-term survivors of leukemia treated in infancy: factors associated with neuropsychologic status. *J Clin Oncol* 1992;10:1095.

299. Waber DP, Urion DK, Tarbell NJ, et al. Late effects of central nervous system treatment of acute lymphoblastic leukemia in childhood are sex-dependent. *Dev Med Child Neurol* 1990;32:238.

300. Aur RJ, Simone JV, Verzosa MS, et al. Childhood acute lymphocytic leukemia: study VIII. *Cancer* 1978;42:2123.

301. Waber DP, Tarbell NJ, Fairclough D, et al. Cognitive sequelae of treatment in childhood acute lymphoblastic leukemia: cranial radiation requires an accomplice. *J Clin Oncol* 1995;13:2490.

302. Copeland DR, Moore BD III, Francis DJ, et al. Neuropsychologic effects of chemotherapy on children with cancer: a longitudinal study. *J Clin Oncol* 1996;14:2826.

303. Filley CM, Kleinschmidt-DeMasters BK. Toxic leukoencephalopathy. *N Engl J Med* 2001;345:425.

304. Sklar C, Mertens A, Walter A, et al. Final height after treatment for childhood acute lymphoblastic leukemia: comparison of no cranial irradiation with 1800 and 2400 centigrays of cranial irradiation. *J Pediatr* 1993;123:59.

305. Didcock E, Davies HA, Didi M, et al. Pubertal growth in young adult survivors of childhood leukemia. *J Clin Oncol* 1995;13:2503.

306. Katz JA, Chambers B, Everhart C, et al. Linear growth in children with acute lymphoblastic leukemia treated without cranial irradiation. *J Pediatr* 1991; 118:575.

307. Voorhess ML, Brecher ML, Glicksman AS, et al. Hypothalamic-pituitary function of children with acute lymphocytic leukemia after three forms of central nervous system prophylaxis. A retrospective study. *Cancer* 1986;57:1287.

308. Stubberfield TG, Byrne GC, Jones TW. Growth and growth hormone secretion after treatment for acute lymphoblastic leukemia in childhood. 18-Gy versus 24-Gy cranial irradiation. *J Pediatr Hematol Oncol* 1995;17:167.

309. Swift PG, Kearney PJ, Dalton RG, et al. Growth and hormonal status of children treated for acute lymphoblastic leukaemia. *Arch Dis Child* 1978;53:890.

310. Halton JM, Atkinson SA, Fraher L, et al. Altered mineral metabolism and bone mass in children during treatment for acute lymphoblastic leukemia. *J Bone Miner Res* 1996;11:1774.

311. Arikoski P, Komulainen J, Voutilainen R, et al. Reduced bone mineral density in long-term survivors of childhood acute lymphoblastic leukemia. *J Pediatr Hematol Oncol* 1998;20:234.

312. Warner JT, Evans WD, Webb DK, et al. Relative osteopenia after treatment for acute lymphoblastic leukemia. *Pediatr Res* 1999;45:544.

313. Brennan BM, Rahim A, Adams JA, et al. Reduced bone mineral density in young adults following cure of acute lymphoblastic leukaemia in childhood. *Br J Cancer* 1999;79:1859.

314. Arikoski P, Komulainen J, Riikonen P, et al. Reduced bone density at completion of chemotherapy for a malignancy. *Arch Dis Child* 1999;80:143.

315. Hanif I, Mahmoud H, Pui CH. Avascular femoral head necrosis in pediatric cancer patients. *Med Pediatr Oncol* 1993;21:655.

316. Thornton MJ, O'Sullivan G, Williams MP, Hughes PM. Avascular necrosis of bone following an intensified chemotherapy regimen including high dose steroids. *Clin Radiol* 1997;52:607.

317. Wei SY, Esmail AN, Bunin N, Dormans JP. Avascular necrosis in children with acute lymphoblastic leukemia. *J Pediatr Orthop* 2000;20:331.

318. Mattano LA Jr, Sather HN, Trigg ME, Nachman JB. Osteonecrosis as a complication of treating acute lymphoblastic leukemia in children: a report from the Children's Cancer Group. *J Clin Oncol* 2000;18:3262.

319. Sorensen K, Levitt G, Bull C, et al. Anthracycline dose in childhood acute lymphoblastic leukemia: issues of early survival versus late cardiotoxicity. *J Clin Oncol* 1997;15:61.

320. Lipshultz SE, Lipsitz SR, Mone SM, et al. Female sex and drug dose as risk factors for late cardiotoxic effects of doxorubicin therapy for childhood cancer. *N Engl J Med* 1995;332:1738.

321. Krischer JP, Epstein S, Cuthbertson DD, et al. Clinical cardiotoxicity following anthracycline treatment for childhood cancer: the Pediatric Oncology Group experience. *J Clin Oncol* 1997;15:1544.

322. Nesbit M, Krivit W, Heyn R, Sharp H. Acute and chronic effects of methotrexate on hepatic, pulmonary, and skeletal systems. *Cancer* 1976;37:1048.

323. Farrow AC, Buchanan GR, Zwiener RJ, et al. Serum aminotransferase elevation during and following treatment of childhood acute lymphoblastic leukemia. *J Clin Oncol* 1997;15:1560.

324. Blatt J, Poplack DG, Sherins RJ. Testicular function in boys after chemotherapy for acute lymphoblastic leukemia. *N Engl J Med* 1981;304:1121.

325. Lendon M, Hann IM, Palmer MK, et al. Testicular histology after combination chemotherapy in childhood for acute lymphoblastic leukaemia. *Lancet* 1978;2:439.

326. Muller HL, Klinkhammer-Schalke M, Seelbach-Gobel B, et al. Gonadal function of young adults after therapy of malignancies during childhood or adolescence. *Eur J Pediatr* 1996;155:763.

327. Green DM, Hall B, Zevon MA. Pregnancy outcome after treatment for acute lymphoblastic leukemia during childhood or adolescence. *Cancer* 1989;64: 2335.

328. Rimm IJ, Li FC, Tarbell NJ, et al. Brain tumors after cranial irradiation for childhood acute lymphoblastic leukemia. A 13-year experience from the Dana-Farber Cancer Institute and the Children's Hospital. *Cancer* 1987;59: 1506.

329. Rosso P, Terracini B, Fears TR, et al. Second malignant tumors after elective end of therapy for a first cancer in childhood: a multicenter study in Italy. *Int J Cancer* 1994;59:451.

330. Walter AW, Hancock ML, Pui CH, et al. Secondary brain tumors in children treated for acute lymphoblastic leukemia at St. Jude Children's Research Hospital. *J Clin Oncol* 1998;16:3761.

331. Pui CH, Behm FG, Raimondi SC, et al. Secondary acute myeloid leukemia in children treated for acute lymphoid leukemia. *N Engl J Med* 1989;321:136.

332. Winick NJ, McKenna RW, Shuster JJ, et al. Secondary acute myeloid leukemia in children with acute lymphoblastic leukemia treated with etoposide. *J Clin Oncol* 1993;11:209.

333. Tucker MA, Meadows AT, Boice JD Jr, et al. Leukemia after therapy with alkylating agents for childhood cancer. *J Natl Cancer Inst* 1987;78:459.

334. Kreissman SG, Gelber RD, Cohen HJ, et al. Incidence of secondary acute myelogenous leukemia after treatment of childhood acute lymphoblastic leukemia. *Cancer* 1992;70:2208.

335. Kimball Dalton VM, Gelber RD, Li F, et al. Second malignancies in patients treated for childhood acute lymphoblastic leukemia. *J Clin Oncol* 1998;16: 2848.

336. Loning L, Zimmermann M, Reiter A, et al. Secondary neoplasms subsequent to Berlin-Frankfurt-Munster therapy of acute lymphoblastic leukemia in childhood: significantly lower risk without cranial radiotherapy. *Blood* 2000;95:2770.

337. Henze G, Fengler R, Hartmann R, et al. Six-year experience with a comprehensive approach to the treatment of recurrent childhood acute lymphoblastic leukemia (ALL-REZ BFM 85). A relapse study of the BFM group. *Blood* 1991;78:1166.

338. Wheeler K, Richards S, Bailey C, Chessells J. Comparison of bone marrow transplant and chemotherapy for relapsed childhood acute lymphoblastic leukaemia: the MRC UKALL X experience. Medical Research Council Working Party on Childhood Leukaemia. *Br J Haematol* 1998;101:94.

339. Gaynon PS, Qu RP, Chappell RJ, et al. Survival after relapse in childhood acute lymphoblastic leukemia: impact of site and time to first relapse—the Children's Cancer Group Experience. *Cancer* 1998;82:1387.

340. Giona F, Testi AM, Rondelli R, et al. ALL R-87 protocol in the treatment of children with acute lymphoblastic leukaemia in early bone marrow relapse. *Br J Haematol* 1997;99:671.

341. Bordigoni P, Esperou H, Souillet G, et al. Total body irradiation-high-dose cytosine arabinoside and melphalan followed by allogeneic bone marrow transplantation from HLA-identical siblings in the treatment of children with acute lymphoblastic leukaemia after relapse while receiving chemotherapy: a Societe Francaise de Greffe de Moelle study. *Br J Haematol* 1998;102:656.

342. Buhrer C, Hartmann R, Fengler R, et al. Peripheral blast counts at diagnosis of late isolated bone marrow relapse of childhood acute lymphoblastic leukemia predict response to salvage chemotherapy and outcome. Berlin-Frankfurt-Munster Relapse Study Group. *J Clin Oncol* 1996;14:2812.

343. Buhrer C, Hartmann R, Fengler R, et al. Superior prognosis in combined compared to isolated bone marrow relapses in salvage therapy of childhood acute lymphoblastic leukemia. *Med Pediatr Oncol* 1993;21:470.

344. Sadowitz PD, Smith SD, Shuster J, et al. Treatment of late bone marrow relapse in children with acute lymphoblastic leukemia: a Pediatric Oncology Group study. *Blood* 1993;81:602.

345. Chessells JM. Relapsed lymphoblastic leukaemia in children: a continuing challenge. *Br J Haematol* 1998;102:423.

346. Rivera GK, Buchanan G, Boyett JM, et al. Intensive retreatment of childhood acute lymphoblastic leukemia in first bone marrow relapse. A Pediatric Oncology Group Study. *N Engl J Med* 1986;315:273.

347. Buchanan GR, Rivera GK, Boyett JM, et al. Reinduction therapy in 297 children with acute lymphoblastic leukemia in first bone marrow relapse: a Pediatric Oncology Group Study. *Blood* 1988;72:1286.

348. Culbert SJ, Shuster JJ, Land VJ, et al. Remission induction and continuation therapy in children with their first relapse of acute lymphoid leukemia. A Pediatric Oncology Group study. *Cancer* 1991;67:37.

349. Belasco JB, Luery N, Scher C. Multiagent chemotherapy in relapsed acute lymphoblastic leukemia in children. *Cancer* 1990;66:2492.

350. Wolfrom C, Hartmann R, Fengler R, et al. Randomized comparison of 36-hour intermediate-dose versus 4-hour high-dose methotrexate infusions for remission induction in relapsed childhood acute lymphoblastic leukemia. *J Clin Oncol* 1993;11:827.

351. Butturini A, Rivera GK, Bortin MM, Gale RP. Which treatment for childhood acute lymphoblastic leukaemia in second remission? *Lancet* 1987;1:429.

352. Barrett AJ, Horowitz MM, Pollock BH, et al. Bone marrow transplants from HLA-identical siblings as compared with chemotherapy for children with acute lymphoblastic leukemia in a second remission. *N Engl J Med* 1994; 331:1253.

353. Uderzo C, Valsecchi MG, Bacigalupo A, et al. Treatment of childhood acute lymphoblastic leukemia in second remission with allogeneic bone marrow transplantation and chemotherapy: ten-year experience of the Italian Bone Marrow Transplantation Group and the Italian Pediatric Hematology Oncology Association. *J Clin Oncol* 1995;13:352.

354. Rivera GK, Hudson MM, Liu Q, et al. Effectiveness of intensified rotational combination chemotherapy for late hematologic relapse of childhood acute lymphoblastic leukemia. *Blood* 1996;88:831.

355. Sanders JE, Thomas ED, Buckner CD, Doney K. Marrow transplantation for children with acute lymphoblastic leukemia in second remission. *Blood* 1987;70:324.

356. Brochstein JA, Kernan NA, Groshen S, et al. Allogeneic bone marrow transplantation after hyperfractionated total-body irradiation and cyclophosphamide in children with acute leukemia. *N Engl J Med* 1987;317:1618.

357. Barrett AJ, Horowitz MM, Gale RP, et al. Marrow transplantation for acute lymphoblastic leukemia: factors affecting relapse and survival. *Blood* 1989;74:862.

358. Dopfer R, Henze G, Bender-Gotze C, et al. Allogeneic bone marrow transplantation for childhood acute lymphoblastic leukemia in second remission after intensive primary and relapse therapy according to the BFM- and CoALL-protocols: results of the German Cooperative Study. *Blood* 1991;78:2780.

359. Weisdorf DJ, Woods WG, Nesbit ME Jr, et al. Allogeneic bone marrow transplantation for acute lymphoblastic leukaemia: risk factors and clinical outcome. *Br J Haematol* 1994;86:62.

360. Torres A, Alvarez MA, Sanchez J, et al. Allogeneic bone marrow transplantation vs chemotherapy for the treatment of childhood acute lymphoblastic leukaemia in second complete remission (revisited 10 years on). *Bone Marrow Transplant* 1999;23:1257.

361. Parsons SK, Castellino SM, Lehmann LE, et al. Relapsed acute lymphoblastic leukemia: similar outcomes for autologous and allogeneic marrow transplantation in selected children. *Bone Marrow Transplant* 1996;17:763.

362. Oakhill A, Pamphilon DH, Potter MN, et al. Unrelated donor bone marrow transplantation for children with relapsed acute lymphoblastic leukaemia in second complete remission. *Br J Haematol* 1996;94:574.

363. Busca A, Anasetti C, Anderson G, et al. Unrelated donor or autologous marrow transplantation for treatment of acute leukemia. *Blood* 1994;83:3077.

364. Davies SM, Wagner JE, Shu XO, et al. Unrelated donor bone marrow transplantation for children with acute leukemia. *J Clin Oncol* 1997;15:557.

365. Schiller G, Feig SA, Territo M, et al. Treatment of advanced acute leukaemia with allogeneic bone marrow transplantation from unrelated donors. *Br J Haematol* 1994;88:72.

366. Saarinen-Pihkala UM, Gustafsson G, Ringden O, et al. No disadvantage in outcome of using matched unrelated donors as compared with matched sibling donors for bone marrow transplantation in children with acute lymphoblastic leukemia in second remission. *J Clin Oncol* 2001;19:3406.

367. Sallan SE, Niemeyer CM, Billett AL, et al. Autologous bone marrow transplantation for acute lymphoblastic leukemia. *J Clin Oncol* 1989;7:1594.

368. Billett AL, Kornmehl E, Tarbell NJ, et al. Autologous bone marrow transplantation after a long first remission for children with recurrent acute lymphoblastic leukemia. *Blood* 1993;81:1651.

369. Schmid H, Henze G, Schwerdtfeger R, et al. Fractionated total body irradiation and high-dose VP-16 with purged autologous bone marrow rescue for children with high-risk relapsed acute lymphoblastic leukemia. *Bone Marrow Transplant* 1993;12:597.

370. Kersey JH, Weisdorf D, Nesbit ME, et al. Comparison of autologous and allogeneic bone marrow transplantation for treatment of high-risk refractory acute lymphoblastic leukemia. *N Engl J Med* 1987;317:461.

371. Maldonado MS, Diaz-Heredia C, Badell I, et al. Autologous bone marrow transplantation with monoclonal antibody purged marrow for children with acute lymphoblastic leukemia in second remission. Spanish Working Party for BMT in Children. *Bone Marrow Transplant* 1998;22:1043.

372. Borgmann A, Schmid H, Hartmann R, et al. Autologous bone-marrow transplants compared with chemotherapy for children with acute lymphoblastic leukaemia in a second remission: a matched-pair analysis. The Berlin-Frankfurt-Munster Study Group. *Lancet* 1995;346:873.

373. George SL, Ochs JJ, Mauer AM, Simone JV. The importance of an isolated central nervous system relapse in children with acute lymphoblastic leukemia. *J Clin Oncol* 1985;3:776.

374. Kun LE, Camitta BM, Mulhern RK, et al. Treatment of meningeal relapse in childhood acute lymphoblastic leukemia. I. Results of craniospinal irradiation. *J Clin Oncol* 1984;2:359.

375. Behrendt H, van Leeuwen EF, Schuwirth C, et al. The significance of an isolated central nervous system relapse, occurring as first relapse in children with acute lymphoblastic leukaemia. *Cancer* 1989;63:2066.

376. Winick NJ, Smith SD, Shuster J, et al. Treatment of CNS relapse in children with acute lymphoblastic leukemia: a Pediatric Oncology Group study. *J Clin Oncol* 1993;11:271.

377. Ritchey AK, Pollock BH, Lauer SJ, et al. Improved survival of children with isolated CNS relapse of acute lymphoblastic leukemia: a Pediatric Ooncology Group study. *J Clin Oncol* 1999;17:3745.

378. Ribeiro RC, Rivera GK, Hudson M, et al. An intensive re-treatment protocol for children with an isolated CNS relapse of acute lymphoblastic leukemia. *J Clin Oncol* 1995;13:333.

379. Borgmann A, Hartmann R, Schmid H, et al. Isolated extramedullary relapse in children with acute lymphoblastic leukemia: a comparison between treatment results of chemotherapy and bone marrow transplantation. BFM Relapse Study Group. *Bone Marrow Transplant* 1995;15:515.

380. Bleyer WA, Poplack DG. Prophylaxis and treatment of leukemia in the central nervous system and other sanctuaries. *Semin Oncol* 1985;12:131.

381. Uderzo C, Grazia Zurlo M, Adamoli L, et al. Treatment of isolated testicular relapse in childhood acute lymphoblastic leukemia: an Italian multicenter study. Associazione Italiana Ematologia ed Oncologia Pediatrica. *J Clin Oncol* 1990;8:672.

382. Wofford MM, Smith SD, Shuster JJ, et al. Treatment of occult or late overt testicular relapse in children with acute lymphoblastic leukemia: a Pediatric Oncology Group study. *J Clin Oncol* 1992;10:624.

383. Finklestein JZ, Miller DR, Feusner J, et al. Treatment of overt isolated testicular relapse in children on therapy for acute lymphoblastic leukemia. A report from the Childrens Cancer Group. *Cancer* 1994;73:219.

384. Novakovic P, Kellie SJ, Taylor D. Childhood leukaemia: relapse in the anterior segment of the eye. *Br J Ophthalmol* 1989;73:354.

385. Heaton DC, Duff GB. Ovarian relapse in a young woman with acute lymphoblastic leukaemia. *Am J Hematol* 1989;30:42.

386. Matthews DC, Appelbaum FR, Eary JF, et al. Develpment of a marrow transplant regimen for acute leukemia using targeted hematopoietic irradiation delivered by 131I-labeled anti-CD45 antibody, combined with cyclophosphamide and total body irradiation. *Blood* 1995;85:1122.

387. Uckun FM, Messinger Y, Chen CL, et al. Treatment of therapy-refractory B-lineage acute lymphoblastic leukemia with an apoptosis-inducing CD19-directed tyrosine kinase inhibitor. *Clin Cancer Res* 1999;5:3906.

388. Cardoso AA, Seamon MJ, Afonso HM, et al. Ex vivo generation of human anti-pre-B leukemia-specific autologous cytolytic T cells. *Blood* 1997;90:549.

389. Cardoso AA, Veiga JP, Ghia P, et al. Adoptive T-cell therapy for B-cell acute lymphoblastic leukemia: preclinical studies. *Blood* 1999;94:3531.

390. Perez-Atayde AR, Sallan SE, Tedrow U, et al. Spectrum of tumor angiogenesis in the bone marrow of children with acute lymphoblastic leukemia. *Am J Pathol* 1997;150:815.

391. Kaspers GJ, Veerman AJ, Pieters R, et al. In vitro cellular drug resistance and prognosis in newly diagnosed childhood acute lymphoblastic leukemia. *Blood* 1997;90:2723.

CHAPTER 26

Chronic Lymphoid Leukemias

Malek M. Safa and Kenneth A. Foon

Leukemia was first described by Velpeau in 1827 (1); in 1844, Donne showed that increased leukocytes were responsible for the clinical features of leukemia (2). The chronic leukemias were first described by Bennett and Virchow in 1847 (3–5). Both splenic and lymphoid types were identified, roughly corresponding to chronic myelogenous leukemia (CML) and chronic lymphoid leukemia (CLL), respectively. At that time, leukemia was thought to originate in the spleen or lymph node. In 1870, however, Neuman showed that blood cells arise from the bone marrow and suggested this as the site of transformation of leukemia (6). The distinction between CML and CLL became clearer in the latter part of the last century, when histochemical stains became available (7). By 1909, current notions of CML and CLL were described in popular medical texts (8). The initial treatment of chronic leukemias involved arsenicals. This was followed by the introduction of radiation therapy in 1902 (9–11). The modern era of chronic leukemia treatment began with the use of nitrogen mustard and radiophosphorus in the 1940s (12,13). In the 1950s, these were gradually replaced with busulfan and chlorambucil.

Many of the current concepts regarding the immunology and biology of CLL were proposed by Dameshek in 1967 (14). Over the past 20 years, a variety of lymphoid malignancies have been distinguished clinically, morphologically, and immunologically from CLL (15). These diseases are summarized in Tables 26-1 and 26-2.

CHRONIC LYMPHOCYTIC LEUKEMIA

CLL is characterized by proliferation and accumulation of mature-appearing but biologically immature B lymphocytes. The National Cancer Institute–Sponsored Working Group (NCISWG) (16) and the International Workshop on Chronic Lymphoid Leukemia (17) have proposed similar criteria for the diagnosis of CLL, which include

- Lymphocytosis (higher than 5×10^9/L) sustained for 4 weeks
- Cells with κ or λ light-chain, low-density surface immunoglobulin (Ig) and CD5 antigen
- Mature lymphocytes with no more than 55% atypical and immature lymphoid cells
- Over 30% bone marrow involvement

Important advances have been made in our understanding of the complex immunology, cytogenetics, cell physiology, and biochemistry associated with CLL.

EPIDEMIOLOGY AND CAUSE

CLL is the most common adult leukemia in Western countries. The average incidence is 2.7 persons with CLL per 100,000 in the United States. Typically, CLL occurs in people over 50 years of age (median age, 60 years), and its incidence is two times higher for men than women. Less than 10% of cases occur in adults under 40 years of age; rare cases have been reported in children. CLL is acquired, and only rarely is there concordance in genetically identical twins. In one set of twins, Ig gene rearrangements in the twins were distinct (18). No reproducible pattern of inheritance has been reported (19).

The cause of CLL is unknown. Environmental factors do not appear to play a major role in the pathogenesis of CLL. Unlike CML and acute leukemias, CLL is not induced by radiation, chemicals, or alkylating agents (20). CLL represents 30% of reported leukemia cases in the West. Ten thousand new cases are diagnosed annually in the United States. In contrast, CLL is rare in Asia, representing less than 5% of all leukemia cases.

Viruses have not been demonstrated to play a role in leukemogenesis. Retroviruses are implicated in some rare forms of lymphoid leukemia. For example, human T-cell leukemia/lymphoma virus type I (HTLV-I) is implicated in the cause of adult T-cell leukemia/lymphoma (ATL) (21–23) (Table 26-2). The mechanism whereby HTLV-I causes ATL is unknown. In addition to ATL, HTLV-I infection has been reported in a chronic form of ATL, persistent T lymphocytosis (24), which resembles but is distinct from CLL.

The possible role of DNA viruses, such as Epstein-Barr virus (EBV) and cytomegalovirus, in CLL is unknown. Direct involvement of EBV seems unlikely. CLL cells can be infected by EBV as indicated by expression of Epstein-Barr nuclear antigen; this does not routinely lead to immortalization (25). One EBV-infected cell line was shown to produce tumors in nude mice (26). However, transformation with EBV has been associated with some cases of Richter transformation.

IMMUNOLOGY

Immune Features

CLL results from malignant transformation of a B lymphocyte; the small proportion of reported cases involving T lympho-

TABLE 26-1. B-Lymphoproliferative Disorders

Disease	Median Age at Diagnosis (yr)	Male/ Female Ratio	Leukocyte Counts × 10^9/L	Lymph Nodes	Spleen (%)	Skin	Morphology (Figure)	Surface Immunoglobulin	Phenotype
Chronic lymphocytic leukemia	60	2:1	10–200	>50	50	<5	3	Weak	DR, CD19, CD20 dim, CD5, CD22 (–5), CD23, CD21, CD11c+/–, CD25+/–, CD43, CD10(–)
Prolymphocytic leukemia	65	4:1	100–500	<25	>90	<5	6	Strong	DR, CD19, CD20 bright, CD5(–), CD23(–), CD10(–), FMC7, CD22
Follicular center	50	2:1	50–200	>90	75	<5	8	Strong	DR, CD10, CD19, CD20, CD21, FMC7, CD22, CD5(–), CD11c(–), CD43(–)
Hairy cell leukemia	50	5:1	1–100	<20	>75	<5	10	Strong	DR, CD19, CD20, CD25, CD11c, CD103, CD5(–), CD22, CD10(–)
Waldenström's macroglobulinemia	50	1:1	5–50	>30	30	<5	7	Strong	DR, CD19, CD20, PCA-1
Mantle cell lymphoma	58	3:1	5–50	>90	>50	<5	9	Strong	DR, CD19, CD20 bright, CD5, CD22, CD23(–), CD10(–), CD43

+/–, variable, more often positive; –, negative; DR, HLA-DR.

cytes most likely represent misdiagnosed cases of one of the chronic T-lymphoid leukemias presented in Table 26-2 or a yet-to-be classified T-cell malignancy. CLL is clonal; the cells express a single Ig light chain on the cell-surface membrane (27,28).

More sophisticated techniques confirm clonality by unique Ig idiotype (29,30), a single pattern of glucose-6-phosphate dehydrogenase (G6PD) activity in heterozygotes (31,32), clonal chromosomal abnormalities (33), and clonal Ig gene rearrangement (34,35).

CLL cells display low-density surface Ig, typically mu or delta and, less commonly, gamma, or no heavy chain. Surface Ig is estimated at approximately 9000 molecules per cell (36). Cytoplasmic Ig is also present (37). Distinct differences between cytoplasmic,

TABLE 26-2. T-Lymphoproliferative Disorders

Disease	Median Age at Diagnosis (yr)	Male/ Female Ratio	Leukocyte Counts × 10^9/L	Lymph Nodes	Spleen (%)	Skin	Morphology (Figure)	Surface Immunoglobulin	Phenotype
Prolymphocytic leukemia	60	4:1	100–500	<25	>90	<10	6	Absent	CD2, CD3, CD4, CD5, CD7, CD8(–)
Adult T-cell leukemia/ lymphoma	40	2:1	5–150	>90	>50	>50	15	Absent	CD2, CD3, CD4, CD5, CD7(–), CD8(–), CD25 bright, DR
T-LGL leukemia	50	2:1	5–300	<10	30	<5	12	Absent	CD2, CD3, CD8, CD4(–), CD7(–), CD5(–), CD56(–), CD57(–), CD25(–), CD16, CD11b
NK-LGL leukemia	40	2:1	5–300	<10	>50	<5	12	Absent	CD2, CD3(–), CD4(–), CD16, CD56, CD8–/+, CD57(–), CD25(–)
Cutaneous T-cell lymphoma	55	2:1	5–150	50	10	100	18	Absent	CD2, CD3, CD4, CD5, CD8(–), CD7+/–, CD25(–)

+/–, variable, more often positive; –/+, variable, more often negative; –, negative; LGL, large granular lymphocytic; NK, natural killer.

surface, and secretory Ig are detected (38). Cells from less than 5% of patients with CLL secrete sufficient levels of IgM to be detected by serum protein electrophoresis. Using high-resolution electrophoresis and immunofixation, circulating monoclonal IgM paraproteins are identified in one-fourth to one-half or more of patients (39–41).

Additional surface features of CLL cells include the B-lymphocyte antigens CD19, CD20, CD21, CD23, and CD24 (15,42–52). In nearly all cases, the cells also express the nominal T-cell–associated antigen CD5, which is identified on a subpopulation of normal B cells (52–54). CD5–B cells are also found in fetal liver and in the blood of bone marrow transplant recipients in the early recovery phase (55,56). Leukemia cells that are CD5 negative generally represent lymphoproliferative diseases other than CLL. Cells from approximately half of patients with CLL express the CD25 activation antigen (57), and most of these patients have soluble CD25 detected in their serum (58). FMC7, CD22, and some myeloid antigens are identified in approximately one-fourth of cases; CD10 and additional T-cell–associated antigens are not found.

The neoplastic B cells in mantle cell lymphoma express many of the same surface antigens as do CLL–B cells, including CD5. However, in contrast to CLL–B cells, mantle cell lymphoma cells generally express CD22 and high levels of CD79a (59), but do not express CD23.

The malignant B lymphocyte that is the usual target of transformation in CLL is an intermediate cell with some, but not all, morphologic features of mature B cells. This cell appears to be arrested in its normal differentiation scheme and does not normally progress to the final stages of B-cell development, although a small proportion of plasma cells from patients with CLL express the same Ig idiotype as the CLL cells, suggesting that they are a component of the malignant clone (60). Incubation of CLL cells *in vitro* with tumor promoters, such as phorbol esters or B-cell mitogens, induces differentiation to activated cells similar to prolymphocytic leukemia (PLL) cells (61), hairy cells (62), or mature plasma cells (63–66). Under these conditions, the cells may begin to actively secrete Ig. Mitogen-induced switching from cell surface IgM to secreted IgG is also reported (67). These data confirm that the malignant B cells typical of CLL are not irreversibly frozen at an immature level of B-cell development.

Immune Function of Chronic Lymphoid Leukemia Cells

Many studies have been done on the immune function of CLL cells. Low levels of surface Ig and impaired Ig capping suggest abnormalities of membrane motility (68). Despite the fact that CLL cells have HLA class II antigens, they show limited or no stimulatory activity in autologous and allogeneic mixed lymphocyte culture (69,70). Other cell activities are also abnormal, including *in vitro* response to B-cell mitogens, such as pokeweed mitogen, lipopolysaccharide, and EBV, and decreased activity in antibody-dependent cellular cytotoxicity (71–74). CLL cells have a decreased proliferative response to B-cell growth factor. This is likely to be secondary to the impaired expression of appropriate cell-surface receptors (75). Cytochalasin B is a potent mitogen for CLL cells (76).

Several studies have used techniques to culture colonies of malignant B cells derived from patients with CLL in semisolid agar (77–79). These techniques may help analyze details of immune function of CLL.

Immune Function of T Lymphocytes and Natural Killer Cells

Increased absolute numbers of T lymphocytes have been reported in untreated patients with CLL. These levels fluctuate during the course of the disease (80). In general, patients with CLL show a marked inversion of the ratio of normal helper T cells (CD4) to suppressor T cells (CD8) in the blood (81–86), with increased suppressor T cells. Additional T-cell surface marker abnormalities include a decreased proportion of cells reactive with the pan-T antiCD3 antibody and the presence of cells that simultaneously express helper T cell–associated and suppressor T cell–associated antigens (87), a characteristic that is normally present on some thymocytes and in a minor population of circulating T lymphocytes (88). These abnormalities of T-cell subsets or levels correlate with disease stage, therapy, or both in some studies (89,90).

Some functional studies of T cells appear normal (91), but proliferative responses to autologous or allogeneic B cells are impaired (74,92). Progenitor T cells, assayed by colony growth in semisolid agar, have been reported as decreased in some studies (93–95). Helper T cell–function is decreased (96), and there may be abnormal suppressor T cells as well. It has also been reported that CLL cells secrete or shed an immune regulatory ganglioside suppressive for lymphocytes (97).

Spontaneous and antibody-dependent cytotoxicity are also decreased in CLL, suggesting an abnormality in natural killer (NK) cells (98,99). Numbers of NK cells detected by reactivity with CD56 and CD57 are increased in CLL; however, studies with CD16, which identifies the crystallizable fragment receptor III typical of NK cells, indicate that cells with this antigen are increased (100,101). These data suggest increased numbers of functionally inactive NK cells in CLL. Some NK-cell functional abnormalities found in CLL are corrected by *in vitro* or *in vivo* exposure to interleukin-2 (IL-2), interferon (IFN), or synthetic thymic polypeptide (102–104).

The origin of T-cell abnormalities in CLL is unknown; it is uncertain whether they are a cause or a consequence of the disease. T cells from patients with CLL are probably not part of the malignant clone. This notion is supported by the lack of chromosomal abnormalities typical of the CLL clone in T cells (105) and by heterozygosity for polymorphic X-linked genetic markers, such as G6PD (106). Most of these studies, however, were performed in patients with CLL of relatively brief duration. The T cells tested may therefore have developed before the onset of leukemia. Consequently, it is not possible to exclude involvement of an immature stem cell with both T- and B-cell differentiation potential as the site of transformation in some cases of CLL. Consistent with this notion is the finding of clonal rearrangement of the T-cell β-receptor in the malignant B cells in approximately 10% of cases of CLL (107). These data are also consistent with the origin of the disease in an immature B cell.

Hypogammaglobulinemia

Hypogammaglobulinemia occurs in patients with CLL. This incidence is time dependent; eventually, almost all CLL patients develop hypogammaglobulinemia. Infections, particularly with encapsulated organisms, as well as gram-negative bacteria, are a frequent cause of morbidity and mortality (108,109). Consistent with their abnormal B- and T-cell function, CLL patients have impaired antibody and cell-mediated immunity to recall antigens (110–112).

The pathogenesis of hypogammaglobulinemia in CLL is controversial and likely reflects several factors. For example, decreased *in vitro* Ig synthesis to polyclonal mitogens or antigens has been reported (113). Regulatory abnormalities of T cells may also be important (84–86,114), including reversal of normal helper/suppressor T cell–ratios. NK cells (CD16+, CD3–) decrease Ig secretion by normal B cells in patients with CLL and hypogammaglobulinemia (115).

Autoimmunity

Many patients with CLL may develop features of autoimmunity of the hematopoietic system. For example, autoimmune hemolytic anemia occurs in approximately 20% of cases sometime during the course of the disease (116). This usually results from IgG antibodies against Rh blood group antigens. These autoantibodies are typically polyclonal and are therefore not produced by the malignant B-cell clone of CLL. Also, approximately 10% of patients with CLL develop thrombocytopenia or neutropenia from autoantibodies to platelets or neutrophils (117,118). Rarely, patients develop a syndrome resembling pure red blood cell (RBC) aplasia (119).

Why patients with CLL develop these autoimmune disorders with such high frequency, particularly in the face of seemingly diminished B-cell function, is unknown. As indicated, clinically important autoantibodies in CLL are directed predominantly to the hematopoietic system. Although there is no increased risk of nonhematologic autoimmune disease in patients with CLL, these diseases seem to be increased in their relatives (120).

Increased numbers of CD5 (Ly-1) B cells are seen in some mice prone to autoimmune disease (121), and some display IgM autoantibodies (122). In humans, CD5 B cells are increased in the human fetus (56) and in patients with rheumatoid arthritis (RA) and other autoimmune disorders (123). In addition, mitogen-stimulated CLL cells secrete Ig that reacts with autoantigens (IgG, single-stranded DNA, double-stranded DNA, but not antinuclear antibody) (123–125). All of these data suggest that the CD5 B cell plays a prominent role in autoimmune diseases. In one study (126), a high proportion of patients with CLL reacted with an antiidiotype antibody raised against an IgM rheumatoid light-chain cross-reacting idiotype. One-fourth of CLL cases expressing light chain reacted with this antibody. This high frequency is related to a conserved variable region gene (V gene) of the IIIb subsubgroup (127). These investigators (128) further demonstrated that 20% of CLL cases studied reacted with an antiidiotype antibody that recognized an antibody heavy-chain–associated, cross-reactive idiotype present on rheumatoid factor paraprotein.

CYTOGENETICS

Specific chromosomal abnormalities have been found to have clinical, prognostic, and pathogenic importance for a variety of hematologic malignancies. Most of this information has been focused on acute leukemias and CML. It has been considerably more difficult to study chromosomes in patients with CLL because of difficulty in obtaining sufficient metaphases for analysis. The cytogenetics of CLL has emerged using a variety of B-cell mitogens, including pokeweed mitogen, cytochalasin B, lipopolysaccharide, phorbol esters, protein A, and EBV. An adequate number of metaphases to evaluate chromosomes is achieved in 50% to 90% of patients (129–139). Among those metaphases that can be evaluated, half are consistently determined to be abnormal.

The most common chromosomal abnormality is del 13q14-23 (Table 26-3). Using a battery of six microsatellite markers from 13q12.3-14.3 between the *BRACA2* gene and the *Rb* gene, deletion in 13q14 was detected in leukemia cells of 29 of 78 CLL patients (37%) (140). However, classic cytogenetics appears less sensitive, as such methods detected the 13q14 deletion in CLL cells in 1%. CLL patients with deletion in 13q14 have a poorer prognosis than do those with normal cytogenetics (140). Nevertheless, patients with 13q14 deletions appear to have a better prognosis than those with trisomy 12 (141).

TABLE 26-3. Common Chromosomal Abnormalities Reported in Patients with Chronic Lymphoid Leukemias

Chromosomal Abnormality	Comments
13q	Most common in chronic lymphocytic leukemia
+12	Chronic lymphocytic leukemia; may also be seen in Waldenstrom's macroglobulinemia, hairy cell leukemia, and B-prolymphocytic leukemia
14q⁺	B-prolymphocytic leukemia, chronic lymphocytic leukemia, hairy cell leukemia, adult T-cell leukemia
11q	Chronic lymphocytic leukemia
6q	Chronic lymphocytic leukemia, B-prolymphocytic leukemia, adult T-cell leukemia, cutaneous T-cell lymphoma
del(3)	B-prolymphocytic leukemia
+3	Adult T-cell leukemia
+7	Adult T-cell leukemia, cutaneous T-cell lymphoma
inv(14)	T-prolymphocytic leukemia, adult T-cell leukemia

The second most common chromosomal abnormality is trisomy 12 (Table 26-3; Fig. 26-1). Approximately one-third of patients have chromosome 12 as the only abnormality. The defect accounting for the association of trisomy 12 and CLL is not known. Earlier studies (142) identified trisomy 12 in the CD34⁺ progenitor cells of the marrow or blood in a subset of patients with CLL. However, a recent analysis (143) at the single-cell level indicated that the subset of CLL patients with genetically aberrant CD34⁺ cells may be extremely rare. Therefore, CLL generally is not associated with genetic defects in the pluripotent stem cell. Instead, trisomy 12 appears to be an acquired genetic defect during disease progression (144). However, a longitudinal study of 41 patients did not find significant changes in the relative proportion of cells with trisomy 12 during a 4-year period, even in patients with disease progression (145).

Approximately 10% to 20% of patients may have leukemia cells with deletions in the long arm of chromosome 11, termed *11q⁻* (146). These patients tend to be younger in age (less than 55 years) and to have more aggressive disease progression. 11q⁻ with breakpoints at 11q21, 11q22, and 11q14 has been identified (139). Potential tumor-suppressor genes within this region include *ATM* and *RDX*. Radixin (RDX) has homology with the neurofibromatosis type-2 gene, tumor-suppressor gene (*NF2*). *ATM*, on the other hand, is the gene mutated in ataxia telangiectasia (147).

The other common chromosomal abnormality is a chromosome 6 deletion at 6q25-27 being detected in 21% of patients with CLL (139,148). The translocations most commonly involving chromosome 14 are at q32 (Ig heavy-chain gene locus), resulting in a 14q⁺ chromosome. A high incidence of trisomy 12 has been reported in patients with small lymphocytic lymphoma, which is the lymphoma counterpart of CLL (149).

In a recently developed cytogenetic method that allows simultaneous analysis of cell morphology, immune phenotype, and karyotype in the same cell, it was demonstrated that trisomy 12 occurs in the neoplastic B cells but not in the presumably normal T cells (104). These investigators propose that this provides the explanation for the common finding of mitosis with normal karyotypes in patients with CLL. The presumed-normal T cells have the normal karyotype, not the malignant B cells, where the karyotype would be expected to be found in all the clonally involved cells. One flaw to this argument is the pos-

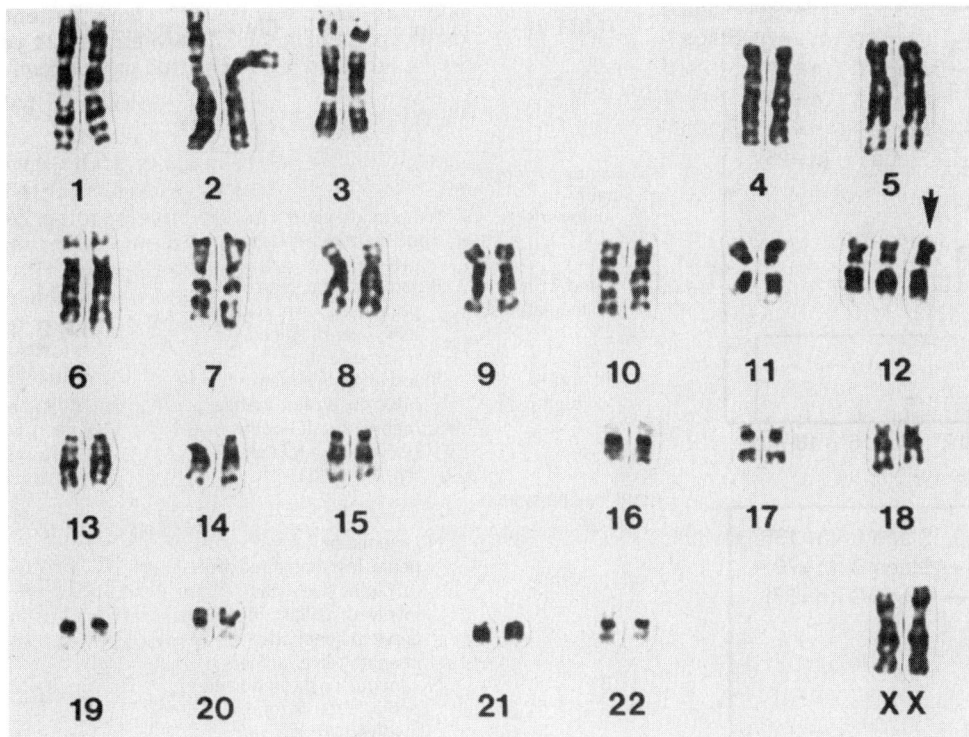

Figure 26-1. Trisomy 12 in a patient with chronic lymphocytic leukemia.

sibility that the T cells studied were long-lived T cells that may have preceded the malignant clone. Investigators have used restriction fragment length polymorphism (RFLP) of genes located on the long arm of chromosome 12 to show that the trisomy consists of a duplication of one of the chromosomes 12, not a triplication of one chromosome 12 with the loss of the other. In addition, using RFLP technology, these investigators demonstrated that the trisomy 12 abnormality was found in all the malignant cells (139).

Important clinical correlations have been gleaned from recent studies. The first important correlation is that an abnormal karyotype is a poor prognostic sign (129,130,132) and that trisomy 12 and possibly 14q⁺ are the least favorable abnormalities (139). In addition, patients with increasing numbers of chromosomal abnormalities do worse. One study reported that in most cases of CLL, the karyotype does not evolve in an individual patient (138). Other studies have clearly demonstrated clonal evolution in selected patients with new chromosomal abnormalities.

ONCOGENES

Several studies have been done on protooncogenes in CLL and related diseases. Most show no specific abnormalities. Unbalanced translocations involving chromosome 17p, where the p53 tumor-suppressor gene is located, are rarely noted in CLL. Two cell lines derived from patients with PLL with the t(11;14)(q13;q32) translocation were studied (150,151). In these cases, a break on chromosome 14 in the J region of the IgH locus was detected. The rearrangement on chromosome 11 involved a postulated protooncogene designated *B-cell lymphoma/leukemia type 1* (*bcl-1*).

Cells from most cases of follicular B-cell lymphoma, a related disorder, have the t(14;18)(q32;q21) translocation (152). Here, the genetic rearrangement on chromosome 18 involves another protooncogene, *bcl-2*. The mechanism of rearrangement between the IgH locus and *bcl-2* probably involves misrecogni-

tion of flanking heptamer–nonamer signal sequences by a normal recombinase involved in IgH recombination. Transgenic mice with a *bcl-2*–IgH locus transgene demonstrate lymphadenopathy and abnormal B-lymphoid infiltrates and suggest a prospective role for the t(14;18) in B-cell growth (153). The *bcl-2* oncogene controls *apoptosis* (programmed cell death). Overexpression of *bcl-2* inhibits apoptosis, leading to a longer cell life.

The t(14;19)(q32;q13) translocation occurs rarely in cells from patients with CLL. The break on chromosome 14 occurs within one of the two switch regions in the Ig heavy-chain locus, and the break on chromosome 19 is upstream of the *bcl-3* gene (154). The complementary DNA from *bcl-3* has been cloned and sequenced. Cells from patients with the t(14;19) have increased *bcl-3* RNA, suggesting a pathogenetic role.

Cases of CLL may be segregated on the basis of whether the leukemia cells express nonmutated versus mutated IgV genes (155,156). Leukemia cells that express nonmutated IgV genes more often may have trisomy 12 and atypical morphology than those that express mutated IgV genes, which, in turn, more frequently tend to have abnormalities involving 13q14 (157). Furthermore, patients with leukemia cells that express mutated IgV genes appear to have a more indolent clinical course than patients with leukemia cells that express nonmutated IgV genes (155,156).

One study analyzing 27 unselected cases of CLL found that more than 75% had low to absent expression of CD79b, an important accessory protein required for expression and signal transduction of surface immunoglobulin (158).

CLINICAL FEATURES

One of the major challenges in CLL is to individualize therapy. The course of CLL is variable. Most patients are older (median age, 60 years) and may have only elevated lymphocytes, asymptomatic lymphadenopathy, or splenomegaly. Others have age-related medical complications. These older patients are unlikely to die from CLL and may require no specific treat-

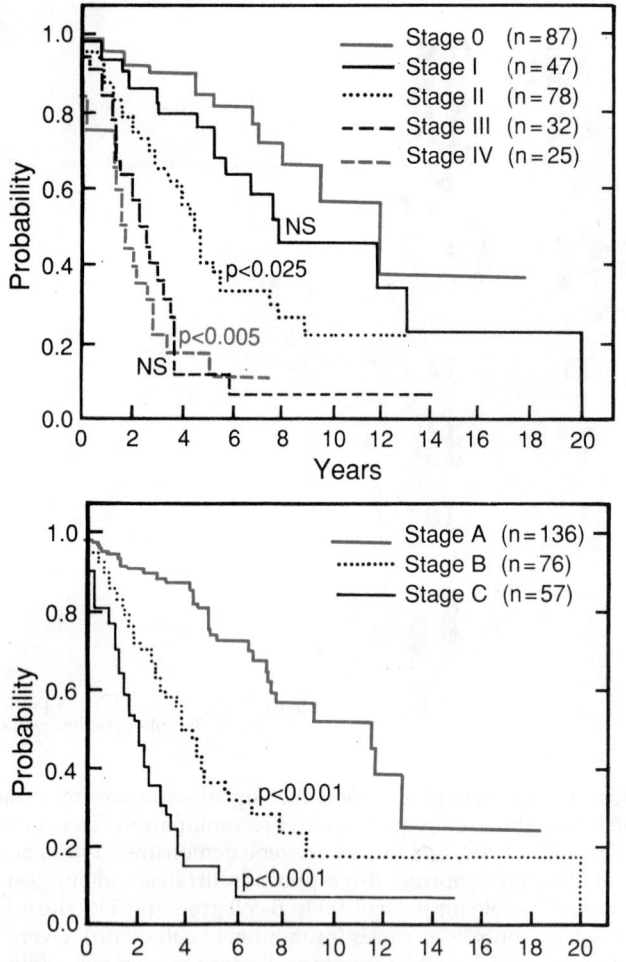

Figure 26-2. Actuarial survival curves of 269 patients classified by the Rai (**A**) and Binet (**B**) staging systems. (From Montserrat E, Rozman C. Prognostic factors in chronic lymphocytic leukemia. In: Polliak A, Catovsky D, eds. *Chronic lymphocytic leukemia.* Chur, Switzerland: Harwood Academic Publishers, 1988:111–122.)

ment. In contrast, some patients with CLL present with severe bone marrow failure, including anemia and thrombocytopenia. They may have a rapid, progressive course, with a median survival of less than 2 years. Most patients with CLL have an intermediate prognosis and do reasonably well for several years without therapy, but eventually require treatment. Rarely, spontaneous remissions are observed in patients with well-documented CLL (159).

Ideally, one would use prognostic factors to select optimal therapy. Several staging systems that reflect grouping of prognostic variables are proposed. The Rai (160) classification (Fig. 26-2A) includes five stages based on lymphocyte levels, lymphadenopathy, splenomegaly or hepatomegaly, and non–immune-related anemia (less than 11 g/dL) and thrombocytopenia (less than 100×10^9/L). This system was simplified into three stages: low risk (stage 0), intermediate risk (stages I and II), and high risk (stages III and IV) (161). These groups constitute approximately 30%, 60%, and 10% of patients, respectively (Table 26-4).

The Binet classification also has three stages (162) (Table 26-4), which are distinguished based on bone marrow failure and the number of abnormal lymphoid areas. Groups A, B, and C account for 60%, 30%, and 10% of patients, respectively (Fig. 26-2B).

TABLE 26-4. Staging Systems for Chronic Lymphocytic Leukemia

	Criteria	Median Survival (yr)
Rai staging system		
Stage[a]		
0 (low-risk)	Lymphocytes >15 × 10⁹/L Bone marrow >40% lymphocytes	>10
I and II (intermediate-risk)	Blood and bone marrow lymphocytosis, lymphadenopathy, liver or spleen enlargement	6
III and IV (high-risk)	Blood and bone marrow lymphocytosis plus anemia (hgb <11 g/dL) or thrombocytopenia (platelets <100 × 10⁹/L)	2
Binet staging system		
Group[a]		
A	No anemia or thrombocytopenia, less than three of the following five areas involved: axillary, inguinal, cervical lymphadenopathy, liver, spleen	9
B	No anemia or thrombocytopenia; three or more involved areas	5
C	Anemia (hgb <10 g/dL) or thrombocytopenia (platelets <100 × 10⁹/L)	2

hgb, hemoglobin.
[a]Autoimmune hemolytic anemia and thrombocytopenia are independent of stage or group.

Several investigators have tested numerous prognostic factors to determine if the course of CLL within a certain stage could be predicted accurately. A short list of these factors, which failed to consistently predict the clinical course of CLL, includes the level of blood lymphocytosis (163,164), proliferative index (165–167), level of deoxythymidine kinase (168), and phenotype (169). Three factors (Table 26-5) stand out as most critical: (a) pattern of bone marrow infiltration (170–173); (b) blood lymphocyte doubling time (174); and (3) chromosome karyotype (130,133,134).

Patients in whom the bone marrow shows diffuse lymphocyte infiltration are more likely to progress than those with a nondiffuse (nodular or interstitial) pattern of lymphocyte infiltration. Likewise, patients who are followed off therapy who have a blood lymphocyte doubling time of less than 12 months tend to do poorer than those with doubling times of greater than 12 months. This criteria cannot be determined at diagnosis.

TABLE 26-5. Prognostic Factors in Chronic Lymphocytic Leukemia

Factor	Favorable	Unfavorable
Bone marrow pattern	Nodular, interstitial	Diffuse
Doubling time of peripheral blood cells	>12 mo	<12 mo
Karyotype	Normal	Abnormal (del 13 or trisomy 12)

Chromosomal analysis is also useful but has limited availability, and most laboratories are successful in these analyses in only half of cases. However, an abnormal karyotype is an independent poor prognostic feature.

An interesting group of patients with Rai stage 0 disease has been reported (175). These patients had normal karyotypes and stable disease for 7 to 24 years. This form of CLL has been termed *benign monoclonal lymphocytosis*.

TRANSFORMATION

CLL typically involves relatively mature-appearing lymphocytes, similar to those observed in small lymphocytic lymphoma in the working formulation (176), or diffuse, well-differentiated lymphocytic lymphoma in the Rappaport classification (177).

The phenotype of CLL is usually stable over months to years, but a small proportion of cases may evolve to a more aggressive form. Several types of transformation have been reported, including diffuse lymphoma (Richter's syndrome), prolymphocytoid transformation, acute lymphoblastic leukemia (ALL), and, possibly, multiple myeloma (178).

Whether transformation of CLL represents clonal evolution or a second malignancy is usually unknown. Although the two neoplastic cell types may express the same light- and heavy-chain Ig isotypes, this is not definitive proof of a common origin. In other instances, the heavy-chain Ig isotypes differ, but this could be due to isotype switching. More precise markers of clonality are now available, including cytogenetics, Ig gene rearrangement, and antiidiotype antibodies.

Evolution to a diffuse large cell lymphoma (Richter's syndrome) has a projected incidence of 3% to 15% of cases (179–183). Development of a diffuse large cell lymphoma in CLL is associated with clinical progression and increasing tumor mass. Whether Richter's syndrome is an independent disease or derived from the CLL clone is controversial, as few cases are carefully studied; when studied, the data suggest some cases are clonal and others represent a second clone (184–189).

PLL is a clinical entity distinct from CLL, with B- and T-cell variants (190–193). A substantial proportion of patients with CLL, however, exhibit some cells that morphologically resemble prolymphocytes. When over 30% of the peripheral blood lymphocytes are prolymphocytes, this is referred to as prolymphocytic transformation of CLL and is distinct from *de novo* PLL (194–198). Although some patients may develop more progressive disease states with resistance to therapy, this is not always the case. The blood usually contains two distinct populations: typical CLL cells and prolymphocytes. The latter have features similar to the CLL cells, including low-intensity, cell-surface membrane Ig and the CD5 antigen. In contrast, cells from *de novo* PLL have high levels of surface Ig and do not express CD5 and CD23, but do express FMC7 and CD22. It is generally assumed that prolymphocytic transformation evolves from the CLL clone.

Another rare form of putative transformation in CLL is development of ALL (199–201). This contrasts with the invariable progression to the acute phase in CML. Most of these cases have the French/American/British classification L2 morphology, with clinical and laboratory features typical of adult ALL. Treatment with antileukemia therapy is usually ineffective, perhaps owing to advanced disease or age. No definitive data indicate that the ALL is derived from the CLL clone. Another complication described in CLL is multiple myeloma. Several cases were studied; in most, the CLL and myeloma were not proved to be related (202–206), and two cases appeared clonal (207,208).

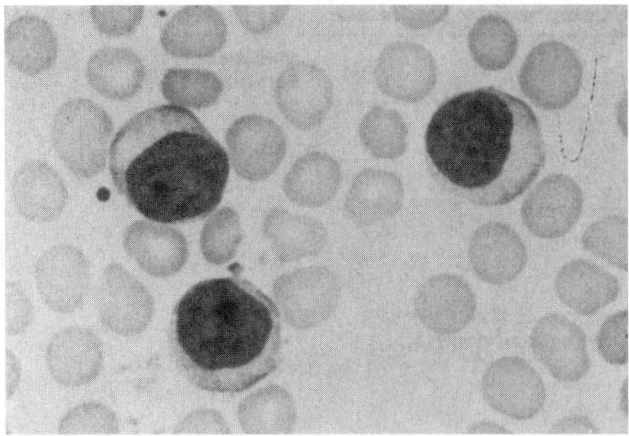

Figure 26-3. Peripheral blood, chronic lymphocytic leukemia (Wright-Giemsa stain; ×400). (See Color Fig. 26-3.)

PATHOLOGY

The typical CLL cell is a mature, well-differentiated lymphocyte with a round, compact nucleus, clumped chromatin, and a distinct nucleolus (Fig. 26-3). These same cells invade the lymph nodes in a diffuse pattern (malignant lymphoma, small lymphocytic), with effacement of the normal architecture (Fig. 26-4).

The marrow is invariably involved with leukemia cells. CLL cells are capable of transendothelial migration (209). They express functional CXCR4 receptors for the stromal cell–derived factor-1 and display chemotaxis toward this chemokine (210). Because marrow stromal cells secrete the stromal cell–derived factor-1, this may account for the observation that CLL cells invariably are present in the marrow. The bone marrow involvement may be diffuse or focal, typically becoming more extensively replaced in advanced disease. Five patterns of infiltration have been described: interstitial, nodular, diffuse involvement, mixed interstitial and nodular, and mixed nodular and diffuse (Fig. 26-5). As previously mentioned, some groups report a correlation between more extensive replacement of bone marrow or a diffuse pattern (or both) with a poor prognosis.

The spleen typically shows a replacement of normal architecture by CLL cells. The proliferation of CLL cells occurs preferentially in the white pulp zone, even in cases in which both the white and red pulp zones are extensively infiltrated (211).

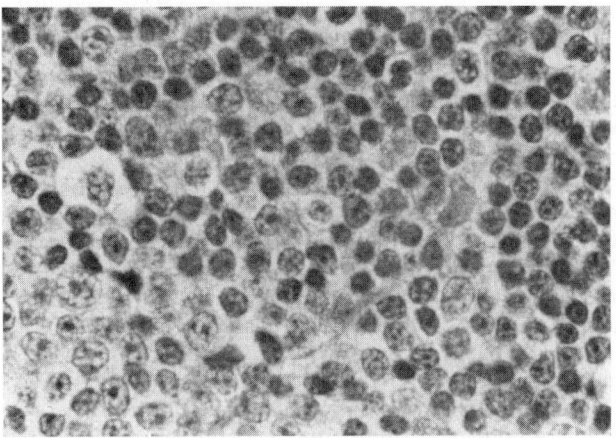

Figure 26-4. Lymph node of patient with malignant small cell lymphocytic lymphoma (hematoxylin and eosin stain; ×100). (See Color Fig. 26-4.)

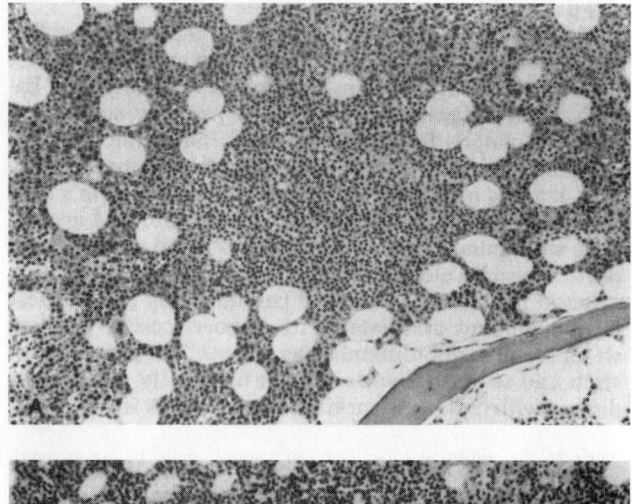

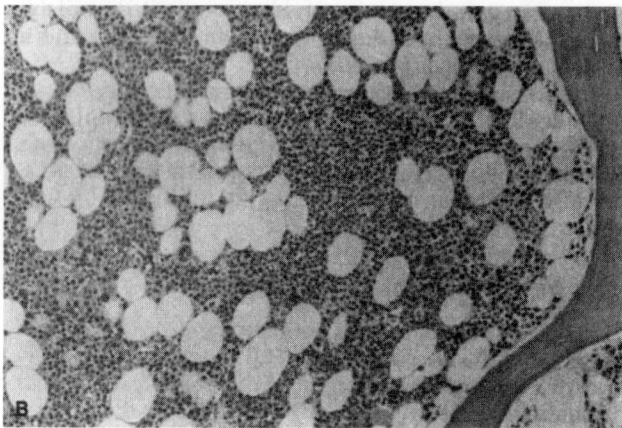

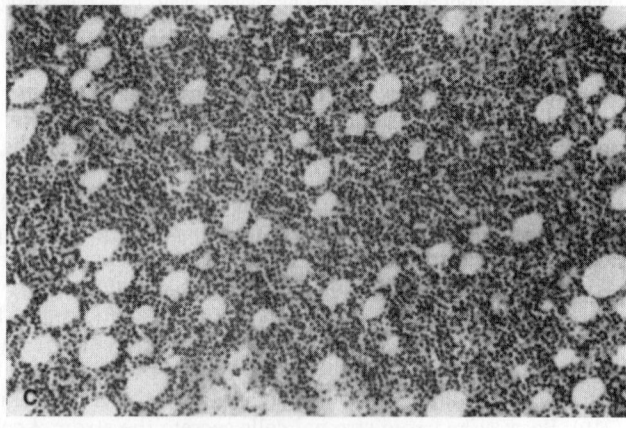

Figure 26-5. Bone marrow of patient with chronic lymphocytic leukemia: nodular (**A**), interstitial (**B**), diffuse (**C**) (hematoxylin and eosin stain; ×160). (See Color Fig. 26-5.)

The liver may be slightly enlarged due to lymphocytic infiltration of periportal tracts, with occasional nodular masses encroaching on the parenchyma. Virtually any other organ site may be infiltrated by CLL cells.

BIOLOGY

Most blood CLL cells are not in the cell mitotic cycle (they are in G_0), as determined by the low incorporation rate of ^{3}H-thymidine by leukemic lymphocytes (212) or by flow cytometric analyses for newly synthesized DNA (213). The low proportion of proliferating cells suggests that the life span of CLL lymphocytes is quite long. Consistent with this, human CLL–B cells can survive for many weeks after transfer into mice with severe combined immune deficiency (214).

CLL cells express high levels of the antiapoptotic protein bcl-2 (215). Although the levels of leukemia cell expression of bcl-2 did not correspond to the extent of tumor mass, higher levels were associated more frequently with aggressive clinical disease or resistance to chemotherapy (216–218).

In addition, the neoplastic B cells of patients with CLL express high levels of another antiapoptotic protein, bcl-x_l, and low levels of the proapoptotic protein bax or bcl-x_s (219). Patients with leukemia cells that contain a high ratio of bcl-2 to bax are resistant to treatment with chlorambucil. Antisense oligonucleotides to BCL-2 can down-modulate expression of messenger RNA encoding this protein in CLL cells in vitro (216), suggesting that such oligonucleotides may be useful therapeutic agents, either alone or in combination with chemotherapy.

Interactions with stroma may enhance leukemia cell resistance to apoptosis. CLL cells express high levels of the $\alpha_4\beta_1$ integrin that can serve as a receptor to fibronectin and facilitates cell-to-cell adhesion and lymphocyte migration (220). CLL cells cultured with fibronectin or the H89 fragment containing the high-affinity ligand CS-1 were found to have increased ratios of bcl-2 to bax and survival times that were greater than that of leukemic cells cultured alone.

DIFFERENTIAL DIAGNOSIS

In contrast to the cell that appears morphologically mature, typical of CLL, B-cell–derived PLL is characterized by larger, less mature-appearing cells with condensed nuclear chromatin, prominent nucleoli (190,191,221) (Fig. 26-6), and surface mark-

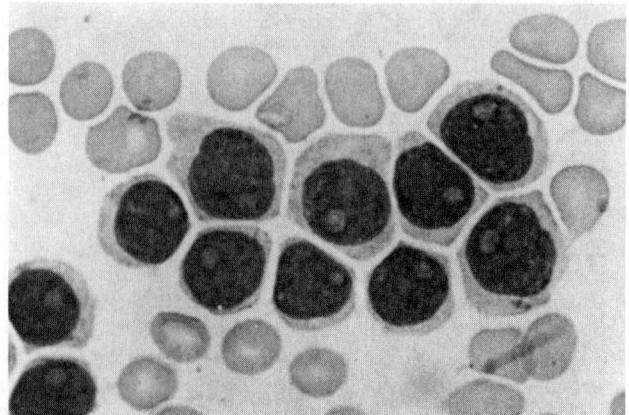

Figure 26-6. Peripheral blood of patient with prolymphocytic leukemia (Wright-Giemsa stain; ×400). (See Color Fig. 26-6.)

TABLE 26-6. Relation between CLL, Prolymphocytic Transformation of CLL (CLL/PLL) and *de novo* PLL

	CLL	CLL/PLL	*de novo* PLL
Age	60	60	70
Leukocyte count (× 10⁹/L)	50–120	>120	>150
PLL(%)	<30	30%–80%	>50%
Spleen	++	+++	++++
Lymph nodes	++++	+++	+
CD5	>80%	>80%	<20%
FMC-7/CD22	<20%	<20%	>80%
Surface-membrane immunoglobulin	Weak	Weak	Strong

CLL, chronic lymphocytic leukemia; PLL, prolymphocytic leukemia; +, minimal; ++, moderate; +++, extensive.

ers distinct from CLL (Table 26-6). Most notable are the presence of FMC7 and CD22 (52,222) and high-density surface Ig and the absence of CD5. Several clinical and laboratory features are also distinctive of B-cell PLL, including extreme leukocytosis (more than 100 × 10⁹/L) and prominent splenomegaly without substantial lymphadenopathy.

The relation between PLL and CLL is complex. At the extremes are classic CLL and classic PLL. The prolymphocytic variant of CLL has features of both diseases. Whereas the cells morphologically appear activated and look like classic PLL cells, they share most immunophenotypic features with CLL cells (223). The clinical course follows the typical pattern of CLL.

Waldenstrom's macroglobulinemia is generally classified as a low-grade lymphoma. The malignant lymphocytes have plasmacytoid features (224–227), often with abundant basophilic cytoplasm (Fig. 26-7). The periodic acid-Schiff (PAS) reaction is frequently positive, indicating the presence of polysaccharide; occasionally, this occurs in globules, leading to the term *grape cells*. Waldenstrom's cells typically have both surface and cytoplasmic IgM and secrete substantial amounts of IgM, resulting in a monoclonal peak on protein electrophoresis. Increased serum viscosity is found in approximately two-thirds of patients; only half of these have symptoms associated with hyperviscosity. Waldenstrom's macroglobulinemia has a peak incidence in the sixth and seventh decades and is frequently an indolent disease with prolonged survival. Bone marrow involvement is invariably seen; most patients have circulating tumor cells, and some have high leukocyte counts. With disease progression,

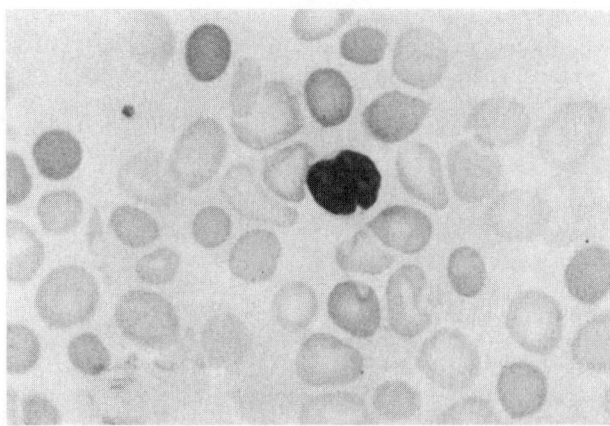

Figure 26-8. Peripheral blood of patient with small cleaved-cell lymphoma (Wright-Giemsa stain; ×400). (See Color Fig. 26-8.)

lymphadenopathy, splenomegaly, and hepatomegaly become prominent, and the clinical pattern resembles a lymphoma. In contrast to multiple myeloma, bone lesions are infrequent. Some investigators prefer to include Waldenström's macroglobulinemia under the broader heading of *lymphoplasmacytic leukemias/lymphomas* (228). This would also include patients without a paraprotein but with other similar morphologic and clinical features of Waldenstrom's macroglobulinemia.

A fourth type of chronic B-cell leukemia (229–231) typically represents the leukemia phase of a follicular small cleaved-cell lymphoma. The typical cells from follicular lymphomas are often pleomorphic, with small, prominent nucleoli (nuclear clefting), a finer chromatin pattern than typical CLL cells, and a high nuclear to cytoplasmic ratio (Fig. 26-8). This disorder typically presents as a lymphoma rather than as leukemia, but up to half of patients have bone marrow involvement at diagnosis. Some patients present with bone marrow and peripheral blood involvement without lymph node involvement; this may be difficult to distinguish from CLL. In the absence of a lymph node biopsy, the diagnosis should be made by morphologic features as well as immunologic features associated with follicular lymphomas, such as lack of mouse erythrocyte rosetting, normal capping, and bright surface-membrane Ig fluorescence (232,233). Unlike CLL, most cases of follicular lymphoma do not express the CD23 and CD5 antigens. Furthermore, most cases of follicular lymphoma express the CD10, CD22, and FMC7 antigens, which are absent in CLL (234).

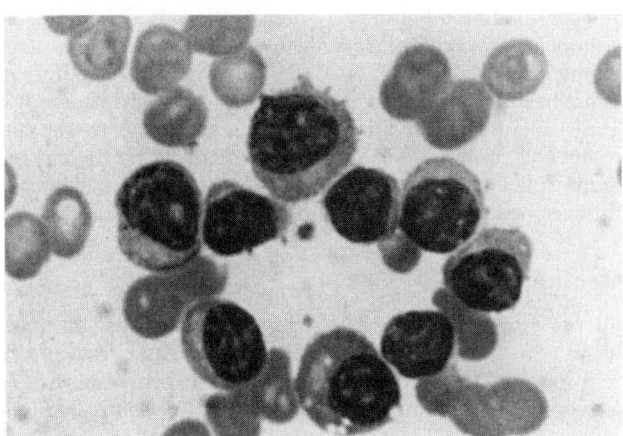

Figure 26-7. Peripheral blood of patient with Waldenström's macroglobulinemia (Wright-Giemsa stain; ×400). (See Color Fig. 26-7.)

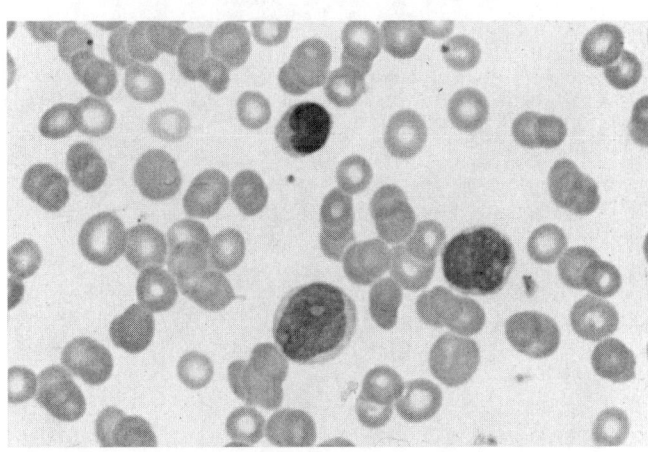

Figure 26-9. Peripheral blood of a patient with mantle cell lymphoma in the leukemic phase (Wright-Giemsa stain; ×400). (See Color Fig. 26-9.)

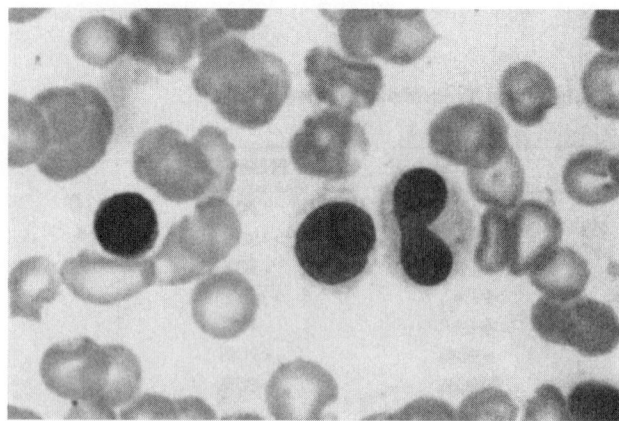

Figure 26-10. Peripheral blood of patient with hairy cell leukemia (Wright-Giemsa stain; ×400). (See Color Fig. 26-10.)

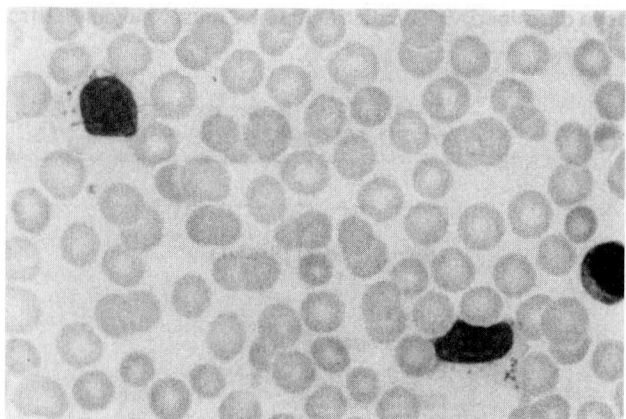

Figure 26-12. Peripheral blood of patient with large granular lymphocytic leukemia (Wright-Giemsa stain; ×400). (See Color Fig. 26-12.)

Splenic lymphoma with villous lymphocytes (SLVL) is a predominately splenic form of lymphoma (235,236). This tends to be an indolent disease. Two-thirds of patients have a small monoclonal band. The leukocyte counts range from 5 to $40 \times 10^9/L$, and the circulating lymphocytes are larger than CLL cells and have short villi, often localized to one pole of the cell. In contrast to hairy cell leukemia, the splenic infiltration is in the white pulp. Surface markers are similar to those in PLL.

The leukemic phase of mantle cell lymphomas is characterized by an aggressive clinical course with a median survival of less than 2 years (237). The blood films show a pleomorphic picture with medium-size lymphocytes with nuclear irregularities and clefts (Fig. 26-9). The membrane phenotype shows intense surface-membrane Ig and reactivity with CD5, CD19, CD20, FMC7, and

CD22. CD10 is positive in half of cases. The lymph nodes show diffuse or a vaguely nodular pattern effacing the nodal architecture, and the bone marrow shows a diffuse pattern of infiltration. The t(11;14)(q13;q32) translocation with rearrangement of the *bcl-1* oncogene is commonly found in mantle cell lymphomas.

Hairy cell leukemia is another form of B-lymphocyte–derived chronic leukemia. The disease is so termed because "hairy" cytoplasmic projections (Fig. 26-10) are sometimes visible by light, phase, or electron microscopy (238–240) (Fig. 26-11). Hairy cell leukemia has a marked male predominance, with pancytopenia and prominent splenomegaly. Although most patients are leukopenic, some have a leukocytosis with a high percentage of hairy cells. This is discussed below in Hairy Cell Leukemia.

A rare disorder termed *large granular lymphocytic* (LGL) *leukemia* or *chronic T-gamma lymphoproliferative disease* has been described (241). The distinguishing morphologic feature is the presence of abundant cytoplasm, usually containing azurophilic granules (241–243) (Fig. 26-12). Immune features include T-cell and NK-cell markers (CD2, CD3, CD8, CD56). Clinical features include relatively low levels of circulating leukocytes and granulocytopenia; recurrent infections are common, whereas lymphadenopathy and skin involvement are typically absent. This is discussed in below in Large Granular Lymphocytic Leukemia.

THERAPY

Immune Cytopenias

Immune-mediated hemolytic anemia, thrombocytopenia, and neutropenia are usually first treated with high-dose corticosteroid therapy (60 to 100 mg/m²/day). The underlying disease does not require treatment (described below under Approach to Therapy by Clinical Stage) unless additional indications for therapy are present Patients who do not respond to corticosteroid therapy may require splenectomy. Intravenous Ig may also be useful but is of unproven benefit for autoimmune complications of CLL (244–248).

Infections

Patients with CLL have increased infections because of numerous factors, including hypogammaglobulinemia, low complement levels (249), altered leukemia-cell expression of major histocompatibility complex class II antigens (250), impaired granulocytic function (251), functional defects in bystander T cells, and altered expression of T-cell receptor V genes (252). Bacterial and viral infections are most common. The risk for infection cor-

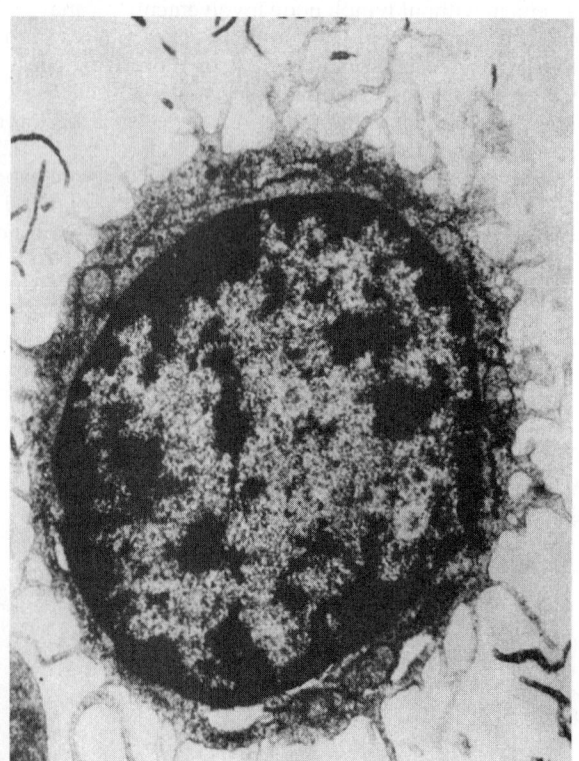

Figure 26-11. Peripheral blood of patient with hairy cell leukemia seen by electron microscopy.

relates inversely with Ig levels. Decreased concentrations of IgG_2 and IgG_4 may be associated with increased susceptibility to infection (253), this possibly reflecting impaired Th1-type immunity. Consequently, several trials have evaluated the role of intravenous Ig in preventing infections in patients with CLL.

A double-blind, randomized study (254) in patients with CLL reported that intravenous Ig (400 mg/kg given every 3 weeks) reduced bacterial infections, particularly infections of moderate severity, by half. The actuarial probability of remaining infection-free and the time to first infection were decreased. The incidence of minor and severe bacterial infections and of all viral infections remained unchanged. Twelve patients completing the trial entered a double-blind crossover study (255) that confirmed the benefit of Ig. The major issue is determining who should receive this treatment. Patients who receive this treatment are likely to have severe hypogammaglobulinemia or a history of serious bacterial infections. Intravenous Ig should also be compared with alternative approaches such as prophylactic antibiotics.

Hyperleukocytosis

Rare patients with peripheral CLL counts exceeding $1000 \times 10^9/L$ may have hyperviscosity-related symptoms and would benefit from leukapheresis (256,257).

Response Criteria

Evaluating therapy has been difficult in CLL because of the lack of uniform response criteria. Recently, the International Workshop (17) and the NCISWG (16) defined *complete remission* (CR) as the resolution of lymphadenopathy and organomegaly, lymphocytes less than $4 \times 10^9/L$, granulocytes more than $1.5 \times 10^9/L$, and platelet counts higher than $100 \times 10^9/L$. The International Workshop (17) includes the resolution of constitutional symptoms and a normal or nondiffuse pattern of bone marrow infiltration. The NCISWG (16) requires fulfillment of the criteria stated earlier for longer than 2 months, after which a bone marrow aspiration and biopsy must show less than 30% lymphocytes. These criteria should provide a basis for comparing results of clinical trials. Their biologic impact has not been tested.

Additional tests to define CRs are used in some studies. These tests may indicate whether serum Ig levels, mouse rosette-forming cell levels, and the ratio of κ to λ light chains normalize and whether chromosomal abnormalities resolve. A more sensitive indicator of CR is the absence of cells expressing the Ig idiotype of the leukemia clone in the blood and bone marrow. Determining this absence requires developing antiidiotype antibodies for each case of CLL. It also has its pitfalls, such as somatic mutation. Another approach is to study DNA from remission cells for clonal rearrangement of Ig heavy- or light-chain genes corresponding to the initial malignant clone by Southern blotting, but this technique is relatively insensitive. The polymerase chain reaction is more sensitive, but its use would require sequencing part of the uniquely rearranged Ig gene sequence for each patient. The ratio of κ to λ light chains (clonal excess) and dual staining for antigen combinations (e.g., CD5 and CD20) are also used to document remission. The latter, however, may not differentiate the small percentage of normal circulating CD5–B cells from CLL cells. CLL cells are likely to persist in all patients considered to have CRs, even if these additional criteria are fulfilled.

Partial response, as defined by the International Workshop (17), is a change from Binet stage C disease to stage A or B, or from stage B to A. The NCISWG (16) defines a partial response as more than a 50% decrease in blood lymphocytes; a 50% decrease in enlarged lymph nodes, the spleen, and the liver; hemoglobin levels higher than 110 g/L (11 g/dL); platelet counts higher than $100 \times 10^9/L$; and granulocytes more than $1.5 \times 10^9/L$; or an improvement of 50% in these values from baseline. The analyses of most clinical studies are flawed by a lack of uniform response criteria. Future clinical trials should use these criteria (16,17).

Approach to Therapy by Clinical Stage

There are no established cures for CLL, and spontaneous remissions, although reported, are extremely rare (258). At first examination, therapy of CLL appears straightforward, but this notion is far from correct, and controversies abound. The prognosis can vary substantially between different patients, depending on the clinical stage and the presence or absence of disease features that have been associated with disease progression or a more adverse clinical outcome. This section considers several issues related to CLL treatment in the context of disease stage.

LOW RISK
In planning strategy for each stage of CLL, it is necessary to consider median survival from diagnosis, likelihood of disease progression, and risk of death from leukemia. For example, patients with low-risk CLL have a median survival of longer than 10 years and are unlikely to die from leukemia. Consequently, the possibility of detecting a benefit of therapy is limited.

The first issue is whether therapy of low-risk CLL should be initiated at diagnosis or only on disease progression. This question has been addressed in a randomized trial comparing immediate versus delayed treatment with chlorambucil. These data suggest no advantage to early treatment (259).

Several issues are unanswered. Would immediate treatment with another approach lead to a different conclusion? Alternative approaches include fludarabine, cladribine (2-chlorodeoxyadenosine), or multidrug chemotherapy, such as the cyclophosphamide, vincristine, and prednisone regimen (CVP) or the cyclophosphamide, hydroxydaunomycin (doxorubicin), vincristine (Oncovin), and prednisone regimen (CHOP). There exsist no data to support the use of any of the drugs, or combinations of drugs, in low-risk patients. The long survival, low likelihood of leukemia progression, and probability of death from leukemia make it unlikely that an impact could be detected. Furthermore, it is difficult to justify use of more intensive therapy under these conditions.

The sum of available data suggests a conservative approach in patients with low-risk CLL. Many affected patients may never need treatment. Others with progressive disease qualify for treatment approaches discussed for patients with intermediate- or advanced-stage CLL.

INTERMEDIATE RISK
Patients with intermediate-risk CLL have a median survival of approximately 5 years. Consequently, evaluating treatment strategies in this setting is easier than in low-stage CLL. The first issue in the therapy of intermediate-risk CLL is that of immediate versus delayed therapy. Patients with only modest symptoms, such as enlarged lymph nodes, may not require immediate therapy. In contrast, patients with severe symptoms or an extremely large tumor mass require immediate treatment. These two situations must be considered separately.

Few data indicate whether it is better to delay treatment of patients with intermediate-risk CLL with a low tumor mass. The difference between this question and the seemingly similar issue discussed in patients with low-risk CLL is the greater likelihood of leukemia progression, briefer survival time, and death from leukemia. Treatments that might be considered in this setting include chlorambucil, fludarabine, cladribine, CVP, or CHOP

(260–265). It is not possible to choose between delaying or initiating therapy. Patients with intermediate-risk CLL and advanced tumor mass need immediate treatment.

HIGH RISK

Patients with high-risk CLL have a median survival of 2 to 4 years, almost always progress, and are likely to die from leukemia. Because of these features, the issue in advanced-stage CLL is *how*, rather than *whether*, to treat affected patients. In addition, patients with progressive disease may benefit from closer follow-up or early therapy. Progressive disease may be associated with the following characteristics:

- A lymphocyte doubling time of less than 12 months
- Atypical morphology (266)
- Elevated serum thymidine kinase levels (267)
- Elevated serum β_2-microglobulin (268)
- High serum levels of soluble CD23 (268)
- A blood leukocyte count of more than $30 \times 10^9/L$
- Any complex karyotype abnormalities, including trisomy 12
- Leukemic cells that express CD38 (156) or nonmutated IgV genes (155,156)

CHEMOTHERAPY

Alkylating Agents

For decades, chlorambucil has been used to treat CLL. Although chlorambucil is useful in the palliative therapy of patients with advanced-stage disease, it does not appear to improve survival and should not be used for asymptomatic patients with early-stage disease (269). Chlorambucil may be administered continuously in a daily dosage of 0.1 mg/kg or intermittently as 0.4 mg/kg every 2 weeks, and these two treatment schedules are of equivalent efficacy, but the intermittent route may produce less myelosuppression (270,271). Overall, the response rates with these regimens is 40% to 60%, with 3% to 10% of patients achieving a CR (270–272).

Prednisone, when combined with chlorambucil, increases the response rate; however, no benefit in terms of survival was demonstrated (273). Thus, steroids are primarily reserved for the treatment of patients with autoimmune hemolytic anemia or thrombocytopenia.

Considerable data suggest that chlorambucil and CVP produce equivalent results (263,264). A randomized study comparing CVP to chlorambucil showed no difference in survival or disease progression at 9 (274) or 53 (275) months.

Several trials have been conducted of alternative therapies for high-risk CLL. One study compared CVP to CHOP in 59 previously untreated patients with Binet stage C disease (276,277). The 3-year survival rates were 28% with CVP and 71% with CHOP, and the median survival times were 22 and 62 months, respectively (277). Other studies (278) failed to confirm that CHOP is superior to CVP. In one study (279), survival of patients receiving chlorambucil or CVP was equivalent to that of the CHOP cohort of the CHOP versus CVP arm, suggesting that the better result with CHOP was due to inferior survival in the CVP arm rather than a benefit of CHOP.

Nucleoside Analogs

Although chlorambucil is still used by many hematologists for initial treatment of patients with CLL, an increasing number of practitioners use fludarabine as front-line therapy for CLL (280). Fludarabine, 25 to 30 mg/m² per day intravenously for 5 days each month, produced an overall response rate of 48% to 58% in previously treated patients, with the CR rates being 13% to 38% (281,282). In untreated patients, the response rate is approximately 70%, with the CR rate being 23% to 27% (272,281). Side effects included myelosuppression, infections, and minor neurologic problems (peripheral neuropathy, muscle weakness, and decreased hearing) (283).

In a randomized intergroup study comparing monthly fludarabine (25 mg/m² intravenously × 5 days) and chlorambucil (40 mg/m² on day 1) in untreated CLL patients, there was a higher response rate, longer duration of response, and improved progression-free survival in patients treated with fludarabine (272). The overall response rate with fludarabine was 70% with a CR of 27%, whereas the response rate with chlorambucil was 43% with the CR rate being 3%. However, no difference in survival was found between the two groups. Also, fludarabine given intravenously has been found effective in the treatment of leukemic cell infiltration of the central nervous system (284).

Autoimmune hemolytic anemia and Evan's syndrome have been reported after treatment with fludarabine (285). Also, fludarabine can induce prolonged immune suppression and depletion of CD4⁻ T cells, leading to an increased risk for opportunistic and nosocomial infections. Nevertheless, the use of fludarabine or related purine analogs has not contributed to an increased risk for secondary malignancies in CLL (286).

Treatment of patients with fludarabine has not been shown to improve overall survival. Therefore, several clinical trials have tested fludarabine in combination with other chemotherapeutic agents. Combinations of fludarabine with either mitoxantrone (287), cisplatin (288), or cytosine arabinoside did not appear to offer significant benefit over single-agent fludarabine. However, combinations of fludarabine, at 30 mg/m² daily for 3 days, and cyclophosphamide, at 300 mg/m² daily for 3 days, resulted in favorable clinical responses in 12 of 13 patients who were extensively pretreated (287). A more recent study using fludarabine at 25 mg/m² daily in combination with cyclophosphamide 250 mg/m² daily for 3 days, repeated every 4 weeks, resulted in similar clinical response rates but reduced myelotoxicity (289).

Pentostatin (2-deoxycoformycin), the oldest of the nucleoside analogs, is also used in CLL. It is usually given as 4 mg/m² intravenously every 2 weeks. Review of some of the studies shows an overall response rate of 25% to 30% with few CRs (290–294). Toxicities included infections, myelosuppression, nausea, vomiting, and pruritus.

A third purine analog is cladribine (2-chlorodeoxyadenosine), a halogenated purine analog, given as 0.1 mg/kg/day by continuous intravenous infusion for 7 days each month or 0.14 mg/kg/day intravenously over 2 hours for 5 days each month. In one study (295,296), 16 of 30 (53%) responses were reported in previously treated patients with advanced CLL. In two studies, cladribine induced complete and partial responses of approximately 70% of previously untreated patients with CLL (297,298). In a prospective, randomized, multicenter trial comparing cladribine plus prednisone versus chlorambucil plus prednisone in previously untreated CLL patients, overall response rate and CR were higher in patients treated with cladribine plus prednisone (87% and 47%) than in patients treated with chlorambucil plus prednisone (57% and 12%) (299). Progression-free survival was also longer in patients treated with cladribine plus prednisone, although overall survival was similar in both groups.

Biotherapy

MONOCLONAL ANTIBODIES

Several studies have been reported using monoclonal antibodies to treat CLL and other chronic lymphoid leukemias (300,301).

Subjects with CLL received an antiCD5 monoclonal antibody reactive with normal and malignant T lymphocytes and CLL cells (302–307). This treatment transiently reduced levels of leukemia cells in the blood with no effect on the leukemia infiltration of bone marrow, lymph nodes, or organs. Side effects were minor. The use of human antibodies and antibodies conjugated to toxins (308,309) or isotopes may prove more effective and are under investigation (310–312).

One interesting therapeutic approach is the use of monoclonal antibodies reactive with the idiotype of the Ig on malignant B cells (antiidiotype) (313,314). These antibodies are operationally tumor specific in CLL. Reproducible responses to antiidiotype antibodies are reported in patients with non-Hodgkin's B-cell lymphomas. A major limitation of such therapy is that antiidiotype antibodies are custom-made for each patient. Some antiidiotype antibodies identify isotypes common in patients with CLL (315). These antiidiotype antibodies were tested against more than 50 cases of CLL (316); one-fourth of the cases reacted with one or more of these antibodies, raising the possibility of using available antiidiotype antibodies for treatment.

Rituximab (IDEC-C2B8) is a humanized monoclonal antibody (mAb) specific for human CD20 that can induce responses in approximately 50% of patients with relapsed follicular lymphoma (317,318). However, CLL–B cells express lower levels of CD20 than do most lymphoma cells and may be less sensitive to treatment with rituximab. Doses higher than 375 mg/m^2 have been used (up to 2500 mg/m^2) to overcome the low expression of CD20 on the surface of B–CLL cells.

Some CLL patients treated with rituximab experienced tumor lysis syndrome. Moreover, patients with leukemia cell counts exceeding 50×10^9/L at the time of treatment have developed a severe cytokine-release syndrome secondary to release of tumor necrosis factor-α and IL-6 (319,320). Clinical symptoms included fever, chills, nausea, vomiting, hypotension, and dyspnea. There was a five- to tenfold increase of liver enzymes, lactic dehydrogenase, and D-dimers, as well as prolongation of the prothrombin time. Lymphocyte and platelet counts dropped to 50% to 75% of baseline within 12 hours after the onset of the infusion. This complication could be mitigated by use of a fractionated dosing schedule with infusion of 50 mg of rituximab on day 1, 150 mg on day 2, and the remainder of the 375 mg/m^2 dose on day 3 (319).

CAMPATH-1H is a genetically engineered mAb that contains the variable region of CAMPATH-1, a CD52 mouse mAb, and the heavy- and light-chain constant regions of human IgG_1 and kappa, respectively. This antibody binds to a surface antigen present on most lymphocytes, including CLL–B cells, and can induce complement-mediated and antibody-dependent cell cytotoxicity. In one study, previously treated patients were given intravenous infusions of 30 mg CAMPATH-1H three times a week for 12 weeks (321). Of the 29 patients to receive such therapy, 38% experienced a partial remission and 4% experienced a CR, with median duration of 12 months. Treatment with CAMPATH-1H causes marked T-cell depletion and immune deficiency. CAMPATH-1H has been approved by the U.S. Food and Drug Administration for the treatment of advanced CLL.

Lym-1 is an IgG_{2a} mouse mAb specific for human B cells that has been used in radioimmunotherapy of CLL (322,323). Conjugated with I^{131}, Lym-1 has been used in phase I and II trials in which patients received ^{I131}–Lym-1 in escalating doses from 1.48 GBq/m^2 to 3.7 GBq/m^2 (40 to 100 mCi/m^2) (324). For patients with splenomegaly, most of the administered radiolabeled antibody localized to the spleen and did not distribute uniformly through other lymphoid tissue. Although the treatment was well tolerated, its efficacy in CLL was lower than that noted for non-Hodgkin's lymphoma.

Interferons

IFN-α induces differentiation and proliferation of CLL cells *in vitro* (325). Whether this occurs *in vivo* and whether it is clinically useful are unknown. IFN-α is not active in patients with intermediate- and high-risk CLL (326,327). The low response rate to IFN-α in patients with advanced CLL contrasts with a 50% rate of response in patients with advanced, low-grade, non-Hodgkin's lymphoma (328–330), a 50% rate of response in patients with cutaneous T-cell lymphoma (CTCL) (331), and a 90% rate of response in patients with hairy cell leukemia (332–335). Recent studies reported greater than 50% responses in patients with previously untreated, low-risk CLL who were treated with low-dose (2×10^6 IU/m^2 three times per week) recombinant IFN-α therapy (336–338). Unfortunately, determining whether this treatment affects survival beneficially will take 10 to 15 years.

Radiation Therapy and Splenectomy

Total body radiation is not recommended for patients with CLL because it causes excessive myelosuppression. In contrast, radiation therapy to bulky lymph nodes or an enlarged spleen may be useful in symptomatic patients, especially when chemotherapy is ineffective. Splenectomy may be of benefit in hypersplenism unresponsive to radiation or chemotherapy (339–341).

Bone Marrow Transplantation

Autologous marrow transplantation has been studied in CLL patients with advanced disease, and marrow purging using monoclonal antibodies was performed in approximately half of these cases (342–344). A high CR rate has been observed, but the follow-up time is too short to assess impact on survival. Transplantation with allogeneic stem cells has been carried out worldwide (345,346). An update of the results on 54 CLL patients less than 60 years old from 30 centers worldwide transplanted between 1984 and 1992 has been published (346). The median age was 41 years (range, 21 to 58 years). Patients received high-dose chemotherapy and radiation, followed by an HLA-matched bone marrow transplant. CR was observed in 70% of patients, and the 3-year survival probability was 46%. Treatment-related mortality was high at 50%, with approximately one-half of these caused by graft-versus-host disease. In single-institute studies, approximately two-thirds of patients with advanced disease achieved a CR, and the incidence of graft-versus-host disease was low (344,346); the latter finding may be related to the fact that many of these patients had received fludarabine, which is a potent immunosuppressive agent. This approach, however, applies to less than 5% of cases of CLL and is associated with high treatment-related morbidity and mortality.

Allogeneic stem cell transplantation with a nonablative preparative regimen (transplant-lite) appears to be most promising in patients with chemotherapy-responsive disease and low tumor burden. This approach produces sufficient immunosuppression to allow engraftment of allogeneic stem cells and induction of graft-versus-leukemia effect. In one study (347), 15 patients (median age, 55; age range, 45 to 71 years) were treated in this fashion, using a regimen consisting of fludarabine and cyclophosphamide before transplantation. Two to three months after transplantation, the patients were infused with donor lymphocytes if they did not have graft-versus-host disease. Eleven patients underwent engraftment of donor cells; of these patients, a complete response was achieved in eight. However, only seven of the 15 treated patients (47%) were alive after a median follow-up of 180 days (range, 90 to 767 days), which indicates that this approach is associated with a high mortality.

PROLYMPHOCYTIC LEUKEMIA

PLL was first described by Galton and coworkers in 1974 (190). The leukocyte count is typically greater than 100×10^9/L and consists predominately of prolymphocytes. Extensive spleen involvement is common, as are hepatomegaly and bone marrow infiltration; lymphadenopathy is usually absent or minimal. The disease is typically aggressive and responds poorly to therapy. PLL may be a disease of B or T cells.

Epidemiology and Cause

The median age of patients with PLL (both B- and T-cell types) is approximately 60 years, with a strong male predominance. The cause is unknown. Data suggest a possible association between HTLV-II and T-cell PLL (348).

Immunology

PLL cells resemble activated lymphocytes. The B-cell variety expresses strong surface Ig staining with either κ or λ light chain, Ia, CD19, CD20, CD21, FMC7, and CD22. The cells exhibit heavy- and light-chain Ig gene rearrangements (349). PLL cells do not have terminal deoxynucleotidyl transferase; PAS staining is typically positive.

Most cases of T-cell PLL are CD4$^+$ and CD8$^-$. The CD8 antigen and combined CD4 and CD8 antigens are seen in a minority of cases (228,350,351). The T-cell variant is typically acid phosphatase–positive and terminal deoxynucleotidyl transferase–negative.

Cytogenetics

Several chromosomal abnormalities are described in B-cell PLL. They include del(3), 6q$^-$, trisomy 6, trisomy 12, and structural abnormalities of chromosome 1. In one study (352), all five patients demonstrated a t(6;12)(q15;p13) translocation. T-cell PLL virtually always demonstrates inv(14)(q11;q32) or other 14q abnormalities (351,353–355).

Clinical Features

Typical presenting features of B-cell PLL are fatigue, weakness, and weight loss (190). Fever unassociated with infection is also common. Some patients experience abdominal pain and early satiety from massive splenomegaly. The outstanding physical sign is splenomegaly; hepatomegaly may also be prominent. Lymphadenopathy is absent or modest. Rare patients have petechiae and purpura from thrombocytopenia. T-cell PLL has similar features, with the addition of skin involvement in 25% of cases and lymphadenopathy in 50% of cases.

Leukocyte counts often exceed 100×10^9/L and are composed predominantly of prolymphocytes. The hemoglobin level is less than 12 g/dL, and platelet counts are less than 150×10^9/L; some patients have granulocytopenia.

Pathology

PLL cells (Fig. 26-6) appear more immature and have more cytoplasm than typical CLL cells and are thought to be activated lymphocytes (221). The cells contain a large, vesicular nucleolus, condensed nuclear chromatin, and moderate cytoplasmic basophilia. PLL–T cells may have nuclear irregularities

and have been referred to as "knobby" cells (228). Ultrastructural studies show coarse chromatin with a large nucleolus. Mitochondria are present, and some cells show strandlike projections (microvilli) from the cytoplasmic border (190).

The bone marrow and spleen are typically diffusely infiltrated by prolymphocytes. Rarely, lymph nodes show diffuse infiltration with effacement of architecture. The liver often shows dense infiltration of the portal tracts and sinusoids (356).

Differential Diagnosis

The distinction among PLL, CLL, SLVL, and the leukemic phase of mantle cell and follicular lymphomas is discussed in the section Chronic Lymphocytic Leukemia. PLL may be confused with ALL; however, patient age and the distinct morphologic features of the cells usually distinguish these diseases. The coarsely clumped nuclear chromatin characteristic of the PLL cell is unlike the typical finely reticulin nuclear chromatin and often inconspicuous nucleoli of the undifferentiated blasts of ALL. In ALL, massive enlargement of the liver and spleen is less common; leukocyte counts are typically higher in PLL than in ALL.

Therapy

PLL typically exhibits a rapid downhill course, but some patients may have more indolent courses. Combination chemotherapy with cyclophosphamide, 750 mg/m^2 intravenously on day 1; doxorubicin, 50 mg/m^2 intravenously on day 1; vincristine, 2 mg intravenously on day 1; and prednisone, 100 mg/day by mouth on days 1 to 5 at 3- to 4-week intervals is often used (357–359). Allopurinol, 300 mg/day, should be administered on the days of chemotherapy. Some CRs have been reported. However, the majority of patients has a short survival (generally few months).

Splenic radiation was also used to treat PLL (360). Twelve patients were treated with weekly doses of 1 Gy to a maximum of 10 Gy; there was little morbidity, and seven patients responded. Splenectomy has been reported to be successful in some instances.

The introduction of purine analogs created an advance in the treatment of patients with PLL. When pentostatin was used to treat patients with PLL, a 40% to 50% response rate was reported (294,351). In another study, nine (45%) of 20 patients treated with pentostatin achieved partial remission, including seven (50%) of 14 with B-cell PLL and two (33%) of six with T-cell PLL (361). No CR was observed, and the median duration of response was 9 months (range, 2–30 months).

Fludarabine was used alone or in combination with prednisone in the treatment of PLL. In one study, 17 patients with PLL were treated with fludarabine alone or with prednisone (362). Three patients (18%) achieved CR, and three (18%) had a partial remission with an overall response rate of 35%.

Information in the literature about the efficacy of cladribine in PLL is sparse (363–365). Among 15 patients treated with one to three courses of cladribine, six (40%) achieved a CR, and most of them had a good response.

Based on the above data, purine analogs should be used as first-line therapy for patients with PLL. It is unknown whether the combination of purine analogs with alkylating agents or monoclonal antibodies will be more effective.

CAMPATH-1H, a human CD52 antibody, produced high response rates in the treatment of prolymphocytic leukemia. In one study, major responses occurred in 11 patients (73%) treated with CAMPATH-1H compared with 40% in those treated with pentostatin (366).

HAIRY CELL LEUKEMIA

Hairy cell leukemia, formerly referred to as *leukemic reticuloendotheliosis*, was first described by Borouncle and coworkers in 1958 (238). Remarkable progress in the diagnosis, biology, immunology, and therapy of this disease has occurred during the past 15 years. Hairy cell leukemia is a B-cell disease; a rare T-cell variant has been reported and occurs in less than 1% of cases.

Epidemiology and Cause

Hairy cell leukemia accounts for 1% to 2% of leukemia cases. It affects males predominantly in a ratio of 5:1. The median age of affected patients is approximately 50 years. In the United States, most patients are white.

HTLV-II has been isolated from cells of rare patients with T-cell–hairy cell leukemia (348). The T-cell variant of hairy cell leukemia is so rare that many investigators question its existence. A viral cause for typical hairy cell leukemia has not been implicated.

Immunology

Surface markers of hairy cell leukemia are consistent with a clonal proliferation of B lymphocytes (367). Surface-membrane Ig with a single light chain confirms the clonality of the disease. B-cell–associated antigens, including CD19, CD20, CD21, FMC7, CD22, and sometimes CD23 and CD24, are also present (368–370). The PCA-1 antigen (371), typical of plasma cells, is present on some hairy cells. These data suggest that hairy cells may be preplasma cells (372). Studies of Ig genes indicate clonal rearrangement of heavy-chain Ig genes and at least one light-chain Ig gene (373,374).

Most cases of hairy cell leukemia demonstrate the CD11c antigen as well as the CD25 antigen (IL-2 receptor) typically identified on malignant and activated T cells (374). Several antigens appear to be restricted to hairy cell leukemia cells, including the CD103 antigen (375–377). Rare cases of hairy cell leukemia with T-cell antigens have been reported (378). Hairy cell leukemia cells contain tartrate-resistant isoenzyme 5 of acid phosphatase (TRAP) (379). The PAS and α-naphthyl acetate esterase tests may be weakly positive, whereas naphthol AS-D-chloroacetate esterase and peroxidase reactions are negative (380).

Some investigators have attempted to predict the course of hairy cell leukemia by Ig light-chain involvement. In one study (381), patients with κ light chains on the cell surface had a favorable prognosis; a second study (382) reached the opposite conclusion. With the new, effective therapies available today, such distinctions are probably unimportant.

Cytogenetics

The most common chromosomal abnormalities in hairy cell leukemia involve chromosome 14 (383). In one study (384), five of 12 cases had a 14q+ chromosome involving band q32. Additional abnormalities included trisomies 7, 12, 18, 22, 12p+, 12q−, monosomy 10 and 17, 6q−, and del(3p21) (383–385).

Clinical Features

The most common presenting complaints are weakness and fatigue (239,386–388). One-third of patients have a bleeding tendency and easy bruising; one-third have recent recurrent infections. Abdominal discomfort from an enlarged spleen is present in one-fourth of cases. A few patients have weight loss, fever,

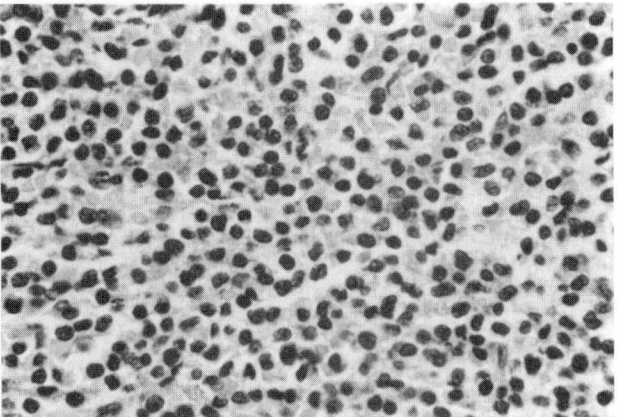

Figure 26-13. Bone marrow of patient with hairy cell leukemia (hematoxylin and eosin stain; ×100). (See Color Fig. 26-13.)

and night sweats. Splenomegaly is the most common physical finding at diagnosis and is found in virtually all patients, over 80% of patients having massive enlargement. Approximately 10% of patients have lymphadenopathy and 20% hepatomegaly with abnormal liver function tests. The serum protein electrophoresis is abnormal in one-fourth of cases; a monoclonal pattern is commonly detected by immunofixation (389). Most patients present with mild to moderate normochromic normocytic anemia secondary to replacement of the bone marrow by leukemia cells and to hypersplenism. Although most patients have hairy cells identifiable on the peripheral smear, only 20% of patients have significantly elevated white blood cell counts. Eighty percent of affected patients have neutropenia; 50% have platelet counts less than 100×10^9/L. Qualitative platelet abnormalities are common (390).

One-third of patients with hairy cell leukemia develop infections during the course of their disease; over half of these involve gram-negative organisms (386). Atypical mycobacteria is common and may require an open-lung biopsy. Disseminated fungal diseases may occur, whereas *Pneumocystis carinii* is rare.

Other complications of hairy cell leukemia include vasculitis and bone lesions (386). Systemic vasculitis is documented by biopsy of skin lesions. The management usually requires high-dose steroids. Long-bone involvement, usually of the femur, can result in lytic lesions and associated pain and pathologic fractures.

Pathology

The typical hairy cell–leukemia cell is an irregular cell with a serrated border (Fig. 26-10). The cytoplasm is sky blue without granules. The nuclear membrane is distinct and the chromatin spongy. Occasionally, a single nucleolus is present. Electron micrographs show pseudopods and long cytoplasmic villi on the surface resembling hairs on the cell (387,388) (Fig. 26-11). The cytoplasm contains abundant oval or round mitochondria with a well-developed Golgi apparatus and free ribosomes and rough endoplasmic reticulum.

The bone marrow cannot be aspirated in more than half of cases because of leukemia infiltration, fibrosis, or both. Core biopsies are usually diagnostic, showing diffuse involvement with hairy cells and increased reticulin (Fig. 26-13). The spleen shows extensive diffuse infiltration of the red pulp, cords, and sinuses (Fig. 26-14). The lymph nodes usually demonstrate diffuse infiltration of the medulla, with neoplastic cells that may extend into the surrounding fat. Obliteration of the lymph node architecture is not typically found. The liver may demonstrate

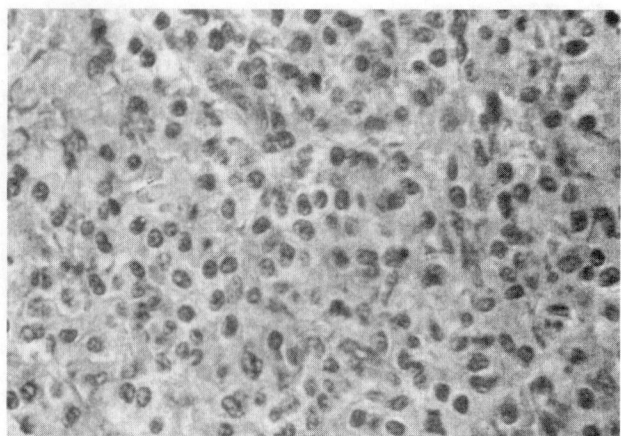

Figure 26-14. Spleen of patient with hairy cell leukemia (hematoxylin and eosin stain; ×400). (See Color Fig. 26-14.)

portal infiltration and diffuse infiltration of the hepatic sinuses with hairy cells.

Differential Diagnosis

Diagnosis of hairy cell leukemia is usually straightforward because of distinct morphologic features of the cells, the typical pattern of the bone marrow involvement, and clinical features. Pancytopenia may be confused with aplastic anemia, but the bone marrow biopsy should be diagnostic. SLVL may be confused with hairy cell leukemia because of the primary splenic involvement, indolent course, and villi on the cells (235,236). The nuclear/cytoplasmic ratio is higher than that in hairy cell leukemia, and the cells do not express CD25 and are TRAP negative. Unlike in hairy cell leukemia, the splenic infiltration in SLVL is in the white pulp. Waldenstrom's macroglobulinemia shares some features with hairy cell leukemia, but the typical IgM monoclonal spike of Waldenstrom's is distinctive, as are morphologic features of the leukemia cells. The distinct features of CLL are discussed in the section Chronic Lymphocytic Leukemia.

Histiocytic disorders, such as histiocytic medullary reticulosis, can resemble hairy cell leukemia. Occasionally, hairy cells demonstrate erythrophagocytosis similar to malignant histiocytes. Histiocytic medullary reticulosis is typically more aggressive than hairy cell leukemia, rarely has marked splenomegaly, and has considerably less blood and bone marrow involvement (388). The circulating cells in histiocytic disorders resemble monoblasts. These typically are nonspecific, esterase positive, and TRAP negative.

A rare variant of hairy cell leukemia has been described (391). The morphologic features of the hairy cell variant are intermediate between those of hairy cell leukemia and PLL, and the clinical course is chronic, with splenomegaly, leukocyte counts higher than 50×10^9/L, and no monocytopenia. Similar to hairy cell leukemia, the variant cells infiltrate the red pulp of the spleen. The cells differ from classic hairy cell leukemia in that they do not express the CD25 antigen.

Therapy

Approximately 10% of patients with hairy cell leukemia never require treatment. These patients are usually elderly, have only modest splenomegaly, and have granulocyte counts higher than 1×10^9/L (386). The remainder ultimately require therapy. Historically, initial therapy for hairy cell leukemia was splenec-

tomy. Spleen size does not predict response to splenectomy (386). Approximately half of cases have normalization of blood counts; this response does not correlate with spleen size, but rather with the degree of bone marrow replacement by hairy cells. Usually a low percentage of hairy cells persists in the peripheral blood. After splenectomy, most patients eventually show disease progression within months to years. Approximately half develop a leukemia phase. In the remaining half of patients, bone marrow failure is the rule. In both groups, the bone marrow is densely infiltrated by hairy cells. When patients with progressive disease received chlorambucil, erythrocyte and platelet count improved, but not the granulocytes. Intensive combination chemotherapy is toxic and rarely effective.

IFN-α at low doses (2 to 3×10^6 IU/m^2) three times weekly induces CR or partial remission in 90% of patients (334,335,392). Because less than 5% of patients become resistant to IFN-α, and 90% have normalization or near normalization of blood counts, most live normal lives without transfusions, bleeding, or infections. Data suggest that approximately 5% of patients develop neutralizing antibody to IFN-α (393). Toxicity is usually restricted to mild fatigue and malaise. Many patients with good partial remission or CR can discontinue IFN-α for periods of 1 to 3 years; they respond again when the disease progresses (394). Interestingly, the variant form of hairy cell leukemia is resistant to IFN-α (395).

Also effective in treating hairy cell leukemia is pentostatin, an adenosine deaminase inhibitor. Treatment with 4 mg/m^2 every 2 weeks produces CR and partial remission in over 90% of cases (396). In fact, pentostatin leads to more rapid and more complete responses than IFN-α. Toxicities include rash, diarrhea, nausea, and vomiting; these are generally mild at these doses. Data suggest that treatment with pentostatin causes a profound decrease in all lymphocyte subsets associated with a marked decrease in proliferative responses to mitogens and alloantigens. Six of 21 patients treated with pentostatin developed localized herpes infections (397).

Cladribine has excellent activity in hairy cell leukemia. Of the first 12 patients treated with 0.1 mg/kg/day by continuous intravenous infusion for 7 days, seven had prior splenectomies, and five had been treated with IFN-α (398); there were 11 complete and 1 partial responses lasting 7 to 46 months. No patient relapsed, and none was treated with maintenance therapy. Toxicity was limited to transient fever and neutropenia. The next 500 patients who were treated with cladribine had similar results to those seen in the first 12 patients.

Long-term outcome after treatment of hairy cell leukemia with pentostatin or cladribine was published. In one study (399), 25 of 28 patients treated with pentostatin achieved CR and three partial remission. Twenty-three patients were alive at a median follow-up duration of 118 months. The relapse-free survival rate was 80% at 5 years and 76% at 10 years. In another long-term follow-up of 49 patients treated with cladribine (400), 37 achieved CR and 12 partial remission, for an overall response rate of 100%. At a median follow-up of 55 months, the relapse-free survival was 80% and overall survival was 95%. Ten patients (20%) have relapsed, and eight were retreated with cladribine and achieved partial remission. There were four patients with a CD25 negative phenotype; all of them relapsed. There was no marked increase in the incidence of second malignancies or late opportunistic infections.

In patients who achieved CR by conventional criteria, minimal residual disease (MRD) detected in bone marrow core biopsies using immunohistochemical techniques was associated with an increased risk of relapse. Five of 39 patients (13%) treated with cladribine had MRD, as compared to seven of 27 patients (26%) treated with pentostatin. In total, six of 12 patients (50%) with MRD have relapsed, whereas three of 54 patients (6%) without MRD have relapsed (401).

In summary, cladribine appears to be the most effective therapy with the least toxicity. Nearly all patients achieve a durable or complete response with one course. It is the treatment of choice for hairy cell leukemia.

ADULT T-CELL LEUKEMIA/LYMPHOMA

ATL is a T-cell lymphoproliferative syndrome first described in Japan in 1977 (402) and later identified in the United States, the Caribbean, and other countries (403–406). ATL is characterized by pleomorphic neoplastic cells with membrane features of mature helper T lymphocytes. Presenting features include lymphadenopathy, hepatomegaly, splenomegaly, cutaneous infiltration, hypercalcemia (with or without lytic bone lesions) and interstitial pulmonary infiltrates. Development of ATL is associated with infection by HTLV-I (22,407,408).

Epidemiology and Cause

Epidemiologic studies of HTLV-I focus on serologic studies of normal populations that might elucidate the distribution of HTLV-I infection. Based on such studies, it is clear that ATL is correlated with HTLV-I infection. Additional data in the United States suggest that patients with the acquired immunodeficiency syndrome and hemophiliacs are often exposed to HTLV-I through blood or blood products. HTLV-I is also associated with a chronic, progressive, spastic, paraparetic, neurologic disease termed *HTLV-I–associated myelopathy and tropical spastic paraparesis* (409). The disease onset is usually insidious, although in some cases, sudden events of illness similar to transverse myelitis occur. Spasticity is usually profound and may overshadow weakness. Motor strength is compromised more in the lower than upper extremities. Bladder and bowel dysfunction are frequent, as are dysesthesia and numbness. Histopathologic changes include mononuclear cell infiltration, lymphocytic perivascular cuffing, capillary proliferation, demyelination, and reactive astrocytosis. The epidemiologic patterns appear to parallel ATL.

When HTLV-I was first isolated from patients in the United States, it was thought that infection was related to mycosis fungoides. Serum specimens from Japanese patients with ATL, however, were positive for HTLV-I (410,411), suggesting that the original U.S. cases were incorrectly diagnosed. This led to testing in the Caribbean, where ATL was endemic; these patients also showed serologic and virologic evidence of infection with HTLV-I (407). A low prevalence of HTLV-I infections has been found in normal individuals in populations where ATL is endemic. For instance, the highest prevalence of ATL in Japan is found in the southern island of Kyushi, where 10% to 15% of the population have the antibody to HTLV-I (410,411). On Japanese islands where ATL is rare, the rate is less than 1%. It is apparent from these and additional data from the Caribbean, the southeastern United States, South America, and Africa that ATL clusters in regions where HTLV-I is prevalent (410–412). It is not known how these regions are linked together, but one hypothesis is that HTLV-I was brought to the Americas from Africa by the slave trade and to the southern islands of Japan by trade with Japan and Africa (410).

Several studies suggest that host susceptibility or a shared environmental exposure, or both, contribute to HTLV-I infection. The prevalence of HTLV-I antibodies in close family members is three to four times higher than in the corresponding normal population (413). In some instances, cell cultures of antibody-positive, clinically normal patients yielded HTLV-I isolates (414).

Retroviruses are a common cause of leukemias and lymphomas in many species; however, evidence of viral leukemogenesis in humans was slow to emerge. In the 1970s, major developments in two animal models rekindled interest in pursuing the search in humans. Retroviruses that cause leukemias in primates (415) and cattle (416) were isolated.

Retroviruses contain a single-stranded RNA genome, usually consisting of three genes. The *gag* gene encodes a precursor peptide that is cleaved to form the major structural protein of the capsid as well as other core proteins. Protease is necessary for maturation of the *gag* polyprotein. The *pol* gene encodes the retroviral nucleic acid enzymatic gene and *env*, which encodes a single precursor peptide that is glycosylated and cleaved into a transmembrane protein and a spike protein (410). The target of a retrovirus infection depends on interaction on the cell surface with the virus envelope. After entry to the cell, retroviral RNA is reverse-transcribed into a DNA provirus by reverse transcriptase; it then integrates into host DNA.

The first isolates of HTLV-I occurred after mature T cells were grown with T-cell growth factor or IL-2 (22). These first isolates contained reverse transcriptase, viral antigens, and high-molecular-weight RNA characteristic of type-C retroviruses. The major core protein, p24, was purified and sequenced (417). Seroepidemiologic studies began using a radioimmunoprecipitate assay with purified p24 and assays using disrupted HTLV-I particles and a monoclonal antibody against another viral core protein, p19 (418). This led to the conclusion that the HTLV-I was endemic chiefly in Japan and the Caribbean. Worldwide isolates of HTLV-I proved similar to the first isolate (410). This is a family of retroviruses in which the most frequently isolated strain is a member of the HTLV-I subgroup. Another subgroup, HTLV-II, with 60% homology to HTLV-I, was initially isolated from a rare case of T-cell–derived hairy cell leukemia (348).

HTLV-I isolates have four common features. These include isolation from and infection of mature T cells, reverse transcriptases with similar biochemical features, and cross-reacting internal core proteins. HTLV-I can infect and immortalize *in vitro* T cells from normal human umbilical cord, blood, and bone marrow (23,419,420). The transfected cells express HTLV-I and resemble neoplastic T cells in that they develop lobulated nuclei, have unregulated growth, have a decreased requirement for IL-2, and express high levels of IL-2 receptors. Interestingly, the cells express foreign class 1 histocompatibility antigens similar to virus-infected tumor cells.

HTLV-I also exerts other biologic effects on T cells that may, in turn, modulate function of hematopoietic cells. HTLV-I–transformed T-cell lines produce several lymphokines, including colony-stimulating factors, IL-2, IL-6, and IFN-γ (421). Some of these factors may be responsible for some secondary features of ATL. For example, hypercalcemia may result from increased osteoclast-activating factors. In addition, the observation that normal IL-2–dependent clones of functional cytotoxic and helper T cells sometimes lose immune function after infection with HTLV-I may explain why HTLV-I–infected patients are immunocompromised and prone to opportunistic infections (422). Evidence also indicates that HTLV-I infection selectively kills self-tolerant cytotoxic T cells (423). It is apparent that HTLV-I may exert profound effects on a spectrum of cells as well as on the immediate target cell. Some seroepidemiologic data indicate that HTLV-I may be indirectly involved in the origin of rare B-cell leukemias in an endemic area of HTLV-I infection, such as Jamaica (411).

Although the *in vitro*–transformed cells provide a model for studying initiation of leukemogenesis by HTLV-I, a second event is likely required for progression to full disease (410). This is suggested by the following observations. First, development of ATL requires long latency periods, whereas HTLV-I transforms cells rapidly (in 4 to 6 weeks). Second, although *in vitro*–transformed cells usually retain a normal karyotype, ATL cells usually exhibit clonal chromosomal abnormalities. No consistent chromosomal abnormality, however, has been identified. Only a minor proportion of patients with HTLV-I infection develop ATL.

Immunology

The malignant cells from patients with ATL typically have the phenotype of mature helper T cells (424,425) and express the CD2, CD3, and CD4 antigens. They also express the CD25 antigen, which is the p55 subunit of the IL-2 receptor. Clonal rearrangements of the T-cell receptor–β chain are present (426–429). Leukemia cells have been reported to suppress B-cell Ig secretion by a complex mechanism involving induction of suppressor cells after activation of normal suppressor cell precursors (424,425).

Cytogenetics

Several cytogenic abnormalities have been reported in patients with ATL (430–437). The most common abnormalities include trisomy or partial trisomy 3q or 6q⁻, 14q, and inv(14). Others include loss of the X chromosome, t(9;21), 5p⁻, 2q⁺, 17q⁺, and trisomy 18. In some studies, survival correlates with karyotype abnormalities (430).

Clinical Features

ATL has various clinical presentations, including an aggressive acute type with leukemia, a lymphoma without lymphocytosis, a chronic type with a modest leukemic phase, and a smoldering type (437). The median age of patients with the aggressive acute type of ATL is approximately 40 years. They typically present with an elevated leukocyte count ranging from 5 to 100×10^9/L (394,403,405), with circulating malignant lymphocytes in most cases. Anemia and thrombocytopenia are uncommon. Onset of symptoms is typically acute, with rapidly developing cutaneous lesions, hypercalcemia, or both. Skin lesions are variable. Some patients have discreet tumor nodules, and others have confluent smaller nodules. Some patients present with plaques, papules, and nonspecific erythematous patches and erythroderma. Patients with hypercalcemia typically have weakness, lethargy, confusion, polyuria, and polydipsia. Radionuclide bone scans show diffusely increased uptake throughout the skeleton, most prominent in the joints and skull. These scans are referred to as *super scans* and are unusual in other patients with malignant lymphomas. Isolated lytic bone lesions may also occur; alkaline phosphatase is typically elevated.

Lymph node enlargement occurs in all patients, although the nodes are initially small in some. Many have generalized lymphadenopathy, and most have retroperitoneal adenopathy. Hilar adenopathy is common, but a mediastinal mass is rare. Bone marrow may be infiltrated with leukemia cells. Additional sites of disease include the lung, liver, skin, gastrointestinal tract, and central nervous system.

Opportunistic infections are common in patients with ATL, even though most have normal serum Ig levels. *P. carinii* infection is common, as is cryptococcal meningitis. Bacterial and fungal infections are also common. A variety of pulmonary problems develops, including infections and leukemic infiltrates.

Patients with the smoldering type of ATL have an indolent course, except for opportunistic infections (403,438). They typi-

cally have a long survival without therapy and without hypercalcemia. Skin lesions are characteristic and occur as erythema, papules, or nodules. The proportion of ATL cells in the blood is low (less than 5%), with minimal lymphadenopathy, hepatosplenomegaly, and bone marrow infiltration. One patient developed aggressive ATL after more than 5 years of illness and another after 13 years. Patients with smoldering ATL are more likely to have a normal karyotype.

Pathology

An important feature is the presence of pleomorphic lymphoid cells in the blood (403) (Fig. 26-15). Although not all cases present with blood involvement, a leukemia phase develops in most at some point. ATL cells have moderately condensed nuclear chromatin, inconspicuous nucleoli, and a markedly irregular nuclear contour that divides the nucleus into several lobes. These cells are characteristic of HTLV-I–associated disease and are readily distinguished from Sézary cells and cells of other mature and immature T-cell malignancies. In approximately 20% of the cases, nuclear irregularities are less extreme; these cells may be difficult to distinguish from Sézary cells.

Pathologic features in lymph nodes and other tissues are more varied. ATL is associated with lymphomas of several histologic subtypes, including diffuse, poorly differentiated small cell; large, mixed small cell; and large cell immunoblastic (406). No apparent correlation exists between clinical course and the histiologic cell type.

Cutaneous involvement occurs in approximately two-thirds of patients with ATL. Focal epidermal infiltration with ATL cells or Pautrier microabscesses is seen in most patients with cutaneous involvement. These abscesses were thought to be pathognomonic of CTCL, and the retrovirus-associated disease was initially reported as CTCL. The acute course and absence of a chronic premycotic phase in most patients with ATL distinguishes it from typical CTCL. Furthermore, serologic studies in cases of CTCL show no association with HTLV-I infection. Rare patients with CTCL are HTLV-I–positive, but this is unusual.

Differential Diagnosis

Smoldering ATL could be confused with CTCL, as the skin lesions and clinical presentation may be similar. The aggressive form of ATL represents a rather unique constellation of clinical and pathologic findings that should be readily distinguished from other leukemias and lymphomas.

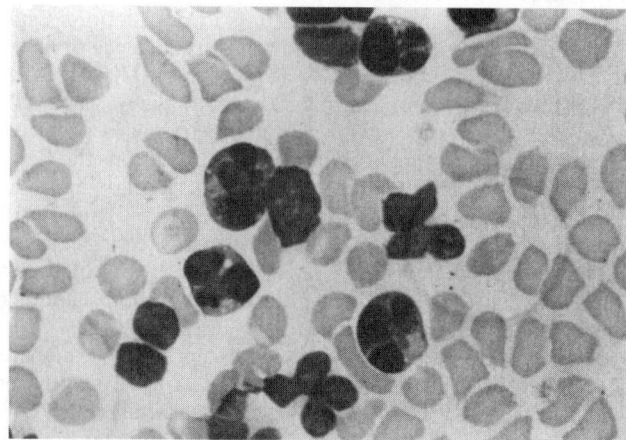

Figure 26-15. Peripheral blood of patient with adult T-cell leukemia (Wright-Giemsa stain; ×400). (See Color Fig. 26-15.)

Therapy

It is standard to treat patients with ATL with combination chemotherapy using a regimen that includes doxorubicin, such as CHOP. Complete and partial responses are attained in most patients. However, most patients experience relapse within 6 to 12 months, and cures are not reported. Encouraging responses have been observed in patients who received passive immunotherapy or radioimmunotherapy using monoclonal antibodies specific for antigens expressed by the neoplastic T cells, such as CD25 (439,440). Other biologic agents, such as IFNs, have had modest effects (441,442). Therapy with the nucleoside pentostatin may benefit some patients with this disease (443). The combination of zidovudine and IFN-α has activity against ATL. Nineteen patients were treated with oral zidovudine and IFN-α (5 to 10 million units subcutaneously each day) (444). Seven of these patients had either relapsed after multiagent chemotherapy or failed to respond to that treatment. Major responses were achieved in 11 (58%) patients, including CR in 5 (26%) patients. Six patients have survived more than 12 months. It is unknown whether the combination of zidovudine, IFN-α, and chemotherapy will be more effective.

CUTANEOUS T-CELL LYMPHOMA

CTCL consists of mycosis fungoides and the Sézary syndrome. These disorders are malignant proliferations of T lymphocytes of the helper phenotype, in which the initial clinical presentation is in the epidermis.

Epidemiology and Cause

CTCL is an uncommon malignancy in the United States, with approximately 1500 new cases reported per year (445). The average annual adjusted mortality rate is approximately 400 to 500 deaths per year (446). CTCL occurs most commonly in males, with a 2:1 ratio; it is less frequent in African Americans. The median age at diagnosis is 55 years. Initial skin lesions are clinically and histologically nonspecific, and it may take many years before the diagnosis is confirmed. Median survival after histologic diagnosis is approximately 10 years.

Although the cause is unknown, recent observations suggest that environmental, infectious, and genetic influences may be important (447). Exposure to toxic chemicals and physical agents and employment in manufacturing, particularly textiles, petrochemicals, and machinery, was reported to be associated with an increased incidence of CTCL, but this remains controversial (445–448). As indicated, HTLV-I was originally isolated in the United States from patients thought to have CTCL (22). Seroepidemiologic studies, however, have suggested that HTLV-I is associated with ATL; and serologic evidence of infection is found in less than 1% of patients with CTCL in the United States (21). In a series of CD25-negative CTCL patients from Italy, a new retrovirus called *HTLV-V* was isolated (449). The significance of this finding is not clear, and it has not been confirmed. Evidence for genetic factors in the cause of CTCL is less impressive. Reports have been made of an increased incidence of lymphoma or leukemia in first-degree relatives of patients with CTCL (445). Data conflict regarding whether there is an increased incidence of CTCL among family members (449).

Immunology

In most cases, the cells express a phenotype associated with mature helper–inducer T lymphocytes that includes CD3, CD5,

TABLE 26-7. Survival by Skin Stage of Cutaneous T-Cell Lymphoma Patients

Skin Stage	Mean Survival	5-yr Survival (%)
Limited plaque (T1)	>9	90
Generalized plaque (T2)	>7	70
Cutaneous tumor (T3)	2.5	35
Generalized erythroderma (T4)	3.5	40

Winkler CF, Bunn PA. Cutaneous T-cell lymphoma: a review. *Crit Rev Oncol Hematol* 1983;1:49.

and CD4 (450–452). These cells can function as helper T lymphocytes in *in vitro* assays (453). The CD7 antigen, which is present on greater than 85% of normal circulating T lymphocytes, is found on mycosis fungoides cells in the skin, but not with circulating Sézary cells (454). The cells are generally negative for markers of T-cell activation, which include Ia antigens and CD25 (IL-2 receptor). Like most malignant T cells, the CTCL cells stain for acid phosphatase, α-naphthyl acetate esterase, and β-glucoronidase. They are generally negative for peroxidase, alkaline phosphatase, and esterase. PAS-positive granules are present in some cases.

Cytogenetics

A wide range of chromosomal abnormalities are described in CTCL (455). Chromosomes 1 and 6 are frequently involved in structural abnormalities, whereas chromosomes 7, 11, 21, and 22 are frequently involved in numeric abnormalities. Rearrangement of chromosome 10 was common in one study (456). Chromosomal abnormalities often correlate with extent of disease and survival.

Clinical Features

Most cases of CTCL progress through distinct stages of skin involvement (Table 26-7). These stages begin with a premycotic, erythematous, or eczematoid stage, progress to an infiltrative plaque stage, and eventuate in the tumor stage (445). Progression is variable but commonly occurs over several years (457).

The premycotic or erythematous stage of CTCL is nonspecific; it is characterized by localized or widespread areas of erythema or dry eczema (445). Lesions may be associated with pruritus. Histologic features are also nonspecific, and a definitive diagnosis is often not possible. This stage may last for months to years before progression. The plaque stage is distinguished by palpable, pruritic, indurated lesions (Fig. 26-16). The tumor stage (Fig. 26-17) is characterized by large lesions; these may develop in previously normal skin or in premycotic lesions or plaques. The lesions occur most often on the face and in body folds, often in a "bathing trunk" distribution. Tumors are often generalized, and ulceration is common. Pruritus is absent.

The erythrodermic form of CTCL is manifested by generalized erythroderma and may precede the appearance of other CTCL lesions by many years. It may also be preceded by premycotic lesions or may appear simultaneously with plaques or tumors. Two common types of erythroderma include exfoliative erythroderma, predominated by intense scaling, and *l'homme rouge* or red man syndrome, in which redness rather than scaling predominates. Transition between forms is common. Lymphadenopathy and alopecia are frequent manifestations.

In 1938, Sézary and Bouvrain (458) described a syndrome of pruritus, generalized exfoliative erythroderma, and abnormal

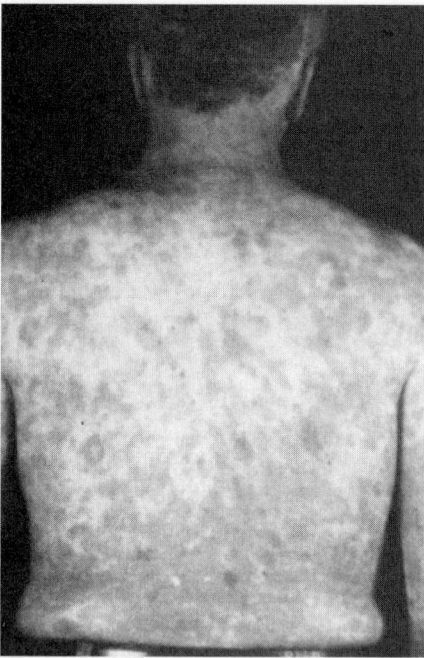

Figure 26-16. Multiple discrete and confluent plaques of cutaneous T-cell lymphoma. (See Color Fig. 26-16.)

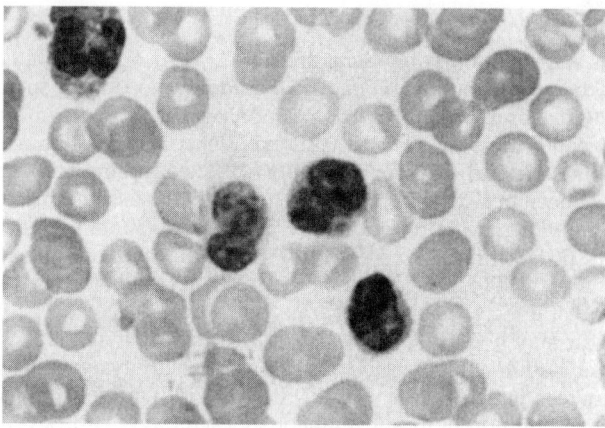

Figure 26-18. Peripheral blood of patient with cutaneous T-cell lymphoma, showing Sézary cells (Wright-Giemsa stain; ×400). (See Color Fig. 26-18.)

hyperconvoluted lymphoid cells in the blood; this is referred to as *Sézary's syndrome.* Sézary's syndrome has biologic features similar to the other forms of mycosis fungoides. Most patients with generalized erythroderma have varying numbers of circulating Sézary cells (Fig. 26-18). One-fourth of those with plaque or tumor stage also have circulating Sézary cells.

Autopsy studies of patients with advanced CTCL show extensive invasion of organs and tissues by malignant T cells. Pulmonary, cardiac, renal, and gastrointestinal involvement are infrequent clinically, but are common autopsy findings (457,459–461). Mediastinal and hilar adenopathy, pleural effusion, parenchymal nodules, and patchy infiltrates also occur. Bony abnormalities are rare, despite bone marrow involvement in 30% to 40% of autopsy cases (457,459). Bony lesions typically occur in long bones, are osteolytic, and may cause pathologic fractures (462,463). CTCL of the cornea, sclera, and lacrimal glands has been reported (464–466). Central and peripheral nervous system involvement by CTCL is documented in 10% of autopsy cases (457,460). Leptomeningitis is common, but infiltrates have been

reported in all areas of the neuroaxis (467,468). Clinical manifestations reflect sites of involvement. Hematologic abnormalities in CTCL are often nonspecific, except for circulating Sézary cells. Bone marrow eosinophilia, monocytosis, and plasmacytosis have been reported, as have elevations of serum Ig, usually IgA and IgE (445).

Fifty percent of deaths of patients with CTCL result from infections. These are usually *Staphylococcus* and *Pseudomonas* related and develop from cutaneous lesions (457,459,469). Septicemia and bacterial pneumonia are common. Herpes infections occur in up to 10% of patients with advanced CTCL (470,471). Progressive CTCL with widespread visceral involvement is the next most common cause of death (457).

Pathology

The initial clinical manifestations of CTCL are nearly always cutaneous, and the diagnosis is usually established by skin biopsy. Early lesions may show polymorphic infiltrations compatible with several benign diseases as well as CTCL. The malignant infiltrate in early CTCL is characteristically epidermotrophic, with exocytosis of single or clusters of convoluted CTCL cells. Epidermal clusters of these cells are termed *Pautrier microabscesses* (Fig. 26-19). The epidermis may also show parakeratosis and acanthosis. A bandlike infiltrate in the upper dermis is composed of lymphocytes, neutrophils, eosinophils, plasma cells, blasts, and histiocytes in early lesions. The atypical, convoluted lymphocytes are present in clusters. In more advanced stages, the infiltrate is less polymorphic, with a predominance of atypical cells extending deeper into the dermis; epidermotrophism may be lost.

Lymph nodes that drain affected areas show partial or complete effacement of normal architecture with a monomorphic infiltrate of CTCL cells. In most lymph nodes, the architecture is not effaced, and dermatopathic changes with varying numbers of atypical lymphocytes in the T-cell paracortical areas of the node are present. The cytologic appearance of the malignant cells in visceral organs is similar to that in the skin (459,460). Lymph node involvement is associated with a poor prognosis (472).

Staging

Cutaneous lesions are defined by using the T staging system. *T1* (limited plaque stage) consists of erythematous patches and plaques covering less than 10% of the body. Plaques covering 10% or more of the skin surface are designated *T2.* Cutaneous

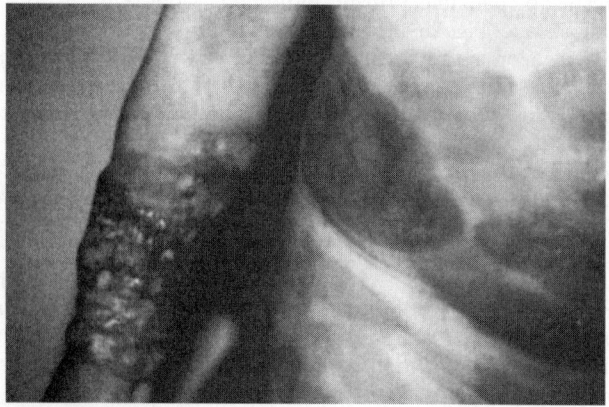

Figure 26-17. Multiple plaques of cutaneous T-cell lymphoma with tumor formation. (See Color Fig. 26-17.)

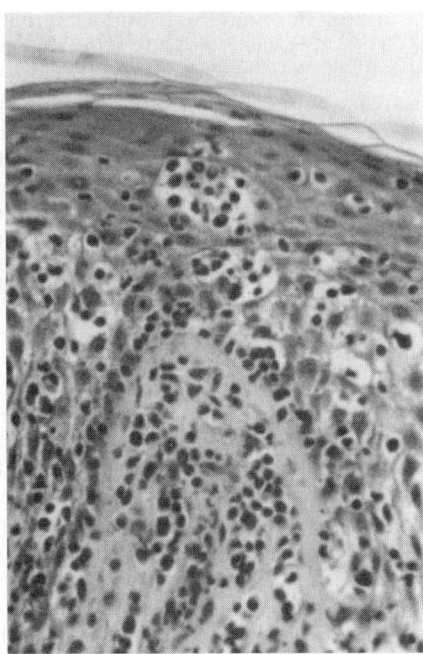

Figure 26-19. Pautrier microabscess (hematoxylin and eosin stain; ×100). (See Color Fig. 26-19.)

tumors are designated *T3* and generalized erythroderma, *T4*. Patients with limited plaque disease have the most favorable prognosis, those with generalized plaques have an intermediate prognosis, and those with tumors or erythroderma have the worst prognosis (472).

As indicated, lymphadenopathy portends a poorer prognosis than disease limited to the skin (457,472–477). Lymphadenopathy is present in approximately half of patients and increases with progressive cutaneous involvement (476,478). Lymphangiograms were used to assess pretreatment involvement of intraabdominal lymph nodes. Computed axial tomographic scans are less invasive, however, and reveal similar information (479,480).

Circulating Sézary cells also increase with advancing disease, which occurs in up to 90% of those with generalized erythroderma. Malignant cells can also be detected using sensitive techniques such as cytogenetics or T-cell receptor gene rearrangement studies. Patients with blood involvement have a higher likelihood of lymphadenopathy, visceral involvement, and shorter survival (481,482). Bone marrow infiltration is infrequently detected by biopsy despite circulating malignant cells; it is identified at autopsy in 30% to 40% of cases (463).

Patients with CTCL with visceral involvement that includes liver, spleen, pleura, and lung have the poorest prognosis; median survival is less than 1 year (457,472,483). Visceral involvement does not appear until late.

Differential Diagnosis

The early diagnosis of CTCL is difficult and can be confused with several benign dermatologic diseases. Often, a definitive diagnosis is delayed for years.

Smoldering ATL has a number of clinical features similar to CTCL, but it can usually be distinguished by the presence of antibodies to HTLV-I and by its regional occurrence. *Pagetoid reticulosis* is a rare skin disorder consisting of solitary or localized cutaneous plaques. The involved areas show a prominent atypical mononuclear cell infiltrate with a hyperplastic epidermis (484). Although this disease is usually indolent and localized, some patients present with a disseminated form referred to as the *Ketron-Goodman variant* (485). Interestingly, recent studies have demonstrated that this is a disease of an activated T lymphocyte that only occasionally expresses the helper T cell–CD4 antigen (486). As is the case in CTCL, gene rearrangement for the β–T-cell receptor is present.

Therapy

Four therapeutic modalities produce remissions in most patients with CTCL: topical nitrogen mustard, photochemotherapy with psoralen and ultraviolet A light (PUVA), radiation therapy (particularly total body electron beam therapy), and systemic chemotherapy. Each induces remission, but cure is uncommon and possible only in early disease.

Topical nitrogen mustard is used predominantly in patients with early cutaneous stages of disease. In more advanced stages, this approach is used to supplement other therapies. The major advantage of topical therapy is that it is relatively nontoxic. Disadvantages include the inconvenience of daily application to large skin surfaces, the allergic reactions in up to half of cases (487), the potential for development of skin cancer (488), and the inability to cure the disease. Nitrogen mustard (10 mg diluted in 60 mL of tap water or 60 g of a water-misable cream or in an anhydrous ointment, which may have less allergic sensitization) is administered daily using a cotton swab or small paint brush. Therapy is continued for up to 12 months in responders. Frequency is then reduced to every other day for an additional 1 to 2 years. Therapy is discontinued after 3 years or when cutaneous lesions disappear completely.

Psoralen is a phototoxic furocoumarin activated by UV-A light. In its active form, it binds covalently and irreversibly to DNA. UV-A light penetrates only the upper part of the dermis. Therefore, psoralen activated by UV-A light affects cells primarily in the epidermis and papillary dermis. A 60% CR rate has been reported with psoralen; patients with generalized erythroderma and tumors have lower response rates than those with plaques (489–491). Psoralen is usually given at a dose of 0.6 mg/kg orally 2 hours before the UV-A light therapy. Treatments are initially given three times weekly. Maintenance therapy may be given every 2 to 4 weeks indefinitely. Adverse effects of PUVA therapy include mild nausea, pruritus, and sunburnlike changes with atrophy and dry skin. PUVA is not cross-resistant with other treatment modalities. Disadvantages are the inability to cure CTCL and expense. Long-term side effects are not yet reported.

Electron beam therapy penetrates only into the upper dermis, and there are minimal systemic effects and an 80% CR rate (492). Twenty percent of patients remain relapse-free at 3 years. Typically, treatment is 4 Gy/week to a total dose of 36 Gy in 8 to 9 weeks. The advantage of electron beam therapy is a high frequency of durable, complete responses without systemic toxicity. Disadvantages are alopecia, atrophy, edema, dermatitis, and high cost (492,493).

Leukapheresis was used to treat patients with CTCL (494,495). Photophoresis or extracorporeal photochemotherapy (ECP) was introduced by Edelson and coworkers in 1985. After the patient ingests psoralen, a pheresed, leukocyte-enriched blood fraction is exposed to UV-A light in an extracorporeal system to photoactivate the psoralen (496). This approach decreased lymphocyte viability by 90%. Edelson et al. were the first to report responses in 27 of 37 patients (64%), with resistant CTCL treated with ECP (496). Subsequent analysis of five large series (496–500) of ECP-treated patients with CTCL (n = 157) demonstrated an objective response (greater than 25% improvement of skin lesions) in 67 of 111 stage-T4 patients (60%), with approximately 20% achieving a CR. A long-term follow-up study of the original 29 patients with erythrodermic CTCL demonstrated a median survival of 60 months (496). As ECP is well tolerated with few complications or adverse effects (496–500), many centers in Europe and the United States have adopted ECP as the first-line treatment for erythrodermic-stage CTCL patients (501). Also, ECP given concurrently with, or immediately after, total-skin electron beam radiation (32–40 Gy) might improve progression-free survival for patients with erythrodermic-stage CTCL compared with total-skin electron beam radiation alone (502).

The largest experience with single-agent chemotherapy is with alkylating agents, including nitrogen mustard, 0.4 mg/kg intravenously every 4 to 6 weeks, cyclophosphamide, and chlorambucil. Response rates of 60%, with 15% CRs, have been reported (503–506). Similar results occur with methotrexate, 2.5 to 10.0 mg/day by mouth; bleomycin, 7.5 to 15.0 mg intramuscularly twice weekly; and doxorubicin (507–513). Single-agent therapy does not cure CTCL. Combination therapy with these and other drugs produces objective responses in more than 80% of patients and complete responses in approximately one-fourth of cases (514–516). Duration of remission varies, with a median of approximately 1 year; no long-term, disease-free survival has been reported.

Randomized trials with whole-body electron beam therapy as a single modality compared with electron beam therapy followed by topical nitrogen mustard suggest a benefit of combined therapy (517). Studies of electron beam therapy combined with chemotherapy suggest an advantage over either alone (518), but cutaneous and hematologic toxicity is increased. In one study (518), combined modality therapy improved disease-free survival in some patients with early-stage disease; those with advanced disease failed to benefit. A report of patients randomized to early intensive therapy with cyclophosphamide, doxorubicin, vincristine, and etoposide combined with either topical nitrogen mustard or 30 Gy of electron beam radiation therapy, versus topical or radiation therapy only, showed no differences (519).

The purine nucleoside analogs have shown activity in CTCL. Pentostatin used in pretreated patients with mycosis fungoides and Sézary's syndrome demonstrated an overall response rate of 41% (range, 15% to 67%), with less than 7% complete responses and short response durations (520–525). Two studies using cladribine to treat 29 patients with mycosis fungoides and Sézary's syndrome demonstrated a response in nine (31%), with 3- to 4-month median duration of response (526,527). Fludarabine alone has shown similar overall responses (528), but in combination with IFNs has demonstrated a higher response rate (51%) and a longer median relapse-free interval of 5.8 months (529).

IFN-α has been extensively studied in CTCL. One study reported a 50% response with high-dose IFN-α (530). In another study, the overall response rate was 52%, with a 17% CR among 207 patients (531). The optimal dose of IFN-α is 3 mouse units (MU) three times a week, based on randomized studies in B-cell indolent lymphoma showing no benefit to higher-dose IFN with respect to response rate or duration (532). Three studies reported a median duration of response to IFN-α: 6 months (533), 8 months (534), and 14 months (535).

The retinoids have been effective in CTCL. They have antiproliferative activity, may induce cellular maturation, and probably modulate immune response. Isotretinoin (13 cis-retinoic acid) and etretinate are the most commonly used oral preparations. Three clinical trials have demonstrated overall objective clinical responses in 66 of 133 patients (58%) treated either with isotretinoin or etretinate and a complete response in 19% (536–538). However, median duration of response ranged from 3 to over 8 months. Another class of retinoids that selectively activates retinoid X receptors has shown promising activity in the treatment of CTCL. Targretin (bexarotene) was evaluated in 152 pretreated patients with advanced and early-stage CTCL in two multicenter clinical studies conducted in North America, Europe, and Australia. At the initial dose of 300 mg/m²/day, 1 (1.6%) and 19 (30%) of 62 patients had a complete and partial responses, respectively. Clinical studies with this new class of retinoids are still going on (539). Therapy with monoclonal antibodies was also studied. Unlabeled monoclonal antibodies had only a minimal transient effect (309–312). In one study (311), I¹³¹-labeled monoclonal antibody produced more prolonged and consistent responses.

Fusion toxin is a novel therapy in CTCL. Conjugation (fusion) of a plant or bacterial toxin gene to a specific receptor ligand can guide the toxin gene to the target cell, where it can be internalized via receptor-mediated endocytosis and translocated into a toxic moiety in the cytosol (540). The IL-2 receptor is present in approximately 60% of tissue in CTCL (541), but not on normal T cells. Two fusion toxins, $DAB_{486}IL$-2 and $DAB_{389}IL$-2, have been used. They consist of the diphtheria toxin conjugated to the human IL-2. In one study (542), 3 of 14 patients with CTCL treated with $DAB_{486}IL$-2 demonstrated an objective response. In another study (543), $DAB_{389}IL$-2–induced clinical responses in 13 of 35 CTCL patients. Denileukin diftitox, which is the $DAB_{389}IL$-2 fusion toxin, has been approved for the treatment of CTCL by the U.S. Food and Drug Administration.

Autologous bone marrow transplantation has been attempted in a small number of patients with CTCL (544,545). Although 5 of 6 patients achieved CR, 3 patients relapsed in 3 months and 2 were alive with no disease at 12 months. Allogeneic, hematopoietic stem cell transplantation for advanced mycosis fungoides was reported to induce a graft-versus-tumor effect (546).

LARGE GRANULAR LYMPHOCYTIC LEUKEMIA

Large granular lymphocytes (LGLs) are a heterogeneous group of thymus-independent cells that are largely responsible for most NK-cell activity and have an important role in antibody-dependent, cell-mediated cytotoxicity. They constitute 10% to 15% of normal peripheral blood mononuclear cells. LGL can be classified into two major lineages: CD3+ LGL, representing in vivo activated cytotoxic T cells, and NK LGL, which lacks CD3 expression (547,548).

LGL leukemia typically follows a chronic course characterized by lymphocytosis with tissue invasion (bone marrow, liver, and spleen), neutropenia, and recurrent infections (241,242,549,550). LGL leukemia could be classified into T-LGL leukemia and NK-LGL leukemia, depending on the cell lineage of the leukemic cells (551).

Immunology

Cells from patients with LGL leukemia usually contain acid phosphatase and β-glucoronidase. T-LGL cells express the pan–T-cell antigens CD2, CD3, and CD5, and the suppressor T-cell–associated antigen CD8. They usually express NK-cell–associated antigens such as CD16 (Fc receptor for IgG), CD56, and CD57. Clonal rearrangement of the β–T-cell receptor has been reported (427,429). NK-LGL cells express only NK-cell–associated antigens, such as CD16, CD56, and CD57, without

T-cell antigens and without rearrangement of the T-cell receptor gene.

The functions of cells from patients with LGL leukemia were studied. In most cases, there is a markedly decreased response to T-cell mitogens and to allogeneic lymphocytes in mixed lymphocyte culture (241). Cells from most patients suppress normal T-cell mitogen responses and Ig production by pokeweed mitogen–stimulated normal B lymphocytes. Most cases studied were positive for antibody-dependent cellular cytotoxicity; only a small proportion showed NK-cell activity. NK-cell activity was induced in one study (552) by incubating leukemia cells overnight at 37°C or in the presence of IFN-β. Because of the granulocytopenia, some subjects were studied for the ability of their leukemia cells to suppress myeloid progenitor cells; no activity was detected. Cells from three patients with this disease and severe RBC aplasia and from one patient with anemia suppressed erythroid progenitor cells (553–555).

Cytogenetics

Few reports have been made of cytogenic analyses in patients with this disorder. Chromosomal abnormalities are often not detected (556); when detected, there are no consistent abnormalities. Trisomies 8 and 14, 6q⁻, and inv(14) have been reported (557).

Pathology

The typical LGL cell is a large lymphocyte with a high cytoplasmic/nuclear ratio and coarse, azurophilic granules (241) (Fig. 26-12). The cells are positive for acid phosphatase and β-glucoronidase and negative for esterase and terminal deoxynucleotidyl transferase. Leukemia cells are found in the peripheral blood and focally infiltrating the bone marrow. The spleen typically shows infiltration of the red pulp; the liver demonstrates sinusoidal infiltration with LGL cells.

Differential Diagnosis

This disease is commonly confused with CLL. In a review of the literature, many cases referred to as T-cell CLL were LGL leukemia (241). This is an important distinction, because the approach to therapy and disease course differ considerably. LGL leukemia is distinguished by its lack of lymph node involvement, limited bone marrow involvement, granulocytopenia disproportionate to lymphocytosis and extent of bone marrow involvement, and characteristic morphologic and immunologic features of the malignant cells.

Hairy cell leukemia has rarely been misdiagnosed as LGL. Both diseases present with splenomegaly and granulocytopenia, but the distinct morphologic and immunologic characteristics permit differential diagnosis.

T–Large Granular Lymphocytic Leukemia

T-LGL leukemia represents 85% of the LGL leukemias. The disease affects principally elderly people with a median age of 60 years (range, 4 to 88 years) without a sex predilection. The typical clinical presentation is that of recurrent bacterial infections, usually secondary to granulocytopenia. Fatigue from anemia is also common. Bleeding is rare; platelet levels are usually normal. Fatigue and "B" symptoms (fever, night sweats, weight loss) are observed in 20% to 30% of cases. One-half of cases have mild to moderate splenomegaly, approximately 20% have hepatomegaly, and less than 10% have lymphadenopathy. A small proportion have hypogammaglobulinemia, and approximately

one-third have hypergammaglobulinemia. Skin infiltration is rare. A particular feature of this lymphoid malignancy is association with other autoimmune diseases (neutropenia, thrombocytopenia, hemolytic anemia, and RA) in 40% of cases (558–560). RA is the most common associated disease, occurring in 25% of patients (559,561–563). It has been suggested that patients with RA and severe granulocytopenia be evaluated for circulating LGLs.

In this disease, the malignant cells infiltrate the bone marrow, blood, spleen, and liver. In half of cases, lymphocyte counts are higher than 10×10^9/L. Bone marrow lymphocytosis ranges from 30% to 75%, and some patients have reduced myelopoiesis. Approximately half of cases have severe granulocytopenia with levels less than 0.5×10^9/L. The mechanism underlying the neutropenia is not clear but could reflect decreased production, increased destruction, or both. There are data suggesting that normal LGLs inhibit myeloid progenitor cells in vitro (564,565). As indicated, this is uncommon in patients with LGL leukemia. Antineutrophil antibodies are rare but were reported in some cases (557).

At least half of patients with this disorder have anemia with hemoglobin levels less than 12 g/dL. The underlying mechanism is unclear. Several mechanisms might operate: (a) bone marrow crowding due to lymphocyte infiltration; (b) direct suppression of erythropoiesis by LGL leukemia, as suggested by in vitro inhibition of erythroid progenitor cells (553–555); (c) reduced levels of erythropoietin; (d) autoantibodies that lyse RBCs by means of complement-dependent or complement-independent mechanisms (557); or (e) erythrophagocytosis (554). The Coombs' test is usually negative, suggesting that anemia is not antibody-mediated. Although the bone marrow of patients with LGL leukemia is usually infiltrated by large numbers of LGLs, this is probably insufficient to explain severe anemia. Several investigators suggested that LGLs may suppress erythroid progenitors.

LGL is typically a chronic disease. Patients often die from bacterial infections secondary to granulocytopenia. Some patients have been reported to develop high-grade lymphomas of LGLs (566,567). Extensive liver and spleen involvement can occur, as can extensive lymphadenopathy. The course of the disease was rapidly progressive, and all patients were treated with high-dose chemotherapy. Similar to LGL leukemia, the lymphocytes from these patients were morphologically and immunologically characterized as LGLs. Whether this disorder is a variant or a phase of LGL leukemia remains to be determined. It may represent a less mature cell of the same lineage.

Most patients do not require therapy, except for transfusions for anemia and antibiotics for infections. Controversial data exist on the benefit of hematopoietic growth factors such as granulocyte-macrophage colony-stimulating factor and granulocyte colony-stimulating factor, which have been tried in few cases; usually the response is partial and transient (568). Some patients respond to prednisone alone with increase of neutrophil count but persistence of LGL clone. Cyclosporin A has occasionally led to good responses, but its toxicity remains a problem for a long treatment (569). Methotrexate, given orally at low dose, was reported to induce CR in 50% of LGL cases (570). In 60% of the responders, a molecular remission was observed. The treatment had to be maintained, as relapse occurred after withdrawal. Recombinant IFN-α was shown to have no benefit in patients with LGL leukemia.

Chemotherapy with single alkylating agents, such as chlorambucil or cyclophosphamide, or combination chemotherapy with alkylating agents, vincristine, and prednisone is used to treat progressive disease. Although chemotherapy is usually not effective and most patients die within 1 year, some cases benefit (241,242,571,572). Some patients were treated by splenectomy or by spleen irradiation without benefit. Minimal data exist on the efficacy of pentostatin, cladribine, and fludarabine.

Because this disease appears to represent a spectrum from almost benign to a more aggressive malignancy, it is not possible to recommend a specific therapeutic approach. Clearly, many patients do not require chemotherapy and can be followed for many years. The first large estimation published in the literature reported 26 deaths among 151 patients after a mean follow-up of 23 months (573). A recent study of 68 patients reported a median survival greater than 10 years (561).

Natural Killer–Large Granular Lymphocytic Leukemia

The clinical presentation of NK-LGL leukemia is more aggressive than in T-LGL leukemia. Patients are younger, with a median age of 39 years. Initial presentation includes "B" symptoms, hepatosplenomegaly, and bone marrow infiltration with fibrosis. RA is never observed. LGL infiltration of the peritoneal and cerebrospinal fluid has been reported. Neutropenia is usually moderate, and anemia and thrombocytopenia are more frequent than in T-LGL cases. EBV infection has been implicated in NK-LGL leukemia in Japan in more than 50% of cases (574).

Most patients have a severe and refractory evolution. Combination chemotherapy is ineffective, and long-term remission has been rarely obtained. Multiorgan failure associated with coagulopathy is the main cause of death. Allogeneic bone marrow transplantation may be considered for young patients having a sibling donor.

REFERENCES

1. Velpeau A. Sur la resorption du pusaet sur l'alteration du sang dans les maladies clinique de persection nenemant: premier observation. *Rev Med* 1827;2:216.
2. Donne A. Del' origine des glubules du sang, de leur mode de formation, de leur fin. *Compt Red Acad De Sci* 1842;14:366.
3. Bennett JH. *Leucocythaemia or white cell blood.* Edinburgh: Sutherland and Knox, 1852.
4. Virchow R. Weisses blut und milztumoren. II. *Med Z* 1847;16:9.
5. Virchow R. Zur pathologischen physiologie des bluts: die bedeutung der nilz- und lymphdrusen-krankheiten fur die blutmischung (leukaemie). *Virchows Arch* 1853;5:43.
6. Neumann E. Ein fall von leukamie mit erkrankung des knochenmarkes. *Arch Heilk* 1870;11:1.
7. Ehrlich P. *Parbenanalytische untersuchungen zur histologie und klinik des blutes.* Berlin: Hirschwald, 1891.
8. Osler W. *Practice of medicine.* New York: Appleton, 1906.
9. Ordway T. Remission in leukemia-produced radium in cases completely resistant to x-ray and benzol treatment. *Boston Med Surg J* 1917;176:490.
10. Pusey WA. Report of cases treated with roentgen rays. *JAMA* 1902;38:911.
11. Rénon D, Dreyfus L. Radium therapie de la leucemia myeloide. *Arch Electric Med* 1933;23:366.
12. Karnofsky DA. Chemotherapy of neoplastic disease. I. Methods of approach. *N Engl J Med* 1948;239:226.
13. Lawrence JH, Dobson RL, Low-Beer BVA, et al. Chronic myelocytic leukemia: study of 129 cases in which treatment was with radioactive phosphorus. *JAMA* 1948;136:672.
14. Dameshek W. Chronic lymphocytic leukemia: an accumulative disease of immunologically incompetent lymphocytes. *Blood* 1967;29:566.
15. Jennings CD, Foon KA. Recent advances in flow cytometry: application to the diagnosis of hematologic malignancy. *Blood* 1997;90(8):2863.
16. Cheson BD, Bennett JM, Rai KR, et al. Guidelines for clinical protocols for chronic lymphocytic leukemia: recommendations of the National Cancer Institute–Sponsored Working Group. *Am J Hematol* 1988;29:152.
17. International Workshop on Chronic Lymphocytic Leukemia. Chronic lymphocytic leukemia: recommendations for diagnosis, staging and response criteria. *Ann Intern Med* 1989;110:236.
18. Brok-Simoni F, Rechavi G, Katzir N, et al. Chronic lymphocytic leukemia in twin sisters: monozygous but not identical. *Lancet* 1987;1:329.
19. Conley CL, Misiti J, Laster AJ. Genetic factors predisposing to chronic lymphocytic leukemia and to autoimmune disease. *Medicine* 1980;5:323.
20. Bizzozero OJ Jr, Johnson KG, Ciocco A, et al. Radiation-related leukemia in Hiroshima and Nagasaki 1946 to 1964. II. Observations on type-specific leukemia survivorship, and clinical behavior. *Ann Intern Med* 1967;66:522.
21. Gallo RC, Kalyanaraman VS, Sarngadharan MG, et al. Association of the human type C retrovirus with a subset of adult T-cell cancers. *Cancer Res* 1983;43:3892.
22. Poiesz BJ, Ruscetti FW, Gazdar AF, et al. Detection and isolation of type-C retrovirus particles from fresh and cultured lymphocytes of a patient with cutaneous T-cell lymphoma. *Proc Natl Acad Sci U S A* 1980;77:7415.
23. Popovic M, Sarin PS, Robert-Guroff M, et al. Isolation and transmission of human retrovirus (human T-cell leukemia virus). *Science* 1983;219:856.
24. Kinoshita K, Amagasaki P, Ikedas S, et al. Preleukemic state of adult T-cell leukemia: abnormal T-lymphocytosis induced by human T-cell leukemia-lymphoma virus. *Blood* 1985;66:120.
25. Rickinson AB, Finerty S, Epstein MA. Interaction of Epstein-Barr virus with leukaemic B cells in vitro. I. Abortive infection and rare cell line establishment from chronic lymphocytic leukaemic cells. *Clin Exp Immunol* 1982;50:347.
26. Ghose T, Lee CL, Faulkner G, et al. Progression of a human B cell chronic lymphocytic leukemia line in nude mide. *Am J Hematol* 1988;28:146.
27. Aisenberg AC, Bloch KJ. Immunoglobulins on the surface of neoplastic lymphocytes. *N Engl J Med* 1976;287:272.
28. Preud'Homme J, Seligmann M. Surface bound immunoglobulins as a cell marker in human lymphoproliferative disease. *Blood* 1972;40:777.
29. Godal T, Funderud S. Human B-cell neoplasms in relation to normal B-cell differentiation maturation processes. *Adv Cancer Res* 1982;36:211.
30. Hamblin TJ, Abdul-Ahad AK, Gordon J, et al. Preliminary experience in treating lymphocytic leukaemia with antibody to immunoglobulin idiotypes on the cell surfaces. *Br J Cancer* 1980;42:495.
31. Fialkow RJ, Najfeld V, Reddy A, et al. Chronic lymphocytic leukemia: clonal origin in a committed B lymphocyte progenitor. *Lancet* 1978;2:444.
32. Solanki DL, McCurdy PR, MacDermott RP. Chronic lymphocytic leukemia: a monoclonal disease. *Am J Hematol* 1982;13:159.
33. Gahrton G, Robert K-H, Friberg K, et al. Nonrandom chromosomal aberrations in chronic lymphocytic leukemia revealed by polyclonal B-cell mitogen stimulation. *Blood* 1980;56:640.
34. Korsmeyer SJ. Hierarchy of immunoglobulin gene rearrangements in B-cell leukemias. *Ann Intern Med* 1985;102:497.
35. Korsmeyer SJ, Heiter PA, Ravetch JV, et al. Developmental hierarchy of immunoglobulin gene rearrangements in human leukemic pre-B-cells. *Proc Natl Acad Sci U S A* 1981;78:7096.
36. Ternynck T, Dighiero G, Follezou J, et al. Comparison of normal and CLL lymphocyte surface Ig determinants using peroxidase-labeled antibodies. I. Detection and quantitation of light chain determinant. *Blood* 1974;43:789.
37. Han T, Ozer H, Blood M, et al. The presence of monoclonal cytoplasmic immunoglobulins in leukemic B cells from patients with chronic lymphocytic leukemia. *Blood* 1982;59:435.
38. Rubartelli A, Sitia R, Zicca A, et al. Differentiation of chronic lymphocytic leukemia cells: correlation between the synthesis and secretion of immunoglobulins and the ultrastructure of the malignant cells. *Blood* 1983;62:495.
39. Deegan MJ, Abraham JP, Sawdy KM, et al. High incidence of monoclonal proteins in the serum and urine of chronic lymphocytic leukemia patients. *Blood* 1984;64:1207.
40. Fitzpatrick J, O'Donnell A, Diloro A, et al. Serum M-proteins in hairy cell leukemia (HCL), chronic lymphocytic leukemia (CLL) and free light chain (FLC) myeloma using high resolution electrophoresis/immunofixation (HRE/IFC). *Blood* 1986;68:208A(abst).
41. Qian GX, Fu SM, Solanki DL, et al. Circulating monoclonal IgM proteins in B-cell chronic lymphocytic leukemia: their identification, characterization and relationship to membrane IgM. *J Immunol* 1984;133:3396.
42. Gupta S, Pahwa R, O'Reilly R, et al. Ontogeny of lymphocyte subpopulations in human fetal liver. *Proc Natl Acad Sci U S A* 1976;73:919.
43. Ross GD, Polley MJ. Specificity of human lymphocyte complement receptors. *J Exp Med* 1975;141:1163.
44. Nadler LM, Anderson KC, Marti G, et al. B4, a human B lymphocyte-associated antigen expressed in normal, mitogen-activated, and malignant B lymphocytes. *J Immunol* 1983;131:244.
45. Stashenko P, Nadler RM, Hardy R, et al. Characterization of a human B lymphocyte specific antigen. *J Immunol* 1980;125:1678.
46. Nadler LM, Stashenko P, Hardy R, et al. Characterization of a human B-cell specific antigen (B2) distinct from B1. *J Immunol* 1981;126:1941.
47. Abramson CS, Kearsey JH, Lebien TW. A monoclonal antibody (BA-1) reactive with cells of human B lymphocyte lineage. *J Immunol* 1981;126:83.
48. Ritz J, Pesando JM, Notis-McConarty J, et al. A monoclonal antibody to human acute lymphoblastic leukemia antigen. *Nature* 1980;283:583.
49. LeBien TW, Bou DR, Bradley G, et al. Antibody affinity may influence antigenic modulation of the common acute lymphoblastic leukemia antigen in vitro. *J Immunol* 1982;129:2287.
50. Faguet GB, Agee JF. Monoclonal antibodies against the chronic lymphatic leukemia antigen cCLLa: characterization and reactivity. *Blood* 1987;70:437.
51. Brooks DA, Beckman I, Bradley J, et al. Human lymphocyte markers defined by antibody derived from somatic cell hybrids. IV. A monoclonal antibody reacting specifically with a subpopulation of human B lymphocytes. *J Immunol* 1980;126:1373.
52. Foon KA, Todd RF III. Immunologic classification of leukemia and lymphoma. *Blood* 1986;68:1.
53. Caligaris-Cappio F, Gobbi M, Bofill M, et al. Infrequent normal B lymphocytes expressed features of B-chronic lymphocytic leukemia. *J Exp Med* 1982;155:623.

54. Gadol N, Ault RA. Phenotypic and functional characterization of human Leu 1 (CD5) B cells. *Immunol Rev* 1986;93:23.

55. Antin JH, Emerson SG, Martin P, et al. Leu 1+ (CD5+) B cells, a major lymphoid subpopulation in human fetal spleen: phenotype and functional studies. *J Immunol* 1986;136:505.

56. Freedman A, Horowitz J, Rosen K, et al. Subpopulations of activated B cells phenotypically resemble B-CLL cells. *Blood* 1986;68[Suppl 1]:245(abst).

57. Freedman AS, Boyd AW, Bieger FR, et al. Normal cellular counterparts of B-cell chronic lymphocytic leukemia. *Blood* 1987;70:418.

58. Kay NE, Burton J, Wagner D, et al. The malignant B cells from B-chronic lymphocytic leukemia patients release TAC-soluble interleukin-2 receptors. *Blood* 1988;72(2):447.

59. Bell PB, Rooney N, Bosanquet AG. CD79a detected by ZL7.4 separates chronic lymphocytic leukemia from mantle cell lymphoma in the leukemic phase. *Cytometry* 1999;38:102.

60. Cooper MD, Bertoli LF, Borzillo GV, et al. Pathogenesis of B-cell malignancies. In: Gale RP, Golde DW, eds. *Leukemia: recent advances in biology and treatment.* New York: Alan R Liss, 1985:453.

61. Robert K-H, Juliusson G, Biberfeld P. Chronic lymphocytic leukemia cells activated in vitro reveal cellular changes that characterize B-prolymphocytic leukaemia and immunocytoma. *Scand J Immunol* 1983;17:397.

62. Caligaris-Cappio F, Pizzolo G, Chilosi M, et al. Phorbol ester induces abnormal chronic lymphocytic leukemia cells to express features of hairy cell leukemia. *Blood* 1985;66:1035.

63. Fu SM, Chiorazzi N, Kunkel HG, et al. Induction of in vitro differentiation and immunoglobulin synthesis of human leukemic B lymphocytes. *J Exp Med* 1978;148:1570.

64. Gordon J, Mellstedt H, Aman P, et al. Phenotypic modulation of chronic lymphocytic leukemia cells by phorbol ester: induction of IgM secretion and changes in the expression of B-cell associated surface antigens. *J Immunol* 1984;132:541.

65. Okamura J, Letarte M, Stein LD, et al. Modulation of chronic lymphocytic leukemia cells by phorbol ester: increase in Ia expression, IgM secretion and MLR stimulatory capacity. *J Immunol* 1982;128:2276.

66. Totterman TH, Nilsson K, Sundstrom C. Phorbol ester–induced differentiation of chronic lymphocytic leukemia cells. *Nature* 1980;288:176.

67. Juliusson G, Robert K-H, Hammerstrom L, et al. Mitogen-induced switching of heavy-chain class secretion in chronic B-lymphocytic leukaemia and immunocytoma cell populations. *Scand J Immunol* 1983;17:51.

68. Slease RB, Wistar R Jr, Scher I. Surface immunoglobulin density on human peripheral mononuclear cells. *Blood* 1979;54:72.

69. Halper JP, Fu SM, Gottlieb AB, et al. Poor mixed lymphocyte reactions stimulatory capacity of leukemic B cells of chronic lymphocytic leukemia patients despite the presence of Ia antigens. *J Exp Med* 1979;64:1141.

70. Wolos JA, Davey FR. B lymphocyte function in B cell chronic lymphocytic leukaemia. *Br J Haematol* 1981;49:395.

71. Gale RP, Zighelboim J, Ossorio RC, et al. A comparison of human lymphoid cells in antibody-dependent cellular cytotoxicity (ADCC). *Clin Immunol Immunopathol* 1975;3:377.

72. Johnstone AP, Jensenius JC, Millard RE, et al. Mitogen-stimulated immunoglobulin production by chronic lymphocytic leukaemic lymphocytes. *Clin Exp Immunol* 1982;47:697.

73. Smith JL, Cowling DC, Barker C. Response of lymphocytes in chronic lymphocytic leukaemia to plant mitogens. *Lancet* 1972;1:229.

74. Smith JB, Knowlton RP, Koons LS. Immunologic studies in chronic lymphocytic leukemia: defective stimulation of T-cell proliferation in autologous mixed lymphocyte culture. *J Natl Cancer Inst* 1977;58:579.

75. Perri RT. Impaired expression of cell surface receptors for B-cell growth factor by chronic lymphocytic leukemia cells. *Blood* 1986;67:943.

76. Larson RA, Yachnin S. Cytochalasin B is a potent mitogen for chronic lymphocytic leukemia cells in vitro. *J Clin Invest* 1983;72:1268.

77. Izaquirre ZA, Minden MD, Howatson AF, et al. Colony formation by normal and malignant human B lymphocytes. *Br J Cancer* 1980;42:430.

78. Perri RT, Kay ME. Monoclonal CLL B-cells may be induced to grow in an in vitro B-cell colony assay system. *Blood* 1982;59:247.

79. Taetle R, Richardson J, To D, et al. Colony-forming assay for circulating chronic lymphocytic leukemia cells. *Leuk Res* 1982;6:335–344.

80. Kay NE, Johnson JD, Stanek R, et al. T-cell subpopulations in chronic lymphocytic leukemia: abnormalities in distribution and in in vitro receptor maturations. *Blood* 1979;54:540.

81. Chiorazzi N, Fu SM, Moutazen G, et al. T cell helper defect in patients with chronic lymphocytic leukemia. *J Immunol* 1979;122:1087.

82. Kay NE. Abnormal T-cell subpopulation function in CLL: excessive suppressor (T) and deficient helper (T) activity with respect to B-cell proliferation. *Blood* 1981;57:418.

83. Kay NE, Oken MM, Perri RT. The influential T cell in B-cell neoplasms. *J Clin Oncol* 1983;8:810.

84. Lauria F, Foa R, Catovsky D. Increase in T gamma lymphocytes in B-cell chronic lymphocytic leukemia. *Scand J Haematol* 1980;24:187.

85. Matutes E, Wechsler A, Gomez R, et al. Unusual T-cell phenotype in advanced B-chronic lymphocytic leukemia. *Br J Haematol* 1981;49:635.

86. Platsoucas CD, Galiniski M, Kempin S, et al. Abnormal T lymphocyte subpopulations in patients with B cell chronic lymphocytic leukemia: an analysis by monoclonal antibody. *J Immunol* 1982;129:2305.

87. Kay NE, Kaplan ME. Defective expression of T cell antigens in chronic lymphocytic leukaemia: relationship to T cell dysfunction. *Br J Haematol* 1984;57:105.

88. Blue M-L, Daley JF, Levine H, et al. Coexpression of T4 and T8 on peripheral blood T cells demonstrated by two-color fluorescence flow cytometry. *J Immunol* 1985;134:2281.

89. Catovsky D, Lauria F, Matutes E, et al. Increase in T gamma lymphocytes and B-cell chronic lymphocytic leukemia. II. Correlation with clinical stage and findings in B-prolymphocytic leukaemia. *Br J Haematol* 1981;47:539.

90. Kay NE, Howe RB, Douglas SD. Effect of therapy on T cell subpopulations in patients with chronic lymphocytic leukemia. *Leuk Res* 1982;6:345.

91. Wybran J, Chantlet S, Fudenberg HH. Isolation of normal T-cells in chronic lymphocytic leukaemia. *Lancet* 1973;2:126.

92. Han T, Bloom ML, Dadly B, et al. Lack of autologous mixed lymphocyte reaction in patients with chronic lymphocytic leukemia: evidence for autoreactive T-cell dysfunction not correlated with phenotype, karyotype, or clinical status. *Blood* 1982;60:1075.

93. Foa R, Catovsky D, Lauria F, et al. Reduced T-colony forming capacity of T-lymphocytes and T-chronic lymphocytic leukemia. *Br J Haematol* 1980;46:623.

94. Foa R, Lauria F, Catovsky D, et al. Reduced T-colony forming capacity in B-chronic lymphocytic leukemia. II. Correlation with clinical stage and findings in B-prolymphocytic leukaemia. *Leuk Res* 1982;6:329.

95. Fernandez LA, Macsween JM, Langley R. Normal T cell colony numbers in untreated patients with chronic lymphocytic leukaemia (CLL). *Br J Haematol* 1984;57:97.

96. Lauria F, Foa R, Mantovani B, et al. T-cell functional abnormality in B-chronic lymphocytic leukaemia: evidence of a defect of the T-helper subset. *Br J Haematol* 1983;54:277.

97. Burton JD, Kay NE. Evidence that malignant chronic lymphocytic leukemia (CLL) B-cells secrete immuno-suppressive ganglioside. *Blood* 1986;68:92A(abst).

98. Platsoucas CD, Fernandes G, Gupta SL, et al. Defective spontaneous and antibody-dependent cytotoxicity mediated by E-rosette–positive and E-rosette–negative cells in untreated patients with chronic lymphocytic leukemia: augmentation by in vitro treatment with interferon. *J Immunol* 1980;125:1216.

99. Zeigler HW, Kay, NE, Zarling JM. Deficiency of natural killer cell activity in patients with chronic lymphocytic leukemia. *Int J Cancer* 1981;27:321.

100. Ziegler-Heitbrock HW, Rumpold H, Kraft D, et al. Patients with a deficiency of natural killer cell activity lack the VEP 13-positive lymphocyte subpopulation. *Blood* 1985;65:65.

101. Foa R, Fierro MT, Lusso P, et al. Reduced natural killer T-cells in B-cell chronic lymphocytic leukaemia identified by three monoclonal antibodies: Leu-11, A10, AB8.28. *Br J Haematol* 1986;62:151.

102. Kay NE, Zarling J. Restoration of impaired natural killer cell activity of B-chronic lymphocytic leukemia patients by recombinant interleukin-2. *Am J Hematol* 1987;24:161.

103. Hokland VP, Ellegaard J. Immunological studies in chronic lymphocytic leukemia. II. Natural killer- and antibody-dependent cellular cytotoxicity potentials of malignant and nonmalignant lymphocyte subsets and the effect of alpha-interferon. *Leuk Res* 1981;5:349.

104. Lauria F, Raspadore D, Tura D. Effect of a thymic factor on T lymphocytes in B cell chronic lymphocytic leukemia: in vitro and in vivo studies. *Blood* 1984;64:667.

105. Knuutila S, Elonen E, Teerenhovi L, et al. Trisomy 12 in B-cells of patients with B-cell chronic lymphocytic leukemia. *N Engl J Med* 1986;314:865.

106. Lucivero G, Prchal JT, Latwon AR, et al. Abnormal T-cell functions in B cell chronic lymphocytic leukemia do not imply T-lymphocyte involvement in the leukemic process: report of a case with demonstrated "polyclonality" of T lymphocytes. *J Clin Immunol* 1983;3:111.

107. O'Connor NTJ, Wainscoat TS, Weatherall DJ, et al. Rearrangement of the T-cell receptor beta-chain gene in the diagnosis of lymphoproliferative disorders. *Lancet* 1985;1:1295.

108. Chapel HM, Bunch C. Mechanisms of infection in chronic lymphocytic leukemia. *Semin Hematol* 1987;24:291.

109. Travade PH, Dusart JD, Cavaroc M, et al. Les infections graves associees a la leucemie lymphoide chronique: 159 episodes infectieux observes chez 60 malades. *Presse Med* 1986;15:1715.

110. Cone L, Uhr JW. Immunologic deficiency disorders associated with chronic lymphocytic leukemia and multiple myeloma. *J Clin Invest* 1964;43:2241.

111. Shaw RK, Szwek C, Boggs DR, et al. Infection and immunity in CLL. *Arch Intern Med* 1960;106:467.

112. Miller DG, Karnofsky DA. Immunologic factors and resistance to infection in CLL. *Am J Med* 1961;31:748.

113. Fauci AS, Pratt KR, Whalen G. Intrinsic B cell defect in the immunoglobulin deficiency of chronic lymphocytic leukemia. *Cancer Res* 1977;25:482(abst).

114. Fernandez LA, Macsween JM, Langley GR. Immunoglobulin secretory function of B cells from untreated patients with chronic lymphocytic leukemia and hypogammaglobulinemia: role of T cells. *Blood* 1983;62:767.

115. Kay NE, Perri RT. Evidence that large granular lymphocytes from B-CLL patients with hypogammaglobulinemia down-regulate B-cell immunoglobulin synthesis. *Blood* 1989;73:1016.

116. Bergsagel DE. The chronic leukemias: a review of disease manifestations and the aims of therapy. *Can Med Assoc J* 1967;96:1615.

117. Ebbe S, Wittels B, Dameshek W. Autoimmune thrombocytopenic purpura ("ITP type") with chronic lymphocytic leukemia. *Blood* 1962;19:23.

118. Rustagi P, Han T, Ziolkowski L, et al. Antigranulocyte antibodies in chronic lymphocytic leukemia and other chronic lymphoproliferative disorders. *Blood* 1983;62:106(abst).

119. Abeloff MD, Waterbury L. Pure red cell aplasia and chronic lymphocytic leukemia. *Arch Intern Med* 1974;134:721.

120. Conley CL, Misiti J, Laster AJ. Genetic factors predisposing to chronic lymphocytic leukemia and to autoimmune disease. *Medicine* 1980;5:323.
121. Hayakawa K, Hardy RR, Parks DR, et al. The "Ly-1 B" cell subpopulation in normal immunodefective, and autoimmune mice. *J Exp Med* 1983;157:202.
122. Hayakawa K, Hardy RR, Honda M, et al. Ly-1 BN cells: functionally distinct lymphocytes that secrete IgM autoantibodies. *Proc Natl Acad Sci U S A* 1984; 81:2492.
123. Hardy RR, Hayakawa K, Shimizu M, et al. Rheumatoid factor secretion from human Leu-1+ B cells. *Science* 1987;236:77.
124. Casali P, Burastero SE, Nakamura M, et al. Human lymphocytes making rheumatoid factor and antibody to ssDNA belong to the Leu-1+ B-cell subset. *Science* 1987;236:75.
125. Sthoeger ZM, Wakai M, Tse DB, et al. Production of autoantibodies by CD5-expressing B lymphocytes from patients with chronic lymphocytic leukemia. *J Exp Med* 1989;169:255.
126. Kipps TJ, Fong S, Tomhave E, et al. High-frequency expression of a conserved kappa light chain variable-region gene in chronic lymphocytic leukemia. *Proc Natl Acad Sci U S A* 1987;84:2916.
127. Kipps TJ, Tomhave E, Chen PP, et al. Autoantibody associated kappa light-chain variable-region gene expressed in chronic lymphocytic leukemia with little or no somatic mutation: implications for etiology and immunotherapy. *J Exp Med* 1988;167:840.
128. Kipps TJ, Robbin BA, Kustar P, et al. Autoantibody associated cross-reactive idiotypes expressed at high frequency in chronic lymphocytic leukemia relative to B-cell lymphomas of follicular center cell origin. *Blood* 1988;72:422.
129. Gahrton G, Robert K-H, Friberg K, et al. Cytogenetic mapping of the duplicated segment of chromosome 12 and lymphoproliferative disorders. *Nature* 1982;297:513.
130. Han T, Ozer H, Sadamor N, et al. Prognostic importance of cytogenetic abnormalities in patients with chronic lymphocytic leukemia. *N Engl J Med* 1984;310:288.
131. Han T, Sadamori N, Ozer H, et al. Cytogenetic studies in 77 patients with chronic lymphocytic leukemia: correlations with clinical immunologic, and phenotypic data. *J Clin Oncol* 1984;2:1121.
132. Han T, Sadamori N, Takeuchi J, et al. Clonal chromosome abnormalities in patients with Waldenström's and CLL-associated macroglobulinemia: significance of trisomy 12. *Blood* 1983;62:525.
133. Juliusson G, Robert K-H, Ost A, et al. Prognostic information from cytogenetic analysis in chronic B-lymphocytic leukemia and leukemic immunocytoma. *Blood* 1985;65:134.
134. Pittman S, Catovsky D. Prognostic significance of chromosome abnormalities in chronic lymphocytic leukaemia. *Br J Haematol* 1984;58:649.
135. Robert K-H, Gahrton G, Friberg K, et al. Extra chromosome 12 and prognosis in chronic lymphocytic leukaemia. *Scand J Haematol* 1982;28:163.
136. Sonnier JA, Buchanan GR, Howard-Peebles PN, et al. Chromosomal translocation involving the immunoglobulin kappa-chain and heavy-chain loci in a child with chronic lymphocytic leukemia. *N Engl J Med* 1983;309:590.
137. Vahdati M, Graafland H, Emberger JM. Karyotype analysis of B lymphocytes transformed by Epstein-Barr virus in 21 patients with B cell chronic lymphocytic leukemia. *Hum Genet* 1983;63:327.
138. Juliusson G, Friberg K, Gahrton G. Consistency of chromosomal aberrations in chronic B-lymphocytic leukemia: a longitudinal cytogenetic study of 41 patients. *Cancer* 1988;62:500.
139. Juliusson G, Gahrton G. Chromosome aberrations in B-cell chronic lymphocytic leukemia: pathogenic and clinical implications. *Cancer Genet Cytogenet* 1990;45:143.
140. Starostik P, O'Brien S, Chung CY, et al. The prognostic significance of 13q14 deletions in chronic lymphocytic leukemia. *Leuk Res* 1999;23:795.
141. Hogan WJ, Tefferi A, Borell TJ, et al. Prognostic relevance of monosomy at the 13q14 locus detected by fluorescence in situ hybridization in B-cell chronic lymphocytic leukemia. *Cancer Genet Cytogenet* 1999;110:77.
142. Liso V, Capalbo S, Lapietra A, et al. Evaluation of trisomy 12 by fluorescence in situ hybridization in peripheral blood, bone marrow and lymph nodes of patients with B-cell chronic lymphocytic leukemia. *Haematologica* 1999;84: 212.
143. Gahn B, Wendenburg B, Troff C, et al. Analysis of progenitor cell involvement in CLL by simultaneous immunophenotypic and genotypic analysis at the single cell level. *Br J Haematol* 1999;105:955.
144. Garcia-Marco JA, Price CM, Catovsky D, et al. Interphase cytogenetics in chronic lymphocytic leukemia. *Cancer Genet Cytogenet* 1997;94:52.
145. Auer RL, Bienz N, Neilson J, et al. The sequential analysis of trisomy 12 in B-cell chronic lymphocytic leukemia. *Br J Haematol* 1999;104:742.
146. Dohner H, Stilgenbauer S, James MR, et al. 11q Deletions identify a new subset of B-cell chronic lymphocytic leukemia characterized by extensive nodal involvement and inferior prognosis. *Blood* 1997;89:2516.
147. Lavin MF, Khanna KK. ATM: the protein encoded by the gene mutated in the radiosensitive syndrome ataxia-telangiectasia. *Int J Radiat Biol* 1999;75:1201.
148. Amiel A, Mulchanov I, Elis A, et al. Detection of 6q21 in chronic lymphocytic leukemia and multiple myeloma detected by fluorescence in situ hybridization. *Cancer Genet Cytogenet* 1999;112:53.
149. Yunis JJ, Oken MM, Kaplan M, et al. Distinctive chromosomal abnormalities in histologic subtypes of non-Hodgkin's lymphoma. *N Engl J Med* 1982;307: 1231.
150. Erikson J, Finan J, Tsujimoto Y, et al. The chromosome 14 breakpoint in neoplastic B cells with the t(11;14) translocation involves the immunoglobulin heavy chain locus. *Proc Natl Acad Sci U S A* 1984;81:41.
151. Tsujimoto Y, Yunis J, Onorato-Showe L, et al. Molecular cloning of the chromosomal breakpoint of B-cell lymphomas and leukemias with the t(11;14) translocation. *Science* 1984;224:1403.
152. Yunis JJ, Frizzera G, Oken MM, et al. Multiple recurrent genomic defects in follicular lymphoma: a possible model for cancer. *N Engl J Med* 1987;316:79.
153. McDonnell TJ, Deane N, Platt FM, et al. bcl-2-Immunoglobulin transgenic mice demonstrate extended B cell survival and follicular lymphoproliferation. *Cell* 1989;57:79.
154. Ohno H, Takimoto G, McKelthan TW. The candidate protooncogene bcl-3 is related to genes implicated in cell lineage determination and cell cycle control. *Cell* 1990;60:991.
155. Hamblin TJ, Davis Z, Gardiner A, et al. Unmutated Ig V-H genes are associated with a more aggressive form of chronic lymphocytic leukemia. *Blood* 1999;94:1848.
156. Damle RN, Wasil T, Fais F, et al. Ig V gene mutation status and CD38 expression as novel prognostic indicators in chronic lymphocytic leukemia. *Blood* 1999;94:1840.
157. Oscier DJ, Thompsett A, Zhu D, et al. Differential rates of somatic hypermutation in V(H) genes among subsets of chronic lymphocytic leukemia defined by chromosomal abnormalities. *Blood* 1997;89:4153.
158. Thompson AA, Do HN, Saxon A, et al. Widespread B29 (CD79b) gene defects and loss of expression in chronic lymphocytic leukemia. *Leuk Lymphoma* 1999;32:561.
159. Han T, Gomez GA, Henderson ES. Spontaneous remission in chronic lymphocytic leukemia. *Blood* 1986;68:199A(abst).
160. Rai KR, Sawitsky A, Cronkite EP, et al. Clinical staging of chronic lymphocytic leukemia. *Blood* 1975;46:219.
161. Rai K. A critical analysis of staging in CLL in chronic lymphocytic leukemia. In: Gale RP, Rai K, eds. *Recent progress and future directions*. New York: Alan R Liss, 1987:253.
162. Binet JL, Auguier A, Dighiero G, et al. A new prognostic classification of chronic lymphocytic leukemia derived from a multivariate survival analysis. *Cancer* 1981;48:198.
163. Baccarani M, Gabol M, Gobbi M, et al. Staging of chronic lymphocytic leukemia. *Blood* 1982;59:1191.
164. Rozman C, Montserrat E, Feliu E, et al. Prognosis of chronic lymphocytic leukemia: a multivariate survival analysis of 150 cases. *Blood* 1982;59:1001.
165. Juliusson G, Robert K-H, Nilsson B, et al. Prognostic value of B-cell mitogen-induced and spontaneous thymidine uptake in vitro in chronic B-lymphocytic leukaemia cells. *Br J Haematol* 1985;60:429.
166. Moayeri H, Sokal JE. In vitro leukocyte thymidine uptake and prognosis in chronic lymphocytic leukemia. *Am J Med* 1979;66:773.
167. Simonsson B, Nilsson K. ^{3}H-thymidine uptake in chronic lymphocytic leukemia cells. *Scand J Haematol* 1980;24:169.
168. Kallander CF, Simonsson B, Hagberg H, et al. Serum deoxthymidine kinase gives prognostic information in chronic lymphocytic leukemia. *Cancer* 1984;54:2450.
169. Baldini L, Mozzana R, Cortelezzezzi A, et al. Prognostic significance of immunoglobulin phenotype in B cell chronic lymphocytic leukemia. *Blood* 1985; 65:340.
170. Bartl R, Frisch B, Burkhardt R, et al. Assessment of marrow trephine in relation to staging in chronic lymphocytic leukaemia. *Br J Haematol* 1982;51:1.
171. Lipshutz MD, Mir R, Rai KR, et al. Bone marrow biopsy and clinical staging in chronic lymphocytic leukemia. *Cancer* 1980;46:1442.
172. Rozman C, Montserrat E, Rodrigues-Fernandez JM, et al. Bone marrow histological pattern: the best single prognostic multivariate survival analysis of 329 cases. *Blood* 1984;64:642.
173. Han T, Barcos M, Enrigh L, et al. Bone marrow infiltration patterns and their prognostic significance in chronic lymphocytic leukemia: correlations with clinical, immunologic, phenotypic, and cytogenetic data. *J Clin Oncol* 1984; 2:562.
174. Montserrat E, Sanchez-Bisoni J, Vinolas N, et al. Lymphocyte doubling time in chronic lymphocytic leukemia: analysis of its prognostic significance. *Br J Haematol* 1986;62:567.
175. Han T, Ozer H, Gavigan M, et al. Benign monoclonal B cell lymphocytosis: a benign variant of CLL–clinical, immunologic, phenotypic and cytogenetic studies in 20 patients. *Blood* 1984;64:244.
176. National Cancer Institute sponsored study of classifications of non-Hodgkin's lymphomas: summary and description of a working formulation for clinical usage. The non-Hodgkin's lymphoma pathologic classification project. *Cancer* 1982;49(10):2112.
177. Pangalis GA, Nathwani BN, Rappaport H. Malignant lymphoma, well differentiated lymphocytic: its relationship with chronic lymphocytic leukemia and macroglobulinemia of Waldenström. *Cancer* 1977;39:999.
178. Foon KA, Thiruvengadam R, Saven A, et al. Genetic relatedness of lymphoid malignancies: transformation of chronic lymphocytic leukemias as a model. *Ann Intern Med* 1993;119:63.
179. Richter MN. Generalized reticular cell sarcoma of lymph nodes associated with lymphatic leukemia. *Am J Pathol* 1928;4:285.
180. Armitage JO, Dick FD, Corder MP. Diffuse histiocytic lymphoma complicating chronic lymphocytic leukemia. *Cancer* 1978;41:422.
181. Dick FR, Maca RD. The lymph node in chronic lymphocytic leukemia. *Cancer* 1978;41:283.
182. Long JC, Aisenberg AC. Richter's syndrome: a terminal complication of chronic lymphocytic leukemia with distinct clinical pathologic features. *Am J Clin Pathol* 1975;63:786.

183. Trump CL, Mann RB, Phelps R, et al. Richter's syndrome: diffuse histiocytic lymphoma in patients with chronic lymphocytic leukemia. *Am J Med* 1980; 68:539.
184. Bertoli LF, Kubagawa H, Borzillo GV, et al. Analysis with anti-idiotype antibody of a patient with chronic lymphocytic leukemia and a large cell lymphoma (Richter's syndrome). *Blood* 1987;70:45.
185. Delsol G, Laurent G, Kuhlein E, et al. Case reports: Richter's syndrome—evidence for the clonal origin of the two proliferations. *Am Soc Clin Pathol* 1981;76:308.
186. Heslop HE, Fitzgerald PH, Beard MEJ. Sustained complete remission in Richter's syndrome. *Cancer* 1987;59:1036.
187. McDonnell JM, Beschorner WE, Staal S, et al. Richter's syndrome with two different B-cell clones. *Cancer* 1986;58:2031.
188. van Dongen JJM, Joojikaas H, Michiels JJ, et al. Richter's syndrome with different immunoglobulin light chains and different heavy chain gene rearrangements. *Blood* 1984;64:571.
189. Splinter TAW, Bom-van Noorloos A, van Heerde P. CLL and diffuse histiocytic lymphoma in one patient: clonal proliferation of two different B cells. *Scand J Haematol* 1978;10:29.
190. Galton DAG, Goldman JM, Wiltshaw E, et al. Prolymphocytic leukemia. *Br J Haematol* 1974;27:7.
191. Katayama I, Aiba M, Pechet L, et al. B-lineage prolymphocytic leukemia as a distinct clinical pathological entity. *Am J Pathol* 1980;99:399.
192. Brouet JC, Flandrin G, Sasportes M, et al. Chronic lymphocytic leukaemia of T-cell origin: immunological and clinical evaluation in 11 patients. *Lancet* 1975;2:890.
193. Catovsky D, Galletto J, Okos A, et al. Prolymphocytic leukaemia of B and T cell type. *Lancet* 1973;2:232.
194. Enno A, Catovsky D, O'Brien M, et al. 'Prolymphocytoid' transformation of chronic lymphocytic leukaemia. *Br J Haematol* 1979;41:9.
195. Stark AN, Limbert HJ, Roberts BE, et al. Prolymphocytoid transformation of CLL: a clinical and immunological study of 22 cases. *Leuk Res* 1986;10:1225.
196. Kjeldsberg CR, Marty J. Prolymphocytic transformation of chronic lymphocytic leukemia. *Cancer* 1981;48:2447.
197. Ghani A, Krause JR, Brody JP. Prolymphocytic transformation of chronic lymphocytic leukemia: a report of three cases and review of the literature. *Cancer* 1986;57:75.
198. Melo JV, Wardle J, Chetty M, et al. The relationship between chronic lymphocytic leukaemia and prolymphocytic leukaemia. *Br J Haematol* 1986;64:469.
199. Miller ALC, Habershaw JA, Dhaliwhal HS, et al. Chronic lymphocytic leukaemia presenting as a blast cell crisis. *Leuk Res* 1984;8:905.
200. Frenkel EP, Ligler FS, Graham MS, Hernandez JA, Kettman JR Jr, Smith RG. Acute lymphocytic leukemic transformation of chronic lymphocytic leukemia: substantiation by flow cytometry. *Am J Hematol* 1981;10:381.
201. Laurent G, Gourdin MF, Flandrin G, et al. Acute blast crisis in a patient with chronic lymphocytic leukemia. *Acta Haematol* 1981;65:60.
202. Pines A, Ben-Bassat I, Selzer G, et al. Transformation of chronic lymphocytic leukemia to plasmacytoma. *Cancer* 1984;54:1904.
203. Brouet JC, Germand JP, Laurent G, et al. The association of chronic lymphocytic leukemia and multiple myeloma: a study of eleven patients. *Br J Haematol* 1985;59:55.
204. Hoffmann KD, Rudders RA. Multiple myeloma and chronic lymphocytic leukemia in a single individual. *Arch Intern Med* 1977;137:232.
205. Jeha MT, Hamblin J, Smith JL. Coincident chronic lymphocytic leukemia and osteosclerotic multiple myeloma. *Blood* 1981;57:617.
206. Pedersen-Bjergaard J, Petersen HD, Thomsen M, et al. Chronic lymphocytic leukemia with subsequent development of multiple myeloma. *Scand J Haematol* 1978;21:256.
207. Fermand JP, James JM, Herait P, et al. Associated chronic lymphocytic leukemia and multiple myeloma: origin from a single clone. *Blood* 1985;66:291.
208. Saltman DL, Ross JA, Banks RE, et al. Molecular evidence for a single clonal origin in biphenotypic concomitant chronic lymphocytic leukemia and multiple myeloma. *Blood* 1989;74:2062.
209. Chen JR, Gu Bj, Dao LP, et al. Transendothelial migration of lymphocytes in chronic lymphocytic leukaemia is impaired and involved down-regulation of both L-selectin and CD23. *Br J Haematol* 1999;105:181.
210. Burger JA, Burger M, Kipps TJ. Chronic lymphocytic leukemia B cells express functional CXCR4 chemokine receptors that mediate spontaneous migration beneath bone marrow stromal cells. *Blood* 1999;94:3658.
211. Lampert IA, Wotherspoon A, Van Noorden S, et al. High expression of CD23 in the proliferation centers of chronic lymphocytic leukemia in lymph nodes and spleen. *Hum Pathol* 1999;30:648.
212. Zimmerman TS, Godwin HA, Perry S. Studies of leukocyte kinetics in chronic lymphocytic leukemia. *Blood* 1968;31:277.
213. Andreeff M, Darzynkiewicz Z, Sharpless TK, et al. Discrimination of human leukemia subtypes by flow cytometric analysis of cellular DNA and RNA. *Blood* 1980;55:282.
214. Kobayashi R, Picchio G, Kirven M, et al. Transfer of human chronic lymphocytic leukemia to mice with severe combined immune deficiency. *Leuk Res* 1992;16:1013.
215. Marschitz R, Tinhofer I, Hittmair A, et al. Analysis of Bcl-2 protein expression in chronic lymphocytic leukemia: a comparison of three semiquantitation techniques. *Am J Clin Pathol* 2000;113:219.
216. Pepper C, Thomas A, Hoy T, et al. Antisense-mediated suppression of Bcl-2 highlights its pivotal role in failed apoptosis in B-cell chronic lymphocytic leukaemia. *Br J Haematol* 1999;107:611.
217. Klein A, Miera O, Bauer O, et al. Chemosensitivity of B-cell chronic lymphocytic leukemia and correlated expression of proteins regulating apoptosis, cell cycle and DNA repair. *Leukemia* 2000;14:40.
218. Stoetzer OJ, Pogrebniak A, Scholz M, et al. Drug-induced apoptosis in chronic lymphocytic leukemia. *Leukemia* 1999;13:1873.
219. Gottardi D, Alfarano A, De Leo AM, et al. In leukaemic CD5+ B cells the expression of Bcl-2 gene family is shifted toward protection from apoptosis. *Br J Haematol* 1996;94:612.
220. de la Fuente MT, Casanova B, Garcia-Gila M, et al. Fibronectin interaction with alpha4beta1 integrin prevents apoptosis in B cell chronic lymphocytic leukemia: correlation with Bcl-2 and Bax. *Leukemia* 1999;3:266.
221. Lampert I, Catovsky D, Mersh GW, et al. Histopathology of prolymphocytic leukaemia with particular reference to the spleen: a comparison with chronic lymphocytic leukaemia. *Histopathology* 1980;4:3.
222. Catovsky D, Cherchi M, Brooks D, et al. Heterogeneity of B-cell leukemias demonstrated by the monoclonal antibody FMC-7. *Blood* 1981;58:406.
223. Melo JV, Catovsky P, Gregory CM, et al. The relationship between chronic lymphocytic leukaemia and prolymphocytic leukaemia. IV. Analysis of survival and prognostic factors. *Br J Haematol* 1987;65:23.
224. Krajny M, Pruzanski W. Waldenströms macroglobulinemia: review of 45 cases. *Can Med Assoc J* 1976;14:899.
225. Preud'Homme J, Seligmann M. Immunoglobulins on the surface of lymphoid cells in Waldenström macroglobulinemia. *J Clin Invest* 1972;551:701.
226. Waldenström J. Incipient myelomatosis or 'essential' hyperglobulinemia with fibrinogenopenia: a new syndrome? *Acta Med Scand* 1974;117:216.
227. MacKenzie MR. Macroglobulinemia. In: Wiernike PH, Canellos GP, Kyle RA, et al, eds. *Neoplastic disease of the blood*. New York: Churchill Livingstone, 1991:501.
228. Bennett JM, Catovsky D, Daniel M-T, et al. Proposals for the classification of chronic (mature) B and T lymphoid leukemias. *J Clin Pathol* 1989;42:567.
229. Isaacs R. Lymphosarcoma cell leukemia. *Ann Intern Med* 1937;11:657.
230. Mintzer DM, Hauptman SP. Lymphosarcoma cell leukemia and other non-Hodgkin's lymphomas in leukemic phase. *Am J Med* 1983;75:110.
231. Zacharski LR, Linman JW. Chronic lymphocytic leukemia versus chronic lymphosarcoma cell leukemia: analysis of 496 cases. *Am J Med* 1969;47:75.
232. Aisenberg AC, Wilkes B. Lymphosarcoma cell leukemia: the contribution of cell surface study to diagnosis. *Blood* 1976;48:707.
233. Koziner B, Filippa DA, Mertelsmann R, et al. Characterization of malignant lymphoma in leukemia phase by multiple differentiation markers on leukemic cells: correlations with clinical features and conventional morphology. *Am J Med* 1977;63:556.
234. Ritz J, Nadler IM, Bhan AK, et al. Expression of common acute lymphoblastic leukemia antigen (CALLA) by lymphomas of B-cell and T-cell lineage. *Blood* 1981;58:648.
235. Melo JV, Hegde U, Parreira A, et al. Splenic B cell lymphoma with circulating villous lymphocytes: differential diagnosis of B cell leukaemias with large spleens. *J Clin Pathol* 1987;40:642.
236. Neiman RS, Sullivan AL, Jaffe R. Malignant lymphoma simulating leukemia reticuloendotheliosis: a clinicopathologic study of ten cases. *Cancer* 1979;43:329.
237. DeOliveira MSP, Jaffe FS, Catovsky D. Leukaemic phase of mantle zone (intermediate) lymphoma: its characterization in 11 cases. *J Clin Pathol* 1989;42:962.
238. Bouroncle BA, Wiseman BK, Doan CA. Leukemic reticuloendotheliosis. *Blood* 1958;13:609.
239. Golomb HM, Catovsky D, Golde DW. Hairy cell leukemia: a clinical review based on 71 cases. *Ann Intern Med* 1978;89:677.
240. Golomb HM, Catovsky D, Golde DW. Hairy cell leukemia: a five-year update on seventy-one patients. *Ann Intern Med* 1983;99:485.
241. Reynold CW, Foon KA. T gamma-lymphoproliferative disorders in man and experimental animals: a review of the clinical, cellular and functional characteristics. *Blood* 1984;64:1146.
242. Newland AC, Catovsky D, Linch D, et al. Chronic T cell lymphocytosis: a review of 21 cases. *Br J Haematol* 1984;58:433.
243. Pandolfi F, Strong MD, Slease RB, et al. Characterization of a suppressor T-cell chronic lymphocytic leukemia with ADCC but not NK activity. *Blood* 1980;56:653.
244. Imbach P, Barandun S, d'Apuzzo V, et al. High-dose intravenous gamma globulin for idiopathic thrombocytopenic purpura in childhood. *Lancet* 1981;1:1228.
245. Carroll RR, Noyes WD, Rosse WF. Kitchens CS. Intravenous immunoglobulin administration in the treatment of severe chronic immune thrombocytopenic purpura. *Am J Med* 1984;76:181.
246. Bussell JB, Pham LC, Aledort L, et al. Maintenance treatment of adults with chronic refractory immune thrombocytopenia purpura using repeated intravenous infusions of gamma globulin. *Blood* 1988;72:121.
247. Bussell JB, Cunningham-Rundles C, Abraham C. Intravenous treatment of autoimmune hemolytic anemia with very high dose gamma globulin. *Vox Sang* 1986;51:264.
248. Besa EC. Use of intravenous immunoglobulin in chronic lymphocytic leukemia. *Am J Med* 1984;76:209.
249. Schlesinger M, Broman I, Lugassy G, et al. The complement system is defective in chronic lymphocytic leukemia patients and in their healthy relatives. *Leukemia* 1996;10:1509.
250. Veenstra H, Jacobs P, Dowdle EB. Abnormal association between invariant chain and HLA class II alpha and beta chains in chronic lymphocytic leukemia. *Cell Immunol* 1996;171:68.
251. Itala M, Vainio O, Remes K. Functional abnormalities in granulocytes predict susceptibility to bacterial infections in chronic lymphocytic leukemia. *Eur J Haematol* 1996;57:46.

252. Rezvany MR, Jeddi-Tehrani M, Osterborg A, et al. Oligoclonal TCRBV gene usage in B-cell chronic lymphocytic leukemia: major perturbations are preferentially seen within the CD4 T-cell subset. *Blood* 1999;94:1063.

253. Aittoniemi J, Miettinen A, Laine S, et al. Opsonising immunoglobulins and mannan-binding lectin in chronic lymphocytic leukemia. *Leuk Lymphoma* 1999;34:381.

254. Intravenous immunoglobulin for the prevention of infection in chronic lymphocytic leukemia. A randomized, controlled clinical trial. Cooperative Group for the Study of Immunoglobulin in Chronic Lymphocytic Leukemia. *N Engl J Med* 1988;319(14):902.

255. Griffiths H, Brennan V, Lea J, et al. Crossover study of immunoglobulin replacement therapy in patients with low-grade B-cell tumors. *Blood* 1989;73:366.

256. Lichtman MA, Rowe JM. Hyperleukocytic leukemias: rheological, clinical, and therapeutic considerations. *Blood* 1982;60:279.

257. Baer MR, Stein RS, Dessypris EN. Chronic lymphocytic leukemia with hyperleukocytosis: the hyperviscosity syndrome. *Cancer* 1985;56:2865.

258. Bernard M, Drenou B, Pangault C, et al. Spontaneous phenotypic and molecular blood remission in a case of chronic lymhocytic leukaemia. *Br J Haematol* 1999;107:213.

259. Effects of chlorambucil and therapeutic decision in initial forms of chronic lymphocytic leukemia (stage A): results of a randomized clinical trial on 612 patients. The French Cooperative Group on Chronic Lymphocytic Leukemia. *Blood* 1990;75(7):1414.

260. Han T, Ezdinli EZ, Shimaoka KS, et al. Chlorambucil vs. combined chlorambucil-corticosteroid therapy in chronic lymphocytic leukemia. *Cancer* 1973;31:5021.

261. Knospe WH, Loeb V Jr, Huguley CM Jr. Bi-weekly chlorambucil treatment of chronic lymphocytic leukemia. *Cancer* 1974;33:555.

262. Sawitsky A, Rai KR, Glidewell O, et al. Comparison of daily versus intermittent chlorambucil and prednisone therapy in the treatment of patients with chronic lymphocytic leukemia. *Blood* 1977;50:1049.

263. French Cooperative Group on Chronic Lymphocytic Leukemia. A randomized clinical trial of chlorambucil versus COP in stage B chronic lymphocytic leukemia. *Blood* 1990;75:1422.

264. Montserrat E, Alcala A, Parody R, et al. Treatment of chronic lymphocytic leukemia in advanced stages: a randomized trial comparing chlorambucil plus prednisone versus cyclophosphamide, vincristine and prednisone. *Cancer* 1985;56:2369.

265. Raphael B, Andersen JW, Silber R, et al. Comparison of chlorambucil and prednisone versus cyclophosphamide, vincristine, and prednisone as initial treatment for chronic lymphocytic leukemia: long-term follow-up of an Eastern Cooperative Oncology Group randomized clinical trial. *J Clin Oncol* 1991;9:770.

266. Criel A, Michaux L, De Wolf-Peeters C. The concept of typical and atypical chronic lymphocytic leukaemia. *Leuk Lymphoma* 1999;33:33.

267. Hallek M, Langenmayer I, Nerl C, et al. Elevated serum thymidine kinase levels identify a subgroup at high risk of disease progression in early, non-smoldering chronic lymphocytic leukemia. *Blood* 1999;93:1732.

268. Molica S, Levato D, Cascavilla N, et al. Clinico-prognostic implications of simultaneous increased serum levels of soluble CD23 and β2-microglobulin in B-cell chronic lymphocytic leukemia. *Eur J Haematol* 1999;62:117.

269. Chemotherapeutic options in chronic lymphocytic leukemia: a meta-analysis of the randomized trials: CLL Trialists' Collaborative Group. *J Natl Cancer Inst* 1999;91:861.

270. Sawitsky A, Rai KR, Glidewell O, et al. Comparison of daily versus intermittent chlorambucil and prednisone therapy in the treatment of patients with chronic lymphocytic leukemia. *Blood* 1977;50:1049.

271. Knospe WH, Loeb V, Huguly CM. Bi-weekly chlorambucil treatment of chronic lymphocytic leukemia. *Cancer* 1974;33:555.

272. Rai KR, Peterson B, Kolitz J, et al. A randomized comparison of fludarabine and chlorambucil for patients with previously untreated chronic lymphocytic leukemia. A CALGB, SWOG, CTG/NCIC-C and ECOG Inter-Group study. *Blood* 1996;88:141a.

273. Han T, Ezdinli EZ, Shimaoka K, et al. Chlorambucil versus combined chlorambucil-corticosteroid therapy in chronic lymphocytic leukemia. *Cancer* 1973;31:502.

274. Prognostic and therapeutic advances in CLL management: the experience of the French Cooperative Group. French Cooperative Group on chronic lymphocytic leukemia. *Semin Hematol* 1987;24(4):275.

275. A randomized clinical trial of chlorambucil versus COP in stage B chronic lymphocytic leukemia. The French Cooperative Group on chronic lymphocytic leukemia. *Blood* 1990;75(7):1422.

276. Effectiveness of "CHOP" regimen in advanced untreated chronic lymphocytic leukaemia. French Cooperative Group on chronic lymphocytic leukaemia. *Lancet* 1986;1(8494):1346.

277. Long-term results of the CHOP regimen in stage C chronic lymphocytic leukaemia. French Cooperative Group on chronic lymphocytic leukaemia. *Br J Haematol* 1989;73(3):334.

278. Hansen MM, Andersen E, Christensen BE, et al. CHOP versus prednisolone + chlorambucil in chronic lymphocytic leukemia (CLL): preliminary results of a randomized multicenter study. *Nouv Rev Fr Hematol* 1988;30(5–6):433.

279. Bennett JM. The use of 'CHOP' in the treatment of CLL. *Br J Haematol* 1990;74(4):546

280. Keating MJ. Chronic lymphocytic leukemia. *Semin Oncol* 1999;26:107.

281. The French Cooperative Group on CLL, Johnson S, Smith AG, Loffler H, et al. Multicentre prospective randomised trial of fludarabine versus cyclophosphamide, doxorubicin, and prednisone (CAP) for treatment of advanced-stage chronic lymphocytic leukaemia. *Lancet* 1996;347:1432.

282. Ross SR, McTavish D, Faulds D. Fludarabine. A review of its pharmacological properties and therapeutic potential in malignancy. *Drugs* 1993;45:737.

283. Keating MJ, O'Brien S, Kantarjian H, et al. Long-term follow-up of patients with chronic lymphocytic leukemia treated with fludarabine as a single agent. *Blood* 1993;81:2878.

284. Elliott MA, Letendre L, Li CY, et al. Chronic lymphocytic leukaemia with symptomatic diffuse central nervous system infiltration responding to therapy with systemic fludarabine. *Br J Haematol* 1999;104:689.

285. Sen K, Kalaycio M. Evan's syndrome precipitated by fludarabine therapy in a case of CLL (letter). *Am J Hematol* 1999;61:219.

286. Cheson BD, Vena DA, Barrett J, et al. Second malignancies as a consequence of nucleoside analog therapy for chronic lymphocytic leukemias. *J Clin Oncol* 1999;17:2454.

287. O'Brien S, Kantarjian H, Beran M, et al. Fludarabine and granulocyte colony-stimulating factor (G-CSF) in patients with chronic lymphocytic leukemia. *Leukemia* 1997;11:1631.

288. Giles FJ, O'Brien SM, Santini V, et al. Sequential cis-platinum and fludarabine with or without arabinosyl cytosine in patients failing prior fludarabine therapy for chronic lymphocytic leukemia: a phase II study. *Leuk Lymphoma* 1999;36:57.

289. Frewin R, Turner D, Tighe M, et al. Combination therapy with fludarabine and cyclophosphamide as salvage treatment in lymphoproliferative disorders. *Br J Haematol* 1999;104:612.

290. Grever M. Investigational chemotherapy of chronic lymphocytic leukemia. In: Gale RP, Rai K, eds. *Chronic lymphocytic leukemia: recent progress and future directions.* New York: Alan R Liss, 1987:399.

291. Dillman RO, Mick R, McIntyre OR. Pentostatin in chronic lymphocytic leukemia: a phase II trial of cancer and leukemia group B. *J Clin Oncol* 1989;7:433.

292. Ho AD, Thaler J, Stryckmans P, et al. Pentostatin in resistant chronic lymphocytic leukemia: a phase II trial of the European organization for research and treatment of cancer. *Proc Am Soc Clin Oncol* 1990;9:206(abst).

293. Dearden C, Catovsky D. Deoxycoformycin in the treatment of mature B-cell malignancies. *Br J Cancer* 1990;62:4.

294. Dearden CE, Matutes E, Catovsky D. Clinical overview of pentostatin (Nipent) use in lymphoid malignancies. *Semin Oncol* 2000;27[2 Suppl 5]:22.

295. Piro LD, Carrera CJ, Beutler E, et al. Chlorodeoxyadenosine: an effective new agent for the treatment of chronic lymphocytic leukemia. *Blood* 1988;72:1069.

296. Saven A, Carrera CJ, Carson DA, et al. Phase II trial update of 2-chlorodeoxyadenosine treatment of advanced chronic lymphocytic leukemia. *Proc Am Soc Clin Oncol* 1990;9:212(abst).

297. Robak T, Blasinska-Morawiec M, Blonski JZ, et al. 2-Chlorodeoxyadenosine (cladribine) in the treatment of elderly patients with B-cell chronic lymphocytic leukemia. *Leuk Lymphoma* 1999;34:151.

298. Robak T, Blonski JZ, Urbanska-Rys H, et al. 2-Chlorodeoxyadenosine (cladribine) in the treatment of patients with chronic lymphocytic leukemia 55 years old and younger. *Leukemia* 1999;13:518.

299. Robak T, Blonski JZ, Kasznicki M, et al. Cladribine with prednisone versus chlorambucil with prednisone as first-line therapy in chronic lymphocytic leukemia: report of a prospective, randomized, multicenter trial. *Blood* 2000;96:2723.

300. Foon KA. Biological response modifiers: the new immunotherapy. *Cancer Res* 1989;49:1621.

301. Dillman RO. Monoclonal antibodies for treating cancer. *Ann Intern Med* 1989;111:592.

302. Foon KA, Schroff RW, Bunn RA, et al. Effects of monoclonal antibody therapy in patients with chronic lymphocytic leukemia. *Blood* 1984;64:1085.

303. Miller RA, Maloney DG, McKillop J, et al. *In vivo* effect of murine hybridoma monoclonal antibody in a patient with T-CLL leukemia. *Blood* 1981;58:78.

304. Dillman RO, Shawler DL, Dillman JB, et al. Therapy of chronic lymphocytic leukemia and cutaneous T-cell lymphoma with T101 monoclonal antibody. *J Clin Oncol* 1984;8:881.

305. Foon KA, Bunn PA, Schroff RW, et al. Monoclonal antibody therapy of chronic lymphocytic leukemia and cutaneous T cell lymphoma: preliminary observations. In: Boss BE, Langman RE, Trowbridge IS, et al, eds. *Monoclonal antibodies and cancer.* Orlando: Academic Press, 1983:39.

306. Miller RA, Levy R. Response of cutaneous T cell lymphoma to therapy with hybridoma monoclonal antibody. *Lancet* 1981;2:226.

307. Miller RA, Oseroff AR, Stratte PT, et al. Monoclonal antibody therapeutic trials in seven patients with T-cell lymphoma. *Blood* 1983;62:988.

308. Hertler AA, Schlossman DM, Borowitz MJ, et al. A phase I study of T101-ricin A chain immunotoxin in refractory chronic lymphocytic leukemia. *J Biol Response Mod* 1988;7:97.

309. Laurent G, Pris J, Farcet JP, et al. Effects of therapy with T101 ricin A-chain immunotoxin in two leukemia patients. *Blood* 1986;67:1680.

310. DeNardo SJ, DeNardo GL, O'Grady LF, et al. Pilot study of radioimmunotherapy of B-cell lymphoma and leukemia using [131]I Lym-1 monoclonal antibody. *Ant Immun Radio* 1988;1:17.

311. Press OW, Eary JR, Badger CC, et al. Treatment of refractory non-Hodgkin's lymphoma with radiolabeled MB-1 (anti-CD37) antibody. *J Clin Oncol* 1989;7:1027.

312. Rosen S, Zimmer AM, Goldman-Neiken R, et al. Radioimmunodetection and radioimmunotherapy of cutaneous T-cell lymphomas using an ^{131}I-labeled monoclonal antibody: an Illinois Cancer Council Study. *J Clin Oncol* 1987;5:562.

313. Miller RA, Maloney DG, Warnke R, et al. Treatment of B-cell lymphoma with monoclonal anti-idiotype antibody. *N Engl J Med* 1982;306:517.

314. Meeker TC, Lowder JN, Maloney DG, et al. A clinical trial of anti-idiotype therapy for B-cell lymphocytic malignancies. *Blood* 1985;65:1349.

315. Miller RA, Hart S, Samoszuk M, et al. Shared idiotypes expressed by human B cell lymphomas. *N Engl J Med* 1989;321:851.
316. Chatterjee M, Barcos M, Han T, et al. Shared idiotype expression by chronic lymphocytic leukemia and B-cell lymphoma. *Blood* 1990;76:1825.
317. Maloney DG, Grillo-Lopez AJ, White CA, et al. IDEC-C2B8 (Rituximab) anti-CD20 monoclonal antibody therapy in patients with relapsed low-grade non-Hodgkin's lymphoma. *Blood* 1997;90:2188.
318. McLaughlin P, Grillo-Lopez AJ, Link BK, et al. Rituximab chimeric anti-CD20 monoclonal antibody therapy for relapsed indolent lymphoma: half of patients respond to a four-dose treatment program. *J Clin Oncol* 1998;16:2825.
319. Winkler U, Jensen M, Manzke O, et al. Cytokine-release syndrome in patients with B-cell chronic lymphocytic leukemia and high lymphocyte counts after treament with an anti-CD20 monoclonal antibody (Rituximab, IDEC-C2B8). *Blood* 1999;94:2217.
320. Lim LC, Koh LP, Tan P. Fatal cytokine release syndrome with chimeric anti-CD20 monoclonal antibody rituximab in a 71-year patient with chronic lymphocytic leukemia (letter). *J Clin Oncol* 1999;17:1962.
321. Osterborg A, Dyer MJ, Bunjes D, et al. Phase II multicenter study of human CD52 antibody in previously treated chronic lymphocytic leukemia: European Study Group of CAMPATH-1H Treatment in Chronic Lynphocytic Leukemia. *J Clin Oncol* 1997;15:1567.
322. Shen S, DeNardo GL, O'Donnell RT, et al. Impact of splenomegaly on therapeutic response and I-131-LYM-1 dosimetry in patients with B-lymphocytic malignancies. *Cancer* 1997;80:2553.
323. DeNardo GL, Lamborn KR, Goldstein DS, et al. Increased survival associated with radiolabeled Lym-1 therapy for non-Hodgkin's lymphoma and chronic lymphocytic leukemia. *Cancer* 1997;80:2706.
324. DeNardo GL, DeNardo SJ, Shen S, et al. Factors affecting ¹³¹I-Lym-1 pharmacokinetics and radiation dosimetry in patients with non-Hodgkin's lymphoma and chronic lymphocytic leukemia. *J Nucl Med* 1999;40:1317.
325. Ostlund L, Einhorn S, Robert KH, et al. Chronic B-lymphocytic leukemia cells proliferate and differentiate following exposure to interferon *in vitro*. *Blood* 1986;67:152.
326. Foon KA, Bottino GC, Abrams PG, et al. Phase II trials of recombinant leukocyte A interferon in patients with advanced chronic lymphocytic leukemia. *Am J Med* 1985;78:216.
327. Roth MS, Foon KA. Alpha interferon in the treatment of hematologic malignancies. *Am J Med* 1986;67:152.
328. Foon KA, Sherwin SA, Abrams PG, et al. Treatment of advanced non-Hodgkin's lymphoma with recombinant leukocyte A interferon. *N Engl J Med* 1984;311:1148.
329. Louie AC, Gallagher JG, Sikora K, et al. Follow-up observations on the effect of human leukocyte interferon on non-Hodgkin's lymphoma. *Blood* 1981;58:712.
330. Merigan TC, Sikora K, Breeden JH, et al. Preliminary observations on the effect of human leukocyte interferon in non-Hodgkin's lymphoma. *N Engl J Med* 1978;299:1449.
331. Bunn PA Jr, Foon KA, Ihde DC, et al. Recombinant leukocyte A interferon: an active agent in advanced cutaneous T-cell lymphomas. *Ann Intern Med* 1984;101:484.
332. Foon KA, Maluish AE, Abrams PG, et al. Recombinant leukocyte A interferon therapy for advanced hairy cell leukemia: therapeutic and immunologic results. *Am J Med* 1986;80:351.
333. Quesada JR, Reuben J, Manning JR, et al. Alpha interferon for induction of remission in hairy-cell leukemia. *N Engl J Med* 1984;301:15.
334. Ratain MJ, Golomb HM, Vardiman JW, et al. Treatment of hairy cell leukemia with recombinant alpha₂ interferon. *Blood* 1985;65:644.
335. Jacobs A, Champlin RE, Golde DW. Recombinant alpha-2-interferon for hairy cell leukemia. *Blood* 1985;65:1017.
336. Rozman C, Montserrat E, Vinolas N, et al. Recombinant alpha-interferon in the treatment of B chronic lymphocytic leukemia in early stages. *Blood* 1988;71:1295.
337. Pangalis GA, Griva E. Recombinant alpha-2b-interferon in untreated stages A and B chronic lymphocytic leukemia: a preliminary report. *Cancer* 1988;61:869.
338. Ziegler-Heltbrock HW, Schlag F, Fleiger D, et al. Favorable response of early stage B CLL patients to treatment with IFN-alpha. *Blood* 1989;73:1426.
339. Adler S, Stutzman L, Sokal JE, et al. Splenectomy for hematology depression in lymphocytic lymphoma and leukemia. *Cancer* 1975;35:521.
340. Merl SA, Theodorakis ME, Goldbert J, et al. Splenectomy for thrombocytopenia in chronic lymphocytic leukemia. *Am J Hematol* 1983;15:153.
341. Thiruvengadam R, Piedmonte M, Barcos M, et al. Survival benefit of splenectomy in advanced chronic lymphocytic leukemia. *Blood* 1989;74:80A(abst).
342. Rabinowe SN, Soiffer RJ, Nadler LE. Innovative treatment strategies for chronic lymphocytic leukemia: monoclonal antibodies, immunoconjugates and bone marrow transplantation. In: Cheson BD, ed. *Chronic lymphocytic leukemia: scientific advances and clinical developments*. New York: Marcel Dekker, 1993:337.
343. Khouri IF, Keating MJ, Vriesendorp H, et al. Autologous and allogeneic bone marrow transplantation for chronic lymphocytic leukemia: preliminary results. *J Clin Oncol* 1994;12:748.
344. Michallet M, Archimbaud E, Juliusson G, et al. Autologous transplants in chronic lymphocytic leukemia: report on 18 cases. *Bone Marrow Transplant* 1995;15[Suppl 2]:S11(abst).
345. Michallet M, Corront B, Molina L, et al. Allogeneic bone marrow transplantation in chronic lymphocytic leukemia: 17 cases—report of the EBMT. *Leuk Lymphoma* 1991;5:127.
346. Michallet M, Archimbaud E, Bandini G, et al. HLA-Identical sibling bone marrow transplantation in younger patients with chronic lymphocytic leukemia. *Ann Intern Med* 1996;124:311.
347. Khouri IF, Keating M, Korbling M, et al. Transplant–lite: induction of graft-versus-malignancy using fludarabine-based nonablative chemotherapy and allogeneic blood progenitor-cell transplantation as treatment for lymphoid malignancies. *J Clin Oncol* 1998;16:2817.
348. Kalyanaraman VS, Sarnagadharan MG, Robert-Guroff M, et al. A new subtype of human T-cell leukemia virus (HTLV-2) associated with a T-cell variant of hairy cell leukemia. *Science* 1982;218:561.
349. Melo JV, Foroni L, Babapulle B, et al. Prolymphocytic leukemia of B cell type: rearranged immunoglobulin (Ig) genes with defective Ig production. *Blood* 1985;66:391.
350. Volk JR, Kjeldsberg CR, Eyre HJ, et al. T-cell prolymphocytic leukemia: clinical and immunologic characterization. *Cancer* 1983;52:2049.
351. Matutes E, Brito-Babapulle V, Swansbury J, et al. Clinical and laboratory features of T-prolymphocytic leukemia. *Blood* 1991;78:3269.
352. Sadamori N, Han T, Minowada J, et al. Possible specific chromosome change in prolymphocytic leukemia. *Blood* 1983;62:729.
353. Ueshima Y, Rowley JD, Variakojis D, et al. Cytogenetic studies in patients with chronic T-cell leukemia/lymphoma. *Blood* 1984;63:1028.
354. Zech L, Cahrton G, Hammarström L, et al. Inversion of chromosome 14 marks human T-cell chronic lymphocytic leukaemia. *Nature* 1984;308:858.
355. Croce CM, Isobe M, Polumbo A, et al. Gene for alpha chain of human T-cell receptor: location on chromosome 14 region involved in T-cell neoplasms. *Science* 1985;227:1044.
356. Polliack A, Leizerowitz R, Berrebi A, et al. Prolymphocytic leukaemia: surface morphology in 21 cases as seen by scanning electron microscopy and comparison with B-type CLL and CLL in prolymphocytoid transformation. *Br J Haematol* 1984;57:577.
357. Taylor HG, Butler WM, Rhoads J, et al. Prolymphocytic leukemia: treatment with combination chemotherapy to include doxorubicin. *Cancer* 1982;49:1524.
358. Konig E, Meusers P, Brittinger G. Efficacy of doxorubicin in prolymphocytic leukaemia. *Br J Haematol* 1979;42:487.
359. Sibbald R, Catovsky D. Complete remission in prolymphocytic leukaemia with the combination chemotherapy CHOP. *Br J Haematol* 1979;42:488.
360. Oscier DG, Catovsky D, Errington RD, et al. Splenic irradiation in B-prolymphocytic leukaemia. *Br J Haematol* 1981;48:577.
361. Dohner H, Ho AD, Thaler J, et al. Pentostatin in prolymphocytic leukemia: phase II trial of the European Organization for Research and Treatment of Cancer Leukemia Cooperative Study Group. *J Natl Cancer Inst* 1993;85:658.
362. Kantarjian HM, Childs C, O'Brien S, et al. Efficacy of fludarabine in patients with prolymphocytic leukemia and the prolymphocytoid variant of chronic lymphocytic leukemia. *Am J Med* 1991;90:223.
363. Lorand-Metze I, Oliveira GB, Aranha FJP. Treatment of prolymphocytic leukemia with cladribine. *Am Hematol* 1998;76:85.
364. Palomera L, Domingo JM, Agullo JA, et al. Complete remission in T-cell prolymphocytic leukemia with 2-chlorodeoxyadenosine. *J Clin Oncol* 1995;13:1284.
365. Barton K, Larson RA, O'Brien S, et al. Rapid response of B-cell prolymphocytic leukemia to 2-chlorodeoxyadenosine. *J Clin Oncol* 1992;10:1821.
366. Pawson R, Dyer MJS, Barge R, et al. Treatment of T-cell prolymphocytic leukemia. *J Clin Oncol* 1997;15:2667.
367. Catovsky D, Pettit JE, Galetto J, et al. The B-lymphocyte nature of the hairy cell of leukemic reticuloendotheliosis. *Br J Haematol* 1974;26:29.
368. Jansen J, LeBien TW, Kersey JH. The phenotype of the neoplastic cells of hairy cell leukemia studies with monoclonal antibodies. *Blood* 1982;59:609.
369. Worman CP, Brooks DA, Hogg N, et al. The nature of hairy cells: a study with a panel of monoclonal antibodies. *Scand J Haematol* 1983;30:223.
370. Divine M, Farcet JP, Gourdin MF, et al. Phenotype study of fresh and cultured hairy cells with the use of immunologic markers and electron microscopy. *Blood* 1984;64:547.
371. Anderson KC, Park EK, Bates MP, et al. Antigens on human plasma cells identified by monoclonal antibodies. *J Immunol* 1983;130:1132.
372. Anderson KA, Boyd AW, Fisher DC, et al. Hairy cell leukemia: a tumor of pre-plasma cells. *Blood* 1985;65:620.
373. Cleary ML, Woods GS, Warnke R, et al. Immunoglobulin gene rearrangements in hairy cell leukemia. *Blood* 1984;64:99.
374. Korsmeyer SJ, Greene WC, Cossman J, et al. Rearrangement and expression of immunoglobulin genes and expression of Tac antigen in hairy cell leukemia. *Proc Natl Acad Sci U S A* 1983;80:4522.
375. Posnett DN, Chiorazzi N, Kunkel HG. Monoclonal antibodies with specificity for hairy cell leukemia cells. *J Clin Invest* 1982;70:254.
376. Foon KA, Robbins BA, Ellison DJ, et al. Immunodiagnosis of lymphoid malignancies. *Adv Oncol Lymphoma* 1991;3:3.
377. Schwarting R, Stein H, Wang CY. The monoclonal antibodies alpha S-HCL1 (alpha Leu- M5) allow the diagnosis of hairy cell leukemia. *Blood* 1985;65:974.
378. Saxon A, Stevens RH, Golde DW. T-lymphocyte variant of hairy-cell leukemia. *Ann Intern Med* 1978;88:323.
379. Li CY, Yam LT, Lam KW. Studies of acid phosphatase isoenzymes in human leukocytes: demonstration of isoenzyme cell specificity. *J Histochem Cytochem* 1970;18:901.
380. Golomb H. Hairy cell leukemia: an unusual lymphoproliferative disease—a study of 24 patients. *Cancer* 1978;42:946.
381. Golomb H, Strehl S, Oleske D, et al. Prognostic significance of immunologic phenotype in hairy cell leukemia: does it exist? *Blood* 1985;66:1358.

382. Jansen J, Schuit HE, Hermans J, et al. Prognostic significance of immunologic phenotype in hairy cell leukemia. *Blood* 1984;63:1241.
383. Ohyashiki K, Ohyashiki JH, Takeuchi J, et al. Cytogenetic studies in hairy cell leukemia. *Cancer Genet Cytogenet* 1987;24:109.
384. Brito-Babapulle V, Pittman S, Melo JV, et al. The 14q+ marker in hairy cell leukaemia: a cytogenetic study of 15 cases. *Leuk Res* 1986;10:131.
385. Ueshima Y, Alimena G, Rowley JD, et al. Cytogenetic studies in patients with hairy cell leukemia. *Hematol Oncol* 1983;1:215.
386. Golomb HM. Hairy cell leukemia: lessons learned in twenty-five years. *J Clin Oncol* 1983;1:652.
387. Bouroncle BA. Leukemic reticuloendotheliosis (hairy cell leukemia). *Blood* 1979;53:3:412.
388. Catovsky D, Pettit JE, Galton DAG, et al. Leukaemic reticuloendotheliosis ('Hairy' cell leukaemia): a distinct clinico-pathological entity. *Br J Haematol* 1974;26:9.
389. Fitzpatrick J, O'Donnell A, DiLoro A, et al. Serum M-proteins in hairy cell leukemia, chronic lymphocytic leukemia and free light chain myeloma causing high resolution electropheresis/immunofixation. *Blood* 1986;69:208A.
390. Rosove MH, Naeim F, Harwig S, et al. Severe platelet dysfunction in hairy cell leukemia with improvement after splenectomy. *Blood* 1980;55:903.
391. Cawley JC, Burns GF, Hayhoe RGH. A chronic lymphoproliferative disorder with distinctive features: a distinct variant of hairy-cell leukemia. *Leuk Res* 1980;4:547.
392. Golomb HM, Jacobs A, Fefer A, et al. Alpha-2 interferon therapy of hairy-cell leukemia: a multicenter study of 64 patients. *J Clin Oncol* 1986:4:900.
393. Steis RG, Smith JW, Urba WJ, et al. Resistance to recombinant interferon alpha 2a in hairy cell leukemia associated with neutralizing antiinterferon antibodies. *N Engl J Med* 1988;318:1409.
394. Ratain MJ, Golomb HM, Bardawil RG, et al. Durability of responses to interferon alfa-2b in advanced hairy cell leukemia. *Blood* 1987;69:872.
395. Sainati L, Matutes E, Mulligan S, et al. A variant form of hairy cell leukemia resistant to alpha-interferon: clinical and phenotypic characteristics of 17 patients. *Blood* 1990;76:157.
396. Spiers SDC, Moore D, Cassileth PA, et al. Hairy cell leukemia: complete remission with pentostatin (2'deoxycoformycin). *N Engl J Med* 1987;316:825.
397. Urba WJ, Baseler MW, Kopp WC, et al. Deoxycoformycin-induced immunosuppression in patients with hairy cell leukemia. *Blood* 1989;73:38.
398. Piro LD, Carrera CJ, Carson DA, et al. Lasting remissions in hairy cell leukemia induced by a single infusion of 2-chlorodeoxyadenosine. *N Engl J Med* 1990;322:117.
399. Johnston JB, Eisenhauer E, Wainman N, et al. Long-term outcome following treatment of hairy cell leukemia with pentostatin: A National Cancer Institute of Canada Study. *Semin Oncol* 2000;27:32.
400. Hoffman MA, Janson D, Rose E, et al. Treatment of hairy cell leukemia with cladribine: response, toxicity, and long-term follow-up. *J Clin Oncol* 1997;15:1138.
401. Tallman MS, Hakimian D, Kopecky KJ, et al. Minimal residual disease in patients with hairy cell leukemia in complete remission treated with 2-chlorodeoxyadenosine or 2-deoxycoformycin and prediction of early relapse. *Clin Cancer Res* 1999;5:1665.
402. Uchiyama T, Yodoi J, Sagawa K, et al. Adult T-cell leukemia: clinical and hematologic features of 16 cases. *Blood* 1977;50:481.
403. Bunn PA, Schechter GP, Jaffe E, et al. Clinical course of retrovirus associated adult T-cell lymphoma in the United States: staging, evaluation and management. *N Engl J Med* 1983;309:257.
404. Catovsky D, Greaves MF, Rose M, et al. Adult T-cell lymphoma/leukaemia in blacks from the West Indies. *Lancet* 1982;1:639.
405. Broder S, Bunn PA Jr, Jaffe ES, et al. NIH conference. T-cell lymphoproliferative syndrome associated with human T-cell leukemia/lymphoma virus. *Ann Intern Med* 1984;100(4):543.
406. Blattner WA, Kalyanaraman VS, Robert-Guroff M, et al. The human type-C retrovirus HTLV, in blacks from the Caribbean region, and relationship to adult T-cell leukemia/lymphoma. *Int J Cancer* 1982;30:257.
407. Posner LE, Robert-Guroff M, Kalyanaraman VS, et al. Natural antibodies to the human T-cell lymphoma virus in patients with T-cell lymphomas. *J Exp Med* 1981;154:333.
408. Kalyanaraman VS, Sarngadharan MG, Bunn PA, et al. Antibodies in human sera reactive against an internal structural protein of human T-cell lymphoma virus. *Nature* 1981;294:271.
409. Greenberg SJ, Tendler CL, Manns A, et al. Altered cellular gene expression in human retroviral-associated leukemogenesis. In: Blattner W, ed. *Current issues in human retrovirology: HTLV-I.* New York: Raven Press, 1990:87.
410. Wong-Staal F, Gallo RC. The family of human T-lymphotropic leukemia viruses: HTLV-I as the cause of adult T-cell leukemia and HTLV-III as the cause of acquired immunodeficiency syndrome. *Blood* 1985;65:253.
411. Blattner WA, Clark JW, Gibbs WN, et al. Human T cell leukemia/lymphoma virus: epidemiology and relationship to human malignancy. In: Gallo RC, Essex M, Gros L, eds. *Human T-cell leukemia/lymphoma virus.* New York: Cold Spring Harbor Laboratory, 1984:267.
412. Saxinger W, Blattner WA, Levine PH, et al. Human T-cell leukemia virus (HTLV-1) antibodies in Africa. *Science* 1984;225:1473.
413. Robert-Guroff M, Kalyanaraman VS, Blattner WA, et al. Evidence for human T-cell lymphoma-leukemia virus infection of family members of human T cell lymphoma-leukemia virus positive T cell leukemia-lymphoma patients. *J Exp Med* 1983;157:248.
414. Sarin PS, Aoki T, Shibata A, et al. High incidence of human type-C retrovirus (HTLV) in family members of a HTLV-positive Japanese T cell leukemia patient. *Proc Natl Acad Sci U S A* 1983;80:2370.
415. Homma T, Kanki PJ, King NW, et al. Lymphoma in macaques: association with virus of human T lymphotropic family. *Science* 1984;225:716.
416. Ferrer JF, Abt DA, Bhatt DM, et al. Studies on the relationship between infection with bovine C-type virus, leukemia and persistent lymphocytes in cattle. *Cancer Res* 1974;34:893.
417. Kalyanaraman VS, Sarngadharan MG, Poiesz BJ, et al. Immunological properties of a type C retrovirus isolated from cultured human T-lymphoma cells and comparison to other mammalian retroviruses. *J Virol* 1981;38:906.
418. Robert-Guroff M, Ruscetti FW, Posner LE, et al. Dectection of the human T-cell lymphoma, virus p19 in cells of some patients with cutaneous T-cell lymphoma and leukemia using a monoclonal antibody. *J Exp Med* 1981;154:1957.
419. Miyoshi I, Kubonishi I, Yoshimoto S, et al. Type C virus particles in a cord T-cell line derived by co-cultivating normal human leukocytes and human leukaemic T cells. *Nature* 1981;294:770.
420. Popovic M, Lange-Wantzin G, Sarin PS, et al. Transformation of human umbilical cord blood T cells by human T-cell leukemia/lymphoma virus. *Proc Natl Acad Sci U S A* 1983;80:5402.
421. Salahuddin SZ, Markham PD, Lindner SG, et al. Lymphokine production by cultured human T-cells transformed by human T-cell leukemia-lymphoma virus-I. *Science* 1984;223:703.
422. Popovic M, Flomenberg N, Volkman DJ, et al. Alteration of T-helper cell functions by infection with HTLV-I and HTLV-II. *Science* 1984;226:459.
423. Mitsuya H, Matis LA, Megson M, et al. Generation of the HLA-restricted cytotoxic T-cell line reactive against cultured tumor cells from a patient infected with human T-cell leukemia/lymphoma virus. *J Exp Med* 1983;158:994.
424. Morimoto C, Matsuyama T, Oshige C, et al. Functional and phenotypic studies of Japanese adult T-cell leukemia cells. *J Clin Invest* 1985;75:836.
425. Waldmann TA, Greene WC, Sarin PS, et al. Functional and phenotypic comparison of human T cell leukemia/lymphoma virus positive adult T cell leukemia with human T cell leukemia/lymphoma virus negative Sézary leukemia, and their distinction using Anti-Tac. *J Clin Invest* 1984;73:1711.
426. Flug F, Pelicci P-G, Bonetti F, et al. T-cell receptor gene rearrangements as markers of lineage and clonality in T cell neoplasms. *Proc Natl Acad Sci U S A* 1985;82:3460.
427. Waldmann TA, David MM, Bongiovanni KF, et al. Rearrangements of genes for the antigen receptor on T cells as markers of lineage and clonality in human lymphoid neoplasms. *N Engl J Med* 1985;313:776.
428. Bertness V, Mirsch I, Hollis G, et al. T-cell receptor gene rearrangements as clinical markers of human T-cell lymphomas. *N Engl J Med* 1985;313:534.
429. Aisenberg AC, Krontiris TG, Mak TW, et al. Rearrangement of the gene for the beta chain of the T-cell receptor in T-cell chronic lymphocytic leukemia and related disorders. *N Engl J Med* 1985;313:530.
430. Sanada I, Tanaka R, Kumagai E, et al. Chromosomal aberrations in adult T cell leukemia: relationship to the clinical severity. *Blood* 1985;65:649.
431. Verma RS, Macera MJ, Krishnamurthy M, et al. Chromosomal abnormalities in adult T-cell leukemia/lymphoma (ATL). *J Cancer Res Clin Oncol* 1987;113(2):892.
432. Miyamoto K, Tomita N, Ishii A, et al. Specific abnormalities of chromosome 14 in patients with acute type of adult T-cell leukemia/lymphoma. *Int J Cancer* 1987;40:461.
433. Shiraishi Y, Taguchi T, Kubonishi I, et al. Chromosome abnormalities, sister chromatid exchanges, and cell cycle analysis in phytohemagglutinin-stimulated adult T cell leukemia lymphocytes. *Cancer Genet Cytogenet* 1985;15:65.
434. Whang-Peng J, Bunn PA, Knutsen T, et al. Cytogenetic studies in human T-cell lymphoma virus (HTLV) positive leukemia-lymphoma in the United States. *J Natl Cancer Inst* 1985;74:357.
435. Shimoyama M, Abe T, Miyamoto K, et al. Chromosome aberrations and clinical features of adult T cell leukemia-lymphoma not associated with human T cell leukemia virus type I. *Blood* 1987;69:984.
436. Brito-Babapulle V, Matutes E, Parreira L, et al. Abnormalities of chromosome 7q and Tac expression in T cell leukemias. *Blood* 1986;67:516.
437. Shimoyama M. Diagnostic criteria and classification of clinical subtypes of adult T-cell leukaemia-lymphoma. A report from the Lymphoma Study Group (1984-87). *Br J Haematol* 1991;79(3):428.
438. Yamaguchi K, Nishimura H, Kohrogi H, et al. A proposal for smoldering adult T-cell leukemia: a clinicopathologic study of five cases. *Blood* 1983;62:758.
439. Waldmann TA, Goldman CK, Bongiovanni KF, et al. Therapy of patients with human T-cell lymphotropic virus I-induced adult T-cell leukemia with anti-Tac, a monoclonal antibody to the receptor for interleukin-2. *Blood* 1988;72:1805.
440. Waldman TA, White JD, Carrasquillo JA, et al. Radioimmunotherapy of interleukin-2R alpha-expressing adult T-cell leukemia with Yttrium-90-labeled anti-Tac. *Blood* 1995;86:4063.
441. Tamura K, Makino S, Araki, Y, et al. Recombinant interferon beta and gamma in the treatment of adult T-cell leukemia. *Cancer* 1987;59:1069.
442. Saigo K, Shiozawa S, Shiozawa K, et al. Alpha-interferon treatment for adult T cell leukemia: low levels of circulating alpha-interferon and its clinical effectiveness. *Blut* 1988;56:83.
443. Daenen S, Rojer RA, Smit JW, et al. Successful chemotherapy with deoxycoformycin in adult T-cell lymphoma-leukemia. *Br J Haematol* 1984;58:723.
444. Gill PS, Harrington W Jr, Kaplan MH, et al. Treatment of adult T-cell leukemia-lymphoma with a combination of interferon alfa and zidovudine. *N Engl J Med* 1995;332(26):1744.

445. Winkler CF, Bunn PA. Cutaneous T-cell lymphoma: a review. *Crit Rev Oncol Hematol* 1983;1:49.

446. Fischmann AB, Bunn PA, Guccion JG, et al. Exposure to chemicals, physical agents and biologic agents in mycosis fungoides and Sézary syndrome. *Cancer Treat Rep* 1979;63:591.

447. Morales Suarez-Varela MM, Llopis Gonzalez A, Marquina Vila A, et al. Mycosis fungoides: review of epidemiological observations. *Dermatology* 2000;201:21.

448. Cohen SR. Mycosis fungoides: clinicopathologic relationships, survival and therapy in 59 patients with observations on occupation as a new prognostic factor. *Cancer* 1980;46:2654.

449. Manzari V, Gismondi A, Barillari G, et al. HTLV-V: a new human retrovirus isolated in a tac-negative T cell lymphoma/leukemia. *Science* 1987;238:1581.

450. Haynes BF, Metzgar RS, Minna JD, et al. Phenotypic characterization of cutaneous T cell lymphoma. *N Engl J Med* 1981;304:1319.

451. Kung PC, Berger CL, Goldstein G, et al. Cutaneous T-cell lymphoma: characterization by monoclonal antibodies. *Blood* 1981;57:261.

452. Schroff RW, Foon KA, Billing RJ, et al. Immunologic classification of lymphocytic leukemias based on monoclonal antibody-defined cell surface antigens. *Blood* 1982;59:207.

453. Broder S, Edelson RL, Lutzner M, et al. The Sézary syndrome: a malignant proliferation of helper T cells. *J Clin Invest* 1976;58:1297.

454. Haynes BF, Hensley LL, Jegasothy BV. Phenotypic characterization of skin-infiltrating T cells in cutaneous T-cell lymphoma: comparison with benign cutaneous T-cell infiltrates. *Blood* 1982;60:463.

455. Whang-Peng J, Bunn PA, Knutsen T, et al. Clinical implications of cytogenetic studies in cutaneous T-cell lymphoma (CTCL). *Cancer* 1982;50:1139.

456. Shapiro PE, Warburton D, Berger CL, et al. Clonal chromosomal abnormalities in cutaneous T-cell lymphoma. *Cancer Genet Cytogenet* 1987;28:267.

457. Epstein EH Jr, Levin DL, Croft JD Jr, et al. Mycosis fungoides: survival, prognostic features, response to therapy, and autopsy findings. *Medicine* 1972;51:61.

458. Sézary A, Bouvrain Y. Etythodermic avec presence de cellules monstrueuses dan le derme et dans le lang circulant. *Bull Soc Fr Dermatol Syph* 1938;45:254.

459. Long JC, Mihm MC. Mycosis fungoides with extracutaneous dissemination: a distinct clinicopathologic entity. *Cancer* 1974;34:1745.

460. Rappaport H, Thomas LB. Mycosis fungoides: the pathology of extracutaneous involvement. *Cancer* 1974;34:1198.

461. Roberts WC, Glancy DL, DeVita VT Jr. Heart in malignant lymphoma (Hodgkin's disease, lymphosarcoma, reticulum cell sarcoma and mycosis fungoides): a study of 196 autopsy cases. *Am J Cardiol* 1968;22:85.

462. Greer KE, Legum LL, Hess CE. Multiple osteolytic lesions in a patient with mycosis fungoides. *Arch Dermatol* 1977;113:1242.

463. O'Reilly GV, Clark TM, Crum CP. Skeletal involvement in mycosis fungoides. *AJR Am J Roentgenol* 1977;129:741.

464. Keltner JL, Fritsch E, Cykiert RC, et al. Mycosis fungoides: intraocular and central nervous system involvement. *Arch Ophthalmol* 1977;95:545.

465. Kitchen CK. Mycosis fungoides keratitis. *Am J Ophthalmol* 1963;55:758.

466. Wolter JR, Leenhouts TM, Hendricks RC. Corneal involvement in mycosis fungoides. *Am J Ophthalmol* 1963;55:317.

467. Lundberg WB, Cadman EC, Skeel RT. Leptomeningeal mycosis fungoides. *Cancer* 1976;38:2149.

468. Hauch TW, Shelbourne JD, Cohen HJ, et al. Meningeal mycosis fungoides: clinical and cellular characteristics. *Ann Intern Med* 1975;82:499.

469. Posner LE, Fossieck BE, Eddy JL, et al. Septicemic complications of the cutaneous T-cell lymphomas. *Arch Dermatol* 1981;71:210.

470. Vonderheid EC, Milstein HJ, Thompson KD, et al. Chronic herpes simplex infection in cutaneous T-cell lymphomas. *Arch Dermatol* 1980;116:1018.

471. Vonderheid EC, Vanvoorstvader PC. Herpes zoster-varicella in cutaneous T-cell lymphomas. *Arch Dermatol* 1980;116:408.

472. Bunn PA, Huberman MS, Whang-Peng J, et al. Prospective staging evaluation of patients with cutaneous T-cell lymphomas: demonstration of high frequency of extra-cutaneous dissemination. *Ann Intern Med* 1980;93:223.

473. Block JB, Edgcomb J, Eisen A, et al. Mycosis fungoides: natural history and aspects of its relationship to other malignant lymphomas. *Am J Med* 1963;34:228.

474. Vonderheid EC, Van Scott EJ, Wallner PE, et al. A 10 year experience with topical mechlorethamine for mycosis fungoides: comparison with patients treated by total-skin electron beam radiation therapy. *Cancer Treat Rep* 1979;63:681.

475. Hoppe RT, Cox RS, Fuks Z, et al. Electron-beam therapy for mycosis fungoides: the Stanford University experience. *Cancer Treat Rep* 1979;63:691.

476. Lamberg SI, Green SB, Byar DP, et al. Status report of 376 mycosis fungoides patients at 4 years: Mycosis Fungoides Cooperative Group. *Cancer Treat Rep* 1979;63:701.

477. Winkelmann RK. Clinical studies of T-cell erythroderma in the Sézary syndrome. *Mayo Clin Proc* 1974;49:519.

478. Green SB, Byar DP, Lamberg SI. Prognostic variables in mycosis fungoides. *Cancer* 1981;47:2671.

479. Castellino RA, Hoppe RT, Blank N, et al. Experience with lymphography in patients with mycosis fungoides. *Cancer Treat Rep* 1979;63:581.

480. Hamminga L, Mulder JD, Evans C, et al. Staging lymphography with respect to lymph node histology, treatment, and follow-up in patients with mycosis fungoides. *Cancer* 1981;47:692.

481. Schechter GP, Bunn PA Jr, Fischmann AB, et al. Blood and lymph node T-lymphocyte in cutaneous T-cell lymphoma: evaluation by light microscopy. *Cancer Treat Rep* 1979;63:571.

482. Moran EM, Walher JR, Aronson IK, et al. Clinical significance of circulating Sézary cells in mycosis fungoides. *Proc AACR ASCO* 1977;18:276.

483. Fuks ZY, Bagshaw MA, Farber EM. Prognostic signs and the management of the mycosis fungoides. *Cancer* 1974;32:1385.

484. Deneau DG, Wood GS, Beckstead J, et al. Woringer-Kolopp disease (Pagetoid reticulosis): four cases with histopathologic ultrastructural, and immunohistologic observations. *Arch Dermatol* 1984;120:1045.

485. Ketron LW, Goodman MH. Multiple lesions of skin apparently of epithelial origin resembling clinically mycosis fungoides: report of a case. *Arch Dermatol Syph* 1931;24:758.

486. Wood GS, Weiss LM, Hu C-H, et al. T-cell antigen deficiencies and clonal rearrangements of T-cell receptor genes in pagetoid recitulosis (Woringer-Kolopp disease). *N Engl J Med* 1988;318:164.

487. Vonderheid EC, Van Scott EJ, Johnson WC, et al. Topical chemotherapy and immunotherapy of mycosis fungoides: intermediate term results. *Arch Dermatol* 1977;113:454.

488. Du Vivier A, Vonderheid EC, Van Scott EJ, et al. Mycosis fungoides, nitrogen mustard and skin cancer. *Br J Dermatol* 1978;99(1):61.

489. Gilchrest BA. Methoxsalen photochemotherapy for mycosis fungoides. *Cancer Treat Rep* 1979;63:633.

490. Roenigk HH. Photochemotherapy for mycosis fungoides: long-term follow-up study. *Cancer Treat Rep* 1979;63:699.

491. Briffa DV, Warin AP, Harrington CI, et al. Photochemotherapy in mycosis fungoides: a study of 73 patients. *Lancet* 1980;2:49.

492. Lo TCM, Salzman FA, Moschella SL, et al. Whole body surface electron irradiation in the treatment of mycosis fungoides: an evaluation of 200 patients. *Radiology* 1979;130:453.

493. Proctor MS, Porice NN, Cox AJ, et al. Subcutaneous mycosis fungoides. *Arch Dermatol* 1978;114:1009.

494. Pineda AA, Winkelmann RN. Leukapheresis in the treatment of Sézary syndrome. *J Am Acad Dermatol* 1981;5:544.

495. Edelson R, Facktor M, Andrews A, et al. Successful management of the Sézary syndrome: mobilization and removal of extravascular neoplastic T-cells by leukapheresis. *N Engl J Med* 1974;291:293.

496. Edelson R, Berger C, Gasparro F, et al. Treatment of cutaneous T-cell lymphoma by extracorporeal photochemotherapy: preliminary results. *N Engl J Med* 1987;316:297.

497. Zic J, Arzubiaga C, Salhany KE, et al. Extracorporeal photopheresis for the treatment of cutaneous T-cell lymphoma. *J Am Acad Dermatol* 1992;27:729.

498. Heald PW, Perez MI, Christensen I, et al. Photophoresis therapy of cutaneous T-cell lymphoma: the Yale-New Haven Hospital experience. *Yale J Biol Med* 1989;62:629.

499. Koh KH, Davis BE, Meola T, et al. Extracorporeal photopheresis for the treatment of 34 patients with cutaneous T-cell lymphoma (CTCL). *J Invest Dermatol* 1994;102:567.

500. Duvic M, Hester JP, Lemark NA, et al. Photopheresis therapy for the treatment of cutaneous T-cell lymphoma. *J Am Acad Dermatol* 1996;35:573.

501. Lim HW, Edelson RL. Photopheresis for the treatment of cutaneous T-cell lymphoma. *Hematol Oncol Clin North Am* 1995;9:1117.

502. Wilson LD, Jones GW, Kim D, et al. Experience with total skin electron beam therapy in combination with extracorporeal photopheresis in the management of patients with erythrodermic (T4) mycosis fungoides. *J Am Acad Dermatol* 2000;43:54.

503. Kierland RR, Watkins CH, Shullenberger CC. The use of nitrogen mustard in the treatment of mycosis fungoides. *J Invest Dermatol* 1947;9/10:195.

504. Van Scott EJ, Grekin DA, Kalmanson JD, et al. Frequent low doses of intravenous mechlorethamine for late-stage mycosis fungoides lymphoma. *Cancer* 1975;36:1613.

505. Van Scott EJ, Auerbach R, Clendenning WE. Treatment of mycosis fungoides with cyclophosphamide. *Arch Dermatol* 1962;85:107.

506. Wright JC, Lyons MM, Walker DB, et al. Observations on the use of cancer chemotherapeutic agents in patients with mycosis fungoides. *Cancer* 1964;17:1045.

507. Haynes HA, Van Scott EJ. Therapy of mycosis fungoides. *Prog Dermatol* 1968;3:1.

508. Wright JC, Gumport SL, Golomb FM. Remissions produced with the use of methotrexate in patients with mycosis fungoides. *Cancer Chemother Rep* 1960;9:11.

509. McDonald CJ, Bertino JR. Treatment of mycosis fungoides lymphomas: effectiveness of infusions of methotrexate followed by oral citovorum factor. *Cancer Treat Rep* 1978;62:1009.

510. Takeda K, Sagawa T, Arakawa T. Therapeutic effect of bleomycin for skin tumors. *Cancer* 1970;61:207.

511. Spigel SC, Coltman CA Jr. Therapy of mycosis fungoides with bleomycin. *Cancer* 1973;32:767.

512. Yogoda A, Mukherji B, Young C, et al. Bleomycin, an anti-tumor antibiotic. *Ann Intern Med* 1972;77:861.

513. Levi JA, Diggs CH, Wiernik PH. Adriamycin therapy in advanced mycosis fungoides. *Cancer* 1977;39:1967.

514. Grozea PN, Jones SE, McKelvey EM, et al. Combination chemotherapy for mycosis fungoides: a Southwest Oncology Group Study. *Cancer Treat Rep* 1979;63:647.

515. Leavell UW Jr, De Simone P. Combined chemotherapy (COP), in treatment of mycosis fungoides: report of four cases. *South Med J* 1976;69:915.

516. Tirelli W, Veronesi A, Galligiani E, et al. Clinical and immunological evaluation of 5 cases of mycosis fungoides in advanced stages. *Tumori* 1979;65:447.

517. Price NK, Hoppe RT, Constantine VS, et al. The treatment of mycosis fungoides: adjuvant topical mechlorethamine after electron beam therapy. *Cancer* 1977;40:2851.

518. Winkler CF, Sausville EA, Ihde DC, et al. Combined modality treatment of cutaneous T cell lymphoma: results of a 6 year follow up. *J Clin Oncol* 1986;4:1094.

519. Kaye F, Eddy J, Ihde DC, et al. Conservative vs aggressive therapy in mycosis fungoides. *Proc ASCO* 1989;8:257.

520. Cummings FJ, Kim K, Neiman RS, et al. Phase II trial of pentostatin in refractory lymphomas and cutaneous T-cell disease. *J Clin Oncol* 1991;9:565.

521. Mercieca J, Matutes E, Dearden C, et al. The role of pentostatin in the treatment of T- cell malignancies: analysis of response rate in 145 patients according to disease subtype. *J Clin Oncol* 1994;12:2588.

522. Monfardini S, Sorio R, Cavalli F, et al. Pentostatin in patients with low grade (B-T-cell) and intermediate- and high-grade (T-cell) malignant lymphomas: phase II study of the EORTC Early Clinical Trials Group. *Oncology* 1996;53:163.

523. Kurzrock R. Pentostatin in T-cell lymphomas. *Semin Oncol* 2000;27:64.

524. Dearden C, Matutes E, Catovsky D. Pentostatin treatment of cutaneous T-cell lymphoma. *Oncology (Huntington)* 2000;4:37.

525. Ho AD, Suciu S, Stryckmans P, et al. Pentostatin in T-cell malignancies. Leukemia Cooperative Group and the European Organization for Research and Treatment of Cancer. *Semin Oncol* 2000;27:52.

526. Kuzel TM, Hurria A, Samuelson E, et al. Phase II trial of 2-chlorodeoxyadenosine for the treatment of cutaneous T-cell lymphoma. *Blood* 1996;87:906.

527. Saven A, Carrera CJ, Carson DA, et al. 2-Chlorodeoxyadenosine: an active agent in the treatment of cutaneous T-cell lymphoma. *Blood* 1992;80:587.

528. Von Hf DD, Dahlberg S, Hartstock RJ, et al. Activity of fludarabine monophosphate in patients with advanced mycosis fungoides: a Southwest Oncology Group Study. *J Natl Cancer Inst* 1990;82:1353.

529. Foss FM, Ihde DC, Linnoila IR, et al. Phase II trial of fludarabine phosphate and interferon alfa-2a in advanced mycosis fungoides/Sezary syndrome. *J Clin Oncol* 1994;12:2051.

530. Bunn PA Jr, Ihde DC, Foon KA. The role of recombinant leukocyte A interferon in the therapy of cutaneous T-cell lymphomas. *Cancer* 1986;57:1315.

531. Bunn PA Jr, Hoffman SJ, Norris D, et al. Systemic therapy of cutaneous T-cell lymphomas (mycosis fungoides and the Sezary syndrome). *Ann Int Med* 1994;121:592.

532. VanderMolen LA, Steis RG, Duffey PL, et al. Low-versus high-dose interferon alfa-2a in relapsed indolent non-Hodgkin's lymphoma. *J Natl Cancer Inst* 1990;82:235.

533. Bunn PA Jr, Foon KA, Ihde DC, et al. Recombinant leukocyte A interferon: an active agent in advanced cutaneous T-cell lymphomas. *Ann Intern Med* 1984;101:484.

534. Kohn EC, Steis RG, Sausville EA, et al. Phase II trial of intermittent high-dose recombinant interferon alfa-2a in mycosis fungoides and the Sezary syndrome. *J Clin Oncol* 1990;8:155.

535. Papa G, Tura S, Mandelli F, et al. Is interferon alpha in cutaneous T-cell lymphoma a treatment of choice? *Br J Haematol* 1991;79:48.

536. Molin K, Thomsen K, Volden G, et al. Oral retinoids in mycosis fungoides and Sezary syndrome: a comparison of isotretinoin and etretinate. A study from the Scandinavian Mycosis Fungoides Group. *Acta Derm Venereol* 1987;67:232.

537. Thomsen K, Molin L, Volden G, et al. 13-cis-Retinoic acid is effective in mycosis fungoides. A report from the Scandinavian Mycosis Fungoides Group. *Acta Derm Venereol* 1984;64:563.

538. Kessler JF, Jones SE, Levine N, et al. Isotretinoin and cutaneous helper T-cell lymphoma (mycosis fungoides). *Arch Dermatol* 1987;123:201.

539. Duvi M, Cather JC. Emerging new therapies for cutaneous T-cell lymphoma. *Dermatol Clin* 2000;18:147.

540. Foss FM, Kuzel TM. Experimental therapies in the treatment of cutaneous T-cell lymphoma. *Hematol Oncol Clin North Am* 1995;9:1127.

541. LeMaistre CF, Kuzel T, Foss F, et al. DAB$_{389}$IL-2 is well tolerated at doses inducing responses in IL-2R expressing lymphomas. *Blood* 1993;82:137a.

542. Foss FM, Borkowski TA, Gilliom M, et al. Chimeric fusion protein toxin DAB$_{486}$IL-2 in advanced mycosis fungoides and the Sezary syndrome: correlation of activity and interleukin-2 receptor expression in a phase II study. *Blood* 1994;84:1765.

543. Mansoor NS, LeMaistre CF, Kuzel TM, et al. Antitumor activity of DAB$_{389}$IL-2 fusion toxin in mycosis fungoides. *J Am Acad Dermatol* 1998;39:63.

544. Bigler RD, Crilley P, Micaily B, et al. Autologous bone marrow transplantation for advanced stage mycosis fungoides. *Bone Marrow Transplant* 1991;7:133.

545. Sterling JC, Marcus R, Burrows NP, et al. Erythrodermic mycosis fungoides treated with total body radiation and autologous bone marrow transplantation. *Clin Exp Dermatol* 1995;20:73.

546. Burt RK, Guitart J, Traynor A, et al. Allogeneic hematopoietic stem cell transplantation for advanced mycosis fungoides: evidence of a graft-versus-tumor effect. *Bone Marrow Transplant* 2000;25:111.

547. Lanier LL, Phillips JH, Hackett J Jr, et al. Natural killer cells: definition of a cell type rather than a function. *J Immunol* 1986;137:2735.

548. McKenna RW, Parkin J, Kersey JH, et al. Chronic lymphoproliferative disorder with unusual clinical, morphologic, ultrastructural and membrane surface marker characteristics. *Am J Med* 1977;62:588.

549. Pandolfi F. T-CLL and allied diseases: new insights into classification and pathogenesis. *Diagn Immunol* 1986;4:61.

550. Loughran TP, Marshall E, Kadin ME, et al. Leukemia of large granular lymphocytes: association with clonal chromosomal abnormalities and autoimmune neutropenia, thrombocytopenia and hemolytic anemia. *Ann Intern Med* 1985;102:169.

551. Loughran TP Jr. Clonal diseases of large granular lymphocytes. *Blood* 1993;82:1.

552. Itoh K, Tsuchikawa K, Awataguchi T, et al. A case of chronic lymphocytic leukemia with properties characteristic of natural killer cells. *Blood* 1983;61:940.

553. Linch DC, Cawley JC, MacDonald SM, et al. Acquired pure red-cell aplasia associated with an increase of T cells bearing receptors for the Fc of IgG. *Acta Haematol* 1981;65:270.

554. Nagasawa T, Abe T, Nakagawa T. Pure red cell aplasia and hypogammaglobulinemia associated with T-cell chronic lymphocytic leukemia. *Blood* 1981;57:1025.

555. Hoffman R, Kopel S, Shu SD, et al. T cell chronic lymphocytic leukemia: presence in bone marrow and peripheral blood of cells that suppress erythropoiesis in vitro. *Blood* 1978;52:255.

556. Dallapicolla B, Alimena G, Chessa L, et al. Chromosome studies in patients with T-CLL chronic lymphocytic leukemia and expansions of granular lymphocytes. *Int J Cancer* 1984;34:171.

557. Loughran TP, Kadin ME, Starkebaum G, et al. Leukemia of large granular lymphocytes: association with clonal chromosomal abnormalities and autoimmune neutropenia, thrombocytopenia, and hemolytic anemia. *Ann Intern Med* 1985;102:169.

558. Wallis WJ, Loughran TP, Kadin ME, et al. Polyarthritis and neutropenia associated with circulating large granular lymphocytes. *Ann Intern Med* 1985;103:357.

559. Barton JC, Prasthofer EF, Egan ML, et al. Rheumatoid arthritis associated with expanded populations of granular lymphocytes. *Ann Intern Med* 1986;104:314.

560. Lamy T, Loughran TP Jr. Pathogenesis of autoimmune diseases in large granular lymphocyte leukemia. *Hematology* 1998;3:17.

561. Dhodapkar MV, Li CY, Lust JA, et al. Clinical spectrum of clonal proliferations of T-large granular lymphocytes: a T-cell clonopathy of undetermined significance? *Blood* 1994;84:1620.

562. Semenzato G, Pandolfi F, Chiesesi T, et al. The lymphoproliferative disease of granular lymphocytes. A heterogenous disorder ranging from indolent to aggressive conditions. *Cancer* 1987;60:2971.

563. Loughran TP, Starkebaum G, Kidd P, et al. Clonal proliferation of large granular lymphocytes in rheumatoid arthritis. *Arthritis Rheum* 1988;31:31.

564. Moretta L, Loretta A, Canonica GW, et al. Receptors for immunoglobulins on resting and activated human T cells. *Immunol Rev* 1981;56:141.

565. Spitzer G, Verma DS, Abramowitz S, et al. Cells with Fc receptors from normal donors suppress granulocyte macrophage colony formation. *Blood* 1982;60:758.

566. Kadin ME, Kamoun N, Lamberg J. Erythrophagocytic T lymphoma: a clinical pathologic entity resembling malignant histiocytosis. *N Engl J Med* 1981;304:648.

567. Pandolfi F, Pezzutto A, DeRossi G, et al. Characterization of two patients with lymphomas of large granular lymphocytes. *Cancer* 1984;53:445.

568. Lamy T, Amiot L, Drenou B, et al. Response to granulocyte-macrophage colony stimulating factor (GM-CSF) but not to G-CSF in a case of agranulocytosis with large granular lymphocyte leukemia. *Blood* 1994;84:2164.

569. Gabor EP, Mishalani S, Lee S. Rapid response to cyclosporin therapy in large granular lymphocyte leukemia. *Blood* 1995;87:1199.

570. Loughran TP, Kidd PG, Starkebaum G. Treatment of large granular lymphocyte leukemia with oral low-dose methotrexate. *Blood* 1994;84:2164.

571. Palutke M, Eisenberg L, Kaplan J, et al. Natural killer and suppressor T-cell chronic lymphocytic leukemia. *Blood* 1983;62:627.

572. Hocking WG, Singh R, Schroff R, et al. Cell mediated inhibition of erythropoiesis and megaloblastic anemia in T-cell chronic lymphocytic leukemia. *Cancer* 1983;51:631.

573. Pandolfi F, Loughran TP, Starkebaum G, et al. Clinical course and prognosis of the lymphoproliferative disease of granular lymphocytes. A multicenter study. *Cancer* 1990;65:341.

574. Kawa-Ha K, Ishihara S, Ninomiya T, et al. CD3-negative lymphoproliferative disease of granular lymphocytes containing Epstein-Barr viral DNA. *J Clin Invest* 1989;84:51.

CHAPTER 27

Hodgkin's Disease

Jonathan W. Friedberg, Jon C. Aster, and George P. Canellos

HISTORIC INTRODUCTION

Hodgkin's disease (HD) is a neoplastic disorder of the lymphoid system characterized by the presence of diagnostic multinucleate giant cells, termed *Reed-Sternberg* (RS) *cells,* in an appropriate mixed inflammatory infiltrate. The enlarged lymph nodes of this condition must be distinguished from those of the other (non-Hodgkin's) malignant lymphomas. Without treatment, HD evolves into a debilitating systemic illness, characterized by fever, night sweats, chills, weight loss, and itching; it leads to death in a few to many years. Radiation therapy and chemotherapy programs developed after World War II now cure most (two-thirds) patients with this disorder (1). Thus, HD represents an outstanding triumph of modern cancer management. Although constituting only 1% of the cancer incidence of developed countries, the disorder has played a pivotal role in the evolution of medical oncology. The youth of the affected patient population (Fig. 27-1), the dramatic clinical picture, and, more recently, the success of treatment, have led to continuing interest within the medical profession and to an extensive literature.

In 1832, Thomas Hodgkin (Fig. 27-2) published a paper in *Medical-Chirurgical Transactions,* entitled "On Some of the Morbid Appearances of the Absorbent Glands and Spleen" (2).

Case 2

September 24th, 1828. Ellenborough King, aged ten years, was admitted to Luke's ward on the 6th of August 1828, under the care of Dr. Bright. He was the youngest of six children, of whom the first five were reported to be all healthy. This child had also been healthy till about thirteen months ago, when his strength, flesh, and healthy appearance began to fail. He was living at that time in the West of England. A tumour was observed in the left hypochondrium in the situation of the spleen, the glandulae concatenatae on the right side were observed to be considerably enlarged, but under the treatment used, these tumours, as well as that in the situation of the spleen, were at times very considerably reduced in size.

It does not appear that he was ever subject to haemorrhage, nor till very lately to dropsical effusion; his appetite was generally good. After admission into the hospital the tumour on the left side was observed to extend considerably below the left hypochondrium, but was reported not to be as large as it had formerly been. The glands on the left side of the neck were swollen, as well as those on the right; the abdomen was somewhat distended, and there was considerable oedema of the scrotum...

The head was not opened.

The glands in the neck had assumed the form of large ovoid masses, connected together merely by loose cellular membrane and minute vessels: when cut into they exhibited a firm cartilaginous structure of a light colour and very feeble vascularity, but with no appearance of softening or suppuration. Glands similarly affected accompanied the vessels into the chest, where the bronchial and mediastinal glands were in the same state and greatly enlarged. There were some old pleuritis adhesions. The substance of the lung was generally healthy. There was a good deal of clear serum in the pericardium, but this membrane, as well as the heart, was quite healthy.

In the peritoneal cavity there was a considerable quantity of clear straw-coloured serum mixed with extensive, recently thin diaphanous films. The mucous membrane of the stomache and intestines was tolerably healthy.

The mesenteric glands were but slightly enlarged, and but little if at all indurated; but those accompanying the aorta, the splenic artery, and the illiacs were in the same state as the glands of the neck.

The liver contained no tubercles, and its structure was quite healthy. The pancreas was rather firm, and the glands situated along its upper edges were, as before stated, greatly enlarged. The spleen was enlarged to at least four times its natural size, its surface sprinkled with tubercles, presenting the same structure as the enlarged glands already described (2).

Hodgkin's astute observation was lost for a generation until Sir Samuel Wilks, working at Guy's Hospital with some of the same pathologic material, independently distinguished the condition from the other causes of chronic lymphadenopathy (carcinoma, tuberculosis, amyloid). When Hodgkin's earlier study came belatedly to Wilks' attention, Wilks generously credited the earlier observation and introduced the eponym by which the disorder is still known (3). Histologic examination of Hodgkin's cases in the present century has verified the nature of three, possibly four, of the original seven cases, including Case 2.

In the late nineteenth century, Greenfield (4), among others, described characteristic giant cells in HD. A full description of the diagnostic cell required Ehrlich's staining methods and awaited the publications of Sternberg in 1898 (5) and, particularly, of Dorothy Reed in 1902 (6). Reed clearly distinguished the process from tuberculosis, a condition that complicated Sternberg's cases.

The first modern approach to HD is found in the Jackson and Parker monograph published in 1947 (7). A conference held in Rye, New York in 1966 provided a simplified version of the Lukes

The authors gratefully acknowledge this introductory history of HD, written for the first edition by Alan Aisenberg, M.D.

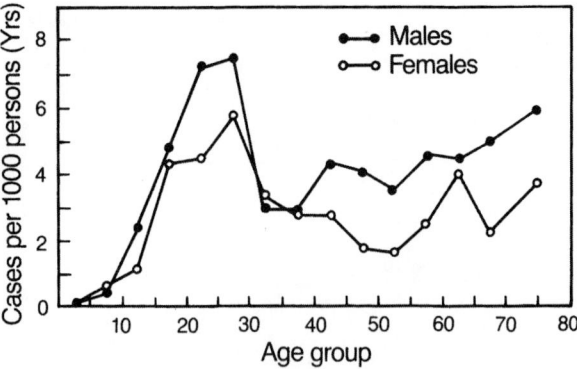

Figure 27-1. Epidemiology of Hodgkin's disease. Age-specific incidence of Hodgkin's disease in the Boston and Worcester standard metropolitan statistical areas from mid-1972 through 1977, according to sex. (From Gutensohn NE, Cole P. Childhood social environment and Hodgkin's disease. *N Engl J Med* 1981;304:135.)

and Butler histologic classification, which remains in use today, and introduced many modern ideas about staging, prognosis, and treatment (8). Successive advances in radiation therapy can be attributed to Rene Gilbert (9),Vera Peters, K. C. H. Middlemiss (10), and Henry Kaplan (11). The landmark use of the MOPP (nitrogen mustard, vincristine, procarbazine, and prednisone) drug combination by Vincent DeVita and colleagues (12) at the National Cancer Institute (NCI) was based on the early laboratory and clinical investigations of Frei, Freireich, Holland, Skipper, Carbone, and Pinkel. The Milan (NCI) group developed a regimen of doxorubicin, bleomycin, vinblastine, and dacarbazine (ABVD), which has evolved to be the more frequently used standard regimen—more from the lack of some of the MOPP-induced toxicities than the induction of superior survival (13).

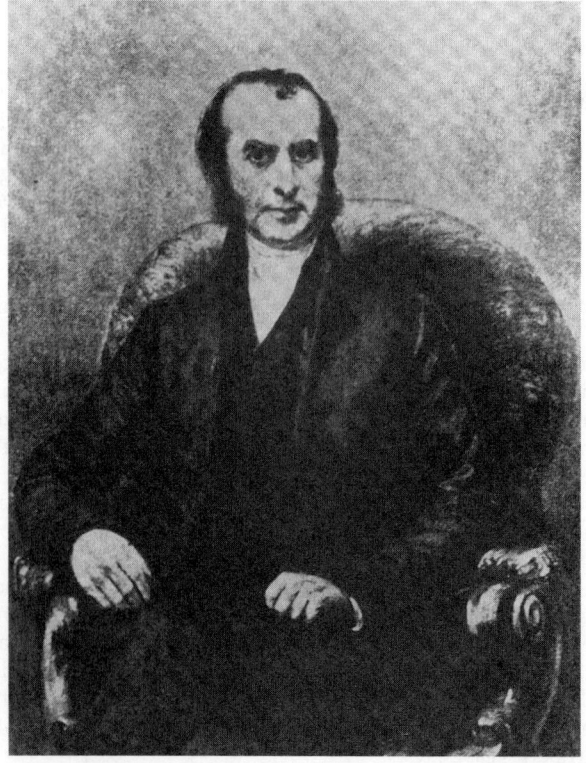

Figure 27-2. Thomas Hodgkin (1798–1866), "a man distinguished alike for scientific attainments, medical skill, and self-sacrificing philanthropy" (epitaph inscribed on Hodgkin's tomb in Jaffa).

PATHOGENESIS AND PATHOBIOLOGY

Few efforts in medical science have produced a more grudging return from the time and resource invested in them than the study of the causes of HD. These difficulties stemmed, in large part, from the relative rarity of the neoplastic cells of HD, the RS cell and variants thereof, which seldom constitute more than 1% of the tumor bulk and frequently constitute less than one-tenth of 1%. Progress awaited the development of single-cell microdissection methods, coupled to sensitive assays that can be applied to a few isolated cells, such as the polymerase chain reaction. Such studies have established recently that, in the large majority of cases, RS cells represent a monoclonal population of B cells. Hence, HD is best considered an unusual form of malignant lymphoma.

The critical clues came from the analysis of the DNA sequences of immunoglobulin (Ig) genes obtained from isolated RS cells and variants (14–16); see review by Stein et al. (17). Such work has shown generally that all of the RS cells within particular cases share the same Ig gene rearrangements. Moreover, the rearranged Ig segments within tumor cells have also undergone somatic hypermutation, an event that is believed to occur only in germinal center B cells. The cell of origin in most cases of HD is thus a neoplastic germinal center or postgerminal center B cell. In a small proportion of cases (1% to 2%), the RS cells lack Ig rearrangements but have T-cell receptor rearrangements (18,19), suggesting that HD may rarely arise from transformed T cells.

Although these molecular studies have settled the issue of cell of origin, many other facets of HD remain poorly understood. These uncertainties are reflected in three central questions relevant to a fuller understanding of the disease: What are the critical genetic events and signals that drive cellular transformation? What is the role of Epstein-Barr virus (EBV)? What are the contributions of the characteristic reactive cellular infiltrate of HD to its biology and response to therapy? These questions are further complicated by the existence of distinct subtypes within the group of entities classified as HD. The mixed-cellularity, nodular-sclerosis, lymphocyte-rich, and lymphocyte-depletion subtypes share similar immunophenotypic features and are grouped together as classic forms of HD. The other well-defined subtype, lymphocyte predominance, is pathologically and biologically distinct from the classic forms.

Genetic and Cytogenetic Aberrations in Hodgkin's Disease

The detection and molecular dissection of recurrent chromosomal translocations have played a central role in understanding the initiating events in many forms of hematopoietic neoplasia. Cytogenetic analysis of RS cells has been challenging due to the paucity of tumor cells, but several themes have emerged from the analysis of cell lines derived from patients, metaphase chromosome preparations obtained from fresh tumor specimens, interphase fluorescence *in situ* hybridization, and comparative genomic hybridization studies.

The tumor cells of classic forms of HD are hyperdiploid, have nonrandom chromosomal breakage, and show a wide variation in chromosomal content from cell to cell in individual tumors, indicating that chromosomal instability is a hallmark of classic HD (20–22). Duplications of chromosomes 1, 2, 5, 12, and 21 have been noted frequently, whereas loss of chromosomes 10, 13, 17, and 22 occurs less often. Rearrangements, especially translocations and deletions, most often involve 1p, 1q, 2q, 6q, 8q, 11p, and 14q. None of the rearrangements involving oncogenes typical of other forms of lymphoma have been clearly demonstrated. Spectral karyotyping has also revealed amplification and ectopic insertion of rRNA genes and subtelomeric repeat regions in a HD cell line (23). It seems that none of these rearrangements are likely to be pathogenetic but may be markers of some underlying problem with DNA repair.

It is likely that the chromosomal instability of RS cells stems from acquired mutations in genes encoding proteins that are involved with the detection and repair of DNA damage. One such protein is P53, which normally functions to maintain genomic stability. Mutations that disrupt P53 function are found in the RS cell in 10% to 25% of HD cases (24–27). When present in a particular case, identical P53 mutations are present in each RS cell (26), providing additional evidence of monoclonal origin. The infrequency of P53 mutation is surprising, based on immunohistochemical data showing that P53 protein, which often accumulates when mutated, is commonly detected in RS cells (28). Whether the accumulation of unmutated P53 in RS cells is truly a marker of diminished function is not known, and the pathogenic events underlying the genomic instability of RS cells in the majority of cases remains to be understood.

The limited cytogenetic data obtained from cases of the lymphocyte-predominance subtype also show evidence of genomic instability. One study of 19 cases detected a high number of genomic imbalances (average, 10.8/case), involving all chromosomes except 19, 22, and Y (29). Recurrent gains of chromosomes 1, 2q, 3, 4q, 5q, 6, 8q, 11q, 12q, and X and loss of chromosome 17 were identified in 36.8% to 68.4% of the cases. Gain of 2q, 4q, 5q, 6, and 11q is rarely observed in other lymphoid malignancies and may be relatively specific for the lymphocyte predominance HD. Rearrangement of the BCL6 gene, which is involved in balanced chromosomal translocations in 30% of diffuse large B-cell lymphomas and a small subset of follicular lymphomas, was detected in approximately 10% of cases.

Role of Nuclear Factor–κB Signaling

A signaling pathway that appears to be activated in the majority of cases of classic HD involves the transcription factor nuclear factor-κB (NF-κB), which has a prominent role in regulation of the normal immune response at the level of gene expression. The NF-κB family includes a number of homo- and heterodimeric transcription factors related in structure to the v-rel oncoprotein. NF-κB is maintained in an inactive state by a family of closely related cytoplasmic polypeptides termed inhibitors of NF-κB (IκBs), which bind and sequester NF-κB in the cytoplasm. Signaling is induced by signals that result in the phosphorylation and degradation of IκB, freeing NF-κB and permitting it to translocate to the nucleus, bind promoter elements, and activate target genes.

Since initial observations of high levels of nuclear NF-κB in multiple HD cell lines (30,31), diverse independent investigations have converged on NF-κB as a possible central player in HD pathogenesis. Analysis of single microdissected RS cells has shown the presence of inactivating mutations in IκB in approximately 20% of cases (32–35). However, even HD cell lines with intact IκB genes have increased nuclear NF-κB (34,36), apparently due to the activation of signaling pathways that degrade IκB. These signals may be mediated through surface receptors that are commonly expressed on RS cells, such as CD30 and CD40, which can trigger signals on activation that result in IκB degradation (37,38). In addition, the best characterized oncoprotein that is encoded in the genome of the EBV, latent membrane protein (LMP)-1, mimics a constitutively active CD40 receptor (39) in activating NF-κB (40–42). Conversely, inhibition of NF-κB leads to the growth inhibition and apoptotic death of HD cell lines (43), supporting its biologic importance and its potential as a therapeutic target. A search is now under way for downstream targets of NF-κB, which appear to include multiple genes encoding apoptosis inhibitors, such as Bfl-1/A1, c-IAP2, TRAF1, and Bcl-x(L) (44).

Interest in antiapoptotic signals, such as those induced by NF-κB, has been further spurred by the observation that the RS cells of classic forms of HD do not express functional Ig receptors and appear to have turned off Ig gene transcription (45). This aberration is highly unusual because normal B cells must express functional Ig receptors to survive, and even the transformed lymphoid cells of B-cell non-Hodgkin's lymphomas, as a rule, also express surface Igs. RS cells have thus been likened to "crippled" B cells that must be rescued from the programmed cell death that would normally be induced by the absence of Ig receptor–mediated survival signals (46). Reed-Sternberg cells down-regulate not only Ig gene transcription but also many other genes normally expressed in germinal center B cells, suggesting that their genesis involves a global change in gene expression to a new pattern that is radically different than that of normal germinal center B cells. This "reprogramming" (the basis of which is not understood) may relieve the dependence of RS cells on Ig receptor–mediated signals for survival and has undoubtedly contributed to the long-standing controversy about the origin of RS cells.

Less is known about the signals that drive the proliferation and survival of RS variants in the lymphocyte-predominance subtype. However, clues come from the recognition that the RS variants in lymphocyte predominance HD usually grow within expanded B-cell follicles, express B-cell markers, and show evidence of ongoing somatic hypermutation (47,48), indicating that they are neoplastic germinal center B cells. Unlike the RS cells of classic forms of HD, the tumor cells in the lymphocyte predominance type express Ig mRNAs and often express Ig proteins (48). Hence, signals that promote the survival of germinal center B cells, such as those mediated through CD40 signaling and the Ig receptor, may be important in the lymphocyte-predominance subtype.

Epstein-Barr Virus in Classic Hodgkin's Disease

EBV has figured prominently as a putative causal agent of classic forms of HD, particularly the mixed-cellularity subtype. Lukes and Tindle first noted the morphologic resemblance of RS cells and EBV-infected B cells (49). Direct evidence for EBV in RS cells was first produced by Poppema and colleagues, who detected EBV antigens in the RS cells of a case of mixed cellularity HD (50). This was expanded on by Weiss et al., who demonstrated the presence of EBV genomes within RS cells in a subset of HD cases (51), an observation that was subsequently replicated in many laboratories. EBV is most highly associated with HD occurring in children (particularly in the developing world), older adults, and acquired immunodeficiency syndrome (AIDS) patients and in the mixed-cellularity and lymphocyte-depletion subtypes. Importantly, the viral genomes isolated from individual EBV+ cases are monoclonal, indicating that the tumor is derived from a single cell infected with EBV before, or at the time of, cellular transformation (51,52). Taken with the ability of EBV to immortalize B cells in culture, it seems likely that EBV has a partial causal role in a subset of cases of HD.

Despite these important associations, many issues relating to the role of EBV remain unclear. A major question is why only a very small number of EBV-infected individuals develop HD. Possible answers include variation in host genotype, acquired clinical or subclinical immune abnormalities that prevent or retard the clearance of EBV-infected cells, or chance acquisition of other unknown genetic aberrations in EBV-infected lymphocytes.

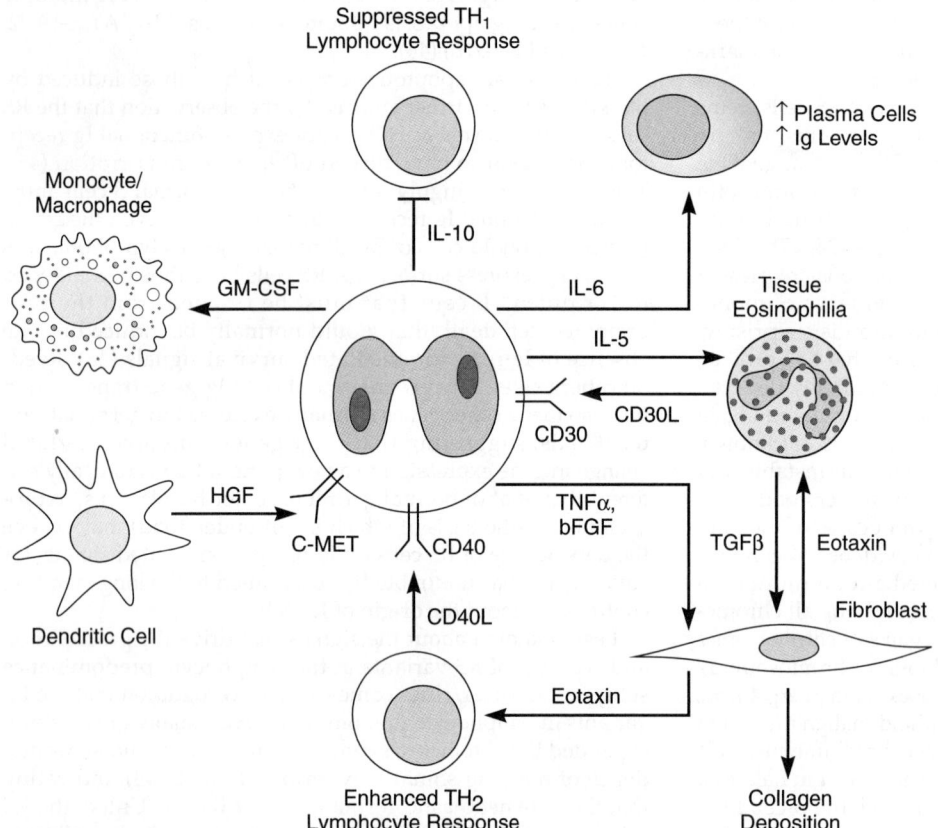

Figure 27-3. Paracrine signaling in Hodgkin's disease. Proposed interactions are shown between a Reed-Sternberg cell and reactive TH-1 and TH-2 T cells, plasma cells, eosinophils, fibroblasts, dendritic cells, and monocyte/macrophages. bFGF, basic fibroblast growth factor; GM-CSF, granulocyte-macrophage colony-stimulating factor; HGF, hepatocyte growth factor; Ig, immunoglobulin; IL, interleukin; TGF, transforming growth factor; TNF, tumor necrosis factor.

Several lines of evidence suggest that abnormal immune responses to EBV have a role in the genesis of HD. Poor nutrition and diminished immunity may be responsible for the high incidence of EBV-related HD in children in the developing world. In the U.S. population, Mueller and co-workers observed that patients who subsequently develop HD had unusually high titers of EBV-specific IgG and IgA antibodies in prediagnostic serum samples (53). Interestingly, in a follow-up study, the presence of EBV+ HD did not correlate with a history of symptomatic mononucleosis, and most patients with abnormal serology did not have EBV+ HD (54). Hence, the relationship between abnormal serologic response to EBV and subsequent HD requires clarification. One scenario would be for EBV to act primarily as an initiator of B-cell proliferation and immortalization but not to be essential for maintenance of established tumors. A case of relapsed HD in which EBV was lost during tumor progression provides a small bit of support for this possibility (55).

More compelling evidence for the importance of immune dysregulation in the risk of developing EBV+ HD comes from studies of AIDS patients. Although the overall risk of HD in AIDS is only modestly elevated, 80% to 100% of AIDS-related cases are EBV associated (56–59), compared to approximately 30% of HD cases in the general U.S. population. It will be of interest to see whether highly active antiretroviral therapy lowers the risk of EBV+ HD in the AIDS population.

A fascinating (although rare) association pointing to the importance of disordered immune function and preexistent genetic aberrations in the genesis of EBV+ HD has been observed in patients with B-cell chronic lymphocytic leukemia. Occasionally, EBV-infected, RS-like cells are observed in lymph nodes or other tissues involved by otherwise typical chronic lymphocytic leukemia (60,61). In some patients, this picture progresses to full-blown EBV+ HD (61,62), and, in such cases, it has been

shown that the RS cells are derived from the preexistent chronic lymphocytic leukemia clone (63,64). Hence, it can be supposed that EBV infection of a cell with preexistent genetic aberrations (e.g., a chronic lymphocytic leukemia cell or clonally related precursor thereof) in the context of altered immune function leads to the outgrowth of RS-like cells. With additional (genetic?) events, full-blown classic HD ensues.

Little is currently known about the role of host genotype in risk of EBV-related HD. A large twin study has demonstrated that genetic factors contribute to risk of HD (65), particularly in young adults, but most concordant cases were of the nodular sclerosis subtype and unassociated with EBV. Alternatively, one small case control study has suggested that there is an excess of the HLA-DPB1*0301 allele in EBV+ HD in young adults (66), and that this risk interacts positively with a history of recent infectious mononucleosis. With the recent development of genome-wide single nucleotide DNA polymorphisms, it should now be possible to study systematically the role of host genotype in HD risk.

The pattern of latent EBV gene expression in the RS cells of HD is restricted to LMP-1, LMP-2A and -2B, Epstein-Barr nuclear antigen–1, and Epstein-Barr virus early regions (67–69), the latter being small nuclear RNAs of unknown function. As mentioned, LMP-1 is a transmembrane protein driving the constitutive activation of NF-κB that is essential for transformation of B lymphocytes by EBV (70). Thus, LMP-1 may serve to rescue cells from programmed cell death by sustaining NF-κB activation.

In addition, LMP-1 signals also lead to activation of AP-1 (a transcription factor that promotes growth) and the JAK/STAT signaling pathway; these events may also be important for cellular transformation (71). Another interesting effect of LMP-1 is its ability to induce the appearance of multinucleated cells resembling diagnostic RS cells in EBV-negative Hodgkin's cell lines (72).

Origin and Significance of the Reactive Cellular Background in Hodgkin's Disease

The histologic hallmark of HD is the presence of characteristic RS cells and variants in the background of abundant reactive nonmalignant cells. Although most work has focused on the tumor cells, the reactive cellular component typically comprises greater than 95% of the tumor mass and undoubtedly plays a critical pathogenic role. Hence, disruption of signaling "crosstalk" between reactive cells and RS cells might be therapeutic if the critical interactions could be identified. It is also likely that factors produced in tissues involved by HD explain its characteristic systemic signs and symptoms, such as leukocytosis, weight loss, night sweats, and pruritus.

Many examples of possible paracrine signaling between classic RS cells and reactive nonmalignant stromal elements have been described (37,73–87). A subset of interactions involving cytokines, chemokines, and their respective cognate receptors that is proposed to produce the characteristic tissue reaction around RS cells, including the accumulation of CD4+ TH-2 subset T cells, eosinophils, macrophages, and plasma cells, often accompanied by collagen deposition, is shown in Figure 27-3. However, instead of an experimental model or therapeutic trials directed against paracrine signals, the contribution of specific signals to the biology of HD remains speculative.

In addition to their local effects, cytokines are also responsible for the systemic symptoms of HD. "B" symptoms may result from elevated levels of tumor necrosis factor-α and interleukin (IL)-6, whereas leukocytosis may stem from elevated granulocyte-macrophage colony-stimulating factor and granulocyte colony-stimulating factor. It is also notable that elevated circulating levels of several cytokines, such as IL-10 (88–91), appear to be independent predictors of outcome.

Relatively little is known about the interactions between the stroma and RS cells in the lymphocyte-predominance subtype. However, signals relevant to the survival and proliferation of normal follicular B cells (e.g., CD40 signaling) are likely important, because the RS-cell variants in this subtype bear a resemblance to germinal center B cells and usually grow in expanded B-cell follicles (92,93).

HISTOPATHOLOGY OF HODGKIN'S DISEASE

As with other lymphomas, the diagnosis of HD requires tissue sampling. Although immunophenotyping plays an important confirmatory role, morphologic identification of RS cells and variants in the appropriate reactive cellular background remains the diagnostic *sine qua non*. Because the tumor cells are in the minority, immunophenotyping is best performed on tissue sections of biopsy material; flow cytometric analysis of disaggregated cells is not helpful. It is possible to make the diagnosis in smears of cells aspirated from enlarged lymph nodes, particularly when immunohistochemical stains are also performed, but this method offers less diagnostic reliability and precision than lymph node biopsy.

Ideally, the surgeon should obtain a large intact lymph node from the center of the disease process. Mediastinoscopy specimens and needle biopsies are often also adequate, particularly if multiple samples or passes are obtained. Diagnostic difficulties arise when the sampled tissues are peripheral to fully involved nodes or only partially involved. In some instances, leveling completely through the embedded tissues may uncover a focus that is diagnostic of involvement, but repeat sampling may be necessary. Another difficult situation arises when patients are treated for concomitant diseases with agents, such as prednisone, that have activity against HD. In such instances, viable RS cells may only be identified in second biopsies obtained after the cessation of drug exposure.

Usually, an unexplained lymph node should be greater than or equal to 2 cm before biopsy is warranted; even then, nodes in the smaller size range should be present for at least 1 month. The initial diagnosis of HD is unlikely to be made from a lymph node not externally visible. Trivial adenopathy is common; HD is not.

Reed-Sternberg Cells and Variants

The criteria originally defined by Lukes and Butler remain the gold standard for morphologic recognition of various types of Hodgkin's cells (94). The diagnostic RS cell is a giant cell with at least two nuclei or distinct nuclear lobes, large eosinophilic inclusion-like nucleoli, a thick, well-defined nuclear membrane, and pale-staining chromatin (Fig. 27-4A, B). The classic cell has two mirror-image nuclei, but cells with more than two nuclei are common, and nuclear lobation may be prominent. RS cells should be identified to make the diagnosis of classic HD, but they may be absent in the lymphocyte-predominance subtype.

Other RS variants are recognized and are highly characteristic of particular subtypes. *Mononuclear variants* are common in the mixed-cellularity subtype (Fig. 27-4C, D). *Lacunar variants* are almost always present in the nodular sclerosis subtype (Fig. 27-4E). Lacunar variants typically have a folded or lobated nucleus, variably conspicuous nucleoli, and abundant pale cytoplasm. When not well fixed, the cytoplasm tears away during tissue sectioning, leaving the nuclei sitting in a partially empty space containing wispy tendrils of residual cytoplasm. Although an artifact, these lacunar variants are highly characteristic and diagnostically helpful when present. The characteristic tumor cell in the lymphocyte-predominance subtype is the *lymphocytic and histiocytic variant*, a large cell with multiple folded or convoluted nuclear contours that sometimes resembles a popcorn kernel (Fig. 27-4F).

Another feature of RS cells is their tendency to undergo a peculiar form of cell death described as *mummification*. Such cells have a shrunken appearance in tissue sections denoted by the presence of dark basophilic nuclei lacking detail and indistinct cytoplasm. Mummified cells do not undergo the usual DNA fragmentation seen in programmed cell death (apoptosis) (95,96), and they are not recognized by tissue macrophages. They are most prominent in the nodular sclerosis and mixed-cellularity subtypes and are diagnostically helpful when present.

Classification of Hodgkin's Disease

The goal of HD pathologic classification is to provide a guide to prognosis and treatment in a disorder of extremely variable natural history. Unlike the non-Hodgkin's lymphomas, the classification of HD has changed relatively little over the past 30+ years. The Rye classification of HD (97) is a four-part system that has prevailed over time. It was developed in 1966 as a simplification of the more complex Lukes and Butler classification (94), which nonetheless provided the specific histologic criteria and terminology for the Rye classification. With the application of immunohistochemistry during the 1980s, it became apparent that lymphocyte predominance HD was distinct from other subtypes. In recognition of this, the Revised European-American Lymphoma (REAL) classification of 1994 (98) divided HD into two broad categories, *classic* and *lymphocyte predominance*, which were defined by the morphology and immunophenotype of the RS cells and variants. A new category of classic HD, *lymphocyte-rich HD*, was also created to subsume

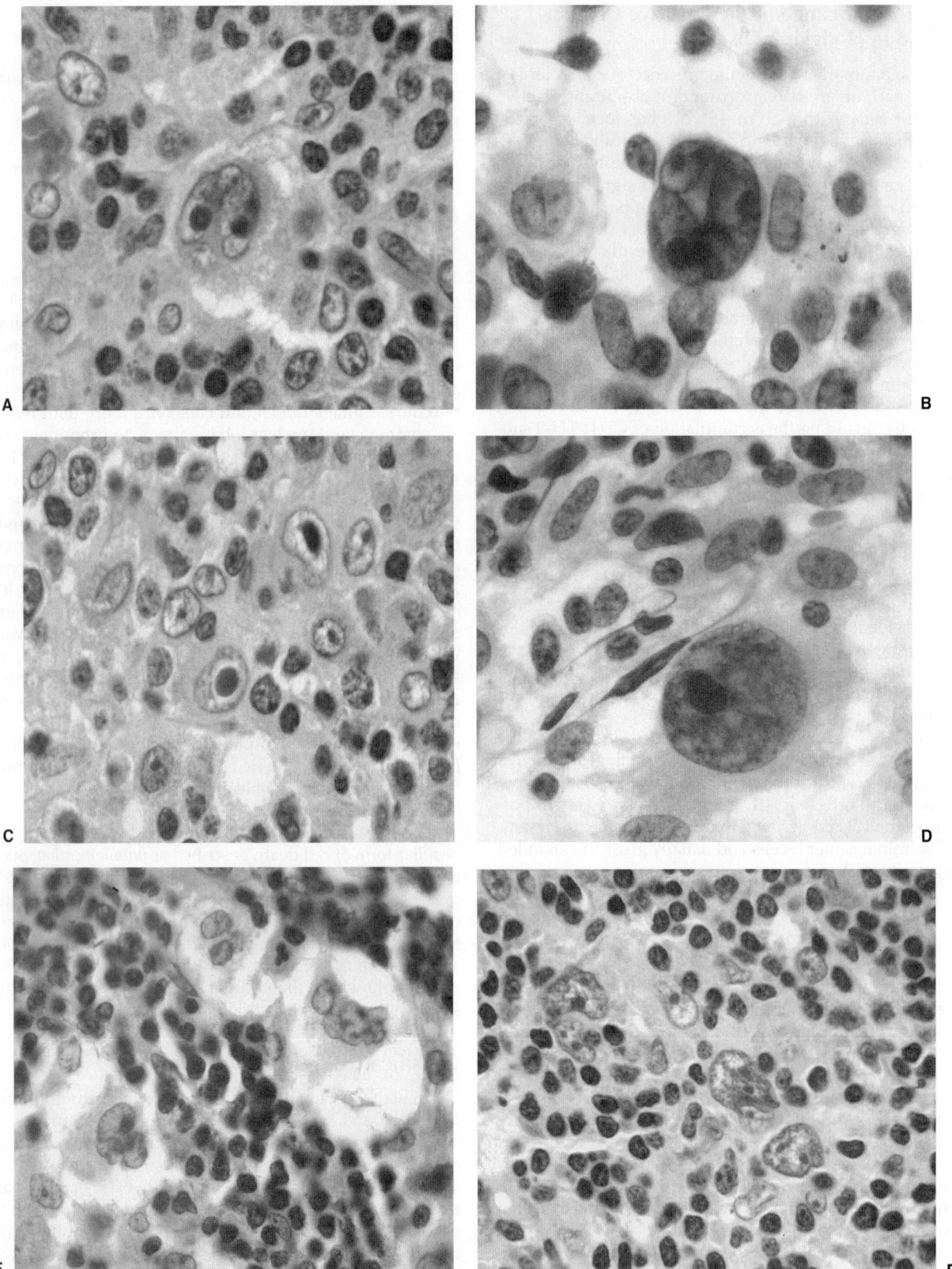

Figure 27-4. Reed-Sternberg cells and variants. All preparations were made from lymph nodes. **A** and **B:** Diagnostic Reed-Sternberg cells in a hematoxylin and eosin (H&E)–stained tissue section and a Giemsa-stained touch preparation, respectively. **C** and **D:** Mononuclear Reed-Sternberg cell variants in an H&E-stained tissue section and a Giemsa-stained touch preparation, respectively. **E:** Lacunar Reed-Sternberg cell variants in an H&E-stained tissue section from a case of nodular sclerosis Hodgkin's disease. **F:** Lymphocytic and histiocytic variants in an H&E-stained tissue section from a case of lymphocyte-predominance Hodgkin's disease.

TABLE 27-1. Histologic Classification of Hodgkin's Disease

Lukes and Butler (1966)	Rye (1971)	REAL (1994), WHO (1997)
Lymphocytic and histiocytic Nodular Diffuse	Lymphocyte-predominance	Lymphocyte-predominance
		Classic Hodgkin's disease Lymphocyte-rich Nodular sclerosis Mixed-cellularity Lymphocyte-depletion
Nodular sclerosis Mixed cellularity Diffuse fibrosis Reticular	Nodular sclerosis Mixed-cellularity Lymphocyte-depletion	

REAL, Revised European-American Lymphoma; WHO, World Health Organization.

those cases in which the RS cells resemble those seen in classic HD, but the background is comprised mainly of small lymphocytes. Many such cases were previously considered to be forms of the lymphocyte-predominance subtype (99). The proposed World Health Organization (WHO) classification (100) leaves the REAL classification unaltered. The relationships of these classification schemes are summarized in Table 27-1, and the clinicopathologic characteristics of currently recognized subtypes are shown in Table 27-2.

Classic Forms of Hodgkin's Disease

These subtypes are united by the presence of RS cells with a characteristic immunophenotype: They are CD15 (101) and CD30 positive (102) (Fig. 27-5A, B) and negative for T-cell markers and CD45 (leukocyte common antigen). In some cases, a subset of tumor cells may stain for the B-cell markers CD20 and CD79, or Bcl-6 protein, which are normally expressed in germinal center B cells. Diagnostic RS cells are always present, although they are most frequent in the mixed-cellularity and lymphocyte-depletion subtypes. In most instances, background lymphocytes are predominantly T cells. Individual subtypes are

distinguished based on the predominant appearance of RS variants and the nature of the cellular reaction.

NODULAR SCLEROSIS SUBTYPE

The most common subtype of HD in the United States, the nodular sclerosis subtype most often arises in the mediastinum or cervical lymph nodes of young women. It is characterized by the presence of frequent lacunar variants (best recognized in formalin-fixed tissue sections) within cellular nodules containing a polymorphous collection of reactive lymphocytes, eosinophils, and macrophages, which are surrounded by well-developed bands of mature collagen that impart a nodular appearance (Fig. 27-6). Diagnostic RS cells can be found but are uncommon. EBV is detected in the tumor cells in a minority of cases.

Several histologic variants of prototypical nodular sclerosis subtype are recognized. In early lymph node involvement, sclerosis may not be well developed, producing a so-called cellular phase that may be confused with the mixed-cellularity type (103). In other cases, RS variants may be numerous within cellular nodules, producing a syncytial appearance (104). In some series (105–108), the syncytial variant of the nodular sclerosis type, as well as cases with unusually pleomorphic RS cells or a paucity of lymphocytes, have been associated with a worse clinical outcome. Based on these observations, a two-tiered grading system for the nodular sclerosis subtype has been proposed. However, the association of "grade II" histology and worse outcome has not been observed in other series (109–111), and its role in patient stratification remains uncertain.

MIXED-CELLULARITY SUBTYPE

This histologic type is characterized by diffuse nodal effacement by a polymorphous cellular infiltrate that includes frequent diagnostic RS cells and mononuclear RS variants. The appearance of the background can be quite varied. Most commonly, it is rich in T lymphocytes and eosinophils mixed with a variable number of macrophages and plasma cells. However, in other cases, epithelioid histiocytes can predominate, and sarcoidal granulomas are sometimes seen. Disorganized fibrosis may also be present, but the well-developed bands of collagen characteristic of the nodular sclerosis type are absent.

The mixed-cellularity subtype is most common in immunosuppressed persons, children, and older male patients and is

TABLE 27-2. Clinicopathologic Features of Hodgkin's Disease Subtypes

	Nodular Sclerosis	Mixed-Cellularity	Lymphocyte-Rich	Lymphocytic-Depletion	Lymphocyte-Predominance
Sex	F > M	M > F	M > F	M > F	M > F
Peak age of onset (yr)	Young adults; unusual at >50	Older adults, children in developing world, immunosuppressed patients of any age	>40	Elderly patients; immunosuppressed patients of any age	25–40
Epstein-Barr virus	~20%	~70%	~40%	>75%	Not present
Typical presentation	Mediastinal mass, cervical nodes	Lymph nodes, above or below diaphragm, ± extranodal sites	Axillary and cervical lymph nodes	Lymph nodes, above or below diaphragm, ± extranodal sites	Axillary and cervical lymph nodes
Reed-Sternberg cells	Lacunar variants; occasional diagnostic forms	Frequent mononuclear variants and diagnostic forms	Frequent mononuclear variants and diagnostic forms	Frequent diagnostic forms and bizarre variants	Lymphocytic and histiocytic variants; diagnostic forms present but rare
Immunophenotype	CD15+, CD30+, CD45−, CD20±, Bcl-6±	CD15+, CD30+, CD45−, CD20±, Bcl±	CD15+, CD30+, CD45−, CD20±, Bcl±	CD15+, CD30+, CD45−, CD20±, Bcl-6±	CD15−, CD30−, CD45+, CD20+, Bcl-6+

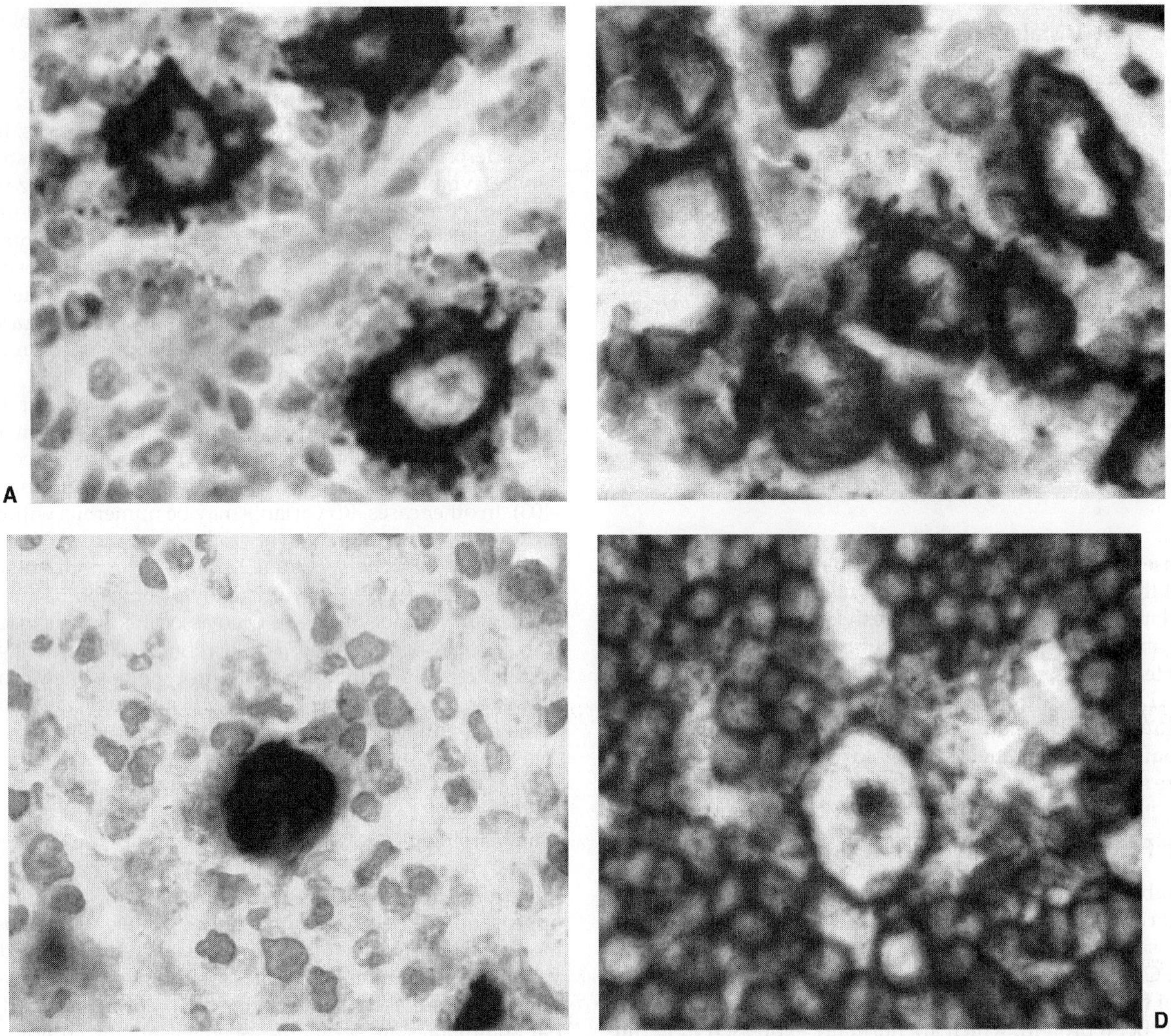

Figure 27-5. Markers useful in characterizing Reed-Sternberg cells. Mononuclear Reed-Sternberg variants are stained with anti-CD15 **(A)** and anti-CD30 **(B)** in a case of classic Hodgkin's disease. In **(C)**, Epstein-Barr virus small nuclear RNAs are detected in the nucleus of a single Reed-Sternberg variant by *in situ* hybridization. In **(D)**, a large lymphocytic and histiocytic variant is stained with anti-CD20; numerous surrounding small reactive B cells are also CD20⁺. In each instance, a method is used that deposits a brown stain on reactive cells.

more likely to present with high stage disease than the nodular sclerosis type. Based on its varied histologic appearance and bimodal age incidence, it has been suggested that this is a pathogenetically heterogeneous group of tumors. One common theme, however, is its strong association with EBV, which is found in the RS cells and variants of mixed cellularity HD in up to 75% of cases. The most sensitive test for the presence of EBV is *in situ* hybridization for EBV-encoded small nuclear RNAs (Fig. 27-5C).

LYMPHOCYTE-RICH SUBTYPE

The lymphocyte-rich subtype constitutes approximately 5% of HD. It was added to the REAL/WHO classification in recognition of cases in which the morphology and phenotype of the RS cells resemble those seen in classic HD, but the reactive cellular background is comprised predominantly of small lymphocytes. Most of these tumors were classified previously as *diffuse lymphocyte-predominance subtype* in the Rye classification.

Most patients with the lymphocyte-rich variant are adult males presenting with asymptomatic axillary or cervical lym-

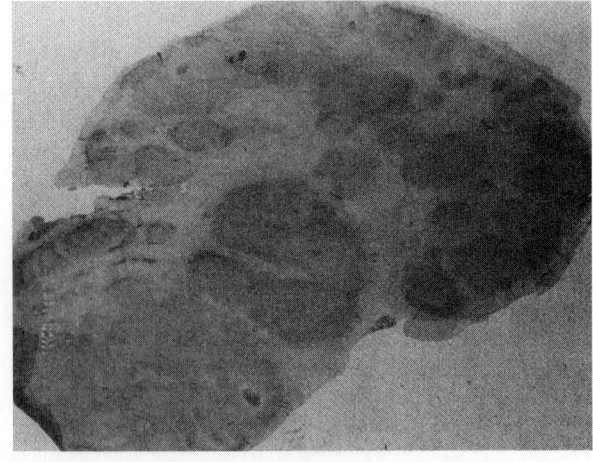

Figure 27-6. Nodular sclerosis. Broad bands of connective tissue and tumor nodules are evident (hematoxylin and eosin, ×8).

phadenopathy without mediastinal involvement (99). The lymph nodes are effaced by small lymphocytes, scattered RS variants, and occasional diagnostic RS cells. Eosinophils are usually sparse. Not uncommonly, RS cells and variants are placed eccentrically about the expanded mantle zones of atrophic germinal centers, producing a nodular appearance that has been referred to as the *follicular variant* (112), although the term *nodular lymphocyte-rich classic HD* is preferred (99). Because of its nodular growth pattern, this variant is frequently misdiagnosed as lymphocyte-predominance subtype and can only be reliably diagnosed through the use of immunohistochemistry (99). Approximately 40% of cases are EBV associated.

LYMPHOCYTE-DEPLETION SUBTYPE

With the application of modern histologic criteria and the advent of routine immunophenotyping, the frequency of the lymphocyte-depletion subtype has decreased to approximately 1% of all HD. Because cases of true lymphocyte-depletion subtype are rare, the diagnosis should be made only when other tumor types have been excluded rigorously by immunophenotyping.

Two histologic variants, originally described by Lukes and Butler, are recognized. The *diffuse fibrosis variant* is characterized by the deposition of disorganized connective tissue that may be fibrillar or amorphous in appearance. The tissue is hypocellular, but foci containing frequent RS variants and diagnostic forms should be found. The *reticular variant* is much more cellular and is marked by the presence of frequent RS variants and diagnostic forms, which may be exceptionally bizarre and pleomorphic. Both patterns may sometimes be seen within different areas of the same lymph node.

RECURRENT CLASSIC HODGKIN'S DISEASE

Although *de novo* lymphocyte depletion HD is rare, other subtypes of classic HD, at recurrence, often demonstrate more numerous, bizarre RS cells in a fibrotic background with few lymphocytes or other reactive elements—an appearance simulating the lymphocyte-depletion subtype. These changes may stem from outgrowth of neoplastic subclones with decreased dependency on reactive elements for growth and survival, and they likely represent a form of tumor progression. In support of this, a comparison of paired newly diagnosed and relapsed HD biopsies has revealed an increased growth fraction and more common expression of P53 in RS cells at relapse (28).

Nonclassic Hodgkin's Disease: Lymphocyte-Predominance Subtype

This lymphocyte-predominance subtype is a distinctive subtype that differs from classic HD in many ways. The characteristic tumor cell, the lymphocytic and histiocytic variant, is positive for CD45 and B-cell markers, such as CD20 (Fig. 27-5D), and negative for CD15 and CD30. This led to the longstanding belief that this is a tumor of B-cell origin (92,113), which has been confirmed by molecular genetic analyses. Diagnostic RS cells are rare (99).

In most instances, lymphocyte-predominance HD involves lymph nodes in a follicular or nodular pattern, as the lymphocytic and histiocytic variants are localized to expanded B-cell follicles that contain follicular dendritic cells and numerous reactive CD20+ small B cells. The tumor cells are often encircled by CD57+ T cells (92), which represent a normal germinal center T-cell subset, and express the Bcl-6 protein (114), which is a reliable marker of germinal center B cells. The tumor cells are also usually positive for epithelial membrane antigen (99) and J chain (115), which can also help to distinguish the tumor from classic forms of HD. In one recent large review, only two-thirds of the cases submitted as lymphocyte-predominance HD were

confirmed, with most of those misdiagnosed being reclassified as lymphocyte-rich classic HD (99). Because of such difficulties, immunophenotyping is essential for accurate diagnosis.

The clinical features of the lymphocyte-predominance subtype also differ from other forms of HD. It presents most commonly in young male patients as low stage disease in the cervical or axillary lymph nodes and is unaccompanied by systemic symptoms. It is sometimes associated with an unusual form of reactive lymphadenopathy, progressive transformation of germinal centers, which may precede or follow lymphocyte predominance HD (116–118). Late recurrences are more common in this subtype in some series (119), but they are usually highly responsive to therapy. As with other indolent B-cell neoplasms, the tumor may transform to diffuse large B-cell lymphoma (120,121), although this occurs in less than 5% of patients and appears to have a better outcome than other large cell transformations.

Usefulness of Hodgkin's Disease Classification

How useful is HD classification in clinical management? Certainly, *stage* (extent of disease; see section Staging and Laboratory Evaluation) is the major prognostic determinant in HD, as opposed to the non-Hodgkin's lymphomas in which *histopathologic subtype* is paramount. One contribution of histopathology is the recognition of the uncommon lymphocyte-predominance subtype, which carries an extremely good prognosis. A second contribution has been to discriminate between the nodular sclerosis and the mixed-cellularity subtypes, although the differences in clinical outcome between these two subtypes have diminished as therapy has improved.

Of more general clinical importance, the widespread use of immunophenotyping has improved the discrimination of HD from other entities with "Hodgkin's-like" features. These "look-alikes" include diffuse large B-cell lymphomas with immunoblastic features (which resemble lymphocyte depletion HD); T-cell–rich diffuse large B-cell lymphomas; anaplastic large cell lymphoma; a variety of other T-cell lymphomas; and solid tumors, which may contain RS-like cells.

Granulomas

Noncaseating sarcoidlike granulomas within the liver, spleen, and lymph nodes are a common finding in patients with HD (122). These granulomas do *not* indicate involvement of that organ with HD and have no adverse prognostic significance.

Spread of Disease

Two mechanisms are involved in the spread of HD. The first is contiguous spread by way of lymphatic channels. This mode of spread accounts for many of the localized presentations of early HD. Contiguous spread is also responsible for the asymmetric and localized distribution of peripheral, mediastinal, and abdominal lymph nodes, which is characteristic of HD.

The multiplicity of lymphatic channels connecting the lymph nodes of the lower neck with those of the mediastinum explains the frequent occurrence of disease in those two areas in the same patient. Pulmonary involvement also follows the lymphatic pathways of the lung, with the process spreading from the nodes of the anterior mediastinum successively to the hilar and bronchopulmonary nodes and then through the lymphatic channels of the bronchovascular bundle into the lung substance and to the pleural surface. Similarly, HD may enter the spinal canal via the lymphatic channels of abdominoaortic lymph nodes overlying the spine.

The second mechanism in HD is hematogenous spread. Characteristically, hematogenous spread is seen first in the spleen and then in the liver and bone marrow. Why hematogenous spread occurs early in one patient and late in another is unknown, but it represents a central event in the evolution of each patient's disease because it mandates systemic therapy.

CLINICAL PRESENTATION

Although the manifestations of HD are varied, the condition evolves in a highly predictable manner. The primary sites of disease are the peripheral and mediastinal lymph nodes (123). Abdominal lymph nodes and spleen may be diseased at the time of diagnosis, but, infrequently, are the only sites of disease. Unlike the non-Hodgkin's lymphomas, HD is rarely of extranodal origin and does not usually compress vascular structures or airways at initial presentation.

Approximately 90% of patients with HD present with painless enlargement of a superficial lymph node (123). In approximately 75% of cases, the first node appreciated is in the neck, usually on the left side. The incidence and distribution of enlargement of the various peripheral lymph nodes at the outset are indicated in Figure 27-7. The enlarged node may fluctuate in size and is usually nontender; on examination, it is firm and rubbery, not hard. Most patients who present without peripheral lymphadenopathy have a mediastinal tumor uncovered on chest x-ray examination that was performed routinely for pulmonary symptoms (usually cough), or, rarely, for intractable itching.

Approximately one-third of HD patients have systemic symptoms, which are also known as "B" symptoms, at the time of diagnosis. Fever is present in approximately 25% of patients at diagnosis (123). Most frequently, the fever initially takes the form of an accentuated diurnal curve. This low-grade pyrexia is usually present in the late afternoon and evening and may progress to debilitating fever, either constant or remitting. *Pel-Ebstein fevers*, classic intermittent fevers recurring at variable intervals of days to weeks, are nearly pathognomonic for HD, but they are not common (124). To be considered a "B" symptom, weight loss should exceed 10% of body weight over the preceding 6-month period.

Pruritus, although no longer considered a "B" symptom, often correlates with disease, and may predate symptomatic lymphadenopathy (125). Pain is rare, but it may occur a few minutes after ingestion of alcohol in sites of bone and nodal involvement of HD (126). Although the symptom has been described in fractures and other benign bone lesions, alcohol-induced pain in lymph nodes is rarely caused by conditions other than HD.

STAGING AND LABORATORY EVALUATION

Staging has an important role in the treatment of all malignancies, but it is critically important in HD. Treatment of HD depends on *stage at presentation*, which is defined by anatomic location of involved sites and presence or absence of specific symptoms. Accurate staging allows optimization of therapy, improving overall survival by decreasing relapse rates. In addition, the unnecessary toxicities of extended-field radiation, laparotomy, or overly aggressive chemotherapy may be avoided with appropriate staging. The risk of secondary malignancies, which exceeds 10% in several series of patients with early stage HD (127), may also be minimized. Patient quality of life during and after therapy may be improved with tailored therapy defined by staging (128).

By defining involved sites of disease, staging not only defines appropriate therapy but also allows comparison of results of treatment among cancer centers, defines entry into clinical trials, and provides prognostic information valuable to both the physician and the patient. Table 27-3 summarizes our current approach to the evaluation of a patient with newly diag-

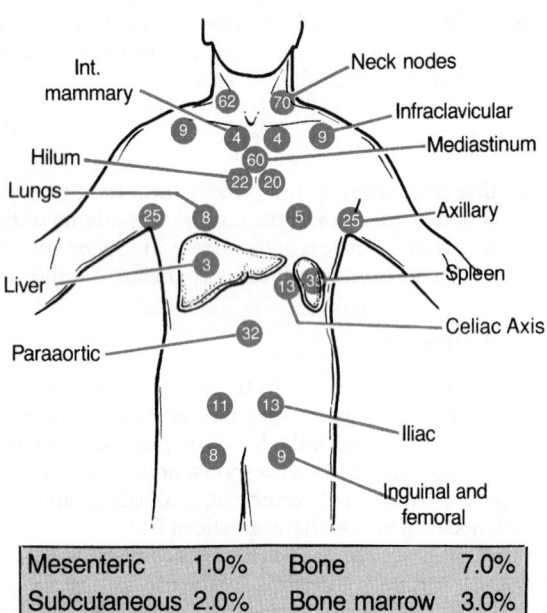

Mesenteric	1.0%	Bone	7.0%
Subcutaneous	2.0%	Bone marrow	3.0%
Epidural	0.4%	Other	4.0%

Figure 27-7. Distribution of Hodgkin's disease in 285 consecutive, untreated patients, 172 of whom had a staging laparotomy and splenectomy. The numbers indicate the percentage of patients with involvement at each site. Int., internal. (From Kaplan HS, Dorfman RF, Nelson TS, et al. Staging laparotomy and splenectomy in Hodgkin's disease: analysis of indications and patterns of involvement in 285 consecutive untreated patients. *NCI Monogr* 1973;36:291.)

TABLE 27-3. Recommended Diagnostic Evaluation for Patients with Newly Diagnosed Hodgkin's Disease

Adequate biopsy sample reviewed by experienced hematopathologist
History and physical examination
    Specific attention to fevers, weight loss, and night sweats and to nodal sites, liver size, spleen size, skin, and sites of bone discomfort
Laboratory studies
    Complete blood cell count, differential, platelet count, erythrocyte sedimentation rate
    Alkaline phosphatase, transaminase evaluation, bilirubin, and albumin
    Renal function testing
    Pregnancy testing (premenopausal female)
    Semen analysis and cryopreservation (males desiring fertility preservation)
Radiographic studies
    Plain chest radiograph
    Computed tomography of chest, abdomen, and pelvis
    Gallium scintigraphy with single photon emission computed tomography imaging or fluorodeoxyglucose positron emission tomography
Bone marrow evaluation
    Only for advanced stages, "B" symptoms, related disease, or abnormal complete blood cell count
Other optional procedures for specific indications (see text)
    Laparotomy with splenectomy and liver biopsy
    Pulmonary function testing
    Echocardiography or radionucleotide ventriculography
    Lymphangiography
    Magnetic resonance imaging
    Bone radiographs or nuclear bone scan

TABLE 27-4. Ann Arbor Staging Classification[a]

Stage	Involvement
I[b]	A single lymph node region or a single extranodal organ or site (I$_E$)
II	Two or more lymph node regions on the same side of the diaphragm or localized involvement of an extranodal organ or site (II$_E$) and of one or more lymph node regions on the same side of the diaphragm
III	Lymph node regions on both sides of the diaphragm, which may also be accompanied by the localized involvement of an extranodal organ or site (III$_E$) or spleen (III$_S$), or both (III$_{SE}$)
IV	Diffuse or disseminated involvement of one or more distant extranodal organs with or without associated lymph node involvement

[a]Clinical staging is based on all clinical and radiologic studies and the initial surgical biopsy. Pathologic staging includes the further surgical removal of tissue including staging laparotomy and splenectomy. Biopsy-documented involvement may be designated by the following symbols: N+, nodes; M+, marrow; H+, liver; L+, lung; P+, pleura; O+, bone; D+, skin.
[b]Fever greater than 38.0°C (100.5°F), night sweats, and weight loss of more than 10% of body weight during the preceding 6 months are systemic symptoms and denoted by the suffix B. Asymptomatic patients are denoted by the suffix A.

nosed HD. Patients with relapsed disease should be staged in a similar fashion to patients presenting *de novo* (129–131).

Staging System: Ann Arbor Guidelines and the Cotswolds Revision

The four-part Ann Arbor Staging classification remains in general use (Table 27-4) (132). The distinction between clinical staging and pathologic staging is a major one. Pathologic stage indicates that the extent of spread has been documented by histologic examination, which is, in practice, the result of a staging laparotomy and splenectomy. Clinical stage is based on all diagnostic procedures except abdominal exploration.

Figure 27-8 illustrates the anatomic definition of separate lymph node regions adopted for staging at the Rye Symposium on HD.

In 1988, a group of experts meeting in the Cotswolds of England suggested that the Ann Arbor Staging classification be modified by (a) the incorporation of the suffix X to denote peripheral or abdominal adenopathy greater than 10 cm or mediastinal adenopathy greater than one-third of the chest diameter, and (b) the subdivision of pathologic stage IIIA into IIIA$_1$ (upper abdominal disease only) and IIIA$_2$ (lower abdominal disease with or without disease in the upper abdomen) (133). The group stressed the importance of recording the number of sites of involvement and the need to recognize how frequently the residual radiographic and tomographic findings constituted an isolated abnormality in patients cured of their disease (131). The general framework of the Ann Arbor classification was maintained; however, computed tomography (CT) scanning was recommended for the detection of intraabdominal disease, and the concept of bulky disease comprising greater than 10 cm or greater than a one-third widening of the mediastinum was introduced. The Cotswolds revision of the Ann Arbor classification continues to be the standard scheme for staging patients with HD and is detailed in Table 27-4.

History and Physical Examination

A detailed history should be obtained, including the presence or absence of the constitutional "B" symptoms of weight loss, night sweats, and fevers. Risk of infection with human immun-

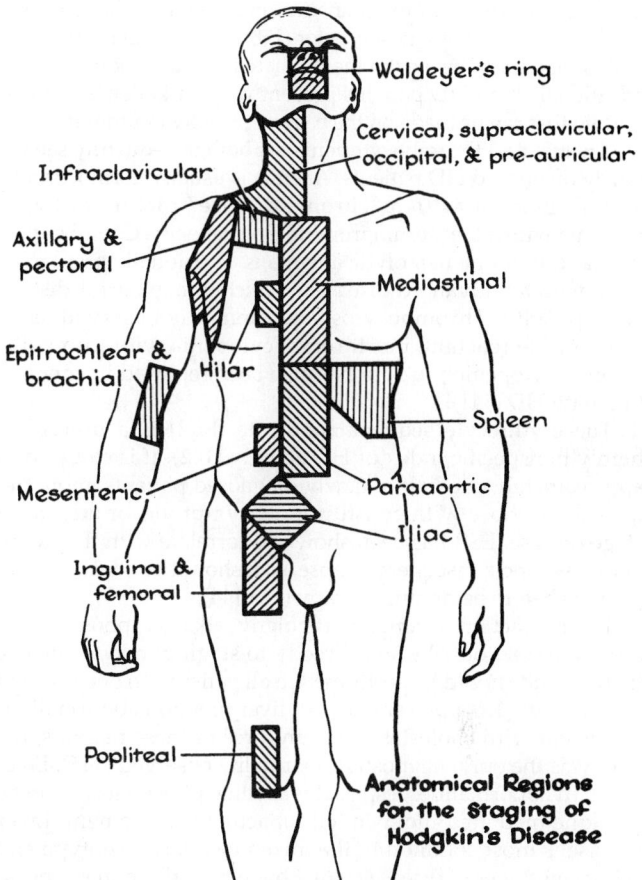

Figure 27-8. Diagram of the anatomic definition of separate lymph node regions adopted for staging purposes at the 1965 Rye Symposium on Hodgkin's Disease. (From Kaplan HS, Rosenberg SA. The treatment of Hodgkin's disease. *Med Clin North Am* 1966;50:1591.)

odeficiency virus should be assessed, as HD appears to be increased in this population, and such history may have important implications on choice of therapy (135,136).

On examination, involved nodes are typically nontender and possess a rubbery consistency on palpation. A measurement of the largest mass in each lymph node region should be recorded. The probability of involvement varies between various lymph node groups (Fig. 27-7). Waldeyer's ring should always be examined and may be involved in up to 5% of patients.

The size of the liver and spleen should also be recorded. Splenomegaly may be present in up to 30% of patients at presentation. Hepatomegaly, although rare, can occur. Skin lesions that have been associated with HD include excoriations from severe pruritus, urticaria, hyperpigmentation, and direct skin infiltration with lymphoma. Cerebellar degeneration and other motor/sensory paraneoplastic syndromes have been reported to occur with HD (137), so all patients should have neurologic assessment on presentation.

Laboratory

A complete blood cell count, differential, and platelet count should be performed on every patient at diagnosis. The routine blood counts are normal in most untreated patients at the time of diagnosis of HD. Nonetheless, they can provide useful information at the onset of disease and, more frequently, in advanced disease. Leukocytosis is seen in 25% of patients at diagnosis, usually with a neutrophil predominance, and, with lymphopenia, it is considered a poor prognostic factor (138). Eosinophilia is common and is thought to be a cytokine-mediated phenomenon (139). An additional 5% of HD patients present with leukopenia, another finding that can be made on the basis of marrow infiltration.

Anemia and thrombocytopenia are both infrequently seen in newly diagnosed HD patients. Anemia is usually normochromic and normocytic with a "chronic-disease" picture of hypoferremia with a low serum iron-binding capacity. Coombs'-positive autoimmune hemolytic anemia is occasionally seen, most often with far-advanced disease in which it may mirror disease activity (140). Thrombocytosis is commonly observed as an acute phase reactant, but thrombocytopenia with idiopathic thrombocytopenic purpura has also been reported in conjunction with HD (141).

The erythrocyte sedimentation rate (ESR) is a useful but highly nonspecific index of HD activity (142). It is elevated in approximately one-half of newly diagnosed patients, more frequently in those with constitutional symptoms or advanced stage disease. ESR has been shown to correlate with the extent of disease and subsequent relapse, so it should be checked in all patients before beginning therapy (143,144).

Liver function testing, particularly alkaline phosphatase, although not contributing directly to staging, may influence therapy and should be performed in all patients. In one series of 421 patients, 1.4% presented with liver function abnormalities consistent with cholestasis, and in three of these patients, the liver was the only diagnostic abnormality observed (145). Liver function abnormalities, especially alkaline phosphatase, can be cytokine mediated independent of actual involvement. Liver disease is most common in the mixed-cellularity subtype and advanced stages of disease (146). Low serum albumin is a negative prognostic factor for advanced stage disease (138) and rarely may be secondary to nephrotic syndrome (147).

Serum calcium may be elevated in advanced disease, or when bone involvement is present, secondary to elevated calcitriol levels, and it should be determined on diagnosis (148,149). Baseline thyroid studies may be helpful in all patients with planned mantle irradiation therapy, because a significant number of these patients develop thyroid abnormalities after therapy (150,151).

Premenopausal female patients should have a pregnancy test and be counseled on the use of birth control. Male patients requiring chemotherapy should undergo semen analysis and discussions regarding sperm cryopreservation. A significant number of these patients have limited viable sperm, which is likely due to disease factors (152,153).

Bone Marrow Biopsy

Bone marrow dissemination is reported in 5% to 15% of patients with newly diagnosed HD (154,155). Spleen involvement almost always accompanies HD in the marrow, and most patients are ill with constitutional symptoms. There is significant controversy and variation in clinical practice over the role of routine unilateral or bilateral bone marrow biopsy in the staging of de novo HD, because it rarely affects choice of therapy (156,157). When performed, aspiration is insufficient to diagnose involvement with HD, so trephine biopsy is required. The German Lymphoma Study Group reported on the role of bone marrow biopsy in over 2000 patients (158). Thirty-two percent of stage IV patients had bone marrow involvement. Marrow involvement had no prognostic relevance with regard to freedom from progression and overall survival, and it did not define a special high-risk group in which a different treatment approach was indicated. For this reason, unilateral marrow biopsy is only advocated for patients with "B" symptoms,

bulky disease, or advanced stage disease, unless the peripheral blood count is abnormal and not easily explained. Patients with recurrent disease, particularly candidates for autologous stem cell transplantation, require a bone marrow biopsy (159).

Laparotomy and Splenectomy

Staging laparotomy was introduced in 1969 by Glatstein and colleagues to elucidate the cause of the high failure rate after radiation therapy and to provide a guide for improving radiation portals (160). The operation has provided major understanding of the evolution of HD within the abdomen, particularly regarding the central role of the spleen (161). Surgical staging with diagnostic laparotomy allows treatment to be tailored to the precise pathologic stage, serving to optimize therapy for an individual patient. Ideally, such tailored therapy should minimize relapses and the long-term effects of overly aggressive therapy. However, the role of laparotomy has significantly decreased over the past decade for several reasons.

A complete staging laparotomy includes splenectomy, liver biopsy, bone marrow biopsy, and a sampling of the following nodal groups: splenic, celiac, hemoptic, portal, and paraaortic. Oophoropexy, or moving the ovaries outside of a potential radiation field, is recommended for women with planned pelvic irradiation (162). Although the mortality of laparotomy is generally low at experienced centers, major immediate complications include infection, hemorrhage, ileus, and pulmonary embolism (163,164). In addition, long-term complications after splenectomy include sepsis from encapsulated bacteria (165,166) and, possibly, an increased risk of secondary malignancies (167–169).

Clinical prognostic factors found to be predictive of a positive staging laparotomy include male gender, presence of "B" symptoms, mixed-cellularity histology, and increased number of involved nodal sites (170). If all of these factors are present, the expected positive laparotomy rate may exceed 80% (171). In contrast, if none of these features are present, the expected positive laparotomy rate is very low (172). In recent years, these factors have limited the patient population who would benefit from laparotomy.

The European Organization for Research and Treatment of Cancer (EORTC) conducted the H6F trial (n = 262), which consisted of randomization to clinical staging plus subtotal nodal irradiation or to staging laparotomy plus treatment adaptation (adjuvant chemotherapy only in the patients with negative laparotomy) (173). In this study, the 6-year freedom from progression rates were similar in the clinical and laparotomy-staged patients. Survival rates were 93% in the clinically staged arm and 89% in the laparotomy-staged arm. The slight increase in mortality in the surgical arm was due to laparotomy-related deaths. The authors concluded that staging laparotomy might be eliminated, even in favorable patients, at no cost to survival or freedom from progression endpoints. However, Ng and colleagues recently constructed a decision-analytic model that addressed the role of laparotomy in patients with early stage, favorable prognosis HD (174). This model included quality of life, as well as recent improvements in both combination chemotherapy and supportive care after surgery. They concluded that the use of laparotomy resulted in a modest net survival gain of 9 months, retaining significance as a beneficial intervention.

Presently, the majority of large centers have abandoned the use of staging laparotomy in the majority of patients. A few centers continue to use this approach in selected patients who are enrolled in a treatment protocol. Laparoscopic staging has been used in some centers, with decreased morbidity; however, the technique has never been prospectively compared with conventional laparotomy in adult patients with HD (175,176). The grow-

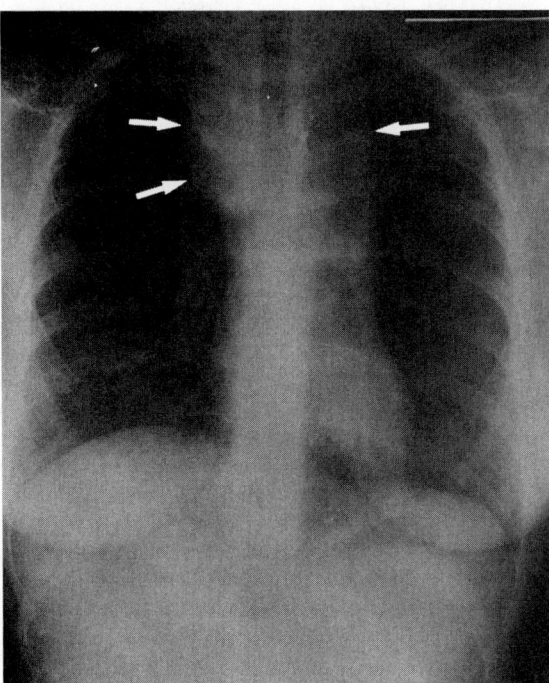

Figure 27-9. Pathologic stage IIA Hodgkin's disease of the nodular sclerosis type. This 11-cm asymptomatic mediastinal mass (*arrows*) in a 28-year-old woman with cervical adenopathy measures more than one-third of the maximum chest diameter (29 cm).

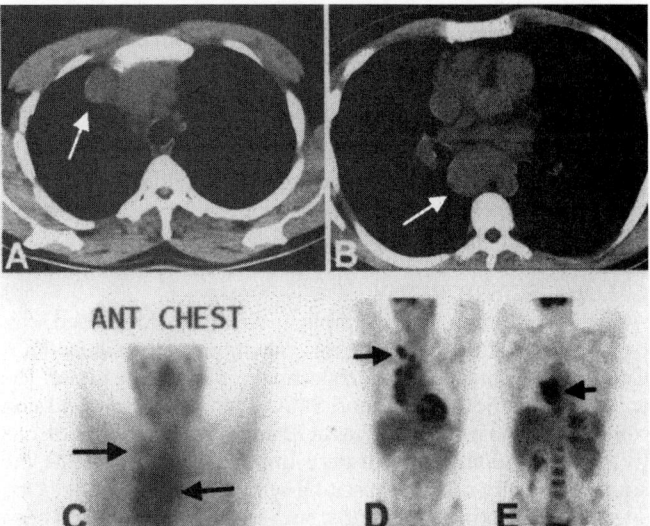

Figure 27-10. Staging studies before the treatment of a 24-year-old man with nodular sclerosing Hodgkin's disease. **A:** Axial computed tomography (CT) image in the upper mediastinum, showing anterior mediastinal adenopathy, with the largest node to the right of midline (*arrow*). **B:** Axial CT image in the lower chest, showing bulky subcarinal adenopathy (*arrow*). **C:** Gallium image of the chest from anterior (ANT CHEST), showing abnormal uptake of radiotracer in both the right superior mediastinal node and subcarinal node (*arrows*). **D:** Coronal image from a fluorodeoxyglucose positron emission tomography (FDG-PET) scan through the level of the myocardium, which shows expected degree of uptake in a fasting patient. The right superior mediastinal node is evident (*arrow*) as are several other mediastinal nodes. **E:** Coronal image from a FDG-PET scan through the posterior mediastinum, showing abnormal uptake in the large subcarinal mass (*arrow*).

ing use of combined modality therapy for patients with early stage disease and effective salvage chemotherapy regimens for patients who do not respond to radiation as initial treatment have limited the value of accurate abdominal staging. However, long-term results from current clinical trials are needed before surgical staging is completely relegated to history (177).

Radiographic Imaging

The staging of HD involves several different radiologic imaging modalities including conventional radiography, CT, sonography and magnetic resonance imaging (occasionally), and radionuclide imaging [predominantly with gallium-67 scintigraphy or positron emission tomography (PET), or both].

EVALUATION OF THE CHEST
Conventional chest radiography is typically the initial radiologic examination obtained in patients with suspected HD (Fig. 27-9) (178–180). HD can affect the pulmonary parenchyma, but at initial presentation, lung disease is nearly always associated with concomitant intrathoracic lymphadenopathy (181). Pulmonary parenchymal involvement, as in non-Hodgkin's lymphoma, presents in one of three radiologic patterns: bronchovascular (or lymphangitic), nodular, or pneumonic (or alveolar).

CT is more sensitive in the assessment of chest disease than conventional chest radiography, and it is considered standard (Fig. 27-10A, B) (178,182). In addition to assessing nodal sites, CT should also evaluate for the presence of pleural effusions (178), which are generally benign pericardial effusions, and chest wall invasion that is typically due to direct extension from contiguous mediastinal or intraparenchymal disease (183).

EVALUATION OF THE ABDOMEN
Data based on staging laparotomy have revealed histologic involvement of the paraaortic lymph nodes and spleen in 34%, the liver in 6%, and the mesenteric lymph nodes in less than 5%

of HD patients at presentation. Of note, mesenteric lymph nodes, when involved, are typically normal in size (184). Historically, bipedal lymphangiography was the procedure of choice for staging abdominal HD. Although lymphangiography is extremely sensitive, specific, and overall accurate in assessing the retroperitoneal and pelvic lymph nodes, CT has supplanted it as the imaging modality of choice for evaluating the abdomen and pelvis due to the expense and considerable expertise required for performance and interpretation of lymphangiography.

Castellino et al., in a study of 121 patients, noted a small but significant increase in the accuracy of lymphangiography over CT scanning in assessing retroperitoneal lymph nodes (185). However, more recent studies have refuted this claim (186); given the evolving treatment patterns with chemotherapy alone or combined chemotherapy and radiotherapy for early stages of disease, the value of lymphangiography is clearly diminishing (187,188).

In addition to assessing retroperitoneal lymph nodes, CT should evaluate for splenic involvement, which typically manifests as subcentimeter nodules (178). The spleen is thus often of normal size despite tumor involvement. Spleen size alone is a poor predictor for the presence or absence of HD. As both splenic and hepatic lesions are typically quite small, they may not be detected by CT.

EVALUATION OF BONE
Bone radiographs are obtained in patients who are symptomatic, and they typically reveal predominantly osteoblastic or mixed lesions; lytic lesions are much less common. In the spine, an "ivory vertebrae" may be seen, which is often associated with an adjacent soft tissue mass (189). Bone scans using technetium 99 bound to pyrophosphate have a very high sensitivity in the detection of lymphomatous involvement and can be used

to follow responses in conjunction with other staging procedures in patients with known bone disease (190).

Nuclear Imaging

Nuclear imaging at diagnosis can clarify findings of uncertain significance on conventional radiographic staging. More importantly, baseline imaging allows accurate response assessment and evaluation of residual masses after therapy.

GALLIUM SCINTIGRAPHY

At present, gallium-67 scintigraphy is the most widely used scintigraphic modality for the staging evaluation of HD (Fig. 27-10C). Gallium-67 citrate binds to transferrin receptors in the tumor. The acquisition of both planar and SPECT (single photon emission computed tomography) images at 72 hours after the injection of 8 to 10 mCi of gallium-67 citrate is important in optimizing the scan. The ability of gallium scintigraphy to disclose undetected sites of disease (predominantly, supradiaphragmatic) has been shown (191,192). However, the overall sensitivity of gallium scanning is fairly low, despite an overall specificity of 98% (193).

Persistent gallium-avid disease during and after treatment is a poor prognostic sign and suggests a high risk of subsequent relapse (193,194). The value of gallium scanning in early stage disease to detect otherwise occult abdominal involvement is currently under investigation; however, normal splenic uptake by gallium limits the sensitivity of this approach. Gallium scintigraphy is especially useful in patients with a residual soft tissue abnormality after the completion of therapy to help differentiate residual disease from fibrosis (195–197).

POSITRON EMISSION TOMOGRAPHY

Several groups have suggested a role for whole-body fluorodeoxyglucose (FDG) PET in predicting relapse in patients with residual masses after therapy for both HD and non-Hodgkin's lymphoma (198). Radiotracers used in PET imaging have been primarily metabolic substrates, such as FDG, that tend to accumulate in malignant cells. These radionuclides are taken up and metabolized by malignant cells. Positrons are emitted in this process, creating a functional image (Fig. 27-10D, E).

FDG-PET appears to accurately assess HD activity, with a sensitivity ranging from 71% to 96% and, importantly, a negative predictive value exceeding 93%. Several studies have shown at least equal sensitivity and increased specificity of PET when compared to CT or magnetic resonance imaging (199–204). Moreover, PET, in contrast to gallium scintigraphy (which is of limited value below the diaphragm), may be useful in detecting splenic involvement as well as bone marrow involvement (205,206).

However, PET does not allow for tumor measurements or exact anatomic locations of disease. Appropriate prospective studies comparing PET to gallium imaging (with SPECT and appropriate radiopharmaceutical dose and time interval) are necessary before PET can be recommended as a standard diagnostic imaging procedure for patients with HD.

Cardiac and Pulmonary Evaluation

Patients with any history of cardiac disease or symptoms or who are older than age 40 to 50 years should undergo evaluation of cardiac function with either a radionucleotide ventriculogram or echocardiogram if therapy is to include chest irradiation or an anthracycline. Patients with abnormal function at baseline require aggressive monitoring to limit the incidence of doxorubicin-associated cardiomyopathy (207).

Complete pulmonary function testing, including diffusing capacity of the lung for carbon monoxide, adjusted for volume and hemoglobin, is recommended if the patient is to receive mantle irradiation or bleomycin as part of a chemotherapy regimen. Although significant controversy exists on the relationship between diffusing capacity of the lung for carbon monoxide and development of bleomycin-induced pulmonary toxicity, patients with significant abnormalities at baseline warrant an aggressive monitoring strategy (208).

CLINICAL PROGNOSTIC FEATURES

The negative influence of female sex, advanced age, unfavorable histology, and advanced stage was described in a series of 1225 patients treated at Stanford with megavoltage radiation and combination chemotherapy (209). The negative influence of male sex, advanced age, unfavorable histology, and advanced stage have been demonstrated in many other studies. Several investigators have looked at constitutional symptoms more closely. Gobbi and associates find the solitary complaint of *sweats* is without negative influence, whereas *severe pruritus* has the same unfavorable significance as fever and weight loss (125). Another study has demonstrated that weight loss plus fever has more importance than either alone, at least in pathologic stage IIB disease (210). Taken together, the two studies suggest that constitutional complaints contribute to poor prognosis in an incremental manner.

Tumor bulk is a second parameter that has been quantitatively linked to HD prognosis. Tumor size was first shown to be prognostically important in the mediastinum. Although the presence of any mediastinal mass reduced the radiation curability of early stage HD (pathologic stages I and II) from 90% to 95% to approximately 80%, several centers reported that the cure was reduced to approximately 50% when the tumor mass exceeded one-third of the maximum chest diameter (211–213). The Danish National Hodgkin's Disease Group has extended the study of the relation of tumor bulk to prognosis; they find that *total tumor burden* (a complex parameter obtained by summation of the tumor bulk of each involved site), not mediastinal mass alone, is the most important factor in predicting disease-free survival of patients in pathologic stages I and II (214). In their multivariate analysis, histology and gender were the only other independent variables.

The EORTC also undertook a multivariate analysis of survival in early (clinical stage I and II) HD treated solely with radiation (215,216). They found that patients with three or more sites of involvement, or with systemic symptoms or a marked elevation of the erythrocyte sedimentation rate, or both, did poorly after irradiation.

Several attempts have been made to apply prognostic criteria to patients with abdominal HD. The markedly unfavorable influence of constitutional complaints in these patients has long been recognized. In addition, several studies have demonstrated markedly inferior disease-free survival and somewhat inferior overall survival in HD patients with disease in the lower abdomen when compared with patients whose disease is restricted to the upper abdomen (217).

Several groups have developed prognostic scoring systems to identify favorable patients at presentation who may benefit from minimization of therapy (218). Age at presentation, stage, bulk of disease, gender, lymphocyte count, anemia, lactic dehydrogenase, and bone marrow involvement have all been predictive in univariate analyses (219–221). More recently, the data from 5141 patients with advanced stage HD was used to develop a parametric model for predicting freedom from disease progression. Seven factors had similar prognostic effects that on multivariate analysis were independent: serum albumin

TABLE 27-5. Alkylating Agent–Containing Regimens Active in the Treatment of Hodgkin's Disease

Regimen	mg/m²	Days	Reference
MOPP			DeVita et al. (12)
Mechlorethamine	6	1, 8	
Vincristine	1.4	1, 8	
Procarbazine	100	1–15	
Prednisone	40	1–15	
ChlVPP			Selby et al. (224)
Chlorambucil	6 (max 10)	1–14	
Vinblastine	6 (max 10)	1, 8	
Procarbazine	100	1–15	
Prednisone	40	1–15	
MVPP			Sutcliffe et al. (225)
Mechlorethamine	6	1, 8	
Vinblastine	100	1, 8	
Procarbazine	100	1–15	
Prednisolone	40	1–15	

max, maximum.

less than 4 g/dL, age older than 45 years, male gender, stage IV disease, leukocytosis greater than 15,000/mL³, and lymphopenia greater than 600/mL³ or less than 8%. Although only 19% of patients had a score of 4 or higher, these patients had a 47% rate of freedom from disease progression at 5 years (138). Beyond simple descriptions of locations of disease, these validated clinical prognostic features should be included in the evaluation of all patients with HD before commencing therapy and, in the future, will help to evaluate the results of clinical trials (222).

THERAPY FOR HODGKIN'S DISEASE

Principles of Therapeutics

Therapeutics in human neoplasia has derived a great deal from the early experiments of combination chemotherapy in the treatment of advanced HD. The 1960s saw the introduction of new drugs that were active in the treatment of lymphoma in general, usually given as single agents in moderate doses to patients previously treated with steroids and radiation therapy. Once antitumor activity was established, it remained to take the next bold step to use them in combination in previously untreated patients with measurable, advanced disease. The precedent was already being set in the treatment of childhood acute lymphoblastic leukemia with encouraging preliminary results. The NCI group pioneered the effective use of combined chemotherapy with the demonstration subsequently that the combination of nitrogen mustard, vincristine, procarbazine, and prednisone, known as *MOPP*, could achieve a high order of response with prolonged duration of complete remission that continued indefinitely in a significant number of patients (223). Table 27-5 is an outline of alkylating agent–containing regimens commonly used in the treatment of HD (12,224,225). These and subsequent variant regimens led to a generation of a series of clinical trials. Initial trials demonstrated that MOPP could cure not only previously untreated patients but also patients in relapse from radiation therapy (226). Maintenance therapy beyond six to eight monthly courses of MOPP did not increase the cure rate. Furthermore, the regimen was possibly as effective as radiation alone in localized disease (227).

The long-term toxicity of alkylating agents in general and MOPP in particular primarily affected bone marrow stem cells resulting in myelodysplasia; leukemia and germ cells resulting in sterilization prompted the need for less toxic but equally

effective treatment (168,228,229). The demonstration that the combination of doxorubicin, bleomycin, vinblastine, and dacarbazine (ABVD), introduced by the NCI Milan group, could provide such a substitute led to its widespread use and may be the current standard in North America. Many of the newer, more intensive regimens are currently being compared to ABVD. A variety of active nonalkylating agent–containing regimens are shown in Table 27-6. They have not been compared to one another and have been confined to mostly phase II trials (13,230–232).

Chemotherapy regimens have been modified to include alternating combinations of active drugs, hybridized regimens, dose intensification per se, and addition of other agents. Hybridized or alternating regimens showed some superiority to MOPP (or variant) alone in response and progression-free survival, but the extensive use of these more toxic regimens remained to be compared to ABVD alone (233–235). There is also a need to replace or diminish the amount of radiation therapy given to young patients at risk for long-term radiation-induced secondary malignancies. The ABVD regimen provided the means to do so

TABLE 27-6. Nonalkylating Combination Chemotherapy Regimens

Regimen	mg/m²	Days	Reference
ABVD			Bonadonna et al. (13)
Doxorubicin	25 i.v.	1, 15	
Bleomycin	10 units	1, 15	
Vinblastine	6	1, 15	
Dacarbazine	375	1, 15	
EVA			Canellos et al. (230)
Etoposide	100	1, 2, 3	
Vinblastine	6	1	
Doxorubicin	50	1 q 28 days	
EVAP			Longo et al. (231)
Etoposide	150 p.o. (200)	1–3	
Vinblastine	6 (10)	1, 8	
Doxorubicin	25	1, 8	
Prednisone	25	1, 8	
NOVP			Hagemeister et al. (232)
Mitoxantrone	10	1	
Vincristine	1.4	8 q 21 days	
Vinblastine	6	1	
Prednisone	100	1–5	

with relative safety as a systemic therapy even for localized presentations. The basis for this was enhanced by many prospective trials that showed a superiority in relapse-free survival for combined modality over radiation therapy alone, although overall survival was not necessarily improved given the ability of chemotherapy to salvage relapse from radiation therapy used as primary treatment (236). Combined modality therapy for localized disease in recent series can be expected to generate a 5-year freedom from progression of 85% with an overall survival greater than 80% (237). The inclusion of chemotherapy in combined modality for localized disease has obviated the need for staging laparotomy. Improvement in radiologic staging also contributed to the abandonment of laparotomy.

The long-term toxicity of radiation therapy has raised the question of the need for radiation therapy in certain early presentations that could be treated with chemotherapy alone. Advances in CT and radionuclide scanning with gallium-67 and PET with fluorodeoxyglucose 19 have contributed to more accurate initial staging and assessment of residual masses (see section Nuclear Imaging).

Nodular lymphocyte-predominant HD represents a special case as far as management is concerned. It has the immunophenotypic and genetic features of a low-grade B-cell lymphoma, often presenting as localized disease. Radiation therapy alone is usually sufficient to control or cure the disease (238). It is the author's experience that, in advanced disease, nonalkylating agent regimens may not have as favorable an outcome as in classic HD. Therefore, alkylating agent–containing regimens may be more effective for advanced stages of this unique, histologic, and biologic group, which represents approximately 5% of patients.

The treatment of advanced disease still requires improvement, given the 30% to 40% likelihood of relapse after six to eight cycles of any of the standard regimens. The challenge to improve therapeutic results has to be tempered by the increased drug-induced toxicity that results from certain agents such as etoposide or alkylating agents, especially when used in higher doses. Dose intensity by means of escalating individual drugs in MOPP or ABVD has not been pursued because of the unique toxicity of the various agents. "Dose intensity" is likely to be relevant because relatively escalated or "intensive" dose regimens tend to have a higher response rate, but whether a survival advantage exists has not yet been shown. Further, escalated doses used with autologous peripheral stem cell or bone marrow transplantation can cure patients who relapse from conventional dose therapy.

MANAGEMENT OF LOCALIZED DISEASE

All randomized trials have shown a consistent superiority of combined modality therapy over extensive irradiation alone in relapse-free survival. Although clinical practice has evolved more to combined modality, several long-term follow-up series of laparotomy-staged patients treated with radiation only have demonstrated a 10-year relapse-free survival of 76% to 83% for stages I or I/II in three series studying 699 patients. The late toxicity of ischemic heart disease (16%) and second tumors (10%) was noted in long-term follow-up. The radiation fields usually included the mantle field of the mediastinum/neck/axillae and extension to the upper paraaortic nodes (Fig. 27-11). The average dose was 35 Gy with a boost to the involved field up to 44 Gy. The dose to uninvolved nodal sites need not exceed 30 Gy. In general, the rate of clinical hypothyroidism is 14%. The in-field disease control rate exceeded 95% (239–241).

Using the EORTC criteria, women younger than 26 years presenting with clinical stage I asymptomatic disease and espe-

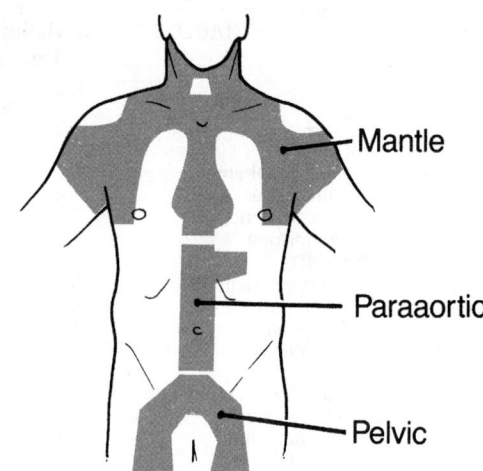

Figure 27-11. Mantle, paraaortic, and pelvic radiation fields.

cially those with lymphocyte-predominant nodular or nodular sclerosis histology can be treated with radiation alone to a mantle field without a laparotomy with excellent outcomes, but the issue of the risk of irradiation-induced breast cancer is expected to be highest in young female patients. The long-term progression-free rate approaches 80% for this subgroup (242). Mantle-only radiation therapy in localized classic HD staged without laparotomy has only a 58% 10-year progression-free survival (243). However, in classic HD, laparotomy staging better selects patients for mantle-only radiation, resulting in a 76% disease-free rate at 10 years (244).

The clinical criteria that define the risk for subsequent dissemination or relapse in patients with unfavorable localized presentations have been presented by the EORTC (Table 27-7) (245). Bulky mediastinal presentations (mass of >10 cm, or >0.33 of the thoracic diameter) have been shown to have at least a 50% chance of recurrence when radiation therapy alone has been used. This has been reduced considerably to ~20% or less with systemic therapy followed by localized irradiation (246). Other unfavorable features include "B" symptoms and an ESR greater than 30 mm or no symptoms, an ESR greater than 50 mm, and more than two nodal areas. These criteria have also been applied in other series (247). The long-term survival of patients in clinical stage IA-IIB treated at the Harvard Joint Center for Radiation Therapy, the vast majority of whom were treated with radiation therapy, is shown in Figure 27-12.

The issue of the elimination of radiation therapy in patients with early stages without bulk disease has been raised based on the preliminary observations that ABVD had a low relapse rate

---

TABLE 27-7. Unfavorable Risk Factors in Localized Disease[a] (EORTC)

Mediastinal mass (≥ 1/3 thoracic diameter)
Age >50 yr
Elevated erythrocyte sedimentation rate
≥4 involved sites with the same side of diaphragm
Mixed-cellularity histology

EORTC, European Organization for Research and Treatment of Cancer.
[a]Unfavorable entails erythrocyte sedimentation rate ≥50 or ≥30 with "B" symptoms. Any one of these factors in clinical stage I/II is unfavorable.
From Tubiana M, Henry-Amar M, Carde P, et al. Toward comprehensive management tailored to prognostic factors of patients with clinical stages I and II in Hodgkin's disease. The EORTC Lymphoma Group Controlled Clinical Trials: 1964–1987. *Blood* 1989;73:47–56.

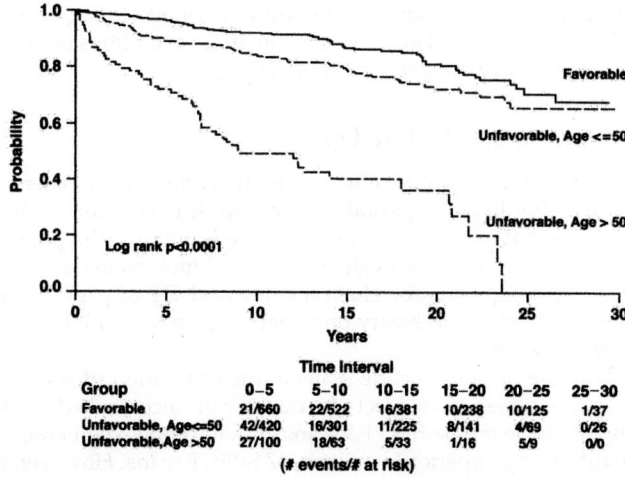

Group	0–5	5–10	10–15	15–20	20–25	25–30
Favorable	21/660	22/522	16/381	10/238	10/125	1/37
Unfavorable, Age<=50	42/420	16/301	11/225	8/141	4/69	0/26
Unfavorable, Age >50	27/100	18/63	5/33	1/16	5/9	0/0

(# events/# at risk)

Figure 27-12. Long-term survival for patients treated at the Joint Center for Radiation Therapy. Overall survival by prognostic groups.

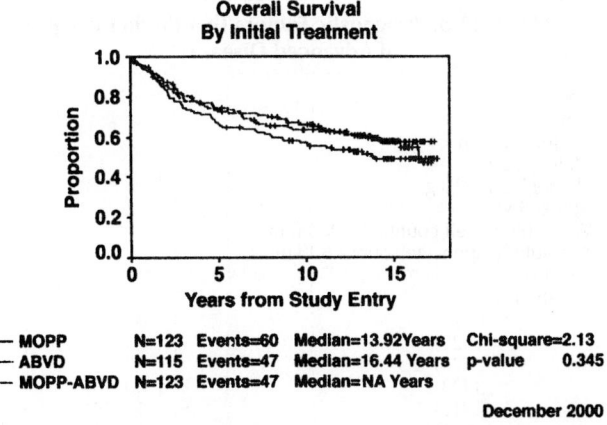

—— MOPP	N=123	Events=60	Median=13.92Years	Chi-square=2.13
—— ABVD	N=115	Events=47	Median=16.44 Years	p-value 0.345
—— MOPP-ABVD	N=123	Events=47	Median=NA Years	

December 2000

Figure 27-13. Long-term progression-free survival of CALGB trial 8251, comparing ABVD (doxorubicin, bleomycin, vinblastine, dacarbuzine) to MOPP (nitrogen mustard, vincristine, procarbazine, prednisone) to 12 months of MOPP alternating with ABVD.

when it was given to such patients in a pilot trial (248). This is the subject of several recent trials and will be the subject of a North American trial. Given the long-term risk of irradiation-induced second tumors in cured young people, the need to explore systemic therapy alone is essential. The long-term risk of second neoplasms exceeds 20% to 25% at 20 to 25 years based on the techniques and doses of radiation used in the past (249–251). These cancers comprise in-field lung cancer, sarcomas, and breast cancer in female patients. Systemic therapy alone or that combined with localized (limited) irradiation is now the approach to most patients with localized disease. Although the approach is in flux, four cycles of ABVD plus involved-field irradiation of at least 30 Gy to the involved field is commonly used for patients presenting with favorable-prognosis localized HD. The general concern for the sterilizing and leukemogenic potential of alkylating agents tends to discourage its use in the setting of localized disease.

Relapse from Localized Disease

Patients with localized disease who are treated with radiation alone have a relapse rate that varies from approximately 20% (for patients without negative prognostic features and carefully staged by laparotomy) to greater than 40% (for clinically staged patients with either bulky mediastinal masses, elevated sedimentation rate, multiple nodal areas, or extranodal extension). The majority of recurrences are detected in extranodal or nodal sites that are not previously irradiated and generally occur within the first 3 years after initiation of irradiation. Late relapses are rare with approximately 5.0% at 4 years and approximately 3.4% at 5 years in two series (252–254).

In general, patients who relapse from primary radiation therapy have an excellent outcome after combination chemotherapy. Patients who were originally in pathologic stage I/IIA can expect a chemotherapy-induced complete response (CR) rate of 80% to 90% with a 60% to 70% 10-year survival (253). Even disseminated recurrence has a second CR rate of approximately 70% with a 58% 10-year survival (255). The current use of combined modality, especially if the full six cycles of chemotherapy are given, has reduced the relapse rate; however, when *early* relapse occurs, there remains the issue of potential drug resistance. Careful planning of second-line therapy is needed, as it is in patients who relapse after chemotherapy alone for stage III or IV disease.

The relapse rate has been reduced in one-half by the use of combined modality compared to radiation alone, although this has necessarily been translated into superior survival because

salvage chemotherapy has been effective in the salvage of relapsed patients.

Management of Advanced Disease

The majority of patients presenting in stage III or IV are treated with combination chemotherapy. In time, the regimens vary in composition and schedules of drugs, and some have been used with radiation therapy. At the time of this writing, the general standard in North America, outside of a clinical trial, is ABVD for six to eight cycles. ABVD has been prospectively (see below) compared to MOPP alone; 12 months of MOPP alternating with ABVD; and MOPP-ABV hybrid (256,257). A long-term follow-up of that trial is presented in Figure 27-13. The progression-free survival continued to show an advantage for ABVD alone for 6 months compared to MOPP. However, the overall survival showed no difference due to the ability of second-line therapy to salvage relapsed patients. In all instances, it was equivalent or superior in progression-free survival without the toxicity of alkylating agents—namely, more profound myelosuppression, sterility, and leukemogenesis. Combination chemotherapy in general, including ABVD used for stage III/IV disease should achieve a clinical CR rate in the 70% to 80% range with an approximately 20% to 30% relapse rate. The outcome is directly proportional to the number of negative prognostic factors (Table 27-8) (138). It is apparent that the majority of patients present with two to three negative factors. Those with five or more have an overall 5-year survival somewhat less than 50%, but they represent only 7% of the total population. In addition to clinical prognostic factors in advanced disease, there are some preliminary biologic factors that correlate with response to chemotherapy. They include the presence of Epstein-Barr viral latent antigen (i.e., LMP-1) exerting a positive impact (258). The presence of tissue eosinophilia and elevated serum IL-10 levels are associated with an inferior failure-free survival (88,259).

It is expected that a salvage rate of 30% to 50% could result in an overall survival at 5 years in the range of 80% and, thus, the potential "cure" rate in the range of 70%. At this time, as far as conventional dose chemotherapy regimens are concerned, the overall survival outcome is likely to be similar regardless of regimen. The major differences in the early follow-up period are in toxicity. Although the North American "standard" is ABVD, it does not preclude continuing investigations into the newer compacted regimens.

TABLE 27-8. Prognostic Factors That Predict Relapse of Advanced Disease[a]

Factors
  Stage IV
  Serum albumin <4 g
  Male gender
  Hemoglobin <10 g
  Age ≥45 yr
  White blood cell count >15,000/mm³
  Absolute lymphocyte count <600/mm³

Number of Factors [Percentage (%) of patients]	Relapse-Free Survival at 6 Yr (%)
0 (7)	85
1 (22)	75–80
2 (29)	65–70
3 (23)	60–65
4 (12)	50–55
≥5 (7)	40–45

[a]Treated with systemic therapy alone or combined with irradiation.
Adapted from Hasenclever D, Diehl V. A prognostic score for advanced Hodgkin's disease. International Prognostic Factors Project on Advanced Hodgkin's Disease. *N Engl J Med* 1998;339:1506–1514.

There are currently two relatively new systemic approaches to advanced disease that are under investigation. The BEACOPP (cyclophosphamide, doxorubicin, vincristine, bleomycin, etoposide, procarbazine, prednisone) regimen developed by the German Hodgkin Group represents a multidrug combination that has a high CR rate. When used in escalated doses, it was indeed more effective and more toxic. The initial results are impressive but require more follow-up to assess whether a survival advantage accrues over ABVD alone. Again, the life-threatening toxicity and quality-of-life comparisons will weigh into the comparison (260). The Stanford V regimen represents more compacted systemic therapy because it is given weekly for 3 months. Again, the preliminary reports from Stanford show an excellent outcome. The program included radiation therapy to nodal sites in the majority of patients; thus, the unique cytotoxic potential compared to ABVD is uncertain (261).

Both regimens are being prospectively compared to ABVD. The higher response rate and progression-free survival of these programs has to be balanced against potential long-term toxicity. It may not result in a better overall survival with improved second-line therapy. As it stands now, 60% to 70% of patients with advanced disease can be rendered into long-term disease-free status with a relative minimum of long-term toxicity or sterilization.

The major toxicity of the ABVD regimen is myelosuppression, but hair loss (a side effect of doxorubicin) is common. Sterility is not common, but sperm banking as an extra precaution could be recommended. The pulmonary toxicity of bleomycin alone or with radiation therapy is usually mild but is a toxic consideration, and monitoring of clinical symptoms as well as periodic carbon monoxide diffusion (diffusing capacity of the lung for carbon monoxide) in selected patients may be warranted. There is often a transient compromise of pulmonary functions as measured by function studies that seems to reverse in time (262). Bleomycin can enhance the severity of radiation pneumonitis. Similarly, cardiac dysfunction in the absence of prior left ventricular irradiation is unusual. Six cycles of the ABVD regimen contain 300 mg/m² of doxorubicin, which is below the known total dose that has the potential for cardiac toxicity. Myelosuppression is reversible in almost all cases, and prolonged myeloid stem cell compromise or myelodysplasia is not seen.

Hybrid regimens with alkylating agents, however, do add the risk of subsequent myelodysplasia/leukemia, the vast majority of which resembles the myelodysplasia/leukemia that occurs with MOPP alone. In the presence of alkylating agent–induced myelodysplasia, chromosomal abnormalities of chromosome 5 and 7 are very common (263).

Evaluation and Follow-Up

The follow-up procedure after successful completion of chemotherapy should entail periodic radiographic evaluation of sites known to have been previously involved. Initially, the patient should undergo clinical evaluation every 3 months in the first 2 years. Radiographs for chest lesions and CT of previously involved sites are necessary on a regular 4- to 6-month basis in the first 3 years.

The role of radionuclide scans in the evaluation of residual disease has been the subject of a number of uncontrolled trials. It is still unclear whether PET scans with fluorodeoxyglucose 18 are ultimately superior to gallium-67 SPECT scans. However, it is known that clinical relapse in irradiated sites is rare, and confirmed in series of posttreatment gallium-67 scans in which only 5% to 10% recurrence was detected. However, unirradiated sites that have become gallium-67 negative post therapy still have an approximately 30% relapse rate. Persistent gallium-67 positivity post therapy should generate a high index of suspicion for relapse (194). Several false-positives post chemotherapy have been noted such as bilateral faint hilar uptake, and, in younger patients, rebound "hyperplasia" in the thymus also yields a false-positive uptake. PET scans are more sensitive and appear to be more likely to detect abdominal disease because gallium-67 has not been particularly useful when the CAT scan shows abdominal abnormalities of uncertain significance (264). Relapsing "large" masses on the CAT scan most likely do not need radionuclide confirmation.

If relapse is to occur in patients treated for stage III/IV disease primarily with systemic therapy, then it usually seen within 3 years and at sites of previous involvement that were not irradiated. Although it is common to add irradiation to bulky sites (usually >5 to 10 cm), even in stage III or some stage IV patients, randomized trials and metaanalysis of many trials have not shown a survival advantage for this approach (265–267). The Southwest Oncology Group trial suggested that patients with nodular sclerosis had a better progression-free survival advantage but overall survival was not affected (268). Dissemination to newer sites and possible resistance to chemotherapy is the major feature of early recurrence in unirradiated visceral or nodal sites of advanced HD relapsing from chemotherapy.

Management of Relapse from Systemic Therapy for Advanced Disease

HD is almost unique among human neoplasia in the ability of second-line therapy to effect long-term control of disease. This is true for those who relapse after primary radiation therapy or chemotherapy. The success of second-line therapy is determined by the stage and duration of first remission (269,270).

The average relapse rate can vary from series to series but is in the range of 30%, with the majority (75%) occurring before 12 months. This includes the average of 5% to 10% of patients who do not achieve an initial CR. The benefit of second-line chemotherapy is enhanced if relapse is localized, asymptomatic, and late occurring beyond 12 months (130,271). One series added histology, suggesting a better salvage rate for nodular sclerosis than mixed cellularity.

Early relapse that occurs at less than 12 months or failure to achieve a complete remission suggests a more aggressive and drug-resistant disease. Current practice would dictate the

TABLE 27-9. Salvage Regimens Published Since 1995 (Conventional Dose)

Regimen	No. of Patients	Response (%)	Duration	Reference (No.)
MiCMA (mitoxantrone, carboplatin, cytarabine, methylprednisolone)	29	86	All to ASCT	Ortu et al. (275)
MINE (mitoguazone, ifosfamide, vinorelbine, etoposide)	100	34 CR	70% to ABMT, 40 pts NED	Fermé et al. (276)
Mini-BEAM (BCNU, etoposide, cytosine arabinoside, melphalan)	44	32	26 pts to ABMT	Colwill et al. (277)
Ifosfamide, vinorelbine	26	77	28% free from progression at 2 yr	Bonfante et al. (278)
VIP (etoposide, ifosfamide, cisplatin)	42	38 CR	28 pts to ABMT	Ribrag et al. (279)

ABMT, autologous bone marrow transplantation; CR, complete response; pts, patients.

prompt use of second-line chemotherapy followed, if possible, by peripheral stem cell or bone marrow harvest and high-dose chemotherapy. In general, patients who relapse from complete remission and are treated with high-dose chemotherapy with autologous peripheral stem cell or bone marrow support have a salvage rate of 35% to 55%, depending on the series and selection criteria for the procedure (272). The German Hodgkin Group study of primary progressive or early relapsing (<3 months) disease showed an overall 17% 5-year freedom from second failure and an overall survival of 26%. Those receiving high-dose therapy had a 5-year freedom from second failure of 31% and a 43% survival. A low Karnofsky score, an age older than 50 years, and failure to achieve a transient remission were very significant negative factors (131) (see Chapter 60).

Patients who relapse late (>12 months) from complete remission represent a slow-growing relapse from a minimal residual state and may not, by definition, be drug resistant. When considering series that omit induction failures and consider only those achieving a CR, then the duration of remission assumes a greater importance in predicting the benefits of second-line therapy. One series of selected patients in relapse generated a prognostic scheme for assessing the benefits of salvage therapy (130). Multivariate analysis identified two negative factors: (a) interval from the end of treatment to relapse of less than 12 months and (b) stage III/IV at relapse. Having any one of these factors suggested, in retrospect, that high-dose therapy is more likely to give a better outcome. However, the same series suggests that late (>12 months) relapse that is nodal and asymptomatic may be salvaged just as well with conventional dose chemotherapy. One retrospective analysis from Stanford suggested that late relapse may have a similar outcome with conventional dose therapy (273). The choice of second-line salvage chemotherapy is empiric (274). Second-line regimens have not been compared to one another. Table 27-9 lists regimens published since 1995 (275–279). Many patients treated with these regimens go on to high-dose therapy so that the independent impact of the regimen is impossible to assess. Some caution is needed in the use of nitrosoureas and excessive quantities of alkylating agents because of the toxic effect on the hemopoietic stem cell reserve, which might limit the quantity of "stem" cells to be used with high-dose therapy.

Complementary radiation therapy to relapsed and not previously irradiated sites is often included. It is difficult to assess whether this is vital but seems reasonable if the relapse site is bulky.

Patients who relapse after high-dose therapy are rarely curable. Allotransplantation has a particularly poor record in such patients (280,281). The majority require palliative chemotherapy, which can be achieved with vinca alkaloids such as vinblastine or vinorelbine or the newly available antimetabolite prodrug gemcitabine (282,283). Some patients may be eligible for new experimental approaches.

New Immune-Based Treatments

Therapeutic progress can be enhanced by the expanding knowledge of the molecular and immunobiology of the malignant cells of HD. Small molecules and inhibitors of activation antigens may have a future role.

There have been some new but experimental treatments in refractory HD that use immunologic therapeutics. They include the testing of monoclonal immunotoxins. The target antigens include CD30 and CD25, the IL-2 receptor. Toxins linked to specific monoclonal antibodies include the ricin-A chain, diphtheria toxin, and saporin-S6, a single-chain ribosome-inactivating protein (284).

Modifications of the monoclonal antibodies to a bispecific combination of anti-CD30 and anti-CD16, which is the Fcγ-receptor extracellular domain in natural killer cells, and mononuclear phagocytes have been associated with antitumor activity (285).

Pilot trials of cellular immunotherapy with infusion of cytotoxic autologous cells raised and sensitized *ex vivo* against Epstein-Barr viral antigens, which may be present on the surface of Hodgkin's cells. Thus far, it has been shown that these cells can survive without host toxicity and infiltrate the tumor (286). A third technique is the use of nonmyeloablative conditioning to suppress host immunity to the point of accepting an allogeneic graft, which is hoped to induce a graft-versus-tumor response (287). The results of all of these trials are preliminary and as yet indeterminate. The ability to achieve second- or third-line salvage with chemotherapy has limited the number of patients eligible for innovative immunotherapeutic manipulations.

REFERENCES

1. Annual cancer statistics review. National Institutes of Health Publication 88-2789. Bethesda, MD: Department of Health and Human Services, National Cancer Institute 1987;II:153.
2. Hodgkin T. On some morbid appearances of the absorbent glands and spleen. *Med Chir Trans* 1832;17:68.
3. Kass AM, Kass EH. *Perfecting the world: the life and times of Dr. Thomas Hodgkin 1798–1866.* Boston: Harcourt Brace Jovanovich, 1988.

4. Greenfield WS. Specimens illustrative of the pathology of lymphadenoma and leucocythemia. *Trans Pathol Soc Lond* 1878;29:272.

5. Sternberg C. Uber eine eigenartige unter dem Bilde der Pseudoleukamie verlaufende Tuberculose des lymphatischen Apparates. *Zeitschr Heilk* 1898; 19:21.

6. Reed DM. On the pathological changes in Hodgkin's disease, with special reference to its relation to tuberculosis. *Johns Hopkins Hosp Rep* 1902;10:133.

7. Jackson H Jr, Parker F Jr. *Hodgkin's disease and allied disorders*. New York: Oxford University Press, 1947.

8. Obstacles to the control of Hodgkin's disease. *Cancer Res* 1966;26:1045.

9. Gilbert R. Radiotherapy in Hodgkin's disease malignant granulomatosis: anatomic and clinical foundations, governing principles, results. *AJR Am J Roentgenol* 1939;41:198.

10. Peters MW, Middlemiss KCH. A study of Hodgkin's disease treated by irradiation. *AJR Am J Roentgenol* 1956;79:114.

11. Kaplan HS. The radical radiotherapy of regionally localized Hodgkin's disease. *Radiology* 1962;78:553.

12. DeVita VT Jr, Serpick A, Carbone PP. Combination chemotherapy in the treatment of advanced Hodgkin's disease. *Ann Intern Med* 1970;73:881.

13. Bonadonna G, Santoro A. ABVD chemotherapy in the treatment of Hodgkin's disease. *Cancer Treat Rev* 1982;9:21–35.

14. Tamaru J, Hummel M, Zemlin M, et al. Hodgkin's disease with a B-cell phenotype often shows a VDJ rearrangement and somatic mutations in the VH genes. *Blood* 1994;84:708–715.

15. Kuppers R, Rajewsky K, Zhao M, et al. Hodgkin's disease: Hodgkin and Reed-Sternberg cells picked from histological sections show clonal immunoglobulin gene rearrangements and appear to be derived from B cells at various stages of development. *Proc Natl Acad Sci U S A* 1994;91:10962–10966.

16. Marafioti T, Hummel M, Foss HD, et al. Hodgkin and Reed-Sternberg cells represent an expansion of a single clone originating from a germinal center B-cell with functional immunoglobulin gene rearrangements but defective immunoglobulin transcription. *Blood* 2000;95:1443–1450.

17. Stein H, Hummel M. Cellular origin and clonality of classic Hodgkin's lymphoma: immunophenotypic and molecular studies. *Semin Hematol* 1999;36: 233–241.

18. Muschen M, Rajewsky K, Brauninger A, et al. Rare occurrence of classical Hodgkin's disease as a T-cell lymphoma. *J Exp Med* 2000;191:387–394.

19. Seitz V, Hummel M, Marafioti T, et al. Detection of clonal T-cell receptor gamma-chain gene rearrangements in Reed-Sternberg cells of classic Hodgkin's disease. *Blood* 2000;95:3020–3024.

20. Weber-Matthiesen K, Deerberg J, Poetsch M, et al. Numerical chromosome aberrations are present within the CD30+ Hodgkin and Reed-Sternberg cells in 100% of analyzed cases of Hodgkin's disease. *Blood* 1995;86:1464–1468.

21. Falzetti D, Crescenzi B, Matteuci C, et al. Genomic instability and recurrent breakpoints are main cytogenetic findings in Hodgkin's disease. *Haematologica* 1999;84:298–305.

22. Pedersen RK, Sorensen AG, Pedersen NT, et al. Chromosome aberrations in adult Hodgkin disease in a Danish population-based study. *Cancer Genet Cytogenet* 1999;110:128–132.

23. MacLeod RA, Spitzer D, Bar-Am I, et al. Karyotypic dissection of Hodgkin's disease cell lines reveals ectopic subtelomeres and ribosomal DNA at sites of multiple jumping translocations and genomic amplification. *Leukemia* 2000; 14:1803–1814.

24. Gupta RK, Patel K, Bodmer WF, et al. Mutation of p53 in primary biopsy material and cell lines from Hodgkin's disease. *Proc Natl Acad Sci U S A* 1993;90:2817–2821.

25. Trumper LH, Brady G, Bagg A, et al. Single-cell analysis of Hodgkin and Reed-Sternberg cells: molecular heterogeneity of gene expression and p53 mutations. *Blood* 1993;81:3097–3115.

26. Inghirami G, Macri L, Rosati S, et al. The Reed-Sternberg cells of Hodgkin disease are clonal. *Proc Natl Acad Sci U S A* 1994;91:9842–9846.

27. Chen WG, Chen YY, Kamel OW, et al. P53 mutations in Hodgkin's disease. *Lab Invest* 1996;75:519–527.

28. Elenitoba-Johnson KS, Medeiros LJ, Khorsand J, et al. P53 expression in Reed-Sternberg cells does not correlate with gene mutations in Hodgkin's disease. *Am J Clin Pathol* 1996;106:728–738.

29. Franke S, Wlodarska I, Maes B, et al. Lymphocyte predominance Hodgkin disease is characterized by recurrent genomic imbalances. *Blood* 2001;97: 1845–1853.

30. Naumovski L, Utz PJ, Bergstrom SK, et al. SUP-HD1: a new Hodgkin's disease-derived cell line with lymphoid features produces interferon-gamma. *Blood* 1989;74:2733–2742.

31. Bargou RC, Leng C, Krappmann D, et al. High-level nuclear NF-kappa B and Oct-2 is a common feature of cultured Hodgkin/Reed-Sternberg cells. *Blood* 1996;87:4340–4347.

32. Wood KM, Roff M, Hay RT. Defective IkappaBalpha in Hodgkin cells lines with constitutively active NF-kappaB. *Oncogene* 1998;16:2131–2139.

33. Cabannes E, Khan G, Aillet F, et al. Mutations in the IkBa gene in Hodgkin's disease suggest a tumour suppressor role for IkappaBalpha. *Oncogene* 1999; 18:3063–3070.

34. Emmerich F, Meiser M, Hummel M, et al. Overexpression of I kappa B alpha without inhibition of NF-kappaB activity and mutations in the I kappa B alpha gene in Reed-Sternberg cells. *Blood* 1999;94:3129–3134.

35. Jungnickel B, Staratschek-Jox A, Brauninger A, et al. Clonal deleterious mutations in the IkappaBalpha gene in the malignant cells in Hodgkin's lymphoma. *J Exp Med* 2000;191:395–402.

36. Krappmann D, Emmerick F, Kordes U, et al. Molecular mechanisms of constitutive NF-kappaB/Rel activation in Hodgkin/Reed-Sternberg cells. *Oncogene* 1999;18:942–953.

37. Russ HJ, Hirschstein D, Wright B, et al. Expression and function of CD30 on Hodgkin and Reed-Sternberg cells and the possible relevance for Hodgkin's disease. *Blood* 1994;84:2305–2314.

38. Duckett CS, Gedrich RW, Gilfillan MC, et al. Induction of nuclear factor kappaB by the CD30 receptor is mediated by TRAF1 and TRAF2. *Mol Cell Biol* 1997;17:1535–1542.

39. Uchida J, Yasui T, Takaoka-Shichijo Y, et al. Mimicry of CD40 signals by Epstein-Barr virus LMP1 in B lymphocyte responses. *Science* 1999;286:300–303.

40. Huen DS, Henderson SA, Croom-Carter D, et al. The Epstein-Barr virus latent membrane protein-1 (LMP1) mediates activation of NF-kappa B and cell surface phenotype via two effector regions in its carboxy-terminal cytoplasmic domain. *Oncogene* 1995;10:549–560.

41. Herrero JA, Mathew P, Paya CV. LMP-1 activates NF-kappa B by targeting the inhibitory molecule I kappa B alpha. *J Virol* 1995;69:2168–2174.

42. Sylla BS, Hung SC, Davidson DM, et al. Epstein-Barr virus-transforming protein latent infection membrane protein 1 activates transcription factor NF-kappaB through a pathway that includes the NF-kappaB-inducing kinase and the IkappaB kinases IKKalpha and IKKbeta. *Proc Natl Acad Sci U S A* 1998;95:10106–10111.

43. Bargou RC, Emmerich F, Krappmann D, et al. Constitutive nuclear factor-kappaB-RelA activation is required for proliferation and survival of Hodgkin's disease tumor cells. *J Clin Invest* 1997;100:2961–2969.

44. Hinz M, Loser P, Mathas S, et al. Constitutive NF-kappaB maintains high expression of a characteristic gene network, including CD40, CD86, and a set of antiapoptotic genes in Hodgkin/Reed-Sternberg cells. *Blood* 2001;97:2798–2807.

45. Stein H, Marafioti T, Foss HD, et al. Down-regulation of BOB, 1/OBF.1 and Oct2 in classical Hodgkin's disease but not in lymphocyte predominant Hodgkin's disease correlates with immunoglobulin transcription. *Blood* 2001; 97:496–501.

46. Kuppers R, Kelin U, Hansmann ML, et al. Cellular origin of human B-cell lymphomas. *N Engl J Med* 1999;341:1520–1529.

47. Braeuninger A, Kuppers R, Strickler JG, et al. Hodgkin and Reed-Sternberg cells in lymphocyte predominant Hodgkin disease represent clonal populations of germinal center-derived tumor B cells. *Proc Natl Acad Sci U S A* 1997; 94:9337–9342.

48. Marafioti T, Hummel M, Anagnostopoulos I, et al. Origin of nodular lymphocyte-predominant Hodgkin's disease from a clonal expansion of highly mutated germinal-center B cells. *N Engl J Med* 1997;337:453–458.

49. Lukes RJ, Tindle BH, Parker JW. Reed-Sternberg-like cells in infectious mononucleosis. *Lancet* 1969;2:1003–1004.

50. Poppema S, van Imhoff G, Torensma R, et al. Lymphadenopathy morphologically consistent with Hodgkin's disease associated with Epstein-Barr viral genomes in Reed-Sternberg cells of Hodgkin's disease. *Am J Clin Pathol* 1985;84:385–390.

51. Weiss LM, Movahed LA, Warnke RA, et al. Detection of Epstein-Barr viral genomes in Reed-Sternberg cells of Hodgkin's disease. *N Engl J Med* 1989; 320:502–506.

52. Gulley ML, Eagan PA, Quintanilla-Martinez L, et al. Epstein-Barr virus DNA is abundant and monoclonal in the Reed-Sternberg cells of Hodgkin's disease: association with mixed-cellularity subtype and Hispanic American ethnicity. *Blood* 1994;83:1595–1602.

53. Mueller N, Evans A, Harris NL, et al. Hodgkin's disease and Epstein-Barr virus. Altered antibody pattern before diagnosis. *N Engl J Med* 1989;320:689–695.

54. Sleckman BG, Mauch PM, Ambinder RF, et al. Epstein-Barr virus in Hodgkin's disease: correlation of risk factors and disease characteristics with molecular evidence of viral infection. *Cancer Epidemiol Biomarkers Prev* 1998;7:1117–1121.

55. Delecluse HJ, Marafioti T, Hummel M, et al. Disappearance of the Epstein-Barr virus in a relapse of Hodgkin's disease. *J Pathol* 1997;182:475–479.

56. Herndier BG, Sanchez HC, Chang KL, et al. High prevalence of Epstein-Barr virus in the Reed-Sternberg cells of HIV-associated Hodgkin's disease. *Am J Pathol* 1993;142:1073–1079.

57. Carbone A, Dolcetti R, Gloghini A, et al. Immunophenotypic and molecular analyses of acquired immune deficiency syndrome-related and Epstein-Barr virus-associated lymphomas: a comparative study. *Hum Pathol* 1996;27:133–146.

58. Dolcetti R, Bioocchi M, Gloghini A, et al. Pathogenetic and histogenetic features of HIV-associated Hodgkin's disease. *Eur J Cancer* 2001;37:1276–1287.

59. Ambinder RF. Epstein-Barr virus associated lymphoproliferations in the AIDS setting. *Eur J Cancer* 2001;37:1209–1216.

60. Hansmann LM, Felbaum C, Hui PK, et al. Morphologic and immunohistochemical investigation of non-Hodgkin's lymphoma combined with Hodgkin's disease. *Histopathology* 1989;15:35–48.

61. Momose H, Jaffe ES, Shin SS, et al. Chronic lymphocytic leukemia/small lymphocytic lymphoma with Reed-Sternberg-like cells and possible transformation to Hodgkin's disease. Mediation by Epstein-Barr virus. *Am J Surg Pathol* 1992;16:859–867.

62. Williams J, Schned A, Cotelingam JD, et al. Chronic lymphocytic leukemia with coexistent Hodgkin's disease. Implications for the origin of the Reed-Sternberg cell. *Am J Surg Pathol* 1991;15:33–42.

63. Ohno T, Smir BN, Weisenburger DD, et al. Origin of the Hodgkin/Reed-Sternberg cells in chronic lymphocytic leukemia with "Hodgkin's transformation." *Blood* 1998;91:1757–1761.

64. Kanzler H, Kuppers R, Helmes S, et al. Hodgkin and Reed-Sternberg-like cells in B-cell chronic lymphocytic leukemia represent the outgrowth of single germinal-center B-cell-derived clones: potential precursors of Hodgkin and Reed-Sternberg cells in Hodgkin's disease. *Blood* 2000;95:1023–1031.

65. Mack TM, Cozen W, Shibata DK, et al. Concordance for Hodgkin's disease in identical twins suggesting genetic susceptibility to the young-adult form of the disease. *N Engl J Med* 1995;332:413–418.

66. Alexander FE, Jarrest RF, Cartwright RA, et al. Epstein-Barr Virus and HLA-DPB1-*0301 in young adult Hodgkin's disease: evidence for inherited susceptibility to Epstein-Barr Virus in cases that are EBV(+ve). *Cancer Epidemiol Biomarkers Prev* 2001;10:705–709.

67. Wu TC, Mann RB, Charache P, et al. Detection of EBV gene expression in Reed-Sternberg cells of Hodgkin's disease. *Int J Cancer* 1990;46:801–804.

68. Herbst H, Steinbrecher E, Niedobitek G, et al. Distribution and phenotype of Epstein-Barr virus-harboring cells in Hodgkin's disease. *Blood* 1992;80:484–491.

69. Deacon EM, Pallesen G, Niedobitek G, et al. Epstein-Barr virus and Hodgkin's disease: transcriptional analysis of virus latency in the malignant cells. *J Exp Med* 1993;177:339–349.

70. Kaye KM, Izumi KM, Kieff E. Epstein-Barr virus latent membrane protein 1 is essential for B-lymphocyte growth transformation. *Proc Natl Acad Sci U S A* 1993;90:9150–9154.

71. Knecht H, Berger C, Rothenberger S, et al. The role of Epstein-Barr virus in neoplastic transformation. *Oncology* 2001;60:289–302.

72. Knect H, McQuain C, Martin J, et al. Expression of the LMP1 oncoprotein in the EBV-negative Hodgkin's disease cell line L-428 is associated with Reed-Sternberg cell morphology. *Oncogene* 1996;13:947–953.

73. Byrne PV, Heit WF, March CJ. Human granulocyte-macrophage colony-stimulating factor purified from a Hodgkin's tumor cell line. *Biochim Biophys Acta* 1986;874:266–273.

74. Samoszuk M, Nansen L. Detection of interleukin-5 messenger RNA in Reed-Sternberg cells of Hodgkin's disease with eosinophilia. *Blood* 1990;75:13–16.

75. Hsu SM, Zie SS, Hsu PL, et al. Interleukin-6, but not interleukin-4, is expressed by Reed-Sternberg cells in Hodgkin's disease with or without histologic features of Castleman's disease. *Am J Pathol* 1992;141:129–138.

76. Kadin M, Butmarc J, Elovic A, et al. Eosinophils are the major source of transforming growth factor-beta 1 in nodular sclerosing Hodgkin's disease. *Am J Pathol* 1993;142:11–16.

77. Herbst H, Foss HD, Samol J, et al. Frequent expression of interleukin-10 by Epstein-Barr virus-harboring tumor cells of Hodgkin's disease. *Blood* 1996;87:2918–2929.

78. Pinto A, Aldinucci D, Gloghini A, et al. Human eosinophils express functional CD30 ligand and stimulate proliferation of a Hodgkin's disease cell line. *Blood* 1996;88:3299–3305.

79. Teruya-Feldstein J, Jaffe ES, Burd PR, et al. Differential chemokine expression in tissues involved by Hodgkin's disease: direct correlation of eotaxin expression and tissue eosinophilia. *Blood* 1999;93:2463–2470.

80. Jundt F, Anagnostopoulos I, Bommert K, et al. Hodgkin/Reed-Sternberg cells induce fibroblasts to secrete eotaxin, a potent chemoattractant for T cells and eosinophils. *Blood* 1999;94:2065–2071.

81. Kapp U, Yeh WC, Patterson B, et al. Interleukin 13 is secreted by and stimulates the growth of Hodgkin and Reed-Sternberg cells. *J Exp Med* 1999;189:1939–1946.

82. Ohshima K, Sugihara M, Suzumiya J, et al. Basic fibroblast growth factor and fibrosis in Hodgkin's disease. *Pathol Res Pract* 1999;195:149–155.

83. Poppema S, van den Berg A. Interaction between host T cells and Reed-Sternberg cells in Hodgkin lymphomas. *Semin Cancer Biol* 2000;10:345–350.

84. Teruya-Feldstein J, Tosato G, Jaffe ES. The role of chemokines in Hodgkin's disease. *Leuk Lymphoma* 2000;38:363–371.

85. Peh SC, Kim LH, Poppema S. Tarc, a cc chemokine, is frequently expressed in classic Hodgkin's lymphoma but not in nlp Hodgkin's lymphoma, T-cell-rich B-cell lymphoma, and most cases of anaplastic large cell lymphoma. *Am J Surg Pathol* 2001;25:925–929.

86. Skinnider BF, Elia AJ, Gascoyne RD, et al. Interleukin 13 and interleukin 13 receptor are frequently expressed by Hodgkin and Reed-Sternberg cells of Hodgkin lymphoma. *Blood* 2001;97:250–255.

87. Teofili L, DeFebo AL, Pierconti F, et al. Expression of the c-met pronto-oncogene and its ligand, hepatocyte growth factor, in Hodgkin disease. *Blood* 2001;97:1063–1069.

88. Sarris AH, Sliche KO, Pethambaram P, et al. Interleukin-10 levels are often elevated in serum of adults with Hodgkin's disease and are associated with inferior failure-free survival. *Ann Oncol* 1999;10:433–440.

89. Bohlen H, Kessler M, Sextro M, et al. Poor clinical outcome of patients with Hodgkin's disease and elevated interleukin-10 serum levels. Clinical significance of interleukin-10 serum levels for Hodgkin's disease. *Ann Hematol* 2000;79:110–113.

90. Viviani S, Notti P, Bonfante V, et al. Elevated pretreatment serum levels of Il-10 are associated with a poor prognosis in Hodgkin's disease, the Milan Cancer Institute experience. *Med Oncol* 2000;17:59–63.

91. Vassilakopoulos TP, Nadali G, Angelopoulou MK, et al. Serum interleukin-10 levels are an independent prognostic factor for patients with Hodgkin's lymphoma. *Haematologica* 2001;86:274–281.

92. Timens W, Visser L, Poppema S. Nodular lymphocyte predominance type of Hodgkin's disease is a germinal center lymphoma. *Lab Invest* 1986;54:457–461.

93. Mason DY, Banks PM, Chan J, et al. Nodular lymphocyte predominance Hodgkin's disease. A distinct clinicopathological entity. *Am J Surg Pathol* 1994;18:526–530.

94. Lukes RJ, Butler JJ. The pathology and nomenclature of Hodgkin's disease. *Cancer Res* 1966;26:1063–1083.

95. Benharroch D, Prinsloo I, Goldstein J, et al. A comparison of distinct modes of tumor cell death in Hodgkin's disease using morphology and in situ DNA fragmentation. *Ultrastruct Pathol* 1996;20:497–505.

96. Lorenzen J, Thiele J, Fischer R. The mummified Hodgkin cell: cell death in Hodgkin's disease. *J Pathol* 1997;182:288–298.

97. Lukes RJ, Craver LF, Hall TC, et al. Report of the nomenclature committee. *Cancer Res* 1966;26:1311.

98. Harris NL, Jaffe ES, Stein H, et al. A revised European-American classification of lymphoid neoplasms: a proposal from the International Lymphoma Study Group. *Blood* 1994;84:1361–1392.

99. Anagnostopoulos I, Hansmann ML, Franssila K, et al. European Task Force on Lymphoma project on lymphocyte predominance Hodgkin disease: histologic and immunohistologic analysis of submitted cases reveals 2 types of Hodgkin disease with a nodular growth pattern and abundant lymphocytes. *Blood* 2000;96:1889–1899.

100. Harris NL, Jaffe ES, Diebold J, et al. World Health Organization classification of neoplastic diseases of the hematopoietic and lymphoid tissues: report of the Clinical Advisory Committee meeting—Airlie House, Virginia, November 1997. *J Clin Oncol* 1999;17:3835–3849.

101. Hsu JL, Jaffe ES. LeuM1 and peanut agglutinin stain the neoplastic cells of Hodgkin's disease. *Am J Clin Pathol* 1984;82:29–32.

102. Schwarting R, Gerdes J, Durkop H, et al. BER-H2 a new anti-Ki-1 (CD30) monoclonal antibody directed at a formol-resistant epitope. *Blood* 1989;74:1678–1689.

103. Colby TV, Hoppe RT, Warnke RA. Hodgkin's disease: a clinicopathologic study of 659 cases. *Cancer* 1982;49:1848–1858.

104. Stickler JG, Michie SA, Warnke RA, et al. The "syncytial variant" of nodular sclerosing Hodgkin's disease. *Am J Surg Pathol* 1986;10:470–477.

105. Haybittle JL, Hayhoe FG, Easterling MJ, et al. Review of British National Lymphoma Investigation studies of Hodgkin's disease and development of prognostic index. *Lancet* 1985;1:967–972.

106. MacLennan KA, Bennett MH, Tu A, et al. Relationship of histopathologic features to survival and relapse in nodular sclerosing Hodgkin's disease: a study of 1659 patients. *Cancer* 1989;64:1686.

107. Wijlhuizen TJ, Vrints LW, Jairam R, et al. Grades of nodular sclerosis (NSI-NSII) in Hodgkin's disease. Are they of independent prognostic value? *Cancer* 1989;63:1150–1153.

108. Ferry JA, Linggood RM, Convery KM, et al. Hodgkin's disease, nodular sclerosis type. Implications of histologic subclassification. *Cancer* 1993;71:457–463.

109. Masih AS, Weisenburger DD, Vose JM, et al. Histologic grade does not predict prognosis in optimally treated, advanced-stage nodular sclerosing Hodgkin's disease. *Cancer* 1992;69:228–232.

110. Hess JL, Bodis S, Pinkus G, et al. Histopathologic grading of nodular sclerosis Hodgkin's disease. Lack of prognostic significance in 254 surgically staged patients. *Cancer* 1994;74:708–714.

111. Van Spronsen DJ, Vrints LW, Hofstra G, et al. Disappearance of prognostic significance of histopathological grading of nodular sclerosing Hodgkin's disease for unselected patients, 1972–92. *Br J Haematol* 1997;96:322–327.

112. Ashton-Key M, Thorpe PA, Allen JP, et al. Follicular Hodgkin's disease. *Am J Surg Pathol* 1995;19:1294–1299.

113. Pinkus GS, Said JW. Hodgkin's disease, lymphocyte predominance type, nodular—a distinct entity? Unique staining profile for L&H variants of Reed-Sternberg cells defined by monoclonal antibodies to leukocyte common antigen, granulocyte-specific antigen, and B-cell-specific antigen. *Am J Pathol* 1985;118:1–6.

114. Falini B, Bigerna B, Pasqualucci L, et al. Distinctive expression pattern of the BCL-6 protein in nodular lymphocyte predominance Hodgkin's disease. *Blood* 1996;87:465–471.

115. Schmid C, Sargent C, Isaacson PG. L and H cells of nodular lymphocyte predominant Hodgkin's disease show immunoglobulin light-chain restriction. *Am J Pathol* 1991;139:1281–1289.

116. Burns BF, Colby TV, Dorfman RF. Differential diagnostic features of nodular L & H Hodgkin's disease, including progressive transformation of germinal centers. *Am J Surg Pathol* 1984;8:253–261.

117. Osborne BM, Butler JJ. Clinical implications of progressive transformation of germinal centers. *Am J Surg Pathol* 1984;8:725–733.

118. Hansmann ML, Fellbaum C, Hui PK, et al. Progressive transformation of germinal center with and without association to Hodgkin's disease. *Am J Clin Pathol* 1990;93:219–226.

119. Regula DP Jr, Hoppe RT, Weiss LM. Nodular and diffuse types of lymphocyte predominance Hodgkin's disease. *N Engl J Med* 1988;318:214–219.

120. Sundeen JT, Cossman J, Jaffe ES. Lymphocyte predominance Hodgkin's disease nodular subtype with coexistent "large cell lymphoma": histologic progression or composite malignancy? *Am J Surg Pathol* 1988;12:599–606.

121. Hansmann ML, Stein H, Fellbaum C, et al. Nodular paragranuloma can transform into high-grade malignant lymphoma of B type. *Hum Pathol* 1989;20:1169–1175.

122. Kadin ME, Donaldson SS, Dorfman RF. Isolated granulomas in Hodgkin's disease. *N Engl J Med* 1970;283:859.

123. Kennedy BJ, Loeb V Jr, Peterson VM, et al. National survey of patterns of care for Hodgkin's disease. *Cancer* 1985;56:2547–2556.

124. Good GR, DiNubile MJ. Images in clinical medicine. Cyclic fever in Hodgkin's disease (Pel-Ebstein fever). *N Engl J Med* 1995;332:436.

125. Gobbi PG, Cavalli C, Gendarini A, et al. Reevaluation of prognostic significance of symptoms in Hodgkin's disease. *Cancer* 1985;56:2874–2880.

126. Atkinson K, Austin DE, McElwain TJ, et al. Alcohol pain in Hodgkin's disease. *Cancer* 1976;37:895–899.

127. Mauch PM, Kalish LA, Marcus KC, et al. Second malignancies after treatment for laparotomy staged IA-IIB Hodgkin's disease: long-term analysis of risk factors and outcome. *Blood* 1996;87:3625–3632.

128. Ng AK, Weeks JC, Mauch PM, et al. Decision analysis on alternative treatment strategies for favorable-prognosis, early-stage Hodgkin's disease. *J Clin Oncol* 1999;17:377–385.

129. Marincek B, Brantschen R, Fuchs WA. Roentgenologic assessment of initial relapse in stage I-III Hodgkin's disease. *Eur J Radiol* 1985;5:285–290.

130. Brice P, Bastion Y, Divine M, et al. Analysis of prognostic factors after the first relapse of Hodgkin's disease in 187 patients. *Cancer* 1996;78:1293–1299.

131. Josting A, Rueffer U, Franklin J, et al. Prognostic factors and treatment outcome in primary progressive Hodgkin lymphoma: a report from the German Hodgkin Lymphoma Study Group. *Blood* 2000;96:1280–1286.

132. Carbone PP, Kaplan HS, Musshoff K, et al. Report of the Committee on Hodgkin's Disease Staging Classification. *Cancer Res* 1971;31:1860–1861.

133. Lister TA, Crowther D, Sutcliffe SB, et al. Report of a committee convened to discuss the evaluation and staging of patients with Hodgkin's disease: Cotswolds meeting [published erratum appears in *J Clin Oncol* 1990;8(9):1602]. *J Clin Oncol* 1989;7:1630–1636.

134. Reference deleted by author.

135. Errante D, Gabarre J, Ridolfo AL, et al. Hodgkin's disease in 35 patients with HIV infection: an experience with epirubicin, bleomycin, vinblastine and prednisone chemotherapy in combination with antiretroviral therapy and primary use of G-CSF. *Ann Oncol* 1999;10:189–195.

136. Levine AM. HIV-associated Hodgkin's disease. Biologic and clinical aspects. *Hematol Oncol Clin North Am* 1996;10:1135–1148.

137. Hammack J, Kotanides H, Rosenblum MK, et al. Paraneoplastic cerebellar degeneration. II. Clinical and immunologic findings in 21 patients with Hodgkin's disease. *Neurology* 1992;42:1938–1943.

138. Hasenclever D, Diehl V. A prognostic score for advanced Hodgkin's disease. International Prognostic Factors Project on Advanced Hodgkin's Disease. *N Engl J Med* 1998;339:1506–1514.

139. Di Biogio E, Sanchez-Borges M, Desenne JJ, et al. Eosinophilia in Hodgkin's disease: a role for interleukin 5. *Int Arch Allergy Immunol* 1996;110:244–251.

140. Levine AM, Thornton P, Forman SJ, et al. Positive Coombs test in Hodgkin's disease: significance and implications. *Blood* 1980;55:607–611.

141. Waddell CC, Cimo PL. Idiopathic thrombocytopenic purpura occurring in Hodgkin's disease after splenectomy: report of two cases and review of the literature. *Am J Hematol* 1979;7:381–387.

142. Tubiana M, Henry-Amar M, Burgers MV, et al. Prognostic significance of erythrocyte sedimentation rate in clinical stages I-II of Hodgkin's disease. *J Clin Oncol* 1984;2:194–200.

143. Specht L. Prognostic factors in Hodgkin's disease. *Semin Radiat Oncol* 1996;6:146–161.

144. Friedman S, Henry-Amar M, Cosset JM, et al. Evolution of erythrocyte sedimentation rate as predictor of early relapse in post-therapy early-stage Hodgkin's disease. *J Clin Oncol* 1988;6:596–602.

145. Cervantes F, Briones J, Bruguera M, et al. Hodgkin's disease presenting as a cholestatic febrile illness: incidence and main characteristics in a series of 421 patients. *Ann Hematol* 1996;72:357–360.

146. Mauch PM, Kalish LA, Kadin M, et al. Patterns of presentation of Hodgkin's disease. Implications for etiology and pathogenesis. *Cancer* 1993;71:2062–2071.

147. Dabbs DJ, Striker LM, Mignon F, et al. Glomerular lesions in lymphomas and leukemias. *Am J Med* 1986;80:63–70.

148. Rieke JW, Donaldson SS, Horning SJ. Hypercalcemia and vitamin D metabolism in Hodgkin's disease. Is there an underlying immunoregulatory relationship? *Cancer* 1989;63:1700–1707.

149. Seymour JF, Gagel RF. Calcitriol: the major humoral mediator of hypercalcemia in Hodgkin's disease and non-Hodgkin's lymphomas. *Blood* 1993;82:1383–1394.

150. Bethge W, Guggenberger D, Bamberg M, et al. Thyroid toxicity of treatment for Hodgkin's disease. *Ann Hematol* 2000;79:114–118.

151. Hancock SL, Cox RS, McDougall IR. Thyroid diseases after treatment of Hodgkin's disease. *N Engl J Med* 1991;325:599–605.

152. Fitoussi, Eghbali H, Tchen N, et al. Semen analysis and cryoconservation before treatment in Hodgkin's disease. *Ann Oncol* 2000;11:679–684.

153. Shekarriz M, Tolentino MV Jr, Ayzman I, et al. Cryopreservation and semen quality in patients with Hodgkin's disease. *Cancer* 1995;75:2732–2736.

154. Myers CE, Chabner BA, DeVita VT, et al. Bone marrow involvement in Hodgkin's disease: pathology and response to MOPP chemotherapy. *Blood* 1974;44:197–204.

155. Rosenberg SA. Hodgkin's disease of the bone marrow. *Cancer Res* 1971;31:1733–1736.

156. Howard MR, Taylor PR, Lucraft HH, et al. Bone marrow examination in newly diagnosed Hodgkin's disease: current practice in the United Kingdom. *Br J Cancer* 1995;71:210–212.

157. Macintyre EA, Vaughan Hudson B, Linch DC, et al. The value of staging bone marrow trephine biopsy in Hodgkin's disease. *Eur J Haematol* 1987;39:66–70.

158. Munker R, Hasenclever D, Brosteanu O, et al. Bone marrow involvement in Hodgkin's disease: an analysis of 135 consecutive cases. German Hodgkin Lymphoma Study Group. *J Clin Oncol* 1995;13:403–409.

159. Chao NJ, Nademanee AP, Long GD, et al. Importance of bone marrow cytogenetic evaluation before autologous bone marrow transplantation for Hodgkin's disease. *J Clin Oncol* 1991;9:1575–1579.

160. Glatstein E, Guernsey JM, Rosenberg SA, et al. The value of laparotomy and splenectomy in the staging of Hodgkin's disease. *Cancer* 1969;24:709–718.

161. Leibenhaut MH, Hoppe RT, Efron B, et al. Prognostic indicators of laparotomy findings in clinical stage I-II supradiaphragmatic Hodgkin's disease. *J Clin Oncol* 1989;7:81–91.

162. Carde P, Glatstein E. Role of staging laparotomy in Hodgkin's disease. In: Mauch P, Armitage J, Diehl V, et al., eds. *Hodgkin's disease*. Philadelphia: Lippincott Williams & Wilkins, 1999:273–293.

163. Taylor MA, Kaplan HS, Nelsen TS. Staging laparotomy with splenectomy for Hodgkin's disease: the Stanford experience. *World J Surg* 1985;9:449–460.

164. Brogadir S, Fialk MA, Coleman M, et al. Morbidity of staging laparotomy in Hodgkin's disease. *Am J Med* 1978;64:429–433.

165. Donaldson SS, Glatstein E, Vosti KL. Bacterial infections in pediatric Hodgkin's disease: relationship to radiotherapy, chemotherapy and splenectomy. *Cancer* 1978;41:1949–1958.

166. Chou MY, Brown AE, Bleveins A, et al. Severe pneumococcal infection in patients with neoplastic disease. *Cancer* 1983;51:1546–1550.

167. Dietrich PY, Henry-Amar M, Cosset JM, et al. Second primary cancers in patients continuously disease free from Hodgkin's disease: a protective role for the spleen? *Blood* 1994;84:1209–1215.

168. Kaldor JM, Day NE, Clarke EA, et al. Leukemia following Hodgkin's disease. *N Engl J Med* 1990;322:7–13.

169. Boivin JF, Hutchinson GB, Zauber AG, et al. Incidence of second cancers in patients treated for Hodgkin's disease. *J Natl Cancer Inst* 1995;87:732–741.

170. Aragon de la Cruz G, Cardenes H, Otero J, et al. Individual risk of abdominal disease in patients with stages I and II supradiaphragmatic Hodgkin's disease. A rule index based on 341 laparotomized patients. *Cancer* 1989;63:1799–1803.

171. Trotter MC, Cloud GA, Davis M, et al. Predicting the risk of abdominal disease in Hodgkin's lymphoma. A multifactorial analysis of staging laparotomy results in 255 patients. *Ann Surg* 1985;201:465–469.

172. Mauch P, Larson D, Osteen R, et al. Prognostic factors for positive surgical staging in patients with Hodgkin's disease. *J Clin Oncol* 1990;8:257–265.

173. Carde P, Hagenbeek A, Hayat M, et al. Clinical staging versus laparotomy and combined modality with MOPP versus ABVD in early-stage Hodgkin's disease: the H6 twin randomized trials from the European Organization for Research and Treatment of Cancer Lymphoma Cooperative Group. *J Clin Oncol* 1993;11:2258–2272.

174. Ng AK, Weeks JC, Mauch PM, et al. Laparotomy versus no laparotomy in the management of early-stage, favorable-prognosis Hodgkin's disease: a decision analysis. *J Clin Oncol* 1999;17:241–252.

175. Lefor AT, Flowers JL, Heyman MR. Laparoscopic staging of Hodgkin's disease. *Surg Oncol* 1993;2:217–220.

176. Beanes S, Emil S, Kosi M, et al. A comparison of laparoscopic versus open splenectomy in children. *Am Surg* 1995;61:908–910.

177. Multani PS, Grossbard ML. Staging laparotomy in the management of Hodgkin's disease: is it still necessary? *Oncologist* 1996;1:41–55.

178. Castellino RA, Blank N, Hoppe RT, et al. Hodgkin disease: contributions of chest CT in the initial staging evaluation. *Radiology* 1986;160:603–605.

179. Diehl LF, Hopper KD, Giguere J, et al. The pattern of intrathoracic Hodgkin's disease assessed by computed tomography. *J Clin Oncol* 1991;9:438–443.

180. Romano M, Libshitz HI. Hodgkin disease and non-Hodgkin lymphoma: plain chest radiographs and chest computed tomography of thoracic involvement in previously untreated patients. *Radiol Med (Torino)* 1998;95:49–53.

181. Berkman N, Breuer R. Pulmonary involvement in lymphoma. *Respir Med* 1993;87:85–92.

182. Hopper KD, Diehl LF, Lesar M, et al. Hodgkin disease: clinical utility of CT in initial staging and treatment. *Radiology* 1988;169:17–22.

183. DiPiro P. The varied manifestations of thoracic lymphoma. *Postgrad Radiol* 1999;36:1–5.

184. Castellino RA. Hodgkin disease: practical concepts for the diagnostic radiologist. *Radiology* 1986;159:305–310.

185. Castellino RA, Hoppe RT, Blank N, et al. Computed tomography, lymphography, and staging laparotomy: correlations in initial staging of Hodgkin disease. *AJR Am J Roentgenol* 1984;143:37–41.

186. Blackledge G, Best JJ, Crowther D, et al. Computed tomography (CT) in the staging of patients with Hodgkin's disease: a report on 136 patients. *Clin Radiol* 1980;31:143–147.

187. Stomper PC, Cholewinski SP, Park J, et al. Abdominal staging of thoracic Hodgkin disease: CT-lymphangiography-GA-67 scanning correlation. *Radiology* 1993;187:381–386.

188. North LB, Wallace S, Lindell MM Jr, et al. Lymphography for staging lymphomas: is it still a useful procedure? *AJR Am J Roentgenol* 1993;161:867–869.

189. Edeiken-Monroe B, Edeiken J, Kim EE. Radiologic concepts of lymphoma of bone. *Radiol Clin North Am* 1990;28:841–864.

190. Anderson KC, Kaplan WD, Leonard RC, et al. Role of 99mTc methylene diphosphonate bone imaging in the management of lymphoma. *Cancer Treat Rep* 1985;69:1347–1351.

191. Delcambre C, Reman O, Henry-Amar M, et al. Clinical relevance of gallium-6f7 scintigraphy in lymphoma before and after therapy. *Eur J Nucl Med* 2000;27:176–184.

192. Blackwell EA, Joshua DE, McLaughlinn AF, et al. Early supradiaphragmatic Hodgkin's disease. High-dose gallium scanning obviates the need for staging laparotomy. *Cancer* 1986;58:883–885.

193. Front D, Israel O. The role of Ga-67 scintigraphy in evaluating the results of therapy of lymphoma patients. *Semin Nucl Med* 1995;25:60–71.

194. Salloum E, Brandt DS, Caride VJ, et al. Gallium scans in the management of patients with Hodgkin's disease: a study of 101 patients. *J Clin Oncol* 1997; 15:518–527.

195. Hagemeister FB, Fesus SM, Lamki LM, et al. Role of the gallium scan in Hodgkin's disease. *Cancer* 1990;65:1090–1096.

196. Wylie BR, Southee AE, Joshua DE, et al. Gallium scanning in the management of mediastinal Hodgkin's disease. *Eur J Haematol* 1989;42:344–347.

197. Gasparini MD, Balzarini L, Castellani MR, et al. Current role of gallium scan and magnetic resonance imaging in the management of mediastinal Hodgkin lymphoma. *Cancer* 1993;72:577–582.

198. Zinzani PL, Magagnoli M, Chierichetti F, et al. The role of positron emission tomography (PET) in the management of lymphoma patients. *Ann Oncol* 1999;10:1181–1184.

199. Wiedmann E, Baican B, Hertel A, et al. Positron emission tomography (PET) for staging and evaluation of response to treatment in patients with Hodgkin's disease. *Leuk Lymphoma* 1999;34:545–551.

200. Jerusalem G, Beguin Y, Fassotte MF, et al. Whole-body positron emission tomography using 18F-fluorodeoxyglucose for post-treatment evaluation in Hodgkin's disease and non-Hodgkin's lymphoma has higher diagnostic and prognostic value than classical computed tomography scan imaging. *Blood* 1999;94:429–433.

201. Bangerter M, Moog F, Buchmann I, et al. Whole-body 2-[18F]-fluoro-2-deoxy-D-glucose positron emission tomography (FDG-PET) for accurate staging of Hodgkin's disease. *Ann Oncol* 1998;9:1117–1122.

202. Moog F, Bangerter M, Diederichs CG, et al. Lymphoma: role of whole-body 2-deoxy-2-[F-18]fluoro-D-glucose (FDG) PET in nodal staging. *Radiology* 1997; 203:795–800.

203. Stumpe KD, Urbinelli M, Steinert HC, et al. Whole-body positron emission tomography using fluorodeoxyglucose for staging of lymphoma: effectiveness and comparison with computed tomography. *Eur J Nucl Med* 1998; 25:721–728.

204. Shah N, Hoskin P, McMillan A, et al. The impact of FDG positron emission tomography imaging on the management of lymphomas. *Br J Radiol* 2000;73: 482–487.

205. Carr R, Barrington SF, Madan B, et al. Detection of lymphoma in bone marrow by whole-body positron emission tomography. *Blood* 1998;91:3340–3346.

206. Bangerter M, Griesshammer M, Binder T, et al. New diagnostic imaging procedures in Hodgkin's disease. *Ann Oncol* 1996;7:55–59.

207. Singal PK, Iliskovic N. Doxorubicin-induced cardiomyopathy. *N Engl J Med* 1998;339:900–905.

208. Comis RL. Bleomycin pulmonary toxicity: current status and future directions. *Semin Oncol* 1992;19:64–70.

209. Kaplan H. *Hodgkin's disease*, 2nd ed. Cambridge, MA: Harvard University Press, 1980.

210. Crnkovich MJ, Leopold K, Hoppe RT, et al. Stage I to IIB Hodgkin's disease: the combined experience at Stanford University and the Joint Center for Radiation Therapy. *J Clin Oncol* 1987;5:1041–1049.

211. Liew KH, Easton D, Horwich A, et al. Bulky mediastinal Hodgkin's disease management and prognosis. *Hematol Oncol* 1984;2:45–59.

212. Mauch P, Gorshein D, Cunningham J, et al. Influence of mediastinal adenopathy on site and frequency of relapse in patients with Hodgkin's disease. *Cancer Treat Rep* 1982;66:809–817.

213. Hoppe RT, Coleman CN, Cox RS, et al. The management of stage I-II Hodgkin's disease with irradiation alone or combined modality therapy: the Stanford experience. *Blood* 1982;59:455–465.

214. Specht L, Nordentoft AM, Cold S, et al. Tumor burden as the most important prognostic factor in early stage Hodgkin's disease. Relations to other prognostic factors and implications for choice of treatment. *Cancer* 1988;61:1719–1727.

215. Tubiana M, Henry-Amar M, van der Werf-Messing B, et al. A multivariate analysis of prognostic factors in early stage Hodgkin's disease. *Int J Radiat Oncol Biol Phys* 1985;11:23–30.

216. Tubiana M, Henry-Amar M, Hayat M, et al. Prognostic significance of the number of involved areas in the early stages of Hodgkin's disease. *Cancer* 1984;54:885–894.

217. Stein RS, Golomb HM, Diggs CH, et al. Anatomic substages of stage III-A Hodgkin's disease. A collaborative study. *Ann Intern Med* 1980;92:159–165.

218. Fermé C, Bastion Y, Brice P, et al. Prognosis of patients with advanced Hodgkin's disease: evaluation of four prognostic models using 344 patients included in the Group d'Etudes des Lymphomes de l'Adulte Study. *Cancer* 1997;80:1124–1133.

219. Wagstaff J, Gregory WM, Swindell R, et al. Prognostic factors for survival in stage IIIB and IV Hodgkin's disease: a multivariate analysis comparing two specialist treatment centres. *Br J Cancer* 1988;58:487–492.

220. Straus DJ, Gaynor JJ, Myers J, et al. Prognostic factors among 185 adults with newly diagnosed advanced Hodgkin's disease treated with alternating potentially noncross-resistant chemotherapy and intermediate-dose radiation therapy. *J Clin Oncol* 1990;8:1173–1186.

221. Proctor SJ, Taylor P, Donnan P, et al. A numerical prognostic index for clinical use in identification of poor-risk patients with Hodgkin's disease at diagnosis. Scotland and Newcastle Lymphoma Group (SNLG) Therapy Working Party. *Eur J Cancer* 1991;27:624–629.

222. Brice P. Prognostic factors in advanced Hodgkin's disease—can they guide therapeutic decisions? *N Engl J Med* 1998;339:1547–1549.

223. DeVita VT Jr, Simon RM, Hubbard SM, et al. Curability of advanced Hodgkin's disease with chemotherapy. Long-term follow-up of MOPP-treated patients at the National Cancer Institute. *Ann Intern Med* 1980;92:587–595.

224. Selby P, Patel P, Milan S, et al. ChlVPP combination chemotherapy for Hodgkin's disease: long term results. *Br J Cancer* 1990;62:279–285.

225. Sutcliffe SB, Wrigley PFM, Peto J, et al. MVPP chemotherapy regimen for advanced Hodgkin's disease. *BMJ* 1978;1:679–683.

226. Canellos GP, Young TC, DeVita VT Jr. Combination chemotherapy for advanced Hodgkin's disease in relapse following extensive radiotherapy. *Clin Pharmacol Ther* 1972;13:750–754.

227. Young RC, Canellos GP, Chabner BA, et al. Maintenance chemotherapy for advanced Hodgkin's disease in remission. *Lancet* 1973;1:1339–1343.

228. Canellos GP, DeVita VT, Arseneau JC, et al. Second malignancies complicating Hodgkin's disease in remission. *Lancet* 1975;1:947–955.

229. Schilsky RL, Lewis BJ, Sherins RJ, et al. Gonadal dysfunction in patients receiving chemotherapy for cancer. *Ann Intern Med* 1980;93(part 1):109–114.

230. Canellos GP, Petroni GR, Barcos M, et al. Etoposide, vinblastine, and doxorubicin: an active regimen for the treatment of Hodgkin's disease in relapse following MOPP. *J Clin Oncol* 1995;13:2005–2011.

231. Longo DL. The use of chemotherapy in the treatment of Hodgkin's disease. *Semin Oncol* 1990;17:716–735.

232. Hagemeister FB, Cabanillas F, Velasquez WS, et al. NOVP: a novel chemotherapeutic regimen with minimal toxicity for treatment of Hodgkin's disease. *Semin Oncol* 1990;17[Suppl 10]:34–40.

233. Bonadonna G, Valagussa P, Santoro A. Alternating non-cross-resistant combination chemotherapy or MOPP in stage IV Hodgkin's disease—a report of 8-year results. *Ann Intern Med* 1986;104:739–746.

234. Hancock BWS, Vaughan-Hudson G, Vaughan-Hudson B, et al. LOPP alternating with EVAP is superior to LOPP alone in the initial treatment of advanced Hodgkin's disease: results of a British National Lymphoma Investigation Trial. *J Clin Oncol* 1992;10:1252–1258.

235. Radford JA, Crowther D, Rohatiner AZS, et al. Results of a randomized trial comparing MVPP chemotherapy with a hybrid regimen, ChlVPP/EVA, in the initial treatment of Hodgkin's disease. *J Clin Oncol* 1995;13:2379–2385.

236. Cosset JM, Fermé C, Noordijk EM, et al. Combined modality treatment for poor prognosis stages I and II Hodgkin's disease. *Semin Radiat Oncol* 1996;6:185–195.

237. Specht L, Gray RG, Clarke MJ, et al. Influence of more extensive radiotherapy and adjuvant chemotherapy on long-term outcome of early-stage Hodgkin's disease: a meta-analysis of 23 randomized trials involving 3,888 patients. *J Clin Oncol* 1998;16:830–843.

238. Bodis S, Kraus MD, Pinkus G, et al. Clinical presentation and outcome in lymphocyte-predominant Hodgkin's disease. *J Clin Oncol* 1997;15:3060–3066.

239. Sears JD, Greven KM, Ferree CR, et al. Definitive irradiation in the treatment of Hodgkin's disease. Analysis of outcome, prognostic factors, and long-term complications. *Cancer* 1997;79:145–151.

240. Vlachaki MT, Ha CS, Hagemeister FB, et al. Long-term outcome of treatment for Ann Arbor stage I Hodgkin's disease: patterns of failure, late toxicity and second malignancies. *Int J Radiat Oncol Biol Phys* 1997;39:609–616.

241. Dühmke E, Franklin J, Pfreundschuh M, et al. Low-dose radiation is sufficient for the noninvolved extended-field treatment in favorable early stage Hodgkin's disease: long-term results of a randomized trial of radiotherapy alone. *J Clin Oncol* 2001;19:2905–2914.

242. Cosset JM, Henry-Amar M, Meerwaldt JH, et al. The EORTC trials for limited stage Hodgkin's disease. *Eur J Cancer* 1992;28A:1847–1850.

243. Wirth A, Chao M, Corry J, et al. Mantle irradiation alone for clinical stage I-II Hodgkin's disease: long-term follow-up and analysis of prognostic factors in 261 patients. *J Clin Oncol* 1999;17:230–240.

244. Jones E, Mauch P. Limited radiation therapy for selected patients with pathological stages IA and IIA Hodgkin's disease. *Semin Radiat Oncol* 1996;6:162–171.

245. Tubiana M, Henry-Amar M, Carde P, et al. Toward comprehensive management tailored to prognostic factors of patients with clinical stages I and II in Hodgkin's disease. The EORTC Lymphoma Group Controlled Clinical Trials: 1964–1987. *Blood* 1989;73:47–56.

246. Colonna P, Jais J-P, Desablens B, et al. Mediastinal tumor size and response to chemotherapy are the only prognostic factors in supradiaphragmatic Hodgkin's disease treated by ABVD plus radiotherapy: ten-year results of the Paris-Ouest-France 81/12 trial, including 262 patients. *J Clin Oncol* 1996;14:1928–1935.

247. Gospodarowicz MK, Sutcliffe SB, Bergsagel DE, et al. Radiation therapy in clinical stage I and II Hodgkin's disease. The Princess Margaret Hospital Lymphoma Group. *Eur J Cancer* 1992;28A:1841–1846.

248. Rueda A, Alba E, Ribelles N, et al. Six cycles of ABVD in the treatment of stage I and II Hodgkin's disease: a pilot study. *J Clin Oncol* 1997;15:1118–1122.

249. Sankila R, Garwicz S, Olsen JH, et al. Risk of subsequent malignant neoplasms among 1,641 Hodgkin's disease patients diagnosed in childhood and adolescence: a population-based cohort study in the five Nordic countries. *J Clin Oncol* 1996;14:1442–1446.

250. Van Leeuwen FE, Klokman WJ, Hagenbeek A, et al. Second cancer risk following Hodgkin's disease: a 20-year follow-up study. *J Clin Oncol* 1994;12:312–325.

251. Bhatia S, Robison LL, Oberlin O, et al. Breast cancer and other second neoplasms after childhood Hodgkin's disease. *N Engl J Med* 1996;334:745–751.

252. Horwich A, Specht L, Ashley S. Survival analysis of patients with clinical stages I or II Hodgkin's disease who have relapsed after initial treatment with radiotherapy alone. *Eur J Cancer* 1997;33:848–853.

253. Bodis S, Henry-Amar M, Bosq J, et al. Late relapse in early-stage Hodgkin's disease patients enrolled on European Organization for Research and Treatment of Cancer protocols. *J Clin Oncol* 1993;11:225–232.
254. Brierley JD, Rathmell AJ, Gospodarowicz MK, et al. Late relapse after treatment for clinical stage I and II Hodgkin's disease. *Cancer* 1997;79:1422–1427.
255. Hoppe RT. The management of Hodgkin's disease in relapse after primary radiation therapy. *Eur J Cancer* 1992;28A:1920–1922.
256. Canellos GP, Anderson JR, Propert KJ, et al. Chemotherapy of advanced Hodgkin's disease with MOPP, ABVD or MOPP alternating with ABVD. *N Engl J Med* 1992;327:1478–1484.
257. Duggan D, Petroni G, Johnson J, et al. MOPP/ABV versus ABVD for advanced Hodgkin's disease—a preliminary report of CALGB 8952 (with SWSOG, ECOG, NCIC). *Proc ASCO* 1997;16:12a.
258. Murray PG, Billingham LJ, Hassan HT, et al. Effect of Epstein-Barr virus infection on response to chemotherapy and survival in Hodgkin's disease. *Blood* 1999;94:442–447.
259. Von Vasielewski, Seth S, Franklin J, et al. Tissue eosinophilia correlates strongly with poor prognosis in nodular sclerosing Hodgkin's disease, allowing for known prognostic factors. *Blood* 2000;95:1207–1213.
260. Diehl V, Franklin J, Hasenclever D, et al. BEACOPP, a new dose-escalated and accelerated regimen, is at least as effective as COPP/ABVD in patients with advanced-stage Hodgkin's lymphoma: interim report from a trial of the German Hodgkin's Lymphoma Study Group. *J Clin Oncol* 1998;16:3810–3821.
261. Bartlett NL, Rosenberg SA, Hoppe RT, et al. Brief chemotherapy, Stanford V, and adjuvant radiotherapy for bulky or advanced stage Hodgkin's disease: a preliminary report. *J Clin Oncol* 1995;13:1080–1088.
262. Horning SJ, Adhikari A, Rizk N, et al. Effect of treatment for Hodgkin's disease on pulmonary function: results of a prospective study. *J Clin Oncol* 1994;12:297–305.
263. LeBeau MM, Albain KS, Larson RA, et al. Clinical and cytogenetic correlations in 63 patients with therapy-related myelodysplastic syndromes and active abnormalities of chromosomes No. 5 and 7. *J Clin Oncol* 1986;4:325–345.
264. Talbot JN, Haioun C, Rain JD, et al. [18F]-FDG positron imaging in clinical management of lymphoma patients. *Crit Rev Oncol Hematol* 2001;38:193–221.
265. Loeffler M, Brosteanu O, Hasenclever D, et al. Meta-analysis of chemotherapy versus combined modality treatment trials in Hodgkin's disease. *J Clin Oncol* 1998;16:818–829.
266. Diehl V, Loeffler M, Pfreundschuh M, et al. Further chemotherapy versus low-dose involved-field radiotherapy as consolidation of complete remission after six cycles of alternating chemotherapy in patients with advanced Hodgkin's disease. *Ann Oncol* 1995;6:901–910.
267. Fermé C, Sebban C, Henniquin C, et al. Comparison of chemotherapy to radiotherapy as consolidation of complete or good partial response after six cycles of chemotherapy for patients with advanced Hodgkin's disease: results of the groupe d'études des lymphomes de l'Adulte H89 trial. *Blood* 2000;95:2246–2252.
268. Fabian CJ, Mansfield CM, Dahlberg S, et al. Low-dose involved field radiation after chemotherapy in advanced Hodgkin disease. A Southwest Oncology Group randomized study. *Ann Intern Med* 1994;120:903–912.
269. Yahalom J. Management of relapsed and refractory Hodgkin's disease. *Semin Radiat Oncol* 1996;6:210–224.
270. Roach M III, Brophy N, Cox R, et al. Prognostic factors for patients relapsing after radiotherapy for early-stage Hodgkin's disease. *J Clin Oncol* 1990;8:623–629.
271. Bonfante V, Santoro A, Viviani S, et al. Outcome of patient with Hodgkin's disease failing after primary MOPP-ABVD. *J Clin Oncol* 1997;15:528–534.
272. Laurence ADJ, Goldstone AH. High-dose therapy with hematopoietic transplantation for Hodgkin's lymphoma. *Semin Hematol* 1999;36:303–312.
273. Yuen AR, Rosenberg SA, Hoppe RT, et al. Comparison between conventional salvage therapy and high-dose therapy with autografting for recurrent or refractory Hodgkin's disease. *Blood* 1997;89:814–822.
274. Canellos GP. Treatment of relapsed Hodgkin's disease: strategies and prognostic factors. *Ann Oncol* 1998;9[Suppl 5]:S91–S96.
275. Ortu La Barbera E, Chiusolo P, Laurenti L, et al. MiCMA: an alternative treatment for refractory or recurrent Hodgkin's disease. *Ann Oncol* 2000;11:867–871.
276. Fermé C, Bastion Y, Lepage E, et al. The MINE regimen as intensive salvage chemotherapy for relapsed and refractory Hodgkin's disease. *Ann Oncol* 1995;6:543–549.
277. Colwill R, Crump M, Couture F, et al. Mini-BEAM as salvage therapy for relapsed or refractory Hodgkin's disease before intensive therapy and autologous bone marrow transplantation. *J Clin Oncol* 1995;13:396–402.
278. Bonfante V, Viviani S, Santoro A, et al. Ifosfamide and vinorelbine: an active regimen for patients with relapsed or refractory Hodgkin's disease. *Br J Haematol* 1998;103:533–535.
279. Ribrag V, Nasr F, Bouhris JH, et al. VIP (etoposide, ifosfamide and cisplatinum) as a salvage intensification program in relapsed or refractory Hodgkin's disease. *Bone Marrow Transplant* 1998;21:969–974.
280. Gajewski JL, Phillips GL, Sobocinski KA, et al. Bone marrow transplants from HLA-identical siblings in advanced Hodgkin's disease. *J Clin Oncol* 1996;14:572–578.
281. Milpied N, Fielding AK, Pearce RM, et al. Allogeneic bone marrow transplant is not better than autologous transplant for patients with relapsed Hodgkin's disease. *J Clin Oncol* 1996;14:1291–1296.
282. Little R, Wittes RE, Longo DL, et al. Vinblastine for recurrent Hodgkin's disease following autologous bone marrow transplant. *J Clin Oncol* 1998;16:584–588.
283. Santoro A, Bredenfeld H, Devizzi, et al. Gemcitabine in the treatment of refractory Hodgkin's disease: results of a multicenter phase II study. *J Clin Oncol* 2000;18:2615–2619.
284. Barth S, Schnell R, Diehl V, et al. Development of immunotoxins for potential clinical use in Hodgkin's disease. *Ann Oncol* 1996;7[Suppl 4]:S135–S141.
285. Hartmann F, Renner C, Jung W, et al. Anti-CD16/CD30 bispecific antibody treatment for Hodgkin's disease: role of infusion schedule and costimulation with cytokines. *Clin Cancer Res* 2001;7:1873–1881.
286. Su Z, Peluso MV, Raffegerst SH, et al. The generation of LMP2a-specific cytotoxic T lymphocytes for the treatment of patients with Epstein-Barr virus-positive Hodgkin disease. *Eur J Immunol* 2001;31:947–958.
287. Anderlini P, Giralt S, Andersson B, et al. Allogeneic stem cell transplantation with fludarabine-based, less intensive conditioning regimens as adoptive immunotherapy in advanced Hodgkin's disease. *Bone Marrow Transplant* 2000;26:615–620.

CHAPTER 28

Non-Hodgkin's Lymphomas

R. Gregory Bociek and James O. Armitage

The illnesses that fall under the category of non-Hodgkin's lymphoma (NHL) represent a diverse group of lymphoid malignancies. They represent a clinical spectrum of disorders ranging from the most indolent neoplasms [e.g., small lymphocytic lymphoma (SLL), follicular small cleaved cell lymphoma] to the most rapidly growing and highly aggressive human tumors (e.g., acute lymphoblastic lymphoma, Burkitt lymphoma). Until the early twentieth century, no distinction was made between NHL and Hodgkin's disease. However, by the 1950s, it was recognized that NHL was an entity separate from Hodgkin's disease and that various subgroups of NHL had differing patterns of clinical behavior.

Burkitt lymphoma was one of the first neoplasms shown to be curable with chemotherapy. It was also the first to be shown to have a consistent chromosomal abnormality (the myc translocation) and the first solid tumor known to be curable by means of autologous bone marrow transplantation. The more common large cell lymphomas were shown to be curable with combination chemotherapy in the 1970s. Observational and correlative studies have added greatly to our knowledge of the relationship between NHLs and the immune system, because these are the solid tumors of the immune system.

EPIDEMIOLOGY

NHL remains largely a disease of older adults, with peak incidence rates seen in individuals older than 60 years. A number of observational studies have suggested an association between NHL and prior exposure to a number of toxins, ionizing radiation, autoimmune diseases, and congenital or acquired immunodeficiencies. An active body of work looking for evidence of specific heritable defects associated with an increased risk of developing NHL is ongoing. Collectively, NHLs are presently the fifth most common tumor diagnosed annually in the United States (1). For reasons largely unknown, their incidence has been continuously on the rise for approximately the past 25 years. Data collected from the Survival, Epidemiology, and End Results project suggest that there has been approximately a twofold rise in incidence (8/100,000 to 16/100,000) between 1973 and 1995 (2). Although it is likely that some of this increase is accounted for by lymphomas associated with acquired immune deficiencies (e.g., human immunodeficiency virus infection, Epstein-Barr virus–associated lymphoproliferative disorders seen in solid organ and allogeneic stem cell transplantation), this accounts for only a small proportion of the total number of increased cases. The observation that mortality rates have risen only by approximately half that of incidence rates suggests (indirectly, at least) that present therapy is improving survival rates for this disease.

CLASSIFICATION OF NON-HODGKIN'S LYMPHOMA

The purpose of any classification system is to provide nomenclature that is both valid and reliable so that entities with similar patterns of clinical behavior can be grouped and treated in a similar fashion by clinicians. However, with time, it has become increasingly evident that neither simple morphologic features nor clinical factors alone are sufficiently discriminative to identify patients whose outcomes will be similar. Present classification schemes have become more sophisticated largely as a result of the increasing availability of evolving techniques such as cytogenetic analysis, flow cytometry, and polymerase chain reaction techniques for the amplification of DNA sequences. The availability of these techniques has forever changed the way pathologists conceptualize lymphomas, and it has added a wealth of information to the modern day diagnosis and classification of lymphomas, as previous systems relied almost solely on morphology for diagnosis. As classification systems in lymphoma move more toward the study and inclusion of the biologic and genetic characteristics unique to particular tumors, it may become possible to exploit such characteristics as part of the development of newer, more directed therapies. A number of classification schemes remain in use in various countries around the world, including the World Health Organization (WHO) classification of malignant lymphomas (3). Some of the more commonly used classification schemes are listed in Table 28-1. It is important to realize that all classification systems are essentially attempting to define the same illnesses using different terms and concepts.

The Rappaport classification (4), published in 1966, was based largely on morphologic criteria. Most tumors within this system were classified on the basis of the appearance of malignant cells within the lymph node (nodular vs. diffuse) and on the appearance of the cells within the node (well differentiated vs. poorly differentiated). Additional descriptive terms (e.g., with or without "plasmacytoid features") were used to further differentiate certain histologic entities. Certain tumors such as Burkitt lymphoma and lymphoblastic lymphoma were defined on the basis of their own unique features. Later classification systems such as

TABLE 28-1. Working Formulation of Non-Hodgkin's Lymphomas for Clinical Usage[a]

Working formulation
  Low grade
    Malignant lymphoma
      Small lymphocytic
        Consistent with chronic lymphocytic leukemia
        Plasmacytoid
    Malignant lymphoma, follicular
      Predominantly small cleaved cell
        Diffuse areas
        Sclerosis
    Malignant lymphoma, follicular
      Mixed, small cleaved, and large cell
        Diffuse areas
        Sclerosis
  Intermediate grade
    Malignant lymphoma, follicular
      Predominantly large cell
        Diffuse areas
        Sclerosis
    Malignant lymphoma, diffuse
      Small cleaved cell
        Sclerosis
    Malignant lymphoma, diffuse
      Mixed, small, and large cell
        Sclerosis
        Epithelioid cell component
    Malignant lymphoma, diffuse
      Large cell
        Cleaved cell
        Noncleaved cell
        Sclerosis
  High grade
    Malignant lymphoma
      Large cell, immunoblastic
        Plasmacytoid
        Clear cell
        Polymorphous
        Epithelioid cell component
    Malignant lymphoma
      Lymphoblastic
        Convoluted cell
        Nonconvoluted cell
    Malignant lymphoma
      Small noncleaved cell
        Burkitt
        Follicular areas
  Miscellaneous
    Composite
    Mycosis fungoides
    Histiocytic
    Extramedullary plasmacytoma
    Unclassifiable
    Other
Rappaport classification
  Nodular
    Lymphocytic, well differentiated
    Lymphocytic, poorly differentiated
    Mixed, lymphocytic and histiocytic
    Histiocytic

  Diffuse
    Lymphocytic, well differentiated without plasmacytoid features
    Lymphocytic, well differentiated with plasmacytoid features
    Lymphocytic, poorly differentiated without plasmacytoid features
    Lymphocytic, poorly differentiated with plasmacytoid features
    Lymphoblastic, convoluted
    Lymphoblastic, nonconvoluted
    Mixed, lymphocytic and histiocytic
    Histiocytic without sclerosis
    Histiocytic with sclerosis
    Burkitt tumor
    Undifferentiated
  Malignant lymphoma, unclassified
  Composite lymphoma
Lukes-Collins classification
  Undefined cell type
  T-cell type, small lymphocytic
  T-cell type, Sézary syndrome/mycosis fungoides (cerebriform)
  T-cell type, convoluted lymphocytic
  T-cell type, immunoblastic sarcoma (T cell)
  B-cell type, small lymphocytic
  B-cell type, plasmacytoid lymphocytic
  Follicular center cell, small cleaved
  Follicular center cell, large cleaved
  Follicular center cell, small noncleaved
  Follicular center cell, large noncleaved
  Immunoblastic sarcoma (B cell)
    Subtypes of follicular center cell lymphomas
      Follicular
      Follicular and diffuse
      Diffuse
      Sclerotic with follicles
      Sclerotic without follicles
  Histiocytic
  Malignant lymphoma, unclassified
Kiel classification
  Low-grade malignancy
    Lymphocytic, chronic lymphocytic leukemia
    Lymphocytic, other
    Lymphoplasmacytoid
    Centrocytic
    Centroblastic—centrocytic, follicular, without sclerosis
    Centroblastic—centrocytic, follicular, with sclerosis
    Centroblastic—centrocytic, follicular and diffuse, without sclerosis
    Centroblastic—centrocytic, follicular and diffuse, with sclerosis
    Centroblastic—centrocytic, diffuse
    Low-grade malignant lymphoma, unclassified
  High-grade malignancy
    Centroblastic
    Lymphoblastic, Burkitt type
    Lymphoblastic, convoluted cell type
    Lymphoblastic, other (unclassified)
    Immunoblastic
    High-grade malignant lymphoma, unclassified
  Malignant lymphoma unclassified (unable to specify as high grade or low grade)
  Composite lymphoma

[a]Represents clinical characteristics of patients in the ten subtypes of the Working Formulation of Non-Hodgkin's Lymphomas for Clinical Usage. Miscellaneous or composite lymphomas are not included.

the Lukes-Collins system (5) attempted to describe lymphomas largely on the basis of their ontogeny (i.e., B cell vs. T cell).

A project undertaken by the National Cancer Institute (NCI) to unify the pathologic diagnosis of NHL led to the development of the Working Formulation for Non-Hodgkin's Lymphoma for Clinical Usage (6,7). This classification was useful because of its simplicity and functionality. Diseases were subclassified by their nodal architecture (i.e., a follicular vs. diffuse pattern) and by the predominant size of malignant cells within the node (small cleaved cells vs. large noncleaved cells vs. mixed populations). Using only these two characteristics, lymphomas could be subclassified into three groups of illnesses (low grade, intermediate

grade, and high grade) on the basis of their natural history, expected response to therapy, and relative prognosis.

The need to update lymphoma classification was driven, in part, by the discovery of a number of more recently recognized or characterized histologic entities not represented within any of these lymphoma classification systems [e.g., mucosa-associated lymphoid tissue (MALT) lymphomas, mantle cell lymphoma, anaplastic large cell lymphoma], as well as by the development of techniques permitting accurate immunophenotyping and cytogenetic analysis. The development of the Revised European-American Lymphoma (REAL) Classification (8) and, subsequently, the WHO classification systems (3) exemplify attempts to characterize

TABLE 28-2. World Health Organization Classification Scheme for Non-Hodgkin's Lymphoma

B-cell neoplasms
  Precursor B-cell neoplasm
    Precursor B-lymphoblastic leukemia/lymphoma
  Mature B-cell neoplasms
    B-cell chronic lymphocytic leukemia/small lymphocytic lymphoma
    B-cell prolymphocytic leukemia
    Lymphoplasmacytic lymphoma
    Splenic marginal zone lymphoma
    Hairy cell leukemia
    Plasma cell myeloma
    Solitary plasma cytoma of bone
    Extraosseous plasmacytoma
    Extranodal marginal zone B-cell lymphoma of MALT type
    Nodal marginal zone B-cell lymphoma
    Follicular lymphoma
    Mantle cell lymphoma
    Diffuse large B-cell lymphoma
    Mediastinal (thymic) large B-cell lymphoma
    Primary effusion lymphoma
    Intravascular large B-cell lymphoma
    Burkitt lymphoma/leukemia
T-cell and NK-cell neoplasms
  Precursor T-cell neoplasms
    Precursor T-lymphoblastic lymphoma/leukemia
    Blastic NK-cell lymphoma
  Mature T-cell and NK-cell neoplasms
    T-cell prolymphocytic leukemia
    T-cell granular lymphocytic leukemia
    Aggressive NK-cell leukemia
    Adult T-cell lymphoma/leukemia (HTLV-1+)
    Extranodal T-cell and NK-cell lymphoma, nasal type
    Enteropathy-type T-cell lymphoma
    Hepatosplenic T-cell lymphoma
    Subcutaneous panniculitis-like T-cell lymphoma
    Mycosis fungoides/Sézary's syndrome
    Primary cutaneous anaplastic large-cell lymphoma
    Anaplastic large-cell lymphoma
    Peripheral T-cell lymphoma unspecified
    Angioimmunoblastic T-cell lymphoma

HTLV-1, human T-cell leukemia virus 1; MALT, mucosa-associated lymphoid tissue; NK, natural killer.

illnesses on the basis of both clinical and pathologic criteria. The use of the term *pathologic criteria* today implies the use of combinations of morphologic criteria, immunophenotypic studies, and cytogenetic analysis. The REAL and WHO classifications have retained and built on key elements of past classification systems, such as the morphologic criteria used in the Working Formulation and the concept of grouping lymphoid malignancies according to their presumed normal counterparts as in the Lukes-Collins classification system. A summary of the most common entities in the proposed WHO classification systems is presented in Table 28-2.

An accurate histologic diagnosis is essential in making clinical decisions in the care of patients with any malignancy. The histologic diagnosis of NHL is among the most difficult tasks that pathologists are asked to perform. Previous classification systems such as the Working Formulation were limited to some extent by both inter- and intraobserver variability (9–13). Simply stated, pathologists could not always agree on uniform diagnoses for the same tissue, and, occasionally, a pathologist would arrive at a different diagnosis on subsequent examination of a malignancy than he or she had rendered previously. Using older classification systems, pathologists can reliably agree on both the identification of a lymphoid malignancy versus other tumors (concordant between 87% and 96% of the time) and the presence of follicularity (concordant between 85% and 95% of the time), but consensus on more specific aspects of diagnosis such as the specific cell type is more difficult to

obtain. A recent study by the Non-Hodgkin's Lymphoma Classification Project (14) demonstrated that expert hematopathologists agreed with a consensus diagnosis 41% to 93% of the time using histologic criteria alone. The addition of immunophenotyping improved diagnostic accuracy substantially for certain tumors (e.g., peripheral T-cell lymphomas, anaplastic large cell lymphoma, and mantle cell lymphoma). Finally in this study, pathologists, on reviewing a case, were able to reproduce their own initial diagnosis or the consensus diagnosis in approximately 85% of cases. Despite a lack of perfect precision in rendering a histologic diagnosis, the clinical significance in certain situations may not be meaningful, particularly when closely related subgroups of illnesses (e.g., low-grade follicular lymphomas) are treated in a similar fashion.

CLINICAL EVALUATION AND STAGING INVESTIGATIONS

The evaluation of patients with NHL requires a meticulous history and physical examination as well as supplemental laboratory and imaging studies. The history should concentrate on the presence or absence of B symptoms (e.g., unexplained fever >38°C, drenching night sweats, or unexplained weight loss of ≥10% of body weight over the preceding 6 months) and unexplained symptoms that could indicate occult involvement in particular organ systems [e.g., gastrointestinal (GI) tract, central nervous system (CNS), or pain in weight-bearing long bones]. Particular attention should be paid to certain factors that could alter staging, treatment, or prognosis (e.g., undiagnosed human immunodeficiency virus infection). Physical examination must concentrate on the reticuloendothelial system, including the examination of Waldeyer's ring as well as the liver and spleen. The history and physical examination should be supplemented with laboratory investigations including a complete blood count, differential, and platelet count as well as serum chemistries [renal function, hepatic function, lactate dehydrogenase (LDH), uric acid, calcium, and phosphate]. Imaging studies should include posteroanterior radiographs of the chest or a computed tomographic (CT) scan of the chest, plus a CT scan of the abdomen and pelvis. Unless patients have specific contraindications to the use of contrast media, contrast scans should be performed, because this improves the detection of abnormal lymphatic tissue in certain regions such as the mediastinum and bowel. The use of gallium scintigraphy is optional but may be of some use in patients with large initial tumor masses. Its sensitivity and specificity are only moderate, but gallium avid lesions at diagnosis can be reimaged at the completion of therapy to help confirm remission status of the patient. The use of positron emission tomography scanning is presently under active investigation in lymphoma. Reported studies suggest that it may be of some value in determining the status of residual masses on CT scans posttherapy (15). A bone marrow aspirate and biopsy are routine parts of initial staging and, in certain cases, should be sent for cytogenetic evaluation (e.g., for the bcl-2 translocation in patients with follicular lymphoma). The use of flow cytometry to assess the marrow for occult involvement that is not visible histologically should be considered for patients on clinical protocols but, based on present recommendations, does not upstage patients when positive in otherwise clinically negative marrows (16). Patients with GI symptomatology or documented involvement of Waldeyer's ring should have additional imaging studies of the GI tract. Patients with aggressive lymphomas in certain anatomic locations (nasopharynx, paranasal sinuses, orbit, paraspinal masses, or testicle) appear to be at higher risk for occult CNS involvement or CNS relapse and should be considered for

TABLE 28-3. Response Criteria for Non-Hodgkin's Lymphoma

Complete response
1. Complete disappearance of all detectable clinical and radiographic evidence of disease; disappearance of all disease-related symptoms if present before therapy; and normalization of any biochemical abnormalities definitely attributable to lymphoma.
2. All lymph nodes and nodal masses ≤1.5 cm in greatest transverse diameter for nodes >1.5 cm before therapy. Previously involved nodes that were 1.1–1.5 cm in their greatest transverse diameter before treatment must be ≤1 cm in their greatest transverse diameter after treatment or have decreased by more than 75% using SPD.
3. The spleen or any other organ considered to be enlarged before therapy due to involvement of lymphoma must have decreased in size and must not be palpable on physical examination. Any macroscopic nodules detected in any organs on imaging techniques should no longer be present.
4. The bone marrow biopsy and aspirate must be negative for disease if involved at study entry.

Complete response/unconfirmed
This includes patients who fulfill criteria 1 and 3 of the complete response, but with one or more of the following features:
1. A residual lymph node mass >1.5 cm in greatest transverse diameter that has regressed by more than 75% in the SPD. Individual nodes that were previously confluent must have regressed by more than 75% in their SPD compared with the size of the original mass.
2. Indeterminate bone marrow (increase number or size of aggregates without cytologic or architectural atypia).

Partial response
1. A decrease in SPD of ≥50% for the six largest dominant nodes or nodal masses.
2. No increase in the size of the other nodes, liver, or spleen.
3. Splenic and hepatic nodules must regress by at least 50% in the SPD.
4. With the exception of splenic and hepatic nodules, involvement of other organs is considered assessable and not measurable disease.
5. No new sites of disease.

Stable disease
This is defined as less than a partial response but not progressive disease.

Relapsed disease
1. Appearance of any new lesion or increase of ≥50% in the size of the previously involved sites (only applies to patients who achieve a complete response or complete response/unconfirmed). The new lesion must be >1.5 cm by radiographic evaluation or >1 cm by physical examination.
2. An increase ≥50% in greatest diameter of any previously identified node >1 cm in its shortest axis or in the SPD of more than one node.

Progressive disease
1. An increase of ≥25% from nadir in the SPD of any previously identified abnormal node for partial responses or nonresponders.
2. The appearance of any new lesion during or at the end of therapy that is >1.5 cm by radiographic evaluation or >1 cm by physical examination.

SPD, sum of the products the greatest diameters.

TABLE 28-4. Ann Arbor Staging System for Lymphomas

Stage[a]	Anatomic Description
I	Involvement of a single lymph node region (I) or a single extralymphatic organ or site (IE)
II	Involvement of two or more lymph node regions on the same side of the diaphragm (II) or localized involvement of an extralymphatic organ or site (IIE)
III	Involvement of lymph node regions on both sides of the diaphragm (III) or with (IIIE) localized involvement of an extralymphatic organ or site
IV	Diffuse involvement of one or more extralymphatic organs or sites, with or without lymphatic involvement

[a]Use of the letter A after the stage description denotes the absence of systemic symptoms (unexplained fevers >38ºC, drenching night sweats, weight loss ≥10% of body weight over previous 6 months). Use of the letter B after the stage description denotes the presence of systemic symptoms.

sions. NHLs continue to be staged using the Ann Arbor staging system (Table 28-4) (19). As this system was originally developed for Hodgkin's disease, it is designed to reflect the process and prognostic importance of the contiguous progression of disease more characteristic of Hodgkin's disease. For staging purposes, lymphatic tissues consist of lymph nodes proper, Waldeyer's ring, Peyer's patches, thymus, and spleen. Other anatomic areas of involvement (e.g., lung, liver, thyroid) are considered extranodal sites of disease. Extranodal sites are classified as such and designated by the letter E for the purposes of staging if they occur in a *localized* fashion anatomically adjacent to an area of lymphatic involvement. For example, a patient with mediastinal and hilar adenopathy and one or more pulmonary nodules localized to a single lobe would be classified as having stage II E disease. A patient, however, with *diffuse* involvement of an extralymphatic tissue or organ [which generally implies hematogenous dissemination (e.g., the presence of pulmonary nodules in multiple lobes)] would be considered to have stage IV disease. For treatment purposes, it is usually sufficient to categorize patients as early stage (nonbulky stage I and II disease) versus advanced stage (the presence of bulky disease or any stage III or IV patient). Before the availability of complex imaging techniques, surgical laparotomy-based staging was often performed. The combination of improvements in anatomic and functional imaging tools, and the ever-broadening range of potential therapies for patients with NHLs has essentially rendered surgical staging obsolete today.

diagnostic lumbar puncture and prophylactic intrathecal chemotherapy (17,18). Sites of disease not detectable by physical examination should be reimaged part of the way through therapy and at completion of therapy to assess remission status. Clinicians should become familiar with the new international response criteria for evaluating NHL (Table 28-3) published by Cheson et al. (16).

STAGING PATIENTS WITH NON-HODGKIN'S LYMPHOMA

Staging systems for any illness are generally designed to serve two purposes. First, they are meant to reproducibly describe the extent of a patient's disease so that clinicians can succinctly communicate with each other. Perhaps more important, staging systems are generally designed to reflect prognosis and to assist the clinician in making treatment deci-

PROGNOSTIC FACTORS IN NON-HODGKIN'S LYMPHOMA

From a therapeutic standpoint, a prognostic factor generally serves two purposes in any illness. First, it gives the clinician some means of estimating treatment outcomes, which can be conferred to the patient. Second, it allows clinicians to consider therapeutic options using a risk-stratified approach. In this way, patients who are likely to do well with standard therapies can be treated as such, and patients with a lower chance of success with standard therapies can be offered participation in studies of investigational therapies. A study published by the International Non-Hodgkin's Lymphoma Prognostic Factors Project in 1993 (20) examined the prognostic significance of various presenting features in a large sample of patients with aggressive subtypes of NHLs (Working Formulation classifications F through H). Using internal validation techniques (performing the analyses on both a training and a validation sample) and step-down multivariate regression analysis, five dichotomous factors were identified as having independent prognostic significance. These were age (≤60 years vs. >60 years); Ann Arbor stage (I or II vs. III or IV); number of extranodal sites (≤1 vs. >1); performance status (0 or 1 vs. ≥2); and serum LDH level (≤normal vs. >normal). Each of these factors was associated with an approximately twofold increase in risk of death. Because the clinical magnitude of each of these factors was similar, a cumulative score was devised to estimate the probability of survival based on the number of risk factors. Five risk groups were identified, referred to as *low risk* (zero to one risk factor), *low intermediate risk* (two risk factors), *high intermediate risk* (three risk factors), and *high risk* (four or five risk factors). An age-adjusted index was also developed for patients older than 60 years of age. This prognostic index has been demonstrated to be of value in a number of other subtypes of aggressive lymphoma, including peripheral T-cell lymphomas (21) and low-grade lymphomas (22), and is a useful tool for risk stratification of patients with respect to treatment options and approaches.

PATHOLOGY, CLINICAL FEATURES, AND TREATMENT OF NON-HODGKIN'S LYMPHOMA

Concept of Indolent versus Aggressive Lymphomas

The concept of indolent versus aggressive lymphomas came about largely as a result of the Working Formulation classification (6). Certain subtypes of lymphoma were characterized as having an indolent (or low-grade) biologic course, collectively accounting for approximately 30% of NHLs. These illnesses are considered to have a relatively slow growth pattern. Although patients with advanced stage disease are generally considered to be incurable, the median survival of such patients treated with standard forms of therapy is generally measured in years. Earlier or more aggressive therapy in patients with advanced indolent lymphomas generally has not been associated with significant alterations in the natural history of the disease. As such, patients with advanced indolent lymphomas are often offered a so-called watch and wait approach, reserving therapy for significant signs of progression. In the Working Formulation, low-grade lymphomas included SLL, follicular small cleaved cell lymphoma, and follicular mixed small cleaved and large cell lymphoma. In the development of the REAL and WHO classification schemes, the functional use of the terms *aggressive* and *indolent* has been abandoned and replaced by the concept that each disease represents a biologic entity with its own unique clinical and pathologic features. Nevertheless, these concepts remain useful as a way to group and understand the collective biology of a number of illnesses with similar clinical patterns of behavior. Using WHO terminology, lymphomas considered to have an indolent course include SLL, lymphoplasmacytic lymphoma, follicular lymphoma grades 1 and 2 (equivalent to follicular small cleaved cell and follicular mixed small cleaved and large cell lymphoma in the Working Formulation), and marginal zone B-cell lymphomas (nodal and extranodal subtypes).

The use of the term *aggressive* with respect to Working Formulation terminology would have referred to lymphomas that were considered to be intermediate grade in their behavior. This group of lymphomas was characterized by a more rapid growth rate and a relatively short survival (e.g., weeks to months) if untreated. This group of illnesses was considered to be curable in a subset of patients if treated with aggressive (i.e., anthracycline-based) combination chemotherapy regimens. In the Work-

ing Formulation, these lymphomas would have included follicular large cell, diffuse small cleaved cell, diffuse mixed small cleaved and large cell, and diffuse large cell lymphoma. Although immunoblastic lymphomas were classified as high-grade lymphomas, their biologic behavior was eventually thought to be similar to diffuse large cell lymphomas. In the REAL and WHO classification systems, the tumor known as *diffuse large B-cell lymphoma* essentially replaces most of the tumors previously designated as intermediate grade or "aggressive" lymphomas in the Working Formulation. Other lymphomas in the WHO classification with a similar pattern of behavior include peripheral T-cell lymphomas and anaplastic large cell lymphomas. Because these are more recently recognized and less common subtypes of NHL, treatment principles tend to follow those used in the treatment of diffuse large B-cell lymphomas (with the exception of the use of anti–B-cell monoclonal antibodies). In comparison with indolent lymphomas, aggressive lymphomas are comparatively more likely to present with localized disease, to present in extranodal sites (e.g., testes, CNS), and to invade adjacent tissues (e.g., bone). Finally, certain subtypes of lymphoma within the WHO and REAL classifications (e.g., mantle cell lymphoma) do not fit either conceptualization well, which demonstrates the functional limitations of the use of these older terms.

A proportion of patients with indolent lymphomas may experience transformation of their illness to a high-grade lymphoma. The occurrence of this event in a patient with chronic lymphocytic leukemia (CLL) was first described by Richter (23). The phenomenon of a high-grade lymphoma developing in patients with indolent lymphoma or CLL is, therefore, often referred to as *Richter's syndrome*. Most frequently, this means the development of a diffuse large B-cell lymphoma. This syndrome occurs in as many as 25% of patients with SLL as seen at autopsy (24). The occurrence of histologic transformation should be suspected in patients with rapid enlargement of one or more lymph node sites, the development of constitutional symptoms, or a rapidly rising LDH. It is most likely that this phenomenon represents a change in the growth rate and differentiation of the original tumor (not a second lymphoma), and similar immunologic characteristics frequently, but not always, may be shared by the two tumors (25,26). Generally, histologic transformation is considered to be associated with a poor prognosis (27–30). However, a proportion of patients treated with a regimen designed for aggressive lymphomas [e.g., CHOP (cyclophosphamide, doxorubicin, vincristine, prednisone)] may experience durable complete remissions. Not surprisingly, patients with limited disease at transformation may have the greatest probability of entering a complete remission (31).

SPECIFIC DISEASE ENTITIES

Small Lymphocytic Lymphoma

SLL accounts for approximately 5% of the lymphomas seen annually in the United States. This tumor represents a neoplasm of small, well-differentiated lymphocytes, which are usually of B-cell origin. In SLL, the lymph node contains a diffuse proliferation of small to medium-sized round lymphocytes. Slight variations in nuclear size and shape may be seen, and as the tumor is slow growing, an absence or paucity of mitotic figures is the rule. This lymphoma is characterized by a diffuse growth pattern, whereas follicular lymphomas have a follicular growth pattern. A vague nodular pattern can be imparted by clusters of large cells with round vesicular nuclei and one or two prominent nucleoli. These clusters are known as *proliferation centers*

TABLE 28-5. Small Lymphocytic Lymphoma

Other names
  Lymphocytic, well differentiated (Rappaport classification)
  Small lymphocytic and plasmacytoid lymphocytic (Lukes-Collins classification)
  Lymphocytic, chronic lymphocytic leukemia, and lymphoplasmacytic/lymphoplasmacytoid (Kiel classification)
  B-cell chronic lymphocytic leukemia[a]/prolymphocytic leukemia/small lymphocytic lymphoma (Revised European-American Lymphoma classification)
  B-cell chronic lymphocytic leukemia[a]/prolymphocytic leukemia/small lymphocytic lymphoma (World Health Organization classification)
Immunophenotype
  Positive: CD19, CD20, CD23, CD79a, CD5
  Negative: CD10
  Surface Ig: IgM faintly positive
  Genetics: Ig heavy and light chains are rearranged trisomy 12, t(11;14)
Differential diagnoses
  Reactive lymphocytosis; reactive lymphadenopathy
  Hairy cell leukemia
Clinical features
  Survival in advanced disease not affected by early therapy; watch-and-wait approach may be appropriate for certain patients
  Repeated relapses with remissions of increasingly shorter duration, eventually refractory disease
  Transformation to a diffuse aggressive lymphoma (most commonly diffuse large B-cell lymphoma)
Initial treatment approaches
  Watch and wait (if no significant symptoms or impaired function related to organ involvement)
  Oral alkylating agents
  Combination chemotherapy (non–anthracycline based, anthracycline based, or nucleoside analog based)

Ig, immunoglobulin.
[a]This malignancy is by convention referred to as *chronic lymphocytic leukemia* when patients present with malignant lymphocytosis of $\geq$5000/mm^3.

(32). Monoclonal immunoglobulins (Igs) (commonly referred to as *paraproteins*) are often present in the serum of patients with SLL. SLL is the nodal morphologic equivalent of CLL. By convention, the term *chronic lymphocytic leukemia* is used when patients present with at least 5000 circulating lymphocytes/mm^3. Lymphoplasmacytic lymphomas are tumors of mature B cells, which are clinically similar to SLL. These lymphomas also often secrete a monoclonal Ig. A lymphoplasmacytic lymphoma which produces monoclonal IgM is known as *Waldenström's macroglobulinemia*. The most salient features of SLL are presented in Table 28-5.

BIOLOGY, CYTOGENETICS, IMMUNOPHENOTYPE, AND DIFFERENTIAL DIAGNOSIS OF SMALL LYMPHOCYTIC LYMPHOMA

The most common chromosomal abnormalities found in patients with SLL involve breakpoints on chromosomes 11 and 14 and the occurrence of an extra entire chromosome (33). These abnormalities have also been reported in patients with CLL (33–36). The breakpoint on chromosome 11 most frequently is located at q22 and on chromosome 14 at q32. The most common translocation reported involves these two breakpoints designated as t(11;14)(q22;q32). Patients with abnormal karyotypes (34), particularly trisomy 12 (36), appear to have a poorer survival rate. The majority of SLLs are B-cell lymphomas, although a small percentage (1% to 5%) are derived from T cells (37). The most common immunophenotype for this tumor is listed in Table 28-5. B-SLLs express usual B-cell antigens (e.g., CD19, CD20), but they also commonly express the pan-T-cell antigen CD5 (Leu-1). This can occasionally be a useful distinction to differentiate this entity from other low-grade lymphomas, especially when the histology is atypical or biopsy material is scant.

The use of other immunologic studies may be of prognostic importance. For example, tumors expressing a high level of the Ki-67 antigen (a marker of cellular proliferation) have been suggested to be associated with a poor prognosis (38,39). In addition, the number of normal T cells infiltrating neoplastic cells in B-SLL has been suggested to be inversely proportional to the severity of disease; that is, patients with small numbers of infiltrating T cells have more aggressive disease (39). The differential diagnosis of SLL includes entities such as mantle cell lymphoma and, occasionally, nodular lymphocyte–predominant Hodgkin's disease.

CLINICAL FEATURES AND EVALUATION OF PATIENTS WITH SMALL LYMPHOCYTIC LYMPHOMA

Common clinical features of patients with SLL are listed in Table 28-5. The median age of patients studied in the Working Formulation was 61 years. This may be younger than the median age that might be seen in the community, because patients from the Working Formulation study came from cancer centers or university teaching hospitals and may reflect some element of referral bias. A slight male predominance was seen, as is true with most subtypes of NHL. Most patients presented with nodal disease, although involvement of bone marrow, liver, and spleen were common (e.g., 71% of patients in the Working Formulation had bone marrow involvement). Staging of patients with SLL should follow the principles outlined previously. Patients with peripheral lymphocytosis should have flow cytometry performed to look for evidence of an abnormal clonal population of lymphocytes. Also, β_2-microglobulin has been advocated as a useful prognostic factor in this illness (40).

SLL commonly presents with advanced stage disease, although patients are generally relatively asymptomatic. This disease follows the pattern of progression characteristic of most indolent lymphomas, which is slow progression of adenopathy and a gradual increase in the number of involved sites over time. Patients with large quantities of circulating IgM in the serum may present with symptoms of hyperviscosity (abnormal bleeding symptoms, evanescent visual or neurologic symptoms, congestive heart failure, and, occasionally, hypercoagulability). Patients with extensive bone marrow involvement may develop thrombocytopenia and anemia. Patients with SLL often have hypogammaglobulinemia. All patients with SLL and all patients with other subtypes of NHL have altered immune function and are at increased risk for infections even before the institution of therapy (41). The combination of hypogammaglobulinemia, altered cellular immunity, and effects of subsequent chemotherapy (42) may increase the risk of developing atypical or opportunistic infections such as *Pneumocystis carinii*, fungal infections, and infections with encapsulated organisms (e.g., *Streptococcus pneumoniae*, *Haemophilus influenzae*, *Neisseria* species). In patients who demonstrate a clinical susceptibility to repeated or unusual infections, periodic use of intravenous Ig may be appropriate.

TREATMENT AND PROGNOSIS OF PATIENTS WITH SMALL LYMPHOCYTIC LYMPHOMA

From a therapeutic standpoint, the distinction between B-SLL, B-CLL, and Waldenström's macroglobulinemia is generally of little significance. One exception to this might be in patients who present with significant symptoms or pathology related to hyperviscosity syndrome associated with the presence of an IgM paraprotein. In these circumstances, the use of plasmapheresis simultaneously with cytotoxic therapy can quickly and temporarily decrease the level of IgM, reducing symptoms associated with hyperviscosity.

TABLE 28-6. Chemotherapy Regimens for Advanced Stage Small Lymphocytic Lymphoma, Grades 1 and 2 Follicular Lymphomas, and Extranodal Marginal Zone B-Cell Lymphomas

Regimen	Drug	Dosage[a]	Administration Day	Frequency (d)
Chlorambucil	Chlorambucil	0.1–0.2 mg/kg p.o.	Daily	Daily
Chlorambucil/prednisone	Chlorambucil	40.0 mg	1, 2	28
	Prednisone	100 mg	1–5	28
CVP	Cyclophospha-mide	400 p.o.	1–5	21
	Vincristine	1.4 i.v. (max 2 mg)	1	
	Prednisone	100 p.o.	1–5	
CHOP	Cyclophospha-mide	750 i.v.	1	21
	Doxorubicin	50 i.v.	1	
	Vincristine	1.4 i.v.	1	
	Prednisone	100 p.o.	1–5	
Fludarabine	Fludarabine	25 i.v.	1–5	28
Fludarabine/mitoxantrone/ dexamethasone	Fludarabine	25 i.v.	1–3	28
	Mitoxantrone	10 i.v.	1	
	Dexamethasone	20 mg i.v. p.o.	1–5	

[a]Dosage is mg/m^2 unless otherwise specified.

Because few patients with SLL present with localized disease (43), few data are available about therapy for stage I disease. The patients who present with disease localized to one nodal or extranodal site seem to have an excellent outlook with radiation therapy; those who present with disease in a single extranodal site have an excellent outlook with surgery with or without subsequent radiation therapy (44). The management of patients with more extensive disease is more controversial. Like other forms of indolent lymphoma, many patients are asymptomatic at the time of presentation. Because the ability to cure or prolong survival in advanced stage patients with earlier or more intense therapy is at best uncertain, watchful waiting with no initial therapy has been proposed for patients who do not have bulky symptomatic disease, autoimmune cytopenias, recurrent infections, or threatened end-organ function (45). After a long follow-up, patients managed in this manner have not had a poorer outlook than patients who received therapy initially (44). For patients requiring therapy, common treatments have included chlorambucil or cyclophosphamide, with or without corticosteroids. In one series, no significant difference was found among patients who received a single alkylating agent or combination chemotherapy as their initial treatment (44). The demonstration of the efficacy of purine analogs in patients with CLL has also made this a popular therapeutic choice for patients with SLL. A phase II European study of single-agent fludarabine in patients with newly diagnosed indolent lymphomas demonstrated response rates of 63% for patients with lymphoplasmacytic lymphoma and 79% for patients with Waldenström's macroglobulinemia (46). The median duration of response was 2.5 years for patients with lymphoplasmacytic lymphoma and greater than 3.0 years for patients with Waldenström's macroglobulinemia. A large randomized trial of patients with previously untreated CLL comparing fludarabine with chlorambucil (employing a crossover design for nonresponders) demonstrated a higher overall response rate (70% vs. 43%) and complete response rate (27% vs. 3%) in patients randomized to initial therapy with fludarabine (47). Progression-free survival was also superior for patients randomized to initial therapy with fludarabine (27 months vs. 17 months; p <.0001). However, no difference in overall survival emerged in this trial. As fludarabine appears to have an extremely high level of activity as a single agent, combination regimens have been developed and tested (42,48,49). Although these

combinations appear to be very active in treating this disease, any effect on prolongation of survival is not known. Examples of treatment regimens for SLL are shown in Table 28-6.

The use of the anti-CD20 monoclonal antibody rituximab (see section Treatment and Prognosis of Patients with Grades 1 and 2 Follicular Lymphomas) in patients with relapsed/resistant SLL appears to induce responses less commonly than in patients with follicular lymphomas (50,51). A multicenter European study of rituximab as single-agent therapy for patients with previously treated SLL (n = 29) demonstrated only a 14% response rate in 28 evaluable patients, with no complete responses being observed (50). The humanized monoclonal antibody CAMPATH-1H is directed against the CD52 antigen, which is expressed on virtually all lymphocytes and monocytes. This antibody has demonstrated efficacy (response rate 42%; median duration 12 months) in patients with previously treated CLL (52) and has recently been approved as a treatment for patients with chemorefractory CLL.

The use of high-dose therapy/autologous hematopoietic stem cell transplantation in this patient population has also demonstrated a high propensity to relapse in comparison with follicular lymphomas (53,54), which has led to ongoing novel studies of *in vivo* purging with agents such as rituximab before stem cell collection. These types of results have also led investigators to explore allogeneic stem cell transplantation (including the use of nonmyeloablative regimens) as a possible means of improving long-term outcome (55–58).

Although the management of patients with SLL is clearly changing, the majority of patients experience progression of their disease at some point in time. In such patients, subsequent therapy obviously needs to be individualized. In many patients, supportive care and radiation to sites of symptomatic involvement are appropriate. Further use of single-agent or combination chemotherapy should be reserved for manifestations of progressive disease that cannot be managed more simply.

Marginal Zone Lymphoma

This lymphoma generally would have been classified as SLL or, occasionally, follicular or diffuse mixed small cleaved and large cell lymphoma in the Working Formulation. These are lymphomas generally of small B cells, described in more recent years.

Marginal zone lymphomas generally have a somewhat heterogeneous cellular appearance, with some cells resembling small cleaved follicle center cells and some cells resembling larger immunoblasts or centroblasts (8). Reactive follicles are usually seen, and the neoplastic cells generally occupy the marginal zone or interfollicular region of the lymph node. When these lymphomas occur in epithelial tissues, they tend to infiltrate the tissue and have been described as *lymphoepithelial lesions*. Marginal zone lymphomas are classified as being either primarily nodal or extranodal depending on their anatomic presentation. Extranodal marginal zone B-cell lymphomas commonly involve mucosal tissues (e.g., GI tract, thyroid, orbit) and in this situation are referred to as *MALT lymphomas*. This group of lymphomas appears to be commonly antigen driven. For example, MALT lymphomas of the thyroid gland commonly arise against a background of Hashimoto's thyroiditis, and gastric MALT lymphomas are often seen in association with gastric *Helicobacter pylori* infection. Nodal marginal zone B-cell lymphomas are also commonly seen in association with the presence of autoimmune disease (e.g., Sjögren's syndrome), and it is possible that these lymphomas represent nodal spread of a MALT lymphoma. Bone marrow involvement may be seen in nodal presentations of this disease.

BIOLOGY, CYTOGENETICS, IMMUNOPHENOTYPE, AND DIFFERENTIAL DIAGNOSIS OF MARGINAL ZONE LYMPHOMA

Extranodal presentations of this lymphoma generally involve mucosal tissues and are therefore referred to as *MALT lymphomas*. This type of lymphoma commonly involves organs such as the orbit, thyroid, and GI tract. Stomach is a particularly common site of presentation.

The immunophenotype of marginal zone lymphomas is generally that of B-cell antigens (CD19, CD20, CD22). They are CD5- and CD10-negative. They commonly express surface Ig. Rearrangement of bcl-1 and -2 is not seen, but trisomy 3 has been reported (59) as well as other chromosomal abnormalities.

The most common differential diagnoses for a pathologist to have to discern with these lesions would be SLL or CLL and mantle cell lymphoma, all of which would be CD5-positive.

CLINICAL FEATURES AND EVALUATION OF PATIENTS WITH MARGINAL ZONE LYMPHOMA

Extranodal marginal zone lymphomas of MALT are generally tumors of adults. It is hypothesized that MALT lymphomas arise as a result of a chronic antigen-driven process. For example, it is not unusual for a MALT lymphoma of the thyroid to arise on a background of Hashimoto's thyroiditis. Gastric MALT lymphomas are commonly accompanied by evidence of chronic gastritis and *H. pylori* infection. It is possible that chronic inflammation caused by such autoimmune or infectious processes eventually leads to the development of a clonal lymphocyte population. Autoimmune diseases are also common in patients with nodal presentations of marginal zone B-cell lymphomas (e.g., Sjögren's syndrome). Localized presentations are relatively common. Nodal presentations of this disease generally are accompanied by bone marrow involvement, and, occasionally, peripheral blood involvement may be seen with nodal presentations. The clinical course of these lymphomas is generally indolent.

TREATMENT AND PROGNOSIS OF PATIENTS WITH MARGINAL ZONE LYMPHOMA

Marginal zone lymphomas are treated in a fashion similar to other low-grade lymphomas. Because they are relatively more recently recognized entities, retrospective series (60,61) have generally been used as a source of information on treatment. Stage I nongastric MALT lymphomas have commonly been

TABLE 28-7. Antibiotic Regimens Used to Treat Helicobacter-Associated Gastric Mucosa–Associated Lymphoid Tissue Lymphomas

Drug	Dosage (mg)	Duration (wk)
Amoxicillin	500 t.i.d.	2
Metronidazole	400 t.i.d.	
Colloidal bismuth	120 q.i.d.	
Amoxicillin	500 t.i.d.	2
Metronidazole	400 t.i.d.	
Omeprazole	20 b.i.d.	
Amoxicillin	1000 b.i.d.	2
Clarithromycin	500 b.i.d.	
Omeprazole	20 b.i.d.	
Amoxicillin	1000 b.i.d.	2
Clarithromycin	500 b.i.d.	
Lansoprazole	40 b.i.d.	

treated with localized radiotherapy. Whether adjuvant chemotherapy adds further benefit to these patients is unknown. Local therapy produces a high probability of long-term disease control. Patients with more advanced stage nongastric MALT lymphomas are likely best treated similar to grades 1 and 2 follicular lymphomas. Examples of treatment regimens for marginal zone lymphomas are shown in Table 28-6.

Gastric MALT lymphomas represent a unique situation with respect to therapy. Patients who have nonbulky stage I disease and who have evidence of *H. pylori* infection have been treated successfully with antibiotic therapy directed at eradicating the organism (Table 28-7) (62). Patients treated in this fashion should be endoscopically restaged after therapy to demonstrate eradication of the organism, as well as to document any treatment effect. Patients who still demonstrate *H. pylori* may be offered second-line antibiotic therapy. Patients who are *H. pylori*–negative may occasionally respond to antibiotic therapy. Such patients can be observed after therapy. Patients with clear evidence of residual disease on biopsy should likely be offered local radiotherapy. Because not all patients with *H. pylori* respond to therapy directed against the organism, it is possible that the antibiotic-responsive cases represent an earlier form of the disease that is antigen driven or antigen dependent. It is conceivable that, over time, the disease may become antigen independent, possibly as further genetic abnormalities occur within the tumor. Large, well-designed longitudinal (cohort) studies of this tumor may help identify the genetic changes that accompany these biologic changes. Patients with advanced stage gastric MALT lymphomas should be treated in a fashion similar to those with advanced stage grades 1 and 2 follicular lymphomas. Patients with aggressive histology (e.g., diffuse large B-cell lymphoma) at diagnosis, or who transform at some further point, should be treated as if they had aggressive lymphomas.

Follicular Lymphomas

Follicular lymphomas include the histologic subtypes follicular small cleaved cell (follicular grade 1), follicular mixed small cleaved and large cell (follicular grade 2), and follicular large cell (follicular grade 3). Follicles are often arranged in a so-called back-to-back pattern within the lymph node. Distinction between subtypes is based on the number of admixed large transformed cells seen in the tumor. In the past, tumors with a large cell component of less than 20% were referred to as *follicular small cleaved cell lymphoma*; tumors with a large cell component of 20% to 50% within the node were termed *follicular mixed lymphoma*; and tumors with greater than 50% large cells were referred to as *follicular large cell lymphomas* (63). More recently,

Mann and Berard (64) proposed that tumors with fewer than five large cells/high-power field be considered *follicular small cleaved lymphomas* (follicular grade 1); tumors with 5 to 15 large cells/high-power field be considered *follicular mixed lymphomas* (follicular grade 2); and tumors with more than 15 cells/high-power field be considered *follicular large cell lymphomas* (follicular grade 3). This comparatively simple and objective approach seems to have excellent clinical correlation and has become an increasingly popular way to classify these tumors. It should be remembered that the cytologic and pathologic features of these lymphomas represent a biologic continuum that has been somewhat artificially separated largely for the purposes of making treatment decisions.

Follicular grade 1 lymphoma is a B-cell neoplasm consisting morphologically of mostly small cleaved lymphocytes originating in follicle center cells. These cells are usually larger than normal lymphocytes and have regular nuclei with prominent indentations and linear cleavage planes. The chromatin pattern is coarse, and nucleoli are small and inconspicuous. Pathologically, the cells are arranged in characteristic follicles of relatively uniform size and shape, which lack a prominent and well-defined lymphoid cuff and compress intervening lymphoid regions. A small number of noncleaved cells are found, and a variable number of large cells with basophilic cytoplasm (centroblasts) are commonly seen scattered among the small cells. As this is a relatively slow-growing tumor, mitotic figures are uncommon. This subtype of lymphoma accounted for approximately 10% of cases in the Non-Hodgkin's Lymphoma Classification Project study (14). There is some evidence to suggest that the incidence of follicular small cleaved cell NHL may be proportionally decreasing (65).

Follicular mixed (follicular grade 2) lymphomas differ from follicular small cleaved cell lymphomas only in the proportion of admixed large transformed lymphoid cells. As described earlier, the criteria of Mann and Berard (64) are perhaps the most widely used today. Using these criteria, tumors with fewer than five large cells/high-power field are considered follicular small cleaved (follicular grade 1), and tumors with 5 to 15 large cells/high-power field are considered follicular mixed (follicular grade 2). This subtype accounted for approximately 6% of cases in the Non-Hodgkin's Lymphoma Classification Project study (14).

In most observational studies, follicular large cell lymphoma (follicular grade 3) appears to have a more aggressive course relative to the other subtypes of follicular lymphoma and as such is generally treated more like diffuse large B-cell lymphoma (66–68). The immunologic and salient clinical features of grades 1 and 2 follicular lymphomas are presented in Table 28-8.

BIOLOGY, CYTOGENETICS, IMMUNOPHENOTYPE, AND DIFFERENTIAL DIAGNOSIS OF GRADES 1 AND 2 FOLLICULAR LYMPHOMAS

Follicular grade 1 and 2 lymphomas are associated with the chromosomal translocation t(14;18)(q32;q21) in 60% to 100% of cases (69–72). This translocation involves the juxtaposition of the Ig heavy chain locus on chromosome 14 with the bcl-2 locus on chromosome 18. It is likely that this chromosomal translocation is involved in the pathogenesis of this subtype of lymphoma, given that constitutive production of bcl-2 protein in cells appears to diminish or abolish normal apoptotic pathways. Thus, the biology of grades 1 and 2 follicular lymphomas is more one of abnormal lymphocytic accumulation rather than excessive growth rates. Even in patients in whom conventional cytogenetic studies do not reveal the t(14;18)(q32;q21) translocation, molecular genetic studies show consistent structural abnormalities (the molecular features of the translocation) within the bcl-2 gene in virtually all cases (73). Indolent follicular lymphomas are tumors of B lymphocytes. The most common immunophenotype seen is listed in

---

TABLE 28-8. Follicular Lymphomas

Other names
  Follicular lymphoma, grade 1: follicular, predominantly small cleaved cell (WF)
  Follicular lymphoma, grade 2: follicular, small cleaved and large cell (WF)
  Follicular lymphoma, grade 3: follicular, predominantly large cell (WF)
Immunophenotype
  Positive: CD10, CD19, CD20, CD22, CD79a, CD5
  Negative: CD5
  Surface Ig: IgM, IgG, IgA
  Genetics: t(14;18)
Differential diagnosis
  Reactive follicular hyperplasia
Clinical features
  Follicular lymphoma grades 1 and 2
    Slow progressive growth or waxing and waning lymphadenopathy
    Survival not likely influenced by earlier or more aggressive therapy in advanced stage disease
    Generally, exquisitely chemosensitive early in course
    Repeated relapses with remissions of increasingly shorter duration; eventually refractory disease
    Transformation to a diffuse aggressive lymphoma (most commonly diffuse large B-cell lymphoma)
  Follicular lymphoma grade 3
    Biology may be closer to diffuse large B-cell lymphoma
Initial treatment approaches
  Follicular lymphoma grades 1 and 2
    Early stage disease
      Radiotherapy
    Advanced stage disease
      Watch and wait (if no significant symptoms or impaired function related to organ involvement)
      Oral alkylating agents
      Combination chemotherapy (non–anthracycline-based, anthracycline-based) single-agent or combination nucleoside analog-based regimens
      Monoclonal antibody therapy
  Follicular lymphoma grade 3
    Early stage disease
      Brief anthracycline-based chemotherapy with involved field radiotherapy
    Advanced stage disease
      Full-course anthracycline-based chemotherapy

Ig, immunoglobulin; WF, working formulation.

Table 28-8. Occasionally, admixtures of normal T cells can infiltrate the tumor so as to obscure the B-cell origin (74,75). This is more likely to be demonstrated when immunophenotyping is performed using flow cytometric analysis. Making a distinction between grade 1 follicular lymphoma and reactive lymphoid hyperplasia may occasionally be difficult. In these situations, the pathologist relies on the ability to demonstrate the presence of clonality, the existence of the t(14;18)(q32;q21) translocation, or the presence of an Ig gene rearrangement.

CLINICAL FEATURES AND EVALUATION OF PATIENTS WITH GRADES 1 AND 2 FOLLICULAR LYMPHOMAS

Patients with grades 1 and 2 follicular lymphomas commonly present with painless lymphadenopathy. The median age of these patients in the Working Formulation was 54 years, but this is probably younger than the median age seen in the community and younger than that seen in a statewide study in Nebraska. A slight male predominance is commonly reported. Approximately 80% of patients present with advanced stage disease. Bone marrow involvement is seen in a relatively high proportion of cases. Occasionally, patients may present with abnormal circulating cells in the peripheral blood. Splenic and hepatic involvement also appear to occur frequently based on imaging studies, but histologic examination of these tissues is performed much less frequently than is bone marrow examination. Constitutional symptoms such as fever, night sweats, and weight loss are relatively uncommon in this subtype of lymphoma. Again, usual staging evaluations should be performed as outlined previously. Grades 1 and 2 follicular lymphomas tend to grow by slowly pushing adjacent tissues and organs out of their way rather than by direct invasion as is more often the case with diseases such as diffuse large B-cell lymphoma. Also, involvement of certain anatomic sites (e.g., CNS, testes) is distinctly uncommon in comparison with diffuse large B-cell lymphomas.

TREATMENT AND PROGNOSIS OF PATIENTS WITH GRADES 1 AND 2 FOLLICULAR LYMPHOMAS

Early Stage Disease. Between 20% and 48% of patients with grade 1 or 2 follicular lymphomas present with early stage (stage I or II) disease (43,76). Based on the results of observational studies with long-term follow-up from centers such as Stanford and the Princess Margaret Hospital (76,77), the most common therapy for the majority of these patients continues to be radiotherapy alone. The series from Stanford (77) contains data on 177 patients with early stage low-grade follicular lymphomas who were treated between 1961 and 1994. With a median follow-up for surviving patients now in excess of 7 years, this study has reported relapse-free survival rates of 44% at 10 years and 37% at 20 years. These authors reported a 64% 10-year probability of survival, and 35% of patients remain alive at 20 years. Very few patients observed for 10 or more years have relapsed. Patients treated with radiotherapy to both sides of the diaphragm experienced a lower probability of relapse, but this did not translate into any improvement in overall survival. Moreover, patients treated on both sides of the diaphragm may have had an increased risk of secondary malignancy (17.0% vs. 6.7%). In multivariate analysis, advanced age was independently associated with an increased risk of both relapse and death. The arguable presence of a plateau on time-to-event curves suggests that some of these patients may be curable with radiotherapy. The apparent increased risk of secondary malignancies suggests that these patients should have life-long oncologic follow-up.

Advanced Stage Disease. The curability of these subtypes of NHLs has been a point of debate for years. Although a proportion of patients who present with truly localized disease appear to be curable, patients who present with advanced stage disease do not appear to be curable with even the most aggressive forms of presently available therapy, including the combined modality use of cytotoxic chemotherapy, radiotherapy, and, more recently, monoclonal antibodies. Despite the appearance of incurability, patients with disseminated disease have tumors that initially tend to be highly responsive to chemotherapy, radiotherapy, and newer monoclonal antibody–based therapy. However, their history is characterized by multiple recurrences with progressively shorter disease-free intervals (78) and, ultimately, refractory untreatable progression. Virtually all types of indolent NHL can be associated with histologic transformation to a higher-grade illness, commonly diffuse large B-cell lymphoma.

Patients with advanced stage disease form the majority of cases in most series. Although advanced stage grades 1 and 2 follicular lymphomas are highly responsive to a number of treatment modalities, virtually all conventional dose therapies are associated with a continuous risk of relapse over time, suggesting that none of these approaches on its own is likely to be curative. As such, it remains difficult today to identify the best single or sequential form of therapy for this disease, and the selection and timing of any therapy for these patients remains a highly charged and controversial area in the treatment of lymphoma. Furthermore, a constantly growing list of new agents

with activity in this disease and the inability to test all of the possible combinations and permutations in appropriately powered randomized trials make it likely that this type of controversy will continue and possibly widen over the coming years. Therapies that have the ability to prolong survival in this illness have been difficult to identify for a number of reasons. First, the long natural history of this disease means that it is necessary to follow large numbers of patients for many years to identify modest survival advantages. Second, because patients are likely to receive multiple therapies (with various associated treatment effects and benefits) during the course of their illness, a small survival advantage conferred by a particular therapy may not be easily identifiable even in a randomized cohort of patients observed over time. In this situation, it is biologically possible that a perceived survival advantage for a particular therapy may actually have been the result of a sequencing effect of prior or subsequent therapies or the result of smaller cumulative benefits of other therapies received, which were by chance unbalanced between the groups being observed and were in part responsible for the improved outcome. For this reason, it may make the most sense for future randomized trials to evaluate the benefit of new therapies using outcomes such as freedom from progression and recurrence, with some attention given to other relevant outcome measures such as economic or quality of life measures associated with a particular therapy. Finally, in helping a patient arrive at the most optimal treatment decision, individual discussions regarding relevant treatment endpoints, toxicity, and duration of delivery of therapy should all be addressed. For example, some patients may accept increased short-term toxicity as a trade-off for a chance to experience more prolonged freedom from disease.

Whether earlier or more aggressive treatment alters significantly the natural history of grades 1 and 2 follicular lymphomas remains unknown. An observational study from Stanford on 83 patients with indolent lymphomas between 1963 and 1984 (79) suggests that patients managed without initial therapy fare as well as patients treated at diagnosis. In this study, the experimental group was compared with 131 protocol patients who were treated at the time of diagnosis. Five-year survival by histologic subtype and the actuarial probability of transformation to a higher-grade lymphoma were nearly identical between the groups. The median survival of the initially untreated group was 11 years, and the median time to institution of therapy was 3 years. Similar findings have been reported by other investigators (80,81). The use of anthracycline-based regimens as initial therapy does not appear to enhance survival and does not produce any evidence of a plateau on survival estimates (82). A small randomized trial by the NCI published in 1988 (83) enrolled 104 patients with low-grade lymphomas and deemed 89 patients appropriate candidates for deferral of immediate therapy. These patients were then randomized either to receive initial combination chemotherapy using ProMACE-MOPP followed by total nodal irradiation or to observation. The 5-year probability of survival was equal for both patient groups, but disease-free survival was longer for patients who were randomized to the initial treatment arm. It is not surprising that earlier treatment produces a longer remission duration (because of a lower tumor burden at the time of treatment), but in the absence of demonstrable survival differences, it remains an appropriate option to observe patients who do not have an overt need for early treatment (i.e., rapidly growing tumor or organ dysfunction caused by lymphoma).

Choices of Therapy for Advanced Stage Disease. Because no one form of therapy has emerged as clearly superior to another, initial therapy for grades 1 and 2 follicular lymphomas should be thought of as a spectrum of choices (Table 28-6). The clinician and patient must take several factors into account including the patient's age and functional status, the cost of therapy, and the toxicity and expected duration of remission associated with a particular approach or specific therapy. Oral alkylating agent therapy (e.g., chlorambucil, cyclophosphamide) is simple to deliver, well tolerated, and, in one small randomized trial, was associated with less toxicity and no survival difference in comparison with CVP (cyclophosphamide, vincristine, prednisone) or radiation (84). Anthracycline-based regimens (e.g., CHOP) have been used frequently presumably because of their effectiveness in treating patients with aggressive lymphomas; but again, there is no evidence to suggest that their inclusion improves outcome compared to less aggressive therapies (85). Similarly, the use of maintenance chemotherapy has not been associated with any demonstrable improvement in outcomes (86).

The use of purine analogs (e.g., fludarabine, 2-chlorodeoxyadenosine, 2-deoxycoformycin) has become popular in recent years, largely based on the results of phase II trials demonstrating a high level of activity in patients with indolent lymphomas (42,87,88). Although promising data have come from these uncontrolled trials, ongoing randomized trials have not reported clear survival advantages associated with the use of these agents alone or in combination compared to more traditional regimens. The most popular combination regimens appear to be fludarabine in combination with mitoxantrone and dexamethasone (42) or with cyclophosphamide (48).

Interferon-α is an agent that has been extensively evaluated in the context of indolent NHLs. Its precise mechanism of action remains elusive but likely includes antiproliferative effects (89), antiangiogenic effects (90), induction of maturation and differentiation in tumor cells (91), induction of apoptosis (92), and activation of nonspecific cellular immune responses (e.g., natural killer cells) (93,94). Early trials of single-agent interferon-α in patients with advanced and often refractory disease demonstrated reasonable levels of activity (93,95–98), and phase II trials, which followed, generally reported response rates in the range of 30% to 50% (99–101). A large number of randomized trials have subsequently been conducted and reported with variable results. One popular way to characterize and compare interferon and chemotherapy trials has been to separate studies into those that used anthracycline-based regimens (e.g., CHOP) and those that did not (e.g., chlorambucil, oral cyclophosphamide, CVP). Trials reporting the use of interferon with non–anthracycline-based regimens have not demonstrated a consistent benefit for interferon (102–105), although two studies comparing CVP with CVP/interferon demonstrated a longer time to progression for patients randomized to CVP/interferon (104,105). The results of interferon in conjunction with anthracycline-based regimens have perhaps more consistently demonstrated a longer time to progression and recurrence for patients receiving interferon as part of their treatment regimen, but consistent overall survival advantages have not been reported. The trial reporting the largest benefit for interferon comes from the Groupe d'Etude des Lymphomes Folliculaires (GELF). This trial compared six cycles of CHVP (cyclophosphamide, doxorubicin, teniposide, prednisone) to six cycles of CHVP plus interferon for 18 months in patients with at least stable disease. This trial has reported a higher response rate for patients randomized to CHVP/interferon (85% vs. 69%) and has consistently reported both an improved median event-free and overall survival advantage for the experimental group (106,107). The final analysis of this trial reported a median progression-free survival of 2.9 years for CHVP/interferon versus 1.5 years for CHVP alone (p = .0002) and a median overall sur-

vival of 5.6 years for CHVP versus not yet reached for CHVP/interferon (p = .008) (107). Not all trials have been able to demonstrate this same advantage for interferon in conjunction with anthracycline-based regimens, however. A large randomized study by the Southwest Oncology Group (SWOG) (108) treated 571 patients with advanced low-grade lymphoma with induction chemotherapy using ProMACE-MOPP followed by involved field radiotherapy for patients achieving only partial remission after chemotherapy. Patients were subsequently randomized to interferon three times weekly for 2 years or no further therapy. This trial was unable to demonstrate any significant difference in outcome between the two treatment groups. The toxicity profile of interferon combined with inconsistent results in randomized trials have led to a decline in the interest for this agent despite the fact that it is one of the agents for which there is an abundance of randomized data suggesting benefit. A metaanalysis of randomized trials using interferon has reported an overall survival advantage for patients who receive interferon in conjunction with anthracycline-based chemotherapy (109). This did not, however, include the data from the SWOG study. Finally, it should be remembered that most of the variability in outcomes of studies using interferon likely comes from differences between these trials in chemotherapy regimens used, interferon preparations and schedules, and the types of patients treated.

In the past several years, a resurgence of interest in monoclonal antibody therapy for lymphoma has been seen largely as a result of the identification of the CD20 surface antigen, which is specific to B lymphocytes. Approximately 85% of NHLs are B-cell tumors, and the CD20 antigen is expressed on the majority of these tumors. Its exact cellular function remains somewhat speculative (110,111), but it is clearly an opportunistic target for the use of monoclonal antibody therapy. The most widely known and utilized monoclonal antibody at the present time is rituximab, which is a chimeric (human-murine) monoclonal anti-CD20 antibody. This combination appears to enhance activity while decreasing autoimmunogenicity. The mechanisms of action of rituximab likely include both antibody- and complement-mediated cytotoxicity, as well as the induction of apoptosis. In phase I trials, it was very well tolerated, without an obvious maximum tolerated dose (112,113). Side effects are generally infusional and may represent manifestations of complement activation (e.g., fever, chills, asthenia). More serious toxicity may occur rarely, including acute bronchospasm, hypotension, and true anaphylaxis. Infusional toxicity appears to lessen in most cases with subsequent infusions. Based on the results of phase I trials, a dose of 375 mg/m^2 was selected as the dose for phase II studies and has generally become the accepted dose in most situations. Numerous phase II studies have now been reported for the use of rituximab in several different clinical situations (114–120). Table 28-9 lists the results of several of these trials, including a demonstration of the efficacy of retreatment of patients who previously responded to rituximab (117). The safety and efficacy of rituximab in conjunction with CHOP has also been demonstrated in a number of studies including a phase II trial of largely previously untreated patients with low-grade or follicular B-cell lymphomas (119). Conjugated monoclonal antibodies such as tositumomab (iodine 131) and ibritumomab (yttrium 90) are also presently being extensively evaluated to define their efficacy and role in the treatment of patients with B-cell lymphomas (121). A number of conventional salvage chemotherapy regimens are also available to patients who do not respond to the previous therapies (Table 28-10). These salvage regimens are used commonly to attempt to reinduce remission before the use of high-dose therapy/hematopoietic stem cell transplantation.

TABLE 28-9. Summary of Rituximab in Indolent Lymphomas

Trial Characteristic	Number of Patients Treated	Response Rate (%)	Median Time to Progression (mo)	Reference
Multidose	37	46	10	114
Pivotal trial	166	48	13	115
8 weekly infusions	37	57	>19	116
Bulky disease	31	43	8	118
Retreatment	58	40	>17	117
CHOP/rituximab	40	95	>29	119
Initial therapy	41	54	82% progression-free at 8 mo	120

CHOP, cyclophosphamide, doxorubicin, vincristine, prednisone.

If monoclonal antibody therapy can be considered a form of passive immunotherapy, then the next obvious level to take this treatment concept to would be that of active immunotherapy, or tumor vaccination. B-cell lymphomas are in some ways ideal tumors to target for vaccine therapy, because they contain on their surfaces an Ig that is a clonal, tumor-specific antigenic determinant known as an *idiotype*. Large quantities of patient-specific idiotype protein can be generated using hybridomas or with recombinant DNA techniques. Because the idiotype is not recognized by the host as immunologically foreign, however, tumor vaccination would seem to have limitations in the magnitude of effect that can likely be induced by attempting to immunize the host against a host-derived protein. One of the present issues is to attempt to find ways to maximize host recognition of an idiotype protein using various forms of chemical or biologic adjuvants. Investigators from Stanford University demonstrated that patients with indolent B-cell lymphomas in remission who were subsequently immunized with idiotype vaccines generated measurable immune responses in approximately 50% of cases. Those patients mounting an immune response experienced longer disease-free survival, and patients in first remission mounting an immune response experienced longer overall survival compared with those who were unable to mount such a response (122). It is, therefore, possible that successful vaccination may be capable of exerting a therapeutic effect in this patient population. It is, however, not possible to rule out the possibility that the ability to demonstrate an immune response to an idiotype vaccine is simply a surrogate marker for patients with intrinsically more functionally intact immune systems who may have done better as a result of their immunologic competence rather than as a result of the therapeutic effect of vaccination. Results from ongoing randomized trials are required to determine the presence of any therapeutic efficacy.

Both allogeneic and autologous hematopoietic stem cell transplantation have been studied in patients with indolent lymphomas, especially in patients with follicular lymphoma. The concept of dose intensification in this disease is an extension of the observation that patients with relapsed aggressive lymphomas have superior disease-free and overall survival when treated with high-dose therapy/autologous hematopoietic stem cell transplantation (123). Pilot and phase II studies of transplantation for patients with refractory and relapsed low-grade lymphoma have reported high complete response rates (124–127) with limited evidence to suggest better freedom from progression when compared to historical controls (124,127). A retrospective analysis of patients who had been enrolled in the GELF 86 trial demonstrated a greater probability of freedom from progression (42% vs. 16%; $p = .0001$) and survival (58% vs. 38%; $p = .0005$) at 5 years for patients receiving high-dose therapy/autologous hematopoietic stem cell transplantation as compared with conventional dose therapy at first relapse (128). Finally, a small randomized trial by Schouten et al. (129), known as the *CUP trial*, treated patients with relapsed follicular lymphoma with three cycles of induction therapy followed by randomization to further conventional chemotherapy, unpurged stem cell transplantation, or purged stem cell transplantation for responding patients. Poor accrual resulted in the randomization of only 89 patients and early closure of the study. However, patients randomized to stem cell transplantation had superior disease-free survival, with a similar trend toward improved overall survival. Despite this small body of evidence suggesting that high-dose chemotherapy/autologous stem cell transplantation offers a higher probability of long-term disease-free survival, there is no convincing evidence of any plateau effect on time-to-event curves for patients treated with this therapy. This makes it difficult to know whether this is curative therapy for many patients with these subtypes of lymphoma.

The use of allogeneic stem cell transplantation is an attempt to exploit a possible immunologically based graft-versus-lymphoma effect, as well as a means to avoid the possibility of reinfusing a graft that contains tumor cells (as is theoretically possible with autologous stem cell products). Comparative studies of allogeneic versus autologous stem cell transplantation suggest that a lower relapse rate is observed with allogeneic transplantation (130), which is indirect evidence for the presence of an immunologic effect of the allogeneic graft, the importance of tumor reinfusion with autologous transplants, or possibly both. Reports of tumor regression in response to the temporal development of graft-versus-host disease (131) are perhaps a more direct suggestion of such a graft-versus-tumor effect. Interestingly, event-free survival curves for patients receiving allogeneic stem cell transplants for indolent lymphomas suggest a relatively high and continuous remission rate (132), suggesting that this therapy may actually be curative for a proportion of patients. However, the increased morbidity and mortality associated with allogeneic transplantation (regimen-related toxicity, infections, and effects of graft-versus-host disease) make it difficult to demonstrate any survival advantage

TABLE 28-10. Common Salvage Regimens for Non-Hodgkin's Lymphoma

Regimen	Agents
DHAP	Cisplatin, cytarabine, dexamethasone
MINE	Ifosfamide, mitoxantrone, etoposide
ESHAP	Etoposide, cisplatin, cytarabine, dexamethasone
ICE	Ifosfamide, carboplatin, etoposide

for this form of therapy and limits its application to younger patients with good functional status and, generally, a matched sibling donor. The use of nonmyeloablative regimens in the setting of allogeneic transplantation may reduce the probability of severe regimen-related toxicity while allowing the eventual development of full donor chimerism required to produce an immunologic benefit from the transplant (58,133). The lower regimen-related morbidity also allows older patients to be considered for this form of allogeneic transplantation. Another approach presently being investigated is to consider the non-myeloablative transplant an immunologic consolidative therapy after autologous transplantation (134).

Grade 3 Follicular Lymphoma

Notwithstanding the acknowledged imperfections in the classification of follicular lymphomas, grade 3 follicular lymphoma is, by most studies, conceptually intermediate in its biology between grades 1 and 2 follicular lymphomas and diffuse large B-cell lymphoma. This is a relatively uncommon subtype of lymphoma, representing approximately 4% of lymphomas in the Working Formulation study (6). Its presentation is similar to diffuse large B-cell lymphoma (67). Like diffuse large B-cell lymphoma, patients who do not achieve complete remission with therapy tend to have a shorter survival relative to those who do (67). Some studies demonstrate the presence of a plateau on freedom-from-progression curves (66), suggesting that this may be a curable lymphoma in certain patients. These types of observations have led most physicians to treat this subtype of lymphoma aggressively with curative intent.

BIOLOGY, CYTOGENETICS, IMMUNOPHENOTYPE, AND DIFFERENTIAL DIAGNOSIS OF GRADE 3 FOLLICULAR LYMPHOMA

The immunophenotype of grade 3 follicular lymphoma is essentially the same as that of other follicular lymphomas (8). These tumors are B-cell lymphomas, and as with other follicular lymphomas, the most common chromosomal abnormality seen in follicular large cell lymphoma is the t(14;18)(q32;q21) translocation. Using traditional cytogenetic techniques, this is found in approximately 50% of the tumors. Other cytogenetic abnormalities have been reported (70,71). Common features of grade 3 follicular lymphoma are presented in Table 28-8.

CLINICAL FEATURES AND EVALUATION OF PATIENTS WITH GRADE 3 FOLLICULAR LYMPHOMA

Although the Working Formulation study found that most patients with grade 3 follicular lymphoma presented with stage IV disease, this has not been the case in all series (67). This may be partially due to differences in exact staging procedures over time in various series. Like other grades of follicular lymphomas, grade 3 follicular lymphoma has a propensity to histologic progression toward diffuse large B-cell lymphoma.

TREATMENT AND PROGNOSIS OF PATIENTS WITH GRADE 3 FOLLICULAR LYMPHOMA

Patients who present with stage I disease can sometimes have durable remissions when treated with radiation therapy with or without combination chemotherapy. For patients who present with more extensive disease, a variety of combination chemotherapy regimens have been employed (Table 28-11). With the use of doxorubicin-based regimens, complete responses have been observed in 49% to 76% of patients (54,67,68). Whether grade 3 follicular lymphoma is curable with combination chemotherapy has been a point of debate in the literature,

because some (66,68) but not all (54,67) series have suggested the presence of a plateau on event-free survival curves. A large series reported by Wendum et al. compared the outcome of 89 patients with grade 3 follicular lymphoma to 1096 patients with diffuse large B-cell lymphoma treated on the same protocol, and they were unable to demonstrate any significant difference in either freedom from progression or overall survival over time. These types of observations leave little doubt about the appropriateness of aggressive therapy in these patients. Patients who experience relapses of their disease are often treated aggressively with salvage therapy to reinduce remission followed by high-dose therapy/autologous hematopoietic stem cell transplantation.

Mantle Cell Lymphoma

In the mid-1970s, Berard et al. (135) described a lymphoma, which commonly displayed a diffuse growth pattern and contained a mixture of cell populations, that was not easily classifiable using existing classification systems. Some of the cells had features consistent with SLL, whereas some had features most consistent with follicular small cleaved cell lymphoma. The term *intermediate* was used to describe these lymphomas. Around this time, Lennert et al. described a tumor with a similar appearance (136). These tumors appear to have origins in the lymphocytes of primary lymphoid follicles and the mantle zones of secondary lymphoid follicles. Over time, these tumors became increasingly well characterized and known as *mantle cell lymphoma*. Variations in the histologic appearance are seen. Most commonly, the lymphocytes are seen growing in a nodular or diffuse pattern. Occasionally, both types of patterns may be seen in a single tumor. The cells are typically small lymphocytes with irregular nuclei. In approximately 20% of cases, larger transformed-appearing (blastic) cells may be seen. Mantle cell lymphoma has been characterized as having the worst features of both indolent and aggressive lymphomas (i.e., the disease appears to be incurable with standard therapies but also has an aggressive course more akin to diffuse large B-cell lymphoma). Mantle cell lymphoma appears to be less responsive to chemotherapy than either indolent or aggressive lymphomas, and patients have a median survival of only approximately 4 to 5 years with conventional therapy (137). There is no evidence to suggest that any form of aggressive conventional-dose combination chemotherapy regimen has curative potential when used to treat this type of lymphoma. Patients may present with peripheral blood involvement and advanced stage disease. Not uncommonly, this subtype of NHL involves the spleen, liver, and GI tract. CNS involvement also occurs occasionally (138–140).

BIOLOGY, CYTOGENETICS, IMMUNOPHENOTYPE, AND DIFFERENTIAL DIAGNOSIS OF MANTLE CELL LYMPHOMA

Mantle cell lymphoma is characterized by the presence of a cytogenetic abnormality, the t(11;14)(q13;q32) translocation. This is seen in the majority of cases (141) but is not entirely specific to mantle cell lymphoma (142). It represents the translocation of a putative oncogene adjacent to *bcl-1* on chromosome 11 into the enhancer region of the Ig heavy chain locus on chromosome 14. The putative oncogene deregulated by this translocation is known as CCND 1 or PRAD 1. The gene encodes for the expression of the protein cyclin D1 and is overexpressed in nearly all cases (138). The means by which this translocation is involved in lymphomagenesis is not yet clear. However, the observation that cyclin D1 appears to be involved in the process of cell cycle regulation makes it likely that the occurrence of this translocation plays a major role in the development of the illness. Mantle cell lymphoma com-

TABLE 28-11. Chemotherapy Regimens for the Treatment of Follicular Large Cell Lymphoma, Diffuse Large B-Cell Lymphoma, Anaplastic Large Cell Lymphoma, and Peripheral T-Cell Lymphoma

Regimen	Drug	Dosage (mg/m²)	Administration Day	Frequency (d)
First generation				
CHOP	Cyclophosphamide	750 i.v.	1	21
	Doxorubicin	50 i.v.	1	
	Vincristine	1.4 i.v.	1	
	Prednisone	100 p.o.	1–5	
CAP-BOP	Cyclophosphamide	650 i.v.	1	21
	Doxorubicin	50 i.v.	1	
	Procarbazine	100 p.o.	1–7	
	Bleomycin	10 U s.c.	15	
	Vincristine	1.4 i.v.	15	
	Prednisone	100 p.o.	15–21	
Second generation				
m-BACOD	Methotrexate	200	8, 15	21
	Bleomycin	4 U i.v.	1	
	Doxorubicin	45 i.v.	1	
	Cyclophosphamide	600 i.v.	1	
	Vincristine	1.4 i.v.	1	
	Dexamethasone	6 p.o.	1–5	
	Leucovorin	10 p.o.	24 hr after methotrexate; q6h × 8 doses	
ProMACE-MOPP[a]	Prednisone	60 p.o.	1–14	
	Methotrexate	1500 i.v.	14	
	Doxorubicin	25 i.v.	1, 8	
	Cyclophosphamide	650 i.v.	1, 8	
	Etoposide	120 i.v.	1, 8	
	Nitrogen mustard	6 i.v.	1, 8	
	Vincristine	1.4 i.v.	1, 8	
	Procarbazine	100 p.o.	1–14	
	Prednisone	50 i.v.	1–14	
	Leucovorin	50 i.v.	24 hr after methotrexate; q6h × 5 doses	
Third generation				
MACOP-B	Methotrexate	400 i.v.	8	28[b]
	Doxorubicin	50 i.v.	1, 15	
	Cyclophosphamide	350 i.v.	1, 15	
	Vincristine	1.4 i.v.	8, 22	
	Prednisone	75[c] p.o.	Daily × 12 wk	
	Bleomycin	10 U i.v.	28	
ProMACE-CytaBOM	Prednisone	60 p.o.	1–14	28
	Doxorubicin	25 i.v.	1	
	Cyclophosphamide	650 i.v.	1	
	Etoposide	60 i.v.	1	
	Cytarabine	300 i.v.	8	
	Bleomycin	5 U i.v.	8	
	Vincristine	1.4 i.v.	8	
	Methotrexate	120 i.v.	8	
	Leucovorin	25 p.o.	q6h × 4 starting 9	

[a]MOPP is given after induction of remission.
[b]MACOP-B is given in three cycles over 12 wk total.
[c]Prednisone is given in a fixed dose of 75 mg.

monly expresses surface IgM and IgD. Its characteristic phenotype is that of the expression of pan-B-cell antigens (CD19, CD20, CD22) and HLA-DR. They are usually CD5 (pan-T-cell antigen)-positive and CD10- and CD23-negative. This immunophenotype is remarkably similar to that seen in SLL and CLL, except for the lack of CD23 expression (which is characteristically present in SLL and CLL). Lymphocytes that are the normal counterparts to mantle cell lymphoma appear to be naïve lymphocytes of primary lymphoid follicles and the mantle zone cells of secondary lymphoid follicles. The differential diagnosis of mantle cell lymphoma includes reactive follicular hyperplasia, angiofollicular lymph node hyperplasia (Castleman's disease), follicular small cleaved lymphoma, and SLL. Occasionally, the blastic form of mantle cell lymphoma may appear similar to B-lymphoblastic lymphoma. In all of

these cases, the clinical history as well as the determination of the presence of clonality, the presence of cyclin D1 overexpression, and the determination of the immunophenotype should make the diagnosis clear. The most common features of mantle cell lymphoma are listed in Table 28-12.

CLINICAL FEATURES AND EVALUATION OF PATIENTS WITH MANTLE CELL LYMPHOMA

Mantle cell lymphoma accounts for approximately 5% of NHLs diagnosed annually in the United States (43). The median age of patients with mantle cell lymphoma is approximately 60 years, and there is a distinct male preponderance to this illness (43,137,138). Approximately 80% of patients present with advanced stage disease (43). Hepatosplenomegaly is common, and GI involvement is seen in approximately 10% to 20% of

TABLE 28-12. Mantle Cell Lymphoma

Other names
  Centrocytic, centroblastic, centrocytoid subtype (Kiel classification)
  Small lymphocytic, plasmacytoid, diffuse small cleaved cell, follicular small cleaved cell, diffuse mixed small cleaved and large cell (Working Formulation)
Immunophenotype
  Positive: CD19, CD20, CD22, CD5
  Negative: CD10, CD23
  Surface Ig: IgM, IgD
  Genetics: Ig heavy and light chains are rearranged; t(11;14)
Differential diagnoses
  Small lymphocytic lymphoma
  Chronic lymphocytic leukemia
  Follicular lymphoma grade 1
Clinical features
  Median age in sixth decade
  Male preponderance
  Hepatosplenomegaly, advanced stage disease, gastrointestinal involvement
  Short remission durations; likely incurable with common combination chemotherapy regimens
Initial treatment approaches
  Combination chemotherapy
  ? Role of early consolidative high-dose therapy/autologous or allogeneic stem cell transplantation

Ig, immunoglobulin.

patients (43,137). Patients with unusual GI symptoms, abnormalities on imaging, or involvement of Waldeyer's ring should be considered for endoscopic evaluation to rule out the possibility of lymphomatous involvement of the GI tract. Lymphomatous polyposis is occasionally seen and should suggest a diagnosis of mantle cell lymphoma. Bone marrow involvement is seen in up to 80% of patients, and elevated LDH is seen in approximately 40% of patients (43,138).

TREATMENT AND PROGNOSIS OF PATIENTS WITH MANTLE CELL LYMPHOMA

The median survival of patients with mantle cell lymphoma is generally between 3 and 4 years (43,138), although one series reported by the British National Lymphoma Investigation group described a median survival of 57 months using non-anthracycline–based chemotherapy regimens (137). Prognostic factors associated with a poor probability of survival include a high International Prognostic Index (IPI) score, a diffuse histologic pattern, a high mitotic index, and p53 overexpression (43,138). Combination chemotherapy used for aggressive lymphomas (e.g., CHOP) can induce a response in approximately 60% of patients (138); however, durability of remissions is invariably rare. The use of agents more commonly seen in the treatment of patients with indolent lymphomas (e.g., fludarabine, 2-chlorodeoxyadenosine) has not been seen as particularly successful (143). Interferon has been used also with limited success, as has the monoclonal antibody rituximab, which in one study had a median time to progression of only 7 months (144). As would be expected, the attainment of a complete remission is associated with a greater probability of long-term survival. Examples of treatment regimens for mantle cell lymphoma are shown in Table 28-13.

The observation that combination agent therapy does not appear to offer much, if any, chance of cure for patients with this disease has led investigators toward the application of high-dose therapy with autologous or allogeneic stem cell transplantation as treatment. The use of high-dose therapy with autologous stem cell transplantation has been associated with a high probability of attaining complete remission (145–

147), but long-term follow-up of patients treated in this fashion has demonstrated a propensity to relapse, with most larger studies reporting median event and progression-free intervals of 8 to 21 months (147–149). As might be expected, factors associated with a longer time to progression include fewer prior therapies (147) and the use of transplantation as part of initial therapy (148,150). Investigators from the M. D. Anderson Cancer Center have evaluated the feasibility and outcome of patients treated with an initial aggressive regimen that alternates a dose-intensified, CHOP-like regimen (hyper-CVAD) with high-dose methotrexate/cytarabine for four cycles followed by high-dose therapy with autologous or allogeneic stem cell transplantation (150). The group receiving autologous transplantation had a 28% probability of event-free survival at 3 years. A historic control group with similar pretreatment characteristics that was treated with CHOP-like regimens between 1986 and 1992 was observed to have the same probability of event-free survival as patients who underwent autologous stem cell transplantation. Studies examining the presence of minimal residual disease in autografts and the effect of purging the autograft before stem cell infusion suggest that autologous grafts may frequently contain evidence of residual disease (151) and that immunologic purging techniques may fail to eradicate evidence of disease in the majority of patients (152). This type of data, with the observation that autologous stem cell transplantation does not produce any apparent plateau on Kaplan-Meier plots of disease-free survival (147–149), suggests that few, if any, patients can be cured using autologous stem cell transplantation.

The use of allogeneic stem cell transplantation offers a potential means to overcome the reinfusion of malignant cells and the ability to provide a possible graft-versus-tumor effect in addition to the cytotoxic effect of the preparative regimen. In the report by Khouri et al. (150) using hyper-CVAD/methotrexate/cytarabine, eight patients received related allogeneic stem cell grafts. In these eight patients, the 3-year probabilities of event-free and overall survival were 73%. However, it is well recognized that selection bias may inadvertently account for some of this apparent improvement in outcome, given that allogeneic transplantation is limited largely to younger patients with good functional status. Nevertheless, this therapy, where feasible, may represent the best chance for long-term freedom from disease for patients with mantle cell lymphoma, and, although still considered experimental, it is becoming a preferred treatment choice in many transplant centers.

Diffuse Large B-Cell Lymphoma

This is generally the most common subtype of NHL and, as such, is the prototype of aggressive lymphoma on which therapy is based for most other forms of aggressive lymphoma. In the Working Formulation, *immunoblastic lymphoma* and *diffuse mixed small cleaved and large cell lymphomas* were considered as separate subtypes. In the more recent classification schemes, these terms have been replaced by this single entity. Diffuse large B-cell lymphoma is a potentially curable disease when treated with aggressive combination chemotherapy regimens.

BIOLOGY, CYTOGENETICS, IMMUNOPHENOTYPE, AND DIFFERENTIAL DIAGNOSIS OF DIFFUSE LARGE B-CELL LYMPHOMA

Diffuse large B-cell lymphoma is composed of large cells that morphologically resemble centroblasts or immunoblasts (8). Occasionally, large cleaved cells (153) and cells identical to those seen in anaplastic large cell lymphoma are visible (8). Immunophenotypically, the cells commonly express surface Ig

TABLE 28-13. Treatment Regimens for Mantle Cell Lymphoma

Regimen	Drug	Dosage (mg/m²)	Administration Day	Frequency (d)
Chlorambucil	Chlorambucil	0.1–0.2 mg/kg p.o.	Daily	Daily
Chlorambucil/	Chlorambucil	40	1, 2	28
prednisone	Prednisone	100 mg	1–5	
CVP	Cyclophosphamide	400 p.o.	1–5	21
	Vincristine	1.4 i.v. (max 2 mg)	1	
	Prednisone	100 p.o.	1–5	
CHOP	Cyclophosphamide	750 i.v.	1	21
	Doxorubicin	50 i.v.	1	
	Vincristine	1.4 i.v.	1	
	Prednisone	100 p.o.	1–5	
Fludarabine	Fludarabine	25 i.v.	1–5	28
Hyper-CVAD[a]	Cyclophosphamide	300 i.v. q12h	1–3	
	Adriamycin	25 i.v.	4–5	
	Vincristine	2 mg i.v.	4, 11	
	Dexamethasone	40 mg	1–4, 11–14	
	G-CSF[b]	5 µg/kg/d	Start 6	
Methotrexate/	Methotrexate	200 i.v.	Bolus 1	
cytarabine[a]	Methotrexate	800 i.v.	24-hr continuous infusion 1	
	Cytarabine[b]	3000 i.v. q12h	2–3	
	Leucovorin	[c]		
	G-CSF[d]			
Rituximab	Rituximab	375 i.v.	Weekly × 4	Weekly × 4

[a]Cycles of hyper-CVAD alternate with cycles of methotrexate/cytarabine.
[b]Consider steroid ophthalmic drops after cytarabine.
[c]Leucovorin given 50 mg p.o. 24 hr after end of methotrexate; then, 15 mg p.o. q6h × eight doses; prophylaxis with twice weekly trimethoprim/sulfamethoxazole recommended. Consider also prophylaxis with antiviral, antifungal, antimicrobial agents.
[d]G-CSF (granulocyte colony-stimulating factor) is given until absolute neutrophil count is >4500.

and B-cell antigens such as CD19, CD20, CD22, and CD45 (8). This entity lacks a unifying genetic abnormality, although the t(14;18) *bcl-2* gene rearrangement is seen in a proportion of cases (154), possibly implying transformation of a previously indolent follicular lymphoma. The most important features of diffuse large B-cell lymphoma are listed in Table 28-14.

CLINICAL FEATURES OF DIFFUSE LARGE B-CELL LYMPHOMA
This illness tends to present with palpable superficial lymphadenopathy, nonspecific symptoms related to deeper lymph nodes (e.g., abdominal pain), or constitutional symptoms (unexplained fevers, weight loss, or profuse night sweats). Patients generally characterize the rate of growth of lymph node masses as having been fairly rapid. Extranodal sites of disease are more common than with follicular lymphomas. Characteristic extranodal sites of disease include bone and bone marrow, stomach, liver, spleen, testes, thyroid, and kidney. The development of the IPI (20) has been helpful in identifying prognostic subgroups in this illness, so that those patients least likely to be curable with standard therapy can be offered new and innovative therapies.

A unique clinicopathologic presentation of this subtype of NHL is seen somewhat more commonly in young females and

is known as *primary mediastinal large B-cell lymphoma*. Patients generally present with signs and symptoms related to massive mediastinal adenopathy (e.g., superior vena cava obstruction, cardiac tamponade) (155). Aberrant expression of β-human chorionic gonadotropin has been reported with this illness (156). The IPI (20) has been demonstrated to have a predictive significance for this illness similar to that of diffuse large B-cell lymphoma (157). Two retrospective series comparing clinical outcomes in primary mediastinal large B-cell lymphoma with diffuse large B-cell lymphoma suggest that this illness behaves in a similar fashion to diffuse large B-cell lymphoma (157,158). Treatment principles for diffuse large B-cell lymphoma should, therefore, guide therapeutic decisions. Because of the large bulk of disease at presentation, most patients have been treated with full-course chemotherapy followed by mediastinal radiotherapy, although no randomized trials comparing chemotherapy to combined modality therapy have been reported.

Anaplastic Large Cell Lymphoma

This subtype of NHL shares many features with diffuse large B-cell lymphoma. Nodal involvement is most common, although

TABLE 28-14. Aggressive Lymphomas

Lymphoma	Other Names	Immunophenotype	Genetic Features
Diffuse large B-cell lymphoma	Diffuse large cell; large cell immunoblastic; diffuse mixed small cleaved and large cell	CD19, CD20, CD22, CD45+	t (14;18) occasionally
Anaplastic large cell lymphoma	Large cell immunoblastic; Ki-1 lymphoma	CD30 (Kiel-1)+; generally, CD45, CD25, CD15, and CD3+; some express neither B nor T antigens	t (2;5)
Peripheral T-cell lymphoma	Diffuse small cleaved; diffuse mixed small cleaved and large cell; diffuse large cell; large cell immunoblastic	Variable CD2, CD3, CD5, CD7+; variable CD4, CD8+	None characteristic

extranodal involvement has also been reported, including in sites such as skin, bone, bone marrow, meninges, pleura, and muscle (159,160). CNS involvement has been reported but appears to be rare (161). The presence of a unique cytogenetic abnormality t(2;5) is characteristic of anaplastic large cell lymphoma.

BIOLOGY, CYTOGENETICS, IMMUNOPHENOTYPE, AND DIFFERENTIAL DIAGNOSIS OF ANAPLASTIC LARGE CELL LYMPHOMA

This subtype of NHL was not a recognized histologic entity in the Working Formulation classification. From a morphologic standpoint, this lymphoma would most likely have been classified as immunoblastic lymphoma and was first described as a separate entity by Flynn and colleagues in 1982 (162). This lymphoma has also been known in the past as *Ki-1 lymphoma*, because it stained with the antibody for Ki-1 (Kiel-1, a Hodgkin's-associated antigen now known as *CD30*). The cells are characteristically large, with pleomorphic nuclei that may be horseshoe shaped (8). Multinucleated cells may be present and appear similar to the Hodgkin-Reed-Sternberg cell. Based on its morphologic appearance and expression of epithelial membrane antigen (163), this lymphoma can be mistakenly diagnosed as an anaplastic carcinoma, illustrating the importance of immunophenotyping in undifferentiated malignancies. Immunophenotypically, the cells usually express CD30 and are variably positive for CD45, CD25, CD15, CD3, and other T-cell antigens (8). The majority of anaplastic large cell lymphomas display T-cell surface antigens, although some express B-cell antigens, and some express neither B- nor T-associated antigens (referred to as the *null cell phenotype*) (8). In 50% to 60% of cases, the T-cell receptor gene rearrangement can be demonstrated. The remainder of cases demonstrate neither T-cell receptor nor Ig gene rearrangements (164,165).

Anaplastic large cell lymphoma is associated with a characteristic translocation, the t(2;5)(166), which results from the fusion of part of the nucleophosmin (NPM) gene on chromosome 5 with the receptor tyrosine kinase gene (ALK) on chromosome 2. The resulting fusion protein is known as the *NPM-ALK protein*. The demonstration of an immunohistochemical reaction to the ALK protein is quite specific for the presence of the t(2;5), because normal lymphoid cells do not express this protein. Experimental models in animals suggest that this translocation could be functionally associated with the development of lymphoma (167).

Because of variability in cellular morphology and expression of ALK, a single gold standard pathologic definition for this disease does not presently exist. The WHO classification has proposed that consideration be given to both morphology and immunophenotype when making this diagnosis, and present recommendations are to use *anaplastic large cell lymphoma* for cases with typical morphology and immunophenotype, classifying them additionally as ALK positive or negative.

The differential diagnoses of anaplastic large cell lymphoma include undifferentiated carcinomas, Hodgkin's disease, and diffuse large B-cell lymphoma. The combination of characteristic large cells, immunophenotype, expression of CD30, and the presence of the characteristic translocation should help resolve the diagnosis in most cases. The most important features of anaplastic large cell lymphoma are listed in Table 28-14.

CLINICAL FEATURES OF ANAPLASTIC LARGE CELL LYMPHOMA

One series has reported this illness to be more common in young males (168). The majority of patients in this study presented with advanced disease and constitutional symptoms. Extranodal disease was seen in approximately 60% of patients.

ALK-negative cases appeared on average to be older and had fewer extranodal sites of disease. ALK-positive patients had a higher complete remission rate (77% vs. 56%) and better overall survival compared to ALK-negative cases (71% vs. 15% at 9 years; *p* = .0007). In the ALK-positive cases, use of the age-adjusted IPI identified a group of patients with an extremely good prognosis (zero to one risk factor; 5-year overall survival, 94%) as compared with cases with greater than or equal to two risk factors (5-year overall survival, 41%). Multivariate analysis identified both ALK positivity and the IPI age-adjusted score as having independent predictive value for survival.

Peripheral T-Cell Lymphoma

In the Working Formulation, this lymphoma would most likely have been classified as a *diffuse small cleaved cell, diffuse mixed small cleaved and large cell,* or *large cell immunoblastic lymphoma.* Being a relatively uncommon subtype, it has yet to be completely classified and understood. In the WHO classification, this entity is known as *peripheral T-cell lymphoma,* which is not otherwise characterized. No subclassification has been proposed, because there does not appear to be clearly defined patterns of immunophenotype or T-cell receptor rearrangements that would assist in further subclassification.

BIOLOGY, CYTOGENETICS, IMMUNOPHENOTYPE, AND DIFFERENTIAL DIAGNOSIS OF PERIPHERAL T-CELL LYMPHOMA

The pathologic feature of this lymphoma is a heterogeneous population of small and large cells. Neoplastic cells are often characterized as having irregular nuclei and, similar to anaplastic large cell lymphoma, may be associated with very large cells resembling Hodgkin-Reed-Sternberg cells (8). Some variability in immunophenotype is seen, but the cells may be positive for CD2, CD3, CD5, and CD7. Expression of either CD4 or CD8 is also variable. This lymphoma does not express B-cell antigens. T-cell receptor gene rearrangement is usually identifiable (8). It is postulated that the normal cellular counterpart to this malignancy would be a T cell in various stages of maturation. Cytogenetic abnormalities appear to be frequent, but no single characteristic abnormality has been described with any particular frequency (169). The most important features of peripheral T-cell lymphomas are listed in Table 28-14.

CLINICAL FEATURES OF PERIPHERAL T-CELL LYMPHOMA

Peripheral T-cell lymphoma is relatively uncommon in the United States, accounting for only 6% of NHL in one series (43). The presence of advanced stage disease at diagnosis is common (43,170), as is the presence of constitutional symptoms, elevated LDH, and sites of bulky disease (43). Extranodal sites of disease are seen frequently, and unusual sites such as prostate have been reported (171). A pooled retrospective analysis was conducted by investigators at the M. D. Anderson Cancer Center from six trials of front-line chemotherapy for aggressive lymphomas. The principal objective of the study was to examine the relative prognostic effect of immunophenotype (172). In comparison with patients with a B-cell immunophenotype, patients with a T-cell phenotype had inferior outcomes independent of both an IPI and an M. D. Anderson Cancer Center prognostic tumor score. A subset of patients with T-cell anaplastic large cell lymphoma demonstrated a trend toward superior overall survival relative to the other subtypes of T-cell lymphoma. A similar study by the Groupe d'Etudes des Lymphomes de l'Adulte demonstrated that unadjusted complete remission rates, 5-year overall survival, and event-free survival were all superior in the subset of patients with a B-cell immunophenotype. Five-year overall sur-

methasone induces G$_1$ growth arrest in myeloma cells, whereas IL-6 facilitates G$_1$ to S phase transition and blocks the effect of dexamethasone. The correlation of changes in p21 expression and cell cycle implicates p21 in the coupling of dexamethasone and IL-6–related signals to cell cycle regulation in myeloma. Finally, murine double minute 2 (MDM2) is constitutively expressed in myeloma cells and may enhance cell cycle progression in tumor cells both by activating E2F-1 and by down-regulating wild-type p53 and p21 (56). Overexpression of MDM2 in myeloma may therefore contribute to the growth and survival of tumor cells, suggesting the potential utility of therapeutic strategies targeting MDM2 in myeloma.

At present, there is also considerable evidence supporting a role for IL-6 in the growth and manifestations of myeloma *in vivo*. Elevated IL-6 serum levels in some studies correlate with poor prognosis and higher tumor cell mass (57,58). In addition, patients with MGUS or indolent or smoldering myeloma have serum IL-6 levels similar to those of healthy individuals, in contrast with those with fulminating myeloma or PCL, who have the highest IL-6 levels. Direct measurement of serum IL-6 levels or of C-reactive protein synthesized in the liver in response to IL-6 may also be a prognostic factor in myeloma (57). IL-6 transgenic mice develop histopathologic changes characteristic of myeloma kidney (59), IL-6 serves as an osteoclast activating factor in myeloma bone disease (60), and anti–IL-6 monoclonal antibody therapy can transiently reverse disease manifestations in patients with myeloma (61). Several studies suggest potential therapeutic utility of inhibiting IL-6 in myeloma. Antihumanized IL-6 receptor and gp 130 antibodies inhibit the growth of IL-6–dependent plasmacytoma cells *in vivo* (62). IL-6 fused to *Pseudomonas* exotoxin or diphtheria toxin effectively and selectively kills myeloma cell lines (63,64). IL-6 receptor superantagonists, which bind IL-6 but do not trigger via gp 130, block IL-6–dependent myeloma cell growth (65–67). Finally, dexamethasone has been shown to inhibit IL-6 and IL-6 receptor gene expression, consistent with another possible mechanism for inhibition of tumor cell growth by corticosteroids (68). Bisphosphonates may also inhibit IL-6 production from myeloma bone marrow stromal cells (66).

Transforming Growth Factor β. Transforming growth factor β (TGF-β) is secreted by myeloma cells and can trigger IL-6 production by BMSCs (55), suggesting that paracine growth via IL-6 may also be induced. TGF-β secreted by myeloma cells likely also contributes to the immunodeficiency characteristic of myeloma by down-regulating B cells, T cells, and natural killer cells without similarly inhibiting the growth of myeloma cells themselves (see Fig. 29-11).

Interleukin-1. Recombinant IL-1α stimulates myeloma cells to produce IL-6, which consequently augments proliferation of myeloma cells (69). IL-1α mRNA is found within myeloma cells, and IL-1 mediates bone-resorbing activity in myeloma (70). These data suggest a possible therapeutic strategy for such antagonists in the treatment of lytic bone disease in myeloma. Serum levels of IL-1 as well as IL-6 were found chronically elevated in patients with polyneuropathy, organomegaly, endocrinopathy, monoclonal protein, and skin changes (POEMS syndrome), consistent with the view that these cytokines may mediate systemic manifestations of this disease (71). Most recently, it has been suggested that IL-1 present in MGUS cells may identify patients likely to progress to myeloma (72).

Other Growth Factors. Peripheral blood mononuclear cells isolated from patients with myeloma cultured with IL-3 and IL-6 for 6 days *in vitro* create a population of proliferating B-cell blasts

that differentiate into idiotypic cytoplasmic Ig+ plasma cells (73). However, the clinical importance of IL-3 in myeloma remains to be defined. Several reports suggest that the bone-resorbing activity produced by cultured human myeloma cells can be mostly blocked by neutralizing antibodies to lymphotoxin (74), indicating that this factor may be involved in bone disease *in vivo*. IL-4 inhibits the growth of myeloma cells *in vitro*, perhaps by blocking endogenous IL-6 synthesis (75), although clinical studies to date are negative. Oncostatin M, leukemia inhibitory factor, and ciliary neurotropic factor induce *in vitro* DNA synthesis by myeloma and plasmacytoma cells using the common gp 130 receptor (76). Granulocyte-macrophage colony-stimulating factor (GM-CSF) has been reported to enhance the IL-6 responsiveness of myeloma cells *in vitro* and has been used to facilitate the development of IL-6–dependent human myeloma lines (77). IL-11, a factor that can support the growth of IL-6–dependent cell lines and promote B-cell differentiation, cannot augment DNA synthesis by purified myeloma cells (78,79). IL-10 is a proliferation factor but not a differentiation factor for human myeloma cells (80). Insulin-like growth factor–1 has been shown to augment myeloma cell growth and survival, and octreotide can inhibit insulin-like growth factor–1 signaling and related tumor cell growth (81). Macrophage inflammatory protein-1α is a potential osteoclast stimulatory factor in MM (82). Autocrine growth mediated by IL-15 has been demonstrated in both myeloma cell lines and patient cells (83). Myeloma cells secrete vascular endothelial growth factor (VEGF), which augments IL-6 secretion in stroma, and IL-6 in turn augments VEGF secretion from tumor cells (84). The presence of Flt-1 on some myeloma cells also suggests autocrine VEGF-mediated myeloma cell growth (85). Long-term engraftment of both myeloma cell lines and freshly isolated cells from myeloma bone marrow has been reported in severe combined immunodeficient (SCID) mice and in SCID mice bearing fetal bone grafts (SCID-hu mice), providing additional models for studying the role of growth factors in the growth of myeloma *in vivo* (86–89).

Kaposi's Sarcoma–Associated Herpes Virus. IL-6 is also a growth factor in other neoplastic diseases, including Kaposi's sarcoma, pleural effusion lymphoma, and multicentric Castleman's disease. Interestingly, Kaposi's sarcoma–associated herpes virus (KSHV) has been detected in cases of these diseases related and unrelated to human immunodeficiency virus (90). A causative role for KSHV is suggested by serologic data that reveal that seroconversion to antibodies against KSHV latent nuclear antigens precedes the development of Kaposi's sarcoma (91). The KSHV genome contains a homolog to human IL-6, viral IL-6 (vIL-6), which retains biologic activity, as demonstrated by its ability to support the growth of the B9 IL-6–dependent murine plasmacytoma cell line (92) as well as a human myeloma cell line (93). It remains controversial whether KSHV genes and antibodies are present in patient bone marrow and peripheral blood samples (94–96). However, KSHV gene sequences have been amplified in myeloma bone marrow stromal cells expressing dendritic lineage antigens (97–101). Further, antibodies to KSHV lytic and latent antigens have recently been detected in 81% and 52% of patients, respectively (102). Ongoing research is now determining the role, if any, of KSHV gene products in the pathogenesis of myeloma. If positive, these studies could provide the basis for novel antiviral therapies as treatment strategies for myeloma.

ROLE OF ADHESION MOLECULES IN MYELOMA

Adhesion molecules mediate both homotypic adhesion of tumor cells and heterotypic adhesion of tumor cells to either extracellular matrix (ECM) proteins or BMSCs (103) (Fig. 29-10).

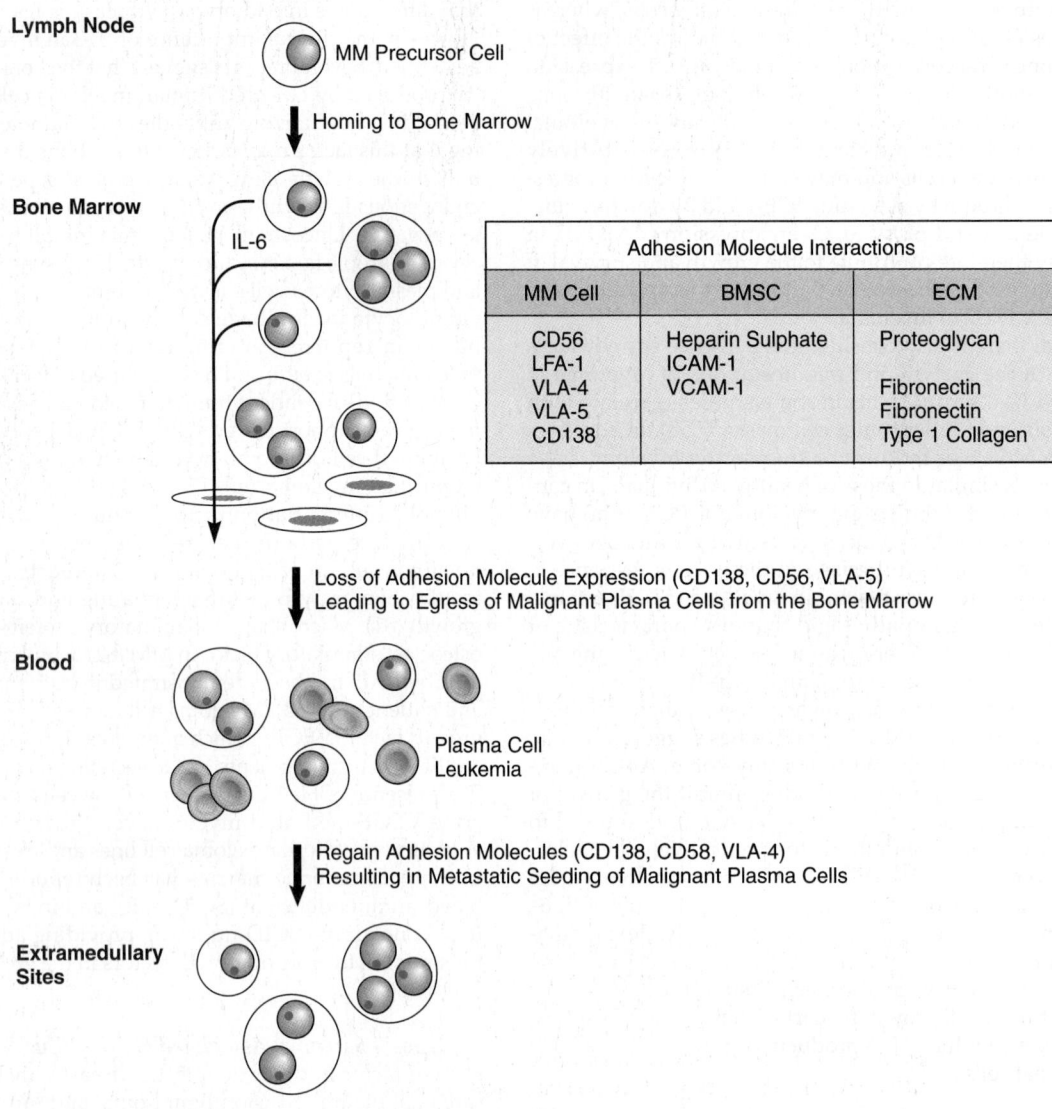

Lymph Node — MM Precursor Cell

Homing to Bone Marrow

Bone Marrow

IL-6

Adhesion Molecule Interactions		
MM Cell	BMSC	ECM
CD56	Heparin Sulphate	Proteoglycan
LFA-1	ICAM-1	
VLA-4	VCAM-1	Fibronectin
VLA-5		Fibronectin
CD138		Type 1 Collagen

Loss of Adhesion Molecule Expression (CD138, CD56, VLA-5)
Leading to Egress of Malignant Plasma Cells from the Bone Marrow

Blood

Plasma Cell
Leukemia

Regain Adhesion Molecules (CD138, CD58, VLA-4)
Resulting in Metastatic Seeding of Malignant Plasma Cells

Extramedullary Sites

Figure 29-10. Role of adhesion molecules in disease pathogenesis. BMSC, bone marrow stromal cell; ECM, extracellular matrix; ICAM, intracellular adhesion molecule; IL, interleukin, LFA, lymphocyte function–associated antigen; MM, multiple myeloma; VCAM, vascular cell adhesion molecule; VLA, very late antigen.

Moreover, they play a critical role in pathogenesis of disease progression. After class switching in the LN, adhesion molecules including CD44, VLA-4, VLA-5, LFA-1, CD56, syndecan-1, and MPC-1 mediate homing of myeloma cells to the bone marrow as well as adhesion to BMSCs and ECM (104–107). Such binding not only localizes tumor cells in the bone marrow microenvironment but also stimulates IL-6 transcription and secretion from BMSCs with related paracrine growth of myeloma cells (41–43). Moreover, triggering via CD40 found on tumor cells induces IL-6 transcription and secretion, with related autocrine myeloma cell growth (40). Syndecan-1 is a multifunctional regulator of tumor cell growth and survival as well as bone cell differentiation. Furthermore, elevated serum syndecan-1 correlates with increased tumor cell mass and decreased metalloproteinase-9 activity (108,109). Studies have shown that adhesion can also induce matrix metalloproteinase-1, which in turn favors bone resorption and tumor invasion (110). In contrast, syndecan-1 is shed from the surface of most myeloma cells and can both induce apoptosis and inhibit the growth of myeloma cells. It also mediates decreased osteoclast and increased osteoblast differentiation, suggesting a complex series of different effects in the process of tumor growth and spread (109). Reflective of these dynamics, disease progression and the development of PCL are characterized by decreased expression of certain adhesion molecules (e.g., CD56, VLA-5, MPC-1, and syndecan-1), which in turn facilitates tumor cell mobilization. Further, the acquisition of other adhesion molecules on PCL cells such as CD11b, CD44, and RHAMM assists transit through endothelium during egress from the bone marrow. Extramedullary spread of MM cells is facilitated by the reappearance of CD56, VLA-5, MPC-1, and syndecan-1.

Because adhesion molecules play a central role in the pathogenesis of myeloma, therapeutic strategies targeting these molecules have been developed and tested in animal models; for example, anti–intracellular adhesion molecule-1 antibodies have been shown to inhibit tumor development in SCID mice (111). Moreover, a model of myeloma in SCID-hu mice (88,89) provides for the first time an *in vivo* model for the evaluation of homing of human MM cells to human BMSCs and ECM proteins. The biologic sequelae of binding as well as the evaluation of novel treatments based on interruption of this process can now be studied. For example, myeloma cells resistant to melphalan and doxorubicin typically overexpress VLA-4, suggesting VLA-4 as a possible target for such strategies in drug-resistant disease (112).

ROLE OF ANGIOGENESIS IN MULTIPLE MYELOMA

Angiogenesis promotes proliferation and metastasis of solid tumors and is of prognostic significance. Angiogenesis has also been found to be important in the context of bone marrow cancers with ready contact with the bloodstream, including leukemia and MM. One study in MM demonstrated that bone marrow neovascularization, plasma cell angiogenic potential, and matrix metalloproteinase-2 secretion parallel progression of human myeloma (113). Other studies have shown that microvessel density is increased in patients with active myeloma compared with patients with asymptomatic myeloma and MGUS. Culture supernatants from patients with active myeloma have demonstrated more angiogenic activity, assessed using the chick embryo chorioallantoic membrane assay; by human umbilical vein endothelial cell proliferation, migration, or monocyte chemotaxis; and by secretion of basic fibroblast growth factor, as compared with patients with inactive myeloma or MGUS. Finally, bone marrow plasma cells from patients with active myeloma express more matrix metalloproteinase-2 mRNA and protein than those with inactive myeloma or MGUS (114). These data suggest that progression of plasma cell tumors is accompanied by an increase in bone marrow neovascularization. In a report of 36 patients treated at the University of Arkansas undergoing tandem stem cell transplantation, low microvessel density was a favorable prognostic feature (115). However, another study examined angiogenesis both before and after high-dose therapy and stem cell transplantation in 13 patients with myeloma, including seven complete and six partial responders (116). Although microvessel density was significantly increased in myeloma compared with normal bone marrow, it remained high even after transplant and did not correlate with clinical response. Given these conflicting observations, further studies are needed to define the importance of angiogenesis in this disease. The fact that KSHV carries three genes (vMIP-1α, KSHV-GPCR, and vIL-6) with potential for angiogenesis and that two of them (vIL-6 and KSHV-GCPR) can up-regulate VEGF expression suggests that angiogenesis and VEGF are important for KSHV biology (117,118). How KSHV contributes to malignant transformation in myeloma remains unproven.

Although the mechanism of action against MM cells is presently unknown, it has a number of properties, including antiangiogenesis, that may mediate anti-MM activity (119,120). The University of Arkansas Cancer Center has evaluated thalidomide as a sole therapeutic agent for advanced and refractory myeloma (121) and extended this experience to approximately 160 patients. Before receiving thalidomide, 85% subjects in this open-label experience underwent at least one cycle of graft-supported high-dose therapy, and 66% had disease relapse or progression after two transplants. The majority of these patients had a number of poor prognostic factors, including IgA subclass of immunoglobulin expression and adverse cytogenetic changes. An analysis of the first 123 patients who had a MM protein concentration greater than 0.3 mg/dL and whose paraprotein concentration increased by more than 10% in the month before thalidomide therapy revealed that 32% of patients responded by Southwest Oncology Group (SWOG) criteria. In most cases in which it was analyzed, the number of bone marrow MM cells declined as the paraprotein concentration decreased. These results suggest that thalidomide

may have a role in treating active MM after high-dose therapy and stem cell transplantation. However, an obvious effect on microvessel density in responding patients was not seen, supporting the notion that, in addition to direct action on tumor-related vascularity, other microenvironmental and stromal effects from thalidomide occur.

MOLECULAR PATHOGENESIS OF MYELOMA

The malignant plasma cells in myeloma are localized to the bone marrow in close association with stromal cells. They are long-lived cells with a very low labeling index (LI, 1%–2%). The rearranged Ig genes are extensively somatically hypermutated in a manner compatible with antigen selection (27) with no evidence that the process of hypermutation is ongoing. However, myeloma cells have a significantly lower rate of Ig secretion than normal plasma cells. Thus it appears that the critical oncogenic events in myeloma cells either occur after most of the normal differentiation process involved in generating a long-lived plasma cell, or do not interfere with it.

By conventional analyses, karyotypic abnormalities are detected in myeloma at a frequency of 30% to 50% in a number of large studies (122–124). The frequency and extent of karyotypic abnormalities correlate with the stage, prognosis, and response to therapy. For example, approximately 20% are abnormal in stage I disease, 60% in stage III patients, and more than 80% in extramedullary tumor. This analysis is dependent on obtaining reliable metaphase preparations and likely underrepresents the extent of DNA alterations in these infrequently dividing cell populations. By interphase fluorescent in situ hybridization analysis, two studies report that at least one chromosome is trisomic in 96% or 89% of myeloma tumor samples, respectively (125,126). Although conventional karyotypes are not routinely reported for MGUS, it appears that a substantial fraction of MGUS plasma cells are aneuploid as well. By fluorescent in situ hybridization analysis, the incidence of trisomy for at least one chromosome was 43% and 53% in two studies of MGUS cells; in the former, 61% of the cells had an aneuploid DNA content by image analysis (125,127). The characteristic numeric abnormalities are monosomy 13 and trisomies of chromosomes 3, 5, 7, 9, 11, 15, and 19. Nonrandom structural abnormalities most frequently involve chromosome 1 with no apparent locus specificity; 14q32(IgH) locus occurs in 20% to 40%; 11q13(Bcl-1 locus) occurs in approximately 20%, mostly translocated to 14q32; 13q14 interstitial deletion occurs in 15%; and 8q24 interstitial deletion occurs in approximately 10%, with approximately half of these involved in a translocation.

The hallmark genetic lesion in many B-lymphocyte tumors involves dysregulation of an oncogene as a consequence of a translocation involving the IgH locus (14q32.3). Less frequently, variant translocations involve one of the IgL loci (2p12, κ, or 22q11, λ). From conventional karyotypic analyses, translocations involving 14q32 appear to occur in approximately 20% to 40% of myeloma with an abnormal karyotype (3). The incidence of these translocations is significantly higher in the extramedullary phase of the disease and in cell lines, perhaps due to a higher number of metaphase spreads that are examined. In approximately 30% of these translocations, the partner chromosomal locus is 11q13 (Bcl-1, cyclin D1), but in most cases the partner is not identified (14q32+). Other recurrent partner loci have been identified infrequently, including 8q24(c-myc) in less than 5%, 18q21(Bcl-2), 11q23(MLL-1), and 6p21.1 (Table 29-5). By combining conventional karyotypic analysis with a comprehensive Southern blot assay that detects translocations involving IgH switch regions, it has become apparent that most myeloma cell lines and one primary tumor fully examined have IgH translocations that mainly involve IgH switch regions (29,128). In six reported cases, translo-

TABLE 29-5. Nonimmunoglobulin Sites for Illegitimate Switch Recombination in Multiple Myeloma

Chromosome	Incidence, % of Patients	Gene	Function
11q13	30	Cyclin D1, others	Induces growth
4q16	25	FGFR3, MMSET	Growth factor
8q24	5	c-myc	Growth/apoptosis
16q23	1	c-maf	Transcription factor
6p25	Rare	IRF4	Transcription factor

FGFR, fibroblast growth factor receptor.
Data from Bergsagel PL, Chesi M, Nardini E, et al. Promiscuous translocations into immunoglobulin heavy chains with regions in multiple myeloma. *Proc Natl Acad Sci U S A* 1996;93:13931–13936; Rajkumar SV, Fonseca R, Witzig TE, et al. Bone marrow angiogenesis in patients achieving complete response after stem cell transplantation for multiple myeloma. *Leukemia* 1999;13:469–472; and Chesi M, Nardini E, Brents LA, et al. Frequent translocation t(4;14)(p16.3;q32.3) in multiple myeloma: association with increased expression and activating mutations of fibroblast growth factor receptor 3. *Nat Genet* 1997;16:260–264.

cation involving 11q13 and overexpression of cyclin D1 occurred. Five additional lines and one primary tumor have been determined to have an IgH switch translocation breakpoint involving the telomeric end of chromosome 4 (i.e., 4p16.3) despite the fact that no karyotypic translocation was detected in five of six of these samples (129). The apparent oncogene dysregulated by the 4;14 translocation is the fibroblast growth factor receptor 3 (FGFR3) gene. It is possible that dysregulated expression of FGFR3, as a result of t(4;14), receives an FGFR3-mediated signal from FGF produced by stromal cells in the bone marrow microenvironment. The t(4;14) translocation in myeloma regulates both FGFR3 and a novel gene, MMSET, resulting in IgH/MMSET hybrid transcripts (130). Finally, there is evidence that elevated expression of c-myc and selective expression of one c-myc allele may occur frequently in myeloma, even though structural genetic changes near c-myc have been identified in only 10% to 20% of tumors (3).

Ras mutations occur in approximately 39% of newly diagnosed myeloma patients, and the frequency of ras mutations increases with disease progression. Mutations of N-ras and K-ras are rarely detected in solitary plasmacytoma and MGUS but occur more frequently in myeloma (9% to 30%) and in the majority of terminal disease or PCL patients (63% to 70%) (131,132). Activating mutations of the ras oncogenes may also result in growth factor independence and suppression of apoptosis in myeloma.

Although translocation (14;18) occurs at a low frequency (0% to 15%) in myeloma, an overexpression of Bcl-2 is seen in the majority of myeloma patients and in myeloma cell lines (133,134). High levels of Bcl-2 protein are likely to mediate the resistance of myeloma cells to apoptosis induced by dexamethasone, IL-6 deprivation, staurosporine, or other drugs (135). In a murine myeloma cell line, Bcl-XL showed a predominant role in preventing apoptosis in response to cycloheximide treatment or IL-6 withdrawal (136). Similarly, overexpression of Bcl-2 or Bcl-XL could prevent apoptosis induced by IL-6 withdrawal in the B-9 IL-6–dependent cell line (137). p53 mutations are infrequent in MM, and a late event in the disease: p53 mutations occur in 5% of inactive MM and in 20% to 40% of acute PCL (138). Thus, p53 mutations may cause a block of plasmablastic apoptosis and differentiation at the final stages of plasma cell maturation.

To date, mutations of the Rb gene or abnormalities in pRb have been described in up to 70% of myeloma patients and 80% of myeloma-derived cell lines (139). Myeloma cells may show a very strong expression of pRb, mostly in its phosphorylated form (52). Furthermore IL-6 induces phosphorylation of pRb, which in turn releases the suppression of IL-6 transcription mediated by dephosphorylated pRb and augments IL-6 mediated myeloma cell growth. In contrast to its effects on normal B cells, TGF-β does not suppress pRb phosphorylation and proliferation of myeloma cells

and in fact stimulates IL-6 secretion from stromal cells (140). The p16^{INK4A} (p16) protein, an inhibitor of cyclin dependent kinases 4 and 6, is expressed in myeloma. Its expression correlates with IL-6 responsiveness of more mature (VLA-5+ MPC-1+) tumor cells, whereas cyclin D1 is more frequent in immature myeloma tumors (VLA-5– MPC-1–) (141). p16 gene hypermethylation occurs more frequently in advanced disease (PCL) and in myeloma cell lines (53,142,143). Germline p16 mutation has recently been implicated in predisposing to MM (144). IL-6 down-regulates and interferon (IFN)-γ up-regulates p21 expression, and this effect correlates with $G_1 \rightarrow S$ transition induced by IL-6 in myeloma cells (55). p21 overexpression in myeloma may induce resistance to apoptosis and slow clinical progression of disease. The overexpression of the MDM2 protein has been reported to enhance cell cycle progression in myeloma (56).

Prognostic Factors

STAGING SYSTEMS

Multiple attempts have been made to define clinical and laboratory parameters that have prognostic significance (145–148). Of the many staging systems, the Durie-Salmon system is most commonly used (146) (Table 29-6). Tumor cell mass for patients in

TABLE 29-6. Durie-Salmon Myeloma Staging System

Stage I, all of the following:
  Hemoglobin value >10 g/dL
  Serum calcium value normal (<12 mg/dL)
  On roentgenogram, normal bone structure (scale) or solitary bone plasmacytoma only
  Low monoclonal component production rates
    IgG value <5 g/dL
    IgA value <3 g/dL
  Urine light chain monoclonal component on electrophoresis <4 g/24 h
Stage II, overall data minimally abnormal as shown for stage I and no single value abnormal as defined for stage III
Stage III, one or more of the following:
  Hemoglobin value <8.5 g/L
  Serum calcium value >12 mg/dL
  Advanced lytic bone lesions (scale 3)
  High monoclonal component production rates
    IgG value >7 g/dL
    IgA value >5 g/dL
  Urine light chain monoclonal component on electrophoresis >12 g/24 h
Subclassification
  a: Relatively normal renal function (serum creatinine value ≤2.0 mg/dL)
  b: Abnormal renal function (serum creatinine ≥2.0 mg/dL)

Ig, immunoglobulin.

stage I is low at less than 0.6×10^{12} cells/m², intermediate for patients with stage II disease at 0.6 to 1.2×10^{12} cells/m², and high for patients with stage III disease with more than 1.2×10^{12} cells/m². In this system, survival duration is 61.2, 54.5, 30.1, and 14.7 months for patients with stage IA, stage IB + IIA + IIB, stage IIIA, and stage IIIB disease, respectively. Gassmann et al. (147) compared the relative value of seven staging systems in 152 patients with myeloma. In their analysis, Cancer and Leukemia Group B and the Southeastern Cancer Study Group divided patients into good-risk and poor-risk groups, with significant (albeit small) differences in survival. In the systems of Durie and Salmon (146), Alexanian et al. (149), Merlini et al. (150), and Carbone (151), some differences in survival were significant and others were not. The British Medical Research Council staging system was best, with median survival times significantly different in stage A (83 months), stage B (52 months), and stage C (26 months) (152). Stages in this system were defined as follows: those patients with blood urea nitrogen less than 8 mmol/L, hemoglobin (Hgb) greater than 10.0 g/L, and minimal symptoms as stage A; those with Hgb less than 7.5 g/L and restricted activity or blood urea nitrogen over 10 mmol/L and restricted activity as stage C; and those patients not in either stage A or stage C as stage B. Interestingly, none of the staging systems was clearly superior to certain single risk factors, especially the presence of anemia (Hgb above or below 8.5 g/L) and renal impairment (creatinine less or more than 177 μmol/L) (147). Bataille et al. (145) examined 147 patients with myeloma using Durie-Salmon, Medical Research Council, and Merlini-Waldenström staging criteria as well as serum β2-microglobulin (β2M) and rate of bone resorption. They found serum β2M to be the most powerful indicator of prognosis, with serum albumin the only variable adding to this prognosis significantly. These two variables were better than any staging systems. Finally, Cavo et al. (153) modified the Durie-Salmon system to include thrombocytopenia, and they demonstrated that platelets above or below 150,000/mm³ can specifically define intermediate risk groups of Durie-Salmon stage II and III patients.

SINGLE RISK FACTORS

Many additional single parameters have been examined for their value as prognostic features.

Morphology. Griepp et al. (154) classified 100 cases of myeloma into mature (28%), intermediate (38%), immature (19%), or plasmablastic (15%) morphology (Fig. 29-5). The median survival of plasmablastic group in this series was 16 months, compared with 35 months for other types. Plasmablastic subtypes had more frequent renal insufficiency and higher plasma cell indices. A study of 453 patients confirmed higher labeling indices, higher serum IL-6 receptor levels, more ras mutations, more aggressive disease, and shortened survival in patients with plasmablast morphology (155).

Serum β2-Microglobulin. Serum β2M represents the light chain of the major histocompatibility complex of the cell membrane. Increased serum β2M results from release by tumors with high growth fraction and cell turnover rates. It is a small protein and is largely excreted in urine; therefore, renal failure can elevate serum β2M. In patients with myeloma and normal renal function, rising serum β2M predicts progression. In patients with myeloma, serum also correlates with clinical stage, as defined by Durie and Salmon, and with response to therapy. For example, Brenning et al. (156) related the pretreatment serum β2M levels to creatinine, clinical stage, and survival in 121 patients with myeloma. Patients in stage III had higher serum β2M levels than patients in stage II or stages I and II. The measure can be used alone or in combination with other variables for

pretreatment stratification (157). For example, of 612 patients who were similarly treated with combination chemotherapy, 322 patients with serum β2M less than 6 mg/L had a significantly longer median survival of 36 months compared with those 225 patients with serum β2M 6 mg/L or less, whose survival was only 23 months ($p < .0001$). Various investigators have chosen different distinct cut-off values for serum β2M, but nonetheless serum β2M retains prognostic importance in most studies.

Labeling Index. The LI, a measure of DNA synthesis by myeloma cells, predicts survival. It is usually low (<1%) at diagnosis, higher at relapse, and lower in MGUS and indolent myeloma. High plasma cell LI correlates with shorter survival time independent of tumor cell mass (148).

Tumor Cell Karyotype. Gould et al. (123) found that hypodiploidy in patients with Bence Jones proteinuria was associated with resistance to therapy. Investigators at the Mayo Clinic found cytogenetic abnormalities in 18% of patients with newly diagnosed myeloma, 63% of patients with aggressive disease, and 40% of those with PCL (122). Survival among newly diagnosed patients was shorter for those with abnormalities than for those without abnormalities. Among all patients, survival from the time of chromosomal analysis was shorter for those in whom a chromosomally abnormal clone was found. In proliferating plasma cells, anomalous 1,11,14 chromosomes and t(11;14)(q13:132) abnormalities were most common. Nonrandom chromosomal rearrangements of 14q13.3 and 19p13.3 and preferential deletion of 1p has been reported in patients with myeloma and PCL (158). The presence of either partial or complete deletions of chromosome 13q14, deletions of 17p13, or abnormalities involving 11q have an adverse influence (159,160). By contrast, trisomies of chromosomes 7, 11, and 15 as well as DNA hyperdiploidy are associated with a favorable outcome (161). Importantly, the presence of any translocation likewise predicts poor outcome after high-dose therapy and autotransplantation (162,163). Monosomy 13 has been associated with the transition from MGUS to overt myeloma (164). Novel nonrandom translocations can be identified using multicolor spectral karyotyping (165) and double-color fluorescent in situ hybridization (166).

Cell Surface Phenotype. Cell surface phenotype has been reported to correlate with disease course. Common acute lymphoblastic leukemia Ag (CD10⁺)-positive myeloma has been reported to have prognostic significance (167). Lactic dehydrogenase, although nonspecific, correlates with tumor mass, as in lymphomas (168). Patients whose myelomas produce only λ light chains have a poorer prognosis than those associated with IgG, IgA, or κ light chains only. Moreover, among those with IgG myeloma, both response rates and median survival are greater in patients with IgG-κ than in those with IgG-λ myeloma. Percentages of peripheral blood CD38 and PCA-1 Ag-bearing lymphocytes were reportedly significantly higher at diagnosis of myeloma compared with MGUS. A further increase has been observed during relapse, suggesting a correlation between plasma cell Ag expression and disease activity (169).

Serum Cytokine/Receptor Levels. Serum IL-2 levels were significantly higher in myeloma patients than in normal controls, and higher serum IL-2 levels were associated with a prolonged actuarial survival (170). Serum IL-6 levels in some studies appear to correlate with both advanced stage of disease and decreased survival (57,58). IL-6 stimulates hepatocytes to produce acute phase proteins, such as C-reactive protein (CRP). CRP may therefore reflect the IL-6 level and proliferative status of bone marrow plasma cells. Indeed, CRP levels are significantly lower in patients with MGUS than in those with myeloma, and survival can be correlated with serum CRP level (171). High levels of serum soluble IL-6 receptor (172), hepatocyte growth factor, (173), and syndecan-1 (174) as well as low serum hyaluronate levels (175) are independent prognostic factors predicting poor outcome.

Peripheral Blood Plasma Cells. The percentage of circulating plasma cells in peripheral blood and their labeling indices are independent prognostic factors for survival in myeloma after both conventional and high-dose therapy (176,177). Of note, plasma cells from primary plasma cell leukemia display singular phenotypic, DNA cell content, and cytogenetic characteristics that lead to a disease evolution different from myeloma (178).

Combinations of Factors. Many of these factors are interrelated and therefore of limited independent value. Using multivariate analysis, several groups have found that the best combination of variables to predict outcome was serum β2M, reflecting both the tumor burden and renal function; and the proliferative activity of plasma cells, evaluated by the LI or number of tumor cells in S phase. Age and performance status also improve the prognostic assessment (179,180). High levels of soluble IL-6 receptor or CRP may also be complementary variables. Nevertheless, it is possible that some of the factors that reflect the intrinsic characteristics of the malignant clone may become even more relevant. For example, the presence of K-ras mutations is associated with a shorter survival (181). More recently, the presence of circulating plasma cells in the peripheral blood stem harvest of patients about to undergo transplant has been associated with poor outcome (176). Conversely, low numbers of circulating CD19+ cells predict poor outcome (182). The identification of more accurate prognostic factors is necessary to select patients for whom more aggressive therapy is indicated, and to provide accurate assessment of the outcome of treatment approaches (183). For example, the presence of any translocation predicts poor outcome after high-dose therapy and autotransplantation (162). Lung resistance–related protein expression predicts for worse outcome after conventional, but not high-dose, therapy (184), demonstrating that certain prognostic factors may vary for specific therapeutic strategies. Future research is needed, particularly as treatment approaches expand.

Complications

Complications of myeloma include bone disease and hypercalcemia, hyperviscosity, recurrent infections, renal failure, and cardiac dysfunction.

BONE DISEASE AND HYPERCALCEMIA
As described in the section Clinical Features, 80% of patients with myeloma present with bone pain. Bone lesions can be isolated, discrete lytic abnormalities or diffuse osteopenia (Fig. 29-4). Bone scans and serum alkaline phosphatase are usually not abnormal. Evaluation with roentgenographs is standard; magnetic resonance imaging is more sensitive and demonstrates bone healing with bisphosphonate therapy. Active osteoclastic bone resorption is usually evident when more than 20% myeloma cells are present, and lytic bone lesions occur when greater than 10^{12} cells are present. Bone resorption leads to increased calcium in extracellular fluid. Although patients with normal renal function can increase urine calcium excretion, those with renal failure develop hypercalcemia. Therefore hypercalcemia is more likely to occur in the setting of Bence

Jones proteinuria, myeloma kidney, chronic infection, or uric acid nephropathy. Overall, hypercalcemia occurs in 20% to 40% of patients with myeloma (185). Osteosclerosis occurs in less than 1% patients and is typically seen in the rare subgroups of patients who have POEMS syndrome (186). It is noteworthy that the differentiation of the POEMS syndrome from osteosclerotic myeloma with peripheral neuropathy appears to have no clinical value, although it is also important to note that a recent series from the Mayo Clinic reports a significantly better prognosis for POEMS patients (with a median overall survival of 77 months) than for patients with myeloma (187).

Pathogenesis. Myeloma cell lines, myeloma cells, and explants of bone containing myeloma cells produce osteoclast activating factor (distinct from parathyroid hormone, prostaglandin E2, vitamin D, and metabolites), which is similar biologically and chemically to bone resorbing activity in normal activated leukocyte culture supernatants (185). Lymphotoxin, tumor necrosis factor (TNF)-α, and IL-1 can also stimulate osteoclastic bone resorption *in vitro*, but their clinical significance remains controversial (70,74). IL-6 can induce TNF-α and IL-1 production in marrow cells and causes bone resorption and hypercalcemia *in vivo*. Macrophage inflammatory protein-1α has been shown to increase osteoclast stimulatory activity in patients with myeloma (82). Osteoprotegerin ligand is an osteoclast differentiation and activation factor, suggesting that osteoprotegerin, which neutralizes osteoprotegerin ligand, may also have a therapeutic application (188). The precise role of these factors in mediating bone resorption and hypercalcemia remains to be determined.

An *in vivo* model of myeloma bone disease has been developed in which SCID mice injected with ARH-77 tumor cells develop radiologically detectable lytic bone lesions. Their marrow plasma contains a bone-resorbing activity that stimulates osteoclastic bone resorption in bone organ cultures and in human and murine marrow cultures (189). It appears that a novel cytokine mediates osteoclast activation in this model. Hjorth-Hansen et al. (190) have used a different human myeloma cell line in this model with similar results. They have identified hepatocyte growth factor as a potential mediator of bone disease.

Treatment. Before the advent of effective bisphosphonate therapy, bone healing in myeloma occurred uncommonly and was delayed in treated patients despite responses to chemotherapy. In this context, a major effort over the last 30 years has been made to either prevent or inhibit further bone resorption in patients with myeloma. A double-blind study of sodium fluoride treatment in patients with myeloma offered neither subjective nor objective benefit in this regard (191). Chloromethylene diphosphonate, an inhibitor of osteoclast activity, decreased urinary excretion of calcium and skeletal pain but to date has not been widely studied or used (192). A double-blind randomized trial of clodronate versus placebo in 350 patients revealed that the proportion of patients with progression of osteolytic lesions was twice as high in the placebo group than in the clodronate-treated group (193). Another randomized trial demonstrated that oral clodronate slowed progressive skeletal disease and associated morbidity but achieved no benefit in survival. The more bioactive intravenous bisphosphonate, pamidronate, has been shown in a prospective randomized trial to reduce skeletal-related events, including pathologic fractures, radiation therapy to bone, and spinal cord compression in patients with Durie-Salmon stage III myeloma and at least one lytic bone lesion (194). This benefit was maintained until 21 months after initiation of therapy (195), and it is now recommended that myeloma patients remain on intravenous bisphosphonates indefinitely to reduce skeletal events and pain regardless of their response to chemotherapy (196). Interestingly, patients in this study who showed no response to first-line chemotherapy also had improved survival, and bisphosphonates are now being evaluated for their antimyeloma activity (197). Recent evidence supports the view that bisphosphonates may down-regulate IL-6 production from bone marrow stromal cells (66) as well as induce apoptosis of both osteoclasts and tumor cells (198). More potent bisphosphonates such as zoledronate are undergoing clinical evaluation, and initial results have been encouraging (199–201).

The treatment of hypercalcemia consists of the treatment of myeloma as well as inhibition of osteoclastic bone resorption with corticosteroids, calcitonin, mithramycin, or bisphosphonates. Corticosteroids may impair formation of new osteoclasts, and mithramycin is toxic to osteoclasts, but it is also nephrotoxic. Calcitonin and corticosteroids are almost always effective for the short term and useful even in the setting of renal failure. Bisphosphonates bind to the bone surface and inhibit osteoclast activity and constitute a mainstay of treatment. Present therapeutic recommendations therefore include initial cytotoxic therapy for myeloma, cautious forced saline diuresis, and bisphosphonate therapy, with the use of calcitonin, prednisone, or mithramycin only for nonresponders to these first-line treatments. A prominent problem exacerbating hypercalcemia is that patients become immobile because of bone pain or other reasons. Therefore an important approach is to keep the patient physically active whenever possible.

HYPERVISCOSITY

Hyperviscosity is characterized clinically by spontaneous bleeding with neurologic and ocular disorders. Hyperviscosity occurred in 4.2% of 238 patients with IgG myeloma and in 22% of 46 patients with serum IgG monoclonal components greater than 5.0 g/dL (202). The IgG3 subclass produces hyperviscosity at lower levels than other IgG paraproteins (203). The severity of the syndrome is not directly related to the serum viscosity. Clinical findings improve with vigorous plasmapheresis, which reduces both myeloma protein concentration and serum viscosity.

RECURRENT INFECTIONS

Patients with myeloma had 15 times more infections than a control group of patients with arteriosclerotic heart disease (204). *Streptococcus pneumoniae* and *Haemophilus* infections usually occur early and typically during response to chemotherapy. Gram-negative infections occur in the settings of refractory, advancing disease; previous antibiotic therapy; instrumentation; immobilization; colonization with hospital flora; myelosuppression secondary to disease; and azotemia. Fatal infections are often acquired during hospitalization, emphasizing the need to minimize indwelling foreign bodies such as catheters in patients with myeloma. Conversely, there is lack of correlation between bacteremia (either gram-negative or gram-positive) and chemotherapy-induced febrile neutropenia. Fungal, herpes, mycobacterial, and *Pneumocystis* infections are only rarely described in myeloma patients. Nonetheless, infection remains the most common cause of death, occurring in between 20% and 50% of patients with active and end-stage disease (21).

The evidence of increased clinical infections in myeloma has led to attempts at prophylaxis. Although myeloma patients have normal rises in antibody titers after pneumococcal vaccination, preimmunization titers are markedly diminished (205). Postimmunization titers are therefore low and considered nonprotective, limiting any benefit for such an approach. Nonetheless, due to its low cost and possible benefit to some patients, the use of pneumococcal vaccination has been recommended.

In a double-blind randomized trial of γ-globulin prophylaxis in patients with myeloma, no benefit of γ-globulin prophylaxis for reducing infection was noted (206). At present γ-globulin is reserved only for those patients with recurrent or life-threatening infections.

The role of prophylactic antibiotics remains controversial (207) and has been evaluated in a recent prospective randomized clinical trial evaluating whether trimethoprim-sulfamethoxazole (TMP/SMX) administered for the first 2 months of chemotherapy can decrease infections during the 3 months from start of chemotherapy (208). Infections occurred in 46% of control patients and 18% of TMP/SMX-treated patients ($p = .04$) and were less severe in the latter group. However, TMP/SMX was discontinued due to nausea or rash in 25% of patients. A larger multiinstitutional randomized study is needed to define better the role of prophylactic antibiotics in patients with myeloma.

RENAL FAILURE

Renal failure in myeloma can predict adverse outcome. One series found that 22% of patients had a serum creatinine greater than 2 mg/dL at diagnosis; renal function normalized with treatment in 50% of those with creatinine greater than 2 but less than 3.9 mg/dL. However, in patients with worse renal dysfunction requiring dialysis, the outcome was poor (209). The causes of renal failure in myeloma are often multifactorial. They include hypercalcemia; myeloma kidney, with distal and proximal tubules obstructed by large laminated casts containing albumin, IgG, and κ and λ light chains surrounded by giant cells; hyperuricemia; toxicity from intravenous urography; dehydration; plasma cell infiltration; pyelonephritis; and amyloidosis. The most important predisposing factor is dehydration; therefore, aggressive hydration is crucial to avoid irreversible renal dysfunction. Otherwise, treatment involves management of the underlying disease and avoidance of inappropriate intravenous urography. Combination chemotherapy incorporating dexamethasone is recommended to achieve a more rapid response than observed with melphalan and prednisone (MP) alone. The type and quantity of proteinuria can distinguish between myeloma kidney, with larger amounts of light chains and less albuminuria; light chain deposition disease, characterized by low levels of both light chains and albumin in urine; and amyloidosis, in which large amounts of albuminuria and less light-chain proteinuria occur (210).

The renal manifestations associated with the production of monoclonal light chains in myeloma, light-chain deposition disease, and amyloidosis result from the deposition of certain Bence Jones proteins as tubular casts, basement-membrane precipitates, or fibrils (211–213). For unknown reasons, the severity of the renal manifestations varies greatly from patient to patient. Bence Jones proteins from 40 patients were injected into mice, and 26 (65%) of 40 were deposited in mouse kidneys as tubular casts, basement-membrane precipitates, or crystals in a pattern similar to those noted in patients (213). This experimental model has potential value for the identification and differentiation of nephrotoxic or amyloidogenic light chains. Further, the development of progressive kidney damage and myeloma kidney has been demonstrated in IL-6–transgenic mice, shedding additional light on the role of IL-6 in the pathogenesis of myeloma (59).

CARDIAC DYSFUNCTION

The mean and median age of patients with myeloma is approximately 60 years, and affected patients are also frequently at risk for cardiovascular disease. However, patients can be uniquely susceptible to cardiac ischemia or congestive heart failure

(CHF) due to myocardial infiltration, with amyloid causing dilated or restricted cardiomyopathy and dysrhythmias, hyperviscosity syndrome, or anemia. Myeloma patients are also susceptible to high-output CHF of unclear etiology (214).

ANEMIA

Anemia in myeloma can be due to a number of factors, including tumor infiltration of the bone marrow, renal impairment, the myelosuppressive effects of chemotherapy, and the decreased production of erythropoietin (EPO) relative to the degree of anemia. Pilot studies demonstrated efficacy of exogenous EPO administration in myeloma (215–217). Osterborg et al. (218) have compared in a randomized study EPO therapy at 10,000 U/day, a titrated dose of EPO starting with 2000 U/day and escalating stepwise until response, and no EPO for 24 weeks. Response was defined as an increase in Hgb greater than 2 g/dL and elimination of transfusion need. Sixty percent of EPO-treated groups responded, including 72% of those with low EPO levels and only 20% of those with normal EPO levels. Ten thousand units subcutaneously three times weekly was reported as an optimal starting dose, although more recently 40,000 units subcutaneously once weekly has become a more widely used approach.

NEUROPATHIES

A variety of malignant and paraproteinemic disorders can be associated with neuropathies (219). In myeloma, a symmetric, distal sensory, or sensorimotor neuropathy is most common, associated with axonal degeneration with or without amyloid deposition. Unfortunately there is no specific therapy other than the treatment of underlying disease. In some cases this treatment is associated with monoclonal antibodies directed against peripheral nerve myelin (220).

ASSOCIATED DISEASES

Myeloma has been described in association with both hematologic disorders and solid tumors. Acute leukemia either is induced by leukemogens such as radiation and alkylating agents or is part of the natural history of myeloma. The mean interval from diagnosis of myeloma to occurrence of acute leukemia is 60 months (range, 17 to 147 months), consistent with either possibility. The occurrence of acute leukemia in untreated myeloma patients suggests that it may be part of the natural history of the disease (221). Furthermore, acute leukemia has been reported in 6 (4.8%) of 125 myeloma patients treated with alkylating agents, significantly higher than the incidence of acute leukemia in ovarian cancer patients treated with irradiation and alkylators (20). Actuarial risk of leukemia in myeloma patients treated with MP or with melphalan, cyclophosphamide, carmustine, and prednisone has been reported as high as 17.4% at 50 months from initiation of therapy (222). Gonzalez et al. (221) described 11 of 476 patients with myeloma who developed myeloid leukemia or sideroblastic anemia. All had received MP for a median of 3 years, and all had major cytogenetic abnormalities. This study suggests that leukemia is predominantly treatment-related. Finally, in 628 patients with myeloma, the incidence and diversity of solid tumors were similar to those observed in otherwise healthy persons of the same age (223).

Treatment. Patients undergoing therapy for myeloma should have clinical and laboratory assessment to ensure safety and efficacy of treatment. Before each course of treatment, a complete blood count including differential and platelets should be performed. Serum chemistries should be measured at least every 3 months, more often if clinically indicated. Concomitantly, monoclonal protein in the serum or urine should be measured by immunoelectrophoresis or preferably, more sensitive immunofixation techniques. A skeletal survey should be performed annually, with bone marrow examination reserved for diagnosis and subsequent change in clinical status, treatment, monoclonal Ig, or hemogram. It is important to remember that reduction of serum or urine monoclonal component as objective evidence of tumor response could reflect increased protein catabolism, decreased protein production, or both. Moreover, nonmonoclonal protein–secreting myeloma clones may emerge during treatment, so even a marked reduction in monoclonal Ig may not correlate with decrease in tumor burden.

Two major definitions of response in myeloma have been widely used: that of the Chronic Leukemia-Myeloma Task Force (224) and that of SWOG (225). The former requires a greater than 50% decrease in monoclonal serum or urine protein, a greater than 50% decrease in cross-sectional areas of plasmacytoma, and some recalcification of bone lesions (without new lesions), whereas the latter requires a 75% or greater reduction in production of myeloma protein to achieve remission. However, the frequencies of response by either definition are similar in previously untreated patients receiving MP. For example, 32% to 53% response rates were noted by SWOG criteria and 33% to 56% by Task Force criteria in the same treatment study. Need for and response to treatment may be a more important determinant of survival than initial tumor stage. For example, a low labeling index may define patients who do not need therapy irrespective of stage. Such patients may have a long course before need for therapy, a gradual response to treatment, and prolonged survival.

Conventional Therapy

INITIAL TREATMENT

Oral administration of MP is a standard form of therapy that produces objective response in as many as 50% to 60% of patients (1,226). Because of the variability of absorption, the dosage of melphalan should be modified if necessary so that some reduction in leukocytes and platelets occurs 3 to 4 weeks after the beginning of each cycle. MP should be given for at least 1 year, until the monoclonal Ig levels in the serum, urine, or both have been stable for at least 6 months (plateau state), then discontinued if the patient has no other evidence of active disease. Typical doses are melphalan 0.15 mg/kg daily for 7 days (8–10 mg/day) and 20 mg prednisone three times daily for the same period. Melphalan must be given before meals because food reduces absorption. Unless the disease progresses rapidly despite adequate therapy, at least three courses of MP should be administered before the drugs are discontinued. It is important to remember that the natural course of MM is one of progression. If the patient's pain is alleviated and there is no evidence of progressive disease, the therapeutic regimen should be considered beneficial despite failure to reach a rapid objective response. In addition, some patients with a low plasma cell proliferative index do not obtain an objective response until the second year. Chemotherapy should thus not be routinely discontinued during the first year unless there is definite evidence of progression of disease or intolerance. Indeed, in a Canadian study of 457 patients treated with MP, the median survival of those patients who responded, had stable disease, or progressed was 48, 49, and 15 months, respectively (227). The prognosis is therefore poor in patients who progress despite MP, and second-line chemotherapy is indicated. However, patients who remain stable should not be switched to other therapy, as they appear to do as well as responders.

The obvious shortcomings of MP have stimulated investigators to use many combinations of chemotherapeutic agents. A major controversy in treatment of myeloma is whether MP is as effective as combination chemotherapy (CCT) (228). Although some studies have demonstrated that CCT was superior to MP (157,225), 10 prospective randomized trials of MP versus a drug combination failed to show clearly that other drug combinations were better than MP (229). Furthermore, improved response rates may not translate into prolonged survival (230). An earlier SWOG study suggested that combinations of vincristine, melphalan, Cytoxan, and prednisone (VMCP) alternating with vincristine, carmustine, adriamycin, and prednisone (VBAP) with or without levamisole were superior to vincristine, Cytoxan, and prednisone with or without levamisole. However, the results of this trial demonstrated only a 54% response rate and a 48-month survival in those receiving VMCP and VBAP without levamisole (231). Similarly, although initial CCT with vincristine, doxorubicin, and dexamethasone (VAD) produced a high response rate (84%) with 28% of all patients having complete response (CR), duration of response was only 18 months (232). Initial therapy with high-dose dexamethasone achieved response rates approximately 15% less than those with VAD and similar to those with MP (233). However, serious complications occurred less than with VAD, and survival was similar. It is also clear that the inclusion of high doses of corticosteroids increases the frequency of response to chemotherapy and may prolong survival in myeloma (234). One of the best-known combinations is the M2 protocol, which includes vincristine, carmustine, melphalan, cyclophosphamide, and prednisone (VBMCP). In an Eastern Cooperative Oncology Group study, 220 evaluable patients were randomized to VBMCP and 221 to MP. The objective response was 72% for VBMCP and 51% for MP, but the median survival was not different at 30 versus 28 months, respectively (235). Elderly bedridden patients had worse survival with VBMCP, but the remaining 85% of patients had a significantly improved survival with the combination of alkylating agents, with the 5-year survival for patients treated with VBMCP at 26% compared with 19% for MP.

In an attempt to determine which patients, if any, do better with more aggressive therapy, Gregory et al. (236) examined published reports of 18 randomized controlled trials comparing MP with CCT in the primary treatment of 3814 patients. The overall results suggested that there was no difference in efficacy between these treatment modalities. Those studies with a high MP 2-year survival rate showed a survival difference in favor of MP, whereas those with a low rate suggested a difference in favor of CCT. The implication of these results is that, rather than there being no difference between MP and CCT, MP is superior for patients with an intrinsically good prognosis and inferior for those patients with a poor prognosis. A second overview of 6633 patients from 27 randomized trials of CCT versus MP confirmed higher response rates to CCT but equivalent mortality and survival (237).

REFRACTORY DISEASE

Almost all patients with MM who initially respond to chemotherapy eventually relapse, and the conventional management of refractory myeloma has been comprehensively reviewed (238). Patients who progress with initial therapy have a 40% response to high-dose or pulsed corticosteroid therapy (239). Patients who relapse during therapy or within 6 months of stopping initial treatment have a 75% response rate to VAD chemotherapy (239–241). Patients who relapse more than 6 months after stopping therapy have a 60% to 70% response rate when initial therapy is reinstituted (226). If no response is achieved, VAD or alternate regimens can be used. Tumor cell associated multidrug resistance cytoplasmic p-glycoprotein (PGP) in aneuploid myeloma cells correlates with resistance to VAD. Verapamil, tamoxifen, cyclosporine, and PSC 833 have been

TABLE 29-7. Potential Mechanisms of Drug Resistance in Myeloma

Gene	Drugs Involved
Mdr1	Anthracyclines, vinca alkaloids, etoposide
MRP	Anthracyclines, vinblastine, etoposide
LRP	Cyclophosphamide, melphalan, anthracyclines
CMOT	Cyclophosphamide
Gdr	Glucocorticoids

evaluated as chemosensitizers for reversing multidrug resistance in such myeloma cells both *in vitro* and in clinical trials (242–244). However, there are multiple mechanisms of drug resistance in myeloma (Table 29-7). Studies have demonstrated that patients who received no previous therapy or cumulative doses of 20 mg vincristine, 340 mg doxorubicin, or both vincristine and doxorubicin had 6%, 50%, 83%, and 100% PGP expression, respectively. This finding suggests that PGP induction is related primarily to therapy (245). Moreover, PGP is functional in refractory myeloma: clinical modulation of multidrug resistance by cyclosporine is mediated through an inhibition of PGP-associated drug efflux, and PGP-expressing plasma cells can be eliminated by combined treatment with VAD and cyclosporine (244). Unfortunately, even in those patients who respond to salvage therapy, the duration of response is limited. For example, a treatment for refractory myeloma consisting of etoposide, cisplatin, cytarabine, and dexamethasone led to a 40% response in patients resistant to MP, VAD, and high-dose melphalan. However, median survival after etoposide, cisplatin, cytarabine, and dexamethasone was only 4.5 months (246). This result may be due to alternative potential mechanisms of drug resistance in myeloma (244). Topotecan has been shown to have activity in resistant and refractory myeloma, achieving partial response (PR) or better in 16% of patients studied (247). Also of interest is the recent observation that cells that are resistant to chemotherapy may be resistant to Fas-mediated apoptosis, suggesting common downstream effectors (51).

A major advance in the treatment of resistant myeloma has been the emergence of thalidomide as an effective therapy (121). Despite its potent teratogenicity, the drug is not mutagenic or carcinogenic. Thalidomide inhibits TNF-α, an angiogenic factor present in the tumor microenvironment. Myeloma bone marrow has abundant neovascularity that can be identified by CD34+ staining, supporting the potential benefit angiogenesis inhibition, as discussed in the section Role of Angiogenesis in Multiple Myeloma. In addition, thalidomide stimulates IL-12 secretion, which in turn induces IFN-γ. IFN-γ has myriad effects, including the induction of IP-10, which decreases neovascularity by inhibiting VEGF synthesis. IFN-γ is also a T-cell stimulant and may stimulate cancer immunity. Thalidomide changes expression of intracellular adhesion molecule and other adhesion molecules, and in the absence of appropriate adhesion molecule binding, myeloma cells undergo apoptosis. Thalidomide modifies extracellular matrix expression and directly inhibits both basic fibroblast growth factor (bFGF) and VEGF expression. Thalidomide inhibits the induction of cyclooxygenase-2, the expression of which is essential for the inhibition of apoptosis in new vessel formation. Preclinical studies of thalidomide and its derivatives have demonstrated significant activity against drug-resistant myeloma cell lines (248). The clinical experience from Arkansas also strongly supports the value of thalidomide in refractory disease with a remarkable response rate of 32% by SWOG criteria and an acceptable toxicity profile in largely posttransplant patients (121).

α-2b Interferon Therapy. The potential mechanisms of action of α-2b IFN (IFN-α) are both direct and indirect. They include direct cytotoxicity on myeloma cells, synergism with chemotherapy, a change in the pharmacokinetics of melphalan, inhibition of IL-6, down-regulation of IL-6 receptor on myeloma cells, down-regulation of activated oncogenes, increase in natural killer cells, increase in tumor cell surface antigens, and expansion of specific cytotoxic T cells (249).

Clinical Studies. Several prospective randomized trials have examined the utility of combined IFN-α and chemotherapy for induction therapy. The largest was from the Nordic Myeloma Study Group which used MP alone or with IFN-α (250). IFN-α prolonged the duration of the plateau phase by 5 to 6 months without a statistically significant increase in median survival. Other trials also found improved response rates and remission duration but no significant prolongation of survival with the addition of IFN-α (251–253). A metaanalysis of 16 randomized trials involving 2286 patients receiving combined IFN-α and chemotherapy for induction treatment yielded higher response rates (CR or PR) in the IFN-α arms, but the average gain was only approximately 10% (251). Similarly, significant but only marginal gains were detected in the IFN-α arms in remission duration (median, 7 months) and survival (median, 5 months).

Mandelli et al. (254) were the first to examine the use of IFN-α maintenance therapy in a randomized trial in patients who had achieved CR, PR, or stable disease after either MP or VMCP/VBAP (254). They treated 202 patients with symptomatic myeloma with 12 monthly courses of either MP or VMCP alternating with VBAP followed by maintenance IFN-α. The median duration of response was 26 months in the patients administered IFN-α and 14 months in the untreated patients (*p* = .0002). Moreover, the median duration of survival (from randomization) was 52 months in the IFN-α group and 39 months in the control group (*p* =.0526). However, subsequent studies did not confirm these positive results. Although remission duration was always longer in the IFN-α arm than in patients without maintenance treatment (255–257), the observed differences reached statistical significance in only a few studies (251,256,257) and were minimal in others (234,258). Substantial increases in survival times were also observed in some trials (251,256,257) but not in others. Metaanalysis of eight trials of 929 patients receiving maintenance IFN-α revealed that both remission duration and survival were significantly longer in the IFN-α arm than in the control arm, but median gains were only 6 and 5 months, respectively (251). It should be noted that patients may develop flulike symptoms and anorexia as well as myelosuppression related to IFN-α therapy, but only a fraction of patients, primarily the elderly, have required either reduction of the dose or discontinuation of IFN-α. A recent survey of patients in the United States found a 6-month risk-benefit trade-off preferred by the majority of interviewed myeloma patients with regard to IFN-α treatment (259). Quality-adjusted time without symptoms or toxicity analysis showed that patients treated with maintenance IFN-α gained an average of 9.8 months without disease relapse (*p* = .001) and 5.8 months of overall survival (*p* = .074) versus the control groups. However, the IFN-α group experienced an average of 4.1 months of moderate or worse toxicity (*p* <.001) (260). At present IFN-α treatment appears to benefit patients who have achieved low tumor burden. However, additional prognostic factors of IFN-α effectiveness are needed to define subgroups of myeloma patients who may benefit from IFN-α treatment, given its potential toxicity.

Radiation Therapy. Radiation therapy for myeloma is used for treatment of localized disease, including plasmacytoma and spinal cord compression syndrome, and is frequently used for palliation. Hemibody radiation therapy has been used either as a consolidation after induction combination chemotherapy or as salvage therapy for chemotherapy-resistant myeloma (261,262). As discussed in the following section, total body irradiation can be used as a component of ablative therapy before hematopoietic stem cell grafting.

High-Dose Therapies. The rationale for the administration of alkylating agents (melphalan, cyclophosphamide, busulfan) in a higher than conventional dose with or without total body irradiation (TBI) followed by transplantation of syngeneic, allogeneic, and autologous bone marrow or peripheral blood progenitor cells (PBPCs) is based on a number of observations: (a) plasma cell dyscrasias remain uniformly fatal, (b) multiple studies document sensitivity of myeloma cells to chemotherapy and radiotherapy, and (c) CRs can be obtained with high-dose therapy, resulting in a possible overall survival benefit.

Allogeneic Stem Cell Transplantation. An encouraging lead for newer treatment approaches in myeloma arose from reports of complete responses after the administration of alkylating agents in higher than conventional doses with or without TBI followed by syngeneic or allogeneic bone marrow transplantation (BMT) (263,264). Reduction in tumor mass in some cases was dramatic, with CR rates commonly in the 40% range and a similar number of PRs. Syngeneic BMT has been performed infrequently, but patients reported from Seattle remain progression-free at long intervals after BMT (265). The European Bone Marrow Transplant Group has reported on allografting in 162 patients with myeloma. Actuarial overall survival (OS) was 32% at 4 years and 28% at 7 years for the 72 (44%) patients who achieved CR after BMT. However, overall progression-free survival was 34% at 6 years, and only 9 patients remain in continuing CR at over 4 years postallograft (266,267). Favorable pre-BMT prognostic factors for both response to and survival after BMT were female sex, IgA myeloma, low serum β2M, stage I disease at diagnosis, one line of previous treatment, and CR before BMT.

Of major concern is the 40% transplant-related mortality (50% in men) in the European Bone Marrow Transplant Group report (268). In an allograft experience reported from Seattle, actuarial probabilities of OS and event-free survival (EFS) for the 36% patients achieving CR were 0.50 ± 0.21 and 43 ± 0.17, respectively, at 4.5 years. Adverse prognostic factors included transplantation greater than 1 year from diagnosis, serum β2M more than 2.5 mg/dL at transplant, female patients transplanted from male donors, more than eight cycles of chemotherapy, and Durie-Salmon stage III disease at presentation. Again toxicity was common, with 35 (44%) patients dying of transplant-related causes within 100 days of BMT (269). Busulfan/cyclophosphamide ablation followed by allogeneic transplantation achieved 4-year disease-free survival of 26% in a report of 19 patients with myeloma, but transplant-related mortality was also 37% (270). Finally, there were 15 deaths among 36 patients within the first 100 days postallograft in an ongoing multigroup randomized trial of high-dose versus conventional therapy for myeloma in the United States. As a result of this excessive toxicity, the allografting arm of this study has been closed and individual academic centers encouraged to develop strategies to achieve and maintain high remission rates while avoiding transplant-related morbidity and mortality.

In an attempt to improve the outcome of allografting in myeloma by avoiding transplant-related toxicity, our center has carried out T (CD6)-depleted allografting using histocompatible sibling donors in 61 patients with myeloma whose disease remained sensitive to conventional chemotherapy (271–274). The patients were 39 men and 22 women with a median age of 44 years. Of the patients, 9, 17, 20, and 11 presented with stages IA, IIA, IIIA, and IIIB disease, respectively, and three presented with plasmacytomas at diagnosis. Median time to white blood cell and platelet engraftment was 12 and 18 days. There were 17 (28%) CRs, 34 (57%) PRs, two (3%) patients with no response and only three (5%) transplant-related deaths. Forty-seven percent of patients did not develop graft-versus-host disease (GVHD), and 36% had grade I GVHD, with only 17% of patients developing a grade II or greater GVHD. Overall survival from time of BMT was a median of 2 years, with approximately 40% of patients surviving beyond 3 years. However, disease-free survival (DFS) after allogeneic BMT was 1 year, with only 20% of patients disease-free beyond 4 years posttransplant. In our series, the OS and DFS do not significantly differ from our outcome after autografting in myeloma (Fig. 29-5).

Graft versus Myeloma Effect. Molecular remissions have been reported to be more common after allografting than after autografting, suggesting the ability of an allogeneic graft-versus-myeloma (GVM) effect to mediate sustained remission (275–278). Data from multiple centers have shown that patients with relapsed hematologic malignancies after allogeneic BMT can achieve marked clinical responses after infusions of lymphocytes collected from the marrow donor (known as *donor lymphocyte infusions*, DLI) (279–281). In the setting of relapsed chronic myelogenous leukemia (CML) after allografting, this therapy is most effective in patients with cytogenetic relapse or those in stable phase (279–281). However, GVHD occurs in 40% to 60% of patients treated with DLI, contributing to a 13% to 18% treatment-related mortality (281). Although many investigators have suggested that DLI induces a graft-versus-leukemia (GVL) effect by the induction of GVHD, some patients can obtain a CR in the absence of clinical GVHD, suggesting that the GVL response may be independent of clinical GVHD. Both T-cell number and CD8+ T cells have been implicated in GVHD, and Champlin et al. (282) have used CD8+ T-cell depletion of donor BM or DLI to avoid GVHD (282). DLI has been used to treat three patients with relapsed myeloma after allografting, providing the first direct evidence of a GVM effect (283,284). In these cases, however, GVHD was observed after DLI. Infusion of thymidine kinase gene-transduced DLI, followed by treatment of the recipient with ganciclovir, has been proposed as a potential strategy to treat DLI-associated GVHD (285).

More recently, we have demonstrated that the GVL effect of DLI can be preserved and GVHD can be abrogated by using CD8-depleted (CD4+) DLI (286). CD4+ DLI was used to treat 15 patients with early relapsed CML, six patients with advanced CML, seven patients with myeloma, and seven patients with other hematologic malignancies that recurred after sibling-histocompatible CD6-depleted allogeneic BMT. Overall, only 8 (25%) of 32 patients evaluable for toxicity developed acute or chronic GVHD. Treatment-related mortality was low (3%), with one death related to infection in the setting of immunosuppression for GVHD. Complete cytogenetic remissions were noted in 11 of 14 patients with early-phase relapsed CML, including 10 molecular remissions. Five of seven patients with myeloma have responded, including three CRs. Overall, 6 of 11 patients with CML developed CRs in the absence of clinical GVHD. Given the high response rates but inevitable relapses observed in the setting of allografting for myeloma (266,267,269,273), CD4+ DLI is now being used at 6 months post–CD6-depleted BM allografting to enhance GVM effect and thereby improve outcome.

Preliminary laboratory data demonstrate that patients who receive DLI have a markedly abnormal T-cell repertoire, detected by molecular analysis of T-cell receptor Vβ gene rearrangements in peripheral T cells (287,288). After infusion of CD4+ DLI, analysis of T-cell receptor use has identified the expansion of clonal and oligoclonal T-cell populations that coincide with the elimination of myeloma cells from marrow and decreases in levels of circulating monoclonal paraprotein. *In vitro* data also suggest that myeloma cells are effective as antigen-presenting cells, as assessed by proliferation of allogeneic cells to irradiated myeloma target cells. Moreover, this response can be augmented by cross-linking CD28 on the cell surface of allogeneic T cells, providing a second signal. Of greatest interest is the observation that triggering myeloma cells *in vitro* via their cell surface CD40 up-regulates expression of adhesion and accessory molecules on the surface of tumor cells, which results in further enhancement of the allogeneic antimyeloma response. This observation suggests the possibility of triggering donor T cells *ex vivo* using CD40 ligand-activated myeloma cells. Finally, attempts are under way to immunize the allogeneic marrow donor to the patient's idiotypic myeloma protein and thereby transfer specific immunity against myeloma at the time of allografting (289). Initial experience demonstrates the transfer of immunity to idiotypic protein, evidenced by the derivation from the patient postallografting of a donor CD4+ T-cell line that proliferates *in vitro* to the immunizing idiotypic protein. Ongoing studies are defining optimal immunization strategies and may vary in distinct clinical settings. For example, Wimperis et al. (290,291) have shown that preimmunization of both bone marrow donors and bone marrow recipients was required to obtain antigen specific responses in recipients at 3 months posttransplantation of T-cell–depleted allogeneic sibling marrows (290,291).

Autologous Stem Cell Transplantation. High-dose chemoradiotherapy followed by transplantation of either autologous bone marrow or PBPCs has also achieved high (40%) CR rates, but the median duration of these responses has typically been 24 to 36 months (263,292). Patients who have sensitive disease and who are less heavily pretreated have the most favorable outcomes. Most importantly, a national French trial of 200 patients with myeloma who received two courses of VMCP alternating with VBAP were then randomized to receive either conventional chemotherapy (eight additional courses of VMCP and VBAP) or high-dose therapy (melphalan and TBI) followed by autologous BMT. They demonstrated significantly higher response rates, EFS, and OS for those patients treated with high-dose therapy compared with those receiving conventional therapy (293) (Fig. 29-11). Response rates in the high-dose and conventional arms were 81% and 57%, respectively. The 5-year probability of EFS and OS was 28% and 52%, in recipients of high-dose therapy and only 10% and 12% in patients treated with conventional therapy. Treatment-related mortality was low and comparable between the two groups. It should be noted that the median survival of patients younger than 65 years who respond to initial chemotherapy is approximately 5 years (294). This finding emphasizes the importance of randomized trials to assess the relative efficacy of high-dose versus conventionally treated groups of similar myeloma patients. A second randomized trial in myeloma examined the relative merits of high-dose therapy early versus late as salvage therapy for relapse after conventional therapy (295). The overall survival was 64 months in both groups, but the quality-adjusted time without symptoms and toxicity analysis strongly favored the early transplant cohort (Table 29-8). A Scandinavian population-based study demonstrated prolonged survival for patients with myeloma younger than 60 years treated with intensive therapy compared with historical controls who received con-

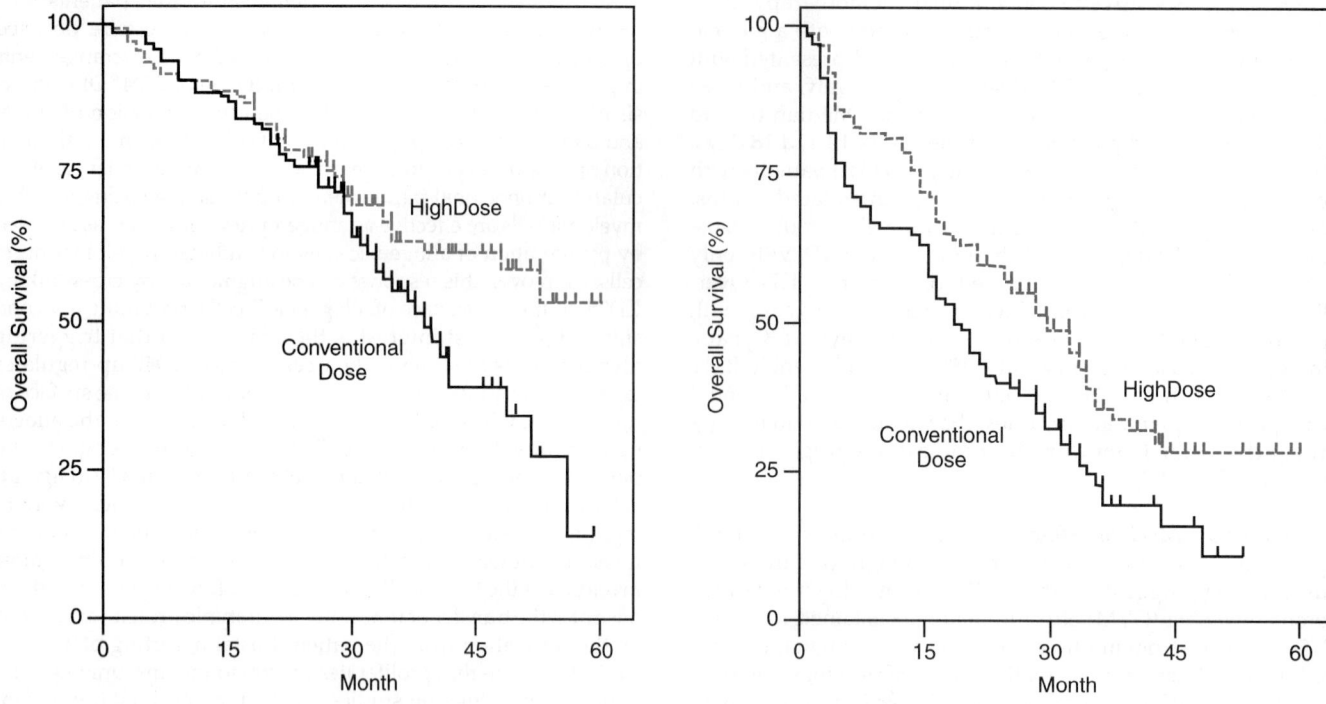

Figure 29-11. French randomized trial of conventional versus high-dose therapy.

ventional therapy (296). Although these studies are encouraging and additional randomized trials in the United States, Scandinavia, Spain, and England are comparing the outcome of conventional therapy versus high-dose therapy and autografting, it is unlikely that patients are cured after a single high-dose and stem cell autografting regimen.

Improving Outcome of Autografting. Attempts to improve the outcome of high-dose therapy followed by autografting include the use of autologous bone marrow or PBPCs either depleted of tumor cells (273,297,298) or processed to select normal hematopoietic progenitor cells by virtue of CD34 expression (299) or multiparameter cell sorting (300). Specifically, we have carried out autografting including monoclonal antibody-purged BM or peripheral blood stem cells (PBSCs) or CD34+ PBSCs in 105 patients with myeloma whose disease remained sensitive to conventional chemotherapy (273,297,298) (Fig. 29-11). These patients were 68 men and 37 women with a median age of 52 years. Of the patients, 18%, 15%, 50%, and 14% presented with stage IA, IIA, IIIA, and IIIB disease, respectively. Median time to white blood cell engraftment was 22 and 11 days in recipients of bone marrow and PBSCs, respectively. Platelet engraftment was at 29 and 13 days in bone marrow and PBSC recipients, respectively. There was a 30% CR rate and a 62% PR rate. Three patients (3%) did not respond, and there was one (1%) toxic death. Median OS from time of BMT was 4.2 years, with 40% patients surviving over 5 years. However, median DFS from BMT was only 2.2 years, with less than 20% of patients remaining disease-free beyond 4 years posttransplant. Therefore, new strategies are needed to treat minimal residual disease (MRD) after autografting, because most patients inevitably relapse.

PBPCs are commonly mobilized for collection using filgrastim after chemotherapy, and one study suggests that stem cell factor and filgrastim enhance yield and reduce the number of phereses required (301). CD34 selection of autologous PBPCs

used to positively select normal hematopoietic progenitors while depleting myeloma cells can achieve up to 5 log depletion of tumor cells (299). However, this finding remains controversial because CD34+ cells in the blood of myeloma patients have been reported to express CD19 and IgH mRNA and have patient-specific IgH VDJ gene rearrangements (302). Moreover, after a median follow-up of 28 months, progression-free survival of 51 patients who underwent high-dose therapy and transplantation of CD34+ PBPCs is only 34% ± 15%, suggesting that the majority of patients are destined to relapse, as in other autografting studies (303). A multicenter trial of 193 patients who received either unpurged or CD34+ selected PBPC autografts after ablative chemotherapy with cyclophosphamide and busulfan therapy assessed hematologic engraftment as well as myeloma burden in the bone marrow and peripheral blood before, at the time of, and after transplantation. Prompt engraftment was noted in both CD34+ and unselected arms. Moreover, in recipients of CD34+ autografts, a median 0.68 and 1.1 log reduction in bone marrow contamination with myeloma was achieved at 100 and 180 days after grafting, respectively. Peripheral blood myeloma burden at 100 and 180 days posttransplant was reduced by a median of greater than 1.8 and 1.9 logs, respectively (304). In

TABLE 29-8. Stem Cell Transplantation as Up-Front versus Rescue Treatment

Measure	PBSCT Early	PBSCT Late
Estimated median overall survival	64.6 mo	64.0 mo
Median event-free survival	39.0 mo	13.0 mo
Quality-adjusted time without symptoms or toxicity	27.8 mo	22.3 mo

PBSCT, peripheral blood stem cell transplantation.

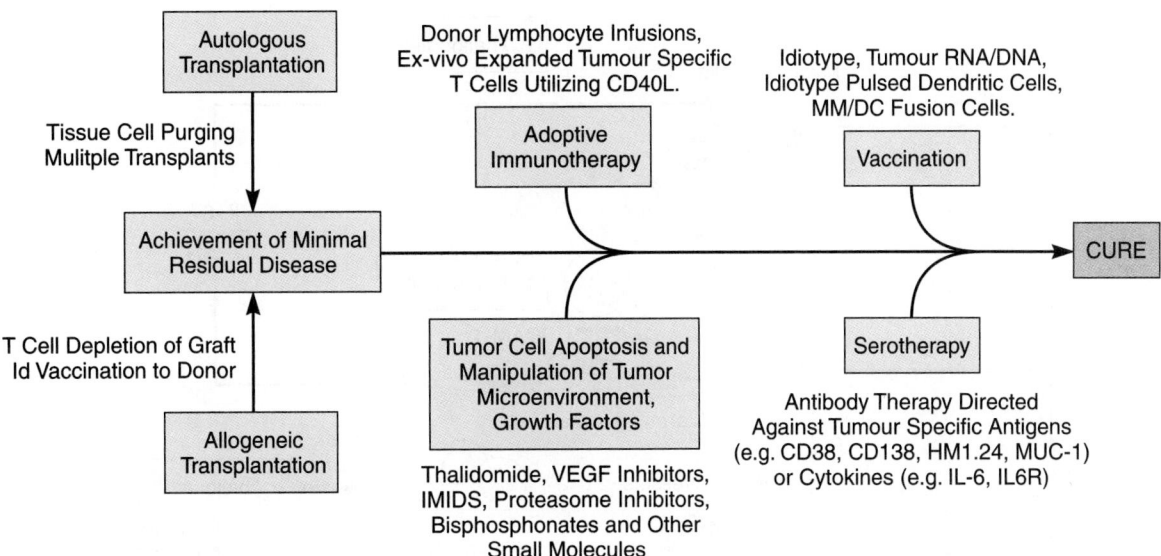

Figure 29-12. Novel treatment approaches to myeloma: from the bench to the bedside. DC, dendritic cell; IL, interleukin; IMIDS, immunomodulatory drugs; MM, multiple myeloma; VEGF, vascular endothelial growth factor.

subsequent analysis of the same study, a median of 3.1 log reduction in myeloma cells within the autografts was achieved (305). Importantly, there was no impact on survival at 2 years (306). A second trial showed that CD34+ selection also had no impact of CD34+ selected autografts on the outcome of either single or tandem high-dose chemotherapy (307). Because residual tumor cells are detectable in the graft as well as in the patient after transplant (303), it would appear that few patients using this approach are likely to be cured.

Several additional strategies are currently under evaluation to improve the outcome of autografting (Fig. 29-12). Barlogie et al. (163,308,309) are performing multiple high-dose therapies and stem cell transplantation. Response rates are higher relative to historically matched controls, but the impact on long-term DFS requires further follow-up. A French randomized trial is comparing single versus double high-dose therapy and stem cell transplantation. Qing et al. (310) have reported on the use of cyclosporine to induce GVHD postautografting in an attempt to generate associated autologous GVM effect. Finally, it may be possible to stimulate autologous immunity to myeloma to treat MRD postautografting and thereby improve outcome. Multiple reports suggest that patients may mount an antimyeloma immune response (311). In one study, five myeloma patients were repeatedly immunized with autologous monoclonal Ig. In three patients, an antiidiotypic specific T-cell response characterized by IFN-γ and IL4 secretion was amplified 1.9-fold to fivefold. B cells secreting antiidiotype Ab also increased during immunization. However, the induced T-cell response was eliminated during repeated immunization (312). In two patients this was associated with a gradual decrease in CD19+ monoclonal B cells. Hsu et al. (313) have investigated the possibility of autologous dendritic cells pulsed *ex vivo* with tumor-specific idiotypic protein to stimulate host antitumor immunity: nine patients developed T-cell–mediated antiidiotype and anti-KLH proliferative responses that were specific for the immunizing Ig. In one case T cells were expanded *in vivo*, a result that specifically lysed autologous tumor. Interestingly, antiidiotypic Abs were not detected, consistent with the view that the idiotype pulsed dendritic cell

induced a T helper 1 rather than a T helper 2 response. Further studies are needed to optimize the immunization schedule to achieve long-lasting T-cell immunity against idiotypic determinants on the myeloma cell and to determine its effect on clinical outcome.

FUTURE DIRECTIONS

Multiple myeloma remains incurable with current therapies, but several new therapeutic options have been derived from recent advances in the understanding of its biology (Fig 29-12). First, multiple lines of evidence suggest that the precursor cell in MM is a cytoplasmic μ-positive B cell that has undergone antigen selection and somatic hypermutation in the lymph node but that has not yet undergone isotype class switching. Chromosomal translocations involving the Ig switch region are common, and multiple partner chromosomes have been described. Given that abnormalities in Ig gene rearrangement, IgH class switching, and DNA damage repair are hallmarks of myeloma, we have undertaken studies of Ku expression and function in human myeloma cells (314). Ku is a heterodimer composed of Ku70 and Ku86 subunits that binds with high affinity to altered DNA and is essential for double-stranded DNA break repair and normal Ig V(D)J recombination. Our studies to date have identified a 69-kd variant of Ku86 in some myeloma cells that neither binds DNA–phosphokinase complexes nor activates kinase activity and therefore may account for decreased DNA repair and increased sensitivity to radiation and chemotherapy. Conversely, Ku86 in myeloma cells confers resistance to therapy and may represent a novel therapeutic target.

Excess plasma cells characteristic of this disease accumulate in the bone marrow microenvironment. Several mechanisms whereby tumor cells specifically adhere to both ECM proteins and BMSCs have been demonstrated. There are also changes in the cell adhesion molecule profile that correlate with egress of tumor cells into the peripheral blood within the context of progressive disease and PCL (107). Adhesion molecules not only localize tumor cells within the bone marrow microenvironment but also have multiple functional sequelae. Adherence to BMSCs confers resistance to apoptosis (112), and agents that

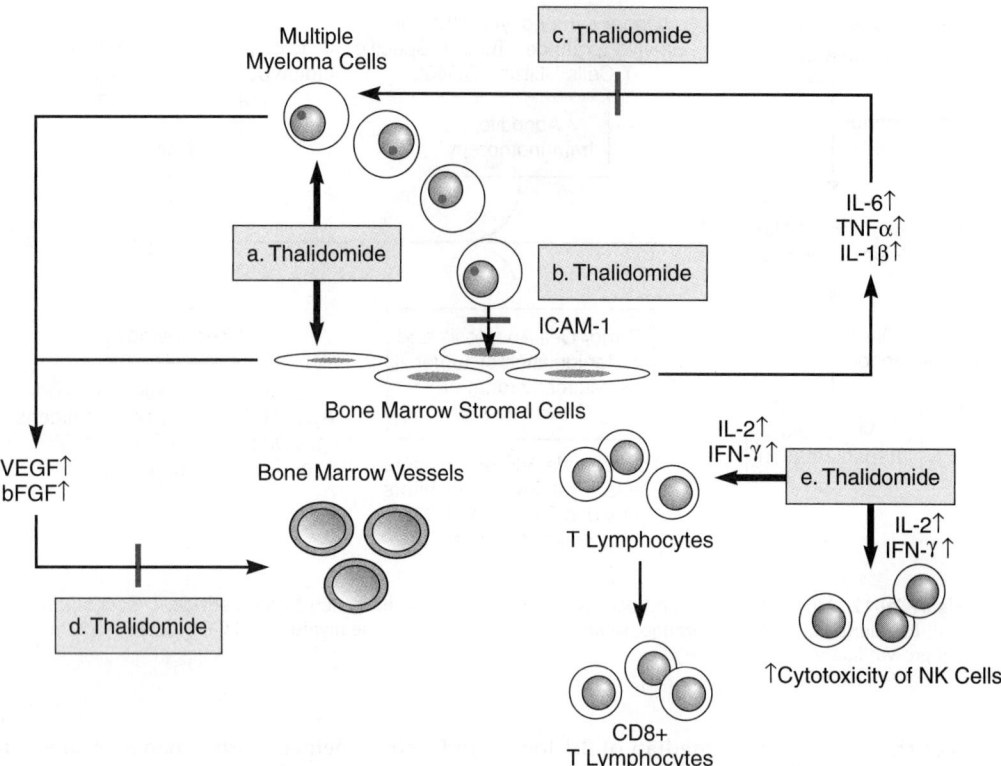

Figure 29-13. Thalidomide: potential mechanisms of antimyeloma activity. (a) Direct effects; (b) antiadhesive action; (c) growth factor inhibition; (d) antiangiogenesis; (e) immunomodulation. bFGF, basic fibroblast growth factor; ICAM, intracellular adhesion molecule; IFN, interferon; IL, interleukin; TNF, tumor necrosis factor; VEGF, vascular endothelial growth factor.

block adhesion, such as bisphosphonates, can confer sensitivity to treatment. Adherence of tumor cells to BMSCs up-regulates nuclear factor (NF)-κB–dependent IL-6 transcription and secretion within BMSCs (41). Moreover, tumor cell secretion of cytokines, including TGF-β within the BM milieu, further enhances IL-6 transcription and secretion in BMSC (140). This finding is of central importance because studies have shown that IL-6 is both a growth and a survival factor for myeloma cells (3). Proteosome inhibitors are novel drugs that inhibit activation of NF-κB (315), and our recent studies show that they both directly induce apoptosis of myeloma cells resistant to conventional therapy and inhibit the NF-κB–dependent up-regulation of IL-6 in BMSCs and related paracrine growth of adherent tumor cells (316). The acceptable toxicity profile and encouraging responses reported in MM patients enrolled in phase I studies of proteosome inhibitors now provide a strong basis for further clinical evaluation to improve outcome.

It may soon be possible to block growth signaling or triggering apoptotic signaling. For example, we have shown that proliferation of myeloma cells triggered by IL-6 is mediated via the MAPK cascade (317), suggesting therapeutic strategies based on blocking this pathway in tumor cells. Apoptosis triggered by γ IR, Fas, and dexamethasone is mediated via distinct signaling cascades. For example, apoptosis induced by dexamethasone (but not IR or Fas) is mediated via activation of RAFTK (48). IL-6 is a survival factor for human myeloma cells, specifically activating SHP2 phosphatase and thereby blocking the activation of RAFTK and related apoptosis in response to dexamethasone (49). Blocking SHP2 activation with small-molecule SHP2 inhibitors may therefore relieve this protective effect. Further delineation of these pathways could provide strategies for triggering

apoptosis, overcoming dexamethasone resistance, and inhibiting survival signals, which will provide the framework for related novel treatment approaches (49).

Our recent studies also suggest that adhesion of myeloma cells to BMSCs up-regulates VEGF secretion by BMSCs and myeloma cells. Therefore, in addition to examining the effect of VEGF on bone marrow angiogenesis, we are evaluating whether VEGF is a growth or survival factor or both for myeloma cells. Preliminary studies suggest that VEGF induces MAPK activation and proliferation of some myeloma cells; thus, VEGF receptor inhibitors may block proliferation of tumor cells and be useful clinically. Based on its antiangiogenic activity, thalidomide has been studied in patients with refractory myeloma, with encouraging results (121). Although thalidomide may be acting in myeloma as an antiangiogenic agent, there are multiple other potential mechanisms of action of thalidomide or its *in vivo* metabolites (Fig. 29-13) (120). First, thalidomide may have a direct effect on the myeloma cell or BMSCs to inhibit their growth and survival. For example, free radical–mediated oxidative DNA damage may play a role in the teratogenicity of thalidomide and may have direct antitumor effects. Second, adhesion of myeloma cells to BMSCs both triggers secretion of cytokines that augment myeloma cell growth and survival and confers drug resistance; thalidomide modulates adhesive interactions and thereby may alter tumor cell growth, survival, and drug resistance. Third, cytokines secreted into the bone marrow microenvironment by myeloma or BMSCs, such as IL-6, IL-1, IL-10, and TNF-α, may augment myeloma cell growth and survival; thalidomide may alter their secretion and bioactivity. Fourth, VEGF and bFGF-2 are secreted by myeloma or BMSCs and may play a role both in tumor cell growth and survival as well as bone marrow angiogenesis. Given its known antiangiogenic activity, thalidomide may inhibit activity of VEGF, bFGF-2, or angiogenesis in myeloma. Finally, thalidomide may be acting against myeloma via its immunomodulatory effects, such as induction of a T helper 1 T-cell response with secretion of IFN and IL-2. Understanding which of these mechanisms mediate antimyeloma activity will be critical both to define its clinical utility optimally and to derive analogs with enhanced potency and fewer side effects. Already two classes of thalidomide analogs have been reported: including selected cytokine inhibitory drugs, which are phosphodiesterase 4 inhibitors and inhibit TNF-α but have little effect on T-cell activation, and immunomodulatory drugs (IMiDs), which are not phosphodiesterase 4 inhibitors but do markedly stimulate T-cell proliferation as well as IFN-γ and IL-2 secretion (119) and inhibit TNF-α. In recent studies, we have delineated mechanisms of antitumor activity of thalidomide and the more potent IMiDs (248). Importantly, these agents act directly to induce apoptosis or G_1 growth arrest in myeloma cell lines and patient myeloma cells that are resistant to melphalan, doxorubicin, and dexamethasone. Moreover, thalidomide and the IMiDs enhance the antimyeloma activity of dexamethasone, with apoptotic signaling triggered by thalidomide and IMiDs associated with activation of RAFTK. Most recent studies suggest that treatment with these drugs may augment myeloma cell adherence to BMSCs and fibronectin but abrogate the up-regulation of IL-6 and VEGF induced by tumor cell binding. Finally, these drugs appear to up-regulate natural killer cell–mediated killing of autologous myeloma cells. These studies establish the framework for the development and testing of thalidomide and the IMiDs in a new treatment paradigm to target both the tumor cell and the microenvironment, overcome classic drug resistance, and achieve improved outcome.

Immune-Based Strategies. Although high response rates can be achieved using high-dose therapy followed by stem cell grafting, patients typically relapse and few, if any, are cured. Major obstacles to cure are the excessive toxicity noted after allografting in myeloma, the contamination of tumor cells in autografts; and the persistence of MRD after high-dose therapy followed by either allogeneic or autologous stem cell transplantation. In this context, improved strategies to treat MRD after high-dose therapy followed by allogeneic or autologous stem cell grafting are being developed. Most important, multiple approaches for the generation and enhancement of allogeneic and autologous antimyeloma immunity *in vitro* and in animal models are being studied. Based on this research, clinical trials are being designed that couple treatments such as transplant to achieve MRD with novel immune-based therapies that target MRD posttransplant in an attempt to achieve long-term DFS and potential cure (Fig. 29-12).

Allografting. Data from our center and others unequivocally demonstrate that DLIs mediate a GVM effect that can effectively treat relapsed myeloma postallografting (286,318). Unfortunately GVHD is a frequent cause of morbidity and mortality after DLI. However, at our center, five of seven patients who had relapsed after CD6-depleted allograft responded (including three CRs) to CD4+ T-cell–enriched DLI, in some cases in the absence of GVHD. This finding raises the possibility that distinct T-cell clones may be mediating GVM versus GVHD. Given the high response rates but inevitable relapses observed in the setting of allografting for myeloma, we are now testing in a clinical protocol whether CD4+ DLI at 6 months after CD6-depleted allografting mediates GVM, effectively treating MRD and improving outcome. To date, 21 patients have undergone CD6-depleted allografting, 18 of whom developed only grades 0 to 1 GVHD. Of these 18 patients, 11 are more than 6 months posttransplant and have received CD4+ DLI. Eight of the eleven patients who received DLI demonstrated further response (including four CRs), suggesting the potential of DLI to treat MRD. These studies already suggest that GVM can be adoptively transferred in this fashion. T-cell repertoire, based on Vβ T-cell receptor gene rearrangement, is being examined to identify those clonal T cells associated with GVM and their target antigens on tumor cells (287,288). It has been shown that T cells mediating GVM can target idiotypic antigens, and ongoing studies are presently identifying other target antigens. The goal of these studies is to characterize, isolate, and expand GVM T-cell clones for antigen-specific adoptive immunotherapy.

Autografting. Although randomized studies convincingly demonstrate a survival advantage for myeloma patients treated with high-dose therapy and autografting compared with those receiving conventional chemotherapy, this treatment is not curative. Two sites of MRD contribute to the failure of autografting: MRD in the autograft, and MRD in the patient after myeloablative therapy. Monoclonal antibodies produced in the laboratory have been used to deplete tumor cells from myeloma autografts (273). CD34 selection techniques have also been evaluated to select normal hematopoietic progenitor cells within autografts (305). However, both these methods deplete only 2 to 3 logs of tumor cells, and over 50% of autografts still contain MRD. Based on our laboratory data that myeloma cells express Muc-1 and adenoviral receptors, we have specifically transduced tumor cells within myeloma autografts with the thymidine kinase gene using an adenoviral vector with a tumor selective (Muc-1) promotor, then purged tumor cells *ex vivo* by treatment with ganciclovir (319). Pilot studies suggest that over 6 to 7 logs of tumor cells can be purged under conditions that do not adversely affect normal hematopoietic progenitor cells, setting the stage for a clinical trial of adenoviral purging before autotransplantation.

We are also attempting to generate and expand antimyeloma specific autologous T cells *ex vivo* for adoptive immunotherapy of MRD in the patient after autotransplant. It is now possible to clone the gene for the patient's specific idiotypic protein, use computer programs to identify gene sequences encoding for peptides predicted to be presented within the groove of class I HLA of a given patient's HLA type, and expand peptide specific T cells *ex vivo* (320). A similar strategy can be used to expand T cells against peptides within shared antigens that are overexpressed on myeloma cells, such as the telomerase catalytic subunit (hTERT) (321), Muc-1 (37), or CYP1B1 (322). Thus, immunologic responses are also being tested to enhance the immunogenicity of the whole tumor cell. As a further example, our laboratory studies have shown that autologous T cells do not proliferate in response to the patient's own tumor cells as targets. However, CD40 activation of myeloma cells up-regulates class I and II HLA, costimulatory, GRP94, and other molecules, and CD40-activated myeloma cells also trigger a brisk autologous T-cell response (323). T cells can, therefore, be harvested from myeloma patients before autografting, expanded *ex vivo* using CD40 activated autologous myeloma cells as a stimulus, and administered as adoptive immunotherapy to treat MRD posttransplant.

We and others are developing and examining the clinical utility of a variety of myeloma vaccines. First, based on our observation that CD40-activated myeloma cells trigger a brisk autologous T-cell response, we are examining the utility of vaccinations of patients with autologous CD40-activated tumor cells. Second, based on our demonstration of the expression of Muc-1 core protein on freshly isolated myeloma cells (37), we are evaluating two vaccines: recombinant vaccinia virus containing the Muc-1 gene, and autologous dendritic cells (DCs) transduced using adenoviral vectors with Muc-1. Of interest, we have recently shown that myeloma cells can be fused to DCs and that the use of the myeloma DC fusion as an antigen-presenting cell presents the entire myeloma cell as foreign. In a syngeneic murine myeloma model, vaccinations with myeloma cell–DC fusions, but not with either myeloma cells or DCs alone, demonstrate both protective and therapeutic efficacy. Most important, we have shown that patient myeloma cells can be fused to autologous DCs, which are readily isolated from either patient bone marrow or peripheral blood (98), and that autologous myeloma cell–DC fusions can trigger specific cytolytic autologous T-cell responses *in vitro* (324). We will therefore translate these findings into clinical trials of myeloma–DC fusion vaccines to assess *in vivo* myeloma-specific T-cell and B-cell responses as well as clinical efficacy. Ultimately, vaccinations can be coupled with adoptive immunotherapy in an attempt to treat MRD after autografting and thereby potentially improve outcome.

Immunization protocols at other centers have already demonstrated a transient anti-Id T-cell response in three of five patients by injection of autologous Id. Moreover, five of five patients injected with autologous Id and GM-CSF had long-lasting major histocompatibility complex class I restricted Id-specific T-cell responses (312,325). Massaia et al. (326) have also shown generation of T-cell–proliferative responses and delayed type hypersensitivity to Id after immunization with Id conjugated to KLH with GM-CSF or IL-2 as immunoadjuvants. Vaccination after autologous PBSC transplantation for MM using idiotype pulsed dendritic cells can achieve idiotype-specific T-cell responses in a minority of patients (327). Other strategies currently under evaluation are immunization with idiotypic DNA vaccines (328) and dendritic cells pulsed with idiotype (313). MAGE antigens (329) and catalytic subunit of telomerase (321) are expressed by myeloma and contain peptides that can be effectively presented by HLA class I molecules to generate autologous specific cytolytic T-cell responses. Myeloma cells that can be efficiently transduced with adenoviral vectors and accessory molecules, including CD80 (330) or GM-CSF (285), are currently being transfected into tumor cells before their use in vaccination.

Serotherapy. A chimeric anti-CD38 antibody (331) has been developed that consists of the Fab portion of the mouse anti-CD38 monoclonal antibody linked by a stable thioether bond to an Fc molecule derived from human IgG$_1$, thereby forming a mouse Fab-human Fc hybrid. In contrast to the parent mouse antibody, the chimeric molecule mediates antibody-dependent cellular cytotoxicity very effectively with human blood mononuclear effector cells, even at low concentration. Daily intravenous injections of anti–IL-6 monoclonal antibody for 2 months led to a dramatic reduction in the percentage of myeloma cells in S phase as well as reduction in serum calcium, serum monoclonal IgG, and CRP levels (61). This finding provides further support for the role of IL-6 in myeloma cell growth *in vivo* and again suggests that strategies designed to interrupt IL-6–mediated growth may provide new treatments for myeloma (65,67,171,332). Several trials of immunotoxin therapy of myeloma have been attempted. Monoclonal antibody (8A) recognizes a plasma cell–associated antigen and has been conjugated to momordin, a ribosome-inactivating protein similar to the ricin A chain (333). Specifically, it may be useful for *ex vivo* purging in autologous marrow grafting in myeloma. A chimeric toxin composed of IL-6 attached to a portion of *Pseudomonas* exotoxin devoid of its own recognition domain has also been produced in *Escherichia coli* (334). This fusion product was cytotoxic to a human myeloma cell line expressing IL-6 receptors, but it had no effect on IL-6 receptor–negative cells. It therefore may be useful in the selective elimination of myeloma cells and other cells with high numbers of IL-6 receptors. Anti-CD19 as well as anti-CD38 monoclonal antibodies have been conjugated to ricin for the *in vivo* elimination of tumor cells but have not shown promise in early studies (335,336). Serotherapy against the plasma cell–specific HM1.24 and other antigens, including CD20 and Muc-1, is also being tested in myeloma (37,337,338).

OTHER PLASMA CELL DYSCRASIAS

Plasmacytomas

CLINICAL CHARACTERISTICS

Plasmacytomas are collections of monoclonal plasma cells originating either in bone (solitary osseous plasmacytoma, SOP) or in soft tissue (extramedullary plasmacytoma, EMP). They comprise less than 10% of plasma cell dyscrasias. Myeloma with plasmacytoma must be excluded before the diagnosis of either SOP or EMP can be made. Magnetic resonance imaging can be useful to show additional marrow abnormalities consistent with myeloma (339). The median age of diagnosis of SOP or EMP is approximately 50 years, nearly 10 years younger than that for myeloma (340–342). Although patients with SOP and EMP can both progress to myeloma, the majority of patients with SOP progress, whereas a maximum of 50% of patients with EMP eventually develop myeloma. The median survival of 86.4 months and 100.8 months for patients with SOP and EMP, respectively, is similar. However, progression-free survival is markedly different, with 16% for SOP patients versus 71% for EMP patients. The persistence of stable monoclonal Ig in serum, urine, or both after primary treatment for plasmacytoma does not necessitate additional therapy because it does not influence survival or DFS (340). In contrast, rising monoclonal Ig levels in a patient with a history of either SOP or EMP should trigger a work-up for either recurrent plasmacytoma or myeloma. It has been suggested, as is true for myeloma, that serum β2M has prognostic value in patients with SOP. Specifically, 17 of 19 patients with elevated serum β2M had transformation to myeloma and shorter survival (at 31 months) than those with normal serum β2M levels (343).

TREATMENT

Treatment for SOP and EMP is local therapy, primarily radiotherapy, with surgery as needed for structural anatomic support (340–342). The benefit of chemotherapy, either alone or in combination with radiotherapy and surgery, as primary therapy for SOP or EMP has not been proven. The benefit of adjuvant chemotherapy to prevent recurrent disease or progression to myeloma is also undefined. One recent report suggests that the disappearance of protein after involved-field radiotherapy predicts long-term DFS and possible cure (344).

Immunoglobulin M Monoclonal Gammopathy

Excess monoclonal IgM in the serum can occur in a variety of diseases. In a Mayo Clinic series of 430 patients in whom a monoclonal IgM protein was identified, 242 (56%) had MGUS, 71 (17%) had Waldenström's macroglobulinemia, 28 (7%) had lymphoma, 21 (5%) had chronic lymphocytic leukemia, 6 (1%) had primary amyloidosis, and 62 (14%) had other malignant lymphoproliferative diseases (345). The median duration of

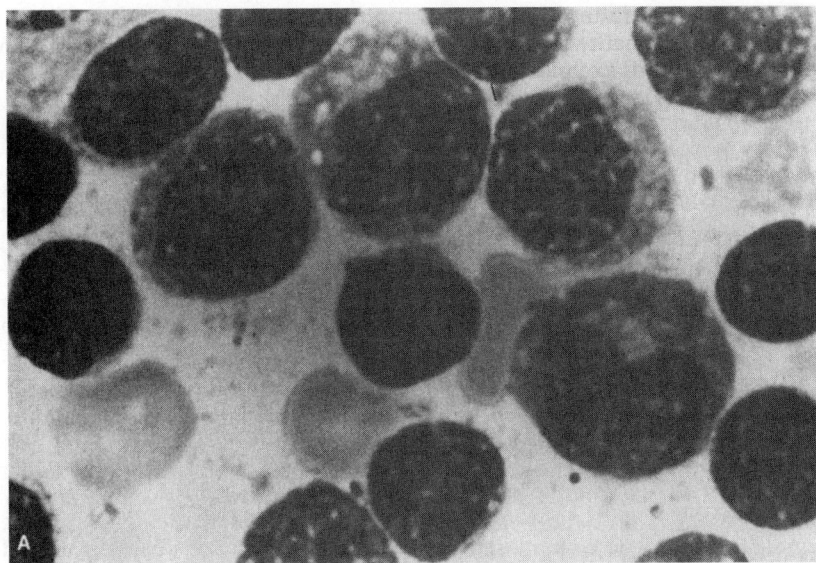

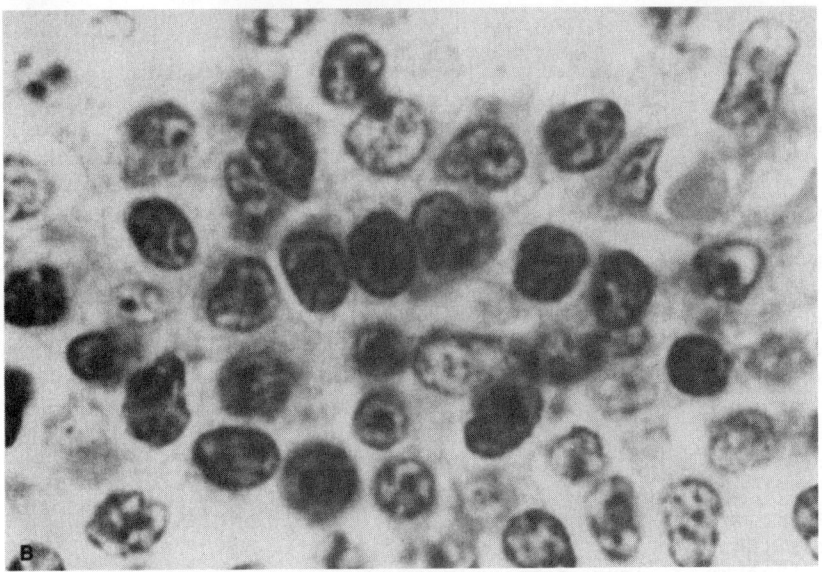

Figure 29-14. Lymphoplasmacytic lymphoma cells of Waldenström's macroglobulinemia. **(A)** Cells on the bone marrow aspirate. **(B)** Aggregates of lymphoma cells on the bone marrow core biopsy. The cells are intermediate in size between small lymphocytes and plasma cells, and the placement of the nucleus in the cells is slightly eccentric.

time from the recognition of the monoclonal protein to the development of a malignant lymphoid disease ranged from 4 to 9 years, suggesting that long-term follow-up of such patients is necessary.

WALDENSTRÖM'S MACROGLOBULINEMIA

The diagnosis of Waldenström's macroglobulinemia (WM) requires an IgM serum level of at least 3.0 g/dL in association with an increase in lymphocytes or plasmacytoid lymphocytes in the marrow (346,347) (Fig. 29-14). It is a distinct clonal disorder of small lymphocytes with maturation to plasma cells producing IgM, whose effects in turn determine most of the clinical features. WM corresponds most closely to lymphoplasmacytic lymphoma under the World Health Organization classification of lymphoid tumors (lymphoplasmacytic lymphoma/immunocytoma under the Revised European American Lymphoma classification). WM accounts for approximately 2% of all hematologic malignancies and is more common in men than women. Its incidence increases with age, and it is more common among whites than blacks (348,349). The etiology of WM is unclear, although genetic factors may contribute to the pathogenesis, given reports of familial aggregation frequently in association with other lymphoproliferative and immunologic disorders

(350). Cytogenetic abnormalities occur in 15% to 90% of cases, and several chromosomal abnormalities have been described in neoplastic cells of patients with WM, but none is specific (351,352). The WM B-cell clone demonstrates intraclonal differentiation, from small lymphocytes with large focal deposits of surface immunoglobulins to lymphoplasmacytic cells and mature plasma cells that contain intracytoplasmic immunoglobulin. This morphologic heterogeneity is reflected by variable expression of phenotypic markers. All WM cells express monoclonal IgM, and most cells are positive for CD19, CD20, CD22, and FMC7. High density of CD38 is also detected with variable intensity of the PCA-1 antigen. CD45 isoform expression is heterogenous, probably reflecting ongoing monoclonal B-cell differentiation. In approximately 20% of cases, CD5 and CD23 expression are seen, but coexpression of both these markers is uncommon (353). Ultimately, clonal B cells are present among circulating B lymphocytes, and their concentration increases in patients who do not respond to therapy or who progress (354). Current data indicate that WM originates from a postgerminal center B cell that has undergone somatic mutations and antigenic selection in the lymphoid follicle (355,356). This cell therefore has the characteristics of an IgM-bearing memory B cell (357).

The median age of onset of WM is 61 years. Symptoms are characteristically vague and nonspecific, with the most common being weakness, anorexia, and weight loss. Symptoms due to peripheral neuropathy and Raynaud's phenomena can precede more serious manifestations. Lymphadenopathy, splenomegaly, or hepatomegaly are present in 30% to 40% of cases, and at least 20% to 25% lymphoplasmacytoid cells are usually present in the marrow. Visceral involvement of small bowel and peripheral nerves can cause the clinical sequelae of malabsorption and neuropathy, respectively. Hemorrhagic complications are common, attributable to abnormal bleeding times, decreased platelet adhesiveness, or direct interference by the IgM protein with the release of platelet factor 3 and with coagulation factors. An important part of the differential diagnosis is the exclusion of the less common entity of IgM MM, which is characterized by lytic bone disease and an absence of organomegaly or lymphocytic involvement; rarely WM can itself progress to IgM myeloma (358). Amyloidosis occurs rarely in WM (359). Hyperviscosity syndrome, described in the section Cardiac Dysfunction as a rare complication in myeloma (202), occurs more commonly in the setting of excess IgM and is characterized by mucosal bleeding and neurologic, ocular, and cardiovascular abnormalities. Therapy with plasmapheresis is more useful to remove excess IgM than it is in the setting of excess IgG monoclonal proteins and related hyperviscosity in myeloma.

Plasmapheresis can be considered only as an adjunctive therapy. Treatment regimens used are similar to those used to treat low-grade lymphomas and myeloma, including chlorambucil, cyclophosphamide, melphalan, and corticosteroids, either as single agents or in combinations (346). As for myeloma, there is no evidence that combined drug regimens are superior to single therapies. The median survival is approximately 50 months, similar to the best reported series of patients with myeloma. In contrast to people with myeloma, however, many individuals with WM have indolent disease requiring no therapy for long periods, with survivals in excess of 20 years. Pretreatment parameters including older age, male sex, general symptoms, and cytopenias define a high-risk population that may benefit from newer therapeutic approaches (360,361). Acute leukemia has developed in patients with WM (362), emphasizing a potential complication of premature and prolonged low-dose therapy with alkylating agents. Nucleoside analogs, including fludarabine and 2-chlorodeoxyadenosine, have been shown effective in newly diagnosed as well as refractory patients with WM and may achieve more rapid cytoreduction than oral chlorambucil (346,363–365). Prospective randomized trials are needed to assess the effect of nucleoside analogs on survival (366).

Several reports describe responses in patients with WM using recombinant γ or α IFN (367,368). Interestingly, patients who had been treated with previous chemotherapy had an equivalent response rate to those who had not. IFN-α may have a role in the treatment of WM, and future studies are needed to assess its effect as a remission therapy or as part of other strategies (369). Although high-dose therapy with autologous stem cell support has been shown effective in many patients with MM or low-grade lymphoma, relatively few patients with WM have undergone transplant. Preliminary data suggest that high-dose therapy is associated with a high CR rate and acceptable toxicity (370). This approach therefore needs further investigation, particularly in younger patients presenting with poor prognostic features. Splenectomy has been reported to be effective in chemotherapy-resistant patients with WM (371,372). Monoclonal antibody therapy with rituximab, a chimeric anti-CD20 monoclonal antibody, produces responses in both treated and untreated patients with low-grade lymphoma. Given that the CD20 antigen is typically present in WM, rituximab has been used to treat patients and achieved response in approximately one third of previously treated patients (373). Studies of this monoclonal antibody, both in combination with other agents and after response has been achieved with chemotherapy, are ongoing.

Heavy-Chain Diseases

Since the original description by Franklin et al. (374) of a patient with malignant lymphoma whose serum and urine contained large amounts of the Fc fragment of IgG, the clinical and immunochemical scope of γ heavy-chain disease (HCD) has broadened. These diseases are characterized by the presence of a portion of the Ig heavy chain in the serum or urine or both. The median age at diagnosis is similar to that for myeloma, approximately 60 years (375). The clinical and laboratory features can be heterogeneous. The most common presenting symptoms include weakness, fatigue, and fever associated with lymphadenopathy and hepatosplenomegaly. In addition to Ig heavy chain in serum or urine, a lymphoplasmacytic marrow infiltrate is noted in most cases. The clinical course can be fulminant and rapidly progressive. Alternatively, the monoclonal heavy chain can persist for years in otherwise asymptomatic patients. Survival is variable, but the median is only 12 months. Treatment options for patients with active disease are similar to those for lymphoma or myeloma, whereas patients with indolent disease should be followed expectantly without therapy. Cases of αHCD, μHCD, and δHCD have also been described. HCD is typically associated with non-Hodgkin's lymphoma, which has a propensity to occur in the gastrointestinal tract. Progression of disease may occur, beginning with plasma cells that produce a heavy chain and aggregate in the intestinal tract, with subsequent transformation into a malignant non-Hodgkin's lymphoma of the immunoblastic type, probably arising from the more mature plasma cells (376). The ideal therapy for an HCD is not known because of its rarity, but intensive chemotherapy including intravenous cyclophosphamide, doxorubicin, vincristine, and oral prednisone appears to offer some patients long-term remissions.

Amyloidosis

Amyloidosis is relatively rare as a clinically significant disease (discussed in Chapter 22). It has been classified into five categories: (a) primary, with or without plasma cell and lymphoid neoplasms, (b) secondary, associated with chronic infections or autoimmune disease, (c) hereditary, associated with familial Mediterranean fever, Portuguese lower limb neuropathy, and others, (d) amyloidosis associated with aging, and (e) amyloidosis of endocrine glands, with medullary thyroid carcinoma and multiple endocrine neoplasia type 2 (359,377). The amyloid found in most cases of amyloidosis can be assigned to one of two types according to whether the fibrils consist mainly of the variable region of Ig light chains (AL, or primary amyloidosis) or protein A (AA, or secondary amyloidosis). Protein A has a molecular weight of 8500 d and consists of 76 amino acids; it is not related to any known immunoglobulin. In AL, amyloid primarily involves the heart, tongue, gastrointestinal tract, and skin, whereas AA primarily results in fibril deposition in liver, kidney, and spleen. A review of 229 patients with AL documented myeloma in 47 (21%) patients (377). Initial presenting symptoms were fatigue and weight loss, with pain more common in those who also had myeloma. Hepatomegaly and macroglossia were present in up to one-third of patients with AL; renal insufficiency was present in one-half of patients, and proteinuria (defined as albuminuria with immune globulin seen only in myeloma) was documented in 82% of patients. Nephrotic syndrome, CHF, orthostatic hypotension, carpal tunnel syndrome, and peripheral neuropathy were all more common in those without myeloma (30% to 70% of patients studied) than persons with myeloma, of whom less than 20% had these features. Overall median survival was 12 months; overall survival was 5 months for those with myeloma and 13 months for those without myeloma.

Although it has been difficult to monitor the distribution and progression of disease, it has been shown that radiolabeled serum amyloid P component, which has specific binding affinity for amyloid fibrils, can be administered intravenously and localizes rapidly and specifically in amyloid deposits (378). This technique may therefore facilitate diagnosis and monitoring of the extent of systemic amyloidosis, including the effects of therapeutic interventions.

Treatment for AL is unsatisfactory. Only 27 (18%) of 153 patients responded to MP, although median survival for responders was prolonged at 89.4 months (359) and only 5% of patients with primary AL survive 10 years or longer (379). A prospective randomized trial has concluded that MP was superior to colchicine when analyzed from time of entry into the study to time of death or progression of disease (380). Other retrospective studies suggest that colchicine is superior to placebo for patients with AL (381). Alkylating agent–based chemotherapy may therefore be beneficial for a subset of patients and result in prolonged survival. One randomized trial of colchicine, MP, or a combination of the three drugs in patients with primary amyloidosis found that therapy with MP results in objective responses and prolonged survival compared with colchicine (382). However, therapy with multiple alkylating agents did not achieve either higher response rate or longer survival time than MP (383).

Early reports suggest that dose-intensive melphalan with blood stem cell support can achieve CRs, with improvement in performance status and clinical remission of organ-specific disease (384). At present, high-dose therapy appears effective at reversing the amyloid deposition but is not without risk (385). Guidelines have been developed for patient selection to maximize benefit and minimize treatment-related mortality. Attempts to improve outcomes for patients with symptomatic and advanced multisystem disease may require both solid and stem cell transplantation as well as the use of less intensive conditioning regimens (386). If outcomes continue to improve, new challenges such as the contamination of autografts with tumor cells will also need to be addressed (387).

REFERENCES

1. Alexanian R, Dimopoulos M. The treatment of multiple myeloma. *N Engl J Med* 1994;330:484–489.
2. Bataille R, Harousseau J-L. Multiple myeloma. *N Engl J Med* 1997;336:1657–1664.
3. Hallek M, Bergsagel PL, Anderson KC. Multiple myeloma: increasing evidence for a multistep transformation process. *Blood* 1998;91:3–21.
4. Kyle RA. Multiple myeloma: review of 869 cases. *Mayo Clin Proc* 1975;50:29–40.
5. Clamp JR. Some aspects of the first recorded case of multiple myeloma. *Lancet* 1967;2:1354–1356.
6. Kyle RA. Multiple myeloma: how did it begin? *Mayo Clin Proc* 1994;69:680–683.
7. Longsworth LG, Shedlovsky T, MacInnes DA. Electrophoretic patterns of normal and pathological human blood serum and plasma. *J Exp Med* 1939;70:399.
8. Grabar P, Williams CA. Methods permettant l'etude conjuguee des proprietes electrophoretiques et immunochimiques d'un melange de protemes: application au serum sanguin. *Biochim Biophys Acta* 1953;10:193.
9. Durie BGM. Staging and kinetics of multiple myeloma. *Semin Oncol* 1986;13:300–309.
10. Kyle RA. "Benign" monoclonal gammopathy—after 20 to 35 years of follow-up. *Mayo Clin Proc* 1993;68:26–36.
11. Dyck PJ, Low PA, Windebank AJ, et al. Plasma exchange in polyneuropathy associated with monoclonal gammopathy of undetermined significance. *N Engl J Med* 1991;325:1482–1486.
12. Bergsagel DE, Wong O, Bergsagel PL, et al. Benzene and multiple myeloma: appraisal of the scientific evidence. *Blood* 1999;94:1174–1182.
13. Bourguet CC, Grufferman S, Delzell E, et al. Multiple myeloma and family history of cancer. *Cancer* 1985;56:2133–2139.
14. Greenlee RT, Murray T, Bolden S, et al. Cancer statistics, 2000. *CA Cancer J Clin* 2000;50:7–33.
15. Herrinton LJ, Weiss NS, Olshan AF. Epidemiology of myeloma. In: Malpas JS, Bergsagel DE, Kyle R, et al., eds. *Myeloma: biology and management.* Oxford: Oxford Medical Publications, 1997:150.
16. Kyle RA, Beard MC, O'Fallon WM, et al. Incidence of multiple myeloma in Olmsted County, Minnesota: 1978 through 1990, with a review of the trend since 1945. *J Clin Oncol* 1994;12:1577–1583.
17. Pruzanski W, Ogryzlo MA. Abnormal proteinuria in malignant diseases. *Adv Clin Chem* 1970;13:335–382.
18. Blade J, Lust JA, Kyle RA. Immunoglobulin D multiple myeloma: presenting features, response to therapy, and survival in a series of 53 cases. *J Clin Oncol* 1994;12:2398–2404.
19. Kyle RA. Long-term survival in multiple myeloma. *N Engl J Med* 1983;308:314–316.
20. Bergsagel DE. Acute leukemia and multiple myeloma: natural history or iatrogenic disease? *Drug Ther* 1977(Oct 9):8–9.
21. Kapadia SB. Multiple myeloma: a clinicopathologic study of 62 consecutively autopsied cases. *Medicine* 1980;59:380–392.
22. Kubagawa H, Vogler LB, Capra JD, et al. Studies on the clonal origin of multiple myeloma: use of individually specific (idiotypic) antibodies to trace the oncogenic event to its earliest point of expression in B cell differentiation. *J Exp Med* 1979;150:792–807.
23. Preud'homme JL, Klein M, Labaume S, et al. Idiotype-bearing and antigen-bearing receptors produced by blood T lymphocytes in a case of human myeloma. *Eur J Immunol* 1977;7:840–846.
24. Epstein J, Xiao HQ, He XY. Markers of multiple hematopoietic-cell lineages in multiple myeloma. *N Engl J Med* 1990;322:664–668.
25. Jensen GS, Grunewald J, Osterborg A, et al. Selective expression of CD45 isoforms defines CALLA+ monoclonal B lineage cells in peripheral blood from myeloma patients as late stage B cells. *Blood* 1991;78:711–719.
26. Bakkus MHC, Heirman C, van Riet I, et al. Evidence that multiple myeloma Ig heavy chain VDJ genes contain somatic mutations but show no intraclonal variation. *Blood* 1992;80:2326–2335.
27. Vescio RA, Cao J, Hong CH, et al. Myeloma Ig heavy chain V region sequences reveal prior antigenic selection and marked somatic mutation but no intraclonal diversity. *J Immunol* 1995;155:2487.
28. Sahota SS, Garand R, Mahroof R, et al. V$_H$ gene analysis of IgM-secreting myeloma indicates an origin from a memory cell undergoing isotype switch events. *Blood* 1999;94:1070–1076.
29. Bergsagel PL, Chesi M, Nardini E, et al. Promiscuous translocations into immunoglobulin heavy chains with regions in multiple myeloma. *Proc Natl Acad Sci U S A* 1996;93:13931–13936.
30. Anderson KC, Bates MP, Slaughenhoupt B, et al. Expression of human B cell associated antigens on leukemias and lymphomas: a model of human B cell differentiation. *Blood* 1984;63:1424–1433.
31. Anderson KC, Park EK, Bates MP, et al. Antigens on human plasma cells identified by monoclonal antibodies. *J Immunol* 1983;130:1132–1138.
32. Epstein J, Barlogie B, Katzmann J, et al. Phenotypic heterogeneity in aneuploid multiple myeloma indicates pre-B cell involvement. *Blood* 1988;71:861–865.
33. Grogan TM, Durie BGM, Lomen C, et al. Delineation of a novel pre-B cell component in plasma cell myeloma: immunochemical, immunophenotypic, genotypic, cytologic, cell culture, and kinetic features. *Blood* 1987;70:932–942.
34. San Miguel JF, Caballero MD, Gonzales M, et al. Immunological phenotype of neoplasms involving the B cell in the last step of differentiation. *Br J Haematol* 1986;62:75–83.
35. Van Camp B, Durie BG, Spier C, et al. Plasma cells in multiple myeloma express natural killer cell-associated antigen: CD56 (NKH-1; Leu-19). *Blood* 1990;76:377–382.
36. Harada H, Kawano MM, Huang N, et al. Phenotypic difference of normal plasma cells from mature myeloma cells. *Blood* 1993;81:2658–2663.
37. Treon SP, Mollick JA, Urashima M, et al. Muc-1 core protein is expressed on multiple myeloma cells and is induced by dexamethasone. *Blood* 1999;93:1287–1298.
38. Klein B, Lu Y, Gaillard JP, et al. Inhibiting IL-6 in human multiple myeloma. *Curr Top Microbiol Immunol* 1992;182:236–243.
39. Kawano MM, Hirano T, Matsuda T, et al. Autocrine generation and requirement of BSF-2/IL-6 for human multiple myeloma. *Nature* 1988;332:83–85.
40. Urashima M, Chauhan D, Uchiyama H, et al. CD40 ligand triggered interleukin-6 secretion in multiple myeloma. *Blood* 1995;85:1903–1912.
41. Chauhan D, Uchiyama H, Akbarali Y, et al. Multiple myeloma cell adhesion-induced interleukin-6 expression in bone marrow stromal cells involves activation of NF-kB. *Blood* 1996;87:1104–1112.
42. Lokhorst HM, Lamme T, de Smet M, et al. Primary tumor cells of myeloma patients induce interleukin-6 secretion in long-term marrow cultures. *Blood* 1994;84:2269–2277.
43. Uchiyama H, Barut BA, Mohrbacher AF, et al. Adhesion of human myeloma-derived cell lines to bone marrow stromal cells stimulates IL-6 secretion. *Blood* 1993;82:3712–3720.
44. Chauhan D, Kharbanda S, Ogata A, et al. Interleukin-6 inhibits Fas-induced apoptosis and stress-activated protein kinase activation in multiple myeloma cells. *Blood* 1997;89:227–234.

45. Chauhan D, Pandey P, Ogata A, et al. Dexamethasone induces apoptosis of multiple myeloma cells in a JNK/SAP kinase independent mechanism. *Oncogene* 1997;15:837–843.

46. Chauhan D, Hideshima T, Treon SP, et al. Functional interaction between retinoblastoma protein and stress activated protein kinase in multiple myeloma cells. *Cancer Res* 1999;59:1192–1195.

47. Chauhan D, Pandey P, Ogata A, et al. Cytochrome-c dependent and independent induction of apoptosis in multiple myeloma cells. *J Biol Chem* 1997;272:29995–29997.

48. Chauhan D, Hideshima T, Pandey P, et al. RAFTK/PYK2-dependent and -independent apoptosis in multiple myeloma cells. *Oncogene* 1999;18:6733–6740.

49. Chauhan D, Anderson KC. Apoptosis in multiple myeloma: therapeutic implications. *Apoptosis* 2001;6:47–55.

50. Catlett-Falcone R, Landowski TH, Oshiro MM, et al. Constitutive activation of STAT3 signaling confers resistance to apoptosis in human U266 myeloma cells. *Immunity* 1999;10:105–115.

51. Landowski TH, Shain KH, Oshiro MM, et al. Myeloma cells selected for resistance to CD95-mediated apoptosis are not cross-resistant to cytotoxic drugs: evidence for independent mechanisms of caspase activation. *Blood* 1999;94:265–274.

52. Urashima M, Ogata A, Chauhan D, et al. Interleukin-6 promotes multiple myeloma cell growth via phosphorylation of retinoblastoma protein. *Blood* 1996;88:2219–2227.

53. Ng MHL, Chung YF, Lo KW, et al Frequent hypermethylation of p16 and p15 genes in multiple myeloma. *Blood* 1997;87:2500.

54. Urashima M, Teoh G, Ogata A, et al. Role of CDK4 and p16^{INK4A} in interleukin-6-mediated growth of multiple myeloma. *Leukemia* 1997;11:1957–1963.

55. Urashima M, Teoh G, Chauhan D, et al. Interleukin-6 overcomes p21^{WAF1} upregulation and G1 growth arrest induced by dexamethasone and interferon-γ in multiple myeloma cells. *Blood* 1997;90:279–289.

56. Teoh G, Urashima M, Ogata A, et al. MDM2 protein overexpression promotes proliferation and survival of multiple myeloma cells. *Blood* 1997;90:1982–1992.

57. Bataille R, Jourdan M, Zhang XG, et al. Serum levels of interleukin-6, a potent myeloma cell growth factor, as a reflection of disease severity in plasma cell dyscrasias. *J Clin Invest* 1989;84:2008–2011.

58. Ludwig H, Nachbaur DM, Fritz E, et al. Interleukin-6 is a prognostic factor in multiple myeloma. *Blood* 1991;77:2794–2795.

59. Fattori E, Della Rocca C, Costa P, et al. Development of progressive kidney damage and myeloma kidney in interleukin-6 transgenic mice. *Blood* 1994;83:2570–2579.

60. Barille S, Collette M, Bataille R, et al. Myeloma cells upregulate IL-6 but downregulate osteocalcin production by osteoblastic cells through cell to cell contact. *Blood* 1995;86:3151–3159.

61. Bataille R, Barlogie B, Yang Z, et al. Biologic effects of anti-interleukin-6 murine monoclonal antibody in advanced multiple myeloma. *Blood* 1995;86:685–691.

62. Ogata A, Nishimoto N, Shima Y, et al. Inhibitory effect of all-trans retinoic acid on the growth of freshly isolated myeloma cells via interference with interleukin-6 signal transduction. *Blood* 1994;84:3040–3046.

63. Chadwick D, Jamal N, Messner HA, et al. Differential sensitivity of human myeloma cell lines and bone marrow colony forming cells to a recombinant diphtheria toxin-interleukin-6 fusion protein. *Br J Haematol* 1993;85:25–36.

64. Kreitman R, Siegall CB, Fitzgerald DJP, et al. Interleukin-6 fused to mutant form of Pseudomonas exotoxin kills malignant cells from patients with multiple myeloma. *Blood* 1992;79:1775–1780.

65. Ehlers M, de Hon FD, Klasse Bos H, et al. Combining two mutations of human interleukin-6 that affect gp130 activation results in a potent interleukin-6 receptor antagonist on human myeloma cells. *J Biol Chem* 1995;270:8158–8163.

66. Savage AD, Belson DJ, Vescio RA, et al. Pamidronate reduces IL-6 production by bone marrow stroma from multiple myeloma patients. *Blood* 1996;88:105a.

67. Sporeno E, Savino R, Ciapponi L, et al. Human interleukin-6 receptor super antagonists with high potency and wide spectrum on multiple myeloma cells. *Blood* 1996;87:4510–4519.

68. Klein B, Zhang XG, Lu XY, et al. Interleukin-6 in human multiple myeloma. *Blood* 1995;85:863–872.

69. Kawano M, Tanaka H, Ishikawa H, et al. Interleukin-1 accelerates autocrine growth of myeloma cells through interleukin-6 in human myeloma. *Blood* 1989;73:2145–2148.

70. Cozzolino F, Torcia M, Aldinucci D, et al. Production of interleukin-1 by bone marrow myeloma cells: its role in the pathogenesis of lytic bone lesions. *Blood* 1989;74:380–387.

71. Gherardi RK, Belec L, Fromont G, et al. Elevated levels of interleukin-1 beta (IL-1 beta) and IL-6 in serum and increased production of IL-1 beta mRNA in lymph nodes of patients with polyneuropathy, organomegaly, endocrinopathy, M protein, and skin changes (POEMS) syndrome. *Blood* 1994;83:2587–2593.

72. Lacy MQ, Donovan DA, Heimbach JH, et al. Comparison of interleukin-1b expression by in situ hybridization in monoclonal gammopathy of undetermined significance and multiple myeloma. *Blood* 1999;93:300–305.

73. Bergui L, Schena M, Gaidano G, et al. Interleukin 3 and interleukin 6 synergistically promote the proliferation and differentiation of malignant plasma cell precursors in multiple myeloma. *J Exp Med* 1989;170:613–618.

74. Garrett IR, Durie BGM, Nedwin GE, et al. Production of lymphotoxin, a bone resorbing cytokine, by cultured human myeloma cells. *N Engl J Med* 1987;317:526–532.

75. Hermann F, Andreff M, Gruss HJ, et al. Interleukin 4 inhibits growth of multiple myeloma by suppressing interleukin 6 expression. *Blood* 1991;78:2070–2078.

76. Chauhan D, Kharbanda S, Ogata A, et al. Oncostatin M induces association of Grb2 with Janus kinase JAK2 in multiple myeloma cells. *J Exp Med* 1995;182:1801–1806.

77. Zhang XG, Bataille R, Jourdan M, et al. Granulocyte-macrophage colony-stimulating factor synergizes with interleukin-6 in supporting the proliferation of human myeloma cells. *Blood* 1990;76:2599.

78. Anderson KC, Morimoto C, Paul SR, et al. Interleukin-11 promotes accessory cell dependent B cell differentiation in man. *Blood* 1992;80:2797–2804.

79. Paul SD, Barut BA, Cochran MA, et al. Lack of a role of interleukin-11 in the growth of multiple myeloma. *Leuk Res* 1992;16:247–252.

80. Lu ZY, Zhang XG, Rodriguez C, et al. Interleukin-10 is a proliferation factor but not a differentiation factor for human myeloma cells. *Blood* 1995;85:2521.

81. Georgii-Hemming P, Stromberg T, Janson ET, et al. The somatostatin analog octreotide inhibits growth of interleukin-6 (IL-6)-dependent and IL-6-independent human multiple myeloma cell lines. *Blood* 1999;93:1724–1731.

82. Choi SJ, Cruz JC, Craig F, et al. Macrophage inflammatory protein 1-alpha is a potential osteoclast stimulatory factor in multiple myeloma. *Blood* 2000;96:671–675.

83. Tinhofer I, Marschitz I, Henn T, et al. Expression of functional interleukin-15 receptor and autocrine production of interleukin-15 as mechanisms of tumor propagation in multiple myeloma. *Blood* 2000;95:610–618.

84. Dankar B, Padro T, Leo R, et al. Vascular endothelial growth factor and interleukin-6 in paracrine tumor-stromal cell interactions in multiple myeloma. *Blood* 2000;95:2630–2636.

85. Bellamy W, Richter L, Frutiger Y, et al. Expression of vascular endothelial growth factor and its receptor in hematological malignancies. *Cancer Res* 1999;59:728–733.

86. Feo-Zuppardi FJ, Taylor CW, Iwato K, et al. Long-term engraftment of fresh human myeloma cells in SCID mice. *Blood* 1992;80:2843–2850.

87. Huang Y-W, Richardson JA, Tong AW, et al. Disseminated growth of a human multiple myeloma cell line in mice with severe combined immunodeficiency disease. *Cancer Res* 1993;53:1392–1396.

88. Urashima M, Chen BP, Chen S, et al. The development of a model for the homing of multiple myeloma cells to human bone marrow. *Blood* 1997;90:754–765.

89. Yaccoby S, Barlogie B, Epstein J. Primary myeloma cells growing in SCID-hu mice: a model for studying the biology and treatment of myeloma and its manifestations. *Blood* 1998;92:2908–2913.

90. Cesarman E, Chang Y, Moore PS, et al. Kaposi's sarcoma-associated herpesvirus-like DNA sequences in AIDS-related body-cavity-based lymphomas. *N Engl J Med* 1995;332:1186–1191.

91. Gao SJ, Kingsley L, Hoover DR, et al. Seroconversion to antibodies against Kaposi's sarcoma-associated herpesvirus-related latent nuclear antigens before the development of Kaposi's sarcoma. *N Engl J Med* 1996;335:233–241.

92. Moore PS, Boshoff C, Weiss RA, et al. Molecular mimicry of human cytokine and cytokine response pathway genes by KSHV. *Science* 1996;274:1739–1744.

93. Burger R, Neipel F, Fleckenstein B, et al. Human herpesvirus type 8 interleukin-6 homologue is functionally active on human myeloma cells. *Blood* 1998;91:1858–1863.

94. Berenson JR, Vescio RA. HHV-8 is present in multiple myeloma patients. *Blood* 1999; 3:3157–3166.

95. Tarte K, Chang Y, Klein B. Kaposi's sarcoma-associated herpesvirus and multiple myeloma: lack of criteria for causality. *Blood* 1999;93:3159–3163.

96. Yi Y, Ekman M, Anton D, et al. Blood dendritic cells from myeloma patients are not infected with Kaposi's sarcoma-associated herpesvirus (KSHV/HHV-8). *Blood* 1998;92:402–404.

97. Chauhan D, Bharti A, Raje N, et al. Detection of Kaposi's sarcoma herpesvirus-8 DNA sequences in multiple myeloma bone marrow stromal cells. *Blood* 1999;93:1482–1486.

98. Raje N, Gong J, Chauhan D, et al. Bone marrow and peripheral blood dendritic cells from patients with multiple myeloma are phenotypically and functionally normal. *Blood* 1999;93:1487–1495.

99. Rettig MB, Ma HJ, Vescio RA, et al. Kaposi's sarcoma-associated herpesvirus infection of bone marrow dendritic cells from multiple myeloma patients. *Science* 1997;276:1851–1854.

100. Said JW, Rettig MR, Heppner K, et al. Localization of Kaposi's sarcoma-associated herpesvirus in bone marrow biopsy samples from patients with multiple myeloma. *Blood* 1997;90:4278–4282.

101. Tisdale JF, Stewart AK, Dickstein B, et al. Molecular and serological examination of the relationship of human herpesvirus 8 to multiple myeloma: orf 26 sequences in marrow stroma are not restricted to myeloma patients and other regions of the genome are not detected. *Blood* 1998;92:2681–2687.

102. Gao S-J, Alsina M, Deng J-H, et al. Antibodies to Kaposi's sarcoma herpesvirus (human herpesvirus 8) in patients with multiple myeloma. *J Infect Dis* 1998;178:846–849.

103. Vidriales MB, Anderson KC. Adhesion of multiple myeloma cells to the bone marrow microenvironment: implications for future therapeutic strategies. *Mol Med Today* 1996;2:425–431.

104. Ahsmann EFM, Lokhorst HM, Dekker HM, et al. Lymphocyte function-associated antigen-1 expression on plasma cells correlates with tumor growth in multiple myeloma. *Blood* 1992;79:2068–2075.

105. Massellis-Smith A, Belch AR, Mant MJ, et al. Hyaluronan-dependent motility of B cells and leukemic plasma cells in blood, but not of bone marrow

plasma cells, in multiple myeloma: alternate use of receptor for hyaluronan-mediated motility (RHAMM) and CD44. *Blood* 1996;87:1891–1899.

106. Ridley RC, Xiao H, Hata H, et al. Expression of syndecan regulates human myeloma plasma cell adhesion to type I collagen. *Blood* 1993;81:767–774.

107. Teoh G, Anderson KC. Interaction of tumor and host cells with adhesion and extracellular matrix molecules in the development of multiple myeloma. *Hematol Oncol Clin North Am* 1997;11:27–42.

108. Dhodapkar MV, Kelly T, Theus A, et al. Elevated levels of shed syndecan-1 correlate with tumour mass and decreased matrix metalloproteinase-9 activity in the serum of patients with multiple myeloma. *Br J Haematol* 1997;99:368–371.

109. Dhodapkar MV, Abe E, Theus A, et al. Syndecan-1 is a multifunctional regulator of myeloma pathobiology: control of tumor cell survival, growth, and bone cell differentiation. *Blood* 1998;91:2679–2688.

110. Barille S, Akhoundi C, Collette M, et al. Metalloproteinases in multiple myeloma: production of metalloproteinase-9 (MMP-9), activation of proMMP-2, and induction of MMP-1 by myeloma cells. *Blood* 1997;90:1649–1655.

111. Huang YW, Richardson JA, Vitetta ES. Anti-CD54 (ICAM-1) has anti-tumor activity in SCID mice with human myeloma cells. *Cancer Res* 1995;55:610–616.

112. Damiano JS, Cress AE, Hazlehurst LA, et al. Cell adhesion mediated drug resistance (CAM-DR): role of integrins and resistance to apoptosis in human myeloma cell lines. *Blood* 1999;93:1658–1667.

113. Ribatti D, Vacca A, Nico B, et al. Bone marrow angiogenesis and mast cell density increase simultaneously with progression of human multiple myeloma. *Br J Cancer* 1999;79:451–455.

114. Vacca A, Ribatti D, Presta M, et al. Bone marrow neovascularization, plasma cell angiogenic potential, and matrix metalloproteinase-2 secretion parallel progression of human multiple myeloma. *Blood* 1999;93:3064–3073.

115. Munshi N, Wilson CC, Penn MJ, et al. Angiogenesis in newly diagnosed multiple myeloma: poor prognosis with increased microvessel density in bone marrow biopsies. *Blood* 1998;92[Suppl]:98a.

116. Rajkumar SV, Fonseca R, Witzig TE, et al. Bone marrow angiogenesis in patients achieving complete response after stem cell transplantation for multiple myeloma. *Leukemia* 1999;13:469–472.

117. Aoki Y, Jaffe ES, Chang Y, et al. Angiogenesis and hematopoiesis induced by Kaposi's sarcoma-associated herpesvirus-encoded interleukin-6. *Blood* 1999;93:4034–4043.

118. Mesri EA. Inflammatory reactivation and angiogenicity of Kaposi's sarcoma-associated herpesvirus/HHV8: a missing link in the pathogenesis of acquired immunodeficiency syndrome-associated Kaposi's sarcoma. *Blood* 1999;93:4031–4033.

119. Corral LG, Haslett PAJ, Muller GW, et al. Differential cytokine modulation and T cell activation by two distinct classes of thalidomide analogues that are potent inhibitors of TNF-a. *J Immunol* 1999;163:380–386.

120. Raje N, Anderson KC. Thalidomide: a revival story. *N Engl J Med* 1999;341:1606–1609.

121. Singhal S, Mehta J, Desikan R, et al. Anti-tumor activity of thalidomide in refractory multiple myeloma. *N Engl J Med* 1999;341:1565–1571.

122. Dewald GW, Kyle RA, Hicks GA, et al. The clinical significance of cytogenetic studies in 100 patients with multiple myeloma, plasma cell leukemia, or amyloidosis. *Blood* 1985;6:380–390.

123. Gould J, Alexanian R, Goodacre A, et al. Plasma cell karyotype in multiple myeloma. *Blood* 1988;71:453–456.

124. Sawyer JR, Waldron JA, Jagannath S, et al. Cytogenic findings in 200 patients with multiple myeloma. *Cancer Genet Cytogenet* 1995;82:41.

125. Drach J, Angerler J, Schuster J, et al. Interphase fluorescence in situ hybridization identifies chromosomal abnormalities in plasma cells from patients with monoclonal gammopathy of undetermined significance. *Blood* 1995;86:3915.

126. Flatctif M, Zandecki M, Lai JL. Interphase fluorescence in situ hybridization (FISH) as a powerful tool for the detection of aneuploidy in multiple myeloma. *Leukemia* 1995;9:2109.

127. Zandecki M, Obein V, Bernardi F, et al. Monoclonal gammopathy of undetermined significance: chromosome changes are a common finding within bone marrow plasma cells. *Br J Haematol* 1995;90:693.

128. Chesi M, Bergsagel PL, Brents LA, et al. Dysregulation of cyclin D1 by translocation into an IgH gamma switch region in two multiple myeloma cell lines. *Blood* 1996;88:674.

129. Chesi M, Nardini E, Brents LA, et al. Frequent translocation t(4;14)(p16.3;q32.3) in multiple myeloma: association with increased expression and activating mutations of fibroblast growth factor receptor 3. *Nat Genet* 1997;16:260–264.

130. Chesi M, Nardini E, Lim RSC, et al. The t(4;14) translocation in myeloma dysregulates both *FGFR3* and a novel gene, *MMSET*, resulting in IgH/MMSET hybrid transcripts. *Blood* 1998;92:3025–3034.

131. Corradini P, Ladetto M, Voena C, et al. Mutational activation of N- and K-ras oncogenes in plasma cell dyscrasias. *Blood* 1993;81:2708–2713.

132. Neri A, Murphy L, Cro L, et al. RAS oncogene mutation in multiple myeloma. *J Exp Med* 1989;170:1715–1725.

133. Ong F, Nieuwkoop JA, de Groot-Swings GM, et al. Bcl-2 protein expression is not related to short survival in multiple myeloma. *Leukemia* 1995;9:1282.

134. Pettersson M, Jernberg-Wiklund H, Larsson LG, et al. Expression of the bcl-2 gene in human multiple myeloma cell lines and normal plasma cells. *Blood* 1992;79:495.

135. Tian E, Gazitt Y. The role of p53, bcl-2 and bax network in dexamethasone induced apoptosis in multiple myeloma cell lines. *Int J Oncol* 1996;8:719.

136. Gauthier ER, Piche L, Lemieux G, et al. Role of bcl-XL in the control of apoptosis in murine myeloma cells. *Cancer Res* 1996;56:1451.

137. Schwarze MMK, Hawley RG. Prevention of myeloma cell apoptosis by ectopic bcl-2 expression or interleukin-6 mediated up-regulation of bcl-XL. *Cancer Res* 1995;55:2262.

138. Portier M, Moles JP, Mazars GR, et al. P53 and RAS gene mutations in multiple myeloma. *Oncogene* 1992;7:2539.

139. Juge-Morineau N, Mellerin MP, Francois S, et al. High incidence of deletions but infrequent inactivation of the retinoblastoma gene in human myeloma cells. *Br J Haematol* 1995;91:664.

140. Urashima M, Ogata A, Chauhan D, et al. Transforming growth factor β1: differential effects on multiple myeloma versus normal B cells. *Blood* 1996;87:1928–1938.

141. Kawano MM, Mahmoud MS, Huang N. Cyclin D1 and p16INK4A are preferentially expressed in immature and mature myeloma cells, respectively. *Br J Haematol* 1997;99:131–138.

142. Tasaka T, Berenson J, Vescio R, et al. Analysis of the p16INKA.P15INK4B and p18INK4C genes in multiple myeloma. *Br J Haematol* 1997;96:98–102.

143. Urashima M, Teoh G, Ogata A, et al. Characterization of p16^{INK4A} expression in multiple myeloma and plasma cell leukemia. *Clin Cancer Res* 1997;3:2173–2179.

144. Dilworth D, Liu L, Stewart AK, et al. Germline *CDKN2A* mutation implicated in predisposition to multiple myeloma. *Blood* 2000;95:1869–1871.

145. Bataille R, Durie BGM, Grenier J, et al. Prognostic factors and staging in multiple myeloma: a reappraisal. *J Clin Oncol* 1986;4:80–87.

146. Durie BGM, Salmon SE. A clinical staging system for multiple myeloma: correlation of measured cell mass with presenting clinical features, response to treatment and survival. *Cancer* 1975;36:842–854.

147. Gassmann W, Pralle H, Haferlach T, et al. Staging systems for multiple myeloma: a comparison. *Br J Haematol* 1985;59:703–711.

148. Greipp PR. Prognosis in myeloma. *Mayo Clin Proc* 1994;69:895–902.

149. Alexanian R, Balcerzak S, Bonnet JD, et al. Prognostic factors in multiple myeloma. *Cancer* 1975;36:1192–1201.

150. Merlini G, Waldenstrom JG, Jayakar SD. A new improved clinical staging system for multiple myeloma based on analysis of 123 patients. *Blood* 1980;55:1011–1019.

151. Carbone PP. A study of the relationship of survival to various clinical manifestations and anomalous protein type in 112 patients. *Am J Med* 1967;42:937–948.

152. Prognostic features in the third MRC myelomatosis trial. Medical Research Council's Working Party on Leukaemia in Adults. *Br J Cancer* 1980;42:831–840.

153. Cavo M, Galieni P, Zuffa E, et al. Prognostic variables and clinical staging in multiple myeloma. *Blood* 1989;74:1774–1780.

154. Greipp PR, Raymond NM, Kyle RA, et al. Multiple myeloma: significance of plasmablastic subtype in morphological classification. *Blood* 1985;65:305–310.

155. Greipp PR, Leong T, Bennett JM, et al. Plasmablastic morphology—an independent prognostic factor with clinical and laboratory correlates: Eastern Cooperative Oncology Group (ECOG) myeloma trial E9486 report by the ECOG myeloma laboratory group. *Blood* 1998;91:2501–2507.

156. Brenning G, Simonsson B, Kallander C, et al. Pretreatment serum beta 2-microglobulin in multiple myeloma. *Br J Haematol* 1986;62:85–93.

157. Durie BGM, Stock-Novack D, Salmon SE, et al. Prognostic value of pretreatment serum beta-2 microglobulin in myeloma: a Southwest Oncology Group study. *Blood* 1990;75:823–830.

158. Taniwaki M, Nishida K, Takashima T, et al. Nonrandom chromosomal rearrangements of 14q32.3 and 19p13.3 and preferential deletion of 1p in 21 patients with multiple myeloma and plasma cell leukemia. *Blood* 1994;84:2283–2290.

159. Zojer N, Konigsberg R, Ackermann J, et al. Deletion of 13q14 remains an independent adverse prognostic variable in multiple myeloma despite its frequent detection by interphase fluorescence *in situ* hybridization. *Blood* 2000;95:1925–1930.

160. Konigsberg R, Zojer N, Ackermann J, et al. Predictive role of interphase cytogenetics for survival of patients with multiple myeloma. *J Clin Oncol* 2000;18:804–812.

161. Tricot G, Barlogie B, Jagannath S, et al. Poor prognosis in multiple myeloma is associated only with partial or complete deletions of Chr 13 or abnormalities involving 11q and not with other karyotype abnormalities. *Blood* 1995;86:4250–4256.

162. Tricot G, Sawyer JR, Jagannath S, et al. Unique role of cytogenetics in the prognosis of patients with myeloma receiving high-dose therapy and autotransplants. *J Clin Oncol* 1997;15:2659–2666.

163. Desikan R, Barlogie B, Sawyer J, et al. Results of high-dose therapy for 1000 patients with multiple myeloma: durable complete remissions and superior survival in the absence of chromosome 13 abnormalities. *Blood* 2000;95:4008–4010.

164. Avet-Loiseau H, Li J-Y, Morineau N, et al. Monosomy 13 is associated with the transition of monoclonal gammopathy of undetermined significance to multiple myeloma. *Blood* 1999;94:2583–2589.

165. Sawyer JR, Lukacs JL, Munshi N, et al. Identification of new nonrandom translocations in multiple myeloma with multicolor spectral karyotyping. *Blood* 1998;92:4269–4278.

166. Finelli P, Fabris S, Zagano S, et al. Detection of t(4;14)(p16.3;q32) chromosomal translocation in multiple myeloma by double-color fluorescent in situ hybridization. *Blood* 1999;94:724–732.

167. Durie BGM, Grogan TM. CALLA-positive myeloma: an aggressive subtype with poor survival. *Blood* 1985;66:229–232.

168. Barlogie B, Smallwood L, Smith T, et al. High serum levels of lactic dehydrogenase identify a high-grade lymphoma-like myeloma. *Ann Intern Med* 1989; 110:521–525.

169. Omede P, Tarella C, Palumbo A, et al. Multiple myeloma: reduced plasma cell contamination in peripheral blood progenitor cell collections performed after repeated high-dose chemotherapy courses. *Br J Haematol* 1997;99:685–691.

170. Cimino G, Avvisati G, Amadori S, et al. High serum IL-2 levels are predictive of prolonged survival in multiple myeloma. *Br J Haematol* 1990;75:373–377.

171. Bataille R, Boccadoro M, Klein B, et al. C-reactive protein and β-2 microglobulin produce a simple and powerful myeloma staging system. *Blood* 1992; 80:733–737.

172. Greipp PR, Gaillard JP, Kalish LA, et al. Independent prognostic value for serum soluble interleukin-6 receptor (sIL-6R) in Eastern Cooperative Oncology Group (ECOG) myeloma trial E9487. *Proc Am Soc Clin Oncol* 1993;12:404.

173. Seidel C, Borset M, Turesson I, et al. Elevated serum concentrations of hepatocyte growth factor in patients with multiple myeloma. *Blood* 1998;91:806–812.

174. Seidel C, Sundan A, Hjorth M, et al. Serum syndecan-1: a new independent prognostic marker in multiple myeloma. *Blood* 2000;95:388–392.

175. Dahl IMS, Turesson I, Holmberg E, et al. Serum hyaluron in patients with multiple myeloma: correlation with survival and Ig concentration. *Blood* 1999;93:4144–4148.

176. Witzig TE, Gertz MA, Lust JA, et al. Peripheral blood monoclonal plasma cells as a predictor of survival in patients with multiple myeloma. *Blood* 1996;88:1780–1787.

177. Rajkumar SV, Fonseca R, Lacy MA, et al. Plasmablastic morphology is an independent predictor of poor survival after autologous stem cell transplantation for multiple myeloma. *J Clin Oncol* 1999;17:1551–1557.

178. Garcia-Sanchez R, Orfao A, Gonzalez M, et al. Primary plasma cell leukemia: clinical, immunophenotypic, DNA ploidy, and cytogenetic characteristics. *Blood* 1999;93:1032–1037.

179. Blade J, Kyle RA, Greipp P. Presenting features and prognosis in 72 patients with multiple myeloma who were younger than 40 years. *Br J Haematol* 1996;93:345–351.

180. San Miguel JF, Caballero MD, Gonzales M, et al. A new staging system for multiple myeloma based on the number of S phase plasma cells. *Blood* 1995; 85:448–455.

181. Liu P, Leong T, Quam L, et al. Activating mutations of N- and K-ras in multiple myeloma show different clinical associations: analysis of the Eastern Cooperative Oncology Group phase III trial. *Blood* 1996;88:2699–2706.

182. Kay NE, Leong T, Kyle RA, et al. Circulating blood B cells in multiple myeloma: analysis and relationship to circulating clonal cells and clinical parameters in a cohort of patients entered on the Eastern Cooperative Oncology Group phase III E9486 clinical trial. *Blood* 1997;90:340–345.

183. Kyle RA. Why better prognostic factors for multiple myeloma are needed. *Blood* 1994;83:1713–1716.

184. Raaijmakers HGP, Izquierdo MAI, Lokhorst HM, et al. Lung-resistance-related protein expression is a negative predictive factor for response to conventional low but not to intensified dose alkylating chemotherapy in multiple myeloma. *Blood* 1998;91:1029–1036.

185. Mundy GR, Bertolini DR. Bone destruction and hypercalcemia in plasma cell myeloma. *Semin Oncol* 1986;13:291–299.

186. Bardwick PA, Zvaifler NJ, Gill GN, et al. Plasma cell dyscrasia with polyneuropathy, organomegaly, endocrinopathy, M protein, and skin changes: the POEMS syndrome: report on two cases and a review of the literature. *Medicine* 1980;59:311–322.

187. Miralles GD, O'Fallon JR, Talley NJ. Plasma-cell dyscrasia with polyneuropathy: the spectrum of POEMS syndrome. *N Engl J Med* 1992;327:1919–1923.

188. Lacey DL, Timms E, Tan HL, et al. Osteoprotegerin ligand is a cytokine that regulates osteoclast differentiation and activation. *Cell* 1998;93:165–176.

189. Alsina M, Boyce BF, Devlin R, et al. Development of an *in vivo* model of human multiple myeloma bone disease. *Blood* 1996;87:1495–1501.

190. Hjorth-Hansen H, Borset M, Seidel C, et al. The JJN-3 cell line gives multiple myeloma with bone disease in SCID mice. *Blood* 1996;88:387a.

191. Harley JB, Schilling A, Glidewell O. Ineffectiveness of fluoride therapy in multiple myeloma. *N Engl J Med* 1972;286:1283–1288.

192. Siris ES, Sherman WH, Baquiran DC, et al. Effects of dichloromethylene diphosphonate on skeletal mobilization of calcium in multiple myeloma. *N Engl J Med* 1980;302:310–315.

193. Lahtinen R, Laasko M, Palva I, et al. Randomised, placebo-controlled multicentre trial of clodronate in multiple myeloma. *Lancet* 1992;340:1049–1052.

194. Berenson J, Lichtenstein A, Porter L, et al. Pamidronate disodium reduces the occurrence of skeletal events in patients with advanced multiple myeloma. *N Engl J Med* 1996;334:488–493.

195. Berenson JR, Lichtenstein A, Porter L, et al. Long-term pamidronate treatment of advanced multiple myeloma patients reduces skeletal events. *J Clin Oncol* 1998;16:593–602.

196. Bloomfield DJ. Should bisphosphonates be part of the standard therapy of patients with multiple myeloma or bone metastases from other cancers? An evidence-based review. *J Clin Oncol* 1998;16:1218–1225.

197. Dhodapkar MV, Singh J, Mehta J, et al. Anti-myeloma activity of pamidronate in vivo. *Br J Haematol* 1998;103:530–532.

198. Hyghes DE, Wright KR, Uy HL. Bisphosphonates promote apoptosis in murine osteoclasts in vitro and in vivo. *J Bone Miner Res* 1995;10:1478–1487.

199. Berenson JR. Phase-1 clinical study of a new bisphosphonate, zoledronate (CGP-42446), in patients with osteolytic bone metastases. *Blood* 1996;88[Suppl 1]:586a.

200. Lipton A. Phase 11 study of the bisphosphonate, zoledronate in patients with osteolytic lesions. In: *Second international conference: cancer-induced bone diseases*. Davos, Switzerland, March 27–29, 1999 (abst 48).

201. Lipton A. The effects of the bisphosphonate, zoledronic acid, when administered as a short intravenous infusion in patients with bone metastases: a phase-1 study. In: *American Society of Clinical Oncology annual meeting*. Denver, CO, May 17–20, 1997 (abst 848).

202. Pruzanski W, Watt JG. Serum viscosity and hyperviscosity syndrome in IgG multiple myeloma. *Ann Intern Med* 1972;77:853–860.

203. Lindsley H, Teller D, Noonan B, et al. Hyperviscosity syndrome in multiple myeloma: a reversible, concentration-dependent aggregation of the myeloma protein. *Am J Med* 1973;54:682–688.

204. Twomey JJ. Infections complicating multiple myeloma and chronic lymphocytic leukemia. *Arch Intern Med* 1973;132:562–565.

205. Jacobsen DR, Zolla-Pazner S. Immunosuppression and infection in multiple myeloma. *Semin Oncol* 1986;13:282–290.

206. Salmon SE, Samal BA, Hayes DM, et al. Role of gammaglobulin for immunoprophylaxis in multiple myeloma. *N Engl J Med* 1967;277:1336–1340.

207. Gilleece MH, Anderson KC. Multiple myeloma: guarding against infection. *Infect Med* 2000;17:500–504.

208. Oken MM, Pomeroy C, Weisdorf D, et al. Prophylactic antibiotics for the prevention of early infection in multiple myeloma. *Am J Med* 1996;100:624–628.

209. Torra R, Blade J, Cases A, et al. Patient with multiple myeloma requiring long term dialysis: presenting features, response to therapy, and outcome in a series of 20 patients. *Br J Haematol* 1995;91:854–859.

210. Stone MJ, Frendel EP. The clinical spectrum of light chain myeloma: a study of 35 patients with special reference to the occurrence of amyloidosis. *Am J Med* 1975;58:601–619.

211. Gallo G, Picken M, Buxbaum J, et al. The spectrum of monoclonal immunoglobulin deposition disease associated with immunocytic dyscrasias. *Semin Hematol* 1989;26:234–245.

212. Gallo G. Renal complications of B cell dyscrasias. *N Engl J Med* 1991;324:1889–1890.

213. Solomon A, Weiss DT, Kattine AA. Nephrotoxic potential of Bence Jones proteins. *N Engl J Med* 1991;324:1845–1851.

214. McBride W, Jackman JD, Gammon RS, et al. High output cardiac failure in patients with multiple myeloma. *N Engl J Med* 1988;319:1651–1653.

215. Beguin Y, Yerna M, Loo M, et al. Erythropoiesis in multiple myeloma: defective red cell production due to inappropriate production. *Br J Haematol* 1992;82:648.

216. Cazzola M, Messinger D, Battistel V, et al. Recombinant human erythropoietin in the anemia associated with multiple myeloma or non Hodgkin's lymphoma: dose finding and identification of prognostic factors. *Blood* 1995;86:4446.

217. Ludwig H, Fritz E, Kotzmann H, et al. Erythropoietin treatment of anemia associated with multiple myeloma. *N Engl J Med* 1990;322:1693–1699.

218. Osterborg A, Boogaerts MÁ, Cimino R, et al. Recombinant human erythropoietin in transfusion-dependent anemic patients with multiple myeloma and non-Hodgkin's lymphoma—a randomized multicenter study. *Blood* 1996;87:2675–2682.

219. Roper AH, Gorson KC. Neuropathies associated with paraproteinemia. *N Engl J Med* 1998;338:1601–1607.

220. Latov N, Sherman WH, Nemni R, et al. Plasma-cell dyscrasia and peripheral neuropathy with a monoclonal antibody to peripheral nerve myelin. *N Engl J Med* 1980;303:618–621.

221. Gonzalez F, Trujillo JM, Alexanian R. Acute leukemia in multiple myeloma. *Ann Intern Med* 1977;86:440–443.

222. Bergsagel DE, Bailey AJ, Langley GR, et al. The chemotherapy of plasma cell myeloma and the incidence of acute leukemia. *N Engl J Med* 1979;301:743–748.

223. Stegman R, Alexanian R. Solid tumors in multiple myeloma. *Ann Intern Med* 1979;90:780–782.

224. Chronic Leukemia-Myeloma Task Force, National Cancer Institute: Proposed guidelines for protocol studies II: plasma cell myeloma. *Cancer Chemother Rep* 1973;4:145–158.

225. Salmon SE, Haut A, Bonnet JD, et al. Alternating combination chemotherapy and levamisole improves survival in multiple myeloma: a Southwest Oncology Group study. *J Clin Oncol* 1983;1:453–461.

226. Kyle RA. Newer approaches to the therapy of multiple myeloma. *Blood* 1990;76:1678–1679.

227. Bergsagel DE. Use a gentle approach for refractory myeloma patients. *J Clin Oncol* 1988;6:757–758.

228. Oken MM. Standard treatment of multiple myeloma. *Mayo Clin Proc* 1996; 69:781–786.

229. Bergsagel DE. Is aggressive chemotherapy more effective in the treatment of plasma cell myeloma? *Eur J Cancer Clin Oncol* 1989;25:159–161.

230. Blade J, San Miguel JF, Alcala A. Alternating combination VCMP/VBAP chemotherapy versus melphalan/prednisone in the treatment of multiple myeloma: a randomized multicentric study of 487 patients. *J Clin Oncol* 1993;11:1165–1171.

231. Durie BGM, Dixon DO, Carter S, et al. Improved survival duration with combination chemotherapy induction for multiple myeloma: a Southwest Oncology Group study. *J Clin Oncol* 1986;4:1227–1237.

232. Samson D, Gaminara E, Newland A, et al. Infusion of vincristine and doxorubicin with oral dexamethasone as first-line therapy for multiple myeloma. *Lancet* 1989;2:882–885.

233. Alexanian R, Dimopoulos MA, Delasalle K, et al. Primary dexamethasone treatment of multiple myeloma. *Blood* 1992;80:887–890.

234. Salmon SE, Crowley JJ, Grogan TM, et al. Combination chemotherapy, glucocorticoids, and interferon alpha in the treatment of multiple myeloma: a Southwest Oncology Group study. *J Clin Oncol* 1994;12:2405–2414.

235. Oken MM, Harrington DP, Abramson N, et al. Comparison of melphalan and prednisone with vincristine, carmustine, melphalan, cyclophosphamide, and prednisone in the treatment of multiple myeloma—results of Eastern Cooperative Oncology Group study E2479. *Cancer* 1997;79:1561–1567.

236. Gregory WM, Richards MA, Malpas JS. Combination chemotherapy versus melphalan and prednisolone in the treatment of multiple myeloma: an overview of published trials. *J Clin Oncol* 1992;10:334–342.

237. Combination chemotherapy versus melphalan plus prednisone as treatment for multiple myeloma: an overview of 6,633 patients from 27 randomized trials. Myeloma Trialists' Collaborative Group. *J Clin Oncol* 1998;16:3832–3842.

238. Buzaid AC, Durie BGM. Management of refractory myeloma: a review. *J Clin Oncol* 1988;6:889–905.

239. Barlogie B, Smith L, Alexanian R. Effective treatment of advanced multiple myeloma refractory to alkylating agents. *N Engl J Med* 1984;310:1353–1356.

240. Monconduit M, Le Loet X, Bernard JF, et al. Combination chemotherapy with vincristine, doxorubicin, dexamethasone for refractory or relapsing multiple myeloma. *Br J Haematol* 1986;63:599–601.

241. Sheehan T, Judge M, Parker AC. The efficacy and toxicity of VAD in the treatment of myeloma and related disorders. *Scand J Haematol* 1986;37:425–428.

242. Salmon SE, Dalton WS, Grogan TM, et al. Multidrug-resistant myeloma: laboratory and clinical effects of verapamil as a chemosensitizer. *Blood* 1991;78:44–50.

243. Sonneveld P, Schoester M, de Leeuw K. Clinical modulation of multidrug resistance in multiple myeloma: effects of cyclosporine on resistant tumor cells. *J Clin Oncol* 1994;12:1584–1591.

244. Sonneveld P. *Drug resistance in myeloma*. Sixth International Workshop on Multiple Myeloma. Boston; 1997.

245. Grogan TM, Spier CM, Salmon SE, et al. P-glycoprotein expression in human plasma cell myeloma: correlation with prior chemotherapy. *Blood* 1993;81:490–495.

246. Barlogie B, Valasquez WS, Alexanian R, et al. Etoposide, dexamethasone, cytarabine, and cisplatin in vincristine, doxorubicin and dexamethasone-refractory myeloma. *J Clin Oncol* 1989;7:1514–1517.

247. Kraut EH, Crowley JJ, Wade JL, et al. Evaluation of topotecan in resistant relapsing multiple myeloma: a Southwest Oncology Group study. *J Clin Oncol* 1998;16:589–592.

248. Hideshima T, Richardson P, Chauhan D, et al. The proteosome inhibitor PS-341 overcomes apoptotic resistance mechanisms in human multiple myeloma cells. *Cancer Res* 2001;61:3071–3076.

249. Portier M, Zhang XG, Caron E, et al. Gamma-interferon in multiple myeloma: inhibition of interleukin 6 dependent myeloma cell growth and downregulation of IL-6 receptor expression in vitro. *Blood* 1993;81:3076–3082.

250. Interferon-alpha 2b added to melphalan-prednisone for initial and maintenance therapy in multiple myeloma: a randomized, controlled trial. The Nordic Myeloma Study Group. *Ann Intern Med* 1996;124:212–222.

251. Ludwig H, Cohen AM, Polliack A, et al. Interferon-alpha for induction and maintenance in multiple myeloma: results of two multicenter randomized trials and summary of other studies. *Ann Oncol* 1995;6:467–476.

252. Montuoro A, De Rosa L, De Blasio A, et al. Alpha-2a-interferon/melphalan/prednisone versus melphalan/prednisone in previously untreated patients with multiple myeloma. *Br J Haematol* 1990;76:365–368.

253. Osterborg A, Bjorkholm M, Bjoreman M, et al. Natural interferon-α in combination with melphalan/prednisone versus melphalan/prednisone in the treatment of multiple myeloma stages II and III: a randomized study from the Myeloma Group of Central Sweden. *Blood* 1993;81:1428–1434.

254. Mandelli F, Avvisati G, Amadori S, et al. Maintenance treatment with recombinant interferon alpha-2b in patients with multiple myeloma responding to conventional induction chemotherapy. *N Engl J Med* 1990;322:1430–1434.

255. Browman GP, Bergsagel DP, Sicheri D, et al. Randomized trial of interferon maintenance in multiple myeloma: a study of the National Cancer Institute of Canada Clinical Trials Group. *J Clin Oncol* 1995;13:2354–2360.

256. Cunningham D, Powles R, Malpas J, et al. A randomized trial of maintenance interferon following high-dose chemotherapy in multiple myeloma: long-term follow-up results. *Br J Haematol* 1998;102:495–502.

257. Westin J. Interferon therapy during the plateau phase of multiple myeloma: an update of a Swedish multicenter study. *Sem Oncol* 1991;18:37–40.

258. Peest D, Deicher H, Coldeway R, et al. Melphalan and prednisone versus vincristine, BCNU, adriamycin, melphalan and dexamethasone induction chemotherapy and interferon maintenance treatment in multiple myeloma: current results of a multicenter trial. *Onkologie* 1990;13:458–460.

259. Ludwig H, Fritz E, Neuda J, et al. Patient preferences for interferon-alpha in multiple myeloma. *J Clin Oncol* 1997;15:1672–1679.

260. Zee B, Cole B, Li T, et al. Quality adjusted time without symptoms or toxicity analysis of interferon maintenance in multiple myeloma. *J Clin Oncol* 1998;16:2834–2839.

261. MacKenzie MR, Wold H, George C, et al. Consolidation hemibody radiotherapy following induction combination chemotherapy in high-tumor-burden multiple myeloma. *J Clin Oncol* 1992;10:1769–1774.

262. Thomas PJ, Daban A, Bontoux D. Double hemibody irradiation in chemotherapy-resistant multiple myeloma. *Cancer Treat Rep* 1984;68:1173–1175.

263. Anderson KC. Who benefits from high dose therapy for multiple myeloma? *J Clin Oncol* 1995;13:1291–1296.

264. Kovasics TJ, Delaly A. Intensive treatment strategies in multiple myeloma. *Sem Hematol* 1997;34[Suppl 1]:49–60.

265. Bensinger WI, Demirer T, Buckner CD, et al. Syngeneic marrow transplantation in patients with multiple myeloma. *Bone Marrow Transplant* 1996;18:527–531.

266. Gahrton G, Tura S, Ljungman P, et al. Allogeneic bone marrow transplantation in multiple myeloma. *N Engl J Med* 1991;325:1267–1273.

267. Gahrton G, Tura S, Ljungman P, et al. Prognostic factors in allogeneic bone marrow transplantation for multiple myeloma. *J Clin Oncol* 1995;13:1312–1322.

268. Bjorkstrand B, Ljungman P, Svensson H, et al. Allogeneic bone marrow transplantation versus autologous stem cell transplantation in multiple myeloma: a retrospective case-matched study from the European Group for Blood and Marrow Transplantation. *Blood* 1996;88:4711–4718.

269. Bensinger WI, Buchner CD, Anasetti C, et al. Allogeneic marrow transplantation for multiple myeloma: an analysis of risk factors on outcome. *Blood* 1996;88:2787–2793.

270. Cavo M, Bandini G, Benni M, et al. High dose busulfan and cyclophosphamide are an effective conditioning regimen for allogeneic bone marrow transplantation in chemosensitive multiple myeloma. *Bone Marrow Transplant* 1998;22:27–32.

271. Schlossman SF, Alyea E, Orsini E, et al. Immune based strategies to improve hematopoietic stem cell transplantation in multiple myeloma. In: Dicke KA, Keating A, eds. *Autologous marrow and blood transplantation.* Charlottesville, VA: Carden Jennings Publishing Co., 1999:207–221.

272. Schlossman RL, Anderson KC. Bone marrow transplantation in multiple myeloma. In: Jones R, ed. *Current opinion in oncology*, vol. 11. Philadelphia: Lippincott Williams & Wilkins, 1999:102–108.

273. Seiden M, Schlossman R, Andersen J, et al. Monoclonal antibody-purged bone marrow transplantation therapy for multiple myeloma. *Leuk Lymphoma* 1995;17:87–93.

274. Soiffer RJ, Murray C, Mauch P, et al. Prevention of graft-versus-host disease by selective depletion of CD6-positive T lymphocytes from donor bone marrow. *J Clin Oncol* 1992;10:1191–1200.

275. Corradini P, Voena C, Tarella C, et al. Molecular and clinical remissions in multiple myeloma: role of autologous and allogeneic transplantation of hematopoietic cells. *J Clin Oncol* 1999;17:208–215.

276. Martinelli G, Terragna C, Zamagni E, et al. Molecular remission after allogeneic or autologous transplantation of hematopoietic stem cells for multiple myeloma. *J Clin Oncol* 2000;18:2273–2281.

277. Cavo M, Terragna C, Martinelli G, et al. Molecular monitoring of minimal residual disease in patients in long-term complete remission after allogeneic stem cell transplantation for multiple myeloma. *Blood* 2000;96:355–357.

278. Willems P, Verhagen O, Segeren C, et al. Consensus strategy to quantitate malignant cells in myeloma patients is validated in a multicenter study. *Blood* 2000;96:63–70.

279. Antin JH. Graft-versus-leukemia: no longer an epiphenomenon. *Blood* 1993;82:2273–2277.

280. Collins R, Shpilberg O, Drobyski W, et al. Donor leukocyte infusions in 140 patients with relapsed malignancy after allogeneic bone marrow transplantation. *J Clin Oncol* 1997;15:433–444.

281. Kolb H-J, Schattenberg A, Goldman JM, et al. Graft-versus-leukemia effect of donor lymphocyte transfusions in marrow grafted patients. *Blood* 1995;86:2041–2050.

282. Champlin R, Ho W, Gajewski J, et al. Selective depletion of CD8+ T lymphocytes for prevention of graft-versus-host disease after allogeneic bone marrow transplantation. *Blood* 1990;76:418–423.

283. Tricot G, Vesole DH, Jagannath S, et al. Graft-versus myeloma effect: proof of principle. *Blood* 1996;87:1196–1198.

284. Verdonck LF, Lokhorst HM, Dekker AW, et al. Graft-versus-myeloma effect in two cases. *Lancet* 1996;347:800–801.

285. Munshi NC, Govindarajan R, Drake R, et al. Thymidine kinase (TK) gene-transduced human lymphocytes can be highly purified, remain fully functional and are killed efficiently with ganciclovir. *Blood* 1997;89:1334–1340.

286. Alyea EP, Soiffer RJ, Canning C, et al. Toxicity and efficacy of defined doses of CD4+ donor lymphocytes for treatment of relapse after allogeneic bone marrow transplant. *Blood* 1998;91:3671–3680.

287. Orsini E, Alyea EP, Schlossman R, et al. Changes in T cell receptor repertoire associated with graft-versus-tumor effect and graft-versus-host disease in patients with relapsed multiple myeloma receiving donor lymphocyte infusions. *Bone Marrow Transplant* 2000;25:623–632.

288. Orsini E, Alyea EP, Chillemi A, et al. Conversion to full donor chimerism following donor lymphocyte infusion is associated with disease response in patients with multiple myeloma. *Biol Blood Marrow Transplant* 2000;6:375–386.

289. Kwak LW, Taub DD, Duffey PL, et al. Transfer of myeloma idiotype-specific immunity from an actively immunized marrow donor. *Lancet* 1995;345:1016–1020.

290. Wimperis JZ, Brenner MK, Prentice HG, et al. Transfer of a functioning humoral immune system in transplantation of T-lymphocyte-depleted bone marrow. *Lancet* 1986;1:339.

291. Wimperis JZ, Brenner MK, Prentice HG, et al. B cell development and regulation after T cell-depleted marrow transplantation. *J Immunol* 1987;138:2445.

292. Harousseau J-L, Attal M. The role of autologous hematopoietic stem cell transplantation in multiple myeloma. *Semin Hematol* 1997;34[Suppl 1]:61–66.

293. Attal M, Harousseau JL, Stoppa AM, et al. Autologous bone marrow transplantation versus conventional chemotherapy in multiple myeloma: a prospective, randomized trial. *N Engl J Med* 1996;335:91–97.

294. Blade J, San Miguel JF, Fontanillas M, et al. Survival of multiple myeloma patients who are potential candidates for early high-dose therapy intensification/autotransplantation and who were conventionally treated. *J Clin Oncol* 1996;14:2167–2173.

295. Fermand J-P, Ravaud P, Chevret S, et al. High-dose therapy and autologous peripheral blood stem cell transplantation in multiple myeloma: up-front or rescue treatment? Results of a multicenter sequential randomized clinical trial. *Blood* 1998;92:3131–3136.

296. Lenhoff S, Hjorth M, Holmberg E, et al. Impact on survival of high-dose therapy with autologous stem cell support in patients younger than 60 years with newly diagnosed multiple myeloma: a population-based study. *Blood* 2000;95:7–11.

297. Anderson KC, Barut BA, Ritz J, et al. Monoclonal antibody purged autologous bone marrow transplantation therapy for multiple myeloma. *Blood* 1991;77:712–720.

298. Anderson KC, Anderson J, Soiffer R, et al. Monoclonal antibody-purged bone marrow transplantation therapy for multiple myeloma. *Blood* 1993;82:2568–2576.

299. Schiller G, Vescio R, Freytes C, et al. Transplantation of CD34 positive peripheral blood progenitor cells following high dose chemotherapy for patients with advanced multiple myeloma. *Blood* 1995;86:390–397.

300. Gazitt Y, Reading CC, Hoffman R, et al. Purified CD34+ Lin– Thy+ stem cells do not contain clonal myeloma cells. *Blood* 1995;86:381–389.

301. Facon T, Harousseau J-L, Maloisel F, et al. Stem cell factor in combination with filgrastim after chemotherapy improves peripheral blood progenitor cell yield and reduces apheresis requirements in multiple myeloma patients: a randomized, controlled trial. *Blood* 1999;94:1218–1225.

302. Szczepek AJ, Bergsagel PL, Axelsson L, et al. CD34+ cells in the blood of patients with multiple myeloma express CD19 and IgH mRNA and have patient-specific IgH VDJ gene rearrangements. *Blood* 1997;89:1824–1833.

303. Schiller G, Vescio R, Lee M, et al. Long-term outcome of a phase II study of autologous CD34+ peripheral blood stem cell transplantation as treatment for multiple myeloma. In: Griffin JD, ed. *American Society of Hematology thirty-eighth annual meeting*. Orlando: American Society of Hematology, 1996:483a.

304. Vescio RA, Schiller GJ, Stewart AK, et al. Quantitative assessment of myeloma peripheral blood and bone marrow tumor burden in patients undergoing autologous transplantation. In: Griffin JD, ed. *American Society of Hematology thirty-eighth annual meeting*. Orlando: American Society of Hematology, 1996:641a.

305. Vescio R, Schiller GJ, Stewart AK, et al. Multicenter phase III trial to evaluate CD34+ selected versus unselected autologous peripheral blood progenitor cell transplantation in multiple myeloma. *Blood* 1999;93:1858–1868.

306. Stewart AK, Vescio R, Schiller G, et al. Purging of autologous peripheral blood stem cells from multiple myeloma patients using CD34+ selection does not improve overall or progression free survival following high dose chemotherapy: results of a multicenter randomized controlled trial *J Clin Oncol* 2001;19:3771–3779.

307. Lemoli RM, Martinelli G, Zamagni E, et al. Engraftment, clinical, and molecular follow-up of patients with multiple myeloma who were reinfused with highly purified CD34+ cells to support single or tandem high-dose chemotherapy. *Blood* 2000;95:2234–2238.

308. Barlogie B, Jagannath S, Desikan KR, et al. Total therapy with tandem transplants for newly diagnosed multiple myeloma. *Blood* 1999;93:55–65.

309. Vesole DH, Tricot G, Jagannath S, et al. Autotransplants in multiple myeloma: what have we learned? *Blood* 1996;88:838–847.

310. Giralt S, Weber D, Colome M, et al. Phase I trial of cyclosporine-induced autologous graft-versus-host disease in patients with multiple myeloma undergoing high-dose chemotherapy with autologous stem-cell rescue. *J Clin Oncol* 1997;15:667–673.

311. Qing Y, Osterborg A. Idiotype-specific T cells in multiple myeloma: targets for an immunotherapeutic intervention? *Med Oncol* 1996;13:1–7.

312. Bergenbrant B, Yiu Q, Osterborg A, et al. Modulation of antiidiotypic immune response by immunization with the autologous M component protein multiple myeloma patients. *Br J Haematol* 1996;92:840–846.

313. Hsu FJ, Benike C, Fagnoni F, et al. Vaccination of patients with B-cell lymphoma using autologous antigen-pulsed dendritic cells. *Nat Med* 1996;2:52–58.

314. Tai YT, Teoh G, Shima Y, et al. Isolation and characterization of human multiple myeloma cell enriched populations. *J Immunol Methods* 2000;235:11–19.

315. Dou Q, Li B. Proteosome inhibitors as potential novel anticancer agents. *Drug Resist Updates* 1999;2:215–223.

316. Hideshima T, Chauhan D, Shima Y, et al. Thalidomide and its analogues overcome drug resistance of human multiple myeloma cells to conventional therapy. *Blood* 2000;96:2943–2950.

317. Ogata A, Chauhan D, Teoh G, et al. Interleukin-6 triggers cell growth via the *ras*-dependent mitogen-activated protein kinase cascade. *J Immunol* 1997;159:2212–2221.

318. Lokhorst HM, Schattenberg JJ, Cornelissen JJ, et al. Donor lymphocyte infusions are effective in relapsed multiple myeloma after allogeneic bone marrow transplantation. *Blood* 1997;90:4206–4211.

319. Teoh G, Chen L, Urashima M, et al. Adenovirus vector-based purging of multiple myeloma cells. *Blood* 1998;92:4591–4601.

320. Trojan A, Schultze JL, Witzens M, et al. Immunoglobulin framework-derived peptides function as cytotoxic T-cell epitopes commonly expressed in B-cell malignancies. *Nat Med* 2000;6:667–672.

321. Vonderheide RH, Hahn WC, Schultze JL, et al. The telomerase catalytic subunit is a widely expressed tumor-associated antigen recognized by cytotoxic T lymphocytes. *Immunity* 1999;10:673–679.

322. Maecker B, Sherr DH, Shen C, et al. Targeting universal tumor antigens with cytotoxic T cells: potential of CYP1B1 for broadly applicable antigen-specific immunotherapy. *Blood* 1999;94[Suppl]:438a.

323. Schultze JL, Anderson KC, Gilleece MH, et al. A pilot study of combined immunotherapy with autologous adoptive tumour-specific T-cell transfer, vaccination with CD40-activated malignant B cells and interleukin 2. *Br J Haematol* 2001;113:455–460.

324. Raje N, Gong J, Chauhan D, et al. Bone marrow and peripheral blood dendritic cells from patients with multiple myeloma are phenotypically and functionally normal despite the detection of Kaposi's sarcoma herpesvirus gene sequences. *Blood* 1999;93:1487–1495.

325. Osterborg A, Yi Q, Henriksson L, et al. Idiotype immunization combined with granulocyte-macrophage colony-stimulating factor in myeloma patients induced type I, major histocompatibility complex-restricted, CD8 and CD4 specific T cell responses. *Blood* 1998;91:2459–2466.

326. Massaia M, Borrione P, Battaglio S, et al. Idiotype vaccination in human myeloma: generation of tumor-specific immune responses after high-dose chemotherapy. *Blood* 1999;94:673–683.

327. Reichardt VL, Okada CY, Liso A, et al. Idiotype vaccination using dendritic cells after autologous peripheral blood stem cell transplantation for multiple myeloma—a feasibility study. *Blood* 1999;93:2411–2419.

328. Stevenson FK, Zhu D, King CA, et al. Idiotypic DNA vaccines against B cell lymphoma. *Immunol Rev* 1995;145:211.

329. Van Baren N, Brasseur F, Godelaine D, et al. Genes encoding tumor-specific antigens are expressed in human myeloma cells. *Blood* 1999;94:1156–1164.

330. Prince HM, Dessureault S, Gallinger S, et al. Efficient adenovirus mediated-gene expression in malignant human plasma cells: relative lymphoid cell resistance. *Exp Hematol* 1998;26:27–36.

331. Stevenson FK, Bell AJ, Cusack R, et al. Preliminary studies for an immunotherapeutic approach to the treatment of human myeloma using chimeric anti-CD38 antibody. *Blood* 1991;77:1071–1079.

332. Ogata A, Anderson KC. Therapeutic strategies for inhibition of interleukin-6 mediated multiple myeloma cell growth. *Leuk Res* 1996;20:303–307.

333. Dinota A, Barbieri L, Gobbi M, et al. An immunotoxin containing momordin suitable for bone marrow purging in multiple myeloma patients. *Br J Cancer* 1989;60:315–319.

334. Siegall CB, Chaudhary VK, Fitzgerald DJ, et al. Cytotoxic activity of an interleukin-6 Pseudomonas exotoxin fusion protein on human myeloma cells. *Proc Natl Acad Sci U S A* 1988;85:9738–9742.

335. Goldmacher VS, Bourret LA, Levine BA, et al. Anti-CD38-blocked ricin: an immunotoxin for the treatment of multiple myeloma. *Blood* 1994;84:3017–3025.

336. Grossbard M, Fidias P, Kinsella J. Anti-B4 blocked ricin: a phase II trial for 7 day continuous infusion in patients with multiple myeloma. *Br J Haematol* 1998;102:509–515.

337. Ozaki S, Kosaka M, Wakatsuki S, et al. Immunotherapy of multiple myeloma with a monoclonal antibody directed against a plasma cell-specific antigen, HM1.24. *Blood* 1997;90:3179–3186.

338. Ozaki S, Kosaka M, Wakahara Y, et al. Humanized anti-HM1.24 antibody mediates myeloma cell cytotoxicity that is enhanced by cytokine stimulation of effector cells. *Blood* 1999;93:3922–3930.

339. Moulopoulos LA, Dimopoulos MA, Weber D, et al. Magnetic resonance imaging in the staging of solitary plasmacytoma of bone. *J Clin Oncol* 1993;11:1311–1315.

340. Frassica DA, Frassica FJ, Schray MF, et al. Solitary plasmacytoma of bone: Mayo Clinic Experience. *Int J Radiat Oncol Biol Phys* 1989;16:43–48.

341. Knowling MA, Harwood AR, Bergsagel DE. Comparison of extramedullary plasmacytomas with solitary and multiple plasma cell tumors of bone. *J Clin Oncol* 1983;1:255–262.

342. Wiltshaw E. The natural history of extramedullary plasmacytoma and its relation to solitary myeloma of bone and myelomatosis. *Medicine* 1976;55:217–238.

343. Aviles A, Huerta J, Zepeda G, et al. Serum beta 2 microglobulin in solitary plasmacytoma. *Blood* 1990;76:1663.

344. Dimopoulos MA, Goldstein J, Fuller L, et al. Curability of solitary bone plasmacytoma. *J Clin Oncol* 1992;10:587–590.

345. Kyle RA, Garton JP. The spectrum of IgM monoclonal gammopathy in 430 cases. *Mayo Clin Proc* 1987;62:719–731.

346. Dimopoulos MA, Alexanian R. Waldenström's macroglobulinemia. *Blood* 1994;83:1452–1459.

347. Kyle RA, Anderson KC. A tribute to Jan Waldenstrom. *Blood* 1997;89:4245–4247.

348. Groves FD, Travis LB, Devesa SS, et al. Waldenström's macroglobulinemia: incidence patterns in the United States, 1988–1994. *Cancer* 1998;82:1078–1081.

349. Herrinton LJ, Weiss NS. Incidence of Waldenström's macroglobulinemia. *Blood* 1993;82:3148–3150.

350. Ogmundsdottir HM, Johannesson GM, Sveinsdottir S, et al. Familial macroglobulinaemia: hyperactive B-cells but normal natural killer function [published erratum appears in *Scand J Immunol* 1995;41:650]. *Scand J Immunol* 1994;40:195–200.

351. Calasanz MJ, Cigudosa JC, Odero MD, et al. Cytogenetic analysis of 280 patients with multiple myeloma and related disorders: primary breakpoints and clinical correlations. *Genes Chromosomes Cancer* 1997;18:84–93.

352. Palka G, Spadano A, Geraci L, et al. Chromosome changes in 19 patients with Waldenström's macroglobulinemia. *Cancer Genet Cytogenet* 1987;29:261–269.

353. Matutes E, Owusu-Ankomah K, Morilla R, et al. The immunological profile of B-cell disorders and proposal of a scoring system for the diagnosis of CLL. *Leukemia* 1994;8:1640–1645.

354. Smith BR, Robert NJ, Ault KA. In Waldenström's macroglobulinemia the quantity of detectable circulating monoclonal B lymphocytes correlates with clinical course. *Blood* 1983;61:911–914.

355. Wagner SD, Martinelli V, Luzzatto L. Similar patterns of V kappa gene usage but different degrees of somatic mutation in hairy cell leukemia, prolymphocytic leukemia, Waldenström's macroglobulinemia, and myeloma. *Blood* 1994;83:3647–3653.

356. Aoki H, Takishita M, Kosaka M, et al. Frequent somatic mutations in D and/or JH segments of Ig gene in Waldenström's macroglobulinemia and chronic lymphocytic leukemia (CLL) with Richter's syndrome but not in common CLL. *Blood* 1995;85:1913–1919.

357. Klein U, Goossens T, Fischer M, et al. Somatic hypermutation in normal and transformed human B cells. *Immunol Rev* 1998;162:261–280.

358. Johansson B, Waldenstrom J, Hasselblom S, et al. Waldenström's macroglobulinemia with the AML/MDS-associated t(1;3)(p36;q21). *Leukemia* 1995;9:1136–1138.

359. Gertz MA, Kyle RA, Noel P. Primary systemic amyloidosis: a rare complication of immunoglobulin M monoclonal gammopathies and Waldenström's macroglobulinemia. *J Clin Oncol* 1993;11:914–920.

360. Facon T, Brouillard M, Duhamel A, et al. Prognostic factors in Waldenström's macroglobulinemia: a report of 167 cases. *J Clin Oncol* 1993;11:1553–1558.

361. Gobbi PG, Bettini R, Montecucco C, et al. Study of prognosis in Waldenström's macroglobulinemia: a proposal for a simple binary classification with clinical and investigational utility. *Blood* 1994;83:2939–2945.

362. Martelli MF, Falini B, Firenze A, et al. Acute leukemia complicating Waldenström's macroglobulinemia. *Haematologica* 1981;66:303–310.

363. Dimopoulos MA, Kantarjian H, Estey E, et al. Treatment of Waldenström macroglobulinemia with 2-chlorodeoxyadenosine. *Ann Intern Med* 1993;118:195–198.

364. Foran J, Rohatiner AZS, Coiffier B, et al. Multicenter phase II study of fludarabine phosphate for patients with newly diagnosed lymphoplasmacytoid lymphoma, Waldenström macroglobulinemia and mantle cell lymphoma. *J Clin Oncol* 1999;17:546–553.

365. Leblond V, Ben-Othman T, Deconinck E, et al. Activity of fludarabine in previously treated Waldenström's macroglobulinemia: a report of 71 cases. *J Clin Oncol* 1998;16:2060–2064.

366. Dimopoulos MA, Panayiotidis P, Moulopoulos LA, et al. Waldenström's macroglobulinemia: clinical features, complications, and management. *J Clin Oncol* 2000;18:214–226.

367. Quesada JR, Alexanian R, Kurzrock R, et al. Recombinant interferon gamma in hairy cell leukemia, multiple myeloma, and Waldenström's macroglobulinemia. *Am J Hematol* 1988;29:1–4.

368. Rotoli B, De Renzo A, Frigeri F, et al. A phase II trial on alpha-interferon (alpha IFN) effect in patients with monoclonal IgM gammopathy. *Leuk Lymphoma* 1994;13:463–469.

369. Legouffe E, Rossi JF, Laporte JP, et al. Treatment of Waldenström's macroglobulinemia with very low doses of alpha interferon. *Leuk Lymphoma* 1995;19:337–342.

370. Desikan R, Dhodapkar M, Siegel D, et al. High-dose therapy with autologous haemopoietic stem cell support for Waldenström's macroglobulinaemia. *Br J Haematol* 1999;105:993–996.

371. Humphrey JS, Conley CL. Durable complete remission of macroglobulinemia after splenectomy: a report of two cases and review of the literature. *Am J Hematol* 1995;48:262–266.

372. Takemori N, Hirai K, Onodera R, et al. Durable remission after splenectomy for Waldenström's macroglobulinemia with massive splenomegaly in leukemic phase. *Leuk Lymphoma* 1997;26:387–393.

373. Byrd JC, White CA, Link B, et al. Rituximab therapy in previously treated Waldenström's macroglobulinemia: preliminary evidence of activity. *Ann Oncol* 1999;10:1525–1527.

374. Franklin EC, Lowenstein J, Bigelow B, et al. Heavy chain disease—a new disorder of serum globulin: report of a case. *Am J Med* 1964;37:332.

375. Kyle RA. The heavy chain diseases. In: Wiernick PH, Canellos GP, Kyle RA, et al., eds. *Neoplastic diseases of the blood*. New York: Churchill Livingstone, 1985:593.

376. Guardia J, Rubies-Prat J, Gallart MT, et al. The evolution of alpha heavy chain disease. *Am J Med* 1976;60:596.

377. Kyle RA, Greipp PR. Amyloidosis (AL)—clinical and laboratory features in 229 cases. *Mayo Clin Proc* 1983;58:665–683.

378. Hawjkins PN, Lavender JP, Pepys MB. Evaluation of systemic amyloidosis by scintigraphy with 123I labelled serum amyloid P component. *N Engl J Med* 1990;323:508–513.

379. Kyle RA, Gertz MA, Greipp PR, et al. Long-term survival (10 years or more) in 30 patients with primary amyloidosis. *Blood* 1999;93:1062–1066.

380. Kyle RA, Greipp PR, Garton JP, et al. Primary systemic amyloidosis: comparison of melphalan/prednisone versus colchicine. *Am J Med* 1985;79:708–716.

381. Cohen AS, Rubinow A, Anderson JJ, et al. Survival of patients with primary (AL) amyloidosis: colchicine-treated cases from 1976 to 1983 compared with cases seen in previous years (1961 to 1973). *Am J Med* 1987;82:1182–1190.

382. Kyle RA, Gertz MA, Greipp PR, et al. A trial of three regimens for primary amyloidosis: colchicine alone, melphalan and prednisone, and melphalan, prednisone, and colchicine. *N Engl J Med* 1997;336:1200–1207.

383. Gertz MA, Lacy MQ, Lust JA, et al. Prospective randomized trial of melphalan and prednisone versus vincristine, carmustine, melphalan, cyclophosphamide, and prednisone in the treatment of primary systemic amyloidosis. *J Clin Oncol* 1999;17:262–267.

384. Comenzo RL, Vosburgh E, Simms RW, et al. Dose-intensive melphalan with blood stem cell support for the treatment of AL amyloidosis: one-year follow-up in five patients. *Blood* 1996;88:2801–2806.

385. Comenzo RL, Vosburgh E, Falk RH, et al. Dose-intensive melphalan with blood stem-cell support for the treatment of AL (amyloid light-chain) amyloidosis: survival and responses in 25 patients. *Blood* 1998;19:3662–3670.

386. Comenzo RL, Vosburgh E, Falk RH, et al. Dose-intensive melphalan with blood stem-cell support for the treatment of AL amyloidosis: survival and responses in 25 patients. *Blood* 1998;91:3662.

387. Comenzo RL, Wally J, Kica G, et al. Stem cell contamination predicts posttransplant survival in AL amyloidosis. *Blood* 1999;94[Suppl 1]:575a.

CHAPTER 30

Histiocytoses and Disorders of the Reticuloendothelial System

Robert J. Arceci and Gregory A. Grabowski

Disorders referred to as *histiocytoses* or *lymphohistiocytoses* represent a heterogeneous and enigmatic collection of disease states. When the description of clinical syndromes precedes our understanding of the biology of disease, nomenclature and classification schemes are often based on anecdotal descriptions associated with historic eponyms. This has been especially true of the histiocytoses. The history of our evolving understanding of these disorders has resulted in discoveries that have gradually linked the treatment of patients to biologically based classifications and more targeted therapies. This chapter focuses on the primary histiocytic disorders but includes lymphohistiocytic syndromes that are related by virtue of their clinical presentation or histopathology.

THE HISTIOCYTE AND THE MONONUCLEAR PHAGOCYTIC SYSTEM: ORIGINS AND OVERVIEW

The generic term *histiocyte* derives from the Latin *histion* meaning "little web" and *kytos* meaning "cell." Thus, histiocytes are resident tissue (i.e., the web) mononuclear phagocytes and represent a heterogeneous group of cell types with some distinct as well as overlapping histologic, biochemical, and functional characteristics. Together, these different cell types comprise the mononuclear phagocytic system, the cellular foundation of innate immunity and a critical part of the phagocytic and antigen-presenting arm of the host's immune system.

After Metchnikov's historic description of the phagocytic reaction of cells in larval starfish in the late 1800s, the groundwork was set for the further conceptualization of what Aschoff termed the *reticuloendothelial system* (RES) (1). *Reticulo* refers to the "lattice or reticulum of cytoplasmic extensions" which the cells comprising this system form. *Endothelial* originally referred to the fact that the RES cells were commonly noted to reside near vascular endothelial cells (2).

Thus, from the beginning, the macrophage has played a central position in the RES. Macrophages, originally described because of their ability to ingest large (hence *macro*, meaning "large" and *phage* meaning "to eat") foreign or excess material, were easily distinguished from polymorphonuclear granulocytes by both morphology and functional characteristics. The functional role of macrophages in antigen presentation would only be discovered later. The heterogeneity of this group of cells became more apparent as additional cell types were added to this lineage, such as peritoneal and alveolar macrophages,

Kupffer's cells, synovial cells, osteoclasts, and microglial cells of the central nervous system (CNS). By the late 1950s, more than two dozen types of cells referred to as *macrophages* had been named, leading Gall to refer to the RES as the "Tower of Babel"(3). In the late 1960s, in an attempt to resolve some of the issues surrounding the proliferation of RES member cells, van Furth introduced the term *mononuclear phagocytic system* (4). This naming was felt to better describe the histologic and functional characteristics of the RES.

When in 1868 Paul Langerhans, then a medical student in Berlin, described epidermal dendritic cells, another critical group of cells was added to the RES or mononuclear phagocytic system (5,6). Although Langerhans' initial description of these cells as neuronal was mistaken, he and others subsequently corrected the incorrect lineage assignment. However, it was only in the 1960s and 1970s that an essential, functional role for these dendritic cells in antigen presentation (especially viral, cancer, and self-antigens) to immunologically naïve T lymphocytes was determined (7,8).

Similarly, additional data demonstrated that macrophages also have the ability to process and present antigens from foreign organisms, especially bacteria, in the context of major histocompatibility complex protein expression to T lymphocytes. This interplay and cross-talk between macrophages and T lymphocytes results in proliferation of both cell types as well as the recruitment of other cell types (e.g., polymorphonuclear granulocytes and eosinophils) along with the release of a wide variety of cytokines. This additional characteristic expanded the role of macrophages to more than just scavenging.

The cellular components of the RES or MPS thus share a closely linked history as well as histologic, biochemical, and functional characteristics, while at the same time maintaining some important distinctions. The clinical importance of the relationships and biologic characteristics of these different cell types is based on their ability to cause or modify disease when they are primary causes of disease or when involved secondarily.

CRITICAL CELL TYPES: LINEAGE AND DISTINGUISHING MARKERS

The wide variety of cell types termed *histiocytes* or cell types belonging to the MPS originate from hematopoietically derived stem cells (9). This is certainly true for the two major groups of

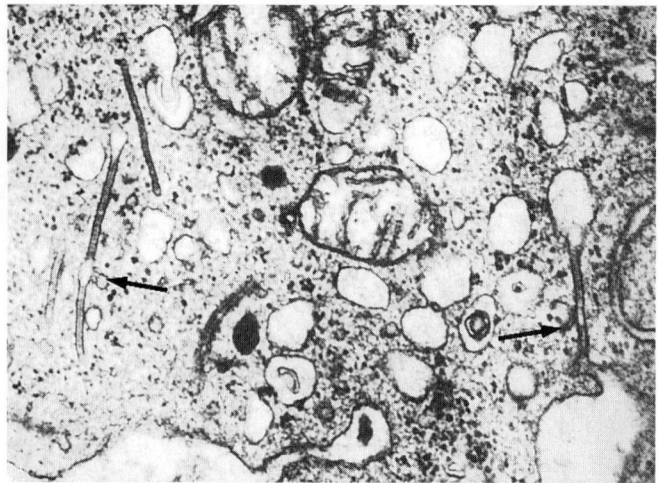

Figure 30-1. Birbeck granules in the cytoplasm of a Langerhans' cell observed at the electron microscopic level. (Courtesy of Dr. Antonio Perez, Department of Pathology, Children's Hospital, Boston.)

cells involved in the histiocytic disorders (i.e., tissue macrophages and dendritic cells, particularly the Langerhans' cell). However, there remain significant areas of controversy, such as whether dermal and follicular dendritic cells are descendents of hematopoietic or soft tissue mesenchymal precursors (9–11). The existence of lymphoid stem cell–derived as well as myeloid-derived dendritic cells has added further complexity to lineage relationships (10). Furthermore, there have been a number of examples in which monocytes or macrophages can be converted into dendritic cells after exposure to different cytokine combinations (12–14). Although such lineage conversions have been primarily described using *in vitro* cell culture methods, *in vivo* examples of cells with intermediate phenotypes have been described (15).

Although macrophages and dendritic cells share many biochemical, immunologic, and functional features, they also express enough significant differences to warrant a more detailed comparison. Such a comparison is not purely academic in that it forms the basis for a pathologic diagnosis and classification of the diverse proliferative histiocytic disorders.

Monocytes and their tissue counterparts, macrophages, are large mononuclear cells with gray-blue cytoplasm characterized by many vacuoles representing their intense lysosomal activity. Langerhans' cells are also large mononuclear cells but usually display a slightly eosinophilic to clear cytoplasm, which contains little vacuolization. They display long cytoplasmic extensions or processes from which the term *dendritic cell* derives. The nucleus of Langerhans' cells is often folded and indented and has an irregular, fine chromatin pattern. Langerhans' cells are located primarily in the skin and buccal, gingival, esophageal, and vaginal mucosa as well as in bone marrow, spleen, thymus, lymph nodes, and other organs.

Ultrastructural analysis of Langerhans' cells has revealed characteristic intracytoplasmic organelles called *Birbeck granules* or *X bodies* (16). These organelles are rarely found in the

TABLE 30-1. Distinguishing Characteristics of Some Histiocyte Cell Types

Marker	Macrophage	Pre-Langerhans'	Langerhans'	Interdigitating DC	Dermal Dendrocyte
Cytoplasmic					
Nonspecific esterase	+	±	±	±	±
AP	+	±	±	±	±
α-Antitrypsin	+	–	–	–	–
S-100	±	+	+	+	–
Lysozyme	±	–	–	–	–
Peanut agglutinin	D/C	?	H/D	H/D	?
Birbeck granule	–	–	+	–	–
Surface					
CD1a	±	+	+	–	–
CMRF-44	±	?	+ to +++	+ to +++	?
CMRF-56	±	?	– to +++	– to +++	?
CD14	+	–	–	–	–
CD68	++	–	±	±	+
CD115 (M-CSF R)	+	–	–	–	–
CD64 (Fc R)	++				
CD32 (Fc R)	++	?	+	+	?
CD16 (Fc R)	+	?	–	–	?
CD40 (Costim.)	+	?	± to ++	± to ++	?
CD80 (Costim.)	+	?	± to ++	± to ++	?
CD86 (Costim.)	+	?	± to ++	± to ++	?
HLA-A,B,C	+ to ++	?	+ to +++	+ to +++	?
HLA-DR	+ to ++	?	+ to ++	+ to ++	?
Factor XIII	–	–	–	–	+
Fascin[a]	–	?	–	+	+
Physiology					
Phagocytic	++++	?	++	++	?
T-cell stimulation	++	?	++++	++++	?

NOTE: This table is not meant to be all-inclusive but rather to highlight some of the more commonly used distinguishing characteristics of several of the important cell types in the reticuloendothelial system related to the histiocytic diseases. The symbols "+" and "–" are shown to indicate a positive or negative reaction. A "?" indicates that insufficient data are available to definitively conclude a positive or negative result. In addition, a "±" sign indicates that variability may exist or that only a subpopulation may express the antigen. A "+ to +++" or "+++ to +" indicates that expression is up-regulated or down-regulated respectively depending on the physiologic conditions.
[a]As discussed in Schmitz L, Favara BE. Nosology and pathology of Langerhans' cell histiocytosis. *Hematol Oncol Clin North Am* 1998;12:221.
AP, acid phosphatase; Costim., costimulatory; D/C, diffuse/cytoplasmic; Fc, fragment; H/D, halo/dot; M-CSF, macrophage colony-stimulating factor; NSE, nonspecific esterase.
Adapted from Arceci RJ. The histiocytoses: the fall of the Tower of Babel. *Eur J Cancer* 1999;35:747–769.

nucleus. Birbeck granules are rod-shaped structures with a central, striated line; they occasionally terminate in a vesicular dilation, giving them a racquet shape (Fig. 30-1). They are variable in length (190–360 nm) with a uniform width of approximately 33 nm. The Birbeck granules arise secondary to the process of receptor-mediated endocytosis, because cell-surface antigens have been localized within them. Monocytes and non-Langerhans' macrophages lack Birbeck granules. Thus, ultrastructural analysis of biopsy specimens can be particularly useful in distinguishing the type of histiocyte present in a lesion.

Unlike other tissue macrophages, Langerhans' cells are negative for lysozyme, α_1-antitrypsin, α_1-antichymotrypsin, aminopeptidase, peroxidase, alkaline phosphatase, α-naphthol-chloroacetate esterase, and β-glucuronidase. Langerhans' cells are positive for adenosine triphosphatase and strongly express α-mannosidase, which is expressed to a much lesser degree by other tissue macrophages (16).

Several other cell markers aid in distinguishing Langerhans' cells from other tissue macrophages when studied in formalin-fixed, paraffin-embedded specimens. The staining pattern for peanut agglutinin (PNA) in Langerhans' cells shows a unique pattern of paranuclear and cell-surface deposition of reaction products, whereas other tissue macrophages show a diffuse reaction (16). Langerhans' cells also show a positive reaction when stained with anti–S-100 antibodies, whereas other tissue macrophages are usually negative (16,17). The Langerhans' cell contains the S-100 β-subunit. Monocytes and macrophages may express the S-100 α-subunit but not the β-subunit (16,17). S-100 is a calcium-binding complex that was initially identified in brain tissue. Most Langerhans' cells are CD1a antigen positive, although this marker is also found on early T lymphocytes in the thymus. Macrophages are negative for CD1a (18–20).

Conversely, monocytes and macrophages are positive for the nonspecific carcinoembryonic cross-reacting antigen, whereas Langerhans' cells are negative (16,17). Most macrophages stain positive for the CD4 antigen, whereas Langerhans' cells are negative or show variable expression. Macrophages are strongly positive for nonspecific esterase and the cell-surface marker, CD11c (Leu-M5). Both the Langerhans' cell and the macrophage usually express class II major histocompatibility molecules, which are involved in the presentation of foreign antigens during an immune response. A comparison of some of the distinguishing features of these different cell types is shown in Table 30-1. Suitable handling of biopsy specimens for both electron microscopic and immunocytochemistry analysis, including frozen tissue sections, is critical in the evaluation of lesions that may represent disorders of the histiocyte. Through a combination of histologic, immunochemical, and immunophenotypic methods performed by experienced pathology laboratory professionals, it is usually possible to discriminate which type of histiocyte is predominantly involved in the disease process. The possibility of further defining lineage type with the use of RNA and DNA microarray methodologies should offer even greater ability to distinguish subsets of these related but distinct cell types.

PATHOPHYSIOLOGY AND CLASSIFICATION OF THE COMMON HISTIOCYTIC DISORDERS

From the shared and distinct characteristics of normal macrophages and dendritic cells, it is possible to understand the varied pathophysiologic consequences and clinical manifestations that result from disorders involving these cell types. For example, the proliferation and activation of macrophages or dendritic cells can result in the swelling and inflammation due to

the release of proinflammatory cytokines and the recruitment of other cell types, such as granulocytes, lymphocytes, and eosinophils. This activation and recruitment of monocytes and macrophages as well as lymphocytes and granulocytes result in a mixture of reactive cells, that is, granuloma formation. Evidence of hemophagocytosis resulting from the interaction of the macrophage Fc receptor for immunoglobulin G (IgG) present on hematopoietic cells. Hemophagocytosis is a relatively nonspecific finding but is frequently observed in histiocytic disorders. The release of cytokines can produce localized tissue damage as well as fever, skin rashes, and hypotension in addition to a variety of alterations in immune responses. For example, bone lesions, usually osteolytic, may result from the secretion of interleukin-1 (IL-1) and prostaglandin E_2 by macrophages (21). The localization and trafficking of these different cell types allows for nearly every organ to be potentially involved in disorders of the MPS.

The proliferative histiocytoses may be the result of the dysregulated response to some as yet unknown inciting agent or antigen. All are characterized by the proliferation of histiocytes as well as other cell types involved in the immune response. The primary type of involved histiocyte may depend on the inciting agent or on where it enters the body, or it may possibly be a result of a cell type–specific lesion in the histiocyte itself or the action of lymphocytes regulating its biologic behavior. Most classification schema for the proliferative histiocytic disorders have been based on the distinctive phenotypic and functional characteristics of the primary cells involved in the pathogenesis of the disease. Thus, the promulgation of classification systems for these disorders has developed along with the improved definition of involved cell types, their function and, more recently, their underlying genetic defects (22). This history also provides for a better understanding of current classification schema.

During the late 1800s and early 1900s, several patients were described who had distinct but overlapping clinical phenotypes (23). In 1865, Smith described what may be the first patient with histiocytosis—an infant with lytic lesions of the skull (24). He did not, however, refer to the disorder as *histiocytosis*. This case was followed by a description by Dr. Alfred Hand from Philadelphia in 1893 of a 3-year-old child with failure to thrive, exophthalmos, hepatosplenomegaly, a generalized scabieslike rash, lymphadenopathy, lytic skull lesions, and diabetes insipidus (25). Similar patients were described in the early 1900s by Drs. Schüller, Christian, and Kay (26–28). In the early 1920s, Dr. Letterer at the University of Wurzburg in Germany described an infant with histiocytosis complicated by diffuse rash, hepatosplenomegaly, anemia, thrombocytopenia, cough, and tachypnea (29). This type of fulminant and fatal disease was further described approximately 10 years later by Dr. Siwe. The diverse presentation of histiocytosis led to descriptions such as *eosinophilic granuloma* for isolated bone lesions and *Hand-Schüller-Christian disease* for young patients with chronic, relapsing disease, characteristically exemplified by exophthalmos, lytic skull lesions, and diabetes insipidus. The fulminant form of the disease was termed *Letterer-Siwe disease*. However, the Boston pathologist Dr. Sidney Farber, made the important conclusion that these different clinical descriptions were all characterized by a similar cellular infiltrate (30). Dr. Lichtenstein proposed that these three different forms of histiocytosis represented different clinical manifestations of the same disease, which he called *histiocytosis X* (31). Dr. Nezelof made the further important observation that the presence of "X bodies" or "Birbeck granules" was observed in the histiocyte accumulating in histiocytosis X as well as in normal Langerhans' cells (32). This sequence of historic events is important in that much of the literature concerning histiocytosis is based on these eponyms as well as the later realization that this disorder was possibly secondary to proliferation and activation of Langerhans' cells.

To this end, the observation made a year before Lichtenstein proposed the name *histiocytosis X*, Farquhar and Clairveaux reported an infant with a familial and rapidly fatal form of histiocytosis closely resembling Letterer-Siwe disease but characterized by profound hemophagocytosis (33). They termed this disease *familial hemophagocytic reticulosis*. Nine years later, in 1961, Nelson reported a similar patient but with the addition of extensive involvement of the CNS (34). In 1963, MacMahon used the term *familial erythrophagocytic lymphohistiocytosis* (FEL) to describe this disorder and distinguish it from Letterer-Siwe disease (35). The macrophage was also noted to be more prominent in the lymphohistiocytic infiltrates than dendritic cells. The first insight into the etiology of FEL, besides the fact that it was often inherited as an autosomal-recessive condition, was the similarity of it to graft-versus-host disease that was pointed out by Miller and Nezelof in the mid-1960s (36). They also made the connection that FEL was likely to be caused by an underlying immunodeficiency. Nonfamilial forms of the disease, often associated with infections (particularly viral illness) as well as malignancies, led to the terms infection-associated hemophagocytic syndrome (IAHS), viral-associated hemophagocytic syndrome (VAHS) and malignancy-associated hemophagocytic syndrome (MAHS).

TABLE 30-2. Classification Schema of Histiocytoses

Dendritic-cell or related disorders
Langerhans' cell histiocytosis
Juvenile xanthogranuloma and related diseases
Solitary histiocytoma (dendritic-cell phenotype)
Secondary dendritic-cell disorders (e.g., association with Hodgkin's
    disease)
Macrophage or related disorders
Hemophagocytic syndromes
    Primary or familial hemophagocytic lymphohistiocytosis
    Secondary or nonfamilial hemophagocytic lymphohistiocytosis
        Infection-associated hemophagocytic syndrome
        Malignancy-associated hemophagocytic syndrome
        Hemophagocytic syndromes associated with miscellaneous causes
            Total parenteral nutrition
            Chemical exposures (e.g., beryllium, zirconium, diphenylhy-
                dantoin)
            Juvenile arthritis
            Immunosuppressive therapy
Sinus histiocytosis with massive lymphadenopathy (Rosai-Dorfman dis-
    ease)
Solitary histiocytoma (macrophage phenotype)
Multicentric reticulohistiocytosis (frequently associated with arthritis)
Generalized eruptive histiocytoma
Malignant disorders
Monocytic leukemia (FAB classification M5)
Monocytic sarcoma
Histiocytic sarcoma
    Dendritic-cell phenotype
    Macrophage cell phenotype
Storage disorders involving the mononuclear phagocytic system
Inherited
    Sphingolipidoses
    Mucopolysaccharidoses
    Mucolipodoses
Acquired
    Associated with high turnover states of hematopoietic cells (e.g.,
        chronic myelogenous leukemia)

Adapted from Favara BE, Feller AC, Pauli M, et al. Contemporary classification of histiocytic disorders. The WHO Committee On Histiocytic/Reticulum Cell Proliferations. Reclassification Working Group of the Histiocyte Society. *Med Pediatr Oncol* 1997;29:157.

The realization that the two major types of histiocytosis were primarily the result of proliferation and activation of Langerhans' cells or macrophages (i.e., non-Langerhans' cells), led the Histiocyte Society to propose a classification schema in 1987 (37). This schema designated these disorders as *class I* or *Langerhans' cell histiocytosis (LCH)*, which included such historic terms as *eosinophilic granuloma, Hand-Schüller-Christian disease*, and *Letterer-Siwe disease*, or *class II* or *non-Langerhans' cell histiocytosis*, primarily represented by hemophagocytic lymphohistiocytoses, such as FEL and IAHS. Class III was termed *malignant histiocytosis*, comprised by malignant disorders of the monocyte or dendritic lineages.

In the lysosomal as well as other types of "storage diseases," the normal phagocytic function of the macrophage is disrupted as a result of an inherited enzymatic defect resulting in abnormal intracellular accumulation of undegraded lysosomal substrates. Such macrophages function poorly and accumulate in multiple organ systems, resulting in displacement of normal organ architecture with subsequent enlargement and dysfunction. These inherited disorders of the histiocyte are referred to as *lysosomal storage diseases* and represent a separate class.

Occasionally, similar overloading of macrophages with lipids can occur in patients with chronic myelogenous leukemia or hemolytic disorders caused by the excessive turnover of hematopoietic precursors and their progeny. This acquired form of lipoidosis results when the ability of the macrophage to metabolize normal phagocytosed material is exceeded and not caused by an inherent defect of the macrophage. Such inherited and acquired storage disorders are not primary proliferative histiocytoses secondary to immune dysregulation. Nevertheless, they result in organ dysfunction caused by the malfunction of the macrophage as well as the disruption of organ architecture and function.

Further scientific investigations have thus extended the classification of these disorders to account for the distinguishing biologic features of the involved histiocytes as well as information concerning the underlying causes and etiology (Table 30-2) (11,22,38). The importance of distinguishing the different types of members of the mononuclear phagocytic system is underscored by recent improvements in outcome due to therapies directed to specific subtypes of these disease classes. This chapter focuses on the primary disorders associated with each category.

LANGERHANS' CELL HISTIOCYTOSIS

Etiology and Pathogenesis

The annual incidence of LCH is approximately 3–7 cases per million people (39–41). Men are more frequently affected than women. Although most cases of LCH have been reported in children, there is a growing realization that this disease can occur at any age (22,42). There have been no significant associations of LCH in terms of seasonal variation or geographic or racial clustering. Such observations have been used to argue against an obvious infectious or genetic etiology for LCH. However, several epidemiology studies have demonstrated some interesting clinical associations in patients with LCH (40,43). For example, a case-control study involving over 450 patients with LCH revealed significant odds ratio for postnatal infections, diarrhea and vomiting, and medication usage in patients with multisystem LCH. Thyroid disease in the patient or in the family of patients was associated with single-system LCH (44). Through retrospective reviews of the literature, a higher association than would be expected by change has been observed for LCH with various malignancies (45–47). For example, LCH has been observed in association with acute lymphoblastic leukemia (ALL), acute myelogenous leukemia (AML), Hodgkin's disease, non-Hodgkin's lymphoma, and a variety of solid tumors. Of interest, LCH often is observed after treatment for ALL, particularly T-lineage leukemia. In contrast, AML has more frequently been observed after treatment for LCH (45–49). These observations have led clinical investigators to propose that patients with LCH may have a predisposition for developing both LCH and various malignancies (45–47). Although such a suggestion is intriguing, there has not been a detailed study of such relations in large populations of people.

Nevertheless, this type of suggestion led to the further investigation of whether there were instances of familial LCH. These studies have identified several sets of identical twins who have had LCH (50–57). These cases usually present when the twins are infants, and there is a close concordance of the onset of LCH between the twins. Several examples of fraternal twins have also been identified, but the disease usually occurs at an older age, and there is much less concordance of the time of onset of LCH in the twins (50). The occurrence of LCH in parents and their children as well as among cousins or other relatives has also been observed (50). The estimated frequency of familial LCH has been proposed to be less than 2% of all cases, although the percentage is not based on a large number of cases (50). The data involving identical twins could be explained by the development of LCH in one twin followed by the transplacental transfer of the disease *in utero*, similar to that which has been observed in congenital leukemia (58–61). An alternative explanation, however, is that there was a common environmental infectious or toxic exposure. However, the development of LCH in fraternal twins or in other different family members suggests that a common genetic (possibly inherited) predisposition could be responsible (62,63). Using the model of Knudsen's hypothesis or "two-hit" model for the development of retinoblastoma, the development of LCH at a young age would suggest that the individual would have possibly inherited a mutant causative gene and then acquired an inactivation of the other allele. Mutations of both alleles of such a predisposing gene would be acquired in older individuals developing LCH.

Such data and their interpretation have led investigators to examine the Langerhans' cell in LCH more closely with the intent of determining whether there was evidence that it represented an activated normal Langerhans' cell, consistent with the concept of LCH being a reactive disorder, or whether the LCH lesional cell was in fact different from its normal counterparts.

Flow cytometry studies of cells from LCH infiltrates or lesions have most consistently demonstrated a diploid DNA content (64). However, using methods to assess clonality based on X chromosome inactivation, several reports have shown that the CD1a+ LCH cells from pathologic lesions are clonal (i.e., derived from a common progenitor) (65–68). This has been demonstrated to be the case in patients with isolated eosinophilic granuloma, multifocal bone disease, isolated skin or nodal involvement, or in the system form of the LCH (65–68). There has been much debate as to whether these results prove that LCH is a malignancy. Clearly, clonality is not sufficient to make the diagnosis of cancer. There are a number of examples, such as dermatologic disorders that are clonal but are not considered cancerous (69,70). Furthermore, LCH does not show the histologic characteristics of cancer. Nevertheless, these data have suggested the possibility that the lesional LCH cell could have acquired somatic mutations in a gene or genes that regulates cell growth, survival, or proliferation. Traditional cytogenetics have not demonstrated any consistently abnormal karyotypic features (64,71), although one intriguing study reported a t(7;12) translocation from a lesion in a patient with LCH (72). This observation is particularly intriguing in that the *tel* gene, originally identified to be involved in a

child with chronic myelomonocytic leukemia, is located in the same region of chromosome 12 (73,74). It remains to be seen whether this observation is observed in other cases of LCH and whether specific genes, such as *tel*, are molecularly altered. More refined approaches to chromosomal analysis using fluorescent *in situ* hybridization have been used but have not yet ascertained any consistent chromosomal alterations (75). Further molecular approaches, possibly using allelotyping methods, may prove useful.

Despite the lack of consistent evidence for genetic alterations in LCH cells, the lesional dendritic cell does demonstrate several phenotypic changes that appear to distinguish it from its normal counterparts. For example, the pattern of staining by the lectin, PNA, is distinct in LCH lesional cells, which demonstrate strong cell-surface and perinuclear staining compared to normal Langerhans' cells, which show a low level of diffuse staining (76). Of interest, the lesional LCH cell PNA pattern is similar to that observed in the pathologic Reed-Sternberg cell of Hodgkin's disease (77,78). LCH lesional cells also express high levels of placental alkaline phosphatase in a constitutive manner compared to normal Langerhans' cells, which transiently induce placental alkaline phosphatase expression after activation (76,79). There is also evidence that the γ-interferon receptor is strongly expressed on LCH lesional cells but is not constitutively expressed on normal Langerhans' cells (76). Similarly, LCH cells constitutively express co-stimulatory receptors such as CD86 and CD80 (76). Relatively high levels of p53 nuclear antigen detection have also been reported, a characteristic commonly observed in tumor cells with p53 mutations or in cells responding to certain genotoxic exposures (80). However, no mutations have been reported in p53 from LCH lesional cells (80). The antigen expression phenotype of the LCH lesional dendritic cells is thus characteristic in many respects as a constitutively activated Langerhans' cell with some aberrant features. When the function of the LCH lesional cells was assessed in terms of antigen presentation and activation of T cells, several investigators reported the surprising results that LCH cells purified from lesions were extremely poor stimulators of T cells (76,81). Langerhans' cells similarly isolated showed potent T-lymphocyte activation capability (76,81). Whether this observation reflects an inherent inability of the LCH cell to stimulate T lymphocytes despite the activated phenotype or whether the abnormal release of immunosuppressive cytokines dampers any immunostimulatory function is currently unknown.

The concept of cytokine release by LCH cells as well as the cells recruited into lesions is another important component of this disease. *In situ* hybridization and immunocytochemical staining methods have been used. The results show a soup of cytokines expressed at high levels in LCH lesions that would be expected to result from or in the activation of T lymphocytes as well as the recruitment of macrophages, eosinophils, and granulocytes (Table 30-3) (82,83). In addition, the accumulation of IL-1 and prostaglandin E_2 and their action on osteoclasts in part explain the propensity of these lesions to result in significant bone loss (21). Patients with LCH have production of immunostimulatory and tissue-damaging cytokines at local sites; it is uncommon for them to have high systemic levels, in contrast to patients with macrophage activation syndromes. Although the expression of these various cytokines in part can be used to explain some of the pathologic and clinical features of LCH as well as providing possible targets for therapeutic interventions, their expression does not explain why wide clinical manifestations of the disease are observed in different age groups.

From epidemiologic, genetic, pathologic, and clinical data, LCH might be considered to be a "clonal proliferative neoplasm with variable clinical manifestations" (22,68). The multitude of

TABLE 30-3. Comparison of Primary Cytokine Expression in Langerhans' Cell Histiocytosis (LCH) and Hemophagocytic Lymphohistiocytosis (HLH)

Cytokine	LCH (lesional)	LCH (serum or plasma levels)	HLH[a,b,c]
IL-1	++++	±	—
IL-2[d]	++++	±	+++
IL-3[e]	++++	±	—
IL-4	++++	±	±
IL-5	–	—	—
IL-6	++++	—	++++
IL-7	—	—	—
IL-8	++++	±	—
IL-9	—	—	—
IL-10	—	—	++++
IL-11	—	—	—
IL-12	—	—	+++
IFN-α	—	—	—
IFN-γ[f]	++++	—	++++
Tumor necrosis factor–α[d]	++++	—	++++
GM-CSF[d,e]	++++	—	—
LIF[d]	++++	—	—
MIP α	—	—	++++
CD40 ligand[b,e]	++++	—	—

±, minimal to absent; +++, very positive; ++++, strongly positive; GM-CSF, granulocyte-macrophage colony-stimulating factor; IFN, interferon; IL, interleukin; LIF, leukemia inhibitory factor; MIP, macrophage inhibitory protein.
[a]All levels are systemic and determined for serum or plasma.
[b]The relative levels for these cytokines are similar in both primary and secondary HLH.
[c]CD40 receptor, soluble IL-2 receptor, soluble CD8, and IL-1 receptor antagonist are all highly expressed systemically in HLH but not in LCH. However, CD40 receptor is expressed locally at high levels by histiocytes in LCH lesions.
[d]Expressed by histiocytes.
[e]Expressed by lymphocytes.
[f]Presence in lesions disputed.
Data are based on references 82 and 83.

reported alterations of immune function in patients with LCH may be a manifestation of the extent to which abnormal Langerhans' cells impact immune regulatory pathways, rather than a primary immunodeficiency.

Diagnosis and Clinical Presentation

The diagnosis of LCH should be based on several pathologic criteria (37). First, as noted, a biopsy specimen of a lesion should have the characteristic reactive infiltrate (Fig. 30-2). In addition, the histiocytes within the lesion should have two or more of the following features: positive staining for adenosine triphosphatase, S-100 protein, α-D-mannosidase, or characteristic binding of peanut lectin. The demonstration of Birbeck granules by electron microscopy lends strong support to the diagnosis of LCH (Fig. 30-1). Positive staining for CD1a in the context of the characteristic histology is sufficient for a definitive diagnosis of LCH (37).

LCH can occur at any age, although it occurs most frequently in children between 1 and 15 years of age. The disease is most often found in patients of northern European descent and rarely in blacks. An association of LCH with the development of various malignant disorders has been suggested (45–47,84–86). A variety of tissues and organs may be affected by the disorder. The signs and symptoms vary according to the site of the lesions. Considerable variability may occur in any one patient during the course of the disease. Historically, LCH has been clinically described as three separate entities: eosinophilic granuloma, Hand-Schüller-Christian disease, and Letterer-Siwe disease. However, a more logical approach to evaluating extent of disease in the context of potentially useful therapeutic interventions is to consider patients to have localized (most commonly involving bone or skin) multifocal bone or multisystem disease.

Localized Langerhans' Cell Histiocytosis

Eosinophilic granuloma is characterized by solitary or multiple bone lesions. Solitary lesions are more common than multifocal disease, especially in older children and adults. Eosinophilic granuloma usually occurs in older children and adults. Prognosis is excellent. The most common site of involvement is the calvaria (87–90). Other commonly involved bones are the femur, scapula, rib, mandible, vertebra, and ilium (87,91,92). Cervical vertebrae are most frequently affected followed by thoracic and lumbar sites (92,93). Vertebral planar is a characteristically observed abnormality and usually represents old lesions that are

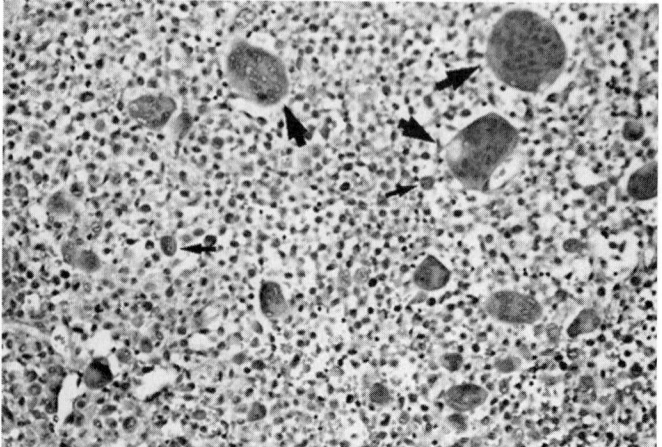

Figure 30-2. Photomicrograph showing a typical infiltrate observed in Langerhans' cell histiocytosis, including numerous dendritic cells, eosinophils, and multinucleated giant cells (*arrows*). (See Color Fig. 30-2.)

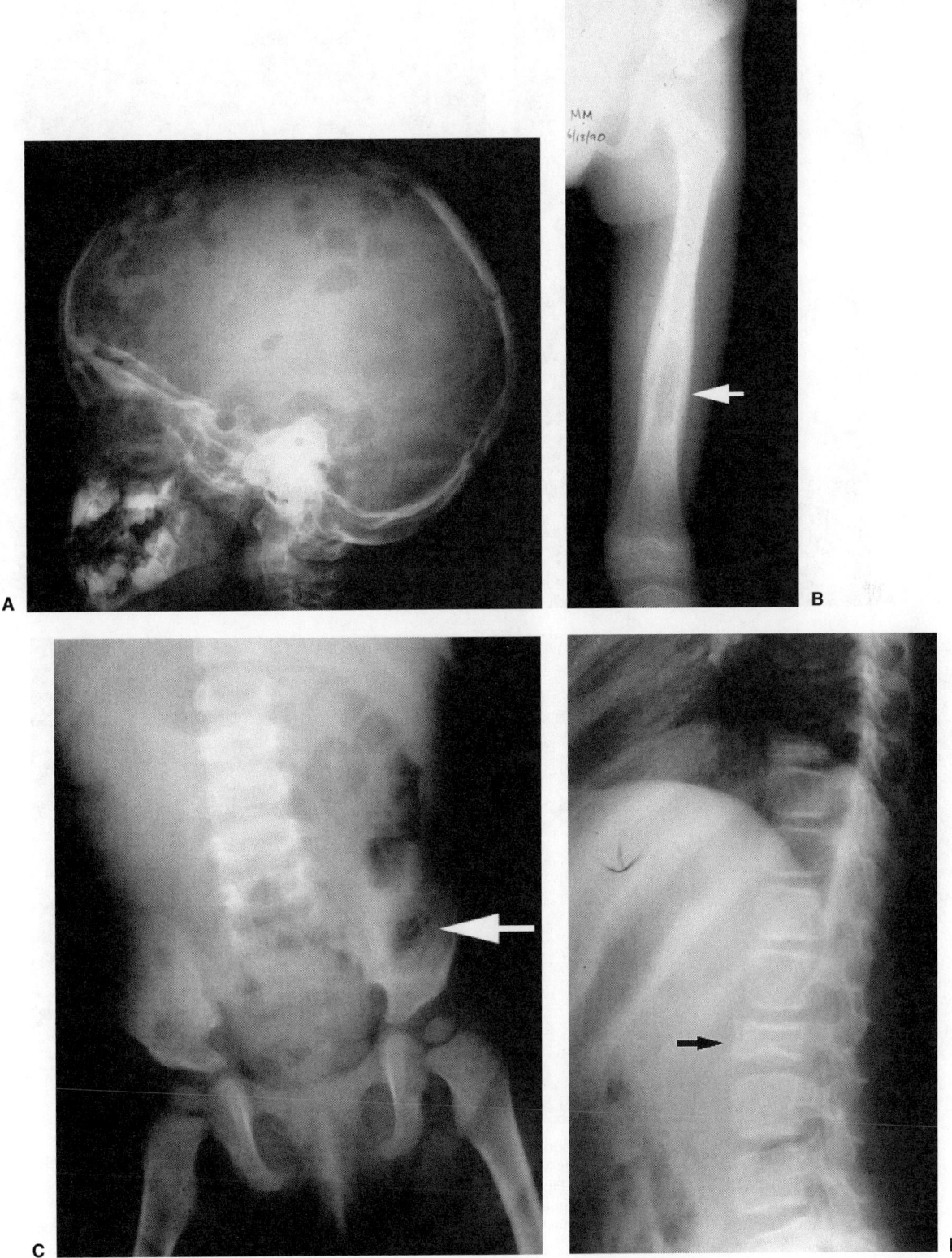

Figure 30-3. Radiographs of bone lesions seen in Langerhans' cell histiocytosis. **A:** Lateral view of skull showing multiple lytic lesions. **B:** Lytic lesion (*arrow*) of distal left femur. **C:** Lesion (*arrow*) of the left side of pelvis. **D:** Lateral views of spine, demonstrating vertebral planar defect (*arrow*). (Courtesy of Children's Hospital Radiology Library Collection, Boston.)

asymptomatic. Although any bone in the body may be affected, the small bones of the hands and feet are rarely involved.

The patient usually presents with a complaint of pain, often associated with soft tissue swelling over the involved site. Limp due to pain associated with weight bearing may occur with ver-

tebral and lower extremity lesions. Young children may refuse to walk. Lesions of the mandible may be associated with pain on chewing. Spinal cord compression can occur with extension of a lesion into the epidural space, resulting in paralysis (92,94). Systemic symptoms are rare.

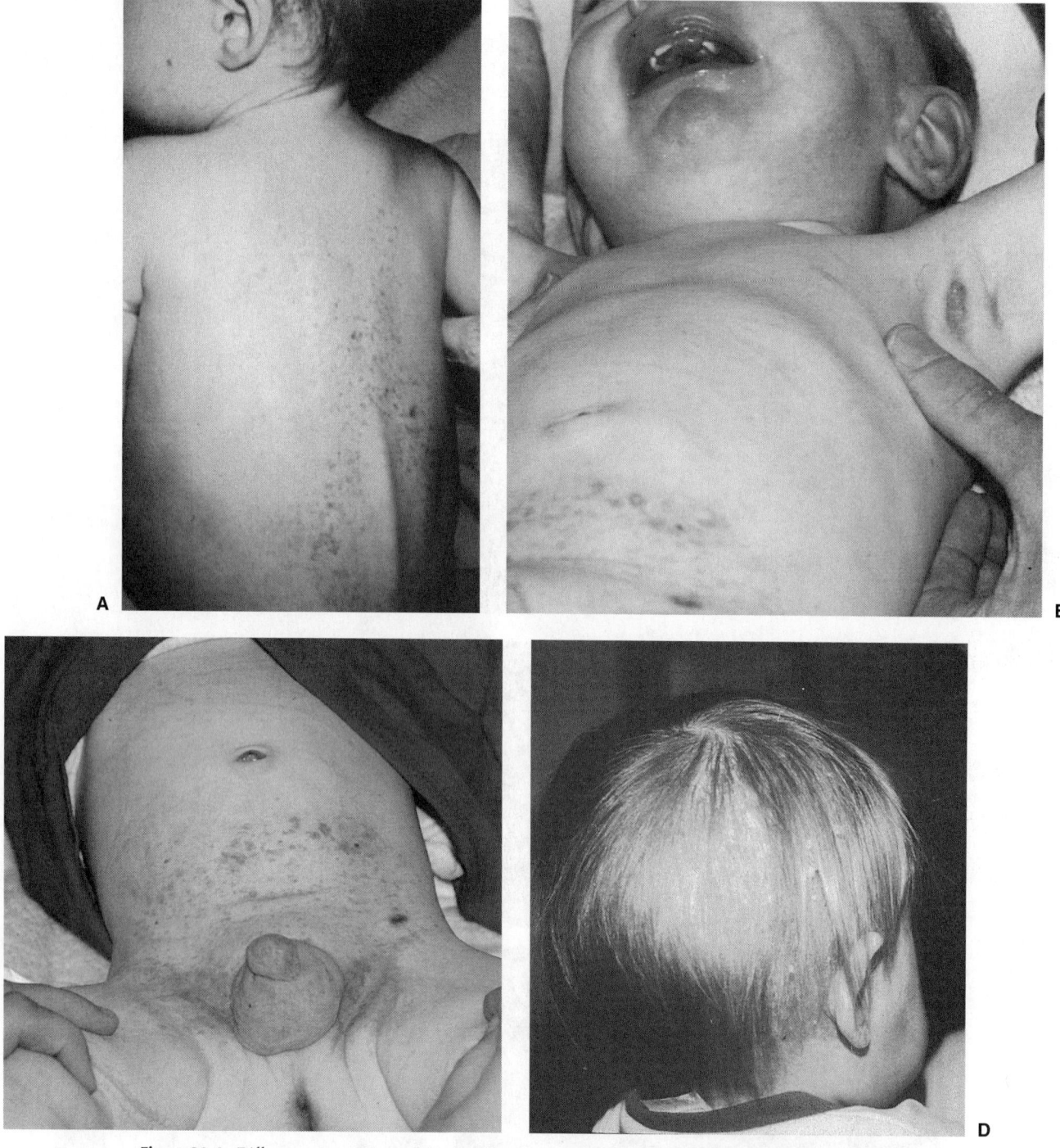

Figure 30-4. Different presentations of skin involvement in Langerhans' cell histiocytosis. **A:** The maculo-papular rash often observed in patients with Letterer-Siwe disease. (Courtesy of Steven Gellis, MD, Department of Dermatology, Children's Hospital, Boston.) **B:** Langerhans' cell histiocytosis involving the lower abdomen, axilla, and upper gum in an infant. **C:** Langerhans' cell histiocytosis involving the abdomen, umbilicus, inguinal, and anal regions in an infant. **D:** Langerhans' cell histiocytosis of the scalp in a toddler. (See Color Fig. 30-4.)

The bone lesions are usually lytic and give rise to a "punched-out" appearance on radiographs, although some lesions may also show a blastic component (Fig. 30-3). A radiographic skeletal survey is believed to be the best way to detect other nonsymptomatic lesions, because most radionuclide isotopes are usually taken up poorly by the lesions. Occasionally, a bone scan may demonstrate involvement in the absence of other radiographic findings (95–97). Hematologic manifestations may be a mild leu-kocytosis and an elevated sedimentation rate. No significant alterations in biochemical parameters are observed.

Patients may also present with localized disease of the skin, manifested by a variety of clinical presentations. The rash may be maculopapular and diffuse, more nodular and eruptive, or even quite erosive when long-standing in the axillary and inguinal regions (Fig. 30-4). Infants commonly present with a "diaper rash" that is refractory to usual treatments. Such rashes have been

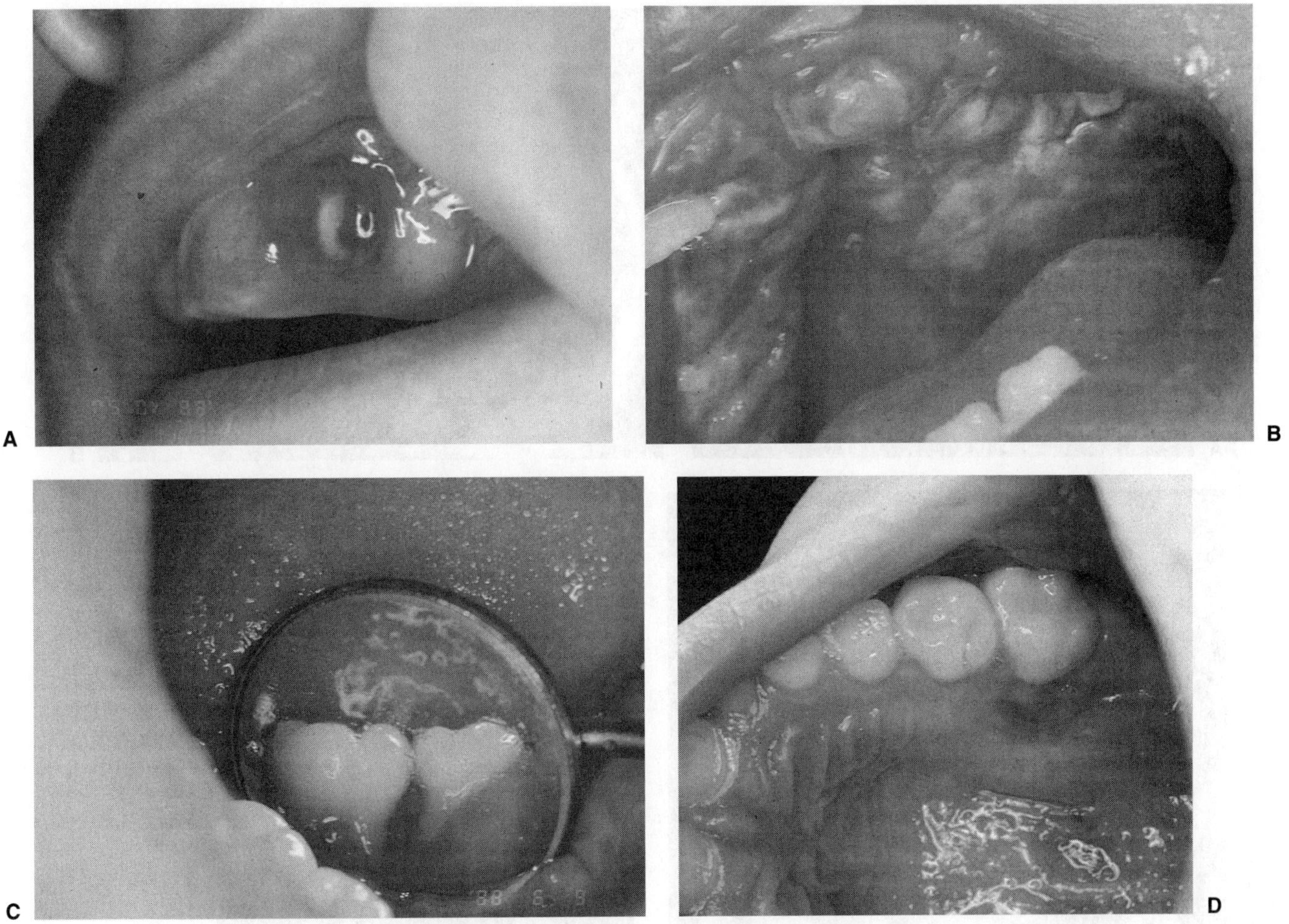

Figure 30-5. Oral lesions observed in Langerhans' cell histiocytosis. **A:** Predentate anterior gum infiltrative lesion. **B:** Severe infiltrative disease of palate in infancy. **C:** Localized bony destruction exposing roots of primary posterior mandibular molars. **D:** Localized palatal lesion in an older child. (See Color Fig. 30-5.) (Courtesy of Dr. Howard Needleman, Department of Dentistry, Children's Hospital, Boston.)

observed to erode through to the muscularis layer of the integument and present a site for serious superinfection and bacteremia.

Multifocal and Multisystem Langerhans' Cell Histiocytosis

Historically, Hand-Schüller-Christian disease was considered most characteristic of multifocal bone disease and classically characterized by the triad of lytic skull lesions, exophthalmos, and diabetes insipidus. However, children with Hand-Schüller-Christian disease can most appropriately be considered to have multifocal Langerhans' cell disease. Young children, usually between 2 and 5 years of age, are most commonly affected, although this type of disease involvement has been described in all age groups. The disease is often chronic, and the patient is likely to experience relapse. Prognosis for survival is good, but these patients will most often benefit from systemic therapy. Long-term sequelae are common, however (90,92,98,99).

The lytic skull lesions are often associated with tender swelling. Exophthalmos develops secondary to orbital bone involvement with soft tissue extension of the reactive infiltrates (87,89). In addition, involvement of the sphenoid bone, sella turcica, mandible, mastoid, and the extremity long bones may be present. Mandibular involvement usually presents as a painful, swollen mass and may lead to eventual diminished height of the mandibular rami as well as displacement and loss of teeth. Maxillary involvement is less common. Temporal and mastoid bone involvement may lead to chronic otitis media with resultant formation of cholesteatomas (100,101). Long-term sequelae include deafness (102).

In addition to the involvement of the osseous aspects of the head, oral cavity disease is frequently present (Fig. 30-5). It is associated with swollen, often hemorrhagic gums and mucosal ulceration (103,104). The periapical region of teeth commonly shows the first signs of involvement, with subsequent erosion of the lamina dura eventually giving rise to the characteristic radiographic picture of teeth floating in their sockets (Fig. 30-6).

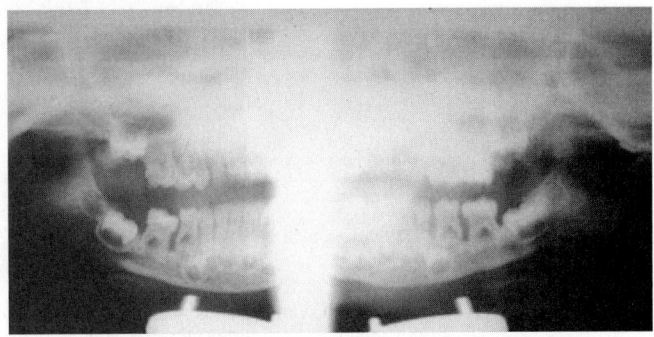

Figure 30-6. Radiograph showing the classic "floating tooth" observed in Langerhans' cell histiocytosis.

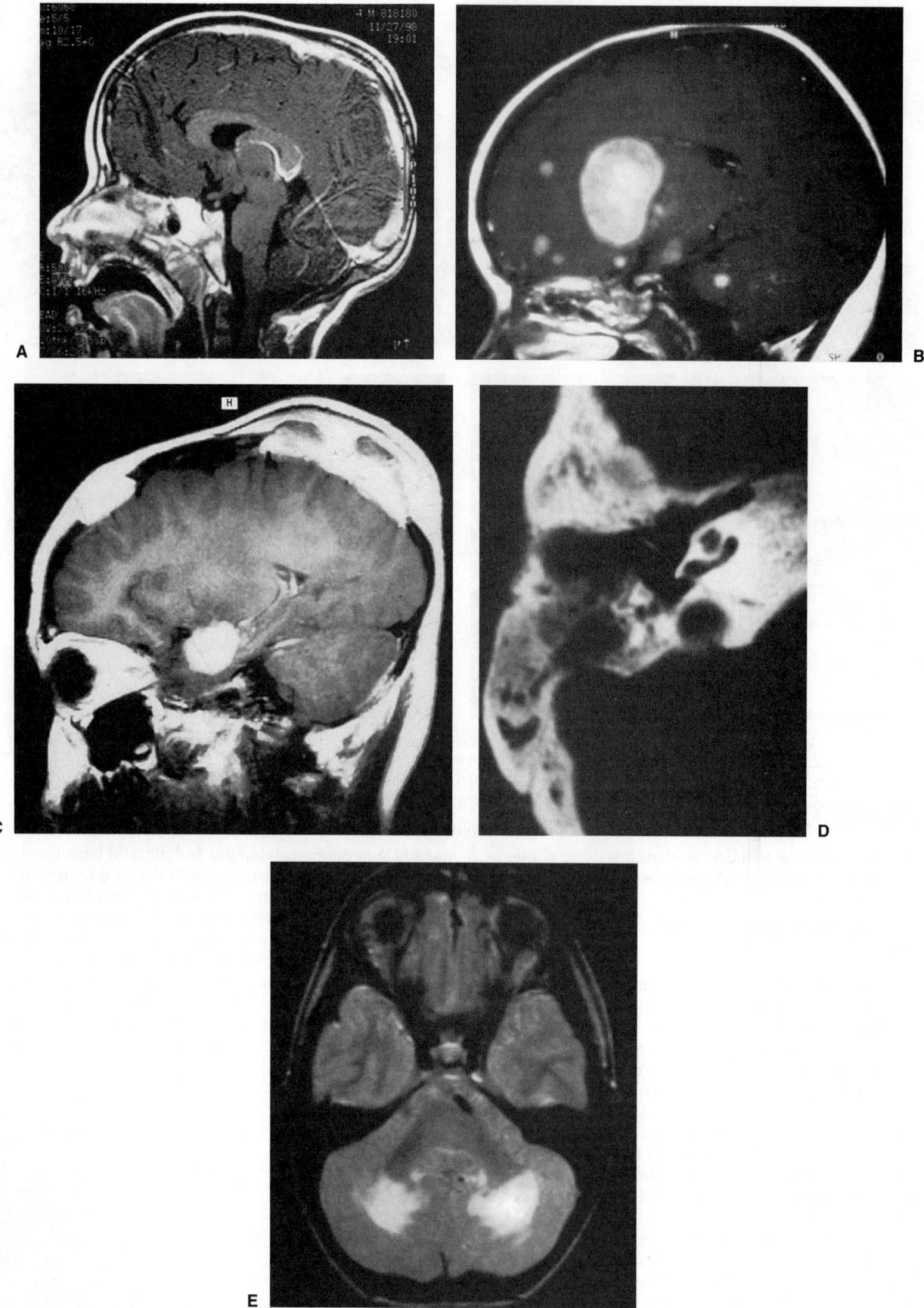

Figure 30-7. Central nervous system involvement by Langerhans' cell histiocytosis. **A:** Widened pituitary stalk from Langerhans' cell histiocytosis resulting in diabetes insipidus. **B:** Parenchymal involvement. **C:** Parenchymal and dural-based skull lesions. **D:** Mastoid erosion and breakthrough to base of temporal lobe. **E:** Bilateral cerebellar involvement characteristic of neurodegenerative disease in Langerhans' cell histiocytosis.

Careful oral examination is therefore critical in evaluating any patient with suspected histiocytosis. Biopsy specimens are easily obtained for diagnosis, thus obviating the need for biopsy of more difficult sites. Cervical adenopathy usually accompanies such oral involvement. The diagnosis of histiocytosis has been made in infants manifesting gingival involvement and premature eruption of teeth (103,105). The course of the disease may often be monitored by following the status of oral involvement, even when other physical signs have regressed.

Diabetes insipidus with polyuria, dehydration, and polydipsia occurs in as much as 20% to 50% of children with multifocal histiocytosis (106–111). It probably results from cellular infiltration of the posterior pituitary fossa (112). Diabetes insipidus usually occurs in patients after the diagnosis of histiocytosis has already been made, often during or after the cessation of treatment (107–111,113,114). In adults, diabetes insipidus may precede other evidence of disease. Laboratory findings establish the diagnosis and reveal hypernatremia and low urine osmolality. After a fluid restriction of several hours, a relative increased serum osmolality and a persistent decreased urine osmolality are observed. In infants and young children, this period of fluid restriction should be done under medical supervision. Radiographic examination by routine film or by computed tomography (CT) may often be negative, although magnetic resonance imaging may reveal hypothalamic or pituitary involvement (115–121).

Involvement of the hypothalamus may result in growth hormone deficiency, which may subsequently result in decreased stature (108,122–124). Affected children may also develop hypogonadism and delayed puberty (106,125). Thyroid involvement with histiocytosis has also been reported (126,127).

Histiocytosis may involve the brain as an eosinophilic granuloma in the multifocal form of the disease or, even more rarely, as an isolated lesion (Fig. 30-7) (121,128,129). Isolated brain involvement occurs more frequently in older children and adults. Neurologic signs and symptoms are headache, vertigo, ataxia, paresis, seizures, dysphagia, nystagmus, and clonus. Focal cranial nerve involvement rarely occurs. Cognitive deficits have also been reported (130,131). Cerebellar involvement may result in ataxia, dysdiadochokinesia, and dysmetria (121).

In addition to problems with otitis media, chronic external otitis media is frequently observed. This is often accompanied by a seborrheic rash of the external ear canal, the posterior auricular region, and the scalp. Adenopathy in nodal groups draining these anatomic areas is common. Occasionally, skin involvement may be limited to intertriginous areas, the penis, or the vulva. Hepatosplenomegaly may be present and associated with mild abnormalities of liver-derived transaminases (102,132,133).

Pulmonary involvement may occur in multifocal or disseminated histiocytosis. Isolated pulmonary involvement is more frequently seen in adolescents and young adults (134–142). When LCH of the lung presents as an isolated disorder, it is often associated with a history of cigarette smoking. In such situations, the disease does not appear to be clonal in all cases, in contrast to other presentations of LCH (143–145). Thus, in a recent study by Yousem et al., only approximately 30% of cases of primary pulmonary histiocytosis were found to be clonal in nature, suggesting that smoking-related pulmonary histiocytosis may be a reactive disorder in many patients and can show improvement with the cessation of smoking (143,146). Findings include cough, dyspnea, pain, hemoptysis, and pneumothoraces (147). Chest radiograph (Fig. 30-8) and chest CT (the preferred imaging modality) reveal micronodular opacities as well as alveolar blebbing (148–152). Pulmonary function tests demonstrate decreased lung compliance and oxygenation. A lung biopsy should be done to confirm pulmonary involvement with histiocytosis. Because the respiratory tract normally contains Langerhans' cells, increased numbers of these cells should be observed to make the diagnosis of histiocytosis involvement (153). Although elevated transaminases are not uncommonly observed in patients with multisystem LCH, liver involvement may also rarely become chronic and result in cirrhosis and sclerosing cholangitis (154–159).

Laboratory tests frequently reveal an elevated sedimentation rate and increased platelet count. Immunologic analysis has not

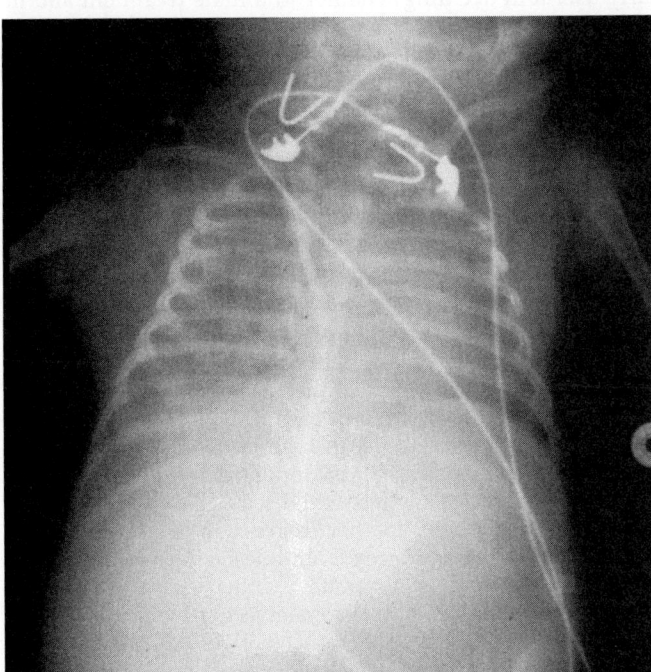
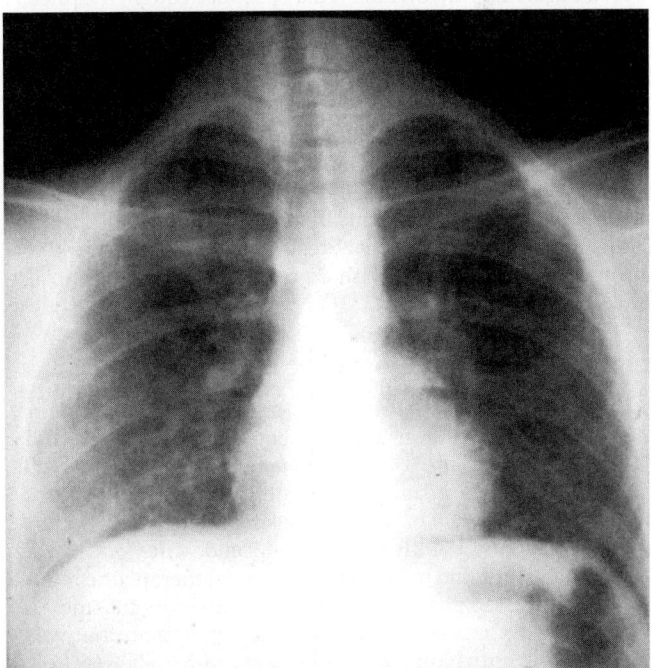

A   **B**

Figure 30-8. Pulmonary involvement in Langerhans' cell histiocytosis. **A:** Complete opacification in an infant with disseminated Langerhans' cell histiocytosis, formerly described as *Letterer-Siwe disease*. **B:** Fibrotic pulmonary involvement with alveolar blebbing as a consequence of Langerhans' cell histiocytosis.

revealed any consistent defect, with most children exhibiting normal B- and T-lymphocyte function (22,133,160,161). Some children have been described as having a deficiency of a suppressor T-lymphocyte population associated with increased numbers of autoreactive cytotoxic T lymphocytes (161,162). These defects resolved with improvement of the disease status. Other studies have not demonstrated such observations, and they remain controversial (163–165).

The extensive systemic clinical manifestation of LCH has been classically referred to as *Letterer-Siwe disease*. Infants younger than 2 years of age are most frequently afflicted, although cases in adults have been reported. Overall prognosis is relatively poor when multiorgan involvement and dysfunction are present, with survival in the 50% to 60% range (166–170).

Letterer-Siwe disease was first described in 1924 by Dr. Erich Letterer in a 6-month-old infant with fever, purpura, otitis media, lymphadenopathy, and hepatosplenomegaly (29). In 1933, Dr. Siwe reported another case and noted the similarities between his patient, that of Dr. Letterer's, and two other patients (171). Abt first referred to the syndrome as *Letterer-Siwe disease* in 1939 (172). Diffuse histiocytic infiltration of involved tissues was observed in all cases.

Patients with Letterer-Siwe disease usually present with intractable fever and a maculopapular or eczematoid, often purpuric rash (Fig. 30-4). The rash is often most severe in its involvement of the scalp and ear canals, but it extends to the trunk and intertriginous areas. Oral involvement is common. The rash frequently becomes denuded and ulcerated, leading to superinfection with microorganisms. The patient has extreme irritability, anorexia, and failure to thrive.

Purulent otitis media and lymphadenopathy are usually present in patients with Letterer-Siwe disease. Hepatosplenomegaly is prominent. Liver involvement may eventually result in extensive fibrosis with associated cholestasis, jaundice, portal hypertension, and esophageal varices as noted above. Liver failure in progressive cases may lead to hypoproteinemia, severe coagulopathy, and hemorrhage. Diarrhea is often secondary to liver disease or histiocytic infiltration of the intestinal lamina propria. Pulmonary involvement may produce cough, dyspnea, tachypnea, hemoptysis, and poor gas exchange. Chest radiograph reveals a micronodular and reticular pattern, which may lead to a honeycomb appearance (Fig. 30-8).

Bone marrow involvement is common in patients with Letterer-Siwe disease and may result in pancytopenia. Decreased blood counts may be secondary to hypersplenism and hemophagocytosis as well as extensive replacement of normal bone marrow hematopoietic elements by histiocytic infiltration. Sepsis and hemorrhage frequently result. Severe hematopoietic compromise is associated with an extremely poor prognosis (166,168–170,173).

Natural History and Prognostic Factors

Assessment of prognostic factors is particularly valuable for guiding therapeutic interventions, counseling patients, and evaluating clinical trials. This is especially true for patients with LCH because of the wide spectrum of disease manifestations and the high incidence of spontaneous remissions and exacerbation. In addition, the disease may wax and wane for several years, thus making the response to any initial therapeutic interventions difficult to interpret in terms of long-term outcome.

Lahey first proposed a scoring or staging system that was predictive of eventual outcome for patients with LCH (166,167). Based on both clinical assessment and laboratory data, the most significant prognostic factors were considered to be age of onset, number of organs involved, and, most important, the presence or absence of dysfunction of the liver, lung, and hematopoietic system. Subsequently, other reports have confirmed and extended these observations, resulting in several staging or grouping systems (133,174,175).

Patients younger than 2 years of age with LCH tend to have a poorer prognosis, whereas those older than 2 years of age have a better prognosis. Patients with localized disease involving four or fewer organ systems have a better prognosis than those with involvement of more than four organ systems. The presence of dysfunction in the hepatic, pulmonary, or hematopoietic system appears to be a critical prognostic variable.

The first international cooperative group study that represented a prospective, randomized chemotherapy trial was LCH I and came to several important conclusions in terms of prognostic variables. First, the response of patients after 6 weeks of therapy was predictive of overall survival. Second, patients who were 2 years of age or older and did not have pulmonary, hepatosplenic, or hematopoietic involvement had a response rate of approximately 90% and a 100% rate of survival. Third, patients who did not show any significant response to therapy during the first six weeks had a particularly poor prognosis with a mortality of nearly 50%. Thus, a young adult with a solitary bone lesion has the best prognosis, whereas an infant with disseminated disease and organ dysfunction has the worst prognosis. Patients with intermediate scores may be predicted to lie between these two extremes but should ultimately do well.

The initial clinical evaluation of patients with biopsy-proven LCH should include a thorough history and physical examination as well as appropriate laboratory investigations to evaluate the different organ systems. The extent of the laboratory studies should be tailored to more detailed examination of those organ systems with suspected involvement from the results of more routine tests.

Treatment Strategies

Staging patients with LCH for the extent of disease is particularly useful in deciding whether to initiate treatment and in deciding what intervention should be used. Evaluating the response to a therapy has also been difficult in patients with these disorders because of the often spontaneously remitting and relapsing course. In addition, the patient may appear to respond well in one site or organ system while simultaneously worsening in another. Therefore, any evaluation of response should include an assessment of each involved site.

Localized Langerhans' Cell Histiocytosis

Localized disease most commonly involves bone or skin. Patients with single bone lesions (and sometimes with multifocal bone lesions) can usually be treated with surgical curettage of a symptomatic and surgically accessible lesion. The surgeon should not necessarily attempt to perform a wide excision or remove a lesion completely as in a cancer operation. Thus, there is no need to put a patient at risk for an orthopedic or cosmetic deformity to remove any residual disease. Simple curettage is sufficient in most cases to effect regression of a symptomatic lesion. In addition, curettage of multiple sites is not indicated.

If a lesion recurs after curettage, other local measures are often effective, such as intralesional injections with corticosteroids or low-dose radiation therapy (156,176–180). It is not clear which approach is more efficacious in easily accessible lesions, because no comparative trials have been performed. The dose of radiation used is usually between 800 and 1200 cGy delivered in 200-rad daily fractions. In the young child, doses between 450 and 600 cGy have proved effective (108,181). In older patients, the lower dose schedule may sometimes result in subsequent local failure. For such patients, an initial dose of 1500 to 2000 cGy has been recommended (178). Radiation therapy is especially indicated when the potential for serious consequences appears imminent, such as in vertebral involvement with signs or symptoms of impending spinal cord compression or in severe exophthalmos. Care should be taken to avoid irradiation of radiosensitive sites, such as the lens of the eye and the thyroid gland (179). Rapid institution of chemotherapy with high-dose steroids or vinblastine may also effect a rapid decrease in the size of such lesions as well as surrounding edema.

The role of radiation therapy in the pituitary in the treatment of new-onset diabetes insipidus remains controversial. Greenberger and associates reported improvement in 8 of 21 such cases treated with radiation therapy (107). The diagnosis of diabetes insipidus in this report was based on clinical findings. Without simultaneous support for the diagnosis from laboratory investigations, it is difficult to interpret these data and thus to recommend such treatment to larger groups of patients (110,111,182). Furthermore, there is the potential for potential long-term sequelae from even low doses of radiation therapy including endocrine dysfunction and secondary malignancies (182). Although the use of magnetic resonance imaging to document hypothalamic or pituitary involvement may prove to be helpful in the diagnosis of diabetes insipidus, chemical documentation of blood and urine electrolytes, osmolality, and vasopressin levels associated with a water deprivation test and followed by documentation of response to 1-desamino-8-D-arginine vasopressin is critical (120,183–185). Many physicians caring for patients with LCH have observed transient episodes of polyuria and polydipsia without frank diabetes insipidus (109).

Treatment for severe skin disease has been accomplished with topical therapy without systemic agents. The first principle in treating areas of involved skin, auditory canals, and gums should be good hygiene. In addition, judicious topical application of nitrogen mustard or corticosteroid creams to limited areas has been successfully used (186,187). Ultraviolet light treatment has been used in older patients (188,189). Both mustine creams and ultraviolet light therapy may predispose the patient to developing cutaneous malignancy.

Multisystem Langerhans' Cell Histiocytosis

For more advanced disease (severe multifocal or disseminated forms), systemic therapy with a variety of agents will usually be beneficial. Over the past 50 years, treatment of advanced histiocytosis with systemic agents has been what might be called a "shotgun" approach to treatment. Depending on what was believed to be the etiology or type of disease process for LCH, patients have been treated with dietary manipulations, arsenic, glycoprotein, corticosteroids, antibiotics, heliotherapy, and a variety of cytotoxic agents to treat malignancies (23). Many of these approaches have by themselves produced significant morbidity and at times have precipitated fatalities. Within the past 20 years, treatment for advanced disease has primarily included a variety of cytotoxic agents. Response rates vary widely, between 25% and 90%, and may reflect the difficulties in discerning true responses from spontaneous regression.

The major controversy regarding systemic chemotherapeutic agents has centered on "how many, how much, and how long." Many studies support a relatively conservative approach to treatment, guided by the philosophy that the therapy should not be worse than the disease and that the intensity of the treatment should be tailored to the severity of the disease

(104,169,190–193). However, other data have been published that would suggest that more intensive therapy followed by longer periods of maintenance therapy might improve overall outcome and reduce the risk of recurrence and adverse long-term sequelae (123,168,170,173).

During the 1980s, two major cooperative trials were performed which based therapy on a "risk group stratification" (113,168,194,195). The AIEOP-CNR-HX 83 study separated patients into two major groups: (a) poor risk (patients with organ dysfunction) and (b) good risk (patients with single-system disease or multisystem disease) (194,195). The poor risk group was treated with multiagent chemotherapy, including prednisone, doxorubicin, vincristine, and cyclophosphamide. The good risk group was treated with thymic extract immunotherapy followed by an escalation schema using single drugs starting with vinblastine for 12 weeks, then progressing to include doxorubicin for four cycles and etoposide for four cycles. This escalation schema depended on the response to therapy. This study demonstrated several important conclusions. First, the use of thymic extract did not show a significant response rate, in contrast to a previous study (196), and thus after 10 patients, this component of the study was stopped. Second, for the monotherapy drugs, the complete response rates were 63% for vinblastine, 43% for doxorubicin, and 88% for etoposide. An important point to consider in evaluating these response rates is the fact that doxorubicin and etoposide were used after treatment with vinblastine or vinblastine then doxorubicin, respectively. Thus, these response rates do not necessarily demonstrate efficacy in chemotherapy naïve patients. Third, relapse or recurrence rates after treatment were 24% for vinblastine, 7% for etoposide, and 67% for doxorubicin. Although these values were not statistically significant, the suggestion that recurrence was not reduced and that the response rates were not superior for doxorubicin led investigators to conclude that the use of this anthracycline was not worthwhile, especially when cardiac toxicity was additionally considered. Fourth, the response rate for patients in the poor risk group was 18%; the mortality was 55%. In contrast, 100% of good risk patients survived.

The DAL-HX 83/90 study from Austria and Germany also directed therapy according to groups of patients stratified according to specific risk factors (113,123,168). Group A patients had multifocal bone disease; Group B patients had soft tissue involvement but no organ dysfunction; Group C patients had organ dysfunction. Initial therapy for all patients included 6 weeks of vinblastine, etoposide (VP-16), and prednisone. After the induction therapy, patients were treated for one year with 6-mercaptopurine, vinblastine, and prednisone (Group A); 6-mercaptopurine, vinblastine, and prednisone plus VP-16 (Group B); and 6-mercaptopurine, vinblastine, and prednisone plus VP-16, and methotrexate (Group C). Complete resolution was achieved in 91% of patients in Groups A and B but in only 67% of Group C patients. In addition, recurrence rates were 12%, 23%, and 42% for patients in Groups A, B, and C, respectively. Although overall mortality for the study was 9%, it was 38% in the highest risk group (Group C).

The results from several smaller, single arm or "escalation" studies have also demonstrated that patients with good prognostic features do well with relatively low intensity treatment, whereas patients with high-risk features have significant morbidity and even mortality despite relatively intense treatment approaches (104,191,197). In each of these studies, overall mortality was in the 15% to 20% range, but mortality in the poor risk groups significantly higher (i.e., in the 35% to 45% range).

The first International Histiocyte Society trial (LCH I) randomized patients with multisystem disease to receive 6 weeks of initial treatment with either vinblastine or VP-16 along with methylprednisolone (169). The initial response was approximately 50% for both the vinblastine and the VP-16 groups. In addition, there was a relatively low response rate when patients who did not respond to one drug were switched to the other regimen. Of further interest was the relatively low response rate in this group of patients with multisystem disease compared, for example, to myeloid malignancies such as AML in which 75% to 85% of patients achieve an initial complete remission (169). The overall mortality for the LCH I randomized patients was 18% with close to 50% of the deaths in the patients who did not show a response to the initial treatment regimen. For patients who were crossed over to the alternative induction regimen, only 34% had a good outcome. Thus, the initial response to therapy in multisystem LCH has proven to be an important prognostic factor.

A comparison of the results from the LCH I and the DAL-HX 83/90 studies shows that although overall survival was not different, the incidence of recurrent disease in patients who had good initial responses to therapy appeared greater on LCH I (68%) compared to DAL-HX 83/90 (43%). In addition, the incidence of diabetes insipidus was 42% on LCH I and only 15% on DAL-HX 83/90. Although such comparisons are complicated and have potentially significant chance for error, these data are intriguing, especially in light of the more aggressive use of methotrexate in the DAL-HX 83/90 study, which may serve to reduce the risk of both systemic and CNS disease (168,173). An LCH II study has recently been completed in which the concept of a more aggressive treatment strategy such as DAL-HX 83/90 results in an improved outcome for patients with multisystem disease. It is too early to be able to report the results of this study. An LCH III trial has also now been initiated that will test whether adding intermediate-dose methotrexate to prednisone and vinblastine during induction therapy will improve outcome. A second important question that this study is asking is whether 6 or 12 months of continuation therapy reduces the risk of recurrence and improves overall outcome.

Although a standard treatment approach for patients with multisystem disease has not yet been achieved, the major trials discussed herein strongly support the need for carefully controlled studies which, in many instances, benefit by their international accrual. Such studies have shown that systemic chemotherapy significantly improves the outcome for patients with multisystem disease and even those with the most severe forms of LCH. Nevertheless, a significant percentage of patients continue to show refractory disease or recurrent disease along with significant adverse sequelae. Thus, improved treatments are needed for patients at the time of diagnosis as well as when the disease is refractory to upfront therapy.

An important lesson learned from LCH I was that patients who had refractory disease during the first 6 weeks of therapy were likely to have a worse prognosis. Alternative treatments are needed for such patients as well as those patients with chronic, recurrent disease. The hypothesis that LCH was the result of an immunodysregulatory process led to the use of immunosuppressive agents for such patients, including such agents as thymic extract, antithymocyte serum, and cyclosporine (156,176). Although some responses have been observed in patients receiving such agents, there has been no consistent or definitive response rate measured to make such approaches appealing in the setting in the refractory or progressive disease. The nucleoside inhibitors, 2-chlorodeoxyadenosine (2CdA) and deoxycoformycin, have proven to have significant activity in patients with relapsed or refractory disease (156,198–207). This agent has several advantages that are likely responsible for its

efficacy, including its profound immunosuppressive ability, its lympholytic and monolytic activity as well as its ability to kill cells at all phases of the cell cycle. It has also proven to be an effective approach to therapy in patients with disorders such as hairy cell leukemia, chronic lymphocytic leukemia, and acute lymphocytic and monocytic leukemia (208,209). Phase II trials have demonstrated significant activity of 2CdA in patients with LCH refractory to conventional therapy in the 30% to 60% range (156,198–207). The combination of 2CdA and cytosine arabinoside has also proven effective in patients with progressive, systemic disease, although insufficient numbers of patients have been treated to know the true response rate of this combination (210). Other agents being tested or in development include thalidomide and other immunosuppressive agents as well as monoclonal antibody targeting of Langerhans' cell-surface antigens, such as CD1a (156,211–219). Although anecdotal reports of successful outcomes of allogeneic transplantation for patients with LCH have been published, the role of hematopoietic stem cell transplantation, whether allogeneic or autologous, has not yet been established but remains a potentially important approach to study (220–227).

Adverse Sequelae

Patients with LCH may have multiple recurrences of their disease over the course of many years. Furthermore, estimates have been published that over half of the patients with multisystem disease will experience adverse sequelae related to LCH (102,104,131,228–231). These sequelae include orthopedic problems, hearing loss, tinnitus, and dental abnormalities as well as scarring of skin.

Patients who develop significant pulmonary involvement are also at risk for progressive pulmonary fibrosis, recurrent pneumothoraces, and insufficiency (138). In the situation in which fibrosis becomes significant, few curative therapeutic options are available, although antiinflammatory agents, such as inhaled or systemic steroids along with bronchodilators, may slow down progression and provide symptomatic relief. Immunosuppressive or antifibroblast activity inhibitors need to be tested (90,156,232–237). Lung transplantation has been performed in patients with end-stage pulmonary fibrosis due to LCH with outcomes similar to those for patients with other causes of fibrosis, although recurrence of LCH in the transplanted lungs has been observed (238–242). Although transient liver involvement may be common, the progressive, sclerosing cholangitis that can occur in patients with LCH is relatively rare (157–159,243–245). However, sclerosing cholangitis can progress to liver failure requiring liver transplantation. A history of LCH should not preclude liver transplantation, as recurrence of LCH in the transplanted liver is not common (154,246–252).

Adverse long-term sequelae involving the CNS include diabetes insipidus and other hypothalamic and pituitary axis deficiencies that can lead to growth retardation and failure to successfully go through puberty (231,253). CNS involvement can also lead to hydrocephalus and seizure disorders. Patients may also develop local proliferative involvement of the CNS with LCH. In addition, often symmetric, primarily gliotic involvement, also termed *neurodegenerative disease*, may develop primarily in the cerebellum and basal ganglia (Fig. 30-7). Signs and symptoms include dysarthria, dysphagia, hyperreflexia, neurocognitive difficulties, and psychologic abnormalities (121,122,254). The etiology of this neurodegenerative syndrome is unclear. A paraneoplastic etiology has been proposed and, in part, helps to explain the often symmetric nature of involvement. Alternatively, active LCH may occur subclinically but set up a pathophysiologic series of events that result in aberrant repair after the initial cellular damage (121–123,255,256). Although an optimal treatment has not been determined for parenchymal brain involvement with LCH, there has been some success using a variety of chemotherapeutic agents, including etoposide, vinblastine, and steroids or 2CdA, as well as radiation therapy in some instances (22,108,110,111,156,182). In contrast, there has been little progress in finding effective treatments for patients with neurodegenerative disease, although agents such as 2CdA, thalidomide, melatonin, and retinoic acid have been used in a few patients with varied results (22,156).

Long-term risk of developing secondary or treatment-related malignancies has also been of concern for patients with LCH. For example, the use of VP-16 has been reported to increase the risk of developing secondary AML, and examples of this have been reported in patients with LCH (257–263). The use of chemotherapeutic agents (e.g., procarbazine) and various alkylating agents (e.g., chlorambucil) should be avoided because of the higher risk of treatment-induced malignancies (264–266). In one report, 5 of 84 patients treated with chemotherapy, including chlorambucil or nitrogen mustard with or without radiation, developed late malignancies (107). Three patients who received such chemotherapy plus radiation developed acute leukemia. One patient developed thyroid carcinoma. Another patient who received chemotherapy alone developed hepatocellular carcinoma. A sixth patient who received only radiation therapy developed a thyroid carcinoma. The time to development of these malignancies varied from 2 to 28 years. Other neoplasms, such as astrocytoma, medulloblastoma, meningioma, and osteogenic sarcoma, have been reported as late complications of treatment in LCH (102).

NON-LANGERHANS' CELL HISTIOCYTOSES

Juvenile Xanthogranulomatous Disease: A Dendritic Cell-Related but Distinct Disorder

Juvenile xanthogranuloma (JXG), first described in 1954 by Helwig and Hackney (267), is a non-LCH for which the cell of origin has been debated. Although a dermal dendrocyte origin has been believed to be the cell of origin based on factor XIIIa expression, this assignment has been questioned based on the analysis of a greater number of antigens as well as the fact that JXG is not always localized to the skin (268–270). For example, in a study of different antigen expression in 27 JXG lesions, Kraus et al. observed that all 27 cases were positive for fascin and CD68 (270). However, positive staining was observed in 26 of the 27 cases for HLA-DR, 25 of 27 for factor XIIIa, 25 of 27 for leukocyte common antigen (LCA), 21 of 27 for CD4, and 8 of 27 for S-100 using a polyclonal antibody demonstrating nuclear and cytoplasmic localization (270). None of the cases were positive for CD1a, CD3, CD34, or CD35. In controls of normal skin, fascin-positive dendritic cells were observed, but these cells were found to be negative for HLA-DR, LCA, CD4, and polyclonal S-100. These observations have led to the conclusion that the cell of origin of JXG lesions is more likely to be a "plasmacytoid monocyte," a dendritic cell precursor. In particular, the CD4 positivity of JXG cells has not been observed on the dermal dendrocyte, thus making it less likely to be the normal counterpart of the JXG cell. In addition, the assignment of the plasmacytoid monocyte as the normal counterpart for JXG helps, in part, to explain the patients with noncutaneous organ involvement (270,271).

The pathology of JXG shows lesions that contain a mixture of foamy macrophages (so-called xanthoma cells), lymphocytes, and scattered Touton giant cells. The foamy macrophages are usually bland in appearance and have varying degrees of xanthomatous changes. These lesions are quite distinct from those of LCH. Dermatofibromas may be considered part of the differential, as they can display xanthomatous features, but these lesions usually occur in older patients and usually include a degree of epidermal hyperplasia along with dermal proliferation of fibroblasts. In addition, unlike JXG lesions, dermatofibromas are negative for HLA-DR, LCA, CD4, and staining with polyclonal S-100 (270,271).

JXG occurs primarily in infants and young children, who present with cutaneous nodular lesions involving the head, extremities, and sometimes the trunk. The lesions are usually nodular and yellow to reddish purple in color. Although the cutaneous lesions are usually only several millimeters to a centimeter in size, some macronodular lesions may be several centimeters in size (Fig. 30-9). Although usually localized to the skin, systemic forms of JXG have been described and can be life-threatening (272–275). Systemic involvement can result in compromised liver and pulmonary function, testicular enlargement, and pericardial disease as well as blindness secondary to ocular and periocular lesions (269,276–284). JXG has also been demonstrated to involve the CNS in which parenchymal, leptomeningeal, and even spinal cord lesions can be observed. Patients can present with seizures, hydrocephalus, and progressive neuromuscular weakness (285–289).

JXG cutaneous lesions require no treatment and usually resolve over the course of several months to years. A related disorder, benign cephalic histiocytosis, usually presents within the first 2 years of life with the development of numerous, small, reddish-brown macules, which primarily involve the scalp but may extend to the shoulders and upper extremities (290–293). The lesions are usually less than 5 mm in diameter and do not display the seborrheic or hemorrhagic manifestations observed in Letterer-Siwe disease. The disease slowly regresses over the course of several months to years, often with residual pigmented macules. No treatment is required.

Although spontaneous regression can also occur in cases of JXG with systemic involvement, in some patients, this is not always the case. In situations in which progressive disease resulting in organ dysfunction occurs, then patients can sometimes benefit from intervention with systemic chemotherapy, similar to that used in LCH. From several anecdotal cases, the use of etoposide has proven to be particularly useful in patients unresponsive to vinblastine or steroids. Patients with isolated CNS involvement may benefit from radiation therapy, and some responses have been observed to 2CdA.

Reticulohistiocytoma

Reticulohistiocytoma usually appears as solitary lesions that occur primarily in adults. These lesions may be dendritic or macrophage derived, thus, in a sense, bridging the classification gap between dendritic and nondendritic histiocytic diseases. They are characterized histologically as having many multinucleated giant cells along with infiltrative mononuclear histiocytes accompanied by fewer lymphocytes and eosinophils. The giant cells usually stain positively for typical macrophage markers and commonly negative for S-100 (294,295). When this type of lesion occurs in multiple cutaneous sites and is associated with polyarthralgias, the term *multicentric reticulohistiocytosis* is used to refer to the disorder (296–298). Surgical excision of single lesions can be curative, but definitive treatment for the multicentric forms has not been established.

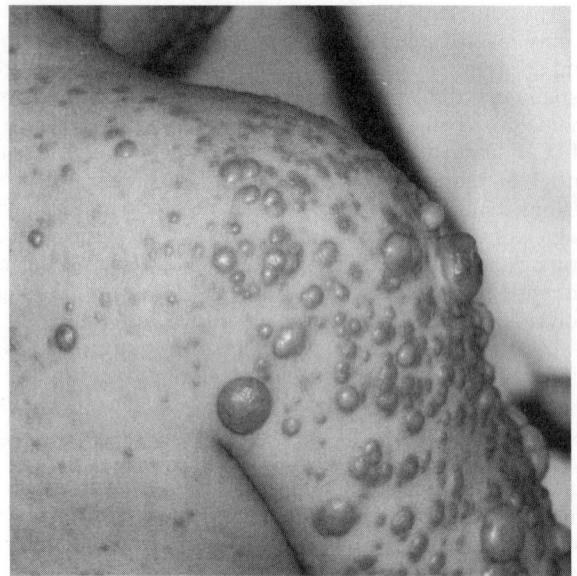
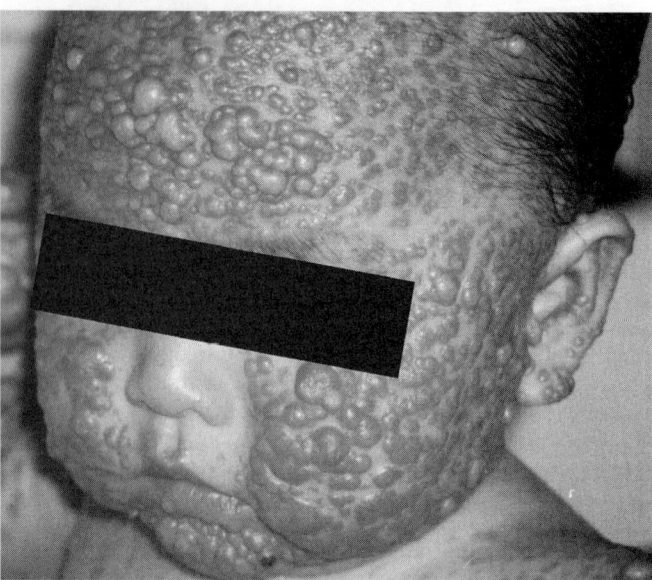
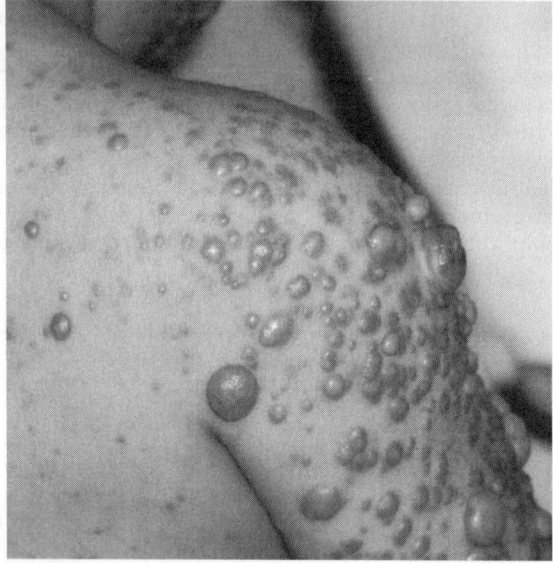

Figure 30-9. Juvenile xanthogranulomatous disease with extensive cutaneous involvement. Such fleshy lesions are usually singular or several in number, although extensive involvement of skin and other organs can occur. **A:** Right shoulder. **B:** Face nearly covered except for sparing of the nose and immediately surrounding eyes (not shown). **C:** Left arm.

MACROPHAGE OR RELATED DISORDERS

Dermatopathic Lymphadenopathies

Paracortical involvement of lymph nodes, usually in the axilla and inguinal regions, can be observed in association with chronic dermatitis. The paracortical region of the lymph node appears microscopically expanded with proliferating histiocytes along with activated lymphocytes. These lesions differ from those of LCH, which usually are sinusoidal in localization, and in which the presence of melanin and hemosiderin are not common cellular inclusions. Histiocytic necrotizing lymphadenitis (Kikuchi's disease) represents a reactive lymphadenopathy (299–302). An inciting agent has not been identified. It appears to be more common in Asian populations and particularly in young females. Subsequent development of systemic lupus erythematosus may be associated (301). Presentation is usually in the form of painless, enlarging cervical and axillary

lymph nodes sometimes associated with low-grade fever and malaise. Lymph node biopsy reveals infiltration with reactive histiocytes and lymphocytes accompanied by areas of focal necrosis. The disorder is self-limited and therapeutic interventions are not required.

Sinus Histiocytosis with Massive Lymphadenopathy (Rosai-Dorfman Disease)

Sinus histiocytosis with massive lymphadenopathy (SHML) was first described by Rosai and Dorfman in 1969 (303). SHML usually is seen during the first decade of life, although cases have been reported in patients older than age 60 years. It occurs in all parts of the world but is observed more frequently in young black patients.

SHML is characterized by massive, painless, cervical lymphadenopathy, although other lymph nodes may also be involved.

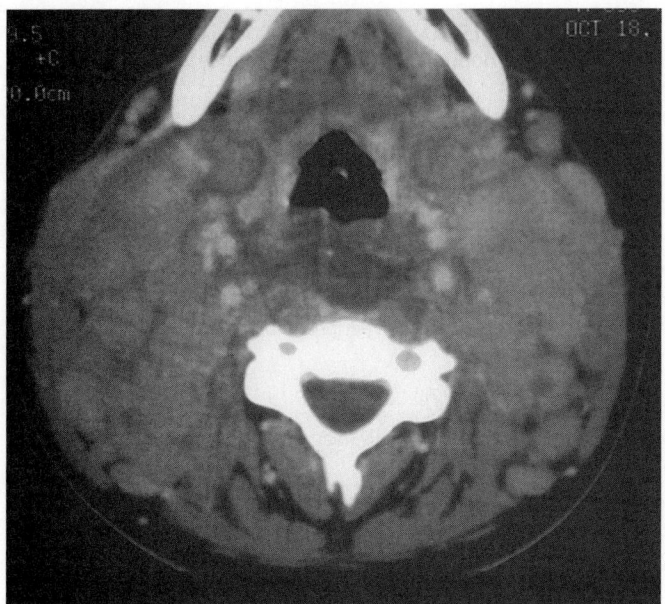

Figure 30-10. Computerized axial tomography scan of the neck showing massive cervical adenopathy in a patient with sinus histiocytosis with massive lymphadenopathy, also known as *Rosai-Dorfman disease.*

Bilateral cervical enlargement is typical (Fig. 30-10). Occasionally, extranodal involvement includes the upper respiratory tract, salivary glands, orbit, bone, testis, and skin (304). A rare finding of epidural involvement resulting in paraplegia has been reported as well as CNS involvement (305–307). Usually chronic, low-grade fevers are present. Laboratory data include leukocytosis with increased granulocytes and a concomitant decreased lymphocyte count. A normochromic anemia may be present. The sedimentation rate is markedly elevated, and a polyclonal hypergammaglobulinemia is frequently observed (303). Several reports have also demonstrated increased titers to Epstein-Barr virus (EBV) as well as to *Klebsiella* antigens (303,308). An exaggerated immune response to rubella virus has been reported (309). Herpesvirus 6 has been detected in involved tissues from several patients (310). The development of SHML in a patient

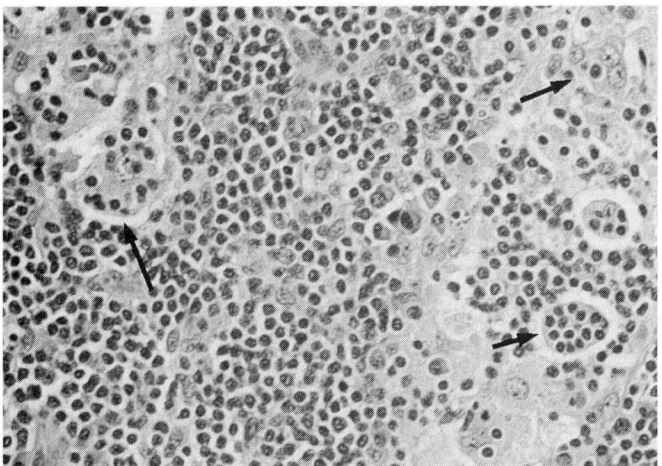

Figure 30-11. Histopathology of a biopsy from a patient (depicted in Fig. 30-10) with sinus histiocytosis with massive lymphadenopathy, or Rosai-Dorfman disease. In addition to the infiltrate and proliferation of reactive histiocytes, the entrapment of lymphocytes by some of the macrophages (termed *empemperiopolesis*) can be seen (*arrows*). (See Color Fig. 30-11.)

previously treated for acute lymphoblastic leukemia has been reported (311). In spite of such associations, the cause of SHML remains unknown. There is evidence that SHML is not a clonal but, instead, a reactive condition (312).

Biopsy of an involved lymph node in SHML reveals sinusoidal dilatation with benign-appearing histiocytes and reactive lymphocytes. The histiocytes may be multinucleated and demonstrate a large amount of foamy cytoplasm (referred to as *Mikulicz's cells*). Leukophagocytosis is extensive, and erythrophagocytosis may be present. S-100–positive histiocytosis demonstrating extensive lymphophagocytosis is pathologically diagnostic of SHML (Fig. 30-11) (313,314).

SHML usually follows a relatively benign course with gradual resolution over several months to years. In rare cases, upper respiratory tract involvement may result in airway compromise (201). In addition, orbital involvement may cause proptosis. Such cases may require a brief course of therapy, either with agents such as prednisone and vinblastine or low-dose radiation therapy (308,315–321). A response to acyclovir has been reported in a single case (322). Because SHML is self-limited and self-resolving, therapeutic interventions are usually not indicated.

Hemophagocytic Lymphohistiocytosis and Macrophage Activation Syndromes

ETIOLOGY AND PATHOGENESIS

Hemophagocytic lymphohistiocytosis (HLH) represents as a diagnostic category a group of disorders best characterized by immune dysregulation due to immunodeficiency and resulting macrophage activation. HLH may be either *familial* (also termed *primary*) or *secondary* (also termed *acquired*). The primary form of HLH was first described by Farquhar and Clairveaux and originally named *familial hemophagocytic reticulosis* but later referred to as *FEL* (33,34,323,324). This disorder was originally thought to be a rapidly fatal familial form of Letterer-Siwe disease. The autosomal nature of FEL was evident from the pattern of inheritance in families as well as the increased incidence in families where consanguinity was present (36,325–327). The incidence of familial form of HLH has been estimated to be approximately 0.12 affected patients per 100,000 children per year (328–330).

The age of onset for the majority of patients with primary HLH is less than 1 year, although some cases have been reported to occur up to age 8 years (329–331). Secondary HLH usually presents in older children and even adults and is usually associated with certain infections (IAHS), particularly viral (VAHS), malignancy (MAHS), or acquired forms of immunodeficiency such as that observed in patients being treated for autoimmune disorders as with juvenile rheumatoid arthritis (22,332–334). The most commonly encountered viruses are those of the herpes group, such as cytomegalovirus, EBV, and varicella zoster, as well as parainfluenza virus and adenovirus (335–337). Bacterial infections associated with IAHS have included both gram-negative and gram-positive bacteria, *Mycobacterium tuberculosis,* syphilis, mycoplasma, listeriosis, typhoid fever, leishmaniasis, and leprosy (338–345). A number of anecdotal cases have also been reported in association with fungal infections, such as histoplasmosis, cryptococcosis, and candidiasis, in addition to parasitic infections, including brucellosis, malaria, toxoplasmosis, leishmaniasis, and babesiosis (339,346). In rare instances, HLH has been associated with exposure to certain drugs such as beryllium, zirconium, and diphenylhydantoin (339). Several reports have observed the development of IAHS in association with various types of malignancies, particularly lymphomas (347–352).

TABLE 30-4. Some Known Genetic Defects in Macrophage Activation Syndromes

Disorder	Inheritance	Gene Defect
Chédiak-Higashi syndrome	AR	Lyst (references 507 and 508)
Griscelli syndrome	AR	Myosin Va (reference 509)
XLP	X	SAP (references 510 and 511)
HLH	AR	Perforin (references 356 and 358–360)

AR, autosomal recessive; X, X-linked; XLP, X-linked lymphoproliferative disease.

Of particular interest, however, is that less than 10% of published cases of HLH in children have been shown to be definitively associated with an underlying immunodeficiency or immunosuppressive treatment (325). This type of data suggests that a common pathway might exist for both primary and secondary HLH, similar to that proposed for a two-hit model of cancer development. For example, it is possible that patients with the primary form of HLH inherit an abnormal allele of a responsible gene, whereas patients with the secondary form are born with two normal alleles but subsequently inactivate both at different times during postnatal life. Alternatively, different defects in the immune system could lead to similar clinical phenotypes by affecting related functional pathways (22,353). This latter possibility has in part been realized by the discovery of different genetic defects that lead to immune dysregulation but often end in a hemophagocytic lymphohistiocytic disorder or macrophage activation syndrome (Table 30-4).

The discovery that at least a portion of cases of HLH are due to a defect in the perforin gene, localized on chromosome, has led to speculation that this defect may result in altered apoptosis and subsequent accumulation of activated lymphocytes and macrophages (354,355). However, it remains unclear how a defect in perforin granule function leads to the hypercytokinemia and lymphohistiocytic proliferation and activation (356–360). Other loci for inherited HLH have also been reported (361–363). Nevertheless, a consistent finding in familial HLH has been the low to absent natural killer (NK) and cytotoxic T lymphocyte function (325,353,364,365). Whether this is a primary and sufficient functional defect to produce HLH is unclear, as some apparently healthy family members of patients with HLH have been reported to have absent NK function (366–372).

Although the exact mechanism by which specific cellular defects contribute to immune dysregulation, HLH and most related syndromes are characterized by hypercytokinemia involving excessive serum levels of IL-2, IL-10, IL-12, and interferon-γ (Table 30-3) (353,373–377). Most of these cytokines are potent activators of both lymphocytes and macrophages. It is unclear what role IL-10 plays in this process, although it is a potent inhibitor of TH1 lymphocyte and NK responses (325,353). Of further interest is that hypercytokinemia is a significant component of the familial and secondary forms of HLH, suggesting that a fundamental imbalance of these and likely other cytokines plays a critical role in the pathophysiology of these activation syndromes (325,353).

DIAGNOSIS AND CLINICAL PRESENTATION OF HEMOPHAGOCYTIC LYMPHOHISTIOCYTOSIS

The diagnosis is made by considering the clinical presentation and histopathology of biopsies, as well as several biochemical and immunologic criteria as shown in Table 30-5. In addition,

TABLE 30-5. Diagnostic Criteria for Hemophagocytic Lymphohistiocytosis

Clinical
Fever[a]
Splenomegaly[a]
Lymphadenopathy
Rash
Jaundice
Edema
Positive family history
Parental consanguinity
Hematologic
Cytopenias (≥2 of 3 lineages in peripheral blood)[a]
 Hemoglobin (<90 g/L)
 Platelets (<100 × 10⁹/L)
 Neutrophils (<1 × 10⁹/L)
Cerebrospinal fluid (CSF)
Pleocytosis of mononuclear cells (macrophages and/or activated T lymphocytes)
Elevated CSF protein
Laboratory
Hypertriglyceridemia (fasting triglycerides ≥2 mmol/L or ≥3 SD above normal)[a]
Increased very-low-density lipoprotein; decreased high-density lipoprotein
Hypofibrinogenemia (≤1.5 g/L or ≤3 SD below normal)[a]
Elevated liver function tests
Hypoproteinemia
Hyperferritinemia
Hyponatremia
Immunologic
Hypercytokinemia (T. 30-6 and 30-7)
Soluble receptors (T. 30-6 and 30-7)
Decreased or absent natural killer cell function
Histopathology
Hemophagocytosis in bone marrow or spleen or lymph nodes without malignancy[a]

SD, standard deviation.
[a]For the diagnosis of hemophagocytic lymphohistiocytosis to be made, at least five of these criteria must be met. A positive family history provides strong evidence in favor of familial hemophagocytic lymphohistiocytosis, and parental consanguinity is suggestive.
Adapted from Henter JI, Elinder G. Familial hemophagocytic lymphohistiocytosis. Clinical review based on the findings in seven children. *Acta Paediatr Scand* 1991;80:269; and Henter J-I, Aricò M, Elinder G, et al. Familial hemophagocytic lymphohistiocytosis. *Hematol Oncol Clin North Am* 1998;12:417.

the demonstration of specific genetic defects is important when available (325,353). Diagnostic biopsies can be obtained from several tissue sources, including lymph nodes, skin, liver, spleen, lungs, and bone marrow. Because of associated coagulopathy, the least invasive biopsy should be attempted. This is often from an involved lymph node, skin, and bone marrow. With proper precautions, a liver biopsy is often useful. Examination reveals a lymphohistiocytic infiltration of portal areas. Langerhans' cells are absent in such biopsies (Fig. 30-12) (378).

FEL usually presents during the first year of life with fever, failure to thrive, hepatosplenomegaly, pancytopenia, hepatic dysfunction, a bleeding diathesis, and, frequently, neurologic manifestations characterized by seizures, disorientation, and stupor (325,353,379). Bone lesions are usually absent. A maculopapular rash is occasionally observed with predilection for the scalp. This rash is red to purple in color and often shows areas of skin breakdown. Lymphadenopathy may occur early in the disease, but eventually lymphoid depletion results. Patients with FEL are acutely ill with multiorgan involvement and require hospitalization, expedient evaluation, and treatment. Although occasional chromosomal abnormalities have been reported in patients with FEL, no consistent finding has been demonstrated (380).

Biochemical features include a marked hyperlipidemia (particularly a hypertriglyceridemia), a profound hypofibrinogene-

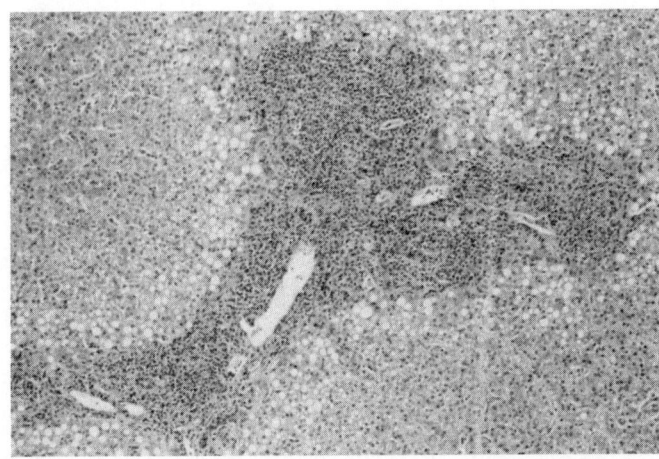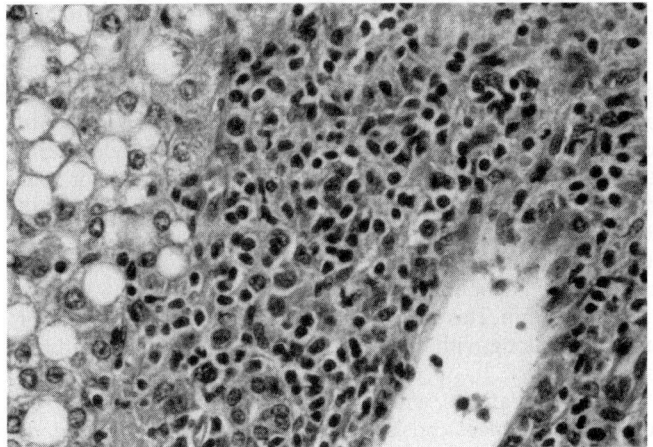

Figure 30-12. Pathologic biopsy specimen of liver, demonstrating low-power **(A)** and high-power **(B)** microscopic views of the lymphohistiocytic infiltrate in portal areas in a patient with familial erythrophagocytic lymphohistiocytosis. (See Color Fig. 30-12.)

mia, elevated hepatic transaminases, and increased bilirubin (325,353,379,381,382). The presence of a plasma inhibitor of lymphocyte mitogenic stimulation has been observed in patients with FEL (383,384).

Hematologically, patients with FEL have pancytopenia secondary to both hepatosplenomegaly and bone marrow involvement. Splenectomy has not had any significant, sustained benefit. In addition to a bone marrow aspirate, a bone marrow biopsy is also useful in establishing cellularity because normal marrow constituents may occasionally be replaced by sheets of invading histiocytes.

CNS involvement is common and is characterized by both meningeal infiltration and focal masses (325,353,379,385–388). A lumbar puncture often reveals a pleocytosis, sometimes with evidence of erythrophagocytosis (Fig. 30-13), and increased protein. A CT scan of the head frequently shows single or multiple foci of parenchyma destruction. Lung involvement may be manifested by increased oxygen requirement secondary to pulmonary infiltrates or pleural effusions. Pulmonary hemorrhage may occur and be fatal.

The presence of a positive family history is often lacking. In the face of a negative family history, it may be difficult to differentiate FEL from infection-associated hemophagocytic syndrome (discussed in Treatment Strategies for Hemophagocytic Lymphohistiocytosis). Thus, in all cases, an exhaustive search for potential infectious agents, particularly viral, should be performed.

TREATMENT STRATEGIES FOR HEMOPHAGOCYTIC LYMPHOHISTIOCYTOSIS

Without early, effective treatment, primary or familial HLH has a uniformly and rapidly fatal course, usually as a result of overwhelming infection or hemorrhagic complications. In an attempt to remove immunosuppressive plasma factors, particularly certain lipids, plasmapheresis was used as one of the early treatments for HLH (383,384). Although clinical improvement was

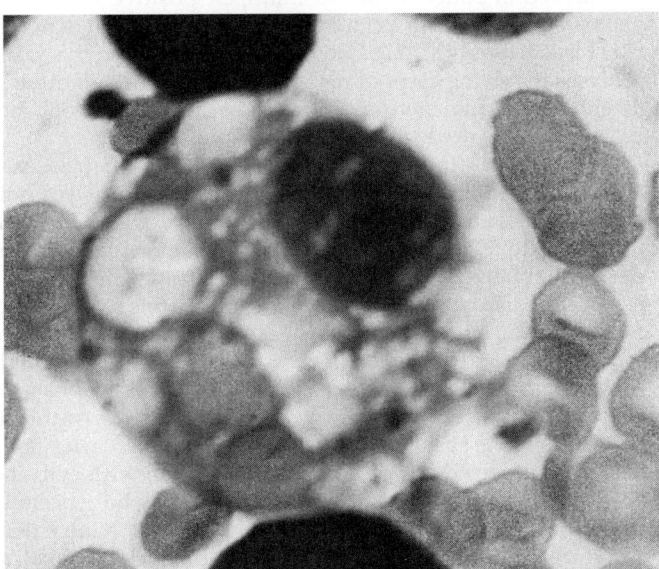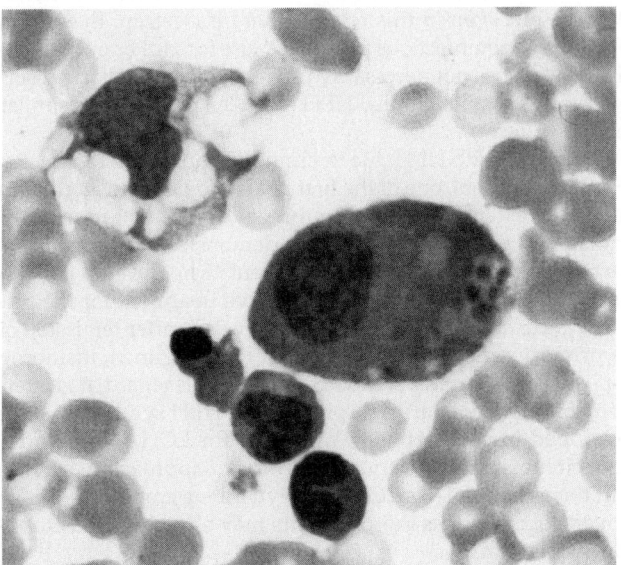

Figure 30-13. Examples of hemophagocytosis in a patient with histiocytic medullary reticulosis. **A:** The macrophage has multiple lysosomal vacuoles with debris from cell fragments as well as evidence for erthyrophagocytosis. **B:** The macrophages in the upper left of the photograph show lysosomal vacuoles with cellular debris, whereas the macrophage in the lower right part of the photograph shows ingestion of red blood cells and platelets. (See Color Fig. 30-13.)

observed in some patients, the effects were quite transient, and this approach was not further developed (384). The treatment of patients with HLH according to treatments designed for children with systemic LCH led to the observation that significant responses could be obtained. The introduction of VP-16 into such regimens, along with high-dose steroids and cyclosporin, resulted in the currently most effective initial therapy for controlling HLH (389–391). The importance of CNS involvement in HLH led to the addition of intrathecal therapy with methotrexate (392). Complete remissions have also been obtained using antithymocyte globulins, steroids, and cyclosporin A (393–395). Experience indicates the initial use of VP-16 with or without prednisone along with treatment of the CNS to obtain an initial remission.

However, patients with familial HLH are not able to be cured with regimens consisting of chemotherapy and immunosuppressive agents alone. Nearly all patients will eventually relapse and die of their disease. The use of allogeneic hematopoietic stem cell transplantation has, however, been shown to be curative for patients with familial HLH, especially for those patients who have an initial excellent response to disease control with chemotherapeutic and immunosuppressive therapy (325,353). The recommended preparative regimen includes myeloablative doses of busulphan, cyclophosphamide and etoposide (325,396–399). In addition, nearly equivalent results have been obtained using matched family or unrelated donors when T-cell depletion is performed and the antigen mismatch is minimal (400,401). Of particular interest has been the observation that even partial chimerism with the donor graft is able to induce long-term remissions in patients with HLH (402). With this type of approach to therapy, more than one-half of patients with familial HLH can be cured. The prognosis remains poor, however, for patients who do not have good responses to the initial therapy or who go to transplantation with active CNS disease (325,403).

Secondary HLH can present with a clinical picture essentially indistinguishable from familial HLH. Although it is considered to be associated with acquired forms of immunosuppression, infection, or malignancy, many patients do not present with obvious initiating conditions. As noted above, patients with secondary forms of HLH are usually older than patients with familial HLH, but even in this regard, there is overlap. Even if an infectious or noninfectious potential cause for HLH can be determined, this does not necessarily prove the etiology of the disorder, as patients with familial HLH can often present with similar findings.

In patients with HLH due to immunosuppressive treatments for other disorders, one of the first goals should be to attempt to reduce the extent of immunosuppressive treatment if possible. Similarly, if a treatable infection is demonstrated, appropriate therapy should be instituted. For patients who develop HLH in conjunction with a malignancy, effective treatment for the primary cancer should be used; if HLH develops after remission of the primary cancer, treatment with a HLH regimen, including etoposide and steroids, should be used. In this regard, it is interesting but not necessarily surprising that HLH syndromes have developed in patients heavily treated for LCH (404). Under these circumstances, alternative treatment approaches, such as with the use of 2CdA or 2CdA and cytarabine arabinoside, have proven successful, as these patients may already be on etoposide and steroids.

If disease-related signs and symptoms do not improve after reduction of immunosuppression, treatment of infection, or remission of a malignancy, treatment with dexamethasone and VP-16 is effective at initially controlling the disease (330,353,405). For patients with HLH believed to be due to infection and who experience a complete response to the initial 8 weeks of therapy, it has been recommended that they be subsequently observed off treatment without proceeding to continuation therapy or transplantation. If their disease reactivates, then further therapy, including transplantation, should be pursued. Of note is that patients with EBV-associated HLH have been shown to have a particularly poor prognosis with greater than 60% mortality (406).

MALIGNANT HISTIOCYTOSES

Malignant histiocytosis is a rare and fulminant disorder affecting mostly older children and young adults, although it has been reported during infancy (407–410). As previously mentioned, some cases of true malignant histiocytosis have been diagnosed as hemophagocytic disorders; the reverse has also occurred (350–352).

Patients usually present with intractable fevers, wasting, lymphadenopathy, and hepatosplenomegaly. Skin infiltration is common. Bone marrow involvement may result in pancytopenia. Diagnosis can be made by lymph node biopsy, which demonstrates infiltration with cytologically malignant histiocytes (410–412). Immunohistochemical identification of the malignant cells as belonging to the histiocytic lineage is important to establish an accurate diagnosis and distinguish malignant histiocytosis from lymphomas (413–417). Circulating malignant cells are rare but have been observed (418).

Cytogenetic analysis of malignant histiocytosis has not definitively delineated a characteristic chromosomal aberration. Several cases have been reported, including hyperdiploid karyotypes, extra C group chromosomes, and a variety of translocations (409,417,419). Of particular note are reports of translocations involving a breakpoint at 5q35, particularly t(2;5)(p23;q35) (420). Located in this distal region of chromosome 5 are the genes encoding macrophage and monocyte colony-stimulating factor and its receptor c-*fms*, which are known to influence the growth and function of specific mononuclear phagocytic cells. This observation of a common chromosomal breakpoint is still controversial in that other reports have presented evidence that this translocation is observed in patients with Ki-1 antigen–positive T-cell lymphoma presenting with a clinical picture similar to that of malignant histiocytosis (412,421). Continued cytogenetic and molecular analyses involving cases of malignant histiocytosis rigorously diagnosed according to clinical, pathologic, and immunophenotypic criteria are needed (422).

The prognosis for patients with malignant histiocytosis has improved significantly over the past decade. Initially a uniformly fatal disease, long-term remissions can be achieved in up to 40% to 50% of cases. Several combination chemotherapeutic regimens have been successfully used. They usually involve the use of cyclophosphamide, vincristine, prednisone, methotrexate, and doxorubicin (422–427). After an intensive induction period to achieve remission, most treatment regimens continue for 1 to 2 years with a maintenance phase of therapy. The need for CNS prophylaxis with intrathecal methotrexate is still controversial. Excellent responses have also been reported with VP-16 in combination with cytosine arabinoside (426). This particular regimen may be especially useful in the patient who has significant hepatic involvement and increased serum bilirubin and in whom the use of doxorubicin might be contraindicated because of its hepatic excretion. Allogeneic bone marrow transplantation after ablative therapy with high-dose VP-16 and cyclophosphamide along with total body irradiation has also been used to treat malignant histiocytosis successfully (428–430).

Histiocytic sarcomas, also referred to as *true histiocytic lymphoma*, are rare malignancies of adulthood. They represent more localized disease than observed in malignant histiocytosis. Patients usually present with lymphadenopathy, although involvement of bone, skin, and gastrointestinal tract has been reported (431–433). An unusual cutaneous form of histiocytic sarcoma that has a more indolent course has been described (432–434). Malignant transformation of Langerhans' cells is exceedingly rare (435,436).

Acute monocytic leukemia and malignant fibrous histiocytoma also represent malignant transformation of cells belonging to the mononuclear phagocytic lineage. In addition, several reports have described neoplastic proliferation of dendrite and interdigitating cells resulting in localized lymphadenopathy (437–440). Lymph node biopsy demonstrates primarily parafollicular involvement of large, S-100 positive, cytologically malignant cells with areas of focal necrosis. Success with chemotherapy has been limited.

LYSOSOMAL STORAGE DISEASES

Concept of the Lysosome

de Duve conceived lysosomes as acid phosphatase–containing cytoplasmic unit-membrane–bound organelles (441). These organelles were originally thought to be the stomach of cells or suicide packages. Confinement of hydrolytic enzymes within lysosomes prevents cellular autodigestion. However, the role of the lysosome has expanded into a dynamic heterogeneous subcellular organelle with tissue and cellular-specific differentiated functions and contents. Specialized lysosomal mechanisms that discharge hydrolytic enzymes into the extracellular microenvironment (osteoclasts and neutrophils) exist in several tissues and are important to host defense, wound healing, and bone remodeling.

Implicit in the lysosomal concept is the need to sort or target proteins and enzymes to that compartment. Similarly, the static view of lysosomal storage disease pathophysiology as architectural distortion had been replaced by a more active role for toxic degradative products (i.e., lysosphingolipids and peptido-glycans) in altering normal cellular function (442). The seminal model of Brown and Goldstein for receptor-mediated endocytosis for the low-density lipoprotein particle (443), and its general implications for the uptake and targeting of proteins to lysosomes, provided the basis for targeted delivery of therapeutic proteins to cells. This together with "cross-corrective factor enzymes" (444) culminated in the characterization of the mannose-6-phosphate (M6P) receptor system by Sly (445), Kornfeld (446–451), von Figura (452), and others. This ligand-mediated system is central to selective uptake and sorting of many lysosomal proteins (447). The concepts of storage, cross-correction, and targeting provided the basis for development of therapeutic interventions for lysosomal storage diseases, including enzyme reconstitution by transplanted tissue or direct enzyme replacement.

Physiology of Lysosomes

Lysosomes do not contain DNA and do not self-replicate. Thus, lysosomal biogenesis is a continuous process that requires synthesis of lysosomal hydrolases, membrane-constitutive proteins, and membrane. Fusion of vesicles from the *trans*-Golgi network (TGN) with late endosomes (multivesicular bodies, MVB) (453,454) provides an intermediate compartment before fusion with existing lysosomes (Fig. 30-14) (455–457). Progres-

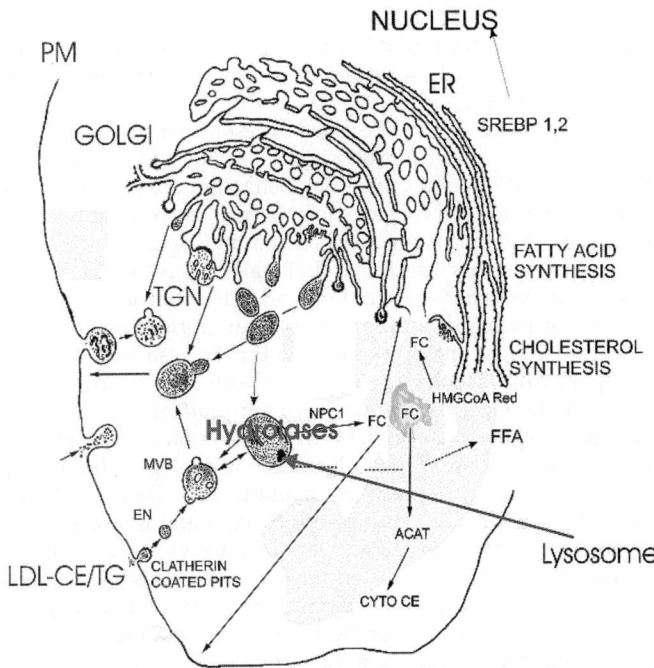

Figure 30-14. Schematic of lysosomal development and interactions with cellular compartments. From the exterior, materials enter the endosome and lysosome system via receptor-mediated endocytosis [e.g., the low-density lipoprotein (LDL) receptor]. The endocytotic vesicles fuse to become the multivesicular body (MVB), in which the small spheroids are topologically equivalent to the exterior of the cell. The lysosome contains acid hydrolases for the degradation and recycling of components or generation of ligands that actively exit the lysosome for interaction with other cellular transducers [e.g., sterol regulatory binding proteins (SREBPs) or peroxisome profilerator-activated receptor γ]. Such ligands and effectors can communicate with the nucleus to modulate metabolism of specific pathways, shown here as fatty acids or cholesterol. From the interior, the lysosomal hydrolases are synthesized in the rough endoplasmic reticulum (ER) and become glycosylated in the Golgi apparatus. Modification of oligosaccharides occurs during transit from the *cis* to *trans* Golgi (TG). In the *trans*-Golgi network (TGN) budding vesicles fuse with preformed lysosomes or endosomes to form increasingly acidic compartments. The lowest pH is within the lysosome (approximately 4.0 to 4.5). Various signals, mannose-6-phosphate or peptide signals, sort the proteins to the lysosome, and the endosomes are recycled to the plasma membrane (PM). Some (approximately 10% to 15%) of soluble lysosomal enzymes are lost to the external surrounding fluid of the cell. ACAT, acyl-cholesterol acyltransferase; CE, converting enzyme; CYTO, cytoplasm; EN, endosome; FC, free cholesterol; FFA, free fatty acid; HMGCoA, hydroxy-methylglutaryl coenzyme A; NPC1, Neimann-Pick C, type 1.

sive vesicular acidification develops as TGN vesicles and endosomes proceed to fusion with MVB or lysosomes. Early endosomes have an internal pH of approximately 6.0 to 6.2, whereas late endosomes and lysosomes have a pH of approximately 5.5 to 6.0 and less than 5, respectively. This gradient facilitates the pH-dependent dissociation of receptors and ligands (e.g., the M6P receptor and M6P–containing oligosaccharides) and the full function of lysosomal hydrolases (446). The development and maintenance of the endosomal-lysosomal compartments requires the complex interaction of over 100 genes, encoding targeting signals, membrane constituents, transport proteins, proton pumps, and tethering proteins (455–457). These proteins and others are essential for the dynamic fusion of preexisting lysosomes with endosomes and reformation of these organelles after mixing and exchanging of their contents (457). Consequently, the view of the lysosome as an end-stage compartment has been replaced by one of dynamic communicating organelles with continuously changing contents, that at least in part, exchange materials with other lysosomes and endosomes in the cell. This implies that the "lysosomal compartment" is a heterogeneous population of similar organelles whose individual contents differ significantly in time and space.

Posttranslational modifications of lysosomal hydrolases are important for specific sorting and targeting of enzymes and their enzymatic activity. Lysosomal enzymes are glycoproteins that are synthesized on ribosomes of the rough endoplasmic reticulum. After cleavage of an N-terminal signal peptide, the lysosomal proteins are co-translationally N-glycosylated. The lysosomal enzymes may undergo additional proteolytic processing or assembly in the endoplasmic reticulum or Golgi apparatus. Most enzymes destined for the lysosome acquire complex oligosaccharide modifications during transport through the Golgi apparatus. Attachment of N-acetylglucosamine-1-phosphate to the sixth position on mannosyl residues of the mannosyl core oligosaccharide occurs before, or coincident with, endoplasmic reticulum or cis-Golgi modifications. This modification can be multivalent and is selective for various oligosaccharide branches. An N-acetylglucosylaminyl-1-phosphotransferase deficiency (458) leads to a severe condition, I-cell disease, in which many soluble lysosomal enzymes are lost by secretion out of the cell (452). A specific hydrolase cleaves the N-acetylglucosamine from the phosphate to expose the M6P residue, the targeting signal for soluble lysosomal proteins. Importantly, many soluble enzymes also use ill-defined M6P–independent intracellular trafficking signals to target the lysosomes.

Lysosomal integral or associated membrane proteins are sorted to the lysosomal membrane by M6P independent trafficking systems. Signals for such trafficking have been identified as strategically located tyrosine residues (YXXN, where N is hydrophobic) near their carboxyl termini (457,459). Some lysosomal proteins also require N- or COOH-terminal proteolytic clipping, phosphorylation, or macromolecular assembly full function within the lysosomal environment.

Although the control of tissue expression of many lysosomal proteins has not been characterized, tissue- and cell-specific expression have been described for prosaposin, acid α-glucosidase, lysosomal acid lipase, and aspartylglucosaminidase (460–463) and probably exists for other lysosomal proteins. These expression patterns may have importance for the variability of the phenotype of these diseases. Most tissues contain similar lysosomal hydrolases for degradation of macromolecules (i.e., mucopolysaccharides, glycoproteins, and glycosphingolipids), because these are essential to cell function. Thus, lysosomal storage disease involvement is apparent in many tissues at the histologic or biochemical levels. However, concordant levels of lysosomal hydrolase activities are not found in all tissues. Lysosomes of neutrophils contain myeloperoxidases that are not in fibroblast lysosomes (464).

Such differential expression allows for extension of the Conzelmann and Sandhoff threshold hypothesis for the development of manifestations of specific lysosomal hydrolase deficiency diseases (465,466). This hypothesis specifies that residual enzymatic activity level is necessary to prevent lysosomal disease manifestations. Disease (in tissues or specific cell type) will be expressed below this threshold, whereas no phenotype will be present above this level. In the simplest form, this formalizes the common-sense notion that less enzyme activity leads to more severe disease, and more enzyme activity results in less severe or delayed disease manifestations. Conceptually, this threshold is important because it carries the implication of a potential for regional and cell type localization of disease manifestations. Also implied is a particular level of enzyme activity needed to normalize each tissue or cellular type. Thus, incremental changes in enzyme activity or substrate flux could have profound effects on disease development and severity.

Importantly, a necessary condition for the development of disease is the relative enzymatic deficiency (i.e., is there sufficient hydrolytic power to cleave the substrate presented at any given time?). Definition of these relative activities also may provide dose and response relationships for treatment of various storage diseases and the evaluation of exogenous enzyme replacement therapy. Once delivered to the tissue and cellular sites of pathology, exogenous enzymes will have finite life spans. Assuming appropriate stoichiometric relationships for components required for intracellular activity, the initial, high hydrolytic rates will decrease to background levels over several half-lives of the supplied enzyme. Thus, large amounts of enzyme, potentially severalfold above threshold levels, may be needed to eliminate the extreme excess tissue burden of substrate. Normal metabolism could then be maintained with pulses or intermittent dosing of lesser amounts of enzyme, presumably at levels slightly above the disease threshold, because only catabolism of new substrate would be required (465).

Therapeutic Approaches and Implications

The threshold hypothesis implies that small amounts of enzymatic activity may be sufficient for prevention of various disease manifestations in the lysosomal diseases. Two major approaches have been exploited to overcome these thresholds and correct the underlying metabolic defects: (a) direct enzyme therapy by delivering a specific, pure, lysosomal enzyme that is missing; and (b) supplying the missing normal enzyme by transplantation of normal organs or cells. Both of these approaches require receptor-mediated endocytosis through specific recognition in the target sites of pathology. This implies the need to correct only specific cell types (e.g., those using the specific receptor system or being derived from bone marrow precursor cells). The normal enzyme could be supplied to deficient cells via partially corrected cell populations (chimerism) or by the administered enzyme. Enzyme therapy or cellular transplantation strategies are thus disease dependent on knowledge of enzyme distribution and intra- and intercellular transport.

Laboratory Features of Lysosomal Storage Diseases

Morphologic and biochemical abnormalities are present in lysosomal storage diseases. Storage cells in biopsy specimens are suggestive of a lysosomal storage disorder. Although frequently referred to as *foam cells*, storage cells is a more generic descriptor of engorged macrophage derivatives. Some have morphologies that are almost unique to specific diseases (Fig. 30-15). These cells are abnormally enlarged (up to 100 μm) macrophages caused by accumulation of lysosomal storage material. Most have eccentric nuclei and in particular diseases (e.g., Gaucher's disease) can be multinucleated. The staining characteristics of foam cells depend on the nature of the undegraded accumulated substrates. Special care is needed for biopsy processing to avoid organic extraction of stored lipids or other materials. Ultrastructural analysis of storage cells may provide characteristic morphologies as clues to the type of lysosomal storage disease (Fig. 30-16). A portion of each biopsy should be frozen for cryosectioning and biochemical analysis and fixed in glutaraldehyde for electron microscopic evaluation. These morphologic studies cannot definitely identify the storage material. Such characterization requires procedures generally available only in research laboratories. Diagnosis of a specific lysosomal storage disease is made by the identification of the specific enzyme deficiency.

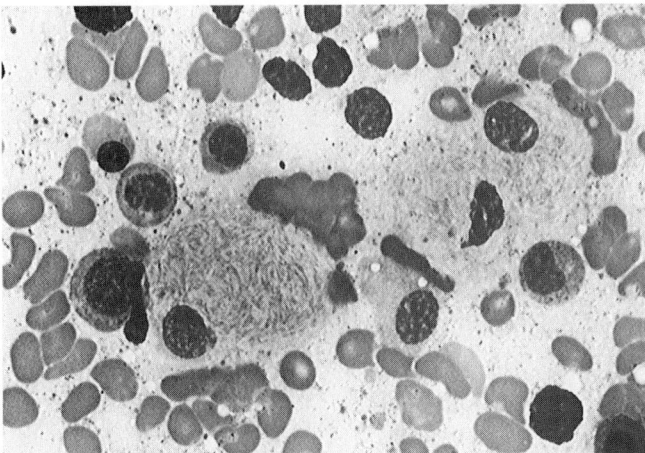

Figure 30-15. Typical Gaucher cells (containing inclusion bodies with an elongated appearance) that fill the cytoplasm. Cells are not "soap-bubble"-like as are Niemann-Pick cells (see Fig. 30-18). Rather, the cells are striated with eccentric nuclei and a delicate nature. (See Color Fig. 30-15.)

Normally, lysosomal enzymes are present in all tissues and most bodily fluids, including amniotic fluid and chorionic villi. Thus, enzyme diagnoses using chromo- or fluorogenic substrates can be made quite handily in specialized laboratories. Sources include serum, plasma, peripheral blood leukocytes, and biopsy specimens, including skin or liver. Carriers with intermediate enzyme activity levels can be identified for many lysosomal storage diseases. However, in some of these diseases (e.g., Gaucher's disease), heterozygotes cannot be reliably determined by enzymatic methods.

Prognosis is dependent on the specific lysosomal disorder affecting the patient. Substantial heterogeneity exists in the presenting signs, symptoms, and clinical course within and among these disorders. Earlier onset of signs and symptoms usually correlates with the more rapid clinical course. Although more slowly progressive clinical courses present later in life, the end result may be equally devastating.

The proven efficacy and safety of regular enzyme infusions in Gaucher's disease type 1 (see Gaucher's Disease) have transformed the outlook for treatment of affected patients with selected lysosomal storage diseases (467,468). Currently, enzyme therapy for Fabry's disease (469,470) is awaiting U.S. Food and Drug Administration approval. Clinical trials with encouraging

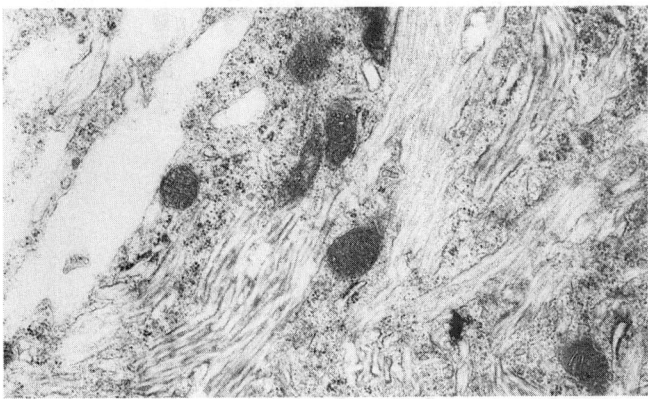

Figure 30-16. Electron micrograph of a typical Gaucher cell. The cytoplasm is filled with unit membrane inclusions that have a twisted tubular appearance typical of the inclusions in Gaucher's disease. These structures, storage bodies, are composed of glucosylceramide, phospholipid, and small amounts of proteins.

biochemical effects are ongoing in Pompe's disease (glycogen storage disease type II) and MPS I S/H and I S (471–474). A trial in MPS II is under way and phase II and III trials are planned for Niemann-Pick (NP) B in the near future. It is likely that the enzyme therapy approaches will provide significant benefit to the visceral manifestations in patients with most lysosomal storage diseases (LSDs). However, the major obstacle to the continuing expansion of effective enzyme therapy for lysosomal diseases is the difficulty in delivering active agents to the CNS. Most of the remaining LSDs without specific treatment have primary CNS degeneration as the major clinical finding and cause of death. Thus, significant advances in CNS delivery of macromolecules will be required to further exploit this therapeutic strategy.

As alternatives to enzyme therapy, cell replacement has been attempted primarily by bone marrow transplantation with significant visceral and variable CNS efficacy (475,476). The recent demonstration of extended plasticity of bone marrow stem cells (i.e., differentiation to CNS neurons) and the potential use of neuronal or embryonic stem cells indicate the need to further explore transplantation and cell replacement strategies for the LSDs. Gene therapy approaches may have similar promise, but will depend on better viral vectors, *in vivo* selection, and improved stem cell isolation techniques for maintenance of pluripotency. For enzyme therapy or other therapeutic approaches, earlier interventions will likely lead to improved outcomes because many or at least some of the major irreversible manifestations in the visceral (i.e., bone) or the CNS might be prevented. The ability to detect LSDs by newborn screening could provide an avenue for such early intervention (477).

For most, LSD prevention remains an important intervention. Most storage disorders are inherited in an autosomal-recessive manner. Either biochemical or genetic analyses can often identify heterozygotic carriers of the abnormal gene. When both parents carry the defective gene, a 25% probability exists that each pregnancy will be affected. The availability of prenatal detection of the homozygous fetus offers the possibility of selective termination and, for some, early intervention. Determination that a fetus is not affected provides a means of avoiding unnecessary termination of a pregnancy and great relief to the families. Mass screening for heterozygotic carriers has been carried out in specific groups of people with a known high incidence of the defective gene (i.e., Tay-Sachs and Gaucher's diseases in the Ashkenazi Jewish population). More general screening for LSD may become practical in time. Discussed in this chapter are the more common forms of lysosomal disorders that made an impact on the reticuloendothelial system. These and some less common disorders are listed in Table 30-6. Extensive reviews are available, and the readers are referred to those for detailed referencing (478).

Gaucher's Disease

Three types of Gaucher's disease have been delineated based on the absence or presence and severity of neuropathic manifestation (479). As shown in Table 30-7, type 1 nonneuronopathic disease has a high frequency in the Ashkenazi Jewish population. Also, a unique variant of type 3 occurs in Swedes of Norbbottnian descent. All types and variants of Gaucher's disease are inherited as autosomal-recessive traits. Over 200 mutations in the acid β-glucosidase gene that encodes a glucocerebrosidase have been found in Gaucher's disease variants. The clinical presentation and signs of Gaucher's disease type 1 are highly variable even among patients with the same acid β-glucosidase genotypes. The characteristics of over 1600 patients with this variant have been summarized (480). Essentially, all patients present at any age with asymptomatic splenomegaly with or without hepatomegaly. As assessed by imaging techniques,

TABLE 30-6. Selected List of Lysosomal Storage Diseases

Disorder (Reference Number)	Enzyme Deficiency	Stored Material	Clinical Types (Onset)	Inheritance	Neurologic	Liver and/or Spleen Enlargement	Skeletal Disease	Hematologic	Major Cell/Tissue Type Involved
Mucopolysaccharidoses (MPS)									
MPS I H, Hurler (136)	α-L-Iduronidase	Dermatan sulfate, heparan sulfate	Infantile	AR	Mental retardation	+++	++++	Vacuolated lymphocytes	Connective tissue, neurons
MPS I H/S, Hurler/Scheie	—	—	Intermediate	—	Mental retardation	—	—	—	—
MPS I S, Scheie	—	—	Adult	—	None	—	—	—	—
MPS II, Hunter (136)	Iduronate sulfatase	Dermatan sulfate, heparan sulfate	Severe infantile, mild juvenile	X-linked	Mental retardation less in mild form	+++	++++	Granulated lymphocytes	—
MPS III A, Sanfilippo A (136)	Heparan-N-sulfatase	Heparan sulfate	Late infantile	AR	Severe mental retardation	+	+	Granulated lymphocytes	Neurons
MPS III B, Sanfilippo B	N-Acetyl-α-glucosaminidase	Heparan sulfate	Late infantile	AR	Severe mental retardation	+	+	Granulated lymphocytes	—
MPS III C, Sanfilippo C	Acetyl-CoA: α-glucosaminide N-acetyltransferase	Heparan sulfate	Late infantile	AR	Severe mental retardation	+	+	Granulated lymphocytes	—
MPS III D, Sanfilippo D	N-Acetylglucosamine-6-sulfate sulfatase	Heparan sulfate	Late infantile	AR	Severe mental retardation	+	+	Granulated lymphocytes	—
MPS IV A, Morquio (136)	N-Acetylgalactosamine-6-sulfate sulfatase	Keratan sulfate, chondroitin-6 sulfate	Childhood	AR	None	+	++++	Granulated neutrophils	Bone, spondyloepiphysial dysplasia
MPS IV B, Morquio (136)	β-Galactosidase	—	Childhood	AR	None	±	++++	—	—
MPS VI, Maroteaux-Lamy (136)	Arylsulfatase B	Dermatan sulfate	Late infantile	AR	None	++	++++	Granulated neutrophils and lymphocytes	Connective tissue, heart valves
MPS VII (136)	β-Glucuronidase	Dermatan sulfate, heparan sulfate	Neonatal, infantile, adult	AR	Mental retardation, absent in some adults	+++	+++	Granulated neutrophils	—
GM₂ gangliosidoses									
Tay-Sachs disease (153)	β-Hexosaminidase A	GM₂ gangliosides	Infantile, juvenile	AR	Mental retardation, seizures, later juvenile form	None	None	None	Neurons
Sandhoff disease (153)	β-Hexosaminidases A and B	GM₂ gangliosides	Infantile	AR	Mental retardation, seizures	++	±	None	Neurons, macrophages
Neutral glycosphingolipidoses									
Fabry's disease (150)	α-Galactosidase A	Globotriaosyl ceramide	Childhood	X-linked	Painful acroparesthesias	None	None	None	Vascular endothelial cells
Gaucher's disease (146)	Acid β-Glucosidase	Glucosylceramide	Type 1, Type 2, Type 3	AR	None, ++++, + →+++	++++, +++, + →+++++	- → +++, +, + →+++++	Gaucher cells in bone marrow, cytopenias	Macrophages
Niemann-Pick disease A and B (144)	Sphingomyelinase	Sphingomyelin	Neuronopathic, type A Nonneuronopathic, type B	AR	Mental retardation and seizures	++++	None, Osteoporosis	Foam cells in bone marrow	Hepatocytes, macrophages
Niemann-Pick disease C (145)	Lysosomal cholesterol transporters	Free cholesterol; sphingolipids	Neuronopathic infantile and juvenile	AR	Mental retardation	+++ (spleen)	None	Occasional foam cells in bone marrow	Hepatocytes, macrophages, neurons

Disease	Enzyme deficiency	Storage material	Age of onset	Inheritance		Neurological		Blood cells	Cells involved
Glycoproteinoses									
Fucosidosis (140)	α-L-Fucosidase	Glycopeptides, oligosaccharides	Infantile; Juvenile	AR	++	Mental retardation	++	Vacuolated lymphocytes, foam cells	Macrophages, hepatocytes, neurons
α-Mannosidosis (140)	α-Mannosidase	Oligosaccharides	Infantile; Milder variant	AR	+++	Mental retardation	++	Vacuolated lymphocytes, granulated neutrophils	—
β-Mannosidosis (140)	β-Mannosidase	Oligosaccharides		AR	—	Seizures, mental retardation	—	Vacuolated lymphocytes, foam cells	—
Aspartylglucosaminuria (141)	Aspartylglucosaminidase	Aspartylglucosamine glycopeptides	Young adult onset	AR	±	Mental retardation	+	Vacuolated lymphocytes, foam cells	—
Sialidosis (140)	Neuraminidase	Sialyloligosaccharides	Type I, congenital; Type II, infantile and juvenile forms	AR	++, less in type I	Myoclonus, mental retardation	++, less in type I	Vacuolated lymphocytes	—
Mucolipidoses									
ML-II, I-cell disease (138)	UDP-N-Acetylglucosamine-1-phosphotransferase	Glycoprotein, glycolipids	Infantile	AR	±	Mental retardation	++++	Vacuolated and granulated neutrophils	Connective tissue, neurons, bone
ML-III, pseudo-Hurler polydystrophy (138)	UDP-N-Acetylglucosamine-1-phosphotransferase	Glycoprotein, glycolipids	Late infantile	AR	None	Mild mental retardation	+++	—	—
Leukodystrophies									
Krabbe's disease (147)	Galactosylceramidase	Galactosylceramide, galactosyl sphingosine	Infantile	AR	None	Mental retardation	None	None	Oligodendrocytes, neurons
Metachromatic leukodystrophy (148)	Arylsulfatase A	Cerebroside sulfate	Infantile; Juvenile; Adult	AR	None	Mental retardation, dementia, and psychosis in adult	None	None	Neurons, oligodendrocytes
Multiple sulfatase deficiency (149)	Active site cysteine to Cα-formylglycine converting enzyme	Sulfatides, mucopolysaccharides	Late infantile	AR	+	Mental retardation	++	Vacuolated and granulated cells	Neurons, macrophages
Disorders of neutral lipids									
Wolman's disease (142)	Lysosomal acid lipase	Cholesteryl esters, triglycerides	Infantile	AR	+++	Mild mental retardation	None	Foam cells	Hepatocytes, macrophages
Cholesteryl ester storage disease (142)	Lysosomal acid lipase	Cholesteryl esters	Childhood	AR	Hepatomegaly	None	None	Foam cells	Macrophages, hepatocytes
Farber's disease (143)	Acid ceramidase	Ceramide	Infantile, juvenile	AR	±	Occasional mental retardation	Arthropathy	Foam cells	—

±, minimal to absent; +, mild; ++, moderate; +++, greatly involved; ++++, massive involvement.

AR, autosomal recessive; ML, mucolipidoses.

NOTE: Numbers in parentheses refer to the chapters in Scriver CR, Beaudet A, Sly W, Valle D, eds. *The metabolic and molecular bases of inherited disease*, Vol. 3, 8th ed. New York: McGraw-Hill, 2001:16.

TABLE 30-7. Types of Gaucher's Disease

Clinical Features	Type 1	Type 2	Type 3
Onset	Childhood/adulthood	Infancy	Childhood
Hepatosplenomegaly	+ → +++	+	+++
Hypersplenism	+ → +++	+	+++
Bone crisis/fractures	+ → +++	—	++
Neurodegenerative course	—	++++	+++
Survival	6–80+ yr	<2 yr	Second to fourth decade
Ethnic predilection	Panethnic (approximately 1/50,000) Ashkenazi Jewish (61/1000)	Panethnic	Northern Swedish

+, slightly positive; ++, positive; +++, very positive; ++++, strongly positive.

splenic volumes were increased 15.2-fold (range, 1.2- to 93.3-fold), and livers were increased twofold (range, 0.5- to 9.9-fold). Over 50% of patients had spleens greater than 15-fold normal size, and the liver and splenic volumes were not necessarily concordant. More than 70% had hemoglobin values less than 12 g/dL, and the median platelet count was 85,000 mm. Over 90% had radiographic evidence of bone disease, including medullary, cortical, or trabecular bone involvement. Chronic pain was present in over 60% of these patients. Extensive destructive bone involvement (Fig. 30-17) is uncommon but not rare. Occasionally, diffuse pulmonary involvement may develop with or without pulmonary hypertension.

The hematologic picture of Gaucher's disease may initially be of a mild normochromic, normocytic anemia secondary to hypersplenism. As the disease progresses, severe pancytopenia develops, resulting from both hypersplenism and bone marrow infiltration with Gaucher cells. Severe episodes of bleeding may develop caused by the thrombocytopenia. Factor IX deficiency has also been reported in Gaucher's disease and may contribute to the bleeding diathesis. Bleeding may occur during the menstrual cycle or rarely may be caused by ruptured esophageal varices secondary cirrhosis and portal hypertension. A leuko-erythroblastic blood smear is indicative of marrow infiltration with Gaucher cells. Increased serum levels of nontartrate-inhibitable acid phosphatase, angiotensin-converting enzyme, and transcobalamin may be present in homozygotes.

Documenting a deficiency of acid β-glucosidase activity in nucleated cells leads to a diagnosis of Gaucher's disease. The enzyme is not present in plasma or red blood cells. Enzyme testing for heterozygosity is unreliable. Mutation identification is useful for heterozygote identification and for genotype and phenotype correlations (Genotype and Phenotype Correla-

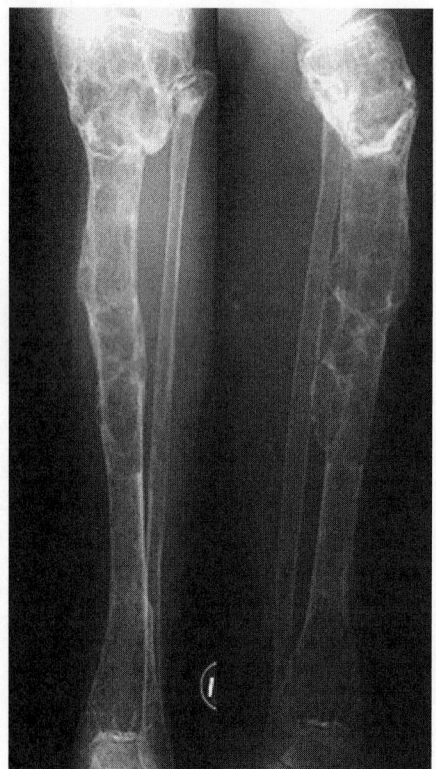
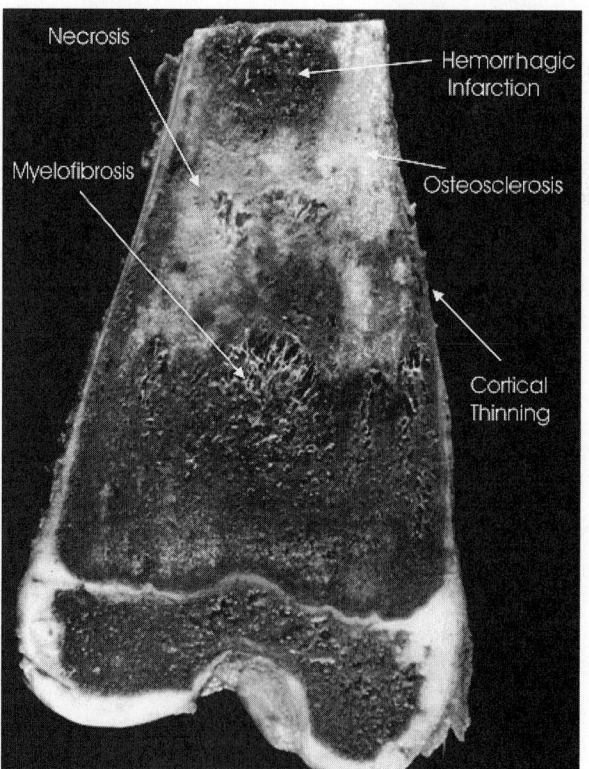

Figure 30-17. Extensive destructive bony lesions of Gaucher's disease. **A:** Massive destruction of the femur and tibia (shown here) in this 50-year-old woman with Gaucher's disease type 1. A "soap bubble" appearance to the bones and cortical thinning are the result of the metabolic effects of Gaucher's disease on the bone and repeated bone infarctions. The interior of the bone is shown in the right panel **(B)** in which the distal femur has been sectioned. The complex lesions of osteosclerosis, osteonecrosis, myelofibrosis, and cortical thinning are present. The classic Erlenmeyer flask deformity of the distal femur also is present. (See Color Fig. 30-17.)

tions). Prenatal diagnosis is available by determining acid β-glucosidase levels in aminocytes or chorionic villus cells.

Type 2 Gaucher's disease is an acute neuropathic infantile variant. Marked hepatosplenomegaly, failure to thrive, and progressive neurologic deterioration, including hypertonia, spasticity, strabismus, dysphagia, laryngeal spasm, and opisthotonic positioning, are seen. Progressive laryngospasm is particularly distressing. The hematologic and laboratory features are similar to those of type 1 disease. The CNS manifestations of this disease are not directly treatable by any current methods.

Type 3 Gaucher's disease is a subacute neuropathic variant. This disease is more highly variable than type 2 and likely represents an extended continuum of the neuronopathic variants. Oculomotor apraxia may appear at 3 months of age and may or may not progress to include additional CNS manifestations. Intractable myoclonic seizures or tonic seizures can occur irrespective of the degree of visceral involvement (481). Death is due to CNS, progressive hepatic cirrhosis, or pulmonary disease. The visceral disease can include massive hepatic and splenic enlargement and failure. Also, severe bony disease with kyphoscoliosis, which leads to restrictive lung disease, occurs with significant frequency. The visceral involvement can and should be treated with enzyme therapy.

GENOTYPE AND PHENOTYPE CORRELATIONS

Of the over 200 mutant alleles of the glucocerebrosidase (GBA) locus found in Gaucher's disease, only approximately six alleles have significant general frequency. Thus, statistics for potential prognostication based on genotype are available only for the N370S(1226G), L444P(14486), and recombinant alleles with multiple point mutations. To date, the N370S allele, either being homoallelic or heteroallelic with another GBA mutant allele is absolutely predictive of type 1 phenotypes. The homozygotes for this allele tend to be more mild when they present for diagnosis, and approximately 50% are thought to have minimal enough signs or symptoms to evade diagnosis (479). The N370S/other mutant allele genotypes lead generally to more severe diseases with clear progression (482). The L444P/L444P genotype is highly associated (>90%) with the neuronopathic variants. However, there appear to be some such homozygotes who may escape neurologic disease at least into their third to fourth decade (483).

ENZYME THERAPY FOR GAUCHER'S DISEASE

The advent of enzyme therapy has revolutionized the care of patients significantly affected with Gaucher's disease type 1 (468). Over the past decade, regular infusions of carbohydrate-modified acid β-glucosidase have proven safe and effective in reducing the visceral and hematologic manifestations of the disease. Over a period of 12 to 24 months, the major hepatic, splenic, and hematologic manifestations are reversed, and most patients are restored to a state of much better health. Bony disease requires more extended (48 months) therapy for measurable effectiveness (484,485), and adjunctive therapy with osteoclast inhibitors, such as bisphosphonates, may be beneficial. To date, enzyme replacement is considered a lifelong therapy (486). IgG antibodies are produced in these cross-reacting immunnologic material–positive patients at a 12% to 15% rate (486) and inhibitory antibodies have been found in less than 2% of patients (487). Adverse events or mild allergic reactions occur in approximately 15% of patients (486). The theoretical basis for enzyme therapy is grounded in the unique involvement of macrophages and their derivatives, accounting for the visceral abnormalities. Human recombinant acid β-glucosidase is overexpressed in CHO cells, and the secreted form is purified from the media. This enzyme has complex N-linked oligosaccharide residues that are subsequently modified *in vivo* to expose the core α-mannosyl residues. This modified enzyme exploits the nearly unique presence the mannose receptor on the macrophage surface (488,489). Preferential *in vivo* uptake of this enzyme into the reticuloendothelial system is probably responsible for the major therapeutic effects (490–492).

Niemann-Pick Diseases A and B

The NP A and B variants are significantly rarer than Gaucher's disease. These disorders are characterized by the infiltration of organs, particularly the reticuloendothelial system, with classic foam cells containing excess sphingomyelin and other phospholipids. The A and B variants are distinguished by the presence of neuronopathic disease in the former and the absence of CNS disease and chronic nature of the latter (493). The hallmark of this disease is the foam cell with a "mulberry" appearance (Fig. 30-18). The diagnosis is established by demonstrating defi-

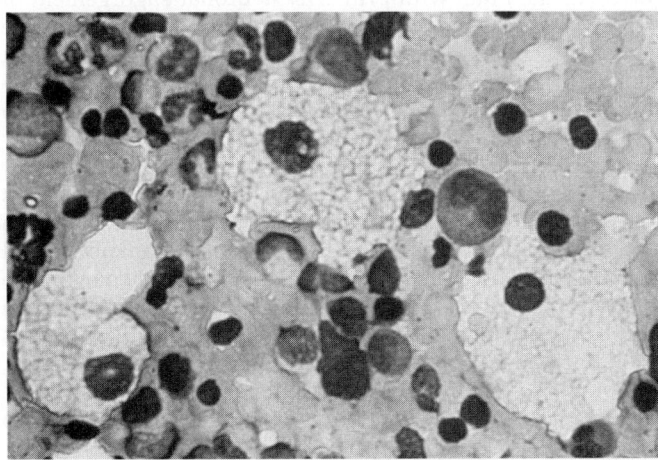
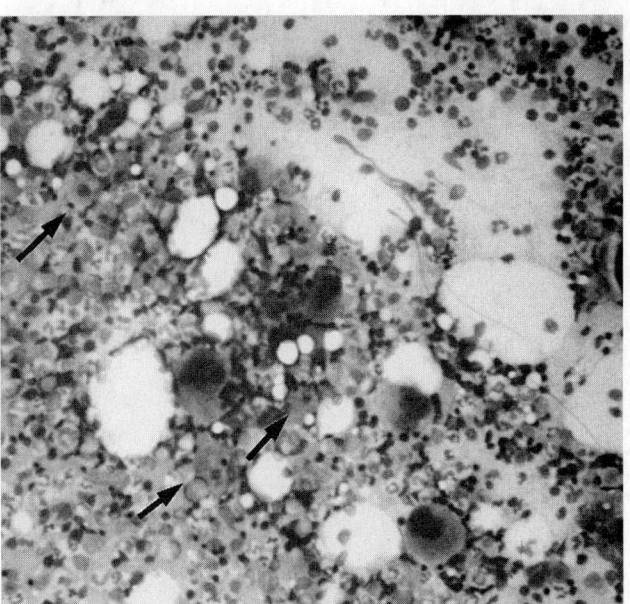

Figure 30-18. Storage cells observed in **(A)** Niemann-Pick disease and **(B)** sea-blue histiocytes (*arrows*). (See Color Fig. 30-18.) (Courtesy of Pearl Levitt, Hematology, Dana Farber Cancer Institute; Dr. Joseph Antin, Hematology Teaching File, Brigham and Women's Hospital.)

cient acid sphingomyelinase in nucleated cells. Numerous mutations at the acid sphingomyelinase locus have been found in NP A or B patients, and some degree of genotype and phenotype correlation has been discerned. NP A and B are inherited in an autosomal-recessive manner. A somewhat higher incidence of NP disease is found among Ashkenazi Jews than in the general population. Scattered foam cells are found in affected tissues in patients with NP A and B hepatocytes, and Kupffer's cells can be involved to similar degrees. These storage cells have a pale yellow to yellow-brown cytoplasm when stained with hematoxylin and eosin. Giemsa staining produces a sea-blue cytoplasm, giving rise to the term *sea-blue histiocyte* (Fig. 30-18). However, enzymatic analysis is critical in making a definitive diagnosis.

NP A disease is an acute neuropathic disease. Patients present during the first few months of life with severe failure to thrive, feeding difficulties, massive hepatosplenomegaly, lymphadenopathy, and neurologic and developmental deterioration. A variant cherry-red spot with a gray halo is observable in the macula of approximately 50% of patients. CNS involvement includes spasticity, blindness, deafness, and severe mental impairment (Fig. 30-19). Death usually occurs before 3 years of age. Preventive measures through genetic counseling and prenatal diagnosis offer the option of having an affected child. Sphingomyelinase activity can be measured in skin fibroblasts and amniotic fluid or trophoblast samples obtained prenatally.

NP B disease is a more chronic progressive reticuloendotheliosis without nervous system involvement. Patients present in childhood with an enlarging abdomen associated with hepatosplenomegaly and infiltration of these organs by foam cells. Although bone deformities may occur, this is less than in Gaucher's disease and is mainly osteoporosis. Bone marrow and lung involvement may be extensive and contribute to death in the second to fourth decades of life. Because this form of NP disease does not involve the CNS, allogeneic bone marrow transplantation or exogenous enzyme replacement offers potentially effective modes of therapy. Enzyme therapy will be in

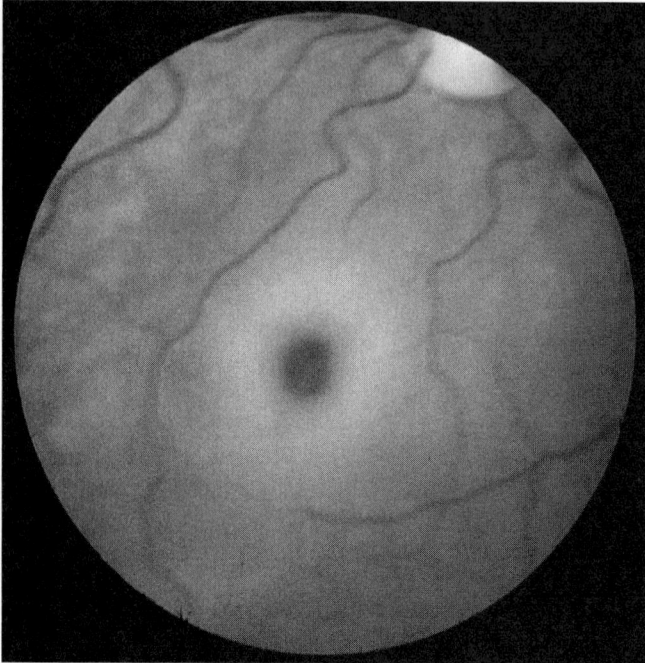

Figure 30-19. Cherry-red macula of Niemann-Pick disease. (See Color Fig. 30-19.) (Courtesy of Dr. Robert Peterson, Department of Ophthalmology, Children's Hospital, Boston.)

clinical trials in the next 2 years. However, targeting of the enzyme must be to the macrophages, hepatocytes, and possibly other cell types. Thus, the delivery will need to exploit the mannose and the M6P receptors. Preliminary findings with bone marrow transplantation are encouraging with evidence of decreased accumulation of sphingomyelin in liver and bone marrow.

Niemann-Pick C disease

NP C was formerly classified with the NP A and B forms of acid sphingomyelinase deficiency because of a similar histology of the foam cells and the accumulation of excess sphingomyelin in tissues. However, genetic studies showed that NP C did not map to the same locus as acid sphingomyelinase and subsequently was shown to be due to a cholesterol transport protein that modulates the egress of cholesterol from lysosomes and probably facilitates the transport of sphingomyelin and other phospholipids out of the lysosome (494–497). There are two variants of NPC, designated NPC1 and NPC2. These two diseases are nonallelic with NPC1 being due to transmembrane cholesterol transporter porter protein and NPC2 being the deficiency of a lysosomal cholesterol-binding protein (498). Phenotypically, the diseases are essentially indistinguishable, but NPC1 is much more frequent than NPC2. NPD was thought to be a unique variant of acid sphingomyelinase deficiency, but it is allelic to NPC1. NPD has some unique phenotypic characteristics that may be due to its genetic isolation in Nova Scotia and in southern Colorado.

The variable hepatosplenomegaly and presence of foam cells or sea-blue histiocytes in the bone marrow and visceral organs have relatively little impact on the overall disease progression, because the major abnormalities are in the CNS. However, pathologically, the major feature is the neurovisceral storage of foam cells and sea-blue histiocytes. Histopathologically, the foam cells, which are macrophages, and the sea-blue histiocytes can be readily distinguished in bone marrow preparations and in the spleen. Sea-blue histiocytes are also present in the tonsils, lymph nodes, liver, and lung. There is more clustering of the storage cells in the spleen in the red pulp and within the sinusoids of the liver, and involvement of hepatocytes with microvacuolization can also be found. Some phenotypes present as a "giant cell hepatitis," and cholestasis can be present. Severe pulmonary disease is rarely present, and the foamy cells are difficult to discern in visceral tissues of adult cases. The remainder of the pathology involves the brain with primarily neuronal engorgement of storage material, including cholesterol or sphingomyelin. The major storage material in the visceral tissues and in the foam cells and sea-blue histiocytes includes unesterified cholesterol, sphingomyelin glucoceramide, bis-(monoacylglycero) phosphate, and glycosphingolipids.

The major pathophysiology of NP C is the inability to transport cholesterol, sphingomyelin, and similar compounds across the lysosomal membrane. Whether additional trafficking within the cell is important to the pathophysiology is unknown, and the exact cause of the neurodegeneration is also unknown. Substantial disruption of intracellular cholesterol metabolism through the sterol regulatory binding protein (SREBP) system is well documented, as are other glycosphingolipid trafficking abnormalities (495). Currently, no therapy is available for the treatment of NP C, but active research programs devoted to these developments are ongoing.

The availability of molecular diagnostics as well as cholesterol trafficking assays provides the ability for diagnosis and of prenatal testing for NPC1 and NPC2. Although rare, approximately 1 in 150,000 live births, NP C may be much more common due to underdiagnosis and confusions with other sea-blue histiocytosis.

Farber's Disease

Farber's disease is a rare autosomal-recessive disorder due to the deficiency of acid ceramidase. The major reason for discussing it here, despite its rarity, is its unique histopathologic findings related to the reticuloendothelial system. This severe disorder has a highly variable phenotype and may have its onset shortly after birth to later in the first year. Typically within a few months after birth, there is painful, progressively deforming joint disease with subcutaneous nodules appearing, particularly near the joints. In addition, a progressive hoarseness secondary to the accumulation of these nodules on the larynx occurs and may lead to stridor and difficulty breathing. Biopsy of the joint and or nodules reveals the presence of granulomas with lipid-laden macrophages. The first histologic finding appears to be the presence of lipid-laden macrophages in the joint or in the area surrounding the joints with eventual development of granulomas. Massive accumulation of lipid-laden macrophages in the liver, spleen, lung, and heart occurs. Furthermore, there can be accumulation of glycosphingolipids, ceramides, and gangliosides in cells of the CNS. In general, the entire reticuloendothelial system is involved with accumulation of these lipid-laden macrophages with granuloma formation. A particularly aggressive variant of Farber's disease includes rapidly progressive massive hepatosplenomegaly with the development of a cherry-red spot in the retina. On ultrastructure, the storage cells contain "Farber's bodies" or "banana bodies" that are comma-shaped curvilinear-tubular structures that contain accumulated stored ceramide. The pathophysiology connecting the storage of ceramide in lysosomes with the development of granulomas (an unusual reaction) is currently unknown. Furthermore, the progressively deforming joint disease as a result of ceramide accumulation of lysosomes or macrophages provides an intriguing research opportunity for understanding the participation of ceramide in joint development.

Farber's disease results from inherited defects in the acid ceramidase gene, and there are several mutations that have been described. These lead to variably defective ceramidase activity that can be detected in any nucleated cell. Thus, diagnosis can be made by measurement of acid ceramidase activity in peripheral blood leukocytes, skin fibroblasts, or other biopsied tissues. In addition, liver biopsies and other tissues contain large amounts of ceramide and of course by ultrastructure the ceramide-containing Farber's bodies. Prenatal diagnosis is also available by ascertainment of acid ceramidase activity in cultured amniotic cells or chorionic villus tissues.

Mucopolysaccharidosis I H and S

Mucopolysaccharidosis (MPS) I H and S represent the phenotypic spectrum of α-L-iduronidase deficiency. These disorders are allelic and lead to variable rates of dumaton and heparan sulfate accumulations in multiple organs. The specific tissues of pathogenesis include connective tissues and the CNS. In addition, MPS I H and S represent the most common MPS diseases, and enzyme and cellular replacement therapies are in the near future.

MPS I H, I H/S and I S span the spectrum of involvement from severe infantile to less severe adolescent disease. In addition, this classification incorporates a continuum from severe CNS, visceral, and skeletal manifestations to moderate involve-

ment to no CNS with primarily skeletal disease (499–501). All are autosomal recessively inherited. MPS I H (Hurler's syndrome) is characterized by onset of skeletal overgrowth, progressive dysmorphia (coarsening facial and physiometry), dysostosis multiplex, macroglossia, hypertrophic gums, contractures of all joints, progressive mental retardation, hydrocephalus, corneal clouding, hepatosplenomegaly, progressive mitral and aortic valvular disease, coronary artery occlusion, and restrictive pulmonary disease (501). Death occurs at 5 to 15 years of age from a combination of progressive heart, pulmonary, and CNS disease. Many patients experience sudden death from cardiac disease. Instability of the cervical spine presents a serious threat to these patients; hyperextension of the neck should be avoided, and cervical fusion may be required (500). Each of these manifestations is less severe in MPS I H/S (Hurler-Scheie disease) and MPS I S (Scheie disease). In Scheie disease, skeletal, cardiac, and pulmonary involvement predominate, and the CNS is spared.

Storage cells and macrophages are present in bone marrow, spleen, liver, and other reticuloendothelial organs. Vacuolated lymphocytes are also plentiful in peripheral blood and lymph nodes. Hypersplenism can occur but is not commonly severe. Skeletal histology displays disorganized cartilaginous and chondrocyte growth. Mucopolysaccharide (proteoglycan) accumulation is also present in the arachnoid granulations, and thickened meninges are found. Clinical and morphologic characteristic findings and the deficiency of α-L-iduronidase activity in all cells establish diagnosis. Prenatal diagnosis can be accomplished by enzyme assays of aminocytes; α-L-iduronidase activity is normally low in chorionic villi, making this a poor source for enzymatic prenatal diagnosis.

Specific therapy has been attempted by bone marrow transplantation with excellent hepatic and splenic response, improvement in cardiopulmonary function, and suggestive positive effects on the CNS (475,499,502). The effects on the skeleton have been disappointing. Enzyme therapy by intravenous infusion of recombinant α-L-iduronidase has provided excellent hepatic and splenic response and suggestive positive effects in cardiopulmonary function (474). These studies were in MPS I H/S patients and were not prolonged enough to assess skeletal or CNS effects. Long-term extension studies currently are under way.

Wolman's Disease and Cholesteryl Ester Storage Disease

These rare disorders result from deficiency of lysosomal acid lipase (503). This enzyme is the key enzyme in the pathway of internalization of circulating cholesteryl esters (CEs) and triglycerides (TGs). Lysosomal acid lipase releases the fatty acid ester bonds of CEs and TGs, freeing cholesterol for exit from the lysosome to participate in the SREBP-mediated pathways of cholesterol and fatty acid synthesis. With deficient activity of lysosomal acid lipase, CEs and TGs accumulate in cells of the liver, spleen, and other reticuloendothelial organs (503,504). In Wolman's disease, the macrophage is the primary cell of accumulation, and these cells are both hypertrophic and hyperplastic; hepatocytes are less involved (505). The liver becomes a greasy yellow to yellow-orange in color, and other reticuloendothelial organs become pale and replaced with engorged macrophages. Adrenal gland calcification develops, and adrenal insufficiency can occur. Steatorrhea and cachexia develop as a result of small intestinal infiltration by lipid-laden macrophages. Death occurs in the first year from cachexia and adrenal insufficiency. CE storage disease is less severe with hepatomegaly and progressive cirrhosis can develop (503). The entire spectrum of CE storage disease has not been determined

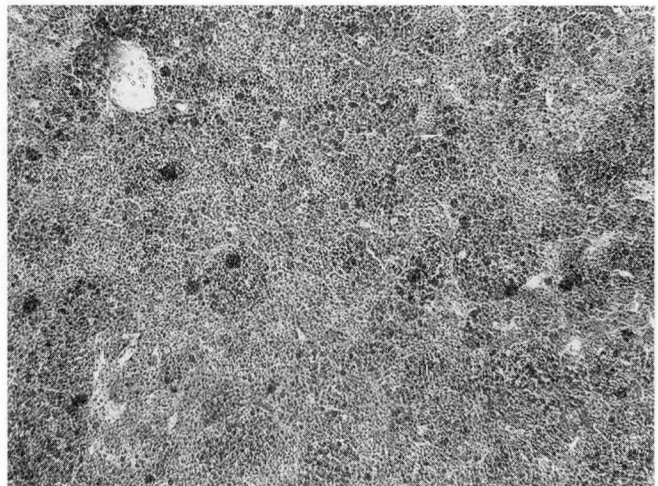

Figure 30-20. Liver biopsy from a Wolman's disease mouse stained with Oil red O for neutral fats. For human and mouse Wolman's disease, the storage cells (macrophages) proliferate within in the liver as islands (potentially of clonal origin). In the mouse, and by analogy in humans, these storage cells express high levels of macrophage colony-stimulating factor. The storage cells stain brightly with Oil red O, indicating the presence of large amounts of neutral fats, cholesteryl esters, cholesterol and triglycerides within the lysosome. With progression, the storage cells can represent over 70% of the cells in the liver. (See Color Fig. 30-20.)

and may include nonspecific fatty infiltration of the liver (hepatic steatosis). Acid lipase deficiency should be excluded on finding foamy macrophages distended with neural fat (Oil red O) accumulation (Fig. 30-20). Enzyme therapy for these diseases seems feasible but has not been definitively tested in clinical trials (506).

REFERENCES

1. Aschoff L. Das reticulo-endotheliale system. *Ergebn Inn Med Kinderhulk* 1924; 26:1.
2. Craddock CG. Defenses of the body: the initiators of defense, the ready reserves, and the scavengers. In: Wintrobe MM, ed. *Blood, pure and eloquent.* New York: McGraw-Hill Book Company, 1980:417.
3. Gall EA. The cytochemical identification and interrelation of mesenchymal cells of lymphoid tissue. *Ann N Y Acad Sci* 1958;73:120.
4. van Furth R. Origin and kinetics of monocytes and macrophages. *Semin Hematol* 1970;7:125.
5. Langerhans P. Über die Nerven der menschlichen Haut. *Virchows Arch* 1868; 44:325.
6. Langerhans P. Berichtigungen. *Archiv Mikroskopische Anatomie* 1882;20:641.
7. Steinman R, Inaba K. Immunogenicity: role of dendritic cells. *Bioessays* 1989; 10:145.
8. Silberberg I, Baer RL, Rosenthal SA. The role of Langerhans cells in contact allergy. I. An ultrastructural study in actively induced contact dermatitis in guinea pigs. *Acta Derm Venereol* 1974;54:321.
9. Thomas C, Donnadieu J, Emile JF, Brousse N. Langerhans' cell histiocytosis. *Arch Pediatr* 1996;3:63.
10. Hart DNJ. Dendritic cells: unique leukocyte populations which control the primary immune response. *Blood* 1997;90:3245.
11. Favara BE, Feller AC, Pauli M, et al. Contemporary classification of histiocytic disorders. The WHO Committee On Histiocytic/Reticulum Cell Proliferations. Reclassification Working Group of the Histiocyte Society. *Med Pediatr Oncol* 1997;29:157.
12. Rosenzwajg M, Canque B, Gluckman JC. Human dendritic cell differentiation pathway from cd334+ hematopoietic precursor cells. *Blood* 1996;87:535.
13. Ryncarz R, Anasetti C. Expression of CD86 on human marrow CD34+ cells identifies immunocompetent committed precursors of macrophages and dendritic cells. *Blood* 1998;91:3892.
14. Mackensen A, Herbst B, Kohler G, et al. Delineation of the dendritic cell lineage by generating large numbers of Birbeck granule-positive Langerhans' cells from human peripheral blood progenitor cells in vitro. *Blood* 1995;86:2699.
15. Klein A, Corazza F, Demulder A, et al. Recurrent viral associated hemophagocytic syndrome in a child with Langerhans' cell histiocytosis. *J Pediatr Hematol Oncol* 1999;21:554.
16. Ishii E, Watanabe S. Biochemistry and biology of the Langerhans' cell. *Hematol Oncol Clin North Am* 1987;1:99.
17. Favara BE, Jaffe R. Pathology of Langerhans' cell histiocytosis. *Hematol Oncol Clin North Am* 1987;1:75.
18. Murphy GF, Bhan AK, Sato S. Characterization of Langerhans' cells by the use of monoclonal antibodies. *Lab Invest* 1981;45:465.
19. Murphy GF, Bhan AK, Sato S, et al. A new immunologic marker for human Langerhans' cells. *N Engl J Med* 1981;304:791.
20. Fithian E, Kung P, Goldstein G. Reactivity of Langerhans' cells with hybridoma antibody. *Proc Natl Acad Sci U S A* 1981;78:2541.
21. Arenzana-Seisdedos F, Barbey S, Virelizier JL, et al. Histiocytosis X. Purified (T6+) cells from bone granuloma produce interleukin 1 and prostaglandin E2 in culture. *J Clin Invest* 1986;77:326.
22. Arceci RJ. The histiocytoses: the fall of the Tower of Babel. *Eur J Cancer* 1999; 35:747.
23. Komp DM. Historical perspectives of Langerhans' cell histiocytosis. *Hematol Oncol Clin North Am* 1987;1:9.
24. Smith T. Skull cap showing congenital deficiency of bone. *Trans Pathol Soc Lond* 1865;2:224.
25. Hand AJ. Polyuria and tuberculosis. *Arch Pediatr* 1893;10:673.
26. Schüller A. Über eigenartige Schädeldefekte im Jugendalter. *Fortschrifte Roentgenstrahlen* 1915;23:12.
27. Christian HA. Defects in membranous bones, exophthalmos and diabetes insipidus; an unusual syndrome of dyspituitarism. *Med Clin North Am* 1919; 3:849.
28. Kay TW. Acquired hydrocephalus with atrophic bone changes, exophthalmos and polyuria (with presentation of patient). *Penn Med* 1905;9:520.
29. Letterer E. Aleukämische Retikulose (Ein Beitrag zu den proliferativen Erkankungen des Retikuloendothelialapparates. *Frankfurter Zeitschrift für Pathologie* 1924;30:377.
30. Farber S. The nature of "solitary or eosiniphilic granuloma" of bone. *Am J Pathol* 1941;17:625.
31. Lichtenstein L. Histiocytosis X: integration of eosiniphilic granuloma of the bone, Letterer-Siwe disease and Schüller-Christian disease as related manifestations of a single nosologic entity. *Arch Pathol* 1953;56:84.
32. Nezelof C, Basset F, Rousseau MF. Histiocytosis X histogenetic arguments for a Langerhans' cell origin. *Biomedicine* 1973;18:365.
33. Farquhar J, Clairveaux A. Familial haemophagocytic reticulosis. *Arch Dis Child* 1952;27:519.
34. Nelson P, Santamaria A, Olson R, et al. Generalized lymphohistiocytic infiltration. A familial disease not previously described and different from Letterer-Siwe and Chédiak-Higashi syndrome. *Pediatrics* 1961;27:931.
35. MacMahon HE, Bedizel M, Ellis C. Familial erythrophagocytic lymphohistiocytosis. *Pediatrics* 1963;32:868.
36. Miller D. Familial reticuloendotheliosis: concurrence of disease in five siblings. *Pediatrics* 1966;38:968.
37. Chu T, D'Angio GJ, Favara BE, et al. Histiocytosis syndromes in children. *Lancet* 1987;2:41.
38. Schmitz L, Favara BE. Nosology and pathology of Langerhans' cell histiocytosis. *Hematol Oncol Clin North Am* 1998;12:221.
39. Carstensen H, Ornvold K. The epidemiology of LCH in children in Denmark, 1975-89. *Med Pediatr Oncol* 1993;21:387.
40. Nicholson HS, Egeler RM, Nesbit ME. The epidemiology of Langerhans' cell histiocytosis. *Hematol Oncol Clin North Am* 1998;12:379.
41. Kaatsch P, Maaf HG, Michalis J, eds. Jahresbericht 1993 des Deutschen Kinderkrebregisters, Vol. 6. Mainz: IMSD Johannes Gutenberg, Universitat Institut fur Medizinishe Statistik und Dokumentation, 1994.
42. Arico M. Langerhans' cell histiocytosis in adults: another orphan disease? *Haematologica* 1999;84:769.
43. Hamre M, Hedberg J, Buckley J, et al. Langerhans' cell histiocytosis: an exploratory epidemiologic study of 177 cases. *Med Pediatr Oncol* 1997;28:92.
44. Bhatia S, Nesbit ME Jr, Egeler RM, et al. Epidemiologic study of Langerhans' cell histiocytosis in children. *J Pediatr* 1997;130:774.
45. Egeler RM, Neglia JP, Arico M, et al. The relation of Langerhans' cell histiocytosis to acute leukemia, lymphomas, and other solid tumors. The LCH-Malignancy Study Group of the Histiocyte Society. *Hematol Oncol Clin North Am* 1998;12:369.
46. Egeler RM, Neglia JP, Puccetti DM, et al. Association of Langerhans' cell histiocytosis with malignant neoplasms. *Cancer* 1993;71:865.
47. Egeler RM, Neglia JP, Arico M, et al. Acute leukemia in association with Langerhans' cell histiocytosis. *Med Pediatr Oncol* 1994;23:81.
48. Horibe K, Matsushita T, Numata S, et al. Acute promyelocytic leukemia with t(15;17) abnormality after chemotherapy containing etoposide for Langerhans' cell histiocytosis. *Cancer* 1993;72:3723.
49. Arico M, Comelli A, Bossi G, et al. Langerhans' cell histiocytosis and acute leukemia: unusual association in two cases. *Med Pediatr Oncol* 1993;21:271.
50. Arico M, Nichols K, Whitlock JA, et al. Familial clustering of Langerhans' cell histiocytosis. *Br J Haematol* 1999;107:883.
51. Kanold J, Vannier JP, Fusade T, et al. Langerhans'-cell histiocytosis in twin sisters. *Arch Pediatr* 1994;1:49.
52. Halton J, Whitton A, Wiernikowski J, Barr RD. Disseminated Langerhans' cell histiocytosis in identical twins unresponsive to recombinant human alpha-interferon and total body irradiation. *Am J Pediatr Hematol Oncol* 1992; 14:269.
53. Katz AM, Rosenthal D, Jakubovic HR, et al. Langerhans' cell histiocytosis in monozygotic twins. *J Am Acad Dermatol* 1991;24:32.

54. Kuwabara S, Takahashi M. Eosinophilic granuloma of the skull in identical twins: case report. *Neurol Med Chir (Tokyo)* 1990;30:1043.

55. Caldarini G. Remarks on a case of Letterer-Siwe disease in a pair of twins. *Clin Pediatr (Bologna)* 1966;48:315.

56. Freundlich E, Amit S, Montag Y, et al. Familial occurrence of Letterer-Siwe disease. *Arch Dis Child* 1972;47:122.

57. Mader I, Stock KW, Radue EW, Steinbrich W. Langerhans' cell histiocytosis in monozygote twins: case reports. *Neuroradiology* 1996;38:163.

58. Bayar E, Kurczynski TW, Robinson MG, et al. Monozygotic twins with congenital acute lymphoblastic leukemia (ALL) and t(4;11)(q21;q23). *Cancer Genet Cytogenet* 1996;89:177.

59. Ford AM, Bennett CA, Price CM, et al. Fetal origins of the TEL-AML1 fusion gene in identical twins with leukemia. *Proc Natl Acad Sci U S A* 1998;95:4584.

60. Ford AM, Pombo-de-Oliveira MS, McCarthy KP, et al. Monoclonal origin of concordant T-cell malignancy in identical twins. *Blood* 1997;89:281.

61. Megonigal MD, Rappaport EF, Jones DH, et al. t(11;22)(q23;q11.2) In acute myeloid leukemia of infant twins fuses MLL with hCDCrel, a cell division cycle gene in the genomic region of deletion in DiGeorge and velocardiofacial syndromes. *Proc Natl Acad Sci U S A* 1998;95:6413.

62. Knudsen AG Jr. Hereditary cancer, oncogenes, and antioncogenes. *Cancer* 1985;45:1437.

63. Egeler RM. Genetic predisposition in Langerhans' cell histiocytosis? An hypothesis (Ph.D. Thesis). In: Haveka BV, ed. Langerhans' cell histiocytosis and other histiocytic disorders. The Netherlands: University of Amsterdam, 1993:181.

64. Ornvold K, Carstensen H, Larsen JK, et al. Flow cytometric DNA analysis of lesions from 18 children with Langerhans cell histiocytosis (histiocytosis x). *Am J Pathol* 1990;136:1301.

65. Yu RC, Chu C, Buluwela L, Chu AC. Clonal proliferation of Langerhans' cells in Langerhans' cell histiocytosis. *Lancet* 1994;343:767.

66. Willman CL, Busque L, Griffith BB, et al. Langerhans'-cell histiocytosis (histiocytosis X)—a clonal proliferative disease. *N Engl J Med* 1994;331:154.

67. Willman CL. Detection of clonal histiocytes in Langerhans' cell histiocytosis: biology and clinical significance. *Br J Cancer Suppl* 1994;23:S29.

68. Willman CL, McClain KL. An update on clonality, cytokines, and viral etiology in Langerhans' cell histiocytosis. *Hematol Oncol Clin North Am* 1998;12:407.

69. Weiss LM, Wood GS, Trela M. Clonal T cell populations in lymphomatoid papulosis: evidence of a lymphoproliferative origin for a clinically benign disease. *N Engl J Med* 1986;315:475.

70. Kurahashi H, Hara J, Yumura-Yagi K. Monoclonal nature of transient abnormal myelopoiesis in Down's syndrome. *Blood* 1991;77:1161.

71. McLelland J, Newton J, Malone M, et al. A flow cytometric study of Langerhans' cell histiocytosis. *Br J Dermatol* 1989;120:485.

72. Betts DR, Leibundgut KE, Feldges A, et al. Cytogenetic abnormalities in Langerhans' cell histiocytosis. *Br J Cancer* 1998;77:552.

73. Golub T, Barker G, Lovett M, Gilliland D. Fusion of PDGF receptor beta to a novel ets-like gene, tel, in chronic myelomonocytic leukemia with t(5;12) chromosomal translocation. *Cell* 1994;77:307.

74. Golub T. TEL gene rearrangements in myeloid malignancy. *Hematol Oncol Clin North Am* 1997;11:1207.

75. Haag MM, Avet-Loiseau H, Favara B, et al. Evaluation of a series of cases of Langerhans' cell histiocytosis by comparative genomic hybridization. 6th International Workshop on Chromosomes in Solid Tumors. Tucson, Arizona; 1991.

76. Chu T, Jaffe R. The normal Langerhans' cell and the LCH cell. *Br J Cancer Suppl* 1994;23:S4.

77. McLelland J. A comparison study of two methods of peanut agglutinin staining with S100 immunostaining in 29 cases of histiocytosis X. *Arch Pathol Lab Med* 1991;115:107.

78. McLelland J, Chu AC. Comparison of peanut agglutinin and S100 stains in the paraffin tissue diagnosis of Langerhans' cell histiocytosis. *Br J Dermatol* 1988;119:513.

79. Hage C, Willman CL, Favara BE, Isaacson PG. Langerhans' cell histiocytosis (histiocytosis X): immunophenotype and growth fraction. *Hum Pathol* 1993; 24:840.

80. Weintraub M, Bhatia KG, Chandra RS, et al. p53 expression in Langerhans' cell histiocytosis. *J Pediatr Hematol Oncol* 1998;20:12.

81. Yu RC, Morris JF, Pritchard J, Chu TC. Defective alloantigen-presenting capacity of 'Langerhans' cell histiocytosis cells.' *Arch Dis Child* 1992;67:1370.

82. Kannourakis G, Abbas A. The role of cytokines in the pathogenesis of Langerhans' cell histiocytosis. *Br J Cancer Suppl* 1994;23:S37.

83. Egeler RM, Favara BE, van Meurs M, et al. Differential in situ cytokine profiles of Langerhans'-like cells and T cells in Langerhans' cell histiocytosis: abundant expression of cytokines relevant to disease and treatment. *Blood* 1999;94:4195.

84. Camargo B, Alves AC, Gorender EF, Bianchi A. Association of malignancy and Langerhans' cell histiocytosis: report of three cases. *Med Pediatr Oncol* 1993;21:451.

85. Mandel M, Toren A, Kende G, et al. Familial clustering of malignant germ cell tumors and Langerhans' histiocytosis. *Cancer* 1994;73:1980.

86. Egeler RM. Acute promyelocytic leukemia with t(15;17) abnormality after chemotherapy containing etoposide for Langerhans' cell histiocytosis. *Cancer* 1995;75:134.

87. Avery ME, McAfee JG, Guild HC. The course and prognosis of reticuloendotheliosis (eosinophilic granuloma), Schüller-Christian disease and Letterer-Siwe disease. A study of 40 cases. *Am J Med* 1957:636.

88. Bartholdy N, Thommesen P. Histiocytosis X. VII. Prognostic significance of skull lesions. *Acta Radiol Oncol* 1983;22:125.

89. Titgemeyer C, Grois N, Minkov M, et al. Pattern and course of single-system disease in Langerhans' cell histiocytosis data from the DAL-X-83- and 90-study. *Med Pediatr Oncol* 2001;37:108.

90. Howarth DM, Gilchrist GS, Mullan BP, et al. Langerhans' cell histiocytosis: diagnosis, natural history, management, and outcome. *Cancer* 1999;85:2278.

91. Oberman HA. Idiopathic histiocytosis; a clinicopathologic study of 40 cases and review of the literature on eosinophilic granuloma of bone, Hand-Schüller-Christian disease and Letterer-Siwe disease. *Pediatrics* 1961;28:307.

92. Berry DH, Becton DL. Natural history of histiocytosis-X. *Hematol Oncol Clin North Am* 1987;1:23.

93. Berry DH, Gresik M, Maybee D, Marcus R. Histiocytosis X in bone only. *Med Pediatr Oncol* 1990;18:292.

94. Cardozo LJ, Bailey IC, Billinghurst JR, Poltera AA. Non-osseous eosinophilic granuloma presenting as acute transverse myelitis. *Br J Surg* 1974;61:747.

95. Crone-Munzebrock W, Brassow F. A comparison of radiographic and bone scan findings in histiocytosis X. *Skeletal Radiol* 1983;9:170.

96. Parker BR, Pinckney L, Etcubanas E. Relative efficacy of radiographic and radionuclide bone surveys in the detection of the skeletal lesions of histiocytosis X. *Radiology* 1980;134:377.

97. Siddiqui AR, Tashjian JH, Lazarus K, et al. Nuclear medicine studies in evaluation of skeletal lesions in children with histiocytosis X. *Radiology* 1981;140:787.

98. Nanduri VR, Jarosz JM, Levitt G, Stanhope R, et al. Basilar invagination as a sequela of multisystem Langerhans' cell histiocytosis. *J Pediatr* 2000;136:114.

99. Berry DH, Gresik MV, Humphrey GB, et al. Natural history of histiocytosis X: a Pediatric Oncology Group Study. *Med Pediatr Oncol* 1986;14:1.

100. Coutte A, Brahe Pedersen C, Bartholdy N, Thommesen P. Histiocytosis X. Recurrent otitis media as a presenting symptom in children with special references to cholesteatoma. *Clin Otolaryngol* 1984;9:111.

101. van Baarle PW. Positive 'fistula sign' with intact ear-drum in a patient with eosinophil granuloma of the mastoid. *J Laryngol Otol* 1976;90:801.

102. Komp DM. Long-term sequelae of histiocytosis X. *Am J Pediatr Hematol Oncol* 1981;3:163.

103. McDonald JS, Miller RL, Bernstein ML, Olson JW. Histiocytosis X: a clinical presentation. *J Oral Pathol* 1980;9:342.

104. Filocoma D, Needleman HL, Arceci R, et al. Pediatric histiocytosis. Characterization, prognosis, and oral involvement. *Am J Pediatr Hematol Oncol* 1993;15:226.

105. Rapidis AD, Langdon JD, Harvey PW, Patel MF. Histiocytosis X. An analysis of 50 cases. *Int J Oral Surg* 1978;7:76.

106. Braunstein GD, Kohler PO. Endocrine manifestations of histiocytosis. *Am J Pediatr Hematol Oncol* 1981;3:67.

107. Greenberger JS, Cassady JR, Jaffe N, et al. Radiation therapy in patients with histiocytosis: management of diabetes insipidus and bone lesions. *Int J Radiat Oncol Biol Phys* 1979;5:1749.

108. Greenberger JS, Crocker AC, Vawter G, et al. Results of treatment of 127 patients with systemic histiocytosis. *Medicine (Baltimore)* 1981;60:311.

109. Dunger DB, Broadbent V, Yeoman E, et al. The frequency and natural history of diabetes insipidus in children with Langerhans'-cell histiocytosis. *N Engl J Med* 1989;321:1157.

110. Broadbent V, Pritchard J. Diabetes insipidus associated with Langerhans' cell histiocytosis: is it reversible? *Med Pediatr Oncol* 1997;28:289.

111. Rosenzweig KE, Arceci RJ, Tarbell NJ. Diabetes insipidus secondary to Langerhans' cell histiocytosis: is radiation therapy indicated? *Med Pediatr Oncol* 1997;29:36.

112. Vawter GF, Greenberger JS, Crocker AC. A retrospective clinico-pathologic analysis of diabetes insipidus in dendritic cell disease. *Med Pediatr Oncol* 1986;14:112.

113. Gadner H, Heitger A, Ritter J, et al. Langerhans' cell histiocytosis in childhood—results of the DAL-HX 83 study. *Klin Padiatr* 1987;199:173.

114. Gadner H, Heitger A, Grois N, et al. Treatment strategy for disseminated Langerhans' cell histiocytosis. DAL HX-83 Study Group. *Med Pediatr Oncol* 1994;23:72.

115. Kaufman A, Bukberg PR, Werlin S, Young IS. Multifocal eosinophilic granuloma ("Hand-Schüller-Christian disease"). Report illustrating H-S-C chronicity and diagnostic challenge. *Am J Med* 1976;60:541.

116. Ober KP, Alexander E Jr, Challa VR, et al. Histiocytosis X of the hypothalamus. *Neurosurgery* 1989;24:93.

117. Graif M, Pennock JM. MR imaging of histiocytosis X in the central nervous system. *AJNR Am J Neuroradiol* 1986;7:21.

118. Jinkins JR. Histiocytosis-X of the hypothalamus: case report and literature review. *Comput Radiol* 1987;11:181.

119. Chiumello G, di Natale B, Pellini C. Magnetic resonance imaging in diabetes insipidus. *Lancet* 1989;4:901.

120. Rosenfield NS, Abrahams J, Komp D. Brain MR in patients with Langerhans' cell histiocytosis: findings and enhancement with Gd-DTPA. *Pediatr Radiol* 1990;20:433.

121. Grois NG, Favara BE, Mostbeck GH, Prayer D. Central nervous system disease in Langerhans' cell histiocytosis. *Hematol Oncol Clin North Am* 1998;12:287.

122. Grois N, Tsunematsu Y, Barkovich AJ, Favara BE. Central nervous system disease in Langerhans' cell histiocytosis. *Br J Cancer Suppl* 1994;23:S24.

123. Grois N, Flucher-Wolfram B, Heitger A, et al. Diabetes insipidus in Langerhans' cell histiocytosis: results from the DAL-HX 83 study. *Med Pediatr Oncol* 1995;24:248.

124. Latorre H, Kenney FM, Lahey ME, Drash A. Short stature and growth hormone deficiency in histiocytosis X. *J Pediatr* 1974;85:813.
125. Sims DG. Histiocytosis X; follow-up of 43 cases. *Arch Dis Child* 1977;52:433.
126. Komp DM. Histiocytosis. *Am J Pediatr Hematol Oncol* 1981;3:43.
127. Zinkham WH. Multifocal eosinophilic granuloma. Natural history, etiology and management. *Am J Med* 1976;60:457.
128. Burn DJ, Watson JD, Roddie M, Chu AC, Legg NJ, Frackowiak RS. Langerhans' cell histiocytosis and the nervous system. *J Neurol* 1992;239:345.
129. Geoffray A. Case of the season. Diagnosis: histiocytosis X of the central nervous system. *Semin Roentgenol* 1984;19:257.
130. Simms S, Warner NJ. A framework for understanding and responding to the psychosocial needs of children with Langerhans' cell histiocytosis and their families. *Hematol Oncol Clin North Am* 1998;12:359.
131. Whitsett SF, Kneppers K, Coppes MJ, Egeler RM. Neuropsychologic deficits in children with Langerhans' cell histiocytosis. *Med Pediatr Oncol* 1999; 33:486.
132. Komp DM. Langerhans' cell histiocytosis. *N Engl J Med* 1987;316:747.
133. Egeler RM, D'Angio GJ. Langerhans' cell histiocytosis. *J Pediatr* 1995;127:1.
134. Marcy TW, Reynolds HY. Pulmonary histiocytosis X. *Lung* 1985;163:129.
135. Basset F, Corrin B, Spencer H, et al. Pulmonary histiocytosis X. *Am Rev Respir Dis* 1978;118:811.
136. Miller WT. Pulmonary Langerhans'-cell histiocytosis. *N Engl J Med* 2000; 343:1656.
137. Khoor A, Myers JL, Tazelaar HD, Swensen SJ. Pulmonary Langerhans' cell histiocytosis presenting as a solitary nodule. *Mayo Clin Proc* 2001;76:209.
138. Arico M, Nichols KE, Danesino C. Pulmonary Langerhans'-cell histiocytosis. *N Engl J Med* 2000;343:1654.
139. O'Regan AW, Brophy MT. Pulmonary Langerhans'-cell histiocytosis. *N Engl J Med* 2000;343:1654.
140. Brown RE. Pulmonary Langerhans'-cell histiocytosis. *N Engl J Med* 2000;343: 1654.
141. Vos LD, Nollen AM, Gooszen HC, Jansen FH. Pulmonary histiocytosis X. *JBR-BTR* 1999;82:132.
142. Callebaut W, Demedts M, Verleden G. Pulmonary Langerhans' cell granulomatosis (histiocytosis X): clinical analysis of 8 cases. *Acta Clin Belg* 1998;53:337.
143. Yousem SA, Colby TV, Chen YY, et al. Pulmonary Langerhans' cell histiocytosis: molecular analysis of clonality. *Am J Surg Pathol* 2001;25:630.
144. Ryu JH, Colby TV, Hartman TE, Vassallo R. Smoking-related interstitial lung diseases: a concise review. *Eur Respir J* 2001;17:122.
145. Bernstrand C, Cederlund K, Ashtrom L, Henter JI. Smoking preceded pulmonary involvement in adults with Langerhans' cell histiocytosis diagnosed in childhood. *Acta Paediatr* 2000;89:1389.
146. Miadonna A, Gibelli S, Tedeschi A, et al. Favourable outcome of a case of pulmonary Langerhans' cell histiocytosis. *Monaldi Arch Chest Dis* 2000;55:3.
147. Okten A, Mocan H, Erduran E, et al. Langerhans' cell histiocytosis associated with recurrent pneumothorax: a case report. *Turk J Pediatr* 1996;38:125.
148. Seely JM, Effmann EL, Muller NL. High-resolution CT of pediatric lung disease: imaging findings. *AJR Am J Roentgenol* 1997;168:1269.
149. Moore AD, Godwin JD, Muller NL, et al. Pulmonary histiocytosis X: comparison of radiographic and CT findings. *Radiology* 1989;172:249.
150. Brauner MW, Grenier P, Mouelhi MM, et al. Pulmonary histiocytosis X: evaluation with high-resolution CT. *Radiology* 1989;172:255.
151. Koh DM, Hansell DM. Computed tomography of diffuse interstitial lung disease in children. *Clin Radiol* 2000;55:659.
152. Soler P, Bergeron A, Kambouchner M, et al. Is high-resolution computed tomography a reliable tool to predict the histopathological activity of pulmonary Langerhans' cell histiocytosis? *Am J Respir Crit Care Med* 2000;162:264.
153. Williams WJ, James DG. Pulmonary Langerhans' cell granulomatosis (LCG). *Sarcoidosis* 1993;10:104.
154. Rand EB, Whitington PF. Successful orthotopic liver transplantation in two patients with liver failure due to sclerosing cholangitis with Langerhans' cell histiocytosis. *J Pediatr Gastroenterol Nutr* 1992;15:202.
155. Mahmoud H, Gaber O, Wang W, et al. Successful orthotopic liver transplantation in a child with Langerhans' cell histiocytosis. *Transplantation* 1991; 51:278.
156. Arceci RJ, Brenner MK, Pritchard J. Controversies and new approaches to treatment of Langerhans' cell histiocytosis. *Hematol Oncol Clin North Am* 1998;12:339.
157. Soua H, Pousse H, Ladeb F, et al. Histiocytosis X and sclerosing cholangitis. *Ann Pediatr (Paris)* 1993;40:316.
158. Thompson HH, Pitt HA, Lewin KJ, Longmire WP Jr. Sclerosing cholangitis and histiocytosis X. *Gut* 1984;25:526.
159. Leblanc A, Hadchouel M, Jehan P, et al. Obstructive jaundice in children with histiocytosis X. *Gastroenterology* 1981;80:134.
160. Newton WA Jr, Hamoudi AB, Shannon BT. Role of the thymus in histiocytosis-X. *Hematol Oncol Clin North Am* 1987;1:63.
161. Osband ME, Lipton JM, Lavin P, et al. Histiocytosis-X. *N Engl J Med* 1981; 304:146.
162. Broadbent V, Pritchard J, Davies EG, et al. Spontaneous remission of multisystem histiocytosis X. *Lancet* 1984;1:253.
163. Shannon BT, Newton WA. Suppressor-cell dysfunction in children with histiocytosis-X. *J Clin Immunol* 1986;6:510.
164. Ceci A, de Terlizzi M, Toma MG, et al. Heterogeneity of immunological patterns in Langerhan's histiocytosis and response to crude calf thymic extract in 11 patients. *Med Pediatr Oncol* 1988;16:111.
165. Zaizov R, Stark B, Friedman I. Cell mediated immunity and activation of macrophages in childhood histiocytoses. *Med Pediatr Oncol* 1986;14:110.
166. Lahey ME. Prognostic factors in histiocytosis X. *Am J Pediatr Hematol Oncol* 1981;3:57.
167. Lahey E. Histiocytosis x: an analysis of prognostic factors. *J Pediatr* 1975; 87:184.
168. Gadner H, Heitger A, Grois N, et al. Treatment strategy for disseminated Langerhans' cell histiocytosis. DAL HX-83 Study Group. *Med Pediatr Oncol* 1994;23:72.
169. Ladisch S, Gadner H, Arico M, et al. LCH-I: a randomized trial of etoposide vs. vinblastine in disseminated Langerhans' cell histiocytosis. The Histiocyte Society. *Med Pediatr Oncol* 1994;23:107.
170. Minkov M, Grois N, Heitger A, et al. Treatment of multisystem Langerhans' cell histiocytosis. Results of the DAL-HX 83 and DAL-HX 90 studies. DAL-HX Study Group. *Klin Padiatr* 2000;212:139.
171. Siwe SA. Die Reticuloendotheliose: ein neues Krankheitsbild unter den Hepatosplenomegalien. *Z Kinderheilk* 1933;55:212.
172. Abt AF, Denenholz EJ. Letterer-Siwe's disease. Splenomegaly associated with wide-spread hyperplasia of nonlipoid-storing macrophages. *Am J Dis Child* 1936;51:499.
173. Gadner H, Grois N, Arico M, et al. A randomized trial of treatment for multisystem Langerhans' cell histiocytosis. *J Pediatr* 2001;138:728.
174. Lavin PT, Osband ME. Evaluating the role of therapy in histiocytosis-X. Clinical studies, staging, and scoring. *Hematol Oncol Clin North Am* 1987;1:35.
175. Broadbent V, Pritchard J. Histiocytosis X—current controversies. *Arch Dis Child* 1985;60:605.
176. Broadbent V, Gadner H. Current therapy for Langerhans' cell histiocytosis. *Hematol Oncol Clin North Am* 1998;12:327.
177. Wirtschafter JD, Nesbit M, Anderson P, McClain K. Intralesional methylprednisolone for Langerhans' cell histiocytosis of the orbit and cranium. *J Pediatr Ophthalmol Strabismus* 1987;24:194.
178. Cassady JR. Current role of radiation therapy in the management of histiocytosis-X. *Hematol Oncol Clin North Am* 1987;1:123.
179. Richter MP, D'Angio GJ. The role of radiation therapy in the management of children with histiocytosis X. *Am J Pediatr Hematol Oncol* 1981;3:161.
180. Egeler RM, Thompson RC Jr, Voute PA, Nesbit ME Jr. Intralesional infiltration of corticosteroids in localized Langerhans' cell histiocytosis. *J Pediatr Orthop* 1992;12:811.
181. Gramatovici R, D'Angio GJ. Radiation therapy in soft-tissue lesions in histiocytosis X (Langerhans' cell histiocytosis). *Med Pediatr Oncol* 1988;16:259.
182. Minehan KJ, Chen MG, Zimmerman D, et al. Radiation therapy for diabetes insipidus caused by Langerhans' cell histiocytosis. *Int J Radiat Oncol Biol Phys* 1992;23:519.
183. Maghnie M, Arico M, Villa A, et al. MR of the hypothalamic-pituitary axis in Langerhans' cell histiocytosis. *AJNR Am J Neuroradiol* 1992;13:1365.
184. Maghnie M, Bossi G, Klersy C, et al. Dynamic endocrine testing and magnetic resonance imaging in the long-term follow-up of childhood Langerhans cell histiocytosis. *J Clin Endocrinol Metab* 1998;83:3089.
185. Tien RD, Newton TH, McDermott MW, et al. Thickened pituitary stalk on MR images in patients with diabetes insipidus and Langerhans cell histiocytosis. *AJNR Am J Neuroradiol* 1990;11:703.
186. Atherton DJ, Broadbent V, Pritchard J. Topical use of mustine hydrochloride in cutaneous histiocytosis-X. *Med Pediatr Oncol* 1986;14:112.
187. Sheehan MP, Atherton DJ, Broadbent V, Pritchard J. Topical nitrogen mustard: an effective treatment for cutaneous Langerhans' cell histiocytosis. *J Pediatr* 1991;119:317.
188. Iwatsuki K, Tsugiki M, Yoshizawa N, et al. The effect of phototherapies on cutaneous lesions of histiocytosis X in the elderly. *Cancer* 1986;57:1931.
189. Sakai H, Ibe M, Takahashi H, et al. Satisfactory remission achieved by PUVA therapy in Langerhans' cell histiocytosis in an elderly patient. *J Dermatol* 1996;23:42.
190. Lipton JM. The pathogenesis, diagnosis, and treatment of histiocytosis syndromes. *Pediatr Dermatol* 1983;1:112.
191. McLelland J, Broadbent V, Yeomans E, et al. Langerhans' cell histiocytosis: the case for conservative treatment. *Arch Dis Child* 1990;65:301.
192. McLelland J, Pritchard J, Chu AC. Current controversies. Histiocytosis-X. *Hematol Oncol Clin North Am* 1987;1:147.
193. Komp DM. Therapeutic strategies for Langerhans' cell histiocytosis. *J Pediatr* 1991;119:274.
194. Ceci A, de Terlizzi M, Colella R, et al. Langerhans' cell histiocytosis in childhood: results from the Italian Cooperative AIEOP-CNR-H.X '83 study. *Med Pediatr Oncol* 1993;21:259.
195. Ceci A, de Terlizzi M, Colella R, et al. Etoposide in recurrent childhood Langerhans' cell histiocytosis: an Italian cooperative study. *Cancer* 1988;62:2528.
196. Osband ME, Lipton JM, Lavin P. Histiocytosis-X: demonstration of abnormal immunity, T cell histamine H_2-receptor deficiency, and successful treatment with thymic extract. *N Engl J Med* 1981;304:146.
197. Egeler RM, de Kraker J, Voute PA. Cytosine-arabinoside, vincristine, and prednisolone in the treatment of children with disseminated Langerhans' cell histiocytosis with organ dysfunction: experience at a single institution. *Med Pediatr Oncol* 1993;21:265.
198. Grau J, Ribera JM, Tormo M, et al. Results of treatment with 2-chlorodeoxyadenosine in refractory or relapsed Langerhans' cell histiocytosis. Study of 9 patients. *Med Clin (Barc)* 2001;116:339.
199. Weitzman S, Wayne AS, Arceci R, et al. Nucleoside analogues in the therapy of Langerhans' cell histiocytosis: a survey of members of the histiocyte society and review of the literature. *Med Pediatr Oncol* 1999;33:476.

200. Betticher DC, Fey MF, von Rohr A, et al. High incidence of infections after 2-chlorodeoxyadenosine (2-CDA) therapy in patients with malignant lymphomas and chronic and acute leukaemias. *Ann Oncol* 1994;5:57.

201. Stine KC, Saylors RL, Williams LL, Becton DL. 2-Chlorodeoxyadenosine (2-CDA) for the treatment of refractory or recurrent Langerhans' cell histiocytosis (LCH) in pediatric patients. *Med Pediatr Oncol* 1997;29:288.

202. Saven A, Piro LD. 2-Chlorodeoxyadenosine: a potent antimetabolite with major activity in the treatment of indolent lymphoproliferative disorders. *Hematol Cell Ther* 1996;38:S93.

203. Dimopoulos MA, Theodorakis M, Kostis E, Papadimitris C, Moulopoulos LA, Anastasiou-Nana M. Treatment of Langerhans' cell histiocytosis with 2 chlorodeoxyadenosine. *Leuk Lymphoma* 1997;25:187.

204. Conias S, Strutton G, Stephenson G. Adult cutaneous Langerhans' cell histiocytosis. *Australas J Dermatol* 1998;39:106.

205. Saven A, Figueroa ML, Piro LD, Rosenblatt JD. 2-Chlorodeoxyadenosine to treat refractory histiocytosis X. *N Engl J Med* 1993;329:734.

206. Saven A, Foon KA, Piro LD. 2-Chlorodeoxyadenosine-induced complete remissions in Langerhans'-cell histiocytosis. *Ann Intern Med* 1994;121:430.

207. McCowage GB, Frush DP, Kurtzberg J. Successful treatment of two children with Langerhans' cell histiocytosis with 2'-deoxycoformycin. *J Pediatr Hematol Oncol* 1996;18:154.

208. Petersen AJ, Brown RD, Gibson J, et al. Nucleoside transporters, bcl-2 and apoptosis in CLL cells exposed to nucleoside analogues in vitro. *Eur J Haematol* 1996;56:213.

209. Lauria F. 2-Chlorodeoxyadenosine, a "novel" agent in the treatment of both lymphoid and myeloid malignancies. *Haematologica* 1992;77:443.

210. Gandhi V, Estey E, Keating MJ, et al. Chlorodeoxyadenosine and arabinosylcytosine in patients with acute myelogenous leukemia: pharmacokinetic, pharmacodynamic, and molecular interactions. *Blood* 1996;87:256.

211. Hirose M, Saito S, Yoshimoto T, Kuroda Y. Interleukin-2 therapy of Langerhans' cell histiocytosis. *Acta Paediatr* 1995;84:1204.

212. Mahmoud HH, Wang WC, Murphy SB. Cyclosporine therapy for advanced Langerhans' cell histiocytosis. *Blood* 1991;77:721.

213. Arico M. Cyclosporine therapy for refractory Langerhans' cell histiocytosis. *Blood* 1991;78:3107.

214. Jakobson AM, Kreuger A, Hagberg H, Sundstrom C. Treatment of Langerhans' cell histiocytosis with alpha-interferon. *Lancet* 1987;2:1520.

215. Albanell J, Salud A, Bellmunt J, et al. Treatment with interferon of systemic Langerhans'-cell histiocytosis in an adult. *Med Clin (Barc)* 1990;94:184.

216. Sato Y, Ikeda Y, Ito E, et al. Histiocytosis X: successful treatment with recombinant interferon-alpha A. *Acta Paediatr Jpn* 1990;32:151.

217. Misery L, Larbre B, Lyonnet S, et al. Remission of Langerhans' cell histiocytosis with thalidomide treatment. *Clin Exp Dermatol* 1993;18:487.

218. Thomas L, Ducros B, Secchi T, et al. Successful treatment of adult's Langerhans' cell histiocytosis with thalidomide. Report of two cases and literature review. *Arch Dermatol* 1993;129:1261.

219. Meunier L, Marck Y, Ribeyre C, Meynadier J. Adult cutaneous Langerhans' cell histiocytosis: remission with thalidomide treatment. *Br J Dermatol* 1995;132:168.

220. Hirose M, Kuroda Y. Successful induction therapy of natural killer/cytotoxic T-lymphocyte cells in the treatment of Langerhans' cell histiocytosis. *Int J Hematol* 1999;69:272.

221. Ringden O, Lonnqvist B, Holst M. 12-year follow-up of allogeneic bone-marrow transplant for Langerhans' cell histiocytosis. *Lancet* 1997;349:476.

222. Ringden O, Ahstrom L, Lonnqvist B, et al. Allogeneic bone marrow transplantation in a patient with chemotherapy-resistant progressive histiocytosis X. *N Engl J Med* 1987;316:733.

223. Stoll M, Freund M, Schmid H. Allogeneic bone marrow transplantation for Langerhans' cell histiocytosis. *Cancer* 1990;66:284.

224. Dehner LP. Allogeneic bone marrow transplantation in a patient with chemotherapy-resistant progressive histiocytosis X. *N Engl J Med* 1987;317:773.

225. Conter V, Reciputo A, Arrigo C, et al. Bone marrow transplantation for refractory Langerhans' cell histiocytosis. *Haematologica* 1996;81:468.

226. Morgan G. Myeloablative therapy and bone marrow transplantation for Langerhans' cell histiocytosis. *Br J Cancer Suppl* 1994;23:S52.

227. A multicentre retrospective survey of Langerhans' cell histiocytosis: 348 cases observed between 1983 and 1993. The French Langerhans' Cell Histiocytosis Study Group. *Arch Dis Child* 1996;75:17.

228. Kusumakumary P, James FV. Permanent disabilities in childhood survivors of Langerhans' cell histiocytosis. *Pediatr Hematol Oncol* 2000;17:375.

229. Cervera A, Madero L, Garcia Penas JJ, et al. CNS sequelae in Langerhans' cell histiocytosis: progressive spinocerebellar degeneration as a late manifestation of the disease. *Pediatr Hematol Oncol* 1997;14:577.

230. Egeler RM, de Kraker J, Voute PA. Langerhans'-cell histiocytosis (histiocytosis X); 20-year experience in the Emma Kinderziekenhuis, 1969-1988. *Ned Tijdschr Geneeskd* 1993;137:955.

231. Nanduri VR, Bareille P, Pritchard J, Stanhope R. Growth and endocrine disorders in multisystem Langerhans' cell histiocytosis. *Clin Endocrinol (Oxf)* 2000;53:509.

232. Hunninghake GW, Kalica AR. Approaches to the treatment of pulmonary fibrosis. *Am J Respir Crit Care Med* 1995;151:915.

233. Zeller B, Storm-Mathisen I, Smevik B, Lie SO. Multisystem Langerhans'-cell histiocytosis with life-threatening pulmonary involvement—good response to cyclosporine A. *Med Pediatr Oncol* 2000;35:438.

234. Brown RE. Bisphosphonates as antialveolar macrophage therapy in pulmonary Langerhans cell histiocytosis? *Med Pediatr Oncol* 2001;36:641.

235. Saven A, Burian C. Cladribine activity in adult Langerhans-cell histiocytosis. *Blood* 1999;93:4125.

236. Mogulkoc N, Veral A, Bishop PW, et al. Pulmonary Langerhans' cell histiocytosis: radiologic resolution following smoking cessation. *Chest* 1999;115:1452.

237. Mapel DW, Samet JM, Coultas DB. Corticosteroids and the treatment of idiopathic pulmonary fibrosis. Past, present, and future. *Chest* 1996;110:1058.

238. Yeatman M, McNeil K, Smith JA, et al. Lung transplantation in patients with systemic diseases: an eleven-year experience at Papworth Hospital. *J Heart Lung Transplant* 1996;15:144.

239. Montoya A, Mawulawde K, Houck J, et al. Survival and functional outcome after single and bilateral lung transplantation. Loyola Lung Transplant Team. *Surgery* 1994;116:712.

240. Arceci RJ. Treatment options—commentary. *Br J Cancer Suppl* 1994;23:S58.

241. Spray TL, Mallory GB, Canter CB, Huddleston CB. Pediatric lung transplantation. Indications, techniques, and early results. *J Thorac Cardiovasc Surg* 1994;107:990.

242. Etienne B, Bertocchi M, Gamondes JP, et al. Relapsing pulmonary Langerhans' cell histiocytosis after lung transplantation. *Am J Respir Crit Care Med* 1998;157:288.

243. Debray D, Pariente D, Urvoas E, et al. Sclerosing cholangitis in children. *J Pediatr* 1994;124:49.

244. Neveu I, Labrune P, Huguet P, et al. Sclerosing cholangitis revealing histiocytosis X. *Arch Fr Pediatr* 1990;47:197.

245. Puel O, Guillard JM. Sclerosing cholangitis in the course of histiocytosis X. *Arch Fr Pediatr* 1990;47:155.

246. Concepcion W, Esquivel CO, Terry A, et al. Liver transplantation in Langerhans' cell histiocytosis (histiocytosis X). *Semin Oncol* 1991;18:24.

247. Hadzic N, Pritchard J, Webb D, et al. Recurrence of Langerhans' cell histiocytosis in the graft after pediatric liver transplantation. *Transplantation* 2000;70:815.

248. Calleja J, Vazquez R, Lopez Baena J, et al. Orthotopic liver transplantation in Langerhans' cell histiocytosis. *Rev Esp Enferm Dig* 1999;91:594.

249. Melendez HV, Dhawan A, Mieli-Vergani G, et al. Liver transplantation for Langerhans' cell histiocytosis—a case report and literature review. *Transplantation* 1996;62:1167.

250. Newell KA, Alonso EM, Kelly SM, et al. Association between liver transplantation for Langerhans' cell histiocytosis, rejection, and development of post-transplant lymphoproliferative disease in children. *J Pediatr* 1997;131:98.

251. Sommerauer JF, Atkison P, Andrews W, et al. Liver transplantation for Langerhans' cell histiocytosis and immunomodulation of disease pre- and posttransplant. *Transplant Proc* 1994;26:178.

252. Zandi P, Panis Y, Debray D, et al. Pediatric liver transplantation for Langerhans' cell histiocytosis. *Hepatology* 1995;21:129.

253. Kaltsas GA, Powles TB, Evanson J, et al. Hypothalamo-pituitary abnormalities in adult patients with Langerhans cell histiocytosis: clinical, endocrinological, and radiological features and response to treatment. *J Clin Endocrinol Metab* 2000;85:1370.

254. Hasegawa K, Mitomi T, Kowa H, et al. A clinico-pathological study of adult histiocytosis X involving the brain. *J Neurol Neurosurg Psychiatry* 1993;56:1008.

255. Goldberg-Stern H, Weitz R, Zaizov R, et al. Progressive spinocerebellar degeneration "plus" associated with Langerhans' cell histiocytosis: a new paraneoplastic syndrome? *J Neurol Neurosurg Psychiatry* 1995;58:180.

256. Saatci I, Baskan O, Haliloglu M, Aydingoz U. Cerebellar and basal ganglion involvement in Langerhans' cell histiocytosis. *Neuroradiology* 1999;41:443.

257. Pui CH, Hancock ML, Raimondi SC. Myeloid neoplasia in children treated for solid tumours. *Lancet* 1991;336:417.

258. Pui CH, Ribeiro RC, Hancock ML. Acute myeloid leukemia in children treated with epipodophyllotoxins for acute lymphoblastic leukemia. *N Engl J Med* 1991;325:1682.

259. Gadner H, Ladisch S, Arico M, et al. VP-16 and the treatment of histiocytosis. *Eur J Pediatr* 1994;153:389.

260. Stine KC, Saylors RL, Sawyer JR, Becton DL. Secondary acute myelogenous leukemia following safe exposure to etoposide. *J Clin Oncol* 1997;15:1583.

261. Haupt R, Fears TR, Heise A, et al. Risk of secondary leukemia after treatment with etoposide (VP-16) for Langerhans' cell histiocytosis in Italian and Austrian-German populations. *Int J Cancer* 1997;71:9.

262. Schiavetti A, Varrasso G, Maurizi P, Castello MA. Two secondary leukemias among 15 children given oral etoposide. *Med Pediatr Oncol* 2001;37:148.

263. Felix CA, Blatt J. Etoposide and Langerhans' cell histiocytosis: second malignancies, a second look. *Pediatr Hematol Oncol* 1999;16:183.

264. Starling KA, Iyer R, Silva-Sosa M, et al. Chlorambucil in histiocytosis X: a Southwest Oncology Group study. *J Pediatr* 1980;96:266.

265. Starling KA. Chemotherapy of histiocytosis-X. *Hematol Oncol Clin North Am* 1987;1:119.

266. Pritchard J. Histiocytosis X: natural history and management in childhood. *Clin Exp Dermatol* 1979;4:421.

267. Helwig EB, Hackney VC. Juvenile xanthogranuloma (nevoxanthoendothelioma). *Am J Pathol* 1954;30:625.

268. Misery L, Boucheron S, Claudy AL. Factor XIIIa expression in juvenile xanthogranuloma. *Acta Derm Venereol* 1994;74:43.

269. Freyer DR, Kennedy R, Bostrom BC, et al. Juvenile xanthogranuloma: forms of systemic disease and their clinical implications. *J Pediatr* 1996;129:227.

270. Kraus MD, Haley JC, Ruiz R, et al. "Juvenile" xanthogranuloma: an immunophenotypic study with a reappraisal of histogenesis. *Am J Dermatopathol* 2001;23:104.

271. Malone M. The histiocytoses of childhood. *Histopathology* 1991;19:105.
272. Amoric JC, Stalder JF, Schmuck C, et al. Ocular complication disclosing juvenile xanthogranuloma. Apropos of a case. *Ann Dermatol Venereol* 1991;118:629.
273. Aref'ev IL, Karmilov VA, Sushchenko IT. Disseminated juvenile xanthogranulomatosis. *Vestn Dermatol Venereol* 1978:61.
274. Cohen DM, Brannon RB, Davis LD, Miller AS. Juvenile xanthogranuloma of the oral mucosa. *Oral Surg Oral Med Oral Pathol* 1981;52:513.
275. Eggli KD, Caro P, Quiogue T, Boal DK. Juvenile xanthogranuloma: non-X histiocytosis with systemic involvement. *Pediatr Radiol* 1992;22:374.
276. Hadden OB. Bilateral juvenile xanthogranuloma of the iris. *Br J Ophthalmol* 1975;59:699.
277. Hamburg A. Juvenile xanthogranuloma of the uvea in an adult. *Ophthalmologica* 1976;172:273.
278. Holland G. Ocular changes in juvenile xantho-granuloma. *Klin Monatsbl Augenheilkd* 1966;149:353.
279. Gallant CJ, From L. Juvenile xanthogranulomas and xanthoma disseminatum—variations on a single theme. *J Am Acad Dermatol* 1986;15:108.
280. Garcia-Pena P, Mariscal A, Abellan C, et al. Juvenile xanthogranuloma with extracutaneous lesions. *Pediatr Radiol* 1992;22:377.
281. Giller RH, Folberg R, Keech RV, et al. Xanthoma disseminatum. An unusual histiocytosis syndrome. *Am J Pediatr Hematol Oncol* 1988;10:252.
282. Mencia-Gutierrez E, Gutierrez-Diaz E, Madero-Garcia S. Juvenile xanthogranuloma of the orbit in an adult. *Ophthalmologica* 2000;214:437.
283. Smith ME, Sanders TE, Bresnick GH. Juvenile xanthogranuloma of the ciliary body in an adult. *Arch Ophthalmol* 1969;81:813.
284. Wertz FD, Zimmerman LE, McKeown CA, et al. Juvenile xanthogranuloma of the optic nerve, disc, retina, and choroid. *Ophthalmology* 1982;89:1331.
285. Borne MJ, Gedde SJ, Augsburger JJ, et al. Juvenile xanthogranuloma of the iris with bilateral spontaneous hyphema. *J Pediatr Ophthalmol Strabismus* 1996;33:196.
286. Bostrom J, Janssen G, Messing-Junger M, et al. Multiple intracranial juvenile xanthogranulomas. Case report. *J Neurosurg* 2000;93:335.
287. Botella-Estrada R, Sanmartin O, Grau M, et al. Juvenile xanthogranuloma with central nervous system involvement. *Pediatr Dermatol* 1993;10:64.
288. Chu AC, Wells RS, MacDonald DM. Juvenile xanthogranuloma with recurrent subdural effusions. *Br J Dermatol* 1981;105:97.
289. Mendez-Martinez OE, Luzardo-Small GD, Cardozo-Duran JJ. Symptomatic bilateral xanthogranulomas of choroid plexus in a child. *Br J Neurosurg* 2000;14:62.
290. Esterly NB, Medenica M. Benign cephalic histiocytosis. *Arch Dermatol* 1985;121:449.
291. Gianotti F, Caputo R, Ermacora E. Singular "infantile histiocytosis with cells with intracytoplasmic vermiform particles." *Bull Soc Fr Dermatol Syphiligr* 1971;78:232.
292. Gianotti F. Histiocytosis with cells containing vermiform intracytoplasmic particles. 2nd case in an infant. *Bull Soc Fr Dermatol Syphiligr* 1972;79:244.
293. Gianotti F, Caputo R. Histiocytic syndromes: a review. *J Am Acad Dermatol* 1985;13:383.
294. Jaffe R, DeVaughn D, Langhoff E. Fascin and the differential diagnosis of childhood histiocytic lesions. *Pediatr Dev Pathol* 1998;1:216.
295. Cobb MW, Barber FA. Solitary papule on the forearm. Solitary reticulohistiocytoma. *Arch Dermatol* 1990;126:667.
296. Perrin C, Lacour JP, Michiels JF, Ortonne JP. Reticulohistiocytomas versus multicentric reticulohistiocytosis. *Am J Dermatopathol* 1995;17:625.
297. Suwabe H, Tsutsumi Y. Reticulohistiocytoma involving the skin, subcutaneous tissue and a regional lymph node. *Pathol Int* 1996;46:531.
298. Zelger BW, Sidoroff A, Orchard G, Cerio R. Non-Langerhans' cell histiocytoses. A new unifying concept. *Am J Dermatopathol* 1996;18:490.
299. Pileri S, Kikuchi M, Helbron D. Histiocytic necrotizing lymphadenitis without granulocytic infiltration. *Virchows Arch* 1982;395:257.
300. Kikuchi M. Lymphadenitis showing focal reticulum cell hyperplasia with nuclear debris and phagocytes: a clinicopathological study. *Nippon Ketsueki Gakkai Zasshi* 1972;35:379.
301. Dorfman RF, Berry GJ. Kikuchi's histiocytic necrotizing lymphadenitis: an analysis of 108 cases with emphasis on differential diagnosis. In: Burke JS, ed. *Seminars in diagnostic pathology*, Vol. 5, 1988:329.
302. Turner RR, Martin J, Dorfman RF. Necrotizing lymphadenitis: a study of 30 cases. *Am J Surg Pathol* 1983;7:115.
303. Rosai J, Dorfman RF. Sinus histiocytosis with massive lymphadenopathy: a pseudolymphomatous benign disorder. Analysis of 34 cases. *Cancer* 1972;30:1174.
304. Remadi S, Anagnostopoulou ID, Jlidi R, et al. Extranodal Rosai-Dorfman disease in childhood. *Pathol Res Pract* 1996;192:1007.
305. Gaetani P, Tancioni F, Di Rocco M, Rodriguez y Baena R. Isolated cerebellar involvement in Rosai-Dorfman disease: case report. *Neurosurgery* 2000;46:479.
306. Kessler E, Srulijes C, Toledo E, Shalit M. Sinus histiocytosis with massive lymphadenopathy and spinal epidural involvement. A case report and review of the literature. *Cancer* 1976;38:1614.
307. Sakai K, Koike G, Seguchi K, Nakazato Y. Sinus histiocytosis with massive lymphadenopathy: a case of multiple dural involvement. *Brain Tumor Pathol* 1998;15:63.
308. Lampert F, Lennert K. Sinus histiocytosis with massive lymphadenopathy: fifteen new cases. *Cancer* 1976;37:783.
309. Sumaya CV, Cherry JD, Gohd R. Exaggerated antibody response following rubella vaccination in a child with sinus histiocytosis with massive lymphadenopathy. *J Pediatr* 1976;89:81.
310. Levine PH, Jahan N, Murari P, et al. Detection of human herpesvirus 6 in tissues involved by sinus histiocytosis with massive lymphadenopathy (Rosai-Dorfman disease). *J Infect Dis* 1992;166:291.
311. Allen MR, Ninfo V, Viglio A, et al. Sinus histiocytosis with massive lymphadenopathy (Rosai-Dorfman disease) in a girl previously affected by acute lymphoblastic leukemia. *Med Pediatr Oncol* 2001;37:150.
312. Paulli M, Bergamaschi G, Tonon L, et al. Evidence for a polyclonal nature of the cell infiltrate in sinus histiocytosis with massive lymphadenopathy (Rosai-Dorfman disease). *Br J Haematol* 1995;91:415.
313. McAlister WH, Herman T, Dehner LP. Sinus histiocytosis with massive lymphadenopathy (Rosai-Dorfman disease). *Pediatr Radiol* 1990;20:425.
314. Wu M, Anderson AE, Kahn LB. A report of intracranial Rosai-Dorfman disease with literature review. *Ann Diagn Pathol* 2001;5:96.
315. Foucar E, Rosai J, Dorfman R. Sinus histiocytosis with massive lymphadenopathy (Rosai-Dorfman disease): review of the entity. *Semin Diagn Pathol* 1990;7:19.
316. Foucar E, Rosai J, Dorfman RF. Sinus histiocytosis with massive lymphadenopathy. An analysis of 14 deaths occurring in a patient registry. *Cancer* 1984;54:1834.
317. Suarez P, el-Naggar AK, Batsakis JG. Intracellular crystalline deposits in lymphoplasmacellular disorders. *Ann Otol Rhinol Laryngol* 1997;106:170.
318. Komp DM. The treatment of sinus histiocytosis with massive lymphadenopathy (Rosai-Dorfman disease). *Semin Diagn Pathol* 1990;7:83.
319. Childs HA, Kim RY. Radiation response of Rosai-Dorfman disease presenting with involvement of the orbits. *Am J Clin Oncol* 1999;22:526.
320. Antonius JI, Farid SM, Baez-Giangreco A. Steroid-responsive Rosai-Dorfman disease. *Pediatr Hematol Oncol* 1996;13:563.
321. Horneff G, Jurgens H, Hort W, et al. Sinus histiocytosis with massive lymphadenopathy (Rosai-Dorfman disease): response to methotrexate and mercaptopurine. *Med Pediatr Oncol* 1996;27:187.
322. Baildam EM, Ewing CI, D'Souza SW, Stevens RF. Sinus histiocytosis with massive lymphadenopathy (Rosai-Dorfman disease): response to acyclovir. *J R Soc Med* 1992;85:179.
323. MacMahon HE, Bedizel M, Ellis CA. Familial erythrophagocytic lymphohistiocytosis. *Pediatrics* 1963;32:868.
324. Nezelhof C, Elizchar E. Familial lymphohistiocytosis: a report of three cases with general review. Possible links with secondary syndromes. *Nouvelle Revue Francaise d Hematologie* 1973;13:319.
325. Henter JI, Arico M, Elinder G, et al. Familial hemophagocytic lymphohistiocytosis. Primary hemophagocytic lymphohistiocytosis. *Hematol Oncol Clin North Am* 1998;12:417.
326. Henter JI, Elinder G. Familial hemophagocytic lymphohistiocytosis. Clinical review based on the findings in seven children. *Acta Paediatr Scand* 1991;80:269.
327. Stark B, Hershko C, Rosen N, et al. Familial hemophagocytic lymphohistiocytosis (FHLH) in Israel. I. Description of 11 patients of Iranian-Iraqi origin and review of the literature. *Cancer* 1984;54:2109.
328. Henter JI, Elinder G, Soder O, Ost A. Incidence in Sweden and clinical features of familial hemophagocytic lymphohistiocytosis. *Acta Paediatr Scand* 1991;80:428.
329. Henter J-I, Aricò M, Elinder G, et al. Familial hemophagocytic lymphohistiocytosis. *Hematol Oncol Clin North Am* 1998;12:417.
330. Henter JI, Arico M, Elinder G, et al. Familial hemophagocytic lymphohistiocytosis. Primary hemophagocytic lymphohistiocytosis. *Hematol Oncol Clin North Am* 1998;12:417.
331. Arico M, Janka G, Fischer A, et al. Hemophagocytic lymphohistiocytosis. Report of 122 children from the International Registry. FHL Study Group of the Histiocyte Society. *Leukemia* 1996;10:197.
332. Henter JI, Elinder G, Ost A. Diagnostic guidelines for hemophagocytic lymphohistiocytosis. The FHL Study Group of the Histiocyte Society. *Semin Oncol* 1991;18:29.
333. Henter JI, Elinder G. Haemophagocytic lymphohistiocytosis: an inherited primary form and a reactive secondary form. *Br J Haematol* 1995;91:774.
334. Majluf-Cruz A, Sosa-Camas R, Perez-Ramirez O, et al. Hemophagocytic syndrome associated with hematological neoplasias. *Leuk Res* 1998;22:893.
335. Risdall RJ, McKenna RW, Nesbit ME, et al. Virus-associated hemophagocytic syndrome: a benign histiocytic proliferation distinct from malignant histiocytosis. *Cancer* 1979;44:993.
336. Wilson ER, Malluh A, Stagno S, Crist WM. Fatal Epstein-Barr virus-associated hemophagocytic syndrome. *J Pediatr* 1981;98:260.
337. Daum GS, Sullivan JL, Ansell J. Virus-associated hemophagocytic syndrome: identification of an immunoproliferative precursor lesion. *Hum Pathol* 1987;18:1071.
338. Campo E, Condom E, Miro MJ, et al. Tuberculosis-associated hemophagocytic syndrome. A systemic process. *Cancer* 1986;58:2640.
339. Risdall RJ, Brunning RD, Hernandez JI, Gordon DH. Bacteria-associated hemophagocytic syndrome. *Cancer* 1984;54:2968.
340. Mallous AA, Saadi AR. Hemophagocytosis with typhoid fever. *Pediatr Infect Dis* 1986;5:720.
341. Fame TM, Engelhard D, Riley HD Jr. Hemophagocytosis accompanying typhoid fever. *Pediatr Infect Dis* 1986;5:367.
342. Udden MM, Banez E, Sears DA. Bone marrow histiocytic hyperplasia and hemophagocytosis with pancytopenia in typhoid fever. *Am J Med Sci* 1986;291:396.
343. Weintraub M, Siegman-Igra Y, Hosiphov J. Histiocytic hemophagocytosis in miliary tuberculosis. *Arch Intern Med* 1984;144:2055.

344. Marom D, Offer I, Tamary H, et al. Hemophagocytic lymphohistiocytosis associated with visceral leishmaniasis. *Pediatr Hematol Oncol* 2001;18:65.
345. Gagnaire MH, Galambrun C, Stephan JL. Hemophagocytic syndrome: a misleading complication of visceral leishmaniasis in children—a series of 12 cases. *Pediatrics* 2000;106:E58.
346. Auerbach M, Haubenstock A, Soloman G. Systemic babesiosis. Another cause of the hemophagocytic syndrome. *Am J Med* 1986;80:301.
347. Yin JAL, Kumaran TO, Marsh GW. Complete recovery of histiocytic medullary reticulosis-like syndrome in a child with acute lymphoblastic leukemia. *Cancer* 1983;51:200.
348. Chen T, Newbit M, McKenna R. Histiocytic medullary reticulosis in acute lymphocytic leukemia of T-cell origin. *Am J Dis Child* 1976;130:1261.
349. Rubin M, Rothenberg SP, Panchacharam P. A histiocytic medually reticulosis-like syndrome as the terminal event in lymphocytic lymphoma. *Am J Med Sci* 1984;287:60.
350. Theodorakis ME, Zamkoff KW, Davey FR, et al. Acute nonlymphocytic leukemia complicated by severe cytophagocytosis of formed blood elements by nonmalignant histiocytes: cause of significant clinical morbidity. *Med Pediatr Oncol* 1983;11:20.
351. Liang DC, Chu ML, Shih CC. Reactive histiocytosis in acute lymphoblastic leukemia and non-Hodgkin's lymphoma. *Cancer* 1986;58:1289.
352. Takasaki N, Kaneko Y, Maseki N, et al. Hemophagocytic syndrome complicating T-cell acute lymphoblastic leukemia with a novel t(11;14)(p15;q11) chromosome translocation. *Cancer* 1987;59:424.
353. Janka G, Imashuku S, Elinder G, et al. Infection- and malignancy-associated hemophagocytic syndromes. Secondary hemophagocytic lymphohistiocytosis. *Hematol Oncol Clin North Am* 1998;12:435.
354. Hasegawa D, Kojima S, Tatsumi E, et al. Elevation of the serum Fas ligand in patients with hemophagocytic syndrome and Diamond-Blackfan anemia. *Blood* 1998;91:2793.
355. Fadeel B, Henter JI, Orrenius S. Apoptosis required for maintenance of homeostasis: familial hemophagocytic lymphohistiocytosis caused by too little cell death. *Lakartidningen* 2000;97:1395.
356. Arico M, Imashuku S, Clementi R, et al. Hemophagocytic lymphohistiocytosis due to germline mutations in SH2D1A, the X-linked lymphoproliferative disease gene. *Blood* 2001;97:1131.
357. Ohadi M, Lalloz MR, Sham P, et al. Localization of a gene for familial hemophagocytic lymphohistiocytosis at chromosome 9q21.3-22 by homozygosity mapping. *Am J Hum Genet* 1999;64:165.
358. Goransdotter Ericson K, Fadeel B, Nilsson-Ardnor S, et al. Spectrum of perforin gene mutations in familial hemophagocytic lymphohistiocytosis. *Am J Hum Genet* 2001;68:590.
359. Zipursky A. Perforin deficiency and familial hemophagocytic lymphohistiocytosis. *Pediatr Res* 2001;49:3.
360. Stepp SE, Dufourcq-Lagelouse R, Le Deist F, et al. Perforin gene defects in familial hemophagocytic lymphohistiocytosis. *Science* 1999;286:1957.
361. Arico M, Bettinelli A, Maccario R, et al. Hemophagocytic lymphohistiocytosis in a patient with deletion of 22q11.2. *Am J Med Genet* 1999;87:329.
362. Dufourcq-Lagelouse R, Pastural E, Barrat FJ, et al. Genetic basis of hemophagocytic lymphohistiocytosis syndrome. *Int J Mol Med* 1999;4:127.
363. Dufourcq-Lagelouse R, Jabado N, Le Deist F, et al. Linkage of familial hemophagocytic lymphohistiocytosis to 10q21-22 and evidence for heterogeneity. *Am J Hum Genet* 1999;64:172.
364. Egeler RM, Shapiro R, Loechelt B, Filipovich A. Characteristic immune abnormalities in hemophagocytic lymphohistiocytosis. *J Pediatr Hematol Oncol* 1996;18:340.
365. Kataoka Y, Todo S, Morioka Y, et al. Impaired natural killer activity and expression of interleukin-2 receptor antigen in familial erythrophagocytic lymphohistiocytosis. *Cancer* 1990;65:1937.
366. Goldberg J, Nezelof C. Lymphohistiocytosis: a multi-factorial syndrome of macrophagic activation clinico-pathological study of 38 cases. *Hematol Oncol* 1986;4:275.
367. Rieux-Laucat F, Le Deist F, Hivroz C, et al. Mutations in Fas associated with human lymphoproliferative syndrome and autoimmunity. *Science* 1995;268:1247.
368. Sullivan KE, Delaat CA, Douglas SD, Filipovich AH. Defective natural killer cell function in patients with hemophagocytic lymphohistiocytosis and in first degree relatives. *Pediatr Res* 1998;44:465.
369. Le Deist F, Emile J, Rieux-Laucat F, et al. Clinical, immunological, and pathological consequences of Fas-deficient conditions. *Lancet* 1996;348:719.
370. Drappa J, Vaishnaw A, Sullivan K, et al. Fas gene mutations in the Canale-Smith syndrome, an inherited lymphoproliferative disorder associated with autoimmunity. *N Engl J Med* 1996;335:1643.
371. Dianzani U, Bragardo M, DiFranco D, et al. Deficiency of the Fas apoptosis pathway without Fas gene mutations in pediatric patients with autoimmunity/lymphoproliferation. *Blood* 1997;89:2871.
372. Bejaoui M, Veber F, Girault D, et al. The accelerated phase of Chediak-Higashi syndrome. *Arch Fr Pediatr* 1989;46:733.
373. Henter JI, Andersson B, Elinder G, et al. Elevated circulating levels of interleukin-1 receptor antagonist but not IL-1 agonists in hemophagocytic lymphohistiocytosis. *Med Pediatr Oncol* 1996;27:21.
374. Osugi Y, Hara J, Tagawa S, et al. Cytokine production regulating Th1 and Th2 cytokines in hemophagocytic lymphohistiocytosis. *Blood* 1997;89:4100.
375. Imashuku S, Hibi S. Cytokines in hemophagocytic syndrome. *Br J Haematol* 1991;77:438.
376. Trinchieri G, Gerosa F. Immunoregulation by interleukin-12. *J Leuk Biol* 1996;59:505.
377. Komp DM, Buckley PJ, McNamara J, van Hoff J. Soluble interleukin-2 receptor in hemophagocytic histiocytoses: searching for markers of disease activity. *Pediatr Hematol Oncol* 1989;6:253.
378. Goldberg JC, Nezelof C. Familial lymphohistiocytosis: the pathologist's view. *Pediatr Hematol Oncol* 1989;6:199.
379. Imashuku S. Differential diagnosis of hemophagocytic syndrome: underlying disorders and selection of the most effective treatment. *Int J Hematol* 1997;66:135.
380. Kletzel M, Gollin SM, Gloster ES, et al. Chromosome abnormalities in familial hemophagocytic lymphohistiocytosis. *Cancer* 1986;57:2153.
381. Wieczorek R, Greco A, McCarthy K. Familial erythrophagocytic lymphohistiocytosis: immunophenotypic, immunohistochemical, and ultrastructural demonstration of the relation to sinus histiocytes. *Hum Pathol* 1986;17:55.
382. Ansbacher LE, Singsen BH, Hosler MW. Familial erythrophagocytic lymphohistiocytosis: an association with serum lipid abnormalities. *J Pediatr* 1983;102:270.
383. Ladisch S. Lipid abnormalities and immunodeficiency in familial erythrophagocytic lymphohistiocytosis. *Pediatr Hematol Oncol* 1989;6:283.
384. Ladisch S, Ho W, Matheson D. Immunologic and clinical effects of repeated blood exchange in familial erythrophagocytic lymphohistiocytosis. *Blood* 1982;60:814.
385. Forbes KP, Collie DA, Parker A. CNS involvement of virus-associated hemophagocytic syndrome: MR imaging appearance. *AJNR Am J Neuroradiol* 2000;21:1248.
386. Munoz Ruano MM, Castillo M. Brain CT and MR imaging in familial hemophagocytic lymphohistiocytosis. *AJR Am J Roentgenol* 1998;170:802.
387. Price DL, Woolsey JE, Rosman NP, Richard EP Jr. Familial lymphohistiocytosis of the nervous system. *Arch Neurol* 1971;24:270.
388. Akima M, Sumi SM. Neuropathology of familial erythrophagocytic lymphohistiocytosis: six cases and review of the literature. *Hum Pathol* 1984;15:161.
389. Alvarado CS, Buchanan GR, Kim TH, et al. Use of VP-16-213 in the treatment of familial erythrophagocytic lymphohistiocytosis. *Cancer* 1986;57:1097.
390. Ambruso DR, Hays T, Zwartjes WJ, et al. Successful treatment of lymphohistiocytic reticulosis with phagocytosis with epipodophyllotoxin VP-16-213. *Cancer* 1980;45:2516.
391. Henter J-I, Elinder G, Finkel Y, Soder O. Successful induction with chemotherapy including teniposide in familial erythrophagocytic lymphohistiocytosis. *Lancet* 1986;13:1402.
392. Fischer A, Virelizier JL, Arenzana-Seiwdedos F, et al. Treatment of four patients with erythrophagocytic lymphohistiocytosis by a combination of epipodophyllotoxin, steroid, intrathecal methotrexate, and cranial irradiation. *Pediatrics* 1985;76:263.
393. Stephan JL, Donadieu J, Ledeist F, et al. Treatment of familial hemophagocytic lymphohistiocytosis with antithymocyte globulins, steroids, and cyclosporin A. *Blood* 1993;82:2319.
394. Bader-Meunier B, Parez N, Muller S. Treatment of hemophagocytic lymphohistiocytosis with cyclosporin A and steroids in a boy with lysinuric protein intolerance. *J Pediatr* 2000;136:134.
395. Loechelt BJ, Egeler M, Filipovich AH, et al. Immunosuppression: preliminary results of alternative maintenance therapy for familial hemophagocytic lymphohistiocytosis (FHL). *Med Pediatr Oncol* 1994;22:325.
396. Durken M, Schneider EM, Blutters-Sawatzki R, et al. Treatment of hemophagocytic lymphohistiocytosis, HLH, with bone marrow transplantation. *Klin Padiatr* 1998;210:180.
397. Blanche S, Caniglia M, Girault D, et al. Treatment of hemophagocytic lymphohistiocytosis with chemotherapy and bone marrow transplantation: a single-center study of 22 cases. *Blood* 1991;78:51.
398. Blanche S, Caniglia M, Fischer A, Griscelli C. Treatment of familial lymphohistiocytosis: chemotherapy or bone marrow transplant? *Pediatr Hematol Oncol* 1989;6:273.
399. Bolme P, Henter JI, Winiarski J, et al. Allogeneic bone marrow transplantation for hemophagocytic lymphohistiocytosis in Sweden. *Bone Marrow Transplant* 1995;15:331.
400. Baker KS, DeLaat CA, Steinbuch M, et al. Successful correction of hemophagocytic lymphohistiocytosis with related or unrelated bone marrow transplantation. *Blood* 1997;89:3857.
401. Jabado N, de Graeff-Meeder ER, Cavazzana-Calvo M, et al. Treatment of familial hemophagocytic lymphohistiocytosis with bone marrow transplantation from HLA genetically nonidentical donors. *Blood* 1997;90:4743.
402. Landman-Parker J, Le Deist F, Blaise A, et al. Partial engraftment of donor bone marrow cells associated with long- term remission of haemophagocytic lymphohistiocytosis. *Br J Haematol* 1993;85:37.
403. Henter JI, Arico M, Egeler RM, et al. HLH-94: a treatment protocol for hemophagocytic lymphohistiocytosis. HLH Study Group of the Histiocyte Society. *Med Pediatr Oncol* 1997;28:342.
404. Hesseling PB, Wessels G, Egeler RM, Rossouw DJ. Simultaneous occurrence of viral-associated hemophagocytic syndrome and Langerhans' cell histiocytosis: a case report. *Pediatr Hematol Oncol* 1995;12:135.
405. Janka GE. Familial hemophagocytic lymphohistiocytosis: therapy in the German experience. *Pediatr Hematol Oncol* 1989;6:227.
406. Imashuku S, Kuriyama K, Teramura T, et al. Requirement for etoposide in the treatment of Epstein-Barr virus-associated hemophagocytic lymphohistiocytosis. *J Clin Oncol* 2001;19:2665.

407. Scott RB, Robb-Smith AHT. Histiocytic medullary reticulosis. *Lancet* 1939; 2:194.
408. Esseltine DW, De Leeuw NK, Berry GR. Malignant histiocytosis. *Cancer* 1983; 52:1904.
409. Schouten TJ, Hustinx TW, Scheres JM, et al. Malignant histiocytosis. Clinical and cytogenetic studies in a newborn and a child. *Cancer* 1983;52:1229.
410. Warnke RA, Kim H, Dorfman RF. Malignant histiocytosis (histiocytic medullary reticulosis). I. Clinicopathologic study of 29 cases. *Cancer* 1975;35:215.
411. Lampert IA, Catovsky D, Bergier N. Malignant histiocytosis: a clinicopathological study of 12 cases. *Br J Haematol* 1978;40:65.
412. Wilson MS, Weiss LM, Gatter KC, et al. Malignant histiocytosis. A reassessment of cases previously reported in 1975 based on paraffin section immunophenotyping studies. *Cancer* 1990;66:530.
413. Weiss LM, Trela MJ, Cleary ML, et al. Frequent immunoglobulin and T-cell receptor gene rearrangements in "histiocytic" neoplasms. *Am J Pathol* 1985; 121:369.
414. Franchino C, Reich C, Distenfeld A, et al. A clinicopathologically distinctive primary splenic histiocytic neoplasm. Demonstration of its histiocyte derivation by immunophenotypic and molecular genetic analysis. *Am J Surg Pathol* 1988;12:398.
415. Kadin ME. T gamma cells: a missing link between malignant histiocytosis and T cell leukemia-lymphoma? *Hum Pathol* 1981;12:771.
416. O'Connor NTJ, Stein H, Gatter KC. Genotypic analysis of large cell lymphomas which express the Ki-1 antigen. *Histopathology* 1987;11:733.
417. Ishii E, Hara T, Okamura J, et al. Malignant histiocytosis in infants: surface marker analysis of malignant cells in two cases. *Med Pediatr Oncol* 1987; 15:102.
418. Lampert IA, Catovsky D, Bergier N. Malignant histiocytosis: a clinico-pathological study of 12 cases. *Br J Haematol* 1978;40:65.
419. Schouten HC, Hopman AH, Haesevoets AM, Arends JW. Large-cell anaplastic non-Hodgkin's lymphoma originating in donor cells after allogenic bone marrow transplantation. *Br J Haematol* 1995;91:162.
420. Benz-Lemoine E, Brizard A, Huret JL, et al. Malignant histiocytosis: a specific t(2;5)(p23;q35) translocation? Review of the literature. *Blood* 1988;72:1045.
421. Kaneko Y, Frizzera G, Edamura S, et al. A novel translocation, t(2;5)(p23;q35), in childhood phagocytic large T- cell lymphoma mimicking malignant histiocytosis. *Blood* 1989;73:806.
422. Kamesaki H, Koya M, Miwa H, et al. Malignant histiocytosis with rearrangement of the heavy chain gene and evidence of monocyte-macrophage lineage. *Cancer* 1988;62:1306.
423. Simon JH, Tebbi CK, Freeman AI, et al. Malignant histiocytosis. Complete remission in two pediatric patients. *Cancer* 1987;59:1566.
424. Ducatman BS, Wick MR, Morgan TW, et al. Malignant histiocytosis: a clinical, histologic, and immunohistochemical study of 20 cases. *Hum Pathol* 1984;15:368.
425. Cabanillas F, Rodriguez V, Freireich EJ. Improvement in complete response rate, duration of response and survival with adriamycin combination chemotherapy for non-Hodgkin lymphoma: a prognostic factor comparison of two regimens. *Med Pediatr Oncol* 1978;4:321.
426. Vera R Jr, Bertino JR, Cadman E, Waldron JA. Malignant histiocytosis. Response to VP-16-213 and cytosine arabinoside. *Cancer* 1984;54:991.
427. Fanin R, Silvestri F, Geromin A, et al. Sequential intensive treatment with the F-MACHOP regimen (+/- radiotherapy) and autologous stem cell transplantation for primary systemic CD30 (Ki-1)—positive anaplastic large cell lymphoma in adults. *Leuk Lymphoma* 1997;24:369.
428. Vowels MR, Lam-Po-Tang PR, Ford D, et al. Bone-marrow transplantation for haematological malignancy in childhood. *Med J Aust* 1986;144:347.
429. Cazin B, Gorin NC, Jouet JP, et al. Successful autologous bone marrow transplantation in second remission of malignant histiocytosis. *Bone Marrow Transplant* 1990;5:431.
430. Kao WY, Hwang WS. Bone marrow transplantation for malignant histiocytosis. *Transplant Proc* 1992;24:1524.
431. Jaffe D, Fleisher G, Grosflam J. Detection of cancer in the pediatric emergency department. *Pediatr Emerg Care* 1985;1:11.
432. Willemze R, Ruiter DJ, Van Vloten WA, Meijer CJ. Reticulum cell sarcomas (large cell lymphomas) presenting in the skin. High frequency of true histiocytic lymphoma. *Cancer* 1982;50:1367.
433. Willemze R, Beljaards RC. Spectrum of primary cutaneous CD30 (Ki-1)-positive lymphoproliferative disorders. A proposal for classification and guidelines for management and treatment. *J Am Acad Dermatol* 1993;28:973.
434. Barron DR, Davis BR, Pomeranz JR, et al. Cytophagic histiocytic panniculitis. A variant of malignant histiocytosis. *Cancer* 1985;55:2538.
435. Goldberg NS, Bauer K, Rosen ST. Histiocytosis-X. *Arch Dermatol* 1986;122:446.
436. Tani M, Ishii N, Kumagai M, et al. Malignant Langerhans' cell tumour. *Br J Dermatol* 1992;126:398.
437. Monda I, Warnke R, Rosai J. A primary lymph node malignancy with features suggestive of dendritic reticulum cell differentiation. A report of 4 cases. *Am J Pathol* 1986;122:562.
438. Feltkamp CA, van Heerde P, Feltkamp-Vroom TM. A malignant tumor arising from interdigitating cells; light microscopical, ultrastructural, immuno- and enzyme-histochemical characteristics. *Virchows Arch* 1981;393:183.
439. Chan WC, Zaatari G. Lymph node interdigitating reticulum cell sarcoma. *Am J Clin Pathol* 1986;85:739.
440. Nakamura S, Hara K, Suchi T. Interdigitating cell sarcoma: a morphologic, immunologic and enzyme histochemical study. *Cancer* 1988;61:562.
441. de Duve C. Lysosomes revisited. *Eur J Biochem* 1983;137:391.
442. Hannun YA, Bell RM. Lysosphingolipids inhibit protein kinase C: implications for the sphingolipidoses. *Science* 1987;235:670.
443. Goldstein JL, Brown MS, Anderson RGW, et al. Receptor mediated endocytosis: concepts emerging from the LDL receptor system. *Annu Rev Cell Biol* 1979;1:1.
444. Fratantoni JC, Hall CW, Neufeld EF. The defect in Hurler and Hunter syndromes II: deficiency of specific factors involved in mucopolysaccharide degradation. *Proc Natl Acad Sci U S A* 1969;64:360.
445. Fisher HD, Gonzalez-Noriega A, Sly WS, Morre DJ. Phosphomannosyl enzyme receptors in rat liver. *J Biol Chem* 1980;255:9608.
446. Dahms NM, Lobel P, Kornfeld S. Mannose 6-phosphate receptors and lysosomal enzyme targeting. *J Biol Chem* 1989;264:12115.
447. Kornfeld S, Mellman I. The biogenesis of lysosomes. *Annu Rev Cell Biol* 1989;5:483.
448. Lobel P, Dahms NM, Breitmeyer J, et al. Cloning of the bovine 215-kDa cation-independent mannose 6-phosphate receptor. *Proc Natl Acad Sci U S A* 1987;84:2233.
449. Lobel P, Dahms NM, Kornfeld S. Cloning and sequence analysis of the cation-independent mannose 6-phosphate receptor. *J Biol Chem* 1988;263:2563.
450. Dahms NM, Lobel P, Breitmeyer J, et al. 46 kd mannose 6-phosphate receptor: cloning, expression, and homology to the 215 kd mannose 6-phosphate receptor. *Cell* 1987;50:181.
451. Kornfeld S. Structure and function of the mannose 6-phosphate/insulin like growth factor II receptors. *Annu Rev Biochem* 1992;61:307.
452. Waheed S, Pohlmann R, Hasilik A, von Figura K. Subcellular location of two enzymes involved in the synthesis of phosphorylated recognition markers in lysosomal enzymes. *J Biol Chem* 1981;256:4150.
453. Greenberg J, Howell KE. Membrane traffic in endocytosis: insights from cell free assays. *Annu Rev Cell Biol* 1989;5:453.
454. Pryer NK, Wuestehube LJ, Schekman R. Vesicle-mediated protein sorting. *Annu Rev Biochem* 1992;61:471.
455. Mullins C, Bonifacino JS. The molecular machinery for lysosome biogenesis. *Bioessays* 2001;23:333.
456. Dell'Angelica EC, Mullins C, Caplan S, Bonifacino JS. Lysosome-related organelles. *FASEB J* 2000;14:1265.
457. Luzio JP, Rous BA, Bright NA, et al. Lysosome-endosome fusion and lysosomal biogenesis. *J Cell Science* 2000;113:1515.
458. Varki A, Kornfeld A. Lysosomal enzyme targeting: N-acetylglucosaminylphosphotransferase selectively phosphorylated native lysosomal enzymes. *J Biol Chem* 1981;256:11977.
459. Braun M, Waheed A, von Figura K. Lysosomal acid phosphatase is transported to lysosomes via the cell surface. *EMBO J* 1989;8:3633.
460. Sun Y, Jin P, Witte DP, Grabowski GA. Tissue preferential expression and promoter analysis of the prosaposin gene in transgenic mice. *Biochem J* 2000;352:549.
461. Aula P, Jalanko A, Peltonen L. Aspartylglucosaminuria. In: Scriver CR, Beaudet A, Sly W, Valle D, eds. *The metabolic and molecular bases of inherited disease*, Vol. 3, 8th ed. New York: McGraw-Hill, 2001:16.
462. Du H, Witte DP, Grabowski GA. Tissue and cellular specific expression of murine lysosomal acid lipase mRNA and protein. *J Lipid Res* 1996;37:937.
463. Uusitalo A, Tenhunen K, Heinonen O, et al. Toward understanding the neuronal pathogenesis of aspartylglucosaminuria: expression of aspartylglucosaminidase in brain during development. *Mol Genet Metabol* 1999;67:294.
464. Nauseef W, Olsson I, Arnljots K. Biosynthesis and processing of myeloperoxidase: a marker for myeloid differentiation. *Eur J Hematol* 1988;40:97.
465. Leinekugel P, Michel S, Conzelmann E, Sandhoff K. Quantitative correlation between the residual activity of beta-hexosaminidase A and arylsulfatase A and the severity of the resulting lysosomal storage disease. *Hum Genet* 1992;88:513.
466. Conzelmann E, Sandhoff K. Partial enzyme deficiencies: residual activities and the development of neurological disorders. *Dev Neurosci* 1983;6:58.
467. Grabowski GA, Leslie N, Wenstrup RJ. Enzyme therapy in Gaucher disease: the first five years. *Blood Rev* 1998;12:115.
468. Grabowski GA, Saal H, Wenstrup RJ, Barton NW. Gaucher disease: a prototype for molecular medicine. *Crit Rev Hematol Oncol* 1996;23:25.
469. Eng CM, Guffon N, Wilcox WR, et al. Safety and efficacy of recombinant human a-galactosidase A–replacement therapy in Fabry's disease. *N Engl J Med* 2001;345:9.
470. Schiffmann R, Kopp JB, Austin HA, et al. Enzyme replacement therapy in Fabry disease: a randomized controlled trial. *JAMA* 2001;285:2743.
471. Van den Hout H RA, Vulto AG, Loonen MC, et al. Recombinant human alpha-glucosidase from rabbit milk in Pompe patients. *Lancet* 2000;356:397.
472. Van den Hout JM RA, de Klerk JB, Arts WF, et al. Enzyme therapy for Pompe disease with recombinant human alpha-glucosidase from rabbit milk. *J Inherit Metab Dis* 2001;24:266.
473. Amalfitano ABA, Morse RP, Majure JM, et al. Recombinant human acid alpha-glucosidase enzyme therapy for infantile glycogen storage disease type II: results of a phase I/II clinical trial. *Genet Med* 2001;3:132.
474. Kakkis ED, Muenzer J, Tiller GE, et al. Enzyme-replacement therapy in mucopolysaccharidosis I. *N Engl J Med* 2001;344:182.
475. Peters C, Shapiro EG, Krivit W. Neuropsychological development in children with Hurler syndrome following hematopoietic stem cell transplantation. *Pediatr Transplant* 1998;2:250.
476. Krivit W, Peters C, Shapiro EG. Bone marrow transplantation as effective treatment of central nervous system disease in globoid cell leukodystrophy, metachromatic leukodystrophy, adrenoleukodystrophy, mannosidosis, fucosi-

dosis, aspartylglucosaminuria, Hurler, Maroteaux-Lamy, and Sly syndromes, and Gaucher disease type III. *Curr Opin Neurol* 1999;12:167.

477. Chang MH, Bindloss CA, Grabowski GA, et al. Saposins A, B, C, and D in plasma of patients with lysosomal storage disorders. *Clin Chem* 2000;46:167.
478. Scriver CR, Beaudet A, Sly W, et al., eds. *The metabolic and molecular bases of inherited disease*, 8th ed. New York: McGraw-Hill, 2001.
479. Beutler E, Grabowski GA. Gaucher disease. In: Scriver CR, Beaudet AL, Sly WS, Valle D, eds. *The metabolic and molecular bases of inherited diseases*, 8th ed. New York: McGraw-Hill, 2001:3635.
480. Charrow J, Andersson HC, Kaplan P, et al. The Gaucher registry: demographics and disease characteristics of 1698 patients with Gaucher disease. *Arch Intern Med* 2000;160:2835.
481. Patterson MC, Di Bisceglie AM, Higgins JJ, et al. The effect of cholesterol-lowering agents on hepatic and plasma cholesterol in Niemann-Pick disease type C. *Neurology* 1993;43:61.
482. Sibille A, Eng CM, Kim SJ, et al. Phenotype/genotype correlations in Gaucher disease type I: clinical and therapeutic implications. *Am J Hum Genet* 1993;52:1094.
483. Dreborg S, Erikson A, Hagberg B. Gaucher disease—Norrbottnian type. I. General clinical description. *Eur J Pediatr* 1980;133:107.
484. Rosenthal DI, Doppelt SH, Mankin HJ, et al. Enzyme replacement therapy for Gaucher disease: skeletal responses to macrophage-targeted glucocerebrosidase. *Pediatrics* 1995;96:629.
485. Elstein D, Hadas-Halpern I, Itzchaki M, et al. Effect of low-dose enzyme replacement therapy on bones in Gaucher disease patients with severe skeletal involvement. *BCMD* 1996;22:101.
486. Rosenberg A, Biesma DH, Sie-Go DM, Slootweg PJ. Primary extranodal CD30-positive T-cell non-Hodgkins lymphoma of the oral mucosa. Report of two cases. *Int J Oral Maxillofac Surg* 1996;25:57.
487. Ponce E, Moskovitz J, Grabowski GA. Enzyme therapy in Gaucher disease type 1: effect of neutralizing antibodies to acid b-glucosidase. *Blood* 1997;90:43.
488. Achord DT, Brot FE, Bell CE, Sly WS. Human beta-glucuronidase: in vivo clearance and in vitro uptake by a glycoprotein recognition system on reticuloendothelial cells. *Cell* 1978;15:269.
489. Stahl PD, Rodman JS, Miller MJ, Schlesinger PH. Evidence for receptor-mediated binding of glycoproteins, glycoconjugates, and lysosomal glycosidases by alveolar macrophages. *Proc Natl Acad Sci U S A* 1978;75:1399.
490. Furbish FS, Steer CJ, Barranger JA, et al. The uptake of native and desialylated glucocerebrosidase by rat hepatocytes and Kupffer cells. *Biochem Biophys Res Commun* 1978;81:1047.
491. Bijsterbosch MK, Donker W, van de Bilt H, et al. Quantitative analysis of the targeting of mannose-terminal glucocerebrosidase. Predominant uptake by liver endothelial cells. *Eur J Biochem* 1996;237:344.
492. Xu Y-H, Ponce E, Sun Y, et al. Turnover and distribution of intravenously administered mannose-terminated human acid beta-glucosidase in murine and human tissues. *Pediatr Res* 1996;39:313.
493. Schuchman RJ. Niemann-Pick disease Types A and B: acid sphingomyelinase deficiencies. In: Scriver CR, Beaudet A, Sly W, Valle D, eds. *The metabolic and molecular bases of inherited disease*, Vol. 3, 8th ed. New York: McGraw-Hill, 2001:22.

494. Carstea ED, Morris JA, Coleman KG, et al. Niemann-Pick C1 disease gene: homology to mediators of cholesterol homeostasis. *Science* 1997;277:228.
495. Loftus SK, Morris JA, Carstea ED, et al. Murine model of Niemann-Pick C disease: mutation in a cholesterol homeostasis gene. *Science* 1997;277:232.
496. Patterson MC, Wanier MT, Suzuki K, et al. Niemann-Pick Disease Type C: a lipid trafficking disorder. In: Scriver CR, Beaudet A, Sly W, Valle D, eds. *The metabolic and molecular bases of inherited disease*, Vol. 3, 8th ed. New York: McGraw-Hill, 2001:24.
497. Watari H, Blanchette-Mackie EJ, Dwyer NK, et al. Niemann-Pick C1 protein: obligatory roles for N-terminal domains and lysosomal targeting in cholesterol mobilization. *Proc Natl Acad Sci U S A* 1999;96:805.
498. Naureckiene S, Sleat DE, Lackland H, et al. Identification of HE1 as the second gene of Niemann-Pick C disease. *Science* 2000;290:2298.
499. Vellodi A, Hobbs JR, O'Donnell NM, et al. Treatment of Niemann-Pick disease type B by allogeneic bone marrow transplantation. *BMJ* 1987;295:1375.
500. Tandon V, Williamson JB, Cowie RA, Wraith JE. Spinal problems in mucopolysaccharidosis I (Hurler syndrome). *J Bone Joint Surg Br* 1996;78:938.
501. Whitley C. The mucopolysaccharidoses. In: Manning S, ed. *Heritable disorders of connective tissue*, 5th ed. St. Louis: Mosby–Year Book, 1993:132.
502. Vellodi A, Young EP, Cooper A, et al. Bone marrow transplantation for mucopolysaccharidosis type I: experience of two British centres. *Arch Dis Child* 1997;76:92.
503. Assmann GS. Acid lipase deficiency: Wolman disease and cholesteryl ester storage disease. In: Scriver CR, Beaudet A, Sly W, Valle D, eds. *The metabolic and molecular bases of inherited disease*, Vol. 3, 8th ed. New York: McGraw-Hill, 2001:22.
504. Du H, Dumanu M, Witte D, Grabowski GA. Targeted disruption of the mouse lysosomal acid lipase gene: a cholesteryl ester storage disease clinical phenotype and Wolman disease biochemistry. *Hum Mol Genet* 1998;7:1347.
505. Du H HM, Duanmu M, Grabowski GA, et al. Lysosomal acid lipase-deficient mice: depletion of white and brown fat, severe hepatosplenomegaly, and shortened life span. *J Lipid Res* 2001;42:489.
506. Du H SS, Levine M, Mishra J, et al. Enzyme therapy for lysosomal acid lipase deficiency in the mouse. *Hum Mol Genet* 2001;10:1639.
507. Faigle W, Raposo G, Tenza D, et al. Deficient peptide loading and MHC class II endosomal sorting in a human genetic immunodeficiency disease: the Chediak-Higashi syndrome. *J Cell Biol* 1998;141:1121.
508. Misumi DJ, Nagle DL, McGrail SH, et al. The physical and genetic map surrounding the Lyst gene on mouse chromosome 13. *Genomics* 1997;40:147.
509. Pastural E, Barrat FJ, Dufourcq-Lagelouse R, et al. Griscelli disease maps to chromosome 15q21 and is associated with mutations in the myosin-Va gene. *Nat Genet* 1997;16:289.
510. Coffey A, Brooksbank R, Brandau O, et al. Host response to EBV infection in X-linked lymphoproliferative disease result from mutations in an SH2-domain encoding gene. *Nat Genet* 1998;20:129.
511. Sayos J, Wu C, Morra M, et al. The X-linked lymphoproliferative-disease gene product SAP regulates signals induced through the co-receptor SLAM. *Nature* 1998;395:462.

CHAPTER 31

Hemostatic System

Stuart E. Lind, Peter W. Marks, and Bruce M. Ewenstein

Blood is a remarkable organ. Like a gas or liquid, it assumes the shape of the vessel that holds it. Unlike either, blood is able to stem its own loss when the integrity of its physiologic container is breached. A multitude of theories of hemostasis have been proposed by a great many scientists and physicians who have labored over several centuries to understand just how this process occurs. Because blood clotting in a patent vessel results in ischemia and necrosis of the tissues that it serves, it is important for the host to have the hemostatic system carefully regulated and coagulation initiated only when necessary and terminated as soon as hemorrhage is brought under control. Study of the hemostatic system has helped to establish many important ideas about physiologic homeostasis, some of which are helpful during the clinical evaluation and treatment of patients. The following are some general principles that should be kept in mind:

1. Hemostasis and thrombosis are opposite sides of the same biologic coin. In general, thrombosis involves the same processes as coagulation but in a different environment. The same principles that govern the activation of platelets, endothelial cells, coagulation, and fibrinolytic proteins are involved in both processes. The major difference between hemorrhage and thrombosis is that in hemorrhage, the inciting stimuli are usually evident, whereas in thrombosis, they often are not.
2. The well-functioning hemostatic system is like a good government: Checks and balances are essential for proper functioning and an imbalance may result in a gradual slide into chaos (Table 31-1).
3. Coagulation proteins and platelets are present in greater concentrations in the normal person than are needed for effective hemostasis. Thus, laboratory abnormalities must be evaluated with knowledge of the natural history of each disorder. The need for prophylactic blood product administration should not be based simply on the desire to generate a normal laboratory value for a particular test. For example, although marked pro-

longations of bleeding or clotting times are often associated with bleeding, less pronounced abnormalities may not be associated with either spontaneous or procedure-related bleeding.
4. Blood coagulation is a complex process involving many participants [platelets, red blood cells (RBCs), white blood cells (WBCs), endothelial cells, coagulation factors, fibrinolytic system proteins, and protease inhibitors], whose contributions wax and wane with time. Readily available clinical assays do not provide a complete picture of the functioning of many of these components.
5. Each of the three major participants in the hemostatic process (platelets, coagulation proteins, fibrinolytic system proteins) interacts with and influences the others.
6. Because concepts of hemostasis have focused either on platelet activation or blood coagulation, the focus traditionally has been on primary (platelet-mediated) and secondary (fibrin-mediated) phases of hemostasis. Clinicians have therefore been taught to obtain a history using a two-component classification system in which defects in primary hemostasis result in immediate bleeding, and defects in secondary hemostasis cause delayed bleeding (Table 31-2). Although effective in analyzing many hemorrhagic events, this formulation tends to downplay the role of late events in hemostasis, such as clot maturation, the action of factor XIII, the involvement of the fibrinolytic system, and the complex interactions among each of the components. Because these components are also difficult to analyze in the clinical laboratory, they can be overlooked unless specifically considered. In some instances, this results in giving too much importance to minor abnormalities in laboratory test results that are not truly linked to clinical events.

The discussion that follows emphasizes three phases of the hemostatic process (Fig. 31-1). Although it is useful to divide this complex system for the sake of discussion and analysis, the temporal involvement described is approximate and based on obser-

TABLE 31-1. Mechanisms of Control of the Hemostatic System

Platelets
Endothelial prostacyclin production
Endothelial and leukocyte membrane adenosine diphosphatase activity
Endothelial nitric oxide production
Protease inhibitors that limit thrombin action
Endothelial cell tissue plasminogen activator release
Coagulation system
Protein-C system
Protein C
Protein S
Thrombomodulin
C_{4b}-binding protein
Circulating antiproteases

Antiproteases	Proteases
Primary inhibitors	
Tissue factor pathway inhibitor	Factor Xa, factor VIIa/tissue factor
Antithrombin III and heparin-like molecules	Thrombin, factors Xa, IXa, XIa, XIIa, kallikrein
C1-esterase inhibitor	Kallikrein, C1, factor XIIa, plasmin
α_2-Macroglobulin	Plasmin, kallikrein, thrombin, factor Xa, protein C_a
Protein C inhibitor	Protein C_a, kallikrein
Secondary inhibitors, or antiproteases of uncertain significance	
α_1-Antitrypsin	Factor XIa, trypsin
Pregnancy zone protein	Plasmin
Heparin cofactor II	Thrombin
Platelet factor XIa inhibitor	Factor XIa
Protease nexin-1	Thrombin
Protease nexin-2/amyloid β-protein precursor	Factor XIa

Fibrinolytic system
α_2-Antiplasmin
Plasminogen activator inhibitor-1
Plasminogen activator inhibitor-2

---

vations of normal subjects. Pathologic conditions or surgical intervention may alter the relative timing or importance of each phase, with resulting clinical consequences.

PRIMARY HEMOSTASIS: PLATELET AND ENDOTHELIAL CELL ACTIVATION

Although the hemostatic system evolved to prevent blood loss after injury to a blood vessel, it can be partially or wholly activated under other circumstances, commonly as a result of trauma, preeclampsia, or the entry of bacteria into the bloodstream. Understanding of these latter events also evolved from an understanding of the hemostatic mechanisms that are activated after physical injury to a blood vessel. Although much of the following discussion of hemostasis is based on biochemical observations, microscopy has played an important role in understanding the sequence of events that accompanies such injury (1).

After injury to the blood vessel, a hemostatic plug is formed that is composed predominantly of platelets. Investigation of platelet function has been directed at determining the sequence of events that is responsible for hemostatic plug formation. Three phases of platelet activation have been described, each of which is associated with one or more clinical bleeding disorders (Fig. 31-2).

Platelet Adhesion

Platelet adhesion is the initial phase of platelet activation whereby a one-cell–thick "carpet" is formed in response to exposure of an appropriate surface. The relevant natural surface *in vivo* is believed to be the subendothelial matrix, which is rich in collagen, fibronectin, von Willebrand's factor (VWF), and other potentially relevant molecules. Artificial surfaces such as vascular grafts also initiate

TABLE 31-2. Clinical Bleeding Syndromes

	Immediate (minutes)	Delayed (hours to days)
Etiology	Platelet defect	Coagulation or fibrinolytic system defect
Common anatomic sites	Skin; mucosal surfaces, including gums, oral mucosa, nose, gastrointestinal tract, endometrium	Skin, muscles, joints
Type of skin bleeding	Petechiae or multiple ecchymoses; after shaving	Large ecchymoses
Common diseases	von Willebrand's disease; drug-induced platelet dysfunction, paraproteins, uremia	Hemophilia A or B, other factor deficiencies; fibrinolytic overactivity
Clinical history	Easy bruising; prolonged menses; excessive bleeding after dental extraction or tonsillectomy	Bleeding after circumcision, surgery, deep hematoma disproportionate to trauma, hemarthroses

---

platelet adherence. Adherence depends largely on the presence of platelet surface glycoproteins that bind VWF as well as adequate plasma or subendothelial concentrations of VWF polymers. Deficiencies in either the glycoprotein platelet receptor for VWF, the glycoprotein (gp) Ib/IX complex, or VWF itself, as seen in von Willebrand's disease (VWD), are most often responsible for defects in platelet adhesion. Direct measurements of platelet adhesion are not available in the clinical laboratory, although the ristocetin cofactor assay is a surrogate for testing the interaction of VWF with gpIb/IX. Platelets also react with subendothelial collagen, primarily through their $\alpha_2\beta_1$ receptors. The relative importance of VWF-

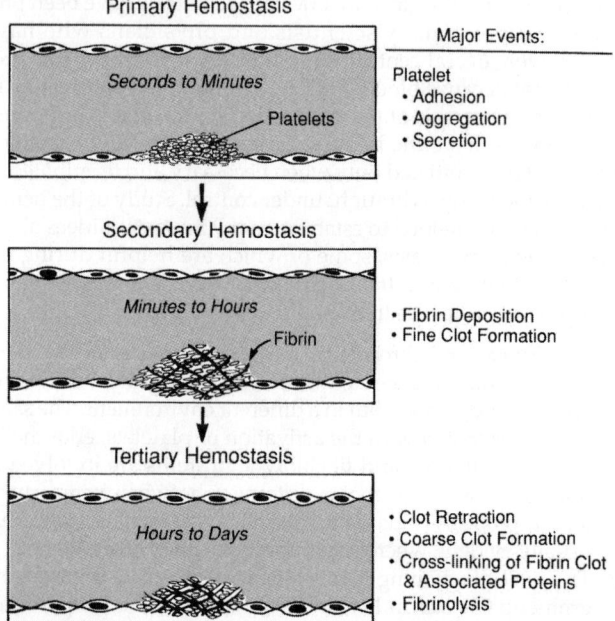

Figure 31-1. Temporal phases of the hemostatic process. The division of this complex process into distinct phases is useful for the sake of illustration and analysis of patient's problems, but it is not physiologically correct insofar as there is significant temporal overlap in the phases. Depending on the anatomic site of the thrombus, there may be ongoing accretion of platelets, fibrin, or both onto the clot (which accounts for clot extension), even as the fibrinolytic system is actively digesting certain of its parts. Not illustrated here is the infiltration of the clot by macrophages and fibroblasts, each of which may release compounds that modify the clot's lifespan.

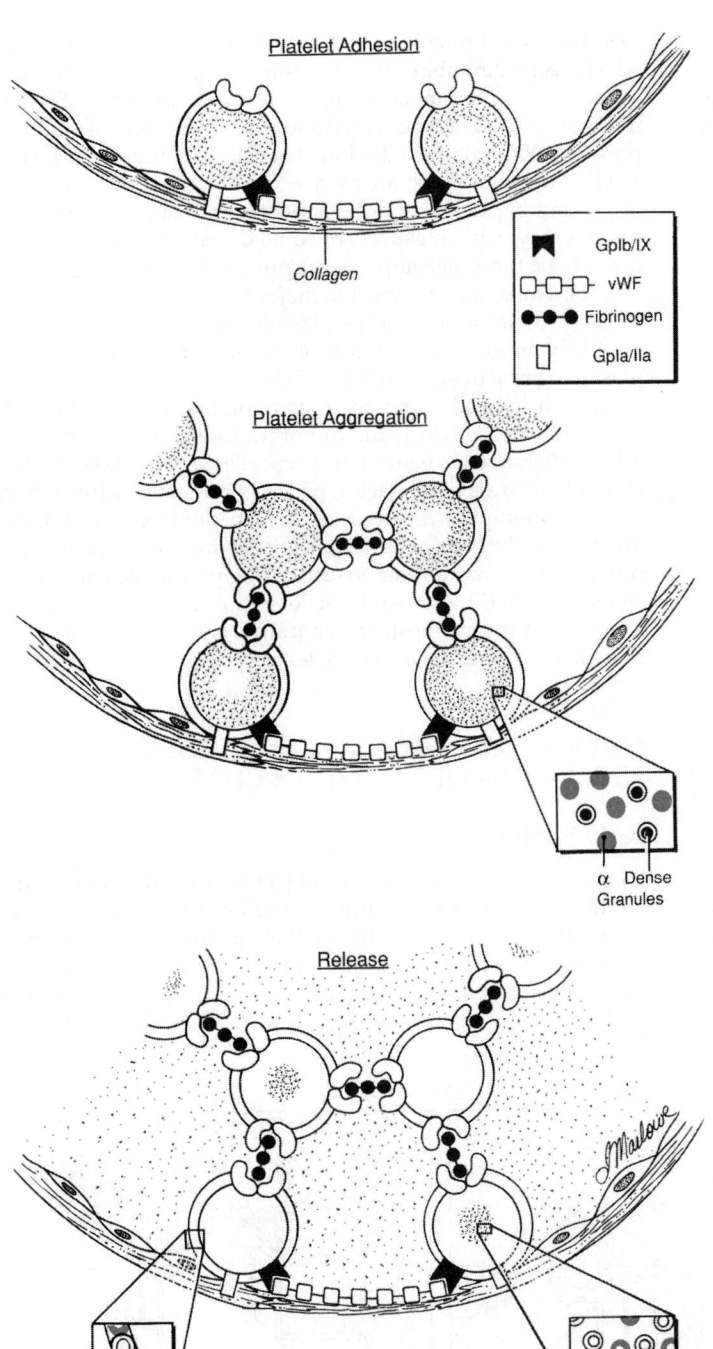

Figure 31-2. Platelet function. *Platelet adhesion* is the process whereby platelets form a one-cell–thick carpetlike monolayer on a blood vessel wall at the site of injury and exposure of the subendothelium because of the interaction of plasma membrane glycoproteins with constituents of the subendothelial matrix. The most important interactions are between the gpIb/IX complex and von Willebrand's factor (VWF) and between the gpIa/IIa complex and collagen. *Platelet aggregation* results when platelet surface receptors for fibrinogen (gpIIb/IIIa complex) become activated, allowing platelet aggregation formation to occur. The *platelet release reaction* results from a series of intracellular signaling events that cause platelet granule membranes to fuse with the invaginations of the plasma membrane known as the *surface-connected canalicular system*, leading to discharge of the granule contents into the extracellular space. The added membrane allows the cell to swell and allows antibodies to bind to proteins originally present in the membranes of the platelet's granules. Some of these proteins (i.e., P-selectin) allow platelets to interact with other cells.

dependent and VWF-independent interactions is a function of local hemodynamic conditions. Adhesion under conditions of high shear requires VWF to "capture" circulating platelets; the binding of $\alpha_2\beta_1$ to collagen serves to stabilize the interaction under conditions of low shear rates, and direct interaction of platelets with collagen is sufficient to support adhesion (1).

Platelet Aggregation

Platelet aggregation is the term used to describe the self-association of platelets into a platelet plug. Platelet aggregation is easily studied clinically and is thus familiar to many clinicians. Platelet aggregation is mediated by the interaction of fibrinogen with glycoprotein receptors on the platelet surface (gpIIb/IIIa complex). The two glycoprotein components of the fibrinogen receptor are held together by the presence of micromolar concentrations of

calcium. Removal of calcium by strong chelating agents such as ethylenediaminetetraacetic acid, which is found in purple top blood-drawing tubes, irreversibly dissociates the complex. Platelet aggregation is usually performed in blood anticoagulated with citrate (found in blue top tubes) because it allows micromolar concentrations of calcium to remain associated with the gpIIb/IIIa complex, thereby maintaining its functional integrity.

Platelet Secretion

Platelet secretion describes the process whereby platelet granules release their contents into the extracellular space. This results in high local concentrations of the contents of the platelets' two major types of granules, many of which contribute to the formation of the stable platelet plug. The platelet-dense granules contain adenosine diphosphate (ADP), serotonin, and Ca^{2+}, whereas the α-granules contain proteins. The release of ADP from a highly responsive subset of platelets following their activation produces a second, and highly important "second wave" of platelet aggregation. Thus, ADP is now recognized as the final common pathway of platelet recruitment and thrombus formation (2). Two α-granule proteins, platelet factor 4 and β-thromboglobulin, are found only in platelets and megakaryocytes. Unlike other α-granule proteins, such as VWF and fibrinogen, which play a role in hemostasis, platelet factor 4 and β-thromboglobulin are not recognized to have a specific hemostatic function. Tests of platelet secretion are generally performed only in specialized hemostasis laboratories.

Platelets also provide a specialized surface on which coagulation and fibrinolytic proteins are activated, a property shared with other cell surfaces (such as those of endothelial cells and monocytes). The importance of the ability of these other membranes to substitute for the platelet surface is evident when one considers that thrombocytopenic patients do not have the same bleeding manifestations as do hemophiliacs. This clinical observation suggests that other membrane surfaces are able to support the formation of a fibrin clot. The ability of phosphatidylserine exposed on the platelet membrane to accelerate coagulation is the basis of the platelet factor 3 availability test, which is no longer performed but may be found in the older literature.

Roles of Endothelial Cells

Endothelial cells play a number of roles in the hemostatic process in addition to binding coagulation factors that lead to thrombin generation and function to prevent, minimize, or terminate the action of platelets and activated coagulation factors. Endothelial cells alter platelet function in several ways. They contain an ecto-ADPase (2), CD39, which destroys ADP and limits platelet activation (3), and they produce two potent antiplatelet compounds, prostacyclin and nitric oxide (NO).

Endothelial cells also modulate the coagulation system and the lifespan of fibrin clots in several ways. First, they contain on their surface a thrombin-binding glycoprotein, thrombomodulin, which keeps thrombin from cleaving fibrinogen and allows it to activate the important anticoagulant protein, protein C. Second, the Weibel-Palade bodies of the endothelial cells are the source of plasma VWF multimers. Endothelial cells in culture secrete large VWF multimers, which are more active than the multimers usually found in plasma, and the appearance of large multimers in plasma may explain aspects of some disease processes such as thrombotic thrombocytopenic purpura (4,5) and sickle cell anemia (6). Third, they release the major intravascular activator of the fibrinolytic system, tissue plasminogen activator (tPA), and are likely an important source of its major regulatory protein, plasminogen activator inhibitor (PAI-1).

Endothelial cells exposed to compounds such as thrombin, endotoxin, interleukin-1, and tumor necrosis factor are known to exhibit alterations in hemostatic properties, as evidenced by their ability to express tissue factor, promote protein C activation, or release fibrinolytic system proteins. Depending on the stimulus involved, endothelial cells may acquire an increased or decreased propensity for promoting or supporting platelet activation and clot formation (7). Although tests of endothelial function are not available in routine hospital laboratories, they may move into clinical use during the next decade.

SECONDARY HEMOSTASIS: COAGULATION AND FORMATION OF THE FIBRIN CLOT

Early Studies

Blood coagulation has been the object of study by a large number of physicians and scientists. Despite many years of study, information continues to emerge that changes our view of how coagulation occurs. In 1905, Morawitz (8) presented an integrated theory of blood coagulation that was based on the work performed up to that time, as shown in Figure 31-3. This view

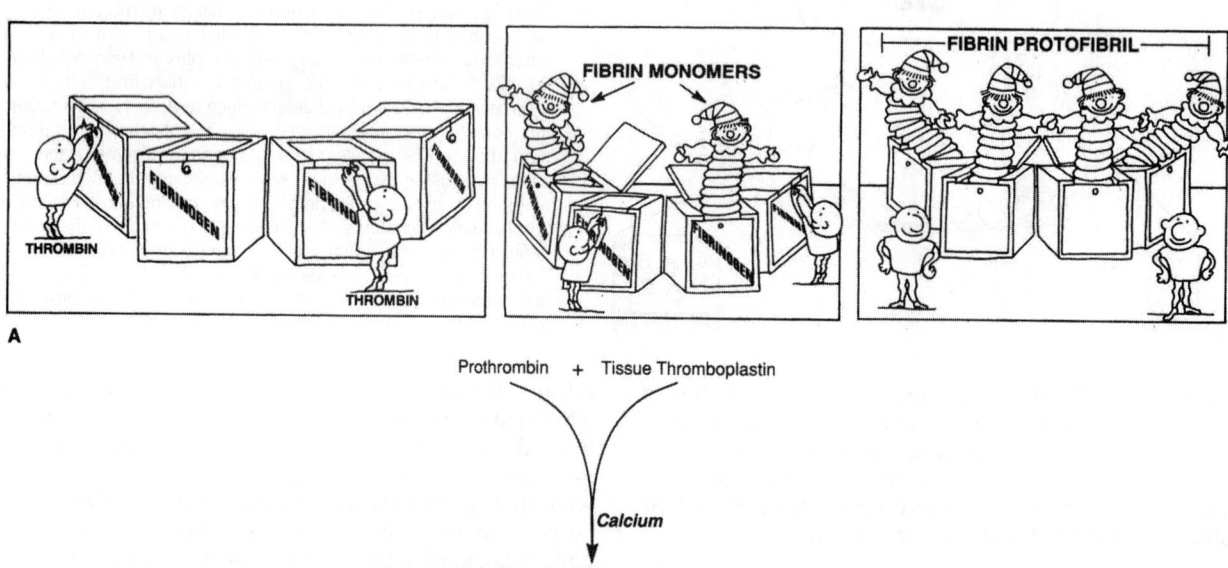

Figure 31-3. Coagulation at the beginning of the 20th century. **A:** Early theories of blood coagulation are thought to have been based on the writings of Plato, who postulated that fibrin was a circulating substance that formed a clot at sites when it left the body and became cooled. By the mid 1800s, it was recognized that blood clotted at physiologic temperatures and resulted from the action of thrombin on fibrinogen. **B:** Morawitz integrated the work of a number of investigators in his theory of coagulation published in 1905. The extract known as *tissue thromboplastin* is now understood to be composed of anionic phospholipids and the membrane-bound glycoprotein, tissue factor. Phospholipids form the surface on which coagulation reactions take place, while tissue factor is the physiologic activator of factor VII. All theories of coagulation recognized the ability of thrombin to clot fibrinogen.

postulated that coagulation was initiated after plasma was exposed to tissue thromboplastin, which is now recognized as being a phospholipid-bearing membrane surface containing the membrane-bound glycoprotein, tissue factor. Only two plasma proteins (prothrombin and fibrinogen) and calcium were believed to be necessary for clot formation. The prothrombin time (PT), which we understand to depend on adequate amounts of factors VII, X, V, and II, was based on this model. Because studies showed adequate levels of fibrinogen in most bleeding patients, it was thought that by adding thromboplastin and calcium to plasma, one could assay for the only other factor required for hemostasis, prothrombin (hence its name) (9). It was not until the 1950s that all the other components of what is now called the *extrinsic pathway* (factors V, VII, and X) were discovered. Thus, for the first half of this century, the initiation of blood coagulation was believed to require the addition of a substance not normally found in blood—thus grew the idea of an extrinsic pathway.

Experiments performed in the late 1940s helped to change thinking about how coagulation was initiated (10). By showing that blood does not clot when placed in a silicone-coated container but does clot when allowed to come into contact with glass, Conley and associates (10) helped to shift the focus of coagulation theories from the extrinsic pathway to one that was intrinsic to the blood itself. Thus, rather than postulate that coagulation resulted from the addition of a tissue factor, it was thought that alterations in the surface at which blood came into contact with its container led to clotting. Recognition of these hemostatic surfaces was found to be mediated by complex interactions of four proteins [factors XI and XII, high-molecular-weight (HMW) kininogen, and prekallikrein] known collectively as the *contact system*.

The rediscovery (11) that blood can clot *in vitro* in the absence of tissue factor suggested to some that it was not necessary to postulate the need for tissue factor to explain clotting *in vivo*, and the intrinsic pathway was viewed as the major physiologic pathway for blood coagulation. This view was reinforced by the fact that *in vitro* clotting of plasma through the addition of tissue factor (as measured by the PT) is normal in patients with hemophilia, whereas clotting initiated by surface activation [as measured by the partial thromboplastin time (PTT)] is prolonged.

Several lessons are worth remembering in this story. First, theories that overlook sound observations can be accepted only as temporary bridges to a more complete understanding. Second, laboratory tests of coagulation are often developed to distinguish a particular group of patients from healthy persons. Although the tests are performed in a manner that makes them most effective in this regard, it is not uncommon for physicians to extrapolate from these results to other groups of patients (or normal physiology), reaching inappropriate conclusions that may take decades to rectify. An example of this is found in the older literature concerning the PT and hemophilia.

The PT was developed in 1935 by Quick (9), who reported that when an excess of thromboplastin is used (conditions still employed in all clinical laboratories), the PT of hemophiliac patients is normal. Five years later, Dam and Venndt (12) noted that when less thromboplastin is added, hemophiliac plasma takes longer to coagulate than does normal plasma. Despite this and later confirmatory observations (13), it was believed for many years that coagulation initiated by tissue factor resulted from a biochemical flow down the extrinsic pathway. Theories of coagulation have since expanded to account for these observations, as discussed in the section Tissue Factor Pathway. Third, the failure of blood to clot in a silicone container serves to point out that stasis by itself is not a physiologic explanation for thrombosis (10).

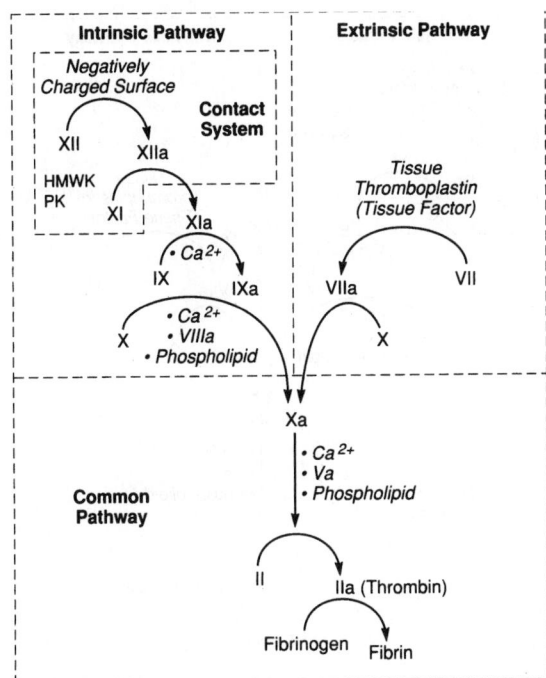

Figure 31-4. Waterfall or cascade scheme of coagulation. Coagulation was viewed in 1964 as a sequence of proteolytic cleavages. Because the intrinsic pathway was believed to be the physiologically important pathway, the extrinsic pathway was not included in the original formulation, although it was added over subsequent years. HMWK, high-molecular-weight kininogen; PK, prekallikrein.

Others have gone on to establish animal models that clearly demonstrate that thrombosis occurs only when stasis is accompanied by a significant change in the biochemical milieu and not simply when blood flow is stopped in a normal vasculature (14).

That the intrinsic pathway was the subject of most thought and attention is evident in the two independent concepts of blood coagulation published in 1964 (15,16), which stressed the sequential nature of blood protein activation. Both the formulation of the "waterfall" (15) and the "cascade" (16) contained diagrams of the intrinsic pathway. In neither paper was the extrinsic pathway specifically shown, although it was later integrated into the coagulation scheme that has been reproduced in many articles, chapters, and lectures about blood coagulation (Fig. 31-4).

Because factor VII deficiency results in a bleeding disorder, activation of the extrinsic pathway was taken to occur under some circumstances. The discovery that the two pathways can interact brought into question the idea that blood coagulation results from activation of one or the other pathway. Because factor VIIa can activate factor IX (17) and factor IXa can activate factor VII (18), many began to think that coagulation could occur through a combination of the two pathways, and a crossover pathway was added to diagrams of the coagulation system (Fig. 31-5).

Tissue Factor Pathway

This development led to a reconsideration of the importance of tissue thromboplastin (or more properly, tissue factor), which was spurred on by several independent lines of thought and investigation. First, the fact that patients lacking proteins found in the initial part of the intrinsic coagulation pathway (factor XII, prekallikrein, and HMW kininogen) do not have a bleeding disorder raised questions about the physiologic importance of this mode of activation (contact pathway). Second, isolation (19) and immunochemical localization (20) of tissue factor caused it

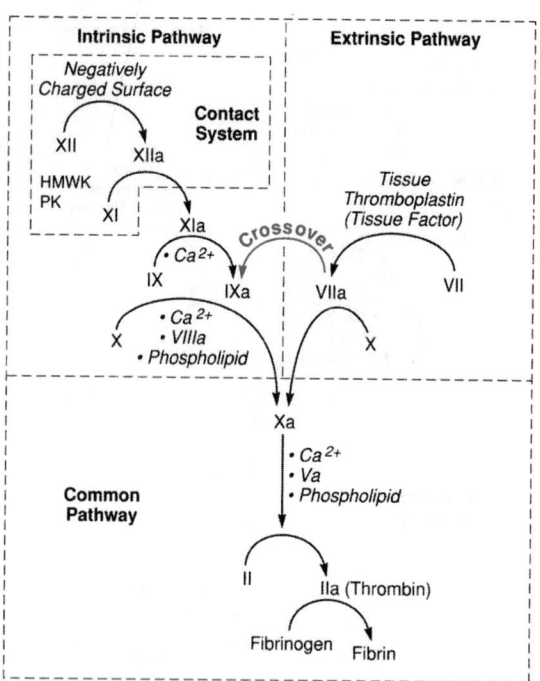

Figure 31-5. Crossover scheme of coagulation. After it was recognized that factor VIIa could activate factor IX, a crossover pathway was added to the coagulation scheme. This pathway allowed physicians to consider how proteins of both the intrinsic and extrinsic pathways might work together to promote physiologic hemostasis and provided a rationale for trials of factor VIIa infusions as therapy for patients with anti–factor VIII antibodies. HMWK, high molecular weight kininogen; PK, prekallikrein.

to be reconsidered as an initiator of coagulation, as did studies showing that it could be induced to appear on the surface of vascular cells by physiologically relevant stimuli (7). Third, the development of immunoassays (21) allowed coagulation system activation to be monitored directly. These assays can detect either small peptides released while clotting factors (or fibrinogen) are activated or complexes of a protease and its regulatory antiprotease, such as thrombin and antithrombin III. By monitoring the pathways of coagulation activation with these assays, it has become clear that the coagulation system is continually being activated in a controlled manner through the tissue factor (extrinsic) pathway (21). Fourth, the ability of thrombin to activate clotting factors other than fibrinogen (such as factors V, VIII, and XI), stimulated consideration of coagulation pathways in which thrombin could provide a positive feedback signal and a degree of amplification not proposed in the classic cascade or waterfall hypothesis. Finally, the isolation and characterization of a lipoprotein-associated inhibitor of the extrinsic pathway [tissue factor pathway inhibitor (TFPI)], helped to focus attention on tissue factor–initiated hemostasis.

The history of TFPI illustrates how biochemical investigation may be driven by observations that have been made many years previously (22). TFPI activity was first detected in plasma in 1947, when it was shown that preincubation of serum with tissue thromboplastin prevented the lethal reaction that occurs if thromboplastin is injected directly into animals (23,24). It was not until the 1980s that TFPI was isolated (25), its complementary DNA cloned (26), and its mechanism of action defined (27,28).

Unlike other antiproteases, TFPI circulates in plasma bound to lipoproteins (and was therefore previously called the *lipoprotein-associated coagulation inhibitor*) and is released in significant quantities by activated platelets. A second pool of TFPI is bound to heparin sulfates on the surface of endothelial cells. TFPI is differ-

ent from other antiproteases, which bind only one protease molecule at a time, insofar as it contains three separate regions capable of binding serine proteases, known as *Kunitz-type domains*. One Kunitz domain binds and inhibits factor Xa, one binds and inhibits the tissue factor–factor VIIa complex, and the function of the third domain is unknown but may be involved in binding to glycosaminoglycans. TFPI is itself under a novel form of regulation. Because it must bind factor Xa before it can inhibit the tissue factor–factor VIIa complex, TFPI's inhibitory activity is not expressed at the first exposure of plasma to tissue factor but only after factor Xa is produced. This ensures that coagulation is initiated before the tissue factor pathway is turned off. If TFPI were able to neutralize tissue factor–factor VIIa complex directly (that is, in the absence of factor Xa), coagulation would not occur until all the TFPI in the microenvironment were saturated, thereby prolonging the onset of clot formation and increasing blood loss. The inability of TFPI to bind factor VIIa in the absence of factor Xa probably explains why activated factor VII is able to circulate in an active form for a relatively long period of time (29) and may explain part of its success as a therapy for patients with factor VIII inhibitors.

Because the tissue factor–VIIa complex is inactivated by TFPI after coagulation has begun, a second mechanism must be responsible for the ongoing generation of factor Xa that is required to ensure complete clot formation. Two theories have been proposed to explain how this may occur, based on recently discovered biochemical interactions (Fig. 31-6). Both postulate that coagulation is initiated by the exposure of plasma to tissue factor, which leads to the generation of factors VIIa and Xa and thrombin. The two theories also agree that additional factor Xa depends on the activation of factors IXa and VIIIa. They differ only with regard to the mechanism responsible for factor IX activation.

One theory is based on a detailed analysis of factor IX activation. Factor IX must be cleaved at two points to become the fully activated protease (factor IXa) capable of cleaving factor X. Contrary to previous conceptions, factor Xa can make the first of these cuts if exposed to factor IX in the presence of a membrane surface (30). It has therefore been postulated that factor Xa, generated by the tissue factor–factor VIIa complex, makes the first cut in factor IX, generating the inactive precursor, factor IXα. The tissue factor–factor VIIa complex makes the second, generating active factor IXa, which in turn activates factor X. The resulting "pulse" of factor Xa is postulated to overcome the local concentrations of TFPI, allowing additional thrombin generation (30,31).

The second theory is based on observations that factor XI can be activated by thrombin in the presence of a negatively charged surface (32,33). It postulates that thrombin's activation of factor XI leads to factor IX activation, as conceived by the waterfall or cascade model. In this model, thrombin is not the last of the proteases generated by the coagulation system but an active participant in an active feed-forward loop. This model can account for activation of factor IX in the presence of uncomplexed TFPI (22).

These models both postulate that coagulation is initiated by the extrinsic pathway, maintained by involvement of factors VIII and IX, and differ only with respect to how factor IX becomes activated. One theory emphasizes the importance of factor XI in blood coagulation; the other theory tries to account for coagulation without implicating it. Neither theory is able to fully explain why some patients with factor XI deficiency bleed and some do not, so neither is a wholly adequate explanation. Both theories may turn out to be true, depending on the circumstances. Because it has not been determined exactly what negatively charged surface is required physiologically for factor XI

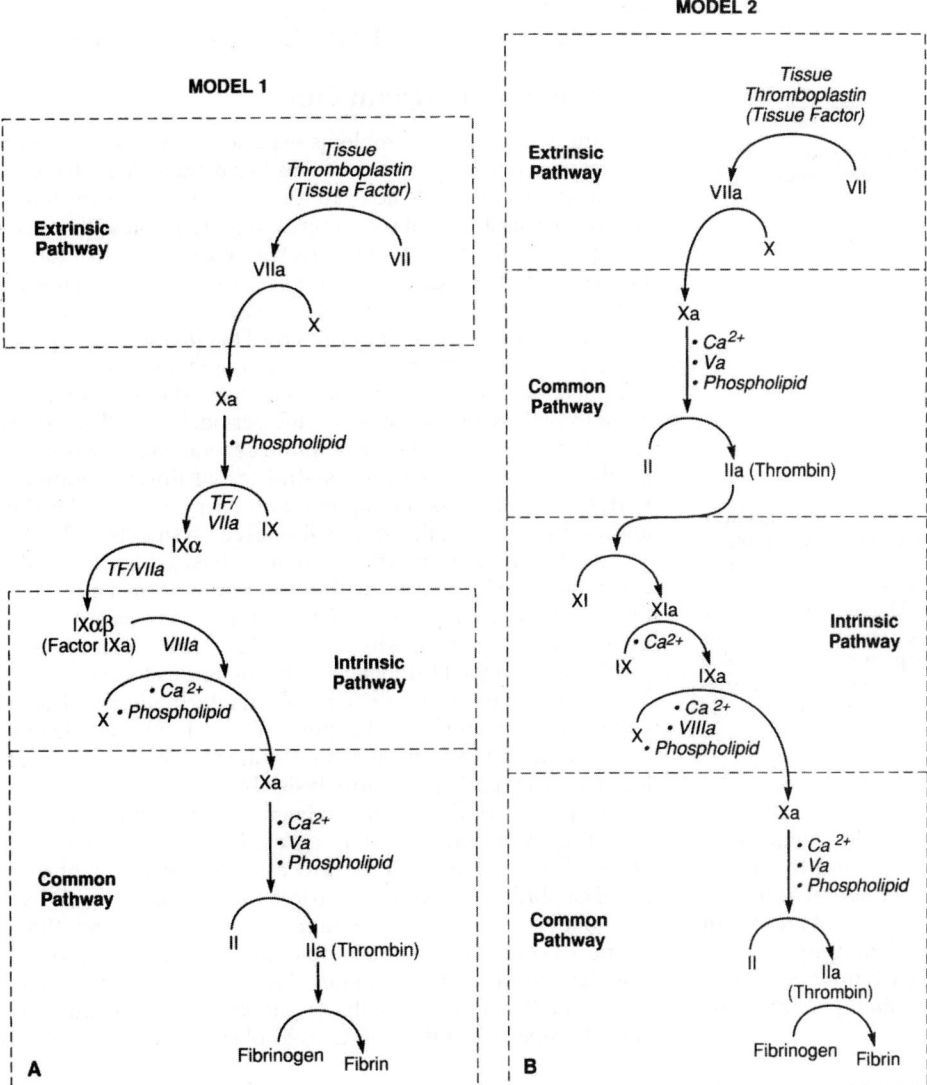

Figure 31-6. Current schemes of coagulation. The use of molecular markers of coagulation system activation and the delineation of tissue factor (TF) have led to new concepts of how the coagulation system functions. Both models are based on the idea that activation of coagulation follows exposure of blood to TF and the generation of factor VII. **A:** Model 1 postulates that membrane-bound factor Xa makes the first of the two cleavages required to activate factor IX, generating the inactive species factor IXα, which then undergoes further cleavage by the TF–factor VIIa complex to form factor IXαβ (also known as factor IXa), which is able to activate factor X in the presence of factor VIIIa. The overall flow, using the terminology of previous schemata, is extrinsic pathway → intrinsic pathway → common pathway → fibrin clot. (From Mann KG, Krishnaswamy S, Lawson JH. Surface-dependent hemostasis. *Semin Hematol* 1992;29:213.) **B:** Model 2 is based on the observation that thrombin, in the presence of a negatively charged surface, can activate factor XI, thereby leading to activation of factor IX. The flow of reactions in this model is extrinsic pathway → common pathway → intrinsic pathway → common pathway → fibrin clot. Although differing in how factor IX becomes activated, the models are similar in their emphasis on the importance of TF-mediated factor VII activation in the initiation of coagulation and the obligatory involvement of factors VIII and IX in the generation of a fibrin clot. (From Broze GJJ. The role of tissue factor pathway inhibitor in a revised coagulation cascade. *Semin Hematol* 1992;29:159.)

to be activated by thrombin, it is possible that this surface is not exposed to plasma under all conditions in which coagulation is required. When such a surface is present, coagulation may proceed via factor XI, and when it is not, via activation of factor IX by membrane-bound factor Xa. Such redundancy may also help to explain the well-recognized lack of close correlation between the degree of factor XI deficiency and clinical bleeding.

Most important, both theories place tissue factor in a primary position with regard to the initiation of hemostasis and view the involvement of factors VIII and IX as obligatory for promoting clot formation. Thus, coagulation is the result of a carefully regulated sequence of events that involves elements of both the intrinsic and extrinsic pathways.

Mechanisms of Control of the Coagulation System

Although activation of the coagulation cascade is crucial, uncontrolled generation of thrombin can lead to disaster. Two major mechanisms are responsible for preventing the generation of thrombin and fibrin from extending beyond the site of injury: limited proteolysis of factors Va and VIIIa by activated protein C (APC) and neutralization of activated coagulation proteases by circulating and endothelial cell-bound antiproteases (Fig. 31-7).

The protein-C system operates on multiple levels (34). First, thrombin binds to the endothelial surface protein, thrombo-

modulin, with a resulting loss of its ability to activate platelets and clot fibrinogen. This is not due to a simple quenching of its proteolytic activity, because thrombin bound to thrombomodulin is able to cleave protein C, a vitamin K–dependent protein. This mechanism represents an unusual example of how a protease's substrate specificity may be changed. The second stage of the protein-C system requires the interaction of APC with its cofactor, protein S, another vitamin K–dependent protein. The principal substrates of this enzyme-cofactor-surface complex are factors Va and VIIIa. In plasma, only approximately 40% of the protein S is unbound and able to carry out its cofactor function. The remainder is bound to C4b-binding protein, which thus serves as an important regulator of the protein-C system. The thrombin-thrombomodulin complex also activates a procarboxypeptidase, TAFI, thrombin-activatable fibrinolysis inhibitor (35), which serves to couple the coagulation and fibrinolytic cascades.

Several antiproteases are involved in the control of the coagulation system, all of which function by binding to or sterically interfering with the enzymatically active site of the relevant protease (Table 31-1). The resulting protease-antiprotease complex can be detected by enzyme-linked immunosorbent assay, using antibodies that bind to each component of the complex. Antithrombin III, the best-known antiprotease, is unusual insofar as it binds poorly to proteases in the

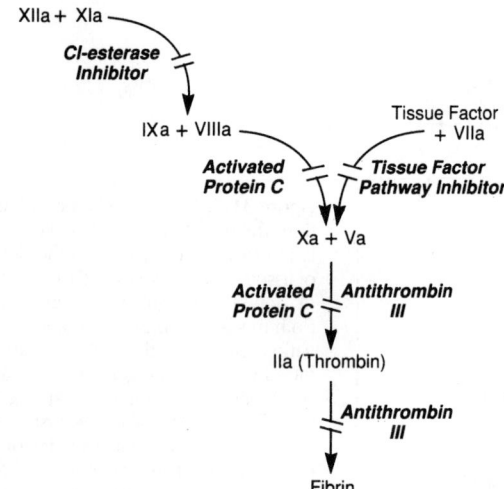

Figure 31-7. Major mechanisms of control of hemostasis. Regulation of the coagulation system is accomplished by the action of plasma proteins that either inhibit activation or terminate ongoing thrombin generation. One means of regulation is through the binding of inhibitors (tissue factor pathway inhibitor, C1-esterase inhibitor, and antithrombin III) to active serine proteases; another means is the proteolysis of required cofactors (factors Va and VIIIa) by activated protein C. Other plasma and endothelial proteins may also play an important role in regulating coagulation reactions. Different control mechanisms operate to regulate the activation and function of platelets and the fibrinolytic system.

absence of a cofactor (heparin or related molecules). Because antithrombin III–heparin complexes are unable to neutralize thrombin (36) or factor Xa (36,37) that are bound to a clot's surface, interest has developed in the clinical use of anticoagulant compounds that can neutralize proteases that are free in solution or bound to a clot surface (38). Examples of such compounds include hirudin (39), bivalirudin (a semisynthetic hirudin derivative), and argatroban (a carboxylic acid derivative).

TERTIARY HEMOSTASIS: CONSOLIDATION AND GRADUAL DISSOLUTION OF THE FIBRIN CLOT

Maturation of the Fibrin Clot

The study of bleeding problems experienced by patients with absent or abnormal plasma proteins has made it clear that clotting tests are not able to account for all abnormalities in clinical hemostasis and thrombosis. Increasing attention is therefore being paid to the molecular events that follow the initial formation of a fibrin clot, because, in some cases, these events are important in determining whether delayed bleeding or thrombosis emerges as a clinical problem. This phase of the hemostatic process is important in determining the lifespan of a clot and therefore the natural history of an injured or occluded vessel, a thrombus, or an embolus. This period, here called *tertiary hemostasis*, may be broken down into several components: formation of a mature clot, cross-linking of fibrin monomers within the clot, cross-linking of auxiliary proteins to the clot, and controlled activation of the fibrinolytic system (Fig. 31-8).

The lifespan of a clot may also be influenced by its cellular composition, which varies with the clinical circumstances. Different cell types may influence the natural history of a clot, including neutrophils, which can release elastase, a protease capable of cleaving fibrinogen and lysing fibrin clots (39); platelets, whose granules release both PAI-1, which inhibits plasmin generation (40) and thrombospondin, which inhibits plasmin (41); and fibroblasts, which can infiltrate clots and deposit collagen, thereby inhibiting fibrinolysis (42).

The process of clot formation begins with the linear association of fibrin monomers first into protofibrils and then into long fibrils. The initial result of this process is the formation of a *fine clot*. The fibrils in the clot are flexible rather than rigid, and are able to move, much as spaghetti moves in boiling water. When the fibrils come into contact with each other, they tend to self-associate, forming thick bundles. The resulting clot is called a *coarse clot*. The bundles scatter light and thereby change the optical properties of the clot. Clotted plasma is transparent ini-

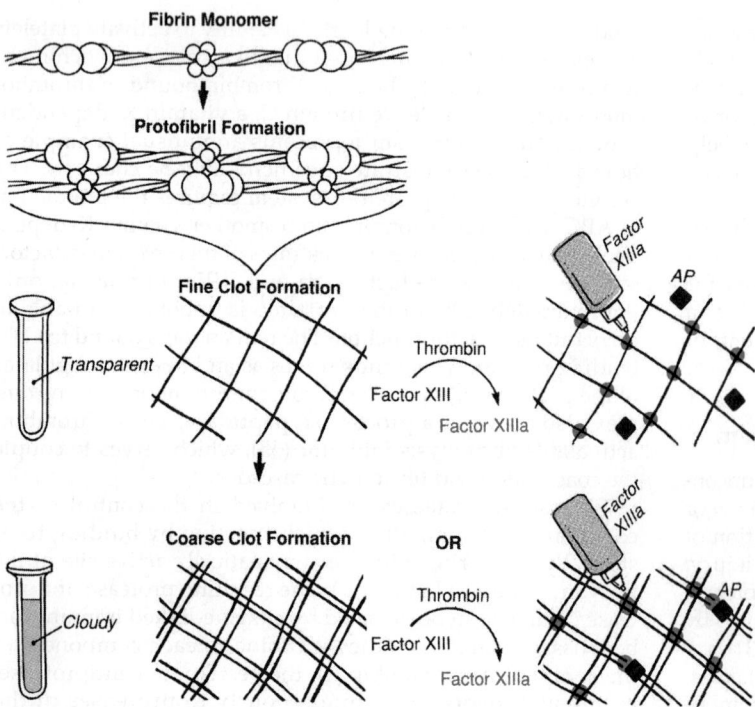

Figure 31-8. Tertiary hemostasis. The fibrin clot is initially transparent because its fibrils are randomly distributed in a fine meshwork. Until the clot becomes cross-linked by factor XIIIa (which takes place over several hours), the fibrils are able to diffuse within the clot and form stable side-to-side associations. The resulting thick fibrin bundles scatter light, rendering the coarse clot opaque or cloudy. Factor XIIIa, a molecular glue, cross-links fibrils to each other and forms covalent bonds between fibrin and key regulatory proteins, such as α_2-antiplasmin (AP). Also part of this phase (not illustrated here) is the initiation of fibrinolysis by tissue plasminogen activator, which is released from endothelial cells in the vicinity of a thrombus.

tially and gradually becomes opaque over the next 10 to 30 minutes, well after clot formation has occurred. In addition to having different optic properties, fine clots are brittle and are easily fractured. This may be of clinical significance, particularly in regions in which the physical demands on the clot are great, such as the alveoli of mechanically ventilated patients.

Two lines of investigation indicate that clot structure is important in determining the clot's susceptibility to lysis (and, hence, its lifespan). First, clots formed in the presence of the radiocontrast agent iopamidol do not exhibit the usual fine-to-coarse transition and are resistant to lysis (43). Second, abnormal fibrinogen molecules have been isolated from patients suffering from recurrent thrombosis that form fine plasmin-resistant clots (44,45). Together, these studies suggest that clot structure may be clinically important in determining susceptibility to lysis.

Although the clot's structure may undergo significant change immediately after it is formed, it is soon locked into a fixed configuration by the action of factor XIIIa, which forms new covalent bonds between adjacent fibrin monomers, thereby cross-linking the clot. The first bonds are formed between two γ chains of adjacent fibrin molecules, whereas later bonds involve the long extensions of α chains. Electrophoretic analysis shows that HMW complexes are formed, indicating the fusion of many α chains. Cross-linking of fibrin clots is important because it enhances their rigidity and increases their resistance to plasmin-induced fibrinolysis. A failure to cross-link fibrin clots or unusually rapid activation of the fibrinolytic system that exposes clots to plasmin before factor XIIIa has cross-linked the clot, results in clinically significant delayed bleeding. A number of proteins are also cross-linked to fibrin's α chains, the most important of which is α_2-antiplasmin, deficiency of which is associated with premature clot lysis and clinically significant bleeding (46).

Activation of the Fibrinolytic System

The fibrinolytic system is generally believed to be activated in concert with the coagulation system, although patients are occasionally seen who have clear evidence of an activated fibrinolytic system in the absence of the usual laboratory markers of coagulation system activation (Fig. 31-9).

There are two physiologic activators of plasminogen, tPA and urokinase. tPA is the major activator of the intravascular space and is released from stimulated endothelial cells. Urokinase is the major activator of the extravascular space and is synthesized by a number of cell types. Also found in neutrophil precursors, urokinase appears to be responsible for bleeding in some patients with acute leukemia, especially promyelocytic leukemia (47). Although activation of the fibrinolytic system is commonly envisioned as taking place on the surface of a clot or in the plasma, fibrinolytic system activation is increasingly recognized as being a cell surface–associated event. For example, a variety of cell types can bind the components of the fibrinolytic system, including plasminogen (48), plasmin (49), urokinase (50), and tPA (51). A cellular receptor for plasmin has also been found on the surface of certain group A streptococci (52), which is an evolutionary testimony to the importance of cell-surface binding of fibrinolytic proteins.

Both plasminogen and plasmin bind to other proteins through specialized domains known as *kringles*, a configuration formed by three disulfide bonds within an 80–amino acid structure. Plasminogen and plasmin have five kringle domains, which bind to certain lysine residues of potential substrates (such as fibrin or fibrinogen) or cellular-binding sites. The lysine-binding sites of the kringles serve as a site of action of two antifibrinolytic drugs,

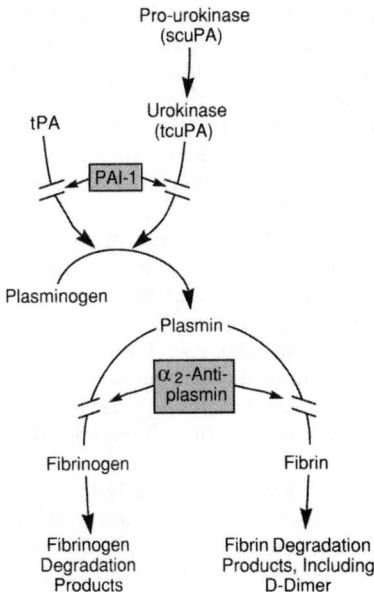

Figure 31-9. Fibrinolytic system pathways. The two major activators of the fibrinolytic system are tissue-type and urokinase-type plasminogen activators (tPA and uPA, respectively). tPA is fully active when secreted and is inhibited by plasminogen activator-1 (PAI-1), an acute phase reactant. uPA is secreted as a single-chain protein (scuPA or prourokinase) that is cleaved by plasmin to the two-chain form (tcuPA), which is used clinically as urokinase. Although both tPA and scuPA are much more effective plasminogen activators in the presence of a fibrin clot, their mechanism of action is different. tcuPA, on the other hand, quickly cleaves plasminogen in the absence of a clot, and its injection quickly leads to the generation of plasmin and fibrinogen degradation products. α_2-Antiplasmin is the major inhibitor of plasmin and can become depleted in states where there is ongoing fibrinolytic system activation.

ε-aminocaproic acid and tranexamic acid. These compounds are lysine analogs and are able to bind the kringle regions. Given in sufficient amounts, ε-aminocaproic acid and tranexamic acid are also able to displace plasmin and plasminogen from fibrin clots, thereby preventing fibrinolysis. Thus, they inhibit proteolysis in an indirect manner.

Another class of plasmin inhibitors, typified by the drug *aprotinin* (also known as *bovine pancreatic trypsin inhibitor* or its European trade name, *Trasylol*), binds directly to plasmin's enzymatically active site and thereby directly inhibits its enzymatic activity. α_2-Antiplasmin, the major circulating plasmin inhibitor, binds to both the kringle and active site regions of plasmin.

Each of the two major plasminogen activators differs from each other and from other serine protease zymogens in important ways. tPA is released by endothelial cells after injury or stimulation. Unlike most serine proteases, it is an active enzyme when secreted and does not require activation by another protease. Its affinity for plasminogen is low, and in the absence of a cofactor protein capable of binding tPA and plasminogen, little plasmin is formed, as when tPA is simply added to plasma. In the presence of an appropriate cofactor, tPA is brought into close contact with plasminogen and is able to make the single cleavage that converts plasminogen to plasmin. Fibrin is the most important of such cofactors, although similar effects are brought about by intracellular and extracellular proteins not normally considered to be part of the fibrinolytic system but that may be present in certain pathologic conditions (53,54).

Urokinase is secreted as a single-chain molecule (called *prourokinase* or *scu-PA*), which is also relatively inactive in the absence of a fibrin clot. Prourokinase is susceptible to cleavage by plasmin, which generates two-chain urokinase (a fully active plasminogen activator) even in the absence of a fibrin clot. Two-chain urokinase is the species found in urine and the form used clinically for several decades. It had been thought that prourokinase is active only after it is cleaved to two-chain urokinase, but evidence indicates that prourokinase itself is active in the presence of a fibrin clot, indicating a unique mechanism of action (55,56).

Two bacterial plasminogen activators, streptokinase and staphylokinase, have been studied in great detail and used clinically. They differ from tPA and urokinase in their mechanism of action in that they are not serine proteases and do not directly cleave plasminogen. Instead, each binds to plasminogen, forming an activator complex that becomes capable of cleaving other plasminogen molecules, generating plasmin. Research suggests that staphylokinase may be more fibrin specific than streptokinase (57).

Like coagulation proteins, fibrinolytic proteins are subject to regulation by specialized circulating antiproteases. The major inhibitor that neutralizes free plasmin is α_2-antiplasmin, whereas the major tPA inhibitor is PAI-1. PAI-1 is released from endotoxin-treated endothelial cells (58) and from the granules of stimulated platelets (59). Fibrinolysis is also attenuated by TAFI, which, in its activated form, potentially attenuates fibrinolysis by removing C-terminal lysine and arginine residues that are important for the binding and activation of plasminogen (60).

Clinically significant bleeding may be associated with the excessive release of plasminogen activators, as occurs during liver transplantation (61), or with the absence of the inhibitors of the fibrinolytic system [such as PAI-1 (62–64) or α_2-antiplasmin (65,66)]. Although some reports have correlated subnormal release of tPA with thrombotic events in certain families (67), this type of measurement has not provide a general approach for the clinical evaluation of patients with thrombotic disorders (68).

High levels of fibrinolytic inhibitors such as PAI-1 have been associated with thrombotic states, such as acute myocardial infarction, in some case-control studies (69). Care must be exercised in studies of this sort because some plasma proteins (including PAI-1) are acute-phase reactants, and their plasma levels may change soon after a clinical event and not correlate with plasma levels drawn in the basal state. These studies are valuable in making initial observations and generating hypotheses that can be tested in prospective studies, which are more rigorous methodologically. Prospective monitoring trials have contributed important information with regard to the relation between plasma levels of coagulation and fibrinolytic proteins and vascular disease. Examples include the confirmation of previously suspected correlations between low plasma fibrinolytic activity (70) or elevations in plasma fibrinogen concentration (71) and myocardial infarction; the failure to confirm observations made by case-control studies that PAI-1 levels are related to the subsequent risk of developing deep venous thrombosis (72); the stimulation of new lines of investigation by revealing important associations not previously well appreciated, such as the relation between the risk of heart disease and plasma levels of tPA (73) or factor VII (74).

In addition to modifying our concepts of risk factors, prospective trials may provide a basis for understanding clinical events. For example, a relation has been described between postoperative levels of plasma PAI-1, postoperative arterial thrombosis, and the type of anesthesia used (general or local) during lower-extremity vascular surgery (75). Additional studies of this sort may lead to an increased understanding of the "fibrinolytic shutdown" that follows surgery and suggest ways that the shutdown might be ameliorated.

CHECKS AND BALANCES IN THE HEMOSTATIC SYSTEM

Although clinical thinking about hemostasis tends to focus on visible initiating events (surgery, trauma, bacteremia) or clinical endpoints (bleeding, embolism, thrombosis), hemostatic homeostasis depends on the appropriate function of relatively invisible control mechanisms (Table 31-1). These controls effectively define thresholds of activation that must be surpassed for cellular or biochemical cascades to begin and define their physical and temporal limitations. If all goes well, they are unseen and unappreciated as they operate behind the clinical scene. Only relatively recently have deficiencies of some of these regulatory proteins been appreciated to cause bleeding or thrombosis. Unfortunately, tests of many of these regulatory proteins are not clinically available on short notice and therefore cannot rapidly influence clinical decision making.

When measuring plasma antiprotease concentrations, be certain of the type of assay (immunologic versus functional) that is being used. Immunologic measurements may not distinguish protease-antiprotease complexes from uncomplexed (free) antiprotease molecules, whereas functional assays measure only the free species. Newer immunoassays have been developed to measure specific protease-antiprotease complexes.

INTERACTIONS AMONG MAJOR MEMBERS OF THE HEMOSTATIC SYSTEM

The frequent division of textbooks into separate chapters discussing coagulation, platelets, or the fibrinolytic system might suggest that these are independent entities, both clinically and academically. Based on both clinical and laboratory observations, it is becoming increasingly clear that this is not true. Three examples are offered to illustrate this point.

Generation of Thrombin at the Cell Surface

Phospholipids have long been known as being necessary for the rapid generation of thrombin. They are not free-floating but are incorporated into the plasma membranes of cells, particularly platelets, endothelial cells, and monocytes, all of which can bind activated clotting factors, the most important of which are factors Va and Xa. Thrombin is thus generated on a surface and not simply in the fluid phase of plasma. This is important not only from the standpoint of how and where clot formation is initiated, but also because thrombin has potent effects on cells and can activate both platelets and endothelial cells to change their shape and release their granules into the extracellular space.

Generation of Plasmin at the Cell Surface

Although hematologic discussions of plasmin focus on its function as a fibrinolytic protein, it actually serves a more fundamental role physiologically and is a major protease of the extracellular space (76). As such, it is able to regulate or influence a number of biologic events. For example, plasmin can cleave procollagenase into collagenase and convert latent transforming growth factor β to an active form. It plays a major role in such diverse biologic processes as tumor cell migration, inflammation, ovulation, and trophoblast invasion (76,77). As previously noted, cellular receptors are recognized for plasminogen, prourokinase, and tPA. Interaction of these proteins with their cellular receptors increases the rate at which plasminogen activators generate plasmin, whereas binding of plasmin to cellular receptors protects it from inactivation by α_2-antiplasmin.

Effects of Fibrinolytic Proteins on Platelet Function

An interaction of plasmin with platelets was first noted 20 years ago (78) and has since been recognized to be of clinical importance. The effects of plasmin on platelets are complex and seemingly paradoxical, for both platelet activation and inhibition have been reported. These disparate findings have been reconciled by following platelet function over time, which reveals that the augmentation and inhibition of platelet function are a function of the plasmin dose and time of exposure to platelets (79). The effects of plasmin are also temperature dependent (80), which may be clinically relevant in explaining differences in blood loss observed when cardiac surgery is conducted at different temperatures (81,82).

Interest in the interaction between plasmin and platelets has been spurred on largely by the renewed interest in thrombolytic therapy for myocardial infarction that developed in the early 1980s and by the observation in the late 1980s that prophylactic administration of aprotinin reduced blood loss after cardiac surgery. The finding that thrombolytic therapy increased plasma levels of fibrinopeptide A, a marker of thrombin generation (83), led to studies that have documented a previously unsuspected interaction of platelets with the coagulation and fibrinolytic systems (84,85). Similarly, efforts to understand why aprotinin reduces blood loss during cardiac surgery (86) have led investigators to consider whether the platelet defect of cardiac surgery might result from the interaction of plasmin with platelets (82,87).

INFLUENCE OF OTHER CELLS OF THE VASCULAR SPACE ON HEMOSTASIS

As emphasized earlier, hemostasis is a complex process that involves the cooperative interactions of many components. Although platelets and proteins of the coagulation and fibrinolytic systems are the most important members of the hemostatic system, they are subject to influence by other cells found in the vascular space, as well as by cells and proteins of the extravascular space. The following are three examples of the multiple interactions that take place between the main members of the hemostatic system and other cell types.

Endothelial Cells

Intact, unstimulated endothelial cells provide a thromboresistant surface through interactions that involve all three major components of the hemostatic system. Endothelial cells help to regulate the duration of coagulation system activation by virtue of the plasma membrane protein, thrombomodulin, which binds thrombin and allows it to activate protein C. Endothelial cell–associated heparin sulfate proteoglycans bind ATIII and TFPI, further reducing procoagulant activity. As previously noted, endothelial cells produce substances (prostacyclin, NO) that directly affect platelet function and can also metabolize prostanoids released by other cells to form prostacyclin (88). Ecto-ADPase on the cell surface degrades ADP released from the dense granules. Finally, the endothelial cell synthesizes, stores, and releases tPA and has receptors for tPA and plasminogen, thereby promoting plasmin formation.

Red Blood Cells

Long considered to be hemostatically inert, RBCs are increasingly recognized as playing a role in the hemostatic process. In 1910, Duke (89) noted that anemia resulted in the prolongation of the bleeding time. The idea that RBCs and platelets interact was strengthened by studies that showed that RBC transfusions shorten the prolonged bleeding time of many uremic patients (90). More than 80 years after Duke's observations, laboratory investigations are beginning to provide explanations for these clinical findings (91,92). Finally, many clinicians have noted that patients with severe anemia have retinal hemorrhages, which is commonly ascribed to tissue hypoxia. It is interesting to speculate that retinal hemorrhage in anemia is due partly to a diminished interaction of erythrocytes and platelets in a particularly vulnerable vasculature.

Although the outer surface of the normal RBC does not support the development of the prothrombinase complex, exposure of plasma to the phospholipids (notably phosphatidylserine) normally found on the inner surface of the RBC membrane accelerates coagulation (93). Exposure of these phospholipids during major transfusions when cells are lysed in the intravascular space may at least partly explain the disseminated intravascular coagulation (DIC) that often accompanies this event. Their presence on the external surface of erythrocytes obtained from patients with sickle cell anemia (94) may explain observations of coagulation system activation in patients with sickle cell disease (95,96).

White Blood Cells

WBCs are able to influence platelets as well as some plasma proteins of importance for hemostasis. They down-regulate platelet function by virtue of an ADPase on their surface (97) as well as their ability to produce NO, a platelet inhibitory substance (98). Neutrophils release potent proteases such as elastase, which can alter the function of platelets (99), endothelial cells (100), TFPI (101), and plasminogen (102). Neutrophils can also metabolize icosanoids derived from platelets (103). DIC is a well-known complication of acute leukemia and results from several distinct effects of immature neoplastic leukocytes on the hemostatic system (104).

LABORATORY TESTS OF HEMOSTASIS

The time it takes for a fibrin clot to form or a bleeding wound to stop bleeding are commonly used endpoints in the laboratory. These endpoints are not readily appreciated as being biologically meaningful values because the normal values of bleeding and clotting time tests may be dramatically changed by alterations in the way the tests are performed. Normal values thus acquire meaning as a result of repeated correlations with clinical events, and errors in clinical judgment are made when seemingly reasonable extrapolations are made.

Many hemostatic tests were either devised for specific groups of patients or initially performed in an arbitrary, rather than clinically significant, manner. For example, the PT performed in the usual manner has long been recognized as being normal in patients with hemophilia (6). It would be understandable to conclude on the basis of this information that tissue factor–initiated coagulation proceeds normally in hemophiliacs, but doing so would be premature. Instead, the conditions of the test should be varied to determine whether the same conclusion can always be reached. (This point is of practical benefit when dealing with a lupus anticoagulant, as discussed in section Detection of Circulating Inhibitors.) In fact, when dilute thromboplastin is used to initiate coagulation, the PT of hemophiliacs is prolonged, a finding taken today to be compatible with the idea that coagulation is initiated by the tissue factor pathway but requires participation of factors IX and VIII

(13,105). It is appropriate not to exclude hemophilia in a patient with a normal PT, because the test as currently performed has been validated by clinical observation and experience. The clinician should keep in mind that many tests, especially functional tests such as bleeding and clotting times, which depend on incompletely defined interactions, may be misinterpreted because of explicit or implicit assumptions that have been forgotten or overlooked.

The PTT was developed (106) and subsequently modified (107) to detect patients with deficiencies of factors VIII, IX, XI, or XII and not to detect those who might bleed during or after surgery. Because the prevalence of these hereditary deficiencies in unselected persons is low (less than 1%), the predictive value of a positive test also is low. It is not surprising that many abnormal preoperative activated PTT (aPTT) determinations are false-positives with regard to this endpoint (108). The aPTT may have value as a predictor of bleeding, if performed in high-risk patients (109), emphasizing the importance of the pretest likelihood of disease in test utilization.

The desire to avoid operative hemorrhage has resulted in the routine use of bleeding and clotting times that were never clinically validated for this purpose, despite long-standing pleas to the contrary (110). For example, it has been known for some time that an abnormal PT does not predict bleeding after surgery or invasive procedures such as thoracentesis or liver biopsy, and some clinicians proceed under these circumstances on the basis of clinical experience. Others are unwilling to do so and give patients plasma transfusions in an attempt to lower the PT, assuming that they will reduce the risk of hemorrhage. The conflict between these views can be resolved only by analyzing clinical outcomes so that the need for transfusion can be assessed objectively. Efforts in this area have documented the inadequacy of tests such as the PT in predicting bleeding (111,112). This is not surprising; although a mild depression of a single clotting factor does not prolong the clotting time, the simultaneous depression of several factors does prolong it (113). This is unlikely to be of clinical significance. In addition, the normal range of the thrombin time is determined by the mean and standard deviation of the test performed on a given number of healthy people and is not a reflection of the normal range associated with good postprocedure hemostasis.

The history and use of the bleeding time are similar in many ways. The Ivy bleeding time, forerunner of the method used today, was developed because investigators wanted to develop a laboratory test that would be abnormal in a clinically defined patient population, much as the developers of the PTT sought to identify hemophiliacs by a laboratory test. Ivy wrote, "some way should be found to make a patient with a hypothetical latent bleeding tendency in jaundice bleed excessively from an ordinary skin puncture, and thus possibly make it manifest" (114).

None of the modifications made over the intervening years was designed specifically to aid in the preoperative evaluation of healthy patients but rather only to improve the reproducibility of the test or its sensitivity to aspirin ingestion. Given this history, it is not surprising that the bleeding time has not been found to be a valid predictor of bleeding when used as a screening test (115–117), although many continue to use it for this purpose.

Commonly Used Tests of the Coagulation System

PROTHROMBIN TIME

The PT test is performed essentially as described by Quick (9) in 1935. It involves the addition of calcium and thromboplastin (a human or rabbit brain extract that provides both a phospholipid surface as well as tissue factor) to the patient's citrated plasma (Fig. 31-10). The amount of thromboplastin used in the test results in a normal value of approximately 11 to 13 seconds and causes a clot to form via the extrinsic pathway. It is sensitive to deficiencies of factors VII, X, V, II, and fibrinogen, as well as circulating inhibitors.

Thromboplastin preparations are widely recognized to differ in their ability to activate coagulation. A strong activator results in a normal PT, even with some degree of depletion of clotting factors. A weak activator is more sensitive to clotting factor depletion, such as that induced by warfarin ingestion, even though it may give the same result as the strong activator when

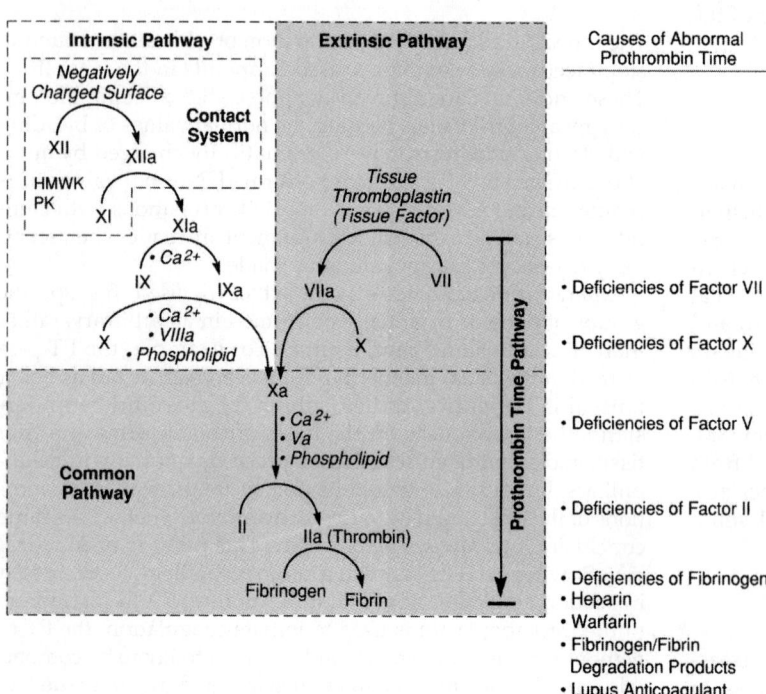

Causes of Abnormal
Prothrombin Time
_____

• Deficiencies of Factor VII

• Deficiencies of Factor X

• Deficiencies of Factor V

• Deficiencies of Factor II

• Deficiencies of Fibrinogen
• Heparin
• Warfarin
• Fibrinogen/Fibrin
  Degradation Products
• Lupus Anticoagulant
• Liver Disease

Figure 31-10. The prothrombin time of plasma was developed by Quick in 1935 and is based on Morawitz's model of coagulation (Fig. 31-3B). Clotting is initiated by the addition of calcium and tissue thromboplastin, an extract containing both phospholipid and the glycoprotein now known as *tissue factor*. Because acquired fibrinogen deficiency was thought to be uncommon and factors V, VII, and X had not been discovered, Quick concluded that a prolongation of prothrombin time was due to prothrombin deficiency. It is now recognized that this test depends on the functional integrity of the entire extrinsic pathway.

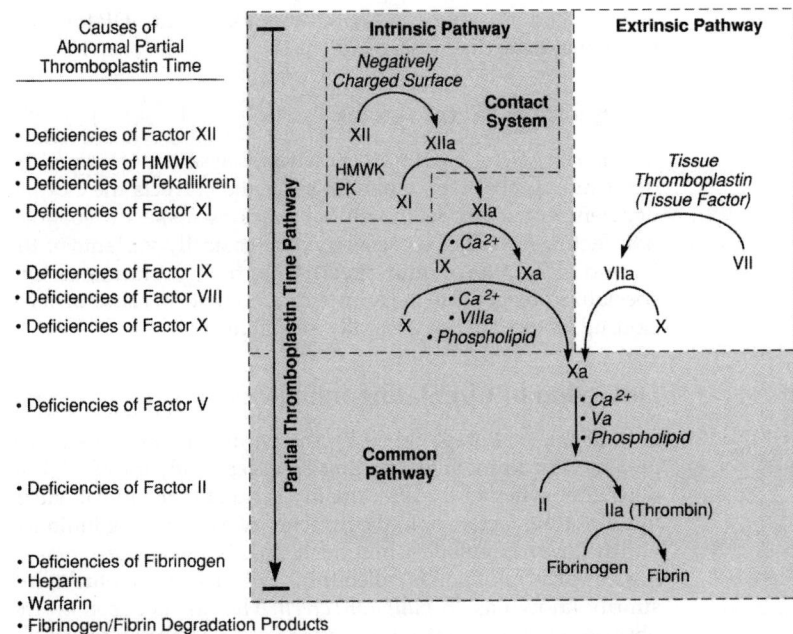

Causes of
Abnormal Partial
Thromboplastin Time

- Deficiencies of Factor XII
- Deficiencies of HMWK
- Deficiencies of Prekallikrein
- Deficiencies of Factor XI

- Deficiencies of Factor IX
- Deficiencies of Factor VIII
- Deficiencies of Factor X

- Deficiencies of Factor V

- Deficiencies of Factor II

- Deficiencies of Fibrinogen
- Heparin
- Warfarin
- Fibrinogen/Fibrin Degradation Products
- Lupus Anticoagulant

- Partially Filled Collection Tube
- Inadequate Citrate in Collection Tube 2° Polycythemia

Figure 31-11. The partial thromboplastin time of plasma was developed in 1953 as a way of differentiating normal subjects from patients with hemophilia. Coagulation is initiated by the addition of calcium and partial thromboplastin, which lacks the tissue factor found in complete tissue thromboplastin. The normal value for the original partial thromboplastin time was 80 to 90 seconds. The test was modified in 1961 to generate what is now known as the *activated partial thromboplastin time* by the addition of an exogenous negatively charged surface (e.g., kaolin, a porcelain clay). This results in more rapid activation of the contact system, whose members include prekallikrein (PK), high-molecular-weight kininogen (HMWK), and factors XII and XI, resulting in a normal value of approximately 30 seconds.

tested with normal plasma. Different PTs can thus be obtained from the same plasma, depending on the thromboplastin preparation being used. Testing in different laboratories may lead to divergent conclusions regarding the adequacy of a patient's anticoagulation therapy, with attendant risks if the therapy is inappropriately modified.

Thus, the PT index (ratio of a patient's PT to a control PT) of different patients cannot be compared unless the same thromboplastin was used for all tests, making clinical trials and reports originating from different centers in Europe and America difficult to compare. As a result, efforts have been undertaken to develop a means whereby the degree of anticoagulation brought about by warfarin therapy may be compared, which depends on a mathematical formulation to correct for differences in thromboplastin preparations. The use of this index, the International Normalized Ratio [INR], is hoped to lead to more uniform (hence, better) patient care. The INR is calculated from the following formula:

$$INR = (PT_{patient}/mean\ PT_{normals})^{ISI}$$

where $PT_{patient}$ is the patient's PT (in seconds), mean $PT_{normals}$ is the mean PT determined in each laboratory using that particular thromboplastin, and ISI is the International Sensitivity Index, a value assigned to each thromboplastin by its manufacturer after it is calibrated against a World Health Association reference thromboplastin.

The INR was devised to aid in the monitoring of patients taking oral anticoagulants (118). The INR should not be used to assess the hemostatic system or thrombotic tendency of patients whose PTs are prolonged for other reasons.

PARTIAL THROMBOPLASTIN TIME

The PTT was originally performed by measuring the time required (usually 80 to 90 seconds) for a clot to form after phospholipid and calcium are added to citrated plasma. Greater sensitivity and reproducibility are obtained when a particulate activator of the intrinsic pathway (which uses factors XII, XI, IX, VIII, X, V, and II, fibrinogen, HMW kininogen, and prekal-

likrein) is used to initiate coagulation (Fig. 31-11). The resulting aPTT is used in almost all laboratories today and is especially sensitive to heparin and levels of factors VIII and IX below 25%. False-normal aPTTs may be seen in patients who are deficient in one clotting factor or have elevated levels of another (often factor VIII, an acute-phase reactant) (119).

THROMBIN TIME

The test for thrombin time is performed by measuring the time required for a citrated plasma sample to clot after the addition of thrombin (Fig. 31-12). The amount of thrombin used—hence, the thrombin time—may differ among laboratories, and there is no standard normal value. The thrombin time may be prolonged by low levels of fibrinogen, abnormal fibrinogen molecules (dysfibrinogenemia), heparin, antibodies, or elevated levels of fibrin degradation products. The *reptilase time* is performed by substituting a snake venom for thrombin in the assay. Because reptilase is not inhibited by heparin, it may be used to confirm the presence of heparin in suspected samples, such as those drawn from intensive care patients with indwelling catheters. Prolonged thrombin times (usually performed using bovine thrombin) have been reported in patients exposed to topical (bovine) thrombin during surgery (120), presumably because of immunization and formation of antibodies (121). In most cases, this is of no clinical importance. There are reports of such patients developing a clinically significant antibody to factor V (human), presumably as the result of cross-reactivity with bovine factor V present in topical thrombin preparations, which may cause significant hemorrhage (122,123).

Fibrinogen

A variety of methods are available for measuring plasma concentrations of fibrinogen, including immunologic techniques that detect the intact molecule as well as degradation products, salt precipitation methods, determination by chemical means of the amount of protein that is clotted by the addition of large doses of thrombin, and measurement of the rate of

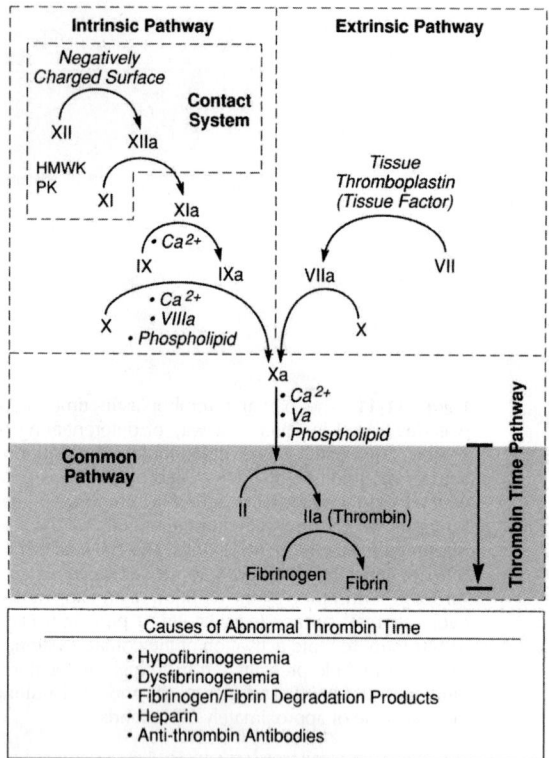

Figure 31-12. Thrombin time. The addition of thrombin (usually of bovine origin) to plasma results in cleavage of fibrinogen and clot formation. The normal value depends on the amount of thrombin added and varies from one laboratory to another. It has been recognized that some patients exposed to topical bovine thrombin during surgery may develop antibodies that prolong the thrombin time. Less frequently, these patients also develop antibodies to factor V and may also have prolonged prothrombin times and activated partial thromboplastin times. HMWK, high-molecular-weight kininogen; PK, prekallikrein.

clotting of diluted plasma treated with thrombin (in quantities sufficient to overcome typical doses of heparin). The latter method (named after its inventor, Clauss) is commonly used but may be affected by the presence of high concentrations of fibrinogen degradation products that can inhibit fibrin fibril polymerization, leading to an underestimation of the true fibrinogen concentration.

TESTS OF FIBRIN AND FIBRINOGEN DEGRADATION PRODUCTS

Several methods have been developed to detect proteolytic degradation products of fibrin or fibrinogen. These tests cannot distinguish fragments derived from fibrin from those derived from fibrinogen and are therefore said to measure FDP/fdp. (*FDP* refers to those species derived from fibrinogen; *fdp* refers to those derived from fibrin.) A commonly used assay for FDP/fdp uses an antibody to fibrinogen to detect fragments that are not removed when the patient's plasma is clotted by measuring the titer of the specimen able to agglutinate latex beads coated with antifibrinogen antibody. Some tests are calibrated so that the reciprocal of the least reacting dilution (titer) is equal to the plasma concentration (in μg/mL) of FDP/fdp.

A more recently developed test, which is being used increasingly more frequently, is the D-dimer assay. This test uses a monoclonal antibody that recognizes the new epitope formed when fibrin is cross-linked by factor XIIIa (Fig. 31-8). Its detection in the circulation is thus taken to indicate the prior production of both thrombin and plasmin in the vascular space. It may

be best used in conjunction with other assays for FDP for seeking to make the diagnosis of DIC (124).

Coagulation Factor Assays

Coagulation factor assays are functional assays performed by determining how well a patient's plasma corrects the clotting deficiency of someone known to be lacking a specific coagulation factor. Although these assays are basically variants of the PT and aPTT, they require precision in their performance and specialized reagents to perform. Immunologic measurements of clotting factors are not generally available.

Detection of Circulating Inhibitors

One of the first steps taken by the clinician confronted by a patient with a prolonged clotting time, especially the aPTT, is to determine whether the abnormality is due to the lack of one or more clotting factors or to the presence of a circulating inhibitor, which slows coagulation. In some hospitals, the key test in making this determination is called the *1:1 plasma mix*; in others, it is simply known as an *inhibitor screen*. The test is based on the observations that clotting times are not prolonged when the level of any one clotting factor is greater than 25% to 30% of normal, and that circulating inhibitors are present in sufficient amounts that they retain their ability to slow coagulation when diluted. The test is performed by mixing equal volumes of the patient's plasma with plasma from a normal donor and then measuring the clotting time (aPTT or PT) of the mixture (Fig. 31-13). In some cases, it is useful to measure the clotting time at various time points after the mixture is prepared (0, 30, 60, 120 min). If the clotting time of the 1:1 mix is normal, the patient's defect is said to have been corrected by the addition of normal plasma, implying a lack of clotting factor as the explanation for the initial abnormally long clotting time. If the clotting time of the mixture is prolonged, the test is interpreted to indicate the presence of a circulating inhibitor able to affect the normal plasma, as well as the patients.

The four major types of circulating inhibitors are heparin (or other anticoagulants such as dermatan sulfate or hirudin), high levels of fibrinogen and fibrin degradation products, antibodies to coagulation factors, and antibodies that react with the phospholipid surface required for coagulation, which is called the *lupus anticoagulant.*

The first two causes of an abnormal inhibitor screen, heparin and elevated levels of fibrinogen and fibrin degradation products, may be determined with routine clotting tests. As previously mentioned, it can be concluded that heparin is present if the thrombin time is abnormal and the simultaneous reptilase time is normal. Antibodies that interfere with specific clotting factors are detected by finding depression of the plasma levels of only one factor. If multiple clotting factors appear to be depressed, the presence of an antibody to a substance (phospholipid) common to all the clotting factor tests must be considered, that is, the lupus anticoagulant.

Lupus anticoagulants are antibodies, usually of the immunoglobulin G (IgG) class, which interfere with coagulation by binding to phospholipids and thereby inhibiting thrombin generation. Despite its name, the lupus anticoagulant is found in many patients who do not have autoimmune diseases and should be considered in everyone with characteristic laboratory test results, regardless of their clinical status. The paradox of the lupus anticoagulant is that although the coagulation times are prolonged, most patients with a lupus anticoagulant do not have excessive spontaneous or postsurgical bleeding. This provides another example of the poor predictive ability of abnor-

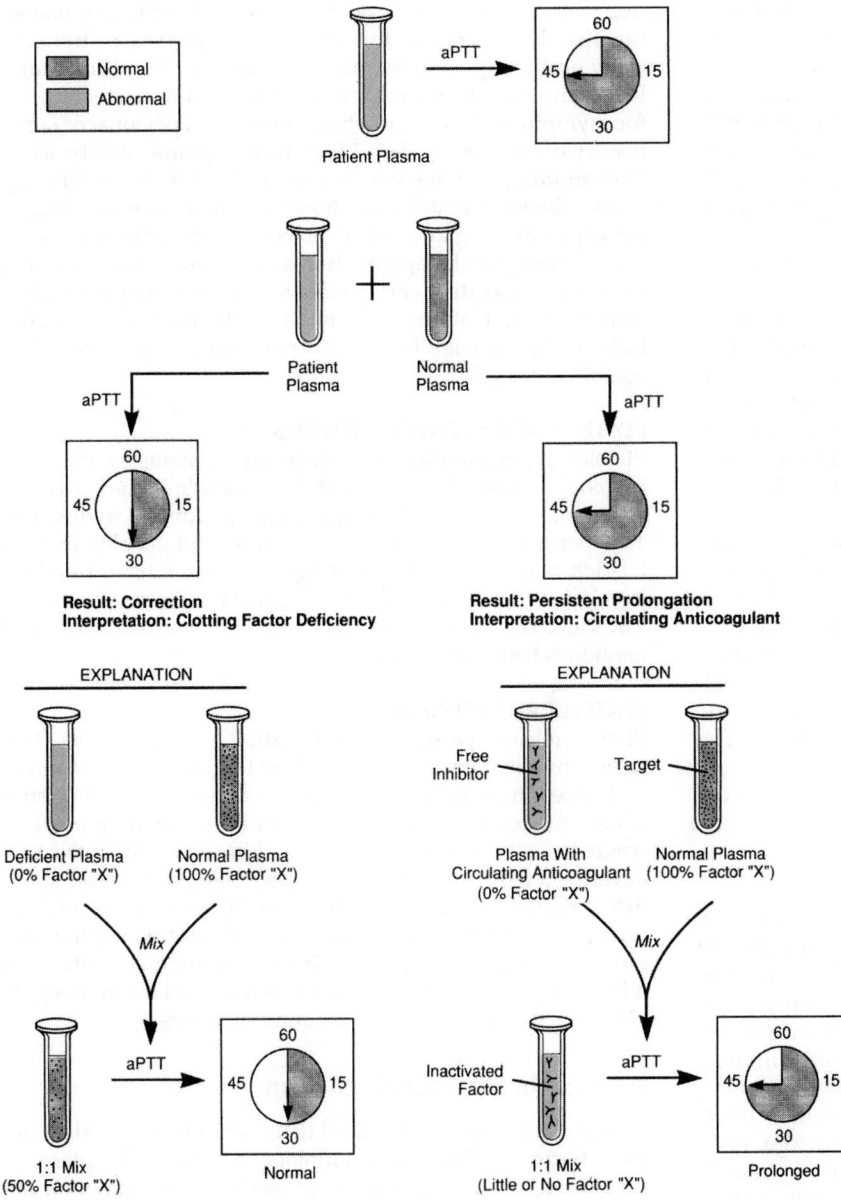

Figure 31-13. Screening for a circulating anticoagulant. Normal plasma contains at least a twofold excess of all coagulation factors, and dilution of plasma with an equal volume of saline does not result in a significantly prolonged clotting time. Thus, if a patient has a long clotting time because of a factor deficiency, the clotting time will correct when a 1:1 mix of patient and normal plasma is tested. Additional testing to identify the missing coagulation factor should be performed. If the patient's plasma contains a circulating anticoagulant (e.g., heparin, fibrin degradation products, a lupus anticoagulant, or a neutralizing antibody that reacts with a specific coagulation protein), the clotting time of the mixture remains prolonged because the inhibitor also inactivates the relevant factor or factors contributed by the normal plasma, and additional tests to identify the circulating anticoagulant should be performed. aPTT, activated partial thromboplastin time.

mal clotting tests for surgical bleeding. Furthermore, patients with lupus anticoagulants appear to have a greater than average risk of suffering from thrombotic disorders, another finding that has been attributed to acquired APC-resistance.

A number of coagulation tests may be used to look for the lupus anticoagulant in the patient with an abnormal inhibitor screen, including the tissue thromboplastin inhibition test, the kaolin clotting time, the dilute Russell viper venom test, and the aPTT (125,126). Neutralization of the antibody's effects by the addition of excess phospholipid is advocated as a means of confirming the diagnosis. This may be accomplished by adding high doses of rabbit brain thromboplastin to the kaolin clotting time (127) or lyophilized platelets (platelet neutralization procedure) (128). The relation of lupus anticoagulants to antiphospholipid or anticardiolipin antibodies is confusing. Strictly speaking, lupus anticoagulants are defined by their property of affecting clotting tests. Because some patients with the lupus anticoagulant have anticardiolipin antibodies and others do not, it seems most appropriate at this time to consider them to be distinct but probably related, especially because many questions remain about their chemistry and mode of action *in vivo* (129).

Antibodies to coagulation factor proteins are rare but clinically important and are usually associated with clinically significant bleeding. These antibodies most often arise in patients with moderate or severe hemophilia as a result of receiving replacement therapy, but they can develop in any patient with a severe plasma protein deficiency exposed to sufficient amounts of that protein. Because factor VIII deficiency is the most common congenital clotting factor deficiency state, antifactor VIII antibodies are the most common antibodies of this class detected in the laboratory. For reasons that have yet to be explained, factor VIII is also the most common antigenic target in nonhemophilic persons who spontaneously develop an antibody to a specific clotting factor. Although anti–factor VIII antibodies have spontaneously developed in normal persons as well as in patients with a variety of autoimmune diseases, they are most commonly present either in the elderly or in women in the postpartum period. These patients usually present with spontaneous, often severe bleeding. Surprisingly, the plasma of these patients may have measurable factor VIII levels (1% to 5%), even though they have moderate or high titer inhibitors (130). Simple modifications of the aPTT allow factor VIII inhibitors to be detected in routine laboratories that are not able to perform the specialized Bethesda inhibitor assays used to quantify factor VIII inhibitors (131).

Use of bovine thrombin as a hemostatic agent during surgery has been associated with the development of antithrombin and anti–factor V antibodies, as mentioned in the previous discussion regarding thrombin time. If the antibody reacts only with bovine thrombin, the patient has an isolated prolongation of thrombin time, because bovine thrombin is used to perform this test. Only when it cross-reacts also with human thrombin are the PT and aPTT prolonged.

In some cases, it may be difficult to distinguish true anticoagulation factor antibodies from the lupus anticoagulant, a situation that may be worsened if decisions must be made at a time when specialized laboratory tests cannot be easily obtained. At such times, the clinician should analyze the situation in terms of the known natural history and associated clinical features that accompany these disorders and arrive at a working diagnosis. Even when the laboratory assistance required to measure clotting factor levels is available, uncertainty about the correct diagnosis may remain, especially if several factors appear to be depressed. Because factor level measurements are based on the same clotting tests that may be affected by the lupus anticoagulant, the clinician must consider whether one mechanism is responsible for all the abnormal tests, whether there are multiple antibodies to different clotting factors, or whether the patient has both a lupus anticoagulant and a specific anticlotting factor antibody.

Several points should be borne in mind that may help in considering this differential diagnosis:

1. Lupus anticoagulant antibodies are common.
2. True antifactor antibodies are rare.
3. The lupus anticoagulant is usually not present in very high concentrations, and its effects are more likely to be affected by diluting the plasma than are most antibodies to clotting factors. Therefore, if multiple clotting factors appear to be depressed, the clinician should call the laboratory and determine whether the levels were determined with relatively low (1:10) dilutions of the patient's plasma and, if so, request that they be determined with plasma diluted at 1:20 or greater. Thus, the effect of the lupus anticoagulant is such that levels of multiple clotting factors appear to increase (in relation to normal persons) as increasingly diluted plasma is assayed.
4. Acquired antifactor VIII antibodies, especially in nonhemophiliacs, do not alter the 1:1 mixing test if the test is performed immediately after mixing, but they do prolong the aPTT if tested after a 1- to 2-hour incubation period at 37°C.

Factor XIII cross-links fibrin monomers to each other after a clot has formed. Because clot formation, rather than cross-linking, is the endpoint of PT, aPTT, and thrombin time, a lack of factor XIII is not detected by these tests, and the clinician must specifically request a test of factor XIII function. The most frequently used tests are performed by placing a clot formed from the patient's plasma in a concentrated salt solution (5 mol/L urea or 1 mol/L monochloroacetic acid). In the absence of cross-linking (covalent bond formation), the fibrin monomers dissociate from each other, and the clot is not visible after 24 hours, whereas a cross-linked clot is stable under such conditions.

Commonly Used Platelet Function Tests (132)

BLEEDING TIME
The test for bleeding time has the longest history of use of any hemostatic test (133). Because it is the only test of platelet func-

tion *in vivo*, it is frequently said to be the best test of platelet function. Unfortunately, this idea has kept physicians from critically evaluating its performance in various clinical conditions. Research suggests that it should not be used as a screening test for asymptomatic persons who do not have a personal or family history of bleeding (115–117,134). Bleeding time may be useful in examining patients whose personal or family history suggests a defect of platelet function (i.e., immediate bleeding). A variety of drugs may affect the bleeding time, but many more drugs affect platelet aggregation studies but not the bleeding time (135). Also, drug combinations may have unique effects on bleeding time. Unfortunately, relatively little information exists to help the clinician faced with patients using specific drug combinations (136).

PLATELET AGGREGATION STUDIES
Platelet aggregation studies have become a mainstay of the clinical coagulation laboratory, but their usefulness has also been called into question (137). Platelet aggregation has traditionally been performed by examining the behavior of platelets in platelet-rich plasma. Whole blood aggregometers have also been developed that examine platelet aggregation without removing RBCs and WBCs. A consensus has not been reached as to which method is better for clinical use.

PLATELET RELEASE REACTION
Platelet release reaction may be studied in several ways. After radioactive serotonin (5-HT) is added to platelets, it is taken up and stored in the cells' dense granules. If the cells are then stimulated, the serotonin is released into the surrounding medium, where it can be assayed. Tests using this observation have been developed to identify patients with storage pool disease and to detect heparin-dependent antibodies. Dense granule secretion can also be monitored by measuring ATP release after the addition of an activating agent. α-Granule secretion results in the release of proteins such as platelet factor 4 and β-thromboglobulin, which can be measured by immunoassays.

Tests of the Fibrinolytic System

The euglobulin lysis time (ELT) determines how quickly a person's fibrin clot dissolves in autologous plasma. The plasma is first treated in a manner that removes fibrinolytic inhibitors and is then clotted. The time required for the resulting clot to lyse (usually 60 to 300 minutes) is proportionate to the concentration of plasminogen activators present in the sample (if there are normal levels of plasminogen and fibrinogen). The test is usually performed with the aim of determining whether a hyperfibrinolytic state is present (i.e., the ELT is short). Hypofibrinogenemia may also result in a short ELT, and the fibrinogen level should be obtained near the time of the test's performance. An alternate evaluation of the fibrinolytic system may be performed by measuring how long a dilute clot takes to lyse.

Activation of the fibrinolytic system results in the production of FDP/fdp or D-dimers. Because activation of the fibrinolytic system is considered to be a physiologic response to fibrin deposition, which occurs normally in many inflammatory states, it may be difficult to differentiate normal from pathologic fibrinolysis with these tests.

An alternative way of assessing the activation of the fibrinolytic system is by performing a functional measurement of α_2-plasmin inhibitor (also called α_2-*antiplasmin*). Congenital deficiencies of α_2-plasmin inhibitor have been described, but the true prevalence either in the general population or among patients with a history of abnormal bleeding is not known (138). Depletion of this antiprotease has also been documented in diseases known to result in a hyperfibrinolytic state (66) and is used in some centers to guide the administration of antifibrinolytic therapy to patients with acute promyelocytic leukemia. Thromboelastography is used to detect excessive fibrinolysis during liver transplantation and to guide the administration of antifibrinolytic agents (139), although it is not widely used in hemostasis laboratories.

CLINICAL BLEEDING SYNDROMES

Immediate Bleeding

Bleeding occurring immediately after a vascular insult suggests a failure of hemostatic plug formation. This is most frequently due to a failure of platelet function but may also be seen in patients with rare disorders in which the ability of the vasculature to support hemostasis is compromised because of a quantitative or qualitative platelet defect.

Delayed Bleeding

Bleeding that becomes evident hours to days after an injury indicates an inability to form a stable clot. The formation of the stable clot requires that (a) clot formation occurs in a timely manner, (b) continued accretion of fibrin into the clot occurs, and (c) the clot is able to resist (appropriately) the action of the fibrinolytic system to dissolve it. This last point is determined by several factors, including cross-linking of fibrin monomers within the clot by factor XIII, the amount of plasminogen activator released in the vicinity of the clot, and the local concentrations of the antiproteases that regulate the fibrinolytic system (α_2-antiplasmin and PAI-1). Thus, delayed bleeding may be due to one or more of the following five conditions: low levels of clotting factors, circulating anticoagulants, decreased amounts of factor XIII, increasing plasminogen activators, or deficiencies of α_2-antiplasmin or PAI-1.

Combined Immediate and Delayed Bleeding

Immediate and delayed bleeding implies the presence of both platelet function defects (or thrombocytopenia) and another factor that promotes bleeding. The clinician should consider VWD as a single cause in patients with a history compatible with a congenital disorder, and liver disease, DIC, or a paraproteinemia as possible acquired causes of this constellation of findings.

PATIENT WORKUP

History

The hemostatic history is a key element of the clinical evaluation of the patient because its findings determine which laboratory tests are ordered by the clinician; it often requires careful interpretation of many subjective impressions or poorly documented clinical events. The areas to be covered may be grouped into several major categories, as shown in Table 31-3.

Many normal persons describe themselves as having suffered from excessive bleeding, whereas many persons with defined bleeding disorders have benign histories, particularly if they have not been exposed to a significant hemostatic stress. Because a hemostatic questionnaire alone is rarely adequate for determining a valid hemostatic history, the patient must be questioned personally by the physician. After the history, the

TABLE 31-3. Hemostatic History

Events associated with hemostatic stresses of daily living
Easy bruising, no recognized precipitating events
Easy bruising in response to minor trauma (note if purpura or ecchymoses)
Hematoma formation or joint bleeding, no recognized precipitating events
Hematoma formation or joint bleeding in response to trauma
Bleeding after shaving
Excessive menstrual bleeding
Epistaxis
Gum bleeding (especially if not associated with gum disease)
Gastrointestinal tract bleeding (with or without telangiectasias)
Urinary tract bleeding
Hemostatic stresses associated with medical procedures or trauma
Procedures associated with good surgical hemostasis
  Most types of surgery
Procedures in which surgical hemostasis may be incomplete
  Childbirth
  Dental extractions
  Abortions
  Tonsillectomy
  Needle biopsies
  Trauma or fractures
  Cardiac surgery
  Circumcision
Associated factors to inquire about if bleeding history is positive
Transfusion history
Medications
Medical history, with particular attention paid to signs, symptoms, and
  laboratory data suggestive of diseases associated with bleeding
  Acute or chronic liver disease
  Renal insufficiency
  Myeloma or paraproteinemia
  Amyloidosis
  Hypercortisolism
  Myelodysplasia
  Myeloproliferative disorders
  Leukemia
  Scurvy
  Connective tissue disorders
  Vasculitis
Family history
Family members believed to be (or to have been) bleeders
  Sex and age of affected and unaffected members
  Evidence for defining a hemorrhagic tendency
  Transfusion history
  Cause of death (if applicable)

physician can decide whether there is a high, low, or indeterminate probability that the patient has a bleeding disorder. This estimation can then be used in deciding which, if any, laboratory tests to obtain.

Physical Examination

The physical examination is usually not helpful in evaluating patients in the preoperative setting, especially if they are asymptomatic. Although bruises are of concern to many patients, extensive workups usually fail to reveal a defined hematologic condition, especially if the patient is female (140). Persons who are seen because of complaints related to skin hemorrhage should be evaluated for signs of vasculitis (palpable purpura); evidence of a coagulation factor, rather than platelet, disorder (as may be suggested by the presence of ecchymoses and not purpura); perifollicular hemorrhage (a sign of scurvy); and bleeding in areas not usually subject to overt or occult trauma. Physical findings of splenic enlargement or hepatic disease may help to focus the subsequent workup.

Evidence of a coagulopathy may be sought in the hospitalized patient by examining the skin overlying the back, flanks, buttocks, and thighs for discoloration, which could suggest a deep site of bleeding, and by examining surgical or traumatic

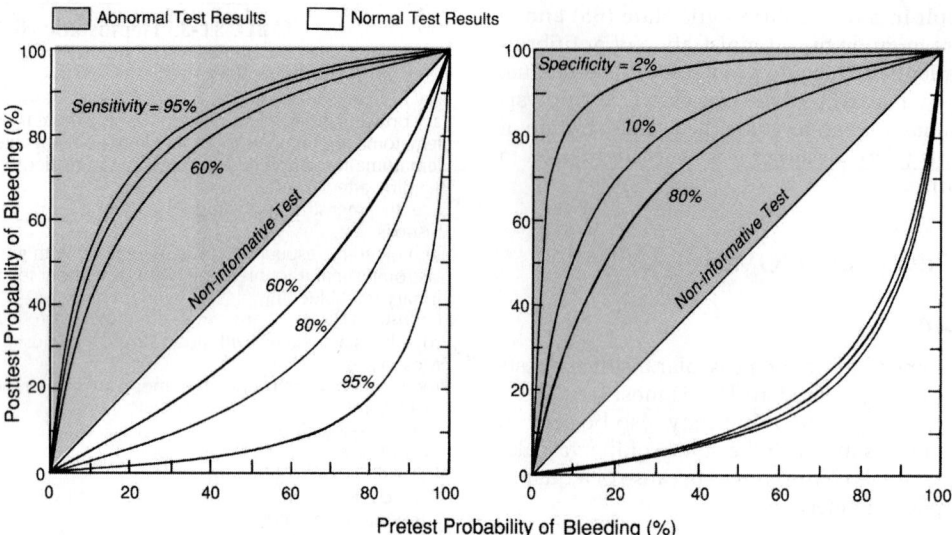

Figure 31-14. Application of Bayes' theorem to the assessment of the likelihood of bleeding in patients with abnormal coagulation test results. Bayes' theorem states that the probability that a disease is present when an abnormal result is obtained depends on the likelihood that the disease (here, excessive bleeding) is present in the patient before the test is performed. Thus, if the physician concludes on the basis of the history and physical examination that the patient has a low probability of having a hemorrhagic tendency, an abnormal result will not raise the probability of such a disorder to greater than 50% unless the test is highly sensitive and specific. The graphs show that the information gained from a test varies with the pretest probability that the disease is present as well as the sensitivity and specificity of the test. The curves above the line of identity (denoting a test that conveys no meaningful information) show the results of abnormal (positive) tests, and those below this line indicate the posttest probabilities if the results are normal (negative). (From Sox HC. Probability theory in the use of diagnostic tests. *Ann Intern Med* 1986;104:60.)

wounds, dressings, sites of catheter insertion, the sputum or stomach suction bottles, and urinary drainage bags.

Laboratory Evaluation

EVALUATION OF PATIENT WITHOUT HISTORY OF BLEEDING

Testing the category of patients with no history of bleeding is appropriately called *screening*. The term *screening test* has acquired two meanings with regard to the hemostatic system. The first indicates that the test itself is a screen for a hemostatic defect but is not specific for a given disorder. Thus, the aPTT is a good screening test for hemophilia because it is able to detect most patients who have the disorder, but it is nonspecific because its prolongation could also be due to poor collection technique, a lupus anticoagulant, vitamin K deficiency, or a specific factor deficiency elsewhere in the intrinsic pathway. The term *screening* is more commonly used by physicians to indicate that one is testing patients who are judged to have a low risk of the disorder in question. A common example is the routine performance of mammography examinations for asymptomatic women.

Use of the expression *screening tests of hemostasis* means one thing to hematologists (who understand the limitations of the tests) but something else to other physicians, surgeons, and anesthesiologists, who are more often dealing with asymptomatic, nonbleeding patients. As a result, discussions by hematologists of screening tests of hemostasis may lead these physicians to conclude that it is appropriate to use these tests in asymptomatic persons. Discussion of this issue often provokes emotional responses, in large part because of the fear of catastrophic bleeding and a failure to consider the relevant clinical epidemiologic issues.

The performance of such routine tests in low-risk patients is to be discouraged for several reasons. First, if the probability of a patient's having a disease is low, then a positive test result has relatively little effect on the probability that the patient has the disease and is more likely to be a false positive than a true positive, even if the test has a high sensitivity and specificity (Fig. 31-14). An abnormal PT, aPTT, or bleeding time result obtained from a patient who has previously undergone surgery uneventfully and has no recent bleeding history or new medical problems is much more likely to be a falsely abnormal result than a sign of a true hemostatic defect.

Although there is usually an explanation for a prolonged clotting time—if only poor blood-drawing technique (141)—the same cannot be said for a prolonged bleeding time, because it is not uncommon to find a prolonged bleeding time on one day and a normal one on the next without obvious cause. Many physicians are surprised to learn that the bleeding time has not proved itself as a predictor of surgical bleeding (115–117). This is not surprising when it is realized that the bleeding time is frequently normal in patients with VWD (142), the most prevalent and carefully studied platelet disorder, and that normal values are simply derived from the mean and standard deviations found in healthy ambulatory persons and not from the study of patients undergoing surgery.

After an abnormal screening test result is obtained, there is inevitably a delay of surgery, worry on the patient's part, and additional expense while consultations and additional laboratory tests are obtained. In some instances, physicians may administer transfusions of blood products in an attempt to correct the abnormal laboratory value. This exposes the patient to the risk of transfusion-transmitted diseases without necessarily decreasing the risk of perioperative hemorrhage.

In general, excessive surgical bleeding is uncommon. Although everyone fears a disastrous, potentially life-threatening hemorrhage, these low-incidence events cannot be avoided simply by ordering enough screening tests. Tonsillectomy, for example, is a procedure that is of concern to physicians because it usually involves children and a mucosal surface where surgical hemostasis may be difficult to attain. One study shows that even when screening tests are used, bleeding occurs in 2% to 3% of patients, comparable to that seen in other published series (143). Thus, screening tests of hemostasis have little overall effect on eliminating operative hemorrhage in the setting in which there is little operative bleeding. Even less usefulness would be anticipated when applied to operations in which all patients lose significant amounts of blood. The importance of detecting mild defects in the hemostatic system is also minimized in operations in which good surgical hemostasis is possible, because one suture is equivalent to many tens of thousands of platelets.

EVALUATION OF PATIENT WITH FAMILY HISTORY OF BLEEDING

Several hemostatic disorders with genetic components warrant specialized evaluation. The most common is VWD, estimated to affect about 1 in 1000 persons (although estimates range widely, from 1 in 100 to 1 in 10,000). Most persons have type I VWD, have only a mild bleeding disorder, and inherit the disease in an autosomal-dominant pattern. Rarely, VWD may be inherited in an autosomal-recessive manner.

Hemophilia A (factor VIII deficiency) accounts for about 85% of the congenital clotting factor deficiencies and affects 1 in 10,000 males. It is generally inherited in a sex-linked manner, and women who are carriers generally (but not invariably) have no symptoms. Hemophilia B (factor IX) deficiency accounts for about 10% of the hereditary coagulopathies and is inherited in a sex-linked manner. It is clinically indistinguishable from factor VIII deficiency. Persons with mild hemophilia (A or B) have levels that are 5% to 25% of normal levels and may not experience any bleeding until they experience surgical or traumatic stresses. Rare cases of apparent autosomal hemophilia have been recognized as well, which appear to be due to a mutation in the VWF gene, which leads to a failure of VWF to bind to factor VIII and protect it from rapid degradation in the circulation.

Factor XI deficiency is usually thought to affect mainly Ashkenazi Jews (whose calculated gene frequency for factor XI deficiency ranges from 2% to 12%, depending on location). Many factor XI–deficient patients are not of Jewish origin (144), and a different ethnic background should not preclude testing for this disorder under appropriate circumstances.

EVALUATION OF PATIENT WITH CLEAR OR QUESTIONABLE BLEEDING HISTORY

The history may clearly indicate a bleeding tendency (clinical estimate of the probability of a bleeding disorder of more than 90%) or may simply raise the probability above the baseline level that one has for previously unstressed patients (less than 5%). In this intermediate range of probabilities, clinical test results have their greatest effects (Fig. 31-14). The same initial laboratory approach should be taken for evaluating both groups of patients. The tests usually obtained include a complete blood count and platelet count, aPTT, PT, thrombin time, and fibrinogen level. If the patient is known to have a disorder associated with DIC, a test for fibrinogen and fibrin degradation products or D-dimer may be useful. If the history is suggestive of a disorder of primary hemostasis, a bleeding time test may be useful as well. If these tests are normal, the clinician must decide whether the history warrants additional testing. Table 31-4 suggests additional testing that may be performed. Referral of the patient or the patient's plasma to a specialized laboratory for additional testing may be advisable.

WORKUP OF COMMON ABNORMALITIES OF HEMOSTATIC SCREENING TESTS

Abnormal Platelet Count

There are many causes of a low platelet count, some of which are shown in Table 31-5. Because platelet counts are no longer

---

TABLE 31-4. Unusual Causes of Bleeding

Platelet defects
Plasma membrane receptor defects
  gpIb/IX—Bernard-Soulier syndrome, pseudo–von Willebrand's disease
  gpIIb/IIIa—Glanzmann's thrombasthenia
Platelet granule deficiencies (storage pool disease)
Hereditary thrombocytopenias, including Alport's syndrome, Fanconi's syndrome, thrombocytopenia with absent radius syndrome
Platelet function defects associated with other congenital abnormalities, including Wiskott-Aldrich syndrome, Hermansky-Pudlak syndrome (albinism), Chédiak-Higashi syndrome, May-Hegglin anomaly, Ehlers-Danlos syndrome
Snake venoms
Coagulation protein defects
Deficiencies of factors II, V, X, VII, XIII
Dysfibrinogenemia
Antibodies to coagulation factors
Amyloidosis
Snake venoms
Excessive fibrinolytic system activation
α_2-Antiplasmin deficiency
Plasminogen activator inhibitor deficiency
Thrombolytic agents
Acute promyelocytic leukemia
Cardiopulmonary bypass
Amyloidosis
Liver disease, liver transplantation

TABLE 31-5. Common Causes of Thrombocytopenia

Immune
Primary
  Idiopathic (autoimmune)
Secondary (immune complex mediated)
  Collagen vascular diseases, especially systemic lupus erythematosus
  Infections, including viruses such as human immunodeficiency virus, parasites, bacteria
  Malignancies
  Drugs
Posttransfusion purpura
Alloimmune thrombocytopenia (in newborns)
Nonimmune
Marrow suppression due to infection
Drugs, including alcohol
Disseminated intravascular coagulation
Thrombotic thrombocytopenic purpura
Hemolytic-uremic syndrome
Hypersplenism
Pregnancy
  Benign thrombocytopenia of pregnancy
  Preeclampsia
  HELLP syndrome (hemolysis, elevated liver enzymes, and low platelet counts)
  Eclampsia
Aplastic anemia
Marrow infiltration (tuberculosis, granulomas, myelofibrosis, leukemia, myeloma, carcinoma)
Myelodysplastic syndrome
Vitamin B_{12} or folate deficiency, rarely iron deficiency
Radiation therapy
Renal transplant rejection
Massive transfusion (dilutional)
Intravascular devices
Pseudothrombocytopenia
Clotting of blood specimen
Platelet-reactive cold agglutinins
Clumping due to antibodies reacting with chelating anticoagulants

TABLE 31-6. Common Causes of a Prolonged Bleeding Time

Thrombocytopenia
von Willebrand's disease
Drugs
    Aspirin
    Nonsteroidal antiinflammatory agents
    High-dose penicillins
    Drug combinations
Uremia
Cirrhosis
Myeloproliferative disorders
Myelodysplastic disorders
Paraproteinemia
Platelet dysfunction syndromes
Chronic disseminated intravascular coagulation

TABLE 31-7. Abnormal Coagulation Tests

Causes of prolonged clotting tests
aPTT
    Clotting factor deficiencies (except factor VII)
    Antibodies to clotting factors
    Lupus anticoagulant
    Heparin
    Elevated fibrin degradation products
    Warfarin or related compounds
PT
    Deficiencies of factors VII, X, V, II, fibrinogen
    Antibodies to clotting factors
    Elevated fibrin degradation products
    Occasionally lupus anticoagulant
    Heparin
    Warfarin or related compounds
Thrombin time
    Low or absent fibrinogen
    Dysfibrinogenemia
    Heparin
    Elevated fibrin degradation products
    Hyperfibrinogenemia
    Antibodies to thrombin
Coagulation abnormalities associated with increased risk of hemorrhage
Prolonged aPTT (other tests normal)
    Factor VIII deficiency
    Factor IX deficiency
    Factor XI deficiency (in some patients)
    von Willebrand's disease
Prolonged PT (other tests normal)
    Warfarin or related compounds
    Vitamin K deficiency (particularly intensive care patients)
    Liver disease
    Factor VII deficiency
Combined prolongation of PT and PTT
    Warfarin or related compounds
    Vitamin K deficiency (particularly intensive care patients)
    Liver disease
    Disseminated intravascular coagulation or excessive fibrinolysis
    Factor X deficiency
    Factor V deficiency
    Factor II (prothrombin) deficiency
    Hypofibrinogenemia
    Heparin
Abnormal inhibitor screening test (1:1 plasma mix)
    Antibody to clotting factor
    Most common: anti–factor VIII, seen both in patients with hemophilia A
        and in previously healthy persons
    Antibodies to factor V in surgical patients exposed to topical thrombin
    Heparin
    Fibrin degradation products
    Lupus anticoagulant in a patient with thrombocytopenia or low factor II
Laboratory abnormalities not associated with increased risk of bleeding
Lupus anticoagulant (unless associated with thrombocytopenia or low
    factor II)
Factor XII deficiency
Prekallikrein deficiency
High-molecular-weight kininogen deficiency
Some patients with prolonged bleeding times

aPTT, activated partial thromboplastin time; PT, prothrombin time.

obtained only on physician request, many asymptomatic patients are incidentally discovered to have thrombocytopenia when screening complete blood counts are obtained. No cause is usually found, and patients are thus accurately classified as having idiopathic thrombocytopenia. Although not well documented, clinical observation suggests that the natural history of patients with low platelet counts is benign. The usefulness of the Coombs' test in diagnosing autoimmune hemolytic anemia has led many to assume that a positive test for antiplatelet antibodies should be obtained before making the diagnosis of idiopathic thrombocytopenia, but there are many reasons for not accepting this as a necessary criterion for making this diagnosis. First, a variety of tests are used in different centers, and cross-center validation of assays is not possible. Second, as many as 15% of clinically diagnosed patients with idiopathic thrombocytopenia may have negative tests, depending on the assay. Third, all platelet-associated IgG is not necessarily antiplatelet antibody, since IgG may be found in the platelet α granules, in the surface-connected canalicular system, or on the plasma membrane, and care must be taken in interpreting these tests (145). This may explain why the positive predictive value of one test measuring platelet-associated IgG was only 46% (146). Furthermore, immune complexes bind to platelet surfaces during viral and bacterial infections (147,148) and may be mistaken for true antiplatelet antibodies.

Abnormal Bleeding Time

There are many reported causes of a prolonged bleeding time (Table 31-6). In many cases, the abnormal test result cannot be duplicated. This may be due to variations in technique, cessation of drugs (or combinations of drugs) that affect the bleeding time, or otherwise unexplained biologic variability of the sort that has been documented to occur in patients with VWD. Although normal upper limits for this test usually range from 9 to 10 minutes, many clinicians believe that minor prolongations (up to 15 minutes) are not associated with a significant bleeding risk. A minor prolongation of the bleeding time should not overshadow a patient's history of successful surgical hemostasis, especially if the surgery involved the creation of irregular mucosal surfaces (as follows tonsillectomy or dental extraction) that are known to be associated with excessive bleeding in patients with VWD.

Persistent or extreme abnormalities in the bleeding time may justify platelet aggregation studies and other specialized tests to determine whether the patient has VWD. Although platelet aggregation studies are frequently ordered, their overall benefit is unclear. Because VWD, renal or liver disease, drug ingestion, and unexplained variability in the bleeding time all are more common causes of a prolonged bleeding time than primary

platelet disorders (storage pool disease, Bernard-Soulier disease, thrombasthenia), a stepped approach to the evaluation of platelet function is warranted (137).

Abnormal Coagulation Tests

Causes of abnormal coagulation tests are shown in Table 31-7. The clinician should know that some plasma protein deficiencies are not associated with an increased risk of bleeding, even though they cause a prolonged clotting time, typically the aPTT.

If the history suggests that the probability of a bleeding disorder is moderate to high, the clinician should consider further testing to determine whether the patient has a factor XIII deficiency or an abnormality affecting proteins of the fibrinolytic system (Table 31-4). Also, patients with mild hemophilia may have clotting factor levels as high as 25% of normal and may exhibit minimal elevations of aPTT. Such patients frequently report that they have experienced little or no bleeding until challenged with surgery, after which they suffer from delayed bleeding. For this reason, a minimally prolonged aPTT in a male patient who has not previously undergone surgery should be followed by measurements of factor VIII and IX levels, even if he has no family history of bleeding.

SUMMARY

Despite many years of study and establishment of the basic principles that define the workings of the hemostatic system, an ongoing rapid evolution is occurring in knowledge concerning this system, which has direct bearing on the clinical management of patients. The ability to evaluate and treat patients with congenital hemostatic defects is relatively well developed. Unfortunately, available laboratory tests are not able to predict with a high degree of accuracy which apparently normal patients will bleed with surgical stress. For this reason, the history, as imperfect as it may be, remains the best tool for determining which patients may be at increased risk for hemorrhage. Extra efforts aimed at obtaining a good history through questioning by the physician and at ensuring good surgical hemostasis are more likely to prevent excessive bleeding than adopting a rigid schedule of screening laboratory tests.

REFERENCES

1. Sixma J, Wester J. The hemostatic plug. *Semin Hematol* 1977;14:265.
2. Marcus AJ, Broekman MJ. The endothelial cell ecto-ADPase responsible for inhibition of platelet function B CD39. *J Clin Invest* 1997;99:1351–1360.
3. Marcus A, et al. Inhibition of platelet function by an aspirin-insensitive endothelial cell ADPase: thromboregulation by endothelial cells. *J Clin Invest* 1991;88:1690.
4. Moake JL, McPherson PD. von Willebrand factor in thrombotic thrombocytopenic purpura and the hemolytic-uremic syndrome. *Transfus Med Rev* 1990;4:163–168.
5. Tsai H-M, et al. The high molecular weight form of endothelial cell von Willebrand factor is released by the regulated pathway. *Br J Haematol* 1991;79:239–245.
6. Wick TM, et al. Unusually large von Willebrand factor multimers increase adhesion of sickle erythrocytes to human endothelial cells under controlled flow. *J Clin Invest* 1987;80:905–910.
7. Rodgers G. Hemostatic properties of normal and perturbed vascular cells. *FASEB J* 1988;2:116.
8. Morawitz P. Die Chemie der Blutgerinnung. *Ergebn Physiol* 1905:307.
9. Quick A, Stanley-Brown M, Bancroft F. A study of the coagulation defect in hemophilia and in jaundice. *Am J Med Sci* 1935;190:501.
10. Conley C, Hartmann R, Worse W. The clotting behavior of human "platelet-free" plasma: evidence for the existence of a "plasma thromboplastin." *J Clin Invest* 1949;28:340.
11. Lister J. On the coagulation of the blood. *Proc R Soc Lond* 1863;12:580.
12. Dam H, Venndt H. Observations on the coagulation of blood plasma in haemophilia. *Lancet* 1940;238:70.
13. Biggs R, Nossel H. Tissue extract and the contact reaction in blood coagulation. *Thromb Haemorrh* 1961;6:1.
14. Wessler S, Reimer S, Sheps M. Biologic assay of a thrombosis-inducing activity in human serum. *J Appl Physiol* 1959;14:943.
15. Davie E, Ratnoff O. Waterfall sequence for intrinsic blood clotting. *Science* 1964;145:1210.
16. MacFarlane RG. An enzyme cascade in the blood clotting mechanism, and its function as a biochemical amplifier. *Nature* 1964;202:498–499.
17. Osterud B, Rapaport S. Activation of factor IX by the reaction product of tissue factor and factor VII: additional pathway for initiating blood coagulation. *Proc Natl Acad Sci U S A* 1977;74:5260.
18. Seligsohn U, et al. Activation of human factor VII in plasma and in purified systems: roles of activated factor IX, kallikrein, and activated factor XII. *J Clin Invest* 1979;64:1056.
19. Bach R, Nemerson Y, Konigsberg W. Purification and characterization of bovine tissue factor. *J Biol Chem* 1981;256:8324.
20. Drake T, Morrisey J, Edgington T. Selective cellular expression of tissue factor in human tissues. *Am J Pathol* 1989;134:1087.
21. Bauer K. Laboratory markers of coagulation activation. *Arch Pathol Lab Med* 1993;117:71.
22. Broze GJ. The role of tissue factor pathway inhibitor in a revised coagulation cascade. *Semin Hematol* 1992;29(3):159–169.
23. Schneider C. The active principle of placental toxin: thromboplastin; its inactivator in blood: antithromboplastin. *Am J Physiol*, 1947;149:123.
24. Thomas L. Studies on the intravascular thromboplastin effect of tissue suspensions in mice. II. A factor in normal rabbit serum which inhibits the thromboplastin effect of the sedimentable tissue component. *Bull Johns Hopkins Hosp* 1947;81:26.
25. Broze G, Miletich J. Isolation of the tissue factor inhibitor produced by HepG2 hepatoma cells. *Proc Natl Acad Sci U S A* 1987;84:1886.
26. Wun T-C, et al. Cloning and characterization of a cDNA coding for the lipoprotein-associated coagulation inhibitor shows that it consists of three tandem Kunitz-type inhibitory domains. *J Biol Chem* 1988;263:6001.
27. Rao L, Rapaport S. Studies of a mechanism inhibiting the initiation of the extrinsic pathway of coagulation. *Blood* 1987;69:645.
28. Broze G, et al. The lipoprotein inhibitor that inhibits the factor VII-tissue factor complex also inhibits factor Xa: insight into its possible mechanism of action. *Blood* 1988;71:335.
29. Seligsohn U, et al. Activated factor VII: presence in factor IX concentrates and persistence in the circulation after infusion. *Blood* 1979;53:828.
30. Lawson J, Mann K. The cooperative activation of human factor IX by the human extrinsic pathway of blood coagulation. *J Biol Chem* 1991;266:11317.
31. Mann K, Krishnaswamy S, Lawson J. Surface-dependent hemostasis. *Semin Hematol* 1992;29:213.
32. Gailani D, Broze G. Factor XI activation in a revised model of blood coagulation. *Science* 1991;253:909.
33. Naito K, Fujikawa K. Activation of human blood coagulation factor XI independent of factor XII: factor XI is activated by thrombin and factor XIa in the presence of negatively charged surfaces. *J Biol Chem* 1991;266:7353.
34. Marlar RA. The protein-C system—how complex is it? *Thromb Haemost* 2001;85:756–757.
35. Bajzar L, et al. TAFI, or plasmaprocarboxy peptidase B, couples the coagulation and fibrinolytic cascades through the thrombin-thrombomodulin complex. *J Biol Chem* 1996;271:16603-16608.
36. Hogg P, Jackson C. Fibrin monomer protects thrombin from inactivation by heparin-antithrombin III: implications for heparin efficacy. *Proc Natl Acad Sci U S A* 1989;86:3619.
37. Eisenberg P, et al. Importance of factor Xa in determining the procoagulant activity of whole-blood clots. *J Clin Invest* 1993;91:1877.
38. Weitz J, et al. Clot-bound thrombin is protected from inhibition by heparin-antithrombin III but is susceptible to inactivation by antithrombin III-independent inhibitors. *J Clin Invest* 1990;86:385.
39. Plow E, Edgington T. An alternative pathway for fibrinolysis. I. The cleavage of fibrinogen by leukocyte proteases at physiologic pH. *J Clin Invest* 1975;56:30.
40. Braaten J, et al. Regulation of fibrinolysis by platelet-released plasminogen activator inhibitor 1: light scattering and ultrastructural examination of lysis of a model platelet-fibrin thrombus. *Blood* 1993;81:1290.
41. Hogg P, Stenflo J, Mosher D. Thrombospondin is a slow tight-binding inhibitor of plasmin. *Biochemistry* 1992;31:265.
42. Mirashahi M, et al. The role of fibroblasts in organization and degradation of fibrin clot. *J Lab Clin Med* 1991;117:274.
43. Gabriel D, Muga K, Boothroyd E. The effect of fibrin structure on fibrinolysis. *J Biol Chem* 1992;267:24259.
44. Carrell N, et al. Hereditary dysfibrinogenemia in a patient with thrombotic disease. *Blood* 1983;62:439.
45. Soria J, Soria C, Caen J. A new type of congenital dysfibrinogenaemia with defective fibrin lysis—Dusard syndrome: possible relation to thrombosis. *Br J Haematol* 1983;53:575.
46. Sakata Y, Aoki N. Significance of cross-linking of 2-plasmin inhibitor to fibrin in inhibition of fibrinolysis and in hemostasis. *J Clin Invest* 1982;69:536.
47. Benett B, et al. The bleeding disorder in acute promyelocytic leukemia: fibrinolysis due to u-PA rather than defibrination. *Br J Haematol* 1989;71:511.
48. Miles L, Plow E. Binding and activation of plasminogen on the platelet surface. *J Biol Chem* 1985;260:4303.
49. Correc P, et al. The presence of plasmin receptors on three mammary carcinoma MCF-7 sublines. *Int J Cancer* 1990;46:745.
50. Vassalli J-D, Baccino D, Belin D. A cellular binding site for the Mr 55,000 form of the human plasminogen activator, urokinase. *J Cell Biol* 1985;100:86.
51. Hajjar K, et al. Binding of tissue plasminogen activator to cultured human endothelial cells. *J Clin Invest* 1987;80:1712.
52. Broder C, et al. Isolation of a prokaryotic plasmin receptor. *J Biol Chem* 1991;266:4922.
53. Stack S, Gonzalez-Gronow M, Pizzo S. Regulation of plasminogen activation by components of the extracellular matrix. *Biochemistry* 1990;29:4966.
54. Lind S, Smith C. Actin accelerates plasmin generation by tissue plasminogen activator. *J Biol Chem* 1991;266:17673.
55. Fleury V, Lijnen H, Angles-Cano E. Mechanism of the enhanced intrinsic activity of single-chain urokinase. *J Biol Chem* 1993;267:15289.
56. Liu J, Pannell R, Gurewich V. A transitional state of prourokinase that has a higher catalytic efficiency against Glu-plasminogen than urokinase. *J Biol Chem* 1993;267:15289.
57. Matsuo O, et al. Thrombolytic properties of staphylokinase. *Blood* 1990;76:925.

58. Keeton M, et al. Cellular localization of type 1 plasminogen activator inhibitor messenger RNA and protein in murine renal tissue. *Am J Pathol* 1993;142:59.

59. Erickson L, Ginsberg M, Loskutoff D. Detection and partial characterization of an inhibitor of plasminogen activation in human platelets. *J Clin Invest* 1984;74:1465.

60. Wang W, et al. A study of the mechanism of inhibition of fibrinolysis by activated thrombin-activatable fibrinolysis inhibitor. *J Biol Chem* 1998;273:27176–27181.

61. Dzik W, et al. Fibrinolysis during liver transplantation in humans: role of tissue-type plasminogen activator. *Blood* 1988;71:1090.

62. Schleef R, et al. Bleeding diathesis due to decreased functional activity of type 1 plasminogen activator inhibitor. *J Clin Invest* 1989;83:1747.

63. Fay W, et al. Complete deficiency of plasminogen-activator inhibitor type 1 due to a frameshift mutation. *N Engl J Med* 1992;327:1729.

64. Lee M, et al. Deficiency of plasma plasminogen activator inhibitor 1 results in hyperfibrinolytic bleeding. *Blood* 1993;81:2357.

65. Saito H. 2-Plasmin inhibitor and its deficiency states. *J Lab Clin Med* 1988;112:671.

66. Williams E. 2-Antiplasmin activity: role in the evaluation and management of fibrinolytic states and other bleeding disorders. *Arch Intern Med* 1989;149:1769.

67. Stead N, et al. Venous thrombosis in a family with defective release of vascular plasminogen activator and elevated plasma factor VIII/von Willebrand's factor. *Am J Med* 1983;74:33.

68. Prins M, Hirsh J. A critical review of the evidence supporting a relationship between impaired fibrinolytic activity and venous thromboembolism. *Arch Int Med* 1991;151:1721.

69. Hamsten A, et al. Increased plasma levels of a rapid inhibitor of tissue plasminogen activator in young survivors of myocardial infarction. *N Engl J Med* 1985;313:1557.

70. Meade T, et al. Fibrinolytic activity, clotting factors, and long-term incidence of ischaemic heart disease in the Northwick Park Heart Study. *Lancet* 1993;342:1076.

71. Wilhelmsen L, et al. Fibrinogen as a risk factor for stroke and myocardial infarction. *N Engl J Med* 1984;311:501.

72. Ridker P, et al. Baseline fibrinolytic state and the risk of future venous thrombosis: a prospective study of endogenous tissue-type plasminogen activator and plasminogen activator inhibitor. *Circulation* 1992;85:1822.

73. Ridker P, et al. Endogenous tissue-type plasminogen activator inhibitor. *Lancet* 1993;341:1165.

74. Meade T, et al. Haemostatic function and cardiovascular death: early results of a prospective study. *Lancet* 1980;1:1050.

75. Rosenfeld B, et al. The effects of different anesthetic regimens on fibrinolysis and the development of postoperative arterial thrombosis. *Anesthesiology* 1993;79:435.

76. Vassalli J-D, Sappino A-P, Belin D. The plasminogen activator/plasmin system. *J Clin Invest* 1991;88:1067.

77. Dano K, et al. Plasminogen activators, tissue degradation, and cancer. *Adv Cancer Res* 1985;44:139.

78. Niewiarowski S, Senyi A, Gillies P. Plasmin-induced platelet aggregation and platelet release reaction. *J Clin Invest* 1973;52:1647.

79. Penny W, Ware J. Platelet activation and subsequent inhibition by plasmin and recombinant tissue-type plasminogen activator. *Blood* 1992;79:91.

80. Lu H, et al. Temperature dependence of plasmin-induced activation or inhibition of human platelets. *Blood* 1991;77:996.

81. Valeri C, et al. Effect of skin temperature on platelet function in patients undergoing extracorporeal bypass. *J Thorac Cardiovasc Surg* 1992;104:108.

82. Boldt J, et al. Platelet function in cardiac surgery: influence of temperature and aprotinin. *Ann Thorac Surg* 1993;55:652.

83. Eisenberg P, Sherman L, Jaffe A. Paradoxic elevation of fibrinopeptide A after streptokinase: evidence for continued thrombosis despite intense fibrinolysis. *J Am Coll Cardiol* 1987;10:527.

84. Winters K, et al. Relative importance of thrombin compared with plasmin-mediated platelet activation in response to plasminogen activation with streptokinase. *Circulation* 1991;84:1552.

85. Aronson D, Chang P, Kessler C. Platelet-dependent thrombin generation after in vitro fibrinolytic treatment. *Circulation* 1992;85:1706.

86. Bidstrup B, et al. Reduction in blood loss and blood use after cardiopulmonary bypass with high dose aprotinin (Trasylol). *J Thorac Cardiovasc Surg* 1989;97:364.

87. van Oeveren W, et al. Aprotinin protects platelets against the initial effect of cardiopulmonary bypass. *J Thorac Cardiovasc Surg* 1990;99:788.

88. Marcus A, Safier L. Thromboregulation: multicellular modulation of platelet reactivity in hemostasis and thrombosis. *FASEB J* 1993;7:516.

89. Duke WW. The relation of blood platelets to hemorrhagic disease. Description of a method for determining the bleeding time and coagulation time and report of three cases of hemorrhagic disease relieved by transfusion. *JAMA* 1910;55:1185.

90. Livio M, et al. Uraemic bleeding: role of anaemia and beneficial effect of red cell transfusions. *Lancet* 1982;2:1013.

91. Luthje J. Extracellular adenine compounds, red blood cells and haemostasis: facts and hypotheses. *Blut* 1989;59:367.

92. Santos M, et al. Enhancement of platelet reactivity and modulation of eicosanoid production by intact erythrocytes. *J Clin Invest* 1991;87:571.

93. Zwaal R, Comfurius P, van Deenen L. Membrane asymmetry and blood coagulation. *Nature* 1977;268:358.

94. Chiu D, et al. Sickled erythrocytes accelerate clotting in vitro: an effect of abnormal membrane lipid asymmetry. *Blood* 1981;58:398–401.

95. Rickles F, O'Leary D. Role of coagulation system in pathophysiology of sickle cell disease. *Arch Intern Med* 1974;133:635.

96. Devine D, et al. Fragment D-dimer levels: an objective marker of vaso-occlusive crisis and other complications of sickle cell disease. *Blood* 1986;68:317.

97. Smith G, Peters T. Subcellular localization and properties of adenosine diphosphatase activity in human polymorphonuclear leukocytes. *Biochim Biophys Acta* 1981;673:234.

98. Wright C, et al. Generation of nitric oxide by human neutrophils. *Biochem Biophys Res Commun* 1989;160:813.

99. Kornecki E, et al. Exposure of fibrinogen receptors in human platelets by surface proteolysis with elastase. *J Clin Invest* 1986;77:750.

100. LeRoy E, Ager A, Gordon J. Effects of neutrophil elastase and other protease on porcine aortic endothelial prostaglandin I2 production, adenine nucleotide release, and responses to vasoactive substances. *J Clin Invest* 1984;74:1003.

101. Higuchi D, et al. The effect of leukocyte elastase on tissue factor pathway inhibitor. *Blood* 1992;79:1712.

102. Machovich R, Owen W. An elastase-dependent pathway of plasminogen activation. *Biochemistry* 1989;28:4517.

103. Valles J, et al. Down-regulation of human platelet reactivity by neutrophils. Participation of lipoxygenase derivatives and adhesive proteins. *J Clin Invest* 1993;92:1357.

104. Tallman M, Kwaan H. Reassessing the hemostatic disorder associated with acute promyelocytic leukemia. *Blood* 1992;79:543.

105. Dam H, Venndt H. Observations on the coagulation of blood plasma in hemophilia. *Lancet* 1940;238:70.

106. Langdell R, Wagner R, Brinkhous K. Effect of antihemophilic factor on one-stage clotting tests; a presumptive test for hemophilia and a simple one-stage antihemophilic factor assay procedure. *J Lab Clin Med* 1953;41:637.

107. Proctor R, Rapaport S. The partial thromboplastin time with kaolin: a simple screening test for the first stage plasma clotting factor deficiencies. *Am J Clin Pathol* 1961;36:212.

108. Eisenberg P, Clarke J, Sussman S. Prothrombin and partial thromboplastin times as preoperative screening tests. *Arch Surg* 1982;117:48.

109. Suchman A, Mushlin A. How well does the activated partial thromboplastin time predict postoperative hemorrhage? *JAMA* 1986;256:750.

110. Diamond L, Porter F. The inadequacies of routine bleeding and clotting times. *N Engl J Med* 1958;259:1025.

111. McVay P, Toy P. Lack of increased bleeding after liver biopsy in patients with mild hemostatic abnormalities. *Am J Clin Pathol* 1990;94:747.

112. McVay P, Toy P. Lack of increased bleeding after paracinesis and thoracentesis in patients with mild coagulation abnormalities. *Transfusion* 1991;31:164.

113. Burns E, Goldberg S, Wenz B. Paradox effect of multiple mild coagulation factor deficiencies on the prothrombin time and activated partial thromboplastin time. *Am J Clin Pathol* 1993;100:94.

114. Ivy A, Shapiro P, Melnick P. The bleeding tendency in jaundice. *Surg Gynecol Obstet* 1935;60:781.

115. Burns ER, Lawrence C. Bleeding time. A guide to its diagnostic and clinical utility. *Arch Pathol Lab Med* 1989;113:1219–1224.

116. Rodgers RP, Levin J. A critical reappraisal of the bleeding time. *Semin Thromb Hemost* 1990;16:1–20.

117. Lind SE. The bleeding time does not predict surgical bleeding. *Blood* 1991;77:2547.

118. Nichols W, Bowie EJ. Standardization of the prothrombin time for monitoring orally administered anticoagulant therapy with use of the international normalized ratio. *Mayo Clin Proc* 1993;68:897.

119. Edson J, Krivit W, White J. Kaolin partial thromboplastin time: high levels of procoagulants producing short clotting times or masking deficiencies of other procoagulants or low concentrations of anticoagulants. *J Lab Clin Med* 1967;70:463.

120. Stricker B, et al. Development of antithrombin antibodies following surgery in patients with prosthetic cardiac valves. *Blood* 1988;72:1375.

121. Flaherty M, Henderson R, Wener M. Iatrogenic immunization with bovine thrombin: a mechanism for prolonged thrombin times after surgery. *Ann Intern Med* 1989;111:631.

122. Berruyer M, et al. Immunization by bovine thrombin used with fibrin glue during cardiovascular operations: development of thrombin and factor V inhibitors. *J Thorac Cardiovasc Surg* 1993;105:892.

123. Cmolik B, et al. Redo cardiac surgery: late bleeding complications from topical thrombin-induced factor V deficiency. *J Thorac Cardiovasc Surg* 1993;105:222.

124. Carr J, McKinney M, McDonagh J. Diagnosis of disseminated intravascular coagulation. *Am J Clin Pathol* 1989;91:280.

125. Lazarchick J, Kizer J. The laboratory diagnosis of lupus anticoagulants. *Arch Pathol Lab Med* 1989;91:280.

126. Triplett D. Coagulation assays for the lupus anticoagulant: review and critique of current methodology. *Stroke* 1992;23(Suppl 1):1–11.

127. Rosove M, et al. Lupus anticoagulants: improved concentrations. *Blood* 1986;68:472.

128. Triplett D, et al. Laboratory diagnosis of lupus inhibitors: a comparison of the tissue thromboplastin inhibition procedure with a new platelet neutralization procedure. *Am J Clin Pathol* 1983;79:678–682.

129. Feinstein D. Lupus anticoagulant, anticardiolipin antibodies, fetal loss, and systemic lupus erythematosus. *Blood* 1992;80:859.

130. Herbst K, et al. Syndrome of an acquired inhibitor of factor VIII responsive to cyclophosphamide and prednisone. *Ann Intern Med* 1981;95:575–578.

131. Lossing T, Kasper C, Feinstein D. Detection of factor VIII inhibitors with partial thromboplastin time. *Blood* 1977;49:793–797.

132. Guidelines on platelet function testing. The British Society for Haematology BCSH Haemostasis and Thrombosis Task Force. *J Clin Pathol* 1988; 41(12): 1322–1330.

133. Bowie EJ, Owen CA Jr. The bleeding time. *Prog Hemost Thromb* 1974;2:249–271.

134. Lind SE. Prolonged bleeding time. *Am J Med* 1984;77:305–312.

135. Lind S. The prolonged bleeding time. *Am J Med* 1984;77:305.

136. Deykin D, Janson P, McMahon L. Ethanol potentiation of aspirin induced prolongation of the bleeding time. *N Engl J Med* 1982;306:852.

137. Remaley A, Kennedy J, Laposata M. Evaluation of the clinical utility of platelet aggregation studies. *Am J Hematol* 1989;31:188.

138. Favier R, Aoki N, de Moerloose P. Congenital alpha(2)-plasmin inhibitor deficiencies: a review. *Br J Haematol* 2001;114(1):4–10.

139. Kang Y, et al. Epsilon-aminocaproic acid for treatment of fibrinolysis during liver transplantation. *Anesthesiology* 1987;66:766.

140. Lackner H, Karpatkin S. On the "easy bruising" syndrome with normal platelet count. *Ann Intern Med* 1975;83:190.

141. Peterson P, Gottfried E. The effects of inaccurate blood sample volume on prothrombin time (PT) and activated partial thromboplastin time (aPTT). *Thromb Hemost* 1982;47:101.

142. Abilgaard CF, et al. Serial studies in von Willebrand's disease: variability versus "variants." *Blood* 1980;56:712–716.

143. Burk C, et al. Preoperative history and coagulation screening in children undergoing tonsillectomy. *Pediatrics* 1992;89:691.

144. Ragni M, et al. Comparison of bleeding tendency, factor XI coagulant activity, and factor XI antigen in 25 factor XI-deficient kindreds. *Blood* 1985; 65:719–724.

145. George J. Platelet immunoglobulin G: its significance for the evaluation of thrombocytopenia and for understanding the origin of the alpha-granule proteins. *Blood* 1990;76:859.

146. Kelton J, Powers P, Carter C. A prospective study of the usefulness of the measurement of platelet-associated IgG for the diagnosis of idiopathic thrombocytopenic purpura. *Blood* 1982;60:1050.

147. Kelton J, et al. Elevated platelet-associated IgG in the thrombocytopenia of septicemia. *N Engl J Med* 1979;300:760.

148. Walsh C, Nardi M, Karpatkin S. On the mechanism of thrombocytopenic purpura in sexually active homosexual men. *N Engl J Med* 1984;311:635.

CHAPTER 32

Platelet Life Cycle: Quantitative Disorders

Theodore E. Warkentin and John G. Kelton

APPROACH TO THE THROMBOCYTOPENIC PATIENT

When assessing a thrombocytopenic patient, the clinician must simultaneously estimate the bleeding risk and determine the cause of the thrombocytopenia.

Many thrombocytopenic patients are not bleeding. The clinician must identify those patients at risk for serious bleeding, however, so that appropriate therapy can be started. Similarly, avoiding inappropriate interventions for the asymptomatic, thrombocytopenic patient prevents treatment-related morbidity.

Unless mimicked by a spurious laboratory result, such as pseudothrombocytopenia, thrombocytopenia is always abnormal. The greatest threat to the patient usually is not the thrombocytopenia itself but the underlying pathologic process, which must be identified and treated.

Estimation of Bleeding Risk

CLINICAL FEATURES

Petechiae and Ecchymoses. Petechiae are the hallmark of thrombocytopenia. These are small (<2 mm) purpura and represent tiny cutaneous or mucosal collections of red blood cells (RBCs) that have leaked from the blood vessels. Petechiae are nonpalpable and typically occur on the dependent regions of the body, especially the legs. Larger subcutaneous collections of blood are called *ecchymoses*. These can be painful and palpable and at times mimic vasculitic lesions.

Clinicians have attempted to estimate the bleeding risk according to the location and extent of petechiae and ecchymoses. In general, the more extensive the purpura, the greater the bleeding risk.

Other types of nonthrombocytopenic purpura must be identified, because these are not associated with bleeding. These lesions include vasculitic purpura, which are frequently palpable, sometimes painful, located on dependent regions, and associated with characteristic histopathologic features; senile purpura, which are caused by subcutaneous fat atrophy and typically occur on the lax skin on the dorsum of the hands; and various pigmented purpuric eruptions (1).

Mucosal and Internal Bleeding. Severe thrombocytopenia can be associated with mucosal bleeding, including bleeding from the mouth, nose, gastrointestinal tract, uterus and vagina, and bladder. Mucous membrane bleeding signifies an even higher risk for serious bleeding than purpura. A useful sign indicating that the patient has a high risk of hemorrhage is the presence of blood blisters inside the mouth. These start as small ($1 cm^2$) mucosal ecchymoses along the bite margins of the inner aspect of the cheek, which can progress to hemorrhagic blisters throughout the mouth and tongue. Although relatively uncommon, spontaneous life-threatening intracranial or visceral hemorrhage can develop in patients with severe thrombocytopenia.

Coexisting Hemostatic Dysfunction. The clinician also should determine if the patient has other hemostatic defects, such as damage to blood vessels (operative procedures), platelet dysfunction (antiplatelet drugs, alcohol, uremia), and coagulopathy (liver disease, vitamin K deficiency, hyperfibrinolysis). Paradoxically, some disorders associated with thrombocytopenia [e.g., heparin-induced thrombocytopenia (HIT), antiphospholipid antibody syndrome] are associated with thrombosis rather than bleeding.

LABORATORY TESTS

The hemostatic risk depends on many factors in addition to the absolute value of the platelet count. Patients with identical platelet counts may or may not bleed when challenged hemostatically (i.e., in surgery). Nevertheless, it is important to estimate bleeding risk so that preventive measures (platelet transfusions) can be considered.

Platelet Count. In general, the lower the platelet count, the greater the risk of bleeding. However, spontaneous bleeding is uncommon if the count is greater than $20 \times 10^9/L$. The hemostatic risk tends to be higher for thrombocytopenic disorders characterized by a low platelet volume. Patients with mild or moderate thrombocytopenia (platelet count above $50 \times 10^9/L$) have a minimal hemostatic risk of bleeding. For patients with intermediate severity of thrombocytopenia who are asymptomatic, however, it may be difficult to estimate the risk of bleeding. In these patients, a bleeding time test may be helpful.

Bleeding Time. The bleeding time test usually is performed using a template-guided blade to make a longitudinal incision on the patient's volar forearm. The time to cessation of bleeding is recorded. Many factors affect the bleeding time, including operator-dependent and operator-independent differences in technique and patient-related factors. Unfortunately, the bleeding time test is neither very sensitive nor specific for platelet-mediated bleeding disorders (2–4). Indeed, the test does not predict bleeding at surgery.

We sometimes use the bleeding time test to help identify those thrombocytopenic patients who require treatment. For example, we do not treat patients with no or only mild symptoms who have stable, moderately severe thrombocytopenia if a normal bleeding time has been documented on different occasions. However, some investigators have questioned the role of the bleeding time test in therapeutic decisions (2–4).

Diagnostic Approach to Thrombocytopenia

Thrombocytopenic disorders are classified into four general groups: increased platelet destruction, platelet sequestration, hemodilution, and decreased platelet production. Although the definitive classification of a patient may require a platelet survival study (Appendix 23), in most circumstances, a patient can be appropriately classified using other information, including history and physical examination, mean platelet volume (MPV), and blood film and bone marrow examination. Although these investigations sometimes provide the diagnosis, more often they suggest one or more diagnostic possibilities, which can be confirmed by specific tests.

HISTORY AND PHYSICAL EXAMINATION

Many patients with thrombocytopenia are identified during routine laboratory investigation or during the investigation of another disorder. For all patients with apparent thrombocytopenia, the first step is the examination of the stained blood film to exclude pseudothrombocytopenic disorders (discussed in the section Spurious Thrombocytosis and Pseudothrombocytopenia).

The focus of the history requires knowing the probable cause of the thrombocytopenia. Consequently, it is helpful to consider the results of the complete blood count. For example, isolated thrombocytopenia is usually caused by increased platelet destruction, whereas a pancytopenia is usually associated with disorders of decreased platelet production, sequestration, or hemodilution.

Identification of Thrombocytopenic Risk Factors. Most thrombocytopenic disorders can affect patients of all ages; however, several are restricted to certain age groups. For example, some disorders only occur in the neonate (e.g., neonatal alloimmune thrombocytopenia). Infants and young children often develop a severe but self-limited thrombocytopenia [acute idiopathic thrombocytopenic purpura (ITP)].

Potentially serious thrombocytopenic disorders that typically begin during late pregnancy or the puerperium include preeclampsia-associated thrombocytopenia; thrombotic microangiopathy; disseminated intravascular coagulation (DIC), which can be secondary to amniotic fluid embolism, abruptio placentae, dead fetus syndrome, retained placenta, or preeclampsia; and puerperal septicemia. However, the most common explanation for mild thrombocytopenia (75×10^9/L to 150×10^9/L) during pregnancy is an entirely benign condition known as *incidental thrombocytopenia of pregnancy* (gestational thrombocytopenia) (5–7). This condition occurs in approximately 7% of pregnant women and is characterized by an absence of a history of maternal thrombocytopenia or bleeding. The thrombocytopenia may be related to increased plasma volume in pregnancy without a compensatory thrombopoietic response (hemodilution) (8). Infants born to these mothers do not develop thrombocytopenia or bleeding complications. Accordingly, no special obstetric maneuvers are indicated for women with incidental thrombocytopenia of pregnancy.

Thrombocytopenia that occurs in a postoperative patient can be caused by hemodilution, septicemia, DIC, drug-induced thrombocytopenia, and, rarely, posttransfusion purpura (PTP). Heparin is by far the most common cause of drug-induced immune thrombocytopenia.

A meticulous drug history should be taken that includes agents purchased without prescription. Particularly for patients with episodic thrombocytopenia of abrupt onset, the physician should inquire about possible exposure to quinine, which is found in many beverages (e.g., tonic water) and can cause quinine-induced thrombocytopenia.

The presence of certain medical disorders, including systemic lupus erythematosus (SLE) and other rheumatic disorders, lymphoproliferative neoplasms, and infection by the human immunodeficiency virus (HIV), suggests an immune-destructive thrombocytopenia. Chronic viral hepatitis causes thrombocytopenia via both hypersplenism and decreased hepatic synthesis of thrombopoietin.

A family history of thrombocytopenia or bleeding tendency should be sought because it suggests hereditary thrombocytopenia.

Temporal Profile of Symptoms. The insidious onset of easy bruising and epistaxis of a duration of several months or years typically occurs in patients with chronic ITP. The abrupt onset of bleeding symptoms suggests acute ITP and immune drug-induced thrombocytopenia.

Physical Examination. The physician should look for physical signs (e.g., fever, lymphadenopathy, splenomegaly, hepatomegaly, rash) suggestive of underlying disorders that can be associated with thrombocytopenia. The presence of intravascular catheters could indicate septicemia or HIT. Arterial or venous thrombotic events that occur in thrombocytopenic patients suggest HIT, antiphospholipid antibody syndrome, neoplasia-associated DIC, or, rarely, paroxysmal nocturnal hemoglobinuria.

PLATELET SIZE

Blood count determinations are obtained using electronic particle counters, which provide the platelet count, MPV, and platelet distribution width (PDW; a marker of platelet heterogeneity). The normal platelet count typically ranges from 150×10^9/L to 450×10^9/L, but this range may be lower in Mediterranean populations (125×10^9/L to 300×10^9/L) with larger platelets (9). There is no normal range for the MPV, because the MPV must be interpreted with the platelet count (10,11). As shown in Figure 32-1, the MPV bears a nonlinear, inverse relation to the platelet count. Thus, the normal MPV for a platelet count of 150×10^9/L is 9 to 12 fL, whereas for a platelet count of 400×10^9/L, it is 7.5 to 10 fL (10).

By correlating the platelet count with the MPV, the clinician can obtain data to help classify the platelet disorder (10,11) (Fig. 32-1). Thrombocytopenia caused by increased platelet destruction with a normal megakaryocyte response is characterized by a larger MPV and more hemostatically effective platelets than disorders characterized by thrombocytopenia due to impaired platelet production or hypersplenism. One pediatric study (12) suggested that the modal platelet size (highest peak of the platelet size histogram) was better than the MPV in distinguishing between platelet destruction and underproduction. Sometimes, however, myeloproliferative and myelodysplastic conditions have large platelets with impaired function.

Increased platelet heterogeneity, measured as increased PDW, has been observed in myeloproliferative disease (13). However, this parameter is not widely used to evaluate thrombocytosis. Our experience is that the MPV and the PDW are only modestly helpful in classifying thrombocytopenic disorders.

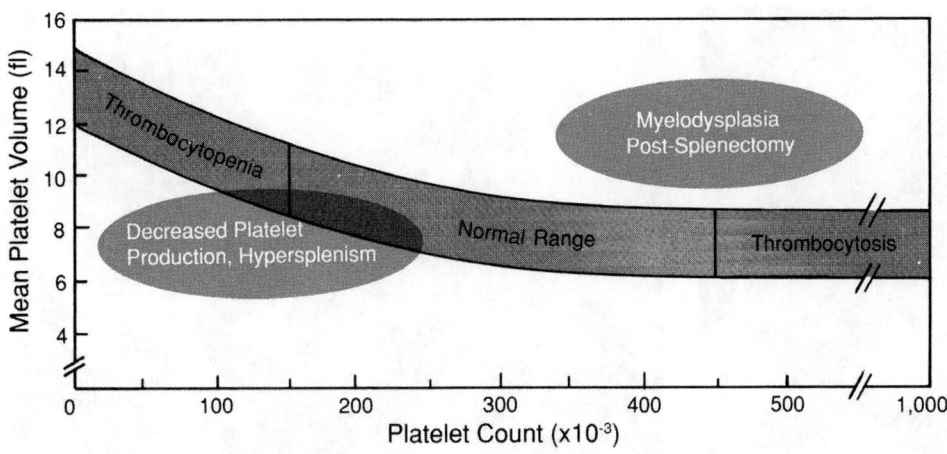

Figure 32-1. Mean platelet volume–platelet count relation in various platelet disorders. (From Bessman JD. Platelets. In: Bessman JD. *Automated blood counts and differentials: a practical guide.* Baltimore: Johns Hopkins University Press, 1986:57; and Bessman JD, Gilmer PR, Gardner FH. Use of mean platelet volume improves detection of platelet disorders. *Blood Cells* 1985;11:127, with permission.)

PERIPHERAL BLOOD FILM AND MARROW EXAMINATION

Peripheral Blood Film. Examination of the peripheral blood film can be helpful in elucidating the cause of unexplained thrombocytopenia. Paradoxically, inspection of the RBCs and leukocytes is usually more helpful than examining the platelets. RBC fragments suggest thrombocytopenia due to microangiopathy. Thrombocytopenia can occur with infiltrating marrow disorders (teardrop and nucleated RBCs), megaloblastic anemia (macrocytes), immune hemolysis (spherocytes), and malaria (protozoal inclusions). Toxic granules, vacuolation, and pale blue cytoplasmic inclusions (Döhle bodies) in leukocytes suggest thrombocytopenia associated with septicemia. Reactive, atypical lymphocytes occur in viral infections, many of which can be complicated by thrombocytopenia. Neoplastic leukocytes suggest thrombocytopenia due to decreased platelet production. Dysplastic leukocytes (e.g., hypogranular, Pelger-Huët anomaly) suggest myelodysplasia, as does red cell macrocytosis with normal B_{12} and folate levels. Abnormal leukocyte inclusions are characteristic of some hereditary thrombocytopenic disorders, such as May-Hegglin, Fechtner, and Sebastian syndromes.

It is important to verify by microscopy a report of a low platelet count, because electronic particle counters can produce erroneous platelet counts in certain situations. For instance, the presence of platelet clumps or platelets adherent to neutrophils and monocytes suggests pseudothrombocytopenia (discussed in the section Spurious Thrombocytosis and Pseudothrombocytopenia). It is preferable to use the electronic determination of the MPV rather than to attempt to judge platelet size morphologically, because platelet heterogeneity ensures that occasional large platelets are present even in the blood films of patients with a small MPV (10). Circulating megakaryocyte fragments can be identified in the blood films of some patients with myeloid neoplastic disorders. Extremely large platelets are observed in some patients with myelodysplasia or myeloid leukemia and are also characteristic of the hereditary macrothrombocytopenic disorders.

Marrow Examination. Megakaryocytes are usually present in normal or increased numbers in thrombocytopenic disorders caused by platelet destruction or sequestration. Depending on the specific pathologic process, megakaryocytes are often reduced or absent (and may be morphologically abnormal) in disorders characterized by decreased platelet production. Sometimes, the bone marrow examination is diagnostic, as in acute leukemia or marrow infiltration by malignancy.

Megakaryocyte ploidy measurements using flow cytometry have been shown to correlate with the mechanism of thrombo-

cytopenia (14). For example, increased megakaryocyte ploidy was a feature of destructive thrombocytopenia in one study (14). This test, although potentially helpful, is seldom performed.

SPURIOUS THROMBOCYTOSIS AND PSEUDOTHROMBOCYTOPENIA

Although platelet count measurements by electronic particle counters are more accurate and less expensive than conventional manual techniques, there is a potential for spurious overestimation or underestimation of the platelet count. For example, abnormal particles similar in size to platelets, such as schistocytes, microspherocytes, leukemic cell fragments, Pappenheimer bodies, and bacteria, can be counted erroneously as platelets and falsely suggest thrombocytosis (10,15–18).

More important is spurious thrombocytopenia, which, if unrecognized, can lead to unnecessary tests or inappropriate therapy. Termed *pseudothrombocytopenia*, this artifact is caused by *in vitro* platelet clumping or platelet adherence to leukocytes, which results in failure of the electronic particle counter to recognize the platelets (Fig. 32-2). Therefore, it is essential that the blood film be examined in every patient with purported thrombocytopenia.

Ethylenediaminetetraacetic Acid–Dependent Pseudothrombocytopenia. Ethylenediaminetetraacetic acid (EDTA) is the anticoagulant used most commonly for determination of the complete blood count. Pseudothrombocytopenia occurs in up to 0.1% of all complete blood counts (19,20) and is usually caused by an EDTA-dependent platelet-agglutinating antibody (21). Platelet clumps usually are seen throughout the blood film and especially in the tail of the blood smear. This phenomenon can persist for decades without signifying any underlying disease (21). *In vivo* platelet counts are normal.

This *in vitro* artifact is caused by EDTA-dependent antibodies directed against a cryptic antigen on the platelet glycoprotein (gp) IIb-IIIa complex that becomes exposed in the presence of EDTA (22,23). The agglutinins can be immunoglobulin (Ig) G, IgM, or IgA, with IgM antibodies most likely to be detected when agglutination also occurs using citrate anticoagulant or at 37°C (21). The phenomenon can be inhibited by RGD peptide and certain gpIIb-IIIa–reactive monoclonal antibodies (22).

Abciximab-Induced Ethylenediaminetetraacetic Acid–Dependent Pseudothrombocytopenia. Approximately 2% of patients treated with abciximab (ReoPro) develop EDTA-dependent pseudothrombocytopenia (24). Rapid assessment of the blood film is required to distinguish this benign condition from true abciximab-induced thrombocytopenia, which can cause bleeding and requires stopping the abciximab.

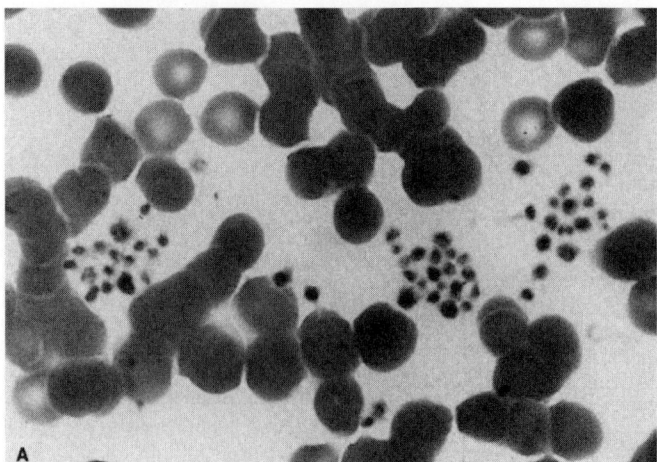 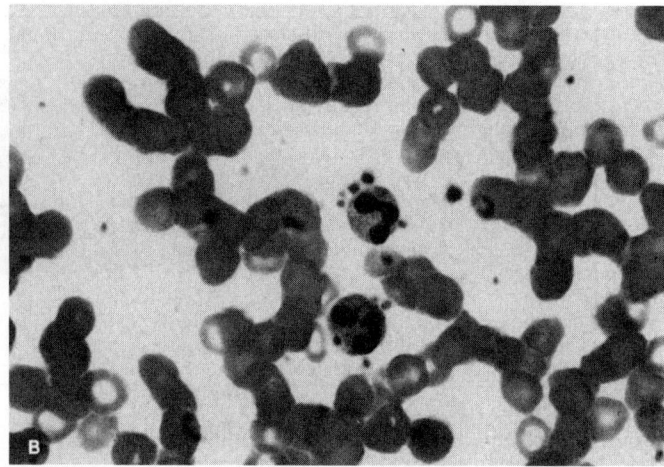

Figure 32-2. Photomicrograph of two types of pseudothrombocytopenia. **A:** Ethylenediaminetetraacetic acid–dependent platelet clumping. **B:** Platelet satellitism.

Platelet Cold Agglutinin. Sometimes, pseudothrombocytopenia is caused by platelet-reactive cold agglutinins that cause platelet clumping in all anticoagulants (25).

Monoclonal Platelet Agglutinin. A patient with anticoagulant-independent and temperature-independent pseudothrombocytopenia caused by a monoclonal IgM paraprotein was described (26). It was impossible to obtain an accurate platelet count in this patient.

Artifacts of Blood Collection. Spurious thrombocytopenia can be caused by technically inadequate blood collection. This problem is usually obvious because clots are seen in the anticoagulated sample. Thrombocytopenia is not present when the platelet count is measured using another blood sample. Overfilling of the vacuum tube can also result in spurious thrombocytopenia (27).

PLATELET SATELLITISM

Platelet satellitism is a rare cause of pseudothrombocytopenia characterized by EDTA-dependent rosetting of platelets around neutrophils or monocytes (28–31). One study showed EDTA-dependent IgG antibodies that interacted with both platelet gpIIb-IIIa and neutrophil FcγIII receptors (31).

PLATELET COUNT DETERMINATION IN PSEUDOTHROMBOCYTOPENIA

Although these platelet agglutinins are usually naturally occurring and without *in vivo* significance, they can make it difficult to determine the platelet count accurately. Sometimes, pseudothrombocytopenia complicates accurate platelet count measurement in a patient with true coexisting thrombocytopenia (32,33).

Several methods can be tried to obtain an accurate platelet count, including the following:

- Collect the blood sample into a different anticoagulant, such as 0.38% sodium citrate [80% success rate (20)].
- Collect the blood sample into a prewarmed tube containing EDTA that is maintained at 37°C until testing [80% success rate (20)].
- For remaining refractory cases, collect the blood into 1% ammonium oxalate and count in a Burker chamber (20).
- Anecdotally, we have had good success by performing a manual (phase-contrast) platelet count using a finger-prick sample that is immediately diluted and counted.

General Approach to Treatment of Thrombocytopenic Patients

WHO SHOULD RECEIVE TREATMENT?

The most important issue is whether the patient requires treatment. For example, many patients with chronic ITP and a platelet count above $20 \times 10^9/L$ do not bleed except under exceptional circumstances. For these patients, the treatment (e.g., corticosteroids) carries higher morbidity than no treatment at all. Thus, factors such as the estimated bleeding risk and natural history of the illness influence the decision to treat.

PREVENTION OF BLEEDING

General Measures. In general, thrombocytopenic patients should not receive intramuscular injections or drugs that interfere with platelet function, such as aspirin. However, an antiplatelet agent could be appropriate if the thrombocytopenia is a sign of a prothrombotic state (e.g., antiphospholipid antibody syndrome).

Prophylactic Platelet Transfusions. The use of platelet transfusion therapy is described elsewhere in this book; only the general use of platelet transfusions in thrombocytopenic patients is discussed here.

Several factors influence the decision to administer *prophylactic* platelet transfusions. One consideration is the general mechanism of the thrombocytopenia. Transfused platelets are usually destroyed rapidly if the thrombocytopenia is caused by increased platelet destruction; therefore, only transient benefit is achieved. Another factor is the probable duration of the thrombocytopenia. Patients with chronic thrombocytopenia (hereditary platelet disorders, aplastic anemia) should not receive prophylactic platelet transfusions because the short-term benefit is outweighed by the risk of developing platelet-reactive alloantibodies, which could jeopardize future use of *therapeutic* platelet transfusions. For these reasons, the best candidates for prophylactic platelet transfusion therapy are patients who have thrombocytopenia caused by underproduction and in whom it is likely that the platelet count will rise to normal levels in a relatively short period (e.g., patients receiving chemotherapeutic agents for leukemia). Prophylactic platelet transfusions sometimes are administered to patients with self-limited, destructive thrombocytopenia if the risk of bleeding on clinical grounds appears to be high (e.g., bacteremia-associated thrombocytopenia, immune drug–induced thrombocytopenia) (34). Prophylactic platelet transfusions should be avoided, if at all possible, in patients with thrombotic thrombocytopenic purpura (TTP) or HIT (35) because the risk of acute platelet-mediated thrombosis theoretically is increased after the platelet transfusion.

Treatment of Bleeding. Platelet transfusions should be administered to all patients with serious or potentially life-threatening bleeding, even if the bleeding is caused by increased platelet destruction, because a transient improvement in hemostasis can be achieved during this critical interval before attaining therapeutic efficacy of other specific therapy.

Although antifibrinolytic therapy (ε-aminocaproic acid or tranexamic acid) is sometimes used to control bleeding in patients with chronic refractory thrombocytopenia (36), the efficacy of this approach remains unproven (37). However, we have found it useful in certain situations such as heavy menses in thrombocytopenic patients.

DESTRUCTIVE THROMBOCYTOPENIA CAUSED BY IMMUNE MECHANISMS

Immune mechanisms usually cause isolated thrombocytopenia. In some disorders, such as chronic ITP, the pathogenic role of the platelet-reactive IgG autoantibodies is well established. In other disorders, such as acute ITP, HIV-associated thrombocytopenia, idiosyncratic drug-induced thrombocytopenia, and PTP, the role of immune platelet destruction is established, but the nature of the platelet–antibody interaction is less well understood.

Platelet–Antibody Interactions

OVERVIEW
IgG can bind to platelets in a number of different ways.

Autoantibody. The Fab regions of IgG can bind to platelet-specific glycoprotein or glycolipid determinants on autologous platelets (e.g., chronic ITP).

Alloantibody. The Fab regions of IgG can bind to platelet-specific glycoprotein determinants on homologous platelets (e.g., neonatal alloimmune thrombocytopenia, passive alloimmune thrombocytopenia). Alloantigens are genetically determined structural differences in proteins or carbohydrates that can be recognized immunologically by certain normal individuals who are exposed to these antigens through pregnancy or transfusion.

Drug-Dependent Antibody. The Fab region of IgG can bind to a drug–platelet glycoprotein complex (e.g., quinidine or sulfa antibiotic-induced immune thrombocytopenia).

In Situ Immune Complex. In HIT, the Fab region of IgG binds to complexes of platelet factor (PF) 4 and heparin that form on the platelet surface (*in situ* immune complex formation); subsequently, the Fc moiety of the IgG binds to platelet Fc receptors, leading to platelet activation.

Antibody-Recognizing Foreign Antigen. The Fab region of IgG can bind to nonplatelet foreign antigens (e.g., microbes) that adsorb to the platelet surface (e.g., malaria-associated thrombocytopenia).

Nonspecific Antibody. IgG can bind to platelets nonspecifically through a poorly defined mechanism (hypergammaglobulinemia).

PLATELET-SPECIFIC GLYCOPROTEINS
Several glycoproteins like the gpIb-IX-V complex or the integrin proteins (e.g., gpIIb-IIIa, gpIa-IIa) occur predominantly on platelets. Although not always unique to platelets (e.g., gpIb can be detected on cultured human endothelial cells [38]), some, like gpIb and gpIIb-IIIa, are called *platelet-specific*. In contrast, there are other glycoproteins (e.g., HLA) and glycolipids (e.g., blood group ABH antigens) that are relatively ubiquitous or that are found in much larger quantities on certain cells other than platelets.

Nonintegrin Adhesive Receptors on Platelet Surfaces. The gpIb-IX-V complex is an important nonintegrin adhesive receptor. There are 20,000 to 30,000 copies on the platelet surface. This receptor is crucial for the initial contact (adhesion) of the platelet to the damaged vessel wall (39). The contact between the platelet gpIb complex and the vessel wall is mediated by a large, multimeric protein known as *von Willebrand's factor* (vWF), which acts as the platelet–vessel wall "glue." Deficiency of gpIb-IX-V characterizes the Bernard-Soulier syndrome (40), a hereditary bleeding disorder discussed in Chapter 30. gpIb-IX-V is also frequently implicated as a target antigen in chronic ITP and some cases of drug-induced immune thrombocytopenia (discussed in the section Drug-Induced Thrombocytopenia). The amino acid polymorphism that defines the Ko alloantigen system has also been localized to the α-subunit of gpIb (41).

Other nonintegrin adhesive receptors found on platelet surfaces (with surface receptor numbers and adhesive ligand in parentheses) include gpIV (25,000 receptors; thrombospondin, collagen), gpVI (receptor number unknown; collagen), platelet endothelial cell adhesion molecule-1 (PECAM-1) (5000 to 10,000 receptors; PECAM-1 on other cells) (42), and P-selectin, also known as *GMP-140* (released onto the surface after platelet activation; P-selectin ligands on other cells). Relevance to immune thrombocytopenia of these receptors includes IgG binding to gpIV in some patients with SLE (43), drug-dependent IgG binding to PECAM-1 in carbimazole-induced thrombocytopenia (44), and expression of P-selectin on platelet surfaces after activation by antibodies that cause HIT (45).

Platelet Integrins. Platelet integrins are a superfamily of integral membrane glycoprotein heterodimers consisting of noncovalently associated α-subunits and β-subunits that are involved in cell-vessel wall and cell–cell contact (46,47). Not all possible αβ pairings exist, however, as there are 22 integrins, rather less than the 128 theoretic combinations than could be formed from the 16 α- and 8 β-subunits. In some instances, the larger α-subunit itself consists of two covalently linked peptide chains, for example, gpIIb (Fig. 32-3), linked to a smaller β-subunit. The integrins are subclassified on the basis of common β-chains. Members of the β_3 and β_1 families are present on platelets. We will use the conventional platelet glycoprotein terminology, with the corresponding integrin terminology given in parentheses.

The platelet β_3-integrins, which are involved in cytoadhesion, are gpIIb-IIIa ($\alpha_{IIb}\beta_3$) and the vitronectin receptor ($\alpha_v\beta_3$). gpIIb-IIIa (40,000 to 80,000 receptors; fibrinogen, vWF, fibronectin, vitronectin) mediates platelet aggregation *in vivo* via binding to adhesive proteins such as fibrinogen and vWF. Inherited deficiency of gpIIb-IIIa is characterized by bleeding resulting from an inability of platelets to bind fibrinogen and to aggregate after agonist stimulation (Glanzmann's thrombasthenia)

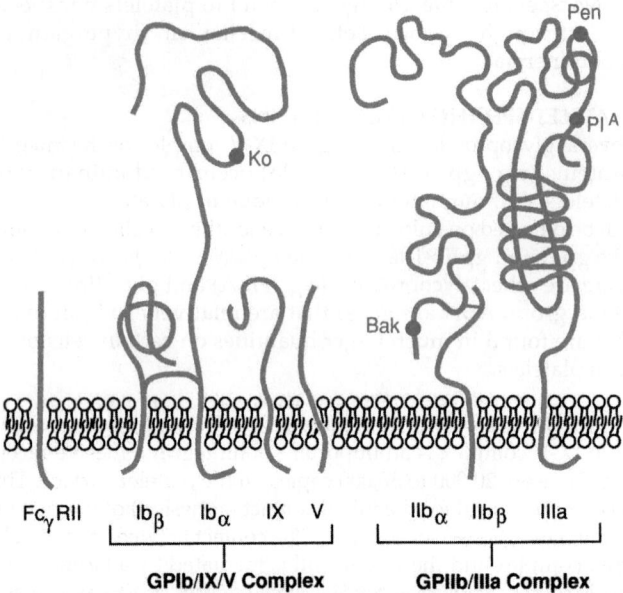

Figure 32-3. Schematic representation of selected platelet alloantigens located on various platelet glycoproteins (GPs).

(48). The platelet β_1-integrins, which are involved in platelet interactions with extracellular matrix proteins, consist of gpIa-IIa ($\alpha_2\beta_1$; 1000 to 10,000 receptors; collagen), gpIc-IIa ($\alpha_5\beta_1$; 1000 receptors; fibronectin), and gpIc'-IIa ($\alpha_6\beta_1$; 1000 receptors; laminin) (49).

Several integrins are implicated in immune thrombocytopenia. For example, the gpIIb-IIIa complex is the most important target autoantigen in chronic ITP (50–52). It can also bind certain drugs, thereby contributing to the antigenic target complex in quinine-dependent or quinidine-dependent immune thrombocytopenia (53). Many of the platelet alloantigen systems are located on gpIIb-IIIa (Fig. 32-3). gpIIIa is the site of the PlA1/A2 (Zwa/b) and Pena/b alloantigen systems. gpIIbα is the site for Baka/b (Leka/b). Several more recently described "private" alloantigens (e.g., Sra, Tua, Moa, Groa, Oea, Laa) are also found on gpIIIa. The Bra/b (Zava/b) system is located on gpIa of the collagen receptor integrin, gpIa-IIa. Table 32-6, which appears later in the section on alloimmune thrombocytopenic disorders, summarizes the platelet alloantigen systems. (Most of the alloantigen systems have more than one designation. In this chapter, we use the names that are most widely accepted; we also indicate alternate names in Table 32-6.)

Molecular Biology of PlA1 System. The PlA1/A2 alloantigen system was the first to be characterized at the molecular level (54). The leucine (Leu) 33/proline (Pro) 33 dimorphism is found on the β_3 integrin of gpIIb-IIIa ($\alpha_{IIb}\beta_3$) and occurs on a small, 13 amino acid loop formed by the pairing of Cys26 to Cys38. Three-dimensional structural constraints imposed by this loop explain why the 13-mer peptide itself is not antigenic (55). Antibodies against PlA1 can inhibit platelet function, presumably via interfering with binding of the fibrinogen ligand (56).

The amino acid dimorphisms reported for other platelet alloantigens are described later in this chapter.

GLYCOPROTEINS EXPRESSED ON PLATELETS AND OTHER CELLS

Human Leukocyte Antigens. Human leukocyte antigens are a highly polymorphic multiallelic system important in the immunologic distinction between self and nonself. HLAs are subdivided into class I (HLA-A, HLA-B, HLA-C) and class II (HLA-DR, HLA-DQ, HLA-DP) antigens. Genes coding for HLA specificity are closely linked on the short arm of chromosome 6 and are inherited in a unit termed the *haplotype.*

HLA class I antigens are located on most cells, including lymphocytes, granulocytes, and platelets, but not RBCs. They are important for the recognition of self by cytotoxic T cells. HLA class II antigens are important in the presentation of antigens by macrophages and B lymphocytes to helper T cells.

HLA class I but not class II antigens are expressed on platelets. HLA class I antigens are intrinsic membrane constituents (57) present in higher densities on platelets than lymphocytes (58). HLA-A and HLA-B antigens are strongly, although variably, expressed (59,60), whereas HLA-C antigens are weakly expressed (61). The HLA system is discussed in greater detail in Chapter 20.

Alloantibodies frequently form against HLA antigens; approximately 20% to 30% of multiparous women and many polytransfused patients have identifiable antibodies against HLA antigens. HLA alloantibodies are important in causing refractoriness to platelet transfusions in some patients. Use of leukocyte-reduced blood products reduces somewhat the risk of HLA alloimmunization (62). Although there have been claims that HLA antibodies might cause neonatal alloimmune thrombocytopenia, this remains unproven (63).

GLYCOLIPIDS AND PHOSPHOLIPIDS EXPRESSED ON PLATELETS AND OTHER CELLS

Red Blood Cell Antigens. The RBC alloantigens ABH, Lewis, Ii, and P are found on platelets (64–71). The ABH and Lewis antigens are glycosphingolipids that are adsorbed to platelets from the plasma (64,67). Additionally, ABH antigens are constitutive platelet membrane components carried on certain glycoproteins (66) and are intrinsic antigens made by megakaryocytes (65,71). These antigens are variably expressed (72).

The importance of group A and B antigens in platelet transfusion incompatibility is debated but can account for a reduced posttransfusion platelet recovery in some patients (73,74). The Lewis, Ii, and P alloantigen systems have no clinical relevance to platelet transfusion.

Other Glycolipids. Glycolipids consist of three basic units—sphingosine, fatty acid, and sugar—and are either neutral or acidic. Acidic glycolipids can be either gangliosides or sulfatides, depending on whether the acidic component is sialic acid or sulfate, respectively. Glycolipids are known to be immunogenic (75) and have been implicated as target autoantigens in some patients with chronic ITP (76,77).

Phospholipids. Many different phospholipids constitute the platelet lipid bilayer membrane, with the most plentiful being phosphatidylcholine, phosphatidylethanolamine, phosphatidylserine, and sphingomyelin (78). These molecules are asymmetrically distributed; most of the sphingomyelin is present in the outer membrane layer, whereas most of the phosphatidylserine is present in the inner membrane layer. Phosphatidylethanolamine and phosphatidylinositol are also more plentiful in the inner membrane layer. These inner membrane phospholipids become exposed during platelet activation (79).

Autoantibodies against phospholipid or phospholipid-protein structures prolong certain clotting tests. These autoantibodies have been called *lupus anticoagulants,* and patients with these autoantibodies can have recurrent arterial and venous thrombosis and recurrent fetal loss (lupus anticoagulant or antiphospholipid syndrome). Thrombocytopenia occurs in 15% to 25% of these patients. In one study (80), anticardiolipin antibodies (cardiolipin is a target antigen in the antiphospholipid syndrome) were detected in 30% of patients with chronic ITP.

Cryptic Antigens and Neoantigens. *Cryptic antigens* are hidden antigens that could become exposed under certain circumstances. *Neoantigens* are antigens that are formed only after changes in molecular conformation (e.g., after platelet activation) (81). It can be difficult to distinguish these two types of antigens.

It is possible that autoantibodies against senescent cryptic antigens or neoantigens are involved in senescent platelet clearance.

Pseudothrombocytopenia caused by EDTA-dependent autoantibodies could be caused by EDTA-induced formation of either cryptic antigens or neoantigens on gpIIb-IIIa.

Acute thrombocytopenia soon after treatment with abciximab (a humanized chimeric Fab fragment of a murine monoclonal antibody against gpIIb-IIIa) could be caused by naturally occurring anti–gpIIb-IIIa autoantibodies that react only after conformational modification of gpIIb-IIIa induced by abciximab.

Binding of heparin to PF4 leads to formation of cryptic autoepitopes on PF4 recognized by the antibodies that cause immune HIT (82).

Adsorbed Nonplatelet Antigens. The platelet has been characterized as a "sponge" capable of adsorbing nonplatelet molecules. For example, both Ig and albumin are present on normal platelets (83,84). Indeed, the quantities of the Ig classes and subclasses on the platelet parallel their plasma concentrations. Ig and albumin are also found within the platelet α-granules (85,86), although it remains uncertain whether incorporation occurs primarily at the megakaryocyte or platelet level (87). Evidence suggests that endocytosis of fibrinogen occurs with both megakaryocytes (88–90) and platelets (90). Other endogenous molecules, such as DNA, can bind to receptors on the platelet surface (91). Finally, foreign substances such as microbes and drugs can be adsorbed to the platelet surface.

Adsorbed autoantigens such as DNA can be involved in the pathogenesis of thrombocytopenia in some autoimmune disorders (92–94).

The thrombocytopenia associated with malaria (95) and drugs such as quinidine (53) is caused by the binding of IgG to these foreign antigens adsorbed to platelets.

Platelet Immunoglobulin Fc Receptors. The platelet IgG Fc receptor is a 40-kd transmembrane receptor that binds with a low affinity to the Cγ2 region of IgG (96–98). The platelet Fc receptor is identical to the FcγIIa IgG receptor found on phagocytic cells. The platelet carries approximately 1500 to 3000 copies of these receptors. The binding of IgG complexes to the platelet FcγIIa receptors initiates platelet aggregation and release and has been implicated in the pathogenesis of HIT (99,100). It remains unproven whether platelet Fc receptors contribute to the pathogenesis of thrombocytopenia in SLE or other immune thrombocytopenic disorders. Platelets also possess IgE Fc receptors that resemble the type I and type II (FcεRI and FcεRII) receptors found on eosinophils (101). It is possible that these platelet IgE Fc receptors play a role in the pathogenesis of thrombocytopenia in IgE-mediated allergic disorders.

Platelet Antibody Testing

Advances in the understanding of immune platelet disorders have resulted from the increasing sophistication and widespread application of *in vitro* platelet antibody tests. The many tests described can be classified into three groups termed *phase I, II,* and *III assays* according to the time of introduction and general technique (Appendix 24). Phase I assays, which were first developed in the 1950s, measure a functional platelet-dependent endpoint, usually platelet activation. Phase II assays detect the presence of Ig or complement on or within the platelet; these assays, first developed in 1975, are often referred to as tests for *platelet-associated IgG* (PAIgG). In 1984, phase III assays were developed that measure the binding of Ig to specific platelet proteins.

Platelets from patients with ITP can carry large amounts of IgG on their surfaces, up to hundreds of thousands of molecules of IgG per platelet (102). Studies from a number of laboratories have shown how technically difficult it is to measure IgG on the surface of the platelets because large amounts of IgG are found within the α-granules of platelets and in the open canalicular system, which communicates with the surface. Presumably, most of the IgG was nonspecifically taken into the platelets at the time of their formation by the megakaryocytes, and unless extraordinary steps are taken during platelet purification and washing, some of this interior or canalicular IgG is measured and incorrectly attributed to the autoantibody that causes immune thrombocytopenia. This possibility could explain why the proportions of platelet immunoglobulin classes and subclasses resembles their respective plasma concentrations (103,104). What remains unexplained is why other nonimmunologic plasma proteins such as albumin are increased on ITP platelets parallel with the increase in IgG (83,84).

Although most platelet–antibody assays were developed to detect platelet antibodies in patients with ITP, modifications permit their use in other clinical situations. For example, platelets of known alloantigen specificity can be used to identify alloantibodies. Also, measurement of drug-dependent antibody binding to platelets can be diagnostic of drug-induced immune thrombocytopenia. Platelet–antibody testing is discussed in detail in Appendix 24.

Idiopathic Thrombocytopenic Purpura

Idiopathic thrombocytopenic purpura, also known as *primary (auto)immune thrombocytopenic purpura*, is a common disorder characterized by accelerated platelet destruction caused by platelet-reactive autoantibodies. ITP is an isolated, destructive thrombocytopenia with no clinically apparent associated conditions or other explanation, such as HIV infection, SLE, lymphoproliferative disorder, myelodysplasia, hypogammaglobulinemia, drug-induced thrombocytopenia, alloimmune thrombocytopenia, or congenital or hereditary thrombocytopenia (105). Until recently, ITP was essentially a diagnosis of exclusion, but newer assays of antiplatelet antibodies now permit the detection of platelet gp-reactive autoantibodies in at least 75% of patients with ITP, with good diagnostic specificity (106,107).

PATHOGENESIS AND CAUSE

Idiopathic thrombocytopenic purpura is caused by the binding of autoantibodies to platelet surface antigens. Thrombocytopenia is a consequence of the premature destruction of the platelets by the reticuloendothelial system.

Platelet-Reactive Autoantibodies. Approximately 40 years ago, Harrington et al. (108) performed a series of experiments that defined the basic pathogenesis of ITP. They self-infused plasma from patients with ITP and documented the development of acute and severe thrombocytopenia. These dramatic experiments demonstrated that ITP is caused by a plasma factor that results in platelet destruction. Subsequent investigators demonstrated that the plasma factor is usually IgG, although in some patients, IgM and IgA platelet-reactive antibodies were identified (103,109,110).

In 1972, McMillan et al. (111) showed that lymphocytes from ITP splenic tissue produced antiplatelet autoantibodies. Subsequent investigations from this group demonstrated that antiplatelet antibody binds to platelets through its Fab terminus (112,113) and that the antibody is capable of depositing complement on the platelets (114). It remains uncertain whether completion of the complement sequence *in vivo* leads to platelet destruction in patients with ITP. β-Thromboglobulin, which is released from activated platelets, is normal in the plasma of patients with ITP (115), arguing against *in vivo* platelet activation or lysis.

Platelet Autoantigens. Usually, the target antigen is on one of the two major platelet glycoprotein complexes, with gpIIb-IIIa implicated more often than gpIb-IX (106,107,116). Indirect evidence that autoantibodies could recognize platelet glycoproteins was first provided by Van Leeuwen et al. (117), who showed that antiplatelet antibody from patients with ITP failed to bind to platelets from patients with Glanzmann's thrombasthenia (lacking gpIIb-IIIa). Further work using several different monoclonal antibodies against the gpIIb-IIIa complex has shown that the anti–gpIIb-IIIa autoantibodies from different patients with ITP react with different epitopes (118). Evidence suggests that platelet glycolipids also can be target antigens in chronic ITP (76,77).

Platelet Kinetics. Initial studies (119,120), which often used chromium-51–labeled homologous platelets, suggested that the platelet lifespan in patients with ITP was uniformly reduced and that platelet turnover was increased. A detailed description of platelet survival methodologies is included in Appendix 23. Studies by several groups of investigators (121–126) using indium-111 (^{111}In)-labeled autologous platelets showed considerable heterogeneity in platelet turnover in chronic ITP. Although the platelet lifespan is often markedly decreased, in some patients the lifespan is only mildly reduced; furthermore, platelet turnover (a measure of platelet production) is frequently subnormal. Overall, approximately 40% of patients with ITP had a reduced platelet turnover (125,126). Low platelet turnover might be the result of megakaryocyte damage by autoantibodies (107) or intramedullary destruction of platelets by marrow monocytes and macrophages. Alternatively, the apparent low platelet turnover could reflect the measurement of a subpopulation of longer-lived platelets.

Both *in vitro* and clinical studies have shown that the spleen is an important site of antibody production (111) and is also the dominant organ for the clearance of IgG-coated platelets (125,126). In a minority of patients, hepatic clearance predominates.

Cause. The fundamental cause of autoantibody formation in ITP is not known. Light chain restriction of platelet-reactive antibodies suggests a clonal (or oligoclonal) origin of autoantibodies in chronic ITP (107). Further, the epitopes involved may be fairly narrow in scope (autoantigen "hot spots"). Abnormalities in T-lymphocyte subpopulations have been reported, as have the presence of autoreactive T lymphocytes in patients with ITP that can be stimulated by tryptic fragments of gpIIb-IIIa (127). It is uncertain whether the autoimmune process occurs *de novo* or whether an antecedent event (e.g., viral infection) is required. Analysis of the VH gene sequences from a human lymphoblastoid cell line derived from an ITP patient with anti-gpIb IgG identified multiple base substitutions when compared with the germline sequence, suggesting that the

autoantibodies were generated by antigen-driven, mature B cells (128).

CLINICAL AND LABORATORY FEATURES

Although chronic ITP can occur at any age and in both sexes, women between 20 and 50 years of age are most commonly affected. The female to male ratio is approximately 3:1.

The onset of bleeding typically is insidious; however, recent aspirin ingestion can cause a patient with asymptomatic chronic ITP to bleed. Most of the bleeding is mucocutaneous and consists of purpura (petechiae and ecchymoses), epistaxis, menorrhagia, oral mucosal bleeding, and gastrointestinal bleeding. Rarely, severe thrombocytopenia can be complicated by spontaneous intracranial hemorrhage. The risk of fatal bleeding is substantially higher in elderly patients with ITP (129). Except for the bleeding symptoms, the patients are asymptomatic.

The complete blood count reveals isolated thrombocytopenia, although anemia of iron deficiency can occur with chronic bleeding. The MPV usually is increased, although in our experience, patients with severe thrombocytopenia may have a normal or even reduced MPV. The bone marrow examination shows normal or increased numbers of megakaryocytes. We do not always perform a bone marrow aspirate if the patient presents with typical ITP, but some hematologists do.

The bleeding time tends to be long if there is marked thrombocytopenia (below 20×10^9/L) (130), although some patients have abnormal platelet function and a prolonged bleeding time despite mild or moderate thrombocytopenia (50 to 150×10^9/L).

Fifteen percent to 25% of patients with otherwise typical ITP have positive antinuclear antibody (ANA) tests (131–134), usually of low titer. It is controversial whether the presence of a high-titer ANA or antibodies against soluble ribonucleoprotein antigens (SS-A/Ro, nuclear RNP) help identify the minority of patients with ITP who subsequently develop SLE. Most likely, however, ANA positivity does not indicate a different clinical outcome compared with ANA-negative patients (134). Other laboratory tests that should be performed in patients with ITP include thyroid function studies because of the association between ITP and immune thyroid dysfunction. Patients with clinical evidence suggesting infectious mononucleosis or HIV infection should have the appropriate serologic tests performed.

Cyclic Thrombocytopenia. Cyclic thrombocytopenia is characterized by regular fluctuations in the platelet count, ranging from severe, symptomatic thrombocytopenia to thrombocytosis. In some women with cyclic thrombocytopenia, platelet count fluctuations parallel the menstrual cycle, with the platelet count nadir coinciding with menstruation (135). Intermittent increased platelet destruction by platelet-reactive autoantibodies may be causative in some instances (135–137), with the platelet count variability attributable to fluctuations either in levels of platelet-reactive autoantibody (136,137) or in reticuloendothelial function (135), perhaps because of fluctuations in cytokine levels (138). In other patients, an underlying marrow disorder is suggested by progression of cyclic platelet count fluctuations to persisting amegakaryocytic thrombocytopenia (139).

OVERVIEW OF TREATMENT

The principles of treatment of ITP in adults are predicated on the following characteristics of the disorder:

1. Most patients with immune thrombocytopenia have hyperfunctional platelets associated with an increased MPV (130,140). Thus, many patients do not need treatment despite moderate or even severe thrombocytopenia.

2. The goal of treatment is to achieve a safe platelet count, not necessarily a normal platelet count.

3. Most adults have chronic ITP. Therefore, the long-term risks of treatment must be balanced against the long-term risk of life-threatening bleeding in patients with chronic hemostatic impairment. Most adult patients are not cured by prednisone. Splenectomy is the preferred treatment of adults with chronic ITP because it offers the best chance for a cure of the thrombocytopenia and avoids the toxicity of medical therapies.

4. Ten percent to 15% of patients fail to respond to corticosteroid therapy and splenectomy, and for them, the treatment options are less satisfactory. It is important to exclude an accessory spleen in these patients. Many treatments have been used, including danazol, vinca alkaloids, cyclophosphamide, azathioprine, intravenous IgG (IVIgG), and Rh immune globulin (anti-D).

5. Patients should avoid drugs that interfere with platelet function, particularly aspirin, other nonsteroidal antiinflammatory agents, and alcohol (141).

CORTICOSTEROIDS

Mechanism of Action. Corticosteroids increase platelet lifespan in ITP (142), possibly by inhibiting both phagocytic activity (143) and autoantibody synthesis (144). Reduction or disappearance of anti–gpIIb-IIIa antibodies has been shown in patients who respond clinically to corticosteroids (145). Investigators (146) using ^{111}In-labeled autologous platelet survival studies concluded that corticosteroids improve marrow platelet production, possibly by inhibiting intramedullary platelet destruction by marrow phagocytic cells. Corticosteroids also reduce capillary leaks, an observation that could explain the reduction in bleeding symptoms that sometimes precedes the rise in the platelet count (147).

Dosage. The standard initial dose of prednisone is 1.0 to 1.5 mg/kg/day, usually administered until the platelet count has risen to safe values (judged clinically, but usually a minimum of 50×10^9/L); regardless of the response, the dose of prednisone is reduced after 14 days (if not sooner), with tapering over several weeks. After the initial platelet count response, we try to administer prednisone on alternate days during tapering, if possible, to minimize side effects. The prednisone should not be continued in large doses for more than 4 weeks in nonresponders because delayed response is unlikely and the risk of adverse effects increases.

Two prospective trials (148,149) compared standard with lower doses of prednisone as induction therapy for acute ITP (1.0 vs. 0.25 mg/kg/day, and 1.5 vs. 0.5 mg/kg/day). There was no difference in the likelihood of remission at 6 months' follow-up in either study. The larger study, however, observed a trend toward an increased frequency of complete remission (46% vs. 35%) in the group receiving the larger dose of prednisone. Moreover, a faster rise in the platelet count was observed in the group receiving the larger dose of prednisone (77% vs. 51% having a platelet count above 50×10^9/L after 14 days of prednisone) (149).

In a small trial (150), prednisone (1 mg/kg/day) resulted in short-term and long-term outcomes at least as good as those achieved with either IVIgG or the combination of both treatments. Whether repeated use of anti-D as initial therapy would provide better outcomes than standard first-line therapy is under investigation.

Very large doses of corticosteroids [e.g., pulse methylprednisolone (1 g over 30 minutes once daily for 3 days) or intermittent high-dose dexamethasone] have also been used for ITP

with variable but not dramatically beneficial results (151–153). Comparative trials with standard-dose prednisone are lacking.

Results of Treatment. Idiopathic thrombocytopenic purpura in adults is usually a chronic disorder. Most patients have a relapse of the thrombocytopenia as the prednisone dose is decreased or during subsequent follow-up observation. Hence, response to prednisone therapy must be related to length of follow-up.

Initial Response. Approximately two-thirds of patients attain a safe platelet count (minimum, 50×10^9/L) while receiving corticosteroids, and most achieve a high platelet count (above 100 to 150×10^9/L) (148,149,154–157).

Early Follow-Up. Several studies (148,149,154–156,158–160) provide information about the likelihood of remission after discontinuation of corticosteroids. The proportion of patients in complete remission (platelet count $>150 \times 10^9$/L) after discontinuation of prednisone therapy is approximately 30%. An additional 20% of patients are in partial remission (platelet count 50 to 150×10^9/L). Thus, approximately half of patients who receive corticosteroids have a safe platelet count after discontinuation of corticosteroid therapy during a relatively brief follow-up period (several months); however, most of the patients will relapse.

Patients with a shorter duration of bleeding symptoms are more likely to respond favorably (155,156,159,160). In one study (160), 94 (39%) of 241 patients with ITP who had symptoms for 6 months or less attained a complete remission, compared with only 19 (14%) of 132 patients who were symptomatic for longer than 6 months. For patients who relapse after an initial complete remission, a repeat course of prednisone can be effective (159).

Late Follow-Up. Studies (155,157,159) describing longer follow-up (minimum 2 years for all patients) indicate that there is continuing risk of relapse in adult patients after initial complete remission with corticosteroid therapy. In one study (159), only 29% of adult patients who had a complete remission remained in remission at 4 years. In summary, only approximately 10% to 15% of all adult patients with ITP who receive prednisone therapy have a durable remission. Consequently, most require either further medical therapy or splenectomy.

Adverse Effects. Two studies (156,160) described the frequency of complications of corticosteroid therapy administered to adult patients with ITP. Common adverse effects (5% to 20% of patients treated) included cushingoid facies, weight gain, nonspecific abdominal symptoms, and acne. Less common (1% to 5%) but important complications included infection, myopathy, diabetes, psychosis, hypertension, and hypokalemia. Osteonecrosis, usually affecting the hips or shoulders, occurs in approximately 5% of patients receiving prolonged corticosteroid treatment, although some patients experience this serious complication after intensive, short-term treatment (161,162).

SPLENECTOMY

Mechanism of Action. Splenectomy is frequently successful because in most patients, the spleen is the major site of both autoantibody production and platelet destruction (111). Platelet survival studies indicate improved platelet lifespan after splenectomy (146).

Perioperative Management. All patients should be vaccinated with polyvalent pneumococcal vaccine, quadrivalent meningococcal polysaccharide vaccine, and *Haemophilus influenzae* type B vaccine (163,164), preferably at least 2 weeks before surgery. This vaccine reduces the risk of overwhelming postsplenectomy infection, which occurred in splenectomized adults (prevaccination era) at a frequency of approximately 1 per 1000 to 1500 patient-years (165). Because most patients who undergo splenectomy have been treated previously with prednisone, perioperative administration of parenteral corticosteroids is usually advised.

Adequate hemostasis usually can be obtained by raising the platelet count perioperatively with corticosteroids, high-dose IVIgG, or anti-D. Despite these maneuvers, many patients are thrombocytopenic at the time of splenectomy; however, most do not have excess bleeding. Accordingly, platelet transfusions should not be administered prophylactically but should be reserved for those patients with intraoperative bleeding. In one study in which platelets were administered only to patients with "marked oozing" at the end of the procedure (157), only 10 (18%) of 55 patients required platelet transfusions. Our own experience is that the number of patients who need platelet transfusions is even lower.

Because thromboembolic complications have been described in these patients after splenectomy (166–169), we would consider prophylactic antithrombotic treatment with heparin as the platelet count rises to normal level if the patient remains immobilized.

Results of Treatment. Approximately 75% of patients enter a complete remission within 4 to 6 weeks after splenectomy (157,160,166–171). In the complete responders, normal platelet counts are reached within 7 days in 90% of patients and within 6 weeks in 98% (170); spontaneous remission rarely occurs thereafter (171).

A partial remission is achieved for approximately 5% to 10% of patients (157,160,166,169), and these patients are asymptomatic. Of the remaining nonresponders, some benefit from low doses of prednisone.

Certain features are associated with a higher probability of response to splenectomy. These include a previous response to corticosteroids (168,172) or IVIgG (173) and younger age (159,167,168,171,174). Some investigators have reported that a predominant splenic clearance of platelets, as shown by radionuclide platelet imaging techniques (146,166,169,171) or normal to increased platelet turnover (125), also predicts a good response to splenectomy; however, not all investigators have reached these conclusions (123,125,146). Measurement of PAIgG levels does not predict response to splenectomy (125,167,171,174). In contrast to results of corticosteroid therapy, patients with a longer duration of thrombocytopenia are not less likely to respond to splenectomy (160).

The risk for a relapse of thrombocytopenia after complete remission postsplenectomy is low (approximately 10% to 15% at 10 years) (169,171).

Accessory Spleens. It is important to search for an accessory spleen both at surgery and in patients who relapse after splenectomy. Accessory spleens are identified at the time of primary splenectomy in approximately 20% of patients (167,170,172). A history that suggests the possibility of an accessory spleen is one in which the patient has an initial response to splenectomy that is later followed by a relapse of ITP. Approximately 50% of these patients have a residual accessory spleen demonstrated with sensitive imaging techniques (159,175,176), and approximately 65% of these patients achieve complete remission after removal of the accessory spleen (159,167,175,176).

It is less certain whether residual accessory splenic tissue accounts for *early* postsplenectomy failure (i.e., persisting or recurrent thrombocytopenia within 6 weeks after splenectomy). In this situation, children often do not respond to the removal of the accessory splenic tissue (177). The results are better for adults; early splenectomy failures can achieve complete remission after removal of an accessory spleen (167,176).

A number of methods can be used to look for an accessory spleen. The presence of typical postsplenectomy changes in the blood film (e.g., Howell-Jolly bodies) does not rule out the possibility of an accessory spleen (159,176). Computed tomography scan, ultrasound, and radionuclide imaging methods have been used successfully. The radionuclide methods include ^{99m}Tc sulfur colloid scans, ^{111}In platelet localization studies, and radiolabeled heat-aggregated RBC studies. We look for accessory splenic tissue by nuclear imaging during the performance of a platelet survival study using ^{111}In. The intraoperative use of a handheld isotope detector probe can help locate an accessory spleen during surgery (167).

Laparoscopic Splenectomy. Splenectomy using the laparoscopic technique is an increasingly popular surgical approach to management of ITP; results are similar to those with open splenectomy (178). A theoretic concern is that residual spleen tissue (accessory spleens) may be overlooked more frequently than with open splenectomy, but to date, this problem does not appear to be occurring. Regardless of the technique used, a careful intraoperative search for accessory spleens is important to reduce the risk of postsplenectomy failure or relapse of the ITP.

Adverse Effects. Perioperative mortality is less than 1%, with most deaths due to thromboembolic complications (157,160,166–170). Morbidity is under 10%, and the most frequent complications are pleuropulmonary (pneumonia, subphrenic abscess, pleural effusion in 4%), followed by major bleeding in 1.5% and thromboembolic complications in 1%. No late deaths due to overwhelming bacterial septicemia were reported in these studies. It is possible that the risk of postsplenectomy septicemia is lower in patients who undergo splenectomy for ITP compared with other reasons for splenectomy (e.g., hematologic neoplasm).

SECOND-LINE THERAPY

In approximately 15% of patients, ITP cannot be controlled by corticosteroid therapy and splenectomy. The large number of therapies that have been used for these treatment failures attests to the difficulty in treating this patient group.

Danazol. **Mechanism of Action.** Danazol is an attenuated androgen with mild virilizing effects that can be used in men and nonpregnant women. It is possible that danazol works by counteracting the effects of estrogens on phagocytic cells. Estrogens increase Fc receptor number and increase the rate of clearance of IgG-sensitized RBCs (179), whereas danazol reduces the number of phagocytic cell Fc receptors (180).

Dosage. Usually, 400 to 1200 mg danazol is administered daily in divided doses, although a report described effectiveness using low doses (50 mg) (181). Response is usually seen within 2 months, although response may take up to 6 months when low doses are used (181).

Results of Treatment. When standard doses are used for a minimum of 2 months to treat adult ITP, danazol produces a sustained increase in the platelet count, above 100×10^9/L, in approximately 30% of patients; an additional 10% of patients have a rise in platelet count to 50 to 100×10^9/L (180–190). However, some studies report essentially negative results (186,187), with sustained benefit shown in less than 10% of patients. Perhaps older women (188) or patients with associated rheumatologic disorders (190) are more likely to respond to treatment. Often, the danazol must be continued to maintain the platelet count, although the clinician periodically should attempt to reduce the dose.

Adverse Effects. Danazol is generally well tolerated. The most frequent adverse effects are fluid retention, persistent nausea, oligomenorrhea and amenorrhea, headache, and hepatitis (182–190). The risk of hepatitis is dose-dependent; therefore, patients treated with higher doses require more careful monitoring of liver enzymes. Rarely encountered side effects include development of multiple cystic blood-filled spaces in the liver or spleen [peliosis (191)] with associated risk of splenic rupture (192), increased fibrinolysis (193), and mild virilization. Concerns about fetal damage precludes the use of danazol during pregnancy (194,195). Rarely, idiosyncratic thrombocytopenia has been described (196).

Vinca Alkaloids. Mechanism of Action. The mechanism of action of vinca alkaloids is uncertain but could be related to inhibition of phagocytic cell function. The vinca alkaloids (vincristine and vinblastine) bind to platelet microtubules (197), which theoretically could help localize the drugs to the platelet-destroying phagocytic cells.

Dosage and Methods of Administration. In adults, the usual dose of vincristine is 1 to 2 mg, and for vinblastine it is 5 to 10 mg. The treatment can be repeated at 5-day to 10-day intervals until response or toxicity is encountered. No more than three doses should be administered if a response is not seen, because subsequent benefit is unlikely and side effects become increasingly problematic.

Usually, the vinca alkaloids are administered by rapid intravenous infusion. However, different methods have been used in an attempt to increase delivery to the phagocytic cells. One method consists of administering the vinca alkaloids by slow infusion (over 4 to 8 hours) (198–203). Another method whereby platelets are incubated in vinblastine or vincristine ("vinca-loaded" platelets) (197,199,204) is seldom used because of toxicity and lack of evidence of superior efficacy (205,206).

Results of Treatment. Summarizing several studies of vincristine for ITP (218,207–212), approximately 65% of patients respond to treatment with a rise in the platelet count to greater than 50×10^9/L. In approximately half of responders, the platelet count entered the normal range. However, only a few patients had a sustained remission (189,207,209,211). In one study (160), none of 19 patients who received vincristine for refractory, chronic ITP had a sustained remission. Concomitant treatment with azathioprine may increase the likelihood of long-term response to vincristine (212,213).

In 1984, Ahn et al. (198) reported the use of vincristine or vinblastine administered by slow infusion for chronic ITP. The platelet count rose to greater than 50×10^9/L in 17 (65%) of 26 patients, and sustained responses (minimum 2 years) were seen in 6 patients. Three other groups subsequently reported their results with slow infusions of vincristine (200,202) or vinblastine (201). Summarizing the results of these three studies in patients with chronic ITP, response was seen in 67% of patients, but sustained complete remission (duration more than 6 months) was seen in only 2 of 21 patients. A randomized trial did not show greater benefit of administering vinblastine by slow rather than rapid infusion (203).

Three studies (200–202) reported the response of adult patients with acute ITP (duration <6 months) to slow infusion of

vinca alkaloids. All 13 patients responded favorably to treatment, and 10 continued in sustained complete remission during a median follow-up of 6 months (range, 2 to 29 months). Our own experience has been much less favorable, and because of their adverse effects, we seldom use vincristine or vinblastine for ITP.

Adverse Effects. Peripheral neuropathy is a common complication of vincristine or vinblastine. Leukopenia and alopecia can complicate vinblastine therapy (198). Fever can occur after repeated injections of vinca by slow infusion (198). Vinca alkaloids are not leukemogenic.

Cyclophosphamide and Azathioprine. Mechanism of Action. Cyclophosphamide and azathioprine are considered together in this section because of their similar immunosuppressive activity, clinical efficacy, and toxicities. Cyclophosphamide is an alkylating agent, whereas azathioprine is metabolized to 6-mercaptopurine, a purine antimetabolite.

Dosage. The usual dosage of both azathioprine and cyclophosphamide is between 50 and 200 mg/day (i.e., approximately 1 to 2 mg/kg/day), with the dose reduced if the patient becomes leukopenic. It usually takes a minimum of 2 to 4 weeks before response to either agent occurs, and sometimes 3 to 6 months of treatment must be administered before a response is seen. Cyclophosphamide also has been administered in intermittent pulses (1.0 to 1.5 g/m^2 every 4 weeks by rapid intravenous infusion) (214,215). Sometimes, cyclophosphamide is combined with other cytotoxic agents in a regimen resembling antineoplasia therapy (216).

Results of Treatment. In 1976, Caplan and Berkman (217) reviewed 28 published reports on the use of immunosuppressive treatments for ITP. Overall, 33% of patients had complete remission after treatment with cyclophosphamide, 21% after treatment with azathioprine. Including patients who had partial benefit from these treatments, approximately two-thirds of all patients responded to cyclophosphamide or azathioprine. Subsequently, the results of a large, multicenter study were reported (160). Sustained complete remissions occurred in approximately 20% of the patients receiving cyclophosphamide or azathioprine (160). Including lesser responses (temporary complete remission, partial remission), between 40% and 60% of patients benefited from these agents (160,189).

Adverse Effects. Toxicities from these drugs are considerable. The most important side effects include leukemogenesis (cyclophosphamide, azathioprine), hemorrhagic cystitis (cyclophosphamide), and marrow suppression (cyclophosphamide, azathioprine). Cases of myeloid leukemia after the use of cyclophosphamide (218) and azathioprine (219) for ITP have been described.

High-Dose Intravenous Immunoglobulin G. There are two general treatments available for ITP that use pooled human antibodies: high-dose IVIgG and Rh immune globulin (anti-D). Table 32-1 compares these two treatments.

High-dose IVIgG has been used to treat ITP since 1981 (220). IVIgG is prepared by ethanol precipitation of pooled plasma followed by techniques to minimize IgG self-aggregation (221). In contrast, immune serum globulin cannot be administered by the intravenous route because of severe adverse reactions, including anaphylactoid reactions, caused by the large amounts of IgG aggregates within these preparations.

More than 95% of IVIgG consists of monomeric IgG. The IgG retains normal Fab and Fc functions required for antigen bind-

TABLE 32-1. Comparison of Intravenous Immunoglobulin G and Anti-D for Treatment of Idiopathic Thrombocytopenic Purpura

Factor	High-Dose Intravenous Immunoglobulin G	Anti-D (Rh immune globulin)
Side effects	Common: headache, hypertension, fever and chills; rare: hemolysis, renal failure, myocardial infarction, stroke	Common: mild, compensated hemolysis; rare: severe hemolysis requiring transfusion or hemodialysis
Response rate	Approximately 80%	Approximately 80%
Response duration	Usually transient	Usually transient
Pattern of platelet increase	Faster increase, higher peak, shorter duration of response	Slower increase, lower peak, longer duration of response
Influence of ABO, Rh type	No influence	Only D-positive patients respond
Influence of splenectomy	Unknown	Minimal response in splenectomized patient
Suitability for emergency treatment of idiopathic thrombocytopenic purpura	Recommended	Not recommended

ing and phagocytic cell interaction, respectively. IgG aggregates, IgA, and other contaminants constitute a negligible fraction. IVIgG has a normal half-life *in vivo*, with a physiologic subclass distribution (221).

Mechanism of Action. A number of models have been proposed to explain the efficacy of IVIgG in ITP (221–226). The two most widely accepted explanations are impairment of phagocytic cell function and suppression of autoantibody synthesis.

Most clinicians think that IVIgG works by reticuloendothelial cell blockade ("medical splenectomy") (Fig. 32-4). The usual total dose of IVIgG (2 g/kg) raises the serum IgG concentration by twofold to fourfold, a level that has been shown to block the clearance of radiolabeled, IgG-sensitized RBCs (227,228). Consistent with this view is the observation that disease-related polyclonal hypergammaglobulinemia also is associated with impaired reticuloendothelial cell function (229). We believe that the monomeric IgG is in equilibrium with the Fc receptor on the phagocytic cells. Even though the binding affinity of Fc receptors for monomeric IgG is low, the high plasma concentration of IgG results in these receptors being occupied (229). It is possible that small quantities of contaminating aggregated IgG could

contribute to phagocytic cell receptor blockade (224). One group (225) has proposed that phagocytic cell inhibition is related to anti-HLA antibodies contained within the Ig preparations. Recent work in a murine model of immune thrombocytopenia suggests that IVIgG might down-regulate immune platelet clearance by inducing surface expression on macrophages of an inhibiting class of Fc receptors (FcγRIIB) (226).

The phagocytic cell blockade theory, however, cannot explain the occasional long-term response that follows treatment with IVIgG, nor the observation that Fc-depleted preparations sometimes are effective in ITP (230). Thus, immune suppression has been invoked as an alternative mechanism of action. In support of this concept is the observation that PAIgG and anti–gpIIb-IIIa levels decline after successful treatment with IVIgG (145,231). The immune suppression could be related to the nonspecific effects of large amounts of IgG, which reduce antibody synthesis, or to specific interaction of certain IgG molecules within the IVIgG preparation with the pathogenic autoantibodies (antiidiotype interactions), thereby blocking autoantibody binding to platelets (232,233). Alterations in lymphocyte subpopulations and reductions in mitogen-stimulated Ig synthesis occur after IVIgG treatment (234,235).

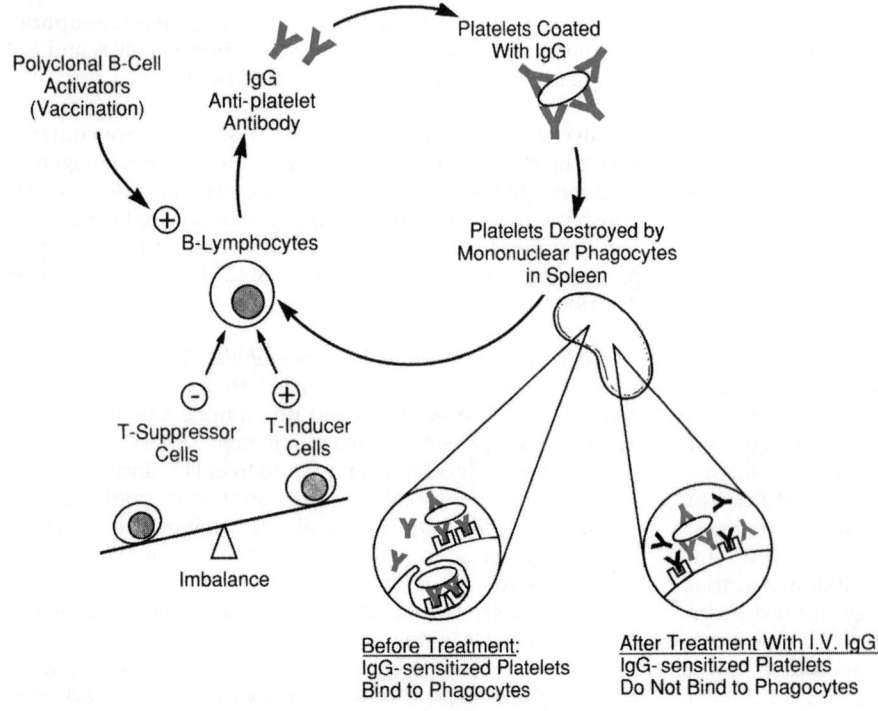

Before Treatment:
IgG-sensitized Platelets
Bind to Phagocytes

After Treatment With I.V. IgG:
IgG-sensitized Platelets
Do Not Bind to Phagocytes

Figure 32-4. Schematic representation of one mechanism of action of high-dose intravenous immunoglobulin (I.V. IgG): occupancy of macrophage Fc receptors by IgG.

Dosage and Preparations. The usual dosage of IVIgG is 2 g/kg administered over 2 to 5 days (i.e., 1 g/kg/day for 2 days, or 0.4 g/kg/day for 5 days). One trial showed no difference between one dose of 1 g/kg versus two doses 1 day apart (236). Thus, one approach is to administer 1 g/kg as a single dose and to repeat the dose 2 days later if no significant increase in platelet count has occurred, possibly avoiding an unneeded second dose. To minimize side effects, the infusion is administered over 6 to 8 hours. Several preparations are available, and there is no evidence that any one of these products offers a major advantage over the others (221).

Results of Treatment. The administration of IVIgG to adults with chronic ITP raises the platelet count above $50 \times 10^9/L$ in approximately 80% of patients. In more than half of responders, the platelet count becomes normal (221,237). Unfortunately, the response is usually transient. The platelet count begins to rise within 1 to 3 days of commencing treatment, peaks at 5 to 10 days, and returns to baseline level by 2 to 6 weeks. There is no difference in response among patients of different ABO or Rh blood groups (238).

Although long-lasting complete remissions in adults with chronic ITP are rare after IVIgG, repeated treatment with IVIgG (maintenance therapy) is sometimes associated with complete or partial remission (236,239). Bussel et al. (239) treated 40 adult patients with chronic ITP with repeated courses of IVIgG. Five patients entered a complete remission, and 11 were classified as "stable without therapy," defined as persisting thrombocytopenia that is asymptomatic or with minor bruising. Thirteen patients required continued maintenance treatment, and the remaining 11 patients became refractory to treatment. However, maintenance therapy with IVIgG is very expensive (240,241) and is rarely used in adults.

In a small randomized trial, IVIgG was not superior to prednisone as initial therapy for adult ITP (150). Thus, its use is usually limited to those patients with ITP in whom a rapid platelet count response is needed, for example, emergency treatment of a bleeding patient or preoperative preparation for surgery.

Adverse Effects. IVIgG is relatively safe. Side effects are infrequent and usually mild (221). Most common are headache, local phlebitis, flushing, and fever at a frequency of 3% to 20%. These symptoms are controlled by briefly stopping or reducing the rate of infusion. Premedication with acetaminophen, antihistamine, or corticosteroids can be helpful. Chest pain, hypertension, hypotension, bronchospasm, and laryngeal edema have been described (242) but are uncommon. These adverse reactions occur with increased frequency in patients with congenital IgA deficiency.

Rare side effects include overwhelming septicemia, hemolysis due to ABO hemolysins contained within the IVIgG (243), acute cryoglobulinemic nephropathy in rheumatoid factor–positive recipients (244), and aseptic meningitis (105). High-dose IVIgG has also been associated with acute myocardial infarction (245) and thrombotic stroke (246), particularly in elderly patients.

Because IVIgG is prepared from the pooled plasma of thousands of donors, there is a potential risk of infection. Although hepatitis C has been transmitted from certain lots (247), this risk is believed to be negligible with currently available products (105).

Other Uses. Although IVIgG is seldom used as a maintenance therapy for adults with chronic ITP, it is frequently used to manage acute immune-mediated thrombocytopenia (discussed in the section Drug-Induced Thrombocytopenia).

Rh Immune Globulin. **Mechanism of Action.** Rh immune globulin (anti-D) has been used to treat Rh(D)-positive patients with ITP since the mid-1980s (248,249). Because effective treatment requires some degree of hemolysis, it is ineffective in Rh(D)-negative individuals. The mechanism of action probably occurs by means of phagocytic cell blockade due to occupancy of the phagocytic cell Fc receptors by the IgG-sensitized RBCs, which prevents the platelets from binding to these receptors. Because a 100-µg dose of anti-D contains between 5 and 200 mg of additional nonspecific IgG (250,251), there is not enough IgG to invoke phagocytic cell blockade by monomeric IgG, as with IVIgG. Interestingly, plasma containing high-titer anti-C has been shown effective in patients carrying this antigen (252). Anti-D therapy is usually ineffective in patients who have undergone splenectomy (253,254).

Dosage. The probability of response increases with the dose administered (255). Successful doses have ranged from 100 µg administered as a single intravenous dose (insufficient to cause a positive direct antiglobulin test) (255) to almost 20 mg administered over 14 days (256). Usually, 25 to 75 µg/kg (total dose) is administered in divided doses over 2 to 5 days (252–262). A common regimen administers 25 µg/kg of anti-D intravenously and repeats the same dose 2 days later if no or minimal response is evident (253). Recent evidence suggests that 75 µg/kg has greater efficacy than 50 µg/kg without more adverse effects (262). Anti-D can be administered safely by intravenous injection over a few minutes. Patients who respond to anti-D often can be maintained with small intermittent maintenance doses of anti-D, perhaps obviating the need for splenectomy (259,260).

Results of Treatment. The frequency of response using optimal, individualized doses of anti-D is similar to that using IVIgG, and, as with IVIgG, the increase in the platelet count usually is transient (2 to 6 weeks) (253–262). Occasional long-term responses can occur. Compared with IVIgG, the peak platelet count tends to be lower, and the time to reach the peak platelet count often is longer. Therefore, a greater interval between maintenance injections may be possible using anti-D. Some patients who fail to respond to IVIgG can still benefit from anti-D, and vice versa; however, patients who have undergone splenectomies have a lower probability of response to anti-D (253,254).

Adverse Effects. A positive direct antiglobulin test and laboratory evidence of hemolysis are present in most patients (249,258). The decline in hemoglobin ranges from 0 to 20 g/L, and most patients do not have to discontinue treatment because of anemia. Response to treatment does not correlate with the degree of hemolysis (258). However, in at least 1 per 1000 recipients, life-threatening acute intravascular hemolysis results that requires transfusion or even hemodialysis (263). Such patients have usually received the U.S. Food and Drug Administration–approved dose of 50 µg/kg, and the explanation for their severe hemolysis is unknown.

The theoretic potential for transmitting infection is illustrated by the epidemic of hepatitis C during 1978 and 1979 in Ireland affecting young mothers who received perinatal anti-D contaminated with this virus from a single infected donor (264). Current availability of solvent-detergent anti-D currently makes this risk of infection negligible.

Other Treatments. Interferon-α (265–269), cyclosporine (270–276), colchicine (277–279), dapsone (280–282), plasma perfusion over staphylococcal protein A columns (283,284), plasmapheresis (285–287), and Fc receptor–blocking (288,289) or B-lymphocyte–

depleting [rituximab (290)] monoclonal antibodies have been used in refractory ITP, but experience is minimal.

For some of these treatments, the initial success has not been confirmed by other studies. For example, after apparent efficacy of interferon-α for refractory ITP (265), others noted absent or only brief responses, with some patients developing worse thrombocytopenia (266,267). However, interferon can increase the platelet count in patients with isolated thrombocytopenia caused by chronic hepatitis C infection (268,269), a disorder that can mimic ITP.

Cyclosporine selectively inhibits adaptive immune responses by blocking T-cell–dependent biosynthesis of lymphokines, particularly interleukin-2, at the level of messenger RNA transcription. Several groups have reported at least transient benefit with cyclosporine for both adults and children with refractory ITP (270–276).

ELDERLY AND HIGH-RISK PATIENTS

Elderly patients may have a lower probability of benefit from splenectomy (167,171). Particularly in poor surgical candidates, splenic irradiation (rather than splenectomy) may raise the platelet count (291,292). Evidence suggests that danazol may be more effective in older patients than in younger female patients (188), and we sometimes try danazol before splenectomy. Dapsone produces oxidant hemolysis and has been used to treat ITP in elderly patients who have not had splenectomies (280), in whom it may work by blocking phagocytic cell function nonimmunologically.

EMERGENCY TREATMENT OF A BLEEDING PATIENT

Intravenous Immunoglobulin G and Platelet Transfusions.
A patient with ITP with life-threatening bleeding should immediately receive platelet transfusions (10 to 20 U). The patient then should receive high-dose IVIgG (1 g/kg over 4 to 6 hours) to block the phagocytic system, followed by further platelet transfusions. This approach almost always raises the platelet count (293). Some physicians have described continuous infusions of IVIgG and platelets for this situation (294). Other treatments to achieve longer-term control of the thrombocytopenia (e.g., corticosteroids) should be commenced simultaneously.

Routine Platelet Transfusions.
Platelet transfusions in patients with ITP often produce a transient rise in the platelet count (295). Consequently, although platelet transfusions are acceptable in certain clinical situations, such as life-threatening or perioperative bleeding, they are not indicated prophylactically because the hazards of platelet transfusion (e.g., risk of alloimmunization, bloodborne infection) outweigh the benefits of a short-lived increase in the platelet count in a chronic disorder.

Preparation for Invasive Procedure.
High-dose IVIgG is usually the treatment of choice for a severely thrombocytopenic patient with ITP who requires urgent surgery or an invasive procedure. Prophylactic platelet transfusions, when deemed necessary, should be administered when maximal hemostasis is required, because the platelet count increment is usually transient. When at least 2 to 3 days are available before the planned procedure, less expensive (and equally effective) options include corticosteroids or anti-D.

Idiopathic Thrombocytopenic Purpura in Pregnancy

IDIOPATHIC THROMBOCYTOPENIC PURPURA VERSUS INCIDENTAL THROMBOCYTOPENIA OF PREGNANCY

Thrombocytopenia during pregnancy is not usually caused by ITP. Rather, a benign condition known as *incidental* or *gestational*

thrombocytopenia is the most likely cause, occurring in approximately 5% to 7% of pregnancies at term (5–7). Newborns of mothers with incidental thrombocytopenia are not at increased risk for neonatal thrombocytopenia. The second most likely cause of thrombocytopenia is pregnancy-induced hypertension (preeclampsia) (discussed in the section Preeclampsia). Immune-mediated thrombocytopenia, whether primary (ITP) or secondary (e.g., SLE, HIV), represents the third most likely explanation for thrombocytopenia in a pregnant woman.

Although relatively uncommon, ITP in pregnancy is an important disorder because of the potential treatment implications for the mother as well as the possibility of fetal or neonatal thrombocytopenia caused by transplacental passage of IgG antiplatelet autoantibodies. Previously, fetuses of mothers with ITP were routinely delivered by cesarian section (296), but this step is not usually taken today, for three reasons. First, the frequency of severe fetal thrombocytopenia (platelet count <20 × 10⁹/L) is now known to be quite low (approximately 4%) (297–300). Moreover, intracranial hemorrhage or other severe bleeding in the thrombocytopenic newborn treated appropriately is uncommon. Second, there is no evidence that cesarian section leads to less intracranial or other bleeding than vaginal delivery. Third, some women with incidental thrombocytopenia misdiagnosed as ITP may undergo an unnecessary intervention.

MANAGEMENT

Many pregnant patients with ITP do not require specific treatment. We treat the mother if the platelet count falls to low levels (<20 to 50 × 10⁹/L) or if the patient has clinical evidence of a hemostatic defect (e.g., petechiae). There are two major treatment options: intermittent high-dose IVIgG and low-dose prednisone. Because of risks of prednisone during pregnancy (teratogenicity in the first trimester, preeclampsia in the second and third trimesters), we generally favor IVIgG as the treatment of choice for ITP in pregnancy. At the time of delivery, patients with thrombocytopenia should not be subjected to a potentially dangerous hemostatic insult such as an epidural analgesic. If the patient has received corticosteroids, increasing the dose at delivery should be considered. Otherwise, no special steps are taken. Platelet transfusions are rarely needed at delivery.

The other patient who must be treated is the fetus. Unfortunately, the fetal platelet count cannot easily be obtained until delivery. A number of maneuvers have been suggested to treat these patients.

Prediction of Neonatal Thrombocytopenia.
The maternal platelet count cannot be used to predict which infants will be thrombocytopenic (301). Indeed, women "cured" of ITP by splenectomy can have thrombocytopenic babies. It is likely that mothers with ITP who have had a previous thrombocytopenic infant are at higher risk for subsequent similar outcomes (302,303). Although both elevated maternal PAIgG (297) and serum platelet-bindable IgG (304) are correlated with increased risk of thrombocytopenia in the neonate, the predictive value of these tests is too low to allow a role in the treatment of pregnant patients with ITP.

Antepartum Maneuvers to Raise Fetal Platelet Count.
It remains uncertain whether administration of low doses of corticosteroids (20 mg/day) to mothers with ITP results in their infants having a higher platelet count (305,306). It also appears unlikely that IVIgG administered to the mother raises the fetal platelet counts (307–309). Regardless of any potential effect on fetal or neonatal platelet counts, we believe that use of IVIgG in pregnancy depends on maternal indications, given the generally favorable natural history in their neonates.

Determination of Fetal Platelet Count by Fetal Cord Sampling (Cordocentesis). Although it is possible to measure the fetal platelet count by sampling umbilical vein blood under ultrasound guidance (310), this procedure has risks of fetal morbidity and mortality and is not justified in this situation (311).

Determination of Fetal Platelet Count by Fetal Scalp Sampling. It is possible to estimate the fetal platelet count shortly before delivery through fetal scalp sampling (312). After the fetal head is engaged and after a spontaneous or an elective rupture of the membranes, the scalp is wiped clean, and a small incision is made using a lancet. A sample of fetal scalp blood is collected, and the count is determined by using a particle counter or by examining a stained blood film. Visual estimation of the platelet count may be preferred, because platelet aggregation can lead to a falsely low measurement by particle counter (313). We have used this approach on a number of patients but have abandoned it for logistic and technical reasons; one reason is that a falsely low platelet count could prompt an unnecessary cesarean section.

Recommended Approach. Our approach is to follow pregnant patients with ITP with frequent platelet counts (every few weeks, depending on their platelet counts). We test for antiphospholipid antibodies (e.g., testing for lupus anticoagulant and anticardiolipin antibodies), which may be an indication for treatment (e.g., corticosteroids, aspirin), especially if previous miscarriages have occurred (314). If treatment for maternal thrombocytopenia is required, we usually give IVIgG. Prednisone is another option, but if more than 20 mg/day is needed, the risk of complications (e.g., preeclampsia) may be increased. It is possible, although unproven, that corticosteroids or IVIgG improves fetal platelet counts. Occasionally, splenectomy may be appropriate during the second trimester, especially if the mother has very severe, refractory thrombocytopenia ($<10 \times 10^9$/L) (105).

Unless a cesarian section is required for unrelated obstetric indications, we recommend spontaneous vaginal delivery for mothers with ITP. An immediate fetal umbilical vein platelet count is obtained at delivery. Relatively severe neonatal thrombocytopenia ($<50 \times 10^9$/L) should be aggressively treated, usually with IVIgG or corticosteroids. It is important to recognize that the platelet count of the newborn infant with passive autoimmune thrombocytopenia will fall, and the platelet count nadir is reached 2 to 5 days after delivery (297). Therefore, daily platelet counts should be obtained until a normal platelet count is documented. For infants who develop significant thrombocytopenia ($<50 \times 10^9$/L), treatment with IVIgG, sometimes combined with corticosteroids or platelet transfusions, raises the platelet count (302,315).

Acute Idiopathic Thrombocytopenic Purpura of Childhood

Acute ITP is a relatively common disorder, with an annual incidence of approximately 1 in 10,000 children. The peak incidence occurs between 2 and 6 years of age, with boys and girls affected equally. Approximately 80% of the children with acute ITP recover completely, usually within 6 months (316). The remainder, who have persistent thrombocytopenia, have chronic ITP, a disorder that probably differs in cause and pathogenesis.

PATHOGENESIS AND CAUSE
It is likely that acute ITP of childhood is a transient autoimmune disorder, because antiplatelet glycoprotein antibodies are usually detected (317,318). Phase II assays show circulating antiplatelet antibodies in at least half of children with acute ITP (319) and elevated levels of PAIgG in at least 85% of children (319–322). Sometimes, only platelet-associated IgM is found (319). PAIgG levels return to normal after resolution of thrombocytopenia and remain normal (321).

The cause of increased IgG binding to platelets is uncertain. Because acute ITP often follows viral infections, the thrombocytopenia could be related to adsorption of virus to platelets or the deposition of virus-containing immune complexes onto platelets. However, thrombocytopenia often occurs weeks after infection, when viremia is no longer apparent. Furthermore, the high incidence of elevated PAIgG and PAIgM, as well as the antiplatelet reactivity of Ig eluted from platelets (319,323), is consistent with an autoimmune process, perhaps resulting from an aberrant immune response to a viral trigger via molecular mimicry (324). Indeed, autoantibodies against gpIIb-IIIa and gpIb-IX have been identified in acute ITP (318,323).

CLINICAL AND LABORATORY FEATURES
The typical clinical presentation of acute ITP is the abrupt onset of bleeding and bruising in a healthy child weeks after a viral infection. Physical examination usually reveals purpura in the absence of lymphadenopathy or organomegaly. Mortality, which is less than 0.5%, usually is due to intracranial hemorrhage.

Laboratory features include thrombocytopenia with elevated MPV and normal RBC and leukocyte counts. The thrombocytopenia usually is severe, and the platelet count usually is less than 10×10^9/L (325). Whether to perform a bone marrow examination remains controversial; however, some physicians do not perform marrow aspirates in patients with typical clinical and laboratory features of acute ITP, as the risk of missing the diagnosis of leukemia is negligible (326). Usually, bone marrow examination reveals normal or increased numbers of megakaryocytes in acute ITP. Sometimes, morphologically distinct lymphoid cells, originally termed *hematogones,* constitute up to half of the marrow cells and may cause diagnostic confusion with acute leukemia (327,328). These nonneoplastic cells are characterized by scant, agranular cytoplasm; homogeneous, condensed nuclei lacking nucleoli; and the surface immunophenotypic profile of immature lymphocytes.

TREATMENT
Fatalities are rare in acute ITP (<1%). Nonetheless, the treatment is to raise the platelet count in patients with very severe thrombocytopenia in an attempt to reduce the small but real risk of intracranial hemorrhage, which has been estimated to occur in approximately 0.5% of children with acute ITP (329). Because such a low incidence of adverse outcomes makes it virtually impossible to perform a clinical trial to determine whether treatment prevents hemorrhagic death, prospective comparative studies have focused on the surrogate endpoint of the time required to raise the platelet count to safe levels (generally, $>20 \times 10^9$/L).

Corticosteroids. Three prospective, randomized clinical trials (330–332) compared prednisone (2 mg/kg/day or 60 mg/m²/day) to no therapy in acute ITP of childhood. Two of the trials (331,332) demonstrated a more rapid increase in platelet count in the corticosteroid-treated group than in the control group, and the third (330) demonstrated a similar trend.

Larger initial doses of corticosteroids have also been used for these children, for example, prednisone (4 to 8 mg/kg/day) (333) or intravenous methylprednisolone (5 to 30 mg/kg/day) (334,335). Almost all the children achieved a platelet count greater than 20×10^9/L within 72 hours of commencing treatment. Side effects, including glycosuria, hypertension, and transient weight gain, were uncommonly encountered. A recent study (336) of 25 consecutive children with severe acute ITP and a brief course of prednisone (4 mg/kg/day for 4 days without tapering) observed platelet count recovery to greater than 20×10^9/L in 83% of patients at 48 hours, although 41% of responding patients did require additional prednisone within 1 month of starting therapy because of recurrent thrombocytopenia.

Intravenous Immunoglobulin G. In 1981, Imbach et al. (220) reported that IVIgG raised the platelet count in children with acute or chronic ITP. Subsequently, these workers reported the results of a prospective, randomized, multicenter trial comparing prednisone (60 mg/m^2/day for 3 weeks) with IVIgG (0.4 g/kg/day for 5 days) as alternate treatment for children with acute ITP (platelet counts $<30 \times 10^9$/L) (337). The study demonstrated that for approximately 60% of the children, either treatment produced a rapid rise in the platelet count to safe levels. For the remainder who were less responsive to treatment, the IVIgG resulted in a faster rise in the platelet count (337). In a Canadian trial (338), both oral prednisone (4 mg/kg/day for 1 week, followed by tapering) and IVIgG (1 g/kg/day for 2 consecutive days) were superior to no therapy; the two treatments were equally effective in reducing the time to platelet count less than 20×10^9/L.

Sometimes, the response to IVIgG is so rapid that only a single dose of IVIgG is required (339). Indeed, the second Canadian trial found no significant differences between IVIgG when 0.8 g/kg was administered once or 1 g/kg/day was administered for 2 consecutive days (340). In contrast, this trial found significantly slower responses in the treatment arm that received anti-D.

Recommended Treatment. The risk of life-threatening bleeding is highest within the first few weeks, so affected children should avoid trauma and restrict physical activity as much as possible. Although most children with acute ITP have a benign clinical course and recover without therapy, it is impossible to identify those who will develop life-threatening bleeding. Consequently, for patients with severe ITP (American Society of Hematology practice guidelines: platelet count $<10 \times 10^9$/L, or $<20 \times 10^9$/L with mucosal hemorrhages), treatment with either IVIgG (1 g/kg) or prednisone (1.5 to 2.0 mg/kg/day for 14 to 21 days, 60 mg/m^2/day for 21 days, or 4 mg/kg/day for 7 days followed by tapering of prednisone until day 21) should be administered (105). Some physicians favor corticosteroids primarily because of the lower cost.

For patients with severe bleeding (e.g., intracranial), combined use of IVIgG and high-dose corticosteroids with platelet transfusions is appropriate. Emergency splenectomy should be considered for the rare patient with life-threatening bleeding who does not respond to platelet transfusions, IVIgG, and high-dose corticosteroid therapy.

Chronic Idiopathic Thrombocytopenic Purpura of Childhood

Thrombocytopenia persists for longer than 6 months (chronic ITP) in approximately 10% to 20% of children with ITP. However, as many as one-third of children with chronic ITP can have a spontaneous remission months or years later (316). Approximately 5% of children with ITP have recurrent ITP, characterized by intermittent episodes of thrombocytopenia followed by lengthy periods of remission.

PATHOGENESIS

The pathogenesis of chronic ITP in children is believed to mimic that in adults. Children with chronic ITP also have detectable autoantibodies reactive with platelet gpIIb-IIIa complex (341,342). However, the serologic profile of these autoantibodies does not distinguish acute from chronic ITP in children (341). Platelet-reactive T-cell clones have been identified in some children with chronic ITP (343).

CLINICAL AND LABORATORY FEATURES

Several clinical and laboratory features are seen more frequently in children with chronic than with acute ITP, although these features are not sufficiently distinctive to be useful in individual patients. Children who develop chronic ITP are more likely to be older than 10 years and female (344); have an insidious onset of bleeding symptoms; lack a viral prodrome; have less severe thrombocytopenia (342); have less marked elevation of the PAIgG (320,321); and have an increased frequency of other immune abnormalities (345), including selective hypogammaglobulinemia, positive ANA (346), and anticardiolipin antibodies (346).

TREATMENT

For many children with chronic ITP, the thrombocytopenia is only moderate, and the symptoms are absent or minimal. For these children, specific treatment is not required. For symptomatic children, the treatment options include maintenance IVIgG or anti-D injections, chronic or intermittent administration of corticosteroids, splenectomy, vinca alkaloids, or immunosuppressive agents (329,347,348).

Corticosteroids. Most children with chronic ITP achieve a safe platelet count on corticosteroid therapy, but the long-term toxicity of this treatment does not justify its prolonged use, except for the rare patient who responds to small doses of alternate-day prednisone. Short courses of corticosteroids can be useful for patients with exacerbations of symptomatic thrombocytopenia or in whom surgical procedures are considered.

Pulse methylprednisolone has been used in patients with severe chronic ITP (349,350). In the largest series (350), approximately half the children maintained a platelet count above 50×10^9/L for a minimum of 1 month after a 3-day course of methylprednisolone (15 mg/kg/day). However, this treatment is used much less often than IVIgG.

Intravenous Immunoglobulin G. Intravenous immunoglobulin G (2 g/kg total dose administered over 2 to 5 days) raises the platelet count in most children with chronic ITP (220,228,351). Because children are at greater risk than adults for overwhelming postsplenectomy sepsis, repeated courses of IVIgG have been used to defer or avoid splenectomy in children with chronic ITP (351). The intervals between the treatment with IVIgG are dictated by symptoms or the platelet count. Most children respond favorably to such maintenance therapy. A few enter a long-term complete or partial remission and require no further therapy, whereas others require intermittent injections of IVIgG to maintain safe platelet counts (351). However, approximately one-fourth of children become refractory to treatment (351). Cost-effectiveness analysis demonstrates a lower cost for young children (<6 years of age) treated with maintenance IVIgG than with splenectomy (352). In recent years, IVIgG has been used when a rapid increase in the platelet count is required, as anti-D has advantages for maintenance therapy of chronic ITP (353).

Anti-D. Anti-D also is effective in raising the platelet count in most Rh-positive children with chronic ITP, and some children have a long-term response. Benefit is usually transient, with a median duration ranging from 3 to 5 weeks (354–356). Anti-D also can be effective as maintenance therapy for chronic

ITP (355–357), thereby avoiding splenectomy (356,357); its advantages over IVIgG for this purpose include comparable efficacy, lower cost, greater ease of administration, and, possibly, less tachyphylaxis.

Splenectomy. Approximately 75% of children have a complete remission after splenectomy (316,344,358). Laparoscopic splenectomy is feasible in infants and children and leads to shorter length of stay (359). The long-term risk of postsplenectomy septicemia (prevaccination era) in children with ITP is approximately 8%, with a case mortality rate of 15% (overall 1% mortality) (360). This risk appears to be even greater in the subgroup of children younger than 3 years (360). Because of the risks of postsplenectomy septicemia, the possibility of late spontaneous remission of the ITP, and the frequent efficacy of intermittent maintenance therapy with IVIgG or anti-D, splenectomy should not be performed in very young children with chronic ITP. Children should receive *H. influenzae* type B vaccine and, if older than 2 years, polyvalent pneumococcal vaccine and quadrivalent meningococcal vaccine at least 2 weeks before elective splenectomy (164,361). Prophylactic oral penicillin V (125 mg twice daily for children younger than 5 years and 250 mg twice daily for children 5 years and older) is also recommended for at least 1 year after splenectomy (361). Although platelet count response to IVIgG and splenectomy are correlated, some children who had poor responses to IVIgG nevertheless have favorable postsplenectomy platelet count responses (362).

Vinca Alkaloids and Immunosuppressive Agents. Treatment results with vinca alkaloids and immunosuppressive agents are variable but generally poor (358,363), and this form of treatment should be restricted to the most severely affected patients.

Systemic Lupus Erythematosus

Thrombocytopenia occurs at some time in 15% to 25% of patients with SLE. Platelet antibodies can be detected in most patients with SLE (364–366), although some patients with increased PAIgG are not thrombocytopenic. Because most nonthrombocytopenic patients with SLE have normal platelet lifespans (367), it is possible that the hypergammaglobulinemia that often complicates SLE impairs phagocytic cell function, preventing the destruction of the IgG-sensitized platelets (229,368).

Mechanisms for thrombocytopenia include platelet glycoprotein-reactive autoantibodies (366), β_2-gpI–containing (and other platelet-reactive) immune complexes (369,370), and hypersplenism, among others. Additionally, the presence of antiphospholipid antibodies, which frequently are found in the sera of SLE patients, has been correlated with thrombocytopenia and thrombosis (371,372). Antiphospholipid antibodies can bind to platelets after perturbation of their membranes, suggesting that these antibodies may bind preferentially to activated platelets (373). Whether such antibodies contribute to *in vivo* platelet activation in SLE or the antiphospholipid antibody syndrome remains uncertain.

Several thrombocytopenic syndromes occur in patients with SLE. In some patients, thrombocytopenia is chronic, mimicking ITP; in others, acute thrombocytopenia complicates systemic flares of the lupus (374). In others with antiphospholipid antibodies, thrombosis rather than bleeding predominates despite thrombocytopenia; sometimes, thrombosis or widespread organ failure suggests the term *catastrophic antiphospholipid antibody syndrome* (375). Rarely, patients with SLE develop an illness that closely resembles TTP and that may be benefited by plasma exchange (376).

MANAGEMENT OF THROMBOCYTOPENIA

Management of thrombocytopenia complicating SLE and ITP is similar, except that in the former, we recommend that danazol be tried before splenectomy. Corticosteroids are the initial therapy. Prednisone usually is effective, but tapering with a view to discontinuing the drug is complicated by the high rate of thrombocytopenic relapse. Long-term use of low doses of corticosteroids may be justified, however, particularly if the drug also achieves control of other symptoms of the SLE.

Splenectomy probably is as effective in achieving platelet count remission in SLE as in ITP (377). However, as there may be a relatively increased risk of postsplenectomy infections in this immunocompromised population (378), and because danazol may be particularly effective in rheumatologic disorders complicated by immune thrombocytopenia (379–381), we prefer a trial of danazol (200 to 1200 mg/day) before splenectomy. Several weeks of treatment may be needed before benefit is seen. However, danazol usually must be continued at least in small doses to maintain the platelet count at safe levels.

For patients refractory to danazol and splenectomy, more aggressive therapies include azathioprine, intermittent pulse cyclophosphamide (382), plasmapheresis synchronized with pulse cyclophosphamide (383), and cyclosporine (384,385). High-dose IVIgG may be useful in a bleeding patient to increase the platelet count transiently.

ANTIPHOSPHOLIPID ANTIBODY SYNDROME

Thrombocytopenia can occur as part of the antiphospholipid antibody syndrome, which also has been termed the *lupus anticoagulant syndrome*. These patients often suffer from recurrent arterial or venous thrombosis rather than bleeding. Other associated abnormalities include recurrent miscarriages, thromboembolic pulmonary hypertension, cardiac valvulitis or cardiomyopathy, adrenal failure, and neurologic disturbances, including strokes and transient ischemic attacks, migraine, and chorea (386,387). Associated dermatologic manifestations include livedo reticularis, Raynaud's phenomenon, leg ulcers, symmetric gangrene of the fingers and toes, and acral microlivedo (nonblanching erythematous or cyanotic macules located on the palms, soles, fingertips, or toes) (388–390). Although frequent in patients with SLE, the antiphospholipid antibody syndrome can occur as a primary disorder (391).

The *sine qua non* of diagnosis is the laboratory demonstration of antiphospholipid antibodies (392). These polyclonal antibodies can often be detected by their ability to prolong phospholipid-dependent clotting tests (lupus anticoagulant), or with solid-phase assays using negatively charged phospholipid target antigens (e.g., anticardiolipin antibody assay), or, sometimes, by a biologic false-positive VDRL result. These antiphospholipid antibodies have been shown to react with negatively charged phospholipids such as cardiolipin or phosphatidylserine in the presence of a plasma protein cofactor, β_2-gpI. The protein cofactor antigen target for antibodies with lupus anticoagulant activity can also be β_2-gpI, as well as prothrombin, protein C, protein S, and other factors (392).

A cross-sectional study showed evidence of elevated baseline thrombin generation in SLE patients with anticardiolipin antibodies (393). Perhaps enhancement of platelet activation by antiphospholipid antibodies contributes to hypercoagulability (394). However, no laboratory features reliably predict thrombosis. Thus, long-term anticoagulant therapy, antiplatelet therapy, or both are recommended for patients who have already developed thrombosis. Corticosteroids may sometimes worsen clinical manifestations in these patients (395).

Thrombocytopenia Complicating Other Immune Disorders

Immune thrombocytopenia can complicate other disorders of immune dysregulation, including autoimmune hemolysis [the combination is called *Evans' syndrome* (396)], rheumatoid arthritis (397,398), dermatomyositis (399), progressive systemic sclerosis (400), localized scleroderma (401), Sjögren's syndrome (402), Graves' disease (403), Hashimoto's thyroiditis (404), pernicious anemia (397), sarcoidosis (405,406), myasthenia gravis (407,408), inflammatory bowel disease (409,410), celiac disease (411), primary biliary cirrhosis (412), autoimmune hyperchylomicronemia (413), and bullous pemphigoid (414). However, antiplatelet autoantibodies using newer glycoprotein-specific assays have been demonstrated in only some of these disorders (407,408).

The approach to treatment should parallel considerations given for the treatment of primary ITP. However, for some of these conditions (e.g., Evans' syndrome), the thrombocytopenia may be less responsive to first-line treatment (corticosteroids and splenectomy) (396).

Neoplasia-Associated Immune Thrombocytopenia

Immune thrombocytopenia can precede, accompany, or follow neoplastic disease (415), particularly the chronic lymphoproliferative syndromes (416–429). Immune thrombocytopenia occurs in 2% to 3% of patients with chronic lymphocytic leukemia (421–423) and in a few with plasma cell disorders (424,425). Conversely, in a series of more than 500 patients with clinical and laboratory evidence for immune thrombocytopenia, 15% had associated neoplastic lymphoproliferative disorders (397). Autoantibodies against the gpIIb-IIIa complex have been demonstrated in patients with lymphoma (408,420).

Immune thrombocytopenia has been estimated to occur in 1% to 2% of patients with Hodgkin's disease (416–418). The immune thrombocytopenia is often not related to the neoplastic disease activity, and the occurrence of immune thrombocytopenia in a patient who is thought to be cured of the Hodgkin's disease does not necessarily mean that the illness has relapsed (418).

Thrombocytopenia occurs commonly in patients with clonal proliferation of large granular lymphocytes (LGLs) (426–430). One such disorder of CD3⁺ T cells, known as *T-LGL leukemia* (formerly *T-chronic lymphocytic leukemia* or *Tγ-lymphoproliferative disease*), is characterized by lymphocytosis, splenomegaly, hepatomegaly, pancytopenia, and associated risk for autoimmune disorders (e.g., rheumatoid arthritis). The clonal proliferation itself is usually indolent, and the major threat to the patient is bacterial infection related to the severity of the neutropenia. Thrombocytopenia may be explained by autoimmune mechanisms, hypersplenism, or both. Much less common is a disorder of natural killer cells (NK-LGL leukemia) that generally exhibits a more acute clinical course, with marked hepatosplenectomegaly, often severe pancytopenia, and frequent multiorgan failure and death within months of diagnosis (429). A more indolent form of this disorder has been reported in association with what otherwise appears to have been typical ITP that failed to respond to splenectomy (430).

TREATMENT OF THROMBOCYTOPENIA
Often, the thrombocytopenia represents less of a risk to the patient than the underlying malignancy, and the first step in the treatment of these patients is management of the underlying disorder. In some patients, the thrombocytopenia resolves as the malignancy responds to therapy, whereas in others, the thrombocytopenia requires specific treatment. The approach to treatment is similar to the treatment of patients with chronic ITP (i.e., corticosteroids followed by splenectomy). One study (416) that reviewed the literature on immune thrombocytopenia complicating Hodgkin's disease concluded that 30% of patients responded to corticosteroids, whereas 75% benefited from splenectomy.

Thrombocytopenia complicating chronic lymphoproliferative disease can also be caused by marrow infiltration with tumor or by effects of therapy. Sometimes, all these processes coexist. A bone marrow examination is often required to determine treatment. Thrombocytopenia occurring in the setting of a nonlymphoproliferative malignancy is much more likely to be caused by nonimmune mechanisms, such as marrow replacement by tumor, marrow suppression by chemotherapy, or DIC.

Human Immunodeficiency Virus–Associated Immune Thrombocytopenia

Thrombocytopenia occurs in approximately 10% to 15% of asymptomatic HIV carriers and 30% to 40% of patients with acquired immune deficiency syndrome. Much less commonly, other retroviruses may also cause thrombocytopenia, for example, infection with human T-cell leukemia virus type I (431).

Increased levels of PAIgG, PAIgM, and platelet-bound complement are present in most cases of HIV-associated thrombocytopenia (432). These levels are often higher than in classic ITP. Two types of platelet antibody have been described: (a) immune complexes consisting of anti-HIV antibodies and anti-F(ab')₂ antibodies (anti-antibodies) (433,434) and (b) platelet-reactive autoantibodies (435). There is evidence (436,437) that some anti-HIV antibodies cross-react with gpIIb-IIIa. Immune complexes containing IgM antiidiotype antibodies may explain the paradox of high levels of PAIgG and PAIgM but low levels of serum platelet-reactive antibodies in this disorder (438).

Besides immune platelet destruction, there are many other ways that infection with HIV can cause thrombocytopenia (439), including impaired platelet production secondary to HIV infection of megakaryocytes, drug-induced myelosuppression (commonly, zidovudine, ganciclovir, and trimethoprim and sulfamethoxazole), HIV-associated thrombotic microangiopathy, hypersplenism, and marrow infiltration by tumor or opportunistic infections. Platelet kinetic studies have revealed a complex interaction of impaired platelet production, increased platelet destruction, and predominant splenic platelet sequestration or destruction (440,441).

Although a reduction in T-helper cells is usually observed, patients with normal lymphocyte numbers and thrombocytopenia have also been described (442). The finding of reduced numbers of T-helper cells is more frequent in adults than in children with HIV-associated thrombocytopenia (443). The occurrence of thrombocytopenia does not increase the risk for progression to a more advanced stage of HIV infection (444), and in some cases, the thrombocytopenia spontaneously disappears.

TREATMENT OF THROMBOCYTOPENIA
Anti-HIV therapy, for example, with the antiretroviral agent zidovudine (also known as *azidothymidine*), increases the platelet count in patients with HIV-associated thrombocytopenia, often within the first 2 weeks of therapy (445–447). For patients refractory to zidovudine, interferon-α can be effective (448). More recently, highly active antiretroviral therapy, typically consisting of two nucleoside analogs in conjunction with an HIT protease inhibitor or a nonnucleoside reverse transcriptase inhibitor, has improved survival of HIV-infected patients (449); such regimens also raise the platelet counts in thrombocytopenic patients (450).

Most patients do not require specific therapy for their thrombocytopenia. For patients with symptomatic thrombocytopenia, however, the treatment approach is similar to that for primary ITP. Approximately 75% of patients respond to a course of corticosteroids, with the platelet count rising above 100×10^9/L in half the responders. However, an adequate platelet count is maintained after tapering or stopping the prednisone in only 20% of the patients (451). Complications of prednisone include oral candidiasis and reactivation of oral and genital herpes. Some physicians avoid using corticosteroids because of the potential risk for infections in this patient population (452).

RE blockade with IVIgG (451,453) or anti-D (252,261) is often effective in transiently raising the platelet count. Particularly in children, HIV-associated thrombocytopenia has been successfully managed for lengthy periods with repeated injections of IVIgG (454) or anti-D (261). As in primary ITP, only Rh-positive, nonsplenectomized individuals respond to anti-D (261).

Splenectomy is as effective in achieving long-term remission for HIV-associated thrombocytopenia as it is in primary ITP (451,455,456). Humoral immunity is impaired in HIV patients, and some physicians administer long-term penicillin prophylaxis (in addition to routine preoperative vaccinations). Splenectomy does not accelerate and may even reduce (457) the rate of progression to acquired immune deficiency syndrome among HIV-infected patients.

Other treatments that occasionally benefit patients with HIV-associated thrombocytopenia include danazol (451) and dapsone (458). There are conflicting data about whether low-dose splenic irradiation is useful in this patient population (459,460).

Transplantation-Associated Immune Thrombocytopenia

Early severe thrombocytopenia caused by marrow ablative therapy is a universal consequence of bone marrow transplantation (BMT). Several syndromes of isolated thrombocytopenia that occur later in the posttransplant course of allogeneic or autologous bone marrow transplantation have been described, including transient benign thrombocytopenia (461); chronic, persistent thrombocytopenia (461,462); and late-onset thrombocytopenia due to autoimmune or alloimmune mechanisms (463–466). Occasionally, dramatic immune thrombocytopenic syndromes occur soon after solid organ transplantation (467–469).

TRANSIENT BENIGN THROMBOCYTOPENIA AFTER BONE MARROW TRANSPLANTATION
In transient benign thrombocytopenia, the platelet count recovery after transplantation is initially normal, with a rise in the platelet count to above 100×10^9/L. These patients then become thrombocytopenic before day 50, with subsequent platelet count recovery before day 70 (461). The incidence of transient benign thrombocytopenia is approximately 15%, and it usually is not serious.

CHRONIC PERSISTENT THROMBOCYTOPENIA AFTER BONE MARROW TRANSPLANTATION
Patients with chronic persistent thrombocytopenia do not develop a platelet count greater than 100×10^9/L during the first 2 to 4 months after transplantation (461). This complication, which has an incidence of approximately 25% (461), is frequently associated with acute or chronic graft-versus-host disease and has a poor prognosis (461,462).

POSTTRANSPLANT AUTOIMMUNE OR ALLOIMMUNE THROMBOCYTOPENIA
Rarely, isolated thrombocytopenia secondary to autoimmune or alloimmune mechanisms can develop several months after BMT or solid organ transplantation. An ITP-like syndrome after BMT could be caused by autoantibodies produced by donor lymphocytes reactive against donor platelets. Pathogenic factors could include transient immune system dysregulation

accompanying donor immune engraftment (463) or graft-versus-host disease (461,462,464). Rarely, late-onset thrombocytopenia is caused by *allo*antibodies, for example, anti-Pl^A1 or anti-Br^a alloantibodies produced by residual host lymphoid cells in a Pl^A1-negative or Br^a-negative recipient that react against the corresponding alloantigen-positive platelets derived from donor cells (465,466).

Rarely, immunocompetent lymphoid cells within a transplanted solid organ cause severe autoimmune (467,468) or alloimmune (469) thrombocytopenia soon after transplantation. For example, all three recipients of solid organs (two kidney, one liver) developed severe alloimmune thrombocytopenia and bleeding within a week after transplantation from a multiparous female donor (469). The two renal transplant recipients' thrombocytopenia was refractory to high-dose IVIgG and platelet transfusions: One patient died, and the other recovered postsplenectomy. The liver transplant recipient developed platelet count recovery when he received a new liver allograft. Even though the platelet donor had normal platelet counts, her serum as well as the posttransplant recipients' sera contained anti-Pl^A1 alloantibodies. Thus, "passenger" immunocompetent lymphoid cells occasionally induce severe alloimmune thrombocytopenia when introduced into an alloincompatible environment.

TREATMENT OF THROMBOCYTOPENIA
Treatment is based on the severity and cause of the thrombocytopenia; therefore, the clinician needs to determine whether the posttransplant thrombocytopenia is caused by drugs [e.g., sulfamethoxazole, trimethoprim (461)], graft rejection (462), relapse of underlying disease (462), or a complicating infection (462). Immune thrombocytopenia could be self-limited (e.g., transient benign thrombocytopenia). Chronic, persistent thrombocytopenia associated with graft-versus-host disease sometimes responds favorably to increased immunosuppressive maneuvers, but most therapy is ineffective (462). Late-onset thrombocytopenia caused by autoimmune or alloimmune mechanisms usually responds to corticosteroids, IVIgG, and splenectomy.

Drug-Induced Thrombocytopenia

Thrombocytopenia is a common and potentially serious complication of drug therapy (470–476). Drugs usually cause thrombocytopenia by impaired platelet production or immune platelet destruction. Miscellaneous causes of drug-induced thrombocytopenia include drug-induced platelet activation [hematin (477), nonimmune heparin-associated thrombocytopenia (478)] or agglutination [ristocetin (479), porcine factor VIII (480)], drug-induced reticuloendothelial sequestration of platelets [protamine sulfate (481)], or drug-induced liver disease with secondary hypersplenism [α-methyldopa, methotrexate, vinyl chloride monomer (482)].

Impaired platelet production most frequently is caused by drugs with predictable, dose-dependent cytotoxicity, such as anticancer chemotherapy. However, some drugs, such as chloramphenicol, phenylbutazone, and gold, cause severe marrow suppression only in susceptible people. Although most drugs that cause thrombocytopenia through marrow suppression damage the hematopoietic stem cell and produce pancytopenia, some agents, such as alcohol, primarily inhibit megakaryocyte production and cause isolated thrombocytopenia.

Approximately 20% to 50% of patients treated with valproic acid (an antiepileptic agent) develop mild thrombocytopenia that was once thought to involve idiosyncratic (immune) mechanisms based on elevated PAIgG levels (483). This mechanism of thrombocytopenia remains unknown but may involved direct effects on the megakaryocyte, because the risk of thrombocytopenia correlates strongly with serum concentrations of a valproic acid metabolite (484). Amrinone (a cardiac inotropic agent) also causes generally mild thrombocytopenia in relation to levels of its metabolite, N-acetylamrinone (485).

Immune mechanisms are an important explanation for thrombocytopenia that occurs unexpectedly and unpredictably in a (usually small) minority of patients who receive the drug (idiosyncratic reaction). Five syndromes with distinct clinical profiles and pathogenesis are discussed here.

1. *HIT* is characterized by mild to moderate thrombocytopenia that typically begins 5 to 10 days after starting heparin and is caused by antibodies (usually IgG) that recognize via their Fab regions complexes of PF4 bound to heparin. The resulting immune complexes composed of IgG–PF4–heparin lead to platelet activation by occupancy of platelet Fc receptors, mediated by the Fc moieties of the HIT-IgG.
2. *Drug-induced immune thrombocytopenic purpura (DITP)* is characterized by the onset of severe thrombocytopenia and mucocutaneous hemorrhage that begins a week or more (sometimes, several weeks, months, or years) after starting the implicated drug. DITP is caused by IgG antibodies that bind via their Fab regions to drug–platelet glycoprotein complex, with platelet clearance effected by removal of IgG-sensitized platelets by the macrophages of the reticuloendothelial system. Many drugs can cause DITP, particularly quinine, quinidine, sulfonamides, rifampin, and vancomycin.
3. *Abciximab and other gpIIb-IIIa inhibitors* can cause abrupt-onset (within hours) severe thrombocytopenia, even in patients who have never previously received one of these agents. The explanation may be that preexisting anti–gpIIb-IIIa autoantibodies become pathogenic when the structure of gpIIb-IIIa is altered by abciximab or another gpIIb-IIIa blocking agent.
4. *Drug-induced autoimmune thrombocytopenia* refers to the onset of a disorder clinically indistinguishable from acute or chronic ITP that is believed to have been initiated by a drug. Agents that may cause this syndrome include gold, procainamide, and the measles–mumps–rubella vaccine.
5. *Drug-induced TTP or hemolytic-uremic syndrome (HUS)* refers to the condition when a drug such as quinine or ticlopidine produces a clinical syndrome that resembles one of the microangiopathic hemolytic disorders.

CRITERIA FOR ESTABLISHING DRUG-INDUCED IMMUNE THROMBOCYTOPENIA
A drug can be implicated definitively as causing idiosyncratic thrombocytopenia if the following criteria are met (470,471): (a) the thrombocytopenia develops while the patient is receiving the drug and resolves after the drug is stopped; (b) the putative drug was the only drug used before onset of thrombocytopenia, or other drugs were continued or reintroduced with a sustained normal platelet count; (c) other causes of thrombocytopenia are excluded; and (d) the thrombocytopenia recurs after readministration of the drug (*in vivo* challenge). Readministration is potentially dangerous, however, and confirmation of the diagnosis is best achieved, if possible, by (e) *in vitro* techniques. However, whereas some tests for drug-induced thrombocytopenia are very useful clinically [e.g., testing for HIT (486)], tests for many other putative drug-induced thrombocytopenic disorders are relatively insensitive, perhaps because the tests are performed without the drug metabolite that actually forms the antigen (487–489).

FREQUENCY AND CLINICAL IMPACT OF DRUG-INDUCED IMMUNE THROMBOCYTOPENIA
The clinical importance of drugs causing immune thrombocytopenia depends on the frequency with which the drug is prescribed, the risk for idiosyncratic thrombocytopenia associated with the drug, and the clinical impact of the thrombocytopenic syndrome, including the temporal course, severity, and complications.

Some drugs cause immune-mediated thrombocytopenia more commonly than others. For example, HIT occurs in 3% to 5% of patients who receive prophylactic-dose unfractionated heparin (UFH) for 1 to 2 weeks after orthopedic surgery (486,490,491). Surprisingly, the risk of this complication is 1% or lower in medical patients receiving heparin (491), possibly because of differences in levels of plasma PF4 (the coantigen of HIT) between medical and surgical patients. Heparins themselves differ in their risk of causing HIT: UFH of bovine lung origin is more immunogenic than UFH derived from porcine intestine (491); low-molecular-weight heparins (LMWHs) are still less immunogenic than UFH (approximately fivefold to tenfold lower risk of HIT) (490,491). Paradoxically, patients with HIT are at greatly increased risk of venous and arterial thrombosis (490,491), despite their thrombocytopenia and their receipt of the anticoagulant, heparin.

In contrast, DITP is generally very rare, occurring, for example, in approximately 1 in 1000 patients who receive quinine or quinidine (492) and in 1 in 15,000 to 25,000 patients treated with trimethoprim and sulfamethoxazole (472,492). Quinine may be taken by nonprescription routes [e.g., tonic water, filler in street drugs (493), and so forth]; therefore, exposure may be difficult to establish by history. In contrast, certain atypical DITP syndromes may be more common. For example, gold-induced (auto)immune thrombocytopenia occurs in 1% to 3% of patients (494). Atypical (abrupt-onset) immune thrombocytopenia occurs in approximately 0.5% to 1.0% of patients treated with the gpIIb-IIIa blocking agent abciximab (476). In contrast to patients with HIT, patients with typical or atypical DITP are at increased risk for bleeding rather than thrombosis.

HEPARIN-INDUCED THROMBOCYTOPENIA
Heparin is a heterogeneous and polydisperse mixture of glycosaminoglycans comprised of alternating substituted uronic acid and glucosamine saccharide units (495). Standard preparations are extracted from bovine lung or porcine intestinal mucosa and have a mean molecular weight ranging from 10 to 20 kd. Low-molecular-weight preparations usually are created by chemical or physical manipulations of the standard preparations.

Heparin acts as an antithrombotic agent by catalyzing the inactivation of several procoagulant serine proteases (e.g., thrombin, factor Xa) by antithrombin (formerly, antithrombin III). Heparin also binds to platelets in a specific and saturable fashion and can cause weak platelet activation and aggregation (478). Heparin also prolongs the bleeding time (496). These nonidiosyncratic interactions of heparin with platelets are of uncertain clinical relevance.

In contrast, a minority of patients who receive heparin develop a syndrome characterized by significant *in vivo* platelet activation that typically begins 5 to 10 days after beginning heparin therapy (497,498). Despite a low (or falling) platelet count and the administration of heparin, at least half of these patients develop venous or arterial thrombosis (490,491,497–499).

Pathogenesis. HIT is caused by platelet-activating IgG that develops during treatment with heparin (99). For most patients, the antigen is composed of multimolecular complexes of PF4 bound to heparin (500–502). Recent studies suggest that HIT antibodies recognize one or more regions on PF4 that have been conformationally modified by being bound to heparin (82,503,504). Two other observations support such a key role for PF4 and a more nonspecific role for heparin: (a) certain nonheparin (but negatively charged) substances, such as polysulfated chondroitin sulfate (Arteparon) (505) or pentosan polysulfate (506), can cause

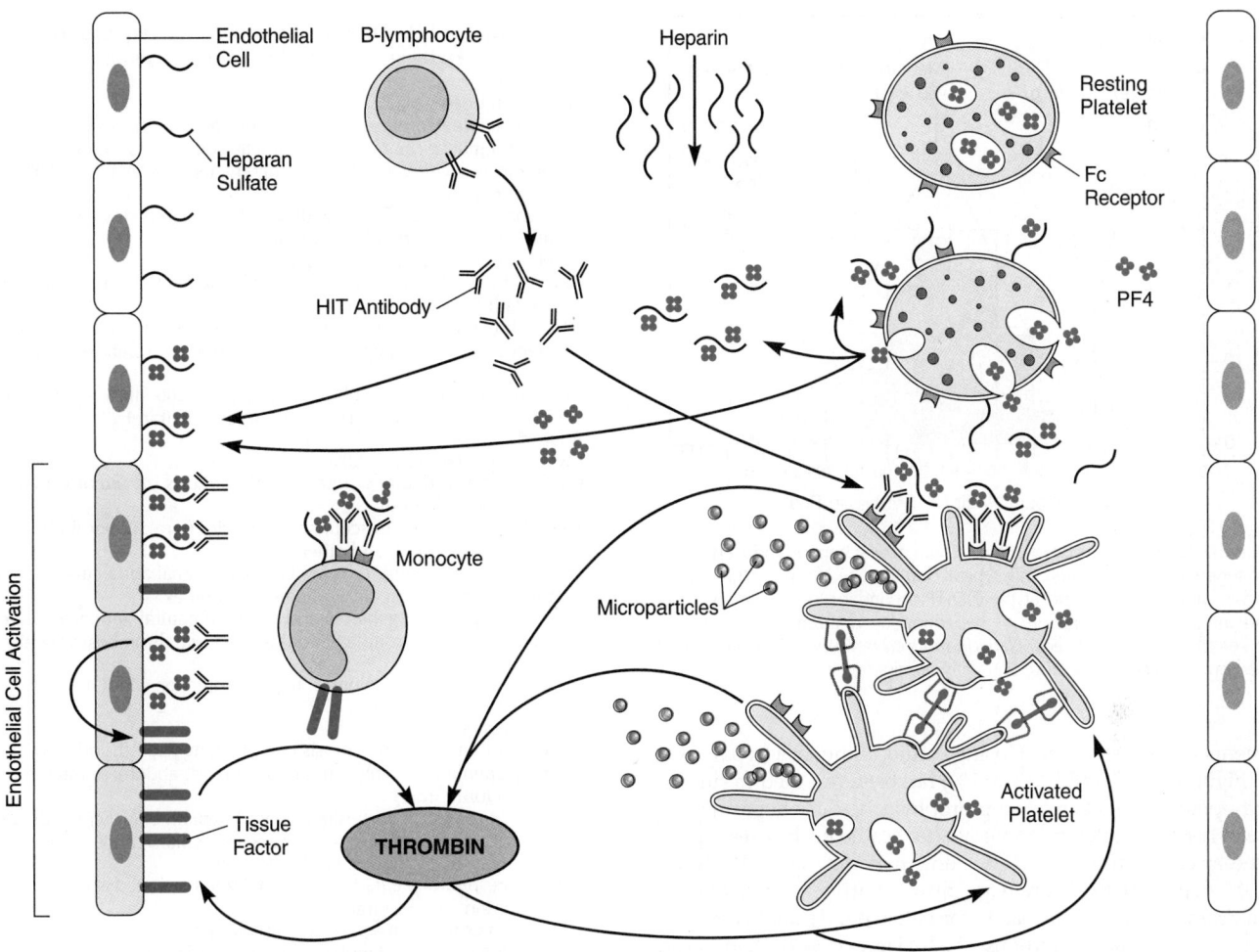

Figure 32-5. Pathogenesis of heparin-induced thrombocytopenia (HIT): a central role for thrombin generation. PF4, platelet factor 4. (From Greinacher A, Warkentin TE. Treatment of heparin-induced thrombocytopenia: an overview. In: Warkentin TE, Greinacher A, eds. *Heparin-induced thrombocytopenia*, 2nd ed. New York: Marcel Dekker, 2001:291, with permission.)

a clinical syndrome identical to HIT, with identical serologic findings, and that will be exacerbated if heparin is administered; and (b) PF4 bound to polyvinylsulfonate (a linear polyanion lacking both the saccharides and sulfate groups characteristic of heparin) can be used to test for HIT antibodies (507).

After formation of PF4–heparin–IgG immune complexes on the platelet surface (*in situ* immune complexes), platelet activation occurs via binding of the IgG Fc moieties to the platelet FcγIIa receptors (99,100). HIT-IgG is a potent platelet activation stimulus, as shown by its ability to effect thromboxane production by platelets (508) and also to cause granule release from washed platelets (99). This is a dynamic process, in which initial small amounts of PF4 release from platelet granules leads to amplification of the platelet activation process (100). Neutralization of heparin's anticoagulant action by PF4 also contributes to the prothrombotic diathesis. Additionally, platelet activation by HIT-IgG stimulates the generation of platelet-derived microparticles with procoagulant activity (509,510). Besides activating platelets, HIT antibodies also can cause activation of endothelial cells (501,511,512) and monocytes (513), with tissue factor expression by these cells. These procoagulant events explain why markers of *in vivo* thrombin generation (e.g., thrombin-antithrombin complexes) are greatly elevated in patients with HIT (514–516) (Fig. 32-5).

Only a minority of patients who form HIT antibodies during heparin therapy develop HIT (486,490,491). Differences in anti-

body titer (517), affinity for PF4 (518), or platelet-activating potential (486,518) could explain differences in antibody pathogenicity. Variability in platelet FcγIIA receptor numbers (519) or an FcγIIa Arg-His polymorphism (520) may explain some of the differences in severity of thrombocytopenia and clinical outcomes as well.

Clinical Features. For approximately 70% of patients, the thrombocytopenia generally begins 5 to 10 days after starting heparin therapy ("typical-onset" of HIT); in the remaining 30% of patients, however, thrombocytopenia is recognized when the platelet count falls abruptly after beginning a course of heparin (497). For this latter group of patients with "rapid-onset" of HIT, there invariably has been recent exposure to heparin, that is, within the past 100 days (497). This temporal profile of HIT likely is explained by the transient nature of HIT antibodies, which tend to become undetectable 50 to 85 days after an episode of HIT, depending on the assay used (497). Thus, rapid onset of HIT occurs when a patient is given heparin who already has circulating HIT antibodies that were formed in relation to use of heparin within the recent past. Otherwise, among patients who do not have detectable HIT antibodies at baseline—regardless of whether they have previously been exposed to heparin—the temporal profile of HIT is the same (i.e., generally, 5 to 10 days after starting heparin).

Although HIT can complicate heparin given in any dose and by any route, the highest risk for HIT antibody formation is in

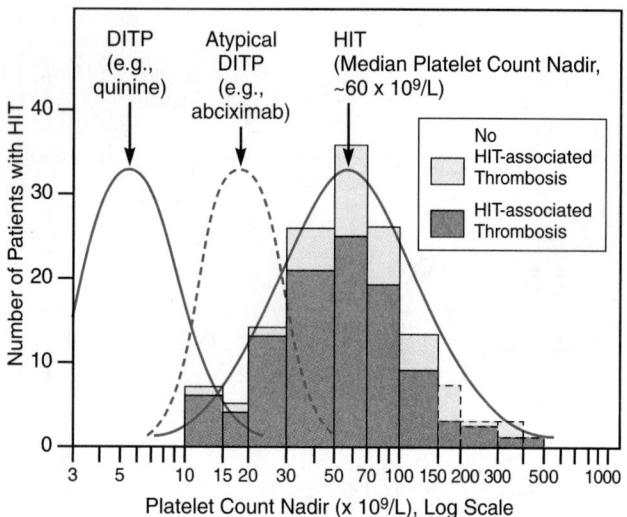

Figure 32-6. A comparison of platelet count nadirs: heparin-induced thrombocytopenia (HIT) compared with typical drug-induced immune thrombocytopenic purpura (DITP) and atypical DITP secondary to abciximab. (From Warkentin TE. Clinical picture of heparin-induced thrombocytopenia. In: Warkentin, Greinacher A, eds. *Heparin-induced thrombocytopenia*, 2nd ed. New York: Marcel Dekker, 2001:43, wtih permission.)

patients after heart surgery using cardiopulmonary bypass, and the highest risk for HIT (3% to 5%) has been reported in surgical (orthopedic) patients receiving prophylactic-dose heparin (486). Use of heparin-coated pulmonary artery catheters has been implicated as contributing to HIT in some patients (491,521). Even a brief, small-dose exposure (e.g., intraoperative "flushing" of an intraarterial catheter) can lead to formation of HIT antibodies with the potential to cause rapid-onset HIT if larger doses of heparin are given 1 or 2 weeks later (522). Rarely, a relatively short exposure to heparin can lead to onset of HIT beginning several days—and potentially presenting with thrombosis and persisting thrombocytopenia several weeks—after discontinuation of heparin (delayed onset of HIT) (523).

In contrast to DITP caused by quinine, quinidine, or sulfa drugs, very severe thrombocytopenia (platelet count below $10 \times 10^9/L$) is rare in HIT (498,499,524) (Fig. 32-6). The median platelet count nadir in patients with HIT is approximately 50 to $60 \times 10^9/L$. For approximately 10% to 15%, the platelet count nadir never falls below $150 \times 10^9/L$, usually because HIT occurred in a postoperative setting already characterized by elevated or rising platelet counts before the episode of HIT (498). Although the risk of HIT-associated thrombosis is approximately 90% in HIT patients with very severe thrombocytopenia, the risk is approximately 50% even in patients with mild thrombocytopenia (524). Indeed, a drop in the platelet count of 50% or more, even when the platelet count nadir remains above $150 \times 10^9/L$, can be associated with thrombotic complications (525,526).

Table 32-2 lists the thrombotic and other clinical sequelae of HIT (498). Venous thromboembolism occurs most commonly: Approximately 25% and 50% of HIT patients develop symptomatic pulmonary embolism and deep venous thrombosis, respectively. Arterial thrombosis is also relatively common (10% to 15% of patients), although the typical localization of arterial thrombosis in HIT (limb artery thrombosis > thrombotic stroke > myocardial infarction) is the converse of that seen in the general population. The nature of thrombotic complications typically depends on other patient-dependent factors. For example, postoperative orthopedic patients have a marked preponderance of venous thrombotic complications, whereas patients with arteriopathy develop arterial and

TABLE 32-2. Thrombotic and Other Sequelae of Heparin-Induced Thrombocytopenia

Venous thrombosis
  DVT (50%): new, progressive, recurrent; lower limb (often bilateral); upper limb (at site of venous catheter); phlegmasia cerulea dolens
  Coumarin-induced venous limb gangrene (approximately 5–10% of DVT treated with warfarin)
  Pulmonary embolism (25%) with or without right-sided cardiac intra-atrial or intraventricular thrombi
  Cerebral dural sinus thrombosis (rare)
  Adrenal hemorrhagic infarction (rare): bilateral (acute or chronic adrenal failure) or unilateral
  DIC with hypofibrinogenemia and acquired natural anticoagulant deficiency causing multiple venous and arterial thromboses (rare)
Arterial thrombosis
  Aortic or iliofemoral thrombosis resulting in acute limb ischemia or infarction (5–10%) or spinal cord infarction (rare)
  Acute thrombotic stroke (3–5%)
  Myocardial infarction (3–5%)
  Cardiac intraventricular or intraatrial thrombosis [*in situ* or via embolization of DVT (rare)]
  Thrombosis involving miscellaneous arteries (rare): upper limb, renal, mesenteric, spinal, and other arteries
  Embolization of thrombus from heart or proximal aorta can also contribute to microvascular ischemic syndromes
  DIC with hypofibrinogenemia and acquired natural anticoagulant deficiency causing multiple venous and arterial thromboses (rare)
Miscellaneous
  Heparin-induced skin lesions at heparin injection sites (10–20%)
    Erythematous plaques
    Skin necrosis
  Coumarin-induced skin necrosis complicating heparin-induced thrombocytopenia involving central sites (breast, abdomen, thigh, leg, and so forth) (rare)
  Acute systemic reactions postintravenous heparin bolus (approximately 25% of sensitized patients who receive an intravenous heparin bolus)
    Inflammatory, e.g., fever, chills, flushing
    Cardiorespiratory, e.g., tachycardia, hypertension, dyspnea; cardiopulmonary arrest (rare)
    Gastrointestinal: nausea, vomiting, diarrhea
    Neurologic: transient global amnesia, headache

DIC, disseminated intravascular coagulation; DVT, deep vein thrombosis.
Reprinted from Warkentin TE. Clinical picture of heparin-induced thrombocytopenia. In: Warkentin TE, Greinacher A, eds. *Heparin-induced thrombocytopenia*, 2nd ed. New York: Marcel Dekker, 2001:43–86, with permission.

venous thrombosis in equal proportions (491). Cerebral vein (dural sinus) thrombosis can complicate HIT (527) and typically presents with persisting headache and progressive neurologic symptoms and signs. Current or recent use of a central venous catheter is an important factor in influencing localization of upper-limb deep vein thrombosis in patients with HIT (528).

Several limb ischemic syndromes can complicate HIT. Limb arterial thrombosis, for example, involving distal aorta or iliofemoral arteries, can cause acute arterial thrombosis with platelet-rich thrombi ("white clots") with a resultant high risk for limb gangrene (498). Also common is the syndrome of warfarin-induced venous limb gangrene: These patients develop progression of deep vein thrombosis to phlegmasia cerulea dolens (an "inflamed, blue, painful" limb) before acral necrosis ranging from distal sloughing of fingers or toes to extensive necrosis leading to above-knee or arm amputation (514). This iatrogenic syndrome is caused by profound imbalance in procoagulant and anticoagulant mechanisms during warfarin therapy—that is, warfarin fails to down-regulate the marked thrombin generation associated with acute HIT, whereas it is able to lead to profound depletion of the vitamin K–dependent natural anticoagulant, protein C (514). Paradoxically, patients with warfarin-induced venous limb gangrene typically have *supra*therapeutic international normalized ratio (INR) values (>4.0) concomitant with onset of limb necrosis, likely because severe reduction in factor VII activity parallels the reduction in protein C (514,529). Rarely, patients with HIT developed "classic" warfarin-induced necrosis—skin necrosis affecting central tissue sites such as breast, abdomen, and thigh (530).

Bleeding is relatively uncommon in patients with HIT, and is usually caused by the anticoagulant therapy used to treat HIT (497,498). There is only one characteristic hemorrhagic manifestation of HIT: adrenal hemorrhagic necrosis (498,531). However, bleeding into the adrenal gland results from preceding adrenal necrosis caused by adrenal vein thrombosis. Bilateral adrenal necrosis can cause acute or chronic adrenal insufficiency; prompt diagnosis and adrenocorticoid replacement can be life-saving. Adrenal necrosis should be suspected in patients with HIT who develop abdominal or flank pain, hypotension, or shock.

Painful skin reactions at heparin injection sites that begin 5 or more days after commencing subcutaneous heparin injections are another clinical manifestation of the HIT syndrome (498,532,533). Ranging from small erythematous plaques to large areas of dermal necrosis, these skin reactions are accompanied by thrombocytopenia in only 25% of patients, even though HIT antibodies can readily be detected even in the absence of thrombocytopenia.

Administration of an intravenous bolus heparin to a patient with circulating HIT antibodies can lead to an acute systemic reaction that begins 5 to 30 minutes after the bolus, accompanied by an abrupt fall in the platelet count (498). Characteristic symptoms and signs include fever, chills, hypertension and tachycardia, dyspnea, flushing, nausea, and vomiting. Sudden death has also been described (534). Transient global amnesia after bolus heparin administration (535) has also been reported.

Diagnostic Tests. Heparin-dependent platelet aggregation using platelet-rich plasma is probably the most common test used to diagnose HIT. However, this assay has low sensitivity and specificity (536,537). Selecting reactive platelet donors can improve test sensitivity (538). However, platelet activation assays to detect HIT antibodies are markedly improved if washed platelets are used, for example, the platelet ^{14}C-serotonin release assay (486,536,539) or the heparin-induced platelet activation assay (540,541). Generation of platelet-derived microparticles is another platelet activation endpoint that can be used (542). A characteristic feature of these assays is platelet activation in the presence of low (0.1 to 0.3 U/mL) heparin concentrations, but inhibition of activation with high heparin levels (100 U/mL) (Fig. 32-7). Diagnostic specificity is increased if an Fc receptor–blocking monoclonal antibody is used to prove that platelet activation by patient serum is mediated via the Fc receptors (536,539). There is considerable variability in the ability of donor platelets to be activated by HIT sera, however, and so quality control should include the use of both strong and weak positive control sera, as well as negative control sera (543). Acute sera from most patients with HIT produce substantial amounts of platelet activation [>80% serotonin release (486)], suggesting that diagnostic interpretation of the assay should take the magnitude of the reaction into account for diagnostic interpretation (536).

Two enzyme-immunoassays are commercially available (536,507,537): One uses PF4 bound to heparin (500), the other PF4 bound to polyvinylsulfonate (507). Although these assays may have greater sensitivity for HIT antibodies, they are more likely to detect clinically insignificant antibodies, and, therefore, have lower diagnostic specificity than the washed platelet activation assays (486,536). A rapid antigen assay that uses agglutination of red cells coated with PF4/heparin complexes is undergoing investigation (544,545).

Prevention of Heparin-Induced Thrombocytopenia. The risk for thrombocytopenia and thrombosis can be reduced by minimizing the duration of heparin exposure; by using porcine instead of

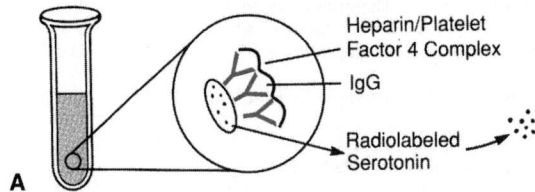

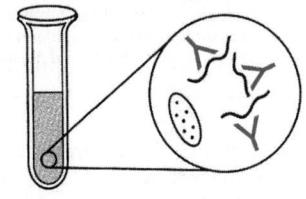

Figure 32-7. Schematic representation of the technique for testing for the presence of heparin-induced thrombocytopenia immunoglobulin G (IgG). **A:** The platelet release of radiolabeled serotonin is triggered by the binding of heparin–platelet factor 4–IgG complexes to platelet Fc receptors. **B:** High heparin concentrations displace the platelet factor 4 and IgG from the platelet surface, preventing platelet Fc receptor occupancy and platelet activation.

bovine heparin (491); and by using LMWH rather than UFH (486,490,491). LMWH is associated with both a reduced risk of formation of HIT antibodies, and possibly also a reduced risk of causing HIT (relative to UFH) when HIT antibodies are present because of preceding UFH use or generated because of use of the LMWH (486). Despite its important advantage in reducing the risk of HIT by 80% to 90%, LMWH is contraindicated as treatment for HIT (discussed subsequently). In the future, newer anticoagulant polysaccharides such as the factor Xa–binding pentasaccharide (546) or specially engineered heparin mimetics (547) may obviate the risk of HIT (495).

Prevention and Treatment of Thrombosis Complicating Heparin-Induced Thrombocytopenia. Despite recommendations that regular platelet count monitoring (at least every other day) be performed in patient populations at relatively high risk for HIT (548), there is no evidence that prompt cessation of heparin reduces the risk of thrombosis (499,549). Indeed, one study (549) showed a trend to a higher thrombotic event-rate among the patients in whom heparin was stopped within 48 hours of developing HIT, compared with patients in whom the heparin was stopped later. Several studies indicate a risk of thrombosis of 38% to 52% (including as many as 5% of patients with sudden death due to pulmonary embolism) over the first month despite stopping heparin, or substitution of heparin with warfarin (499,549). Thus, it is now recommended that physicians consider anticoagulating patients who are suspected to have "isolated HIT" (550–552), generally using an alternative anticoagulant in therapeutic doses (552). Indeed, the U.S. Food and Drug Administration approved a novel anticoagulant in 2000 (argatroban), both for the prevention and treatment of thrombosis complicating HIT; the identical (therapeutic-dose) regimen is recommended for both indications (552).

Regarding alternative anticoagulants (see Table 32-3 for doses) to prevent or treat thrombosis complicating HIT, treat-

TABLE 32-3. Anticoagulants Used to Treat Heparin-Induced Thrombocytopenia (HIT)[a]

Drug	Indications	Dose	Maintenance
Danaparoid	Therapeutic dose Prophylactic dose[d]	Loading: 2250 U bolus[b] 750 U q8h to q12h s.c.	150–200 U/h (target anti-Xa level, 0.5 to 0.8 U/mL)[c]
Lepirudin	Therapeutic dose	Loading: 0.4 mg/kg i.v. bolus	0.15 mg/kg/h i.v., adjusted to keep aPTT 1.5–2.5 × the median of the laboratory normal range[e]
Argatroban	Therapeutic dose[f]	Initial infusion rate (no bolus): 2 µg/kg/min	Infusion rate adjusted to keep aPTT 1.5–3.0 × the baseline value (not to exceed 100 sec)[e]

aPTT, activated partial thromboplastin time.

[a]Other protocols and specialized situations such as dosing in renal failure are discussed elsewhere (551–555).

[b]Adjust loading dose based on weight: 1500 U if <50 kg, 3000 U if 75 to 90 kg, 3750 U if >90 kg. After the initial bolus, some investigators administer danaparoid for 400 U/h for 4 h, then 300 U/h for 4 h before continuing at the maintenance rate (150 to 200 U/h).

[c]If preferred, after initial i.v. bolus, danaparoid can be administered s.c. (generally, 1500 U q8h to q12h); if anti-Xa measurements not available, danaparoid can still be administered safely for most patients, as there is a high probability of achieving the target anticoagulant range with this regimen and bleeding is uncommon. However, anti-Xa monitoring is recommended for very small and large patients, patients with renal failure, and patients with life-threatening or limb-threatening thrombosis.

[d]The dose indicated is most appropriate for patients with previous HIT who require prophylactic anticoagulation; for patients with acute HIT, therapeutic-dose danaparoid may be more appropriate to prevent HIT-associated thrombosis (551,552).

[e]Although aPTT monitoring is readily available, care should be taken that the patient's aPTT reflects the anticoagulant effect (e.g., the recommended aPTT range may not be appropriate if the patient's baseline aPTT is prolonged due to warfarin or liver disease).

[f]The identical dosing regimen is approved for both treatment and prevention of HIT-associated thrombosis (555).

ment options depend on availability. For example, danaparoid was withdrawn from the U.S. market in April 2002, although it remains available elsewhere (550–555).

Danaparoid sodium (Orgaran, formerly Org 10172) is a mixture of anticoagulant glycosaminoglycans (predominantly low-sulfated heparan sulfate) with predominant anti–factor Xa activity that has been used for over a decade for management of HIT (553,556). Although weak *in vitro* cross-reactivity of HIT antibodies against one or more constituents of danaparoid [most likely, dermatan sulfate (478)] can be detected in 15% to 40% of patients (556,557), this does not predict *in vivo* cross-reactivity, which appears to be rare (<3% of patients). Clinical evaluation of danaparoid has shown superior efficacy compared with dextran-70 [randomized trial (558)] and ancrod [retrospective study (559)] and had similar efficacy (with less bleeding) compared with lepirudin (retrospective study) (560). Danaparoid has been approved for treatment of HIT in Canada, the European Union, and New Zealand (553). In the United States, danaparoid has been approved for prophylaxis against thrombosis in postoperative orthopedic patients, and until recently, was available for "off-label" treatment and prevention of thrombosis in HIT (553). Danaparoid does not interfere with the INR, and has a long half-life (anti–factor Xa activity, 25 hours). Thus, we find it to be useful in patients with venous thromboembolism complicating HIT in whom a gradual transition to warfarin is desired for long-term anticoagulant management (discussed subsequently).

Lepirudin (Refludan) is a recombinant derivative of hirudin (antithrombin produced by the medicinal leech), and is a 65–amino acid polypeptide of approximately 7 kd (554,561). Lepirudin forms noncovalent, but irreversible, 1:1 complexes with thrombin and inhibits both soluble and clot-bound thrombin. Based on historically controlled clinical trials (562–564), lepirudin has been approved for treatment of thrombosis complicating HIT in the European Union, the United States, and Canada. Although monitoring of lepirudin's action can be performed readily using the activated partial thromboplastin time, this may not be ideal in certain situations [e.g., patients with abnormal baseline activated partial thromboplastin time values; high doses of lepirudin are required if used for cardiopulmonary bypass (565)]. The ecarin clotting time may provide superior monitoring in these situations but is not widely available. Two other drawbacks of lepirudin include the substantial risk for drug accumulation and bleeding in renal failure, as well as the high risk for formation of antilepirudin xenoantibodies (although these are usually not clinically significant) (566). With no normal function, its half-life is approximately 80 minutes.

Argatroban is a synthetic, small-molecule direct thrombin inhibitor that was shown in historically controlled trials to be effective for treatment of thrombosis complicating HIT, as well as prevention of thrombosis in patients with "isolated HIT" (567), and it has been approved for both of these indications in the United States. The half-life is only 40 to 50 minutes, and anticoagulant monitoring is achieved using the aPTT (Table 32-3) (555). Argatroban prolongs the INR, however, and thus during overlapping anticoagulation with warfarin, a target INR of >4.0 is usually necessary (568) (after discontinuation of argatroban, however, the standard target of INR between 2.0 and 3.0 then becomes applicable). Argatroban is also used to anticoagulate patients with HIT undergoing percutaneous coronary intervention (FDA-approved indication) (569).

Treatment Caveats. There are several counterintuitive treatment caveats for managing HIT, including use of prophylactic platelet transfusions, warfarin anticoagulation, and use of LMWH (551,552).

Prophylactic platelet transfusions should be avoided, even in severely thrombocytopenic patients, as this therapy may contribute to risk of thrombosis (550,551). Patients with HIT generally do not have petechiae, and spontaneous bleeding is uncommon (498). Platelet transfusions are appropriate in a bleeding patient, however, or in a severely thrombocytopenic patient in whom the diagnosis remains uncertain.

Low-molecular-weight heparin should not be used to treat acute HIT (550–552), even though these agents are less likely to cause HIT than UFH when given to nonsensitized patients. However, in a patient who already has formed HIT antibodies, the risk of persistent or recurrent thrombocytopenia during LMWH treatment is approximately 50% (*in vivo* cross-reactivity) (570). Indeed, using sensitive washed platelet activation assays, there is virtually 100% *in vitro* cross-reactivity of HIT serum for LMWH (490). As better treatment options exist, we do not recommend LMWH as treatment for HIT.

Warfarin and other coumarins should not be used as monotherapy for acute HIT (550–552). One reason is that warfarin therapy during acute HIT is associated with a high risk of thrombosis (499). Another reason is that warfarin plays a key role in the pathogenesis of venous limb gangrene complicating HIT (514,530). This syndrome is characterized by progression of deep venous thrombosis to distal limb necrosis even though the arterial pulses remain palpable or identifiable by Doppler signals. A characteristic feature is a supratherapeutic INR, generally greater than 4.0, which has been linked to acquired depletion of the natural anticoagulant, protein C. Despite the elevated INR, the warfarin has failed to control thrombin generation in such patients, as shown by elevated levels of thrombin-antithrombin complexes (a marker of *in vivo* thrombin generation) (514). For longer-term control of thrombosis, therefore, we recommend initiating warfarin anticoagulation only after the platelet count has recovered to $100 \times 10^9/L$ or greater, and only once adequate anticoagulation and clinical improvement have been reached with an alternate anticoagulant such as danaparoid, lepirudin, or argatroban.

Adjunctive Treatments. Sometimes, limb-salvaging procedures such as surgical thromboembolectomy (571) might be appropriate in selected patients. Plasmapheresis might benefit patients with HIT, possibly by removing pathogenic IgG as well as correcting acquired coagulation disturbances (514). High-dose IVIgG can inhibit platelet activation by HIT antibodies *in vitro* and may be appropriate as a treatment adjunct in patients with severe HIT (572). We believe that antiplatelet agents such as aspirin and dextran are relatively ineffective treatments for HIT, although they could be used as adjunctive therapy in a patient with acute HIT and arteriopathy. Although ancrod (a defibrinogenating agent derived from the Malaysian pit viper) has provided anecdotal success in some patients with HIT (573), it does not inhibit thrombin generation (515) and has been associated with treatment failure in patients with DIC complicating HIT (523).

Heparin Reexposure. HIT antibodies usually become undetectable within a few weeks or months after an episode of acute HIT (497). In such patients, there is increasing evidence that HIT antibodies do not usually recur, particularly if only a brief course of heparin is given. This means that a brief course of heparin can be considered for patients with previous HIT who require cardiac or vascular surgery (497,565,574). If this treatment is considered, we recommend that HIT antibodies be excluded using one or more sensitive assays, and that a brief exposure to heparin be used to permit surgery. Postoperative anticoagulation with an alternative agent can then be given.

Special Situations. HIT can occur in patients who require hemodialysis or urgent cardiac surgery. Alternative anticoagulants such as danaparoid or lepirudin have been used for these situations (553,554,565,575,576), but each approach has certain problems, and no single ideal treatment exists. The metabolism of argatroban is not affected by renal insufficiency (555), and so this agent has advantages in patients with significant azotemia.

DRUG-DEPENDENT FAB BINDING OF IMMUNOGLOBULIN G TO PLATELETS: DRUG-INDUCED IMMUNE THROMBOCYTOPENIC PURPURA

Table 32-4 lists drugs that have been implicated in causing DITP (470–476,577–604). However, a definite causal role has

TABLE 32-4. Drugs Implicated in Immune Thrombocytopenia[a]

Drug	Platelet Count Nadir $<20 \times 10^9/L$	*In Vivo* Challenge	*In Vitro* Challenge	Selected References[c]
Acetaminophen	+	+	++	489,577
Acetazolamide	+	–	+	—
Acetylsalicylic acid	+	+	+	—
Actinomycin D	+	+	–	578
Allylisopropylcarbamide (Sedormid)	+	+	+	—
Alprenolol	+	+	–	—
Aminoglutethimide	+	+	–	—
Amiodarone	+	+	–	—
Amitriptyline	+	+	–	—
Ampicillin	+	–	+	—
Amrinone	–	–	+[b]	485
Antazoline	+	+	+	—
Apalcillin	+	–	–	—
Atorvastatin	+	+	–	—
Captopril	+	–	–	—
Carbamazepine	+	+	+	489,579
Carbimazole	–	–	++	44
Cefamandole	+	–	+	—
Cefotetan	+	–	+	580
Ceftazidime	+	—	—	—
Cephalothin	+	+	+	—
Chlorpheniramine	+	+	+	—
Chlorpropamide	+	–	–	—
Chlorthalidone	–	–	+	—
Chlorthiazide	+	+	+	—
Cimetidine	+	+	+	—
Ciprofloxacin	–	+	–	—
Clarithromycin	+	–	–	—
Clonazepam	—	–	–	—
Cocaine	+	+	–	—
Danazol	+	+	–	—
Desferrioxamine	–	+	–	—
Desipramine	–	–	+	—
Diatrizoate	+	+	–	—
Diazepam	+	+	+	—
Diazoxide	–	+	–	—
Diclofenac	+	+	+	489,581
Difluoromethylornithine	–	+	–	—
Diflunisal	+	–	+	—
Digitoxin	–	+	+	—
Digoxin	–	+	+	—
Doxepin	+	–	–	—
Etretinate	–	–	–	—
Ethchlorvynol	+	+	+	—

(continued)

TABLE 32-4. (*continued*)

Drug	Platelet Count Nadir <20 ×10^9/L	*In Vivo* Challenge	*In Vitro* Challenge	Selected References[c]
Fenoprofen	+	–	–	—
Fluconazole	+	–	–	582
Furosemide	+	+	+	—
Fusidic acid	+	+	++	583
Gentamicin	+	+	+	—
Gold salts	+	+	+	494,584
Glibenclamide (glyburide)	+		–	—
Heparin	Unique pathogenesis and clinical manifestations (see text)			
Heroin	+	+	–	—
Hydrochlorothiazide	+	–	+	—
Ibuprofen	+	–	+	489
Imipramine	–	–	+	—
Indomethacin	+	–	–	—
Interferon	+	+	+[b]	—
Ipodate (sodium)	+	+	+	—
Iocetamic acid	+	–	–	—
Iopanoic acid	+	+	+	—
Irinotecan	+	+	+	585
Isoniazid	–	–	–	—
Isotretinoin	+	+	–	—
Levamisole	–	+	–	—
Lidocaine	+	+	+	—
Lincomycin	–	–	–	—
Meclofenamate	+	+	–	—
Mefenamic acid	+	–	+	—
Methicillin	+	+	+	—
Methyldopa	+	+	+	—
Mezlocillin	+	–	+	—
Mianserin	+	+	+	—
Minoxidil	–	+	+	—
Morphine	+	–	+	—
Nalidixic acid	+	+	–	—
Naproxen	+	–	++	577
Nimesulide	–	+	–	—
Nomifensine	+	–	+	489
Novobiocin	–	+	+	—
Oxyphenbutazone	+	–	–	—
Oxprenolol	+	+	–	—
Oxytetracycline	+	+	–	—
Papaverine	+	+	+	—
Paraaminosalicylic acid	+	+	+	—
Penicillin	+	+	+	586
Pentagastrin	–	+	–	—
Pentamidine	+	–	++	587
Phenylbutazone	–	–	+	—
Phenytoin	+	+	–	588
Piperacillin	+	+	–	—
Pirenzepine	–	+	–	—
Piroxicam	+	–	–	—
Primidone	–	–	–	—
Procainamide	+	+	+	589,590
Quinidine	+	+	++	489,591–596
Quinine	+	+	++	489,493,591–596
Ranitidine	+	–	++	489,597
Rifampin	+	+	++	489,598
Spironolactone	+	–	+	—
Stibophen, sodium stibogluconate	+	+	+	—
Sulfamethoxazole	+	–	++	599
Sulfamethoxypyridazine	+	–	–	—
Sulfasalazine	+	+	–	—
Sulfisoxazole	+	+	++	599
Sulindac	–	–	+	—
Suramin	+	–	+	600
Tamoxifen	–	+	+	601
Teicoplanin	+	+	+	602
Ticlopidine	–	–	+	—
Tobramycin	–	–	–	—
Tolbutamide	–	–	–	—
Tolmetin	+	+	–	—
Toluene diisocyanate	+	–	–	—
Trimethoprim–sulfamethoxazole	+	+	++	488,489,599
Valproic acid	+	+	+[b]	484
Vancomycin	+	+	++	489,603,604

[a]Evidence supporting immune drug-induced destruction is indicated by + if the following were demonstrated: platelet count nadir less than 20 × 10^9/L, recurrent thrombocytopenia on *in vivo* challenge, or drug-dependent platelet–antibody test (*in vitro* challenge) using phase I assay, phase II assay, or both; ++ indicates drug-dependent platelet–antibody test using a phase III assay. A minus sign indicates that the feature listed has not been reported.
[b]Elevated platelet-associated immunoglobulin G was found in these patients, but *in vitro* drug-dependent increase in platelet-associated immunoglobulin G was not reported.
[c]Other references can be found in the first edition of this book and elsewhere (474,476).

only been established for relatively few drugs. For example, for less than a dozen drugs (e.g., quinine, quinidine, sulfa antibiotics, acetaminophen, fusidic acid, rifampin, vancomycin) has DITP been established based on the constellation of severe thrombocytopenia, recurrent thrombocytopenia on drug rechallenge, and *in vitro* testing confirming drug-dependent and platelet glycoprotein–dependent reactivity.

Clinical Features. Abrupt onset of severe thrombocytopenia with purpura and mucosal hemorrhage is characteristic, especially in a patient who has been previously sensitized to the agent. For patients who develop DITP during their initial exposure to the drug, the onset usually occurs 1 week or more (sometimes, several months) after beginning its administration. For quinine, it may be difficult to establish a history of drug ingestion (605) because quinine is present in many tonics and beverages and can contaminate illicit heroin preparations (493).

The platelet count nadir typically is less than $20 \times 10^9/L$. Generally mild thrombocytopenia has been reported in patients receiving valproic acid and amrinone; however, despite elevated PAIgG levels in these patients, there is evidence that the thrombocytopenia may be caused by decreased platelet production (484,485). Rarely, mild to moderate thrombocytopenia can be caused by immune mechanisms; for example, in a report of five patients with carbimazole-induced thrombocytopenia, the median platelet count nadir was $60 \times 10^9/L$ (44). The unusual clinical picture was believed to be caused by the unique target platelet glycoprotein recognized by the drug-dependent IgG, namely PECAM-1 (44).

Usually, the platelet count returns to normal within several days of discontinuing the drug, although thrombocytopenia persisting for several weeks is sometimes observed (594). Rarely, there is concomitant immune hemolysis or neutropenia; in such patients, distinct drug-dependent antibodies are responsible for the different cytopenias observed (606,607).

Pathogenesis. In past years, several models have been proposed to explain DITP (475). In the *hapten model*, antibodies recognize a drug epitope, which then can bind to the platelet if the drug itself binds to the platelet. However, except possibly for penicillin (586), such a mechanism has not been demonstrated. In the *immune complex model*, it was suggested that complexes of drug (or drug–protein) and IgG form in circulation, then bind to platelets. However, platelets have only low-affinity Fcγ receptors. Moreover, studies have shown that drug-dependent antibodies bind to platelets via their Fab moieties (593,608).

Currently, it is believed that DITP is caused by formation of *ternary complexes* that consist of drug, platelet glycoprotein, and the pathogenic IgG. In this model, the Fab moiety of the IgG binds to a complex of drug (or drug metabolite) and a specific region of one of the major glycoprotein complexes, either gpIb-IX or gpIIb-IIIa. Nevertheless, heterogeneity among patient sera exists. For example, studies of various patients with quinine-induced or quinidine-induced thrombocytopenia show variability both in the affinity and saturability of IgG for drug and platelet (609,610). Furthermore, the drug epitopes differ: Some sera recognize both quinidine and quinine, and other sera recognize only one drug. For quinine-induced or quinidine-induced thrombocytopenia, the IgG–drug interaction often involves the platelet gpIb-IX complex (606,610), which can explain absence of reactivity against Bernard-Soulier platelets (which lack this glycoprotein complex) (592).

The orientation of binding of the IgG to the platelet is mediated by the Fab region of the IgG molecule, as shown by two observations: The drug-dependent binding of (Fab')$_2$ is similar to that observed using intact IgG (593), and staphylococcal protein A beads can bind to platelets containing IgG–drug complexes (608). The initial event appears to be formation of a labile drug–IgG complex that is stabilized by binding to the platelet surface (611). Other platelet glycoproteins may also be involved in some instances, such as gpIIb-IIIa for sulfa antibiotics (599), pentamidine (587), and a minority of patients with quinine-induced or quinidine-induced thrombocytopenia (53,594,595) and PECAM-1 for carbimazole-induced DITP (44).

In some patients, the thrombocytopenia persists for several weeks after discontinuation of the drug. Drug-independent antibodies have been demonstrated in some of these patients, suggesting that formation of an antiplatelet autoantibody can follow drug-induced thrombocytopenia (609,612).

Diagnostic Test. Many *in vitro* assays are suitable for the diagnosis of DITP, such as flow cytometry to demonstrate drug-dependent and patient serum–dependent increase in PAIgG (613), and the monoclonal antibody–specific immobilization of platelet antigens (MAIPA; which also permits identification of the target platelet glycoprotein) (489,614). A practical source of drug metabolite is the patient's own (pH-buffered) urine (488). It is critical that all reaction media—including wash buffers—have the drug (or drug metabolite) present in the appropriate concentration to prevent loss of antibody binding and that appropriate controls are used (489). No assay has been prospectively evaluated, and the clinical usefulness remains uncertain.

Treatment. The responsible drug should be discontinued. For bleeding patients or those judged, on clinical grounds, to be at high risk of life-threatening hemorrhage, treatment should include platelet transfusions and IVIgG (588). Corticosteroids are often administered, but their efficacy has not been proven. Drug-dependent antibodies can persist for years, and sensitivity is presumed to be life-long (contrast HIT).

GLYCOPROTEIN IIB-IIIA RECEPTOR–INDUCED THROMBOCYTOPENIA

Several gpIIb-IIIa receptor antagonists are now available, such as abciximab, eptifibatide, and tirofiban, for treating coronary heart disease (615,616). Abciximab (c7E3, or ReoPro) is a humanized chimeric Fab fragment of a murine monoclonal antibody (7E3) directed against gpIIb-IIIa, whereas eptifibatide is a peptide, and tirofiban a peptidomimetic, gpIIb-IIIa receptor antagonist. In excess of approximately 0.5% to 1.8% of patients (compared with controls) developed a platelet count fall to less than $50 \times 10^9/L$ within several hours of treatment with abciximab (615–618), with a much lower frequency for eptifibatide and tirofiban (615). Perhaps surprisingly, given the severity of the thrombocytopenia and use of a potent platelet inhibitor, many patients do not experience petechiae or bleeding (619) (although fatal bleeding has been reported). Bleeding occurs most often at the percutaneous puncture site.

Intravenous immunoglobulin G is usually not effective (620,621). Platelet transfusions usually lead to a rapid and sustained platelet count increase and are the treatment of choice for a bleeding patient (620,621). Abciximab has a very high affinity—and low dissociation constant—for gpIIb-IIIa (615), and redistribution of abciximab to the transfused platelets is minimal; thus, a single platelet transfusion usually suffices. However, eptifibatide and tirofiban have a much lower affinity for gpIIb-IIIa (615), have higher plasma levels, and will bind to transfused platelets. Thus, a repeat platelet transfusion after 4 to 6 hours, after much of these agents have cleared, may be helpful (476). Patients with severe abciximab-induced thrombocytopenia have been described who developed no platelet count falls with subsequent treatment with tirofiban (622) or eptifibatide (623).

The mechanism of the thrombocytopenia is uncertain, although the abrupt onset of severe thrombocytopenia suggests an immune pathogenesis, perhaps by naturally occurring and preexisting anti–gpIIb-IIIa antibodies that recognize conformational modifications induced by these drugs—ligand-induced binding sites (475). Although approximately 5% of patients treated with abciximab develop antibodies against the human part of this chimeric antibody, this phenomenon does not appear to be correlated with thrombocytopenia (476).

Pseudothrombocytopenia. In 15% to 30% of patients with apparent thrombocytopenia after treatment with abciximab, examination of the blood film shows platelet clumping, suggesting pseudothrombocytopenia (24,476). Such patients are not at risk for bleeding and do not need treatment. Indeed, inappropriate platelet transfusions and cessation of antithrombotic therapy could lead to increased thrombotic risk.

DRUG-INDUCED AUTOIMMUNE THROMBOCYTOPENIA

Some drugs may induce the generation of platelet-reactive autoantibodies, analogous to the generation of RBC autoantibodies by α-methyldopa. For example, this mechanism has been ascribed to procainamide in one patient who was shown to have antibodies reactive with gpIb and gpV (589). The measles–mumps–rubella vaccine can produce an illness that clinically resembles acute ITP of childhood beginning within 6 weeks' postvaccination (624,625).

Gold-Induced Thrombocytopenia. Approximately 1% to 3% of patients who receive gold injections develop immune thrombocytopenia, usually within the first 20 weeks of administration. Thrombocytopenia has also been described with the newer orally administered preparations (584). There are two unique temporal features of gold-induced thrombocytopenia: The thrombocytopenia can persist for several weeks, months, or even years, despite stopping the gold; and, rarely, gold-induced thrombocytopenia can occur as long as 18 months after the gold injections were discontinued (626). It is possible that both of these unusual temporal features are caused by otherwise typical drug-dependent platelet-reactive antibodies (584,609) that destroy platelets long after discontinuation of the drug because of the prolonged mobilization of gold from tissue storage sites. Alternatively, other investigators have proposed that gold causes autoimmune thrombocytopenia (627). In keeping with immune-mediated platelet destruction, megakaryocytes are either normal or increased in number, in contrast to the less common—and more serious—syndrome of idiosyncratic gold-induced marrow aplasia.

As many as 85% of patients with gold-induced thrombocytopenia carry the HLA-DR3 alloantigen (494), whereas the prevalence of this HLA antigen in the general population is approximately 22%. However, because most patients who possess this HLA phenotype gene do not develop gold-induced thrombocytopenia, the practical value of this marker is uncertain. The risk for severe gold-induced thrombocytopenia or pancytopenia can be reduced by monitoring the complete blood count before each injection to ensure that there has been no drop in the platelet count or other cellular elements. If cytopenia develops, the gold must be discontinued. For patients with symptomatic thrombocytopenia, additional treatment is required. Corticosteroids are frequently effective (628) and are the first-line treatment. For patients with persisting symptomatic thrombocytopenia inadequately controlled with prednisone, other treatments include IVIgG (629), immunosuppression (630), and splenectomy (628). Chelating agents (e.g., dimercaprol, *N*-acetylcysteine) may be useful to promote gold excretion (626,631).

DRUG-INDUCED THROMBOTIC THROMBOCYTOPENIC PURPURA/HEMOLYTIC-UREMIC SYNDROME

Rarely, drugs can produce a syndrome of microangiopathic hemolysis and thrombocytopenia that closely resembles TTP or HUS. For example, quinine-induced HUS has been associated with quinine-dependent antibodies panreactive against platelets, endothelial cells, and neutrophils (632). Ticlopidine (633,634) and clopidogrel (635) are two antiplatelet agents that can cause TTP within a few weeks after initiating treatment. This complication occurs in approximately 1 of 2000 to 5000 patients who receive ticlopidine postcoronary stenting (636) but is believed to complicate less than 1 of 20,000 patients treated with clopidogrel (635). The mortality is high, although patients can respond to stopping the drug and treatment with plasmapheresis. Autoantibodies against vWF-cleaving metalloproteinase have been identified in clopidogrel-induced TTP (637). Other causes of drug-induced microangiopathy include certain antineoplastic agents [especially mitomycin C (638)], immunosuppressive agents [cyclosporine (638), FK506 (tacrolimus) (638)], and possibly others [simvastatin (639), penicillamine, penicillin, oral contraceptives]. TTP and HUS are discussed in the section Thrombotic Microangiopathic Disorders.

Alloimmune Thrombocytopenic Disorders

Five alloimmune thrombocytopenic disorders have been described (Table 32-5). The two classic alloimmune thrombocytopenic syndromes are neonatal alloimmune thrombocytopenia and PTP. Two less common syndromes are passive alloimmune thrombocytopenia (PAT) and transplantation-associated alloimmune thrombocytopenia. Although refractoriness to platelet transfusions is usually caused by patient morbidity (e.g., septicemia) or HLA alloantibodies, platelet-specific alloantibodies may be important in occasional patients. Table 32-6 lists the platelet-specific alloantibody systems that have been described (640–728), which are also reviewed elsewhere (729–732).

Neonatal Alloimmune Thrombocytopenia

Neonatal alloimmune thrombocytopenia (NAT) is a transient but potentially life-threatening thrombocytopenic disorder limited to fetal and neonatal life. It is caused by maternal IgG alloantibodies that cross the placenta and result in the premature destruction of platelets bearing paternally derived platelet alloantigens (analogous to hemolytic disease of the newborn). NAT occurs in approximately 1 to 1.5 per 1000 live births (733–736).

PATHOGENESIS

Most cases of NAT are caused by anti-Pl[A1] (anti-Zw[a]), anti-Br[a] (anti-Zav[a]), and, possibly, anti-Gov[a] alloantibodies (718,737). Other alloantigens that have been implicated in the syndrome include Pl[A2], Bak[a], Bak[b], Pen[a], Pen[b], Ko[a], and Br[b] (Table 32-6). In addition, several low-frequency or even "private" (i.e., identified so far in only one family) alloantigens have been implicated in causing NAT (Table 32-6). In a large series of NAT patients

---

TABLE 32-5. Five Alloimmune Thrombocytopenic Syndromes

Classic alloimmune thrombocytopenic syndromes
    Neonatal alloimmune thrombocytopenia
    Posttransfusion purpura
Other alloimmune thrombocytopenic syndromes
    Passive alloimmune thrombocytopenia
    Transplantation-associated thrombocytopenia
    Platelet transfusion refractoriness

TABLE 32-6. Platelet-Specific Alloantigen Systems[a]

HPA Nomenclature	Original Designations	White Genotype Frequency	White Phenotype Frequency	Japanese Genotype Frequency	Japanese Phenotype Frequency	Clinical Alloimmune Syndromes	Glycoprotein Localization (Amino Acid Polymorphism)	Comments	References
HPA-1a -1b	Zw^a, Pl^{A1} Zw^b, Pl^{A2}	0.85 0.15	0.98 0.27	0.98 0.02	>0.999 0.04	NAT, PTP, PAT, TAT, PTR NAT, PTP, PTR	IIIa Leu$_{33}$ Pro$_{33}$	Anti-HPA-1a is the most frequent cause of severe alloimmune thrombocytopenia in whites: alloimmunization associated with HLA-DR3	54,55,465,469,640–657
HPA-2a -2b	Ko^b Ko^a, Sib^a	0.911 0.089	0.992 0.169	0.864 0.136	0.982 0.254	?NAT, ?PTR NAT, PTR	Ibα Thr$_{145}$ Met$_{145}$	Usually immunoglobulin M alloantibodies; NAT appears to be very rare; anti-HPA has been reported to cause PTR in Japan	41, 658–664
HPA-3a -3b	Bak^a, Lek^a Bak^b, Lek^b	0.61 0.39	0.85 0.66	0.54 0.46	0.79 0.71	NAT, PTP NAT, PTP, PTR	IIbα Ile$_{843}$ Ser$_{843}$	Although less common, NAT and PTP caused by anti-HPA-3 alloantibodies are usually as severe as those observed in the HPA-1 system	641,665–675
HPA-4a -4b	Pen^a, Yuk^b Pen^b, Yuk^a	>0.99 <0.01	>0.999 <0.001	0.9917 0.0083	>0.999 0.017	NAT, PTP NAT	IIIa Arg$_{143}$ Gln$_{143}$	More frequent alloimmune syndromes in Japanese than whites because of higher frequency of homozygous HPA-4b phenotype	676–685
HPA-5a -5b	Br^b, Zav^b Br^a, Zav^a, Hc^a	0.89 0.11	0.99 0.21	— —	— —	NAT, ?PTP, PTR NAT, PTP, PAT, TAT, PTR	Ia Glu$_{505}$ Lys$_{505}$	Can only be detected by sensitive methods; less severe alloimmune thrombocytopenic syndromes, compared with those involving glycoprotein IIb-IIIa; first and second most common cause of NAT in Japanese and white populations, respectively	466,686–699
HPA-6b	Tu^a, Ca	~0.003	~0.007	0.027	—	NAT	IIIa (Arg$_{489}$/Gln$_{489}$)	Low-frequency antigen found in a few unrelated families	700–704
HPA-7b	Mo^a	~0.001	~0.002	<0.0015	—	NAT	IIIa (Pro$_{407}$/Ala$_{407}$)	"Private" alloantigen system	705
HPA-8b	Sr^a	<0.003	<0.01	<0.0015	—	NAT	IIIa (Arg$_{636}$/Cys$_{636}$)	"Private" alloantigen system	706,707
HPA-9b	Max^a	0.003	0.007	—	—	NAT	IIb (Val$_{837}$/Met$_{837}$)	Max^a occurs only with HPA-3b, i.e., the Max^a mutation occurred after the HPA-3a/b polymorphism established	708
HPA-10b	La^a	<0.01	—	—	—	NAT	IIIa (Arg$_{62}$/Gln$_{62}$)	"Private" alloantigen system located near site of HPA-8b (Sr^a) mutation	709
HPA-11b	Gro^a	<0.001	—	—	—	NAT	IIIa (Arg$_{633}$/His$_{633}$)		710,711
HPA-12b	Iy^a	0.002	—	—	—	NAT	Ibb (Gly$_{15}$/Glu$_{15}$)	Low-frequency antigen	712,713
HPA-13b	Sit^a	0.0025	—	—	—	NAT	Ia (Thr$_{799}$/Met$_{799}$)	Low-frequency antigen; Sit^a-platelets show decreased aggregation to collagen	714
	Gov^a Gov^b	0.53 0.47	0.81 0.74	— —	— —	NAT, ?PTP NAT, ?PTR	CD109	Relatively common cause of mild NAT	715–718
	Va^a	<0.002	<0.004	—	—	NAT	IIb-IIIa	"Private" alloantigen system	719
	Oe^a	<0.005	0.01	—	—	NAT	IIIa		720
	Dy^a	<0.01	—	—	—	NAT	38 kd		721
	Nak^a	0.94	0.9966	0.7	0.96	NAT?, PTP?, PTR	IV (CD36)	Severe neonatal thrombocytopenia Anti-Nak^a isoantibodies can form in polytransfused glycoprotein IV-deficient patients	722–726

HPA, human platelet antigen; NAT, neonatal alloimmune thrombocytopenia; PAT, passive alloimmune thrombocytopenia; PTP, posttransfusion purpura; PTR, platelet transfusion refractoriness; TAT, transplantation-associated thrombocytopenia.

[a] Platelet alloantigens implicated in platelet alloimmune syndromes. The HPA system was proposed to systemize platelet alloantigen nomenclature (727). A drawback of this system, however, is that it implies the existence of alleles, such as HPA-6a, HPA-7a, and HPA-8a, which in fact are all identical at the molecular level with HPA-1a/HPA-4a (728). For alleles HPA-6b through HPA-13b (inclusive), the second of the two amino acids shown indicates the low-frequency/private allele. Note that anti-Nak^a are isoantibodies, i.e., they are formed by individuals deficient in glycoprotein IV (4% of the Japanese population lacks glycoprotein IV. Platelet alloantigens are also discussed elsewhere in review articles (729–732).

with serologic confirmation, anti-Pl^{A1} was found in 75% of the cases, anti-Br^a in approximately 20%, and remaining specificities in less than 5% (737). A more recent study (718) suggested that anti-Gov^a and anti-Gov^b alloantibodies (detectable only by sensitive assays such as the MAIPA) may be as common an explanation for NAT as alloantibodies of the $Br^{a/b}$ system. Serologic evidence for alloantibodies is lacking in approximately 60% of possible cases of NAT identified using clinical criteria (737).

Because the frequency of the Pl^{A1}-negative phenotype is approximately 2%, approximately 1 in 50 newborns is theoretically at risk for NAT. The actual risk is much lower, however, because only a minority of susceptible women exposed to heterologous platelets during pregnancy form antiplatelet antibodies (733). Further, the observed ratio of NAT caused by anti-Pl^{A1}/anti-Pl^{A2} alloantibodies (144:1) (737) is almost 1000 times greater than predicted based on the observed gene frequencies (729). Indeed, immunogenetics (648–651) is a major factor determining alloimmunization against Pl^{A1}: There is a strong association between formation of anti-Pl^{A1} and HLA-DRB3*0101 and HLA-DQB1*0201 (odds ratio, 25 and 40, respectively) (648). In contrast, no HLA association exists for immunization against Pl^{A2} (650). Thus, it appears that individuals with certain HLA genotypes are much more likely to generate an alloimmune response when gpIIIa bears the Leu33 substitution that determines the Pl^{A1} phenotype.

Overall, based on the observed allelic frequencies, the expected theoretic ratio of NAT for anti-Br^a, compared with anti-Br^b, should be approximately 8. A similar ratio (47:3, or approximately 16) has been observed (687). However, although the expected and observed ratios are similar (contrast the $Pl^{A1/A2}$ system), a role for immunogenetics and alloimmunization also exists for the $Br^{a/b}$ system (692,693).

CLINICAL AND LABORATORY FEATURES

Neonatal alloimmune thrombocytopenia typically presents with unexpected isolated, severe thrombocytopenia in an otherwise healthy neonate, particularly when fetomaternal incompatibility involves an alloantigen on gpIIb-IIIa. Petechiae are found in 90%; gastrointestinal tract hemorrhage in 30%; and hemoptysis, hematuria, and retinal bleeding in less than 10% of patients (737). Approximately 10% to 20% of affected neonates have intracranial hemorrhage (737). Serious sequelae of fetal and neonatal intracranial bleeding include hydrocephalus, porencephalic cysts (676), and epilepsy. First-born offspring constitute approximately half of cases, suggesting that, unlike hemolytic disease of the newborn, sensitization can occur early during the first pregnancy (737). Subsequent affected siblings are usually thrombocytopenic to a similar or greater extent (738).

The thrombocytopenia usually is severe, with the platelet count falling to 10×10^9/L or lower, but is transient, and the platelet count returns to normal within several weeks after birth. Bone marrow examination reveals normal or increased megakaryocyte numbers. Anemia and hyperbilirubinemias can occur from extravasation and resorption of blood (737).

SEROLOGIC INVESTIGATION

The evaluation of possible NAT involves three steps. The first is to have a high index of suspicion in any thrombocytopenic infant. Isolated thrombocytopenia in an otherwise well infant must be assumed to be NAT until proven otherwise. The second step is to type maternal platelets to see if the mother lacks certain platelet alloantigens that often are associated with alloimmune thrombocytopenia. For example, maternal homozygous $Pl^{A2/A2}$ ("Pl^{A1}-negative") status confers risk for NAT caused by anti-Pl^{A1} alloantibodies. The third step is to determine whether the mother has antiplatelet alloantibodies in her serum. Not infrequently, no alloantibodies can be detected in the mother's

serum despite severe neonatal thrombocytopenia. Approximately one-fourth of Pl^{A1}-negative mothers suspected to have had infants with NAT cannot be shown to have anti-Pl^{A1} alloantibodies (737). The potential role of low-incidence platelet-specific alloantigens indicates the importance of testing maternal serum against paternal platelets whenever possible.

DIFFERENTIAL DIAGNOSIS OF NEONATAL THROMBOCYTOPENIA

Differential diagnosis of neonatal thrombocytopenia is discussed in the section Fetal and Neonatal Thrombocytopenia.

TREATMENT

Neonatal thrombocytopenia is much more severe, and the bleeding symptoms more prominent, than the thrombocytopenia in neonates with passive autoimmune thrombocytopenia caused by maternal ITP. For this reason, we treat mothers with ITP conservatively and do not favor invasive procedures such as percutaneous umbilical blood sampling. In contrast, the frequently unfavorable outcome of infants with NAT supports a more aggressive approach to diagnosis and intervention. The explanation for the increased risk is not known but may be related to the more severe thrombocytopenia that characterizes alloimmune thrombocytopenia. Severe thrombocytopenia and serious bleeding is much less frequently caused by alloantibodies of the $Br^{a/b}$ and $Gov^{a/b}$ alloantigen systems, possibly because the platelet glycoproteins bearing these alloantigens are present in lower quantities than gpIIb-IIIa.

Prenatal Management. In approximately half of cases, NAT is suspected during the prenatal period. Usually, NAT is suspected because the mother previously had an affected infant. Sometimes, the diagnosis of NAT is first suspected *in utero* because a fetal ultrasound reveals cerebral hemorrhage, hydrocephalus, or hydrops fetalis (739). If the father is heterozygous for the implicated alloantigen system (which occurs in 25% and 20% of instances involving the Pl^A and Br systems, respectively), then fetal platelet allotyping using genetic methods is important, because a homozygous fetus will not develop NAT, obviating need for any subsequent therapy. For at-risk pregnancies, the potential for intracranial hemorrhage during the fetal period has led to attempts to prevent *in utero* bleeding.

General approaches to prevent bleeding (738,739) are regular administration of high-dose IVIgG to the mother, repeated *in utero* platelet transfusions, or both. The first step is to obtain a fetal platelet count between 20 and 24 weeks' gestation using percutaneous umbilical vein sampling (PUBS). This procedure requires that maternal platelets be available on hand for transfusion to minimize risk for fetal exsanguination. Then, IVIgG can be given at a dose of 1 g/kg/week starting within 1 week of documented fetal thrombocytopenia, with repeat PUBS 4 to 6 weeks later to determine fetal platelet count response to IVIgG therapy. Corticosteroid salvage (prednisone, 60 mg/day) can be administered if no platelet count improvement is observed (740). However, this treatment is not always successful (740–742).

Another approach, used more commonly in Europe, has been to administer regular intrauterine platelet transfusions by PUBS until shortly before delivery (743,744). This therapy appeared effective compared with outcomes of previously affected siblings. Because each fetal transfusion entails some risk of fetal hemorrhage and death, whether such an approach is warranted depends considerably on the experience of the fetomaternal unit.

Delivery of infants with NAT should be by cesarean section. Although cesarean section itself is unlikely to protect thrombocytopenic neonates compared with vaginal delivery, it does allow for an organized approach to the peripartum care of the newborn.

Postnatal Management. The cornerstone of treatment is the immediate administration of washed, irradiated maternal platelets to the thrombocytopenic neonate (745,746). The platelets are obtained using pheresis and should be washed to remove the maternal alloantibody and irradiated to prevent graft-versus-host disease, which could be caused by maternal lymphocytes. In some centers (e.g., National Blood Service, United Kingdom), Pl^{A1}-negative and Br^a-negative platelets (theoretically effective in >95% of affected neonates) can be obtained on request (739). In an emergency, immediate administration of random donor platelets may be of some benefit to a bleeding infant. Administration of IVIgG to the infant (1 g/kg/day for 2 consecutive days) is effective in raising the platelet count (746) and should be given along with platelet transfusions.

Posttransfusion Purpura

PTP is a very rare disorder characterized by the abrupt onset of severe thrombocytopenia that begins approximately 5 to 10 days after receiving a blood transfusion, most often red cell concentrates (729,747,748). Invariably, high-titer, platelet-specific alloantibodies are found in the patient's serum or plasma. Although the platelet-specific alloantibodies are causative, the pathogenesis remains obscure, and the conundrum is why autologous platelets are destroyed.

PATHOGENESIS

Three hypotheses have been developed that relate to the pathogenesis of PTP (748):

Immune-complex platelet destruction: autologous platelets are destroyed by immune complexes consisting of alloantibodies interacting with allogeneic platelet antigens (747).

Conversion of antigen-negative to antigen-positive platelets: allogeneic platelet antigens are absorbed onto autologous platelets, rendering them susceptible to alloimmune destruction (749).

Alloantibodies cross-reactive with antigen-positive and antigen-negative platelets (pseudospecificity): the pathogenic alloantibodies recognize the autologous platelet determinants in addition to the foreign alloantigen (750). Perhaps in support of this view, it has been observed that panreactive anti–gpIIb-IIIa antibodies are readily detected during, but not after, an episode of PTP; in contrast, alloantibody reactivity usually persists for several years (751).

Although Pl^{A1} is the alloantigen most frequently implicated in PTP, other alloantigens have been described in PTP, including Pl^{A2}, Bak^a, Bak^b, Pen^a, Br^a, and Br^b (Table 32-6). Sometimes, more than one type of platelet-specific alloantibody can be identified in the patient's serum (688,752). As in NAT, the HLA-DR3 antigen is found in most Pl^{A1}-negative patients with PTP (649).

CLINICAL AND LABORATORY FEATURES

The disease usually occurs in middle-aged or older women who have been pregnant. A literature survey of PTP demonstrated that 95% of patients were women and 85% were between the ages of 40 and 80 (748). Almost always, there is a history of previous pregnancy, although in a few patients, the initial sensitization is believed to have occurred through previous blood transfusion.

Typically, the onset of bleeding and thrombocytopenia occurs 5 to 10 days after the transfusion of RBCs, which presumably results in resensitization by the contaminating platelets. Rarely, plasma transfusions cause the syndrome (753). Although the thrombocytopenia usually lasts from 1 to 4 weeks, the duration can be as short as 3 days to as long as 4 months or more (754,755). The thrombocytopenia is severe, usually less than 10×10^9/L (729,748). Cutaneous, mucosal, and postoperative wound bleeding are encountered frequently, and fatal outcome has been reported.

TREATMENT

High-dose IVIgG was reported in 1983 to be effective treatment for PTP (756), and it remains the treatment of choice today. More than 90% of patients respond favorably, with an average of 4 days before attaining a platelet count above 100×10^9/L (757). Corticosteroids are frequently administered but probably do not influence the natural history and should be considered as possible adjunct rather than primary therapy. Splenectomy (758) can be considered for the rare patient refractory to IVIgG, corticosteroids, and matched platelet transfusions.

Random donor platelets should not be administered because they usually are ineffective and can cause severe febrile or even anaphylactoid reactions (751,759). Pl^{A1}-negative platelets may provide benefit when PTP is caused by anti-Pl^{A1} alloantibodies (760–762). Red cell concentrates should be washed (763) or filtered (762) before administration to remove contaminating platelet antigens.

FUTURE PRECAUTIONS

PTP theoretically can recur if the patient receives future blood products containing the incriminated platelet alloantigen. Not every patient will have a recurrence (764), however, suggesting that residual high-titer alloantibodies can protect against recurrence by destroying the transfused incompatible platelet antigens. Regardless, patients with a history of PTP should receive only washed or autologous RBCs and platelet alloantigen-compatible plasma or platelet products (748). Patients who have recovered from PTP must not donate blood because their plasma could trigger thrombocytopenia.

Passive Alloimmune Thrombocytopenia

Passive alloimmune thrombocytopenia is characterized by abrupt onset of thrombocytopenia within a few hours of transfusing a blood product (usually plasma) that contains high-titer, platelet-specific alloantibodies (652–655,699). This syndrome is clinically distinct from PTP, however, because the thrombocytopenia immediately follows the transfusion, and the duration of thrombocytopenia is shorter (several hours to a few days). Although the platelet-specific alloantibody can be detected in the donor's plasma and on the recipient's platelets, it is not detectable in the recipient's plasma, suggesting that virtually 100% of the transfused alloantibodies bind soon after transfusion. PAT caused by anti-Pl^{A1} typically has more severe thrombocytopenia than that caused by anti-Br^a alloantibodies (729). It is important to investigate cases of possible PAT; because of the potential for multiple recipients to develop this syndrome, the responsible blood donor must not donate blood in the future.

Transplantation-Associated Alloimmune Thrombocytopenia

The very rare syndrome of transplantation-associated alloimmune thrombocytopenia, which can occur either very soon (469) or very long (465,466) after transplantation with a solid organ (469) (kidney, liver) or allogeneic bone marrow (465,466), respectively, was described in the section Posttransplant Autoimmune or Alloimmune Thrombocytopenia. Both anti-Pl^{A1} and anti-Br^a alloantibodies have been implicated (465,466,469) (Table 32-6).

Alloimmune Platelet Transfusion Refractoriness

Platelet transfusion refractoriness (PTR) is defined as an unexpectedly poor platelet count increment to transfused platelets (discussed in Chapter 20). Nonimmune, patient-dependent factors are usually involved; thus, poor platelet count recoveries can persist even when HLA alloimmunization is prevented by using leukocyte-depleted blood products or when HLA-compatible or ABO-compatible platelets or both are administered.

There is anecdotal evidence, however, that platelet-specific alloantibodies sometimes cause PTR (641,663). In a prospective study, Novotny et al. (765) found that even when HLA alloantibody formation was largely prevented using prestorage-filtered blood products, platelet-specific alloantibodies at most explained 4 (5%) of 79 patients with PTR. Nevertheless, there are occasions when the transfusion service needs to provide HLA-specific and platelet-specific antigen-compatible platelet products to manage difficult situations of alloimmune PTR (766).

THROMBOCYTOPENIA CAUSED BY THROMBIN (DISSEMINATED INTRAVASCULAR COAGULATION)

DIC is defined as excess of thrombin generation within the vasculature, resulting in generalized derangement of the hemostatic mechanism (767–770). Dysregulated thrombin production leads to increased consumption of coagulation factors, such as fibrinogen; depletion of coagulation factors can lead to bleeding. There is also consumption of natural anticoagulants, such as protein C and antithrombin. Protein C depletion in particular is associated with microvascular thrombosis. In addition to thrombin generation, there usually is parallel production of plasmin and formation of products of fibrinolysis, including fibrin and fibrinogen degradation products.

Increased platelet turnover is a universal feature of DIC, resulting in thrombocytopenia in almost all patients. Platelet destruction may be related to direct activation by thrombin, which is the most potent of all physiologic platelet agonists. Indeed, concentrations of α-thrombin as low as 0.15 nmol/L can activate platelets without any effect on fibrin generation (771). Thrombin-induced platelet activation is associated with generation of procoagulant platelet-derived microparticles (772), suggesting that platelet activation plays an important role in promoting the consumption of the coagulation factors in DIC.

The clinical spectrum of DIC is wide and ranges from laboratory abnormalities without clinical sequelae, to severe bleeding caused by depletion of coagulation factors and platelets, to organ dysfunction and skin necrosis resulting from microvascular thrombosis and to thrombosis involving large veins and arteries. The course of DIC can be acute, fulminant, and rapidly fatal. Alternatively, the process can be chronic and compensated, with increased factor production leading to maintenance of adequate levels of coagulation factors and platelets (767–770).

MISCELLANEOUS DESTRUCTIVE THROMBOCYTOPENIA

Several thrombocytopenic disorders, such as the thrombocytopenia of infections (viral, bacterial, fungal, protozoal), TTP and HUS, and preeclampsia-associated thrombocytopenia are discussed together. Although these disorders have different inciting events and disease associations, they all are characterized by thrombocytopenia caused by increased platelet destruction. However, clinically significant DIC is usually not present, and the pathogenesis of the platelet destruction remains unresolved. Although elevated PAIgG is found in many patients, this feature does not necessarily indicate that an immune pathogenesis is responsible for the thrombocytopenia. The section also considers other miscellaneous disorders believed to be associated, at least in part, with increased platelet destruction, including

thrombocytopenia associated with allergy and anaphylaxis, glomerulonephritis, renal transplantation rejection, extracorporeal circulation, intravascular catheters and prostheses, cardiopulmonary bypass surgery, cardiovascular disease, severe bleeding requiring massive transfusion support, and administration of fatty acids.

Thrombocytopenia of Infection

THROMBOCYTOPENIA COMPLICATING BACTEREMIA AND FUNGEMIA

Thrombocytopenia is a frequent and sometimes early sign of systemic bacterial or fungal infections. The frequency of thrombocytopenia ranges from 15% to 35% for patients with clinical evidence for infection (773,774), to 45% to 75% for patients with positive blood cultures (775–778), to 90% to 95% for patients with evidence of septic shock or DIC (779–781).

Usually, the thrombocytopenia is moderately severe, with the platelet counts averaging from 50 to 100×10^9/L. Occasionally, it can be severe, with platelet counts falling below 10×10^9/L. Blood cultures should be performed in patients in whom the diagnosis is suspected. Coagulation tests also should be performed, although decompensated DIC is relatively uncommon.

Disseminated Intravascular Coagulation. In one prospective study using sensitive and specific markers for thrombin activation, including fibrinopeptide A levels and fibrinogen gel chromatography for detection of fibrin and fibrinogen multimers, most patients with mild to moderate thrombocytopenia complicating bacteremia had no evidence of DIC. However, DIC was found in most patients with a platelet count below 50×10^9/L (777). A large retrospective study found evidence for DIC in only 20% of thrombocytopenic patients with gram-negative bacteremia (778).

In contrast, severe DIC is a major factor in explaining the syndrome of systemic microvascular thrombosis, especially involving the acral regions of the limbs (purpura fulminans), and most frequently complicates bacteremia with certain organisms, including *Neisseria meningitidis*, *H. influenzae*, and *Streptococcus pneumoniae*, particularly in the postsplenectomy patient. Internal organ damage also can be caused by microvascular thrombosis—for example, bilateral adrenal hemorrhagic necrosis complicating meningococcemia (i.e., Waterhouse-Friderichsen syndrome) (782). Sometimes the systemic effects of the hypercoagulable state are vividly apparent, such as the syndrome of symmetric peripheral gangrene (783). Particularly in patients with meningococcemia, the severity of peripheral tissue necrosis parallels the severity of depletion of the natural anticoagulant, protein C (784). Congenital abnormalities in the natural anticoagulant pathways may explain such severe complications in some infected patients (785,786).

Microbe-Induced Activation of Hemostasis and Host Response. Some bacteria cause platelet activation by means of endotoxin (787,788) or other toxins (789–791). Further, thrombocytopenia could result from endotoxin-induced release of endogenous mediators, such as platelet-activating factor (792,793). Various proinflammatory cytokines produced during the host response (e.g., tumor necrosis factor-α, interleukin-1β) activate coagulation by increasing intravascular tissue factor production and by causing impairment of protein C activation by endothelium (794). Interleukin-6 leads to increased platelet production with increased sensitivity of the platelets to activation by thrombin (794).

Endothelial Damage. Microbe-induced endothelial damage may cause thrombocytopenia by exposing subendothelial tissues to the flowing blood. Thrombocytopenia, purpuric rash, and multiorgan dysfunction are common in Rocky Mountain spotted fever, the result of endothelial invasion by the pathogenic *Rickettsia rickettsii* (795), probably generating procoagulant tissue factor on endothelium (796).

Hypersplenism. Reticuloendothelial cell hyperplasia can contribute to thrombocytopenia in some chronic infections, such as subacute bacterial endocarditis and malaria.

THROMBOCYTOPENIA COMPLICATING VIRAL INFECTIONS

Acute ITP can develop weeks after infection with rubella, rubeola, varicella (797), live virus vaccines (624,625), or, most frequently, an unidentified viral upper respiratory tract infection (798). Thrombocytopenia also occurs during the active phase of viral infections, especially infections caused by the herpesviruses [Epstein-Barr virus (799), cytomegalovirus, herpes simplex] but also with varicella, mumps, rubella, measles, parvovirus (800), and hantavirus (801) infection. Although the frequency of thrombocytopenia with acute viral infection is not known, it may be high. For example, in one study, approximately 75% of patients with Epstein-Barr virus-induced infectious mononucleosis developed mild to moderate thrombocytopenia during the second week of illness (799). When thrombocytopenia occurs during the acute phase of the viral infection, reduced numbers of megakaryocytes and hypersplenism sometimes contribute to the pathogenesis of thrombocytopenia. However, particularly when thrombocytopenia occurs days or weeks after infection, virus-induced immune mechanisms predominate.

Viral hepatitis causes thrombocytopenia, usually because of cirrhosis (hypersplenism). However, impaired hepatic thrombopoietin production also contributes to decreased platelet production (802), which may explain why interferon treatment sometimes raises the platelet count in chronic hepatitis C (268,269). On the other hand, interferon also can exacerbate thrombocytopenia in some patients (802,803). The antiviral agent ribavirin may lead to platelet count improvement and even permit reintroduction of interferon (803).

Pancytopenia also can occur in children who develop the life-threatening syndrome of virus-associated hemophagocytic lymphohistiocytosis. This syndrome is characterized by constitutional symptoms, lymphadenopathy, hepatomegaly, splenomegaly, and coagulopathy (804–808). Histologically benign histiocytes exhibiting erythrophagocytosis can be demonstrated in marrow aspirates, liver, or lymph node biopsy specimens. The syndrome occurs most frequently in association with Epstein-Barr virus, herpesvirus-6, cytomegalovirus, or adenovirus infections. This syndrome may represent an aberrant T-cell response to infection (809–811).

THROMBOCYTOPENIA COMPLICATING PROTOZOAL INFECTIONS

Malaria is a common and well-studied parasitic infection that often causes thrombocytopenia. Thrombocytopenia is caused by increased platelet destruction (812,813), possibly due to immune mechanisms, because specific antimalaria IgG can bind to malarial antigens adsorbed to the platelet membrane (95,814). The severity of thrombocytopenia shows an inverse relation with macrophage colony-stimulating factor levels in malaria, suggesting that this mediator could produce increased macrophage-mediated platelet destruction (815).

MANAGEMENT

The general approach to all infection-induced thrombocytopenia is the same: treat the underlying infection, evaluate the hemostatic risk, and treat the hemostatic dysfunction.

The diagnosis of thrombocytopenia complicating bacteremia or fungemia requires a high index of suspicion. Often, the thrombocytopenia precedes other evidence for infection, including fever and leukocytosis. Hence, we consider isolated thrombocytopenia in a patient at risk as presumptive evidence of an infection.

The most important step is to start appropriate antimicrobial treatment. For patients with severe thrombocytopenia (platelet count $<20 \times 10^9/L$), we often administer prophylactic platelet transfusions (34). Even though the transfused platelets are cleared rapidly, they can prevent life-threatening bleeding during the short period of risk before onset of antibiotic efficacy. Platelet transfusions also are administered to patients with higher platelet counts if bleeding occurs.

The role of heparin therapy in DIC complicating septicemia is debated. Heparin can improve the coagulation indices, although no impact on survival has been demonstrated (779). For patients with clinical evidence of microvascular thrombosis, including acral ischemia, livedo reticularis, or purpura fulminans, heparin therapy should be considered because it may reduce the thrombin generation that can lead to microvascular fibrin deposition. Activated protein C concentrates can reduce mortality in sepsis (816), perhaps by reducing inflammation, microvascular thrombosis, or both in septicemia-associated DIC. Antithrombin concentrates are another potential therapy that showed a trend to reduced mortality in one study (817).

Thrombotic Microangiopathic Disorders

Thrombotic microangiopathy (also known as *microangiopathic hemolytic anemia*) is defined as the triad of Coombs'-negative microangiopathic hemolytic anemia, destructive thrombocytopenia, and microvascular platelet thrombi (818,819). Patients with the syndrome have laboratory evidence of schistocytic hemolysis and thrombocytopenia. Often there is organ dysfunction caused by microvascular thrombosis.

The prototypic illness is TTP. Patients with TTP always have thrombocytopenia and schistocytic hemolysis and often have central nervous system and renal impairment, presumably caused by ischemia. HUS is a related condition in which the microangiopathic process is usually limited to the kidneys. Sometimes, the distinction between the syndromes is blurred. Renal dysfunction can be prominent in TTP, and focal neurologic deficits can occur in otherwise typical HUS (820,821).

TTP usually is a primary illness, but secondary disease associations have been described (633–639,822–840) (Table 32-7). In contrast, many episodes of HUS are accompanied by secondary disorders (632,832,834,840–860), such as concomitant gastrointestinal infection by verotoxin-producing *Escherichia coli* (Table 32-7). Approximately 5% to 10% of patients with *E. coli* O157:H7 infection develop HUS; children and elderly patients are at the highest risk.

Although TTP and HUS share the common pathologic feature of intraluminal platelet thrombus formation, it remains uncertain whether a common pathogenesis exists. These disorders can also be confused with other illnesses that can produce schistocytic hemolysis and thrombocytopenia, such as DIC associated with septicemia or adenocarcinoma, malignant hypertension, or HIT (819).

THROMBOTIC THROMBOCYTOPENIC PURPURA

Pathogenesis. For two decades, research interest in TTP has focused on the presence of platelet-aggregating factors and abnormalities in high-molecular-weight (HMW) multimeric forms of vWF in patients with TTP. More recently, several laboratories have reported deficiency of an enzyme that proteo-

TABLE 32-7. Secondary Causes of Thrombotic Microangiopathy

Thrombotic thrombocytopenic purpura
  Infections
    Viral (822,823), including human immunodeficiency virus (824–826) and human T-cell leukemia virus type I (826)
    Bacteria (828,829) (overlap with hemolytic-uremic syndrome)
    Other (830,831)
  Pregnancy and the postpartum period (832)
  Drugs (633–639,833,834), e.g., ticlopidine, clopidogrel, simvastatin, atorvastatin, tacrolimus (FK506), penicillamine
  Collagen vascular disorders (835–838)
  Familial (839,840)
Hemolytic-uremic syndrome
  Infections
    Enteric pathogens
      Verotoxin-producing *Escherichia coli* (841–845)
      Shigella dysenteriae (846,847)
      Campylobacter (848,849)
      Yersinia (850)
    Streptococcus pneumoniae (851)
    Human immunodeficiency virus (825,826)
  Pregnancy and the postpartum period (832)
  Drugs (632,834,852–855), e.g., quinine, mitomycin C, cyclosporine, deoxycoformycin, gemcitabine, tacrolimus (FK506)
  Allogeneic bone marrow transplant recipients (856–858) (overlap with thrombotic thrombocytopenic purpura)
  Familial (840,859,860)

lyzes vWF as well as a factor that produces endothelial cell apoptosis. A unifying explanation for all of these disparate features remains elusive.

In 1979, a platelet-aggregating factor (861,862) was identified in the plasma of patients with TTP. Subsequently, abnormalities in the HMW multimeric forms of vWF were reported in patients with chronic relapsing TTP and in HUS (863,864). Another group of investigators (865) found that the activity of a platelet-aggregating factor in TTP serum could be enhanced by large multimers of vWF, perhaps indicating a synergistic role between platelet-aggregating factor and vWF. The aggregating factor was subsequently identified (866–869) as a proteolytic enzyme termed *calcium-dependent cysteine protease* (calpain). Other workers have identified a cathepsin-like cysteine protease activity in blood from patients with TTP (870).

In the late 1990s, investigators reported deficiency of a vWF-cleaving protease in patients with congenital (chronic relapsing) TTP (871,872) and acute idiopathic TTP (873,874); inhibitory antiprotease IgG was identified in this latter group of patients (873,874). Because cleavage of the endothelium-derived, unusually large vWF multimers occurs physiologically in the plasma by a vWF metalloproteinase in a shear-dependent manner (875), the concept arose that deficient proteolysis of these large vWF multimers might contribute to TTP.

These observations have led to the following hypotheses: *Idiopathic TTP* is caused by an IgG autoantibody directed against the vWF-cleaving metalloproteinase, leading to platelet-vWF aggregates under conditions of high shear (microcirculatory thrombosis) (873,874); *congenital, recurrent TTP* represents a constitutional deficiency in the vWF-cleaving metalloproteinase that predisposes patients to recurrent episodes of TTP (871,872) [indeed, mutations in a newly discovered member of the ADAMTS family of zinc metalloproteinase genes (ADAMTS13) were recently found in patients with congenital TTP (876)]; *hemolytic-uremic syndrome* is not characterized by absence of the metalloproteinase (873), and, thus, it has a distinct pathogenesis. However, questions remain about the specificity of the abnormalities of vWF multimers observed in patients with TTP (819,877,878). Finally, endothelial injury by one or more plasma factors may also contribute to the pathogenesis of TTP (879,880).

Clinical and Laboratory Features. TTP is a rare disease with an annual incidence of approximately 1 in 1 million people (881,882). There is a slight female preponderance (3:2), and most patients are young or middle-aged adults, although patients of all ages have been affected.

Symptoms and signs of organ dysfunction are frequent, with neurologic dysfunction (confusion, headache, focal neurologic defects, coma) relatively common. Dramatic recovery from profound neurologic dysfunction, including coma, is possible with treatment, although neuroradiologic abnormalities may persist (883). Other clinical features that have been described include abdominal pain, visual complaints, heart failure, cardiac arrhythmia, and pulmonary edema. Nonspecific symptoms, including fever, can be prominent. Although hematuria, proteinuria, and mild renal dysfunction are frequent, oliguria and severe renal failure are uncommon.

Thrombocytopenia caused by increased platelet destruction characterizes TTP. Although the thrombocytopenia can be severe and can be accompanied by platelet dysfunction, bleeding symptoms are uncommon. Anemia due to microangiopathic hemolysis is common, but severe anemia is rare. Schistocytes and polychromatophilia are observed in the stained blood film, and nucleated RBCs can be seen. Laboratory signs of hemolysis include reticulocytosis, free plasma hemoglobin, decreased plasma haptoglobin, elevated lactate dehydrogenase of RBC origin, and unconjugated hyperbilirubinemia. The direct antiglobulin test is negative. Coagulation changes of DIC are occasionally encountered in patients with severe TTP. Hyperamylasemia is sometimes seen.

The characteristic pathologic lesions are disseminated arteriolar and capillary hyaline thrombi made of platelet aggregates enmeshed in fibrinogen and vWF (884). Adjacent endothelial swelling is often observed. *In vitro* assays of vWF-cleaving protease may prove useful in distinguishing TTP from HUS and in distinguishing among subtypes of TTP (885).

Treatment. Without therapy, TTP often is fulminant and fatal, with a mortality rate as high as 95% (886). At least 50% to 80% of patients recover with plasma therapy delivered by infusion or exchange (887,888). The efficacy of exchange transfusion with whole blood was first reported in 1959 (889); subsequently, fresh frozen plasma (FFP) administered by infusion (890) or apheresis (819,891) became commonly used. A randomized trial showed that plasma is most effective for TTP when administered by exchange (887).

Antiplatelet agents, including aspirin (325 to 1300 mg/day) and dipyridamole (200 to 600 mg/day), often are used as an adjunct to plasma therapy (887,892). Many physicians administer high-dose corticosteroid therapy (e.g., prednisone 200 mg/day) for patients with TTP (893).

Platelet transfusions are relatively contraindicated because they can result in clinical deterioration (894). Similarly, patients can die suddenly after an initial response to treatment, suggesting that increased platelet numbers are hazardous if the platelet-aggregating process remains unchecked (894).

The major recommended treatment is FFP administered by apheresis (generally, 1 plasma volume per exchange) (819). Patients who do not respond within a few days to plasmapheresis should receive larger volume plasma exchanges [e.g., 1.5 plasma volumes per exchange or two 1-plasma volume exchanges per day (819)] or have (vWF-depleted) cryosupernatant substituted for FFP (818,895–897). Unfortunately, major complications of plasma exchange therapy, especially related to the central venous catheter (e.g., pneumothorax, hemorrhage, infection, venous thrombosis), occur in 30% of patients (898). Although patience and persistence with plasma exchange is probably most important, sometimes other treatments are introduced for severe, refractory disease [e.g., splenectomy (899), vincristine (900)]. High-dose IVIgG appears to be ineffective and may even exacerbate TTP (901).

Early or late relapse is relatively common in patients who have recovered from TTP (888,899). Some physicians administer antiplatelet drugs for several months after remission, but it is unknown whether this treatment reduces the risk of relapse. Splenectomy may be helpful to reduce risk of relapse in patients with recurrent TTP (902).

HEMOLYTIC-UREMIC SYNDROME

HUS occurs most frequently in infants and young children and represents the most common cause of acute renal failure in this age group. The annual incidence of HUS in children younger than 5 years is approximately 1 in 100,000 and may be increasing (903,904). HUS can also occur in adults, particularly in the aged, suggesting that susceptibility to HUS is greatest at the extremes of age.

Pathogenesis. It was first recognized in 1977 that certain strains of *E. coli* produce a toxin active on vero cells, a cell line derived from African green monkey kidney cells (905). In 1983, Karmali et al. (841) described a striking association between HUS and evidence of infection by this organism. These workers (906) found that 75% of Canadian children with HUS had been infected by toxin-producing *E. coli*. A recent prospective U.S. study found that 80% of patients with HUS had recent infection with toxin-producing *E. coli* (844).

Formerly called *verotoxins* or *verocytotoxins*, these toxins are now known as *Shiga toxins* (907). The toxin consists of two distinct subunits: Subunit A is homologous to ricin and is cytotoxic because it inhibits protein synthesis; subunit B binds to endothelial receptors. Although several strains of *E. coli* can produce these toxins and thus cause HUS, most frequently, *E. coli* O157:H7 has been implicated (908,909).

It is uncertain how the Shiga toxin produces HUS, although binding of Shiga toxin to glycosphingolipid receptors on platelets (910), the gastrointestinal tract, and kidney may be important. Intravenous injection of Shiga toxin into baboons causes thrombocytopenia, hemolytic anemia, and renal thrombotic microangiopathy (911).

The possible involvement of the complement pathway is suggested by the discovery that a mutation that results in defective production of complement factor H (a down-regulating factor of the alternative pathway of complement) occurs in some patients with familial HUS (859,860).

Clinical and Laboratory Features. HUS commonly follows an acute diarrheal episode. Hemorrhagic colitis, usually caused by Shiga toxin–producing *E. coli*, is frequent, but HUS has been associated with other dysenteric syndromes, including those caused by *Shigella*, *Salmonella*, and *Campylobacter jejuni* (Table 32-7). The risk of developing HUS is *increased* with use of antibiotics to treat a diarrheal prodrome (odds ratio, 14) (912). The gastrointestinal symptoms can range from mild and nonspecific to severe and life-threatening. Abdominal pain and vomiting are common. Less commonly, the prodrome consists of upper or lower respiratory tract symptoms (atypical HUS). The prognosis may be worse for patients with atypical HUS. HUS can occur as an inheritable form (either autosomal recessive or dominant) beginning in early childhood (859,860).

Anemia and thrombocytopenia tend to be less severe than in TTP. At presentation, the platelet count is greater than $100 \times 10^9/L$ in half of patients (913). As in TTP, bleeding is uncommon. Nonspecific neurologic symptoms attributable to the metabolic effects

of azotemia are frequent. In a minority of patients, focal neurologic symptoms and signs indicative of thrombosis are seen (820,821).

Oliguria or anuria usually is present. Hyperkalemia secondary to hemolysis and renal impairment also is commonly encountered. Laboratory evidence for DIC is usually not present but can occur. HUS associated with *Shigella* infections may be more likely to lead to DIC (914).

Stool cultures may be positive for the pathogenic organism. Other diagnostic techniques include demonstration of Shiga toxin or specific bacterial DNA in stool extracts, or a rise in the titer of specific antibodies (844,906).

Renal histopathology reveals a preglomerular and glomerular thrombotic microangiopathy. The colon in verotoxin-associated HUS is hemorrhagic and edematous, without inflammation or ulceration (915).

Treatment. Despite appropriate treatment, as many as 10% of children with HUS die from the disease. A further 10% have severe, irreparable renal damage, and 10% are left with some degree of renal impairment (916). The mortality rate is greater in the elderly (908).

Supportive care, including attention to fluid and electrolyte balance, control of hypertension, transfusion for anemia, and dialysis when necessary for renal failure, is the mainstay of treatment (917). Experimental therapies include the use of agents designed to bind Shiga toxin in the gastrointestinal tract (917).

Children with epidemic diarrhea-associated HUS are usually not treated with plasmapheresis, as most recover (819). In contrast, plasma infusion or exchange probably is beneficial in adults with HUS after *E. coli* O157:H7 infection (918). In addition, plasma therapy can benefit children with atypical (nondiarrheal) HUS (919) or familial HUS (920).

Renal transplantation has been effective for many patients with chronic renal failure after HUS, but recurrence of the HUS after transplantation has been described in some recipients (921,922).

Preeclampsia

Preeclampsia is a common hypertensive disorder of pregnancy defined by hypertension and proteinuria that begins between 20 weeks of gestation and 4 weeks postpartum (923). Preeclampsia complicates approximately 7% to 10% of pregnancies and is most common in primigravida women. Thrombocytopenia occurs in approximately 10% to 20% of preeclamptic women and in approximately half of women with severe preeclampsia or eclampsia (924–927). A subgroup of thrombocytopenic, preeclamptic women with associated microangiopathic hemolysis and elevated liver enzymes, termed the *HELLP syndrome* (*h*emolysis, *e*levated *l*iver enzymes, *l*ow *p*latelets), has been described, which may confer a greater risk of maternal and fetal morbidity or mortality than preeclampsia alone (928–930).

The thrombocytopenia is caused by increased platelet destruction (924,931). Furthermore, in some patients, platelet dysfunction is evidenced by a bleeding time that is disproportionately prolonged (924,932,933), as well as defective *in vitro* thromboxane synthesis in preeclamptic patients' platelets (924).

The pathogenesis of the thrombocytopenia in preeclampsia is unknown. Placental ischemia resulting from abnormal cytotrophoblast invasion of spiral arterioles leads to activation of maternal vascular endothelium, increased formation of endothelin and thromboxane, and decreased formation of vasodilators such as nitric oxide and prostacyclin (934). In addition, thrombin (i.e., subclinical or overt DIC) may contribute to the thrombocytopenia (935,936). Low antithrombin levels are used by some investigators as a marker for DIC in preeclampsia. A randomized controlled trial of antithrombin concentrates for preeclampsia showed higher D-dimer levels in patients receiving placebo (937). Sometimes, overt DIC in preeclampsia indicates an underlying complication such as placental abruption (938).

An important question for the clinician is whether the presence of maternal thrombocytopenia with or without microangiopathic hemolysis or liver dysfunction indicates a worse prognosis or a different treatment approach for preeclamptic women. Many physicians regard isolated thrombocytopenia or elevated liver enzymes as evidence of severe preeclampsia regardless of the degree of hypertension and advise aggressive treatment, usually prompt delivery (928,929). Thrombocytopenic preeclamptic or eclamptic women usually do not have serious bleeding at the time of delivery, and routine platelet transfusions are not recommended.

Pharmacologic agents, such as aspirin have not clearly been shown to reduce the risk of preeclampsia (939). Although dexamethasone might be helpful in treating severe preeclampsia or HELLP syndrome (940,941), delivery is the mainstay of therapy.

Allergy and Anaphylaxis

Allergic and anaphylactic reactions in people sensitized to various allergens, including foods, can be accompanied by thrombocytopenia (942–946). Food antigen–containing immune complexes can be demonstrated after ingestion (947), and it is possible that platelet destruction is caused by platelet IgG Fc receptors interacting with the circulating immune complexes. A role for platelet IgE Fc receptors is unproven. Animal studies suggest that inflammatory mediators such as platelet-activating factor may play a role in the thrombocytopenia of anaphylaxis (948).

Glomerulonephritis

Rarely, poststreptococcal (949,950) or other forms of glomerulonephritis (951) are complicated by thrombocytopenia. Decreased platelet survival in the absence of thrombocytopenia also occurs in glomerulonephritis (952).

Thrombocytopenia Associated with Renal Transplantation

Intermittent thrombocytopenia can occur with normally functioning renal allografts (953) and during rejection episodes (954). It is possible that platelet activation and deposition in the renal vessels contributes to the rejection process (955). Thrombocytopenia also can complicate medical therapy of renal transplant rejection, such as the use of antithymocyte globulin (956) or sirolimus (957).

Platelets in Contact with Foreign Materials

EXTRACORPOREAL PERFUSION (CARDIOPULMONARY BYPASS)
During cardiopulmonary bypass, there is extensive contact between heparin-anticoagulated blood and the synthetic surfaces of the extracorporeal perfusion device (blood oxygenator). Excess bleeding is a frequent problem in these patients. Many patients receive blood transfusions, and approximately 5% require urgent reoperation for postoperative bleeding (958,959).

Thrombocytopenia and transient platelet dysfunction are observed in virtually every patient. Typically, the platelet count falls by 33% to 50%, primarily due to hemodilution, but also secondary to losses within the extracorporeal perfusion device (960). The bleeding time rises markedly during heart surgery (>30 minutes) but usually improves to less than 15 minutes shortly after surgery and to normal several hours later. By contrast, the throm-

bocytopenia persists for 3 to 4 days, followed by recovery of the platelet count to values exceeding the preoperative baseline (peak at days 12 to 14).

The pathogenesis and clinical significance of the hemostatic defect in these patients remain uncertain, but the defect is probably multifactorial. Studies have described transient, *intrinsic* defects in platelet function (958–962). These include decreased *in vitro* platelet aggregation, decreased platelet surface membrane proteins (963), selective depletion of platelet α-granules (964), and evidence of *in vivo* platelet activation (965) and platelet vesiculation (965). The platelet dysfunction in heart surgery is also attributable to an *extrinsic* platelet defect resulting from thrombin inhibition by the high doses of heparin (966). Further, an important role for hyperfibrinolysis in the pathogenesis of bleeding is shown by elevated D-dimer levels in bleeding patients (967) as well as the efficacy of antifibrinolytic agents (968,969) in the prevention and treatment of heart surgery–associated bleeding. Other factors in some patients include residual heparin effect postbypass [including heparin rebound (970)] and preoperative use of aspirin, clopidogrel, or other antiplatelet agents.

HEMODIALYSIS
Uremic patients often have mild thrombocytopenia due to decreased platelet production (971). Thrombocytopenia can also be caused by hemodialysis, probably because of platelet consumption in the dialyzer membrane (972–974). This condition only rarely causes significant bleeding (975). HIT with extracorporeal circuit thrombosis can also occur in some patients, usually approximately 1 to 2 weeks after commencing acute hemodialysis (575).

APHERESIS
Mild thrombocytopenia occurs frequently in patients undergoing apheresis procedures, especially with continuous flow systems (976). *In vitro* platelet dysfunction has also been demonstrated (977). Bleeding is uncommon.

CATHETERS AND PROSTHESES
The platelet lifespan is reduced in patients with prosthetic heart valves, arterial catheters, Dacron vascular grafts, arteriovenous Silastic cannulas, balloon-tipped pulmonary artery (Swan-Ganz) catheters, and ventriculojugular shunts (978–981). Thrombocytopenia is rare, however, because of compensatory increases in platelet production. The platelet lifespan improves over time, presumably because of progressive endothelialization of the implanted foreign material (980–982). In some instances, thrombocytopenia and thrombosis associated with use of invasive catheters are related to coadministration of heparin (i.e., HIT) (498,521,522).

Thrombocytopenia Associated with Cardiovascular Disease

CONGENITAL CYANOTIC HEART DISEASE
Thrombocytopenia caused by a decrease in platelet lifespan occurs in many patients with cyanotic congenital heart disease, particularly when there is marked arterial hypoxemia (oxygen saturation <60%) and polycythemia (hematocrit >0.6) (983–987). In some patients, increased platelet destruction may be caused by DIC triggered by hyperviscosity and venous stasis. Bleeding can be related to thrombocytopenia, platelet function defects (983,988,989), coagulopathy (990,991), and hyperfibrinolysis (992). Some of the hemostatic defects described, however, could be secondary to *in vitro* artifacts, and care should be taken to adjust the amount of anticoagulant for the high hematocrit to reduce the likelihood of spurious results. Reducing the hematocrit *in vivo* using phlebotomy with plasma infusion can improve hemostasis (991,993).

VALVULAR HEART DISEASE

Mild thrombocytopenia occurs in some patients with valvular heart disease (994,995), perhaps because of increased platelet consumption. However, bleeding in patients with severe aortic stenosis is more often caused by isolated deficiency of the largest multimers of vWF (996–999) rather than by thrombocytopenia.

PULMONARY HYPERTENSION

Primary pulmonary hypertension can be accompanied by thrombocytopenia (1000,1001). Platelet survival is diminished in most patients with pulmonary hypertension, but the pathogenesis is uncertain (995). Thrombocytopenia occurs in infants with elevated pulmonary artery pressures related to aortopulmonary transposition with an intact ventricular septum. Improvement in the platelet count after corrective surgery despite persisting pulmonary hypertension suggests that hypoxemia and polycythemia are more important in the pathogenesis of thrombocytopenia than the degree of pulmonary hypertension (985).

PULMONARY EMBOLISM

Thrombocytopenia can complicate severe pulmonary embolism, possibly because of DIC associated with clot-bound thrombin (1002–1004). When a patient develops pulmonary embolism and thrombocytopenia in association with heparin use, testing for HIT antibodies may be needed to determine whether HIT or pulmonary embolism *per se* explains the thrombocytopenia (1004).

Bleeding and Hemodilution

Bleeding patients who require massive transfusion support often develop thrombocytopenia. Thrombocytopenia occurs because of platelet consumption and DIC and by hemodilution resulting from administration of fluid and blood products. Platelet counts typically fall to approximately $100 \times 10^9/L$ after replacement of one blood volume and remain reduced for 2 to 3 days (1005,1006). Prophylactic platelet transfusions are usually not indicated in massive transfusion (1007) but may be appropriate in patients at high risk for bleeding (e.g., trauma patients, postoperative patients), especially if the platelet count has fallen below $50 \times 10^9/L$.

Fatty Acid–Induced Thrombocytopenia

Intravenous administration of fat emulsions over several weeks can cause thrombocytopenia. In one study, decreased platelet lifespan was documented, and sea-blue histiocytes exhibiting hemophagocytosis were evident on marrow examination. It was proposed that increased platelet destruction occurs as a result of fat emulsion–induced reticuloendothelial system hyperactivation (1008). Dietary therapy of adrenoleukodystrophy with Lorenzo's oil (contains 4:1 mixture of glycerol trioleate and trierucate) alters platelet composition and biology (1009) and can cause thrombocytopenia (1010,1011) and platelet dysfunction (1012).

Fetal and Neonatal Thrombocytopenia

In a retrospective study of 5194 consecutive fetuses who underwent fetal blood sampling for various indications, 247 (4.8%) were thrombocytopenic (defined as a platelet count $<150 \times 10^9/L$) (1013). The most common explanations included congenital infection (toxoplasmosis, rubella, cytomegalovirus; evidence for DIC was found in some patients), platelet-specific alloantibodies or autoantibodies, and chromosomal abnormalities (e.g., trisomy 18).

Healthy full-term and premature infants have the same normal platelet count range as adults (150 to $450 \times 10^9/L$) (1014). Thrombocytopenia is frequently encountered in the sick neonate (1014,1015). In one prospective study (1016), 22% of 807 consecu-

tive infants admitted to a neonatal intensive care unit developed thrombocytopenia within the first week of life. Radionuclide platelet survival studies indicated that platelet destruction was the predominant mechanism for the thrombocytopenia, with platelet sequestration playing a contributory role in some neonates (1016,1017). DIC was identified in 20% of thrombocytopenic neonates. In 12%, exchange transfusion was the explanation for the thrombocytopenia. In the remaining neonates, the pathogenesis was undefined (although many had elevated PAIgG, of uncertain relevance). However, increased thrombin generation indicative of DIC may occur in newborns without abnormalities in the platelet count or screening coagulation assays (1018).

Almost all the causes of neonatal thrombocytopenia are due to increased platelet destruction. For convenience, however, neonatal thrombocytopenic disorders caused by hemodilution (exchange transfusion) and decreased platelet production (erythroblastosis fetalis, some congenital infections, congenital infiltrative marrow disorders) are discussed here as well.

ASPHYXIA

Birth asphyxia, as assessed by 5-minute Apgar scores, was found in 70% of neonates with thrombocytopenia, compared with 32% of a control group of sick, nonthrombocytopenic neonates (1016). The etiologic role for this thrombocytopenic risk factor remains uncertain. Thrombocytopenia is frequently encountered in infants with intrauterine growth retardation, which could reflect increased platelet consumption associated with placental dysfunction and chronic hypoxia.

FETAL AND NEONATAL INFECTIONS

Infection is a common cause of thrombocytopenia in the newborn and can be related to infections acquired *in utero* or during the neonatal period (e.g., cytomegalovirus, rubella, herpesvirus, echovirus, toxoplasmosis, syphilis) (1013,1019–1023). Purpura accompanied by jaundice, hepatosplenomegaly, intracranial calcifications, neurologic defects, and congenital heart disease suggests the possibility of a congenital infection.

In many septicemic infants, the platelet count is markedly reduced (1023). Although increased platelet destruction is the most frequent mechanism of thrombocytopenia (1016,1017), in some infections (e.g., congenital rubella syndrome), decreased numbers of megakaryocytes suggest decreased platelet production (1019). In a recent study, thrombopoietin levels were inversely correlated with platelet counts in neonates with septicemia, with thrombopoietin levels falling to normal with platelet count recovery (1024).

DISORDERS ASSOCIATED WITH PREMATURITY

Thrombocytopenia occurs frequently in premature infants and may be secondary to respiratory distress syndrome (1025,1026), perinatal aspiration (1027), necrotizing enterocolitis (1028,1029), and hyperbilirubinemia requiring phototherapy (1030). One group identified mechanical ventilation as an independent factor in contributing to thrombocytopenia (1026). Among children with necrotizing enterocolitis, thrombocytopenia usually indicates a poor prognosis (1029). In a rabbit model, phototherapy led to reduced platelet survival (1030).

EXCHANGE TRANSFUSIONS

Exchange transfusion therapy, which is used in the management of alloimmune hemolytic disease of the newborn, is another cause of thrombocytopenia in the neonatal intensive care unit (1016). Dilutional thrombocytopenia occurs because the transfused RBCs and plasma do not contain viable platelets. The platelet count begins to rise in affected infants within 3 days and reaches preexchange levels by day 7 (1014).

MATERNAL PREECLAMPSIA

Transient neonatal thrombocytopenia is sometimes encountered in the offspring of preeclamptic mothers (1031–1033). It is likely that the thrombocytopenia reflects prematurity and comorbid illnesses in these infants.

THROMBOCYTOPENIA ASSOCIATED WITH HEMANGIOMAS (KASABACH-MERRITT SYNDROME)

Kasabach-Merritt syndrome (KMS) refers to the association between one or more hemangiomas in infancy and thrombocytopenia accompanied by consumptive coagulopathy (DIC) (1034,1035). For unknown reasons, less than 1% of infants with hemangiomas develop KMS. Although solitary, cutaneous hemangiomas involving the proximal extremities, trunk, or neck are most common, expanding visceral hemangiomas involving liver, spleen, or bone often have a more severe clinical course. In some series, one-third of children die from hemorrhage (e.g., massive intrahepatic bleeding) (1035). Although older studies described capillary or cavernous hemangiomas, recent reports have emphasized the presence of kaposiform hemangioendothelioma and tufted angiomas (formerly angioblastomas) in histopathology of KMS hemangiomas (1036).

Rarely, a congenital hemangioma triggers DIC during adulthood in relation to surgery or pregnancy (1037). Sometimes, KMS is associated with hemangiomas that occur as part of a recognized syndrome, such as Klippel-Trénaunay syndrome (macular vascular nevus, skeletal or soft-tissue hypertrophy, venous and lymphatic anomalies such as visceral and facial hemangiomas), blue rubber bleb nevus syndrome (multiple cavernous hemangiomas), or Gorham-Stout disease ("vanishing bone disease," i.e., osteolysis followed by replacement of bony matrix by proliferating thin-walled vascular channels); in such patients, risk for developing hemorrhagic manifestations of KMS remains life-long (1035).

Laboratory studies usually reveal a platelet count below 20×10^9/L, with schistocytic RBCs. Coagulation abnormalities include hypofibrinogenemia and elevated fibrin degradation, consistent with DIC related to localized consumption of platelets and fibrinogen within the abnormal tumor vasculature (1038).

Some children have no or minimal bleeding symptoms, and eventual spontaneous tumor regression usually occurs. For bleeding patients, supportive treatment includes platelets, FFP, and sometimes cryoprecipitate (1035). Antifibrinolytic (1039) or antiplatelet therapy might also be useful in some bleeding patients. Treatment for the hemangioma itself must be individualized (1035), and can include tumor excision, ligation, compression, or embolization (1040) (for localized disease), corticosteroids, local irradiation, α-interferon [possible antiangiogenesis action (1041)], or single-agent or combination chemotherapy (1035).

Rarely, placental vascular tumors are responsible for transient neonatal thrombocytopenia (1042,1043).

NEONATAL ALLOIMMUNE THROMBOCYTOPENIA

Neonatal alloimmune thrombocytopenia was discussed in the section Alloimmune Thrombocytopenic Disorders.

TRANSIENT PASSIVE AUTOIMMUNE THROMBOCYTOPENIA

Transient neonatal immune thrombocytopenia can also be caused by the transplacental passage of maternal autoantibodies, as found in ITP (1044) and SLE (1045,1046). This condition is discussed in the section Idiopathic Thrombocytopenic Purpura in Pregnancy.

MATERNAL DRUGS

Rarely, transplacental passage of drug and drug-dependent antibodies can result in both maternal and neonatal thrombocytopenia, as has been documented for quinine (1047). Maternal ingestion of thiazide diuretics (1048), hydralazine (1049), and tolbutamide (1050) has been implicated in neonatal thrombocytopenia, but the evidence is circumstantial and is sometimes disputed (1051,1052). Neonatal platelets are not adversely affected by the low doses of aspirin sometimes administered to prevent preeclampsia (1053).

NEONATAL THROMBOSIS

Thrombocytopenia in some neonates has been attributed to platelet consumption secondary to thrombosis at the site of an indwelling plastic catheter (1054,1055). Thrombocytopenia is frequently encountered in sick neonates with umbilical catheters [76% in one study (1016)], so an association with catheter-related thrombosis remains speculative. Thrombocytopenia can also occur in neonates developing renal vein or inferior vena caval thrombosis (1056,1057). The possibility that thrombosis and thrombocytopenia in certain neonates might be secondary to immune HIT (1058) remains open.

POLYCYTHEMIA

Polycythemic neonates with a hematocrit greater than 0.70 are commonly thrombocytopenic, particularly if they have associated cyanotic heart disease (1059,1060). The platelet count rises after phlebotomy (991).

CONGENITAL THROMBOCYTOPENIA AND MICROANGIOPATHIC HEMOLYSIS

Sometimes, recurrent thrombocytopenia and microangiopathic hemolysis that responds to plasma infusion begins in early infancy (867,1061–1064). Some of these patients have abnormal circulating HMW multimers of vWF (1064).

HOMOZYGOUS PROTEIN C DEFICIENCY

Thrombocytopenia can be a prominent feature of homozygous protein C deficiency, which can present as neonatal purpura fulminans syndrome with DIC (1065).

FATTY ACID–INDUCED THROMBOCYTOPENIA

Thrombocytopenia temporally related to the parenteral administration of lipid emulsions has been described in the neonate (1066). In some children, this condition may be related to cholestasis associated with total parenteral nutrition (1067). Platelet activation by administered fatty acids (1068) may be responsible for the thrombocytopenia as well as for the intimal vascular lesions that neonates receiving parenteral lipid preparations can develop (1069,1070). Alternatively, enhanced platelet destruction by reticuloendothelial cells has been described (1008). However, other studies suggest that thrombocytopenia is not a common complication of fat emulsions (1071).

INHERITED METABOLIC DISORDERS

Inherited metabolic disorders associated with thrombocytopenia include methylmalonic acidemia (1072), ketotic hyperglycinemia secondary to propionic acidemia (1073), mevalonic aciduria (1074,1075), holocarboxylase synthetase deficiency (1076), and isovaleric acidemia (1077,1078). Sometimes there is pancytopenia associated with hepatosplenomegaly (1074,1075). Pancytopenia associated with isovaleric acidemia likely results from toxicity of elevated isovaleric acid levels on marrow progenitor cells (1077,1078).

ERYTHROBLASTOSIS FETALIS

Thrombocytopenia and neutropenia can complicate Rh hemolytic disease of the newborn. The findings of a low MPV and reduced numbers of megakaryocyte progeny generated *in vitro* from circulating multipotent progenitor cells suggest reduced platelet production (1079). Other potential contributory factors include hypersplenism in hydropic infants and exchange transfusion using platelet-poor concentrated RBC preparations.

HEREDITARY THROMBOCYTOPENIC DISORDERS

Both the hereditary hypomegakaryocytic (e.g., thrombocytopenia and absent radii syndrome, Fanconi's anemia, congenital amegakaryocytic thrombocytopenia) and hereditary ineffective thrombopoiesis disorders (e.g., Wiskott-Aldrich syndrome) are discussed in the section on decreased platelet production.

CONGENITAL INFILTRATIVE MARROW DISORDERS

Thrombocytopenia in association with depression of both myeloid and erythroid elements during the neonatal period can be the consequence of congenital infiltrative marrow disorders such as acute leukemia (1080,1081), stage IV congenital neuroblastoma (1082), osteopetrosis (1083), and histiocytosis X (1084,1085). Sometimes children with trisomy 21 (Down's syndrome) present with marked leukocytosis mimicking acute leukemia (leukemoid reaction), which spontaneously resolves (1081).

THROMBOCYTOPENIA CAUSED BY PLATELET SEQUESTRATION

Hypersplenism

Hypersplenism is defined as a reduction in one or more of the peripheral blood counts caused by increased blood cell sequestration by the spleen. The spleen is enlarged and almost always palpable. Table 32-8 lists the causes of hypersplenism. The hematologic cytopenias of hypersplenism can be cured by splenectomy, although this procedure is rarely indicated.

PATHOGENESIS

The spleen normally pools approximately one-third of the platelets (see section on platelet distribution). This physiologic splenic pooling (sequestration) is related to the splenic blood flow and the comparatively lengthy transit time of the blood cells through the spleen, approximately 10 minutes for platelets and leukocytes and 2 minutes for RBCs.

The pathogenesis of the hematologic cytopenias in hypersplenism is multifactorial (1086) but is predominantly related to increased pooling within an enlarged spleen. Increased blood flow to a larger spleen results in increased pooling of blood cells within the spleen, even if the transit time is unchanged (1087). Increased cell destruction also contributes to the thrombocytopenia of hypersplenism. This condition may be the result of the longer splenic transit time, allowing the cells to interact with phagocytic cells. In addition, patients with hypersplenism typically have an increased plasma volume (1088), which contributes to the cytopenia by a dilutional effect. Finally, it is also possible that some patients with hypersplenism underproduce one or more of the cellular elements, such as reduced thrombopoietin in patients with hypersplenism secondary to cirrhosis (1089).

DIAGNOSIS

The diagnosis of hypersplenism is usually one of exclusion. Typically, the patient has thrombocytopenia and leukopenia, with anemia being less severe, although a disproportionate reduction in any single cell line can occur. The patient has an enlarged spleen, which is almost always sufficiently enlarged to be palpable. In patients in whom it is technically difficult to palpate the spleen, an accurate determination of spleen size can be obtained using radionuclide scanning techniques or ultrasonography (1090).

The diagnosis of hypersplenic thrombocytopenia can be confirmed by a radiolabeled platelet lifespan study (Appendix 23). Patients with hypersplenism have a dramatically reduced platelet recovery. The normal percentage of recovery of autologous platelets is approximately 70%, whereas the percentage of platelet

---

TABLE 32-8. Causes of Hypersplenism

Congestive splenomegaly
  Cirrhosis
  Budd-Chiari syndrome (hepatic vein thrombosis)
  Portal vein obstruction or thrombosis
  Chronic passive congestion secondary to cardiac failure or constrictive pericarditis
  Hepatic schistosomiasis
Acute and chronic infections
  Viral illnesses[a] (especially infectious mononucleosis and acute hepatitis)
  Malaria[a]
  Tuberculosis
  Typhoid fever
  Bacterial endocarditis[a]
  Leishmaniasis
  Brucellosis
  Trypanosomiasis
  Echinococcosis
  Leprosy
Inflammatory conditions
  Sarcoidosis[a]
  Systemic lupus erythematosus[a]
  Felty's syndrome
  Rheumatoid arthritis associated with proliferation of large granular lymphocytes
  Vasculitis
Chronic hemolytic disorders
  Congenital hemolytic disorder
  Acute splenic sequestration crisis
Hematologic neoplasms
  Myeloproliferative syndromes (polycythemia rubra vera, chronic myeloid leukemia, agnogenic myeloid metaplasia)
  Lymphoproliferative disorders (Hodgkin's and non-Hodgkin's lymphoma, chronic lymphocytic leukemia, hairy cell leukemia)
  Histiocytosis X
Nonhematologic neoplasms
  Metastatic carcinoma
  Sarcoma
  Hemangioma
  Lymphangioma
Storage pool disorders
  Gaucher's disease
  Niemann-Pick disease
  Amyloidosis
  Sea-blue histiocytosis
  Diabetic lipemia
  Tangier disease
  Hurler's syndrome
  Hunter's syndrome
Miscellaneous
  Primary splenic hyperplasia (tropical and nontropical)
  Thyrotoxicosis
  Splenic cysts
  Hamartoma
  Amyloidosis
  Hereditary hemorrhagic telangiectasia
  "Wandering spleen"

[a]Thrombocytopenia in these disorders may be more frequently caused by immune platelet destruction than by hypersplenism.

---

recovery in a hypersplenic patient is often much less than 50%. Platelet survival is normal or only mildly reduced (1091,1092).

TREATMENT

It is rare for a patient with cytopenia caused by hypersplenism to require treatment for the cytopenia. Although the platelets are reduced in patients with hypersplenism, the thrombocytopenia is not severe, and the platelet count typically ranges from 50 to 150 $\times 10^9$/L. Consequently, these patients do not bleed because of the thrombocytopenia. Similarly, the leukopenia and anemia tend to be mild and asymptomatic. The definitive treatment of hypersplenism is splenectomy, and although splenectomy can be performed as a treatment for hypersplenism, it is more frequently performed for other reasons.

Sometimes, a procedure other than a splenectomy has therapeutic benefit. For example, the most common cause of hypersplenism in North America and Europe is alcoholic cirrhosis. In these patients, the hypersplenism is caused by portal hypertension, and death is much more likely to result from variceal hemorrhage than from complications of the hypersplenic cytopenias. Decompressive procedures, either surgical [e.g., distal splenorenal shunt (1093,1094)] or radiologic [e.g., transjugular intrahepatic portasystemic shunt (1095)], that are used to prevent recurrent variceal hemorrhage can also improve the cytopenias. However, these procedures are usually used for indications other than thrombocytopenia *per se* (1094,1095).

Investigators (1096,1097) have described the deliberate infarction of a proportion of the spleen by splenic arterial embolization. Although long-term benefits can result, sometimes efficacy is relatively transient, and the procedure has many complications. Thus, this procedure should be restricted to highly selected patients in whom the procedure is performed by experienced physicians.

Gaucher's disease is a storage disease caused by deficiency in glucocerebrosidase. Deposition of glucocerebroside occurs in the reticuloendothelial organs, and enlargement of the spleen up to 20 times normal is typical (1098). Bleeding manifestations may relate to platelet dysfunction (1099), as thrombocytopenia is rarely severe. Although splenectomy can cure hypersplenism, it is contraindicated because subsequent bone destruction and liver failure can arise from increased deposition of glucocerebroside in those organs postsplenectomy. Thus, partial splenectomy (1100) and partial splenic embolization (1101) have been used in selected patients. More recently, the hematologic abnormalities of Gaucher's disease have been treated effectively by replacement of glucocerebrosidase obtained from placentas (alglucerase) or by recombinant technology (imiglucerase) (1102).

Splenectomy is frequently effective in treating the cytopenias associated with hairy cell leukemia or other chronic lymphoproliferative disorders (1103). In addition to correction of hypersplenism, splenectomy removes a large tumor burden and reduces the neoplastic cell-associated humoral suppression of normal hematopoiesis (1104). Early splenectomy may also improve survival in patients with chronic lymphoid leukemia and severe thrombocytopenia (platelet count $< 50 \times 10^9/L$) (1105). Patients with agnogenic myeloid metaplasia frequently benefit from splenectomy not only because of improvement in the cytopenias but also because of control of pain and discomfort caused by the enlarged spleen (1106).

Idiopathic splenomegaly (primary splenic hyperplasia) is a rare cause of hypersplenism that is associated with an increased risk of lymphoma (1107). Primary splenic lymphoma is a rare condition that can present as hypersplenism (1108).

Rarely, thrombocytopenia secondary to hypersplenism is associated with an enlarged, ectopic spleen located in the lower abdomen or pelvis ("wandering spleen") (1109,1110). More often, the diagnosis is made because of an acute surgical abdomen resulting from torsion of the elongated splenic pedicle.

COMPLICATIONS OF SPLENECTOMY

The complications of splenectomy were discussed in the section Idiopathic Thrombocytopenic Purpura and consist of early postoperative complications (pleuropulmonary, infections, embolism) and late risk of overwhelming postsplenectomy septicemia. The complication rate is reported to be highest in patients with myeloproliferative syndromes (1111).

Hypothermia

Observations in experimental and hibernating animals as well as in humans cooled for surgery indicate that hypothermia is frequently accompanied by mild to moderate thrombocytopenia (1112–1115). Thrombocytopenia has also been observed in accidental hypothermia both in infants (1116) and in the elderly (1117–1121), as well as in infants (1122) or adults (1123) suffering from hypothalamic dysfunction and temperature dysregulation. The thrombocytopenia is transient and corrects with rewarming. In some patients, bleeding symptoms were attributed to the thrombocytopenia (1117,1122). Platelet kinetic studies in cooled dogs demonstrated reversible hepatic and splenic platelet sequestration (1112,1124,1125). Indirect evidence suggests that decreased platelet production may play a contributory role (1117,1122).

Red Blood Cell Transfusions

It has been observed (1126–1128) that platelet count reductions averaging 33% to 40% occur over 72 hours in patients receiving 2 to 5 U packed RBCs. Radionuclide studies revealed that this phenomenon was associated with splenic platelet sequestration. Accordingly, this phenomenon is not observed in asplenic patients (1128). Removal of microaggregate debris by filtration or washing of the packed RBCs markedly reduces the extent of platelet count decrease (1126,1127).

THROMBOCYTOPENIA CAUSED BY DECREASED PLATELET PRODUCTION

Thrombocytopenia often is caused by decreased platelet production, which can be divided into three categories: acquired, generalized marrow disorders; acquired, isolated megakaryocytic disorders; and hereditary thrombocytopenic disorders.

By far the most common cause of decreased platelet production is acquired, generalized marrow disorders. The pathologic process disturbs all cell lines, and pancytopenia typically results. Occasionally, however, isolated thrombocytopenia is the first abnormality detected during the early stages of a panmyelopathy.

Except for alcohol-induced thrombocytopenia, acquired disorders restricted to megakaryocytes are uncommon.

The hereditary thrombocytopenic disorders also are relatively rare. They can be broadly considered in two categories: hypomegakaryocytic thrombocytopenia and ineffective thrombopoiesis. The hypomegakaryocytic thrombocytopenic disorders are characterized by absent or markedly reduced megakaryocyte numbers. They usually present in infancy, and associated nonhematologic phenotypic abnormalities are frequent. The hereditary disorders of ineffective thrombopoiesis are a heterogeneous group ranging from isolated, clinically insignificant thrombocytopenia to severe, symptomatic thrombocytopenia associated with nonhematologic abnormalities, such as immune deficiency (Wiskott-Aldrich syndrome). Megakaryocyte numbers are usually normal.

Acquired, Generalized Marrow Disorders

Acquired, generalized marrow disorders are discussed in detail elsewhere in this book and, except for myelodysplasia-associated thrombocytopenia, are summarized here in outline form.

NONNEOPLASTIC HYPOPROLIFERATIVE STEM CELL DISORDERS

Thrombocytopenia accompanies aplastic anemia, chemotherapy-induced pancytopenia, and idiosyncratic drug-induced aplastic anemia. Sometimes, isolated thrombocytopenia is a precursor of aplastic anemia.

NEOPLASTIC STEM CELL DISORDERS, INCLUDING MYELODYSPLASIA

Thrombocytopenia is common with primary neoplastic disorders of the bone marrow. These include neoplasms of the myeloid series, such as acute myeloid leukemia, myelodysplasia (MDS), myeloproliferative syndromes, and paroxysmal nocturnal hemoglobinuria. Lymphoid neoplasms include acute lymphoid leukemia and many chronic lymphoproliferative disorders, such as chronic lymphoid leukemia, hairy cell leukemia, non-Hodgkin's lymphoma, adult T-cell leukemia and lymphoma, multiple myeloma, and Waldenström's macroglobulinemia.

Isolated, refractory thrombocytopenia is the initial presentation in 1% to 3% of patients with MDS and can be confused with ITP (1129–1131). Sometimes, serious bleeding complications occur, especially as there may be coexisting defects in platelet function (1132,1133).

Peripheral blood examination often reveals giant platelets, which sometimes are hypogranular. Marrow examination reveals dysmegakaryocytopoiesis in half of cases. Typically, the megakaryocytes are abnormally small, but large mononuclear and abnormal segmented megakaryocytes are found in some patients (1131). Megakaryocyte numbers are usually normal, but increased megakaryocytes (resembling ITP) (1131) or amegakaryocytic thrombocytopenia (1130) have also been observed.

Treatment includes supportive care and, in selected cases, chemotherapy. Corticosteroids are generally ineffective. In a minority of patients, androgens such as danazol (600 to 800 mg/day) (1134–1137) or fluoxymesterone (1 mg/kg/day) (1137) result in a platelet count increase, possibly by reduced platelet destruction resulting from lower monocyte Fcγ receptor numbers (1135). One group (1138) reported benefit from splenectomy in a small subset of thrombocytopenic patients with MDS shown to have shortened platelet survival.

INFILTRATIVE MARROW DISORDERS

Thrombocytopenia can be secondary to infiltration of the bone marrow by nonhematologic metastatic malignancies, infectious organisms, storage-cell disorders, myelofibrosis, and osteopetrosis.

MEGALOBLASTIC ANEMIA

Megaloblastic anemia, which usually is caused by vitamin B_{12} or folic acid deficiency, is often associated with thrombocytopenia. Vitamin deficiency–induced defective DNA synthesis results in megakaryocytes of low ploidy, which produce small platelets (1139). Thus, the combination of large, heterogeneous red cells together with small platelets (low MPV) suggests megaloblastic anemia, although it also can be seen in some patients with primary marrow disorders.

Acquired Megakaryocytic Disorders

ALCOHOL-INDUCED THROMBOCYTOPENIA

Thrombocytopenia is a common complication of alcohol abuse, occurring in approximately one-fourth of alcoholic patients admitted to the hospital (1140). Severe thrombocytopenia and bleeding are uncommon, although platelet counts as low as 10×10^9/L have been described (1141). Consequently, a bleeding patient should be investigated for local causes of bleeding (esophageal varices, gastritis, peptic ulcers) and other types of hemostatic impairment (coagulopathy, platelet dysfunction of cirrhosis). Other causes of thrombocytopenia, including hypersplenism and folate deficiency, should also be considered. Alcohol itself causes platelet dysfunction (1141,1142).

Alcohol-induced thrombocytopenia can occur in the absence of liver disease or nutrient deficiency (1143–1146). In one study (1144), administration of alcohol and normal calorie and nutrient supplementation caused an isolated fall in the platelet count in half the volunteers after 3 to 5 weeks of daily alcohol consumption. In two other studies (1145,1146), in which hospitalized patients were allowed alcohol *ad libitum*, thrombocytopenia developed within 11 to 15 days. The platelet count begins to rise 2 to 3 days after cessation of alcohol consumption and reaches normal values usually within 1 week. The maximal platelet count, which often reaches supernormal values, usually occurs 10 to 18 days after stopping alcohol (1143–1146). Rebound thrombocytosis after alcohol cessation can also occur in the absence of preceding thrombocytopenia, a phenomenon that may contribute to increased risk of thrombotic stroke among alcoholics (1147,1148).

Besides thrombocytopenia, the complete blood cell count often reveals red cell macrocytosis produced by alcohol (1149). The bone marrow examination usually shows normal megakaryocyte morphology, although normoblast and promyelocyte vacuolations frequently are evident (1143,1144). Reduced megakaryocyte numbers can occur and may be associated with slower recovery of platelet counts (1150).

Platelet kinetic data (1151), recovery patterns from plateletpheresis (1152), MPV studies (1153), and marrow culture studies (1150,1154) all indicate that the platelet production is impaired by alcohol. The *in vitro* studies, both in humans (1150) and rodents (1154), suggest that alcohol decreases platelet production by suppressing the maturing megakaryocytes, with little effect on the progenitor colony-forming unit-megakaryocyte. Other effects of alcohol include moderate reduction in platelet lifespan (1151) and platelet ultrastructural alterations.

ACQUIRED AMEGAKARYOCYTIC THROMBOCYTOPENIA

Acquired amegakaryocytic thrombocytopenia is a rare, acquired disorder characterized by isolated thrombocytopenia associated with a total or marked reduction in megakaryocytes. Sometimes, there is associated RBC macrocytosis, and progression to aplastic anemia or myelodysplasia can occur (1130,1155–1157). The disorder also has been described in association with SLE (1158) or a positive direct Coombs' test (1159) or as an idiosyncratic drug reaction (1160). Cyclic amegakaryocytic thrombocytopenia also has been observed in a few patients (1161–1163).

The pathogenesis is heterogeneous, and four different mechanisms have been implicated: (a) an intrinsic stem cell defect, as evidenced by defective growth of megakaryocyte precursors (1156); (b) cytotoxic IgG autoantibody against megakaryocyte precursors (1156,1164); (c) T-cell–mediated suppression of megakaryocyte development (1158); and (d) IgG autoantibody inhibiting the responsiveness of megakaryocyte progenitor cells to granulocyte-macrophage colony-stimulating factor (1161). Levels of thrombopoietin are much higher than in patients with ITP (1165).

Standard-dose corticosteroids, androgens, lithium, 6-mercaptopurine, vincristine, and splenectomy are generally ineffective (1155,1156). Partial or complete responses to antithymocyte globulin (1166,1167), high-dose corticosteroids (1158,1168), or both (1157) have been reported. Case reports have described benefit from cyclosporine (1162,1169,1170), danazol (1159,1163,1171), vinblastine (1164), and cyclophosphamide (1172). Allogeneic BMT from an HLA-matched sibling was successful in one patient (1173).

IRON DEPLETION AND REPLETION

Although iron deficiency is usually associated with normal or increased numbers of platelets (1174), thrombocytopenia can accompany severe iron deficiency anemia (1175–1183), with evidence for reduced numbers of megakaryocytes (1176,1178–1180). Some patients with iron deficiency anemia and normal or elevated platelet counts develop transient thrombocytopenia after iron replacement therapy, with platelet count nadirs noted 6 to 12 days after institution of iron repletion (1181–1183). Thrombocytopenia in iron depletion or after iron repletion may result from competition between erythroid and megakaryocytic precursors (1183,1184). For example, rats given high levels of erythropoietin together with iron supplements initially develop thrombocytosis, followed by thrombocytopenia, likely because increasing erythropoiesis limits thrombocytopoiesis (1185).

Hereditary Thrombocytopenic Disorders

Hereditary thrombocytopenic disorders are believed to be uncommon, although they probably are underdiagnosed. Sometimes, they can be recognized by characteristic nonhematologic syndromic features (e.g., absent radii, deafness, nephritis) (1186,1187). However, if the thrombocytopenia is an isolated finding that is first recognized later in life, it may be misdiagnosed as ITP. Hereditary thrombocytopenia is primarily categorized based on whether megakaryocytes are absent or reduced (hypomegakaryocytic) or there is ineffective thrombopoiesis with adequate megakaryocyte numbers (Table 32-9).

Hereditary Hypomegakaryocytic Thrombocytopenia

Multiple congenital malformations, most frequently absent radii, can accompany hereditary hypomegakaryocytic thrombocytopenia. Sometimes, isolated thrombocytopenia heralds the onset of pancytopenia in patients with a hereditary aplastic anemia, such as Fanconi's anemia or dyskeratosis congenita.

THROMBOCYTOPENIA WITH ABSENT RADII
The autosomal-recessive syndrome of hypomegakaryocytic thrombocytopenia with bilateral absent radii (TAR) usually presents with severe thrombocytopenia and bleeding during the first weeks or months of life; rarely, patients do not develop thrombocytopenia until adult age (1187,1188). Usually, thrombocytopenia is most severe during the first year of life and gradually improves, so that most patients become asymptomatic (1189). Bone marrow examination shows absent or markedly reduced numbers of megakaryocytes that appear immature. The thrombocytopenia in TAR appears to be due to an intrinsic defect that prevents certain megakaryocyte progenitor cells from maturing normally (1190).

Skeletal defects involving intercalary (nonterminal) bones of the upper and lower extremities are common (1189–1191). Thus, in contrast to Fanconi's anemia, the thumb and fingers are present, but they may be hypoplastic. Approximately 20% of patients also have cardiac anomalies. A leukemoid reaction, sometimes accompanied by eosinophilia, is common during the neonatal period and usually subsides spontaneously within a few months. Chromosomal abnormalities have not been described.

Although the syndrome of thrombocytopenia and absent radii is an autosomal-recessive disorder, consanguinity is uncommon, suggesting that affected patients may be heterozygous for two distinct genetic defects (1192). These patients have approximately a 25% risk for future affected offspring. Prenatal diagnosis is possible by radiography or ultrasonography (1193,1194) with fetal blood sampling (1195).

Corticosteroids and splenectomy are not usually effective. Bone marrow transplantation is not indicated because of the favorable natural history. Patients with bleeding may require platelet transfusions and fibrinolytic inhibitors (1189). Orthopedic procedures to improve upper limb function or appearance are best postponed until after infancy, when the platelet counts are improved.

TABLE 32-9. Hereditary (Congenital) Thrombocytopenic Disorders[a]

Hypomegakaryocytic
  Plus skeletal abnormalities
    Thrombocytopenia with absent radii
    Miscellaneous disorders, e.g., amegakaryocytic thrombocytopenia and radioulnar synostosis
  Isolated thrombocytopenia
    Congenital amegakaryocytic thrombocytopenia
  Hereditary aplastic anemia
    Fanconi's anemia
    Miscellaneous disorders, e.g., dyskeratosis congenita
Ineffective thrombopoiesis (usually autosomal dominant)
  Macrothrombocytopenia
    Isolated macrothrombocytopenia (nonsyndromic)
      Mediterranean macrothrombocytopenia
    Plus leukocyte inclusions: May-Hegglin anomaly, Sebastian syndrome, Fechtner syndrome
    Plus hearing or renal impairment[b]: Epstein syndrome, isolated hearing loss, Fechtner syndrome
  Macrothrombocytopenia with thrombocytopathy
    Platelet glycoprotein (gp) abnormalities
      Bernard-Soulier syndrome (absence of gpIb-IX-V complex) (AR)
      Velocardiofacial syndrome (reduced gpIbβ)
      X-linked macrothrombocytopenia with dyserythropoiesis (reduced gpIbα)
      gpIV abnormality
      Mitral valve insufficiency (reduced gpIa, Ic, IIa) (AR)
    Miscellaneous disorders
      Gray platelet syndrome
      Paris-Trousseau thrombocytopenia
      Montreal platelet syndrome
      "Swiss-cheese" platelets
      Impaired platelet procoagulant activity
      Increased megakaryocyte ploidy
  Normal-sized platelets
    Isolated thrombocytopenia (nonsyndromic)
    Miscellaneous disorders
      Familial platelet disorder with predisposition to acute myeloid leukemia
      Quebec platelet disorder
      Platelet-type vWD and vWD-2B
      X-linked thrombocytopenia with thalassemia
  Microthrombocytopenia with thrombocytopathy (X-linked inheritance)
    Wiskott-Aldrich syndrome
      X-linked microthrombocytopenia (variant Wiskott-Aldrich syndrome)

AR, autosomal recessive; vWD, von Willebrand's disease.
[a]Usually autosomal dominant, unless otherwise indicated.
[b]Alport's syndrome refers to duad of glomerulonephritis and sensorineural deafness.

MISCELLANEOUS SYNDROMIC HYPOMEGAKARYOCYTIC THROMBOCYTOPENIA
Although congenital hypomegakaryocytic thrombocytopenia usually occurs with bilateral absent radii, it can be associated with other congenital abnormalities. These include trisomy 18 (1196–1198), microcephaly (1199,1200), multiple malformations and neurologic dysfunction (1201), and elevated fetal hemoglobin (1202). An autosomal-dominant syndrome of amegakaryocytic thrombocytopenia associated with radioulnar synostosis (i.e., proximal fusion of the ulna and radius) has been associated with mutation in a homeobox gene (HOXA11) (1203). This finding is consistent with the known function of homeobox genes to encode regulatory proteins involved in bone morphogenesis and hematopoiesis.

CONGENITAL AMEGAKARYOCYTIC THROMBOCYTOPENIA
Congenital amegakaryocytic thrombocytopenia is a very rare, autosomal-recessive disorder characterized by isolated, severe thrombocytopenia with near absence of megakaryocytes during infancy that often exhibits progressive bone marrow failure involving other cell lines. No skeletal or other congenital abnor-

malities are found. Defective expression of c-Mpl (thrombopoietin receptor) due to mutations in *c-mpl* have been implicated (1204,1205). Because thrombopoietin also has an antiapoptotic influence on hematopoietic progenitor cells (1204–1206), this defect also can explain progression of isolated thrombocytopenia to marrow failure and pancytopenia over time. Allogeneic transplantation of marrow or peripheral stem cells can cure this disorder (1207,1208).

HEREDITARY APLASTIC ANEMIA

Fanconi's Anemia. Fanconi's anemia is an autosomal-recessive disorder characterized by aplastic anemia, usually beginning between the ages of 5 and 10 years. Approximately two-thirds of patients have extrahematologic abnormalities, which include growth retardation, skeletal malformations (especially dysplasia or absence of the thumbs, sometimes with absent radii), neurologic abnormalities, hyperpigmentation, and genitourinary abnormalities (1209–1212). These patients are also at increased risk for developing acute myeloid leukemia. Multiple, spontaneous chromosomal breaks are characteristic (1213).

Isolated thrombocytopenia usually precedes the pancytopenia. Thus, a patient with Fanconi's anemia and absent radii who presents with thrombocytopenia during infancy may be thought to have TAR syndrome. Distinct from TAR syndrome, however, the thumbs are lacking in Fanconi's anemia if the radii are absent. The chromosomal and hemoglobin findings characteristic of Fanconi's anemia also aid in differentiating these disorders. Treatment of Fanconi's anemia is discussed in Chapter 8.

Other Hereditary Aplastic Anemias. Other patients that initially present with congenital hypomegakaryocytic thrombocytopenia can subsequently develop aplastic anemia (1211,1212). For example, isolated thrombocytopenia can precede or accompany the development of dyskeratosis congenita (reticular skin pigmentation, nail dystrophy, mucosal leukokeratosis), a hereditary disorder frequently associated with onset of aplastic anemia in childhood (1214,1215). Approximately 50% of patients with Pearson's syndrome (refractory sideroblastic anemia, exocrine pancreatic insufficiency, plus other abnormalities) also have neutropenia and thrombocytopenia (1212).

A syndrome of X-linked congenital amegakaryocytic thrombocytopenia with elevated fetal hemoglobin progressing to aplastic anemia has been described (1216). A syndrome of bone marrow failure occurring either in childhood (1217) or adulthood (1218) associated with proximal fusion of the radius and ulna has been observed in several unrelated families. Thrombocytopenia and macrocytosis preceded the development of pancytopenia in some of the patients. Inheritance is autosomal-dominant, and the chromosomes are normal. Other autosomal-dominant disorders that can manifest thrombocytopenia and upper limb abnormalities (among other malformations) include the oculootoradial (also called *IVIC*) and WT syndromes (1219–1222).

Hereditary Thrombocytopenia with Ineffective Thrombopoiesis

Hereditary thrombocytopenia with ineffective thrombopoiesis is characterized by thrombocytopenia with normal or increased numbers of megakaryocytes and normal RBC and leukocyte counts (1186,1187). Although decreased platelet survival is found in some patients (1223), normal platelet survival and reduced platelet turnover suggest that ineffective thrombopoiesis is the predominant abnormality (1224,1225).

INEFFECTIVE THROMBOPOIESIS WITH MACROTHROMBOCYTES

Most patients with hereditary ineffective thrombopoiesis have large platelets, and the mode of inheritance usually is autosomal dominant (1186,1187,1225,1226). Defective thrombopoiesis in an animal model of congenital macrothrombocytopenia (Wistar-Furth rat) has been described (1227,1228). Both nonsyndromic and syndromic forms are recognized.

Isolated Macrothrombocytopenia (Nonsyndromic). Many families have been identified with chronic thrombocytopenia transmitted in an autosomal-dominant fashion, large platelets, normal platelet survival, adequate numbers of megakaryocytes, and absence of other clinical abnormalities (1225,1226). PAIgG levels are often elevated, but this elevation reflects the large platelet size, as glycoprotein-specific platelet antibody assays are normal (1226).

It has been reported that among Mediterranean patients, the reference platelet count range may be relatively low (125 to 300 vs. 150 to 400×10^9/L) (9). In general, patients with lower platelet counts tend to have larger platelet size. It remains uncertain whether "Mediterranean macrothrombocytopenia" reflects the inclusion of individuals who might otherwise be classified as having hereditary isolated macrothrombocytopenia.

Several distinct clinical syndromes are recognized:

Macrothrombocytopenia with leukocyte inclusions or renal or hearing abnormalities (May-Hegglin anomaly, Sebastian's syndrome, Fechtner's syndrome, Epstein's syndrome): Several macrothrombocytopenic syndromes with autosomal-dominant inheritance have been observed. Three of these are also characterized by leukocyte inclusions. The *May-Hegglin anomaly* is characterized by giant platelets and blue, spindle-shaped inclusions within granulocytes and monocytes (1229–1232). By ultrastructural analysis, these inclusions consist of parallel rows of ribosomes interspersed between intermediate filaments (1230). Many patients have mild thrombocytopenia, although the platelet count may appear considerably lower by particle counter (1231,1232). Bleeding symptoms are often only mild or moderate. Platelet function is usually normal. Platelet transfusions are appropriate for treating bleeding episodes, although desmopressin appeared effective in one severely affected patient (1232). Recently, mutations in the nonmuscle myosin heavy-chain type A gene have been identified in the May-Hegglin anomaly as well as the Fechtner's and Sebastian syndromes (1233,1234).

In *Fechtner's syndrome* and *Sebastian's syndrome*, leukocyte inclusions are composed of dispersed (nonparallel) filament, ribosomes, and endoplasmic reticulum in a pattern thus ultrastructurally distinct from those of Döhle bodies and May-Hegglin inclusions (1230,1235–1238). Whereas abnormalities in Sebastian's syndrome are limited to macrothrombocytopenia and the leukocyte inclusions (1230,1237,1238), patients with Fechtner's syndrome also have the duad of glomerulonephritis and deafness (Alport's syndrome), sometimes accompanied by cataracts (1235,1236,1239).

In contrast, leukocyte inclusions are not observed in *Epstein's syndrome*, which is characterized by macrothrombocytopenia and Alport's syndrome (1240–1243). Platelet aggregation abnormalities are observed in some families (1241). Thrombocytopenia occurs in infancy, but progressive albuminuria, hematuria, and renal insufficiency as well as sensorineural hearing impairment predominantly affecting high-pitched tones develops in childhood or early adulthood. Sometimes, macrothrombocytopenia and hearing loss without renal abnormalities occur (1244,1245).

Macrothrombocytopenia with Platelet Glycoprotein Deficiency. Several hereditary macrothrombocytopenic disorders have platelet glycoprotein abnormalities. *Bernard-Soulier syn-*

drome (1246) is an autosomal-recessive disorder characterized by thrombocytopenia, giant platelets, and prolonged bleeding time associated with complete or partial absence of the gpIb-IX-V membrane complex (39,40,1247,1248). Desmopressin infusion can correct the prolonged bleeding times in these patients (1249). A variant disorder characterized by macrothrombocytopenia and reduced sialic acid on gpIb has also been described (1250). In addition, giant platelets and mild thrombocytopenia have been reported in patients with velocardiofacial syndrome (velopharyngeal insufficiency, conotruncal heart disease, learning disability), which is caused by a deletion in chromosome 22q11 that also contains the coding region for gpIbβ (1251–1253).

X-linked macrothrombocytopenia with dyserythropoiesis secondary to mutations in the X-linked *GATA1* gene has been described in two families (GATA1 is transcription factor essential for normal erythropoiesis and megakaryocyte differentiation) (1254,1255). Deficiency in gpIbα (but not gpIbβ) has been observed (1255).

A family with asymptomatic chronic macrothrombocytopenia and autosomal-dominant inheritance has been described in whom decreased glycosylation of platelet gpIV was detected (1256). Another family with mitral valve insufficiency and macrothrombocytopenia was reported with autosomal-recessive inheritance and deficiency in glycoproteins Ia, Ic, and IIa (1257).

Miscellaneous Macrothrombocytopenic Disorders. The *gray platelet syndrome* is an inherited disorder characterized by large, agranular, gray-appearing platelets on the stained blood film (1258,1259). Usually, the thrombocytopenia and bleeding symptoms are mild. There is a virtual absence of α-granules in platelets and megakaryocytes caused by a defect in targeting of endogenously synthesized proteins to these granules (1260): Thus, these platelets are not activated by HIT antibodies (which recognize the α-granule glycoprotein, PF4) (1261).

Paris-Trousseau thrombocytopenia is characterized by giant α-granules that do not release their contents after thrombin stimulation (1262,1263). A minority of the platelets are increased in size. A deletion of the distal part of chromosome 11 is seen in this disorder (1262,1263).

The *Montreal platelet syndrome* is a hereditary giant-platelet syndrome disorder characterized by bleeding, thrombocytopenia, spontaneous platelet aggregation, and hypervolumetric shape change on platelet activation (1264,1265). The abnormal platelet aggregation is not mediated by fibrinogen and calcium. A defect in platelet calpain has been identified in this syndrome (1266).

The designation *"Swiss-cheese" platelets* has been used to describe platelets from certain patients with generally mild bleeding tendencies, macrothrombocytopenia, various platelet function abnormalities, and dilatation of the open canalicular system demonstrated ultrastructurally (1267,1268). These morphologic findings probably can result from both hereditary platelet metabolic disturbances and certain acquired thrombocytopathies, such as myelodysplasia and pernicious anemia (1269).

Impaired platelet procoagulant activity (decreased PF3) has been reported in several families with macrothrombocytopenia (1270,1271). However, neither large platelet size nor thrombocytopenia is seen in the phospholipid scrambling disorder known as *Scott's syndrome* (1272,1273). In contrast, in patients with *Stormorken's syndrome*, thrombocytopenia with large platelets is observed with constitutional expression of a membrane phospholipid profile consistent with the activated platelet state (1273,1274).

Increased megakaryocyte ploidy was a feature of one family with an autosomal-dominant bleeding disorder also characterized by macrothrombocytopenia, abnormal platelet aggregation, and platelet arachidonic acid deficiency (1275).

INEFFECTIVE THROMBOPOIESIS WITH NORMAL-SIZED PLATELETS

Isolated Normothrombocytopenia (Nonsyndromic). Two large kindreds with autosomal-dominant thrombocytopenia (mean, 43 to 62×10^9/L) and normal MPV have been reported in which the disease gene locus has been identified on the short arm of chromosome 10 (1276–1278). Megakaryocyte numbers are generally normal or mildly reduced, but micromegakaryocytes with reduced ploidy are seen; progression to marrow aplasia is not seen. Increased numbers of colony-forming unit-megakaryocyte progenitors suggest a defect in maturation of megakaryocytes (1276). Other families with autosomal-dominant thrombocytopenia and normal-sized platelets have also been reported (1279–1281); some patients exhibit platelet function abnormalities (1279,1280).

Miscellaneous Normothrombocytopenia. *Familial platelet disorder with predisposition to acute myeloid leukemia* has been observed in several unrelated families (1282–1286) and is characterized by autosomal-dominant thrombocytopenia, normal MPV, impaired platelet secretion, and a lifetime propensity to develop acute myeloid leukemia estimated at approximately 30% (1284). Haploinsufficiency of the hematopoietic transcription factor *CBFA2* has been identified in this disorder (1286).

Quebec platelet disorder (formerly, Quebec factor V) is an autosomal-dominant disorder reported in two large pedigrees in Quebec and is characterized by thrombocytopenia and delayed onset of bleeding after trauma (1287–1289). Although the platelets are structurally normal, many proteins within α-granules are proteolyzed, including factor V, vWF, fibrinogen, multimerin, and plasminogen. The recent report of a 100-fold increase in platelet urokinase levels in Quebec platelet disorder (1289) may explain why bleeding episodes are benefited by antifibrinolytic agents but not by platelet transfusions.

Platelet-type von Willebrand's disease (pseudo-vWD) is an autosomal-dominant disorder characterized by mild intermittent thrombocytopenia, mild bleeding, absence of HMW multimers of vWF, and increased ristocetin-induced platelet aggregation. The defect resides not within the vWF molecule but within the platelet membrane, which has enhanced reactivity to vWF (1290). *Type 2B vWD* is clinically similar; however, abnormal vWF with increased platelet reactivity causes intermittent thrombocytopenia, particularly during pregnancy (1291,1292) and the postoperative state (1293). The usual mode of inheritance is autosomal dominant, but patients with an autosomal-recessive inheritance have been described (1293). For both disorders, desmopressin is contraindicated because thrombocytopenia is exacerbated (1294).

X-linked thrombocytopenia with thalassemia is characterized by moderate thrombocytopenia, splenomegaly, reticulocytosis, and unbalanced hemoglobin chain synthesis resembling β-thalassemia minor. Platelet size is normal (1295,1296).

INEFFECTIVE THROMBOPOIESIS WITH MICROTHROMBOCYTES

Wiskott-Aldrich Syndrome. Wiskott-Aldrich syndrome (WAS) consists of thrombocytopenia (platelet count usually below 70×10^9/L) with microthrombocytes (MPV usually <5 fL), eczema, and an impaired immune system manifest as increased susceptibility to viral and bacterial infections (1297–1299). The illness is often fatal by 10 years of age because of infection (44%), bleeding (23%), or lymphoreticular malignancy (26%) (1298). The immune defects can be profound, with impairment of both cellular and humoral immunity. There is progressive decline in lymphocyte number during early childhood and reduced lymphocyte response to mitogens, allogeneic cells, and polysaccharide antigens (1300). Immune dysregulation can also manifest as autoimmune hemolysis, vasculitis, inflammatory bowel disease, and allergy to cow milk and other foods (1299).

WAS is inherited in an X-linked recessive fashion and is caused by mutation in the α gene located in the short arm of the X chromosome that encodes a 502–amino acid protein known as WASp (1301). This intracellular protein is expressed only in hematopoietic cells and is a member of a family of more widely expressed proteins involved in signal transduction from cell-surface receptors to the actin cytoskeleton (1299). Interestingly, platelets produced *in vitro* by WAS megakaryocytes have normal size but abnormal cytoarchitecture (1302). Perhaps the structural abnormalities lead to splenic remodeling of the WAS platelets, because splenectomy generally corrects both thrombocytopenia and MPV in these patients (1303).

Platelet survival is reduced by approximately 50% (1300) and is related to the intrinsic platelet abnormalities, because homologous platelets have normal survival in patients with WAS (1304). Platelet production is decreased, however, despite adequate megakaryocyte numbers (ineffective thrombopoiesis) (1300). The marked reduction (approximately 50%) in platelet size is sufficiently unique (1300,1305) that electronic platelet sizing of fetoscopically obtained blood has been used for prenatal diagnosis (1305) (although genetic methods are now preferred). Despite the small platelets, PAIgG levels are strikingly elevated (1306).

Splenectomy usually raises the platelet count to normal (1307,1308), a feature that is unique among the hereditary thrombocytopenias. Splenectomy also appears to improve patient survival and has been used as a primary treatment option for children with WAS (1308). However, the only curative therapy is BMT (1308,1309). For children transplanted at younger than 5 years, survival is at least 80% and appears to be similar whether an HLA-identical sibling or an HLA-matched unrelated donor is used (1299); however, for older children, transplantation with HLA-matched siblings is superior.

The cellular immune deficiency makes these patients susceptible to graft-versus-host disease caused by transfused lymphocytes, and platelets and other blood products must be irradiated before administration. These children also must receive antibiotic prophylaxis after splenectomy in addition to vaccination before splenectomy (1308).

X-Linked Thrombocytopenia (Variant Wiskott-Aldrich Syndrome). Hereditary thrombocytopenia inherited in an X-linked recessive fashion has been described in several families (1310–1314). Atopic symptoms (1310,1312–1314), laboratory immunologic abnormalities (1310,1311,1313,1314), reduced MPV (1312,1314), and elevated PAIgG (1314) in some affected thrombocytopenic patients suggest a forme fruste relation to WAS that has been confirmed by genetic studies (1315). Indeed, a mutation in the WASp gene or absent WASp mRNA or protein should be sought in male patients with congenital thrombocytopenia characterized by small platelets (1299,1316). A large study (1317) suggested that missense mutations in the first three exons of the WASp gene are generally associated with reduced (but not absent) production of WASp and, thus, less severe disease. As in classic WAS, thrombocytopenia improves with splenectomy (1310–1313).

Miscellaneous X-Linked Thrombocytopenia. Other families with X-linked thrombocytopenia have been described with normal (1318) or elevated (1255) MPV values. Some represent distinct clinical syndromes, such as X-linked thrombocytopenia

with thalassemia (1296), X-linked dyskeratosis congenita (1319), and chronic idiopathic intestinal pseudoobstruction (1320). The genetic bases for these disorders are distinct from WAS and variant WAS (1296,1321).

REFERENCES

1. Sherertz EF. Pigmented purpuric eruptions. *Semin Thromb Hemost* 1984;10:90.
2. Rodgers RPC, Levin J. A critical reappraisal of the bleeding time. *Semin Thromb Hemost* 1990;16:1.
3. Lind SE. The bleeding time does not predict surgical bleeding. *Blood* 1991;77:2547.
4. Gewirtz AS, Miller ML, Keys TF. The clinical usefulness of the preoperative bleeding time. *Arch Pathol Lab Med* 1996;120:353–356.
5. Burrows RF, Kelton JG. Incidentally detected thrombocytopenia in healthy mothers and their infants. *N Engl J Med* 1988;319:142.
6. Burrows RF, Kelton JG. Thrombocytopenia at delivery: a prospective survey of 6715 deliveries. *Am J Obstet Gynecol* 1990;162:731.
7. Shehata N, Burrows R, Kelton JG. Gestational thrombocytopenia. *Clin Obstet Gynecol* 1999;42:327–334.
8. Rinder HM, Bonan JL, Anandan S, et al. Noninvasive measurement of platelet kinetics in normal and hypertensive pregnancies. *Am J Obstet Gynecol* 1994;170:117.
9. Lozano M, Narváez J, Faúndez A, et al. Recuento de plaquetas y volumen plaquetario medio en la población española. *Med Clin (Barc)* 1998;110:774–777.
10. Bessman JD. Platelets. In: Bessman JD, ed. *Automated blood counts and differentials: a practical guide.* Baltimore: Johns Hopkins University Press, 1986:57.
11. Bessman JD, Gilmer PR, Gardner FH. Use of mean platelet volume improves detection of platelet disorders. *Blood Cells* 1985;11:127.
12. Niethammer AG, Forman EN. Use of the platelet histogram maximum in evaluating thrombocytopenia. *Am J Hematol* 1999;60:19–23.
13. Osselaer JC, Jamart J, Scheiff JM. Platelet distribution width for differential diagnosis of thrombocytosis. *Clin Chem* 1997;43:1072–1076.
14. Tomer A, Friese P, Conklin R, et al. Flow cytometric analysis of megakaryocytes from patients with abnormal platelet counts. *Blood* 1989;74:594.
15. Gloster ES, Strauss RA, Jiminez JF, et al. Spurious elevated platelet counts associated with bacteremia. *Am J Hematol* 1985;18:329.
16. Akwari AM, Ross DW, Stass SA. Spuriously elevated platelet counts due to microspherocytosis. *Am J Clin Pathol* 1982;77:220.
17. Morton BD, Orringer EP, Lattart LA, et al. Pappenheimer bodies: an additional cause for a spurious platelet count. *Am J Clin Pathol* 1980;74:310.
18. Stass SA, Holloway ML, Peterson V, et al. Cytoplasmic fragments causing spurious platelet counts in the leukemic phase of poorly differentiated lymphocytic leukemia. *Am J Clin Pathol* 1979;71:125.
19. Bartels PC, Schoorl M, Lombarts AJ. Screening for EDTA-dependent deviations in platelet counts and abnormalities in platelet distribution histograms in pseudothrombocytopenia. *Scand J Clin Lab Invest* 1997;57:629–636.
20. Bizzaro N. EDTA-dependent pseudothrombocytopenia: a clinical and epidemiological study of 112 cases, with 10-year follow-up. *Am J Hematol* 1995;50:103–109.
21. Pegels JG, Bruynes ECE, Engelfriet CP, et al. Pseudothrombocytopenia: an immunologic study on platelet antibodies dependent on ethylene diamine tetra-acetate. *Blood* 1982;59:157.
22. Casonato A, Bertomoro A, Pontara E, et al. EDTA dependent pseudothrombocytopenia caused by antibodies against the cytoadhesive receptor of platelet gpIIB-IIIA. *J Clin Pathol* 1994;47:625–630.
23. Fiorin F, Steffan A, Pradella P, et al. IgG platelet antibodies in EDTA-dependent pseudothrombocytopenia bind to platelet membrane glycoprotein Iib. *Am J Clin Pathol* 1998;110:178–183.
24. Sane DC, Damaraju LV, Topol EJ, et al. Occurrence and clinical significance of pseudothrombocytopenia during abciximab therapy. *J Am Coll Cardiol* 2000;36:75–83.
25. Cunningham VL, Brandt JT. Spurious thrombocytopenia due to EDTA-independent cold-reactive agglutinins. *Am J Clin Pathol* 1992;97:359.
26. Hoyt RH, Durie BGM. Pseudothrombocytopenia induced by a monoclonal IgM kappa platelet agglutinin. *Am J Hematol* 1989;31:50.
27. Pewarchuk W, VanderBoom J, Blajchman MA. Pseudopolycythemia, pseudothrombocytopenia, and pseudoleukopenia due to overfilling of blood collection vacuum tubes. *Arch Pathol Lab Med* 1992;116:90.
28. Bizzaro N. Platelet satellitosis to polymorphonuclears: cytochemical, immunological, and ultrastructural characterization of eight cases. *Am J Hematol* 1991;36:235.
29. Cohen AM, Lewinski UH, Klein B, et al. Satellitism of platelets to monocytes. *Acta Hematol* 1980;64:61.
30. Shahab N, Evans ML. Images in clinical medicine: platelet satellitism. *N Engl J Med* 1998;338:591.
31. Bizzaro N, Goldschmeding R, von dem Borne AE. Platelet satellitism is Fc gamma RIII (CD16) receptor-mediated. *Am J Clin Pathol* 1985;103:740.
32. Forscher CA, Sussman II, Friedman EW, et al. Pseudothrombocytopenia masking true thrombocytopenia. *Am J Hematol* 1985;18:313.
33. Mori M, Kudo H, Yoshitake S, et al. Transient EDTA-dependent pseudothrombocytopenia in a patient with sepsis. *Intensive Care Med* 2000;26:218–220.

34. Kelton JG, Ali AM. Platelet transfusions: a critical appraisal. *Clin Oncol* 1983;2:549.

35. Contreras M. The appropriate use of platelets: an update from the Edinburgh Consensus Conference. *Br J Haematol* 1998;101[Suppl 1]:10–12.

36. Bartholomew JR, Salgia R, Bell WR. Control of bleeding in patients with immune and nonimmune thrombocytopenia with aminocaproic acid. *Arch Intern Med* 1989;149:1959.

37. Fricke W, Alling D, Kimball J. Lack of efficacy of tranexamic acid in thrombocytopenic bleeding. *Transfusion* 1991;31:345.

38. Konkle BA, Shapiro SS, Asch AS, et al. Cytokine-enhanced expression of glycoprotein Ib in human endothelium. *J Biol Chem* 1990;265:19833.

39. Andrews RK, Shen Y, Gardiner EE, et al. The glycoprotein Ib-IX-V complex in platelet adhesion and signaling. *Thromb Haemost* 1999;82:357–364.

40. Hayashi T, Suzuki K. Molecular pathogenesis of Bernard-Soulier syndrome. *Semin Thromb Hemost* 2000;26:53–59.

41. Murata M, Furihata K, Ishida F, et al. Genetic and structural characterization of an amino acid dimorphism in glycoprotein Ib alpha involved in platelet transfusion refractoriness. *Blood* 1992;79:3086.

42. Newman PJ. The biology of PECAM-1. *J Clin Invest* 1997;99:3–8.

43. Macchi L, Rispal P, Clofent-Sanchez G, et al. Anti-platelet antibodies in patients with systemic lupus erythematosus and the primary antiphospholipid antibody syndrome: their relationship with the observed thrombocytopenia. *Br J Haematol* 1997;98:336–341.

44. Kroll H, Sun QH, Santoso S. Platelet endothelial cell adhesion molecule-1 (PECAM-1) is a target glycoprotein in drug-induced thrombocytopenia. *Blood* 2000;96:1409–1414.

45. Chong BH, Murray B, Berndt MC, et al. Plasma P-selectin is increased in thrombotic consumptive platelet disorders. *Blood* 1994;83:1535–1541.

46. Ruoslahti E. Integrins. *J Clin Invest* 1991;87:1.

47. Kunicki TJ. Platelet immunology. In: Colman RW, Hirsh J, Marder VJ, et al., eds. *Hemostasis and thrombosis: basic principles & clinical practice*, 4th ed. Philadelphia: Lippincott Williams & Wilkins, 2001:461–477.

48. George JN, Caen JP, Nurden AT. Glanzmann's thrombasthenia: the spectrum of clinical disease. *Blood* 1990;75:1383–1395.

49. Ruggeri ZM. Platelet-vessel wall interactions in flowing blood. In: Colman RW, Hirsh J, Marder VJ, et al., eds. *Hemostasis and thrombosis: basic principles & clinical practice*, 4th ed. Philadelphia: Lippincott Williams & Wilkins, 2001:683–698.

50. Van Leeuwen EF, Van der Ven JTM, Engelfriet CP, et al. Specificity of autoantibodies in autoimmune thrombocytopenia. *Blood* 1982;59:23.

51. Kiefel V, Freitag E, Kroll H, et al. Platelet autoantibodies (IgG, IgM, IgA) against glycoproteins IIb/IIIa and Ib/IX in patients with thrombocytopenia. *Ann Hematol* 1996;72:280–285.

52. Brighton TA, Evans S, Castaldi PA, et al. Prospective evaluation of the clinical usefulness of an antigen-specific assay (MAIPA) in idiopathic thrombocytopenic purpura and other immune thrombocytopenias. *Blood* 1996;88:194–201.

53. Christie DJ, Mullen PC, Aster RH. Quinine and quinidine platelet antibodies can react with GPIIb/IIIa. *Br J Haematol* 1987;67:213.

54. Newman PJ, Derbes RS, Aster RH. The human platelet alloantigens, PlA1 and PlA2, are associated with a leucine33/proline33 amino acid polymorphism in membrane glycoprotein IIIa, and are distinguishable by DNA typing. *J Clin Invest* 1989;83:1778.

55. Flug F, Espinola R, Liu LX, et al. A 13-mer peptide straddling the leucine33/proline33 polymorphism in glycoprotein IIIa does not define the PlA1 epitope. *Blood* 1991;77:1964–1969.

56. Val Leeuwen E, Leeksma O, van Mourik J, et al. Effect of the binding of anti-Zwa antibodies on platelet function. *Vox Sang* 1984;47:280–289.

57. Santoso S, Mueller-Eckhardt G, Santoso S, et al. HLA antigens on platelet membranes: in vitro and in vivo studies. *Vox Sang* 1986;51:327.

58. Haynes WDG, Jones JV, Cumming JCO. HLA-antigens on circulating platelets: ultrastructural demonstration. *Transplantation* 1974;18:81.

59. Pereira J, Cretney C, Aster RH. Variation of class I HLA antigen expression among platelet density cohorts: a possible index of platelet age? *Blood* 1988;71:516.

60. Aster RH, Szatkowski N, Liebert M, et al. Expression of HLA-B12, HLA-B8, w4 and w6 on platelets. *Transplant Proc* 1977;9:1695.

61. Mueller-Eckhardt G, Hauck M, Kayser W, et al. HLA-C antigens on platelets. *Tissue Antigens* 1980;16:91.

62. Legler TJ, Fischer I, Dittmann J, et al. Frequency and causes of refractoriness in multiply transfused patients. *Ann Hematol* 1997;74:185–189.

63. Taaning E. HLA antibodies and fetomaternal alloimmune thrombocytopenia: myth or meaningful. *Transfus Med Rev* 2000;14:275–280.

64. Kelton JG, Hamid C, Aker S, et al. The amount of blood group A substance on platelets is proportional to the amount in the plasma. *Blood* 1982;59:980.

65. Dunstan RA, Simpson MB, Knowles RW, et al. The origin of ABH antigens on human platelets. *Blood* 1985;65:615.

66. Santoso S, Kiefel V, Mueller-Eckhardt C. Blood groups A and B determinants are expressed on platelet glycoproteins IIa, IIIa and Ib. *Thromb Haemost* 1991;65:196.

67. Dunstan RA, Simpson MB, Rosse WF. Lea blood group antigen on human platelets. *Am J Clin Pathol* 1985;83:90.

68. Dunstan RA, Simpson MB, Rosse WF. The presence of the Ii blood group system on human platelets. *Am J Clin Pathol* 1984;82:74.

69. Dunstan RA, Simpson MB, Rosse WF. Presence of P blood group antigens on human platelets. *Am J Clin Pathol* 1985;83:731.

70. Dunstan RA, Simpson MB, Rosse WF. Erythrocyte antigens on human platelets: absence of Rh, Duffy, Kell, Kidd and Lutheran antigens. *Transfusion* 1984;24:243.

71. Mollicone R, Caillard T, Le Pendu J, et al. Expression of ABH and X (Lex) antigens on platelets and lymphocytes. *Blood* 1988;71:1113.

72. Dunstan RA, Simpson MB. Heterogeneous distribution of antigens on human platelets demonstrated by fluorescence flow cytometry. *Br J Haematol* 1985;61:603.

73. Heal JM, Blumberg N, Masel D. An evaluation of crossmatching, HLA, and ABO matching for platelet transfusions to refractory patients. *Blood* 1987;70:23.

74. Lee EJ, Schiffer CA. ABO compatibility can influence the results of platelet transfusions: results of a randomized trial. *Transfusion* 1989;29:384.

75. Marcus DM, Schwarting GA. Immunochemical properties of glycolipids and phospholipids. *Adv Immunol* 1976;23:203.

76. Van Vliet HHDM, Kappers-Klunne MC, Van der Hel JWB, et al. Antibodies against glycosphingolipids in sera of patients with idiopathic thrombocytopenic purpura. *Br J Haematol* 1987;67:103.

77. Koerner TAW, Weinfeld HM, Bullard LSB, et al. Antibodies against platelet glycosphingolipids: detection in serum by quantitative HPTLC-autoradiography and association with autoimmune and alloimmune processes. *Blood* 1989;74:274.

78. Marcus AJ, Ullman HL, Safier LB. Lipid composition of subcellular particles of human blood platelets. *J Lipid Res* 1969;10:108.

79. Zwaal RF, Schroit AJ. Pathophysiologic implications of membrane phospholipid asymmetry in blood cells. *Blood* 1997;89:1121.

80. Arfors L, Winiarski J, Lefvert AK. Prevalence of antibodies to cardiolipin in chronic ITP and reactivity with platelet membranes. *Eur J Haematol* 1996;56:230.

81. Nugent DJ, Kunicki TJ, Berglund C, et al. A human monoclonal autoantibody recognizes a neoantigen on glycoprotein IIIa expressed on stored and activated platelets. *Blood* 1987;70:16.

82. Newman PM, Chong BH. Further characterization of antibody and antigen in heparin-induced thrombocytopenia. *Br J Haematol* 1999;107:303.

83. Kelton JG, Steeves K. The amount of platelet-bound albumin parallels the amount of IgG on washed platelets from patients with immune thrombocytopenia. *Blood* 1983;62:924.

84. George JN, Saucerman S. Platelet IgG, IgM, and albumin: correlation of platelet and plasma concentrations in normal subjects and in patients with ITP or dysproteinemia. *Blood* 1988;72:362.

85. George JN, Saucerman S, Levine SP, et al. Immunoglobulin G is a platelet alpha granule-secreted protein. *J Clin Invest* 1985;76:2020.

86. Sixma JJ, Van den Berg A, Schiphorst M, et al. Immunocytochemical localization of albumin and factor XIII in thin cryo sections of human blood platelets. *Thromb Haemost* 1984;51:388.

87. Hughes M, Hayward CP, Horsewood P, et al. Measurement of endogenous and exogenous alpha-granular platelet proteins in patients with immune and nonimmune thrombocytopenia. *Br J Haematol* 1999;106:762.

88. Cramer EM, Debili N, Martin JF, et al. Uncoordinated expression of fibrinogen compared with thrombospondin and von Willebrand factor in maturing human megakaryocytes. *Blood* 1989;73:1123.

89. Handagama PJ, Shuman MA, Bainton DF. Incorporation of intravenously injected albumin, immunoglobulin G, and fibrinogen in guinea pig megakaryocyte granules. *J Clin Invest* 1989;84:73.

90. Harrison P, Wilbourn B, Debili N, et al. Uptake of plasma fibrinogen into the alpha granules of human megakaryocytes and platelets. *J Clin Invest* 1989;84:1320.

91. Clejan L, Menahem M. Binding of deoxyribonucleic acid to the surface of human platelets. *Acta Haematol* 1977;58:84.

92. Asano T, Furie BC, Furie B. Platelet binding properties of monoclonal lupus autoantibodies produced by human hybridomas. *Blood* 1985;66:1254.

93. Jacob L, Lety MA, Louvard D, et al. Binding of a monoclonal anti-DNA autoantibody to identical protein(s) present at the surface of several human cell types involved in lupus pathogenesis. *J Clin Invest* 1985;75:315.

94. Rauch J, Meng QH, Tannenbaum H. Lupus anticoagulant and antiplatelet properties of human hybridoma autoantibodies. *J Immunol* 1987;139:2598.

95. Kelton JG, Keystone J, Moore J, et al. Immune-mediated thrombocytopenia of malaria. *J Clin Invest* 1983;71:832.

96. Rosenfeld SI, Looney RJ, Leddy JP, et al. Human platelet Fc receptor for immunoglobulin G: identification as a 40,000 molecular-weight membrane protein shared by monocytes. *J Clin Invest* 1985;76:2317.

97. Kelton JG, Smith JW, Santos AV, et al. Platelet IgG Fc receptor. *Am J Hematol* 1987;25:299.

98. Denomme GA. The platelet Fc receptor in heparin-induced thrombocytopenia. In: Warkentin TE, Greinacher A, eds. *Heparin-induced thrombocytopenia.* New York: Marcel Dekker, 2000:175.

99. Kelton JG, Sheridan D, Santos A, et al. Heparin-induced thrombocytopenia: laboratory studies. *Blood* 1988;72:925.

100. Newman PM, Chong BH. Heparin-induced thrombocytopenia: new evidence for the dynamic binding of purified anti-PF4-heparin antibodies to platelets and the resultant platelet activation. *Blood* 2000;96:182.

101. Hasegawa S, Pawankar R, Suzuki K, et al. Functional expression of the high affinity receptor for IgE (FcεRI) in human platelets and its intracellular expression in human megakaryocytes. *Blood* 1999;93:2543.

102. Kelton JG, Murphy WG, Lucarelli A, et al. A prospective comparison of four techniques for measuring platelet-associated IgG. *Br J Haematol* 1989;71:97.

103. Von dem Borne AEGK, Helmerhorst FM, Van Leeuwen EF, et al. Autoimmune thrombocytopenia: detection of platelet autoantibodies with the suspension immunofluorescence test. *Br J Haematol* 1980;45:319.

104. Rosse WF, Adams JP, Yount WJ. Subclasses of IgG antibodies in immune thrombocytopenic purpura (ITP). *Br J Haematol* 1980;46:109.

105. George JN, Woolf SH, Raskob GE, et al. Idiopathic thrombocytopenic purpura: a practice guideline developed by explicit methods for the American Society of Hematology. *Blood* 1996;88:3.

106. Warner MN, Moore JC, Warkentin TE, et al. A prospective study of protein-specific assays used to investigate idiopathic thrombocytopenic purpura. *Br J Haematol* 1999;104:442.

107. McMillan R. Autoantibodies and autoantigens in chronic immune thrombocytopenic purpura. *Semin Hematol* 2000;37:239–248.

108. Harrington WJ, Minnich V, Hollingsworth JW, et al. Demonstration of a thrombocytopenic factor in the blood of patients with thrombocytopenic purpura. *J Lab Clin Med* 1951;38:1.

109. Hegde UM, Ball S, Zuiable A, et al. Platelet associated immunoglobulins (PAIgG and PAIgM) in autoimmune thrombocytopenia. *Br J Haematol* 1985;59:221.

110. Cines DB, Wilson SB, Tomaski A, et al. Platelet antibodies of the IgM class in immune thrombocytopenic purpura. *J Clin Invest* 1985;75:1183.

111. McMillan R, Longmire RL, Yelenosky R, et al. Immunoglobulin synthesis in vitro by splenic tissue in idiopathic thrombocytopenic purpura. *N Engl J Med* 1972;286:681.

112. McMillan R, Mason D, Tani P, et al. Evaluation of platelet surface antigens: localization of the Pl^A1 alloantigen. *Br J Haematol* 1982;51:297.

113. Mason D, McMillan R. Platelet antigens in chronic idiopathic thrombocytopenic purpura. *Br J Haematol* 1984;56:529.

114. McMillan R, Martin M. Fixation of C3 to platelets in vitro by anti-platelet antibody from patients with immune thrombocytopenic purpura. *Br J Haematol* 1981;47:251.

115. Han P, Turpie AGG, Genton E. Plasma β-thromboglobulin: differentiation between intravascular and extravascular platelet destruction. *Blood* 1979;54:1192.

116. Kiefel V, Santoso S, Katzmann E, et al. Autoantibodies against platelet glycoprotein Ib/IX: a frequent finding in autoimmune thrombocytopenic purpura. *Br J Haematol* 1991;79:256.

117. Van Leeuwen EF, Van der Ven JTH, Engelfriet CP, et al. Specificity of autoantibodies in autoimmune thrombocytopenia. *Blood* 1982;59:23.

118. Tsubakio T, Tani P, Woods VL Jr, et al. Autoantibodies against platelet GPIIb/IIIa in chronic ITP react with different epitopes. *Br J Haematol* 1987;67:345.

119. Aster RH, Keene WR. Sites of platelet destruction in idiopathic thrombocytopenic purpura. *Br J Haematol* 1969;16:61.

120. Harker LA. Thrombokinetics in idiopathic thrombocytopenic purpura. *Br J Haematol* 1970;19:95.

121. Grossi A, Vannucchi AM, Casprini P, et al. Different patterns of platelet turnover in chronic idiopathic thrombocytopenic purpura. *Scand J Haematol* 1983;31:206.

122. Schmidt KG, Rasmussen JW. Kinetics and distribution in vivo of ^111In-labelled autologous platelets in idiopathic thrombocytopenic purpura. *Scand J Haematol* 1985;34:47.

123. Heyns A du P, Lotter MG, Badenhorst PN, et al. Kinetics and sites of destruction of 111-indium-oxine–labeled platelets in idiopathic thrombocytopenic purpura: a quantitative study. *Am J Hematol* 1982;12:167.

124. Ballem PJ, Segal GM, Stratton JR, et al. Mechanisms of thrombocytopenia in chronic autoimmune thrombocytopenic purpura: evidence of both impaired platelet production and increased platelet clearance. *J Clin Invest* 1987;80:33.

125. Siegel RS, Rae JL, Barth S, et al. Platelet survival and turnover: important factors in predicting response to splenectomy in immune thrombocytopenic purpura. *Am J Hematol* 1989;30:206.

126. Louwes H, Zeinali Lathori OA, Vellenga E, et al. Platelet kinetic studies in patients with idiopathic thrombocytopenic purpura. *Am J Med* 1999;106:430.

127. Kuwana M, Kaburaki J, Ikeda Y. Autoreactive T cells to platelet GPIIb-IIIa in immune thrombocytopenic purpura: role in production of anti-platelet autoantibody. *J Clin Invest* 1998;102:1393.

128. Hiraiwa A, Nugent DJ, Milner EB. Sequence analysis of monoclonal antibodies derived from a patient with idiopathic thrombocytopenic purpura. *Autoimmunity* 1990;8:107.

129. Cohen YC, Djulbegovic B, Shamai-Lubovitz O, et al. The bleeding risk and natural history of idiopathic thrombocytopenic purpura in patients with persistent low platelet counts. *Arch Intern Med* 2000;160:1630.

130. Harker LA, Slichter SJ. The bleeding time as a screening test for evaluation of platelet function. *N Engl J Med* 1972;287:155.

131. Anderson MJ, Peebles CL, McMillan R, et al. Fluorescent anti-nuclear antibodies and anti-SS-A/Ro in patients with immune thrombocytopenia subsequently developing systemic lupus erythematosus. *Ann Intern Med* 1985;103:548.

132. Kurata Y, Miyagawa S, Kosugi S, et al. High-titer antinuclear antibodies, anti-SSA/Ro antibodies and anti-nuclear RNP antibodies in patients with idiopathic thrombocytopenic purpura. *Thromb Haemost* 1994;71:184.

133. Panzer S, Penner E, Graninger W, et al. Antinuclear antibodies in patients with chronic idiopathic autoimmune thrombocytopenia followed 2–30 years. *Am J Hematol* 1989;32:100.

134. Vantelon JM, Godeau B, André C, et al. Screening for autoimmune markers is unnecessary during follow-up of adults with autoimmune thrombocytopenic purpura and no autoimmune markers at onset. *Thromb Haemost* 2000;83:42–45.

135. Tomer A, Schreiber AD, McMillan R, et al. Menstrual cyclic thrombocytopenia. *Br J Haematol* 1989;71:519.

136. Menitove JE, Pereira J, Hoffman R, et al. Cyclic thrombocytopenia of apparent autoimmune etiology. *Blood* 1989;73:1561.

137. Yanabu M, Nomura S, Fukuroi T, et al. Periodic production of antiplatelet autoantibody directed against GPIIIa in cyclic thrombocytopenia. *Acta Haematol* 1993;89:155.

138. Kimura F, Nakamura Y, Sato K, et al. Cyclic change of cytokines in a patient with cyclic thrombocytopenia. *Br J Haematol* 1996;94:171.

139. Balduini CL, Stella CC, Rosti V, et al. Acquired cyclic thrombocytopenia-thrombocytosis with periodic defect of platelet function. *Br J Haematol* 1993;85:718.

140. Rinder HM, Tracey JB, Recht M, et al. Differences in platelet alpha-granule release between normals and immune thrombocytopenic patients and between young and old platelets. *Thromb Haemost* 1998;80:457–462.

141. Rubin R, Rand ML. Alcohol and platelet function. *Alcohol Clin Exp Res* 1994;18:105.

142. Branehog I, Weinfeld A. Platelet survival and platelet production in idiopathic thrombocytopenic purpura (ITP) before and during treatment with corticosteroids. *Scand J Haematol* 1974;12:69.

143. Handin RI, Stossel TP. Effect of corticosteroid therapy on the phagocytosis of antibody-coated platelets by human leukocytes. *Blood* 1978;51:771.

144. McMillan R, Longmire R, Yelenosky R. The effect of corticosteroids on human IgG synthesis. *J Immunol* 1976;116:1592.

145. Berchtold P, Wenger M. Autoantibodies against platelet glycoproteins in autoimmune thrombocytopenic purpura: their clinical significance and response to treatment. *Blood* 1993;81:1246.

146. Gernsheimer T, Stratton J, Ballem PJ, et al. Mechanisms of response to treatment in autoimmune thrombocytopenic purpura. *N Engl J Med* 1989;320:974.

147. Kitchens CS. Amelioration of endothelial abnormalities by prednisone in experimental thrombocytopenia in the rabbit. *J Clin Invest* 1977;60:1129.

148. Mazzucconi MG, Francesconi M, Fidani P, et al. Treatment of idiopathic thrombocytopenic purpura (ITP): results of a multicentric protocol. *Haematologica (Pavia)* 1985;70:329.

149. Bellucci S, Charpak Y, Chastang C, et al. Low doses v conventional doses of corticoids in immune thrombocytopenic purpura (ITP): results of a randomized clinical trial in 160 children, 223 adults. *Blood* 1988;71:1165.

150. Jacobs P, Woods L, Novitzky N. Intravenous gammaglobulin has no advantages over oral corticosteroids as primary therapy for adults with immune thrombocytopenia: a prospective randomized clinical trial. *Am J Med* 1994;97:55–59.

151. von dem Borne AEGK, Vos JJE, Pegels JG, et al. High dose intravenous methylprednisolone or high dose intravenous gammaglobulin for autoimmune thrombocytopenia. *BMJ* 1988;296:249.

152. Andersen JC. Response of resistant idiopathic thrombocytopenic purpura to pulsed high-dose dexamethasone therapy. *N Engl J Med* 1994;330:1560.

153. Warner M, Wasi P, Couban S, et al. Failure of pulse high-dose dexamethasone in chronic idiopathic immune thrombocytopenia. *Am J Hematol* 1997;54:267.

154. Thompson RL, Moore RA, Hess CE, et al. Idiopathic thrombocytopenic purpura: long-term results of treatment and the prognostic significance of response to corticosteroids. *Arch Intern Med* 1972;130:730.

155. Ikkala E, Kivilaakso E, Kotilainen M, et al. Treatment of idiopathic thrombocytopenic purpura in adults: long-term results in a series of 41 patients. *Ann Clin Res* 1978;10:83.

156. Kochupillai V, Nundy S, Sharma S. Idiopathic thrombocytopenic purpura in adults: response to corticosteroids and splenectomy. *J Assoc Physicians India* 1986;34:555.

157. Jacobs P, Wood L, Dent DM. Results of treatment in immune thrombocytopenia. *QJM* 1986;58:153.

158. Jiji RM, Firozvi T, Spurling CL. Chronic idiopathic thrombocytopenic purpura: treatment with steroids and splenectomy. *Arch Intern Med* 1973;132:380.

159. DiFino SM, Lachant NA, Kirshner JJ, et al. Adult idiopathic thrombocytopenic purpura: clinical findings and response to therapy. *Am J Med* 1980;69:430.

160. Pizzuto J, Ambriz R. Therapeutic experience on 934 adults with idiopathic thrombocytopenic purpura: multicentric trial of the Cooperative Latin American Group on Hemostasis and Thrombosis. *Blood* 1984;64:1179.

161. Mankin HJ. Nontraumatic necrosis of bone (osteonecrosis). *N Engl J Med* 1992;326:1473.

162. McKee MD, Waddell JP, Kudo PA, et al. Osteonecrosis of the femoral head in men following short-course corticosteroid therapy: a report of 15 cases. *CMAJ* 2001;164:205–206.

163. Gardner P, Schaffner W. Immunization of adults. *N Engl J Med* 1993;328:1252.

164. Centers for Disease Control and Prevention. Recommendations of the Advisory Committee on Immunization Practices (ACIP): use of vaccines and immune globulins in patients with altered immunocompetence. *MMWR Recomm Rep* 1993;42:1.

165. Styrt B. Infection associated with asplenia: risks, mechanisms, and prevention. *Am J Med* 1990;88:5N–33N.

166. Cola B, Tonielli E, Sacco S, et al. Surgical treatment of chronic idiopathic thrombocytopenic purpura: results in 107 cases. *Int Surg* 1986;71:195.

167. Akwari OE, Itani KM, Coleman RE, et al. Splenectomy for primary and recurrent immune thrombocytopenic purpura (ITP): current criteria for patient selection and results. *Ann Surg* 1987;206:529.

168. Coon WW. Splenectomy for idiopathic thrombocytopenic purpura. *Surg Gynecol Obstet* 1987;164:225.

169. Russo D, Gugliotta L, Mazzucconi MG, et al. Long-term results of splenectomy in adult chronic idiopathic thrombocytopenic purpura. *Haematologica* 1987;72:445.
170. Schwartz SI, Hoepp LM, Sachs S. Splenectomy for thrombocytopenia. *Surgery* 1980;88:497.
171. Fenaux P, Caulier MT, Hirschauer MC, et al. Reevaluation of the prognostic factors for splenectomy in chronic idiopathic thrombocytopenic purpura (ITP): a report on 181 cases. *Eur J Haematol* 1989;42:259.
172. Mintz SJ, Petersen SR, Cheson B, et al. Splenectomy for immune thrombocytopenic purpura. *Arch Surg* 1981;116:645.
173. Law C, Marcaccio M, Tam P, et al. High-dose intravenous immune globulin and the response to splenectomy in patients with idiopathic thrombocytopenic purpura. *N Engl J Med* 1997;336:1494.
174. Fabris F, Zanatta N, Casonato A, et al. Response to splenectomy in idiopathic thrombocytopenic purpura: prognostic value of the clinical and laboratory evaluation. *Acta Haematol* 1989;30:206.
175. Ambriz P, Munoz R, Quintanar E, et al. Accessory spleen compromising response to splenectomy for idiopathic thrombocytopenic purpura. *Radiology* 1985;155:793.
176. Gibson J, Rickard KA, Bautovich G, et al. Management of splenectomy failures in chronic immune thrombocytopenic purpura: role of accessory splenectomy. *Aust N Z J Med* 1986;16:695.
177. Reid MM, Saunders PWG, Fenwick JD, et al. Splenunculectomy in thrombocytopenic purpura. *Arch Dis Child* 1986;61:192.
178. Marcaccio MJ. Laparoscopic splenectomy in chronic idiopathic thrombocytopenic purpura. *Semin Hematol* 2000;37:267–274.
179. Friedman D, Netti F, Schreiber AD. Effect of estradiol and steroid analogues on the clearance of immunoglobulin G-coated erythrocytes. *J Clin Invest* 1985;75:162.
180. Schreiber AD, Chien P, Tomaski A, et al. Effect of danazol in immune thrombocytopenic purpura. *N Engl J Med* 1987;316:503.
181. Ahn YS, Mylvaganam R, Garcia RO, et al. Low-dose danazol therapy in idiopathic thrombocytopenic purpura. *Ann Intern Med* 1987;107:177.
182. Ahn YS, Harrington WJ, Simon SR, et al. Danazol for the treatment of idiopathic thrombocytopenic purpura. *N Engl J Med* 1983;308:1396.
183. Ambriz-Fernandez R, Chavez-Sanchez G, Pizzuto-Chavez J, et al. Danazol in refractory autoimmune thrombocytopenic purpura (ATP): a new therapeutic sequence. *Arch Invest Med (Mex)* 1985;16:295.
184. Buelli M, Cortelazzo S, Viero P, et al. Danazol for the treatment of idiopathic thrombocytopenic purpura. *Acta Haematol* 1985;74:97.
185. Heyd J, Hershko C. Use of danazol in the management of chronic idiopathic thrombocytopenic purpura. *Isr J Med Sci* 1985;21:418.
186. McVerry BA, Auger M, Bellingham AJ. The use of danazol in the management of chronic immune thrombocytopenic purpura. *Br J Haematol* 1985;61:145.
187. Mazzucconi MG, Francesconi M, Falcione E, et al. Danazol therapy in refractory chronic immune thrombocytopenic purpura. *Acta Haematol* 1987;77:45.
188. Ahn YS, Rocha R, Mylvaganam R, et al. Long-term danazol therapy in autoimmune thrombocytopenia: unmaintained remission and age-dependent response in women. *Ann Intern Med* 1989;111:723.
189. Schiavotto C, Castaman G, Rodeghiero F. Treatment of idiopathic thrombocytopenic purpura (ITP) in patients with refractoriness to or with contraindication for corticosteroids and/or splenectomy with immunosuppressive therapy and danazol. *Haematologica* 1993;78[Suppl 2]:29.
190. Blanco R, Martinez-Taboada VM, Rodriguez-Valverde V, et al. Successful therapy with danazol in refractory autoimmune thrombocytopenia associated with rheumatic diseases. *Br J Rheumatol* 1997;36:1095.
191. Nesher G, Dollberg L, Zimran A, et al. Hepatosplenic peliosis after danazol and glucocorticoids for ITP. *N Engl J Med* 1985;312:242.
192. Javier Penalver F, Somolinos N, Villanueva C, et al. Splenic peliosis with spontaneous splenic rupture in a patient with immune thrombocytopenia treated with danazol. *Haematologica* 1990;83:646.
193. Ford I, Li TC, Cooke ID, et al. Changes in haematological indices, blood viscosity and inhibitors of coagulation during treatment of endometriosis with danazol. *Thromb Haemost* 1994;72:218.
194. Wentz AC. Adverse effects of danazol in pregnancy. *Ann Intern Med* 1982;96:672.
195. Brunskill PJ. The effects of fetal exposure to danazol. *Br J Obstet Gynaecol* 1992;99:212.
196. Yamamoto K, Hoshiai H, Tsubaki K, et al. Danazol induced thrombocytopenia. *Tohoku J Exp Med* 1997;182:249.
197. Ahn YS, Harrington WJ, Mylvaganam R. Use of platelets as drug carriers for the treatment of hematologic diseases. *Methods Enzymol* 1987;149:312.
198. Ahn YS, Harrington WJ, Mylvaganam R. Slow infusion of vinca alkaloids in the treatment of idiopathic thrombocytopenic purpura. *Ann Intern Med* 1984;100:192.
199. Ahn YS, Harrington WJ. Clinical uses of macrophage inhibitors. *Adv Intern Med* 1980;25:453.
200. Manoharan A. Slow infusion of vincristine in the treatment of idiopathic thrombocytopenic purpura. *Am J Hematol* 1986;21:135.
201. Simon M, Jouet JP, Fenaux P, et al. The treatment of adult idiopathic thrombocytopenic purpura: infusion of vinblastine in ITP. *Eur J Haematol* 1987;39:193.
202. Linares M, Cervero A, Sanchez M, et al. Slow infusion of vincristine in the treatment of refractory thrombocytopenic purpura. *Acta Haematol* 1988;80:173.
203. Facon T, Caulier MT, Wattel E, et al. A randomized trial comparing vinblastine in slow infusion and by bolus i.v. injection in idiopathic thrombocytopenic purpura: a report on 42 patients. *Br J Haematol* 1994;86:678.
204. Ahn YS, Byrnes JJ, Harrington WJ, et al. The treatment of idiopathic thrombocytopenia with vinblastine-loaded platelets. *N Engl J Med* 1978;298:1101.
205. Kelton JG, McDonald JWD, Barr RM, et al. The reversible binding of vinblastine to platelets: implications for therapy. *Blood* 1981;57:431.
206. Rosse WF. Whatever happened to vinca-loaded platelets? *N Engl J Med* 1984;310:1051.
207. Ahn YS, Harrington WJ, Seelman RC, et al. Vincristine therapy of idiopathic and secondary thrombocytopenias. *N Engl J Med* 1974;291:376.
208. Burton IE, Roberts BE, Child JA, et al. Responses to vincristine in refractory idiopathic thrombocytopenic purpura [Letter]. *BMJ* 1976;2:918.
209. Tangun Y, Atamer T. More on vincristine in treatment of ITP [Letter]. *N Engl J Med* 1977;297:894.
210. Cervantes F, Montserrat E, Rozman C, et al. Low-dose vincristine in the treatment of corticosteroid-refractory idiopathic thrombocytopenic purpura (ITP) in non-splenectomized patients. *Postgrad Med J* 1980;56:711.
211. Cervantes F, Montserrat E, Rozman C. Treatment of idiopathic thrombocytopenic purpura [Letter]. *N Engl J Med* 1981;305:830.
212. Kueh YK. Vincristine therapy in refractory chronic idiopathic thrombocytopenic purpura. *Ann Acad Med Singapore* 1982;11:290.
213. Van Zyl-Smit R, Jacobs P. The use of vincristine in refractory auto-immune thrombocytopenic purpura. *S Afr Med J* 1974;48:2039.
214. Weinerman B, Maxwell I, Hryniuk W. Intermittent cyclophosphamide treatment of autoimmune thrombocytopenia. *Can Med Assoc J* 1974;111:1100.
215. Reiner A, Gernsheimer T, Slichter SJ. Pulse cyclophosphamide therapy for refractory autoimmune thrombocytopenic purpura. *Blood* 1995;85:351.
216. Figueroa M, Gehlsen J, Hammond D, et al. Combination chemotherapy in refractory immune thrombocytopenic purpura. *N Engl J Med* 1993;328:1226.
217. Caplan SN, Berkman EM. Immunosuppressive therapy of idiopathic thrombocytopenic purpura. *Med Clin North Am* 1976;60:971.
218. Krause JR. Chronic idiopathic thrombocytopenic purpura (ITP): development of acute non-lymphocytic leukemia subsequent to treatment with cyclophosphamide. *Med Pediatr Oncol* 1982;10:61.
219. Fukuda M, Horibe K, Miyajima Y, et al. [Chronic myelomonocytic leukemia developed 9 years after the diagnosis of idiopathic thrombocytopenic purpura in a child.] *Rinsho Ketsueki* 1994;35:609.
220. Imbach P, Barandun S, d'Appuzo V, et al. High-dose intravenous gammaglobulin for idiopathic thrombocytopenic purpura in childhood. *Lancet* 1981;1:1228.
221. Boshkov LK, Kelton JG. Use of intravenous gammaglobulin as an immune replacement and an immune suppressant. *Transfus Med Rev* 1989;3:82.
222. Imbach P, Jungi TW. Possible mechanisms of intravenous immunoglobulin treatment in childhood idiopathic thrombocytopenic purpura (ITP). *Blut* 1983;46:117.
223. Bussel JB, Hilgartner MW. The use and mechanism of action of intravenous immunoglobulin in the treatment of immune haematologic disease. *Br J Haematol* 1984;56:1.
224. Saleh M, Court W, Huster W, et al. Effect of commercial immunoglobulin G preparation on human monocyte Fc-receptor dependent binding of antibody coated platelets. *Br J Haematol* 1988;68:47.
225. Neppert J, Clemens M, Mueller-Eckhardt C. Immune phagocytosis inhibition by commercial immunoglobulins. *Blut* 1986;52:67.
226. Samuelsson A, Towers TL, Ravetch JV. Anti-inflammatory activity of IVIG mediated through the inhibitory Fc receptor. *Science* 2001;291:484.
227. Fehr J, Hofmann V, Kappeler U. Transient reversal of thrombocytopenia in idiopathic thrombocytopenic purpura by high-dose intravenous gammaglobulin. *N Engl J Med* 1982;306:1254.
228. Bussel JB, Kimberly RP, Inman RD, et al. Intravenous gammaglobulin treatment of chronic idiopathic thrombocytopenic purpura. *Blood* 1983;62:480.
229. Kelton JG, Singer J, Rodger C, et al. The concentration of IgG in the serum is a major determinant of Fc-dependent reticuloendothelial function. *Blood* 1985;66:490.
230. Burdach SEG, Evers KG, Geursen RG. Treatment of acute idiopathic thrombocytopenic purpura of childhood with intravenous immunoglobulin G: comparative efficacy of 7S and 5S preparations. *J Pediatr* 1986;109:770.
231. Winiarski J, Kreuger A, Ejderhamn J, et al. High dose intravenous IgG reduces platelet associated immunoglobulins and complement in idiopathic thrombocytopenic purpura. *Scand J Haematol* 1983;31:342.
232. Sultan Y, Kazatchkine MD, Maisonneuve P, et al. Anti-idiotypic suppression of autoantibodies to factor VIII (antihaemophilic factor) by high-dose intravenous gammaglobulin. *Lancet* 1984;2:765.
233. Berchtold P, Dale GL, Tani P, et al. Inhibition of autoantibody binding to platelet glycoprotein IIb/IIIa by anti-idiotypic antibodies in intravenous gammaglobulin. *Blood* 1989;74:2414.
234. Macey MG, Newland AC. CD4 and CD8 subpopulation changes during high dose intravenous immunoglobulin treatment. *Br J Haematol* 1990;76:513.
235. Tsubakio T, Kurato Y, Katageri S, et al. Alteration of T cell subsets and immunoglobulin synthesis in vitro during high dose gamma-globulin therapy in patients with idiopathic thrombocytopenic purpura. *Clin Exp Immunol* 1983;53:607.
236. Godeau B, Lesage S, Divine M, et al. Treatment of adult chronic autoimmune thrombocytopenic purpura with repeated high-dose intravenous immunoglobulin. *Blood* 1993;82:1415.
237. Bussel JB, Pham LC. Intravenous treatment with gammaglobulin in adults with immune thrombocytopenic purpura: review of the literature. *Vox Sang* 1987;52:206.

238. Sturgill MG, Nagabandi SR, Drachtman RA, et al. The effect of ABO and Rh blood type on the response to intravenous immune globulin (IVIG) in children with immune thrombocytopenic purpura (ITP). *J Pediatr Hematol Oncol* 1997;19:523.

239. Bussel JB, Pham LC, Aledort L, et al. Maintenance treatment of adults with chronic refractory immune thrombocytopenic purpura using repeated intravenous infusions of gammaglobulin. *Blood* 1988;72:121.

240. Simpson KN, Coughlin CM, Eron J, et al. Idiopathic thrombocytopenia purpura: treatment patterns and an analysis of cost associated with intravenous gammaglobulin and anti-D therapy. *Semin Hematol* 1998;35:58.

241. Sandler SG, Novak SC, Roland B. The cost of treating immune thrombocytopenic purpura using intravenous Rh immune globulin versus intravenous immune globulin. *Am J Hematol* 2000;63:156.

242. Lederman HM, Roifman CM, Lavi S, et al. Corticosteroids for prevention of adverse reactions to intravenous immune serum globulin infusions in hypogammaglobulinemic patients. *Am J Med* 1986;81:443.

243. Kim HC, Park CL, Cowan JH III, et al. Massive intravascular hemolysis associated with intravenous immunoglobulin in bone marrow transplant recipients. *Am J Pediatr Hematol Oncol* 1988;10:69.

244. Barton JC, Herrera GA, Galla JH, et al. Acute cryoglobulinemic renal failure after intravenous infusion of gamma globulin. *Am J Med* 1987;82:624.

245. Elkayam O, Paran D, Milo R, et al. Acute myocardial infarction associated with high dose intravenous immunoglobulin for autoimmune disorders: a study of four cases. *Ann Rheum Dis* 2000;59:77.

246. Woodruff RK, Grigg AP, Firkin FC, et al. Fatal thrombotic events during treatment of autoimmune thrombocytopenia with intravenous immunoglobulin in elderly patients [Letter]. *Lancet* 1986;2:217.

247. Lever AML, Webster ADB, Brown D, et al. Non-A, non-B hepatitis occurring in agammaglobulinaemic patients after intravenous immunoglobulin. *Lancet* 1984;2:1062.

248. Salama A, Mueller-Eckhardt C, Kiefel V. Effect of intravenous immunoglobulin in immune thrombocytopenia: competitive inhibition of reticuloendothelial system function by sequestration of autologous red blood cells? *Lancet* 1983;2:193.

249. Salama A, Kiefel V, Amberg R, et al. Treatment of autoimmune thrombocytopenic purpura with rhesus antibodies (anti-Rh₀ [D]). *Blut* 1984;49:29.

250. Friesen AD, Bowman JM, Price HW. Column ion exchange preparation and characteristics of an Rh immune globulin (WinRho) for intravenous use. *J Appl Biochem* 1981;3:164.

251. Contreras M, Mollison PL. Anti-Rh(D) immunoglobulin for immune thrombocytopenic purpura [Letter]. *Lancet* 1986;2:49.

252. Oksenhendler E, Bierling P, Brossard Y, et al. Anti-RH immunoglobulin therapy for human immunodeficiency virus-related immune thrombocytopenic purpura. *Blood* 1988;71:1499.

253. Bussel JB, Graziano JN, Kimberly RP, et al. Intravenous anti-D treatment of immune thrombocytopenic purpura: analysis of efficacy, toxicity, and mechanism of effect. *Blood* 1991;77:1884.

254. Salama A, Kiefel V, Mueller-Eckhardt C. Effect of IgG anti-Rh₀(D) in adult patients with chronic autoimmune thrombocytopenia. *Am J Hematol* 1986;22:241.

255. Boughton BJ, Chakraverty R, Baglin TP, et al. The treatment of chronic idiopathic thrombocytopenia with anti-D (Rho) immunoglobulin: its effectiveness, safety and mechanism of action. *Clin Lab Haematol* 1988;10:275.

256. Durand JM, Harle JR, Verdot JJ, et al. Anti-Rh(D) immunoglobulin for immune thrombocytopenic purpura. *Lancet* 1986;2:49.

257. Mueller-Eckhardt C, Salama A. Anti-Rh(D) immunoglobulin for immune thrombocytopenic purpura [Letter]. *Lancet* 1986;2:50.

258. Panzer S, Grumayer ER, Haas OA, et al. Efficacy of rhesus antibodies (anti-Rh₀[D]) in autoimmune thrombocytopenia: correlation with response to high dose IgG and the degree of haemolysis. *Blut* 1986;52:117.

259. Waintraub SE, Brody JI. Use of anti-D in immune thrombocytopenic purpura as a means to prevent splenectomy: case reports from two university hospital medical centers. *Semin Hematol* 2000;37[Suppl 1]:45.

260. Scaradavou A. Splenectomy-sparing, long-term maintenance with anti-D for chronic immune (idiopathic) thrombocytopenic purpura: the New York Hospital experience. *Semin Hematol* 2000;37[Suppl 1]:42.

261. Scaradavou A, Woo B, Woloski BMR, et al. Intravenous anti-D treatment of immune thrombocytopenic purpura: experience in 272 patients. *Blood* 1997;89:2689.

262. Newman GC, Novoa MV, Fodero EM, et al. A dose of 75 mg/kg/d of i.v. anti-D increases the platelet count more rapidly and for a longer period of time than 50 mg/kg/d in adults with immune thrombocytopenic purpura. *Br J Haematol* 2001;112:1076.

263. Gaines AR. Acute onset hemoglobinemia and/or hemoglobinuria and sequelae following Rh₀(D) immune globulin intravenous administration in immune thrombocytopenic purpura patients. *Blood* 2000;95:2523.

264. Kenny-Walsh E, for the Irish Hepatology Research Group. Clinical outcomes after hepatitis C infection from contaminated anti-D immune globulin. *N Engl J Med* 1999;340:1228.

265. Proctor SJ, Jackson G, Carey P, et al. Improvement of platelet counts in steroid-unresponsive idiopathic immune thrombocytopenic purpura after short-course therapy with recombinant 166 2b interferon. *Blood* 1989;74:1894.

266. Sekreta CM, Baker DE. Interferon alpha therapy in adults with chronic idiopathic thrombocytopenic purpura. *Ann Pharmacother* 1996;30:1176.

267. Stern SCM, Asagba GO, Hegde UM. Prolonged thrombocytopenia following alpha-interferon for refractory immune thrombocytopenic purpura. *Clin Lab Haematol* 1994;16:183.

268. Lee CA, Kernoff PBA, Karayiannis P, et al. Interferon therapy for chronic non-A non-B and chronic delta liver disease in haemophilia. *Br J Haematol* 1989;72:235.

269. Garcia-Suárez J, Burgaleta C, Hernanz N, et al. HCV-associated thrombocytopenia: clinical characteristics and platelet response after recombinant α2b-interferon therapy. *Br J Haematol* 2000;110:98.

270. Kelsey PR, Schofield KP, Geary CG. Refractory idiopathic thrombocytopenic purpura (ITP) treated with cyclosporine. *Br J Haematol* 1985;60:197.

271. Velu TJ, Debusscher L, Stryckmans PA. Ciclosporine for the treatment of refractory idiopathic thrombocytopenic purpura [Letter]. *Eur J Haematol* 1987;38:95.

272. Matsumura O, Kawashima Y, Kato S, et al. Therapeutic effect of cyclosporine in thrombocytopenia associated with autoimmune disease. *Transplant Proc* 1988;20:317.

273. Schultz KR, Strahlendorf C, Warrier I, et al. Cyclosporin A therapy of immune-mediated thrombocytopenia in children. *Blood* 1995;85:1406.

274. Emilia G, Messora C, Longo G, et al. Long-term salvage treatment by cyclosporin in refractory autoimmune haematological disorders. *Br J Haematol* 1996;93:341–344.

275. Shirota T, Yamamoto H, Fujimoto H, et al. Cyclic thrombocytopenia in a patient treated with cyclosporine for refractory idiopathic thrombocytopenic purpura. *Am J Hematol* 1997;56:272.

276. Moskowitz IPG, Gaynon PS, Shahidi NT, et al. Low-dose cyclosporin A therapy in children with refractory immune thrombocytopenic purpura. *J Pediatr Hematol Oncol* 1999;21:77.

277. Strother SV, Zuckerman KS, LoBuglio AF. Colchicine therapy for refractory idiopathic thrombocytopenic purpura. *Arch Intern Med* 1984;144:2198.

278. Jim RTS. Therapeutic use of colchicine in thrombocytopenia. *Hawaii Med J* 1986;45:221.

279. Bonnotte B, Gresset AC, Chvetzoff G, et al. Efficacy of colchicine alone or in combination with vinca alkaloids in severe corticoid-resistant thrombocytopenic purpura: six cases [Letter]. *Am J Med* 1999;107:645.

280. Durand JM, Lefevre P, Hovette P, et al. Dapsone for idiopathic autoimmune thrombocytopenic purpura in elderly patients. *Br J Haematol* 1991;78:459.

281. Radaelli F, Calori R, Goldaniga M, et al. Adult refractory chronic idiopathic thrombocytopenic purpura: can dapsone be proposed as second-line therapy? [Letter] *Br J Haematol* 1999;104:641.

282. Le Louet H, Ruivart M, Bierling P, et al. Lack of relevance of the acetylator status on dapsone response in chronic autoimmune thrombocytopenic purpura. *Am J Hematol* 1999;62:251.

283. Snyder HW Jr, Cochran SK, Balint JP Jr, et al. Experience with protein A-immunoadsorption in treatment-resistant adult immune thrombocytopenic purpura. *Blood* 1992;79:2237.

284. Cahill MR, Macey MG, Cavenagh JD, et al. Protein A immunoadsorption in chronic refractory ITP reverses increased platelet activation but fails to achieve sustained clinical benefit. *Br J Haematol* 1998;100:358.

285. Marder VJ, Nusbacher J, Anderson FW. One-year follow-up of plasma exchange therapy in 14 patients with idiopathic thrombocytopenic purpura. *Transfusion* 1981;21:291.

286. Blanchette VS, Hogan VA, McCombie NE, et al. Intensive plasma exchange in ten patients with idiopathic thrombocytopenic purpura. *Transfusion* 1984;24:388.

287. Bussel JB, Saal S, Gordon B. Combined plasma exchange and intravenous gammaglobulin in the treatment of patients with refractory immune thrombocytopenic purpura. *Transfusion* 1988;28:38.

288. Clarkson SB, Bussel JB, Kimberly RP, et al. Treatment of refractory immune thrombocytopenic purpura with an anti-Fcγ-receptor antibody. *N Engl J Med* 1986;314:1236.

289. Soubrane C, Tourani JM, Andrieu JM, et al. Biologic response to anti-CD16 monoclonal antibody therapy in a human immunodeficiency virus-related immune thrombocytopenic purpura patient. *Blood* 1993;81:15.

290. Ratanatharathorn V, Carson E, Reynolds C, et al. Anti-CD20 chimeric monoclonal antibody treatment of refractory immune-mediated thrombocytopenia in a patient with chronic graft-versus-host disease. *Ann Intern Med* 2000;133:275.

291. Calverley DG, Jones GW, Kelton JG. Splenic irradiation as a potential treatment for corticosteroid resistant immune thrombocytopenia. *Ann Intern Med* 1992;116:977.

292. Caulier MT, Darloy F, Rose C, et al. Splenic irradiation for chronic autoimmune thrombocytopenic purpura in patients with contra-indications to splenectomy. *Br J Haematol* 1995;91:208.

293. Baumann MA, Menitove JE, Aster RH, et al. Urgent treatment of idiopathic thrombocytopenic purpura with single-dose gamma-globulin infusion followed by platelet transfusion. *Ann Intern Med* 1986;104:808.

294. Chandramouli NB, Rodgers GM. Prolonged immunoglobulin and platelet infusion for treatment of immune thrombocytopenia. *Am J Hematol* 2000;65:85.

295. Carr JM, Kruskall MS, Kaye JA, et al. Efficacy of platelet transfusions in immune thrombocytopenia. *Am J Med* 1986;80:1051.

296. Territo M, Finklestein J, Oh W, et al. Management of autoimmune thrombocytopenia in pregnancy and in the neonate. *Obstet Gynecol* 1973;41:579.

297. Kelton JG, Inwood MJ, Barr RM, et al. The prenatal prediction of thrombocytopenia in infants of mothers with clinically diagnosed immune thrombocytopenia. *Am J Obstet Gynecol* 1982;144:449.

298. Burrows RF, Kelton JG. Pregnancy in patients with idiopathic thrombocytopenic purpura: assessing the risks for the infant at delivery. *Obstet Gynecol Surv* 1993;48:781.

299. Burrows RF, Kelton JG. Low fetal risks in pregnancies associated with idiopathic thrombocytopenic purpura. *Am J Obstet Gynecol* 1990;163:1147.
300. Burrows RF, Kelton JG. Fetal thrombocytopenia and its relation to maternal thrombocytopenia. *N Engl J Med* 1993;329:1463.
301. Barbui T, Cortelazzo S, Viero P, et al. Idiopathic thrombocytopenic purpura and pregnancy: maternal platelet count and antiplatelet antibodies do not predict the risk of neonatal thrombocytopenia. *La Ricerca Clin Lab* 1985; 15:139.
302. Bussel JB. Immune thrombocytopenia in pregnancy: autoimmune and alloimmune. *J Reprod Immunol* 1997;37:35.
303. Christiaens GC, Nieuwenhuis HK, Bussel JB. Comparison of platelet counts in first and second newborns of mothers with immune thrombocytopenic purpura. *Obstet Gynecol* 1997;90:546.
304. Cines DB, Dusak B, Tomaski A, et al. Immune thrombocytopenic purpura and pregnancy. *N Engl J Med* 1982;306:826.
305. Karpatkin M, Porges RF, Karpatkin S. Platelet counts in infants of women with autoimmune thrombocytopenia: effects of steroid administration to the mother. *N Engl J Med* 1981;305:936.
306. al-Mofada SM, Osman ME, Kides E, et al. Risk of thrombocytopenia in the infants of mothers with idiopathic thrombocytopenia. *Am J Perinatol* 1994; 11:423.
307. Barton JC, Saleh MN, Stedman CM, et al. Case report: immune thrombocytopenia: effects of maternal gamma globulin infusion on maternal and fetal serum, platelet, and monocyte IgG. *Am J Med Sci* 1987;293:112.
308. Bessho T, Ida A, Minagawa K, et al. Effects of maternally administered immunoglobulin on platelet counts of neonates born to mothers with autoimmune thrombocytopenia: re-evaluation. *Clin Exp Obstet Gynecol* 1997; 24:53.
309. Sacher RA, King JC. Intravenous gamma-globulin in pregnancy: a review. *Obstet Gynecol Surv* 1989;44:25.
310. Daffos F, Capella-Pavlovsky M, Forestier F. Fetal blood sampling during pregnancy with use of a needle guided by ultrasound: a study of 606 consecutive cases. *Am J Obstet Gynecol* 1985;153:655.
311. Christiaens GC. Immune thrombocytopenic purpura in pregnancy. *Baillieres Clin Haematol* 1998;11:373.
312. Scott JR, Cruikshank DP, Kochenour NK, et al. Fetal platelet counts in the obstetric management of immunologic thrombocytopenic purpura. *Am J Obstet Gynecol* 1980;136:495.
313. Adams DM, Bussel JB, Druzin ML. Accurate intrapartum estimation of fetal platelet count by fetal scalp samples smear. *Am J Perinatol* 1994;11:42.
314. Caruso A, De Carolis S, Di Simone N. Antiphospholipid antibodies in obstetrics: new complexities and sites of action. *Hum Reprod Update* 1999;5:267.
315. Ballin A, Andrew M, Ling E, et al. High-dose intravenous gamma-globulin therapy for neonatal autoimmune thrombocytopenia. *J Pediatr* 1988;112:789.
316. Hoyle C, Darbyshire P, Eden OB. Idiopathic thrombocytopenia in childhood: Edinburgh experience 1962–82. *Scott Med J* 1986;31:174.
317. Winiarski J. Mechanisms in childhood idiopathic thrombocytopenic purpura. *Acta Paediatr Suppl* 1998;424:54.
318. Taub JW, Warrier I, Holtkamp C, et al. Characterization of autoantibodies against the platelet glycoprotein antigens IIb/IIIa in childhood idiopathic thrombocytopenia purpura. *Am J Hematol* 1995;48:104.
319. Van Leeuwen EF, Von dem Borne AEGK, Van der Plas-Van Dalen C, et al. Idiopathic thrombocytopenic purpura in children: detection of platelet autoantibodies by immunofluorescence. *Scand J Haematol* 1981;26:285.
320. Lightsey AL Jr, Koenig HM, McMillan R, et al. Platelet-associated immunoglobulin G in childhood idiopathic thrombocytopenic purpura. *J Pediatr* 1979;94:201.
321. Ware R, Kinney TR, Friedman HS, et al. Prognostic implications for direct platelet-associated IgG in childhood idiopathic thrombocytopenic purpura. *Am J Pediatr Hematol Oncol* 1986;8:32.
322. Cheung NKV, Hilgartner MW, Schulman I, et al. Platelet-associated immunoglobulin G in childhood idiopathic thrombocytopenic purpura. *J Pediatr* 1983;102:366.
323. Winiarski J. IgG and IgM antibodies to platelet membrane glycoprotein antigens in acute childhood idiopathic thrombocytopenic purpura. *Br J Haematol* 1989;73:88.
324. Rand ML, Wright JF. Virus-associated idiopathic thrombocytopenic purpura. *Transfus Sci* 1998;19:253.
325. Zeller B, Helgestad J, Hellebostad M, et al. Immune thrombocytopenic purpura in childhood in Norway: a prospective, population-based registration. *Pediatr Hematol Oncol* 2000;17:551.
326. Calpin C, Dick P, Poon A, et al. Is bone marrow aspiration needed in acute childhood idiopathic thrombocytopenic purpura to rule out leukemia? *Arch Pediatr Adolesc Med* 1998;152:345.
327. Longacre TA, Foucar K, Crago S, et al. Hematogones: a multiparameter analysis of bone marrow precursor cells. *Blood* 1989;73:543.
328. Cornelius AS, Campbell D, Schwartz E, et al. Elevated common acute lymphoblastic leukemia antigen expression in pediatric immune thrombocytopenic purpura. *Am J Pediatr Hematol Oncol* 1991;13:57.
329. Blanchette V, Carcao M. Approach to the investigation and management of immune thrombocytopenic purpura in children. *Semin Hematol* 2000;37:299.
330. Buchanan GR, Holtkamp CA. Prednisone therapy for children with newly diagnosed idiopathic thrombocytopenic purpura: a randomized clinical trial. *Am J Pediatr Hematol Oncol* 1984;6:355.
331. Dunn NL, Maurer HM. Prednisone treatment of acute idiopathic thrombocytopenic purpura of childhood. *Am J Pediatr Hematol Oncol* 1984;6:159.
332. Sartorius JA. Steroid treatment of idiopathic thrombocytopenic purpura in children: preliminary results of a randomized cooperative study. *Am J Pediatr Hematol Oncol* 1984;6:165.
333. Suarez CR, Rademaker D, Hasson A, et al. High-dose steroids in childhood acute idiopathic thrombocytopenia purpura. *Am J Pediatr Hematol Oncol* 1986;8:111.
334. Jayabose S, Patel P, Inamdar S, et al. Use of intravenous methylprednisolone in acute idiopathic thrombocytopenic purpura. *Am J Pediatr Hematol Oncol* 1987;9:133.
335. Van Hoff J, Ritchey AK. Pulse methylprednisolone therapy for acute childhood idiopathic thrombocytopenic purpura. *J Pediatr* 1988;113:563.
336. Carcao MD, Zipursky A, Butchart S, et al. Short-course oral prednisone therapy in children presenting with acute immune thrombocytopenic purpura. *Acta Paediatr* 1998;87[Suppl 424]:71.
337. Imbach P, Wagner HP, Berchtold W, et al. Intravenous immunoglobulin versus oral corticosteroids in acute immune thrombocytopenic purpura in childhood. *Lancet* 1985;2:464.
338. Blanchette VS, Luke B, Andrew M, et al. A prospective, randomized trial of high-dose intravenous immune globulin G therapy, oral prednisone therapy, and no therapy in childhood acute immune thrombocytopenic purpura. *J Pediatr* 1993;123:989.
339. Bussel JB, Goldman A, Imbach P, et al. Treatment of acute idiopathic thrombocytopenic purpura of childhood with intravenous infusions of gammaglobulin. *J Pediatr* 1985;106:886.
340. Blanchette V, Imbach P, Andrew M, et al. Randomised trial of intravenous immunoglobulin G, intravenous anti-D, and oral prednisone in childhood acute immune thrombocytopenic purpura. *Lancet* 1994;344:703.
341. Berchtold P, McMillan R, Tani P, et al. Autoantibodies against platelet membrane glycoproteins in children with acute and chronic immune thrombocytopenic purpura. *Blood* 1989;74:1600.
342. Taub JW, Warrier I, Holtkamp C, et al. Characterization of autoantibodies against the platelet glycoprotein antigens IIb/IIIa in childhood idiopathic thrombocytopenia purpura. *Am J Hematol* 1995;48:104.
343. Ware RE, Howard TA. Phenotypic and clonal analysis of T lymphocytes in childhood immune thrombocytopenic purpura. *Blood* 1993;82:2137.
344. Simons SM, Main CA, Yaish HM, et al. Idiopathic thrombocytopenic purpura in children. *J Pediatr* 1975;87:16.
345. McIntosh S, Johnson C, Hartigan P, et al. Immunoregulatory abnormalities in children with thrombocytopenic purpura. *J Pediatr* 1981;99:525.
346. Zimmerman SA, Ware RE. Clinical significance of the antinuclear antibody test in selected children with idiopathic thrombocytopenic purpura. *J Pediatr Hematol Oncol* 1997;19:297.
347. Tarantino MD. Treatment options for chronic immune (idiopathic) thrombocytopenia purpura in children. *Semin Hematol* 2000;37[Suppl 1]:35.
348. Lilleyman JS. Chronic childhood idiopathic thrombocytopenic purpura. *Baillieres Clin Haematol* 2000;13:469.
349. Menichelli A, Del Principe D, Rezza E. Intravenous pulse methylprednisolone in chronic idiopathic thrombocytopenia. *Arch Dis Child* 1984;59:777.
350. Del Principe D, Menichelli A, Mori PG, et al. Phase II trial of methylprednisolone pulse therapy in childhood chronic thrombocytopenia. *Acta Haematol* 1987;77:226.
351. Bussel JB, Schulman I, Hilgartner MW, et al. Intravenous use of gammaglobulin in the treatment of chronic immune thrombocytopenic purpura as a means to defer splenectomy. *J Pediatr* 1983;103:651.
352. Hollenberg JP, Subak LL, Ferry JJ Jr, et al. Cost-effectiveness of splenectomy versus intravenous gamma globulin in treatment of chronic immune thrombocytopenic purpura in childhood. *J Pediatr* 1988;112:530.
353. Bussel JB, Szatrowski TP. Uses of intravenous gammaglobulin in immune hematologic disease. *Immunol Invest* 1995;24:451.
354. Becker T, Kuenzlen E, Salama A, et al. Treatment of childhood idiopathic thrombocytopenic purpura with rhesus antibodies (anti-D). *Eur J Pediatr* 1986;145:166.
355. Andrew M, Blanchette VS, Adams M, et al. A multicenter study of the treatment of childhood chronic idiopathic thrombocytopenic purpura with antiD. *J Pediatr* 1992;120:522.
356. Scaradavou A. Splenectomy-sparing, long-term maintenance with anti-D for chronic immune (idiopathic) thrombocytopenic purpura: the New York Hospital experience. *Semin Hematol* 2000;37[Suppl 1]:42.
357. Bennett CL, Weinberg PD, Golub RM, et al. The potential for treatment of idiopathic thrombocytopenic purpura with anti-D to prevent splenectomy: a predictive cost analysis. *Semin Hematol* 2000;37[Suppl 1]:26.
358. Den Ottolander GJ, Gratama JW, De Konig J, et al. Long-term follow-up study of 168 patients with immune thrombocytopenia: implications for therapy. *Scand J Haematol* 1984;32:101.
359. Rescorla FJ. Laparoscopic splenectomy. *Semin Pediatr Surg* 1998;7:207.
360. Konigswieser H. Incidence of serious infections after splenectomy in children. *Prog Pediatr Surg* 1985;18:173.
361. Infectious Diseases and Immunization Committee, Canadian Paediatric Society. Prevention and therapy of bacterial infections for children with asplenia or hyposplenia. *Pediatr Child Health* 1999;4:417.
362. Hemmila MR, Foley DS, Castle VP, et al. The response to splenectomy in pediatric patients with idiopathic thrombocytopenic purpura who fail high-dose intravenous immune globulin. *J Pediatr Surg* 2000;35:967.
363. Joseph A, Evans DI. Immunosuppressive treatment of idiopathic thrombocytopenic purpura in children. *Acta Paediatr Scand* 1982;71:467.
364. Karpatkin S, Strick N, Karpatkin MB, et al. Cumulative experience in the detection of antiplatelet antibody in 234 patients with idiopathic thrombocy-

topenic purpura, systemic lupus erythematosus and other clinical disorders. *Am J Med* 1972;52:776.

365. Mueller-Eckhardt C, Kayser W, Mersch-Baumert K, et al. The clinical significance of platelet associated IgG: a study on 298 patients with various disorders. *Br J Haematol* 1980;46:123.

366. Macchi L, Rispal P, Clofent-Sanchez G, et al. Anti-platelet antibodies in patients with systemic lupus erythematosus and the primary antiphospholipid antibody syndrome: their relationship with the observed thrombocytopenia. *Br J Haematol* 1997;98:336.

367. Bergstrom AL, Olsson LB, Kutti J. Platelet survival and platelet production in systemic lupus erythematosus (SLE). *Scand J Rheum* 1980;9:209.

368. Kelton JG, Carter CJ, Rodger C, et al. The relationship among platelet-associated IgG, platelet lifespan, and reticuloendothelial cell function. *Blood* 1984;63:1434.

369. Kurata Y, Hayashi S, Kosugi S, et al. Elevated platelet-associated IgG in SLE patients due to anti-platelet autoantibody: differentiation between autoantibodies and immune complexes by ether elution. *Br J Haematol* 1993;85:723.

370. George J, Gilburd B, Langevitz P, et al. β2 glycoprotein I containing immune-complexes in lupus patients: association with thrombocytopenia and lipoprotein (a) levels. *Lupus* 1999;8:116.

371. Kalunian KC, Peter JB, Middlekauff HR, et al. Clinical significance of a single test for anti-cardiolipin antibodies in patients with systemic lupus erythematosus. *Am J Med* 1988;85:602.

372. Nojima J, Suehisa E, Kuratsune H, et al. High prevalence of thrombocytopenia in SLE patients with a high level of anticardiolipin antibodies combined with lupus anticoagulant. *Am J Hematol* 1998;58:55.

373. Khamashta MA, Harris EN, Sharavi AE, et al. Immune mediated mechanism for thrombosis: antiphospholipid antibody binding to platelet membranes. *Ann Rheum Dis* 1988;47:849.

374. Miller MA, Urowitz MB, Gladman DD. The significance of thrombocytopenia in systemic lupus erythematosus. *Arthritis Rheum* 1983;26:1181.

375. Triplett DA, Asherson RA. Pathophysiology of the catastrophic antiphospholipid syndrome (CAPS). *Am J Hematol* 2000;65:154.

376. Nesher G, Hanna VE, Moore TL, et al. Thrombotic microangiopathic hemolytic anemia in systemic lupus erythematosus. *Semin Arthritis Rheum* 1994;24:165.

377. Hakim AJ, Machin SJ, Isenberg DA. Autoimmune thrombocytopenia in primary antiphospholipid syndrome and systemic lupus erythematosus: the response to splenectomy. *Semin Arthritis Rheum* 1998;28:20.

378. Rivero SJ, Alger M, Alarcon-Segovia D. Splenectomy for hemocytopenia in systemic lupus erythematosus: a controlled appraisal. *Arch Intern Med* 1979;139:773.

379. Agnello V, Pariser K, Gell J, et al. Preliminary observations on danazol therapy of systemic lupus erythematosus: effects on DNA antibodies, thrombocytopenia and complement. *J Rheumatol* 1983;10:682.

380. West SG, Johnson SC. Danazol for the treatment of refractory autoimmune thrombocytopenia in systemic lupus erythematosus. *Ann Intern Med* 1988;108:703.

381. Blanco R, Martinez-Taboada VM, Rodriguez-Valverde V, et al. Successful therapy with danazol in refractory autoimmune thrombocytopenia associated with rheumatic diseases. *Br J Rheumatol* 1997;36:1095–1099.

382. Boumpas DT, Barez S, Klippel JH, et al. Intermittent cyclophosphamide for the treatment of autoimmune thrombocytopenia in systemic lupus erythematosus. *Ann Intern Med* 1990;112:674.

383. Hanly JG, Hong C, Zayed E, et al. Immunomodulating effects of synchronised plasmapheresis and intravenous bolus cyclophosphamide in systemic lupus erythematosus. *Lupus* 1995;4:457.

384. Manger K, Kalden JR, Manger B. Cyclosporin A in the treatment of systemic lupus erythematosus: results of an open clinical study. *Br J Rheumatol* 1996;35:669–675.

385. Sugiyama M, Ogasawara H, Kaneko H, et al. Effect of extremely low dose cyclosporine treatment on the thrombocytopenia in systemic lupus erythematosus. *Lupus* 1998;7:53.

386. Chartash EK, Lans DM, Paget SA, et al. Aortic insufficiency and mitral regurgitation in patients with systemic lupus erythematosus and the antiphospholipid syndrome. *Am J Med* 1989;86:407.

387. McCroskey RD, Phillips A, Mott F, et al. Antiphospholipid antibodies and adrenal hemorrhage. *Am J Hematol* 1991;36:60.

388. Asherson RA, Mavou SC, Merry P, et al. The spectrum of livedo reticularis and anticardiolipin antibodies. *Br J Dermatol* 1989;120:215.

389. Grob JJ, San Marco M, Aillaud MF, et al. Unfading acral microlivedo: a discrete marker of thrombotic skin disease associated with anti-phospholipid antibody syndrome. *J Am Acad Dermatol* 1991;24:53.

390. Naldi L, Locati F, Marchesi L, et al. Cutaneous manifestations associated with antiphospholipid antibodies in patients with suspected primary antiphospholipid syndrome: a case-control study. *Ann Rheum Dis* 1993;52:219.

391. Asherson RA, Khamashta MA, Gil A, et al. Cerebrovascular disease and antiphospholipid antibodies in systemic lupus erythematosus, lupus-like disease, and the primary antiphospholipid syndrome. *Am J Med* 1989;86:391.

392. Schultz DR. Antiphospholipid antibodies: basic immunology and assays. *Semin Arthritis Rheum* 1997;26:724.

393. Ginsberg JS, Demers C, Brill-Edwards P, et al. Increased thrombin generation and activity in patients with systemic lupus erythematosus and anticardiolipin antibodies: evidence for a prothrombotic state. *Blood* 1993;81:2958.

394. Martinuzzo ME, Maclouf J, Carreras LO, et al. Antiphospholipid antibodies enhance thrombin-induced platelet activation and thromboxane formation. *Thromb Haemost* 1993;70:667.

395. Davies GE, Triplett DA. Corticosteroid-associated blue toe syndrome: role of antiphospholipid antibodies. *Ann Intern Med* 1990;113:893.

396. Mathew P, Chen G, Wang W. Evans syndrome: results of a national survey. *J Pediatr Hematol Oncol* 1997;19:433.

397. Hegde UM, Zuiable A, Ball S, et al. The relative incidence of idiopathic and secondary autoimmune thrombocytopenia: a clinical and serological evaluation in 508 patients. *Clin Lab Haematol* 1985;7:7.

398. Sheehan NJ, Stanton-King K. Polyautoimmunity in a young woman. *Br J Rheumatol* 1993;32:254.

399. Cooper C, Fairris G, Cotton DWK, et al. Dermatomyositis associated with idiopathic thrombocytopenia. *Dermatologica* 1986;172:173.

400. Pettersson T, Von Bonsdorff M. Auto-immune haemolytic anaemia and thrombocytopenia in scleroderma. *Acta Haematol* 1988;80:179.

401. Neucks SH, Moore TL, Lichtenstein JR, et al. Localised scleroderma and idiopathic thrombocytopenia. *J Rheumatol* 1980;7:741.

402. Schattner A, Friedman J, Klepfish A, et al. Immune cytopenias as the presenting finding in primary Sjogren's syndrome. *QJM* 2000;93:825.

403. Bizzaro N. Familial association of autoimmune thrombocytopenia and hyperthyroidism. *Am J Hematol* 1992;39:294.

404. Segal BM, Weintraub MI. Hashimoto's thyroiditis, myasthenia gravis, idiopathic thrombocytopenic purpura [Letter]. *Ann Intern Med* 1976;85:761.

405. Guzzi LM, Kucera RF, Lillis P, et al. Human gammaglobulin use in the treatment of severe thrombocytopenia associated with sarcoidosis. *Am J Med Sci* 1991;301:331.

406. Chakrabarti S, Behera D, Varma S, et al. High-dose methyl prednisolone for autoimmune thrombocytopenia in sarcoidosis. *Sarcoidosis Vasc Diffuse Lung Dis* 1997;14:188.

407. Anderson MJ, Woods VL Jr, Tani P, et al. Autoantibodies to platelet glycoprotein IIb/IIIa and to the acetylcholine receptor in a patient with chronic idiopathic thrombocytopenic purpura and myasthenia gravis. *Ann Intern Med* 1984;100:829.

408. Berchtold P, Harris JP, Tani P, et al. Autoantibodies to platelet glycoproteins in patients with disease-related immune thrombocytopenia. *Br J Haematol* 1989;73:365.

409. Boyne MS, Dye KR. Crohn's colitis and idiopathic thrombocytopenic purpura. *Postgrad Med J* 2000;76:299.

410. Bauer WM, Litchtin A, Lashner BA. Can colectomy cure immune thrombocytopenic purpura in a patient with ulcerative colitis? *Dig Dis Sci* 1999;44:2330.

411. Kahn O, Fiel ML, Janowitz HD. Celiac sprue, idiopathic thrombocytopenic purpura, and hepatic granulomatous disease: an autoimmune linkage? *J Clin Gastroenterol* 1996;23:214.

412. Mizukami Y, Ohhira M, Matsumoto A, et al. Primary biliary cirrhosis associated with idiopathic thrombocytopenic purpura. *J Gastroenterol* 1996;31:284.

413. Kihara S, Matsuzawa Y, Kubo M, et al. Autoimmune hyperchylomicronemia. *N Engl J Med* 1989;320:1255.

414. Taylor G, Venning V, Wojnarowska F. Bullous pemphigoid and associated autoimmune thrombocytopenia: two case reports. *J Am Acad Dermatol* 1993;29:900.

415. Schwartz KA, Slichter SJ, Harker LA. Immune-mediated platelet destruction and thrombocytopenia in patients with solid tumors. *Br J Haematol* 1982;51:17.

416. Sonnenblick M, Kramer MR, Hershko C. Corticosteroid responsive immune thrombocytopenia in Hodgkin's disease. *Oncology* 1986;43:349.

417. Bradley SJ, Hudson GV, Linch DC. Idiopathic thrombocytopenic purpura in Hodgkin's disease: a report of eight cases. *Clin Oncol (R Coll Radiol)* 1993;5:355.

418. Bachmeyer C, Audouin J, Bouillot JL, et al. Immune thrombocytopenic purpura as the presenting feature of gastric MALT lymphoma. *Am J Gastroenterol* 2000;95:1599.

419. Kaden BR, Rosse WF, Hauch TW. Immune thrombocytopenia in lymphoproliferative diseases. *Blood* 1979;53:545.

420. Kubota T, Tanoue K, Murohashi I, et al. Autoantibody against platelet glycoprotein IIb/IIIa in a patient with non-Hodgkin's lymphoma. *Thromb Res* 1989;53:379.

421. Hamblin TJ, Oscier DG, Young BJ. Autoimmunity in chronic lymphocytic leukaemia. *J Clin Pathol* 1986;39:713.

422. Duhrsen U, Augener W, Zwingers T, et al. Spectrum and frequency of autoimmune derangements in lymphoproliferative disorders: analysis of 637 cases and comparison with myeloproliferative diseases. *Br J Haematol* 1987;67:235.

423. Kipps TJ, Carson DA. Autoantibodies in chronic lymphocytic leukemia and related systemic autoimmune diseases. *Blood* 1993;81:2475.

424. Gupta V, Hegde UM, Parameswaran R, et al. Multiple myeloma and immune thrombocytopenia. *Clin Lab Haematol* 2000;22:239.

425. Yasuda K, Yatomi Y, Matsushima T, et al. A case of POEMS syndrome with thrombocytopenia and biliverdinaemia. *Br J Haematol* 1994;86:389.

426. Barton JC, Prasthofer EF, Egan ML, et al. Rheumatoid arthritis associated with expanded populations of granular lymphocytes. *Ann Intern Med* 1986;104:314.

427. Loughran TP Jr, Kadin ME, Starkebaum G, et al. Leukemia of large granular lymphocytes: association with clonal chromosomal abnormalities and autoimmune neutropenia, thrombocytopenia, and hemolytic anemia. *Ann Intern Med* 1985;102:169.

428. Akashi K, Shibuya T, Taniguchi S, et al. Multiple autoimmune haemopoietic disorders and insidious clonal proliferation of large granular lymphocytes. *Br J Haematol* 1999;107:670.

429. Bartlett NL, Longo DL. T-small lymphocyte disorders. *Semin Hematol* 1999;36:164.
430. Garcia-Suarez J, Prieto A, Reyes E, et al. Persistent lymphocytosis of natural killer cells in autoimmune thrombocytopenic purpura (ATP) patients after splenectomy. *Br J Haematol* 1995;89:653.
431. Matsuoka T, Tamura H, Fujishita M, et al. Thrombocytopenic purpura in a carrier of human T-cell leukemia virus type I. *Am J Hematol* 1988;27:142.
432. Walsh CM, Nardi MA, Karpatkin S. On the mechanism of thrombocytopenic purpura in sexually active homosexual men. *N Engl J Med* 1984;311:635.
433. Karpatkin S, Nardi M, Lennette ET, et al. Anti-human immunodeficiency virus type 1 antibody complexes on platelets of seropositive thrombocytopenic homosexuals and narcotic addicts. *Proc Natl Acad Sci U S A* 1988; 85:9763.
434. Yu J-R, Lennette ET, Karpatkin S. Anti-F(ab')₂ antibodies in thrombocytopenic patients at risk for acquired immunodeficiency syndrome. *J Clin Invest* 1986;77:1756.
435. Bettaieb A, Oksenhendler E, Fromont P, et al. Immunochemical analysis of platelet autoantibodies in HIV-related thrombocytopenic purpura: a study of 68 patients. *Blood* 1989;73:241.
436. Bettaieb A, Fromont P, Louache F, et al. Presence of cross-reactive antibody between human immunodeficiency virus (HIV) and platelet glycoproteins in HIV-related immune thrombocytopenic purpura. *Blood* 1992;80:162.
437. Gonzalez-Conejero R, Rivera J, Rosillo MC, et al. Association of autoantibodies against platelet glycoproteins Ib/IX and IIb/IIIa, and platelet-reactive anti-HIV antibodies in thrombocytopenic narcotic addicts. *Br J Haematol* 1996;93:464.
438. Nardi M, Karpatkin S. Antiidiotype antibody against platelet anti-GPIIIa contributes to the regulation of thrombocytopenia in HIV-1-ITP patients. *J Exp Med* 2000;191:2093.
439. Coyle TE. Hematologic complications of human immunodeficiency virus infection and the acquired immunodeficiency syndrome. *Med Clin North Am* 1997;81:449.
440. Cole JL, Marzec UM, Gunthel CJ, et al. Ineffective platelet production in thrombocytopenic human immunodeficiency virus-infected patients. *Blood* 1998;91:3239.
441. Van Wyk V, Kotzé HF, Heyns AP. Kinetics of indium-111-labelled platelets in HIV-infected patients with and without associated thrombocytopaenia. *Eur J Haematol* 1999;62:332.
442. Shannon KM, Ammann AJ. Acquired immune deficiency syndrome in childhood. *J Pediatr* 1985;106:332.
443. Falloon J, Eddy J, Wiener L, et al. Human immunodeficiency virus infection in children. *J Pediatr* 1989;114:1.
444. Holzman RS, Walsh CM, Karpatkin S. Risk for the acquired immunodeficiency syndrome among thrombocytopenic and nonthrombocytopenic homosexual men seropositive for the human immunodeficiency virus. *Ann Intern Med* 1987;106:383.
445. Swiss Group for Clinical Studies on the Acquired Immunodeficiency Syndrome (AIDS). Zidovudine for the treatment of thrombocytopenia associated with human immunodeficiency virus (HIV): a prospective study. *Ann Intern Med* 1988;109:718.
446. Rarick MU, Espina B, Montgomery T, et al. The long-term use of zidovudine in patients with severe immune-mediated thrombocytopenia secondary to infection with HIV. *AIDS* 1991;5:1357.
447. Landonio G, Cinque P, Nosari A, et al. Comparison of two dose regimens of zidovudine in an open, randomized, multicentre study for severe HIV-related thrombocytopenia. *AIDS* 1993;7:209–212.
448. Marroni M, Gresele P, Landonio G, et al. Interferon-α is effective in the treatment of HIV-1-related, severe, zidovudine-resistant thrombocytopenia: a prospective, placebo-controlled, double-blind trial. *Ann Intern Med* 1994; 121:423.
449. Palella FJ Jr, Delaney KM, Moorman AC, et al. Declining morbidity and mortality among patients with advanced human immunodeficiency virus infection. HIV Outpatient Study Investigators. *N Engl J Med* 1998;338:853–860.
450. Aboulafia DM, Bundow D, Waide S, et al. Initial observations on the efficacy of highly active antiretroviral therapy in the treatment of HIV-associated autoimmune thrombocytopenia. *Am J Med Sci* 2000;320:117.
451. Oksenhendler E, Bierling P, Farcet JP, et al. Response to therapy in 37 patients with HIV-related thrombocytopenic purpura. *Br J Haematol* 1987;66:491.
452. Shafer RW, Offit K, Macris NT, et al. Possible risk of steroid administration in patients at risk for AIDS [Letter]. *Lancet* 1985;1:934.
453. Jahnke L, Applebaum S, Sherman LA, et al. An evaluation of intravenous immunoglobulin in the treatment of human immunodeficiency virus-associated thrombocytopenia. *Transfusion* 1994;34:759–764.
454. Kurtzberg J, Friedman HS, Kinney TR, et al. Management of human immunodeficiency virus–associated thrombocytopenia with intravenous gamma globulin. *Am J Pediatr Hematol Oncol* 1987;9:299.
455. Lord RVN, Coleman MJ, Milliken ST. Splenectomy for HIV-related immune thrombocytopenia: comparison with results of splenectomy for non-HIV immune thrombocytopenic purpura. *Arch Surg* 1998;133:205–210.
456. Aboulian A, Ricci M, Shapiro K, et al. Surgical treatment of HIV-related immune thrombocytopenia. *Int Surg* 1999;84:81.
457. Tsoukas MC, Bernard BF, Abrahamowicz M, et al. Effect of splenectomy on slowing human immunodeficiency virus disease progression. *Arch Surg* 1998;133:25.
458. Godeau B, Oksenhendler E, Bierling P. Dapsone for autoimmune thrombocytopenic purpura. *Am J Hematol* 1993;44:70.
459. Needleman SW, Sorace J, Poussin-Rosillo H. Low-dose splenic irradiation in the treatment of autoimmune thrombocytopenia in HIV-infected patients. *Ann Intern Med* 1992;116:310.
460. Marroni M, Sinnone MS, Landonio G, et al. Splenic irradiation versus splenectomy for severe, refractory HIV-related thrombocytopenia: effects on platelet counts and immunological status. *AIDS* 2000;14:1664–1667.
461. First LR, Smith BR, Lipton J, et al. Isolated thrombocytopenia after allogeneic bone marrow transplantation: existence of transient and chronic thrombocytopenic syndromes. *Blood* 1985;65:368.
462. Anasetti C, Rybka W, Sullivan KM, et al. Graft-v-host disease is associated with autoimmune-like thrombocytopenia. *Blood* 1989;73:1054.
463. Minchinton RM, Waters AH, Malpas JS, et al. Platelet- and granulocyte-specific antibodies after allogeneic and autologous bone marrow grafts. *Vox Sang* 1984;46:125.
464. Chan EY, Lawton JW, Lie AK, et al. Autoantibody formation after allogeneic bone marrow transplantation: correlation with the reconstitution of CD5+ B cells and occurrence of graft-versus-host disease. *Pathology* 1997;29:184.
465. Panzer S, Kiefel V, Bartram CR, et al. Immune thrombocytopenia more than a year after allogeneic marrow transplantation due to antibodies against donor platelets with anti-Pl^A1 specificity: evidence for a host-derived immune reaction. *Br J Haematol* 1989;71:259.
466. Bierling P, Pignon JM, Kuentz M, et al. Thrombocytopenia after bone marrow transplantation caused by a recipient origin Br^a allo-antibody: presence of mixed chimerism 3 years after the graft without hematologic relapse. *Blood* 1994;83:274–279.
467. Friend PJ, McCarthy LJ, Filo RS, et al. Transmission of idiopathic (autoimmune) thrombocytopenic purpura by liver transplantation. *N Engl J Med* 1990;323:807.
468. Kita Y, Harihara Y, Hirata M, et al. Splenectomy for idiopathic thrombocytopenic purpura after living-related liver transplantation [Letter]. *Transplantation* 2000;70:553.
469. West KA, Anderson DR, McAlister VC, et al. Alloimmune thrombocytopenia after organ transplantation. *N Engl J Med* 1999;341:1504.
470. Hackett T, Kelton JG, Powers P. Drug-induced platelet destruction. *Semin Thromb Hemost* 1982;8:116.
471. George JN, Raskob GE, Shah SR, et al. Drug-induced thrombocytopenia: a systematic review of published case reports. *Ann Intern Med* 1998;129:886.
472. Kaufman DW, Kelly JP, Johannes CB, et al. Acute thrombocytopenic purpura in relation to the use of drugs. *Blood* 1993;82:2714.
473. Pedersen-Bjergaard U, Andersen M, Hansen PB. Drug-induced thrombocytopenia: clinical data on 309 cases and the effect of corticosteroid therapy. *Eur J Clin Pharmacol* 1997;52:183.
474. Warkentin TE, Kelton JG. Thrombocytopenia due to platelet destruction and hypersplenism. In: Hoffman R, Benz EJ Jr, Shattil SJ, et al., eds. *Hematology: basic principles and practice*, 3rd ed. New York: Churchill Livingstone, 1999:2138–2154.
475. Aster RH. Drug-induced immune thrombocytopenia: an overview of pathogenesis. *Semin Hematol* 1999;36[Suppl 1]:2.
476. Greinacher A, Eichler P, Lubenow N, et al. Drug-induced and drug-dependent immune thrombocytopenias. *Rev Clin Exp Hematol* 2001;5:166–200.
477. Neely SM, Gardner DV, Reynolds N, et al. Mechanism and characteristics of platelet activation by haematin. *Br J Haematol* 1984;58:305.
478. Horne MK III. Non-immune heparin-associated thrombocytopenia. In: Warkentin TE, Greinacher A, eds. *Heparin-induced thrombocytopenia*, 2nd ed. New York: Marcel-Dekker, 2001:123–136.
479. Gangarosa EJ, Johnson TR, Ramos HS. Ristocetin-induced thrombocytopenia: site and mechanism of action. *Arch Intern Med* 1960;105:83.
480. Green D, Tuite GF Jr. Declining platelet counts and platelet aggregation during porcine VIII:C infusions. *Am J Med* 1989;86:222.
481. Heyns A du P, Lotter MG, Badenhorst PN, et al. Kinetics and in vivo redistribution of ¹¹¹indium-labelled human platelets after intravenous protamine sulphate. *Thromb Haemost* 1980;44:65.
482. Blendis LM, Smith PM, Lawrie BW, et al. Portal hypertension in vinyl chloride monomer workers: a hemodynamic study. *Gastroenterology* 1978;75:206.
483. Barr RD, Copeland SA, Stockwell ML, et al. Valproic acid and immune thrombocytopenia. *Arch Dis Child* 1982;57:681.
484. Delgado MR, Riela AR, Mills J, et al. Thrombocytopenia secondary to high valproate levels in children with epilepsy. *J Child Neurol* 1994;9:311.
485. Ross MP, Allen-Webb EM, Pappas JB, et al. Amrinone-associated thrombocytopenia: pharmacokinetic analysis. *Clin Pharmacol Ther* 1993;53:661.
486. Warkentin TE, Sheppard JI, Horsewood P, et al. Impact of the patient population on the risk for heparin-induced thrombocytopenia. *Blood* 2000;96:1703.
487. Eisner EV, Shahidi NT. Immune thrombocytopenia due to a drug metabolite. *N Engl J Med* 1972;287:376.
488. Kiefel V, Santoso S, Schmidt S, et al. Metabolite-specific (IgG) and drug-specific antibodies (IgG, IgM) in two cases of trimethoprim-sulfamethoxazole-induced immune thrombocytopenia. *Transfusion* 1987;27:262.
489. Kiefel V. Differential diagnosis of acute thrombocytopenia. In: Warkentin TE, Greinacher A, eds. *Heparin-induced thrombocytopenia*, 2nd ed. New York: Marcel Dekker, 2001:19.
490. Warkentin TE, Levine MN, Hirsh J, et al. Heparin-induced thrombocytopenia in patients treated with low-molecular-weight heparin or unfractionated heparin. *N Engl J Med* 1995;332:1330.
491. Lee DH, Warkentin TE. Frequency of heparin-induced thrombocytopenia. In: Warkentin TE, Greinacher A, eds. *Heparin-induced thrombocytopenia*, 2nd ed. New York: Marcel Dekker, 2001:87.

492. Danielson DA, Douglas SW III, Herzog P, et al. Drug-induced blood disorders. *JAMA* 1984;252:3257.

493. Christie DJ, Walker RH, Kolins MD, et al. Quinine-induced thrombocytopenia following intravenous use of heroin. *Arch Intern Med* 1983;143:1174.

494. Adachi JD, Bensen WG, Kassam Y, et al. Gold-induced thrombocytopenia: 12 cases and a review of the literature. *Semin Arthritis Rheum* 1987;16:287.

495. Alban S, Greinacher A. Role of sulfated polysaccharides in the pathogenesis of heparin-induced thrombocytopenia. In: Warkentin TE, Greinacher A, eds. *Heparin-induced thrombocytopenia*, 2nd ed. New York: Marcel Dekker, 2001:167.

496. Kelton JG. Heparin-induced thrombocytopenia. *Haemostasis* 1986;16:173.

497. Warkentin TE, Kelton JG. Temporal aspects of heparin-induced thrombocytopenia. *N Engl J Med* 2001;344:1286.

498. Warkentin TE. Clinical picture of heparin-induced thrombocytopenia. In: Warkentin TE, Greinacher A, eds. *Heparin-induced thrombocytopenia*, 2nd ed. New York: Marcel Dekker, 2001:43.

499. Warkentin TE, Kelton JG. A 14-year study of heparin-induced thrombocytopenia. *Am J Med* 1996;101:502.

500. Amiral J, Bridey F, Dreyfus M, et al. Platelet factor 4 complexed to heparin is the target for antibodies generated in heparin-induced thrombocytopenia [Letter]. *Thromb Haemost* 1992;68:95.

501. Greinacher A, Pötzsch B, Amiral J, et al. Heparin-associated thrombocytopenia: isolation of the antibody and characterization of a multimolecular PF4-heparin complex as the major antigen. *Thromb Haemost* 1994;71:247.

502. Kelton JG, Smith JW, Warkentin TE, et al. Immunoglobulin G from patients with heparin-induced thrombocytopenia binds to a complex of heparin and platelet factor 4. *Blood* 1994;83:3232–3239.

503. Ziporen L, Li ZQ, Park KS, et al. Defining an antigenic epitope on platelet factor 4 associated with heparin-induced thrombocytopenia. *Blood* 1998;92:3250.

504. Suh JS, Aster RH, Visentin GP. Antibodies from patients with heparin-induced thrombocytopenia/thrombosis recognize different epitopes on heparin:platelet factor 4. *Blood* 1998;91:916.

505. Greinacher A, Michels I, Schafer M, et al. Heparin-associated thrombocytopenia in a patient treated with polysulphated chondroitin sulphate: evidence for immunological crossreactivity between heparin and polysulphated glycosaminoglycans. *Br J Haematol* 1992;81:252.

506. Tardy-Poncet B, Tardy B, Grelac F, et al. Pentosan polysulfate-induced thrombocytopenia and thrombosis. *Am J Hematol* 1994;45:252.

507. Visentin GP, Moghaddam M, Beery SE, et al. Heparin is not required for detection of antibodies associated with heparin-induced thrombocytopenia/thrombosis. *J Lab Clin Med* 2001;138:22–31.

508. Chong BH, Pitney WR, Castaldi PA. Heparin-induced thrombocytopenia: association of thrombotic complications with heparin-dependent IgG antibody that induces thromboxane synthesis and platelet aggregation. *Lancet* 1982;2:1246.

509. Warkentin TE, Hayward CPM, Boshkov LK, et al. Sera from patients with heparin-induced thrombocytopenia generate platelet-derived microparticles with procoagulant activity: an explanation for the thrombotic complications of heparin-induced thrombocytopenia. *Blood* 1994;84:3691.

510. Hughes M, Hayward CPM, Warkentin TE, et al. Morphological analysis of microparticle generation in heparin-induced thrombocytopenia. *Blood* 2000;96:188.

511. Cines DB, Tomaski A, Tannenbaum S. Immune endothelial-cell injury in heparin-associated thrombocytopenia. *N Engl J Med* 1987;316:581.

512. Visentin GP, Ford SE, Scott JP, et al. Antibodies from patients with heparin-induced thrombocytopenia/thrombosis are specific for platelet factor 4 complexed with heparin or bound to endothelial cells. *J Clin Invest* 1994;93:81.

513. Pouplard C, Iochmann S, Renard B, et al. Induction of monocyte tissue factor expression by antibodies to heparin-platelet factor 4 complexes developed in heparin-induced thrombocytopenia. *Blood* 2001;97:3300.

514. Warkentin TE, Elavathil LJ, Hayward CPM, et al. The pathogenesis of venous limb gangrene associated with heparin-induced thrombocytopenia. *Ann Intern Med* 1997;127:804.

515. Warkentin TE. Limitations of conventional treatment options for heparin-induced thrombocytopenia. *Semin Hematol* 1998;35[Suppl 5]:17.

516. Greinacher A. Recombinant hirudin for the treatment of heparin-induced thrombocytopenia. In: Warkentin TE, Greinacher A, eds. *Heparin-induced thrombocytopenia*, 2nd ed. New York: Marcel Dekker, 2001:349.

517. Suh JS, Malik MI, Aster RH, et al. Characterization of the humoral immune response in heparin-induced thrombocytopenia. *Am J Hematol* 1997;54:196.

518. Amiral J, Pouplard C, Vissac AM, et al. Affinity purification of heparin-dependent antibodies to platelet factor 4 developed in heparin-induced thrombocytopenia: biological characteristics and effects on platelet activation. *Br J Haematol* 2000;109:336.

519. Chong BH, Pilgrim RL, Cooley MA, et al. Increased expression of platelet IgG Fc receptors in immune heparin-induced thrombocytopenia. *Blood* 1993;81:988.

520. Denomme GA. The platelet Fc receptor in heparin-induced thrombocytopenia. In: Warkentin TE, Greinacher A, eds. *Heparin-induced thrombocytopenia*, 2nd ed. New York: Marcel Dekker, 2001:189.

521. Laster J, Silver D. Heparin-coated catheters and heparin-induced thrombocytopenia. *J Vasc Surg* 1988;7:667.

522. Ling E, Warkentin TE. Intraoperative heparin flushes and subsequent acute heparin-induced thrombocytopenia. *Anesthesiology* 1998;89:1567.

523. Warkentin TE, Kelton JG. Delayed-onset heparin-induced thrombocytopenia and thrombosis. *Ann Intern Med* 2001;135:502.

524. Warkentin TE. Clinical presentation of heparin-induced thrombocytopenia. *Semin Hematol* 1998;35[Suppl 5]:9.

525. Phelan BK. Heparin-associated thrombosis with thrombocytopenia. *Ann Intern Med* 1983;99:637.

526. Risch L, Pihan H, Zeller C, et al. ET gets HIT–thrombocytotic heparin-induced thrombocytopenia (HIT) in a patient with essential thrombocythemia (ET). *Blood Coagul Fibrinolysis* 2000;11:663.

527. Calhoun BC, Hesser JW. Heparin-associated antibody with pregnancy: discussion of two cases. *Am J Obstet Gynecol* 1987;156:964.

528. Warkentin TE, Hong AP. Frequency of upper limb deep venous thrombosis (UL-DVT) in relation to central venous catheter (CVC) use in patients with heparin-induced thrombocytopenia (HIT): evidence for interaction of systemic (HIT) and local (CVC) prothrombotic risk factors. *Blood* 1998;92[Suppl 1]:500a(abst).

529. Warkentin TE. Venous limb gangrene during warfarin treatment of cancer-associated deep venous thrombosis. *Ann Intern Med* 2001;135:589.

530. Warkentin TE, Sikov WM, Lillicrap DP. Multicentric warfarin-induced skin necrosis complicating heparin-induced thrombocytopenia. *Am J Hematol* 1999;62:44.

531. Bleasel JF, Rasko JEJ, Rickard KA, et al. Acute adrenal insufficiency secondary to heparin-induced thrombocytopenia-thrombosis syndrome. *Med J Aust* 1992;157:192.

532. Platell CFE, Tan EGC. Hypersensitivity reactions to heparin: delayed onset thrombocytopenia and necrotizing skin lesions. *Aust N Z J Surg* 1986;56:621.

533. Warkentin TE. Heparin-induced skin lesions. *Br J Haematol* 1996;92:494.

534. Ansell JE, Clark WP Jr, Compton CC. Fatal reactions associated with intravenous heparin. *Drug Intell Clin Pharm* 1986;20:74.

535. Warkentin TE, Hirte HW, Anderson DR, et al. Transient global amnesia associated with acute heparin-induced thrombocytopenia. *Am J Med* 1994;97:489.

536. Warkentin TE. Laboratory testing for heparin-induced thrombocytopenia. *J Thromb Thrombolysis* 2001;10:35.

537. Warkentin TE, Greinacher A. Laboratory testing for heparin-induced thrombocytopenia. In: Warkentin TE, Greinacher A, eds. *Heparin-induced thrombocytopenia*, 2nd ed. New York: Marcel Dekker, 2001:231.

538. Chong BH, Burgess J, Ismail F. The clinical usefulness of the platelet aggregation test for the diagnosis of heparin-induced thrombocytopenia. *Thromb Haemost* 1993;69:344.

539. Sheridan D, Carter C, Kelton JG. A diagnostic test for heparin-induced thrombocytopenia. *Blood* 1986;67:27.

540. Greinacher A, Michels I, Kiefel V, et al. A rapid and sensitive test for diagnosing heparin-associated thrombocytopenia. *Thromb Haemost* 1991;66:734.

541. Greinacher A, Amiral J, Dummel V, et al. Laboratory diagnosis of heparin-associated thrombocytopenia and comparison of platelet aggregation test, heparin-induced platelet activation test, and platelet factor 4/heparin enzyme-linked immunosorbent assay. *Transfusion* 1994;34:381.

542. Lee DH, Warkentin TE, Denomme GA, et al. A diagnostic test for heparin-induced thrombocytopenia: detection of platelet microparticles using flow cytometry. *Br J Haematol* 1996;95:724.

543. Warkentin TE, Hayward CPM, Smith CA, et al. Determinants of donor platelet variability when testing for heparin-induced thrombocytopenia. *J Lab Clin Med* 1992;120:371.

544. Meyer O, Salama A, Pittet N, et al. Rapid detection of heparin-induced platelet antibodies with particle gel immunoassay (ID-HPF4). *Lancet* 1999;354:1525.

545. Eichler P, Raschke R, Lubenow N, et al. The new ID-heparin/PF4 antibody test for rapid detection of heparin-induced antibodies in comparison with functional and antigenic assays. *Br J Haematol* 2002;116:887.

546. Turpie AG, Gallus AS, Hoek JA, for the Pentasaccharide Investigators. A synthetic pentasaccharide for the prevention of deep-vein thrombosis after total hip replacement. *N Engl J Med* 2001;344:619.

547. Herbert JM, Hérault JP, Bernat A, et al. SR123781A, a synthetic heparin mimetic. *Thromb Haemost* 2001;85:852.

548. Warkentin TE. Platelet count monitoring and laboratory testing for heparin-induced thrombocytopenia. Recommendations of the College of American Pathologists. *Arch Pathol Lab Med* 2002;126:in press.

549. Wallis DE, Workman DL, Lewis BE, et al. Failure of early heparin cessation as treatment for heparin-induced thrombocytopenia. *Am J Med* 1999;106:629.

550. Hirsh J, Warkentin TE, Shaughnessy SG, et al. Heparin and low-molecular-weight heparin: mechanisms of action, pharmacokinetics, dosing, monitoring, efficacy, and safety. *Chest* 2001;119[Suppl]:64S.

551. Greinacher A, Warkentin TE. Treatment of heparin-induced thrombocytopenia: an overview. In: Warkentin TE, Greinacher A, eds. *Heparin-induced thrombocytopenia*, 2nd ed. New York: Marcel Dekker, 2001:291.

552. Warkentin TE. Heparin-induced thrombocytopenia: yet another treatment paradox? *Thromb Haemost* 2001;85:947.

553. Chong BH, Magnani HN. Danaparoid for the treatment of heparin-induced thrombocytopenia. In: Warkentin TE, Greinacher A, eds. *Heparin-induced thrombocytopenia*, 2nd ed. New York: Marcel Dekker, 2001:323.

554. Greinacher A. Recombinant hirudin for the treatment of heparin-induced thrombocytopenia. In: Warkentin TE, Greinacher A, eds. *Heparin-induced thrombocytopenia*, 2nd ed. New York: Marcel Dekker, 2001:349.

555. Lewis BE, Hursting MJ. Argatroban therapy in heparin-induced thrombocytopenia. In: Warkentin TE, Greinacher A, eds. *Heparin-induced thrombocytopenia*, 2nd ed. New York: Marcel Dekker, 2001:381.

556. Chong BH, Ismail F, Cade J, et al. Heparin-induced thrombocytopenia: studies with a new low molecular weight heparinoid, Org 10172. *Blood* 1989;73:1592.

557. Newman PM, Swanson RL, Chong BH. Heparin-induced thrombocytopenia: IgG binding to PF4-heparin complexes in the fluid phase and cross-reactivity with low molecular weight heparin and heparinoid. *Thromb Haemost* 1998;80:292.

558. Chong BH, Gallus AS, Cade JF, et al. Prospective randomised open-label comparison of danaparoid with dextran 70 in the treatment of heparin-induced thrombocytopenia with thrombosis: a clinical outcome study. *Thromb Haemost* 2001;86:1170.

559. Warkentin TE. Danaparoid (Orgaran®) for the treatment of heparin-induced thrombocytopenia (HIT) and thrombosis: effects on *in vivo* thrombin and cross-linked fibrin generation, and evaluation of the clinical significance of *in vitro* cross-reactivity (XR) of danaparoid for HIT-IgG. *Blood* 1996;88[Suppl 1]:626a(abst).

560. Farner B, Eichler P, Kroll H, et al. A comparison of lepirudin and danaparoid for heparin-induced thrombocytopenia. *Thromb Haemost* 2001;85:950.

561. Greinacher A, Lubenow N. Recombinant hirudin in clinical practice: focus on lepirudin. *Circulation* 2001;103:1479.

562. Greinacher A, Völpel H, Janssens U, et al. Recombinant hirudin (lepirudin) provides safe and effective anticoagulation in patients with the immunologic type of heparin-induced thrombocytopenia: a prospective study. *Circulation* 1999;99:73.

563. Greinacher A, Janssens U, Berg G, et al. Lepirudin (recombinant hirudin) for parenteral anticoagulation in patients with heparin-induced thrombocytopenia. Heparin-Associated Thrombocytopenia Study (HAT) Investigators. *Circulation* 1999;100:587.

564. Greinacher A, Eichler P, Lubenow N, et al. Heparin-induced thrombocytopenia with thromboembolic complications: meta-analysis of 2 prospective trials to assess the value of parenteral treatment with lepirudin and its therapeutic aPTT range. *Blood* 2000;96:846.

565. Poetzsch B, Madlener K. Management of cardiopulmonary bypass anticoagulation in patients with heparin-induced thrombocytopenia. In: Warkentin TE, Greinacher A, eds. *Heparin-induced thrombocytopenia*, 2nd ed. New York: Marcel Dekker, 2001:429.

566. Eichler P, Friesen HJ, Lubenow N, et al. Antihirudin antibodies in patients with heparin-induced thrombocytopenia treated with lepirudin: incidence, effects on aPTT, and clinical relevance. *Blood* 2000;96:2373.

567. Lewis BE, Wallis DE, Berkowitz M, et al. Argatroban anticoagulant therapy in patients with heparin-induced thrombocytopenia. *Circulation* 2001;103:1838.

568. Sheth SB, DiCicco RA, Hursting MJ, et al. Interpreting the International Normalized Ratio (INR) in individuals receiving argatroban and warfarin. *Thromb Haemost* 2001;85:435.

569. Lewis BE, Iaffaldano R, McKiernan TL, et al. Report of successful use of argatroban as an alternative anticoagulant during coronary stent implantation in a patient with heparin-induced thrombocytopenia and thrombosis syndrome. *Cathet Cardiovasc Diagn* 1996;38:206.

570. Ranze O, Eichler P, Lubenow N, et al. The use of low-molecular-weight heparins in heparin-induced thrombocytopenia (HIT): a cohort study. *Ann Hematol* 2000;79[Suppl 1]:P198(abst).

571. Sobel M, Adelman B, Szentpetery S, et al. Surgical management of heparin-associated thrombocytopenia: strategies in the treatment of venous and arterial thromboembolism. *J Vasc Surg* 1988;8:395.

572. Greinacher A, Liebenhoff U, Kiefel V, et al. Heparin-associated thrombocytopenia: the effects of various intravenous IgG preparations on antibody mediated platelet activation—a possible new indication for high dose i.v. IgG. *Thromb Haemost* 1994;71:641.

573. Demers C, Ginsberg JS, Brill-Edwards P, et al. Rapid anticoagulation using ancrod for heparin-induced thrombocytopenia. *Blood* 1991;78:2194.

574. Pötzsch B, Klövekorn WP, Madlener K. Use of heparin during cardiopulmonary bypass in patients with a history of heparin-induced thrombocytopenia [Letter]. *N Engl J Med* 2000;343:515.

575. Fischer KG. Hemodialysis in heparin-induced thrombocytopenia. In: Warkentin TE, Greinacher A, eds. *Heparin-induced thrombocytopenia*, 2nd ed. New York: Marcel Dekker, 2001:409.

576. Warkentin TE, Dunn GL, Cybulsky IJ. Off-pump coronary artery bypass grafting for acute heparin-induced thrombocytopenia. *Ann Thorac Surg* 2001;72:1730.

577. Bougie D, Aster R. Immune thrombocytopenia resulting from sensitivity to metabolites of naproxen and acetaminophen. *Blood* 2001;97:3846.

578. Yu LC, Warrier RP, Gaumer R, et al. Actinomycin-induced immune thrombocytopenia. *Clin Pediatr (Phila)* 1990;29:196.

579. Ishikita T, Ishiguro A, Fujisawa K, et al. Carbamazepine-induced thrombocytopenia defined by a challenge test. *Am J Hematol* 1999;62:52.

580. Christie DJ, Lennon SS, Drew RL, et al. Cefotetan-induced immunologic thrombocytopenia. *Br J Haematol* 1988;70:423.

581. Kim HL, Kovacs MJ. Diclofenac-associated thrombocytopenia and neutropenia. *Ann Pharmacother* 1995;29:713.

582. Mercurio MG, Elewski BE. Thrombocytopenia caused by fluconazole therapy. *J Am Acad Dermatol* 1995;32:525.

583. El-Kassar N, Kalfon P, Fromont P, et al. Fusidic acid induced acute immunologic thrombocytopenia. *Br J Haematol* 1996;93:427.

584. Kosty MP, Hench PK, Tani P, et al. Thrombocytopenia associated with auranofin therapy: evidence for a gold-dependent immunologic mechanism. *Am J Hematol* 1989;30:236.

585. Bozec L, Bierling P, Fromont P, et al. Irinotecan-induced immune thrombocytopenia. *Ann Oncol* 1998;9:453.

586. Murphy MF, Riordan T, Minchinton RM, et al. Demonstration of an immune-mediated mechanism of penicillin-induced neutropenia and thrombocytopenia. *Br J Haematol* 1983;55:155.

587. Christie DJ, Sauro SC, Cavanaugh AL, et al. Severe thrombocytopenia in an acquired immunodeficiency syndrome patient associated with pentamidine-dependent antibodies specific for glycoprotein IIb/IIIa. *Blood* 1993;82:3075.

588. Holtzer CD, Reisner-Keller LA. Phenytoin-induced thrombocytopenia. *Ann Pharmacother* 1997;31:435.

589. Devine DV, Currie MS, Rosse WF, et al. Pseudo–Bernard-Soulier syndrome: thrombocytopenia caused by autoantibody to platelet glycoprotein Ib. *Blood* 1987;70:428.

590. Landrum EM, Siegert EA, Hanlon JT, et al. Prolonged thrombocytopenia associated with procainamide in an elderly patient. *Ann Pharmacother* 1994;28:1172.

591. Bolton FG, Young RV. Observations on cases of thrombocytopenic purpura due to quinine, sulphamezathine, and quinidine. *J Clin Pathol* 1953;6:320.

592. Kunicki TJ, Johnson MM, Aster RH. Absence of the platelet receptor for drug-dependent antibodies in the Bernard-Soulier syndrome. *J Clin Invest* 1978;62:716.

593. Smith ME, Reid DM, Jones CE, et al. Binding of quinine- and quinidine-dependent drug antibodies to platelets is mediated by the Fab domain of the immunoglobulin G and is not Fc dependent. *J Clin Invest* 1987;79:912.

594. Visentin GP, Newman PJ, Aster RH. Characteristics of quinine- and quinidine-induced antibodies specific for platelet glycoproteins IIb and IIIa. *Blood* 1991;77:2668.

595. Pfueller SL, Bilston RA, Logan D, et al. Heterogeneity of drug-dependent platelet antigens and their antibodies in quinine- and quinidine-induced thrombocytopenia: involvement of glycoproteins Ib, IIb, IIIa, and IX. *Blood* 1988;72:1155.

596. Lopez JA, Li CQ, Weisman S, et al. The glycoprotein Ib-IX complex-specific monoclonal antibody SZ1 binds to a conformation-sensitive epitope on glycoprotein IX: implications for the target antigen of quinine/quinidine-dependent autoantibodies. *Blood* 1995;85:1254.

597. Gentilini G, Curtis BR, Aster RH. An antibody from a patient with ranitidine-induced thrombocytopenia recognizes a site on glycoprotein IX that is a favored target for drug-induced antibodies. *Blood* 1998;92:2359.

598. Pereira J, Hidalgo P, Ocqueteau M, et al. Glycoprotein Ib/IX complex is the target in rifampicin-induced immune thrombocytopenia. *Br J Haematol* 2000;110:907.

599. Curtis BR, McFarland JG, Wu GG, et al. Antibodies in sulfonamide-induced immune thrombocytopenia recognize calcium-dependent epitopes on the glycoprotein IIb/IIIa complex. *Blood* 1994;84:176.

600. Tisdale JF, Figg WD, Reed E, et al. Severe thrombocytopenia in patients treated with suramin: evidence for an immune mechanism in one. *Am J Hematol* 1996;51:152.

601. Yao JC, Thomakos N, McLaughlin P, et al. Tamoxifen-induced thrombocytopenia. *Am J Clin Oncol* 1999;22:529.

602. Veldman RG, van der Pijl JW, Claas FHJ. Teicoplanin-induced thrombocytopenia. *Nephron* 1996;73:721.

603. Mizon, P, Kiefel V, Mannessier L, et al. Thrombocytopenia induced by vancomycin-dependent platelet antibody. *Vox Sang* 1997;73:49.

604. Howard CE, Adams LA, Admire JL, et al. Vancomycin-induced thrombocytopenia: a challenge and rechallenge. *Ann Pharmacother* 1997;31:315.

605. Reid DM, Shulman NR. Drug purpura due to surreptitious quinidine intake. *Ann Intern Med* 1988;108:206.

606. Chong BH, Berndt MC, Koutts J, et al. Quinidine-induced thrombocytopenia and leukopenia: demonstration and characterization of distinct antiplatelet and antileukocyte antibodies. *Blood* 1983;62:1218.

607. Hou M, Horney E, Stockelberg D, et al. Multiple quinine-dependent antibodies in a patient with episodic thrombocytopenia, neutropenia, lymphocytopenia, and granulomatous hepatitis. *Blood* 1997;90:4806.

608. Christie DJ, Mullen PC, Aster RH. Fab-mediated binding of drug-dependent antibodies to platelets in quinidine- and quinine-induced thrombocytopenia. *J Clin Invest* 1985;75:310.

609. Kelton JG, Meltzer D, Moore J, et al. Drug-induced thrombocytopenia is associated with increased binding of IgG to platelets both in vivo and in vitro. *Blood* 1981;58:524.

610. Christie DJ, Aster RH. Drug-antibody-platelet interaction in quinine and quinidine-induced thrombocytopenia. *J Clin Invest* 1982;70:989.

611. Christie DJ, Weber RW, Mullen PC, et al. Structural features of the quinidine and quinine molecules necessary for binding of drug-induced antibodies to human platelets. *J Lab Clin Med* 1984;104:730.

612. Nieminen U, Kekomäki R. Quinidine-induced thrombocytopenic purpura: clinical presentation in relation to drug-dependent and drug-independent platelet antibodies. *Br J Haematol* 1992;80:77

613. Visentin GP, Wolfmeyer K, Newman PJ, et al. Detection of drug-dependent, platelet-reactive antibodies by antigen-capture ELISA and flow cytometry. *Transfusion* 1990;30:694.

614. Kiefel V, Santoso S, Weisheit M, et al. Monoclonal antibody-specific immobilization of platelet antigens (MAIPA): a new tool for the identification of platelet-reactive antibodies. *Blood* 1987;70:1722.

615. Tcheng JE. Clinical challenges of platelet glycoprotein IIb/IIIa receptor inhibitor therapy: bleeding, reversal, thrombocytopenia, and retreatment. *Am Heart J* 2000;139:S38.

616. Kereiakes DJ, Runyon JP, Broderick TM, et al. IIb's are not IIb's. *Am J Cardiol* 2000;85:23C.

617. Berkowitz SD, Harrington RA, Rund MM, et al. Acute profound thrombocytopenia after C7E3 Fab (abciximab) therapy. *Circulation* 1997;95:809.

618. Berkowitz SD, Sane DC, Sigmon KN, et al. Occurrence and clinical significance of thrombocytopenia in patients undergoing high-risk percutaneous

coronary revascularisation: Evaluation of c7E3 for the Prevention of Ischemic Complications (EPIC) Study Group. *J Am Coll Cardiol* 1998;32:311.

619. Dasgupta H, Blankenship JC, Wood GC, et al. Thrombocytopenia complicating treatment with intravenous glycoprotein IIb/IIIa receptor inhibitors: a pooled analysis. *Am Heart J* 2000;140:206.

620. Kereiakes DJ, Essell JH, Abbottsmith CW, et al. Abciximab-associated profound thrombocytopenia: therapy with immunoglobulin and platelet transfusion. *Am J Cardiol* 1996;78:1161.

621. Jubelirer SJ, Koenig BA, Bates MC. Acute profound thrombocytopenia following C7E3 Fab (abciximab) therapy: case reports, review of the literature and implications for therapy. *Am J Hematol* 1999;61:205.

622. Desai M, Lucore CL. Uneventful use of tirofiban as an adjunct to coronary stenting in a patient with a history of abciximab-associated thrombocytopenia 10 months earlier. *J Invasive Cardiol* 2000;12:109.

623. Rao JR, Mascarenhas DA. Successful use of eptifibatide as an adjunct to coronary stenting in a patient with abciximab-associated acute profound thrombocytopenia. *J Invasive Cardiol* 2001;13:471.

624. Nieminen U, Peltola H, Syrjälä MT, et al. Acute thrombocytopenic purpura following measles, mumps and rubella vaccination: a report on 23 patients. *Acta Paediatr* 1993;82:267.

625. Miller E, Waight P, Farrington P, et al. Idiopathic thrombocytopenic purpura and MMR vaccine. *Arch Dis Child* 2001;84:227.

626. Stafford BT, Crosby WH. Late onset of gold-induced thrombocytopenia: with a practical note on the injections of dimercaprol. *JAMA* 1978;239:50.

627. Von dem Borne AEGK, Pegels JG, Van der Stadt RJ, et al. Thrombocytopenia associated with gold therapy: a drug-induced autoimmune disease? *Br J Haematol* 1986;63:509.

628. Coblyn JS, Weinblatt M, Holdsworth D, et al. Gold-induced thrombocytopenia: a clinical and immunogenetic study of twenty-three patients. *Ann Intern Med* 1981;95:178.

629. Goldstein R, Blanchette VS, Huebsch LB, et al. Treatment of gold-induced thrombocytopenia by high-dose intravenous gamma globulin. *Arthritis Rheum* 1986;29:426.

630. Kozloff M, Votaw M, Penner JA. Gold-induced thrombocytopenia responsive to cyclophosphamide. *South Med J* 1979;72:1490.

631. Godfrey NF, Peter A, Simon TM, et al. IV N-acetylcysteine treatment of hematologic reactions to chrysotherapy. *J Rheumatol* 1982;9:519.

632. Gottschall JL, Neahring B, McFarland JG, et al. Quinine-induced immune thrombocytopenia with hemolytic uremic syndrome: clinical and serological findings in nine patients and review of literature. *Am J Hematol* 1994;47:283.

633. Page Y, Tardy B, Zeni F, et al. Thrombotic thrombocytopenic purpura related to ticlopidine. *Lancet* 1991;337:774.

634. Bennett CL, Weinberg PD, Rozenberg-Ben-Dror K, et al. Thrombotic thrombocytopenic purpura associated with ticlopidine: a review of 60 cases. *Ann Intern Med* 1998;128:541.

635. Bennett CL, Connors JM, Carwile JM, et al. Thrombotic thrombocytopenic purpura associated with clopidogrel. *N Engl J Med* 2000;342:1773.

636. Steinhubl SR, Tan WA, Foody JM, et al., for the EPISTENT Investigators. Incidence and clinical course of thrombotic thrombocytopenic purpura due to ticlopidine following coronary stenting. *JAMA* 1999;281:806.

637. Tsai HM, Rice L, Sarode R, et al. Antibody inhibitors to von Willebrand factor metalloproteinase and increased binding of von Willebrand factor to platelets in ticlopidine-associated thrombotic thrombocytopenic purpura. *Ann Intern Med* 2000;132:794.

638. Moake JL, Byrnes JJ. Thrombotic microangiopathies associated with drugs and bone marrow transplantation. *Hematol Oncol Clin North Am* 1996;10:485.

639. McCarthy LJ, Porcu P, Fausel C, et al. Thrombotic thrombocytopenic purpura and simvastatin [Letter]. *Lancet* 1998;352:1284.

640. Van der Weerdt CM, Veenhoven-von Riesz LE, Nijenhuis LE, et al. The Zw blood group system in platelets. *Vox Sang* 1963;8:513.

641. Langenscheidt F, Kiefel V, Santoso S, et al. Platelet transfusion refractoriness associated with two rare platelet-specific alloantibodies (anti-Bak^a and anti-Pl^{A2}) and multiple HLA antibodies. *Transfusion* 1988;28:597.

642. Gabriel A, Lassnigg A, Kurz M, et al. Post-transfusion purpura due to HPA-1a immunization in a male patient: response to subsequent multiple HPA-1a-incompatible red-cell transfusions. *Transfus Med* 1995;5:131.

643. Taaning E, Morling N, Ovesen H, et al. Posttransfusion purpura and anti-Zw^b (-Pl^{A2}). *Tissue Antigens* 1985;26:143.

644. Jaegtvik S, Husebekk A, Aune B, et al. Neonatal alloimmune thrombocytopenia due to anti-HPA-1a antibodies: the level of maternal antibodies predicts the severity of thrombocytopenia in the newborn. *BJOG* 2000;107:691–694.

645. Mueller-Eckhardt C, Becker T, Weisheit M, et al. Neonatal alloimmune thrombocytopenia due to fetomaternal Zw^b incompatibility. *Vox Sang* 1986;50:94.

646. Winters JL, Jennings CD, Desai NS, et al. Neonatal alloimmune thrombocytopenia due to anti-HPA-1b (Pl^{A2}, Zw^b): a case report and review. *Vox Sang* 1998;74:256.

647. Mueller-Eckhardt C, Mueller-Eckhardt G, Willen-Ohff H, et al. Immunogenicity of and immune response to the human platelet antigen Zw^a is strongly associated with HLA-B8 and DR3. *Tissue Antigens* 1985;26:71.

648. L'Abbé D, Tremblay L, Filion M, et al. Alloimmunization to platelet antigen HPA-1a (Pl^{A1}) is strongly associated with both HLA-DR3 *0101 and HLA-DQB1*0201. *Hum Immunol* 1992;34:107.

649. De Waal LP, Van Dalen CM, Engelfriet CP, et al. Alloimmunization against the platelet-specific Zw^a antigen, resulting in neonatal thrombocytopenia or posttransfusion purpura, is associated with the supertypic DRw52 antigen including DR3 and DRw6. *Hum Immunol* 1986;17:45.

650. Kuippers RWAM, von dem Borne AEGK, Kiefel V, et al. Leucine^{33}-proline^{33} substitution in human platelet glycoprotein IIIa determine HLA-DRw52a(Dw24) association of the immune response against HPA-1a (Zw^a/Pl^{A1}) and HPA-1b (Zw^b/Pl^{A2}). *Hum Immunol* 1992;34:253.

651. Cobos E, Gandara DR, Geier LJ, et al. Post-transfusion purpura and isoimmune neonatal thrombocytopenia in the same family. *Am J Hematol* 1989;32:235.

652. Ballem PJ, Buskard NA, Decary F, et al. Post-transfusion purpura secondary to passive transfer of anti-Pl^{A1} by blood transfusion. *Br J Haematol* 1987;66:113.

653. Scott EP, Moilan-Bergeland J, Dalmasso AP. Posttransfusion thrombocytopenia associated with passive transfusion of a platelet-specific antibody. *Transfusion* 1988;28:73.

654. Nijjar TS, Bonacosa IA, Israels LG. Severe acute thrombocytopenia following infusion of plasma containing anti Pl^{A1}. *Am J Hematol* 1987;25:219.

655. Brunner-Bolliger S, Kiefel V, Horber FF, et al. Antibody studies in a patient with acute thrombocytopenia following infusion of plasma containing anti-Pl^{A1}. *Am J Hematol* 1997;56:119.

656. Roy V, Verfaillie CM. Refractory thrombocytopenia due to anti-PLA1 antibodies following autologous peripheral stem cell transplantation: case report and review of literature. *Bone Marrow Transplant* 1996;17:115.

657. Kickler T, Kennedy SD, Braine HG. Alloimmunization to platelet-specific antigens on glycoproteins IIb-IIIa and Ib/IX in multiply transfused thrombocytopenic patients. *Transfusion* 1990;30:622.

658. Marcelli-Barge A, Poirier JC, Dausset J. Allo-antigens and alloantibodies of the Ko system, serological and genetic study. *Vox Sang* 1973;24:1.

659. Kuijpers RWAM, Ouwehand WH, Bleeker PMM, et al. Localisation of the platelet-specific HPA-2 (Ko) alloantigens on the N-terminal globular fragment of platelet glycoprotein Ib alpha. *Blood* 1992;79:283.

660. Kuijpers RWAM, van den Anker JN, Baerts W, et al. A case of severe neonatal thrombocytopenia with schizencephaly associated with anti-HPA-1b and anti-HPA-2a. *Br J Haematol* 1994;87:576.

661. Bizzaro N, Dianese G. Neonatal alloimmune amegakaryocytosis: case report. *Vox Sang* 1988;54:112.

662. Kroll H, Muntean W, Kiefel V, et al. Anti Ko^a as a cause of neonatal alloimmune thrombocytopenia. *Beitr Infusionsther Transfusionsmed* 1994;32:244.

663. Saji H, Maruya E, Fujii H, et al. New platelet antigen, Sib^a, involved in platelet transfusion refractoriness in a Japanese man. *Vox Sang* 1989;56:283.

664. Tazzari PL, Ricci F, Tassi C, et al. Alloimmunization against human platelet antigen 2 (HPA2) in a series of multitransfused beta-thalassemia patients. *Haematologica* 1998;83:765.

665. Von dem Borne AEGK, Von Riesz E, Verheugt FWA, et al. Bak^a, a new platelet-specific antigen involved in neonatal allo-immune thrombocytopenia. *Vox Sang* 1980;39:113.

666. McGrath K, Minchinton R, Cunningham I, et al. Platelet anti-Bak^b antibody associated with neonatal alloimmune thrombocytopenia. *Vox Sang* 1989;57:182.

667. Boehlen F, Kaplan C, de Moerloose P. Severe neonatal alloimmune thrombocytopenia due to anti-HPA-3a. *Vox Sang* 1998;74:201.

668. Glade-Bender J, McFarland JG, Kaplan C, et al. Anti-HPA3A induces severe neonatal alloimmune thrombocytopenia. *J Pediatr* 2001;138:862.

669. Kiemowitz RM, Collins J, Davis K, et al. Post-transfusion purpura associated with alloimmunization against the platelet-specific antigen, Bak^a. *Am J Hematol* 1986;21:79.

670. Von dem Borne AEGK, Van der Plas-van Dalen CM. Bak^a and Lek^a are identical antigens [Letter]. *Br J Haematol* 1986;62:404.

671. Kickler TS, Herman JH, Furihata K, et al. Identification of Bak^b, a new platelet-specific antigen associated with posttransfusion purpura. *Blood* 1988;71:894.

672. Kiefel V, Santoso S, Glockner WM, et al. Posttransfusion purpura associated with an anti-Bak^b. *Vox Sang* 1989;56:93.

673. Lyman S, Aster RH, Visentin GP, et al. Polymorphism of human platelet membrane glycoprotein IIb associated with the Bak^a/Bak^b alloantigen system. *Blood* 1990;75:2343.

674. Take H, Tomiyama Y, Shibata Y, et al. Demonstration of the heterogeneity of epitopes of the platelet-specific alloantigen, Bak^a. *Br J Haematol* 1990;76:395.

675. Goldberger A, Kolodziej M, Poncz M, et al. Effect of single amino acid substitutions on the formation of the Pl^A and Bak alloantigenic epitopes. *Blood* 1991;78:681.

676. Friedman JM, Aster RH. Neonatal alloimmune thrombocytopenic purpura and congenital porencephaly in two siblings associated with a "new" maternal antiplatelet antibody. *Blood* 1985;65:1412.

677. Shibata Y, Matsuda I, Miyaji T, et al. Yuk^a, a new platelet antigen involved in two cases of neonatal alloimmune thrombocytopenia. *Vox Sang* 1986;50:177.

678. Matsui K, Ohsaki E, Goto A, et al. Perinatal intracranial hemorrhage due to severe neonatal alloimmune thrombocytopenic purpura (NAITP) associated with anti-Yuk^b (HPA-4a) antibodies. *Brain Dev* 1995;17:352.

679. Morel-Kopp MC, Blanchard B, Kiefel V, et al. Anti-HPA-4b (anti-Yuk^a) neonatal alloimmune thrombocytopenia: first report in a Caucasian family. *Transfus Med* 1992;2:273.

680. Puig J, Muniz-Diaz E, Monteagudo E, et al. A second case of neonatal alloimmune thrombocytopenia by anti-HPA-4b (anti-Yuk^a) in a Caucasian family. *Transfus Med* 1993;3:164.

681. Shibata Y, Miyaji T, Ichikawa Y, et al. A new platelet antigen system, Yuk^a/Yuk^b. *Vox Sang* 1986;51:334.

682. Simon TL, Collins J, Kunicki TJ, et al. Posttransfusion purpura associated with alloantibody specific for the platelet antigen, Pen^a. *Am J Hematol* 1988;29:38.

683. Santoso S, Shibata Y, Kiefel V, et al. Identification of the Yuk[b] allo-antigen on platelet glycoprotein IIIa. Vox Sang 1987;53:48.

684. Furihata K, Nugent DJ, Bissonette A, et al. On the association of the platelet-specific alloantigen, Pen[a], with glycoprotein IIIa: evidence for heterogeneity of glycoprotein IIIa. J Clin Invest 1987;80:1624.

685. Wang R, Furihata K, McFarland JG, et al. An amino acid polymorphism within the RGD binding domain of platelet membrane glycoprotein IIIa is responsible for the formation of the Pen[a]/Pen[b] alloantigen system. J Clin Invest 1992;90:2038.

686. Kiefel V, Santoso S, Katzmann B, et al. A new platelet-specific alloantigen Br[a]: report of 4 cases with neonatal alloimmune thrombocytopenia. Vox Sang 1988;54:101.

687. Santoso S, Kiefel V, Mueller-Eckhardt C. Immunochemical characterization of the new platelet alloantigen system Br[a]/Br[b]. Br J Haematol 1989;72:191.

688. Smith JW, Kelton JG, Horsewood P, et al. Platelet specific alloantigens on the platelet glycoprotein Ia/IIa complex. Br J Haematol 1989;72:534.

689. Woods VL Jr, Pischel KD, Avery ED, et al. Antigenic polymorphism of human very late activation protein-2 (platelet glycoprotein Ia-IIa): platelet alloantigen Hc[a]. J Clin Invest 1989;83:978.

690. Santoso S, Kalb R, Walka M, et al. The human platelet alloantigens Br[a] and Br[b] are associated with a single amino acid polymorphism on glycoprotein Ia (integrin subunit 211 2). J Clin Invest 1993;92:2427.

691. Covas DT, Bíscaro TA, Nasciutti DC, et al. Gene frequencies of the HPA-3 and HPA-5 platelet antigen alleles among the Amerindians. Eur J Haematol 2000;65:128.

692. Mueller-Eckhardt C, Kiefel V, Kroll H, et al. HLA-DRw6, a new immune response marker for immunization against the platelet alloantigen Br[a]. Vox Sang 1989;57:90.

693. Semana G, Zazoun T, Alizadeh M, et al. Genetic susceptibility and anti-human platelet antigen 5b alloimmunization: role of HLA Class II and TAP genes. Hum Immunol 1996;46:114.

694. Bettaieb A, Fromont P, Rodet M, et al. Br[b], a platelet alloantigen involved in neonatal alloimmune thrombocytopenia. Vox Sang 1991;60:230.

695. Kurz M, Stöckelle E, Eichelberger B, et al. IgG titer, subclass, and light-chain phenotype of pregnancy-induced HPA-5b antibodies that cause or do not cause neonatal alloimmune thrombocytopenia. Transfusion 1999;39:379.

696. Ohto H, Yamaguchi T, Takeuchi C, et al. Anti-HPA-5b-induced neonatal alloimmune thrombocytopenia: antibody titre as a predictor. Br J Haematol 2000;110:223.

697. Christie DJ, Pulkrabek S, Putnam JL, et al. Posttransfusion purpura due to an alloantibody reactive with glycoprotein Ia/IIa (anti-HPA-5b). Blood 1991;77:2785.

698. Anolik JH, Blumberg N, Snider J, et al. Posttransfusion purpura secondary to an alloantibody reactive with HPA-5a (Br[b]). Transfusion 2001;41:633.

699. Warkentin TE, Smith JW, Hayward CPM, et al. Thrombocytopenia caused by passive transfusion of anti-glycoprotein Ia/IIa alloantibody (anti-HPA-5b). Blood 1992;79:2480.

700. Kekomäki R, Jouhikainen T, Ollikainen J, et al. A new platelet alloantigen, Tu[a], on glycoprotein IIIa associated with neonatal alloimmune thrombocytopenia in two families. Br J Haematol 1993;83:306.

701. McFarland JG, Blanchette V, Collins J, et al. Neonatal alloimmune thrombocytopenia due to a new platelet-specific alloantibody. Blood 1993;81:3318.

702. Wang R, McFarland JG, Kekomäki R, et al. Amino acid 489 is a mutational "hot spot" on the β3 integrin chain: the CA/Tu human platelet alloantigen system. Blood 1993;82:3386.

703. Westman P, Hashemi-Tavoularis S, Blanchette V, et al. Maternal DRB1*1501, DQA1*0102, DQB1*0602 haplotype in fetomaternal alloimmunization against human platelet alloantigen HPA-6b (GPIIIa-Gln489). Tissue Antigens 1997;50:113.

704. Tanaka S, Taniue A, Nagao N, et al. Genotype frequencies of the human platelet antigen, Ca/Tu, in Japanese, determined by a PCR-RFLP method. Vox Sang 1996;70:40.

705. Kuijpers RWAM, Simsek S, Faber NM, et al. Single point mutation in human glycoprotein IIIa is associated with a new platelet-specific alloantigen (Mo) involved in neonatal alloimmune thrombocytopenia. Blood 1993;81:70.

706. Kroll H, Kiefel V, Santoso S, et al. Sr[a], a private platelet antigen on glycoprotein IIIa associated with neonatal alloimmune thrombocytopenia. Blood 1990;76:2296.

707. Santoso S, Kalb R, Kroll H, et al. A point mutation leads to an unpaired cysteine residue and a molecular weight polymorphism of a functional platelet β3 integrin subunit: the Sr[a] alloantigen system of GPIIIa. J Biol Chem 1994;269:8439.

708. Noris P, Simsek S, de Bruijne-Admiraal LG, et al. Maxa, a new low-frequency platelet-specific antigen localized on glycoprotein IIb, is associated with neonatal alloimmune thrombocytopenia. Blood 1995;86:1019.

709. Peyruchaud O, Bourre F, Morel-Kopp MC, et al. HPA-10w[b] (La[a]): genetic determination of a new platelet-specific alloantigen on glycoprotein IIIa and its expression in COS-7 cells. Blood 1997;89:2422.

710. Simsek S, Goldschmeding R, Kuijpers RWAM, et al. A new private platelet alloantigen, Gro[a], localized on GP IIIa involved in neonatal alloimmune thrombocytopenia. Vox Sang 1994;67:302.

711. Simsek S, Folman C, van der Schoot CE, et al. The Arg633His substitution responsible for the private platelet antigen Gro[a] unravelled by SSCP analysis and direct sequencing. Br J Haematol 1997;97:330.

712. Kiefel V, Vicariot M, Giovangrandi Y, et al. Alloimmunization against Iy, a low-frequency antigen on platelet glycoprotein Ib/IX as a cause of severe neonatal alloimmune thrombocytopenic purpura. Vox Sang 1995;69:250.

713. Sachs UJ, Kiefel V, Böhringer M, et al. Single amino acid substitution in human platelet glycoprotein Ibbeta is responsible for the formation of the platelet-specific alloantigen Iy[a]. Blood 2000;95:1849.

714. Santoso S, Amrhein J, Hofmann HA, et al. A point mutation Thr$_{799}$Met on the alpha(2) integrin leads to the formation of a new human platelet alloantigen Sit[a] and affects collagen-induced aggregation. Blood 1999;94:4103.

715. Kelton JG, Smith JW, Horsewood P, et al. The Gov[a/b] alloantigen system on human platelets. Blood 1990;75:2172.

716. Smith JW, Hayward CPM, Horsewood P, et al. Characterization and localization of the Gov[a/b] alloantigens to the glycosylphosphatidylinositol-anchored protein CDw109 on human platelets. Blood 1995;86:2807.

717. Bordin JO, Kelton JG, Warner MN, et al. Maternal immunization to Gov system alloantigens on human platelets. Transfusion 1997;37:823.

718. Berry JE, Murphy CM, Smith GA, et al. Detection of Gov system antibodies by MAIPA reveals an immunogenicity similar to the HPA-5 alloantigens. Br J Haematol 2000;110:735.

719. Kekomäki R, Raivio P, Kero P. A new low-frequency platelet alloantigen, Va[a], on glycoprotein IIb/IIIa associated with neonatal alloimmune thrombocytopenia. Transfus Med 1992;2:27.

720. Kroll H, Santoso S, Böhringer M, et al. Neonatal alloimmune thrombocytopenia caused by immunization against Oe[a], a new low frequency alloantigen on platelet glycoprotein IIIa. Blood 1995;86[Suppl 1]:540a(abst).

721. Smith JW, Horsewood P, McCusker PJ, et al. Severe neonatal alloimmune thrombocytopenia due to a novel low-frequency alloantigen, Dy[a]. Blood 1998;90[Suppl 1]:180a(abst).

722. Ikeda H, Mitani T, Ohnuma M, et al. A new platelet-specific antigen Nak[a] involved in the refractoriness of HLA-matched platelet transfusion. Vox Sang 1989;57:212.

723. Tomiyama Y, Take H, Ikeda H, et al. Identification of the platelet-specific alloantigen, Nak[a], on platelet membrane glycoprotein IV. Blood 1990;75:684.

724. Yamamoto N, Ikeda H, Tandon NN, et al. A platelet membrane glycoprotein (GP) deficiency in healthy blood donors: Nak[a-] platelets lack detectable GPIV (CD36). Blood 1990;76:1698.

725. Bierling P, Godeau B, Fromont P, et al. Posttransfusion purpura-like syndrome associated with CD36 (Naka) isoimmunization. Transfusion 1995;35:777.

726. Kankirawatana S, Kupatawintu P, Juji T, et al. Neonatal alloimmune thrombocytopenia due to anti-Nak[a]. Transfusion 2001;41:375.

727. Von dem Borne AEG, Décary F, and the ICSH/ISBT Expert Panel on Serology Working Party on Platelet Serology. Nomenclature of platelet specific antigens. Br J Haematol 1990;74:239.

728. Newman PJ. Nomenclature of human platelet alloantigens: a problem with the HPA system? Blood 1994;83:1447.

729. Warkentin TE, Smith JW. The alloimmune thrombocytopenic syndromes. Transfus Med Rev 1997;11:296.

730. Santoso S, Kiefel V. Human platelet-specific alloantigens: update. Vox Sang 1998;74[Suppl 2]:249.

731. Kroll H, Kiefel V, Santoso S. Clinical aspects and typing of platelet alloantigens. Vox Sang 1998;74[Suppl 2]:345.

732. Lucas GF, Metcalfe P. Platelet and granulocyte glycoprotein polymorphisms. Transfus Med 2000;10:157.

733. Blanchette VS, Chen L, Salomon de Friedber Z, et al. Alloimmunization to the PI[A1] platelet antigen: results of a prospective study. Br J Haematol 1990;74:209.

734. Dreyfus M, Kaplan C, Verdy E, et al. Frequency of immune thrombocytopenia in newborns: a prospective study. Blood 1997;89:4402.

735. Williamson LM, Hackett G, Rennie J, et al. The natural history of feto-maternal alloimmunisation to the platelet-specific antigen HPA-1a (PI[A1], Zw[a]) as determined by antenatal screening. Blood 1998;92:2280–2287.

736. Sainio S, Järvenpää AL, Renlund M, et al. Thrombocytopenia in term infants: a population-based study. Obstet Gynecol 2000;95:441.

737. Mueller-Eckhardt C, Kiefel V, Grubert A, et al. 348 cases of suspected neonatal alloimmune thrombocytopenia. Lancet 1989;1:363.

738. Bussel JB, Zabusky MR, Berkowitz RL, et al. Fetal alloimmune thrombocytopenia. N Engl J Med 1997;337:22.

739. Ouwehand WH, Smith G, Ranasinghe E. Management of severe alloimmune thrombocytopenia in the newborn. Arch Dis Child Fetal Neonatal Ed 2000;82:F173.

740. Bussel JB, Berkowitz RL, Lynch L, et al. Antenatal management of alloimmune thrombocytopenia with intravenous γ-globulin: a randomized trial of the addition of low-dose steroid to intravenous γ-globulin. Am J Obstet Gynecol 1996;174:1414.

741. Kroll H, Kiefel V, Giers G, et al. Maternal intravenous immunoglobulin treatment does not prevent intracranial haemorrhage in fetal alloimmune thrombocytopenia. Transfus Med 1994;4:293–296.

742. Sainio S, Teramo K, Kekomäki R. Prenatal treatment of severe fetomaternal alloimmune thrombocytopenia. Transfus Med 1999;9:321–330.

743. Murphy MF, Pullon HWH, Metcalfe P, et al. Management of fetal alloimmune thrombocytopenia by weekly in utero platelet transfusions. Vox Sang 1990;58:45.

744. Murphy MF, Waters AH, Doughty HA, et al. Antenatal management of fetomaternal alloimmune thrombocytopenia—report of 15 affected pregnancies. Transfus Med 1994;4:281–292.

745. Kelton JG, Blanchette VS, Wilson WE, et al. Neonatal thrombocytopenia due to passive immunization: prenatal diagnosis and distinction between maternal platelet alloantibodies and autoantibodies. N Engl J Med 1980;302:1401.

746. Blanchette VS, Johnson J, Rand M. The management of alloimmune neonatal thrombocytopenia. *Baillieres Clin Haematol* 2000;13:365.
747. Shulman NR, Aster RH, Leitner A, et al. Immunoreactions involving platelets. V. Post-transfusion purpura due to a complement-fixing antibody against a genetically controlled platelet antigen: a proposed mechanism for thrombocytopenia and its relevance in "autoimmunity." *J Clin Invest* 1961;40:1597.
748. Kunicki TJ, Beardsley DS. The alloimmune thrombocytopenias: neonatal alloimmune thrombocytopenic purpura and post-transfusion purpura. *Prog Hematol* 1989;9:203.
749. Kickler TS, Ness PM, Herman JH, et al. Studies on the pathophysiology of posttransfusion purpura. *Blood* 1986;68:347.
750. Mueller-Eckhardt C. Post-transfusion purpura. *Br J Haematol* 1986;64:419.
751. Taaning E, Tønnesen F. Pan-reactive platelet antibodies in post-transfusion purpura. *Vox Sang* 1999;76:120.
752. Chapman JF, Murphy MF, Berney SI, et al. Post-transfusion purpura associated with anti-Bak[a] and anti-Pl[A2] platelet antibodies and delayed haemolytic transfusion reaction. *Vox Sang* 1987;52:313.
753. Cimo PL, Aster RH. Post-transfusion purpura: successful treatment by exchange transfusion. *N Engl J Med* 1972;287:290.
754. Lillicrap DP, Ford PM, Giles AR. Prolonged thrombocytopenia in posttransfusion purpura (PTP) associated with changes in the crossed immunoelectrophoretic pattern of von Willebrand factor (vWF), circulating immune complexes and endothelial cell cytotoxicity. *Br J Haematol* 1986;62:37.
755. Chong BH, Cade J, Smith JA, et al. An unusual case of posttransfusion purpura: good transient response to high-dose immunoglobulin. *Vox Sang* 1986; 51:182.
756. Mueller-Eckhardt C, Kuenzlen E, Thilo-Korner D, et al. High-dose intravenous immunoglobulin for post-transfusion purpura [Letter]. *N Engl J Med* 1983;308:287.
757. Mueller-Eckhardt C, Kiefel V. High-dose IgG for post-transfusion purpura: revisited. *Blut* 1988;57:163.
758. Cunningham CC, Lind SE. Apparent response of refractory posttransfusion purpura to splenectomy. *Am J Hematol* 1989;30:112.
759. Walker WS, Yap PL, Kilpatrick DC, et al. Post-transfusion purpura following open heart surgery: management by high dose intravenous immunoglobulin infusion. *Blut* 1988;57:323.
760. Lippman SM, Lizak GE, Foung SKH, et al. The efficacy of Pl[A1]-negative platelet transfusion therapy in posttransfusion purpura. *West J Med* 1988;148:86.
761. Win N, Peterkin MA, Watson WH. The therapeutic value of HPA-1a-negative platelet transfusion in post-transfusion purpura complicated by life-threatening haemorrhage. *Vox Sang* 1995;69:138.
762. Win N, Matthey F, Slater GP. Blood components–transfusion support in post-transfusion purpura due to HPA-1a immunization. *Vox Sang* 1996;71:191.
763. Gabriel A, LaBnigg A, Kurz M, et al. Post-transfusion purpura due to HPA-1a immunization in a male patient: response to subsequent multiple HPA-1a-incompatible red-cell transfusions. *Transfus Med* 1995;5:131.
764. Lau P, Sholtis CM, Aster RH. Post-transfusion purpura: an enigma of alloimmunization. *Am J Hematol* 1980;9:331.
765. Novotny VMJ, van Doorn R, Witvliet MD, et al. Occurrence of allogeneic HLA and non-HLA antibodies after transfusion of prestorage filtered platelets and red cells: a prospective study. *Blood* 1995;85:1736–1741.
766. Kekomäki S, Volin L, Koistinen P, et al. Successful treatment of platelet transfusion refractoriness: the use of platelet transfusions matched for both human leucocyte antigens (HLA) and human platelet alloantigens (HPA) in alloimmunized patients with leukaemia. *Eur J Haematol* 1998;60:112.
767. Warkentin TE. Diagnosis and treatment of disseminated intravascular coagulation. In: Ginsberg JS, Kearon C, Hirsh J, eds. *Critical decisions in thrombosis and hemostasis*. Hamilton: BC Decker, 1998:322–329.
768. Levi M, ten Cate H. Disseminated intravascular coagulation. *N Engl J Med* 1999;341:586.
769. De Jong E, Levi M, Stoutenbeek CP, et al. Current drug treatment strategies for disseminated intravascular coagulation. *Drugs* 1998;55:767.
770. Bick RL, Arun B, Frenkel EP. Disseminated intravascular coagulation: clinical and pathophysiological mechanisms and manifestations. *Haemostasis* 1999;29:111.
771. Jamieson GA. The activation of platelets by thrombin: a model for activation by high and moderate affinity receptor pathways. *Prog Clin Biol Res* 1988; 283:137.
772. Sims PJ, Wiedmer T, Esmon CT, et al. Assembly of the platelet prothrombinase complex is linked to vesiculation of the platelet plasma membrane: studies in Scott syndrome—an isolated defect in platelet procoagulant activity. *J Biol Chem* 1989;264:17049.
773. Goldenfarb PB, Zucker S, Corrigan JJ Jr, et al. The coagulation mechanism in acute bacterial infection. *Br J Haematol* 1970;18:643.
774. Svanbom M. A prospective study on septicemia, II. Clinical manifestations and complications, results of antimicrobial treatment and a report of a follow-up study. *Scand J Infect Dis* 1980;12:189.
775. Corrigan JJ Jr. Thrombocytopenia: a laboratory sign of septicemia in infants and children. *J Pediatr* 1974;85:219.
776. Kelton JG, Neame PB, Gauldie J, et al. Elevated platelet-associated IgG in the thrombocytopenia of septicemia. *N Engl J Med* 1979;300:760.
777. Neame PB, Kelton JG, Walker IR, et al. Thrombocytopenia in septicemia: the role of disseminated intravascular coagulation. *Blood* 1980;56:88.
778. Kreger BE, Craven DE, McCabe WR. Gram-negative bacteremia, IV. Re-evaluation of clinical features and treatment in 612 patients. *Am J Med* 1980; 68:344.
779. Corrigan JJ Jr, Jordan CM. Heparin therapy in septicemia with disseminated intravascular coagulation: effect on mortality and on correction of hemostatic defects. *N Engl J Med* 1970;283:778.
780. Milligan GF, MacDonald JAE, Mellon A, et al. Pulmonary and hematologic disturbances during septic shock. *Surg Gynecol Obstet* 1974;138:43.
781. Oppenheimer L, Hryniuk WM, Bishop AJ. Thrombocytopenia in severe bacterial infections. *J Surg Res* 1976;20:211.
782. Varon J, Chen K, Sternbach GL. Rupert Waterhouse and Carl Friderichsen: adrenal apoplexy. *J Emerg Med* 1998;16:643.
783. Knight TT Jr, Gordon SV, Canady J, et al. Symmetrical peripheral gangrene: a new presentation of an old disease. *Am Surg* 2000;66:196.
784. Fijnvandraat K, Derkx B, Peters M, et al. Coagulation activation and tissue necrosis in meningococcal septic shock: severely reduced protein C levels predict a high mortality. *Thromb Haemost* 1995;73:15.
785. Inbal A, Kenet G, Zivelin A, et al. Purpura fulminans induced by disseminated intravascular coagulation following infection in 2 unrelated children with double heterozygosity for factor V Leiden and protein S deficiency. *Thromb Haemost* 1997;77:1086.
786. Kondaveeti S, Hibberd ML, Booy R, et al. Effect of the factor V Leiden mutation on the severity of meningococcal disease. *Pediatr Infect Dis J* 1999;18:893.
787. MacIntyre DE, Allen AP, Thorne KJI, et al. Endotoxin-induced platelet aggregation and secretion, I. Morphological changes and pharmacological effects. *J Cell Sci* 1977;28:211.
788. Salat A, Murabito M, Boehm D, et al. Endotoxin enhances in vitro platelet aggregability in whole blood. *Thromb Res* 1999;93:145.
789. Arvand M, Bhakdi S, Dahlbäck B, et al. Staphylococcus aureus alpha-toxin attack on human platelets promotes assembly of the prothrombinase complex. *J Biol Chem* 1990;265:14377.
790. Bryant AE, Chen RY, Nagata Y, et al. Clostridial gas gangrene, II. Phospholipase C-induced activation of gpIIb/IIIa mediates vascular occlusion and myonecrosis in Clostridium perfringens gas gangrene. *J Infect Dis* 2000; 182:808.
791. Karpman D, Papadopoulou D, Nilsson K, et al. Platelet activation by Shiga toxin and circulatory factors as a pathogenetic mechanism in the hemolytic uremic syndrome. *Blood* 2001;97:3100.
792. Lopez Diez F, Nieto ML, Fernandez-Gallardo S, et al. Occupancy of platelet receptors for platelet-activating factor in patients with septicemia. *J Clin Invest* 1989;83:1733.
793. Ono S, Mochizuki H, Tamakuma S. A clinical study on the significance of platelet-activating factor in the pathophysiology of septic disseminated intravascular coagulation in surgery. *Am J Surg* 1996;171:409.
794. Esmon CT. Possible involvement of cytokines in diffuse intravascular coagulation and thrombosis. *Baillieres Clin Haematol* 1999;12:343.
795. Helmick CG, Bernard KW, D'Angelo LJ. Rocky Mountain spotted fever: clinical, laboratory, and epidemiological features of 262 cases. *J Infect Dis* 1984;150:480.
796. Courtney MA, Haidaris PJ, Marder VJ, et al. Tissue factor mRNA expression in the endothelium of an intact umbilical vein. *Blood* 1996;87:174.
797. Wright JF, Blanchette VS, Wang H, et al. Characterization of platelet-reactive antibodies in children with varicella-associated acute immune thrombocytopenic purpura (ITP). *Br J Haematol* 1995;95:145.
798. Ben-Yehuda D, Gillis S, Eldor A. Clinical and therapeutic experience in 712 Israeli patients with idiopathic thrombocytopenic purpura. Israeli ITP Study Group. *Acta Haematol* 1994;91:1.
799. Carter RL. Platelet levels in infectious mononucleosis. *Blood* 1965;25:817.
800. Yoto Y, Kudoh T, Suzuki N, et al. Thrombocytopenia induced by human parvovirus B19 infections. *Eur J Haematol* 1993;50:255.
801. Nolte KB, Feddersen RM, Foucar K, et al. Hantavirus pulmonary syndrome in the United States: a pathological description of a disease caused by a new agent. *Hum Pathol* 1995;26:110.
802. Peck-Radosavljevic M, Wichlas M, Pidlich J, et al. Blunted thrombopoietin response to interferon alpha-induced thrombocytopenia during treatment for hepatitis C. *Hepatology* 1998;28:1430.
803. Jiménez-Sáenz M, Rojas M, Piñar A, et al. Sustained response to combination therapy in a patient with chronic hepatitis C and thrombocytopenia secondary to α-interferon. *J Gastroenterol Hepatol* 2000;15:561.
804. Risdall RJ, McKenna RW, Nesbit ME, et al. Virus-associated hemophagocytic syndrome: a benign histiocytic proliferation distinct from malignant histiocytosis. *Cancer* 1979;44:993.
805. Watson HG, Goulden NJ, Manson LM, et al. Virus-associated haemophagocytic syndrome: further evidence for a T-cell mediated disorder. *Br J Haematol* 1994;86:213.
806. Kikuta H, Sakiyama Y, Matsumoto S, et al. Fatal Epstein-Barr virus-associated hemophagocytic syndrome. *Blood* 1993;82:3259.
807. Chen RL, Lin KH, Lin DT, et al. Immunomodulation treatment for childhood virus-associated haemophagocytic lymphohistiocytosis. *Br J Haematol* 1995; 89:282.
808. De Kerguenec C, Hillarie S, Molinie V, et al. Hepatic manifestations of hemophagocytic syndrome: a study of 30 cases. *Am J Gastroenterol* 2001;96:852.
809. Aricò M, Danesino C, Pende D, et al. Pathogenesis of haemophagocytic lymphohistiocytosis. *Br J Haematol* 2001;114:761.
810. Hill GJ II, Knight V, Jeffery GM. Thrombocytopenia in vivax malaria. *Lancet* 1964;1:240.
811. Beale PJ, Cormack JD, Oldrey TBN. Thrombocytopenia in malaria with immunoglobulin (IgM) changes. *BMJ* 1972;1:345.
812. Skudowitz RB, Katz J, Lurie A, et al. Mechanisms of thrombocytopenia in malignant tertial malaria. *BMJ* 1973;2:515.

813. Horstmann RD, Dietrich M, Bienzle U, et al. Malaria-induced thrombocytopenia. *Blut* 1981;42:157.
814. Grau GE, Piguet PF, Greterner D, et al. Immunopathology of thrombocytopenia in experimental malaria. *Immunology* 1988;65:501.
815. Lee SH, Looareesuwan S, Chan J, et al. Plasma macrophage colony-stimulating factor and P-selectin levels in malaria-associated thrombocytopenia. *Thromb Haemost* 1997;77:289.
816. Bernard GR, Vincent JL, Laterre PF, et al. Efficacy and safety of recombinant human activated protein C for severe sepsis. *N Engl J Med* 2001;344:699.
817. Fourrier F, Chopin C, Huart JJ, et al. Double-blind, placebo-controlled trial of antithrombin III concentrates in septic shock with disseminated intravascular coagulation. *Chest* 1993;104:882.
818. Rock GA. Management of thrombotic thrombocytopenic purpura. *Br J Haematol* 2000;109:496.
819. George JN. How I treat patients with thrombotic thrombocytopenic purpura–hemolytic uremic syndrome. *Blood* 2000;96:1223.
820. Trevathan E, Dooling EC. Large thrombotic strokes in hemolytic-uremic syndrome. *J Pediatr* 1987;111:863.
821. Hahn JS, Havens PL, Higgins JJ, et al. Neurological complications of hemolytic-uremic syndrome. *J Child Neurol* 1989;4:108.
822. Wasserstein A, Hill G, Goldfarb S, et al. Recurrent thrombotic thrombocytopenic purpura after viral infection: clinical and histologic simulation of chronic glomerulonephritis. *Arch Intern Med* 1981;141:685.
823. Kok RH, Wolfhagen MJ, Klosters G. A syndrome resembling thrombotic thrombocytopenic purpura associated with human parvovirus B19 infection. *Clin Infect Dis* 2001;32:311.
824. Rarick MU, Espina B, Mocharnuk R, et al. Thrombotic thrombocytopenic purpura in patients with human immunodeficiency virus infection: a report of three cases and review of the literature. *Am J Hematol* 1992;40:103.
825. Sutor GC, Schmidt RE, Albrecht H. Thrombotic microangiopathies and HIV infection: report of two typical cases, features of HUS and TTP, and review of the literature. *Infection* 1999;27:12.
826. Ucar A, Fernandez HF, Byrnes JJ, et al. Thrombotic microangiopathy and retroviral infections: a 13-year experience. *Am J Hematol* 1994;45:304.
827. Bar Meir E, Amital H, Levy Y, et al. Mycoplasma pneumoniae-induced thrombotic thrombocytopenic purpura. *Acta Haematol* 2000;103:112.
828. Jaeschke R, Irvine EJ, Moore J, et al. Campylobacter jejuni and thrombotic thrombocytopenic purpura. *Can J Gastroenterol* 1990;4:154.
829. Kovacs MJ, Roddy J, Grégoire S, et al. Thrombotic thrombocytopenic purpura following hemorrhagic colitis due to Escherichia coli O157:H7. *Am J Med* 1990;88:177.
830. Tarantolo SR, Landmark JD, Iwen PC, et al. Bartonella-like erythrocyte inclusions in thrombotic thrombocytopenic purpura. *Lancet* 1997;350:1602.
831. Modi KS, Dahl DC, Berkseth RO, et al. Human granulocytic ehrlichiosis presenting with acute renal failure and mimicking thrombotic thrombocytopenic purpura: a case report and review. *Am J Nephrol* 1999;19:677.
832. Dashe JS, Ramin SM, Cunningham FG. The long-term consequences of thrombotic microangiopathy (thrombotic thrombocytopenic purpura and hemolytic uremic syndrome) in pregnancy. *Obstet Gynecol* 1998;91:662.
833. Au WY, Lie AKW, Lam CCK, et al. Tacrolimus (FK 506)-induced thrombotic thrombocytopenic purpura after ABO mismatched second liver transplantation: salvage with plasmapheresis and prostacyclin. *Haematologica* 2000;85:659.
834. Kwaan HC. Miscellaneous secondary thrombotic microangiopathy. *Semin Hematol* 1987;24:141.
835. Musio F, Bohen EM, Yuan CM, et al. Review of thrombotic thrombocytopenic purpura in the setting of systemic lupus erythematosus. *Semin Arthritis Rheum* 1998;28:1.
836. Brunner HI, Freedman M, Silverman ED. Close relationship between systemic lupus erythematosus and thrombotic thrombocytopenic purpura in childhood. *Arthritis Rheum* 1999;42:2346.
837. Ter Borg EJ, Houtman PM, Kallenberg CGM, et al. Thrombocytopenia and hemolytic anemia in a patient with MCTD due to thrombotic thrombocytopenic purpura. *J Rheumatol* 1988;15:1174.
838. Campbell GN, Gallo JH. Relapsing thrombotic thrombocytopenic purpura (TTP) in Sjogren's syndrome [Letter]. *Aust N Z J Med* 1998;28:214.
839. Daghistani D, Jimenez JJ, Moake JL, et al. Familial infantile thrombotic thrombocytopenic purpura. *J Pediatr Hematol Oncol* 1996;18:171.
840. Galbusera M, Noris M, Rossi C, et al. Increased fragmentation of von Willebrand factor, due to abnormal cleavage of the subunit, parallels disease activity in recurrent hemolytic uremic syndrome and thrombotic thrombocytopenic purpura and discloses predisposition in families. *Blood* 1999;94:610.
841. Karmali MA, Steele BT, Petric M, et al. Sporadic cases of haemolytic-uraemic syndrome associated with faecal cytotoxin and cytotoxin-producing *Escherichia coli* in stools. *Lancet* 1983;1:619.
842. Chart H, Smith HR, Scotland SM, et al. Serological identification of Escherichia coli O157:H7 infection in haemolytic uraemic syndrome. *Lancet* 1991;337:138.
843. Besser RE, Griffin PM, Slutsker L. *Escherichia coli* O157:H7 gastroenteritis and the hemolytic uremic syndrome: an emerging infectious disease. *Annu Rev Med* 1999;50:355.
844. Banatvala N, Griffin PM, Greene KD, et al. The United States National Prospective Hemolytic Uremic Syndrome Study: microbiologic, serologic, clinical, and epidemiologic findings. *J Infect Dis* 2001;183:1063.
845. Flores FX, Jabs K, Thorne GM, et al. Immune response to Escherichia coli O157:H7 in hemolytic uremic syndrome following salmonellosis. *Pediatr Nephrol* 1997;11:488.
846. Raghupathy P, Date A, Shastry JCM, et al. Haemolytic-uraemic syndrome complicating Shigella dysentery in South Indian children. *BMJ* 1978;1:1518.
847. Bhimma R, Coovadia HM, Adhikari M, et al. Re-evaluating criteria for peritoneal dialysis in "classical" (D+) hemolytic uremic syndrome. *Clin Nephrol* 2001;55:133.
848. Denneberg T, Friedberg M, Holmberg L, et al. Combined plasmapheresis and hemodialysis treatment for severe hemolytic-uremic syndrome following *Campylobacter* colitis. *Acta Paediatr Scand* 1982;71:243.
849. Delans RJ, Biluso JD, Saba SR, et al. Hemolytic uremic syndrome after Campylobacter-induced diarrhea in an adult. *Arch Intern Med* 1984;144:1074.
850. Chart H, Cheasty T, Cope D, et al. The serological relationship between Yersinia enterocolitica O9 and Escherichia coli O157 using sera from patients with yersiniosis and haemolytic uraemic syndrome. *Epidemiol Infect* 1991;107:349.
851. Krysan DJ, Flynn JT. Renal transplantation after Streptococcus pneumoniae associated hemolytic uremic syndrome. *Am J Kidney Dis* 2001;37:E15.
852. Gordon LI, Kwaan HC. Thrombotic microangiopathy manifesting as thrombotic thrombocytopenic purpura hemolytic uremic syndrome in the cancer patient. *Semin Thromb Hemost* 1999;25:217.
853. Zarifian A, Meleg-Smith S, O'Donovan R, et al. Cyclosporine-associated thrombotic microangiopathy in renal allografts. *Kidney Int* 1999;55:2457.
854. Leach JW, Pham T, Diamandidis D, et al. Thrombotic thrombocytopenic purpura-hemolytic uremic syndrome (TTP-HUS) following treatment with deoxycoformycin in a patient with cutaneous T cell lymphoma (Sezary syndrome): a case report. *Am J Hematol* 1999;61:268.
855. Fung MC, Storniolo AM, Nguyen B, et al. A review of hemolytic uremic syndrome in patients treated with gemcitabine therapy. *Cancer* 1999;85:2023.
856. Sarode R, McFarland JG, Flomenberg N, et al. Therapeutic plasma exchange does not appear to be effective in the management of thrombotic thrombocytopenic purpura/hemolytic uremic syndrome following bone marrow transplantation. *Bone Marrow Transplant* 1995;16:271.
857. Fuge R, Bird JM, Fraser A, et al. The clinical features, risk factors and outcome of thrombotic thrombocytopenic purpura occurring after bone marrow transplantation. *Br J Haematol* 2001;113:58.
858. Roy V, Rizvi MA, Vesely SK, et al. Thrombotic thrombocytopenic purpura-like syndromes following bone marrow transplantation: an analysis of associated conditions and clinical outcomes. *Bone Marrow Transplant* 2001;27:641.
859. Noris M, Ruggenenti P, Perna A, et al. Hypocomplementemia discloses genetic predisposition to hemolytic uremic syndrome and thrombotic thrombocytopenic purpura: role of factor H abnormalities. *J Am Soc Nephrol* 1999;10:281.
860. Ying L, Katz Y, Schlesinger M, et al. Complement factor H gene mutation associated with autosomal recessive atypical hemolytic uremic syndrome. *Am J Hum Genet* 1999;65:1538.
861. Lian EC, Harkness DR, Byrnes JJ. Presence of a platelet aggregating factor in the plasma of patients with thrombotic thrombocytopenic purpura (TTP) and its inhibition by normal plasma. *Blood* 1979;53:333.
862. Siddiqui FA, Lian ECY. Novel platelet-agglutinating protein from a thrombotic thrombocytopenic purpura plasma. *J Clin Invest* 1985;76:1330.
863. Moake JL, Rudy CK, Troll JH, et al. Unusually large plasma factor VIII: von Willebrand factor multimers in chronic relapsing thrombotic thrombocytopenic purpura. *N Engl J Med* 1982;307:1432.
864. Moake JL, McPherson PD. Abnormalities of von Willebrand factor multimers in thrombotic thrombocytopenic purpura and the hemolytic-uremic syndrome. *Am J Med* 1989;87:9N–15N.
865. Kelton JG, Moore J, Santos A, et al. Detection of a platelet-agglutinating factor in thrombotic thrombocytopenic purpura. *Ann Intern Med* 1984;101:589.
866. Kelton JG, Moore JC, Murphy WG. Studies investigating platelet aggregation and release initiated by sera from patients with thrombotic thrombocytopenia purpura. *Blood* 1987;69:924.
867. Murphy WG, Moore JC, Kelton JG. Calcium-dependent cysteine protease activity in the sera of patients with thrombotic thrombocytopenic purpura. *Blood* 1987;70:1683.
868. Moore JC, Murphy WG, Kelton JG. Calpain proteolysis of von Willebrand factor enhances its binding to platelet membrane glycoprotein IIb/IIIa: an explanation for platelet aggregation in thrombotic thrombocytopenic purpura. *Br J Haematol* 1990;74:457.
869. Kelton JG, Warkentin TE, Hayward CPM, et al. The calpain activity in patients with thrombotic thrombocytopenic purpura is associated with platelet microparticles. *Blood* 1992;80:2246.
870. Falanga A, Consonni R, Ruggenenti P, et al. A cathepsin-like cysteine proteinase proaggregating activity in thrombotic thrombocytopenic purpura. *Br J Haematol* 1991;79:474.
871. Furlan M, Robles R, Solenthaler M, et al. Deficient activity of von Willebrand factor-cleaving protease in chronic relapsing thrombotic thrombocytopenic purpura. *Blood* 1997;89:3097.
872. Allford SL, Harrison P, Lawrie AS, et al. Von Willebrand factor-cleaving protease activity in congenital thrombotic thrombocytopenic purpura. *Br J Haematol* 2000;111:1215.
873. Furlan M, Robles R, Galbusera M, et al. Von Willebrand factor-cleaving protease in thrombotic thrombocytopenic purpura and the hemolytic-uremic syndrome. *N Engl J Med* 1998;339:1578.
874. Tsai HM, Lian ECY. Antibodies to von Willebrand factor-cleaving protease in acute thrombotic thrombocytopenic purpura. *N Engl J Med* 1998;339:1585.
875. Tsai HM. Physiologic cleavage of von Willebrand factor by a plasma protease is dependent on its conformation and requires calcium ion. *Blood* 1996;87:4235.

876. Levy GG, Nichols WC, Lian EC, et al. Mutations in a member of the ADAMTS gene family cause thrombotic thrombocytopenic purpura. *Nature* 2001;413:488.

877. Moore JC, Hayward CPM, Warkentin TE, et al. Decreased von Willebrand factor protease activity associated with thrombocytopenic disorders. *Blood* 2001;98:1842.

878. Mannucci PM, Canciani MT, Forza I, et al. Changes in health and disease of the metalloprotease that cleaves von Willebrand factor. *Blood* 2001;98:2730.

879. Dang CT, Magid MS, Weksler B, et al. Enhanced endothelial cell apoptosis in splenic tissues of patients with thrombotic thrombocytopenic purpura. *Blood* 1999;93:1264.

880. Jiminez JJ, Jy W, Mauro LM, et al. Elevated endothelial microparticles in thrombotic thrombocytopenic purpura: findings from brain and renal microvascular cell culture and patients with active disease. *Br J Haematol* 2001;112:81.

881. Kwaan HC. Clinicopathologic features of thrombotic thrombocytopenic purpura. *Semin Hematol* 1987;24:71.

882. Petitt RM. Thrombotic thrombocytopenic purpura: a thirty-year review. *Semin Thromb Hemost* 1980;6:350.

883. Gruber O, Wittig I, Wiggins CJ, et al. Thrombotic thrombocytopenic purpura: MRI demonstration of persistent small cerebral infarcts after clinical recovery. *Neuroradiology* 2000;42:616.

884. Asada Y, Sumiyoshi A, Hayashi T, et al. Immunohistochemistry of vascular lesion in thrombotic thrombocytopenic purpura, with special reference to factor VIII related antigen. *Thromb Res* 1985;38:469.

885. Gerritsen HE, Turecek PL, Schwarz HP, et al. Assay of von Willebrand factor (vWF)-cleaving protease based on decreased collagen binding affinity of degraded vWF. *Thromb Haemost* 1999;82:1386.

886. Amorosi EL, Ultmann JE. Thrombotic thrombocytopenic purpura: report of 16 cases and review of the literature. *Medicine (Baltimore)* 1966;45:139.

887. Rock GA, Shumak KH, Buskard NA, et al. Comparison of plasma exchange with plasma infusion in the treatment of thrombotic thrombocytopenic purpura. *N Engl J Med* 1991;325:393.

888. Hayward CPM, Sutton DMC, Carter WH Jr, et al. Treatment outcomes in patients with adult thrombotic thrombocytopenic purpura-hemolytic uremic syndrome. *Arch Intern Med* 1994;154:982.

889. Rubinstein MA, Kagan BM, MacGillviray MH, et al. Unusual remission in a case of thrombotic thrombocytopenic purpura syndrome following fresh blood exchange transfusions. *Ann Intern Med* 1959;51:1409.

890. Byrnes JJ, Khurana M. Treatment of thrombotic thrombocytopenic purpura with plasma. *N Engl J Med* 1977;297:1386.

891. Blitzer JB, Granfortuna JM, Gottlieb AJ, et al. Thrombotic thrombocytopenic purpura: treatment with plasmapheresis. *Am J Hematol* 1987;24:329.

892. Del Zoppo GJ. Antiplatelet therapy in thrombotic thrombocytopenic purpura. *Semin Hematol* 1987;24:130.

893. Bell WR, Braine HG, Ness PM, et al. Improved survival in thrombotic thrombocytopenic purpura-hemolytic uremic syndrome: clinical experience in 108 patients. *N Engl J Med* 1991;325:398.

894. Gordon LI, Kwaan HC, Rossi EC. Deleterious effects of platelet transfusions and recovery thrombocytosis in patients with thrombotic microangiopathy. *Semin Hematol* 1987;24:184.

895. Byrnes JJ, Moake JL, Klug P, et al. Effectiveness of the cryosupernatant fraction of plasma in the treatment of refractory thrombotic thrombocytopenic purpura. *Am J Hematol* 1990;34:169.

896. Molinari E, Costamagna L, Perotti C, et al. Refractory thrombotic thrombocytopenic purpura: successful treatment by plasmapheresis with plasma cryosupernatant. *Haematologica* 1993;78:389.

897. Rock G, Shumak KH, Sutton DMC, et al., and the Canadian Apheresis Group. Cryosupernatant as replacement fluid for plasma exchange in thrombotic thrombocytopenic purpura. *Br J Haematol* 1996;94:383–386.

898. Rizvi MA, Vesely SK, George JN, et al. Complications of plasma exchange in 71 consecutive patients treated for clinically suspected thrombotic thrombocytopenic purpura–hemolytic-uremic syndrome. *Transfusion* 2000;40:896.

899. Onundarson PT, Rowe JM, Heal JM, et al. Response to plasma exchange and splenectomy in thrombotic thrombocytopenic purpura: a 10-year experience at a single institution. *Arch Intern Med* 1992;152:791.

900. O'Connor NT, Bruce-Jones P, Hill LF. Vincristine therapy for thrombotic thrombocytopenic purpura. *Am J Hematol* 1992;39:234.

901. Durand JM, Lefevre P, Kaplanski G, et al. Deleterious effects of intravenous immunoglobulin in a patient with thrombotic thrombocytopenic purpura [Letter]. *Am J Hematol* 1993;44:214.

902. Crowther MA, Heddle N, Hayward CPM, et al. Splenectomy done during hematologic remission to prevent relapse in patients with thrombotic thrombocytopenic purpura. *Ann Intern Med* 1996;125:294.

903. Tarr PI, Neill MA, Allen J, et al. The increasing incidence of the hemolytic-uremic syndrome in King County, Washington: lack of evidence for ascertainment bias. *Am J Epidemiol* 1989;129:582.

904. Martin DL, MacDonald KL, White KE, et al. The epidemiology and clinical aspects of the hemolytic uremic syndrome in Minnesota. *N Engl J Med* 1990;323:1161.

905. Konowalchuk J, Speirs JI, Stavric S. Vero response to a cytotoxin of Escherichia coli. *Infect Immunol* 1977;18:775.

906. Karmali MA, Petric M, Lim C, et al. The association between idiopathic hemolytic uremic syndrome and infection by verotoxin-producing *Escherichia coli*. *J Infect Dis* 1985;151:775.

907. Calderwood SB, Auclair F, Donohue-Rolfe A, et al. Nucleotide sequence of the *Shiga*-like toxin genes of *Escherichia coli*. *Proc Natl Acad Sci U S A* 1987;84:4364.

908. Carter AO, Borczyk AA, Carlson JAK, et al. A severe outbreak of *Escherichia coli* O157:H7-associated hemorrhagic colitis in a nursing home. *N Engl J Med* 1987;317:1496.

909. Rowe PC, Orrbine E, Lior H, et al. Risk of hemolytic uremic syndrome after sporadic *Escherichia coli* O157:H7 infection: results of a Canadian collaborative study. *J Pediatr* 1998;132:777.

910. Cooling LL, Walker KE, Gille T, et al. Shiga toxin binds human platelets via globotriaosylceramide (Pk antigen) and a novel platelet glycosphingolipid. *Infect Immun* 1998;66:4355.

911. Siegler RL, Pysher TJ, Tesh VL, et al. Response to single and divided doses of Shiga toxin-1 in a primate model of hemolytic uremic syndrome. *J Am Soc Nephrol* 2001;12:1458.

912. Wong CS, Jelacic S, Habeeb RL, et al. The risk of the hemolytic-uremic syndrome after antibiotic treatment of *Escherichia coli* O157:H7 infections. *N Engl J Med* 2000;342:1930.

913. Neild G. The haemolytic uraemic syndrome: a review. *QJM* 1987;63:367.

914. Badami KG, Srivastava RN, Kumar R, et al. Disseminated intravascular coagulation in post-dysenteric haemolytic uraemic syndrome. *Acta Paediatr Scand* 1987;76:919.

915. Richardson SE, Karmali MA, Becker LE, et al. The histopathology of the hemolytic uremic syndrome associated with verocytotoxin-producing *Escherichia coli* infections. *Hum Pathol* 1988;19:1102.

916. Van Dyck M, Proesmans W, Depraetere M. Hemolytic uremic syndrome in childhood: renal function ten years later. *Clin Nephrol* 1988;29:109.

917. Trachtman H, Christen E. Pathogenesis, treatment, and therapeutic trials in hemolytic uremic syndrome. *Curr Opin Pediatr* 1999;11:162.

918. Dundas S, Murphy J, Soutar RL, et al. Effectiveness of therapeutic plasma exchange in the 1996 Lanarkshire *Escherichia coli* O157:H7 outbreak. *Lancet* 1999;354:1327.

919. Siegler RL, Pavia AT, Hansen FL, et al. Atypical hemolytic-uremic syndrome: a comparison with postdiarrheal disease. *J Pediatr* 1996;128:505.

920. Landau D, Shalev H, Levy-Finer G, et al. Familial hemolytic uremic syndrome associated with complement H deficiency. *J Pediatr* 2001;138:303.

921. Kaplan BS, Leonard MB. Autosomal dominant hemolytic uremic syndrome: variable phenotypes and transplant results. *Pediatr Nephrol* 2000;14:464.

922. Lahlou A, Lang P, Charpentier B, et al. Hemolytic uremic syndrome. Recurrence after renal transplantation. *Medicine (Baltimore)* 2000;79:90.

923. Higgins JR, de Swiet M. Blood-pressure measurement and classification in pregnancy. *Lancet* 2001;357:131.

924. Burrows RF, Hunter DJS, Andrew M, et al. A prospective study investigating the mechanism of thrombocytopenia in preeclampsia. *Obstet Gynecol* 1987;70:334.

925. Gibson B, Hunter D, Neame PB, et al. Thrombocytopenia in preeclampsia and eclampsia. *Semin Thromb Hemost* 1982;8:234.

926. Metz J, Cincotta R, Francis M, et al. Screening for consumptive coagulopathy in preeclampsia. *Int J Gynaecol Obstet* 1994;46:3.

927. Cincotta R, Ross A. A review of eclampsia in Melbourne: 1978–1992. *Aust N Z J Obstet Gynaecol* 1996;36:264.

928. Weinstein L. Syndrome of hemolysis, elevated liver enzymes, and low platelet count: a severe consequence of hypertension in pregnancy. *Am J Obstet Gynecol* 1982;142:159.

929. Murray D, O'Riordan M, Geary M, et al. The HELLP syndrome: maternal and perinatal outcome. *Ir Med J* 2001;94:16.

930. Vigil-de Gracia P. Pregnancy complicated by pre-eclampsia–eclampsia with HELLP syndrome. *Int J Gynaecol Obstet* 2001;72:17.

931. Stubbs TM, Lazarchick J, Van Dorsten JP, et al. Evidence of accelerated platelet production and consumption in nonthrombocytopenic pre-eclampsia. *Am J Obstet Gynecol* 1986;155:263.

932. Kelton JG, Hunter DJS, Neame PB. A platelet function defect in pre-eclampsia. *Obstet Gynecol* 1985;65:107.

933. Ramanathan J, Sibai BM, Vu T, et al. Correlation between bleeding times and platelet counts in women with preeclampsia undergoing cesarian section. *Anesthesiology* 1989;71:188.

934. Granger JP, Alexander BT, Bennett WA, et al. Pathophysiology of pregnancy-induced hypertension. *Am J Hypertens* 2001;14:178S.

935. Kobayashi T, Terao T. Preeclampsia as chronic disseminated intravascular coagulation: study of two parameters: thrombin-antithrombin III complex and D-dimers. *Gynecol Obstet Invest* 1987;24:170.

936. Cadroy Y, Grandjean H, Pichon J, et al. Evaluation of six markers of haemostatic system in normal pregnancy and pregnancy complicated by hypertension or pre-eclampsia. *Br J Obstet Gynaecol* 1993;100:416.

937. Maki M, Kobayashi T, Terao T, et al. Antithrombin therapy for severe preeclampsia: results of a double-blind, randomized, placebo-controlled trial. *Thromb Haemost* 2000;84:583.

938. Sibai BM, Spinnato JA, Watson DL, et al. Pregnancy outcome in 303 cases with severe preeclampsia. *Obstet Gynecol* 1984;64:319.

939. Dekker G, Sibai B. Primary, secondary, and tertiary prevention of pre-eclampsia. *Lancet* 2001;357:209.

940. Mecacci F, Carignani L, Cioni R, et al. Time course of recovery and complications of HELLP syndrome with two different treatments: heparin or dexamethasone. *Thromb Res* 2001;102:99.

941. Isler CM, Barrilleaux PS, Magann EF, et al. A prospective, randomized trial comparing the efficacy of dexamethasone and betamethasone for the treatment of antepartum HELLP (hemolysis, elevated liver enzymes, and low platelet count) syndrome. *Am J Obstet Gynecol* 2001;184:1337.

942. Storck H, Hoigne R, Koller F. Thrombocytes in allergic reactions. *Int Arch Allergy Appl Immunol* 1955;6:372.

943. Caffrey EA, Sladen GE, Isaacs PET, et al. Thrombocytopenia caused by cow's milk [Letter]. *Lancet* 1981;2:316.
944. Bousquet J, Huchard G, Michel FB. Toxic reactions induced by Hymenoptera venom. *Ann Allergy* 1984;52:371.
945. Kolecki P. Delayed toxic reaction following massive bee envenomation. *Ann Emerg Med* 1999;33:114.
946. Martinez E, Collazos J, Mayo J. Hypersensitivity reactions to rifampin. Pathogenetic mechanisms, clinical manifestations, management strategies, and review of the anaphylactic-like reactions. *Medicine (Baltimore)* 1999;78:361.
947. Paganelli R, Levinsky RJ, Atherton DJ. Detection of specific antigen within circulating immune complexes: validation of the assay and its application to food antigen-antibody complexes formed in healthy and food-allergic subjects. *Clin Exp Immunol* 1981;46:44.
948. Choi IH, Ha TY, Lee DG, et al. Occurrence of disseminated intravascular coagulation (DIC) in active systemic anaphylaxis: role of platelet-activating factor. *Clin Exp Immunol* 1995;100:390.
949. Medani CR, Pearl PL, Hall-Craggs M. Acute renal failure, hemolytic anemia, and thrombocytopenia in poststreptococcal glomerulonephritis. *South Med J* 1987;80:370.
950. Muguruma T, Koyama T, Kanadani T, et al. Acute thrombocytopenia associated with post-streptococcal acute glomerulonephritis. *J Paediatr Child Health* 2000;36:401.
951. Krause I, Garty BZ, Davidovits M, et al. Low serum C3, leukopenia, and thrombocytopenia: unusual features of Henoch-Schonlein purpura. *Eur J Pediatr* 1999;158:906.
952. George CRP, Slichter SJ, Quadracci LJ, et al. A kinetic evaluation of hemostasis in renal disease. *N Engl J Med* 1974;291:1111.
953. Landis TF, Von Felten A, Berchtold H. Thrombocytopenic episodes in patients with well-functioning renal allografts: inverse relationship between platelet count and platelet size pointing to intermittent platelet destruction. *Acta Haematol* 1979;61:2.
954. Bunting RW, Quay SC. Case records of the Massachusetts General Hospital. *N Engl J Med* 1979;300:1262.
955. Leithner C, Sinzinger H, Schwarz M. Treatment of chronic kidney transplant rejection with prostacyclin: reduction of platelet deposition in the transplant: prolongation of platelet survival and improvement of transplant function. *Prostaglandins* 1981;22:783.
956. Madaio MP, Spiegel JE, Levey AS. Life-threatening thrombocytopenia complicating antithymocyte globulin therapy for acute kidney transplant rejection: evidence of in situ immune complex formation on the platelet surface. *Transplantation* 1988;45:647.
957. Kelly PA, Gruber SA, Behbod F, et al. Sirolimus, a new, potent immunosuppressive agent. *Pharmacotherapy* 1997;17:1148.
958. Woodman RC, Harker L. Bleeding complications associated with cardiopulmonary bypass. *Blood* 1990;76:1680.
959. Bevan DH. Cardiac bypass haemostasis: putting blood through the mill. *Br J Haematol* 1999;104:208.
960. Hope AF, Heyns A du P, Lotter MG, et al. Kinetics and sites of sequestration of indium 111-labeled human platelets during cardiopulmonary bypass. *J Thorac Cardiovasc Surg* 1981;81:880.
961. Holloway DS, Summaria L, Sandesara J, et al. Decreased platelet number and function and increased fibrinolysis contribute to postoperative bleeding in cardiopulmonary bypass patients. *Thromb Haemost* 1988;59:62.
962. Tabuchi N, Tigchelaar I, van Oeveren W. Shear-induced pathway of platelet function in cardiac surgery. *Semin Thromb Hemost* 1995;21[Suppl 2]:66.
963. Rinder CS, Mathew JP, Rinder HM, et al. Modulation of platelet surface adhesion receptors during cardiopulmonary bypass. *Anesthesiology* 1991;75:563.
964. Harker LA, Malpass TW, Branson HE, et al. Mechanism of abnormal bleeding in patients undergoing cardiopulmonary bypass: acquired transient platelet dysfunction associated with selective alpha-granule release. *Blood* 1980;56:824.
965. Abrams CS, Ellison N, Budzynski AZ, et al. Direct detection of activated platelets and platelet-derived microparticles in humans. *Blood* 1990;75:128.
966. Kestin AS, Valeri CR, Khuri SF, et al. The platelet function defect of cardiopulmonary bypass. *Blood* 1993;82:107.
967. Gelb AB, Roth RI, Levin J, et al. Changes in blood coagulation during and following cardiopulmonary bypass: lack of correlation with clinical bleeding. *Am J Clin Pathol* 1996;106:87–99.
968. Davis R, Whittington R. Aprotinin: a review of its pharmacology and therapeutic efficacy in reducing blood loss associated with cardiac surgery. *Drugs* 1995;49:954.
969. Katsaros D, Petricevic M, Snow NJ, et al. Tranexamic acid reduces postbypass blood use: a double-blinded prospective, randomized study of 210 patients. *Ann Thorac Surg* 1996;61:1131.
970. Teoh KH, Young E, Bradley CA, et al. Heparin binding proteins: contribution to heparin rebound after cardiopulmonary bypass. *Circulation* 1993;88:II420.
971. Gafter U, Bessler H, Malachi T, et al. Platelet count and thrombopoietic activity in patients with chronic renal failure. *Nephron* 1987;45:207.
972. Docci D, Turci F, Del Vecchio C, et al. Hemodialysis-associated platelet loss: study of the relative contribution of dialyzer membrane composition and geometry. *Int J Artif Organs* 1984;7:337.
973. Hakim RM, Schafer AI. Hemodialysis-associated platelet activation and thrombocytopenia. *Am J Med* 1985;78:575.
974. Schmitt GW, Moake JL, Rudy CK, et al. Alterations in hemostatic parameters during hemodialysis with dialyzers of different membrane composition and flow design: platelet activation and factor VIII-related von Willebrand factor during hemodialysis. *Am J Med* 1987;83:411.
975. Vicks SL, Gross ML, Schmitt GW. Massive hemorrhage due to hemodialysis-associated thrombocytopenia. *Am J Nephrol* 1983;3:30.
976. Bick RL. Hemostasis defects associated with cardiac surgery, prosthetic devices, and other extracorporeal circuits. *Semin Thromb Hemost* 1985;11:249.
977. Smith DA, Monaghan WP, Hann WD, et al. Evaluation of in vivo platelet adhesiveness during discontinuous-flow centrifugal thrombocytopheresis. *Plasma Ther Transfus Technol* 1983;4:37.
978. Harker LA, Slichter SJ. Studies of platelet and fibrinogen kinetics in patients with prosthetic heart valves. *N Engl J Med* 1970;283:1302.
979. Harker LA, Slichter SJ. Platelet and fibrinogen consumption in man. *N Engl J Med* 1972;287:999.
980. Harker LA, Slichter SJ, Sauvage LR. Platelet consumption by arterial prostheses: the effects of endothelialization and pharmacologic inhibition of platelet function. *Ann Surg* 1977;186:594.
981. Neumann I, Meisl FT, Kopriva G, et al. ^{111}In-labelled platelets for assessment of thrombogenicity of new haemodialysis vascular access. *Nucl Med Commun* 1999;20:445.
982. Stratton JR, Thiele BL, Ritchie JL. Natural history of platelet deposition on Dacron aortic bifurcation grafts in the first year after implantation. *Am J Cardiol* 1983;52:371.
983. Goldschmidt B. Platelet functions in children with congenital heart disease. *Acta Paediatr Scand* 1974;63:271.
984. Waldman JD, Czapek EE, Paul MH, et al. Shortened platelet survival in cyanotic heart disease. *J Pediatr* 1975;87:77.
985. Terai M, Nakazawa M, Takao A, et al. Thrombocytopenia in patients with aortopulmonary transposition and an intact ventricular septum. *Br Heart J* 1987;57:371.
986. Komp DM, Sparrow AW. Polycythemia in cyanotic heart disease: a study of altered coagulation. *J Pediatr* 1970;76:231.
987. Ihenacho HN, Fletcher DJ, Breeze GR, et al. Consumption coagulopathy in congenital heart disease. *Lancet* 1973;1:231.
988. Maurer HM, McCue CM, Caul J, et al. Impairment in platelet aggregation in congenital heart disease. *Blood* 1972;40:207.
989. Ekert H, Dowling SV. Platelet release abnormality and reduced prothrombin levels in children with cyanotic congenital heart disease. *Aust Paediatr J* 1977;13:17.
990. Henriksson P, Värendh G, Lundstrom NR. Haemostatic defects in cyanotic congenital heart disease. *Br Heart J* 1979;41:23.
991. Wedemeyer AL, Lewis JH. Improvement in hemostasis following phlebotomy in cyanotic patients with heart disease. *J Pediatr* 1973;83:46.
992. Ekert H, Sheers M. Pre and postoperative studies of fibrinolysis and prothrombin in cyanotic congenital heart disease. *Haemostasis* 1974;3:158.
993. Maurer HM, McCue CM, Robertson LW, et al. Correction of platelet dysfunction and bleeding in cyanotic congenital heart disease by simple red cell volume reduction. *Am J Cardiol* 1975;35:831.
994. Jacobson RJ, Rath CE, Perloff JK. Intravascular haemolysis and thrombocytopenia in left ventricular outflow obstruction. *Br Heart J* 1973;35:849.
995. Steele PP, Weily HS, Davies H, et al. Platelet survival in patients with rheumatic heart disease. *N Engl J Med* 1974;290:537.
996. Gill JC, Wilson AD, Endres-Brooks J, et al. Loss of the largest von Willebrand factor multimers from the plasma of patients with congenital cardiac defects. *Blood* 1986;67:758.
997. Warkentin TE, Moore JC, Morgan DG. Aortic stenosis and bleeding gastrointestinal angiodysplasia: is acquired von Willebrand's disease the link? *Lancet* 1992;340:35.
998. Anderson RP, McGrath K, Street A. Reversal of aortic stenosis, bleeding gastrointestinal angiodysplasia, and von Willebrand syndrome by aortic valve replacement [Letter]. *Lancet* 1994;347:689.
999. Warkentin TE, Moore JC, Morgan DG. Resolution of bleeding from gastrointestinal angiodysplasia and type IIA von Willebrand's syndrome after aortic-valve replacement [Letter]. *N Engl J Med* 2002;347.
1000. Wang Y, From AHL, Krivit W, et al. Disseminated pulmonary arterial thrombosis associated with thrombocytopenia: occurrence in identical twins. *Circulation* 1965;31:215.
1001. Edwards BS, Weir EK, Edwards WD, et al. Coexistent pulmonary and portal hypertension: morphologic and clinical features. *J Am Coll Cardiol* 1987;10:1233.
1002. Stahl RL, Javid JP, Lackner H. Unrecognized pulmonary embolism presenting as disseminated intravascular coagulation. *Am J Med* 1984;76:772.
1003. Mustafa MH, Mispireta LA, Pierce LE. Occult pulmonary embolism presenting with thrombocytopenia and elevated fibrin split products. *Am J Med* 1989;86:490.
1004. Warkentin TE. Pseudo-heparin-induced thrombocytopenia. In: Warkentin TE, Greinacher A, eds. *Heparin-induced thrombocytopenia*, 2nd ed. New York: Marcel Dekker, 2001:271.
1005. Noe DA, Graham SM, Luff R, et al. Platelet counts during rapid massive transfusion. *Transfusion* 1982;22:392.
1006. Hewson JR, Neame PB, Kumar N, et al. Coagulopathy related to dilution and hypotension during massive transfusion. *Crit Care Med* 1985;13:387.
1007. Reed RL II, Heimbach DM, Counts RB, et al. Prophylactic platelet administration during massive transfusion: a prospective, randomized, double-blind clinical study. *Ann Surg* 1986;203:40.

1008. Goulet O, Girot R, Maier-Redelsperger M, et al. Hematologic disorders following prolonged use of intravenous fat emulsions in children. *JPEN J Parenter Enteral Nutr* 1986;10:284.

1009. Kickler TS, Zinkham WH, Moser A, et al. Effect of erucic acid on platelets in patients with adrenoleukodystrophy. *Biochem Mol Med* 1996;57:125.

1010. Zierz S, Schröder R, Unkrig CJ. Thrombocytopenia induced by erucic acid therapy in patients with X-linked adrenoleukodystrophy. *Clin Invest* 1993;71:802.

1011. Crowther MA, Barr RD, Kelton J, et al. Profound thrombocytopenia complicating dietary erucic acid therapy for adrenoleukodystrophy [Letter]. *Am J Hematol* 1995;48:132.

1012. Chai BC, Etches WS, Stewart MW, et al. Bleeding in a patient taking Lorenzo's oil: evidence for a vascular defect. *Postgrad Med J* 1996;72:113.

1013. Hohlfeld P, Forestier F, Kaplan C, et al. Fetal thrombocytopenia: a retrospective sampling of 5,194 fetal blood samplings. *Blood* 1994;84:1851.

1014. Andrew M, Kelton J. Neonatal thrombocytopenia. *Clin Perinatol* 1984;11:359.

1015. George D, Bussel JB. Neonatal thrombocytopenia. *Semin Thromb Hemost* 1995;21:276.

1016. Castle V, Andrew M, Kelton J, et al. Frequency and mechanism of neonatal thrombocytopenia. *J Pediatr* 1986;108:749.

1017. Castle V, Coates G, Kelton JG, et al. 111In-oxine platelet survivals in thrombocytopenic infants. *Blood* 1987;70:652.

1018. Schmidt B, Vegh P, Johnston M, et al. Do coagulation screening tests detect increased generation of thrombin and plasmin in sick newborn infants? *Thromb Haemost* 1993;69:418.

1019. Cooper LZ, Green RH, Krugman S, et al. Neonatal thrombocytopenic purpura and other manifestations of rubella contracted in utero. *Am J Dis Child* 1965;110:416.

1020. Hanshaw JB. Congenital and acquired cytomegalovirus infection. *Pediatr Clin North Am* 1966;13:279.

1021. Whitaker JA, Sartain P, Shaheedy M. Hematological aspects of congenital syphilis. *J Pediatr* 1965;66:629.

1022. Jones MJ, Kolb M, Votava JH, et al. Intrauterine echo-virus type 11 infection. *Mayo Clin Proc* 1980;55:509.

1023. Zipursky A, Jaber HM. The haematology of bacterial infections in newborn infants. *Clin Haematol* 1978;7:175.

1024. Colarizi P, Fiorucci P, Caradonna A, et al. Circulating thrombopoietin levels in neonates with infection. *Acta Paediatr* 1999;88:332.

1025. Mehta P, Vasa R, Neumann L, et al. Thrombocytopenia in the high risk infant. *J Pediatr* 1980;97:791.

1026. Ballin A, Koren G, Kohelet D, et al. Reduction of platelet counts induced by mechanical ventilation in newborn infants. *J Pediatr* 1987;111:445.

1027. Segall ML, Goetzman BW, Schick JB. Thrombocytopenia and pulmonary hypertension in the perinatal aspiration syndromes. *J Pediatr* 1980;96:727.

1028. Tudehope DI, Yu VYH. The haematology of neonatal necrotizing enterocolitis. *Aust Paediatr J* 1977;13:193.

1029. Ververidis M, Kiely EM, Spitz L, et al. The clinical significance of thrombocytopenia in neonates with necrotizing enterocolitis. *J Pediatr Surg* 2001;36:799.

1030. Maurer HM, Frakin M, McWilliams MB. Effects of phototherapy on platelet counts in low-birthweight infants and on platelet production and life span in rabbits. *Pediatrics* 1976;57:506.

1031. Kleckner HB, Giles HR, Corrigan JJ Jr. The association of maternal and neonatal thrombocytopenia in high-risk pregnancies. *Am J Obstet Gynecol* 1977;128:235.

1032. Brazy JE, Grimm JK, Little VA. Neonatal manifestations of severe maternal hypertension occurring before the thirty-sixth week of pregnancy. *J Pediatr* 1982;100:265.

1033. Pritchard JA, Cunningham FG, Pritchard SA, et al. How often does maternal preeclampsia-eclampsia incite thrombocytopenia in the fetus? *Obstet Gynecol* 1987;69:292.

1034. Kasabach HH, Merritt KK. Capillary hemangioma with extensive purpura: report of case. *Am J Dis Child* 1940;59:1063.

1035. Hall GW. Kasabach–Merritt syndrome: pathogenesis and management. *Br J Haematol* 2001;112:851.

1036. Enjolras O, Mulliken JB, Wassef M, et al. Residual lesions after Kasabach–Merritt syndrome phenomenon in 41 patients. *J Am Acad Dermatol* 2000;42:225.

1037. Singh G, Rajendran C. Kasabach-Merritt syndrome in two successive pregnancies. *Int J Dermatol* 1998;37:690.

1038. Schmidt RP, Lentle BC. Hemangioma with consumptive coagulopathy (Kasabach-Merritt syndrome): detection by indium-111-oxine labeled platelets. *Clin Nucl Med* 1984;9:389.

1039. Shulkin BL, Argenta LC, Cho KJ, et al. Kasabach–Merritt syndrome: treatment with epsilon-aminocaproic acid and assessment by indium 111 platelet scintigraphy. *J Pediatr* 1990;117:746.

1040. Sato Y, Frey EE, Wicklund B, et al. Embolization therapy in the management of infantile hemangioma with Kasabach Merritt syndrome. *Pediatr Radiol* 1987;17:503.

1041. Ezekowitz RAB, Mulliken JB, Folkman J. Interferon alfa-2a therapy for life-threatening hemangioma of infancy. *N Engl J Med* 1992;326:1456.

1042. Froehlich LA, Housler M. Neonatal thrombocytopenia and chorangioma. *J Pediatr* 1971;78:516.

1043. Bauer CR, Fojaco RM, Bancalar E, et al. Microangiopathic hemolytic anemia and thrombocytopenia in a neonate associated with a large placental chorioangioma. *Pediatrics* 1978;62:574.

1044. Valat AS, Caulier MT, Devos P, et al. Relationships between severe neonatal thrombocytopenia and maternal characteristics in pregnancies associated with autoimmune thrombocytopenia. *Br J Haematol* 1998;103:397.

1045. Hanada T, Saito K, Nagasawa T, et al. Intravenous gammaglobulin therapy for thromboneutropenic neonates of mothers with systemic lupus erythematosus. *Eur J Haematol* 1987;38:400.

1046. Watson R, Kang JE, May M, et al. Thrombocytopenia in the neonatal lupus syndrome. *Arch Dermatol* 1988;124:560.

1047. Mauer AM, DeVaux LO, Lahey MD. Neonatal and maternal thrombocytopenic purpura due to quinine. *Pediatrics* 1957;19:84.

1048. Rodriguez SU, Leikin SL, Hiller MC. Neonatal thrombocytopenia associated with ante-partum administration of thiazide drugs. *N Engl J Med* 1964;270:881.

1049. Widerlov E, Karlman I, Storsater J. Hydralazine-induced neonatal thrombocytopenia [Letter]. *N Engl J Med* 1980;303:1235.

1050. Schiff D, Aranda JV, Stern L. Neonatal thrombocytopenia and congenital malformations associated with administration of tolbutamide to the mother. *J Pediatr* 1970;77:457.

1051. Merenstein GB, O'Loughlin EP, Plunket DC. Effects of maternal thiazides on platelet counts of newborn infants. *J Pediatr* 1970;76:766.

1052. Jerkner K, Kutti J, Victorin L. Platelet counts in mothers and their newborn infants with respect to ante-partum administration of oral diuretics. *Acta Med Scand* 1973;194:473.

1053. Louden KA, Broughton Pipkin F, Heptinstall S, et al. Neonatal platelet reactivity and serum thromboxane B2 production in whole blood: the effect of maternal low dose aspirin. *Br J Obstet Gynecol* 1994;101:203.

1054. Wigger HJ, Bransilver BR, Blanc WA. Thromboses due to catheterization in infants and children. *J Pediatr* 1970;76:1.

1055. Nachman RL, Thomas M, Patel D, et al. Thrombocytopenia as evidence of local thrombus: the umbilical arterial catheter [Letter]. *Pediatrics* 1972;50:825.

1056. Renfield ML, Kraybill EN. Consumptive coagulopathy with renal vein thrombosis. *J Pediatr* 1973;82:1054.

1057. Hawker RE, Celermajer JM, Cartmill TB, et al. Thrombosis of the inferior vena cava following balloon septostomy in transposition of the great arteries. *Am Heart J* 1971;82:593.

1058. Spadone D, Clark F, James E, et al. Heparin-induced thrombocytopenia in the newborn. *J Vasc Surg* 1992;15:306.

1059. Rivers RPA. Coagulation changes associated with a high haematocrit in the newborn infant. *Acta Paediatr Scand* 1975;64:449.

1060. Katz J, Rodriguez E, Mandani G, et al. Normal coagulation findings, thrombocytopenia, and peripheral hemoconcentration in neonatal polycythemia. *J Pediatr* 1982;101:99.

1061. Monnens LAH, Retera RJM. Thrombotic thrombocytopenic purpura in a neonatal infant. *J Pediatr* 1967;71:118.

1062. Upshaw JD Jr. Congenital deficiency of a factor in normal plasma that reverses microangiopathic hemolysis and thrombocytopenia. *N Engl J Med* 1978;298:1350.

1063. Sartori PC, Enayat MS, Darbyshire PJ. Congenital microangiopathic haemolytic anemia: a variant of thrombotic thrombocytopenic purpura? *Pediatr Hematol Oncol* 1993;10:271.

1064. Chintagumpala MM, Hurwitz RL, Moake JL, et al. Chronic relapsing thrombotic thrombocytopenic purpura in infants with large von Willebrand factor multimers during remission. *J Pediatr* 1992;120:49.

1065. Peters C, Casella JF, Marlar RA, et al. Homozygous protein C deficiency: observations on the nature of the molecular abnormality and the effectiveness of warfarin therapy. *Pediatrics* 1988;81:272.

1066. Lipson AH, Pritchard J, Thomas G. Thrombocytopenia after intralipid infusion in a neonate [Letter]. *Lancet* 1974;2:1462.

1067. Colomb V, Jobert-Giraud A, Lacaille F, et al. Role of lipid emulsion in cholestasis associated with long-term parenteral nutrition in children. *JPEN J Parenter Enteral Nutr* 2000;24:345.

1068. Spragg RG, Abraham JL, Loomis WH. Pulmonary platelet deposition accompanying acute oleic acid-induced pulmonary injury. *Am Rev Resp Dis* 1982;126:553.

1069. Dahms BB, Halpin TC Jr. Pulmonary arterial lipid deposit in newborn infants receiving intravenous lipid infusion. *J Pediatr* 1980;97:800.

1070. Wakely PE, Hug G. Intralipid vasculopathy [Letter]. *Lancet* 1981;2:1416.

1071. Spear ML, Spear M, Cohen AR, et al. Effect of fat infusions on platelet concentration in premature infants. *JPEN J Parenter Enteral Nutr* 1990;14:165.

1072. Morrow G III, Barness LA, Auerbach VH, et al. Observations on the coexistence of methylmalonic acidemia and glycinemia. *J Pediatr* 1969;74:680.

1073. Branksi D, Gale R, Gross-Kieselstein E, et al. Propionic acidemia and anorectal anomalies in three siblings. *Am J Dis Child* 1977;131:1379.

1074. De Klerk JB, Duran M, Dorland L, et al. A patient with mevalonic aciduria presenting with hepatosplenomegaly, congenital anaemia, thrombocytopenia and leukocytosis. *J Inherit Metab Dis* 1988;11:233.

1075. Hinson DD, Rogers ZR, Hoffmann GF, et al. Hematological abnormalities and cholestatic liver disease in two patients with mevalonate kinase deficiency. *Am J Med Genet* 1998;78:408.

1076. Roth KS, Yang W, Foreman JW, et al. Holocarboxylase synthetase deficiency: a biotin-responsive organic acidemia. *J Pediatr* 1980;96:845.

1077. Kelleher JF Jr, Yudkoff M, Hutchinson R, et al. The pancytopenia of isovaleric acidemia. *Pediatrics* 1980;65:1023.

1078. Gilbert-Barness E, Barness LA. Isovaleric acidemia with promyelocytic myeloproliferative syndrome. *Pediatr Dev Pathol* 1999;2:286.

1079. Koenig JM, Christensen RD. Neutropenia and thrombocytopenia in infants with Rh hemolytic disease. *J Pediatr* 1989;114:625.

1080. Sande JE, Arceci RJ, Lampkin BC. Congenital and neonatal leukemia. *Semin Perinatol* 1999;23:274.

1081. Zipursky A, Rose T, Skidmore M, et al. Hydrops fetalis and neonatal leukemia. *Pediatr Hematol Oncol* 1996;13:81.

1082. Shown TE, Durfee MF. Blueberry muffin baby: neonatal neuroblastoma with subcutaneous metastases. *J Urol* 1970;104:193.

1083. Shapiro F. Osteopetrosis: current clinical considerations. *Clin Orthop* 1993;294:34.

1084. Hertz CG, Hambrick GW Jr. Congenital Letterer-Siwe disease: a case treated with vincristine and corticosteroids. *Am J Dis Child* 1968;116:553.

1085. Nezelof C, Frileux-Herbet F, Cronier-Sachot J. Disseminated histiocytosis X: analysis of prognostic factors based on a retrospective study of 50 cases. *Cancer* 1979;44:1824.

1086. Sills RH. Hypersplenism. In: Pochedly C, Sills RH, Schwartz AD, eds. *Disorders of the spleen: pathophysiology and management.* New York: Marcel Dekker, 1989;167.

1087. Wadenvik H, Denfors I, Kutti J. Splenic blood flow and intrasplenic platelet kinetics in relation to spleen volume. *Br J Haematol* 1987;67:181.

1088. Todd D, Chan TK. Abnormalities of blood volume in disorders of the spleen. In: Bowdler AJ, ed. *The spleen: structure, function and clinical significance.* London: Chapman and Hall, 1990:191.

1089. Peck-Radosavljevic M. Thrombocytopenia in liver disease. *Can J Gastroenterol* 2000;14(Suppl D):60D.

1090. Shah SH, Hayes PC, Allan PL, et al. Measurement of spleen size and its relation to hypersplenism and portal hemodynamics in portal hypertension due to hepatic cirrhosis. *Am J Gastroenterol* 1996;91:2580.

1091. Schmidt KG, Rasmussen JW, Bekker C, et al. Kinetics and in vivo distribution of ^{111}In-labelled autologous platelets in chronic hepatic disease: mechanisms of thrombocytopenia. *Scand J Haematol* 1985;34:39.

1092. Hill-Zobel RL, McCandless B, Kang SA, et al. Organ distribution and fate of human platelets: studies of asplenic and splenomegalic patients. *Am J Hematol* 1986;23:231.

1093. Henderson JM, Warren WD. Selective variceal decompression: current status and recent advances. *Adv Surg* 1984;18:81.

1094. Shilyansky J, Roberts EA, Superina RA. Distal splenorenal shunts for the treatment of severe thrombocytopenia from portal hypertension in children. *J Gastrointest Surg* 1999;3:167.

1095. Sanyal AJ. The use and misuse of transjugular intrahepatic portasystemic shunts. *Curr Gastroenterol Rep* 2000;2:61.

1096. Watanabe Y, Todani T, Noda T. Changes in splenic volume after partial splenic embolization in children. *J Pediatr Surg* 1996;31:241.

1097. Sangro B, Bilbao I, Herrero I, et al. Partial splenic embolization for the treatment of hypersplenism in cirrhosis. *Hepatology* 1993;18:309.

1098. Charrow J, Andersson HC, Kaplan P, et al. The Gaucher registry: demographics and disease characteristics of 1698 patients with Gaucher disease. *Arch Intern Med* 2000;160:2835.

1099. Gillis S, Hyam E, Abrahamov A, et al. Platelet function abnormalities in Gaucher disease patients. *Am J Hematol* 1999;61:103.

1100. Rubin M, Yampolski I, Lambrozo R, et al. Partial splenectomy in Gaucher's disease. *J Pediatr Surg* 1986;21:125.

1101. Thanopoulos BD, Frimas CA, Mantagos SP, et al. Gaucher disease: treatment of hypersplenism with splenic embolization. *Acta Paediatr Scand* 1987;76:1003.

1102. Morales LE. Gaucher's disease: a review. *Ann Pharmacother* 1996;30:381.

1103. Coad JE, Matutes E, Catovsky D. Splenectomy in lymphoproliferative disorders: a report on 70 cases and review of the literature. *Leuk Lymphoma* 1993;10:245.

1104. Lindemann A, Ludwig WD, Oster W, et al. High-level secretion of tumor necrosis factor-alpha contributes to hematopoietic failure in hairy cell leukemia. *Blood* 1989;73:880.

1105. Cusack JC Jr, Seymour JF, Lerner S, et al. Role of splenectomy in chronic lymphocytic leukemia. *J Am Coll Surg* 1997;185:237.

1106. Brenner B, Nagler A, Tatarsky I, et al. Splenectomy in agnogenic myeloid metaplasia and postpolycythemic myeloid metaplasia: a study of 34 cases. *Arch Intern Med* 1988;148:2501.

1107. Dacie JV, Brain MC, Harrison CV, et al. "Non-tropical idiopathic splenomegaly" ("primary hypersplenism"): a review of ten cases and their relationship to malignant lymphomas. *Br J Haematol* 1969;17:317.

1108. Gobbi PG, Grignani GE, Pozzetti U, et al. Primary splenic lymphoma: does it exist? *Haematologica* 1994;79:286.

1109. Moll S, Igelhart JD, Ortel TL. Thrombocytopenia in association with a wandering spleen. *Am J Hematol* 1996;53:259.

1110. Benoist S, Imbaud P, Veyrieres M. Reversible hypersplenism after splenopexy for wandering spleen. *Hepatogastroenterology* 1998;45:2430.

1111. Malmaeus J, Akre T, Adami HO, et al. Early postoperative course following elective splenectomy in haematological disease: a high complication rate in patients with myeloproliferative disorders. *Br J Surg* 1986;73:720.

1112. Villalobos TJ, Adelson E, Riley PA Jr, et al. A case of thrombocytopenia and leucopenia that occurs in dogs during deep hypothermia. *J Clin Invest* 1958;37:1.

1113. Bjork VO, Hultquist G. Brain damage in children after deep hypothermia for open-heart surgery. *Thorax* 1960;15:284.

1114. Reddick RL, Poole BL, Penick GD. Thrombocytopenia of hibernation: mechanism of induction and recovery. *Lab Invest* 1973;28:270.

1115. Shenaq SA, Yawn DH, Saleem A, et al. Effect of profound hypothermia on leukocytes and platelets. *Ann Clin Lab Sci* 1986;16:130.

1116. Cohen IJ, Amir J, Gedaliah A, et al. Thrombocytopenia of neonatal cold injury. *J Pediatr* 1984;104:620.

1117. O'Brien H, Amess JA, Mollin DL. Recurrent thrombocytopenia, erythroid hypoplasia and sideroblastic anaemia associated with hypothermia. *Br J Haematol* 1982;51:451.

1118. Easterbrook PJ, Davis HP. Thrombocytopenia in hypothermia: a common but poorly recognized complication. *BMJ* 1985;291:23.

1119. Vella MA, Jenner C, Betteridge DJ, et al. Hypothermia-induced thrombocytopenia. *J R Soc Med* 1988;81:228.

1120. Chan KM, Beard K. A patient with recurrent hypothermia associated with thrombocytopenia. *Postgrad Med J* 1993;69:227.

1121. Balcombe NR. The chilling tale of a patient with thrombocytopenia. *Postgrad Med J* 1999;75:621.

1122. Holm IA, McLaughlin JF, Feldman K, et al. Recurrent hypothermia and thrombocytopenia after severe neonatal brain infection. *Clin Pediatr* 1988; 27:326.

1123. White KD, Scoones DJ, Newman PK. Hypothermia in multiple sclerosis. *J Neurol Neurosurg Psychiatry* 1996;61:369.

1124. Pina-Cabral JM, Amaral I, Pinto MM, et al. Hepatic and splenic platelet sequestration during deep hypothermia in the dog. *Haemostasis* 1974;2:235.

1125. Hessel EA II, Schmer G, Dillard DH. Platelet kinetics during deep hypothermia. *J Surg Res* 1980;28:23.

1126. Bareford D, Chandler ST, Hawker RJ, et al. Splenic platelet-sequestration following routine blood transfusion is reduced by filtered/washed blood products. *Br J Haematol* 1987;67:177.

1127. Lim S, Boughton BJ, Bareford D. Thrombocytopenia following routine blood transfusion: microaggregate blood filters prevent worsening thrombocytopenia in patients with low platelet counts. *Vox Sang* 1989;56:40.

1128. Hart S, Bareford D, Smith N, et al. Post-transfusion thrombocytopenia: its duration in splenic and asplenic individuals [Letter]. *Vox Sang* 1990;59:123.

1129. Tricot G, Criel A, Verwilghen RL. Thrombocytopenia as presenting symptom of preleukaemia in 3 patients. *Scand J Haematol* 1982;28:243.

1130. Hallett JM, Martell RW, Sher C, et al. Amegakaryocytic thrombocytopenia with duplication of part of the long arm of chromosome 3. *Br J Haematol* 1989;71:291.

1131. Menke DM, Colon-Otero G, Cockerill KJ, et al. Refractory thrombocytopenia: a myelodysplastic syndrome that may mimic immune thrombocytopenic purpura. *Am J Clin Pathol* 1992;98:502.

1132. Berndt MC, Kabral A, Grimsley P, et al. An acquired Bernard-Soulier-like platelet defect associated with juvenile myelodysplastic syndrome. *Br J Haematol* 1988;68:97.

1133. Mittelman M, Zeidman A. Platelet function in the myelodysplastic syndromes. *Int J Hematol* 2000;71:95.

1134. Buzaid AC, Garewal HS, Lippman SM, et al. Danazol in the treatment of myelodysplastic syndromes. *Eur J Haematol* 1987;39:346.

1135. Stadtmauer EA, Cassileth PA, Edelstein M, et al. Danazol treatment of myelodysplastic syndromes. *Br J Haematol* 1991;77:502.

1136. Hebbar M, Kaplan C, Caulier MT, et al. Low incidence of specific anti-platelet antibodies detected by the MAIPA assay in the serum of thrombocytopenic MDS patients and lack of correlation between platelet autoantibodies, platelet lifespan and response to danazol therapy. *Br J Haematol* 1996;94:112.

1137. Wattel E, Cambier N, Caulier MT, et al. Androgen therapy in myelodysplastic syndromes with thrombocytopenia: a report on 20 cases. *Br J Haematol* 1994;87:205.

1138. Bourgeois E, Caulier MT, Rose C, et al. Role of splenectomy in the treatment of myelodysplastic syndromes with peripheral thrombocytopenia: a report on six cases. *Leukemia* 2001;15:950.

1139. Bessman JD. The relation of megakaryocyte ploidy to platelet volume. *Am J Hematol* 1984;16:161.

1140. Cowan DH. Effect of alcoholism on hemostasis. *Semin Hematol* 1980;17:137.

1141. Post RM, Desforges JF. Thrombocytopenia and alcoholism. *Ann Intern Med* 1968;68:1230.

1142. Haut MJ, Cowan DH. The effect of ethanol on hemostatic properties of human blood platelets. *Am J Med* 1974;56:22.

1143. Lindenbaum J, Hargrove RL. Thrombocytopenia in alcoholics. *Ann Intern Med* 1968;68:526.

1144. Lindenbaum J, Lieber CS. Hematologic effects of alcohol in man in the absence of nutritional deficiency. *N Engl J Med* 1969;281:333.

1145. Ryback R, Desforges J. Alcoholic thrombocytopenia in three inpatient drinking alcoholics. *Arch Intern Med* 1970;125:475.

1146. Cowan DH, Hines JD. Thrombocytopenia of severe alcoholism. *Ann Intern Med* 1971;74:37.

1147. Haselager EM, Vreeken J. Rebound thrombocytosis after alcohol abuse: a possible factor in the pathogenesis of thromboembolic disease. *Lancet* 1977;1:774.

1148. Numminen H, Hillbom M, Juvela S. Platelets, alcohol consumption, and onset of brain infarction. *J Neurol Neurosurg Psychiatry* 1996;61:376.

1149. Savage DG, Ogundipe A, Allen RH, et al. Etiology and diagnostic evaluation of macrocytosis. *Am J Med Sci* 2000;319:343.

1150. Gewirtz AM, Hoffman R. Transitory hypomegakaryocytic thrombocytopenia: aetiological association with ethanol abuse and implications regarding regulation of human megakaryocytopoiesis. *Br J Haematol* 1986;62:333.

1151. Cowan DH. Thrombokinetic studies in alcohol-related thrombocytopenia. *J Lab Clin Med* 1973;81:64.

1152. Sullivan LW, Adams WH, Liu YK. Induction of thrombocytopenia by thrombopheresis in man: patterns of recovery in normal subjects during ethanol ingestion and abstinence. *Blood* 1977;49:197.

1153. Sahud MA. Platelet size and number in alcoholic thrombocytopenia. *N Engl J Med* 1972;286:355.

1154. Levine RF, Spivak JL, Meagher RC, et al. Effect of ethanol on thrombopoiesis. *Br J Haematol* 1986;62:345.

1155. Stoll DB, Blum S, Pasquale D, et al. Thrombocytopenia with decreased mega-karyocytes: evaluation and prognosis. *Ann Intern Med* 1981;94:170.

1156. Hoffman R, Bruno E, Elwell J, et al. Acquired amegakaryocytic thrombocytopenic purpura: a syndrome of diverse etiologies. *Blood* 1982;60:1173.

1157. Chan DKY, O'Neill B. Successful trial of antithymocyte globulin therapy in amegakaryocytic thrombocytopenic purpura [Letter]. *Med J Aust* 1988;148:602.

1158. Nagasawa T, Sakurai T, Kashiwagi H, et al. Cell-mediated amegakaryocytic thrombocytopenia associated with systemic lupus erythematosus. *Blood* 1986;67:479.

1159. Koduri PR. Amegakaryocytic thrombocytopenia with a positive direct Coombs' test. *Am J Hematol* 1993;44:68.

1160. Font J, Nomdedeu B, Martinez-Orozco F, et al. Amegakaryocytic thrombocytopenia and an analgesic [Letter]. *Ann Intern Med* 1981;95:783.

1161. Hoffman R, Briddell RA, Van Besien K, et al. Acquired cyclic amegakaryocytic thrombocytopenia associated with an immunoglobulin blocking the action of granulocyte-macrophage colony-stimulating factor. *N Engl J Med* 1989;321:97.

1162. Telek B, Kiss A, Pecze K, et al. Cyclic idiopathic pure acquired amegakaryocytic thrombocytopenic purpura: a patient treated with cyclosporin A. *Br J Haematol* 1989;73:128.

1163. Kashyap R, Choudhry CP, Pati HP. Danazol therapy in cyclic acquired amegakaryocytic thrombocytopenic purpura: a case report. *Am J Hematol* 1999;60:225.

1164. Hoffman R, Zaknoen S, Yang HH, et al. An antibody cytotoxic to megakaryocyte progenitor cells in a patient with immune thrombocytopenic purpura. *N Engl J Med* 1985;312:1170.

1165. Mukai HY, Kojima H, Todokoro K, et al. Serum thrombopoietin (TPO) levels in patients with amegakaryocytic thrombocytopenia are much higher than those with immune thrombocytopenic purpura. *Thromb Haemost* 1996;76:675.

1166. Faldt R. Remission of amegakaryocytic thrombocytopenia induced by anti-lymphocyte globulin (ALG). *Br J Haematol* 1986;63:205.

1167. Trimble MS, Glynn MFX, Brain MC. Amegakaryocytic thrombocytopenia of 4 years duration: successful treatment with antithymocyte globulin. *Am J Hematol* 1991;37:126.

1168. Smeets REH, Hillen HFP. Acquired amegakaryocytic thrombocytopenic purpura: treatment with high-dose dexamethasone pulse therapy and review of the literature. *Neth J Med* 1988;32:27.

1169. Hill W, Landgraf R. Successful treatment of amegakaryocytic thrombocytopenic purpura with cyclosporine [Letter]. *N Engl J Med* 1985;312:1060.

1170. Peng CT, Kao LY, Tsai CH. Successful treatment with cyclosporin A in a child with acquired pure amegakaryocytic thrombocytopenic purpura. *Acta Paediatr* 1994;83:1222.

1171. Kayser W, Euler HH, Schmitz N, et al. Danazol in acquired amegakaryocytic thrombocytopenic purpura: a case report. *Blut* 1985;51:401.

1172. El Saghir NS, Geltman RL. Treatment of acquired amegakaryocytic thrombocytopenic purpura with cyclophosphamide. *Am J Med* 1986;81:139.

1173. Lonial S, Bilodeau PA, Langston AA, et al. Acquired amegakaryocytic thrombocytopenia treated with allogeneic BMT: a case report and review of the literature. *Bone Marrow Transplant* 1999;24:1337.

1174. Schloesser LL, Kipp MA, Wenzel FJ. Thrombocytosis in iron deficiency anemia. *J Lab Clin Med* 1967;66:107.

1175. Gross S, Keefer V, Newman AJ. The platelets in iron-deficiency anemia. I. The response to oral and parenteral iron. *Pediatrics* 1964;34:315.

1176. Lopas H, Rabiner SF. Thrombocytopenia associated with iron deficiency anemia: a report of five cases. *Clin Pediatr* 1966;5:609.

1177. Dincol K, Aksoy M. On the platelet levels in chronic iron deficiency anemia. *Acta Haematol* 1969;41:135.

1178. Scher H, Silber R. Iron responsive thrombocytopenia [Letter]. *Ann Intern Med* 1976;84:571.

1179. Michaeli J, Admon D, Lugassy G, et al. Idiopathic thrombocytopenic purpura presenting as iron-responsive thrombocytopenia. *Haemostasis* 1987;7:105.

1180. Berger M, Brass LF. Severe thrombocytopenia in iron deficiency anemia. *Am J Haematol* 1987;24:425.

1181. Knizley H Jr, Noyes WD. Iron deficiency anemia, papilledema, thrombocytosis, and transient hemiparesis. *Arch Intern Med* 1972;129:483.

1182. Soff GA, Levin J. Thrombocytopenia associated with repletion of iron in iron deficiency anemia. *Am J Med Sci* 1988;295:35.

1183. Go RS, Porrata LF, Call TG. Thrombocytopenia after iron dextran administration in a patient with severe iron deficiency anemia [Letter]. *Ann Intern Med* 2000;132:925.

1184. Beguin Y. Erythropoietin and platelet production. *Haematologica* 1999;84:541.

1185. Loo M, Beguin Y. The effect of recombinant human erythropoietin on platelet counts is strongly modulated by the adequacy of iron supply. *Blood* 1999;93:3286.

1186. Bellucci S. Megakaryocytes and inherited thrombocytopenias. *Ballieres Clin Haematol* 1997;10:149.

1187. Mhawech P, Saleem A. Inherited giant platelet disorders: classification and literature review. *Am J Clin Pathol* 2000;113:176.

1188. Hall JG, Levin J, Kuhn JP, et al. Thrombocytopenia with absent radius (TAR). *Medicine (Baltimore)* 1969;48:411.

1189. Hedberg VA, Lipton JM. Thrombocytopenia with absent radii: a review of 100 cases. *Am J Pediatr Hematol Oncol* 1988;10:51.

1190. Letestu R, Vitrat N, Massé A, et al. Existence of a differentiation blockage at the stage of a megakaryocyte precursor in the thrombocytopenia and absent radii (TAR) syndrome. *Blood* 2000;95:1633.

1191. Christensen CP, Ferguson RL. Lower extremity deformities associated with thrombocytopenia and absent radius syndrome. *Clin Orthop* 2000;375:202.

1192. Aldenhoff P, von Muhlendahl KE, Waldenmaier C. Das EEC-Syndrom: Fall-bericht und Uberlegungen zur pathogenese. *Monatsschr Kinderheilkd* 1978;126:575.

1193. Luthy DA, Mack L, Hirsch J, et al. Prenatal ultrasound diagnosis of thrombocytopenia with absent radii. *Am J Obstet Gynecol* 1981;141:350.

1194. Donnenfeld AE, Wiseman B, Lavi E, et al. Prenatal diagnosis of thrombocytopenia absent radius syndrome by ultrasound and cordocentesis. *Prenat Diagn* 1990;10:29.

1195. Labrune P, Pons JC, Khalil M, et al. Antenatal thrombocytopenia in three patients with TAR (thrombocytopenia with absent radii) syndrome. *Prenat Diagn* 1993;13:463.

1196. Christodoulou C, Werner B. A girl with 18-trisomy and thrombocytopenia. *Acta Genet* 1967;17:77.

1197. Rabinowitz JG, Moseley JE, Mitty HA, et al. Trisomy 18, esophageal atresia, anomalies of the radius and congenital hypoplastic thrombocytopenia. *Radiology* 1967;89:488.

1198. Becerra M, Moya F, Lacassie Y, et al. Clinico-pathological conference: a pre-term infant with multiple congenital anomalies. *Am J Med Genet* 1992;44:503.

1199. Eisenstein EM. Congenital amegakaryocytic thrombocytopenic purpura. *Clin Pediatr* 1966;5:143.

1200. Hoyeraal HM, Lamvik J, Moe PJ. Congenital hypoplastic thrombocytopenia and cerebral malformations in two brothers. *Acta Paediatr Scand* 1970;59:185.

1201. Gardner RJM, Morrison PS, Abbott GD. A syndrome of congenital thrombocytopenia with multiple malformations and neurologic dysfunction. *J Pediatr* 1983;102:600.

1202. Van Oostrom CG, Wilms RHH. Congenital thrombocytopenia, associated with raised concentrations of haemoglobin F. *Helv Paediatr Acta* 1978;33:59.

1203. Thompson AA, Nguyen LT. Amegakaryocytic thrombocytopenia and radio-ulnar synostosis are associated with HOXA11 mutation. *Nat Genet* 2000;26:397.

1204. Van den Oudenrijn S, Bruin M, Folman CC, et al. Mutations in the thrombopoietin receptor, Mpl, in children with congenital amegakaryocytic thrombocytopenia. *Br J Haematol* 2000;110:441.

1205. Ballmaier M, Germeshausen M, Schulze H, et al. *c-mpl* mutations are the cause of congenital amegakaryocytic thrombocytopenia. *Blood* 2001;97:139.

1206. Borge OJ, Ramsfjell V, Cui L, et al. Ability of early acting cytokines to directly promote survival and suppress apoptosis of human primitive CD34+CD38-bone marrow cells with multilineage potential at the single-cell level: key role of thrombopoietin. *Blood* 1997;90:2282.

1207. Lackner A, Basu O, Bierings M, et al. Haematopoietic stem cell transplantation for amegakaryocytic thrombocytopenia. *Br J Haematol* 2000;109:773.

1208. Yeşilipek MA, Hazar V, Küpesiz A, et al. Peripheral stem cell transplantation in a child with amegakaryocytic thrombocytopenia. *Bone Marrow Transplant* 2000;26:571.

1209. Fanconi G. Familial constitutional panmyelocytopathy: Fanconi's anemia (F.A.). *Semin Hematol* 1967;4:233.

1210. Gordon-Smith EC, Rutherford TR. Fanconi anaemia: constitutional, familial aplastic anaemia. *Baillieres Clin Haematol* 1989;2:139.

1211. Alter BP, Young NS. The bone marrow failure syndromes. In: Nathan DG, Orkin HS, eds. *Hematology of infancy and childhood*. Philadelphia: WB Saunders, 1998:237–335.

1212. Sieff CA, Nisbet-Brown E, Nathan DG. Congenital bone marrow failure syndromes. *Br J Haematol* 2000;111:30.

1213. Joenje H, Patel KJ. The emerging genetic and molecular basis of Fanconi anaemia. *Nat Rev Genet* 2001;2:446.

1214. De Boeck K, Degreef H, Verwilghen R, et al. Thrombocytopenia: first symptom in a patient with dyskeratosis congenita. *Pediatrics* 1981;67:898.

1215. Juneja HS, Elder FFB, Gardner FH. Abnormality of platelet size and T-lymphocyte proliferation in an autosomal recessive form of dyskeratosis congenita. *Eur J Haematol* 1987;39:306.

1216. Griffiths AD. Constitutional aplastic anemia: a family with a new X linked variety of amegakaryocytic thrombocytopenia. *J Med Genet* 1983;20:361.

1217. Thompson AA, Woodruff K, Feig SA, et al. Congenital thrombocytopenia and radio-ulnar synostosis: a new familial syndrome. *Br J Haematol* 2001;113:866.

1218. Dokal I, Ganly P, Riebero I, et al. Late onset bone marrow failure associated with proximal fusion of radius and ulna: a new syndrome. *Br J Haematol* 1989;71:277.

1219. Arias S, Penchaszadeh VB, Pinto-Cisternas J, et al. The IVIC syndrome: a new autosomal dominant complex pleiotropic syndrome with radial ray hypoplasia, hearing impairment, external ophthalmoplegia, and thrombocytopenia. *Am J Med Genet* 1980;6:25.

1220. Sammito V, Motta D, Capodieci G, et al. IVIC syndrome: report of a second family. *Am J Med Genet* 1988;29:875.

1221. Czeizel A, Göblyös P, Kodaj I. IVIC syndrome: report of a third family [Letter]. *Am J Med Genet* 1989;33:282.

1222. Gonzalez CH, Durkin-Stamm MV, Geimer NF, et al. The WT syndrome—a "new" autosomal dominant pleiotropic trait of radial/ulnar hypoplasia with high risk of bone marrow failure and/or leukemia. *Birth Defects Original Article Series* 1977;13:31.

1223. Law IP, Deveny A, Meiser RJ. Case report: familial thrombocytopenia in seven members of three generations. *Postgrad Med* 1978;63:136.

1224. Slichter SJ, Harker LA. Thrombocytopenia: mechanisms and management of defects in platelet production. *Clin Haematol* 1978;7:523.

1225. Najean Y, Lecompte T. Genetic thrombocytopenia with autosomal dominant transmission: a review of 54 cases. *Br J Haematol* 1990;74:203.

1226. Fabris F, Cordiano I, Salvan F, et al. Chronic isolated macrothrombocytopenia with autosomal dominant transmission: a morphological and qualitative platelet disorder. *Eur J Haematol* 1997;58:40.

1227. Jackson CW, Hutson NK, Steward SA, et al. The Wistar Furth rat: an animal model of hereditary macrothrombocytopenia. *Blood* 1988;71:1676.

1228. Leven RM, Tablin F. Megakaryocyte and platelet ultrastructure in the Wistar Furth rat. *Am J Pathol* 1988;132:417.

1229. Hegglin R. Gleichzeitige konstitutionelle Veranderungen an Neutrophilen und Thrombozyten. *Helv Med Acta* 1945;12:439.

1230. Greinacher A, Mueller-Eckhardt C. Hereditary types of thrombocytopenia with giant platelets and inclusion bodies in the leukocytes. *Blut* 1990;60:53.

1231. Greinacher A, Bux J, Kiefel V, et al. May-Hegglin anomaly: a rare cause of thrombocytopenia. *Eur J Pediatr* 1992;151:668.

1232. Noris P, Spedini P, Belletti S, et al. Thrombocytopenia, giant platelets, and leukocyte inclusion bodies (May-Hegglin anomaly): clinical and laboratory findings. *Am J Med* 1998;104:355.

1233. Seri M, Cusano R, Gangarossa S, et al. Mutations in MYH9 result in the May-Hegglin anomaly, and Fechtner and Sebastian syndromes. The May-Hegglin/Fechtner Syndrome Consortium. *Nat Genet* 2000;26:103.

1234. Kelley MJ, Jawien W, Ortel TL, et al. Mutation of MUH9, encoding non-muscle myosin heavy chain A, in May-Hegglin anomaly. *Nat Genet* 2000; 26:106.

1235. Peterson LC, Rao VK, Crosson JT, et al. Fechtner syndrome: a variant of Alport's syndrome with leukocyte inclusions and macrothrombocytopenia. *Blood* 1985;65:397.

1236. Heynen MJ, Blockmans D, Verwilghen RL, et al. Congenital macrothrombocytopenia, leucocyte inclusions, deafness and proteinuria: functional and electron microscopic observations on platelets and megakaryocytes. *Br J Haematol* 1988;70:441.

1237. Greinacher A, Nieuwenhuis HK, White JG. Sebastian platelet syndrome: a new variant of hereditary macrothrombocytopenia with leukocyte inclusions. *Blut* 1990;61:282.

1238. Young G, Luban NLC, White JG. Sebastian syndrome: case report and review of the literature. *Am J Hematol* 1999;61:62.

1239. Gershoni-Baruch R, Baruch Y, Viener A, et al. Fechtner syndrome: clinical and genetic aspects. *Am J Med Genet* 1988;31:357.

1240. Epstein CJ, Sahud MA, Piel CF, et al. Hereditary macrothrombocytopathia, nephritis and deafness. *Am J Med* 1972;52:299.

1241. Eckstein DJ, Filip DJ, Watts JC. Hereditary thrombocytopenia, deafness, and renal disease. *Ann Intern Med* 1975;82:639.

1242. Hansen MS, Behnke O, Tinggaard Pedersen N, et al. Megathrombocytopenia associated with glomerulonephritis, deafness and aortic cystic medianecrosis. *Scand J Haematol* 1978;21:197.

1243. Standen GR, Saunders J, Michael J, et al. Epstein's syndrome: case report and survey of the literature. *Postgrad Med J* 1987;63:573.

1244. Brodie HA, Chole RA, Griffin GC, et al. Macrothrombocytopenia and progressive deafness: a new genetic syndrome. *Am J Otol* 1991;13:507.

1245. Gilman AL, Sloand E, White JG, et al. A novel hereditary macrothrombocytopenia. *J Pediatr Hematol Oncol* 1995;17:296.

1246. Bernard J, Soulier JP. Sur une nouvelle variete de dystrophie thrombocytaire hemorrhagique congenitale. *Semin Hop Paris* 1948;24:3217.

1247. Drouin J, McGregor JL, Parmentier S, et al. Residual amounts of glycoprotein Ib concomitant with near-absence of glycoprotein IX in platelets of Bernard-Soulier patients. *Blood* 1988;72:1086.

1248. Ware J, Russell S, Ruggeri ZM. Generation and rescue of a murine model of platelet dysfunction: the Bernard-Soulier syndrome. *Proc Natl Acad Sci U S A* 2000;97:2803.

1249. Greinacher A, Potzsch B, Kiefel V, et al. Evidence that DDAVP transiently improves hemostasis in Bernard-Soulier syndrome independent of von Willebrand factor. *Ann Hematol* 1993;67:149.

1250. Aakhus AM, Stavem P, Hovig T, et al. Studies on patients with thrombocytopenia, giant platelets and a platelet membrane glycoprotein Ib with reduced amount of sialic acid. *Br J Haematol* 1990;74:320.

1251. Budarf LM, Konkle AB, Ludlow BL, et al. Identification of a patient with Bernard-Soulier syndrome and a deletion in the DiGeorge/Velo-cardio-facial chromosomal region in 22q11.2. *Hum Mol Genet* 1995;4:763.

1252. Ludlow LB, Schick BP, Budarf ML, et al. Identification of a mutation in a GATA binding site of the platelet glycoprotein Ibbeta promoter resulting in the Bernard-Soulier syndrome. *J Biol Chem* 1996;271:22076.

1253. Van Geet C, Devriendt K, Eyskens B, et al. Velocardiofacial syndrome patients with a heterozygous chromosome 22q11 deletion have giant platelets. *Pediatr Res* 1998;44:607.

1254. Nichols KE, Crispino JD, Poncz M, et al. Familial dyserythropoietic anaemia and thrombocytopenia due to an inherited mutation in GATA1. *Nat Genet* 2000;24:266.

1255. Freson K, Devriendt K, Matthijs G, et al. Platelet characteristics in patients with X-linked macrothrombocytopenia because of a novel *GATA1* mutation. *Blood* 2001;98:85.

1256. Yufu Y, Ideguchi H, Narishige T, et al. Familial macrothrombocytopenia associated with decreased glycosylation of platelet membrane glycoprotein IV. *Am J Hematol* 1990;33:271.

1257. Becker SP, Clavell AL, Beardsley DS. Giant platelets with abnormal surface glycoproteins: a new familial disorder associated with mitral valve insufficiency. *J Pediatr Hematol Oncol* 1998;20:69.

1258. Raccuglia G. Gray platelet syndrome: a variety of qualitative platelet disorder. *Am J Med* 1971;51:818.

1259. Drouin A, Favier R, Masse JM, et al. Newly recognized cellular abnormalities in the gray platelet syndrome. *Blood* 2001;98:1382.

1260. Smith MP, Cramer EM, Savidge GF. Megakaryocytes and platelets in alpha-granule disorders. *Baillieres Clin Haematol* 1997;10:125.

1261. Horne MK III, Alkins BR. Importance of PF4 in heparin-induced thrombocytopenia: confirmation with gray platelets [Letter]. *Blood* 1995;85:1408.

1262. Breton-Gorius J, Favier R, Guichard J, et al. A new congenital dysmegakaryopoietic thrombocytopenia (Paris-Trousseau) associated with giant platelet alpha-granules and chromosome 11 deletion at 11q23. *Blood* 1995;85:1805.

1263. Krishnamurti L, Neglia JP, Nagarajan R, et al. Paris-Trousseau syndrome platelets in a child with Jacobsen's syndrome. *Am J Hematol* 2001;66:295.

1264. Milton JG, Frojmovic MM. Shape-changing agents produce abnormally large platelets in a hereditary "giant platelets syndrome" (MPS). *J Lab Clin Med* 1979;93:154.

1265. Milton JG, Frojmovic MM, Tang SS, et al. Spontaneous platelet aggregation in a hereditary giant platelet syndrome (MPS). *Am J Pathol* 1984;114:336.

1266. Okita JR, Frojmovic MM, Kristopeit S, et al. Montreal platelet syndrome: a defect in calcium-activated neutral proteinase (calpain). *Blood* 1989;74:715.

1267. Smith TP, Dodds WJ, Tartaglia AP. Thrombasthenic-thrombopathic thrombocytopenia with giant, "Swiss-cheese" platelets: a case report. *Ann Intern Med* 1973;79:828.

1268. Green D, Ts'ao CH, Cohen I, et al. Haemorrhagic thrombocytopathy associated with dilatation of the platelet–membrane complex. *Br J Haematol* 1981;48:595.

1269. Maldonado JE. "Swiss-cheese" platelets [Letter]. *Ann Intern Med* 1974;81:860.

1270. Cullum C, Cooney DP, Schrier SL. Familial thrombocytopenia thrombocytopathy. *Br J Haematol* 1967;13:147.

1271. Kurstjens R, Bolt C, Vossen M, et al. Familial thrombopathic thrombocytopenia. *Br J Haematol* 1968;15:305.

1272. Weiss HJ, Vicic WJ, Lages BA, et al. Isolated deficiency of platelet procoagulant activity. *Am J Med* 1979;67:206.

1273. Solum NO. Procoagulant expression in platelets and defects leading to clinical disorders. *Arterioscler Thromb Vasc Biol* 1999;19:2841.

1274. Stormorken H, Holmsen H, Sund R, et al. Studies on the hemostatic defect in a complicated syndrome: an inverse Scott syndrome platelet membrane abnormality? *Thromb Haemost* 1995;74:1244.

1275. Greaves M, Pickering C, Martin J, et al. A new familial "giant platelet syndrome" with structural, metabolic and functional abnormalities of platelets due to a primary megakaryocyte defect. *Br J Haematol* 1987;65:429.

1276. Drachman JG, Jarvik GP, Mehaffey MG. Autosomal dominant thrombocytopenia: incomplete megakaryocyte differentiation and linkage to human chromosome 10. *Blood* 2000;96:118.

1277. Iolascon A, Perrotta S, Amendola G, et al. Familial dominant thrombocytopenia: clinical, biologic, and molecular studies. *Pediatr Res* 1999;46:548.

1278. Savoia A, Del Vecchio M, Totaro A, et al. An autosomal dominant thrombocytopenia gene maps to chromosomal region 10p. *Am J Hum Genet* 1999;65:1401.

1279. Sheth NK, Prankerd TAJ. Inherited thrombocytopenia with thrombasthenia. *J Clin Pathol* 1968;21:154.

1280. Danielsson L, Jelf E, Lundkvist L. A new family with inherited thrombocytopenia. *Scand J Haematol* 1980;24:427.

1281. Tonelli R, Strippoli P, Grossi A, et al. Hereditary thrombocytopenia due to reduced platelet production: report on two families and mutational screening of the thrombopoietin receptor gene (c-mpl). *Thromb Haemost* 2000;83: 931.

1282. Dowton SB, Beardsley D, Jamison D, et al. Studies of a familial platelet disorder. *Blood* 1985;65:557.

1283. Gerrard JM, Israels ED, Bishop AJ, et al. Inherited platelet-storage pool deficiency associated with a high incidence of acute myeloid leukaemia. *Br J Haematol* 1991;79:246.

1284. Ho CY, Otterud B, Legare RD, et al. Linkage of a familial platelet disorder with a propensity to develop myeloid malignancies to human chromosome 21q22.1-22.2. *Blood* 1996;87:5218.

1285. Arepally G, Rebbeck TR, Song W, et al. Evidence for genetic homogeneity in a familial platelet disorder with predisposition to acute myelogenous leukemia (FPD/AML) [Letter]. *Blood* 1998;92:2600.

1286. Song W-J, Sullivan MG, Legare RD, et al. Haploinsufficiency of CBFA2 causes familial thrombocytopenia with propensity to develop acute myelogenous leukaemia. *Nat Genet* 1999;23:166.

1287. Tracy PB, Giles AR, Mann KG, et al. Factor V (Quebec): a bleeding diathesis associated with a qualitative platelet factor V deficiency. *J Clin Invest* 1984; 74:1221.

1288. Hayward CPM, Rivard GE, Kane WH, et al. An autosomal dominant, qualitative platelet disorder associated with multimerin deficiency, abnormalities in platelet factor V, thrombospondin, von Willebrand factor, and fibrinogen and an epinephrine aggregation defect. *Blood* 1996;87:4967.

1289. Kahr WHA, Zheng S, Sheth PM, et al. Platelets from patients with the Quebec platelet disorder contain and secrete abnormal amounts of urokinase-type plasminogen activator. *Blood* 2001;98:257.

1290. Weiss HJ, Meyer D, Rabinowitz R, et al. Pseudo-von Willebrand's disease: an intrinsic platelet defect with aggregation by unmodified human factor VIII/von Willebrand factor and enhanced adsorption of its high-molecular-weight multimers. *N Engl J Med* 1982;306:326.

1291. Giles AR, Hoogendoorn H, Benford K. Type IIB von Willebrand's disease presenting as thrombocytopenia during pregnancy. *Br J Haematol* 1987;67: 349.

1292. Hultin MB, Sussman II. Postoperative thrombocytopenia in type IIB von Willebrand disease. *Am J Hematol* 1990;33:64.

1293. Donner M, Holmberg L, Nilsson IM. Type IIB von Willebrand's disease with probable autosomal recessive inheritance and presenting as thrombocytopenia in infancy. *Br J Haematol* 1987;66:349.

1294. Holmberg L, Nilsson IM, Borge L, et al. Platelet aggregation induced by 1-desamino-8-D-arginine vasopressin (DDAVP) in type IIB von Willebrand's disease. *N Engl J Med* 1983;309:816.

1295. Thompson AR, Wood WG, Stamatoyannopoulos G. X-linked syndrome of platelet dysfunction, thrombocytopenia, and imbalanced globin chain synthesis with hemolysis. *Blood* 1997;50:303.

1296. Raskind WH, Niakan KK, Wolff J, et al. Mapping of a syndrome of X-linked thrombocytopenia with thalassemia to band Xp11-12: further evidence of genetic heterogeneity of X-linked thrombocytopenia. *Blood* 2000;95:2262.

1297. Aldrich RA, Steinberg AG, Campbell DC. Pedigree demonstrating a sex-linked recessive condition characterized by draining ears, eczematoid dermatitis and bloody diarrhea. *Pediatrics* 1954;13:133.

1298. Sullivan KE, Mullen CA, Blaese RM, et al. A multi-institutional survey of the Wiskott–Aldrich syndrome. *J Pediatr* 1994;125:876.

1299. Thrasher AJ, Kinnon C. The Wiskott-Aldrich syndrome. *Clin Exp Immunol* 2000;120:2.

1300. Ochs HD, Slichter SJ, Harker LA, et al. The Wiskott-Aldrich syndrome: studies of lymphocytes, granulocytes, and platelets. *Blood* 1980;55:243.

1301. Derry JM, Ochs HD, Francke U. Isolation of a novel gene mutated in Wiskott–Aldrich syndrome. *Cell* 1994;78:635.

1302. Haddad E, Cramer E, Riviere C, et al. The thrombocytopenia of Wiskott–Aldrich syndrome is not related to a defect in proplatelet formation. *Blood* 1999;94:509.

1303. Nathan DG. Splenectomy in the Wiskott-Aldrich syndrome. *N Engl J Med* 1980;302:916.

1304. Krivit W, Yunis E, White JG. Platelet survival studies in Aldrich syndrome. *Pediatrics* 1966;37:339.

1305. Holmberg L, Gustavii B, Jonsson A. A prenatal study of fetal platelet count and size with application to fetus at risk for Wiskott-Aldrich syndrome. *J Pediatr* 1983;102:773.

1306. Corash L, Shafer B, Blaese M. Platelet-associated immunoglobulin, platelet size, and the effect of splenectomy in the Wiscott-Aldrich syndrome. *Blood* 1985;65:1439.

1307. Lum LG, Tubergen DG, Corash L, et al. Splenectomy in the management of the thrombocytopenia of the Wiskott-Aldrich syndrome. *N Engl J Med* 1980;302:892.

1308. Mullen CA, Anderson KD, Blaese RM. Splenectomy and/or bone marrow transplantation in the management of the Wiskott-Aldrich syndrome: long-term follow-up of 62 cases. *Blood* 1993;82:2961.

1309. Parkman R, Rappeport J, Geha R, et al. Complete correction of the Wiskott-Aldrich syndrome by allogeneic bone-marrow transplantation. *N Engl J Med* 1978;298:921.

1310. Vestermark B, Vestermark S. Familial sex-linked thrombocytopenia. *Acta Paediatr Scand* 1964;53:365.

1311. Canales L, Mauer AM. Sex-linked hereditary thrombocytopenia as a variant of Wiskott-Aldrich syndrome. *N Engl J Med* 1967;277:899.

1312. Murphy S, Oski FA, Naiman JL, et al. Platelet size and kinetics in hereditary and acquired thrombocytopenia. *N Engl J Med* 1972;286:499.

1313. Weiden PL, Blaese RM. Hereditary thrombocytopenia: relation to Wiskott-Aldrich syndrome with special reference to splenectomy. *J Pediatr* 1972; 80:226.

1314. Donner M, Schwartz M, Carlsson KU, et al. Hereditary X-linked thrombocytopenia maps to the same chromosomal region as the Wiskott-Aldrich syndrome. *Blood* 1988;72:1849.

1315. Villa A, Notarangelo L, Macchi P, et al. X-linked thrombocytopenia and Wiskott-Aldrich syndrome are allelic diseases with mutations in the WASP gene. *Nat Genet* 1995;9:414.

1316. Qasim W, Gilmour KC, Heath S, et al. Protein assays for diagnosis of Wiskott–Aldrich syndrome and X-linked thrombocytopenia. *Br J Haematol* 2001;113:861.

1317. Zhu Q, Watanabe C, Liu T, et al. Wiskott–Aldrich syndrome/X-linked thrombocytopenia: WASP gene mutations, protein expression, and phenotype. *Blood* 1997;90:2680.

1318. Knox-Macaulay HHM, Bashawri L, Davies KE. X linked recessive thrombocytopenia. *J Med Genet* 1993;30:968.

1319. Heiss NS, Knight SW, Vulliamy TJ, et al. X-linked dyskeratosis congenital is caused by mutations in a highly conserved gene with putative nucleolar functions. *Nat Genet* 1998;19:32.

1320. FitzPatrick DR, Strain L, Thomas AE, et al. Neurogenic chronic idiopathic intestinal pseudo-obstruction, patent ductus arteriosus, and thrombocytopenia segregating as an X linked recessive disorder. *J Med Genet* 1997;34:666.

1321. Oda A, Ochs HD. Wiskott–Aldrich syndrome protein and platelets. *Immunol Rev* 2000;178:111.

CHAPTER 33

Life of the Blood Platelet

John H. Hartwig and Joseph E. Italiano, Jr.

Platelets are reproducible, anucleate, cytoplasmic particles absolutely required for normal blood hemostasis. After vascular injury, platelets work together in concert to form a plug on the vessel wall that prevents further leakage. In humans, 10^{11} platelets must be released each day from megakaryocytes to maintain the normal platelet count of 2 to 3×10^8/mL, as an equivalent number of senescent platelets are removed daily by the macrophages of the liver and spleen. This chapter discusses the structure, organization, and function of the resting platelet and how this structure is altered after platelet activation. It also discusses new aspects of platelet production and death.

STRUCTURE OF THE PLATELET IN CIRCULATION

Originally believed to be little more than amorphic bags of membrane-bound cytoplasm, platelets are highly structured subcellular fragments that are released from megakaryocytes. The fundamental structure of the resting platelet is invariable, although platelets are heterogeneous in size as a population, due to small variations in construction or to changes in size as they age. Platelets have discoid shapes with flat, featureless surfaces that are interrupted only by numerous pitlike openings. These demarcate openings to an anastomosing internal system of membrane-bound tubes called either the *open canalicular system* (OCS) or *the surface-connected canalicular system* (SCCS). The OCS permeates the cytoplasmic space of the platelet and functions both as a reservoir of plasma membrane to be used when the cell activates, as these cells lack external redundant membrane, and as a conduit to the external world into which the intracellular cytoplasmic granules release their contents after activation.

A small, thin zone of cytoplasm (Fig. 33-1) separates the plasma membrane of the resting platelet from a marginal microtubule coil and the general intracellular space, which contains all inclusion bodies. Although this peripheral zone appears featureless when thin sections of resting platelets are viewed in the electron microscope, specialized techniques that reveal cytoskeletal elements show that this zone is filled with a planar membrane skeleton (Fig. 33-1B). Beneath this zone sits a microtubule coil, followed by cytoplasmic space replete with filaments of actin that embed granules, organelles, the OCS, and other specialized membrane systems, such as smooth endoplasmic reticulum.

INTRACELLULAR COMPONENTS OF THE RESTING PLATELET

Granules

One of the main functions of activated platelets is to recruit other bloodborne cells to areas of vascular damage. The enlistment of additional blood cells is accomplished by the release of preformed mediators, packaged in intracellular granules that initiate secondary hemostatic interactions, and through the expression of a "sticky" apical surface after the platelets adhere. In the resting platelet, granules that contain these mediators sit juxtaposed to one another and near the membranes of the OCS. The release reaction of platelet granules differs from that of other cells, as these granules rarely fuse with the plasma membrane and instead exocytose into the OCS. One accepted reason for this difference is that, in the activated platelet, granules have difficulty approaching the plasma membrane of the activated cell, because actin assembly densely fills the cortical cytoplasm with filaments. This assembly reaction compresses the cellular granules and organelles into the cell center, where they can release only by fusing with the OCS. Actin filaments thus form an extensive barrier that prevents granule movements to, and fusion with, the plasma membrane.

Platelets have three types of granules: α, dense, and lysosomal (Table 33-1). α-Granules, 200 to 500 nm in size, are the most abundant in the cell and contain proteins that enhance the adhesive process, promote cell–cell interactions, and stimulate vascular repair. Critical molecules for adhesion include fibrinogen, fibronectin, vitronectin, von Willebrand's factor (vWf), and thrombospondin. Growth factors contained in the α-granules are necessary to stimulate the growth of endothelial cells at areas of erosion and for the normal maintenance of endothelial integrity within the vascular system. One symptom of thrombocytopenic patients is their tendency to develop leaky vessels because of the loss of this cross-talk mechanism between platelets and endothelial cells.

P-selectin, vWf receptor (vWfR), and integrin molecules are also embedded in the membranes of the α-granules. Of all of these molecules, only P-selectin is not expressed on the surface of the resting platelet. However, once inserted into the plasma membrane, P-selectin can recruit neutrophils through the counter-receptor, the P-selectin glycoprotein (GP) ligand. *Dense granules* (or *dense bodies*), 250 nm in size, identified in electron micrographs by virtue of their electron-dense cores, contain small molecules and function primarily to recruit additional platelets to sites of injury. Critical platelet-activating components released from the dense granules on cell activation include serotonin and adenosine diphosphate (ADP). ADP is a potent platelet agonist, stimulating platelet shape change, the granule release reaction, and aggregation.

Lysosomes

Less obvious in sections but identifiable after specific cytologic staining procedures are lysosomes and peroxisomes. Platelet peroxisomes are small organelles that contain the enzyme catalase. Lysosomes are also small in number compared to their counterparts in nucleated cells. They contain, however, the usual assortment of degradative enzymes, including acid phosphatases, aryl sulfatase, β-glucuronidase, cathepsin, and β-galactosidase. These organelles function in the degradation of materials ingested by pinocytosis or phagocytosis, and recent studies have shown that the contents of lysosomes can also be exocytosed by the cell.

Organelles

Platelets contain a few mitochondria, which are easily identified under the electron microscope by their internal system of membrane cisternae. These provide a necessary energy source for the platelet, and mitochondria inhibitors adversely affect specific platelet functions.

MEMBRANE COMPARTMENTS

Open Canalicular System

The OCS is an extensive system of internal membrane conduits. One function of the OCS is to serve as a passageway to the outside world, into which granular contents are released. The second function of the OCS is to serve as a reservoir of plasma membrane, membrane receptors, and proteins. For example, approximately 30% of the thrombin receptors are localized in the OCS of the resting cell, awaiting movement to the surface of the activated cells. Membrane receptors are also removed from the cell surface into this membrane reservoir, a process that has been termed *down-regulation*, after cell activation. The best-studied surface GP in this regard is the vWfR. After activation of platelets in suspension, a centrifugal flow of surface GPIbαβ/IX/V into the cell center and OCS ensues. Although contiguous with the plasma membrane, not all proteins on the cell surface can enter the OCS. Factors controlling movement into the OCS remain to be defined but depend on the actin cytoskeleton. Entry restriction, however, occurs at the necks of the OCS infoldings; for example, immunoglobulin G (IgG) molecules that label both surface and OCS proteins fail to penetrate into the OCS. The third function of the OCS is to serve as a source of redundant plasma membrane for cell spreading. OCS membrane is initially disgorged to the surface after cell activation. When cells are activated in solution, much

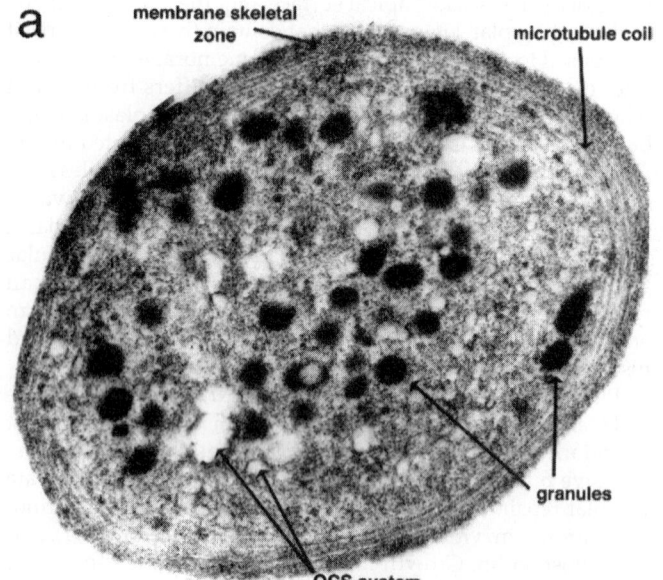
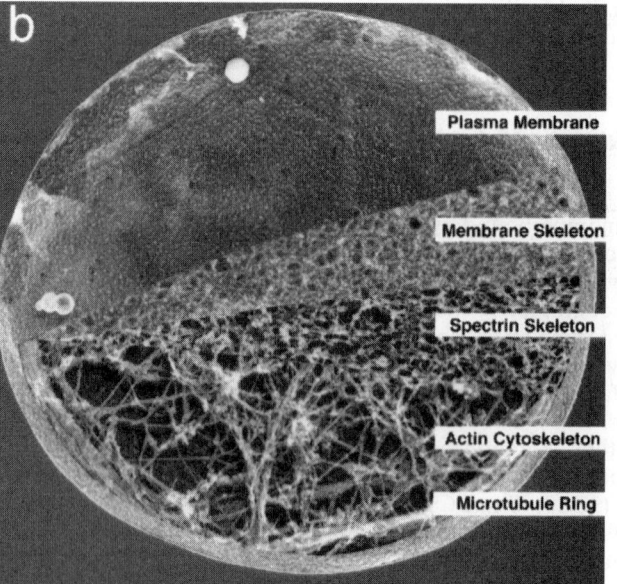

Figure 33-1. Structure of the resting platelet. **A:** Electron micrograph of a resting platelet. This platelet was sectioned through its flat axis. This cut plane shows the coiling of the microtubule around the cell periphery in this axis. The microtubule coil is separated from the plasma membrane by a 50- to 100-nm–thick rim of cytoplasm. Below the microtubule coil is the general cytoplasmic space of the platelet. The cytoplasm embeds mitochondria, granules, and the other membrane systems of the cell. OCS, open canalicular system. **B:** Structure of the resting platelet cytoskeleton. The cytoskeleton is revealed by removing membranes with detergents, followed by fixation, freezing at liquid helium temperatures, freeze drying, and metal coating. This figure is a composite of micrographs taken from different specimens. The resting cell has a surface that is interrupted only by the OCS infoldings of the plasma membrane. These appear as holes in these preparations. A fibrous membrane skeleton that is directly coupled to the underlying actin filaments supports the plasma membrane. The dense form of the membrane skeleton retains the bulk of associated platelet surface glycoproteins. When stripped of these glycoproteins, the fundamental structure of the membrane skeleton is revealed. It is composed of 200-nm–long spectrin strands that are interconnected by actin filaments. These filaments arrive at the plasma membrane from the cell interior, where they are cross-linked into a rigid network by filamin, α-actinin, and other proteins. (*continued*)

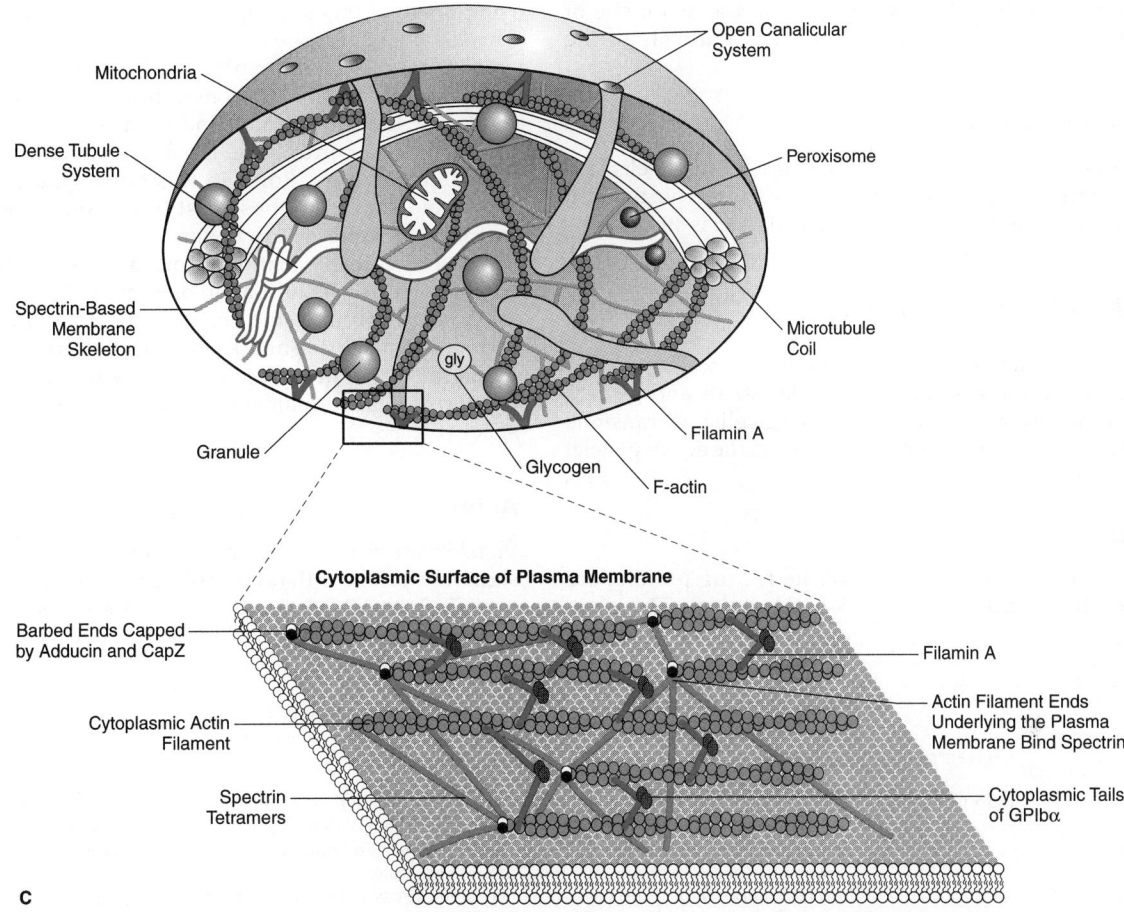

Figure 33-1. (*continued*) **C:** Diagram illustrating the key features of the resting platelet cytoskeleton. The arrangement and connections between the various cytoskeletal elements are depicted. Actin filaments, originating in the cytoplasmic space, arrive and end near the plasma membrane. The cytoplasmic side of the plasma membrane is coated with a two-dimensional lattice of spectrin. Spectrin molecules bind to these ends and thereby link the membrane skeleton to filamin A–GPIbα connections.

of this membrane is subsequently reabsorbed into the remnants of the OCS.

Endoplasmic Reticulum/Dense Tubular System

The dense tubular system (DTS) is a membranous compartment that is randomly woven through the cytoplasmic volume. It is believed to be analogous in function to the smooth endoplasmic reticular system and serves as the major calcium storage system in the platelet. The membranes forming the DTS have inwardly directed Ca^{2+}-pumps [Ca^{2+}/Mg^{2+} adenosine triphosphatase (ATPase)]. Their pumps maintain cytosolic calcium concentrations in the nanomolar range in resting cells. Calcium pumped from the cytoplasm is bound in the cavity of the DTS by the calcium-binding protein, calreticulin. The DTS also contains ligand-responsive calcium gates. Calcium is released by the soluble messenger inositol 1,4,5-trisphosphate (IP_3), which binds to a special receptor in

TABLE 33-1. Platelet Granule Contents

Protein	α-Granule	Dense Granule
Adhesion—soluble	Fibrinogen, fibronectin, vibronectin, thrombospondin, vWf	—
Adhesion—membrane bound	P-selectin, vWfR, αIIbβ3, CD36, CD9	P-selectin, granulophysin
Procoagulants	Factor V, PF4	—
Enzymes and inhibitors	Plasminogen, α_2-antiplasmin	—
Growth factors	PDGF, TGF-α, TGF-β, GGF, ECGF	—
Activating agents	Guanine nucleotides	ADP, ATP, serotonin, guanine nucleotides
Bactericidal	β-Lysin	—
Other	Mg^{2+}	Mg^{2+}, Ca^{2+}, pyrophosphate

ADP, adenosine diphosphate; ATP, adenosine triphosphate; CD, cluster of differentiation; ECGF, endothelial cell growth factor; GGF, glial growth factor; PDGF, platelet-derived growth factor; PF4, platelet factor 4; TGF-α, transforming growth factor α; TGF-β, transforming growth factor β; vWfR, von Willebrand's factor receptor.

the membrane of the DTS. The DTS is also the major site of prostaglandin and thromboxane (TXA$_2$) synthesis in the platelet.

Cytoplasmic Inclusions

The only major cytoplasmic inclusions observed in platelets are glycogen particles. This material serves as a reservoir that can be mobilized to release glucose when the platelet is stimulated.

CYTOSKELETAL COMPONENTS

Resting blood platelets contain well-defined cytoskeletons. In the resting cell, this system of molecular struts and girders maintains the discoid shape of the resting cell and transmits mechanical forces to the plasma membrane in the active platelet to confer shape change.

Spectrin

The plasma membrane and OCS of the resting platelet are supported by an elaborate cytoskeletal system. The main component of this system is a planar spectrin network (1–3). This network is composed of spectrin strands cross-linked by actin filaments (2). It laminates the cytoplasmic surface of both the plasma and OCS membrane systems. In this network, the spectrin strands bind to the ends of actin filaments to assemble a continuous meshlike structure beneath the plasma membrane. Pores in this network are triangular in shape and similar to those first described in the erythrocyte membrane skeleton. However, the organization of actin is somewhat different than that found in the erythrocyte (4–6). Instead of binding short actin oligomers, the platelet spectrin strands are bound to the ends of long actin filaments. These actin filaments arrive at the cytoplasmic surface of the plasma membrane from the cytoplasm, where they are the struts of a rigid, cross-linked filament network that fills the cytoplasmic space (Fig. 33-1).

Actin

Platelets are rich in actin and in actin-associated proteins and signaling proteins that control actin assembly and architecture (7). Table 33-2 lists the proteins associated with the plate-

TABLE 33-2. Platelet Cytoskeletal and Cytoskeletal Signaling Proteins

Protein	Concentration	Function	References
Actin	0.55 mM	42-kd protein that reversibly assembles into polarized filaments. In platelets and other cells, assembly occurs only at the end of the filament having the higher affinity for actin monomer (the barbed end of S1-labeled filaments). The barbed end is capped, except when the cell is experiencing net filament assembly.	—
Filamin A, filamin B	3.0 μM, 0.3 μM	560-kd homodimeric actin cross-linking protein. Cross-links actin filaments in the platelet cytoplasm into rigid networks. Attaches the cytoplasmic tails of GPIbα to underlying actin filaments. Two isoforms are expressed in platelets. Molar ratio of filamin A to F-actin is 6:1 in the resting platelet.	10–12, 69, 265, 266
α-Actinin	3 μM	200-kd homodimeric protein that cross-links actin filaments into loose bundles. Subunits assemble into small bipolar rods, 35 nm in length. α-Actinin has been reported to bind to the cytoplasmic tails of the β1 integrins.	9, 267–274
α,γ Adducing	3 μM	Barbed end capping protein that caps many of the ends of actin filaments in the resting cell. Adducin is released from the cytoskeleton after platelet activation. Negatively regulated by phosphorylation, polyphosphoinositides, and calcium-calmodulin.	Barkalow in prep
ARP2/3 complex	9 μM	Complex of seven polypeptides, including the actin-related proteins 2 and 3 and five novel components: ARC16, ARC20, ARC21, ARC34, and ARC41. Approximately 30% of the Arp2/3 complex is bound to the resting cytoskeleton. Activation I increases the amount of Arp2/3 in the cytoskeleton to 70–80% of the total. Positively regulated by polyphosphoinositides, the small GTPase cdc42, and the WASp family of proteins.	Falet in prep
β4-Thymosin	0.5 mM	5-kd (44 amino acids) constitutive actin monomer binding protein present at equal molar ratio to actin. Binding affinity (k$_d$) for ATP-actin monomer of 0.2–1.0 μM.	44–46, 275, 276
capZ	5 μM	Heterodimer composed of 36- and 32-kd subunits. Constitutively binds to the barbed ends of actin filaments. In the resting cell, capZ caps many of the barbed filament ends.	51, 53
cdc42	0.2 μM	Small GTPase that binds to the cytoskeleton of the activated and/or aggregated platelet. Is believed to stimulate the growth of filopodia and activate the WASp family of proteins.	104, 115, 116, 277
Cofilin	30 μM	Small actin binding protein (20 kd) that accelerates the depolymerization rate of actin filaments by accelerating the dissociation of monomers from the pointed filament end. Preferentially binds to ADP-actin. Negatively regulated by phosphorylation and ppls.	278–280
Dynein	?	Large microtubule-associated motor protein known to power microtubule sliding and granule movement over microtubules.	—
Dystrophin (skeleton)	?	Large, elongated protein believed to cross-link actin filaments and link them to membranes. It has been identified by immunohistochemistry as a component of the resting membrane skeleton. Its function is unknown. Present at very low concentrations.	281
Flightless 1	0.5 μM	Barbed end capping protein. Participates in capping the filaments of the resting cell and helps cap filaments assembled after cell stimulation.	282
Gelsolin	5 μM	80-kd calcium-activated actin filament severing protein. Gelsolin activation converts the resting discoid shape into a spheric shape. Is negatively regulated by ppls and LPA.	56, 60, 68, 283
GPIbαβ/IX/V	6 μM	Multicomponent membrane receptor for vWf that is also a critical structural component of the resting cytoskeleton. The link between actin filaments and the α-chain of this receptor stabilizes the resting spectrin-based membrane skeleton.	13, 15, 265, 266

(continued)

TABLE 33-2. (*continued*)

Protein	Concentration	Function	References
$\alpha_{IIb}\beta_3$	6–12 μM	Major platelet integrin receptor. This receptor links to the cytoskeleton of the activated cell and is used to mechanically connect the actin cytoskeleton to matrix components.	125
MARCKS	?	PKC substrate recently identified in platelets. Has been postulated to function in granule secretion.	284
Moesin	?	Protein of the erzin family that is involved in the connection of actin filaments to membrane primarily in filopodia.	285, 286
Myosin II	3 μM	500-kd hexameric contractile protein (2 × 200 kd heavy chain, 2 × 20 and 2 × 15 kd light chains). Reversibly assembles into bipolar filaments, 300 nm in length, containing 28 myosin molecules. Component of the membrane skeleton of the resting cell. Required for the centralization of GPIb/IX on the surface of the activated cell.	130
Profilin	20–50 μM	Actin monomer sequestration and ATP-charging protein for actin. Actin interaction inhibited by phosphoinositides.	287–290
Spectrin	0.5 μM	Large elongated tetrameric protein that forms the strands of the membrane skeleton.	1, 2, 291
Talin	3 μM	Adhesion site protein involved in attaching integrin receptors to the cytoskeleton. Has been reported to directly bind actin.	126, 292–294
Tensin	?	Actin capping protein of adhesion sites. Expressed at low abundance in platelets. Function ill-defined.	295
Tropomyosin	?	Protein that binds along actin filaments. Each molecule binds along six actin subunits of the filament. Amplifies myosin II actin-activated ATPase activity. Other functions unclear in nonmuscle cells.	—
α,β Tubulin		Tubulin dimers reversibly assemble into a single long microtubule coil in the resting platelet. This microtubule coil is reorganized into many microtubules after activation. β1 is the major tubulin β-chain isoform and the most diverse. Deletion of β1 from mice leads to altered resting morphology.	251
VASP	?	50-kd protein component of the spatial actin monomer delivery system. Is believed to self-associate into tetramers. Each subunit has four profilin binding sites. VASP binds to vinculin and zyxin.	296–300
Vinculin	?	130-kd protein of adhesion sites. Although its precise function is unclear, vinculin is involved in attaching actin filaments to adhesion sites. Vinculin contains a cryptic actin binding site in its N-terminal head domain. It also has PPI and VASP binding sites.	301
WASP	?	Protein mutated or lacking in myeloid cells from patients having Wiskott-Aldrich syndrome. Is known to bind the small GTPase Cdc42. WASp contains a pH domain and polyproline rich domains.	111, 113, 114, 302–304
WIP	?	Recently identified protein that is directly associated with WASp. Highly enriched in polyproline domains.	305, 306
Zyxin	?	Protein of adhesion sites. Contains binding site for VASP.	296, 307, 308
14-3-3		Small adaptor protein associated with the cytoplasmic tails of the vWf receptor. Has been reported to be involved in actin assembly in platelets stimulated with collagen.	309, 310
Calpain		Calpain cleavage of cytoskeletal proteins has been suggested to be involved in certain aspects of platelet shape change.	311–314
GEFs		Critical intermediates between trimeric GTPases and small GTPases, although the precise proteins remain to be identified. May include VAV, SOS, Trio, and others.	315–320
PI-3 kinase		Family of enzymes that phosphorylate phosphoinositides in the D3 position. Platelets have at least two forms of this enzyme. One is regulated by trimeric G proteins (βγ-p110). The other is activated by interacting with tyrosine kinase receptors (p85/p110). Rho has been reported to also activate the latter form of the kinase.	100, 321–325
PI-5 kinase Iα		Kinase that phosphorylates PI_4P in the D3 position. This enzyme has been shown to bind to both the rac and rho GTPases. This kinase is also activated by phosphatidic acid.	107, 108, 326
Pleckstrin		Adaptor protein involved in the coupling of different signaling cascades in the platelet. Contains two pH domains. These domains bind either PIP_2 or G-protein subunits. On platelet activation, pleckstrin is phosphorylated in three positions by PKCs.	98–103, 118, 321, 327, 328
rac	2–3 μM	Small GTPase that directs the assembly of lamellipods and ruffles. In platelets, this protein leads to the activation of PI-5 kinase.	104
rala		Small GTPase that binds to filamin A in platelets and is involved in the formation of filopodia.	329, 330
rap1b		Small GTPase involved in either the regulation of GPIIb/IIIa or connecting this receptor to other signaling cascades.	331
rho		Small GTPase that initiates stress fiber and adhesion site formation.	123
Trimeric G proteins		Critical family of signaling proteins that couples serpentine receptors to cellular functions.	78–81

ADP, adenosine diphosphate; ATP, adenosine triphosphate; GEF, guanine exchange factor; GP, glycoprotein; GTPase, guanosine triphosphatase; LPA, lysophosphatidic acid; PI, phosphoinositide; PI_4P, phosphatidylinositol 4-phosphate; $PI_{4,5}P_2$, phosphatidylinositol 4,5-bisphosphate; PKC, protein kinase C; PPI, polyphosphoinositide; VASP, vasodilator-stimulated phosphoprotein; vWf, von Willebrand's factor; WASp, Wiskott-Aldrich Syndrome protein.

let cytoskeleton. The concentration of actin in the resting cell is 0.55 mM, of which 40% is assembled into filaments, sufficient to assemble approximately 2000 to 5000 filaments/platelet, each 1 μm in length. Underlying the cytoplasmic surface of the plasma membrane is a planar network assembled from approximately 2000 spectrin strands. The molar ratio of spectrin to actin filaments is, therefore, near equality. Each spectrin molecule, 200 nm in length, is a bipolar assembly of two αβ-dimers. Elongated dimers are composed of antiparallel and intertwined α- and β-chains that have self-association and actin-binding sites on opposing ends. Spectrin interconnects into a network by binding to the ends of the underlying

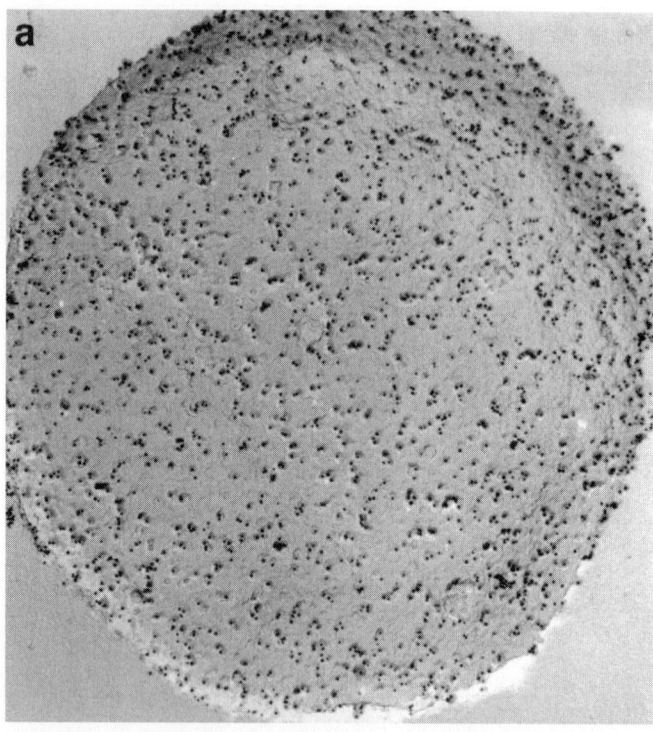

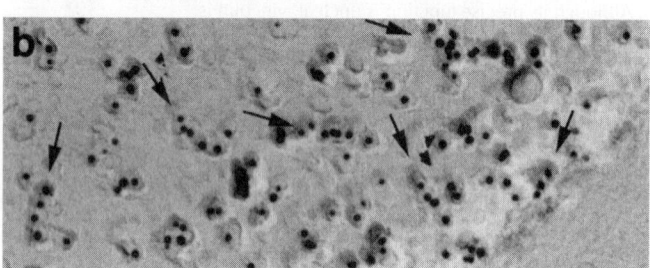

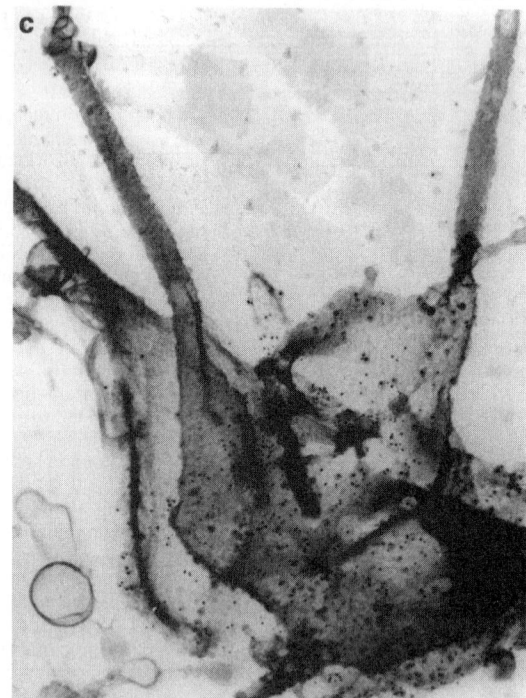

Figure 33-2. Distribution of GPIbα on the surface of resting and active platelets. **A,B:** Distribution of GPIbα on the surface of a resting platelet. The von Willebrand's factor receptor (vWfR) is linearly arrayed on the surface of the platelet at rest. Anti-GPIbα–coated 10-nm gold particles label the vWfR on the cell surface. **B:** High magnification showing the alignment of the receptor into rows (*arrows*). Because the vWfR is connected to actin via filamin, this arrangement reflects the organization of actin filaments beneath the plasma membrane. **C:** Distribution of GPIbα on the surface of the active platelet. GPIbα is restricted from filopods and lamellae.

actin filaments that extend from the cytoplasm of the cell, where they are interconnected into a rigid network by the major actin filament cross-linking proteins of the platelet, filamin and α-actinin (8,9). Both proteins are expressed at 5 μM concentrations, considerably higher levels than those of spectrin, making each sixfold in excess of the number of actin filaments. At least two isoforms of filamin are expressed in platelets: filamin A [X chromosome, also called *ABP-280* (10,11)] and filamin B [chromosome 3 (12)]. Filamin A, however, accounts for 95% of the filamin in the platelet. In addition to linking actin filaments together, filamin molecules also attach the actin network to the plasma membrane. Filamin is an elongated bipolar dimer in solution. Each subunit has a binding site for actin at its amino terminus and a self-association site at its carboxyl terminus. The binding site for the α-chain of the GPIbαβ/IX/V complex that binds vWf is located between repeats 17 and 20, near the carboxyl end of the subunit (13). Biochemical experiments have shown that the bulk of filamin is stably complexed to GPIbα in the platelet (14,15). This interaction not only links the vWfR to actin, but also rigidifies the spectrin membrane skeleton as the filamin-GPIbα links sit in the pores of the spectrin network, where they restrict its lateral movement. Hence, this laminate of the membrane skeleton and cytoplasmic actin network confines the movement of membrane GPs and serves as a scaffold onto which membrane proteins and cytoplasmic signaling proteins attach. Attachment of GPIbα to actin filaments by filamin

aligns the vWfR into linear rows on the surface of the resting platelet (Fig. 33-2).

Tubulin

Perhaps the most distinguishing cytoskeletal feature of the resting platelet is its marginal microtubule coil (16). Like actin, tubulin dimers reversibly assemble into microtubule polymers under physiologic ionic conditions, and in the resting platelet, tubulin is equally divided between polymer and monomer fractions. Microtubules are long, stiff, hollow polymers that transmit the force for movement in many cellular functions, including organelle transport and mitotic chromosome segregation. The microtubule ring in the resting platelet is formed from a single tubule polymer that grows to a length of approximately 100 μm and is rolled 8 to 12 times to fit inside the boundary of the platelet (17–19). Platelets also express the microtubule motor proteins, kinesin and dynein, which bind to microtubules to exert force (20,21). Although it has been suggested (as discussed in Cytoskeletal Components) that the primary function of the microtubule coil is to create and maintain the discoid shape of the platelet (18), microtubules may serve as tracks to shuttle platelet organelles and granules inside the cytoplasmic space of the activated cell. Certainly, after platelet activation and shape change, the microtubule coil can be converted into a number of individual microtubules. In many cases, these microtubules spiral out from the cell center into filopods that are extended during cell activation and spreading. Whether the microtubule ring plays the major role in defining the structure of the resting platelet or is simply the residue of the process that buds platelets off the ends of proplatelets is unknown.

PLATELET FORMATION

The mechanism by which blood platelets are produced has been actively studied for close to 100 years. In 1906, Wright (22) discovered that platelets derive from giant precursor cells called *megakaryocytes*. Many theories have been proposed over the years to explain how megakaryocytes produce platelets. Early microscopists recognized that the maturing cells became filled with membranes, called *demarcation membranes*, and postulated that this membrane system defined fields in which the individual platelets were formed and became mature (23). Release was postulated to occur by a massive fragmentation of the megakaryocyte into the individual platelets. Subsequently, it was observed that megakaryocytes protrude long processes called *proplatelets* whose shafts decorate with platelet-sized swellings. The "proplatelet theory" was first introduced by Becker and De Bruyn (24), who proposed that these proplatelet processes elaborated by megakaryocytes fracture into platelets. Radley and Haller (25) later developed the "flow model," which postulated that platelets derived from the beadlike structures connected along the shaft of these proplatelets. Proplatelets have been observed across species, and the bulk of the experimental evidence now supports the involvement of proplatelets in platelet formation. Although the general concept that proplatelets give rise to platelets is correct, the precise mechanism of platelet release has only recently been determined. Platelets release only from the ends of long, thin megakaryocyte processes called *proplatelets* (Fig. 33-3).

Megakaryocytes use an elaborate process to form platelets and release them into the circulation. As megakaryocytes mature, they become polyploid (4X-32XN) through repeated cycles of DNA replication without cell division (26). This process, called *endomitosis*, is not just a lack of mitosis, but rather a shortened mitosis caused by a block in anaphase (27,28). These highly specialized cells increase in size until they are approximately 100 to 150 μm in diameter. As they enlarge, their cytoplasmic space, except for the most cortical regions, becomes densely filled with membranes. This unique internal membrane system was initially referred to as the *demarcation membrane system* (DMS) and was once proposed to play a role in defining preformed "platelet territories" within the megakaryocyte cytoplasm (23). This theory of cytoplasmic fragmentation as a mechanism for platelet formation has lost support because of several observations. For example, platelet fields within the megakaryocyte cytoplasm lack the marginal microtubule coil, the most characteristic feature of platelet structure (29). In addition, there is no direct evidence that platelet fields shatter into mature, functional platelets. Although the role of the DMS in platelet formation has yet to be defined, it may function as a reservoir that continuously provides membrane for the growth of proplatelets. During this period of development, cells fill with contractile proteins and platelet-specific proteins such as vWfR and the $\alpha_{IIb}\beta_3$ integrin. When the cell reaches a yet-to-be-ascertained state of preparedness, platelet production begins.

The discovery of thrombopoietin (30) and the development of megakaryocyte cultures that faithfully reconstitute platelet formation (31,32) have provided systems to study megakaryocytes in the act of making platelets *in vitro* (Fig. 33-4A–C). The erosion of one pole of the megakaryocyte cytoplasm (Fig. 33-4A) first distinguishes platelet production. Thick pseudopodia are initially formed that subsequently elongate to yield thin tubules. These slender tubules in turn develop periodic densities along their length that impart the beaded appearance of proplatelets. As this process gains momentum, more and more of the megakaryocyte is spooled out into these proplatelets. The extension of the proplatelet processes from the cortex of megakaryocytes is driven by a microtubule-based mechanism. As discussed in the section Tubulin, tubulin exists in solution as $\alpha\beta$-dimers that, like actin, reversibly polymerize into microtubules. Although little is known concerning the mechanism of microtubule dynamics in megakaryocytes, it has been determined that microtubules consolidate into bundles that fill the shafts of the proplatelet processes, and agents that prevent microtubules from assembling inhibit the elaboration of proplatelets (33). The most curious feature displayed by the microtubules occurs at the bulbous proplatelet end. Microtubule bundles running along the shaft make a U-turn at the end of the process and reenter the shaft, forming teardrop-shaped structures (Fig. 33-4). This arrangement of microtubules suggests

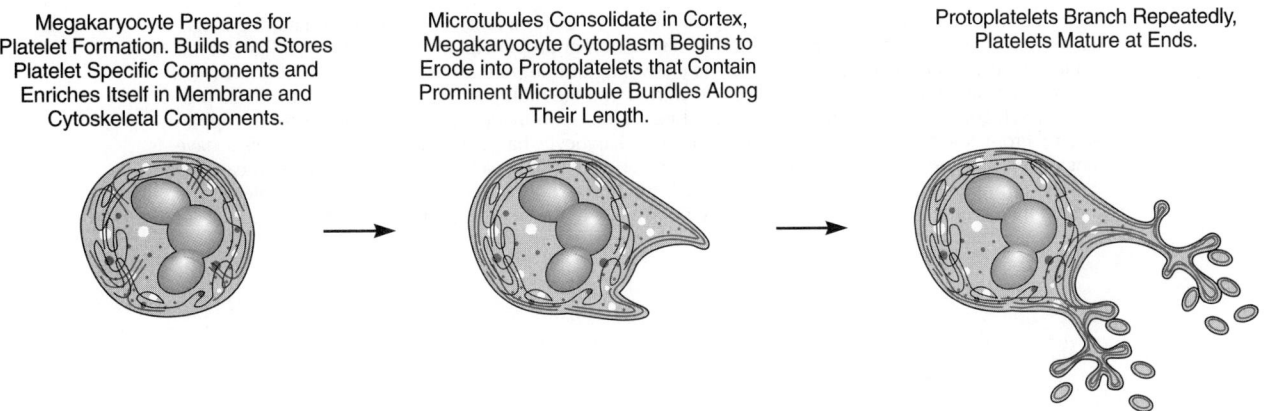

| Megakaryocyte Prepares for Platelet Formation. Builds and Stores Platelet Specific Components and Enriches Itself in Membrane and Cytoskeletal Components. | Microtubules Consolidate in Cortex, Megakaryocyte Cytoplasm Begins to Erode into Protoplatelets that Contain Prominent Microtubule Bundles Along Their Length. | Protoplatelets Branch Repeatedly, Platelets Mature at Ends. |

Figure 33-3. Model for the formation and release of platelets by megakaryocytes. In a microtubule-driven reaction, proplatelet processes elaborate from mature megakaryocytes. Platelets mature and release only at the ends of these proplatelet processes. Process ends are amplified by an actin-based mechanism that first bends, then bifurcates, the individual proplatelet processes. Packets of platelet inclusions are delivered to the proplatelet ends along the microtubules that core the proplatelets. Platelet release occurs when a single microtubule rolls into a coil at the end of a proplatelet and after the intracellular inclusions deliver into this budding process.

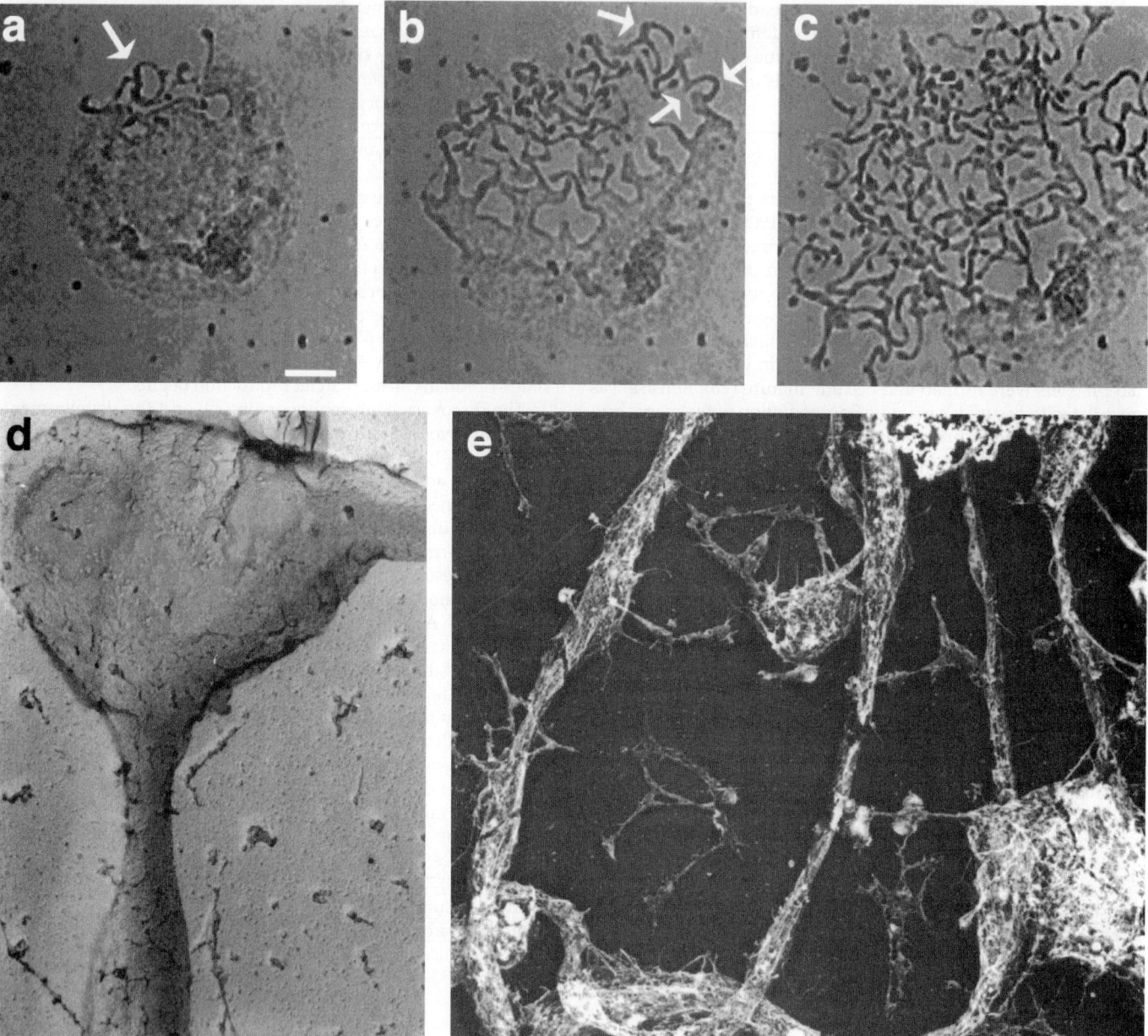

Figure 33-4. Formation of platelets by megakaryocytes. **A–C:** Time-lapse sequence of a maturing mega-karyocyte, showing the events that lead to the elaboration of proplatelet process *in vitro*. **A:** Platelet formation begins when the megakaryocyte starts unraveling at one pole (*arrow*). The bar is 25 µm. **B:** The bulk of megakaryocyte cytoplasm has been converted into the multiple proplatelet processes. These processes are highly dynamic. Bends (*arrows*) and bifurcations in individual proplatelet processes are apparent. **C:** Proplatelets grow until the bulk of the megakaryocyte has been consumed. Proplatelets have lengthened and become highly branched. **D:** Appearance of proplatelets. Proplatelets lack open canalicular system openings, and bends appear as bulbous structures. **E:** Cytoskeleton of the proplatelet. The plasma membrane of the proplatelet tube is supported by a fibrous membrane skeleton that is similar in structure to the membrane skeleton of mature platelets. (*continued*)

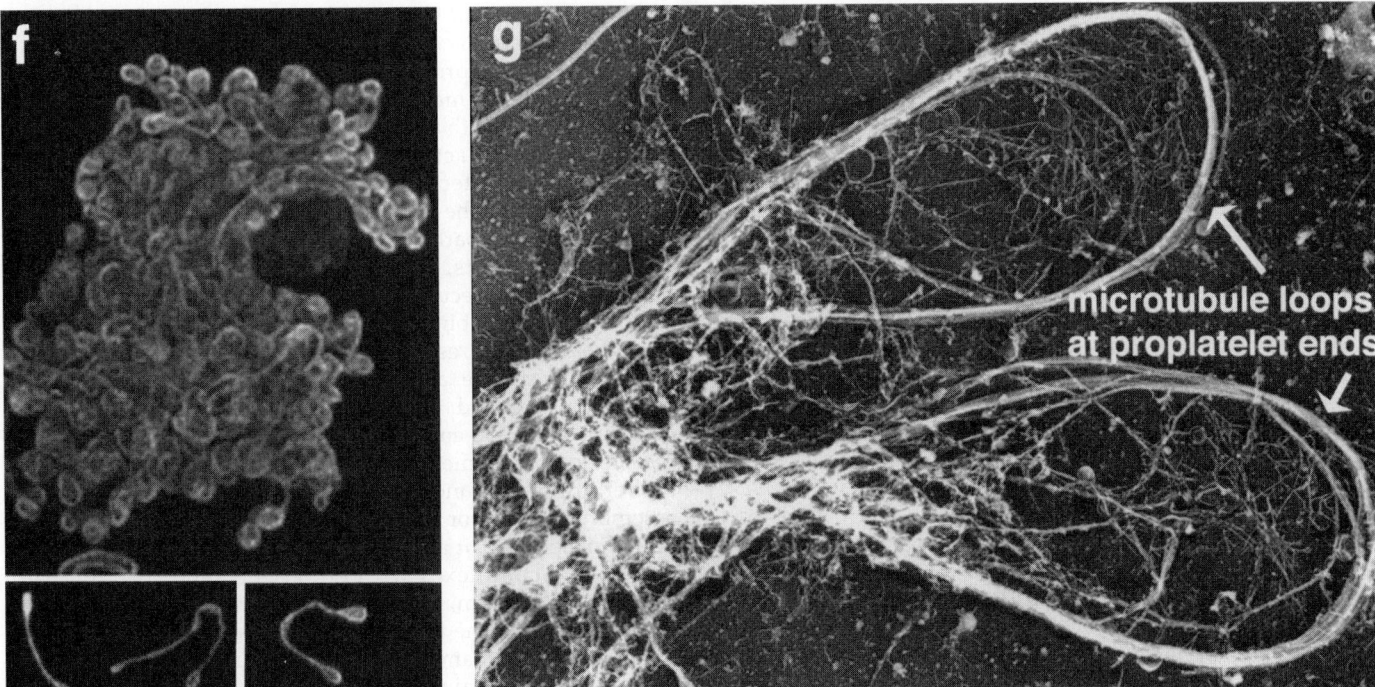

Figure 33-4. (*continued*) **F:** Platelets form only at the ends of proplatelets. This megakaryocyte has been stained with antitubulin antibodies to reveal the organization of its microtubules. Microtubules form coils only at the ends of the proplatelet processes. Many of the particles released are dumbbell shapes that appear to be maturing into two platelets. **G:** Organization of microtubules in the proplatelet ends. Microtubules are aligned into bundles in the shaft of the proplatelet. At the proplatelet tips, these microtubule bundles loop and reenter the proplatelet shaft.

that the elongation of the processes does not occur by the growth of microtubules at the end of the process, as it lacks free microtubule ends. Images have also shown that the shaft can elongate while the end is fixed in space, suggesting a role for microtubule sliding in this process. Microtubule bundles are very thick near the body of the megakaryocyte as they enter the proplatelet shaft, but progressively thin throughout the shaft such that only five to ten microtubules remain at the end of the proplatelet. Packets of material have been observed to translocate along the proplatelet shaft, and the linear arrays of microtubules lining the proplatelet shaft may also serve as tracks for the transport of membrane, organelles, and granules into assembling platelets (34).

The microtubule cytoskeleton undergoes a massive reorganization during proplatelet formation and ultimately reorganizes into hundreds of microtubule coils that can be observed at the end of each proplatelet protruded by megakaryocytes in culture (Fig. 33-4F). Many of the proplatelets released into these cultures remain connected by thin cytoplasmic strands (Fig. 33-4F). The most abundant particles released are barbell forms composed of two plateletlike enlargements at the ends that are connected by a thin cytoplasmic strand containing a microtubule bundle. Maturation of platelets occurs only at the ends of proplatelets (34). The ends are the only parts of proplatelets where a single microtubule can roll into a coil having dimensions similar to the microtubule coil of the released platelet. The mechanism of coiling remains to be determined. Because the maturation of the platelet is limited to these sites, efficient platelet production requires that a large number of ends be generated by the megakaryocyte. Proplatelet ends are

amplified by a dynamic mechanical process that first bends the shaft of an elongating proplatelet. Subsequently, a new branch grows out of the bend, creating a new proplatelet process, and the end is added to the megakaryocyte. Whereas proplatelet growth is accomplished through microtubules, bending and branching are mediated by actin filaments. Actin filament assemblies decorate branch points, and agents that disrupt actin assembly, such as the cytochalasins, abolish proplatelet branching.

Although *in vitro* systems have provided many insights into understanding platelet production, the exact location of platelet formation *in vivo* is still highly debated. Megakaryocytes are produced in the bone marrow and may undergo fragmentation into platelets at this location (35). Bone marrow megakaryocytes situated on the abluminal side of sinus endothelial cells have been observed extending proplatelets through junctions in the endothelial lining, where they have been hypothesized to be released into circulation and undergo further fragmentation into individual platelets. However, megakaryocytes can also circulate and have been identified in intravascular sites within the lung, leading to a theory that platelets are formed predominantly in the pulmonary circulation (36). Additionally, Behnke and Forer have proposed an interesting model suggesting that the formation of individual platelets occurs exclusively in the blood. This theory is based on the observation that megakaryocyte processes and proplatelets circulate in blood and make up 5% to 20% of the platelet-rich plasma (17). Based on the number of megakaryocytes in bone marrow, the number of circulating platelets in circulation, and their turnover times, each megakaryocyte must be capable of producing and releasing hundreds, if not thousands, of platelets (37–40).

THE ACTIVE PLATELET

In response to vascular damage, platelets undergo rapid shape change, secrete the contents of their α- and dense granules, and up-regulate the expression and ligand-binding activity of adhesion receptors. Platelets are activated by soluble agonists, including thrombin, ADP, and TXA$_2$, and also by the tethered agonists, such as collagen and vWf. When soluble vWf binds to collagen exposed by vascular damage, cryptic epitopes are exposed that initiate the hemostatic reaction. The shape-change reaction is considered first, followed by the ligand-receptor pairs that mediate activation.

Shape Change

Platelets respond both temporally and spatially to specific stimuli by changing shape. Tethered agonists cause platelets to bind, become round, extend filopodia, and then flatten using large lamellipodia (Fig. 33-5). To accomplish these feats, whereby the apparent surface area of the cell is greatly increased, the cytoskeleton of the resting platelet is rapidly remodeled. Remodeling is driven by mechanisms that first fragment the existing actin filaments of the resting cell and then assemble cytoplasmic actin into filaments using actin-filament barbed ends that are formed/exposed during activation (41). Activation doubles the actin filament content of the platelet from a resting concentration of 0.22 mM (subunits in filaments) to 0.44 mM (80% of the total) (42,43). To assemble cytoplasmic actin, actin stored as monomeric complex with β4-thymosin and profilin is converted into filaments. β4-thymosin is equal molar with actin in platelets. It binds to actin monomers with an affinity of approximately 1 µM, sufficient to sequester actin from the pointed filament end but insufficient to protect it from the barbed end, which has a higher affinity for the actin monomer (44–46). Actin assembly occurs only at the barbed ends of actin filaments. Actin forms polarized filaments, first recognized by the stereospecific binding of the molecular motor myosin to the filaments (47). As a myosin head binds to an actin subunit in the filament, arrowhead structures are formed that can be seen with the electron microscope, allowing the definition of a pointed and barbed filament end. This definition has been useful in indicating that the two ends of the filament have different affinities for actin monomer, with the barbed end having a tenfold higher affinity for monomer (48). This situation biases the assembly reaction for the barbed end of the growing filament (49). Furthermore, it appears that the storage forms of actin, one-to-one complexes with either the small protein β4-thymosin or profilin, interact solely with the barbed ends of filaments (50). In the resting cell, the binding and capping of the barbed actin filament ends by adducin and capZ prevent the addition and maintain the pool (51–53). Actin, an ATPase, binds to the adenosine nucleotides ADP and ATP. Barbed-end bias actin assembly, however, as it occurs in cells, requires energy derived from the hydrolysis of ATP bound to actin. Actin monomer is maintained in an ATP state by profilin (54), a protein that can both exchange ADP for ATP and promote ATP-actin transfer to the barbed filament end (55).

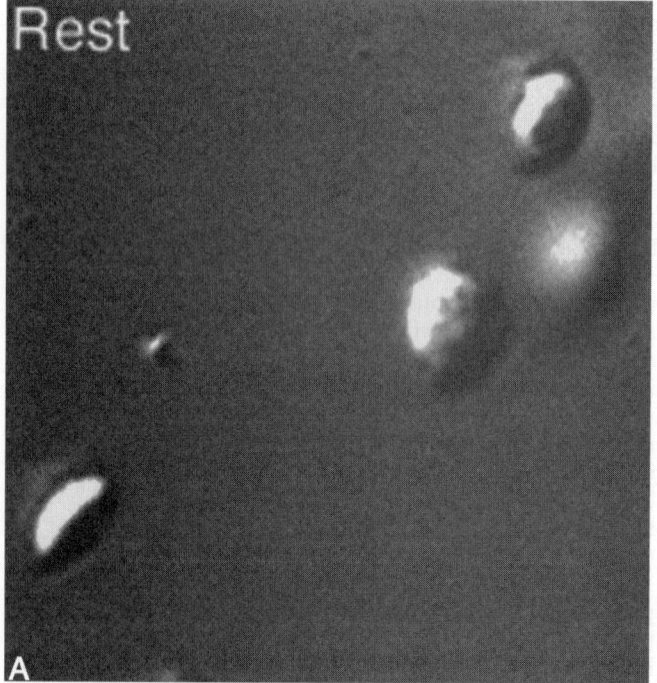

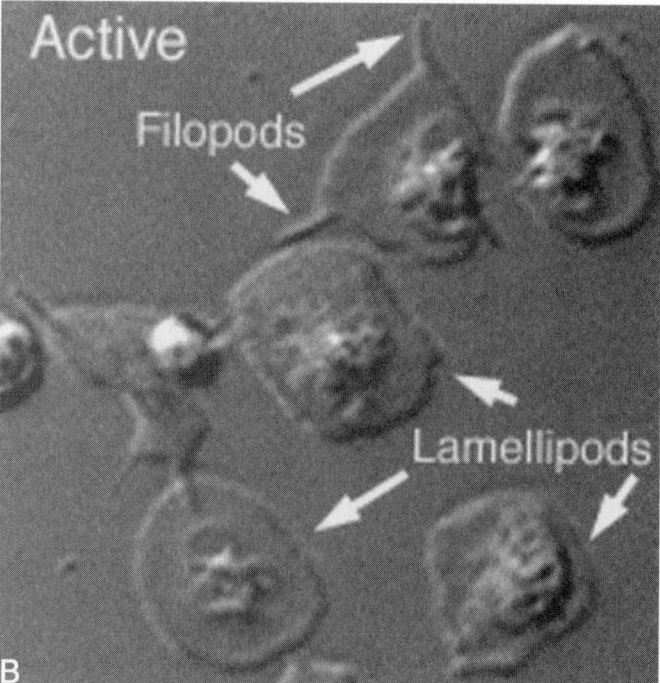

Figure 33-5. The resting to active transition of platelets. **A,B:** Differential interference contrast micrographs comparing **(A)** discoid resting platelets in solution to platelets activated by contact to a surface **(B)**. As platelets activate on a surface, they grow long filopodia and spread over the surface using lamellipodia. (*continued*)

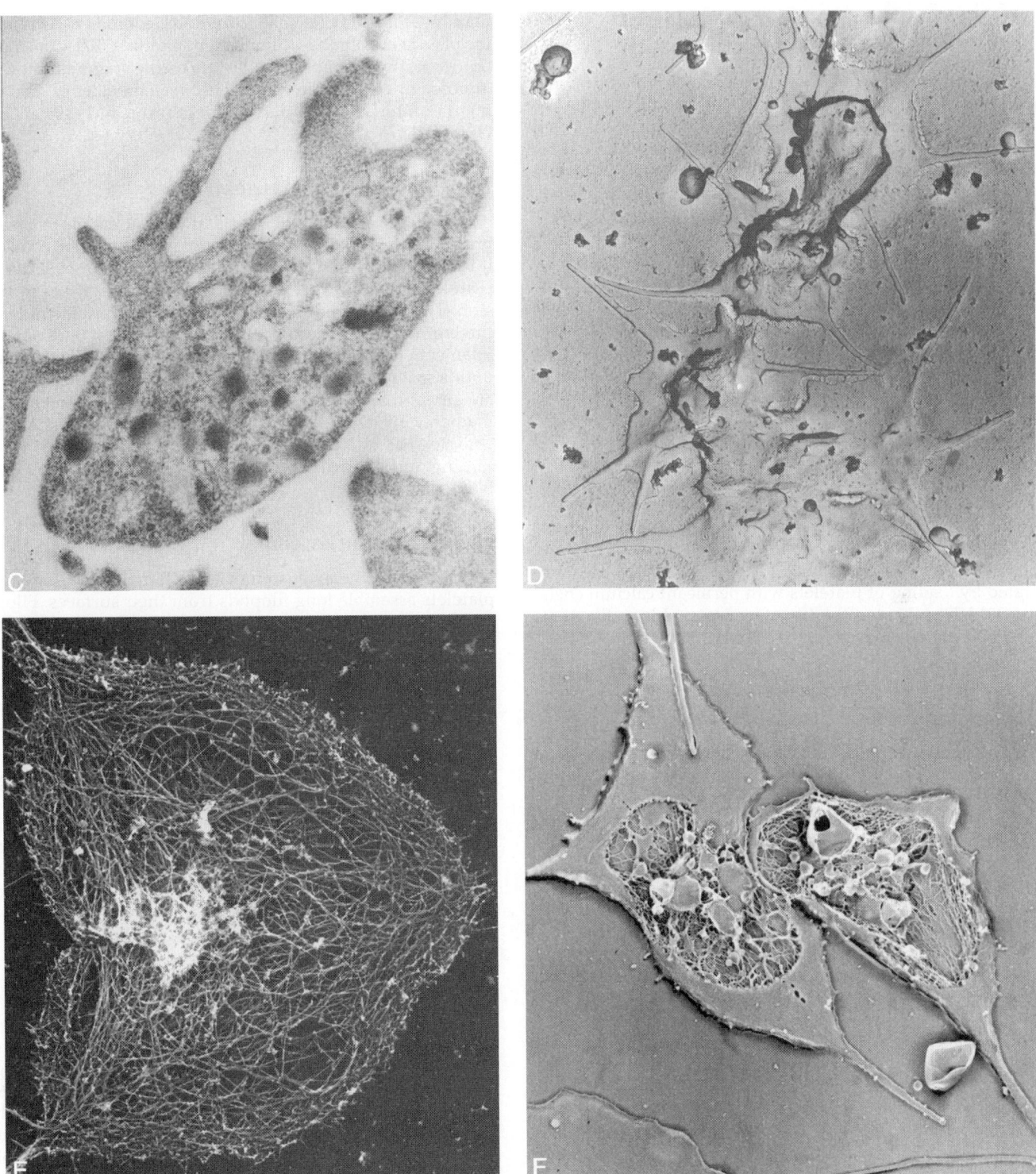

Figure 33-5. (*continued*) **C–F:** Structure of the active platelet. **C:** Activation leads to the growth of irregular projections from the platelet surface. **D:** Remodeling of the platelet is best appreciated as the cells activate on a surface. Surface-activated platelets protrude filopodia, 3–5 μm in length. Once filopodia have been extended, flat sheets of membrane called *lamellipodia* are used to fill between them, flattening the cell on the surface. **E:** Remodeling of the platelet cytoskeleton after surface activation. Filopods and cortical lamellipods are densely filled with actin filaments. Long actin filaments core the filopodia. These filaments originate in the cell center and coalesce into bundles in the filopodia. A three-dimensional network of short actin filaments supports the lamellipods. Removing the bulk of cellular membranes with the detergent Triton X-100 revealed the platelet cytoskeleton. **F:** Granules and internal cell membranes are aggregated into the cell center of the activated cell. The internal organization of membranes was revealed by mechanical removal of the apical cell membrane.

Actin Filament Fragmentation: Rounding of the Platelet (Disc-to-Sphere Transformation)

To stimulate the disc-to-sphere transformation that precedes actin polymerization, a receptor-driven rise in cytosolic calcium is used to activate a calcium-dependent filament-severing reaction. The protein responsible for actin filament severing in the platelet is gelsolin, as platelets from gelsolin-null mice lack the severing response after activation (56). Severing of the actin filaments that underlie the plasma membrane by gelsolin releases the constraints imposed by the filamin vWfR on the membrane skeleton, allowing for the outward flow of membrane in its underlying spectrin skeleton (57). After severing the actin filaments, gelsolin remains tightly attached (K_d ~ nM) to the barbed ends of the filament fragments (58,59). The requirement for filament severing was first revealed in experiments using cytochalasin B to inhibit actin assembly, allowing actin assembly–independent changes in the cell cytoskeleton to be visualized (57). In these experiments, it was observed that the long actin filaments of the resting cell disappeared after agonist treatment and that, in their place, numerous short filament fragments appeared (57). In the resting platelet, more than 95% of the total gelsolin is not bound to actin (inactive) and is therefore available to participate (activate) in calcium-elicited filament severing (60). The calcium dependence of this reaction was demonstrated by loading of platelets with permeant calcium chelators, which prevented the transformation of long filaments into short ones.

Actin Filament Assembly: Protrusion of Filopods and Lamellae

The formation of filopods and platelet spreading requires actin filament assembly, and the filament-severing reaction is temporally followed by the formation/exposure of nuclei that initiate the assembly of new actin filaments beneath the plasma membrane. This actin polymerization provides the mechanical force that forms membrane-bound protrusions. As discussed earlier, actin assembly occurs only onto the barbed end of filaments. In platelets, actin assembly begins, therefore, when (a) gelsolin and/or other proteins that can cap the barbed filament end are dissociated from preexisting filaments, providing free barbed ends (51), and/or (b) when a complex of proteins called the *Arp2/3 complex* (61–67) is activated to generate barbed ends *de novo*. Barbed ends are sufficient to initiate assembly, because they have a higher affinity for actin monomers than do the proteins that complex with the monomer. After a rapid burst of assembly, filaments are again recapped on their barbed ends, stopping the assembly process.

Actin assembly mediated by uncapping of preexisting filaments has been clearly established using platelets from transgenic mice that lack gelsolin (56,68). The mice have increased bleeding times and the platelets display defects *in vitro*. In particular, shape change is blunted, and the ability of these cells to assemble actin in response to different stimulatory ligands is markedly reduced. In addition, these cells have a marked inability to form large thrombi in high shear arteries, and the thrombi that do form are unstable (Wagner, personal communication, 2001). Severing not only reorganizes the resting platelet cytoskeleton but also participates in the exposure of the filament templates (nuclei) that drive the formation of actin filaments in lamellipodia: The short actin filaments derived from calcium-dependent fragmentation can be uncapped to generate nuclei. Because the resultant filament fragments are held together by filamin crosslinks, also linked to the membrane via

filamin-GPIbαβ/IX/V connections, lamellipods expand from the plasma membrane–actin filament interface (57). Constraints on the resting membrane skeleton before fragmentation are imposed by connections running between the sides of actin filaments underlying the plasma membrane and GPs such as GPIbαβ/IX/V (15,69).

Lamellipodial Actin Assembly

Although the assembly of actin filaments at the plasma membrane drives the membrane outward, resulting in protrusion, it is the organization of the actin filaments assembled during platelet activation that determines the shape of the protrusion. The lamellipodia of spread platelets contains a dense, three-dimensional meshwork of cross-linked actin filaments. Filament cross-linking by filamin establishes the architecture of this space-filling filament network. Filamin binds actin filaments into orthogonal networks *in vitro* and organizes actin filaments into these arrays in the platelet cortex. The Arp2/3 complex has also been proposed to play a role in the cross-linking and dendritic branching of newly assembled actin filaments.

Filopodial Actin Assembly

In addition to the extension of large lamellipods, activated platelets assemble long filopods from their surfaces. Filopodial projections contain tight bundles of long actin filaments, and the roots of these bundles originate near the cell center. Bundles begin as a loose connection of filaments, which are then zipped together into tight bundles nearer to the cell periphery. The actin-assembly reaction that generates filopodia is different from that which forms lamellipodia. The former requires a spatial collection of filament nucleating sites and/or proteins to cross-link filaments into the tight bundles. It does not require a prior filament fragmentation per se. Tight attachment to substratum prohibits directed cell movement, such as chemotaxis, by platelets. Instead, filopodia grown by platelets are used to locate other platelets and fibrin fibers. Platelets rigorously wave and rotate filopodia around their periphery as part of the seeking process (68). Filopodia are also used to apply myosin-based contractile force within fibrin gels.

Signaling and Platelet Activation

As discussed earlier, platelets circulate in blood as discs until localized damage of the vascular system is detected. Damage, in most cases, de-endothelializes the vessel wall, exposing the underlying fibrils of collagen that compose the subendothelial basement membrane. The loss of continuous endothelial layer shifts the hemostatic equilibrium of the endothelial-platelet interaction from nonthrombogenic to thrombogenic. Normally, the continuous endothelial layer generates antithrombogenic properties, as endothelial cells produce and secrete a number of platelet-relaxing factors. These factors include (a) prostacyclin (PGI_2), an eicosanoid that increases the cytosolic concentrations of cyclic adenosine monophosphate (cAMP) in platelets, which antagonizes factors that activate platelets; (b) nitrous oxide; and (c) an ectoADPase that degrades extracellular ADP, a potent platelet agonist.

Exposure of the subendothelial basement membrane begins a cascade of events that leads to platelet adherence, activation, and spreading. De-endothelialization of the vessel wall is first detected by circulating platelets. Responding platelets begin to roll over the damaged area, then bind tightly, activate, and spread over the damaged area. The initial adhesion event, particularly when it occurs in high shear vessels, is mediated by vWf. Soluble vWf binds to exposed fibers of collagen in the basement membrane. This interaction linearizes the vWf molecule and/or causes it to undergo a conformational change, allowing it to be recognized by the GPIbαβ/IX/V receptor complex (70). Engagement of vWf by GPIbαβ/IX/V on the platelet surface begins the rolling process (71,72). GPIbαβ/IX/V, abundant on the platelet surface, has both high on and off binding rate constants for vWf, causing it to repeatedly bind and release from vWf. The cyclic nature of this interaction causes platelets to repeatedly bind, release, and roll under flow from tethered vWf. Ligation of the α-chain of GPIbαβ/IX/V under flow leads to the generation of cytoplasmic signals that increase cytoplasmic calcium levels (73), activate $\alpha_{IIb}\beta_3$, induce actin assembly and shape change (74), and cause secretion, TXA_2 production, thrombin generation, and ultimately the aggregation of platelets into large multicellular plugs. $\alpha_{IIb}\beta_3$ Receptor activation is required to tightly adhere platelets to the collagen-vWf surface by binding to an RGD motif present in vWf and collagen. Thrombin, generated by the cleavage of the inactive prothrombin by enzymes of the clotting cascade, and ligation of the collagen receptors α2β1 and GPVI cooperate to maximally activate, adhere, and effect spreading of platelets (Fig. 33-6). Activated $\alpha_{IIb}\beta_3$ expressed on the surface of adherent platelets binds soluble fibrinogen, and these $\alpha_{IIb}\beta_3$-fibrinogen-$\alpha_{IIb}\beta_3$ crossbridges recruit platelets from the circulation to grow the thrombus. P-selectin inserted into the plasma membrane during exocytosis of α-granules captures leukocytes to the growing thrombus. Outside-in signals are subsequently generated by $\alpha_{IIb}\beta_3$ that rigidify the platelet-adherence reaction.

Whether ligation of GPIbαβ/IX/V alone (74) or synergy between multiple released ligands and receptor systems is required to initiate signals leading to platelet activation remains to be defined. There is precedent for the synergistic action of combined ligands to stimulate platelets under conditions in which the concentration of each agonist is insufficient to activate alone. For synergy, different signaling pathways intersect in common downstream pathways. Platelet activation or inhibition is initiated through the binding of extracellular ligands to specific receptors on the platelet surface. Key ligands leading to platelet activation include collagen, vWf, fibrin, thrombin, ADP, and TXA_2. Epinephrine is a weak agonist usually used as a coactivating stimulus. Inhibitory agents are the prostaglandins and nitric oxide. Receptor ligation activates complex and intertwined biochemical pathways that direct the subsequent platelet responses of shape change and cytoskeletal rearrangement, secretion, receptor avidity regulation, and production of bioactive lipids. The signals and responses generated after ligation depend on the class of receptor involved and on the cytoplasmic effector proteins to which the pathways lead.

Activation of platelets occurs primarily by coupling receptors to signaling pathways using either G proteins or kinases/phosphatases. G proteins bind guanine nucleotides, either guanosine triphosphate (GTP) or guanosine diphosphate (GDP), and GTP charging couples serpentine receptor–ligand complexes to cytoplasmic signaling events (75).

G Proteins

Platelets express a large family of trimeric G proteins and small GTPases. As shown in Figure 33-7, serpentine receptors couple directly to G proteins (76). Platelets express at least ten different Gα proteins (Fig. 33-8), whose functions have been clarified by studying platelets from patients with bleeding abnormalities, by applying inhibitors of G proteins to platelets (77), and, most recently, by studying the responses of platelets isolated from mice engineered to lack a specific G protein (78–82). These include the pertussis toxin–inhibited family of G_i ($G_{i1\alpha}$, $G_{i2\alpha}$, $G_{i3\alpha}$, and $G_{z\alpha}$), the G_q family ($G_{q\alpha}$ and $G_{16\alpha}$) and the G_{12} family ($G_{12\alpha}$ and $G_{13\alpha}$). The G_q and G_i family couple their receptors to phospholipase Cβ (PLC). G_q family members are potent activators of phospholipase C (PLC), whereas G_i members, which couple to PLC using the Gβγ heterodimer, are less potent. G_i couples not only to PLC but also to adenylate cyclase, the activity of which it inhibits, thereby potentiating the activating effects of other receptors also signaling through it. Adenylate cyclase is also coupled to the serpentine receptor for PGI_2. Ligation of this receptor by PGI_2 increases the activity of adenylate cyclase to decrease the responsiveness of platelets. The linkage between the production of cAMP and decreased responsiveness is, however, poorly understood (83,84). The treatment of platelets with cAMP analogs results in the phosphorylation of many platelet cytoskeletal components (85,86), a process that is believed to contribute to down-regulation of platelet function. G proteins also couple to phospholipase A_2 (PLA_2) to produce arachadonic acid and thereby stimulate TXA_2 production.

G proteins are receptor-coupled trimeric complexes composed on α, β, and γ subunits (75). G proteins cycle between an inactive heterotrimer (αβγ) and active, dissociated subunits. When the receptor is off (not complexed to its ligand), GDP is tightly bound to the α subunit, and all three subunits are locked into a tight complex with one another and the cytoplasmic domain of the receptor (Fig. 33-7). Ligation of the receptor stimulates its guanine-exchange activity, and GDP on the α subunit is exchanged for GTP, an event that dissociates the α subunit from the βγ subunits. Both the GTP-bound α subunit and the βγ subunits release from the receptor into the cytoplasm, where they can interact with appropriate downstream target proteins such as PLC, phosphoinositide 3-kinase (PI-3K), and adenylate cyclase. Receptor signaling terminates when the GTP bound to the α subunit is hydrolyzed by its intrinsic GTPase activity, allowing the inactive holoprotein (αβγ complex) to reassemble.

A second family of small GTPases posits at the critical branch points of platelet signaling cascades. The activities of the small GTPases, like those of heterotrimeric G proteins, are positively regulated by GTP charging (87–90). Small GTPases are cytoplasmic in their off state, stoichiometrically bound to sequestering proteins, such as GDI and GDP. After cell activation, guanine exchange factors (GEFs) charge these proteins with GTP, leading to their activation. GTP loading releases them from sequestering partners and, in most cases, facilitates their movement to the plasma membrane or to other membrane-bound targets via their covalently attached lipid moieties, where they interact with effector proteins. Inactivation is effected by endogenous GTPase activity, a process stimulated by GTPase activating proteins. In platelets, small GTPases include the rho family of GTPases (rhoA, rac, and cdc42), the ras family (ras, rap1b), and the rabs. Small GTPases are activated downstream of signals initiated from both heterotrimeric G-protein receptors and tyrosine kinase–regulated receptors that contain immunoreceptor tyrosine-based activation motif (ITAM) domains in their cytoplasmic domains, such as the GPVI/Fcγ complexes and FcγRIIa. Intermediate targets of both pathways are proteins that function as GTPase-activating proteins for the small GTPases and replace GDP with GTP. GEFs, which play critical roles in platelets, include VAV1 and VAV2. Small GTPases regulate the activity of lipases (PLC,

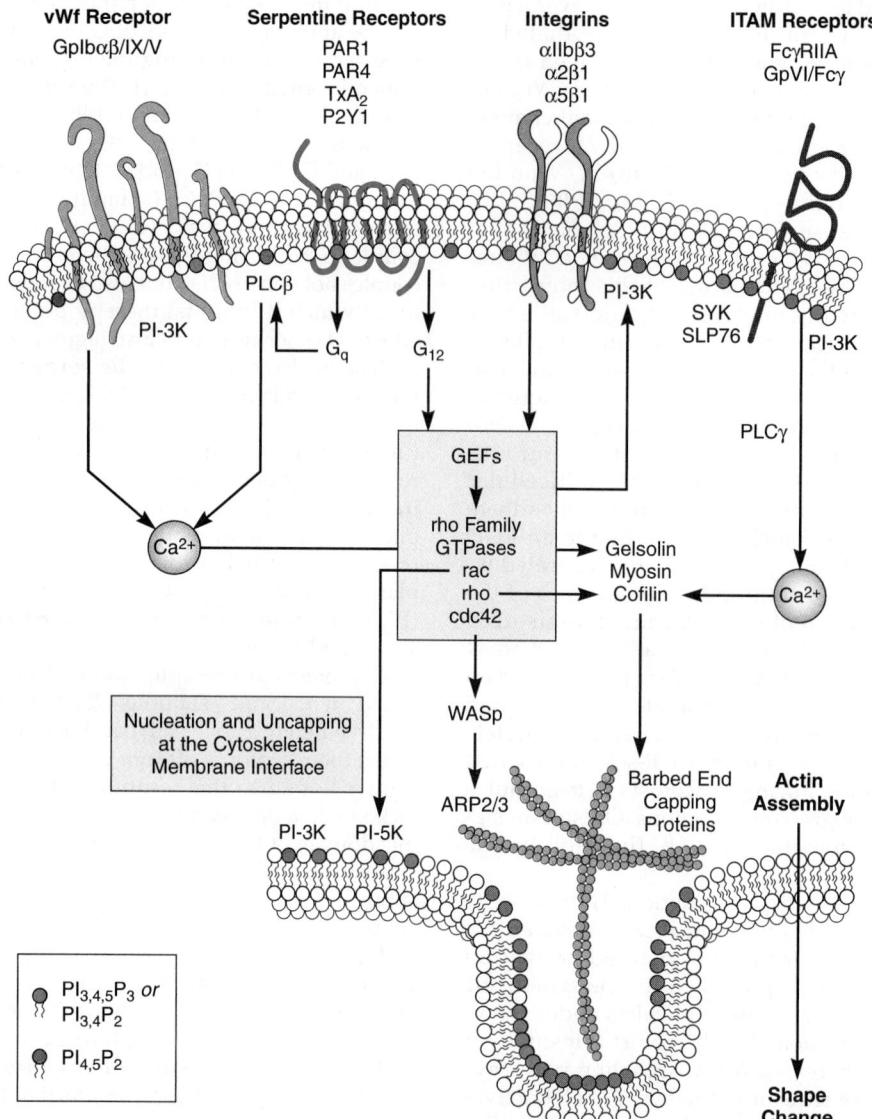

Figure 33-6. Signaling from platelet receptors to actin. Actin assembly from platelet receptors is integrated at the level of calcium release, guanosine triphosphatases (GTPases), and polyphosphoinositide synthesis. The best-understood signaling receptors to actin are the serpentine receptor family that includes thrombin, the protease activated receptors 1 and 4 (PARs) and thromboxane (TxA_2) and adenosine diphosphate (P2Y1) receptors. These receptors initially connect to downstream effectors through trimeric G proteins. Stimulation of PAR-1, for example, leads to G_q and the activation of phospholipase Cβ (PLCβ), the hydrolysis of membrane phosphatidylinositol 4,5-bisphosphate ($PI_{4,5}P_2$) to inositol 1,4,5-trisphosphate (IP_3) and diacylglycerol (DAG). IP_3 binds to receptors on the smooth endoplasmic reticulum to release calcium into the cytosol. Micromolar calcium activates gelsolin to fragment the actin filaments of the resting cytoskeleton and also mediates the activation of myosin II via myosin light chain kinase. Simultaneous with calcium mobilization, the trimeric GTPase G_{12} is activated, leading to the stimulation of the activity of cytoplasmic guanine exchange factors (GEFs). This leads to the GTP-charging and activation of small GTPases of the rhoA family. Small GTPases are central in the regulation of cellular actin assembly and architecture. GTP-rac activates downstream effectors, including the lipid kinases phosphoinositide 5-kinase (PI-5K) and phosphoinositide 3-kinase (PI-3K) and members of the SCAR/WAVE protein family (263,264). GTP-cdc42 binds Wiskott-Aldrich syndrome protein (WASp) family members, and this also potentiates the nucleation activity of the Arp2/3 complex. Phospholipid production in the plasma membrane stimulates actin filament assembly by coactivating the Arp2/3 complex and by dissociating actin capping proteins from the barbed filament ends, targeting all new actin assembly to the membrane-cytoskeletal interface. Stimulation of the immunoreceptor tyrosine-based activation motif (ITAM)–containing receptors (FcγRIIA and GpVI/Fcγ) significantly increases the tyrosine phosphorylation of these receptors, the protein tyrosine kinase Syk, SLP76, and PLCγ. Phosphorylation of PLCγ activates it to hydrolyze $PI_{4,5}P_2$, release IP_3, and mobilize calcium. PI-3K is also activated, helping to induce lipid hydrolysis by PLCγ. The lipid products of this enzyme, phosphatidylinositol-3,4 bisphosphate ($PI_{3,4}P_2$) or phosphatidylinositol-3,4,5 trisphosphate ($PI_{3,4,5}P_3$), also directly promote actin assembly reactions. Connections of this receptor leading to GTPases remain unexplored. Signals generated by the von Willebrand's factor (vWf) receptor and by integrin receptors that lead to actin assembly are less well defined. Outside-in signaling from $\alpha_{IIb}\beta_3$ has been shown to lead to the GTP-charging of the small GTPases rac and rho, which provides one entrance to pathways leading to actin assembly. PI-3K has also been shown to be involved in both the integrin and vWf receptor signaling pathway, based on inhibitor studies.

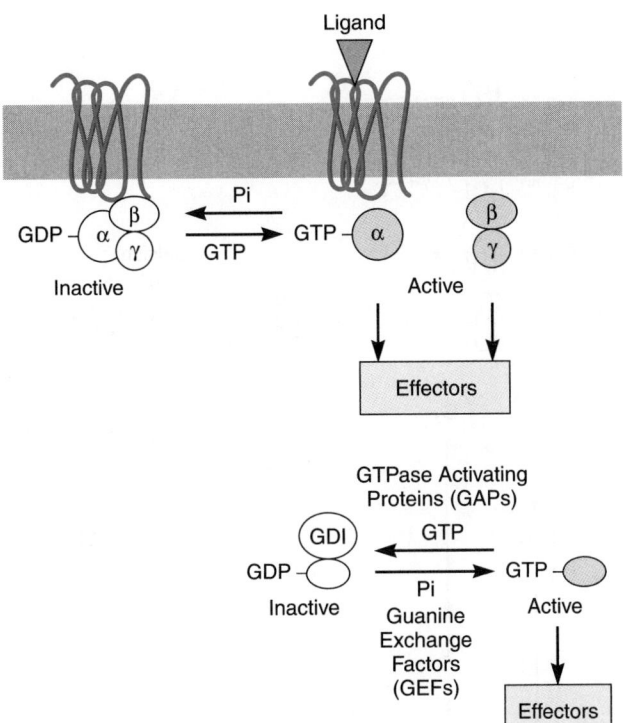

Figure 33-7. Signaling from serpentine receptors through guanosine triphosphate (GTP)-binding proteins. Serpentine receptors of platelets couple to downstream effector proteins through heterotrimeric G proteins and small GTPases. Ligation of the receptor triggers it to exchange guanosine diphosphate (GDP) on the α-subunit of the trimeric complex for GTP. This process dissociates the complex and releases the α and βγ components to activate downstream proteins such as phospholipase C and phosphoinositide 3-kinase. Hydrolysis of GTP to GDP and inorganic phosphate (Pi) results in loss of activity and reaggregation into a trimeric complex. In pathways that are not defined, signals arrive at cytoplasmic guanine exchange proteins such as VAV1, VAV2, and SOS that lead to the activation of small GTPases. These, in turn, activate effector proteins that amplify the initial signaling event.

PLD) and lipid kinases [PI-3K, phosphoinositide 5-kinase Iα (PI-5K Iα)] as well as binding to and activating cytoskeletal effector proteins.

Phospholipase C

Central for all platelet responses after activation by agonists is the metabolism of membrane phosphoinositides and calcium release. The membrane-bound phospholipids regulate calcium release (through PLC), shape change, and the activation and targeting of various proteins to the plasma membrane. They have also been implicated in the secretion reaction of platelets and other cells. Phospholipase Cβ is activated by the βγ subunits of trimeric G proteins coupling it to agonist–serpentine receptor function (91,92). Phospholipase Cγ is activated by phosphorylation by ITAM-dependent protein kinases such as syk, src, fyn, and lck (93–97). Major pathways leading to platelet activation converge at the level of PLC activation. This family of enzymes, activated by receptor occupancy, breaks down membrane phosphatidylinositol 4,5-bisphosphate ($PI_{4,5}P_2$) into the two potential intracellular messengers IP_3 and diacylglycerol (DAG). IP_3 is soluble and free to diffuse to a specialized intracellular membrane-bound compartment derived from the remnants of smooth endoplas-

mic reticulum (also called *calciosomes*) that serve as the storage site for calcium in platelets. Binding of IP_3 to its receptor embedded in the membranes of these organelles stimulates calcium release into the cytoplasm, elevating cytoplasmic calcium into μM levels. Calcium influx may also be stimulated from the extracellular fluid, as specific calcium channels may be opened in the plasma membrane to increase cytosolic calcium to greater than 10-μM levels. Although catalysis of $PI_{4,5}P_2$ diminishes the pool of membrane $PI_{4,5}P_2$, synthesis of phosphoinositides is also activated immediately after receptor ligation. Mobilization of cytoplasmic calcium in activated platelets leads to secretion and the release of granule contents. Released ADP and serotonin, in turn, activate and recruit additional platelets. Signals are generated by these receptors to also activate platelet integrins, particularly $α_{IIb}β_3$. These inside-out signals lead to conformational changes in the surface integrins facilitating ligand binding, leading to the binding of fibrinogen/fibrin to initiate novel and additional intracellular signals. Biochemical pathways are activated that lead to the production of TXA_2 and either stimulate or inhibit the production of cAMP and cyclic guanosine monophosphate (cGMP), which in turn modulate the activation process.

DAG, on the other hand, is a potent activator of protein kinase C (PKC), which regulates many platelet functions through serine/threonine phosphorylation. Although there are many targets of PKC, one major target is pleckstrin, which is phosphorylated at three internal sites. Phosphorylation activates pleckstrin, facilitating its movement to the cytoplasmic surface of the plasma membrane. Phosphopleckstrin has been shown to be intimately involved in the integration of cytoskeletal dynamics (98–103).

Role of Phosphatidylinositol-4,5 Bisphosphate Metabolism

Resting platelets maintain high, approximately 200 μM, concentrations of phosphatidylinositol 4-phosphate (PI_4P) and $PI_{4,5}P_2$ although very little, if any, phosphatidylinositol 3-phosphate, phosphatidylinositol-3,4 bisphosphate, or phosphatidylinositol-3,4,5 trisphosphate is present. After cell activation, there is a rapid hydrolysis of $PI_{4,5}P_2$ by PLC as discussed earlier. This reaction is extremely robust and produces IP_3 and DAG in amounts far in excess of that which is accounted for by the $PI_{4,5}P_2$ mass of the resting platelet, demonstrating that, although $PI_{4,5}P_2$ is posited to be rapidly hydrolyzed by pathways that activate PLCs, activation of cells leads rapidly to the enzymes that synthesize $PI_{4,5}P_2$. Estimates based on the amount of IP_3 produced indicate that the membrane mass of $PI_{4,5}P_2$ must turn over approximately five times after platelet activation. In the first second after ligation of the thrombin receptor, the net degradation rate exceeds the synthetic rate despite the stimulation of the lipid kinases, and the mass content of $PI_{4,5}P_2$ drips to a low value of approximately 160 μM. Mass levels of $PI_{4,5}P_2$, however, are rapidly restored and actually exceed the resting values to reach a maximum of approximately 280 μM 30 to 60 seconds after ligation of protease activated receptor 1 (PAR-1). The membrane concentrations of PI_4P, which is the primary substrate for the production of $PI_{4,5}P_2$ and is synthesized from PI by PI-4 kinase, follow similar biphasic kinetics as those of $PI_{4,5}P_2$. The activity of PI-3K is also markedly stimulated after cell activation. There are two forms of this enzyme, one that is activated downstream from heterotrimeric G proteins and another downstream of tyrosine kinase activity. Because phosphoinositides phosphorylated in the 3 position of the inositol ring are not cleaved by PLC, they accumulate rapidly after platelet activation. PI_4P is first phos-

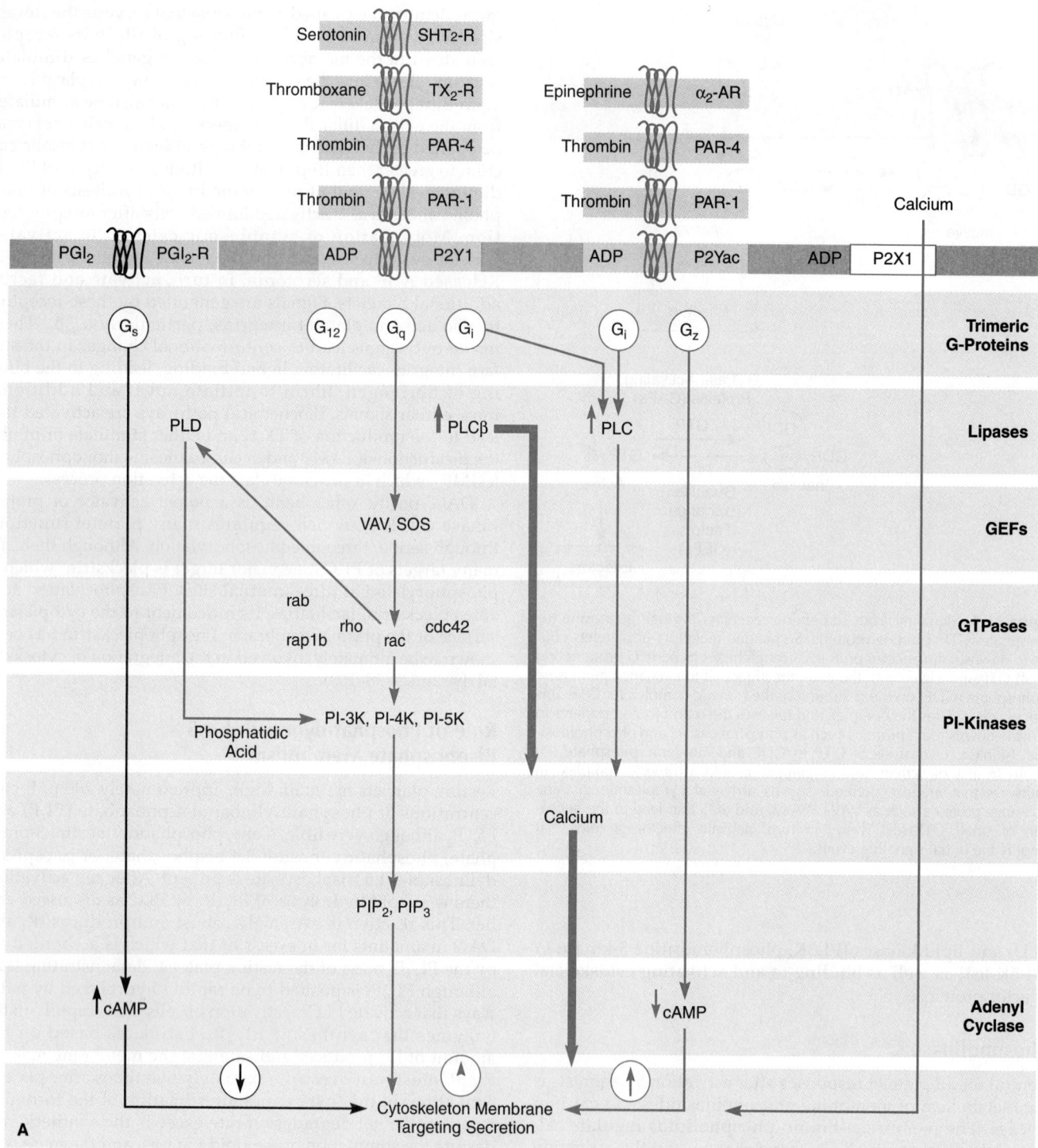

Figure 33-8. A: Signaling pathways from serpentine receptors. (*continued*)

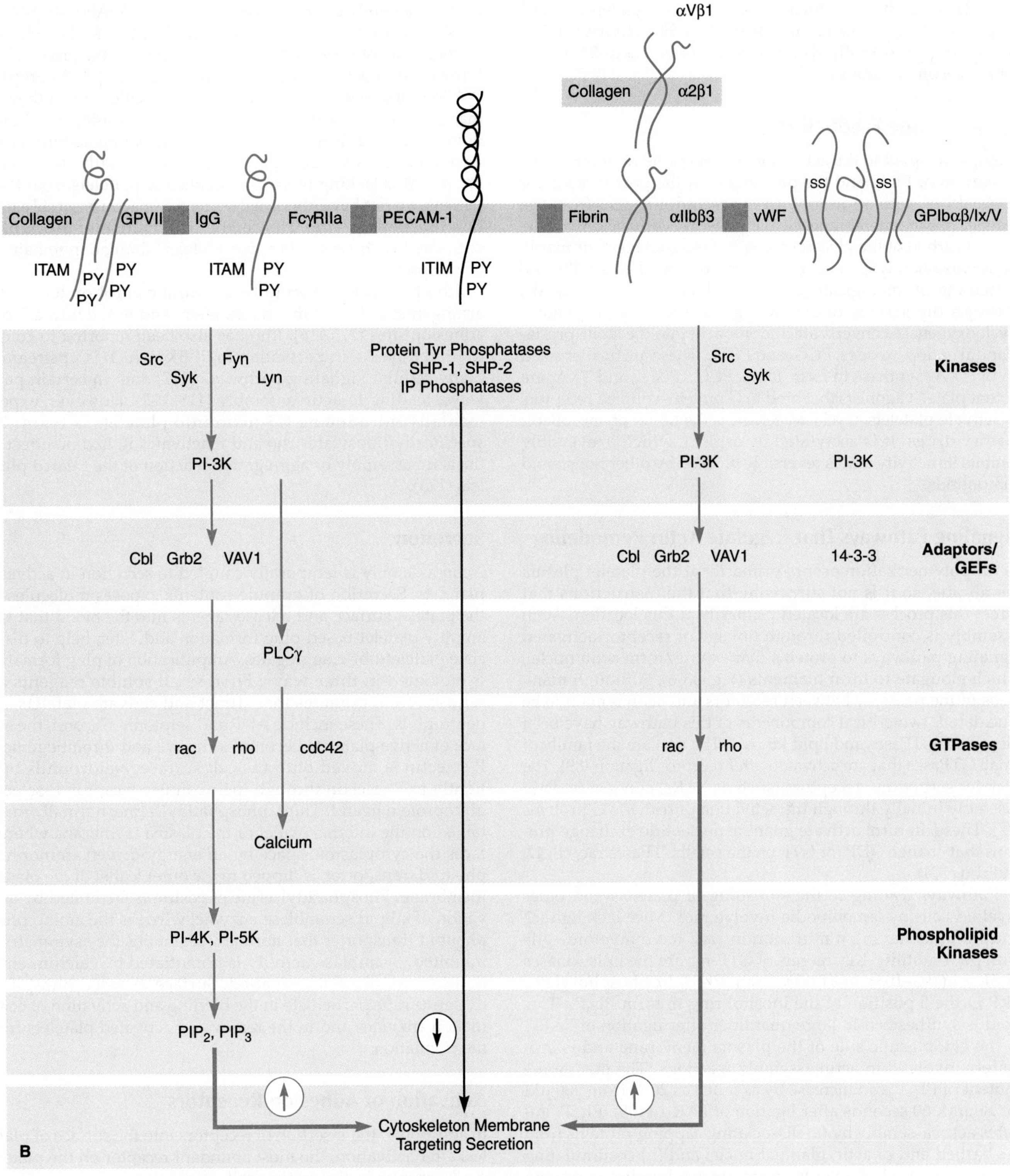

Figure 33-8. (*continued*) B: Signaling pathways from kinase/phosphatase coupled receptors. Certain signaling events have been unraveled in platelets. This figure summarizes the current state of knowledge. It is organized in layers corresponding to the order of reactants in the signaling pathways. Positive regulation is indicated with upward arrows, negative with downward arrows. The strength of the signal is denoted by the thickness of the arrow. ADP, adenosine diphosphate; cAMP, cyclic adenosine monophosphate; FcγRIIA, Fc receptor; GEF, guanine exchange factor; GP, glycoprotein; GTPase, guanosine triphosphatase; ITAM, immunoreceptor tyrosine-based activation motif; ITIM, immunoreceptor tyrosine-based inhibitory motif; PAR, protease activated receptor; PI-3K, phosphoinositide 3-kinase; PI-4K, phosphoinositide 4-kinase; PI-5K, phosphoinositide 5-kinase; $PI_{4,5}P_2$, phosphatidylinositol 4,5-bisphosphate; $PIP_{3,4,5}$, phosphatidylinositol 3,4,5-trisphosphate; PLC, phospholipase C; PY, phosphotyrosine; Tx2, thromboxane; vWf, von Willebrand's factor.

phorylated to $PI_{3,4}P_2$, which is then phosphorylated by the 5 kinase to $PI_{3,4,5}P_3$. Even at the peak of PI-3K activity, the D3-containing phospholipids account for only 1% to 2% of the total phosphoinositides.

Thromboxane Production

Strongly coupled to the activation of serpentine receptors is the activation of PLA_2 and the production of the potent mediator TXA_2. PLA_2 activation mobilizes arachidonic acid from the platelet plasma membrane, cleaving the free fatty acid from the second carbon of the glycerol phospholipid backbone, primarily from phosphatidylcholine. Free arachidonic acid is rapidly converted into its biologically active metabolites, the eicosanoids, through the actions of cyclooxygenase and lipoxygenase. Cyclooxygenase converts arachidonic acid into the labile prostaglandin endoperoxides, PGG_2 and PGH_2. These are further acted on by TXA_2 synthase to form TXA_2. PGG_2, PGH_2, and TXA_2 are potent platelet agonists that bind to G protein–coupled receptors to activate platelets. Cyclooxygenase is the target of antiinflammatory drugs. It is acetylated by aspirin, which irreversibly inhibits its activity and is reversibly blocked by other nonsteroid compounds.

Signaling Pathways That Regulate Actin Remodeling

Actin polymerization occurs primarily at the platelet plasma membrane, so it is not surprising that the instructions that direct this process are located primarily at this location. Actin assembly is controlled through linkage of receptor-activated signaling pathways to proteins that expose/form actin nuclei, which elongate to form filaments (Fig. 33-6). Although many steps in the pathway between receptors and actin remain to be elucidated, two critical components of this pathway have been identified: GTPases and lipid kinases. The first are the family of small GTPases that are activated after receptor ligation (89). The platelet serpentine receptors, such as PARs, connect to actin assembly initially through the activation of trimeric G proteins (77). These, in turn, activate guanine nucleotide exchange proteins that change GDP for GTP on the small GTPases rac, cdc42, and rho (104).

Pathways leading to the spreading of platelets and other myeloid cells by lamellipodia involve rac1. Mice lacking rac2 and humans having a mutation in rac2 have myeloid cells with poor motility. Key targets of GTP-rac are the lipid kinases PI-5K Iα (105–108) and PI-3K (109). PI-5K Iα phosphorylates PI_4P in the 5 position of the inositol ring to form $PI_{45}P_2$. This lipid is synthesized in large quantities after ligation of PAR-1 in the cytoplasmic side of the plasma membrane and is intimately involved in actin assembly reactions. The membrane content of $PI_{4,5}P_2$ can increase by as much as 20%, from 200 μM to 280 μM, 60 seconds after ligation of PAR-1 (105). $PI_{4,5}P_2$ initiates actin assembly by (a) dissociating capping proteins from the barbed end of actin filament nuclei and (b) costimulating along with cdc42 platelet Wiskott-Aldrich Syndrome protein (WASp) family members. Active WASp, in turn, binds to the Arp2/3 complex, making it complementary to nucleate actin filament assembly. Because $PI_{4,5}P_2$ is formed only in membranes, all actin assembly reactions begin at these critical interfaces.

Signaling to filopodial actin assembly in nucleated cells is believed to involve the cdc42 GTPase. One platelet protein that has been reported to bind to cdc42 is the WASp, which belongs to a family of intermediate proteins discovered in a group of patients with thrombocytopenia and lymphocytopenia. The myeloid cells from these patients lack WASp (110). This protein is one of a family of proteins that includes N-WASp (the ubiquitously expressed form), WAVE, and SCAR (111–114). Human platelets do not express the N-WASp variant of the protein. This family couples GTPases and lipids to the Arp2/3 complex. WASp molecules exist in a closed conformation when they are inactive. Binding of activators opens them, exposing a carboxyl-domain that binds and activates the nucleation activity of the Arp2/3 complex. Although WASp was initially discovered because it is lacking in WAS patients, the platelets from these patients do not have abnormal structure or actin assembly reaction functions in vitro. Hence, the contribution of the Arp2/3 pathway to actin assembly after platelet stimulation remains to be deciphered.

Rho has been shown to be a central control protein in the arrangement of actin into stress fibers and in the formation of adhesion sites (115,116). Rho has also been reported to couple to lipid kinases, in particular, to PI-3K, which is upstream in many cellular signaling pathways (117) and, in certain pathways, leading to actin assembly (118–122). However, experimentally introducing C3-toxin into platelets, a toxin that specifically ribosylates rho and inactivates it, had no effect on the actin assembly or aggregation reaction of the treated platelets (123).

Secretion

Actin assembly is temporally coupled to secretion in activated platelets. Secretion of granule contents exposes molecules on the platelet surface and releases agents into the blood that first amplify platelet-based plug formation and, later, help to dissociate platelet-fibrin aggregates. Amplification of plug formation is mediated in three ways. First, small soluble reagents are released from granules that attract and activate platelets and neutrophils. These include ADP and serotonin. Second, the surface of active platelets becomes adhesive and thrombogenic as P-selectin is moved onto the cell surface. Neutrophils bind tightly to P-selectin through their counter-receptor, P-selectin glycoprotein ligand. Third, phosphatidylserine, normally maintained on the internal leaflet of the plasma membrane where it faces the cytoplasmic space by an energy-driven aminophospholipid transporter, is flipped to the outer leaflet of the plasma membrane. Phosphatidylserine exposure is facilitated by activation of a lipid scramblase enzyme, whereas the amino phospholipid transporter that normally maintains the asymmetry is inhibited. Scamblase activity is potentiated by calcium entry that follows platelet activation. Surface-exposed phosphatidylserine rafts participate in the binding and activation of coagulation enzymes and in the removal of activated platelets from the circulation.

Activation of Adhesion Receptors

In addition to the insertion of receptors into the surface of platelets after activation, the most abundant receptor on the platelet $\alpha_{IIb}\beta_3$, cryptic in the resting cell, undergoes a conformational change that allows it to bind fibrinogen. This conformational change, imparted by the cytoplasmic tail of the α-chain, has been widely studied and is reviewed in another chapter. This receptor promotes platelet–platelet interactions through the binding ligand fibrin and participates in adhering rolling platelets into tightly attached plugs.

Platelet Inhibition

Platelet activation is blunted, and in some cases reversed, by the activation of certain platelet biochemical processes. Normally, these pathways are thought to function to maintain platelets in their discoid shapes as they circulate through blood vessels. Pathways that activate adenylate cyclase, and, hence, lead to the production of cAMP, are the most important of these processes. cAMP is an important inhibitory second messenger molecule in the platelet, and as its concentration increases, activation capacity is diminished. These pathways are coupled to specific inhibitory receptors (Fig. 33-8), in particular, the PGI_2 receptor that couples to adenylate cyclase through trimeric G-protein G_s and the epinephrine receptor that couples through G_z. cAMP has been shown to negatively affect calcium mobilization and PKC activation through direct effects on PLC activity. cAMP also modulates the release of arachidonic acid by PLA_2 and dampens cytoskeletal mobilization, shape change and actin assembly, and the activation of myosin II that is normally mediated by myosin light chain kinase. cGMP also has an inhibitory role in the platelet, once again primarily through effects on the activity of PLC. Nitric oxide, a potent inhibitory agent, elevates cGMP levels by increasing guanylate cyclase activity. Both cAMP and cGMP can act synergistically to block platelet functions.

Contraction of Clots

In addition to providing a surface onto which fibrin is assembled, platelets become embedded in fibrin networks and function to contract or collapse them. Contractile tension is applied to fibrin by actomyosin through linkage of the $\alpha_{IIb}\beta_3$ integrin: Linkage of approximately 20% of the $\alpha_{IIb}\beta_3$ integrin to underlying actin filaments occurs after engagement of $\alpha_{IIb}\beta_3$ (124,125). Linkage requires the assembly of a multicomponent bridge complex between actin and $\alpha_{IIb}\beta_3$. On one hand, $\alpha_{IIb}\beta_3$ has been reported to bind directly to talin (126), α-actinin (127), and vinculin. On the other hand, ligation of $\alpha_{IIb}\beta_3$ results in the activation of kinases that have been associated with focal adhesion sites in many cell types. The list includes the tyrosine kinases pp60[c-src], pp62[c-yes], fyn, and pp125[fak]; lipid kinases PI-3K, PI-4K, and PI-5K; PKC, PLC; and small GTPases, rap, rho, and rac. Although the precise details are currently under intense study, evidence so far shows that these proteins interact to tightly connect actin filaments in the platelet cytoplasm to fibrin in the extracellular environment. This process allows force to be transmitted across platelets.

The motor for this contraction is actomyosin. Platelets, like other cells, express a number of different myosin types. The myosin type associated with clot contraction is myosin II (128). Platelet activation greatly increases the amount of myosin II associated with the platelet cytoskeleton (129). This protein, a large hexamer composed of two heavy chains and two pairs of light chains, can reversibly assemble into bipolar myosin filaments 300 nm in length in platelets (130). Regulation of myosin filament assembly and the ATPase activity of myosin, which both provide the force to move actin filaments, occurs through two different signaling pathways. The first myosin II activation pathway discovered links myosin activity to cytoplasmic calcium release. Myosin light chain kinase phosphorylates ser-19 of the 20 kd regulatory light chains of myosin II, promoting both filament assembly and ATPase activity (131). Myosin II light chain kinase is positively regulated by calcium-calmodulin complex. The second pathway is calcium insensitive and activates myosin through the small GTPase rho (79). GTP-rho binds to and activates rho kinase that phosphorylates ser-19 of the myosin light chain as well as the inhibitory phosphatase (132). Phosphorylation of the phosphatase is inhibitory, amplifying myosin activation.

REMOVAL OF PLATELETS

Platelets circulate in humans for approximately 7 days, after which they are removed from the blood (Fig. 33-9). Clearance occurs primarily in the spleen and liver by macrophages that recognize phagocytic signals expressed on the platelet surface. Studies have begun to address the nature of some of the signals that can lead to platelet clearance. One pathway that is involved in the clearance of damaged platelets is the macrophage scavenger receptor system. For example, platelets manipulated *in vitro* to express high levels of phosphatidylserine on their surfaces are rapidly ingested by macrophages (133). Phosphatidylserine expression is known to occur in cells induced to undergo apoptosis, but apoptotic proteases need not be activated in these platelets. Phosphatidylserine expression also occurs after activation of platelets with certain agonists, particularly collagen. Whether phosphatidylserine expression increases as platelets age in the circulatory system has not been established.

Changes in Platelet Function with Age

Studies have revealed that platelets are a heterogeneous collection of sizes in blood, and it has been postulated that size is related to age. In particular, it has been suggested, based on the ability of platelets to vesiculate into microparticles *in vitro*, that size decreases with age via membrane shedding. Whether such shedding plays a role in clearance is unknown, although conditions that lead to microvesiculation also lead to the activation of platelet calpain and promote the up-regulation of phosphatidylserine to the cell surface. How microparticles are cleared has not been investigated.

EVALUATION OF PLATELET FUNCTION

Bleeding Times

Historically, measurements of bleeding time have been used to assess platelet function in patients. To perform bleeding times, uniform small incisions are made on a specific area of the skin (usually the forearm), and the time required for cessation of bleeding is measured. The extent to which blood continues to leak from the cut is determined by the periodic blotting of the wound with filter paper. Cut size is standard, and blood pressure is maintained at 40 mm Hg with a blood pressure cuff.

Bleeding times depend on three variables: (a) platelet count; (b) platelet physiologic function; and (c) vascular integrity. Platelet count is the most critical variable, and studies have shown that patients with counts lower than 100,000 µL have extended bleeding times. Bleeding times increase in proportion to diminished platelet counts until the count is below approximately 15,000 to 20,000 µL, a range where further decrease is without effect (Fig. 33-10). Long bleeding times are measured with functional platelet defects in platelet-vascular interactions such as those in Glanzmann's disease, in which the platelets lack $\alpha_{IIb}\beta_3$. Particularly long bleeding times occur in thrombocytopenic patients also having platelets with profound functional defects, such as Bernard-Soulier platelets that lack the vWf receptor, and in WAS platelets. Immune diseases such as idiopathic thrombocytopenic purpura, which involves the increased removal of older platelets, create a thrombocytopenia composed of relatively young platelets and, surprisingly, short bleed times relative to the low platelet count. Bleeding times can also be lowered by vascular disease and by abnormalities in the clotting cascade.

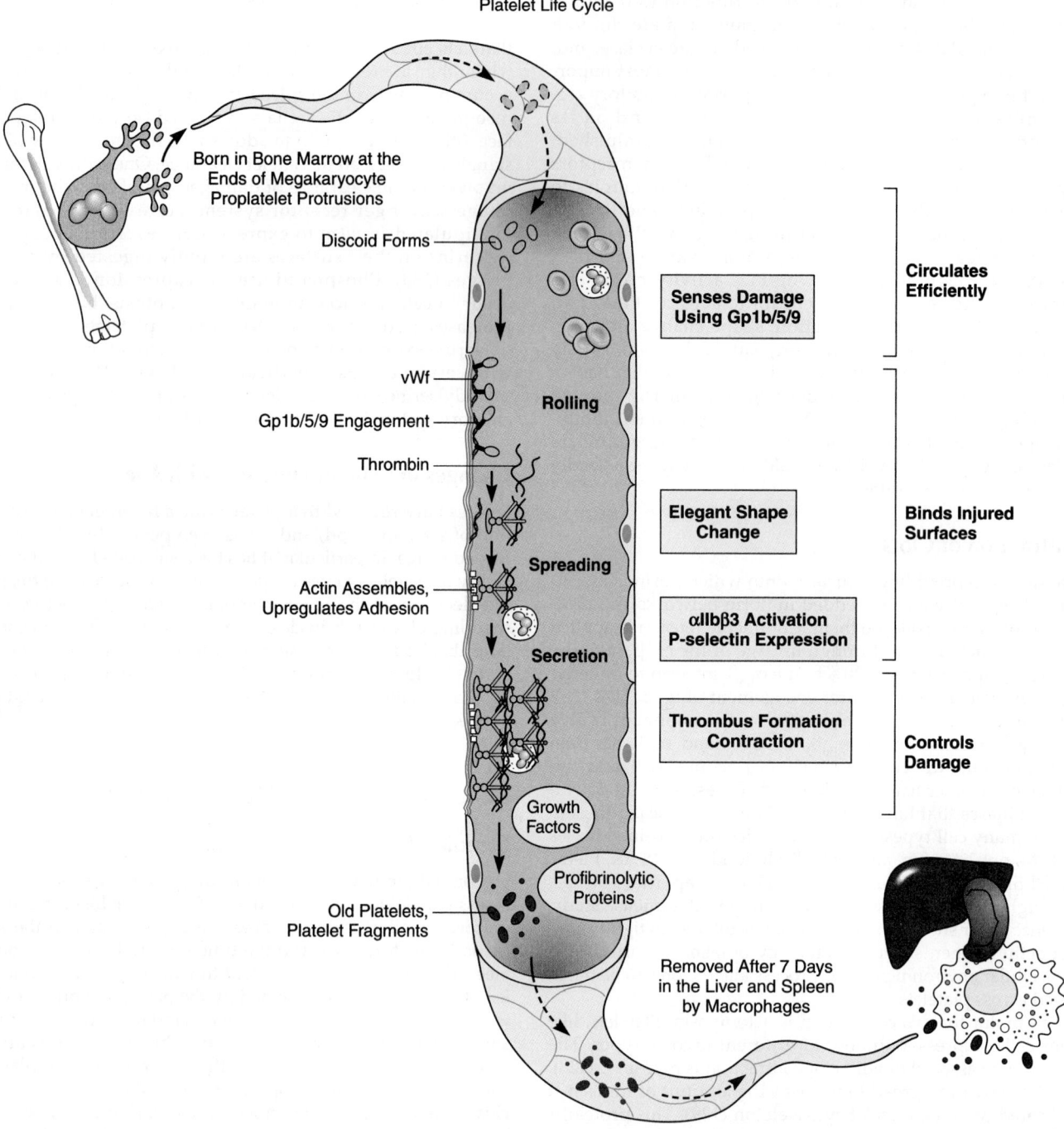

Figure 33-9. The life cycle of the platelet. Platelets are released from megakaryocytes living primarily in bone marrow. Discs enter the circulation and circulate for a maximum of 7 days, after which they are removed by liver and spleen macrophages. If damage is encountered, von Willebrand's factor receptor (vWfR) is presented to the platelet to begin the activation process. Ligation of vWfR by vWf promotes calcium release, exocytosis, shape change, and integrin activation. These events result in thrombi plug formation, in which both platelets and neutrophils are incorporated. Gp, glycoprotein.

Evaluation of Hemostasis *In Vitro*

Devices have been developed that have gained some acceptance for the measurement of platelet-based hemostasis in whole blood *in vitro*. The PFA100 is a device in which anticoagulated whole blood is drawn by capillary onto a membrane that is coated with certain platelet agonists. The membrane is coated with collagen and either ADP or epinephrine. The membrane contains a small hole, and blood is pumped through it until a

platelet plug forms and blocks the flow. An analyzer records the time taken for the hole to be plugged. This method for evaluating hemostasis, like bleeding time *in situ*, is dependent on the platelet count, the shear rate, and the hematocrit.

Evaluation of Platelet Function *In Vitro*

A variety of tests for platelet function have been used in clinical and laboratory settings. Once low platelet count has been

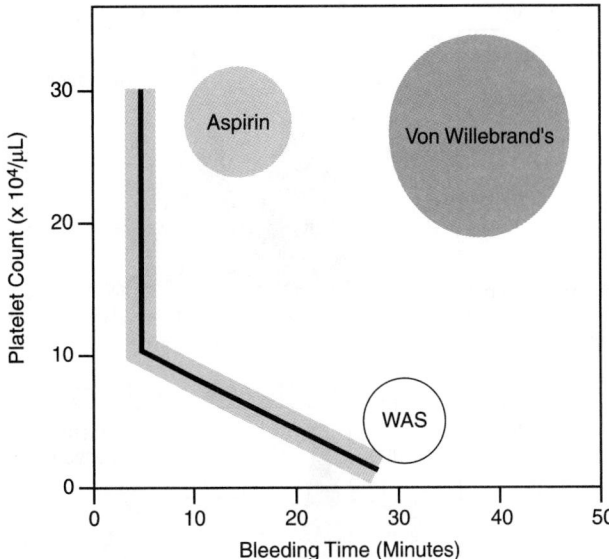

Figure 33-10. Relationship of bleeding time to platelet count in normal and impaired platelet function. Bleeding times are relatively insensitive to platelet counts above 100,000 µL. Below this count, there is an inverse relationship between count and bleeding time. Patients with Bernard-Soulier syndrome (von Willebrand's disease) have diminished platelet counts but, relative to the count, bleed profusely. Wiskott-Aldrich syndrome (WAS) patients have extreme thrombocytopenia, but the function of these platelets is normal. Aspirin shifts bleeding times to the right.

eliminated as the source for bleeding problems, specific platelet functional deficiencies must be considered. These include abnormalities or deficiencies in platelet surface GPs, particularly in the vWf and $\alpha_{IIb}\beta_3$ receptors, storage pool diseases, and hyperreactivity of circulating platelets.

Integrin Activation and Aggregation

Agonist-induced platelet aggregation has been classically used as the main test for platelet function (Fig. 33-11). Aggregation is usually measured in the turbidimetric assay of Born (134). Platelet-enriched plasma is first prepared from citrated blood by centrifugation, placed in siliconized tubes in an aggregometer apparatus at 37°C, and stirred. Because the discoid shape of the platelets imparts turbidity to plasma, the aggregation of platelets induced by the addition of agonists decreases the turbidity of the solution. Most apparatus convert the turbidity data into light transmission, generating positive data instead of negative. A continuous recording of light transmission is measured, generating the aggregometer profiles seen in the literature.

Clinical laboratories routinely test a panel of agonists on platelet responsiveness (Fig. 33-11). Agonists used include ADP, thrombin, collagen, epinephrine, ristocetin, and arachidonate. ADP at concentrations of 2.5 to 5.0 µM and epinephrine are weak agonists that induce biphasic responses for instances in which there is an initial aggregation response that is followed by a second, more robust response. The secondary response depends entirely on platelet secretion to release additional platelet agonists into the medium. Therefore, either of these agonists can be used to evaluate, in a qualitative sense, the ability of platelets to release their granule contents. In the absence of secretion, the initial aggregation response reverses with time. Higher concentrations of ADP, or the addition of strong agonists such as thrombin, collagen, and arachidonate, cause only a single robust and irreversible aggregation reaction. The addition of ristocetin, an agent that induces the

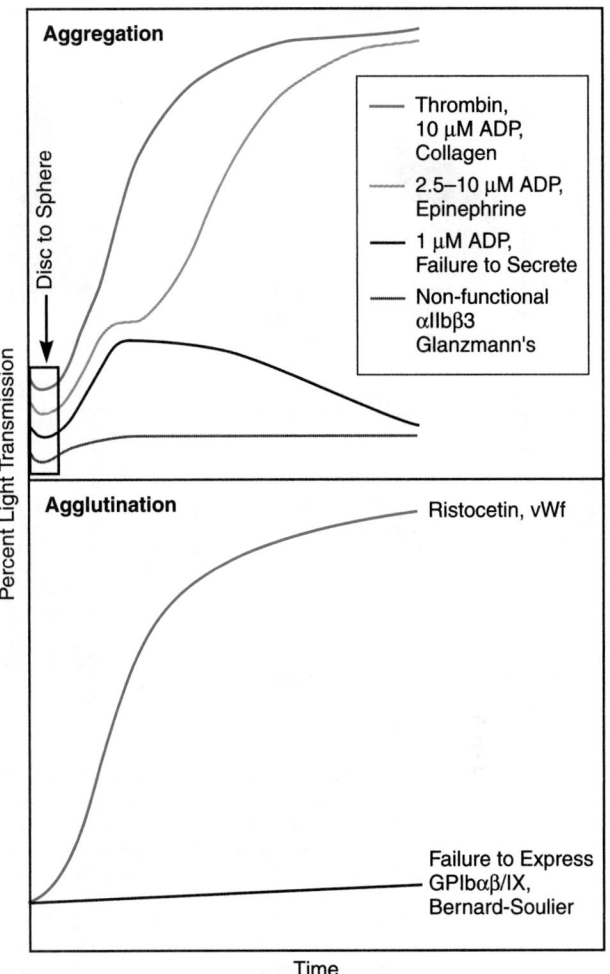

Figure 33-11. Platelet aggregation/agglutination measured in an aggregometer. One of the most widely used clinical tests for platelet function is aggregometry. In this assay, platelet-enriched plasma is stirred in a small siliconized tube and activated with a panel of agonists. The initial platelet shape change as platelets convert from discs to spheres causes an initial dip in the light transmission. Strong agonists, such as thrombin, collagen, and lower-than-10-µM adenosine diphosphate (ADP), cause a single wave of irreversible aggregation. Epinephrine and ADP at concentrations of 2.5 to 10.0 mm produce biphasic aggregation curves. The first wave indicates reversible aggregation, and the second wave corresponds to irreversible aggregation due to the granule release reaction. Low concentrations of ADP induce only the first wave of aggregation that is reversible. Agglutination is mediated by cross-linking of GPIbαβ/IX/V by von Willebrand's factor (vWf). This process is facilitated *in vitro* by the addition of ristocetin.

binding of soluble vWf to the vWfR, also induces a single-phase, aggregation-like response. Because this response occurs by a different mechanism and is used to diagnose von Willebrand's and Bernard-Soulier diseases, this response is termed *agglutination*. Aggregation to all of these reagents, with the exception of ristocetin, requires activation of the major platelet integrin $\alpha_{IIb}\beta_3$ to bind fibrinogen, and requires fibrinogen crosslinks to be formed between platelets. Failure to aggregate, therefore, is indicative of Glanzmann's thrombasthenia, in which patients lack surface expression of $\alpha_{IIb}\beta_3$. The amount of fibrinogen in plasma can also include the extent of the aggregation reaction.

The activation state of $\alpha_{IIb}\beta_3$ receptors on the platelet surface can now be routinely assayed by flow cytometry in the clinical laboratory (Fig. 33-12). Because the $\alpha_{IIb}\beta_3$ receptor's binding site for

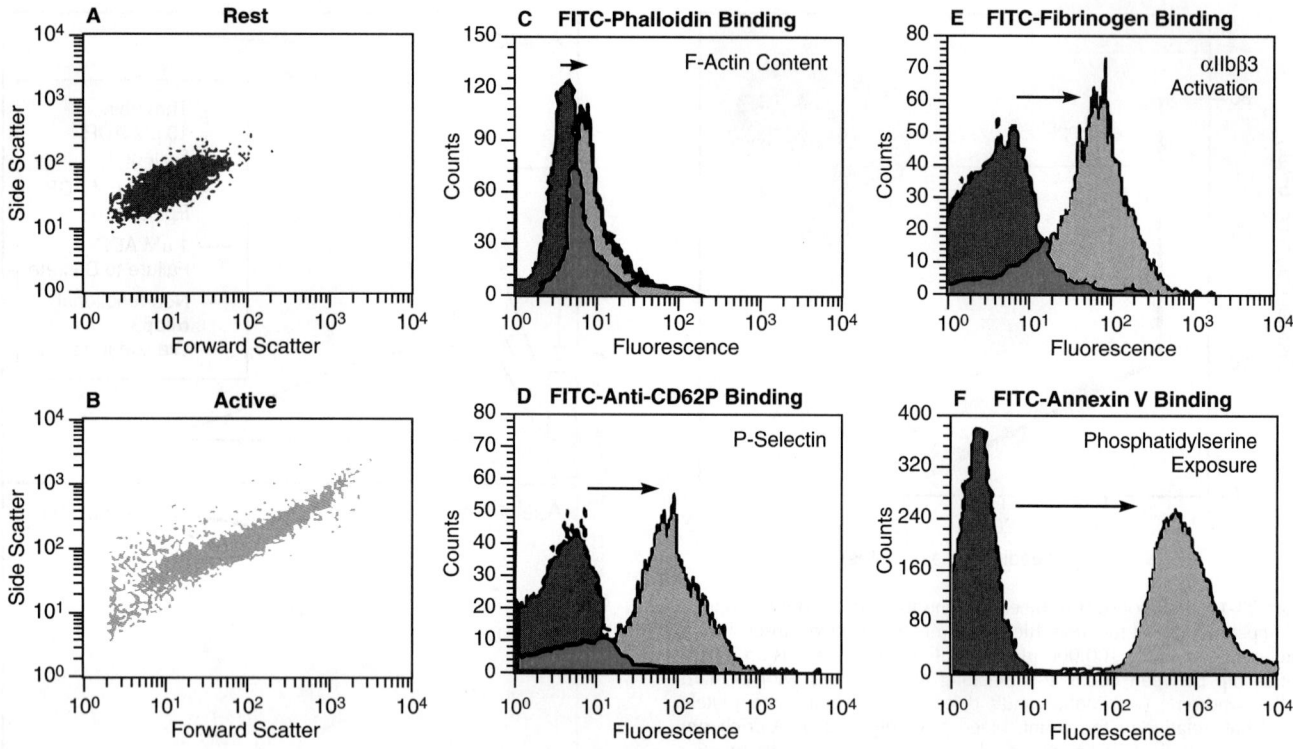

Figure 33-12. Analysis of platelet function by flow cytometry. **A,B:** Dot plot of side light scatter versus forward light scatter of isolated platelets at rest (**A**) or after addition of a strong agonist such as thrombin (**B**). Activation shifts scatter up and to the right as the discoid shape is lost. **C:** Increase in F-actin content after treatment with agonists. Actin content is measured using fluorescent-phalloidins, which are commercially available from Sigma. The resting distribution of F-actin in platelets is shown in gray. Approximately 40% of the actin is filamentous in the resting platelet. Activation shifts the distribution to the right (*light blue*). Dark blue represents the shared distribution. **D:** Surface expression of P-selectin in the resting and active platelet. Resting platelets have very little P-selectin expressed on their surfaces. P-selectin is stored in the membranes of granules. Activation results in secretion of these granules and a large increase in the binding of antibodies against P-selectin. **E:** Conversion of αIIbβ3 to its ligand binding form after platelet activation. This conversion can be detected using fluorescent-fibrinogen as shown here or with the PAC-1 IgM antibody. **F:** Exposure of phosphatidylserine after platelet activation. In this experiment, platelets were treated with the ionophore A23187, which induces maximal expression of phosphatidylserine in platelets. Phosphatidylserine is detected using fluorescent-annexin V, which binds tightly to it. FITC, fluorescein isothiocyanate.

the RGDS sequence is cryptic in the resting cell, assays that measure the exposure of a fibrinogen binding site detect large increases in the binding of fluorescently tagged reagents (Fig. 33-12E). Two types of reagents are used: fluorescein isothiocyanate–fibrinogen or fluorescein isothiocyanate–labeled antibodies specific for the open state of the receptor, e.g., the fibrinogen binding site. The most widely used antibody for this process is a site-mimic IgM-monoclonal antibody called *PAC-1*, developed by Shattil (135). Because the flow cytometry assay measures fluorescence associated with individual cells, these experiments are performed without stirring and at sufficiently low cell concentrations that cell–cell interactions are minimal. The binding of either reagent is also limited to unfixed platelets with fixation used after labeling, if desired.

Shape Change and Actin Assembly

Shape change requires the net assembly of actin filaments. Shape change can be evaluated qualitatively in the light microscope and in the aggregometer. In the aggregometer, there is an initial dip in the light transmission as platelets convert from discoid shape to a more spheric shape (Fig. 33-11A,B). However, to quantify the ability of platelets to change shape, the most reliable test is to measure actin filament content. The filamentous content of platelets can easily be measured by flow cytometry using fluorescently tagged

phalloidins (Fig. 33-12C). Phalloidin, a toxin from mushrooms of the *Amanita* genus (136–138), binds with high affinity to actin subunits when assembled into a filament, but not to monomeric actin. There is one phalloidin binding site exposed per actin subunit in the filaments (370 subunits/μm filament). Binding stabilizes the filaments and prevents disassembly. Various fluorescent versions of phalloidin are commercially available.

To assay for F-actin content, dilute resting or agonist-treated platelets are fixed by the addition of 3.7% formaldehyde for 1 hour. After the fixation period, the platelets are permeabilized with a final concentration of 0.1%, containing 1 to 2 μM of the tagged phalloidin. Fluorescence is then quantified per cell by flow cytometry after a minimum time of 30 minutes. The typical shift to the right in fluorescence after the activation of platelets through ligation of PAR-1 (25 μM TRAP peptide) is shown in Figure 33-12B. In the same experiment, measurements of side versus forward light scatter can be used to also qualitatively observe shape change, as the scattergram generated by activated platelets shifts in a characteristic fashion from the more symmetric resting profile.

Surface Expression of P-Selectin and Secretion

In the resting platelet, P-selectin is carried embedded in the membranes of intracellular secretory granules. Activating agonists that lead to secretion effect the movement of P-selectin to the cell surface, where it can be detected with anti–P-selectin antibodies. Once again, the appearance of this receptor can be easily detected and quantified by flow cytometry (Fig. 33-12D).

Secretion can also be evaluated by loading platelets with radiolabeled serotonin *in vitro* and measuring release of radiolabel after the addition of agonists.

Phosphatidylserine Exposure

Flow cytometry can also be used to evaluate phosphatidylserine exposure in activated platelets (Fig. 33-12F). Phosphatidylserine on the cell surface serves as a procoagulant substrate.

DISORDERS OF PLATELET ADHESION TO THE VESSEL WALL

Bernard-Soulier Syndrome

Bernard-Soulier syndrome (BSS) is a rare, autosomal-recessive bleeding disorder caused by impaired adhesion of platelets to the vessel wall during the initial stage of hemostasis (139–142). BSS is characterized by thrombocytopenia, giant spherical platelets, and prolonged bleeding time with normal clot retraction. The platelet count ranges from approximately 30 to 200 $\times$ 10^9/L, and the platelet lifespan is shortened to approximately 50% of normal. Although platelet aggregation in response to ADP, collagen, and arachidonic acid is normal in BSS patients, ristocetin-dependent agglutination is defective and cannot be rescued with the addition of normal plasma, as observed in von Willebrand's disease. The platelets of Bernard-Soulier patients exhibit impaired adhesion to the subendothelium under high shear rates observed during rapid blood flow (143,144).

The molecular basis of BSS arises from a dysfunction or the absence of the vWfR, which, by binding to activated vWf, initiates hemostasis by triggering the rolling and adhesion of platelets over the injured vascular surface (145). This receptor, a member of the leucine-rich family, is a surface membrane complex composed of four GPs: $GPIb_\alpha$, $GPIb_\beta$, GPIX, and GPV (146–148). $GPIb_\alpha$, $GPIb_\beta$, and GPIX assemble into a complex with equal stoichiometry. Two of each GPIbα, GPIbβ: GPIX subunits are further linked together by a single GPV to form a complete vWfR complex $(GPIb_{\alpha\beta}/IX)_2V$ (149). Each polypeptide chain in the complex is the product of a separate gene. Forced expression studies have demonstrated that all subunit components of the complex with the exception of GPV are required for stable expression on the surface of cells (147,149,150). Several individual patients heterozygous for BSS mutations do not exhibit the severe bleeding phenotype but do have platelets with GPIbα levels of approximately 50% of the normal, suggesting that GPIbα may be the rate-limiting component of the complex (151,152). Most of the defects reported for BSS patients occur from deletion, missense, or nonsense mutations of the GPIbα (141,153) and GPIX genes (154–156). Mutations in the GPIbα gene typically lead to either a synthesis defect, in which only small quantities of GPIbα are expressed, or to a functional defect, which generates a complex that fails to bind vWf.

Recent studies have demonstrated that the binding of vWf to the GPIb/IX/V complex stimulates signal transduction pathways that lead to platelet shape change, lamellipodia and filopodia assembly, secretion, and activation of the fibrinogen receptor (73,157–159). GPIb/IX/V complex also binds α-thrombin and appears to aid the activation of platelets by thrombin at low concentrations (160–163). In addition to functioning as an adhesion molecule, the GPIb/IX/V complex is also an important structural component of the resting platelet cytoskeleton that functions as the major membrane-actin filament linkage in platelets. The importance of this linkage is demonstrated by the abnormal morphology and extreme fragility of platelets observed in BSS (164,165). Morphologic studies of megakaryocytes from BSS patients show increased volume and ploidy, an abnormal distribution of the DMS, a nonhomogeneous distribution of granules, and randomly distributed microtubules (166). These observations are consistent with both a defect in platelet formation and dysfunction of platelets (167,168). Recently, a GPIbα-deficient mouse has been generated that recapitulates the human phenotype of BSS, providing further evidence that the GPIb/IX/V-filamin-actin linkage may play a crucial role in platelet morphogenesis (169).

von Willebrand's Disease and Pseudo–von Willebrand's Disease

VON WILLEBRAND'S DISEASE

von Willebrand's disease is a heterogeneous bleeding disorder that is also caused by a defect in the adhesion of platelets to the vessel wall. The disorder was first described in 1926 by Erik von Willebrand and is characterized by severe to moderate bleeding with epistaxis and mucosal and gastrointestinal hemorrhage (170). (Basic aspects of vWf and von Willebrand's disease are summarized here. These topics are covered more extensively in Chapter 35.) von Willebrand's disease is the most prevalent inherited bleeding disorder in humans (171–173) and is attributed to a deficiency or abnormality in the vWf protein, which plays an essential role in the adhesion of platelets to the subendothelium (174,175). Aggregation with ristocetin is lacking in vWf disease, but, in contrast to BSS, the defect can be corrected by the infusion of normal factor VIII (i.e., frozen plasma or cryoprecipitate), demonstrating that the defect is in the plasma and not intrinsic to the platelets (176). Subtypes of von Willebrand's disease are divided into either quantitative (type 1 or type 3) or qualitative (type 2) defects in vWf protein. All mutations that have been identified occur in the vWf gene (174,177,178). Type 1 von Willebrand's disease is the most common and makes up approximately 70% of the cases (172,179–181). Patients typically have mild to modest bleeding and decreased (30% to 50%) levels of vWf with normal multimer distribution. Type 1 von Willebrand's disease is inherited as an autosomal-dominant disorder. Type 2 von Willebrand's disease accounts for 20% to 30% of the cases, distinguished by a defect in vWf function and often by an altered plasma vWf multimer pattern (172,179–182). Type 2 von Willebrand's disease is typically inherited in an autosomal-dominant pattern and includes subtypes 2A, 2B, 2M, and 2N. Type 3 von Willebrand's disease is rare, inherited in an autosomal-recessive pattern, and characterized by severe bleeding.

PSEUDO–VON WILLEBRAND'S DISEASE

Pseudo–von Willebrand's disease, or platelet-type von Willebrand's disease, is a familial platelet disorder with autosomal-dominant inheritance characterized by prolonged skin bleeding time, sporadic thrombocytopenia, and reduced levels of high-molecular-weight vWf multimers (183–186). There is a distinct reduction in the level of high-molecular-weight vWf multimers and also decreased adhesion of platelets to the subendothelium at high shear rates (184). Platelets isolated from patients with pseudo–von Willebrand's disease show increased sensitivity to ristocetin-dependent agglutination and aggregate when exposed to vWf without the addition of ristocetin (183,184). Although pseudo–von Willebrand's disease is similar in some aspects to type 2A and type 2B von Willebrand's disease, pseudo–von Willebrand's disease is attributed to an intrinsic defect in the vWfR and not by plasma vWf (187). The genetic defect appears to be caused by a single amino acid substitution in the carboxyl terminal of the GPIbα gene (188,189). This mutation increases the adhesion of the GPIb/IX/V complex to vWf and results in the clearance of multimers from the plasma. The depletion of vWf multimers from plasma most likely causes the poor adhesion of platelets observed at high shear rates.

DISORDERS OF PLATELET SECRETION (RELEASE)

Storage Pool Deficiency

Storage pool deficiencies (SPDs) are a heterogeneous group of disorders characterized by deficiencies in platelet granule contents. The SPDs are subdivided into deficiencies of dense granules (δ-SPD), α-granules (α-SPD, or gray platelet syndrome), and deficiencies of both dense and α-granules.

δ-SPD

δ-SPD is defined as a mild bleeding disorder in which there is a complete absence or deficiency of dense bodies in the platelets and megakaryocytes (190,191). δ-SPD is transmitted as an autosomal-dominant trait, and clinical manifestations include prolonged bleeding time with normal platelet count and normal platelet morphology. Megakaryocytes and platelets from patients with δ-SPD contain normal amounts of α-granules but are clearly lacking dense bodies (192–195) and contain decreased levels of dense body components (190). In normal platelets, dense bodies harbor ADP, ATP, serotonin, and other essential components secreted during platelet activation. Therefore, it is not surprising that δ-SPD platelets lack the second-wave response to agonists, which is dependent on dense granule release and secretion. Although it is unclear which missing specific α-granule components contribute to the molecular pathogenesis of δ-SPD, there appears to be a direct correlation between ADP content and bleeding times in these patients. δ-SPD platelets exhibit reduced thrombus assembly at high shear rates in proportion to the degree of dense body deficiency (144). δ-SPD is sometimes associated with other inherited bleeding disorders. Hermansky-Pudlak syndrome is an autosomal-recessive disorder of tyrosinase-positive oculocutaneous albinism and progressive pulmonary disease with deposits of ceroidlike pigments throughout the reticuloendothelial system. Inflammatory enteritis and pulmonary fibrosis appear to result from accumulations of pigment-loaded macrophages in the lungs and intestine (196–200). Although the extent of dense body deficiency in platelets and bleeding time varies among Hermansky-Pudlak patients, most patients exhibit clinical manifestations similar to those observed with δ-SPD. Hermansky-Pudlak syndrome has been well characterized in Puerto Rican and Swiss cohorts, and the gene has been mapped to chromosome segment 10q23.1–q23.3 (201,202). Patients are deficient in a 40-kd dense granule membrane protein that has been identified as CD63 (203,204). Other hereditary bleeding disorders that are accompanied by δ-SPD include Chédiak-Higashi syndrome, WAS (205), and thrombocytopenia and absent radii syndrome. Chédiak-Higashi syndrome is an autosomal-recessive syndrome associated with defective leukocytes and abnormal granules in a variety of cell types (206–208). The molecular defect appears to be due to a marked reduction of lysosomes (209,210). The gene for Chédiak-Higashi has been localized to chromosome segment 1q42–44 (211,212).

α-SPD (GRAY PLATELET SYNDROME)

Gray platelet syndrome, first described by Raccuglia in 1971 (213), is a very rare bleeding disorder characterized by mild thrombocytopenia, prolonged bleeding, and giant platelets. Both megakaryocytes and platelets from these patients have an agranular appearance after Wright-Giemsa staining of blood and bone marrow smears, due to a lack of α-granules. An autosomal-dominant mode of inheritance has been observed with some sporadic cases. The platelet counts have been reported to range from a low of $2 \times 10^4/\mu L$ to normal values, but a prolonged bleeding time is observed even in the patients with normal platelet counts, suggesting a defect in platelet function. Although platelet aggregation in response to thrombin and collagen is decreased, aggregation in response to ADP is normal. Ristocetin-dependent aggregation is also reduced to normal (214–216).

Gray platelet syndrome platelets typically contain unusually large vacuoles, and very few, if any, α-granules. Normal numbers of dense bodies, mitochondria, and lysosomes are present in these platelets (217,218). Electron microscopy studies of gray platelet syndrome megakaryocytes have revealed small granules up to 100 μm in diameter that may represent the precursors of α-granules (218). Biochemical studies show the platelets and megakaryocytes to be deficient in the α-granule contents of vWf, fibronectin PF4, fibrinogen, and thrombospondin (219–221), although these proteins are found at normal or elevated levels in plasma. The defect of gray platelet syndrome, therefore, appears to be caused by the failure of megakaryocytes to normally package secretory proteins into α-granules during platelet development (217,219,220). This defect results in premature discharge of α-granule components from the megakaryocyte. Newly synthesized proteins that are normally packaged into α-granules appear to leak out into the marrow. Both platelet-derived growth factor and PF4 are α-granule proteins that leak out into the marrow and appear to cause the myelofibrosis seen in many patients. The bleeding observed in gray platelet syndrome may be caused by the shortened platelet lifespan (216), sequestering of platelets in the spleen, or one of several possible defects in platelet function. Because α-granule contents play crucial roles in platelet adhesion to the vessel wall, platelet aggregation, and thrombin generation, these processes may be suboptimal in these α-granule–deficient gray platelets (183).

αδ-SPD

αδ-SPD, like δ-SPD, is defined by a marked reduction in platelet dense bodies (192). However, the platelets of patients with αδ-SPD also have a heterogeneous reduction in α-granules. Therefore, αδ-SPD platelets may also exhibit the same light gray appearance after Wright-Giemsa staining as those observed in the gray platelet syndrome. In contrast to gray platelets, the amount of P-selectin in αδ-SPD platelets is also reduced (222). Platelet thrombus assembly is also decreased in αδ-SPD platelets relative to gray platelets (144). The clinical manifestations of defects in platelet function are similar to those observed in gray platelet syndrome (192).

DISORDERS OF PLATELET–PLATELET INTERACTIONS (AGGREGATION)

Glanzmann's Thrombasthenia

Glanzmann's thrombasthenia, first described by Glanzmann in 1918, is a rare bleeding disorder characterized by prolonged bleeding after lacerations and surgery, with normal platelet count and discoid morphology (223–226). Platelets adhere normally to the subendothelium (227) and change shape (lamellipodia and filopodia formation) in response to platelet agonists (228). However, the platelets from patients with Glanzmann's thrombasthenia do not aggregate in response to agonists such as thrombin, collagen, epinephrine, and ADP. They do, however, undergo ristocetin-dependent agglutination, demonstrating that the interaction between the GPIb/IX/V complex and vWf is normal (192). The molecular lesion in Glanzmann's thrombasthenia is due to a qualitative or quantitative abnormality in the platelet membrane glycoprotein $\alpha_{IIb}\beta_3$ complex, the platelet fibrinogen receptor (145,229). In activated platelets, the $\alpha_{IIb}\beta_3$ complex undergoes a conformational change that induces fibrinogen binding. Fibrinogen serves as the cross-link between platelets, mediating the aggregation reaction. Glanzmann's platelets cannot use this mechanism and are unable to bind fibrinogen after stimulation because the $\alpha_{IIb}\beta_3$ receptor is either absent, highly reduced, or nonfunctional (230). Platelets from type I Glanzmann's thrombasthenia have very low levels (1% to 5% of the normal) of the $\alpha_{IIb}\beta_3$ complex on their surface and exhibit an obvious defect in aggregation and clot retraction. Type I Glanzmann's thrombasthenic platelets have greatly reduced levels of α-granule fibrinogen, suggesting that the $\alpha_{IIb}\beta_3$-mediated uptake of plasma fibrinogen into α-granules of megakaryocytes and platelets is defective. Type I Glanzmann's thrombasthenia appears to be caused by a wide variety of molecular defects consisting of point mutations, deletions, and insertions in the genes that encode both the GPIIb and GPIIIa subunits. Type II Glanzmann's thrombasthenia appears as a milder form of the disease. The level of $\alpha_{IIb}\beta_3$ on the surface is detectable but still reduced by 80% to 90% of the normal (231). Type II Glanzmann's thrombasthenic platelets contain normal levels of α-granule fibrinogen and can still form small aggregates after stimulation, but are unable to form large aggregates (225,232). There are also several variant forms of Glanzmann's thrombasthenia that contain reduced to normal levels of $\alpha_{IIb}\beta_3$ that have functional defects in binding fibrinogen (233–236).

Afibrinogenemia

Afibrinogenemia is an extremely rare bleeding disorder characterized by abnormal platelet aggregation due to a severe deficiency of plasma fibrinogen. Afibrinogenemia is characterized by epistaxis, prolonged bleeding time, and excessive hemorrhage after trauma or surgery. The disorder has an autosomal mode of inheritance. Levels of fibrinogen in plasma and α-granules are undetectable or very low (237,238). Surprisingly, the platelet aggregation defects in afibrinogenemia are not as severe as those observed in patients who have absent or nonfunctional fibrinogen receptors (Glanzmann's thrombasthenia). Platelets from afibrinogenemic patients undergo normal aggregation after stimulation with thrombin and only slightly abnormal aggregation after ADP stimulation. These results suggest that only small amounts of fibrinogen may be necessary for platelet aggregation. Other plasma molecules, such as vWf, may also provide a mechanism of platelet aggregation in the absence of fibrinogen (237,238).

MODEL SYSTEMS AND HUMAN DISEASES TO STUDY PLATELET FORMATION

Transcription Factors

GATA-1
The zinc-finger protein GATA-1 is a transcription factor that plays a critical role in driving the expression of genes essential for megakaryocyte maturation. GATA proteins were initially thought to regulate erythrocyte maturation, because genetic disruption of the GATA-1 gene in mice results in embryonic lethality due to a block in erythropoiesis (239). However, several observations also implicate GATA-1 as an important regulator of megakaryocyte development. First, forced expression of GATA-1 in the early myeloid cell line 416b induced megakaryocyte differentiation of these cells (240). Second, Shivdasani and colleagues used targeted mutagenesis of regulatory elements within the GATA-1 locus to generate mice with a selective loss of GATA-1 in the megakaryocyte lineage (241). These knockdown mice express sufficient levels of GATA-1 in erythroid cells to overcome the embryonic lethality caused by anemia. GATA-1 deficiency in megakaryocytes leads to severe thrombocytopenia. Platelet counts are reduced to approximately 15% of normal, and the small number of circulating platelets are typically round and significantly larger than usual. These mice have an increased number of small megakaryocytes that exhibit an increased rate of proliferation. The small cytoplasmic volume of GATA-1–deficient megakaryocytes typically contains an excess of rough endoplasmic reticulum, very few platelet-specific granules, and an underdeveloped or disorganized DMS, suggesting that maturation of megakaryocytes is arrested in GATA-1–deficient megakaryocytes (242).

A human family with X-linked dyserythropoietic anemia and thrombocytopenia due to a mutation in GATA-1 has been described (243). A single nucleotide substitution in the amino terminal zinc finger of GATA-1 inhibits the interaction of GATA-1 with its essential cofactor, Friend of GATA-1 (FOG). Although the megakaryocytes in affected family members are abundant, they are unusually small and exhibit several abnormal features, including an abundance of smooth endoplasmic reticulum, an underdeveloped DMS, and a lack of granules. These observations suggest an essential role for the FOG-1/GATA-1 interaction in thrombopoiesis. Genetic elimination of FOG in mice unexpectedly resulted in specific ablation of the megakaryocyte lineage, suggesting a GATA-1–independent role for FOG in early stages of megakaryocyte development (244).

NUCLEAR FACTOR-ERYTHROID 2
NF-E2 is a basic leucine zipper transcription factor that appears to play a crucial role in megakaryocyte maturation and platelet biogenesis. NF-E2 is a protein composed of a ubiquitously expressed p18 subunit and two p45 subunits found only in the erythroid and megakaryocytic lineages (245). NF-E2 was initially thought to be a transcription factor that specifically drove the expression of genes essential for erythropoiesis, but mice lacking p45 NF-E2 do not exhibit defects in erythropoiesis. Instead, p45 NF-E2–deficient mice die from hemorrhage shortly after birth due to a complete lack of circulating platelets (246). These megakaryocytes undergo normal endomitosis and proliferate in response to Tpo. NF-E2–deficient mice produce increased numbers of megakaryocytes that are larger than normal, contain fewer granules, exhibit a highly disorganized DMS, and fail to produce proplatelets *in vitro* (247), a phenotype indicative of a late block in megakaryocyte maturation. Mice lacking the p18 subunit of NF-E2, called *mafG*, also exhibit abnormal megakaryocyte development with accompanying thrombocytopenia (248). NF-E2 appears to control the transcription of a limited number of genes involved in cytoplasmic maturation and platelet formation. Shivdasani and colleagues have generated a subtracted cDNA library that is enriched in transcripts down-regulated in NF-E2 knock-out megakaryocytes. This approach has begun to identify the downstream targets of NF-E2 and has allowed analysis of their precise role in the final stages of megakaryocyte differentiation (247).

Cytoskeletal Proteins

β1 TUBULIN

The importance of β1 tubulin in platelet biogenesis has been established by several observations. Immunofluorescence studies show β1 tubulin to be the major component of the pro-platelet microtubule cytoskeleton (249,250). β1 tubulin is expressed exclusively in platelets and megakaryocytes during late stages of megakaryocyte development. Reorganization of the megakaryocyte microtubule cytoskeleton and the assembly of the marginal microtubule coil are important steps in platelet formation. mRNA subtraction between wild-type and NF-E2–deficient megakaryocytes demonstrates that β1 tubulin is a downstream effector of the transcription factor NF-E2. β1 tubulin protein and mRNA are practically absent from NF-E2–deficient megakaryocytes (250). Genetic elimination of β1 tubulin in mice results in thrombocytopenia (251). β1 tubulin–deficient mice have circulating platelet counts below 50% of normal. This reduction in platelet number appears to be due to a defect in generating proplatelets, as megakaryocytes from β1 tubulin knock-out mice fail to form proplatelets *in vitro*. β1 tubulin–deficient platelets are spherical in shape, and this appears to be due to defective marginal bands with fewer microtubule coilings. Whereas normal platelets possess a marginal band that consists of 8 to 12 coils, β1 tubulin knock-out platelets contain only two to three coils (251).

NONMUSCLE MYOSIN HEAVY CHAIN A

May-Hegglin anomaly (MHA), the most common form of the inherited giant platelet disorders, was first described by May in 1909 (252) and later by Hegglin in 1945 (253). This rare autosomal-dominant disorder is characterized by giant platelets, thrombocytopenia, leukocyte inclusions, and mild bleeding tendency. The giant platelets have a dispersed organization of microtubules. The disease appears to arise from a mutation in the MYH9 gene encoding nonmuscle myosin heavy chain A, a 224-kd polypeptide that makes up 2% to 5% of the total platelet protein (254–256). Myosin II is an ATPase motor molecule that binds to actin filaments and generates force for contraction. Each myosin has two heads and a long, rodlike tail. The major function of the rodlike tail of myosin II is to permit the molecules to assemble into bipolar filaments. This assembly is crucial for the function of myosin II and the hematologic phenotype of MHA may be due to a block in the polymerization of myosin II into filaments during megakaryocyte development and platelet formation. Mutations in MYH9 are also responsible for Fechtner's and Sebastian syndromes, which are similarly autosomal-dominant disorders characterized by thrombocytopenia, leukocyte inclusions, and giant platelets (256,257). In contrast to MHA, Fechtner's syndrome is associated with cataracts, nephritis, and hearing disability (258). Sebastian syndrome can be differentiated from MHA by ultrastructural leukocyte inclusion properties (259).

Rab Geranylgeranyl Transferase

Gunmetal mice have a coat color mutation along with prolonged bleeding, macrothrombocytopenia, and a deficiency in α- and dense granule contents. Megakaryocytes are increased in number in gunmetal mice and have an abnormal intracellular membrane system. Platelet synthesis is decreased (260,261). The molecular basis for these defects is a mutation in the α-subunit of the Rab geranylgeranyl transferase, an enzyme that transfers geranylgeranyl groups to Rab GTPase proteins (262). This modification is essential for membrane localization. Rab proteins are small, Ras-related GTPases that are typically involved in aspects of vesicle transport in the secretory and endocytic pathways. Impaired prenylation of Rab geranylgeranyl substrates in gunmetal mice may prevent specific Rab proteins from associating with membranes and possibly inhibit membrane remodeling and granule packaging during megakaryocyte development.

REFERENCES

1. Fox J, Reynolds C, Morrow J, et al. Spectrin is associated with membrane-bound actin filaments in platelets and is hydrolyzed by the Ca²⁺-dependent protease during platelet activation. *Blood* 1987;69:537.
2. Hartwig J, DeSisto M. The cytoskeleton of the resting human blood platelet: structure of the membrane skeleton and its attachment to actin filaments. *J Cell Biol* 1991;112:407.
3. Burridge K, Kelly T, Mangeat P. Nonerythrocyte spectrins: actin-membrane attachment proteins occurring in many cell types. *J Cell Biol* 1982;95:478.
4. Liu SC, Windisch P, Kim S, et al. Oligomeric states of spectrin in normal erythrocyte membranes: biochemical and electron microscopic studies. *Cell* 1984;37:587.
5. McGough A, Josephs R. On the structure of erythrocyte spectrin in partially expanded membrane skeletons. *Proc Natl Acad Sci U S A* 1990;87:5208.
6. Morrow J. The spectrin membrane skeleton: emerging concepts. *Curr Opin Cell Biol* 1989;1:23.
7. Nachmias VT, Yoshida KI. The cytoskeleton of the blood platelet: a dynamic structure. *Adv Cell Biol* 1988;2:181.
8. Rosenberg S, Stracher A, Lucas R. Isolation and characterization of actin and actin-binding protein from human platelets. *J Cell Biol* 1981;91:201.
9. Rosenberg S, Stracher A, Burridge K. Isolation and characterization of a calcium-sensitive a-actinin-like protein from human platelet cytoskeletons. *J Biol Chem* 1981;256:12986.
10. Gorlin J, Yamin R, Egan S, et al. Human endothelial actin-binding protein (ABP-280, non-muscle filamin): a molecular leaf spring. *J Cell Biol* 1990;111:1089.
11. Gorlin J, Henske E, Warren S, et al. Actin-binding protein (ABP-280) filamin gene (FLN) maps telomeric to the color vision locus (R/GCP) and centromeric to G6PD in Xq28. *Genomics* 1993;17:496.
12. Takafuta T, Wu G, Murphy G, et al. Human β-filamin is a new protein that interacts with the cytoplasmic tail of glycoprotein 1bα. *J Biol Chem* 1998;273:17531.
13. Meyer S, Zuerbig S, Cunningham C, et al. Identification of the region in actin-binding protein that binds to the cytoplasmic domain of glycoprotein Ibα. *J Biol Chem* 1997;272:2914.
14. Kovacsovics T, Hartwig J. Thrombin-induced GPIb-IX centralization on the platelet surface requires actin assembly and myosin II activation. *Blood* 1996;87:618.
15. Ezzell R, Kenney D, Egan S, et al. Localization of the domain of actin-binding protein that binds to membrane glycoprotein Ib and actin in human platelets. *J Biol Chem* 1988;263:13303.
16. White J. Influence of taxol on the response of platelets to chilling. *Am J Pathol* 1982;108:184.
17. Behnke O, Forer A. From megakaryocytes to platelets: platelet morphogenesis takes place in the bloodstream. *Eur J Haematol* 1998;60:3.
18. Kenney D, Linck R. The cytoskeleton of unstimulated blood platelets: structure and composition of the isolated marginal microtubular band. *J Cell Sci* 1985;78:1.
19. White J. Effects of colchicine and vinca alkaloids on human platelets. *Am J Pathol* 1968;53:281.
20. Sheetz M. Microtubule motor complexes moving membranous organelles. *Cell Struct Funct* 1996;21:369.
21. Rothwell S, Calvert V. Activation of human platelets causes post-translational modifications to cytoplasmic dynein. *Thromb Haemost* 1997;78:910.
22. Wright J. The origin and nature of blood platelets. *Boston Med Surg J* 1906;154:643.
23. Yamada F. The fine structure of the megakaryocyte in the mouse spleen. *Acta Anat* 1957;29:267.
24. Becker RP, DeBruyn PP. The transmural passage of blood cells into myeloid sinusoids and the entry of platelets into the sinusoidal circulation; a scanning electron microscopic investigation. *Am J Anat* 1976;145:1046.
25. Radley JM, Scurfield G. The mechanism of platelet release. *Blood* 1980;56:996.
26. Ebbe S. Biology of megakaryocytes. *Prog Hemost Thromb* 1976;3:211.
27. Nagata Y, Muro Y, Todokoro K. Thrombopoietin-induced polploidization of bone marrow megakaryocytes is due to a unique regulatory mechanism in late mitosis. *J Cell Biol* 1997;139:449.
28. Vitrat N, Cohen-Solal K, Pique C, et al. Endomitosis of human megakaryocytes are due to abortive mitosis. *Blood* 1998;91:3711.
29. Radley JM, Haller CJ. The demarcation membrane system of the megakaryocyte: a misnomer? *Blood* 1982;60:213.
30. Kaushansky K. Thrombopoietin: the primary regulator of platelet production. *Blood* 1995;85:419.
31. Choi E, Nichol JL, Hokom MM, et al. Platelets generated in vitro from proplatelet-displaying human megakaryocytes are functional. *Blood* 1995;85:402.

32. Cramer E, Norol F, Guichard J, et al. Ultrastructure of platelet formation by human megakaryocytes cultured with the Mpl ligand. *Blood* 1997;89:2336.

33. Tablin F, Castro M, Leven R. Blood platelet formation in vitro. The role of the cytoskeleton in megakaryocyte fragmentation. *J Cell Sci* 1990;97:59.

34. Italiano J Jr, Lecine P, Shivdasani R, et al. Blood platelets are assembled principally at the ends of proplatelet processes produced by differentiated megakaryocytes. *J Cell Biol* 1999;147:1299.

35. Behnke O. An electron microscope study of the rat megakaryocyte. II. Some aspects of platelet release and microtubules. *J Ultrastruct Res* 1969;26:111.

36. Trowbridge E, Martin J, Slater D. Evidence for a theory of physical fragmentation of megakaryocytes implying that all platelets are produced in the pulmonary circulation. *Thromb Res* 1982;28:461.

37. Kaufman RM, Airo R, Pollack S, et al. Circulating megakaryocytes and platelet release in the lung. *Blood* 1965;26:720.

38. Trowbridge EA, Martin JF, Slater DN, et al. The origin of platelet count and volume. *Clin Phys Physiol Meas* 1984;5:145.

39. Stenberg PE, Levin J. Mechanisms of platelet production. *Blood Cells* 1989; 15:23.

40. Harker LA, Finch CA. Thrombokinetics in man. *J Clin Invest* 1969;48:963.

41. Fox JEB, Phillips DR. Inhibition of actin polymerization in blood platelets by cytochalasins. *Nature* 1981;292:650.

42. Carlsson L, Markey F, Blikstad I, et al. Reorganization of actin in platelets stimulated by thrombin as measured by the DNase I inhibition assay. *Proc Natl Acad Sci U S A* 1979;76:6376.

43. Markey F, Persson T, Lindberg U. Characterization of platelet extracts before and after stimulation with respect to the possible role of profilactin as microfilament precursor. *Cell* 1981;23:145.

44. Safer D, Nachmias V. Beta thymosins as actin binding peptides. *Bioessays* 1994;16:473.

45. Nachmias V, Cassimeris L, Golla R, et al. Thymosin beta 4 (Tβ4) in activated platelets. *Eur J Cell Biol* 1993;61:314.

46. Nachmias V. Small actin-binding proteins: the β-thymosin family. *Curr Opin Cell Biol* 1993;5:56.

47. Huxley H. Electron microscopic studies on the structure of natural and synthetic protein filaments from striated muscle. *J Mol Biol* 1963;3:281.

48. Pollard TD, Weeds AG. The rate constant for ATP hydrolysis by polymerized actin. *FEBS Lett* 1984;170:94.

49. Woodrum DI, Rich SA, Pollard TD. Evidence for biased unidirectional polymerization of actin filaments using heavy meromyosin by an improved method. *J Cell Biol* 1975;67:231.

50. Carlier MF, Didry D, Erk I, et al. Tβ4 is not a simple G-actin sequestering protein and interacts with F-actin at high concentration. *J Biol Chem* 1996; 271:9231.

51. Barkalow K, Witke W, Kwiatkowski D, et al. Coordinated regulation of platelet actin filament barbed ends by gelsolin and capping protein. *J Cell Biol* 1996;134:389.

52. Barkalow K, Hartwig J. The role of actin filament barbed-end exposure in cytoskeletal dynamics and cell motility. *Biochem Soc Trans* 1995;23:451.

53. Nachmias V, Golla R, Casella J, et al. Cap Z, a calcium insensitive capping protein in resting and activated platelets. *FEBS Lett* 1996;378:258.

54. Goldschmidt-Clermont PJ, Furman MI, Wachsstock D, et al. The control of actin nucleotide exchange by thymosin b4 and profilin. A potential regulatory mechanism for actin polymerization in cells. *Mol Biol Cell* 1992;3:1015.

55. Carlier M, Pantaloni D. Actin assembly in response to extracellular signals: role of capping proteins, thymosin beta 4 and profilin. *Semin Cell Biol* 1994; 5:183.

56. Witke W, Sharpe A, Hartwig J, et al. Hemostatic, inflammatory, and fibroblast responses are blunted in mice lacking gelsolin. *Cell* 1995;81:41.

57. Hartwig J. Mechanism of actin rearrangements mediating platelet activation. *J Cell Biol* 1992;118:1421.

58. Yin H, Hartwig J, Marayama K, et al. Ca²⁺ control of actin filament length. Effect of macrophage gelsolin on actin polymerization. *J Biol Chem* 1981; 256:9693.

59. Yin HL, Albrecht J, Fattoum A. Identification of gelsolin, a Ca2+-dependent regulatory protein of actin gel sol transformation. Its intracellular distribution in a variety of cells and tissues. *J Cell Biol* 1981;91:901.

60. Lind SE, Janmey PA, Chaponnier C, et al. Reversible binding of actin to gelsolin and profilin in human platelet extracts. *J Cell Biol* 1987;105:833.

61. Mullins R, Heuser J, Pollard T. The interaction of Arp2/3 complex with actin: nucleation, high affinity pointed end capping, and formation of branched networks of filaments. *Proc Natl Acad Sci U S A* 1998;95:6181.

62. Mullins R, Pollard T. Rho-family GTPases require the Arp2/3 complex to stimulate actin polymerization in *Acanthamoeba* extracts. *Curr Biol* 1999;9:405.

63. Rohatgi R, Ma L, Miki H, et al. The interaction between N-WASP and the Arp2/3 complex links Cdc42-dependent signals to actin assembly. *Cell* 1999;97:221.

64. Welch M, Rosenblatt J, Skoble J, et al. Interaction of human Arp2/3 complex and the *Listeria monocytogenes* ActA protein in actin filament nucleation. *Science* 1998;281:105.

65. Welch M, DePace A, Verma S, et al. The human Arp2/3 complex is composed of evolutionarily conserved subunits and is localized to cellular regions of dynamic actin filament assembly. *J Cell Biol* 1997;138:375.

66. Welch M, Mitchison T. Purification and assay of the platelet Arp2/3 complex. *Methods Enzymol* 1998;298:52.

67. Machesky L, Gould K. The Arp2/3 complex: a multifunctional actin organizer. *Curr Opin Cell Biol* 1999;11:117.

68. Falet H, Barkalow K, Pivniouk V, et al. Roles of SLP-76, phosphoinositide 3-kinase, and gelsolin in the platelet shape changes initiated by the collagen receptor GPVI/FcR γ-chain complex. *Blood* 2000;96:3786.

69. Fox J. Identification of actin-binding protein as the protein linking the membrane skeleton to glycoproteins on platelet plasma membrane. *J Biol Chem* 1985;260:11970.

70. Siedlecki C, Lestini B, Kottke-Marchant K, et al. Shear-dependent changes in the three-dimensional structure of human von Willebrand factor. *Blood* 1996;88:2939.

71. Savage B, Shattil S, Ruggeri Z. Modulation of platelet function through adhesion receptors. A dual role for glycoprotein IIb-IIIa (integrin αIIbβ3) mediated by fibrinogen and glycoprotein Ib-von Willebrand factor. *J Biol Chem* 1992;267:11300.

72. Ruggeri ZM. Von Willebrand factor and fibrinogen. *Curr Opin Cell Biol* 1993; 5:898.

73. Kroll M, Harris T, Moake J, et al. von Willebrand factor binding to platelet GP1b initiates signals for platelet activation. *J Clin Invest* 1991;88:1568.

74. Yuan Y, Kulkarni S, Ulsemer P, et al. The von Willebrand factor-glycoprotein Ib/V/IX interaction induces actin polymerization and cytoskeletal reorganization in rolling platelets and glycoprotein Ib/V/IX-transfected cells. *J Biol Chem* 1999;274:36241.

75. Neer EJ, Clapham DE. Roles of G protein subunits in transmembrane signalling. *Nature* 1988;333:129.

76. Brass LF, Manning DR, Cichowski K, et al. Signaling through G proteins in platelets: to the integrin and beyond. *Thromb Haemost* 1997;78:581.

77. Brass LF, Laposata M, Banga HS, et al. Regulation of the phosphoinositide hydrolysis pathway in thrombin-stimulated platelets by a pertussis toxin-sensitive guanine nucleotide-binding protein. Evaluation of its contribution to platelet activation and comparisons with protein Gi. *J Biol Chem* 1986; 261:16838.

78. Brass LF. More pieces of the platelet activation puzzle slide into place. *J Clin Invest* 1999;104:1663.

79. Klages B, Brandt U, Simon M, et al. Activation of G12/G13 results in shape change and rho/rho kinase-mediated myosin light chain phosphorylation in mouse platelets. *J Cell Biol* 1999;144:745.

80. Offermanns S, Hu YH, Simon M. Gα12 and Gα13 are phosphorylated during platelet activation. *J Biol Chem* 1996;271:26044.

81. Offermanns S, Toombs CF, Hu YH, et al. Defective platelet activation in Gaq-deficient mice. *Nature* 1997;389:183.

82. Offermanns S. New insights into the in vivo function of heterotrimeric G-proteins through gene deletion studies. *Naunyn Schmiedebergs Arch Pharmacol* 1999;360:5.

83. van Willigen G, Akkerman J. Protein kinase C and cyclic AMP regulate reversible exposure of binding sites for fibrinogen on the glycoprotein IIb-IIIa complex of human platelets. *Biochem J* 1991;273:115.

84. van Willigen G, Ackerman J-W. Protein kinase C and cyclic AMP regulate reversible exposure of fibrinogen binding sites on the glycoprotein IIb-IIIa complex of human platelets. *Biochem J* 1991;273:115.

85. Chen N, Stracher A. In situ phosphorylation of platelet actin-binding protein by cAMP-dependent protein kinase stabilizes it against proteolysis by calpain. *J Biol Chem* 1989;264:14282.

86. Yada Y, Okano Y, Nozawa Y. Enhancement of GTP γ-S-binding by cAMP-dependent phosphorylation of a filamin-like 250 kDa membrane protein in human platelets. *Biochem Biophys Res Commun* 1990;172:256.

87. Schmidt A, Hall M. Signaling to the actin cytoskeleton. *Annu Rev Cell Dev Biol* 1998;14:305.

88. Hall A. Ras related proteins. *Curr Opin Cell Biol* 1993;5:265.

89. Hall A. Small GTP-binding proteins and the regulation of the actin cytoskeleton. *Annu Rev Cell Dev Biol* 1994;10:31.

90. Kjøller L, Hall A. Signaling to rho GTPases. *Exp Cell Res* 1999;253:166.

91. Baldassare JJ, Fisher GJ. Regulation of membrane-associated and cytosolic phospholipase C activities in human platelets by guanosine triphosphate. *J Biol Chem* 1986;261:11942.

92. Vouret-Craviari V, Obberghren-Schilling EV, Rasmussen U, et al. Synthetic a-thrombin receptor peptides activate G-protein-coupled signaling pathways but are unable to induce mitogenesis. *Mol Biol Cell* 1992;3:95.

93. Pasquet JM, Bobe R, Gross B, et al. A collagen-related peptide regulates phospholipase Cγ2 via phosphatidylinositol 3-kinase in human platelets. *Biochem J* 1999;342:171.

94. Pasquet JM, Gross B, Quek L, et al. LAT is required for tyrosine phosphorylation of phospholipase Cγ2 and platelet activation by the collagen receptor GPVI. *Mol Biol Cell* 1999;19:8326.

95. Watson SP, Gibbins J. Collagen receptor signalling in platelets: extending the role of the ITAM. *Immunol Today* 1998;19:260.

96. Poole A, Gibbins J, Turner M, et al. The Fc receptor γ-chain and the tyrosine kinase Syk are essential for activation of mouse platelets by collagen. *EMBO J* 1997;16:2333.

97. Gross BS, Melford SK, Watson SP. Evidence that phospholipase C-γ2 interacts with SLP-76, Syk, Lyn, LAT and the Fc receptor γ-chain after stimulation of the collagen receptor glycoprotein VI in human platelets. *Eur J Biochem* 1999;263:612.

98. Ma A, Brass L, Abrams C. Pleckstrin associates with plasma membrane and induces the formation of membrane projections: requirements for phosphorylation and the NH2-terminal PH domain. *J Cell Biol* 1997;136:1071.

99. Ma A, Abrams C. Pleckstrin induces cytoskeletal reorganization via a rac-dependent pathway. *J Biol Chem* 1999;274:28730.

100. Abrams C, Zhang J, Downes C, et al. Phosphopleckstrin inhibits Gβγ-activable platelet phosphatidylinositol-4,5-bisphosphate 3-kinase. *J Biol Chem* 1996; 271:25192.

101. Abrams C, Zhao W, Brass L. A site of interaction between pleckstrins pH domains and Gβγ. *Biochim Biophys Acta* 1996;1314:233.

102. Abrams C, Zhao W, Belmonte E, et al. Protein kinase C regulates pleckstrin by phosphorylation of sites adjacent to the N-terminal pleckstrin homology domain. *J Biol Chem* 1995;270:23317.

103. Auethavekiatt V, Abrams C, Majerus P. Phosphorylation of platelet pleckstrin activates inositol polyphosphate 5-phosphatase I. *J Biol Chem* 1997;272: 1786.

104. Azim A, Barkalow K, Chou J, et al. Activation of the small GTPases, rac and cdc42, following ligation of the platelet PAR-1 receptor. *Blood* 2000;95:959.

105. Hartwig J, Bokoch G, Carpenter C, et al. Thrombin receptor ligation and activated Rac uncap actin filament barbed ends through phosphoinositide synthesis in permeabilized human platelets. *Cell* 1995;82:643.

106. Hartwig J, Kung S, Kovacsovics T, et al. D3 Phosphoinositides and outside-in integrin signaling by GPIIb/IIIa mediate platelet actin assembly and Filopodial extension induced by phorbol 12-myristate 13-acetate. *J Biol Chem* 1996;271:32986.

107. Tolias K, Cantley L, Carpenter C. Rho family GTPases bind to phosphoinositide kinases. *J Biol Chem* 1995;270:17656.

108. Tolias K, Hartwig J, Ishihara H, et al. Type Ia phosphatidylinositol-4-phosphate 5-kinase mediates Rac-dependent actin assembly. *Curr Biol* 2000;10:153.

109. Kovacsovics T, Bachelot C, Toker A, et al. Phosphoinositide 3-kinase inhibition spares actin assembly in activating platelets, but reverses platelet aggregation. *J Biol Chem* 1995;270:11358.

110. Derry J, Ochs H, Francke U. Identification of a novel gene mutated in Wiskott-Aldrich syndrome. *Cell* 1994;78:635.

111. Kolluri R, Tolias K, Carpenter C, et al. Direct interaction of the Wiskott-Aldrich syndrome protein with the GTPase, Cdc42. *Proc Natl Acad Sci U S A* 1996;93:5615.

112. Machesky L, Insall RH. Scar1 and the related Wiskott-Aldrich syndrome protein, WASP, regulate the actin cytoskeleton through the Arp2/3 complex. *Curr Biol* 1998;8:1347.

113. Aspenstrom P, Lindberg U, Hall A. The two GTPases, Cdc42 and Rac, bind directly to a protein implicated in the immunodeficiency disorder Wiskott-Aldrich syndrome. *Curr Biol* 1996;6:70.

114. Symons M, Derry J, Karlak B, et al. Wiskott-Aldrich syndrome protein, a novel effector for the GTPase CDC42Hs, is implicated in actin polymerization. *Cell* 1996;84:723.

115. Nobes C, Hall A. Rac, rho, and cdc42 GTPase regulate the assembly of multimolecular focal complexes associated with actin stress fibers, lamellipodia, and filopodia. *Cell* 1995;81:53.

116. Nobes C, Hall A. Rho GTPases control polarity, protrusion, and adhesion during cell movement. *J Cell Biol* 1999;144:1235.

117. Zhang J, Zhang J, Benovic JL, et al. Sequestration of the G-protein βγ subunit or ADP-ribosylation of rho can inhibit thrombin-induced activation of platelet phosphoinositide 3-kinase. *J Biol Chem* 1995;270:6589.

118. Ma A, Metjian A, Bagrodia S, et al. Cytoskeletal reorganization by G protein-coupled receptors is dependent on phosphoinositide 3-kinase γ, a rac guanosine exchange factor, and rac. *Mol Cell Biol* 1998;18:4744.

119. Pasquet J, Gross B, Gratacap MP, et al. Thrombopoietin potentiates collagen receptor signaling in platelets through a phosphatidylinositol 3-kinase-dependent pathway. *Blood* 2000;95:3429.

120. Saci A, Pain S, Rendu F, et al. Fc receptor-mediated platelet activation is dependent on phosphatidylinositol 3-kinase activation and involves p120cbl. *J Biol Chem* 1999;274:1898.

121. Gibbins JM, Briddon S, Shutes A, et al. The p85 subunit of phosphatidylinositol 3-kinase associates with the Fc receptor γ-chain and linker for activator of T cells (LAT) in platelets stimulated by collagen and convulxin. *J Biol Chem* 1998;273:34437.

122. Jackson S, Schoenwaelder S, Yuan Y, et al. Adhesion receptor activation of phosphatidylinositol 3-kinase. von Willebrand factor stimulates the cytoskeletal association and activation of phosphatidylinositol 3-kinase and pp60^c-src in human platelets. *J Biol Chem* 1994;269:27093.

123. Leng L, Kashiwagi H, Ren XD, et al. RhoA and the function of platelet integrin αIIbβ3. *Blood* 1998;91:4206.

124. Bertagnolli M, Beckerle M. Evidence for the selective association of a subpopulation of GPIIb-IIa with the actin cytoskeletons of thrombin-activated platelets. *J Cell Biol* 1993;121:1329.

125. Fox J, Shattil S, Kinlough-Rathbone R, et al. The platelet cytoskeleton stabilizes the interaction between αIIbβ3 and its ligand and induces selective movement of ligand-occupied integrin. *J Biol Chem* 1996;271:7004.

126. Knezevic I, Leisner T, Lam ST. Direct binding of the platelet integrin αIIbβ3 (GPIIb-IIIa) to talin. *J Biol Chem* 1996;271:16416.

127. Otey C, Pavalko F, Burridge K. An interaction between α-actinin and the β₁ integrin subunit in vitro. *J Cell Biol* 1990;111:721.

128. Tanaka K, Onji T, Okamoto K, et al. Reorganization of contractile elements in the platelet during clot retraction. *J Ultrastruct Res* 1984;89:98.

129. Nachmias VT. Reversible association of myosin with the platelet cytoskeleton. *Nature* 1985;313:70.

130. Niederman R, Pollard T. Human platelet myosin II. In vitro assembly and structure of myosin filaments. *J Cell Biol* 1975;67:72.

131. Adelstein RS, Conti MA. Phosphorylation of platelet myosin increases actin activated myosin ATPase activity. *Nature* 1975;256:597.

132. Essler M, Amano M, Kruse HJ, et al. Thrombin inactivates myosin light chain phosphatase via rho and its target rho kinase in human endothelial cells. *J Biol Chem* 1998;273:21867.

133. Brown S, Clarke M, Magowan L, et al. Constitutive death of platelets leading to scavenger receptor-mediated phagocytosis. A caspase independent program. *J Biol Chem* 2000;275:5987.

134. Born G. Quantitative investigations into the aggregation of blood platelets. *J Physiol* 1962;162:67.

135. Shattil SJ, Cunningham M, Hoxie J. Detection of activated platelets in whole blood using activation-dependent monoclonal antibodies and flow cytometry. *Blood* 1987;70:307.

136. Vanderkerckhove J, Deboben A, Nassal M, et al. The phalloidin binding site of F-actin. *EMBO J* 1985;4:2815.

137. Wieland T. Poisonous principles of mushrooms of the genus *Amanita*. *Science* 1968;159:946.

138. Wieland T. Phallotoxins. In: *Peptides of poisonous Amanita mushrooms*. New York: Springer-Verlag New York, 1986:69.

139. Bernard J, Soulier J. Sur une nouvelle variété de dystrophie thrombocytaire hemorragique congenitale. *Semaine des Hopitaux de Paris* 1948;24:3217.

140. Berndt M, Fournier D, Castaldi P. Bernard-Soulier syndrome. *Baillieres Clin Haematol* 1989;2:585.

141. Miller J, Lyle V, Cunningham D. Mutation of leucine-57 to phenylalanine in a platelet glycoprotein Ib alpha leucine rich tandem repeat occurring in patients with an autosomal dominant variant of Bernard-Soulier disease. *Blood* 1992;79:439.

142. Nurden A. Polymorphisms of human platelet membrane glycoproteins: structure and clinical significance. *Thromb Haemost* 1995;74:345.

143. Weiss H, Tschopp T, Baumgartner H. Effect of shear rate on platelet interaction with subendothelium in citrated and native blood. Shear-dependent decrease of adhesion in von Willebrand's disease and Bernard-Soulier syndrome. *J Lab Clin Med* 1978;92:750.

144. Weiss H, Turitto V, Baumgartner H. Platelet adhesion and thrombus formation on subendothelium in platelets deficient in glycoproteins IIb-IIa, Ib and storage granules. *Blood* 1986;67:322.

145. Nurden A, Caen J. Specific roles for platelet surface glycoproteins in platelet function. *Nature* 1975;255:720.

146. Lanza F, Morales M, de la Salle C, et al. Cloning and characterization of the gene encoding the human platelet glycoprotein V. A member of the leucine-rich glycoprotein family cleaved during thrombin-induced platelet activation. *J Biol Chem* 1993;268:20801.

147. Lopez J. The platelet glycoprotein-IX complex. *Blood Coagul Fibrinolysis* 1994; 5:97.

148. Andrews R, Lopez J, Berndt M. Molecular mechanisms of platelet adhesion and activation. *Int J Biochem Cell Biol* 1997;21:91.

149. Modderman P, Admiraal L, Sonnenberg A. Glycoproteins V and IX form a noncovalent complex in the platelet membrane. *J Biol Chem* 1992;267:364.

150. Lopez J, Leung B, Reynolds C, et al. Efficient plasma membrane expression of a functional platelet glycoprotein Ib-IX complex requires the presence of its three subunits. *J Biol Chem* 1992;267:12851.

151. Ware J, Russell S, Vicente V, et al. Nonsense mutation in the glycoprotein Ibα coding sequence associated with Bernard-Soulier syndrome. *Proc Natl Acad Sci U S A* 1990;87:2026.

152. Hourdille P, Heilmann E, Combrie R, et al. Thrombin induces a rapid redistribution of glycoprotein Ib-IX complexes with the membrane systems of activated human platelets. *Blood* 1990;76:1503.

153. Li C, Pasquale D, Roth G. Bernard-Soulier syndrome with severe bleeding: absent platelet glycoprotein Ib alpha due to a homozygous one-base deletion. *Thromb Haemost* 1996;76:670.

154. Clemetson J, Kyrle P, Brenner B, et al. Variant Bernard-Soulier syndrome associated with homozygous mutation in the leucine-rich domain of glycoprotein IX. *Blood* 1994;84:1124.

155. Noda M, Fujimura K, Takafuta T, et al. Heterogeneous expression of glycoprotein Ib, IX and V in platelets from two patients with Bernard-Soulier syndrome caused by different genetic abnormalities. *Thromb Haemost* 1995;74:1411.

156. Wright S, Michaelides K, Johnson D. Double heterozygosity for mutations in the platelet glycoprotein IX gene in three siblings with Bernard-Soulier syndrome. *Blood* 1993;81:2339.

157. Ikeda Y, Handa M, Kamata T, et al. Transmembrane calcium influx associated with von Willebrand factor binding to GP Ib in the initiation of shear-induced platelet aggregation. *Thromb Haemost* 1993;69:496.

158. Ozaki Y, Satoh K, Yatomi Y. Protein tyrosine phosphorylation in human platelets induced by interaction between glycoprotein Ib and von Willebrand factor. *Biochim Biophys Acta* 1995;1243:482.

159. Clemetson K. Platelet activation: signal transduction via membrane receptors. *Thromb Haemost* 1995;69:496.

160. Greco N, Jamieson G. High and moderate affinity pathways for α-thrombin-induced platelet activation. *Proc Soc Exp Biol Med* 1991;198:792.

161. Connolly TM, Condra C, Feng DM, et al. Species variability in platelet and other cellular responsiveness to thrombin receptor-derived peptides. *Thromb Haemost* 1994;72:627.

162. Berndt M, Gregory C, Dowden G, et al. Thrombin interactions with platelet membrane proteins. *Ann N Y Acad Sci* 1986;485:374.

163. Harmon J, Jamieson G. The glycocalicin portion of platelet glycoprotein Ib expresses both high and moderate affinity receptor sites for thrombin. A soluble radio-receptor assay for the interaction of thrombin with platelets. *J Biol Chem* 1986;261:13224.

164. Clemetson K, McGregor J, James E, et al. Characterization of the platelet membrane glycoprotein abnormalities in Bernard-Soulier syndrome and comparison with normal by surface-labeling techniques and high-resolution two-dimensional gel electrophoresis. *J Clin Invest* 1982;70:304.

165. Lopez JA, Andrews RK, Afshar-Kharghan V, et al. Bernard-Soulier Syndrome. *Blood* 1998;91:4397.

166. Tomer A, Scharf R, McMillan R, et al. Bernard-Soulier syndrome: quantitative characterization of megakaryocytes and platelets by flow cytometric and platelet kinetic measurements. *Eur J Haematol* 1994;52:193.

167. Nurden P, Nurden A. Giant platelets, megakaryocytes and the expression of glycoprotein Ib-IX complexes. *CR Acad Sci III* 1996;319:717.

168. Kass L, Leichtman D, Beals T. Megakaryocytes in the giant platelet syndrome: a cytochemical and ultrastructural study. *Thromb Haemost* 1977;38:652.

169. Ware J, Russell S, Ruggeri Z. Generation and rescue of a murine model of platelet dysfunction: the Bernard-Soulier syndrome. *Proc Natl Acad Sci U S A* 2000;97:2803.

170. von Willebrand E. Hereditar pseudohemofili. *Finska Lakarsallskapetes Handl* 1926;67:7.

171. Nilsson I. von Willebrand's disease: fifty years old. *Acta Med Scand* 1977;201:497.

172. Nilsson I. In memory of Erik Jorpes. von Willebrand's disease from 1926–1983. *Scand J Haematol Suppl* 1984;40:21.

173. Mammen E. von Willebrand's disease: history, diagnosis and management. *Semin Thromb Hemost* 1975;2:61.

174. Nichols W, Ginsburg D. von Willebrand disease. *Medicine* 1997;76:1.

175. Alexander B, Goldstein R. Dual hemostatic defect in pseudohemophilia. *J Clin Invest* 1953;32:551.

176. Nilsson I, Blomback M, Jorpes E. von Willebrand's disease and its correction with human plasma fraction 1-0. *Acta Med Scand* 1957;164:179.

177. Sadler J. von Willebrand disease. In: Scriver C, Beaudet A, Sly W, et al., eds. *The metabolic basis of inherited disease.* New York: McGraw-Hill, 1995:3269.

178. Gralnick H, Ginsburg D. von Willebrand disease. In: Beutler E, Lichtman M, Coller B, et al., eds. *Williams hematology.* New York: McGraw-Hill, 1994:1458.

179. Nilsson I, Blomback M, Blomback B. von Willebrand's disease in Sweden: its pathogenesis and treatment. *Acta Med Scand* 1959;164:263.

180. Holmberg L, Nilsson I. von Willebrand's disease. *Eur J Haematol* 1992;48:127.

181. Miller C, Graham J, Goldin L, et al. Genetics of classic von Willebrand's disease. I. Phenotypic variation within families. *Blood* 1979;54:117.

182. Hoyer L, Rizza C, Tuddenham E, et al. von Willebrand factor multimer patterns in von Willebrand's disease. *Br J Haematol* 1983;55:493.

183. George J, Nurden A, Phillips D. Molecular defects in interactions of platelets with the vessel wall. *N Engl J Med* 1984;311:1084.

184. Weiss H, Meyer D, Rabinowitz E, et al. Pseudo-von Willebrand's disease: an intrinsic platelet defect with aggregation by unmodified human factor VIII/von Willebrand factor and enhanced absorption of its high-molecular weight multimers. *N Engl J Med* 1982;306:326.

185. Miller J, Castella A. Platelet-type von Willebrand's disease: characterization of a new bleeding disorder. *Blood* 1982;60:790.

186. Miller J, Kupinsi J, Castella A, et al. von Willebrand factor binds to platelets and induces aggregation in platelet-type but not type IIb von Willebrand disease. *J Clin Invest* 1983;72:1532.

187. Miller J, Ruggeri Z, Lyle V. Unique interactions of asialo von Willebrand factor with platelets in platelet-type von Willebrand disease. *Blood* 1987;70:1804.

188. Miller J, Cunningham D, Lyle V. Mutation in the gene encoding the α-chain of platelet glycoprotein Ib in the platelet type von Willebrand disease. *Proc Natl Acad Sci U S A* 1991;88:4761.

189. Takahashi H, Murata M, Moriki T, et al. Substitution of Val for Met at residue 239 of platelet glycoprotein Ibα in Japanese individuals with platelet-type von Willebrand disease. *Blood* 1995;85:727.

190. Weiss H, Witte L, Kaplan K, et al. Heterogeneity in storage pool deficiency: studies on granule-bound substances in 18 individuals including variants deficient in alpha-granules, platelet factor 4, β-thromboglobulin and platelet derived growth factor. *Blood* 1979;54:1296.

191. Holmsen H, Weiss H. Further evidence of a deficient storage pool of adenine nucleotides in platelets from individuals with thrombocytopathia: "storage pool disease." *Blood* 1972;39:179.

192. Coller B. Platelets and their disorders. In: Ratnoff O, Forbes C, eds. *Disorders of haemostasis.* Orlando: Grune & Stratton, 1984:73.

193. Weiss H, Ames R. Ultrastructural findings in storage pool disease and aspirin like defects of platelets. *Am J Pathol* 1973;71:447.

194. White J, Edson J, Desnick S, et al. Studies of platelets in a variant of the Hermansky-Pudlak syndrome. *Am J Pathol* 1971;63:319.

195. Bellucci S, Tobelem G, Caen J. Inherited platelet disorders. *Prog Hematol* 1983;13:223.

196. Hermansky F, Pudlak P. Albinism associated with hemorrhagic diathesis and unusual pigmented reticular cells in the bone marrow: report of two cases with histochemical studies. *Blood* 1959;14:162.

197. Hardisty R. Hereditary disorders of platelet function. *Clin Haematol* 1983;12:153.

198. Davies B, Tuddenham E. Familial pulmonary fibrosis associated with oculocutaneous albinism and platelet function defect. A new syndrome. *QJM* 1976;45:219.

199. Garay S. Hermansky-Pudlak syndrome. Pulmonary manifestations of a ceroid storage disorder. *Am J Med* 1979;66:737.

200. White J. Inherited abnormalities of the platelet membrane and secretory granules. *Hum Pathol* 1987;18:123.

201. Wildenberg S, Oetting W, Almodovar C, et al. A gene causing Hermansky-Pudlak syndrome in a Puerto Rican population maps to chromosome 10q2. *Am J Hum Genet* 1995;57:755.

202. Fukai K, Oh J, Frenk E, et al. Linkage disequilibrium mapping of the gene for Hermansky-Pudlak syndrome to chromosome 10q23.1-q23.3. *Hum Mol Genet* 1995;4:1665.

203. Gerrard J, Lint D, Sims P, et al. Identification of a platelet dense granule membrane protein that is deficient in an individual with Hermansky-Pudlak syndrome. *Blood* 1991;77:101.

204. Nishori M, Cham B, McNicol A, et al. The protein CD63 is in platelet dense granules, is deficient in an individual with Hermansky-Pudlak syndrome, appears identical to granulophysin. *J Clin Invest* 1993;91:1775.

205. Parkman R, Reynold-O'Donnell E, Kenney D, et al. Surface protein abnormalities in lymphocytes and platelets from individuals with Wiskott-Aldrich syndrome. *Lancet* 1981;2:1387.

206. Buchanan G, Handin R. Platelet function in the Chediak-Higashi syndrome. *Blood* 1976;47:941.

207. Costa J, Fauci A, Wolff S. A platelet abnormality in the Chediak-Higashi syndrome of man. *Blood* 1976;48:517.

208. Apitz-Castro R, Cruz MR, Ledezema C, et al. The storage pool deficiency in platelets from humans with the Chediak-Higashi syndrome: study of six patients. *Br J Haematol* 1985;59:471.

209. Baetz K, Isaaz S, Griffiths G. Loss of cytotoxic T lymphocyte function in the Chediak-Higashi syndrome arises from a secretory defect that prevents lytic granule exocytosis. *J Immunol* 1995;154:6122.

210. Ballard R, Tier R, Nohria V, et al. The Chediak-Higashi syndrome: CT and MR findings. *Pediatr Radiol* 1994;24:266.

211. Barrat F, Auloge L, Pastural E, et al. Genetic and physiological mapping of the Chediak-Higashi syndrome on chromosome 1q42-43. *Am J Hum Genet* 1996;59:625.

212. Fukai K, Oh J, Karim M, et al. Homozygosity mapping of the gene for Chediak-Higashi syndrome to chromosome 1q42-44 in a segment conserved synteny that includes the mouse beige locus (bg). *Am J Hum Genet* 1996;59:620.

213. Raccuglia G. Gray platelet syndrome: a variety of qualitative platelet disorders. *Am J Med* 1971;51:881.

214. Mori K, Suzuki S, Sugai K. Electron microscopic and functional studies on platelets in gray platelet syndrome. *Tohoku J Exp Med* 1984;143:261.

215. Jantunen E, Hanninen A, Naukkarinen A, et al. Gray platelet syndrome with splenomegaly and signs of extramedullary hematopoiesis: a case report with review of the literature. *Am J Hematol* 1994;46:218.

216. Kohler M, Hellstern P, Morgenstern E, et al. Gray platelet syndrome: selective alpha-granule deficiency and thrombocytopenia due to increased platelet turnover. *Blut* 1985;50:331.

217. White J. Ultrastructural studies of the gray platelet syndrome. *Am J Pathol* 1979;95:45.

218. Cramer E, Vainchenker W, Vinci G, et al. Gray platelet syndrome: immunoelectron microscopic localization of fibrinogen and von Willebrand factor in platelets and megakaryocytes. *Blood* 1985;66:1309.

219. Gerrard J, Phillips D, Rao G, et al. Biochemical studies of two patients with gray platelet syndrome: selective deficiency of platelet alpha granules. *J Clin Invest* 1980;66:102.

220. Levy-Toledano S, Caen J, Breton-Gorius J, et al. Gray platelet syndrome: alpha granule deficiency—its influence on platelet function. *J Lab Clin Med* 1981;98:831.

221. Nurden A, Kunicki T, Dupuis D, et al. Specific protein and glycoprotein deficiencies in platelets isolated from two patients with gray platelet syndrome. *Blood* 1982;59:709.

222. Lages B, Shattil S, Bainton D, et al. Decreased content and surface expression of alpha-granule membrane protein GMP-140 in one of two types of platelet ad-storage pool deficiency. *J Clin Invest* 1991;87:919.

223. Glanzmann E. Hereditare hamorrhagische thrombasthenie. Ein beitrag znr pathologie der blutplattchen. *Jahr Kinderheilk* 1918;88:1.

224. Bray P. Inherited diseases of platelet glycoproteins: considerations for rapid molecular characterization. *Thromb Haemost* 1994;72:492.

225. Caen J. Glanzmann's thrombasthenia. *Baillieres Clin Haematol* 1989;2:609.

226. Berndt M, Caen J. Platelet glycoproteins. *Prog Hemost Thromb* 1984;7:111.

227. Tschopp T, Weiss H, Baumgartner H. Interaction of platelets with subendothelium in thrombasthenia: normal adhesion, impaired aggregation. *Experientia* 1975;31:113.

228. Caen J, Castaldi P, Leclerc J, et al. Congenital bleeding disorders with long bleeding time and normal platelet count. I. Glanzmann's thrombasthenia (report of fifteen patients). *Am J Med* 1966;41:4.

229. Phillips D, Jenkins C, Luscher E, et al. Molecular differences of exposed surface proteins on thrombasthenic platelet plasma membranes. *Nature* 1975;257:559.

230. Kunicki T, Nurden A, Ridard D, et al. Characterization of human platelet glycoprotein antigens giving rise to individual immunoprecipitates in crossed-immunoelectrophoresis. *Blood* 1981;58:1190.

231. George J, Caen J, Nurden A. Glanzmann's thrombasthenia: the spectrum of clinical disease. *Blood* 1990;75:1383.

232. Burgess-Wilson M, Cockbill S, Johnston G, et al. Platelet aggregation in whole blood from individuals with Glanzmann's thrombasthenia. *Blood* 1987;69:38.

233. Loftus J, O'Toole T, Plow E, et al. A b3 integrin mutation abolishes ligand binding and alters divalent cation-dependent conformation. *Science* 1990;249:915.

234. Fournier D, Kabral A, Castaldi P, et al. A variant of Glanzmann's thrombasthenia characterized by abnormal glycoprotein IIb-IIIa complex formation. *Thromb Haemost* 1989;62:977.
235. Ginsberg M, Lightsey A, Kunicki T, et al. Divalent cation regulation of the surface orientation of platelet membrane glycoprotein I. Correlation with fibrinogen binding and definition of a novel variant of Glanzmann's thrombasthenia. *J Clin Invest* 1986;78:1103.
236. Ginsberg M, Frelinger A, Lam S, et al. Analysis of platelet aggregation disorders based on flow cytometric analysis of membrane glycoprotein IIb-IIIa with conformation-specific monoclonal antibodies. *Blood* 1990;76:2017.
237. Weiss H, Rogers J. Fibrinogen and platelets in the primary arrest of bleeding: studies in two patients with congenital afibrinogenemia. *N Engl J Med* 1971;285:369.
238. Gugler E, Luscher E. Platelet function in congenital afibrinogenemia. *N Engl J Med* 1965;14:361.
239. Pevny L, Simon M, Robertson E, et al. Erythroid differentiation in chimaeric mice blocked by a targeted mutation in the gene for transcription factor GATA-1. *Nature* 1991;349:.
240. Visvader J, Elefanty A, Strasser A, et al. GATA-1 but not SCL induces megakaryocytic differentiation in an early myeloid line. *EMBO J* 1992;11:4557.
241. Shivdasani R, Fujiwara Y, McDevitt M, et al. A lineage-selective knockout establishes the critical role of transcription factor GATA-1 in megakaryocyte growth and platelet development. *EMBO J* 1997;16:3965.
242. Vyas P, Ault K, Jackson C, et al. Consequences of GATA-1 deficiency in megakaryocytes and platelets. *Blood* 1999;93:2867.
243. Nichols K, Crispino J, Poncz M, et al. Familial dyserythropoietic anaemia and thrombocytopenia due to an inherited mutation in GATA1. *Nat Genet* 2000;24:266.
244. Tsang A, Fujiwara Y, Hom D, et al. Failure of megakaryopoiesis and arrested erythropoiesis in mice lacking the GATA-1 transcriptional cofactor FOG. *Genes Dev* 1998;12:1176.
245. Andrews N, Erdjument-Bromage H, Davidson M, et al. Erythroid transcription factor NF-E2 is a hematopoietic-specific basic-leucine zipper protein. *Nature* 1993;362:722.
246. Shivdasani RA, Rosenblatt MF, Zucker-Franklin D, et al. Transcription factor NF-E2 is required for platelet formation independent of the actions of thrombopoietin/MGDF in megakaryocytes. *Cell* 1995;81:695.
247. Lecine P, Villeval J, Vyas P, et al. Mice lacking transcription factor NF-E2 provide in vivo validation of the proplatelet model of thrombocytopoiesis and show a platelet production defect that is intrinsic to megakaryocytes. *Blood* 1998;92:1608.
248. Shavit J, Motohashi H, Onodera K, et al. Impaired megakaryopoiesis and behavioral defects in mafG-null mutant mice. *Genes Dev* 1998;12:2164.
249. Wang D, Villasante A, Lewis S, et al. The mammalian B-tubulin repertoire: hematopoietic expression of a novel B-tubulin isotype. *J Cell Biol* 1985;103:1903.
250. Lecine P, Italiano J, Kim S, et al. Hematopoietic-specific β1 tubulin participates in a pathway of platelet biogenesis dependent on the transcription factor NF-E2. *Blood* 2000;96:1366.
251. Schwer H, Lecine P, Tiwari S, et al. A lineage-restricted and divergent β-tubulin isoform is essential for the biogenesis, structure and function of blood platelets. *Curr Biol* 2001;11:579.
252. May R. Leokozyteneinschlusse. *Deutsch Arch Klin Med* 1909;96:1.
253. Hegglin R. Gleichzeitige konstitutionelle veranderungen an neurtophilen und thrombocyten. *Helv Med Acta* 1945;12:439.
254. Kelley M, Jawien W, Ortel T, et al. Mutation of MYH9, encoding non-muscle myosin heavy chain A, in May-Hegglin anomaly. *Nat Genet* 2000;26:106.
255. Kunishima S, Kojima T, Matsushita T, et al. Mutations in the NMMHC-A gene cause autosomal dominant macrothrombocytopenia with leukocyte inclusions (May-Hegglin anomaly/Sebastian syndrome). *Blood* 2001;97:1147.
256. Seri M, Savino M, (The May-Hegglin/Fechtner Syndrome Consortium). Mutations in MYH9 result in May-Hegglin anomaly, and Fechtner and Sebastian syndromes. *Nat Genet* 2000;26:103.
257. Kunishima S, Kojima T, Matsushita T, et al. Mutations in the NMMHC-A gene cause autosomal dominant macrothrombocytopenia with leukocyte inclusions (May-Hegglin anomaly/Sebastian syndrome). *Blood* 2001;97:1147.
258. Peterson L, Rao K, Crosson J, et al. Fechtner syndrome: a variant of Alport's syndrome with leukocyte inclusions and macrothrombocytopenia. *Blood* 1985;65:397.
259. Greinacher A, Nieuwenhuis H, White J. Sebastian platelet syndrome: a new variant of the hereditary macrothrombocytopenia with leukocyte inclusions. *Blut* 1990;61:282.
260. Novak E, Reddington M, Zhen L, et al. Inherited thrombocytopenia caused by reduced platelet production in mice with the gunmetal pigment gene mutation. *Blood* 1995;85:1781.
261. Swank R, Jiang S, Reddington M, et al. Inherited abnormalities in platelet organelles and platelet formation and associated altered expression of low molecular weight guanosine triphosphate-binding proteins in the mouse pigment mutant gunmetal. *Blood* 1993;81:2626.
262. Detter J, Zhang Q, Mules E, et al. Rab geranylgeranyl transferase alpha mutation in the gunmetal mouse reduces Rab prenylation and platelet synthesis. *Blood* 2000;97:4144.
263. Miki H, Yamaguchi H, Suetsugu S, et al. IRSp53 is an essential intermediate between rac and WAVE in the regulation of membrane ruffling. *Nature* 2000;408:732.
264. Miki H, Suetsugu S, Takenawa T. WAVE, a novel WASP-family protein involved in actin reorganization induced by Rac. *EMBO J* 1998;17:6932.
265. Andrews R, Fox J. Interaction of purified actin-binding protein with the platelet membrane glycoprotein Ib-IX complex. *J Biol Chem* 1991;266:7144.
266. Andrews R, Fox J. Identification of a region in the cytoplasmic domain of the platelet membrane glycoprotein Ib-IX complex that binds to purified actin-binding protein. *J Cell Biol* 1992;267:18605.
267. Izaguirre G, Aguirre L, Ji P, et al. Tyrosine phosphorylation of α-actinin in activated platelets. *J Biol Chem* 1999;274:37012.
268. Burn P, Rotman A, Meyer RK, et al. Diacylglycerol in large α-actinin/actin complexes and in the cytoskeleton of activated platelets. *Nature* 1985;314:469.
269. Landon F, Olomucki A. Isolation and physio-chemical properties of blood platelet α-actinin. *Biochim Biophys Acta* 1983;742:129.
270. Langer BG, Gonnella PA, Nachmias VT. Alpha actinin and vinculin in normal and thrombasthenic platelets. *Blood* 1984;63:606.
271. Pho DB, Desbruyeres E, Terrossian ED, et al. Cytoskeletons of ADP- and thrombin-stimulated blood platelets. Presence of a caldesmon-like protein, α-actinin and gelsolin at different steps of the stimulation. *FEBS Lett* 1986;202:117.
272. Sixma J, van den Berg A, Jockusch B, et al. Immunoelectron microscopic localization of actin, α-actinin, actin-binding protein and myosin in resting and activated human blood platelets. *Eur J Cell Biol* 1989;48:271.
273. Gache Y, Landon F, Touitou H, et al. Susceptibility of platelet alpha-actinin to a Ca2+-activated neutral protease. *Biochem Biophys Res Commun* 1984;124:877.
274. Landon F, Gache Y, Touitou H, et al. Properties of two isoforms of human blood platelet α-actinin. *Eur J Biochem* 1985;153:231.
275. Safer D, Golla R, Nachmais V. Isolation of a 5-kilodalton actin-sequestering peptide from human blood platelets. *Proc Natl Acad Sci U S A* 1990;87:2536.
276. Safer D, Elzinga M, Nachmias VT. Thymosin β4 and Fx, an actin-sequestering peptide, are indistinguishable. *J Biol Chem* 1991;266:4029.
277. Dash D, Aepfelbacher M, Siess W. Integrin αIIbβ3-mediated translocation of CDC42Hs to the cytoskeleton in stimulated human platelets. *J Biol Chem* 1995;270:17321.
278. Carlier MF, Laurent V, Santolini J, et al. Actin depolymerizing factor (ADF/cofilin) enhances the rate of filament turnover: implication in actin-based motility. *J Cell Biol* 1997;136:1307.
279. Carlier M, Ressad F, Pantaloni D. Control of actin dynamics in cell motility. Role of ADF/Cofilin. *J Biol Chem* 1999;274:33824.
280. Davidson M, Haslam R. Dephosphorylation of cofilin in stimulated platelets roles for GTP-binding protein and Ca2+. *Biochem J* 1994;301:41.
281. Earnest J, Santos G, Zuerbig S, et al. Dystrophin-related protein in platelet membrane skeleton. *J Biol Chem* 1995;270:27259.
282. Claudianos C, Campbell H. The novel flightless-I gene brings together two gene families, actin-binding proteins related to gelsolin and leucine-rich-repeat proteins involved in ras signal transduction. *Mol Biol Evol* 1995;12:405.
283. Janmey P, Stossel T. Modulation of gelsolin function by phosphatidylinositol 4,5-bisphosphate. *Nature* 1987;325:362.
284. Elzagallaai A, Rose S, Trifaro J. Platelet secretion induced by phorbol esters stimulation is mediated through phosphorylation of MARCKS: a MARCKS-derived peptide blocks MARCKS phosphorylation and serotonin release without affecting pleckstrin phosphorylation. *Blood* 2000;95:894.
285. Nakamura F, Huang L, Pestonjamasp K, et al. Regulation of F-actin binding to platelet moesin in vitro by both phosphorylation of threonine 558 and polyphosphatidylinositides. *Mol Biol Cell* 1999;10:2669.
286. Shcherbina A, Kenney D, Bretscher A, et al. Dynamic association of moesin with the membrane skeleton of thrombin-activated platelets. *Blood* 1999;93:2128.
287. Goldschmidt-Clermont P, Machesky L, Baldassare J, et al. The actin-binding protein profilin binds to PIP2 and inhibits its hydrolysis by phospholipase C. *Science* 1990;247:1575.
288. Goldschmidt-Clermont P, Kim J, Machesky L, et al. Regulation of phospholipase C-γ1 by profilin and tyrosine phosphorylation. *Science* 1991;251:1231.
289. Markey F, Lindberg U, Eriksson L. Human platelets contain profilin, a potential regulator of actin polymerizability. *FEBS Lett* 1978;88:75.
290. Lassing I, Lindberg U. Specific interaction between phosphatidylinositol 4,5-bisphosphate and profilactin. *Nature* 1985;318:472.
291. Fox J, Boyles J, Berndt M, et al. Identification of a membrane skeleton in platelets. *J Cell Biol* 1988;106:1525.
292. Beckerle M, Miller D, Bertagnolli M, et al. Activation-dependent redistribution of the adhesion plaque protein, talin, in intact human platelets. *J Cell Biol* 1989;109:3333.
293. Muguruma M, Matsumura S, Fukazawa T. Direct interactions between talin and actin. *Biochem Biophys Res Commun* 1990;171:1217.
294. O'Halloran T, Beckerle MC, Burridge K. Identification of talin as a major cytoplasmic protein implicated in platelet activation. *Nature* 1985;317:449.
295. Lo S, An Q, Bao S, et al. Molecular cloning of chick cardiac muscle tensin: full-length cDNA sequence, expression and characterization. *J Biol Chem* 1994;269:22310.
296. Reinhard M, Tripier D, Walter U. Identification, purification and characterization of a zyxin-related protein that binds the focal adhesion and microfilament protein VASP (vasodilator-stimulated phosphoprotein). *Proc Natl Acad Sci U S A* 1995;92:7956.
297. Reinhard M, Rudiger M, Jockusch B, et al. VASP interaction with vinculin: a recurring theme of interactions with proline-rich motifs. *FEBS Lett* 1996;399:103.
298. Reinhard M, Giehl K, Abel K, et al. The proline-rich focal adhesion and microfilament protein VASP is a ligand for profilins. *EMBO J* 1995;14:1583.

299. Reinhard M, Halbrügge M, Scheer U, et al. The 46/50 kDa phosphoprotein VASP purified from human platelets is a novel protein associated with actin filaments and focal contacts. *EMBO J* 1992;11:2063.

300. Abel K, Mieskes G, Walter U. Dephosphorylation of the focal adhesion protein VASP in vitro and in intact human platelets. *FEBS Lett* 1995;370:184.

301. Rosenfeld G, Hou D, Dingus J, et al. Isolation and partial characterization of human platelet vinculin. *J Cell Biol* 1985;100:669.

302. Aspenström P. Effectors for the Rho GTPases. *Cur Opin Cell Biol* 1999;11:95.

303. Lal AA, Korn ED, Brenner SL. Rate constants for actin polymerization in ATP determined using cross-linked actin trimers as nuclei. *J Biol Chem* 1984;259:8794.

304. Snapper S, Rosen F, Mizoguchi E, et al. Wiskott-Aldrich syndrome protein-deficient mice reveal a role for WASP in T but not B cell activation. *Immunity* 1998;9:81.

305. Ramesh N, Antón I, Martínez-Quiles N, et al. Waltzing with WASP. *Trends Cell Biol* 1999;9:15.

306. Ramesh N, Anton I, Hartwig J, et al. WIP, a protein associated with Wiskott-Aldrich syndrome protein, induces actin polymerization and redistribution in lymphoid cells. *Proc Natl Acad Sci U S A* 1997;94:14671.

307. Reinhard M, Zumbrunn J, Jaquemar D, et al. An α-actinin binding site for zyxin is essential for subcellular zyxin localization and α-actinin recruitment. *J Biol Chem* 1999;274:13410.

308. Crawford A, Michelsen J, Beckerle M. An interaction between zyxin and alpha-actinin. *J Cell Biol* 1992;116:1381.

309. Wardell M, Reynolds C, Berndt M, et al. Platelet glycoprotein Ibβ is phosphorylated on serine 166 by cyclic AMP-dependent kinase. *J Biol Chem* 1989;264:15656.

310. Du X, Fox J, Pei S. Identification of a binding sequence for the 14-3-3 protein within the cytoplasmic domain of the adhesion receptor, platelet glycoprotein Ibα. *J Biol Chem* 1996;267:18605.

311. Schoenwaelder S, Yuan Y, Cooray P, et al. Calpain cleavage of focal adhesion proteins regulates the cytoskeletal attachment of integrin αIIbβ3 (platelet glycoprotein IIb/IIIa) and the cellular retraction of fibrin clots. *J Biol Chem* 1996;272:1694.

312. Schoenwaelder S, Burridge K. Evidence for a calpeptin-sensitive protein-tyrosine phosphatase upstream of the small GTPase Rho. *J Biol Chem* 1999; 274:14359.

313. Fox J, Reynolds C, Austin C. The role of calpain in stimulus-response coupling: evidence that calpain mediates agonist-induced expression of procoagulant activity in platelets. *Blood* 1990;76:2510.

314. Fox J, Taylor R, Taffarel M, et al. Evidence that activation of platelet calpain is induced as a consequence of binding of adhesive ligand to the integrin, glycoprotein IIb-IIIa. *J Cell Biol* 1993;120:1501.

315. Bellanger JM, Lazaro JB, Diriong S, et al. The two guanine nucleotide exchange domains of Trio link the rac1 and the rhoA pathways in vivo. *Oncogene* 1998;16:147.

316. Abe K, Rossman K, Liu B, et al. Vav2 is an activator of cdc42, rac1, and rhoA. *J Biol Chem* 2000;275:10141.

317. Cichowski K, Brugge J, Brass L. Thrombin receptor activation and integrin engagement stimulate tyrosine phosphorylation of the proto-oncogene product, p95^{vav}, in platelets. *J Biol Chem* 1996;271:7544.

318. Fischer KD, Kong YY, Nishina H, et al. Vav is a regulator of cytoskeletal reorganization mediated by the T-cell receptor. *Curr Biol* 1998;8:554.

319. Holsinger L, Graef I, Swat W, et al. Defects in actin-cap formation in Vav-deficient mice implicate an actin requirement for lymphocyte signal transduction. *Curr Biol* 1998;8:563.

320. Miranti C, Leng L, Maschberger P, et al. Identification of a novel integrin signaling pathway involving the kinase Syk and the guanine nucleotide exchange factor Vav1. *Curr Biol* 1998;8:1289.

321. Zhang J, Falck J, Reddy K, et al. Phosphatidylinositol (3,4,5)-trisphosphate stimulates phosphorylation of pleckstrin in human platelets. *J Biol Chem* 1995;270:22807.

322. Zhang J, King W, Dillon S, et al. Activation of platelet phosphatidylinositide 3-kinase requires the small GTP-binding protein rho. *J Biol Chem* 1993;268:22251.

323. Zhang J, Zhang J, Shattil S, et al. Phosphoinositide 3-kinase γ and p85/phosphoinositide 3-kinase in platelets. Relative activation by thrombin receptor or β-phorbol myristate acetate and roles in promoting the ligand-binding function of $\alpha_{IIb}\beta_3$ integrin. *J Biol Chem* 1996;271:6265.

324. Vemuri G, Zhang J, Huang R, et al. Thrombin stimulates wortmannin-inhibitable phosphoinositide 3-kinase and membrane blebbing in CHRF-288 cells. *Biochem J* 1996;314:805.

325. Zhang J, Fry M, Waterfield M, et al. Activated phosphoinositide 3-kinase associates with membrane skeleton in thrombin-exposed platelets. *J Biol Chem* 1992;267:4686.

326. Chong L, Traynor-Kaplan A, Bokoch G, et al. The small GTP-binding protein rho regulates a phosphatidylinositol 4-phosphate 5-kinase in mammalian cells. *Cell* 1994;79:507.

327. Abrams C, Wu H, Zhao W, et al. Pleckstrin inhibits phosphoinositide hydrolysis initiated by g-protein-coupled and growth factor receptors: a role for pleckstrins pH domains. *J Biol Chem* 1995;270:14485.

328. Hu M, Bauman E, Roll R, et al. Pleckstrin 2, a widely expressed paralog of pleckstrin involved in actin rearrangement. *J Biol Chem* 1999;274:21515.

329. Ohta Y, Suxuki N, Nakamura S, et al. The small GTPase RalA targets filamin to induce filopodia. *Proc Natl Acad Sci U S A* 1999;96:2122.

330. Wolthuis R, Franke B, van Treiest M, et al. Activation of the small GTPase Ral in platelets. *Mol Cell Biol* 1998;18:2486.

331. Franke B, Akkerman JW, Bos J. Rapid Ca^{2+}-mediated activation of Rap1 in human platelets. *EMBO J* 1997;16:252.

CHAPTER 34

Platelet Membrane Proteins and Their Disorders

Mark L. Kahn, Joel S. Bennett, Lawrence F. Brass, and Mortimer Poncz

Although platelets may contribute to one's inflammatory response, their central role is in hemostasis, interacting with components of the blood vessel wall and linking together to form multicellular aggregates. The platelet is designed to function much like a sophisticated "sea mine" that can detect a disturbance in its natural environment and react to that disturbance almost instantaneously. They must be able to react rapidly to perturbations in the vascular bed, for they are rapidly flowing by the site of injury, and it does an organism little good if platelet activation occurs downstream of the injury. To accomplish this task, the platelet "sea mine" is equipped with multiple types of sophisticated receptors on its surface to detect perturbations in its environme   nt, an intracellular series of pathways to rapidly transmit the signal internally, and a series of organelles to release an explosion of procoagulant agents. In addition, the platelet contributes to the development of a thrombus by having a number of surface receptors that become activated by "inside-out" signaling pathways, so that previously quiescent receptors now have high affinity for their ligands and cross-link platelets to each other and to their environment. This chapter reviews the structure and function of the principal platelet membrane proteins and the disorders caused by their loss or dysfunction.

CLASSIFICATION OF THE PLATELET MEMBRANE GLYCOPROTEINS

Over the past 15 years, many of the membrane receptors have been cloned. Initially, many of these protein receptors had been classified by their electrophoretic mobility and molecular mass and numbered sequentially. Now, it is clear that many of these proteins are members of several large families of receptors. These include the integrin αβ heteroduplexes, the leucine-rich receptor glycoprotein (gp) Ibα-Ibβ-IX-V (the gpIb-IX complex), the seven-transmembrane membrane, the G protein–coupled receptors (GPCRs), and the superimmunoglobulin family. Such a classification takes advantage of the common structure and, often, the common function of members of these families. Further, family members share common pathways by which they interact with the intracellular environment. Table 34-1 lists the members of these families of receptors that are found on platelets, as well as several receptors that do not belong to any of these families. Many of these receptors have other historic names, and these names as well as their

cluster differentiation (CD) antigen nomenclature are noted in Table 34-1. Below, we present a detailed description of many of these receptors, their biologic function, and their clinical implications.

INTEGRIN RECEPTORS IN PLATELET AGGREGATION AND ADHESION

Integrins are members of a ubiquitous family of receptors that mediate cell–cell and cell–matrix interactions involved in processes as diverse as tissue migration during embryogenesis, cellular adhesion, lymphocyte-helper and killer cell functions, and thrombosis (1). Integrins are noncovalent heterodimers of α and β subunits and have been grouped into subfamilies based on the type of β subunit. More than 20 different integrins have been identified in mammalian cells. Approximately one-half of the known receptors can be inhibited by peptides containing an RGD sequence (1). Platelets express five integrins that support platelet adhesion to the subendothelial matrix and mediate platelet aggregation.

Integrins Mediating Platelet Adhesion

The *vascular endothelium* is a barrier that separates platelets from adhesive substrates in the subendothelial connective tissue matrix. When trauma or disease disrupts this barrier, platelets adhere to components of the subendothelial matrix. At lower shear rates, the integrins $\alpha_2\beta_1$, $\alpha_5\beta_1$, and $\alpha_6\beta_1$ mediate platelet adherence to collagen, fibronectin, and laminin, respectively (2). However, at the higher shear rates present in the arterial and microcirculation, platelet adhesion requires binding of the nonintegrin GPIb-IX complex to vWF (3).

$\alpha_2\beta_1$

The integrin $\alpha_2\beta_1$ is a Mg^{2+}-dependent receptor for collagen in many cells, including platelets (4). In platelets, collagen not only serves as an adhesive substrate, but also functions as an agonist for platelet aggregation. As discussed below with reference to GPVI and other potential collagen receptors, $\alpha_2\beta_1$'s role as an agonist receptor may be complex. Two patients with histories of bleeding have been reported whose platelets did not respond normally to collagen and lacked $\alpha_2\beta_1$ (5,6), as well as a patient with a myeloproliferative disorder whose platelets were both unresponsive to collagen and lacked $\alpha_2\beta_1$ (7). In addition, anti-

TABLE 34-1. Major Receptors Described on the Human Platelet Surface

Class of Receptor	Receptor	Other Names	Number of Receptors/Platelet	Ligand
Integrins				
Adhesion	$\alpha_2\beta_1$	CD49b	~2000	Collagen
	$\alpha_5\beta_1$	CD49e	~4000	Fibronectin
	$\alpha_6\beta_1$	CD49f		Laminin
Aggregation	αIIbβ3	GPIIb-IIIa; CD41b	~80,000	Fibrinogen; vWF
	αvβ3		~500	Vitronectin; osteopontin
Leucine-rich repeats receptor	GPIb-IX	CD42a,b,c	~25,000	vWF; thrombin; P-selectin
G protein–coupled receptors	PAR-1		~2000	Thrombin
	PAR-4		Low	Thrombin
	P2Y1			ADP
	P2X1			ADP
	P2Y12			ADP
	α_{2A}		~700	Epinephrine
	TP		~1000	Thromboxane
	IP			Prostaglandin I$_2$
	CXCR1 and R2		~2000 each	Interleukin-8
	CXCR4		~2000	Stromal-derived factor 1
	CCR4		~2000	Macrophage-derived chemokine
Immunoglobulin superfamily	GPVI	GMP-140; PADGEM	1–3000	Collagen
receptors	P-selectin	CD31	~10,000	P-selectin glycoprotein-1PECAM-
	PECAM-1	CD32	1600–4600	1Immune complexes
	FcγRIIA			
Others	GPIV	CD36	~25,000	Collagen
	p65			Collagen

ADP, adenosine diphosphate; CD, cluster differentiation; GMP, granule membrane glycoprotein; GP, glycoprotein; PAR, protease-activated receptor; PADGEM, platelet activation–dependent granule-external membrane protein; PECAM-1, platelet-endothelial cell adhesion molecule-1; vWF, von Willebrand's factor.

$\alpha_2\beta_1$ monoclonal antibodies have been reported that block the collagen-stimulated phosphorylation of phospholipase C (PLC) γ_2 and the tyrosine kinase Syk (8). Thus, these data suggest that collagen binding to $\alpha_2\beta_1$ is a necessary component of collagen-induced signaling.

There is substantial variability in the density of $\alpha_2\beta_1$ on the surface of platelets from different individuals (9). These differences in $\alpha_2\beta_1$ expression are associated with the presence of three α2 alleles defined by combinations of eight linked nucleotide polymorphisms in the α2 gene (10). Studies *in vitro* indicate that increased density of $\alpha_2\beta_1$ increases the rate of platelet attachment to type 1 collagen under high shear condition (10), and some (11,12), but not all (13), epidemiologic surveys suggest that increased $\alpha_2\beta_1$ density is a risk factor for nonfatal myocardial infarction and stroke in younger individuals. On the other hand, an increased prevalence of the lower $\alpha_2\beta_1$ density allele has been reported in patients with type 1 von Willebrand's disease, suggesting that this allele may contribute to bleeding symptoms in these patients (14).

$\alpha_5\beta_1$ AND A$_6\beta_1$

Studies *in vitro* demonstrate that $\alpha_5\beta_1$ mediates platelet adhesion and spreading on surfaces coated with fibronectin under both static and flow conditions (15,16), whereas $\alpha_6\beta_1$ mediates platelet adhesion—but not spreading—on surfaces coated with laminin (17,18). Nevertheless, the physiologic roles of these receptors for platelet adhesion *in vivo* are not clear.

Integrins Mediating Platelet Aggregation

αIIbβ3

The integrin αIIbβ3 (GPIIb-IIIa) mediates the aggregation of agonist-stimulated platelets by binding soluble macromolecular ligands such as fibrinogen or vWF (19). αIIbβ3-bound fibrinogen or vWF then cross-links platelets into a hemostatic plug

or thrombus. αIIbβ3 is the most prevalent protein on the platelet surface (Table 34-1), with approximately 80,000 αIIbβ3 molecules on the surface of platelets (20). Additional molecules, which are present in the membrane of the platelet α-granules, can be translocated to the platelet surface after platelet activation (21). αIIbβ3 is a calcium-dependent noncovalent heterodimer composed of two type I transmembrane proteins: αIIb (GPIIb, CD41) and β3 (GPIIIa, CD61) (Fig. 34-1). *αIIb* is a disulfide-linked two-chain molecule composed of a 136-kd heavy chain and a 23-kd light chain (22). The latter anchors the molecule in the platelet membrane via a single carboxyl-terminal transmembrane domain. The amino terminal half of the αIIb heavy chain consists of seven tandem repeats; computer modeling of the repeats suggests that this portion of αIIb may fold into a β-propeller configuration (23). Crystallographic studies of αvβ3 support this organization (23a). Each of the carboxyl terminal four repeats contains a 12–amino acid stretch homologous to the Ca^{2+}-binding loops of Ca^{2+}-binding proteins such as calmodulin and parvalbumin (24). Measurements of Ca^{2+} binding to polypeptides containing this region of αIIb and the homologous region of integrin subunit α5 indicate that the region contains four Ca^{2+}-binding sites, two with a kd of 30 µM and two with a kd of 120 µM (25,26). The αIIb fifth repeat also contains a site that can be chemically cross-linked to peptides corresponding to the carboxyl terminus of the fibrinogen γ-chain. β3 is a single chain of 110 kd under reducing conditions that is notable for the presence of 28 disulfide bonds, many of which are concentrated in a protease-resistant core (27,28). Chemical cross-linking experiments suggest that peptides containing the sequence Arg-Gly-Asp (RGD) bind to β3 in the vicinity of amino acids 109 to 171 (29). β3 is anchored in the platelet membrane by a single carboxyl-terminal transmembrane domain. Electron micrographs of the purified heterodimer reveal that it consists of a 12- by 8-nm globular head with two 18-nm tails extending from one side (30). Each tail contains

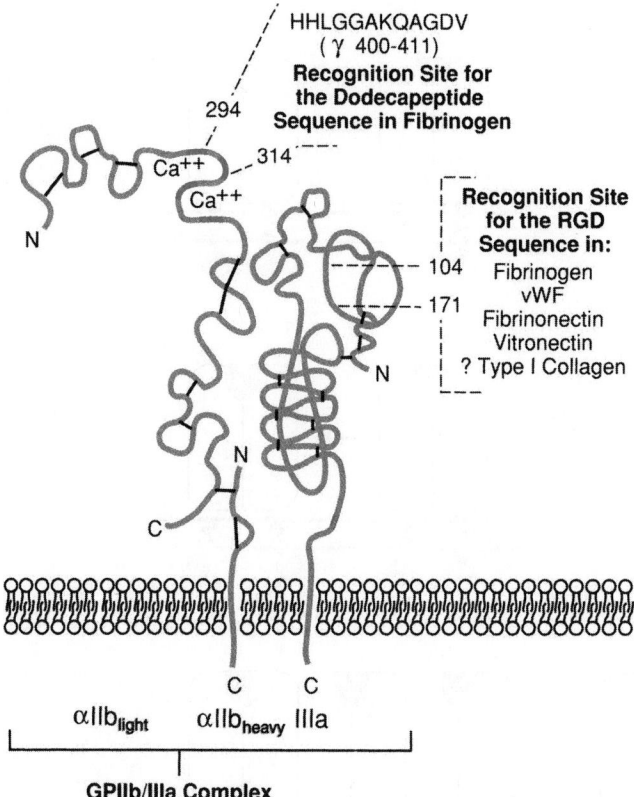

HHLGGAKQAGDV
(γ 400-411)
**Recognition Site for
the Dodecapeptide
Sequence in Fibrinogen**

**Recognition Site
for the RGD
Sequence in:**
Fibrinogen
vWF
Fibrinonectin
Vitronectin
? Type I Collagen

Figure 34-1. Structure of the αIIbβ3 complex. αIIb is synthesized as a single precursor, which is cleaved to produce αIIbα and αIIbβ. αIIbβ anchors the protein in the lipid bilayer of the membrane and is disulfide-bonded to αIIbα. αIIb contains four calcium-binding domains. β3 is a single-chain polypeptide that contains a cysteine-rich sequence just distal to the plasma membrane. RGD, arginine-glycine-aspartic acid; vWF, von Willebrand's factor.

the carboxyl terminus of one subunit, and the ligand-binding site is located on the globular head on the side opposite of the tails. In the presence of Ca²⁺ chelators, the αIIbβ3 dissociates into comma-shaped monomers consisting of a small globular head and a single 24- to 27-nm tail.

αIIb and β3 are the products of separate genes located 1.3 cm apart on the long arm of human chromosome 17 at q21 (31) and are assembled into heterodimers in the Ca²⁺-rich environment of the endoplasmic reticulum (32). Like many oligomeric proteins, neither αIIb nor β3 can exit the endoplasmic reticulum in the absence of heterodimer formation (33). Consequently, mutations that impair the synthesis of either αIIb or β3 result in the inherited platelet disorder Glanzmann's thrombasthenia (GT) by preventing αIIbβ3 expression on the platelet surface. In the Golgi complex, the asparagine-linked carbohydrates of αIIb are remodeled, and αIIb is cleaved into heavy and light chains on the carboxyl side of the dibasic sequence Arg[837]-Arg[838] by an enzyme of the furin family of endoproteases (34). Why αIIb undergoes cleavage is not clear.

The affinity of αIIbβ3 for its ligands is tightly regulated to avoid spontaneous—and potentially deleterious—platelet aggregation. Thus, αIIbβ3 on the surface of circulating platelets is inactive (Fig. 34-2) but is rapidly activated by platelet agonists such as thrombin, adenosine diphosphate (ADP), and collagen (19). Because activation occurs without an increase in the number of αIIbβ3 complexes on the platelet surface, it is assumed to result from a conformational change in αIIbβ3 (Fig. 34-2) (35,36). The sequence of biochemical reactions regulating αIIbβ3 affinity

remains uncertain. Platelet stimulation activates PLC, generating diacylglycerol and inositol 1,4,5-triphosphate from phosphatidylinositol 4,5-bisphosphate (37). Diacylglycerol, in turn, activates protein kinase C (PKC), whereas inositol 1,4,5-triphosphate increases intracellular calcium, facilitating the activation of phospholipase A₂ and the release of arachidonic acid from membrane phospholipids. Phorbol esters activate PKC and are potent platelet agonists, suggesting that PKC plays an important role in inside-out signaling in platelets. However, agonists can activate αIIbβ3 despite the presence of PKC inhibitors, implying that platelets contain both PKC-dependent and PKC-independent activation pathways (38). Platelets also contain high concentrations of the protein tyrosine kinase Src; the Src family members Fyn, Lyn, Hck, and Yes; and the protein kinase Syk (37). Moreover, platelet activation results in the phosphorylation of a number of intracellular proteins on serine, threonine, and tyrosine residues. Which, if any, of these phosphorylated proteins is involved in αIIbβ3 activation is not known.

Tyrosine phosphorylation in platelets occurs in three waves (39). The first wave occurs within seconds of agonist stimulation and results in the phosphorylation of pp60[src], cortactin, pp72[syk], p21[ras]GAP, and proteins of 59 kd and 68 kd. It could be involved in regulating αIIbβ3 affinity. The second and third waves of phosphorylation, in contrast, require αIIbβ3 occupation by ligands (40,41). The second wave, which is likely the result of αIIbβ3 clustering (Fig. 34-2E), produces phosphorylation of proteins of 140 kd and 50 to 68 kd and pp72[syk]. The third wave results from platelet aggregation and induces the phosphorylation of proteins such as pp125[FAK] as well as proteins of 95 to 97 kd. Concurrent with the second and third waves of Tyr phosphorylation, αIIbβ3 activation results in reorganization of the platelet cytoskeleton.

Glanzmann's Thrombasthenia

GT, a rare congenital platelet disorder characterized by a prolonged bleeding time, a normal platelet count, and absent macroscopic platelet aggregation, results from deficiency or dysfunction of αIIbβ3 (Table 34-2) (42). In addition, the amount of α-granule fibrinogen is decreased or absent in thrombasthenic platelets (43), the retraction of clots containing thrombasthenic platelets is either reduced or absent (44), and thrombasthenic platelets are unable to spread normally on the subendothelial matrix (45,46).

MOLECULAR ABNORMALITIES

GT is inherited as an autosomal-recessive disorder (47) and historically has been classified into three types (43). In type I, platelets contain less than 5% of the normal amount of αIIbβ3, and clot retraction and α-granule fibrinogen are absent. In type II, platelets contain 10% to 20% of the normal amount of αIIbβ3, clot retraction is decreased, and α-granule fibrinogen is present. "Variant" thrombasthenia is a qualitative rather than a quantitative disorder; platelets contain 50% or more of the normal amount of αIIbβ3 but still do not aggregate.

As the genetic defects underlying the thrombasthenic phenotype have become defined, the rationale for maintaining these three traditional categories of GT becomes less convincing, and, alternatively, more complicated classifications have been proposed that are based on surface expression or on the fate of αIIb and β3 subunits as they traffic through the cell to reach the plasma membrane (46). Currently, the most common method used for determining the levels of αIIbβ3 on thrombasthenic platelets involves flow cytometry (47) and Western blot (immunoblot) analysis (48).

Nearly 200 individuals with GT have been described in the literature. To date, more than 60 of these have been solved at the

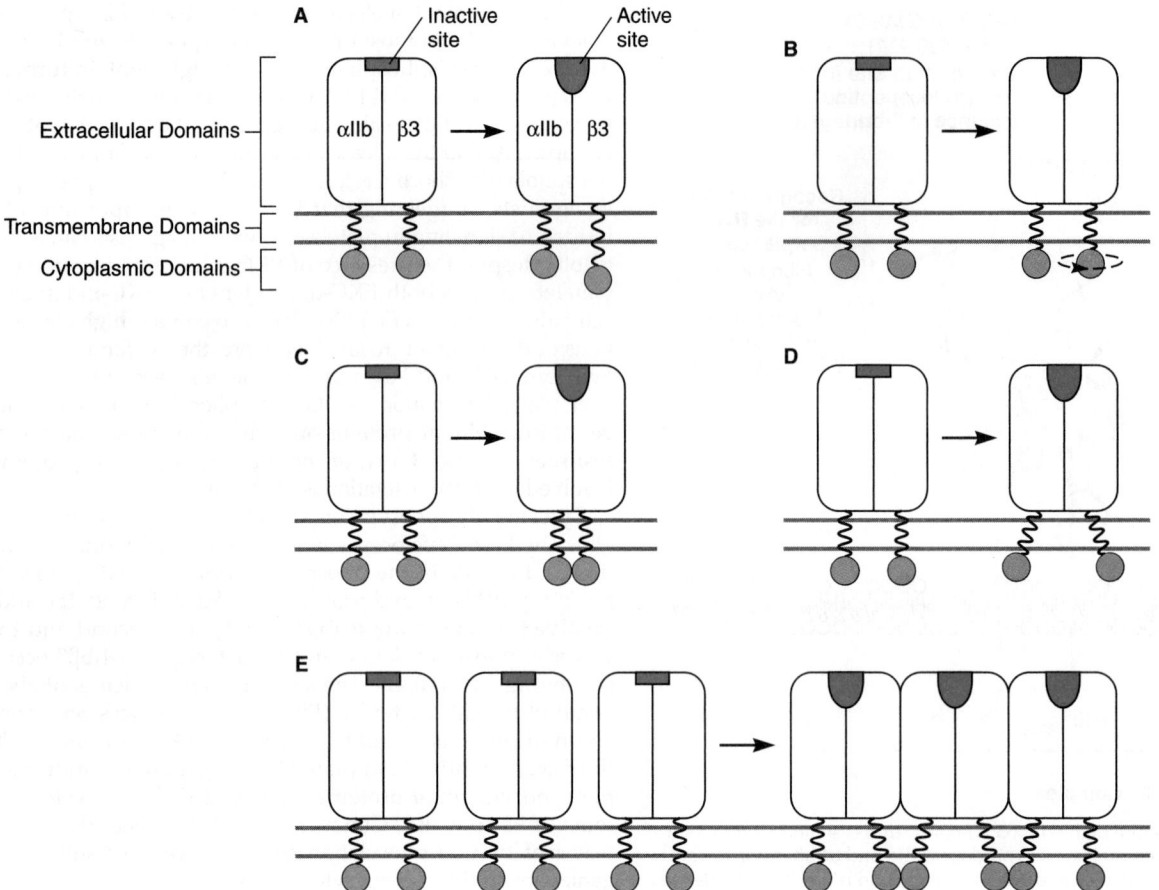

Figure 34-2. Possible mechanisms of αIIbβ3 activation. αIIbβ3 resides in the platelet membrane and is represented in this figure as two boxes with extracellular, transmembrane, and cytoplasmic domains. αIIbβ3 is represented as being in the inactive form and is activated by signals that interact with its cytoplasmic domains, inducing a conformation change in its extracellular domain that exposes its ligand-binding active site. Possible mechanisms of αIIbβ3 activation are illustrated. One transmembrane helix could be displaced in a vertical direction in relation to the other (**A**); one transmembrane domain could rotate in the plane of the membrane in relation to the other (**B**); signal-induced release of intracellular constraints could allow the transmembrane or cytoplasmic domains (or both) of αIIb and β3 to bind to each other (**C**) or move away from each other (**D**), or it could induce αIIbβ3 clustering (**E**).

molecular level (Table 34-3). As in most genetic disorders, the molecular abnormalities have been found to range from major deletions and inversions to single point mutations identified by nucleotide sequence analysis of genomic DNA or platelet mRNA-derived polymerase chain reaction products (for review, see reference 49 and http://med.mssm.edu/glanzmanndb). *In vitro* studies have indicated that production of both protein subunits is required for proper surface expression and function (49), and this concept has been nicely corroborated at the level of human biology through the molecular biologic analysis of GT defects. The mutations that have been identified in the αIIb and β3 genes result in qualitative or quantitative abnormalities, or both, of the platelet membrane proteins (49–52), and the molecular characterization of GT in patients and their families has permitted DNA-based carrier detection and prenatal diagnoses to be performed (53,54). Some of the better-characterized subgroups of mutations are described later and in Table 34-3.

The earliest and largest group of thrombasthenic mutations described did not express αIIbβ3 on the cell surface. Several of these patients had major deletions or inversions in their αIIb or β3 genes. In addition, a number of point mutations or small deletions in the αIIb or β3 genes have been described that block surface expression of complex. Here both chains are formed

intracellularly and complex to each other, but do not undergo further intracellular processing and do not reach the cell surface (Table 34-3). These result in a type I form of thrombasthenia. One major subgroup of these patients has missense mutations in the N-terminal β-propeller repeats of αIIb near the proposed Ca^{2+}-binding sites on its lower surface (55,56).

This last group of mutations is of interest because mutations in the same β-propeller region have a different phenotype—but at sites that are modeled to be present on the upper surface.

TABLE 34-2. Clinical Criteria for the Diagnosis of Thrombasthenia

Autosomal-recessive inheritance.
Epistaxis, ecchymoses, gingival bleeding beginning in infancy.
Menorrhagia, gastrointestinal bleeding, posttraumatic hemorrhage.
Prolonged bleeding time.
Normal platelet count and size.
Platelets fail to aggregate with any agonists and do not bind fibrinogen.
Agglutination with ristocetin and binding of von Willebrand's factor is normal.
Absence (type I) or reduction (type II) of the αIIbβ3 complex or presence of dysfunctional proteins that cannot bind fibrinogen.

TABLE 34-3. Glanzmann's Thrombasthenia Mutations Involving Either Point Mutations or Small Deletions

Class of Mutations	Mutation	Mutation Phenotype	Amino Acid Substitution
Mutations with no surface expression (type I)			
αIIb	818G→A	Missense	$G^{242}D$
	1063G→A	Missense	$E^{324}K$
	1787T→C	Missense	$I^{565}T$
	1073G→A	Missense	$R^{327}H$
	1346G→A	Missense	$G^{418}D$
	1366–1371 deletion	Deletion	$V^{425}D^{426}$ deletion
β3	428T→G	Missense	$L^{117}W$
	847 deletion GC	Premature termination	—
Mutations with decreased surface expression but no ligand binding (type II)			
αIIb	620C→T	Missense	$T^{176}I$
	641T→C	Missense	$L^{183}P$
	526C→G	Missense	$P^{145}A$
	527C→T	Missense	$P^{145}L$
Mutations with near-normal surface expression but no ligand binding (variant)			
β3	433G→T	Missense	$D^{119}Y$
	433G→A	Missense	$D^{119}N$
	718C→T	Missense	$R^{214}W$
	719G→A	Missense	$R^{214}Q$
	725G→A	Missense	$R^{216}Q$
	2248C→T	Missense	$R^{724}X$
	2332T→C	Missense	$S^{752}P$

Data taken from French DL, Coller BS. Hematologically important mutations: Glanzmann thrombasthenia. *Blood Cells Mol Dis* 1996;23:39; http://med.mssm.edu/glanzmanndb.

These mutations are located within the α-chain β-propeller in the vicinity of the third blade (W3) of the β-propeller, a region located close to a predicted β-turn structure that has been implicated in the ligand binding of αIIbβ3 and other integrin receptors (57,58). Several missense mutations have been identified. The $L^{183}P$ and $P^{145}A$ mutations have been shown to result in both a quantitative and a qualitative defect of the receptor complex, resulting in a type II version of thrombasthenia. Independent support for the functional importance of this region has been shown by the $D^{224}V$ mutation (59), located within the connecting strand between the third and fourth blades of the propeller. This mutation was identified from *in vitro*–generated mutant αIIbβ3 receptors expressed in CHO cells (60) and disrupts the ligand-binding function of the receptor.

Another early recognized group of thrombasthenic defects was characterized by having significant levels of αIIbβ3 surface expression, although the complex is not able to interact with its natural ligands (Table 34-3). In contrast to the platelets of patients having integrin maturational defects, the binding of many αIIbβ3 complex-specific antibodies is normal in this group, indicating that subunit association and intracellular trafficking are largely unaffected by the nature of the mutation. That the αIIbβ3 complex is not normal is indicated by the fact that divalent-cation–dependent regulation of its conformation can be affected, and the complex may be easily dissociable by chelation of external calcium ions with ethylenediaminetetraacetic acid (patient Cam, $D^{119}Y$ mutation) (61). Many of these missense mutations have been identified within the cation-binding metal ion–dependent adhesion site (MIDAS) . The importance of these sites is reinforced by the identification of a group of *in vitro*–generated mutant αIIbβ3 receptors expressed in CHO cells (60). The mutations $D^{119}N$, $R^{214}W$, $D^{198}N$, $E^{220}Q$, and $E^{220}K$ were identified as functional defects providing independent support for the importance of the MIDAS domain in ligand binding.

Another group of mutations with normal levels of surface αIIbβ3 receptors have mutations in the cytoplasmic domain of β3, demonstrating the importance of this domain for integrin

activation and regulation of ligand binding (147–149). Two GT mutations have been identified in this region. One is a $R^{724}X$ nonsense mutation (patient RM) (62) that deletes the carboxy-terminal 39 residues of β3, and the other is a $S^{752}P$ missense mutation (patient P or Paris I) (63–65). These mutations do not affect surface expression of platelet αIIbβ3 complexes, but mutant receptors are unresponsive to agonist stimulation. Mammalian cell expression studies show normal adhesion to immobilized fibrinogen but abnormal cell spreading. Cells expressing the $S^{752}P$ mutant receptors have reduced focal adhesion plaque formation, and cells expressing the $R^{724}X$ mutant receptors have undetectable tyrosine phosphorylation of focal adhesion kinase pp125[FAK]. These mutations provide compelling evidence for the role of the β3 cytoplasmic tail in the function of the αIIbβ3 receptor complex.

CLINICAL COURSE

Thrombasthenia typically presents in neonates and infants with mucocutaneous bleeding (Table 34-2) (50). Spontaneous petechiae are common, often unusually large, and diffusely scattered over the patient's body. Severe and recurrent nosebleeds and gum oozing occur. Occult gastrointestinal blood loss requires patients to be monitored for the development of iron deficiency, especially during infancy and childhood. Menorrhagia can be severe and require hormonal suppression of menses. Pregnancy and birth are also periods of greater risk to the female patient, especially if she has developed resistance to platelet transfusions. Joint bleeds and intracranial bleeds, although rare, do occur and may be more problematic to treat than in patients with hemophilia. More than 95% of patients reach adulthood. It is noteworthy that the severity of the hemostatic defect in a given thrombasthenic patient is not predictable and does not correlate with the extent of the αIIbβ3 deficiency.

TREATMENT

Platelet transfusion is the gold standard of care in thrombasthenia but has many drawbacks. The major issue is the eventual development of resistance to platelet transfusions, although the strict use of white cell–poor platelets may reduce the incidence of this complication. Therefore, aggressive local management should be pursued to limit exposure to transfused platelets. Proper local compression, topical thrombin, and the use of local vasoconstrictors may control most nosebleeds. Oral contraceptives can control menorrhagia in these patients, and the adjunctive use of fibrinolytic inhibitors, such as epsilon aminocaproic acid, may be useful in controlling bleeding, particularly after dental extractions. Corticosteroids are not effective in managing bleeding in thrombasthenic patients, and DDAVP is not likely to be useful (50). A number of reports have suggested that administration of recombinant factor VIIa may prevent or control bleeding in thrombasthenic patients (66,67), although a number of agents were often given simultaneously to these patients, so that the efficacy and safety of recombinant factor VIIa administration to bleeding patients with thrombasthenia remains to be clarified (68).

$\alpha IIb\beta 3$ Antagonists

Platelet aggregation is responsible for the intravascular thrombi responsible for the morbidity and mortality of arterial vascular disease (69). Because ligand binding to $\alpha IIb\beta 3$ is a prerequisite for platelet aggregation, $\alpha IIb\beta 3$ antagonists have been developed to inhibit arterial thrombosis. Three intravenous $\alpha IIb\beta 3$ antagonists have been approved for use in the setting of acute coronary artery disease: abciximab, eptifibatide, and tirofiban.

Abciximab (c7E3, ReoPro) is the Fab fragment of a human-murine chimeric monoclonal antibody that inhibits platelet aggregation by preventing fibrinogen binding to $\alpha IIb\beta 3$ (70). Abciximab also binds to the vitronectin receptor $\alpha v\beta 3$ and to the leukocyte integrin $\alpha M\beta 2$ (71). Four large clinical trials [EPIC (72), CAPTURE (73), EPILOG (74), and EPISTENT (75)] have shown that administration of abciximab to patients undergoing percutaneous coronary intervention in the setting of acute coronary disease decreased the incidence of death, acute myocardial infarction, and urgent intervention at 30 days by 29% to 57%. Nonetheless, there is little evidence for a beneficial effect beyond the acute period, except perhaps for patients with diabetes (76). Despite its ability to antagonize $\alpha IIb\beta 3$, abciximab can be administered without excessive bleeding (74). Abciximab administration has been associated with thrombocytopenia (77,78). Abciximab-induced thrombocytopenia generally can be reversed immediately by platelet transfusion, and it reverses spontaneously over several days after the drug is stopped. Because abciximab is a human-murine chimera, it is immunogenic (79). Nonetheless, it has been readministered to more than 300 patients without hypersensitivity reactions or loss of efficacy (79).

Eptifibatide (Integrilin), a synthetic RGD-related cyclic heptapeptide based on the snake venom disintegrin barbourin, binds exclusively to $\alpha IIb\beta 3$ (80). In both the IMPACT-II (81) and PURSUIT (82) trials, eptifibatide was modestly beneficial for patients with acute coronary artery disease, although in the former study, the effect was not statistically significant. In the ESPIRIT trial, higher eptifibatide doses improve the outcome of nonurgent coronary artery stent implementation (82a). Tirofiban (MK-0383, Aggrastat) is an RGD-based peptidomimetic analog of tyrosine that binds specifically to $\alpha IIb\beta 3$ (83). After intravenous administration to healthy subjects, its half-life in plasma ranges from 1 to 2 hours. Its efficacy in patients undergoing percutaneous coronary intervention was tested in the RESTORE trial (84) and in patients with unstable angina and non–Q-wave myocardial infarction in the PRISM (85) and PRISM-PLUS (86) trials. In each of these trials, tirofiban offered significant protection against early cardiac events such as death, refractory ischemia, and myocardial infarction.

Nine oral $\alpha IIb\beta 3$ antagonists have been developed to potentially extend the beneficial effects of the intravenous agents (87). All but two of the antagonists are prodrugs that must be metabolically converted to active forms, and all have limited bioavailability and steep dose-response curves. There have been four large trials testing the efficacy and safety of these agents. In the SYMPHONY (88) and EXCITE (89) trials, neither sibrafiban nor xemilofiban decreased the incidence of death, nonfatal, or urgent revascularization, but they did increase the incidence of mucocutaneous bleeding. Both the OPUS-TIMI 16 (90) and BRAVO (91) trials were halted early because preliminary analysis indicated that orbofiban and lotrafiban, respectively, did not reduce clinical events and may have been associated with excess in early mortality. Thus, a role of oral $\alpha IIb\beta 3$ antagonists in the management of patients with chronic coronary artery disease is currently uncertain.

$\alpha v\beta 3$

Platelets express 50- to 500-fold fewer copies of $\alpha v\beta 3$ compared to $\alpha IIb\beta 3$ on the platelet surface (93). Although $\alpha v\beta 3$ is generally considered to reside on the surface of most cells in a constitutively active state, $\alpha v\beta 3$ on platelets resides on the cell surface in an inactive state and can be induced to interact with ligands by conventional platelet agonists (94). *In vitro* studies indicate that $\alpha v\beta 3$ can mediate RGD-dependent platelet adhesion to surfaces coated with the matrix proteins osteopontin and vitronectin (95). Although both of these proteins are present in the matrix of atherosclerotic plaques, a contribution of $\alpha v\beta 3$ to physiologic and pathologic platelet adhesion remains to be determined.

LEUCINE-RICH REPEATS RECEPTOR IN PLATELET ADHESION

Structure and Function of the GPIb-IX Receptor

Whereas the $\alpha IIb\beta 3$ integrin receptor is the predominant receptor on the platelet surface and has a major role in platelet aggregation, the GPIb-IX receptor has a predominant role in the initial sticking of platelets to a site of injury, especially under high flow conditions (96,97). This process is called *platelet adhesion* and is especially important in arterioles and in the microcirculation, where high shear rates are present. After this initial adhesion event, additional platelets aggregate to the site of injury, forming the platelet plug.

Adhesion through the GPIb-IX complex involves vWF binding to the subendothelium. Platelet membranes contain two binding sites for vWF (98). One of these sites requires prior platelet activation and is located on the platelet membrane $\alpha IIb\beta 3$ complex. The second binding site involves the GPIb-IX complex, and it is this membrane complex that is crucial for initial attachment and proper adhesion to the extracellular matrix of a damaged vessel wall (Fig. 34-3) (99). The GPIb-IX complex represents the second most common receptor on the platelet membrane surface, with approximately 25,000 copies/platelet (99). As shown in Figure 34-3, this complex actually consists of four different proteins. All of these proteins have an N-terminal signal peptide and a hydrophobic transmembrane domain near the C-terminus. Each of the four proteins also contains one or more leucine-rich repeats, which is comprised of a 24–amino acid motif that contains seven conserved leucine residues. Other proteins have been described with this leucine-rich repeat, but the biologic significance of this structure is unknown, as the proteins have disparate functions such as a hormone receptor (lutropin-choriogonadotropin receptor) (100), a photoreceptor

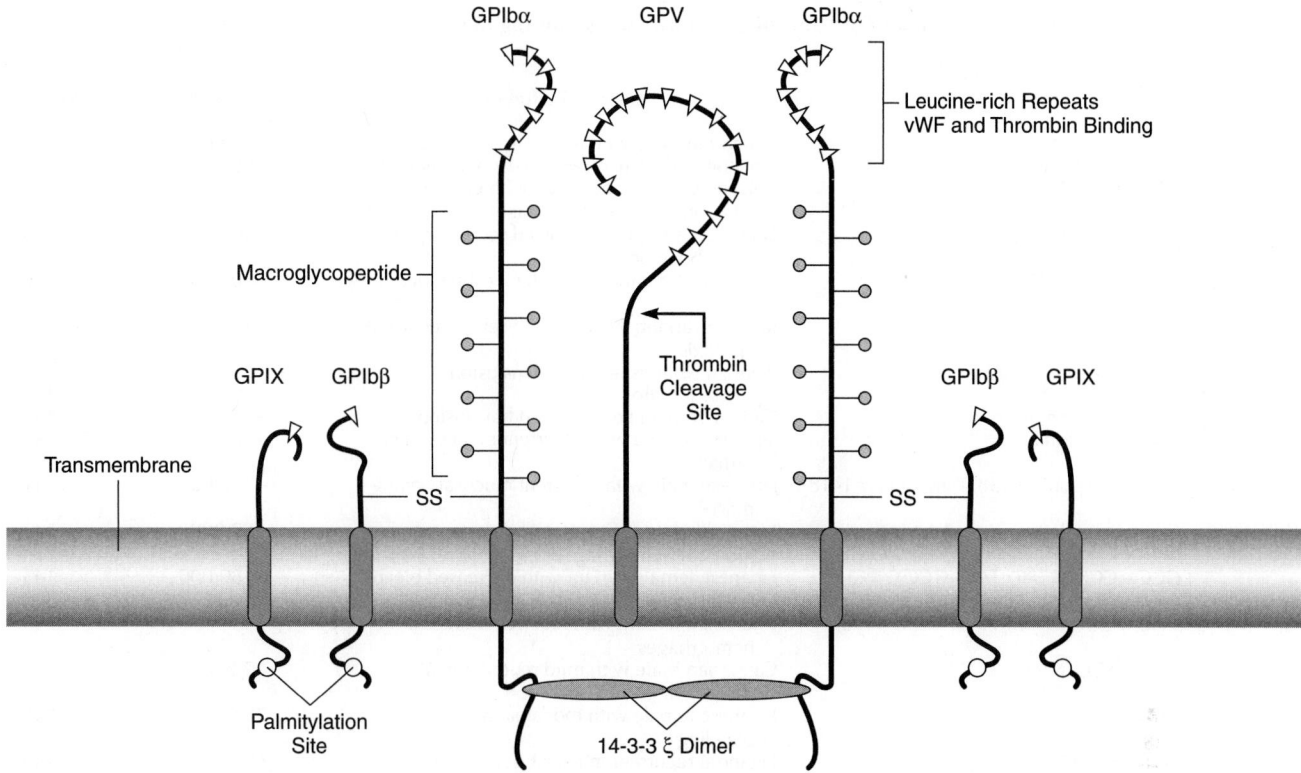

Figure 34-3. This receptor consists of the four proteins glycoprotein (GP) Ibα, GPIbβ, GPIX, and GPV in a 2:2:2:1 stoichiometric ratio, respectively. Structural features found in this receptor complex are depicted, including the leucine-rich repeats found in each protein, the O-linked carbohydrate-rich region of GPIbα, the thrombin cleavage site in GPIbα, the disulfide bond linking GPIbα and GPIbβ, the thrombin- and von Willebrand's factor–binding domain of GPIbα, and some of the intracellular interaction sites, as well as the 14-3-3 ζ-intracytoplasmic dimer. SS, single strand.

(chaoptin) (101), and adenylate cyclase (102). In addition, these repeats have some similarity with the DNA-binding leucine zipper proteins (103–105). These repeats may contribute to vWF binding (11) by the multiprotein GPIb-IX receptor. Finally, it should be pointed out that the GPIb-IX complex may also bind to other ligands, including P-selectin (106).

GPIbα is the largest subunit (135 kd, 610 amino acids) with seven leucine repeats (107). It is susceptible to cleavage by trypsin or by calpain, giving rise to a water-soluble, heavily glycosylated 135-kd N-terminal fragment known as *glycocalicin* (108). In addition to containing the binding site for vWF, the glycocalicin portion of GPIbα may also bind thrombin (109,110). The biologic role of the thrombin-binding site is unclear, because enzymatic cleavage of the GPIb complex, although leading to a loss of vWF-mediated platelet agglutination, does not significantly affect the ability of human platelets to respond to thrombin (111). These data may be explained by the cloning of the protease-activated receptor (PAR) discussed in Thrombin Receptors.

In between the leucine-rich domains and an O-linked glycosylation domain on GPIbα is a region from amino acid residues 220 to 310 that contains the vWF and thrombin-binding regions. Studies with peptide inhibitors suggest that amino acids 269 to 301 contain two charged domains that represent the major binding site for vWF (112,113). *In vivo*, plasma vWF does not bind to the GPIb complex, and it is likely that changes in vWF conformation occur once it has bound to components of the subendothelium or has become subject to shear that enables it to then interact with its platelet receptor (97). In clinical assays, the antibiotic ristocetin or the venom-derived

protein botrocetin is used to mimic this effect, inducing conformational changes in vWF that promote binding to GPIb in stirred platelet-rich plasma (114).

All four chains of the GPIb complex are glycosylated. GPIbα has four potential N-glycosylation sites, whereas GPIbβ and GPIX each have a single N-glycosylation site. In GPIbα, O-linked carbohydrates are associated with a series of five nine–amino acid repeats in a heavily glycosylated region of glycocalicin (115). Thus, members of the GPIb complex contain carbohydrate moieties ending with sialic acid residues, contributing significantly to the negative charge of the platelet surface. This O-linked sugar-rich domain is highly polymorphic with one to four repeats in various individuals (116). Each repeat extends the N-terminal globular region out approximately 45 nm from the cell surface. The thrombophilic implications of this polymorphism are not clear.

GPIbα is disulfide-bonded to GPIbβ (25 kd, 181 amino acids) (117) through a single cysteine residue located in each subunit near the transmembrane domains of GPIbα and GPIbβ. This peptide has only one leucine repeat. The cytoplasmic tail of GPIbβ contains a potential serine phosphorylation site that may be important in tethering the receptor to the cytoskeleton after agonist stimulation (118). The disulfide-bound GPIbα-β is noncovalently associated with platelets GPIX and GPV (119). GPIX is the smallest member of the GPIb complex (22 kd, 160 amino acids) with only one leucine repeat (120). GPV (82 kd, 344 amino acids) is a transmembrane protein with 15 leucine repeats (121). This protein is susceptible to digestion by calpain, and it is a proteolytic substrate for thrombin, releasing a 69-kd soluble fragment

TABLE 34-4. Summary of Molecular Abnormalities Causing Bernard-Soulier Syndrome[a]

Patient	Molecular Defect (Amino Acid Substitution)	Clinical Features	Platelet Count (/mm³)	Reference
GPIbα	TGG→TGA (W[343]X)	Caucasian male with epistaxis	~30,000	131
	CTC→TTC (L[57]F)	Autosomal dominant; Caucasian with epistaxis	~80,000	133
	GCT→GTT (A[156]V)	Bolzano variant; Caucasian with epistaxis and fatal intracranial hemorrhage	~80,000	134
	TGC→AGC (C[209]S)	Spanish male splenectomized secondary to thrombocytopenia	~30,000	135
	CTC→CCC (L[129]P)	African-American, mucosal, menstrual hemorrhage	~80,000	136
	TGG→TGA (W[498]X)	Karlstad variant; Swedish with severe recurrent epistaxis	~10,000	137
	2-base deletion at AA[654]	German siblings required transfusion	~70,000	138
	TCA→TAA (S[444]X)	Japanese female	~20,000	139
	1-base deletion at AA[76]	Caucasian with epistaxis and transfusions	~40,000	140
	2-base deletion at AA[294]	Japanese female with recurrent mucosal hemorrhages	~60,000	141
	1-base deletion at 1438; T insertion at 1418	Japanese male with recurrent mucosal hemorrhages	~30,000	141
GP1bβ	GATA site deletion; gene deletion	Male with velo-facial-cranial defects and mucosal hemorrhages	~80,000	142
	GCC→CCC (A[108]P); TAC→TCC (Y[88]C)	Japanese female variant with decreased bleeding as adult	~180,000	143
GP1X	GAC→GGC (D[21]G); AAC→AGC (N[45]S)	Caucasian female with recurrent mucosal hemorrhages	???	143
	ACC→AGC (N[45]S)	Caucasian male with mild mucosal hemorrhage	60,000	144
	TGG→TGA (W[126]X)	Japanese female with moderate mucosal bleeding	75,000	145
	TGT→TAT (C[73]Y)	Japanese recurrent mucosal, sometimes fatal hemorrhages	???	146
	TTT→TCT (F[55]S)	Male with moderate mucosal hemorrhages	50,000	147

GP, glycoprotein.
[a]Many of the patients have homozygous mutations.

(122). GPV is interesting in that the other three components of the complex are present as two copies/complex, but GPV is only present as a single copy/complex. Further, its biologic role may be antithrombotic because it prevents signaling by thrombin bound to GPIbα from activating the platelet until thrombin cleaves GPV and leads to its removal (123). Thus, the GPV knock-out mouse appears to have a mild prothrombotic state (124).

Binding of activated vWF to the GPIb complex activates platelets (125) and operates through an arachidonic acid metabolite–dependent activation of PLC. This signal results in the mobilization of PKC, promotes platelet secretion, and potentiates platelet aggregation. The GPIb-IX complex also appears to activate the cell through two unusual mechanisms: (a) GPIbα binds to the cytoskeleton protein 14-3-3ζ (126) that, in turn, binds Raf-1 (127), and (b) the GPIb-IX complex interacts with the FcγRIIA receptor on platelets, which activates an intracellular tyrosine-based activation motif (ITAM) receptor pathway leading through Fyn and Lyn to platelet activation (128).

Bernard-Soulier Syndrome

Bernard-Soulier syndrome represents the second most recognized inherited platelet disorder. Bernard-Soulier syndrome was first described in 1948 in a 5-month-old infant with a prolonged bleeding time, giant platelets, and a sibling who had died from hemorrhagic complications (129). Since this original description, additional patients with the combination of mucocutaneous bleeding; enlarged platelets; normal platelet aggregation with ADP, collagen, and epinephrine with a delayed

response to thrombin; and absent platelet aggregation with human vWF and ristocetin or with bovine vWF alone have been described (for review, see reference 130).

MOLECULAR ABNORMALITIES

There are more than 55 cases of Bernard-Soulier syndrome published, and 18 molecular defects have been defined (Table 34-4). In general, these disorders can be classified by whether any complex reaches the platelet membrane and by the specific subunit that is affected. The first described mutation was found within the coding sequence of the GPIbα gene (131), in which a TGG→TGA mutation resulted in the conversion of Thr[343]Stop. The resulting GPIbα chain lacks a portion of the extracellular domain and the entire transmembrane and cytoplasmic domains, providing a likely explanation for the absence of GPIb complex expression on the platelet surface. In the Balzano variant, an Ala[156]Val substitution within the leucine-rich repeat domain of GPIbα was identified (132) and was shown to be responsible for the defect because a recombinant GPIbα protein containing this substitution, when reconstituted into an otherwise normal GPIb complex, was shown to have impaired binding to vWF but normal thrombin binding. Several dominant variants of Bernard-Soulier syndrome have been defined in which surface expression of the GPIb complex is approximately 50% of normal (133).

It is clear that Bernard-Soulier syndrome can also be due to mutations of the GPIbβ and GPIX genes (Table 34-4). Because these two genes and GPV have been more recently cloned than GPIbα, it is unclear what the relative importance of each is to the appearance of the Bernard-Soulier syndrome phenotype. In

---

TABLE 34-5. Clinical Criteria for the Diagnosis of Bernard-Soulier Syndrome

Autosomal-recessive inheritance (usually)
Epistaxis, ecchymoses, gingival bleeding beginning in infancy
Menorrhagia, gastrointestinal bleeding, posttraumatic hemorrhage
Prolonged bleeding time
Variable, moderate to severe thrombocytopenia
Large (lymphocytoid) platelets
Failure of platelets to agglutinate with ristocetin, but otherwise normal
No correction with added von Willebrand's factor
Absence of the glycoprotein Ib-IX complex by electrophoresis and flow cytometry or presence of a dysfunctional complex

---

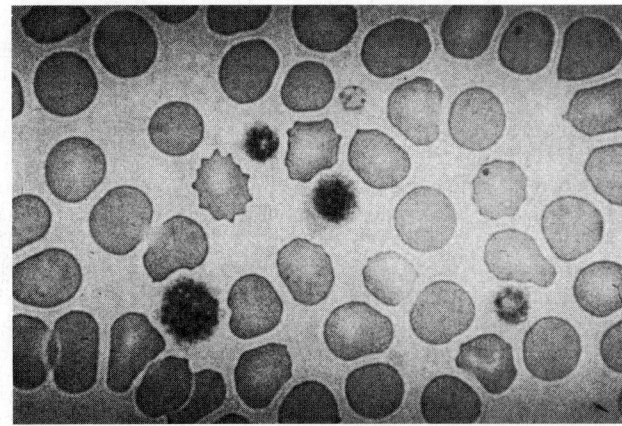

Figure 34-4. Peripheral blood smear of a patient with Bernard-Soulier syndrome. Although reduced in number, platelets are large and can approach the size of mature lymphocytes.

the first described GPIbβ case, the patient was heterozygous for a large deletion on one chromosome, resulting in the velo-cranial-facial syndrome as well as Bernard-Soulier syndrome (142). This patient is also of interest because her remaining GPIbβ gene has the first demonstrated naturally occurring mutation in a GATA-binding site, providing important evidence for the role of the GATA-1 transcription factor in the regulated expression of a megakaryocyte-specific gene. The other GPIbβ mutation occurred in a Japanese patient and resulted in a mild bleeding diathesis (148), with normal activation by either botrocetin- or ristocetin-activated vWF *in vitro* and normal levels of surface GPIb-IX complex. The patient had large platelets, and it was proposed that the defect involved a GPIbα-GPIbβ disulfide linkage and intracellular signaling.

Mutations in the gene for GPIX also occur, demonstrating that this chain is important for normal receptor expression and function. The first described defects were missense mutations in the leucine-rich repeats (Table 34-4) (149,150). Expression studies in culture demonstrated that these mutations prevented complex formation with GPIbα and GPIbβ, suggesting that the leucine-rich repeats may have a role in subunit interactions.

TREATMENT

The bleeding manifestations of these patients are similar to those of other patients who have platelet dysfunction and centers of mucocutaneous bleeding with purpuric skin bleeding, epistaxis, gastrointestinal hemorrhage, and menorrhagia (Table 34-5) (130,151). Platelet transfusions can control the bleeding manifestations. Alloantibodies to components of the GPIb-IX-V complex can develop after platelet transfusions, and, thereby, secondary complications from their refractoriness to platelet therapy can develop (130,151,152). In addition to local forms of therapy such as proper pressure and topical thrombin, platelet transfusion therapy, and hormonal management of menses, there have been several reports that have suggested that the synthetic vasopressin homolog DDAVP (1-deamino-8-D-arginine vasopressin) may be useful in the treatment of Bernard-Soulier syndrome (153). These studies have demonstrated improved bleeding times in these patients after DDAVP therapy, although the improvement did not correlate with the ability of the DDAVP to increase the level of circulating vWF. Furthermore, there are anecdotal reports that recombinant factor VIIa may be useful in the treatment of qualitative platelet defects (154).

LABORATORY EVALUATION

Bernard-Soulier syndrome patients are thrombocytopenic to some degree, with some patients having platelet counts as low as 20,000/mL (Table 34-5) (130,155). The platelets tend to be increased in size, with a mean diameter ranging from 3 to 20 times larger than normal (Fig. 34-4). Other cell types appear normal. Megakaryocytes in this disorder appear normal in size

and morphology on light microscopic examination. However, on electron microscopy, a striking feature in these cells is the variable and intermittent nature of the demarcation system, which is often vacuolar (156). The relationship between this structural feature in the megakaryocyte and the giant platelet is not fully understood. It is believed that the absence of interactions between the GPIb-IX complex and the platelet cytoskeleton underlies both the morphologic abnormality seen in the megakaryocyte and the size of the platelets.

Bleeding times are prolonged in these patients, but the distinctive abnormality of Bernard-Soulier syndrome platelets is the failure of agglutination in the presence of ristocetin, an abnormality that cannot be corrected by the addition of normal plasma (157). Aggregation by other agonists such as ADP, collagen, and epinephrine are normal, although the response to low-dose thrombin may be delayed.

DIFFERENTIAL DIAGNOSIS

Several other syndromes are characterized by large platelets and thrombocytopenia, but Bernard-Soulier syndrome is the only disorder in which ristocetin-induced platelet agglutination is defective. For example, giant platelets, thrombocytopenia, and Döhle bodies in leukocytes are the classic findings in May-Hegglin anomaly. May-Hegglin platelets, however, function normally, and there is no abnormality in any of the identified membrane proteins (158,159). Bleeding is unusual in May-Hegglin patients and has been observed, only occasionally, in patients with marked thrombocytopenia (160). Patients with Epstein's syndrome—autosomal-dominant hereditary nephritis and sensorineural deafness—may also have thrombocytopenia and large platelets (161). There are some reports of a functional abnormality in these patients characterized by decreased aggregation and secretion in response to ADP, collagen, and epinephrine (161–163). The Montreal platelet syndrome is a disorder with giant platelets, thrombocytopenia, a prolonged bleeding time, and normal aggregation in response to agonists but spontaneous aggregation when platelets are stirred at 37°C (164,165). In contrast to Bernard-Soulier syndrome, it is inherited as an autosomal-dominant trait. Membrane GP patterns are normal, but calcium-activated protease activity is reduced (166).

Acquired forms of this relatively rare inherited disorder are even more infrequent. A small number of patients with idiopathic or autoimmune thrombocytopenia have antibodies that recognize epitopes on the GPIb-IX complex. In a few cases, binding of these antibodies to the platelet has produced a syndrome that resembles Bernard-Soulier syndrome (167,168). These patients had thrombocytopenia and platelets that did not agglutinate with ristocetin; however, the platelets were of normal size, and there was no family history of the disease. In addition, the antibody can be detected in plasma or eluted from the patient's platelets. A patient with a lymphoproliferative disorder was reported who had an immunoglobulin (Ig) G antibody that inhibited ristocetin-dependent platelet agglutination (169). The patient had a prolonged bleeding time, normal platelet morphology, and a normal platelet count. The antibody appeared to interact with a 210-kd platelet protein, which is larger than any of the components of the GPIb-IX complex. There was also one case of childhood myelodysplasia with bleeding, in which there was a population of large platelets that did not react with ristocetin (170). Further examination showed that the platelets lacked the GPIb-IX complex.

G PROTEIN–COUPLED RECEPTORS IN PLATELET ACTIVATION

In this section and the next section, we discuss the families of receptors that are most involved in platelet activation. In addition to adhering to a damaged vessel site through vWF, platelets can adhere to collagen through the $\alpha_2\beta_1$ integrin and GPVI receptors (see below). Platelets that have adhered to collagen change their shape, spreading along the fibrils and releasing into the circulation thromboxane A_2 (TxA$_2$) and ADP. The released TxA$_2$ and ADP recruit additional platelets, causing them to stick to each other and to the platelets directly adhering to collagen. Collagen, ADP, and TxA$_2$ are not alone in their ability to activate platelets. Vascular injury and inflammation expose tissue factor as well as collagen, and formation of the tissue factor/factor VIIa complex leads to the local generation of thrombin from prothrombin. Thrombin is a potent agonist that activates platelets by cleaving receptors on the platelet surface. Platelets facilitate this process by providing procoagulant phospholipids that accelerate thrombin generation. As a result, platelet activation and fibrin deposition are intimately linked, maximizing the growth and strength of the hemostatic plug. Human platelets express two related GPCRs that can be cleaved and activated by thrombin, and these are described below. Activation of these receptors is modulated to some extent by the binding of thrombin to a high-affinity site on GPIbα (96). The requirement for cleavage accounts for the long-established observation that only proteolytically active thrombin can activate platelets.

Platelet agonists initiate platelet activation by binding to receptors on the platelet surface. Most of these receptors are GPCRs that are comprised of a single polypeptide chain with seven transmembrane domains and an extracellular N-terminus. The sites for interactions with agonists and antagonists are located in the extracellular and transmembrane domains. The cytoplasmic domains specify which G proteins interact with which receptors. G proteins are molecular switches consisting of a GTP-binding α subunit plus a βγ heterodimer. G proteins are inactive when GDP is bound to the α subunit and active when GTP is bound. Activated receptors known as *guanine nucleotide exchange factors* promote the replacement of GDP with GTP and switch on the G protein. GPCRs typically have a limited duration of activity after which they are turned off by phosphorylation and, in some cases, cleared from the cell surface by endocytosis. The sites involved in phosphorylation and endocytosis are usually in the cytoplasmic tail of the receptor. Agonists whose receptors fall into this category include thrombin, TxA$_2$, ADP, and epinephrine (Fig. 34-5). In several cases, human platelets express more than one GPCR for a particular agonist. For example, there are at least three different PAR family members

that can respond to thrombin and at least two receptors for ADP. The number of copies of each receptor/platelet at first glance appears small, but, given the limited surface area of human platelets, the density of the receptors is actually substantial.

Platelet agonists are sometimes classified as strong or weak. Strong agonists, such as thrombin and collagen, can trigger granule secretion even when aggregation is prevented. Weak agonists, such as ADP and epinephrine, require aggregation for secretion to occur. Presumably, the real differences between strong and weak agonists reflect differences in the sets of intracellular effectors that are coupled to their receptors. Strong agonists potently stimulate phosphoinositide hydrolysis and are relatively unaffected by inhibitors of cyclooxygenase such as aspirin. The weaker agonists, on the other hand, have little or no ability to cause phosphoinositide hydrolysis and are more dependent on TxA$_2$ formation for their effects. Both strong and weak agonists can inhibit adenyl cyclase, promoting platelet activation by lowering basal cyclic adenosine monophosphate (cAMP) levels.

Thrombin Receptors

Thrombin is arguably the most potent activator of platelets *in vivo*. When added to platelets *in vitro*, it causes phosphoinositide hydrolysis, TxA$_2$ formation, protein phosphorylation, and an increase in (Ca^{2+})$_i$ concentration, as well as shape change, granule secretion, and aggregation. These responses can be detected at thrombin concentrations as low as 0.1 nM. Thrombin also suppresses cAMP synthesis in platelets by inhibiting adenylyl cyclase (171). All of these effects require thrombin to be proteolytically active. In 1991, two laboratories independently cloned thrombin receptors from the human megakaryoblastic DAMI cell line (172) and from hamster fibroblasts (173). The predicted sequence includes a cleavage site for thrombin between residues Arg^{41} and Ser^{42} in the N-terminus (Fig. 34-6A) (174). Mutations at this site prevent receptor activation by thrombin, and synthetic peptides containing the first residues beyond the cleavage site (SFLLRN) can mimic the effects of thrombin by activating the receptor. These and subsequent observations suggest that thrombin receptors are activated by cleavage at a specific site, exposing a new N-terminus (the "tethered ligand") that interacts with residues in the second extracellular loop and a proximal N-terminus of the receptor initiating signaling (Fig. 34-6B) (172,174). Once activated, each receptor generates signals for a brief period before it is turned off and desensitized by the phosphorylation of serine and threonine residues located in the cytoplasmic domains of the receptor. The kinases responsible are members of the family of G protein receptor kinases (175).

The first thrombin receptor that was cloned is now known as *PAR-1* to distinguish it from three subsequently described receptors, *PAR-2* (176), *PAR-3* (177), and *PAR-4* (178). PAR-1 is expressed on human platelets, endothelial cells, vascular smooth muscle cells, fibroblasts, and neurons. Knockouts of the PAR-1 gene in mice are notable for the death *in utero* of one-half of the homozygous (–/–) mice at approximately the ninth day of gestation—a point at which intravascular pressure begins to rise (179,180). This is also the point at which deletion of coagulation proteins needed for the local generation of active thrombin also has lethal effects. The surviving PAR-1 (–/–) mice appear normal. However, although their fibroblasts lack the ability to respond to thrombin, their platelets do not—an observation that led to the eventual identification of PAR-3 and PAR-4, which appear to be the principal thrombin receptors on mouse platelets. PAR-2 is the second PAR family member that was identified. PAR-2 is expressed on human endothelial cells,

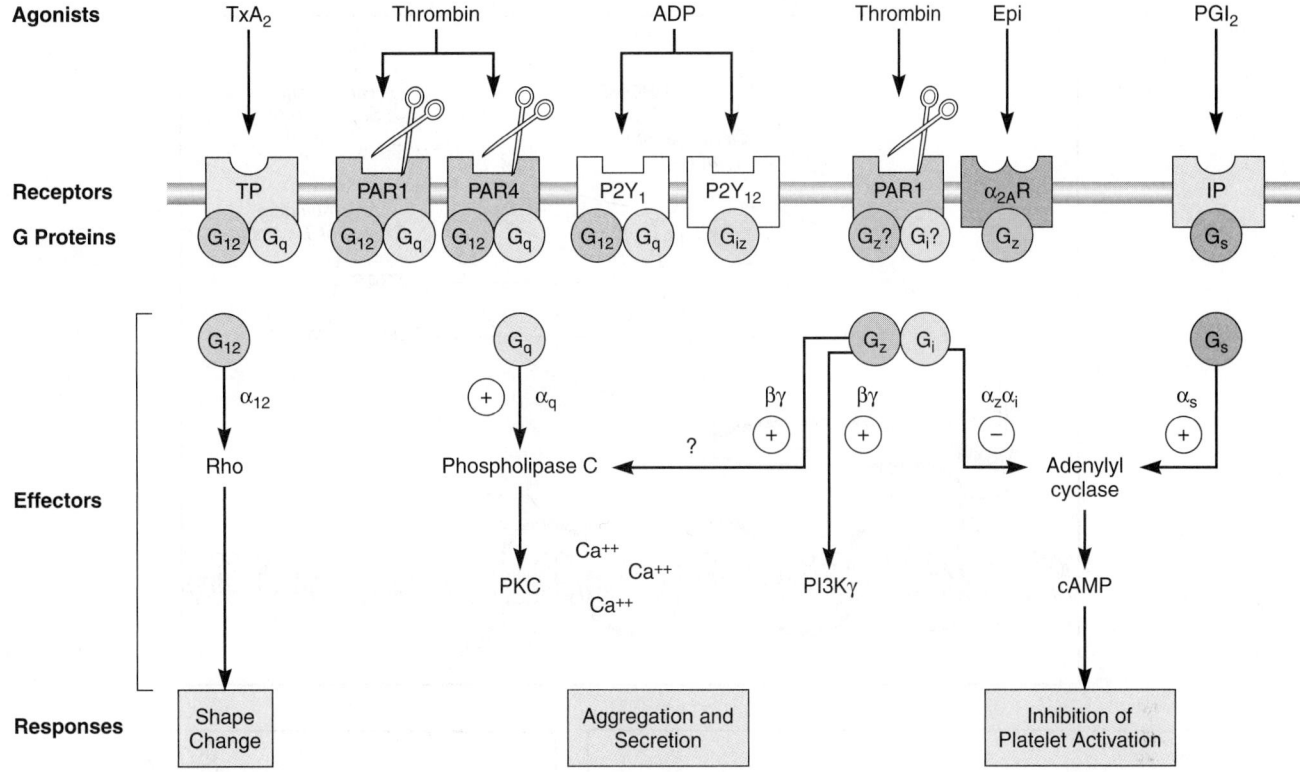

Figure 34-5. Schematic of signaling through seven transmembrane receptors on the surface of platelets. According to current models, platelet receptors for thrombin, adenosine diphosphate (ADP), and thromboxane A_2 (TxA$_2$) are coupled to G$_q$ and G$_{12}$, activating phospholipase C (PLC) and Rho family members to produce shape change, aggregation, and secretion. ADP, epinephrine (Epi), and thrombin are also coupled via one or more G$_i$ family members to the inhibition of cyclic adenosine monophosphate (cAMP) formation and (via Gβγ derived from G$_i$ family members) to the activation of PLC and PI 3-kinase γ (PI3Kγ). The assignment of particular G proteins to particular responses is based, in part, on results from studies with platelets from mice lacking one or more G protein α subunits. PAR, protease-activated receptor; PGI$_2$, prostaglandin I$_2$.

keratinocytes, vascular smooth muscle, and gastrointestinal epithelium. It is not expressed on human platelets and is not activated by thrombin (181). In contrast, PAR-3 and PAR-4, like PAR-1, are thrombin receptors. PAR-3 is expressed in mouse and rat platelets [which do not express PAR-1 (177)]. mRNA that encodes PAR-3 has been detected in human platelets, but it appears to be expressed at very low levels (182). PAR-4 is also expressed on human platelets (183). PAR-4 requires higher thrombin concentrations than PAR-1 and PAR-3 for activation (178). PAR-1 activates PLC via Gq and Gi family members and inhibits cAMP via Gi family members (Fig. 34-5). PAR-4 activates PLC in a similar manner, but it does not inhibit adenyl cyclase (Fig. 34-5) (184). Peptide agonists corresponding to the tethered ligand domain of PAR-4 activate the receptor, but the concentrations required are approximately two orders of magnitude higher than those required for activation of PAR-1 by SFLLRN. Peptides corresponding to the tethered ligand domain of PAR-3 do not activate PAR-3 at any concentration that has been reported. Finally, it has been known for a long time that GPIbα has a high-affinity binding site for thrombin. Recent evidence suggests that interaction with this site accelerates cleavage of PAR-1 (185).

Based on expression level and sensitivity to thrombin, PAR-1 appears to be the primary thrombin receptor on human platelets at low thrombin concentrations. There are approximately 2000 copies of it on the surface of human platelets (186) (Table 34-1). Additional PAR-1 is initially located in the surface-connecting membrane system and becomes exposed when platelets are acti-

vated (187). Cleavage of PAR-1 can be detected with antibodies directed N-terminal to the cleavage site (188) or with assays for the released N-terminal fragment (189). Because platelets synthesize very little protein, platelets usually respond to thrombin only once. This is in contrast to endothelial cells, which possess a large intracellular pool of PAR-1 that can replace cleaved receptors over 2 to 3 hours (190).

Adenosine Diphosphate Receptors

ADP is stored in platelet-dense granules and released on platelet activation. When added to platelets *in vitro*, ADP causes TxA$_2$ formation, protein phosphorylation, an increase in cytosolic Ca^{2+}, shape change, aggregation, and secretion. ADP also inhibits cAMP formation. These responses are half-maximal at approximately 1 μM of ADP. However, ADP is a weak activator of PLC in human platelets (191). At least two patients with bleeding defects have been described whose platelets show greatly diminished responsiveness to ADP and reduced numbers of binding sites for ADP analogs (192), a phenotype not dissimilar from that produced by ADP antagonists such as ticlopidine. Recent efforts to identify ADP receptors show that human platelets express P2Y1, P2Y12, and P2X1 (193–196). P2Y1 is a GPCR that interacts with Gq family members to activate PLCβ (Fig. 34-5). P2Y12 is coupled to Gi family members and inhibits cAMP formation by adenyl cyclase. P2X1 is a ligand-gated nonspecific cation channel that may contribute to the influx of extracellular Ca^{2+} that occurs in response to ADP,

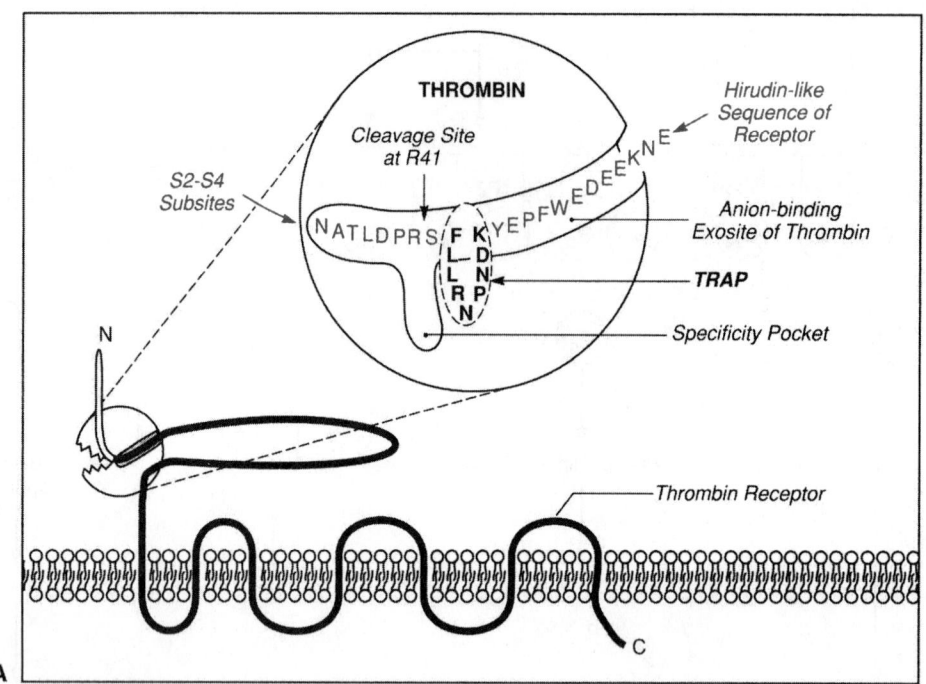

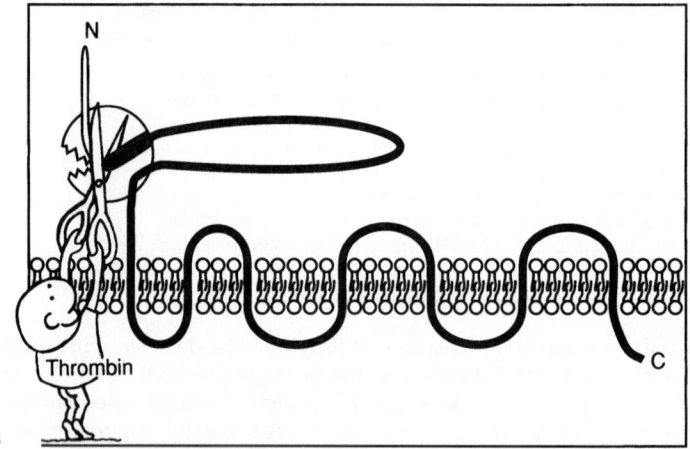
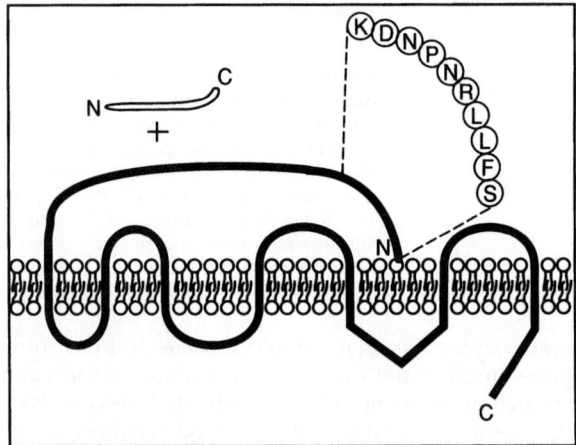

Figure 34-6. A: Interactions between thrombin and the platelet thrombin receptor. Thrombin binds to the receptor and activates it by a specific proteolytic cleavage at Arg[41] (R41). The thrombin receptor contains an amino terminal sequence that binds to the S2-S4 subsite of thrombin and a hirudin-like sequence that fits into the anion exosite of thrombin. **B:** Mechanism of thrombin activation of the thrombin receptor. Cleavage at arginine 41 of the receptor produces a new amino terminal sequence, which can fold over and activate the receptor. The sequence acts as a "tethered ligand."

although recent studies suggest that P2X1 may actually prefer ATP to ADP.

Epinephrine Receptor

In several respects, epinephrine is unique among platelet agonists because it causes aggregation and secretion but not the cytoskeletal reorganization that underlies shape change. PLC activation by epinephrine appears to be dependent on TxA_2 formation and can be suppressed with aspirin (Fig. 34-5) (197). Aspirin also blocks second-wave, or secretion-dependent, platelet aggregation in response to epinephrine. This gives rise to a characteristic aggregometer tracing in which epinephrine-induced primary aggregation is followed by disaggregation of the initially formed platelet clumps. Dependence on TxA_2 formation does not adequately account for epineph-

rine's ability to aggregate platelets, however, because epinephrine can still cause fibrinogen receptor expression in aspirin-treated platelets (198). These observations suggest that there are other, unknown mechanisms involved in platelet responses to epinephrine. What might those be? Epinephrine, like thrombin, is a potent inhibitor of cAMP formation, but it does not appear that this alone can trigger platelet activation. Epinephrine has also been reported to increase the rate of Na^+/H^+ exchange across the platelet plasma membrane (199), although this may not occur until after fibrinogen receptor exposure (200). Platelet responses to epinephrine are mediated by α_2-adrenergic receptors (201) and are notoriously labile. In fact, some otherwise normal platelets do not respond to epinephrine or do so only after a prolonged delay (202). There are reports of families in which a mild bleeding disorder was associated with impaired epinephrine-induced aggregation and reduced numbers of α_2-adrenergic receptors (203). Many patients with myeloproliferative disorders, especially essential thrombocytosis, selectively lose their ability to aggregate with epinephrine (204). Their platelets are also missing α_2-adrenergic receptors when assessed by radioligand-binding assays and coupling to adenylate cyclase (205,206). The clinical significance of this abnormality is unclear. In addition, platelets from up to 10% of apparently normal people might not aggregate when challenged with epinephrine (207). Recent studies on mouse platelets show that deletion of the gene encoding the α subunit of Gz (a member of the Gi family) greatly impairs the ability of epinephrine to inhibit cAMP formation (208).

Thromboxane A$_2$ Receptor

TxA$_2$ is produced from arachidonate in platelets by the aspirin-sensitive cyclooxygenase pathway. A number of stable endoperoxide/thromboxane analogs have been synthesized, including U46619. When added to platelets *in vitro*, U46619 causes shape change, aggregation, secretion, phosphoinositide hydrolysis, protein phosphorylation, and an increase in (Ca^{2+})$_i$, while having little effect on cAMP formation that is not mediated by secreted ADP (Fig. 34-5). Similar responses occur when platelets are incubated with exogenous arachidonate (209). Because the effects of arachidonate can be inhibited with aspirin, they are thought to be largely due to thromboxane formation (210). Once formed, TxA$_2$ can diffuse across the plasma membrane and activate other platelets (211). Like ADP, this amplifies the initial stimulus for platelet activation and helps to recruit additional platelets. This process is effective locally, but it is limited by the brief (approximately 30 seconds) half-life of TxA$_2$ in solution, helping to confine the spread of platelet activation to the original area of injury.

Platelets express the thromboxane prostanoid receptor TP, a GPCR for TxA$_2$ (212). There are two C-terminal cytoplasmic isoforms of this receptor, and the α form predominates in platelets (213). Platelets also contain a receptor for prostacyclin (PGI$_2$), an endothelial cell prostaglandin that is a potent platelet inhibitor. Binding of PGI$_2$ to this receptor stimulates adenylate cyclase activity and inhibits platelet function (214). A few patients have been described who have a mild bleeding disorder due to a congenital absence of the TxA$_2$ receptor. Two Japanese patients have had their mutations defined and were found to have a common R^{60}L substitution in the first cytoplasmic loop of TxA$_2$ (215). There are no known clinical disorders ascribed to the PGI$_2$ receptor, but deletion of the gene in mice increases their risk of thrombosis after arterial injury (216).

Chemokine Receptors

Beginning in 1989, it was recognized that a family of small inflammatory proteins, termed *chemokines*, influenced megakaryocyte development when platelet factor 4 was shown to be a negative *in vitro* autocrine for megakaryopoiesis (217). Since then, receptors for a number of chemokines, including stromal-derived factor 1 and macrophage-derived chemokine, were found on the surface of megakaryocytes and platelets; some of these chemokines can behave as weak agonists, suggesting a role in thrombus development at sites of inflammation and vasculitis (218). Whether the role of these chemokines and their receptors is during megakaryocyte development or platelet biology remains to be determined. Certainly, the presence of CXCR4, the receptor for stromal-derived factor 1 on the surface of developing megakaryocytes and on platelets, may contribute to the development of

thrombocytopenia during human immunodeficiency virus infections (219).

IMMUNOGLOBULIN SUPERFAMILY RECEPTORS

There are a number of important platelet receptors that fall into the class of Ig superfamily receptors. First recognized in 1984, these receptors share a common motif of repeating disulfide-bound globular domains that are closely related in three-dimensional structure to IgV or IgC domains (220). These receptors include GPVI, an important collagen receptor; FcγRIIA, an important receptor for immune complex–dependent thrombocytopenia; and PECAM-1 and P-selectin, which are involved in the overlapping processes of thrombosis and inflammation. A number of these receptors also signal by common intracellular pathways.

Glycoprotein VI and Other Collagen Receptors

As mentioned above, there is more than one receptor that recognizes vWF—the αIIbβ3 receptor and the GPIb-IX complex. These receptors have overlapping but distinct roles in thrombus formation because neither can be lost without having a significant bleeding diathesis. Whereas the GPIb-IX complex binds thrombin, the thrombin receptors are distinct from this receptor complex and involve closely related members of the PAR family that activate platelets by slightly different pathways. ADP appears to involve a series of distantly related purinergic receptors that actually activate distinct intracellular pathways. It should, therefore, not be surprising that collagen activates platelets by several distinct receptor systems. The present model of collagen signaling in platelets is significant because it provides an excellent model for the evolution of cooperativity between platelet surface receptors to accomplish both adhesion and signaling by a single ligand.

Exposed collagen initiates two essential platelet functions: adhesion of circulating platelets to the site of injury and activation of platelet signaling, which stimulates thrombus growth. Platelet adhesion to collagen occurs both indirectly via binding of platelet GPIb-IX to plasma vWF, which binds exposed collagen (221), and directly via interaction with the platelet integrin $\alpha_2\beta_1$ (222), GPVI (223), and, perhaps, other collagen receptors. Activation of platelets by collagen has been observed for more than 30 years (224). Collagen remains the sole matrix protein, which has been demonstrated to directly activate platelets.

A large number of receptors have been proposed as platelet collagen receptors, including $\alpha_2\beta_1$ (222), GPIV (225), GPVI (223), and p65 (226), but the only receptors for which demonstrated roles exist are $\alpha_2\beta_1$ and GPVI. A recently proposed model for collagen activation of platelets is a two-receptor, two-step model in which platelets adhere to collagen via the high-affinity integrin receptor $\alpha_2\beta_1$ and subsequently signal in response to collagen through the lower-affinity receptor GPVI (227) (Fig. 34-7). This model is based on the pharmacologic studies outlined below as well as on several individual human deficiency states (228–231), which have not yet been characterized at the molecular level.

Below is a brief description of the known roles of these collagen receptors for adhesion and signal transduction by collagen.

$\alpha_2\beta_1$

The integrin $\alpha_2\beta_1$ is the most studied collagen receptor on platelets and is established as the major platelet receptor for adhesion to collagen. This receptor is discussed in greater detail above among the integrin receptors.

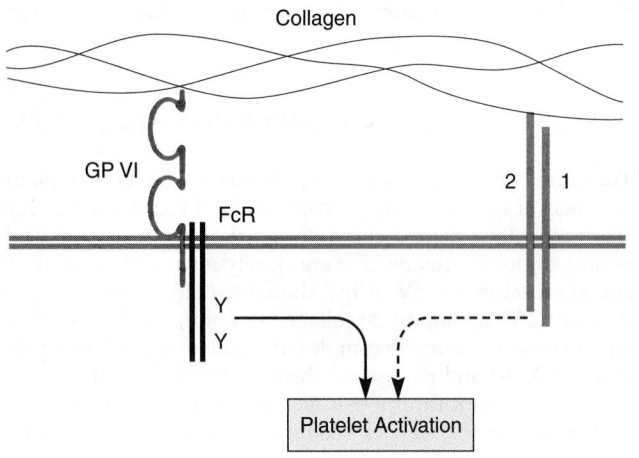

Figure 34-7. Collagen activation of platelets. Direct interaction of platelets with collagen is mediated by two receptor complexes, the integrin $\alpha_2\beta_1$ and the nonintegrin glycoprotein (GP) VI-FcRγ. Clustering of GPVI-FcRγ by collagen activates platelets through the immunoreceptor signaling pathway (*solid arrow*). $\alpha_2\beta_1$ is an important adhesive receptor for collagen, but its role in platelet activation is not defined (*dashed arrow*). Y indicates the FcRγ tyrosines, which are phosphorylated during signaling by GPVI.

GLYCOPROTEIN VI

This receptor is a recently cloned 62-kd surface protein (232,233) that was first identified by iodination of platelet surface GPs (223). GPVI is 339 amino acids and includes a putative 23–amino acid signal sequence and a 19–amino acid transmembrane domain between residues 247 and 265. GPVI belongs to the Ig superfamily, and its sequence is closely related to FcαR and to the natural killer receptors. Its extracellular chain has two IgC2-like domains formed by disulfide bridges. An arginine residue is found in position 3 of the transmembrane portion, which should permit association with FcRγ with its immunoreceptor tyrosine-based activation motif via a salt bridge. Thus, GPVI is a type I transmembrane protein whose deduced amino acid sequence identifies it as an Ig domain that contains a receptor homologous to the Fc and natural killer receptors, which are known to signal via the signaling adaptor FcRγ (234), and suggests that GPVI signals via the known associated Syk/SLP76/PLCγ intracellular signaling pathway (235), perhaps in a manner similar to that of the GPIb-IX receptor discussed above.

GPVI was proposed as a signaling receptor for collagen after the description of individuals with mild bleeding disorders whose platelets could not be activated by fibrillar collagen types I and III and lacked GPVI despite having normal levels of the platelet integrin $\alpha_2\beta_1$ (220). Unlike $\alpha_2\beta_1$, significant direct evidence suggests that GPVI-collagen interaction initiates intracellular signaling, resulting in platelet activation. Antisera from transfused GPVI-deficient individuals recognize GPVI and are capable of activating normal platelets, whereas Fab fragments specifically inhibit collagen activation of platelets, suggesting a clustering mechanism of signal initiation (236). Collagen-related peptides (peptides containing glycine-proline-hydroxyproline repeats whose cross-linked structure resembles that of triple-helical collagen) are potent activators of platelets whose activation is not inhibited by $\alpha_2\beta_1$-inactivating monoclonal antibodies (237) and cannot activate GPVI-deficient platelets (238). Finally, convulxin, a snake venom protein isolated from a South American rattlesnake, is also a potent activator of platelets that is capable of desensitizing platelets specifically to collagen and has been demonstrated to bind specifically to GPVI (239). Thus, studies using three distinct ligands as well as a human deficiency state support the hypoth-

esis that GPVI–collagen binding is necessary and sufficient for collagen-induced platelet activation.

GLYCOPROTEIN IV

GPIV was proposed as a platelet collagen receptor based on the ability of anti-GPIV antibodies to interfere with aggregation and adhesion of platelets to collagen (240). Subsequent studies, however, have demonstrated that up to 5% of the Japanese population lacks surface GPIV but demonstrates normal collagen responses (241). Thus, GPIV does not appear necessary for collagen signaling in platelets, and the contribution of GPIV to collagen signaling remains to be defined.

P65

p65 is a platelet surface protein distinct from GPVI, which has been proposed as a collagen receptor (226), for which significant functional data has yet to be reported. The role of this protein for collagen signaling in platelets is unknown.

Lectin Receptor

P-selectin (Table 34-1) is a member of the selectin family of receptors (see review in reference 242) that is unique because it is not on the surface of quiescent platelets, and it is involved in protein–carbohydrate interactions rather than protein–protein interactions. In 1989, two groups described P-selectin as an α-granule membrane protein (243,244). In addition, P-selectin was found on the surface of Weibel-Palade bodies of endothelial cells (245). After platelet activation, it is rapidly redistributed to the platelet membrane and also to the surface of endothelial cells. In addition to P-selectin, the selectin family includes L-selectin (found on white cells) and E-selectin (found on endothelial cells). All of these receptors are cysteine-rich proteins with multiple extracellular domains, including a "lectin" region; an "EGF" domain; nine tandem consensus repeats related to those in complement-binding proteins, making them part of the Ig superfamily of receptors; a transmembrane domain; and a short cytoplasmic tail.

Whereas P-selectin becomes exposed on the surface of platelets and endothelial cells after fusion of their specific granules with the surface membranes, the other selectins reach the cell surface by a different mechanism. For example, E-selectin becomes expressed on the surface of endothelial cells after protein synthesis in activated endothelial cells (246,247). Whereas P-selectin becomes available almost instantaneously, E-selectin is a slower response. Certainly, there are advantages to having a fast and slow response system *in vivo*, which are being detailed by studies of P- and E-selectin and the double knock-out mice.

The selectins bind to negatively charged carbohydrate side chains of membrane proteins (248). These side chains tend to be carbohydrate determinants related to sialyl Le(x) antigens on neutrophil and monocyte surfaces. In particular, P-selectin has a specific high affinity for a particular GP: P-selectin GP-1 (249). These reactions appear to be critical for attachment of platelets and leukocytes to injured endothelial cells. P-selectin is critical for activated platelets to "roll" on injured endothelial cells (250) and for leukocytes to "roll" on a platelet surface before coming to a halt (251).

Targeted disruption of P-selectin has provided additional insights into the biology of this receptor (250). The P-selectin knockout has defective rolling of leukocytes on a platelet surface (250) and has an increased susceptibility to bacterial infections (252). Furthermore, P-selectin is important for appropriate thrombosis because the targeted knock-out animals have prolonged bleeding times and develop unusually large thrombi at sites of inflammation (253). Further, it appears that P-selectin deficiency results in delayed atherosclerotic development (254). Whether these biologic effects are due to the P-selectin on the platelet or on the endothelial lining (or both) still needs to be determined.

Platelet-Endothelial Cell Adhesion Molecule-1

Platelet-endothelial cell adhesion molecule (PECAM)–1 is a 130-kd protein expressed on the surface of circulating cells such as platelets, monocytes, and neutrophils and on endothelial cells. Although cloned more than a decade ago (255), the function of PECAM-1 in platelets is only now being appreciated, and strong evidence suggests that this protein may serve as a negative signaling receptor in platelets while performing more classic adhesive functions in other cell types such as endothelial cells (reviewed in references 256,257).

PECAM-1 is encoded by a complex gene and is subject to significant splice variation affecting the intracellular tail of the receptor, with the result that several forms of this receptor are expressed. It is likely that different PECAM splice variants have different functional properties, although the biologic importance of this observation is not known. PECAM-1 has a 574–amino acid extracellular domain, which contains six Ig domains (255). The PECAM-1 intracellular tail is 118 amino acids long and contains numerous potential signaling motifs—the most important of which is the presence of an immunoreceptor tyrosine-based inhibitory motif (ITIM) (discussed below) (257).

There is ample evidence that PECAM-1/PECAM-1 interaction mediates cellular adhesion between neighboring endothelial cells and between circulating leukocytes and the vascular endothelium (258). PECAM-1 binds strongly to itself, and there is not yet evidence of binding to another ligand. PECAM-1–mediated cellular adhesion plays a demonstrated role in the extravasation of leukocytes from the circulation (258). The intercellular borders between endothelial cells are sites of extremely dense PECAM-1 expression, but the importance of PECAM expression at these sites is not yet clear. It is possible that platelet PECAM-1 also serves an important adhesive function between platelets and other circulating cells or platelets and endothelial cells, but this has not yet been demonstrated, although a recent report of prolonged bleeding times in PECAM-1–deficient mice supports this idea (259).

The recent identification of a consensus ITIM sequence in the intracellular tail of PECAM-1 has generated the hypothesis that PECAM-1 is an inhibitory receptor on platelets in a manner analogous to inhibitory immune receptors (257). Phosphorylation of the tyrosine residues in ITIMs enables recruitment and activation of cellular phosphates such as SHP-1, SHP-2, and SHIP, which oppose the action of cellular tyrosine kinases activated by ITAM domain–containing receptors such as GPVI (discussed above). Given the recent discovery of the importance of ITAM-mediated cell signaling for collagen activation of platelets as well as signaling through FcγRIIa, the existence of opposing inhibitory receptors is attractive. In a preliminary report, this balance between platelet activation through ITAM-based pathways and inhibition through ITIM-based pathways may underlie the observation that platelets from PECAM-1–deficient mice are more strongly activated by collagen than normal mice, because they lack the balancing influence of the ITIM pathway through PECAM-1 (260). Two groups have now shown, however, that cross-linking PECAM-1 before activation of GPVI results in the inhibition of GPVI signaling (260), and that the PECAM-1 knockout has exaggerated responses to collagen (261). Mutation of the critical tyrosine residue in the putative PECAM-1 ITIM eliminates the inhibition, supporting the notion

that the PECAM-1 ITIM is functional (257). The *in vivo* importance of inhibitory signaling by PECAM-1 remains undefined, however, and whether platelet PECAM-1 responds primarily to endothelial PECAM-1, to PECAM-1 on other circulating cells, or to an as yet unidentified ligand is unknown. Finally, it is intriguing to consider that other ITIM-containing receptors may exist, which regulate platelet responsiveness.

FcγRIIA

Human platelets express a low-affinity Fc receptor for IgG, FcγRIIA (reviewed in 262). The extracellular domain of FcγRIIA is homologous to the high-affinity Fc receptors for IgG, FcγRI, and FcγRIII. Unlike these receptors and GPVI, however, FcγRIIA has an intracellular C tail, which contains a functional ITAM domain. FcγRIIA can, therefore, signal independently of the ITAM-containing adaptor, FcRγ. In considering the roles of FcγRIIA in platelets, it is important to note that no FcγRIIA is found on mouse platelets, and we cannot, therefore, study the loss of function of FcγRIIA in the mouse to guide studies of human biology. Interestingly, human FcγRIIA has been successfully expressed in mouse platelets, where it couples efficiently to downstream signaling effectors and is capable of activating platelets and enhancing immune clearance of platelets (263).

FcγRIIA is expressed on leukocytes as well as platelets and, in these cells, clearly serves as an immune receptor where it responds to IgG_2-coated targets. Whether platelet FcγRIIA plays a role in natural immune responses remains unclear, but a role for FcγRIIA in pathologic immune responses has been demonstrated. FcγRIIA cross-linking and platelet activation have been implicated in heparin-induced thrombocytopenia type II, and the density of FcγRIIA receptors correlates with the platelet response and disease severity. The importance of FcγRIIA in the development of heparin-induced thrombocytopenia has recently been shown using double-transgenic mice that express both human platelet factor 4 and FcγRIIA (264).

Several groups have demonstrated a physical association between FcγRIIA and the platelet GPIb-IX receptor (265,266). This has led to the suggestion that FcγRIIA may function as a signaling adaptor like the FcRγ chain. This is an intriguing hypothesis, especially in light of the evidence for GPIb signal transduction discussed above, and FcγRIIA phosphorylation has been demonstrated to follow platelet exposure to vWF (265,266). The biologic importance of this observation, however, remains unknown. The lack of a mouse FcγRIIA ortholog suggests either that such a function is dispensable for hemostasis *in vivo* or that mouse platelets use a distinct adaptor for GPIb signaling. Further studies of GPIb and FcγRIIA in mouse knock-out and transgenic models is likely to prove informative in this regard.

PLATELET REGULATION OF COAGULATION REACTIONS

In addition to their important role in primary hemostasis, platelets are one of the principal sites for plasma coagulation reactions. The plasma membrane of activated platelets provides a surface on which coagulation factor complexes assemble. There is evidence that both the "Xase" complex (factors IXa, VIIIa, and X) and the "prothrombinase" complex (factors Xa and Va and prothrombin) assemble on the platelet surface (267). The platelet surface accelerates these important reactions several thousand–fold by increasing the proximity and

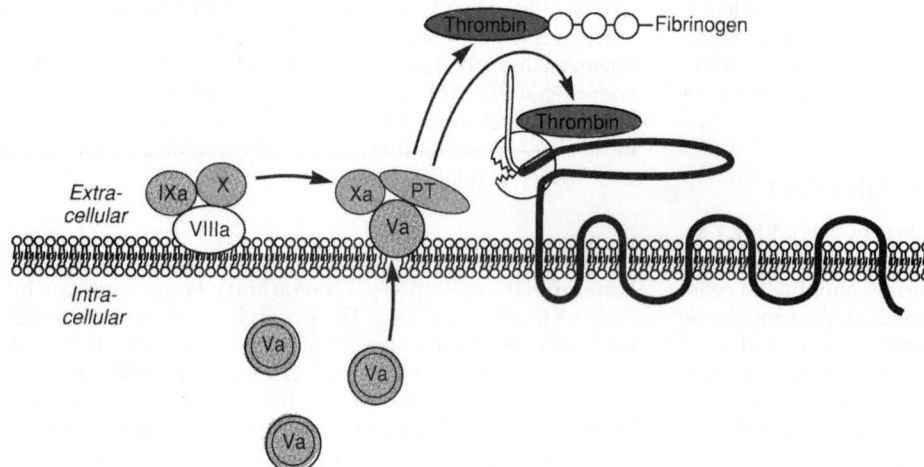

Figure 34-8. Role of the platelet in accelerating plasma coagulation reactions. The assembly of the "Xase" and the "prothrombinase" complexes both require phospholipid that is supplied by the platelet membrane. Factor VIIIa, derived from plasma, binds to platelet membrane phospholipids and then binds factors IXa and X. Factor Xa generated from the complex then assembles with prothrombin and factor Va to form the prothrombinase complex. Factor Va is derived from plasma and platelet granules. Thrombin generated from the complex can bind to the platelet thrombin receptor and other cells or generate fibrin from fibrinogen.

concentration of the reactants and providing the appropriate phospholipid moieties needed for both reactions. This property of activated platelets was formerly referred to as platelet factor 3 activity. The Xase and prothrombinase complexes also bind to artificial micelles made up of anionic phospholipids (267,268) (Fig. 34-8). Although there is little anionic phospholipid in the outer leaflet of the unactivated platelet, activation by agonists like thrombin or collagen is thought to reorient membrane phospholipids and bring the appropriate anionic phospholipid to the outer leaflet. Alternately, activation may induce membrane vesiculation and the production of platelet microparticles with procoagulant activity (Fig. 34-9) (269).

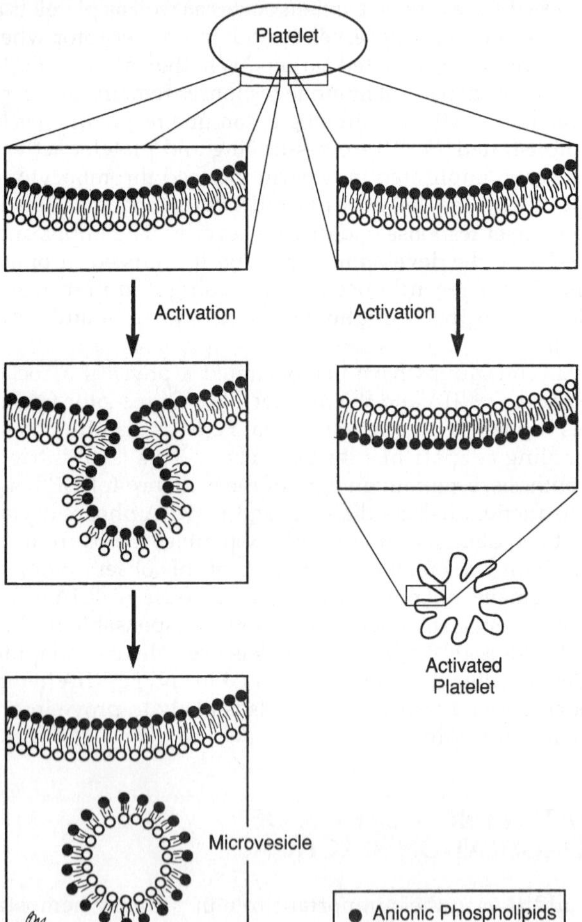

A selective deficiency in platelet coagulant activity is a rare clinical event but has been described (269–273). This phenomenon has been referred to as *Scott's syndrome* after the propositus of one well-studied family. The patient had prolonged bleeding after dental extractions, bleeding after surgical procedures, and a spontaneous retroperitoneal hematoma (Table 34-6) (274). The patient has been carefully studied and is the subject of several papers. The patient secreted a normal quantity of factor Va, a platelet α-granule constituent, but had only 20% to 25% of the normal number of factor Xa-binding sites on activated platelets (275). Moreover, when platelets were challenged with the agonists thrombin and collagen, fewer anionic phospholipid-binding sites were translocated to the platelet surface (273). In addition, the formation of microparticles is defective in patients with Scott's syndrome (269). This is important because platelet-binding sites for factor Va appear on the microparticles generated after platelet activation.

These fairly well-defined biochemical abnormalities produce a distinct set of laboratory abnormalities. Although this is a platelet defect, patients with Scott's syndrome have a normal bleeding time and normal platelet aggregation and secretion (Table 34-6). In addition, standard screening tests for plasma coagulation such as the prothrombin time and partial thromboplastin time, which use artificial lipid micelles, are normal. The diagnostic abnormality is a shortened serum prothrombin time owing to reduced prothrombin consumption. This is due to the inability to generate normal platelet procoagulant activity. Patients can be readily treated with platelet transfusions, which improve hemostasis and reduce postoperative blood loss.

Figure 34-9. The generation of a platelet membrane surface that supports coagulation reactions and potential defects in Scott's syndrome. The platelet membrane alters its natural phospholipid asymmetry by redistributing anionic phospholipids to the outer leaflet of the plasma membrane or to buds of microvesicles that have anionic phospholipids on their outer surface. Inability to carry out either function may result in defective platelet procoagulant activity (Scott's syndrome).

Table 34-6. Clinical Criteria for the Diagnosis of Scott's Syndrome

History of mild to moderate bleeding
Normal bleeding time and platelet aggregation
Autosomal-recessive inheritance
Reduced prothrombin consumption and short serum prothrombin time
Platelet procoagulant activity decreased
Reduced factor Xa binding to platelets

CONCLUSION

During the past few years, there has been an explosion of new information about the structure and function of platelet membrane proteins and their role in hemostasis. With this information, the molecular basis of platelet membrane disorders like Bernard-Soulier syndrome and Glanzmann's thrombasthenia have been defined. In addition, low copy number receptors, which bind important ligands like thrombin, catecholamines, ADP, and collagen, have been identified and characterized. New receptor families with potential roles in platelet development and biology, such as the chemokine receptors, have been shown to be present and active on platelets. Interaction and the thrombotic counterbalance between distinct receptors such as FcγRIIA and the GPIb-IX receptor complex are beginning to be appreciated. The power of combining insights from clinical medicine with the techniques of modern genetics and molecular and cellular biology is nicely demonstrated by the progress that has been made in understanding the platelet membrane and its disorders.

REFERENCES

1. Hynes RO. Integrins: versatility, modulation, and signaling in cell adhesion. *Cell* 1991;69:11.
2. Hemler ME, Crouse C, Takada Y, et al. Multiple very late antigen (VLA) heterodimers on platelets. Evidence for distinct VLA-2, VLA-5 (fibronectin receptor), and VLA-6 structures. *J Biol Chem* 1988;263:7660.
3. Turrito VT, Weiss HJ, Zimmerman TS, et al. Factor VIII/von Willebrand factor in subendothelium mediates platelet adhesion. *Blood* 1985;65:823.
4. Staatz WD, Rajpara SM, Wayner EA, et al. The membrane glycoprotein Ia-IIa (VLA-2) complex mediates the Mg⁺⁺-dependent adhesion of platelets to collagen. *J Cell Biol* 1989;108:1917.
5. Nieuwenhuis HK, Akkerman JWN, Houdijk WPM, et al. Human blood platelets showing no response to collagen fail to express surface glycoprotein Ia. *Nature* 1985;318:470.
6. Kehrel B, Balleisen L, Kokott R, et al. Deficiency of intact thrombospondin and membrane glycoprotein Ia in platelets with defective collagen-induced aggregation and spontaneous loss of disorder. *Blood* 1988;71:1074.
7. Handa M, Watanabe K, Kawai Y, et al. Platelet unresponsiveness to collagen: involvement of glycoprotein Ia-IIa (alpha 2 beta 1 integrin) deficiency associated with a myeloproliferative disorder. *Thromb Haemost* 1995;73:521.
8. Keely PJ, Parise LV. The α2β1 integrin is a necessary co-receptor for collagen-induced activation of Syk, and the subsequent phosphorylation of PLCγ 2 in platelets. *J Biol Chem* 1996;271:26668.
9. Kunicki TJ, Orchekowski R, Annis D, et al. Variability of integrin α2β1 activity on human platelets. *Blood* 1993;82:2693.
10. Kritzik M, Savage B, Nugent DJ, et al. Nucleotide polymorphisms in the alpha2 gene define multiple alleles that are associated with differences in platelet alpha2 beta1 density. *Blood* 1998;92:2382.
11. Santoso S, Kunicki TJ, Kroll H, et al. Association of the platelet glycoprotein Ia C807T gene polymorphism with nonfatal myocardial infarction in younger patients. *Blood* 1999;93:2449.
12. Carlsson LE, Santoso S, Spitzer C, et al. The alpha2 gene coding sequence T807/A873 of the platelet collagen receptor integrin alpha2beta1 might be a genetic risk factor for the development of stroke in younger patients. *Blood* 1999;93:3583.
13. Corral J, Gonzalez-Conejero R, Rivera J, et al. Role of the 807 C/T polymorphism of the alpha2 gene in platelet GP Ia collagen receptor expression and function—effect in thromboembolic diseases. *Thromb Haemost* 1999;81:951.
14. Di Paola J, Federici AB, Mannucci PM, et al. Low platelet α2β1 levels in type 1 von Willebrand disease correlate with impaired platelet function in a high shear stress system. *Blood* 1999;93:3578.
15. Piotrowicz RS, Orchekowski RP, Nugent DJ, et al. Glycoprotein Ic-IIa functions as an activation-independent fibronectin receptor on human platelets. *J Cell Biol* 1988;106:1359–1364.
16. Nievelstein PF, Sixma JJ. Glycoprotein IIb-IIIa and RGD(S) are not important for fibronectin-dependent platelet adhesion under flow conditions. *Blood* 1988;72:82.
17. Ill CR, Engvall E, Ruoslahti E. Adhesion of platelets to laminin in the absence of activation. *J Cell Biol* 1984;99:2140.
18. Hindriks G, Ijsseldijk MJW, Sonnenberg A, et al. Platelet adhesion to laminin: role of Ca²⁺ and Mg²⁺ ions, shear rate, and platelet membrane glycoproteins. *Blood* 1992;79:928.
19. Bennett JS. Structural biology of glycoprotein IIb-IIIa. *Trends Cardiovasc Med* 1996;16:31.
20. Wagner CL, Mascelli MA, Neblock DS, et al. Analysis of GPIIb/IIIa receptor number by quantitation of 7E3 binding to human platelets. *Blood* 1996; 88:907.

21. Niiya K, Hodson E, Bader R, et al. Increased surface expression of the membrane glycoprotein IIb/IIIa complex induced by platelet activation. Relationship to the binding of fibrinogen and platelet aggregation. *Blood* 1987;70:475.
22. Poncz M, Eisman R, Heidenreich R, et al. Structure of the platelet membrane glycoprotein IIb. *J Biol Chem* 1987;262:8476.
23. Springer TA. Folding of the N-terminal, ligand-binding region of integrin alpha-subunits into a beta-propeller domain. *Proc Natl Acad Sci U S A* 1997;94:65.
23a. Xiong JP, Stehle T, Diefenbach B, et al. Crystal structure of the extracellular segment of integrin alpha V beta 3. *Science* 2001;294:339.
24. Strynadka NCJ, James MNG. Crystal structures of the helix-loop-helix calcium-binding proteins. *Ann Rev Biochem* 1989;58:951.
25. Gulino D, Boudignon C, Zhang L, et al. Ca²⁺-binding properties of the platelet glycoprotein IIb ligand-interacting domain. *J Biol Chem* 1992;267: 1001.
26. Baneres JL, Roquet F, Green M, et al. The cation-binding domain from the alpha5 subunit of integrin alpha5 beta1 is a minimal domain for fibronectin recognition. *J Biol Chem* 1998;273:24744.
27. Zimrin AB, Eisman R, Vilaire G, et al. Structure of platelet glycoprotein IIIa. *J Clin Invest* 1988;81:1470.
28. Calvete JJ, Henschen A, Gonzalez-Rodriguez J. Assignment of disulphide bonds in human platelet GPIIIa. A disulphide pattern for the beta-subunits of the integrin family. *Biochem J* 1991;274:63.
29. D'Souza SE, Ginsberg MH, Burke TA, et al. Localization of an Arg-Gly-Asp recognition site within an integrin adhesion receptor. *Science* 1988;242:91.
30. Weisel JW, Nagaswami C, Vilaire G, et al. Examination of the platelet membrane glycoprotein IIb/IIIa complex and its interaction with fibrinogen and other ligands by electron microscopy. *J Biol Chem* 1992;267:16637.
31. Thornton MA, Poncz M, Korostishevsky M, et al. The human platelet alphaIIb gene is not closely linked to its integrin partner beta3. *Blood* 1999;94: 2039.
32. Kolodziej MA, Vilaire G, Rifat S, et al. Effect of deletion of glycoprotein IIb exon 28 on the expression of the platelet glycoprotein IIb/IIIa complex. *Blood* 1991;78:2344.
33. O'Toole TE, Loftus JC, Plow EF, et al. Efficient surface expression of platelet GPIIb-IIIa requires both subunits. *Blood* 1989;74:14.
34. Kolodziej MA, Vilaire G, Gonder D, et al. Study of the endoproteolytic cleavage of platelet glycoprotein IIb using oligonucleotide-mediated mutagenesis. *J Biol Chem* 1991;266:23499.
35. Shattil SJ, Hoxie JA, Cunningham M, et al. Changes in the platelet membrane glycoprotein IIb-IIIa complex during platelet activation. *J Biol Chem* 1985; 260:11107.
36. Sims PJ, Ginsberg MH, Plow EF, et al. Effect of platelet activation on the conformation of the plasma membrane glycoprotein IIb-IIIa complex. *J Biol Chem* 1991;266:7345.
37. Shattil SJ, Kashiwagi H, Pampori N. Integrin signaling: the platelet paradigm. *Blood* 1998;91:2645.
38. Paul BZ, Jin J, Kunapuli SP. Molecular mechanism of thromboxane A₂-induced platelet aggregation. Essential role for p2ₜₐc and alpha₂ₐ receptors. *J Biol Chem* 1999;274:29108.
39. Clark EA, Shattil SJ, Brugge JS. Regulation of protein tyrosine kinases in platelets. *Trends Biochem Sci* 1994;19:464.
40. Lipfert L, Haimovich B, Schaller MD, et al. Integrin-dependent phosphorylation and activation of the protein tyrosine kinase pp125ᶠᴬᴷ in platelets. *J Cell Biol* 1992;119:905.
41. Huang M-M, Lipfert L, Cunningham M, et al. Adhesive ligand binding to integrin αIIbβ3 stimulates tyrosine phosphorylation of novel protein substrates before phosphorylation of pp125ᶠᴬᴷ. *J Cell Biol* 1993;122:473.
42. George JN, Nurden AT, Phillips DR. Molecular defects in interactions of platelets with the vessel wall. *N Engl J Med* 1984;311:1084.
43. Caen J. Glanzmann thrombasthenia. *Clin Haematol* 1972;1:383.
44. Caen JP, Castaldi PA, Leclerc JC, et al. Congenital bleeding disorders with long bleeding time and normal platelet count. 1. Glanzmann's thrombasthenia (report of fifteen cases). *Am J Med* 1966;41:4.
45. Reference deleted by author.
46. Kato A, Yamamoto K, Aoki N. Classification of Glanzmann's thrombasthenia based on the intracellular transport pathway of GPIIb-IIIa. *Thromb Haemost* 1992;68:615.
47. Jennings LK, Ashmun RA, Wang WC, et al. Analysis of human platelet glycoproteins IIb-IIIa and Glanzmann's thrombasthenia in whole blood by flow cytometry. *Blood* 1986;68:173.
48. Nurden AT, Didry D, Kieffer N, et al. Residual amounts of glycoproteins IIb and IIIa may be present in the platelets of most patients with Glanzmann's thrombasthenia. *Blood* 1985;65:1021.
49. French DL, Coller BS. Hematologically important mutations: Glanzmann thrombasthenia. *Blood Cells Mol Dis* 1996;23:39.
50. George JN, Caen JP, Nurden AT. Glanzmann's thrombasthenia: the spectrum of clinical disease. *Blood* 1990;75:1383.
51. French DL. The molecular genetics of Glanzmann's thrombasthenia. *Platelets* 1998;9:5.
52. Newman PJ. Platelet GPIIb-IIIa: molecular variations and alloantigens. *Thromb Haemost* 1991;66:111.
53. Seligsohn U, Mibashan RS, Rodeck CH, et al. Prenatal diagnosis of Glanzmann's thrombasthenia. *Lancet* 1985;2:1419.
54. French DL, Coller BS, Usher S, et al. Prenatal diagnosis of Glanzmann thrombasthenia using the polymorphic markers BRCA1 and THRA1 on chromosome 17. *Br J Haematol* 1998;102:582.

55. Grimaldi CM, Chen FP, Wu CH, et al. Glycoprotein IIb Leu[214]Pro mutation produces Glanzmann thrombasthenia with both quantitative and qualitative abnormalities in GPIIb/IIIa. *Blood* 1998;91:1562.
56. Basani RB, French L, Vilaire G, et al. A platelet αIIb mutation site defines a region involved in ligand binding by the fibrinogen receptor. *Blood* 2000;95:180.
57. Irie A, Kamata T, Puzon-McLaughlin W, et al. Critical amino acid residues for ligand binding are clustered in a predicted β-turn of the third N-terminal repeat in the integrin α4 and α5 subunits. *EMBO J* 1995;14:5550.
58. Kamata T, Irie A, Tokuhira M, et al. Critical residues of integrin αIIb subunit for binding of αIIbβ3 (glycoprotein IIb-IIIa) to fibrinogen and ligand-mimetic antibodies (PAC-1, OP-G2, and LJ-CP3). *J Biol Chem* 1996;271:18610.
59. Tozer EC, Baker E, Ginsberg MH, et al. A mutation in the α subunit of the platelet integrin αIIbβ3 identifies a novel region important for ligand binding. *Blood* 1999;93:918.
60. Baker EK, Tozer EC, Pfaff M, et al. A genetic analysis of integrin function: Glanzmann thrombasthenia *in vitro. Proc Natl Acad Sci U S A* 1997;94:1973.
61. Loftus JC, O'Toole TE, Plow EF, et al. A β3 integrin mutation abolishes ligand binding and alters divalent cation-dependent conformation. *Science* 1990;249: 915.
62. Wang R, Shattil SJ, Ambruso DR, et al. Truncation of the cytoplasmic domain of β3 in a variant form of Glanzmann thrombasthenia abrogates signaling through the integrin αIIbβ3 complex. *J Clin Invest* 1997;100:2393.
63. Chen YP, Djaffar I, Pidard D, et al. Ser[752]Pro mutation in the cytoplasmic domain of integrin β3 subunit and defective activation of platelet integrin αIIbβ3 (glycoprotein IIb-IIIa) in a variant of Glanzmann thrombasthenia. *Proc Natl Acad Sci U S A* 1992;89:10169.
64. Ylanne J, Chen Y, O'Toole TE, et al. Distinct functions of integrin α and β subunit cytoplasmic domains in cell spreading and formation of focal adhesions. *J Cell Biol* 1993;122:223.
65. Chen YP, O'Toole TE, Ylanne J, et al. A point mutation in the integrin β3 cytoplasmic domain (S752P) impairs bidirectional signaling through αIIbβ3 (platelet glycoprotein IIb-IIIa). *Blood* 1994;84:1857.
66. d'Oiron R, Menart C, Trzeciak MC, et al. Use of recombinant factor VIIa in 3 patients with inherited type I Glanzmann's thrombasthenia undergoing invasive procedures. *Thromb Haemost* 2000;83:644.
67. Poon MC, Demers C, Jobin F, et al. Recombinant factor VIIa is effective for bleeding and surgery in patients with Glanzmann thrombasthenia. *Blood* 1999;94:3951.
68. Aledort LM. Recombinant factor VIIa is a pan-hemostatic agent? *Thromb Haemost* 2000;83:637.
69. Lefkovits J, Plow E, Topol E. Platelet glycoprotein IIb/IIIa receptors in cardiovascular medicine. *N Engl J Med* 1995;332:1553.
70. Coller BS. A new murine monoclonal antibody reports an activation-dependent change in the conformation and/or microenvironment of the platelet glycoprotein IIb-IIIa complex. *J Clin Invest* 1985;76:101.
71. Coller BS. Binding of abciximab to αVβ3 and activated αMβ2 receptors: with a review of platelet-leukocyte interactions. *Thromb Haemost* 1999;82:326.
72. EPIC Investigators. Use of a monoclonal antibody directed against the platelet glycoprotein IIb/IIIa receptor in high-risk coronary angioplasty. *N Engl J Med* 1994;330:956.
73. CAPTURE Investigators. Randomised placebo-controlled trial of abciximab before and during coronary intervention in refractory unstable angina: the CAPTURE Study. *Lancet* 1997;349:1429.
74. EPILOG Investigators. Platelet glycoprotein IIb/IIIa receptor blockade and low-dose heparin during percutaneous coronary revascularization. *N Engl J Med* 1997;336:1689.
75. Randomised placebo-controlled and balloon-angioplasty-controlled trial to assess safety of coronary stenting with use of platelet glycoprotein-IIb/IIIa blockade. The EPISTENT Investigators. Evaluation of Platelet IIb/IIIa Inhibitor for Stenting. *Lancet* 1998;352:87.
76. Marso SP, Lincoff AM, Ellis SG, et al. Optimizing the percutaneous interventional outcomes for patients with diabetes mellitus: results of the EPISTENT diabetic substudy. *Circulation* 1999;100:2477.
77. Madan M, Berkowitz SD. Understanding thrombocytopenia and antigenicity with glycoprotein IIb-IIIa inhibitors. *Am Heart J* 1999;138:317.
78. Berkowitz SD, Harrington RA, Rund MM, et al. Acute profound thrombocytopenia after C7E3 Fab (abciximab) therapy. *Circulation* 1997;95:809.
79. Tcheng JE, Kereiakes DJ, Braden GA, et al. Readministration of abciximab: interim report of the ReoPro readministration registry. *Am Heart J* 1999;138:S33.
80. Scarborough RM. Development of eptifibatide. *Am Heart J* 1999;138:1093.
81. IMPACT-II Investigators. Randomised placebo-controlled trial of effect of eptifibatide on complications of percutaneous coronary intervention: IMPACT-II. *Lancet* 1997;349:1422.
82. The PURSUIT Investigators. Inhibition of platelet glycoprotein IIb/IIIa with eptifibatide in patients with acute coronary syndromes. *N Engl J Med* 1998;339: 436.
82a. O'Shea JC, Buller CE, Cantor WJ, et al. ESPIRIT Investigators. Long-term efficacy of platelet glycoprotein IIb/IIIa integrin blockade with eptifibatide in coronary stent intervention. *JAMA* 287(5):618–621,2001.
83. Cook JJ, Bednar B, Lynch JL Jr, et al. Tirofiban (Aggrastat®). *Cardiovasc Drug Rev* 1999;17:199.
84. RESTORE Investigators. Effects of platelet glycoprotein IIb/IIIa blockade with tirofiban on adverse cardiac events in patients with unstable angina or acute myocardial infarction undergoing coronary angioplasty. *Circulation* 1997;96: 1445.
85. PRISM Investigators. A comparison of aspirin plus tirofiban with aspirin plus heparin for unstable angina. *N Engl J Med* 1998;338:1498.
86. PRISM-PLUS Investigators. Inhibition of the platelet glycoprotein IIb/IIIa receptor with tirofiban in unstable angina and non-Q-wave myocardial infarction. *N Engl J Med* 1998;338:1488.
87. Kereiakes DJ. Oral blockade of the platelet glycoprotein IIb/IIIa receptor: fact or fancy? *Am Heart J* 1999;138:S39.
88. SYMPHONY Investigators. Comparison of sibrafiban with aspirin for prevention of cardiovascular events after acute coronary syndromes: a randomized trial. *Lancet* 2000;355:337–345.
89. O'Neill WW, Serruys P, Knudtson M, et al. Long-term treatment with a platelet glycoprotein-receptor antagonist after percutaneous coronary revascularization. *N Engl J Med* 2000;342:1316.
90. Ferguson JJ. Meeting highlights. Highlights of the 48th scientific sessions of the American College of Cardiology. *Circulation* 1999;100:570.
91. SoRelle R. SmithKline Beecham halts tests of lotrafiban, an oral glycoprotein IIb/IIIa inhibitor. *Circulation* 2001;103:E9001.
92. Reference deleted by author.
93. Coller BS, Cheresh DA, Asch E, et al. Platelet vitronectin receptor expression differentiates Iraqi-Jewish from Arab patients with Glanzmann thrombasthenia in Israel. *Blood* 1991;77:75.
94. Bennett JS, Chan C, Vilaire G, et al. Agonist-activated αvβ3 on platelets and lymphocytes binds to the matrix protein osteopontin. *J Biol Chem* 1997;272:8137.
95. Helluin O, Chan C, Vilaire G, et al. The activation state of αvβ3 regulates platelet and lymphocyte adhesion to intact and thrombin-cleaved osteopontin. *J Biol Chem* 2000;275:18337.
96. Roth GJ. Developing relationships: arterial platelet adhesion, glycoprotein Ib, and leucine-rich glycoproteins. *Blood* 1991;77:5.
97. Ruggeri ZM. Mechanisms initiating platelet thrombus formation. *Thromb Haemost* 1997;78:611.
98. Ruggeri ZM, De Marco L, Gatti L, et al. Platelets have more than one binding site for von Willebrand factor. *J Clin Invest* 1983;72:1.
99. Coller BS, Peerschke EL, Scudder IE, et al. Studies with a murine monoclonal antibody that abolishes ristocetin-induced binding of von Willebrand factor to platelets: additional evidence in support of GPIb as a platelet receptor for von Willebrand factor. *Blood* 1983;61:99.
100. McFarland KC, Sprengel R, Phillips HS, et al. Lutropin-choriogonadotropin receptor: an unusual member of the G protein-coupled receptor family. *Science* 1989;245:494.
101. Reinke R, Krantz DE, Yen D, et al. Chaoptin, a cell surface glycoprotein required for Drosophila photoreceptor cell morphogenesis, contains a repeat motif found in yeast and human. *Cell* 1988;52:291.
102. Kataoka T, Broek D, Wigler M. DNA sequence and characterization of the *S. cerevisiae* gene encoding adenylate cyclase. *Cell* 1985;43:493.
103. Landschultz WH, Johnson OF, McKnight SL. The leucine zipper: a hypothetical structure common to a new class of DNA binding proteins. *Science* 1990;240:1759.
104. Bohmann D, Bos TJ, Admon A, et al. Human proto-oncogene c-jun encodes a DNA binding protein with structural and functional properties of transcription factor AP-1. *Science* 1987;238:1386.
105. Setoyama C, Frunzio R, Liau G, et al. Transcription activation encoded by the v-fos gene. *Proc Natl Acad Sci U S A* 1986;83:3213.
106. Romo GM, Dong JF, Schade AJ, et al. The glycoprotein Ib-IX-V complex is a platelet counterreceptor for P-selectin. *J Exp Med* 1999;190:803.
107. Lopez JA, Chung DW, Fujikawa K, et al. The alpha and beta chains of human platelet glycoprotein Ib are both transmembrane proteins containing a leucine-rich amino acid sequence. *Proc Natl Acad Sci U S A* 1988;85: 2135.
108. Okumura T, Lombart C, Jamieson GA. Platelet glycocalicin II. Purification and characterization. *J Biol Chem* 1976;251:5950.
109. Handa M, Titani K, Holland LZ, et al. The von Willebrand factor-binding domain of platelet membrane glycoprotein Ib. *J Biol Chem* 1986;261:12579.
110. Wicki AN, Clemetson KJ. Structure and function of platelet membrane glycoprotein Ib and V. Effects of leucocyte elastase and other proteases on platelet response to von Willebrand factor and thrombin. *Eur J Biochem* 1985; 153:1.
111. Berndt MC, Gregory C, Dowden G, et al. Thrombin interactions with platelet membrane proteins. *Ann NY Acad Sci* 1986;485:374.
112. Vicente V, Houghten RA, Ruggeri ZM. Identification of a site in the alpha chain of platelet glycoprotein Ib that participates in von Willebrand factor binding. *J Biol Chem* 1990;265:274.
113. Handin RI, Peterson E. Production of recombinant glycoprotein Ibalpha fragments and delineation of the von Willebrand factor binding site. *Blood* 1989;74:4777.
114. Howard MA, Firkin BG. Ristocetin—a new tool in the investigation of platelet aggregation. *Thromb Diath Haemorrh* 1971;26:362.
115. Pepper DS, Jamieson GA. Isolation of a macroglycopeptide from human platelets. *Biochemistry* 1970;9:3706.
116. Lopez JA, Ludwig EH, McCarthy BJ. Polymorphism of human glycoprotein Ibα results from a variable number of tandem repeats of a 13-amino acid sequence in the mucin-like macroglycopeptide region. Structure/function implications. *J Biol Chem* 1992;267:10055.
117. Fox JEB, Aggerbeck LP, Berndt MC. Structure of the glycoprotein Ib-IX complex from platelet membranes. *J Biol Chem* 1988;263:4882.
118. Fox JE, Berdnt MC. Cyclic AMP-dependent phosphorylation of glycoprotein GPIb inhibits collagen-induced polymerization on platelets. *J Biol Chem* 1989;264:9520.
119. Modderman PW, Admiraal LG, Sonnenberg A, et al. Glycoprotein-V and glycoprotein-Ib-IX form a noncovalent complex in the platelet membrane. *J Biol Chem* 1992;267:364.

120. Hickey MJ, Williams SA, Roth GJ. Human platelet glycoprotein IX: an adhesive prototype of leucine-rich glycoproteins with flank-center-flank structures. *Proc Natl Acad Sci U S A* 1989;86:6773.

121. Clemetson KJ, Shimomura T, Phillips DR. Cloning and characterization of the gene encoding the human platelet glycoprotein V. A member of the leucine-rich glycoprotein family cleaved during thrombin-induced platelet activation. *J Biol Chem* 1993;268:20801.

122. Zafar RS, Walz DA. Platelet membrane glycoprotein V: characterization of the thrombin-sensitive glycoprotein from human platelets. *Thromb Res* 1989;53:31.

123. Ramakrishnan V, DeGuzman F, Bao M, et al. Thrombin receptor function for platelet glycoprotein Ib-IX unmasked by cleavage of glycoprotein V. *Proc Natl Acad Sci U S A* 2001;98:1823.

124. Ni H, Ramakrishnan V, Papalia JM, et al. Increased thrombogenesis and embolus formation in mice lacking glycoprotein V. *Blood* 2000;96:812a.

125. Yuan Y, Kulkarni S, Ulsemer P, et al. The von Willebrand factor-glycoprotein Ib/V/IX interaction induces actin polymerization and cytoskeletal reorganization in rolling platelets and glycoprotein Ib/V/IX-transfected cells. *J Biol Chem* 1999;274:36241.

126. Du X, Harris SJ, Tetaz TJ, et al. Association of the phospholipase A_2 (14-3-3ζ) with the platelet glycoprotein Ib-IX complex. *J Biol Chem* 1994;269:18287.

127. Muslin AJ, Tanner JW, Allen PM, et al. Interaction of 14-3-3 with signaling proteins is mediated by the recognition of phosphoserine. *Cell* 1996;84:889.

128. Falati S, Edmead CE, Poole AW. Glycoprotein Ib-V-IX, a receptor for von Willebrand factor, couples physically and functionally to the Fc receptor gamma-chain, Fyn, and Lyn to activate human platelets. *Blood* 1999;94:1648.

129. Bernard J, Soulier JP. Sur une nouvele variete de dystrophie thrombocytaire haemoragipare congenitale. *Semin Hop Paris* 1948;24:3217.

130. Lopez JA, Andrews RK, Afshar-Kharghan V, et al. Bernard-Soulier syndrome. *Blood* 1998;91:4397.

131. Ware J, Russell SR, Vicente V, et al. Nonsense mutation in the glycoprotein Ib alpha coding sequence associated with Bernard-Soulier syndrome. *Proc Natl Acad Sci U S A* 1990;87:2026.

132. De Marco L, Mazzucato M, Fabris F, et al. Variant Bernard-Soulier syndrome type bolzano. A congenital bleeding disorder due to a structural and functional abnormality of the platelet glycoprotein Ib-IX complex. *J Clin Invest* 1990;86:25.

133. Miller JL, Lyle VA, Cunningham D. Mutation of leucine-57 to phenylalanine in a platelet glycoprotein Ib alpha leucine tandem repeat occurring in patients with an autosomal dominant variant of Bernard-Soulier disease. *Blood* 1992;79:439.

134. Ware J, Russell SR, Marchese P, et al. Point mutation in a leucine-rich repeat of platelet glycoprotein Ib alpha resulting in the Bernard-Soulier syndrome. *J Clin Invest* 1993;92:1213.

135. Simsek S, Noris P, Lozano M, et al. Cys[209]Ser mutation in the platelet membrane glycoprotein Ibα gene is associated with Bernard-Soulier syndrome. *Br J Haematol* 1994;88:839.

136. Li C, Martin S, Roth G. The genetic defect in two well-studied cases of Bernard-Soulier syndrome: a point mutation in the fifth leucine-rich repeat of platelet glycoprotein Ibα. *Blood* 1996;86:3805.

137. Holmberg L, Karpman D, Nilsson I, et al. Bernard-Soulier syndrome Karlstad: Trp498→Stop mutation resulting in a truncated glycoprotein Ib alpha that contains part of the transmembrane domain. *Br J Haematol* 1997;98:57.

138. Afshar-Kharghan V, Lopez JA. Bernard-Soulier syndrome caused by a dinucleotide deletion and frameshift in the region encoding the glycoprotein Ibα transmembrane domain. *Blood* 1997;90:2634.

139. Kunishima S, Miura H, Fukutani H, et al. Bernard-Soulier syndrome Kagoshima: Ser444→stop mutation of glycoprotein (GP) Ib alpha resulting in circulating truncated GPIb alpha and surface expression of GPIb beta and GPIX. *Blood* 1994;84:3356.

140. Simsek S, Admiraal LG, Modderman PW, et al. Identification of a homozygous single base pair deletion in the gene coding for the human platelet glycoprotein Ibα causing Bernard-Soulier syndrome. *Thromb Haemost* 1994;72:444.

141. Kanaji T, Okamura T, Kuroiwa M, et al. Molecular and genetic analysis of two patients with Bernard-Soulier syndrome: identification of new mutations in glycoprotein Ibα gene. *Thromb Haemost* 1997;77:1055.

142. Budarf ML, Konkle BA, Ludlow LB, et al. Identification of a patient with Bernard-Soulier syndrome and a deletion in the DiGeorge/Velo-cardio-facial chromosomal region in 22q11.2. *Hum Mol Genet* 1995;4:763.

143. Kunishima S, Lopez JA, Kobayashi S, et al. Missense mutations of the glycoprotein (GP) Ibβ gene impairing the GPIbα/β disulfide linkage in a family with giant platelet disorder. *Blood* 1997;89:2404.

144. Wright SD, Michaelides K, Johnson DJ, et al. Double heterozygosity for mutations in the platelet glycoprotein IX gene in three siblings with Bernard-Soulier syndrome. *Blood* 1993;81:2339.

145. Noda M, Fujimura K, Takafuta T, et al. Heterogeneous expression of glycoprotein Ib, IX and V in platelets from two patients with Bernard-Soulier syndrome caused by different genetic abnormalities. *Thromb Haemost* 1995;74:1411.

146. Noda M, Fujimura K, Takafuta T, et al. A point mutation in glycoprotein IX coding sequence (Cys73(TGT) to Tyr(TAT)) causes impaired surface expression of GPIb/IX/V complex in two families with Bernard-Soulier syndrome. *Thromb Haemost* 1996;74:874.

147. Noris P, Simsek S, Stibbe J, et al. A phenylalanine-55 to serine amino acid substitution in the human glycoprotein IX leucine-rich repeat is associated with Bernard-Soulier syndrome. *Br J Haematol* 1997;97:312.

148. Kunishima S, Lopez JA, Kobayashi S, et al. Missense mutations of the glycoprotein (GP) Ibβ gene impairing the GPIbα/β disulfide linkage in a family with giant platelet disorder. *Blood* 1997;89:2404.

149. Wright SD, Michaelides K, Johnson DJ, et al. Double heterozygosity for mutations in the platelet glycoprotein IX gene in three siblings with Bernard-Soulier syndrome. *Blood* 1993;81:2339.

150. Clemetson JM, Kyrle PA, Brenner B, et al. Variant Bernard-Soulier syndrome associated with a homozygous mutation in the leucine-rich domain of glycoprotein IX. *Blood* 1994;84:1124.

151. Blanchette VS, Sparling C, Turner C. Inherited bleeding disorders. *Baillieres Clin Haematol* 1991;4:291.

152. Saade G, Homsi R, Seoud M. Bernard-Soulier syndrome in pregnancy: a report of four pregnancies in one patient and review of the literature. *Eur J Obstet Gynecol Reprod Biol* 1991;40:149.

153. Cuthbert RJG, Watson HH, Handa SI, et al. DDAVP shortens the bleeding time in Bernard-Soulier syndrome. *Thromb Res* 1988;49:649.

154. Poon MC, d'Oiron R. Recombinant activated factor VII (NovoSeven) treatment of platelet-related bleeding disorders. International Registry on Recombinant Factor VIIa and Congenital Platelet Disorders Group. *Blood Coagul Fibrinolysis* 2000;11:S55.

155. Bithell TC, Parekh SJ, Strong RR. Platelet-function studies in the Bernard-Soulier syndrome. *Ann N Y Acad Sci* 1972;201:145.

156. Hourdille P, Pico M, Jandrot-Perrus M, et al. Studies on the megakaryocytes of a patient with the Bernard-Soulier syndrome. *Br J Haematol* 1990;76:521.

157. Howard MA, Hutton RA, Hardisty RM. Hereditary giant platelet syndrome: a disorder of a new aspect of platelet function. *BMJ* 1973;2:586.

158. Coller BS, Zarrabi MH. Platelet membrane studies in the May-Hegglin anomaly. *Blood* 1981;58:279.

159. Epstein CJ, Sahud MA, Piel CF, et al. Hereditary macrothrombocytopathia, nephritis, deafness. *Am J Med* 1972;52:299.

160. Godwin HA, Ginsburg AD. May-Hegglin anomaly: a defect in megakaryocyte fragmentation? *Br J Haematol* 1974;26:117.

161. Eckstein JD, Filip DJ, Watts JC. Hereditary thrombocytopenia, deafness, and renal disease. *Ann Intern Med* 1975;82:639.

162. Peterson LC, Rao KV, Crosson JT, et al. Fechtner syndrome—a variant of Alport's syndrome with leukocyte inclusions and macrothrombocytopenia. *Blood* 1985;65:397.

163. Bernheim J, Dechavanne M, Bryon PA, et al. Thrombocytopenia, macrothrombocytopathia, nephritis and deafness. *Am J Med* 1976;61:145.

164. Milton JG, Frojmovic MM. Shape-changing agents produce abnormally large platelets in a hereditary "giant platelet syndrome (MPS)." *J Lab Clin Med* 1979;93:154.

165. Frojmovic MM, Milton JG. Physical, chemical and functional changes following platelet activation in normal and "giant" platelets. *Blood Cells* 1983;9:359.

166. Okita JR, Frojmovic MM, Fristopeit S, et al. Montreal platelet syndrome: a defect in calcium-activated protease (Calpain). *Blood* 1989;74:715.

167. Stricker RB, Wong D, Saks SR, et al. Acquired Bernard-Soulier syndrome: evidence for the role of a 210,000-molecular weight protein in the interaction of platelets with von Willebrand factor. *J Clin Invest* 1985;76:1274.

168. Szatkowski NS, Kunicki TJ, Aster RH. Identification of glycoprotein Ib as a target for auto antibody (autoimmune) thrombocytopenic purpura. *Blood* 1986;67:310.

169. Devine DV, Currie MS, Rosse WF, et al. Pseudo-Bernard Soulier syndrome: thrombocytopenia caused by autoantibody to platelet glycoprotein Ib. *Blood* 1987;70:428.

170. Berndt MC, Kabral A, Grimsley P, et al. An acquired Bernard-Soulier-like platelet defect associated with juvenile myelodysplastic syndrome. *Br J Haematol* 1988;68:97.

171. Aktories K, Jakobs KH. N_i-mediated inhibition of human platelet adenylate cyclase by thrombin. *Eur J Biochem* 1984;145:333.

172. Vu T-KH, Hung DT, Wheaton VI, et al. Molecular cloning of a functional thrombin receptor reveals a novel proteolytic mechanism of receptor activation. *Cell* 1991;64:1057.

173. Rasmussen UB, Vouret-Craviari V, Jallat S, et al. cDNA cloning and expression of a hamster α-thrombin receptor coupled to Ca^{2+} mobilization. *FEBS Lett* 1991;288:123.

174. Burnham MR, Harte MT, Richardson A, et al. The identification of p130[cas]-binding proteins and their role in cellular transformation. *Oncogene* 1996;12:2467.

175. Ishii K, Chen J, Ishii M, et al. Inhibition of thrombin receptor signaling by a G-protein coupled receptor kinase. Functional specificity among G-protein coupled receptor kinases. *J Biol Chem* 1994;269:1125.

176. Nystedt S, Emilsson K, Wahlestedt C, et al. Molecular cloning of a potential proteinase activated receptor. *Proc Natl Acad Sci U S A* 1994;91:9208.

177. Ishihara H, Connolly AJ, Zeng D, et al. Protease-activated receptor 3 is a second thrombin receptor in humans. *Nature* 1997;386:502.

178. Xu W-F, Andersen H, Whitmore TE, et al. Cloning and characterization of human protease-activated receptor 4. *Proc Natl Acad Sci U S A* 1998;95:6642.

179. Connolly AJ, Ishihara H, Kahn ML, et al. Role of the thrombin receptor in development and evidence for a second receptor. *Nature* 1996;381:516.

180. Darrow AL, Fung-Leung WP, Ye RD, et al. Biological consequences of thrombin receptor deficiency in mice. *Thromb Haemost* 1996;76:860.

181. Molino M, Barnathan ES, Numerof R, et al. Interactions of mast cell tryptase with thrombin receptors and PAR-2. *J Biol Chem* 1997;272:4043.

182. Brass LF, Vassallo RR Jr, Belmonte E, et al. Structure and function of the human platelet thrombin receptor: studies using monoclonal antibodies

against a defined epitope within the receptor N-terminus. *J Biol Chem* 1992;267:13795.

183. Kahn ML, Nakanishi-Matsui M, Shapiro MJ, et al. Protease-activated receptors 1 and 4 mediate activation of human platelets by thrombin. *J Clin Invest* 1999;103:879.

184. Faruq TR, Weiss EJ, Shapiro MJ, et al. Structure-function analysis of protease-activated receptor 4 tethered ligand properties: determinants of specificity and utility in assays of receptor function. *J Biol Chem* 2000:275: 19728.

185. De Candia E, Hall SW, Rutella S, et al. Binding of thrombin to glycoprotein Ib accelerates the hydrolysis of Par-1 on intact platelets. *J Biol Chem* 2001;276:4692.

186. Norton KJ, Scarborough RM, Kutok JL, et al. Immunologic analysis of the cloned platelet thrombin receptor activation mechanism: evidence supporting receptor cleavage, release of the N-terminal peptide, and insertion of the tethered ligand into a protected environment. *Blood* 1993;82:2125.

187. Molino M, Bainton DF, Hoxie JA, et al. Thrombin receptors on human platelets: initial localization and subsequent redistribution during platelet activation. *J Biol Chem* 1997;272:6011.

188. Brass LF, Pizarro S, Ahuja M, et al. Changes in the structure and function of the human thrombin receptor during activation, internalization and recycling. *J Biol Chem* 1994;269:2943.

189. Ramachandran R, Klufas AS, Molino M, et al. Release of the thrombin receptor N-terminus from the surface of human platelets activated by thrombin. *Thromb Haemost* 1997;78:1119.

190. Woolkalis MJ, DeMelfi TM, Blanchard N, et al. Regulation of thrombin receptors on human umbilical vein endothelial cells. *J Biol Chem* 1995;270:9868.

191. Fisher GJ, Bakshian S, Baldassare JJ. Activation of human platelets by ADP causes a rapid rise in cytosolic free calcium without hydrolysis of phosphatidylinositol-4,5-bisphosphate. *Biochem Biophys Res Commun* 1985;129:958.

192. Cattaneo M, Lecchi A, Randi AM, et al. Identification of a new congenital defect of platelet function characterized by severe impairment of platelet responses to adenosine diphosphate. *Blood* 1992;80:2787.

193. Léon C, Hechler B, Vial C, et al. The P2Y$_1$ is an ADP receptor antagonized by ATP and expressed in platelets and megakaryoblastic cells. *FEBS Lett* 1997;403:26.

194. Hollopeter G, Jantzen H-M, Vincent D, et al. Molecular identification of the platelet ADP receptor targeted by antithrombotic drugs. *Nature* 2001;409:202.

195. Zhang FL, Luo L, Gustafson E, et al. ADP is the cognate ligand for the orphan G protein-coupled receptor SP1999. *J Biol Chem* 2001;276(11):8608–8615.

196. McKenzie AB, Mahout-Smith MP, Sage SO. Activation of receptor-operated channels via P2X1 not P2T purinoreceptors in human platelets. *J Biol Chem* 1996;271:2879.

197. Siess W, Weber PC, Lapetina EG. Activation of PLC is dissociated from arachidonate metabolism during platelet shape change induced by thrombin or platelet-activating factor. Epinephrine does not induce PLC activation or platelet shape change. *J Biol Chem* 1984;259:8286.

198. Bennett JS, Vilaire G, Burch JW. A role for prostaglandins and thromboxanes in the exposure of platelet fibrinogen receptors. *J Clin Invest* 1981;68:981.

199. Sweatt JD, Connolly TM, Cragoe EJ, et al. Evidence that Na$^+$/H$^+$ exchange regulates receptor-mediated phospholipase A$_2$ activation in human platelets. *J Biol Chem* 1986;261:8667.

200. Banga HS, Simons ER, Brass LF, et al. Activation of phospholipases A and C in human platelets exposed to epinephrine: role of glycoproteins IIb/IIIa and dual role of epinephrine. *Proc Natl Acad Sci U S A* 1986;83:9197.

201. Kaywin P, McDonough M, Insel PA, et al. Platelet function in essential thrombocythemia: decreased epinephrine responsiveness associated with a deficiency of platelet alpha-adrenergic receptors. *N Engl J Med* 1978;299: 505.

202. Scrutton MC, Clare KC, Hutton RA, et al. Depressed responsiveness to adrenaline in platelets from apparently normal human donors: a familial trait. *Br J Haematol* 1981;49:303.

203. Rao AK, Willis J, Kowalska MA, et al. Differential requirements for platelet aggregation and inhibition of adenylate cyclase by epinephrine. Studies of a familial platelet α$_2$-adrenergic receptor defect. *Blood* 1988;71:494.

204. Spaet TH, Lejnieks I. Studies on the mechanism whereby platelets are clumped by adenosine diphosphate. *Thromb Diath Haemorrh* 1966;15:36.

205. Cooper B, Handin RJ, Young LH, et al. Agonist regulation of the human platelet alpha-adrenergic receptor. *Nature* 1978;271:703.

206. Cooper B, Shafer AI, Puchalsky D, et al. Platelet resistance to PGD2 in patients with myeloproliferative disorders. *Blood* 1978;52:618.

207. Scrutton MC, Clare KA, Hutton RA, et al. Depressed responsiveness to adrenaline in platelets from apparently normal human donors: a familial trait. *Br J Haematol* 1981;49:303.

208. Yang J, Wu J, Kowalska MA, et al. Loss of signaling through the G protein, Gz, results in abnormal platelet activation and altered responses to psychoactive drugs. *Proc Natl Acad Sci U S A* 2000;97:9984.

209. Gerrard JM, Carroll RC. Stimulation of protein phosphorylation by arachidonic acid and endoperoxide analog. *Prostaglandins* 1981;22:81.

210. Siess W, Siegel FL, Lapetina EG. Arachidonic acid stimulates the formation of 1,2-diacylglycerol and phosphatidic acid in human platelets. Degree of PLC activation correlates with protein phosphorylation, platelet shape change, serotonin release, and aggregation. *J Biol Chem* 1983;258:11236.

211. FitzGerald GA. Mechanisms of platelet activation: thromboxane A$_2$ as an amplifying signal for other agonists. *Am J Cardiol* 1991;68:11B.

212. Hirata M, Hayashi Y, Ushikubi F, et al. Cloning and expression of cDNA for a human thromboxane A$_2$ receptor. *Nature* 1991;349:617.

213. Habib A, FitzGerald GA, Maclouf J. Phosphorylation of the thromboxane receptor α, the predominant isoform expressed in human platelets. *J Biol Chem* 1997;274:2645.

214. Schafer AI, Cooper B, O'Hara D, et al. Identification of platelet receptors for prostaglandin I2 and D2. *J Biol Chem* 1979;254:2914.

215. Higuchi W, Fuse I, Hattori A, et al. Mutations of the platelet thromboxane A$_2$ (TXA$_2$) receptor in patients characterized by the absence of TXA$_2$-induced platelet aggregation despite normal TXA$_2$ binding activity. *Thromb Haemost* 1999;82:1528.

216. Murata T, Ushikubi F, Matsuoka T, et al. Altered pain perception and inflammatory response in mice lacking prostacyclin receptor. *Nature* 1997;388:678.

217. Gewirtz AM, Calabretta B, Rucinski B, et al. Inhibition of human megakaryocytopoiesis in vitro by platelet factor 4 (PF4) and a synthetic COOH-terminal PF4 peptide. *J Clin Invest* 1989;83:1477.

218. Kowalska MA, Ratajczak M, Majka M, et al. SDF-1 and MDC: complementary chemokines at the crossroads between inflammation and thrombosis. *Blood* 2000;96:50.

219. Kowalska MA, Ratajczak J, Hoxie J, et al. Platelets and megakaryocytes express the HIV co-receptor CXCR4 on their surface: response to stromal-derived factor-1 (SDF-1). *Br J Haematol* 1999;104:220.

220. Williams AF. The immunoglobulin superfamily takes shape [news]. *Nature* 1984;308:12.

221. Savage B, Almus-Jacobs F, Ruggeri ZM. Specific synergy of multiple substrate-receptor interactions in platelet thrombus formation under flow. *Cell* 1998;94:657.

222. Santoro SA. Identification of a 160,000 dalton platelet membrane protein that mediates the initial divalent cation-dependent adhesion of platelets to collagen. *Cell* 1986;46:913.

223. Clemetson KJ, McGregor JL, James E, et al. Characterization of the platelet membrane glycoprotein abnormalities in Bernard-Soulier syndrome and comparison with normal by surface-labeling techniques and high-resolution two-dimensional gel electrophoresis. *J Clin Invest* 1982;70:304.

224. Wilner GD, Nossel HL, LeRoy EC. Aggregation of platelets by collagen. *J Clin Invest* 1968;47:2616–2621.

225. Nakamura T, Jamieson GA, Okuma M, et al. Platelet adhesion to native type I collagen fibrils. Role of GPVI in divalent cation-dependent and -independent adhesion and thromboxane A2 generation. *J Biol Chem* 1998;273:4338–4344.

226. Chiang TM, Rinaldy A, Kang AH. Cloning, characterization, and functional studies of a nonintegrin platelet receptor for type I collagen. *J Clin Invest* 1997;100:514.

227. Barnes MJ, Knight CG, Farndale RW. The collagen-platelet interaction. *Curr Opin Hematol* 1998;5:314.

228. Nieuwenhuis HK, Akkerman JW, Houdijk WP, et al. Human blood platelets showing no response to collagen fail to express surface glycoprotein Ia. *Nature* 1985;318:470.

229. Sugiyama T, Okuma M, Ushikubi F, et al. A novel platelet aggregating factor found in a patient with defective collagen-induced platelet aggregation and autoimmune thrombocytopenia. *Blood* 1987;69:1712.

230. Moroi M, Jung SM, Okuma M, et al. A patient with platelets deficient in glycoprotein VI that lack both collagen-induced aggregation and adhesion. *J Clin Invest* 1989;84:1440.

231. Arai M, Yamamoto N, Moroi M, et al. Platelets with 10% of the normal amount of glycoprotein VI have an impaired response to collagen that results in a mild bleeding tendency. *Br J Haematol* 1995;89:124.

232. Clemetson JM, Polgar J, Magnenat E, et al. The platelet collagen receptor glycoprotein VI is a member of the immunoglobulin superfamily closely related to FcalphaR and the natural killer receptors. *J Biol Chem* 1999;274:29019.

233. Jandrot-Perrus M, Busfield S, Lagrue AH, et al. Cloning, characterization, and functional studies of human and mouse glycoprotein VI: a platelet-specific collagen receptor from the immunoglobulin superfamily. *Blood* 2000;96:1798.

234. Morton HC, van den Herik-Oudijk IE, Vossebeld P, et al. Functional association between the human myeloid immunoglobulin A Fc receptor (CD89) and FcR gamma chain. Molecular basis for CD89/FcR gamma chain association. *J Biol Chem* 1995;270:29781.

235. Gross BS, Melford SK, Watson SP. Evidence that PLC-gamma2 interacts with SLP-76, Syk, Lyn, LAT and the Fc receptor gamma-chain after stimulation of the collagen receptor glycoprotein VI in human platelets. *Eur J Biochem* 1999; 263:612.

236. Moroi M, Okuma M, Jung SM. Platelet adhesion to collagen-coated wells: analysis of this complex process and a comparison with the adhesion to matrigel-coated wells. *Biochim Biophys Acta* 1992;1137:1.

237. Morton LF, Hargreaves PG, Farndale RW, et al. Integrin alpha 2 beta 1-independent activation of platelets by simple collagen-like peptides: collagen tertiary (triple-helical) and quaternary (polymeric) structures are sufficient alone for alpha 2 beta 1-independent platelet reactivity. *Biochem J* 1995;306:337.

238. Kehrel B, Wierwille S, Clemetson KJ, et al. Glycoprotein VI is a major collagen receptor for platelet activation: it recognizes the collagen-activating quaternary structure of collagen, whereas CD36, glycoprotein IIb/IIIa, and von Willebrand factor do not. *Blood* 1998;91:491.

239. Jandrot-Perrus M, Lagrue AH, Okuma M, et al. Adhesion and activation of human platelets induced by convulxin involve glycoprotein VI and integrin alpha2beta1. *J Biol Chem* 1997;272:27035.

240. Tandon NN, Kralisz U, Jamieson GA. Identification of glycoprotein IV (CD36) as a primary receptor for platelet-collagen adhesion. *J Biol Chem* 1989;264:7576.

241. Daniel JL, Dangelmaier C, Strouse R, et al. Collagen induces normal signal transduction in platelets deficient in CD36 (platelet glycoprotein IV). *Thromb Haemost* 1994;71:353.

242. Cummings RD, Smith DF. The selectin family of carbohydrate-binding proteins: structure and importance of carbohydrate ligands for cell adhesion. *Bioessays* 1992;14:849.

243. Johnston GI, Cook RG, McEver RP. Cloning of GMP-140, a granule membrane protein of platelets and endothelium: sequence similarity to proteins involved in cell adhesion and inflammation. *Cell* 1989;56:1033.

244. Yeo E, Furie BC, Furie B. PADGEM protein in human erythroleukemia cells. *Blood* 1989;73:722.

245. Bonfanti R, Furie BC, Furie B, et al. PADGEM (GMP140) is a component of Weibel-Palade bodies of human endothelial cells. *Blood* 1989;73:1109.

246. Bevilacqua MP, Stengelin S, Gimbrone MA Jr, et al. Endothelial leukocyte adhesion molecule 1: an inducible receptor for neutrophils related to complement regulatory proteins and lectins. *Science* 1989;243:1160.

247. Montgomery KF, Osborn L, Hession C, et al. Activation of endothelial-leukocyte adhesion molecule 1 (ELAM-1) gene transcription. *Proc Natl Acad Sci U S A* 1991;88:6523.

248. Brandley BK, Swiedler SJ, Robbins PW. Carbohydrate ligands of the LEC cell adhesion molecules. *Cell* 1990;63:861.

249. Yang J, Furie BG, Furie B. The biology of P-selectin glycoprotein ligand-1: its role as a selectin counterreceptor in leukocyte-endothelial and leucocyte-platelet interaction. *Thromb Haemost* 1999;81:1.

250. Frenette PS, Johnson RC, Hynes RO, et al. Platelets roll on stimulated endothelium in vivo: an interaction mediated by endothelial P-selectin. *Proc Natl Acad Sci U S A* 1995;92:7450.

251. Dore M, Korthuis RJ, Granger DN, et al. P-selectin mediates spontaneous leukocyte rolling in vivo. *Blood* 1993;82:1308.

252. Munoz FM, Hawkins EP, Buffard DC, et al. Host defense against systemic infection with *Streptococcus pneumoniae* is impaired in E-P- and E-/P-selectin deficient mice. *J Clin Invest* 1997;100:2099.

253. Subramaniam M, Frenette PS, Saffaripour S, et al. Defects in hemostasis in P-selectin-deficient mice. *Blood* 1996;87:1238.

254. Johnson RC, Chapman SM, Dong ZM, et al. Absence of P-selectin delays fatty streak formation in mice. *J Clin Invest* 1997;99:1037.

255. Newman PJ, Berndt MC, Gorski J, et al. PECAM-1 (CD31) cloning and relation to adhesion molecules of the immunoglobulin gene superfamily. *Science* 1990;247:1219.

256. Newman PJ. The biology of PECAM-1. *J Clin Invest* 1997;99:3.

257. Newman PJ. Switched at birth: a new family for PECAM-1. *J Clin Invest* 1999;103:5.

258. Piali L, Hammel P, Uherek C, et al. CD31/PECAM-1 is a ligand for alpha v beta 3 integrin involved in adhesion of leukocytes to endothelium. *J Cell Biol* 1995;130:451.

259. Mahooti S, Graesser D, Patil S, et al. PECAM-1 (CD31) expression modulates bleeding time in vivo. *Am J Pathol* 2000;157:75.

260. Cicmil M, Thomas JM, Sage T, et al. PECAM-1: a negative regulator of platelet activation? *Blood* 2000;96;245a.

261. Patil S, Newman DK, Newman PJ. PECAM-1 serves as an inhibitory receptor that modulates platelet responses to collagen. *Blood* 2000;96:446a.

262. Anderson CL, Chacko GW, Osborne JM, et al. The Fc receptor for immunoglobulin G (Fc gamma RII) on human platelets. *Semin Thromb Hemost* 1995; 21:1.

263. McKenzie SE, Taylor SM, Malladi P, et al. The role of the human Fc receptor Fc gamma RIIA in the immune clearance of platelets: a transgenic mouse model. *J Immunol* 1999;162:4311.

264. Reilly MP, Taylor SM, Hartman NK, et al. Heparin-induced thrombocytopenia/thrombosis in a transgenic mouse model demonstrates the requirement for human platelet factor 4 and platelet activation through FcγRIIA. *Blood* 2000;96:221a.

265. Sullam PM, Hyun WC, Szollosi J, et al. Physical proximity and functional interplay of the glycoprotein Ib-IX-V complex and the Fc receptor FcgammaRIIA on the platelet plasma membrane. *J Biol Chem* 1998;273:5331.

266. Torti M, Bertoni A, Canobbio I, et al. Rap1B and Rap2B translocation to the cytoskeleton by von Willebrand factor involves FcgammaII receptor-mediated protein tyrosine phosphorylation. *J Biol Chem* 1999;274:13690.

267. Rosing J, van Rijn JLML, Bevers EM, et al. The role of activated human platelets in prothrombin and factor X activation. *Blood* 1985;65:319.

268. Zwall RFA, Comfurius P, van Deenen LLM. Membrane asymmetry and blood coagulation. *Nature* 1977;268:358.

269. Sims PJ, Wiedmer T, Esmon CT, et al. Assembly of the platelet prothrombinase complex is linked to vesiculation of the platelet plasma membrane. Studies in Scott syndrome: an isolated defect in platelet procoagulant activity. *J Biol Chem* 1989;264:17049.

270. Weiss HJ, Vicic WJ, Lages BA, et al. Isolated deficiency of platelet procoagulant activity. *Am J Med* 1979;67:206.

271. Minkoff M, Wu KK, Walasek J, et al. Bleeding disorder due to an isolated platelet factor 3 deficiency. *Arch Intern Med* 1980;140:366.

272. Miletich JP, Kane WH, Hofmann SL, et al. Deficiency of factor Xa-factor V binding sites on the platelets of a patient with a bleeding disorder. *Blood* 1979;54:1015.

273. Rosing J, Bevers EM, Comfurius P, et al. Impaired factor X and prothrombin activation associated with decreased phospholipid exposure in platelets from a patient with a bleeding disorder. *Blood* 1985;65:1557.

274. Weiss HJ, Vicic WJ, Lages BA, et al. Isolated deficiency of platelet procoagulant activity. *Am J Med* 1979;67:206.

275. Miletich JP, Kane WH, Hofmann SL, et al. Deficiency of factor Xa-factor V binding sites on the platelets of a patient with a bleeding disorder. *Blood* 1979;54:1015.

von Willebrand's Disease

Robert I. Handin and Bruce M. Ewenstein

von Willebrand's disease (vWD), the most common inherited coagulopathy, is best defined as a group of autosomally inherited bleeding disorders that are caused by quantitative or qualitative abnormalities in von Willebrand's factor (vWF). vWF has two roles in normal hemostasis. First, vWF provides a molecular bridge between platelets and the exposed subendothelium in damaged blood vessels (1) (Fig. 35-1). Second, vWF serves as an intravascular carrier for factor VIII, the procoagulant protein with which it is noncovalently complexed in the plasma (2). Thus, abnormalities in vWF may produce defects in primary and secondary hemostasis.

The definition of vWD as a clinical entity dates back to 1924, when Professor Eric von Willebrand evaluated a 5-year-old girl who was brought to a Helsinki hospital from her native Föglö Island in the Åland archipelago of Finland. She and many of her siblings had severe bleeding symptoms, and four died of hemorrhagic complications. After studying a total of 66 family members, Dr. von Willebrand concluded that the affected patients were experiencing a previously undescribed disorder, which now bears his name.

PATHOGENESIS

vWD was shown to differ from classic hemophilia in three important ways (3,4). First, the inheritance pattern was autosomal dominant and not X-linked. Second, the bleeding primarily involved mucous membranes, and hemarthroses, which are common in classic hemophilia, were absent in this family. Third, unlike hemophiliacs, patients with vWD had prolonged bleeding times. Descriptions of similar patients appeared in the late 1920s in American clinical literature (5,6). In 1953, several reports appeared that described a bleeding disorder that was characterized by an increased bleeding time and decreased factor VIII coagulant activity (7–9). The similarity between this disorder and the condition that was uncovered almost three decades earlier was discovered when the original Åland archipelago pedigree was reinvestigated, and these patients also were shown to have diminished levels of plasma factor VIII (10,11).

The pathophysiology of vWD was first suggested by the early studies of von Willebrand. Prompted by his clinical observations, von Willebrand developed a glass capillary apparatus to measure platelet function *in vitro* and found a delay in thrombus formation in blood from the affected members of this pedigree but not in blood from patients with hemophilia (12).

Modified forms of this test, which use glass beads, were reintroduced in the 1960s and were found to be sensitive ways to detect vWD (13,14). Later, model systems were developed to evaluate the role of vWF in platelet–subendothelial matrix interactions in flowing blood (15). Rabbit blood vessels that were denuded of subendothelium were perfused with blood under varying flow rates and shear stresses. Under conditions of high shear stress, the interactions between platelets and subendothelium required the plasma factor that was missing in vWD.

The common feature of diminished plasma factor VIII levels in vWD and classic hemophilia suggested a relation between these disorders, despite differences in their clinical presentation and mode of inheritance. In the late 1950s and early 1960s, a series of publications confirmed that the defect in vWD resided in the plasma (16–21). The prolonged bleeding time in vWD patients could be corrected by plasma and plasma-derived concentrates but not by platelets from normal donors (16,22–24). Conversely, platelets from patients with vWD improved hemostasis in patients with severe thrombocytopenia secondary to aplastic anemia. Plasma infusion had different effects in these two conditions. The infusion of plasma into a patient with hemophilia A resulted in an immediate peak, followed by a rapid decline, in factor VIII levels. In contrast, infusion of hemophilic plasma into a patient with vWD produced a delayed but sustained increase in factor VIII levels (24,25). Finally, after infusion of the more highly purified concentrates of factor VIII that became available in the 1970s, there was a clear dissociation between the elevation of factor VIII, the correction of the bleeding time, and the control of clinical bleeding (26,27).

Further elucidation of the relation between factor VIII and vWD was achieved after the development of immunologic reagents (28,29). Using the immunoelectrophoretic technique of Laurell (30), Zimmerman et al. (28) observed a diminished quantity of factor VIII–related antigen in patients with vWD but not in patients with hemophilia A. In the same year, Howard and Firkin (31) observed that the previously described agglutination of normal platelets by the antibiotic ristocetin was absent in some patients with vWD (32). Later, it was shown that the reduced ristocetin-induced platelet agglutination could be corrected by plasma or purified vWF (33).

vWF is synthesized by endothelial cells and megakaryocytes and circulates in plasma as a heterogeneous series of multimers that are assembled from a 220-kd subunit polypeptide. Plasma vWF multimers vary in size from 440 to $10 \times 10,000$ kd, with

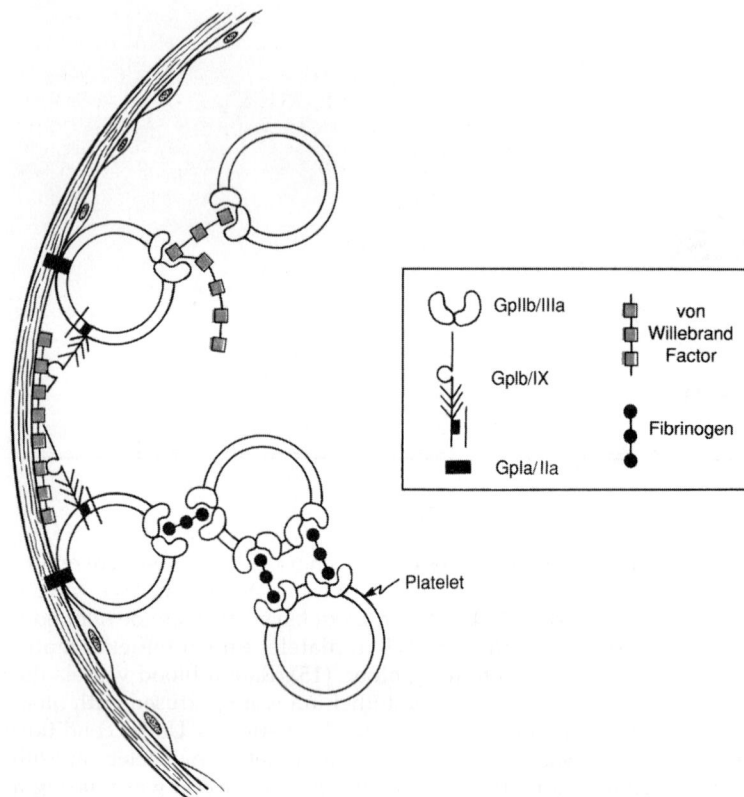

Figure 35-1. Role of von Willebrand's factor (vWF) in platelet adhesion and aggregation. Platelets adhere directly to collagen via a specific collagen receptor on the glycoprotein (gp) Ia/IIa complex. vWF adheres to constituents in vascular subendothelium, primarily collagen, and to the platelet gpIb/IX complex. This interaction stabilizes adherent platelets and prevents their detachment during high-flow or high-shear stress. Adherent activated platelets then bind fibrinogen to the gpIIb/IIIa complex and form aggregates. In addition, some component of adhesion is due to an interaction between vWF and gpIIb/IIIa (not shown).

even larger multimers noted within endothelial cell storage organelles. Studies from multiple laboratories have demonstrated a close relation between multimer size and the hemostatic effectiveness of vWF (34,35). The ability of vWF to support shear-induced platelet aggregation is dependent on multimer size (36). As further proof of this relation, in disorders like thrombotic thrombocytopenic purpura (TTP), in which there is unregulated secretion of large vWF multimers from endothelial cells, patients develop thrombocytopenia and platelet thrombi (37). Conversely, in some forms of vWD, in which a selective loss of high-molecular-weight (HMW) vWF multimers and a normal plasma level of vWF are seen, patients have defective hemostasis and clinical bleeding.

vWF has been purified to homogeneity, and its complete amino acid sequence has been determined by both classic protein chemistry (38) and molecular cloning techniques (39–42). The defects that cause vWD are beginning to be defined at the molecular level, producing some unifying theories and at the same time raising new issues (43). Despite the rapidity of recent progress, our knowledge of the molecular and cellular basis of most cases of vWD remains imperfect. Moreover, the wide variety of defects, which together are termed *vWD*, and the variable expression of vWD phenotypes have made it difficult to establish clear-cut diagnostic criteria.

STRUCTURE OF VON WILLEBRAND'S FACTOR

The primary vWF translation product is a protein that contains 2813 amino acids that have a predicted molecular weight of 309 kd (44–48). Based on direct protein sequencing, the amino terminal of the mature vWF subunit can be located at codon 764 (38). The first 763 amino acids consist of a 22–amino acid hydrophobic signal peptide and a large propeptide that is identical with a protein that is found in plasma and is called

von Willebrand's antigen II (vW AgII) (49,50). The vWF propeptide is cleaved from the mature subunit between codons 763 and 764 after a pair of basic amino acids (Lys-Arg). Cleavage is presumed to be mediated by a member of a newly discovered enzyme family, with specificity for pairs of basic amino acids, which thus is given the acronym *PACE* (*p*aired *a*mino acid *c*leaving *e*nzyme) (51). They are members of a subtilisin-related family of endoproteases and are homologous to the yeast enzyme Kex2 (52,53). Site-specific mutagenesis of the vWF Lys-Arg sequence abolishes cleavage of the propolypeptide, without disrupting vWF multimer assembly or function (54,55). Persons have been described whose circulating vWF multimers are made up of an approximately equal mix of cleaved and uncleaved pro-vWF subunits (56). It is presumed, but has not been proven, that they have mutations in the PACE recognition sequence. Despite the retention of the prosequence, hemostatic function is completely normal. In contrast, removal of the propeptide sequence from the vWF complementary DNA (cDNA) abolishes multimer formation, thus suggesting that at least one important function of the propeptide is to direct the assembly of vWF dimers into multimers (54,55).

vWF is almost entirely composed of four types of homologous repeated sequences (Fig. 35-2). The D repeats, which contain most of the 233 cysteine residues that are found in each subunit, are repeated twice in the propeptide and again in the amino- and carboxy-terminal portions of each mature subunit. These cysteine-rich D repeats form large globular domains that are readily visible by molecular level electron microscopy (57). The A repeats, which contain relatively few cysteine residues, are located in an extended filamentous region in the central one-third of each subunit.

The ligand interaction sites in vWF have been localized to specific repeats in the vWF polypeptide. The vWF-A1 repeat, which extends from residues 449 to 728 of the mature vWF sub-

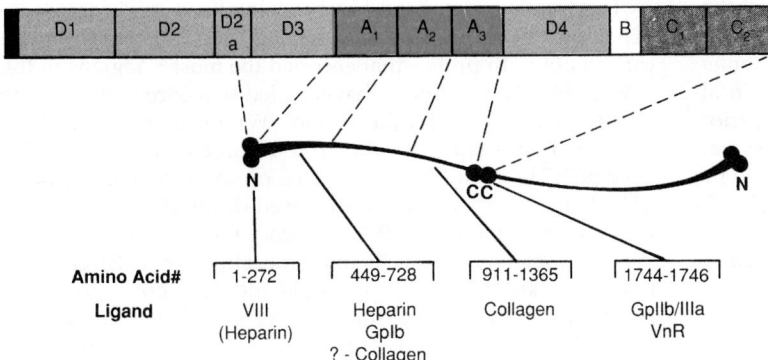

Figure 35-2. Organization of von Willebrand's factor (vWF) complementary deoxyribonucleic acid and subunit polypeptide. The vWF complementary deoxyribonucleic acid encodes a series of homologous repeats. The D repeats encode much of the propolypeptide and the globular amino- and carboxy-terminal domains of the mature vWF subunit polypeptide. The triplicated A domains encode a filamentous extended region in the central one-third of each subunit. The A1 and A3 domains contain ligand binding sites of vWF interactions with collagen and heparin, as depicted. The binding site for factor VIII is located at the amino terminal of each subunit, and the glycoprotein (gp) IIb/IIIa interaction site is located near the carboxy terminal.

unit, mediates vWF binding to the platelet glycoprotein (gp)–Ib/IX receptor (58,59), as well as to sulfated glycosaminoglycans, including heparin (60–62), and to sulfatides (63). Data that were derived from competitive inhibition binding studies with tryptic fragments of polymeric vWF and chemically synthesized peptides suggested, initially, that collagen binding sites were in the A1 and A3 repeats (64–67). More recent studies that used purified recombinant proteins that encode the A1 and A3 domains have shown that the principal collagen binding site in the mature vWF subunit is in the A3 domain between amino acids 911 and 1365 (68). The A2 repeat, which is made up of residues 729 to 910, has no known binding function, although, as is discussed in the following text, it contains a protease-sensitive region that is important in the pathogenesis of some forms of type IIA vWD. The factor VIII binding site of vWF has been localized to the amino terminal 272–amino acid residues of the mature vWF subunit. Although the sequence that spans residues Thr78 to Thr96 was originally proposed as the entire factor VIII binding site (69,70), subsequent experience with mutant

forms of vWF that cannot bind factor VIII suggests that additional sites are important for the regulation of factor VIII binding that occurs outside of this sequence.

The crystal structures of the vWF-A1 and -A3 repeats have recently been solved, and the three-dimensional structure of the domains is now known with some precision. The domains are made up of a series of short, alternating, α-helical and β-pleated sheet sequences that form a compact globular domain with a central cleft. The overall structure is similar to that previously reported in nucleotide binding proteins and in the inserted or I domain of the leukocyte integrin protein $\alpha_2\beta_1$ (71–74). The hydrophobic β sheets form the central core of each domain, and the charged α helices are aligned around the outside of the domain, as shown in Figure 35-3. Site-specific mutagenesis of critical residues, coupled with the accurate three-dimensional structure that is afforded by the crystal structure, have allowed the partial localization of the gpIb binding region of the vWF-A1 domain and the collagen interaction site of vWF-A3. It has also been possible to localize residues, which cause some of the variant forms of vWD

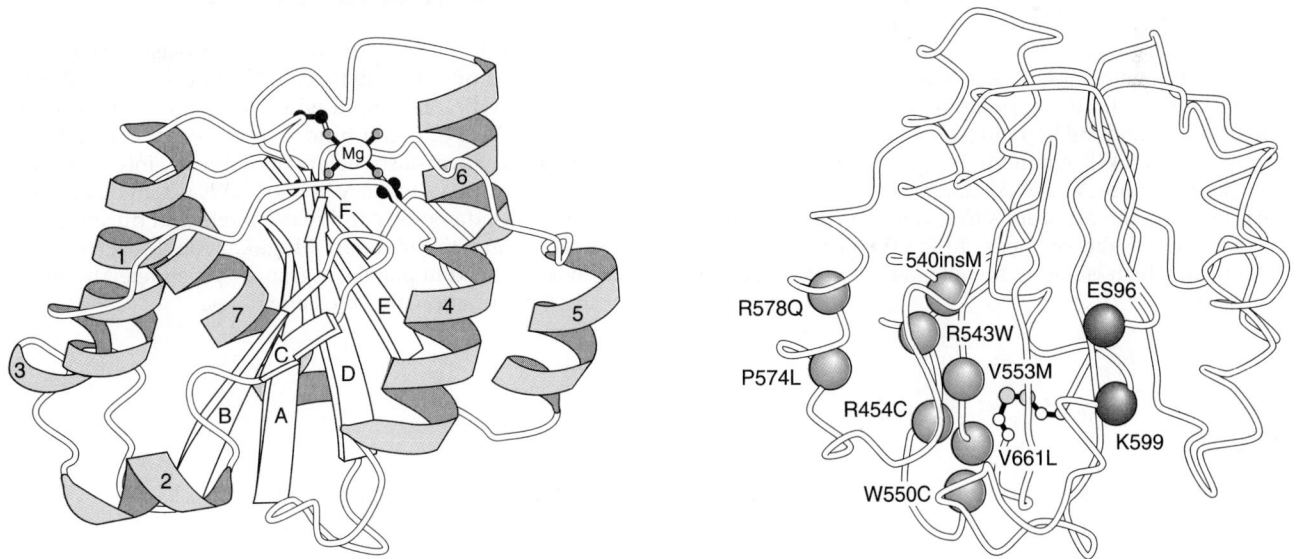

Figure 35-3. The overall structure of the von Willebrand's factor (vWF) A domains is shown in the left-hand panel, and the location of some of the mutations that cause types IIb and IIM von Willebrand's disease (vWD) are shown in the right-hand panel. The vWF A domains are made up of a series of alternating α helices (labeled 1–7) and β pleated sheets (labeled A–E). The charged hydrophilic α helices make up the outer surface of the domain, and the hydrophobic β sheets constitute the interior or core of the domain. Residues that are implicated in type IIb vWD are marked in blue, and two of the residues that are implicated in type IIM vWD are marked in gray. The type IIb and IIM mutations are distant from the glycoprotein Ib binding region of the domain, which is on the upper anterior face of the molecule. [From Sadler JE. vWF and platelet adhesion. *Blood* 2001;98(6):cover art, with permission. Copyright American Society of Hematology.]

when they are mutated, on the three-dimensional map of the vWF-A1 domain.

The gpIb interaction site has been localized to the upper anterior face of the vWF-A1 domain, whereas residues that are critical to the binding of vWF-A3 to collagen are located on the inferior face of the domain (75,76). By site-specific mutagenesis, several residues in α3β4 and α1β2 loops of vWF-A3 were found to be critical for their interaction with collagen. Residues H1023, R963, and R1016 were particularly critical. This interaction site is distinct from the collagen interaction site that has been defined in the cellular membrane integrin receptor $\alpha_2\beta_3$ (73,77,78).

The binding of factor VIII to vWF prevents its interaction with phospholipids (79). Infusion of vWF into patients with severe vWD results in a prolonged supranormal elevation of factor VIII levels (80), suggesting that vWF influences factor VIII biosynthesis or secretion (81). This contention is supported by more recent experiments that demonstrate that vWF promotes the association of the light and heavy chains of factor VIII (82,83) and enhances recombinant factor VIII production by transfected mammalian cells (84).

Two RGD consensus adhesion recognition sequences are in the primary pro-vWF transcript. The RGD sequence is present in a number of adhesive glycoproteins and mediates their binding to cellular integrin receptors (85). The importance of the RGD in the vWF propeptide is unclear. The second RGD sequence, at residues 1744 to 1746, is critically important for vWF binding to platelet gpIIb/IIIa (86,87). Monoclonal antibodies that recognize epitopes in this region, as well as high concentrations of the tetrapeptide RGDs, inhibit vWF binding to activated platelets (88,89). In addition, point mutations in the vWF RGD sequence selectively abolish vWF binding to platelet gpIIb/IIIa (90). Thus, each vWF subunit contains the information necessary to mediate all known vWF interactions. Despite the presence of functional binding sites in the vWF polypeptide subunit, the ability of vWF to mediate platelet adhesion depends on the assembly of multiple subunits into a large multimeric structure (91).

The vWF gene contains 52 exons that span 178 kilobases (kb) of DNA on chromosome 12 (92) (Fig. 35-4). The gene is so large that it encompasses 0.1% of the chromosome 12 DNA. Individual exons vary considerably in size, ranging from 40 base pairs to 1.4 kb. In general, little correlation exists between intron/exon boundaries and the homologous repeats that were previously noted in the vWF subunit polypeptide. Exon 28, the largest, encodes the entire A1 and A2 domains. This is of particular interest, because the mutations that cause types IIA and IIB vWD are located in this segment of the vWF gene. In contrast, the A3 repeat, which is highly homologous, is encoded by five separate exons.

The human vWF gene has been localized to chromosome 12p12-pter (93,94). The original gene localization studies were carried out with probes that encoded the most 5' regions of the vWF cDNA. When probes that encoded sequence in the middle of the cDNA were used, a second vWF locus was identified, which was subsequently shown to be an incomplete pseudogene (95). The pseudogene is located on chromosome 22q11.22–q11.23 and represents a nonprocessed duplication of exons 23 through 34 (96). It shares 97% sequence identity with the corresponding region of the authentic gene, although it also contains multiple translational stop signals and does not encode any protein product (97). The human vWF pseudogene appears to be of relatively recent origin, because it is not present in the genome of a number of other mammalian species (98,99). The presence of the pseudogene and the high degree of sequence identity between it and the authentic gene have complicated the analysis of vWF mutations, particularly in patients with type IIA and IIB vWD.

A large number of polymorphisms have been discovered in the vWD gene that have been used to study linkage between various vWD phenotypes and the vWF gene (100–110). In addition, a useful number-variable tandem repeat, with at least eight allelic forms, has been identified in intron 40 (111). The high degree of heterozygosity at this marker has made it informative in the study of families with various forms of vWD.

Little information is available on potential regulatory elements in the vWF gene. The translational start site has been mapped. Although there is a typical TATA box at position –30, no CCAAT or GC box elements have been described to date (92,99,112). The paucity of information regarding vWF promoter elements may be due to the difficulty of transfecting the two relevant cell types—endothelial cells and megakaryocytes.

BIOSYNTHESIS, STORAGE, AND SECRETION OF VON WILLEBRAND'S FACTOR

Although vWF is usually thought of as a plasma protein, four distinct pools of vWF exist. Endothelial cell–derived vWF is secreted into the plasma, in which it circulates in a complex with factor VIII and can bind to exposed subendothelium. Endothelial cells can also secrete vWF directly into subendothelium and contain a secretory pool of vWF, which is sequestered in Weibel-Palade bodies and may be released during primary and secondary hemostasis. Megakaryocyte-derived vWF, which is localized in platelet α granules, is secreted by platelets during the formation of hemostatic plugs.

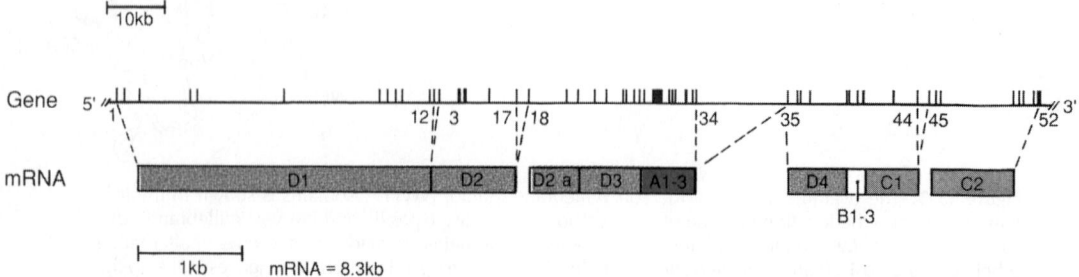

Figure 35-4. Organization of the von Willebrand's factor gene and its primary translation product. The gene is composed of 52 exons, which vary in size from 40 to 1400 base pairs. The single, large exon 28 encodes the entire A1 and A2 repeats and is the location of the mutations that cause type IIA and IIB von Willebrand's disease. The von Willebrand's factor gene is located on chromosome 12, and the incomplete pseudogene, which encompasses exons 23 to 34, is located on chromosome 22. kb, kilobase; mRNA, messenger RNA.

Endothelial Cells

vWF can be localized to endothelial cells within vascular tissue sections (113,114) and is readily detected in cultured endothelial cells (115–119). The ability to establish and passage endothelial cells in culture has permitted a detailed understanding of vWF biosynthesis (115,120). Although these processes have been chiefly characterized in human umbilical vein endothelial cells, more limited studies of endothelial cells that are derived from a number of adult vessels (121) and megakaryocytes (122) indicate that the umbilical vein is a representative model of vWF biosynthesis.

The precursor pro-vWF subunits first form covalently linked dimers in the endoplasmic reticulum through an unknown number of disulfide bonds in the COOH-terminal regions of adjacent subunits (123,124). The addition of high-mannose carbohydrate is required for dimerization of vWF, because inhibition of Asn-linked glycosylation by pretreatment with tunicamycin prevents dimer formation and subsequent secretion (125). The high-mannose carbohydrate is then processed to a more complex form in the Golgi apparatus, yielding an approximately 600-kd dimer. Each subunit has 12 Asn-linked glycosylation sites, all but one of which contains the consensus Asn-X-Thr/Ser sequence (38). A limited number of these Asn-linked oligosaccharides are also sulfated (126,127). Complex carbohydrate formation is apparently not critical for subsequent molecular processing, because inhibition of the Golgi enzyme mannosidase II by swainsonine does not prevent secretion of vWF (128). Ten O-linked glycosylation sites (eight threonine and two serine residues) are also present in the vWF sequence (38), and it may be presumed that these amino acids are glycosylated in the Golgi apparatus. Eight of these sites are clustered in the A1 domain, flanking a disulfide loop that is created by cysteines 509 and 695. Mature vWF contains 18.7% carbohydrate (129).

The formation of larger multimers from pro-vWF dimers begins in the *trans*-Golgi and is completed in secretory vesicles. In this process, dimeric units are linked in a head-to-head fashion through disulfide bonds, which are located within the D region (D3) of the NH_2 terminal to form expanding multimeric complexes (123,124). Strong evidence suggests that the vWF propeptide mediates N-terminal polymerization of dimers into multimers. First, a truncated form of recombinant vWF that lacks the propeptide sequence fails to form large multimers when it is expressed in heterologous cells (54,55). Multimerization is restored by the coexpression of the vWF propeptide, even when it is not expressed *cis* to the mature vWF subunit (55). This suggests that free propeptide may transiently link to the mature vWF subunit and provide proper alignment of adjacent pro-vWf dimers (130). Recent evidence suggests that the presence of vicinal cysteines in each of the D domains in the propolypeptide is also needed for proper multimer assembly (131). Cleavage of the 741–amino acid propolypeptide is one of the last steps in vWF biosynthesis, and the cleaved prosequence is co-localized and secreted along with mature vWF in platelets (132) and endothelial cells (133,134). In plasma, the propeptide circulates independently of vWF as a noncovalently linked homodimer of 100-kd subunits. Although it binds to collagen and inhibits platelet-collagen interactions, no specific biologic function has been ascribed to the circulating vWF propeptide (135,136).

STORAGE POOLS

Weibel-Palade Bodies. The endothelial cell vWF storage organelle is the Weibel-Palade body, a rod-shaped structure that is unique to endothelium. First described in large blood vessels, Weibel-Palade bodies have since been found in virtually all vascular and lymphatic endothelial cells (137). Their abundance appears to be proportional to the diameter of the blood vessel (138) and may be increased in neovascular tissue that surrounds certain tumors (139–141). In the electron microscope, Weibel-Palade bodies are 0.1 μm in diameter and up to 4 μm in length and are surrounded by a unit membrane. Within the organelle are longitudinally arranged tubules that are 150 Å in diameter and embedded in an electron-dense matrix. From electron microscopic studies, Weibel-Palade bodies appear to originate from the *trans*-Golgi apparatus and eventually distribute throughout the endothelial cytoplasm (142,143).

The presence of vWF within the Weibel-Palade body was first demonstrated by immunoelectron microscopy (116–119) and later confirmed by cell fractionation techniques (134,144). Fully processed vWF (subunit of 220 kd) and its propeptide (vW AgII) are the only secreted proteins that have been identified within the organelle so far (134,144,145). Sodium dodecyl sulfate (SDS)–agarose analysis of Weibel-Palade body vWF has shown that it consists of an unusually large size distribution of multimeric forms (134). The unique morphology of the Weibel-Palade body most likely is a result of the highly polymerized state of its principal secretory product. The precise conditions within the organelle that facilitate multimerization are not known, but high protein concentration (146) and acidic conditions (147) promote vWF polymerization *in vitro* and are likely to contribute to the process. This contention is supported by the finding that multimer formation is inhibited by weak bases, such as ammonium chloride or chloroquine, which disrupt the normally acidic conditions that are present within secretory organelles (125).

Clinical Relevance. Clinical evidence shows that a sizable portion of the body stores of vWF exists in a rapidly mobilized storage pool. This accounts for the rapid rise in plasma vWF levels after exercise (148) or the injection of agents, such as adrenalin (148), vasopressin, nicotinic acid, and a vasopressin analog, 1-deamino-8-D-arginine-vasopressin (DDAVP) (149). Vascular endothelium is thought to be the principal source of the increased plasma vWF that is observed under these conditions. vWF is also secreted by platelets that are stimulated by a variety of physiologic agonists, including thrombin, collagen, adenosine diphosphate, and epinephrine, although much of this protein remains associated with the platelet surface (150).

SECRETION

Endothelial cells, in culture, secrete vWF along constitutive and regulated pathways (151). The constitutive pathway is responsible for the basal secretion of smaller multimers. This pathway is directly linked to protein synthesis, because basal secretion can be blocked by cycloheximide, an inhibitor of protein synthesis (152). In contrast, secretion by the regulated pathway, which requires exogenous stimulation of the endothelium, results in the release of unusually large vWF multimers and is unaffected by cycloheximide. In cultured endothelial cells, 5% of newly synthesized vWF is targeted for the regulated pathway, whereas the remainder is constitutively secreted (153). The relative contribution of these two pathways to the plasma and subendothelial pools of vWF is unknown.

The basal rate of vWF secretion in cultured endothelial cells is regulated by genetic and extragenic factors. Endothelial cells that are cultured from the umbilical vein of neonates who are subsequently diagnosed with type I vWD endothelial cells constitutively secrete less vWF and contain less vWF messenger RNA (mRNA) than their normal counterparts (154–156). Harrison and McKee (157) demonstrated a significant increase in constitutive secretion of vWF in cultured endothelial cells in response to 17β-estradiol, a finding that mirrors the elevation of vWF plasma levels

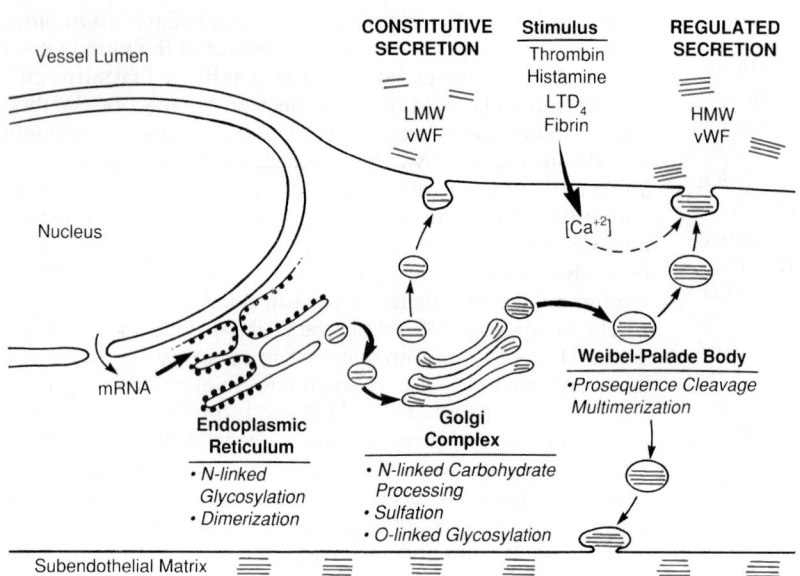

Figure 35-5. Biosynthesis and secretion of von Willebrand's factor (vWF) in endothelial cells (see text for details). This model is based principally on *in vitro* data, and the relative contributions of the constitutive and regulated pathway in the formation of the plasma vWF multimeric pattern are not known. HMW, high molecular weight; LMW, low molecular weight; LTD_4, leukotriene D_4; mRNA, messenger RNA.

that is observed in pregnancy and in response to oral contraceptive medications (158–160). Plasma vWF levels are also elevated during the course of bacterial, viral, and parasitic infections. It has been proposed that these acute, transient elevations are mediated by circulating mediators of the acute phase response, such as interleukin-1 and tumor necrosis factor (161). There have been conflicting reports on the effects of these cytokines on vWF secretion *in vitro* (162–166).

Cultured endothelial cells rapidly secrete vWF in response to a number of naturally occurring agonists, including thrombin (167,168), histamine (169), leukotriene D4 (170), platelet-activating factor, vascular permeability factor, fibrin (171,172), and the terminal components of complement (173) (Fig. 35-5). In contrast, vasopressin analogs such as DDAVP, which cause rapid and marked elevations of vWF *in vivo* (see the previous section, Clinical Relevance), do not directly stimulate vWF secretion in cultured endothelial cells (174,175). Rather, they appear to act independently by stimulating monocyte production of one or more endothelial cell agonists (176).

Elevation of $[Ca^{2+}]_i$ in response to agonist is thought to be the critical second messenger that regulates vWF secretion in endothelial cells (115,152,169,177–179). In contrast to that which occurs in platelets, elevation of intracellular cyclic adenosine monophosphate levels in endothelial cells does not inhibit thrombin- or calcium ionophore–induced vWF secretion (152).

After agonist stimulation, Weibel-Palade bodies are rapidly translocated to the cell surface (180). Fusion of organelle and plasma membranes occurs rapidly after agonist addition and is maximal within 10 minutes (173). Release of vWF within the granules takes longer, and release patches of vWF, which are noted by immunofluorescence, can persist for several hours (153,171). In contrast, vW AgII, which co-localizes with vWF in the Weibel-Palade body, does not remain associated with the cells after release (130). The association of vWF with the external surface of the endothelial cell may be mediated by the endothelial vitronectin receptor (181,182), the gpIb receptor (183,184), or a constituent of the Weibel-Palade body itself that has yet to be identified.

Plasma von Willebrand's Factor

ORIGIN AND PHYSICAL CHARACTERISTICS

The plasma concentration of vWF is approximately 10 μg/mL. Although vWF is synthesized in endothelial cells and megakaryocytes, clinical observations and animal models suggest that most of the plasma vWF is derived from vascular endothelial cells. First, patients with severe thrombocytopenia secondary to bone marrow failure (e.g., aplastic anemia, congenital amegakaryocytosis) have normal plasma vWF levels. Second, transplantation of normal bone marrow into a pig with severe vWD fails to elevate the plasma vWF levels, despite normalization of platelet vWF content (185).

One of the hallmarks of vWF is its propensity to form extremely large polymers (multimers) that are made up of integral numbers of dimeric units, each of which, in turn, contain two identical 220-kd subunits. A series of such multimers, which range in size from 450 to 20,000 kd, is normally found in plasma (186,187). The relative contribution of the constitutive and regulated pathways of endothelial cell secretion to the spectrum of plasma multimers remains controversial (153,188,189). Even under normal circumstances, a small fraction of subunits consists of uncleaved precursor or proteolytically degraded forms that give rise to satellite bands on high-resolution SDS-agarose gels.

Our understanding of the processing of vWF multimers has grown enormously with the discovery and characterization of a vWF cleaving protease that is present in plasma. The enzyme has been postulated to exist for some time, and bioassays were developed to measure its activity. Recently, however, the enzyme has been carefully defined by molecular genetic and biochemical techniques (190–192). The vWF cleaving protease is ADAMTS13, a member of a large family of metalloproteinases. ADAMTS13 cleaves a specific sequence in the vWF-A2 domain, which produces a distinct 176-kd polypeptide from the backbone 220-kd vWF subunit. The enzyme is present in plasma and is constitutively active. It appears to selectively cleave vWF that has been partially unfolded by shear stress or denaturing agents. It has been postulated that the ultra-HMW vWF forms that are secreted from endothelial cells are readily unfolded by shear stress and are then cleaved to produce the heterogeneous spectrum of multimers that is detected in plasma by SDS-agarose gel electrophoresis (Fig. 35-6).

The definitive proof of the importance of the enzyme in normal physiology is the observation that individuals who lack this enzyme have a TTP illness, the Upshaw-Schulman syndrome, which is characterized by recurrent episodes of thrombocytopenia and microangiopathic hemolytic anemia that can be aborted by infusion of normal plasma (192–196). In addition, patients with the more common acquired form of TTP have an inhibitor of

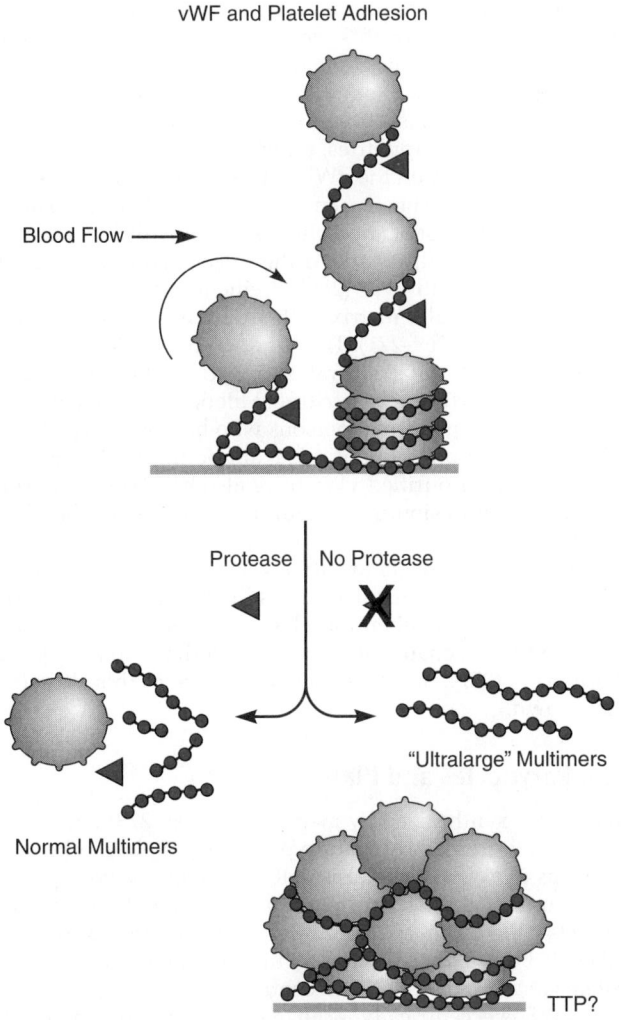

vWF and Platelet Adhesion

Blood Flow →

Protease | No Protease

"Ultralarge" Multimers

Normal Multimers

TTP?

Figure 35-6. The role of the von Willebrand's factor (vWF) cleaving protease (ADAMTS13) in normal physiology and in the pathogenesis of thrombotic thrombocytopenic purpura (TTP) is depicted here. Ordinarily, the enzyme cleaves ultra–high molecular weight (HMW) vWF into the spectrum of multimers that are present in plasma. These multimers do not bind to or agglutinate platelets. In the absence of the enzyme, ultra-HMW vWF persists in the circulation and spontaneously binds to and agglutinates platelets, thus causing the changes that are seen in TTP.

the ADAMTS13 vWF-cleaving activity. This explains why patients with TTP usually respond to a combination of plasmapheresis to reduce inhibitor titer and plasma infusion to raise the ADAMTS13 level in plasma.

The broader implications of the vWF regulatory system are just being explored, and we do not yet know whether changes in ADAMTS13 levels or activity result in thrombotic or hemorrhagic disorders. There are some intriguing preliminary reports that show that certain types of thromboembolism are associated with lowered vWF-cleaving protease activity. Also, there are studies that show that some patients with TTP have normal amounts of vWF-cleaving protease activity (197–200). The limitations of these studies are that they have relied on rather crude bioassays to measure activity. With the molecular cloning of ADAMTS13 and ascertainment of its primary structure, it may be possible to devise more precise assays. For example, with genetic tests, one could determine with precision whether heterozygosity for one of the known ADAMTS13 inactivating mutations increases the risk of thromboembolism. Finally, although we equate ADAMTS13 with vWF-cleaving

activity, we do not know whether the enzyme may have other proteolytic substrates and whether vWF multimers are its only cleavage products.

In plasma, vWF circulates in a noncovalent complex with factor VIII with a stoichiometry of approximately 50:1 (vWF to factor VIII) by weight. This association serves to stabilize plasma factor VIII activity that is otherwise lost because of proteolysis (2,201,202) and to facilitate factor VIII activation by thrombin (203).

EXTRAGENIC MODULATION OF PLASMA LEVELS

Influence of Blood Type. The influence of the ABO blood group locus on plasma levels of the factor VIII/vWF complex was first noted by Preston and Barr (204) and has been confirmed and extended in several subsequent studies. Blood group type O has been universally associated with lower factor VIII (205–209) and vWF (206–211) levels, although some disagreement exists on possible differences among individuals with the A, B, and AB blood group types. In one carefully performed study of 158 monozygotic and dizygotic twin pairs, Orstavik et al. (207) concluded that the effect on factor VIII was secondary to the effect on vWF and that 30% of the genetic variance of the level of vWF was due to the ABO blood type. Moreover, these investigators determined that the level of vWF varied inversely with the amount of plasma H substance, with the lowest levels in group O, intermediate levels in group A_2 and the highest levels in group A_1, B, and AB individuals. This conclusion was further supported by the finding that, among persons who belong to blood group O, patients who were found to be secretors (Lewis phenotype [Le(a–b+)]) and thus were known to have the highest levels of plasma H substance (212) also had the lowest levels of vWF and factor VIII (213).

The mechanism by which the ABO locus influences vWF levels is unknown. The association is clearly not the result of genetic linkage between ABO and vWF genes, because the gene for ABO is on chromosome 9 (214), whereas the gene for vWF is on chromosome 12 (39). Blood group antigens A, B, and H are present on vWF (215,216). It has been postulated that these oligosaccharide structures influence the biosynthesis, secretion, or catabolism of the protein. Because removal of terminal sialic acid residues from vWF oligosaccharides shortens the survival of the protein, the catabolism of the protein may be influenced by ABO-related carbohydrate moieties (215).

Age. Both factor VIII and vWF levels are moderately low in preterm infants and then rise above adult norms at term (217). The stress of the delivery itself may be at least partially responsible for the elevation of the factor VIII/vWF complex. For this reason, the diagnosis of vWD may be missed in the newborn period (218). Fetal and neonatal plasma contain unusually large vWF multimers that are similar to those that are found in endothelial Weibel-Palade bodies and platelet α granules (219–221). Among persons who are 10 to 70 years of age, plasma concentrations of factor VIII (205,207,222,223) and vWF (207) increase with age. Although Graham et al. (208) and Gill et al. (209) found the increase in vWF levels to be linear over the entire period that was studied, Jeremic et al. (205) noted that the increase was more marked in the later years. As is true for the effects of blood group antigens, the effect of age on factor VIII is due to its primary effect on vWF levels (207).

Hormonal Influences. Increased levels of vWF have been reported in healthy pregnant women and women who are taking oral contraceptives (160,224,225). Similar findings have been reported in most (158,159,226–229) but not all (226,230) patients with vWD. vWF levels rise incrementally throughout pregnancy and, in type I vWD patients, often reach normal levels at term (229). This spontaneous correction in vWF during pregnancy obviates the need for specific therapy in the normal delivery of most patients, although postpartum hemorrhage may occur owing to the rapid fall of vWF and factor VIII levels that follows delivery (226,228,231). Pregnancy-associated increases in plasma levels of abnormal vWF with hyperaffinity to platelets in patients with type IIB vWD may lead to profound thrombocytopenia (232,233).

Thyroid hormone also influences vWF levels (234), and hypothyroidism may induce mild acquired vWD with clinical bleeding (235–238). In all reported cases, plasma vWF returned to normal after correction of the hormonal deficiency. Moreover, hyperthyroidism and the administration of thyroxine to euthyroid subjects increase vWF levels (234,239). The mechanism by which thyroid hormone controls vWF plasma levels is not known but has been postulated to result from nonspecific effects on mRNA and protein synthesis (236).

Physical Activity. A rapid increase in plasma factor VIII activity after exercise was first noted by Rizza (240) and was confirmed later in a number of independent studies (241,242). Exercise also induces a rapid but slightly smaller increase in plasma vWF:Ag and vWF:ristocetin cofactor (RCoF) activity (242–245). It is not known whether the disproportionate increase in factor VIII activity is due to preferential release of factor VIII from a separate storage site, enhancement of factor VIII activity (243), or an increase in factor VIII binding to vWF after exercise. Prior treatment with the calcium channel blocker verapamil (but not nicardipine) blunts the rise in exercise-induced vWF:Ag release (246).

EXTRACELLULAR MATRIX

The vWF that is present in vascular subendothelium is predominantly derived from the overlying endothelial cell layer (247,248). vWF binds to the subendothelium in an unsaturable manner that does not require calcium (249,250). Binding is principally to types I, III, and VI collagen (251–255), although binding to fibronectin (256) and heparin (257) may also be important. vWF can bind to fibrillar and nonfibrillar type III collagen, whereas nonfibrillar type I collagen binds vWF poorly (253). All three chains of type VI collagen, which is abundant in extracellular matrices (258), contain regions that are homologous to the vWF A domains and to platelet gpIb, which could play a role in binding (259). The binding of vWF to immobilized collagen fibrils is saturable and reversible and is of moderately high affinity (260).

vWF in the extracellular cellular matrix consists of extremely HMW multimers that contain fully processed 225-kd subunits (261). Although HMW forms of vWF bind most avidly to subendothelium (254,262,263), lower-molecular-weight forms of vWF are also capable of supporting platelet adhesion (264).

The role of subendothelial matrix–vWF interactions in primary hemostasis has been inferred, chiefly from perfusion experiments. In 1973, Baumgartner (15) described a technique that was performed with blood in which an annular device with a central core contained an everted segment of rabbit aorta that had been previously denuded of endothelial cells by balloon catheterization. Experiments have used everted segments of human renal or umbilical artery (249,265). Blood is passed over the vessel segments under controlled conditions of temperature and flow, permitting detailed rheologic analysis (266,267). After perfusion, the number of platelets bound or bound to and spread on the subendothelial surface, as well as any platelet

thrombi, can be determined by using standard histologic methods. A modification of this technique permits perfusion of unanticoagulated venous blood (268).

In these perfusion models, which are performed at high shear rates that correspond to those that are encountered in small arteries and capillaries, platelet–subendothelial matrix interactions depend on the vWF that is bound to the subendothelial matrix (268). Thus, when plasma vWF is bound to subendothelium, and the subendothelium subsequently is exposed to reconstituted blood, platelet adherence correlates with the amount of prebound vWF (249). Preincubation of vessel segments or extracellular matrix with antibodies to vWF reduces platelet adhesion (269–271). The adhesion of platelets to subendothelium at arterial shear rates (500 to 1000 per second) is reduced after perfusion with citrated blood from patients with vWD (272) or from normal persons who had been depleted of vWF by adsorption with anti-vWF antibodies (273). Immobilized fractions of purified vWF have also been shown to support platelet adhesion in parallel plate perfusion chambers (274–276).

Adhesion of platelets to native vWF occurs only when the vWF is bound to a surface. It has been proposed that the binding of vWF to subendothelial proteins or to other substrates induces a change in confirmation that supports platelet adhesion (277), but the molecular nature of this alteration is unknown.

Megakaryocytes and Platelets

vWF is also synthesized by megakaryocytes (278) and stored within the α granules of mature platelets (279–284). The complex steps of vWF biosynthesis in the megakaryocyte appear to be similar to those that were previously noted in the endothelial cells (114). Platelet α granules are membrane-limited spherical bodies (0.3 to 0.5 μm in diameter) that contain numerous other proteins in addition to vWF. In contrast to other α-granule proteins, vWF is eccentrically localized within the organelle and forms tubular structures that are reminiscent of those seen in Weibel-Palade bodies (285). Many α-granule constituent proteins are not synthesized by the megakaryocyte or the platelet but enter the megakaryocyte endocytosis and are then transported to the α granule (286). Although megakaryocytes synthesize vWF in culture (278), the possibility that some fraction of the platelet-associated vWF might be derived from the plasma pool cannot be excluded.

Platelet vWF content is between 0.25 and 0.80 U/10⁹ platelets, as measured by electroimmunoassay (EIA) and immunoradiometric assay (IRMA), and accounts for approximately 20% of the blood pool of vWF (28,287,288). Platelet-associated vWF, like the Weibel-Palade body pool of endothelial cell vWF, contains an increased proportion of large multimeric species and an increased ratio of vWF:RCoF activity to vWF:Ag, when compared to that contained in plasma (288,289). On stimulation, vWF is secreted along with the other granule contents. Approximately 65% of the α-granule pool of vWF remains associated with the platelet (150,289–291).

The physiologic relevance of platelet vWF is underscored by a number of clinical and experimental observations. First, the prolonged bleeding time in subsets of patients with type I vWD can be best correlated with the amount of platelet-associated vWF (292,293). Second, when they are resuspended in normal plasma, platelets that are obtained from type III vWD patients adhere less well to collagen fibrils or rabbit subendothelium than do normal platelets (294,295). Third, patients with severe vWD who are treated with normal platelets and cryoprecipitate have a more pronounced shortening of the bleeding time than patients who are treated with cryoprecipitate alone (296).

Heterologous Expression

Although vWF biosynthesis is normally restricted to endothelial cells and megakaryocytes, vWF cDNA can be transfected into a variety of heterologous cells to produce functional vWF multimers. The original transfections were carried out in COS and CHO cells but have been extended to a variety of other cultured cell lines (44,54,131,297–300). In each case, vWF multimers are constitutively secreted into the conditioned medium. In contrast, in endothelial cells and megakaryocytes, much or all of the vWF is packaged into secretory organelles like the Weibel-Palade body and the α granule. Packaging of vWF for secretion has also been achieved in a heterologous cell model. The transfection of vWF cDNA into AtT20 cells, a pituitary cell line that secretes adrenocorticotropic hormone, results in the assembly and packaging of vWF multimers in granules (297,300). These studies suggest that all the information that is needed for the assembly of multimeric vWF and its sorting into granules is derived from its primary sequence. In addition, they suggest that the tissue-specific expression is regulated by *cis* and *trans* regulatory elements in the vWF promoter region.

CLINICAL DESCRIPTION

Presentation

Most patients with vWD have clinical symptoms that are consistent with a primary hemostatic defect. Mucocutaneous bleeding, including epistaxis, easy bruising, and gingival bleeding, was reported in 35% to 60% of patients who were observed in two large studies (24,301). Menorrhagia, often severe, is reported in approximately one-third of women with vWD. Postsurgical bleeding, especially after dental extraction or tonsillectomy, is common and is often the event that leads to the initial diagnosis. Gastrointestinal bleeding, sometimes associated with colonic angiodysplasia or telangiectasia, is seen in approximately 10% of patients. Hemarthroses and muscle bleeding are decidedly rare, except in severely affected patients with factor VIII levels of less than 5%.

Prevalence

Generally, vWD is claimed to be the most common inherited bleeding disorder. Previously cited incidences of between 4 and 7 per population of 100,000 are likely to be underestimates (302,303). In an epidemiologic investigation of more than 1200 schoolchildren in northern Italy, vWD, as defined by a low vWF level in combination with a family history of low vWF levels or a personal or family history of clinically significant bleeding, was diagnosed in 1% of the children who were studied (304). The incidence of severe type III vWD varies from 0.11 to 0.55 per one million persons in most of Europe to approximately 3.1 per one million persons in Sweden and 5.3 per one million persons in Israel (305–307). Overall, mild type I vWD accounts for 75% to 80% of all cases, with the remainder of cases classified principally to one of the type II varieties (308,309).

LABORATORY EVALUATION

In severe cases with unequivocal quantitative or qualitative vWF abnormalities, the diagnosis of vWD is straightforward. In contrast, the diagnosis in mild cases can be problematic. The bleeding time, factor VIII, and vWF:Ag and vWF:RCoF activity have become the standard screening tests for vWD. Based on these conventional laboratory tests, it has been estimated that the penetrance of the vWD genotype varies from 60% to 90% (310,311). Yet, in a study of affected persons from two extended families, only 15% had abnormal results on all four tests, and 50% of patients who carry a vWD allele by pedigree analysis had only one abnormal test result (310,311). Thus, the sensitivity and specificity of laboratory tests for the vWD phenotype are lower than those observed in other common disorders. In light of the pronounced intraindividual variability of different hemostatic variables, most clinicians recommend repeated testing of a person who is at risk, before excluding the diagnosis of vWD (312,313). Although the use of discriminant analysis improves the diagnosis of the heterozygous vWD phenotype, this approach is not commonly used (311).

Bleeding Time

Bleeding time is regarded by many clinicians as the most reliable *in vivo* indicator of primary hemostatic function. Although, when carefully analyzed, measurement of bleeding time is not generally useful for the preoperative screening of patients without a personal or family bleeding history (314–316), bleeding time remains an important tool in the diagnosis of vWD. The method of Duke (which dates to 1910), which measures the duration of bleeding from small incisions in the ear lobe, was the technique used in the earliest descriptions of vWD (317). This method is relatively insensitive and difficult to quantitate and may induce uncontrollable hemorrhage and hematomas in patients with severe vWD.

In most hospitals, bleeding times are performed using a modification (318,319) of the Ivy technique (320). This involves making an incision on the volar aspect of the forearm, while venous pressure is maintained at 40 mm Hg with a blood pressure cuff. Tests based on Ivy methodology are more sensitive than those that are based on the older Duke ear lobe method for detection of vWD (321,322). Tests for bleeding time remain difficult to standardize, are notoriously dependent on the experience of the person administering the test, and may be produce normal results in a large percentage of mildly affected patients (310,311,323,324). It had been suggested that the sensitivity of bleeding time for the diagnosis of vWD could be increased by first treating patients with low doses of aspirin (325,326). A third technique, which involves the puncture of the tip of a finger with a surgical blade, was shown to be as sensitive as the Ivy method (327). Although this method enjoys the advantage of not producing a scar at the site of incision, it is not widely used.

Despite these limitations, the judicious use of the bleeding time in patients with an established diagnosis of vWD provides some measure of the severity of the bleeding diathesis. Similarly, the bleeding time can be used, in certain circumstances, to help to judge the effectiveness of treatment.

Factor VIII

As discussed, factor VIII biosynthesis, secretion, and plasma stability are regulated by vWF. Thus, a diminution of plasma vWF:Ag levels is usually accompanied by a parallel reduction in factor VIII (308). However, reduction of factor VIII is not a universal finding in mild vWD, and increased factor VIII to vWF:Ag ratios are not uncommon (324,328). Because factor VIII levels are only moderately reduced in most forms of vWD, the activated partial thromboplastin time may remain in the normal range. Thus, a normal activated partial thromboplastin time does not exclude the diagnosis of vWD.

In Vitro Assays of von Willebrand's Factor

IMMUNOLOGIC MEASUREMENTS

Immunologic measurements of vWF (vWF:Ag) may be performed by EIA (28), IRMA (329–333), or enzyme-linked immunosorbent assay (ELISA) (334–337). In EIA (30), plasma samples undergo electrophoresis through agarose gels that contain polyspecific anti-vWF antibodies. The resulting precipitin line appears as a rocket, whose height depends on the concentration of vWF that is present in the original plasma sample. Increased sensitivity can be achieved by using radiolabeled anti-vWF antibodies in the agarose gel (338). IRMA and ELISA of vWF offer greater sensitivity. Important methodologic differences exist between EIA, which measures the number of vWF molecules, and IRMA and ELISA, which measure the number of antigenic sites on vWF. Thus, vWF:Ag levels appear higher in vWD subtypes with a reduced concentration of large multimers when they are measured by EIA than when they are analyzed by IRMA or ELISA methods. This discrepancy is often so pronounced that it has been suggested as a means of identifying subtypes of vWD that lack the HMW vWF multimers in the plasma (339).

MULTIMERIC ANALYSIS

Crossed Immunoelectrophoresis. One of the earliest methods that was devised to analyze the multimeric composition of vWF was crossed immunoelectrophoresis. vWF multimers are first separated by electrophoresis in agarose and then are subjected to immunoelectrophoresis in a second direction through agarose that contains anti-vWF antibodies. The resultant precipitin line reflects the partial separation of vWF multimers in the first dimension. Thus, samples that are deficient in the multimers with the highest molecular weights, like those found in the plasma of patients with type II vWD, lack the most cathodal portion of the normal protein arc.

Sodium Dodecyl Sulfate–Agarose Electrophoresis. More recently, electrophoretic methods have been developed that more clearly separate each of the many multimeric forms of vWF. In this method, vWF multimers are separated on agarose gels in the presence of SDS. Resolution in the regions of the multimeric spectrum with the highest or lowest molecular weights can be optimized by varying the concentration and gelling characteristics of the agarose and the length of the gel (187,287,340). The multimers are then visualized by incubation of the gel with ^{125}I-labeled (287) or enzyme-linked antibodies (341) to vWF. Alternatively, the separated multimers of vWF

may be transferred to nitrocellulose and detected with one of several enzyme-linked antibody systems (342–346). Each of these electrophoretic methods permits a direct and clear comparison among several samples in a single run and has provided potentially important insights into the molecular basis of the abnormalities that underlie type II vWD. For example, in the regions of the gel with the lowest molecular weight, high-resolution SDS-agarose electrophoresis has demonstrated that each multimeric band is actually composed of a predominant species that is accompanied by two to four satellite components with slightly different electrophoretic mobilities (187,347). The satellite components are thought to represent proteolytic fragments of the predominant species. Several of the type II vWD subtypes (see the section Type II Variants) have been defined, based on differences in the electrophoretic patterns that are produced by these fragments. Typical electrophoretic patterns are shown in Figures 35-7 through 35-10.

Functional Assays of von Willebrand's Factor

BACKGROUND

Early studies by von Willebrand and Juergens (12) demonstrated that, in contrast to platelets that were derived from normal persons or from patients with classic hemophilia, platelets from patients with vWD did not agglutinate normally in a capillary thrombometer. A number of laboratory techniques are available to demonstrate abnormal vWF-platelet interactions in vWD. Perhaps the most relevant are those that analyze platelet–subendothelial matrix interactions under defined conditions of temperature and flow rate (272). Although such studies have provided valuable insights into vWF physiology, they require highly sophisticated equipment and are technically difficult to perform. Similarly, assays that are based on the retention of platelets on glass beads (13,348,349) are sensitive indicators of vWF dysfunction, even when other laboratory tests are equivocal (24). Some investigators have found this test inconsistent and nonspecific, and it is rarely used today (350). In contrast, assays that are based on the interaction of the antibiotic ristocetin with vWF and platelets are relatively simple to perform and have become the predominant clinical laboratory test of vWF function.

RISTOCETIN-BASED ASSAYS

Ristocetin is an antibiotic that is isolated from *Nocardia lurida*, which has a molecular structure and spectrum of activity that are similar to those of vancomycin. It was withdrawn soon after its introduction in the 1950s, because it caused thrombocytope-

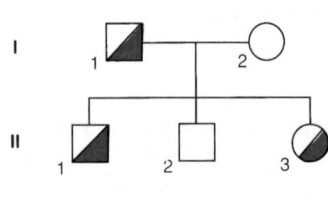

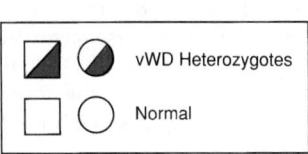

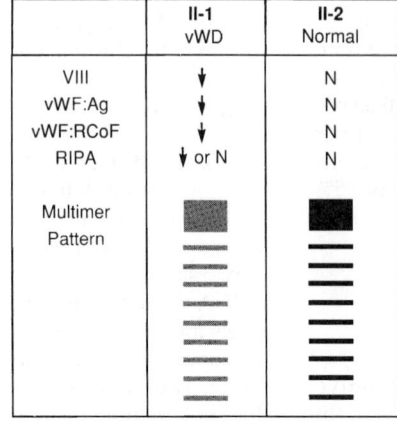

Figure 35-7. Inheritance and laboratory abnormalities in type I von Willebrand's disease (vWD). Typically, there is a proportional decrease (↓) in factor VIII, von Willebrand's factor antigen (vWF:Ag), and vWF–ristocetin cofactor (RCoF) activity. Ristocetin-induced platelet aggregation (RIPA) is most often normal (N). All multimeric forms are present, albeit in reduced abundance. Incomplete penetrance of the vWD phenotype is common, and direct linkage of type I vWD to the vWF gene has been established in only a few pedigrees.

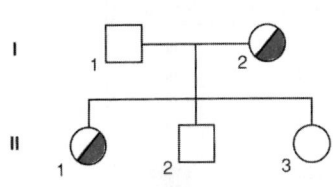

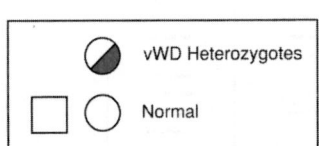

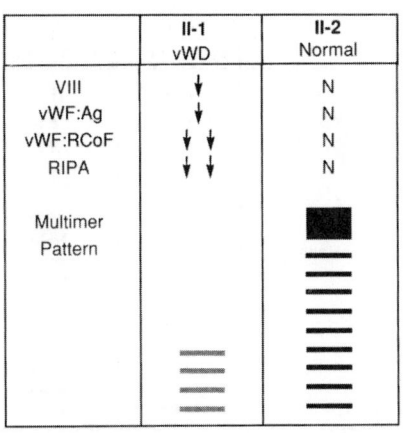

Figure 35-8. Inheritance pattern and expected laboratory abnormalities in type IIA von Willebrand's disease (vWD). A disproportionate reduction in von Willebrand's factor (vWF)–ristocetin cofactor (RCoF) activity is typical, and vWF antigen (Ag) and factor VIII levels may be in the low (↓) to normal (N) range. Large- and intermediate-sized multimers are absent in the plasma but may be present in the platelet. Similar laboratory abnormalities are seen in other forms of type II vWD and can be distinguished only by high-resolution agarose gel electrophoretic patterns. RIPA, ristocetin-induced platelet aggregation.

nia and macroscopic aggregation of platelets *in vitro* (32). The link between this deleterious side effect and vWF was made by Howard and Firkin (31), who observed that ristocetin induced platelet aggregation in platelet-rich plasma from normal persons but not in that from vWD patients.

The molecular basis of the ristocetin-mediated binding of vWF to the platelets has been partially elucidated. Ristocetin-induced platelet aggregation (RIPA) is known to be mediated by the passive binding of vWF to platelet gpIb/IX and subsequent platelet activation through a poorly defined signal transduction pathway (351,352). The essential role of gpIb/IX in the process is demonstrated by the fact that ristocetin fails to induce the aggregation of platelets from patients with Bernard-Soulier syndrome, who lack the gpIb/IX receptor complex (33,353,354). Platelets that are treated with proteolytic enzymes that partially degrade gpIb and platelets that have been treated with monoclonal antibodies to gpIb do not agglutinate with ristocetin (355,356). Although, in the presence of vWF, appropriate concentrations of ristocetin can induce metabolically active platelets to aggregate with activation of the gpIIb/IIIa receptor, the binding of vWF to gpIb/IX and the initial wave of agglutination constitute a passive process and occur even with formalin-fixed platelets.

The mechanism by which ristocetin induces vWF-mediated platelet agglutination is complex and incompletely understood. Ristocetin binds to platelets and reduces their electrostatic surface charge, which could promote the binding of vWF to gpIb/IX (357). Other cationic compounds, such as Polybrene, can also promote vWF-dependent platelet agglutination (358–360). Ristocetin can also bind to vWF and may reduce its net negative charge and alter its confirmation. Similarly, modified vWF, in which negatively charged sialic acid residues have been enzy-

matically removed (asialo vWF), induces platelet aggregation in the absence of ristocetin (361–363).

Evidence also exists that ristocetin-mediated platelet agglutination depends most heavily on the largest multimeric forms of vWF. First, ristocetin-mediated platelet agglutination is diminished out of proportion to vWF:Ag in those vWD subtypes in which HMW vWF multimers are missing (287,364,365). Second, pools of HMW vWF show enhanced binding to gpIb/IX and increased ristocetin-dependent platelet agglutination (34,366,367). Whether the requirement of HMW forms of vWF for optimal ristocetin-dependent platelet-vWF interactions is related to the increased number of potential platelet receptor binding sites or simply to an increase in the size of the vWF molecule is unknown.

RISTOCETIN-INDUCED PLATELET AGGREGATION

In the RIPA assay, final concentrations of 0.3 to 1.2 mg/mL of ristocetin are added to platelet-rich plasma in an aggregometer. Despite attempts to make the test semiquantitative by careful titration of pH and standardization of mixing conditions, the test remains qualitative (368). Most clinical laboratories simply report the minimum concentration of ristocetin that is capable of inducing a preestablished degree of aggregation, usually a 30% increase in light transmission. The RIPA test is relatively insensitive, is not abnormal until the vWF:Ag level falls to less than 30%, and thus fails to detect many patients with mild to moderate vWD (33,369). The RIPA test is easy to perform in conjunction with other platelet aggregation studies and is essential to the diagnosis of those vWD variants with enhanced responsiveness to ristocetin, such as type I (*New York*) (370), type IIB (371), and pseudo-vWD (372). Patients whose defects

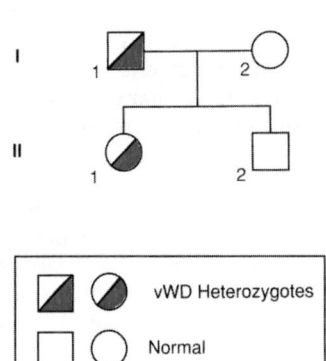

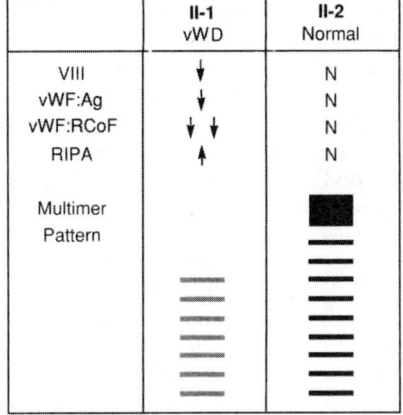

Figure 35-9. Inheritance pattern and laboratory abnormalities in type IIB von Willebrand's disease (vWD). Hypersensitivity to ristocetin in the ristocetin-induced platelet aggregation (RIPA) assay is diagnostic of this (or a related) subtype. The largest multimer species are typically lacking in plasma but are present in the platelet pool. ↓, decrease; ↑, increase; Ag, antigen; N, normal; RCoF, ristocetin cofactor; vWF, von Willebrand's factor.

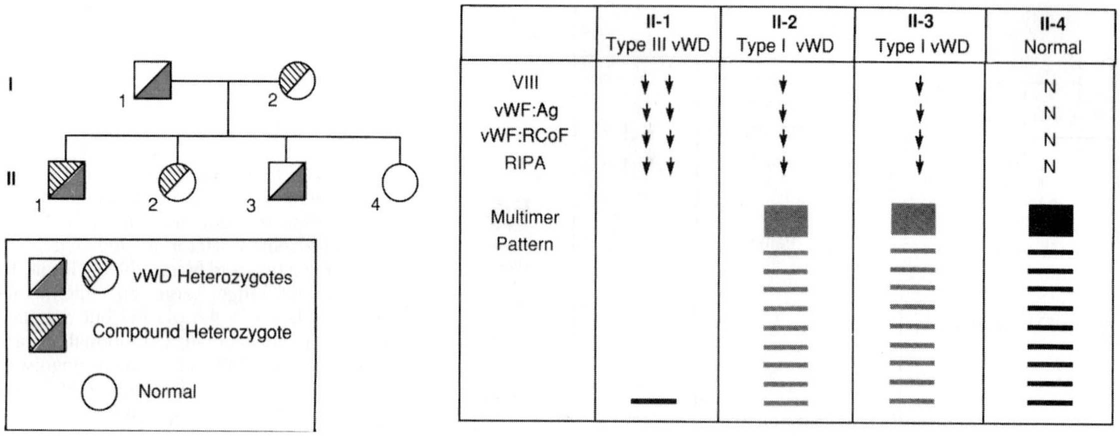

Figure 35-10. The inheritance pattern and expected laboratory abnormalities in type III von Willebrand's disease (vWD). Typically, von Willebrand's factor antigen (vWF:Ag) and vWF ristocetin cofactor (RCoF) are undetectable, and factor VIII levels are measurable but low (↓) (less than 5 U/dL) in type III vWD patients. Obligate heterozygotes often appear as type I vWD patients but are sometimes clinically normal (N) and may even exhibit normal laboratory parameters. RIPA, ristocetin-induced platelet aggregation.

reside in the vWF molecule (e.g., vWD type IIB) can also be distinguished from those with abnormal platelets (pseudo-vWD) by comparing the response of washed normal platelets in the presence of patient plasma to that of washed patient platelets in the presence of normal plasma.

RISTOCETIN COFACTOR ACTIVITY

RCoF activity assays are designed to obtain information about the function of the plasma vWF. Dilutions of patient plasma are tested for their ability to induce the agglutination of washed normal platelets (25) or paraformaldehyde fixed platelets (351) in the presence of a fixed concentration of ristocetin (usually 1 mg/mL). The availability of lyophilized fixed platelets has allowed standardization among clinical laboratories (373). The vWF:RCoF activity can be quantified by measuring the maximal rate of agglutination or the time to visible agglutination (374). In type I vWD, the reduction in vWF:RCoF activity parallels that of vWF:Ag. In many of the subtypes in which HMW multimers are absent or reduced in the plasma, vWF:RCoF activity may be decreased disproportionately. This test correlates moderately well with the bleeding time and clinical bleeding (25,308,375).

PLATELET RETENTION ON GLASS BEADS

In the assay of platelet retention on glass beads, citrated blood is passed over a column of glass beads, and the difference between the afferent and efferent platelet count is recorded to calculate platelet adhesiveness or retention (13,348,349,376). Net retention on the column is dependent on initial adhesion of platelets to the beads, which is largely dependent on fibrinogen, and subsequent platelet–platelet interactions and aggregate formation, which are dependent on vWF and released adenosine diphosphate. A number of important variables that can affect the assay have been identified, including the presence or absence of red cells, the temperature, the contact time of blood with the glass beads, the type of anticoagulant, and the type of plastic used in the column (377). The assay is technically difficult and has been supplanted by the ristocetin-based tests.

COLLAGEN-BASED ADHESION ASSAYS

As described previously, ristocetin-induced platelet agglutination and RCoF activity have achieved wide acceptance as surrogate tests for vWF-mediated platelet adhesion. An alternative

test that examines the collagen binding activity of vWF, a function that is mediated largely by sequences in the vWF-A3 domain, has been proposed to be a superior clinical test. Although not yet widely adapted, it is available commercially and may be adopted in the future by clinical laboratories. The collagen binding assays (378–381) have been compared to ristocetin-based assays, and there are some promising results as well as some technical difficulties. For example, there is evidence that a collagen binding assay might be superior to conventional assays in the detection of various forms of type II vWD (types IIA, IIb, and IIM). There are technical issues relating to the sources and concentration of collagen that are used in the assays that need to be worked out before the tests gain full acceptance, but the tests are interesting and promising.

CLASSIFICATION

More than 20 distinct variants of vWD have been described (382). Although a complete classification of vWD requires a fuller understanding of the molecular basis of the disease, it has been possible to establish a working classification system that is based on clinical and laboratory criteria. As in other genetic disorders, the present classification first seeks to differentiate between quantitative and qualitative abnormalities (Table 35-1).

Quantitative Disorders of von Willebrand's Factor

The quantitative group includes subtypes with a reduction in plasma vWF but, with few exceptions, no obvious abnormalities in vWF structure or function. This group may be broadly divided on the basis of vWF:Ag levels into mild (5 to 35 U/dL) and severe (less than 5 U/dL) categories. Characteristically, there is a concordant reduction of vWF:Ag levels, vWF:RCoF activity, and factor VIII levels.

TYPE I

Mild or type I vWD accounts for 60% to 70% of all cases of vWD (365,383). Affected patients manifest highly variable clinical symptoms, but the bleeding diathesis is rarely life-threatening. Characteristically, there is a concordant reduction of vWF:Ag, vWF:RCoF activity, and factor VIII levels (Fig. 35-7). A full range of vWF multimers is exhibited on SDS-agarose gels,

TABLE 35-1. Summary of Inherited von Willebrand's Disease (vWD) Phenotypes

Subtype	Clinical Features	Mode of Inheritance	Laboratory Diagnosis	Comments
Quantitative				
Type I (classic)	Mild to moderate bleeding	Autosomal dominant (incomplete penetrance ≈60%)	Concordant reduction of plasma vWF:Ag, vWF:RCoF, factor VIII (5–40 U/dL)	Subtypes may be defined based on analysis of platelet vWF; represents 60–70% of all vWD
Type III	Moderate to severe bleeding, including mucosal and deep tissues	Autosomal recessive (usually compound heterozygotes)	Marked reduction in vWF:Ag, vWF:RCoF, and factor VIII (<5 U/dL)	—
Qualitative				
Diminished RIPA activity				
Type I variants	Mild to moderate bleeding	Autosomal dominant	Plasma studies are similar to type I but with decreased vWF:RCoF to vWF:Ag ratio; all multimers are present; relative abundance of high-molecular-weight multimers may be abnormal; abnormal satellite subbands may be present	Subtypes include type IB ("platelet discordant") and IC; patients often exhibit a poor response to DDAVP
Type IIA	Mild to moderate bleeding	Autosomal dominant	Variable reduction in vWF:Ag and factor VIII; marked reduction in vWF:RCoF; large- and intermediate-sized multimers are absent; prominent satellite bands	Subdivision is possible, based on *in vitro* studies; large multimers may be present in the platelet
Type IIC	Mild to moderate bleeding	Autosomal recessive	Similar to type IIa, except satellite bands are absent	May represent compound heterozygotes
Type IID-1	Mild to moderate bleeding	Autosomal dominant	Similar to type IIA, but with unique electrophoretic patterns on high-resolution gels	Type IID is described in several independent pedigrees; other subtypes represent single families
Type II *Buffalo*				
Type B				
Enhanced RIPA activity				
Type I *New York* and other variants	Mild to moderate bleeding	Autosomal dominant	Similar to type I (classic), but with increased sensitivity to ristocetin in RIPA	Described in three pedigrees
Type IIB and other variants	Mild to moderate bleeding	Autosomal dominant, with a few exceptions	Plasma studies are similar to type IIA; hypersensitivity in RIPA (aggregation at ristocetin ≤0.5 mg/mL); high-molecular-weight multimers are absent in the plasma; all multimers are present in the platelet	Patients usually exhibit mild to moderate thrombocytopenia that is exacerbated by stresses, such as pregnancy or surgery
Platelet-type vWD (pseudo-vWD)	Mild to moderate bleeding	Autosomal dominant	Similar to type IIB	Defect lies within the platelet glycoprotein Ib receptor; laboratory differentiation from type IIB by mixing studies with normal platelets and plasma
Other				
Factor VIII binding defects	Variable bleeding of the hemophilic type	Autosomal recessive (heterozygotes may be mildly affected)	Marked reduction in factor VIII to vWF:Ag ratio	Distinguished from mild hemophilia A by specialized binding studies and mode of inheritance

Ag, antigen; DDAVP, 1-deamino-8-D-arginine-vasopressin; RCoF, ristocetin cofactor; RIPA, ristocetin-induced platelet aggregation; vWF, von Willebrand's factor.

although the intensities of high-, intermediate-, and low-molecular-weight forms may not always be normal.

The molecular basis of most forms of type I vWD has not been elucidated. Perhaps most perplexing is the fact that the phenotypic expression of the severe vWD genotype is variable. Thus, gene deletions or nonsense mutations, when present in the homozygous form, markedly reduce vWF levels and cause severe clinical disease and may produce mild bleeding, modest laboratory abnormalities, or a totally normal phenotype in heterozygotes (95,305,384–386). This variability in the phenotypic expression in heterozygotes is probably due to the influences of factors that are intrinsic to the vWD gene and to a variety of extragenic influences that may affect the biosynthesis, intracellular storage, and secretion of vWF. Many patients with autosomal-dominant type I vWD are likely to carry alleles that

function in a dominant-negative manner and interfere with the expression of the normal vWF allele (43).

Platelet-Associated von Willebrand's Factor. Patients with type I vWD can be subdivided on the basis of the platelet vWF content. By comparing platelet and plasma vWF levels, Weiss et al. (339) identified three distinct vWD subgroups. In patients who were classified as having type I-1, a parallel reduction was found in plasma and platelet vWF:Ag content. In contrast, five unrelated patients who were classified as having type I-2 had moderately decreased plasma vWF levels (33 to 57 U/dL) but normal levels of platelet vWF (58 to 130 U/dL). Finally, two patients, who were classified as having type I-3, were described in whom platelet vWF, but not plasma vWF, was reduced. One of these patients was the asymptomatic father of a severely affected vWD patient.

An alternative subdivision of type I vWD patients on the basis of platelet vWF content was proposed by Mannucci et al. (292), who described six patients from four kindreds with severe reductions in plasma vWF:Ag (4 to 11 U/dL) and vWF:RCoF (less than 7 U/dL) levels and normal platelet levels of vWF. These patients were classified as *platelet-normal* to distinguish them from *platelet-low* patients, in whom similar reductions in plasma and platelet vWF:Ag and vWF:RCoF activity were noted. It has been hypothesized that platelet-low vWD results from defective production of vWF, whereas platelet-normal vWD arises from the impaired release of vWF from cellular compartments. Importantly, the bleeding time in platelet-normal patients is normal or modestly prolonged, despite the striking reduction in plasma vWF levels (292). A highly significant inverse relation between bleeding time and the level of platelet (but not plasma) vWF in type I vWD patients was also noted by Gralnick et al. (293). Moreover, platelet-normal patients have a better response to DDAVP infusions when the response is judged by the increase in plasma vWF levels and reduction in bleeding time. The molecular and cellular basis of the discordance between plasma and platelet vWF has not been established.

von Willebrand's Disease Vicenza. Two kindreds have been identified in which plasma vWF contains a set of larger-than-normal (supranormal) vWF multimers, similar to those present in plasma after desmopressin infusion (see later discussion) (387). In this subtype, which is termed *vWD Vicenza*, although plasma factor VIII, vWF:Ag, and vWF:RCoF activity levels are low, the bleeding time is slightly prolonged and bleeding manifestations are mild. The relatively mild clinical symptoms that are associated with this subtype are thought to be due to normal levels of platelet vWF (388). The genetic defect has been localized close to or within the vWF gene (389).

TYPE III

Type III vWD is characterized by marked reductions in vWF:Ag (less than 4 U/dL), vWF:RCoF (less than 5 U/dL), and factor VIII (less than 20 U/dL) levels (305,390) (Fig. 35-10). In some patients, plasma vWF:Ag is undetectable by sensitive radioimmunoassays, with sensitivity down to 0.01 U/dL (331). vWF is also markedly decreased or absent in platelets (391) and in vascular endothelial cells (392). Factor VIII levels are always depressed, although they are still measurable (1 to 5 U/dL), even in patients in whom the vWF:Ag activity is undetectable (384,390). Clinically, patients are severely affected and experience frequent mucocutaneous bleeding episodes. Because factor VIII is also severely diminished, patients may experience classic hemophilic symptoms, including hemarthroses and deep hematomas.

The inheritance of type III vWD is usually recessive and carriers (who are identified by restriction fragment length polymorphism or gene deletion analysis) of the type III vWD trait may be asymptomatic and have normal laboratory tests. In a number of cases, carriers have subnormal vWF:Ag or vWF:RCoF activity levels, similar to type I vWD patients (305,384). Patients with type III vWD and with consanguineous parents have been identified as homozygous for complete (95,384) or partial gene deletions (385). This subset of patients appears to be at the greatest risk of developing inhibitors to vWF after exposure to blood products. Other patients have been described who are heterozygous for a vWF gene deletion (87,384) or in whom no gross genetic alteration could be detected (393). Recently, Nichols et al. (386) demonstrated defective vWF mRNA expression from maternal and paternal alleles in one type III vWD pedigree by comparing genomic DNA and platelet vWF mRNA (by using the polymerase chain reaction technique).

Qualitative Disorders of von Willebrand's Factor

There are a large number of vWD subtypes with a structural or functional abnormality in vWF. Affected patients have a reduced ratio of vWF:RCoF to vWF:Ag and a reduction or a complete loss of HMW and intermediate-molecular-weight plasma multimers. These qualitative disorders may be further subdivided into two clinically important subgroups. The first subgroup comprises those subtypes (IB, IC, IIA, and IIC through II-I) in which the characteristic plasma findings are also reflected in platelet vWF and the RIPA response is lost or markedly reduced. The second subgroup comprises those subtypes [IIB, IIB *Tampa*, and type I (*New York*)] in which HMW forms of vWF are present in platelets, and a heightened RIPA response is present. These two different responses in the RIPA assay have important clinical implications for diagnosis and treatment.

More recently, patients have been identified in whom vWF levels are modestly reduced but who exhibit a disproportionate reduction in factor VIII levels as a result of abnormal binding of the factor VIII molecule to its vWF carrier (394,395). Finally, there is a rare platelet disorder, platelet-type vWD (pseudo-vWD), which is clinically indistinguishable from most forms of type IIB vWD.

SUBTYPES WITH DIMINISHED RISTOCETIN-INDUCED PLATELET AGGREGATION ACTIVITY

Type I Variants. Two type I variants have been described in which there is the full range of vWF multimers but functional abnormalities. The inheritance pattern in each of these subtypes is autosomal dominant.

Type IB (Platelet Discordant). In 1983, Hoyer et al. (365) characterized a variant of vWD, which they termed *type IB*. Although all multimeric species were present, a relative reduction in the largest forms was seen. This variant was not uncommon and was detected in 15 of 47 families that were studied. The patients had clinical bleeding, moderately prolonged bleeding times, and reduced vWF:RCoF activity. A similar variant was described in four patients from three kindreds by Mannucci et al. (292) and termed *platelet discordant* to reflect the discordance between vWF:RCoF and vWF:Ag levels in the platelet. They also noted a decreased ratio of plasma vWF:RCoF to vWF:Ag that was accentuated after treatment with DDAVP. Type IB patients had markedly prolonged bleeding times and poor clinical responses to DDAVP.

Type IC. Five persons from two unrelated families have been described with mild bleeding symptoms; in these patients, all plasma multimers are present, but an abnormal satellite pattern is seen by high-resolution SDS-agarose electrophoresis (340). Despite normal vWF:Ag levels, most affected members of these families had a prolonged bleeding time and reduced vWF:RCoF activity. This disorder is transmitted as an autosomal-dominant trait.

Type II Variants. Type II variants are characterized by the absence of the large- and intermediate-sized multimers in the plasma and a decreased vWF:RCoF to vWF:Ag ratio. They are a heterogeneous group with autosomal-dominant and recessive inheritance patterns, variable clinical manifestations, and a variety of electrophoretic abnormalities. In some variants, a reproducible increase of a 176-kd proteolytic fragment (type IIA) is found, and, in others, proteolytic fragments of vWF are reduced (types IIE, IIF, IIH, II-I) or undetectable (types IIC and IID).

Type IIA. *Type IIA vWD* may be defined as a group of molecular defects that produce markedly reduced vWF:RCoF and

RIPA activity and a characteristic electrophoretic pattern that consists chiefly of the five smallest oligomers of vWF with an increased abundance of the fastest migrating band in the triplet structure (287) (Fig. 35-8). Clinical symptoms range from mild to severe bleeding. The structural abnormalities were first suggested by increased anodal mobility in cross-immunoelectrophoresis and are thought to arise in some kindreds from enhanced proteolysis of circulating vWF (94,364,396). In this variant, plasma vWF:Ag levels may be normal or reduced, with values that are obtained by Laurell EIA consistently higher than those that are determined by IRMA (339). Factor VIII levels and vWF:Ag levels are usually concordant. Platelet vWF also lacks the large forms of vWF, although intermediate-sized forms are present, and a few patients (termed *type II-3*) have been described in which the platelet vWF electrophoretic pattern appears normal (339).

Heterogeneity within the IIA subtype was first suggested by a variable degree of susceptibility to *in vitro* proteolysis (397,398) and a variable response to DDAVP, as judged by the appearance of large multimeric forms in the plasma and correction of the bleeding time (398–400). The inheritance pattern has been reported to be autosomal dominant in all (287,365,401,402) but one (403) of the large number of kindreds that have been studied.

Compelling evidence suggests that decreased secretion or increased proteolysis of the HMW forms of vWF may give rise to the type IIA variants (404,405). In the first instance, it has been suggested that point mutations lead to defects in intracellular transport or degradation within the endothelial cell, thus resulting in the preferential retention of the largest forms of vWF. In the second mechanism, vWF with a normal multimeric distribution is secreted but is unusually susceptible to subsequent proteolysis (406). The collection of blood from patients who carry these mutations into protease inhibitors results in a variable and incomplete restoration of the larger vWF multimers, which suggests that the proteolysis is an *in vivo* phenomenon (397,398). The enzyme or enzymes that are responsible for the proteolysis of vWF *in vivo* are not known. Although a number of proteases, including calpain I (407), elastase (408), and plasmin (409,410), can cleave vWF *in vitro*, epitope mapping of the resultant fragments has shown that they are derived from different regions of the vWF subunit than the 176-kd fragment that is present in normal persons or patients with type IIA vWD (411,412).

Genetic linkage studies first established that the type IIA phenotype was tightly linked to the vWD gene (413). Subsequently, point mutations were identified in the vWF gene in a number of type IIA patients. Fourteen missense mutations have been identified in 17 families (43,382,404,405,414) (Fig. 35-11). All but two of these mutations fall within the vWF A2 domain between residues 742 and 875, and at least three mutations are close to the previously identified site of proteolysis within vWF, which produces the normally observed 176-kd fragment (415). It is interesting that one of these mutations (Arg 834 → Trp) has been identified in six unrelated type IIA patients (43). Expression of recombinant vWF that contains several of the identified type IIA mutations in heterologous cells has resulted in the production of mutant vWF that is devoid of the largest multimers (404,405). In addition, an endothelial cell culture that was derived from the umbilical vein of a patient who carried the Ser 850 → Pro mutation produced vWF with decreased amounts of large multimers and an increase in rapidly migrating satellite species (416,417).

Type IIC. The type IIC variant is characterized by a unique electrophoretic pattern that shows the loss of large- and intermediate-sized multimers from plasma and platelets. There is a relative increase in the smallest oligomer and an absence of satellite bands and triplet structure (365,418–420). When analyzed under reducing conditions by SDS–polyacrylamide gel electrophoresis, the normal 176- and 140-kd proteolytic fragments are missing, which suggests markedly decreased or absent proteolysis of circulating vWF (406). However, the addition of protease inhibitors during blood collection enhanced the structural differences that were noted between plasma and platelet pools of vWF in one family (398,421). vWF:RCoF activity is markedly reduced, and the bleeding time is significantly prolonged. Clinical symptoms range from mild to severe, and the response to DDAVP is poor.

Although the inheritance of type IIC variant was classically described as autosomal recessive (418,420), an increased bleeding

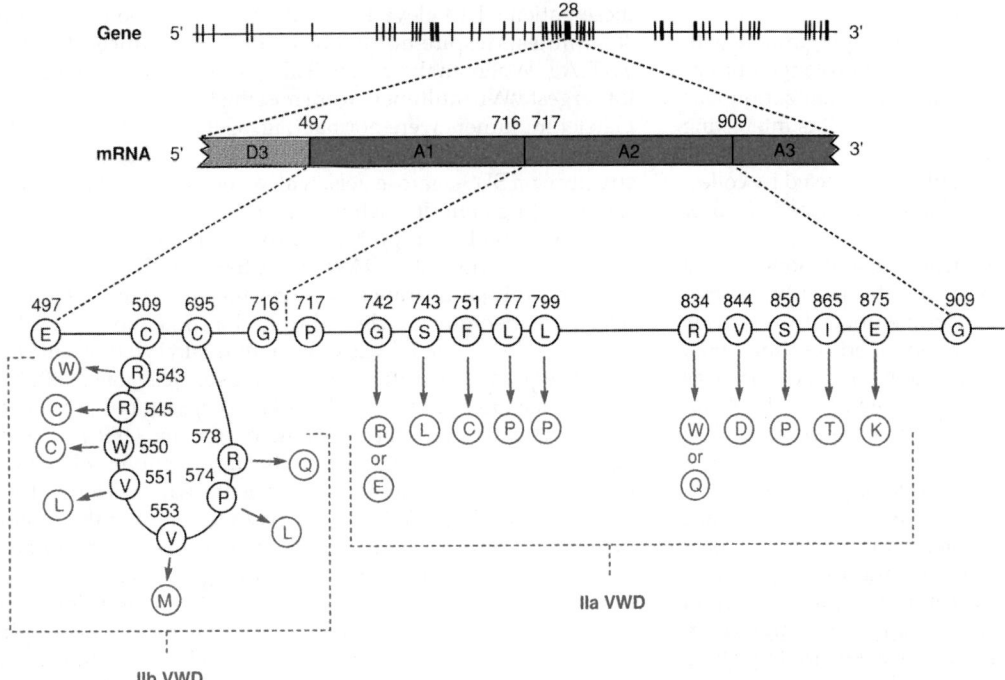

Figure 35-11. Schematic representation of some of the known mutations in the A1 and A2 domains of von Willebrand's factor that cause, respectively, types IIB and IIA von Willebrand's disease (vWD). The A1 and A2 domains are encoded by exon 28 in the von Willebrand's factor gene (382). mRNA, messenger RNA.

time and mild clinical symptoms have been described in heterozygotes in several kindreds (422,423). Moreover, unaffected members of these families may have crossed immunoelectrophoretic or SDS-agarose multimer patterns that are intermediate between normal and type IIC individuals. vWD type IIC patients probably are compound heterozygotes (420,422,423).

Type IID. In the type IID subtype, the normal satellite pattern that is observed on high-percentage agarose gels is replaced by a unique complex of bands. Similar electrophoretic patterns have been reported in four unrelated families from Japan, Sweden, England, and Scotland (292,424–426), which suggests that this variant may not be rare. vWF:Ag and factor VIII:C levels are unusually normal, but the vWF:RCoF is moderately or severely reduced. RIPA is reduced, and the response to DDAVP appears to be modest (426). As in type IIC, the normal triplet structure is absent in type IID plasma (406).

Other Variants. Several variants of type II vWD, types IIE through II-I, have been reported in which there is a selective loss of the large multimeric forms of plasma vWF and unique electrophoretic abnormalities on high-resolution SDS-agarose gels. In general, they are associated with mild to moderate bleeding and decreased vWF:RCoF to vWF:Ag ratios.

The type IIE variant was described in two members of a single family (406). The multimeric pattern appears similar to type IIC, except that the dominance of the smallest oligomer is not seen, and the inheritance pattern is autosomal dominant. Similar to types IIC and IID, there is a reduction in the circulating 176-kd proteolytic fragment, although it is not reduced to the same extent as in these other variants.

Type IIF was described in a single patient with a life-long bleeding tendency and a markedly prolonged bleeding time (347). Plasma vWF from this variant is characterized by the absence of large multimers and the presence of a unique satellite banding pattern. In contrast, platelet vWF levels are not reduced, and the electrophoretic pattern of this vWF pool is indistinguishable from that seen in normal platelets. Although DDAVP was found to elevate vWF:Ag and vWF:RCoF activity, the bleeding time remained prolonged, and the clinical response was poor. The inheritance pattern could not be formally evaluated but appeared to be recessive.

Type IIG was likewise described in a single patient with moderate clinical symptoms and a markedly prolonged bleeding time. A uniquely abnormal multimeric organization was found in vWF from plasma and platelets (397). It is interesting that the electrophoretic pattern that is found in the platelet pool, but not in the plasma pool, of vWF could be corrected by collection of blood directly into ethylenediaminetetraacetic acid or protease inhibitors.

Type IIH was discovered in a patient with a life-long history of bleeding whose initial diagnosis was obscured by normal measurements of vWF:Ag and borderline normal vWF:RCoF activity in the presence of a prolonged bleeding time (367). RIPA was abnormal, and an electrophoretic pattern that was similar to, but distinct from, type IIC was noted on high-resolution agarose gels. A short-lived correction of the bleeding time occurred after DDAVP infusion.

Type II-I vWD was described in two family members with life-long histories of severe bleeding and a unique electrophoretic pattern on high-resolution gels. Similar to that which occurs in some type IIA variants, the platelet vWF multimeric structure was normal. However, unlike that seen in previously reported type IIA patients, no increase in the quantity of proteolytic fragments of vWF in the plasma was seen. Unlike type IIF, the inheritance pattern of type II-I appears to be dominant (427).

Type II *Buffalo* was described in three members of a single family and is characterized by a low vWF:RCoF to vWF:Ag ratio and a multimeric pattern that is similar to type IIA vWD. Administration of DDAVP-induced platelet agglutination and thrombocytopenia are similar to that observed in type IIB patients. However, unlike type IIB vWD, there was no hypersensitivity to ristocetin (428).

Type B vWD was described in a single patient with undetectable vWF:RCoF activity, despite normal levels of vWF:Ag and factor VIII. It is of interest that normal platelet aggregation was observed with botrocetin, which also induces vWF binding to gpIb (429). Multimer analysis revealed a unique electrophoretic pattern. A single amino acid substitution, Gly 561 → Ser, in the A1 domain of vWF is responsible for this unique phenotype (430).

SUBTYPES WITH HEIGHTENED RESPONSIVENESS TO RISTOCETIN

The vWD variants that are considered in this section are characterized by a heightened interaction between platelets and vWF manifesting as hyperresponsiveness to ristocetin in RIPA assays or spontaneous platelet aggregation.

Type I New York. Three independent kindreds have been reported in whom there is a mild to moderate bleeding diathesis with increased RIPA and a normal distribution of vWF multimers (370,431,432). Mixing studies that use washed platelets and platelet-poor plasma from affected patients and normal persons distinguish this condition from pseudo-vWD, whereas the normal multimeric pattern distinguishes this from type IIB vWD (see the section Type IIB). vWF binds to platelet gpIb/IX and gpIIb/IIIa in an abnormal manner, and the sialic content of the vWF appears normal (370). Note that DDAVP shortens the prolonged bleeding time that is found in some of these patients, without inducing the thrombocytopenia that is usually associated with the use of this drug in type IIB patients (431).

Type IIB. The type IIB vWD variant was first recognized in a study of 20 patients from five unrelated families who, in contrast to other vWD patients who were studied at that time, demonstrated platelet aggregation in the presence of reduced concentrations of ristocetin (less than 0.6 mg/mL) (371). Most of these patients had elevated bleeding times (some greater than 30 minutes) despite normal or moderately reduced levels of vWF:Ag. When analyzed by SDS-agarose gel electrophoresis, the largest vWF multimers were missing from plasma, although platelet multimers were normal (Fig. 35-9). As in type IIA vWF, plasma vWF from type IIB variants has an abnormal triplet structure on SDS-agarose gels, with an enhancement of the fastest migrating band in each oligomeric group and an increased quantity of the 176-kd proteolytic fragment (406).

Administration of DDAVP to patients with type IIB produces a rapid appearance of larger multimers in the plasma which are then quickly cleared from the circulation (399). This process is due to the release of an abnormal vWF molecule and its subsequent adsorption on platelet surfaces (399,433). The splenic clearance of the resultant platelet aggregates produces a transient but often profound thrombocytopenia (169,434). Similarly, transient or even chronic thrombocytopenia has been found in subsets of type IIB vWD patients, which is termed *type IIB Tampa* (232,362,435–440), and may worsen with the physiologic increase in circulating vWF that is seen in pregnancy (232,233), normal aging (441), or after surgery (442).

In most pedigrees, type IIB vWD is dominantly inherited, although a few cases have been reported with a recessive phenotype (443,444). A total of nine amino acid substitutions and one insertion have been identified in patients with type IIB

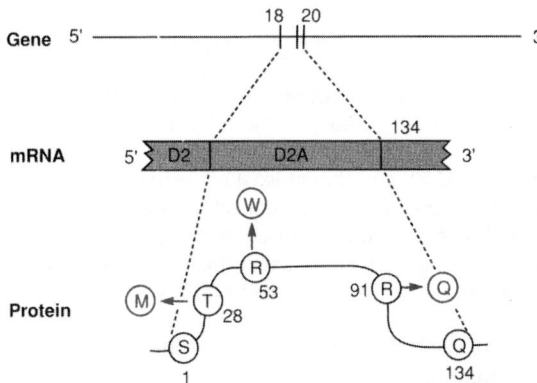

Figure 35-12. Schematic representation of some of the mutations that cause autosomal hemophilia, the variant form of von Willebrand's disease in which factor VIII binding to von Willebrand's factor is perturbed. All mutations described as of 2002 arose in exons 18 to 20 of the von Willebrand's factor gene (382). mRNA, messenger RNA.

vWD (382,445–449), and four of these mutations account for 90% of the families that have been studied as of 2002 (43). Several of these mutations have been reported in more than one pedigree as a result of what is presumed to be independent genetic events (445). All but three of these mutations are located between amino acid residues 540 and 578 in the A1 domain (Fig. 35-11). This region of vWF, between amino acid residues Val 449 and Lys 728, had previously been demonstrated to contain the platelet gpIb binding site (450,451). Normally, vWF binding to this receptor requires prior activation of vWF, which may be produced by the binding of vWF to collagen, or a reduction in net negative charge by agents such as ristocetin. The single amino acid substitutions, which have been described in type IIB patients, are presumed to facilitate vWF binding to platelet gpIb/IX by introducing conformational changes that mimic the effects of collagen or ristocetin. Full-length recombinant vWF that contains some of the described mutations has been expressed and has been shown to bind spontaneously to platelets (445,452–456).

VARIANTS WITH DEFECTIVE FACTOR VIII BINDING

In most vWD variants, the level of plasma factor VIII is decreased in a rough proportion to the decreased level of plasma vWF. Pedigrees have been described, however, in which factor VIII deficiency was autosomally inherited without a proportionate reduction in plasma vWF levels (457–459). This led to the hypothesis that mutations in vWF could reduce factor VIII binding capacity. Three mutations within the N-terminal region of vWF, which reduce or eliminate factor VIII binding *in vitro* and decrease factor VIII to vWF ratios in the plasma of affected persons, have been described in eight apparently unrelated families (394,395,460–467) (Fig. 35-12). The most frequently observed mutation is Arg 91 → Gln. This mutation lies within the region of vWF (residues 78 to 96) that was previously shown to be critical for factor VIII binding by using monoclonal antibodies (69,70). At least three of the four affected individuals are compound heterozygotes and carry the Arg 91 → Gln mutation and a type I vWD allele. Because recombinant vWF that contains this mutation has a markedly decreased capacity for factor VIII binding (463,465), there may be partial compensation by the incorporation of low levels of the other allelic product into vWF multimers. A second mutation, Thr 28 → Met, has been identified in two families and produces severe factor VIII deficiency with variable vWF protein levels in the homozygous state (461,468). A substitution of Arg 53 → Trp has been detected

in two persons with low factor VIII levels and normal vWF protein levels. One of these persons also carried the Arg 91 → Gln mutation (462). A second double mutation, Arg 19 → Trp and His 54 → Gln, has also been described (464). The frequency of these mutations is unknown, but they may account for a significant proportion of patients who were previously diagnosed with mild hemophilia A.

ACQUIRED VON WILLEBRAND'S DISEASE

Acquired vWD comprises a heterogeneous group of disorders in which previously normal individuals develop a mucosal bleeding disorder and decreased levels of vWF. The clinical presentation is similar to that seen in other vWD patients, except that the patients are generally elderly and have no family or previous personal history of bleeding. Epistaxis and easy bruising are the most common presenting complaints. Laboratory features of acquired vWD are identical with those that are seen in congenital vWD and include reduced plasma levels of factor VIII, vWF:Ag, and vWF:RCoF. In some cases, selective depletion of the largest forms of vWF occurs, which results in a plasma multimeric distribution that is similar to that seen in congenital type II vWD (469,470).

At least three distinct mechanisms that cause acquired vWD have been described. In some patients, diminished vWF levels result from the presence of a circulating inhibitor, usually an antibody of the immunoglobulin G or immunoglobulin M class (471). These inhibitors may be associated with monoclonal gammopathies (472), multiple myeloma (472), lymphoproliferative diseases such as chronic lymphocytic leukemia (471), poorly differentiated lymphocytic lymphoma (473), hairy cell leukemia (474), and autoimmune diseases such as systemic lupus erythematosus (475) and mixed connective tissue disease (476). The presence of the circulating inhibitor can sometimes be detected by the loss of vWF:RCoF activity and, sometimes, by decreased factor VIII activity in mixtures of normal and patient plasmas (471,477–479). In other cases, nonneutralizing antibodies may form immune complexes with vWF that lead to increased clearance in the reticuloendothelial cells (480,481).

Acquired vWD may also result from the absorption of vWF onto the surface of malignant cells, such as lymphoid tumors (473), Waldenström's macroglobulinemia (90,482), multiple myeloma (483), Wilms' tumor (129,484,485), and other solid tumors (486–488). In such cases, there is often a selective loss of the largest vWF multimers with a consequent loss of RCoF activity that is out of proportion to the vWF:Ag. In some cases, internalization of vWF by the tumor cells could be demonstrated (483,488). Acquired vWD may also be seen in patients with myeloproliferative diseases (489,490). In such patients, selective loss of the largest multimeric forms of vWF may result from increased proteolysis, which is suggested by abnormal satellite banding patterns on SDS-agarose gels (490).

PLATELET-TYPE VON WILLEBRAND'S DISEASE

Platelet-type vWD, or pseudo-vWD, is a rare autosomal disorder with a clinical phenotype that most closely resembles type IIB vWD (372,491,492). Large vWF multimers are absent in the plasma but are present in platelet lysates. Plasma vWF:RCoF activity is decreased, but responsiveness to ristocetin in RIPA assays is heightened. In contrast to other variants of vWD with hyperresponsiveness to ristocetin, the defect that is responsible for platelet-type vWD lies within the platelet itself, within the gpIb/IX complex. As of 2002, two point mutations with the α-chain of gpIb have been described (493,494). Laboratory differentiation between platelet-type vWD and type IIB and similar variants involves the addition of normal cryoprecipitate or purified vWF to washed patient platelets (372,492,495). A less cumbersome assay that takes advantage of the hyperaffinity of type IIB vWF, but not vWF from platelet-type vWD patients, for formalin-fixed platelets has been described (496).

TREATMENT

General Considerations

Few controlled studies are available to guide the clinician with respect to intensity or duration of treatment in vWD. In most vWD patients, factor VIII levels are high enough to support normal thrombin generation, and bleeding is primarily of the mucosal type. Because laboratory tests are often imprecise measures of the hemostatic defect in vWD, treatment is often empiric, with the efficacy judged by clinical endpoints. In certain situations, such as high-risk surgery, therapy should be monitored by measuring the bleeding time. Although the Duke bleeding time is more easily corrected than the template modification of the Ivy bleeding time, correction of the Duke bleeding time correlates with improved hemostasis (322,497).

In patients with severe vWD, who can develop hemophilic-type bleeding, the aim of therapy is to increase plasma factor VIII levels to 30 to 50 U/dL, as well as to correct the defect in primary hemostasis. The duration of treatment is determined by the severity of hemorrhage and clinical response. Life-threatening hemorrhage (e.g., intracranial bleeding), which is exceedingly rare in vWD, may raise the factor VIII level to 100 U/dL. When patients with vWD are treated with vWF-containing products, the elevation in plasma factor VIII levels lasts longer than it does in hemophilia A patients (19).

Therapeutic Modalities

DESMOPRESSIN

Desmopressin acetate (also known as *DDAVP*) is a synthetic analog of the antidiuretic hormone L-arginine vasopressin with enhanced antidiuretic potency but little pressor activity. Infusion of a standard dose of 0.3 µg/kg desmopressin into healthy volunteers results in a two- to threefold increase in vWF antigenic levels and a five- to sixfold increase in factor VIII levels (149,498,499). Peak responses are usually seen 30 to 60 minutes after infusion and persist for as long as 6 hours. Desmopressin is almost always administered intravenously, although subcutaneous (500–502) or intranasal (503,504) administration of more concentrated forms of the drug are equally effective.

Desmopressin is effective for only 6 to 12 hours, and tachyphylaxis may be observed after as few as two or three doses (505). In such cases, effective hemostasis may require infusion of an exogenous source of vWF. The duration of responsiveness to DDAVP varies, and repeated responses have been documented over several days (506). A single daily dose, which may be sufficient in some clinical settings, reduces the likelihood of tachyphylaxis (507).

Desmopressin generally causes only minor side effects, which include facial flushing and, less frequently, nausea and headache. A reduction of the rate of infusion usually obviates these difficulties. More serious side effects have also been reported. First, through its antidiuretic effect, desmopressin may produce clinically significant water intoxication and hyponatremia, which may be profound enough to precipitate seizures (508–510). Infancy, frequent dosing, and the concomitant use of narcotics appear to be additional risk factors for hyponatremia. Frequent monitoring of serum sodium and careful fluid management may be necessary in high-risk patients. Second, desmopressin has been associated with thrombosis and myocardial infarction in anecdotal reports (511,512). However, a statistical examination of these reports

failed to establish causality (513). Finally, it is widely believed that the use of DDAVP in patients with type IIB vWD is contraindicated, because the release of HMW forms of the abnormal vWF that is found in these patients may worsen the often present thrombocytopenia (433,434). Although more recent reports suggest that some type IIB patients are clinically improved by treatment with DDAVP and that at least some instances of decreased platelet counts may be a blood collection artifact (pseudothrombocytopenia), the routine use of DDAVP in type IIB vWD cannot be advocated at this time. Similarly, the use of DDAVP is not recommended in patients with platelet-type vWD.

EXOGENOUS SOURCES OF VON WILLEBRAND'S FACTOR

The treatment of vWD patients who do not respond to desmopressin or who have experienced tachyphylaxis to the drug depends on exogenous sources of vWF. In the past, cryoprecipitate has been the preferred blood product, because it contains the full range of vWF multimers. Typically used dosages of cryoprecipitate are 1 U/10 kg every 12 to 24 hours. The duration of therapy depends on the clinical circumstances but is usually 48 to 72 hours. Although most factor VIII concentrates contain significant quantities of vWF, they are typically deficient in the HMW multimers that are found normally in plasma and are not effective in correcting the primary hemostatic defect that is present in vWD patients (514). At least one such concentrate, Humate-P (Research Laboratories of Behringwerke AG, Marburg, Germany; Armour Pharmaceutical Company, Collegeville, PA, USA), has a significant fraction of the higher-molecular-weight forms of vWF that are found normally in plasma (515,516), can correct the laboratory abnormalities, and improves hemostasis in patients with type I, type II, and severe (type III) vWD (93,515–518). Because Humate-P is produced by a process that includes viral inactivation by heat treatment in the wet state (pasteurization), the risk of human immunodeficiency virus and viral hepatitis transmission is low (518,519). Typically, empiric dosages of 40 U of factor VIII per kilogram are given every 12 to 24 hours. A high-purity, virally attenuated, vWF concentrate, which contains HMW vWF multimers and a high specific activity of RCoF activity, has been introduced in Europe. The clinical efficacy of this product is still under investigation but appears to show promising results in a limited number of patients (516,520,521). The use of this product in severe vWD patients may be limited by the expected delay in the achievement of therapeutic factor VIII levels. Other intermediate- and high-purity factor VIII concentrates are under investigation for the treatment of vWD.

ADJUNCTIVE THERAPY

In addition to specific therapy that is aimed at increasing plasma vWF levels, a number of adjunctive measures are often useful in the treatment of vWD. Oral cavity bleeding is effectively treated with the antifibrinolytic drugs, ε-aminocaproic acid or tranexamic acid, which block plasminogen activation (522). Each drug may be given intravenously, orally, or topically as an oral rinse; they are particularly useful in preventing bleeding after dental surgery and tonsillectomy (523). Severe menorrhagia may require hormonal therapy with oral contraceptives, which reduce menstrual blood loss and increase vWF levels in mildly affected patients. High doses of conjugated estrogens may be required in unusually severe cases. The use of brief courses of conjugated estrogens has been proposed as treatment for women who undergo elective surgery (524).

Treatment Strategies

The choice of the therapeutic strategy depends primarily on the subtype of vWD and the nature of the bleeding diathesis (Table 35-2).

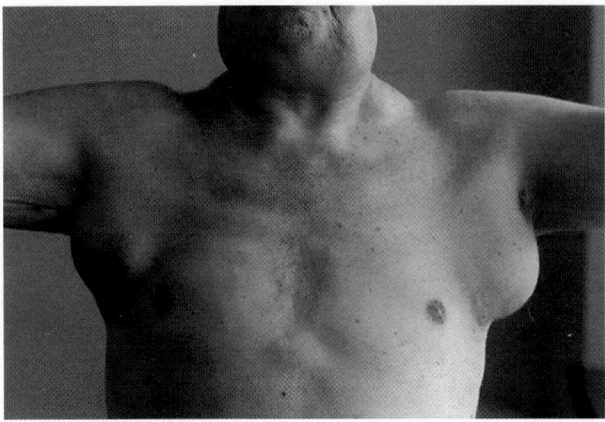

Color Figure 1-2. Malignant adenopathy of lymphoma. The nodes are larger than 2 cm in diameter, multiple, rubbery, and nontender.

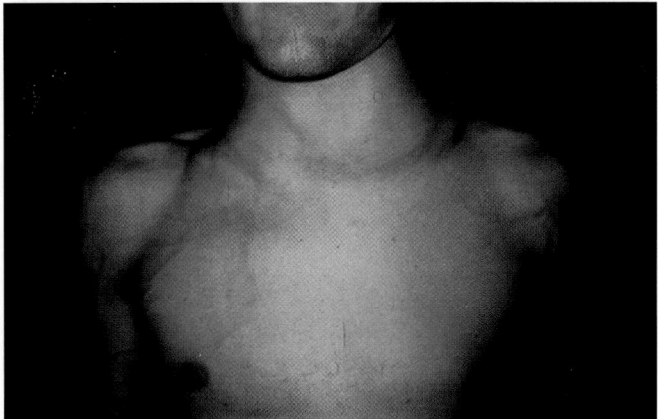

Color Figure 1-3. Venous engorgement secondary to superior vena cava obstruction.

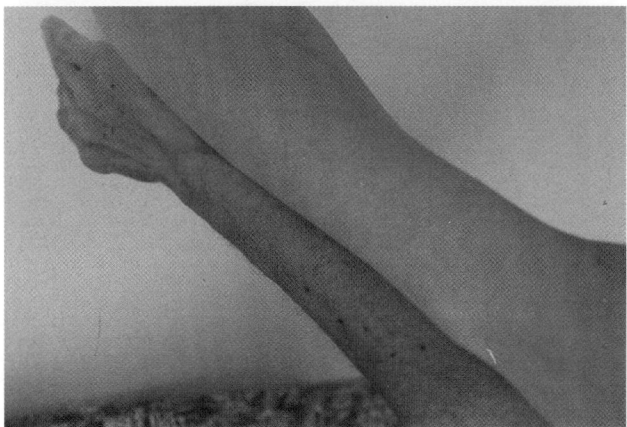

Color Figure 1-4. Slate gray discoloration of the skin of a patient with hemachromatosis, compared with normal coloration.

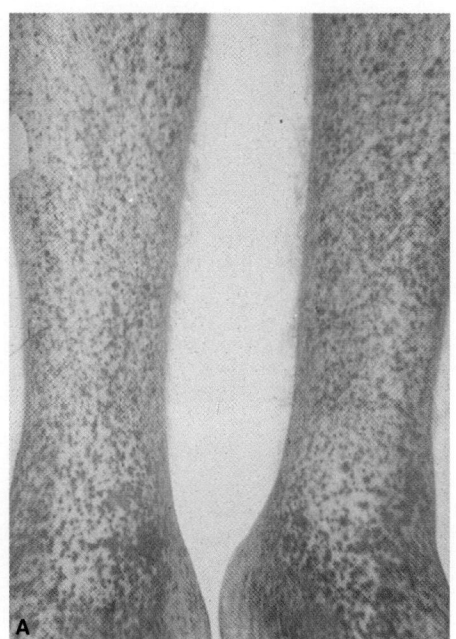

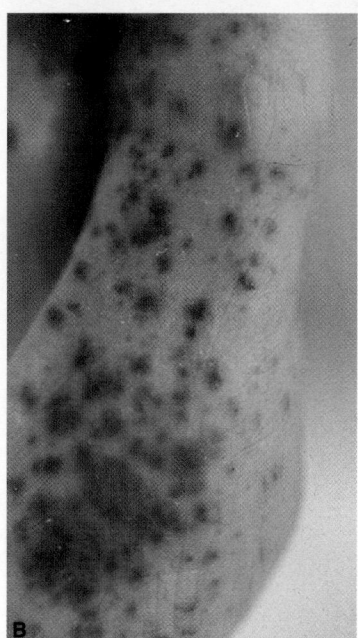

Color Figure 1-5. A: Showers of petechiae and purpura on the legs of a thrombocytopenic patient. **B:** Close-up of same patient.

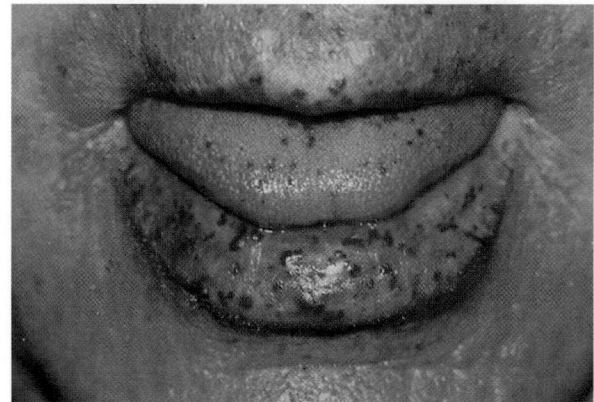

Color Figure 1-6. Mucosal telangiectasias in a patient with Rendu-Osler-Weber disease.

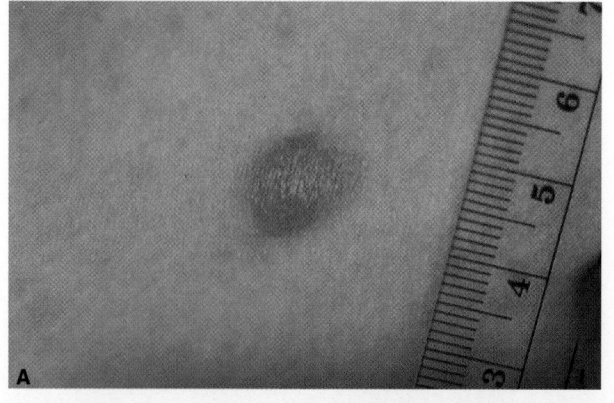

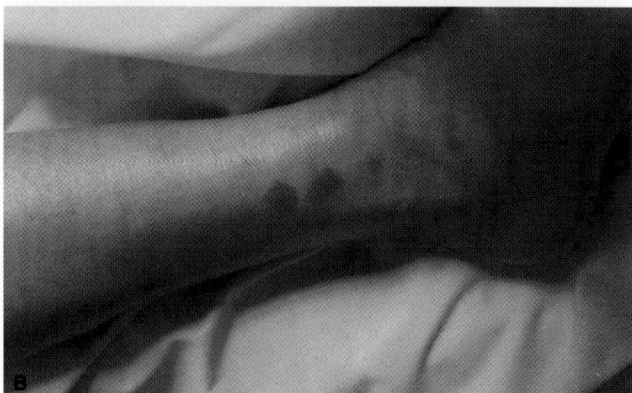

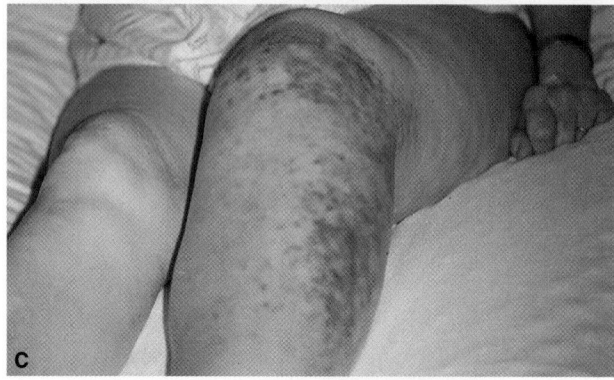

Color Figure 1-7. Leukemia cutis. **A:** Small salmon-colored nodules. **B:** Larger purplish subcutaneous lesions. **C:** Massive cutaneous infiltration by leukemia.

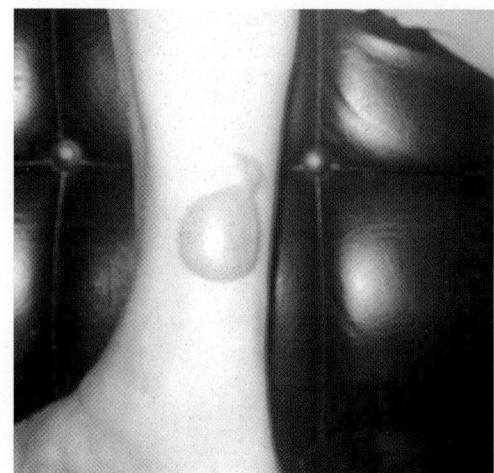

Color Figure 1-8. Exaggerated response to mosquito bite in a patient with chronic lymphocytic leukemia.

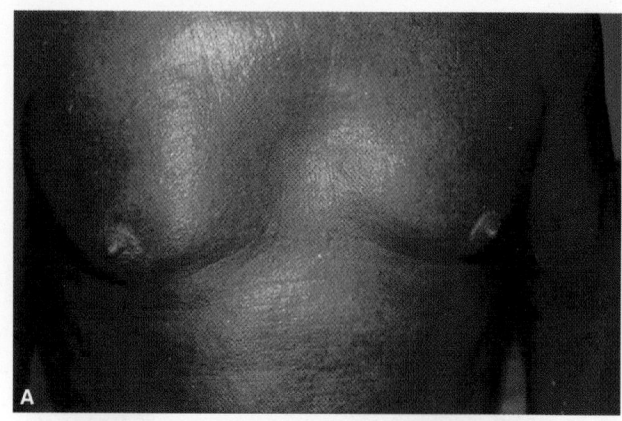

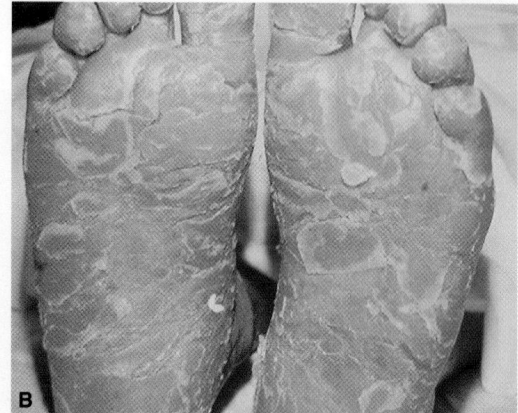

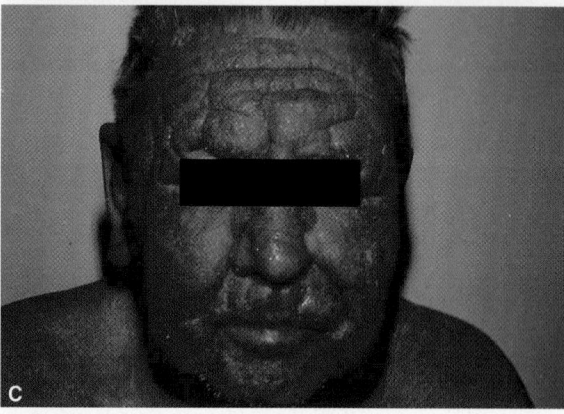

Color Figure 1-9. Sézary's syndrome. **A:** *L'homme rouge.* **B:** Hyperkeratosis with fissuring. **C:** Leonine facies. (From Wieselthier JS, Koh HK. Sézary's syndrome: diagnosis, prognosis and critical review of treatment options. *J Am Acad Dermatol* 1990;22:381, with permission.)

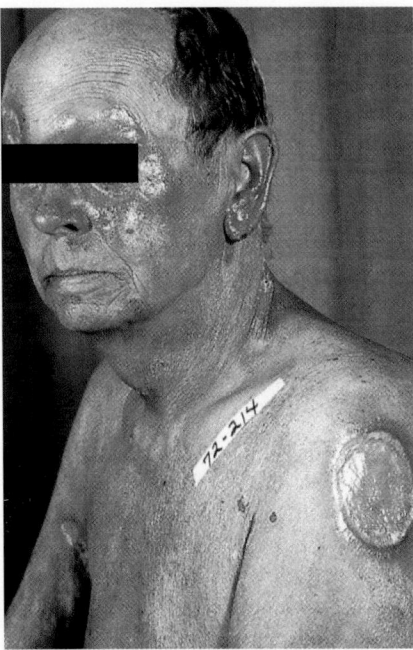

Color Figure 1-10. Mycosis fungoides. Note plaques and ulcerative nodules.

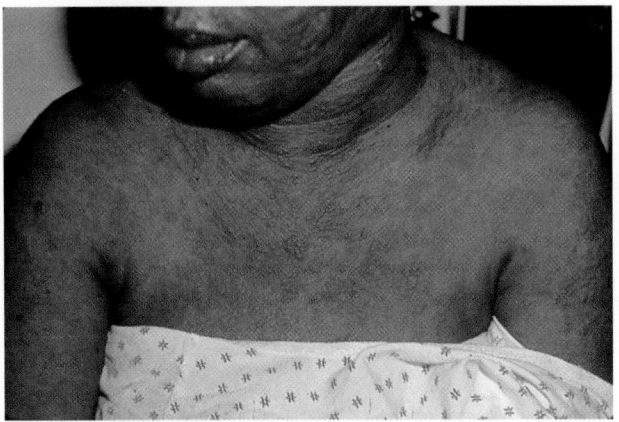

Color Figure 1-11. Erythematous, nonpruritic nodular infiltrate in a patient with adult T-cell leukemia-lymphoma.

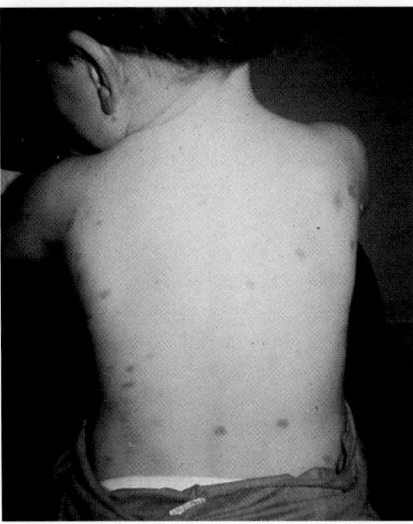

Color Figure 1-12. Multiple reddish-brown nodules in a patient with urticaria pigmentosa.

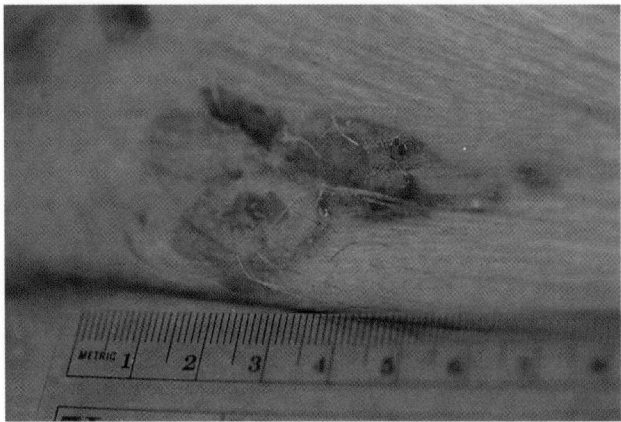

Color Figure 1-13. Necrosis of the skin after warfarin administration in a patient with protein-C deficiency.

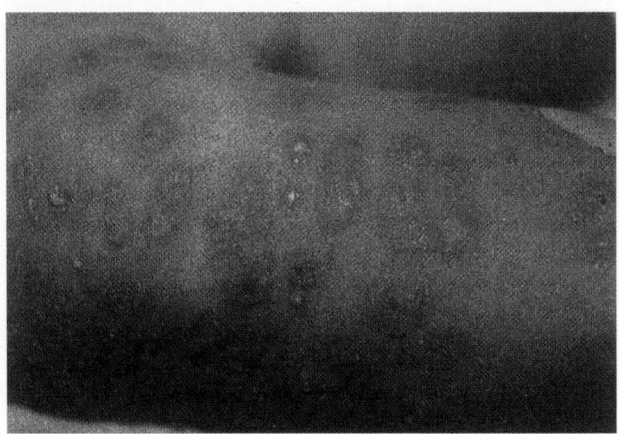

Color Figure 1-14. Patient with Sweet's syndrome. (From Dover JS. Case records of the Massachusetts General Hospital. Weekly clinicopathologic exercises. Case 30-1990. A 47-year-old man with a rash, fever, and headaches. *N Engl J Med* 1990;323:254, with permission.)

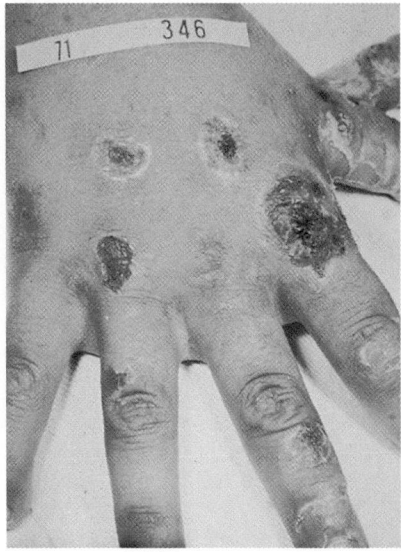

Color Figure 1-15. Necrotic ulcerations in a patient with erythropoietic porphyria.

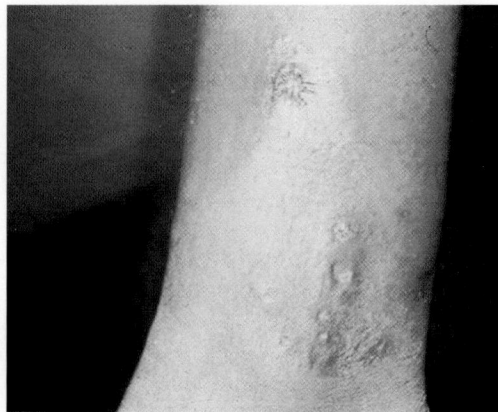

Color Figure 1-16. Scars with hyperpigmented borders due to recurrent ulceration in a patient with sickle cell anemia.

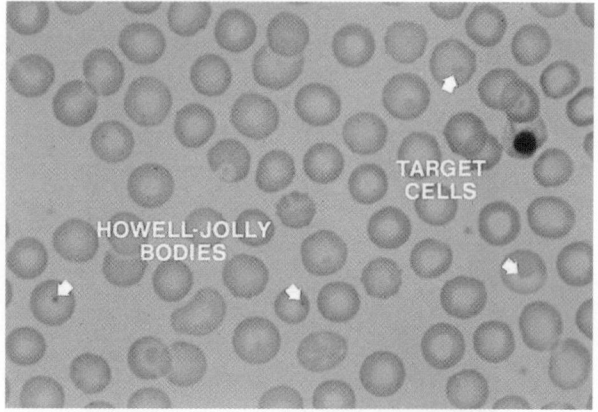

Color Figure 2-6. Peripheral blood smear from an infant with congenital asplenia. Note the presence of increased numbers of target cells (*arrows*) and the small round darkly staining cellular inclusions [Howell-Jolly bodies (*arrows*)]. A nucleated red blood cell is also present in the field. The Howell-Jolly bodies represent retained nuclear material that has not been removed because of lack of splenic function.

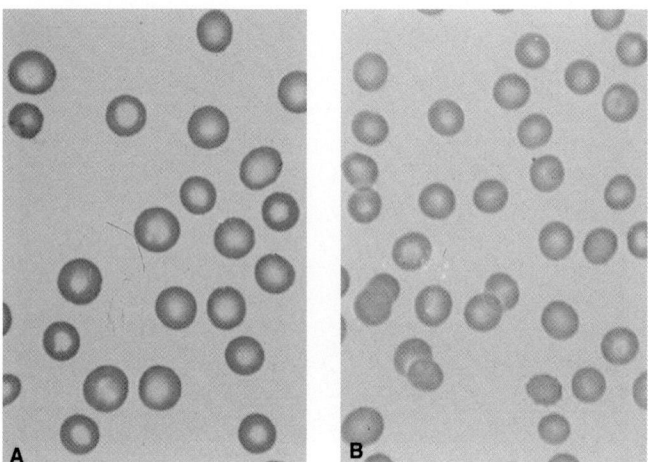

Color Figure 2-1. Thin peripheral blood smear from a newborn infant (**A**) and an adult (**B**). Note the adequate preservation of central pallor. The mean corpuscular volume of the newborn blood is 108 fL, whereas that of the adult blood is 92 fL. This difference is not perceptible on the peripheral smear.

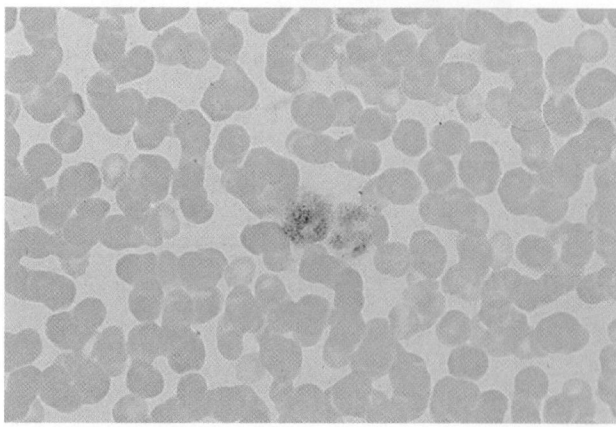

Color Figure 2-7. Leukocyte alkaline phosphatase stain. Note the presence of variable numbers of dark blue granules in the cytoplasm of two mature polymorphonuclear leukocytes.

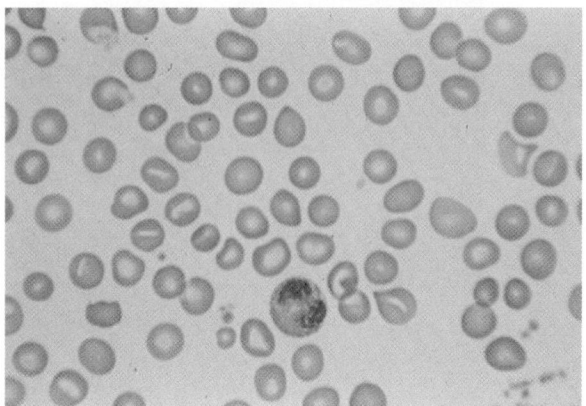

Color Figure 2-2. Peripheral smear with adequate preservation of central pallor. Platelets and a single polymorphonuclear leukocyte are present. Red blood cells vary in size and shape.

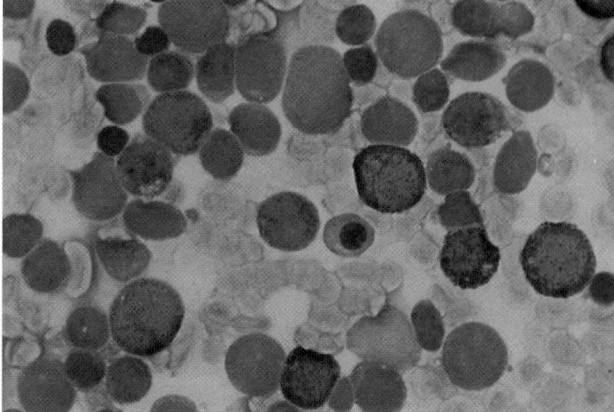

Color Figure 2-8. Myeloperoxidase stain. Granules containing myeloperoxidase stain an intense red-orange. Some cells contain only a few positive granules, and others are intensely positive.

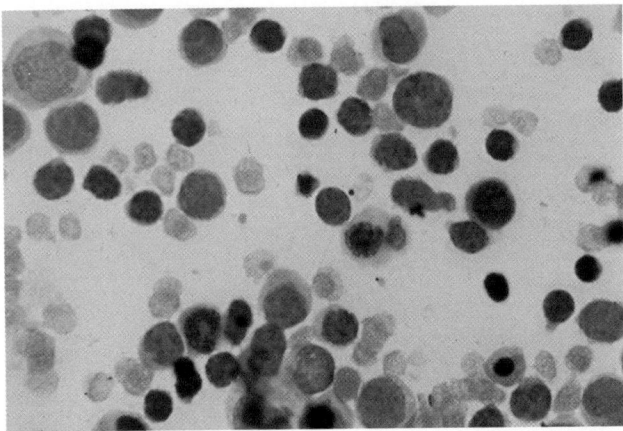

Color Figure 2-9. Chloracetate esterase stain. Two immature band neutrophil cells demonstrate intense cytoplasmic staining.

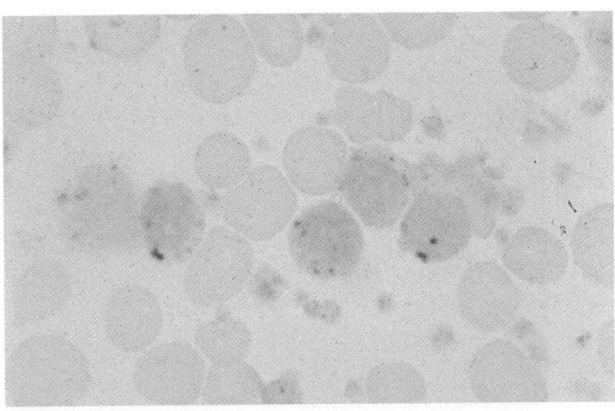

Color Figure 2-11. Tartrate-resistant acid phosphatase stain. Abnormal lymphoid cells from a patient with leukemic reticuloendotheliosis (hairy cell leukemia) are stained with acid phosphatase in the presence of tartrate.

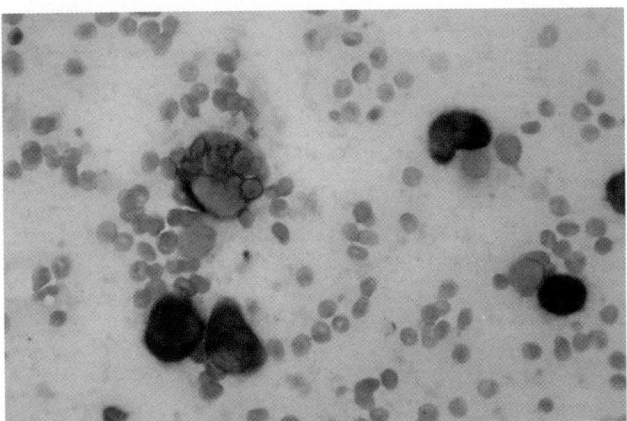

Color Figure 2-10. Nonspecific esterase stain. The butyrate substrate was used to demonstrate a positive reaction in this case of acute monoblastic leukemia (French-American-British M-5a).

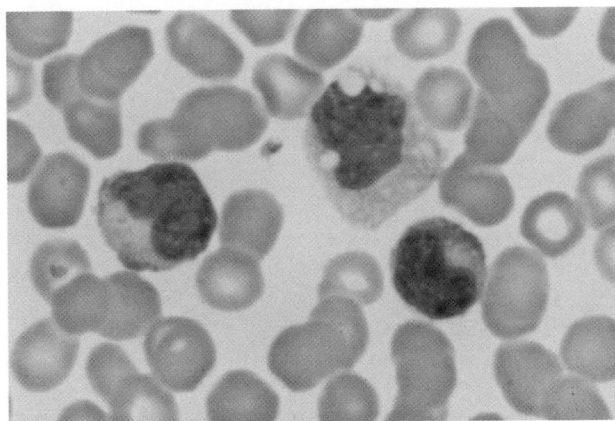

Color Figure 2-19. Examples of variant lymphocytes obtained from the blood of a patient with infectious mononucleosis. Large mononuclear cells with open nuclear chromatin can be seen.

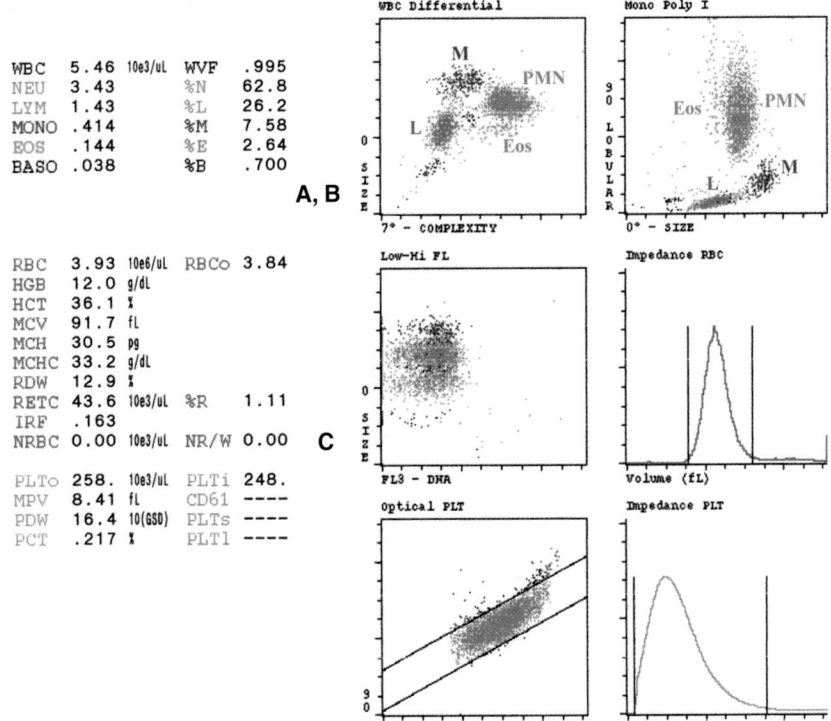

WBC	5.46	10e3/uL	WVF	.995	
NEU	3.43		%N	62.8	
LYM	1.43		%L	26.2	
MONO	.414		%M	7.58	
EOS	.144		%E	2.64	
BASO	.038		%B	.700	

A, B

RBC	3.93	10e6/uL	RBCo	3.84	
HGB	12.0	g/dL			
HCT	36.1	%			
MCV	91.7	fL			
MCH	30.5	pg			
MCHC	33.2	g/dL			
RDW	12.9	%			
RETC	43.6	10e3/uL	%R	1.11	
IRF	.163				
NRBC	0.00	10e3/uL	NR/W	0.00	**C**

PLTo	258.	10e3/uL	PLTi	248.	
MPV	8.41	fL	CD61	----	
PDW	16.4	10(GSD)	PLTs	----	
PCT	.217	%	PLT1	----	

Color Figure 2-24. Results and histogram display from the Abbott Cell-Dyn 4000. **A,B:** The white blood cell (WBC) differential is based on 0-degree, 7-degree, and 90-degree light scatter characteristics. Cell classes are indicated as follows: Eos, eosinophils; L, lymphocytes; M, monocytes; and PMN, neutrophils. **C:** Histogram plotting cell size (y-axis) and fluorescence due to a DNA binding dye on the x-axis. If nonviable leukocytes or nucleated red cells are present, the cell populations are shifted to the right. BASO, basophils; HCT, hematocrit; HGB, hemoglobin; IRF, immature reticulocyte fraction; MCH, mean corpuscular hemoglobin; MCHC, mean corpuscular hemoglobin concentration; MCV, mean corpuscular volume; MPV, mean platelet volume; PCT, platelet "crit"; PDW, platelet distribution width; PLT, platelet; RBC, red blood cell; RDW, red cell distribution width; RETC, reticulocyte count; WVF, WBC viability fraction.

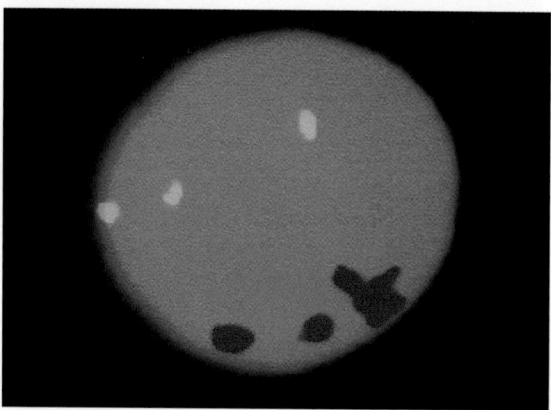

Color Figure 2-32. Fluorescence *in situ* hybridization using centrimeric probes for chromosomes 6 (*red*) and 21 (*green*) in a pediatric patient with acute lymphoblastic leukemia. The leukemia shows trisomy for chromosomes 6 and 21. (Photograph courtesy of Dr. K. Richkind, Genzyme Genetics, Santa Fe, NM.)

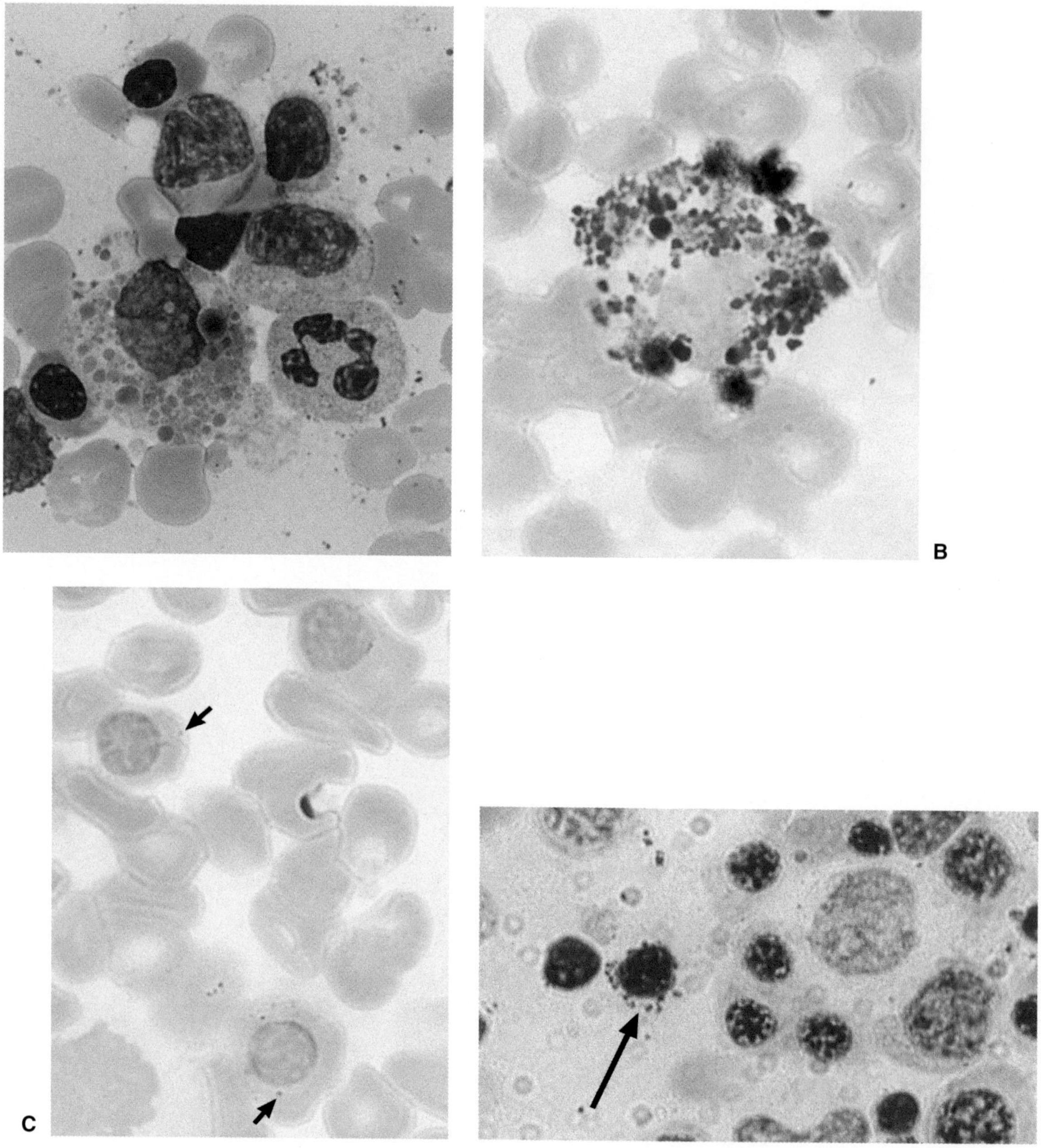

A

B

C

D

Color Figure 3-6. Siderophage (Wright-Giemsa, aspirate) **(A)**, siderophage **(B)**, sideroblast **(C)** (*arrows*), and ringed sideroblasts **(D)** (*arrow*). **B–D**: Prussian blue aspirates. **A–D**: ×1000.

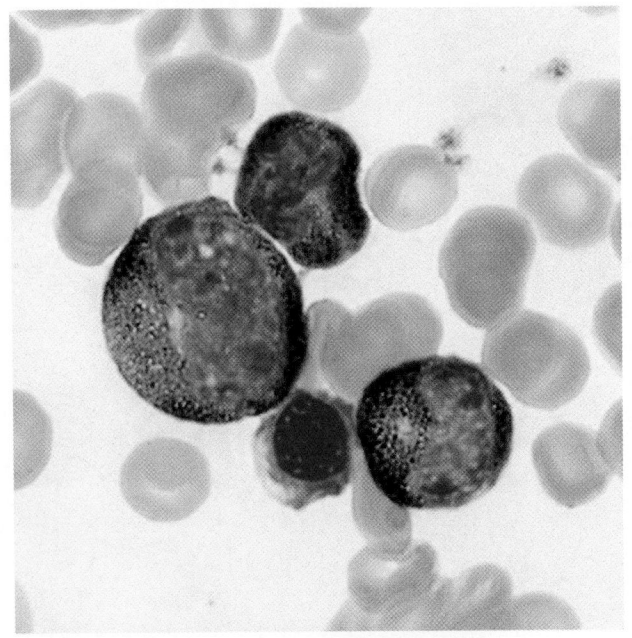

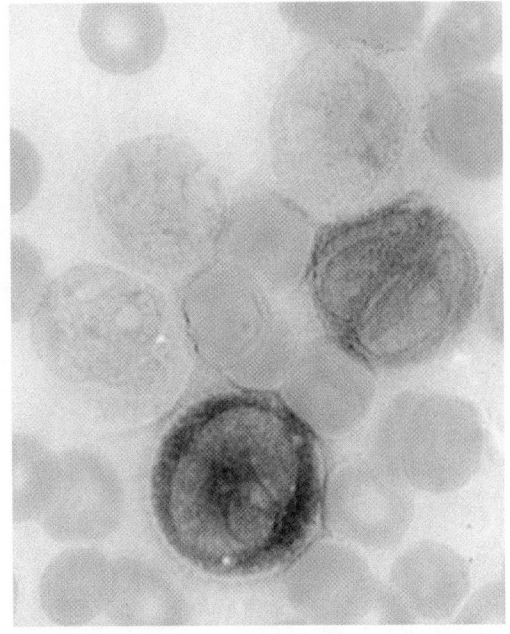

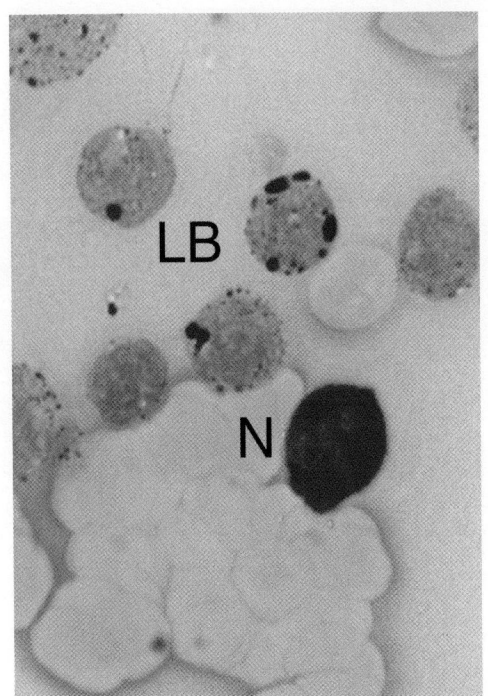

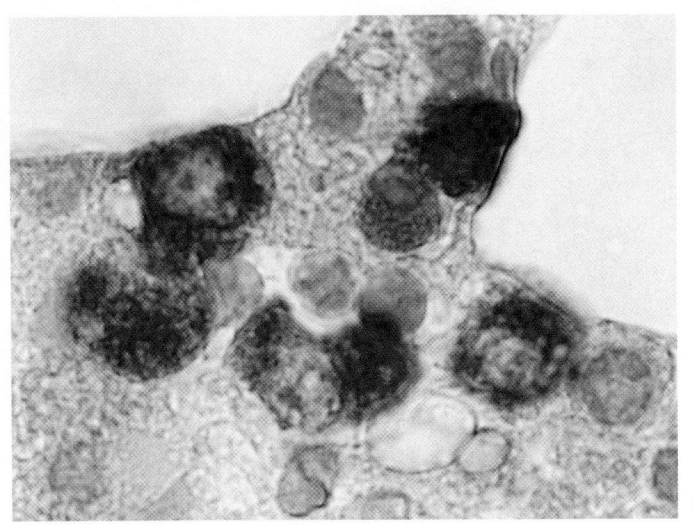

Color Figure 3-7. Histochemical stains. Granulocytes and myeloblasts positive for myeloperoxidase (myeloperoxidase; aspirate) **(A)**. Monocyte precursors positive for nonspecific esterase (nonspecific esterase; aspirate) **(B)**. Diffuse positivity of neutrophil (N) and block positivity of lymphoblast (LB) on periodic acid-Schiff stain (periodic acid-Schiff; aspirate) **(C)**. Neutrophilic myeloid precursors positive for chloroacetate esterase (chloroacetate esterase; biopsy) **(D)**. **A–D:** ×1000.

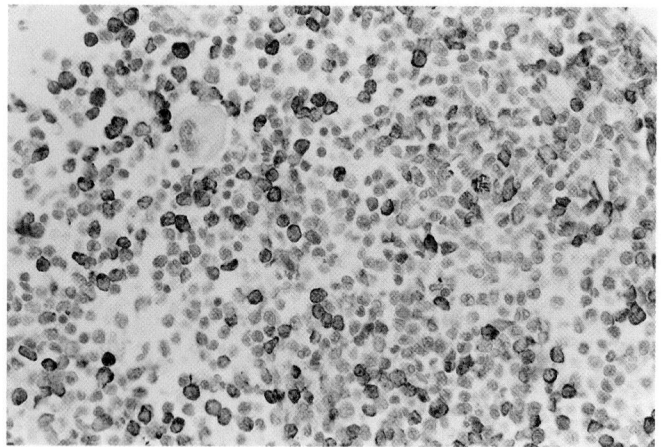

Color Figure 3-8. Immunohistochemical staining for CD34 in a case of acute myelogenous leukemia with 35% blasts (CD34; biopsy; ×200).

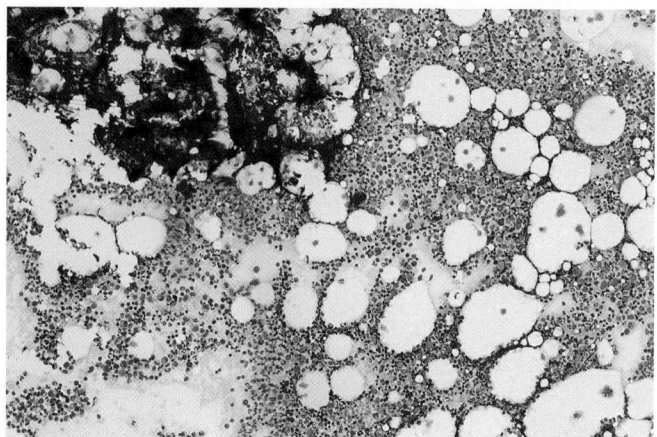

Color Figure 3-9. Normocellular bone marrow aspirate (Wright-Giemsa; aspirate; ×200).

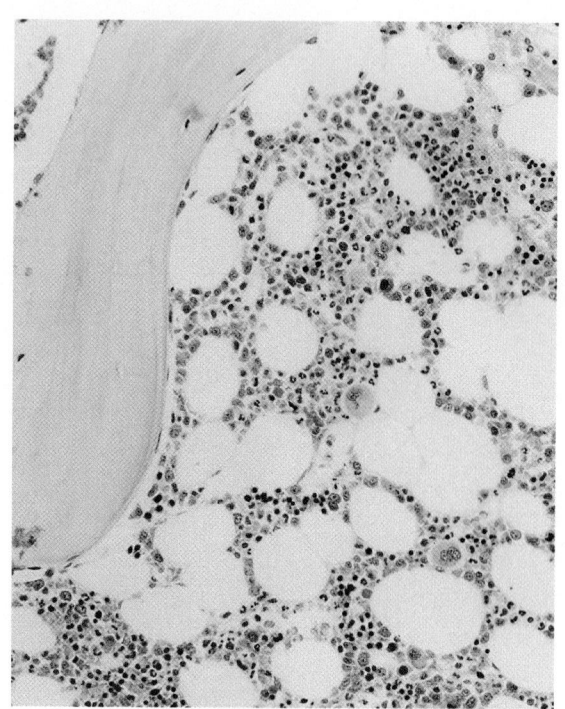

A

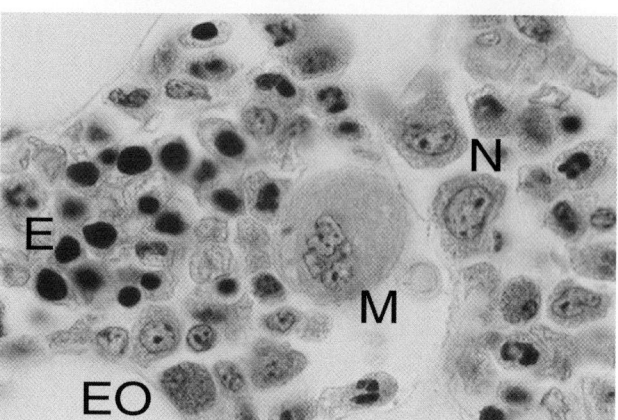

B

Color Figure 3-10. Normal bone marrow biopsy, showing distribution of hematopoietic cells, fat, and trabecular bone: erythroid precursors (E), neutrophil precursors (N), eosinophil precursor (EO), megakaryocyte (M). [Giemsa; biopsies; ×250 **(A)** and ×1000 **(B)**.]

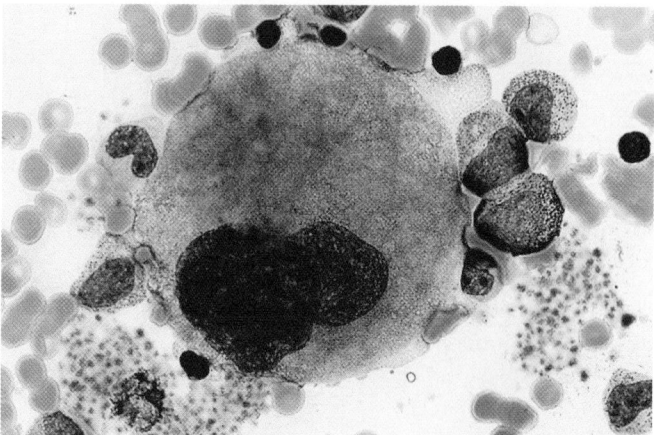

Color Figure 3-11. Megakaryocyte (Wright-Giemsa; aspirate; ×1000).

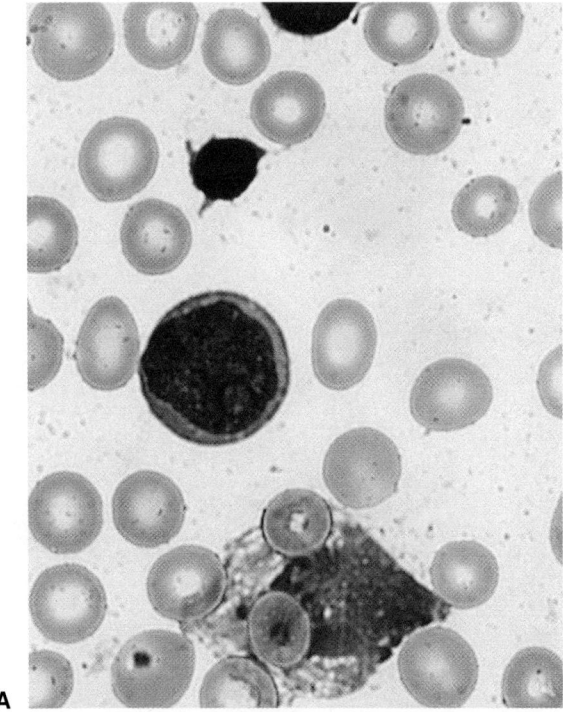

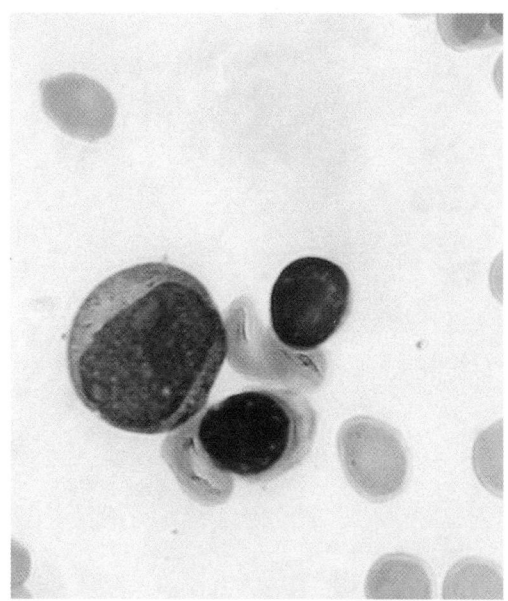

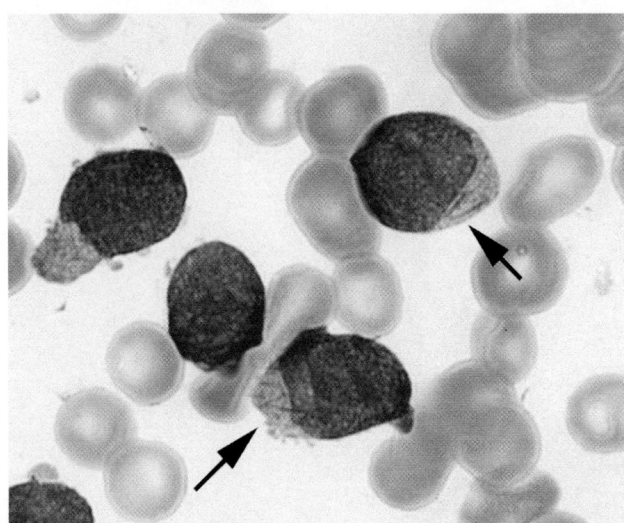

Color Figure 3-12. Myeloblasts in normal **(A, B)** and neoplastic **(C)** marrows. Note Auer rods (*arrows*). (Wright-Giemsa; aspirates; ×1000.)

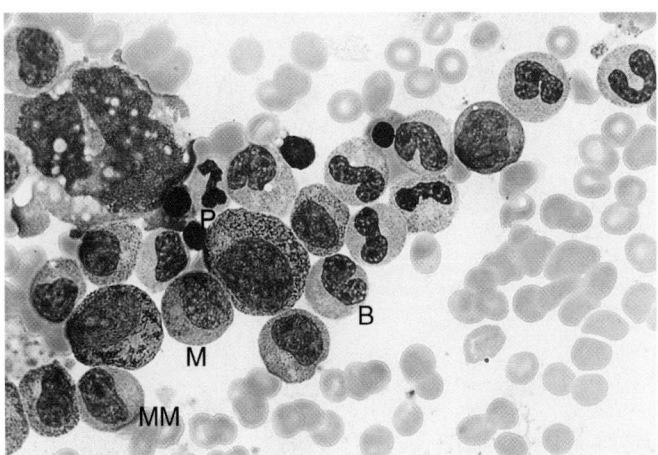

Color Figure 3-13. Neutrophilic maturation: promyelocyte (P), neutrophilic myelocyte (M), neutrophilic metamyelocyte (MM), band neutrophil (B). (Wright-Giemsa; aspirate; ×1000.)

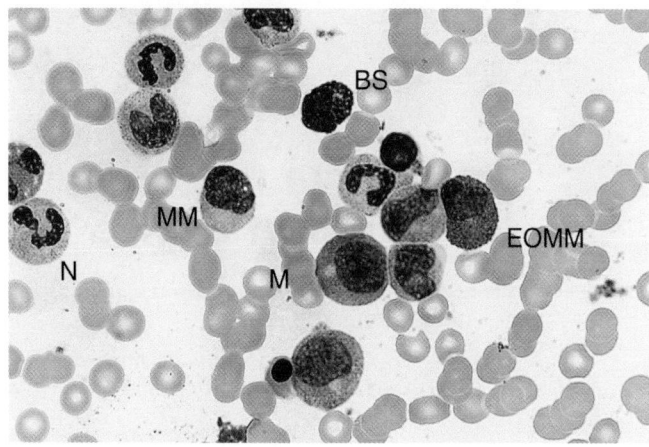

Color Figure 3-14. Myeloid maturation: neutrophilic myelocyte (M), neutrophilic metamyelocyte (MM), band neutrophil, segmented neutrophil (N), eosinophilic metamyelocyte (EOMM), basophil (BS). (Wright-Giemsa; aspirate; ×1000.)

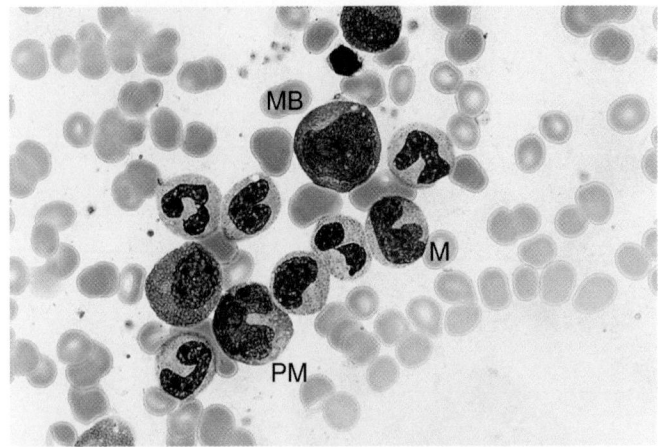

Color Figure 3-15. Monoblast (MB), promonocyte (PM), and monocyte (M) (Wright-Giemsa; aspirate; ×1000).

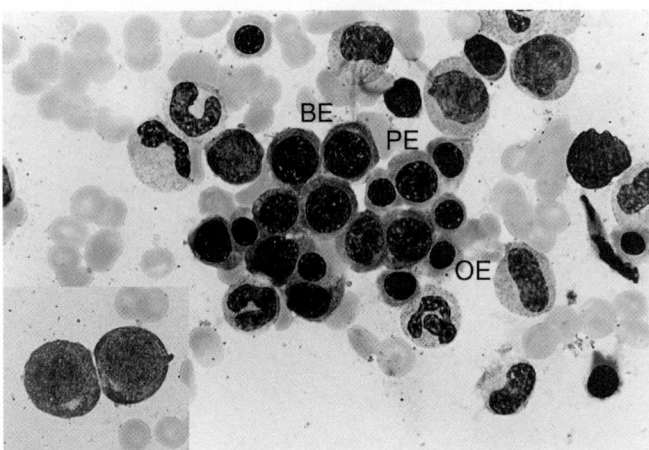

Color Figure 3-16. Erythroid maturation: proerythroblasts **(inset)**, basophilic erythroblast (BE), polychromatophilic erythroblasts (PE), and orthochromatic erythroblasts (OE) (Wright-Giemsa; aspirate; ×1000).

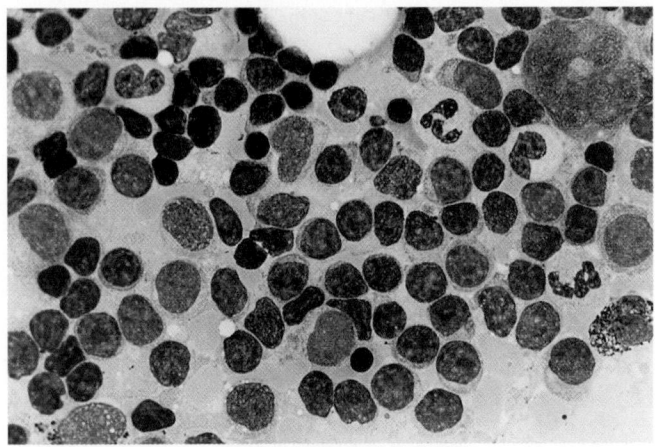

Color Figure 3-17. Reactive lymphoid aggregate (Wright-Giemsa; aspirate; ×1000).

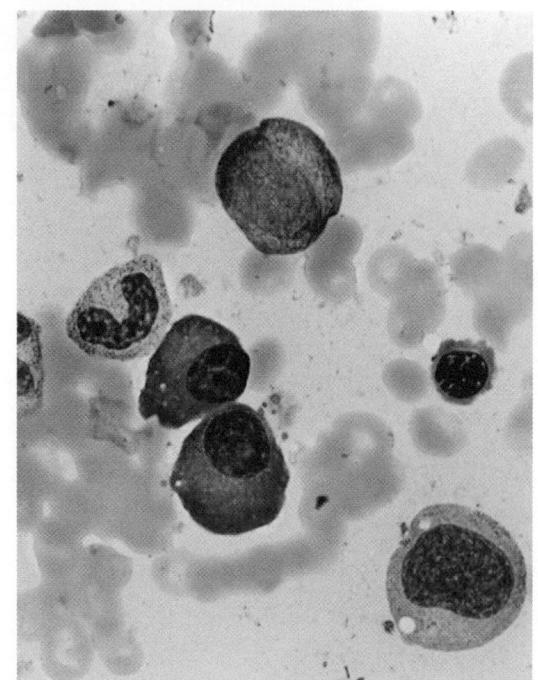

A

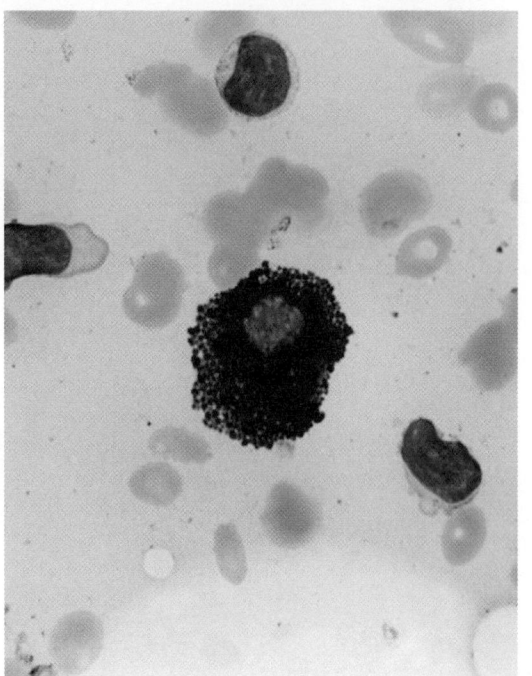

B

Color Figure 3-18. Plasma cells **(A)** and mast cell **(B)** (Wright-Giemsa; aspirates; ×1000).

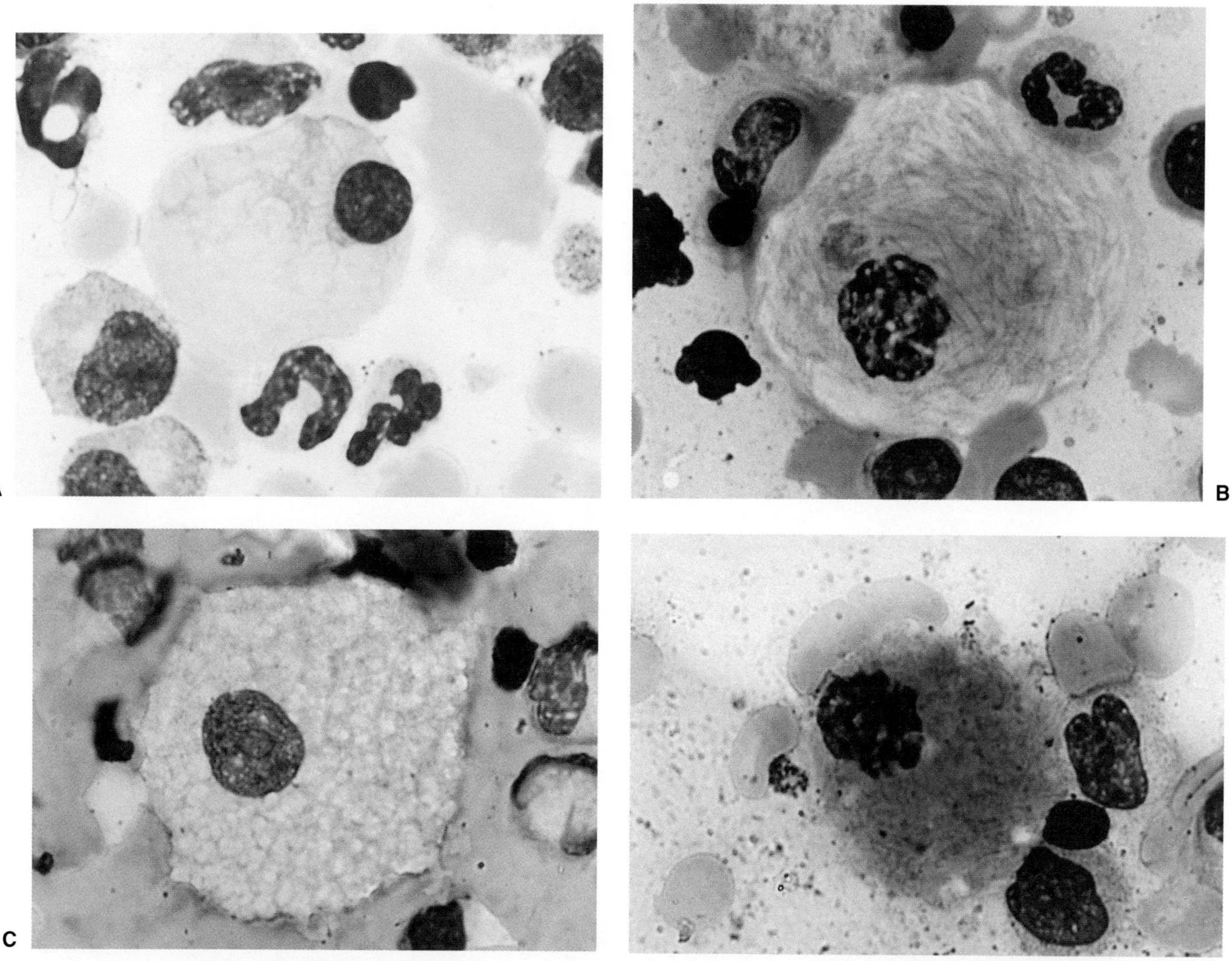

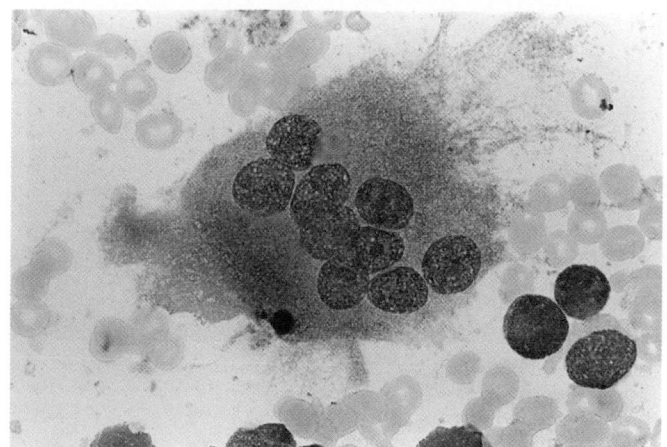

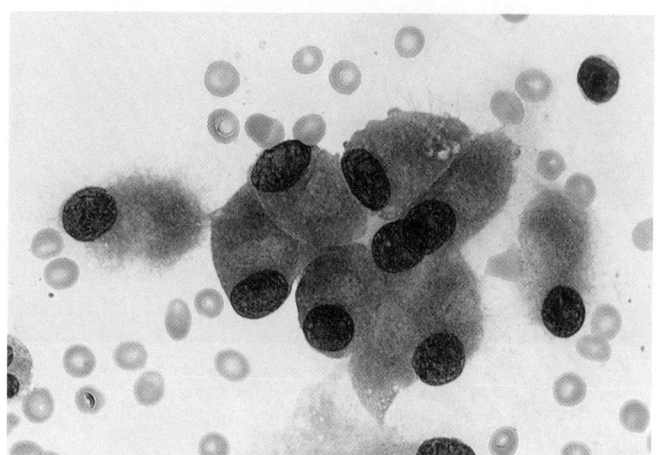

Color Figure 3-19. Histiocytes/macrophages: histiocyte **(A)**, Gaucher cell **(B)**, Niemann-Pick cell **(C)**, sea-blue histiocyte **(D)** (Wright-Giemsa; aspirates; ×1000).

Color Figure 3-20. Osteoclast (Wright-Giemsa; aspirate; ×1000).

Color Figure 3-21. Osteoblasts (Wright-Giemsa; aspirate; ×1000).

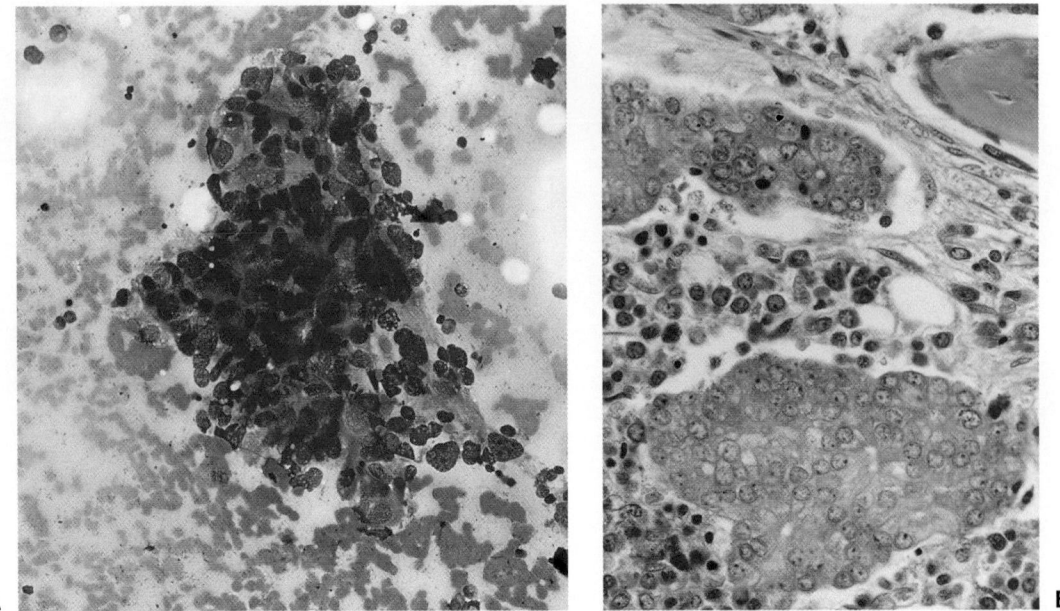

Color Figure 3-22. Metastatic prostate carcinoma aspirate (Wright-Giemsa; aspirate; ×400) **(A)** and biopsy (Giemsa; biopsy; ×400) **(B)**.

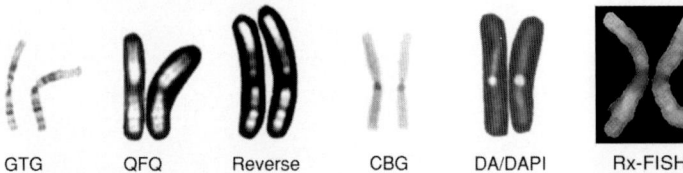

GTG QFQ Reverse CBG DA/DAPI Rx-FISH

Color Figure 5-3. Chromosome 1 shown after various banding techniques: GTG, QFQ, reverse, CBG, DA/DAPI, and cross-species color banding (Rx-fluorescence *in situ* hybridization).

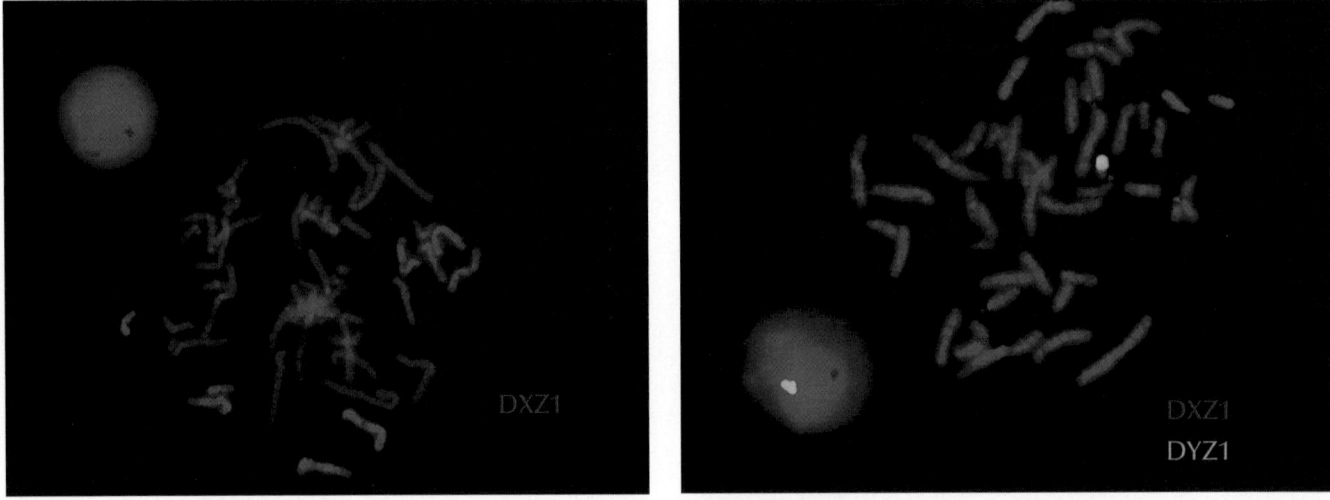

Color Figure 5-6. Interphase nuclei hybridized with probes for the X and Y chromosomes reveal disomy for the X chromosome (i.e., two red signals), designated nuc ish Xcen(DXZ1x2) **(A)** and monosomy for both the X and the Y chromosomes (i.e., one red and one green signal), designated nuc ish Xcen(DXZ1x1),Yq11.2(DYZ1x1) **(B)**.

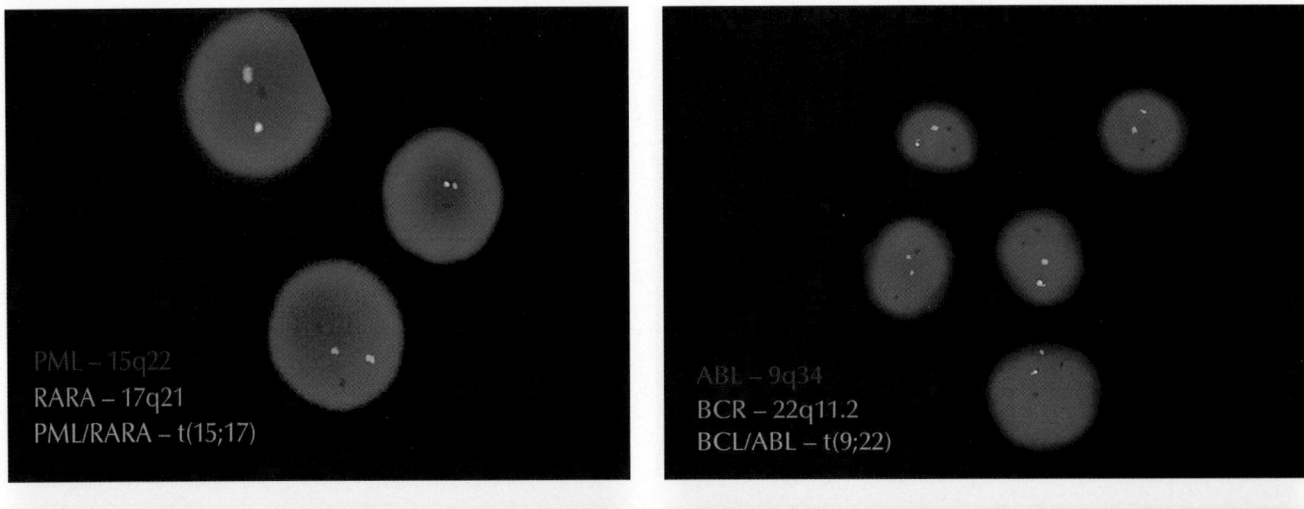

Color Figure 5-7. Locus-specific probes reveal recurrent breakpoints by fluorescence *in situ* hybridization. A single fusion probe is shown in **(A)** for detection of the *PML/RARA* fusion from a t(15;17)(q22;q21); this result is described as nuc ish 15q22(PMLx2),17q21(RARAx2)(PML con RARAx1). The *BCR/ABL* fusion from a t(9;22)(q34;q11.2) is detected by an extra-signal probe in **(B)**; this result is described as nuc ish 9q34(ABLx2),22q12(BCRx2)(ABL con BCRx1). A dual fusion probe is visualized in **(C)** for an *IGH/BCL2* fusion from a t(14;18)(q32;q21); this result is described as nuc ish 14q32(IGHx2)(IGH con BCL2x1),18q21(BCL2x2)(BCL2 con IGHx1). A break-apart probe reveals a rearrangement in the *MLL* gene **(D)**; this result is described as nuc ish 11q23(MLLx2)(5'MLL sep 3'MLLx1).

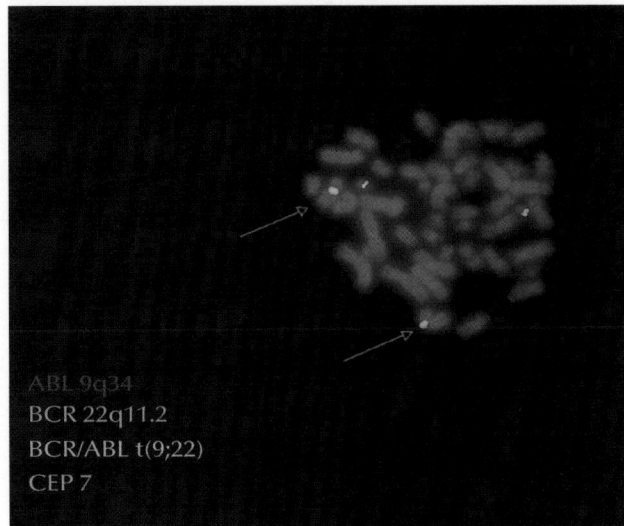

Color Figure 5-9. Fluorescence *in situ* hybridization studies reveal a *BCR/ABL* fusion in one copy of chromosome 22 and a deletion of *ABL* sequences on the der(9) detectable by the extra-signal probe for *ABL* that spans the breakpoint in *ABL*. This karyotype is described as 46,XY,t(7;8)(q22;q13).ish 9q34(ABLx1),22q11(BCRx2)(BCR con ABLx1).

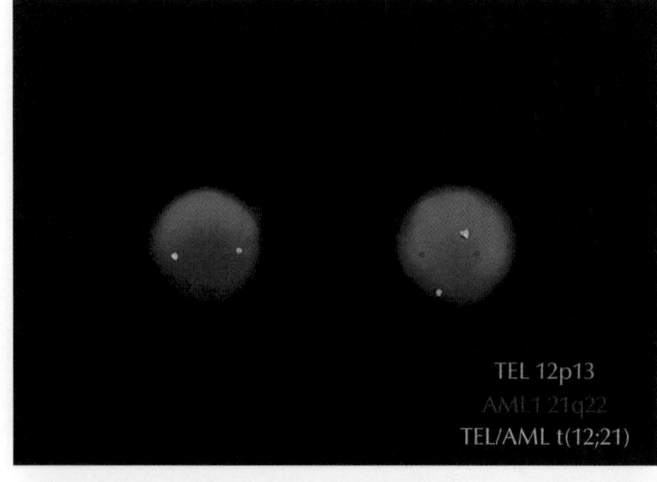

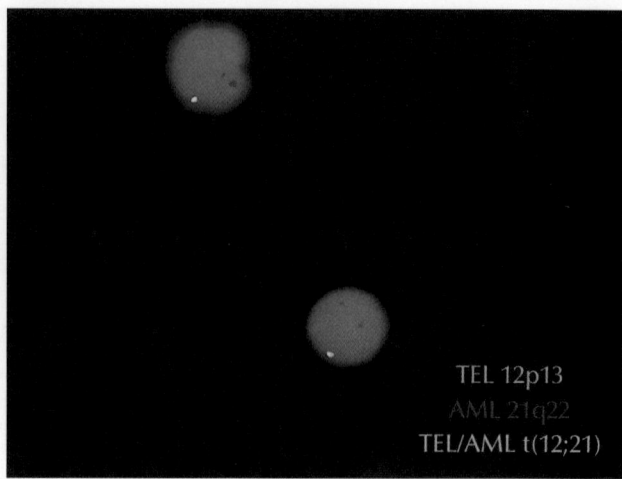

TEL 12p13
AML1 21q22
TEL/AML t(12;21)

A

TEL 12p13
AML 21q22
TEL/AML t(12;21)

B

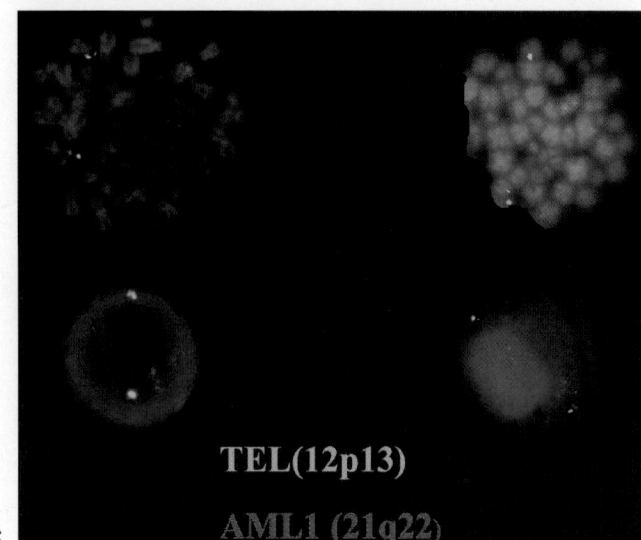

TEL(12p13)

AML1 (21q22)

C

Color Figure 5-12. Interphase nuclei hybridized with the *TEL/AML1* probe: *TEL* is indicated in green and *AML1* in red. A typical rearrangement is detected in **(A)** and is described using the International System for Human Cytogenetic Nomenclature 1995 as nuc ish 12p13(TELx2),21q22(AML1x2)(TEL con AML1x1). A hybridization pattern is observed in **(B)**, indicating a fusion between chromosomes 12 and 21 (yellow signal) and a deletion of the other copy of *TEL* (no green signal). One of the red signals representing the translocated copy of *AML1* is diminished in size due to a portion of the probe residing in the fusion signal. This fluorescence *in situ* hybridization result is described as nuc ish 12p13(TELx1), 21q22(AML1x2)(TEL con AML1x1). In **(C)**, multiple red signals are present, representing amplification of *AML1*, and this finding is described as nuc ish 21q22(AML1amp).

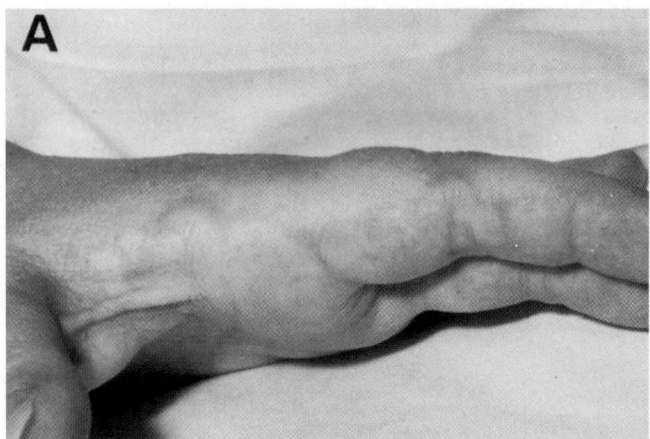

A

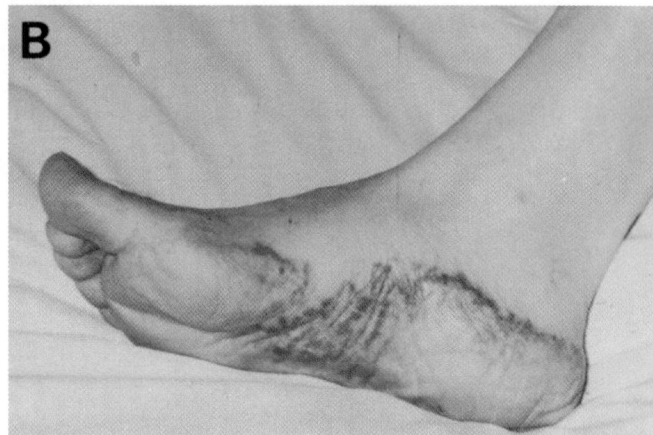

B

Color Figure 9-8. Serum sickness rash of the hand **(A)** and foot **(B)**. If the patient has severe thrombocytopenia, petechiae may etch the serpiginous margin between volar and dorsal surfaces.

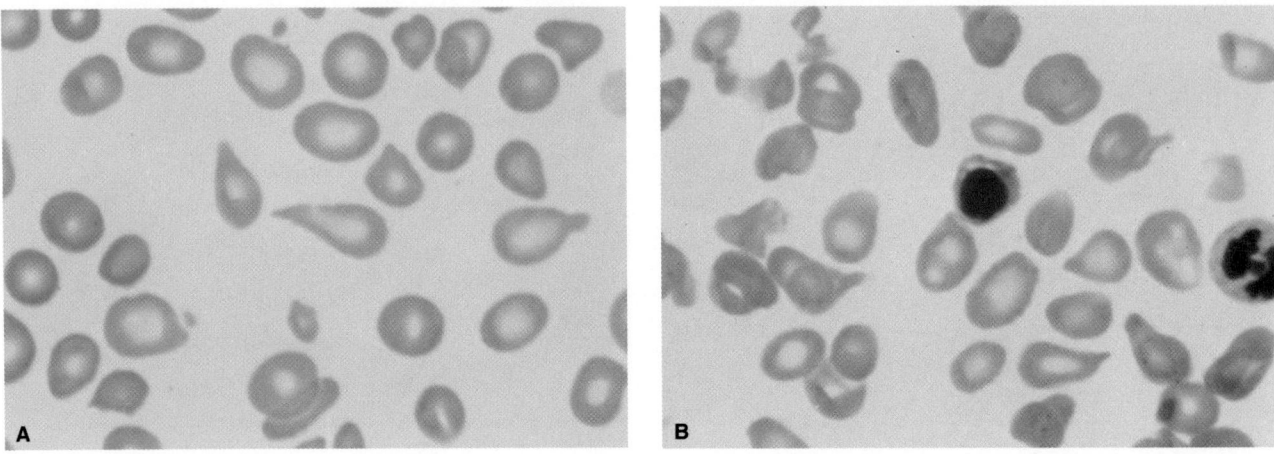

Color Figure 12-14. Teardrop-shaped red blood cells (RBCs), poikilocytes (**A** and **B**), and a nucleated RBC (**B**) from the blood of a patient with myofibrosis (Wright's stain, ×1000).

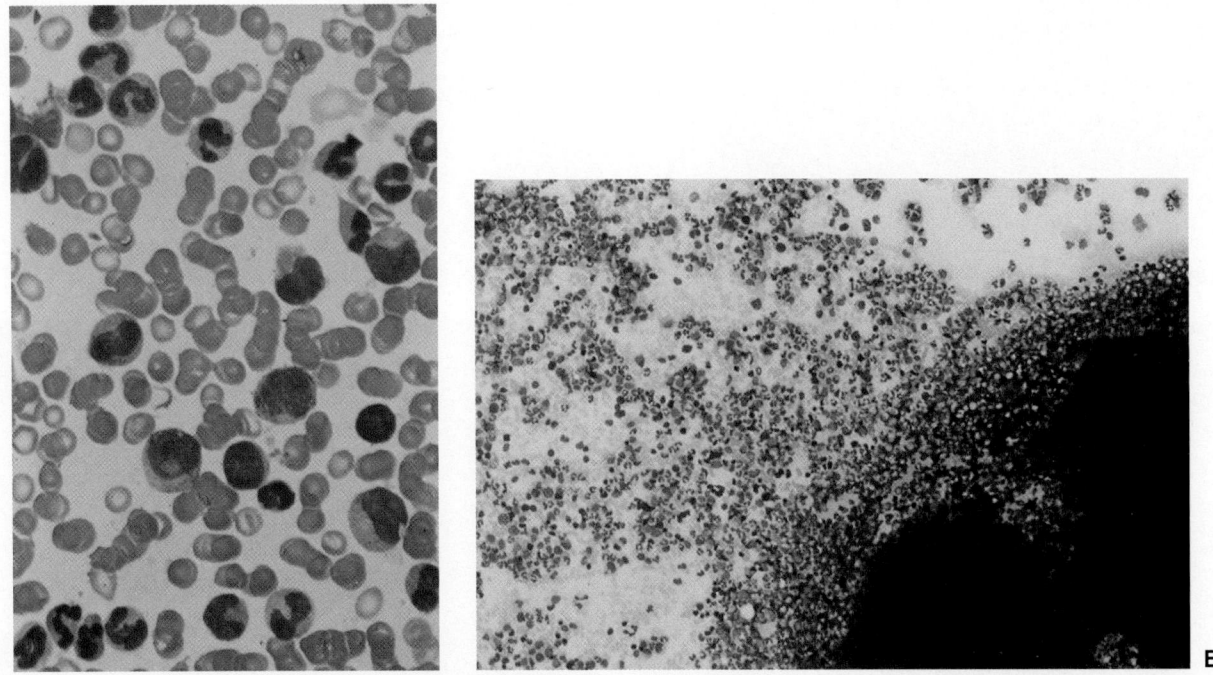

Color Figure 13-3. Photomicrographs of a blood peripheral smear (**A**) and bone marrow aspiration (**B**) from a patient with chronic myelogenous leukemia. The peripheral blood smear reveals the presence of multiple mature and immature myeloid forms and an increased number of eosinophils and basophils. Bone marrow is hypercellular, with excess myeloid precursors, megakaryocytes, and mild fibrosis.

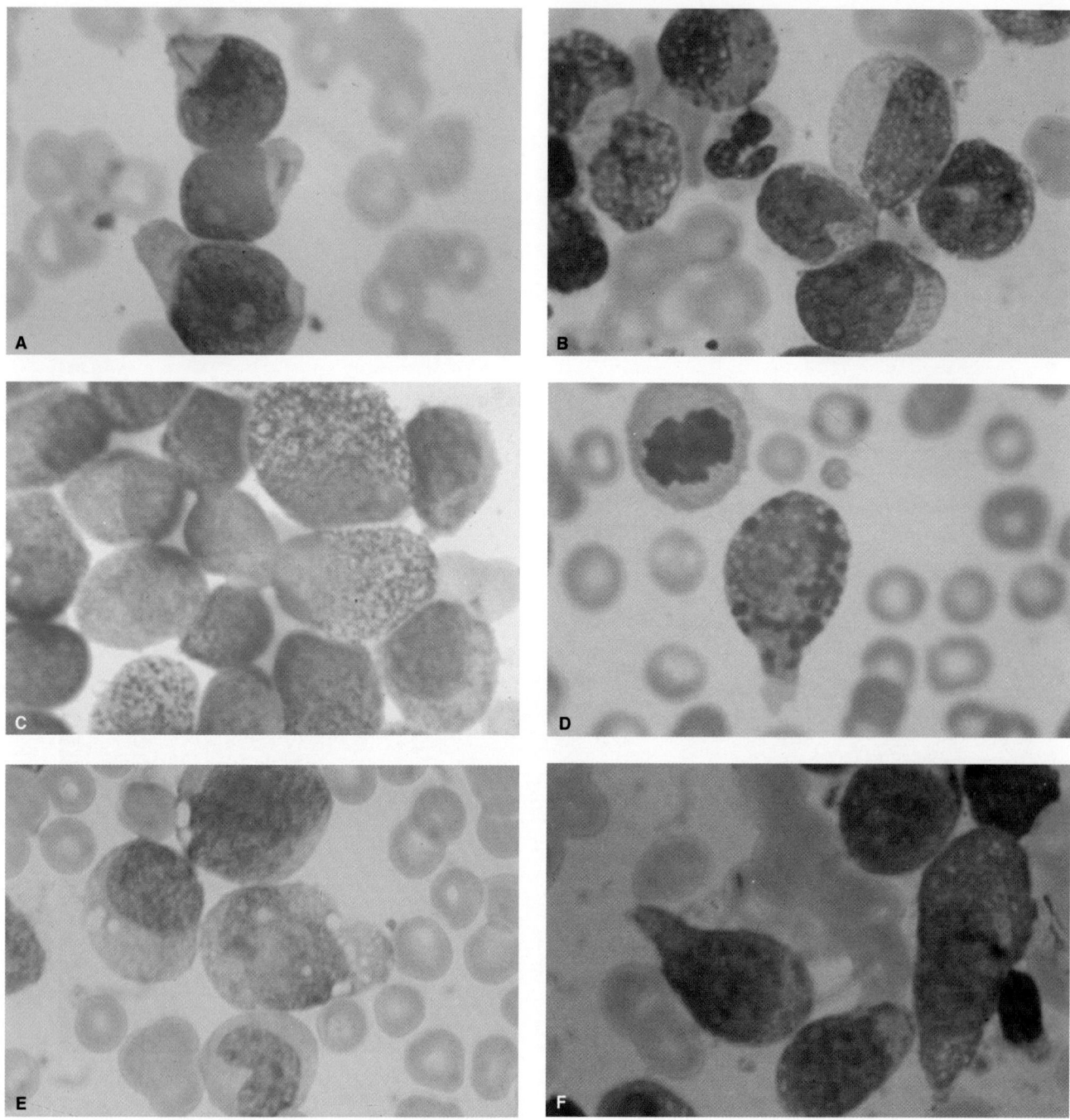

Color Figure 15-1. Morphologic appearance of bone marrow in Wright-Giemsa–stained films for each French/American/British type of acute myelogenous leukemia. **A:** M1: myeloblastic without maturation; the blasts contain Auer rods. **B:** M2: myeloblastic with maturation. **C:** M3: hypergranular promyelocytic. **D:** M4: myelomonocytic. **E:** M4Eo: myelomonocytic with abnormal eosinophilic and basophilic granules. **F:** M5: monocytic. (*continued*)

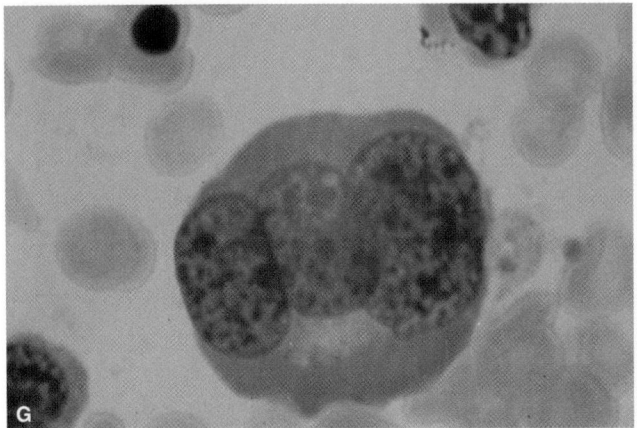

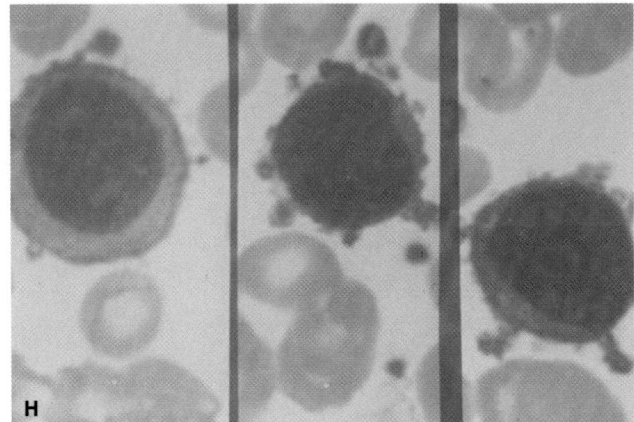

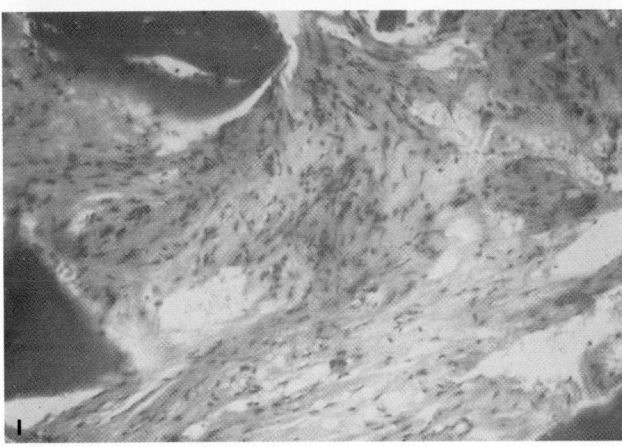

Color Figure 15-1. (*continued*) **G:** M6: erythroleukemic. **H:** M7: megakaryoblastic. **I:** M7: myelofibrotic. (Courtesy of Pearl Leavitt and Dr. Arthur Skarin, Dana-Farber Cancer Institute, Boston.)

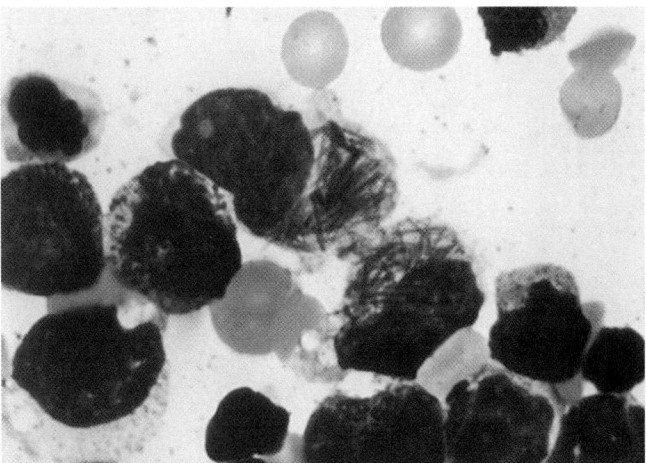

Color Figure 15-2. Fagot cell containing numerous Auer rods in the bone marrow aspirate from a patient with acute promyelocytic leukemia (French/American/British M3). (Courtesy of Dr. Martin Tallman, Northwestern University Medical School, Chicago.)

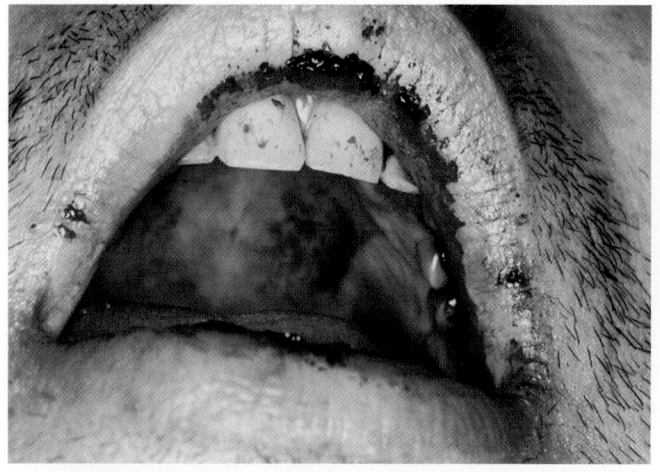

A

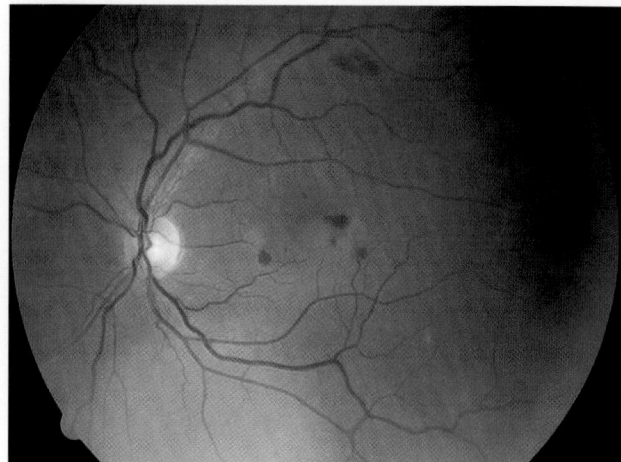

B

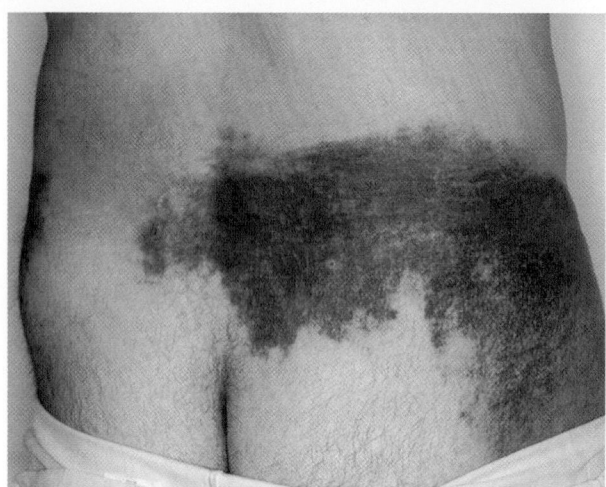

C

Color Figure 15-6. Various hemorrhagic complications at presentation in patients with acute promyelocytic leukemia, including **(A)** oral mucosal bleeding, **(B)** retina hemorrhages, and **(C)** extensive subcutaneous bleeding.

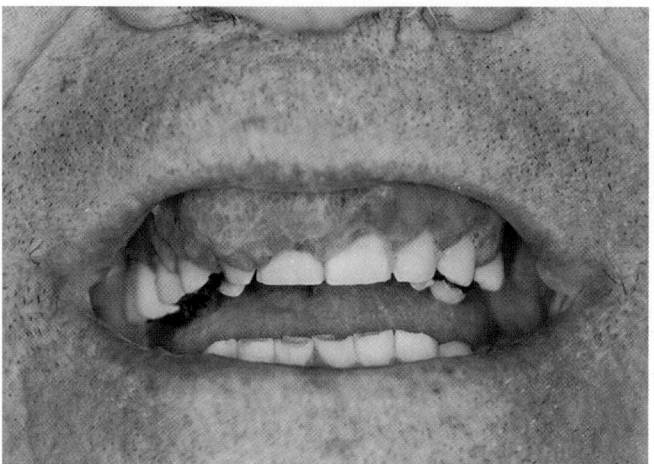

Color Figure 15-7. Gingival hypertrophy in a patient with French/American/British M5. (Courtesy of Dr. Martin Tallman, Northwestern University Medical School, Chicago.)

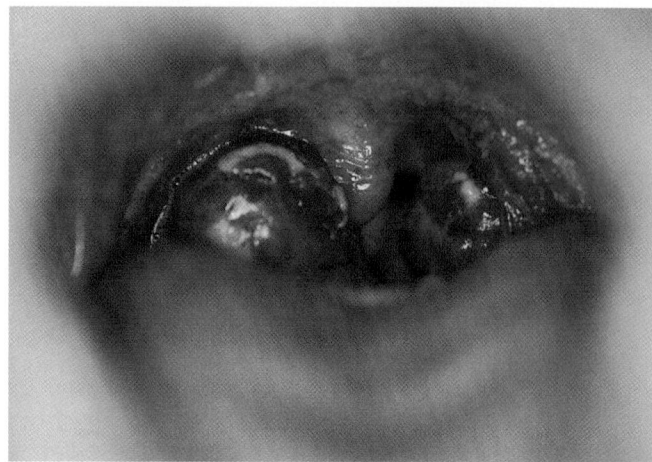

Color Figure 15-8. Bilateral tonsillar enlargement and skin rash in a patient with M5a. (Courtesy of Dr. Martin Tallman, Northwestern University Medical School, Chicago.)

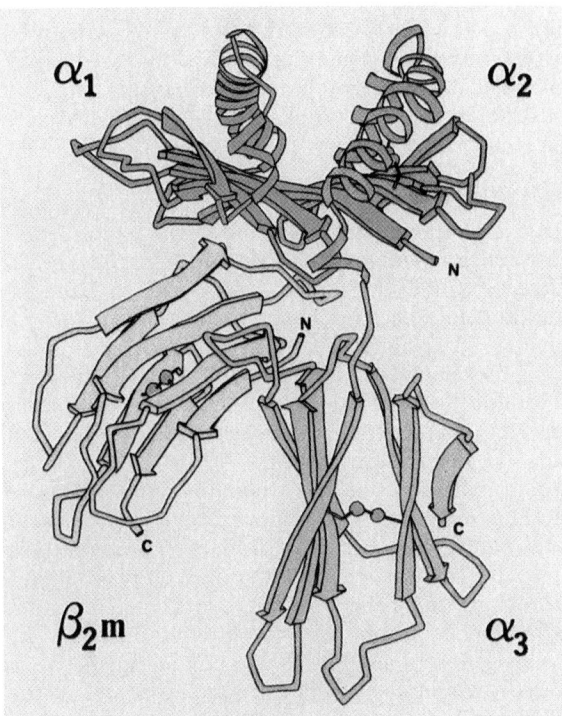

Color Figure 19-4. Schematic representation of an HLA class I molecule. Ribbon diagram of a class I molecule showing the four domains. The α_3- and β_2-microglobulin domains proximal to the cell membrane are shown at the bottom, and the polymorphic α_1 and α_2 domains are shown at the top. The β strands are indicated as wide arrows, whereas α-helical portions are shown as coiled ribbons. N, N-terminus; C, C-terminus.

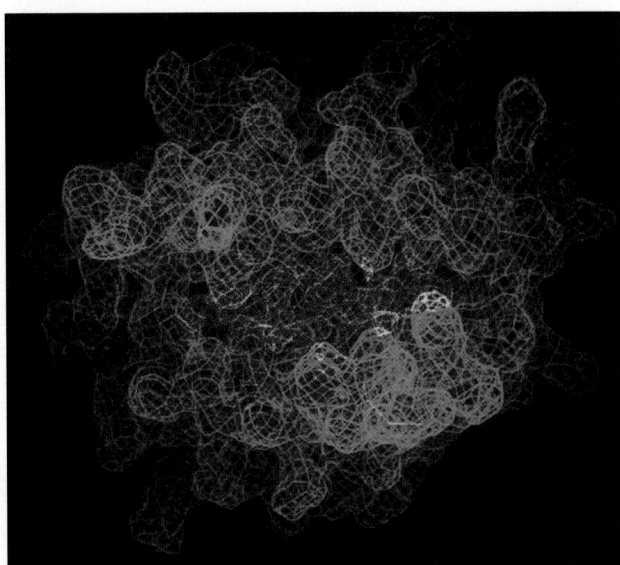

Color Figure 19-6. Electron density map of an HLA-A2 molecule. van der Waals surface representation of the top of an HLA-A2 molecule (*blue*), showing the antigen-binding groove and electron dense material (*pink*) representing bound peptide. (Reprinted from Bjorkman PJ, Saper MA, Samrowi B, et al. Structure of the human class I histocompatibility antigen, HLA-A2. *Nature* 1987;329:506–512. http://www. nature.com, with permission.)

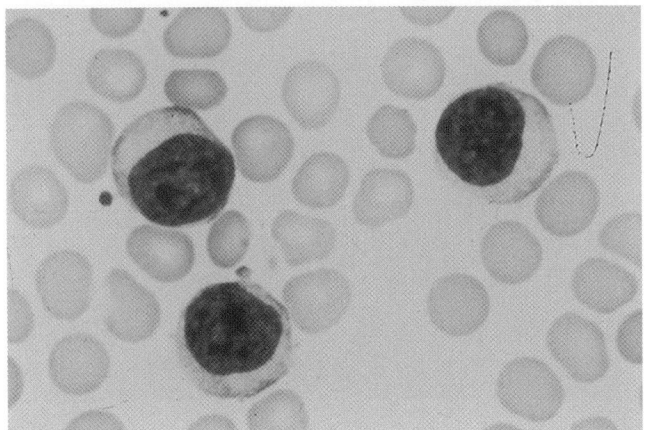

Color Figure 26-3. Peripheral blood, chronic lymphocytic leukemia (Wright-Giemsa stain; ×400).

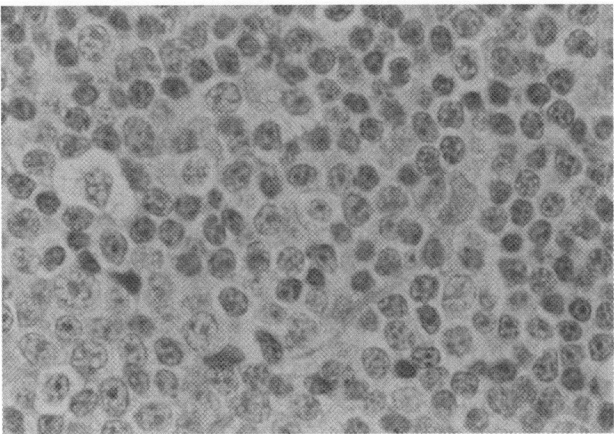

Color Figure 26-4. Lymph node of patient with malignant small cell lymphocytic lymphoma (hematoxylin and eosin stain; ×100).

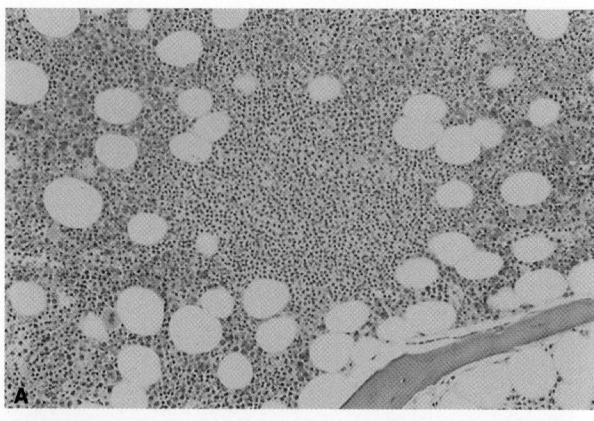

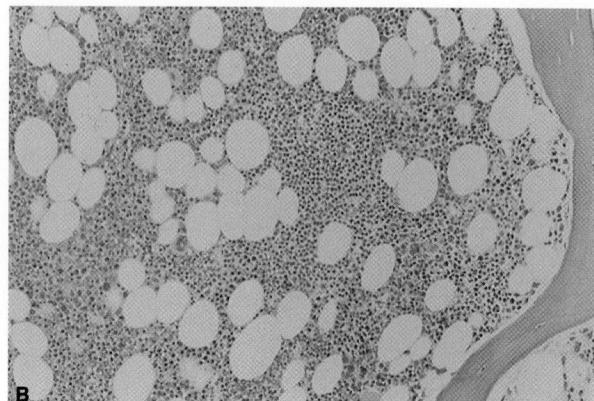

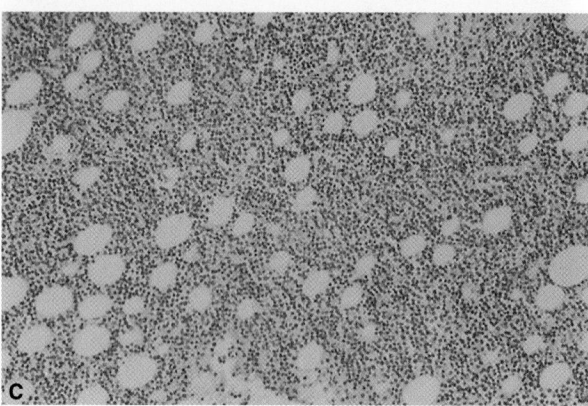

Color Figure 26-5. Bone marrow of patient with chronic lymphocytic leukemia: nodular **(A)**, interstitial **(B)**, diffuse **(C)** (hematoxylin and eosin stain; ×160).

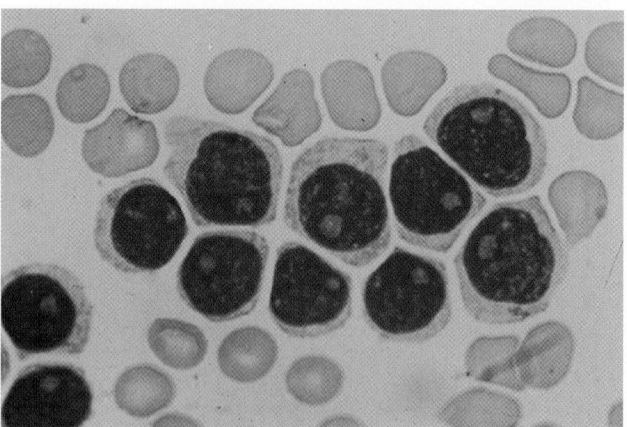

Color Figure 26-6. Peripheral blood of patient with prolymphocytic leukemia (Wright-Giemsa stain; ×400).

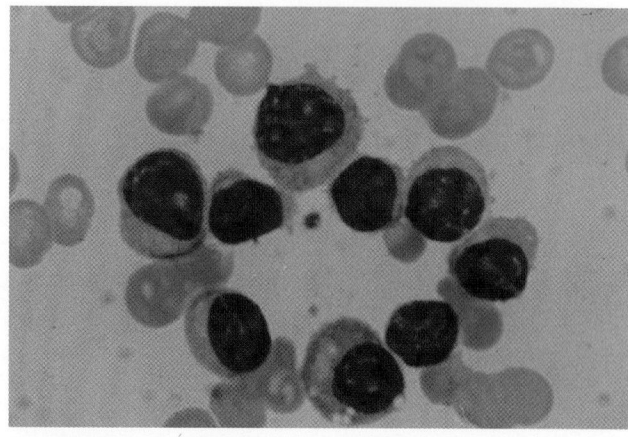

Color Figure 26-7. Peripheral blood of patient with Waldenström's macroglobulinemia (Wright-Giemsa stain; ×400).

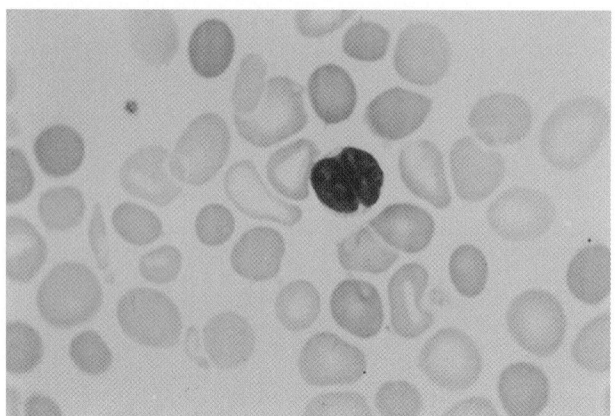

Color Figure 26-8. Peripheral blood of patient with small cleaved-cell lymphoma (Wright-Giemsa stain; ×400).

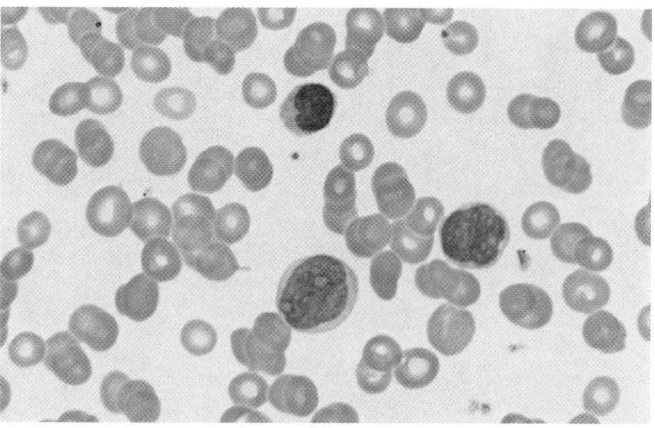

Color Figure 26-9. Peripheral blood of a patient with mantle cell lymphoma in the leukemic phase (Wright-Giemsa stain; ×400).

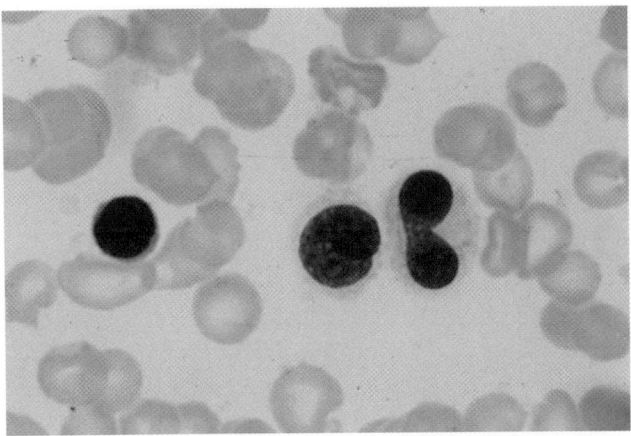

Color Figure 26-10. Peripheral blood of patient with hairy cell leukemia (Wright-Giemsa stain; ×400).

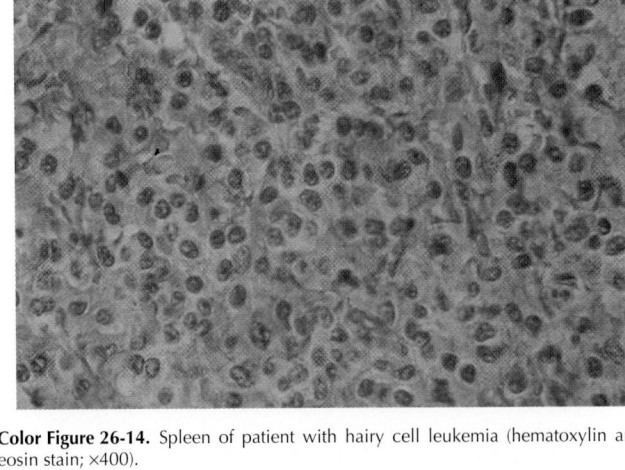

Color Figure 26-14. Spleen of patient with hairy cell leukemia (hematoxylin and eosin stain; ×400).

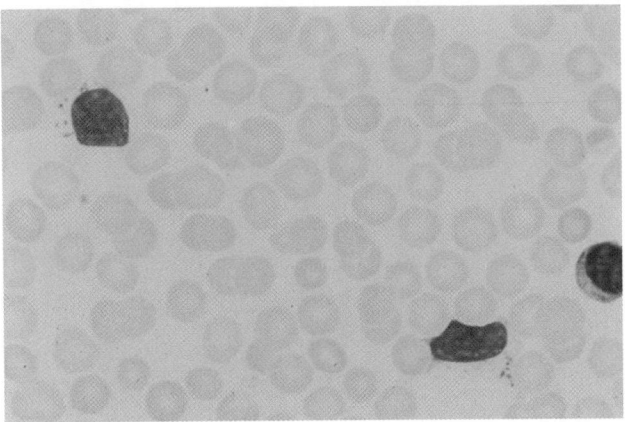

Color Figure 26-12. Peripheral blood of patient with large granular lymphocytic leukemia (Wright-Giemsa stain; ×400).

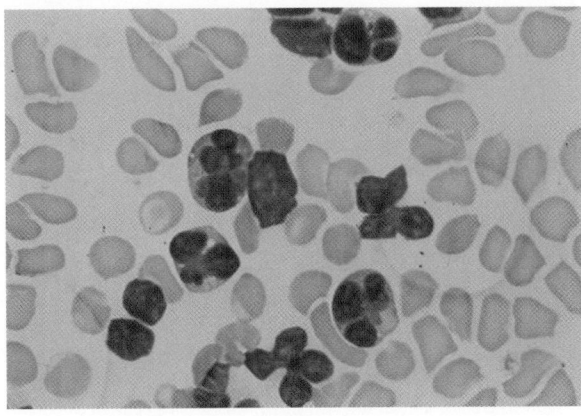

Color Figure 26-15. Peripheral blood of patient with adult T-cell leukemia (Wright-Giemsa stain; ×400).

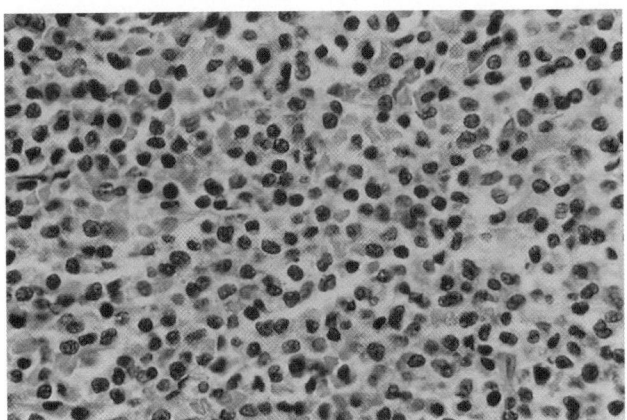

Color Figure 26-13. Bone marrow of patient with hairy cell leukemia (hematoxylin and eosin stain; ×100).

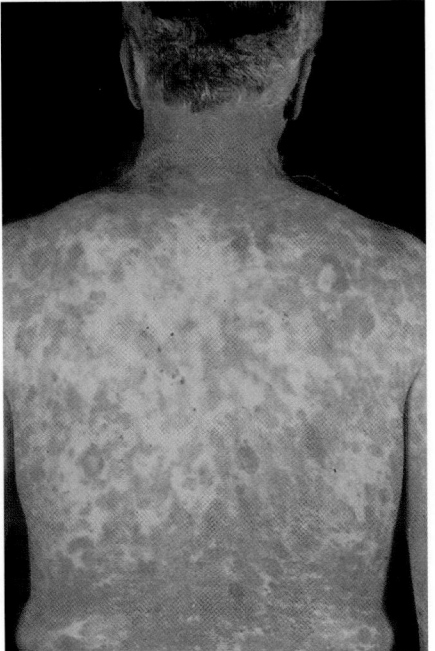

Color Figure 26-16. Multiple discrete and confluent plaques of cutaneous T-cell lymphoma.

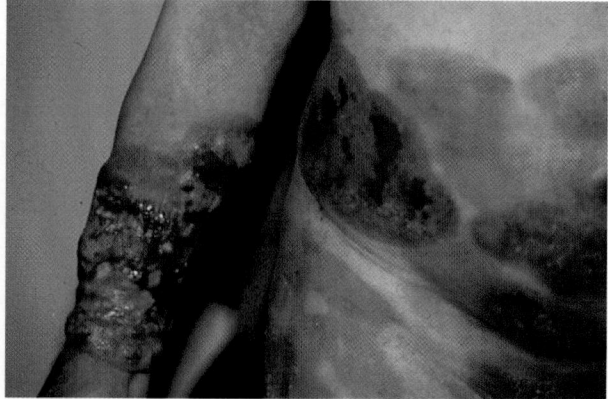

Color Figure 26-17. Multiple plaques of cutaneous T-cell lymphoma with tumor formation.

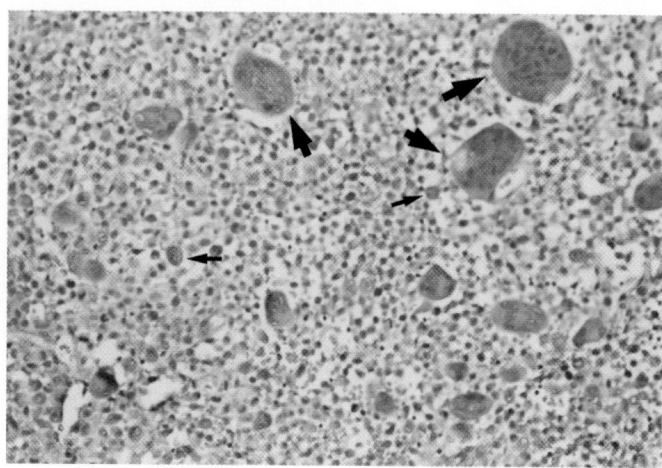

Color Figure 30-2. Photomicrograph showing a typical infiltrate observed in Langerhans' cell histiocytosis, including numerous dendritic cells, eosinophils, and multinucleated giant cells (*arrows*).

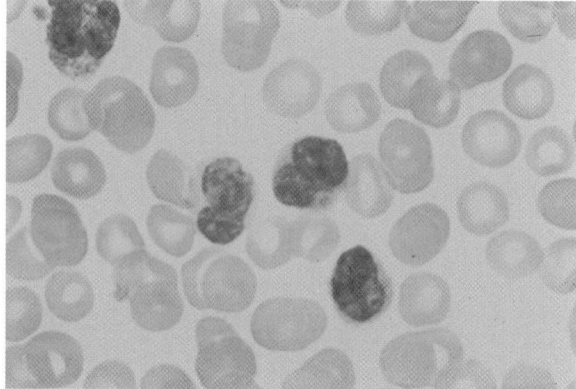

Color Figure 26-18. Peripheral blood of patient with cutaneous T-cell lymphoma, showing Sézary cells (Wright-Giemsa stain; ×400).

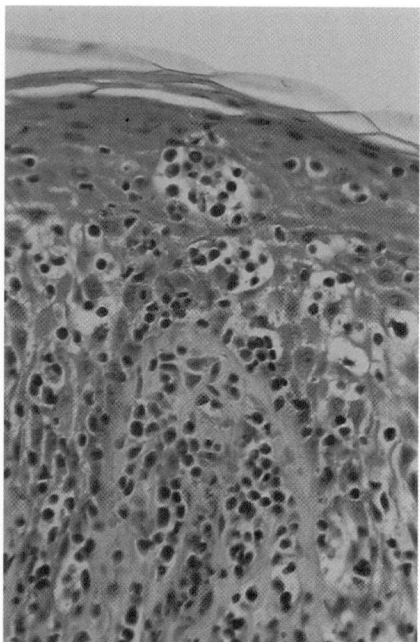

Color Figure 26-19. Pautrier microabscess (hematoxylin and eosin stain; ×100).

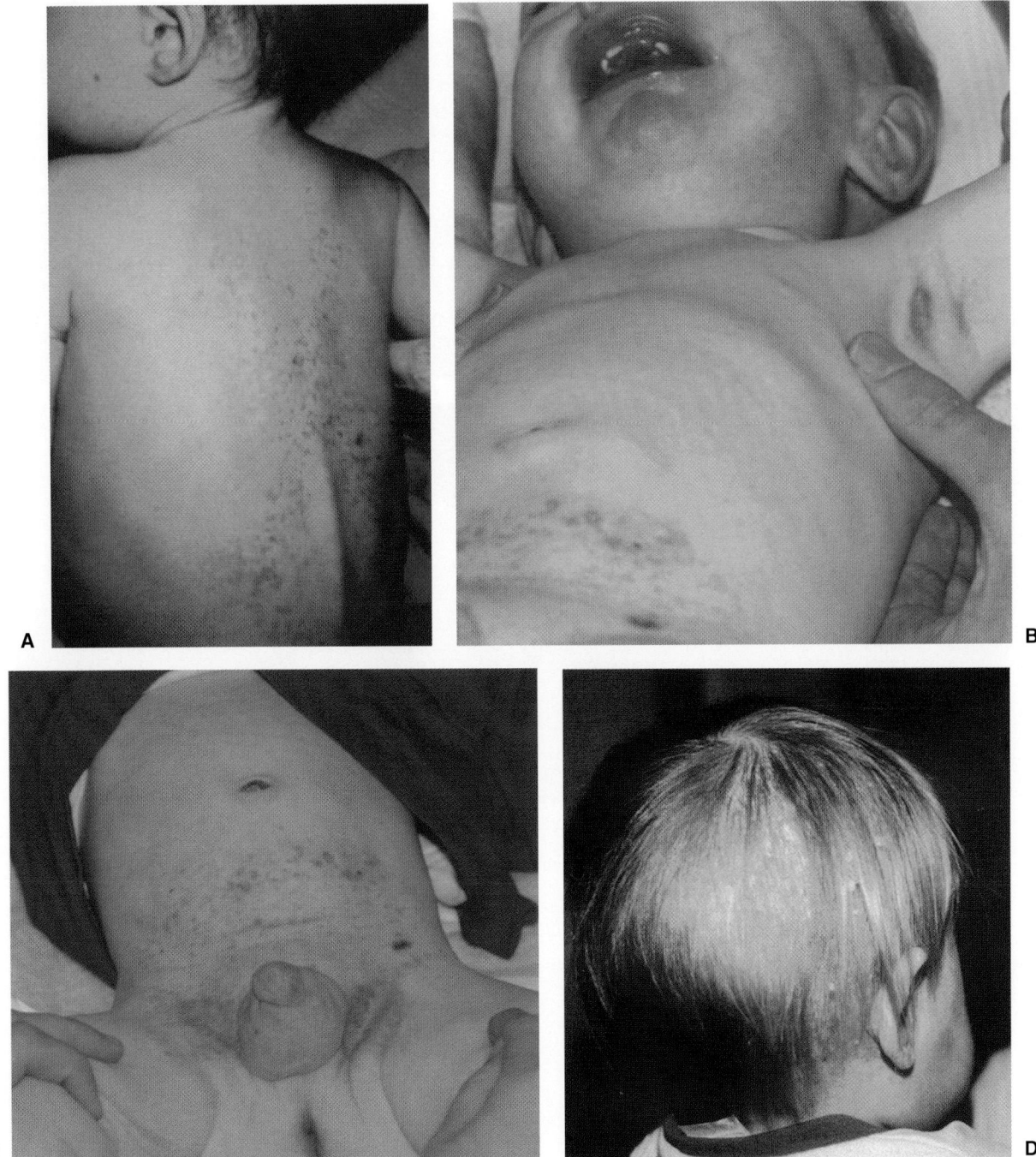

Color Figure 30-4. Different presentations of skin involvement in Langerhans' cell histiocytosis. **A:** The maculopapular rash often observed in patients with Letterer-Siwe disease. (Courtesy of Steven Gellis, MD, Department of Dermatology, Children's Hospital, Boston.) **B:** Langerhans' cell histiocytosis involving the lower abdomen, axilla, and upper gum in an infant. **C:** Langerhans' cell histiocytosis involving the abdomen, umbilicus, inguinal, and anal regions in an infant. **D:** Langerhans' cell histiocytosis of the scalp in a toddler.

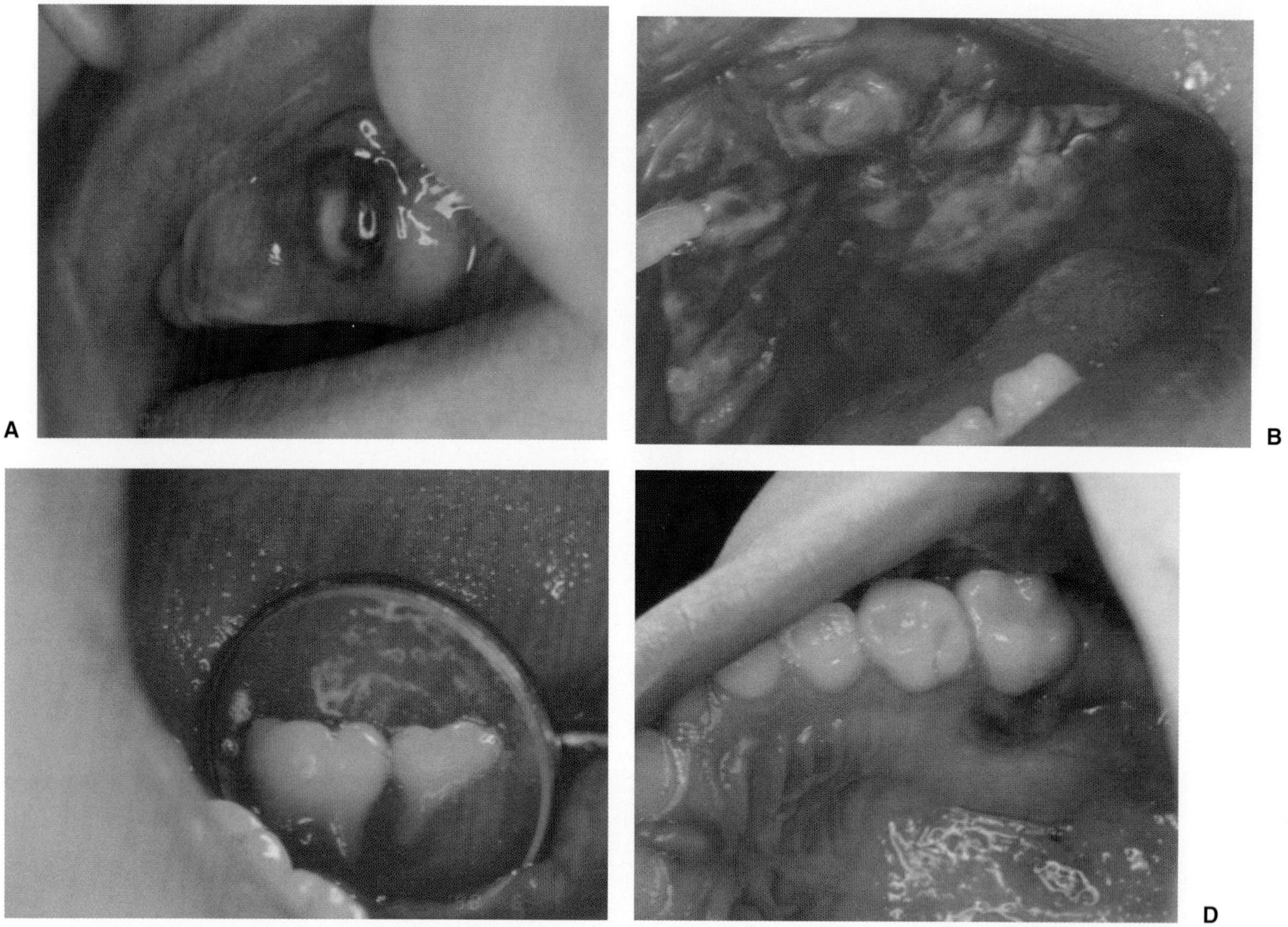

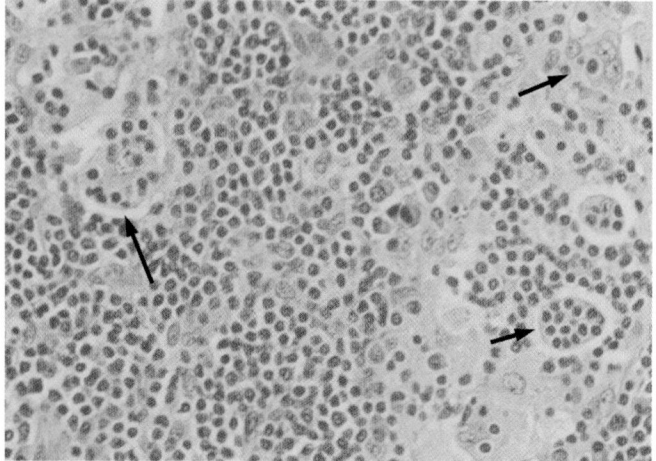

Color Figure 30-5. Oral lesions observed in Langerhans' cell histiocytosis. **A:** Predentate anterior gum infiltrative lesion. **B:** Severe infiltrative disease of palate in infancy. **C:** Localized bony destruction exposing roots of primary posterior mandibular molars. **D:** Localized palatal lesion in an older child. (Courtesy of Dr. Howard Needleman, Department of Dentistry, Children's Hospital, Boston.)

Color Figure 30-11. Histopathology of a biopsy from a patient (depicted in Fig. 30-10) with sinus histiocytosis with massive lymphadenopathy, or Rosai-Dorfman disease. In addition to the infiltrate and proliferation of reactive histiocytes, the entrapment of lymphocytes by some of the macrophages (termed *emperiopolesis*) can be seen (*arrows*).

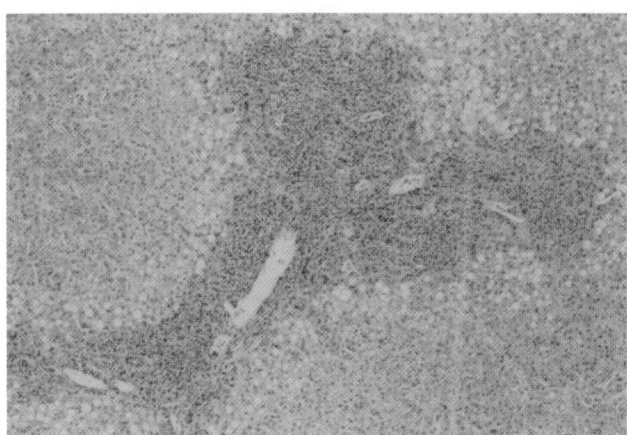

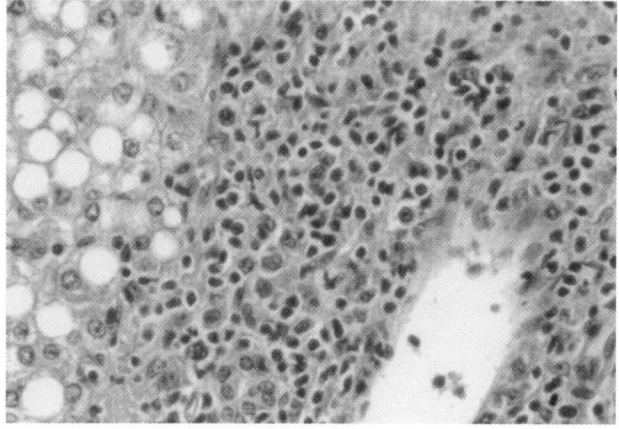

Color Figure 30-12. Pathologic biopsy specimen of liver, demonstrating low-power (**A**) and high-power (**B**) microscopic views of the lymphohistiocytic infiltrate in portal areas in a patient with familial erythrophagocytic lymphohistiocytosis.

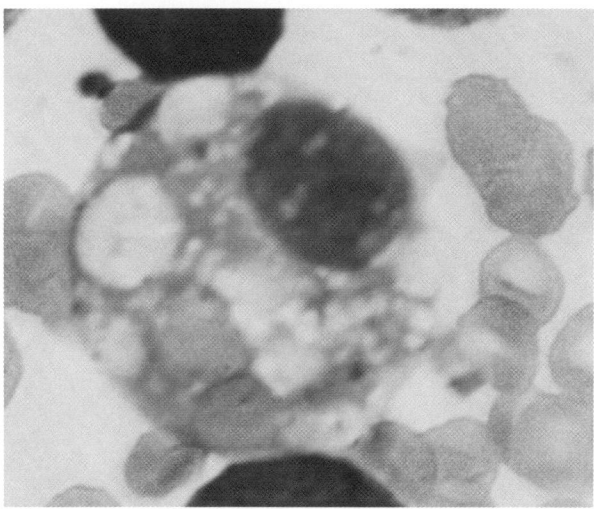

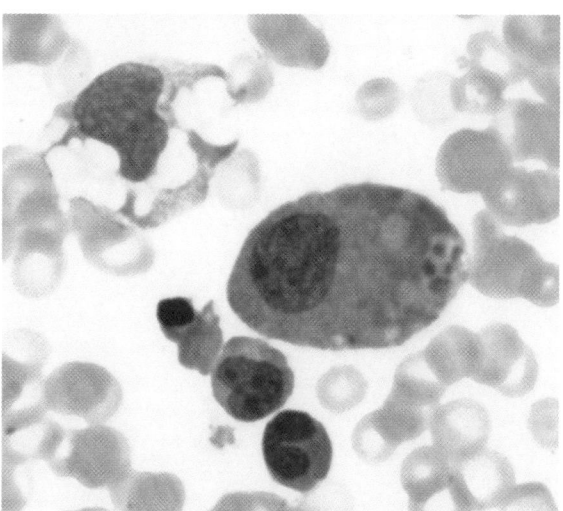

Color Figure 30-13. Examples of hemophagocytosis in a patient with histiocytic medullary reticulosis. **A:** The macrophage has multiple lysosomal vacuoles with debris from cell fragments as well as evidence for erythrophagocytosis. **B:** The macrophages in the upper left of the photograph show lysosomal vacuoles with cellular debris, whereas the macrophage in the lower right part of the photograph shows ingestion of red blood cells and platelets.

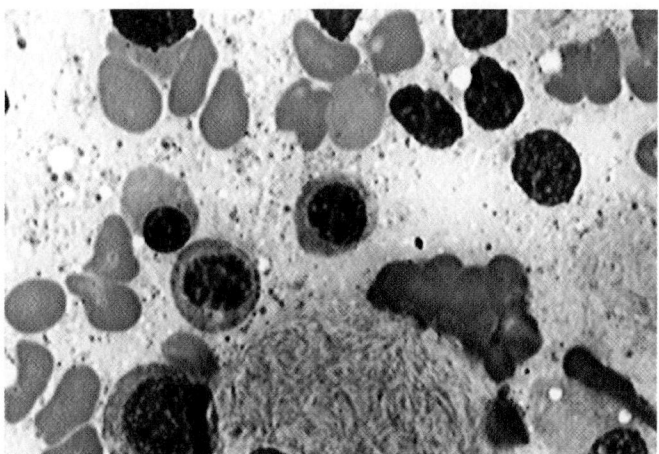

Color Figure 30-15. Typical Gaucher cells (containing inclusion bodies with an elongated appearance) that fill the cytoplasm. Cells are not "soap-bubble"-like as are Niemann-Pick cells (see Fig. 30-18). Rather, the cells are striated with eccentric nuclei and a delicate nature.

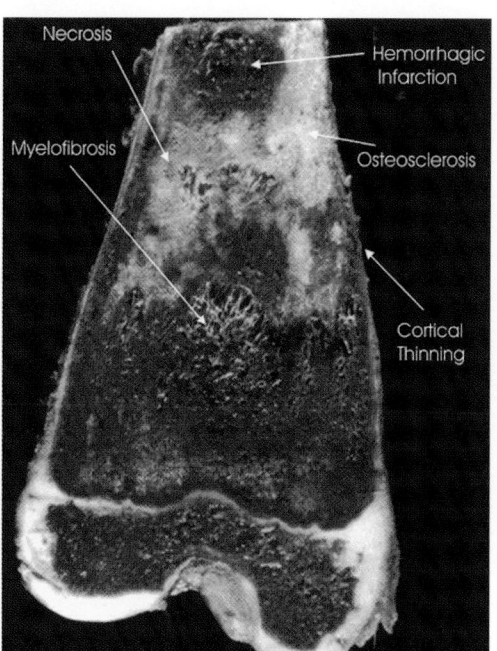

Color Figure 30-17B. The interior of the bone is shown in (**B**) in which the distal femur has been sectioned. The complex lesions of osteosclerosis, osteonecrosis, myelofibrosis, and cortical thinning are present. The classic Erlenmeyer flask deformity of the distal femur also is present.

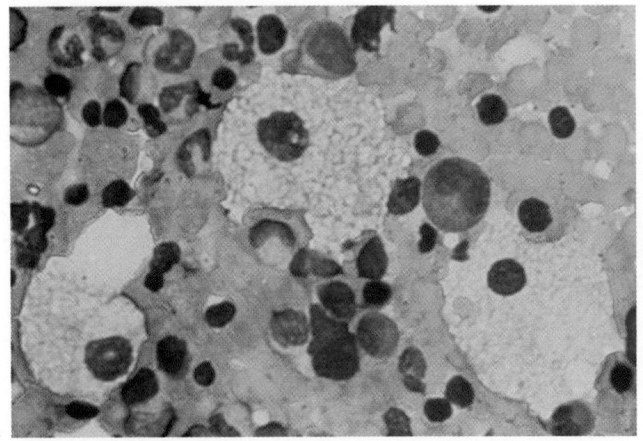

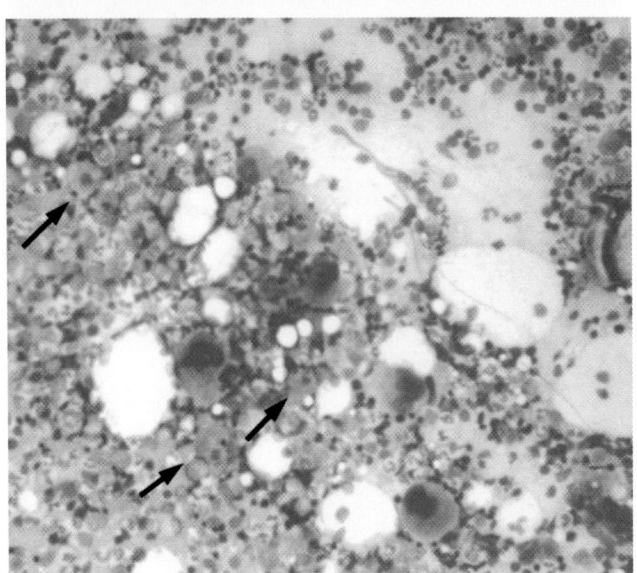

Color Figure 30-18. Storage cells observed in **(A)** Niemann-Pick disease and **(B)** sea-blue histiocytes (*arrows*). (Courtesy of Pearl Levitt, Hematology, Dana Farber Cancer Institute; Dr. Joseph Antin, Hematology Teaching File, Brigham and Women's Hospital.)

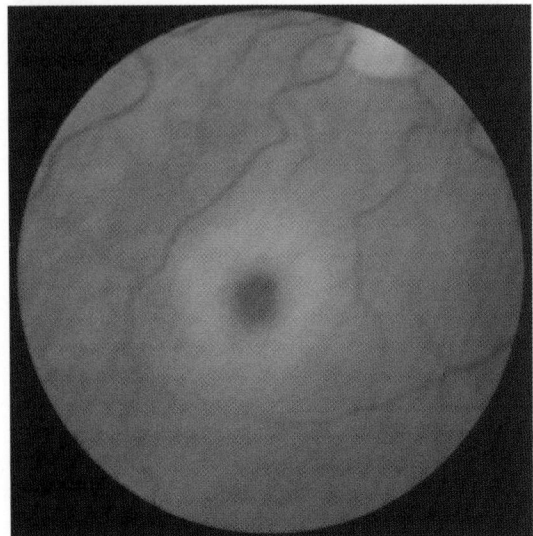

Color Figure 30-19. Cherry-red macula of Niemann-Pick disease. (Courtesy of Dr. Robert Peterson, Department of Ophthalmology, Children's Hospital, Boston.)

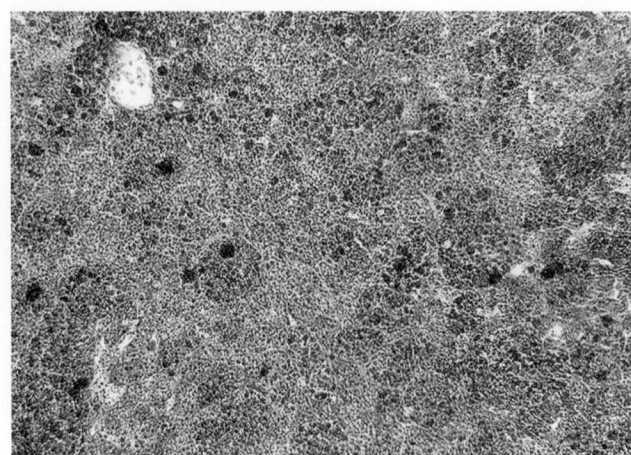

Color Figure 30-20. Liver biopsy from a Wolman's disease mouse stained with Oil red O for neutral fats. For human and mouse Wolman's disease, the storage cells (macrophages) proliferate within the liver as islands (potentially of clonal origin). In the mouse, and by analogy in humans, these storage cells express high levels of macrophage colony-stimulating factor. The storage cells stain brightly with Oil red O, indicating the presence of large amounts of neutral fats, cholesteryl esters, cholesterol and triglycerides within the lysosome. With progression, the storage cells can represent over 70% of the cells in the liver.

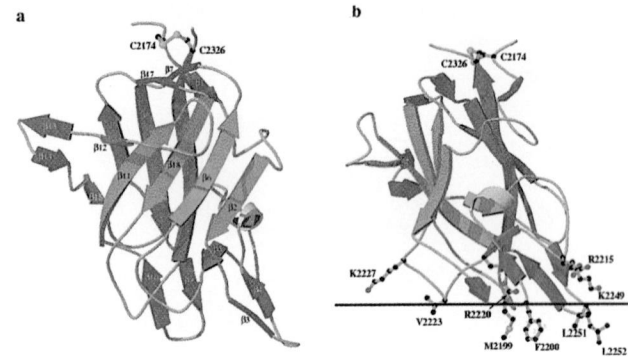

Color Figure 38-4. Ribbon diagram of factor VIII C2 and proposed membrane-binding mode. **A:** The structure consists of 19 β-strands, including an eight-stranded β-sandwich core. Two of the three β-hairpins and an additional loop extend beyond the core fold. These regions, which are predominantly hydrophobic, flank a pair of positively charged clefts. **B:** The putative membrane-binding surface includes M2199 and F2200 from the first turn, L2251 and L2252 from the second turn, and V2223 from the adjacent loop. These hydrophobic residues and a belt of basic residues partition on either side of the horizontal gray line, which indicates the putative polar-nonpolar boundary of a phospholipid bilayer surface.

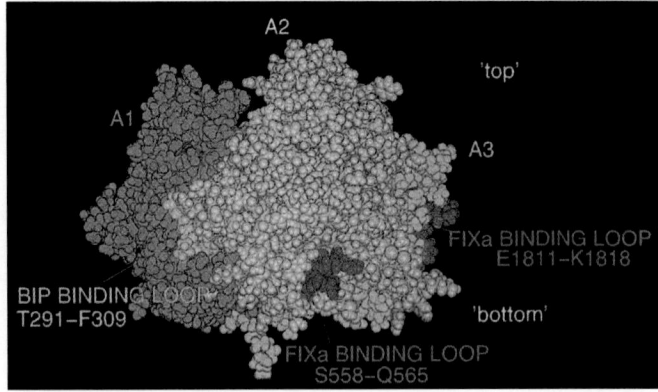

Color Figure 38-5. Factor VIII A domains. BIP, binding protein; FIXa, factor IXa.

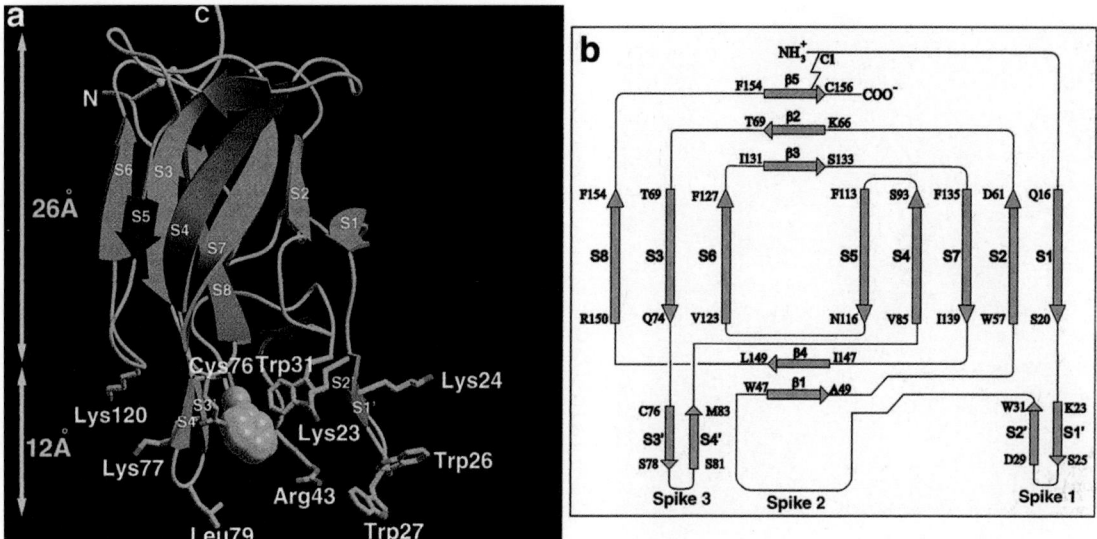

Color Figure 38-6. Structure of factor V C2 domain. **A:** Ribbon plot of the open crystal form in the reference orientation, which highlights the major secondary structure elements. Several noticeable side chains and the Cys 1–Cys 156 disulfide bridge are displayed. The phenyl mercury molecule (space-filling model) that is used for structure determination is shown covalently attached to Cys 76. **B:** Topology diagram that shows the arrangement of secondary-structure elements.

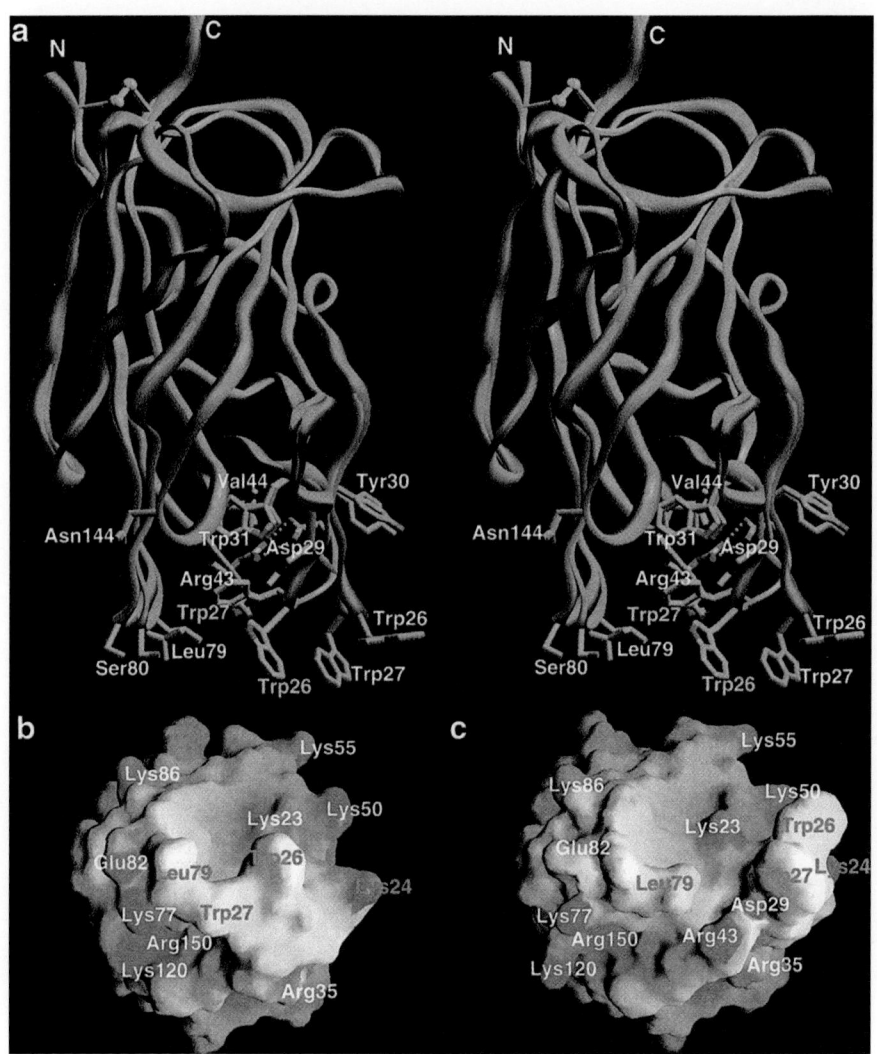

Color Figure 38-7. Conformational flexibility in the hydrophobic spike region of the factor V C2 domain. **A:** Stereo view of the factor V C2 structures, superimposed in the same orientation as in Fig. 38-2. The open form is shown in green. The closed form is displayed in yellow, with several side chains that are color-coded (carbon, yellow; oxygen, red; nitrogen, blue). **B,C:** GRASP 30 surface representations of the electrostatic potential (red, negative; blue, positive) of factor V C2 in the closed (**B**) and in the open (**C**) crystal form. The view is from the apparent membrane-binding site.

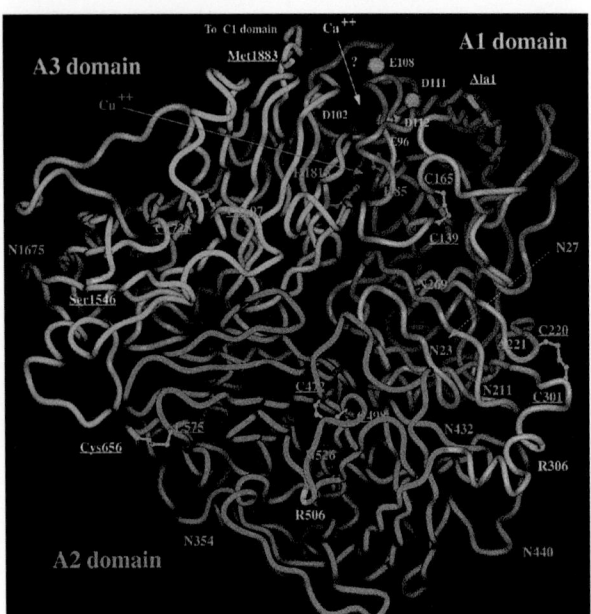

Color Figure 38-8. Homology model of the three A domains of factor V based on ceruloplasmin structure. The model is viewed down the pseudo-threefold axis. The disulfide bridges (ball and stick model) are shown in orange; R306 and R506 (cleavage sites for activated protein C) are in yellow; the N-terminus of the A1 domain and C-terminus of the A2 domain are in white, the N-terminus and C-terminus of the A3 domain are also shown in white; the two histidines (H85 and H1815), which are most likely involved in copper binding, are in magenta (ball and stick model); potential residues (E96, D102, E108, D111, D112) that are involved in calcium binding are shown as creatine phosphokinase spheres (*yellow*).

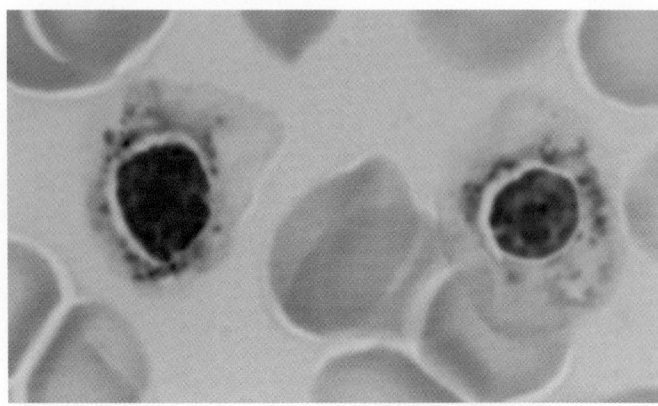

A

Color Figure 47-7A. Microscopic view of ring sideroblasts. Note the perinuclear localization of iron-laden mitochondria, which are visualized by Prussian blue staining. Large granules with stainable iron, which are termed *siderosomes,* in the abnormal erythroblasts surround the nucleus of the cells like a ring. The findings are most marked in the mature erythroblasts with the most active heme biosynthesis, whereas siderosomes are much less marked in immature erythroblasts.

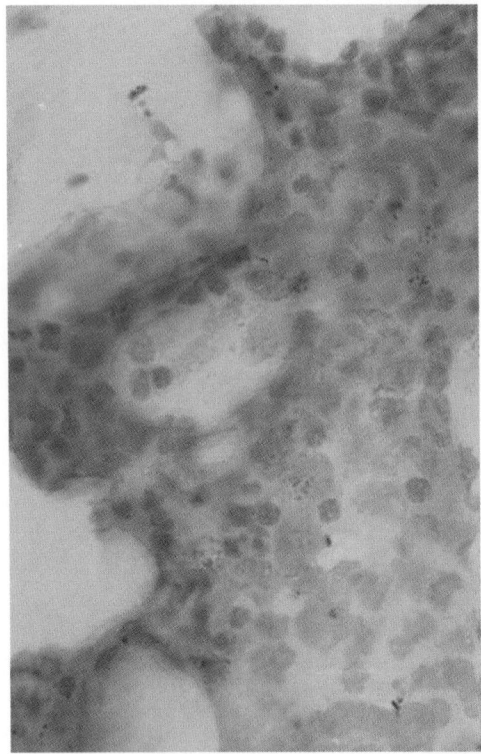

Color Figure 46-8. Perls' Prussian blue staining of bone marrow macrophages. Granular blue deposits of iron are abundant in macrophages in this bone marrow sample from a patient who has recently received intravenous iron dextran.

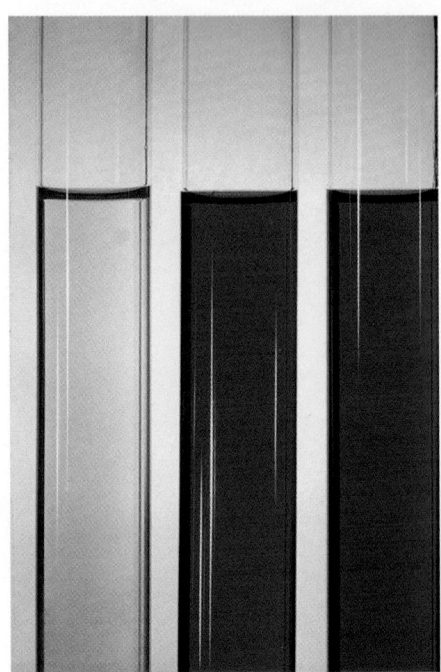

Color Figure 47-13. Appearance of urine samples from a healthy patient and a patient with acute intermittent porphyria. **Left:** Normal urine. **Center:** Acute intermittent porphyria urine. **Right:** Red wine that has been diluted with water.

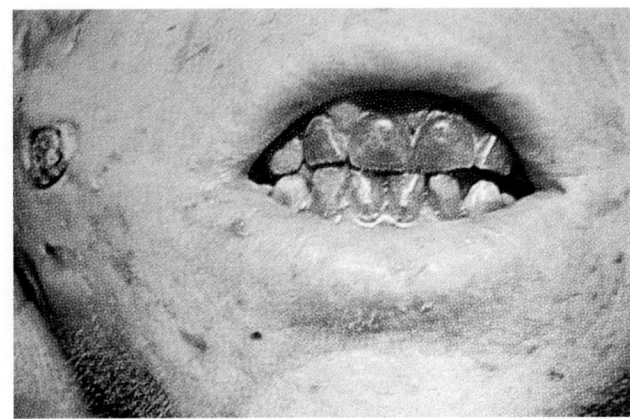
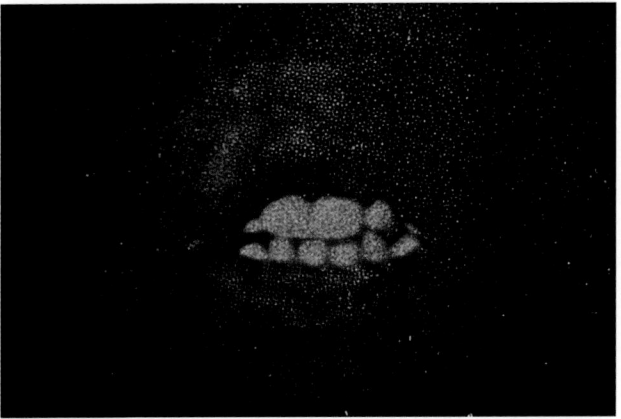

A **B**

Color Figure 47-18. Erythrodontia of a patient with congenital erythropoietic porphyria. **A:** Normal view. Note the brownish discoloration of teeth by uroporphyrin deposition, the atrophic changes in the lip at the corner of the mouth, the deformed healing of erosion on the right cheek, and the pigmentation and discoloration of the skin. **B:** Fluorescent view. When viewed under ultraviolet light, the teeth show intense red fluorescence due to uroporphyrin.

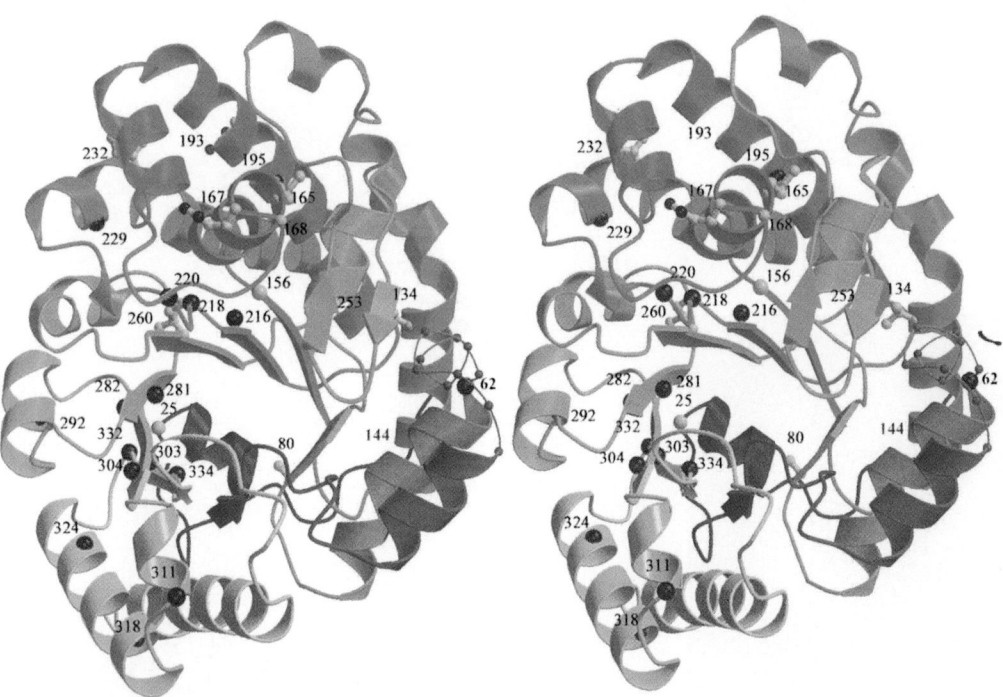

Color Figure 47-20. The crystal structure of human uroporphyrinogen decarboxylase (UROD), and the location of mutations in the UROD structure. Stereodiagram of the structure of a UROD monomer, from blue to green to yellow, along the amino acid sequence. The disordered loop is shown as a thin blue line with spheres on the Ca positions. Numbers indicate the positions of mutant residues. Mutated amino acids that have been identified in porphyria cutanea tarda or hepatoerythropoietic porphyria are depicted either as yellow or pink spheres. (From Phillips JD, Parker TL, Schubert HL, et al., *Blood* 2001;98: 3179, with permission.)

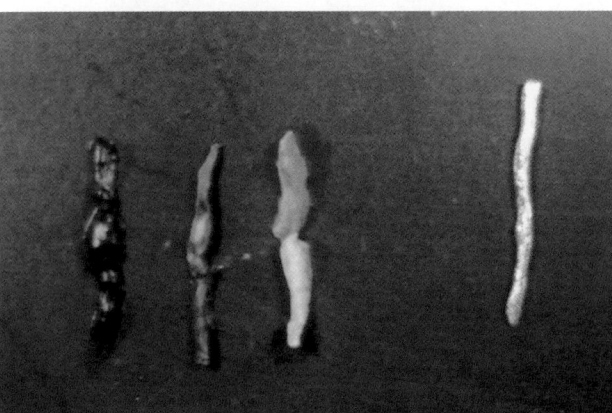

Color Figure 47-23. Liver biopsy sample from a patient with hepatoerythropoietic porphyria that shows various degrees of fluorescence (*far right*), whereas samples from nonporphyric subjects do not.

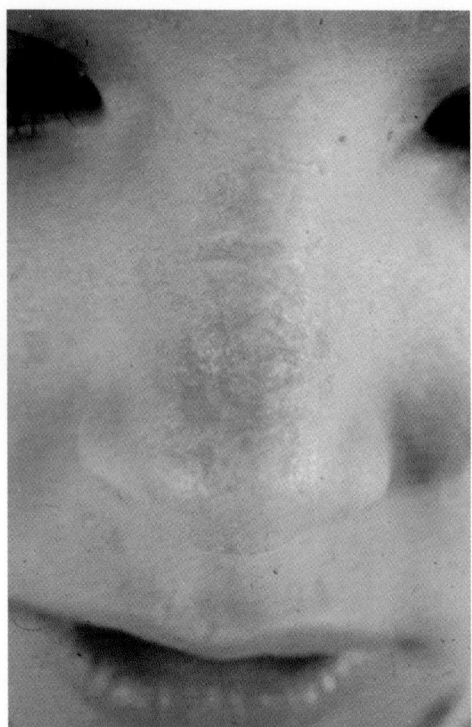

Color Figure 47-26. Typical shallow, elliptical scars over the nose in a child with erythropoietic protoporphyria. (From Poh-Fitzpatrick MB. Porphyrin-sensitized cutaneous photosensitivity: pathogenesis and treatment. *Clin Dermatol* 1985;3:41, with permission.)

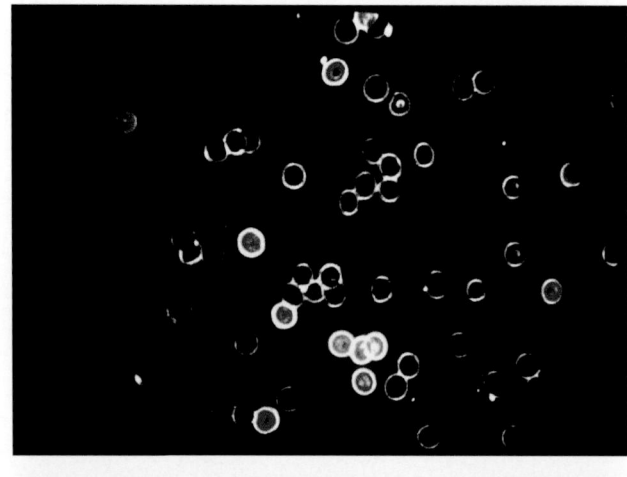

A

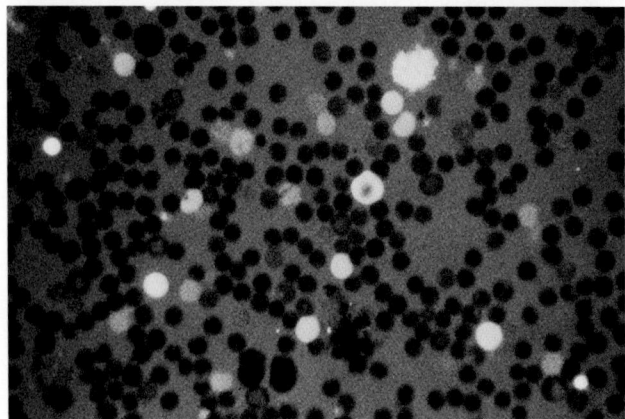

B

Color Figure 47-27. Fluorescent erythrocytes and erythroblasts in a patient with erythropoietic protoporphyria. **A:** Peripheral blood smear. Some cells contain a large amount of protoporphyrin, but others do not. **B:** Bone marrow smear. Some erythroblasts contain a large amount of protoporphyrin. Dimorphic distribution of fluorocytes in blood and of fluoroblasts in the bone marrow is characteristic of erythropoietic protoporphyria.

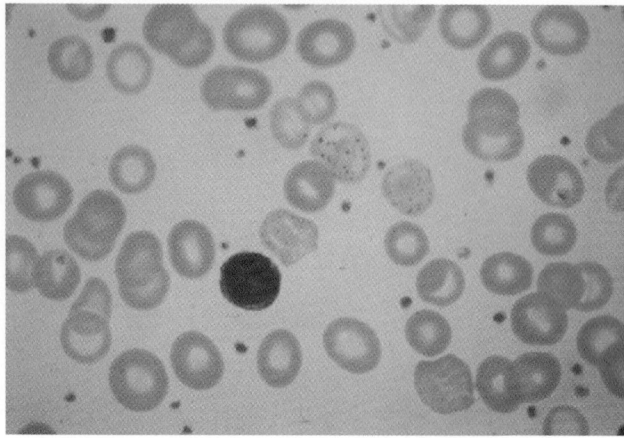

Color Figure 47-33. Basophilic stippling of erythrocytes in lead poisoning. (Courtesy of Dr. F. H. Bunn.)

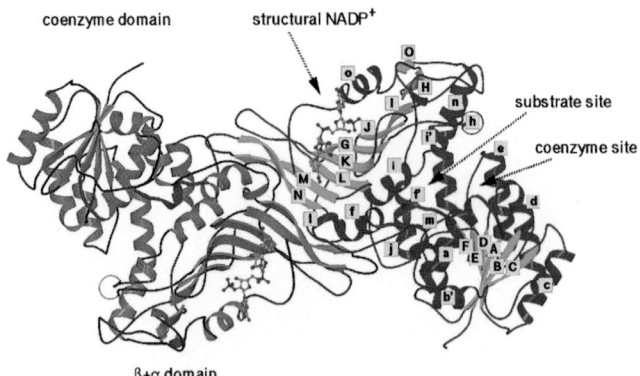

Color Figure 54-4. NADP+, oxidized form of nicotinamide adenine dinucleotide phosphate. The three-dimensional structure of human glucose-6-phosphate dehydrogenase. The active dimer is shown, with the alpha helices and beta sheets labeled on one subunit. [Modified from Au SW, Gover S, Lam VM, et al. Human glucose-6-phosphate dehydrogenase: the crystal structure reveals a structural NADP(+) molecule and provides insights into enzyme deficiency. *Structure* 2000;8:293–303; provided courtesy of Dr. S. Gover and Prof. M. Adams.]

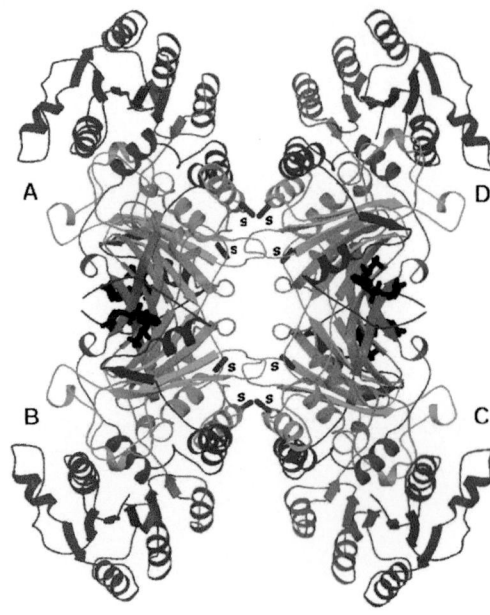

Color Figure 54-5. The human glucose-6-phosphate dehydrogenase tetramer. This is a dimer of dimers. The shading is ramped from the C to the N terminus in each of the four subunits. [Modified from Au SW, Gover S, Lam VM, et al. Human glucose-6-phosphate dehydrogenase: the crystal structure reveals a structural NADP(+) molecule and provides insights into enzyme deficiency. *Structure* 2000;8:293–303; provided courtesy of Dr. S. Gover and Prof. M. Adams.]

TABLE 35-2. Treatment Strategies in von Willebrand's Disease (vWD)

vWD Variant	Primary Therapy	Secondary Therapy
Type I	Desmopressin	Factor concentrate[a] Cryoprecipitate
Type IIA (and related subtypes)	Desmopressin	Factor concentrate[a] Cryoprecipitate
Type IIB	Factor concentrate[a] Cryoprecipitate	?? Desmopressin
Type III	Factor concentrate[a] Cryoprecipitate	Platelet transfusion Desmopressin
Autosomal hemophilia (vWD Normandy)	Factor concentrate[a]	Desmopressin
Acquired vWD[b]	Desmopressin	Platelet transfusion Factor concentrate[a]

[a]Refers to intermediate-purity factor VIII concentrates (see text). These products are not yet licensed in the United States for the treatment of vWD.
[b]Refers to therapy of acute bleeding manifestations. Long-term management is best achieved by treatment of the underlying disease.

SUBTYPES

Type I. Most patients with type I vWD respond to desmopressin, with a marked rise in all components of the vWF–factor VIII complex and a shortening or normalization of the bleeding time. DDAVP has become the mainstay of treatment for most of these patients. A small subset of patients with diminished levels of platelet-associated vWF do not have a significant rise in vWF or fail to show any improvement in hemostasis (292). Responses to desmopressin among type I patients are inconsistent enough to warrant a test infusion to help to predict the likelihood of a response (525). After the response to DDAVP has been demonstrated, treatment can usually be instituted, when it is needed at a later date.

As discussed, the goal of treatment in type I vWD patients in the postoperative period requires adequate primary hemostasis for 48 to 72 hours. Although this may be achieved with DDAVP alone, it is advisable to have exogenous sources of vWF available, especially for patients who undergo high-risk surgical procedures or in whom rapid tachyphylaxis has been observed.

Type II. Highly variable responses to desmopressin have been observed in patients with type II vWD. Thus, although most type II patients have a significant increase in vWF:Ag and factor VIII (526,527), normalization of the vWF multimeric pattern and improvement in bleeding time are not consistently observed (399,400). Infusion of desmopressin in patients with type IIB vWD results in the transient appearance of HMW forms of the vWF, which are then rapidly cleared from the plasma (399,433). Desmopressin is said to be contraindicated in type IIB patients, because it exacerbates the thrombocytopenia that is seen in this subtype (433). Two reports (528,529) suggest that the decrease in platelet count after DDAVP administration to type IIB vWD patients is artifactual (pseudothrombocytopenia) and that the drug has clinical benefit.

Type III. Patients with type III vWD do not increase vWF:Ag or factor VIII levels after DDAVP infusion. The use of desmopressin in conjunction with cryoprecipitate shortens the bleeding time more effectively than does the use of cryoprecipitate alone, thus suggesting an additional action of desmopressin that is independent of its effect on vWF secretion (530). In addition, platelet transfusion may provide an important additional source of vWF for severe vWD patients who fail to respond to exogenous vWF alone (296,531). Platelet transfusion may be especially helpful in treating type III vWD patients who have

developed alloantibodies to vWF as a result of previous treatment with exogenous vWF preparations.

Autosomal Hemophilia. Treatment of patients with autosomal hemophilia requires an exogenous source of vWF. The infusion of intermediate-purity factor VIII concentrates produces an immediate correction of factor VIII levels and a prolonged elevation of factor VIII that is due to the stimulation of endogenous biosynthesis and enhanced plasma stability (460,532).

Acquired Disease. The treatment of acquired vWD is often problematic. Treatment of the underlying condition, if possible, often leads to the disappearance of the vWD manifestations (474,475,485,488,490). Amelioration of acute bleeding manifestations can sometimes be achieved with DDAVP or large amounts of exogenous vWF. Platelet transfusions may also be useful in patients who fail to respond to other measures.

SPECIAL CONSIDERATIONS

Surgery. In preoperative patients, it is necessary to ensure a factor VIII level that is greater than 50 U/dL and to raise the RCoF activity and shorten the bleeding time. Although little specific evidence supports this point, most clinicians attempt to achieve RCoF activity levels of at least 50 U/dL and to partially correct the template Ivy bleeding time (507). For patients with more severe defects, or when surgery results in mucosal bleeding, more careful attention to the bleeding time and the RCoF levels is recommended. For the typical vWD patient with an adequate level of factor VIII, the defect is predominantly one of primary hemostasis. Thus, treatment can often be limited to the first 48 to 72 hours after surgery. Although this may be achievable in some patients with DDAVP alone, it is generally advisable to consider the use of exogenous sources of vWF, especially in patients who undergo high-risk surgical procedures or in whom rapid tachyphylaxis has been observed. In unusually severe type I vWD patients, further therapy may be required to maintain factor VIII levels of greater than 30 U/dL for an additional 4 to 7 days. When appropriate therapy is instituted, the operative risk in vWD is not increased (533). As in other patients with bleeding disorders, antiplatelet drugs, particularly aspirin, should be avoided.

Pregnancy. The management of vWD in pregnancy is a commonly encountered clinical problem that deserves special consideration. Pregnancy induces a significant increase in factor

VIII, vWF:Ag, and vWF:RCoF in most type I vWD patients, although the Ivy bleeding time may remain prolonged (224). The likelihood of hemorrhage at the time of delivery is acceptably small, so long as the factor VIII level is greater than 50 U/dL, as is true in most vWD patients at the time of delivery (231,534). Although there is less evidence on this point, it appears that even cesarean section can be safely performed without specific therapy in most vWD patients (439). Because plasma vWF may rapidly return to baseline levels in the postpartum period, careful monitoring for excessive mucosal bleeding is warranted. Special consideration should also be given to those women with other subtypes of vWD in whom correction of the hemostatic defects is less predictable. In women with type IIB and similar vWD variants, thrombocytopenia may result from increased plasma levels of the abnormal vWF protein (233,437). When treatment is required, first consideration should be given to the use of DDAVP, especially in patients with a previously documented history of a favorable response. Documentation of the efficacy of DDAVP in the peripartum period is highly limited, and the need for exogenous vWF replacement must be individually evaluated.

REFERENCES

1. Meyer D, Baumgartner HR. Role of von Willebrand factor in platelet adhesion to the subendothelium. Br J Haematol 1983;54:1.
2. Weiss HJ, Sussman II, Hoyer LW. Stabilization of factor VIII in plasma by the von Willebrand factor: studies on posttransfusion and dissociated factor VIII and in patients with von Willebrand's disease. J Clin Invest 1977;60:390.
3. von Willebrand EA. Hereditär pseudohemofili. Finska Läkaresällskapets Handlingar 1926;67:7.
4. von Willebrand EA. Ueber hereditaere pseudohaemophilie. Acta Med Scand 1931;76:521.
5. Minot GR. A familial hemorrhagic condition associated with prolongation of bleeding times. Am J Med Sci 1928;175:301.
6. Buckman TE. Atypical pathologic hemorrhage in early life. Am J Med Sci 1928;175:307.
7. Alexander B, Goldstein R. Dual hemostatic defect in pseudohemophilia. J Clin Invest 1953;32:551.
8. Quick AJ, Hussey CV. Hemophilic condition in the female. J Lab Clin Med 1953;42:929.
9. Larrieu MJ, Soulier JP. Deficit en facteur antihémophilique a chez une fille associé a un trouble saignement. Rev Hematol 1953;8:361.
10. Nilsson IM, Blombäck M, von Francken I. On an inherited autosomal hemorrhagic diathesis with antihemophilic globulin (AHG) deficiency and prolonged bleeding time. Acta Med Scand 1957;159:35.
11. Juergens R, Lehmann W, Wegelius O, et al. Antihemophilic globulin factor (factor VIII) deficiency in Aland (Willebrand-Juergens) thrombopathy. Thromb Diath Haemorrh 1957;1:257.
12. von Willebrand EA, Juergens R. Ueber ein neue bluterkrankheit, die konstitutionelle thrombopathie. Klin Wochenschr 1933;12:414.
13. Salzman EW. Measurement of platelet adhesiveness: a simple in vitro technique demonstrating an abnormality in von Willebrand's disease. J Lab Clin Med 1963;62:724.
14. Bowie EJ, Owen CA Jr, Thompson JH Jr, et al. Platelet adhesiveness in von Willebrand's disease. Am J Clin Pathol 1969;52:69.
15. Baumgartner HR. The role of blood flow in platelet adhesion, fibrin deposition and formation of mural thrombi. Microvasc Res 1973;5:167.
16. Nilsson IM, Blomback M, Jorpes E, et al. von Willebrand's disease and its correction with human plasma fraction I-0. Acta Med Scand 1957;159:179.
17. Nilsson IM, Blombäck M, Blombäck B. von Willebrand's disease in Sweden: its pathogenesis and treatment. Acta Med Scand 1959;164:263.
18. Weiss HJ. The use of plasma and plasma fractions in the treatment of a patient with von Willebrand's disease. Vox Sang 1962;7:267.
19. Biggs R, Matthews JM. The treatment of haemorrhage in von Willebrand's disease and the blood level of factor VIII (AHG). Br J Haematol 1963;9:203.
20. Cornu P, Larrieu MJ, Caen JP, et al. Transfusion studies in von Willebrand's disease: effect on bleeding time and factor VIII. Br J Haematol 1963;9:189.
21. Perkins HA. Correction of the hemostatic defects in von Willebrand's disease. Blood 1967;30:375.
22. Bennett E, Dormandy K. Pool's cryoprecipitate and exhausted plasma in the treatment of von Willebrand's disease and factor XI deficiency. Lancet 1966;2:731.
23. Weiss HJ, Rogers J. Correction of the platelet abnormality in von Willebrand's disease by cryoprecipitate. Am J Med 1972;53:734.
24. Larrieu MJ, Caen JP, Meyer DO, et al. Congenital bleeding disorders with long bleeding time and normal platelet count II von Willebrand's disease (report of thirty-seven patients). Am J Med 1968;45:354.
25. Weiss HJ, Rogers J, Brand H. Defective ristocetin-induced platelet aggregation in von Willebrand's disease and its correction by factor VIII. J Clin Invest 1973;52:2697.
26. Green D, Potter EV. Failure of AHF concentrate to control bleeding in von Willebrand's disease. Am J Med 1976;60:357.
27. Blatt PM, Brinkhous KM, Culp HR, et al. Antihemophilic factor concentrates therapy in von Willebrand's disease: dissociation of bleeding-time factor and ristocetin-cofactor activities. JAMA 1976;236:2770.
28. Zimmerman TS, Ratnoff OD, Powell AE. Immunologic differentiation of classic hemophilia (factor VIII deficiency) and von Willebrand's disease, with observations on combined deficiencies of antihemophilic factor and proaccelerin (factor V) and an acquired circulating anticoagulant against antihemophilic factor. J Clin Invest 1971;50:244.
29. Stites DP, Hershgold EJ, Perlman JD, et al. Factor VIII detection by hemagglutination inhibition: hemophilia A and von Willebrand's disease. Science 1971;171:196.
30. Laurell CB. Quantitative estimation of proteins by electrophoresis in agarose gel containing antibodies. Anal Biochem 1966;15:45.
31. Howard MA, Firkin BG. Ristocetin: a new look in the investigation of platelet aggregation. Thromb Haemost 1971;26:362.
32. Gangarosa EJ, Johnson TR, Ramos HS. Ristocetin-induced thrombocytopenia: site and mechanism of action. Arch Intern Med 1960;105:83.
33. Howard MA, Sawers RJ, Firkin BG. Ristocetin: a means of differentiating von Willebrand's disease into two groups. Blood 1973;41:687.
34. Doucet-deBruine MH, Sixma JJ, Over J, et al. Heterogeneity of human factor VIII. II. Characterization of forms of factor VIII binding to platelets in the presence of ristocetin. J Lab Clin Med 1978;92:96.
35. Martin SE, Marder VJ, Francis CW, et al. Structural studies on the functional heterogeneity of von Willebrand protein polymers. Blood 1981;57:313.
36. Moake JL, Turner MA, Stathopoulos NA, et al. Involvement of large plasma von Willebrand factor (vWF) multimers and unusually large vWF forms derived from endothelial cells in shear stress-induced platelet aggregation. J Clin Invest 1986;78:1456.
37. Moake JL. von Willebrand factor and the pathophysiology of thrombotic thrombocytopenia: from human studies to a new animal model. Lab Invest 1988;59:415.
38. Titani K, Kumar S, Takio K, et al. Amino acid sequence of human von Willebrand factor. Biochemistry 1986;25:3171.
39. Ginsburg D, Handin RI, Bonthron DT, et al. Human von Willebrand factor (vWF): isolation of complementary DNA (cDNA) clones and chromosomal localization. Science 1985;228:1401.
40. Lynch DC, Zimmerman TS, Collins CJ, et al. Molecular cloning of cDNA for human von Willebrand factor: authentication by a new method. Cell 1985;41:49.
41. Sadler JE, Shelton-Inloes BB, Sorace JM, et al. Cloning and characterization of two cDNAs coding for human von Willebrand factor. Proc Natl Acad Sci U S A 1985;82:6394.
42. Verweij CL, de Vries CJ, Distel B, et al. Construction of cDNA coding from human von Willebrand factor using antibody probes from colony-screening and mapping of the chromosomal gene. Nucleic Acids Res 1985;13:4699.
43. Ginsburg D, Bowie EJW. Molecular genetics of von Willebrand disease. Blood 1992;79:2507.
44. Bonthron DT, Handin RI, Kaufman RJ, et al. Structure of pre-pro-von Willebrand factor and its expression in heterologous cells. Nature 1986;324:270.
45. Bonthron DT, Orr EC, Mitsock LM, et al. Nucleotide sequence of pre–pro-von Willebrand factor cDNA. Nucleic Acids Res 1986;14:7125.
46. Shelton-Inloes BB, Broze GR Jr, Miletich JP, et al. Evaluation of human von Willebrand factor: cDNA sequence polymorphisms, repeated domains, and relationship to von Willebrand antigen II. Biochem Biophys Res Commun 1987;144:657.
47. Shelton-Inloes BB, Titani K, Sadler JE. cDNA sequences for human von Willebrand factor reveal five types of repeated domains and five possible protein sequence polymorphisms. Biochemistry 1986;25:3164.
48. Verweij CL, Diergaarde PJ, Hart M, et al. Full length von Willebrand factor (vWF) cDNA encodes a highly repetitive protein considerably larger than the mature vWF subunit. EMBO J 1986;5:1839.
49. Fay PJ, Kawai Y, Wagner DD, et al. Propolypeptide of von Willebrand factor circulates in blood and is identical to von Willebrand antigen II. Science 1986;232:995.
50. Montgomery RR, Zimmerman TS. von Willebrand's disease antigen II. J Clin Invest 1978;61:1498.
51. Wise RJ, Barr PJ, Wong PA, et al. Expression of a human proprotein processing enzyme: correct cleavage of the von Willebrand factor precursor at a paired basic amino acid site. Proc Natl Acad Sci U S A 1990;87:9378.
52. Barr PJ. Mammalian subtilisins: the long-sought dibasic processing endoproteases. Cell 1991;66:1.
53. Smeekens SP. Processing of protein precursors by a novel family of subtilisin-related mammalian endoproteases. Biotechnology 1993;11:182.
54. Verweij CL, Hart M, Pannekoek H. Expression of variant von Willebrand factor (vWF) cDNA in heterologous cells: requirement of the pro-polypeptide in vWF multimer formation. EMBO J 1987;6:2885.
55. Wise RJ, Pittman DD, Handin RI, et al. The propeptide of von Willebrand factor independently mediates the assembly of von Willebrand multimers. Cell 1988;52:229.
56. Montgomery RR, Dent J, Schmidt W, et al. Hereditary persistence of circulating pro von Willebrand factor (pro-vWF). Circulation 1986;74[Suppl]:406.

57. Slayter H, Loscalzo J, Bockenstedt PL, et al. Native conformation of human von Willebrand protein: analysis by electron microscopy and quasielastic light scattering. *J Biol Chem* 1985;260:8559.

58. Mohri H, Fujimura Y, Shima M, et al. Structure of the von Willebrand factor domain interacting with glycoprotein Ib. *J Biol Chem* 1988;263:17901.

59. Berndt MC, Ward CM, Booth WJ, et al. Identification of aspartic acid 514 through glutamic acid 542 as a glycoprotein Ib-IX complex receptor recognition sequence in von Willebrand factor: mechanism of modulation of von Willebrand factor by ristocetin and botrocetin. *Biochemistry* 1992;31:11144.

60. Mohri H, Yoshioka A, Zimmerman TS, et al. Isolation of the von Willebrand factor domain interacting with platelet glycoprotein Ib, heparin, and collagen and characterization of its three distinct functional sites. *J Biol Chem* 1989;264:17361.

61. Fujimura Y, Titani K, Holland LZ, et al. A heparin-binding domain of human von Willebrand factor: characterization and localization of a tryptic fragment extending from amino acid residue Val449 to Lys728. *J Biol Chem* 1987;262:1734.

62. Sixma JJ, Schiphorst ME, Verweij CL, et al. Effect of deletion of the A1 domain of von Willebrand factor on its binding to heparin, collagen and platelets in the presence of ristocetin. *Eur J Biochem* 1991;196:369.

63. Christophe O, Obert B, Meyer D, et al. The binding domain of von Willebrand factor to sulfatides is distinct from those interacting with glycoprotein Ib, heparin, and collagen and resides between amino acid residues Leu512 and Lys673. *Blood* 1991;78:2310.

64. Pareti FI, Niiya K, McPherson JM, et al. Isolation and characterization of two domains of human von Willebrand factor that interact with fibrillar collagen types I and III. *J Biol Chem* 1987;262:13835.

65. Mohri H, Fujimura Y, Shima M, et al. Isolation of the von Willebrand factor domain interacting with platelet glycoprotein Ib, heparin, and collagen and characterization of its three distinct functional sites. *J Biol Chem* 1989;264:17361.

66. Roth GJ, Titani K, Hoyer LW, et al. Localization of binding sites within human von Willebrand factor for monomeric type III collagen. *Biochemistry* 1986;25:8357.

67. Kalafatis M, Takahashi Y, Girma JP, et al. Localization of a collagen-interactive domain of human von Willebrand factor between amino acid residues Gly 911 and Glu 1365. *Blood* 1987;70:1577.

68. Cruz MA, Handin RI, Wise RJ. The interaction of the von Willebrand factor–A1 domain with platelet glycoprotein Ib/IX: the role of glycosylation and disulfide bonding in a monomeric recombinant A1 domain protein. *J Biol Chem* 1993;268:21238.

69. Bahou WF, Ginsburg D, Sikkink R, et al. A monoclonal antibody to von Willebrand factor (vWF) inhibits factor VIII binding. *J Clin Invest* 1989;84:56.

70. Ginsburg D, Bockenstedt PL, Allen EA, et al. Fine mapping of monoclonal antibody epitopes on human von Willebrand factor using a recombinant peptide library. *Thromb Haemost* 1991;67:166.

71. Cruz MA, Diacovo TG, Emsley J, et al. Mapping the glycoprotein Ib-binding site in the von Willebrand factor A1 domain. *J Biol Chem* 2000;275:19098–19105.

72. Emsley J, Cruz M, Handin R, et al. Crystal structure of the von Willebrand factor A1 domain and implications for the binding of platelet glycoprotein Ib. *J Biol Chem* 1998;273:10396–10401.

73. Emsley J, King SL, Bergelson JM, et al. Crystal structure of the I domain from integrin alpha2beta1. *J Biol Chem* 1997;272:28512–28517.

74. Bienkowska J, Cruz M, Atiemo A, et al. The von Willebrand factor A3 domain does not contain a metal ion-dependent adhesion site motif. *J Biol Chem* 1997;272:25162–25167.

75. Romijn RA, Bouma B, Wuyster W, et al. Identification of the collagen-binding site of the von Willebrand factor A3-domain. *J Biol Chem* 2001;276:9985–9991.

76. Huizinga EG, Martijn van der Plas R, Kroon J, et al. Crystal structure of the A3 domain of human von Willebrand factor: implications for collagen binding. *Structure* 1997;5:1147–1156.

77. Kamata T, Liddington RC, Takada Y. Interaction between collagen and the alpha(2) I-domain of integrin alpha(2)beta(1). Critical role of conserved residues in the metal-ion-dependent adhesion site (MIDAS) region. *J Biol Chem* 1999;274:32108–32111.

78. Smith C, Estavillo D, Emsley J, et al. Mapping the collagen-binding site in the I domain of the glycoprotein Ia/IIa (integrin alpha(2)beta(1)). *J Biol Chem* 2000;275:4205–4209.

79. Fay PJ, Coumans JV, Walker FJ. von Willebrand factor mediates protection of factor VIII from activated protein C–catalyzed inactivation. *J Biol Chem* 1991;266:2172.

80. Tuddenham EG, Lane RS, Rotblat F, et al. Response to infusions of polyelectrolyte fractionated human factor VIII concentrate in human hemophilia A and von Willebrand disease. *Br J Haematol* 1982;52:259.

81. Kaufman RJ. Biological regulation of factor VIII activity. *Annu Rev Med* 1992;43:325.

82. Fay PJ. Reconstitution of human factor VIII from isolated subunits. *Arch Biochem Biophys* 1988;262:525.

83. Wise RJ, Dorner AJ, Krane M, et al. The role of von Willebrand factor multimers and propeptide cleavage in binding and stabilization of factor VIII. *J Biol Chem* 1991;266:21948.

84. Kaufman RJ, Wasley LC, Dorner AJ. Synthesis, processing and secretion of recombinant human factor VIII expressed in mammalian cells. *J Biol Chem* 1988;263:6352.

85. Ruoslahti E, Pierschbacher MD. New perspectives in cell adhesion: RGD and integrins. *Science* 1987;238:491.

86. Ruggeri ZM, DeMarco L, Gatti L, et al. Platelets have more than one binding site for von Willebrand factor. *J Clin Invest* 1983;72:1.

87. Sakariassen KS, Nievelstein PF, Coller BS, et al. The role of platelet membrane glycoproteins Ib and IIb-IIIa in platelet adherence to human artery subendothelium. *Br J Haematol* 1986;63:681.

88. Berliner S, Niiya K, Roberts Jr, et al. Generation and characterization of peptide-antibodies that inhibit von Willebrand factor binding to glycoprotein IIb-IIIa without interacting with other adhesive molecules. *J Biol Chem* 1988;263:7500.

89. Parker RI, Gralnick HR. Inhibition of platelet-von Willebrand factor binding to platelets by adhesion site peptides. *Blood* 1989;74:1226.

90. Brody JI, Haidar ME, Rossman RE. A hemorrhagic syndrome in Waldenström's macroglobulinemia secondary to immunoadsorption of factor VIII: recovery after splenectomy. *N Engl J Med* 1979;300:408.

91. Sixma JJ, Sakariassen KS, Beeser-Visser NH, et al. Adhesion of platelets to human artery subendothelium: effect of factor VIII–von Willebrand factor of various multimeric composition. *Blood* 1984;63:128.

92. Mancuso DJ, Tuley EA, Westfield LA, et al. Structure of the gene for human von Willebrand factor. *J Biol Chem* 1989;264:19514.

93. Fukui H, Nishino M, Terada S, et al. Hemostatic effect of a heat-treated factor VIII concentrate (Haemate P) in von Willebrand's disease. *Blut* 1988;56:171.

94. Peake IR, Bloom AL, Giddings JC. Inherited variants of factor VIII-related protein in von Willebrand's disease. *N Engl J Med* 1974;291:113.

95. Shelton-Inloes BB, Chelab FF, Mannucci PM, et al. Gene deletions correlate with the development of alloantibodies in von Willebrand disease. *J Clin Invest* 1987;79:1459.

96. Patracchini P, Calzolari E, Aiello V, et al. Sublocalization of von Willebrand factor pseudogene to 22q11.22-q11.23 by in situ hybridization. *Hum Genet* 1989;83:264.

97. Mancuso DJ, Tuley EA, Westfield LA, et al. Human von Willebrand factor gene and pseudogene: structural analysis and differentiation by polymerase chain reaction. *Biochemistry* 1991;30:253.

98. Bahou WF, Bowie EJ, Fass DN, et al. Molecular genetic analysis of porcine von Willebrand disease: tight linkage to the von Willebrand factor locus. *Blood* 1988;72:308.

99. Collins CJ, Underdahl JP, Levene RB, et al. Molecular cloning of the human gene for von Willebrand factor and identification of the transcription initiation site. *Proc Natl Acad Sci U S A* 1987;84:4393.

100. Verweij CL, Hofker M, Quadt R, et al. RFLP for a human von Willebrand factor cDNA clone, pvWF1100. *Nucleic Acids Res* 1985;13:8289.

101. Nishino K, Lynch DC. A polymorphism of the human von Willebrand factor gene with BamHI. *Nucleic Acids Res* 1986;14:4697.

102. Quadt R, Verweij CL, DeVries CJ, et al. A polymorphic Xba I site within the human von Willebrand factor gene identified by a vWF cDNA clone. *Nucleic Acids Res* 1986;14:7139.

103. Bernardi J, Marchetti G, Bertagnolo V, et al. Two TaqI RFLPs in the human von Willebrand factor gene. *Nucleic Acids Res* 1987;15:1347.

104. Iannuzzi MC, Konkle BA, Ginsburg D, et al. RsaI RFLP in the human von Willebrand factor gene. *Nucleic Acids Res* 1987;15:5909.

105. Konkle BA, Kim S, Iannuzzi MC, et al. SacI RFLP in the human von Willebrand factor gene. *Nucleic Acids Res* 1987;15:6766.

106. Lavergen JM, Bahnak BR, Verweij CL, et al. A second Xba I polymorphic site within the human von Willebrand factor gene. *Nucleic Acids Res* 1987;15:9099.

107. Lavergen JM, Bahnak BR, Assouline Z, et al. A Taq I polymorphism in the 5' [region of the von Willebrand factor gene. *Nucleic Acids Res* 1988;16:2742.

108. Lindstedt M, Anvret M. An EcoRI polymorphism of the human von Willebrand factor cDNA. *Nucleic Acids Res* 1989;17:2882.

109. Inbal A, Handin RI. Two TaqI polymorphisms in the 5' region of the von Willebrand factor gene. *Nucleic Acids Res* 1989;17:10143.

110. Sadler JE, Ginsburg D. A database of polymorphisms in the von Willebrand factor gene and pseudogene. *Thromb Haemost* 1993;69:185.

111. Peake IR, Bowen D, Bignell P, et al. Family studies and prenatal diagnosis is severe von Willebrand's disease by polymerase chain reaction amplification of a variable repeat region of the von Willebrand factor gene. *Blood* 1990;76:555.

112. Bonthron D, Orkin SH. The human von Willebrand factor gene: structure of the 5' region. *Eur J Biochem* 1988;171:51.

113. Bloom AL, Giddings JC, Wilk CJ. Factor VIII on the vascular intima: possible importance in hemostasis and thrombosis. *Nat New Biol* 1973;241:217.

114. Hoyer LW, de los Santo RP, Hoyer JR. Antihemophilic factor antigen. Localization in endothelial cells by immunofluorescent microscopy. *J Clin Invest* 1973;52:2737.

115. Jaffe EA, Hoyer LW, Nachman RL. Synthesis of antihemophilic factor antigen by cultured human endothelial cells. *J Clin Invest* 1973;52:2757.

116. Wagner DD, Olmsted JB, Marder VJ. Immunolocalization of von Willebrand protein in Weibel-Palade bodies of human endothelial cells. *J Cell Biol* 1982;95:355.

117. Hormia M, Lehto VP, Virtanen I. Factor VIII-related antigen: a pericellular matrix component of culture human endothelial cells. *Exp Cell Res* 1983;149:483.

118. Kagawa H, Fujimoto S, Ueda H, et al. Immunocytochemical localization of factor VIII-related antigen in human umbilical vein. *J UOEH* 1985;7:365.

119. Warhol MJ, Sweet JM. The ultrastructural localization of von Willebrand factor in endothelial cells. *Am J Pathol* 1984;117:310.

120. Gimbrone MA Jr. Culture of vascular endothelium. In: Spaet TH, ed. *Progress in hemostasis and thrombosis*, vol. 3. New York: Grune & Stratton, 1973:1.

121. van Wachem PB, Reinders JH, van Buul-Wortelboer MF, et al. von Willebrand factor in cultured human vascular endothelial cells from adult and umbilical cord arteries and veins. *Thromb Haemost* 1986;56:189.

122. Sporn LA, Chavin SI, Marder VJ, et al. Biosynthesis of von Willebrand protein by human megakaryocytes. *J Clin Invest* 1985;76:1102.

123. Fretto LJ, Fowler WE, Darrell DR, et al. Substructure of human von Willebrand factor: proteolysis by V8 and characterization of two functional domains. *J Biol Chem* 1986;261:15679.

124. Wagner DD, Lawrence SO, Ohlsson-Wilhelm BM, et al. Topology and order of formation of interchain disulfide bonds in von Willebrand factor. *Blood* 1987;69:27.

125. Wagner DD, Mayadas T, Marder VJ. Initial glycosylation and acidic pH in the Golgi apparatus are required for multimerization of von Willebrand factor. *J Cell Biol* 1986;102:1320.

126. Browning PJ, Ling EH, Zimmerman TS, et al. Sulfation of von Willebrand factor by human umbilical vein endothelial cells. *Blood* 1983;62:281a.

127. Carew JA, Browning PJ, Lynch DC. Sulfation of von Willebrand factor. *Blood* 1990;76:2530.

128. Wagner DD, Mayadas T, Urban-Pickering M, et al. Inhibition of disulfide bonding of vW protein by monensin results in small, functionally defective multimers. *J Cell Biol* 1985;101:112.

129. Chopek MW, Girma JP, Fujikawa K, et al. Human von Willebrand factor: a multivalent protein composed of identical subunits. *Biochemistry* 1986;25:3146.

130. Wagner DD, Fay PJ, Sporn LA, et al. Divergent fates of von Willebrand factor and its propolypeptide (von Willebrand antigen II) after secretion from endothelial cells. *Proc Natl Acad Sci U S A* 1987;84:1955.

131. Mayadas TN, Wagner DD. Vicinal cysteines in the prosequence play a role in von Willebrand factor multimer assembly. *Proc Natl Acad Sci U S A* 1992;89:3531.

132. Scott JP, Montogomery RR. Platelet von Willebrand's antigen II: active release by aggregating agents and a marker of platelet release in vivo. *Blood* 1981;58:1075.

133. McCarroll DR, Levin EG, Montgomery RR. Endothelial cell synthesis of von Willebrand antigen II, von Willebrand factor, and von Willebrand factor/von Willebrand antigen II complex. *J Clin Invest* 1985;75:1089.

134. Ewenstein BM, Warhol MJ, Handin RI, et al. Composition of the vWF storage organelle (Weibel-Palade body) isolated from cultured human umbilical vein endothelial cells. *J Cell Biol* 1987;104:1423.

135. Takagi J, Sekiya F, Kasahara K, et al. Inhibition of platelet-collagen interaction by propolypeptide of von Willebrand factor. *J Biol Chem* 1989;264:6017.

136. Takagi J, Kasahara K, Sekiya F, et al. A collagen-binding glycoprotein from bovine platelets is identical to the propolypeptide of von Willebrand factor. *J Biol Chem* 1989;264:10425.

137. Weibel ER, Palade GC. New cytoplasmic components in arterial endothelia. *J Cell Biol* 1964;23:101.

138. Fuchs A, Weibel ER. Morphometrische untersuchung der verterlung liner spezifischen cytoplasmatischen organelle in endothelzellen der ratte. *Z Zellforsch* 1966;73:1.

139. Kumar P, Kumar S, Marsden HB, et al. Weibel-Palade bodies in endothelial cells as a marker for angiogenesis in brain tumors. *Cancer Res* 1980;40:2010.

140. Kumar P, Erroi A, Sattar A, et al. Weibel-Palade bodies as a marker for neovascularization induced by tumor and rheumatoid angiogenesis factors. *Cancer Res* 1985;45:4339.

141. Ho KL. Ultrastructure of cerebellar capillary hemangioblastoma. 1. Weibel-Palade bodies and stroma cell histogenesis. *J Neuropathol Exp Neurol* 1984;43:592.

142. Matsuda H, Sugiura S. Ultrastructure of "tubular body" in endothelial cells of the ocular blood vessels. *Invest Ophthalmol* 1970;9:919.

143. Sengel A, Stoebner P. Golgi origin of tubular inclusions in endothelial cells. *J Cell Biol* 1970;44:223.

144. Reinders JH, de Groot PG, Gonsalves MD, et al. Isolation of a storage and secretory organelle containing vW protein from cultured human endothelial cells. *Biochim Biophys Acta* 1984;844:306.

145. Reinders JH, de Groot PG, Dawes J, et al. Comparison of secretion and subcellular localization of von Willebrand protein with that of thrombospondin and fibronectin in cultured human vascular endothelial cells. *Biochim Biophys Acta* 1985;844:306.

146. Loscalzo J, Fisch M, Handin RI. Solution studies of the quaternary structure and assembly of human von Willebrand factor. *Biochemistry* 1985;24:4468.

147. Mayadas TN, Wagner DD. In vitro multimerization of von Willebrand factor is triggered by low pH. Importance of the propolypeptide and free sulfhydryls. *J Biol Chem* 1989;264:13497.

148. Prentice CR, Forbes CD, Smith SM. Rise of factor VIII after exercise and adrenalin infusion measured by immunological and biological techniques. *Thromb Res* 1972;1:493.

149. Mannucci PM, Aberg M, Nilsson IL, et al. Mechanism of plasminogen activator and factor VIII increase after vasoactive drugs. *Br J Haematol* 1975;30:81.

150. Koutts J, Walsh PN, Plow EF, et al. Active release of human platelet factor VIII-related antigen by adenosine diphosphate, collagen and thrombin. *J Clin Invest* 1978;62:1255.

151. Kelly RB. Pathways of protein secretion in eukaryotes. *Science* 1985;230:25.

152. Loesberg C, Gonsalves MD, Zanderbergen J, et al. The effect of calcium on the secretion of factor VIII-related antigen by cultured endothelial cells. *Biochim Biophys Acta* 1983;763:160.

153. Sporn LA, Marder VJ, Wagner DD. Inducible secretion of large, biologically potent von Willebrand factor multimers. *Cell* 1986;46:185.

154. Booyse FM, Quarfoot AJ, Chediak J, et al. Characterization and properties of cultured human von Willebrand umbilical vein endothelial cells. *Blood* 1981;58:788.

155. Ewenstein BM, Inbal A, Pober JS, et al. Molecular studies of von Willebrand's disease: reduced von Willebrand factor biosynthesis, storage and release in endothelial cells derived from patients with type I von Willebrand's disease. *Blood* 1990;75:1466.

156. Federici AB, de Groot PG, Moia M, et al. Type I von Willebrand disease, subtype "platelet low": decreased platelet adhesion can be explained by low synthesis of von Willebrand factor in endothelial cells. *Br J Haematol* 1992;83:88.

157. Harrison RL, McKee PA. Estrogen stimulates von Willebrand factor production by cultured endothelial cells. *Blood* 1984;63:657.

158. Strauss HS, Diamond LK. Elevation of factor VIII (antihemophilic factor) during pregnancy in normal persons and in a patient with von Willebrand's disease. *N Engl J Med* 1963;269:1251.

159. Leone G, Moneta E, Paparatti G, et al. von Willebrand's disease in pregnancy. *N Engl J Med* 1975;293:456.

160. Crowell EB, Clatanoff DV, Kiekhofer W. The effect of oral contraceptive on factor VIII levels. *J Lab Clin Med* 1971;77:551.

161. Pottinger BE, Read RC, Paleolog EM, et al. von Willebrand factor is an acute phase reactant in man. *Thromb Res* 1989;53:389.

162. Schorer AE, Moldow CF, Rick ME. Interleukin 1 or endotoxin increases the release of von Willebrand factor from human endothelial cells. *Br J Haematol* 1987;67:193.

163. Giddings JC, Shall L. Enhanced release of von Willebrand factor by human endothelial cells in culture in the presence of phorbol myristate acetate and interleukin 1. *Thromb Res* 1987;47:259.

164. de Groot PG, Verweij CL, Nawrath PP, et al. Interleukin 1 inhibits the synthesis of von Willebrand factor in endothelial cells which results in a decreased reactivity of their matrix towards platelets. *Arteriosclerosis* 1987;7:605.

165. Zavoico GB, Ewenstein BM, Schafer AI, et al. IL-1 and related cytokines enhance thrombin stimulated PGI2 production in cultured endothelial cells without affecting thrombin-stimulated von Willebrand factor secretion or platelet-activating factor biosynthesis. *J Immunol* 1989;142:3993.

166. Paleolog EM, Crossman DC, McVey JH, et al. Differential regulation by cytokines of constitutive and stimulated secretion of von Willebrand factor from endothelial cells. *Blood* 1989;75:688.

167. Levine JD, Harlan JM, Harker LA, et al. Thrombin-mediated release of factor VIII antigen from human umbilical vein endothelial cells in culture. *Blood* 1982;60:531.

168. de Groot PG, Gonsalves MD, Loesberg C, et al. Thrombin-induced release of von Willebrand factor from endothelial cells is mediated by phospholipid methylation. Prostacyclin synthesis is independent of phospholipid methylation. *J Biol Chem* 1984;259:13329.

169. Hamilton KK, Sims PJ. Changes in cytosolic Ca2+ associated with von Willebrand factor release in endothelial cells exposed to histamine. *J Clin Invest* 1987;79:600.

170. Ewenstein BM, Jacobson BC, Romano M, et al. Peptide-leukotrienes stimulate von Willebrand factor release from human endothelial cells. *Blood* 1991;78:69a.

171. Ribes JA, Francis CW, Wagner DD. Fibrin induces release of von Willebrand factor from endothelial cells. *J Clin Invest* 1987;79:117.

172. Ribes JA, Ni F, Wagner DD, et al. Mediation of fibrin-induced release of von Willebrand factor from cultured endothelial cells by the fibrin beta chain. *J Clin Invest* 1989;84:435.

173. Hattori R, Hamilton KK, McEver RP, et al. Complement proteins C5b-9 induce secretion of high molecular weight multimers of endothelial von Willebrand factor and translocation of granule membrane protein GMP140 to the cell surface. *J Biol Chem* 1989;264:9053.

174. Booyse FM, Osilowicz G, Feder S. Effects of various agents on ristocetin-Willebrand factor activity in long term cultures of vWF and normal human umbilical vein endothelial cells. *Thromb Haemost* 1981;46:668.

175. Tuddenham EG, Lazarchich J, Hoyer LW. Synthesis and release of factor VIII by cultured human endothelial cells. *Br J Haematol* 1981;47:617.

176. Hashemi S, Tackaberry ES, Palmer DS, et al. DDAVP-induced release of von Willebrand factor from endothelial cells in vitro: the effect of plasma and blood cells. *Biochim Biophys Acta* 1990;1052:63.

177. Hallam TJ, Jacob R, Merritt JE. Evidence that agonists stimulate bivalent-cation influx into human endothelial cells. *Biochem J* 1988;255:179.

178. Rotrosen D, Gallin JI. Histamine type I receptor occupancy increases endothelial cytosolic calcium, reduces F-actin, and promotes albumin diffusion across cultured endothelial monolayers. *J Cell Biol* 1986;130:2379.

179. Birch KA, Pober JS, Zavoico GB, et al. Calcium/calmodulin transduced thrombin-stimulated secretion: studies in intact and minimally permeabilized human umbilical vein endothelial cells. *J Cell Biol* 1992;118:1501.

180. McNiff JM, Gil J. Secretion of Weibel-Palade bodies observed in extraalveolar vessels of rabbit lung. *J Appl Physiol* 1983;54:1284.

181. Fitzgerald LA, Charo IF, Philips DR. Human and bovine endothelial cells synthesize membrane proteins similar to human platelet glycoproteins IIb and IIIa. *J Biol Chem* 1985;260:10893.

182. Beacham DA, Wise RJ, Turci SM, et al. Selective inactivation of the Arg-Gly-Asp-Ser (RGDS) binding site in von Willebrand factor by site-directed mutagenesis. *J Biol Chem* 1992;267:3409.

183. Sprandio JD, Shapiro SS, Thiagarjan P, et al. Cultured human vein endothelial cells contain a membrane glycoprotein immunologically related to platelet glycoprotein Ib. *Blood* 1988;71:234.

184. Konkle BA, Shapiro SS, Asch AS, et al. Cytokine-enhanced expression of glycoprotein Ib in human endothelium. *J Biol Chem* 1990;265:19838.

185. Bowie EJ, Solberg LA, Fass DN, et al. Transplantation of normal bone marrow into a pig with severe von Willebrand's disease. *J Clin Invest* 1986;78:26.

186. Hoyer LW, Shainoff JR. Factor VIII-related protein circulates in normal human plasma as high molecular weight multimers. *Blood* 1980;55:1056.

187. Ruggeri ZM, Zimmerman TS. The complex multimeric composition of factor VIII/von Willebrand factor. *Blood* 1981;57:1140.

188. Zheng X, Chung D, Takayama TK, et al. Structure of von Willebrand factor-cleaving protease (ADAMTS13), a metalloproteinase involved in thrombotic thrombocytopenic purpura. *J Biol Chem* 2001;276:41059.

189. Reference deleted.

190. Levy GG, Nichols WC, Lian EC, et al. Mutations in a member of the ADAMTS gene family cause thrombotic thrombocytopenic purpura. *Nature* 2001;413:488–494.

191. Remuzzi G, Galbusera M, Noris M, et al. von Willebrand factor cleaving protease (ADAMTS13) is deficient in recurrent and familial thrombotic thrombocytopenic purpura and hemolytic uremic syndrome. *Blood* 2002;100:778–785.

192. Bianchi V, Robles R, Alberio L, et al. von Willebrand factor-cleaving protease (ADAMTS13) in thrombocytopenic disorders: a severely deficient activity is specific for thrombotic thrombocytopenic purpura. *Blood* 2002;100:710–713.

193. Kokame K, Matsumoto M, Soejima K, et al. Mutations and common polymorphisms in ADAMTS13 gene responsible for von Willebrand factor-cleaving protease activity. *Proc Natl Acad Sci U S A* 2002;99:11902–11907.

194. Zheng X, Majerus EM, Sadler JE. ADAMTS13 and TTP. *Curr Opin Hematol* 2002;9:389–394.

195. Park YD, Yoshioka A, Kawa K, et al. Impaired activity of plasma von Willebrand factor-cleaving protease may predict the occurrence of hepatic veno-occlusive disease after stem cell transplantation. *Bone Marrow Transplant* 2002;29:789–794.

196. Mannucci PM, Canciani MT, Forza I, et al. Changes in health and disease of the metalloprotease that cleaves von Willebrand factor. *Blood* 2001;98:2730–2735.

197. He S, Cao H, Magnusson CG, et al. Are increased levels of von Willebrand factor in chronic coronary heart disease caused by decrease in von Willebrand factor cleaving protease activity? A study by an immunoassay with antibody against intact bond 842Tyr-843Met of the von Willebrand factor protein. *Thromb Res* 2001;103:241–248.

198. Pimanda J, Hogg P. Control of von Willebrand factor multimer size and implications for disease. *Blood Rev* 2002;16:185.

199. Sporn LA, Marder VJ, Wagner. Differing polarity of the constitutive and regulated secretory pathways for von Willebrand factor in endothelial cells. *J Cell Biol* 1989;108:1283.

200. Tsai HM, Nagel RL, Hatcher VB, et al. The high molecular weight form of endothelial cell von Willebrand factor is released by the regulated pathway. *Br J Haematol* 1991;79:239.

201. Koedam JA, Meijers JC, Sixma JJ, et al. Inactivation of human factor VIII by activated protein C. Cofactor activity of protein S and protective effect of von Willebrand factor. *J Clin Invest* 1988;82:1236.

202. Fay PJ, Coumans JV, Walker FJ. von Willebrand factor mediates protection of factor VIII from activated protein C-catalyzed inactivation. *J Biol Chem* 1991;266:2172.

203. Hamer RJ, Koedam JA, Beeser-Visser NH, et al. The effect of thrombin on the complex between factor VIII and von Willebrand factor. *Eur J Biochem* 1987;167:253.

204. Preston AE, Barr A. The plasma concentration of factor VIII in the normal population: the effects of age, sex and blood groups. *Br J Haematol* 1964;10:238.

205. Jeremic M, Weisert O, Gedde-Dahl TW. Factor VIII (AHG) levels in 1016 regular blood donors: the effects of age, sex and ABO blood groups. *Scand J Clin Lab Invest* 1976;36:461.

206. McCallum CJ, Peake IR, Newcombe RG, et al. Factor VIII levels in blood group antigens. *Thromb Haemost (Stuttg)* 1983;50:757.

207. Orstavik KH, Magnus P, Reisner H, et al. Factor VIII and factor IX in a twin population: evidence for a major effect of ABO locus on factor VIII level. *Am J Hum Genet* 1985;37:89.

208. Graham JB, Rizza CR, Chediak J, et al. Carrier detection in hemophilia A: a cooperative international study. I. The carrier phenotype. *Blood* 1986;67:1554.

209. Gill JC, Endres-Brooks J, Bauer PJ, et al. The effect of ABO blood group on the diagnosis of von Willebrand disease. *Blood* 1987;69:1691.

210. Stormorken H, Erikssen J. Plasma antithrombin III and factor VIII antigen in relation to angiographic findings, angina and blood groups in middle-aged men. *Thromb Haemost (Stuttg)* 1977;38:874.

211. Wahlberg TB, Savidge GF, Blombäck M, et al. Influence of age, sex and blood groups on 15 blood coagulation laboratory variables in a reference material composed of 80 blood donors. *Vox Sang* 1980;39:301.

212. Rouger P, Riveau D, Salmon C. Detection of the H and I blood group antigens in normal plasma. *Vox Sang* 1979;37:78.

213. Orstavik KH, Kornstad L, Reisner H, et al. Possible effect of secretor locus on plasma concentrations of factor VIII and von Willebrand factor. *Blood* 1989;73:990.

214. Van Cong N, Weil D, Finaz C, et al. Assignment of the ABO-Np-Akl linkage group to chromosome 9 in man-hamster hybrids. *Cytogenet Cell Genet* 1976;16:241.

215. Sodetz JM, Paulson JC, McKee PA. Carbohydrate composition and identification of blood groups A, B and H oligo-saccharide structures of human factor VIII/von Willebrand factor. *J Biol Chem* 1979;254:10754.

216. Mazurier C, Samor B, Mannessier L, et al. Blood group A and B activity associated with factor VIII/von Willebrand factor. *Blood Transfusion Immunohaematol* 1981;24:289.

217. Johnson SS, Montgomery RR, Hathaway WE. Newborn factor VIII complex: elevated activities in term infants and alterations in electrophoretic mobility related to illness and activated coagulation. *Br J Haematol* 1981;47:597.

218. Weinger RS, Cecalupo AJ, Olson JD, et al. Neonatal von Willebrand's disease: diagnostic difficulty at birth. *Am J Dis Child* 1980;134:793.

219. Weinstein MJ, Blanchard R, Moake JL, et al. Fetal and neonatal von Willebrand factor (vWF) is unusually large and similar to the vWF in patients with thrombotic thrombocytopenic purpura. *Br J Haematol* 1989;72:68.

220. Katz JA, Moake JL, McPherson PD, et al. Relationship between human development and disappearance of unusually large von Willebrand factor multimers from plasma. *Blood* 1989;73:1851.

221. Maruzier C, Daffos F, Forestier F. Electrophoretic and functional characteristics of the von Willebrand factor in human fetal plasma. *Br J Haematol* 1992;81:263.

222. Cooperberg AA, Teitelbaum J. The concentration of antihemophilic globulin (AHG) related to age. *Br J Haematol* 1960;6:281.

223. Pitney WR, Kvik RL, Arnold BJ, et al. Plasma antihaemophilic factor (factor VIII) concentrations in normal families. *Br J Haematol* 1962;8:421.

224. Kasper CK, Hoag MS, Aggeler PM, et al. Blood clotting factor in pregnancy: factor VIII concentrates in normal and AHF-deficient women. *Obstet Gynecol* 1964;24:242.

225. Bennett B, Ratnoff OD. Changes in antihemophilic factor (AHF, factor VIII) procoagulant activity and AHF-like antigen in normal pregnancy, and following exercise and pneumoencephalography. *J Lab Clin Med* 1972;80:256.

226. Noller KL, Bowie EJ, Kempers RD, et al. von Willebrand's disease in pregnancy. *Obstet Gynecol* 1973;41:865.

227. Bennett B, Oxnard SC, Douglas AS, et al. Studies on antihemophilic factor (AHF, factor VIII) during labor in normal women, in patients with premature separation of the placenta, and in a patient with von Willebrand's disease. *J Lab Clin Med* 1974;84:851.

228. Krishnamurthy M, Miotti AB. von Willebrand's disease and pregnancy. *Obstet Gynecol* 1977;49:244.

229. Chediak JR, Alban GM, Maxey B. von Willebrand's disease and pregnancy: management during delivery and outcome of offspring. *Am J Obstet Gynecol* 1986;155:618.

230. Adashi EY. Lack of improvement in von Willebrand's disease during pregnancy. *N Engl J Med* 1980;303:1178.

231. Punnonen R, Nyman D, Grönroos M, et al. von Willebrand's disease and pregnancy. *Acta Obstet Gynecol Scand* 1981;60:507.

232. Rick ME, Williams SB, Sacher RA, et al. Thrombocytopenia associated with pregnancy in a patient with type IIB von Willebrand's disease. *Blood* 1987;69:786.

233. Giles AR, Hoogendoorn H, Benford K. Type IIB von Willebrand's disease presenting as thrombocytopenia during pregnancy. *Br J Haematol* 1987;67:349.

234. Rogers JS II, Shane SR, Jencks FS. Factor VIII activity and thyroid function. *Ann Intern Med* 1982;97:713.

235. Egeberg O. Influence of thyroid function on the blood clotting system. *Scand J Clin Lab Invest* 1963;15:1.

236. Dalton RG, Dewar MS, Savidge GF, et al. Hypothyroidism and von Willebrand's disease. *Lancet* 1987;1:1007.

237. MacCallum PK, Rodgers M, Taberner DA. Hypothyroidism and von Willebrand's disease. *Lancet* 1987;1:1314.

238. Smith SR, Auger MJ. Hypothyroidism and von Willebrand's disease. *Lancet* 1987;1:1314.

239. Rogers JS II, Shane SR. Factor VIII activity in normal volunteers receiving oral thyroid hormone. *J Lab Clin Med* 1983;102:444.

240. Rizza CR. Effect of exercise on the level of antihaemophilic globulin in human blood. *J Physiol (Lond)* 1961;156:128.

241. Egeberg O. On the nature of blood and antihemophilic A factor (AHA-FVIII) increase associated with muscular exercise. *Scand J Clin Lab Invest* 1963;15:202.

242. Stibbe J. Effect of exercise on FVIII complexes: proportional increase of ristocetin cofactor (von Willebrand factor) and FVIII-AGN, but disproportional increase of FVIII-AHF. *Thromb Res* 1977;10:163.

243. Brown JE, Baugh RF, Hougie C. Effector of exercise on the factor VIII complex: correlation of the von Willebrand antigen and factor VIII coagulant antigen increase. *Thromb Res* 1979;15:61.

244. Wheeler ME, Davis GL, Gillespie WJ, et al. Physiological changes in hemostasis associated with acute exercise. *J Appl Physiol* 1986;60:986.

245. Andrew M, Carter C, O'Brodovich H, et al. Increases in factor VIII complex and fibrinolytic activity are dependent on exercise intensity. *J Appl Physiol* 1986;60:1917.

246. Musemeci V, Cardillo C, Baroni S, et al. Effects of calcium channel blockers on the endothelial release of von Willebrand factor after exercise in healthy subjects. *J Lab Clin Med* 1989;113:525.

247. Rand JH, Sussman II, Gordon RE, et al. Localization of factor VIII-related antigen in human vascular subendothelium. *Blood* 1980;55:752.

248. Sussman II, Rand JR. Subendothelial deposition of von Willebrand factor requires the presence of endothelial cells. *J Lab Clin Med* 1982;100:526.

249. Sakariassen KS, Bolhuis PA, Sixma JJ. Human blood platelet adhesion to artery subendothelium is mediated by factor VIII-von Willebrand factor bound to the subendothelium. *Nature* 1979;279:636.

250. Sakariassen KS, Ottenhof-Rovers M, Sixma JJ. Factor VIII-von Willebrand factor requires calcium for facilitation of platelet adherence. *Blood* 1984;63:996.

251. Scott DM, Griffin B, Pepper DS, et al. The binding of purified factor VIII/von Willebrand factor to collagens of different type and forms. *Thromb Res* 1981;24:467.

252. Santoro SA. Adsorption of von Willebrand factor/VIII by the genetically distinct interstitial collagens. *Thromb Res* 1981;21:689.

253. Morton LF, Griffin B, Pepper DS, et al. The interaction between collagens and factor VIII/von Willebrand factor: investigation of the structural requirements for interaction. *Thromb Res* 1983;32:545.

254. Kessler CM, Floyd CM, Rick ME, et al. Collagen-factor VIII/von Willebrand factor protein interaction. *Blood* 1984;63:1291.

255. Rand JH, Patel ND, Schwartz E, et al. 150-kD von Willebrand factor binding protein extracted from human vascular subendothelium is type VI collagen. *J Clin Invest* 1991;88:253.

256. Wagner DD, Urban-Pickering M, Marder VJ. von Willebrand protein binds to extracellular matrices independently of collagen. *Proc Natl Acad Sci U S A* 1984;81:471.

257. Madaras F, Bell WR, Castaldi PA. Isolation and insolubilisation of human F-VIII by affinity chromatography. *Haemostasis* 1978;7:321.

258. Trueb B, Schreier T, Bruckner P, et al. Type VI collagen represents a major fraction of connective tissue collagens. *Eur J Biochem* 1987;166:699.

259. Bonaldo P, Colombatti A. The carboxyl terminus of the chicken alpha 3 chain of collagen VI is a unique mosaic structure with glycoprotein Ib-like, fibronectin type III, and Kunitz modules. *J Biol Chem* 1989;264:20235.

260. Bockenstedt P, McDonagh J, Handin RI. Binding and covalent cross-linking of purified von Willebrand factor to native monomeric collagen. *J Clin Invest* 1986;78:551.

261. Tannenbaum SH, Rick ME, Shafer B, et al. Subendothelial matrix of cultured endothelial cells contains fully processed high molecular weight von Willebrand factor. *J Lab Clin Med* 1989;113:372.

262. Santoro SA. Preferential binding of high molecular weight forms of von Willebrand factor to fibrillar collagen. *Biochim Biophys Acta* 1983;756:123.

263. Sporn LA, Marder VJ, Wagner DD. von Willebrand factor released from Weibel-Palade bodies binds more avidly to extracellular matrix than that secreted constitutively. *Blood* 1987;69:1531.

264. Sixma JJ, Sakariassen KS, Beeser-Visser NH, et al. Adhesion of platelets to human artery subendothelium: effect of factor VIII-von Willebrand factor of various multimeric compositions. *Blood* 1984;63:128.

265. Tschopp TB, Baumgartner HR, Silberbauer K, et al. Platelet adhesion and platelet thrombus formation on subendothelium of human arteries and veins exposed to flowing blood in vitro. A comparison with rabbit aorta. *Haemostasis* 1979;8:19.

266. Turitto VT, Baumgartner HR. Platelet deposition on subendothelium exposed to flowing blood: mathematical analysis of physical parameters. *Trans Am Soc Artif Intern Organs* 1975;21:593.

267. Turitto VT, Baumgartner HR. Rheological factors influencing platelet interaction with vessel surfaces. *J Rheology* 1979;23:735.

268. Weiss HJ, Turitto VT, Baumgartner HR. Effect of shear rate on platelet interaction with subendothelium in citrated and native blood. Shear-rate dependent decrease of adhesion in von Willebrand's disease and the Bernard-Soulier syndrome. *J Lab Clin Med* 1978;92:750.

269. Stel HV, Sakariassen KS, de Groot PG, et al. von Willebrand factor in the vessel wall mediates platelet adherence. *Blood* 1985;65:85.

270. Turitto VT, Weiss HJ, Zimmerman TS, et al. Factor VIII/von Willebrand factor in subendothelium mediates platelet adhesion. *Blood* 1985;65:823.

271. Baruch D, Denis C, Mareaux C, et al. Role of von Willebrand factor associated to extracellular matrices in platelet adhesion. *Blood* 1991;77:519.

272. Tschopp TB, Weiss HJ, Baumgartner HR. Decreased adhesion of platelets to subendothelium in von Willebrand's disease. *J Lab Clin Med* 1974;83:296.

273. Baumgartner HR, Turitto VT, Weiss HJ. Effect of shear rate on platelet interaction with subendothelium in citrated and native blood. II. Relationships among platelet adhesion, thrombus dimensions and fibrin formation. *J Lab Clin Med* 1980;95:208.

274. Sakariassen KS, Aarts PA, de Groot PD, et al. A perfusion chamber to investigate platelet interaction in flowing blood with human vessel wall cells, their extracellular matrix and purified components. *J Lab Clin Med* 1983;102:522.

275. Sixma JJ, Nievelstein PF, Houdijk WP, et al. Adhesion of blood platelets to isolated components of the vessel walls. *Ann N Y Acad Sci* 1987;509:103.

276. Olson JD, Zaleski A, Herrman D, et al. Adhesion of platelets to purified solid-phase von Willebrand factor: effects of walls shear rate, ADP, thrombin and ristocetin. *J Lab Clin Med* 1989;114:6.

277. Furlan M. Factor VIII/von Willebrand factor: a multivalent ligand binding to platelets and collagen. *Blut* 1986;52:329.

278. Nachman RL, Levine R, Jaffe EA. Synthesis of factor VIII antigen by cultured guinea pig megakaryocytes. *J Clin Invest* 1977;60:914.

279. Howard MA, Montgomery DC, Hardisty RM. Factor VIII related antigen in platelets. *Thromb Res* 1974;4:617.

280. Nachman RL, Jaffe EA. Subcellular platelet factor VIII antigen and von Willebrand factor. *J Exp Med* 1975;141:1101.

281. Slot JW, Bouma BN, Montgomery R, et al. Platelet factor VIII-related antigen: immunofluorescent localization. *Thromb Res* 1978;13:871.

282. Zucker MB, Broekman MJ, Kaplan KL. Factor VIII-related antigen in human blood platelets. *J Lab Clin Med* 1979;94:675.

283. Wencel-Drake JD, Painter RG, Zimmerman TS, et al. Ultrastructural localization of human platelet thrombospondin, fibrinogen and fibronectin and vW factor in frozen thin section. *Blood* 1985;65:929.

284. Jeanneau C, Avner P, Sultan Y. Use of monoclonal antibody and colloidal gold in E.M. localization of von Willebrand factor in megakaryocytes and platelets. *Cell Biol Int Rep* 1984;8:841.

285. Cramer EM, Meyer D, Le Menn R, et al. Eccentric localization of vW factor in an internal structure of platelet-granule resembling that of Weibel-Palade bodies. *Blood* 1985;66:710.

286. Harrison P, Savidge GF, Cramer EM. The origin and physiological relevance of alpha-granule adhesive proteins. *Br J Haematol* 1990;74:125.

287. Ruggeri ZM, Zimmerman TS. Variant von Willebrand's disease: characterization of two subtypes by analysis of multimeric composition of factor VIII/von Willebrand factor in plasma and platelets. *J Clin Invest* 1980;65:1318a.

288. Gralnick HR, Williams SB, McKeown LP, et al. Platelet von Willebrand factor: comparison with plasma von Willebrand factor. *Thromb Res* 1985;38:623.

289. Fernandez MF, Ginsburg MH, Ruggeri ZM, et al. Multimeric structure of platelet factor VIII/von Willebrand factor: the presence of larger multimers and their reassociation with thrombin-stimulated platelets. *Blood* 1982;60:1132.

290. George JN, Onofre AR. Human platelet surface binding of endogenous secreted factor VIII-von Willebrand factor and platelet factor 4. *Blood* 1982;59:194.

291. Parker RI, Rick ME, Gralnick HR. Effect of calcium on the availability of platelet von Willebrand factor. *J Lab Clin Med* 1985;106:336.

292. Mannucci PM, Lombardi R, Bader R, et al. Heterogeneity of type I von Willebrand disease: evidence for a subgroup with an abnormal von Willebrand factor. *Blood* 1985;66:796.

293. Gralnick HR, Rick ME, McKeown LP, et al. Platelet von Willebrand factor: an important determinant of the bleeding time in type I von Willebrand's disease. *Blood* 1986;68:58.

294. Fressinaud E, Baruch D, Rothschild C, et al. Platelet von Willebrand factor: evidence for its involvement in platelet adhesion to collagen. *Blood* 1987;70:1214.

295. Castillo R, Escolar G, Monteagudo J, et al. Role for platelet von Willebrand factor in supporting platelet-vessel wall interactions in von Willebrand disease. *Am J Hematol* 1989;31:153.

296. Castillo R, Monteagudo J, Escolar G, et al. Hemostatic effect of normal platelet transfusion in severe von Willebrand disease patients. *Blood* 1991;77:1901.

297. Voorberg J, Fonjijn R, Calafat J, et al. Biogenesis of von Willebrand factor-containing organelles in heterologous transfected CV-1 cells. *EMBO J* 1993;12:749.

298. Kramer W, Drutsa V, Jansen HW, et al. The gapped duplex DNA approach to oligonucleotide-directed mutation construction. *Nucleic Acids Res* 1984;12:9441.

299. Meulien P, Nishino M, Mazurier C, et al. Processing and characterization of recombinant von Willebrand factor expressed in different cell types using a vaccinia virus vector. *Thromb Haemost* 1992;67:154.

300. Wagner DD, Saffaripour S, Bonfanti R, et al. Induction of specific organelles by von Willebrand factor propolypeptide. *Cell* 1991;64:403.

301. Silwer J, Nilsson IM. On a Swedish family with 51 members affected by von Willebrand's disease. *Acta Med Scand* 1964;175:627.

302. Bloom AL. The von Willebrand syndrome. *Semin Hematol* 1980;17:215.

303. Bachman F. Diagnostic approach to mild bleeding disorders. *Semin Hematol* 1980;17:292.

304. Rodeghiero F, Castman G, Dini E. Epidemiological investigation of the prevalence of von Willebrand's disease. *Blood* 1987;69:454.

305. Berliner SA, Seligsohn U, Zivelin A, et al. A relatively high frequency of severe (type III) von Willebrand's disease in Israel. *Br J Haematol* 1986;62:535.

306. Weiss HJ, Ball AP, Mannucci PM. Incidence of severe von Willebrand's disease. *N Engl J Med* 1982;307:127.

307. Mannucci PM, Bloom AL, Larrieu MJ, et al. Atherosclerosis and von Willebrand factor: prevalence of severe von Willebrand's disease in western Europe and Israel. *Br J Haematol* 1984;57:163.

308. Italian Working Group. Spectrum of von Willebrand's disease: a study of 100 cases. *Br J Haematol* 1977;35:101.

309. Holmber L, Nilsson IM. von Willebrand's disease. *Eur J Haematol* 1992;48:127.

310. Miller CH, Graham JB, Goldin LR, et al. Genetics of classic von Willebrand's disease. I. Phenotypic variation within families. *Blood* 1979;54:117.

311. Miller CH, Graham JB, Goldin LR, et al. Genetics of classic von Willebrand's disease. II. Optimal assignment of the heterozygous genotype (diagnosis) by discriminant analysis. *Blood* 1979;54:137.

312. Blombäck M, Eneroth P, Landgren BM, et al. On the intraindividual and gender variability of haemostatic components. *Thromb Haemost* 1992;67:70.

313. Blombäck M, Eneroth P, Andersson O, et al. On laboratory problems in diagnosing mild von Willebrand's disease. *Am J Hematol* 1992;40:117.

314. Lind SE. Prolonged bleeding time. *Am J Med* 1984;77:305.

315. Burns ER, Lawrence C. Bleeding time. A guide to its diagnostic and clinical utility. *Arch Pathol Lab Med* 1989;113:1219.

316. Rodgers RP, Levin J. A critical reappraisal of the bleeding time. *Semin Thromb Haemost* 1990;16:1.

317. Bowie EJ, Didisheim P, Thompson JH, et al. von Willebrand's disease: a critical review. *Hematol Rev* 1968;1:1.

318. Mielke CH, Kaneshiro MM, Maher IA, et al. The standardized normal Ivy bleeding time and its prolongation by aspirin. *Blood* 1969;34:204.

319. Kumar R, Ansell JE, Canoso RT, et al. Clinical trials of a new bleeding time device. *Am J Clin Pathol* 1978;70:642.

320. Ivy AC, Shapiro PF, Melnich P. The bleeding tendency in jaundice. *Surg Gynecol Obstet* 1935;60:357.
321. Nilsson IM, Magnusson S, Borchgrevink C. The Duke and Ivy methods for determination of the bleeding time. *Thromb Diath Haemorrh* 1963;10:223.
322. Borchgrevink CF, Egeberg O, Godal HC, et al. The effect of plasma and Cohn's fraction I on the Duke and Ivy bleeding times in von Willebrand's disease. *Acta Med Scand* 1963;173:235.
323. Pitney WR, Arnold BJ. Laboratory findings in families of patients suffering from von Willebrand's disease. *Br J Haematol* 1960;6:81.
324. Abildgaard CF, Suzuki Z, Harrison J, et al. Serial studies in von Willebrand's disease: variability versus "variants." *Blood* 1980;56:712.
325. Quick AJ. Salicylates and bleeding: the aspirin tolerance test. *Am J Med Sci* 1967;252:265a.
326. Quick AJ. The Minot-von Willebrand syndrome. *Am J Med Sci* 1967;253:520.
327. Ratnoff OD, Bennett B. Clues to the pathogenesis of bleeding in von Willebrand's disease. *N Engl J Med* 1973;289:1182.
328. Lian EC, Deykin D. In vivo dissociation of factor VIII (AHF) activity and factor VIII-related antigen in von Willebrand's disease. *Am J Hematol* 1976;1:71.
329. Hoyer LW. Immunological studies on antihemophilia factor (AHF, factor VIII). IV. Radioimmunoassay of AHF antigen. *J Lab Clin Med* 1972;80:822.
330. Counts RB. Solid-phase immunoradiometric assay of factor-VIII protein. *Br J Haematol* 1975;31:429.
331. Ruggeri ZM, Mannucci PM, Jeffcoate SL, et al. Immunoradiometric assay of factor VIII related antigen, with observations in 32 patients with von Willebrand's disease. *Br J Haematol* 1976;33:221.
332. Green D, Reynolds N. Double-antibody radioimmunoassay for factor VIII-related antigen. *Clin Chem* 1977;23:1648.
333. Girma JP, Ardaillou N, Meyer D, et al. Fluid-phase immunoradiometric assay for the detection of qualitative abnormalities of factor VIII/von Willebrand factor in variants of von Willebrand's disease. *J Lab Clin Med* 1979;93:926.
334. Bartlett A, Dormandy KM, Hawkey CM, et al. Factor VIII-related antigen: measurement by enzyme immuno-assay. *BMJ* 1976;1:994.
335. Mazurier C, Parquet-Gernez A, Goudemand M. Dosage de l'antigène lié au facteur VIII par la technique ELISA: intérêt dans l'étude de la maladie de Willebrand. *Pathol Biol* 1977;25[Suppl]:18.
336. Yorde LD, Hussey CV, Yorde DE, et al. Competitive enzyme-linked immunoassay for factor VIII antigen. *Clin Chem* 1979;25:1924.
337. Short PE, Williams CE, Picken AM, et al. Factor VIII related antigen: an improved enzyme immunoassay. *Med Lab Sci* 1982;39:351.
338. Batlle J, Lopez-Fernandez MF. Laboratory assays for von Willebrand factor. In: Zimmerman TS, Ruggeri ZM, eds. *Coagulation and bleeding disorders.* New York: Marcel Dekker Inc, 1989:325.
339. Weiss HJ, Pietu G, Rabinowitz R, et al. Heterogenous abnormalities in the multimeric structure, antigenic properties, and plasma-platelet content of factor VIII/von Willebrand factor in subtypes of classic (type I) and variant (type IIA) von Willebrand's disease. *J Lab Clin Med* 1983;101:411.
340. Ciavarella G, Ciavarella N, Antoncecchi S, et al. High-resolution analysis of von Willebrand factor multimeric composition defines a new variant of type I von Willebrand disease with aberrant structure but presence of all size multimers (type IC). *Blood* 1985;66:1423.
341. Aihara M, Sawada Y, Ueno K, et al. Visualization of von Willebrand factor multimers by immunoenzymatic stain using avidin-biotin peroxidase complex. *Thromb Haemost* 1986;55:263.
342. Miller MA, Pascak JE, Thompson MR, et al. A modified SDS agarose gel method for determining factor VIII von Willebrand factor multimers using commercially available reagents. *Thromb Res* 1983;39:777.
343. Chow R, Savidge GF. Enzyme linked antibody system for the visualization of FVIII multimers. *Thromb Haemost* 1985;54:75a.
344. Bukh A, Ingerslev J, Stenbjerg S, et al. The multimeric structure of plasma FVIII: Ag studies by electroelution and immunoperoxidase detection. *Thromb Res* 1986;43:579.
345. Lombardi R, Gelfi C, Righetti P, et al. Electroblot and immunoperoxidase staining for rapid screening of the abnormalities of the multimeric structure of von Willebrand factor in von Willebrand's disease. *Thromb Haemost* 1986;55:246.
346. Brosstad F, Kjoennisksen I, Roenning B, et al. Visualization of von Willebrand factor multimers by enzyme-conjugated secondary antibodies. *Thromb Haemost* 1986;55:276.
347. Mannucci PM, Lombardi R, Federici AB, et al. A new variant of type II von Willebrand disease with aberrant multimeric structure of plasma but not platelet von Willebrand factor (type IIF). *Blood* 1986;68:269.
348. Zucker MB. In vitro abnormality of the blood in von Willebrand's disease correctable by normal plasma. *Nature* 1963;197:601.
349. O'Brien JR, Heywood JB. Some interactions between human platelets and glass: von Willebrand's disease compared with normal. *J Clin Pathol* 1967;20:56.
350. Weiss HJ. von Willebrand's disease: diagnostic criteria. *Blood* 1968;32:668.
351. Allain JP, Cooper HA, Wagner RH, et al. Platelets fixed with paraformaldehyde: a new reagent for assay of von Willebrand factor and platelet aggregating factor. *J Lab Clin Med* 1975;85:318.
352. Kroll MH, Harris TS, Moake JL, et al. von Willebrand factor binding to platelet GpIb initiates signals for platelet activation. *J Clin Invest* 1991;88:1568.
353. Jenkins CS, Phillips DR, Clemetson KJ, et al. Platelet membrane glycoproteins implicated in ristocetin-induced aggregation. *J Clin Invest* 1976;57:112.
354. Moake JL, Olson JD, Troll JH, et al. Binding of radioiodinated human von Willebrand factor to Bernard-Soulier, thrombasthenic and von Willebrand's disease platelets. *Thromb Res* 1980;19:21.
355. Ruan C, Tobelem G, McMichael AJ, et al. Monoclonal antibody to human platelet glycoprotein I. II. Effects on human platelet function. *Br J Haematol* 1981;49:511.
356. Coller BS, Peerschke EI, Scudder LE, et al. Studies with a murine monoclonal antibody that abolished ristocetin-induced binding of von Willebrand factor to platelets: additional evidence in support of Gp Ib as a platelet receptor for von Willebrand factor. *Blood* 1983;61:99.
357. Coller BS. The effects of ristocetin and von Willebrand factor on platelet electrophoretic mobility. *J Clin Invest* 1977;61:1168.
358. Rosborough TK, Swaim WR. Abnormal polybrene-induced platelet agglutination in von Willebrand's disease. *Thromb Res* 1978;12:937.
359. Rosborough TK. von Willebrand factor, polycations, and platelet aggregation. *Thromb Res* 1980;17:481.
360. Coller BS. Polybrene-induced agglutination and reduction in electrophoretic mobility: enhancement by von Willebrand factor and inhibition by vancomycin. *Blood* 1980;55:276.
361. De Marco L, Shapiro SS. Properties of human asialo-factor VIII: a ristocetin-independent platelet-aggregating agent. *J Clin Invest* 1981;68:321.
362. Gralnick HR, Williams SB, McKeown LP, et al. von Willebrand's disease with spontaneous platelet aggregation induced by an abnormal plasma von Willebrand factor. *J Clin Invest* 1985;76:1522.
363. De Marco L, Grolami A, Russell S, et al. Interaction of asialo von Willebrand factor with glycoprotein Ib induces fibrinogen binding to the glycoprotein IIb/IIIa complex and mediates platelet aggregation. *J Clin Invest* 1985;75:1198.
364. Gralnick HR, Sultan Y, Coller BS. von Willebrand's disease: combined qualitative and quantitative abnormalities. *N Engl J Med* 1977;296:1024.
365. Hoyer LW, Rizza CR, Tuddenham EG, et al. von Willebrand factor multimer patterns in von Willebrand's disease. *Br J Haematol* 1983;55:493.
366. Gralnick HR, Williams SB, Morisato DK. Effect of the multimeric structure of the factor VIII/von Willebrand factor protein on binding to platelets. *Blood* 1981;58:387.
367. Federici AB, Mannucci PM, Lombardi R, et al. Type IIH von Willebrand disease: new structural abnormality of plasma and platelet von Willebrand factor in a patient with prolonged bleeding time and borderline levels of ristocetin cofactor activity. *Am J Hematol* 1989;32:287.
368. Coller BS, Franza B Jr, Gralnick HR. The pH dependence of quantitative ristocetin-induced platelet aggregation: theoretical and practical implications: a new device for maintenance of platelet-rich plasma pH. *Blood* 1976;47:841.
369. Weiss HJ. Abnormalities of factor VIII and platelet aggregation—use of ristocetin in diagnosing the von Willebrand syndrome. *Blood* 1975;45:403.
370. Weiss HJ, Sussman II. A new von Willebrand factor variant (type I, New York): increased ristocetin-induced platelet aggregation and plasma von Willebrand factor containing all vWF multimers. *Blood* 1986;68:149.
371. Ruggeri ZM, Pareti FI, Mannucci PM, et al. Heightened interaction between platelets and factor VIII/von Willebrand factor in a new subtype of von Willebrand's disease. *N Engl J Med* 1980;302:1047b.
372. Weiss HJ, Meyer D, Rabinowitz R, et al. Pseudo–von Willebrand's disease: an intrinsic platelet defect with aggregation by unmodified factor VIII/von Willebrand factor and enhanced adsorption of its high-molecular-weight multimers. *N Engl J Med* 1982;306:326.
373. Brinkhous KM, Read MS. Preservation of platelet receptors for platelet aggregating factor/von Willebrand factor by air drying, freezing or lyophilization: new stable platelet preparations for von Willebrand factor assays. *Thromb Res* 1978;13:591.
374. Sarji KE, Stratton RD, Wagner RH, et al. Nature of von Willebrand factor: a new assay and a specific inhibitor. *Proc Natl Acad Sci U S A* 1974;71:2937.
375. Weiss HJ. Relation of von Willebrand factor to bleeding time [Letter]. *N Engl J Med* 1974;291:420.
376. Hellem AJ. Platelet adhesiveness in von Willebrand disease: a study with a new modification of the glass bead filter method. *Scand J Haematol* 1970;7:374.
377. Bowie EJ, Owen CA Jr. Some factors influencing platelet retention in glass bead columns, including the influence of plastics. *Am J Clin Pathol* 1971;56:479.
378. Favaloro EJ. Collagen binding assay for von Willebrand factor (VWF:CBA): detection of von Willebrand's disease (VWD), and discrimination of VWD subtypes, depends on collagen source. *Thromb Haemost* 2000;83:127–135.
379. Favaloro EJ, Henniker A, Facey D, et al. Discrimination of von Willebrand's disease (VWD) subtypes: direct comparison of von Willebrand factor:collagen binding assay (VWF:CBA) with monoclonal antibody (MAB) based VWF-capture systems. *Thromb Haemost* 2000;84:541–547.
380. Casonato A, Pontara E, Bertomoro A, et al. von Willebrand factor collagen binding activity in the diagnosis of von Willebrand disease: an alternative to ristocetin co-factor activity? *Br J Haematol* 2001;112:578–583.
381. Federici AB, Canciani MT, Forza I, et al. Ristocetin cofactor and collagen binding activities normalized to antigen levels for a rapid diagnosis of type 2 von Willebrand disease—single center comparison of four different assays. *Thromb Haemost* 2000;84:1127–1128.
382. Ginsburg D, Sadler JE. von Willebrand disease: a database of point mutations, insertions, and deletions. *Thromb Haemost* 1993;69:177.
383. Nilsson IM. von Willebrand's disease from 1926. *Scand J Haematol* 1984;33:21.
384. Ngo KY, Glotz VT, Koziol JA, et al. Homozygous and heterozygous deletions of the von Willebrand factor gene in patients and carriers of severe von Willebrand disease. *Proc Natl Acad Sci U S A* 1988;85:2753.
385. Peake IR, Liddell MB, Moodie P, et al. Severe type III von Willebrand's disease caused by deletion of exon 42 of the von Willebrand factor gene: family studies that identify carriers of the condition and a compound heterozygous individual. *Blood* 1990;75:654.

386. Nichols WC, Lyons SE, Harrison JS, et al. Severe von Willebrand disease due to a defect at the level of von Willebrand factor mRNA expression: detection by exonic PCR-restriction fragment length polymorphism analysis. *Proc Natl Acad Sci U S A* 1991;88:3857.

387. Mannucci PM, Lombardi R, Castaman G, et al. von Willebrand disease "Vicenza" with larger-than-normal (supranormal) von Willebrand factor multimers. *Blood* 1988;71:65.

388. D'Alessio PA, Castaman G, Rodeghiero F, et al. In vivo experiments indicate that relatively high platelet deposition in von Willebrand's disease "Vicenza" is caused by normal platelet-VWF levels rather than by high VWF-multimers in plasma. *Thromb Res* 1992;65:221.

389. Randi AM, Sacchi E, Castaman GC, et al. The genetic defect of type I von Willebrand disease "Vicenza" is linked to the von Willebrand factor gene. *Thromb Haemost* 1993;69:173.

390. Zimmerman TS, Ruggeri ZM, Fulcher CA. Factor VIII/von Willebrand factor. *Prog Hematol* 1983;13:279.

391. Ruggeri ZM, Mannucci PM, Bader R, et al. Factor VIII-related properties in platelets from patients with von Willebrand's disease. *J Lab Clin Med* 1978;91:132.

392. Holmberg L, Mannucci PM, Turesson I, et al. Factor VIII antigen in the vessel walls in von Willebrand's disease and haemophilia A. *Scand J Haematol* 1974;13:33.

393. Bernardi F, Guerra S, Paracchini P, et al. von Willebrand disease investigated by two novel RFLPs. *Br J Haematol* 1988;68:243.

394. Nishino M, Girma JP, Rothschild C, et al. New variant of von Willebrand disease with defective binding to factor VIII. *Blood* 1989;74:1591.

395. Mazurier C, Dieval J, Jorieux S, et al. A new von Willebrand factor (vWF) defect in a patient with factor VIII (FVIII) deficiency but with normal levels and multimeric patterns of both plasma and platelet vWF: characterization of abnormal vWF/FVIII interaction. *Blood* 1990;75:20.

396. Kernoff PB, Gruson R, Rizza CR. A variant of factor VIII related antigen. *Br J Haematol* 1974;26:435.

397. Gralnick HR, Williams SB, McKeown LP, et al. A variant of type II von Willebrand disease with an abnormal triplet structure and discordant effects of protease inhibitors on plasma and platelet von Willebrand factor structure. *Am J Hematol* 1987;24:259.

398. Batlle J, Lopez-Fernandez MF, Campos M, et al. The heterogeneity of type IIA von Willebrand's disease: studies with protease inhibitors. *Blood* 1986;68:1207.

399. Ruggeri ZM, Mannucci PM, Lombardi R, et al. Multimeric composition of factor VIII/von Willebrand factor following administration of DDAVP: implications for pathophysiology and therapy of von Willebrand's disease subtypes. *Blood* 1982;59:1272.

400. Gralnick HR, Williams SB, McKeown LP, et al. DDAVP in type IIA von Willebrand's disease. *Blood* 1986;67:465.

401. Sultan Y, Simeon J, Caen JP. Electrophoretic heterogeneity of normal factor VIII/von Willebrand protein and abnormal electrophoretic mobility in patients with von Willebrand disease. *J Lab Clin Med* 1976;87:185.

402. Hill FG, Enayat MS, George AJ. Investigation including VIII R:Ag multimeric analysis of a large kindred with type II A von Willebrand's disease showing a dominant inheritance and a similar gene expression in four generations. *Thromb Haemost* 1983;50:735.

403. Asakura A, Harrison J, Gomperts E, et al. Type IIA von Willebrand disease with apparent recessive inheritance. *Blood* 1987;69:1419.

404. Ginsburg D, Konkle BA, Gill JC, et al. Molecular basis of human von Willebrand disease: analysis of platelet von Willebrand factor mRNA. *Proc Natl Acad Sci U S A* 1989;86:3723.

405. Lyons SE, Bruck ME, Bowie EJ, et al. Impaired intracellular transport produced by a subset of type IIA von Willebrand mutations. *J Biol Chem* 1992;267:4424.

406. Zimmerman TS, Dent JA, Ruggeri ZM, et al. Subunit composition of plasma von Willebrand factor: cleavage is present in normal individuals, increased in IIA and IIB von Willebrand disease, but minimal in variants with aberrant structure of individual oligomers (types IIC, IID, and IIE). *J Clin Invest* 1986;77:947.

407. Kunicki TJ, Montgomery RR, Shullek J. Cleavage of human von Willebrand factor by platelet calcium-activated protease. *Blood* 1985;66:352.

408. Thompson EA, Howard MA. Proteolytic cleavage of human von Willebrand factor induced by enzyme(s) released from polymorphonuclear cells. *Blood* 1986;67:1281.

409. Federici AB, Elder JH, De Marco L, et al. Carbohydrate moiety of von Willebrand factor is not necessary for maintaining multimeric structure and ristocetin cofactor activity but protects from proteolytic degradation. *J Clin Invest* 1984;74:2049.

410. Hamilton KK, Fretto LJ, Grierson DS, et al. Effects of plasmin on von Willebrand multimers: degradation in vitro and stimulation of release in vivo. *J Clin Invest* 1985;76:261.

411. Berkowitz SD, Dent J, Roberts J, et al. Epitope mapping of the von Willebrand factor subunit distinguishes fragments present in normal and type IIA von Willebrand disease from those generated by plasmin. *J Clin Invest* 1987;79:524.

412. Berkowitz SD, Nozaki H, Titani K, et al. Evidence that calpains and elastase do not produce the von Willebrand factor fragments present in normal plasma and IIA von Willebrand disease. *Blood* 1988;72:721.

413. Verweij CL, Quadt R, Briet E, et al. Genetic linkage of two intragenic restriction fragment length polymorphisms with von Willebrand's disease type IIA. Evidence for a defect in the von Willebrand factor gene. *J Clin Invest* 1988;81:1116.

414. Iannuzzi MC, Hidaka N, Boehnke ML, et al. Analysis of the relationship of von Willebrand disease (vWD) and hereditary hemorrhagic telangiectasia and identification of a potential type IIA vWD mutation. *Am J Hum Genet* 1991;48:757.

415. Dent JA, Berkowitz SD, Ware J, et al. Identification of a cleavage site directing the immunochemical detection of molecular abnormalities in type IIA von Willebrand factor. *Proc Natl Acad Sci U S A* 1990;87:6306.

416. Levene RB, Booyse FM, Chediak J, et al. Expression of abnormal von Willebrand factor by endothelial cells from a patient with type IIA von Willebrand disease. *Proc Natl Acad Sci U S A* 1987;84:6550.

417. Chang HY, Chen YP, Chediak JR, et al. Molecular analysis of von Willebrand factor produced by endothelial cell strains from patients with type IIA von Willebrand disease. *Blood* 1989;74:131(abst).

418. Ruggeri ZM, Nilsson IM, Lombardi R, et al. Aberrant multimeric structure of von Willebrand factor in a new variant of von Willebrand's disease (type IIC). *J Clin Invest* 1982;70:1124.

419. Armitage H, Rizza CR. Two populations of factor VIII-related antigen in a family with von Willebrand's disease. *Br J Haematol* 1979;55:493.

420. Mannucci PM, Lombardi R, Pareti FI, et al. A variant of von Willebrand's disease characterized by recessive inheritance and missing triplet structure of von Willebrand factor multimers. *Blood* 1983;62:1000.

421. Batlle J, Lopez-Fernandez MF, Fernandez Villamor A, et al. Multimeric pattern discrepancy between platelet and plasma von Willebrand factor in type IIC von Willebrand disease. *Am J Hematol* 1986;22:87.

422. Batlle J, Lopez-Fernandez MF, Lasierra J, et al. von Willebrand disease type IIC with different abnormalities of von Willebrand factor in the same sibship. *Am J Hematol* 1986;21:177.

423. Mazurier C, Mannucci PM, Parquet-Gernez A, et al. Investigation of a case of subtype IIC von Willebrand disease: characterization of the variability of this subtype. *Am J Hematol* 1986;22:301.

424. Lamme S, Wallmark A, Holmberg L, et al. The use of monoclonal antibodies in measuring factor VIII/von Willebrand factor. *Scand J Clin Lab Invest* 1985;15:17.

425. Hill FG, Enayat MS, George AJ. Investigation of a kindred with a new autosomal dominantly inherited variant type von Willebrand's disease (possibly type IID). *J Clin Pathol* 1985;38:665.

426. Thomas N, O'Callaghan U, Lowe GD, et al. Response to desmopressin in type IID von Willebrand's disease. *Clin Lab Haematol* 1989;11:189.

427. Castaman G, Rodeghiero F, Lattuada A, et al. A new variant of von Willebrand disease (type II I) with a normal degree of proteolytic cleavage of von Willebrand factor. *Thromb Res* 1991;65:343.

428. Sweeney JD, Hoernig LA, Behrens AN, et al. von Willebrand's variant (type II Buffalo). *Am J Clin Pathol* 1990;93:522.

429. Fujimura Y, Holland LZ, Ruggeri ZM, et al. The von Willebrand factor domain-mediating botrocetin-induced binding to glycoprotein Ib lies between Val449 and Lys728. *Blood* 1987;70:985.

430. Rabinowitz I, Tuley EA, Mancuso DJ, et al. von Willebrand disease type B: a missense mutation selectively abolishes ristocetin-induced von Willebrand factor binding to platelet glycoprotein Ib. *Proc Natl Acad Sci U S A* 1992;89:9846.

431. Holmberg L, Berntorp E, Donnér M, et al. von Willebrand's disease characterized by increased ristocetin sensitivity and the presence of all von Willebrand factor multimers in plasma. *Blood* 1986;68:668.

432. Wylie B, Gibson J, Urh E, et al. von Willebrand's disease characterized by increased ristocetin sensitivity and the presence of all von Willebrand factor multimers in plasma: a new subtype. *Pathology* 1988;62:63.

433. Holmberg L, Nilsson IM, Borge L, et al. Platelet aggregation induced by 1-desamino-8-D-arginine vasopressin (DDAVP) in type IIB von Willebrand's disease. *N Engl J Med* 1983;309:816.

434. Kyrle PA, Niessner H, Dent J. IIB von Willebrand's disease: pathogenetic and therapeutic studies. *Br J Haematol* 1988;69:55.

435. Rivard GE, Daviault M, Brault N, et al. von Willebrand's disease associated with thrombocytopenia and a fast migrating factor VIII related antigen. *Thromb Res* 1977;11:507.

436. Andes A. Thrombocytopenia in von Willebrand's disease. *Thromb Res* 1983;30:391.

437. Giles AR. Type IIB von Willebrand's disease presenting as a lifelong bleeding diathesis associated with chronic thrombocytopenia and spontaneous platelet aggregation. *Thromb Haemost* 1985;54:1126.

438. Saba HI, Saba SR, Dent J, et al. Type IIB Tampa: a variant of von Willebrand disease with chronic thrombocytopenia, circulating platelet aggregates, and spontaneous platelet aggregation. *Blood* 1985;66:282.

439. Conti M, Mari D, Conti E, et al. Pregnancy in women with different types of von Willebrand disease. *Obstet Gynecol* 1986;68:282.

440. De Marco L, Mazzuccato M, Del Ben MG, et al. Type IIb von Willebrand factor with normal sialic content induces platelet aggregation in the absence of ristocetin. *J Clin Invest* 1987;80:475.

441. Mazurier C, Parquet-Gernez A, Goudemand J, et al. Investigation of a large kindred with type IIB von Willebrand's disease, dominant inheritance and age-dependent thrombocytopenia. *Br J Haematol* 1988;69:499.

442. Hultin MB, Sussman II. Postoperative thrombocytopenia in type IIB von Willebrand disease. *Am J Hematol* 1990;33:64.

443. Federici AB, Mannucci PM, Bader R, et al. Heterogeneity in type IIB von Willebrand disease: two unrelated cases with no family history and mild abnormalities of ristocetin-induced interaction between von Willebrand factor and platelets. *Am J Hematol* 1986;23:381.

444. Donnér M, Holmberg L, Nilsson IM. Type IIB von Willebrand's disease with probable autosomal recessive inheritance and presenting as thrombocytopenia in infancy. *Br J Haematol* 1987;66:349.

445. Cooney KA, Nichols WC, Bruck ME, et al. The molecular defect in type IIB von Willebrand disease: identification of four potential missense mutations within the putative GpIb binding domain. *J Clin Invest* 1991;87:1227.

446. Randi AM, Rabinowitz I, Mancuso DJ, et al. Molecular basis of von Willebrand disease type IIb. Candidate mutation cluster in one disulfide loop between proposed platelet glycoprotein Ib binding sequences. *J Clin Invest* 1991;87:1220.

447. Ware J, Dent JA, Azuma H, et al. Identification of a point mutation in type IIB von Willebrand disease illustrating the regulation of von Willebrand factor affinity for the platelet membrane glycoprotein Ib-IX receptor. *Proc Natl Acad Sci U S A* 1991;88:2946.

448. Cooney KA, Lyons SE, Ginsburg D. Functional analysis of a type IIB von Willebrand disease missense mutation: increased binding of large von Willebrand factor multimers to platelets. *Proc Natl Acad Sci U S A* 1992;89:2869.

449. Murray EW, Giles AR, Lillicrap D. Germ-line mosaicism for a valine-to-methionine substitution at residue 553 in the glycoprotein Ib-binding domain of von Willebrand factor, causing type IIB von Willebrand disease. *Am J Hum Genet* 1992;50:199.

450. Fujimura Y, Titani K, Holland LZ, et al. von Willebrand factor: a reduced and alkylated 52/48-kDa fragment beginning at amino acid residue 449 contains the domain interacting with platelet glycoprotein Ib. *J Biol Chem* 1986;261:381.

451. Mohri H, Fujimura Y, Shima M, et al. Structure of the von Willebrand factor domain interacting with glycoprotein Ib. *J Biol Chem* 1988;263:17901.

452. Rabinowitz I, Randi AM, Shindler KS, et al. Type IIB mutation His505→Asp implicates a new segment in the control of von Willebrand factor binding to platelet glycoprotein Ib. *J Biol Chem* 1993;268:20497.

453. Hilbert L, Gaucher C, de Romeuf C, et al. Leu697→Val mutation in mature von Willebrand factor is responsible for type IIB von Willebrand disease. *Blood* 1994;83:1542.

454. Kroner PA, Kluessendorf ML, Scott JP, et al. Expressed full-length von Willebrand factor containing missense mutations linked to type IIB von Willebrand disease shows enhanced binding to platelets. *Blood* 1991;79:2048.

455. Randi AM, Jorieux S, Tuley EA, et al. Recombinant von Willebrand factor Arg578→Gln. *J Biol Chem* 1992;267:21187.

456. Ribba AS, Voorberg J, Meyer D, et al. Characterization of recombinant von Willebrand factor corresponding to mutations in type IIA and type IIB von Willebrand disease. *J Biol Chem* 1992;267:23209.

457. Veltkamp JJ, van Tilburg NH. Autosomal hemophilia: a variant of von Willebrand's disease. *Br J Haematol* 1974;26:141.

458. Graham JB, Barrow ES, Roberts HR, et al. Dominant inheritance of hemophilia A in three generations of women. *Blood* 1975;46:175.

459. Montgomery RR, Hathaway WE, Johnson J, et al. A variant of von Willebrand's disease with abnormal expression of factor VIII procoagulant activity. *Blood* 1982;60:201.

460. Mazurier C, Gaucher C, Jorieux S, et al. Evidence for a von Willebrand factor defect in factor VIII binding in three members of a family previously misdiagnosed as mild haemophilia A and haemophilia A carriers: consequences for therapy and genetic functional sites. *Br J Haematol* 1990;76:372.

461. Gaucher C, Jorieux S, Mercier B, et al. The "Normandy" variant of von Willebrand factor: characterization of a point mutation in the von Willebrand factor gene. *Blood* 1991;77:1937.

462. Gaucher C, Mercier B, Jorieux S, et al. Identification of two point mutations in the von Willebrand factor gene of three families with the "Normandy" variant of von Willebrand disease. *Br J Haematol* 1991;78:506.

463. Kroner PA, Friedman KD, Fahs SA, et al. Abnormal binding of factor VIII is linked with the substitution of glutamine for arginine 91 in von Willebrand factor in a variant form of von Willebrand disease. *J Biol Chem* 1991;266:19146.

464. Kroner PA, Fahs SA, Vokac EA, et al. Novel missense mutations in von Willebrand factor (vWF) associated with defective vWF/factor VIII interaction in a patient with type I von Willebrand disease. *Blood* 1991;78:178a.

465. Cacheris PM, Nichols WC, Ginsburg D. Molecular characterization of a unique von Willebrand disease variant: a novel mutation affecting von Willebrand factor/factor VIII interaction. *J Biol Chem* 1991;266:13499.

466. Tuley EA, Gaucher C, Jorieux S, et al. Expression of von Willebrand factor "Normandy," an autosomal mutation that mimics hemophilia A. *Proc Natl Acad Sci U S A* 1991;88:6377.

467. Jorieux S, Tuley EA, Gaucher C, et al. The mutation Arg(53)→Trp [causes von Willebrand disease Normandy by abolishing binding to factor VIII: studies with recombinant von Willebrand factor. *Blood* 1992;79:563.

468. Wise RJ, Ewenstein BM, Gorlin J, et al. Autosomal recessive transmission of hemophilia A due to a von Willebrand factor mutation. *Hum Genet* 1993;91: 367.

469. Meyer D, Frommel D, Larrieu MJ, et al. Selective absence of large forms of factor VIII/von Willebrand factor in acquired von Willebrand's syndrome: response to transfusion. *Blood* 1979;54:600.

470. Ball J, Malia RG, Greaves M, et al. Demonstration of abnormal factor VIII multimers in acquired von Willebrand's disease associated with a circulating inhibitor. *Br J Haematol* 1987;65:95.

471. Handin RI, Martin V, Moloney WC. Antibody-induced von Willebrand's disease: a newly defined inhibitor syndrome. *Blood* 1976;48:393.

472. Mannucci PM, Lombardi R, Bader R, et al. Studies of the pathophysiology of acquired von Willebrand's disease in seven patients with lymphoproliferative disorders or benign monoclonal gammopathies. *Blood* 1984;64:614.

473. Joist JH, Cowan JF, Zimmerman TS. Acquired von Willebrand's disease: evidence for a quantitative and qualitative factor VIII disorder. *N Engl J Med* 1978;298:988.

474. Roussi JH, Houbouyan LL, Alterescu R, et al. Acquired von Willebrand's syndrome associated with hairy cell leukaemia. *Br J Haematol* 1980;46:503.

475. Simone JV, Cornet JA, Abildgaard CF. Acquired von Willebrand's syndrome in systemic lupus erythematosus. *Blood* 1968;31:806.

476. Yoshida H, Arai K, Wakashin M. Development of acquired von Willebrand's disease after mixed connective tissue disease. *Am J Med* 1988;85:445.

477. Stableforth P, Tamagnini GL, Dormandy KM. Acquired von Willebrand's syndrome and thrombopathy in patient with chronic lymphocytic leukemia. *Scand J Haematol* 1970;16:128.

478. Gazengel C, Prieur AM, Jacques C, et al. Antibody induced von Willebrand's syndrome: inhibition of VIII-vWF and VIII-Agn with sparing of VIII-Ahf by the autoantibody. *Am J Hematol* 1978;5:355.

479. Gouault-Heilmann M, Dumont MD, Intrator L, et al. Acquired von Willebrand's syndrome with IgM inhibitor against von Willebrand factor. *J Clin Pathol* 1979;32:1030.

480. Zettervall O, Nilsson IM. Acquired von Willebrand's disease caused by a monoclonal antibody. *Acta Med Scand* 1978;204:521.

481. Gan TE, Sawers RJ, Koutts J. Pathogenesis of antibody induced acquired von Willebrand syndrome. *Am J Hematol* 1980;9:363.

482. Bovill EG, Ershler WB, Golden EA, et al. A human myeloma-produced monoclonal protein directed against the active subpopulation of von Willebrand factor. *Am J Clin Pathol* 1986;85:115.

483. Richard C, Cuadrado MA, Prieto M, et al. Acquired von Willebrand disease in multiple myeloma secondary to absorption of von Willebrand factor by plasma cells. *Am J Hematol* 1990;35:114.

484. Noronha PA, Hruby MA, Maurer HS. Acquired von Willebrand disease in a patient with Wilms' tumor. *J Pediatr* 1979;95:997.

485. Scott JP, Montgomery RR, Tubergen DG, et al. Acquired von Willebrand's disease in association with Wilms' tumor: regression following treatment. *Blood* 1981;58:665.

486. Holland L, Adamson A, Ingram GI, et al. Acquired von Willebrand syndrome. *Br J Haematol* 1980;45:161.

487. Sampson BM, Greaves M, Malia RG, et al. Acquired von Willebrand's disease: demonstration of a circulating inhibitor to the factor VIII complex in four cases. *Br J Haematol* 1983;54:233.

488. Facon T, Caron C, Courtin P, et al. Acquired type II von Willebrand's disease associated with adrenal cortical carcinoma. *Blood* 1992;80:488.

489. Budde U, Schaefer G, Mueller N, et al. Acquired von Willebrand's disease in the myeloproliferative syndrome. *Blood* 1984;64:981.

490. Budde V, Dent JA, Berkowitz SC, et al. Subunit composition of plasma von Willebrand factor in patients with the myeloproliferative syndrome. *Blood* 1986;68:1213.

491. Takahasi H. Studies on the pathophysiology and treatment of von Willebrand's disease. IV. Mechanism of increased ristocetin-induced platelet aggregation in von Willebrand's disease. *Thromb Res* 1980;19:857.

492. Miller JL, Castella A. Platelet-type von Willebrand's disease: characterization of a new bleeding disorder. *Blood* 1982;60:790.

493. Miller JL, Cunningham D, Lyle VA, et al. Mutation in the gene encoding the alpha chain of platelet glycoprotein Ib in platelet-type von Willebrand disease. *Proc Natl Acad Sci U S A* 1991;88:4761.

494. Russell SD, Roth GJ. A mutation in the platelet glycoprotein (GP) Ib alpha gene associated with pseudo–von Willebrand disease. *Blood* 1991;78:281.

495. Miller JL, Kupinski JM, Castella A, et al. von Willebrand factor binds to platelets and induces aggregation in platelet-type but not type IIb von Willebrand disease. *J Clin Invest* 1983;72:1532.

496. Scott JP, Montgomery RR. The rapid differentiation of type IIb von Willebrand's disease from platelet-type (pseudo-) von Willebrand's disease by the "neutral" monoclonal antibody binding assay. *Am J Clin Pathol* 1991;96:723.

497. Bowie EJ, Owen CA Jr. The bleeding time. *Prog Hemost Thromb* 1974;2:249.

498. Cash JD, Gader AM, Da Costa J. Release of plasminogen activator and factor VIII in response to LVP, AVP, DDAVP, angiotensin II and oxytocin in man. *Br J Haematol* 1974;27:363.

499. Mannucci PM, Canciani MT, Rota L, et al. Response of factor VIII/von Willebrand factor to DDAVP in healthy subjects and patients with haemophilia A and von Willebrand's disease. *Br J Haematol* 1981;47:283.

500. Köhler M, Hellstern P, Reiter B, et al. The subcutaneous administration of the vasopressin analogue 1-desamino-8-D-arginine vasopressin in patients with von Willebrand's disease and hemophilia. *Klin Wochenschr* 1984;62:543.

501. De Sio L, Mariani G, Muzzucconi MG, et al. Comparison between subcutaneous and intravenous DDAVP in mild and moderate hemophilia. *Thromb Haemost* 1985;54:387.

502. Mannucci PM, Vicente V, Alberca I, et al. Intravenous and subcutaneous administration of desmopressin (DDAVP) to hemophiliacs: pharmacokinetics and factor VIII responses. *Thromb Haemost* 1987;58:1037.

503. Lethagen S, Harris AS, Nilsson IM. Intranasal desmopressin (DDAV) by spray in mild hemophilia A and von Willebrand's disease type I. *Blut* 1990; 60:187.

504. Rose EH, Aledort LM. Nasal spray desmopressin (DDAVP) for mild hemophilia A and von Willebrand disease. *Ann Intern Med* 1991;114:563.

505. Theiss W, Schmidt G. DDAVP in von Willebrand's disease: repeated administration and the behaviour of the bleeding time. *Thromb Res* 1978;13:1119.

506. Isola L, Forster A, Aledort LM. Deamino-D-arginine vasopressin and bleeding time in von Willebrand's disease. *Ann Intern Med* 1984;101:719.

507. Aledort LM. Treatment of von Willebrand's disease. *Mayo Clin Proc* 1991;66:841.

508. Smith TJ, Gill JC, Ambruso DR, et al. Hyponatremia and seizures in young children given DDAVP. *Am J Hematol* 1989;31:199.

509. Sheperd LL, Hutchinson RJ, Worden EK, et al. Hyponatremia and seizures after intravenous administration of desmopressin acetate for surgical hemostasis. *J Pediatr* 1989;144:470.

510. Weinstein RE, Bona RD, Altman AJ, et al. Severe hyponatremia after repeated intravenous administration of desmopressin. *Am J Hematol* 1989;32:258.

511. O'Brien JR, Green PJ, Salmon G, et al. Desmopressin and myocardial infarction. *Lancet* 1989;1:664.

512. Byrnes JJ, Larcada A, Moake JL. Thrombosis following desmopressin for uremic bleeding. *Am J Hematol* 1988;28:63.

513. Mannucci PM, Lusher JM. Desmopressin and thrombosis. *Lancet* 1989;2:675.

514. Nilsson IM, Hedner U. Characteristics of various factor VIII concentrates used in treatment of hemophilia. *Br J Haematol* 1977;37:543.

515. Berntorp E, Nilsson IM. Biochemical, in vivo properties of commercial virus-inactivated factor VIII concentrates. *Eur J Haematol* 1988;48:205.

516. Mannucci PM, Tenconi PM, Castaman G, et al. Comparison of four virus-inactivated plasma concentrates for treatment of severe von Willebrand disease: a cross-over randomized trial. *Blood* 1992;79:3130.

517. Köhler M, Hellstern P, Wenzel E. The use of heat-treated factor VIII-concentrates in von Willebrand's disease. *Blut* 1985;50:25.

518. Schimpf K, Mannucci PM, Kreutz W, et al. Absence of hepatitis after treatment with a pasteurized factor VIII concentrate in patients with hemophilia and no previous transfusions. *N Engl J Med* 1987;316:918.

519. Fukui H, Nishino M, Terada S, et al. Hemostatic effect of a heat-treated factor VIII concentrate (Haemate-P) in von Willebrand's disease. *Blut* 1988;56:171.

520. Mazurier C, Jorieux S, de Romeuf C, et al. In vitro evaluation of a very-high-purity solvent/detergent-treated, von Willebrand factor concentrate. *Vox Sang* 1991;61:1.

521. Rothschild C, Fressinaud E, Wolf M, et al. Unexpected results following treatment of patients with von Willebrand disease with a new highly purified von Willebrand factor concentrate. *Thromb Haemost* 1991;65:1126.

522. Ogston D. *Antifibrinolytic drugs: chemistry, pharmacology and clinical usage.* Chichester, UK: John Wiley and Sons, 1984.

523. Sindet-Pedersen S, Ramstrom G, Bernvil S, et al. Hemostatic effect of tranexamic acid mouthwash in anticoagulant-treated patients undergoing oral surgery. *N Engl J Med* 1989;320:840.

524. Alperin JB. Estrogens and surgery in women with von Willebrand's disease. *Am J Med* 1982;73:367.

525. Rodeghiero F, Castaman G, di Bona E, et al. Consistency of responses to repeated DDAVP infusions in patients with von Willebrand's disease and hemophilia A. *Blood* 1989;74:1997.

526. De la Fuente B, Kasper CK, Rickles FR, et al. Response of patients with mild and moderate hemophilia A and von Willebrand's disease to treatment with desmopressin. *Ann Intern Med* 1985;103:6.

527. Mannucci PM. Desmopressin (DDAVP) for treatment of disorders of hemostasis. In: Coller BS, ed. *Progress in hemostasis and thrombosis*, vol. 8. Philadelphia: Grune & Stratton, 1986:19.

528. Casonato A, Sartori T, deMarco L, et al. 1-Desamino-8-D-arginine vasopressin (DDAVP) infusion in type IIB von Willebrand's disease: shortening of bleeding time and induction of a variable pseudothrombocytopenia. *Thromb Haemost* 1990;64:117.

529. Feigert JM, Wolf DJ, Schleider MA. Porcine factor (PF) VIII controls severe bleeding in acquired von Willebrand's disease (AVWD) by supplying von Willebrand's factor (vWF). *Blood* 1987;58:371.

530. Cattaneo M, Moia M, Valle PD, et al. DDAVP shortens the prolonged bleeding times of patients with severe von Willebrand disease treated with cryoprecipitate: evidence for a mechanism of action independent of released von Willebrand factor. *Blood* 1989;74:1972.

531. Boda Z, Pfliegler G, Harsfalvi J, et al. Successful treatment of a severe bleeding episode in type III von Willebrand's disease by simultaneous administration of cryoprecipitate and platelet concentrate. *Thromb Haemost* 1991;65:1125.

532. Lopez-Fernandez MF, Blanco-Lopez MJ, Castiñeira MP, et al. Further evidence for recessive inheritance of von Willebrand disease with abnormal binding of von Willebrand factor to factor VIII. *Am J Hematol* 1992;40:20.

533. Blombäck M, Johansson G, Johnsson H, et al. Surgery in patients with von Willebrand's disease. *Br J Surg* 1989;76:398.

534. Telfer MC, Checiak J. Factor VIII–related disorders and their relationship to pregnancy. *J Reprod Med* 1977;19:211.

CHAPTER 36

Contact System and Its Disorders

Allen P. Kaplan and Michael Silverberg

When blood is drawn into a clean glass tube, it rapidly clots. If the tube is coated with silicone or is made of plastic, clotting is delayed. This interaction of a group of plasma proteins with the negatively charged surface of clean glass to initiate blood coagulation is known as *contact activation*. The coagulation pathway activated by this mechanism is termed *intrinsic* because all of the protein factors required for clotting are found in the plasma; this is in contrast to the extrinsic pathway, which requires the exposure of plasma to cell-surface tissue factor for clotting to occur. Factor X activation is conventionally depicted as the site of the branch point between the intrinsic and extrinsic coagulation pathways. A new picture has emerged in recent years, however, in which the distinction between intrinsic and extrinsic pathways of clotting *in vivo* is largely eliminated. Rather, there are two processes distinguished by time rather than pathway: an initial phase triggered by the tissue factor–factor VIIa complex followed by a maintenance phase involving factor XI. In this phase, factor XI is apparently activated by the relatively small amounts of thrombin produced during the early phase. More discussion of the role of factor XI in clotting is found in the section Relation of Contact Factor Deficiencies to Hemostasis.

Despite the apparent uninvolvement of the contact system in clotting *in vivo*, the protein components of the contact system have been identified through the discovery of individuals with abnormal clotting times that resulted from a deficiency of one of them. The pathway has been shown to comprise a complex loop of interactions in which two zymogens—factor XII (Hageman factor) and prekallikrein (Fletcher factor)—become activated to trypsinlike proteases in the presence of the nonenzymatic cofactor high-molecular-weight kininogen (HMWK) and an appropriate surface (Fig. 36-1). This complex trimolecular reaction is the first step in the intrinsic coagulation cascade, and all three proteins are clotting factors *in vitro*. Clotting is then initiated through the action of activated factor XII on factor XI. As a result, factor XI becomes activated, and a series of additional conversions of proenzyme to enzyme leads to the formation of thrombin and the conversion of fibrinogen to fibrin to form a clot.

In addition, kallikrein, which is also formed during the contact phase, generates bradykinin by digestion of HMWK; *bradykinin* is a nine amino acid vasoactive peptide that is an important component of the body's inflammatory response. Other activities that are dependent on the activation of factor XII have also been identified. These are weak fibrinolytic activity, the activation of prorenin to renin, interactions with the complement system, and cellular components of the blood.

Although all of these pathways have been described and characterized *in vitro*, the physiologic functioning of the contact activation system remains obscure in several aspects. Thus, despite profound prolongation of the activated partial thromboplastin time (APTT), none of the persons described with deficiencies had a bleeding diathesis except those with a deficiency of factor XI. This deficit causes a variable but usually mild form of hemophilia. Other mechanisms of factor XI activation independent of factor XII activation may explain this phenomenon. Similarly, the role of bradykinin in the inflammatory process is still being defined.

The application of the methods of modern molecular biology has resulted in the determination of the amino acid sequences of all of the proteins of the contact system as well as elucidation of their gene structures. The most surprising aspect of these results has been the close evolutionary relationship between the enzymes of the contact system and the fibrinolytic enzymes urokinase and tissue plasminogen activator (TPA).

FACTOR XII

Biochemistry

PROPERTIES OF ZYMOGEN

Factor XII (Hageman factor) circulates as a single-chain zymogen with no detectable enzymatic activity. The zymogen migrates as a β-globulin, and its apparent molecular weight is 80 kd on sodium dodecyl sulfate (SDS) gel electrophoresis (1). When a reducing agent is omitted, the apparent molecular weight is lower, implying that the intact disulfide bonds maintain the protein in a more compact, perhaps globular, structure. Hageman factor is synthesized in the liver and circulates in normal plasma at a concentration of 30 to 35 µg/mL (1). This number implies that the specific clotting activity of purified factor XII, referred to normal plasma defined as having one unit/mL, should be approximately 28 to 35 U/mg. In practice, investigators have reported values ranging from 40 to as high as 80 U/mg. The reason for this discrepancy is not known. Other physical and chemical data are listed in Table 36-1.

MECHANISM OF ACTIVATION

Factor XII zymogen has no enzymatic activity against synthetic oligopeptide substrates, nor does it react with specific inhibitors (2). During contact activation of normal human plasma, it is converted into a functional serine protease by kallikrein in the presence of HMWK (3–5). This reaction is contingent on the introduction of a polyanionic substance (see section High-

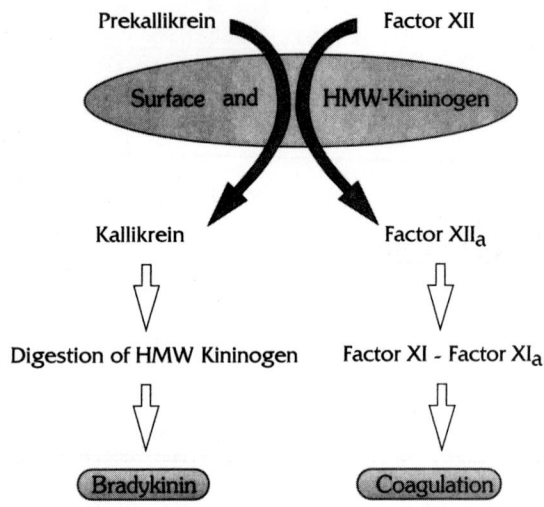

Figure 36-1. The factor XII–dependent pathways of contact activation. HMW, high molecular weight.

Molecular-Weight Kininogen). Purified factor XII can be activated by kallikrein *in vitro* in the absence of HMWK (6). The rate of this reaction is accelerated by polyanionic substances, apparently through the induction of a favorable conformation for cleavage by the binding of the factor XII zymogen to the polyanion (7,8).

A second reaction observed *in vitro* is the autoactivation of factor XII, which occurs as the polyanion catalyzes activation of factor XII zymogen by factor XIIa (9). This reaction is much slower than the activation by kallikrein (8) but may be responsible for the increase of the clotting activity of prekallikrein-deficient plasma when the contact time is prolonged.

Activation of factor XII by kallikrein gives a series of active enzymes formed by successive cleavages. The first cleavage to produce factor XIIa from factor XII occurs within a disulfide bond to yield a two-chain disulfide-linked molecule with the new amino-terminal sequence of Val-Val-Gly (10). The newly formed factor XIIa retains the 80,000 molecular weight of the zymogen but on reduced SDS gels is seen to comprise a heavy chain of 50 kd and a light chain of 28 kd. The light chain contains the catalytic domain and is derived from the carboxy-terminal region of the zymogen, whereas the heavy chain, which contains the surface-binding region, is derived from the amino terminal region (11). Further cleavage can occur in the heavy chain to produce a series of fragments of activated factor XII, all of which retain enzymatic activity (12,13).

The most prominent cleavage product of factor XIIa is the 30-kd species termed *factor XIIf*. Careful examination of the bands obtained on SDS gel electrophoresis in the absence of reducing agent indicated a doublet; the band of higher molecular weight was in time converted to one of lower molecular weight at approximately 28.5 kd (13). Reduced gels of high acrylamide content show that these species are comprised of the light chain of factor XIIa and a very small fragment of the original heavy chain.

A minor cleavage product formed from factor XIIa is a 40-kd species that represents cleavage of factor XIIa into two half molecules. The C-terminal half comprises the 28-kd serine protease moiety linked to an approximately 12- to 15-kd portion by a disulfide bridge. When the activation is accomplished by factor XIIa (autoactivation), the 40-kd fragments are produced in much greater proportion than when factor XII is digested by kallikrein (13).

FUNCTION OF ACTIVATED FACTOR XII

The activated forms of factor XII are trypsinlike serine proteases. When assayed with low-molecular-weight (LMW) substrates, they show a strong preference for cleavage at the carboxy terminal of arginine residues. Kinetic data have been obtained with a number of tri- and tetrapeptide substrates and inhibitors (14). In all cases, factor XIIa and factor XIIf show identical kinetics with LMW compounds.

The major macromolecular substrates for factor XIIa are prekallikrein and factor XI. In addition, factor XII is a substrate in the autoactivation reaction (9), and because prolonged incubation gives rise to the series of fragments described above (12), factor XIIa must be able to further cleave the heavy chain. Factor XIIf cleaves prekallikrein in the fluid phase (15–17) but does not readily cleave factor XI (18) and thus is not a procoagulant enzyme. In clotting assays, factor XIIf has only 2% to 4% of the activity of factor XIIa (19). Similarly, factor XIIf does not activate factor XII zymogen (9). The lack of activity against these two substrates must reflect the absence of the surface-binding site that is found in the heavy chain. We can envisage, therefore, that during contact activation, surface-bound factor XIIa becomes cleaved to factor XIIf, which, free of the surface-binding domain, can diffuse away and promote kinin generation via activation of prekallikrein at sites distant from the original activation site (11). Perhaps the heavy chain is left to compete for binding to the surface and could serve to limit further activation.

Factor XIIf can also activate the first component of complement (20) and factor VII, a critical component of the intrinsic pathway (21). In addition, factor XIIa has been reported to aggregate neutrophils and cause degranulation (22). The physiologic significance, if any, of these activities is not known.

The role of plasma inhibitors in regulating the activity of activated factor XII is discussed in the section Inhibition and Regulation of the Contact Activation System. Several inhibitors have been found useful for *in vitro* studies; these are listed in Table 36-2.

TABLE 36-1. Physical and Chemical Data

Protein	Factor XII	Prekallikrein	Factor XI	High-Molecular-Weight Kininogen
Molecular weight (d; calculated)	80,427	79,545	140,000	116,643
Carbohydrate (w/w)	16.8%	15%	5%	40%
Isoelectric point	6.3	8.7	8.6	4.7
Extinction coefficient ($E^{1\%}_{280/nm}$)	14.2	11.7	13.4	7.0
Plasma concentration				
µg/mL	30–45	35–50	4–6	70–90
nmol/L (average)	400	534	36	686

TABLE 36-2. Inhibitors Useful in Studies of Contact Activation[a]

Inhibitor	Factor XIIa	Kallikrein
Pancreatic or lung trypsin inhibitor (aprotinin)	−	+
Soybean trypsin inhibitor	−	+
Lima bean trypsin inhibitor	+	−
Corn inhibitor	+	−
Peptide chloromethyl ketones[b]		
phe-phe-arg	+	+++
phe-pro-arg	+	+
pro-phe-arg	+	++
dansyl-glu-gly-arg	+	−
p-Amidino phenylmethylsulfonyl fluoride	+	+
Diisopropyl fluorophosphate	+	+

[a]Kinetic constants are not given because even when known, they depend on conditions of buffer, ionic strength, pH, etc.
[b]Chloromethyl ketones are listed in order of reactivity with factor XIIa.[14] Where quantitative measurements[14] have indicated that kallikrein is much more reactive than factor XIIa, it is indicated by ++ or +++.

Structure

PROTEIN

The primary structure of factor XII is known from analysis of complementary DNA (cDNA) isolated from human liver cDNA libraries (23,24) and from direct protein sequence data (10,25). The mature protein has a sequence of 596 amino acids; the molecular weight is 66,915 d, excluding carbohydrate. Together with the measured carbohydrate content of 16.8%, the total predicted molecular weight is 80,427 d.

The amino-terminal heavy-chain region of the protein shows extensive homologies with other proteins. In particular, distinct domains are found that bear strong homology with characteristic domains of fibronectin, plasminogen, and plasminogen activators (Fig. 36-2). The immediate amino-terminal region is homologous to the type II "finger" region of fibronectin; residues 13 to 69 share approximately 40% homology with the two fibronectin sequences. These sequences in fibronectin are probably involved in collagen binding. There are two regions (residues 79 to 111 and 159 to 190) of the sequence that are homologous to epidermal growth factor sequences found in a number of proteins, including TPA and several other clotting factors. These regions are separated by a region (residues 116 to 151) bearing limited homology to the type I "finger" region of fibronectin. The final recognizable domain of the heavy-chain region is an 83-residue "kringle" (193 to 276) as found in prothrombin, plasminogen, and the plasminogen activators. This structure is characterized by six invariant half-cystines, giving a characteristic pattern of three disulfide bridges. The kringle region of the sequence is followed by a region (residues 279 to 330) that connects the heavy chain with the catalytic serine protease domain. This connecting region has 17 prolines in 52 residues and also bears the proposed attachment sites of six O-linked carbohydrate chains.

The C-terminal residues from 354 to 596 make up the catalytic domain of the factor XII sequence. This light-chain region is homologous with the pancreatic serine proteases, trypsin, chymotrypsin, and elastase. The cleavage by kallikrein to form factor XIIa occurs at Arg[353] to Val[354] (Figs. 36-2 and 36-3) (23,25). The sequence data also account for the observations of two forms of factor XIIf (13). Thus, cleavage at Arg[334] produces a disulfide-linked two-chain molecule comprising the serine protease moiety linked to a 19 amino acid peptide. A second cleavage occurs at Arg[343] to leave a nine-residue peptide linked through the disulfide bond to the serine protease (Fig. 36-3). The catalytic domain bears an average 36% homology with the pancreatic serine proteases, which is similar to the 41% figure for their homology among themselves. In addition, five of the

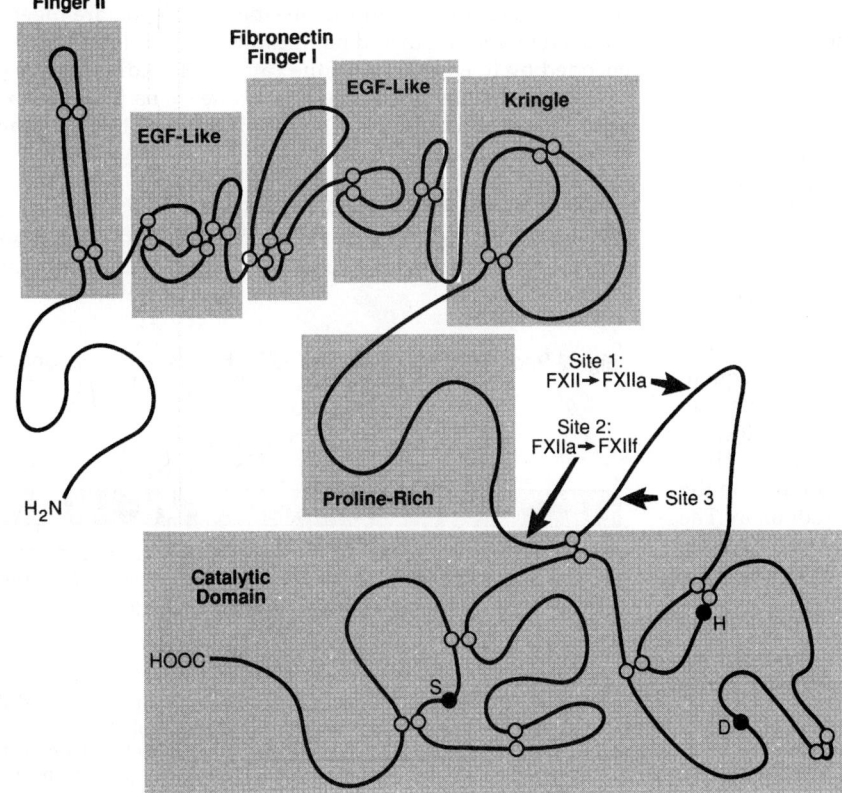

Figure 36-2. Schematic diagram of the protein chain of factor XII, showing the structural domains inferred from sequence homologies. The catalytic triad residues are shown by solid circles, half cystines are indicated by open circles, and the cleavage sites leading to activation (site 1) and the two forms of factor XIIf (sites 2 and 3) are marked with arrows. The domains are fibronectin type II, growth factor–like (EGF–Like), fibronectin type I, kringle, and proline-rich. (Adapted from Cool DE, Edgell CS, Louie GV, et al. Characterization of human blood coagulation factor XII cDNA. *J Biol Chem* 1985;25:13666.)

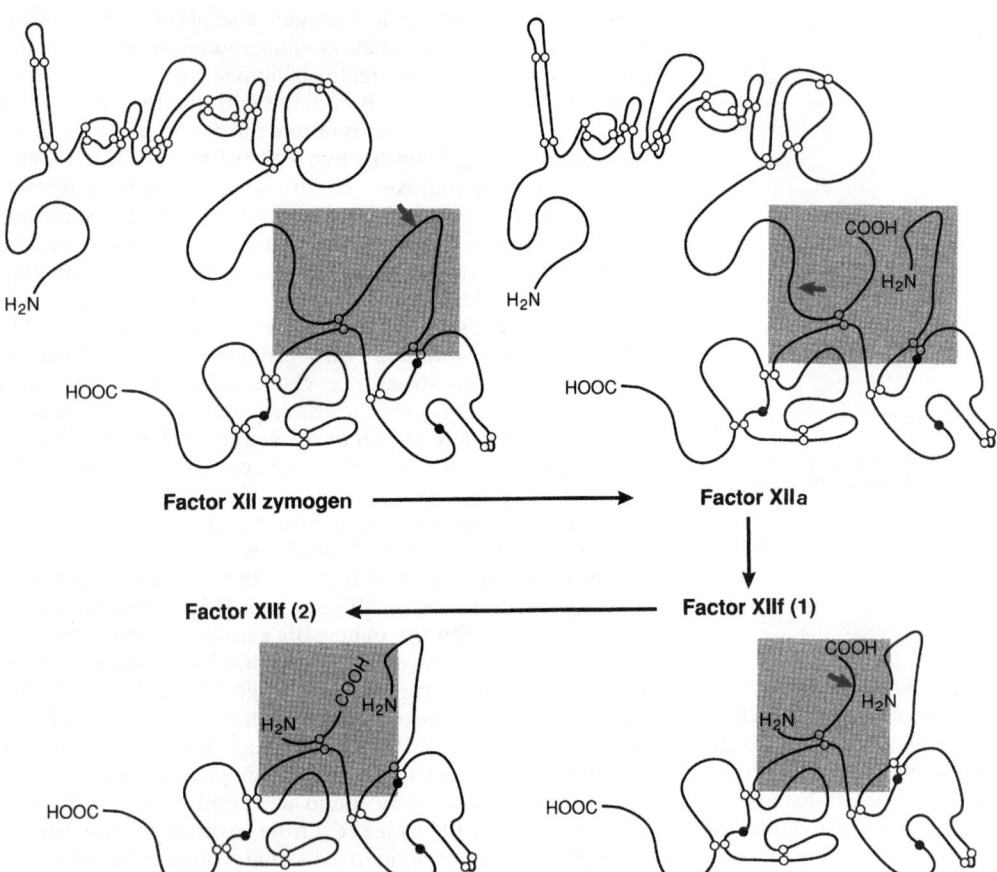

Factor XII zymogen ⟶ **Factor XIIa**

Factor XIIf (2) ⟵ **Factor XIIf (1)**

Figure 36-3. Diagram of the activation of factor XII to factor XIIa and the sequential production of the two forms of factor XIIf.

seven disulfide bridges of the factor XII light chain occur in similar positions in trypsin or chymotrypsin. This makes it likely that the tertiary structure of the catalytic domain is closely homologous with that of the serine proteases. The members of the catalytic triad of factor XIIa are His[40], Asp[89], and Ser[191], numbering from the amino terminus of the light chain (residue 354 of the zymogen).

Apart from the catalytic domain, the relationship of structure to function of factor XII remains largely unknown. The most important known property of the heavy chain is its ability to bind to negatively charged surfaces during contact activation. Data in the literature derived from studies with monoclonal antibodies and synthetic peptides identified two separate regions that appeared to be involved with in the binding of factor XII to the surface. Initial studies suggested that an epitope comprising residues 134 to 153, located in the fibronectin type I–like domain, was the surface-binding site (26). A subsequent publication, however, reported that the epitope that reacts with monoclonal antibodies that inhibit surface binding was located in the immediate N-terminal sequence of factor XII (27). Thus, the primary surface-binding site appears to be located in the first domain of factor XII—the fibronectin type II domain. The initial results may indicate, however, that there is at least one secondary binding site that contributes to surface binding.

GENE

Studies with cDNA hybridization probes (28,29) have shown that the gene is found on chromosome 5, it has been localized to the 5q33-qter region of the chromosome (29), and its complete structure has been determined (30). The gene encompasses approximately 12 kilobase pairs (kbp) of DNA in which there are 14 exons and 13 introns (Fig. 36-4). Twelve of the exons are

located within a stretch of 4.2 kbp. The first exon at the 5' end codes for a putative 19-residue signal peptide. Subsequent exons code for the discrete domains described in the preceding section. The kringle- and the proline-rich region are together encoded by the eighth and ninth exons. The catalytic domain is encoded by five exons, with the catalytic histidine, aspartate, and serine residues all located in separate exons. The final exon is the largest and includes 150 bp corresponding to the untranslated 3' end of the mRNA.

HOMOLOGIES WITH OTHER PROTEINS

As described earlier, the domain structure of factor XII has been defined on the basis of sequence homologies with correspond-

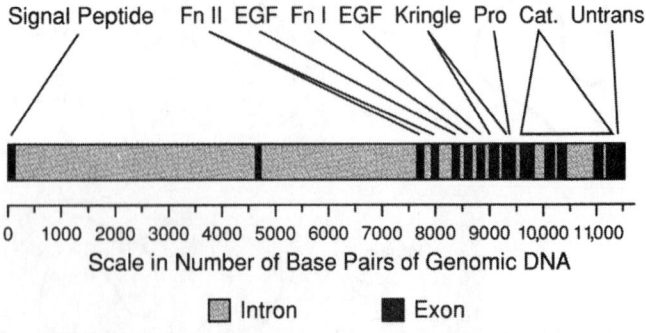

Signal Peptide Fn II EGF Fn I EGF Kringle Pro Cat. Untrans

Scale in Number of Base Pairs of Genomic DNA

▨ Intron ■ Exon

Figure 36-4. Structure of the factor XII gene, showing introns and the exons coding for the domains shown in Figure 36-2. EGF, external growth factor. (Data from Cool DE, MacGillivray RT. Characterization of the human blood coagulation factor XII gene: intron/exon gene organization and analysis of the 5-flanking region. *J Biol Chem* 1987;262:13662.)

ing domains of fibronectin, plasmin, plasminogen inhibitors, and pancreatic serine proteases. For some of the domains, such as the kringle and catalytic domains, it has been possible to extend the analysis of homologies.

A detailed study of the homologies of the kringles in plasmin, prothrombin, TPA, urokinase, and factor XII has been made (31). The factor XII sequence shows the closest homologies with TPA kringle 2; 41 residues are conserved when one gap of three residues is inserted into the factor XII sequence. Other close homologies are with urokinase (39 residues) and TPA kringle 1 (35 residues). In contrast, the widest separation in sequence homology was between factor XII and prothrombin kringle 5, which still had 27 residues conserved. This high sequence homology between the kringles of factor XII and other proteins does not necessarily translate into close structural homology. Secondary structure prediction showed a marked difference between the predicted structures of the factor XII and urokinase kringles despite their close sequence homologies. These differences arise from significant single amino acid substitutions.

In the case of the catalytic domain, however, there appears to be good reason for proposing close structural homologies with other serine proteases. The 36% sequence homology with the pancreatic serine proteases is similar to the 41% average homology among themselves. The latter homology translates to highly homologous (approximately 85%) tertiary structures. Thus, a tentative tertiary structure of the catalytic domain has been proposed (23), which allows the insertions in the sequence relative to the pancreatic enzymes to be accommodated at the surface of the molecule.

Knowing the sequence of the factor XII gene also allows the analysis of homology in terms of intron and exon structure (30). The exons coding for the fibronectin type I, the growth factor domain, and the kringle in factor XII are also all found in TPA and urokinase, but the proline-rich region of factor XII is unique. In the serine protease region, the factor XII gene is also more closely related to the plasminogen activators than to the clotting factors or the pancreatic enzymes.

Overall, the results of analysis of both the DNA and protein sequences show that TPA is the protein most closely related to factor XII. Other close homologies are with urokinase and plasmin. The clotting factors such as prothrombin show relatively little homology in either sequence or gene structure.

PREKALLIKREIN

Biochemistry

Like factor XII, prekallikrein is a zymogen without detectable activity that is converted to a functional serine protease during contact activation (16). On SDS gel electrophoresis, purified prekallikrein always yields two bands at 85 kd and 88 kd. Activation is accomplished in plasma by either factor XIIa or factor XIIf and results in a disulfide-linked two-chain form comprising a heavy chain of 56 kd and a light chain bearing the catalytic center. The heterogeneity shown by the zymogen is reflected in the light chain; upon reduction, a pair of bands at 33 kd and 36 kd is seen, each of which contains a diisopropylfluorophosphate (DFP)-inhibitable active site (16,32). Physical and chemical data for human plasma prekallikrein are found in Table 36-1.

Prekallikrein binds to HMWK through a site on its heavy chain with a dissociation constant of 12 to 15 nm (33,34). This value, which is unchanged by conversion to kallikrein, is such that at plasma concentrations of HMWK and prekallikrein, approximately 80% to 90% of the prekallikrein circulates bound to HMWK in 1:1 complex. Thus, it is the prekallikrein-

HMWK complex that participates in surface-induced contact activation, and the binding of prekallikrein to the surface is mediated through the HMWK. The dissociation of 10% to 20% of the kallikrein into the fluid phase may serve to propagate both the activation of factor XII and the generation of bradykinin (35,36).

Most of the measurable proteolytic activity evolved in normal human plasma as a result of contact activation is due to kallikrein. It is responsible for most of the factor XII activation that takes place in plasma, and it converts factor XIIa to factor XIIf (12,13). Kallikrein also digests HMWK to liberate the vasoactive peptide bradykinin. Kallikrein shows preference for cleaving peptide bonds carboxy-terminal to arginine residues, and cleaves HMWK and factor XII at a number of different arginine-containing sequences. In the case of the liberation of bradykinin, however, the second cleavage to liberate the bradykinin from the carboxy-terminal end of the kininogen-heavy chain occurs at the sequence Leu-Met-Lys. Apparently, the quaternary structure of the substrate HMWK must be present to induce kallikrein to cleave this bond (37). Kallikrein is active in the factor XII–dependent fibrinolytic pathway in two ways. It can directly convert plasminogen to plasmin (38,39), and it also converts plasma prourokinase to urokinase (40–42).

Kallikrein possesses other functions that may have a role in inflammation. It is chemotactic for human neutrophils (43) and monocytes (44), and it causes neutrophil aggregation (45) and secretion of elastase (46). There is, however, controversy regarding these functions among different laboratories (47). Kallikrein also can destroy the first component of complement (48) and activate factor B of the alternative complement pathway (49). Finally, kallikrein can convert plasma prorenin to renin, and it is responsible for the neutral phase of acid-induced prorenin activation (50,51).

Kallikrein is inhibited in plasma mainly by C1 inhibitor (C1 INH) and by α_2-macroglobulin (52–54). The role of these inhibitors in regulating contact activation is described in the section Initiation and Regulation of the Contact Activation System. Table 36-2 indicates nonphysiologic inhibitors that are of experimental importance.

Structure

The entire amino acid sequence of the protein has been determined by a combination of direct protein sequencing and amino acid sequence prediction from cDNA isolated from a λ gt-11 expression library (55). The gene is found on chromosome 4 and is composed of 15 exons and 14 introns, with a total length of approximately 30 kb (56). The signal peptide of 19 residues is followed by the sequence of the mature plasma prekallikrein molecule, which has 619 amino acids with a calculated molecular weight of 69,710 d; together with 15% carbohydrate, the total predicted molecular weight is 79,545 d. Five asparagine residues have been identified as attachment sites for carbohydrate—three in the light chain and two in the heavy chain. The molecular weight heterogeneity seen on SDS gel electrophoresis is not explained by any sequence heterogeneity and may, therefore, be due to variations in glycosylation.

The site of the cleavage that generates kallikrein from prekallikrein is at Arg^{371}-Ile^{372}, generating a light chain of 248 amino acid residues with the new amino-terminal sequence Ile-Val-Gly. The catalytic triad is comprised of His^{415}, Asp^{464}, and Ser^{559}. The amino acid sequence of the heavy chain is unusual and has little homology with other serine proteases of the coagulation cascade, with the exception of factor XI. In place of the heterogeneous

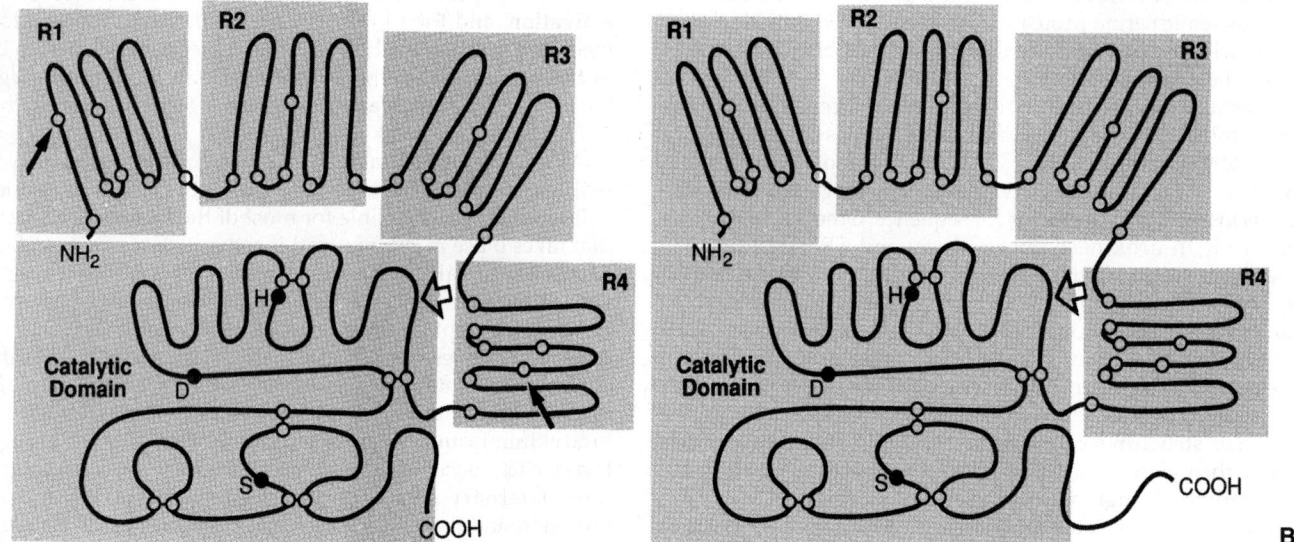

Figure 36-5. Schematic diagram of the protein chains of factor XI (**A**) and prekallikrein (**B**), showing the structural domains inferred from sequence homologies. The catalytic triad residues are shown by solid circles. Half cystines are indicated by open circles, and the cleavage sites leading to activation by activated factor XII are marked with open arrows. The solid arrows indicate the unmatched half-cystines that might be involved in interchain disulfide bonds. (Adapted from Fujikawa K, Chung DW, Hendrickson LE, et al. Amino acid sequence of human factor XI: a blood coagulation factor with four tandem repeats that are highly homologous with plasma prekallikrein. *Biochemistry* 1986;25:2417.)

domain structure found in factor XII, the heavy chain sequence of prekallikrein comprises four tandem repeats, each of which contains approximately 90 to 91 amino acids (Fig. 36-5). The presence of six conserved one-half cystines per repeat suggests a repeating structure with three disulfide loops (Fig. 36-5). The two carbohydrate sites found in the heavy chain are found in the second and fourth repeats. It is postulated that a gene segment coding for the ancestor of the repeat sequence duplicated and then the entire segment duplicated again to give the present structure.

FACTOR XI

Biochemistry

Similar to factor XII and prekallikrein, factor XI is a zymogen that is activated to a serine protease during contact activation. Factor XI is unique among the clotting factors in that the circulating zymogen consists of two identical subunits that are linked by disulfide bonds; the dimer has an apparent molecular weight of 160 kd on SDS gel electrophoresis (57,58). Factor XI is activated by factor XIIa in the presence of an anionic surface and HMWK; other enzymes produced during contact activation, including the LMW forms of activated factor XII, are not efficient activators of factor XI. Thrombin has also been shown to activate factor XI, and an autoactivation reaction can occur (59,60). The physiologic significance of these reactions is discussed further in the section on hemostasis.

The activation of factor XI follows the familiar pattern of cleavage of a peptide bond within a disulfide linkage to yield an amino-terminal heavy chain and a disulfide-linked light chain. Because both precursor subunits can be cleaved, and each resulting light chain bears a functional active site, factor XIa is a four-chain protein with two active sites. Physical and chemical data for human factor XI are found in Table 36-1.

Factor XI circulates with a plasma concentration of only 4 to 6 µg/mL. The heavy chain of factor XIa, like that of kallikrein,

binds to the light chain of HMWK. Thus, factor XI and HMWK also circulate as a complex (61); the dissociation constant is approximately 70 nm (62), which is high enough to ensure that approximately 90% of the factor XI is complexed. The molar ratio of the complex can be either one or two molecules of HMWK/factor XI because of the dimeric nature of factor XI (63). The binding site for HMWK on the factor XI heavy chain has been localized to the first (amino-terminal) tandem repeat (64).

Although it is possible to activate prekallikrein in the fluid phase by factor XIIf—bound or not bound to HMWK—factor XI activation requires interaction with the surface (18), and HMWK is an obligate cofactor (4,65,66). Thus, both factor XII and HMWK interact with the initiating surface, and HMWK facilitates factor XI cleavage by factor XIIa.

The primary function of factor XIa is to activate the next protein in the intrinsic coagulation cascade (i.e., to convert factor IX to IXa). This next step is the first one involving a vitamin K–dependent clotting factor, and the reaction is accelerated by calcium ions. In the later reactions of the clotting pathway, the vitamin K–dependent factors, factor X and prothrombin, are activated by calcium-dependent surface assemblies of enzyme (factor IXa or Xa, respectively) and a protein cofactor (factor VIII or V, respectively). By contrast, the activation of factor IX by factor XIa does not require a protein cofactor. However, the presence of a binding site on the heavy chain of factor XI for factor IXa has been inferred from studies with monoclonal antibodies (67). This site is distinct from the catalytic center on the light chain and appears to interact with factor IX only in the presence of calcium ions (68). Thus, in a sense, the heavy chain of factor XIa may function as an intrinsic "protein cofactor." The binding of HMWK to factor XIa does not affect the reaction with factor IX. Thus, the HMWK-factor XIa complex activates factor IX, and activation may take place on the contact surface.

Factor XIa also makes a small contribution to factor XII–dependent fibrinolysis by its ability to directly convert plasminogen to plasmin (16). Its potency is approximately equal to that of kallikrein (39), but it makes a lesser contribution because kallikrein is generated in greater quantities. As discussed below, the feedback by thrombin appears to initiate a factor XI–dependent inhibition of clot lysis, which appears to be more significant *in vivo* than the fibrinolytic action of factor XI (69,70).

Receptors for both factor XI and factor XIa are found on platelets (71,72), and these may be involved in a platelet-dependent but factor XII–independent pathway for factor XI activation (73). Whether such binding is relevant to physiologic factor IX activation is not clear.

Structure

PROTEIN
The amino acid sequence of human factor XI has been determined by translation of a cDNA insert obtained from a λ gt-11 cDNA library prepared from human liver poly(A) RNA (74). An 18–amino acid leader peptide is followed by a 607–amino acid sequence for each of the two subunits of the mature protein. The calculated molecular weight of the two polypeptide chains totals 135,979 d, and with the addition of 5% carbohydrate, the total molecular weight would be approximately 140 kd. Five potential N-glycosylation sites have been identified in each subunit, three in the heavy chain and two in the light chain portions of the sequence.

Conversion of factor XI to factor XIa occurs by cleavage between Arg^{369} and Ile^{370}, giving a light chain of 238 amino acids with a new N-terminal sequence of Ile-Val-Gly-Gly. The light chain has the characteristic features of the trypsinlike serine proteases, the catalytic triad being comprised of His^{44}, Asp^{93}, and Ser^{188}. The sequence of heavy chain of factor XIa, like that of kallikrein, contains four tandem repeats of approximately 90 amino acids, including six conserved one-half cystines, suggesting that each repeat forms a domain containing three internal disulfide bridges (Fig. 36-5). The domains, labeled *A1* through *A4*, have been shown to mediate distinct interactions of factor XI (75); the A1 domain contains binding sites for HMWK and thrombin, the A2 domain binds factor IX, the A3 domain is responsible for the binding to platelets, and the A4 domain binds factor XIIa as well as providing site for dimer formation (76).

GENE
The gene for factor XI spans 23 kbp and is divided into 15 exons and 14 introns (77). Each tandem repeat found in the protein-heavy chain sequence is demarcated by an intron at its amino-terminal end, and each contains one intron in essentially the same position. The catalytic domain is coded by five exons arranged identically to the exon structure of TPA and urokinase.

HOMOLOGIES WITH OTHER PROTEINS
The amino acid sequence of factor XI shows a striking degree of homology with prekallikrein. Thus, the complete sequence of factor XI has 58% identity with that of prekallikrein, and, if homologous amino acids are included, the degree of homology is 67% (74). Thirty-four out of 36 one-half cystines are in matching positions, whereas the remaining two are believed to be involved in the interchain disulfide bonds as described earlier. The carboxy terminal sequence of 88 amino acids, which includes the active site serine residue and the substrate-binding pocket, has 81% identity. These data show that both proteins are very likely to have evolved from a common ancestor.

Both prekallikrein and factor XI have five potential sites for Asn-linked carbohydrate. Three sites are identical in the two proteins (one in the heavy chain and two in the light chain), but the carbohydrate content of factor XI is only 5% compared to approximately 15% in prekallikrein. Whether the difference is accounted for by fewer attached chains or shorter ones is undetermined.

The structure of the gene for the active site domain of factor XI is very similar to those for TPA, urokinase, and factor XII. The heavy-chain region, however, is quite different from the strings of kringles and growth factor–like regions described for factor XII. The structure of the gene for prekallikrein is very similar to that for factor XI (56).

HIGH-MOLECULAR-WEIGHT KININOGEN

Biochemistry

HMWK [also abbreviated HK (78)] circulates as a single-chain glycoprotein with an apparent molecular weight of 200 kd by gel filtration (33) and 115 kd by SDS gel electrophoresis under reducing conditions (79). HMWK circulates at a plasma concentration of 70 to 90 µg/mL (80–83) and forms a noncovalent complex with prekallikrein (33) with a dissociation constant of 15 nm (34,84) and a similar complex with factor XI (61) with a dissociation constant of 70 nm (62). Other physical and chemical data are given in Table 36-1.

During contact activation, plasma kallikrein digests HMWK and leaves a disulfide-linked heterodimer, consisting of an amino-terminal heavy chain (65 kd) and initially a carboxy-terminal light chain of 56 to 62 kd. A subsequent cleavage reduces the light chain to 45 to 49 kd (84–88). The digestion of HMWK by kallikrein releases bradykinin (NH_2-Arg-Pro-Pro-Gly-Phe-Ser-Pro-Phe-Arg-COOH), which is a potent vasoactive peptide with multiple effects in inflammation (79,89,90). Bradykinin is discussed in more detail in the section Assessment of Contact Activation in Human Disease. HMWK is also cleaved by tissue kallikrein* to form the heterodimer of the heavy chain and the 56- to 62-kd light chain; the additional cleavage made by plasma kallikrein in the light chain is not made by the tissue enzyme (87,88,91).

The complexes of HMWK with prekallikrein and factor XI are formed with the light chain region, and the isolated reduced and alkylated light chain of HMWK forms these complexes with the same dissociation constants as the whole molecule (34,62,84,92). Calculations of the proportion of plasma HMWK that circulates as complexes with prekallikrein and factor XI give results in the range of 80% to 90%.

Secondary structure prediction from the sequence of the light chain suggests a low degree of α-helix and a very flexible structure (93). This is in accord with the experimental observation that light chain isolated after reduction, alkylation, and gel filtration in guanidine hydrochloride retains full functional activity (90).

Kallikrein first cleaves HMWK at the carboxy-terminal of the bradykinin sequence, leaving the bradykinin attached to the carboxy-terminal end of the heavy chain of cleaved HMWK (37,86,87). The sequence Leu-Met-Lys-Arg is cleaved at the Lys-Arg bond to liberate bradykinin from the heavy chain (Fig. 36-6).

As described above, HMWK binds to negatively charged surfaces through the histidine-rich region of the light chain. The ability to bind to a surface and simultaneously complex factor XI or prekallikrein is responsible for its cofactor activity in contact activation (35). When a surface such as a glass slide is intro-

---

*Tissue kallikrein: There is another enzyme that is a kallikrein (i.e., it can release kinin from kininogen). This enzyme is released from tissue as an active enzyme, not a zymogen, and is also found in urine. Tissue or urinary kallikrein is not related to plasma kallikrein immunologically and has somewhat different substrate specificity when assayed with peptide substrates. The primary substrate of tissue kallikrein is LMW kininogen (LMWK), which it cleaves to release lysyl-bradykinin (kallidin). The pharmacologic properties of kallidin are very similar to those of bradykinin; a plasma aminopeptidase converts kallidin to bradykinin.

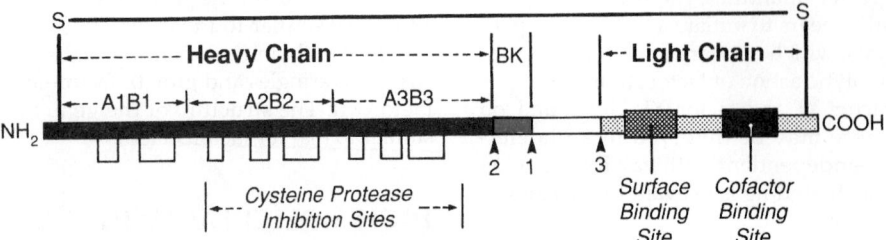

Figure 36-6. The structure of high-molecular-weight kininogen. The heavy-chain region consists of three homologous domains—A1B1, A2B2, and A3B3—of which the latter two are sulfhydryl protease inhibition sites. The small rectangles under the heavy-chain region represent the eight intra–heavy-chain disulfide bonds. The light-chain region of high-molecular-weight kininogen, which contains the binding sites for surface and prekallikrein or factor XI, is located toward the C-terminal end of the protein. The heavy and light chains are held together by the ninth disulfide bond. The arrowheads labeled 1, 2, and 3 indicate the sites and the order in which plasma kallikrein cleaves high-molecular-weight kininogen. BK, bradykinin.

duced into plasma, it is first coated with fibrinogen, but this is then rapidly displaced by HMWK (94–96). The mechanism of this effect is not fully understood. HMWK also binds to heparin and may influence thereby the inhibition of clotting by antithrombin III (ATIII) in heparinized plasma (97). The manner in which HMWK functions as a cofactor in contact activation will be discussed in detail in the section Role of High-Molecular-Weight Kininogen.

Structure

PROTEIN
The complete amino acid sequence of HMWK has been determined from cDNA as well as by direct sequence analysis of purified protein (98–101). HMWK contains a total of 626 amino acid residues with a calculated molecular weight of 69,896 d, which, together with 40% carbohydrate, gives a total molecular weight close to that observed. The heavy chain of 362 residues, which is derived from the N-terminus, is followed by the nine-residue bradykinin sequence and then the light-chain sequence of 255 residues (Fig. 36-6). The mature protein has a blocked N-terminal amino acid (pyroglutamic acid). There are three glycosidic linkage sites on the heavy chain and nine on the light chain. Interestingly, all the glycosidic bonds on the heavy chain are N-linked, and those on the light chain are O-linked.

The heavy chain contains three contiguous sequences that are homologous to each other: Domain 1 comprises residues 1 to 116, domain 2 residues 117 to 238, and domain 3 residues 239 to 360 (Fig. 36-6). Of the 17 one-half cystines, one is near the N-terminal and forms a disulfide bond with the light chain; the others form a linear arrangement of eight consecutive disulfide loops aligned with the sequence repeats (98). These three domains share considerable homology with a family of small (12 to 13 kd) cysteine protease inhibitors called *cystatins*, and domains 2 and 3, but not 1, exhibit cysteine protease inhibitor activity (102–105). It has been shown by limited proteolytic digestion that protease-sensitive sites on the heavy chain map to its inter-domain junctions, and it was suggested that cleavage at these sites may occur in plasma to release the inhibitory domains under certain pathologic conditions. The isolated heavy chain has greater cysteine protease inhibitor activity than native HMWK and is able to bind two molecules of papain (104).

The procoagulant properties of HMWK are all resident in the light-chain portion of HMWK (90,92). The light chain is divided into a basic amino-terminal portion, which binds to activating surfaces (90,92,106), and an acidic carboxy-terminal portion, which bears the binding sites for prekallikrein and factor XI (62,107). The surface-binding region spanning residues 91 to

121 of the light chain is called the *histidine-rich* region, because 24 out of 91 residues are histidines and a further 11 residues are lysine. Interestingly, this histidine-rich region also exhibits three internally homologous sequences of approximately 30 residues each, and each sequence, in turn, contains further internally homologous sequences. It is speculated that the entire histidine-rich region may have evolved by repeated duplication of the sequence Gly-His (or His-Gly) (100). The sole one-half cystine found in the light chain forms a disulfide bond with the heavy chain. No homologies with any protein except for other kininogens have been recognized.

The prekallikrein binding site of HMWK maps to residues 194 to 224 of the light chain (31 amino acids) (62,107). A corresponding synthetically prepared peptide has been shown to bind prekallikrein with the same affinity as the intact light chain. Factor XI also bound to the same region of HMWK but, in this case, optimal binding required a 58-amino acid peptide spanning residues 185 to 242 of the light chain (62).

RELATIONSHIP TO LOW-MOLECULAR-WEIGHT KININOGEN
There is another circulating protein that is also a kininogen; because it has a molecular weight of only 68 kd, it is termed *LMWK*. Like HMWK, LMWK is digested by tissue kallikrein to a two-chain form from which bradykinin has been excised (108,109). This digestion yields a 65-kd amino-terminal heavy chain disulfide linked to a light chain of 4 kd (98,110,111). In contrast to HMWK, LMWK is not cleaved by plasma kallikrein. The sequences of LMWK and HMWK are identical from the amino-terminus through the bradykinin sequence and the next twelve amino acids (110). Studies of the cDNA show that the identity persists through the 18 residue signal peptide and the 5' untranslated region of the mRNA (99).

KININOGEN GENES
Both HMWK and LMWK are produced from a single gene (27 kbp in size) that is thought to have originated by two successive duplications of a primordial kininogen gene (99). As schematically represented in Figure 36-7, this gene consists of a total of 11 exons. Of these, the first nine exons code for the kininogen heavy chain; each of the three domains indicated by the protein sequence is coded by a set of three exons. The tenth exon codes for bradykinin and the light chain of HMWK, whereas the light chain of LMWK is coded for by exon 11. The mRNAs for HMWK and LMWK are produced from this single gene by alternative splicing which includes the sequences for the heavy chain and bradykinin in both protein products but provides HMWK and LMWK with different light-chain moieties (Fig. 36-7).

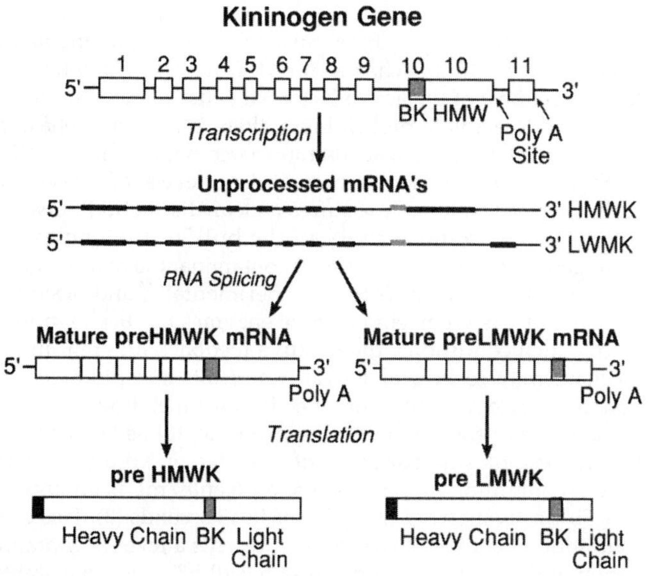

Kininogen Gene

Figure 36-7. The gene for high-molecular-weight kininogen (HMWK). The boxes labeled 1 to 9 represent the exon coding for the heavy chain of both HMWK and low-molecular-weight kininogen (LMWK). Exon 10 codes for the bradykinin (BK) sequence and the light chain of HMWK, whereas exon 11 codes for the light chain of LMWK. The mature messenger RNAs (mRNAs) are assembled by alternative splicing events in which the light-chain sequences are attached to the 3' end of the 12–amino acid common sequence C terminal to BK.

INITIATION AND REGULATION OF THE CONTACT ACTIVATION SYSTEM

Initiation of the intrinsic coagulation pathway via the contact activation system occurs when a negatively charged surface is introduced into plasma containing the full complement of protease zymogens [factor XII, prekallikrein (6,15)] and protein

cofactors [HMWK (3)]. Contact with the surface induces the formation of the active enzymes—factor XIIa and kallikrein as depicted in Figure 36-1. The second step, separated rather arbitrarily, can be viewed as the activation of factor XI by factor XIIa (Figs. 36-1 and 36-8); the roles of prekallikrein and HMWK, viewed from a coagulation point of view, are to accelerate conversion of factor XII to factor XIIa. If we are to explain initiation and regulation of contact activation, therefore, we have to understand how the activation of factor XII is triggered by the introduction of a surface and why it does not occur before then. The first question is concerned with the interactions among the proteins and with the surface, the second involves the influence of other plasma proteins, most notably the various protease inhibitors.

Interactions of Proteins and Surfaces in the Initiation of Contact Activation

CHARACTER OF THE "SURFACE"

Contact activation was originally observed by the interaction of blood with glass surfaces (112); subsequently, finely divided kaolin was used extensively as an experimental surface and for coagulation assays (113). Both of these materials are ill-defined in terms of their interactions with plasma proteins, and, of course, neither bears any obvious relationship to physiologic substances. The first apparently soluble activator of contact activation was the tanninlike substance ellagic acid (114), which has also been used as a component of commercial assay systems. It has been since shown, however, that ellagic acid is only effective when it can form large sedimentable aggregates in the presence of traces of contaminant-heavy metal ions (115); ellagic acid must therefore also be considered a particulate activator.

Dextran sulfate (116,117) and sulfatide (117) were subsequently introduced for studies of contact activation. Sulfatide is a naturally occurring sphingolipid bearing a galactose sulfate group. It is normally found in small quantities in nerve tissue, where it is too diluted by other lipids to be a likely physiologic

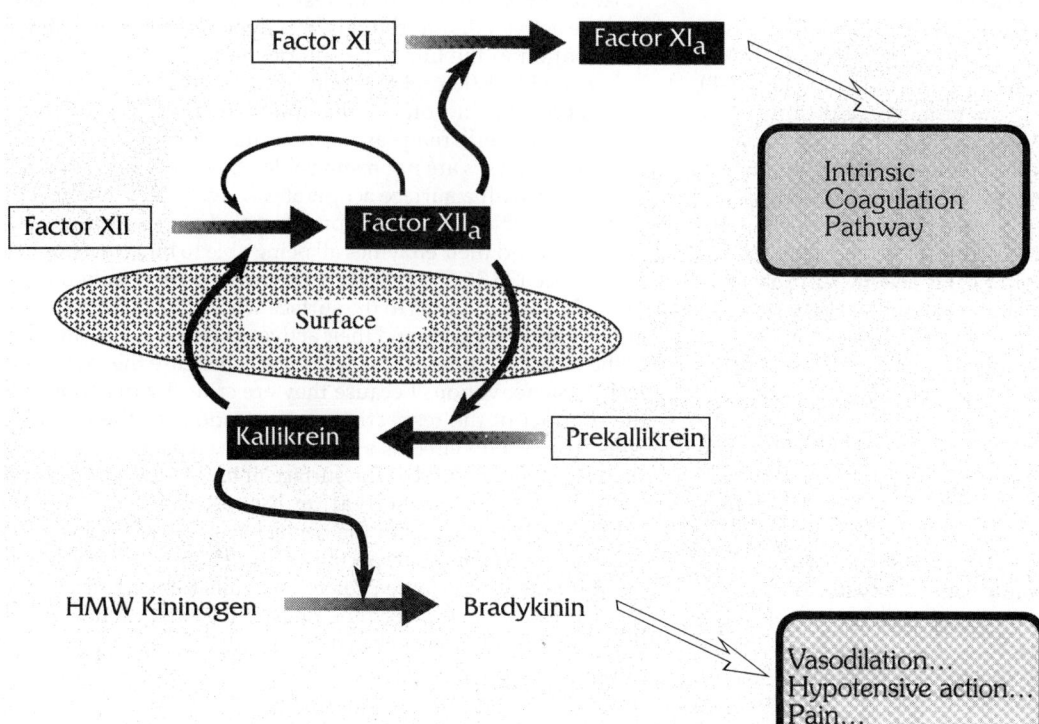

Figure 36-8. The pathways of contact activation. Open boxes, zymogens; black boxes, proteases; graded arrows, activation reactions; solid arrows, catalytic activities. HMW, high molecular weight.

activator. Purified sulfatide, however, can form micelles with a highly charged surface of sulfate groups; such micelles are very efficient activators of the contact system (118,119).

Dextran sulfate is a truly soluble activator and a close homolog of naturally occurring sulfated polysaccharides. Initially, high-molecular-weight preparations (500-kd nominal molecular weight) were found to support the activation of factor XII and prekallikrein (2,8,117). However, in a study of factor XII autoactivation, much smaller fractions were found to be capable of supporting the reaction (120). When the dependence of the rate of autoactivation on the size of the dextran sulfate was examined, there was a low but definite reaction with molecular weights as low as 5 kd. The rate increased markedly above 10 kd, in which range the theoretical number of binding sites/particle increased from one to two. Very similar results were obtained with heparin (120), thus indicating that this naturally occurring polysaccharide could support contact activation by a similar mechanism to dextran sulfate. Other studies of natural sulfated polysaccharides have found that only highly sulfated species, such as heparin or chondroitin sulfate E, were active (121,122). This requirement for a high density of strong negative charges was also suggested by the finding of a relationship between the rate of factor XII autoactivation and the sulfate content of a series of dextran sulfate preparations (123).

Although it is very attractive to consider that substances rich in sulfated polysaccharides, such as basement membrane of endothelial cell matrix, may support contact activation, this remains a theoretical possibility and has not been demonstrated. On the other hand, the surfaces of endothelial cells or platelets may indeed be the physiologic locus of activation (see section Interaction with Cells). One pathophysiologic substance that is very likely to initiate contact activation *in vivo* is endotoxin (124–126). As discussed below, there is good reason to believe that the contact system is activated in gram-negative septicemia and that in septic shock, the observed symptoms are due, at least in part, to the generation of bradykinin.

SURFACE-INDUCED ACTIVATION OF FACTOR XII AND PREKALLIKREIN

The most striking feature of the contact activation pathway is its cyclic or reciprocal form (6) in which the activator of prekallikrein is factor XIIa and that of factor XII is kallikrein (Fig. 36-8). This feature gives the pathway the property of positive feedback, which ensures an accelerating reaction once initiation has occurred (2,8). Similarly, the autoactivation of factor XII is also a mechanism with positive feedback (9), although with slower kinetics (8).

The mechanism by which initiation occurs is of interest because all of the components are present in plasma as zymogens (factor XII and prekallikrein) or as a nonenzymatic cofactor (HMWK). No reaction takes place until a negatively charged surface or polyanion is added; because such substances do not have intrinsic enzymatic activity, some further explanation is required.

The simplest explanation would be that one of the zymogens possesses a small level of enzymatic activity that can initiate activation in the presence of a surface. Because prekallikrein-deficient plasma eventually clots after the addition of surface, it must be possible for factor XII to activate and generate factor XI. Indeed, the plasminogen activators closely homologous to factor XII—TPA and prourokinase—do possess measurable enzymatic activity in their single-chain forms. This was confirmed by site-specific mutagenesis at their cleavage sites to produce uncleavable molecules (127–130). In the case of TPA, fibrinogen or fibrin may be able to substitute for the new amino-terminal formed by cleavage of trypsinogen or chymotrypsinogen. In contrast, studies of factor XII indicated that all the observable activity is kinetically indistinguishable from authentic factor XIIa or factor XIIf (2). When factor XII is treated with inhibitors to remove most of the active factor XIIa and this preparation is then used to activate prekallikrein, there is a distinct phase of acceleration before the reaction rate matches that of factor XIIf.

Experimental demonstration of low levels of enzymatic activity in the zymogen requires a clear distinction between intrinsic enzymatic activity in the bulk of the uncleaved zymogen molecules and traces of contaminant-activated factor XII. This is very difficult to do experimentally, and often the presence of a few percent of active enzymes has been ignored. Under such conditions, the positive feedback inherent in the mechanism of reciprocal activations results in rapid acceleration of the rate of generation of active enzyme, thus obscuring the kinetics of the initiation. For example, it has been shown that mixing plasma concentrations of factor XII and prekallikrein containing just one active molecule/mL is enough to give 50% activation of both proteins in 13 seconds (8). This concentration of activated enzymes represents a level of contamination of the purified zymogens of 5×10^{-13}%. Also, the ability of factor XIIa to activate factor XII (autoactivation) was not appreciated. Thus, activity generated in pure preparations of factor XII after exposure to surfaces was ascribed to the zymogen (131) when it was almost certainly due to the generation of factor XIIa by autoactivation.

A more reasonable explanation that is consistent with the data is that the contact activation reactions are proceeding continuously at a low rate in plasma, thereby maintaining a low steady-state concentration of the enzymes factor XIIa and kallikrein (2,123) but controlled by the reaction of the enzymes with the plasma inhibitors (132). The introduction of a surface or other polyanionic substance would then induce "activation" by accelerating many thousand-fold the baseline turnover of factor XII and prekallikrein, rapidly generating significant quantities of factor XIIa and kallikrein.

Factor XII can also be slowly activated by plasmin (19). It is thus possible that under circumstances such as the release of TPA, factor XII and then the rest of the contact system could become activated. Interestingly, this hypothesis has received little attention in the literature, although the activation of factor XII or the HMWK-prekallikrein complex by cell-derived proteases might be a potent inflammatory mechanism. Clearly, however, in cell-free plasma in contact with surfaces, cell-derived proteases are not responsible for contact activation.

Contact with a surface accelerates activation by two mechanisms. The first is a localization effect that comes from the two zymogens and their enzymes all being able to bind reversibly to the surface (35,36,65,119,123). This creates a local milieu in the fluid phase contiguous to the surface where the local concentrations of the zymogens and their activated forms are greater than in the bulk fluid phase. This will greatly increase the rates of the reciprocal activations because they are critically dependent on the product of the respective concentrations of the two reactants. The second effect is a conformational change in factor XII such that when bound to the surface, it becomes more susceptible to cleavage and activation by various proteases (7). Although the reactants of the contact system are bound to the surface, the inhibitors, especially C1 INH, are not, so that surface binding offers some protection against inactivation (133). Thus, the balance between the rates of the activation reactions and the inactivation reactions is profoundly changed at the fluid-surface interface.

Whether the surface-bound zymogens are activated by neighboring surface-bound enzyme molecules or by fluid phase enzymes is not clear. In a study of the effect of molecular size of dextran sulfate on the rate of factor XII autoactivation (120), the maximum rate varied with the size of the polyanion but always occurred at the same relative concentrations of factor XII and factor XII binding sites, implying an optimal ratio of free to bound factor XII. Also, activation occurred with molecular weights of dextran sulfate that probably had only one binding site for factor XII/particle, implying that activation of bound factor XII by fluid phase factor XIIa was occurring. In studies of the activation of factor XII by kallikrein, enhancements of 3000- (134) to 12,000-fold (8) have been found when surface was added. This enhancement must include a component ascribable to the binding of factor XII to the surface and also a component ascribable to the binding of kallikrein to the surface. The isolated, active, light chain of kallikrein (which lacks the surface-binding site) is far less effective than intact kallikrein; in the presence of surface, it digested factor XII only 30 times faster than it did in the fluid phase (134). Thus, the kallikrein-surface interaction may have a 100-fold kinetic effect. This could be the result of localization effects or of a requirement for bound enzyme to cleave bound substrate. In a different study, however, the authors concluded that surface-bound factor XII was activated by fluid-phase kallikrein (119), so the localization effect may be the prime mechanism by which the surface enhances the rate of factor XII activation by kallikrein.

In the reciprocal reaction (i.e., the activation of prekallikrein by activated factor XII) the surface appears to play a smaller role. Thus the effect of dextran sulfate was to increase by 70-fold the rate of prekallikrein activation by factor XIIa (8). Factor XIIf, the final cleavage product of factor XII activation, cleaved prekallikrein at a similar rate to that of factor XIIa in solution, but since factor XIIf does not have surface-binding sites, its activation of prekallikrein is unaffected by the presence of surface. This result indicates that, in contrast to factor XII, the binding of prekallikrein to the surface does not cause a change in its properties as a substrate. In the presence of HMWK, however, the situation may be different, as described below.

Whatever the mechanism by which factor XII activation is initiated, once some kallikrein has been formed by the action of factor XIIa on prekallikrein, it rapidly digests surface-bound factor XII, thus creating the positive feedback kinetics characteristic of the contact activation pathway. The activation of surface-bound factor XII by kallikrein is approximately 2000-fold more rapid than the rate of factor XII autoactivation, so that when factor XII activation is considered quantitatively, the major activator is kallikrein (8). It has been shown that plasma that is congenitally deficient in prekallikrein (Fletcher trait plasma) has an *in vitro* clotting defect that is unique. Its PTT is abnormal, but it autocorrects as the time of incubation with the surface is increased from 2 minutes to 10 minutes before the addition of calcium (4,135–137). During this time, sufficient factor XIIa is formed to activate factor XI normally. We believe this autocorrection results from the factor XII autoactivation pathway.

ROLE OF HIGH-MOLECULAR-WEIGHT KININOGEN

If purified factor XII and prekallikrein are mixed in the presence of a substance such as dextran sulfate or sulfatide, the reciprocal activations previously described generate the active forms of both proteins. In plasma, however, the involvement of a third protein was indicated by the discovery of persons who were not deficient in either prekallikrein or factor XII but whose plasma had very long APTTs and who generated no bradykinin (138). This phenomenon was explained by the identification of HMWK as a nonenzymatic cofactor in contact activation (3,139,140). Initial observations suggested that HMWK accelerated the activations of both factor XII and prekallikrein as well as that of factor XI (4,5,65,66).

It was subsequently demonstrated that both prekallikrein (33) and factor XI (61) form specific complexes with HMWK. By analogy with the mechanism for cofactor activity in the activation of factor X and prothrombin, one might predict that HMWK would also interact with factor XII, thus forming a ternary activation complex on the surface. In fact, no evidence has been adduced for such a complex, and, as we have described previously, in buffer systems, when dextran sulfate or sulfatides are used as initiators of contact activation, both factor XII and prekallikrein can be rapidly activated even in the absence of HMWK. Indeed, under some experimental conditions, high concentrations of HMWK relative to the surface cause inhibition of contact activation reactions (141). This is almost certainly due to competition between HMWK and factor XII for the same binding sites on the surface (142).

As described in preceding sections, the magnitudes of the dissociation constants and the plasma concentrations of the three proteins are such that approximately 90% of the factor XI and prekallikrein circulate bound to HMWK. Thus, the substrates for factor XIIa during contact activation are prekallikrein and factor XI bound to the surface via HMWK (35,66) (Fig. 36-9). It appears that the function of the HMWK is to present the substrates for factor XIIa in a conformation that facilitates their activation (35). Thus, prekallikrein was found to bind to kaolin in the absence of HMWK but was not subsequently activated by factor XII. Peptides bearing the carboxy-terminal sequence of the HMWK light chain inhibited HMWK-dependent coagulant activity of normal plasma by competitively interfering with the binding of prekallikrein to the light chain of HMWK, thereby preventing its activation by activated factor XII (62). Similarly, a monoclonal antibody directed against the prekallikrein binding site of HMWK inhibited coagulation and the activation of prekallikrein in plasma (143). Thus, HMWK appears to catalyze conversion of prekallikrein to kallikrein either by altering the

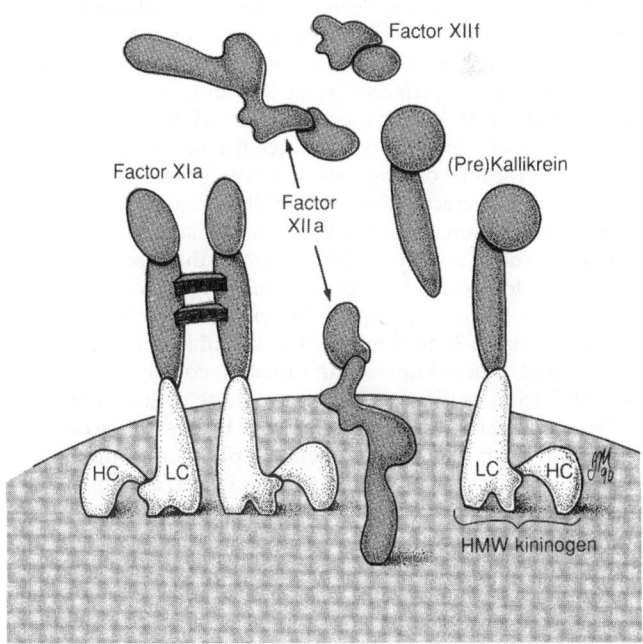

Figure 36-9. Illustration of the interactions between the proteins and the surface in contact activation. Prekallikrein and factor XI are shown bound to the surface by the light chain (LC) of high-molecular-weight (HMW) kininogen. Factor XII binds directly to the surface. (No distinction is made in the figure between the zymogens and their disulfide-linked two-chain activated forms.) Factor XI1 prekallikrein and factor XIIf are also found in the fluid phase. HC, heavy chain.

conformation of prekallikrein or by preventing the formation of an unfavorable conformation when prekallikrein binds directly to the surface. For some surfaces, the presence of HMWK also increases the amount of prekallikrein that is bound (35,66), although this may be of lesser importance. Factor XI activation is almost totally dependent on the formation of surface-binding complexes with HMWK (65,66).

HMWK can augment the rate of factor XII activation in plasma (5,66), although it does not augment the activity of kallikrein directly against synthetic substrates or fluid phase factor XII; rather, its effects appear to be largely indirect. First, HMWK is required for efficient generation of kallikrein in surface-activated plasma. Further, because the kallikrein-HMWK complex has a dissociation constant of 15 nm (34), at plasma concentrations approximately 10% of the kallikrein dissociates; kallikrein formed on the surface can thereby dissociate and interact with surface-bound factor XII on other particles, thus disseminating the reaction (35,36). As a result, the effective concentration ratio of kallikrein/factor XII is increased in the presence of HMWK and may account for the augmentation seen. Finally, in plasma, HMWK is able to displace other adhesive glycoproteins, such as fibrinogen, from the surface (95).

Plasma that lacks HMWK is found to have a relative absence of prekallikrein, thus factor XII activation is very slow and dependent largely on autoactivation. The factor XIIa generated then does not convert factor XI to XIa because factor XI binding to HMWK and attachment of the complex to surfaces is also required for normal factor XI activation (4,66) (Fig. 36-9). Consequently, the plasma has a profoundly prolonged APTT that is almost as abnormal as that of factor XII deficiency.

Regulation of Contact Activation

INHIBITION OF CONTACT ACTIVATION

Regulation of factor XII–dependent pathways occurs by both intrinsic and extrinsic controls. Cleavage of factor XIIa to XIIf is one example of an intrinsic control. The factor XIIf produced is not surface bound and is a very poor activator of factor XIa. At the same time, the heavy-chain moiety, which has no enzymatic activity, retains the surface-binding site and can compete with factor XII and HMWK for the surface. Thus, the conversion of factor XIIa to factor XIIf will reduce the rate of the surface-dependent reactions of coagulation, whereas bradykinin generation via fluid-phase activation of prekallikrein continues. Similarly, digestion of kinin-free HMWK by factor XIa has been reported to limit its coagulant activity (144), although, in this case, the kinetics appear to be too slow to be of physiologic importance (88).

Extrinsic controls are provided by plasma inhibitors for each enzyme. Table 36-3 indicates the major inhibitors of each active enzyme and, where known, their relative contributions to the total inhibition in plasma. Inhibition of the contact activation proteases is clearly different from that of the rest of the coagulation pathways in that ATIII appears to play only a minor role. Instead, contact activation appears to be limited mainly by C1 INH, which is not active against any other of the clotting factors except for a weak inhibition of factor XI. C1 INH is a monovalent inhibitor that is cleaved by the protease it inhibits but remains at the active site in a covalent complex. It may remain in a stable form of the acyl enzyme intermediate found in the normal serine protease mechanism (145). Thus, after a protease has reacted with C1 INH, it cannot digest protein substrates or hydrolyze small synthetic substrates, and the reaction of the active site serine with DFP is abolished.

C1 INH is the only major plasma inhibitor of factor XIIa and factor XIIf (146–149). Although ATIII can inhibit activated factor XII (148,150,151), its contribution to factor XIIa inhibition in

TABLE 36-3. Plasma Inhibitors of Enzymes of Contact Activation: Relative Contributions to Inhibition in Normal Human Plasma

Inhibitor	Enzyme			
	Factor XIIa	Factor XIIf	Kallikrein	Factor XIa
C1 inhibitor	91.3	93	52 (84)[a]	8
Antithrombin III[b]	1.5	4	nd	16
α_2-Macroglobulin	4.3	—	35 (16)[a]	—
α_1-Protease inhibitor	—	—	nd	68
α_2-Antiplasmin	3.0	3	nd	8

nd, not determined separately.
[a]Data obtained from generation of kallikrein *in situ*.
[b]Data are for results obtained in the absence of added heparin.

plasma is apparently only a few percent of that due to C1 INH (148,149). Disagreement exists over the effect of heparin on the inhibition of activated factor XII by ATIII. Some investigators have observed little enhancement of the rate of factor XIIa inhibition (152), whereas others have observed a significant increase (150,151). Heparin can act as an activating surface for contact activation, and factor XII and factor XIIa can bind to it (120,121). This binding is a factor in the inhibition by ATIII since inhibition of factor XIIf, which lacks the surface-binding site, is not augmented in the presence of heparin as much as that of factor XIIa (151). Curiously, α_2-macroglobulin, although thought of as a "universal" protease inhibitor (153), does not significantly inhibit either form of activated factor XII.

The two major inhibitors of plasma kallikrein are C1 INH and α_2-macroglobulin (52,154,155). Together they account for over 90% of the kallikrein inhibitory activity of plasma, with the remainder contributed by ATIII (53,54). When kallikrein is added to plasma, approximately one-half is bound to C1 INH and one-half to α_2-macroglobulin (53,54,156). α_2-Macroglobulin does not bind to the active site of kallikrein but appears to trap the protease within its structure so as to sterically interfere with its ability to cleave large protein substrates (153). The degree of inhibition is greater than 95%, but the residual activity is detectable when assayed for lengthy incubation periods. In contrast, digestion of small synthetic substrates is much less affected, and approximately one-third of the starting activity is retained. When a surface such as kaolin is added to plasma so that kallikrein is generated *in situ* close to 70% or 80% of it is bound to C1 INH (156). The reason for the difference between the patterns of inhibition of added kallikrein and of endogenously produced kallikrein is unknown. Interestingly, at low temperatures, most of the inhibition of added kallikrein is accounted for by α_2-macroglobulin (156); C1 INH appears to be ineffective in the cold (151), and this may underlie the phenomenon of cold activation. The inhibition of kallikrein by ATIII is also enhanced by heparin (157) and may become significant in heparinized plasma.

The inhibition profile of factor XI is complicated by the involvement of several factors. In kinetic studies of purified components, a 1-antiproteinase inhibitor (a 1-antitrypsin) appears to be the most significant inhibitor of factor Xia (158,159), which is not typical of enzymes of the coagulation cascade. When the generation of irreversible enzyme inhibitor complexes was assessed in plasma, however, C1 INH was found to be the key inhibitor (160), with approximately equal contributions by α_2-antiplasmin and a 1-antiproteinase inhibitor (Table 36-3). ATIII is also an inhibitor with potential for augmentation by heparin, the magnitude of which is uncertain (161,162). Physiologic glycosaminoglycans also augment inhibition by C1 INH (160,163). The combined effects of ATIII and C1 INH may therefore be most significant at the surfaces where these substances are plentiful. Finally, platelets secrete protease nexin-2 (a soluble form of amyloid beta-protein precursor), which is an efficient but reversible inhibitor of factor XIa. This may be more important than the irreversible inhibitors in the regulation of factor XIa activity when first generated, although the protective effect of HMWK against inactivation may also be important (164,165).

The predominant role of C1 INH in the regulation of contact activation in human plasma is underscored by the fact that it alone is an efficient inhibitor of activated factor XII, kallikrein, and factor XIa. In plasma from patients with hereditary angioedema (HAE), in which C1 INH is absent, the amount of dextran sulfate required to produce activation is reduced tenfold compared to normal plasma (151); similar results are obtained in cold plasma. Because some surface was still required for activation under these conditions, we may surmise that the other inhibitors that are active against the contact factors do serve to limit their reactions, but that in normal plasma it is inhibition by C1 INH that forms the barrier to the initiation of contact activation. The plasma concentration of C1 INH is approximately 2 μmol/L, and it is remarkable that its inhibition is ever overcome. That surfaces are able to induce activation must reflect the protection of the proteases at the surface from inhibition. It has also been proposed that kallikrein bound to HMWK is protected from inactivation by C1 INH (166,167) and α₂-macroglobulin (167,168) and that factor XIa is similarly protected from a 1-antiproteinase inhibitor (159); this mechanism has been ruled out in the case of kallikrein and C1 INH (54,169), however, and may not be an important factor.

INACTIVATION OF BRADYKININ

Bradykinin is an exceedingly potent vasoactive peptide that can cause venular dilatation, activation of arterial endothelial cells, increased vascular permeability, hypotension, constriction of uterine and gastrointestinal smooth muscle, constriction of the coronary and pulmonary vasculature, bronchoconstriction, and activation of phospholipase A₂ to augment arachidonic acid metabolism. Its regulation is of prime importance, and a variety of enzymes in plasma contribute to kinin degradation. Carboxypeptidase N (170) removes the C-terminal Arg from bradykinin to leave an octapeptide, des-arg⁹ bradykinin (171), which is then digested by angiotensin-converting enzyme (ACE), acting as tripeptidase, to separate the tripeptide, Ser-Pro-Phe, from the pentapeptide Arg-Pro-Pro-Gly-Phe (172). Enzymes that have not been characterized rapidly digest Ser-Pro-Phe to individual amino acids and more slowly convert the pentapeptide to Arg-Pro-Pro plus Gly and Phe. The final products of bradykinin degradation are the peptide Arg-Pro-Pro, plus one mole each of Gly, Ser, Pro, and Arg, and two moles of Phe (173). The initial change of bradykinin to des-Arg⁹ bradykinin by carboxypeptidase N is fast, whereas the other steps are slower when assessed *in vitro*. It is of interest that the des-Arg⁹ bradykinin formed by this initial cleavage retains some but not all the various activities of bradykinin (174). It can, for example, interact with B₁ receptors induced by inflammation in the vasculature and cause hypotension, but bradykinin's activities on the skin and the contraction of other smooth muscles are abolished. Bradykinin interacts with constitutively expressed B₂ receptors to mediate all its functions. Selective B₂ receptor antagonists have been synthesized (175–177).

When blood is clotted and serum is studied, all of the reactions for bradykinin degradation occur as described, but the rate of the initial Arg removal is accelerated fivefold compared to plasma (173). This is probably due to the action of thrombin activatable fibrinolysis inhibitor—see section Relation of Contact Factor Deficiencies to Hemostasis. It should also be noted that bradykinin degradation *in vivo* occurs largely along the pulmonary vasculature and that endothelial cells there have carboxypeptidase as well as angiotensin-converting enzyme activities. In the pulmonary circulation, the initial cleavage may occur by angiotensin-converting enzyme acting as a dipeptidase to first remove Phe-Arg, then Ser-Pro (each of which is next cleaved to free amino acids), leaving the pentapeptide Arg-Pro-Pro-Gly-Phe. This is then metabolized further as described. The cough, wheeze, and angioedema sometimes associated with the use of ACE inhibitors for treatment of hypertension or heart failure may be due to inhibition of kinin metabolism leading to increased levels of bradykinin (178). Because bradykinin is a peripheral vasodilator, it has been considered to be a counterbalance to the vasopressor effects of angiotensin II. It is clear that the two peptides are also related in terms of metabolism, because ACE cleaves His-Leu from the C-terminal of angiotensin I, a decapeptide, to leave the octapeptide angiotensin II. Thus, ACE creates a vasoconstrictor and inactivates a vasodilator.

RELATION OF THE CONTACT FACTORS TO OTHER SYSTEMS

Intrinsic Fibrinolytic Cascade

A factor XII–dependent pathway leading to the conversion of plasminogen to plasmin was described in the 1960s and early 1970s (179–181), and a defect in this pathway has been observed in plasma deficient in either factor XII, prekallikrein, or HMWK (3,135–137,139,140). The factor XII–dependent fibrinolytic activity is relatively weak and difficult to demonstrate in whole plasma because large quantities of a potent plasminogen activator are not formed. Relatively little plasmin is generated, and this is rapidly inactivated by plasma inhibitors (α₂-antiplasmin, α₂-macroglobulin). Most studies have therefore used diluted, acidified plasma (182) or chloroform-treated plasma (180) in which inhibition of contact activation and plasmin is minimized, or have studied a euglobulin preparation that concentrates the plasma enzymes and cofactors but limits inhibition (183), or have added organic compounds that destroy α₂-antiplasmin and C1 INH (40,184,185). In comparison, such measures are not needed to study blood coagulation or the liberation of bradykinin.

Plasminogen can be activated by kallikrein (38) and factor XIa (16,39). When purified preparations are compared, kallikrein and factor XIa are equipotent as direct plasminogen activators (39). The plasma concentration of prekallikrein is approximately tenfold higher than that of factor XI, however, and in addition, factor XIIf can readily convert prekallikrein to kallikrein in the fluid phase (15,17), whereas it has minimal activity on factor XI (19). Furthermore, kallikrein can dissociate from surfaces and act in the fluid phase, whereas factor XIa cannot. For these reasons, kallikrein is more important in this pathway; nevertheless, it is possible to demonstrate a fibrinolytic abnormality in factor XI–deficient plasma (186).

Activated factor XII (XIIa or XIIf) can also convert plasminogen to plasmin (187), but its activity is only 5% of that of kallikrein. These are all weak reactions in that the potencies of kallikrein and factor XIa as plasminogen activators are thousands of times lower than that of urokinase (39,188,189). Thus, it can be argued that plasminogen is not a significant substrate for any of them. Although each of these proteins is capable of converting plasminogen to plasmin, the other blood clotting enzymes—

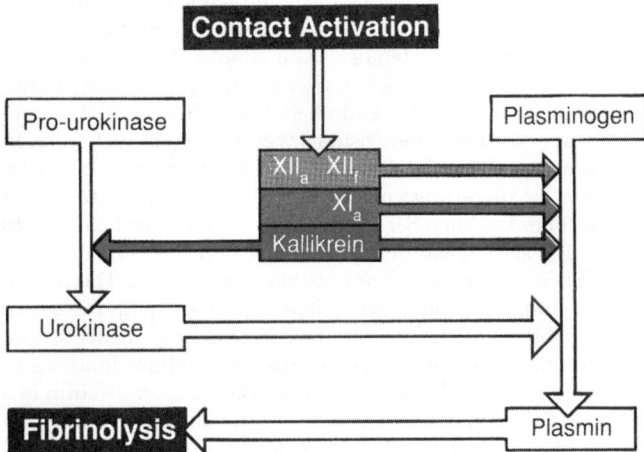

Figure 36-10. Pathways of factor XII–dependent fibrinolysis.

factors IXa, Xa, VIIa, and thrombin—have no such activity, which argues against this activity's being a contingent epiphenomenon.

More recent studies of contact-activated fibrinolysis indicate that kallikrein activates the trace quantity of prourokinase in plasma (41,190) and that urokinase is the main plasminogen activator of plasma (191) (Fig. 36-10). Inhibition by antiurokinase antisera supports this notion (40) as do zymographic gel studies using plasma euglobulin preparations (42). Other workers have suggested a role for plasma urokinase in factor XII–independent fibrinolysis (192). Although urokinase is clearly a much more potent plasminogen activator than any of the enzymes associated with contact activation, the quantities of urokinase generated are very small. If the effects of α_2-antiplasmin and C1 INH are abrogated by addition of flufenamic acid derivatives, contact activation results in the formation of approximately 35 ng/mL of plasmin (185), which represents activation of 0.05% of plasma plasminogen. Of particular interest are recent studies in which kinetically favorable prourokinase activation occurred at the surface of platelets or endothelial cells on addition of activated factor XII, HK, and prekallikrein (193,194). Although the role *in vivo* of this cascade as a pathway for fibrinolysis is not clear, patients with abnormalities of contact activation proteins such as factor XII have died of thrombosis.

An alternative interaction between the kallikrein-kinin system and *in vivo* fibrinolysis is suggested by the observation that bradykinin is a potent stimulator of the release of TPA from endothelial cells (195).

Regulation of Blood Pressure

The possible relationship of the contact system to blood pressure regulation is an intriguing question. As already seen, ACE creates the hypertensive peptide, angiotensin II, and plays a major role in inactivating the hypotensive product of contact activation, bradykinin. An unfortunate circumstance has dramatized the kinin-forming capacity of factor XIIf; trauma patients given plasma protein fractions as plasma expanders that were contaminated with factor XIIf showed profound hypotension (196,197). The mechanism by which infused factor XIIf causes hypotension has been demonstrated to involve bradykinin formation rather than prostaglandins (198).

A much more tenuous connection also exists between blood pressure regulation and the contact system in the factor XII–dependent activation of plasma prorenin. Prorenin is activated to renin by cold treatment of plasma or acidification to pH 3.3.

With acid treatment, most of the renin activity is produced after reneutralization; this alkaline phase activation is mediated by kallikrein (50,51), as is the cold-induced activation (199). Kallikrein is able to activate purified prorenin (200), but when added to plasma, it does not cause prorenin activation in the absence of an acidification step. Although it has been supposed that the acid treatment serves to destroy kallikrein inhibitors, prorenin is not activated in plasma deficient in C1 INH or α_2-macroglobulin (201). Thus, some other unknown event must occur upon acidification. The physiologic significance of this reaction is uncertain.

Interaction with Other Plasma Proteases

Factor XIIf has been reported to activate factor VII (21,202) and thereby initiate the extrinsic coagulation pathway. This reaction contributes minimally to the kaolin-activated PTT as usually performed, but it is responsible for the shortened clotting time seen when plasma is exposed to the cold (203,204). This is accentuated in women who use oral contraceptives containing estrogen, apparently owing to an increased concentration of factor XII (205–207). It is theorized that this pathway might contribute to the increased incidence of thrombosis reported as a complication of oral contraceptive use.

Factor XIIf (but not factor XIIa) can enzymatically activate the first component of complement when it is incubated with purified C1 or added to plasma (208) (Fig. 36-7). C1 activation is due to cleavage of the C1r subcomponent (20) by factor XIIf. Little complement activation is seen when kaolin is incubated with whole plasma, and significant complement activation may be seen only in conditions that result in substantial conversion of factor XIIa to factor XIIf. One such circumstance is C1 INH deficiency (i.e., HAE), in which factor XII activation may contribute to complement consumption (209,210). Kallikrein can also cleave C1 subcomponents, but the net result is destruction rather than activation. On the other hand, kallikrein can activate factor B of the alternative complement pathway and thereby substitute for factor D (49).

Interactions with Cells

Three different modes of interaction of the contact system with cells have been described: the assembly and activation of the pathway on cell surfaces; the effects of contact proteins, activated or not, on cells; and the effects of the product of the pathway, bradykinin, on cells.

Recent data have described the assembly of the contact system on the endothelial cell surface (Fig. 36-11) which may, therefore, be a locus of bradykinin formation in health and disease. HMWK can bind directly to vascular endothelial cells by its heavy- and light-chain moieties (211–213). More recently, three receptors for HMWK have been described: cytokeratin 1 (214), gC1qR (215,216), and the urokinase plasminogen-activated receptor (217). HMWK binds to each of these in a zinc-dependent reaction. However, experiments using HMWK affinity chromatography of solubilized cell membranes isolated only cytokeratin 1 and gC1qR, and antibodies to cytokeratin 1 and to gC1qR eliminated virtually all of this independent binding of HMWK to the cell surface, suggesting that urokinase plasminogen-activated receptor is of lesser importance as a receptor (218). However, it readily binds HMWK that has been cleaved to bradykinin. The light chain of HMWK binds preferentially to gC1qR, although it appears capable of binding to cytokeratin 1 as well, whereas the heavy chain of HMWK binds exclusively to cytokeratin 1.

Factor XII also binds to the cell surface in a zinc dependent fashion, and HMWK and factor XII can compete with each

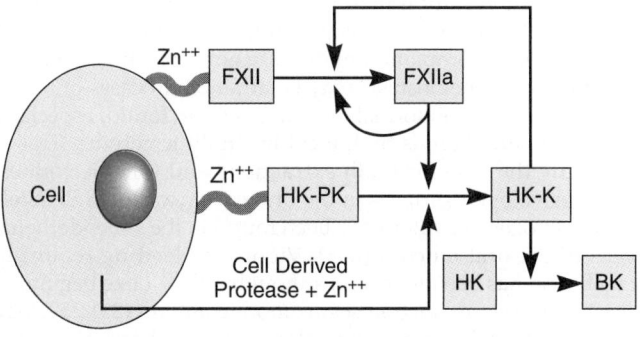

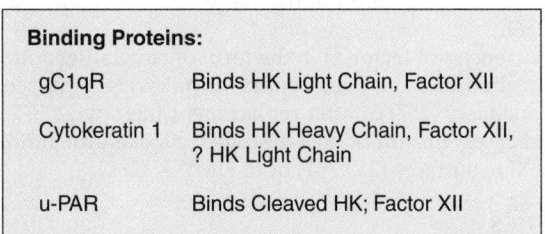

Binding Proteins:

gC1qR   Binds HK Light Chain, Factor XII

Cytokeratin 1   Binds HK Heavy Chain, Factor XII,
                 ? HK Light Chain

u-PAR   Binds Cleaved HK; Factor XII

Figure 36-11. Diagrammatic representation of the binding of factor XII, high-molecular-weight kininogen (HK), and prekallikrein (PK) to endothelial cells indicating the contributions of gC1qR, cytokeratin 1, and urokinase plasminogen-activated receptor (u-PAR). Also shown are two possible initiation mechanisms; one by autoactivation of factor XII and the second, activation of the HK-PK complex by a cell-derived protease. BK, bradykinin.

other for binding to the cell surface via gC1qR (219); and it appears to bind to cytokeratin 1 and u-PAR as well.

There is no separate prekallikrein receptor, but it is bound to the cell surface by virtue of its ability to bind to the light chain of HMWK (220). Endothelial cell-bound HMWK was also able to bind factor XI and promoted the activation of factor IX, suggesting that the interaction of HMWK with endothelial cells may participate in the initiation of blood coagulation at sites of vascular injury (221).

The entire cascade can be activated at the surface of the cell with gC1qR as an initiator capable of catalyzing factor XII autoactivation; C1 INH can inhibit all of these reactions at the cell surface. It has also been shown that endothelial cells possess an enzyme that can bypass factor XII and activate the HMWK-PK complex (220,222). However, the kinetics of this factor XII–independent reaction in plasma is much slower than the factor XII dependent activation (Joseph K and Kaplan A; unpublished observations, 2002) so that if a cell-derived enzyme were to activate some prekallikrein in the presence of factor XII, the subsequent reciprocal activations of factor XII and prekallikrein by kallikrein and factor XIIa, respectively, would become kinetically dominant. Thus, the factor XII–dependent and –independent processes become virtually identical.

The components of the contact activation system also interact with platelets. Apparently, plasma factor XI and factor XIa have separate platelet receptors (71). Platelets also have an intrinsic protein with factor XI activity which cross-reacts with plasma factor XI immunologically but differs from it in molecular weight and isoelectric point. It has been demonstrated that this protein is produced from the factor XI gene by alternative splicing so as to lack exon 5 (223). This activity is present in patients who are deficient in plasma factor XI (224,225). Platelet-associated factor XI can be activated by factor XII–dependent and factor XII–independent mechanisms (73). The membrane of activated platelets may also provide a surface on which factor

XII can be activated in the presence of prekallikrein and HMWK (73) so that bound factor XI is then activated.

HMWK has been shown to be present within the alpha granules of platelets (226) and to become available during platelet activation (227). HMWK exhibits zinc-dependent (228) binding to the platelet surface (226,229) and augments binding of factor XIa (71). The binding of HMWK to platelets involves both the heavy and light chains (230). The cell receptor for HMWK is glycoprotein 1b (231,232). The domain 3 site on the heavy chain, in particular, inhibits thrombin binding to platelets (233), inhibits thrombin-induced platelet aggregation (234), and is the site of interaction with gp1b (231). A domain 4 bradykinin-derived N-terminal pentapeptide interferes with thrombin activation of protease-activated receptor-1 by binding to both the active site of thrombin as well as protease-activated receptor-1 (235,236).

Despite the demonstrated interactions of contact factors with platelets, it is clear that platelets are not requisite for contact activation, as they are for later steps in coagulation. Thus, contact activation proceeds normally in platelet-poor plasma, and the addition of platelets provides little or no augmentation. In fact, there is evidence that platelets may actually inhibit prekallikrein and factor XII activation by secretion of β-thromboglobulin (237,238). Nevertheless, it is possible that platelet activation in peripheral tissues due to injury or localized thrombosis may contribute to contact activation and local kinin formation. In some circumstances, the platelets may also provide a factor XII bypass in contact activation (239).

Kallikrein has been reported to interact with human leukocytes in a variety of ways. It is a chemotactic factor for neutrophils (43) and monocytes (44), and it has been shown to cause neutrophil aggregation (45) and release of elastase (46). In a rabbit model, kallikrein stimulation of chemotaxis appeared to require cleavage of C5 and release of C5a chemotactic factor (47). Therefore, C5 bound to the surface of neutrophils can possibly be cleaved in the aforementioned reactions. Anti-kallikrein serum was inhibitory, whereas anti-C5 serum had no effect; the authors therefore concluded that the effect of kallikrein on human neutrophils is independent of complement. Furthermore, a degraded form of kallikrein (β-kallikrein), in which the heavy chain is partially digested, is enzymatically active on kininogen to form kinin, but possesses a markedly attenuated reactivity with neutrophils (240). Factor XIIa has also been shown to stimulate neutrophils; because factor XIIf did not do this, a requirement for a binding site in the heavy chain was inferred (22). No studies have demonstrated either a cell-surface receptor for these enzymes or required cleavage of surface components. In each instance, the active site of the enzyme is required, and the proenzyme or DFP-treated enzyme is inactive (43,45).

The interaction of HMWK with endothelial cells and the subsequent generation of bradykinin from cell-bound HMWK (241) may also be physiologically significant. Bradykinin stimulates the production of endothelium-derived relaxing factor (chemically related to nitric oxide) in these cells, which has profound effects on the vascular tone (242,243). Bradykinin has also been shown to stimulate the release of prostaglandin I_2 and thromboxane A_2 from cultured endothelial cells (244,245) and has been identified as a powerful stimulant of the release of TPA from endothelial cells (195,246).

DEFICIENCIES OF PROTEINS OF THE CONTACT ACTIVATION SYSTEM

Historically, the proteins of the contact system, like other coagulation proteins, have each been discovered as a consequence of the identification of individuals whose plasma was found to give abnormal clotting times in *in vitro* assays. Deficiencies of each of the proteins of the contact system are well recognized and are characterized by abnormal results in tests of the intrinsic coagulation pathway and in some cases by clinical bleeding.

Deficiency of any of the contact factors may be suspected when a coagulation profile reveals prolongation of the APTT with a normal prothrombin time. It is most important to rule out the possibility of factor VIII or factor IX deficiency, because these deficiencies result in serious defects of hemostasis. Generally, patients with these deficiencies will present with a major bleeding diathesis, and often they or their male relatives (they are X-linked traits) have a history of repeated bleeding. If these factors are specifically assayed and found to be normal, a defect in one of the early components (factor XII, prekallikrein, HMWK, or factor XI) would be likely. The plasma in question can be assayed for each of these by testing its ability to correct the APTT of plasmas that are selectively deficient in each component; such plasmas are commercially available. If a functional defect of any of the components is seen, one can then determine whether the protein is absent or whether a defective protein has been synthesized. This is done by quantitative immunoassays using monospecific antisera.

The degree of prolongation of the clotting time varies with the particular protein deficiency. There is no correlation, however, between the severity of any of the defects of *in vitro* coagulation and clinical sequelae. Of the contact factor deficiencies, only factor XI deficiency has been associated with a bleeding diathesis. In factor XI deficiency, kinin formation is normal; conversely, plasmas deficient in factor XII, prekallikrein, or HMWK do not generate any bradykinin on the addition of a surface. Thus, we will consider factor XI deficiency separately from that of the latter proteins that comprise the kinin-forming pathways.

Deficiency of Factor XI

CLINICAL MANIFESTATIONS

Of all the contact system proteins, factor XI is the only one for which a deficiency is associated with a hemophiliac syndrome (247,248). It is characterized in this case by the variability in its clinical picture. Approximately one-half of identified factor XI–deficient patients have experienced postoperative or post-trauma bleeding. Other patients are frequently identified by abnormal APTTs with no history of bleeding. When APTTs were not a standard preoperative procedure, the deficiency was not always recognized until excessive postoperative hemorrhage occurred (249). Even with routine APTT screens, there is no close correlation between the severity of bleeding, if any, and the measured level of factor XI activity or factor XI antigen. Even the distinction of heterozygotes (with 15% to 62% factor XI activity) from homozygotes (with <15% activity) does not divide bleeders from nonbleeders, because equal frequencies of bleeding are found in each group (250).

Although no cases of bleeding into joints have been reported, there have been reports of mild spontaneous bleeding in the form of nosebleeds, hematuria, menorrhagia, and one case of retinal hemorrhage (251). Little or no spontaneous bruising and little abnormal bruising even in response to severe trauma have been reported (252). Some women, however, have reported episodes of spontaneous bruising, sometimes associated with heavy menstrual bleeding for up to 2 weeks (253).

A characteristic of factor XI deficiency is that the same patient may have great variability in the tendency to bleed in response to different surgical procedures at different times (253,254). The reason for this variability is not known; suggestions (251) of fluctuation with time of the residual plasma levels of factor XI have not been supported by long-term studies, and

the apparent variation may in fact be a response to varying degrees of hemostatic challenge. To the extent that major surgery is often accompanied by transfusions of whole blood or plasma, normal hemostasis may be attained. In cases of minor surgery, however, abnormal bleeding is often found, especially in areas where there is high local fibrinolytic activity. This is especially the case for tooth extractions and tonsillectomies, which leave open surfaces in the oral cavity where high levels of plasminogen activator have been found in the subendothelial areas of the oral mucosa (255). Vigorous bleeding requiring transfusion has been reported, although a slow ooze beginning 3 to 4 days after extraction seems more common (251,252,254). Surgical procedures of the urologic system have also been found to cause problems for factor XI–deficient patients (249,256).

Deficiencies of factor XI in the form of circulating anticoagulant antibodies have been reported that were acquired both spontaneously (257) or after replacement therapy (258–260). In several cases, the antibodies described blocked the binding of factor XI to surfaces (259,261) or to HMWK (260).

GENETICS

Factor XI deficiency was originally described as a rare autosomal-dominant trait (248) with a frequency of 1 in 100,000. Subsequent work indicated that factor XI deficiency is transmitted by an incompletely recessive autosomal gene so that heterozygotes may have factor XI levels of 20% to 60% of normal (251,252).

Factor XI deficiency is largely found in the Ashkenazi Jewish population, in which it has a frequency of 0.15% to 0.30% (262); the frequency of heterozygotes is in the range of 5% to 11%. Among the Ashkenazi population, there is no evidence of a regional localization in eastern Europe, but the gene appears to be distributed through the whole Ashkenazi population. Two alleles have been identified, one of which is specific to Ashkenazi Jews and another that can be found at low frequency in non-Ashkenazi Jews and Arabs and may have arisen before the divergence of the populations (263).

Initially, only a handful of cases of factor XI deficiency were described in which Jewish descent was improbable. More recently, two studies (250,264), comprising a total of 105 factor XI–deficient kindreds, found that 82 were Jewish, and the remaining kindreds included members of a variety of ethnic groups. There have been scattered reports of individuals from various ethnic backgrounds with unique mutations (265–267). There appears to be some statistically significant difference between the "Jewish" factor XI deficiency and the non-Jewish syndrome. Thus, a higher proportion of Jewish propositi have factor XI levels below 15% and are classified as homozygotes (264). Within the respective homozygote and heterozygote populations, however, Jewish propositi have higher mean factor XI:C levels (250). The significance, if any, of these observations remains unknown.

One study found that the likelihood of bleeding or not bleeding, although not correlated with factor XI levels, was consistent within families (264). Thus, in 12 families in which the propositus was a nonbleeder, no other factor XI–deficient family member was found to bleed, whereas in 13 families in which the propositus was a bleeder, other family members were also bleeders.

In all studies of multiple kindreds, the level of cross-reacting antigen (cross-reacting material, CRM) was closely correlated with the level of factor XI activity, although a very few individuals have been found to be CRM+. In this respect, factor XI deficiency differs from deficiencies of other clotting factors, where CRM+ variants are commonly found.

THERAPY

The absence of significant spontaneous bleeding or bruising in factor XI deficiency means that maintenance therapy is not usually required. Surgical patients with factor XI deficiency, however, need careful management to reduce the risk of postoperative hemorrhage. Generally, the circulating level of factor XI needs to be raised to 20% to 30% of normal (249,268) using fresh whole blood or plasma or fresh frozen plasma [banked whole blood loses 80% of its factor XI content during the first week of storage (269)]. Cryoprecipitate supernatant, if available, may also be used, because it retains most of the factor XI activity (270). The half-life of infused factor XI is 60 to 80 hours (268), and hemostasis is normally achieved with 10 to 20 mL plasma/kg/day (249,254). The progress of the treatment can be monitored with APTT or specific factor XI assays.

Deficiencies of Proteins Involved in Kinin Formation

FACTOR XII

Several hundred cases of factor XII deficiency (Hageman trait) have been identified. The APTT is markedly prolonged in factor XII deficiency. In a manual assay using kaolin, clotting times of 200 to 300 seconds are found compared with less than 50 seconds for controls. If the second stage is performed at room temperature, a clot may not form for 20 minutes. Automated commercial APTT systems give clotting times of approximately 100 seconds.

In spite of the profound defect of *in vitro* functioning of the intrinsic pathway, no bleeding disorder is seen, nor is there protection against thrombotic disease. In fact, Mr. Hageman, the propositus case of factor XII deficiency, died of a pulmonary embolus (271), and several other cases have suffered myocardial infarction (272–274).

The gene for factor XII has been localized to chromosome 5 (28,29). Most cases have no antigenic material in the circulation, but CRM+ persons have been described. In one study of factor XII deficiency, there was frequent occurrence of a mutation in the second intron of the gene such that homozygotes were markedly deficient, and heterozygotes had a partial deficiency (275). This was seen in four of five unrelated Italian subjects with factor XII deficiency from different regions of the country. No deletions were identified. Other mutations have been identified in the promoter region (276) or at a splice site (277) to yield a truncated fragment. Another mutation, designated factor XII Tenri, appears to be largely degraded intracellularly (278).

In general, patients appear to have some predisposition to thrombosis (279–283), suggesting that the inhibition of intrinsic fibrinolysis in factor XII deficiency may have clinical significance. Factor XII deficiency has also been found in association with factor V Leiden and von Willebrand's disease (284–286).

PREKALLIKREIN

Prekallikrein deficiency (135) (Fletcher trait) is known to occur in approximately 30 families. The APTT of prekallikrein-deficient plasma is unique in that the final clotting time after recalcification shortens as the length of the activation step is prolonged (4,135–137). This autocorrection implies that the role of kallikrein in the activation of the intrinsic clotting pathway is to accelerate the activation of factor XII. In the former's absence, factor XII becomes activated much more slowly, but eventually enough factor XIIa accumulates to activate factor XI at a normal rate. The slow activation of factor XII in prekallikrein-deficient plasma may be achieved through the autoactivation reaction and possibly a positive feedback by factor XIa. Prekallikrein-deficient plasma does not generate bradykinin on activation (136).

Like Hageman trait, Fletcher trait is not characterized by any observable hemostatic abnormalities (287), and cases of prekallikrein deficiency with myocardial infarction (288) and multiple episodes of cerebral thrombosis (289) have been reported.

Nonfunctional antigenic species of prekallikrein have been found in several cases of Fletcher trait (290). In one family described (291), three children had 35% antigen and 80% function; others had twice as much antigenic content and no function. A nonfunctional variant protein that had no clotting activity was isolated; it was cleaved by activated factor XII at 0% to 5% of the normal rate, but the product was functionless. The 80-kd protein was immunologically indistinguishable from normal prekallikrein, and it complexed normally with HMWK. Isoelectric focusing suggested a unit charge difference, thus a single amino acid substitution is implied.

HIGH-MOLECULAR-WEIGHT KININOGEN

HMWK deficiency was discovered almost simultaneously in three different patients—Fitzgerald (292), Williams (3), and Flaujeac (139)—and has been named after all three. Other cases have since been reported, although the total number known remains small, probably fewer than 20. The APTT is markedly prolonged but not so much as in factor XII deficiency; manual clotting times with kaolin are in the range of 100 to 200 seconds, and automated instruments can give times less than 100 seconds (compared to <40 seconds for controls). As with factor XII or prekallikrein deficiency, deficiencies of HMWK do not cause apparent defects in normal hemostasis.

HMWK deficiency can occur as a complete absence of HMW and LMWK (Williams) or lack only the HMW species (Fitzgerald). Because the mRNA for the two proteins are transcribed from the same gene (Fig. 36-7), these phenotypic variants might represent defects in either the heavy chain sequence or the sequence coding for the light chain of HMWK, respectively. Molecular characterization of total kininogen deficiency in Japanese patients has been characterized, and they have heavy-chain abnormalities leading to neither high nor LMWK synthesis (293).

Relation of Contact Factor Deficiencies to Hemostasis

The contrast between the role of contact activation in *in vitro* clotting assays and its apparent irrelevance *in vivo* has long been a striking enigma. The longest clotting times are found in factor XII deficiency, followed by deficiency of HMWK, whereas the clotting times of factor XI–deficient plasmas are much shorter. In apparent contradiction to these *in vitro* results, the clinical data are that deficiency of factor XI causes a hemostatic abnormality, whereas those of the other proteins of the contact system do not. A further complication is that the hemophilia associated with factor XI deficiency is both mild and variable, in marked contrast to the deficiencies of factors VIII and IX, and no apparent correlation exists between the measured factor XI clotting activity and the degree of clinical hemophilia.

These paradoxical results have long fueled speculation that an alternative mechanism or pathway must exist for the activation of factor XI which does not require the activation of factor XII.

Two reports that described the activation of purified factor XI by thrombin or by autoactivation (59,60) offered a solution to the enigma posed by the requirement for factor XI but not factor XII for normal hemostasis. Although the activation of a substantial fraction of factor XIa in plasma is contingent on the presence of factor XII and a surface (294), studies with very sensitive assays showed that small amounts of factor XIa are formed and can activate factor IX (295).

Since those reports, a consensus has developed around a new model of clotting *in vivo* which does not involve the participation of the contact pathway (296,297). Factor XI is activated by the small amounts of thrombin formed in the initial phase of clot formation. The factor XIa so formed then initiates, via factor IX and X, the generation of the large amounts of thrombin that are formed after initial clot formation (298). The high concentrations of thrombin formed at the surface of the clot are able to activate thrombin-activatable fibrinolysis inhibitor and thus protect the clot from lysis. This mechanism neatly accounts for the predilection of factor XI–deficient patients to bleed, especially from sites of high local fibrinolytic activity. The function of factor XI as an antifibrinolytic factor *in vivo* has been demonstrated in an experimental thrombosis model in rabbits in which antibodies to factor XI caused increased thrombolysis (299).

Clearly, defects in *in vitro* clotting assays do not necessarily imply clinical bleeding, and the interaction of soluble proteins with cell surfaces, platelets, or fibrin clots allow for many potential pathways of activation and inhibition. Currently, there is general agreement that factor XII and prekallikrein are not required for coagulation *in vivo*, although the participation of the contact activation pathway in fibrinolysis seems important *in vivo* (300) and may be responsible for the higher incidence of thromboembolism in factor XII deficiency (301). It remains to be seen if there is a reduced incidence of thromboembolism among factor XI–deficient patients, which the current model of coagulation would appear to predict.

ASSESSMENT OF CONTACT ACTIVATION IN HUMAN DISEASE

As described in the preceding section, the factor XII–dependent pathways do not appear to contribute to thrombosis. Thus, although activation of factor XII leads to *in vitro* clot formation, in most thrombotic disorders, activation of the extrinsic (tissue factor) pathway initiates clotting. Certainly, there is no thrombosis associated with HAE, a disorder in which contact activation is prominent. Similarly, patients deficient in factor XII, prekallikrein, and HMWK have no obvious bleeding diathesis, and the bleeding disorder in factor XI–deficient patients is highly variable and often mild (see previous section). Most evidence suggests that the importance of the cascade relates to the pathogenesis of inflammatory reactions, the local control of blood flow (in which bradykinin functions as a hormone), and perhaps control of blood pressure.

HAE has received considerable attention because C1 INH is absent, and there is simultaneous activation of the factor XII–dependent pathways and the classic complement pathways. Aside from HAE, there is a relatively large literature describing activation of the factor XII–dependent pathways in plasma or serum in a wide variety of inflammatory disorders, and in some disorders, activation is coincident with the patients' symptoms. There are no data, however, that prove that the consequences of such activation lead to disease manifestations or conversely, that inhibition of the pathway will ameliorate symptoms. These should be viewed as promising associations and are important areas for future investigation. The reader is referred to Table 36-4 for a list of these; some of them will be briefly described below.

Assay Methods

To assess the factor XII–dependent pathways in human disease, ideally one should measure the concentrations of each active enzyme, determine the extent of HMWK cleavage, and assay bradykinin. These measurements are difficult because the

TABLE 36-4. Disorders Associated with Contact Activation

Disease	Reference Number
Adult respiratory distress syndrome	357
Carcinoid syndrome	358,359
Cirrhosis	See text
Disseminated intravascular coagulation	See text
Hereditary angioedema	See text
Nephrotic syndrome	See text
Postgastrectomy dumping syndrome	360
Polycythemia vera	361
Rocky Mountain spotted fever	362
Sepsis (septic shock)	See text
Transfusion reactions	See text
Typhoid fever	363
Type II hyperlipidemia	364

enzymes are rapidly inactivated, and bradykinin is rapidly degraded. Thus, often only the level of residual proenzyme can be determined. One can quantitate factor XII, prekallikrein, or HMWK in plasma by coagulant assay (113), immunologic determination of antigen levels (302–304), or by *in vitro* activation and assay of evolved enzymatic activity (116,305–308). Shifts in electrophoretic mobility indicate complex formation between enzymes and their inhibitors and provide qualitative evidence that activation has occurred. Thus far, monoclonal antibodies that react solely with the active site of enzymes have not been developed, although monoclonal antibodies have been described (309,310) that react with neoantigens in C1 INH that has formed complexes with plasma enzymes.

The previously described assays are useful if sufficient activation has occurred to cause significant depletion of substrate. But if only a small amount of each factor is converted, it may be missed. Assays have recently been developed for enzyme-inhibitor complexes based on the assay for plasmin–α_2-antiplasmin complexes by Harpel (311). These include double-antibody enzyme-linked immunosorbent assay methods for factor XIIa–C1 INH (312), kallikrein–C1 INH (313), and kallikrein–α_2-macroglobulin complexes (156), which can detect as little as 1% activation of any of the components. A radioimmunoassay based on a monoclonal antibody to a neodeterminant in complexed or cleaved C1 INH has been reported to detect 0.05% activation of factor XII or prekallikrein (314). Bradykinin (315) and des-Arg^9 bradykinin (316) can also be determined by radioimmunoassay.

Finally, assays using immunoblotting (Western blotting) can detect cleaved HMWK in plasma (88), and this can be used to develop a quantitative assay (83). These latter assays have just begun to be applied to disease states; most of the literature refers to results obtained with earlier methods describing depletion of contact factors, particularly prekallikrein, associated with particular conditions.

Hereditary Angioedema

HAE is the disease state associated with a deficiency of C1 INH. Patients present with episodic swelling occurring virtually anywhere in the body, attacks of severe abdominal pain due to edema of the bowel wall, and laryngeal edema. These symptoms are now known to be mediated by bradykinin and not by activation of the complement pathway (317–319). This is confirmed by the discovery of one family in which a form of C1 INH circulates that is inactive in the complement cascade but inhibits factor XIIa and kallikrein normally; none of the members of this family have symptoms of angioedema (320).

During attacks of angioedema, there is depletion of prekallikrein and HMWK (321), and blisters induced in the skin of patients are found to have elevated plasma kallikrein levels (322). The formation of bradykinin (323) and cleaved HMWK (324) have been detected. The complement activation appears due to autoactivation of C1 (specifically C1r) in the absence of C1 INH (325,326), but this may be augmented by factor XIIf (20,208), particularly during acute attacks of swelling.

Sepsis and Disseminated Intravascular Coagulation

Severe infections with gram-negative organisms leading to septic shock carry a poor prognosis and a high mortality rate. The pooling of fluid into body cavities, the intravascular volume depletion, and the hypotension seen may be caused by release of bradykinin. Activation of factor XII can be induced by the lipid A component of endotoxin (124,125,327), and contact activation proteins are depleted in endotoxic shock (328–331). In patients hospitalized because of trauma, the onset of sepsis has been shown to be associated with kininogen depletion. Determination of serial kininogen levels had prognostic value (329) because a drop in the kininogen level to near zero usually indicated a lethal outcome, as did lower prekallikrein levels (332). Enzyme–C1 INH complexes may be difficult to detect in sepsis, however, even when factor XII and prekallikrein levels are reduced, because of rapid clearance (314). Using a sensitive assay for factor XI activation in a model of low-grade endotoxemia, factor XII–independent activation of factor XI was seen (333).

In patients with disseminated intravascular coagulation (DIC) due to endothelial injury or endotoxemia (including gram-negative sepsis, gram-positive sepsis, or viremia), decreased levels of plasma factor XII and prekallikrein and kallikrein inhibitory activity are seen (334,335). These changes were not observed in DIC associated with leukemia, carcinoma, or abortion. The data suggest activation of the factor XII–dependent pathways. A case has also been reported of DIC in preeclampsia in which activation of the contact system was seen (336).

In a baboon model of sepsis, studies with a monoclonal antibody to factor XII showed that the contact system contributed significantly to the development of irreversible hypotension but not to DIC (337,338).

Other Disorders with Associated Contact Activation

Contact activation may occur during allergic diseases such as allergic rhinitis. Nasal washings from patients who have been challenged with antigen contain lysyl bradykinin, bradykinin, kininogen, and kallikreins derived from mast cells and from plasma (339–342). The latter may represent contact activation on a surface altered by the initial inflammation or possibly induced by negatively charged macromolecules in mucosal secretions or by mast cell heparin (121,122,343). Although we routinely use dextran sulfates as model compounds on which factor XII activation can occur, other sulfated mucopolysaccharides may serve similar functions in vivo (344).

The synovial fluid of patients with rheumatoid arthritis has been shown to contain plasma kallikrein, which has been shown to activate procollagenase to collagenase (345). Uric acid and pyrophosphate crystals can act as surfaces for contact activation and may contribute to the inflammation of gout and pseudogout (346,347). A role for the contact activation system in inflammatory arthritis is therefore possible and may involve other functions of the enzymes formed in addition to any effects of kinins. It should be noted, however, that at least one case of gout (274) and one of rheumatoid arthritis (348) associated with factor XII deficiency have been reported.

In some patients with nephrotic syndrome, a diminution of factor XII has been reported (349) that could not be explained simply by a loss of proteins in the urine (350). Immunoreactive but nonfunctional factor XII was found in the plasma (351,352), which suggested that activation of factor XII in the nephrotic kidney might be occurring. There is disagreement over whether prekallikrein is also diminished in nephrotic syndrome.

Cirrhosis, as might be anticipated, is associated with diminished levels of plasma prekallikrein, HMWK, and to a lesser degree, factor XII, which seems to be caused by a diminished rate of protein synthesis (305,353,354). A similar depression of prekallikrein level apparently related to liver dysfunction has been noted in dengue fever (355).

In experimental models of inflammatory arthritis and enterocolitis, activation of the kinin system occurs, and the disease is modulated by a kallikrein inhibitor (356).

Other associations of contact activation with disease states are listed in Table 36-3. Finally, the severe facial angioedema seen due to ACE inhibitors is due to bradykinin (365).

SUMMARY AND CONCLUSIONS

The contact system is unusual among proteolytic pathways in its self-contained cyclic nature. Rather than being activated by an extrinsic activity, it is able to "switch itself on," converting two zymogens to proteases—factor XIIa and kallikrein. The process is initiated by surface activation and characterized by extreme positive feedback. Once formed, the proteases can participate in the initiation of a number of pathways, especially blood coagulation, fibrinolysis, and the formation of bradykinin. It is a paradox that despite these multiple activities, deficiencies of contact activation do not have any obvious clinical consequences. This may reflect the observed parallelism in the pathways that maintain homeostasis. The symptoms of HAE, however, a disease associated with deficiency of C1 INH, are clearly caused by the production of bradykinin via the contact pathway. A number of other disease states are associated with activation of the contact system, including endotoxic shock and allergic and inflammatory reactions, although there is no unequivocal attribution of symptoms to the products of contact activation. Thus, the role of the contact system in normal homeostasis remains elusive. Nevertheless, if mutations leading to deficiencies of contact system proteins were truly neutral, one would expect them to be common, whereas to date, they have been found relatively infrequently. Taken together, these observations suggest that the role of the contact system may be more critical in host defense mechanisms and the pathogenesis of inflammation than in hemostasis. These questions will be more amenable to study as clinically useful antagonists to bradykinin and to the contact system enzymes become available.

REFERENCES

1. Revak SD, et al. Structural changes accompanying enzymatic activation of human Hageman factor. *J Clin Invest* 1974;54:619.
2. Silverberg M, Kaplan AP. Enzymatic activities of activated and zymogen forms of human Hageman factor (factor XII). *Blood* 1982;60:64.
3. Colman RW, et al. Williams trait: human kininogen deficiency with diminished levels of plasminogen proactivator and prekallikrein associated with abnormalities of the Hageman factor–dependent pathways. *J Clin Invest* 1975;56:1650.
4. Meier HL, et al. Activation and function of human Hageman factor. The role of high molecular kininogen and prekallikrein. *J Clin Invest* 1977;60:18.
5. Revak SD, Cochrane CG, Griffin JH. The binding and cleavage characteristics of human Hageman factor during contact activation: a comparison of normal plasma with plasma deficient in factor XI, prekallikrein or high molecular weight kininogen. *J Clin Invest* 1977;58:1167.

6. Cochrane CG, Revak SD, Wuepper KD. Activation of Hageman factor in solid and fluid phases. *J Exp Med* 1973;138:1564.
7. Griffin JH. Role of surface in surface-dependent activation of Hageman factor (blood coagulation factor XII). *Proc Natl Acad Sci U S A* 1978;75:1998.
8. Tankersley DL, Finlayson JS. Kinetics of activation and autoactivation of human factor XII. *Biochemistry* 1984;23:273.
9. Silverberg M, et al. Autoactivation of human Hageman factor. *J Biol Chem* 1980;255:7281.
10. Fujikawa K, McMullen BA. Amino acid sequence of human b-factor XIIa. *J Biol Chem* 1983;258(18):10924.
11. Revak SD, Cochrane CG. The relationship of structure and function in human Hageman factor. *J Clin Invest* 1977;57:852.
12. Dunn JT, Silverberg M, Kaplan AP. The cleavage and formation of activated Hageman factor by autodigestion and by kallikrein. *J Biol Chem* 1982;275:1779.
13. Dunn JT, Kaplan AP. Formation and structure of human Hageman factor fragments. *J Clin Invest* 1982;70:627.
14. Silverberg M, Kaplan AP. Human Hageman factor and its fragments. *Methods Enzymol* 1988;163:68.
15. Kaplan AP, Austen KF. A pre-albumin activator of prekallikrein. *J Immunol* 1970;105(4):802.
16. Mandle RJJ, Kaplan AP. Hageman factor substrates. II. Human plasma prekallikrein. Mechanism of activation by Hageman factor and participation in Hageman factor-dependent fibrinolysis. *J Biol Chem* 1977;252:6097.
17. Tankersley DL, Fournel MA, Schroeder DD. Kinetics of activation of prekallikrein by prekallikrein activator. *Biochemistry* 1980;19(14):3121.
18. Revak SD, et al. Surface and fluid phase activities of two forms of activated Hageman factor produced during contact activation of plasma. *J Exp Med* 1978;147:719.
19. Kaplan AP, Austen KF. A prealbumin activator of prekallikrein II. Derivation of activators of prekallikrein from active Hageman factor by digestion with plasmin. *J Exp Med* 1971;133(4):696.
20. Ghebrehiwet B, et al. Mechanism of activation of the classical pathway of complement by Hageman factor fragment. *J Clin Invest* 1983;71:1450.
21. Radcliffe R, et al. Activation of factor VII by Hageman factor fragments. *Blood* 1977;59:611.
22. Wachtfogel YT, et al. Purified plasma factor XIIa aggregates human neutrophils and causes degranulation. *Blood* 1986;67(6):1731.
23. Cool DE, et al. Characterization of human blood coagulation factor XII cDNA. *J Biol Chem* 1985;25:13666.
24. Que BG, Davie EW. Characterization of a cDNA coding for human factor XII (Hageman factor). *Biochemistry* 1986;8:1525.
25. McMullen BA, Fujikawa K. Amino acid sequence of the heavy chain of human a-factor XIIa (activated Hageman factor). *J Biol Chem* 1985;260(9):5328.
26. Pixley RA, et al. A monoclonal antibody recognizing an icosapeptide sequence in the heavy chain of human factor XII inhibits surface-catalyzed activation. *J Biol Chem* 1987;262(21):10140.
27. Clarke BJ, et al. Mapping of a putative surface-binding site of human coagulation factor XII. *J Biol Chem* 1989;264(19):11497.
28. Citarella F, et al. Assignment of human coagulation factor XII (fXII) to chromosome 5 by cDNA hybridization to DNA from somatic cell hybrids. *Hum Genet* 1988;80:397.
29. Royle NJ, et al. Structural gene encoding human factor XII is located at 5q33-qter. *Somat Cell Mol Genet* 1988;14:217.
30. Cool DE, MacGillivray RT. Characterization of the human blood coagulation factor XII gene. Intron/exon gene organization and analysis of the 5'-flanking region. *J Biol Chem* 1987;262:13662.
31. Castellino FJ, Beals JM. The genetic relationships between the kringle domains of human plasminogen, prothrombin, tissue plasminogen activator, urokinase, and coagulation factor XII. *J Mol Evol* 1987;26:358.
32. Bouma BN, et al. Human plasma prekallikrein. Studies of its activation by activated factor XII and of its inactivation by diisopropyl phosphofluoridate. *Biochemistry* 1980;19:1151.
33. Mandle RJ, Colman RW, Kaplan AP. Identification of prekallikrein and high molecular weight kininogen as a complex in plasma. *Proc Natl Acad Sci U S A* 1976;73:4179.
34. Bock PE, et al. Protein-protein interactions in contact activation of blood coagulation. Binding of high molecular weight kininogen and the 5-(iodoacetamido) fluorescein-labeled kininogen light chain to prekallikrein, kallikrein, and the separated kallikrein heavy and light chains. *J Biol Chem* 1985;260:12434.
35. Silverberg M, Nicoll JE, Kaplan AP. The mechanism by which the light chain of cleaved HMW-kininogen augments the activation of prekallikrein, factor XI, and Hageman factor. *Thromb Res* 1980;70:173.
36. Cochrane CG, Revak SD. Dissemination of contact activation in plasma by plasma kallikrein. *J Exp Med* 1980;152:608.
37. Bouma BN, Easton E, van Iwaarden F. *Thromb Haemost* 1985;54:228(abstr).
38. Colman RW. Activation of plasminogen by plasma kallikrein. *Biochem Biophys Res Commun* 1969;351:273.
39. Mandle RJJ, Kaplan AP. Hageman factor dependent fibrinolysis. Generation of fibrinolytic activity by the interaction of human activated factor XI and plasminogen. *Blood* 1979;54:850.
40. Miles LA, Rothschild Z, Griffin JH. Dextran sulfate stimulated fibrinolytic activity in whole human plasma. Dependence on the contact activation system and a urokinase-related antigen. *Thromb Haemost* 1981;46:211.
41. Ichinose A, Fujikawa K, Suyama T. The activation of pro-urokinase by plasma kallikrein and its inactivation by thrombin. *J Biol Chem* 1986;261:3486.
42. Hauert J, et al. Plasminogen activators in dextran sulfate-activated euglobulin fractions: a molecular analysis of factor XII- and prekallikrein-dependent fibrinolysis. *Blood* 1989;73(4):994.
43. Kaplan AP, Kay AB, Austen KF. A prealbumin activator of prekallikrein III. Appearance of chemotactic activity for human neutrophils by the conversion of human prekallikrein to kallikrein. *J Exp Med* 1972;135:81.
44. Gallin JI, Kaplan AP. Mononuclear cell chemotactic activity of kallikrein and plasminogen activator and its inhibition by C1 INH and α_2 macroglobulin. *J Immunol* 1974;113:1928.
45. Schapira M, et al. Purified human plasma kallikrein aggregates human blood neutrophils. *J Clin Invest* 1982;69:1199.
46. Wachtfogel YT, et al. Human plasma kallikrein releases neutrophil elastase activity during blood coagulation. *J Clin Invest* 1983;22:1672.
47. Wiggins RC, Giglas PC, Henson PM. Chemotactic activator generated from the fifth component of complement by plasma kallikrein of the rabbit. *J Exp Med* 1981;153:1391.
48. Cooper NR, Miles LA, Griffin JH. Effects of plasma kallikrein and plasmin on the first complement component. *J Immunol* 1980;124:1517.
49. DiScipio RG. The activation of the alternative pathway C3 convertase by human plasma kallikrein. *Immunol* 1982;45:587.
50. Derkx FHM, et al. An intrinsic factor XII-prekallikrein-dependent pathway activates the human plasma renin-angiotensin system. *Nature* 1979;280:315.
51. Sealey JE, et al. Initiation of plasma prorenin activation by Hageman factor-dependent conversion of plasma prekallikrein to kallikrein. *Proc Natl Acad Sci U S A* 1979;76:5914.
52. Harpel PC. Circulatory inhibitors of human plasma kallikrein. In: Pisano JJ, Austen KF, eds. *Chemistry and biology of the Kallikrein-Kinin system in health and disease.* Washington: US Government Printing Office, 1974:169.
53. Schapira M, Scott CF, Colman RW. Contribution of plasma protease inhibitors to the inactivation of kallikrein in plasma. *J Clin Invest* 1982;69:462.
54. van der Graaf F, Koedam JA, Bouma BN. Inactivation of kallikrein in human plasma. *J Clin Invest* 1983;71:149.
55. Chung DW, et al. Human plasma prekallikrein, a zymogen to a serine protease that contains four tandem repeats. *Biochemistry* 1986;25(9):2410.
56. Yu H, et al. Genomic structure of the human plasma prekallikrein gene, identification of allelic variants, and analysis in end-stage renal disease. *Genomics* 2000;69(2):225.
57. Bouma BN, Griffin JH. Human blood coagulation factor XI: purification, properties, and mechanism of activation by factor XII. *J Biol Chem* 1977;252:6432.
58. Kurachi K, Davie EW. Activation of human factor XI (plasma thromboplastin antecedent) by factor XII (activated Hageman factor). *Biochemistry* 1977;16:5831.
59. Gailani D, Broze GJ. Factor XI activation in a revised model of blood coagulation. *Science* 1991;253(5022):909.
60. Naito K, Fujikawa K. Activation of human blood coagulation factor XI independent of factor XII. Factor XI is activated by thrombin and factor XIa in the presence of negatively charged surfaces. *J Biol Chem* 1991;266(12):7353.
61. Thompson RE, Mandle RJ, Kaplan AP. Association of factor XI and high molecular weight kininogen in human plasma. *J Clin Invest* 1977;60:1376.
62. Tait J, Fujikawa K. Primary structure requirements for the binding of human high molecular weight kininogen to plasma prekallikrein and factor XI. *J Biol Chem* 1987;262:11651.
63. Warn-Cramer BJ, Bajaj SP. Stoichiometry of binding of high molecular weight kininogen to factor XI/XIa. *Biochem Biophys Res Commun* 1985;133:417.
64. Baglia FA, Sinha D, Walsh PN. Functional domains in the heavy-chain region of factor XI: a high molecular weight kininogen-binding site and a substrate binding site for factor IX. *Blood* 1989;74(1):244.
65. Griffin JH, Cochrane CG. Mechanisms for the involvement of high molecular weight kininogen in surface-dependent reactions of Hageman factor. *Proc Natl Acad Sci U S A* 1976;73:2554.
66. Wiggins RC, et al. Role of high molecular weight kininogen in surface binding and activation of coagulation factor XI and prekallikrein. *Proc Natl Acad Sci U S A* 1977;77:4636.
67. Sinha D, et al. Functional characterization of human blood coagulation factor XIa using hybridoma antibodies. *J Biol Chem* 1985;260(19):10714.
68. Sinha D, Seaman FS, Walsh PN. Role of calcium ions and the heavy chain of factor XIa in the activation of human coagulation factor IX. *Biochemistry* 1987;26(13):3768.
69. von dem Borne PA, et al. Thrombin-mediated activation of factor XI results in a thrombin-activatable fibrinolysis inhibitor-dependent inhibition of fibrinolysis. *J Clin Invest* 1997;99(10):2323.
70. von dem Borne PA, Meijers JC, Bouma BN. Feedback activation of factor XI by thrombin in plasma results in additional formation of thrombin that protects fibrin clots from fibrinolysis. *Blood* 1995;86(8):3035.
71. Sinha D, et al. Blood coagulation factor XIa binds specifically to a site on activated human platelets distinct from that for factor XI. *J Clin Invest* 1984;73:1550.
72. Greengard JS, et al. Binding of coagulation factor XI to washed human platelets. *Biochemistry* 1986;25(13):3884.
73. Walsh PN, Griffin JH. Contributions of human platelets to the proteolytic activation of blood coagulation factors XII and XI. *Blood* 1981;57(1):106.
74. Fujikawa K, et al. Amino acid sequence of human factor XI, a blood coagulation factor with four tandem repeats that are highly homologous with plasma prekallikrein. *Biochemistry* 1986;25(9):2417.

75. Baglia FA, Walsh PN. A binding site for thrombin in the apple 1 domain of factor XI. *J Biol Chem* 1996;271(7):3652.

76. Meijers JC, et al. Apple four in human blood coagulation factor XI mediates dimer formation. *Biochemistry* 1992;31(19):4680.

77. Asakai R, Davie EW, Chung DW. Organization of the gene for human factor XI. *Biochemistry* 1987;26(23):7221.

78. Colman RW, Muller-Esterl W. Nomenclature of kininogens. *Thromb Haemost* 1988;60:340.

79. Keribiriou DM, Griffin JH. Human high molecular weight kininogen: studies of structure-function relationships and of proteolysis of the molecule occurring during contact activation of plasma. *J Biol Chem* 1979;245:12020.

80. Proud D, Pierce JV, Pisano JJ. Radioimmunoassay of human high molecular weight kininogen in normal and deficient plasma. *J Lab Clin Med* 1980;95:563.

81. Adam A, et al. Human kininogens of low and high molecular mass: quantification by radioimmunoassay and determination of reference values. *Clin Chem* 1985;31:423.

82. Berrettini M, et al. Detection of in vitro and in vivo cleavage of high molecular weight kininogen in human plasma by immunoblotting with monoclonal antibodies. *Blood* 1986;68:455.

83. Reddigari SR, Kaplan AP. Quantification of human high molecular weight kininogen by immunoblotting with a monoclonal anti-light chain antibody. *J Immunol Meth* 1989(119):19.

84. Bock PE, Shore JD. Protein-protein interaction of blood coagulation. Characterization of a fluorescein-labeled human high molecular weight kininogen light chain as a probe. *J Biol Chem* 1983;258:15079.

85. Schiffman S, Mannhalter C, Tynerk D. Human high molecular weight kininogen. Effects of cleavage by kallikrein on protein structure and procoagulant activity. *J Biol Chem* 1980;255:6433.

86. Mori K, Nagasawa S. Studies on human high molecular weight (HMW) kininogen. II. Structural change in HMWK by the action of human plasma kallikrein. *J Biochem* 1981;89:1465.

87. Mori K, Sakamoto W, Nagasawa S. Studies on human high molecular weight (HMW) kininogen III. Cleavage of HMW kininogen by the action human salivary kallikrein. *J Biochem* 1981;90:503.

88. Reddigari SR, Kaplan AP. Cleavage of high molecular weight kininogen by purified kallikreins and upon contact activation of plasma. *Blood* 1988;71:1334.

89. Nakayasa T, Nagasawa S. Studies on human kininogen I. Isolation, characterization, and cleavage by plasma kallikrein of high molecular weight kininogen. *J Biochem* 1979;85:249.

90. Thompson RE, Mandle RJ, Kaplan AP. Characterization of human high molecular weight kininogens: procoagulant activity associated with the light chain of kinin-free high molecular weight kininogen. *J Exp Med* 1978;147:488.

91. Maier M, Austen KF, Spragg J. Characterization of the procoagulant chain derived from high molecular weight kininogen (Fitzgerald factor) by tissue kallikrein. *Blood* 1983;62:457.

92. Thompson RE, Mandle RJ, Kaplan AP. Studies of the binding of prekallikrein and factor XI to high molecular weight kininogen and its light chain. *Proc Natl Acad Sci U S A* 1979;79:4862.

93. Villanueva GB, et al. Conformation of high molecular weight kininogen: effects of kallikrein and factor XIa cleavage. *BBRC* 1989;158:72.

94. Vroman L, et al. Interaction of high molecular weight kininogen, factor XII and fibrinogen in plasma at interfaces. *Blood* 1980;55(156).

95. Schmaier AH, et al. The effects of high molecular weight kininogen on surface-adsorbed fibrinogen. *Thromb Res* 1984;33:51.

96. Brash JL, et al. Mechanism of transient adsorption of fibrinogen from plasma to solid surfaces: role of the contact and fibrinolytic systems. *Blood* 1988;71:932.

97. Bjork I, et al. Binding of heparin to human high molecular weight kininogen. *Biochemistry* 1989;28(3):1213.

98. Kellermann J, et al. Completion of the primary structure of human high molecular weight kininogen. The amino acid sequence of the entire heavy chain and evidence for its evolution by gene triplication. *Eur J Biochem* 1986;154:471.

99. Kitamura N, et al. Structural organization of the human kininogen gene and a model for its evolution. *J Biol Chem* 1985;260:8610.

100. Lottspeich F, et al. The amino acid sequence of the light chain of human high molecular mass kininogen. *Eur J Biochem* 1985;152:307.

101. Takagaki Y, Kitamura N, Nakanishi S. Cloning and sequence analysis of cDNAs for high molecular weight and low molecular weight prekininogens. *J Biol Chem* 1985;260:8601.

102. Gounaris AD, Brown MA, Barrett AJ. Human plasma α₁-cystein proteinase inhibitor. Purification by affinity chromatography, characterization, and isolation of an active fragment. *Biochem J* 1984;221:445.

103. Muller-Esterl W, et al. Human plasma kininogens are identical with α₂-cysteine protease inhibitors. Evidence from immunological, enzymological, and sequence data. *FEBS Lett* 1985;182:310.

104. Higashiyama S, et al. Human high molecular weight kininogen as a thiol protease inhibitor: presence of the entire inhibition capacity in the native form of heavy chain. *Biochemistry* 1986;25:1669.

105. Ishiguro H, et al. Mapping of functional domains of human high molecular weight and high molecular weight kininogens using murine monoclonal antibodies. *Biochemistry* 1987;26:7021.

106. Ikari N, et al. The role of bovine high molecular weight kininogen in contact-mediated activation of bovine factor XII: interaction of HMW kininogen with kaolin and plasma prekallikrein. *J Biochem* 1981;89:1699.

107. Tait J, Fujikawa K. Identification of the binding site plasma prekallikrein in human high molecular weight kininogen. *J Biol Chem* 1986;261:15396.

108. Jacobsen S, Kritz M. Some data on two purified kininogens from human plasma. *Br J Pharmacol* 1967;29:25.

109. Lottspeich F, et al. Human low-molecular-mass kininogen. Amino-acid sequence of the light chain; homology with other protein sequences. *Eur J Biochem* 1984;142:227.

110. Muller-Esterl W, et al. Limited proteolysis of human low-molecular mass kininogen by tissue kallikrein. Isolation and characterization of the heavy and light chains. *Eur J Biochem* 1985;149:15.

111. Johnson DA, et al. Rapid isolation of human kininogens. *Thromb Res* 1987;48:187.

112. Margolis J. Activation of plasma by contact with glass: evidence for a common reaction which releases plasma kinin and initiates coagulation. *J Physiol* 1958;144:1.

113. Proctor RR, Rapaport SJ. The partial thromboplastin time with kaolin: a simple screening test for first stage clotting deficiencies. *Am J Clin Pathol* 1961;35:212.

114. Ratnoff OD, Crum JD. Activation of Hageman factor by solutions of ellagic acid. *J Lab Clin Med* 1964;63(3):359.

115. Bock PE, Srinivasan KR, Shore JD. Activation of intrinsic blood coagulation by ellagic acid: insoluble ellagic acid metal ion complexes are the activating species. *Biochemistry* 1981;20:7258.

116. Kluft C. Determination of prekallikrein in human plasma: optimal conditions for activating prekallikrein. *J Lab Clin Med* 1978;91:83.

117. Fujikawa K, et al. Activation of bovine factor XII (Hageman factor) by plasma kallikrein. *Biochemistry* 1980;19:1322.

118. Tans G, Griffin JH. Properties of sulfatides in factor XII dependent contact activation. *Blood* 1982;59:69.

119. Griep MA, Fujikawa K, Nelsestuen GL. Binding and activation properties of human factor XII, prekallikrein and derived peptides with acidic lipid vesicles. *Biochemistry* 1985;24:4124.

120. Silverberg M, Diehl SV. The autoactivation of factor XII (Hageman factor) induced by low Mr heparin and dextran sulphate. *Biochem J* 1987;248:715.

121. Hojima Y, et al. In vitro activation of the contact (Hageman factor) system of plasma by heparin and chondroitin sulfate E. *Blood* 1984;63(6):1453.

122. Brunnee T, et al. Mast cell derived heparin activates the contact system: a link to kinin generation in allergic reactions. *Clin Exp Allergy* 1997;27(6):653.

123. Silverberg M, Diehl SV. The activation of the contact system of human plasma by polysaccharide sulfates. *Ann N Y Acad Sci* 1987;516:268.

124. Morrison DC, Cochrane CG. Direct evidence for Hageman factor (factor XII) activation by bacterial lipopolysaccharides (endotoxins). *J Exp Med* 1974;140:787.

125. Pettinger MA, Young R. Endotoxin-induced kinin (bradykinin) formation: activation of Hageman factor and plasma kallikrein in human plasma. *Life Sci* 1970;9:313.

126. Roeise O, et al. Dose dependence of endotoxin-induced activation of the plasma contact system: an in vitro study. *Circ Shock* 1988;26:419.

127. Tate KM, et al. Functional role of proteolytic cleavage at arginine-275 of human tissue plasminogen activator as assessed by site-directed mutagenesis. *Biochemistry* 1987;26:338.

128. Petersen LC, et al. The effect of polymerised fibrin on the catalytic activities of one-chain tissue-type plasminogen activator as revealed by an analogue resistant to plasmin cleavage. *Biochim Biophys Acta* 1988;952:245.

129. Nelles L, et al. Characterization of recombinant human single chain urokinase-type plasminogen activator mutants produced by site-specific mutagenesis of lysine 158. *J Biol Chem* 1987;262(12):5682.

130. Lijnen HR, et al. Characterisation of a mutant recombinant human single chain urokinase-type plasminogen activator (scu-PA), obtained by substitution of Arginine 156 and Lysine 158 with Threonine. *Fibrinolysis* 1988;2:85.

131. Ratnoff OD, Saito H. Amidolytic properties of single chain activated Hageman factor. *Proc Natl Acad Sci U S A* 1979;76:1411.

132. Weiss R, Silverberg M, Kaplan AP. The effect of C1 inhibitor upon Hageman factor autoactivation. *Blood* 1986;68:239.

133. Pixley R, Schmaier A, Colman RW. Effect of negatively charged activating compounds on inactivation of factor XIIa by CI inhibitor. *Arch Biochem Biophys* 1987;256:490.

134. Rosing J, Tans G, Griffin JH. Surface-dependent activation of human factor XII by kallikrein, and its light chain. *Eur J Biochem* 1985;151:531.

135. Wuepper KD. Prekallikrein deficiency in man. *J Exp Med* 1973;138:1345.

136. Weiss AS, Gallin JI, Kaplan AP. Fletcher factor deficiency. A diminished rate of Hageman factor activation caused by absence of prekallikrein with abnormalities of coagulation, fibrinolysis, chemotactic activity and kinin generation. *J Clin Invest* 1974;53:622.

137. Saito H, Ratnoff D, Donaldson VH. Defective activation of clotting, fibrinolytic and permeability-enhancing systems in human Fletcher trait. *Circ Res* 1974;34:641.

138. Schiffman S, Lee P. Preparation, characterization and activation of a highly purified factor XI. Evidence that hitherto unrecognised plasma activating factor participates in the interaction of factors XI and XII. *Br J Haematol* 1974;27:101.

139. Wuepper KD, Miller DR, LaCombe MJ. Flaujeac trait. Deficiency of human plasma kininogen. *J Clin Invest* 1975;56:1663.

140. Donaldson VH, Glueck HI, Miller MA. Kininogen deficiency in Fitzgerald trait: role of high molecular weight kininogen in clotting and fibrinolysis. *J Lab Clin Med* 1976;89:327.

141. Espana F, Ratnoff OD. The role of prekallikrein and high molecular weight kininogen in the contact activation of Hageman factor (factor Xll) by sulfatides and other agents. *J Lab Clin Med* 1983;102:487.

142. Shimada T, et al. Interaction of factor XII, high molecular weight kininogen and prekallikrein with sulfatide: analysis by fluorescence polarization. *J Biochem* 1985;97:1637.

143. Reddigari SR, Kaplan AP. Monoclonal antibody to human high molecular weight kininogen recognizes its prekallikrein binding site and inhibits its coagulant activity. *Blood* 1989;74:695.

144. Scott CF, et al. Cleavage of human high molecular weight kininogen by factor XIa in vitro. Effect on structure and function. *J Biol Chem* 1985; 260:10856.

145. Travis J, Salvesen GS. Human plasma proteinase inhibitors. *Annu Rev Biochem* 1983;52:655.

146. Forbes CO, Pensky J, Ratnoff OD. Inhibition of activated Hageman factor and activated plasma thromboplastin antecedent by purified Cl inactivator. *J Lab Clin Med* 1970;76:809.

147. Schreiber AD, Kaplan AP, Austen KF. Inhibition by C 1 INH of Hageman factor fragment activation of coagulation, fibrinolysis, and kinin generation. *J Clin Invest* 1973;52:1402.

148. de Agostini A, et al. Inactivation of factor Xll active fragment in normal plasma. Predominant role of Cl-inhibitor. *J Clin Invest* 1984;73:1542.

149. Pixley R, Schapira AM, Colman RW. The regulation of human factor XII by plasma proteinase inhibitors. *J Biol Chem* 1985;260:1723.

150. Stead N, Kaplan AP, Rosenberg RD. Inhibition of activated factor XII by antithrombin-heparin cofactor. *J Biol Chem* 1976;251:6481.

151. Cameron CL, et al. Studies on contact activation: effects of surfaces and inhibitors. *Med Prog Technol* 1989;15:53.

152. Pixley RA, Colman RW. Effect of heparin in the inactivation of human factor XIIa by antithrombin III. *Blood* 1985;66:198.

153. Barrett AJ, Starkey PM. The interaction of α_2-macroglobulin with proteinases. *Biochem J* 1973;133:709.

154. Gigli I, et al. Interaction of plasma kallikrein with Cl inhibitor. *J Immunol* 1970;104:574.

155. McConnell DJ. Inhibitors of kallikrein in human plasma. *J Clin Invest* 1972; 51:1611.

156. Harpel PC, Lewin MF, Kaplan AP. Distribution of plasma kallikrein between C1 inactivator and α_2-macroglobulin-kallikrein complexes. *J Biol Chem* 1985: 4257.

157. Vennerod AM, et al. Inactivation and binding of human plasma kallikrein by antithrombin III. *Thromb Res* 1976;9:457.

158. Heck LW, Kaplan AP. Substrates of Hageman factor: I. Isolation and characterization of human factor Xl (PTA) and inhibition of the activated enzyme by α_1- antitrypsin. *J Exp Med* 1974;140:1615.

159. Scott CF, et al. Inactivation of factor Xla by plasma protease inhibitors. Predominant role of α_1-protease inhibitor and protective effect of high molecular weight kininogen. *J Clin Invest* 1982;69:844.

160. Wuillemin WA, et al. Inactivation of factor XIa in human plasma assessed by measuring factor XIa-protease inhibitor complexes: major role for C1-inhibitor. *Blood* 1995;85(6):1517.

161. Scott CF, Schapira M, Colman RW. Effect of heparin on the inactivation of human factor XIa by antithrombin III. *Blood* 1982;60:940.

162. Beeler DL, et al. Interaction of factor Xla and antithrombin in the presence and absence of heparin. *Blood* 1985;67(5):1488.

163. Wuillemin WA, et al. Modulation of contact system proteases by glycosaminoglycans. Selective enhancement of the inhibition of factor XIa. *J Biol Chem* 1996;271(22):12913.

164. Zhang Y, et al. The mechanism by which heparin promotes the inhibition of coagulation factor XIa by protease nexin-2. *J Biol Chem* 1997;272(42):26139.

165. Scandura JM, et al. Progress curve analysis of the kinetics with which blood coagulation factor XIa is inhibited by protease nexin-2. *Biochemistry* 1997;36 (2):412.

166. Schapira M, Scott CF, Colman RW. Protection of human plasma kallikrein from inactivation by C1 inhibitor and other protease inhibitors. The role of high molecular weight kininogen. *Biochemistry* 1981;20:2738.

167. Schapira M, et al. High molecular weight kininogen or its light chain protects human plasma kallikrein from inactivation by plasma protease inhibitors. *Biochemistry* 1982;21:567.

168. van der Graaf F, et al. Interaction of human plasma kallikrein and its light chain with α_2-macroglobulin. *Biochemistry* 1984;23(8):1760.

169. Silverberg M, Longo J, Kaplan AP. Study of the effect of high molecular weight kininogen upon the fluid phase inactivation of kallikrein by C1-inhibitor. *J Biol Chem* 1986;261:14965.

170. Erdos EG, Sloane GM. An enzyme in human plasma that inactivates bradykinin and kallidins. *Biochem Pharmacol* 1962;11:585.

171. Sheikh IA, Kaplan AP. Studies of the digestion of bradykinin, lysylbradykinin and kinin degradation products by carboxypeptidases A, B and N. *Biochem Pharmacol* 1986;35:1957.

172. Sheikh IA, Kaplan AP. Studies of the digestion of bradykinin, lysylbradykinin and des-arg9 bradykinin by angiotensin converting enzyme. *Biochem Pharmacol* 1986;35:1951.

173. Sheikh IA, Kaplan AP. The mechanism of digestion of bradykinin and lysylbradykinin (kallidin) in human serum: the role of carboxy-peptidase, angiotensin converting enzyme, and determination of final degradation products. *Biochem Pharmacol* 1989;38(6):993.

174. Marceau F, et al. Pharmacology of kinins: their relevance to tissue injury and inflammation. *Gen Pharmacol* 1983;14:209.

175. Vavrek RJ, Stewart JM. Competitive antagonists of bradykinin. *Peptides* 1985;6:1610164.

176. Beierwaltes WH, et al. Competitive analog antagonist of bradykinin in the canine hindlimb. *Proc Soc Exp Biol Med* 1987;186:79.

177. Stewart JM, et al. Bradykinin antagonists: present progress and future prospects. [Review] [29 refs]. *Immunopharmacology* 1999;43(2-3):155.

178. Nussberger J, et al. Plasma bradykinin in angio-oedema. *Lancet* 1998;351 (9117):1693.

179. Iatridis PG, Ferguson JH. Active Hageman factor. A plasma lysokinase of the human fibrinolytic system. *J Clin Invest* 1962;41:1277.

180. Ogston D, et al. Studies on a complex mechanism for the activation of plasminogen by kaolin and by chloroform. The participation of Hageman factor and additional cofactors. *J Clin Invest* 1967;48:1786.

181. McDonagh JS, Ferguson JH. Studies on the participation of Hageman factor in fibrinolysis. *Thromb Haemost* 1970;24:1.

182. Ogston D, et al. The assay of a plasma component necessary for the generation of a plasminogen activator in the presence of Hageman factor (Hageman factor cofactor). *Br J Haematol* 1971;20:209.

183. Kluft C. Occurrence of C1-inhibitor and other proteinase inhibitors in euglobulin fractions and their influence on fibrinolytic activity. *Haemostasis* 1976;5:136.

184. Kluft C. Elimination of inhibition of euglobulin fibrinolysis by use of flufenamate: involvement of C1-inactivator. *Haemostasis* 1977;6:351.

185. Miles L, Rothschild AZ, Griffin JH. Dextran sulfate dependent fibrinolysis in whole human plasma. *J Lab Clin Med* 1983;101:214.

186. Saito H. The participation of plasma thromboplastin antecedent (factor Xl) in contact-activated fibrinolysis. *Proc Soc Exp Biol Med* 1980;164:153.

187. Goldsmith G, Saito H, Ratnoff OD. The activation of plasminogen by Hageman factor (factor Xll) and Hageman factor fragments. *J Clin Invest* 1978; 12:54.

188. Miles LA, Greengard JS, Griffin JH. A comparison of the abilities of plasma kallikrein, factor XIIa, factor Xla, and urokinase to activate plasminogen. *Thromb Res* 1983;29:407.

189. Jorg M, Binder BR. Kinetic analysis of plasminogen activation by purified plasma kallikrein. *Thromb Res* 1985;39:323.

190. Hauert J, Bachmann F. Prourokinase activation in euglobulin fractions. *Thromb Haemost* 1985;54:122.

191. Huisveld IA, et al. Contribution of contact activation factors to urokinase-related fibrinolytic activator in whole plasma. *Thromb Haemost* 1985;54:102.

192. Kluft C, Wijngaards G, Jie AFH. Intrinsic plasma fibrinolysis: involvement of urokinase-related activity in the factor Xll independent plasminogen proactivator pathway. *J Lab Clin Med* 1984;103:408.

193. Lenich C, Pannell R, Gurewich V. Assembly and activation of the intrinsic fibrinolytic pathway on the surface of human endothelial cells in culture. *Thromb Haemost* 1995;74(2):698.

194. Loza JP, et al. Platelet-bound prekallikrein promotes pro-urokinase-induced clot lysis: a mechanism for targeting the factor XII dependent intrinsic pathway of fibrinolysis. *Thromb Haemost* 1994;71(3):347.

195. Smith D, Gilbert M, Owen WG. Tissue plasminogen activator release in vivo in response to vasoactive agents. *Blood* 1985;66(4):835.

196. Alving BM, et al. Hypotension associated with prekallikrein activator (Hageman factor fragments) in plasma protein fraction. *N Engl J Med* 1978;229:66.

197. Alving BM, et al. Contact activation factors: contaminants of immunoglobulin preparations with coagulant and vasoactive properties. *J Lab Clin Med* 1980;96(2):334.

198. Waeber G, et al. Hypotensive effect of the active fragment derived from factor XII is mediated by an activation of the plasma kallikrein-kinin system. *Circ Shock* 1988;26(4):375.

199. Brown CF, Osmond DH. Factor XII and prekallikrein-kallikrein-kinin in the cryoactivation of human plasma prorenin. *Clin Sci* 1984;66:533.

200. Yokosawa N, et al. Isolation of completely inactive plasma prorenin and its activation by kallikreins. *Biochim Biophys Acta* 1979;569:211.

201. Purdon AD, et al. Prorenin activation by plasma kallikrein in inhibitor deficient plasma. *J Lab Clin Med* 1985;105:694.

202. Seligsohn U, et al. Activation of human factor VII by Hageman factor fragments. *J Clin Invest* 1979;64:1056.

203. Gjonnaess H. Cold promoting activation of factor VII. III. Relation to the kallikrein system. *Thromb Diath Haemorrh* 1972;28:182.

204. Laake K, et al. Cold-promoted activation of factor VII in human plasma: studies on the associated acyl-arginine esterase activity. *Thromb Res* 1974; 4:769.

205. Gordon EM, et al. Rapid fibrinolysis, augmented Hageman factor (factor XII) titers and decreased C1 esterase inhibitor titers in women using oral contraceptives. *J Lab Clin Med* 1980;96:762.

206. Gordon E, Douglas MJ, Ratnoff OD. Influence of augmented Hageman factor (factor XII) titers on the cryoactivation of plasma prorenin in women using oral contraceptives. *J Clin Invest* 1983;72:1833.

207. Jesperson J, Kluft C. Increased euglobulin potential in women on oral contraceptives low in oestrogen-levels of extrinsic and intrinsic plasminogen activators, prekallikrein, factor XII and C1-inactivator. *Thromb Haemost* 1985; 54:454.

208. Ghebrehiwet B, Silverberg M, Kaplan AP. Activation of the classical pathway of complement by Hageman factor fragment. *J Exp Med* 1981;153:665.

209. Donaldson VH. Mechanism of activation of C1 esterase in hereditary angioneurotic edema in vitro. The role of Hageman factor, a clot promoting agent. *J Exp Med* 1967;127:411.

210. Fields T, Ghebrehiwet B, Kaplan AP. Kinin formation in hereditary angioedema plasma: evidence against kinin derivation from C2 and in support of "spontaneous" formation of bradykinin. *J Allergy Clin Immunol* 1983;72:54.

211. Schmaier AH, et al. The expression of high molecular weight kininogen on human umbilical vein endothelial cells. *J Biol Chem* 1988;31:16327.

212. van Iwaarden F, de Groot PG, Bouma BN. The binding of high molecular weight kininogen to cultured human endothelial cells. *J Biol Chem* 1988;263 (10):4698.

213. Reddigari SR, et al. Human high molecular weight kininogen binds to human umbilical vein endothelial cells via its heavy and light chains. *Blood* 1993;81(5):1306.

214. Hasan AA, Zisman KT, Schmaier AH. Identification of cytokeratin 1 as a binding protein and presentation receptor for kininogens on endothelial cells. *Proc Natl Acad Sci U S A* 1998;95(7):3615.

215. Herwald H, et al. Isolation and characterization of the kininogen-binding protein p33 from endothelial cells. Identity with the gC1q receptor. *J Biol Chem* 1996;271(22):13040.

216. Joseph K, et al. Identification of the zinc-dependent endothelial cell binding protein for high molecular weight kininogen and factor XII: identity with the receptor that binds to the globular "heads" of C1q (gC1q-R). *Proc Natl Acad Sci U S A* 1996;93(16):8552.

217. Colman RW, et al. Binding of high molecular weight kininogen to human endothelial cells is mediated via a site within domains 2 and 3 of the urokinase receptor. *J Clin Invest* 1997;100(6):1481.

218. Joseph K, Ghebrehiwet B, Kaplan AP. Cytokeratin 1 and gC1qR mediate high molecular weight kininogen binding to endothelial cells. *Clin Immunol* 1999;92(3):246.

219. Reddigari SR, et al. Human Hageman factor (factor XII) and high molecular weight kininogen compete for the same binding site on human umbilical vein endothelial cells. *J Biol Chem* 1993;268(16):11982.

220. Motta G, et al. High molecular weight kininogen regulates prekallikrein assembly and activation on endothelial cells: a novel mechanism for contact activation. *Blood* 1998;91(2):516.

221. Berrettini M, et al. Assembly and expression of an intrinsic factor IX activator complex on the surface of cultured human endothelial cells. *J Biol Chem* 1992;267(28):19833.

222. Rojkjaer R, et al. Factor XII does not initiate prekallikrein activation on endothelial cells. *Thromb Haemost* 1998;80(1):74.

223. Hsu TC, et al. Molecular cloning of platelet factor XI, an alternative splicing product of the plasma factor XI gene. *J Biol Chem* 1998;273(22):13787.

224. Lipscomb MS, Walsh PN. Human platelets and factor XI. Localization in platelet membranes of factor XI-like activity and its functional distinction from that of factor XI. *J Clin Invest* 1979;63:1006.

225. Tuszynski GP, et al. Factor XI antigen and activity in human platelets. *Blood* 1982;59:1148.

226. Schmaier AH, et al. High molecular weight kininogen: a secreted platelet protein. *J Clin Invest* 1983;71:1477.

227. Schmaier AH, et al. High molecular weight kininogen: localization in unstimulated and activated platelets and activation by a platelet calpain(s). *Blood* 1986;67:119.

228. Gustafson EJ, et al. High molecular weight kininogen binds to unstimulated platelets. *J Clin Invest* 1986;78:310.

229. Greengard J, Griffin JH. Receptor for high molecular kininogen on stimulated washed human platelets. *Biochemistry* 1984;23:6863.

230. Meloni FJ, Gustafson EJ, Schmaier AH. High molecular weight kininogen binds to platelets by its heavy and light chains and when bound has altered susceptibility to kallikrein cleavage. *Blood* 1992;79(5):1233.

231. Bradford HN, et al. Human kininogens regulate thrombin binding to platelets through the glycoprotein Ib-IX-V complex. *Blood* 1997;90(4):1508.

232. Joseph K, et al. Platelet glycoprotein Ib: a zinc-dependent binding protein for the heavy chain of high-molecular-weight kininogen. *Mol Med* 1999;5(8):555.

233. Jiang YP, Muller-Esterl W, Schmaier AH. Domain 3 of kininogens contains a cell-binding site and a site that modifies thrombin activation of platelets. *J Biol Chem* 1992;267(6):3712.

234. Puri RN, et al. High molecular weight kininogen inhibits thrombin-induced platelet aggregation and cleavage of aggregin by inhibiting binding of thrombin to platelets. *Blood* 1991;77(3):500.

235. Hasan A, Amenta AS, Schmaier AH. Bradykinin and its metabolite, Arg-Pro-Pro-Gly-Phe, are selective inhibitors of alpha-thrombin-induced platelet activation [published erratum appears in *Circulation* 1996 Oct 1;94(7):1794]. *Circulation* 1996;94(3):517.

236. Hasan AA, et al. The mechanisms of thrombostatin's inhibition of thrombin-induced platelet aggregation. *Circulation* 1998;Suppl 1:I.

237. Scully M, Weerasinghe FK, Kakhar VV. Inhibition of contact activation by platelet factor 4. *Thromb Res* 1980;20:461.

238. Kodania K, Kato H, Iwanaga S. Isolation of bovine platelet cationic proteins which inhibit the surface-mediated activation of factor XII and prekallikrein. *J Biochem* 1985;97:139.

239. Walsh PN. The effects of collagen and kaolin on the intrinsic coagulant activity of platelets. Evidence for an alternative pathway in intrinsic coagulation not requiring factor XII. *Br J Haematol* 1972;22:393.

240. Colman RW. Effect of cleavage of the heavy chain of human plasma kallikrein on its functional properties. *Blood* 1985;65:311.

241. Nishikawa K, et al. Generation of vasoactive peptide bradykinin from human umbilical vein endothelium-bound high molecular weight kininogen by plasma kallikrein. *Blood* 1992;80(8):1980.

242. Palmer RM, Ferrige AG, Moncada S. Nitric oxide release accounts for the biological activity of endothelium-derived relaxing factor. *Nature* 1987;327 (6122):524.

243. Pelc LR, Gross GJ, Warltier DC. Mechanism of coronary vasodilation produced by bradykinin. *Circulation* 1991;83(6):2048.

244. Hong SL. Effect of bradykinin and thrombin on prostacyclin synthesis in endothelial cells from calf and pig aorta and human umbilical cord vein. *Thromb Res* 1980;18:787.

245. Crutchly DJ, et al. Bradykinin induced release of prostacyclin and thromboxanes from bovine pulmonary artery endothelial cells. *Biochim Biophys Acta* 1983;751:99.

246. Brown NJ, Nadeau JH, Vaughan DE. Selective stimulation of tissue-type plasminogen activator (t-PA) in vivo by infusion of bradykinin. *Thromb Haemost* 1997;77(3):522.

247. Rosenthal RH, Dreskin OH, Rosenthal N. New hemophiliac-like disease caused by a deficiency of a third plasma thromboplastin factor. *Proc Soc Exp Biol Med* 1953;82:171.

248. Rosenthal RL, Dreskin OH, Rosenthal N. Plasma thromboplastin antecedent (PTA) deficiency: clinical coagulation, therapeutic and hereditary aspects of a new hemophilia-like disease. *Blood* 1955;10:120.

249. Sidi A, et al. Factor XI deficiency: detection and management during urological surgery. *J Urol* 1978;119:528.

250. Saito H, et al. Failure to detect variant (CRM+) plasma thromboplastin antecedent (factor XI) molecules in hereditary plasma thromboplastin antecedent deficiency: a study of 125 patients of several ethnic backgrounds. *J Lab Clin Med* 1985;106(6):718.

251. Leiba H, Ramot B, Many A. Hereditary and coagulation studies in ten families with factor XI (plasma thromboplastin antecedent) deficiency. *Br J Haematol* 1965;11:654.

252. Rapaport SI, et al. The mode of inheritance of PTA deficiency: evidence for the existence of major PTA deficiency and minor PTA deficiency. *Blood* 1961;18:149.

253. Rimon A, et al. Factor XI activity and factor XI antigen in homozygous and heterozygous factor XI deficiency. *Blood* 1976;48:165.

254. Schwartz HC, Stone JD. Hereditary factor XI deficiency. *J Oral Surg* 1967; 34:453.

255. Megquier RJ. Fibrinolytic activity in human dental sockets after extractions. *J Oral Surg* 1971;29:321.

256. Kaufmann JM. Prostatectomy in factor XI deficiency. *J Urol* 1977;117:75.

257. Reece EA, et al. Spontaneous factor XI inhibitors. Seven additional cases and a review of the literature. *Arch Intern Med* 1984;144:525.

258. Stern DM, Nossel HL, Owen J. Acquired antibody to factor XI in a patient with congenital factor XI deficiency. *J Clin Invest* 1982;69:1270.

259. Morgan K, Schiffman S, Feinstein D. Acquired factor XI inhibitors in two patients with hereditary factor XI deficiency. *Thromb Haemost* 1984;51(3):371.

260. De La Cadena RA, et al. Naturally occurring human antibodies against two distinct functional domains in the heavy chain of FXI/FXIa. *Blood* 1988;72(5):1748.

261. Chediak J, et al. Studies on a circulating anticoagulant inhibiting factor XI in a patient with congenital deficiency and carcinoma of the prostate. *Br J Haematol* 1986;63(1):123.

262. Seligsohn U. High gene frequency of factor XI (PTA) deficiency in Ashkenazi Jews. *Blood* 1978;51:1223.

263. Peretz H, et al. The two common mutations causing factor XI deficiency in Jews stem from distinct founders: one of ancient Middle Eastern origin and another of more recent European origin. *Blood* 1997;90(7):2654.

264. Ragni MV, et al. Comparison of bleeding tendency, factor XI coagulant activity, and factor XI antigen in 25 factor XI-deficient kindreds. *Blood* 1985;65 (3):719.

265. Sato E, et al. A novel mutation that leads to a congenital factor XI deficiency in a Japanese family. *Am J Hematol* 2000;63(4):165.

266. Alhaq A, et al. Identification of a novel mutation in a non-Jewish factor XI deficient kindred. *Br J Haematol* 1999;104(1):44.

267. Martincic D, et al. Identification of mutations and polymorphisms in the factor XI genes of an African American family by dideoxyfingerprinting. [erratum appears in *Blood* 1999 Mar 1;93(5):1786]. *Blood* 1998;92(9):3309.

268. Nossel HL, Niemetz J, Sawitsky A. Blood PTA (factor XI) levels following plasma infusion. *Proc Soc Exp Biol Med* 1964;115:896.

269. Horowitz HI, Fujimoto MM. Survival of factor XI in vitro and in vivo. *Transfusion* 1965;5:539.

270. Bennett E, Dormandy K. Pool's cryoprecipitate and exhausted plasma in the treatment of von Willebrand's disease and factor XI deficiency. *Lancet* 1966; 2:731.

271. Ratnoff OD, Busce FJ, Sheon RP. The demise of John Hageman. *N Engl J Med* 1968;279:760.

272. Hoak JC, Swenson LW, Warner ED. Myocardial infarction associated with severe factor XII deficiency. *Lancet* 1966;2:884.

273. Goodnough LT, Saito H, Ratnoff OD. Thrombosis or myocardial infarction in congenital clotting factor abnormalities and chronic thrombocytopenia: a report of 21 patients and a review of 50 previously reported cases. *Medicine* 1983;62:248.

274. Londino A, Luparello FJ. Factor XII deficiency in a man with gout and angio-immunoblastic lymphadenopathy. *Arch Intern Med* 1984;144:1497.

275. Bernardi F, et al. A frequent factor XII gene mutation in Hageman trait. *Hum Genet* 1993;80:149.

276. Hofferbert S, et al. A novel 5'-upstream mutation in the factor XII gene is associated with a TaqI restriction site in an Alu repeat in factor XII-deficient patients. *Hum Genet* 1996;97(6):838.

277. Schloesser M, et al. The novel acceptor splice site mutation 11396(G→A) in the factor XII gene causes a truncated transcript in cross-reacting material negative patients. *Hum Mol Genet* 1995;4(7):1235.

278. Kondo S, et al. Factor XII Tenri, a novel cross-reacting material negative factor XII deficiency, occurs through a proteasome-mediated degradation. *Blood* 1999;93(12):4300.

279. Castaman G, et al. Thrombosis in patients with heterozygous and homozygous factor XII deficiency is not explained by the associated presence of factor V Leiden [letter]. *Thromb Haemost* 1996;76(2):275.

280. Cornudella R, et al. Deficit congenito de factor XII y trombosis venosa espontanea tratada con urokinasa. *Sangre* 1995;40(3):219.

281. Helft G, et al. Factor XII deficiency associated with coronary stent thrombosis [letter]. *Am J Hematol* 2000;64(4):322.

282. Yamada J, et al. Activation of the kallikrein-kinin system in Rocky Mountain spotted fever. *Ann Intern Med* 1978;88:764.

283. Zeerleder S, et al. Reevaluation of the incidence of thromboembolic complications in congenital factor XII deficiency—a study on 73 subjects from 14 Swiss families. *Thromb Haemost* 1999;82(4):1240.

284. Zeitler P, Meissner N, Kreth HW. Combination of von Willebrand disease type 1 and partial factor XII deficiency in children: clinical evidence for a diminished bleeding tendency. *Acta Paediatr* 1999;88(11):1233.

285. Bux-Gewehr I, et al. Combined von Willebrand factor deficiency and factor XII deficiency [letter]. *Thromb Haemost* 2000;83(3):514.

286. Girolami A, et al. Symptomatic combined homozygous factor XII deficiency and heterozygous factor V Leiden. luscaber@tin.it. *J Thromb Thrombol* 2000;9(3):271.

287. Sollo DG, Saleem A. Prekallikrein (Fletcher factor) deficiency. *Ann Clin Lab Sci* 1985;15(4):279.

288. Currimbhoy Z, et al. Fletcher factor deficiency and myocardial infarction. *Am J Clin Pathol* 1976;65(6):970.

289. Harris MG, et al. Multiple cerebral thrombosis in Fletcher factor (prekallikrein) deficiency: a case report. *Am J Hematol* 1985;19(4):387.

290. Saito H, et al. Heterogeneity of human prekallikrein deficiency (Fletcher trait): evidence that 5 of 18 cases are positive for cross-reacting material. *N Engl J Med* 1981;305(16):910.

291. Bouma BN, et al. Characterization of a variant prekallikrein, prekallikrein Long Beach, from a family with mixed cross-reacting material-positive and cross-reacting material-negative prekallikrein deficiency. *J Clin Invest* 1986;78(1):170.

292. Saito H, et al. Fitzgerald trait. Deficiency of a hitherto unrecognized agent, Fitzgerald factor, participating in surface-mediated reactions of clotting, fibrinolysis, generation of kinins, and the property of diluted plasma enhancing vascular permeability. *J Clin Invest* 1975;55:1082.

293. Ishimaru F, et al. Molecular characterization of total kininogen deficiency in Japanese patients. *Int J Hematol* 1999;69(2):126.

294. Brunnee T, et al. Activation of factor XI in plasma is dependent on factor XII. *Blood* 1993;81(3):580.

295. von dem Borne PA, et al. Surface independent factor XI activation by thrombin in the presence of high molecular weight kininogen. *Thromb Haemost* 1994;72(3):397.

296. Minnema MC, Ten Cate H, Hack CE. The role of factor XI in coagulation: a matter of revision. [Review] [143 refs]. *Thromb Haemost* 1999;25(4):419.

297. Bouma BN, Meijers JC. Role of blood coagulation factor XI in downregulation of fibrinolysis. [Review] [58 refs]. *Curr Opin Hematol* 2000;7(5):266.

298. Rand MD, et al. Blood clotting in minimally altered whole blood. *Blood* 1996;88(9):3432.

299. Minnema MC, et al. Enhancement of rabbit jugular vein thrombolysis by neutralization of factor XI. In vivo evidence for a role of factor XI as an antifibrinolytic factor. [erratum appears in *J Clin Invest* 1998 Feb 15;101(4):917]. *J Clin Invest* 1998;101(1):10.

300. Levi M, et al. Reduction of contact activation related fibrinolytic activity in factor XII deficient patients. Further evidence for the role of the contact system in fibrinolysis in vivo. *J Clin Invest* 1991;88(4):1155.

301. Lammle B, et al. Thromboembolism and bleeding tendency in congenital factor XII deficiency—a study on 74 subjects from 14 Swiss families. *Thromb Haemost* 1991;65(2):117.

302. Bouma BN, et al. Immunological studies of prekallikrein, kallikrein and high molecular weight kininogen in normal and deficient plasmas and in normal plasma after cold dependent activation. *J Lab Clin Med* 1980;96:693.

303. Mancini G, Carbonara AO, Heremans JF. Immunochemical quantification of antigens by single radial immunodiffusion. *Immunochemistry* 1965;2:235.

304. Laurell CB. Quantitative estimate of proteins by electrophoresis in agarose gel containing antibodies. *Anal Biochem* 1966;15:45.

305. Fisher CA, et al. Assay of prekallikrein in human plasma: comparison of amidolytic, esterolytic, coagulation and immunochemical assays. *Blood* 1982;59:963.

306. Tankersley DL, Alving BM, Finlayson JS. Activation of factor XII by dextran sulfate. The basis for an assay of factor XII. *Blood* 1983;62:448.

307. Alving BM, Tankersley DL, Mason BL. Plasma prekallikrein: quantitative determination by direct activation with Hageman factor fragment (beta-XIIa). *J Lab Clin Med* 1983;101(2):226.

308. Gallimore MJ. Chromogenic substrate assays for studying components of the plasma kallikrein system in health and disease. In: Fritz HJ, et al, eds. *Kinins III—Part A. Advances in experimental medicine and biology.* New York: Plenum, 1983:225.

309. de Agostini A, et al. Human plasma kallikrein and C I inhibitor form a complex possessing an epitope that is not detectable on the parent molecules: demonstration using a monoclonal antibody. *Proc Natl Acad Sci U S A* 1985;82:5190.

310. de Agostini A, et al. A common neoepitope is created when the reactive center of C1-inhibitor is cleaved by plasma kallikrein, activated factor XII fragment, C1 esterase, or neutrophil elastase. *J Clin Invest* 1988;82:700.

311. Harpel PC. α₂-Plasmin inhibitor and α₂-macroglobulin plasmin complexes in plasma. Quantitation by an enzyme-linked differential antibody immunosorbent assay. *J Clin Invest* 1981;68:46.

312. Kaplan AP, Gruber B, Harpel PC. Assessment of Hageman factor activation in human plasma. Quantification of activated Hageman factor-CI inactivator complexes by an enzyme-linked differential antibody immunosorbent assay. *Blood* 1985;66:636.

313. Lewin MF, Kaplan AP, Harpel PC. Studies of CI inactivator-plasma kallikrein complexes in purified systems and in plasma. Quantification by enzyme-linked differential antibody immunosorbent assay. *J Biol Chem* 1983;258:6415.

314. Nuijens JH, et al. Quantification of plasma factor XIIa-C1-inhibitor and kallikrein-C1-inhibitor complexes in sepsis. *Blood* 1988;72(6):1841.

315. Shimamoto K, et al. A sensitive radioimmunoassay method for urinary kinins in man. *J Lab Clin Med* 1978;91:721.

316. Odya CE, et al. Development of a radioimmunoassay for des-Arg⁹-bradykinin. *Biochem Pharmacol* 1983;32:337.

317. Cugno M, et al. Activation of factor XII and cleavage of high molecular weight kininogen during acute attacks in hereditary and acquired C1-inhibitor deficiencies. *Immunopharmacology* 1996;33(1-3):361.

318. Shoemaker LR, et al. Hereditary angioneurotic oedema: characterization of plasma kinin and vascular permeability-enhancing activities. *Clin Exp Immunol* 1994;95(1):22.

319. Nussberger J, et al. Local bradykinin generation in hereditary angioedema. *J Allergy Clin Immunol* 1999;104(6):1321.

320. Zahedi R, et al. Unique C1 inhibitor dysfunction in a kindred without angioedema. II. Identification of an Ala443→Val substitution and functional analysis of the recombinant mutant protein. *J Clin Invest* 1995;95(3):1299.

321. Schapira M, et al. Prekallikrein activation and high molecular weight kininogen consumption in hereditary angioedema. *N Engl J Med* 1985;3:1050.

322. Curd JG, Prograis LJJ, Cochrane CG. Detection of active kallikrein in induced blister fluids of hereditary angioedema patients. *J Exp Med* 1980;152:242.

323. Talamo RC, Haber E, Austen KF. A radioimmunoassay for bradykinin in plasma and synovial fluid. *J Lab Clin Med* 1969;74:816.

324. Lämmle B, et al. Detection and quantitation of cleaved and uncleaved high molecular weight kininogen in plasma by ligand blotting with radiolabeled plasma prekallikrein or factor XI. *Thromb Haemost* 1988;59(2):151.

325. Ziccardi RJ. Spontaneous activation of the first component of human complement (C I) by an intramolecular autocatalytic mechanism. *J Immunol* 1982;128:2500.

326. Cooper NR. Activation and regulation of the first component of complement. *Fed Proc* 1983;42:134.

327. Kimball HR, Melmon KL, Wolff SM. Endotoxin-induced kinin production in man. *Proc Soc Exp Biol Med* 1972;139:1078.

328. Mason JW, et al. Plasma kallikrein and Hageman factor in gram-negative bacteremia. *Ann Intern Med* 1970;73:545.

329. Hirsch EF, et al. Kinin-system responses in sepsis after trauma in man. *J Surg Res* 1974;17:147.

330. Robinson JA, et al. Endotoxin, prekallikrein, complement, and systemic vascular resistances. Sequential measurement in man. *Am J Med* 1975;59:61.

331. O'Donnell TF, et al. Kinin activation in the blood of patients with sepsis. *Surg Gynecol Obstet* 1976;143:539.

332. Martinez-Brotóns F, et al. Plasma kallikrein-kinin system in patients with uncomplicated sepsis and septic shock—comparison with cardiogenic shock. *Thromb Haemost* 1987;4(2):709.

333. Minnema MC, et al. Activation of clotting factor XI without detectable contact activation in experimental human endotoxemia. *Blood* 1998;92(9):3294.

334. Mason JN, Colman RW. The role of Hageman factor in disseminated intravascular coagulation induced by sepsis, neoplasia, or liver disease. *Thromb Diath Haemorrh* 1971;26:325.

335. Lämmle B, et al. Plasma prekallikrein, factor XII, antithrombin III, C1-inhibitor and α₂-macroglobulin in critically ill patients with suspected disseminated intravascular coagulation (DIC). *Am J Clin Pathol* 1984;82:396.

336. Vaziri ND, et al. Activation of intrinsic coagulation pathway in pre-eclampsia. *Am J Med* 1986;80(1):103.

337. Pixley RA, et al. The contact system contributes to hypotension but not disseminated intravascular coagulation in lethal bacteremia. In vivo use of a monoclonal anti-factor XII antibody to block contact activation in baboons. *J Clin Invest* 1993;91(1):61.

338. Pixley RA, et al. Activation of the contact system in lethal hypotensive bacteremia in a baboon model. *Am J Pathol* 1992;140(4):897.

339. Naclerio RM, et al. Mediator release after nasal airway challenge with allergen. *Am Rev Respir Dis* 1983;128:597.

340. Proud D, et al. Kinins are generated in vivo following nasal airway challenge of allergic individuals with allergen. *J Clin Invest* 1983;72:1678.

341. Naclerio RM, et al. Inflammatory mediators in late antigen-induced rhinitis. *N Engl J Med* 1985;313:65.

342. Baumgarten CR, et al. Influx of kininogens into nasal secretions after antigen challenge of allergic individuals. *J Clin Invest* 1985;76:191.

343. Noga O, et al. Heparin, derived from the mast cells of human lungs is responsible for the generation of kinins in allergic reactions due to the activation of the contact system. *Int Arch Allergy Immunol* 1999;120(4):310.

344. Moskowitz RW, et al. Generation of kinin-like agents by chondroitin sulfate, heparin, chitin sulfate, and human articular cartilage: possible pathophysiologic implications. *J Lab Clin Med* 1970;76:790.

345. Nagase H, et al. Identification of plasma kallikrein as an activator of latent collagenase in rheumatoid synovial fluid. *Biochim Biophys Acta* 1982;707:133.

346. Kellermeyer RW, Breckenridge RT. The inflammatory process in acute gouty arthritis, I. Activation of Hageman factor by sodium urate crystals. *J Lab Clin Med* 1965;63:307.

347. Ginsberg M, et al. Urate crystal dependent cleavage of Hageman factor in human plasma and synovial fluid. *J Lab Clin Med* 1980;95:497.

348. Donaldson VH, Glueck HI, Fleming T. Rheumatoid arthritis in a patient with Hageman trait. *N Engl J Med* 1972;386:528.

349. Honig GR, Lindley A. Deficiency of Hageman factor (factor XII) in patients with the nephrotic syndrome. *J Pediatr* 1971;78:633.

350. Lange LGI, et al. Activation of Hageman factor in the nephrotic syndrome. *Am J Med* 1974;56:565.

351. Hruby MA, Honig GR, Shapira E. Immunoquantitation of Hageman factor in urine and plasma of children with nephrotic syndrome. *J Lab Clin Med* 1980;96(3):501.

352. Saito H, et al. Urinary excretion of Hageman factor (factor XII) and the presence of nonfunctional factor in the nephrotic syndrome. *Am J Med* 1981;70:531.

353. Wong P, et al. Kallikrein bradykinin system in chronic alcoholic liver disease. *Ann Intern Med* 1972;77:205.

354. van Vliet ACM, et al. Plasma prekallikrein and endotoxemia in liver cirrhosis. *Thromb Haemost* 1981;45(1):65.

355. Edelman R, et al. Evaluation of the plasma kinin system in dengue hemorrhagic fever. *J Lab Clin Med* 1975;86(3):410.

356. Colman RW, et al. The plasma kallikrein-kinin system in sepsis, inflammatory arthritis, and enterocolitis. [Review] [44 refs]. *Clin Rev Allergy Immunol* 1998;16(4):365.

357. Carvalho AC, DeMarinis S, Scott CF, et al. Activation of the contact system of plasma proteolysis in the adult respiratory distress syndrome. *J Lab Clin Med* 1988;112:270.

358. Oates JA, Pettinger WA, Doctor RB. Evidence for the release of bradykinin in carcinoid syndrome. *J Clin Invest* 1966;45:173.

359. Melmon KL, Lovenberg W, Sjoerdsma A. Characteristics of carcinoid tumor kallikrein: identification of lysyl-bradykinin as a peptide it produces *in vitro*. *Clin Chim Acta* 1965;12:292.

360. Wong PY, Talamo RC, Colman RW. Kallikrein-kinin system in post-gastrectomy dumping syndrome. *Ann Intern Med* 1974;80:577.

361. Carvalho AC, Ellman L. Activation of the coagulation system in polycythemia vera. *Blood* 1976;47:669.

362. Yamada J, Herber P, Pettit GW, et al. Activation of the kallikrein-kinin system in Rocky Mountain spotted fever. *Ann Intern Med* 1978;88:764.

363. Colman RW, Edelman R, Scott CF, Gilman RH. Plasma kallikrein activation and inhibition during typhoid fever. *J Clin Invest* 1978;61:287.

364. Carvalho AC, Lees RS, Vaillancourt RA, et al. Activation of the kallikrein system in hyperbetalipoproeinemia. *J Lab Clin Med* 1978;91:117.

365. Nussberger J, Cugno M, Amstutz C, et al. Plasma bradykinin in angioedema. *Lancet* 1998;352:1693–1697.

Vitamin K–Dependent Blood Coagulation Proteins: Normal Function and Clinical Disorders

Bruce Furie, Barbara C. Furie, and David A. Roth

BACKGROUND AND HISTORY

The vitamin K–dependent blood coagulation proteins were discovered sequentially over a 60-year period. The most abundant protein of this class, prothrombin, was identified more than 100 years ago by Alexander Schmidt (1), who postulated that thrombin could not circulate freely in the blood but must exist in a precursor form. Based on the classic theory of blood coagulation, Morawitz (2) proposed that prothrombin was converted to thrombin by a hypothetic enzyme, thrombokinase. Prothrombin was subsequently purified and extensively characterized, with the earliest work dominated by Seegers (3). As with many of the plasma proteins, the discovery of most of the vitamin K–dependent blood coagulation proteins was associated with the observation of "an experiment of nature": a hereditary coagulation disorder due to a deficiency of an unknown clotting activity. Based on the observation that mixing of two hemophiliac plasmas from unrelated patients sometimes led to a correction of the clotting time of the mixed plasma, Aggeler et al. (4) and Schulman and Smith (5) identified the protein known as *factor IX* in 1952. This protein is missing or defective in patients with hemophilia B, but it is distinct from factor VIII, the protein absent in hemophilia A. Factor VII was identified in 1951 after the evaluation of a patient with a hereditary clotting disorder (6). Factor X was discovered simultaneously by Telfer et al. (7) and Hougie et al. (8) by detailed investigation of the plasma of patients with inherited hemorrhagic disorders due to absence of factor X. Proteins that require vitamin K for their synthesis are presented in Table 37-1. The positions of the vitamin K–dependent proteins in the coagulation cascade were proposed independently by Ratnoff and Davie (9) and Macfarlane (10). An updated version of the 1964 model of blood coagulation is presented in Figure 37-1. Considerable confusion arose from the original claim that the activities of "autoprothrombin III" (factor X), "cothromboplastin" (factor VII), and "autoprothrombin II" (factor IX) were derived from a single precursor "prothrombin" molecule (11). Subsequent characterization of these plasma components led to their identification as distinct proteins derived as separate gene products but with structural homology to prothrombin.

As part of his investigation of cholesterol metabolism, Dam (12) observed in 1929 that chickens fed a diet depleted of fat-soluble components developed a hemorrhagic disorder. One of these components, Koagulations vitamin—or vitamin K—was subsequently isolated from alfalfa (13,14). The chemical structure of vitamin K was determined by Doisy et al. (15) (Fig. 37-2). Dam and Doisy shared the Nobel Prize in Medicine in 1943 for their pioneering work on vitamin K. The vitamin K antagonists, including warfarin, were discovered independently. A hemorrhagic disease of cattle plaguing farmers in the Great Plains in the 1920s was found to be associated with the ingestion of spoiled sweet clover hay (16,17). Campbell and Link (18) isolated bishydroxycoumarin (dicoumarol) from bacteria contaminating the hay and demonstrated that this material was the cause of hypoprothrombinemia in the cattle herds. This compound became the model for warfarin and for other coumarin compounds used as rodenticides and as anticoagulants for the treatment of human thrombotic disease.

BIOSYNTHESIS

The vitamin K–dependent plasma proteins required for normal blood clotting are synthesized in the liver (19–21). The properties of these proteins are summarized in Table 37-2 and Figure 37-3. Posttranslational γ-carboxylation occurs in the endoplasmic reticulum. These proteins, including prothrombin and factors IX, X, and VII, circulate in the blood as trace components. Although the protein concentration of plasma is approximately 70 mg/mL, the concentrations of prothrombin and factors IX, X, and VII are 110, 5, 10, and 0.5 μg/mL, respectively. These proteins are synthesized in the hepatocyte in a precursor form and undergo extensive posttranslational modification during transit through the cell to the plasma (22). The vitamin K–dependent proteins are synthesized with a signal peptide sequence and a propeptide sequence that are subsequently cleaved before the mature protein is secreted (22,23). The propeptide is positioned between the signal peptide and the mature amino-terminus of the vitamin K–dependent protein (23). Posttranslational modifications of these proteins include glycosylation, signal peptide and propeptide cleavage, and disulfide bond formation. In addition, because they are members of a unique class of calcium-binding proteins that contain γ-carboxyglutamic acid (24,25), the posttranslational synthesis of γ-carboxyglutamic acid from specific glutamic acid (Glu) residues in these proteins occurs in the hepatocyte (Fig. 37-4). With the single exception of prothrombin, the vitamin K–dependent blood coagulation proteins also undergo β-hydroxylation of specific Asp residues in certain epidermal growth factor (EGF)-like domains (26,27).

TABLE 37-1. Vitamin K–Dependent Proteins

Blood coagulation proteins
    Prothrombin
    Factor IX
    Factor X
    Factor VII
Regulatory proteins in blood coagulation
    Protein C
    Protein S
Bone Proteins
    Osteocalcin (bone Gla protein)
    Matrix Gla protein

ROLE OF VITAMIN K: BIOSYNTHESIS OF γ-CARBOXYGLUTAMIC ACID

Posttranslational modification of Glu to γ-carboxyglutamic acid and regeneration of the active cofactor, vitamin KH_2, requires a series of linked enzyme reactions. The carboxylation reaction includes as substrates a reduced form of vitamin K (vitamin KH_2), molecular oxygen, carbon dioxide, and the protein precursor containing Glu residues (28,29). The vitamin K–dependent carboxylase, isolated in near homogeneous form from bovine liver, has a molecular mass of approximately 94 kd (30). This enzyme was reported to be an integral membrane protein situated on the luminal side of the rough endoplasmic reticulum (31–33). The cDNA for

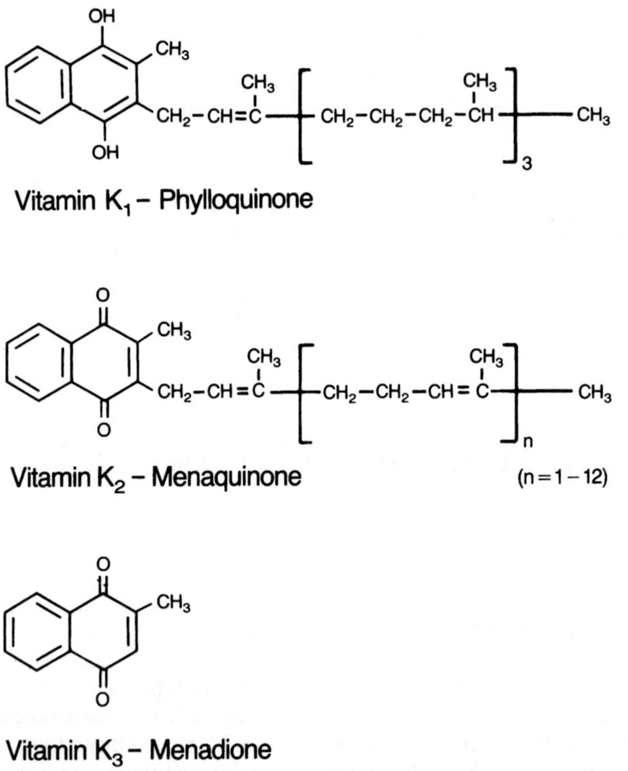

Figure 37-2. Chemical structure of vitamin K. Several forms of vitamin K are found in nature. Vitamin K_1 is a component of plants, and vitamin K_2 is produced by bacteria. Vitamin es to the length of the terpine carbon chain.

the human carboxylase has been cloned and shown to be a single-chain protein of 758 amino acids with several transmembrane regions whose boundaries remain uncertain (34–36). The human carboxylase gene is localized to chromosome 2 at 2p12 (37). The gene is 13 kilobases (kb) in length and contains 15 exons (38). Two cases of missense mutations in the carboxylase leading to combined congenital deficiency of vitamin K–dependent coagulation factors have been reported: Arg 394→Leu and Trp 501→Ser (39,40). γ-Glutamyl carboxylase has been cloned in full or in part from a variety of other species including cow, rat, mouse, whale, fish, chicken, hagfish, cone snail, horseshoe crab, and fruit fly (34,35,41–43). These studies emphasize the marked sequence homology of this enzyme in the animal kingdom.

The reaction catalyzed by the γ-carboxylase leads to the removal of a hydrogen from the γ-carbon of Glu residues on the protein and to the addition of a carboxyl group at this same position with concurrent conversion of vitamin K from the hydroquinone to the epoxide (Fig. 37-5A). Although early studies showed that vitamin K epoxidase activity and glutamyl carboxylase activity are closely linked (44–47), cloning and expression of the vitamin K–dependent carboxylase demonstrated that these two reactions are carried out by the same enzyme (34,35). Previous data suggested vitamin K hydroquinone (vitamin KH_2) may activate a hydrogen at the γ-position of a glutamyl residue (48) and that this hydrogen extraction likely generates a carbanion rather than a free radical at the γ-carbon (49,50). It is likely that a more basic species is required for hydrogen abstraction. Increasing evidence supports the model in which an active oxygenated species of vitamin K abstracts the hydrogen from the γ-carbon of Glu (Fig. 37-5B). The activated vitamin K then collapses to vitamin K epoxide, and carbon dioxide is added to the γ-carbon (51–53).

This model suggests that the initiation of formation of the active oxygenated vitamin K species occurs through abstraction

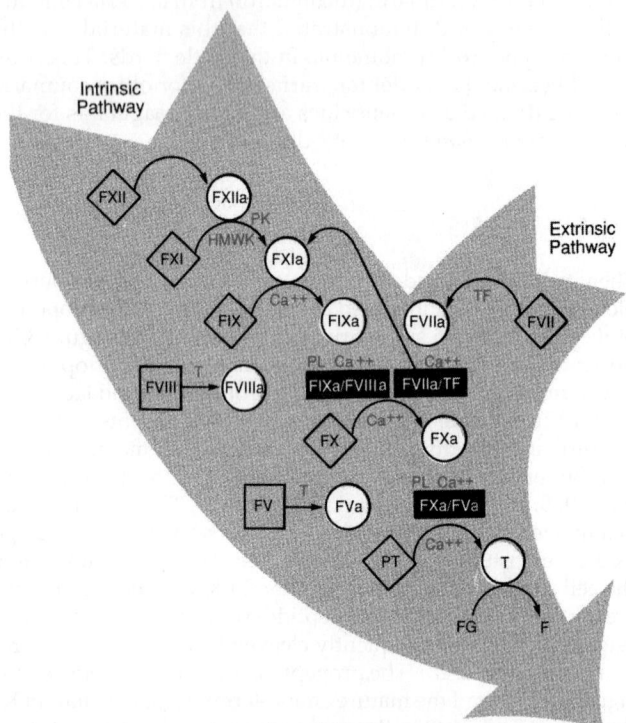

Figure 37-1. Role of the vitamin K–dependent proteins in blood coagulation. The blood coagulation cascade involves the intrinsic and the extrinsic pathways. The vitamin K–dependent proteins (*squares*) circulate in the blood in an inactive, proenzyme form. On activation of blood coagulation, they are converted to their active, procoagulant form (*circles*). These proteins have the special property of displaying maximal enzyme activity on membrane surfaces. F, fibrin; FG, Fibrinogen; FIX, factor IX; FV, factor FV; FVII, factor VII; FX, factor X; FXI, factor XI; FXII, factor XII. HMWK, high-molecular-weight kinnogen; PK, prekalleKrein; PL, phospholipid; PT, prothrombin; T, thrombin; TF, tissue factor. (From Furie B, Furie BC. Molecular basis of blood coagulation. *Cell* 1988;53:505.)

TABLE 37-2. Properties of the Genes, Messenger RNAs, and Gene Products of the Vitamin K–Dependent Blood Coagulation Proteins

Protein	Molecular Weight	Gene (kb)	Chromosome	Messenger RNA (kb)	Exon	Plasma Concentration (µg/mL)	Function
Prothrombin	72,000	21	11p11–q12	2.1	14	100	Protease zymogen
Factor X	56,000	22	13q34	1.5	8	10	Protease zymogen
Factor IX	56,000	34	Xq26–27.3	2.8	8	5	Protease zymogen
Factor VII	50,000	13	13q34	2.4	8	0.5	Protease zymogen

Modified from Furie B, Furie BC. Molecular basis of blood coagulation. *Cell* 1988;53:505.

of a hydrogen from vitamin K by the sulfhydryl group of a cysteine residue in the active site of the carboxylase. Indeed, the importance of free sulfhydryl groups in the carboxylase is well recognized (28,54,55). Two well-conserved cysteines have been identified as important for carboxylase activity (56).

Vitamin KH_2 is the active cofactor required for carboxylase activity (57–59). During the course of the carboxylase reaction, vitamin KH_2 is converted to vitamin K epoxide. Furthermore, vitamin K from dietary sources (15) or gut flora (60) takes the quinone form. Thus, a mechanism is required for generating the active cofactor either from vitamin K quinone or vitamin K epoxide. Two different enzymes can reduce vitamin K quinone to vitamin KH_2: DT diaphorase and vitamin K epoxide reductase (61,62). Of these, only the latter can reduce vitamin K epoxide to vitamin KH_2 (63).

Vitamin K epoxide reductase recycles vitamin K epoxide in a two-step process that goes through the quinone form of vitamin K and uses a dithiol as a cofactor (64–66). The vitamin K epoxide reductase works at low concentrations of vitamin K epoxide and vitamin K quinone and is likely the physiologically important enzyme for recycling vitamin K. This is the enzyme that is inhibited by warfarin, resulting in insufficient vitamin K hydroquinone to support full carboxylation of the vitamin K–dependent blood coagulation proteins (67). The vitamin K epoxide reductase is believed to be an enzyme complex residing in the membrane of the endoplasmic reticulum. Two components of this complex have been identified: microsomal epoxide hydrolase and a glutathione S-transferase. A summary of the vitamin K cycle is shown in Figure 37-5 (68,69). A genetic defect in the vitamin K epoxide reductase complex is suspected in two families with congential deficiency of the vitamin K–dependent coagulation factors (70).

The DT-diaphorase, an oxidoreductase that requires nicotinamide adenine dinucleotide phosphate, also requires high concentrations of vitamin K and likely does not play a role in vitamin K recycling at physiologic tissue concentrations of the vitamin (67). Vitamin K antagonists used as oral anticoagulants such as warfarin (Fig. 37-6) prevent the γ-carboxylation of the vitamin K–dependent proteins. The des-γ-carboxy (abnormal) forms of the vitamin K–dependent proteins are functionally inert and circulate in the blood in place of the active, carboxylated blood-clotting proteins. Warfarin inhibits both the reduction of vitamin K epoxide and vitamin K quinone by the epoxide reductase, preventing recycling of the vitamin to its active form (71). The nicotinamide adenine dinucleotide phosphate–dependent reduction of vitamin K quinone to the hydroquinone is affected only minimally by warfarin and related compounds (71). This enzyme may play an important role when vitamin K in the quinone form is used to overcome warfarin intoxication. Dithiothreitol reduces vitamin K to vitamin K hydroquinone *in vitro* (72,73).

SUBSTRATE SPECIFICITY

γ-Carboxyglutamic acid is synthesized by a vitamin K–dependent posttranslational carboxylation of specific Glu residues in the intracellular precursor of the vitamin K–dependent proteins. These intracellular prothrombin precursors were first demonstrated in 1971 by Shah and Suttie (74). When vitamin K was administered to vitamin K–deficient rats in the presence of an inhibitor of protein synthesis, cycloheximide, prothrombin activity increased rapidly despite the absence of *de novo* protein synthesis. The prothrombin released into the circulation on administration of vitamin K was

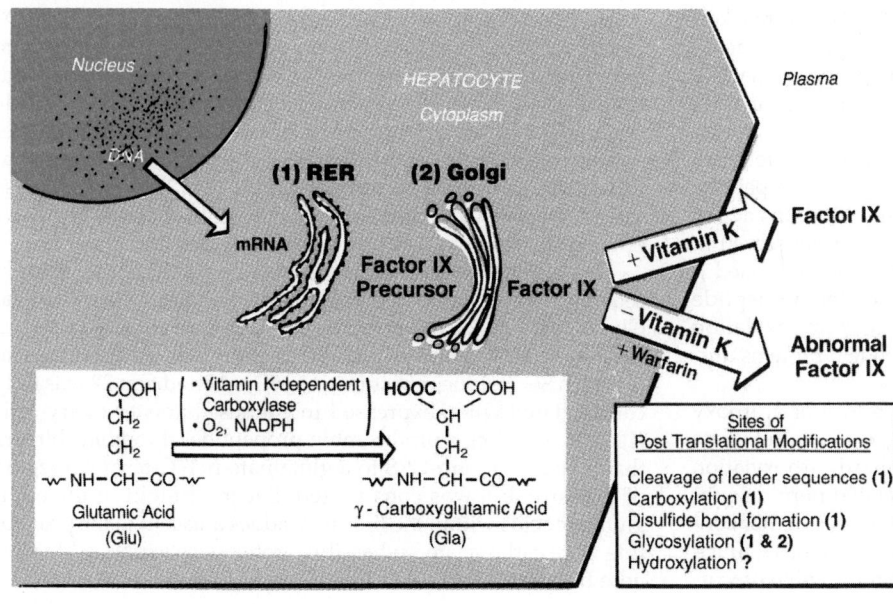

Figure 37-3. Biosynthesis of the vitamin K–dependent proteins. Factors IX, X, and VII and prothrombin are synthesized in the liver in a precursor, prozymogen form. The vitamin K–dependent carboxylase modifies this prozymogen posttranslationally, converting some N-terminal Glu residues to γ-carboxyglutamic acid. This reaction requires vitamin K in its reduced form, carbon dioxide, and oxygen. After subsequent cleavage of the propeptide, the zymogen is secreted into the plasma.

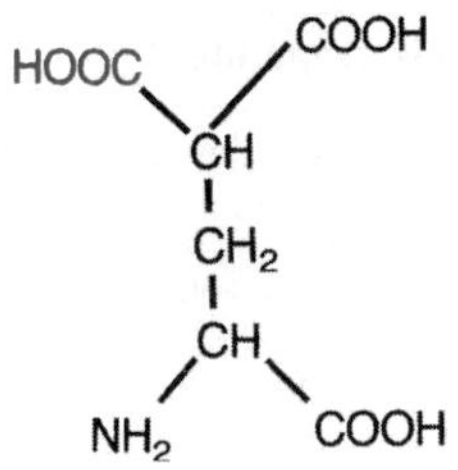

Figure 37-4. Chemical structure of γ-carboxyglutamic acid. γ-Carboxyglutamic acid is synthesized from Glu residues in proteins. The additional carboxyl group is substituted for a γ-hydrogen in a reaction catalyzed by the vitamin K–dependent carboxylase.

derived from a precursor pool. This prothrombin precursor, like des-γ–carboxy (abnormal) prothrombin, contains an intact thrombin domain but cannot be activated by factor Xa, presumably because of the absence of γ-carboxyglutamic acid residues (75). These observations demonstrate that the vitamin K–dependent step in the synthesis of prothrombin is the posttranslational modification of a hepatic prothrombin precursor.

Two prothrombin precursors have been isolated from rat liver (76,77), and other forms have been observed (78,79). These precursors are functionally distinct from des-γ–carboxy (abnormal) prothrombin (80,81), the secreted form of prothrombin that is deficient in γ-carboxyglutamic acid, in that they are excellent substrates for the carboxylase. This observation indicates that there must be recognition sites on the prothrombin precursor that direct carboxylation in the liver; these sites are not present on the secreted forms of the protein (82). In support of this hypothesis, the carboxylase activity in solubilized liver microsomes is bound to an endogenous precursor (83). The carboxylase binds to a site on the protein substrate, the carboxylation recognition site (84), adjacent to the region that becomes carboxylated. This recognition element is located on the propeptide of the vitamin K–dependent proteins, a region of the precursor protein that is cleaved and discarded during the final stages of protein synthesis (23).

Diuguid et al. (85) determined the size of the propeptide of factor IX by analysis of a mutant factor IX, termed *factor IX Cambridge*. This mutant factor IX has an 18-residue NH$_2$-terminal extension due to the mutation of Arg −1 to a Ser, precluding propeptide cleavage by a propeptidase with trypsinlike specificity. Factor IX Cambridge and factor IX San Dimas (86), a mutant identical to factor IX Oxford 3 (87), are incompletely carboxylated, indicating a link between a propeptide point mutation and vitamin K–dependent carboxylation. These data and the marked sequence homology of this domain in γ-carboxyglutamic acid–containing proteins (88) (Fig. 37-7) led to the proposal that the propeptide targeted protein precursors for subsequent γ-carboxylation. Using site-specific mutagenesis and a heterologous mammalian expression system, Jorgensen et al. (84) and Rabiet et al. (89) demonstrated that factor IX lacking the 18-residue propeptide was not carboxylated *in vivo*. Similarly, point mutations at −16 (Phe→Ala) or −10 (Ala→Glu), two positions highly conserved in the propeptides of the vitamin K–dependent proteins, inhibited γ-carboxylation. These results demonstrated that the propeptide contains a recognition element, designated the γ-carboxylation recognition site, that flags the vitamin K–dependent proteins during hepatic biosynthesis for γ-carboxylation.

A synthetic peptide comprising residues 5 to 9 of acarboxy bovine prothrombin (Phe-Leu-Glu-Glu-Val) serves as a substrate for ^{14}C-bicarbonate incorporation by a solubilized carboxylation system (90). Studies of this substrate and related peptide substrates demonstrate that their carboxylation requires higher concentrations of vitamin K and that this pentapeptide has a much higher K$_m$ than carboxylation of endogenous prothrombin precur-

sors (90–92). Also, only the first of two adjacent Glu residues in these synthetic peptides is carboxylated (93). These results suggest that substrate properties, other than the sequence immediately surrounding the glutamic acids that are destined to be carboxylated, are required for efficient carboxylation by the vitamin K–dependent carboxylase.

Ulrich et al. (94) have shown that the vitamin K–dependent carboxylase recognizes the γ-. A 28-residue synthetic peptide based on residues −18 to +10 in prothrombin (the propeptide and the first ten residues of the mature form of prothrombin) is efficiently carboxylated, with a K$_m$ of 3 μM. In contrast, synthetic peptides lacking the complete γ-CRS were not efficiently carboxylated. These peptides included the pentapeptide substrate FLEEL (K$_m$ of 2200 μM) (90), a 20-residue peptide analogous to residues −10 to +10 in prothrombin, and a 10-residue peptide analogous to residues +1 to +10 in prothrombin. Recombinant protein C expressed in *Escherichia coli* incorporated ^{14}CO$_2$ into γ-carboxyglutamic acid only slightly better when the protein substrate also included a segment (residues −10 to −1) of the propeptide (95). Given that the propeptide of protein C extends from −24 to −1 (96), these results and those of Ulrich et al. (94) indicate the importance of the intact γ-CRS for efficient carboxylation both *in vivo* and *in vitro*.

Further characterization of the γ-CRS has better defined the requirements for recognition by the carboxylase. Mutagenesis of the propeptide of prothrombin indicated that a molecular surface of approximately five amino acids located within the propeptide, including residues −18, −17, −16, −15, and −10, define a carboxylation recognition site (97). Although Phe is preferred at residue −16, Leu, Val, and Lys at this position also support carboxylation (98). Based on affinities of the propeptides of a variety of vitamin K–dependent proteins for the carboxylase (99) and in subsequent mutagenesis studies, a consensus propeptide, AVFLSREQAN-QVLQRRRR, was identified that has higher affinity for carboxylase than any naturally occurring propeptide (100). In addition to those previously identified, this peptide illustrates the importance of residues at −6 and −9.

Two naturally occurring propeptide mutants of factor IX, Ala −10 to Thr or Val, have been described in humans. The phenotype and factor IX levels in the patients with these mutations were normal unless they were exposed to a vitamin K antagonist. Individuals with these mutations are extremely sensitive to coumarin-type anticoagulants, and these mutations are associated with severe inhibition of carboxylation in excess of that observed with the other vitamin K–dependent proteins (101,102).

Based on the predicted structure of the propeptide of factor X, Knobloch and Suttie (103) have proposed that an 18-residue peptide plays a regulatory role in carboxylation as an allosteric modifier of the vitamin K–dependent carboxylase. This peptide stimulates the carboxylation of a small synthetic substrate, but similar peptides inhibit the longer synthetic substrates that include the carboxylation recognition site (94). These results raise the possibility that the propeptide may be an allosteric regulator of the carboxylase as well as a recognition element.

An additional consensus sequence within the mature sequence of vitamin K–dependent proteins, Glu 16-Xaa-Xaa-Xaa-Glu 20-Xaa-Cys 22, has been proposed as a carboxylase recognition site (104). However, a double point mutant of prothrombin in which Ser residues substituted for Cys 17 and Cys 22 was fully carboxylated when expressed in Chinese hamster ovary cells (105). In addition, a prothrombin propeptide/thrombin chimera that juxtaposes the γ-CRS to a glutamate-rich C-terminal region of prothrombin was constructed. Seven or eight of the eight glutamic acids within the first 40 residues adjacent to the propeptide were carboxylated when this protein was expressed in Chinese hamster ovary cells (105). Except for the requirement that

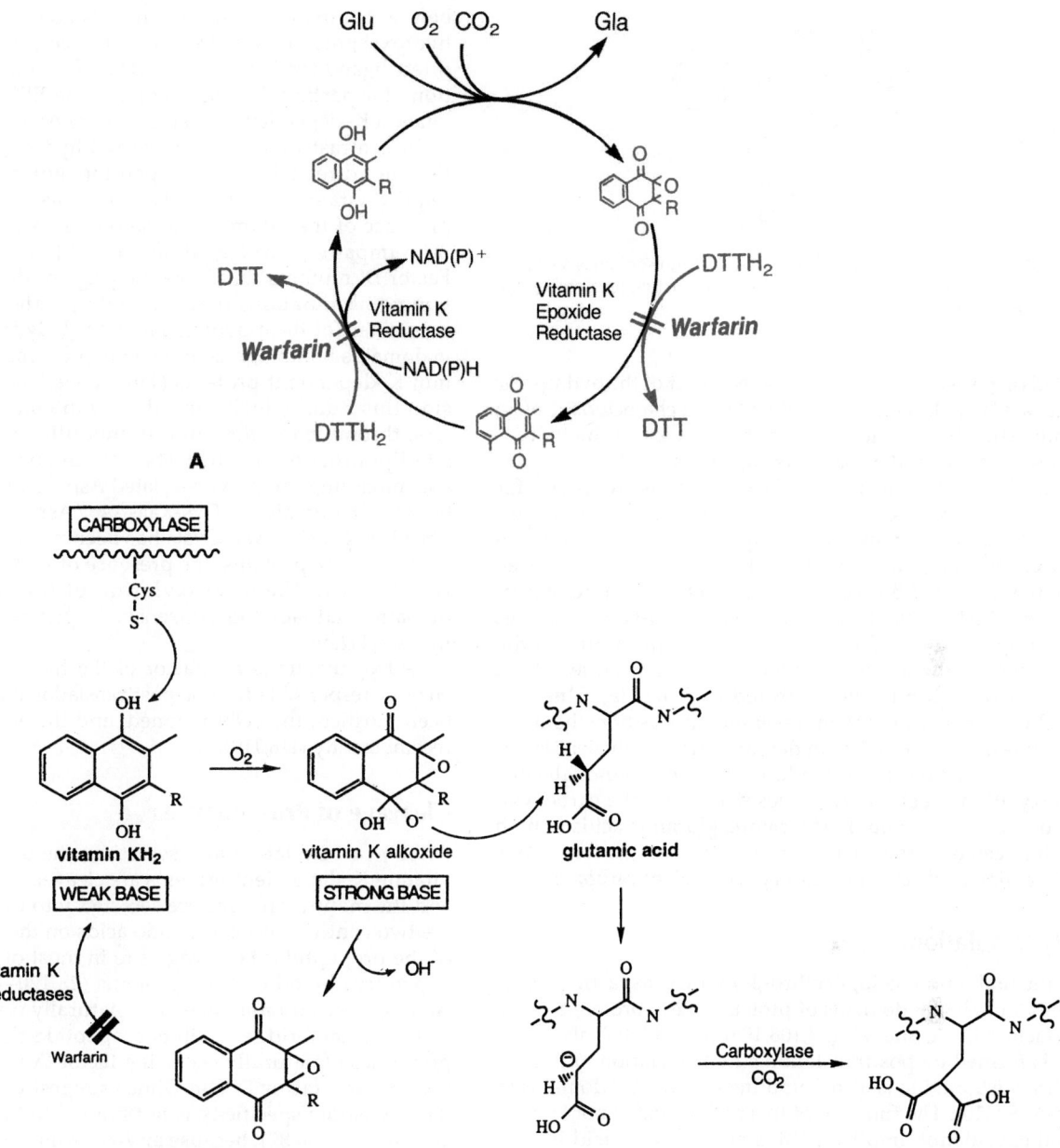

Figure 37-5. A: Vitamin K cycle. Vitamin K is an essential metabolite and can be considered a limited resource. Therefore, it is recovered in an altered form after carboxylation and recycled to its original chemical form. Vitamin K is reduced to vitamin KH_2. The vitamin K epoxide is formed by the vitamin K epoxidase that is closely linked to the vitamin K–dependent carboxylase. The vitamin K epoxide is then converted to vitamin K. **B:** Biosynthetic pathway for vitamin K–dependent production of γ-carboxyglutamic acid. It has been hypothesized that a free cysteine residue in the carboxylase converts vitamin KH_2 into a "strong base" of sufficient basicity to abstract a hydrogen from the γ-carbon of Glu. Subsequently, CO_2 is added to the γ-carbon of glutamic acid to form γ-carboxyglutamic acid. The activated vitamin K species collapses into vitamin K eposide and is recycled back to vitamin KH_2 after the action of two vitamin K reductases, one of which is sensitive to warfarin. (**B** from Furie B, Bouchard BA, Furie BC. Vitamin K–dependent biosynthesis of γ-carboxyglutamic acid. *Blood* 1999;93:1789, with permission.)

Glu residues are in close proximity to the γ-carboxylation recognition site, there is no compelling evidence that a consensus sequence or a unique amino acid sequence adjacent to the glutamic acids that are to be carboxylated is required for carboxylation. Within the 28-residue synthetic peptide representing –18 to +10 of the proprothrombin sequence, substitution of Ala or Asp for one of the two glutamic acids does not interfere with the carboxylation of the remaining Glu (106). Although the Asp or Ala residues do not become carboxylated, their presence does not inhibit carboxylation of the adjacent Glu. Furthermore, homologous synthetic peptides based on the primary structure of the propeptide and the first ten residues of factor IX are also efficiently carboxylated. These results suggest similar chemical surfaces on the propeptides of prothrombin and on factor IX despite the absence of perfect sequence homology in these structures. Analysis of the propeptide's structure suggests that the polypeptide backbone assumes an α helical structure (107). Propeptide models indicate that most of the hydrophobic amino acids are

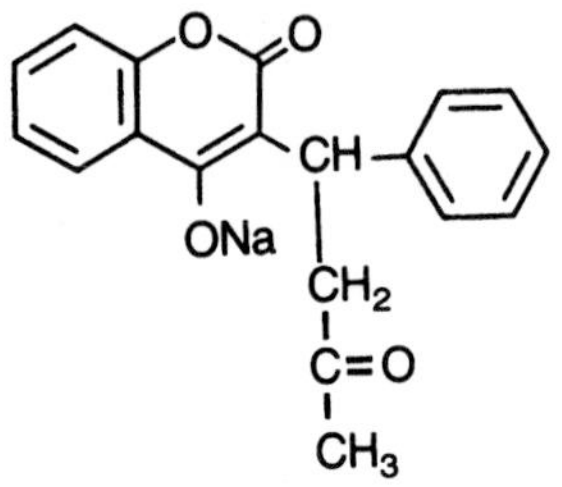

Figure 37-6. Chemical structure of warfarin. Warfarin sodium is a vitamin K antagonist that is used as an anticoagulant. Its structure reassembles the essential elements of vitamin K.

located on one side of the helix, whereas most of the hydrophilic amino acids are located on the other side, a characteristic of an amphipathic helix. The hydrophobic surface of the helix is assumed to be the carboxylation recognition site.

The vitamin K–dependent carboxylase is highly specific for Glu residues. Using small synthetic peptides, Asp residues can be β-carboxylated at approximately 10% of the rate of the γ-carboxylation of glutamic acids. Hubbard et al. (106), however, have not observed β-carboxylation of Asp in synthetic peptides that include the propeptide. When Glu-Glu sequences (homologous to residues 6 and 7 in prothrombin) in the 28-residue synthetic peptide (homologous to residues −18 to +10 in prothrombin) were altered to Glu-Ala, Glu-Asp, Ala-Glu, or Asp-Glu glutamyl residues at positions homologous to residues 6 and 7, both demonstrated equivalent kinetics of carboxylation. These results confirm that, although not a carboxylation substrate, Asp does not inhibit the carboxylation of an adjacent Glu. Furthermore, glutamic acids at both positions can be carboxylated. The presence of two contiguous acidic amino acids is not necessary for efficient carboxylation.

β-Hydroxylation

An unusual amino acid, erythro-β–hydroxyaspartic acid, is located in the EGF domains of protein C (26), protein S (108), and factors IX, X, and VII (27,108,109) (Fig. 37-8). This amino acid is formed by posttranslational hydroxylation of Asp. β-Hydroxyasparagine is also found in several EGF domains in protein S (110). The function of this amino acid is not known. Initial speculation implicated this novel amino acid in Ca^{2+} binding in the EGF domains (111,112). Although the two sequence motifs that determine calcium ion binding and β-hydroxylation of Asp or Asn appear to be coupled phylogenetically in Ca^{2+}-binding EGF modules, there are exceptions, such as the first EGF module of protein S, which contains the hydroxylation motif but lacks the Ca^{2+} consensus sequence

before the first Cys residue. There is no evidence that the β-hydroxyl group of β-hydroxyaspartic acid/asparagine forms a direct ligand for Ca^{2+} binding (113). The role of β-hydroxylation of aspartic acid/asparagine in the EFG domains of the vitamin K–dependent proteins remains obscure.

In contrast to γ-carboxylation, β-hydroxylation of factor IX is not directed by the propeptide, nor does this reaction require vitamin K. Similarly, synthesis of factor IX in the presence of the vitamin K antagonists such as sodium warfarin impairs γ-carboxylation but not β-hydroxylation (89). Factor IX mutants that have the propeptide deleted or contain point mutations that eliminate γ-carboxylation remain substrates for the β-hydroxylase (89). β-Hydroxylation occurs in domains homologous to the EGF precursor in certain vitamin K–dependent proteins (110) as well as in proteins outside this family, including the complement proteins C1r, C1s, thrombomodulin, and uromodulin, and the low-density lipoprotein receptor (114–116). A consensus sequence encompassing the β-hydroxylated Asp residue within a number of EGF domains, NCys-Xaa-Asp/Asn-Xaa-Xaa-Xaa-Xaa-Phe/Tyr-Xaa-Cys-Xaa-CysC has been noted by Stenflo et al. (110). In some proteins, the presence of an Asn in place of an Asp leads to the hydroxylation of the Asn (110). EGF domains that lack this consensus sequence do not undergo hydroxylation.

2-Oxoglutarate is a cofactor of the hydroxylase (117). The enzyme responsible for this posttranslational modification has been purified, the cDNA cloned, and the enzyme expressed recombinantly (118,119).

Cleavage of Prosequences

After γ-carboxylation and secretion, the propeptides of the vitamin K–dependent proteins are cleaved in the *trans*-Golgi, and the mature proteins are secreted into the plasma. There are two contiguous basic amino acids on the N-terminal side of the propeptidase cleavage site in most of the vitamin K–dependent blood clotting proteins (23,120–124) (Fig. 37-7). An Arg→Ser mutation at −1 in a naturally occurring mutant, factor IX Cambridge, inhibits propeptide cleavage (85). The properties of naturally occurring factor IX mutants, factor IX Oxford, and factor IX San Dimas suggest that the propeptidase substrate specificity is not limited to the basic residues at −1 and −2 (86,87), because an Arg→Gln substitution at residue −4 in the propeptide completely inhibits propeptide cleavage. Deletion mutations in protein C further emphasize the role of the four COOH-terminal amino acids of the propeptide (96). Furin has been implicated in the cleavage of the propeptide from factor IX (125). However, there is a large family of related proconvertases involved in cleavage of

Protein	−24	−23	−22	−21	−20	−19	−18	−17	−16	−15	−14	−13	−12	−11	−10	−9	−8	−7	−6	−5	−4	−3	−2	−1	+1
Factor IX							Thr	Val	Phe	Leu	Asp	His	Glu	Asn	Ala	Asn	Lys	Ile	Leu	Asn	Arg	Pro	Lys	Arg	Tyr
Prothrombin	Ser	Leu	Val	His	Ser	Gln	His	Val	Phe	Leu	Ala	Pro	Gln	Gln	Ala	Arg	Ser	Leu	Leu	Gln	Arg	Val	Arg	Arg	Ala
Factor X	Leu	Leu	Leu	Leu	Gly	Glu	Ser	Leu	Phe	Ile	Arg	Arg	Glu	Gln	Ala	Asn	Asn	Ile	Leu	Ala	Arg	Val	Thr	Arg	Ala
Protein C	Thr	Pro	Ala	Pro	Leu	Asp	Ser	Val	Phe	Ser	Ser	Ser	Glu	Arg	Ala	His	Gln	Val	Leu	Arg	Ile	Arg	Lys	Arg	Ala
Factor VII	Trp	Lys	Pro	Gly	Pro	His	Arg	Val	Phe	Val	Thr	Glu	Glu	Glu	Ala	His	Gly	Val	Leu	His	Arg	Arg	Arg	Arg	Ala
Protein S	Val	Leu	Pro	Val	Leu	Glu	Ala	Asn	Phe	Leu	Ser	Arg	Gln	His	Ala	Ser	Gln	Val	Leu	Ile	Arg	Arg	Arg	Arg	Ala
Bone Gla protein	Ser	Gly	Ala	Glu	Ser	Ser	Lys	Ala	Phe	Val	Ser	Lys	Gln	Glu	Gly	Ser	Glu	Val	Val	Lys	Arg	Pro	Arg	Arg	Tyr

Figure 37-7. Sequence homologies of the propeptide regions of the vitamin K–dependent proteins. The factor IX propeptide is 18 residues long. The γ-carboxylation recognition site is located on the propeptides of the vitamin K–dependent proteins. (From Furie B, Furie BC. Molecular basis of blood coagulation. *Cell* 1988;53:505.)

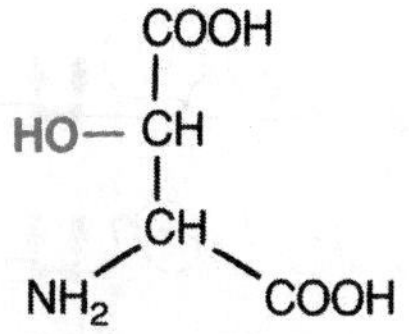

Figure 37-8. Chemical structure of β-hydroxyaspartic acid. This amino acid is observed in some epidermal growth factor domains of the vitamin K–dependent proteins. It is also observed in proteins that do not require vitamin K for their synthesis.

propeptides that contain Arg or Lys at the –2 position and Arg at –1. The actual procovertase that removes the propeptides of the vitamin K–dependent proteins is not known (126). Removal of the propeptide occurs late in the processing pathway (127). γ-Carboxylated extracellular vitamin K–dependent proteins bind to acidic membranes in the presence of calcium ions. It appears that the presence of the propeptide at the amino-terminus of the γ-carboxylated protein prevents the binding to the endoplasmic reticulum membrane where the calcium ion concentration is high enough to support binding of a mature γ-carboxylated vitamin K–dependent protein.

ROLE OF γ-CARBOXYGLUTAMIC ACID

γ-Carboxyglutamic acid residues (24,25), essential for biologic activity of these proteins, confer metal-binding properties on the vitamin K–dependent proteins and allow interaction with calcium ions and subsequent binding to phospholipid or membrane surfaces (81,128–131). The N-terminal sequences of the vitamin K–dependent proteins, including the distribution and spacing of the γ-carboxyglutamic acid residues, are homologous across species (e.g., bovine and human) and to each other (132–138). Studies of the γ-carboxyglutamic acid-metal complex in solution using nuclear magnetic resonance paramagnetic relaxation techniques (139) suggest that the metal is bound by one or both of the γ-carboxyl groups. The γ-carboxyl oxygens are coordinated to half the primary coordination sphere of the metal ion, leaving the other half available to interact with another γ-carboxyglutamic acid residue or another metal ligand. The metal ion therefore serves as an intramolecular bridge to link a γ-carboxyglutamic acid in one region of a protein to a γ-carboxyglutamic acid in another region (140).

The interaction of metal ions with γ-carboxyglutamic acid provides insight into the nature of the metal-binding sites of γ-carboxyglutamic acid-containing proteins like the vitamin K–dependent coagulation proteins. The proteins contain both high-affinity and low-affinity metal-binding sites (141–148). Occupancy of these sites by a variety of metal ions causes a conformational transition demonstrated by circular dichroism (149), fluorescence spectroscopy (150,151), and immunochemical studies using conformation-specific antibodies (152–156). This conformational transition has been localized to the N-terminal of prothrombin (157), and it is required to obtain the functionally active conformer capable of binding to membranes containing negatively charged phospholipid. The structure of the Gla domain and first kringle domain of prothrombin in the presence of calcium ions has been determined by x-ray crystallography (158). This structure showed that the Gla domain is highly structured and that most of the γ-carboxyglutamic acid side chains point inward to a linear array of internal calcium ions. Several of these calcium ions are com-

pletely sequestered inside the core of the Gla domain and not exposed to solvent.

COMMON FEATURES OF VITAMIN K–DEPENDENT BLOOD CLOTTING PROTEINS

The vitamin K–dependent plasma proteins involved in blood coagulation include the zymogens of four serine proteases: prothrombin and factors X, IX, and VII. As determined by amino acid sequence analysis (133–135,137,138,157,159,160) or by prediction of the amino acid sequence from the DNA sequence (23,121,123,124), these four proteins show marked homology to each other. They are composed of structural units or domains that are common to many other proteins. One commonality is that these proteins are zymogens (proenzymes) of serine proteases, which use catalytic mechanisms that involve a Ser in the active site (161).

The N-terminals of the vitamin K–dependent blood clotting proteins contain 10 to 12 γ-carboxyglutamic acid (Gla) residues within the first 42 amino acids (132–138). These amino acids bind calcium ions (139,140,162–165), forming a noncovalent intramolecular bridge between regions of the polypeptide backbone. This bond stabilizes the tertiary structure of this region of the protein (157). On binding calcium, the proteins undergo two conformational changes that expose a membrane-binding site (150,151,156,166,167). Although the Gla domain is required for these conformational transitions, it had been uncertain whether some of the γ-carboxyglutamic acids directly bind to membrane surfaces through calcium ion bridges (168) or whether metal binding to γ-carboxyglutamic acid in the Gla domain alters the structure of adjacent domains, exposing a membrane-binding surface (158,169,170). Recent x-ray crystallography studies of prothrombin fragment 1 bound to phospholipid have revealed that the interaction of the Gla domain with phospholipid membranes includes elements of both models. The group of amino acids that define the hydrophobic patch insert into the membrane (171), whereas the phosphoserine headgroup interacts with Arg 10 and Arg 16 and with a calcium ion bound to Gla 21 in bovine prothrombin (172).

The *aromatic amino acid stack*, a short linking segment that contains the sequence Phe-Trp-Xaa-Xaa-Tyr, is present in all the vitamin K–dependent blood coagulation proteins. Although hydrophobic, this region is on the surface of prothrombin fragment 1. This region is in fact an integral component of the Gla domain, a phospholipid-binding domain, because residues 1–42 of factor IX do not interact with phospholipid membranes, whereas residues 1–47 do (172a).

With the exception of prothrombin, the vitamin K–dependent blood coagulation proteins contain two EGF domains homologous to a domain in the EGF precursor (173). This domain is a 53–amino acid peptide containing three disulfide bonds that bind other proteins to specific cell-surface receptors (174,175). The EGF domains in the vitamin K–dependent proteins are involved in protein complex formation. The EGF domains may be responsible for the high-affinity interaction of some proteins with binding domains on other proteins, such as the cofactors factor VIII and factor V.

There are two *kringle domains* on prothrombin, each approximately 100 amino acids long (176). This domain contains three disulfide bonds. Its three-dimensional structure resembles an eccentric oblate ellipsoid, and its folding is defined by close contacts between the sulfur atoms of two of the disulfide bridges, which form a sulfur cluster in the center of the kringle (177).

Internal amino acids are well conserved among various proteins containing kringles. Differences in the molecular surfaces probably distinguish functional properties among proteins that contain kringle domains besides prothrombin, such as tissue plasminogen activator (178), factor XII (179), prourokinase (180), and plasminogen (181). These domains contain recognition elements important for protein assembly on membrane surfaces.

The *serine protease domain* is common to all of the vitamin K–dependent blood coagulation proteins. The structure and organization of genes among the serine proteases emphasize that the evolution of new protein function occurs via gene duplication, gene modification, and exon shuffling (182,183). Each of the exons may be considered a module coding for a homologous domain in each protein (Fig. 37-9). Evidence suggests that the three-dimensional structure of the polypeptide backbone of these domains is nearly identical. Substitutions in the amino acid side chains on the protein surfaces define the unique properties of substrate recognition, cofactor binding, or membrane interaction (184). The serine protease family as a whole, and the blood coagulation proteases in particular, remain a prime example of a family of proteins with diverse functional properties but common, unified structural elements.

The vitamin K–dependent blood clotting proteins circulate in the plasma in their proenzyme form (9,10). Each of these proteins is converted to its active enzyme by the cleavage of one or two peptide bonds. Like trypsin and other serine proteases, they contain the catalytic triad of a Ser, histidine (His), and Asp in the active enzyme site. In the blood clotting enzymes, the domain with marked sequence homology and presumed three-dimensional structural homology (184) with trypsin is known as the *catalytic domain*. The blood clotting serine proteases have an active site and an internal core that is nearly identical to trypsin; however, the different molecular surfaces that surround the enzyme active site provide substrate-binding sites and are responsible for the unique substrate specificities of these enzymes.

PROTHROMBIN

Gene Structure

The human (161) and bovine (185) prothrombin genes are partially homologous to those encoding the other vitamin K–dependent proteins (Fig. 37-10). The human prothrombin gene is located in chromosome 11 (186); it includes approximately 24 kb of DNA and contains 14 exons. As shown in Figure 37-10, exon I encodes the signal peptide. Exon II encodes the propeptide (including the γ-carboxylation recognition site) (84,96) and the Gla domain. Exon III encodes the aromatic amino acid stack domain. Exons I, II, and III are homologous in structure and organization to the same exons in the factor IX gene family, which includes factors IX, X, and VII and protein C (187–190). Exons IV, V, VI, and VII encode the two kringle regions. These domains are not parallel with structures in the factor IX family but are observed in other proteins involved in hemostasis, including tissue plasminogen activator (178), plasminogen (181), prourokinase (180), and factor XII (179). Exons VIII and IX encode for the sites of proteolytic cleavage by factor Xa, which converts prothrombin to thrombin. The catalytic domain of thrombin is responsible for enzyme catalysis and substrate specificity; it is encoded by exons X, XI, XII, XIII, and XIV.

Despite the structural homologies of the catalytic domains in the vitamin K–dependent proteins, this portion of the gene's organization differs from the coding for the analogous domains in the factor IX gene family (191). In prothrombin, the amino acids that form the catalytic triad of serine proteases are

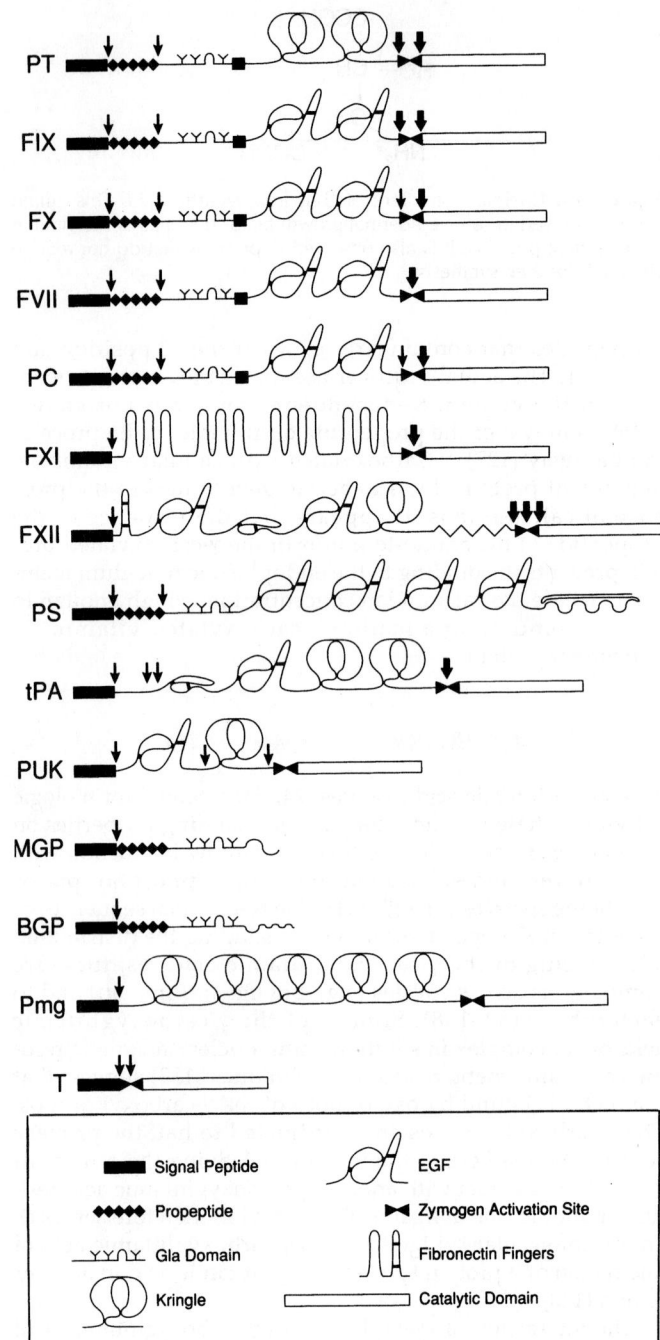

Figure 37-9. Domain structure of the vitamin K–dependent proteins and other proteins that are structurally or functionally related. Domains indicated include the signal peptide, the propeptide, the Gla domain, the epidermal growth factor (EGF) domain, the repeat sequences, the kringle region, the fibronectin (type I and II) domains, the aromatic amino acid stack, the zymogen activation region, and the catalytic domain. The sites of proteolytic cleavage associated with synthesis of the mature protein are indicated by thin arrows. The sites of proteolytic cleavage associated with zymogen activation are indicated by the thick arrows. BGP, bone Gla protein; FIX, factor IX; FVII, factor VII; FX, factor X; FXI, factor XI; FXII, factor XII; MGP, matrix Gla protein; PC, protein C; Pmg, plasminogen; PS, protein S; PT, prothrombin; PUK, prourokinase; T, trypsin; tPA, tissue-type plasminogen activator. (From Furie B, Furie BC. Molecular basis of blood coagulation. *Cell* 1988;53:505.)

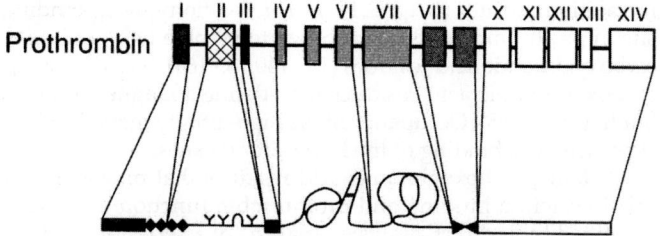

Figure 37-10. Gene structure of human prothrombin. Exons are shown schematically according to scale. Introns, indicated by double lines, are not drawn to scale. (From Furie B, Furie BC. Molecular basis of blood coagulation. *Cell* 1988;53:505.)

encoded in a separate exon, with His in exon X, Asp in exon XI, and Ser in exon XIII.

Protein Structure

The amino acid sequence of human prothrombin is diagrammed in Figure 37-11 (133,159). The sequences of the signal peptide and propeptide are also presented in Figure 37-11 (121,192). Human prothrombin is composed of a single polypeptide chain made up of 579 amino acids. Prothrombin is a glycoprotein; approximately 10% of its mass is carbohydrate. *N*-Asparagine–linked carbohydrate is attached to Asn 78, Asn 100, and Asn 373 in bovine prothrombin (193). Human prothrombin likely contains carbohydrate in analogous posi-

tions because these Asn residues are conserved in the bovine and human prothrombin sequences. Bovine prothrombin contains complex Asn-linked oligosaccharides that include NeuAcα2→3Galβ1→3(NeuAcα2→6)GlcNAc components in the outer chain. The structure of these complex carbohydrates is known and includes Galβ1→3GlcNAc (193).

The ten γ-carboxyglutamic acid residues, located near the amino terminal of the protein, are found at positions 6, 7, 14, 16, 19, 20, 25, 26, 29, and 32 in human prothrombin (133). Individual mutation of most of these γ-carboxyglutamic acid residues interferes with stabilization of protein structure, phospholipid binding, or both (194). This γ-carboxyglutamic acid–rich domain contains the calcium-binding sites of prothrombin (141,157). This region is responsible for the membrane-binding properties of prothrombin and also interacts with factor V during formation of the complex of prothrombin with the prothrombinase complex (195). Abnormal prothrombin lacks γ-carboxyglutamic acid residues and does not interact with calcium (80,81,131,196). This interaction is critical for calcium-dependent prothrombin–membrane interaction (130).

Prothrombin contains two kringle domains, each composed of 79 amino acid residues (191). These structures have a characteristic distribution of cysteines that form a cluster of disulfide bonds in the center of each kringle. The three-dimensional structure of this region has been determined by x-ray crystallography (177). The kringles play a role in protein assembly, interacting with the cofactor, factor V (197,198).

The serine protease domain stretches for approximately 250 amino acids and is homologous to the prototypic serine protease,

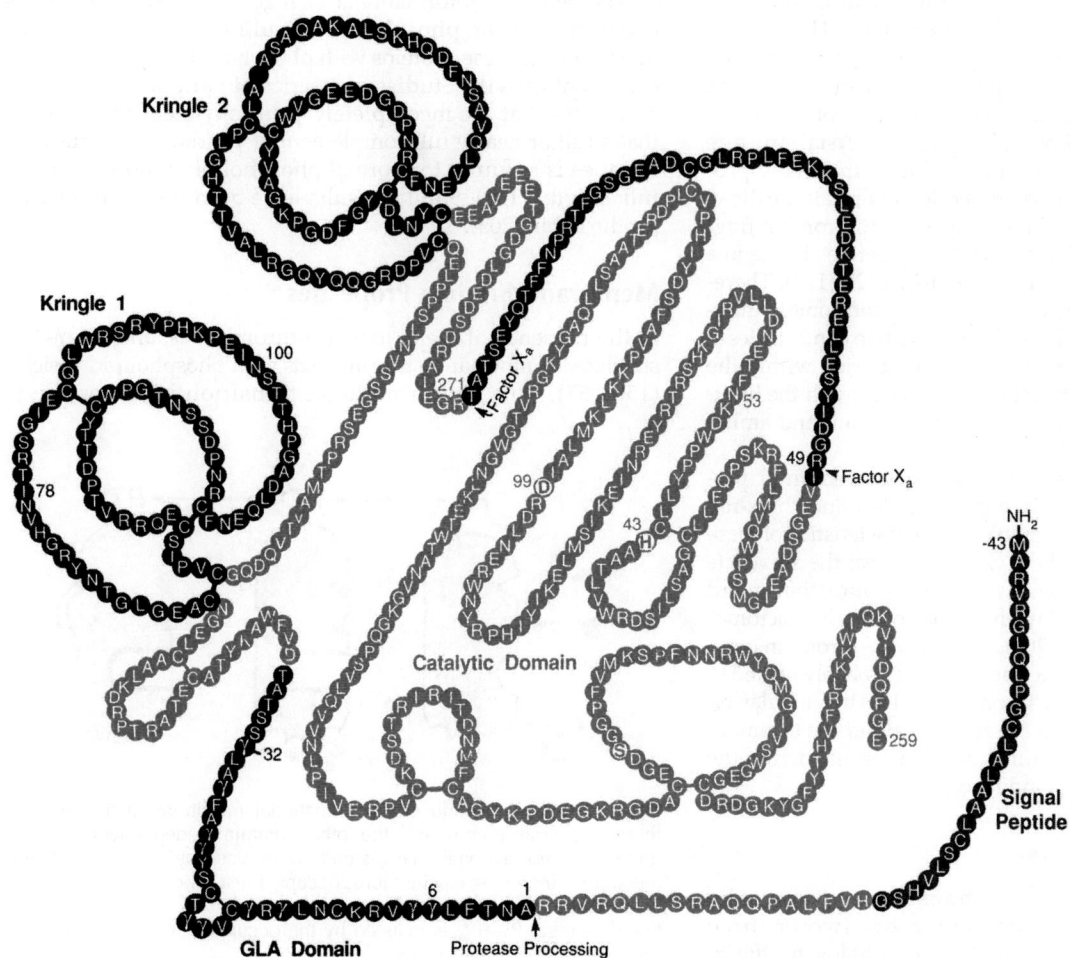

Figure 37-11. Amino acid sequence of human prothrombin.

trypsin (161). Approximately 33% of this region, representing the enzyme thrombin, demonstrates marked sequence homology to trypsin (159). The cleavage of two peptide bonds in the activation region of the serine protease domain converts the zymogen prothrombin to the enzyme thrombin. In the absence of crystallographic studies, a computer model of thrombin provided a first approximation of the three-dimensional structure of this enzyme (184). This model was based on the assumption that the marked sequence homology of trypsin to thrombin predicts homology of the tertiary structure. It also emphasizes the similarity of trypsin to thrombin in the internal core and in the complete preservation of the active site. Thrombin has now been crystallized and its structure determined. The differences lie in the unique molecular surfaces of thrombin and trypsin that impart unique functional properties to these proteins. This surface defines unique substrate specificity for the macromolecular substrate by use of an extended substrate-binding site around the active site.

Although intact prothrombin has not been crystallized, the structure of individual domains of prothrombin have been determined by x-ray crystallography. The N-terminal 156 amino acids of prothrombin, known as *fragment 1*, includes the Gla domain. This region, specifically the Gla domain, is responsible for the membrane-binding properties of prothrombin. This fragment has been crystallized in the presence of calcium ions and its three-dimensional structure determined (199). The structure of the Gla domain–calcium ion complex reveals that the calcium ions are internal in the structure, and most are not exposed to the external solvent. These calcium ions are chelated by multiple γ-carboxyglutamic acid residues that form a coordinated calcium–carboxylate network. By stabilizing the polypeptide backbone of the metal-dependent conformer, calcium induces a structural transition that leads to the exposure of three hydrophobic residues on the surface that form a hydrophobic patch. The specificity of the calcium-stabilized form of fragment 1 for phospholipid membranes that include phosphatidylserine can be understood by analysis of the structure of the ternary complex of prothrombin fragment 1, calcium, and phospholipid. The crystal structure of the complex of lysophosphatidylserine with bovine prothrombin fragment 1 in the presence of calcium reveals the direct interaction between phosphatidylserine and prothrombin fragment 1. The head groups of lysophosphatidylserine chelate to a specific calcium ion, which is anchored to Gla 21 (172). Therefore, it would appear that the Gla domain of prothrombin interacts with acidic phospholipid membranes via two contact sites: a hydrophobic cluster of amino acids that are buried within the membrane, and the ionic interactions associated with the binding of the phosphoserine head group with calcium and amino acid side chains of prothrombin.

The structure of thrombin, the enzyme derived from prothrombin via limited proteolysis, has been determined by x-ray crystallography. The B chain resembles the characteristic polypeptide fold of serine proteases. The A chain folds near the active site of the enzyme. Several protuberances, unique to thrombin, guard the active site and probably play an important role in macromolecular substrate recognition (200). The hirudin–thrombin complex shows many contact sites, a feature that is probably related to the high affinity of hirudin for thrombin (201). The globular N-terminal domain interacts with the region around the thrombin active site. An extended C-terminal domain reaches across the thrombin surface to the anion-binding exosite.

Calcium-Binding Properties

The metal-binding properties of prothrombin are conferred by γ-carboxyglutamic acids. Prothrombin has two or three high-affinity metal-binding sites and four to eight lower-affinity

metal-binding sites (141,142,144). A high-affinity metal-binding site in prothrombin has been shown to involve two or three γ-carboxyglutamic acid residues (139,140,163,164), but only two γ-carboxyglutamic acid residues may define a magnesium ion-binding site (165). Occupancy of the high-affinity metal-binding sites facilitates binding of the lower-affinity sites.

Certain γ-carboxyglutamic acid residues that play a critical role in calcium binding and prothrombin function have been identified by indirect analysis. Analysis of a series of partially carboxylated prothrombins from a patient with a hereditary defect in carboxylation suggests that Gla 16 plays a special role in calcium binding and is the high-affinity metal-binding site in prothrombin (196,202). This observation is consistent with earlier spectroscopic results that suggested that this residue might be involved in high-affinity metal binding (140).

Metal-Induced Conformational Transitions

The addition of metal ions, including most divalent cations, induces an alteration in the conformation of prothrombin. This conformational change can be monitored by the quenching of the intrinsic fluorescence of the protein (150,151), by perturbation of the structure of the polypeptide backbone as monitored by circular dichroism measurements (149), or by the expression of new antigenic determinants on the metal-stabilized conformer (152–156). Only calcium ions, however, convert prothrombin to the active conformer that can bind to membrane surfaces. It appears that calcium also induces a second metal-dependent conformational transition, as has been observed by immunochemical techniques (156). Both conformational transitions are induced by only calcium ions (Fig. 37-12).

The second conformational change is associated with the expression of the phospholipid-binding sites necessary for interaction of these proteins with phospholipid surfaces and for coagulant activity. Studies of a series of variant prothrombin molecules that are incompletely γ-carboxylated demonstrate that a full or nearly full complement of γ-carboxyglutamic acid residues is required for normal phospholipid binding and for full activity (196). Similar results have been found for bovine prothrombin (203).

Membrane-Binding Properties

In the presence of metal ions, prothrombin assumes a metal-stabilized conformation that interacts with phospholipid vesicles (150,167). This conformational transition involves the γ-

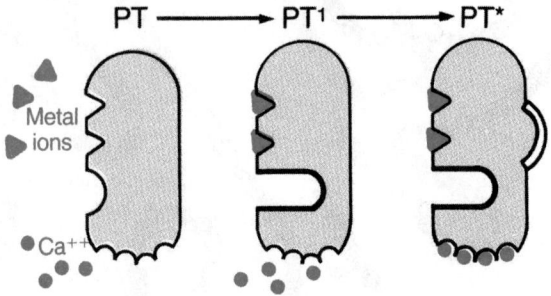

Figure 37-12. Metal-induced conformational transitions in human prothrombin. Prothrombin and the other vitamin K–dependent proteins undergo conformational changes that are induced by metal ions. Many metal ions, including calcium ions, occupy a first set of binding sites that leads to an initial conformational change, PT→P¹. A second conformational change, P¹→P*, is induced by the occupancy of a second set of metal-binding sites by calcium.

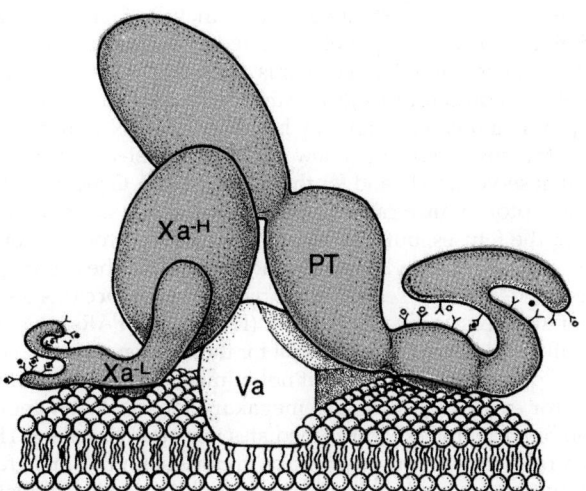

Figure 37-13. A model for protein complex formation associated with zymogen activation. The proteins involved in blood coagulation assemble on membrane surfaces. The interaction of calcium ions with the γ-carboxyglutamic acids on the vitamin K–dependent proteins stabilizes a conformer of the protein that expresses a membrane binding site. This assembly facilitates enzyme–substrate interaction. The protein cofactor may have a regulatory role in this complex. Open and filled circles, calcium ions; dark patch, lipid binding sites; PT, prothrombin substrate; Va, cofactor; Xa-H, heavy-chain enzyme; Xa-L, light-chain enzyme; Y, γ-carboxyglutamic acid. (From Furie B, Furie BC. Molecular basis of blood coagulation. *Cell* 1988;53:505.)

carboxyglutamic acid residues (161). Prothrombin has a strong preference for phospholipid vesicles composed of acidic phospholipids, specifically phosphatidylserine (167). Interaction of prothrombin with phospholipid vesicles containing phosphatidylserine and phosphatidylcholine requires calcium ions; a binding constant (K_d) of 2.3 μM describes this interaction (204–206). The phospholipid-binding properties of prothrombin are resident in the Gla domain.

Assembly of the Prothrombinase Complex

The activation of prothrombin requires the assembly of the enzyme, factor Xa, and the active cofactor, factor Va, on phospholipid vesicles in the presence of calcium ions (Fig. 37-13). This macromolecular assembly—called the *prothrombinase complex*—efficiently cleaves prothrombin to thrombin (207,208). A mathematic model of this process has been developed to simulate the kinetics of prothrombin activation by the prothrombinase complex (209). If factor Va or phospholipid membranes are deleted from the system, the relative rate of conversion of prothrombin decreases from 100% to 0.13% and 0.008%, respectively. If both factor Va and phospholipid membranes are removed from the activation mixture, the relative rate of prothrombin activation is decreased from 100% to 0.0007%. Factor Xa alone activates prothrombin at a relative rate of 0.0003%. Therefore, formation of the complete prothrombinase complex enhances the rate of factor Xa activation of prothrombin to thrombin approximately 300,000 times.

Although prothrombin alone does not bind to cells, the prothrombinase complex assembles on cell surfaces. Prothrombinase activity has been detected on platelets, endothelial cells (210,211), monocytes, leukocytes (212,213), and diseased aorta (214). Platelets bind approximately 1000 factor Va molecules with high affinity (178). These high-affinity sites are not accessible to factor V, which binds to lower-affinity sites. Once bound, factor Va provides the receptor for factor Xa interaction

(215,216). Although the liver is the primary site of synthesis for factor V, factor V is also synthesized in megakaryocytes and stored in platelet α granules along with other proteins. On platelet stimulation and activation, platelet factor V is secreted and immediately binds to the plasma membrane in an active form (factor Va) (217).

Activation of Prothrombin

The proteolytic events leading to *in vitro* activation of prothrombin have been well characterized (Fig. 37-14). Prothrombin is converted to thrombin by the action of the enzyme factor Xa in a reaction that requires calcium ions and is greatly accelerated by factor Va and phospholipid vesicles (207). Activation requires the sequential cleavage of at least two peptide bonds (214,218–224). The cleavage of the Arg 271-Thr 272 bond yields prothrombin fragment 1β2 and prethrombin 2. The cleavage of the Arg 322-Ile 323 bond in prethrombin 2 then yields fully active thrombin that contains two chains, A and B, connected by a disulfide bond (225). The precursor, prethrombin 2, has no enzymatic activity. Cleavage of prothrombin instead of prethrombin 2 at the Arg 322-Ile 323 bond generates meizothrombin, a form of thrombin that has enzymatic activity toward small synthetic substrates but that does not proteolyze macromolecular substrates (226). Specifically, meizothrombin does

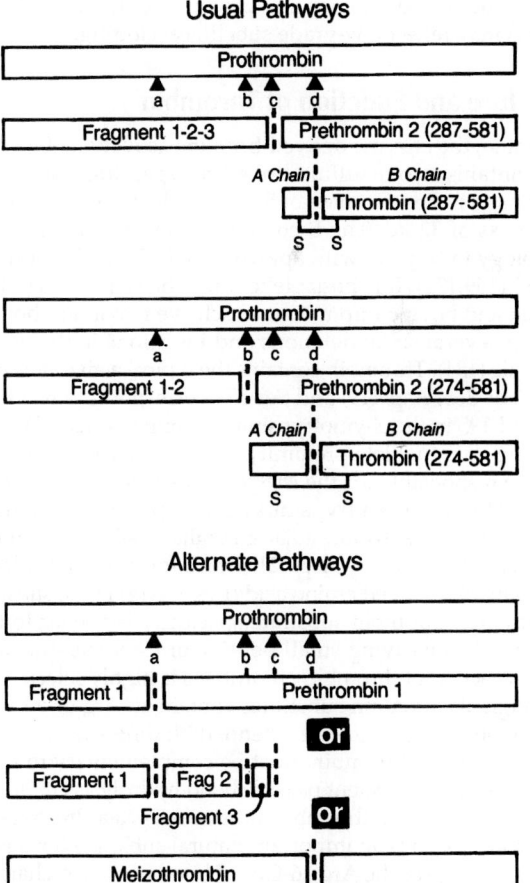

Figure 37-14. Activation pathways of human prothrombin. Prothrombin is cleaved at up to four sites (*arrowheads*) during activation to thrombin. Cleavage sites d and either b or c are required for thrombin formation. The intermediates that are generated depend on the conditions of the reaction. In plasma, it appears that the cleavage of bonds c and d occur without the cleavage at a and b.

not convert fibrinogen to fibrin. *In vitro*, thrombin generated during the activation of prothrombin can cleave the Arg 155-Ser 156 bond in prothrombin to yield fragment 1 (residues 1 to 155) and prethrombin 1, or the Arg 155-Ser 156 bond in fragment 1·2 to yield fragment 1 and fragment 2 (227).

During prothrombin activation in plasma, fragments 1 and 2 are not generated, indicating that the Arg 155-Ser 156 bond is not cleaved by thrombin under physiologic conditions (228). When human prothrombin is activated in plasma, fragment 1·2·3 and a shortened form of prethrombin 2 are formed by the cleavage of Arg 284-Thr 286 (229). Under these conditions, cleavage of the Arg 271-Thr 272 bond observed *in vitro* is not seen. The precise activation pathway for the *in vivo* generation of thrombin is not certain. Antibodies that detect fragment 1·2 cross-react with fragment 1·2·3 (230). Therefore, of the four bonds in prothrombin that potentially could be cleaved during prothrombin activation, two (Fig. 37-14, bonds c and d) are definitely cleaved, one (bond b) may be cleaved, and one (bond a) is not cleaved.

The *in vivo* activation of prothrombin can be monitored by the appearance of circulating fragment 1·2/fragment 1·2·3 (231). Given the pathways described, the generation of each thrombin molecule generates either a fragment 1·2 or fragment 1·2·3 molecule. Thus, the plasma fragment 1·2 level accurately reflects the *in vivo* activation of prothrombin. The measurement of prothrombin activation by this methodology offers considerable insight into hypercoagulable states (232). Studies with this technique have shown elevation of fragment 1·2 in patients with antithrombin III deficiency and protein C deficiency. These elevations may reflect low-grade subclinical clotting.

Structure and Function of Thrombin

Thrombin, the enzyme derived from the activation of prothrombin, contains two disulfide-linked polypeptide chains. The A chain has a molecular mass of 5 kd, and the B chain has a molecular mass of 32 kd. The B chain shows remarkable sequence homology to trypsin, with approximately 70% of residues conserved (159,191). It is possible to align the sequences of bovine trypsin and bovine thrombin and achieve maximum homology placing several small deletions and insertions in the thrombin molecule (184). Thrombin contains the typical active site catalytic triad. His 365, Asp 419, and Ser 527 correspond to residues 57, 102, and 195 in the chymotrypsin numbering system. These residues are in immediate proximity to each other in the active site and are responsible for the *charge relay system* in all serine proteases. Thrombin is a trypsinlike serine protease, requiring an Arg or Lys in the substrate adjacent to the sessile bond. Thrombin specificity is defined by Asp 521, which forms a salt bridge with the positively charged amino acid (Lys or Arg) in the substrate.

Although thrombin substrate specificity is similar to that of trypsin when cleaving small peptide or ester substrates (233–235), the action of thrombin on proteins is highly selective (236). Although all thrombin substrates contain an Arg or a Lys adjacent to the sessile bond, the extended binding site surrounding the active site of thrombin must be complementary to the protein substrate for efficient peptide bond hydrolysis (184). A common cleavage site in thrombin substrates is Xaa-Pro-Arg-↓–Xaa (236). Fibrinogen is an important natural substrate for thrombin (236). Cleavage of the Arg 16-Gly 17 bond in the Aα chain leads to the release of fibrinopeptide A and the polymerization of fibrin. Cleavage of the Arg 14-Gly 15 bond in the Bβ chain leads to the release of fibrinopeptide B. Thrombin also cleaves two critical bonds in factor VIII, both adjacent to Arg 372 and to Arg 1689, leading to the expression of factor VIIIa activity (237). Similarly, thrombin cleaves two critical bonds in factor V, leading to the expression of the active cofactor, factor Va (238,239). Other

physiologically important substrates include factor XIII (240) and glycoprotein V on platelets cleared by thrombin (241).

The platelet thrombin receptor is a member of the seven transmembrane domain receptor family. Thrombin activates this receptor in a unique manner by hydrolyzing an N-terminal fragment, thereby producing a new amino terminal–activating peptide that serves as a ligand for the receptor (242). Gene deletion of this receptor in mice causes embryonic death in approximately half of the fetuses, but the remaining embryos produce normal adult mice without a bleeding tendency (243). These data provided evidence for a second thrombin receptor. Since this discovery of a protease-activated receptor (PAR), other PARs have been identified (244). PAR1 is important for thrombin-mediated activation of platelets in humans but not in mice; PAR3 is a thrombin receptor expressed in mouse megakaryocytes. PAR4, another thrombin-activating receptor, mediates thrombin signaling. Thus, a two-receptor system appears to be important for thrombin function on platelets and relates blood coagulation to inflammation and blood vessel development (245).

Thrombin also serves as a substrate. α-Thrombin undergoes limited autodigestion *in vitro*, with hydrolysis of the B chain from a molecular mass of 32 to 28 kd (246). This reaction produces β-thrombin, which cannot convert fibrinogen to fibrin but which retains hydrolytic activity toward small synthetic substrates. Autolysis of β-thrombin to γ-thrombin is associated with further reduction of the B chain to a molecular mass of 15 kd and total loss of enzymatic activity.

After activation, thrombin circulates only briefly in plasma. Several proteins inhibit thrombin function. Antithrombin III, also known as *heparin cofactor*, forms a complex with thrombin that completely inhibits coagulant activity (247,248). The formation kinetics of this complex are greatly accelerated by heparin (249). Antithrombin III plays a critical role in regulating blood coagulation by scavenging active thrombin molecules that have wandered from tissue injury and bleeding sites. Other plasma inhibitors of thrombin that are of possible physiologic importance include α₂-macroglobulin (250) and α₁-antiprotease (251). Measurement of the thrombin–antithrombin complex may be a useful quantitative marker of thrombin generation (232,252,253).

Hirudin is a potent anticoagulant found in leeches (254) that binds to thrombin and inhibits thrombin function. Recombinant hirudin is an important anticoagulant agent, particularly in cases in which heparin can not be used (255). The globular N-terminal domain interacts with the region around the thrombin active site. An extended C-terminal domain reaches across the thrombin surface to the anion-binding exosite.

Physiology of Prothrombin

Prothrombin is synthesized exclusively in the liver within the hepatocyte (19–21). Although the control mechanisms that regulate prothrombin gene expression and biosynthesis are unknown, the prothrombin level in plasma is tightly controlled at 100 μg/mL (256,257). A biologic activity known as *coagulopoietin II* has been described (258,259). This material activity increases the level of prothrombin. Under normal conditions, prothrombin does not form a complex with other plasma proteins but circulates free in the blood in its zymogen form. The basal conversion rate of prothrombin to thrombin is low in the absence of tissue injury. Even in the event of localized clot formation, the prothrombin level does not change measurably, indicating that minimal amounts of prothrombin are consumed while generating physiologically relevant quantities of thrombin (260). The plasma half-life of prothrombin is approximately 3 days.

Inactivation of the prothrombin gene by targeted gene disruption in mice leads to partial embryonic lethality. More than half of the prothrombin null embryos died between embryonic days 9.5 and 11.5 due to bleeding into the yolk sac cavity and varying degrees of tissue necrosis. Approximately one-quarter of the homozygous null mice survived to term but developed fatal hemorrhage and died within a few days of birth. These observations demonstrate that prothrombin, or the thrombin derived from prothrombin, is important in maintaining vascular integrity during development as well as hemostasis in postnatal life (261).

Warfarin sodium and other vitamin K antagonists inhibit the posttranslational γ-carboxylation of prothrombin (80,81). Warfarin also inhibits synthesis of prothrombin antigen, as shown by a 30% decrease in total prothrombin antigen in the plasma of patients treated with warfarin (257).

FACTOR X

Gene Structure

The factor X gene is 22 kb long and is located on the long arm of chromosome 13 at 13q34. The coding region is found on eight separate exons (187) (Fig. 37-15). Exon I encodes the signal peptide. Exon II encodes the propeptide and Gla domain. Exon III codes for the aromatic amino acid stack domain. Exons IV and V each code the EGF-like regions of factor X. Exon VI encodes the activation domain of factor X, whereas exons VII and VIII encode the catalytic domain. The organization of the factor X gene is nearly identical to that of factors IX and VII and protein C. After transcription, a factor X message is generated that is approximately 1.5 kb long (124). This messenger RNA includes a short 3' untranslated region of 10 nucleotides that follow the stop codon TGA. The polyadenylation site is embedded in the 3' end of the coding sequence.

Protein Structure

Factor X (molecular weight 56,000) is synthesized as a single chain (122,124) but is converted to a two-chain zymogen that circulates in the plasma. The heavy chain of bovine and human factor X has a molecular mass of approximately 380 kd (160,262,263); the light chain is approximately 18 kd (134,135). The primary structure of human factor X, extrapolated from the cDNA of factor X (122,124), is shown in Figure 37-16. The three amino acids Arg-Lys-Arg at residues 139 to 141 are removed from the single chain by cleavage of the Arg 139-Lys 140 bond and of the Arg 141-Ser 142 bond. This generates the light chain (residues 1 to 139) and the heavy chain (residues 142 to 445) (124). This segment may be removed within the cell, but the presence of some single-chain factor X circulating in the plasma suggests that cleavage is inefficient or that the process is also extracellular.

The light chain of human factor X includes 11 γ-carboxyglutamic acid residues, and the first EGF domain includes a single β-hydroxyaspartic acid at residue 63 (27,128). γ-Carboxyglutamic acid residues are found at positions 6, 7, 14, 16, 19, 20, 25, 26, 29, 32, and 39 (136). The activation peptide is cleaved from the heavy chain during activation of factor X by the factor IXa–factor VIIIa complex or by the factor VIIa–tissue factor complex to yield the enzyme factor Xa (264,265). It remains closely associated with factor Xa (266). The remaining portion of the heavy chain contains the catalytic region that is homologous to trypsin. Nonphysiologic activation of factor X by the coagulant protein of Russell viper venom yields the same reaction products (266,267). The catalytic triad characteristic of the serine proteases includes Ser 233, His 93, and Asp 138 in bovine factor X (268). The process of factor X activation involves functionally significant but structurally subtle conformational changes in factor X (269).

Bovine factor X contains both Asn-linked carbohydrate of Asp 36 and Thr-linked carbohydrate at Thr 300 (270). The complex Asn-linked oligosaccharides have NeuAcα2→3Galβ1→3 (NeuAcα2→6)GlcNAc components in the outer chain.

Three-Dimensional Structure

The three-dimensional structure of factor Xa lacking the Gla domain has been determined by x-ray crystallography (271,272). Although the first EGF domain is flexible, the second EGF domain makes contact with the catalytic domain. The polypeptide backbone of the catalytic domain has a fold characteristic of Ser proteases.

Assembly of Factor X on Membrane Surfaces

Factor X is a metal-binding protein that contains two or three high-affinity sites and multiple lower-affinity sites (143,148). Factor X undergoes a conformational transition during metal binding that leads to the expression of both lipid-binding sites and new antigenic determinants (166,204,206,273,274). The concentration of calcium that induces the half-maximal transition is approximately 200 μM. Factor X binds to phospholipid vesicles in the presence of calcium ions with a preference for acidic phospholipids (e.g., phosphatidylserine) that is characteristic of the vitamin K–dependent proteins (206).

Factor Xa is the enzyme component of the prothrombinase complex. This complex includes factor Xa and factor Va and assembles on phospholipid surfaces in the presence of calcium ions.

Factor Xa also binds tightly to platelet membranes in the presence of factor Va, catalyzing the conversion of prothrombin to thrombin (216,275). Thrombin-activated platelets express approximately 300 factor Xa–binding sites, whereas resting platelets do not bind to factor Xa. The interaction of factor Xa and activated platelets is of high affinity, with a binding constant of 3×10^{-11} M determined (216,275). The factor Xa–binding site appears to be defined by factor V (215,276), and activation

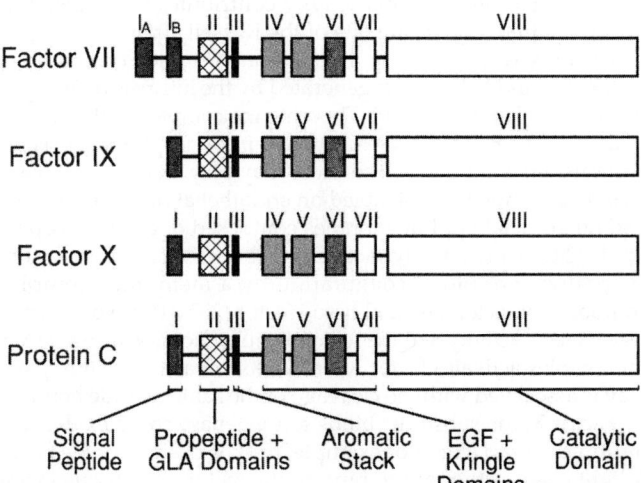

Figure 37-15. Gene structure of human factor X, factor VII, factor IX, and protein C. Exons are shown schematically according to scale. Introns, indicated by double lines, are not drawn to scale. EGF, epidermal growth factor. (From Furie B, Furie BC. Molecular basis of blood coagulation. *Cell* 1988;53:505.)

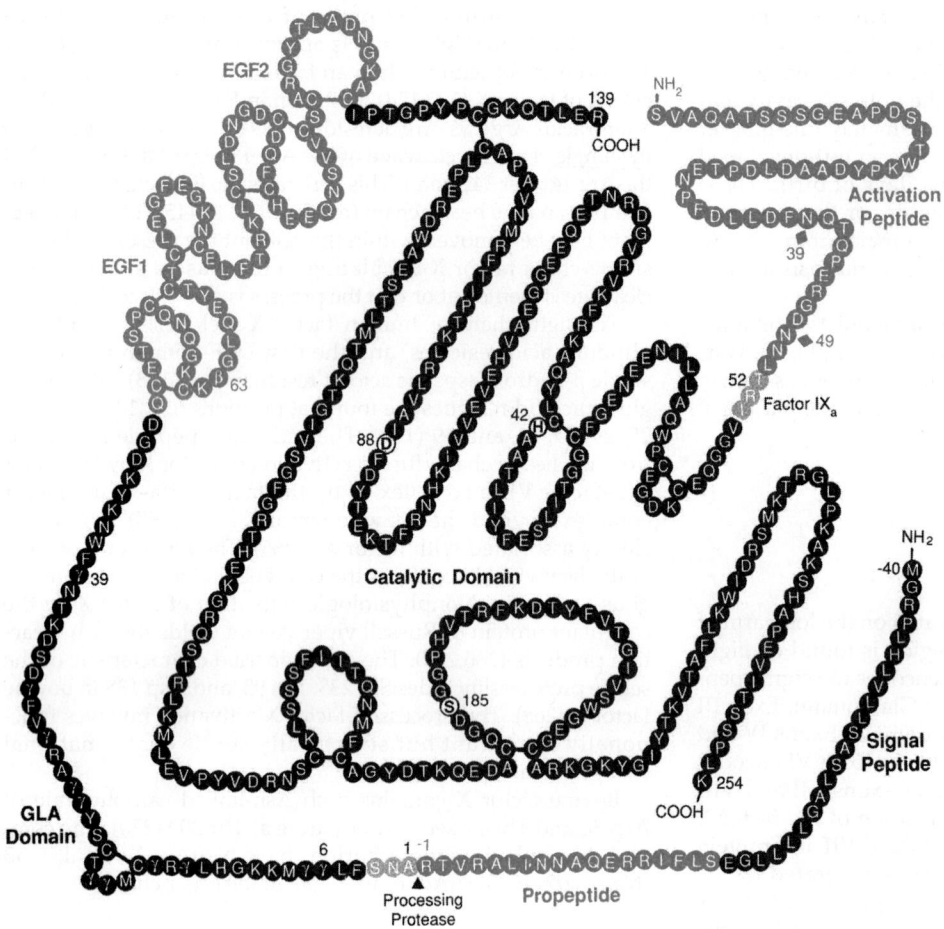

Figure 37-16. Amino acid sequence of human factor X.

of platelets leads to the secretion of factor Va from the α granules. Patients with factor V deficiency lack the expression of factor Xa–binding sites (217).

Activation of Factor X

Factor X is activated by the cleavage of a single peptide bond between Arg 51 and Ile 52 on the heavy chain (267,268) (Fig. 37-17). The activation peptide (1 to 51) remains noncovalently associated with factor Xa (266). Cleavage of a peptide bond near

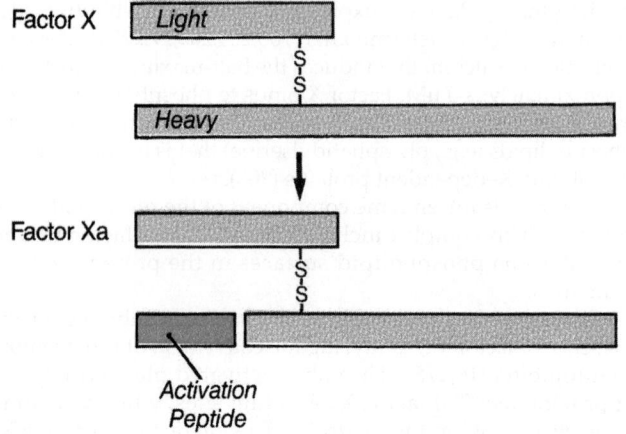

Figure 37-17. Activation of factor X. Factor X is activated to factor Xa by the factor IXa–factor VIII complex or the factor VIIa–tissue factor complex. A single bond is cleaved, generating an activation peptide.

the carboxy terminal is considered a side reaction with no functional consequences (265). Several proteases are physiologically important activators of factor X, including factors IXa and VIIa. Other factor X activators play a pathologic role. For example, activation of factor X by trypsin may occur under pathologic conditions, as in severe pancreatitis. A factor X activator has been isolated from lung carcinoma tissue (277,278). Furthermore, the coagulant protein in Russell viper venom activates factor X (266,268,279). This activity contributes to the bleeding syndrome that follows the bite of the Russell viper.

Factor X is activated by a membrane complex composed of factors IXa and VIIIa that is generated by the intrinsic pathway of blood coagulation (267,280). This enzyme complex is also known as the *tenase complex*. This reaction requires phospholipid vesicles and calcium, although cell surfaces may play an essential role *in vivo*. This complex is assembled on endothelial cell surfaces (281) and on artificial lipid membranes composed of acidic phospholipids (282). Alternatively, factor X can be activated by the extrinsic pathway of blood coagulation by a membrane complex composed of factor VIIa and tissue factor (283). The expression of tissue factor activity and the formation of a factor VIIa–tissue factor complex activates factor X. Factor X activated by either pathway is associated with the cleavage of the same peptide bond.

Factor X, the substrate, binds to the tenase complex through multiple contact sites. For example, the Gla domain of the factor X light chain is thought to bind to the factor VIIa–tissue factor complex near the membrane surface, whereas the Gla domain of factor VIIa binds to factor X (284). Indeed, substrate recognition of factor X by the extrinsic tenase complex of factor VIIa and tissue factor involves an extended protein substrate-binding site far removed from the active site of factor VIIa (285).

Regulation of Factor X

The plasma concentration of factor X is maintained at approximately 10 µg/mL. The regulation of the factor X concentration is precise, but its molecular basis is uncertain. Coagulopoietin X, a heat stable material that is able to increase the plasma concentration of factor X, might play a role in this process (286).

Factor Xa is inhibited by three of the major plasma protease inhibitors in the absence of heparin: antithrombin III, α_1-antitrypsin, and α_2-macroglobulin (248,287,288). Although *in vitro* experiments have suggested that antithrombin III and α_1-proteinase inhibitor play a dominant role in the inhibition of factor Xa (287), *in vivo* experiments suggest that α_2-macroglobulin is a major physiologic regulator of factor Xa (288).

Protein Z is a vitamin K–dependent protein with a molecular weight of 62,000. The N-terminal half of protein Z is homologous to the vitamin K–dependent blood clotting proteins, and the Gla domain supports membrane binding. However, the sequence of the C-terminal half, albeit homologous to the serine proteases, lacks components of the catalytic triad, indicating that protein Z is not a proteinase. Protein Z is a cofactor involved in inhibition of factor Xa activity. Protein Z–dependent plasma protease inhibitor is a plasma protein with a molecular weight of 72,000 (289). The complex of protein Z and protein Z inhibitor inhibits factor Xa in the presence of calcium ions and phospholipid membranes.

Protein Z plays a physiologic role in hemostasis because the absence of protein Z increases the thrombotic tendency in factor V Leiden–deficient mice. Homozygous protein Z-null mice, when bred with mice that represent an animal model of factor V Leiden, yield offspring with a dramatically increased severity of the prothrombotic phenotype of factor V Leiden (290).

Targeted disruption of the factor X gene results in partial embryonic lethality, with approximately one-third of the homozygous null mouse embryos dying at approximately embryonic day 12 of massive bleeding (291). No histologic defects in the vasculature were observed. The remaining animals die of bleeding during the immediate postnatal period.

FACTOR X CELL RECEPTOR

The presence of a factor X cell receptor remains controversial. Originally described as a novel cell-surface receptor for factor Xa, this effector cell protease receptor-1 is composed of 337 amino acids, a large extracellular domain, a transmembrane domain, and a Ser-rich cytoplasmic tail (292). This receptor binds tightly to factor Xa. The absence of this cDNA in the human or mouse genome and the homology to survivin cDNA, except in the opposite orientation, have led to questions about effector cell protease receptor-1 (293).

FACTOR VII

Gene Structure

The factor VII gene spans 13 kb (189) and is located on the long arm of chromosome 13 at 13q34, adjacent to the factor X gene (294). The coding region is located on nine separate exons. Two alternate forms of preprofactor VII have been identified. One form, incorporating exon I, arises from a gene analogous to the factor X, factor IX, and protein C genes. The second form arises from a gene containing a ninth exon, exon Ia, which codes for a polypeptide extension of the NH_2-terminal that elongates the prepropeptide from 38 to 60 residues. The significance of these two preprofactor VII forms is unknown. Exon II encodes the propeptide and Gla domain. Exon III codes for the aromatic amino acid stack domain, a short linking segment common to

all of the vitamin K–dependent proteins. Exons IV and V each code the EGF-like regions of factor VII. Exon VI encodes the activation domain of factor VII, whereas exons VII and VIII code the catalytic domain. The organization of the factor VII gene is nearly identical to that of factors IX and X and protein C. After transcription, a factor VII message is generated that is approximately 2.4 kb (123) and contains a 3' untranslated region of 1 kb and poly(A) tail after the stop codon. This untranslated region also contains the polyadenylation sequence.

Protein Structure

Factor VII is a component of the extrinsic pathway of blood coagulation. This protein circulates in the blood as a single-chain zymogen (295,296) with a molecular mass of approximately 50 kd. Human factor VII contains 406 amino acids (123), whereas bovine factor VII is composed of 407 amino acids (138) (Fig. 37-18). These two factor VII forms show 71% sequence identity. Activation of factor VII occurs after the cleavage of an Arg 152-Ile 153 bond, leading to a two-chain form: factor VIIa, with a light chain and heavy chain linked by a disulfide bond (297–299). The light chain contains 152 amino acids, and the heavy chain contains 254 amino acids. The NH_2-terminal domain of factor VII, identical to the light chain of factor VIIa, contains 11 γ-carboxyglutamic acid residues at positions 6, 7, 14, 16, 19, 20, 25, 26, 29, 34, and 35 in the bovine sequence (138). As observed in factor IX, the Asp in the first EGF domain, located at residue 63, is only 20% to 30% β-hydroxylated. The heavy chain contains the catalytic domain, homologous in structure and function to trypsin.

Factor VII, a glycoprotein, contains 13% carbohydrate by weight. One carbohydrate chain is linked to Asn 145 in the light chain. Another carbohydrate chain is linked to Asn 203 in the heavy chain (138). The precise structure of the carbohydrate in factor VII is not known.

Factor VII is activated to factor VIIa by thrombin, factor Xa, or factor XIIa (297,299). Factor VIIa, in a complex with tissue factor, activates factor X.

Assembly of Factor VII on Membranes

Tissue factor is a receptor protein expressed on cell membranes that is required for the activation of the extrinsic pathway of blood coagulation. Tissue factor is expressed constitutively on many extravascular cells; in addition, monocytes (300,301) and endothelial cells (281,302,303) can be induced to express tissue factor. Neoplastic cells can also express tissue factor (304). This protein, which contains both lipid and carbohydrate, has an estimated molecular mass of 45 kd (301,305,306) and forms a calcium-dependent complex with factor VII on cell surfaces (307). This tissue factor–factor VII complex then activates factor X to factor Xa, and factor IX to factor IXa (308,309). The structure of tissue factor has recently been determined (310,311). Tissue factor is a transmembrane protein composed of 263 amino acids. The largest domain, containing the NH_2-terminal, is extracellular and oriented toward the blood. A domain containing 23 amino acids, most with hydrophobic properties, spans the cell membrane. A small, 21–amino acid cytoplasmic domain includes the COOH terminal. This tail contains two fatty acids, palmitate and stearate, bound by a thioester bond to a free Cys (312).

Substrates of Tissue Factor–Factor VIIa Complex

Both factor VII and factor VIIa bind to tissue factor on cell surfaces, but the mechanism by which the initial factor VIIa is generated remains uncertain. One speculation is that factor VII is

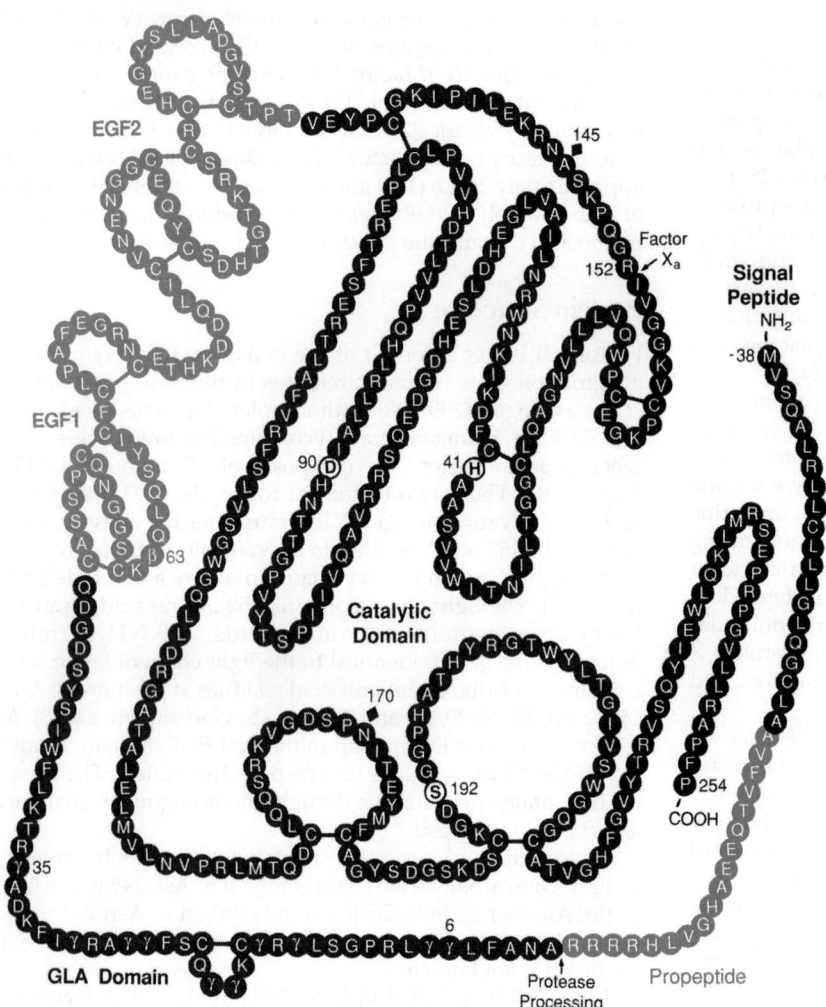

Figure 37-18. Amino acid sequence of human factor VII.

an active enzyme but considerably less active than factor VIIa (300). The tissue factor–factor VII complex activates factor X to factor Xa. Factor Xa can then catalyze the conversion of factor VII to factor VIIa, increasing the efficiency of factor X activation (313). The control of tissue factor–factor VII initiation of blood coagulation remains a major unresolved question.

The tissue factor–factor VIIa complex has been solved by x-ray crystallography to reveal at the atomic level the interactions between domains of both proteins (314). The most remarkable feature of this complex is the significant complementary surfaces at the interface of these proteins.

The tissue factor–factor VII complex has two physiologically important substrates. Although this reaction has traditionally been viewed as a critical event in thrombin generation in the extrinsic pathway, the complex also activates factor IX in the intrinsic pathway to factor IXa (308,309) (Fig. 37-19). The rate of factor IX activation by this pathway is approximately six times slower than the rate of factor X activation by the tissue factor–factor VIIa complex (315). Studies by Bauer et al. (253) suggest that the dominant basal mechanism *in vivo* is the activation of factor X by the factor VIIa-tissue factor complex.

Regulation of Factor VII

The plasma concentration of factor VII, 500 ng/mL, is the lowest of the vitamin K–dependent blood coagulation proteins. Unlike the other serine proteases involved in blood coagulation, factor VIIa is not inhibited by antithrombin III (316). The recent

discovery of a lipoprotein-associated coagulation inhibitor that inhibits the tissue factor–factor VII complex suggests a regulatory role for this protein (317–320). This protein, tissue factor pathway inhibitor or LACI, first forms a complex with factor Xa, which in turn forms a complex with tissue factor–factor VII in the presence of calcium ions (321).

Tissue Factor Pathway Inhibitor

The activity of the tissue factor–factor VIIa complex is regulated by tissue factor pathway inhibitor (TFPI) and antithrombin III (322,323). TFPI is a plasma protein but is also released from platelets during their activation and degranulation. TFPI inhibits the tissue factor–factor VIIa complex but requires the presence of factor Xa (324,325). An inactive complex forms between

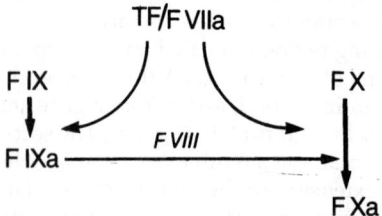

Figure 37-19. Alternate pathways of activation of blood coagulation by factor VIIa (FVII). The factor VIIa–tissue factor (TF) complex can activate factor X (FX) or factor IX (FIX).

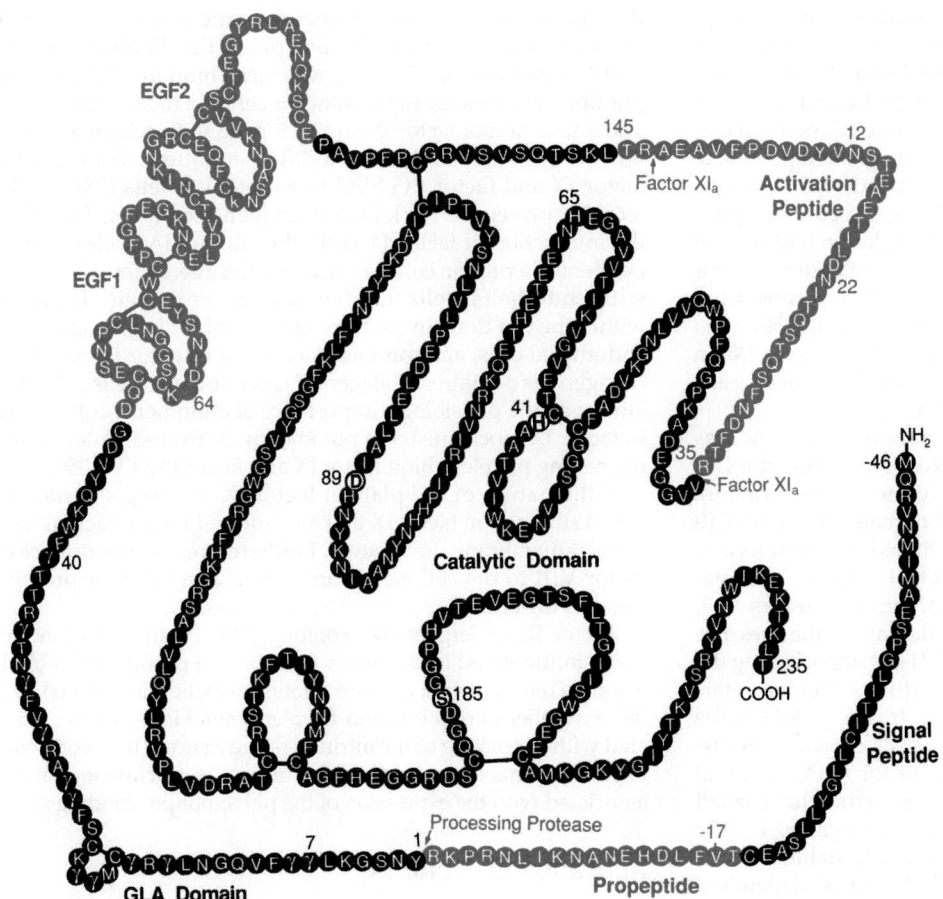

Figure 37-20. Amino acid sequence of human factor IX.

tissue factor, factor VIIa, factor Xa, and TFPI. Although antithrombin III does not inhibit factor VIIa, it does inhibit the active factor VIIa–tissue factor complex.

FACTOR IX

Gene Structure

The factor IX gene is 34 kb, but only a limited amount of this DNA codes for the factor IX protein. The seven introns range in size from 188 nucleotides to almost 10 kb (188). The gene is found on the tip of the long arm of the X chromosome, Xq26-27.3 (326). The coding region is found on eight separate exons (Fig. 37-15). The first exon, exon I, codes for the signal peptide. The second exon, exon II, codes for the propeptide and Gla domain of factor IX. Exon III codes for a short linking segment common to all of the vitamin K–dependent proteins. Exons IV and V, separated by a large intron, each code the EGF-like regions of factor IX. Exon VI codes for the activation domain of factor IX, whereas exons VII and VIII code the catalytic domain. In the factor IX gene, the entire catalytic domain is encoded by two exons, unlike prothrombin, in which five exons encode the homologous domain (161,185). This observation suggests that the factor IX gene was derived ancestrally from a precursor of the prothrombin gene (190). Reorganization of the gene by intron deletion led to consolidation of the exons encoding the serine protease domain. The gene organization of factor IX is nearly identical to that of factors X and VII and protein C. The relationship of this gene family to the prothrombin gene is shown by comparing Figures 37-10 and 37-15. After transcription, a factor IX message

is generated that is approximately 2.8 kb (23,120). This messenger RNA includes a 5' untranslated region and a long 3' untranslated region of 1.4 kb. The polyadenylation sequence is near the poly(A) tail. An androgen-sensitive element in the promoter is responsible for the phenotype of factor IX Leiden (327,328). Mutations in the factor IX promoter that are associated with factor IX Leiden include –6 (329) and –21 (330). Furthermore, disruption of the C/EPB-binding site leads to severe hemophilia B (331), and a mouse deficient in the C/EPB gene expresses low levels of factor IX (332).

Protein Structure

Human factor IX is a single-chain protein composed of 415 amino acids (23,120,137) (Fig. 37-20). It is a glycoprotein containing approximately 17% carbohydrate, and both bovine and human factor IX have a molecular mass of 56 kd (333,334). The NH_2-terminal Gla domain includes 12 γ-carboxyglutamic acid residues at residues 7, 8, 15, 17, 20, 21, 26, 27, 30, 33, 36, and 40 (128,129). A small loop formed by Cys residues at residues 18 and 23 is common to all of the vitamin K–dependent blood clotting proteins. The Gla domain defines some of the metal-binding properties of factor IX, although the EGF domain also contains metal-binding sites (335). After a short linking segment, factor IX contains two adjacent EGF domains. These EGF domains are characterized by a segment of 53 amino acids and a pattern of disulfide-bonded Cys residues, but their function is unknown. The first of the two EGF domains contains an unusual amino acid, β-hydroxyaspartic acid, at residue 64 (27). This modified amino acid is formed by posttranslational modification of Asp. β-Hydroxyaspartic acid and β-hydroxyasparagine are found in the EGF domains of all the vitamin K–dependent proteins except prothrombin, which lacks EGF domains, as well as in other proteins (26,117). From the cDNA derived for factor IX (23,120), factor X (124), protein C (336,337), protein S (338), and factor VII (123), it is apparent that specific Asp or Asn residues in precursor forms of these proteins undergo β-hydroxylation posttranslationally. The function of β-hydroxyaspartic acid remains unknown. Indeed, recombinant factor IX expressed in the presence of 2-ketoglutarate to inhibit β-hydroxylation had normal specific coagulant activity *in vitro* (339). The remainder of factor IX demonstrates marked sequence homology to zymogens of serine proteases, such as trypsin. This region is almost 250 amino acids long and contains the enzymatic activity of factor IXa in latent form. The cleavage of two peptide bonds in factor IX leads to the generation of the enzyme factor IXa.

The structure of factor IX in the absence of metal ions was solved by x-ray crystallography (340). However, the Gla domain was sufficiently disordered that most of its structure could not be determined. The first EGF domain shows flexibility, whereas the second EGF domain is linked such that its axis is approximately 110 degrees to the first EGF domain. The catalytic domain has the fold characteristic of serine proteases.

To establish the structure of the Gla domain in the presence and absence of metal ions, a peptide FIX (1-47), representing the entire Gla domain, was synthesized and its structure determined by nuclear magnetic resonance spectroscopy (341). In the absence of metal ions, the structure of the Gla domain was disordered, as in the x-ray structure, except for the C-terminal helix (342). On binding to calcium ions, a structure that formed is remarkably similar to that of prothrombin fragment 1 (343). However, magnesium ions, which can partially stabilize structure but can not support interaction of vitamin K–dependent proteins with phospholipid membrane surfaces, stabilize residues 12 to 47, but the ω-loop (residues 1 to 12) is disordered (344). These results identify the ω-loop as a critical component of the phospholipid-binding site of factor IX.

Calcium-Binding Properties of Factor IX

Factor IX in its carboxylated form binds to metal ions. There are two classes of metal-binding sites: one with high affinity for divalent cations and one with low affinity for divalent cations (146). Although the Gla domain contains some of these metal-binding sites (335), a highly conserved series of Asp residues in the first EGF domain form another calcium-binding site (112). For example, factor IX that is chemically modified by the removal of the Gla domain retains calcium-binding properties (335). The γ-carboxyglutamic acid–rich domain is responsible for the metal-dependent interaction of these proteins with membranes (22). The β–hydroxyaspartic acid–containing EGF domain may also be important for cell membrane recognition. Rees and Brownlee (112) have suggested that Asp 64 in factor IX may be part of a calcium-binding site and that mutation of Asp 64 inactivates factor IX. These results suggest that Asp 64 in the EGF domain may define a metal-binding site and that the EGF domain may be critical for protein–cell membrane interaction.

Membrane-Binding Properties of Factor IX

The interaction of factor IX and factor IXa with phospholipid membranes has been studied using phosphatidylserine-phosphatidylcholine vesicles (166,345). Factor IX binds to vesicles in the presence of Ca(II) but not in the presence of Mg(II) or EDTA. Furthermore, des-γ–carboxy factor IX, prepared from warfarinized plasma, does not interact with phospholipid vesicles even in the presence of Ca(II) (166). These results emphasize

the importance of the γ-carboxyglutamic acid-rich region in defining the phospholipid-binding properties. Furthermore, factor IX Alabama (Asp 47→Gly), which can bind to artificial phospholipid vesicles, does not bind to cellular membranes (345). The interaction of factor IX and factor IXa with cell membranes, however, is characterized by a different pattern. For example, factor IX and factor IXa bind to endothelial cells (281), and a receptor protein of 140 kd has been identified (346). Therefore, the interaction of factor IX with phospholipid vesicles is independent of a protein cofactor, whereas the interaction of factor IX with endothelial cells involves a receptor protein. Residues within the Gla domain are responsible for binding a receptor on endothelial cells, and this endothelial cell receptor is within the collagenous domain of collagen IV on endothelial cells (347,348). However, the physiologic importance of endothelial collagen IV to factor IX biochemistry is not known. Activated platelets, but not resting platelets, bind factor IX and factor IXa (349,350). Neither the nature of the platelet factor IX–binding site nor the actual surfaces on factor IX that are required for interaction with platelet membranes are known. Furthermore, the importance of factor VIII to the cell membranes (e.g., as a receptor protein) remains uncertain.

Factor IX undergoes two conformational transitions that are metal-induced and lead to the expression of a phospholipid-binding site (166). The first conformational transition is induced by a large number of divalent and trivalent metal ions and is associated with quenching of the intrinsic fluorescence. The second conformational transition is induced primarily by calcium ions and is associated with the expression of the phospholipid-binding site.

Activation of Factor IX

The activation of factor IX by factor IXa is highly metal-selective (146,351), with optimal activation achieved only in the presence of Ca(II); suboptimal activation occurs in the presence of Sr(II). Although the proteolytic activity of factor XIa is present on the light chain, the heavy chain of factor XIa may be necessary for the Ca(II)-dependent acceleration of factor IX activation (352–354). Because the factor IX–phospholipid interaction is inhibited by antifactor IX:Ca(II)–specific antibodies and the metal requirements parallel those for activation by factor XIa, a chemical similarity between a domain of factor XIa that interacts with factor IX and phospholipid vesicles in the presence of Ca(II) has been suggested (166). On the basis of antibody inhibition studies using both antibodies for factor XIa (354) and factor IX (166), the heavy chain of factor XIa is implicated in the specific binding of the phospholipid-binding site of factor IX in the presence of Ca(II).

Factor IX is converted to its enzyme form, factor IXa, by factor XIa (Fig. 37-21). This reaction requires calcium ions but takes place in solution. In contrast to the activation of other vitamin K–dependent blood clotting proteins, membrane surfaces (including phospholipid vesicles or cell surfaces) do not enhance factor IX activation. Activation of factor IX requires the cleavage of two peptide bonds, one located at Arg 145-Ala 146, the other at Arg 180-Val 181 (355,356). With the release of the internal carbohydrate-rich activation fragment from residues 146 to 180, the factor IXa light chain (molecular weight 17,000) and heavy chain (molecular weight 28,000) remain bound by a single disulfide bond. The serine protease activity is associated with the heavy chain.

Once generated, factor IXa forms a complex with factor VIIIa on membrane surfaces in an interaction that is calcium-dependent. This enzyme complex on the membrane is required for activation of factor X at rates that are physiologically significant (357). In contrast to the solution phase activation of factor IX by factor XIa, factor X is converted to its enzyme form, factor Xa, by fac-

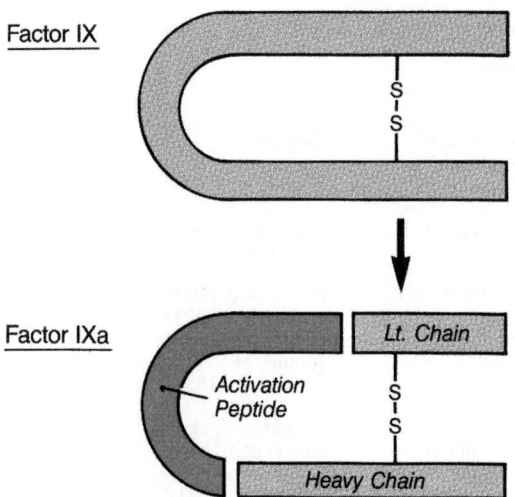

Figure 37-21. Activation of factor IX. Factor IX is activated by factor XIa or by the tissue factor–factor VIIa complex in a reaction that requires calcium ions. Factor IX requires the cleavage of two peptide bonds to generate factor IXa. An internal activation peptide is released during activation and a two-chain factor IXa results from proteolytic activation.

tor IXa in complex with factor VIIIa on membrane surfaces. This reaction also requires calcium ions. Either phospholipid vesicles or cell surfaces are required for significant factor X activation. Whereas factor IX does not require membrane surface for activation, factor IXa requires a membrane surface to express its enzymatic activity. These proteins may have two distinct binding domains, one related to zymogen activation and the other to macromolecular assembly of the enzyme in complex with the specific cofactor.

Factor X is the physiologic substrate for factor IXa. Some evidence suggests, however, that factor IXa can activate factor VII and factor VIII (358,359). As with all the trypsinlike serine proteases, factor IXa cleaves at peptide bonds adjacent to the Arg residues.

Regulation of Factor IX

The plasma concentration of factor IX is maintained at 5 µg/mL, but the molecular basis of regulation is not known. With the sequencing of the factor IX gene, several possible regulatory elements have been noted (188). A TATA box, coded as TGTA, is located 27 nucleotides upstream from a proposed initiation site, which is located 29 nucleotides upstream from the initiator methionine. Other possible TATA sequences are located further upstream. Studying the transcription of factor IX after site-specific mutagenesis of these regions has led to the identification of important regulatory elements. The C/EBP transcription factor is important for factor IX expression. Deletion of the C/EBP gene results in significantly reduced factor IX transcription (360). Mutations in the promoter give rise to a curious form of hemophilia B in which males are born with a severe form of factor IX deficiency that corrects spontaneously during puberty (361–363).

Plasma factor IXa is regulated by the protease inhibitors that modulate the other active blood clotting enzymes. For example, antithrombin III inhibits factor IXa activity (364,365).

CLINICAL DISORDERS OF VITAMIN K– DEPENDENT PROTEINS

A bleeding tendency is associated with the decrease in biologic activities of the vitamin K–dependent blood coagulation pro-

teins. The extent of this tendency correlates closely with the severity of the deficiency in these protein activities. Some deficiencies in the vitamin K–dependent blood clotting proteins are hereditary. That is, inherited genetic defects that interfere in the synthesis, processing, or normal lifespan of a protein can cause a bleeding disorder. Other disorders of the vitamin K–dependent proteins are acquired, not inherited. Diseases that interfere with the synthesis of the vitamin K–dependent blood clotting proteins in the liver or defects in the availability or use of vitamin K represent prime examples of these disorders.

Inherited Disorders Involving Vitamin K– Dependent Blood Clotting Proteins

A rare inherited defect in the synthesis of the vitamin K–dependent proteins was initially reported in four families, and additional examples of this defect continue to be observed (366–368). Deficiency of factor IX, factor X, factor VII, and prothrombin activities was observed in two patients (366,367). These defects were associated with marked prolongation of the partial thromboplastin time and prothrombin time and clinical bleeding manifestations. Partial correction of this coagulation defect was observed with high doses of vitamin K. However, another patient with mild combined deficiency of the vitamin K–dependent proteins did not correct on administration of high doses of vitamin K (369). In these cases, a defect in vitamin K–dependent carboxylation could be associated with a defect either in vitamin K metabolism (e.g., vitamin K absorption and transport, vitamin K reduction) or in the vitamin K carboxylase itself. The discovery of two siblings with a combined carboxylation defect limited to prothrombin and factor X suggests a carboxylation abnormality and not a defect in vitamin K metabolism (370). The mechanisms for such defects are beginning to be elucidated. Recent studies associated missense mutations in the vitamin K–dependent carboxylase gene with the autosomal-recessive inheritance of combined deficiency of all vitamin K–dependent blood coagulation proteins (371,372). The genetic heterogeneity of this rare clinical disorder is further emphasized by an analysis of two affected families with normal carboxylase gene sequences and increased vitamin K epoxide levels, suggesting a defect in the vitamin K epoxide reductase multienzyme complex (373). Future molecular analyses of such patients will undoubtedly contribute greatly to our understanding of this complex inherited bleeding disorder and the biochemistry of vitamin K metabolic pathways.

Given the similarity of the carboxylation recognition site on the propeptides of the vitamin K–dependent proteins (84,88), it remains unclear how a defect in the carboxylase can alter the posttranslational processing of some vitamin K–dependent proteins but not others. Recently, a novel missense mutation in the propeptide sequence of factor IX (Ala 10→Thr) was shown to decrease selectively the affinity of the carboxylase for the mutant propeptide in factor IX, resulting in a novel mechanism for increased warfarin sensitivity (374). The role of similar mutations in other vitamin K–dependent proteins is possible and may contribute to the pathogenesis of bleeding associated with decreased vitamin K–dependent protein function. Alternatively, the possibility of a family of carboxylating enzymes has not been ruled out. However, the vitamin K–dependent carboxylase itself is represented as a single copy in the genome, making this an unlikely possibility (375).

DISORDERS OF FACTOR IX

Genetic defects in the vitamin K–dependent blood coagulation proteins may be associated with hemophilia, a disease characterized by increased bleeding connected with trauma or, in its most severe form, spontaneous bleeding. Defects in factor IX (hemo-

TABLE 37-3. Molecular Defects Caused by Point Mutations Known to Cause Hemophilia B

Defect	Location	Phenotype	Study
Propeptide point mutations			
Factor IX Cambridge	Arg –1→Ser	Severe hemophilia B	Diuguid et al. (85)
Factor IX Oxford3	Arg –4→Gln	Severe hemophilia B	Bentley et al. (87)
Factor IX San Dimas	Arg –4→Gln	Severe hemophilia B	Ware et al. (86)
Point mutations that interfere with macromolecular assembly			
Factor IX Alabama	Asp 47→Gly	Moderate hemophilia B	Davis et al. (384)
Factor IX Durham	Gly 60→Ser	Mild hemophilia B	Denton et al. (386)
Point mutations that interfere with zymogen activation			
Factor IX Chapel Hill	Arg 145→His	Mild hemophilia B	Noyes et al. (389a)
Factor IX Hilo	Arg 180→Gln	Hemophilia B$_M$	Huang et al. (381)
Factor IX Chicago II	Arg 145→His	Severe hemophilia B	Diuguid et al. (379)
Factor IX Albuquerque	Arg 145→Cys	Severe hemophilia B	Toomey et al. (380)
Factor IX Kashihara	Val 182→Phe	Hemophilia B	Sakai et al. (383)
Point mutations that alter enzyme activity and substrate binding			
Factor IX Angers	Gly 396→Arg	Moderate hemophilia B	Vidaud et al. (391)
Factor IX Lake Elsinore	Ala 390→Val	Severe hemophilia B$_M$	Spitzer et al. (390)
Factor IX Eagle Rock	Gly 363→Val	Hemophilia B$_M$	Geddes et al. (389)
Factor IX Vancouver	Ile 397→Thr	Moderate hemophilia B	Ware et al. (387)
Factor IX Long Beach	Ile 397→Thr	Moderate hemophilia B	
Factor IX Los Angeles	Ile 397→Thr	Moderate hemophilia B	Spitzer et al. (388)

philia B) account for approximately 20% of cases of hemophilia in the United States (376). Correlation of the gene's structural defect to the protein's functional activity has contributed to our understanding of structure–function relation in these proteins and to our knowledge of the molecular basis of hemophilia B.

Hemophilia B is due to either a diminished factor IX antigen or functionally defective factor IX. In approximately one-third of cases, the defective factor IX antigen includes a point mutation (377). This mutant protein circulates in the blood, although its reduced biologic activity precludes normal participation in the blood clotting process. In other forms of hemophilia B, factor IX is not synthesized because of major defects in its gene structure, or an unstable factor IX is synthesized that is rapidly destroyed. A comprehensive listing of all known factor IX mutations is accessible on the Internet (378). The database currently includes 1918 patient entries. There are point mutations that result in amino substitutions, deletions, addition mutations, or a combination of these and nearly 700 unique molecular events probably causing the disease. Mutations have been localized to protein coding sequences and all gene regulatory regions with the exception of the factor IX polyadenylation sequence. Mutations in 9 of the 12 γ-carboxyglutamic acid residues have been reported, confirming their critical role for the calcium-dependent membrane binding and function of factor IX. Amino acid substitutions have also been found in each of the 22 cysteines, emphasizing the importance of disulfide bridges that contribute to the structure of factor IX. Selected factor IX mutants illustrate important examples.

Point Mutations in Factor IX. As discussed in the section Factor IX, factor IX has a series of domains that carry out specific functions of the factor IX molecule. A point mutation in any of these domains may interfere with factor IX function. *A priori,* it is reasonable to assume one of the following:

1. A defect in the posttranslational process or a defect in the Gla domain may inhibit membrane binding.
2. A defect in the EGF domains may interfere with protein assembly on membrane surfaces and the interaction with factor VIII.
3. A defect in the activation domain may interfere in the zymogen activation of factor IX to factor IXa.

4. A defect in the active site or the extended substrate-binding site may alter the ability of the mutant factor IX to recognize or to cleave physiologically important substrates (Table 37-3).

Factor IX Chapel Hill (Arg 145→His) is the prototype for mutant zymogens that cannot be activated to their enzyme form because of mutation of the Arg adjacent to the sessile bond (311,312). This mutant was the first hemophiliac factor IX to be characterized at the molecular level and the first identification of a specific point mutation. More recently, factor IX Chicago II and factor IX Albuquerque, discovered in unrelated patients, have a similar molecular defect (379,380). In this mutant form, the Arg adjacent to the cleavage site between the activation peptide and the light chain of factor IXa is substituted so that the sessile bond cannot be cleaved. Cleavage of this bond is necessary for the generation of activated factor IXa, which can act on factor X. In factor IX Hilo, the sessile bond between the activation peptide and the heavy chain cannot be cleaved because of mutation of Arg to Gln (381,382). In this mutant, the enzyme cannot be formed because this critical proteolytic event is analogous to the peptide bond cleaved to generate trypsin from trypsinogen. Similarly, factor IX Kashihara (Val 182→Phe) has a substitution that interferes with the cleavage of the peptide bond between residues 180 and 181, yielding an inactive factor IX (383).

Factor IX Cambridge (Arg –1→Ser) (85), factor IX Oxford 3 (Arg –4→Gln) (87), and factor IX San Dimas (Arg –4→Gln) (86) contain point mutations in the propeptide domain of the factor IX precursor, profactor IX. In these factor IX mutants, a mutation at position –1 or –4 prevents proteolytic removal of the propeptide by a propeptidase. Failure to cleave the propeptide partially inhibits γ-carboxylation, leading to a protein that cannot bind to phospholipid vesicles or exhibit coagulant activity. Factor IX Cambridge does not undergo the metal-induced conformational change characteristic of factor IX, but factor IX San Dimas does undergo this conformational transition. These results suggest that the distribution of γ-carboxyglutamic acid residues differs in the partially carboxylated factor IX Cambridge and factor IX San Dimas (86).

Factor IX Alabama (Asp 47→Gly) probably lacks coagulant activity because it fails to bind to cell membrane surfaces (384). However, this mutant with its intact Gla region binds normally to

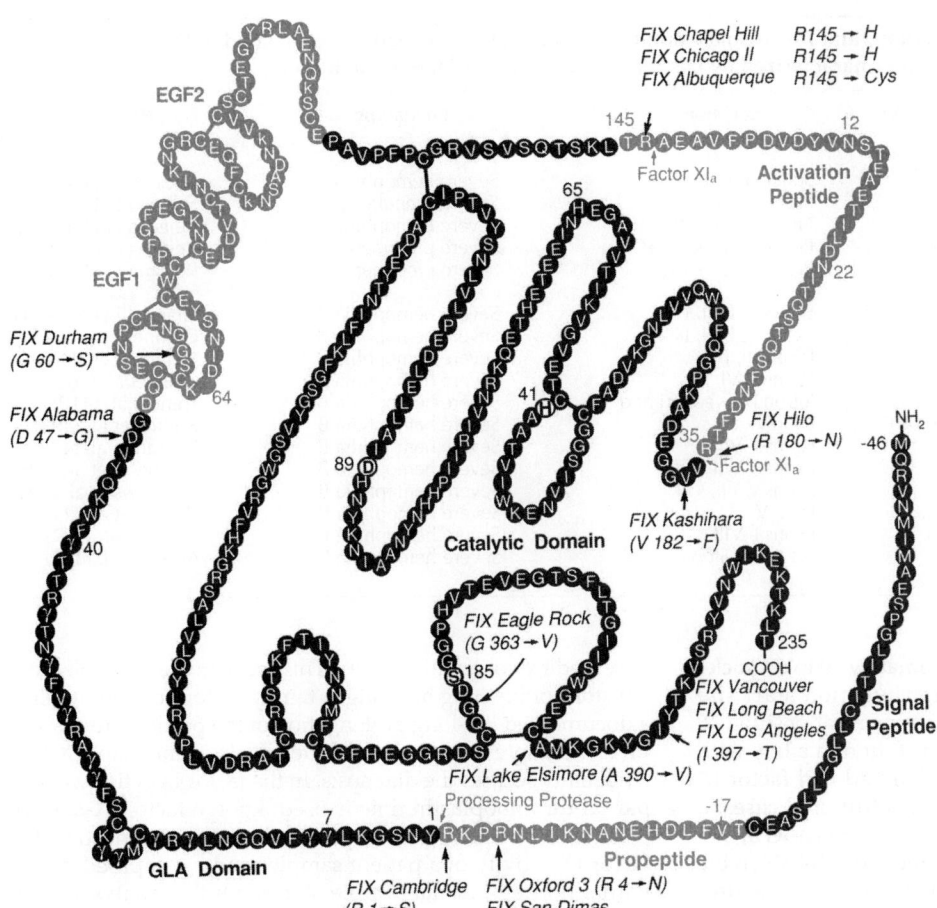

Figure 37-22. Molecular defects in mutant factor IX (FIX). The point mutations identified in FIX are indicated by the solid circles. Mutations have been identified in the propeptide, epidermal growth factor domain, activation domain, and catalytic domain.

phospholipid vesicles (345). Alternatively, evidence suggests that this mutant does not bind to factor VIII (385). Factor IX Durham (Gly 60→Ser) has been isolated from two presumably unrelated patients with a mild form of hemophilia B (386). These mutants represent defects in the first EGF domain, but a complete understanding of their functional implications is unavailable.

Point mutations in the catalytic domain have been described in mutant factor IXs isolated from patients with hemophilia B. Factor IX Vancouver (Ile 397→Thr), factor IX Long Beach (Ile 397→Thr), and factor IX Los Angeles (Ile 397→Thr) share the same point mutation (387–389). Residue 397 is near but not in the active site of the factor IXa. The precise mechanism by which this substitution inhibits coagulant activity is unknown. Factor IX Lake Elsinore (Ala 390→Val) (390) and factor IX Angers (Gly 396→Arg) (391,392) disrupt enzymatic activity. Factor IX Eagle Rock (Gly 363→Val) contains a substituted amino acid adjacent to the active site Ser 365, eliminating enzyme activity of the mutant factor IXa (388). Factor IX London 2 includes a Gln substituted for an Arg at position 333 (393). A summary of selected point mutations in hemophilia B is compiled in Figure 37-22.

Other factor IX mutants have been purified and characterized, but the precise point mutations are unknown. Factor IX Deventer cannot be activated by the coagulant protein of Russell viper venom, suggesting a defect in zymogen activation (394). Factor IX Zutphen contains an extra peptide of 33 kd that is cross-linked to the factor IX molecule through a disulfide bond (395). This mutant factor IX has impaired calcium-binding properties.

Of the 11 factor IX mutants described, three groups have identical mutations: (1) factor IX Oxford 3 and factor IX San Dimas; (2) factor IX Chapel Hill, factor IX Chicago II, and factor IX Albuquerque; and (3) factor IX Vancouver, factor IX Los

Angeles, and factor IX Long Beach. In patients with mutant plasma proteins, the mutation of Arg to another amino acid appears to be a developing theme. The CG sequence, a component of four of the six Arg codons, as a mutational hot spot may represent an important cause for the development of spontaneous point mutations (396,397). Because internal point mutations are likely to destabilize protein structure and lead to markedly diminished circulating protein levels, patients preselected for circulating mutant protein antigen are likely to contain amino acid substitutions on the protein surface. Arginines, located on the protein surface, are used by proteases of the trypsin family to hydrolyze adjacent bonds during protein processing and zymogen activation. Given the importance of arginines, it would appear that their mutation leads to phenotypically obvious defects in protein function.

Thus, as summarized in Figure 37-21, there are examples of factor IX mutants that interfere with posttranslational processing, factor IX cell interaction, factor IX zymogen activation, and enzyme activity or normal substrate-binding properties. In the past few years, 425 different amino acid substitution mutations have been described (378).

Factor IX Gene Defects. Little or no factor IX antigen may circulate in the blood of some patients with hemophilia B. A particularly curious form of hemophilia B has been described in which male children are severely afflicted with factor IX deficiency, but factor IX approaches normal levels after puberty (361). This form, factor IX Leyden, appears to involve alterations in the promoter region of the factor IX gene that are sensitive to sex hormones (362,363). Several mutations have been found within the "Leyden-specific region" of the factor IX pro-

TABLE 37-4. Point Mutations and Partial and Complete Factor IX Gene Deletions Associated with Hemophilia and Characterized by Decreased Factor IX Antigen in the Blood

Defect	Size (kb)	Location	Phenotype	Reference
Defects in splicing and promotor (factor IX Leyden)				
Point mutation	—	Splice 3' of exon VI	Severe hemophilia B	Rees et al. (404)
Point mutation	—	Promoter (G −6→A)	Severe prepuberty	Fahner et al. (362)
Point mutation	—	Promoter (T −20→AP)	Severe hemophilia B	Reitsma et al. (363)
Point mutation	—	Promoter (A +13→G)	Severe prepuberty	Reitsma et al. (363)
Deletion	—	Promoter (A +13)	Severe prepuberty	Reitsma et al. (363)
Partial and complete gene deletions				
Deletion	18	Exons I, II, III, IV–?	Severe hemophilia B	Giannelli et al. (401)
Deletion	18	Exons I, II, III, IV–?	Severe hemophilia B	Giannelli et al. (401)
Deletion	9	Exons III, IV–?	Severe hemophilia B	Giannelli et al. (401)
Deletion	10	Exons V, VI	Severe hemophilia B	Chen et al. (402)
Deletion/insertion	—	Intron between VI and VII	Severe hemophilia B	Trent et al. (410)
Deletion/frameshift	0.001	Exon V	Severe hemophilia B	Schach et al. (405)
Deletion	41	Exons I–VII	Severe hemophilia B	Hassan et al. (409)
Deletion	114	Exons I–VIII	Severe hemophilia B	Matthews et al. (408)
Deletion	77	Exons V, VII, VIII	Severe hemophilia B	Matthews et al. (408)
Deletion	2.8	Exon V	Severe hemophilia B	Vidaud et al. (412)
Deletion	120	Exons I–VIII	Severe hemophilia B	Peake et al. (407)
Nonsense	—	Lys 411→Stop	Severe hemophilia B	Attree et al. (392)

moter, a region that encompasses approximately 40 to 60 nucleotides around the major factor IX transcription start site (398,399). A mutation of adenosine for guanosine at position −6 relative to the transcription start site was found in a boy with factor IX deficiency and in his uncle, who had had factor IX deficiency before puberty (362). In three additional cases, a T→A mutation at −20, an A deletion at +13, and an A→G at +13 is associated with the factor IX Leyden phenotype (400) (Table 37-4). It appears that disruption of a naturally occurring androgen response element in this region of the factor IX gene plays an important role in the phenotypic correction of hemophilia B Leyden. However, the identity of the transcription factors involved in the recovery mechanism in response to testosterone, the androgen response element, or both remain uncertain.

Hemophilia B can also result from gene deletions, abnormal splicing of the factor IX transcript, or nonsense mutations that terminate translation (401,402) (Table 37-2). In the study by Chen et al. (402), the 5' end of the gene is intact, and a truncated expression product of 36 kd is secreted but cleared from the blood into the urine (403). In the abnormality described by Rees et al. (404), a point mutation (G→T) is located at base 21,165 within the obligatory GT of a splice junction at the 3' site of exon VI. The change from GT to TT interferes with splicing, causing a severe defect in transcription. In factor IX Seattle (405), an A at position 17,699 in the gene is deleted. This deletion causes a frameshift, leading to the coding of a Val at residue 85 and a stop codon at position 86. Similarly, the factor IX Bordeaux gene codes for a stop sequence in place of Lys 411, terminating synthesis (406). Deletion of the entire factor IX gene has been described by Peake et al. (407) and Matthews et al. (408), and nearly complete factor IX gene deletions have been described by Hassan et al. (409).

A novel mechanism of hemophilia B involves the deletion and insertion of DNA between exons VI and VII (410). Other partial and complete gene deletions have been identified and partially characterized (411–417). These examples emphasize the heterogeneity of hemophilia B, particularly the form of hemophilia B in which defective factor IX does not circulate in the blood. A single base deletion and frameshift mutation, a point mutation in the splice junction, and partial or gross gene deletions have been described.

Laboratory Diagnosis of Hemophilia B. Hemophilia B is suspected when an isolated deficiency in plasma factor IX activity is observed by coagulation assay. This measurement coupled with a history of life-long bleeding, a family history of hemophilia B, a documented life-long prolongation of the partial thromboplastin time, or previous documentation of deficient factor IX activity usually secures the diagnosis. In the factor IX activity assay, a partial thromboplastin time is used; known factor IX-deficient plasma is corrected with test plasma from the patient so that the factor IX activity of a patient sample can be compared directly with a normal plasma sample. Although this analysis is adequate to assess the factor IX activity level of a patient, other ancillary assays are of interest. For example, measurement of the plasma factor IX antigen distinguishes between patients that have improperly functioning circulating factor IX in their blood (e.g., point mutations) and those who do not have circulating factor IX in their blood because of large gene deletions.

The evaluation of the factor IX level in family members provides insight into the pattern of inheritance and potential severity of hemophilia B. As a rule, the level of the factor IX deficiency in hemophilia B is consistent among members of a hemophilia family, presumably because the genetic defect is identical in all afflicted family members and each genetic defect is associated with a specific level of plasma factor IX activity. In other words, a specific genotype should manifest itself with a characteristic phenotype. Evaluation of the propositus often identifies other family members afflicted with this disorder and demonstrates transmission of the inherited defective factor IX gene from generation to generation. Carrier analysis of female members of hemophilia B families can be important for genetic counseling. Although the expression of excess factor IX antigen compared to activity (e.g., ratio of factor IX activity to factor IX antigen in plasma) has been previously used to identify the carrier state (418), these methods have limited predictive value because of random inactivation of the X chromosome in somatic cells and the variability of factor IX levels in normal individuals. For these reasons, direct genetic analysis using restriction fragment length polymorphisms has been used for accurate carrier state diagnosis and antenatal diagnosis (419). Six intragenic and three closely linked extragenic polymorphisms have been described for factor IX in the white population (326,419–423). On this basis, approximately 80% of families can be evaluated for a hemophilia B gene with approximately 99% accuracy (421). The intragenic polymorphisms can be observed with a number of restriction enzymes. A BamH1 polymorphism due to polymorphism at nucleotide −587 occurs in approximately 6% of subjects (420). The DdeI polymorphism due to a deletion at nucleotide position 5505 to 5554 is observed in 24% of subjects, the XmnI polymorphism due to a G→C at 7076 has a frequency of 29% (419), and the TaqI polymorphism due to alteration at nucleotide 11,111 has a frequency of 35% (326,423). MspI (altered near 16,000) and OP1 (due to G→A at 20,422) have frequencies of 22% and 33%, respectively (422). Three closely linked extragenic polymorphisms have been observed with SstI and TaqI (424–426). One of the factor IX polymorphisms, Thr or Ala at residue 148, can be detected immunochemically (427,428); this method has also been explored for carrier detection.

Clinical Diagnosis of Hemophilia B. Hemophilia B is a sex-linked disease seen in males, with rare exception (429,430). On the basis of symptoms and physical examination, hemophilia B is indistinguishable from hemophilia A, which is due to factor VIII deficiency. The clinical presentation of hemophilia is described in detail in Chapter 39. Ten percent of patients with hemophilia have factor IX deficiency. The severity of this disorder closely correlates with the level of factor IX activity in the plasma, although rare examples of a lack of concordance do exist. Patients with low levels of factor IX may be clinically normal; they may even proceed through surgery without special therapy or even the recognition of factor IX deficiency state. Other patients with factor IX levels that should correlate with mild hemophilia may have severe bleeding manifestations.

Patients with severe manifestations of hemophilia B usually have a factor IX activity that is less than 1% of the normal plasma level. These patients are characterized by recurrent, spontaneous bleeding episodes. Moderate hemophilia B is associated with plasma factor IX activity levels of 1% to 4% and is less commonly associated with spontaneous bleeding. In the more mild forms of hemophilia B, the factor IX activity is above 4%. These patients often show little or no spontaneous bleeding and require attention only during surgery or after trauma.

Except in its most mild forms, hemophilia B is usually diagnosed in early childhood. If excessive bleeding from the umbilical cord or after circumcision goes unnoticed, ecchymoses during the minor trauma of the toddler phase may clue the parents to an underlying clotting disorder. Families with a history of hemophilia B are particularly alert to these bleeding abnormalities and often request a plasma assay of factor IX during the first month or two after birth.

The laboratory diagnosis of factor IX requires measurement of the plasma factor IX activity. Because neonates have 50% of the adult level of the vitamin K–dependent proteins (431), even when vitamin K replete, a low factor IX (e.g., 30%) needs to be interpreted with caution before it is assumed that the child has hemophilia B. Because of the difficulties in sample handling and factor IX assay, clinical laboratories with considerable experience in the measurement of this protein should be used to obtain reliable results.

Clinical Manifestations of Hemophilia B. The clinical manifestations of hemophilia B and hemophilia A are indistinguishable. Depending on the severity of the disease, patients are characterized by spontaneous hemarthroses, hematomas, ecchymoses, and, rarely, spontaneous central nervous system bleeding. Hematuria is not uncommon, and gastrointestinal bleeding may also be observed. The most common problem by far involves hemarthroses, either spontaneous or associated with minor trauma. Hemorrhage into the ankle, knee, shoulder, or elbow is associated with severe pain, discomfort, or irritability. Long before there is clinical evidence for bleeding, patients easily identify the pain and inflammation of ongoing bleeding

into the joint. The proper treatment is to stop bleeding as soon as possible. If indicated, factor IX replacement therapy can be instituted. The joint is immobilized by bed rest or splinting. Some orthopedists advocate casting the limb for complete immobilization, but care must be exercised to assure that there is adequate room to accommodate tissue swelling associated with inflammation. As a compromise, a bivalve case allows immobilization with the ease of routine observation of the joint. With effective therapy, the patient may observe the cessation of bleeding in 12 to 24 hours. Treatment should be continued for several days. Afterward, a physical therapy program should be instituted with factor IX coverage. Unlike other forms of arthritis, there is no need to tap the joint even if an effusion is present unless a septic arthritis complicates the hemarthrosis.

Chronic debilitating arthritis remains a serious problem for the patient with severe hemophilia. Chronic pain, limitations of joint motion, and disfiguration of the joint are common problems in severe hemophilia. With chronic crippling hemarthroses, patients are often restricted in their abilities to perform certain tasks. Specifically, persons with hemophilia with limited range of motion in their knees have difficulty in walking, standing from a seated position, and descending stairs.

In patients with the most crippling arthritis, orthopedic surgery, including joint fusion and joint replacement, may be considered. Chronic pain may be minimized with an ankle fusion, but movement in the joint is lost with the procedure. Prosthetic joints have been used successfully but are recommended only in instances in which the patient is extremely disabled, and orthopedic surgery and hematology expertise is available to allow an ample repair without significant surgical risk. The patient must also be willing and able to participate in an extended, aggressive postsurgical physical rehabilitation program; otherwise, the patient risks an unfavorable outcome.

The onset of back or flank pain may be the initial presentation of retroperitoneal bleeding. Significant bleeding can usually be diagnosed radiographically by observation of the loss of the psoas shadow. With large hematoma formation, ureteral deviation or obstruction can occur. Bed rest and full factor IX replacement therapy are indicated.

Superficial hematomas, lacerations, and ecchymoses may not require more than conservative, supportive therapy. However, large hematomas such as those that are formed in the closed space of the quadriceps can significantly compromise the distal circulation. Urgent aggressive therapy is required.

Infection with or without abscess formation, a general complication of hematoma formation, is occasionally observed as a further complication of hemophilia B. Treatment with antibiotic therapy and surgical drainage are important considerations.

Treatment of Hemophilia B. Replacement therapy in hemophilia B includes the infusion of factor IX concentrate or fresh frozen plasma. Cryoprecipitate, factor VIII concentrate, and desmopressin acetate, important for use in the treatment of factor VIII deficiency or hemophilia A, have no role in the treatment of hemophilia B. Despite significant advances that have improved the safety of currently available blood products, there is still a risk of bloodborne pathogens. Therefore, the indications for infusion must be weighted against the exposure history of the patient. A patient with severe hemophilia who has been transfused multiple times with human plasma–derived factor IX concentrate with evidence of exposure to the hepatitis viruses, human immunodeficiency virus (HIV), or both may be considered differently from patients with mild hemophilia who may have had little or no previous exposure to human plasma–derived blood products. Every effort should be made to reduce the risks of transmission of bloodborne pathogens. If conservative treatment measures are insufficient and replacement therapy is necessary, we recommend the use of recombinant DNA–derived factor IX concentrates, particularly in previously untreated or minimally treated patients. This replacement product, in contrast to human plasma–derived factor IX concentrates, has no risk of transmission of human bloodborne pathogens. Recombinant factor IX is manufactured and formulated without any animal or human plasma–derived protein supplements (432,433). In emergency situations in which recombinant factor IX is unavailable, plasma-derived factor IX concentrates, which have an excellent viral safety record, or fresh frozen plasma, with low risks of hepatitis transmission and HIV transmission, may be used after consideration of the immediate risks of withholding therapy.

Factor IX has a plasma half-life of approximately 24 hours and rapidly equilibrates between the intravascular and extravascular space. Therefore, after an initial loading dose, factor IX can be administered once daily. Recombinant factor IX has an approximately 30% lower recovery than human plasma–derived factor IX, so a higher dose may be required to achieve the same target levels after intravenous injection, particularly in children younger than 15 years or in patients known to have no circulating factor IX antigen. Because the half-life of recombinant factor IX is the same as human plasma–derived factor IX, similar dosing intervals may be used. The target level of plasma factor IX depends on the bleeding problem. For treatment of a mild hemarthrosis, a factor IX level of 30% to 40% is adequate. For major abdominal surgery or a central nervous system or retroperitoneal hemorrhage, normalization of the factor IX level to 100% is indicated. The factor IX dose, using factor IX concentration, can be calculated from the patient's body weight and the factor IX target level. For a 50-kg man in whom a 50% (0.5 IU/mL) plasma factor IX level is desired, 2000 units of factor IX must be transfused (Fig. 37-23). This calculation is derived by multiplying the estimated plasma volume of 2000 mL (50 kg × 40 mL/kg) by the desired factor IX level (0.5 IU/mL), then multiplying by 2, given the volume of distribution or the dilution of factor IX equally between the intravascular and extravascular space. Because the elimination half-life of factor IX is approxi-

mately 24 hours, infusion of 1000 units of factor IX every 24 hours should maintain a plasma factor IX level between 50% (after the infusion) and 25% (before the next infusion). These calculations provide useful predictions of the plasma factor IX level, but these estimates should be confirmed by direct monitoring of the factor IX activity level to ensure adequate therapy.

Factor IX therapy is administered in several clinical settings. Patients with severe hemophilia B are treated in home maintenance programs. In such programs, factor IX concentrate is refrigerated until needed, then infused by either the patient or a trained family member after the initiation of a bleeding episode. These programs have been highly successful in developing the medical independence of the patient and family (434). Furthermore, the cost of medical care has been significantly reduced. When patients with hemophilia, including those on home treatment programs, develop significant bleeding problems that are beyond the scope of their training in routine care, outpatient care is sought in hospitals in which medical professionals skilled in the treatment of hemophilia may assist the patient. Often, satisfactory treatment can be initiated in the emergency room or in the outpatient clinic. More serious problems, however, require inpatient admission for maintenance of replacement therapy.

Complications of Therapy. Factor IX concentrate carries attendant risks in addition to viral hepatitis (435). Although the molecular basis is not clear, the intermediate-purity factor IX concentrates cause a hypercoagulable state (436–439). Patients who receive an excessive quantity of the factor IX concentrates can develop deep venous thrombosis and pulmonary embolism (436). This remains a particular problem in those receiving considerable amounts of intermediate-purity factor IX concentrate, such as those undergoing major surgery (439). The quality of these factor IX concentrates has improved greatly, with highly purified factor IX currently available. The risk of HIV has been eliminated since the introduction of a heat-treatment step to the production of factor IX concentrate (440,441). All low-purity or high-purity human plasma–derived factor IX concentrates that are currently available for human use in the United States are either heat-treated, solvent-detergent–treated, or immunoaffinity-purified with monoclonal antibodies and subjected to ultrafiltration to eliminate viral infectious risks. Recombinant DNA–derived factor IX is also ultrafiltered to provide an added layer of viral safety.

Some patients with hemophilia B develop antibodies to factor IX as an immunologic reaction to a foreign protein. The incidence of this complication in patients with hemophilia B (approximately 1% to 3%) is lower than the analogous complication of developing antibodies to factor VIII in patients with hemophilia A (approximately 20%). In all patients with hemophilia B, the development of factor IX antibodies is most frequently observed in those with severe factor IX deficiency. Because many patients with severe hemophilia B have partial or complete gene deletions, it is suspected that the absence of factor IX antigen in the blood may predispose these patients to the production of antifactor IX antibodies (401). But many factor IX antigen–negative patients with gene deletions do not have circulating inhibitors against factor IX (414). The development of factor IX antibodies has a significant impact on the therapy of these patients. Factor IX replacement therapy is usually withheld to allow the titer of the antifactor IX antibody to fall to low levels. Only conservative, supportive measures are taken to avoid reexposure to factor IX. When a life-threatening bleed develops, factor IX concentrate can be administered and the plasma factor IX level maintained transiently at normal levels before the amnestic response leads to a rise in factor IX antibody titer. During this brief period, bleeding can be controlled. Although immunosuppressive techniques have not in general

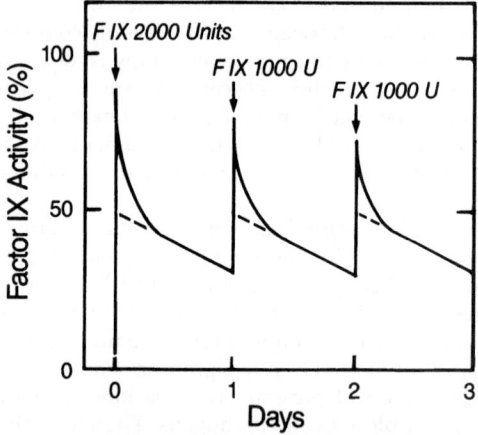

Figure 37-23. Factor IX (FIX) infusion therapy in the treatment of hemophilia B. FIX, administered in the form of FIX concentrate of intermediate purity, is infused initially at 2000 U. Because of equilibration between the intravascular and extravascular space over several hours, the FIX level achieved is only approximately half that expected if all of the FIX remains in the intravascular space. With a FIX half-life of 24 hours, repeated infusions of factor IX are required on a daily basis. Evidence that a satisfactory FIX level has been obtained should be established by the performance of a FIX assay or, at a minimum, correction of the partial thromboplastin time.

been effective, several approaches for eradicating inhibitors by inducing immunologic tolerance have been attempted (442). In contrast to hemophilia A inhibitor patients, hemophilia B inhibitor patients are at risk of anaphylaxis after replacement therapy (443). It appears that complete factor IX gene deletions confer the highest risk for development of this rare complication. Additional complications experienced by hemophilia B patients during immune tolerance induction include the development of nephrotic syndrome as well as other allergic reactions to factor IX protein infusions (444,445).

Patients with hemophilia B who were treated with factor IX concentrate between 1979 and 1984 have a high risk of exposure to HIV (446). A majority of these patients have been exposed to HIV and have developed acquired immunodeficiency syndrome (AIDS). This syndrome is the same as in patients who acquired AIDS by other routes. However, it is not uncommon for HIV-positive hemophilia patients to have a long latency period between exposure and development of AIDS. Immunoaffinity purification techniques have been applied to the purification of factor IX from plasma (447–449). Subsequently, recombinant factor IX was expressed in active form in mammalian cells (450–453). Improvements in the technology related to posttranslational processing of recombinant factor IX, specifically optimizing the efficiency of factor IX propeptide cleavage and γ-carboxylation, have resulted in a commercial source of recombinant factor IX. The application of recombinant DNA technology to the treatment of inherited bleeding disorders continues to benefit patients and provides great hope to patients with hemophilia B. In particular, recent advances and developments in basic and preclinical gene therapy studies have been made with a specific focus on the treatment of hemophilia (454). A recent human clinical investigation to assess the safety of factor IX gene therapy reported preliminary evidence for factor IX gene transfer and expression in the skeletal muscle of hemophilia B patients after intramuscular injection of an adeno-associated viral vector (455). These early findings represent the first promising observations in a rapidly growing field of investigation. It is a general hope that steady progress in the field of molecular biology and its application to gene therapy for hemophilia will result in novel therapeutic approaches in the near future to treat factor IX deficiency.

DISORDERS OF PROTHROMBIN

Mutant Prothrombins. Hereditary defects in the plasma prothrombin activity are rare, commensurate with the autosomal inheritance of mutant prothrombins and with the absence of clinical symptoms and signs in patients heterozygous for a mutant prothrombin. These patients have prothrombin levels approximately 50% of the normal level. Patients with hereditary prothrombin deficiency have a clinical bleeding disorder closely related to the quantity of prothrombin coagulant activity in the plasma and to the nature of the molecular defect. Therefore, only patients with homozygous prothrombin deficiency would be expected to be severely affected, and only a few cases have been described (456). Patients with heterozygous prothrombin deficiency have been more commonly identified.

As in factor IX deficiency, hereditary hypoprothrombinemia is a heterogeneous disorder. Some patients have low prothrombin activity levels despite normal prothrombin antigen levels. These patients are likely to have point mutations that give rise to dysprothrombinemias, mutant prothrombins with defective function circulating in the plasma. Other patients may not synthesize prothrombin and thus have a parallel deficiency of prothrombin activity and prothrombin antigen. These patients have aprothrombinemia.

In 1971, Josso et al. (457) reported one of the first cases of a congenital dysprothrombinemia, *prothrombin Barcelona*. This defect was characterized by the low level of thrombin generated from the mutant prothrombin during activation with factor Xa. The plasma prothrombin antigen level was normal, however. Family studies suggested that the propositus and three siblings were homozygous, and that the parents were heterozygous for mutant forms of prothrombin. Prothrombin Barcelona is characterized by a defect in zymogen activation in which cleavage of the Arg 271-Thr 272 bond is precluded (458). A second peptide bond is cleaved normally, however, generating an active enzyme with activity toward small synthetic substrates but not generating physiologically important substrates such as fibrinogen (459). The defect in this protein is due to a mutation of Arg271 to a Cys (460). Factor Xa is specific for peptide bonds adjacent to Arg; the conversion of this Arg to a Cys precludes peptide bond hydrolysis and zymogen activation of prothrombin.

A second, unrelated patient with similar clinical symptoms had a mutant prothrombin known as *prothrombin Madrid* (379,461). This mutant (Arg 271→Cys) is identical to prothrombin Barcelona. From a functional point of view, these defects are analogous to those of factor IX Chapel Hill and factor IX Chicago II.

Two mutant prothrombins contain defects in the thrombin portion of the molecule. The defects interfere with the ability of these thrombins to convert fibrinogen to fibrin. Prothrombin Tokushima (Arg 418→Trp) is defective at a site adjacent to the Asp in the catalytic triad of the serine protease (462,463). This enzyme is defective in catalytic activity against large and small substrates. The catalytic domain is also defective in prothrombin Quick I and prothrombin Quick II. Both proteins, isolated from the plasma of a single patient with severe hypoprothrombinemia (less than 2% prothrombin activity), represent gene products of two mutant prothrombin genes (464). In prothrombin Quick I, a Cys is substituted for an Arg at residue 382 (465). This enzyme is defective in the binding and conversion of fibrinogen. The molecular defect in prothrombin Quick II involves replacement of Gly 558 with Val. This mutant does not hydrolyze small substrates based on Arg but instead has substrate specificity resembling elastase.

Other prothrombin mutants have been purified and partially characterized, but prothrombin Barcelona, prothrombin Tokushima, prothrombin Quick I, and prothrombin Quick II are the only mutant prothrombins to be characterized at the level of the molecular defect (Fig. 37-24 and Table 37-5). Prothrombin Cardeza (466) and prothrombin Clamart (467) cannot be converted to thrombin by factor Xa, indicating a defect in zymogen activation. Prothrombin Metz (468), prothrombin Salakta (469,470), and prothrombin Molise (471) have defects in their catalytic domains.

In aprothrombinemia, the prothrombin activity and prothrombin antigen are both low. The causes of hereditary aprothrombinemia are not known, but it is assumed that these cases are due to partial or complete deletions of the prothrombin gene or to structural alterations in the expressed prothrombin that lead to rapid clearance of the mutant prothrombin.

Clinical Aspects. As an autosomal-recessive disorder, prothrombin deficiency in its heterozygous form is usually clinically silent. A careful family history may provide a clue to diagnosis. The prothrombin time and the partial thromboplastin time may be prolonged, but the extent of prolongation depends on the level of prothrombin activity deficiency. A direct prothrombin assay in prothrombin-deficient plasma allows determination of the plasma prothrombin coagulant activity. Immunoassay based on antiprothrombin antibodies permits the measurement of the plasma prothrombin antigen.

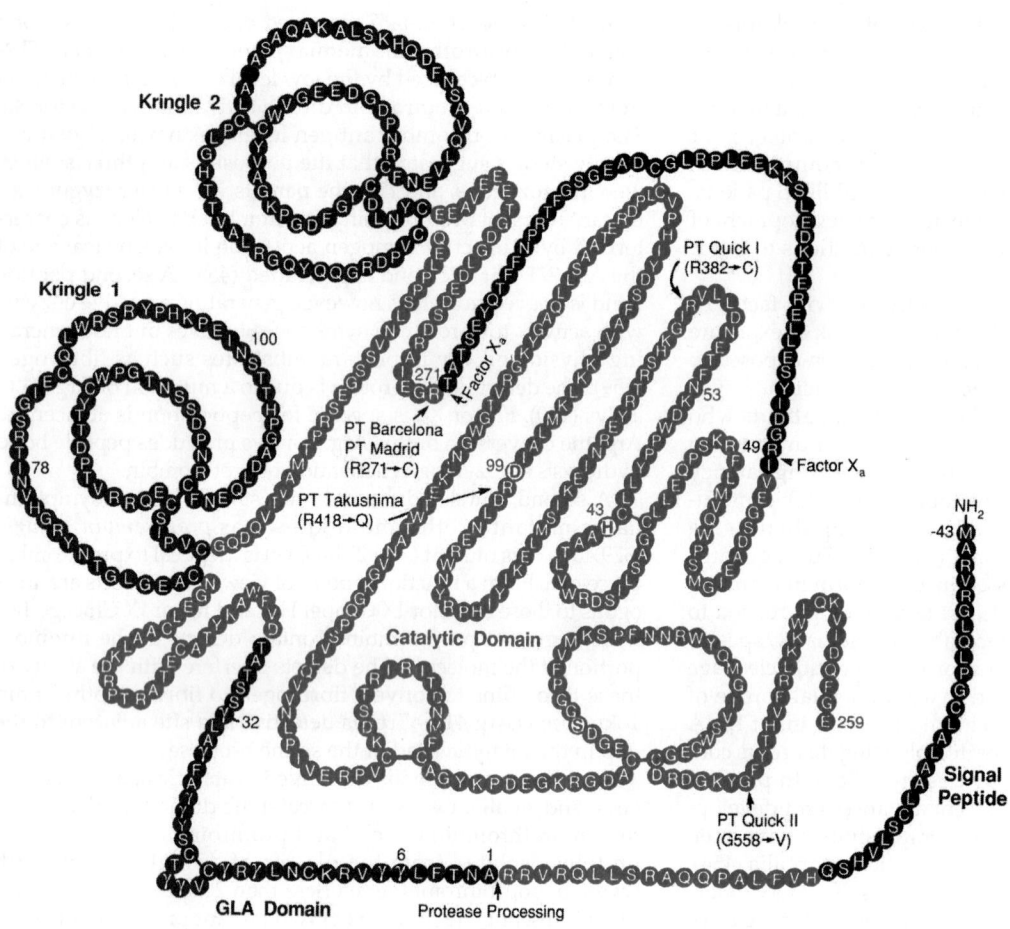

Figure 37-24. Molecular defects in mutant prothrombins (PTs). The point mutations identified in PT are indicated by the solid circles. Mutations have been identified in the activation and catalytic domains. EGF, epidermal growth factor.

Even in the homozygous form, prothrombin deficiency causes only a moderate bleeding tendency because at least a small amount of coagulant activity occurs. The clinical manifestations do not distinguish prothrombin deficiency from other hereditary clotting factor deficiencies. Hereditary prothrombin deficiency is treatable with the prothrombin contained in fresh frozen plasma or intermediate-purity factor IX concentrates, which contain prothrombin. As described, low-purity factor IX concentrates are associated with thromboembolic complications, hepatitis, and the transmission of other viral diseases. For patients without chronic need for replacement therapy, fresh frozen plasma offers therapy without a high risk of the transmission of viral diseases. The plasma half-life of prothrombin is approximately 3 days. Therefore, intermittent therapy is sufficient for the treatment of bleeding episodes. Vitamin K therapy has no role in the treatment of congenital prothrombin deficiency.

TABLE 37-5. Molecular Defects Associated with Dysprothrombinemia

Defect	Location	Reference
Point mutations that interfere with zymogen activation		
Prothrombin Barcelona	Arg 271→Cys	Rabiet et al. (460)
Prothrombin Madrid	Arg 271→Cys	Diuguid et al. (379)
Point mutations that alter enzyme activity and substrate binding		
Prothrombin Quick I	Arg 382→Cys	Henriksen and Mann (465)
Prothrombin Takushima	Arg 418→Trp	Miyata et al. (463)
Prothrombin Quick II	Gly 558→Val	Henriksen and Mann (465a)

DISORDERS OF FACTOR X

Mutant Factor X. Hereditary factor X deficiency is a rare autosomal-recessive disorder estimated to occur in fewer than 1 in 500,000 people. Mutant factor X molecules have been isolated from patients with hereditary factor X deficiency and their gene defects characterized. The majority of reported factor X gene mutations are point mutations resulting in amino acid substitutions; however, at least one report attributes congenital factor X deficiency to a mutation in an intron that results in a factor X messenger RNA splicing abnormality (472). Although the molecular basis of hereditary factory X deficiency is certainly less well understood than that of hereditary factor IX deficiency, it appears that factor X deficiencies are heterogeneous at the molecular level and that they have the same pattern of defects associated with factor IX and prothrombin deficiency. Several mutant factor X molecules (including the two original families, Stuart and Prower) have been studied with biochemical and immunochemical techniques. Both factor X activity and antigen are low in Stuart plasma, whereas Prower plasma has low factor X activity and normal factor X antigen (7,8). Factor X Friuli plasma is characterized by normal factor X antigen but a factor X activity of 5% (473). The prothrombin time and partial thromboplastin time are abnormal, but activation of factor X Friuli by the coagulant protein in Russell viper venom is normal. This defect is due to a point mutation (474). Approximately 50 cases of factor X deficiency have been described, but complete description of the biochemical defects is lacking (475,476). Factor X Roma and factor X Padua are among these variant factor X molecules that have been partially characterized (477–479) and are likely to yield to detailed structural analyses.

The factor X gene is located on the long arm of chromosome 13, closely linked to the factor VII gene (294,405). Some patients with defects on chromosome 13 have associated factor X deficiency (480). Combined deficiency of factor X and VII also has been associated with deletion of chromosome 13 (481). Factor X deficiency associated with partial 4q duplication due to inherited der(13),t(4;13)(q26;q34)mat in a girl has been described (482).

Clinical Characteristics. As discussed, hereditary factor X deficiency is inherited as an autosomal-recessive disorder. Approximately one-third of these patients have a deficiency in factor X antigen and factor X activity; in the remaining patients, factor X activity is low despite normal antigen levels (475,476). The severity of the clinical manifestations of factor X deficiency parallel the degree of factor X deficiency. Heterozygotes are usually asymptomatic and may go undetected. Their prothrombin times and partial thromboplastin times are usually marginally prolonged. In homozygotes, bleeding may be associated with surgery or trauma. Patients occasionally have sufficiently severe factor X deficiency to cause spontaneous bleeding. The pattern of the bleeding disorder does not distinguish it from other forms of hemophilia.

Hereditary factor X deficiency is treated with fresh frozen plasma or intermediate-purity factor IX concentrate, which contains factor X. Therapy with prothrombin complex concentrates has been effective for the treatment of hemorrhage as well as for prevention of hemorrhage, as reported for a patient with severe factor X deficiency (483). For patients who do not need chronic replacement therapy, fresh frozen plasma is a therapy without a high risk of transmitting viral diseases or inducing thromboembolic complications.

DISORDERS OF FACTOR VII

Mutant Factor VII. Hereditary factor VII deficiency is an extremely rare, autosomal-recessive disorder estimated to occur in 1 of 500,000 live births. A total of 238 individuals have been described with mutations in their factor VII genes (484). A database of known factor VII gene mutations can be found on the Internet (484a). The database demonstrates mutations in the 5' flanking region of the gene that disrupt transcription factor binding to important promoter elements. The majority of mutations correspond to single amino acid substitutions throughout functionally important regions of factor VII. Splice site mutations in introns and frameshift mutations that result in global disruption of the protein are also present. The heterogeneity of documented mutations is similar to that of the other vitamin K–dependent protein genes.

Clinical Characteristics. The clinical manifestations of factor VII deficiency are highly variable and do not correlate closely with the measured plasma factor VII activity using routinely available reagents. The total absence of factor VII in plasma leads to hemorrhagic death shortly after birth. Most patients with factor VII defects are asymptomatic or remain undiagnosed unless a laboratory evaluation of a prolonged prothrombin time is pursued. Severe bleeding is most commonly observed in individuals with factor VII activity levels less than 2% of normal (e.g., patients who are homozygous for factor VII gene mutations). Some patients with severe deficiency have severe bleeding problems, including intracranial hemorrhage (485). Other patients have typical musculoskeletal bleeding and hemarthroses (486). Others are asymptomatic, even when subjected to surgical procedures (487). Still others have disorders complicated by deep venous thrombosis and pulmonary embo-

lism (488). One study suggests that the major determinant of clinical bleeding in factor VII deficiency is racial origin, because none of nine evaluated black patients with factor VII deficiency had a history of bleeding, whereas all of the white patients in this study bled (489). Treatment with prothrombin complex concentrates or plasma-derived factor VII concentrates has been used with success. The development of recombinant DNA–derived factor VIIa has been used successfully as a bypassing agent for the treatment of hemophilia A and B patients with inhibitors (490) and has demonstrated safety and efficacy in the treatment of congenital factor VII deficiency (491).

Acquired Disorders of Vitamin K–Dependent Proteins

Any process that interferes with protein synthesis in the liver or impairs the availability of vitamin K can alter the level of activity of the vitamin K–dependent blood coagulation proteins. Deficiency of these proteins may also occur by overuse of the vitamin K–dependent proteins, as in intravascular coagulation, or by enhanced clearance mechanisms, as has been observed in the factor X deficiency associated with amyloidosis.

IMPAIRED PROTEIN SYNTHESIS OF VITAMIN K–DEPENDENT PROTEINS DUE TO VITAMIN K DEFICIENCY

Factor VII, factor IX, factor X, and prothrombin are part of a unique class of calcium-binding proteins that contain γ-carboxyglutamic acid (24,25). A posttranslational processing step requires vitamin K. In its reduced form, vitamin K is an essential cofactor for a liver carboxylase (28). In the absence of vitamin K or in the presence of vitamin K antagonists, γ-carboxylation of selected Glu residues is blocked, and the resulting proteins have no or decreased amounts of γ-carboxyglutamic acid (196,492,493). The γ-carboxyglutamic acid–deficient forms do not bind to phospholipid or calcium ions normally and have no biologic activity (130,131). The sole known clinical manifestation of vitamin K deficiency in both children and adults is a reduction in the activity of the vitamin K–dependent proteins. Depending on the degree of vitamin K deficiency, the coagulant activities of these proteins may vary from only a laboratory abnormality to serious bleeding.

Food, especially fresh green leafy vegetables (14), represents the primary nutritional source of vitamin K. Colonic bacteria produce vitamin K_2 (494), but it remains uncertain whether this source of vitamin K supplements the dietary intake, because bacteria are located in the large intestine and vitamin K absorption takes place in the ileum. Controversy remains about whether retrograde movement of vitamin K proximally to the ileum and passive absorption of vitamin K in the colon are important mechanisms. The daily dietary requirement for vitamin K is less than 1 μg/kg (495) as measured by a prolongation of the prothrombin time. The daily vitamin K requirement may be closer to 2 to 3 μg/kg, however, if the appearance of abnormal (des-γ–) carboxyprothrombin is used to monitor this requirement (294).

Patients who are severely malnourished, especially those receiving antibiotics, are more prone to vitamin K deficiency. In these cases, both the dietary and bacterial sources of vitamin K are considerably reduced or eliminated (496). Although vitamin K deficiency in the absence of antibiotics is unusual, bulimia can depress vitamin K–dependent protein activity (497). Clinically, significant vitamin K deficiency can appear in a healthy individual in 1 or 2 weeks. In a typical example, a patient undergoes elective surgery and requires parenteral antibiotics and intravenous fluid. Within a week, the patient develops a prolonged prothrombin time. Patients with marginal vitamin K reserves, such as those with end-stage malignancy, may also develop severe vitamin K deficiency within a week. Vitamin K deficiency in the postsurgical patient is sufficiently common that this diagnosis is usually made by the surgical staff. Any medical or surgical patients who require parenteral nutrition should receive a vitamin K supplement. Patients with severe, protracted vomiting may develop vitamin K deficiency, especially if they are treated with antibiotics. Vitamin K deficiency may also be a component of malabsorption syndromes such as sprue, kwashiorkor, or cholestasis.

Because both the intrinsic pathway and extrinsic pathway of blood coagulation involve vitamin K–dependent proteins, deficiency in the coagulation activity of these proteins prolongs both the prothrombin time and partial thromboplastin time. The diagnosis of vitamin K deficiency is confirmed by normalization of the prothrombin time 12 to 24 hours after the administration of 10 mg vitamin K_1. Vitamin K can be administered by subcutaneous or intravenous injection. Partial or complete correction indicates a component of vitamin K deficiency as a cause of the prolonged prothrombin time. Although the prothrombin time and the partial thromboplastin time are both prolonged by vitamin K deficiency, the prothrombin time is routinely used to evaluate vitamin K deficiency. Because prolongation of the prothrombin time may be associated with numerous other disorders and is not specific for vitamin K deficiency, the diagnosis of vitamin K deficiency cannot be made unless vitamin K administration significantly reduces a prolonged prothrombin toward the normal value.

Specific immunoassay of plasma abnormal (des-γ–carboxy) prothrombin is approximately 1000 times more sensitive than the prothrombin time in the detection of vitamin K deficiency (257,498). Because normal subjects do not have any circulating abnormal prothrombin in the plasma, the appearance of abnormal prothrombin in plasma can be readily detected by immunoassay. If the abnormal prothrombin appears because of a deficiency of vitamin K, administration of vitamin K leads to the disappearance of abnormal prothrombin in the plasma (499,500) (Fig. 37-25). A comparison of thrombin generation by factor Xa and by *Echis carinatus* venom also permits detection of vitamin K deficiency, but this approach is considerably less sensitive than the immunologic approach. Comparison of these assays before and after the administration of vitamin K allows the diagnosis of vitamin K deficiency over other conditions associated with a prolonged prothrombin time, such as liver disease (501). Direct assay of vitamin K in serum based on high-performance liquid chromatography has also been used to define vitamin K deficiency (502).

Vitamin K deficiency is treated with vitamin K_1 in a water-soluble preparation. The absorption of oral vitamin K is variable and unpredictable, particularly in patients with cholestasis and malabsorption. For this reason, the diagnosis and treatment of vitamin K deficiency should involve the administration of parenteral vitamin K_1. Hematomas can form after intramuscular injection in a patient with severe vitamin K deficiency. Therefore, intramuscular injection should be avoided. The definitive treatment of vitamin K deficiency involves the infusion of 10 to 15 mg vitamin K_1 intravenously. Because anaphylactic reactions can be associated with intravenous vitamin K administration, albeit rarely, care should be taken when this route of administration is used. This therapy should be used only in a hospital setting, with epinephrine available for the treatment of emergent allergic reactions. The prothrombin time usually corrects in 12 to 24 hours after vitamin K infusion. Patients with a serious bleeding disorder, such as intraabdominal or intracranial hemorrhage, who require urgent treatment of their vitamin K deficiency, should be treated with fresh frozen plasma to replace vitamin K–dependent proteins. Fresh frozen plasma carries the risk of viral infection, which must be balanced against the severity of the bleeding episode. Intermediate-purity prothrombin complex concentrates, previously used to treat hemophilia B, contain all of the vitamin K–dependent proteins. In available forms, however, they nearly guarantee the transmission of hepatitis to a patient without immunity to hepatitis. Therefore, these agents are contraindicated. Improvements in the large-scale preparation of purified vitamin K–dependent proteins may offer new agents that prove useful (447–449).

HEMORRHAGIC DISEASE OF THE NEWBORN

Hemorrhagic disease of the newborn is a bleeding disorder arising immediately after birth because of vitamin K deficiency (503–505). Bleeding usually begins between days 2 and 7 after birth and is clinically demonstrated by hematomas, bleeding from mucous membranes, hemorrhage after circumcision, and bleeding from venipuncture sites. In its most severe form, this disorder can cause internal bleeding, intracranial hemorrhage, and death (506). Before the introduction of prophylactic vitamin K, approximately 1 of 100 neonates bled from this syndrome; approximately 25% of these infants died. As many as 25% of all untreated, asymptomatic newborns have a prothrombin time and partial thromboplastin time consistent with hemorrhagic disease of the newborn (507). Using the abnormal (des-γ–carboxy) prothrombin as a sensitive serum marker of vitamin K deficiency, essentially all newborns have evidence of vitamin K deficiency at birth, as do approximately 30% of their mothers (508).

This hemorrhagic disorder is due to insufficient intake of vitamin K during the newborn period. This deficiency state is reversed on the colonization of the intestine with vitamin K–producing bacteria and the ingestion of vitamin K–containing food (505). Breast-fed neonates are susceptible to vitamin K deficiency (506,509,510) because human milk contains only 15 g/L vitamin K (505,511).

As in all vitamin K–deficient states, infants with hemorrhagic disease of the newborn have a prolonged partial thromboplastin time and prothrombin time. Because the synthesis of the vitamin K–dependent proteins is decreased in the neonate and the levels of these proteins are only half of adult levels (431), impaired car-

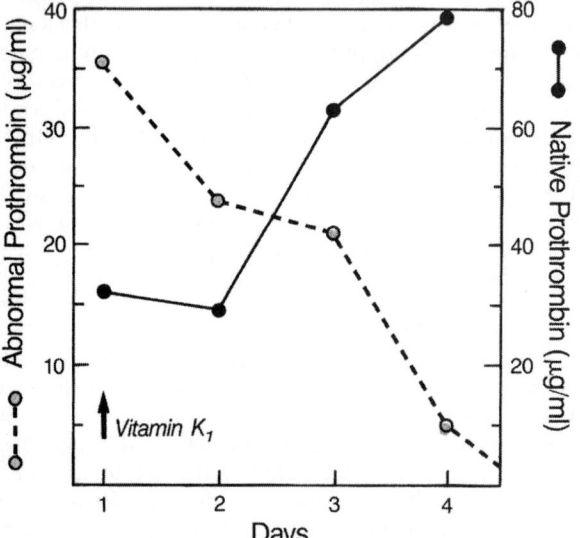

Figure 37-25. Vitamin K deficiency. Changes in the prothrombin time, native prothrombin antigen, and abnormal prothrombin antigen following treatment with vitamin K. (From Blanchard RA, Furie BC, Jorgensen MJ, et al. Acquired vitamin K-dependent carboxylation deficiency in liver disease. *N Engl J Med* 1981;305:242.)

boxylation of these proteins due to concomitant vitamin K deficiency exaggerates the potential bleeding risk. The syndrome is reversed with the administration of vitamin K, but fresh frozen plasma, despite the risk of infection, is justified in patients with life-threatening hemorrhage. A single dose of vitamin K (100 μg) is sufficient to correct the bleeding tendency.

To prevent hemorrhagic disease of the newborn, all hospital-born infants in the United States are prophylactically treated with vitamin K at birth by the subcutaneous injection of vitamin K (511). The usual dosage used is 100 μg to 1 mg (511). Larger doses should be avoided because vitamin K can interfere with the conjugation of bilirubin in the liver or cause hemolytic anemia (512,513).

DEFICIENCY OF VITAMIN K–DEPENDENT PROTEIN DUE TO VITAMIN K ANTAGONISTS

Reduced vitamin K is required as a cofactor for vitamin K–dependent carboxylation. In the metabolic pathway that recovers and recycles vitamin K, reduced vitamin K is converted to the vitamin K epoxide in a reaction that is thought to be linked to the carboxylation process. Under the action of the vitamin K epoxide reductase, vitamin K epoxide is then converted to vitamin K. The vitamin K reductase converts vitamin K to reduced vitamin K, completing the vitamin K cycle. Sodium warfarin inhibits vitamin K–dependent carboxylation by inhibiting the vitamin K reductase and vitamin K epoxide reductase (28). Because sodium warfarin is widely used clinically as an oral anticoagulant and is sold both as a pharmacologic agent and as a rodenticide, it is a frequent cause of reduced vitamin K–dependent protein activity. Some patients directed to take warfarin as an oral anticoagulant have bleeding complications despite careful monitoring of the prothrombin time (514–520). With the introduction of lower intensity warfarin therapy (514,516,521), the percentage of patients treated with warfarin who develop bleeding complications has decreased.

The accidental ingestion of warfarin or related agents can also lead to a deficiency of the vitamin K–dependent blood clotting proteins because rat poisons, or rodenticides, contain vitamin K antagonists. Children can come in contact with poorly placed bait and ingest the bait; severe bleeding can ensue within 48 hours to 1 week. Most of the first-generation rodenticides include warfarin as an active ingredient. The new superwarfarins, targeted at the warfarin-resistant rat populations, are fat-soluble and long-acting. These agents, such as brodifacoum, can cause prolongation of the prothrombin time for more than 6 months after a single ingestion (522–524). Patients poisoned with these second-generation rodenticides require treatment with high doses of vitamin K_1 (100 mg/day) by the oral route. Therapy must be extended until the residual vitamin K antagonist is depleted.

The surreptitious ingestion of vitamin K antagonists can lead to a bleeding disorder, factitious purpura (525–527). A severe psy-

chologic disorder often leads to ingestion. Covert anticoagulant abuse is most often seen in individuals associated with the medical profession, such as medical students, nurses, and medical technologists. In addition, those with relatives of patients taking warfarin may use warfarin covertly. Treatment of covert warfarin ingestion or over-dosage is identical in these patients and patients requiring anticoagulant therapy. Factitious superwarfarin ingestion, including brodifacoum, is particularly difficult to diagnose (528) (Fig. 37-26). The serum warfarin levels are undetectable despite a markedly prolonged prothrombin time and partial thromboplastin time. Patients who ingest these agents have marked prolongation of the prothrombin time for many months after a single exposure. Diagnosis is complicated by the fact that serum assays for these agents are not readily available. High doses of vitamin K_1 (e.g., 100 mg/day by the oral route) administered chronically can titrate the effects of brodifacoum.

Acetylsalicylic acid in toxic doses is known to induce a vitamin K deficient–like state (529). At high doses, acetylsalicylic acid likely oxidizes vitamin K so that it cannot be used in vitamin K–dependent carboxylation. This disorder responds to treatment with vitamin K. Certain antibiotics, including moxalactam, cause vitamin K deficiency (520–532). The inhibition of the vitamin K–dependent carboxylase by moxalactam and other antibiotics has been proposed (533). The precise structural moiety responsible for inhibition of vitamin K–dependent carboxylation is not known.

Treatment of warfarin toxicity or vitamin K inhibition depends on the severity of the clinical presentation. Furthermore, the clinical indication for oral anticoagulation must be weighed in the treatment plan. In the absence of clinically significant bleeding, warfarin may be discontinued, then restarted when the prothrombin time is in the therapeutic range. The prothrombin time gradually normalizes, particularly if a normal diet is continued. If necessary, the depletion of the vitamin K–dependent proteins can be reversed by the administration of vitamin K. These patients are refractory to further oral anticoagulant therapy for some time, however. When a bleeding disorder is serious and rapid replacement of the vitamin K–dependent proteins is indicated, fresh frozen plasma can be administered. Intermediate-purity factor IX concentrates should not be used because of the high incidence of viral infection.

DEFICIENCY OF VITAMIN K–DEPENDENT PROTEIN SECONDARY TO LIVER DISEASE

The liver is the site of synthesis of the vitamin K–dependent blood coagulation proteins (19–21). Parenchymal diseases of the liver (cirrhosis and hepatitis), infiltrative diseases involving the liver (metastatic neoplasms), and primary liver neoplasms (primary hepatocellular carcinoma) can all interfere with the normal synthesis of the vitamin K–dependent blood coagulation proteins (534–536). Some patients may not demonstrate

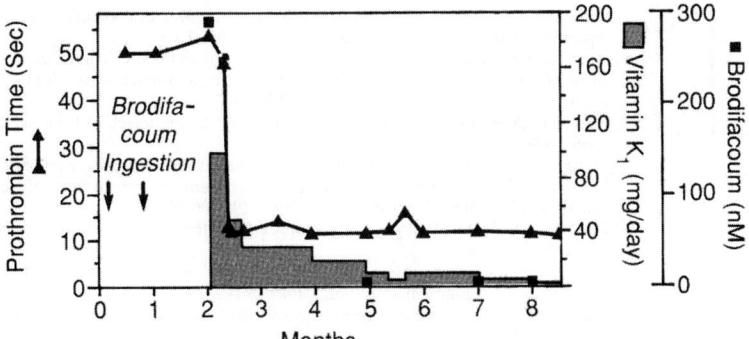

Figure 37-26. Deficiency of the vitamin K–dependent proteins due to ingestion of brodifacoum, a potent rodenticide. (From Weitzel JN, Sadowski JA, Furie BC, et al. Hemorrhagic disorder caused by surreptitious ingestion of a long-acting vitamin K antagonist/rodenticide, brodifacoum. *Blood* 1990;76:2555.)

increased bleeding tendencies, but their prolonged prothrombin time is secondary to impaired synthesis of the vitamin K–dependent proteins. Prolongation of the prothrombin time is observed in moderate to severe cases of liver disease. Most often, the hemostatic abnormalities of liver disease are without overt clinical manifestations. Although des-γ–carboxy forms of prothrombin in the plasma of patients with liver disease serve as a diagnostic marker of impaired γ-carboxylation, the minor defect in the vitamin K–dependent carboxylation does not contribute significantly to the hemostatic disorder (257). It is the generalized decreased synthesis of the vitamin K–dependent proteins, as measured by decreased plasma prothrombin antigen (257,537), that causes the laboratory abnormalities.

These hemostatic abnormalities often are diagnosed when significant bleeding occurs in a patient with liver disease or when a preoperative bleeding evaluation is requested before liver biopsy. In liver disease patients with poor dietary intake and a history of alcohol abuse, the coagulation abnormalities may only partially arise from vitamin K deficiency. Therefore, the prothrombin time and partial thromboplastin time usually do not normalize with administration of vitamin K. The absence of at least partial correction of the prothrombin time 24 hours after administration of vitamin K_1 (10 to 15 mg) intravenously indicates a hemostatic abnormality other than vitamin K deficiency. Fresh frozen plasma in adequate quantity partially corrects the plasma levels of the vitamin K–dependent proteins and decreases the bleeding tendency during surgery (538). Intermediate-purity factor IX concentrates, which are associated with the development of thromboembolic disease and transmission of hepatitis, are contraindicated in the treatment of severe liver disease (436,539). This material induces a hypercoagulable state and is compounded by the acquired antithrombin III deficiency that characterizes severe liver disease.

Most patients with hepatitis and cirrhosis as well as those with primary hepatocellular carcinoma have a defect in vitamin K–dependent carboxylation (257,540). In fact, abnormal (des-γ–carboxy) prothrombin can be used as a marker for hepatocellular carcinoma (540–542) and can supplement the α-fetoprotein assay (Fig. 37-27).

ACQUIRED FACTOR X DEFICIENCY AND AMYLOIDOSIS

Rarely, primary amyloidosis is associated with an acquired coagulation disorder characterized by factor X deficiency (543–545). These patients have bleeding complications in addition to the clinical manifestations of amyloidosis. This disorder is due to the removal of factor X from the plasma. Factor X is immobilized along the amyloid-infiltrated vasculature and distributed in the reticuloendothelial system (545). Factor X has a curious affinity for amyloid fibrils (546).

These patients do not respond to the infusion of factor X in fresh frozen plasma, intermediate-purity factor IX concentrates, or large-volume plasmapheresis and plasma exchange (545,547). Splenectomy, with removal of a large burden of amyloid, has been associated with the rapid normalization of plasma factor X levels in two reported cases (548,549). Chemotherapy with antimyeloma agents, such as cyclophosphamide and prednisone, has been successful in one case (550), but most patients with amyloidosis who receive this therapy are not responsive. A recent report of the use of recombinant factor VIIa offers a new approach to the treatment of life-threatening bleeding or prophylaxis for splenectomy (551).

MISCELLANEOUS ACQUIRED DEFECTS OF VITAMIN K–DEPENDENT PROTEINS

The lupus anticoagulant causes a prolongation of the partial thromboplastin time due to the inhibition of the assay by antiphospholipid antibodies. In a small percentage of cases, however, this antibody cross-reacts with prothrombin and leads to the rapid clearance of prothrombin from the blood (552). The induced hypoprothrombinemia can cause significant bleeding in contrast to the absence of bleeding problems associated with the lupus anticoagulant.

A deficiency of factor IX has been reported in association with the nephrotic syndrome (553–555). This diagnosis is often made in patients under evaluation before renal biopsy. Although the presence of factor IX deficiency correlates with the extent of proteinuria, the mechanism of the factor IX deficiency is unknown.

REFERENCES

1. Schmidt A. *Zur Blutlehre*. Leipzig: Vogel, 1892.
2. Morawitz P. *Die Chemie der Blutzgerinnung. Ergio Physiol* 1905;4:307.
3. Seegers WH. *Prothrombin*. Cambridge, MA: Harvard University Press, 1962.
4. Aggeler PM, White SG, Glendenning MB, et al. Plasma thromboplastin component (PTC) deficiency: a new disease resembling hemophilia. *Proc Soc Exp Biol Med* 1952;79:692.
5. Schulman I, Smith CH. Hemorrhagic disease in an infant due to deficiency of a previously undescribed clotting factor. *Blood* 1952;7:794.
6. Alexander B, Godstein R, Landwehr G, et al. Congenital SPCA deficiency: a hitherto unrecognized coagulation defect with hemorrhage rectified by serum and serum fractions. *J Clin Invest* 1951;30:596.
7. Telfer TP, Denson KW, Wright DR. A "new" coagulation defect. *Br J Haematol* 1956;2:308.
8. Hougie E, Barrow EM, Graham JB. Stuart clotting defect, I. Segregation of an hereditary hemorrhagic state from the heterogeneous group heretofore called "stable factor" deficiency. *J Clin Invest* 1957;36:485.
9. Ratnoff OD, Davie EW. Waterfall sequence for intrinsic blood clotting. *Science* 1964;145:1310.
10. Macfarlane RG. An enzyme cascade in the blood clotting mechanism and its function as a biochemical amplifier. *Nature* 1964;202:498.
11. Seegers WH. Blood clotting mechanisms: three basic reactions. *Annu Rev Physiol* 1969;31:269.

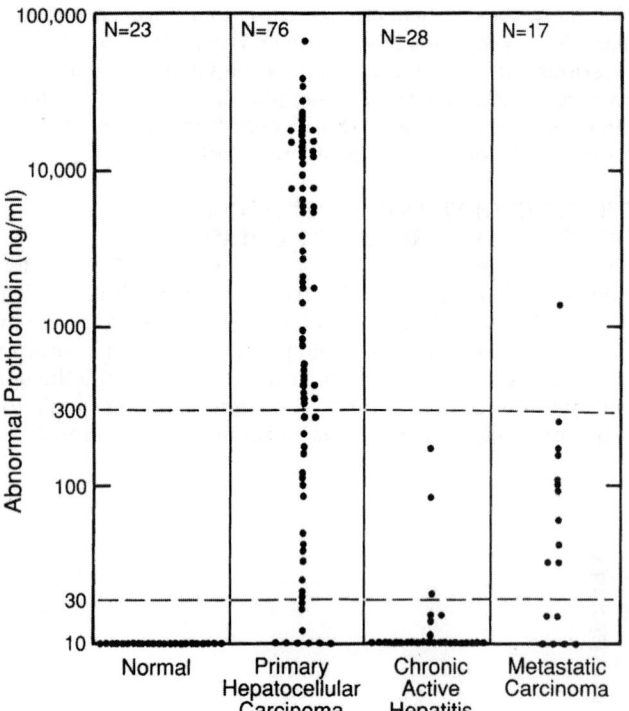

Figure 37-27. Impaired vitamin K–dependent carboxylation. Abnormal prothrombin is a marker of primary hepatocellular carcinoma. [After Liebman HA, Furie BC, Tong MJ, et al. Des-γ-carboxy (abnormal) prothrombin as a serum marker of primary hepatocellular carcinoma. *N Engl J Med* 1984;310:1427.]

12. Dam H. Cholesterinstoffwechsel in Huhnereiern und Huhnchen. *Biochem Zeitschr* 1929;215:475.

13. Dam H. The antihaemorrhagic vitamin of the chick: occurrence and chemical nature. *Nature* 1935;135:652.

14. Almquist HJ. Purification of the antihemorrhagic vitamin. *J Biol Chem* 1936;114:241.

15. Doisy EA, MacCorquodale DW, Thayer SA, et al. The isolation, constitution, and synthesis of vitamin K_1. *Science* 1939;90:407.

16. Schofield FW. A brief account of a disease in cattle simulating hemorrhagic septicemia due to feeding sweet clover. *Can Vet Rec* 1922;3:74.

17. Roderick LM. A problem in the coagulation of the blood "sweet clover" disease of cattle. *Am J Physiol* 1931;96:413.

18. Campbell HA, Link KP. Studies on the hemorrhagic sweet clover disease: IV. the isolation and crystallization of the hemorrhagic agent. *J Biol Chem* 1941;138:21.

19. Mann FD, Shonyo ES, Mann FC. Effect of removal of the liver on blood coagulation. *Am J Physiol* 1951;164:111.

20. Pool J, Robinson J. In vitro synthesis of coagulation factors by rat liver slices. *Am J Physiol* 1959;196:423.

21. Olson JP, Miller LL, Troup SB. Synthesis of clotting factors by the isolated perfused rat liver. *J Clin Invest* 1966;45:690.

22. Furie B, Furie BC. Molecular basis of blood coagulation. *Cell* 1988;53:505.

23. Kurachi K, Davie EW. Isolation and characterization of a cDNA coding for human factor IX. *Proc Natl Acad Sci U S A* 1982;79:6461.

24. Stenflo J, Fernlund P, Egan W, et al. Vitamin K dependent modifications of glutamic acid residues in prothrombin. *Proc Natl Acad Sci U S A* 1974;71:2730.

25. Nelsestuen GL, Zytkovicz TH, Howard JB. The mode of action of vitamin K: identification of γ-carboxyglutamic acid as a component of prothrombin. *J Biol Chem* 1974;249:6347.

26. Drakenberg T, Fernlund P, Roepstorff P, et al. β–Hydroxyaspartic acid in vitamin K–dependent protein C. *Proc Natl Acad Sci U S A* 1983;80:1802.

27. McMullen BA, Fujikawa K, Kisiel W. The occurrence of β–hydroxyaspartic acid in the vitamin K-dependent blood coagulation zymogens. *Biochem Biophys Res Commun* 1983;115:8.

28. Suttie JW. Mechanism of action of vitamin K: synthesis of gamma-carboxyglutamic acid. *CRC Crit Rev Biochem* 1980;8:191.

29. Furie B, Bouchard BA, Furie BC. Vitamin K-dependent biosynthesis of γ-carboxyglutamic acid. *Blood* 1999;93:1789.

30. Wu S-M, Morris DP, Stafford DW. Identification and purification to near homogeneity of the vitamin K-dependent carboxylase. *Proc Natl Acad Sci U S A* 1991;88:2236.

31. Helgeland L. The submicrosomal site for the conversion of prothrombin precursor to biologically active prothrombin in rat liver. *Biochim Biophys Acta* 1977;499:181.

32. Wallin R, Prydz H. Studies on a subcellular system for vitamin K-dependent carboxylation. *Thromb Haemost* 1979;41:529.

33. Carlisle TL, Suttie JW. Vitamin K-dependent carboxylase: subcellular location of the carboxylase and enzymes involved in vitamin K metabolism in rat liver. *Biochemistry* 1980;19:1161.

34. Wu S-M, Cheung W-F, Frazier DF, et al. Cloning and expression of the cDNA for human γ-glutamyl carboxylase. *Science* 1991;254:1634.

35. Rehemtulla A, Roth DA, Wasley L, et al. In vitro and in vivo functional characterization of bovine vitamin K-dependent γ-carboxylase expressed in Chinese hamster ovary cells. *Proc Natl Acad Sci U S A* 1993;90:4611.

36. Tie J, Wu S-M, Jin D, et al. A topological study of the human gamma-glutamyl carboxylase. *Blood* 2000;96:978.

37. Kuo WL, Stafford DW, Cruces M, et al. Chromosomal localization of the γ-glutamyl carboxylase gene at 2p12. *Genomics* 1994;25:746.

38. Wu S-M, Stafford DW, Frazier LD, et al. Genomic sequence and transcription start site for the human γ-glutamyl carboxylase gene. *Biochem Biophys Res Commun* 1997;89:4058.

39. Brenner B, Sanchez-Vega B, Wu S-M, et al. A missense mutation in gamma-glutamyl carboxylase gene causes combined deficiency of all vitamin K-dependent blood coagulation factors. *Blood* 1998;92:4554.

40. Spronk HM, Farah RA, Buchanan GR, et al. Novel mutation in the gamma-glutamyl carboxylase gene resulting in congenital combined deficiency of all vitamin K-dependent blood coagulation factors. *Blood* 2000;96:3650.

41. Romero EE, Deo R, Velazquez-Estades LJ, et al. Cloning, structural organization, and transcriptional regulation of the rat vitamin K-dependent–glutamyl carboxylase gene. *Biochem Biophys Res Commun* 1998;248:783.

42. Begley GS, Furie BC, Czerwiec E, et al. A conserved motif within the vitamin K-dependent carboxylase gene is widely distributed across animal phyla. *J Biol Chem* 2000;46:36245.

43. Li T, Yang CT, Jin D, et al. Identification of a Drosophila vitamin K-dependent gamma-glutamyl carboxylase. *J Biol Chem* 2000;275:18291.

44. Wallin R, Suttie JW. Vitamin K-dependent carboxylase: evidence for cofraction of carboxylase and epoxidase activities, and for carboxylation of a high molecular weight microsomal protein. *Arch Biochem Biophys* 1982;214:155.

45. Suttie JW, Larson AE, Canfield LM, et al. Relationship between vitamin K-dependent carboxylation and vitamin K epoxidation. *Fed Proc* 1978;37:2605.

46. Sadowski JA, Schnoes HK, Suttie JW. Vitamin K epoxidase: properties and relationship to prothrombin synthesis. *Biochemistry* 1977;16:3856.

47. Suttie JW, Geweke LO, Martin SL, et al. Vitamin K epoxidase: dependence of epoxidase activity on substrates of the vitamin K-dependent carboxylation reaction. *FEBS Lett* 1980;109:267.

48. Friedman PA, Shia MA, Gallop PM, et al. Vitamin K-dependent gamma-carbon hydrogen bond cleavage and nonmandatory concurrent carboxylation of peptide-bound glutamic acid residues. *Proc Natl Acad Sci U S A* 1979;76:3126.

49. McTigue JJ, Suttie JW. Vitamin K-dependent carboxylase: demonstration of a vitamin K- and O_2-dependent exchange of ^3H from ^3H_2O into glutamic acid residues. *J Biol Chem* 1983;258:12129.

50. Anton DL, Friedman PA. Fate of the activated γ–carbon-hydrogen bond in the uncoupled vitamin K-dependent γ–glutamyl carboxylation reaction. *J Biol Chem* 1983;258:14084.

51. Dowd P, Hershline R, Ham SW, et al. Vitamin K and energy transduction: a base strength amplification mechanism. *Science* 1995;269:1684.

52. Dowd P, Ham SW, Hershline R. Role of oxygen in the vitamin K-dependent carboxylation reaction: incorporation of a second atom of ^{18}O from molecular oxygen-$^{18}O_2$ into vitamin K during carboxylase activity. *J Am Chem Soc* 1992;114:7613.

53. Kuliopulos A, Hubbard BR, Lam Z, et al. Dioxygen transfer during vitamin K-dependent carboxylase catalysis. *Biochemistry* 1992;31:7722.

54. Morris DP, Soute BAM, Vermeer C, et al. Characterization of the purified vitamin K-dependent γ-glutamyl carboxylase. *J Biol Chem* 1993;268:8735.

55. Bouchard BA, Furie B, Furie BC. Glutamyl substrate-induced exposure of a free cysteine residue in the vitamin K-dependent γ-glutamyl carboxylase is critical for vitamin K epoxidation. *Biochemistry* 1999;38:9517.

56. Pudota BN, Miyagi M, Hallgren KW, et al. Identification of the vitamin K-dependent carboxylase active site: Cys-99 and Cys-450 are required for both epoxidation and carboxylation. *Proc Natl Acad Sci U S A* 2000;97:13033.

57. Giradot J-M, Mack DO, Floyd RA, et al. Evidence for vitamin K semiquinone as the functional form of vitamin K in the liver vitamin K-dependent protein carboxylation reaction. *Biochem Biophys Res Commun* 1976;70:655.

58. Friedman PA, Shia M. Some characteristics of a vitamin K-dependent carboxylating system from rat liver microsomes. *Biochem Biophys Res Commun* 1976;70:647.

59. Esmon CT, Suttie JW. Vitamin K-dependent carboxylase: solubilization and properties. *J Biol Chem* 1976;251:6238.

60. Pennock JF. Occurrence of vitamin K and related quinones. *Vitam Horm* 1966;24:307.

61. Wallin R. No strict coupling of vitamin K_1 (2-methyl-3-phytyl-1,4-naphthaquinone)-dependent carboxylation and vitamin K_1 epoxidation in detergent-solubilized microsomal fractions from rat liver. *Biochem J* 1979;178: 513.

62. Wallin R, Hutson S. Vitamin K-dependent carboxylation: evidence that at least two microsomal dehydrogenases reduce vitamin K_1 to support carboxylation. *J Biol Chem* 1982;57:1583.

63. Wallin R, Gabhardt O, Prydz H. NAD(P)H dehydrogenase and its role in the vitamin K (2-methyl-3-phytyl-1,4-napthaquinone)-dependent carboxylation reaction. *Biochem J* 1978;169:95.

64. Matschiner JT, Zimmerman A, Bell RG. The influence of warfarin on vitamin K epoxide reductase. *Thromb Diath Haemorrh* 1974;57[Suppl]:45.

65. Zimmerman A, Matschiner JT. Biochemical basis of hereditary resistance to warfarin in the rat. *Biochem Pharmacol* 1974;23:1033.

66. Sherman PA, Sander EG. Vitamin K epoxide reductase: evidence that vitamin K dihydroquinone is a product of vitamin K epoxide reduction. *Biochem Biophys Res Commun* 1981;103:997.

67. Wallin R, Martin LF. Warfarin poisoning and vitamin K antagonism in rat and human liver: design of a system that mimics the system in vivo. *Biochem J* 1987;241:389.

68. Guenthner TM, Cai D, Wallin R. Co-purification of microsomal epoxide hydrolase with the warfarin-sensitive vitamin K1 oxide reductase of the vitamin K cycle. *Biochem Pharmacol* 1998;55:169.

69. Cain D, Hutson SM, Wallin R. Assembly of the warfarin sensitive vitamin K 2,3-epoxide reductase enzyme complex in the endoplasmic reticulum membrane. *J Biol Chem* 1997;272:29068.

70. Oldenburg J, von Brederlow B, Fregin A, et al. Congenital deficiency of vitamin K dependent coagulation factors in two families presents as a genetic defect of the vitamin K-epoxide-reductase-complex. *Thromb Haemost* 2000;84:937.

71. Fasco MJ, Hildebrandt EF, Suttie JW. Evidence that warfarin anticoagulant action involves two distinct reduction activities. *J Biol Chem* 1982;257:11210.

72. Whitlon DS, Sadowski JA, Suttie JW. Mechanism of coumarin action: significance of vitamin K epoxide reductase inhibition. *Biochemistry* 1978;17:1371.

73. Fasco MJ, Principe LM. Vitamin K_1 hydroquinone formation catalyzed by a microsomal reductase system. *Biochem Biophys Res Commun* 1980;97:1487.

74. Shah DV, Suttie JW. Mechanism of action of vitamin K: evidence for the conversion of a precursor protein to prothrombin in the rat liver. *Proc Natl Acad Sci U S A* 1971;68:1653.

75. Suttie JW. Mechanism of action of vitamin K: demonstration of a liver precursor of prothrombin. *Science* 1973;179:192.

76. Esmon CT, Sadowski JA, Suttie JW. A new carboxylation reaction: the vitamin K-dependent incorporation of H_2CO_3 into prothrombin. *J Biol Chem* 1975;250:4744.

77. Grant GA, Suttie JW. Rat liver prothrombin precursors: purification of a second, more basic form. *Biochemistry* 1976;24:5387.

78. Graves GB, Brabau GG, Olson RE, et al. Immunochemical isolation and electrophoretic characterization of precursor prothrombins in H-35 rat hepatoma cells. *Biochemistry* 1980;19:266.

79. Swanson JC, Suttie JW. Prothrombin biosynthesis: characterization of processing events in rat liver microsomes. *Biochemistry* 1985;24:3890.

80. Ganrot PO, Nilehn JE. Plasma prothrombin during treatment with dicumarol: demonstration of an abnormal prothrombin fraction. *Scand J Clin Invest* 1968;22:23.

81. Nelsestuen GL, Suttie JW. The purification and properties of an abnormal prothrombin protein provided by dicumarol-treated cows. *J Biol Chem* 1972;247:8176.

82. Shah DV, Swanson JC, Suttie JW. Vitamin K-dependent carboxylase: effect of detergent concentrations, vitamin K status and added protein precursors on activity. *Arch Biochem Biophys* 1983;222:216.

83. DeMetz M, Vermeer C, Soute BAM, et al. Partial purification of bovine liver vitamin K-dependent carboxylase by immunospecific adsorption onto anti-factor X. *FEBS Lett* 1981;123:215.

84. Jorgensen MJ, Cantor AB, Furie BC, et al. Recognition site directing vitamin K-dependent γ-carboxylation resides on the propeptide of factor IX. *Cell* 1987;48:185.

85. Diuguid DL, Rabiet M-J, Furie BC, et al. Molecular basis of hemophilia B: a defective enzyme due to an unprocessed propeptide is caused by a point mutation in the factor IX precursor. *Proc Natl Acad Sci U S A* 1986;83:5803.

86. Ware J, Diuguid DL, Liebman HA, et al. Factor IX San Dimas: substitution of glutamine for arginine –4 in the propeptide leads to incomplete γ-carboxylation and altered phospholipid binding properties. *J Biol Chem* 1989;264:11401.

87. Bentley AK, Rees DJG, Rizza C, et al. Defective propeptide processing of blood clotting factor IX caused by mutation of arginine to glutamine at position –4. *Cell* 1986;45:343.

88. Pan LC, Price PA. The propeptide of rat bone gamma-carboxyglutamic acid protein shares homology with other vitamin K-dependent protein precursors. *Proc Natl Acad Sci U S A* 1985;82:6109.

89. Rabiet MJ, Jorgensen MJ, Furie B, et al. Effect of propeptide mutations on posttranslational processing of factor IX: evidence that β-hydroxylation and γ-carboxylation are independent events. *J Biol Chem* 1987;262:14895.

90. Suttie JW, Hageman JM. Vitamin K-dependent carboxylase: development of a peptide substrate. *J Biol Chem* 1976;251:5827.

91. Suttie JW, Lehrman SR, Geweke LO, et al. Vitamin K-dependent carboxylase: requirement for carboxylation of soluble peptide substrates and substrate specificity. *Biochem Biophys Res Commun* 1979;86:500.

92. Rich DH, Lehrman SR, Kawai M, et al. Synthesis of peptide analogues of prothrombin precursor sequence 5-9: substrate specificity of vitamin K-dependent carboxylase. *J Med Chem* 1981;24:706.

93. Decottignies-Le Marechal P, Rikong-Adie H, Azerad R. Vitamin K-dependent carboxylation of synthetic substrates: nature of the products. *Biochem Biophys Res Commun* 1979;90:700.

94. Ulrich M, Furie B, Jacobs M, et al. Vitamin K-dependent carboxylation: a synthetic peptide based upon the γ-carboxylation recognition site sequence of the prothrombin propeptide is an active substrate for the carboxylase in vitro. *J Biol Chem* 1988;263:9697.

95. Suttie JW, Hoskins JA, Engelke J, et al. Vitamin K-dependent carboxylase: possible role of the substrate "propeptide" as an intracellular recognition site. *Proc Natl Acad Sci U S A* 1987;84:2730.

96. Foster DC, Rudinski MS, Schach BG, et al. Propeptide of human protein C is necessary for γ-carboxylation. *Biochemistry* 1987;26:7003.

97. Huber P, Schmitz T, Griffin J, et al. Identification of amino acids in the γ-carboxylation recognition site on the propeptide of prothrombin. *J Biol Chem* 1990;265:12467–12473.

98. Tward JD, Furie BC, Bouchard BA, et al. Other amino acids than phenylalanine at position –16 in the carboxylation recognition site in the prothrombin propeptide can support γ-carboxylation. *Blood* 1997;90:291a.

99. Stanley TB, Jin D-Y, Lin P-J, et al. The propeptides of the vitamin K-dependent proteins possess different affinities for the vitamin K-dependent carboxylase. *J Biol Chem* 1999;274:16940.

100. Stanley TB, Humphries J, High KA, et al. Amino acids responsible for reduced affinities of vitamin K-dependent propeptides for the carboxylase. *Biochemistry* 1999;38:15681.

101. Chu K, Wu S-M, Stanley T, et al. A mutation in the propeptide of factor IX leads to warfarin sensitivity by a novel mechanism. *J Clin Invest* 1996;98:1619.

102. Oldenburg J, Quenzel E-M, Harbrecht U, et al. Missense mutation at Ala –10 in the factor IX propeptide: an insignificant variant in normal life but a decisive cause of bleeding during oral anticoagulant therapy. *Br J Haematol* 1997;98:240.

103. Knobloch JE, Suttie JW. Vitamin K-dependent carboxylase: control of enzyme activity by the "propeptide" region of factor X. *J Biol Chem* 1987;262:15334.

104. Price PA, Fraser JD, Metz-Virca G. Molecular cloning of matrix Gla protein: implications for substrate recognition by the vitamin K-dependent γ-carboxylase. *Proc Natl Acad Sci U S A* 1987;84:8335.

105. Furie BC, Ratcliffe J, Tward J, et al. The γ-carboxylation recognition site is sufficient to direct vitamin K-dependent carboxylation on an adjacent glutamate-rich region of thrombin in a propeptide-thrombin chimera. *J Biol Chem* 1997;272:28258.

106. Hubbard B, Jacobs M, Ulrich M, et al. Vitamin K-dependent carboxylation: in vitro modification of synthetic peptides containing the γ-carboxylation recognition site. *J Biol Chem* 1989;264:14145.

107. Sanford DG, Kanagy C, Sudmeir JL, et al. Structure of the propeptide of prothrombin containing the γ-carboxylation recognition site determined by two-dimensional NMR spectroscopy. *Biochemistry* 1991;30:9835.

108. Fernlund P, Stenflo J. Beta-hydroxyaspartic acid in vitamin K-dependent proteins. *J Biol Chem* 1983;258:12509.

109. McMullen BA, Fujikawa K, Kisiel W, et al. Complete amino acid sequence of the light chain of human blood coagulation factor X: evidence for identification of residue 63 as β-hydroxyaspartic acid. *Biochemistry* 1983;22:2875.

110. Stenflo J, Lundwall A, Dahlback B. β-Hydroxyasparagine in domains homologous to the epidermal growth factor precursor in the vitamin K-dependent protein S. *Proc Natl Acad Sci U S A* 1987;84:368.

111. Ohlin A-K, Landes G, Bourdon P, et al. β-Hydroxyaspartic acid in the first epidermal growth factor-like domain of protein C: its role in Ca²⁺ binding and biological activity. *J Biol Chem* 1988;263:19240.

112. Rees DJG, Jones IM, Handford PA, et al. The role of β-hydroxyaspartate and adjacent carboxylate residues in the first EGF domain of human factor IX. *EMBO J* 1988;7:2053.

113. Sunnerhagen MS, Persson E, Dahlqvist I, et al. The effect of aspartate hydroxylation on calcium binding to epidermal growth factor-like modules in coagulation factors IX and X. *J Biol Chem* 1993;268:23339.

114. Arlaud GJ, Van Dorsselaer A, Bell A, et al. Identification of erythro-β-hydroxyasparagine in the EGF-like domain of human C1r. *FEBS Lett* 1987;222:129.

115. Stenflo J, Onlin A-K, Owen WG, et al. β-Hydroxyaspartic acid or β-hydroxyasparagine in bovine low density lipoprotein receptor and in bovine thrombomodulin. *J Biol Chem* 1988;263:21.

116. Przysiecki CT, Staggers JE, Ramjit HG, et al. Occurrence of β-hydroxylated asparagine residues in non-vitamin K-dependent proteins containing epidermal growth factor-like domains. *Proc Natl Acad Sci U S A* 1987;84:7856.

117. Stenflo J, Holme E, Lindstedt S, et al. Hydroxylation of aspartic acid in domains homologous to the epidermal growth factor precursor is catalyzed by a 2-oxoglutarate-dependent dioxygenase. *Proc Natl Acad Sci U S A* 1989;86:444.

118. Gronke RS, Welsch DJ, VanDusen WJ, et al. Partial purification and characterization of bovine liver aspartyl beta-hydroxylase. *J Biol Chem* 1990;265:8558.

119. Jia S, VanDusen WJ, Diehl RE, et al. cDNA cloning and expression of bovine aspartyl (asparaginyl) beta-hydroxylase. *J Biol Chem* 1992;267:14322.

120. Choo KH, Gould KG, Rees DJG, et al. Molecular cloning of the gene for human anti-haemophilic factor IX. *Nature* 1982;299:178.

121. Degen SJ, MacGillivrey RT, Davie EW. Characterization of the cDNA and gene coding for human prothrombin. *Biochemistry* 1983;22:2087.

122. Fung MR, Hay CW, MacGillivray RTA. Characterization of an almost full-length cDNA coding for human factor X. *Proc Natl Acad Sci U S A* 1985;82:3591.

123. Hagen FS, Gray CL, O'Hara P, et al. Characterization of the cDNA coding for human factor VII. *Proc Natl Acad Sci U S A* 1986;83:2412.

124. Leytus SP, Chung DW, Kisiel W, et al. Characterization of a cDNA coding for human factor X. *Proc Natl Acad Sci U S A* 1984;81:3699.

125. Wasley LC, Rehemtulla A, Bristol JA, et al. PACE/furin can process the vitamin K-dependent profactor IX precursor within the secretory pathway. *J Biol Chem* 1993;268:8458.

126. Bristol JA, Furie BC, Furie B. Propeptide processing during factor IX biosynthesis: effect of point mutations adjacent to the propeptide cleavage site. *J Biol Chem* 1993;268:7577.

127. Bristol JA, Ratcliffe JV, Roth DA, et al. Biosynthesis of prothrombin: intracellular localization of the vitamin K-dependent carboxylase and the sites of γ-carboxylation. *Blood* 1996;88:2585.

128. Bucher D, Nebelin E, Thomsen J, et al. Identification of γ-carboxyglutamic acid residues in bovine factors IX and X, and in a new vitamin K-dependent protein. *FEBS Lett* 1976;68:293.

129. Fryklund L, Borg H, Andersson L-O. Amino terminal sequence of human factor IX: presence of a γ-carboxyglutamic acid residues. *FEBS Lett* 1976;65:187.

130. Esmon CT, Suttie JW, Jackson CM. The functional significance of vitamin K action: difference in phospholipid binding between normal and abnormal prothrombin. *J Biol Chem* 1975;250:4095.

131. Stenflo J, Ganrot P-O. Vitamin K and the biosynthesis of prothrombin: identification and purification of a dicoumarol-induced abnormal prothrombin from bovine plasma. *J Biol Chem* 1972;247:8160.

132. Magnusson S, Sottrup-Jenssen L, Petersen TE, et al. Primary structure of the vitamin K-dependent part of prothrombin. *FEBS Lett* 1974;44:189.

133. Walz DA, Hewett-Emmett D, Seegers WH. Amino acid sequence of human prothrombin fragments 1 and 2. *Proc Natl Acad Sci U S A* 1977;74:1969.

134. Enfield DL, Ericsson LE, Walsh KA, et al. Bovine factor X₁ (Stuart factor), primary structure of the light chain. *Proc Natl Acad Sci U S A* 1975;72:16.

135. McMullen B, Fujikawa K, Kisiel W, et al. Complete amino acid sequence of the light chain of human blood coagulation factor X: evidence for identification of residue 63 as β-hydroxyaspartic acid. *Biochemistry* 1983;22:2875.

136. Morris HR, Dell A, Petersen TE, et al. Mass spectrometric identification and sequence location of the ten residues of the new amino acid (β-carboxyglutamic acid) in the N-terminal region of prothrombin. *Biochem J* 1976;153:663.

137. Katayama K, Ericsson L, Enfield D, et al. Comparison of amino acid sequence of bovine coagulation factor IX (Christmas factor) with that of other vitamin K-dependent proteins. *Proc Natl Acad Sci U S A* 1979;76:4990.

138. Takeya H, Kawabata S-I, Nakagawa K, et al. Bovine factor VII: its purification and complete amino acid sequence. *J Biol Chem* 1988;263:14868.

139. Sperling R, Furie BC, Blumenstein M, et al. Metal binding properties of γ-carboxyglutamic acid. *J Biol Chem* 1978;253:3898.

140. Furie BC, Blumenstein M, Furie B. Metal binding sites of a γ-carboxyglutamic acid-rich fragment of bovine prothrombin. *J Biol Chem* 1979;254:12521.

141. Bajaj SP, Butkowski RJ, Mann KG. Prothrombin fragments, Ca²⁺ binding and activation kinetics. *J Biol Chem* 1975;250:2150.

142. Benarous R, Elion J, Labie D. Ca^{2+} binding properties of human prothrombin. *Biochemistry* 1976;38:391.

143. Furie BC, Furie B. Interaction of lanthanide ions with bovine factor X and their use in the affinity chromatography of the venom coagulant protein of *Vipera russelli. J Biol Chem* 1975;250:601.

144. Furie BC, Mann KG, Furie B. Substitution of lanthanide ions for calcium ions in the activation of bovine prothrombin by activated factor X: high affinity metal binding sites of prothrombin and the derivatives of prothrombin activation. *J Biol Chem* 1976;251:3235.

145. Nelsestuen GL, Broderius M, Zytkovicz TH, et al. On the role of γ–carboxyglutamic acid in calcium and phospholipid binding. *Biochem Biophys Res Commun* 1975;65:233.

146. Amphlett GW, Byrne R, Castellino FJ. The binding of metal ions to bovine factor IX. *J Biol Chem* 1978;253:6774.

147. Henriksen RA, Jackson CM. Cooperative calcium binding by the phospholipid binding region of prothrombin: a requirement for intact disulfide bridges. *Arch Biochem Biophys* 1975;170:149.

148. Robertson P Jr, Hiskey RG, Koehler KA. Calcium and magnesium binding to γ–carboxyglutamic acid-containing peptides via metal ion nuclear magnetic resonance. *J Biol Chem* 1978;253:5880.

149. Bloom JW, Mann KG. Metal ion-induced conformational transitions of prothrombin and prothrombin fragment 1. *Biochemistry* 1978;17:4430.

150. Nelsestuen GL. Role of gamma-carboxyglutamic acid: an unusual transition required for calcium-dependent binding of prothrombin to phospholipid. *J Biol Chem* 1976;251:5648.

151. Prendergast FG, Mann KG. Differentiation of metal ion-induced transitions of prothrombin fragment 1. *J Biol Chem* 1977;252:840.

152. Furie B, Provost K, Blanchard RA, et al. Antibodies directed against a γ–carboxyglutamic acid-rich region of bovine prothrombin: preparation, isolation and characterization. *J Biol Chem* 1978;253:8980.

153. Furie B, Furie BC. Conformation-specific antibodies as probes of the γ–carboxyglutamic acid-rich region of bovine prothrombin: studies of metal-induced structural changes. *J Biol Chem* 1979;254:9766.

154. Tai MM, Furie BC, Furie B. Conformation-specific antibodies directed against the bovine prothrombin-calcium complex. *J Biol Chem* 1980;255:2790.

155. Madar DA, Hall TJ, Reisner HM, et al. The interaction of bovine prothrombin fragment 1 with metal ions: an immunological approach to kinetic and equilibrium studies. *J Biol Chem* 1980;255:8599.

156. Borowski M, Furie BC, Bauminger S, et al. Prothrombin requires two sequential metal-dependent conformational transitions to bind phospholipid. *J Biol Chem* 1986;261:14969.

157. Tai MM, Furie BC, Furie B. Localization of the metal-induced conformational transition of bovine prothrombin. *J Biol Chem* 1984;259:4162.

158. Soriano-Garcia M, Padmanabhan K, de Vos AM, et al. The Ca^{2+} ion and membrane binding structure of the Gla domain of Ca-prothrombin fragment 1. *Biochemistry* 1992;31:2554.

159. Butkowski RJ, Elion J, Downing MR, et al. Primary structure of human prothrombin 2 and thrombin. *J Biol Chem* 1977;252:4942.

160. Titani K, Fujikawa K, Enfield DL, et al. Bovine factor X$_1$ (Stuart factor): amino acid sequence of heavy chain. *Proc Natl Acad Sci U S A* 1975;72:3082.

161. Friezner Degen SJ, Davie EW. Nucleotide sequence of the gene for human prothrombin. *Biochemistry* 1987;26:6165.

162. Soriano-Garcia M, Padmanabhan K, de Vos AM, et al. The Ca^{2+} ion and membrane binding structure of the Gla domain of Ca-prothrombin fragment 1. *Biochemistry* 1992;31:2554.

163. Bajaj SP, Price PA, Russell WA. Decarboxylation of γ–carboxyglutamic acid residues in human prothrombin. *J Biol Chem* 1982;257:3726.

164. Bajaj SP, Saini R, Katz A, et al. Metal ion blockage of tritium incorporation into γ–carboxyglutamic acid of prothrombin. *J Biol Chem* 1988;263:9725.

165. Lewis MR, Deerfield DW II, Hoke RA, et al. Studies on Ca(II) binding to γ–carboxyglutamic acid. *J Biol Chem* 1988;263:1358.

166. Liebman HA, Furie BC, Furie B. The factor IX phospholipid-binding site is required for calcium-dependent activation of factor IX by factor XIa. *J Biol Chem* 1987;262:7605.

167. Nelsestuen GL, Broderius M, Martin G. Role of γ–carboxyglutamic acid: cation specificity of prothrombin and factor X-phospholipid interaction. *J Biol Chem* 1976;251:6886.

168. Mann KG, Nesheim ME, Tracy PB, et al. Assembly of the prothrombinase complex. *Biophys J* 1982;37:106.

169. Christiansen WT, Jalbert LR, Robertson RM, et al. Hydrophobic amino acid residues of human anticoagulation protein C that contribute to its functional binding to phospholipid vesicles. *Biochemistry* 1995;34:10376–10382.

170. Freedman SJ, Blostein MD, Baleja JD, et al. Identification of the phospholipid binding site in the vitamin K-dependent blood coagulation protein factor IX. *J Biol Chem* 1996;271:16227–16236.

171. Falls L, Furie BC, Jacobs M, et al. The ω-loop region of the human prothrombin Gla domain penetrates phospholipid membranes to a depth of 7.0 A. *J Biol Chem* 2001;276:23895.

172. Huang M, Huang G, Furie B, et al. Molecular basis of vitamin K–dependent protein-membrane interaction: x-ray structure of prothrombin-phospholipid at 2.0 Å. *Blood* 2000;96:1928(abst.)

172a. Jacobs M, Freedman SJ, Furie BC, et al. Membrane binding properties of the factor IX gamma-carboxyglutamic acid-rich domain prepared by chemical synthesis. *J Biol Chem* 1994;269:25494–25501.

173. Cooke RM, Wilkinson AJ, Baron M, et al. The solution structure of human epidermal growth factor. *Nature* 1987;327:339.

174. Appella E, Robinson EA, Ullrich SJ, et al. The receptor-binding sequence of urokinase. *J Biol Chem* 1987;262:4437.

175. Heath WF, Merrifield RB. A synthetic approach to structure-function relationships in the murine epidermal growth factor molecule. *Proc Natl Acad Sci U S A* 1986;83:6367.

176. Magnusson S, Petersen TE, Sottrup-Jensen L, et al. Complete primary structure of prothrombin: isolation, structure and reactivity of ten carboxylated glutamic acid residues and regulation of prothrombin activation by thrombin. In: Reich E, Rifkin DB, Shaw E, eds. *Proteases and biological control.* Cold Spring Harbor, NY: Cold Spring Harbor Laboratory, 1973:123.

177. Park CH, Tulinsky A. Three-dimensional structure of the kringle sequence: structure of prothrombin fragment 1. *Biochemistry* 1986;25:3977.

178. Ny T, Elgh F, Lund B. The structure of the human tissue-type plasminogen activator gene: correlation of intron and exon structures to functional and structural domains. *Proc Natl Acad Sci U S A* 1984;81:5355.

179. Cool DE, Edgell CJS, Louie GV, et al. Characterization of human blood coagulation factor XII cDNA. *J Biol Chem* 1985;260:13666.

180. Holmes WE, Pennica D, Blaber M, et al. Cloning and expression of the gene for prourokinase in E coli. *Biotechnology* 1985;3:923.

181. Malinowski DP, Sadler JE, Davie EW. Characterization of a complementary deoxyribonucleic acid coding for human and bovine plasminogen. *Biochemistry* 1984;23:4243.

182. Gilbert W. Why genes in pieces? *Nature* 1978;271:501.

183. Patthy L. Evolution of the proteases of blood coagulation and fibrinolysis by assembly from modules. *Cell* 1985;41:657.

184. Furie B, Bing DH, Feldmann RJ, et al. Computer-generated models of blood coagulation factor Xa, factor IXa, and thrombin based upon structural homology with other serine proteases. *J Biol Chem* 1982;257:3875.

185. Irwin DM, Ahern KG, Pearson GD. Characterization of the bovine prothrombin gene. *Biochemistry* 1985;24:6854.

186. Royle NJ, Irwin DM, Koschinsky ML, et al. Human genes encoding prothrombin and ceruloplasmin map to 11p11-q12 and 3q21-24 respectively. *Somat Cell Mol Genet* 1987;13:285.

187. Leytus SP, Foster DC, Kurachi K, et al. Gene for human factor X: a blood coagulation factor whose gene organization is essentially identical with that of factor IX and protein C. *Biochemistry* 1986;25:5098.

188. Yoshitake S, Schach BG, Foster DC, et al. Nucleotide sequence of the gene for human factor IX. *Biochemistry* 1985;24:3736.

189. O'Hara PJ, Grant FJ, Haldeman BA, et al. Nucleotide sequence of the gene coding for human factor VII, a vitamin K-dependent protein participating in blood coagulation. *Proc Natl Acad Sci U S A* 1987;84:5158.

190. Foster DC, Yoshitake S, Davie EW. The nucleotide sequence of the gene for human protein C. *Proc Natl Acad Sci U S A* 1985;82:4673.

191. Irwin DM, Robertson KA, MacGillivray RTA. Structure and evolution of the bovine prothrombin gene. *J Mol Biol* 1988;200:31.

192. Jorgensen MJ, Cantor AB, Furie BC, et al. Expression of completely γ–carboxylated recombinant human prothrombin. *J Biol Chem* 1987;262:6729.

193. Mizuochi T, Yamashita K, Fujikawa K, et al. The carbohydrate of bovine prothrombin: occurrence of Gal-β 1-3GlcNAc grouping in asparagine-linked sugar chains. *J Biol Chem* 1979;254:6419.

194. Ratcliffe J, Furie B, Furie BC. The importance of specific γ–carboxyglutamic acid residues in prothrombin: evaluation by site-specific mutagenesis. *J Biol Chem* 1993;268:24339–24345.

195. Blostein M, Rigby A, Jacobs M, et al. The Gla domain of prothrombin binds to factor Va. *J Biol Chem* 2000;275:38120–38126.

196. Borowski M, Furie B, Goldsmith GH, et al. Metal and phospholipid binding properties of partially carboxylated variant prothrombins. *J Biol Chem* 1985;260:9258.

197. Kotkow K, Dietcher S, Furie B, et al. The second kringle domain of prothrombin promotes factor V-mediated prothrombin activation by prothrombinase. *J Biol Chem* 1995;270:4551–4557.

198. Deguchi H, Takeya H, Gabazza EC, et al. Prothrombin kringle 1 domain interacts with factor Va during the assembly of prothrombinase complex. *Biochem J* 1997;321:729–735.

199. Soriano-Garcia M, Padmanabhan K, de Vos AM, et al. The Ca2+ ion and membrane binding structure of the Gla domain of Ca-prothrombin fragment 1. *Biochemistry* 1992;31:2554–2566.

200. Bode W, Mayr I, Baumann U, et al. The refined 1.9 A crystal structure of human alpha-thrombin: interaction with D-Phe-Pro-Arg chloromethylketone and significance of the Tyr-Pro-Pro-Trp insertion segment. *EMBO J* 1989;8:3467–3475.

201. Rydel TJ, Ravichandran KG, Tulinsky A, et al. The structure of a complex of recombinant hirudin and human alpha-thrombin. *Science* 1990;249:277–280.

202. Borowski M, Furie BC, Furie B. Distribution of γ–carboxyglutamic acid residues in partially carboxylated prothrombins. *J Biol Chem* 1986;261:1624.

203. Wright SF, Berkowitz P, Deerfield DW II, et al. Chemical modification of bovine prothrombin fragment 1 in the presence of Tb^{3+} ions. *J Biol Chem* 1986;261:10598.

204. Nelsestuen GL, Lim TK. Equilibria involved in prothrombin- and blood clotting factor X-membrane binding. *Biochemistry* 1977;16:4164.

205. Bajaj SP, Butkowski RJ, Mann KG. Prothrombin fragments: calcium binding and activation kinetics. *J Biol Chem* 1975;250:2150.

206. Nelsestuen GL, Broderius M. Interaction of prothrombin and blood clotting factor X with membranes. *Biochemistry* 1977;16:4172.

207. Mann KG, Jenny RJ, Krishnaswamy S. Cofactor proteins in the assembly and expression of blood clotting enzyme complexes. *Annu Rev Biochem* 198;57:915.

208. Rosing J, Tans G, Govers-Riemslag JWP, et al. The role of phospholipids and factor Va in the prothrombinase complex. *J Biol Chem* 1980;255:274.

209. Nesheim ME, Tracy RP, Mann KG. Clotspeed, a mathematical simulation of the functional properties of prothrombinase. *J Biol Chem* 1984;259:1447.

210. Maruyama I, Salem H, Majerus PW. Coagulation factor Va binds to human umbilical vein endothelial cells (HUVE) and accelerates protein C activation. *J Clin Invest* 1984;73:654.

211. Rodgers GM, Shuman MA. Prothrombin is activated on vascular endothelium by factor Xa and calcium. *Proc Natl Acad Sci U S A* 1983;80:7001.

212. Tracy P, Rohrbach MS, Mann KG. Functional prothrombinase complex assembly on isolated monocytes and lymphocytes. *J Biol Chem* 1983;258:7264.

213. Tracy P, Eide LL, Mann KG. Human prothrombinase complex assembly and function on isolated peripheral blood cell populations. *J Biol Chem* 1985;260:2119.

214. Rodgers GM, Kane WH, Pitas RE. Formation of factor Va by atherosclerotic rabbit aorta mediates factor Xa-catalyzed prothrombin activation. *J Clin Invest* 1988;81:1911.

215. Kane WH, Lindhout MJ, Jackson CM, et al. Factor Va-dependent binding of factor Xa to platelets. *J Biol Chem* 1980;255:1170.

216. Miletich JP, Jackson CM, Majerus PW. Interaction of coagulation factor Xa with human platelets. *Proc Natl Acad Sci U S A* 1977;74:4033.

217. Miletich JP, Jackson CM, Majerus PW. Patients with congenital factor V deficiency have decreased factor Xa binding sites on their platelets. *J Clin Invest* 1978;62:824.

218. Stenn KS, Blout ER. Mechanism of bovine prothrombin activation by an insoluble preparation of bovine factor Xa (thrombokinase). *Biochemistry* 1972;11:4502.

219. Rosenberg JS, Beeler DL, Rosenberg RD. Activation of human prothrombin by highly purified human factors V and Xa in the presence of human antithrombin. *J Biol Chem* 1975;250:1607.

220. Esmon CT, Jackson CM. The conversion of prothrombin to thrombin, V. The activation of prothrombin by factor Xa in the presence of phospholipid. *J Biol Chem* 1974;249:7798.

221. Esmon CT, Jackson CM. The conversion of prothrombin to thrombin, III. The factor Xa catalyzed activation of prothrombin. *J Biol Chem* 1974;249:7782.

222. Heldebrant CM, Butkowski RJ, Bajaj SP, et al. The activation of prothrombin, II. Partial reactions, physical and chemical characterization of the intermediates of activation. *J Biol Chem* 1973;248:7149.

223. Downing MR, Butkowski RJ, Clark MM, et al. Human prothrombin activation. *J Biol Chem* 1975;250:1607.

224. Nesheim ME, Mann KG. Kinetics and cofactor dependence of the two cleavages involved in prothrombin activation. *J Biol Chem* 1984;258:5386.

225. Rosing J, Zwaal RFA, Tans G. Formation of meizothrombin as intermediate in factor Xa-catalyzed prothrombin activation. *J Biol Chem* 1986;261:4222.

226. van Rijn JLML, Govers-Riemslag JWP, Zwaal RFA, et al. Kinetic studies of prothrombin activation: effect of factor Va and phospholipids on the formation of the enzyme-substrate complex. *Biochemistry* 1984;23:4557.

227. Esmon CT, Owen WG, Jackson CM. The conversion of prothrombin to thrombin, II. Differentiation between thrombin and factor Xa-catalyzed proteolysis. *J Biol Chem* 1974;249:606.

228. Aronson DL, Stevan L, Ball AP, et al. Generation of the combined prothrombin activation peptide (F1.2) during the clotting of blood and plasma. *J Clin Invest* 1977;60:1410.

229. Rabiet MJ, Blashill A, Furie B, et al. Prothrombin fragment 1.2.3, a major product of prothrombin activation in human plasma. *J Biol Chem* 1986;261:13210.

230. Teitel JM, Bauer KA, Lau HK, et al. Studies of the prothrombin activation pathway utilizing radioimmunoassays for the F2/F1+2 fragment and thrombin-antithrombin complex. *Blood* 1982;59:1086.

231. Lau HK, Rosenberg JS, Beeler DL, et al. The isolation and characterization of a specific antibody population directed against the prothrombin activation fragments F2 and F1+2. *J Biol Chem* 1979;254:8751.

232. Bauer KA, Rosenberg RD. The pathophysiology of the prethrombotic state in humans: insights gained from studies using markers of hemostatic system activation. *Blood* 1987;70:343.

233. Sherry S, Troll W. The action of thrombin on synthetic substrates. *J Biol Chem* 1954;208:95.

234. Chase T Jr, Shaw E. Comparison of the esterase activities of trypsin, plasmin and thrombin on guanidinobenzoate esters. *Biochemistry* 1969;8:2212.

235. Morita T, Kato H, Iwanaga S, et al. New fluorogenic substrates for alpha-thrombin, factor Xa, kallikreins and urokinase. *J Biochem* 1977;82:1495.

236. Blomback B, Blomback M, Hessel B, et al. Structure of N-terminal fragments of fibrinogen and specificity of thrombin. *Nature* 1967;215:1445.

237. Pittman D, Kaufman R. Proteolytic requirements for thrombin activation of anti-hemophilic factor (factor VIII). *Proc Natl Acad Sci U S A* 1988;85:2429.

238. Esmon CT. The subunit structure of thrombin-activated factor V: isolation of activated factor V: separation of subunits and reconstitution of biological activity. *J Biol Chem* 1979;254:964.

239. Nesheim ME, Mann KG. Thrombin-catalyzed activation of single-chain bovine factor V. *J Biol Chem* 1979;254:10952.

240. Schwartz ML, Pizzo SV, Hill RL, et al. Human factor XIII from plasma and platelets. *J Biol Chem* 1973;248:1395.

241. McGowan EB, Ding A-H, Detwiler TC. Correlation of thrombin-induced glycoprotein V hydrolysis and platelet activation. *J Biol Chem* 1983;258:11243.

242. Vu TK, Hung DT, Wheaton VI, et al. Molecular cloning of a functional thrombin receptor reveals a novel proteolytic mechanism of receptor activation. *Cell* 1991;64:1057–1068.

243. Connolly AJ, Ishihara H, Kahn ML, et al. Role of the thrombin receptor in development and evidence for a second receptor. *Nature* 1996;381:516–519.

244. Kahn ML, Zheng YW, Huang W, et al. A dual thrombin receptor system for platelet activation. *Nature* 1998;394:690–694.

245. Coughlin SR. Thrombin signaling and protease-activated receptors. *Nature* 2000;407:258–264.

246. Boissel JP, Le Bonnier B, Rabiet MJ, et al. Covalent structures of beta and gamma autolytic derivatives of human alpha-thrombin. *J Biol Chem* 1984;259:5691.

247. Abildgaard U. Binding of thrombin to antithrombin III. *Scand J Clin Lab Invest* 1969;24:89.

248. Damus PS, Hicks M, Rosenberg RD. Anticoagulant action of heparin. *Nature* 1973;246:355.

249. Rosenberg RD, Damus PS. The purification and mechanism of action of human antithrombin-heparin cofactor. *J Biol Chem* 1973;248:6490.

250. Downing MR, Bloom JW, Mann KG. Comparison of the inhibition of thrombin by three plasma protease inhibitors. *Biochemistry* 1978;17:2649.

251. Matheson NR, Travis J. Inactivation of human thrombin in the presence of human alpha 1-proteinase inhibitor. *Biochem J* 1976;159:495.

252. Lau HK, Rosenberg RD. The isolation and characterization of a specific antibody population directed against the thrombin-antithrombin complex. *J Biol Chem* 1980;255:5885.

253. Bauer KA, Broekmans AW, Bertina RM, et al. Hemostatic enzyme generation in the blood of patients with hereditary protein C deficiency. *Blood* 1988;71:1418.

254. Markwardt F. Hirudin as an inhibitor. *Methods Enzymol* 1970;19:924.

255. Rydel TJ, Ravichandran KG, Tulinsky A, et al. The structure of a complex of recombinant hirudin and human alpha-thrombin. *Science* 1990;249:277–280.

256. Josso F, Lavergne JM, Weilland C, et al. Etude immunologique de la prothrombine et de la thrombine humaines. *Thromb Diath Haemorrh* 1967;18:311.

257. Blanchard RA, Furie BC, Jorgensen MJ, et al. Acquired vitamin K-dependent carboxylation deficiency in liver disease. *N Engl J Med* 1981;305:242.

258. Karpatkin M, Karpatkin S. Humoral factor that specifically regulates prothrombin (factor II) levels (coagulopoietin II). *Proc Natl Acad Sci U S A* 1979;76:491.

259. Shah DV, Nyari LJ, Swanson JC, et al. Effect of a humoral factor on plasma prothrombin and vitamin K-dependent liver carboxylase levels in the rat. *Thromb Res* 1980;19:111.

260. Shapiro SS, Martinez J. Human prothrombin metabolism in normal man and in hypocoagulable subjects. *J Clin Invest* 1969;48:1292.

261. Sun WY, Witte DP, Degen JL, et al. Prothrombin deficiency results in embryonic and neonatal lethality in mice. *Proc Natl Acad Sci U S A* 1998;95:7597–7602.

262. Jackson CM. Characterization of two glycoprotein variants of bovine factor X and demonstration that the factor X zymogen contains two polypeptide chains. *Biochemistry* 1972;11:4873.

263. Fujikawa K, Legaz ME, Davie EW. Bovine factors X_1 and X_2 (Stuart factor): isolation and characterization. *Biochemistry* 1972;11:4882.

264. Radcliffe RD, Barton PD. Comparisons of the molecular forms of activated bovine factor X. *J Biol Chem* 1973;248:6788.

265. Jesty J, Spencer AK, Nemerson Y. The mechanism of activation of factor X. *J Biol Chem* 1974;249:5614.

266. Furie BC, Furie B, Gottlieb AJ, et al. Activation of bovine factor X by the venom coagulant protein of Vipera russelli: complex formation of the activation fragments. *Biochim Biophys Acta* 1974;365:121.

267. Fujikawa K, Coan MH, Legaz ME, et al. The mechanism of activation of bovine factor X (Stuart factor) by intrinsic and extrinsic pathways. *Biochemistry* 1974;13:5290.

268. Fujikawa K, Legaz ME, Davie EW. Bovine factor X_1 (Stuart factor): mechanism of activation by protein from Russell's viper venom. *Biochemistry* 1972;11:4892.

269. Furie B, Furie BC. Spectral changes in bovine factor X associated with activation by the venom coagulant protein of Vipera russelli. *J Biol Chem* 1976;251:6807.

270. Mizuochi T, Yamashita K, Fujikawa K, et al. The structures of the carbohydrate moieties of bovine blood coagulation factor X. *J Biol Chem* 1980;255:3526.

271. Padmanabhan K, Padmanabhan KP, Tulinsky A, et al. Structure of human des(1-45) factor Xa at 2.2 A resolution. *J Mol Biol* 1993;232:947–966.

272. Brandstetter H, Kuhne A, Bode W, et al. X-ray structure of active site-inhibited clotting factor Xa: implications for drug design and substrate recognition. *J Biol Chem* 1996;271:29988.

273. Lim TK, Bloomfield VA, Nelsestuen GL. Structure of the prothrombin- and blood clotting factor X-membrane complex. *Biochemistry* 1977;16:4177.

274. Keyt B, Furie BC, Furie B. Structural transitions in bovine factor X associated with metal binding and zymogen activation: studies using conformation-specific antibodies. *J Biol Chem* 1982;257:8687.

275. Dahlback B, Stenflo J. Binding of bovine coagulation factor Xa to platelets. *Biochemistry* 1978;17:4938.

276. Kane WH, Lindhout MJ, Jackson CM, et al. Factor Va-dependent binding of factor Xa to human platelets. *J Biol Chem* 1979;257:3963.

277. Gordon SG, Cross BA. A factor X-activating cysteine protease from malignant tissue. *J Clin Invest* 1981;67:1665.

278. Falanga A, Gordon SG. Isolation and characterization of cancer pro-coagulant: a cysteine proteinase from malignant tissue. *Biochemistry* 1985;24:5558.

279. Williams WJ, Esnouf MP. The fractionation of Russell's viper (Vipera russelli) venom with special reference to the coagulant protein. *Biochem J* 1962;84:52.

280. Hultin M, Nemerson Y. Activation of factor X by factors IXa and VIII: a specific assay for factor IXa in the presence of thrombin-activated factor VIII. *Blood* 1978;52:928.

281. Stern D, Nawroth P, Handley D, et al. An endothelial cell-dependent pathway of coagulation. *Proc Natl Acad Sci U S A* 1985;82:2523.
282. Neuenschwander P, Jesty J. A comparison of phospholipid and platelets in the activation of human factor VIII by thrombin and factor Xa, and in the activation of factor X. *Blood* 1988;72:1761.
283. Silverberg SA, Nemerson Y, Zur M. Kinetics of the activation of bovine coagulation factor X by components of the extrinsic pathway: kinetic behavior of two-chain factor VII in the presence and absence of tissue factor. *J Biol Chem* 1977;252:8481.
284. Ruf W, Shobe J, Rao SM, et al. Importance of factor VIIa Gla-domain residue Arg-36 for recognition of the macromolecular substrate factor X Gla-domain. *Biochemistry* 1999;38:1957–1966.
285. Baugh RJ, Dickinson CD, Ruf W, et al. Exosite interactions determine the affinity of factor X for the extrinsic Xase complex. *J Biol Chem* 2000;275:28826.
286. Trauber D, Hawkins K, Karpatkin M, et al. Humoral factor that specifically regulates factor X levels in rabbits (coagulopoietin-X). *J Clin Invest* 1979;64:1713.
287. Gitel SN, Medina VM, Wessler S. Inhibition of human activated factor X by antithrombin III and alpha 1-proteinase inhibitor in human plasma. *J Biol Chem* 1984;259:6890.
288. Fuchs HE, Pizzo SV. Regulation of factor Xa in vitro in human and mouse plasma and in vivo in mouse: role of the endothelium and plasma proteinase inhibitors. *J Clin Invest* 1983;72:2041.
289. Han X, Fiehler R, Broze GJ Jr. Isolation of a protein Z-dependent plasma protease inhibitor. *Proc Natl Acad Sci U S A* 1998;95:9250–9255.
290. Yin Z-F, Huang Z-F, Cui J, et al. Prothrombotic phenotype of protein Z deficiency. *Proc Natl Acad Sci U S A* 2000;97:6734–6738.
291. Dewerchin M, Liang Z, Carmeliet P, et al. Blood coagulation factor X deficiency causes partial embryonic lethality and fatal neonatal bleeding in mice. *Thromb Haemost* 2000;83:185–190.
292. Altieri DC. Molecular cloning of effector cell protease receptor-1, a novel cell surface receptor for the protease factor Xa. *J Biol Chem* 1994;269:3139–3142.
293. Zaman GJ, Conway EM. The elusive factor Xa receptor: failure to detect transcripts that correspond to the published sequence of EPR-1. *Blood* 2000;96:145–148.
294. Gilgenkrantz S, Briquel ME, Andre E, et al. Structural genes of coagulation factors VII and X located on 13q34. *Ann Genet* 1986;29:32.
295. Broze GJ, Majerus PW. Purification and properties of human coagulation factor VII. *J Biol Chem* 1980;255:1242.
296. Radcliffe R, Nemerson Y. Activation and control of factor X and thrombin: isolation and characterization of a single chain form of factor VII. *J Biol Chem* 1974;250:388.
297. Kisiel W, Fujikawa K, Davie EW. Activation of bovine factor VII (pro-convertin) by factor XIIa (activated Hageman factor). *Biochemistry* 1977;16:4189.
298. Radcliffe R, Nemerson Y. Mechanism of action of bovine factor VII: products of cleavage by factor Xa. *J Biol Chem* 1976;251:4797.
299. Radcliffe R, Bagdassarian A, Colman R, et al. Activation of bovine factor VII by Hageman factor fragments. *Blood* 1977;50:611.
300. Niemetz J. Coagulant activity of leukocytes: tissue factor activity. *J Clin Invest* 1972;51:307.
301. Levy GA, Edgington TS. Lymphocyte cooperation is required for amplification of macrophage procoagulant activity. *J Exp Med* 1980;151:1232.
302. Colucci M, Balconi G, Lounzet R, et al. Cultured human endothelial cells generate tissue factor in response to endotoxin. *J Clin Invest* 1983;71:1893.
303. Rodgers GM, Greenberg CS, Shuman MA. Characterization of the effects of cultured vascular cells on the activation of blood coagulation. *Blood* 1983;61:1155.
304. Ploplis VA, Edgington TS, Fair DS. Initiation of the extrinsic pathway of coagulation: association of factor VIIa with a cell line expressing tissue factor. *J Biol Chem* 1987;262:9503.
305. Guha A, Bach R, Konigsberg W, et al. Affinity purification of human tissue factor: interaction of factor VII and tissue factor in detergent micelles. *Proc Natl Acad Sci U S A* 1986;83:299.
306. Bach R, Nemerson Y, Konigsberg W. Purification and characterization of bovine tissue factor. *J Biol Chem* 1981;256:8324.
307. Fair DS, MacDonald MJ. Cooperative interaction between factor VII and cell surface-expressed tissue factor. *J Biol Chem* 1987;262:11692.
308. Zur M, Nemerson Y. Kinetics of factor IX activation via the extrinsic pathway. *J Biol Chem* 1980;255:5703.
309. Osterud B, Rapaport SI. Activation of factor IX by the reaction product of tissue factor and factor VII: additional pathway for initiating blood coagulation. *Proc Natl Acad Sci U S A* 1977;74:5260.
310. Spicer EK, Horton R, Bloem L, et al. Isolation of cDNA clones coding for human tissue factor: primary structure of the protein and cDNA. *Proc Natl Acad Sci U S A* 1987;84:5148.
311. Morrissey JH, Fakhrai H, Edgington TS. Molecular cloning of the cDNA for tissue factor, the cellular receptor for the initiation of the coagulation protease cascade. *Cell* 1987;50:129.
312. Bach R, Konigsberg WH, Nemerson Y. Human tissue factor contains thioester-linked palmitate and stearate on the cytoplasmic half-cystine. *Biochemistry* 1988;27:4227.
313. Zur M, Radcliffe RD, Oberdick J, et al. Dual role of factor VII in blood coagulation. *J Biol Chem* 1982;257:5623.
314. Banner DW, D'Arcy A, Chene C, et al. The crystal structure of the complex of blood coagulation factor VIIa with soluble tissue factor. *Nature* 1996;380:41–46.
315. Jesty J, Silverberg SA. Kinetics of the tissue factor-dependent activation of coagulation factors IX and X in a bovine plasma system. *J Biol Chem* 1979;254:12337.
316. Kondo S, Kisiel W. Regulation of factor VIIa activity in plasma: evidence that antithrombin III is the sole plasma protease inhibitor of human factor VIIa. *Thromb Res* 1987;46:325.
317. Broze GJ Jr, Miletic JP. Isolation of the tissue factor inhibitor by HepG2 hepatoma cells. *Proc Natl Acad Sci U S A* 1987;84:1886.
318. Sanders NL, Bajaj SP, Zivelin A, et al. Inhibition of tissue factor/factor VIIa activity in plasma requires factor X and an additional plasma factor. *Blood* 1985;66:204.
319. Rao LV, Rapaport SI. Studies of a mechanism inhibiting the initiation of the extrinsic pathway of coagulation. *Blood* 1987;69:645.
320. Rapaport SI. Inhibition of factor VIIa/tissue factor-induced blood coagulation: with particular emphasis upon a factor Xa-dependent inhibitory mechanism. *Blood* 1989;73:359.
321. Broze GJ Jr, Warren LA, Novotny WF, et al. The lipoprotein-associated coagulation inhibitor that inhibits the factor VII-tissue factor complex also inhibits factor Xa: insight into its possible mechanism of action. *Blood* 1988;71:335.
322. Rao LV, Rapaport SI. Studies of a mechanism inhibiting the initiation of the extrinsic pathway of coagulation. *Blood* 1987;69:645–651.
323. Wun TC, Kretzmer KK, Girard TJ, et al. Cloning and characterization of a cDNA coding for the lipoprotein-associated coagulation inhibitor shows that it consists of three tandem Kunitz-type inhibitory domains. *J Biol Chem* 1988;263:6001–6004.
324. Rapaport SI. The extrinsic pathway inhibitor: a regulator of tissue factor-dependent blood coagulation. *Thromb Haemost* 1991;66:6–15.
325. Broze GJ Jr. The role of tissue factor pathway inhibitor in a revised coagulation cascade. *Semin Hematol* 1992;29:159–169.
326. Camerino G, Grzeschik KH, Jaye M, et al. Regional localization on the human X chromosome and polymorphism of the coagulation factor IX gene (hemophilia B locus). *Proc Natl Acad Sci U S A* 1984;81:498.
327. Crossley M, Ludwig M, Stowell KM, et al. Recovery from hemophilia B Leyden: an androgen-responsive element in the factor IX promoter. *Science* 1992;257:377–379.
328. Morgan GE, Rowley G, Green PM, et al. Further evidence for the importance of an androgen response element in the factor IX promoter. *Br J Haematol* 1997;98:79–85.
329. Nguyen P, Cornillet P, Potron G. A new case of severe hemophilia B Leyden, associated with a G to C mutation at position –6 of the factor IX promoter. *Am J Hematol* 1995;49:259–260.
330. Reijnen MJ, Peerlinck K, Maasdam D, et al. (Hemophilia B Leyden: substitution of thymine for guanine at position –21 results in a disruption of a hepatocyte nuclear factor 4 binding site in the factor IX promoter. *Blood* 1993;82:151–158.
331. Crossley M, Brownlee GG. Disruption of a C/EBP binding site in the factor IX promoter is associated with haemophilia B. *Nature* 1990;345:444–446.
332. Davies N, Austen DE, Wilde MD, et al. Clotting factor IX levels in C/EBP alpha knockout mice. *Br J Haematol* 1997;99:578–579.
333. Fujikawa K, Thompson AR, Legaz ME, et al. Isolation and characterization of bovine factor IX (Christmas factor). *Biochemistry* 1973;12:4938.
334. DiScipio RG, Hermodson MA, Yates SG, et al. A comparison of human prothrombin, factor IX (Christmas factor), factor X (Stuart factor) and protein S. *Biochemistry* 1977;16:698.
335. Morita T, Isaacs BS, Esmon CT, et al. Derivatives of blood coagulation factor IX contain a high affinity Ca^{2+} binding site that lacks γ–carboxyglutamic acid. *J Biol Chem* 1984;259:5698.
336. Beckmann RJ, Schmidt RJ, Santerre RF, et al. The structure and evolution of a 461 amino acid human protein C precursor and its messenger RNA, based upon the DNA sequence of cloned human liver cDNAs. *Nucleic Acids Res* 1985;13:5233.
337. Long GL, Belagaje RM, MacGillivray RTA. Cloning and sequencing of liver cDNA coding for bovine protein C. *Proc Natl Acad Sci U S A* 1984;81:5653.
338. Lundwall A, Dackowski W, Cohen E, et al. Isolation and sequence of the cDNA for human protein S, a regulator of blood coagulation. *Proc Natl Acad Sci U S A* 1986;83:6716.
339. Derian CK, VanDusen W, Przysiecki CT, et al. Inhibitors of 2-ketoglutarate-dependent dioxygenases block aspartyl beta-hydroxylation of recombinant human factor IX in several mammalian expression systems. *J Biol Chem* 1989;264:6615–6618.
340. Brandstetter H, Bauer M, Huber R, et al. X-ray structure of clotting factor IXa: active site and module structure related to Xase activity and hemophilia B. *Proc Natl Acad Sci U S A* 1995;92:9796–9800.
341. Jacobs, M, Freedman SJ, Furie BC, et al. Membrane binding properties of the factor IX γ-carboxyglutamic acid-rich domain prepared by chemical synthesis. *J Biol Chem* 1994;269:25494–25501.
342. Freedman SJ, Furie B, Furie BC, et al. Structure of the metal-free γ-carboxyglutamic acid-rich membrane binding region of factor IX by 2D NMR spectroscopy. *J Biol Chem* 1995;270:7980–7987.
343. Freedman SJ, Furie BC, Furie B, et al. Structure of the factor IX Gla domain bound to calcium ions. *Biochemistry* 1995;34:12126–12137.
344. Freedman SJ, Blostein MD, Baleja JD, et al. Identification of the phospholipid binding site in the vitamin K-dependent protein factor IX. *J Biol Chem* 1996;271:16227–16236.
345. Jones ME, Griffity MJ, Monroe DM, et al. Comparison of lipid binding and kinetic properties of normal, variant, and γ–carboxyglutamic acid modified human factor IX and factor IXa. *Biochemistry* 1985;24:8064.

346. Rimon S, Melamed R, Savion N, et al. Identification of a factor IX/IXa binding protein on the endothelial cell surface. *J Biol Chem* 1987;262:6023.

347. Cheung WF, van den Born J, Kuhn K, et al. Identification of the endothelial cell binding site for factor IX. *Proc Natl Acad Sci U S A* 1996;93:11068–11073.

348. Wolberg AS, Stafford DW, Erie DA. Human factor IX binds to specific sites on the collagenous domain of collagen IV. *J Biol Chem* 1997;272:16717–16720.

349. Rawala R, Ahmad SS, Walsh PN. Factor IXa binding to activated human platelets promotes factor X activation. *Blood* 1987;70:393a.

350. Ahmad SS, Rawala-Sheikh RR, Walsh PN. Comparative interactions of factor IX and factor IXa with human platelets. *J Biol Chem* 1989;264:3244.

351. Byrne R, Amphlett GW, Castellino FJ. Metal ion specificity of the conversion of bovine factors IX, IX alpha, and IXa alpha to bovine factor IXa beta. *J Biol Chem* 1980;255:1430.

352. van der Graaf F, Greengard JS, Bouma BN, et al. Isolation and functional characterization of the active light chain of activated human blood coagulation factor XI. *J Biol Chem* 1983;258:9669.

353. Sinha D, Koshy A, Seaman FS, et al. Functional characterization of human blood coagulation factor XIa using hybridoma antibodies. *J Biol Chem* 1985;260:10714.

354. Sinha D, Seaman FS, Walsh PN. Role of calcium ions and the heavy chain of factor IXa in the activation of human coagulation factor IX. *Biochemistry* 1987;26:3884.

355. DiScipio RG, Kurachi K, Davie EW. Activation of human factor IX (Christmas factor). *J Clin Invest* 1978;61:1528.

356. Lindquist PA, Fujikawa K, Davie EW. Activation of bovine factor IX (Christmas factor) by factor XIa (activated plasma thromboplastin antecedent) and a protease from Russell's viper venom. *J Biol Chem* 1978;254:1902.

357. van Dieigen G, Tans G, Rosing J, et al. The role of phospholipid and factor VIIIa in the activation of bovine factor X. *J Biol Chem* 1981;256:3433.

358. Masys DR, Bajaj SP, Rapaport SI. Activation of factor VII by activated factors IX and X. *Blood* 1982;60:1143.

359. Rick ME. Activation of factor VIII by factor IXa. *Blood* 1982;60:744.

360. Davies N, Austen DE, Wilde MD, et al. Clotting factor IX levels in C/EBP alpha knockout mice. *Br J Haematol* 1997;99:578–579.

361. Briet E, Bertina RM, van Tilberg NH, et al. Hemophilia B Leyden. *N Engl J Med* 1982;306:788.

362. Fahner JB, Salier JP, Landa L, et al. Defective promoter structure in a human factor IX Leyden. *Blood* 1988;72[Suppl 1]:295a.

363. Reitsma PH, Bertina RM, Ploos van Amstel JK, et al. The putative factor IX gene promoter in hemophilia B Leyden. *Blood* 1988;72:1074.

364. Rosenberg J, McKenna P, Rosenberg RD. Inhibition of human factor IXa by human antithrombin. *J Biol Chem* 1975;250:8883.

365. Kurachi K, Fujikawa K, Schmer G, et al. Inhibition of bovine factor IXa and factor Xa by antithrombin III. *Biochemistry* 1976;15:373.

366. McMillan CW, Roberts HR. Congenital combined deficiency of coagulation factors II, VII, IX, X. *N Engl J Med* 1979;274:1313.

367. Chung KS, Bezeaud A, Goldsmith JC, et al. Congenital deficiency of blood clotting factors II, VII, IX and X. *Blood* 1979;53:776.

368. Vicente V, Maia R, Alberca I, et al. Congenital deficiency of vitamin K-dependent coagulation factors and protein C. *Thromb Haemost* 1984;51:343.

369. Johnson CA, Chung HS, McGrath KM, et al. Characterization of a variant prothrombin in a patient congenitally deficient in factor II, VII, IX and X. *Br J Haematol* 1980;44:461.

370. Goldsmith GH Jr, Pence RE, Ratnoff OD, et al. Studies on a family with combined functional deficiencies of vitamin K-dependent coagulation factors. *J Clin Invest* 1982;69:1253.

371. Brenner B, Sanchez-Vega B, Wu SM, et al. A missense mutation in gamma-glutamyl carboxylase gene causes combined deficiency of all vitamin K-dependent blood coagulation factors. *Blood* 1998;92:4554–4559.

372. Spronk HM, Farah RA, Buchanan GR, et al. Novel mutation in the gamma-glutamyl carboxylase gene resulting in congenital combined deficiency of all vitamin K-dependent blood coagulation factors. *Blood* 2000;96:3650–3652.

373. Oldenburg J, von Brederlow B, Fregin A, et al. Congenital deficiency of vitamin K dependent coagulation factors in two families presents as a genetic defect of the vitamin K-epoxide-reductase-complex. *Thromb Haemost* 2000;84:937–941.

374. Chu K, Wu SM, Stanley T, et al. A mutation in the propeptide of factor IX leads to warfarin sensitivity by a novel mechanism. *J Clin Invest* 1996;98:1619–1625.

375. Romero EE, Deo R, Velazquez-Estades LJ, et al. Cloning, structural organization, and transcriptional activity of the rat vitamin K-dependent gamma-glutamyl carboxylase gene. *Biochem Biophys Res Commun* 1998;248:783–788.

376. Soucie JM, Evatt B, Jackson D. Occurrence of hemophilia in the United States. Hemophilia Surveillance System Project Investigators. *Am J Hematol* 1998;59:288–294.

377. Kasper CK, Osterud B, Minami JY, et al. Hemophilia B: characterization of genetic variants and detection of carriers. *Blood* 1977;50:351.

378. Green PM, Giannelli F, Sommer SS, et al. Haemophilia B: database of point mutations and short additions and deletions, v9.0. Available at: http://www.kcl.ac.uk/ip/petergreen/haemBdatabase.html.

379. Diuguid DL, Rabiet MJ, Furie BC, et al. Molecular defects of factor IX Chicago-2 (Arg 145—His) and prothrombin Madrid (Arg 271→Cys): arginine mutations that preclude zymogen activation. *Blood* 1989;74:193.

380. Toomey JR, Stafford D, Smith K. Factor IX Albuquerque (arginine 145 to cysteine) is cleaved slowly by factor XIa and has reduced coagulant activity. *Blood* 1988;72[Suppl 1]:312a.

381. Huang MN, Kasper CK, Roberts HR, et al. Molecular defect in factor IX Hilo,

382. Monroe DM, McCord DM, High KA, et al. Functional consequences of an Arg 180 to Gln mutation in factor IX Hilo. *Blood* 1988;72[Suppl 1]:304a.

383. Sakai T, Fujimura Y, Yoshioka A, et al. Blood clotting factor IX Kasihara: amino acid substitution of valine 182 by phenylalanine. *Blood* 1988;72[Suppl 1]:304a.

384. Davis LM, McGraw RA, Ware JL, et al. Factor IX Alabama: a point mutation in a clotting protein results in hemophilia B. *Blood* 1987;69:140.

385. McCord DM, Monroe DM, Roberts HR. Characterization of the functional defect in factor IX Alabama: a mutation near the first EGF-like domain results in defective interaction with factor VIIIa. *Blood* 1988;72[Suppl].302a.

386. Denton PH, Fowlkes DM, Lord ST, et al. Hemophilia B Durham: a mutation in the first EGF-like domain of factor IX that is characterized by polymerase chain reaction. *Blood* 1988;72:1407.

387. Ware J, Davis L, Frazier D, et al. Genetic defect responsible for the dysfunctional protein: factor IX Long Beach. *Blood* 1988;72:820.

388. Spitzer SG, Warn-Cramer BJ, Kasper CK, et al. Replacement of isleucine-397 by threonine in the clotting proteinase factor IXa (Los Angeles and Long Beach variants) affects macromolecular catalysis but not L-tosylarginine methyl ester hydrolysis. Lack of correction between the ox brain prothrombin time and the mutation site in the variant proteins. *Biochem J* 1990;265:219–225..

389. Geddes VA, LeBonniec BF, Louie GV, et al. A moderate form of hemophilia B is caused by a novel mutation in the protease domain of factor IX Vancouver. *J Biol Chem* 1989;264:4689.

389a. Noyes CM, Griffith MJ, Roberts HR, et al. Identification of the molecular defect in factor IX Chapel Hill: substitution of histidine for arginine at position 145. *Proc Natl Acad Sci U S A* 1983;80:4200–4202.

389b. Bajaj SP, Spitzer SG, Welsh WJ, et al. Experimental and theoretical evidence supporting the role of Gly363 in blood coagualtion factor IXa (Gly193 in chymotrypsin) for proper activation of the proenzyme. *J Biol Chem* 1990;265:2956–2961.

390. Spitzer SG, Pendurthi UR, Kasper CK, et al. Molecular defect in factor IX$_{Bm}$ Lake Elsinore. *J Biol Chem* 1988;263:10545.

391. Vidaud M, Attree O, Schaad O, et al. Self-inhibition of factor IX by a Gly to Arg mutation at the substrate binding pocket is linked to severe hemophilia B. *Blood* 1988;72[Suppl 1]:313a.

392. Attree O, Vidaud D, Vidaud M, et al. Rapid characterization of mutations in the catalytic domain of human coagulation factor IX. *Blood* 1988;72[Suppl 1]:289a.

393. Tsang TC, Bentley DR, Mibashan RS, et al. A factor IX mutation, verified by direct genomic sequencing, causes haemophilia B by a novel mechanism. *EMBO J* 1988;7:3009.

394. Bertina RM, van der Linden IK. Factor IX Deventer: evidence for the heterogeneity of hemophilia B$_M$. *Thromb Haemost* 1985;54:120a.

395. Bertina RM, van der Linden IK. Factor IX Zutphen: a genetic variant of blood coagulation factor IX with an abnormally high molecular weight. *J Lab Clin Med* 1982;100:695–704.

396. Gitschier J, Wood WI, Shuman MA, et al. Identification of a missense mutation in the factor VIII gene of a mild hemophiliac. *Science* 1986;232:1415.

397. Youssoufian H, Kazazian HH Jr, Phillips DG, et al. Recurrent mutations in haemophilia A give evidence for CpG mutation hotspots. *Nature* 1986;324: 380.

398. Picketts DJ, Mueller CR, Lillicrap D. Transcriptional control of the factor IX gene: analysis of five cis-acting elements and the deleterious effects of naturally occurring hemophilia B Leyden mutations. *Blood* 1994;84:2992–3000.

399. Kurachi S, Furukawa M, Salier JP, et al. Regulatory mechanism of human factor IX gene: protein binding at the Leyden-specific region. *Biochemistry* 1994;33:1580–1591.

400. Reitsma PH, Mandalaki T, Kasper CK, et al. Novel point mutations correlate with an altered developmental expression of blood coagulation factor IX (hemophilia B Leyden phenotype). *Blood* 1989;73:743.

401. Giannelli F, Choo KH, Rees DJG, et al. Gene deletions in patients with haemophilia B and anti-factor IX antibodies. *Nature* 1983;303:181.

402. Chen S-H, Yoshitake S, Chance PF, et al. An intragenic deletion of the factor IX gene in a family with hemophilia B. *J Clin Invest* 1985;76:2161.

403. Bray GL, Thompson AR. Partial factor IX protein in a pedigree with hemophilia B due to a partial gene deletion. *J Clin Invest* 1986;77:1194.

404. Rees DJG, Rizza CR, Brownlee GG. Haemophilia B caused by a point mutation in a donor splice junction of the human factor IX gene. *Nature* 1985;316:643.

405. Schach BG, Yoshitake S, Davie EW. Hemophilia B factor IX (Seattle 2) due to a single nucleotide deletion in the gene for factor IX. *J Clin Invest* 1987;80:1023.

406. Attree O, Vidaud D, Vidaud M, et al. Mutations in the catalytic domain of human coagulation factor IX. *Genomics* 1989;4:266.

407. Peake IR, Furlong BL, Bloom AL. Carrier detection by direct gene analysis in a family with haemophilia B (factor IX deficiency). *Lancet* 1984;1:242.

408. Matthews RJ, Anson DS, Peake IR, et al. Heterogeneity of the factor IX locus in nine hemophilia B inhibitor patients. *J Clin Invest* 1987;79:746.

409. Hassan HJ, Leonardi JA, Guerriero R, et al. Hemophilia B with inhibitor: molecular analysis of the subtotal deletion of the factor IX gene. *Blood* 1985;66:728.

410. Trent RJ, Wallace RC, Rickard KA. Deletion/insertion of DNA in an intron of the factor IX gene produces severe hemophilia B. *Blood* 1988;72[Suppl 1]:312a.

411. Poon MC, Chui DH, Patterson M, et al. Hemophilia B (Christmas disease) variants and carrier detection analyzed by DNA probes. *J Clin Invest* 1987;79:1204.

412. Vidaud M, Chabret C, Gazengel C, et al. A de novo intragenic deletion of the potential EGF domain of the factor IX gene in a family with severe hemophilia B. *Blood* 1986;68:961.

413. Bernard F, del Senno L, Barbieri R, et al. Gene deletion in an Italian hemophilia B subject. *J Med Genet* 1985;22:305.

414. Wadelius C, Blomback M, Pettersson U. Molecular studies of haemophilia B

in Sweden: identification of patients with total deletion of the factor IX gene and without inhibitory antibodies. *Hum Genet* 1988;81:13.

415. Anson DS, Blake DJ, Winship PR, et al. Nullisomic deletion of the mcf.2 transforming gene in two haemophilia B patients. *EMBO J* 1988;7:2795.

416. Tanimoto M, Kojima T, Kamiya T, et al. DNA analysis of seven patients with hemophilia B who have anti-factor IX antibodies: relationship to clinical manifestations and evidence that the abnormal gene was inherited. *J Lab Clin Med* 1988;112:307.

417. Taylor SA, Lillicrap DP, Blanchette V, et al. A complete deletion of the factor IX gene and new TaqI variant in a hemophilia B kindred. *Hum Genet* 1988;79: 273.

418. Kasper CK, Osterud B, Minami JY, et al. Hemophilia B: characterization of genetic variants and detection of carriers. *Blood* 1977;50:351.

419. Winship PR, Anson DS, Rizza CR, et al. Carrier detection in hemophilia B using two further intragenic restriction fragment length polymorphisms. *Nucleic Acids Res* 1984;12:8861.

420. Hay CW, Robertson KA, Yong S-L, et al. Use of a BamHI polymorphism in the factor IX gene for the determination of hemophilia B carrier status. *Blood* 1986;67:1508.

421. Winship PR, Brownlee GG. Diagnosis of haemophilia B carriers using intragenic oligonucleotide probes. *Lancet* 1986;2:218.

422. Freedenberg DL, Chen S-H, Kurachi K, et al. MspI polymorphic site within the factor IX gene. *Hum Genet* 1987;76:262.

423. Giannelli F, Choo KH, Winship PR, et al. Characterization and use of an intragenic polymorphic marker for detection of carriers of haemophilia B (factor IX deficiency). *Lancet* 1984;1:239.

424. Mulligan L, Holden JJA, White BN. A DNA marker closely linked to the factor IX (haemophilia B) gene. *Hum Genet* 1987;75:381.

425. Drayna D, Davies K, Hartley D, et al. Genetic mapping of the human X chromosome by using restriction fragment length polymorphisms. *Proc Natl Acad Sci U S A* 1984;81:2836.

426. Arveiler B, Oberle I, Vincent A, et al. Genetic mapping of the Xq27-q28 region: new RFPL markers useful for diagnostic applications in fragile-X and hemophilia B families. *Am J Hum Genet* 1988;42:380.

427. Thompson AR, Chen SH, Smith KJ. Diagnostic role of an immunoassay-detected polymorphism of factor IX for potential carriers of hemophilia B. *Blood* 1988;72:1633.

428. Smith KJ, Thompson AR, McMullen BA, et al. Carrier testing in hemophilia B with an immunoassay that distinguishes a prevalent factor IX dimorphism. *Blood* 1987;70:1006.

429. Lusher JM, McMillan CW. Hemophilia study group: severe factor VIII and factor IX deficiency in females. *Am J Med* 1978;65:637.

430. Nisen P, Stamberg J, Ehrenpreis R, et al. The molecular basis of severe hemophilia B in a girl. *N Engl J Med* 1986;315:1139.

431. Corrigan JJ Jr, Kryc JJ. Factor II (prothrombin) levels in cord blood: correlation of coagulant activity with immunoreactive protein. *J Pediatr* 1980;97:979.

432. Harrison S, Adamson S, Bonam D, et al. The manufacturing process for recombinant factor IX. *Semin Hematol* 1998;35[Suppl 2]:4–10.

433. Bush L, Webb C, Bartlett L, et al. The formulation of recombinant factor IX: stability, robustness, and convenience. *Semin Hematol* 1998;35[Suppl 2]:18–21.

434. Levine PH. Efficacy of self-therapy in hemophilia: a study of 72 patients with hemophilia A and B. *N Engl J Med* 1974;291:1381.

435. Faria R, Fiumara NJ. Hepatitis B associated with Konyne. *N Engl J Med* 1972; 287:358.

436. Blatt PM, Lundblad RL, Kingdon HS, et al. Thrombogenic materials in prothrombin complex concentrates. *Ann Intern Med* 1974;81:766.

437. Cederbaum AI, Blatt PM, Roberts HR. Intravascular coagulation with use of human prothrombin complex concentrates. *Ann Intern Med* 1976;84:683.

438. Kasper CK. Clinical use of factor IX concentrates: report on thromboembolic complications. *Thromb Diath Haemorrh* 1975;33:642.

439. Kasper CK. Postoperative thrombosis in hemophilia B. *N Engl J Med* 1973; 289:610.

440. Ragni MV, Winkelstein A, Kingsley L, et al. 1986 update of HIV sero-prevalence, seroconversion, AIDS incidence and immunologic correlates of HIV infection in patients with hemophilia A and B. *Blood* 1987;70:786.

441. Brettler DB, Brewster F, Levine PH, et al. Immunologic aberrations, HIV seropositivity and seroconversion rates in patients with hemophilia B. *Blood* 1987;70:276.

442. Hedner U. Treatment of patients with factor VIII and factor IX inhibitors with special focus on the use of recombinant factor VIIa. *Thromb Haemost* 1999;82:531–539.

443. Thorland EC, Drost JB, Lusher JM, et al. Anaphylactic response to factor IX replacement therapy in haemophilia B patients: complete gene deletions confer the highest risk. *Haemophilia* 1999;5:101–105.

444. Tengborn L, Hansson S, Fasth A, et al. Anaphylactoid reactions and nephrotic syndrome—a considerable risk during factor IX treatment in patients with haemophilia B and inhibitors: a report on the outcome in two brothers. *Haemophilia* 1998;4:854–859.

445. Warrier I, Lusher JM. Development of anaphylactic shock in haemophilia B patients with inhibitors. *Blood Coagul Fibrinolysis* 1998;9[Suppl 1]:S125–S128.

446. Stehr Green JK, Holman RC, Jason JM, et al. Hemophilia-associated AIDS in the United States, 1981 to September 1987. *Am J Public Health* 1988;78:439.

447. Liebman HA, Limentani SA, Furie BC, et al. Immunoaffinity purification of factor IX (Christmas factor) using conformation-specific antibodies directed against the factor IX-metal complex. *Proc Natl Acad Sci U S A* 1985;82:3879.

448. Limentani SA, Furie BC, Poiesz BJ, et al. Separation of human plasma factor IX from HTLV-I or HIV by immunoaffinity chromatography using conformation-specific antibodies. *Blood* 1987;70:1312.

449. Smith KJ. Immunoaffinity purification of factor IX from commercial concentrates and infusion studies in animals. *Blood* 1988;72:1269.

450. Anson DS, Austen DEG, Brownlee GG. Expression of active human clotting factor IX from recombinant DNA clones in mammalian cells. *Nature* 1985;315:683.

451. Busby S, Kumar A, Joseph M, et al. Expression of active human factor IX in transfected cells. *Nature* 1985;316:271.

452. de la Salle H, Alterburger W, Elkaim R, et al. Active γ-carboxylated human factor IX expressed using recombinant DNA techniques. *Nature* 1985;316:268.

453. Kaufman R, Wasley L, Furie BC, et al. Expression, purification, and characterization of recombinant γ-carboxylated human factor IX. *J Biol Chem* 1986;261:9622.

454. Kaufman RJ. Advances toward gene therapy for hemophilia at the millennium. *Hum Gene Ther* 1999;10:2091–2107.

455. Kay MA, Manno CS, Ragni MV, et al. Evidence for gene transfer and expression of factor IX in haemophilia B patients treated with an AAV vector. *Nat Genet* 2000;24:257–261.

456. Girolami A, Scarano L, Saggiorato G, et al. Congenital deficiencies and abnormalities of prothrombin. *Blood Coagul Fibrinolysis* 1998;9:557–569.

457. Josso F, Monasterio de Sanchez J, Lavergne JM, et al. Congenital abnormality of the prothrombin molecule (factor II) in four siblings: prothrombin Barcelona. *Blood* 1971;38:9.

458. Rabiet MJ, Benarous R, Labie D, et al. Abnormal activation of a human prothrombin variant: prothrombin Barcelona. *FEBS Lett* 1978;87:132.

459. Rabiet MJ, Elion J, Benarous R, et al. Activation of prothrombin Barcelona: evidence for active high molecular weight intermediates. *Biochim Biophys Acta* 1979;584:66.

460. Rabiet MJ, Furie BC, Furie B. Molecular defect of prothrombin Barcelona. *J Biol Chem* 1986;261:15045.

461. Guillin M-C, Bezeaud A. Characterization of a variant of human prothrombin: prothrombin Madrid. *Ann N Y Acad Sci* 1981;370:414.

462. Inomoto T, Shirakami A, Kawauchi S, et al. Prothrombin Tokushima: characterization of dysfunctional thrombin derived from a variant of human prothrombin. *Blood* 1987;69:565.

463. Miyata T, Morita T, Inomoto T, et al. Prothrombin Tokushima, a replace of arginine 418 by tryptophan that impairs the fibrinogen clotting activity of derived thrombin Tokushima. *Biochemistry* 1987;26:1117.

464. Henriksen RA, Owen WG, Nesheim ME, et al. Identification of a congenital dysthrombin, thrombin Quick. *J Clin Invest* 1980;66:934.

465. Henriksen RA, Mann KG. Identification of the primary structural defect in the dysthrombin thrombin Quick I: substitution of cysteine for arginine 382. *Biochemistry* 1988;27:9160.

465a. Henriksen RA, Mann KG. Substitution of valine for glycine-558 in the congenital dysthrombin thrombin Quick II alters primary substrate specificity. *Biochemistry* 1989;28:2078–2082.

466. Shapiro SS, Martinez J, Holburn RR. Congenital dysprothrombinemia: an inherited structural disorder of human prothrombin. *J Clin Invest* 1969;48:2251.

467. Huisse M-G, Dreyfus M, Guillin M-C. Prothrombin Clamart: prothrombin variant with defective Arg 320-Ile cleavage by factor Xa. *Thromb Res* 1986; 44:11.

468. Rabiet MJ, Jandrot-Perrus M, Boissel JP, et al. Thrombin Metz: characterization of the dysfunctional thrombin derived from a variant of human prothrombin. *Blood* 1984;63:927.

469. Bezeaud A, Drouet L, Soria C, et al. Prothrombin Salakta: an abnormal prothrombin characterized by a defect in the active site of thrombin. *Thromb Res* 1984;34:507.

470. Bezeaud A, Elion J, Guillin M-C. Functional characterization of thrombin Salakta: an abnormal thrombin derived from a human prothrombin variant. *Blood* 1988;71:556.

471. Girolami A, Coccheri G, Palaretti G, et al. Prothrombin Molise: a "new" congenital dysprothrombinemia, double heterozygosis with an abnormal prothrombin and "true" prothrombin deficiency. *Blood* 1978;52:115.

472. Hayashi T, Yahagi A, Suzuki K, et al. Molecular abnormality observed in a patient with coagulation factor X (FX) deficiency: a novel three-base-pair (CTT) deletion within the polypyrimidine tract of the FX intron D. *Br J Haematol* 1998;102:926–928.

473. Girolami A, Molaro G, Lazzarin M, et al. A new congenital haemorrhagic condition due to the presence of an abnormal factor X (factor X Friuli): study of a large kindred. *Br J Haematol* 1970;19:179.

474. James HL, Girolami A, Fair DS. Molecular defect in coagulation factor X Friuli results from a substitution of serine for proline at position 343. *Blood* 1991;77:317–323.

475. Fair DS, Plow EF, Edgington TS. Combined functional and immunochemical analysis of normal and abnormal human factor X. *J Clin Invest* 1979;64:884.

476. Fair DS, Edgington TS. Heterogeneity of hereditary and acquired factor X deficiencies by combined immunochemical and functional analyses. *Br J Haematol* 1985;59:235.

477. De Stefano V, Leone G, Ferrelli R, et al. Factor X Roma: a congenital factor X variant defective at different degrees in the intrinsic and extrinsic activation. *Br J Haematol* 1988;69:387.

478. Nora RE, Bell WR, Noe DA, et al. Novel factor X deficiency: normal partial thromboplastin time and associated spindle cell thymoma. *Am J Med* 1985;79:122.

479. Girolami A, Vicarioto M, Ruzza G, et al. Factor X Padua: a new congenital factor X abnormality with a defect only in the extrinsic system. *Acta Haematol* 1985;73:31.

480. Scamgler PJ, Williamson R. The structural gene for human coagulation factor X is located on chromosome 13q34. *Cytogenet Cell Genet* 1985;39:231.

481. Pfeiffer RA, Ott R, Gilgendrantz S, et al. Deficiency of coagulation factors VII and X associated with deletion of a chromosome 13 (q34). *Hum Genet* 1982;62:358.

482. Stoll C, Roth MP. Partial 4q duplication due to inherited der(13),t(4;13)(q26;q34) in a girl with a deficiency of factor X. *Hum Genet* 1980;53:303.

483. Kouides PA, Kulzer L. Prophylactic treatment of severe factor X deficiency with prothrombin complex concentrate. *Haemophilia* 2001;7:220–223.

484. McVey JH, Boswell E, Mumford AD, et al. Factor VII deficiency and the FVII mutation database. *Hum Mutat* 2001;17:3–17.

484a. Available at: http://europium.csc.mrc.ac.uk.

485. Matthay KK, Koerper MA, Ablin AR. Intracranial hemorrhage in congenital factor VII deficiency. *J Pediatr* 1979;94:413.

486. Kuzel T, Green D, Stulberg SD, et al. Arthropathy and surgery in congenital factor VII deficiency. *Am J Med* 1988;84:771.

487. Yorke AJ, Mant MJ. Factor VII deficiency and surgery: is preoperative replacement therapy necessary? *JAMA* 1977;238:424.

488. Gershwin ME, Gude JK. Deep vein thrombosis and pulmonary embolism in congenital factor VII deficiency. *N Engl J Med* 1973;288:141.

489. Triplett DA, Brandt JT, Batard MAM, et al. Hereditary factor VII deficiency: heterogeneity defined by combined functional and immunochemical analysis. *Blood* 1985;66:1284.

490. Hedner U. Recombinant coagulation factor VIIa: from the concept to clinical application in hemophilia treatment in 2000. *Semin Thromb Hemost* 2000;26:363–366.

491. Mariani G, Testa MG, Di Paolantonio T, et al. Use of recombinant, activated factor VII in the treatment of congenital factor VII deficiencies. *Vox Sang* 1999;77:131–136.

492. Friedman PA, Rosenberg RD, Hauschka PV, et al. A spectrum of partially carboxylated prothrombin in the plasma of coumarin-treated patients. *Biochem Biophys Acta* 1977;494:271.

493. Esnouf MP, Prowse CV. The gamma-carboxyglutamic acid content of human and bovine prothrombin following warfarin treatment. *Biochim Biophys Acta* 1977;490:471.

494. McKee RW, Binkley SB, Thayer SA, et al. The isolation of vitamin K_2. *J Biol Chem* 1939;131:327.

495. Frick PG, Riedler G, Brogli H. Dose response and minimal daily requirement for vitamin K in man. *J Appl Physiol* 1967;23:387.

496. Ansell JE, Kumar R, Deykin D. The spectrum of vitamin K deficiency. *JAMA* 1977;237:40.

497. Niiya K, Kitagawa T, Fujishita M, et al. Bulimia nervosa complicated by deficiency of vitamin K-dependent coagulation factors. *JAMA* 1983;250:792.

498. Blanchard RA, Furie BC, Kruger SF, et al. Immunoassays of human prothrombin species which correlate with functional coagulant activities. *J Lab Clin Med* 1983;101:242.

499. Krasinski SD, Russell RM, Furie BC, et al. The prevalence of vitamin K deficiency in chronic gastrointestinal disorders. *Am J Clin Nutr* 1985;41:639.

500. Kaplan MM, Elta GH, Furie B, et al. Fat soluble vitamin nutriture in primary biliary cirrhosis. *Gastroenterology* 1988;95:787.

501. Bertina RM, Van der Marel-van Nieuwkoop W, Dubbeldam J, et al. New method for the rapid detection of vitamin K deficiency. *Clin Chem Acta* 1980;105:93.

502. Mummah-Schendel LL, Suttie JW. Serum phylloquinone concentrations in a normal adult population. *Am J Clin Nutr* 1986;44:686.

503. Brinkhous KM, Smith HP. Plasma prothrombin level in normal infancy and in hemorrhagic disease of the newborn. *Am J Med Sci* 1937;193:475.

504. Dam H, Tage-Hansen E. Vitamin K lack in normal and sick infants. *Lancet* 1939;2:1157.

505. Dam H, Dyggve H. Relation of vitamin K deficiency to hemorrhagic disease of the newborn. *Adv Pediatr* 1952;5:129.

506. Sutherland JM, Glueck HI, Glesser G. Hemorrhagic disease of the newborn. *Am J Dis Child* 1967;113:524.

507. Wefring KW. Hemorrhage in the newborn and vitamin K prophylaxis. *J Pediatr* 1962;61:686.

508. Shearer MJ, Rahim S, Stimmler L, et al. Plasma vitamin K_1 in mothers and their newborn babies. *Lancet* 1982;2:460.

509. Keenan WJ, Jewett T, Glueck HI. Role of feeding and vitamin K in hypoprothrombinemia of the newborn. *Am J Dis Child* 1971;121:271.

510. Schneider DL, Fluckiger HB, Manes JD. Vitamin K content of infant formula products. *Pediatrics* 1974;53:273.

511. Committee on Nutrition, American Academy of Pediatrics. Vitamin K supplementation for infants receiving milk substitute infant formulas and for those with fat malabsorption. *Pediatrics* 1972;48:483.

512. Bound JP, Telfer JP. Effect of vitamin K dosage on plasma bilirubin levels in premature infants. *Lancet* 1956;1:720.

513. Allison AC. Danger of vitamin K to newborn. *Lancet* 1955;1:669.

514. Hull R, Hirsh J, Jay R, et al. Different intensities of oral anticoagulant therapy in the treatment of proximal vein thrombosis. *N Engl J Med* 1982;307:1676.

515. Hull R, Delmore T, Carter C, et al. Adjusted subcutaneous heparin versus warfarin sodium in the long-term treatment of venous thrombosis. *N Engl J Med* 1982;306:189.

516. Turpie AGG, Gunstensen J, Hirsh J, et al. Randomised comparison of two intensities of oral anticoagulant therapy after tissue heart valve replacement. *Lancet* 1988;1:1242.

517. Forfar JC. Prediction of hemorrhage during long-term oral coumarin anticoagulation by excessive prothrombin ratio. *Am Heart J* 1982;103:445.

518. Coon WW, Willis PW. Hemorrhagic complications of anti-coagulant therapy. *Arch Intern Med* 1974;133:386.

519. Coon WW, Willis PW. Thromboembolic complications during anti-coagulant therapy. *Arch Surg* 1972;105:209.

520. Levine MN, Raskob G, Hirsh J. Hemorrhagic complications of long-term anticoagulant therapy. *Chest* 1986;89[Suppl 2]:16.

521. Hirsh J, Deykin D, Poller L. "Therapeutic range" for oral anticoagulant therapy. *Chest* 1986;89[Suppl 2]:11.

522. Lipton RA, Klass EM. Human ingestion of a "superwarfarin" rodenticide resulting in a prolonged anticoagulant effect. *JAMA* 1984;252:3004.

523. Jones EC, Growe GH, Naiman SC. Prolonged anticoagulation in rat poisoning. *JAMA* 1984;252:3005.

524. Chong LL, Chau WK, Ho CH. A case of "superwarfarin" poisoning. *Scand J Haematol* 1986;36:314.

525. O'Reilly RA, Aggeler PM. Covert anticoagulant ingestion: study of 25 patients and review of world literature. *Medicine* 1976;55:389.

526. O'Reilly RA, Aggeler PM, Gibbs JO. Hemorrhagic state due to surreptitious ingestion of bishydroxycoumarin. *N Engl J Med* 1962;267:19.

527. Bowie EJW, Todd M, Thompson JH Jr, et al. Anticoagulant malingerers ("the dicoumarol-eaters"). *Am J Med* 1965;39:855.

528. Weitzel JN, Sadowski JA, Furie BC, et al. Hemorrhagic disorder caused by surreptitious ingestion of a long-acting vitamin K antagonist/rodenticide, brodifacoum. *Blood* 1990;76:2555.

529. Goldsweig HG, Kapusta M, Schwartz J, et al. Bleeding, salicylates, and prolonged prothrombin time: three case reports and a review of the literature. *J Rheumatol* 1976;3:37.

530. Uotila L, Suttie JW. Inhibition of vitamin K-dependent carboxylase in vitro by cefamanadole and its structural analogs. *J Infect Dis* 1983;148:571.

531. Bang NU, Tessler SS, Heidenreich RO, et al. Effects of moxalactam on blood coagulation and platelet function. *Rev Infect Dis* 1982;4:S546.

532. Barza M, Furie B, Brown AE, et al. Defects in vitamin K-dependent carboxylation associated with moxalactam treatment. *J Infect Dis* 1986;153:1166.

533. Lipksy JJ. Mechanism of the inhibition of the γ–carboxylation of glutamic acid by N-methylthiotetrazole-containing antibiotics. *Proc Natl Acad Sci U S A* 1984;81:2893.

534. Ratnoff OD. Hemostatic mechanisms in liver disease. *Med Clin North Am* 1963;47:721.

535. Rapaport SI, Ames SB, Mikkelsen S, et al. Plasma clotting factors in chronic hepatocellular disease. *N Engl J Med* 1960;263:278.

536. Donaldson GWK, Davies SH, Darg A, et al. Coagulation factors in chronic liver disease. *J Clin Pathol* 1969;22:199.

537. Corrigan JJ, Earnest DL. Factor II antigen in liver disease and warfarin-induced vitamin K deficiency. *Am J Hematol* 1980;8:249.

538. Spector I, Corn M, Ticktin HE. Effect of plasma transfusions on the prothrombin time and clotting factors in liver disease. *N Engl J Med* 1966;275:1032.

539. Green G, Dymock IW, Poller L, et al. Use of factor VII-rich prothrombin complex concentrate in liver disease. *Lancet* 1975;1:1311.

540. Liebman HA, Furie BC, Tong MJ, et al. Des-γ–carboxy(abnormal)prothrombin as a serum marker of primary hepatocellular carcinoma. *N Engl J Med* 1984;310:1427.

541. Fujiyama S, Morishita T, Hashiguichi O, et al. Plasma abnormal prothrombin (des-γ–carboxy prothrombin) as a marker of hepatocellular carcinoma. *Cancer* 1988;61:1621.

542. Fujiyama S, Morishita T, Sagara K, et al. Clinical evaluation of plasma abnormal prothrombin (PIVKA-II) in patients with hepatocellular carcinoma. *Hepatogastroenterology* 1986;33:201.

543. Howell M. Acquired factor X deficiency associated with systemic amyloidosis. *Blood* 1963;21:739.

544. Pechet L, Kastrul JJ. Amyloidosis associated with factor X (Stuart) deficiency. *Ann Intern Med* 1964;61:316.

545. Furie B, Greene E, Furie BC. Syndrome of acquired factor X deficiency and systemic amyloidosis. *N Engl J Med* 1977;297:81.

546. Furie B, Voo L, McAdam KPWJ, et al. Mechanism of factor X deficiency in systemic amyloidosis. *N Engl J Med* 1981;304:827.

547. Spero JA, Lewis JH, Hasiba V, et al. Treatment of amyloidosis associated factor X deficiency. *Thromb Haemost* 1976;35:377.

548. Greipp PR, Kyle RA, Bowie EJW. Factor X deficiency in primary amyloidosis. *N Engl J Med* 1979;301:1018.

549. Rosenstein ED, Itzkowitz SH, Penziner AS, et al. Resolution of factor X deficiency in primary amyloidosis following splenectomy. *Arch Intern Med* 1983;143:597.

550. Camoriano JK, Greipp PR, Bayer GK, et al. Resolution of acquired factor X deficiency and amyloidosis with melphalan and prednisone therapy. *N Engl J Med* 1987;316:1133.

551. Boggio L, Green D. Recombinant human factor VIIa in the management of amyloid-associated factor X deficiency. *Br J Haematol* 2001;112:1074–1075.

552. Bajaj SP, Rapaport SI, Barclay S, et al. Acquired hypoprothrombinemia due to non-neutralizing antibodies to prothrombin: mechanism and management. *Blood* 1985;65:1538.

553. Handley DA, Lawrence JR. Factor IX deficiency in the nephrotic syndrome. *Lancet* 1967;1:1079.

554. Natelson EA, Lynch EC, Hettig RA, et al. Acquired factor IX deficiency in the nephrotic syndrome. *Ann Intern Med* 1970;73:373.

555. Vaziri ND, Branson HE, Ness R. Changes in coagulation factors IX, VIII, VII, X and V in nephrotic syndrome. *Am J Med Sci* 1980;280:167.

CHAPTER 38

Coagulation Factors V and VIII: Normal Function and Clinical Disorders

Gilbert C. White and Gary E. Gilbert

Factors V and VIII are structurally and functionally homologous proteins that play a central role in blood coagulation, acting as cofactors in the conversion of prothrombin to thrombin and factor X to Xa, respectively. In contrast to other blood-clotting proteins, factors V and VIII are not active enzymes but function as cofactors, which promote the assembly of enzyme and substrate on surfaces. In doing so, they increase the rate of substrate activation. Thus, factor V promotes the interaction of factor Xa with prothrombin on phospholipid surfaces to form the *prothrombinase complex* that leads to the generation of thrombin. Similarly, factor VIII promotes the interaction of factor IXa with factor X on phospholipid surfaces to form the *tenase complex* that leads to the generation of activated factor Xa.

Deficiency of factor VIII results in hemophilia A, a severe X-linked bleeding disorder that is characterized by recurrent joint and soft-tissue bleeding that results in crippling hemarthroses and organ damage. In contrast, a deficiency of factor V results in a disorder called *parahemophilia*. This is a somewhat milder bleeding disorder than hemophilia A, with primarily mucous membrane and cutaneous bleeding and less tendency to joint and organ bleeding. The inheritance of parahemophilia is autosomal.

The purposes of this chapter are to present what is known of the structure, function, and genetics of factors VIII and V and to describe and compare the associated clinical deficiency syndromes, as well as the syndromes of excessive activity. The reader is also referred to several reviews (1–7).

HISTORICAL OVERVIEW

Clinical bleeding disorders were described in antiquity—the first recorded reference, probably classical hemophilia, is from the Babylonian Talmud from the second century A.D. Rabbi Judah the Patriarch, redactor of the Mishneh, the second century compilation of Jewish law, wrote, "If she circumcised her first child and he died, and a second one also died, she must not circumcise her third child." This is a clear and remarkably accurate description that infers the severity of the bleeding defect and the X-linked pattern of inheritance, as well as a rational approach to prevention. Although the clinical description of bleeding disorders continued through the Middle Ages into the

early part of the twentieth century, the identification of the missing factors and characterization of those factors did not come until much later, when advances in biochemistry made purification of the proteins feasible and molecular biology techniques permitted characterization of the genes and *in vitro* production of large quantities of the protein.

The discovery of factor V is attributed to Owren (8) in 1947, when he reported a rare, autosomal-recessive bleeding disorder that was characterized by a prolonged prothrombin time (PT) but normal levels of prothrombin and fibrinogen. Subsequent characterization showed that factor V was labile in plasma, readily adsorbed to glass or plastic during purification, and easily degraded. Purification and characterization of human factor V was accomplished by three groups (9–11). The complementary deoxyribonucleic acid (DNA) for factor V was cloned by Kane et al. (12) and by Jenny et al. (13) in 1987.

Factor VIII was initially identified by Patek and Taylor (14), who described properties of the "factor" from normal plasma that corrected the coagulation defect of hemophilic blood. Early on, it was shown by Brinkhous that a deficiency of factor VIII resulted in delayed thrombin generation (14a) and that bleeding was related to the defect in thrombin formation. Factor VIII was distinguished from factor IX by Pavlovsky (15), who presented evidence in 1947 that plasma from one hemophiliac could correct the clotting defect from another, which was evidence that there were two forms of hemophilia. Factor VIII and von Willebrand's factor (vWF) were first separated by Owen and Wagner (16) and Weiss et al. (16a), providing the first biochemical basis for the separation of these two disorders. The technique of monoclonal antibody affinity chromatography that was developed by Zimmerman et al. (16b) led to the first purification of factor VIII and was later used by Fass et al. (17) to immunopurify porcine factor VIII. The amino acid sequences that were obtained by Fass et al. contributed in part to the subsequent cloning of factor VIII and the elucidation of the full-length sequence and activation mechanism (18,19). Recombinant factor VIII was first synthesized for clinical use in 1987 (20).

STRUCTURES OF FACTORS V AND VIII

The gene that codes for factor VIII is at the tip of the long arm of the X chromosome, near the genes for glucose-6-phosphate

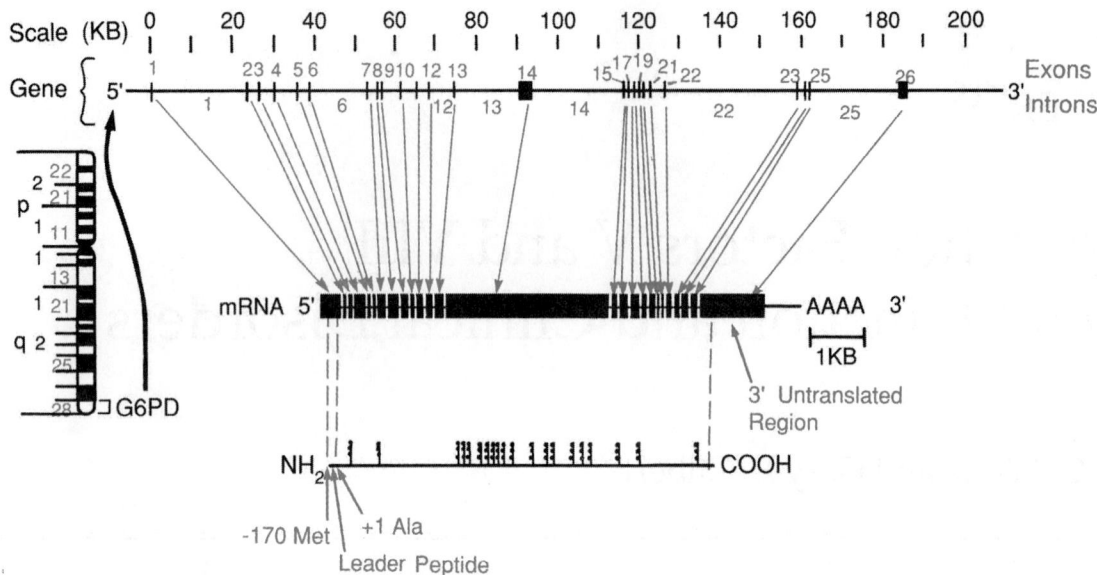

Figure 38-1. Map of human factor VIII gene. The factor VIII gene is at the tip of the long arm of the X chromosome, near the gene for glucose-6-phosphate dehydrogenase (G6PD). The gene (*top line*) spans 186 kilobases (kb) and consists of 26 exons or coding regions (*filled boxes*). The messenger ribonucleic acid (mRNA) transcription product (*middle line*) is approximately 9 kb and codes for the 2351–amino acid factor VIII protein (*bottom line*). The curved lines on the protein indicate sites of potential N-linked glycosylation. (From White GC, Shoemaker CB. Factor VIII gene and hemophilia A. *Blood* 1989;73:1–12, with permission.)

dehydrogenase and color vision (Fig. 38-1). It is made up of nearly 186,000 base pairs (bp) and constitutes approximately 0.1% of the X chromosome (21,22). The gene is organized into 26 separate exons that range in size from 69 to 3106 bp and are separated by 25 intervening regions (introns), which range in size from 207 to 32,400 bp. The complete gene consists of approximately 9 kilobase (kb) of exon and 177 kb of intron.

The factor VIII messenger RNA (mRNA) encodes a precursor protein of 2351 amino acids, which is composed of a 19 amino acid hydrophobic signal peptide (removed during secretion) and the mature factor VIII protein. Analysis of the predicted amino acid sequence of mature human factor VIII reveals a complex protein with two types of internal homology (23,24) (Fig. 38-2). Three A domain repeats are present, each approximately 350 amino acids in length with approximately 30% amino acid homology between repeats. The first repeat begins at the amino terminus of the mature protein and is separated from the second repeat by 36 largely acidic amino acids. After the second A domain repeat, the completion of the heavy chain of mature plasma factor VIII is a stretch of 983 amino acids, which is rich in potential asparagine-linked glycosylation sites but, unlike the rest of factor VIII, contains few cysteines. This region, known as the B domain, is encoded entirely by a single large exon (which also encodes parts of the A2 and A3 repeats) and is presumed to be an ancient insertion into an existing gene. Of the 25 potential

N-linked glycosylation sites (Asn–X–Thr/Ser) that are present in the mature protein, 19 are found in the B domain. The third A domain repeat is found at the amino terminus of the light chain of mature plasma factor VIII, immediately after another short segment of 41, predominantly acidic, amino acids. This acidic region contains the putative binding site for vWF (25,26) and is the site of tyrosine sulfation in factor VIII (27).

The second internal homology is the C domain, which occurs as a contiguous tandem repeat at the carboxyl terminus of the molecule. Both copies are approximately 150 amino acids in length, with 37% homology between repeats. The third A domain and the two C-domain repeats make up the light chain of mature plasma factor VIII, whereas the A1, A2, and B domains make up the heavy chain.

The A domains show striking homology with similar repeats in ceruloplasmin, a blue copper-containing oxidase in human plasma. Like factor VIII, ceruloplasmin contains a triplicated repeat, each analogous to the A domain of factor VIII (28). Copper binding occurs in the carboxyl terminal portion of each repeat. A total of six copper atoms are bound per mole of ceruloplasmin: four in the active site, each bound by different mechanisms (types I, II, III, and IV, based on kinetic characteristics), and two elsewhere. The residues that are believed to be involved in binding copper atoms are also present in factor VIII. As predicted by the ceruloplasmin homology, factor VIII binds at least

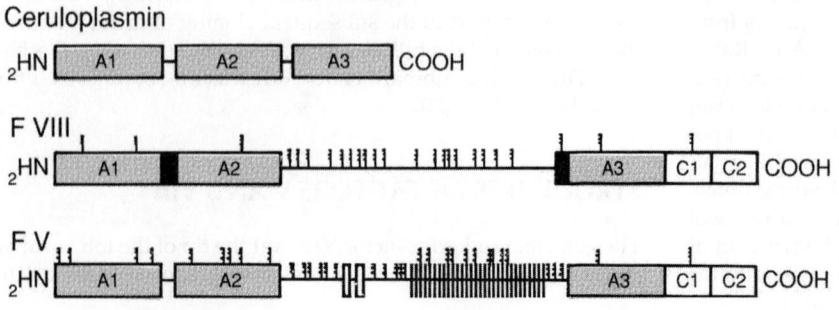

Figure 38-2. Domain structure of ceruloplasmin and human factors (Fs) V and VIII. The colored boxes indicate the three A-domain repeats (A1, A2, A3) in each protein. The white boxes indicate the two C-domain repeats (C1 and C2) in Fs V and VIII. The A2 and A3 domains of Fs V and VIII are separated by nonhomologous connecting regions, which contain most of the potential N-linked glycosylation sites. The acidic regions between the A1 and A2 domains and between the B and A3 domains in F VIII are shown as filled boxes. Potential N-linked glycosylation sites are indicated by the wavy line.

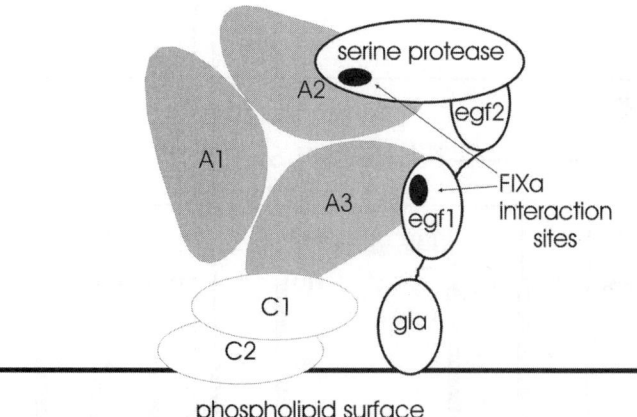

Figure 38-3. Model of membrane-bound activated factor VIII that is bound to factor IXa (FIXa), the factor Xase complex. egf, epidermal growth factor; gla, γ-carboxyglutamic acid.

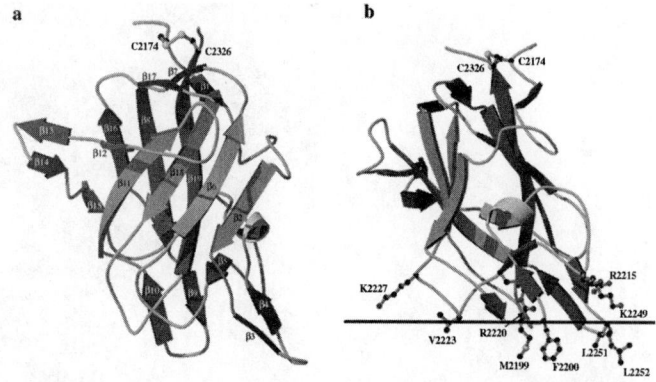

Figure 38-4. Ribbon diagram of factor VIII C2 and proposed membrane-binding mode. **A:** The structure consists of 19 β-strands, including an eight-stranded β-sandwich core. Two of the three β-hairpins and an additional loop extend beyond the core fold. These regions, which are predominantly hydrophobic, flank a pair of positively charged clefts. **B:** The putative membrane-binding surface includes M2199 and F2200 from the first turn, L2251 and L2252 from the second turn, and V2223 from the adjacent loop. These hydrophobic residues and a belt of basic residues partition on either side of the horizontal gray line, which indicates the putative polar-nonpolar boundary of a phospholipid bilayer surface. (See Color Fig. 38-4.)

two copper ions with high affinity (29). Although factor VIII retains partial function when the copper ions are removed, the ions enhance function approximately 1.5-fold. In the absence of copper ions, calcium ions apparently substitute for the same sites. The C domain of factor VIII shares homology with milk fat globule protein (30) and with discoidin I, a phospholipid- and galactose-binding lectin from the slime mold *Dictyostelium discoideum*. The second C domain contains the major phospholipid-binding motif of factor VIII (31–33).

Although synthesized as a single polypeptide chain, factor VIII undergoes proteolytic processing before secretion, such that plasma factor VIII circulates as a two-chain, metal, ion-stabilized complex that consists of a variable heavy chain of 90 to 210 kd and a 80-kd light chain (34–36).

A model of the three-dimensional structure of factor VIII and the way it interacts with factor IXa has emerged from x-ray crystallographic studies, distance measurements, and analysis of mutations that cause loss of function. One version of the model is depicted in Figure 38-3 (37). Factor VIII is depicted as bound to a phospholipid membrane by the C2 domain. The B domain is absent, because it is cleaved in the course of factor VIII activation. The A domains are arranged symmetrically around an axis that is approximately parallel to the membrane, so that the A2 domain is farther from the membrane than the A3 domain. Identified sites on the A2 and A3 domains of factor VIII that interact with the factor IXa protease domain and epidermal growth factor (EGF) 1 and EGF2 regions, respectively, are aligned vertically on one surface of the protein. The distance from the membrane to the factor IXa active site is approximately 8 nm.

The C2 domains of factor V and factor VIII have been crystallized and the structures solved. Overall, they share a high degree of structural homology as β barrels and have similar motifs that appear to be good candidates for membrane binding. The β-barrel core and protruding β-strand loops of the factor VIII C2 domain are illustrated in Figure 38-4. The membrane-binding function is hypothesized to be mediated via five solvent-exposed hydrophobic amino acids that extend from the lower surface of the domain. These are illustrated as penetrating a hydrophobic membrane plane in Figure 38-4B. Site-directed mutagenesis studies have confirmed that four of the hydrophobic residues—Met2199, Phe2200, Leu2251, and Leu2252—participate in binding to phospholipid membranes and vWF (38).

The crystal structure of ceruloplasmin has provided a template from which the triplicated A domains of factor VIII and factor V have been modeled. The three domains are arranged in

a triangle. The models appear correct in the placement of amino acids that are known to bind other proteins on the surface rather than in the core. The model of the factor VIII A domains is depicted in Figure 38-5, with each A domain colored differently (37). The side perspective illustrates that the identified amino acids within the A2 domain and A3 domain that bind factor IXa are aligned along a tangent to the outer edge of the triangle. The peptide that is recognized by BiP, a chaperone protein that decreases cellular secretion of factor VIII, is colored yellow.

The factor V gene is located on chromosome 1 in humans (39) and contains 25 exons, which range in size from 72 to 2820 bp (40). The structure of the gene for factor V is similar to that for the gene for factor VIII. Of the 24 intron-exon boundaries in the factor V gene, 21 occur at the same location as in the factor VIII gene, after the amino acid sequences of the two proteins are aligned.

The mRNA for factor V contains 6903 bp and consists of 76 nucleotides of 5' untranslated sequence, 6672 nucleotides of coding sequence, and 155 nucleotides of 3' untranslated sequence that contains an AATAAA polyadenylation signal that is 9 bp upstream from the poly(A)+ tail (41–43). The protein that is encoded by the factor V mRNA is composed of a hydropho-

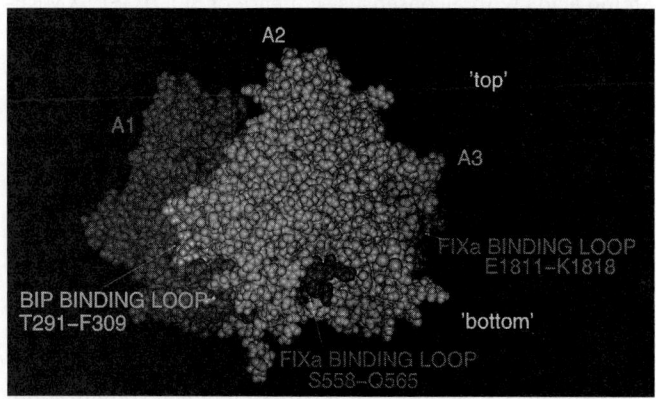

Figure 38-5. Factor VIII A domains. BIP, immunoglobulin binding protein; FIXa, factor IXa. (See Color Fig. 38-5.)

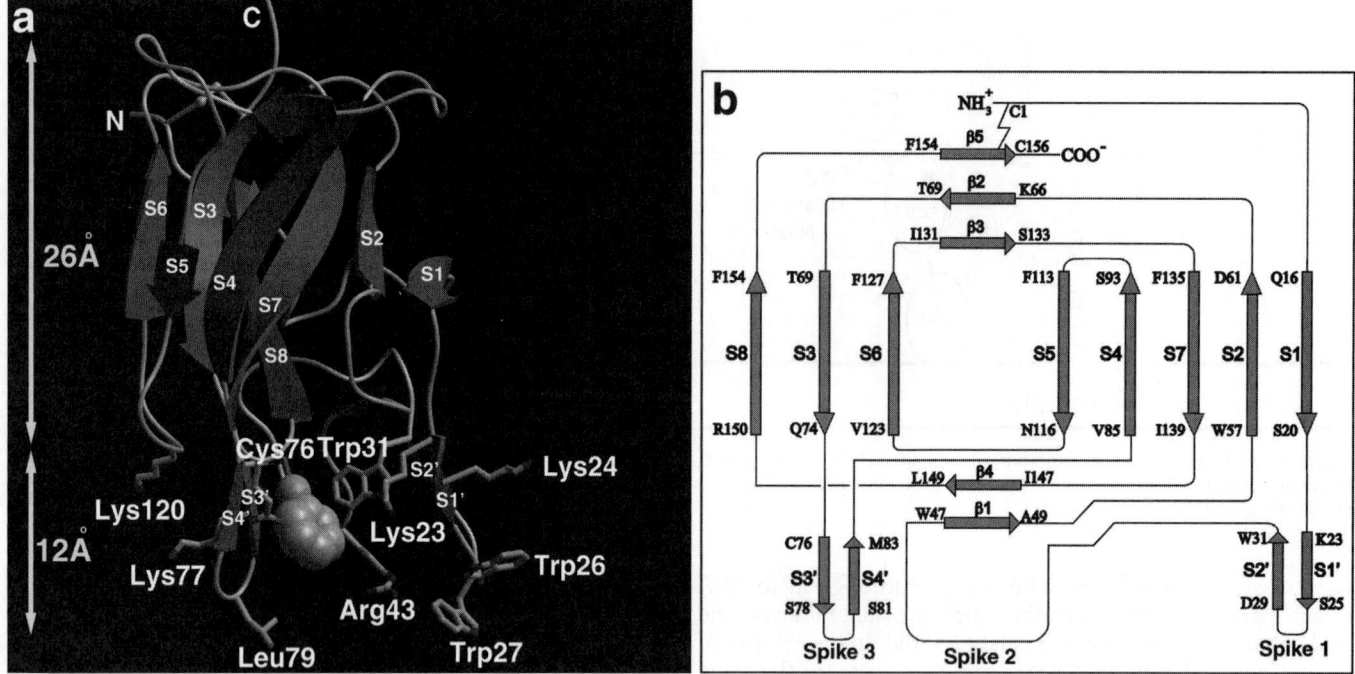

Figure 38-6. Structure of factor V C2 domain. **A:** Ribbon plot of the open crystal form in the reference orientation, which highlights the major secondary structure elements. Several noticeable side chains and the Cys 1–Cys 156 disulfide bridge are displayed. The phenyl mercury molecule (space-filling model) that is used for structure determination is shown covalently attached to Cys 76. **B:** Topology diagram that shows the arrangement of secondary-structure elements. (See Color Fig. 38-6.)

bic leader peptide, which is 28 amino acids in length and is cleaved off during the secretion process, and a mature factor V protein that is 2196 amino acids in length.

Factor V contains triplicated A-domain repeats that are homologous with those of factor VIII and ceruloplasmin (41,44) (Fig. 38-2). Like factor VIII, factor V binds copper, apparently via a type II binding site at the interface between the A1 and A3 domains (45). The function, if any, of copper binding in factor V is unknown. The arrangement of A repeats in factor V is similar to the arrangement in factor VIII (A1–A2–connecting region–A3). One important difference between factor V and factor VIII is that the acidic regions between the A1 and A2 domains and the B and A3 domains of factor VIII are not present in factor V. The connecting region of factor V is approximately 836 residues in length and bears no sequence homology with the B domain of factor VIII. The primary structural features of the connecting region of factor V are the presence of two tandem repeats of 17 amino acids with a consensus sequence of SQDTGSPSXMRP-WEDXP, followed by 31 tandem repeats of nine amino acids with a consensus sequence of [T,N,P]LSPDLSQT. Like the B domain of factor VIII, the connecting region of factor V is a major site of potential carbohydrate attachment. Of the 37 potential N-linked oligosaccharide attachment sites (Asn-X-Ser/Thr) in factor V, 25 are in the connecting region. Also, like factor VIII, the connecting region is not needed for factor V coagulant activity. Factor V contains two segments that are homologous with the C-domain repeats of factor VIII. The overall amino acid sequences of factor V and factor VIII are approximately 30% homologous.

The mature factor V protein is a single-chain polypeptide with an estimated molecular weight of 286 kd (46–48). It is approximately 13% carbohydrate by weight and contains both N-linked and O-linked carbohydrate chains (49). Removal of sialic acid has little effect on factor V function, but removal of

the penultimate galactose residues destroys factor V activity (50,51). Physical characterization of the purified bovine protein indicates that it is highly asymmetric with a rodlike structure (47,48,52), whereas electron microscopy of bovine and human factor V demonstrates a globular structure (53).

A three-dimensional model of factor V shares the major features of the factor VIII model with regard to arrangement of the A domains and contact of the membrane by the C2 domain. The folding scheme of the factor V C2 domain is depicted in Figure 38-6B, and a ribbon diagram of the folded structure is depicted in Figure 38-6A (54). Like the factor VIII C2 domain, the factor V C2 domain displays two hydrophobic spikes on the lower end of the β sandwich. The first spike of factor V has consecutive tryptophan residues instead of the methionine and phenylalanine in factor VIII. The consecutive leucines in the second loop of factor VIII have been replaced by a single leucine. Site-directed mutagenesis studies have confirmed that the two consecutive tryptophans contribute to membrane-binding affinity (55). Thus, the available data indicate that similar hydrophobic spikes are present in factors V and VIII and participate in membrane binding for factors V and VIII. Fortuitously, the factor V C2 domain was crystallized in two different conformations (Fig. 38-7). This has led to a hypothetical membrane-binding mechanism in which factor V circulates in plasma in the closed form, with the two hydrophobic spikes collapsed toward one another. On contact with a phospholipid bilayer that displays phosphatidylserine, the hydrophobic spikes separate and point outward, exposing the phospho-L-serine binding motif. Further studies are required to demonstrate whether the leucine hydrophobic spike contributes to membrane binding and whether the putative phospho-L-serine site is correct.

Figure 38-8 illustrates the symmetric arrangement of the three A domains of factor V (56). The model shows the cleavage

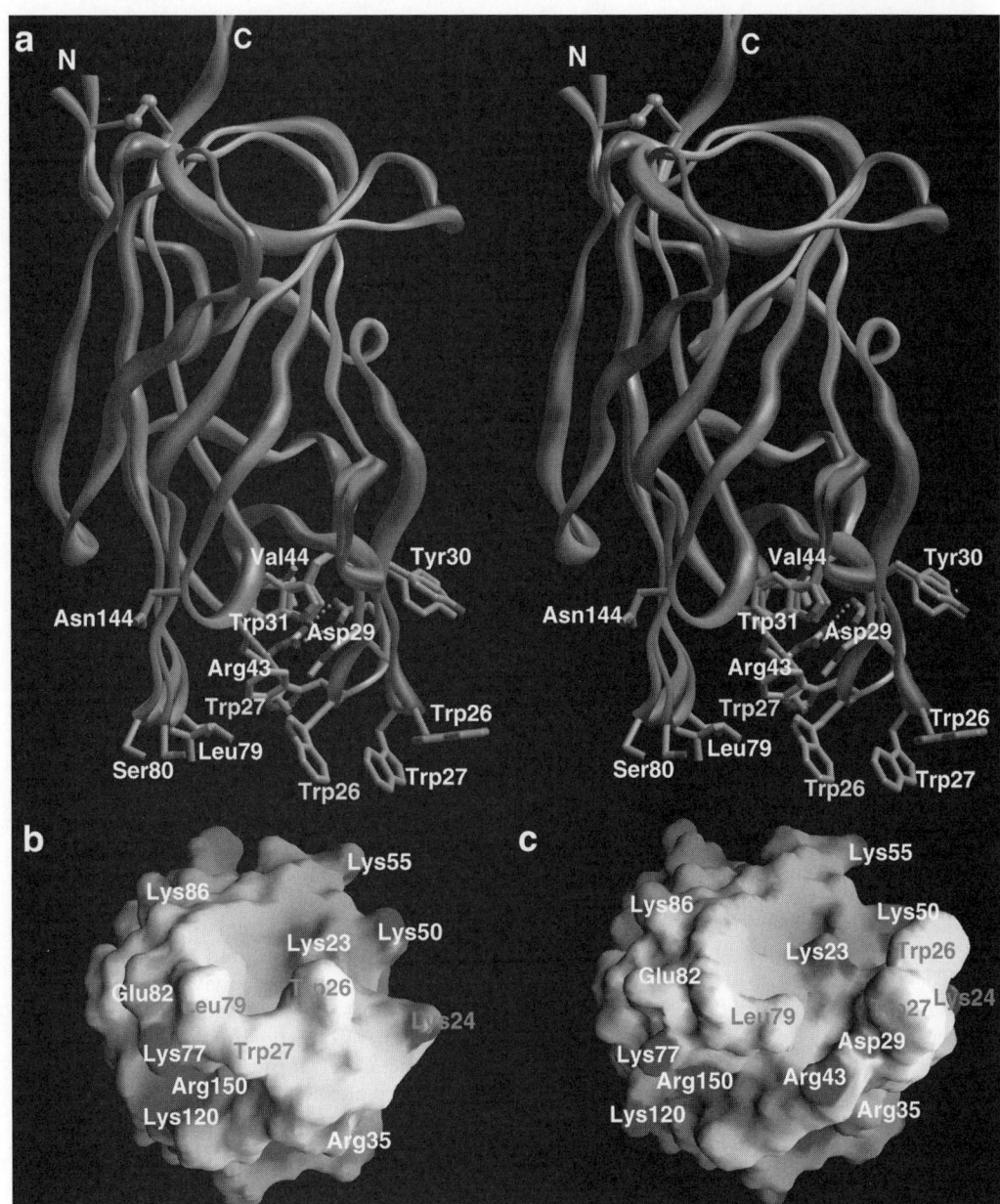

Figure 38-7. Conformational flexibility in the hydrophobic spike region of the factor V C2 domain. **A:** Stereo view of the factor V C2 structures, superimposed in the same orientation as in Figure 38-6. The open form is shown in green. The closed form is displayed in yellow, with several side chains that are color-coded (carbon, yellow; oxygen, red; nitrogen, blue). **B,C:** Surface representations of the electrostatic potential (red, negative; blue, positive) of factor V C2 in the closed **(B)** and in the open **(C)** crystal form. The view is from the apparent membrane-binding site. (See Color Fig. 38-7.)

sites for activated protein C on the surface and a copper binding site at the interface between the A1 and A3 domains. The model suggests that the B domain extends, rodlike (57), from one side of the triangle and that its cleavage in the course of factor V activation does not have a large impact on the triangular structure.

BIOSYNTHESIS OF FACTORS V AND VIII

Both factors V and VIII are secretory proteins that are synthesized and glycosylated on membrane-bound polysomes in the rough endoplasmic reticulum and then transported by a guanosine-triphosphate–dependent mechanism to the Golgi apparatus, where sulfation occurs, and where the oligosaccharides are further processed to complex-type units that contain sialic acid. From there, factors V and VIII are transported to secretory granules or vesicles from which the proteins are secreted. The signal peptide provides a crucial recognition site that targets the protein for secretion.

Factors VIII and V are accompanied by chaperone proteins, including BiP (immunoglobulin binding protein), in their transit

through the Golgi apparatus. ERGIC-53 (Endoplasmic Reticulum Golgi Intermediate Compartment, M_r 53,000), a lectin from the late Golgi apparatus, processes both factors VIII and V. The function of ERGIC-53 was illuminated by study of a rare autosomal-recessive bleeding disorder, with plasma levels of factors VIII and V reduced to the 5% to 30% range (58,59). Positional cloning implicated null mutations in ERGIC-53 as the cause of the deficiency. ERGIC-53 binds factors VIII and V via branched carbohydrates that are linked to the respective B domains (60). The hypothesized function is to retain misfolded protein for degradation while directing properly folded protein to the Golgi apparatus for secretion. ERGIC-53 had previously been identified as a ubiquitous protein of the late Golgi compartment with unknown function. Surprisingly, the patients who lack functional ERGIC-53 have no apparent health problems and no evident protein deficiencies, other than partial deficiency of factor VIII and factor V. Although the majority of patients with deficiencies of factor VIII and factor V have mutations in the ERGIC-53 gene, several do not (61,62). This raises the possibility that additional, unidentified proteins process factors VIII and V.

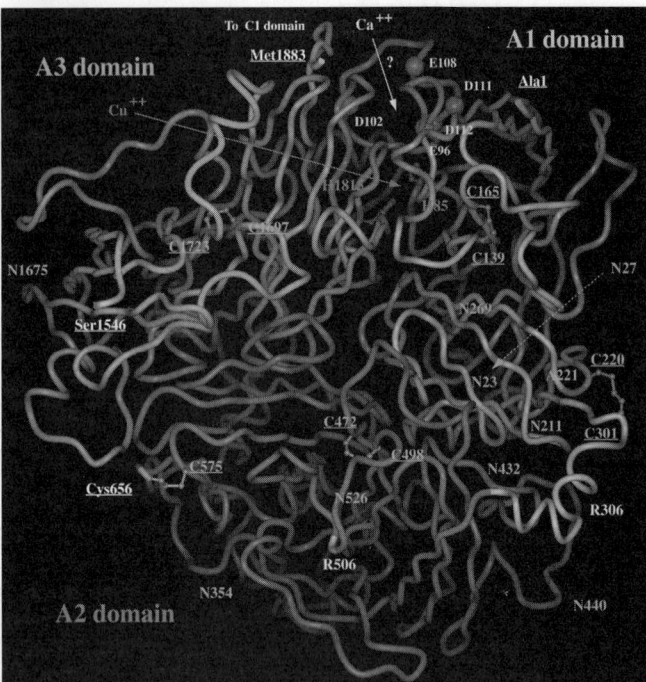

Figure 38-8. Homology model of the three A domains of factor V, based on the ceruloplasmin structure. The model is viewed down the pseudo-three-fold axis. The disulfide bridges (ball and stick model) are shown in orange; R306 and R506 (cleavage sites for activated protein C) are in yellow; the N-terminus of the A1 domain and C-terminus of the A2 domain are in white; the N-terminus and C-terminus of the A3 domain are also shown in white; the two histidines (H85 and H1815), which are most likely involved in copper binding, are in magenta (ball and stick model); potential residues (E96, D102, E108, D111, D112) that are involved in calcium binding are shown as creatine phosphokinase spheres (yellow). (See Color Fig. 38-8.)

Early studies undertaken to identify the tissue of origin of factor VIII involved transplantation of selected organs into hemophilic animals (63). These studies showed that transplantation of normal livers into hemophilic animals induced factor VIII production, whereas the transplantation of hemophilic livers into normal animals resulted in reduced, but adequate, factor VIII levels. These studies provided an early clue that factor VIII synthesis occurred in, but was not exclusive to, the liver. Recent reports of liver transplantation in hemophiliacs with end-stage liver disease have confirmed these animal studies and support the role of the liver in factor VIII synthesis (64,65). With identification of the gene for factor VIII and the development of probes that are specific to mRNA coding for factor VIII, it has become possible to look for factor VIII expression in a variety of cell types. Wion et al. (66) have used such probes to identify factor VIII mRNA in liver, spleen, kidney, and lymphocytes, thus confirming the existence of multiple potential sites of factor VIII synthesis. Fractionation of liver revealed mRNA in the hepatocyte fraction and not in the sinusoidal fraction. At the same time, monoclonal antibodies to factor VIII have been used to localize factor VIII production (67–69). With the use of colloidal gold-labeled antibody to factor VIII, immunoreactive factor VIII has been demonstrated in normal hepatocytes, especially the rough endoplasmic reticulum and Golgi apparatus, but not in hemophilic hepatocytes or in other cells in the liver. Based on the available studies, the major source of factor VIII appears to be the hepatocyte, but other sites of production exist and may play an important role in production of factor VIII in patients with liver disease. Endothelial cells, which synthesize vWF, do not synthesize factor VIII but may provide a storage site for factor VIII (69,70).

Control of factor VIII synthesis is poorly understood, although hormonal influences may be important. Vasopressin and its analogs can increase plasma levels of factor VIII in normal persons and those with mild hemophilia (71,72) by a mechanism that can be blocked by propranolol, which suggests involvement of β-adrenergic receptors (73). Whether vasopressin acts at the level of transcription, translation, secretion, or sites of storage is unknown, but the rapidity of response to vasopressin suggests that the vasopressin effect is posttranslational. Like fibrinogen, factor VIII is an acute-phase reactant, and levels of factor VIII increase in states of chronic infection and inflammation (74). There also appears to be a relation between factor VIII levels and blood type, with factor VIII levels decreased most in persons with blood group O (75–78). Among persons belonging to blood group O, those who were secretors of ABH substances had the lowest factor VIII levels (79).

An important question relates to how and where factor VIII, which is synthesized as a single polypeptide chain, is converted to the two-chain molecule that is found in plasma. Several lines of evidence suggest that the two-chain structure results from intracellular processing and not from plasma proteolysis. First, the structural heterogeneity of factor VIII persists when human plasma is collected in the presence of a variety of protease inhibitors. Under these conditions, factor VIII is a heterogeneous two-chain molecule with a variable heavy chain of 210 to 90 kd and a light chain of 80 kd, which is similar to factor VIII when it is isolated in the absence of inhibitors (34–36). Second, multiple forms of active factor VIII, similar to those found in plasma, have been observed in the supernatants of cultured cells that express recombinant factor VIII (80,81). Third, pulse-chase studies in Chinese hamster ovary cells that express recombinant factor VIII demonstrate an immunoreactive 80-kd light chain in Golgi-enriched cellular fractions but not in fractions that are enriched with rough endoplasmic reticulum, which indicates that processing to a two-chain form had occurred within the Golgi apparatus (81). This intracellular processing was not inhibited by the addition of serum as a source of vWF, although vWF may promote secretion of factor VIII (81). The protease that is responsible for the intracellular processing of factor VIII has not been identified.

After it is secreted, factor VIII forms a noncovalent complex with plasma vWF and circulates while bound in an approximate stoichiometry of one factor VIII molecule per vWF multimer (82–84), although each vWF monomer has a high-affinity binding site for vWF (85). The biologic half-life of factor VIII after transfusion into healthy persons or patients with hemophilia is 8 to 12 hours (Table 38-1). In contrast, the half-life of purified factor VIII in patients with severe von Willebrand's disease is 1.0 to 2.4 hours, suggesting that the *in vivo* association with vWF protects factor VIII from biologic degradation (86,87). Interestingly, humans who lack vWF (type III von Willebrand's disease) have five to tenfold lower concentrations of plasma factor VIII than animals that lack vWF. For example vWF-deficient dogs have 50% (88),

TABLE 38-1. Characteristics of Factors VIII and V

Parameter	Factor VIII	Factor V
Molecular weight (kd)	286	330
Specific activity (U/mg)	3500	2000
Site of synthesis	Liver, other	Liver, megakaryocyte
Plasma concentration (µg/mL)	0.05	7
Carrier protein	von Willebrand's factor	None
Biologic half-life (h)	8–12	12–15

pigs have 40% (89), and mice have 20% (90) of normal factor VIII concentration compared to humans who have 4% of the normal concentration (91). These data suggest that the factor VIII clearance pathway is tenfold more efficient in humans or that free human factor VIII is tenfold more susceptible to the clearance pathway than free factor VIII of other mammals.

One pathway of factor VIII clearance is via the lipoprotein-related protein receptor that is found on hepatocytes, macrophages, and other cell types (92,93). This receptor recognizes the phospholipid and vWF-binding C2 domain of factor VIII, as well as a site on the A2 domain of activated factor VIII. Clearance via this pathway is blocked when the C2 domain binding site is blocked by vWF (93). One possible explanation for the rapid clearance of human factor VIII is a higher affinity for the lipoprotein-related protein.

Unlike factor VIII, factor V is found in the plasma and the platelets (94,95). Production of plasma factor V appears to occur primarily in the liver, although other cells have been shown to produce factor V, including bovine aortic, but not human umbilical vein, endothelial cells and rabbit alveolar macrophages (96–98). Early studies that implicated the liver as the source of plasma factor V consisted of whole-organ perfusion experiments that showed factor V production by the liver. Biosynthesis of factor V that is structurally, functionally, and immunologically indistinguishable from plasma factor V has been demonstrated in a human hepatocellular carcinoma cell line, HepG2, suggesting that the hepatocyte is the site of synthesis within the liver (97). Factor V produced by HepG2 cells is a single-chain protein, and the rate of production of factor V by HepG2 cells in culture was approximately 5 ng/10^6 cells per hour.

Another major site of factor V production is the megakaryocyte (99,100). Human megakaryocytes that are cultured in factor V–deficient medium synthesize immunoreactive factor V. Despite inclusion of protease inhibitors, most of the factor V that was detected was a multichain form that is similar to the thrombin-activated form of plasma factor V. Immunoreactive factor V was also associated with small mononuclear cells that contained platelet membrane glycoproteins IIb and IIIa and platelet factor 4, suggesting that megakaryocyte precursors may also contain factor V. The subcellular localization of factor V within megakaryocytes is unknown, but its location in platelets has been the subject of several studies. By immunofluorescence microscopy, most of the platelet factor V colocalizes with platelet fibrinogen and is therefore believed to be in the α granules (101,102). Within the α granule, factor V binds to multimerin, a large multimeric platelet protein of unknown function (103). The concentration of factor V in platelets is approximately 1.1 μg/2.5 × 10^8 platelets, which constitutes almost 18% to 25% of the factor V in whole blood (102).

Platelet factor V has been isolated and characterized. In contrast to plasma factor V, which is a single-chain protein, platelet factor V is present in multiple forms, which range in size from 330 to 115 kd (104). Platelet factor V, as well as plasma factor V, are capable of binding multimerin and multimerin is secreted from platelets together with factor V (103). Multimerin is also secreted constitutively from endothelial cells (105). However, the role of multimerin in the processing and function of factor V remains unknown. The mechanism of platelet factor V processing remains to be elucidated, but recent reports have suggested that factor V is a substrate for the platelet calcium-activated protease (106,107).

BIOCHEMISTRY OF FACTORS V AND VIII

Factors VIII and V function as cofactors for enzymes. Both proteins are pro-cofactors, which means that cleavage of specific peptide bonds by thrombin is necessary before cofactor function is enabled. The thrombin-activated forms of factor VIII and factor V are designated *factor VIIIa* and *factor Va*. Factor VIIIa forms a complex with the serine proteinase, factor IXa, which cleaves factor X to the active form, factor Xa. Factor Va forms a complex with the serine proteinase, factor Xa, which cleaves prothrombin to form thrombin. Thrombin is the most essential effector of hemostasis and thrombosis. Further cleavage by activated protein C inactivates each protein, thus providing a mechanism for controlling the coagulation process.

Factor VIII and factor IX, when bound together on a membrane, form an enzyme complex that is remarkably efficient (Table 38-2). This complex, which is called the *factor Xase complex* (Xase complex, tenase complex), can activate sufficient factor X to saturate all possible prothrombinase complexes in a volume of blood in 20 seconds, assuming assembly of the Xase complex at the plasma concentration of factor VIII. Because of the remarkable efficiency of the assembled complex, compared to activated factor IX (factor IXa) alone, it is possible that Xase activity may be modulated physiologically by assembly of the complex, rather than by proteolytic activation of factor IX. This possibility, together with the challenge of understanding the mechanisms of enzymatic efficiency, motivates detailed studies of enzyme complex assembly.

The cofactor and the enzyme of the Xase complex, factor VIII and factor IX, are homologous with factor V and factor X, respectively, of the prothrombinase complex. Likewise, assembly of the Xase complex is analogous to assembly of the prothrombinase complex (108,109). Furthermore, the substrate of the Xase complex, factor X, becomes the enzyme in the prothrombinase complex after activation, so that these enzyme complexes function sequentially. Similarities in the membrane

TABLE 38-2. Effect of Complex Assembly on Enzymatic Efficiency of the Xase and Prothrombinase Complexes

Component	K_m (M × 10^{-6})	k_{cat} (min^{-1})	k_{cat}/K_m (M^{-1} min^{-1})
Factor Xase (reference 367)			
IXa	180	0.01	0.015
IXa + PSPC[a]	0.4	0.02	13.8
IXa + VIIIa + PSPC	0.06	500	2.3 × 10^6
Prothrombinase (reference 368)			
Xa	80	0.7	2.5
Xa + PSPC	0.4	4	2.8 × 10^3
Xa + Va + PSPC	0.2	20,000	2.8 × 10^6

k_{cat}, catalytic rate constant; K_m, affinity constant; PSPC, phosphatidylserine:phosphatidylcholine.
NOTE: All values reported are in the presence of millimolar calcium ions.
[a]The membrane source was sonicated vesicles of phosphatidylserine:phosphatidylcholine 1:3.

TABLE 38-3. Proteins of the Factor Xase and Prothrombinase Complexes

Component	Molecular Weight (d)	Function	Plasma Concentration (nmol/L)
Factor Xase			
Factor VIII[a]	280,000[b]	Cofactor	0.4[c]
Factor IX[d]	56,000	Protease	90
Factor X	56,000	Substrate-zymogen	180
Prothrombinase			
Factor V[a]	330,000	Cofactor	30
Factor X[d]	56,000	Protease	180
Prothrombin	72,000	Substrate-zymogen	1400

[a]Factors VIII and V are procofactors and are proteolytically activated to species with lower molecular weight before function.
[b]Plasma factor VIII is heterogeneous in molecular weight, ranging from 210,000 to 280,000 d, as illustrated in Figure 38-9.
[c]Total factor VIII concentration, nearly all of which is complexed with von Willebrand's factor.
[d]Factors IX and X are zymogens and are proteolytically activated before function.

receptor characteristics indicate that both complexes may function on adjacent receptors of the same cell membrane. For these reasons, the properties of the Xase and the prothrombinase complexes are compared.

How does assembly of a ternary complex lead to an increase in efficiency of greater than one million–fold? Enzyme complex assembly leads to improved substrate binding (detected as a decrease in the Michaelis constant) and increased substrate cleavage rate [detected as increased catalytic rate constant (k_{cat})] (Table 38-2). These gains result from allosteric activation of factor IXa (factor Xase) and factor Xa (prothrombinase) and also from condensation of enzyme complexes and substrates on a membrane surface. Allosteric activation indicates a change in conformation of factor IXa and is a classic mechanism of enzyme activation. Surface condensation refers to concentration of the enzyme and substrate on the same membrane and also encompasses alignment of enzyme and substrate, because the corresponding domains are anchored to the same membrane. This mechanism of enzyme acceleration is less common among well-characterized enzymes.

Factor VIIIa has two identified contact sites that interact with factor IXa. The first is localized within the A2 domain and interacts with the catalytic domain of factor IXa (110). This interaction causes a conformational change in the extended substrate-binding cleft of factor IXa, which is detected by a change in fluorescence of a suicide substrate that occupies the active site cleft (110,111). This interaction enhances the k_{cat} 100-fold, even when the other domains of factor VIIIa are not engaged. The second contact site, which is localized to the A3 domain (112), may interact with a hinge region between the two EGF domains of factor IXa (113). This interaction does not occur effectively, unless the entire factor VIIIa–factor IXa complex binds to a phosphatidylserine-containing membrane. This results in further enhancement of the k_{cat} (114). It is possible that factor VIIIa further improves binding of the substrate, factor X, by providing a factor X contact surface. For this mechanism, factor VIIIa functions as an extension to the extended substrate-binding site of factor IXa. In the prothrombinase complex, factor Va provides this function for the substrate, prothrombin (115).

Substrate delivery to the prothrombinase complex and, presumably, to the Xase complex is enhanced by the fact that the substrate, as well as the enzyme complex, bind to the same phosphatidylserine-containing membrane. Apparently, lateral diffusion on the membrane is sufficiently rapid so that the more concentrated, but slower-moving, membrane-bound molecules have more collisions than those in bulk solution (116). Membrane binding is expected to affect substrate delivery further by anchoring corresponding portions of the enzyme and substrate, thereby allowing only rotational and lateral motion of the

enzyme active site and substrate target peptide within a single plane that is parallel to the membrane (117,118).

The forces that govern the assembly of the Xase and prothrombinase complexes may be thought of in terms of interactions between individual components of the complex. Comparison of the component protein concentrations in Table 38-3 shows that factor VIII is present at the lowest concentration and that components of the Xase complex are present at lower concentrations than components of the prothrombinase complex. The increasing concentrations of the Xase and prothrombinase complex components, with the prothrombin concentration highest, are consistent with the general scheme that was proposed by McFarlane (119) and by Davie and Ratnoff (120) in which the overall effect of both enzyme complexes, functioning sequentially, is the amplification of a low-level stimulus to produce substantial quantities of thrombin. Assembly and function of the Xase and prothrombinase complexes on a phospholipid membrane are depicted in Figure 38-8. Most measurements of the individual interactions that contribute to formation of the Xase and prothrombinase complexes have been made with synthetic membranes that are composed of phosphatidylserine and phosphatidylcholine (Table 38-4). The cofactors, factor VIIIa and factor Va; the enzymes, factor IXa and factor Xa; and the substrates, factor X and prothrombin, all bind to phosphatidylserine-containing membranes. Only the final product, thrombin, does not bind to such membranes and is efficiently released into bulk plasma.

Although the affinity of factors VIII and V for phosphatidylserine-containing membranes is high, comparable to interactions between ligands and protein receptors, the membrane affinities of factor IXa, Xa, and prothrombin are 100 to 1000 times lower. The low affinity of factor Xa for factor Va in the absence of a phosphatidylserine-containing membrane indicates that this interaction is not likely to be of consequence *in vivo*. The corresponding interaction between factor VIIIa and factor IXa has a much higher affinity but is still too low to make physiologic relevance likely. However, the affinity of factor IXa for membrane-bound factor VIIIa is high. It is likely that the apparently high affinity of factor IXa for factor VIIIa is the result of cumulative interactions between factor IXa and factor VIIIa and between factor IXa and the membrane.

The order in which components of the Xase complex are assembled has not been investigated. However, kinetic studies indicate that factor VIII, like factor V, binds rapidly to phosphatidylserine-containing membrane sites (121,122). In the prothrombinase complex, factor Xa binds to factor Va, only after factor Va has bound to the membrane, as predicted by equilibrium binding affinities (123). The approach of factor Xa includes adherence to the membrane and then lateral migration to encounter factor Va (123,124).

TABLE 38-4. Equilibrium Interactions of the Xase and Prothrombinase Complexes

Reactant 1	Reactant 2	Dissociation Constant (nmol/L)	Stoichiometry (Reactant 2/Reactant 1)	Reference
Factor Xase				
Factor VIII/VIIIa[a]	PSPC membrane sites[b]	4	180[c]	371,372
Factor IX/IXa	PSPC membrane sites	300–2000	35[d]	373–375
Factor IXa	Factor VIIIa	46	1	369
Factor IXa	Factor VIIIa–PSPC[e]	2	1	376
Prothrombinase				
Factor V	PSPC membrane sites	4	130[c]	371,377
Factor Va	PSPC membrane sites	3	42[f]	378
Factor Xa	PSPC membrane sites	100–600	35[d]	373,378
Factor Xa	Factor Va	8000	1	379
Factor Xa	Factor Va:PSPC sites	1	1	380,381

PSPC, phosphatidylserine:phosphatidylcholine.

[a]Proteolytic activation of factor VIII releases it from von Willebrand's factor, which allows it to bind to phospholipid membranes (372). It is likely that *in vivo* factor VIII is activated by thrombin before membrane binding.

[b]Phospholipid molecules are assumed to function as independent clusters, so that the membrane is a collection of discreet, independent binding sites. This assumption may be inadequate, as equilibrium binding constants between factor VIII and phospholipid membranes and between factor V and phospholipid membranes do not predict kinetic association and dissociation data (370,371).

[c]Reflects the protein to phospholipid ratio for small unilamellar vesicles of composition phosphatidylserine:phosphatidylcholine 1:4.

[d]For small unilamellar vesicles of composition phosphatidylserine:phosphatidylethanolamine:phosphatidylcholine 1:1:1.

[e]Factor IXa is reported to bind to membrane-bound factor VIII before and after activation by thrombin. The affinity was unaltered by thrombin activation.

[f]Reflects the protein to phospholipid ratio for small unilamellar vesicles of composition phosphatidylserine:phosphatidylcholine 1:3.

Platelet membranes are believed to provide the primary physiologic site at which the prothrombinase and factor Xase complexes assemble and function. Resting platelets do not display binding sites for factor VIII or factor V. However, after stimulation by strong agonists, for example, thrombin and fibrin ligation to GPIIb-IIIa, platelets display high-affinity binding sites for factor VIII (125,126) and factor V (127). The number of high-affinity, specific binding sites that are exposed under these conditions is relatively small, 300 to 1500 sites per platelet. It is believed that exposure of these sites correlates to translocation of a small fraction of the phosphatidylserine and phosphatidylethanolamine from the inner leaflet to the outer leaflet of the plasma membranes. However, in contrast to apoptosis of nucleated cells (128) or platelets (129), the quantity of phosphatidylserine that is exposed is insufficient to detect with phosphatidylserine-binding proteins, such as annexin V. Thus, some uncertainty remains as to whether phospholipid determinants define the binding sites or whether protein receptors are also involved (125).

Phospholipid is a critical component of the factor Xase and prothrombinase complexes. The phospho-L-serine motif of phosphatidylserine interacts with stereoselective sites on factor VIII (130) and factor V (131). Interaction with this motif is critical for the specific high-affinity binding (132) that allows these proteins to recognize specific phospholipid sites, even in the presence of plasma (133). Phosphatidylethanolamine is also critical in membranes that have a physiologic content of phosphatidylserine (134). It may function to decrease lateral pressure at the surface of the membrane, thus allowing penetration of specific phospholipid-binding peptides. In addition to providing binding motifs, which anchor factors VIII and V to a suitable membrane, phospholipid molecules contribute to activation of the factor Xase (114) and prothrombinase complex (135). The activating properties are best illustrated by experiments with water-soluble phosphatidylserine that contains 6-carbon acyl chains. This reagent causes improved affinity of the factor VIIIa–factor IXa complex for factor X and also enhances the k_{cat} of the assembled factor VIIIa–factor IXa complex (136). For the factor VIIIa–factor IXa complex, binding to phosphatidylserine causes engagement of contact sites that are located on the A3 domain and the first acidic peptide with factor IXa and factor X, respec-

tively (137). Only the contact site within the A2 domain of factor VIIIa is engaged with factor IXa in the absence of phospholipid.

Although mature factor VIII may have some activity, the catalytic efficiency of factor VIII is greatly increased by activation by thrombin or factor Xa (34,36,138–143). The cleavage fragments of both the 90-kd heavy chain and 80-kd light chain are necessary for factor VIIIa activity. Although neither chain alone is active, factor VIIIa activity can be reconstituted from the three isolated subunits by recombination in the presence of Mn^{2+} or Ca^{2+} (144,145). Gene deletion studies have shown that the B domain is not needed for the procoagulant activity of factor VIII (146–149). Factor VIIIa is inactivated by further exposure to thrombin or by activated protein C (150).

Activation and subsequent inactivation of factor VIII by thrombin has been correlated with a sequence of proteolytic cleavages (22,23,35,81,151–153). Thrombin initially cleaves an arginine (Arg)–Ser bond at position 740 of the mature protein, which results in conversion of the variable-sized heavy chain to a uniform 90-kd heavy chain (Fig. 38-9). Subsequent processing by thrombin cleaves two bonds: the first at position 372, the junction between the first acidic region and the second A domain, and the second at position 1689, the junction between the second acidic region and the third A domain. As a result, the 90-kd heavy chain is converted to 50-kd and 43-kd polypeptides, and the 80-kd light chain is converted to a 73-kd polypeptide. When the activated factor VIII is subjected to gel filtration chromatography, all three polypeptides comigrate, unless the activated factor VIII is treated with calcium chelating agents (81).

To assess the relative importance of each proteolytic site in factor VIII activation, arginine residues at positions 740, 372, and 1689 were selectively mutated to isoleucine residues, and the procoagulant function of the altered factor VIII molecules was examined (154). Modification of the arginine at position 740 inhibited cleavage at that site but had little or no effect on *in vitro* procoagulant activity or activation of factor VIII by thrombin. In contrast, modification of the arginine at position 372 or 1689 inhibited thrombin cleavage at the modified site, as well as activation by thrombin, although residual basal *in vitro* procoagulant activity was present. From this work, it appears that cleavage at positions 372 and 1689 is required for activation of factor VIII, whereas the initial cleavage at position 740 is not

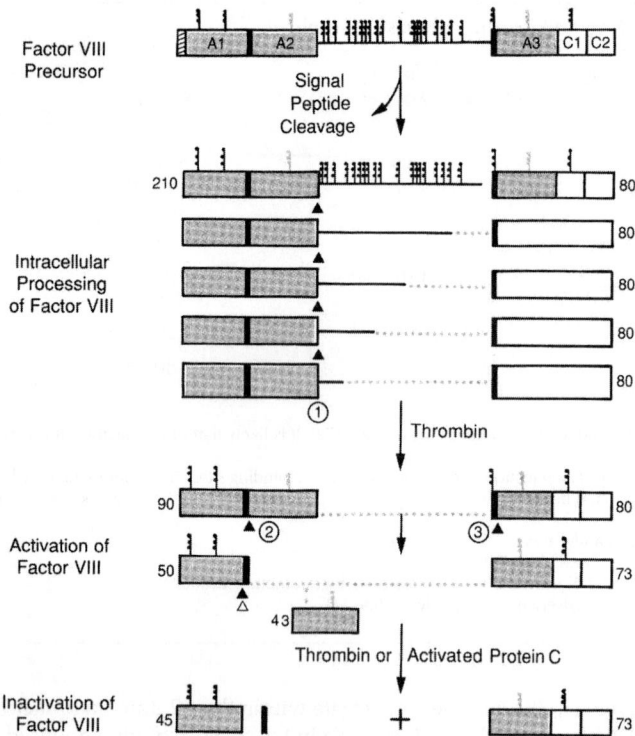

Factor VIII
Precursor

Signal
Peptide
Cleavage

Intracellular
Processing
of Factor VIII

Thrombin

Activation of
Factor VIII

Thrombin or Activated Protein C

Inactivation of
Factor VIII

Figure 38-9. Factor VIII processing. Factor VIII is processed intracellularly and circulates in multiple active forms, with variable heavy chains of between 90 and 210 kd and a light chain of 80 kd. Activation of factor VIII by thrombin occurs through a series of proteolytic cleavages. The factor VIII heavy chain is cleaved at the junction of the A2 and B domains to form a uniform 90-kd heavy chain. A second cleavage occurs in the heavy chain at the junction of the acidic region and the A2 domain to convert the heavy chain to 50- and 45-kd polypeptides. The light chain is cleaved at the junction of the acidic region and the A3 domain to form a 73-kd light chain. Activated factor VIII is inactivated by further processing by thrombin or activated protein C through cleavage of the heavy chain between the A1 domain and the acidic region. Solid arrowheads, sites of thrombin cleavage; open arrowhead, site of protein C cleavage. (From White GC, Shoemaker CB. Factor VIII gene and hemophilia A. *Blood* 1989;73:1–12, with permission.)

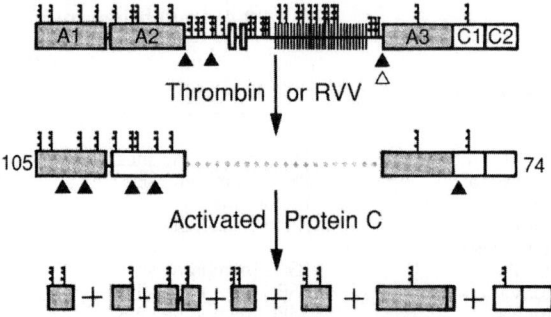

Thrombin   or RVV

Activated   Protein C

Figure 38-10. Factor V processing. Factor V circulates as a single polypeptide chain. On activation by thrombin, factor V is cleaved at the junction between the A2 and B domains and the junction between the B and A3 domains. A thrombin cleavage site is also present in the connecting region. As a result of these cleavages, factor V is converted to a two-chain–activated factor V that consists of a 105-kd heavy chain and a 74-kd light chain. Factor V can also be activated by Russell viper venom (RVV) through a single cleavage (*open arrowhead*) at the junction between the B and A3 domains. Factor V is inactivated by activated protein C. Multiple cleavage sites (*solid arrowheads*) for activated protein C are present in factor V.

required. This conclusion is supported by two additional observations. First, studies showed that monoclonal antibodies against the two acidic regions inhibit factor VIII cofactor activity (155,156). Second, a report indicated that a patient with severe hemophilia had a mutation of the thrombin cleavage site at position 1689 (157). The patient had normal antigenic levels of factor VIII in plasma, but the factor VIII was functionally inactive.

On longer exposure to thrombin, factor VIII is inactivated (35,52,138–143). Inactivation correlates with cleavage at the C-terminus of the first A domain of an Arg-Ser bond at position 336, which releases the first acidic region. As a result, the 50-kd fragment is converted to a 45-kd fragment. Modification of the Arg at position 336 results in enhanced activity of factor VIII under basal conditions (154). Activation of the modified factor VIII by thrombin occurs normally.

Thrombin-activated factor VIII is also susceptible to inactivation through proteolytic cleavage by activated protein C. The proposed site of cleavage by activated protein C is also at the Arg-Ser bond at position 336, and results in the release of the 36-residue acidic peptide that separates the first two A domain repeats (150,153,154). Thus, activation of factor VIII appears to involve release of the acidic peptide at the amino terminus of the light chain and separation of the first two A domain repeats,

whereas inactivation occurs with the subsequent release of the second acidic peptide.

Activation of factor V by thrombin is achieved through a series of proteolytic cleavages (Fig. 38-10). Cleavage sites for thrombin are present at position 709, which is between the A2 domain and the connecting peptide; at position 1018 in the connecting peptide; and at position 1545, which is between the connecting peptide and the A3 domain (41–43). As a result of these cleavages, single-chain precursor factor V is converted to a two-chain, metal ion-linked molecule, activated factor V, which consists of a 115-kd heavy chain and a 73-kd light chain.

Factor V can also be activated by a number of other enzymes, including factor Xa and an enzyme in Russell viper venom (49,158–160). Russell viper venom cleaves factor V at only one site, position 1545, between the connecting peptide and the A3 domain, which is the same site that is cleaved by thrombin (41). Because factor V that is activated by Russell viper venom is functionally indistinguishable from thrombin-activated factor V, it can be concluded that cleavage of the Arg-Ser bond at position 1545, but not the cleavages at positions 709 and 1018, is required for activation of factor V by thrombin.

The relative roles of plasma and platelet factor V in the formation of the prothrombinase complex remain to be determined. Studies in patients with congenital deficiency of plasma factor V have shown that the bleeding tendency correlates with the platelet levels of factor V, which suggests that platelet factor V can be active in the formation of the prothrombin complex (161). Further support for the importance of platelet factor V is provided by studies of a patient with a mild bleeding disorder who was found to have severely reduced levels of platelet factor V, only slightly reduced levels of plasma factor V, and normal binding of exogenous plasma factor V to the patient's platelets (162). The bleeding tendency in this defect, which is called *factor V Quebec*, was attributed to the abnormal platelet factor V. Finally, Nesheim et al. (163) has reported a patient with an inhibitor to factor V who has less than 1% plasma factor V but normal platelet factor V and no bleeding tendency.

Activated factor V is inactivated by activated protein C in a surface-dependent reaction that requires calcium ions and a nonenzymatic cofactor, protein S (164–168). The initial cleavage by activated protein C is in the heavy chain and correlates with inactivation of factor Va. Several potential cleavage sites for activated protein C are present in human factor V. Based on the analogy with bovine factor V, the heavy chain of human factor Va appears to be cleaved at position 506 and results in 70-kd and 20-kd fragments (169). The light chain of activated factor V is cleaved more slowly than the heavy chain and results in 50-kd and 25-kd fragments. The probable site of human light-chain cleavage, based on the bovine model, is at position 1765 (169).

Factor V may also function as a cofactor for the degradation of factor VIIIa and factor Va by activated protein C (170). Abnormalities of factor V that interfere with this cofactor activity may result in resistance to activated protein C and a thrombotic tendency termed *factor V Leiden*.

INCIDENCE AND MODE OF INHERITANCE OF FACTOR V AND VIII DEFICIENCY

Hemophilia A is one of the most common inherited bleeding disorders, occurring in approximately 20 of 100,000 men (171,172). The disease is geographically dispersed and occurs approximately equally in all races. It is inherited in an X-linked recessive manner (173,174). Thus, hemophilia is expressed in men, who inherit a hemophilic gene (X_h) from the mother and a male chromosome (Y) from the father; it is carried by females, who inherit a hemophilic gene (X_h) from one parent and a normal gene (X) from the other parent. As illustrated in Figure 38-11, all the daughters of a hemophilic man are obligate carriers, whereas the sons are normal. The sons of a carrier woman have a 50% chance of having hemophilia, and daughters have a 50% chance of being carriers.

In as many as one-third of cases, no family history of hemophilia is found. In some instances, this may be the result of a sporadic mutation in the factor VIII gene. A hemophilic gene is able to pass through several generations of women before it becomes expressed in a man. Thus, in cases in which no family history of hemophilia exists, it can be difficult to determine whether hemophilia is the result of a spontaneous mutation or of inheritance, a distinction that may be of importance in genetic counseling. Previous estimates that are based on population genetics have suggested that sporadic mutations may account for the defect in as many as 25% of hemophiliacs (175). With the development of new genetic probes, it has become possible to estimate the mutation rate more accurately (176).

Factor VIII deficiency may be expressed in women in certain situations, such as genetic mosaicism (46, XX/XO), testicular feminization, Turner's syndrome (45, XO), double heterozygotes (X_hX_h), lyonized carriers (see the section Genetic Counseling in Hemophilia A), and rare forms of autosomal inheritance, such as combined deficiency of factors V and VIII and Normandy-type von Willebrand's disease (177–181).

The diagnosis of hemophilia A is based on the demonstration by specific assay of factor VIII deficiency. Screening coagulation tests typically reveal a prolonged partial thromboplastin time (PTT) and normal PT and thrombin time. The prolongation of the PTT is proportional to the degree of factor VIII deficiency and may be normal in patients with mild hemophilia A. In general, the PTT is prolonged, with factor VIII levels of less than 20%, and normal, with factor VIII levels of more than 30%. Assays for vWF and factor V should be performed in persons with mild to moderate factor VIII deficiency to rule out von Willebrand's disease and combined factor V-VIII deficiency (see the following section, Molecular Genetics of Factor V and VIII Deficiency).

Compared with hemophilia A, factor V deficiency or parahemophilia is an uncommon bleeding disorder, with probably fewer than 500 patients affected worldwide and an incidence of less than one in one million. The inheritance of factor V deficiency is autosomal (Fig. 38-11) and usually recessive, but dominant and recessive forms have been described (182).

Factor V deficiency is diagnosed by specific factor V assay. Because factor V acts as a cofactor in intrinsic and extrinsic coagulation pathways, screening tests typically reveal a prolonged PTT and PT and a normal thrombin time. The bleeding time has been prolonged in some patients with congenital factor V deficiency.

MOLECULAR GENETICS OF FACTOR V AND VIII DEFICIENCY

Phenotypically, patients with hemophilia are deficient in factor VIII. This deficiency is highly variable, with levels of less than 1% to 60% (with a normal range from 60% to 140%). Some patients have no detectable factor VIII activity and normal levels of immunoreactive factor VIII. These patients have cross-reacting material (CRM) and are said to be *CRM-positive*. Others have reduced levels of immunoreactive factor VIII, but levels that are in excess of functional factor VIII. These patients are said to be *CRM-reduced*. Patients with levels of immunoreactive factor VIII that are similar to levels of functional protein are CRM-negative. The presence of CRM was first shown by Hoyer and Breckenridge (183) and by Denson et al. (184), who found that some hemophilia A plasmas with no factor VIII activity were able to neutralize alloantibodies against factor VIII. This has been examined further by Reisner et al. (185) by using an immunoradiometric assay to quantify factor VIII antigen (VIII:Ag) in hemophilic plasma. In a series of 43 arbitrarily chosen subjects who were studied by Reisner et al., 18 demonstrated VIII:Ag in excess of factor VIII activity; that is, 18 were CRM-positive or CRM-reduced.

Knowledge of the factor VIII gene and the availability of probes for the factor VIII gene have led to the identification of the molecular defects in a number of cases of hemophilia. More than 1000 patients with hemophilia A have been examined by recombinant DNA analysis to screen for the defects that cause factor VIII deficiency (157,186–205). In moderate to mild hemophilia A, most defects are single amino acid missense mutations within functional regions of the factor VIII protein. The result is a reduction in factor VIII coagulant activity. In severe hemophilia A, a variety of molecular defects have been demon-

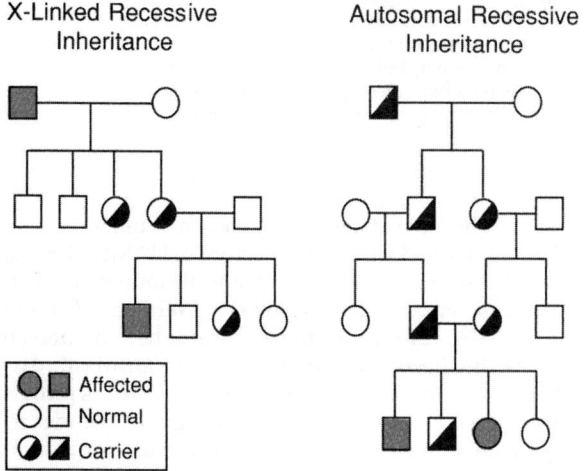

Figure 38-11. Genetic inheritance patterns of hemophilia A and factor V deficiency. Hemophilia A is inherited in a sex-linked recessive manner, whereas factor V deficiency is an autosomal-recessive (or dominant) disorder.

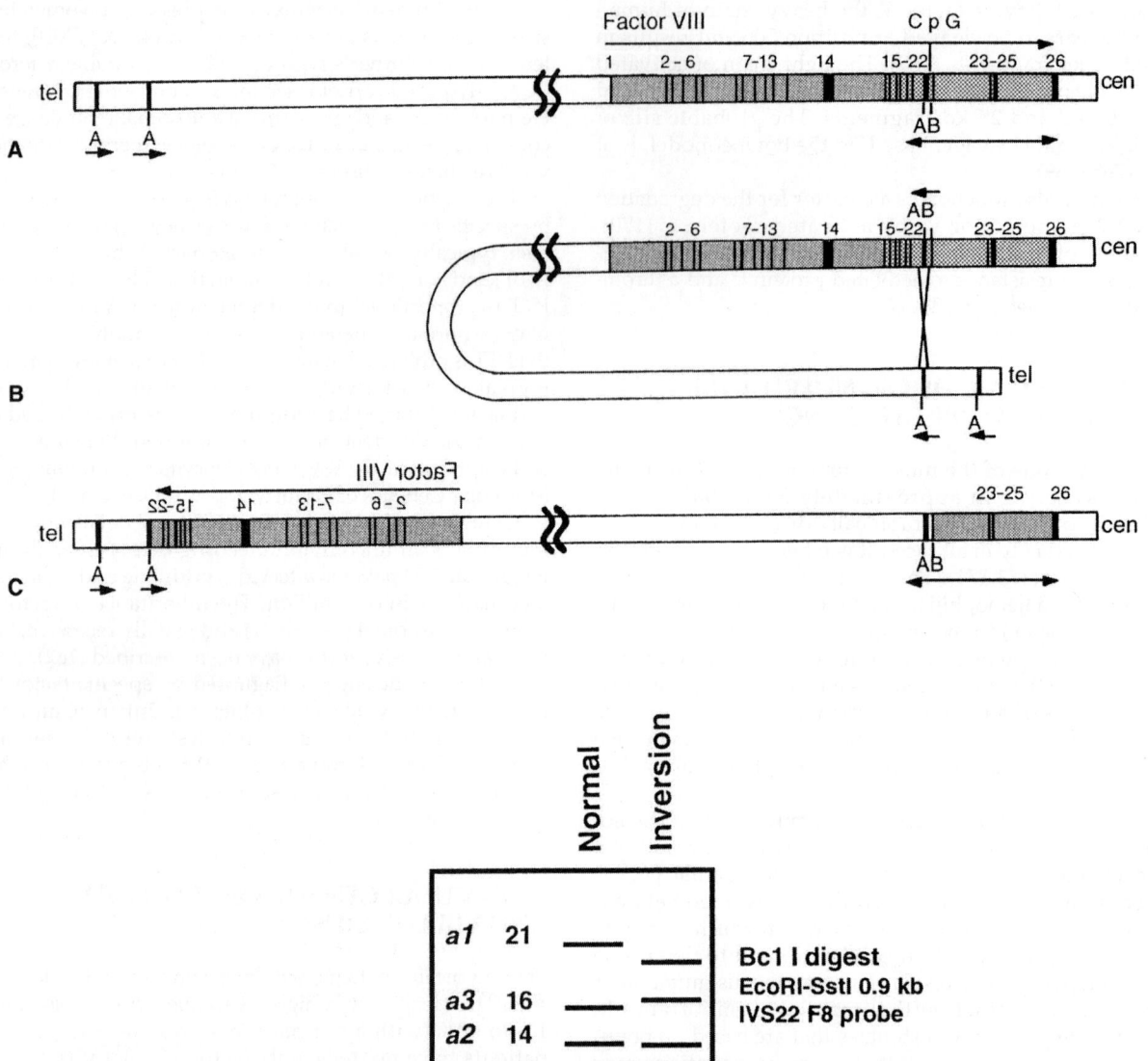

Figure 38-12. Diagram of the factor VIII gene and illustration of the inversion model. **A:** The q28 region of the X chromosome, with the telomere (tel) to the left and centromere (cen) to the right, showing the factor VIII gene and exons 1 to 26. Three copies of an intronless gene that is termed *A* are shown, one in intron 22 of the factor VIII gene and two upstream of factor VIII. The B gene is also shown in intron 22. The arrows indicate the direction of transcription of the factor VIII and internal A and B genes. The direction of the upstream A genes is hypothesized to be as shown. **B:** Homologous recombination between the intron 22 copy of gene A and one of the two upstream copies. **C:** A crossover between these two identical regions, which is oriented as shown, would result in an inversion of sequence between the two recombined A genes. Recombination could involve either of the upstream A genes, but only one is presented. The crossover could occur anywhere in the region of homology, which includes the A genes. (From Lakich D, Kazazian HH Jr, Antonarakis SE, et al. Inversions disrupting the factor VIII gene are a common cause of severe haemophilia A. *Nat Genet* 1993;5:236, with permission.)

strated. The most prevalent defect, accounting for nearly one-half of cases, is a partial inversion of the factor VIII gene that is due to homologous recombination between a small intronless "gene within a gene" in intron 22 of the factor VIII gene and one of two similar intronless genes at the tip of the X chromosome that is more than 400 kb distant (206,207). As a result, the factor VIII gene, up to and including exon 22, is inverted and separated from the 3' end of factor VIII by 400 kb (Fig. 38-12). This disrupts factor VIII transcription and produces truncated, nonfunctional forms of the molecule. Along with deletions and insertions, point mutations that result in nonsense defects, splice variants, or missense mutations account for most of the rest of the defects in patients with severe hemophilia.

A comprehensive database of known mutations is maintained at the Internet site with the acronym HAMSTeRS (Hemophilia A Mutation, Structure, Test, and Resource Site: http://europium.csc.mrc.ac.uk/usr/WWW/WebPages/main.dir/main.htm). Several things are clear from the data presented. First, as with the thalassemias and hemophilia B, diverse defects give rise to the same clinical disorder that is recognized as hemophilia. Their distribution throughout the factor VIII gene indicates no evidence for a single mutational site that causes hemophilia. Second, although it has been suggested that hemophilic patients with inhibitors may represent a subset of patients with significant deletions, the data suggest that patients with large deletions, even deletion of the entire factor

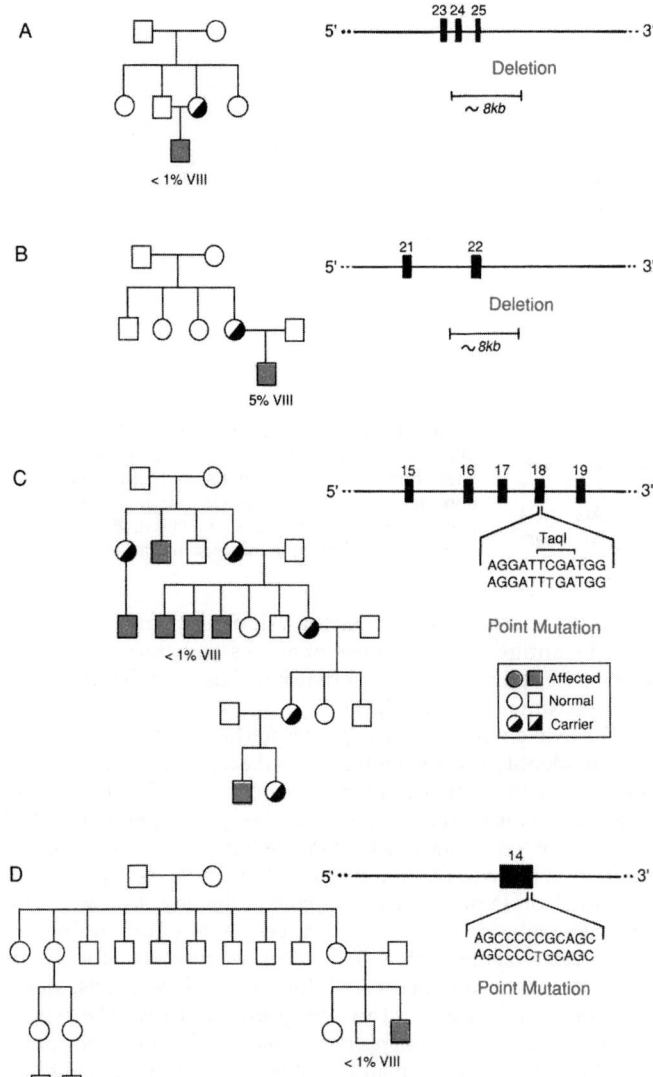

Figure 38-13. Genetic defects in hemophilia. **A:** An 8-kilobase (kb) frameshift deletion that encompasses exons 24 and 25 and results in severe hemophilia. **B:** An 8-kb in-frame deletion that encompasses exon 22 and results in moderately severe hemophilia. **C:** A nonsense mutation at a *Taq* I site in exon 18 that results in severe hemophilia. **D:** A point mutation in exon 14 that results in an arginine to cysteine substitution and severe hemophilia.

VIII gene, do not necessarily develop inhibitors. Furthermore, among patients with the same gene defect, some may develop an inhibitor, and the others may not. Finally, many of the point mutations that have been described to date in hemophilia have involved sites that are recognized by the restriction enzyme, Taq I. The recognition sequence for this nuclease, TCGA, contains the dinucleotide CpG, the most common site of methylation in human DNA and a possible site of increased mutation owing to deamination of cytosine that leads to C to T transitions (208). Evidence for this as a mutational hot spot in hemophilia has been presented (189).

Figures 38-13 and 38-14 show the molecular details of some of the defects that result in hemophilia. In Figure 38-13A, the defect is a 7-kb deletion that encompasses exons 24 and 25. This deletion results in a frameshift, so that the normal translation reading frame is altered. As a result, not only are exons 24 and 25 lost, but exon 26 is not translated or makes a nonsense protein. Thus, a large portion of the C domain (which constitutes

most of the light chain of activated factor VIII) is abnormal. In Figure 38-13B, a 5.5-kb deletion encompasses exon 22. In contrast to the preceding example, this is an in-frame deletion; that is, the normal translation reading frame is not altered. In this case, amino acids that are encoded by exon 22 are not present, but exons 23 to 26 are translated and expressed. The result is production of a molecule with decreased but detectable clotting activity.

In Figure 38-13C, the defect is a point mutation at nucleotide 62 in exon 18. The nucleotide sequence AGGATTCGATGG is mutated to AGGATTTGATGG. As a result, CGA, which codes for an arginine residue in the mature protein, is changed to TGA, a signal to stop translation (called a *stop codon*). The result is premature termination of translation at amino acid 1940 and production of a shortened, nonfunctional factor VIII. In Figure 38-13D, the defect is a point mutation in exon 14. Instead of the normal nucleotide sequence CAGAGCCCCCGCAGCTTTC, the sequence is CAGAGCCCCTGCAGCTTTC. In this instance, codon 1689 is mutated from an arginine residue to a cysteine residue, which results in the loss of the thrombin cleavage site between the second acidic region and the third A domain. Thus, in the patient, factor VIII antigenic levels are normal, which indicates that synthesis and secretion of factor VIII is normal, but factor VIII cannot be activated by thrombin and is associated with a severe form of hemophilia.

Figure 38-14 shows how two distinct point mutations within a single codon can produce hemophilia of different severity. In Figure 38-14A, a CGA in exon 26, which codes for an arginine, is mutated to TGA, which is a stop codon. The resulting factor VIII molecule is significantly truncated and is associated with a severe hemorrhagic diathesis with less than 1% functional factor VIII. The defect that is illustrated in Figure 38-14B involves the same codon, but the mutation is CGA to CAA, which codes for a glutamine. The resulting factor VIII molecule is a full-length molecule with a single amino acid change; this is associated with a mild hemorrhagic diathesis with 9% functional factor VIII activity.

Kazazian et al. (209) have reported a novel mechanism for mutation of the factor VIII gene as a cause of hemophilia. They described two unrelated patients, both with severe hemophilia A, who had nonviral insertions of 3.8 and 2.3 kb, respectively, in exon 14. In both patients, the insertion contained the 3' portion of the human L1 sequence, which is a family of long, interspersed repeats that are present throughout the human genome and may function as retrotransposons. It was postulated that, in both cases, the insertion of the L1 sequence occurred through base-pairing of the poly(T) tail of L1 complementary DNA with an A-rich region in exon 14 of factor VIII.

Much less is known about the molecular defects that result in factor V deficiency. This is partly because factor V deficiency is an uncommon disorder. Most cases of factor V deficiency appear to be CRM-negative and were originally presumed to represent disorders in which synthesis of factor V was decreased (210–213). Subsequent studies showed that, in some CRM-negative patients, nonfunctional antigenic material was in their platelets, which suggests that a dysfunctional factor V molecule was produced. A series of CRM-positive patients has been described, with less than 10% coagulant activity and factor V antigen levels of 45% to 70% (214). Thus, factor V deficiency, like factor VIII deficiency, appears to constitute a spectrum of genetic defects. Definition of these defects at the molecular level should provide important insight into the function of factor V.

Factor V Quebec is a variant form of factor V deficiency that is characterized by plasma factor V levels of 40% to 60%, plasma factor V antigen levels of 65% to 75%, platelet factor V activity of 2% to 4%, and platelet factor V antigen levels of 70% to 80%

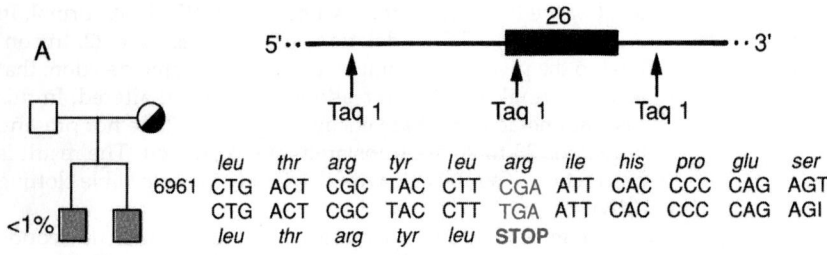

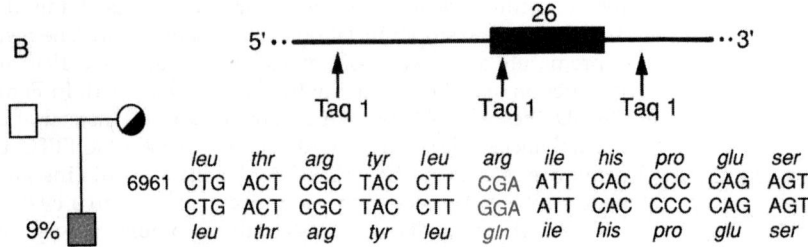

Figure 38-14. Genetic defects in hemophilia. Examples of point mutations within a single codon in exon 26 that cause hemophilia of different severity. The *Taq* I restriction sites are indicated by arrows. **A:** Severe hemophilia that results from a nonsense mutation. **B:** Mild hemophilia that results from a missense mutation.

(162). In the kindred reported, the factor V defect was inherited as an autosomal-dominant trait. This appears to be the first description of a qualitative abnormality of platelet factor V. The defect is a consequence of excess urine plasminogen activator in platelet alpha granules. The active enzyme degrades factor V together with other alpha granule proteins (C. Hayward, personal communication, 2002).

Factor V deficiency may also be seen in association with factor VIII deficiency (215–233). Combined factor V-VIII deficiency is inherited in an autosomal-recessive manner. Levels of factor V and VIII are commensurately reduced and range from 5% to 25%. Antigenic levels of factors V and VIII may be normal or may be concordant with activity levels. Using positional cloning methods, Nichols and co-workers have identified a 53-kd lectin from the endoplasmic reticulum–Golgi intermediate compartment that is deficient in many cases of combined factor V-VIII deficiency (58,59). In the absence of this protein, termed *ERGIC-53*, factors V and VIII fail to transit the Golgi and are not secreted, leading to deficiency. Recently, a second gene associated with combined factor V-VIII deficiency was identified. *CFD2* is an EF-band protein that interacts with ERGIC-53 in a calcium-dependent manner.

Genetic Counseling in Hemophilia A

Standard methods of carrier detection in hemophilia A have been based on assays for factor VIII biologic activity. Although a female carrier possesses two X chromosomes ($X_h X$), only one of the X chromosomes is expressed in a given somatic cell. Inactivation of the second X chromosome occurs by a process that is known as *lyonization* (named after Dr. Mary Lyon, who first described the process) and is a random event. Thus, in a carrier, some factor VIII–producing cells (those with an active X chromosome) express normal amounts of factor VIII, and other cells (those with an active X_h chromosome) express no factor VIII. Because of lyonization, only one-half of the potential factor VIII–producing cells in a carrier produce factor VIII. On the average, factor VIII levels in a carrier are one-half of the average level of factor VIII in normal women. Also, factor VIII activity in a large population of carrier females assumes a gaussian curve that overlaps with the gaussian curve that is obtained from a normal population. Because of this overlap, results of carrier testing that are based on factor VIII activity are always probabilistic (238). The accuracy of carrier testing can be increased by

using bivariate analysis of factor VIII activity and von Willebrand's antigen. With the use of assays and statistical refinements, the error rate in carrier detection has been determined to be approximately 10% (77,239).

The availability of genetic probes for factor VIII makes it possible to identify carriers with increased accuracy. In general, two approaches to carrier detection have been used. The first, which depends on the direct recognition of the specific genomic defect, is used when the gene defect in the pedigree that is under investigation is known. Detection of the defect may be by a labeled oligonucleotide probe that is specific to the defect or by restriction site analysis, if the defect involves the recognition site for a restriction enzyme, such as Taq I. This approach has the advantage of not requiring pedigree information, if the precise defect has been established in the family under study. The second approach, which is called *restriction fragment length polymorphism (RFLP) analysis*, takes advantage of RFLPs that are linked to the factor VIII gene. The DNA probes that are used in this approach identify independently segregating restriction polymorphisms that are close to or in the factor VIII gene. With this technique, it is not necessary to know the specific genomic defect in a given family, but it requires a male who is affected to establish which allele contains the mutant X chromosome. It also requires that the mother be heterozygous for the polymorphism.

Numerous reports of DNA probes that are being used for carrier testing and prenatal diagnosis have appeared since 1984, when the factor VIII gene was cloned. Initial studies described a Bgl II RFLP that was detected with an X-chromosome–specific probe, DXS15 (DX13) (240). No crossovers between the hemophilia A locus and the DXS15 locus were observed. Oberle et al. (241) described a Taq I RFLP that was detected with DXS52 (St14), another X-chromosome–specific probe that was extragenic to the factor VIII gene. Reports of crossover between Bgl II–DXS15 or Taq I–DXS52 and the factor VIII gene have appeared (242–245). Although this may limit the usefulness of these markers, they remain valuable probes for some patients.

RFLPs within the factor VIII gene provide more accurate carrier detection and prenatal diagnosis. To identify intragenic markers, Gitschier et al. (246) screened the factor VIII gene for polymorphisms with 37 restriction enzymes. One enzyme, Bcl I, revealed a polymorphic site that lies 3' to exon 18; this has proved useful for carrier detection and antenatal diagnosis (247,248). Additional intragenic polymorphisms with Bgl I, Xba I, Msp I, and Hind III have subsequently been described (187,

TABLE 38-5. DNA Polymorphisms for Diagnosis of Hemophilia

Probe	Enzyme	Number of Alleles	Heterozygosity (%)	Polymorphic Site	Fragment Size (kilobase)	Allelic Incidence (%)	Reference
Extragenic polymorphisms							
DXS15	Bgl II	2	50	—	—	—	232
DXS52	Taq I	10	90	—	—	—	233
	Msp I	3					
Intragenic polymorphisms							
Factor VIII (p114.12)	Bcl I	—	—	Intron 18	1.2	29	238
					0.8	71	
Factor VIII (p114.12)	Hind III	—	—	Intron 19	2.7	82	243,244
					2.6	18	
Factor VIII (p482.6)	Xba I	—	—	Intron 22	6.2	41	241
					4.8	59	
Factor VIII (C)	Bgl I	—	—	Intron 25	20	10	178
					5	90	
Factor VIII (p625.3)	Msp I	—	—	3' flank	7.5	68	242
					4.3	32	
(CA)n	—	—	91	Intron 13	—	—	253

249–252). In addition to these polymorphic restriction sites, the factor VIII gene also contains a polymorphic hypervariable (CA)n dinucleotide repeat that can be used for carrier analysis (253). Table 38-5 summarizes polymorphic restriction sites that have been useful in the genetic diagnosis of hemophilia.

Carrier detection can be enhanced by using multiple DNA probes. Janco et al. (254) have compared the usefulness of three intragenic polymorphisms (Bcl I–F8IVS18,* Xba I–F8IVS22, and Bgl I–F8IVS25) and one extragenic polymorphism (Taq I–DXS52) for carrier detection. The intragenic polymorphisms alone were informative in 32% to 58% of women who were tested. Bgl I–F8IVS25 and Bcl I–F8IVS18 were in apparent linkage disequilibrium and provided no additional information. Using Bcl I–F8IVS18 and Xba I–F8IVS22, accurate information was obtained in 64% of women who were tested. In the remaining women, who were uninformative with any intragenic probe, all were informative with the extragenic Taq I–DXS52 polymorphism. Because a significant risk of recombination between Taq I–DXS52 and the factor VIII gene exists, Janco et al. (254) recommended first testing with Xba I–F8IVS22 or Xba I–F8IVS22 and Bcl I–F8IVS18. In a similar study, Pecorara et al. (255) showed that the combination of Bcl I–F8IVS18 and Taq I–DXS52 was informative in 91% of carriers, whereas Bcl I–F8IVS18, Taq I–DXS52, and Bgl II–DXS15 were informative in 96% of carriers.

Genetic probes have also been used to estimate the rate of spontaneous mutations in hemophilia. In two studies, families with isolated or sporadic cases of hemophilia were studied by RFLP analysis (176,255). The origin of the mutation was inferred from the RFLP pattern and coagulation studies. In 13 of 20 families, the mutation was derived from the normal maternal grandfather. Although both studies were small, the combined results indicate a higher mutation rate in men than in women and confirm previous studies that are based on segregation analysis and coagulation studies (256).

A newer method that has proven to be useful in genetic diagnosis is the technique of gene amplification with the polymerase chain reaction method, which was described by Saiki et al. (257). This technique uses repeated cycles of DNA denaturation, primer reannealing, and DNA synthesis to amplify specific DNA sequences as much as several hundred-thousand times. The advantages of this method are that it is rapid, and it provides an alternate method to Southern blot, which is expen-

sive. Instead of radioactive detection, amplified sequences can be restricted and visualized by ultraviolet fluorescence after staining with ethidium bromide. Kogan et al. (258) used this technique to successfully perform carrier detection and prenatal diagnosis in two families with hemophilia A.

Given the prevalence of the partial inversion, a rational approach to genetic counseling in families with severe hemophilia is to first screen for the inversion with simple Southern blotting procedures by using F8IVS22 probes after digestion with Bcl I. If this is unrevealing, and the molecular defect in the family is unknown, the next step is to analyze for polymorphic markers, perhaps starting with the hypervariable (CA)n repeat.

Prenatal Testing in Hemophilia A

Prenatal testing also has been based on factor VIII detection, but it uses immunologic assays for VIII:Ag because of the small sample obtained. When a known or potential carrier woman presents for prenatal evaluation, first discuss frankly and openly the goals of testing and her feelings and the family's feelings about termination of pregnancy. Why does she want prenatal testing? Does she understand the genetics of hemophilia? How strong are her feelings for or against abortion? The risks and accuracy of the procedures must be explained.

After these issues have been satisfactorily addressed, the first step in prenatal diagnosis is amniocentesis. This can be done between weeks 13 and 16 of pregnancy. Amniocentesis has a 0.5% morbidity rate, and it reveals the sex of the fetus. In addition, amniocentesis can provide DNA for analysis by using the various techniques that were previously described. DNA can be obtained earlier in the pregnancy (between 9 and 12 gestational weeks) by chorionic villus sampling. The risk of this procedure is also approximately 0.5%. If amniocentesis indicates that the fetus is a male, and DNA studies fail to establish a diagnosis, the next step is fetal blood sampling by ultrasound-guided needle aspiration or by fetoscopy. In this procedure, umbilical vein blood is sampled, and VIII:Ag is determined. Obviously, measurement of VIII:Ag is diagnostic only in a CRM-negative family and cannot be used in CRM-positive families.

Often, sufficient fetal blood can be obtained by ultrasound-guided needle aspiration to permit measurement of factor VIII activity. This provides a useful alternative for CRM-positive families or families in whom no affected member is available. Fetal blood sampling is done between gestational weeks 18 and 20 and has a 1% morbidity rate.

---

*The nomenclature that is used for polymorphisms specifies the restriction enzyme and the location of the polymorphic site. Thus, Bcl I–F8IVS18 denotes a polymorphic Bcl I site in intron (IVS) 18 of the factor VIII gene.

Graham et al. (238) and Lillicrap et al. (259) have reviewed the advantages of phenotypic and genotypic assays in carrier detection and prenatal diagnosis. Their conclusion is that genetic assays undoubtedly improve the accuracy of carrier detection and prenatal diagnosis, but there are still many instances in which, because of the paucity of polymorphisms, DNA methods cannot be applied. Combining phenotypic and genotypic assays increases the certainty of diagnosis. The advantage of genotypic studies is that they are independent of lyonization and, when the marker is intragenic, the results are nonprobabilistic.

CLINICAL MANIFESTATIONS OF FACTOR VIII DEFICIENCY

The primary clinical manifestations of hemophilia patients result from bleeding and the complications of replacement therapy with plasma-derived blood products. The incidence and severity of bleeding are related to plasma levels of functional factor VIII (Table 38-6). Patients with less than 1% activity have a severe hemorrhagic tendency that is characterized by recurrent joint and soft-tissue bleeding that may occur as often as two to four times per month. Hemorrhage after trauma may be life-threatening, and surgical bleeding, if not treated, is severe and may be complicated by delayed hemorrhage that occurs 7 to 14 days postoperatively. Patients with factor VIII levels of 1% to 5% have moderately severe hemophilia. Spontaneous hemorrhage may occur, especially in previously damaged joints, but it is much less common than in severe hemophilia. In contrast, bleeding after trauma or surgery is often severe and may be indistinguishable from that seen in patients with severe hemophilia. Patients with factor VIII levels that are higher than 5% have mild hemophilia. Spontaneous bleeding is rare. Surgery and other procedures may be performed with little or no bleeding on some occasions, but may be associated with excessive bleeding on other occasions. Many patients with mild hemophilia are completely asymptomatic and are diagnosed only incidentally.

Hemarthroses, which are joint hemorrhages, are the most characteristic and among the most disabling of the hemorrhages that occur in hemophilia (260–262). They account for 75% to 85% of bleeding episodes in patients with severe disease. Two types of joint involvement are encountered: the acute manifestation of hemorrhage into the joint and the chronic changes in the joint that occur as a result of recurrent hemarthroses.

In acute hemarthroses, the initial observation, as described by most patients, is a "bubbling" or "tingling" sensation in the joint, which may last several hours. As bleeding into the joint continues, distention of the joint capsule and pain develop. If bleeding in the joint is allowed to persist, the joint may become swollen and visibly distended. Range of motion in the affected joint may become severely limited. Treatment with factor VIII generally stops the bleeding and relieves the symptoms. The earlier that treatment is started, the more rapidly the symptoms resolve. The proclivity for joint bleeding is characteristic of hemophilia and is not a feature of any blood-clotting factor deficiency other than factor IX and, possibly, factor VII deficiency.

The reason for this peculiar distribution is unknown and is one of the great mysteries in the field.

With recurrent bleeding in the joint, damage to the synovial tissue occurs and progressive joint destruction produces the characteristic hemophilic arthropathy, which is the major disabling lesion in hemophilia. Initially, chronic synovitis with synovial hypertrophy develops. The joint becomes chronically swollen and boggy. A mild joint effusion may be present that, if tapped, is hemorrhagic. Arnold and Hilgartner (263) termed this stage *subacute hemarthropathy*. Because of the vascularity of the hypertrophic synovium, such joints often bleed more frequently and become target joints. Later, more chronic changes occur. Loss of the synovium, erosion of cartilage, destruction of the joint space, and articulation of bone on bone occur. Severe limitation of motion results, which further stresses the joint and causes muscular atrophy. Deformities may further affect joint function. A vicious cycle ensues in which the damaged joint is more prone to bleeding, which further damages the joint. Chronic pain becomes more prominent. The changes that occur in the hemophilic joint can be visualized and graded radiologically (Fig. 38-15) (263–265), although the correlation between radiologic grade and joint function is only approximate. Magnetic resonance imaging may also be useful in the evaluation of hemophilic arthropathy and is being evaluated for correlation with joint function and surgical outcome (266).

The pathophysiology of these destructive changes is uncertain but may involve mechanisms that are similar to those that are involved in the joint destruction that is seen in rheumatoid arthritis (263,267–269). Blood breakdown products, including iron from erythrocytes and various proteases, growth factors, cytokines, and other inflammatory mediators from leukocytes and platelets, are released into the joint space. With repeated episodes of bleeding, the synovium becomes inflamed and thickened. Histologically, villous hypertrophy and a marked increase in vascularity are found. Iron particles are found in the synoviocytes along the villous processes, and foci of chronic inflammation are present throughout the synovium. Later in the course of joint damage, the synovium becomes replaced by fibrous tissue and disintegrates. This scarring is associated with a loss of joint motion.

In addition, after the protective synovium is lost, the articular cartilage becomes the target of attack. The chondrocyte is especially susceptible to damage by iron. Cartilaginous erosion occurs. Initially, the joint space is preserved, but as uneven wearing of the articular surface occurs, the joint space becomes narrowed and deformities begin to develop. Osteoporosis and bone cysts are prominent features later in the course of hemophilic arthropathy. In the advanced hemophilic joint, the joint space collapses, and the joint range of motion becomes severely limited. At this stage, bleeding usually becomes infrequent because of limited joint motion and loss of vascular tissue in the joint.

In older hemophiliacs, arthritis is often a major complaint. Treatment with nonsteroidal antiinflammatory agents is beneficial in some patients. First generation agents may impair platelet function and increase the incidence and severity of joint bleeding and other bleeding in the hemophiliac (270,271). Peptic ulceration and gastritis with gastrointestinal bleeding that is secondary to nonsteroidal antiinflammatory agents may be especially dangerous in the hemophiliac. These risks are reduced with newer nonsteroidal antiinflammatory agents. In patients in whom antiinflammatory agents do not relieve pain or cannot be used because of complications, stronger, potentially addicting, pain medications are frequently used. A major dilemma in hemophilia care is treading the fine line between pain relief and narcotic addiction. Psychological consultation, biofeedback, and transcutaneous nerve stimulators are part of the armamentarium of the physician who cares for hemophiliacs with chronic pain.

TABLE 38-6. Clinical Classification of Hemophilia A

Symptoms	Factor VIII%
Severe	<1
Moderate	1–5
Mild	>5

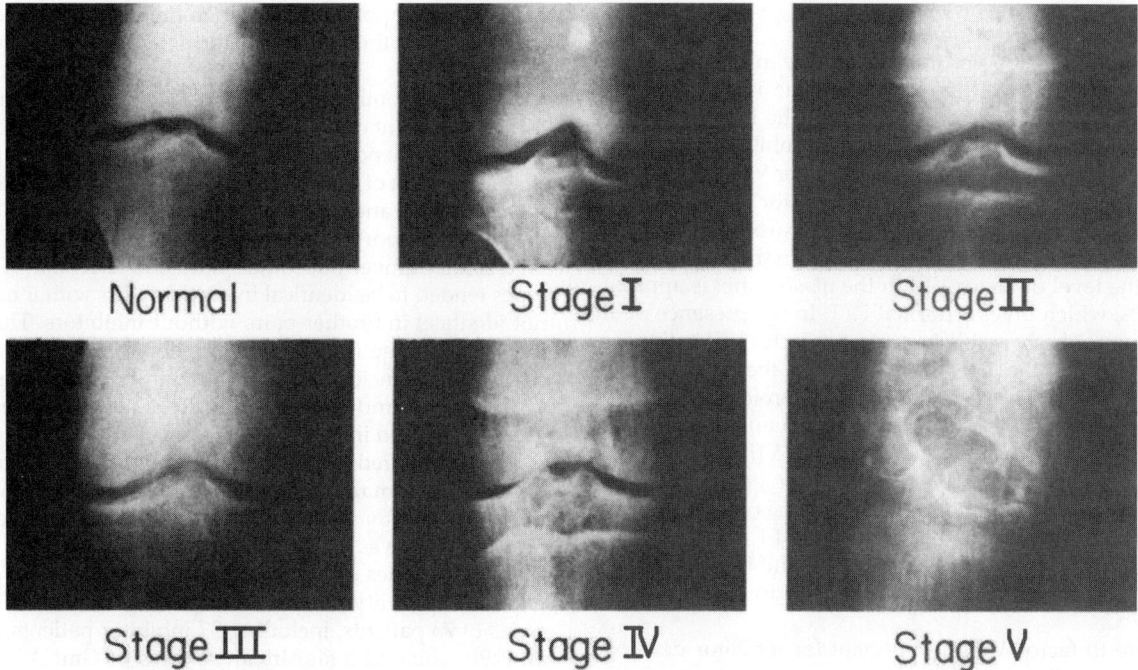

Figure 38-15. Radiologic knee joint changes in hemophilia A, illustrating the various changes of hemophilic arthropathy. **Stage I:** No skeletal abnormalities; soft tissue swelling due to bleeding in and around the joint. **Stage II:** Osteoporosis and epiphyseal overgrowth; joint space intact; no bone cysts. **Stage III:** Subchondral cysts; minor irregularities of the joint surface; joint space preserved. **Stage IV:** Cysts and joint surface irregularities are more prominent; joint space is narrowed as a result of cartilage damage. **Stage V:** Loss of joint space; marked epiphyseal overgrowth. (Courtesy of Bonner Guilford. From White GC II. Disorders of blood coagulation. In: Stein JH, ed. *Internal medicine.* Boston: Little, Brown and Company, 1987:1012, with permission.)

Muscle hematomas occur less frequently than joint bleeds in patients with hemophilia, but the consequences may be more acute. Expansion of a hematoma in a muscle compartment may lead to vascular or neurologic compromise with acute and permanent loss of function. Retroperitoneal bleeding into the iliopsoas or iliacus muscles is especially prone to neurologic complications, because the femoral nerve and iliopsoas traverse the ischial ramus together (272–274). Extension of an iliopsoas or iliacus bleed inferiorly may result in compression of the femoral nerve. Clinically, patients with retroperitoneal hematomas present with lower abdominal and back pain that may mimic renal colic. The leg is typically held in flexion at the hip, and extension of the leg or rotation of the hip accentuates the pain. Dysesthesias in the distribution of the lateral cutaneous femoral nerve may be the first clue to incipient femoral nerve damage. Hematuria is not present. Computed tomography of the abdomen usually reveals a characteristic mass lesion in the retroperitoneal tissues.

Hemophilic cysts or *pseudotumors* are tense, blood-filled cysts that can mimic osteogenic sarcomas radiologically (275,276). Pseudotumors are found most frequently in the pelvis and thigh but have been reported in the calves, feet, arms, and hands. They usually occur in patients with severe hemophilia but may also be seen in those with mild hemophilia. Aspiration of the cyst, which is fraught with danger, yields dark-brown fluid. The wall of the pseudotumor is thick, fibrous tissue. The origin of the pseudotumor is probably a hematoma with incomplete resolution. The encapsulated collection of blood breaks down and begins to expand from recurrent bleeds and increased oncotic pressure. As the encapsulated blood expands, it produces pressure on surrounding tissues and leads to pressure necrosis. The patient presents with a painless mass, 10 to 20 years after the initial bleeding episode. Destruction of bone may be evident radiologically.

Before acquired immunodeficiency syndrome (AIDS) became a widespread disease, intracranial bleeds accounted for nearly 25% of the deaths in patients with hemophilia (274,277,278). These include intracerebral, subarachnoid, subdural, and intraspinal bleeds. The symptoms are similar to intracranial bleeds in patients without hemophilia and include headache, nausea, seizures, nuchal rigidity, and progressive neurologic impairment. Although many patients have a history of significant trauma, almost one-half of patients have no antecedent trauma (278). A major goal of home treatment in hemophiliacs is early treatment after head trauma or after onset of a severe headache that is associated with a spontaneous intracranial bleed.

Hematuria occurs frequently in patients with hemophilia. As many as 83% of patients with severe hemophilia can expect to experience at least one episode of hematuria in their lifetime (279). Most episodes are spontaneous, last 2 to 3 days, and resolve without treatment. Anemia due to hematuria in the hemophiliac is unusual. A careful history to exclude other causes of hematuria, such as recent streptococcal infections, nephrolithiasis, urinary tract infection, and trauma, must be obtained. Despite the bleeding tendency, extravasated blood in the urinary tract can clot and lead to obstructive symptoms. If hematuria persists, evaluation should include intravenous pyelography. This often shows abnormalities of the collecting system, with filling defects due to clots. These may persist long after the hematuria has resolved.

Hemorrhage in other sites may also occur in hemophilia. Epistaxis may be prominent in children. Gastrointestinal bleeding is typically secondary to an intestinal lesion and should stimulate a complete gastrointestinal evaluation. Intramural hematomas in the intestine may occur in hemophiliacs and cause pain that can mimic acute appendicitis, acute cholecystitis, or other acute abdominal syndromes.

Inhibitors

Inhibitors are alloantibodies that specifically inhibit the procoagulant activity of factor VIII. Inhibitors occur in approximately 15% of persons with severe hemophilia. The first clue that a patient with hemophilia has developed an inhibitor is a failure to respond to replacement therapy with factor VIII. The diagnosis is confirmed by clotting assay. The inhibitor may be evident on a routine mixing assay, in which equal parts of patient and normal plasma are mixed and then clotted. In the absence of an inhibitor, the level of factor VIII in the plasma mix is approximately 50%, which gives a normal PTT. In the presence of an inhibitor, the antibody is able to neutralize factor VIII in the normal plasma so that the level of factor VIII in the plasma mix is low, 1% or 2%, and the PTT is prolonged. A prolonged PTT mix is seen in some patients with hemophilia A and an inhibitor, but, in contrast to other inhibitors, the factor VIII inhibitor may be manifest only by incubation at 37°C for 2 hours. This curious property of factor VIII inhibitors forms the basis of the Bethesda assay, which is a standardized incubated PTT mix (280). *One Bethesda unit* is defined as the amount of inhibitor that inactivates one-half of the factor VIII in 1 mL of normal plasma in 2 hours at 37°C.

Exposure to factor VIII is important for inhibitor development. A hemophiliac who does not receive transfusions rarely develops an inhibitor, and a hemophiliac who is treated on more than 250 occasions rarely develops an inhibitor (281,282). The typical inhibitor is an IgG (immunoglobulin G) antibody, predominantly IgG4 or mixtures of IgG1 and IgG4 (283,284). Light-chain typing has revealed a single light-chain type, κ or λ, in many cases. Thus, inhibitors to factor VIII appear to be restricted polyclonal antibodies.

Fulcher et al. (285) and Scandella et al. (286,287) have analyzed the epitopes on factor VIII against which the inhibitor antibodies are directed. Although antibodies recognize epitopes from all domains of factor VIII, most of the inhibitory antibodies recognize a site on the A2 domain or a site on the C2 domain. Antibodies against the A2 domain prevent a contact with factor IXa that causes a conformational change that is associated with an accelerated k_{cat} (Fig. 38-16).

Preliminary studies in patients with hemophilia B have suggested that inhibitors occur in patients with gene deletions. As previously discussed in the section Molecular Genetics of Factor V and VIII Deficiency, studies on hemophilia A do not support this association. Of a total of 20 hemophilia A subjects with gene deletions, only eight have inhibitors. Conversely, of the 83 subjects with inhibitors, only 20 have detectable deletions. Why, then, do only 15% of hemophiliacs develop inhibitors? The location of the deletion may be important. A deletion that involves some antigenic hot spot may be more likely to predispose to inhibitor formation. Correlation with CRM status

may also be important. Further studies are needed to correlate the location of the deletion with the tendency to inhibitor formation.

In addition, other genetic host factors may be important in the development of inhibitors. Several studies have reported an increased incidence of inhibitors in brother pairs (281,288). The first suggestion of a possible link between the immune response in hemophilia and human leukocyte antigen (HLA) determinants was a report from Frommel and Allain (289). Their study on a small number of brother pairs indicated that HLA haplotypes tended to be identical in brother pairs with inhibitors and not identical in brother pairs without inhibitors. This was followed by a large multicenter cooperative inhibitor study that compared the incidence of HLA-A and HLA-B alleles in hemophiliacs with and without inhibitors (288). The results suggested a reduced incidence of HLA-A1 and HLA-B8 in inhibitor patients compared to that in noninhibitor patients, but the sample size was small and the HLA-DR locus, which has been shown to directly influence the antibody response to a variety of substances, was not analyzed.

The Gm series of γ-chain allotypes has also been associated with susceptibility to a variety of autoimmune disorders. In a series of 73 patients, including 37 inhibitor patients, Reisner et al. (290) showed a significant excess of Gm(a) in inhibitor patients compared to that in noninhibitor patients.

From a clinical perspective, two types of inhibitors are found (291). *High-response inhibitors* are antibodies that exhibit an anamnestic response to administration of factor VIII. This response can be dramatic, with increases from 1 or 2 Bethesda units to more than 9000 Bethesda units. Several patterns of response may be seen. In the typical, high-response person, the antibody rises to a level of 200 to 300 Bethesda units, beginning 4 to 7 days after administration of factor VIII. The inhibitor titer peaks, then begins to fall. If no further factor VIII is administered, the level may return to its original level after 3 to 5 months, only to increase after subsequent factor VIII infusion. In other hemophiliacs, the inhibitor may remain at high levels, even in the absence of treatment. *Low-response inhibitors* are antibodies that do not exhibit anamnesis after factor VIII administration. Inhibitor levels remain below 10 Bethesda units, despite repeated exposure to factor VIII. Patients with low-response inhibitors can be treated with factor VIII. In time, some low-response inhibitors convert to high-response inhibitors, and some go away.

Psychosocial Issues

Suicide is frequent in hemophilia. This is related partly to the high financial cost of hemophilia, a poor self-image that results from crippling hemarthropathy, life-long chronic pain and abuse of narcotic pain medications, and family psychodynamics during childhood and adolescence (292). The cost of care for a hemophilia patient can be staggering. The average hemophiliac uses approximately 50,000 U of factor VIII per year. At an average cost of $0.65/U, this can amount to $30,000 to $40,000 per year for replacement therapy alone. If hospitalization is required, the cost may increase to $50,000 or more per year. For patients with inhibitors, replacement therapy is even more expensive. Insurance caps are often reached and exceeded. Because of chronic joint disease, the hemophiliac is often unable to work and becomes dependent on social programs. Hemophilia assistance programs are active in some states but are unavailable in others, and they fail to reflect the recent increases in the cost of replacement therapy in others. Comprehensive hemophilia clinics have been developed to deal partly with these complex issues.

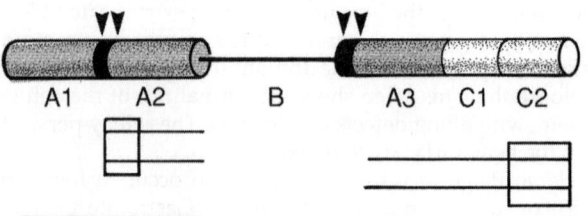

Figure 38-16. Factor VIII epitopes that are recognized by human alloantibodies. Horizontal lines show domains that are recognized by human factor VIII inhibitor antibodies. Boxes indicate antibodies that were studied further by synthesis of peptides and localized to the boxed regions. Arrowheads indicate thrombin cleavage sites.

CLINICAL MANIFESTATIONS OF FACTOR V DEFICIENCY

The clinical manifestations of factor V deficiency are variable but are generally milder than those of factor VIII deficiency. The severity of symptoms depends, in part, on the plasma and platelet levels of factor V. Hemarthroses may occur in patients with severe factor V deficiency but are uncommon, and the chronic sequelae of hemarthroses that are typical of severe hemophilia are not seen in patients with factor V deficiency. The following are major clinical manifestations:

Ecchymoses: Patients with severe factor V deficiency bruise easily. Spontaneous and trauma-associated ecchymoses are common.

Epistaxis: Epistaxis is common in patients with factor V deficiency, but its rate of occurrence may decrease with age.

Menorrhagia: One of the most common symptoms in women with factor V deficiency, menorrhagia may be severe and may cause anemia and iron deficiency. Usually, this can be controlled by administration of a progesterone preparation, such as medroxyprogesterone (Provera).

Inhibitors: Inhibitors to factor V may arise in patients with factor V deficiency. Like inhibitors to factor VIII, these are alloantibodies that specifically inhibit factor V clotting activity. The antibody is typically an IgG antibody. Antibodies to factor V neutralize factor V activity in a time- and temperature-dependent manner; therefore, diagnosis of a factor V inhibitor requires demonstration of an abnormal, incubated PTT mix (see the previous section Inhibitors).

TREATMENT FOR FACTOR VIII DEFICIENCY

Treatment for hemophilia consists of replacement of the deficient clotting factor with preparations of factor VIII. In developed countries, this is usually accomplished with commercial lyophilized concentrates of factor VIII derived from plasma or with recombinant factor VIII concentrates (293). Factor VIII concentrates are prepared from donors who are screened for human immunodeficiency virus (HIV) and hepatitis viruses. In addition, all factor VIII concentrates are processed to reduce viral contaminants in the final product. Some concentrates are extracted with various solvents and detergents to lyse lipid-coated viruses. Others are pasteurized to destroy virus. Affinity chromatography with monoclonal antibodies to factor VIII

or vWF has been used to purify factor VIII and has also been shown to reduce viral contamination in factor VIII concentrates. Some of the products that are available are listed in Table 38-7.

The normal level of factor VIII in plasma is 1 U/mL (where *U* is defined as the amount of factor VIII present in 1 mL of normal plasma). Replacement with factor VIII is based on the following formula:

$$VIII_i = (VIII_f - VIII_s) = P_V$$

where VIII_i equals the amount of factor VIII to be infused in units, VIII_f equals the desired peak VIII level in units per milliliter, VIII_s equals the initial VIII level in units per milliliter and P_V equals the plasma volume in milliliters.

Plasma volume is estimated as 5% of the body weight in kilograms. Thus, a 60-kg person has a plasma volume of 60×0.05, or 3 L. To raise the factor VIII level in a 60-kg person with less than 1% (less than 0.01 U/mL) factor VIII to 30% (0.3 U/mL) would require infusion of $0.3 - 0.01 \times 3000$ or 900 U of factor VIII. Most manufacturers provide lyophilized factor VIII concentrates in vials that contain approximately 250, 500, and 1000 U, which can be reconstituted in as little as 30 to 50 mL of diluent. To raise this theoretical 60-kg subject to 30% of factor VIII, a 1000-U vial could be reconstituted in 30 to 50 mL of diluent and infused as a bolus.

Most joint and simple muscle bleeds can be treated with a single bolus of factor VIII that is estimated to raise the factor VIII level to 30% (Table 38-8). Because the biologic half-life of factor VIII is 8 to 12 hours (294), treatment with a single dose to 30% of factor VIII provides hemostatic levels of greater than 5% for more than 24 hours. Sometimes, a severe joint or muscle bleed may require a second treatment. In general, the faster that a bleed is treated, the smaller the amount of factor that is required to stabilize it. For this reason, early treatment is encouraged. Occasionally, bleeds recur in a single joint and require treatment two to four times per month. Such a joint is called a *target joint*. Initial treatment of a target joint should be aimed at the prevention of bleeding by prophylactic use of factor VIII. A typical prophylactic regimen for target joints is treatment to 30% of factor VIII three times a week for 3 weeks, followed by treatment twice a week for 3 weeks. If this does not stop bleeding in the joint, or if breakthrough bleeding occurs on prophylaxis, surgical intervention should be considered. In HIV-seropositive hemophiliacs, persistent joint pain may also be caused by septic arthritis.

TABLE 38-7. Therapeutic Concentrates in Hemophilia A

Concentrate	Volume to 100%	Ease of Use	Risk of Hepatitis	Risk of Acquired Immunodeficiency Syndrome	Risk of Hemolysis
Intermediate purity	50	4+	−	−	+
Monoclonal	50	4+	−	−	−
Recombinant	50	4+	−	−	−
Recombinant-AF	50	4+	−	−	−

± to 4+, degree of increasing risk or ease of use with each product; −, no risk; AF, albumin-free recombinant factor VIII.
NOTE: Intermediate purity concentrates are solvent- and detergent-extracted to remove coated viruses, including HIV-1 and hepatitis viruses. Monoclonal factor VIII concentrates are ultrapure products that are prepared by using affinity chromatography and viral inactivation steps. Recombinant factor VIII is a synthetic product that is prepared in Chinese hamster ovary cells or baby hamster kidney cells.

TABLE 38-8. Treatment of Bleeding Episodes in Hemophilia A

Site	Level (%)	Treatment Length
Joint	30	1 dose
Muscle	30	1 dose
Hematuria	30	1 dose
Retroperitoneal	50	5–7 d
Gastrointestinal	50	5–7 d
Neck	100	7–10 d
Intracranial	100	10–14 d

For retroperitoneal, gastrointestinal, intracranial, neck, and muscle bleeding with incipient nerve compression, more prolonged treatment with factor VIII is needed (Table 38-8). This can be done in one of two ways. One way is to infuse factor VIII at 12-hour intervals. For example, a 60-kg person with retroperitoneal hemorrhage requires an initial infusion of 1500 U to raise the factor VIII level to 50%. Twelve hours later, when the level has fallen to 25%, a bolus of 750 U would raise the level to 50%. The disadvantage of this method is that, although a level of 50% is achieved, the plasma factor VIII can drop to an unacceptably low level at times. It is also inconvenient to have to time a blood sample to check a factor VIII level. Another method to maintain treatment levels is to give a continuous infusion of factor VIII. In the same patient with retroperitoneal hemorrhage, an initial infusion of 1500 U is given and is immediately followed by 750 U that is infused over the next 12 hours. Blood for factor VIII levels can be drawn at any time, and no peaks and troughs should occur.

1-Deamino-8-D-Arginine Vasopressin

After observations that epinephrine and stress increase levels of factor VIII in normal persons, studies were undertaken to evaluate the effect of a vasopressin analog on factor VIII in patients with hemophilia (71,72). The analog, 1-deamino-8-D-arginine vasopressin (DDAVP) (also known as *desmopressin acetate*) has the same effect on factor VIII as vasopressin, with less than 1% of the pressor effect of the parent compound.

DDAVP can be administered intravenously or subcutaneously with essentially equivalent results (295). The response in hemophiliacs with factor VIII levels greater than 2% is a reproducible two- or threefold increase in factor VIII activity. For hemophiliacs with a basal factor VIII level of 2% to 5%, this rise is generally not sufficient to permit invasive procedures, and factor VIII concentrates may be needed. For hemophiliacs with basal levels greater than 5% to 7%, the increase in response to DDAVP is sufficient for dental work and other minor procedures. The dose is 0.3 µg/kg administered intravenously in a volume of 100 mL over 30 minutes. For subcutaneous administration of DDAVP, the intravenous preparation is used at the same dose with subcutaneous injection of no more than 1.5 mL per site. (A single treatment may require three to four subcutaneous injections.) Intranasal preparations of DDAVP that are suitable for treating patients with hemophilia are available and are most commonly used.

The response to DDAVP that is given on successive days diminishes (Fig. 38-17), presumably because of exhaustion of endothelial stores of vWF or factor VIII. For this reason, operative patients who receive DDAVP should be watched closely for signs of bleeding on the second to fourth postoperative days. The response returns to normal after several days. Water intoxication with hyponatremia is a rare complication of DDAVP use.

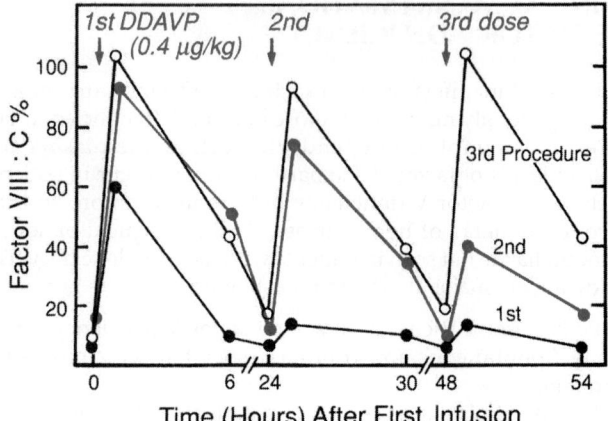

Figure 38-17. Response to repeated infusions of 1-deamino-8-D-arginine vasopressin (DDAVP). Repeated infusions of DDAVP were administered to a mild hemophiliac who underwent dental procedures that were several weeks apart. (From Mannucci PM, Ruggeri ZM, Pareti FI, et al. 1-Deamino-8-D-arginine vasopressin: a new pharmacological approach to the management of hemophilia and von Willebrand's disease. *Lancet* 1977;1:869, with permission.)

Home Therapy

Many patients with hemophilia treat themselves at home. Lyophilized concentrates can be stored at room temperature and transported on trips; they are easy to reconstitute. Home treatment may be life-saving in intracranial bleeding. Studies indicate that progression of joint deterioration may be retarded in patients on home treatment (296–298).

Many children with hemophilia A are treated prophylactically with regular doses of factor VIII. The goal of primary prophylaxis is to prevent the development of hemorrhages and progressive joint destruction through the maintenance of continuous clotting factor levels. Current standards for prophylaxis are 50 U/kg three times weekly, which, given the 12-hour half-life of factor VIII, is calculated to maintain factor VIII levels of at least 1.5%. Numerous studies have demonstrated the effectiveness of this approach, but the cost is high, and primary prophylaxis is currently used predominantly in children, typically those who are younger than 12 years of age. In children older than 12 years of age, because of their size, prophylaxis becomes too expensive. Secondary prophylaxis may be given at any age and is used to treat so-called *target joints*, joints that become inflamed and bleed in recurrent manner. Dosages of 30 to 50 U/kg two to three times a week for 4 to 6 weeks are typically used.

Gene Therapy

There are a number of factors that make hemophilia a good target for gene therapy: It is a monogenic disorder, so correction of the single gene defect results in beneficial clinical effects; excellent small and large animal models of hemophilia exist for preclinical testing; factor VIII is well characterized, and sensitive assays for both antigenic and functional activity are available; and any level of factor VIII achieved would be likely to change the course of the disease. Several phase I clinical trials that use *ex vivo* gene transfer and *in vivo* gene transfer, using retrovirus, adeno-associated virus, and adenovirus-based vectors, have been undertaken and demonstrate the initial safety of gene transfer in hemophilia.

Orthopedic Management

The indications for surgical treatment of joint disease in hemophilia are intractable bleeding that responds poorly to medical therapy and advanced joint destruction with disabling joint dysfunction. The decision to undertake surgery is a complicated one that must include a careful consideration of these indications but must also take into account the HIV status of the patient, his or her life expectancy, and his or her quality of life without surgery.

Initially, intractable bleeding should be treated medically with factor VIII and immobilization. Treatment to 30% levels with factor VIII two to three times per week for as long as 6 weeks often stops the bleeding, and the patient can then resume normal demand therapy. In a number of patients, this fails to stop the bleeding or bleeding recurs after therapy is stopped. In such patients, when the bleeding appears to be caused by hypertrophied, vascularized synovium, synovectomy should be considered. Some centers, including our own, use radiologic staging to predict surgical response to synovectomy. In general, joints that are radiologic grade I or II appear to respond well to synovectomy, whereas joints that are grade III, IV, or V respond poorly, if at all, to synovectomy. Usually, synovectomy stops the recurrent bleeding in the joint, but loss of motion, which may be as much as 45 to 50 degrees, may occur in the joint after synovectomy (299,300). Radiation synovectomy, called *synoviorthesis*, is an alternative in some patients (301).

Joint deformity may occur as a result of chronic arthropathy and may contribute to intractable bleeding and pain through biomechanical mechanisms. Osteotomy can lead to a more normal distribution of load, thereby relieving stress on the joint and resulting in symptomatic improvement (302).

Joint replacement has been successfully performed in patients with hemophilia. Knee and hip replacements have been most frequently performed, but elbow and shoulder replacements have been described. Because the lifespan of replaced joints is finite, these operations should be most strongly considered for patients who are older than 40 years of age and who have advanced joint disease, as evidenced by chronic pain, significantly decreased joint range of motion, and advanced radiographic grade (stage IV, V, or VI). On the other hand, if the joint disease is sufficiently advanced that the joint is fixed and muscle atrophy has occurred, the long-term outcome of the replacement may be less favorable. Thus, the timing of joint replacement is important and requires orthopedic evaluation.

Finally, arthrodesis relieves symptoms of pain and bleeding but may produce secondary changes in other joints (303).

Inhibitors

The treatment of bleeding episodes in patients with inhibitors is determined by the titer of the antibody at the time that treatment is required, the antibody response to administration of factor VIII, and the severity of the bleed. Patients with low-response inhibitors can be treated with factor VIII for all bleeding episodes, although doses of as much as 4000 U or more may be needed to achieve factor VIII levels of 30%. Some patients with inhibitor titers of 1 to 2 Bethesda units can be maintained on home treatment, after the appropriate dose of factor VIII is determined.

In patients with high-response, high-titer inhibitors, it is impossible to infuse sufficient factor VIII to achieve hemostasis. For these persons, several alternate treatment modalities are available, including porcine factor VIII, activated prothrombin complex concentrates (PCCs), plasmapheresis, recombinant factor VIIa, and immunosuppressive agents, although none work as well as factor VIII in patients without inhibitors. The treatment of

choice for a life- or limb-threatening bleed in patients with high-response, high-titer inhibitors is porcine factor VIII (304,305). Porcine and human factor VIII are functionally similar, but enough difference in primary structure is present that many alloantibodies do not recognize the porcine protein. By substituting porcine factor VIII for normal plasma in the Bethesda assay, the cross-reaction of the inhibitor for the porcine molecule can be determined. Doses of 5000 to 15,000 U are administered as a bolus. If an adequate level of factor VIII is achieved, treatment is continued. Complications of porcine factor VIII are allergic and pyrogenic reactions and mild thrombocytopenia. Anamnestic responses to porcine factor VIII may occur.

For a bleed that is not threatening to life or limb, the treatment of choice is more complicated and involves doing nothing or using activated or nonactivated PCCs or recombinant factor VIIa (306,307). Two activated PCCs are available: Autoplex (NABI, Boca Raton, FL) and FEIBA (Baxter Bioscience, Deerfield, IL). A double-blind, controlled trial comparing FEIBA to a nonactivated PCC in the treatment of joint and muscle bleeds showed FEIBA to be 64% effective compared to a 52% response to the nonactivated PCC (251). Subjective improvement, as well as objective improvement in joint range of motion, was observed. The active principle in PCCs may be activated factor VII or X (308,309). Intravenous IgG has been used in acquired factor VIII inhibitors but is usually not efficacious in hemophilic inhibitors.

Patients with high-response, low-titer inhibitors can be treated with factor VIII, but this treatment is likely to result in an anamnestic increase in inhibitor titer. For this reason, use of factor VIII in these patients is often reserved for life-threatening bleeding episodes. For other hemorrhages, such as joint bleeds or hematuria, treatment with PCCs is sometimes effective but is less likely to produce an anamnestic increase in inhibitor titer (310).

CASE REPORT

A 21-year-old male hemophiliac with a high-response inhibitor presented to the emergency department with headache, lethargy, and early papilledema. His last inhibitor titer, which was administered 1 month before presentation to the emergency department, was 4 Bethesda units. The last time he was treated with factor VIII, his inhibitor level rose from 10 to 349 Bethesda units. In the emergency department, the patient was given a bolus of 5000 U of factor VIII concentrate, as soon as it was prepared, and he was sent for a computed tomography scan of the head, which revealed an intracerebral hematoma. A postinfusion factor VIII level of 59% was obtained. He was given another 3000 U of factor VIII, and a continuous infusion of 250 U/hour was started. His factor VIII level after the second bolus was 88%. He was seen by a neurosurgeon, and an angiogram revealed no aneurysm. The patient remained on factor VIII with levels between 90% and 130% until 5 days later, when his morning factor VIII was 16%. A second sample was obtained, and the factor VIII level was 2%. Another bolus of 5000 U was administered, after which the factor VIII level was 4%, which indicated that anamnesis had occurred. To provide an additional 5 to 7 days of hemostasis for intracranial bleeding, the patient was given activated PCC, 75 U/kg every 8 hours. Recovery was uneventful, and the patient was neurologically intact at discharge.

Three months later, the patient returned with spontaneous bleeding in the left knee. His inhibitor titer was 150 Bethesda units. He was admitted and treated with recombinant activated factor VIII (NovoSeven, Novo Nordisk, Copenhagen), 90 to 120 µg/kg every 2 hours, for a total of three doses. Joint pain resolved gradually, and range of motion improved. The patient's inhibitor level at the end of treatment was 135 Bethesda units.

The approaches outlined here are intended to treat acute hemorrhagic episodes. Several methods have been proposed to eradicate inhibitors. Many of these, such as steroids, plasmapheresis, and cytotoxic agents, have not been uniformly successful. In 1977, Brackmann and Gormsen (311) described a protocol that used high doses of factor VIII over prolonged periods of time. In their protocol, treatment with 100 U/kg is given twice a day for as long as 1 to 3 years. In the typical patient, the inhibitor titer rises over the first month, then starts to fall, despite continued administration of factor VIII, and continues to fall to undetectable levels. It has been suggested that treatment with large doses of factor VIII induces a state of immune tolerance. Although the average cost of this treatment may be as high as $1,000,000, it may be cost-effective in the inhibitor patient who is admitted many times a year (312).

TREATMENT OF FACTOR V DEFICIENCY

Although factor V deficiency is a milder disorder than hemophilia A, patients with factor V deficiency may sometimes require replacement therapy. Treatment is usually with fresh frozen plasma, because no commercial concentrates of factor V are available. Recent studies indicate that platelet concentrates may also provide hemostasis in patients with factor V deficiency and in patients with inhibitors to factor V.

Plasma contains one unit of factor V per milliliter. Thus, replacement of factor V can be calculated by the same method that was described for factor VIII replacement. For example, a 60-kg person with severe factor V deficiency with an estimated plasma volume of 3000 mL requires infusion of 900 U of factor V to raise the plasma factor V level to 30%. Because fresh frozen plasma is provided in bags of approximately 250 mL, and plasma contains 1 U of factor V per mL, nearly 1000 mL (four bags) of fresh frozen plasma would be needed to achieve a factor V level of 30%. Estimation of replacement with platelet concentrates is more difficult, because the number of platelets that are harvested may vary from donor to donor and from blood bank to blood bank. A gross rule of thumb that is based on the specific activity of factor V and the estimated concentration of factor V in platelets is 1500 to 3000 U per unit of apheresis platelets.

Because factor V deficiency is a milder bleeding disorder than hemophilia A, and because large volumes of fresh frozen plasma are required to raise factor V levels to greater than 40%, most bleeding episodes in patients with factor V deficiency can be treated with sufficient fresh frozen plasma to raise the plasma factor V level to 30%. Menorrhagia is best controlled hormonally.

COMPLICATIONS OF THERAPY

Hepatitis and Chronic Liver Disease

Transfusion-associated hepatitis occurs in a large percentage of hemophiliacs who receive replacement therapy. The incidence of acute hepatitis, as manifested by jaundice and elevated liver enzymes, is between 10% and 26% in most series (313–316). Acute fulminant hepatitis in hemophilia is rare. When followed up for several years, nearly 80% of hemophiliacs who have multiple transfusions demonstrate at least intermittent abnormali-

ties of liver function tests, and as many as 30% of patients demonstrate persistently abnormal liver function.

To evaluate the causes of liver dysfunction in hemophilia, several centers have performed liver biopsies in patients with persistently abnormal liver enzymes, which are defined as elevations of at least two times the normal for more than 6 months (317–320). Of a total of 35 biopsies that were performed, 17 showed chronic active hepatitis, and 16 showed chronic persistent hepatitis. These studies provided the first concrete evidence that severe forms of liver disease could occur in hemophilia. The patients who underwent biopsies in these studies were generally the most abnormal in each center. To more accurately gauge the liver disease that characterized most hemophiliacs, biopsies were performed on the livers of 18 randomly chosen hemophiliacs with mild or intermittent liver dysfunction (321). Of the 18 patients, only one patient was found to have chronic active hepatitis. The remainder had chronic persistent hepatitis or mild portal inflammation. Thus, most hemophiliacs with multiple transfusions appear to have nonprogressive forms of liver disease.

All forms of transfusion-associated hepatitis have been reported in hemophilia. Approximately 80% of hemophiliacs who require replacement therapy have serologic evidence of exposure to hepatitis B virus (HBV). Antibody to HBV (HBsAb) is present in 60% to 80% of patients, and 10% to 15% of patients are chronic carriers of HBsAg. Because most hemophiliacs have been immunized by exposure to HBV, acute HBV infection is rare in this population. Hepatitis C is now the most common cause of jaundice and acute liver disease in hemophiliacs. Delta hepatitis has also been reported in hemophiliacs.

Hepatitis B vaccine should be given to patients who have never been treated before or who demonstrate negative hepatitis B serology.

Hemolysis

Antibodies to red-cell blood group substances may be present in intermediate purity preparations of factor VIII (322) and can cause red-cell hemolysis in intensively treated patients with blood type A, B, or AB (322,323). Newer ultrapure concentrates are generally free of these antibodies, and hemolysis has not been reported with these products.

Acquired Immunodeficiency Syndrome

Prior to the development of viral inactivation methods, patients with hemophilia were also at risk to develop AIDS (324–333). The source of infection was through the use of clotting factor concentrates that were contaminated with HIV. Retrospective studies suggest that concentrates were contaminated with HIV from approximately 1978 until 1984 or 1985 (329,330), when HIV antibody donor screening and viral inactivation steps during concentrate manufacture were instituted (334–336). HIV infection is more prevalent in patients who received factor VIII concentrates than in those who received factor IX concentrates (332,333). In the United States, 75% to 85% of severe hemophiliacs are infected with HIV.

AIDS in hemophilia is similar to AIDS in other risk groups, except that Kaposi's sarcoma is extremely rare in hemophiliacs. Progression to AIDS in HIV-infected hemophiliacs occurs more rapidly in adults than in children (337). Predictive markers for the development of AIDS are the percentage of CD4+ lymphocytes and viral antigenemia (337–342). *Pneumocystis carinii* pneumonia, cryptococcal meningitis, toxoplasmosis, *Mycobacterium avium*-intracellulare infection, and disseminated cytomegalovirus infection are among the infections that are reported in

HIV-infected hemophiliacs. In addition, septic arthritis, especially in hemophiliacs with joint replacements, and bacterial sinusitis occur more frequently (343).

Recommendations for treatment of HIV-infected patients have been established and are similar to recommendations for other groups.

Excess Activity of Factor V and Factor VIII That Is Associated with Thrombophilia

The most common inherited procoagulant defect in peoples of European descent has recently been identified as a point mutation in the factor V gene, G1691→A, which causes an Arg506→Gln mutation in the A2 domain of mature factor V (347). The defect can be identified in 25% to 60% of patients who are evaluated for unexplained thrombosis. The mutation has a prevalence of 2% to 16% in unselected populations from various regions. Heterozygosity confers a sevenfold increased risk for thrombosis and an 80-fold increased risk for homozygosity (348).

The disorder was discovered as resistance to the anticoagulant action of activated protein C resistance in the plasma of patients with familial thrombosis (349). The biochemical explanation for the thrombotic risk relates to resistance of factor V Leiden to degradation by activated protein C. Arg506 represents one of three activated protein C cleavage sites within factor Va. Cleavage at Arg506 is insufficient to inactivate the molecule. However, this site is the most susceptible of the three sites to initial cleavage by protein C, and its cleavage promotes more rapid cleavage at the other two activated protein C cleavage sites, Arg306 and Arg679 (350). Thus, the length of time that any factor Va molecule can contribute to an active prothrombinase complex is increased. In addition, factor V, together with protein S, serves as a cofactor for inactivation of factor VIIIa by activated protein C (170,351). This cofactor activity of factor V is localized to the C terminal portion of the B domain (352). Because this portion of the molecule is removed in the course of factor V activation by thrombin, factor Va has no cofactor activity toward factor VIIIa degradation. The factor V Leiden mutation ablates the factor V cofactor activity toward degradation of factor VIIIa by activated protein C (353).

Although the most common sites of thrombosis are the deep veins of the lower extremity, factor V Leiden is also associated with increased risk of thrombosis in superficial veins (354), the cerebral veins (355), and, probably, the portal and mesenteric veins. Thrombosis of small superficial veins, such as occurs in patients who lack protein C and are treated with warfarin (Coumadin), is not a frequent thrombotic manifestation. The risk of thrombosis that is conferred by factor V Leiden is substantially increased by other risk factors, such as protein C deficiency (356,357), protein S deficiency (358,359), and the prothrombin 20210A allele. The relationship between arterial thrombosis, particularly in the coronary and cerebral circulation, has been studied extensively. No definite relationship has been identified between the factor V Leiden mutation and arterial thrombosis (360).

The treatment of thrombosis that is associated with factor V Leiden does not differ from the treatment of idiopathic thrombosis, because the risk of subsequent thrombosis is similar (361). Therapy is initiated with heparin, and patients are subsequently managed with warfarin. The duration of warfarin therapy is probably best determined by the clinical setting in which thrombosis occurred. Patients who developed thrombosis without an identifiable predisposing cause, such as immobilization, injury, or surgery, should receive warfarin for at least 1 year and, probably, for the indefinite future, unless bleeding complications occur. In contrast, thrombosis in the setting of immobilization, injury, or surgery may require warfarin therapy for only 6 months, so long as the thrombosis was not life threatening.

Factor VIII and Thrombophilia

Elevated plasma levels of factor VIII are associated with an elevated risk of venous thrombosis (362). In patients of European descent, an elevated factor VIII level may be present in 25%, whereas normal individuals may have a prevalence of 10%. The relative risk of a factor VIII concentration of greater than 150% of normal is two- to fivefold. Although less common than the factor V Leiden mutation, elevated factor VIII is apparently one of the most common thrombophilia-associated coagulation abnormalities. One source of variation in the factor VIII level is variation in the vWF level. The elevated factor VIII levels in pregnancy and inflammatory states are thought to be a consequence of the elevated vWF level. Likewise, the factor VIII level varies with vWF in different blood groups, presumably due to the variable rates of clearance of the carbohydrate antigens (363). The elevated risk of thrombosis in these conditions is apparently related to the elevated factor VIII level, but this association is not easily distinguished from other changes in pregnancy and inflammation. However, factor VIII levels vary within the range of 60% to 250% of the mean (1 unit factor VIII/mL), independent of vWF (364,365). The established risk of thrombosis correlates with this variation, which is not directly related to changes in the vWF level.

The cause of variation in factor VIII levels has not been identified. However, in many of the patients, the association pattern suggests a genetic component (366). No risk of arterial thrombosis has yet been clearly linked to an elevated plasma factor VIII level. Treatment of thrombosis that is associated with elevated plasma factor VIII is governed by the same considerations as idiopathic venous thrombosis or thrombosis that is associated with factor V Leiden.

REFERENCES

1. Kane WH, Davie EW. Blood coagulation factors V and VIII: structural and functional similarities and their relationship to hemorrhagic and thrombotic disorders. *Blood* 1988;71:539–555.
2. Mann KG, Jenny RJ, Krishnaswamy S. Cofactor proteins in the assembly and expression of blood clotting enzyme complexes. *Annu Rev Biochem* 1988; 57:915–956.
3. White GC, Shoemaker CB. Factor VIII gene and hemophilia A. *Blood* 1989;73:1–12.
4. Pittman DD, Kaufman RJ. Structure-function relationships of factor VIII elucidated through recombinant DNA technology. *Thromb Haemost* 1989;61:161–165.
5. Fay PJ. Regulation of factor VIIIa in the intrinsic factor Xase. *Thromb Haemost* 1999;82:193–200.
6. Kaufman RJ, Pipe SW. Regulation of factor VIII expression and activity by von Willebrand factor. *Thromb Haemost* 1999;82:201–208.
7. Spiegel PC Jr, Jacquemin M, Saint-Remy JR, et al. Structure of a factor VIII C2 domain-immunoglobulin G4κ Fab complex: identification of an inhibitory antibody epitope on the surface of factor VIII. *Blood* 2001;98:13–19.
8. Owren PA. The coagulation of blood: investigations of a new clotting factor. *Acta Med Scand* 1947;128[Suppl]:1.
9. Dahlback B. Human coagulation factor V purification and thrombin-catalyzed activation. *J Clin Invest* 1980;66:583–591.
10. Kane WH, Majerus PW. Purification and characterization of human coagulation factor V. *J Biol Chem* 1981;256:1002–1007.
11. Katzmann JA, Nesheim ME, Hibbard LS, et al. Isolation of functional human coagulation factor V by using a hybridoma antibody. *Proc Natl Acad Sci U S A* 1981;78:162–166.
12. Kane WH, Ichinose A, Hagen FS, et al. Cloning of cDNAs coding for the heavy chain region and connecting region of human factor V, a blood coagulation factor with four types of internal repeats. *Biochemistry* 1987;26:6508–6514.
13. Jenny RJ, Pittman DD, Toole JJ, et al. Complete cDNA and derived amino acid sequence of human factor V. *Proc Natl Acad Sci U S A* 1987;84:4846–4850.
14. Patek A, Taylor F. Hemophilia. II. Some properties of a substance obtained from normal human plasma effective in accelerating the coagulation in hemophilic blood. *J Clin Invest* 1937;16:113.

14a. Brinkhous K. A study of the clotting defect in hemophilia: the delayed formation of thrombin. *Am J Med Sci* 1939;198:509.

15. Pavlovsky A. Contribution to the pathogenesis of hemophilia. *Blood* 1947; 2:185–191.

16. Owen WG, Wagner RH. Antihemophilic factor: separation of an active fragment following dissociation by salts or detergents. *Thromb Diath Haemorrh* 1972;27:502–515.

16a. Weiss H, Phillips L, Rosner W. Separation of subunits of antihemophilic factor (AHF) by agarose gel chromatography. *Thrombos Diath Haemorrh* 1972;27: 212.

16b. Zimmerman TS, Edgington T. Molecular immunology of factor VIII. *Annu Rev Med* 1974;25:303.

17. Fass D, Knutson G, Katzmann J. Monoclonal antibodies to porcine factor VIII coagulant and their use in the isolation of active coagulant protein. *Blood* 1982;59:594–600.

18. Toole JJ, Knopf JL, Wozney JM, et al. Molecular cloning of a cDNA encoding human antihemophilic factor. *Nature* 1984;312:342–347.

19. Vehar G, Keyt B, Eaton D, et al. Structure of human factor VIII. *Nature* 1984;312:337–342.

20. White GC II, McMillan CW, Kingdon HS, et al. Use of recombinant antihemophilic factor in the treatment of two patients with classic hemophilia. *N Engl J Med* 1989;320:166–170.

21. Gitschier J, Wood WI, Goralka TM, et al. Characterization of the human factor VIII gene. *Nature* 1984;312:326.

22. Toole JJ, Knopf JL, Wozney JM, et al. Molecular cloning of a cDNA encoding human antihaemophilic factor. *Nature* 1984;312:342.

23. Truett MA, Blacher R, Burke RL, et al. Characterization of the polypeptide composition of human factor VIII:C and the nucleotide sequence and expression of the human cDNA. *DNA* 1986;4:333.

24. Vehar GA, Keyt B, Eaton D, et al. Structure of human factor VIII. *Nature* 1984;312:337.

25. Hamer RJ, Koedam JA, Beeser-Visser NH, et al. Factor VIII binds to von Willebrand factor via its Mr 80,000 light chain. *Eur J Biochem* 1987;166:37.

26. Foster PA, Fulcher CA, Houghten RA, et al. An immunogenic region within residues Val1670-Glu1684 of factor VIII light chain induces antibodies which inhibit binding of factor VIII to von Willebrand factor. *J Biol Chem* 1988;263:5230.

27. Pittman DD, Wasley LC, Murray BL, et al. Analysis of structural requirements for factor VIII function using site directed mutagenesis. *Thromb Haemost* 1987;58:344(abst).

28. Rydén L, Björk I. Reinvestigation of some physicochemical and chemical properties of human ceruloplasmin (ferroxidase). *Biochemistry* 1976;15:3411.

29. Sudhakar K, Fay PJ. Effects of copper on the structure and function of factor VIII subunits: evidence for an auxiliary role for copper ions in cofactor activity. *Biochemistry* 1998;37:6874–6882.

30. Stubbs J, Lekutis C, Singer K, et al. cDNA cloning of a mouse mammary epithelial cell surface protein reveals the existence of epidermal growth factor-like domains linked to factor VIII-like sequences. *Proc Natl Acad Sci U S A* 1990;87:8417–8421.

31. Bloom JW. The interaction of rDNA factor VIII, factor VIIIdes979–1562 and factor VIIIdes979–1562-derived peptides with phospholipid. *Thromb Res* 1987; 48:439.

32. Arai M, Scandella D, Hoyer LW. Molecular basis of factor VIII inhibiting human antibodies: antibodies that bind to the factor VIII light chain prevent the interaction of factor VIII with phospholipid. *J Clin Invest* 1989;83:1978.

33. Foster PA, Fulcher CA, Houghten RA, et al. Synthetic factor VIII peptides with amino acid sequences contained within the C2 domain of factor VIII inhibit factor VIII binding to phosphatidylserine. *Thromb Haemost* 1989;62:34(abst).

34. Vehar GA, Davie EW. Preparation and properties of bovine factor VIII. *Biochemistry* 1980;19:401.

35. Fass DN, Knutson GJ, Katzmann JA. Monoclonal antibodies to porcine factor VIII coagulant and their use in the isolation of active coagulant protein. *Blood* 1982;59:594.

36. Fulcher CA, Zimmerman TS. Characterization of the human factor VIII procoagulant protein with a heterologous precipitating antibody. *Proc Natl Acad Sci U S A* 1982;79:1648.

37. Pemberton S, Lindley P, Zaitsev V, et al. A molecular model for the triplicated A domains of human factor VIII based on the crystal structure of human ceruloplasmin. *Blood* 1997;89:2413–2421.

38. Gilbert GE, Kaufman RJ, Arena AA, et al. Four hydrophobic amino acids in the factor VIII C2 domain are constituents of the membrane-binding and von Willebrand factor-binding motif. *J Biol Chem* 2002;277:6374–6381.

39. Dahlbäck B, Hansson C, Islam MQ, et al. Assignment of gene for coagulation factor V to chromosome 1 in man and chromosome 13 in rat. *Somat Cell Mol Genet* 1988;14:509.

40. Cripe LD, Moore KD, Kane WH. Structure of the gene for human coagulation factor V. *Biochemistry* 1992;31:3777.

41. Kane WH, Davie EW. Cloning of a cDNA coding for human factor V: a blood coagulation factor homologous to factor VIII and ceruloplasmin. *Proc Natl Acad Sci U S A* 1986;83:6800.

42. Jenny RJ, Pittman DD, Toole JJ, et al. Complete cDNA and amino acid sequence of human factor V. *Proc Natl Acad Sci U S A* 1987;84:4846.

43. Kane WH, Ichinose A, Hagen FS, et al. Cloning of cDNAs coding for the heavy chain region and connecting region of human factor V: a blood coagulation factor with four types of internal repeats. *Biochemistry* 1987;26:6508.

44. Fass DN, Hewick RM, Knutson GJ, et al. Internal duplication and sequence homology in factors V and VIII. *Proc Natl Acad Sci U S A* 1985;82:1688.

45. Mann KG, Lawler CM, Vehar GA, et al. Coagulation factor V contains copper ions. *J Biol Chem* 1984;259:12949.

46. Saraswathi S, Rawala R, Colman RW. The subunit structure of bovine factor V: influence of proteolysis during blood coagulation. *J Biol Chem* 1978;253: 1024.

47. Esmon CT. The subunit structure of thrombin-activated factor V. *J Biol Chem* 1979;254:964.

48. Nesheim ME, Myrmel KH, Hibbard L, et al. Isolation and characterization of single chain bovine factor V. *J Biol Chem* 1979;254:508.

49. Kane WH, Majerus PW. Isolation and characterization of human coagulation factor V. *J Biol Chem* 1981;256:1002.

50. Gumprecht JG, Colman RW. Roles of sialic acid in the function of bovine factor V. *Arch Biochem Biophys* 1975;169:278.

51. Saraswathi S, Colman RW. Role of galactose in bovine factor V. *J Biol Chem* 1975;250:8111.

52. Mann KG, Nesheim ME, Tracy PB. Molecular weight of undegraded factor V. *Biochemistry* 1981;20:28.

53. Dahlbäck B. Bovine coagulation factor V visualized with electron microscopy: ultrastructure of the isolated activated forms and of the activation fragments. *J Biol Chem* 1986;261:9495.

54. Macedo-Ribeiro S, Bode W, Huber R, et al. Crystal structures of the membrane-binding C2 domain of human coagulation factor V. *Nature* 1999;402: 434–439.

55. Kim SW, Quinn-Allen MA, Camp JT, et al. Identification of functionally important amino acid residues within the C2-domain of human factor V using alanine-scanning mutagenesis. *Biochemistry* 2000;39:1951–1958.

56. Villoutreix BO, Dahlback B. Structural investigation of the A domains of human blood coagulation factor V by molecular modeling. *Protein Sci* 1998;7:1317–1325.

57. Mosesson MW, Fass DN, Lollar P, et al. Structural model of porcine factor VIII and factor VIIIa molecules based on scanning transmission electron microscope (STEM) images and STEM mass analysis. *J Clin Invest* 1990;85: 1983–1990.

58. Nichols WC, Seligsohn U, Zivelin A, et al. Linkage of combined factors V and VIII deficiency to chromosome 18q by homozygosity mapping. *J Clin Invest* 1997;99:596–601.

59. Nichols WC, Seligsohn U, Zivelin A, et al. Mutations in the ER-Golgi intermediate compartment protein ERGIC-53 cause combined deficiency of coagulation factors V and VIII. *Cell* 1998;93:61–70.

60. Moussalli M, Pipe SW, Hauri HP, et al. Mannose-dependent endoplasmic reticulum (ER)–Golgi intermediate compartment-53-mediated ER to Golgi trafficking of coagulation factors V and VIII. *J Biol Chem* 1999;274:32539–32542.

61. Neerman-Arbez M, Johnson KM, Morris MA, et al. Molecular analysis of the ERGIC-53 gene in 35 families with combined factor V-factor VIII deficiency. *Blood* 1999;93:2253–2260.

62. Nichols WC, Terry VH, Wheatley MA, et al. ERGIC-53 gene structure and mutation analysis in 19 combined factors V and VIII deficiency families. *Blood* 1999;93:2261–2266.

63. Webster WP, Zukoski CF, Hutchin P, et al. Plasma factor VIII synthesis and control as revealed by canine organ transplantation. *Am J Physiol* 1971;220:1147.

64. Bontempo FA, Lewis JH, Gorenc TJ, et al. Liver transplantation in hemophilia A. *Blood* 1987;69:1721.

65. Gibas A, Dienstag JL, Schafer AI. Cure of hemophilia A by orthotopic liver transplantation. *Gastroenterology* 1988;95:192.

66. Wion KL, Kelly D, Summerfield JA, et al. Distribution of factor VIII mRNA and antigen in human liver and other tissues. *Nature* 1985;317:726.

67. Zelechowska MG, van Mourik JA, Brodniewicz-Proba T. Ultrastructural localization of factor VIII procoagulant antigen in human liver hepatocytes. *Nature* 1985;317:729.

68. van der Kwast TH, Stel HV, Cristen E, et al. Localization of factor VIII-procoagulant antigen: an immunohistochemical survey of the human body using monoclonal antibodies. *Blood* 1986;67:222.

69. Kadhom N, Wolfrom C, Gautier M, et al. Factor VIII procoagulant antigen in human tissues. *Thromb Haemost* 1988;59:289.

70. Wood WI, Capon DJ, Simonsen CC, et al. Expression of active human factor VIII from recombinant DNA clones. *Nature* 1984;312:330.

71. Mannucci PM, Ruggeri ZM, Pareti FI, et al. 1-Deamino-8-D-arginine vasopressin: a new pharmacological approach to the management of hemophilia and von Willebrand's disease. *Lancet* 1977;1:869.

72. de la Fuente B, Kasper CK, Rickles FR, et al. Response of patients with mild and moderate hemophilia A and von Willebrand's disease to treatment with desmopressin. *Ann Intern Med* 1985;103:6.

73. Ingram GI, Vaughan-Jones R. The rise in clotting factor VIII induced in man by adrenaline: effect of α- and β-blockers. *J Physiol* 1966;187:447–454.

74. Holmberg L, Nilsson IM. AHF related protein in clinical practice. *Scand J Haematol* 1974;12:221.

75. Preston AE, Barr A. The plasma concentration of factor VIII in the normal population: the effects of age, sex and ABO blood groups. *Br J Haematol* 1965; 10:238.

76. McCallum CJ, Peake IR, Newcombe RG, et al. Factor VIII levels and blood group antigens. *Thromb Haemost* 1983;50:757.

77. Graham JB, Rizza CR, Chediak J, et al. Carrier detection in hemophilia A: a cooperative international study. I. The carrier phenotype. *Blood* 1986;67:1554.

78. Gill JC, Endress-Brooks J, Bauer PJ, et al. The effect of ABO blood group on the diagnosis of von Willebrand disease. *Blood* 1987;69:1691.

79. Orstavik KH, Kornstad L, Reisner HM, et al. Possible effect of secretor locus on plasma concentrations of factor VIII and von Willebrand factor. *Blood* 1989;73:990.

80. Eaton DL, Hass PE, Riddle L, et al. Characterization of recombinant human factor VIII. *J Biol Chem* 1987;262:3285.

81. Kaufman RJ, Wasley LC, Dorner AJ. Synthesis, processing, and secretion of recombinant human factor VIII expressed in mammalian cells. *J Biol Chem* 1988;263:6352.

82. Tuddenham E, Lane R, Rotblat F, et al. Response to infusions of polyelectrolyte fractionated human factor VIII concentrate in human hemophilia A and von Willebrand's disease. *Br J Haematol* 1982;52:259.

83. Over J, Sixma J, Doucet-de-Bruine M, et al. Survival of 125iodine-labeled factor VIII in normals and patients with classic hemophilia. *J Clin Invest* 1978;62:223.

84. Weiss H, Sussman I, Hoyer L. Stabilization of factor VIII in plasma by the von Willebrand factor. Studies on posttransfusion and dissociated factor VIII and in patients with von Willebrand's disease. *J Clin Invest* 1977;60:390–404.

85. Lollar P, Parker CG. Stoichiometry of the porcine factor VIII–von Willebrand factor association. *J Biol Chem* 1987;262:17572.

86. Tuddenham EG, Lane RS, Rotblat F, et al. Responses to infusions of polyelectrolyte fractionated human factor VIII concentrate in human haemophilia A and von Willebrand's disease. *Br J Haematol* 1982;52:259.

87. Brinkhous KM, Sandberg H, Garris JR, et al. Purified human factor VIII procoagulant protein: comparative hemostatic response after infusions into hemophilic and von Willebrand disease dogs. *Proc Natl Acad Sci U S A* 1985;82:8752.

88. Turecek PL, Gritsch H, Pichler L, et al. In vivo characterization of recombinant von Willebrand factor in dogs with von Willebrand disease. *Blood* 1997;90:3555–3567.

89. Sawada Y, Fass DN, Katzmann JA, et al. Hemostatic plug formation in normal and von Willebrand pigs: the effect of the administration of cryoprecipitate and a monoclonal antibody to Willebrand factor. *Blood* 1986;67:1229–1239.

90. Denis C, Nassia M, Rayburn H, et al. Generation and characterization of von Willebrand factor-deficient mice. *Blood* 1997;90:429(abst).

91. Morfini M, Mannucci PM, Tenconi PM, et al. Pharmacokinetics of monoclonally purified and recombinant factor VIII in patients with severe von Willebrand disease. *Thromb Haemost* 1993;70:270–272.

92. Saenko EL, Yakhyaev AV, Mikhailenko I, et al. Role of the low density lipoprotein-related protein receptor in mediation of factor VIII catabolism. *J Biol Chem* 1999;274:37685–37692.

93. Lenting PJ, Neels JG, van den Berg BM, et al. The light chain of factor VIII comprises a binding site for low density lipoprotein receptor-related protein. *J Biol Chem* 1999;274:23734–23739.

94. Tracy PB, Eide LL, Bowie EJW, et al. Radioimmunoassay of factor V in human plasma and platelets. *Blood* 1982;60:59.

95. Tracy PB, Eide LL, Mann KG. Human prothrombinase complex assembly and function on isolated peripheral blood cell populations. *J Biol Chem* 1985;260:2119.

96. Cerveny TJ, Fass DN, Mann KG. Synthesis of coagulation factor V by cultured aortic endothelium. *Blood* 1984;63:1467.

97. Wilson DB, Salem HH, Mruk JS, et al. Biosynthesis of coagulation factor V by a human hepatocellular carcinoma cell line. *J Clin Invest* 1984;73:654.

98. Rothberger H, McGee MP. Generation of coagulation factor V activity by cultured rabbit alveolar macrophages. *J Exp Med* 1984;160:1880.

99. Gewirtz AM, Keefer M, Doshi K, et al. Biology of megakaryocyte factor V. *Blood* 1986;67:1639.

100. Nichols WL, Hewick RM, Knutson GJ, et al. Identification of human megakaryocyte coagulation factor V. *Blood* 1985;65:1396.

101. Wencel-Drake JD, Dahlbäck B, White JG, et al. Ultrastructural localization of coagulation factor V in human platelets. *Blood* 1986;68:244.

102. Chesney CM, Pifer DD, Colman RW. Subcellular localization and secretion of factor V from human platelets. *Thromb Res* 1983;29:75.

103. Hayward CP, Furmaniak-Kazmierczak E, Cieutat AM, et al. Factor V is complexed with multimerin in resting platelet lysates and colocalizes with multimerin in platelet alpha-granules. *J Biol Chem* 1995;270:19217–19224.

104. Viskup RW, Tracy PB, Mann KG. The isolation of human platelet factor V. *Blood* 1987;69:1188.

105. Hayward CP, Cramer EM, Song Z, et al. Studies of multimerin in human endothelial cells. *Blood* 1998;91:1304–1317.

106. Rodgers GM, Cong J, Goll DE, et al. Activation of coagulation factor V by calcium-dependent protease. *Biochim Biophys Acta* 1987;929:263.

107. Bradford HN, Annamalai A, Doshi K, et al. Factor V is activated and cleaved by platelet calpain: comparison with thrombin proteolysis. *Blood* 1988;71:388.

108. Mann KG, Nesheim ME, Church WR, et al. Surface-dependent reactions of the vitamin K–dependent enzyme complexes. *Blood* 1990;76:1–16.

109. Kane WH, Davie EW. Blood coagulation factors V and VIII: structural and functional similarities and their relationship to hemorrhagic and thrombotic disorders. *Blood* 1988;71:539–555.

110. Fay PJ, Koshibu K. The A2 subunit of factor VIIIa modulates the active site of factor IXa. *J Biol Chem* 1998;273:19049–19054.

111. Duffy E, Parker E, Mutucumarana V, et al. Binding of factor VIIIa and factor VIII to factor IXa on phospholipid vesicles. *J Biol Chem* 1992;267:17006–17011.

112. Lenting PJ, van de Loo JW, Donath MJ, et al. The sequence Glu1811-Lys1818 of human blood coagulation factor VIII comprises a binding site for activated factor IX. *J Biol Chem* 1996;271:1935–1940.

113. Christophe OD, Lenting PJ, Kolkman JA, et al. Blood coagulation factor IX residues Glu78 and Arg94 provide a link between both epidermal growth factor-like domains that is crucial in the interaction with factor VIII light chain. *J Biol Chem* 1998;273:222–227.

114. Gilbert GE, Arena AA. Activation of the factor VIIIa–factor IXa enzyme complex of blood coagulation by membranes containing phosphatidyl-L-serine. *J Biol Chem* 1996;271:11120–11125.

115. Armstrong S, Husten J, Esmon C, et al. The active site of membrane-bound meizothrombin: a fluorescence determination of its distance from the phospholipid surface and its conformational sensitivity to calcium and factor Va. *J Biol Chem* 1990;265:6210–6218.

116. Giesen P, Willems G, Hermens W. Production of thrombin by the prothrombinase complex is regulated by membrane-mediated transport of prothrombin. *J Biol Chem* 1991;266:1379–1382.

117. Husten E, Esmon C, Johnson A. The active site of blood coagulation factor Xa. *J Biol Chem* 1987;262:12953–12961.

118. Mutucumarana V, Duffy E, Lollar P, et al. The active site of factor IXa is located far above the membrane surface and its conformation is altered upon association with factor VIIIa: a fluorescence study. *J Biol Chem* 1992;267:17012–17021.

119. McFarlane R. An enzyme cascade in the blood clotting mechanism and its function as a biochemical amplifier. *Nature* 1964;202:498.

120. Davie E, Ratnoff O. Waterfall sequence for intrinsic blood coagulation. *Science* 1964;145:1310.

121. Pusey ML, Mayer LD, Wei GJ, et al. Kinetic and hydrodynamic analysis of blood clotting factor V-membrane binding. *Biochemistry* 1982;21:5262.

122. Bardelle C, Furie B, Furie BC, et al. Kinetic studies of factor VIII binding to phospholipid membranes indicate a complex binding process. *J Biol Chem* 1993;268:8815–8824.

123. Krishnaswamy S, Jones K, Mann K. Prothrombinase complex assembly: kinetic mechanism of enzyme assembly on phospholipid vesicles. *J Biol Chem* 1988;263:3823–3834.

124. Higgins D, Callahan P, Prendergast F, et al. Lipid mobility in the assembly and expression of the activity of the prothrombinase complex. *J Biol Chem* 1985;260:3604–3612.

125. Nesheim ME, Furmaniakkazmierczak E, Henin C, et al. On the existence of platelet receptors for factor-V(a) and factor-VIII(a). *Thromb Haemost* 1993;70:80–86.

126. Phillips JE, Rooney MM, Lord ST, et al. Expression of factor VIII binding sites on thrombin-stimulated platelets is enhanced by fibrin. *Blood* 1998;92[Suppl]:30a.

127. Tracy P, Peterson J, Nesheim M, et al. Interaction of coagulation factor V and factor Va with platelets. *J Biol Chem* 1979;254:10345.

128. Fadok VA, Voelker DR, Campbell PA, et al. Exposure of phosphatidylserine on the surface of apoptotic lymphocytes triggers specific recognition and removal by macrophages. *J Immunol* 1992;148:2207–2216.

129. Dachary-Prigent J, Freyssinet JM, Pasquet JM, et al. Annexin V as a probe of aminophospholipid exposure and platelet membrane vesiculation: a flow cytometry study showing a role for free sulfhydryl groups. *Blood* 1993;81:2554–2565.

130. Gilbert GE, Drinkwater D. Specific membrane binding of factor VIII is mediated by O-phospho-L-serine, a moiety of phosphatidylserine. *Biochemistry* 1993;32:9577–9585.

131. Comfurius P, Smeets EF, Willems GM, et al. Assembly of the prothrombinase complex on lipid vesicles depends on the stereochemical configuration of the polar head group of phosphatidylserine. *Biochemistry* 1994;33:10319–10324.

132. Gilbert GE, Furie BC, Furie B. Binding of human factor VIII to phospholipid vesicles. *J Biol Chem* 1990;265:815–822.

133. Gilbert GE, Drinkwater D, Barter S, et al. Specificity of phosphatidylserine-containing membrane binding sites for factor VIII: studies with model membranes supported by glass microspheres (liposphères). *J Biol Chem* 1992;267:15861–15868.

134. Gilbert GE, Arena AA. Phosphatidylethanolamine induces high affinity binding sites for factor VIII on membranes containing phosphatidyl-L-serine. *J Biol Chem* 1995;270:18500–18505.

135. Kung C, Hayes E, Mann KG. A membrane-mediated catalytic event in prothrombin activation. *J Biol Chem* 1994;269:25838–25848.

136. Gilbert GE, Arena AA. Partial activation of the factor VIIIa–factor IXa enzyme complex by dihexanoic phosphatidylserine at submicellar concentrations. *Biochemistry* 1997;36:10768–10776.

137. Gilbert GE, Brahmavar AS. Phospholipid membranes alter the configuration of the factor VIIIa–Factor IXa complex. *Blood* 1999;94:456a.

138. van Dieijen G, Tans G, Rosing J, et al. The role of phospholipid and factor VIIIa in the activation of bovine factor X. *J Biol Chem* 1987;256:3433.

139. Rapaport SI, Shiffman S, Patch MJ, et al. The importance of activation of antihemophilic globulin and proaccelerin by traces of thrombin in the generation of intrinsic prothrombinase activity. *Blood* 1963;21:221.

140. Knutson GJ, Fass DN. Porcine factor VIII:C prepared by affinity interaction with von Willebrand factor and heterologous antibodies: sodium dodecyl sulfate polyacrylamide gel analysis. *Blood* 1982;59:615.

141. Hoyer LW, Trabold NC. The effect of thrombin on human factor VIII. Cleavage of the factor VIII procoagulant protein during activation. *J Lab Clin Med* 1981;97:50.

142. Griffith MJ, Reisner HM, Lundblad RL, et al. Measurement of human factor IXa activity in an isolated factor X activation system. *Thromb Res* 1982;27:289.

143. Hultin MB, Jesty J. The activation and inactivation of human factor VIII by thrombin: effect of inhibitors of thrombin. *Blood* 1981;57:476.

144. Nordfang O, Ezban M. Generation of active coagulation factor VIII from isolated subunits. *J Biol Chem* 1988;263:1115.

145. Fay PJ. Reconstitution of human factor VIII from isolated subunits. *Arch Biochem Biophys* 1988;262:525.

146. Toole JJ, Pittman DD, Orr EC, et al. A large region (95 kDa) of human factor VIII is dispensable for in vitro procoagulant activity. *Proc Natl Acad Sci U S A* 1986;83:5939.

147. Eaton DL, Wood WI, Eaton D, et al. Construction and characterization of an active factor VIII variant lacking the central one-third of the molecule. *Biochemistry* 1986;25:8343.

148. Pavirani A, Meulien P, Harrer H, et al. Two independent domains of factor VII co-expressed using recombinant vaccinia viruses have procoagulant activity. *Biochem Biophys Res Commun* 1987;145:234.

149. Burke RL, Pachl C, Quiroga M, et al. The functional domains of coagulation factor VIII:C. *J Biol Chem* 1986;261:12574.

150. Fulcher CA, Gardiner JE, Griffin JH, et al. Proteolytic inactivation of human factor VIII procoagulant protein by activated protein C and its analogy with factor V. *Blood* 1984;63:486.

151. Fulcher CA, Roberts JR, Zimmerman TS. Thrombin proteolysis of purified factor VIII procoagulant protein: correlation of activation with generation of a specific polypeptide. *Blood* 1983;61:807.

152. Fay P, Anderson MT, Chavin SI, et al. The size of human factor VIII heterodimers and the effects produced by thrombin. *Biochim Biophys Acta* 1986;871:268.

153. Eaton D, Rodriguez H, Vehar GA. Proteolytic processing of human factor VIII: correlation of specific cleavages by thrombin, factor Xa, and activated protein C with activation and inactivation of factor VIII coagulant activity. *Biochemistry* 1986;25:505.

154. Pittman DD, Kaufman RJ. Proteolytic requirements for thrombin activation of anti-hemophilic factor (factor VIII). *Proc Natl Acad Sci U S A* 1988;85:2429.

155. Ware JA, Toomey JR, Stafford DW. Localization of a factor VIII-inhibiting antibody epitope to a region between residues 338 and 362 of factor VIII heavy chain. *Proc Natl Acad Sci U S A* 1988;85:3165.

156. Shima M, Fulcher CA, de Graf Mahoney S, et al. Localization of the binding site for a factor VIII activity neutralizing antibody to amino acid residues Asp1663-Ser1669. *J Biol Chem* 1988;263:10198.

157. Gitschier J, Kogan S, Levinson B, et al. Mutations of the factor VIII cleavage sites in hemophilia A. *Blood* 1988;72:1022.

158. Smith CM, Hanahan DJ. The activation of factor V by factor Xa or alpha-chymotrypsin and comparison with thrombin and RVV-V action: an improved factor V isolation procedure. *Biochemistry* 1976;15:1830.

159. Esmon CT. The use of proteolytic enzymes in establishing the structure and activation pathways of factor V. In: Mann KG, Taylor FB, eds. *The regulation of coagulation*. New York: Elsevier Science, 1980:137.

160. Suzuki K, Dahlbäck B, Stenflo J. Thrombin-catalyzed activation of human coagulation factor V. *J Biol Chem* 1982;257:6556.

161. Miletich JP, Majerus DW, Majerus PW. Patients with congenital factor V deficiency have decreased factor Xa binding sites on their platelets. *J Clin Invest* 1978;62:824.

162. Tracy PB, Giles AR, Mann KG, et al. Factor V (Quebec): a bleeding diathesis associated with a qualitative platelet factor V deficiency. *J Clin Invest* 1984;74:1221.

163. Nesheim ME, Nichols WL, Cole TL, et al. Isolation and study of an acquired inhibitor of human coagulation factor V. *J Clin Invest* 1986;77:405.

164. Tucker MM, Foster WB, Katzmann JA, et al. A monoclonal antibody which inhibits the factor Va:factor Xa interaction. *J Biol Chem* 1983;258:1210.

165. Tucker MM, Nesheim ME, Mann KG. Differentiation of enzyme and substrate binding in the prothrombinase complex. *Biochemistry* 1983;22:4540.

166. Guinto ER, Esmon CT. Loss of prothrombin and of factor Xa-factor Va interactions upon inactivation of factor Va by activated protein C. *J Biol Chem* 1984;259:13986.

167. Walker FJ, Sexton PW, Esmon CT. The inhibition of blood coagulation by activated protein C through the selective inactivation of activated factor V. *Biochim Biophys Acta* 1979;571:333.

168. Suzuki K, Stenflo J, Dahlbäck B, et al. Inactivation of human factor V by activated protein C. *J Biol Chem* 1983;258:1914.

169. Odegaard B, Mann KG. Proteolysis of factor Va by factor Xa and activated protein C. *J Biol Chem* 1987;262:11233.

170. Dahlbäck B, Hildebrand B. Inherited resistance to activated protein C is corrected by anticoagulant cofactor activity found to be a property of factor V. *Proc Natl Acad Sci U S A* 1994;91:1396.

171. Department of Health, Education, and Welfare: National Heart, Lung, and Blood Institute study to evaluate the supply-demand relationships for AHF and PTC through 1980. Washington: US Government Printing Office, 1977.

172. Ramgren O. A clinical and medico-social study of haemophilia in Sweden. *Acta Med Scand* 1962;171:759.

173. Graham JB. Biochemical genetics of blood coagulation. *Am J Hum Genet* 1956;8:63.

174. Kerr CB. Genetics of human blood coagulation. *J Med Genet* 1965;2:254.

175. Biggs R, Rizza CR. The sporadic case of hemophilia A. *Lancet* 1979;2:431.

176. Bernardi F, Marchetti G, Bertagnolo V, et al. RFLP analysis in families with sporadic hemophilia A: estimate of the mutation ratio in male and female gametes. *Hum Genet* 1987;76:253.

177. Holmberg L. Genetic studies in a family with testicular feminization, haemophilia and color blindness. *Clin Genet* 1972;3:253.

178. Andrejev YN, Korenevskaya MI, Rutbert RA, et al. Haemophilia A in a patient with testicular feminization. *Thromb Diath Haemorrh* 1965;14:332.

179. Bithell TC, Pizzaro A, Macdiarmid WD. Variant of factor IX deficiency in females with 45X Turner's syndrome. *Blood* 1970;36:169.

180. Gilchrist GS, Hammond D, Mecnyk J. Hemophilia A in a phenotypically normal female with XX/XO mosaicism. *N Engl J Med* 1965;273:1402.

181. Piétu G, Thomas-Maison N, Sié P, et al. Haemophilia A in a female: study of a family using intragenic and extragenic restriction site polymorphism. *Thromb Haemost* 1988;60:102.

182. Kingsley CS. Familial factor V deficiency: the pattern of heredity. *QJM* 1954;23:323.

183. Hoyer LW, Breckenridge RT. Immunologic studies of antihemophilic factor (AHF, factor VIII): cross-reacting material in a genetic variant of hemophilia A. *Blood* 1968;32:962.

184. Denson KW, Biggs RG, Haddon ME, et al. Two types of haemophilia (A+ and A-): a study of 48 cases. *Br J Haematol* 1969;17:163.

185. Reisner HM, Price WA, Blatt PM, et al. Factor VIII coagulant antigen in hemophilic plasma: a comparison of five alloantibodies. *Blood* 1980;56:615.

186. Gitschier J, Wood WI, Tuddenham EG, et al. Detection and sequence of mutations in the factor VIII gene of haemophiliacs. *Nature* 1985;315:425.

187. Antonarakis SE, Waber PG, Kittur SD, et al. Hemophilia A: detection of molecular defects and of carriers by DNA analysis. *N Engl J Med* 1985;313:842.

188. Gitschier J, Wood WI, Shuman MA, et al. Identification of a missense mutation in the factor VIII gene of a mild hemophiliac. *Science* 1986;232:1415.

189. Youssoufian H, Kazazian HH Jr, Phillips DG, et al. Recurrent mutations in haemophilia A give evidence for CpG mutation hotspots. *Nature* 1986;324:380.

190. Youssoufian H, Antonarakis SE, Aronis S, et al. Characterization of five partial deletions of the factor VIII gene. *Proc Natl Acad Sci U S A* 1987;84:3772.

191. Youssoufian H, Antonarakis SE, Bell W, et al. Nonsense and missense mutations in hemophilia A: estimation of the relative mutation rate at CG dinucleotides. *Am J Hum Genet* 1988;42:718.

192. Higuchi M, Kochhan L, Schwab R, et al. Detection of mutations of hemophilia A. *Thromb Haemost* 1987;58:336.

193. Levinson B, Janco RL, Phillips J III, et al. A novel missense mutation in the factor VIII gene identified by analysis of amplified hemophilia DNA sequences. *Nucleic Acids Res* 1987;15:9797.

194. Antonarakis SE. Hemophilia A persistence and gene mutational vulnerability. *Hosp Pract* 1987;22:93.

195. Youssoufian H, Wong C, Aronis S, et al. Moderately severe hemophilia A resulting from Glu→Gly substitution in exon 7 of the factor VIII gene. *Am J Hum Genet* 1988;42:867–871.

196. Mikami S, Nishimura T, Naka H, et al. Nonsense mutation in factor VIII gene of a severe hemophiliac patient with anti-factor VIII antibody. *Jpn J Hum Genet* 1988;33:409.

197. Inaba H, Fujimaki M, Kazazian HH. Mild hemophilia A resulting from Arg-to-Leu substitutions in exon 26 of the factor VIII gene. *Hum Genet* 1989;81:335.

198. Bernardi F, Volinia S, Patracchini P, et al. A recurrent missense mutation (Arg→Glu) and a partial deletion in factor VIII gene causing severe hemophilia A. *Br J Haematol* 1989;71:271–276.

199. Din N, Schwartz M, Kruse T, et al. Factor VIII gene-specific probes used to study heritage and molecular defects in hemophilia A. *Res Clin Lab* 1986;16:182.

200. Casarino L, Pecorara M, Mori PG, et al. Molecular basis for hemophilia A in Italians. *Res Clin Lab* 1986;16:227.

201. Bardoni B, Sampietro M, Romano M, et al. Characterization of a partial deletion of the factor VIII gene in a haemophiliac with inhibitor. *Hum Genet* 1988;79:86.

202. Lillicrap D, Taylor SA, Grover H, et al. Genetic analysis in hemophilia A: identification of a large F. VIII gene deletion in a patient with high titre antibodies to human and porcine F. VIII. *Blood* 1986;68:337a.

203. Youssoufian H, Patel A, Phillips D, et al. Hemophilia A: recurrent mutations and an unusual deletion. *Pediatr Res* 1987;21:296A.

204. Mikami S, Nishimura T, Naka H, et al. A deletion involving intron 13 and exon 14 of factor VIII gene in a haemophiliac with anti-factor VIII antibody. *Jpn J Hum Genet* 1988;33:401.

205. Youssoufian H, Kasper CK, Phillips DG, et al. Restriction endonuclease mapping of six novel deletions of the factor VIII gene in hemophilia A. *Hum Genet* 1988;80:143.

206. Lakich D, Kazazian HH Jr, Antonarakis SE, et al. Inversions disrupting the factor VIII gene are a common cause of severe haemophilia A. *Nat Genet* 1993;5:236.

207. Naylor J, Brinke A, Hassock S, et al. Characteristic mRNA abnormality found in half the patients with severe haemophilia A is due to large DNA inversions. *Hum Mol Genet* 1993;2:1773.

208. Barker D, Schafer M, White R. Restriction sites containing CpG show a higher frequency of polymorphism in human DNA. *Cell* 1984;36:131.

209. Kazazian HH Jr, Wong C, Youssoufian H, et al. Haemophilia A resulting from de novo insertion of L1 sequences represents a novel mechanism for mutation in man. *Nature* 1988;332:164.

210. Seeler RA. Parahemophilia: factor V deficiency. *Med Clin North Am* 1972;56:119.

211. Feinstein DI, Rapaport SI, McGehee WG, et al. Factor V anticoagulants: clinical, biochemical and immunological observations. *J Clin Invest* 1970;49:1578.

212. Fratantoni JW, Hilgartner MW, Nachman RL. Nature of the defect in congenital factor V deficiency: study in a patient with acquired circulating anticoagulant. *Blood* 1972;39:751.

213. Giddings JC, Shearn SA, Bloom AL. The immunological localization of factor V in human tissue. *Br J Haematol* 1975;29:57.

214. Chiu HC, Whitaker E, Colman RW. Heterogeneity of human factor V deficiency: evidence for the existence of an antigen-positive variance. *J Clin Invest* 1983;72:493.
215. Hultin MD, Eyster ME. Combined factor V-VIII deficiency: a case report with studies of factor V and VIII activation by thrombin. *Blood* 1981;58:983.
216. Seligsohn U, Zivelin A, Zwang E. Combined factor V and factor VIII deficiency among non-Ashkenazi Jews. *N Engl J Med* 1982;307:1191.
217. Girolami A, Violante M, Cella G, et al. Combined deficiency of factor V and factor VIII: a report of another case. *Blut* 1976;32:415.
218. Girolami A, Brunetti A, de Mario L. Congenital combined factor V and factor VIII deficiency in a male born from brother-sister incest. *Blut* 1974;28:33.
219. Cimo PL, Moake JL, Gonzalez MF, et al. Inherited combined deficiency of factor V and factor VIII: report of a case with normal factor VIII antigen and ristocetin-induced platelet aggregation. *Am J Hematol* 1977;2:385.
220. Oeri J, Matter M, Isenschmid H. Angeborener mangel an factor V (parahemophilie) verbunden mit echter haemophilia A bie zwei brüdern. *Bibl Pediatr* 1954;58:575.
221. Iverson T, Bastrup-Madsen P. Congenital familial deficiency of factor V (parahemophilia) combined with deficiency of anti-hemophilic globulin. *Br J Haematol* 1956;2:265.
222. Seibert RH, Margolius A, Ratnoff OD. Observation on hemophilia, parahemophilia and co-existent hemophilia and parahemophilia. *J Lab Clin Med* 1958;52:449.
223. Jones JM, Rizza CR, Hardisty RM, et al. Combined deficiency of factor V and factor VIII (antihemophilic globulin): a report of three cases. *Br J Haematol* 1962;8:120.
224. Parr D, Egli H, Christians JM, et al. Kongenitaler mangel von faktor V and faktor VIII. *Thromb Diath Haemorrh* 1967;17:194.
225. Gobbi F, Ascari E, Barbieri U. Congenital combined deficiency of factor VIII (AHF) and factor V (proaccelerin) in two siblings. *Thromb Diath Haemorrh* 1967;17:194.
226. DeVries JT. Hemorragische diathese dorr tekort aan faktor V (proaccelerine). *Ned Tijdschr Geneeskd* 1968;12:741.
227. Ménaché D, Hakin S. Un nouveau cas de deficit associé en facteur VIII et V. *Pathol Biol* 1968;16:969.
228. Saito H, Shioya H, Koie K, et al. Congenital combined deficiency of factor V and factor VIII: a case report and the effect transfusion of normal plasma and hemophilic blood. *Thromb Diath Haemorrh* 1969;22:316.
229. Seligsohn U, Ramot B. Combined factor V and factor VIII deficiency: report of four cases. *Br J Haematol* 1969;16:475.
230. Smit-Sibinga CT, Gökemeyer JD, ten Kate LP, et al. Combined deficiency of factor V and factor VIII: report of a family and genetic analysis. *Br J Haematol* 1972;23:467.
231. Ciavarella H, Petronelli M, Wierdis T, et al. Su di un raro caso de deficit combinato de fattore V et di fattore VIII. *Haematologica* 1973;58:778.
232. Kleinmans M, Kordich L, Vizcorgúenga MI. Deficiencia congenita combinade de factores V y VIII. *Sangre* 1975;30:505.
233. Girolami A, Gastaldi G, Patrussi G, et al. Combined congenital deficiency of factor V and factor VIII: a report of a further case with some considerations on the hereditary transmission of this disorder. *Acta Haematol* 1976;55:234.
234. Reference deleted.
235. Reference deleted.
236. Reference deleted.
237. Reference deleted.
238. Graham JB, Green PP, McGraw RA, et al. Application of molecular genetics to prenatal diagnosis and carrier detection in the hemophilias: some limitations. *Blood* 1985;66:759.
239. Green PP, Mannucci PM, Briet E, et al. Carrier detection in hemophilia A: a cooperative international study. II. The efficiency of linear discriminants. *Blood* 1986;67:1560.
240. Harper K, Winter RM, Pembrey ME, et al. A clinically useful DNA probe closely linked to haemophilia A. *Lancet* 1984;2:6.
241. Oberle I, Camerino G, Heilig R, et al. Genetic screening for hemophilia A (classic hemophilia) with a polymorphic DNA probe. *N Engl J Med* 1985;312:682.
242. Winter RM, Harper K, Goldman E, et al. First trimester prenatal diagnosis and detection of carriers of haemophilia A using the linked DNA probe DX13. *BMJ* 1985;291:765.
243. Peake IR, Lillicrap DP, Liddell MB, et al. Linked and intragenic probes for haemophilia A. *Lancet* 1985;2:1003.
244. Lehesjoki A-E, de la Chapelle A, Rasi V. Haemophilia A: two recombinations detected with probe St14. *Lancet* 1986;2:280.
245. Driscoll MC, Miller CH, Goldberg JD, et al. Recombination between factor VIII:C gene and St14 locus. *Lancet* 1986;2:279.
246. Gitschier J, Drayna D, Tuddenham EGD, et al. Genetic mapping and diagnosis of haemophilia A achieved through a BclI polymorphism in the factor VIII gene. *Nature* 1985;314:738.
247. Gitschier J, Lawn RM, Rotblat F, et al. Antenatal diagnosis and carrier detection of haemophilia A using factor VIII gene probe. *Lancet* 1985;1:1093.
248. Din N, Schwartz M, Kruse T, et al. Factor VIII gene specific probe for prenatal diagnosis of haemophilia A. *Lancet* 1985;1:1446.
249. Wion KL, Tuddenham EG, Lawn RM. A new polymorphism the factor VIII gene for prenatal diagnosis of hemophilia A. *Nucleic Acids Res* 1986;14:4535.
250. Youssoufian H, Phillips DG, Kazazian HH Jr, et al. MspI polymorphism in the 3' flanking region of the human factor VIII gene. *Nucleic Acids Res* 1987;15:6312.
251. Ahrens P, Kruse TA, Schwartz M, et al. A new Hind III restriction fragment length polymorphism in the hemophilia A locus. *Hum Genet* 1987;26:127.
252. Bernardi F, Legnani C, Volinia S, et al. A Hind III RFLP and a gene lesion in the coagulation factor VIII gene. *Hum Genet* 1988;78:359.
253. Lalloz MR, McVey JH, Pattinson JK, et al. Haemophilia A diagnosis by analysis of a hypervariable dinucleotide repeat within the factor VIII gene. *Lancet* 1991;338:207.
254. Janco RL, Phillips JA III, Orlando PJ, et al. Detection of hemophilia A carriers using intragenic factor VIII:C DNA polymorphisms. *Blood* 1987;69:1539.
255. Pecorara M, Casarino L, Mori PG, et al. Hemophilia A: carrier detection and prenatal diagnosis by DNA analysis. *Blood* 1987;70:531.
256. Vogel F, Rathenberg R. Spontaneous mutation in men. In: Harris H, Hirschhorn K, eds. *Advances in human genetics.* New York: Plenum Publishing, 1975:223.
257. Saiki RK, Scharf S, Faloona F. Enzymatic amplification of β-globin genomic sequences and restriction site analysis for diagnosis of sickle cell anemia. *Science* 1985;230:1350.
258. Kogan SC, Doherty M, Gitschier J. An improved method for prenatal diagnosis of genetic diseases by analysis of amplified DNA sequences: application to hemophilia A. *N Engl J Med* 1987;317:985.
259. Lillicrap D, Holden JJ, Giles AR, et al. Carrier detection strategy in haemophilia: the benefits of combined DNA marker analysis and coagulation testing in sporadic haemophilic families. *Br J Haematol* 1988;70:321.
260. Ahlberg A. Haemophilia in Sweden. VIII. Incidence, treatment and prophylaxis of arthropathy and other musculoskeletal manipulations of haemophilia A and B. *Acta Orthop Scand* 1965;77:5.
261. Gilbert MS. Musculoskeletal manifestations of hemophilia. *Mt Sinai J Med* 1977;44:339.
262. Hilgartner MW. Hemophilic arthropathy. *Adv Pediatr* 1975;21:139.
263. Arnold WD, Hilgartner MW. Hemophilic arthropathy. Current concepts of pathogenesis and management. *J Bone Joint Surg* 1977;59:287.
264. Schreiber RR. Musculoskeletal system: radiologic findings. In: Brinkhous KM, Hemker HC, eds. *Handbook of hemophilia.* Part I. New York: Elsevier Science, 1975:333.
265. Pettersson H, Ahlberg A, Nilsson IM. A radiologic classification of hemophilic arthropathy. *Clin Orthop* 1980;149:153.
266. Kulkarni MV, Drotshagen LE, Kaye JJ, et al. Imaging of hemophilic arthropathy. *J Comput Assist Tomogr* 1986;10:445.
267. Mainardi C, Levine PH, Werb Z, et al. Proliferative synovitis in hemophilia: biochemical and morphological observations. *Arthritis Rheum* 1978;21:137.
268. Harris ED Jr, Parker HG, Radin EL, et al. Effects of proteolytic enzymes on structural and mechanical properties of cartilage. *Arthritis Rheum* 1972;15:497.
269. Swanton MW. Hemophilic arthropathy in dogs. *Lab Invest* 1959;8:1269.
270. White GC II, Blatt PM, McMillan CW, et al. Use of analgesic and anti-inflammatory drugs in the haemophilias. In: Seligsohn U, Rimon A, Horoszowski H, eds. *Haemophilia.* Kent, England: Castle House, 1981:231.
271. Thomas P, Hepburn B, Kim HC, et al. Nonsteroidal anti-inflammatory drugs in the treatment of hemophilic arthropathy. *Am J Hematol* 1982;12:131.
272. Tallroth A. Hemophilia with spontaneous hemorrhage in the iliopsoas muscle followed by injury to the femoral nerve. *Acta Chir Scand* 1941;84:124.
273. Silverstein A. Neuropathy in hemophilia. *JAMA* 1964;190:162.
274. van Trotsenburg L. Neurological complications of hemophilia. In: Brinkhous KM, Hemker HC. *Handbook of hemophilia.* Part I. New York: Elsevier Science, 1975:389.
275. Gilbert MS. Characterizing the hemophilic pseudotumor. *Ann N Y Acad Sci* 1975;240:311.
276. Brant EE, Jordan HH. Radiologic aspects of hemophilic pseudotumors in bone. *Am J Roentgenol Radium Ther Nucl Med* 1972;115:525.
277. Silverstein A. Intracranial bleeding in hemophilia. *Arch Neurol* 1960;3:141.
278. Eyster ME, Gill FM, Blatt PM, et al. Central nervous system bleeding in hemophiliacs. *Blood* 1978;51:1179.
279. Prentice CR, Lindsay RD, Barr RD, et al. Renal complications in hemophilia and Christmas disease. *QJM* 1971;40:47.
280. Kasper CK, Aledort LM, Counts RB, et al. A more uniform measurement of factor VIII inhibitors. *Thromb Diath Haemorrh* 1975;34:869.
281. White GC II, McMillan CW, Blatt PM, et al. Factor VIII inhibitors: an overview. *Am J Hematol* 1982;13:335.
282. McMillan CW, Shapiro SS, Whitehurst D, et al. The natural history of factor VIII:C inhibitors in patients with hemophilia A: a national cooperative study. II. Observations on the initial development of factor VIII:C inhibitors. *Blood* 1988;71:344.
283. Hultin MB, London FS, Shapiro SS, et al. Heterogeneity of factor VIII antibodies: further immunochemical and biologic studies. *Blood* 1977;49:807.
284. Hoyer LW, Gawryl MS, de la Fuente B. Immunochemical characterization of factor VIII inhibitors. *Prog Clin Biol Res* 1984;150:73.
285. Fulcher CA, de Graf Mahoney S, Roberts JR, et al. Localization of human factor FVIII inhibitor epitopes to two polypeptide fragments. *Proc Natl Acad Sci U S A* 1985;82:7728.
286. Scandella D, Mattingly M, de Graf Mahoney S, et al. Localization of epitopes for human factor VIII inhibitor antibodies by immunoblotting and antibody neutralization. *Blood* 1989;74:1618.
287. Scandella D, de Graf Mahoney S, Mattingly M, et al. Epitope mapping of human factor VIII inhibitor antibodies by deletion analysis of factor VIII fragments expressed in *Escherichia coli. Proc Natl Acad Sci U S A* 1988;85:6152.

288. Shapiro SS. Genetic predisposition to inhibitor formation. In: Hoyer LW, ed. *Factor VIII inhibitors.* New York: Alan R. Liss, 1984:45.

289. Frommel D, Allain JP. Genetic predisposition to develop factor VIII antibody in chronic hemophilia. *Clin Immunol Immunopathol* 1977;8:34.

290. Reisner HM, Reisner EA, Kostyu DD, et al. Possible association of HLA and Gm with the alloimmune response to FVIII. *Thromb Haemost* 1987;58:338 (abst).

291. Allain JP, Frommel D. Antibodies to factor VIII. V. Patterns of immune response to factor VIII in hemophilia. *Blood* 1976;47:973.

292. Hurt CH. Psychological and social aspects. In: Boone DC, ed. *Comprehensive management of hemophilia.* Philadelphia: FA Davis Co, 1977:117.

293. Brettler DB, Levine PH. Factor concentrates for treatment of hemophilia: which one to choose? *Blood* 1989;73:2067.

294. Biggs R, Denson KW. The fate of prothrombin and factor VIII, IX, and X transfused to patients deficient in these factors. *Br J Haematol* 1963;9:532.

295. de Sio L, Mariani G, Muzzoccon MG, et al. Comparison between subcutaneous and intravenous DDAVP in mild and moderate hemophilia A. *Thromb Haemost* 1985;54:387.

296. Levine PH. Efficacy of home therapy in hemophilia: a study of 72 patients with hemophilia A and B. *N Engl J Med* 1974;291:1381.

297. Brettler D, Forsberg AD, O'Connell FD, et al. A long term study of hemophilic arthropathy of the knee joint in a program of factor VIII replacement at time of each hemarthrosis. *Am J Hematol* 1985;18:13.

298. Guenther EE, Hilgartner MW, Miller CH, et al. Hemophilic arthropathy: effect of home care on treatment patterns and joint disease. *J Pediatr* 1980;97:378.

299. Storti E, Ascari E. Long-term evaluation of synovectomy in the treatment of recurrent hemophilic hemarthrosis. In: Brinkhous KM, Hemker HC, eds. *Handbook of hemophilia.* Part II. New York: Elsevier Science, 1975:727.

300. Kay L, Stainsby D, Buzzard B, et al. The role of synovectomy in the management of recurrent haemarthroses in haemophilia. *Br J Haematol* 1981;49:53.

301. Gamba G, Grignani G, Ascari E. Synoviorthesis versus synovectomy in the treatment of recurrent haemophilic haemarthrosis: long-term evaluation. *Thromb Haemost* 1981;45:127.

302. Smith MS, Urquhart DR, Savidge GF. The surgical management of varus deformity in haemophilia arthropathy of the knee. *J Bone Joint Surg* 1981;63:261.

303. Houghten GR, Duthie B. Orthopaedic problems in haemophilia. *Clin Orthop* 1979;138:197.

304. Mayne EE, Madden M, Crothers IS, et al. Highly purified porcine factor VIII in haemophilia A with inhibitors to factor VIII. *BMJ* 1981;282:318.

305. Kernoff PB, Thomas ND, Lilley PA, et al. Clinical experience with polyelectrolyte-fractionated porcine factor VIII concentrate in the treatment of hemophiliacs with antibodies to factor VIII. *Blood* 1984;63:31.

306. Lusher JM, Shapiro SS, Palascak JE, et al. Efficacy of prothrombin complex concentrates in hemophiliacs with antibodies to factor VIII: a multicenter therapeutic trial. *N Engl J Med* 1980;303:421.

307. Samsjoedin LJ, Heijnen L, Mauser-Bunschoten EP, et al. The effect of activated prothrombin complex concentrate (FEIBA) on joint and muscle bleeding in patients with hemophilia A and antibodies to factor VIII: a double-blind clinical trial. *N Engl J Med* 1981;305:717.

308. White GC II, Roberts HR, Kingdon HS, et al. Prothrombin complex concentrates: potentially thrombogenic materials and clues to the mechanism of thrombosis in vivo. *Blood* 1977;49:159.

309. Hultin MB. Studies of factor IX concentrate therapy in hemophilia. *Blood* 1983;62:677.

310. Kasper CK. Effect of prothrombin complex concentrates on factor VIII inhibitor levels. The Hemophilia Study Group. *Blood* 1979;54:1358.

311. Brackmann HH, Gormsen J. Massive factor-VIII infusion in haemophiliacs with factor-VIII inhibitor, high response. *Lancet* 1972;2:933.

312. White GC II, Taylor RE, Blatt PM, et al. Treatment of a high titer antifactor VIII antibody by continuous factor VIII administration: report of a case. *Blood* 1983;62:141.

313. Mannucci PM, Capitanio A, del Ninno E, et al. Asymptomatic liver disease in haemophiliacs. *J Clin Pathol* 1974;28:620.

314. Hasiba UW, Spero JA, Lewis JH. Chronic liver dysfunction in multitransfused hemophiliacs. *Transfusion* 1977;17:490.

315. Cederbaum AI, Blatt PM, Levine PM. Abnormal serum transaminase levels in patients with hemophilia A. *Arch Intern Med* 1982;142:481.

316. Rizetto M, Morello C, Mannucci PM, et al. Delta infection and liver disease in hemophilic carriers of hepatitis B surface antigen. *J Infect Dis* 1982;145:18.

317. Lesesne HR, Morgan JE, Blatt PM, et al. Liver biopsy in hemophilia A. *Ann Intern Med* 1977;86:703.

318. Spero JA, Lewis JH, van Thiel DH, et al. Asymptomatic structural liver disease in hemophilia. *N Engl J Med* 1978;298:1373.

319. Preston FE, Triger DR, Underwood JC, et al. Percutaneous liver biopsy and chronic liver disease in haemophiliacs. *Lancet* 1978;2:592.

320. Mannucci PM, Rhonchi G, Rota L, et al. A clinicopathologic study of liver disease in hemophilia. *J Clin Pathol* 1978;31:779.

321. White GC II, Zeitler KD, Lesesne HR, et al. Chronic hepatitis in patients with hemophilia A: histologic studies in patients with intermittently abnormal liver function tests. *Blood* 1982;60:1259.

322. Seeler RA, Telischi M, Langehennig PL, et al. Comparison of anti-A and anti-B titers in factor VIII and IX concentrates. *J Pediatr* 1976;89:87.

323. Orringer EO, Koury MJ, Blatt PM, et al. Hemolysis caused by factor VIII concentrates. *Arch Intern Med* 1976;136:1018.

324. Centers for Disease Control. *Pneumocystis carinii* pneumonia among persons with hemophilia. *MMWR Morb Mortal Wkly Rep* 1982;31:365.

325. Barre-Sinoussi F, Chermann JC, Rey F, et al. Isolation of a T-lymphotropic retrovirus from a patient at risk for acquired immunodeficiency syndrome. *Science* 1983;220:868.

326. Gallo RC, Salahuddin SZ, Popovic M, et al. Frequent detection and isolation of cytopathic retroviruses (HTLV-III) from patients with AIDS and at risk for AIDS. *Science* 1984;224:500.

327. Evatt BL, Ramsey RB, Lawrence MD, et al. The acquired immunodeficiency syndrome in patients with hemophilia. *Ann Intern Med* 1984;100:499.

328. Kitchen LW, Barin F, Sullivan JL, et al. Aetiology of AIDS: antibodies to human T-cell leukaemia virus (type III) in haemophiliacs. *Nature* 1984;312:367.

329. Geodert JJ, Sarngadharan MG, Eyster ME, et al. Antibodies reactive with human T-cell leukemia viruses (HTLV-III) in the sera of hemophiliacs receiving factor VIII concentrate. *Blood* 1985;65:492.

330. Evatt BL, Gomperts ED, McDougal JS, et al. Coincidental appearance of LAV1/HTLV-III antibodies in hemophiliacs and the onset of the AIDS epidemic. *N Engl J Med* 1985;312:483.

331. Levine PH. The acquired immunodeficiency syndrome in persons with hemophilia. *Ann Intern Med* 1985;103:723.

332. Ragni MV, Tegtmeier GE, Levy JA, et al. AIDS retrovirus antibodies in hemophiliacs treated with factor VIII or factor IX concentrates, cryoprecipitate, or fresh frozen plasma: prevalence, seroconversion, and clinical correlations. *Blood* 1986;67:592.

333. Jason J, McDougal JS, Holman RC, et al. Human T-lymphotropic retrovirus type III/lymphadenopathy-associated virus antibody. Association with hemophiliacs' immune status and blood component usage. *JAMA* 1985;253:3409.

334. McDougal JS, Martin LS, Cort SP, et al. Thermal inactivation of the acquired immunodeficiency syndrome virus, human T-lymphotropic virus-III/lymphadopathy-associated virus, with special reference to antihemophilic factor. *J Clin Invest* 1985;76:875.

335. Levy JA, Mitra GA, Wong MF, et al. Inactivation by wet and dry heat of AIDS-associated retroviruses during factor VIII purification from plasma. *Lancet* 1985;1:1456.

336. Piszkiewicz D, Bourret L, Lieu M, et al. Heat inactivation of human immunodeficiency virus in lyophilized factor VIII and factor IX concentrates. *Thromb Res* 1987;47:235.

337. Goedert JJ, Kessler CM, Aledort LM, et al. A prospective study of human immunodeficiency virus type I infection and the development of AIDS in subjects with hemophilia. *N Engl J Med* 1989;321:1141.

338. Jones P, Hamilton PJ, Bird G, et al. AIDS and haemophilia: morbidity and mortality in a well defined population. *BMJ* 1985;291:695.

339. Kreiss JK, Kitchen LW, Prince EH, et al. Human T cell leukemia virus type III antibody, lymphadenopathy, and acquired immunodeficiency syndrome in hemophiliac subjects. *Am J Med* 1986;80:345.

340. Eyster ME, Gail MH, Ballard JO, et al. Natural history of human immunodeficiency virus infections in hemophiliacs: effects of T cell subsets, platelet counts, and age. *Ann Intern Med* 1987;107:1.

341. Allain JP, Laurian Y, Paul DA, et al. Long-term evaluation of HIV antigen and antibodies to p24 and gp41 in patients with hemophilia: potential clinical importance. *N Engl J Med* 1987;317:1114.

342. Eyster ME, Ballard JO, Gail MH, et al. Predictive markers for the acquired immunodeficiency syndrome (AIDS) in hemophiliacs: persistence of p24 antigen and low T4 cell count. *Ann Intern Med* 1989;110:963.

343. Pappo AS, Buchanan GR, Johnson A. Septic arthritis in children with hemophilia. *Am J Dis Child* 1989;143:1226.

344. Reference deleted.

345. Reference deleted.

346. Reference deleted.

347. Bertina RM, Koeleman BP, Koster T, et al. Mutation in blood coagulation factor V associated with resistance to activated protein C [See comments]. *Nature* 1994;369:64–67.

348. Rosendaal FR, Koster T, Vandenbroucke JP, et al. High risk of thrombosis in patients homozygous for factor V Leiden (activated protein C resistance) [See comments]. *Blood* 1995;85:1504–1508.

349. Dahlback B, Carlsson M, Svensson PJ. Familial thrombophilia due to a previously unrecognized mechanism characterized by poor anticoagulant response to activated protein C: prediction of a cofactor to activated protein C [See comments]. *Proc Natl Acad Sci U S A* 1993;90:1004–1008.

350. Kalafatis M, Haley PE, Lu D, et al. Proteolytic events that regulate factor V activity in whole plasma from normal and activated protein C (APC)-resistant individuals during clotting: an insight into the APC-resistance assay. *Blood* 1996;87:4695–4707.

351. Shen L, Dahlback B. Factor V and protein S as synergistic cofactors to activated protein C in degradation of factor VIIIa. *J Biol Chem* 1994;269:18735–18738.

352. Thorelli E, Kaufman RJ, Dahlback B. The C-terminal region of the factor V B-domain is crucial for the anticoagulant activity of factor V. *J Biol Chem* 1998;273:16140–16145.

353. Varadi K, Rosing J, Tans G, et al. Factor V enhances the cofactor function of protein S in the APC-mediated inactivation of factor VIII: influence of the factor VR506Q mutation. *Thromb Haemost* 1996;76:208–214.

354. de Moerloose P, Wutschert R, Heinzmann M, et al. Superficial vein thrombosis of lower limbs: influence of factor V Leiden, factor II G20210A and overweight. *Thromb Haemost* 1998;80:239–241.

355. Martinelli I, Landi G, Merati G, et al. Factor V gene mutation is a risk factor for cerebral venous thrombosis [See comments]. *Thromb Haemost* 1996;75:393–394.

356. Koeleman BP, Reitsma PH, Allaart CF, et al. Activated protein C resistance as an additional risk factor for thrombosis in protein C-deficient families. *Blood* 1994;84:1031–1035.

357. Brenner B, Zivelin A, Lanir N, et al. Venous thromboembolism associated with double heterozygosity for R506Q mutation of factor V and for T298M mutation of protein C in a large family of a previously described homozygous protein C-deficient newborn with massive thrombosis. *Blood* 1996; 88:877–880.

358. Koeleman BP, van Rumpt D, Hamulyak K, et al. Factor V Leiden: an additional risk factor for thrombosis in protein S deficient families? *Thromb Haemost* 1995;74:580–583.

359. Zoller B, Berntsdotter A, Garcia de Frutos P, et al. Resistance to activated protein C as an additional genetic risk factor in hereditary deficiency of protein S. *Blood* 1995;85:3518–3523.

360. Bertina RM. Molecular risk factors for thrombosis. *Thromb Haemost* 1999; 82:601–609.

361. Eichinger S, Pabinger I, Stumpflen A, et al. The risk of recurrent venous thromboembolism in patients with and without factor V Leiden. *Thromb Haemost* 1997;77:624–628.

362. Koster T, Blann AD, Briet E, et al. Role of clotting factor VIII in effect of von Willebrand factor on occurrence of deep-vein thrombosis. *Lancet* 1995;345: 152–155.

363. Wautrecht JC, Galle C, Motte S, et al. The role of ABO blood groups in the incidence of deep vein thrombosis [Letter]. *Thromb Haemost* 1998;79:688–689.

364. O'Donnell J, Tuddenham EG, Manning R, et al. High prevalence of elevated factor VIII levels in patients referred for thrombophilia screening: role of increased synthesis and relationship to the acute phase reaction. *Thromb Haemost* 1997;77:825–828.

365. O'Donnell J, Mumford AD, Manning RA, et al. Elevation of FVIII: C in venous thromboembolism is persistent and independent of the acute phase response [See comments]. *Thromb Haemost* 2000;83:10–13.

366. Kamphuisen PW, Lensen R, Houwing-Duistermaat JJ, et al. Heritability of elevated factor VIII antigen levels in factor V Leiden families with thrombophilia. *Br J Haematol* 2000;109:519–522.

367. Gilbert GE, Arena AA. Activation of the factor VIIIa–factor IXa enzyme complex of blood coagulation by membranes containing phosphatidyl-L-serine. *J Biol Chem* 1996;271:11120–11125.

368. Bardelle C, Furie B, Furie BC, et al. Kinetic studies of factor VIII binding to phospholipid membranes indicate a complex binding process. *J Biol Chem* 1993;268:8815–8824.

369. van Dieijen G, Tans G, Rosing J, et al. The role of phospholipid and Factor VIIIa in the activation of bovine factor X. *J Biol Chem* 1981;256:3433–3442.

370. Rosing J, Tans G, Govers-Riemslag J, et al. The role of phospholipids and factor Va in the prothrombinase complex. *J Biol Chem* 1980;255:274–283.

371. Gilbert GE, Furie BC, Furie B. Binding of human factor VIII to phospholipid vesicles. *J Biol Chem* 1990;265:815–822.

372. Gilbert GE, Drinkwater D, Barter S, et al. Specificity of phosphatidylserine-containing membrane binding sites for factor VIII: studies with model membranes supported by glass microspheres (lipospheres). *J Biol Chem* 1992;267: 15861–15868.

373. Burri B, Edgington T, Fair D. Molecular interactions of the intrinsic activation complex of coagulation: binding of native and activated human factors IX and X to defined phospholipid vesicles. *Biochim Biophys Acta* 1987;923: 176–186.

374. Jones M, Griffith M, Monroe D, et al. Comparison of lipid binding and kinetic properties of normal, variant, and γ-carboxyglutamic acid modified human factor IX and factor IXa. *Biochemistry* 1985;24:8064–8069.

375. Beals J, Castellino F. The interaction of bovine factor IX, its activation intermediate, factor IXa, and its activation products, factor IXaa and factor IXab, with acidic phospholipid vesicles of various compositions. *Biochem J* 1986; 236:861–869.

376. Duffy E, Parker E, Mutucumarana V, et al. Binding of factor VIIIa and factor VIII to factor IXa on phospholipid vesicles. *J Biol Chem* 1992;267:17006–17011.

377. Bloom J, Nesheim M, Mann K. Phospholipid-binding properties of bovine factor V and factor Va. *Biochemistry* 1979;18:4419–4425.

378. Krishnaswamy S, Mann K. The binding of factor Va to phospholipid vesicles. *J Biol Chem* 1988;263:5714–5723.

379. Pryzdial EL, Mann KG. The association of coagulation factor Xa and factor Va. *J Biol Chem* 1991;266:8969–8977.

380. Nesheim M, Kettner C, Shaw E, et al. Assembly of the prothrombinase complex in the absence of prothrombin. *J Biol Chem* 1981;256:9874–9882.

381. Krishnaswamy S. Prothrombinase complex assembly: contributions of protein-protein and protein-membrane interactions toward complex formation. *J Biol Chem* 1990;265:3708–3718.

CHAPTER 39

Biology and Disorders of Fibrinogen and Factor XIII

Charles S. Greenberg, Thung-S. Lai, Robert A. S. Ariëns,
John W. Weisel, and Peter J. Grant

The conversion of fibrinogen to a fibrin gel must be carefully regulated to prevent thrombosis. Failure to generate a critical mass of protease-resistant fibrin will not prevent blood loss or promote wound healing. Factor XIII, once activated, is responsible for catalyzing the covalent coupling of fibrin molecules to generate a blood clot that is resistant to mechanical and proteolytic disruption. Fibrin controls its own metabolism by regulating its stabilization and degradation by controlling plasmin formation, fibrinolysis, and factor XIII activation. The failure by fibrin to regulate fibrinolysis and factor XIIIa formation can produce either bleeding or thrombotic disorders. In this chapter, the structure and function of fibrinogen and factor XIII are reviewed, then the diagnosis and treatment of congenital and acquired disorders of fibrinogen and factor XIII are discussed. Disorders of fibrinogen and factor XIII, although rare, offer investigators the opportunity to discover the specific function(s) of various domains within these proteins. Recent advances regarding the genetic polymorphism of these proteins illustrate the importance they play in the clinical manifestation of bleeding, thrombotic, and atherosclerotic diseases.

FIBRINOGEN STRUCTURE

The fibrinogen molecule is a large, disulfide-bonded glycoprotein that is composed of two half-molecules, each containing three distinct polypeptide chains, designated $A\alpha$, $B\beta$, and γ (Fig. 39-1) (1–3). The human fibrinogen molecule is 340 kd and folded to form a trinodular structure. The $A\alpha$-, $B\beta$-, and γ-chains are 63.5, 56.0, and 47.0 kd, respectively, and are assembled intracellularly in hepatocytes with multiple disulfide bonds before secretion (1–3).

Electron microscopy provided the first images of fibrinogen molecules folding into a trinodular structure (4–7). The two larger D-regions are separated from the central E-region by a linear coiled-coil domain. More detailed x-ray crystallography studies have verified the folding pattern of individual protein chains in fibrinogen (8,9). The fibrinogen molecule is 45 nm long and has a slightly sigmoidal shape (8,9) (Fig. 39-2). The central E-region contains the N-terminal ends of all six-polypeptide chains and forms a structure designated as a *disulfide knot* (4–6) (Fig. 39-1). The fibrinopeptides A and B are located in the central E-region. The two D-regions are made of the C-terminal two-thirds of the $B\beta$- and γ-chains (8,9). The $B\beta$- and γ-chain segments in the D-region play an important role in fibrin polymerization and are oriented diagonally along the long axis of the molecule (Fig. 39-1) (8–10). An additional globular domain representing the carboxy-terminus of the α-chain, designated αC *domain*, can be detected in highly purified fibrinogen associated with the D- and E-regions (11) (Fig. 39-2).

The E- and D-regions are separated from each other by a stretch of 111 to 112 amino acids to form the three- or four-stranded α-helical coiled-coil structure (Figs. 39-1 and 39-2) (1–3). The coiled-coil region is supported on either side by a set of disulfide bonds called *disulfide rings* (Fig. 39-1). These disulfide bonds must form to guarantee that the protein is folded properly and then secreted (Fig. 39-1) (12–15). The disulfide rings in the coiled-coil region also provide mechanical stability to the molecule. Recent studies have shown that the coiled-coil domain is flexible, allowing the molecule to bend during fibrin polymerization (9).

The fibrinogen molecule is cleaved by plasmin, the serine protease that regulates fibrinolysis in a very specific pattern. Plasmin first removes the αC domains, producing the clottable fragment X molecules with a molecular weight of 240 to 260 kd (Fig. 39-3) (16,17). Fragment X molecules can have either one or both αC domains cleaved. Fragment X is then cleaved at one of the two coiled-coil regions, producing fragment D, which is approximately 100 kd, and fragment Y, which is approximately 150 kd. Fragment Y is then cleaved, yielding another fragment D and a fragment E that is approximately 45 kd (Fig. 39-3).

DNA and amino acid sequencing established the complete primary structure for each of the fibrinogen chains (18–25). The primary sequence of the polypeptide chains demonstrates homology, suggesting a common ancestral gene (26). The $A\alpha$-chain, which is usually 610 amino acids long, can be divided into three sections (21). The N-terminus amino acids 1 to 194 are linked by disulfide bonds to both the $B\beta$- and the γ-chains. The amino acids 195 to 239, in the midsection, represent a protease-sensitive domain that has multiple prolines and four plasmin cleavage sites (thick dark arrow, Fig. 39-1) (1–3). The $A\alpha$-chain from amino acid 240 to 424 is very rich in polar amino acids, with ten tandem repeats, each 13 amino acids long (21). Two glutamine residues at amino acid 328 and 366 function as inter-

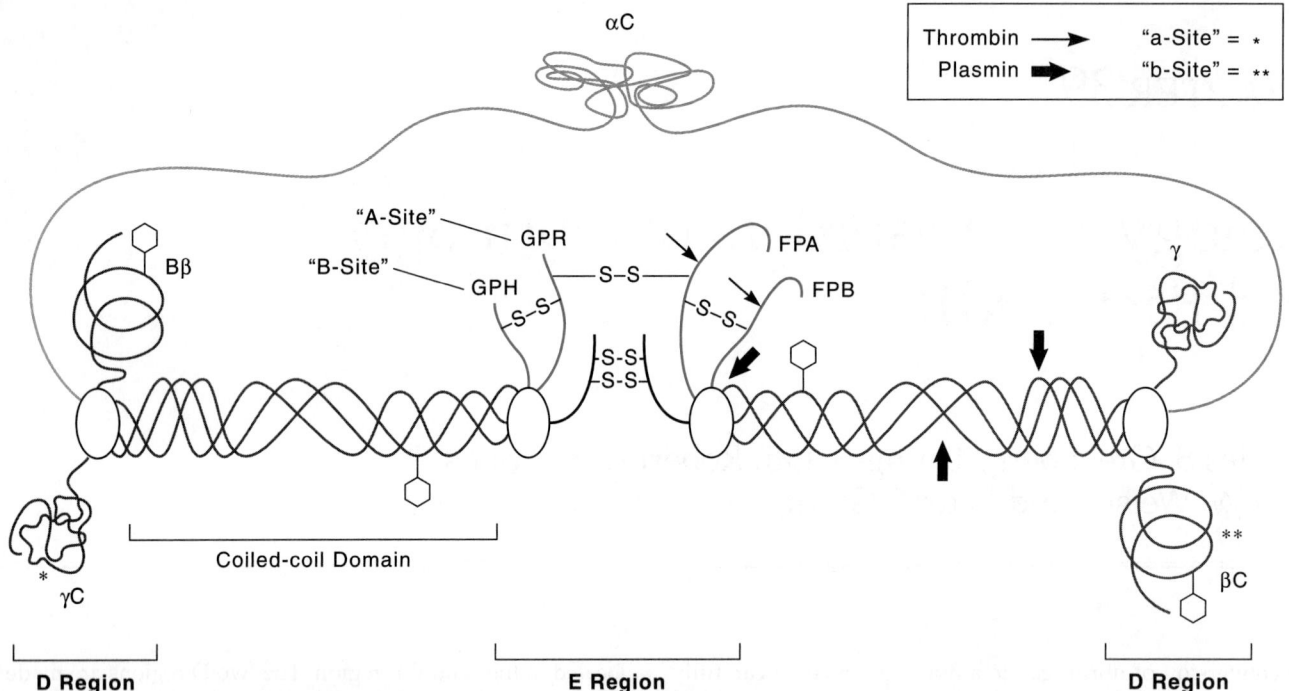

Figure 39-1. Model structure of fibrinogen. The fibrinogen model is a large glycoprotein that forms a trinodular structure. Three distinct polypeptide chains, designated Aα, Bβ, and γ, are disulfide bonded to produce two symmetric half molecules. The entire molecule is 45 nm long and 9 nm in diameter. The two D-regions form the outer nodules and are made up of the carboxyterminal two-thirds of the Bβ- and γ-chains. X-ray diffraction studies suggest that the D-region has two subdomains, formed by the independent folding of the C-termini of the Bβ- and γ-chains, designated βC and γC, respectively. These subdomains are located diagonally from the long axis. Within the carboxyterminal γ-chain domain (γC), there exist the glutamine and lysine cross-linking sites, calcium binding site, and a platelet and factor XIII binding domain. The central E-region nodule is 5 nm in diameter and is formed by disulfide bonding the six aminotermini of each polypeptide chain (designated *disulfide knot*). The D- and E-regions are separated from each other by a set of disulfide bonds called *disulfide rings* and a stretch of amino acids called the *coiled-coil domain*. Plasmin sequentially degrades the molecule by cleaving the Bβ-chain, then the Aα and four sites in the coiled-coil region (*thick dark arrows*). Thrombin cleaves fibrinopeptides A and B from the aminotermini from the Aα- and Bβ-chains (*thin arrows*) to expose GPR "a-site" and GPH "b-site," respectively. The GPR and GHR binding sites are indicated by "a-site" and "b-site," respectively. The "a-site" and "b-site" that promote fibrin polymerization are also indicated as "*" and "* *," respectively. FPA, fibrinopeptide A; FPB, fibrinopeptide B. (Modified from Mosesson MW. Fibrin polymerization and its regulatory role in hemostasis. *J Lab Clin Med* 1990;116:8.)

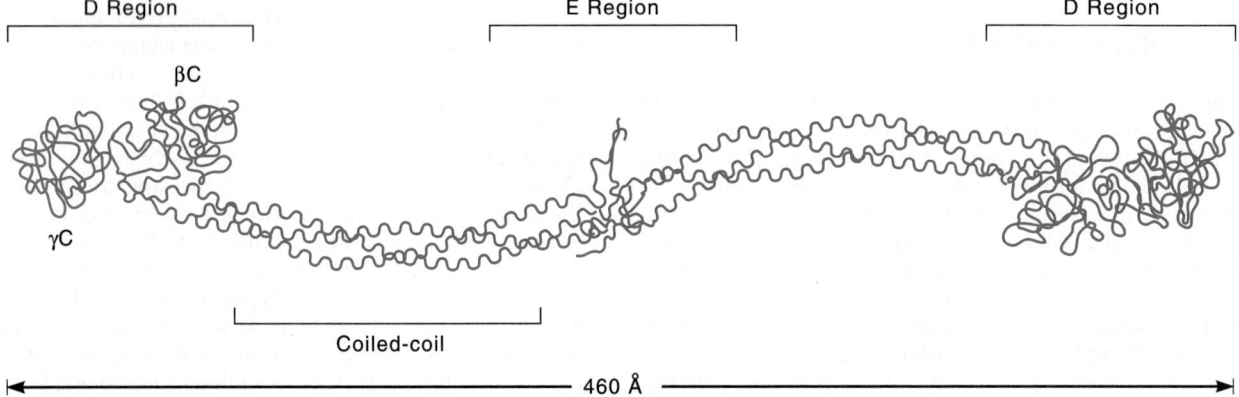

Figure 39-2. Crystal structure of chicken fibrinogen: a model of native chicken fibrinogen. This figure depicts the model derived from analyzing chicken fibrinogen. Note the trinodular appearance and location of D- and E-regions separated by the coiled-coil region that appears sigmoidal in shape. This model is similar to the structure obtained for bovine fibrinogen and used the method of molecular replacement using the human fragment D-structure in the search model. Note in this model the αC domain is not shown, as chicken fibrinogen does not have this domain, making it easier to form x-ray crystals.

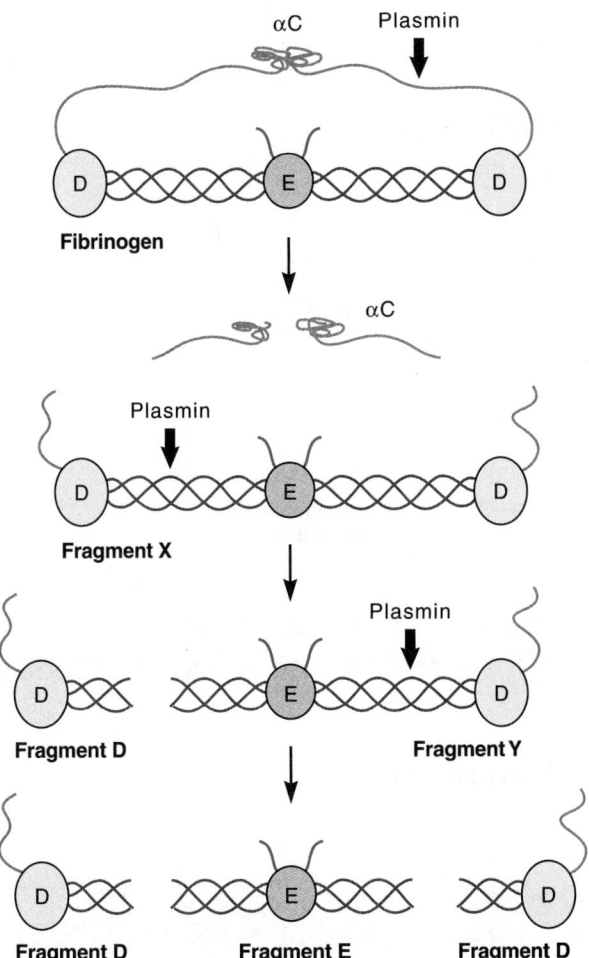

Figure 39-3. Model of fibrinogen degradation. Fibrinogen and fibrin molecules are shown as trinodular structures. The central E-regions are shown as closed ovals. Plasmin digests fibrinogen at specific lysyl-X and arginyl-X bonds to produce small, soluble degradation products. The first step involves the removal of the αC domains to produce fragment X. Fragment X (240 kd) is then converted to an asymmetric intermediate, fragment Y (155 kd), and an equimolar amount of fragment D (83 kd). Fragment Y is further converted to fragment E (50 kd) and another fragment D.

molecular Aα-chain cross-linking sites (21). The C-terminal domain of the Aα-chain forms a globular domain, designated αC, which associates with the central fragment E-region and is linked to the distal end of the coiled-coil via a connector strand. During fibrin polymerization (11), the αC-domain undergoes a conformational change and is released from the central region, after which it is free to interact with the Aα-chain in adjacent protofibrils to promote lateral aggregation (Fig. 39-4) (11). The fibronectin (27) and α2-antiplasmin (28) cross-linking sites are located in the C-terminus of the Aα-chain (21).

The Bβ-chain, which is 461 amino acids long, can also be subdivided into three sections. The first 80 amino acids are approximately 15% identical to the Aα-chain and are held together by disulfide bonds with the N-termini of the other chains to form the central E-region, or N-terminal disulfide knot and part of the coiled-coil (Fig. 39-1). The midsection (amino acids 81 to 192) contains the two sets of disulfide rings that define the linear coiled-coil segment (Fig. 39-1). The C-terminus (amino acids 193 to 461) folds to form a subsection of the D-region, designated βC, and contains the site that binds GHRP (b-site) (Fig. 39-1) (1,2). This β-chain GHRP-binding site may interact with the newly exposed amino acid after thrombin cleaves fibrinopeptide B from frag-

ment E (designated *b-site*) and promote lateral aggregation of protofibrils (8,9). This intermolecular interaction (B-b) may help to regulate the thickness of fibrin fibers (Fig. 39-5).

The γ-chain, which is only 411 amino acids long, is also readily subdivided into thirds. The N-terminus is just 18 amino acids long, followed by amino acids 19 to 129, which contain the disulfide rings and subsequent residues forming the coiled-coil region (11). The final third of the γ-chain, amino acids 130 to 411, forms the globular segment of the D-region (Fig. 39-1) (1–3). The C-terminal contains the amino acids that participate in factor XIIIa–mediated cross-linking (27). The carboxyl-terminus of the γ-chain also contains the sequences for staphylococcal clumping, cell adhesion, and platelet aggregation (Fig. 39-1) (1–3). The C-terminal γ-chain site folds to form the fibrin polymerization site involved in binding the GPR sequence that gets exposed after release of fibrinopeptide A (8,9). The GPR site (designated *a-site*) is the site that promotes fibrin polymerization and D-E contact (8,9). The carboxy-terminal γ-chain domain also contains the sites that promote end-to-end association of fibrin monomers, designated the *D-D contact site* (8,9). The D-D site encourages the end-to-end association of fibrin monomers during fibrin polymerization.

Calcium ions control the structure and function of fibrinogen and fibrin molecules (29). There are several calcium binding sites within the fibrinogen molecule (29–31). Sites are located within residues 311 to 336 of the γ-chains in the D-region, which is homologous to the calcium binding site in calmodulin. When calcium ions occupy this site, the γ-chain is protected from plasmin degradation. There is also a calcium binding site located in the E-region (30). The calcium binding sites have sufficient affinity for calcium so they are occupied at physiologic plasma concentrations (1.5 mM free calcium). Calcium ions modulate fibrin polymerization by enhancing lateral association of protofibrils to form fibrin strands (29). The location of the binding sites for GPRP and calcium have been directly visualized in x-ray crystals of fragment D (2). The calcium binding site must be intact for the proper functioning of the GPR binding site (A-site).

The carbohydrates attached to both the β- and γ-chains can play a role in fibrin polymerization (32–34). The carbohydrates are linked to fibrinogen by N-glycosidic bonds to asparagines with the sequence Asn-X-Thr (33). Removal of all carbohydrate from fibrinogen results in fibrin clots made up of very thick fibers with few branch points and large pores (35). Deglycosylation of fibrinogen accelerates polymerization and increases lateral aggregation of fibrin fibers (36), whereas removal of only sialic acid residues leads to clots made up of slightly thinner fibers. Fibrinogen sialic acid residues are low-affinity calcium binding sites that influence fibrin assembly. These results suggest that the carbohydrate moieties play an important role in the regulation of clot structure through modulation of the degree of lateral aggregation. Defective fibrin polymerization occurs when abnormal carbohydrates, especially the negatively charged sialic acid molecules, are added to fibrinogen, as occurs in cirrhosis and hepatomas (37).

There are two very distinct molecular forms of the γ-chain in the human plasma fibrinogen molecule. These γ-chains are distinguished by both their size and charge. The γ-chain, present in approximately 85% of the plasma fibrinogen molecules, is shorter and more positively charged than the longer, more negatively charged γ'-chain. These two forms of the γ-chain are always present in human fibrinogen (6,39). The human γ chain is formed by alternative polyadenylation of the last intron (40). A polyadenylation signal in the last intron causes it to remain unspliced in approximately 15% of the transcripts producing γ' messenger RNA (mRNA). The C-terminal extension does not modify fibrin

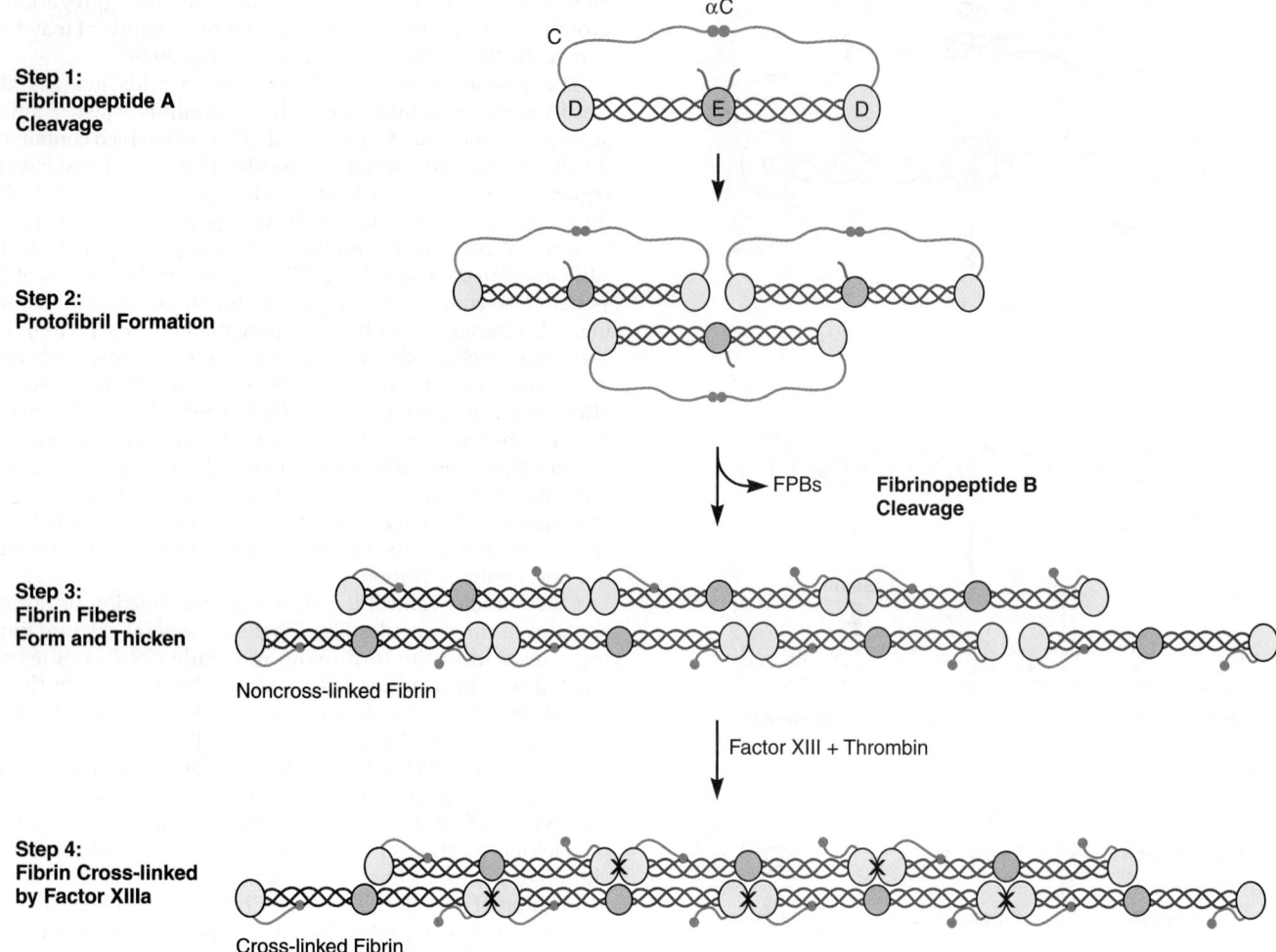

Figure 39-4. Models of fibrin polymerization and cross-linking. Fibrinogen and fibrin molecules are shown as trinodular structures. The central E-regions are shown as a closed ovals. In this model of fibrinogen polymerization, the fibrinopeptide A is cleaved first, which leads to formation of protofibril. At this stage of fibrin polymerization, the αC domain remains associated with the central fragment E domain. Once the fibrinopeptides B (FPBs) are cleaved, the αC domains dissociate and can then contribute to intermolecular binding, which holds protofibrils together by lateral aggregation. In the presence of factor XIII and thrombin, fibrin fibers can be cross-linked. The cross-linking site is between D-D contact and is marked as X.

cross-linking but does interfere with platelet aggregation (41,42). Platelets exclusively contain γ'-chains in their α-granules, and they may be selectively imported into the platelet (41). Recent studies indicate that the γ'-chain is a carrier for the zymogen of factor XIII in circulating blood (43). The γ'-chain also binds thrombin and functions to limit thrombin's action within fibrin (1).

There has been a great deal of interest in the structure of the C-terminus of the γ-chain of fibrinogen because this domain binds to platelets, promotes fibrin polymerization, binds calcium, and contains the cross-linking site for factor XIIIa (1–3). Patients with molecular defects in this portion of fibrinogen can have either bleeding or thrombotic problems and are discussed in the section Clinical Disorders of Fibrinogen (44).

FIBRIN FORMATION

There are three major steps needed to occur to produce a stable fibrin-based blood clot. They are the following: (a) thrombin cleavage of fibrinopeptides A and B, (b) fibrin polymerization, and (c) fibrin cross-linking. In the first phase of fibrin formation, thrombin cleaves two specific Arg-Gly bonds in the amino ter-

mini of the Aα- and Bβ-chains of fibrinogen, releasing fibrinopeptides A and B, respectively (Figs. 39-1 and 39-5) (1–3). Release of fibrinopeptide A (Aα 1 to 16) initiates the process by which fibrin assembles into a gel composed of interconnecting fibrin strands. Release of fibrinopeptide A exposes the amino acid sequence GPR, which is designated the *A-site* (Figs. 39-1 and 39-4). Release of fibrinopeptide B exposes amino acid sequence GPH, which is designated the *B-site*. Exposure of the "A" and "B" sites promote fibrin polymerization (Figs. 39-1 and 39-4).

In the second phase, thrombin-catalyzed release of fibrinopeptides A and B exposes intermolecular binding sites (A and B sites) (Figs. 39-4 and 39-5) in the central E-region, the resulting fibrin monomers molecule self associates (Figs. 39-4 and 39-5) (1–3). The newly exposed "A site" in the central E-region will interact with a complementary polymerization site (a-site) in the γ-chain of the D-region of adjacent fibrin monomers (Figs. 39-4 and 39-5) (1–3) to form a D-E contact site (Figs. 39-4 and 39-5) (1–3). The D-E contacts provide stability to fibrin protofibrils composed of overlapping fibrin molecules (Figs. 39-4 and 39-5) (45,46).

X-ray crystallography studies demonstrate that the fibrin polymerization a-site in the C-γ-chain forms a small hole that binds GPR residues of the a-site (Fig. 39-1). The complementary

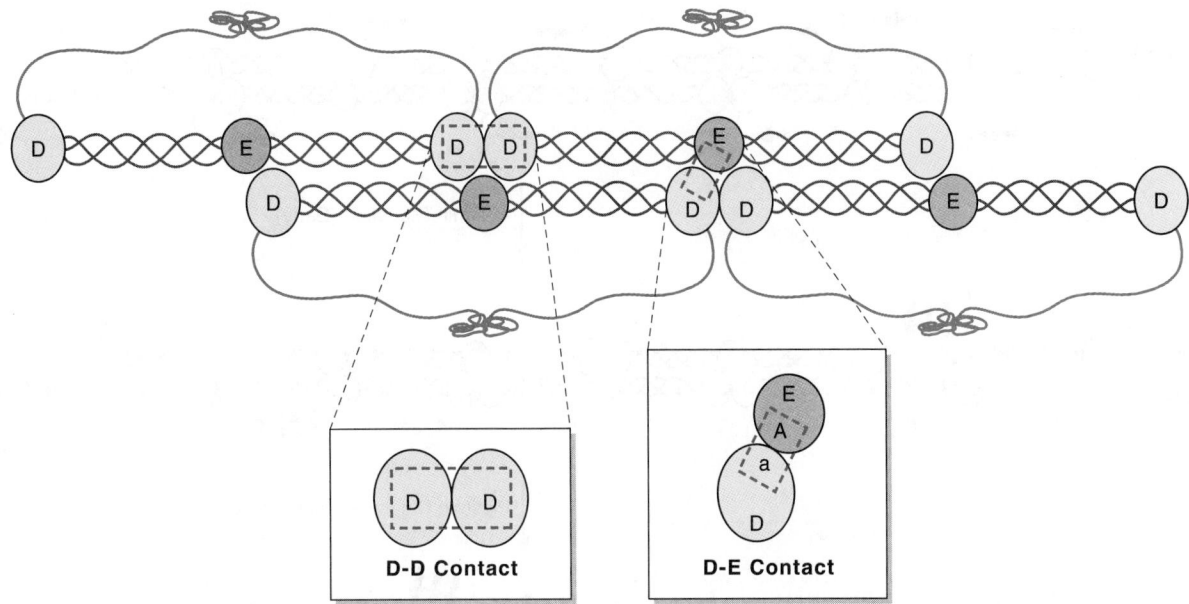

Figure 39-5. A model of the interactions in D-D and D-E. Fibrinogen and fibrin molecules are shown as trinodular structures. The central E domains are shown as closed ovals. In this model, there are interactions in the D-D and D-E on adjacent protofibrils. The sites of interactions are called "A-a" and "B-b" sites. The interactions contribute to the stabilization of protofibrils.

GPR sequence, A-site, is located in the N-terminus of the Aα-chain in the region exposed after thrombin releases fibrinopeptide A (47,48). The a-sites in the D-region are always exposed, allowing even fibrinogen molecules to form D-E contacts, producing fibrinogen/fibrin complexes. Synthetic peptides mimicking the new N-terminus sequence GPR binds to fibrinogen and inhibits fibrin polymerization (47,48). The half-staggered overlapping molecules elongate to form a trimeric structure with the addition of another monomer, forming a D-D contact as well as another D-E contact (Figs. 39-4 and 39-5) (1–3). The three-dimensional structure of the D-D site was recently revealed by x-ray crystallography (32). A two-stranded protofibril is formed as this elongation process continues (Fig. 39-5) (1–3). After long protofibrils form, they assemble into thicker fibers of fibrin (1–3). The protofibrils associate with other protofibrils through lateral associations that are held together by another set of interactions. These noncovalent interactions are distinct from the D-E contacts and are sensitive to changes in pH, ionic strength, and temperature (1–3,49–51). These sites (B-sites) in the C-terminus of the β-chain may enhance the lateral association of fibrin. Cleavage of only A or only B fibrinopeptides results in the formation of clots made up of normal-looking fibers, suggesting that the B-b interactions are not absolutely necessary for lateral aggregation of protofibrils to form fibers (52), but release of the negatively charged fibrinopeptide B exposes the B-site, enhancing the rate and extent of fibrin fiber formation (Fig. 39-5) (1–3,49,50). Conformational change in the αC domain is also required for fibrin polymerization to be optimum. Normally, in fibrinogen, the αC domains are associated with the central region of the molecule, but on cleavage of the B fibrinopeptides, the αC domains are released, so they can interact intermolecularly to enhance lateral aggregation (53–55). During fibrin polymerization, factor XIIIa covalently attaches adjacent D-regions, producing a very insoluble and protease-resistant fibrin clot.

When plasmin attacks factor XIIIa cross-linked fibrin molecules, a large variety of different size of fragments appear (Fig. 39-6). Some of these fragments are released from the fibrin after it has formed a gel, whereas others are degraded when fibrin polymers are still soluble (56). The final breakdown product of cross-linked fibrin is designated the *DDE complex* (Fig. 39-6) (56). Specific monoclonal antibodies have been made to factor XIIIa cross-linked fibrin degradation products that can be used to detect deep venous thrombosis and other intravascular thrombotic conditions where intravascular fibrin has formed (57).

FIBRINOGEN SYNTHESIS

Several laboratories (58–60) have expressed human fibrinogen from mammalian cells. The ability to express fibrinogen provides a means to study the synthesis, secretion, and function of various sites in individual fibrinogen chains. Site-directed mutagenesis of cysteine residues involved in the disulfide bonding between fibrinogen chains has established the steps in fibrinogen assembly (59). There is a progression from single chains to 2-chain complexes and then trimeric half-molecules. The Aα βγ half-molecule then dimerizes to form intact fibrinogen.

Recombinant fibrinogens were also used to determine which domains are involved in cell adhesion and platelet aggregation. Fibrinogen binds to both platelets and endothelial cells, and multiple binding sites were proposed for regulating these events. The Aα-chain of fibrinogen contains the RGD cellular adhesion sequence (61) at both residues Aα95 to 97 and Aα572 to 574. The γ-chain of fibrinogen contains another potential binding site, the dodecapeptide sequence at the carboxyterminus of the γ-chain, γ 400 to 411 (62–64). Platelet aggregation is supported by the γ-chain site (65,66), and endothelial cell adhesion relies on the RGD domain at Aα 572 to 574 (67) in human fibrinogen. Another study using mutant recombinant fibrinogen demonstrated that the γ-chain domain (42) is not required for clot retraction (68), implying that other domains are important for this process (69).

The synthesis of the fibrinogen molecule is complex, which leads to substantial heterogeneity in the structure of the secreted plasma protein. The fibrinogen genes are located in a cluster in the distal third of chromosome 4, bands q23-q32 (70). The gene

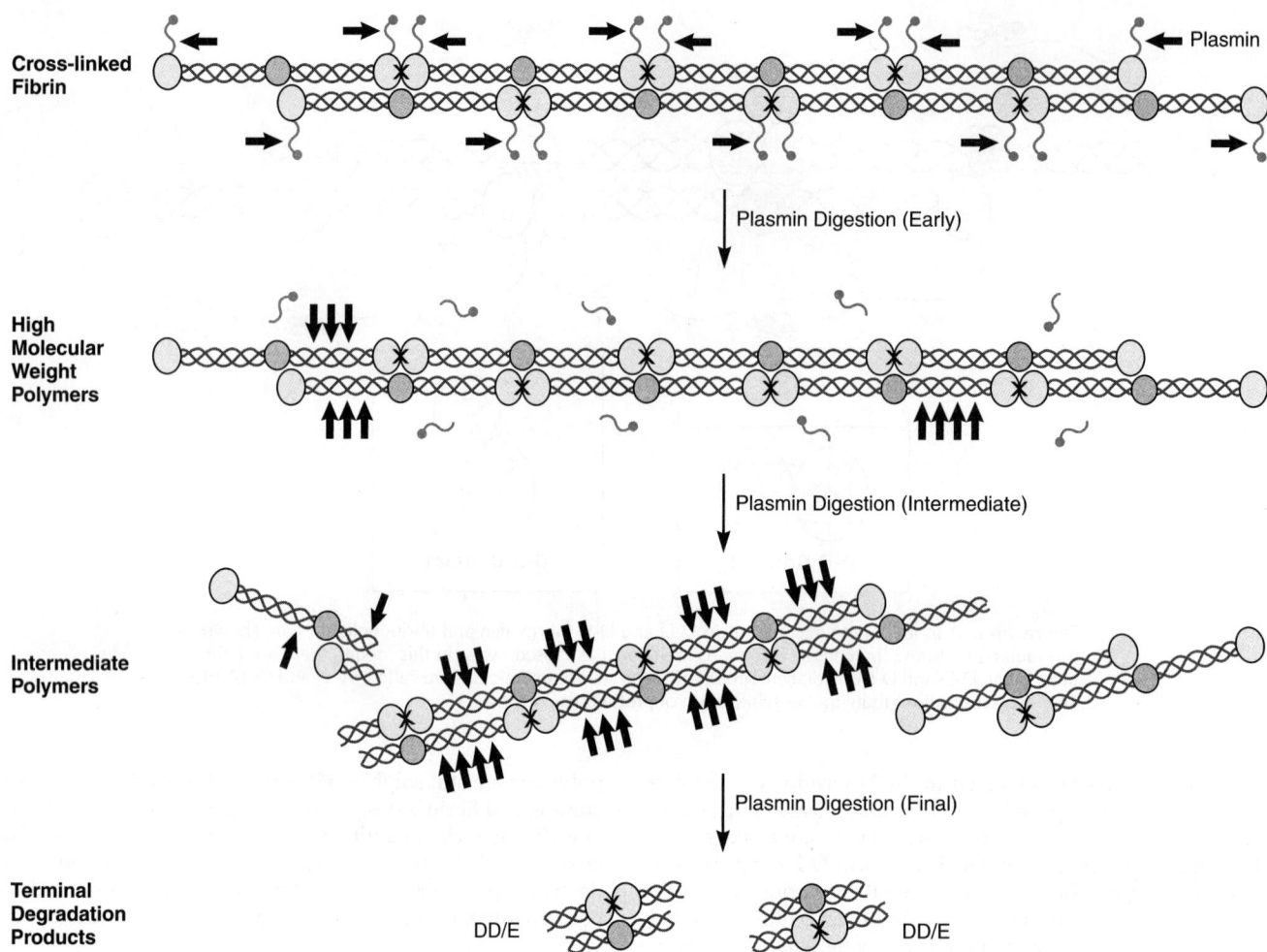

Figure 39-6. Model of cross-linked fibrin degradation. Degradation of cross-linked fibrins. After the factor XIIIa cross-linking reaction, the degradation of cross-linked fibrins by plasmin can be separated into early, intermediate, and late stages. The final degradation product is DD/E. The arrows in the figure indicate the plasmin cleavage.

for the fibrinogen Aα-chain consists of five exons, which code for a mature protein of 625 amino acids (65.5 kd), and is located in the center of the fibrinogen gene cluster (70). Alternative splicing of the mRNA leads to the inclusion of a sixth exon and the transcription of an extended alpha EC domain (4). Approximately 1% of the fibrinogen molecules in an adult have the alpha EC domain, leading to a protein with a molecular weight of 420 kd, called *fibrinogen-420*. The gene for the Bβ-chain is located 13 kb downstream of the Aα gene and is transcribed in the opposite direction of the Aα and γ genes (70). The Bβ gene contains eight exons coding a 461–amino acid polypeptide of 52 kd (1–3). The third gene of the fibrinogen cluster, that of the γ-chain, is located 10 kb upstream of the Aα gene (70). This gene consists of ten exons, which code for a mature protein of 411 amino acids (46.5 kd). Alternative processing of the γ-chain transcript leads to a read-through of the exon IX/intron I splice junction, which causes the formation of the γ'-chain that contains a 20 amino acid–extension at the C-terminus (38). The γ' extension is negatively charged and is present in approximately 10% to 15% of the plasma fibrinogen molecules.

There are several posttranslational modifications of fibrinogen. Approximately 3% of fibrinogen's mass is carbohydrate, linked to specific asparagine residues in the Bβ- and γ-chains. In addition, there are phosphorylation and sulfation (71–76) reactions, which appear to regulate some fibrinogen functions. Molecular genetic

defects in the synthesis and assembly of the fibrinogen molecule can produce low plasma levels that cause serious bleeding problems, afibrinogenemia, or hypodysfibrinogenemia, discussed in the section Clinical Disorders of Fibrinogen.

GENETIC POLYMORPHISMS IN FIBRINOGEN

Most of the polymorphisms in the fibrinogen genes occur in the noncoding regions of the locus. Two recent reviews regarding the fibrinogen polymorphisms and their effects on circulating fibrinogen levels were published (77,78). The main polymorphisms in the noncoding regions of the genes are at a Taq1 site in the Aα gene and a BclI, –148 C/T and –455 G/A polymorphism in the Bβ gene (78). No polymorphism is reported in the γ-chain gene. The noncoding fibrinogen polymorphism at –455 G/A of fibrinogen Bβ locus has been studied the most because it is located close to an interleukin-6-responsive element and an HNF 1 element, which is the rate-limiting step in fibrinogen biosynthesis. The –455 A/G polymorphism was associated with changes in plasma fibrinogen levels (79), and the changes were influenced by exercise and smoking (80–83). The lipid-lowering drug pravastatin changed fibrinogen levels in patients with coronary artery disease, and the changes were associated with the –455G/A polymorphism (84). These studies suggest that the effect of –455A/G on fibrinogen levels are dependent on environmental and acute phase reactions. Two studies have investigated the effects of the –455 A/G polymorphism on the promoter function of the 5' flanking region of the fibrinogen Bβ-chain gene. They concluded that the –455G/A and –854G/A could explain approximately 11% of the variation in plasma fibrinogen levels (85).

There are only two common polymorphisms that cause a change in the amino acid sequence of fibrinogen. One is in the fibrinogen Aα gene, which causes a change from threonine to alanine at residue 312, with an allele frequency of approximately 0.23 (85). The other is in the Bβ gene, which changes arginine to lysine at residue 448, with an allele frequency of 0.15 (85,86). The Aα Thr312Ala polymorphism occurs close to glutamine 328, which is involved in α-α cross-links and the site where α₂-antiplasmin is cross-linked to the Aα-chain (lysine 303). This proximity to functional cross-linking sites suggests that the polymorphism could affect the factor XIII cross-linking and the clot's plasmin-resistant structure.

FACTOR XIII STRUCTURE

Factor XIII was discovered approximately 15 years before the first case of congenital factor XIII deficiency was reported in 1960 (87). Factor XIIIa, a transglutaminase, is designated an *R-glutaminyl-peptide: amine γ-glutamyltransferase* (EC 2.3.2.13). The remarkable specificity and reaction mechanism of this enzyme is detailed in the literature (88–95). The ability of factor XIIIa to covalently couple fibrin molecules to each other and to proteins in plasma and the extracellular matrix is important for normal hemostasis. Fibrin is the major substrate for factor XIIIa in blood and is formed as fibrin polymerizes at sites of vascular injury. The fibrin clot is initially stabilized by the factor XIIIa that is generated by thrombin cleavage of plasma factor XIII before fibrin forming a visible thrombus. In blood, 50% of the total factor XIII is inside the platelet, and this can also serve as a source of additional factor XIIIa during wound healing.

The A- and B-chain protein sequences were derived from isolating the genes and determining the cDNA sequence (96–101). The three-dimensional structure of the recombinant A-chain was determined by x-ray crystallography (101–104). Mutant forms of the A-chain protein were expressed and provide investigators with new insights into the structure and function of this protein in hemostasis and thrombosis. Molecular modeling of mutations in congenital factor XIII deficiency has also been helpful in elucidating the structure and function of factor XIII (105).

Plasma Factor XIII Structure

The plasma factor XIII molecule circulates in blood as a 325.8-kd tetramer composed of two A-chains of 83.2 kd and two B-chains of 79.7 kd (106–109). In addition, 50% of the total factor XIIIa activity in blood is inside the platelet as a dimer composed of A-chains (110). The A-chains function as the catalytic domain, whereas the B-chains serve as carrier molecules that stabilize the protein and allow it to associate with fibrinogen (111–114). Liver and bone marrow transplantation established that the A-chains are derived from both the liver and the bone marrow (115). The B-chains are synthesized by the liver and secreted as a monomer that binds to the A-chains in plasma (114).

X-ray crystallography of recombinant A-chains demonstrates that each chain is folded into four domains, designated the β-*sandwich*, the *catalytic core, barrel 1*, and *barrel 2* (Fig. 39-7) (102,116). The 37 amino acid long activation peptide inhibits substrates from entering the active site pocket that contains cysteine 314 (102). The activation peptide from one chain crosses the opening to the active site pocket on the other A-chain. A portion of the activation peptide structure is stabilized by multiple hydrogen bonds and salt bridges between the β-sandwich and the catalytic core domain within the dimer. X-ray crystallography studies of thrombin-cleaved factor XIII A-chain molecules reveal that the activation peptides stay associated with the protein in the absence of a substrate (117). Fibrin polymers (118,119) enhance thrombin cleavage of the activation peptide, suggesting fibrin can have an allosteric effect on this segment of the protein. Further studies are required to determine how fibrin enhances either the release or reorientation of the activation peptides.

The A-chain contains six potential asparagine-linked glycosylation sites, but no carbohydrates were detected by mass spectrometry (109). In contrast, carbohydrates contribute approximately 8.5% of the factor XIII B-chain molecular weight (120). The B-chain is composed of ten repeated Sushi or GP-1 domains (98,121), with each Sushi domain containing two disulfide bonds that maintain the tertiary structure. There are a total of 40 cysteine residues and 20 disulfide bonds in the B-chain. The functions of the B-chain include regulating the plasma half-life and the binding of plasma factor XIII to fibrinogen. However, there is an excess of B-chains in plasma, and additional functions may exist (114).

ACTIVATION OF FACTOR XIII MOLECULES

The A-chains must be cleaved to activate the plasma factor XIII. In contrast, there are thrombin-dependent and nonproteolytic mechanisms to activate dimeric platelet factor XIII (122,123). Several serine proteases can attack the Arg37-Gly38 peptide, making it feasible that other serine proteases can activate factor XIII. The endogenous platelet acid protease (123) and calpain (124) were reported to activate factor XIII.

Thrombin cleaves plasma factor XIII very slowly and requires a cofactor for factor XIIIa to be generated in a timely fashion to aid hemostasis. Fibrin polymers serve as the cofactor to rapidly generate factor XIIIa (118,119,125–128). A complex between thrombin, fibrin polymers, and plasma factor XIII accelerates the cleavage of the A-chains. Because factor XIII will not be activated until a critical mass of fibrin polymerizes, this restricts factor XIIIa formation to a time when factor XIIIa is needed. The generation of factor XIIIa in plasma can be triggered when only 1% to 2% of fibrinogen is converted to fibrin polymers. However, because at least 20% of the fibrinogen must be cleaved by thrombin before a fibrin clot forms, factor XIIIa begins stabilizing fibrin polymers before a visible thrombus appears. The plasma concentrations of the factor XIII A-chain and fibrinogen are approximately 15 μg/mL and 3 mg/mL, respectively. Thus, the molar ratio of factor XIII to fibrinogen in plasma is in excess of 1:100. The large excess of fibrinogen facilitates the conversion of factor XIII to factor XIIIa by fibrin polymers.

Platelet factor XIII is more rapidly activated by thrombin than plasma factor XIII (129). This lag phase of plasma factor XIII activation represents the time it takes for the B-chains to dissociate (119,130,131). Dissociation of the B-chains from the A-chains is necessary to expose the active site cysteine in plasma factor XIII (Fig. 39-8). There are no B-chains bound to fibrin, and this suggests the B-chains dissociate before fibrin gels (132). The αC-domain of fibrin (residues 242 to 424) was identified as regulating the dissociation of the B-chains (133). More than 90% of the A-chains remain bound to fibrin, localizing the catalytic chain to the fibrin gel.

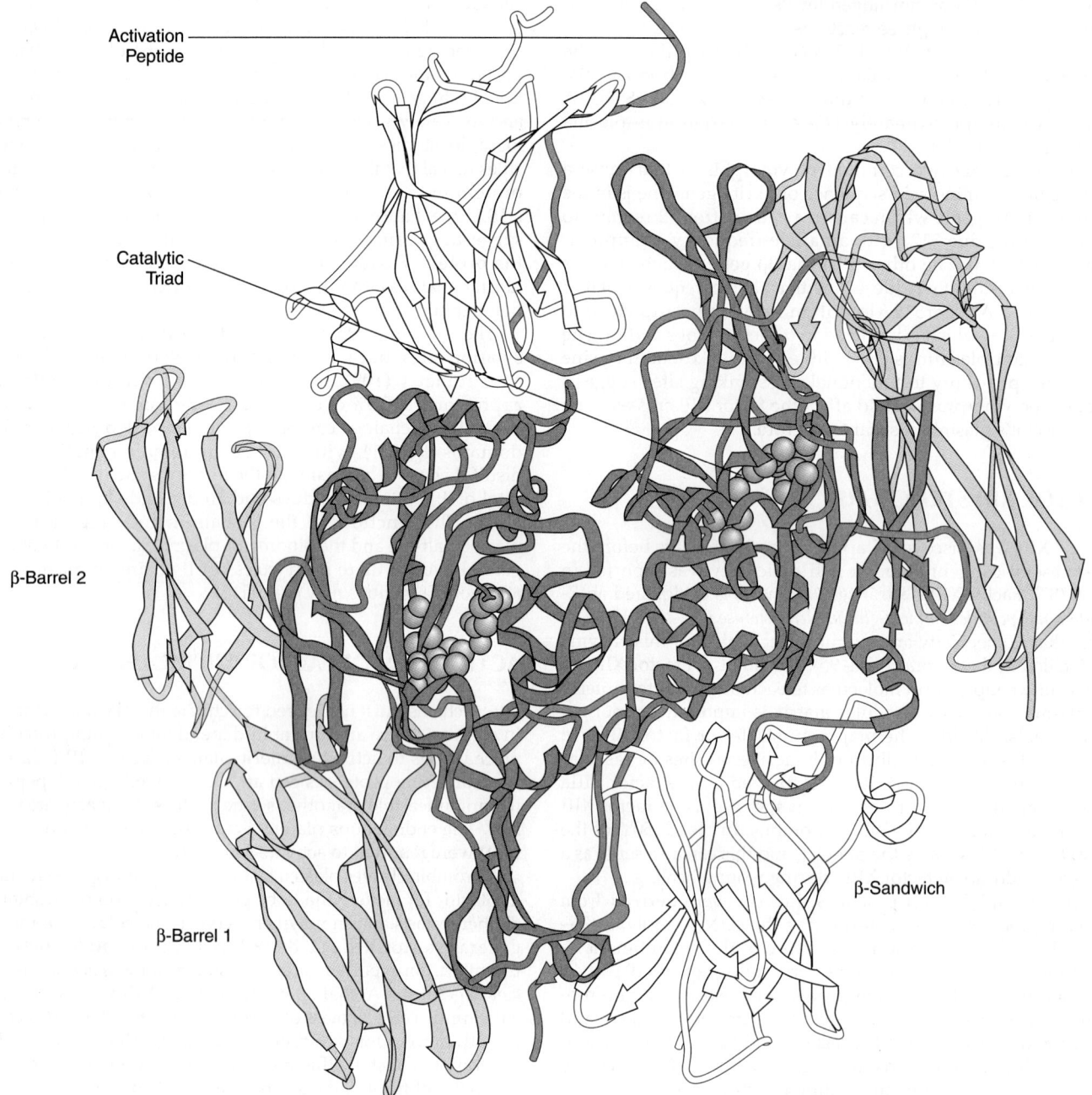

Activation Peptide

Catalytic Triad

β-Barrel 2

β-Sandwich

β-Barrel 1

Figure 39-7. Factor XIII. A-chain structure. Four distinct domains make up the factor XIII monomer: the β-sandwich, residues 43-184; the catalytic core, residues 185-515; barrel 1, residues 516-628; and barrel 2, residues 629-727. The secondary structure of the β-sandwich, barrel 1 and barrel 2 domains, is predominantly β-sheet, whereas the catalytic core is a mixture of β-sheet and α-helix. Thrombin-cleaved factor XIII A-chains acquire catalytic activity after calcium ions induce exposure of the active site C_{314}. The catalytic triad is composed of residues C314, H373, and D396. A three-dimensional model of factor XIII highlights the domains characterized from the resolved crystal structure. This image was created using the atomic coordinates of the x-ray crystal structure of factor XIII deposited in the Protein Data Bank at Brookhaven National Laboratory and the graphics program, Sybyl 6.7 (Tripos, Inc., St. Louis, MO).

INTERACTION BETWEEN FACTOR XIII AND FIBRIN

Serum factor XIII levels are more than 90% lower than plasma levels (134,135). Plasma factor XIII binds to both fibrinogen and fibrin (132). Thrombin-cleaved factor XIII binds to fibrin through an interaction with sites in the αC-domains of fibrinogen (136). The plasma factor XIII zymogen does not compete for fibrin-binding sites with factor XIIIa, establishing that the zymogen and factor XIIIa bind to distinct and noninteracting domains.

In addition, the zymogen does not interfere with the ability of fibrinogen to promote B-chain dissociation from thrombin-cleaved plasma factor XIII (126). The portion of the fibrinogen molecule that binds the plasma factor XIII zymogen was only recently defined. Plasma factor XIII binds to fibrinogen through interactions between the B-chain and the γ' region of fibrinogen

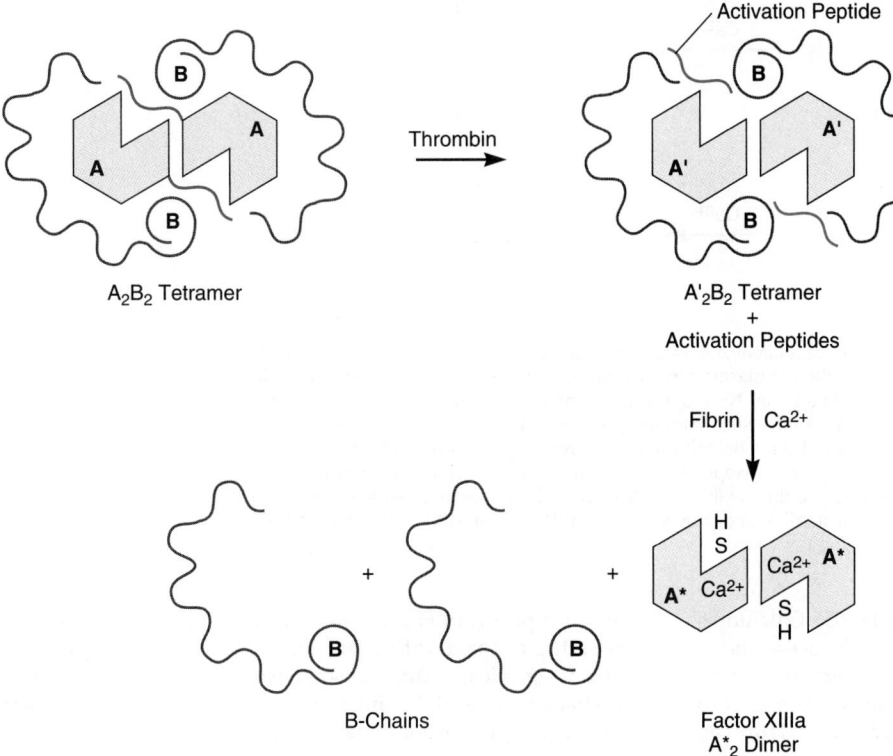

Figure 39-8. Factor XIII tetrameric structure and activation. Plasma factor XIII is a heterologous tetramer consisting of two A-subunits and two B-subunits. The A-subunits contain the enzyme's active site, and the B-subunits serve a carrier function of the hydrophobic A-subunit in the aqueous environment of human plasma. Activation of factor XIII involves cleavage of the activation peptides from the A-subunit, which then may or may not dissociate from the complex. In a second step, calcium and fibrin induce the dissociation of the B-subunits from A to expose the active site's thiol group. The B-chains bind to the γ'-chain of fibrinogen and serve to promote the formation of plasma factor XIII-fibrinogen complex in plasma.

(137). This binding plays a role in localizing factor XIIIa to the fibrin clot. The localization of factor XIIIa to the fibrin clot is a complex process and suggests that both the zymogen and factor XIIIa can interact with fibrinogen as well as fibrin.

Thrombin Cleavage of Factor XIII

Serine proteases often use an exosite to orient the substrate and facilitate proteolysis. Recent studies suggest that a site outside of the factor XIII activation peptide domain that is involved in thrombin binding may exist (138). The B-chain may also sterically interfere with the cleavage of the A-chains, because they can inhibit the proteolysis of the activation peptide of platelet factor XIII (119,131). Further studies are needed to define the structural domain(s) responsible for thrombin cleavage of plasma factor XIII. A model where plasma factor XIII binds to the γ' site allows thrombin bound to the fragment E-region to react with plasma factor XIII during fibrin polymerization. The process of fibrin polymerization may also realign the B-chains to promote thrombin cleavage of plasma factor XIII A-chains.

Catalytic Mechanism of Factor XIIIa

The enzymology of the plasma and tissue transglutaminases was extensively studied, and the molecular mechanism very well defined (88). Recent x-ray crystallography data established that a catalytic triad that was formed by Cys314, His373, and Asp396 participated in the formation of the isopeptide bond (102,116). The first step in catalysis was the binding of a select glutamine residue to form an enzyme substrate complex (88,89). The cysteine in the active site pocket forms a thioester bond that releases ammonia from glutamine (Fig. 39-9) (88,89). The second step involves the binding of the enzyme-substrate complex to a primary amine, which is a protein-bound lysine, polyamine, or other primary amine (i.e., serotonin, histamine) and has limited substrate specificity. The thioester intermediate is extremely reactive and will rapidly form an isopeptide bond (Fig. 39-9) (91,93,95,139). The enzyme-substrate complex will also react with water, releasing the enzyme and converting the glutamine to glutamic acid if there are no primary amines available in the active site pocket (88,89). In the case of fibrin, the lysine residues in the γ-chains are aligned to promote γ-γ-chain cross-linking.

When x-ray crystals of factor XIII were analyzed at high resolution (104), it was discovered that there were also nonproline cis-bonds present in the molecule at amino acids Arg310-Tyr311 and Gln425-Phe426. The conversion of these nonproline cis-peptide bonds to the trans-configuration could provide a conformational change to expose the active site to protein substrates (104). When site-directed mutagenesis of either Arg310 or Tyr311 to Ala occurred, the mutant factor XIII molecules were inactive (140). These findings suggest that catalysis cannot occur when this nonproline cis-peptide bond is disrupted.

The stereospecific orientation of specific glutamine and lysine residues in the active site is just beginning to be investigated by site-directed mutagenesis. Mutagenesis of amino acid residues on either side of the active site cysteine caused substantial loss of enzymatic activity but did not change the binding to fibrin (140). This suggests that the sites used for fibrin binding are different or less susceptible to disruption by point mutations around the active site cysteine (amino acid residues 310 to 317). Further studies are needed to establish the nature of the fibrin binding sites in factor XIIIa.

Calcium and Factor XIIIa Function

Calcium ions are required for plasma factor XIII to be enzymatically active after thrombin cleavage (141–143). Calcium induces the B-chain to dissociate from thrombin-cleaved plasma factor XIII by a poorly understood process. Calcium ions are also required for the first step of catalysis, which is protein-bound glutamine substrate recognition. The catalytic triad is close to the calcium-binding domain and could indirectly reg-

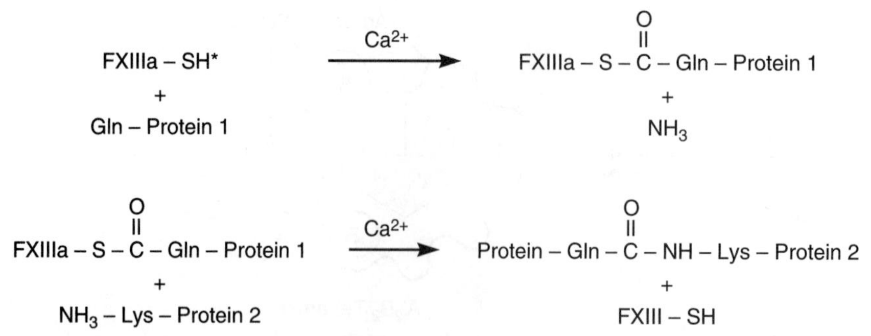

$$\text{FXIIIa} - \text{SH}^* \ + \ \text{Gln} - \text{Protein 1} \quad \xrightarrow{\text{Ca}^{2+}} \quad \overset{\overset{\textstyle O}{\|}}{\text{FXIIIa} - \text{S} - \text{C} - \text{Gln} - \text{Protein 1}} \ + \ \text{NH}_3$$

$$\overset{\overset{\textstyle O}{\|}}{\text{FXIIIa} - \text{S} - \text{C} - \text{Gln} - \text{Protein 1}} \ + \ \text{NH}_3 - \text{Lys} - \text{Protein 2} \quad \xrightarrow{\text{Ca}^{2+}} \quad \overset{\overset{\textstyle O}{\|}}{\text{Protein} - \text{Gln} - \text{C} - \text{NH} - \text{Lys} - \text{Protein 2}} \ + \ \text{FXIII} - \text{SH}$$

Figure 39-9. Formation of factor XIIIa-catalyzed isopeptide bond. Factor XIIIa recognizes glutamine-containing side chains in several different plasma proteins. In this diagram, two separate fibrin molecules are aligned in an antiparallel configuration. Note opposite orientation of amino- and carboxy termini of the individual proteins. Factor XIIIa's active site cysteine (Cys$_{314}$) will form a calcium-dependent thioester complex with the glutamine residue. Then a neighboring lysine residue, aligned by fibrin polymerization, will serve as an electron acceptor, and an isopeptide γ-glutaminyl, ε-lysyl bond will form between the proteins. Ammonia is released during the catalytic process from the glutamine residue. Intermolecular covalent bonds provide structural stability and prevent fibrin proteolysis and the chemical and physical disruption of hemostatic plugs.

ulate the conformation of the active site pocket (103). Calcium is actually serving as a cofactor for the enzymatic process and is not directly involved in the catalytic events. Calcium-dependent proteases, such as the calpains, also use calcium ions to align the enzyme and substrate for efficient catalysis (116). The transglutaminase reaction and active site pocket have many of the same properties as calpain, although they form covalent bonds and do not hydrolyze them (116).

Although biochemical analysis of factor XIIIa's reaction suggest that a conformational change is expected to occur when calcium is bound, the x-ray crystal structure reveals no major structural change in factor XIII with calcium (117). This suggests that other factors, such as substrate binding, are necessary for conformational change to occur in the active site pocket.

Factor XIII has a very low affinity for calcium, and several sites were reported as calcium-binding domains. X-ray crystallography of recombinant factor XIII A-chain bound to divalent ligands revealed that the major calcium-binding ligands were at Glu485, Glu490, Asp436, and Asn438 (103,144). Point mutations at Glu485 and Glu490 increased the Kact for calcium by 25-fold, indicating that they modulate the calcium requirement for the enzyme (145).

Platelet factor XIII A-chain dimers are more rapidly cleaved by thrombin and activated at lower calcium concentrations (1 mM) than plasma factor XIII. Calcium ion concentrations greater than 10 mM are required for full expression of plasma factor XIIIa activity (141–143). These plasma factor XIII calcium concentrations are higher than plasma levels, suggesting that a cofactor must exist to promote the rapid activation of plasma factor XIII. Fibrinogen binding to thrombin-cleaved plasma factor XIII becomes fully active at plasma calcium concentrations of 1 mM. Fibrinogen promotes the dissociation of the B-chains from thrombin-cleaved plasma factor XIII in the presence of calcium ions (146). Calcium binding also protects factor XIIIa from degradation by preventing the exposure of additional serine protease cleavage sites that exist in the C-terminus and would inactivate the enzyme if cleaved.

The calcium binding site is physically close to the β-barrels and is folded in an immunoglobulin-like β-pleated sheet in the C-terminus. The β-barrels prevent glutamine and lysine substrates from entering the active site pocket (102). A conformational change in the β-barrel domains must occur to allow the substrate to react with the catalytic triad. This change in conformation is not dependent on protease cleavage or release of the

activation peptide. High concentrations of calcium ions can induce the autoactivation of platelet factor XIII, suggesting there are significant effects of solvents on protein conformation. It has been proposed that intracellular platelet factor XIII is activated by this protease-independent pathway (123).

Other Factors Regulating Factor XIIIa Activity

Nitric oxide influences a number of biologic processes, including platelet activation, regulation of vascular tone, and blood pressure. Nitric oxide can exert its biologic action by nitrosylation of reactive thiol groups in proteins. Nitric oxide donors can inhibit factor XIII activity by S-nitrosylation of the active-site cysteine of factor XIIIa (147). Regulation of factor XIII activity by nitric oxide at sites of vascular injury could influence local stability of a clot. The ability of nitric oxide to modulate factor XIII activity may provide an inhibitory mechanism to prevent protein cross-linking. Factor XIIIa does not have any other natural inhibitor in human plasma.

Substrate Specificity

The mechanism by which transglutaminases recognize their protein substrates remains unknown. Most of the existing information on the molecular basis of substrate specificity was established using low-molecular-weight molecules and not the typical macromolecular plasma protein substrates with the enzyme (148,149). Recombinant chimeras of factor XIII and tissue transglutaminase demonstrated that some of the properties required for the transglutaminases to recognize protein substrates reside in the amino acid residues within the exon that defines the active site pocket (150). Exchanging the active site exon of factor XIII for the tissue transglutaminase sequence produced a recombinant enzyme that cross-linked fibrin in a pattern more characteristic of the tissue enzyme. Other regions outside the active site pocket must be important for protein substrate recognition, because these chimeras were less active than the native enzyme (151). A stringent stereospecificity for γ-chain cross-linking can be inferred by looking at the x-ray crystal structure of cross-linked fibrin (2). Any change in the active site pocket would reduce the ability of factor XIIIa to react with the γ-chains during fibrin polymerization.

The reactivity of a glutamine residue requires that the glutamine be surface-exposed, and there are very specific structural requirements within the enzyme's active site pocket (152,153). When a 13 amino acid peptide was modeled after the sequence surrounding the glutamine in the fibrin γ-chain, it was found to be a poor substrate for factor XIIIa (152). This suggests that an exosite with additional secondary and tertiary structures regulates fibrin γ-chain cross-linking. An exosite in the N-terminus of keratinocyte transglutaminase was found to regulate substrate specificity for this homologous enzyme (154).

Although the second part of the cross-linking reaction involves a primary amine and is not as specific, there are steric restrictions placed on protein-bound lysines. The amino acid residue that precedes the lysine modulates the recognition of this cross-linking site (155,156). Additional studies are needed to establish how three large proteins (factor XIIIa and two fibrin monomer molecules) can bind to rapidly produce an intermolecular ε-(γ-glutamyl) lysine bond.

The process of fibrin polymerization influences the cross-linking process by aligning the molecule to enhance intermolecular catalysis. A double-headed Gly-Pro-Arg-Pro ligand mimicked the fragment E-domain by joining two D-fragments and allowing for γ-chain cross-linking to occur (157). In the absence of the double-headed ligand (or the E-region) intermolecular cross-linking takes place very slowly between two D-fragments. These studies show that polymerization of the fibrin monomers modulates the formation of the γ-γ cross-linking reaction within fibrin.

Because factor XIIIa contains two cysteines in distinctly folded active site pockets formed independently by each A-chain, factor XIIIa must be oriented such that the molecule does not have to move substantially to generate the two isopeptide bonds at the D-region interface. X-ray crystal structure of the D-dimer reveals that the isopeptide bonds are situated between molecules that are aligned along the same plane (158). This alignment is designated the *cis-configuration*, as opposed to the trans-configuration, which was based on the detection of γ-chain trimers and tetramers. Because the D-dimer domain interface is not completely resolved by x-ray crystallography and appears flexible, other configurations could be established at branch points in the fibrin gel structure, producing γ-chain trimers and tetramers (1).

BIOLOGIC SUBSTRATES OF FACTOR XIII

Fibrin γ-Chain Cross-Linking

Six isopeptide bonds can be formed between one fibrin molecule and its neighbor (89,95). These covalent bonds strengthen the fibrin clot and make it resistant to mechanical, chemical, and enzymatic degradation, compared with the non–cross-linked polymer (159–162). The cross-linking allows the isopeptide bond to be placed in an antiparallel orientation (163). The initial fibrin cross-linking reaction involves Lys406 in the carboxy tail of the γ-chain with either Gln398 or Gln399 in the γ-chain of a second fibrin molecule (164,165).

Fibrin α-Chain Cross-Linking

The cross-linking of the α-chains of fibrin occurs much more slowly than the cross-linking of the γ-chains (166). Each α-chain has at least two glutamine acceptor sites located at amino acid residues 328 and 366 and five potential lysine sites between residues 518 and 584 (161,167). A highly complex and intricate cross-linking forms along the coiled-coil region of the fibrin clot. The α-chain cross-linking plays a very important role in regulating fibrinolysis (168–172) and determines the deformability of fibrin. The α-chain functions to stabilize the intermolecular

assembly of protofibrils into thick fibers with high tensile strength. The α-chain cross-linked network appears to form a protective barrier to prevent plasmin from degrading the sites in the coiled-coil domain. Plasmin must degrade fibrin within the coiled-coil region to cause fibrin to completely lose its structural integrity (173–176).

Covalent cross-linking by factor XIIIa between the α- and γ-chains of fibrin has also been described (177). The α-γ cross-link is promoted by the formation of γ-γ cross-links. The function of α-γ cross-linking is still unknown; however, it could play an important role in the stabilization of clot structure. Direct sequence analysis of the amino acids participating in this cross-linking reaction remains to be established. There has been some analysis of the sequences that are cross-linked in this reaction (178). Factor XIIIa will cross-link fibrinogen in the same pattern as fibrin, with γ-chain dimers occurring first, followed by Aα-chain polymer formation. Factor XIIIa can also cross-link soluble fibrinogen to fibrin before it has formed an insoluble fibrin clot (179). Soluble fibrinogen-fibrin cross-linked complexes were demonstrated to be present *in vivo* (180–182).

α₂-Antiplasmin and Other Important Cross-Linking Reactions

Factor XIIIa rapidly cross-links α_2-antiplasmin, the fast acting plasmin inhibitor, to the α-chain of fibrin (183,184). This cross-linking reaction occurs between Gln2 in the N-terminus of α_2-antiplasmin (185) and Lys303 in the fibrin α-chain (183). The α_2-antiplasmin functions as a plasmin inhibitor when covalently cross-linked to fibrin and can play a major role in the fibrinolysis of the fibrin clot (186,187). Individuals congenitally deficient in α_2-antiplasmin experience a serious bleeding disorder similar to that of patients with congenital factor XIII deficiency (188).

There are other adhesive glycoproteins that are cross-linked to fibrin and are important reactions *in vivo*. Fibronectin can be cross-linked to both itself and collagen through Gln3 at the amino terminal end of the molecule (189). However, when fibrin is present, fibronectin-fibrin complexes are the preferred cross-linked products (190). Fibronectin is cross-linked to the α-chain of the fibrin molecule (190,191). Even though both fibronectin and α_2-antiplasmin are cross-linked to the α-chain of fibrin, fibronectin cross-linking does not modify α_2-antiplasmin incorporation (192). Cross-linking of fibronectin to fibrin clots can alter the mechanical properties (192) of the clot and promote cell adhesion and migration of cells into the fibrin clot (193). This reaction could be important to facilitate the wound healing process.

The early clinical studies on defective wound healing in factor XIII–deficient individuals provided the first evidence that factor XIIIa plays an essential role in forming the provisional matrix necessary for tissue repair (87,194). During vascular injury, fibrin clots may be covalently attached to collagen in the vessel wall by factor XIIIa. This reaction may prevent the clot from being dislodged from the vessel wall. Collagen types I, II, III, and V can be cross-linked to fibronectin by factor XIIIa (195). Collagen provides the lysine residues necessary to form an isopeptide bond with Gln3 in fibronectin. The cross-linking of both fibronectin and collagen to fibrin suggests that these reactions could stabilize the extracellular matrix that forms at sites of tissue injury.

von Willebrand factor can be cross-linked by factor XIIIa to fibrin or other extracellular matrix molecules, including collagen (196,197). Cross-linked complexes of von Willebrand's factor also bind noncovalently to cross-linked fibrin (198) and could promote platelet adhesion and aid the hemostasis response. Vitronectin is also a substrate for factor XIIIa (199), with the glutamine cross-linking site localized to glutamine 93 (200). Thrombospondin is also another factor XIIIa substrate that becomes covalently incorporated into fibrin during fibrin polymerization (201). Factor V is also a substrate for factor XIIIa (202,203). As factor V plays an important role in thrombin-generation, this reaction could provide a means for localizing thrombin generation.

Actin can be cross-linked to the α-chain of fibrin (204,205), and myosin isolated from platelets and skeletal muscle can form high-molecular-weight complexes when incubated with factor XIIIa. Vinculin (206) and the fibrinogen receptor on platelets (glycoprotein IIb/IIIa) (207) are also substrates for factor XIIIa. The physiological significance of this reaction is not entirely clear, but it is likely that covalent cross-links between fibrinogen, glycoprotein IIb/IIIa, and cytoskeletal proteins may increase the structural integrity of the platelet-fibrin plug during hemostasis. The cross-linking of platelet proteins to fibrin may also play an important role in clot retraction (208).

PLATELET FACTOR XIII

Platelet factor XIII is predominantly in the platelet cytoplasm and composed of two A-chains (106). Plasma factor XIIIa binds to glycoprotein IIb/IIIa on platelets, and this binding site can be cleaved by plasmin (209). Recent studies indicate that normal platelets resuspended in factor XIII–free plasma cross-link fibrin to each other and cross-link α_2-antiplasmin to fibrin (210). Therefore, some platelet factor XIII must get surface-exposed or secreted to stabilize fibrin clots (211). Platelets also provide a surface for accelerating the cross-linking of fibrin polymers. Platelet membrane-associated factor XIII is a marker of platelet activation (212). Recently, the ability of platelet factor XIII to cross-link serotonin to platelet proteins provides a way for platelets to bind these proteins and localize them using serotonin receptors (213). Further investigations are required to determine the precise role of platelet factor XIII in the clot stabilization process and fibrinolysis.

FACTOR XIII GENES

Factor XIII A-chain belongs to the transglutaminase gene family. The best-characterized members of this gene family are factor XIII, keratinocyte, tissue, and epidermal transglutaminases (214–216). The factor XIII A-chain gene has been localized to chromosome 6 bands p24-p25 and shows linkage with the major histocompatibility complex (214–216). The A-chain gene encodes for a mature protein of 731 amino acids and has 15 exons separated by 14 introns and is more than 160 kb in size (214–216).

The factor XIII B-chain gene encodes for a mature protein of 641 amino acids, is 28 kb in size and is composed of 12 exons separated by 11 introns (214–216). It is located on chromosome 1 bands q32-q32.1 (214–216). The B-chain contains a structural feature of ten short consensus repeat units also known as *Sushi domains* (105,214–216). Sushi domains are a common structural feature of proteins associated with the regulation of the complement system (105,214–216). This family of proteins includes five complement control proteins: factor H, C4 binding protein, CR1, decay-accelerating factor, and the membrane cofactor proteins. The genes for other Sushi domain proteins are located in the same locus at band q32 on chromosome 1 (105,214–216). Gene duplication may have played a role in the evolutionary development of the factor XIII B-chain.

GENETIC POLYMORPHISMS IN FACTOR XIIIA

A vast body of research on factor XIII exists from forensic scientists and population geneticists regarding genetic polymor-

phisms. Polymorphisms in the A-chain were first described using agarose gel electrophoresis (217–221). There were two main factor XIII A-chain alleles, A*1 and A*2, with allele frequencies at 0.8 and 0.2, respectively. The frequencies of these two alleles are not different between races (217–221). In addition, less frequent variations in the factor XIII A-chain gene were also described including alleles A*3, A*4, and A*5, with the last two alleles having population-specific differences (217–221).

New subtypes of each of the two major factor XIII A alleles were found by isoelectric focusing in polyacrylamide gels supplemented with 2M urea and were named A*1A, A*1B, A*2A, and A*2B. Population-specific differences in frequency were found for the A*1A allele, and this allele was nearly absent in Brazilian Indians (217–221).

The molecular basis for the four factor XIII A-chain alleles was reported in 1994 (217–221). A Pro564Leu substitution in barrel 1 of the mature factor XIII A-chain protein was responsible for discriminating A*1A and 1B (217–221). A Val650Ile substitution and a Glu651Gln in barrel 2 of the A-chain are responsible for the differences between the A*1A and 2A and between A*1B and 2B, respectively (217–221). Varying combinations of these three polymorphisms can explain all four alleles that have been described by isoelectric focusing.

In addition to the coding polymorphisms Pro564Leu, Val650Ile, and Glu651Gln detected by isoelectric focusing, four other silent polymorphisms in the coding region of the factor XIII A-chain gene were identified. The polymorphisms that induce an amino acid change are depicted in Table 39-1, with their approximate allele frequencies in the general population listed in the legend of the table. Investigators studying the molecular basis of factor XIII deficiency (217–221) identified a common G/T transition in codon 34 of the factor XIII A-chain, leading to a substitution of valine with leucine. This transition was not associated with the factor XIII deficiency state, but did change factor XIII function. A tyrosine-to-phenylalanine polymorphism was identified at residue 204 in the central domain of the factor XIII A-chain (217–221). Tyr204Phe has the lowest frequency in the general population of the main five coding polymorphisms with a frequency of 0.01 to 0.03 and was associated with an increased risk for recurrent miscarriage in pregnant women (217–221). Finally, two silent base changes that do not alter the amino acid sequence were identified in codons 331 (exon 5) and 567 (exon 12) (217–221).

There are two polymorphisms identified in the promoter region of the factor XIII A-chain gene. One is at –246 G to A transition (210–214), close to SP-1 and MZF-1 bindings sites (217–221). The effects of this polymorphism on protein expression and factor XIII levels have not been reported. The other polymorphism in the promoter is a short tandem repeat (AAAG)n, approximately 800 to 900 base pairs upstream of the transcription start site (217–221). This tetranucleotide repeat occurs close to a GATA-1 binding site (217–221), and its functional effect on expression has not been reported. Genetic polymorphisms can play important roles on disease susceptibility, and recent work has established a role for factor XIII polymorphism in bleeding and thrombotic disease.

Factor XIIIA Val34Leu Polymorphism

Research into factor XIII polymorphisms and human disease increased after the discovery of the Val34Leu polymorphism (219,220). This polymorphism occurs in the activation peptide of factor XIII, only three amino acids away from the thrombin cleavage site between argine37 and glycine38 (Fig. 39-7, Table 39-1). Val34Leu is common, with an allele frequency of approximately 0.25 to 0.30 in the Caucasian population (Table 39-1) (222–224). Its allele frequency varies significantly among differ-

TABLE 39-1. Relationship between the Factor XIIIA Val34Leu Polymorphism and Disease

Disease	Association with Disease	Number of Subjects	Origin of Subjects	Odds Ratio	Author (and Reference Number)
MI	+	398; 196 controls	Northern UK	0.67 (0.54–0.85)	Kohler (222)
MI	+	470	Finland	0.59 (0.38–0.93)	Wartiovaara (226)
MI	+	150; 150 controls	Brazil	0.6 (0.4–0.9)	Franco (230)
MI	–	201; 244 controls	Southern France	NA	Canavy (298)
MI	–	191	UK Asians	NA	Warner (206)
MI, DVT, CVD	–, –, –	101,97,104	Southern Spain	NA	Corral (232)
MI, ICH, BI+TIA	+,+,+	120,130,120+120 and matched controls	Northern Italy	0.59, 1.74, 0.60	Gemmati (237)
DVT	+	226; 254 controls	Northern UK	0.63 (0.38–0.82)	Catto (229)
DVT	+	189; 189 controls	Brazil	0.16 (0.05–0.50) for homozygous Leu	Franco (230)
DVT	+	154; 308 controls	Austria	0.7 (0.5–1.0)	Renner (231)
DVT	–	273; 288 controls	Hungary	NA	Balogh (267)
DVT	–	427; 1045 controls	Southern Italy	NA	Margaglione (233)
ICH	+	612; 436 controls	Northern UK	–	Catto (229)
BI	+	456; 456 controls	France	0.58 (0.44–0.75)	Elbaz (236)
ICH	–	201; 201 controls	Southern Spain	NA	Corral (235)

BI, brain infarction; CVD, cerebrovascular disease; DVT, deep vein thrombosis; ICH, intracranial hemorrhage; MI, myocardial infarction; NA, not applicable; TIA, transient ischemic attack; UK, United Kingdom.

ent populations. The frequency of the leucine34 allele is highest in Caucasians (0.25 to 0.30) and American Indians (0.29), with a maximum of 0.40 in the population of Pima Indians (Table 39-1) (223,224). In Asian Indians and African populations, however, frequency of the leucine34 allele is less at approximately 0.13 and 0.17, respectively (Table 39-1) (223,224), and it reaches its lowest point in the Japanese, with an average of 0.01 (224).

The valine to leucine change is relatively conservative, with an additional CH2-group present in the leucine side chain. The polymorphism affects the rates of activation rather than cross-linking activity *per se* (225). The activation of the leucine34 variant by thrombin proceeds more rapidly than that of the valine34 protein (225–228). This effect persists in the presence or absence of the B-chains (226). The catalytic efficiency of thrombin cleavage is increased approximately 2.5-fold from 0.2 µM-1sec-1 for the Val34 peptide to 0.5 µM-1sec-1 for the Leu34 peptide (225). The difference between thrombin cleavage of the two forms of the factor XIII activation peptide is even greater when a segment of the factor XIII polypeptide surrounding the cleavage site is taken into consideration.

The mechanism causing the substitution of Val34 with leucine to accelerate thrombin cleavage is not established, but studies suggest that this is a site where there is an interaction between factor XIII and thrombin during proteolysis of the activation peptide.

An important factor involved in the regulation of factor XIII activity is fibrin. Activation of factor XIII is a complex reaction, which is enhanced by the presence of polymerizing fibrin, but this enhancing effect is lost once the fibrin is cross-linked (118,119,123–128). Formation of factor XIII cross-linking activity therefore proceeds only efficiently in the presence of its polymerizing, non–cross-linked substrate. In the presence of polymerizing fibrin, the catalytic efficiencies of thrombin cleavage of the activation peptide were increased approximately tenfold, but activation of factor XIII Leu34 remains faster than that of Val34, with a catalytic efficiency of 4.8 µM-1sec-1, compared with 2.2 µM-1sec-1 (225).

The cleavage of the Leu34 activation peptide proceeds with a rate similar to fibrinopeptide A, whereas the Val34 peptide cleavage rate is similar to that of fibrinopeptide B (225). These data suggest that factor XIII Leu34 is activated during the for-

mation of des-A fibrin formation, whereas Val34 factor XIII is activated when des-AB fibrin is formed.

The alteration in factor XIII activation kinetics induced by the Val34Leu polymorphism appears to change fibrin's structure. The early covalent cross-linking acting to fix the thinner des-A fibrin structure inhibits lateral aggregation of the fibrin fibers. Fibrin clots formed in the presence of Leu34 factor XIII were found to have thinner fibers, smaller pores, and altered permeation characteristics compared to clots formed with Val34 variant (225).

FACTOR XIII POLYMORPHISMS AND DISEASES

Factor XIII Val34Leu and Coronary Artery Disease

Thrombosis is one of the major causes of morbidity and mortality in the developed world. Several studies have been undertaken to investigate the relationship between factor XIII Val34Leu and risk of myocardial infarction (MI). The results demonstrated a highly significant underrepresentation of the Leu34 allele in subjects with a history of MI compared with subjects with no history of MI and with controls (222). These results suggested that possession of the Leu allele was protective against MI. A study from Finland confirmed the protective association of factor XIII Leu34 in a combined postmortem and coronary angiography (226). Two further published studies have reported a protective effect of Leu34 against MI (230,237). The first, from Brazil, was carried out in 150 young survivors of MI compared to 150 controls and reported an odds ratio of 0.6 (0.4 to 0.9). Some publications also reported no association between Leu34 and risk of MI. However, there has been an insufficient number of patients enrolled in these studies for the results to be statistically significant.

Factor XIII Val34Leu and Venous Thrombotic Disorders

A total of six studies have investigated the relationship between factor XIII Val34Leu and venous thrombosis. Three of these have shown significant protective associations similar to those described for MI (229–231), whereas the others had no association (222,223). A metaanalysis of the available studies suggests that the protective effect of factor XIII Val34Leu is weak. Two studies have addressed the question as to whether interactions occur between factor XIII Val34Leu and factor V Leiden, and none were detected (230,234).

Factor XIII Val34Leu and Cerebrovascular Disease

The original paper demonstrated a higher prevalence of the Leu 34 allele in subjects with primary intracranial hemorrhage and no association with ischemic stroke. The findings in relation to intracranial hemorrhage were not confirmed by a much larger study from Spain (235). A large case control study of cerebral infarction reported a major protective effect of Leu34, with interactions with smoking that modified risk of stroke (236). These findings were supported by a smaller study from Italy (237).

GENETIC POLYMORPHISMS IN FACTOR XIII B-CHAIN

The factor XIII B-chain shows three distinct alleles, and the frequency of each allele changes in each population studied. The B*2 allele, which is rare in Asian and white populations, is more common in African-Americans (237). The molecular basis of the three most common B-chain alleles remains unknown (237).

CLINICAL DISORDERS OF FIBRINOGEN

Although fibrinogen defects are rare, they represent important examples of critical structure-function relationships in the protein (238,239). The term *dysfibrinogenemia* refers to molecules that have abnormal function but are present in normal amounts as determined by an antigen assay. The combination of a low clottable fibrinogen value by a functional assay with higher values determined by antigenic assays are diagnostic features of the dysfibrinogenemias. Detailed biochemical analysis of dysfibrinogen molecules established that amino acid substitutions, deletions, or insertions in the DNA of the individual fibrinogen chains were the cause of these abnormalities. A comprehensive listing of these defects is now published and made available on the Internet (http://www.geht.org/pages/database_fibrino_uk.html, entitled Fibrinogen Variants). There are also changes in the nature and composition of the carbohydrates in some inherited and acquired dysfibrinogenemia. The molecular basis for dysfibrinogenemia is discussed later.

Heterogeneity in the clinical expression of the fibrinogen defects is often difficult to explain. There are several potential explanations for this variability including (a) the laboratory tests to establish the diagnosis are not standardized, (b) there may be coexisting conditions that alter fibrinogen levels, and (c) there may exist other genes that compensate for or alter the genetic expression of the fibrinogen defect.

CONGENITAL DYSFIBRINOGENEMIA

There are more than 270 cases of congenital dysfibrinogens recorded in the central database cataloging these abnormalities (http://www.geht.org/pages/database_fibrino_uk.html, entitled Fibrinogen Variants). Comprehensive reviews have been reported, and there is an ever-growing number of cases described (238–240). The true prevalence of dysfibrinogens is not well established because discovering them requires that specific tests of fibrinogen function and antigen levels be performed simultaneously. These disorders are typically found in individuals who experience bleeding or thrombotic problems. However, more than one-half of the dysfibrinogens also get discovered as part of routine laboratory testing. A large number of mutations, affecting most of the known functional properties of fibrinogen, are reported.

The dysfibrinogens are named after the city where they were originally discovered, and there are cases reported with the same molecular defect. The dysfibrinogenemias are inherited in an autosomal-dominant pattern. In Table 39-1, representative cases are listed for specific functional defects. Homozygous expression is reported in several patients (238), although most are heterozygous with expression of an equal quantity of normal and mutant fibrinogen chains. Because most of the laboratory tests of fibrinogen rely on thrombin cleavage of the fibrinopeptides and fibrin polymerization, these defects are the most commonly reported abnormalities (238). In the following section, a brief description of each of the mutations in individual fibrinogen chains is discussed, along with the major functional defects they produce. Functional defects are reported at sites that control (a) cleavage of fibrinopeptides, (b) fibrin polymerization, (c) fibrin cross-linking, or (d) fibrinolysis. Most of the point mutations influence either the thrombin cleavage site alone or the γ-chain polymerization sites (A-site).

Alpha-Chain Abnormalities: Abnormal Cleavage of Fibrinopeptide A

Thrombin releases both fibrinopeptides A and B from the Aα- and B-beta chains, respectively, whereas reptilase releases only fibrinopeptide A (241,242). Because the substrate specificities for these proteases are different, dysfibrinogens may have defective release of fibrinopeptide A with either one or both enzymes. Reptilase is not influenced by the heparin–antithrombin III complex and should always be used to be certain that heparin or a heparin-like molecule is not causing a prolongation in the thrombin time.

High-pressure liquid chromatography (HPLC) methods allow the quantitative determination of fibrinopeptide A and B release by thrombin and other proteases and require a research laboratory to purify the fibrinogen and analyze the protein. In addition, qualitative abnormalities in the fibrinogen may be detected by this method because a mutant peptide may cause a change in the peptide's migration during HPLC analysis. Several different amino acid substitutions in the Aα-chain that alter fibrinopeptide A release are reported (243). These mutations are present at amino acid positions 7, 11, 12, 16, 17, 18, and 19 of the Aα-chain. The Glu 11 residue in fibrinopeptide A forms a salt bridge with Arg 173 residue in thrombin, so any mutation of this residue disrupts thrombin's recognition of fibrinogen.

Replacement of Arg16 with a histidine in the Aα-chain, the site of thrombin cleavage, is the most commonly observed mutation in fibrinogen. Thrombin cleavage is reduced several hundred-fold, and reptilase does not cleave this bond. Fibrinogens Bicêtre I (244) and Giessen I (245) are homozygous for this mutation, and these fibrinogens also do not clot with reptilase (246). All the other patients known to have fibrinogens with Arg16–His mutations are heterozygous, with approximately equal amounts of normal and abnormal molecules. These fibrinogens are characterized by long clotting times with both thrombin and reptilase. Some patients experience bleeding problems, whereas others are asymptomatic.

Substitution of cysteine for Arg16 was detected in several fibrinogen variants. Fibrinogen Metz is a homozygous mutation (247), whereas the other cases are heterozygous for this cysteine substitution at Arg16 (244,246). Fibrinopeptide A cleavage with either thrombin or reptilase does not occur when a cysteine is present at Arg16. Blood will clot very slowly in the fibrinogen Metz patient, although no fibrinopeptide A is released. This occurs because fibrinopeptide B release assists in polymerization in the absence of fibrinopeptide A release (248) to produce an abnormal fibrin gel. These patients have a history of moderately severe bleeding, with the most serious bleeding complications after any surgery or dental extraction (247). The other cases with abnormalities reported in the release of the fibrinopeptide A have variable clinical severity and have either spontaneous abortions, postpartum bleeding, thrombosis, or remain asymptomatic (238). The cysteine residue also binds to albumin and displays abnormalities in fibrinolysis (238).

Aα-Chain Defects with Defective Fibrinopeptide Release and Abnormal Fibrin Polymerization

Residues 17 to 20 in the alpha-chain form part of the newly exposed polymerization domain that regulates D-E contact and contain the "A-site" that binds the reciprocal "a-site" in the γ-chain (238). Substitutions in these amino acids cause abnormal fibrin polymerization and reduce the release of fibrinopeptide A. In fibrinogen Detroit, the first abnormal fibrinogen in which a protein sequence determination was made, Arg19 is replaced by serine (249). All clotting assays of the patients' plasma are greatly prolonged, and the purified fibrinogen does not clot with thrombin. Only after sufficient fibrinopeptide B gets released will a fibrin clot form. Reptilase also cleaves fibrinopeptide A normally; however, no fibrin polymer is formed (249–251). The fibrin monomer prepared from fibrinogen Detroit will not bind normal fibrinogen because it cannot form D-E contacts. This is in contrast to normal fibrin monomer, which has a high affinity for fibrinogen. Normal fibrin monomer also binds fibrinogen Detroit (252) because the polymerization site (a-site) in the D-region is normal in fibrinogen Detroit. These data indicate that the polymerization site ("A-site") in the E-region is defective. Other mutations in this Aα-chain polymerization domain are reported in patients that are heterozygous. In the heterozygotes, the rate of fibrinopeptide A cleavage from fibrinogen is reduced, and nonclottable fibrinogen can be found in the serum. Fibrin polymerization is markedly abnormal even when one-half of the fibrinogen is normal, because the abnormal fibrinogen acts as an inhibitor of fibrin polymerization, and clotting times are greatly prolonged.

Aα-Chain Defect: Normal Fibrinopeptide Release and Defective Polymerization

An unusual abnormality in the alpha chain was reported in fibrinogen Lima, where an Arg141 to Ser substitution leads to glycosylation at aspartic acid 139. The presence of negatively charged carbohydrates in this region of the protein interfered with lateral aggregation of fibrin fibers and inhibited fibrin formation. These patients had no symptoms, although they had abnormalities in fibrin polymerization and normal fibrinopeptide release (238).

Aα-Chain Defects and Abnormal Fibrinolysis

There are several abnormal fibrinogens reported with an Arg554 to Cys substitution. Fibrinogen Dusart, Chapel Hill III, and Paris V, with Arg554 substituted by Cys, are associated with thrombosis. This molecule has impaired fibrinolysis from thin fibers that display abnormal plasminogen binding and

resistance to plasmin. The Cys residue is covalently bound to albumin. Normal fibrin enhances the activity of tissue plasminogen activator (tPA), but in fibrinogen Dusart, the fibrin that is formed is slowly lysed by the tPA-activated fibrinolytic system (253), probably because it is made up of very thin, highly branched fibers that are lysed very slowly. This may explain the thromboembolic diathesis observed in the affected kindreds. Fibrinogen Chapel Hill III, which has the same structural defect as fibrinogen Dusart (Arg554 to Cys), is also resistant to plasmin degradation (254). These variant molecules have normal fibrinopeptide release and defective fibrin assembly. The abnormal fibrin fibers are very thin and rigid, making them resistant to plasmin. The plasmin cleavage site in the C-terminus of the Aα-chain is modified by this mutation, which may also delay other steps in plasmin cleavage.

In fibrinogen Marburg, there is an alpha-chain mutation at Lys461, which leads to a stop codon, producing an alpha chain that cannot be disulfide bonded. The cysteine that is left free binds albumin and interferes with lateral aggregation, making very thin fibrin fibers. The clinical symptoms of fibrinogen Marburg include bleeding and thrombotic problems (238).

Defects in the Bβ-Chain

Defects in the Bβ-chain are the least common reported abnormality in fibrinogen. In fibrinogen Ise, there is a Gly15 to Cys substitution that slows thrombin cleavage of fibrinopeptide B, and there is a prolongation of the thrombin time and a delay in fibrin polymerization. This mutation did not cause any clinical problems (238).

Fibrinogen New York I (255) is a heterozygous condition, and one-half of the fibrinogen molecules are missing the Bβ 9 to 72 sequence, which contains the thrombin cleavage and fibrin polymerization sites. Fibrin cross-linking is also defective, probably as a result of the disordered fibrin fiber assembly. The amino acid sequences that are deleted correspond to exon 2 of the fibrinogen gene (256). Although the Aα-chain is structurally normal, fibrinopeptide A cleavage is markedly reduced with thrombin and reptilase. The abnormal fibrinogen does not clot after the removal of fibrinopeptide A, but it does in the presence of Ca^{2+}. Cys65 of the Bβ-chain forms a disulfide bond with Cys36 of the Aα-chain (257), and this is missing in fibrinogen New York I. Therefore, a significant conformational change in the N-terminus occurs that causes a defect in thrombin cleavage, and fibrin polymerization occurs. Fibrinogen New York I is associated clinically with thrombosis, and there were multiple episodes of venous thrombosis and pulmonary embolism. Fibrin derived from fibrinogen New York I also fails to support activation of plasminogen by tPA. The plasminogen activation rate by this molecule is 50 times slower than normal fibrin (258). Although fibrin is slow to form, the fibrinolysis rate may be impaired to a greater extent, which then favors a thrombotic disorder.

γ-Chain Defects: Abnormal Fibrin Polymerization and Normal Fibrinopeptide Release

When a defect in fibrin polymerization is suspected, the process of fibrin polymerization must be studied under conditions where fibrinopeptide A and B release is completed. This requires specialized testing in a laboratory interested in characterizing dysfibrinogens (238). Fibrinopeptide A cleavage must occur to expose the functional polymerization sites (GPR–"A-sites") in the E-region. The rate and magnitude of fibrin polymerization is monitored by an increase in the optical density of a solution containing purified fibrin monomer. Abnormal polymerization occurs whenever there is a mutation in the C-terminal regions of the D fragment, which makes the γ-chain polymerization site (a-site) defective. The γ-chain dysfibrinogens have normal release of fibrinopeptide A and B (238). A recent review of the γ-chain dysfibrinogens details the advances made concerning the structure and function of the γ-chain (240). One interesting aspect of the γ-chain dysfibrinogens is the fact that they often are associated with thrombosis and not bleeding disorders.

γ-Chain Defects and Calcium Binding Site Mutations

The calcium ion forms specific bonds with the side chains of D318 and D320 and with the oxygen in the backbone of F322 and G324 (240). Calcium ions promote fibrin polymerization, and a single amino acid substitution can affect the calcium-dependent conformation that enhances fibrin polymerization (240). A thrombotic tendency is reported in the dysfibrinogens that directly alter calcium binding. The deletion of N319 and D320 in fibrinogen Vlissingen and the D318G substitution in fibrinogen Giessen IV are associated with thrombotic problems. Mutations within residues 275 to 375 (exons VII and VIII) all have abnormal fibrin polymerization (240).

γ-Chain Defects with Abnormalities in D-E Interactions

The side chain of D364 forms a salt bridge with the charged residues in the α-chain sequence GPR in the E-region during fibrin polymerization. Substitutions with D364H in fibrinogen Matsumoto and D364V in fibrinogen Melun I cause abnormal fibrin polymerization. There are other mutations that influence the D:E interaction and directly or indirectly alter the "a-site" and inhibit D:E interactions, including fibrinogens Nagoya I (Q329R), Milano I (D330V), Kyoto III (D330Y), Bern I (N337L), and Osaka V(R375G) (254).

γ-Chain Defects with Alterations in D-D Interactions

Mutations at Arg275 is the most commonly observed mutation in the γ-chain (240,259,260). The side chain of R 275 plays a role in D-D interactions during fibrin polymerization and cross-linking (240). The following substitutions were reported for Arg275: R275C, R275H, and R275S (240). In addition, R275 interacts with G309 and N308, which stabilizes the structure of this critical polymerization pocket. Dysfibrinogens caused by mutations at amino acids 308 and 310 are reported and provide further evidence concerning the structural importance of this segment of the γ-chain (240,261). In fibrinogen Kyoto I (262), asparagine in position 308 of the γ-chain is replaced by a lysine with defective fibrin polymerization.

γ-Chain Defects in Factor XIIIa Cross-Linking Site

Molecular defects in the stabilization of fibrin are not reported for the specific sites known to be factor XIIIa cross-linking sites: Q398, Q399, or K406. This suggests that alteration in any of these sites alone is insufficient to produce a non–cross-linked clot (240). Fibrinogen Paris I has γ-chain insertion of 15 amino acids at amino acid position 350 caused by abnormal splicing of mRNA transcripts. The Paris I γ-chains do not undergo covalent cross-linking by factor XIIIa. Paris I γ-chains cannot incorporate a lysine analog into the glutamine acceptor sites. In addition, fibrin polymerization of Paris I is also abnormal due to the major impact that an insertion of 15 amino acids has on this domain. Specific mutation at Gln's 397 and 398 has not been reported (240).

PLATELET FIBRINOGEN AND CONGENITAL DYSFIBRINOGENEMIA

Platelet fibrinogen is synthesized by megakaryocytes, but an exchange between the plasma pool and the platelet can occur by endocytosis. The normal γ'-chain variant is not present in the platelet (263,264). The absence of γ'-chain variant in platelets suggests a different mechanism for regulating fibrinogen synthesis in hepatocytes and megakaryocytes. There is no consistent finding and limited analysis of platelet fibrinogen in the dysfibrinogenemic patients. The observation that platelet fibrinogen may be normal when plasma fibrinogen is defective may partly explain why some patients with dysfibrinogenemia are asymptomatic.

ACQUIRED DYSFIBRINOGENEMIA

Acquired disorders of fibrinogen are commonly found in liver disease. It has been reported that more than 80% of patients with cirrhosis, chronic active hepatitis, or liver failure have abnormal fibrinogen function (265). An increase in the carbohydrate content of the fibrinogen in cirrhosis or hepatoma is well established (266) with 1.5 to 3.5 times the amount of sialic acid/fibrinogen molecule. These acquired dysfibrinogens are characterized by prolonged thrombin clotting times, normal fibrinopeptide A cleavage, and delayed aggregation of fibrin monomers. When the excess sialic acid is removed by neuraminidase, fibrinogen function is restored to normal (266,267). The mechanism appears to be due to increased sialyltransferase activity in hepatocytes undergoing hepatocellular regeneration (267). The negative charge of sialic acid has an effect on one or more of the polymerization domains involved in the association of fibrin monomers, such that very thin fibers are formed (268).

DIAGNOSIS OF DYSFIBRINOGENEMIA

To determine whether the fibrinogen molecule functions properly, testing should include a fibrinogen concentration measured by functional and immunochemical assays, a thrombin clotting time, and either a reptilase or ancrod clotting time. A functional fibrinogen assay is based on the rate of fibrin formation and polymerization and is performed with bovine thrombin. Immunologically detectable fibrinogen antigen is measured by radial immunodiffusion or other immunologic assays. Most dysfunctional fibrinogens have low clottable fibrinogen, normal fibrinogen antigen levels, and a prolongation of thrombin or snake venom clotting times (reptilase or ancrod). The prothrombin time (PT) and partial thromboplastin time (PTT) may be normal. The presence of low or discordant fibrinogen levels combined with an abnormal clotting time are sufficient for a diagnosis of fibrinogen dysfunction as long as there is no evidence of disseminated intravascular coagulation. A heparinlike substance in the patient plasma can also prolong the thrombin time, and a normal reptilase time will exclude this as a possibility. In addition, paraproteins that alter the nature of the fibrin clot can also cause a prolongation of the clotting times, and a serum protein electrophoresis will be useful. The simplest way to prove that an abnormality is congenital is to determine the presence of the defect in a family member. Testing of family members will determine whether they also have the same abnormality. A specific molecular genetic defect needs to be defined to make a definitive diagnosis. This requires a specialized laboratory interested in studying the structure and function of the abnormal purified protein.

The cleavage rates of fibrinopeptides A and B can be determined by reverse-phase HPLC. A structural mutation in one of the peptides is apparent from the aberrant migration on the chromatogram (244). Polymerization of fibrin monomers can be monitored by light scattering as change in turbidity due to the growth of the fibers (269,270). Direct sequencing of the DNA will verify the molecular genetic basis of any abnormality.

THERAPY OF DYSFIBRINOGENS

Treatment of the patient with dysfibrinogenemia depends on many factors, including prior history of bleeding or thrombosis, family history of bleeding and thrombosis, and nature and location of any surgery. If the patient is actively bleeding and has a procedure where bleeding would be life threatening or cause serious morbidity, replacement of the fibrinogen with cryoprecipitate is indicated. Normal hemostasis can be obtained by raising the fibrinogen levels to approximately 100 mg/dL plasma. The *in vivo* half-life of the infused fibrinogen is 3 to 4 days (271–274).

One unit of cryoprecipitate raises the fibrinogen level 10 mg/dL. Doses of fibrinogen to be infused can be calculated and a fibrinogen assay performed to verify normal functional fibrinogen levels after infusion. The infusion of fibrinogen preparations can lead to allergic reactions (275) and, in rare instances, to the formation of fibrinogen antibodies. Antibodies to fibrinogen have been described in two afibrinogenemic patients after multiple transfusions (275,276).

If the patient has a thrombotic abnormality, then anticoagulation is indicated. It is advisable to correct the clottable fibrinogen level as well if the patient has had any bleeding history. Duration of anticoagulation will depend on the other risk factors, both genetic and clinical, that could alter the duration of the treatment. Because thrombosis can be caused by intraluminal bleeding in the vessel wall, correcting the clottable fibrinogen defect followed by anticoagulation may be indicated (277). If the patient is asymptomatic and there is a negative family history, then no replacement therapy is indicated. However, if there is a strong family history of bleeding or thrombosis, the clinician may have to make a decision regarding the risk and benefit of any intervention after discussing the matter with the patient.

CONGENITAL AFIBRINOGENEMIA AND HYPOFIBRINOGENEMIAS

The congenital absence of plasma fibrinogen (afibrinogenemia) has been reported in more than 150 cases (278). There also exist some families that have levels that are measurable but are lower than normal (designated *hypofibrinogenemia*). In some of these cases, the fibrinogen molecule does not have normal function, and these cases are designated *hypodysfibrinogenemias* (278). Plasma fibrinogen is synthesized in hepatocytes. Low levels of plasma fibrinogen could result from alterations in either biosynthesis or catabolism; however, all cases reported to date are due to a defect in the synthesis and secretion of the protein. The clinical manifestations of low fibrinogen levels can be quite variable. Patients with no detectable fibrinogen by clotting assays often have minimal bleeding. However, the majority suffer a lifelong bleeding disorder with bleeding into the gums, into the soft tissues, after surgery, after trauma, and into the central nervous system, all of which can cause serious morbidity and mortality. The afibrinogenemia patients do not bleed as often into their joint spaces as hemophiliacs. Because platelets require fibrinogen for aggregation, they experience many of the same bleeding manifestations as individuals with platelet function defects. Women who are deficient in fibrinogen have recurrent miscarriages and require replacement therapy. In the absence of plasma

fibrinogen, other adhesion molecules may aid hemostasis, as observed in transgenic mice where both fibrinogen and von Willebrand's factor function are completely eliminated (278). There must exist other pathways that allow platelets to form hemostatic plugs in individuals that do not have any detectable fibrinogen. It is quite remarkable that human development can proceed normally *in utero* in the absence of fibrinogen.

The pathogenesis and inheritance of congenital afibrinogenemia is beginning to be defined (278). The disease is inherited as an autosomal-recessive trait with a reduced level of fibrinogen in plasma and platelets. The most common defect is a point mutation in one of the three fibrinogen genes, which causes a severe truncation and leads to impaired secretion of fibrinogen. When some of these truncation mutants were studied, it was found that the truncated mRNA was not degraded, as commonly occurs in other disease states (278). The truncated Aα-chain was transcribed, and the protein produced a mutant fibrinogen molecule that could not get secreted (278). The majority of the truncation mutants are in the coiled-coil region of the Aα-chain. This portion of the Aα-chain is known to play an important role in the initial phase of fibrinogen synthesis (278). Additional studies are needed to establish whether any of these truncated molecules are retained in the hepatocytes and trigger inclusion body formation and hepatocellular injury. In several families, a hereditary defect in fibrinogen synthesis has been observed, characterized by immunochemically detectable deposits of fibrinogen-related material in hepatocytes, low levels of circulating fibrinogen, and slightly elevated serum transaminase levels. These findings have been interpreted as a defect in fibrinogen secretion (279).

Diagnosis of afibrinogen is made by the fact that all blood coagulation tests are abnormal, including the PT and PTT, thrombin time, and reptilase times. These abnormalities are corrected by adding normal plasma. The diagnosis is readily confirmed by immunologic assay of fibrinogen, which does not detect any fibrinogen-related antigen in plasma. These patients also have abnormal platelet aggregation, which is corrected by the addition of fibrinogen. Approximately 20% of patients have a borderline low platelet count. In hypofibrinogenemias, the fibrinogen levels may vary from 10 to 50 mg%, and the immunologic assays will correlate with clottable assays. In contrast with the hypodysfibrinogen cases, the immunologic assay will be higher than the clottable assay. Replacement therapy is indicated in hypofibrinogenemic patients, and levels of 100 mg need to be maintained to achieve normal hemostasis following traumatic injury or surgery.

The treatment of this disease requires that patients receive cryoprecipitate as a source of fibrinogen whenever they experience trauma or surgery. All bleeding episodes require rapid treatment. Each bag of cryoprecipitate has approximately 300 mg of fibrinogen in a volume of 30 to 50 mL. Approximately 25% of the fibrinogen is distributed extravascularly, and this must be taken into consideration when calculating the dose based on plasma volume. Levels of 100 mg% are required to obtain normal hemostasis. Because each day 25% of the fibrinogen is catabolized, it is recommended that patients receive one-third of the initial dose daily until healing has thoroughly occurred. The duration of the treatment depends on the magnitude of the injury and how quickly the wound heals. In the pregnant patient, prophylactic replacement therapy is required for the duration of the pregnancy (to prevent loss of the fetus) and into the postpartum period to aid recovery.

FACTOR XIII DEFICIENCY STATES

Severe bleeding into soft tissues or the central nervous system following trauma, poor wound healing, and recurrent miscarriages characterizes deficiency of the plasma factor XIII molecule. This is a rare disease, but more than 250 cases have been reported worldwide. Factor XIII deficiency can be caused by mutations and deletions in the A-chain gene, leading to the absence of activity from both plasma and platelets, or by mutations and deletions in the B-chain gene. In the case of B-chain defects, plasma factor XIII activity is reduced but present in platelets. The bleeding diathesis of B-chain deficiency is usually milder than that of factor XIII A-chain deficiency. The B-chains appear to function to regulate the half-life of the A-chains in plasma (214–216). Factor XIII A-chain deficiency can be caused by many different molecular genetic mechanisms which have been reviewed recently (221). To date, point mutations in critical residues, deletions, mRNA splicing defects, frameshifts, and stop codons have been described (217–221). Factor XIII B-chain deficiency is a very rare autosomal-recessive disorder with only a few reported cases in the literature, recently reviewed (217–221).

CONGENITAL DEFICIENCY OF FACTOR XIII

Congenital factor XIII deficiency is rare and is inherited in an autosomal-recessive pattern with a high incidence of consanguinity in families expressing this disorder (280–282). The first patient congenitally deficient in factor XIII was described in 1960, more than 15 years after the protein was identified (281). Undetectable levels of factor XIII A-chain in plasma characterize the most common form of congenital factor XIII deficiency. The homozygous factor XIII–deficient patients have approximately 50% of the B-chain levels in their plasma (283). Patients who are plasma factor XIII–deficient are also deficient in platelet and monocyte factor XIII. The phenotypic expression of factor XIII deficiency is variable and may result in mild to life-threatening hemorrhage. The etiology of this variability is not well established, although the presence of other transglutaminase genes in the blood vessels and tissues could contribute to this phenomenon (214–216). The heterozygous factor XIII–deficient individuals display approximately 50% to 60% of normal A-chain levels, and B-chain levels are approximately 80% of normal.

The molecular defect is known for more than 30 factor XIII–deficient cases, as recently reviewed (217,284). There does not appear to be any one area where the mutation defects occur in the A-chain. Missense mutations are reported in the catalytic core and β-barrel 1 and 2 domains (217,284). Many of the mutations produce unstable proteins that have only been studied by molecular modeling approaches (217,284). The deletion events appear to be clustered around exons II, III, and XI, suggesting that specific sequences surrounding this area account for this process (217,284). There are limited data regarding the molecular genetic basis of the few cases of factor XIII B-chain deficiency. Defects producing a protein that can be secreted and bind factor XIII A-chain are reported (217,221,284).

CLINICAL MANIFESTATIONS OF FACTOR XIII DEFICIENCY

Factor XIII deficiency is characterized clinically by delayed bleeding after tissue injury. Typically, the hemostatic response is normal, but as fibrin gets deposited, it is rapidly degraded, and bleeding recurs (285). Bleeding can stop and restart multiple times, producing large hematomas until factor XIII replacement therapy is infused (85). All forms of bleeding can occur after minor trauma, including bleeding into the brain or spinal cord,

either spontaneously or following trauma. The central nervous system bleeding is common and the most serious problem causing significant morbidity and mortality (280). Central nervous system complications are documented in approximately 35% of patients and are the cause of death in 50% of the reported cases (286). These findings warrant prophylactic therapy in the factor XIII–deficient patient.

Factor XIII–deficient women who become pregnant will spontaneously abort unless they are treated (217,221,284). It is not clear why the mother must have plasma factor XIII for a successful pregnancy. However, recent studies in animals deficient in plasma fibrinogen suggest a stable fibrin clot is required to aid implantation and growth of the fetus (287). Factor XIIIa cross-linking may be necessary for placental adherence or to prevent uterine or placental hemorrhage. The first reported case of factor XIII deficiency also had some degree of abnormal wound healing (281), and fibroblasts would not grow normally in the fibrin clots derived from the patient's plasma (288). Only approximately 15% of factor XIII–deficient patients experience abnormalities in wound healing (286). Again, the other forms of the transglutaminases in endothelial cells, fibroblasts, and epidermis may compensate for the deficiency of factor XIII (216).

Treatment of factor XIII requires that a safe and effective form of plasma factor XIII be infused intravenously. The long half-life (8 to 14 days) of plasma factor XIII and the observation that low levels, approximately 5%, of factor XIII are sufficient to stop and prevent bleeding (289,290) make the treatment and prevention feasible by using a plasma product containing plasma factor XIII. There was extensive clinical experience with a placental concentrate (291), and more recently a pasteurized plasma product with the same clinical efficacy was produced. This product, designated *Fibrogrammin-P* (Aventis), is not routinely available in the United States but can be obtained by compassionate use protocols and is available in other countries. The data regarding its half-life and dosage for treatment have been reported recently (284) and are available from the manufacturer.

Initial levels of factor XIII after treatment should be in the range of approximately 50% and levels kept elevated for at least 2 weeks to allow for adequate healing. To prevent recurrence of bleeding and to aid hemostasis, prophylactic treatment is usually given every 4 to 6 weeks. The factor XIII level should probably not fall below 5% to 10%. It is useful to document the half-life of the product used for treatment in a particular patient because this will assist in minimizing the exposure of the patient to blood product.

Although some would argue that the phenotypic expression of factor XIII is quite variable, it is not necessary to give prophylactic treatment and not justified to expose the patient to a life-threatening risk of central nervous system bleeding when there exists a form of therapy that is safe and effective. It is important that, after the mildest trauma, the patient always be treated aggressively. Dental extractions also pose a threat to a factor XIII–deficient patient as is the case in any hemophiliac. These patients should be treated with factor XIII infusion or with a fibrinolytic inhibitor drug (292).

DIAGNOSIS OF CONGENITAL FACTOR XIII DEFICIENCY

Patients who are factor XIII–deficient have normal PT, PTT, thrombin clotting time, bleeding time, platelet aggregation, and α_2-plasmin inhibitor levels. The clinical screening test that is abnormal is clot solubility in 5 mol/L urea or 1% monochloroacetic acid. This test is based on the observation that solubility of fibrin in these solvents correlates with the degree of fibrin cross-linking (293,294). The clot solubility test is a widely used screen for factor XIII deficiency, and it differentiates those patients who have less than 1% plasma factor XIII levels. Test results may not be positive for those patients who have factor XIII levels from 5% to 10%, but this patient population represents less than 5% of factor XIII–deficient patients. Clot solubility testing cannot differentiate heterozygotes from normal individuals. The other disadvantage of the clot solubility test is that it is not entirely specific. Patients with low levels of fibrinogen, α_2-antiplasmin deficiency, or antibodies to factor XIII or fibrin cross-linking sites could also have positive clot solubility tests. However, this is a useful screening test that can be performed in most laboratories and is the first step in establishing a diagnosis of factor XIII deficiency.

ACQUIRED DEFICIENCY OF FACTOR XIII

There are a number of reports that plasma factor XIII is decreased in various diseases, but the significance of this with respect to hemorrhagic risk is unclear. Diseases with activation of the clotting system (disseminated intravascular coagulation, deep vein thrombosis) result in a decrease in plasma factor XIII levels (295–297). There are several reports of decreased plasma factor XIII in leukemia; this may be associated with disseminated intravascular coagulation or with a release of circulating elastase (295,297–299).

There are anecdotal reports of treatment with factor XIII of patients with Henoch-Schönlein purpura with good results (300,301). There are also a number of reports that treatment of patients with systemic scleroderma may result in improvement of cutaneous symptoms (288,302,303). This might be because of the effects of factor XIII on wound healing and its interaction with collagen, but the specific reason is not known. Recent data suggest that factor XIIIa can alter vascular permeability, and this could have a beneficial influence (304). There are also many anecdotal reports on the efficacy of treating inflammatory bowel disease (particularly ulcerative colitis and Crohn's disease) with factor XIII concentrates (305). The fact that factor XIII is incorporated into fibrin may explain its decrease in various disorders associated with intravascular fibrin formation. In addition, the action of factor XIIIa within intravascular fibrin may also contribute to organ damage in the disseminated intravascular coagulation (DIC) syndromes. Animals depleted of factor XIII did not experience the same degree of organ damage as those that had normal factor XIII levels after DIC was induced (306). Future studies using agents that alter factor XIIIa function could have an impact on the morbidity and mortality caused by the DIC syndrome.

Replacement of reduced levels of plasma factor XIII after coronary artery bypass surgery are promising if they are confirmed to reduce postoperative bleeding complications (307). Large-scale clinical trials that are double-blinded are needed to establish a role of replacement therapy in these conditions.

ANTIBODIES TO FACTOR XIII

Antibody inhibitors to fibrin cross-linking are extremely rare. Several antibodies were reported to develop in factor XIII–deficient patients (308,309). An unusual antibody to the thrombin-cleaved form of the A-chain and factor XIIIa developed in an elderly woman who was taking procainamide. This antibody specifically inhibited the binding site factor XIIIa to fibrinogen and fibronectin. The antibody inhibited cross-linking of fibrin and blocked formation of fibrin-fibronectin complexes. However, the antibody did not inhibit alpha 2–plasmin inhibitor cross-linking to fibrin alpha-chains (310).

The other reported factor XIII inhibitors developed spontaneously in individuals who had previously normal plasma factor XIII levels. These patients typically presented with massive bleeding and no previous history of a coagulopathy. Like most of the other autoimmune coagulation inhibitors, these patients are difficult to treat. Frequently, the antibody titer is high and hard to overcome by infusing factor XIII concentrates. In approximately one-half of these patients, the inhibitor will spontaneously regress, whereas the other half dies from bleeding. The inhibitors are antibodies that are directed at several epitopes on factor XIII. Antibodies to plasma factor XIII, thrombin-cleaved plasma factor XIII, and factor XIIIa, as well as to cross-linking sites on fibrin, are reported (308–312). All of these antibodies result in defective fibrin cross-linking. Several of the antibodies to factor XIII developed after patients were treated with isoniazid. Isoniazid can be a substrate for factor XIIIa, and it is thought that this may induce antibodies in some patients (312). Some of the other inhibitor patients were treated with penicillin and diphenylhydantoin. Treatment with these drugs is also associated with formation of other coagulation inhibitors.

REFERENCES

1. Mosesson MW, Siebenlist KR, Meh DA. The structure and biological features of fibrinogen and fibrin. *Ann New York Acad Sci* 2001;936:11–30.
2. Doolittle RF, Yang Z, Mochalkin I. Crystal structure studies on fibrinogen and fibrin. *Ann N Y Acad Sci U S A* 2001;936:31–43.
3. Blomback B. Fibrinogen: evolution of the structure-function concept. Keynote address at fibrinogen 2000 congress. *Ann N Y Acad Sci U S A* 2001;936:1–10.
4. Hall CE, Slayter HS. The fibrinogen molecule: its size, shape and mode of polymerization. *J Biophys Biochem Cytol* 1959;5:11–15.
5. Weisel JW, Phillips GN Jr, Cohen C. A model from electron microscopy for the molecular structure of fibrinogen and fibrin. *Nature* 1981;289:263–267.
6. Fowler WE, Erickson HP. Trinodular structure of fibrinogen. Confirmation by both shadowing and negative stain electron microscopy. *J Mol Biol* 1979;134:241–249.
7. Mosesson MW, Hainfeld J, Wall J, et al. Identification and mass analysis of human fibrinogen molecules and their domains by scanning transmission electron microscopy. *J Mol Biol* 1981;153:695–718.
8. Brown J, Volkmann N, Jun G, et al. The crystal structure of modified bovine fibrinogen. *Proc Natl Acad Sci U S A* 2000;97:85–90.
9. Yang Z, Mochalkin I, Veerapandian L. Crystal structure of native fibrinogen at 5.5A resolution. *Proc Natl Acad Sci U S A* 2000;97:3507–3912.
10. Weisel JW, Stauffacher CV, Bullitt E, et al. A model for fibrinogen: domains and sequence. *Science* 1985;230:1388–1391.
11. Weisel JW, Medved L. The structure and function of the alpha C domains of fibrinogen. *Ann N Y Acad Sci* 2001;936:312–327.
12. Gardlund B, Hessel B, Marguerie G, et al. Primary structure of human fibrinogen. Characterization of disulfide-containing cyanogen-bromide fragments. *Eur J Biochem* 1977;77:595–610.
13. Blomback B, Blomback M, Henschen A, et al. N-terminal disulphide knot of human fibrinogen. *Nature* 1968;218:130–134.
14. Blomback B, Hessel B, Hogg D. Disulfide bridges in nh2-terminal part of human fibrinogen. *Thromb Res* 1976;8:639–658.
15. Bouma H, Takagi T, Doolittle RF. The arrangement of disulfide bonds in fragment D from human fibrinogen. *Thromb Res* 1978;13:557–562.
16. Marder VJ, Budzynski AZ. The structure of the fibrinogen degradation products. *Prog Hemost Thromb* 1974;2:141–174.
17. Gaffney PJ. The biochemistry of fibrinogen and fibrin degradation products. In: Ogston D, Bennett B, eds. *Haemostasis: biochemistry, physiology and pathology.* London: John Wiley, 1977;105–168.
18. Lottspeich F, Henschen A. Amino acid sequence of human fibrin. Preliminary note on the completion of the gamma-chain sequence. *Hoppe Seylers Z Physiol Chem* 1977;358:935–938.
19. Henschen A, Lottspeich F. Amino acid sequence of human fibrin. Preliminary note on the completion of the beta-chain sequence. *Hoppe Seylers Z Physiol Chem* 1977;358:1643–1646.
20. Watt KW, Takagi T, Doolittle RF. Amino acid sequence of the beta chain of human fibrinogen: homology with the gamma chain. *Proc Natl Acad Sci U S A* 1978;75:1731–1735.
21. Doolittle RF, Watt KW, Cottrell BA, et al. The amino acid sequence of the alpha-chain of human fibrinogen. *Nature* 1979;280:464–468.
22. Chung DW, Chan WY, Davie EW. Characterization of a complementary deoxyribonucleic acid coding for the gamma chain of human fibrinogen. *Biochemistry* 1983;22:3250–3256.
23. Chung DW, Que BG, Rixon MW, et al. Characterization of complementary deoxyribonucleic acid and genomic deoxyribonucleic acid for the beta chain of human fibrinogen. *Biochemistry* 1983;22:3244–3250.

24. Rixon MW, Chan WY, Davie EW, et al. Characterization of a complementary deoxyribonucleic acid coding for the alpha chain of human fibrinogen. *Biochemistry* 1983;22:3237–3244.

25. Chung DW, Rixon MW, MacGillivray RT, et al. Characterization of a cDNA clone coding for the beta chain of bovine fibrinogen. *Proc Natl Acad Sci U S A* 1981;78:1466–1470.

26. Crabtree GR, Comeau CM, Fowlkes DM, et al. Evolution and structure of the fibrinogen genes. Random insertion of introns or selective loss? *J Mol Biol* 1985;185:1–19.

27. Mosher DF. Cross-linking of cold-insoluble globulin by fibrin-stabilizing factor. *J Biol Chem* 1975;250:6614–6621.

28. Kimura S, Aoki N. Cross-linking site in fibrinogen for alpha 2-plasmin inhibitor. *J Biol Chem* 1986;261:15591–15595.

29. Hardy JJ, Carrell NA, McDonagh J. Calcium ion functions in fibrinogen conversion to fibrin. *Ann N Y Acad Sci* 1983;408:279–287.

30. Nieuwenhuizen W, Haverkate F. Calcium-binding regions in fibrinogen. *Ann N Y Acad Sci* 1983;408:92–96.

31. Dang CV, Ebert RF, Bell WR. Localization of a fibrinogen calcium binding site between gamma-subunit positions 311 and 336 by terbium fluorescence. *J Biol Chem* 1985;260:9713–9719.

32. Everse SJ, Spraggon G, Veerapandian L, et al. Crystal structure of fragment double-D from fibrin with two different bound ligands. *Biochemistry* 1998; 37:8637–8642.

33. Nickerson JM, Fuller GM. Modification of fibrinogen chains during synthesis: glycosylation of B beta and gamma chains. *Biochemistry* 1981;20:2818–2821.

34. Townsend RR, Hilliker E, Li YT, et al. Carbohydrate structure of human fibrinogen. Use of 300-MHz 1H-NMR to characterize glycosidase-treated glycopeptides. *J Biol Chem* 1982;257:9704–9710.

35. Langer BG, Weisel JW, Dinauer PA, et al. Deglycosylation of fibrinogen accelerates polymerization and increases lateral aggregation of fibrin fibers. *J Biol Chem* 1988;263(29):15056–15063.

36. Dang CV, Shin CK, Bell WR, et al. Fibrinogen sialic acid residues are low affinity calcium binding sites that influence fibrin assembly. *J Biol Chem* 1989;264(25):15104–15108.

37. Martinez J, Palascak JE, Kwasniak D. Abnormal sialic acid content of the dysfibrinogenemia associated with liver disease. *J Clin Invest* 1978;61:535–538.

38. Mosesson MW. Fibrinogen heterogeneity. *Ann N Y Acad Sci* 1983;408:97–113.

39. Francis CW, Kraus DH, Marder VJ. Structural and chromatographic heterogeneity of normal plasma fibrinogen associated with the presence of three gamma-chain types with distinct molecular weights. *Biochim Biophys Acta* 1983;744:155–164.

40. Fornace AJ Jr, Cummings DE, Comeau CM, et al. Structure of the human gamma-fibrinogen gene. Alternate mRNA splicing near the 3' end of the gene produces gamma A and gamma B forms of gamma-fibrinogen. *J Biol Chem* 1984;259:12826–12830.

41. Mosesson MW, Homandberg GA, Amrani DL. Human platelet fibrinogen gamma chain structure. *Blood* 1984;63:990–995.

42. Hettasch JM, Bolyard MG, Lord ST. The residues AGDV of recombinant gamma chains of human fibrinogen must be carboxyterminal to support human platelet aggregation. *Thromb Haemost* 1992;68:701–706.

43. Siebenlist KR, Meh DA, Mosesson MW. Plasma factor XIII binds specifically to fibrinogen molecules containing gamma chains. *Biochemistry* 1996;35:10448–10453.

44. Cote HCF, Lord ST, Pratt KP. Gamma-chain dysfibrinogenemias—molecular structure–function relationship of naturally occurring mutation in the γ chain of human fibrinogen. *Blood* 1998;92:2195–2212.

45. Ferry JD. The mechanism of polymerization of fibrinogen. *Proc Natl Acad Sci U S A* 1952;38:566–569.

46. Madrazo J, Brown JH, Litvenovich S, et al. Crystal structure of the central region of bovine fibrinogen at 1.4 Å resolution. *Proc Natl Acad Sci U S A* 2001;98:11967–11972.

47. Laudano AP, Doolittle RF. Synthetic peptide derivatives that bind to fibrinogen and prevent the polymerization of fibrin monomers. *Proc Natl Acad Sci U S A* 1978;75:3085–3089.

48. Laudano AP, Doolittle RF. Studies on synthetic peptides that bind to fibrinogen and prevent fibrin polymerization. Structural requirements, number of binding sites, and species differences. *Biochemistry* 1980;19:1013–1019.

49. Shen LL, Hermans J, McDonagh J, et al. Role of fibrinopeptide B release: comparison of fibrins produced by thrombin and Ancrod. *Am J Physiol* 1977; 232:H629–H633.

50. Wiltzius P, Dietler G, Kanzig W, et al. Fibrin aggregation before sol-gel transition. *Biophys J* 1982;38:123–132.

51. Shainoff JR, Dardik BN. Fibrinopeptide B and aggregation of fibrinogen. *Science* 1979;204:200–202.

52 Weisel JW. Fibrin assembly. Lateral aggregation and the role of the two pairs of fibrinopeptides. *Biophys J* 1986;50(6):1079–1093.

53 Veklich YI, Gorkun OV, Medved LV, et al. Carboxyl-terminal portions of the alpha chains of fibrinogen and fibrin. Localization by electron microscopy and the effects of isolated alpha C fragments on polymerization. *J Biol Chem* 1993;268(18):13577–13585.

54 Gorkun OV, Veklich YI, Medved LV, et al. Role of the alpha C domains of fibrin in clot formation. *Biochemistry* 1994;33(22):6986–6997.

55. Weisel JW, Medved L. The structure and function of the alpha C domains of fibrinogen. *Ann N Y Acad Sci* 2000;936:312–327.

56. Gaffney PJ. Fibrin degradation products. A review of structures found in vitro and in vivo. *Ann N Y Acad Sci* 2001; 936:594–610.

57. Pfitzner SA, Dempfle CE, Matsuda M, Heene DL. Fibrin detected in plasma of patients with disseminated intravascular coagulation by fibrin-specific antibodies consists primarily of high molecular weight factor xiiia-cross-linked and plasmin-modified complexes partially containing fibrinopeptide a. *Thromb Haematol* 1997;78:1069–1078.

58. Roy SN, Procyk R, Kudryk BJ, et al. Assembly and secretion of recombinant human fibrinogen. *J Biol Chem* 1991;266:4758–4763.

59. Zhang JZ, Kudryk B, Redman CM. Symmetrical disulfide bonds are not necessary for assembly and secretion of human fibrinogen. *J Biol Chem* 1993;268:11278–11282.

60. Huang S, Mulvihill ER, Farrell DH, et al. Biosynthesis of human fibrinogen. Subunit interactions and potential intermediates in the assembly. *J Biol Chem* 1993;268:8919–8926.

61. Ruoslahti E, Pierschbacher MD. New perspectives in cell adhesion: rGD and integrins. *Science* 1987;238:491–497.

62. Kloczewiak M, Timmons S, Hawiger J. Localization of a site interacting with human platelet receptor on carboxyterminal segment of human fibrinogen gamma chain. *Biochem Biophys Res Commun* 1982;107:181–187.

63. Kloczewiak M, Timmons S, Hawiger J. Recognition site for the platelet receptor is present on the 15-residue carboxyterminal fragment of the gamma chain of human fibrinogen and is not involved in the fibrin polymerization reaction. *Thromb Res* 1983;29:249–255.

64. Kloczewiak M, Timmons S, Lukas TJ, et al. Platelet receptor recognition site on human fibrinogen. Synthesis and structure-function relationship of peptides corresponding to the carboxyterminal segment of the gamma chain. *Biochemistry* 1984;23:1767–1774.

65. Farrell DH, Thiagarajan P, Chung DW, et al. Role of fibrinogen alpha and gamma chain sites in platelet aggregation. *Proc Natl Acad Sci U S A* 1992;89: 10729–10732.

66. Farrell DH, Thiagarajan P. Binding of recombinant fibrinogen mutants to platelets. *J Biol Chem* 1994;269:226–231.

67. Thiagarajan P, Rippon AJ, Farrell DH. Alternative adhesion sites in human fibrinogen for vascular endothelial cells. *Biochemistry* 1996;35:4169–4175.

68. Rooney MM, Parise LV, Lord ST. Dissecting clot retraction and platelet aggregation. Clot retraction does not require an intact fibrinogen gamma chain C terminus. *J Biol Chem* 1996;271:8553–8555.

69. Rooney MM, Farrell DH, Van Hemal BM, et al. The contribution of the three hypothesized integrin–binding sites in fibrinogen to platelet-mediacted clot retraction. *Blood* 1998;92:2374–2381.

70. Furlan M. Structure of fibrinogen and fibrin. In: Francis JL, ed. *Fibrinogen, fibrin stabilization, and fibrinolysis.* Chichester, England: Ellis Horwood, 1988:17.

71. Seydewitz HH, Witt I. Increased phosphorylation of human fibrinopeptide A under acute phase conditions. *Thromb Res* 1985;40:29.

72. Hirose S, Oda K, Ikehara Y. Tyrosine O-sulfation of the fibrinogen γB chain in primary cultures of rat hepatocytes. *J Biol Chem* 1988;263:7426.

73. Hortin GL. Sulfation of a gamma-chain variant of human fibrinogen. *Biochem Int* 1989;19(6):1355–1362.

74. Binnie CG, Hettasch JM, Strickland E, Lord ST. Characterization of purified recombinant fibrinogen: partial phosphorylation of fibrinopeptide A. *Biochemistry* 1992;32(1):107–113.

75. Maurer MC, Peng JL, An SS, et al. Structural examination of the influence of phosphorylation on the binding of fibrinopeptide A to bovine thrombin. *Biochemistry* 1998;37(17):5888–5902.

76. Seydewitz HH, Kaiser C, Rothweiler H, Witt I. The location of a second in vivo phosphorylation site in the A alpha-chain of human fibrinogen. *Thromb Res* 1984;33(5):487–498.

77. Humphries SE, Luong LA, Montgomery HE, et al. Gene-environment interaction in the determination of levels of plasma fibrinogen. *Thromb Haemost* 1999;82:818–825.

78. Lane DA, Grant PJ. Role of hemostatic gene polymorphisms in venous and arterial thrombotic disease. *Blood* 2000;95:1517–1532.

79. Humphries SE, Cook M, Dubowitz M, et al. Role of genetic variation at the fibrinogen locus in determination of plasma fibrinogen concentrations. *Lancet* 1987;27:1452–1455.

80. Thomas AE, Green FR, Kelleher CH, et al. Variation in the promoter region of the beta fibrinogen gene is associated with plasma fibrinogen levels in smokers and non-smokers. *Thromb Haemost* 1991;65:487–490.

81. Humphries SE, Ye S, Talmud P, et al. European atherosclerosis research study: genotype at the fibrinogen locus (G-455-A beta gene) is associated with differences in plasma fibrinogen levels in young men and women from different regions in Europe. Evidence for gender-genotype-environment interaction. *Arterioscler Thromb Vasc Biol* 1995;15:96–104.

82. Montgomery HE, Clarkson P, Nwose OM, et al. The acute rise in plasma fibrinogen concentration with exercise is influenced by the G-453-A polymorphism of the beta-fibrinogen gene. *Arterioscler Thromb Vasc Biol* 1996;16:389–391.

83. Thomas AE, Green FR, Humphries SE. Association of genetic variation at the beta-fibrinogen gene locus and plasma fibrinogen levels; interaction between allele frequency of the G/A-455 polymorphism, age and smoking. *Clin Genet* 1996;50:184–190.

84. de Maat MP, Kastelein JJ, Jukema JW. -455G/A polymorphism of the beta-fibrinogen gene is associated with the progression of coronary arterosclerosis in symptomatic men: proposed role for an acute-phase reaction pattern of fibrinogen. REGRESS group. *Arterioscler Thromb Vasc Biol* 1998;18:265–271.

85. Van 't Hooft FM, von Bahr SJ, Silveira A, et al. Two common, functional polymorphisms in the promoter region of the beta-fibrinogen gene contribute to

regulation of plasma fibrinogen concentration. *Arterioscler Thromb Vasc Biol* 1999;19:30636–30700.

86. Baumann RE, Henschen AH. Human fibrinogen polymorphic site analysis by restriction endonuclease digestion and allele-specific polymerase chain reaction amplification: identification of polymorphisms at positions A alpha 312 and B beta 448. *Blood* 1993;82:2117–2124.

87. Duckert F, Jung E, Shmerling DH. A hitherto undescribed congenital hemorrhagic diathesis probably due to fibrin stabilizing factor deficiency. *Thromb Diath Haemorrh* 1960;5:179–186.

88. Folk JE. Mechanism and basis for specificity of transglutaminase-catalyzed epsilon-(gamma-glutamyl) lysine bond formation. *Adv Enzymol Relat Areas Mol Biol* 1983;54:1–56.

89. Folk JE, Finlayson JS. The epsilon-(gamma-glutamyl)lysine cross-link and the catalytic role of transglutaminases. *Adv Protein Chem* 1977;31:1–133.

90. Lorand L, Konishi K, Jacobsen A. Transpeptidation mechanism in blood clotting. *Nature* 1962;194:1148–1149.

91. Matacic S, Loewy AG. The identification of isopeptide cross-links in insoluble fibrin. *Biochem Biophys Res Commun* 1968;30:356–362.

92. Matacic S, Loewy AG. Transglutaminase activity of the fibrin cross-linking enzyme. *Biochem Biophys Res Commun* 1966;24:858–866.

93. Loewy AG, Matacic S, Darnell JH. Transamidase activity of the enzyme responsible for insoluble fibrin formation. *Arch Biochem Biophys* 1966;113:435–438.

94. Loewy AG. Fibrinase (Factor XIII). *Haemorrh Suppl* 1964;13:109–114.

95. Pisano JJ, Finlayson JS, Peyton MP. Cross-link in fibrin polymerized by factor 13: epsilon-(gamma-glutamyl)lysine. *Science* 1968;160:892–893.

96. Grundmann U, Amann E, Zettlmeissl G, Kupper HA. Characterization of cDNA coding for human factor XIIIa. *Proc Natl Acad Sci U S A* 1986;83:8024–8028.

97. Ichinose A, Hendrickson LE, Fujikawa K, Davie EW. Amino acid sequence of the a subunit of human factor XIII. *Biochemistry* 1986;25:6900–6906.

98. Ichinose A, McMullen BA, Fujikawa K, Davie EW. Amino acid sequence of the b subunit of human factor XIII, a protein composed of ten repetitive segments. *Biochemistry* 1986;25:4633–4638.

99. Takahashi N, Takahashi Y, Putnam FW. Primary structure of blood coagulation factor XIIIa (fibrinoligase, transglutaminase) from human placenta. *Proc Natl Acad Sci U S A* 1986;83:8019–8023.

100. Ichinose A, Davie EW. Characterization of the gene for the a subunit of human factor XIII (plasma transglutaminase), a blood coagulation factor. *Proc Natl Acad Sci U S A* 1988;85:5829–5833.

101. Grundmann U, Nerlich C, Rein T, Zettlmeissl G. Complete cDNA sequence encoding the B subunit of human factor XIII. *Nucleic Acids Res* 1990;18:2817–2818.

102. Yee VC, Pedersen LC, Le Trong I, et al. Three-dimensional structure of a transglutaminase: human blood coagulation factor XIII. *Proc Natl Acad Sci U S A* 1994;91:7296–7300.

103. Yee VC, Le Trong I, Bishop PD, et al. Structure and function studies of factor XIIIa by x-ray crystallography. *Semin Thromb Hemost* 1996;22:377–384.

104. Weiss MS, Metzner HJ, Hilgenfeld R. Two non-proline cis peptide bonds may be important for factor XIII function. *FEBS Lett* 1998;423:291–296.

105. Muszbek L, Yee VC, Hevessy Z. Coagulation factor XIII: structure and function. *Thromb Res* 1999;94(5):271–305.

106. Schwartz ML, Pizzo SV, Hill RL, McKee PA. Human Factor XIII from plasma and platelets. Molecular weights, subunit structures, proteolytic activation, and cross-linking of fibrinogen and fibrin. *J Biol Chem* 1973;248:1395–1407.

107. Folk JE, Chung SI. Blood coagulation factor XIII: relationship of some biological properties to subunit structure. In: Reich E, ed. *Proteases and biological control*. Cold Spring Harbor, Cold Spring Harbor Laboratory 2, 1975:150–174.

108. Chung SI, Lewis MS, Folk JE. Relationships of the catalytic properties of human plasma and platelet transglutaminases (activated blood coagulation factor XIII) to their subunit structures. *J Biol Chem* 1974;249:940–950.

109. Ashcroft AE, Grant PJ, Ariëns RAS. A study of human coagulation factor XIII A-subunit by electrospray ionization mass spectrometry. *Rapid Commun Mass Sp* 2000;14:1607–1611.

110. McDonagh J, McDonagh RP Jr, Delage JM, Wagner RH. Factor XIII in human plasma and platelets. *J Clin Invest* 1969;48:940–946.

111. Weisberg LJ, Shiu DT, Conkling PR, Shuman MA. Identification of normal human peripheral blood monocytes and liver as sites of synthesis of coagulation factor XIII a-chain. *Blood* 1987;70:579–582.

112. Muszbek L, Ádány R, Kavai M, et al. Monocytes of patients congenitally deficient in plasma factor XIII lack factor XIII subunit a antigen and transglutaminase activity. *Thromb Haemost* 1988;59:231–235.

113. Ádány R, Nemes Z, Muszbek L. Characterization of factor XIII containing-macrophages in lymph nodes with Hodgkin's disease. *Br J Cancer* 1987;55:421–426.

114. Nagy JA, Kradin RL, McDonagh J. Biosynthesis of factor XIII A and B subunits. *Adv Exp Med Biol* 1988;231:29–49.

115. Wölpl A, Lattke H, Board PG, et al. Coagulation factor XIII A and B subunits in bone marrow and liver transplantation. *Transplantation* 1987;43:151–153.

116. Pedersen LC, Yee VC, Bishop PD, et al. Transglutaminase factor XIII uses proteinase-like catalytic triad to cross-link macromolecules. *Protein Sci* 1994;3:1131–1135.

117. Yee VC, Pedersen LC, Bishop PD, et al. Structural evidence that the activation peptide is not released on thrombin cleavage of factor XIII. *Thromb Res* 1995;78:389–397.

118. Greenberg CS, Miraglia CC, Rickles FR, Shuman MA. Cleavage of blood coagulation factor XIII and fibrinogen by thrombin during in vitro clotting. *J Clin Invest* 1985;75:1463–1470.

119. Greenberg CS, Achyuthan KE, Fenton JW. Factor XIIIa formation promoted by complexing of alpha-thrombin, fibrin, and plasma factor XIII. *Blood* 1987;69:867–871.

120. Bohn H, Haupt H, Kranz T. Die molekulare Struktur der fibrinstabilisierenden Faktoren des Menschen. *Blut* 1972;25:235–248.

121. Bottenus RE, Ichinose A, Davie EW. Nucleotide sequence of the gene for the b subunit of human factor XIII. *Biochemistry* 1990;29:11195–11209.

122. Takagi T, Doolittle RF. Amino acid sequence studies on factor XIII and the peptide released during its activation by thrombin. *Biochemistry* 1974;13:750–756.

123. Lynch GW, Pfueller SL. Thrombin-independent activation of platelet factor XIII by endogenous platelet acid protease. *Thromb Haemost* 1988;59:327–372.

124. Ando Y, Imamura S, Yamagata Y, et al. Platelet factor XIII is activated by calpain. *Biochem Biophys Res Commun* 1987;144:484–490.

125. Lewis SD, Janus TJ, Lorand L, Shafer JA. Regulation of formation of factor XIIIa by its fibrin substrates. *Biochemistry* 1985;24:6772–6777.

126. Hornyak TJ, Shafer JA. Interactions of factor XIII with fibrin as substrate and cofactor. *Biochemistry* 1992;31:423–429.

127. Naski MC, Lorand L, Shafer JA. Characterization of the kinetic pathway for fibrin promotion of alpha-thrombin-catalyzed activation of plasma factor XIII. *Biochemistry* 1991;30:934–941.

128. Janus TJ, Lewis SD, Lorand L, Shafer JA. Promotion of thrombin-catalyzed activation of factor XIII by fibrinogen. *Biochemistry* 1983;22:6269–6272.

129. Hornyak TJ, Bishop PD, Shafer JA. Alpha-thrombin-catalyzed activation of human platelet factor XIII: relationship between proteolysis and factor XIIIa activity. *Biochemistry* 1989;28:7326–7332.

130. Lorand L, Gray AJ, Brown K, et al. Dissociation of the subunit structure of fibrin stabilizing factor during activation of the zymogen. *Biochem Biophys Res Commun* 1974;56:914.

131. Chung SI, Folk JE. Kinetic studies with transglutaminases. The human blood enzymes activated coagulation factor 13 and the guinea pig hair follicle enzyme. *J Biol Chem* 1972;247:2798–2807.

132. Greenberg CS, Dobson JV, Miraglia CC. Regulation of plasma factor XIII binding to fibrin in vitro. *Blood* 1985;66:1028–1034.

133. Matsuda M. Structure and function of fibrinogen inferred from hereditary dysfibrinogens. *Int J Hematol* 2000;72:436–447.

134. Israels ED, Paraskevas F, Israels LG. Immunological studies of coagulation factor XIII. *J Clin Invest* 1973;52:2398–2403.

135. Skrzynia C, Reisner HM, McDonagh J. Characterization of the catalytic subunit of factor XIII by radioimmunoassay. *Blood* 1982;60:1089–1095.

136. Procyk R, Bishop PD, Kudryk B. Fibrin-recombinant human factor XIII A-subunit association. *Thromb Res* 1993;71:127–138.

137. Siebenlist KR, Meh DA, Mosesson MW. Plasma factor XIII binds specifically to fibrinogen molecules containing gamma chains. *Biochemistry* 1996;35:10448–10453.

138. Achyuthan KE. Characterization of the reciprocal binding sites on human α-thrombin and factor XIII A-chain. *Mol Cell Biochem* 1998;178:289–297.

139. Lorand L, Ong HH, Lipinski B, et al. Lysine as amine donor in fibrin cross-linking. *Biochem Biophys Res Commun* 1966;25:629–637.

140. Hettasch JM, Greenberg CS. Analysis of the catalytic activity of human factor XIIIa by site-directed mutagenesis. *J Biol Chem* 1994;269:28309–28313.

141. Hornyak TJ, Shafer JA. Role of calcium ion in the generation of factor XIII activity. *Biochemistry* 1991;30:6175–6182.

142. Credo RB, Curtis CG, Lorand L. Ca2+-related regulatory function of fibrinogen. *Proc Natl Acad Sci U S A* 1978;75:4234–4237.

143. Curtis CG, Brown KL, Credo RB, et al. Calcium-dependent unmasking of active center cysteine during activation of fibrin stabilizing factor. *Biochemistry* 1974;13:3774–3780.

144. Fox BA, Yee VC, Pedersen LC, et al. Identification of the calcium binding site and a novel ytterbium site in blood coagulation factor XIII by x-ray crystallography. *J Biol Chem* 1999;274:4917–4923.

145. Lai TS, Slaughter TF, Peoples KA, Greenberg CS. Site-directed mutagenesis of the calcium binding site of blood coagulation factor XIIIa. *J Biol Chem* 1999;274:24953–24958.

146. Credo RB, Curtis CG, Lorand L. Alpha-chain domain of fibrinogen controls generation of fibrinoligase (coagulation factor XIIIa). Calcium ion regulatory aspects. *Biochemistry* 1981;20:3770–3778.

147. Catani MV, Bernassola F, Rossi A, Melino G. Inhibition of clotting factor xiii activity by nitric oxide. *Biochem Biol Res Comm* 1998;249(1):275–278.

148. Gross M, Whetzel NK, Folk JE. Amine binding sites in acyl intermediates of transglutaminases. Human blood plasma enzyme (activated coagulation factor XIII) and guinea pig liver enzyme. *J Biol Chem* 1977;252:3752–3759.

149. Schrode J, Folk JE. Stereochemical aspects of amine substrate attachment to acyl intermediates of transglutaminases. Human blood plasma enzyme (activated coagulation factor XIII) and guinea pig liver enzyme. *J Biol Chem* 1979;254:653–661.

150. Hettasch JM, Peoples KA, Greenberg CS. Analysis of factor XIII substrate specificity using recombinant human factor XIII and tissue transglutaminase chimeras. *J Biol Chem* 1997;272:25149–25156.

151. Gorman JJ, Folk JE. Structural features of glutamine substrates for human plasma factor XIIIa (activated blood coagulation factor XIII). *J Biol Chem* 1980;255:419–427.

152. Gorman JJ, Folk JE. Structural features of glutamine substrates for transglutaminases. Specificities of human plasma factor XIIIa and the guinea pig liver enzyme toward synthetic peptides. *J Biol Chem* 1981;256:2712–2715.

153. Gorman JJ, Folk JE. Structural features of glutamine substrates for transglutaminases. Role of extended interactions in the specificity of human

plasma factor XIIIa and of the guinea pig liver enzyme. *J Biol Chem* 1984;259: 9007–9010.

154. Kim SY, Kim IG, Chung SI, Steinert PM. The structure of the transglutaminase 1 enzyme. Deletion cloning reveals domains that regulate its specific activity and substrate specificity. *J Biol Chem* 1994;269:27979–27986.

155. Groenen PJ, Smulders RH, Peters RF, et al. The amine-donor substrate specificity of tissue-type transglutaminase. Influence of amino acid residues flanking the amine-donor lysine residue. *Eur J Biochem* 1994;220:795–799.

156. Grootjans JJ, Groenen PJ, de Jong WW. Substrate requirements for transglutaminases. Influence of the amino acid residue preceding the amine donor lysine in a native protein. *J Biol Chem* 1995;270:22855–22858.

157. Lorand L, Parameswaran KN, Murthy SN. A double-headed Gly-Pro-Arg-Pro ligand mimics the functions of the E domain of fibrin for promoting the end-to-end cross-linking of gamma chains by factor XIIIa. *Proc Natl Acad Sci U S A* 1998;95:537–541.

158. Spraggon G, Everse SJ, Doolittle RF. Crystal structures of fragment D from human fibrinogen and its cross-linked counterpart from fibrin. *Nature* 1997;389:455–462.

159. Shen LL, Hermans J, McDonagh J, et al. Effects of calcium ion and covalent cross-linking on formation and elasticity of fibrin cells. *Thromb Res* 1975;6: 255–265.

160. Gerth C, Roberts WW, Ferry JD. Rheology of fibrin clots. II. Linear viscoelastic behavior in shear creep. *Biophys Chem* 1974;2:208–217.

161. Cottrell BA, Strong DD, Watt KW, Doolittle RF. Amino acid sequence studies on the alpha chain of human fibrinogen. Exact location of cross-linking acceptor sites. *Biochemistry* 1979;18:5405–5410.

162. Laki K, Lorand L. On the solubility of fibrin clots. *Science* 1948;108:280.

163. Hoeprich PD Jr, Doolittle RF. Dimeric half-molecules of human fibrinogen are joined through disulfide bonds in an antiparallel orientation. *Biochemistry* 1983;22:2049–2055.

164. Chen R, Doolittle RF. γ-γ cross-linking sites in human and bovine fibrin. *Biochemistry* 1971;10:4487–4491.

165. Purves L, Purves M, Brandt W. Cleavage of fibrin-derived D-dimer into monomers by endopeptidase from puff adder venom (Bitis arietans) acting at cross-linked sites of the gamma-chain. Sequence of carboxy-terminal cyanogen bromide gamma-chain fragments. *Biochemistry* 1987;26:4640–4646.

166. Schwartz ML, Pizzo SV, Hill RL, McKee PA. The effect of fibrin-stabilizing factor on the subunit structure of human fibrin. *J Clin Invest* 1971;50:1506–1513.

167. Fretto LJ, Ferguson EW, Steinman HM, McKee PA. Localization of the alpha-chain cross-link acceptor sites of human fibrin. *J Biol Chem* 1978;253:2184–2195.

168. Shen LL, McDonagh RP, McDonagh J, Hermans J. Early events in the plasmin digestion of fibrinogen and fibrin. Effects of plasmin on fibrin polymerization. *J Biol Chem* 1977;252:6184–6189.

169. Gaffney PJ, Whitaker AN. Fibrin cross-links and lysis rates. *Thromb Res* 1979;14:85–94.

170. Rampling MW. Factor XIII cross-linking and the rate of fibrinolysis induced by streptokinase and urokinase. *Thromb Res* 1978;12:287–295.

171. McDonagh RP Jr, McDonagh J, Duckert F. The influence of fibrin cross-linking on the kinetics of urokinase-induced clot lysis. *Br J Haematol* 1971;21:323–332.

172. Gaffney PJ, Lane DA, Kakkar VV, Brasher M. Characterisation of a soluble D dimer-E complex in cross-linked fibrin digests. *Thromb Res* 1975;7:89–99.

173. Muller MF, Ris H, Ferry JD. Electron microscopy of fine fibrin clots and fine and coarse fibrin films. Observations of fibers in cross-section and in deformed states. *J Mol Biol* 1984;174:369–384.

174. Francis CW, Marder VJ, Barlow GH. Plasmic degradation of cross-linked fibrin. Characterization of new macromolecular soluble complexes and a model of their structure. *J Clin Invest* 1980;66:1033–1043.

175. Murthy SN, Wilson JH, Lukas TJ, et al. Transglutaminase-catalyzed cross-linking of the A alpha and gamma constituent chains in fibrinogen. *Proc Natl Acad Sci U S A* 2000;97(1):44–48.

176. Pizzo SV, Taylor LM Jr, Schwartz ML, et al. Subunit structure of fragment D from fibrinogen and cross-linked fibrin. *J Biol Chem* 1973;248:4584–4590.

177. Gaffney PJ, Brasher M. Subunit structure of the plasmin–induced degradation products of cross-linked fibrin. *Biochim Biophys Acta* 1973;295:308–313.

178. Shainoff JR, Urbanic DA, DiBello PM. Immunoelectrophoretic characterizations of the cross-linking of fibrinogen and fibrin by factor XIIIa and tissue transglutaminase. Identification of a rapid mode of hybrid alpha-/gamma-chain cross-linking that is promoted by the gamma-chain cross-linking. *J Biol Chem* 1991;266:6429–6437.

179. Procyk R, Blomback B. Factor XIII-induced cross-linking in solutions of fibrinogen and fibronectin. *Biochim Biophys Acta* 1988;967:304–313.

180. von Hugo R, Hafter R, Stemberger A, Graeff H. Complex formation of cross-linked fibrin oligomers with agarose-coupled fibrinogen and fibrin. *Hoppe Seylers Z Physiol Chem* 1977;358:1359–1563.

181. Shainoff JR, Page IH. Cofibrins and fibrin-intermediates as indicators of thrombin activation in vivo. *Circ Res* 1960;8:1013–1019.

182. Kierulf P. Studies on soluble fibrin in plasma. V. Isolation and characterization of the clottable proteins obtained from patient plasmas on gelation with ethanol. *Thromb Res* 1974;4:183–187.

183. Kimura S, Aoki N. Cross-linking site in fibrinogen for alpha 2-plasmin inhibitor. *J Biol Chem* 1986;261:15591–15595.

184. Sakata Y, Aoki N. Cross-linking of alpha 2-plasmin inhibitor to fibrin by fibrin-stabilizing factor. *J Clin Invest* 1980;65:290–297.

185. Kimura S, Tamaki T, Aoki N. Acceleration of fibrinolysis by the N-terminal peptide of alpha 2-plasmin inhibitor. *Blood* 1985;66:157–160.

186. Mimuro J, Kimura S, Aoki N. Release of alpha 2-plasmin inhibitor from plasma fibrin clots by activated coagulation factor XIII. Its effect on fibrinolysis. *J Clin Invest* 1986;77:1006–1013.

187. Sakata Y, Aoki N. Significance of cross-linking of alpha 2-plasmin inhibitor to fibrin in inhibition of fibrinolysis and in hemostasis. *J Clin Invest* 1982;69: 536–542.

188. Aoki N, Saito H, Kamiya T, et al. Congenital deficiency of alpha 2-plasmin inhibitor associated with severe hemorrhagic tendency. *J Clin Invest* 1979;63:877–884.

189. Mosher DF, Schad PE, Vann JM. Cross-linking of collagen and fibronectin by factor XIIIa. Localization of participating glutaminyl residues to a tryptic fragment of fibronectin. *J Biol Chem* 1980;255:1181–1188.

190. Procyk R, Adamson L, Block M, Blomback B. Factor XIII catalyzed formation of fibrinogen-fibronectin oligomers—a thiol enhanced process. *Thromb Res* 1985;40:833–852.

191. Niewiarowska J, Cierniewski CS. Inhibitory effect of fibronectin on the fibrin formation. *Thromb Res* 1982;27:611–618.

192. Tamaki T, Aoki N. Cross-linking of alpha 2-plasmin inhibitor and fibronectin to fibrin by fibrin-stabilizing factor. *Biochim Biophys Acta* 1981;661:280–286.

193. Barry EL, Mosher DF. Factor XIIIa-mediated cross-linking of fibronectin in fibroblast cell layers. Cross-linking of cellular and plasma fibronectin and of amino-terminal fibronectin fragments. *J Biol Chem* 1989;264:4179–4185.

194. Duckert F. Documentation of the plasma factor XIII deficiency in man. *Ann N Y Acad Sci* 1972;202:190–199.

195. Mosher DF, Schad PE. Cross-linking of fibronectin to collagen by blood coagulation Factor XIIIa. *J Clin Invest* 1979;64:781–787.

196. Hada M, Kaminski M, Bockenstedt P, McDonagh J. Covalent cross-linking of von Willebrand factor to fibrin. *Blood* 1986;68:95–101.

197. Bockenstedt P, McDonagh J, Handin RI. Binding and covalent cross-linking of purified von Willebrand factor to native monomeric collagen. *J Clin Invest* 1986;78:551–556.

198. Ribes JA, Francis CW. Multimer size dependence of von Willebrand factor binding to cross-linked or noncross-linked fibrin. *Blood* 1990;75:1460–1465.

199. Sane DC, Moser TL, Pippen AM, et al. Vitronectin is a substrate for transglutaminases. *Biochem Biophys Res Commun* 1988;157:115–120.

200. Skorstengaard K, Halkier T, Hojrup P, Mosher D. Sequence location of a putative transglutaminase cross-linking site in human vitronectin. *FEBS Lett* 1990;262:269–274.

201. Bale MD, Westrick LG, Mosher DF. Incorporation of thrombospondin into fibrin clots. *J Biol Chem* 1985;260:7502–7508.

202. Francis RT, McDonagh J, Mann KG. Factor V is a substrate for the transamidase factor XIIIa. *J Biol Chem* 1986;261:9787–9792.

203. Huh MM, Schick BP, Schick PK, Colman RW. Covalent cross-linking of human coagulation factor V by activated factor XIII from guinea pig megakaryocytes and human plasma. *Blood* 1988;71:1693–1702.

204. Mui PT, Ganguly P. Cross-linking of actin and fibrin by fibrin-stabilizing factor. *Am J Physiol* 1977;233:H346–H349.

205. Cohen I, Blankenberg TA, Borden D, et al. Factor XIIIa-catalyzed cross-linking of platelet and muscle actin. Regulation by nucleotides. *Biochim Biophys Acta* 1980;628:365–375.

206. Asijee GM, Muszbek L, Kappelmayer J, et al. Platelet vinculin: a substrate of activated factor XIII. *Biochim Biophys Acta* 1988;954:303–308.

207. Cohen I, Lim CT, Kahn DR, et al. Disulfide-linked and transglutaminase-catalyzed protein assemblies in platelets. *Blood* 1985;66:143–151.

208. Cohen I, Gerrard JM, White JG. Ultrastructure of clots during isometric contraction. *J Cell Biol* 1982;93:775–787.

209. Cox AD, Devine DV. Factor XIIIa binding to activated platelets is mediated through activation of glycoprotein IIb-IIIa. *Blood* 1994;83:1006–1016.

210. Hevessy Z, Haramura G, Boda Z, et al. Promotion of the cross-linking of fibrin and alpha 2-antiplasmin by platelets. *Thromb Haemost* 1996;75:161–167.

211. Devine DV, Bishop PD. Platelet-associated factor XIII in platelet activation, adhesion, and clot stabilization. *Semin Thromb Hemost* 1996;22:409–413.

212. Devine DV, Andestad G, Nugent D, Carter CJ. Platelet-associated factor XIII as a marker of platelet activation in patients with peripheral vascular disease. *Arterioscler Thromb* 1993;13:857–862.

213. Dale GL, Friese P, Batar P, et al. Stimulated platelets use serotonin to enhance their retention of procoagulant proteins on the cell surface. *Nature* 2002;415 (6868):175–179.

214. Greenberg CS, Birckbichler PJ, Rice RH. Transglutaminases: multifunctional cross-linking enzymes that stabilize tissues. *FASEB J* 1991;5:3071–3077.

215. Aeschlimann D, Mosher D, Paulsson M. Tissue transglutaminase and factor XIII in cartilage and bone remodeling. *Semin Thromb Hemost* 1996;22(5):437–443.

216. Ichinose A. Physiopathology and regulation of factor XIII. *Thromb Haemost* 2001;86(1):57–65.

217. Ichinose A, Souri M, Izumi T, Takahashi N. Molecular and genetic mechanisms of factor XIII A subunit deficiency. *Semin Thromb Hemost* 2000;26(1):5–10.

218. Castle SL, Board PG. An extended survey of the genetic polymorphism at the human coagulation factor XIII A subunit structural locus. *Hum Hered* 1985; 35:101–106.

219. Mikkola H, Syrjälä M, Rasi V et al. Deficiency in the A-subunit of coagulation factor XIII: two novel point mutations demonstrate different effects on transcript levels. *Blood* 1994;84:517–525.

220. Anwar R, Stewart AD, Miloszewski KJ, et al. Molecular basis of inherited factor XIII deficiency: identification of multiple mutations provides insights into protein function. *Br J Haematol* 1995;91:728–735.

221. Board PG, Losowsky MS, Miloszewski KJA. Factor xiii—inherited and acquired deficiency. *Blood* 1993;7(4):229–242.

222. Kohler HP, Stickland MH, Ossei-Gerning N, et al. Association of a common polymorphism in the factor XIII gene with myocardial infarction. *Thromb Haemost* 1998;79:8–13.

223. McCormack LJ, Kain K, Catto AJ, et al. Prevalence of FXIII V34L in populations with different cardiovascular risk [letter]. *Thromb Haemost* 1998;80:523–524.

224. Attié-Castro FA, Zago MA, Lavinha J, et al. Ethnic heterogeneity of the factor XIII Val34Leu polymorphism. *Thromb Haemost* 2000;84:601–603.

225. Ariëns RAS, Philippou H, Nagaswami C, et al. The factor XIII V34L polymorphism accelerates thrombin activation of factor XIII and affects cross-linked fibrin structure. *Blood* 2000;96:988–995.

226. Wartiovaara U, Mikkola H, Szôke G, et al. Effect of Val34Leu polymorphism on the activation of the coagulation factor XIII-A. *Thromb Haemost* 2000;84:595–600.

227. Balogh I, Szôke G, Kárpáti L, et al. Val34Leu polymorphism of plasma factor XIII: biochemistry and epidemiology in familial thrombophilia. *Blood* 2000;96:2479–2486.

228. Trumbo TA, Maurer MC. Examining thrombin hydrolysis of the factor XIII activation peptide segment leads to a proposal for explaining the cardioprotective effects observed with the factor XIII V34L mutation. *J Biol Chem* 2000;275:20627–20631.

229. Catto AJ, Kohler HP, Coore J, et al. Association of a common polymorphism in the factor XIII gene with venous thrombosis. *Blood* 1999;93:906–908.

230. Franco RF, Reitsma PH, Lourenço D, et al. Factor XIII Val34Leu is a genetic factor involved in the aetiology of venous thrombosis. *Thromb Haemost* 1999;81:676–679.

231. Renner W, Köppel H, Hoffmann C, et al. Prothrombin G20210A, factor V Leiden, and factor XIII Val34Leu: common mutations of blood coagulation factor and deep vein thrombosis in Austria. *Thromb Res* 2000;99:35–39.

232. Corral J, González-Conejero R, Iniesta JA, et al. The FXIIIVal34Leu polymorphism in venous and arterial thromboembolism. *Haematologica* 2000;85:293–297.

233. Margaglione M, Bossone A, Brancaccio V, et al. Factor XIII Val34Leu polymorphism and risk of deep vein thrombosis. *Thomb Haemost* 2000;84:1118–1119.

234. Morange PE, Henry M, Brunet D, et al. Factor XIIIV34L is not an additional genetic risk factor for venous thrombosis in factor V Leiden carriers [letter]. *Blood* 2001;97:1894–1895.

235. Corral J, Iniesta JA, Gónález-Conejero R, et al. Polymorphisms of clotting factor modify the risk for primary intracranial hemorrhage. *Blood* 2001;97:2979–2982.

236. Elbaz A, Poirier O, Canaple S, et al. The association between the Val34Leu polymorphism in the factor XIII gene and brain infarction. *Blood* 2000;95:586–591.

237. Gemmati D, Serino ML, Ongaro A, et al. A common mutation in the gene for coagulation factor XIII-A (Val34Leu): a risk factor for primary intracerebral hemorrhage is protective against atherothrombotic diseases. *Am J Hematol* 2001;67:183–188.

238. Roberts HR, Stinchcombe TE, Gabriel DA. The dysfibrinogenaemias. *Br J Haematol* 2001;114(2):249–257.

239. Mosesson MW. Dysfibrinogenemia and thrombosis. *Semin Thromb Hemost* 1999;25(3):311–319.

240. Cote HCF, Lord ST, Pratt KP. Gamma-chain dysfibrinogenemias: molecular structure–function relationships of naturally occurring mutations in the gamma chain of human fibrinogen. *Blood* 1998;92(7):2195–2212.

241. Bilezikian SB, Nossel HL, Butler VP Jr, Canfield RE. Radioimmunoassay of human fibrinopeptide B and kinetics of fibrinopeptide cleavage by different enzymes. *J Clin Invest* 1975;56:438.

242. Stocker K, Fischer H, Meier J. Thrombin-like snake venom proteinases. *Toxicon* 1982;20:265.

243. McDonagh J. Dysfibrinogenemia and other disorders of fibrinogen structure and function, chapter 53. In: Colman R, Hirsh J, Marder V, et al., eds. *Hemostasis and thrombosis: basic principles and clinical practice*. Philadelphia: Lippincott, 2000:855–892.

244. Southan C, Henschen A, Lottspeich F. The search for molecular defects in abnormal fibrinogens. In: Henschen A, Graeff H, Lottspeich F, eds. *Fibrinogen: recent biochemical and medical aspects*. Berlin: Walter de Gruyter, 1982:133.

245. Alving BM, Henschen A. Fibrinogen Giessen I: a congenital homozygously expressed dysfibrinogenemia with Aα 16 Arg—His substitution. *Am J Hematol* 1987;25:479.

246. Kehl M, Lottspeich F, Henschen A. Genetically abnormal fibrinogens releasing abnormal fibrinopeptides as characterized by high-performance liquid chromatography. In: Haverkate F, Henschen A, Nieuwenhuizen W, Straub PW, eds. *Fibrinogen: structure, functional aspects, metabolism*. Berlin: Walter de Gruyter, 1983:183.

247. Soria J, Soria C, Samama M, et al. Fibrinogen Troyes- fibrinogen Metz: two new cases of congenital dysfibrinogenemia. *Thromb Diath Haemorrh* 1972;27:619.

248. Miyata T, Terukina S, Matsuda M, et al. Fibrinogens Kawaguchi and Osaka: an amino acid substitution of Aα arginine to cysteine which forms an interchain disulfide between the two Aα chains. *J Biochem (Tokyo)* 1987; 102:93.

249. Blombäck M, Blombäck B, Mammen EF, Prasad AS. Fibrinogen "Detroit": a molecular defect in the N-terminal disulfide knot of human fibrinogen? *Nature* 1968;218:134.

250. Blombäck B, Hessel B, Hogg D, Therkildsen L. A two-step fibrinogen–fibrin transition in blood coagulation. *Nature* 1978;275:501.

251. Mammen EF, Prasad AS, Barnhart MI, Au CC. Congenital dysfibrinogenemia: fibrinogen Detroit. *J Clin Invest* 1969;48:235.

252. Kudryk B, Blombäck B, Blombäck M. Fibrinogen Detroit: an abnormal fibrinogen with non-functional NH₂-terminal polymerization domain. *Thromb Res* 1976;9:25.

253. Lee MH, Kaczmarek E, Chin DT, et al. Fibrinogen Ledyard (AαArg16—Cys): biochemical and physiologic characterizaiton. *Blood* 1991;78:1744.

254. Carrell N, Gabriel DM, Carr ME, et al. Hereditary dysfibrinogenemia in a patient with thrombotic disease. *Blood* 1983;62:439.

255. Liu CY, Koehn JA, Morgan FJ. Characterization of fibrinogen New York I: a dysfunctional fibrinogen with a deletion of Bβ(9–72) corresponding exactly to exon 2 of the gene. *J Biol Chem* 1985;260:4390.

256. Liu CY, Morgan FJ. Fibrinogen New York I: a deletion in the Bβ chain corresponding to exon 2 of the gene. *Circulation* 1984;70:II351.

257. Blombäck B, Hessel B, Hogg D. Disulfide bridges in NH₂-terminal part of human fibrinogen. *Thromb Res* 1976;8:639.

258. Liu CY, Wallen P. Fibrinogen New York I: defective fibrin potentiation of plasminogen activation by tissue plasminogen activator. *Circulation* 1983;70:II366.

259. Laudano AP, Doolittle RF. Studies on synthetic peptides that bind to fibrinogen and prevent fibrin polymerization: structural requirements, number of binding sites, and specific differences. *Biochemistry* 1980;19:1013.

260. Yamazumi K, Terukina S, Onohara S, Matsuda M. Normal plasmic cleavage of the γ-chain variant of "fibrinogen Saga" with an Arg-275 to His substitution. *Thromb Haemost* 1988;60:476.

261. Grailhe P, Boyerneumann C, Haverkate F, et al. The mutation in fibrinogen bicetre-ii (gamma-asn308-lys) does not affect the binding of t-pa and plasminogen to fibrin. *Blood Coagul Fibrinolysis* 1993;4(5):679–687.

262. Yoshida N, Terukina S, Okuma M, et al. Characterization of apparently lower molecular weight γ-chain variant in fibrinogen Kyoto I. *J Biol Chem* 1988;263:13848.

263. Martinez J, Keane PM, Gilmon PB, Palascak JE. The abnormal carbohydrate composition of the dysfibrinogenemia associated with liver disease. *Ann N Y Acad Sci* 1983;408:388.

264. Carrell N, McDonagh J. Functional defects in abnormal fibrinogens. In: Henschen A, Hessel B, McDonagh J, Saldeen T, eds. *Fibrinogen: structural variants and interaction*. Berlin: Walter de Gruyter, 1985:155.

265. Francis JL, Armstrong DJ. Acquired dysfibrinogenemia in liver disease. *J Clin Pathol* 1982;35:667.

266. Martinez J, MacDonald KA, Palascal JE. The role of sialic acid in the dysfibrinogenemia associated with liver disease: distribution of sialic acid on the constituent chains. *Blood* 1983;61:1196.

267. Francis JL, Armstrong DJ. Sialic acid and sialyltransferase in the pathogenesis of acquired dysfibrinogenemia. In: Haverkate F, Henschen A, Nieuwenhuizen W, Straub PW, eds. *Fibrinogen: structure, functional aspects, metabolism*. Berlin: Walter de Gruyter, 1982:195.

268. Dang CV, Shin CK, Bell WR, Nagaswami C, Weisel JW. Fibrinogen sialic acid residues are low affinity calcium binding sites that influence fibrin assembly. *J Biol Chem* 1989;264(25):15104–15108.

269. Gralnick HR, Givelber HM, Shainoff JR, Finlayson JS. Fibrinogen Bethesda: a congenital dysfibrinogenemia with delayed fibrinopeptide release. *J Clin Invest* 1971;50:1819.

270. Latallo ZS, Fletcher AP, Alkjaersig N, Sherry S. Influence of pH, ionic strength, neutral ions, and thrombin on fibrin polymerization. *Am J Physiol* 1962;202:675.

271. Collen D, Tytgat GN, Claeys H, et al. Metabolism and distribution of fibrinogen. I. Fibrinogen turnover in physiological conditions in humans. *Br J Haematol* 1972;22:681.

272. Gitlin D, Borges WH. Studies on the metabolism of fibrinogen in two patients with congenital afibrinogenemia. *Blood* 1953;8:697.

273. Mason DY, Ingram GIC. Management of the hereditary coagulation disorders. *Semin Hematol* 1971;8:158.

274. Tytgat GN, Collen D, Vermylen J. Metabolism and distribution of fibrinogen. II. Fibrinogen turnover in polycythemia, thrombocytosis, haemophilia A, congenital afibrinogenemia and during streptokinase therapy. *Br J Haematol* 1972;22:701.

275. Lane DA, Scully MF, Thomas DP, et al. Acquired dysfibrinogenemia in acute and chronic liver disease. *Br J Haematol* 1977;35:301.

276. de Vries A, Rosenberg T, Kochwa S, Boss JH. Precipitating antifibrinogen antibody appearing after fibrinogen infusions in a patient with congenital afibrinogenemia. *Am J Med* 1961;30:486.

277. Martinez J. Congenital dysfibrinogenemia. *Curr Opin Hematol* 1997;4(5):357–365.

278. Asselta R, Duga S, Spena S, et al. Congenital afibrinogenemia: mutations leading to premature termination codons in fibrinogen A alpha-chain gene are not associated with the decay of the mutant mRNAs. *Blood* 2001;98(13):3685–3692.

279. Blombäck B, Blombäck M, Henschen A, et al. The N-terminal disulphide knot of human fibrinogen. *Nature* 1968;218:130.

280. Duckert F. Documentation of the plasma factor XIII deficiency in man. *Ann N Y Acad Sci* 1972;202:190.

281. Duckert F, Jung E, Shmerling DH. A hitherto undescribed congenital hemorrhagic diathesis probably due to fibrin stabilizing factor deficiency. *Thromb Diath Haemorrh* 1960;5:179.

282. McDonagh J, McDonagh RP Jr, Duckert F. Genetic aspects of factor XIII deficiency. *Ann Hum Genet* 1971;35:195.

283. Ikematsu S, McDonagh RP, Reisner HM, et al. Immunochemical studies of human factor XIII: radioimmunoassay for the carrier subunit of the zymogen. *J Lab Clin Med* 1981;97:662.

284. Anwar R, Miloszewski KJA. Factor XIII deficiency. *Br J Haematol* 1999;107(3): 468–484.

285. Hantgan RR, Francis CW, Marder VJ. Fibrinogen, structure and physiology. In: Colman RV, Hirsh J, Marder VJ, Salzman EW, eds. *Hemostasis and thrombosis: basic principles and clinical practice*, ed 3. Philadelphia: JB Lippincott, 1994:277.

286. Miloszewski KJA, Losowsky MS. Fibrin stabilisation and factor XIII–deficiency. In: Francis JL, ed. *Fibrinogen, fibrin stabilisation and fibrinolysis*. Chichester, England: Ellis Horwood, 1988:175.

287. Iwaki T, Sandoval-Cooper MJ, Paiva M, et al. Fibrinogen stabilizes placental-maternal attachment during embryonic development in the mouse. *Am J Pathol* 2002;160(3):1021–1034.

288. Beck E, Duckert F, Ernst M. The influence of fibrin-stabilizing factor on the growth of fibroblasts in vitro and wound healing. *Thromb Diath Haemorrh* 1961;6:485.

289. Winkelman L, Sims GE, Haddon ME, et al. A pasteurised concentrate of human plasma factor XIII for therapeutic use. *Thromb Haemost* 1986;55:402.

290. Daly HM, Haddon ME. Clinical experience with a pasteurised human plasma concentrate in factor XIII–deficiency. *Thromb Haemost* 1988;59:171.

291. Karges HE, Clemens R. Factor XIII: enzymatic and clinical aspects. *Behring Inst Mitt* 1988;82:43.

292. Suzuki H, Kaneda T. Tooth extraction in two patients who had congenital deficiency of factor XIII. *J Oral Maxillofac Surg* 1985;43:221.

293. Elms MJ, Bunce IH, Bundesen PG, et al. Rapid detection of cross-linked fibrin degradation products in plasma using monoclonal antibody-coated latex particles. *Am J Clin Pathol* 1986;85:360.

294. Francis JL. Detection and measurement of factor XIII. In: Francis JL, ed. *Fibrinogen, fibrin stabilisation, and fibrinolysis*. Chichester, England: Ellis Horwood, 1988:203.

295. Ballerini G, Guerra S, Rodeghiero F, Castaman G. A contribution to the pathology of acquired plasma factor XIII–deficiency. *Semin Thromb Hemost* 1985; 11:357.

296. Adany R, Belkin A, Vasilevskaya T, Muszbek L. Identification of blood coagulation factor XIII in human peritoneal macrophages. *Eur J Cell Biol* 1985; 38:171.

297. Duswald KH, Jochum M, Schramm W, Fritz H. Released granulocytic elastase: an indicator of pathobiochemical alterations in septicemia after abdominal surgery. *Surgery* 1985;98:892.

298. Galloway MJ, Mackie MJ, McVerry BA. Elastase-α 1 antitrypsin complexes in acute leukaemia. *Thromb Res* 1985;38:311.

299. Anders O, Gross EW, Ernst B, Konrad H. Detection of factor XIII–deficiency in acute leukemia with resonance thrombography. *Folia Haematol (Leipz)* 1987; 114:670.

300. Kamitsuji H, Tani K, Yasui M, et al. Activity of blood coagulation factor XIII as a prognostic indicator in patients with Henoch-Schönlein purpura: efficacy of factor XIII substitution. *Eur J Pediatr* 1987;146:519.

301. Henriksson P, Hender U, Nilsson IM. Factor XIII (fibrin stabilising factor) in Henoch-Schönlein's purpura. *Acta Paediatr Scand* 1977;66:273.

302. Guillevin L, Chouvet B, Mery C, et al. Treatment of progressive systemic sclerosis using factor XIII. *Pharmatherapeutica* 1985;4:76.

303. Grivoux M, Pieron R. Brochiolo-alveolar carcinoma complicating systemic scleroderma under long-term treatment with factor XIII. *Rev Pneumol Clin* 1987;43:102.

304. Noll T, Wozniak G, McCarson K, et al. Effect of factor XIII on endothelial barrier function. *J Exp Med* 1999;189(9):1373–1382.

305. Lorenz R, Heinmüller M, Classen M, et al. Substitution of factor XIII: a therapeutic approach to ulcerative colitis. *Haemostasis* 1991;21:5.

306. Lee SY, Chang SK, Lee IH, et al. Depletion of plasma factor XIII prevents disseminated intravascular coagulation-induced organ damage. *Thromb Haemost* 2001;85(3):464–469.

307. Godje O, Haushofer M, Lamm P, Reichart B. The effect of factor XIII on bleeding in coronary surgery. *Thorac Cardiovasc Surg* 1998;46(5):263–267.

308. Lorand L, Urayama T, De Kiewiet JWC, Nossel HL. Diagnostic and genetic studies on fibrin-stabilizing factor with a new assay based on amine incorporation. *J Clin Invest* 1969;48:1054.

309. Henriksson P, McDonagh J, Villa M. Type I autoimmune inhibitor of factor XIII in a patient with congenital factor XIII deficiency. *Thromb Haemost* 1983;50:272.

310. Fukue H, Anderson K, McPhedran P, Clyne, et al. A unique factor XIII inhibitor to a fibrin-binding site on factor XIIIA. *Blood* 1992;79:65.

311. Lorand L, Losowsky MS, Miloszewski KJM. Human factor XIII: fibrin stabilizing factor. In: Spaet TH, ed. *Progress in hemostasis and thrombosis*, vol 5. New York: Grune & Stratton, 1980:245.

312. Lorand L, Jacobsen A. Isonicotinic acid hydrazide as an inhibitor of transpeptidation: relevance for blood coagulation. *Nature* 1967;216:508.

CHAPTER 40

Fibrinolytic System and Its Disorders

Roger H. Lijnen and Désiré Collen

Mammalian blood contains an enzymatic system called the *fibrinolytic* (or *plasminogen-plasmin*) *system* that is capable of dissolving blood clots. This system (Fig. 40-1) comprises an inactive proenzyme (plasminogen) that can be converted to the active enzyme (plasmin) that degrades fibrin into soluble fibrin-degradation products. Two immunologically distinct types of physiologic plasminogen activators have been identified: *tissue-type plasminogen activator* (t-PA) and *urokinase-type plasminogen activator* (u-PA). t-PA–mediated plasminogen activation is mainly involved in the dissolution of fibrin in the circulation (1). u-PA binds to a specific cellular receptor (u-PAR) resulting in enhanced activation of cell-bound plasminogen. The main role of u-PA appears to be in the induction of pericellular proteolysis via the degradation of matrix components or via activation of latent proteases or growth factors (2–4). A u-PAR–independent function of u-PA has also been demonstrated in fibrin clearance (5) and in arterial neointima formation (4). Inhibition of the fibrinolytic system may occur either at (a) the level of the plasminogen activators by plasminogen activator inhibitor-1 (PAI-1) and plasminogen activator inhibitor-2 (PAI-2) or (b) the level of plasmin, by α_2-antiplasmin or α_2-macroglobulin. The physicochemical properties of these main components of the fibrinolytic system are summarized in Table 40-1. Plasminogen activation may also be induced by an intrinsic pathway involving several proteins, such as factor XII, high-molecular-weight kininogen, and prekallikrein. Kallikrein, generated from prekallikrein by the action of factor XII and high-molecular-weight kininogen, may convert single-chain u-PA (scu-PA) to two-chain u-PA (tcu-PA).

This chapter discusses t-PA– and u-PA–mediated fibrinolysis. Normal hemostasis requires precise regulation and control of the fibrinolytic system and depends on specific molecular interactions between its main components. Impaired fibrinolysis can cause thrombotic complications; excessive activation of the fibrinolytic system can cause a bleeding tendency (6–9).

Circumstantial evidence has been provided for a role of the fibrinolytic system in a variety of other biologic phenomena, including reproduction, embryogenesis, cell invasion, angiogenesis, brain function, thrombosis, restenosis, atherosclerosis, neoplasia, metastasis, and chronic lung or kidney inflammatory disorders (1,2,4). Recently, the generation of transgenic mice over- or underexpressing components of the plasminogen-plasmin system has allowed investigators to establish its causal role in several of these biologic processes (4,10). Furthermore, several interactions between the fibrinolytic and matrix metalloproteinase (MMP) systems, suggest that both systems may cooperate in achieving extracellular matrix degradation (11).

COMPONENTS INVOLVED IN ACTIVATION OF THE FIBRINOLYTIC SYSTEM

Tissue-Type Plasminogen Activator

SOURCES

Many reports on the purification and characterization of t-PA are culled from various sources, including pig heart, hog ovaries, postmortem vascular perfusates, and postexercise blood. The first satisfactory purification of human t-PA was from uterine tissue (12). Using an antiserum raised against uterine plasminogen activator, it was shown that t-PA, vascular plasminogen activator, and blood plasminogen activator are immunologically identical but distinct from urokinase. The major plasminogen activator found in blood is vascular plasminogen activator, which is synthesized and secreted by endothelial cells and is called *t-PA* (13).

t-PA was purified from the culture fluid of a stable human melanoma cell line (Bowes, RPMI-7272) in sufficient amounts to study its biochemical and biologic properties (14). t-PA for clinical use (alteplase) is presently produced by recombinant DNA technology [Actilyse, Boehringer Ingelheim GmbH].

STRUCTURAL PROPERTIES

t-PA is a serine (Ser) proteinase of approximately 70 kd and is composed of a single polypeptide chain of 527 amino acids, with Ser as the NH_2-terminal amino acid (15). Its primary structure—deduced from complementary DNA (cDNA) cloning—is illustrated in Figure 40-2. Native t-PA contains an NH_2-terminal extension of three additional amino acids [glycine (Gly)-alanine (Ala)-arginine (Arg)]. The molecule has 17 disulfide bonds and an additional free cysteine (Cys) at position 83. t-PA is converted by plasmin to a two-chain form by hydrolysis of the Arg275-isoleucine (Ile)276 peptide bond (numbering based on a total of 527 residues). The NH_2-terminal region is composed of several domains with homologies to other proteins: Residues 1 to 43 are homologous to the finger domains (F) in fibronectin, residues 44 to 91 are homologous to human epidermal growth factor (E), and residues 92 to 173 (K_1) and 180 to 262 (K_2) are homologous to the kringle regions of plasminogen. The region comprising resi-

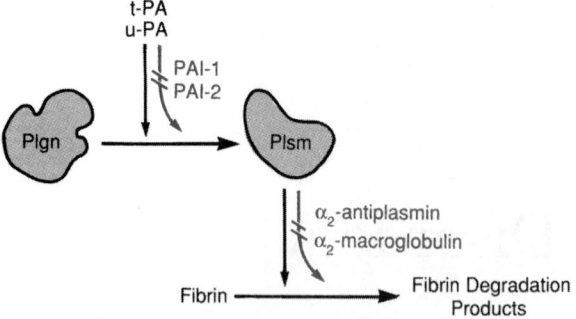

Figure 40-1. Schematic representation of the fibrinolytic system. PAI-1, plasminogen activator inhibitor-1; PAI-2, plasminogen activator inhibitor-2; Plgn, plasminogen; Plsm, plasmin; t-PA, tissue-type plasminogen activator; u-PA, urokinase-type plasminogen activator.

dues 276 to 527 is homologous to that of other Ser proteinases and contains the catalytic site, which is composed of histidine (His)322, aspartic acid (Asp)371, and Ser478 (15).

Melanoma t-PA exists as two variants (types I and II) that differ in carbohydrate content. Type I t-PA contains N-linked glycans at residues asparagine (Asn)117, -184, and -448, whereas the type II t-PA lacks the glycan at position 184. Both forms contain a high-mannose oligosaccharide at position 117 (16). Recombinant t-PA contains approximately 7% carbohydrate by weight, consisting of a high-mannose oligosaccharide at position 117 and complex fucosylated oligosaccharides at Asn184 and Asn448 (17).

The distinct domains in t-PA appear to be involved in several enzyme functions, including its binding to fibrin, rapid clearance *in vivo*, plasminogen activating activity with fibrin specificity (enzymatic properties), and binding to endothelial cell receptors. As discussed later, characterization of deletion mutants lacking one or more of these domains has allowed a detailed study of structure-function relationships of t-PA.

BINDING TO FIBRIN

t-PA has a moderately high affinity for fibrin. The dissociation constant of the t-PA–fibrin complex is estimated to be 0.14 µmol/L in the presence of plasminogen (18). The stoichiometry of binding is approximately 1 mol of t-PA per 1 mol of fibrin monomer. Scatchard analysis of iodine-125–t-PA binding to fibrin in the absence of plasminogen suggests the existence of a single class of binding sites with K_a of 1.65×10^6 L/mol (which would correspond to a K_d of 0.6 µmol/L) and a maximum molar binding ratio of 0.88 mol t-PA per 1 mol of fibrin (19).

The structures involved in fibrin binding of t-PA are localized within the heavy chain (A chain), evidenced by the intact fibrin-affinity of the A chain. The finger domain of t-PA is involved in the fibrin binding of the enzyme, as shown by the finding that a deletion mutant of t-PA consisting only of the finger and Ser protease domains binds to fibrin (20). Evidence obtained with additional deletion mutants suggests that binding of t-PA to fibrin is mediated via both the finger domain and the second kringle region (K_2) (21). A lysine (Lys)-binding site is involved in the interaction of the K_2 domain with fibrin. This interaction is abolished by the Lys analog 6-aminohexanoic acid. A Lys-binding site is not involved, however, in the interaction of the finger domain with fibrin (20). The presence of a weaker Lys-binding site in K_2, similar to the AH site observed in plasminogen, is also suggested. This AH site would interact with internal Lys residues in the fibrin matrix, whereas the Lys-binding site would interact with carboxyl-terminal Lys residues exposed on initial plasmic digestion of fibrin (21).

ENZYMATIC PROPERTIES

The structures required for enzymatic activity of t-PA are localized in the light chain (B chain), because the isolated B chain retains full enzymatic activity. The plasminogen-activating activity of the isolated B chain is not stimulated by the presence of fibrin.

The activation of plasminogen by t-PA—in both the presence and absence of fibrin—follows Michaelis-Menten kinetics. Hoylaerts and associates (18) found that the Michaelis constant (K_m) was 65 µmol/L, and the catalytic rate constant (k_{cat}) was 0.05 s⁻¹ in the absence of fibrin. In the presence of fibrin, the K_m decreased to 0.16 µmol/L with only a minor change in k_{cat}. The catalytic efficiency (k_{cat}/K_m) of t-PA for the activation of plasminogen thus increases approximately 1500 times in the presence of fibrin. Lys residue 157 in the Aα-chain of fibrinogen was identified as the residue involved in fibrin-induced stimulation of plasminogen activation by t-PA (22). Rijken and coworkers (23), using a system in which lysis of fibrin was prevented by an excess of aprotinin (a potent inhibitor of plasmin), found a K_m of 1.1 µmol/L. These changes and differences in K_m in the presence of fibrin are explained by the exposure of a strong plasminogen-binding site on initial fibrin degradation (24). Although single-chain t-PA is less active with regard to low-molecular-weight (LMW) substrates and inhibitors, it is now generally accepted that its activity with regard to plasminogen is comparable to that of the two-chain form. On the basis of conformational similarities between single-chain and two-chain t-PA, it was postulated that the activity of single-chain t-PA would involve an equilibrium between an active and a proenzyme or zymogenic confor-

TABLE 40-1. Physicochemical Properties of the Main Components of the Fibrinolytic System

	M_r (kd)	Carbohydrate Content (%)	Number of Amino Acids	Catalytic Triad	Reactive Site	Plasma Concentration (mg/L)
Plasminogen	92	2	791	—	—	200
Plasmin	85	2	±715	His603, Asp646, Ser741	—	—
t-PA	68	7	527	His322, Asp371, Ser478	—	0.005
u-PA	54	7	411	His204, Asp255, Ser356	—	0.008
u-PAR	55–60	± 35	313	—	—	—
α₂-antiplasmin	67	13	464	—	Arg376-Met377	70
PAI-1	52	ND	379	—	Arg346-Met347	0.05
PAI-2	47	ND	393	—	Arg358-Thr359	<0.005

Arg, arginine; Asp, aspartic acid; His, histidine; PAI-1, plasminogen activator inhibitor-1; PAI-2, plasminogen activator inhibitor-2; Met, methionine; ND, not determined; Ser, serine; Thr, threonine; t-PA, tissue-type plasminogen activator; u-PA, urokinase-type plasminogen activator; u-PAR, u-PA receptor.

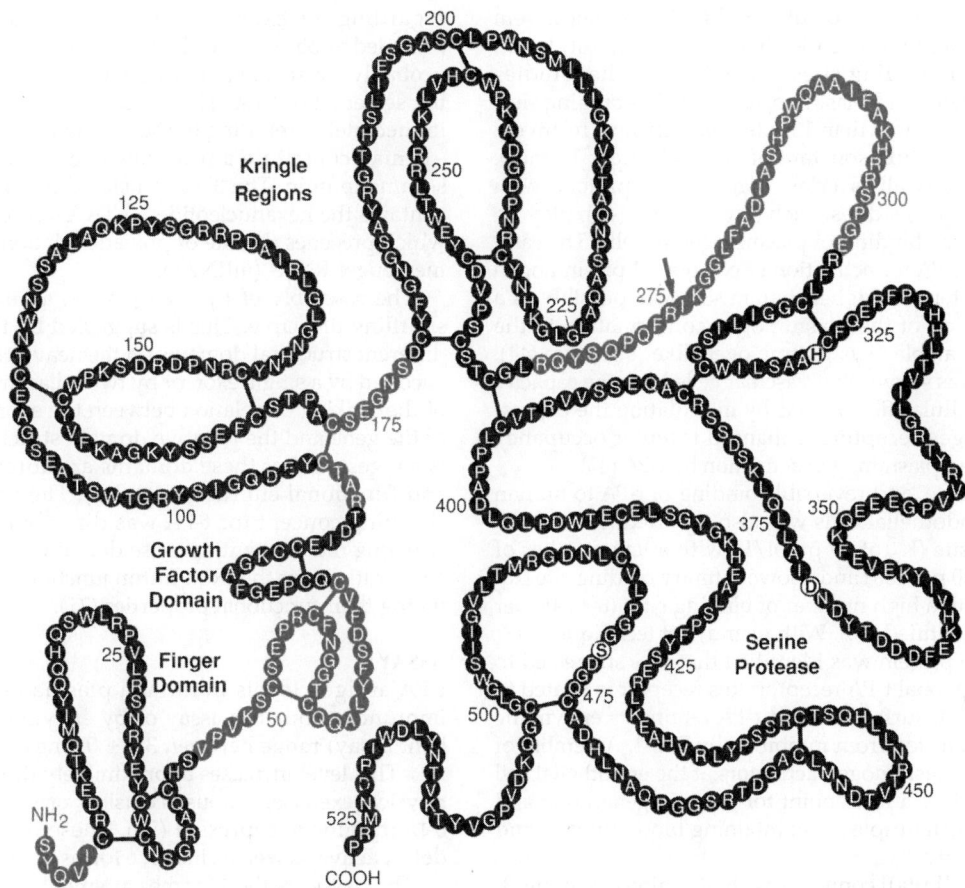

Figure 40-2. Schematic representation of the primary structure of tissue-type plasminogen activator. The arrow indicates the cleavage site for plasmin. The active site residues are indicated by white circles.

mation, which would be shifted to the active conformation on substrate binding (25). Alternatively, mutational analysis suggested that Lys156 contributes directly to the enzymatic activity of single-chain t-PA, by forming a salt bridge with Asp194 that selectively stabilizes the active conformation (26). This observation was confirmed by the x-ray crystal structure of the catalytic domain of recombinant human single-chain t-PA (27).

Deletion mutants of t-PA have been used to identify the domains that are involved in the stimulation of plasminogen-activating potential by fibrin. t-PA mutants lacking the finger domain are stimulated by fibrin to the same degree as intact t-PA, whereas mutants lacking the K_2 structure but retaining the finger domain show significantly reduced stimulation. This suggests that the interaction of the K_2 domain with fibrin may regulate fibrin stimulation (21).

Conversely, Kalyan and associates (28) reported that a deletion mutant of t-PA lacking both the finger and growth factor domains (t-PA–ΔFE) was less stimulated by fibrin than wild-type t-PA. This contrasts with the similar mutants described by Gething and colleagues (29) and by Larsen and associates (30), which showed no change in stimulation by fibrin. This difference may be due to conformational changes (caused by deletion) in the other domains of the heavy chain. Several additional reports on the fibrin affinity of t-PA deletion mutants added to the existing confusion.

Some studies conclude that the presence of the finger domain is sufficient for fibrin stimulation of t-PA; others report that deletion of K_1 and K_2 reduces fibrin stimulation, K_1 and K_2 are equivalent in their ability to stimulate catalytic activity by fibrin, or only K_2 and not K_1 is relevant (21).

On the basis of these studies with deletion mutants, a recombinant t-PA variant, consisting only of K_2 and the proteinase domain (K_2P, reteplase), has been developed for clinical use as a thrombolytic agent (31). The plasminogenolytic activities of reteplase and wild-type t-PA are comparable in the absence of a stimulator, but the activity of reteplase in the presence of fibrin(ogen) fragments is fourfold lower, and its binding to fibrin is fivefold lower (32,33). The affinity of reteplase for endothelial cell and monocyte receptors is also reduced. These differences are probably the consequence of the domain deletions.

There is a striking analogy between the role of fibrin and that of cell surfaces in plasminogen activation. Many cell types bind plasminogen activators and plasminogen, resulting in enhanced plasminogen activation (34–37) and protection of bound plasmin from inhibition by α_2-antiplasmin (38,39). Miles and Plow (36) have shown that platelets bind plasminogen, and platelet-bound plasminogen is more sensitive to activation by t-PA. Stricker and associates (40) found that incubation of normal, washed human platelets with plasminogen at physiologic concentrations and t-PA at concentrations achieved during thrombolytic therapy resulted in a ten- to 50-fold increase in plasmin activity relative to that obtained without platelets. These results suggest that platelets may also provide a surface for activation of plasminogen by pharmacologic concentrations of t-PA.

The kinetics of plasminogen activation by t-PA are also influenced by the presence of lipids: Negatively charged lipids lower the K_m value six- to 20-fold, whereas neutral lipids raise the K_m. This finding suggests that plasminogen activation by cell-associated t-PA may be influenced by the net charge of membrane lipids (41).

Binding of plasminogen to cultured human umbilical vein endothelial cells was reported with a K_D of 310 nmol/L and approximately 10^6 binding sites per cell (35). Other studies report that most cells bind plasminogen via its Lys binding sites with a high capacity (more than 10^7 sites per cell) but a relatively low affinity (dissociation constant of approximately 1 μmol). Gangliosides (42), as well as a class of membrane proteins with COOH-terminal Lys residues, such as α-enolase (43), play an important role in the binding of plasminogen to cells. The catalytic efficiency of t-PA for activation of cell-bound plasminogen is approximately tenfold higher than in solution, possibly as a result of conversion of the plasminogen conformation to the more readily activatable "Lys-plasminogen–like" structure (44). Alternatively, it was shown that vascular cells have the capacity to regulate pericellular fibrinolysis by modulating the expression of plasminogen receptors; enhanced receptor occupancy results in enhanced plasminogen activation by t-PA (45).

Specific, saturable, and reversible binding of t-PA to human umbilical vein endothelial cells was also reported (34). A high affinity binding site (K_D of 29 pmol/L) with a low number of binding sites (3700 per cell) and a lower affinity binding site (K_D of 18 nmol/L) with a high number of binding sites (800,000 per cell) have been identified (46). With ligand blot techniques a M_r 40,000 membrane protein was identified that was suggested to represent the functional t-PA receptor; this receptor is related to annexin II (47). Cell surface–bound t-PA retains its enzymatic activity and is protected from inhibition by PAI-1. Assembly of plasminogen and plasminogen activators at the endothelial cell surface thus provides a focal point for plasmin generation and may play an important role in maintaining blood fluidity and non-thrombogenicity.

Lipoprotein (a) [Lp(a)] competes with plasminogen for binding to endothelial cells, resulting in down-regulated activation of cell surface–bound plasminogen by t-PA. Thus, Lp(a) may also play a role in the regulation of fibrinolysis at the endothelial cell surface (48).

GENE STRUCTURE

The gene encoding human t-PA was localized to chromosome 8. The t-PA gene localization (chromosome 8, bands 8p12 ™q11.2) coincides with a translocation breakpoint observed in myeloproliferative disorders (49). A total of 36,594 base pairs (bp) were sequenced (including 32,720 bp from the transcription initiation site to the polyadenylation site), in addition to 3530 bp of 5' and 344 bp of 3' flanking DNA. Thirteen intervening sequences (30,068 bp) divide the gene into 14 coding regions; the exons range from 43 to 914 bp, and the introns range in size from 111 bp to 14,257 bp (50). The transcription initiation site is an A residue with a TATA box nearby upstream (TATAAAAA at positions −22 to −29) and a CAAT box further upstream (CAATG at positions −112 to −116). The polyadenylation signal (AATAAA) is found at positions 32,688 to 32,693.

The proximal promoter sequences also contain potential recognition sequences for transcription factors (e.g. AP1, NF1, SP1, AP2) (51,52). Consensus sequences of a cyclic adenosine monophosphate (cAMP)–responsive element and of a AP2-binding site have been identified, which may have a cooperative effect on constitutive t-PA gene expression (53). Allelic dimorphism has been observed in the human t-PA gene as a result of an Alu insertion-deletion event that occurred early in evolution (54).

The complete 2530-bp cDNA sequence of mature t-PA contains a single reading frame that begins with the ATG codon at nucleotides 85 to 87. This ATG probably serves as the site of translation initiation and is followed (562 codons later) by a TGA termination triplet at nucleotides 1771 to 1773. The Ser residue originally designated as the NH_2-terminal amino acid (dis-

regarding the extension of 3 amino acids in native t-PA) is preceded by 35 amino acids, 20 to 23 of which (residues −35 to −13) probably constitute a hydrophobic signal peptide involved in the secretion of t-PA. The remaining hydrophobic amino acids immediately preceding the start of mature t-PA (residues −14 to −1) may constitute a pro sequence similar to that found for serum albumin. The 3' untranslated region of 759 nucleotides contains the hexanucleotide AATAAA (positions 2496 to 2501), which precedes the site of polyadenylation in many eukaryotic messenger RNAs (mRNAs).

The assembly of the t-PA gene is an example of the exon-shuffling principle. This is suggested by the findings that the different structural domains on the heavy chain (F, E, K_1, K_2) are encoded by a single exon or by two adjacent exons (55). Because of the striking correlation between the exon-intron distribution of the gene and the putative domain structure of the protein, it is suggested that these domains are autonomous, structural, and functional entities (modules). The validity of this exon-shuffling concept for t-PA was directly investigated by constructing mutants with precise domain deletions, insertions, or substitutions (at the exon-intron junction of the gene) and evaluating their functional properties (21).

ASSAY

t-PA antigen levels in human plasma at rest (measured by immunoradiometric assay or by enzyme-linked immunosorbent assay) range between 3.4 ± 0.8 ng/mL and 6.6 ± 2.9 ng/mL. This level increases approximately threefold by exhaustive physical exercise, venous occlusion, or infusion of 1-desamino-8-D-arginine vasopressin (56). These immunologic methods detect active as well as inactive forms of antigen, however.

The classic method for measurement of fibrinolytic activity is the fibrin-plate method (57), using euglobulin fractions. This assay is nonspecific, because both intrinsic and extrinsic plasminogen activators are measured. It is used to express the activity of t-PA in International Units (IU). An International Reference Preparation for t-PA was established in 1985 in which 1 IU corresponds to 2 ng of protein (58). This preparation was replaced by a second international standard for t-PA, coded 86/670 (59).

Methods for measuring the functionally active level of t-PA were developed based on the stimulation of the activation of plasminogen by t-PA in the presence of fibrin or fibrin fragments. Ranby and others (60) developed a sensitive parabolic rate assay in which plasminogen, t-PA, fibrin monomer, and a plasmin-sensitive chromogenic substrate are incubated together. This method was adapted for euglobulin fractions, using cyanogen bromide–digested fibrinogen as a stimulator (61). Plasma in which proteinase inhibitors are neutralized by acidification was used in combination with fibrin monomer as stimulator (62). Using an enzyme-linked immunosorbent assay based on a specific monoclonal antibody, detectable levels (4.5 ± 0.8 ng/mL) of free, single-chain t-PA were found in plasma of six to ten health subjects; this level increased to 7.6 ± 3.1 ng/mL after venous occlusion (63).

Urokinase-Type Plasminogen Activator

SOURCES

tcu-PA, a trypsinlike Ser proteinase composed of two polypeptide chains (20 and 34 kd), was isolated from human urine and from cultured human embryonic kidney cells. Several groups have isolated a single-chain form of urokinase (scu-PA) from urine, plasma, or conditioned cell culture media. It was also obtained by recombinant DNA technology and prepared from the translation product in Escherichia coli of an expression plasmid coding for human urokinase (64,65). In addition to the 54-kd scu-PA, a previously unrecognized LMW form (32 kd) of

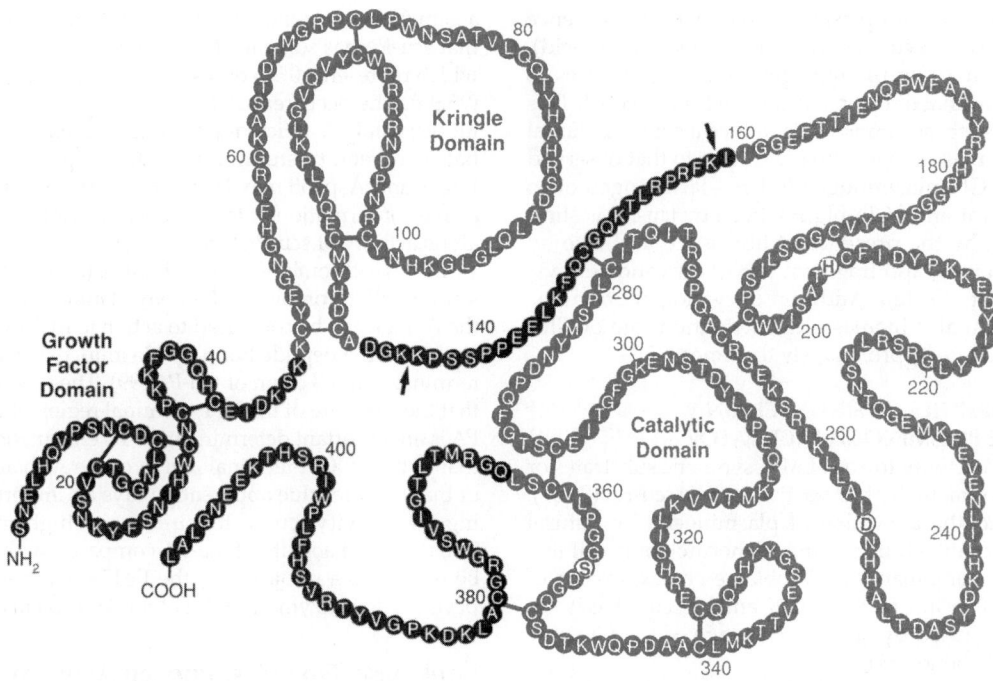

Figure 40-3. Schematic representation of the primary structure of single-chain urokinase-type plasminogen activator. The arrows indicate the cleavage sites for plasmin. The active site residues are indicated by white circles.

scu-PA (scu-PA–32k) was purified from the conditioned medium of CALU-3 cells (human lung adenocarcinoma) (66). This scu-PA–32k was subsequently produced by recombinant DNA technology (67).

STRUCTURAL PROPERTIES

scu-PA is a single-chain glycoprotein of 54 kd containing 411 amino acids (64) (Fig. 40-3). On limited hydrolysis by plasmin, kallikrein, trypsin, cathepsin B, human T-cell–associated Ser proteinase 1, or thermolysin of the Lys158-Ile159 peptide bond, the molecule is converted to a two-chain derivative. The light chain (A chain; NH2-terminal) contains 158 amino acids and the heavy chain (B chain) 253; both chains are connected by a Cys148-Cys279 interchain disulfide bond. Commercial, highly purified tcu-PA, however, often has phenylalanine instead of Lys as COOH-terminal amino acid of the light chain. The catalytic center is located in the carboxyl-terminal chain and is composed of Asp255, His204, and Ser356. The amino-terminal chain contains regions homologous to human epidermal growth factor (residues 5 to 49) and one region homologous to the plasminogen kringles. A single carbohydrate moiety is attached to Asn302, and threonine (Thr)18 is fucosylated. A LMW (33 kd) tcu-PA can be generated with plasmin by hydrolysis of the Lys135-Lys136 peptide bond after previous cleavage of the Lys158-Ile159 bond (68). scu-PA–32k is generated by specific proteolytic cleavage of the Glu143–leucine 144 peptide bond in scu-PA by MMPs (MMP-3 and MMP-7) (69). Thrombin cleaves the Arg156–phenylalanine 157 peptide bond in scu-PA, resulting in an inactive tcu-PA molecule (70). This inactivation is strongly enhanced in the presence of thrombomodulin and is dependent on the O-linked glycosaminoglycan of thrombomodulin (71).

A single-chain urokinase species was purified by chromatography on fibrin-celite, suggesting a specific fibrin affinity (72–74). In other studies, however, direct fibrin binding of scu-PA (75,76) or of scu-PA–32k (66,67) has not been observed.

GENE STRUCTURE

The cDNA of u-PA was isolated and the nucleotide sequence determined (64,77,78). The cDNA sequence contains an open reading frame that starts with ATG at nucleotide positions 77 to 79 and extends for 1293 nucleotides until a TGA stop codon is reached at positions 1370 to 1372 (64). The open reading frame is preceded by at least 76 nucleotides of 5' untranslated mRNA, which are extremely rich in G/C nucleotides (83%). Beyond the termination codon, the cDNA extends for another 932 nucleotides. The sequence includes two poly (A) adenylation signals (positions 2271 to 2276 and 2284 to 2289), preceding the polyadenylation site at position 2304. The human u-PA gene is 6.4 kilobases (kb) long and located on chromosome 10. It contains 11 exons, and the exon-intron organization of the gene closely resembles that of the t-PA gene. Exons III, VIII, and IX of t-PA are totally missing, however, and exon IV is partially missing in the u-PA gene; this accounts for the absence of a finger domain and a K2 in u-PA. Exon II of the u-PA gene codes for a signal peptide consisting of 20 amino acids, exons III and IV code for the growth factor domain, and exons V and VI code for the kringle region. The 5' region of exon VII, which codes for the peptide connecting the light and the heavy chain, is 39 bp longer than the corresponding exon X of the t-PA gene. The 3' regions of exon VII and exons VIII to XI code for the heavy chain.

ENZYMATIC PROPERTIES OF TWO-CHAIN UROKINASE-TYPE PLASMINOGEN ACTIVATOR

The activation of plasminogen by tcu-PA obeys Michaelis-Menten kinetics. For the activation of native (Glu) plasminogen by urokinase in a purified system, kinetic parameters were reported ranging between 1.4 and 200 µmol/L for the K_m and between 0.26 and 1.48 s^{-1} for the k_{cat}. This yields second-order rate constants (k_{cat}/K_m) between 0.0074 and 0.5 µmol^{-1}.L.s^{-1} (79,80), probably depending on the quality of the plasminogen preparation and on the experimental conditions used. Activation of Lys-plasminogen by tcu-PA appears to be three to ten times faster than that of Glu-plasminogen (81). In the presence of certain ω-aminocarboxylic acids (e.g., 6-aminohexanoic acid), the rate of activation of Glu-plasminogen by tcu-PA increases 10 to 20 times, whereas that of Lys-plasminogen is unaffected. This is probably because these amino acids induce a conformational change in the Glu-plasminogen moiety similar to that observed on conversion of Glu-plasminogen to Lys-plasminogen or to plasmin (82). Activation of Glu-plasminogen by tcu-PA is stimulated somewhat by the presence of fibrin (83) and also by fibrinogen, fragment D, and fragment E (84); activation of Lys-plasminogen is not affected. Addition of cyanogen bromide–digested fibrinogen also increases the activation rate of Glu-plasminogen by tcu-PA approximately ten times (85).

ENZYMATIC PROPERTIES OF SINGLE-CHAIN UROKINASE-TYPE PLASMINOGEN ACTIVATOR

scu-PA has a low reactivity toward LMW synthetic substrates or active-site titrants that are highly reactive toward tcu-PA (86,87).

We investigated the activation of plasminogen by natural scu-PA purified from the human lung adenocarcinoma cell line CALU-3 (75); by recombinant scu-PA obtained by expression of cDNA in *E. coli* (88) or in CHO cells (89); and by scu-PA–32k, an LMW scu-PA generated by specific cleavage of the Glu143–leucine 144 peptide bond (66,67).

These kinetic studies revealed that in mixtures of scu-PA and plasminogen, tcu-PA and plasmin are quickly generated. Addition of plasmin inhibitors prohibits the conversion of scu-PA to tcu-PA but not the activation of plasminogen to plasmin, suggesting that scu-PA activated plasminogen directly (76). Kinetic analysis reveals that the conversion of scu-PA and plasminogen to tcu-PA and plasmin, respectively, can be described by a sequence of three reactions that each obey Michaelis-Menten kinetics (88,90). In a first reaction, scu-PA directly activates plasminogen to plasmin; in the second reaction, plasmin then converts scu-PA to tcu-PA; plasminogen is activated by tcu-PA in the third reaction.

Activation of Lys-plasminogen occurs with comparable affinity but with a higher k_{cat}, resulting in more efficient activation by scu-PA (approximately tenfold) (91). This high affinity is not mediated via the high-affinity Lys-binding site of plasminogen (located in kringles 1 to 3), nor via the low-affinity Lys-binding site comprised within kringle 4, as evidenced by the comparable K_m of scu-PA for native and LMW plasminogen (a derivative lacking these structures) (91). The similar kinetic constants obtained with scu-PA–32k and scu-PA, furthermore, indicate that the plasminogen activating properties are independent of the NH_2-terminal 143 amino acids of scu-PA (66,67).

To further investigate the significance of the conversion of scu-PA to tcu-PA for the activation of plasminogen, mutants of recombinant scu-PA were constructed by site-specific mutagenesis of Lys158 to glycine 158 or Glu158, thereby destroying the plasmic cleavage site for conversion to tcu-PA (89). At the plasminogen concentrations used to measure the kinetic parameters for activation by scu-PA (around 1 μmol/L), no significant activation is observed with these mutants. When higher plasminogen concentrations are used (10 to 100 μmol/L), concentration-dependent activation of plasminogen is observed, after Michaelis-Menten kinetics. The kinetic constants show that the mutants activate plasminogen with a k_{cat} that is approximately five times higher than that of rscu-PA, but with a K_m that is 60 to 80 times higher. The catalytic efficiency (k_{cat}/K_m) of both mutants is therefore 10 to 20 times lower than that of wild rscu-PA. From these experiments, we conclude that scu-PA has some intrinsic plasminogen activating potential. A low intrinsic plasminogen activating potential of scu-PA is confirmed by others (92), whereas some authors claim that scu-PA has no enzymatic activity and is

a genuine proenzyme (93,94). Taken together, most data indicate that scu-PA has some intrinsic plasminogen activating potential, which represents 0.5% or less of the catalytic efficiency of tcu-PA (95,96). The occurrence of a transitional state of scu-PA with a higher catalytic efficiency for native plasminogen than tcu-PA has also been postulated (97). A charge interaction between Ile159 and Asp355 may be the primary force for stabilizing the active conformation of tcu-PA and determining the intrinsic catalytic activity of scu-PA (98).

Inactive thrombin-derived tcu-PA (obtained by treatment of scu-PA with thrombin) with phenylalanine 157 as NH_2-terminal of the B chain can be converted to active tcu-PA by hydrolysis of the Lys158-Ile159 peptide bond by plasmin, exposing Ile159 as NH_2-terminal of the B chain of tcu-PA (99). These observations suggest that the structure of the NH_2-terminal region of the B chain of tcu-PA is an important determinant for its enzymatic activity, whereas that of the COOH-terminal region of the A chain is not. Exposure of the Ile159 residue apparently plays an important role, converting low-activity scu-PA to tcu-PA with high enzymatic activity. The increased activity of tcu-PA compared with scu-PA may thus be related to a refolding of the Ile159 residue into the binding pocket of the enzyme, as with other Ser proteinases.

Urokinase-Type Plasminogen Activator Receptor

The specific cell-surface receptor for u-PA is a heterogeneously glycosylated protein of 50 to 60 kd, synthesized as a 313 amino acid polypeptide, which is anchored to the plasma membrane by a glycosyl-phosphatidylinositol moiety attached at amino acids 282, 283, or 284. The u-PAR molecule is composed of three distantly related structural domains, of which the NH_2-terminal domain is involved in binding u-PA; it binds all forms of u-PA containing an intact growth factor domain (see reference 100). Most of the residues of u-PA required for interaction with u-PAR are located within loop B (amino acids 20–30) (101).

The binding of u-PA to its receptor at the cell surface is believed to be crucial for its activity under physiologic conditions. Binding results in a strongly enhanced plasmin generation, owing to effects on both the activation of plasminogen (102) and on the feedback activation of scu-PA to tcu-PA by generated plasmin (103). Both of these effects are also critically dependent on the cellular binding of plasminogen. Cell-associated plasmin is protected from rapid inhibition by $α_2$-antiplasmin, which further favors the activation of receptor-bound scu-PA. This system can, however, be efficiently inhibited by PAI-1 and PAI-2 (104). The observation that direct anchorage of u-PA to the cell surface (using a glycosyl-phosphatidylinositol–anchored u-PA mutant) leads to a potentiation of plasmin generation equivalent to that observed in the presence of u-PAR suggests that u-PAR mainly functions to localize u-PA at the cell surface (105). Assembly of u-PAR–mediated plasminogen activation complexes also requires direct interactions between u-PA and plasminogen not involving the active site (106). Concentration of proteolytic activity at the cell surface may also occur via vitronectin, trapping soluble u-PAR–u-PA complexes (107). Both u-PA and u-PAR have been found in a complex with $β_1$-, $β_2$-, and $β_3$-integrins, thereby allowing mutual interactions and regulatory processes between cell adhesion and proteolysis [reviewed by May and colleagues (108)].

Plasminogen

PHYSICOCHEMICAL PROPERTIES

Human plasminogen is a single-chain glycoprotein of 92 kd, containing approximately 2% carbohydrate. The complete primary structure of the molecule was elucidated by amino acid

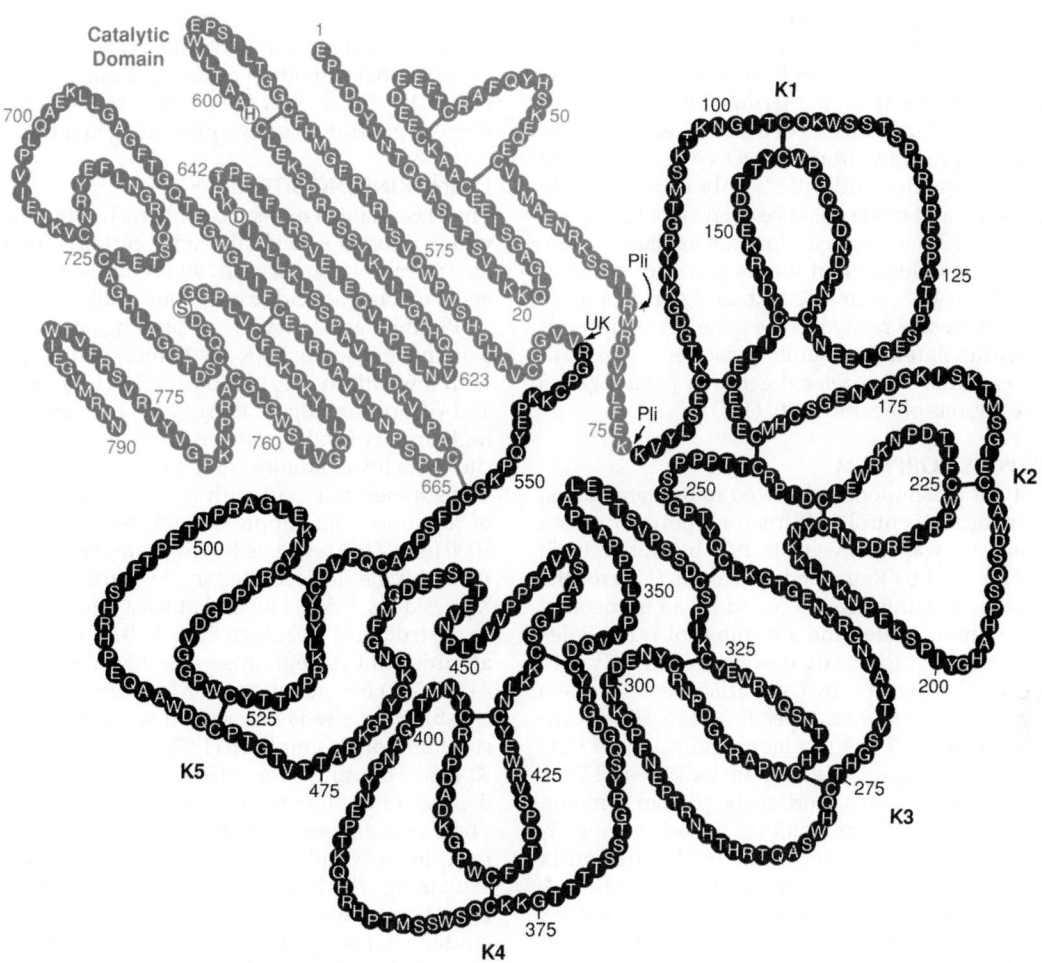

Figure 40-4. Schematic representation of the primary structure of plasminogen. Pli, plasma cleavage sites for conversion of Glu-plasminogen to Lys-plasminogen; UK, cleavage site for plasminogen activators, yielding plasmin.

and cDNA sequencing (109,110). The plasminogen molecule consists of 791 amino acids; it contains 24 disulfide bridges and five homologous triple-loop structures or kringles. The covalent structure of plasminogen is represented in Figure 40-4.

Plasminogen can be determined in plasma using immunologic methods or by complex formation with streptokinase and measuring the plasminogen-streptokinase complex with a chromogenic substrate (111). The normal plasma concentration is approximately 1.5 to 2.0 µmol/L. Native plasminogen has NH_2-terminal glutamic acid (Glu-plasminogen) but is easily converted by limited plasmic digestion to modified forms having NH_2-terminal Lys, valine (Val), or methionine (Met), commonly designated *Lys-plasminogen*. This conversion occurs by hydrolysis of the Arg68-Met69, Lys77-Lys78, or Lys78-Val79 peptide bonds. Native plasminogen may adopt distinct conformations, involving two intramolecular interactions: one mediated by regions of the NH_2-terminal peptide and kringle 5 and the other between kringles 3 and 4 (112).

The method of choice for purifying human plasminogen is affinity chromatography on insolubilized Lys, a method introduced by Deutsch and Mertz (113). Glu-plasminogen and Lys-plasminogen forms can be separated by chromatography on diethylaminoethyl-Sephadex.

The Glu-plasminogen occurring in human blood displays at least two types of microheterogeneity. Affinity chromatography on Lys-Sepharose, using gradient elution with 6-aminohexanoic acid, separates plasminogen into two fractions (called *type I* and *type II* in the order of their elution from Lys-Sepharose) (114). Differences in carbohydrate and amino acid composition were invoked to explain this heterogeneity (115,116). Each of these two fractions can be separated into approximately six forms having different isoelectric points (pI), as a result of differences in sialic acid content. All 12 molecular forms appear to be present in single-donor plasma (115). Hayes and Castellino (117–119) have shown that type I plasminogen contains a glucosamine-based carbohydrate chain on Asn288 and a galactosamine-based carbohydrate chain on Thr345; type II plasminogen has only the latter. These differences in carbohydrate composition play a role in the interaction with α_2-antiplasmin and fibrin, with type II showing the strongest interaction with both (120).

The turnover of Glu-plasminogen and Lys-plasminogen labeled with radioiodine was studied in healthy subjects (121). Glu-plasminogen had a plasma half-life of 2.20 ± 0.29 days and a fractional catabolic rate of 0.55 ± 0.10 of the plasma pool per day; Lys-plasminogen disappeared with a half-life of approximately 0.8 days. The two forms of Glu-plasminogen with different affinity for Lys-Sepharose have similar turnover characteristics in humans. The turnover of plasminogen increased during reptilase (Defibrase) treatment in patients with liver cirrhosis and in several clinical conditions associated with intravascular coagulation.

GENE STRUCTURE

A 2.7-kb insert of a cDNA clone for human plasminogen containing the complete coding region was sequenced. A 5' noncoding region of 64 bp and a 3' noncoding region of 253 bp are present in the full-length clone. A consensus AATAAA sequence is located at a position 46 nucleotides upstream of the polyadenylation site. The coding region contains an amino-terminal sequence of 19 amino acids having the characteristics of a signal sequence. The amino acid sequence predicted from this cDNA is close to the published protein sequence and differs only in four amide assignments (Glx, Asx) and in the presence of an extra Ile at position 65, giving a total of 791 amino acids for human plasminogen.

The *plasminogen* gene, located on the long arm of chromosome 6 at band q26 or q27, spans 52.5 kb and consists of 19 exons (122,123). It is closely related to the gene of apolipoprotein (a); the 5' untranslated and flanking sequences of both genes and of at least four other related genes or pseudogenes contain extensive regions of near identity (124).

PLASMINOGEN POLYMORPHISM

The heterogeneity of plasminogen observed in human plasma appears to be genetically controlled. Structural polymorphism of human plasminogen was discovered in 1979 by Hobart (125) for the native protein and by Raum and colleagues (126) for the desialylated protein. Plasminogen is coded by an autosomal gene with two common alleles and a number of rare alleles (125–127). Plasminogen variants are designated according to the relative direction of their pI, by comparison with the two common types. The two common types found in all investigated races are designated PLG A (for more acidic pI) and PLG B (for more basic pI); the respective alleles are indicated PLG* A and PLG* B. Rare variants with a more acidic pI than common PLG A or a more basic pI than common PLG B receive a numerical suffix for the relative direction of their pI shift (suffix increases from basic to acidic direction of pI shift for PLG A variants and from acidic to basic direction for PLG B variants). The variants between common PLG A and PLG B are designated as PLG M1, PLG M2, PLG M3, and so forth (suffix increases from basic to acidic direction of pI shift) (126).

The allele frequencies differ substantially in various racial groups but are fairly constant within one race. In the European populations, the distribution is roughly as follows: common PLG* A, 0.70; common PLG* B, 0.28; and rare PLG*, 0.020. The PLG B variant found in Japanese (allele frequency 0.022) had a normal antigen level but activity was reduced to 40% of normal (128). A direct correlation with thrombotic tendency was suggested but could not be established. The occurrence of a silent allele (PLG°) was reported in a Swiss family (129).

MECHANISM OF ACTIVATION TO PLASMIN

Lys-plasminogen is converted to plasmin by cleavage of a single Arg-Val peptide bond corresponding to the Arg561-Val562 bond (130). The two-chain plasmin molecule is composed of a heavy chain (A chain) originating from the NH_2-terminal part of plasminogen and of a light chain (B chain) constituting the COOH-terminal part. The B chain contains (a) an active site similar to that of trypsin, composed of a His residue sensitive to tosyl-Lys chloromethyl ketone, and (b) a Ser residue reactive toward diisopropyl-phosphofluoridate (131). The active site of plasmin is composed of His603, Asp646, and Ser741.

Activation of Glu-plasminogen to plasmin by urokinase in a purified system occurs approximately 20 times slower than activation of Lys-plasminogen, but Lys-plasmin is formed in either case. In view of the great sensitivity of the Arg68-Met69 bond to plasmin, it was suggested that the major pathway for activation of plasminogen is via Lys-plasminogen generated by plasmic cleavage of Glu-plasminogen (132). Activation of Glu-plasminogen in the presence of the physiologic plasmin inhibitor α_2-antiplasmin generates inhibited Glu-plasmin, however (133).

Investigation of the activation pathways of plasminogen with the use of monoclonal antibodies specific for Lys-plasminogen revealed that activation of Glu-plasminogen in human plasma occurs by direct cleavage of the Arg561-Val562 peptide bond without generation of Lys-plasminogen intermediates (134).

LYSINE-BINDING SITES

The plasminogen molecule contains Lys-binding site structures, which interact specifically with certain amino acids, such as Lys, 6-aminohexanoic acid, and *trans*-4-amino-methylcyclohexane-1-carboxylic acid (tranexamic acid).

Plasminogen contains one binding site with high affinity for 6-aminohexanoic acid (K_d of 9 µmol/L) and approximately four with low affinity (K_d of 5 mmol/L) (135). For tranexamic acid and Glu-plasminogen, these K_d values are 1.1 µmol/L for the high-affinity binding site and 750 µmol/L for the four or five sites with lower affinity (136). Lys-plasminogen has one site that binds tranexamic acid with K_d of 2.2 µmol/L, one site with K_d of 36 µmol/L, and approximately two or three sites with K_d of 1000 µmol/L. These Lys-binding sites are located in the plasmin A chain. One site is located in the fourth triple-loop structure or K_4 (residues 355 to 440) and at least one in the first three triple-loop structures (residues 80 to 338 or to 354), shown by their affinities to Lys-Sepharose. The LMW plasminogen (residues 443 to 791) has no affinity for Lys-Sepharose. The high-affinity Lys-binding site is comprised within the first three kringle structures of plasminogen (137), and is most probably located in K_1 (138). Binding of ω-aminocarboxylic acids to isolated K_4 is dependent on the presence of Arg70 and Asp56 residues (139). These essential residues are preserved in homologous positions in K_1 but are replaced by neutral amino acids in K_5, possibly explaining why K_5 has no ω-aminocarboxylic acid binding site. From nuclear magnetic resonance studies on K_4, it was also concluded that several aromatic residues may be lining the ω-aminocarboxylic acid binding site (140).

Plasminogen can specifically bind to fibrin through its Lys-binding sites. In both purified systems and in plasma, Lys-plasminogen has a higher affinity for fibrin than Glu-plasminogen (141). The differences in binding of Glu-plasminogen and Lys-plasminogen to fibrin might be due to an intramolecular interaction of one of the Lys-binding sites, with a specific site in the NH_2-terminal region of Glu-plasminogen that is no longer present in Lys-plasminogen. The presence of 6-aminohexanoic acid prohibits the adsorption of plasminogen to fibrin in the purified system and in the plasma system. Thus, one of the functions of the Lys-binding sites in plasminogen is to mediate its interaction with fibrin. In addition, Glu-plasminogen, Lys-plasminogen, and LMW plasminogen contain a weak Lys-binding site, termed the *AH site*; this site preferably interacts with ligands not carrying a free carboxylate function and, therefore, may bind proteins via Lys side chains. It was suggested that the initial binding of plasminogen to fibrin is mainly determined by the AH site (142).

The Lys-binding sites of plasmin(ogen) also mediate its interaction with α_2-antiplasmin, as discussed later. On the basis of these interactions, it is suggested that the Lys-binding sites play a crucial role in the regulation of fibrinolysis (143,144).

Glu-plasminogen also binds in a specific and saturable manner to unstimulated human platelets, and this binding is enhanced fivefold by thrombin stimulation (40). Both phenomena occur through different pathways involving either glycoprotein IIb-IIIa or fibrin(ogen) for binding to unstimulated or stimulated platelets, respectively (145). The region comprising the first three kringles appears to be the primary recognition site for plasminogen binding to both thrombin-stimulated and unstimulated platelets. K_4 and LMW plasminogen contribute differently to binding to stimulated and unstimulated platelets,

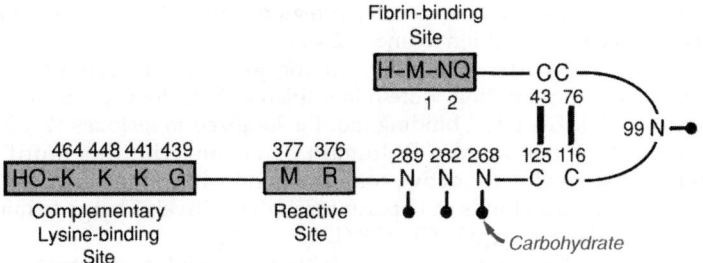

Figure 40-5. Schematic representation of the primary structure of α_2-antiplasmin.

confirming the occurrence of two distinct mechanisms (146). Platelets thus apparently have the potential to enhance fibrinolysis by localizing plasminogen in a thrombus and enhancing its activation.

COMPONENTS INVOLVED IN INHIBITION OF THE FIBRINOLYTIC SYSTEM

Inhibition of the fibrinolytic system may occur at the level of plasmin or at the level of plasminogen activators. For a long time, it was accepted that there were essentially two functionally important plasmin inhibitors in plasma: one immediately reacting inhibitor and one slower reacting inhibitor identical to α_2-macroglobulin and α_1-antitrypsin, respectively. Approximately 25 years ago, another plasmin inhibitor, α_2-antiplasmin, was identified in human plasma. On activation of plasminogen in plasma, plasmin is preferentially bound by this inhibitor. The complete activation of plasminogen (concentration, approximately 2 μmol/L), resulting in saturation of this plasmin inhibitor (concentration, approximately 1 μmol/L), must occur before the excess plasmin is neutralized by α_2-macroglobulin. Inhibition of the physiologic plasminogen activators t-PA and u-PA in human plasma occur mainly by PAI-1 and PAI-2.

α_2-Antiplasmin

PHYSICOCHEMICAL CHARACTERIZATION

α_2-Antiplasmin is a single-chain glycoprotein of 70 kd containing approximately 13% carbohydrate. The molecule consists of 464 amino acids and contains two disulfide bridges (147,148) (Fig. 40-5). Subsequently, it has been suggested that α_2-antiplasmin contains only one Cys-Cys disulfide bond and two unpaired Cys (149). α_2-Antiplasmin belongs to the Ser protease inhibitor protein family (serpins). Two molecular forms were detected in approximately equal amounts in purified preparations of the inhibitor: a native 464 residue long inhibitor with NH$_2$-terminal Met (Met^1-α_2-antiplasmin) and a 12–amino acid shorter form with NH$_2$-terminal Asn (Asn^{13}-α_2-antiplasmin) (150). It is not known whether Asn^{13}-α_2-antiplasmin is present in the circulating blood or whether it is generated *in vitro*. The NH$_2$-terminal Gln^{14}-residue of α_2-antiplasmin can cross-link to Aα-chains of fibrin in a process that requires Ca^{2+} and is catalyzed by activated coagulation factor XIII (151). Asn^{13}-α_2-antiplasmin appears to be more efficiently cross-linked to fibrin than Met^1-α_2-antiplasmin (152).

The concentration of the inhibitor in normal plasma is approximately 7 mg/dL (approximately 1 μmol/L) (153). The half-life of purified biologically intact iodine-labeled α_2-antiplasmin is 2.6 days, whereas the plasmin-α_2-antiplasmin complex disappears from plasma with a half-life of approximately half a day (154). The inhibitor in normal plasma is heterogeneous and consists of functionally active and inactive material. Complete activation of the plasminogen present in

normal plasma converts only approximately 70% of the antigen material into a complex with plasmin; 30% of the inhibitor-related antigen appears to be functionally inactive. Human plasma contains two forms of the inhibitor that differ in binding to plasminogen. The form that does not bind remains an active plasmin inhibitor (155) but reacts much slower with plasmin. This form lacks a 26-residue peptide from the carboxyl-terminal end of α_2-antiplasmin (156). This peptide inhibits the interaction of α_2-antiplasmin with plasmin, which suggests that it contains the plasminogen-binding site. Wiman and coworkers (157) measured the ratio of these forms in the plasma of pregnant women subjected to extensive plasmapheresis, and they concluded that the plasminogen-binding form of α_2-antiplasmin is primarily synthesized, and it becomes partly converted to the non-plasminogen–binding form in the circulating blood.

MECHANISMS OF INTERACTION WITH PLASMIN

In purified systems and in plasma, α_2-antiplasmin forms a 1:1 stoichiometric complex with plasmin that is devoid of protease or esterase activity. α_2-Antiplasmin, like many other plasma proteinase inhibitors, has a broad *in vitro* inhibitory spectrum, but its physiologic role as an inhibitor of proteinases other than plasmin seems negligible.

Kinetic studies of the inhibition of human plasmin by α_2-antiplasmin revealed that the disappearance of plasmin activity after addition of excess α_2-antiplasmin does not follow first-order kinetics (158–160). Although most of the plasmin is rapidly inactivated, the process slowly proceeds toward completion. This time course of the reaction is compatible with a kinetic model composed of two successive reactions: a fast, reversible second-order reaction followed by a slower, irreversible first-order transition. The model can be represented by the following:

$$P + A \underset{k_{-1}}{\overset{k_1}{\rightleftharpoons}} PA \overset{k_2}{\rightarrow} PA'$$

where:
P = plasmin, A = α_2-antiplasmin, PA = reversible inactive complex, and PA' = irreversible inactive complex.

The second-order rate constant (k_1) is 2 to 4×10^7 mol^{-1}.L.s^{-1}. This is among the fastest protein-protein reactions described. Such rate constants approach the theoretical values for a diffusion-controlled process. The dissociation constant of the reversible complex is 2×10^{-10} mol/L. The half-life of the first-order transition, PA $\rightarrow$ PA', is 166 seconds, corresponding to a k_2 value of 4.2×10^{-3}.s^{-1}. Christensen and Clemmensen (158) reported a value of 6.5×10^{-3}.s^{-1} for k_2.

Plasmin molecules with a synthetic substrate bound to their active site or with 6-aminohexanoic acid bound to their Lys-binding sites do not react or only react slowly with α_2-antiplasmin (155,159). The first step of the process thus clearly depends on the presence of a free Lys-binding site and active site in the plasmin molecule. This was further substantiated by studying the kinetics of the reaction between α_2-antiplasmin and a LMW form of plasmin (LMW plasmin) lacking Lys-binding sites (160). The reaction scheme is identical to that observed with normal plasmin, but the rate constant of the first step is approximately 60 times smaller and is only slightly inhibited by 6-aminohexanoic acid. These findings show that the first reversible step in the reaction between plasmin and α_2-antiplasmin can be divided into two parts: (a) a reaction between the Lys-binding sites in the plasmin A chain and the corresponding site in the α_2-antiplasmin molecule and (b) a reaction between the active site of plasmin and a reactive site in α_2-antiplasmin. Because the reaction rate is strongly dependent on the availability of free Lys-binding sites, the main pathway is probably a consecutive reaction in this order. From competition experiments between plasminogen fragments containing Lys-binding sites and plasmin for binding of α_2-antiplasmin, it was concluded that the high-affinity Lys-binding sites situated in K_1 to K_3 of the plasmin A chain are mainly responsible for the interaction with α_2-antiplasmin (137).

Plasmin and α_2-antiplasmin form a stoichiometric 1:1 complex of approximately 140 kd by interaction between the B chain of plasmin and the inhibitor. A nondisulfide-bonded peptide (8 kd) is released concomitantly with complex formation. On disulfide bond reduction, the complex is dissociated in two parts: (a) an intact plasmin A chain (60 kd) and (b) a stable complex between the plasmin B chain and α_2-antiplasmin (80 kd), provided the complex formation is performed in excess α_2-antiplasmin (133). The reactive-site peptide bond in α_2-antiplasmin cleaved by plasmin consists of Arg376-Met377. A bond is formed between the active-site seryl residue in plasmin and a specific arginyl residue in the inhibitor. The reaction rate between plasmin and α_2-antiplasmin in plasma may be reduced by the presence of plasma proteins, such as His-rich glycoprotein (161) or fibrinogen (137), which interfere with the reaction. The half-life of plasmin molecules on the fibrin surface is estimated to be two to three orders of magnitude longer than that of free plasmin (143).

GENE STRUCTURE
The gene for human α_2-antiplasmin, located on chromosome 17p13 (162), is approximately 16 kb and contains 10 exons (163). The NH$_2$-terminal region of the protein, comprising the fibrin cross-linking site, is encoded by exon IV, whereas both the reactive site and the plasminogen-binding site in the COOH-terminal region are encoded by exon X.

Plasminogen Activator Inhibitor-1
PHYSIOCHEMICAL CHARACTERIZATION
PAI-1 was first identified in conditioned media of cultured human endothelial cells and subsequently in plasma, platelets, placenta and conditioned media of fibrosarcoma cells, and hepatocytes (164,165). In healthy individuals, highly variable plasma levels of both PAI activity and PAI-1 antigen have been observed. PAI activity ranges from 0.5 to 47.0 U/mL (t-PA neutralizing units, 1 mg active PAI-1 corresponds to 700,000 U) with 80% of the values below 6 U/mL. PAI-1 antigen ranges between 6 and 85 ng/mL (geometric mean, 24 ng/mL). PAI-1 levels are strongly elevated in several thromboembolic disease states (see Pathophysiology of Fibrinolysis). PAI-1 is a single-chain glycoprotein of approximately 52 kd, consisting of 378 amino acids. The cDNA sequence revealed that PAI-1 is a member of the serpin family with reactive site peptide bond Arg346-Met347 (166,167). Saturation mutagenesis of PAI-1 indicated that a basic amino acid was required at P1 for significant inhibitory activity, whereas all substitutions, except Pro, were tolerated at P'1 (168). The *PAI-1* gene, located on chromosome 7, bands q21.3-q22, is approximately 12.2 kb, and consists of nine exons (169). As a result of alternative polyadenylation yielding

an additional 3' untranslated region, a mRNA species of 3.2 kb occurs in addition to one of 2.4 kb.

PAI-1 is stabilized by binding to a plasminogen activator inhibitor binding protein identified as S-protein or vitronectin (170). The PAI-1 binding motif is localized to residues 12–30 of the somatomedin B domain of vitronectin; this motif is anchored in the active conformation by disulfide bonds (171). PAI-1 also binds to heparin through positively charged amino acids in the region 65 to 88 (172).

PAI-1 occurs as an active inhibitory form that spontaneously converts to a latent form that can be partially reactivated by denaturing agents (173). Positive charges in the turn connecting s4C with s3C are essential for the functional stability of PAI-1 (174,175). The structural basis of the latency in PAI-1 has been resolved by determination of the structure by single-crystal x-ray diffraction. Part of the reactive center loop is inserted in the major β-sheet of PAI-1 and is therefore not accessible to the target enzyme (locked conformation). Reactivation of latent PAI-1 by denaturants results in partial elimination of this insertion (176). Another molecular form of intact PAI-1 has been isolated that does not form stable complexes with t-PA but is cleaved at the P1-P1' peptide bond ("substrate PAI-1") (177). By point mutations in the reactive site loop, PAI-1 could be converted from an inhibitor into a substrate (178). The x-ray structure of the cleaved substrate variant shows that it has a new β-strand (s4A) formed by insertion of the NH$_2$-terminal portion of the reactive site loop into β-sheet A subsequent to cleavage (179). Thus, inhibitory PAI-1 may not only convert to latent PAI-1, which can be reactivated, but also to substrate PAI-1, which is irreversibly degraded by its target proteinases. This observation may thus have implications for the regulation of the fibrinolytic system.

MECHANISM OF ACTION
PAI-1 reacts very rapidly with single-chain and two-chain t-PA and with tcu-PA, with second-order inhibition rate constants of the order of 10^7 mol^{-1}.L.s^{-1}, and it does not react with scu-PA (165,180).

Like other serpins, PAI-1 inhibits its target proteinases by formation of a 1:1 stoichiometric reversible complex, followed by covalent binding between the hydroxylgroup of the active site Ser residue of the proteinase and the carboxylgroup of the P1 residue at the Arg346-Met347 reactive center ("bait region") of the serpin. The rapid inhibition of both t-PA and u-PA by PAI-1 involves a reversible high-affinity second-site interaction that does not depend on a functional active site (181). Modeling approaches suggest that sequence 350-355 of PAI-1, which contains three negatively charged amino acids, interacts with highly positively charged regions in t-PA (residues 296-304) (182) or in u-PA (residues 179-184) (183). In the presence of fibrin, single-chain t-PA is protected from rapid inhibition by PAI-1 (181). It has, however, also been reported that PAI-1 binds to fibrin and that fibrin-bound PAI-1 may inhibit t-PA–mediated clot lysis (184,185).

In the presence of vitronectin, PAI-1 displays a 200-fold accelerated thrombin inhibition, as a result of a conformational effect of vitronectin binding on the reactive site loop of PAI-1 (186,187). This may be relevant for the control of extravascular proteolysis (188,189). By high affinity binding to vitronectin, PAI-1 may compete with u-PAR–dependent or integrin-dependent binding of cells to the extracellular matrix (190–194). Thereby, PAI-1 may play a role in cell adhesion and/or migration via a mechanism independent of its antiproteolytic activity.

Plasminogen Activator Inhibitor-2
PAI-2 levels in plasma are very low but are drastically elevated during pregnancy (195). PAI-2 exists in two different forms with

comparable inhibitory properties that are derived from a single mRNA: an intracellular nonglycosylated form of 47 kd and pI 5.0 and a secreted glycosylated form of 60 kd and pI 4.4. PAI-2 extracted from placenta is essentially nonglycosylated, whereas circulating PAI-2 observed during pregnancy is glycosylated. The function of intracellular PAI-2 is unclear, because its main target enzyme (u-PA) occurs extracellularly. It may constitute a storage pool from which PAI-2 can be secreted on cell injury (196). The precise (patho)physiologic role of PAI-2 remains to be determined.

PAI-2 is a serpin of 393 amino acids with reactive site peptide bond Arg358-Thr359. The *PAI-2* gene, located on chromosome 18 bands q21-23, spans 16.5 kb and contains 8 exons. The structure of the gene is different from that of the *PAI-1* gene, but is similar to that of the chicken ovalbumin gene (197). PAI-2 inhibits tcu-PA with a second-order rate constant (k_1) of 9×10^5 mol^{-1}.L.s^{-1}, which is approximately tenfold slower than PAI-1. PAI-2 also efficiently inhibits two-chain t-PA ($k_1 = 2 \times 10^5$ mol^{-1}.L.s^{-1}) and, less efficiently, single-chain t-PA ($k_1 = 9 \times 10^3$ mol^{-1}.L.s^{-1}), but it does not inhibit scu-PA. Secretion of PAI-2 is regulated by endotoxin and by phorbol esters, which stimulate the gene transcription more than 50-fold.[165]

MECHANISM OF PHYSIOLOGIC FIBRINOLYSIS

Mechanism of Action of Tissue-Type Plasminogen Activator

t-PA is a poor enzyme in the absence of fibrin, but the presence of fibrin strikingly enhances the activation rate of plasminogen (18). The kinetic data support a mechanism where fibrin provides a surface to which t-PA and plasminogen adsorb in a sequential and ordered way, yielding a cyclic ternary complex. The presence of fibrin increases the local plasminogen concentration by creating an additional interaction between t-PA and its substrate. The high affinity of t-PA for plasminogen in the presence of fibrin thus allows efficient activation on the fibrin clot, whereas plasminogen activation by t-PA in plasma occurs very slowly. Plasmin formed on the fibrin surface has both its Lys-binding sites and active site occupied and is only slowly inactivated by α_2-antiplasmin (half-life of approximately 10 to 100 seconds); free plasmin, when formed, is rapidly inhibited by α_2-antiplasmin (half-life of approximately 0.1 second) (159). The fibrinolytic process thus seems to be triggered by and confined to fibrin. It was proposed that initial binding of t-PA to fibrin is governed by the finger domain and, after partial degradation of fibrin, newly exposed carboxyl-terminal Lys residues result in enhanced binding of t-PA via K_2 (20). Higgins and Vehar (198) confirmed that when fibrin is degraded by plasmin, new t-PA binding sites with markedly lower dissociation constants (two to four orders of magnitude) are formed. During fibrinolysis, fibrinogen and fibrin itself are continuously modified by cleavage with thrombin or plasmin, yielding a diversity of reaction products (199). Thrombin-catalyzed formation of desA-fibrin monomer, and a certain degree of desA-fibrin polymerization are essential for stimulation of plasminogen activation by t-PA. Optimal stimulation is only obtained after early plasmin-cleavage in the COOH-terminal Aα-chain and the NH$_2$-terminal Bβ-chain of fibrin, yielding fragment X-polymer. The increase in fibrin stimulation after formation of fibrin X-polymers is associated with enhanced binding of t-PA and plasminogen. This increased and altered binding of both enzyme and substrate to fibrin is mediated in part by COOH-terminal Lys residues generated by plasmin-cleavage. Interaction of these COOH-terminal Lys with Lys binding sites on t-PA and plasminogen may allow an improved alignment, as well as

allosteric changes of the t-PA and plasminogen moieties, thus enhancing the rate of plasminogen activation (199).

During lysis of a fibrin clot, single-chain t-PA is converted to two-chain t-PA on the fibrin surface. This conversion is probably of little physiologic relevance, because the activity of single-chain t-PA and two-chain t-PA is enhanced to the same extent in the presence of fibrin or fragment X-polymer (200).

Proteins that compete with plasminogen for binding to fibrin may have an antifibrinolytic action. Thus, Lp(a), a protein with multiple copies of a plasminogen kringle 4–like domain, a single copy of a kringle 5–like domain, and an inactive proteinase domain (201), binds to fibrin via its Lys-binding domains. As for plasminogen, binding of Lp(a) to fibrin is enhanced by partial proteolytic degradation of the fibrin surface (202). Thereby, the fibrin-dependent enhancement of plasminogen activation by t-PA is reduced (203–205), although kinetic studies suggest that the effect of Lp(a) on plasminogen activation by t-PA is only very limited (206).

Alternatively, proteins that remove Lys residues from the fibrin surface, such as the thrombin activatable fibrinolysis inhibitor (TAFI) may have an antifibrinolytic action. TAFI is a 60-kd single-chain protein, identical to plasma procarboxypeptidase B, occurring at a concentration of 75 nmol/L (207,208). Thrombin, trypsin, or plasmin converts the protein to an active carbopeptidase B. Activated TAFI suppresses fibrinolysis, most likely by removing COOH-terminal Lys residues from (partially degraded) fibrin, thereby preventing additional binding of plasminogen and/or t-PA (209).

Mechanism of Action of Urokinase-Type Plasminogen Activator

tcu-PA has no specific affinity for fibrin, and activates fibrin-bound and circulating plasminogen relatively indiscriminately. Extensive plasminogen activation and depletion of α_2-antiplasmin may occur after treatment of thromboembolic diseases with tcu-PA, leading to degradation of several plasma proteins, including fibrinogen, factor V, and factor VIII. scu-PA, in contrast to tcu-PA, has significant fibrin specificity.

In plasma, in the absence of fibrin, scu-PA is stable and does not activate plasminogen; in the presence of a fibrin clot, it induces fibrin-specific clot lysis (95). scu-PA does not bind to a significant extent to fibrin, but its intrinsic activity toward fibrin-bound plasminogen may contribute to its fibrin-specificity. In addition, plasma α_2-antiplasmin prevents conversion of scu-PA to tcu-PA outside the clot and thus preserves fibrin-specificity (210). Fibrin fragment E-2 selectively promotes the activation of plasminogen by scu-PA, mainly by enhancing the k_{cat} of the activation (211). scu-PA is an inefficient activator of plasminogen bound to internal Lys residues on intact fibrin but has a higher activity toward plasminogen bound to newly generated COOH-terminal Lys residues on partially degraded fibrin (212). Thus, the fibrin-specificity of scu-PA does not require its conversion to tcu-PA but is mediated by enhanced binding of plasminogen to partially digested fibrin (213).

PATHOPHYSIOLOGY OF FIBRINOLYSIS

The physiologic importance of the fibrinolytic system is demonstrated by the association between abnormal fibrinolysis and a tendency toward bleeding or thrombosis. Impaired fibrinolysis is a commonly observed hemostatic abnormality in patients with thrombosis. It may be due to defective synthesis and/or release of t-PA from the vessel wall, a deficiency or functional defect in the plasminogen molecule, or increased levels of inhibitors of t-PA and plasmin. On the other hand, excessive fibrinolysis due to increased levels of t-PA or to α_2-antiplasmin or PAI-1 deficiency may result in accelerated clot lysis and bleeding.

α_2-Antiplasmin Deficiency and Bleeding

CONGENITAL α_2-ANTIPLASMIN DEFICIENCY

The first case of congenital homozygous α_2-antiplasmin deficiency was described in a patient who presented with a hemorrhagic diathesis (214). Several cases of heterozygosity have been described with no or only mild bleeding symptoms (6). The α_2-antiplasmin levels in all heterozygotes described thus far are consistently between 40% and 60% of normal. Antigen and activity levels usually correspond well, suggesting that the deficiency is due to decreased synthesis of a normal α_2-antiplasmin molecule. The bleeding tendency in these patients may be due to premature lysis of hemostatic plugs, because, in the absence of α_2-antiplasmin, the half-life of plasmin molecules generated on the fibrin surface may be considerably prolonged.

The molecular defect in α_2-antiplasmin Okinawa was identified as a trinucleotide deletion in exon VII, leading to deletion of Glu137 in the protein (215). In α_2-antiplasmin Nara, insertion of a cytidine nucleotide in exon X leads to a shift in the reading frame of the mRNA, resulting in deletion of the COOH-terminal 12 amino acids of native α_2-antiplasmin and replacement with 178 unrelated amino acids (216). These mutations may lead to the deficiency by causing folding of the protein into a nonnative configuration and, thereby, blocking its intracellular transport from the endoplasmatic reticulum to the Golgi complex (215).

Generation of α_2-antiplasmin–deficient mice revealed that they develop and reproduce normally. They also have an enhanced endogenous fibrinolytic capacity without overt bleeding. The absence of a bleeding phenotype in these mice, in contrast to humans, may reflect the fact that the coagulation system adequately prevents bleeding if the fibrinolytic system is not dramatically challenged (217).

ACQUIRED α_2-ANTIPLASMIN DEFICIENCY

Increased fibrinolysis in liver disease, especially in cirrhosis, is a well-known phenomenon. The serum level of α_2-antiplasmin is significantly decreased in liver cirrhosis and in several other liver diseases. Teger-Nilsson and coworkers (218) reported a mean value of 73% ± 15% for liver cirrhosis (controls, 100% ± 8%), and Aoki and Yamanaka found values of 4.24 ± 0.87 mg/dL and 2.56 ± 0.87 mg/dL for compensated and decompensated liver cirrhosis, respectively (controls, 6.2 ± 0.8 mg/dL) (219). Thus, the decreased level of α_2-antiplasmin appears to be an important factor in the increased fibrinolytic activity observed in liver cirrhosis. Moreover, it is likely that the liver is the organ of synthesis or storage of α_2-antiplasmin (220).

Decreased levels of α_2-antiplasmin also have been reported in patients having disseminated intravascular coagulation and some forms of renal disease (221). α_2-Antiplasmin levels may be significantly reduced in patients undergoing thrombolytic therapy as a result of systemic activation of the fibrinolytic system. After intravenous infusion of either recombinant t-PA or streptokinase in patients with acute myocardial infarction, the decrease of α_2-antiplasmin is significantly greater in the streptokinase group (222).

DYSFUNCTIONAL α_2-ANTIPLASMIN

An abnormal α_2-antiplasmin associated with a serious bleeding tendency was found in two siblings in a Dutch family; it is referred to as α_2-antiplasmin Enschede. These individuals have 3% of normal functional activity and 100% of normal antigen levels (223). Their apparently heterozygous parents have 50%

functional activity and 100% antigen levels. The ability of the protein to reversibly bind plasmin or plasminogen was not affected, but the abnormal α_2-antiplasmin is converted from an inhibitor of plasmin to a substrate. The molecular defect of α_2-antiplasmin Enschede was revealed by sequencing of cloned genomic DNA fragments (224). It consists of the insertion of an extra Ala residue (GCG insertion) 7 to 10 positions on the amino-terminal side of the P_1 residue (Arg376) in the reactive site of α_2-antiplasmin. This 3-bp, in-frame insertion within the gene of α_2-antiplasmin was identified in two true heterozygotes and in their two homozygous children.

Plasminogen Activator Inhibitor Activity and Thrombosis

SYNTHESIS AND SECRETION OF PLASMINOGEN ACTIVATOR INHIBITOR-1

PAI-1 mRNA has been demonstrated in a large variety of tissues, suggesting that a cell common to these tissues, such as endothelial or smooth muscle cells (SMCs), may be the site of production (225). PAI-1 is found in plasma, platelets, placenta, and in the extracellular matrix. Except for platelets, which contain an inactive form of PAI-1, PAI-1 is not stored within cells but is rapidly and constitutively secreted after synthesis. For unknown reasons, PAI-1 exhibits a circadian variation; its plasma concentration is highest in the morning and lowest in the late afternoon and evening, whereas t-PA exhibits an opposite diurnal variation (7).

Synthesis and secretion of PAI-1 can be modulated by various agonists such as hormones, growth factors, endotoxin, cytokines, and phorbolesters (225,226). Although posttranscriptional regulation of PAI-1 mRNA levels has been suggested (227–229), most studies on the regulation of PAI-1 expression demonstrate an effect at the transcriptional level (230–234). Alterations in mRNA stability may also contribute to increased PAI-1 levels in some cells (225). In endothelial cells, PAI-1 gene expression is stimulated by lipopolysaccharide (228,235–238), interleukin 1 (237–239), tumor necrosis factor-α (228,240,241), transforming growth factor β (TGF-β) (242), basic fibroblast growth factor (242), phorbol esters (234,243–245), thrombin (246–248), very-low-density lipoprotein (VLDL) (249), Lp(a) (250), insulin (233) or proinsulin (251), glucose (252), unsaturated fatty acids (253), recombinant human erythropoietin (254), and angiotensin II (255,256). Angiotensin II–induced PAI-1 expression in cultured endothelial cells is mediated via angiotensin receptors (255,257). Captopril, an inhibitor of the angiotensin-converting enzyme, reduces PAI-1 expression in the vessel wall *in vivo* by blocking the receptor pathways (258). Studies on the mechanism of the induction of PAI-1 synthesis by phorbol esters suggested that it is mediated by two regulatory DNA sequences in the proximal promoter of the PAI-1 gene, which are called *Box A* (–65 to –50) and *Box B* (–82 to –65) (259). Recently, the DNA encoding a novel transcription factor that selectively interacts with Box B and that is also involved in basal expression was characterized. This factor presents conserved helicase and RING finger domains, and is called *helicase-like transcription factor* (260).

Several *cis*-responsive elements in the *PAI-1* promoter may be involved in the regulation of *PAI-1* gene transcription. The 5'-flanking region of the human *PAI-1* gene contains a major TGF-β–responsive element and a minor element upstream from the cap site, both of which are active in HepG2 cells (261). Two transcription factors, a CCAAT-binding transcription factor–nuclear factor 1 and an ubiquitous factor of the β-helix-loop-helix family bind to sequences in the major TGF-β–responsive element and are important for the TGF-β response (262). There are four putative AP-1–like binding sites that closely resemble the consensus phorbol myristate acetate (PMA)–responsive element, TGAgcTCA, in the 5'-flanking region of the human *PAI-1* gene: two proximal sites and two distal sites (259,263,264). Two proximal sites are required for PMA response (264), whereas the two distal sites are involved in the induction of PAI-1 by TGF-β (261). Binding of the c-Jun homodimer to a PMA-responsive element is important in basal activity and PMA induction of the *PAI-1* promoter in HeLa cells (259), HepG2 cells (265), and in some human breast carcinoma cells (264). p53, a tumor suppressor, transactivates the human *PAI-1* gene promoter by binding to a region that is highly similar to the p53 consensus binding sequence, whereas p53 represses transcription from the enhancer and promoter of the human *u-PA* and *t-PA* gene through a non-DNA binding mechanism (266).

In endothelial cells juxtaposed to thrombi, in SMCs adjacent to the neointima, and in macrophages, PAI-1 mRNA is increased and PAI-1 protein is detectable. This augmented arterial wall expression of PAI-1 induced by thrombosis may shift the local balance between fibrinolysis and thrombosis towards the latter (267).

Only a few studies have reported down-regulation of PAI-1 synthesis in endothelial cells, either by forskolin, by endothelial cell growth factor combined with heparin, or by gemfibrozil (a lipid-lowering drug) (243,268–270).

RELATION WITH THROMBOSIS

Several lines of evidence suggest that increased PAI-1 levels may promote fibrin deposition *in vivo*. When endotoxin-treated rabbits, with a markedly increased plasma PAI-1 level, are infused with the defibrinogenating snake venom ancrod, renal fibrin deposits are produced, whereas, in normal rabbits, ancrod infusion causes hypofibrinogenemia without fibrin deposition (271). In an experimental rabbit model of jugular vein thrombosis, inhibition of PAI-1 with the use of a monoclonal antibody resulted in promotion of endogenous thrombolysis and inhibition of thrombus extension (272). Mice, transgenic for the human PAI-1 gene, develop venous thrombosis at the tip of the tail within 3 days after birth but no arterial thrombosis (273). Furthermore, transgenic mice, which totally lack functional PAI-1, lyse experimental pulmonary emboli at a faster rate than controls (274). In humans, increased levels of PAI activity resulting in a decreased fibrinolytic capacity have been reported in several thrombotic disease states, including venous thromboembolism, obesity, sepsis, coronary artery disease, and acute myocardial infarction (275–279). It should be noticed that in some cases of familial thrombophilia associated with increased PAI-1 levels and decreased fibrinolytic activity, concomitant protein-S deficiency may be the main cause of thrombosis (280,281). In addition, resistance to activated protein C is a strong risk factor for venous thrombosis and may explain a significant portion of previously unexplained cases of thrombophilia (see Chapter 42) (282).

Evidence has been provided for transcriptional regulation of PAI-1 synthesis. Genetic variation at a polymorphic locus of the PAI-1 gene is associated with differences in plasma PAI-1 levels (283), and a single guanosine insertion/deletion (4G/5G) polymorphism in the PAI-1 promoter region may play an important role in the regulation of *PAI-1* gene expression (284). The 5G allele contains an additional binding site for a DNA-binding protein that may function as a transcriptional repressor (284). There is an association between the 4G/5G polymorphism and plasma PAI-1 activity, with the 4G allele, which occurs at a frequency of approximately 0.56 and higher PAI-1 levels in asymptomatic young adults; in young Swedish patients with myocardial infarction (283,284); in both myocardial infarction patients and healthy controls (French and Irish)

of the Etude Cas-Temoins sur l'Infarctus du Myocarde (ECTIM) study (285); and in an Italian population (286). The 4G allele of this polymorphism was claimed to be a risk factor for myocardial infarction (287), although this was not confirmed in the ECTIM study (285). Thus, the homozygous form of the 4G allele is associated with increased PAI-1 antigen levels, but the relation to thrombotic disease remains to be established. Four other polymorphisms were identified by single-strand conformational polymorphism analysis followed by sequencing. These polymorphisms were investigated in relation to PAI-1 levels in a sample of 256 healthy men, aged 50 to 59 years, from France and Northern Ireland. Two G/A substitutions were detected at positions –844 and +9785. The former is in strong positive linkage disequilibrium with the previously described 4G/5G polymorphism at position –675. Two polymorphisms in the 3' untranslated region were identified. One corresponds to a T/G substitution at position +11,053 and is in negative linkage disequilibrium with the G/A substitution (+9785). The other is a 9-nucleotide insertion-deletion located between nucleotides +11,320 and 11,345 in a threefold-repeated sequence. This polymorphism is in strong positive linkage disequilibrium with the G/A substitution (+9785). The overall heterozygosity provided by the five PAI-1 polymorphisms (including the four new variants and the 4G/5G polymorphism) was 0.77. No significant association was found between PAI-1 activity and genotypes; furthermore, the well-known associations between PAI activity and body mass index, serum triglycerides, or insulin were homogeneous according to PAI-1 genotypes (288). Possibly gene-environment interactions complicate this association, as suggested by different correlations of PAI-1 activity and triglyceride levels among the 4G/5G genotypes in patients with non-insulin–dependent diabetes mellitus (289,290), or in dyslipidemic patients (286).

The relative contribution of both metabolic factors involved in the insulin resistance (IR) syndrome and polymorphisms of the PAI-1 gene to plasma levels of PAI-1 was investigated in 228 healthy white families from the Stanislas Cohort. Variables related to IR included body mass index, waist to hip ratio, fasting insulin, triglyceride, and high-density lipoprotein cholesterol. Five PAI-1 gene polymorphisms were studied, including a newly described G+12,078A substitution in the 3' region. A sex difference was observed, with fathers exhibiting higher IR state and PAI-1 levels and stronger correlations between PAI-1 and IR variables than mothers. Such a difference was not observed in offspring. Family correlations were of similar magnitude for fibrinolytic parameters and IR variables. The PAI-1 genotypes, A-844G, –675 4G/5G, and G+12,078A polymorphisms, which were in strong linkage disequilibrium, were associated with plasma PAI-1 levels. In multivariate analysis, IR explained a major part of PAI-1 variability (49% in fathers, 29% in mothers), whereas polymorphisms had only a minor contribution, explaining 3% of variability in women and having no significant effect in men (291,292).

VLDLs induce transcription by the human PAI-1 promoter in endothelial cells. A VLDL responsive element is located at residues –672 to –657 in the promoter region, and its activity is influenced by the common 4G/5G polymorphism located adjacent to and upstream of the binding site of the VLDL-inducible transcription factor. These findings may provide a molecular explanation for the link between VLDL and enhanced plasma PAI-1 activity and for the interaction between the 4G/5G polymorphism and plasma levels of triglycerides (293).

Plasminogen Activator Inhibitor-1 and Venous Thrombosis.
Defective fibrinolysis in patients with venous thrombosis may be due to a low concentration of t-PA or to an increased level of PAI-1 (277). In 35% of patients with spontaneous or recurrent

deep vein thrombosis, a poor fibrinolytic response to venous occlusion was observed, which was due to deficient t-PA release in 25% and increased PAI-1 levels in 75% of these cases (278). In six studies with healthy subjects as controls, an impaired fibrinolytic capacity after venous occlusion was observed in patients with thrombotic episodes (294), whereas, in one study with a control group of patients with clinically suspected venous thrombosis, no differences in t-PA or PAI-1 levels between controls and cases were observed before or after 1-desamino-8-D-arginine vasopressin administration (295). Grimaudo et al. (296) reported increased PAI-1 levels in patients with a history of idiopathic deep vein thrombosis and/or pulmonary embolism as compared to healthy controls, but this difference was no longer evident after adjustment for body mass index. In the Physician's Health Study (297), PAI-1 levels in patients who developed venous thrombosis during a 5-year follow-up were not different from controls. The association between enhanced PAI-1 levels and symptomatic venous thrombosis is not consistent and requires further study.

Plasminogen Activator Inhibitor-1 and Atherothrombosis.
High plasma PAI-1 levels in patients with acute myocardial infarction or unstable angina were found to be predictive for recurrent (within 3 years) myocardial infarction in some studies (298,299) but not in others (300,301). In a prospective study in patients with angina pectoris, high basal levels of t-PA antigen but not PAI activity were associated with an increased risk of myocardial infarction (302,303). In the Physician's Health Study (304), increased t-PA antigen levels were predictive for myocardial infarction within the 5-year follow-up period, but this association disappeared after adjustment for body mass index, high-density lipoprotein cholesterol, and blood pressure. In the ARIC (Atherosclerosis Risk in Communities) study (305), high baseline PAI-1 levels were correlated with vessel wall thickness, suggesting a relationship between PAI-1 levels and the severity of vessel wall damage. Local high concentrations of PAI-1 have also been observed in coronary arteries with atherogenic lesions and may contribute to the development of vessel wall damage (306–308). However, enhanced local expression of plasminogen activators was observed within the atherosclerotic plaque, which may contribute to destabilization and rupture of the plaque (309,310).

In the prospective ECAT (European Concerted Action on Thrombosis) study, ten fibrinolytic variables were measured in 3043 patients with angina pectoris recruited from 18 European centers (311,312). A first analysis after adjustment for other nonfibrinolytic coronary risk factors (body mass index, triglyceride levels, diabetes, systolic blood pressure), revealed that an increased risk of coronary events within 2 years was associated with higher baseline concentrations of t-PA antigen but not of PAI-1 activity and antigen levels. However, several studies, including the ECAT study, have reported strong correlations between t-PA and PAI-1 antigen levels, in healthy populations as well as in patients with coronary heart disease (313,314). Therefore, it was surprising that in the ECAT study only t-PA antigen and not PAI-1 was identified as a predictive risk factor for coronary heart disease. The prognostic value of the fibrinolytic variables determined in the ECAT study was recently re-examined after separate adjustment for clusters of markers of IR, inflammation, or endothelial cell damage (315). These adjustments affected the prognostic value of PAI-1 and t-PA levels differently. Factors involved in the IR syndrome strongly affected PAI-1 and, to a lesser extent, t-PA antigen. The latter was primarily influenced by inflammation and endothelial cell damage. Thus, t-PA antigen levels may constitute a biologic marker of coronary heart disease, influenced by a variety of pathophysiologic pathways, including inflammation. In contrast, PAI levels that determine fibrinolytic activity and that are mainly dependent on the metabolic status emerge as risk factors predictive for the future development of atherothrombosis.

Plasminogen Activator Inhibitor-1 and Insulin Resistance.
Increased levels of PAI-1 were observed in the IR syndrome, and a significant correlation was found between plasma PAI-1 levels and body mass index, triglyceride levels, insulin levels, and systolic blood pressure (316). Modulation of IR with diet, exercise, or oral antidiabetic drugs, such as methformin, results in a decrease in plasma PAI-1 and has a beneficial effect on IR. In patients with IR syndrome, interventions aimed at improving the lipid profile also enhanced fibrinolytic activity. Thus, treatment with gemfibrozil reduces the risk for coronary events (317); it induces an improvement of the lipid profile, associated with enhanced fibrinolytic activity as a result of reduced PAI-1 levels (318,319). Increased insulin sensitivity as a result of dietary interventions in obese women is associated with an improvement of the lipid profile (lower total cholesterol and triglyceride levels) and enhanced fibrinolytic activity due to reduced PAI-1 activity (320).

The mechanisms by which enhanced PAI-1 levels are linked with the IR syndrome are not well understood. *In vitro* data indicate that PAI-1 synthesis by endothelial cells and hepatocytes could be affected by insulin, proinsulin, and atherogenic lipoproteins (308,321–323). Production of PAI-1 by murine adipocytes was observed and was enhanced in response to cytokines or TGF-β, which may explain the high PAI-1 levels in insulin-resistant obese patients (324–327). In humans, a significant correlation was observed between the visceral fat area and plasma PAI-1 levels (328,329). PAI-1 secretion from adipose tissue was more pronounced with visceral fat (330) and also related to cell lipid content and volume of fat cells (331). Furthermore, PAI-1 expression in human adipose tissue is controlled by insulin and glucocorticoids that may contribute to enhanced PAI-1 levels in patients with android obesity (332). Studies in obese mice confirmed that elevated PAI-1 levels associated with obesity result in part from insulin induction of PAI-1, specifically by adipocytes within the fat itself (333). Studies on the role of PAI-1 in the relation between the adipocyte and the hemostatic balance in obesity were recently reviewed (292,326,334).

Plasminogen Deficiency and Thrombosis

CONGENITAL PLASMINOGEN DEFICIENCY
The plasma concentration of plasminogen antigen in full-term newborns is approximately one-half that of adults, whereas the functional activity is comparable or lower than expected on the basis of antigen concentration.

Plasminogen deficiency as a cause of thrombosis, characterized by a parallel decrease of functional and immunoreactive plasminogen, was reported in only a few cases [see Lijnen and Collen (6)]. Hasegawa and others (335) report three unrelated families with inherited low levels of plasminogen and recurrent pulmonary embolism and deep venous thrombosis. Ten Cate and associates (336) report isolated plasminogen deficiency in a woman with recurrent thrombophlebitis and pulmonary embolism, characterized by a reduction of plasminogen antigen and activity to 45%. Lottenberg and colleagues (337) identified a patient with pulmonary hypertension, a history of venous thrombosis, and severe plasminogen deficiency (30% of normal antigen and activity). All functional properties of the isolated plasminogen were normal, and no evidence for increased plasminogen activation or increased turnover was found. The authors concluded that this patient had a deficiency of normally functioning plasminogen, probably due to decreased synthesis.

This abnormality was also found in two siblings and family members, but inheritance of the deficiency could not be established. Mannucci and others (338) reported a case of a young man having a history of venous thrombotic disease with a reduction of both antigenic and functional plasminogen to 50% of normal. This deficiency was inherited as an autosomal trait, and the propositus and his sister were heterozygotes. Administration of the anabolic steroid stanozolol transiently normalized the plasminogen level. A case of heterozygous plasminogen deficiency (50% of normal antigen and activity) was also observed in a mother (55 years) and daughter (10 years) and was found to be inherited autosomally (339). The mother showed a lifelong thrombotic tendency.

In all these cases, other investigated hemostatic parameters were normal; thus, they apparently represent true isolated plasminogen deficiencies (activity and antigen level between 30% and 50% of normal) that are associated with severe thromboembolic complications.

Homozygous plasminogen deficiency has recently been described in patients with ligneous conjunctivitis, a rare and unusual form of chronic pseudomembranous conjunctivitis caused by massive fibrin deposition within the extravascular space of mucous membrane (340). In several patients, a homozygous point mutation was identified as a probable cause of the deficiency (341,342). Replacement therapy with Lys-plasminogen was shown to be successful (342). The finding that plasminogen-deficient mice also develop ligneous conjunctivitis supports a causal role of plasminogen in the disease (343).

Two independent studies have shown that disruption of the plasminogen gene in mice causes a severe thrombotic phenotype but is compatible with relative normal fetal development and subsequent reproduction (344,345). Plasminogen deficiency, indeed, did not appear to compromise embryonic development and viability of the mice and did not drastically affect male fertility. This is surprising, in view of the presumed role of the plasminogen system in spermatocyte migration and fertilization. Homozygous plasminogen-deficient mice display a greatly reduced spontaneous lysis of pulmonary plasma clots, and young animals develop multiple spontaneous thrombotic lesions in liver, stomach, colon, rectum, lung pancreas, and other tissues (344,345). Restoration of normal plasminogen levels in these mice by bolus administration of plasminogen resulted in normalization of the thrombolytic potential toward experimentally induced pulmonary emboli and in removal of endogenous fibrin deposits in the liver (346), thus establishing conclusively that *in vivo* fibrin dissolution is critically dependent on the plasminogen-plasmin system. Interestingly, delayed but not absent clot lysis (later than 24 hours) was observed in plasminogen-deficient mice (344), as well as in mice with combined deficiency of t-PA and u-PA (347). Lysis may be mediated by plasminogen-independent proteinases such as leucocyte-derived cathepsins or elastase or the Mac glycoprotein-dependent fibrin clearance pathway. An increased incidence of gastric ulcerations in plasminogen-deficient mice suggests that the plasminogen system plays a role in the prevention and/or healing of damaged tissue (344,345).

A surprising finding, considering the well-established linkage between plasmin and the proteolytic activation of plasminogen activators, is that the level of active u-PA in urine remains unaffected. Therefore, plasminogen appears to play a pivotal role in fibrinolysis and hemostasis but not to be essential for activation of scu-PA, development, or growth to sexual maturity (345). Removal of fibrin(ogen) from the extracellular environment (mice with combined deficiency of plasminogen and fibrinogen) alleviates the diverse spontaneous pathologies associated with plasminogen deficiency (348).

ACQUIRED PLASMINOGEN DEFICIENCY

Reduced levels of plasminogen have been observed in several clinical conditions, including liver disease (349) and sepsis (25% to 45% of normal activity) (350). Possible mechanisms for acquired plasminogen deficiency in severe liver disease are depressed synthesis and/or increased consumption. Degradation of plasminogen into LMW plasminogen by leukocyte elastase is a possible explanation for the reduction observed in septic patients. In the plasma of some septic patients, a LMW plasminogen-like molecule has indeed been identified (350). Human plasma contains at least two proteins—α_2-antiplasmin and His-rich glycoprotein (HRG)—that bind to the Lys-binding sites of plasminogen and thereby counteract plasminogen binding to fibrin. For the interaction of α_2-antiplasmin (137) or HRG (161) with plasminogen, dissociation constants of 4 or 1 μmol/L, respectively, were determined in purified systems. In the absence of other interactions in plasma, 50% of the plasminogen would be expected to circulate reversibly bound to HRG and 15% to circulate reversibly bound to α_2-antiplasmin. Jespersen and colleagues (351) found consistently higher concentrations of HRG in 34 patients with acute myocardial infarction associated with deep venous thrombosis. In a more extensive study, however, no significant change in the plasma level of HRG was found in a group of 40 patients with arterial thrombosis or in 152 patients with venous thrombosis (352). Increased HRG levels, apparently associated with thrombosis, were observed only in a few families.

DYSPLASMINOGENEMIA

Abnormalities in the plasminogen molecule, resulting in defective activation to plasmin, have been described by several authors (6). In 1978, Aoki and coworkers (353) identified a patient with recurrent thrombosis over a 15-year period who had abnormally low plasminogen activity (approximately 50% of normal) but a normal level of plasminogen antigen. This antigen was a mixture of normal and abnormal molecules in approximately equal amounts. Studies of the patient's family members suggest that the molecular abnormality was inherited in an autosomal-dominant pattern. One of the family members was a homozygote having virtually no plasminogen activity but normal antigen level. Functional analysis of this plasminogen [Tochigi (354)] revealed that (a) it forms a complex with streptokinase, but this complex does not incorporate the active-site titrant diisopropyl fluorophosphate; (b) it is converted to an inactive two-chain plasmin molecule by urokinase; and (c) the Lys-binding sites are functionally intact. An additional characteristic is the gel electrofocusing pattern of the purified plasminogen from the heterozygotes, which consists of ten normal bands and ten abnormal bands, each having a slightly higher pI than the respective corresponding normal component. The gel electrofocusing pattern of the homozygote plasminogen consists of abnormal bands only. Miyata and associates (355) demonstrated that the absence of proteolytic activity in plasminogen Tochigi is due to a single amino acid substitution (Ala601 to Thr) near the His603 residue of the active site. The genetic change responsible for this substitution is a G to A transition in the first nucleotide (5' terminal) of the Ala601 codon. This Ala to Thr substitution in the plasmin light chain may affect the side chain of the Asp646 or His603 active-site residues and thereby disturb the active-site charge relay system, leading to loss of enzymatic activity.

In this and several other cases, the propositus suffered from thrombotic complications, whereas other family members with the same plasminogen abnormality usually had not presented with clinical symptoms of thrombosis.

Wohl and coworkers characterized three human plasminogen variants (Chicago I, II, and III) identified in young males

**TABLE 40-2. Characterization of Dysplasminogenemia
(See References 6–8)**

Molecular Defect	Antigen Level	Functional Level (% Normal)	Thrombosis Propositus	Thrombosis Relatives
Active site Ala600–Thr substitution	Normal	40	Yes	No
Lower affinity for activators	Normal	40	Yes	?
Lower affinity for activators + impaired cleavage of Arg561-Val562	Normal	80	Yes	?

Ala, alanine; Arg, arginine; Thr, threonine; Val, valine.

with a history of recurring deep venous thrombosis (356,357). No clear inheritance pattern was observed. Homozygote plasminogens Chicago I and II have an activation defect characterized by a high K_m and impaired plasminogen activator binding, but normal cleavage of the Arg561-Val562 peptide bond. The homozygote plasminogen Chicago III has impaired affinity for plasminogen activators and impaired cleavage of the Arg561-Val562 peptide bond.

Characteristic of all these dysplasminogenemias is a low ratio of functional to immunoreactive plasminogen, ranging from 0.2 (plasminogen Tokyo) to 0.88 (plasminogen Chicago II) (Table 40-2).

Plasminogen Activator Deficiency and Thrombosis

RELEASE AND INHIBITION OF UROKINASE-TYPE PLASMINOGEN ACTIVATOR

Whereas t-PA synthesis occurs mainly in endothelial cells, immunocytochemical staining of tissues with antibodies directed against u-PA reveals that many different cells produce u-PA (358).

Many cells contain a receptor that is specific for scu-PA and for high-molecular-weight tcu-PA, but does not bind LMW tcu-PA. The amino acid sequence spanning residues 18 to 30 in the growth factor domain of human u-PA is probably involved in binding to this receptor. The dissociation constant of the interaction of u-PA with its receptor is 10^{-9} to 10^{-10} mol/L; approximately 50,000 binding sites are present in the monocyte-like U-937 cell. Membrane-bound u-PA retains its plasminogen-activating potential and is protected, to some extent, from extracellular inhibitors. The presence of u-PA receptors on many normal and malignant cells may constitute a mechanism to remodel the extracellular matrix. PMA treatment of U-937 cells induces an increase in synthesis and a decrease in affinity of the u-PA receptor, which results in increased u-PA binding to other substrates. This effect of PMA may be mediated by protein kinase C (359).

tcu-PA is slowly inhibited in human plasma by several protease inhibitors including α_2-macroglobulin, α_1-antitrypsin, antithrombin III, α_2-antiplasmin, and plasminogen activator inhibitor-3 (PAI-3), which is identical to the inhibitor of activated protein C. More specific and rapid inhibition occurs by PAI-1 and PAI-2. Urokinase inhibitor assays based on clot lysis depend strongly on the presence of plasmin inhibitors and therefore are not specific. Assayed with such clot lysis methods, the half-life of tcu-PA was 9 to 16 minutes *in vivo* but 27 to 61

minutes *in vitro* (360); this suggests that clearing of the enzyme from the blood is important.

RELEASE AND INHIBITION OF TISSUE-TYPE PLASMINOGEN ACTIVATOR

Vascular endothelial cells synthesize and secrete t-PA into the circulating blood. Stimulation of vascular endothelium by venous occlusion, infusion of 1-desamino-8-D-arginine vasopressin or epinephrine, and physical exercise results in a rapid release (within minutes) of t-PA (361). This response is too rapid to represent increased synthesis and may reflect release from cellular storage pools, although these have not been conclusively defined. Agents, such as thrombin, that stimulate the release of t-PA from endothelial cells, also stimulate the secretion of PAI-1 (246,247). Dexamethasone increases t-PA antigen levels in hepatoma cells moderately (1.5-fold) but increases PAI-1 antigen levels to a greater extent (four- to fivefold), resulting in inhibition of t-PA activity (362).

A variety of agents increase the synthesis of t-PA by cultured endothelial cells. These include thrombin (246,247), histamine (247), butyrate (363), PMA (364), basic fibroblast growth factor (365), activated protein C (366), butanol and alcohol derivatives (367), and retinoids (368). However, only histamine, butyrate, or a combination of cAMP with protein kinase C agonists selectively stimulates t-PA synthesis without affecting PAI-1 synthesis.

The mechanisms by which these agents increase t-PA synthesis are different and are now being gradually elucidated. Recently, a functional retinoic acid (RA) response element, which consists of a direct repeat of the GGTCA motif spaced by 5 nucleotides (DR5), has been localized 7.3 kb upstream of the transcription start site of the human *t-PA* gene. This element mediates the direct regulation by RA in human fibrosarcoma, endothelial, and neuroblastoma cells (369). This t-PA/DR5–RA response element is part of a multihormone responsive enhancer covering an upstream fragment, which contains a complex glucocorticoid responsive unit composed of four binding sites for the receptor (370). Induction of t-PA synthesis by RA in human umbilical vein endothelial cells involves a two-step mechanism, requiring induction of RA receptor β_2 via RA receptor α_1, followed by induction of t-PA synthesis via RA receptor β_2 (371). Vasoactive substances, such as histamine and thrombin, bind to specific receptors and activate phospholipase C, which acts on phosphatidylinositol bisphosphate to produce diacylglycerol. Diacylglycerol activates membrane-bound protein kinase C, which plays an important role in the regulation of t-PA synthesis. This is suggested by the findings that direct activation of protein kinase C by phorbol esters induces t-PA synthesis, whereas suppression of protein kinase C impairs the increase in t-PA synthesis by histamine and PMA (372). The increase in t-PA induced by histamine, thrombin, and PMA in endothelial cells is paralleled by increased levels of mRNA, as a result of enhanced transcription of the t-PA gene (373). Very little is known, however, about the regulation of human *t-PA* gene transcription. Two *cis* elements (a cAMP responsive element in the proximal promoter and an activator protein-2 binding site in exon 1) have been identified, which are involved in basal expression and induction of human *t-PA* gene transcription by cAMP and phorbol esters (53). *In vivo* footprinting analysis revealed that specificity protein 1 (*Sp1*) binds the t-PA promoter at two proximal sites, one of which overlaps with the activator protein-2 site in exon 1 (374). Interestingly, plasmin inhibits the biosynthesis of t-PA antigen by human umbilical vein endothelial cells in a dose-dependent manner, possibly through the signal transduction pathway involving one or more protein kinases (375).

The mechanisms involved in removal of t-PA from the blood are multiple. A main one is clearance by the liver, which results in a half-life of a few minutes in animals and humans. t-PA occurs in plasma in a free active form and in complexes with α_2-antiplasmin, α_1-antitrypsin, and C_1-inhibitor. Its main rapid-reacting inhibitor is PAI-1, which is present in normal human plasma at a low concentration or at a higher concentration in many clinical conditions, including thromboembolic disease.

Cellular receptors may not only be important for the localization of proteolytic activity at the cell surface, but may also play a role in the rapid clearance of t-PA from the circulation. Circulating t-PA (half-life of 5 to 6 minutes in humans) may interact with several receptor systems in the liver. Liver endothelial cells possess a mannose receptor that recognizes the high mannose-type carbohydrate on K_1. Liver parenchymal cells contain a calcium-dependent receptor that interacts with F- and/or E-domains of t-PA (376). Parenchymal cells also contain a high affinity receptor for the uptake and degradation of t-PA–PAI-1 complexes, which also binds free t-PA albeit with lower affinity; this receptor, termed *low-density lipoprotein receptor-related protein* is identical to the α_2-macroglobulin receptor (377). The lipoprotein receptor-related protein-binding site on PAI-1 is exposed only when in complex with a proteinase and is located within the previously identified heparin-binding domain (378).

PATHOPHYSIOLOGY OF IMPAIRED FIBRINOLYTIC ACTIVITY

Impairment of fibrinolysis due to deficient synthesis and/or release of t-PA from the vessel wall may be associated with a tendency to thrombosis. Defective release of t-PA from the vessel wall during venous occlusion and/or a decreased t-PA content in walls of superficial veins is found in approximately 70% of patients with idiopathic recurrent venous thrombosis (379). As discussed earlier, a deficient fibrinolytic response may be caused by a deficient release of t-PA from the vessel wall, but also by an increased rate of neutralization (277,278).

To date, genetic deficiencies of t-PA or u-PA have not been reported in humans. Thus, inactivation of the t-PA or u-PA genes in mice might have been anticipated to result in a lethal phenotype. However, single- and double-deficient mice are normal at birth, suggesting that neither t-PA nor u-PA, individually or in combination, is required for normal embryonic development. Double-deficient mice are able to reproduce but are significantly less fertile than wild-type mice or mice with a single deficiency of t-PA or u-PA; this may be due to the poor general health of these animals or to the presence of large fibrin deposits in their gonads. These findings suggest that proteinases other than t-PA and u-PA may be more essential in reproduction and embryonic development than previously suspected (347). Furthermore, data obtained in these gene-deficient mice suggest a divergent and specific role of t-PA and u-PA in fibrinolysis and macrophage function. The role of plasminogen activators in clearing fibrin deposits is supported by the observation that t-PA–deficient and t-PA:u-PA–deficient mice have virtually no endogenous spontaneous thrombolytic potential, and u-PA–deficient and t-PA:u-PA–deficient mice suffer occasional or extensive spontaneous fibrin deposition, respectively. Interestingly, mice with a combined deficiency of t-PA and u-PAR do not display excessive fibrin deposits, suggesting that sufficient plasmin proteolysis can occur in the absence of u-PA binding to u-PAR (5). The observed increased occurrence of venous thrombosis after endotoxin injection and the abnormal fibrin deposition in liver, skin, and intestine in u-PA– and t-PA:u-PA–deficient mice may be explained by impaired fibrin dissolution by u-PA–deficient macrophages. The almost total lack of endogenous lysis of a iodine-125–fibrin labeled plasma clot, the more severe thrombotic phenotype, and the more severely retarded growth and reduced fertility and survival in the double-deficient mice further support the notion that u-PA and t-PA cooperate in a variety of biologic phenomena, possibly related to fibrin degradation, matrix remodeling, and/or growth factor activation (347).

Excess Tissue-Type Plasminogen Activator Levels and Bleeding

Excessive fibrinolysis due to increased t-PA activity levels may be associated with a bleeding tendency. A lifelong hemorrhagic disorder associated with enhanced fibrinolysis due to increased levels of circulating plasminogen activator has been described in only a few patients (380,381).

Alternatively, excessive fibrinolysis due to decreased PAI-1 levels has been reported in a few cases and was apparently associated with bleeding complications (382,383). A complete deficiency of PAI-1 has been reported in a 9-year-old girl who had several episodes of major hemorrhage, all in response to trauma or surgery (384). DNA sequence analysis revealed a 2-bp insertion at the 3' end of exon 4. This mutation results in a shift in the reading frame after the codon for amino acid 210, resulting in a new stop codon. The predicted protein thus lacks the 169 COOH-terminal amino acid region of mature PAI-1, which includes the Arg346-Met347 reactive-site peptide bond.

Recently, the effect of PAI-1 gene disruption on organ development and reproduction, hemostasis, thrombosis, and thrombolysis has been investigated in mice. Surprisingly, PAI-1–deficient mice are viable and fertile and have no significant organ abnormalities, demonstrating that reproduction and development can proceed normally in the absence of PAI-1. Possibly, other proteinase inhibitors, which are able to reduce plasminogen activation and/or plasmin activity, might compensate for PAI-1 deficiency, or PAI-1 deficiency in mice may induce only a mild hyperfibrinolytic state (274). Lysis of a pulmonary plasma clot was significantly faster in homozygous PAI-1–deficient mice when compared to wild-type mice, consistent with an inhibitory role of PAI-1 on plasminogen activation *in vivo*. Homozygous PAI-1–deficient mice developed significantly less frequently venous thrombi than wild-type mice after local injection of endotoxin in the footpad, although a similar extent of inflammation was observed. Thus, these findings support a causal role for PAI-1 in the development of venous thrombosis. Spontaneous bleeding or delayed rebleeding was not observed after partial amputation of the tail or of the cecum in PAI-1–deficient mice. This is in contrast with the delayed rebleeding observed after trauma or surgery in patients with reduced or absent PAI-1 levels. This difference in phenotype between mice and humans may be due to the approximately fivefold lower basal plasma levels of active PAI-1 in wild-type mice than in humans, but species-dependent differences in the plasma levels of t-PA and possibly of other components of the fibrinolytic system might also contribute to this phenotypic dissimilarity.

PATHOPHYSIOLOGIC RELEVANCE OF INTERACTIONS BETWEEN THE FIBRINOLYTIC AND MATRIX METALLOPROTEINASE SYSTEM

Several interactions between the plasminogen-plasmin and MMP systems suggest that both systems may cooperate in extracellular matrix degradation (10). The degradation of matrix is a requirement for cell migration and tissue remodeling and may play an essential role in many (patho)physiologic processes.

MMPs constitute a tightly regulated family of enzymes that degrade most components of the extracellular matrix. They are classified on the basis of substrate specificity. Collagenases (MMP-1, interstitial collagenase; MMP-8, neutrophil collagenase; MMP-13, collagenase-3) degrade connective tissue collagens; gelatinases (MMP-2, gelatinase A; MMP-9, gelatinase B) degrade collagen types IV, V, VII, and X; elastin; and denatured collagens; stromelysins (MMP-3, stromelysin-1; MMP-10, stromelysin-2) and matrilysin (MMP-7) degrade the proteoglycan core proteins, laminin, fibronectin, elastin, gelatin, and nonhelical collagen, whereas stromelysin-3 (MMP-11) does not degrade any of the major extracellular matrix components; macrophage metalloelastase (MMP-12) degrades insoluble elastin, collagen IV, fibronectin, laminin, entactin, and proteoglycans. More than 20 members of the MMP family have been identified, among which at least four are membrane-type MMPs.

MMPs are generally secreted as zymogens that are extracellularly activated by organomercurial compounds, several proteinases (including plasmin, trypsin, chymotrypsin, kallikrein, cathepsin G, or neutrophil elastase), oxygen radicals, or association with the cell surface. Active MMPs are inhibited by specific tissue inhibitors (TIMPs) via formation of a noncovalent stoichiometric complex. Four members of the TIMP family have been identified, of which TIMP-1, synthesized by most types of connective tissue cells as well as by macrophages, acts against all members of the collagenase, stromelysin, and gelatinase classes (see reference 11).

Restenosis

Vascular interventions for the treatment of atherothrombosis induce restenosis of the vessel within 3 to 6 months in 30% to 50% of treated patients. Arterial stenosis may result from remodeling of the vessel wall and/or from accumulation of cells and extracellular matrix in the intimal layer. Proteinases from the plasminogen-plasmin and the metalloproteinase system participate in the proliferation and migration of SMC and in matrix remodeling during arterial wound healing (385,386). Of the MMPs, only MMP-2 is expressed in quiescent SMC, whereas expression of MMP-3, MMP-7, MMP-9, MMP-12, and MMP-13 is induced in injured, transplanted, or atherosclerotic arteries (387–393). In a balloon-injured rat carotid artery model, a correlation was observed between changes in plasminogen activators (394–396) or MMPs (397,398) and SMC migration. Increased levels of PAI-1 and TIMP-2 in this model suggested that changes in the proteolytic balance play a role in SMC migration after arterial injury (399). This is supported by the findings that *in vivo* SMC migration in the rat was inhibited by administration of the plasmin inhibitor tranexamic acid (399) or of MMP inhibitors (397,400) and by overexpression of TIMP-1 (401). Adenovirus-mediated gene transfer of the human TIMP-1 gene inhibits SMC migration and neointimal formation in the human saphenous vein (402). Furthermore, SCM migration in baboon aortic explants requires plasminogen activators, MMP-2, MMP-9, basic fibroblast growth factor, and platelet-derived growth factor (403,404). Platelet-derived growth factor–induced migration of SMC was found to depend on MMP-2, whereas basic fibroblast growth factor–induced migration depended on both MMP-2 and MMP-9 (403). Studies in balloon-injured rabbit carotid arteries suggested that MMP-2 facilitates migration of SMC from the media to the intima and does not affect replication (405).

To assess the role of the plasminogen-plasmin system in neointima formation, a perivascular electric injury model was applied to mice with targeted inactivation of the main components of the system (406). These studies revealed that the degree and the rate of arterial neointima formation up to 6 weeks after injury was sig-

nificantly reduced in u-PA–deficient and plasminogen-deficient mice, as compared to wild-type and t-PA–deficient mice (406–408). Impaired migration of SMCs and leukocytes from the uninjured border into the central injured region in u-PA and in plasminogen-deficient mice was a significant cause of reduced neointima formation in these genotypes. These data substantiate a physiologic role for u-PA–mediated plasmin proteolysis in SMC migration and neointima formation. Additional studies indicate that the temporal and topographic expression pattern of MMPs (MMP-2, MMP-3, MMP-9, MMP-12, and MMP-13) after vascular injury is compatible with a role in extracellular matrix degradation and SMC migration. The consistently lower MMP expression in u-PA–deficient mice as compared to wild-type mice may contribute to reduced vascular remodeling (409).

Arterial neointima formation after vascular injury was also studied in mice with deficiency of TIMP-1 (410). At 1 to 3 weeks after injury, the intimal areas were significantly larger in TIMP-1–deficient mice as compared to wild-type mice, whereas the medial areas were comparable, resulting in significantly higher intima-media ratios in the TIMP-1–deficient mice. These data thus confirm a physiologic role of TIMP-1 in vascular remodeling, most likely via monitoring of MMP activity.

Atherosclerosis

A potential role for increased proteolysis by plasmin or MMPs in atherosclerosis is suggested by the enhanced expression of t-PA, u-PA, and several MMPs in plaques (387,392,411,412). Proteolysis might indeed participate in neovascularization and rupture of plaques or in ulceration and rupture of aneurysms. A causative role of the fibrinolytic and/or MMP system in these processes has, however, not been conclusively demonstrated. Therefore, atherosclerosis was studied in mice deficient in apolipoprotein E (apoE) (413) singly or combined deficient in t-PA or u-PA (414). No differences in the size or the predilection site of early fatty streaks and more advanced plaques were observed between mice with a single deficiency of apoE or with a combined deficiency of apoE and t-PA or of apoE and u-PA, suggesting that plasmin is not essential for subendothelial infiltration by macrophages. However, destruction of the media with resultant erosion, transmedial ulceration, necrosis of medial SMC, aneurysmal dilatation, and rupture of the vessel wall were more frequent and severe in mice lacking apoE or apoE and t-PA than in mice lacking apoE and u-PA (414). Elastin fibers were eroded, fragmented, and completely degraded, whereas collagen bundles and glycoprotein-rich matrix were disorganized and scattered in apoE-deficient and in apoE:t-PA–deficient mice but not in apo-E:u-PA–deficient mice, which were virtually completely protected. A dramatic increase of free u-PA activity was generated by infiltrating plaque macrophages in the apoE and apoE:t-PA–deficient mice. Because plasmin by itself is unable to degrade insoluble elastin or fibrillar collagen, it most likely activated MMPs. Macrophages in murine atherosclerotic plaques indeed abundantly expressed MMP-3, MMP-9, MMP-12, and MMP-13 (414). In addition, wild-type and t-PA–deficient but not u-PA–deficient cultured macrophages activated secreted proMMP-3, proMMP-9, proMMP-12, and proMMP-13 but only in the presence of plasminogen, indicating that u-PA–generated plasmin was responsible for the activation. These MMPs co-localized with u-PA in plaque macrophages, suggesting that plasmin is a likely activator of these pro-MMPs *in vivo*. Studies in plasminogen-deficient mice indicated that plasmin proteolysis plays a major role in allograft arteriosclerosis by mediating elastin degradation, macrophage infiltration, media remodeling, medial SMC migration, and neointima formation. In this model, expression of u-PA, t-PA, MMP-3, MMP-9, MMP-12, and MMP-13 were significantly increased within 2 weeks of transplantation, when cells actively migrate (393). Recently, it was shown that overexpression of TIMP-1 reduced atherosclerotic lesions in apoE-deficient mice (415) and prevented aortic aneurysm degeneration and rupture in a rat model (416), thus further substantiating a functional role of MMPs.

Taken together, these data implicate u-PA in maintaining the structural integrity of the atherosclerotic vessel wall, likely via triggering activation of MMPs, and suggest that increased u-PA levels are a risk factor for aneurysm formation and progression.

PROSPECTIVE EPIDEMIOLOGIC STUDY WITH MYOCARDICAL INFARCTION

The early tests to measure overall plasma fibrinolytic activity, such as euglobulin lysis time and the fibrin plate method using euglobulin fractions, were insensitive and aspecific. More recently, specific and quantitative assays have become available to measure antigen and activity levels of most components of the fibrinolytic system, including t-PA, PAI-1, plasminogen, α_2-antiplasmin, and TAFI. Application of such assays is, however, complicated by the requirement to collect blood samples under well-defined standard conditions and by the known diurnal variation of, for example, PAI-1 and t-PA levels. Although many studies (as discussed earlier) have reported a correlation between hypofibrinolysis as a result of increased PAI-1 or decreased t-PA levels and thrombotic events, it is still not established whether hypofibrinolysis is cause or consequence. For patients with venous thrombosis, recent studies seem to suggest that fibrinolytic assays are not useful, as they have no predictive value and no influence on application of anticoagulant therapy (417–420). Studies in patients with coronary heart disease have suggested that t-PA antigen levels may represent a biologic marker, which is, however, influenced by many pathophysiologic processes, including inflammation. PAI-1 levels appeared mainly dependent on the metabolic status and emerged as a risk factor predictive for development of atherothrombosis (311–316,421).

The paradoxic association between cardiovascular risk and increased levels of the profibrinolytic enzyme t-PA may be the result of assay methods that do not discriminate between free active t-PA and t-PA complexed by PAI-1. However, Wiman et al. (422) recently observed a strong correlation between t-PA–PAI-1 complexes and both PAI-1 activity and t-PA antigen [Stockholm Heart Epidemiology Program (SHEEP study)]. Patients with t-PA–PAI-1 complex (or von Willebrand factor) higher than the seventy-fifth percentile of the controls had a reinfarction risk that was increased by 80% (or 130%) (422). These findings are in line with the study, in which more than 10,000 male participants provided epidemiologic evidence for a role of fibrinogen and PAI-1 in the pathogenesis of coronary heart disease (423). The true clinical impact of these findings remains uncertain, because it is not proved that more intensive or different secondary prophylaxis would result in fewer reinfarctions in this subpopulation (424). It, thus, remains to be shown to what extent measurement of these fibrinolytic parameters may be useful to identify patients at elevated cardiovascular risk and whether this may have therapeutic consequences (424).

Several studies have shown that determinations of D-dimer and of fibrin monomer—markers of ongoing fibrinolysis—can be used for the exclusion of pulmonary embolism in symptomatic outpatients (425,426).

Taken together, it appears that at present these fibrinolytic assays are of limited value to the clinician in treating individual patients. Epidemiologic data will, however, contribute to understanding of the etiology of thromboembolic disease. Alternatively, prothrombotic abnormalities such as factor V Leiden or enhanced

TAFI levels may represent an enhanced risk of venous thrombosis. The clinical value of these assays also remains to be studied in more detail.

REFERENCES

1. Collen D, Lijnen HR. Basic and clinical aspects of fibrinolysis and thrombolysis. *Blood* 1991;78:3114.
2. Blasi F. Urokinase and urokinase receptor: a paracrine/autocrine system regulating cell migration and invasiveness. *Bioessays* 1993;15:105.
3. Bachmann F. The plasminogen-plasmin enzyme system. In: Colman RW, Hirsch J, Marder VJ, Salzman EW, eds. *Hemostasis and thrombosis: basic principles and clinical practice*, 3rd ed. Philadelphia: J.B. Lippincott, 1993:1592.
4. Carmeliet P, Collen D. Gene manipulation and transfer of the plasminogen and coagulation system in mice. *Semin Thromb Hemost* 1996;22:525.
5. Bugge TH, Flick MJ, Danton MJS, et al. Urokinase-type plasminogen activator is effective in fibrin clearance in the absence of its receptor or tissue-type plasminogen activator. *Proc Natl Acad Sci U S A* 1996;93:5899.
6. Lijnen HR, Collen D. Congenital and acquired deficiencies of components of the fibrinolytic system and their relation to bleeding or thrombosis. *Fibrinolysis* 1989;3:67.
7. Wiman B, Hamsten A. The fibrinolytic enzyme system and its role in the etiology of thromboembolic disease. *Semin Thromb Hemost* 1990;16:207.
8. Declerck PJ, Juhan-Vague I, Felez J, et al. Pathophysiology of fibrinolysis. *J Intern Med* 1994;236:425.
9. Wiman B. Predictive value of fibrinolytic factors in coronary heart disease. *Scand J Clin Lab Invest* 1999;59 (Suppl 230):23.
10. Carmeliet P, Collen D. Development and disease in proteinase-deficient mice: role of the plasminogen, matrix metalloproteinase and coagulation system. *Thromb Res* 1998;91:255.
11. Lijnen HR. Interactions between the fibrinolytic and matrix metalloproteinase systems and their role in arterial neointima formation after vascular injury. *Thromb Haemost* 1999;82:837.
12. Rijken DC, Wijngaards G, Zaal-De Jong M, et al. Purification and partial characterization of plasminogen activator from human uterine tissue. *Biochim Biophys Acta* 1979;580:140.
13. Collen D, Lijnen HR, Todd PA, et al. Tissue-type plasminogen activator. A review of its pharmacology and therapeutic use as a thrombolytic agent. *Drugs* 1989;38:346.
14. Rijken DC, Collen D. Purification and characterization of the plasminogen activator secreted by human melanoma cells in culture. *J Biol Chem* 1981;256:7035.
15. Pennica D, Holmes WE, Kohr WJ, et al. Cloning and expression of human tissue-type plasminogen activator cDNA in E coli. *Nature* 1983;301:214.
16. Pohl G, Einarsson M, Nilsson B, et al. The size heterogeneity in melanoma tissue plasminogen activator is caused by carbohydrate differences. *Thromb Res* 1985;50:163.
17. Vehar GA, Spellman MW, Keyt BA, et al. Characterization studies of human tissue-type plasminogen activator produced by recombinant DNA technology. In: *Cold Spring Harbor Symposia on Quantitative Biology*, vol LI. Cold Spring Harbor, NY, 1986:551.
18. Hoylaerts M, Rijken DC, Lijnen HR, et al. Kinetics of the activation of plasminogen by human tissue plasminogen activator: role of fibrin. *J Biol Chem* 1982;257:2912.
19. Liu CY, Wallen P. The binding of tissue plasminogen activator by fibrin. *Circulation* 1984;70(Suppl II):365.
20. van Zonneveld AJ, Veerman H, Pannekoek H. On the interaction of the finger and kringle-2 domain of tissue-type plasminogen activator with fibrin. *J Biol Chem* 1986;261:14214.
21. Lijnen HR, Collen D. Strategies for the improvement of thrombolytic agents. *Thromb Haemost* 1991;66:88.
22. Voskuilen M, Vermond A, Veeneman GH, et al. Fibrinogen lysine residue Aα157 plays a crucial role in the fibrin-induced acceleration of plasminogen activation, catalyzed by tissue-type plasminogen activator. *J Biol Chem* 1987;262:5944.
23. Rijken DC, Hoylaerts M, Collen D. Fibrinolytic properties of one-chain and two-chain human extrinsic (tissue-type) plasminogen activator. *J Biol Chem* 1982;257:2920.
24. Suenson E, Lützen O, Thorsen S. Initial plasmin-degradation of fibrin as the basis of a positive feed-back mechanism in fibrinolysis. *Eur J Biochem* 1984;140:513.
25. Nienaber VL, Young SL, Birktoft JJ, et al. Conformational similarities between one-chain and two-chain tissue plasminogen activator (t-PA): implications to the activation mechanism on one-chain t-PA. *Biochemistry* 1992;31:3852.
26. Tachias K, Madison EL. Converting tissue type plasminogen activator into a zymogen. *J Biol Chem* 1997;272:28.
27. Renatus M, Engh RA, Stubbs MT, et al. Lysine 156 promotes the anomalous proenzyme activity of tPA: x-ray crystal structure of single-chain human tPA. *EMBO J* 1997;16:4797.
28. Kalyan NK, Lee SG, Wilhelm J, et al. Structure-function analysis with tissue-type plasminogen activator. Effect of deletion of NH₂-terminal domains on its biochemical and biological properties. *J Biol Chem* 1988;263:3971.

29. Gething MJ, Adler B, Boose JA, et al. Variants of human tissue-type plasminogen activator that lack specific structural domains of the heavy chain. *EMBO J* 1988;7:2731.
30. Larsen GR, Henson K, Blue Y. Variants of human tissue-type plasminogen activator: fibrin binding, fibrinolytic, and fibrinogenolytic characterization of genetic variants lacking the fibronectin finger-like and/or the epidermal growth factor domains. *J Biol Chem* 1988;263:1023.
31. The GUSTO-III investigators. A comparison of reteplase with alteplase for acute myocardial infarction. *N Engl J Med* 1997;337:1118.
32. Kohnert U, Rudolph R, Verheijen JH, et al. Biochemical properties of the kringle 2 and protease domains are maintained in the refolded t-PA deletion variant BM 06.022. *Protein Eng* 1992;5:93.
33. Stürzebecher J, Neumann U, Kohnert U, et al. Mapping of the catalytic site of CHO-t-PA and the t-PA variant BM 06.022 by synthetic inhibitors and substrates. *Protein Sci* 1992;1:1007.
34. Hajjar KA, Hamel NM, Harpel PC, et al. Binding of tissue plasminogen activator to cultured human endothelial cells. *J Clin Invest* 1987;80:1712.
35. Hajjar KA, Harpel PC, Jaffe EA, et al. Binding of plasminogen to cultured human endothelial cells. *J Biol Chem* 1986;261:11656.
36. Miles LA, Plow EF. Binding and activation of plasminogen on the platelet surface. *J Biol Chem* 1985;260:4303.
37. Stephens RW, Pöllänen J, Tapiovaara H, et al. Activation of pro-urokinase and plasminogen on human sarcoma cells: a proteolytic system with surface-bound reactants. *J Cell Biol* 1989;108:1987.
38. Miles LA, Plow EF. Plasminogen receptors: ubiquitous sites for cellular regulation of fibrinolysis. *Fibrinolysis* 1988;2:61.
39. Plow EF, Freaney DE, Plescia J, et al. The plasminogen system and cell surfaces: evidence for plasminogen and urokinase receptors on the same cell type. *J Cell Biol* 1986;103:2411.
40. Stricker RB, Wong D, Shiu DT, et al. Activation of plasminogen by tissue plasminogen activator on normal and thrombasthenic platelets: effects on surface proteins and platelet aggregation. *Blood* 1986;68:275.
41. Soeda S, Kakiki M, Shimeno H, et al. Some properties of tissue-type plasminogen activator reconstituted onto phospholipid and/or glycolipid vesicles. *Biochem Biophys Res Commun* 1987;146:94.
42. Miles LA, Dahlberg CM, Levin EG, et al. Gangliosides interact directly with plasminogen and urokinase and may mediate binding of these fibrinolytic components to cells. *Biochemistry* 1989;28:9337.
43. Miles LA, Dahlberg CM, Plescia J, et al. Role of cell-surface lysines in plasminogen binding to cells: identification of alpha-enolase as a candidate plasminogen receptor. *Biochemistry* 1991;30:1682.
44. Hajjar KA, Nachman RL. Endothelial cell-mediated conversion of Glu-plasminogen to Lys-plasminogen. Further evidence for assembly of the fibrinolytic system on endothelial cell surface. *J Clin Invest* 1988;82:1769.
45. Félez J, Miles LA, Fàbregas P, et al. Characterization of cellular binding sites and interactive regions within reactants required for enhancement of plasminogen activation by t-PA on the surface of leukocytic cells. *Thromb Haemost* 1996;76:577.
46. Barnathan ES, Kuo A, Van der Keyl H, et al. Tissue-type plasminogen activator binding to human endothelial cells. Evidence for two distinct binding sites. *J Biol Chem* 1988;263:7792.
47. Hajjar KA, Jacovina AT, Chacko J. An endothelial cell receptor for plasminogen/tissue plasminogen activator. I. Identity with annexin II. *J Biol Chem* 1994;269:21191.
48. Nachman RL, Hajjar KA. Endothelial cell fibrinolytic assembly. *Ann N Y Acad Sci* 1991;614:240.
49. Yang-Feng TL, Opdenakker G, Volckaert G, et al. Human tissue-type plasminogen activator gene located near chromosomal breakpoint in myeloproliferative disorder. *Am J Hum Genet* 1986;39:79.
50. Degen SJF, Rajput B, Reich E. The human tissue plasminogen activator gene. *J Biol Chem* 1986;261:6972.
51. Feng P, Ohlsson M, Ny T. The structure of the TATA-less rat tissue-type plasminogen activator gene. Species-specific sequence divergences in the promoter predict differences in regulation of gene expression. *J Biol Chem* 1990; 265:2022.
52. Kooistra T, Bosma PJ, Toet K, et al. Role of protein kinase C and cyclic adenosine monophosphate in the regulation of tissue-type plasminogen activator, plasminogen activator inhibitor-1, and platelet-derived growth factor mRNA levels in human endothelial cells. Possible involvement of protooncogenes c-jun and c-fos. *Arterioscler Thromb* 1991;11:1042.
53. Medcalf RL, Rueegg M, Schleuning WD. A DNA motif related to the cAMP-responsive element and an exon-located activator protein-2 binding site in the human tissue-type plasminogen activator gene promoter cooperate in basal expression and convey activation by phorbol ester and cAMP. *J Biol Chem* 1990;265:14618.
54. Ludwig M, Wohn KD, Schleuning WD, et al. Allelic dimorphism in the human tissue-type plasminogen activator (tPA) gene as a result of an Alu insertion/deletion event. *Hum Genet* 1992;88:388.
55. Patthy L. Evolution of the proteases of blood coagulation and fibrinolysis by assembly from modules. *Cell* 1985;41:657.
56. Rijken DC, Juhan-Vague I, De Cock F, et al. Measurement of human tissue-type plasminogen activator by a two-site immunoradiometric assay. *J Lab Clin Med* 1983;101:274.
57. Astrup T, Müllertz S. Fibrin plate method for estimating fibrinolytic activity. *Arch Biochem Biophys* 1952;40:346.
58. Gaffney PJ, Curtis AD. A collaborative study of a proposed international standard for tissue plasminogen activator (t-PA). *Thromb Haemost* 1985;53:134.
59. Gaffney PJ, Curtis AD. A collaborative study to establish the 2nd International Standard for Tissue Plasminogen Activator (t-PA). *Thromb Haemost* 1987;58:1085.
60. Ranby M, Norrman B, Wallen P. A sensitive assay for tissue plasminogen activator. *Thromb Res* 1982;27:743.
61. Verheijen JH, Mullaert E, Chang GTG, et al. A simple, sensitive spectrophotometric assay for extrinsic (tissue-type) plasminogen activator applicable to measurement in plasma. *Thromb Haemost* 1982;48:266.
62. Wiman B, Mellbring G, Ranby M. Plasminogen activator release during venous stasis and exercise as determined by a new specific assay. *Clin Chim Acta* 1983;127:279.
63. Holvoet P, Boes J, Collen D. Measurement of free, one-chain tissue-type plasminogen activator in human plasma with an enzyme-linked immunosorbent assay based on an active site-specific murine monoclonal antibody. *Blood* 1987;69:284.
64. Holmes WE, Pennica D, Blaber M, et al. Cloning and expression of the gene for pro-urokinase in Escherichia coli. *Biotechnology* 1985;3:923.
65. Winkler ME, Blaber M, Bennett GL, et al. Purification and characterization of recombinant urokinase from Escherichia coli. *Biotechnology* 1985;3:990.
66. Stump DC, Lijnen HR, Collen D. Purification and characterization of a novel low molecular weight form of single-chain urokinase-type plasminogen activator. *J Biol Chem* 1986;261:17120.
67. Lijnen HR, Nelles L, Holmes W, et al. Biochemical and thrombolytic properties of a low molecular weight form (comprising Leu^{144} through Leu^{411}) of recombinant single-chain urokinase-type plasminogen activator. *J Biol Chem* 1988;263:5594.
68. Lijnen HR, Stump DC, Collen D. Single-chain urokinase-type plasminogen activator: mechanism of action and thrombolytic properties. *Semin Thromb Haemost* 1987;13:152.
69. Ugwu F, Van Hoef B, Bini A, et al. Proteolytic cleavage of urokinase-type plasminogen activator by stromelysin-1 (MMP-3). *Biochemistry* 1998;37:7231.
70. Ichinose A, Fujikawa K, Suyama T. The activation of pro-urokinase by plasma kallikrein and its inactivation by thrombin. *J Biol Chem* 1986;261:3486.
71. de Munk GA, Parkinson JF, Groeneveld E, et al. Role of the glycosaminoglycan component of thrombomodulin in its acceleration of the inactivation of single-chain urokinase-type plasminogen activator by thrombin. *Biochem J* 1993;290:655.
72. Husain SS, Gurewich V, Lipinski B. Purification and partial characterization of a single-chain high-molecular-weight form of urokinase from human urine. *Arch Biochem Biophys* 1983;220:31.
73. Kohno T, Hopper P, Lillquist JS, et al. Kidney plasminogen activator: a precursor form of human urokinase with high fibrin affinity. *Biotechnology* 1984;2:628.
74. Sumi H, Maruyama M, Matsuo O, et al. Higher fibrin-binding and thrombolytic properties of single polypeptide chain-high molecular weight urokinase. *Thromb Haemost* 1982;47:297.
75. Stump DC, Lijnen HR, Collen D. Purification and characterization of single-chain urokinase-type plasminogen activator from human cell cultures. *J Biol Chem* 1986;261:1274.
76. Lijnen HR, Zamarron C, Blaber M, et al. Activation of plasminogen by pro-urokinase: I. Mechanism. *J Biol Chem* 1986;261:1253.
77. Verde P, Stoppelli MP, Galeffi P, et al. Identification and primary sequence of an unspliced human urokinase poly(A)$^+$ RNA. *Proc Natl Acad Sci U S A* 1984;81:4727.
78. Riccio A, Grimaldi G, Verde P, et al. The human urokinase-plasminogen activator gene and its promoter. *Nucleic Acids Res* 1985;13:2759.
79. Christensen U. Kinetic studies of the urokinase-catalysed conversion of NH$_2$-terminal glutamic acid plasminogen to plasmin. *Biochim Biophys Acta* 1977;481:638.
80. Wohl RC, Sinio L, Summaria L, et al. Comparative activation kinetics of mammalian plasminogens. *Biochim Biophys Acta* 1983;745:20.
81. Christensen U, Müllertz S. Kinetic studies on the urokinase catalysed conversion of NH$_2$-terminal lysine plasminogen to plasmin. *Biochim Biophys Acta* 1977;480:275.
82. Castellino FJ, Brockway WJ, Thomas JK, et al. Rotational diffusion analysis of the conformational alterations produced in plasminogen by certain antifibrinolytic amino acids. *Biochemistry* 1973;12:2787.
83. Camiolo SM, Thorsen S, Astrup T. Fibrinogenolysis and fibrinolysis with tissue plasminogen activator, urokinase, streptokinase-activated human globulin, and plasmin. *Proc Soc Exp Biol Med* 1971;138:277.
84. Lucas MA, Straight DL, Fretto LJ, et al. The effects of fibrinogen and its cleavage products on the kinetics of plasminogen activation by urokinase and subsequent plasmin activity. *J Biol Chem* 1983;258:12171.
85. Lijnen HR, Van Hoef B, Collen D. Influence of cyanogen-bromide-digested fibrinogen on the kinetics of plasminogen activation by urokinase. *Eur J Biochem* 1984;144:541.
86. Wun TC, Ossowski L, Reich E. A proenzyme form of human urokinase. *J Biol Chem* 1982;257:7262.
87. Nielsen LS, Hansen JG, Skriver L, et al. Purification of zymogen to plasminogen activator from human glioblastoma cells by affinity chromatography with monoclonal antibody. *Biochemistry* 1982;21:6410.
88. Collen D, Zamarron C, Lijnen HR, et al. Activation of plasminogen by pro-urokinase. II. Kinetics. *J Biol Chem* 1986;261:1259.
89. Nelles L, Lijnen HR, Collen D, et al. Characterization of recombinant human single chain urokinase-type plasminogen activator mutants produced by site-specific mutagenesis of lysine 158. *J Biol Chem* 1987;262:5682.

90. Lijnen HR, Van Hoef B, Collen D. Comparative kinetic analysis of the activation of human plasminogen by natural and recombinant single-chain urokinase-type plasminogen activator. *Biochim Biophys Acta* 1986;884:402.

91. Lijnen HR, Zamarron C, Collen D. Characterization of the high-affinity interaction between human plasminogen and pro-urokinase. *Eur J Biochem* 1985;150:141.

92. Ellis V, Scully MF, Kakkar VV. Plasminogen activation by single-chain urokinase in functional isolation: a kinetic study. *J Biol Chem* 1987;262:14998.

93. Petersen LC, Lund LR, Nielsen LS, et al. One-chain urokinase-type plasminogen activator from human sarcoma cells is a proenzyme with little or no intrinsic activity. *J Biol Chem* 1988;263:11189.

94. Husain SS. Single-chain urokinase-type plasminogen activator does not possess measurable intrinsic amidolytic or plasminogen activator activities. *Biochemistry* 1991;30:5797.

95. Gurewich V, Pannell R, Louie S, et al. Effective and fibrin-specific clot lysis by a zymogen precursor form of urokinase (pro-urokinase). A study in vitro and in two animal species. *J Clin Invest* 1984;73:1731.

96. Lijnen HR, Van Hoef B, Nelles L, Collen D. Plasminogen activation with single-chain urokinase-type plasminogen activator (scu-PA). Studies with active site mutagenized plasminogen (Ser740 → Ala) and plasmin-resistant scu-PA (Lys158 → Glu). *J Biol Chem* 1990;265:5232.

97. Liu JN, Pannell R, Gurewich V. A transitional state of pro-urokinase that has a higher catalytic efficiency against Glu-plasminogen than urokinase. *J Biol Chem* 1992;267:15289.

98. Sun Z, Liu BF, Chen Y, et al. Analysis of the forces which stabilize the active conformation of urokinase-type plasminogen activator. *Biochemistry* 1998;37:2935.

99. Lijnen HR, Van Hoef B, Collen D. Activation with plasmin of two-chain urokinase-type plasminogen activator derived from single-chain urokinase-type plasminogen activator by treatment with thrombin. *Eur J Biochem* 1987;169:359.

100. Lijnen HR, Bachmann F, Collen D, et al. Mechanisms of plasminogen activation. *J Intern Med* 1994;236:415.

101. Magdolen V, Rettenberger P, Koppitz M, et al. Systematic mutational analysis of the receptor-binding region of the human urokinase-type plasminogen activator. *Eur J Biochem* 1996;237:743.

102. Ellis V, Behrendt N, Dano K. Plasminogen activation by receptor-bound urokinase. A kinetic study with both cell-associated and isolated receptor. *J Biol Chem* 1991;266:12752.

103. Ellis V, Scully MF, Kakkar VV. Plasminogen activation initiated by single-chain urokinase-type plasminogen activator. Potentiation by U937 monocytes. *J Biol Chem* 1989;264:2185.

104. Ellis V, Wun TC, Behrendt N, et al. Inhibition of receptor-bound urokinase by plasminogen-activator inhibitors. *J Biol Chem* 1990;265:9904.

105. Lee SW, Ellis V, Dichek DA. Characterization of plasminogen activation by glycosylphosphatidylinositol-anchored urokinase. *J Biol Chem* 1994;269:2411.

106. Ellis V, Whawell SA, Werner F, et al. Assembly of urokinase receptor-mediated plasminogen activation complexes involves direct, non-active-site interactions between urokinase and plasminogen. *Biochemistry* 1999;38:651.

107. Chavakis T, Kanse SM, Yutzy B, et al. Vitronectin concentrates proteolytic activity on the cell surface and extracellular matrix by trapping soluble urokinase receptor-urokinase complexes. *Blood* 1998;91:2305.

108. May AE, Kanse SM, Chavakis T, et al. Molecular interactions between the urokinase receptor and integrins in the vasculature. *Fibrinolysis Proteolysis* 1998;12:205.

109. Sottrup-Jensen L, Petersen TE, Magnusson S. Plasminogen Sequence In: Dayhoff MO, ed. *Atlas of protein sequence and structure*, vol. 5, suppl 3. Washington, DC: National Biomedical Research Foundation, 1978:91.

110. Forsgren M, Raden B, Israelsson M, et al. Molecular cloning and characterization of a full-length cDNA clone for human plasminogen. *FEBS Lett* 1987;213:254.

111. Friberger P, Knos M. Plasminogen determination in human plasma. In: Scully MF, Kakkar VV, eds. *Chromogenic peptide substrates*. Edinburgh: Churchill Livingstone, 1979:128.

112. Marshall JM, Brown AJ, Ponting CP. Conformational studies of human plasminogen and plasminogen fragments: evidence for a novel third conformation of plasminogen. *Biochemistry* 1994;33:3599.

113. Deutsch DG, Mertz ET. Plasminogen: purification from human plasma by affinity chromatography. *Science* 1970;170:1095.

114. Brockway WJ, Castellino FJ. Measurement of the binding of antifibrinolytic amino acids to various plasminogens. *Arch Biochem Biophys* 1972;151:194.

115. Collen D, De Maeyer L. Molecular biology of human plasminogen: I. physicochemical properties and microheterogeneity. *Thromb Diath Haemorrh* 1975;34:396.

116. Castellino FJ, Siefring GE Jr, Sodetz IM, et al. Amino terminal amino acid sequences and carbohydrate of the two major forms of rabbit plasminogen. *Biochem Biophys Res Commun* 1973;53:845.

117. Hayes ML, Castellino FJ. Carbohydrate of the human plasminogen variants. I. Carbohydrate composition, glycopeptide isolation and characterization. *J Biol Chem* 1979;254:8768.

118. Hayes ML, Castellino FJ. Carbohydrate of the human plasminogen variants. II. Structure of the asparagine-linked oligosaccharide unit. *J Biol Chem* 1979;254:8772.

119. Hayes ML, Castellino FJ. Carbohydrate of the human plasminogen variants. III. Structure of the O-glycosidically linked oligosaccharide unit. *J Biol Chem* 1979;254:8777.

120. Lijnen HR, Van Hoef B, Collen D. On the role of the carbohydrate side chains of human plasminogen in its interaction with α_2-antiplasmin and fibrin. *Eur J Biochem* 1981;120:149.

121. Collen D, Verstraete M. Molecular biology of human plasminogen: II. Metabolism in physiological and some pathological conditions in man. *Thromb Diath Haemorrh* 1975;34:403.

122. Murray JC, Buetow KH, Donovan M, et al. Linkage disequilibrium of plasminogen polymorphisms and assignment of the gene to human chromosome 6q26-6q27. *Am J Hum Genet* 1987;40:338.

123. Petersen TE, Martzen MR, Ichinose A, et al. Characterization of the gene for human plasminogen, a key proenzyme in the fibrinolytic system. *J Biol Chem* 1990;265:6104.

124. Wade DP, Clarke JG, Lindahl GE, et al. 5'control regions of the apolipoprotein(a) gene and members of the related plasminogen gene family. *Proc Natl Acad Sci U S A* 1993;90:1369.

125. Hobart MJ. Genetic polymorphism of human plasminogen. *Ann Hum Genet* 1979;42:419.

126. Raum D, Marcus D, Alper CA. Genetic polymorphism of human plasminogen. *Am J Genet* 1980;32:681.

127. Skoda U, Bertrams J, Dykes D, et al. Proposal for the nomenclature of human plasminogen (PLG) polymorphism. *Vox Sang* 1986;51:244.

128. Kera Y, Nishimukai H, Yamasawa K, et al. Comparative study of phenotypes on activity and plasma concentration in the genetic system of plasminogen. *Hum Hered* 1983;33:52.

129. Brandt-Casadevall C, Dimo-Simonin N, et al. A plasminogen silent allele detected in a Swiss family. *Hum Hered* 1987;37:389.

130. Robbins KC, Summaria L, Hsieh B, et al. The peptide chains of human plasmin: mechanism of activation of human plasminogen to plasmin. *J Biol Chem* 1967;242:2333.

131. Groskopf WR, Summaria L, Robbins KC. Studies on the active center of human plasmin: partial amino acid sequence of a peptide containing the active center serine residue. *J Biol Chem* 1969;244:3590.

132. Violand BN, Castellino FJ. Mechanism of the urokinase-catalyzed activation of human plasminogen. *J Biol Chem* 1976;251:3906.

133. Wiman B, Collen D. On the mechanism of the reaction between human α_2-antiplasmin and plasmin. *J Biol Chem* 1979;254:9291.

134. Holvoet P, Lijnen HR, Collen D. A monoclonal antibody specific for Lys-plasminogen: application to the study of the activation pathways of plasminogen in vivo. *J Biol Chem* 1985;260:12106.

135. Markus G, DePasquale JL, Wissler FC. Quantitative determination of the binding of ε-aminocaproic acid to native plasminogen. *J Biol Chem* 1978;253:727.

136. Markus G, Priore RL, Wissler FC. The binding of tranexamic acid to native (Glu) and modified (Lys) human plasminogen and its effect on conformation. *J Biol Chem* 1979;254:1211.

137. Wiman B, Lijnen HR, Collen D. On the specific interaction between the lysine-binding sites in plasmin and complementary sites in a$_2$-antiplasmin and in fibrinogen. *Biochim Biophys Acta* 1979;579:142.

138. Vali Z, Patthy L. Location of the intermediate and high affinity omega-aminocarboxylic acid-binding sites in human plasminogen. *J Biol Chem* 1982;257:2104.

139. Trexler M, Vali Z, Patthy L. Structure of the omega-aminocarboxylic acid-binding sites of human plasminogen: arginine 70 and aspartic acid 56 are essential for binding of ligand by kringle 4. *J Biol Chem* 1982;257:7401.

140. Trexler M, Banyai L, Patthy L, et al. The solution structure of kringle 4: NMR studies on native and several chemically modified kringle 4 species of human plasminogen. *FEBS Lett* 1983;154:311.

141. Rakoczi I, Wiman B, Collen D. On the biological significance of the specific interaction between fibrin, plasminogen and antiplasmin. *Biochim Biophys Acta* 1978;540:295.

142. Christensen U. The AH-site of plasminogen and two C-terminal fragments: a weak lysine-binding site preferring ligands not carrying a free carboxylate function. *Biochem J* 1984;223:413.

143. Wiman B, Collen D. Molecular mechanism of physiological fibrinolysis. *Nature* 1978;272:549.

144. Collen D. On the regulation and control of fibrinolysis. *Thromb Haemost* 1980;43:77.

145. Miles LA, Ginsberg MH, White JG, et al. Plasminogen interacts with human platelets through two distinct mechanisms. *J Clin Invest* 1986;77:2001.

146. Miles LA, Dahlberg CM, Plow EF. The cell-binding domains of plasminogen and their function in plasma. *J Biol Chem* 1988;263:11928.

147. Holmes WE, Nelles L, Lijnen HR, Collen D. Primary structure of human α_2-antiplasmin, a serine protease inhibitor (serpin). *J Biol Chem* 1987;262:1659.

148. Lijnen HR, Holmes WE, Van Hoef B, et al. Amino-acid sequence of human α_2-antiplasmin. *Eur J Biochem* 1987;166:565.

149. Christensen S, Berglund L, Sottrup-Jensen L. Primary structure of bovine alpha-2-antiplasmin. *FEBS Lett* 1994;343:223.

150. Bangert K, Johnsen AH, Christensen U, et al. Different N-terminal forms α_2-plasmin inhibitor in human plasma. *Biochem J* 1993;291:623.

151. Kimura S, Aoki N. Cross-linking site in fibrinogen for α_2-plasmin inhibitor. *J Biol Chem* 1986;261:15591.

152. Sumi Y, Ichikawa Y, Nakamura Y, et al. Expression and characterization of pro α_2-plasmin inhibitor. *J Biochem* (Tokyo) 1989;106:703.

153. Wiman B, Collen D. Purification and characterization of human antiplasmin, the fast-acting plasmin inhibitor in plasma. *Eur J Biochem* 1977;78:19.

154. Collen D, Wiman B. Turnover of antiplasmin, the fast-acting plasmin inhibitor of plasma. *Blood* 1979;53:313.

155. Christensen U, Clemmensen I. Purification and reaction mechanisms of the primary inhibitor of plasmin from human plasma. *Biochem J* 1978;175:635.
156. Sugiyama N, Sasaki T, Iwamoto M, et al. Binding site of α_2-plasmin inhibitor to plasminogen. *Biochim Biophys Acta* 1988;952:1.
157. Wiman B, Nilsson T, Cedergren B. Studies on a form of α_2-antiplasmin in plasma which does not interact with the lysine-binding sites in plasminogen. *Thromb Res* 1982;28:193.
158. Christensen U, Clemmensen I. Kinetic properties of the primary inhibitor of plasmin from human plasma. *Biochem J* 1977;163:389.
159. Wiman B, Collen D. On the kinetics of the reaction between human antiplasmin and plasmin. *Eur J Biochem* 1978;84:573.
160. Wiman B, Boman L, Collen D. On the kinetics of the reaction between human antiplasmin and a low-molecular-weight form of plasmin. *Eur J Biochem* 1978;87:143.
161. Lijnen HR, Hoylaerts M, Collen D. Isolation and characterization of a human plasma protein with affinity for the lysine binding sites in plasminogen: role in the regulation of fibrinolysis and identification as histidine-rich glycoprotein. *J Biol Chem* 1980;255:10214.
162. Kato A, Hirosawa S, Toyota S, et al. Localization of the human alpha2-plasmin inhibitor gene (PLI) to 17 p 13. *Cytogenet Cell Genet* 1993;62:190.
163. Hirosawa S, Nakamura Y, Miura O, et al. Organization of the human α_2-plasmin inhibitor gene. *Proc Natl Acad Sci U S A* 1988;85:6836.
164. Kruithof EKO, Tran-Thang C, Ransijn A, et al. Demonstration of a fast-acting inhibitor of plasminogen activators in human plasma. *Blood* 1984;64:907.
165. Kruithof EKO. Plasminogen activator inhibitors—a review. *Enzyme* 1988;40:113.
166. Ny T, Sawdey M, Lawrence D, et al. Cloning and sequence of a cDNA coding for the human β-migrating endothelial-cell-type plasminogen activator inhibitor. *Proc Natl Acad Sci U S A* 1986;83:6776.
167. Pannekoek H, Veerman H, Lambers H, et al. Endothelial plasminogen activator inhibitor (PAI): a new member of the serpin gene family. *EMBO J* 1986;5:2539.
168. Sherman PM, Lawrence DA, Yang AY, et al. Saturation mutagenesis of the plasminogen activator inhibitor-1 reactive center. *J Biol Chem* 1992;267:7588.
169. Klinger KW, Winqvist R, Riccio A, et al. Plasminogen activator inhibitor type 1 gene is located at region q21.3-q22 of chromosome 7 and genetically linked with cystic fibrosis. *Proc Natl Acad Sci U S A* 1987;84:8548.
170. Declerck PJ, De Mol M, Alessi MC, et al. Purification and characterization of a plasminogen activator inhibitor-1 binding protein from human plasma. Identification as a multimeric form of S protein (Vitronectin). *J Biol Chem* 1988;263:15454.
171. Deng G, Royle G, Wang S, et al. Structural and functional analysis of the plasminogen activator inhibitor-1 binding motif in the somatomedin B domain of vitronectin. *J Biol Chem* 1996;271:12716.
172. Ehrlich HJ, Gebbink RK, Keijer J, et al. Elucidation of structural requirements on plasminogen activator inhibitor 1 for binding to heparin. *J Biol Chem* 1992;267:11606.
173. Hekman CM, Loskutoff DJ. Endothelial cells produce a latent inhibitor of plasminogen activators that can be activated by denaturants. *J Biol Chem* 1985;260:11581.
174. Gils A, Lu J, Aertgeerts K, et al. Identification of positively charged residues contributing to the stability of plasminogen activator inhibitor 1. *FEBS Lett* 1997;415:192.
175. Gils A, Declerck PJ. Structure-function relationships in serpins: current concepts and controversies. *Thromb Haemost* 1998;80:531.
176. Mottonen J, Strand A, Symersky J, et al. Structural basis of latency in plasminogen activator inhibitor-1. *Nature* 1992;355:270.
177. Declerck PJ, De Mol M, Vaughan DE, Collen D. Identification of a conformationally distinct form of plasminogen activator inhibitor-1, acting as a non-inhibitory substrate for tissue-type plasminogen activator. *J Biol Chem* 1992;267:11693.
178. Audenaert A-M, Knockaert I, Collen D, Declerck PJ. Conversion of plasminogen activator inhibitor-1 from inhibitor to substrate by point mutations in the reactive-site loop. *J Biol Chem* 1994;269:19559.
179. Aertgeerts K, De Bondt HL, De Ranter CJ, et al. Mechanisms contributing to the conformational and functional flexibility of plasminogen activator inhibitor-1. *Nat Struct Biol* 1995;2:891.
180. Thorsen S, Philips M, Selmer J, et al. Kinetics of inhibition of tissue-type and urokinase-type plasminogen activator by plasminogen-activator inhibitor type 1 and type 2. *Eur J Biochem* 1988;175:33.
181. Chmielewska J, Ranby M, Wiman B. Kinetics of the inhibition of plasminogen activators by the plasminogen-activator inhibitor. Evidence for 'second site' interactions. *Biochem J* 1988;251:327.
182. Madison EL, Goldsmith EJ, Gerard RD, et al. Serpin-resistant mutants of human tissue-type plasminogen activator. *Nature* 1989;339:721.
183. Adams DS, Griffin LA, Nachajko WR, et al. A synthetic DNA encoding a modified human urokinase resistant to inhibition by serum plasminogen activator inhibitor. *J Biol Chem* 1991;266:8476.
184. Wagner OF, de Vries C, Hohmann C, et al. Interaction between plasminogen activator inhibitor type 1 (PAI-1) bound to fibrin and either tissue-type plasminogen activator (tPA) or urokinase-type plasminogen activator (u-PA). *J Clin Invest* 1989;84:647.
185. Reilly CF, Hutzelmann JE. Plasminogen activator inhibitor-1 binds to fibrin and inhibits tissue-type plasminogen activator-mediated fibrin dissolution. *J Biol Chem* 1992;267:17128.
186. Fa M, Karolin J, Aleshkov S, et al. Time-resolved polarized fluorescence spectroscopy studies of plasminogen activator inhibitor type 1: conformational

changes of the reactive center upon interactions with target proteinases, vitronectin and heparin. *Biochemistry* 1995;34:13833.
187. Gibson A, Baburaj K, Day DE, et al. The use of fluorescent probes to characterize conformational changes in the interaction between vitronectin and plasminogen activator inhibitor-1. *J Biol Chem* 1997;272:5112.
188. Naski MC, Lawrence DA, Mosher DF, et al. Kinetics of inactivation of alpha-thrombin by plasminogen activator inhibitor-1. Comparison of the effects of native and urea-treated forms of vitronectin. *J Biol Chem* 1993;268:12367.
189. Ehrlich HJ, Klein GR, Preissner KT, et al. Alteration of serpin specificity by a protein cofactor. Vitronectin endows plasminogen activator inhibitor-1 with thrombin inhibitory properties. *J Cell Biol* 1991;115:1773.
190. Deng G, Curriden SA, Wang SJ, et al. Is plasminogen activator inhibitor-1 the molecular switch that governs urokinase receptor-mediated cell adhesion and release? *J Cell Biol* 1996;134:1563.
191. Kanse SM, Kost C, Wilhelm OG, et al. The urokinase receptor is a major vitronectin-binding protein on endothelial cells. *Exp Cell Res* 1996;224:344.
192. Stefansson S, Lawrence DA. The serpin PAI-1 inhibits cell migration by blocking integrin $\alpha_v\beta_3$ binding to vitronectin. *Nature* 1996;383:441.
193. Kjoller L, Kanse SM, Kirkegaard T, et al. Plasminogen activator inhibitor-1 represses integrin- and vitronectin-mediated cell migration independently of its function as an inhibitor of plasminogen activation. *Exp Cell Res* 1997;232:420.
194. Waltz DA, Natkin LR, Fujita RM, et al. Plasmin and plasminogen activator inhibitor type 1 promote cellular motility by regulating the interaction between the urokinase receptor and vitronectin. *J Clin Invest* 1997;100:58.
195. Kruithof EKO, Gudinchet A, Bachmann F. Plasminogen activator inhibitor 1 and plasminogen activator inhibitor 2 in various disease states. *Thromb Haemost* 1988;59:7.
196. Belin D. Biology and facultative secretion of plasminogen activator inhibitor-2. *Thromb Haemost* 1993;70:144.
197. Ye RD, Ahem SM, Le Beau MM, et al. Structure of the gene for human plasminogen activator inhibitor-2. The nearest mammalian homologue of chicken ovalbumin. *J Biol Chem* 1989;264:5495.
198. Higgins DL, Vehar GA. Interaction of one-chain and two-chain tissue plasminogen activator with intact and plasmin-degraded fibrin. *Biochemistry* 1987;26:7786.
199. Thorsen S. The mechanism of plasminogen activation and the variability of the fibrin effector during tissue-type plasminogen activator-mediated fibrinolysis. *Ann N Y Acad Sci* 1992;667:52.
200. Andreasen PA, Petersen LC, DanØ K. Diversity in catalytic properties of single-chain and two-chain tissue-type plasminogen activator. *Fibrinolysis* 1991;5:207.
201. McLean JW, Tomlinson JE, Kuang WJ, et al. cDNA sequence of human apolipoprotein(a) is homologous to plasminogen. *Nature* 1987;330:132.
202. Harpel PC, Gordon BR, Parker TS. Plasmin catalyzes binding of lipoprotein (a) to immobilized fibrinogen and fibrin. *Proc Natl Acad Sci U S A* 1989;86:3847.
203. Fleury V, Anglés-Cano E. Characterization of the binding of plasminogen to fibrin surfaces: the role of carboxy-terminal lysines. *Biochemistry* 1991;30:7630.
204. Loscalzo J, Weinfeld M, Fless GM, et al. Lipoprotein(a), fibrin binding and plasminogen activation. *Arteriosclerosis* 1990;10:240.
205. Edelberg JM, Gonzales-Gronow M, Pizzo SV. Lipoprotein(a) inhibition of plasminogen activation by tissue-type plasminogen activator. *Thromb Res* 1990;57:155.
206. Liu JN, Harpel PC, Pannell R, et al. Lipoprotein(a): a kinetic study of its influence on fibrin-dependent plasminogen activation by prourokinase or tissue plasminogen activator. *Biochemistry* 1993;32:9694.
207. Bajzar L, Manuel R, Nesheim ME. Purification and characterization of TAFI, a thrombin-activable fibrinolysis inhibitor. *J Biol Chem* 1995;270:14477.
208. Eaton DL, Malloy BE, Tsai SP, et al. Isolation, molecular cloning, and partial characterization of a novel carboxypeptidase B from human plasma. *J Biol Chem* 1991;266:21833.
209. Nesheim M, Wang W, Boffa M, et al. Thrombin, thrombomodulin and TAFI in the molecular link between coagulation and fibrinolysis. *Thromb Haemost* 1997;78:386.
210. Declerck PJ, Lijnen HR, Verstreken M, et al. Role of alpha 2-antiplasmin in fibrin-specific clot lysis with single-chain urokinase-type plasminogen activator in human plasma. *Thromb Haemost* 1991;65:394.
211. Liu JN, Gurewich V. Fragment E-2 from fibrin substantially enhances pro-urokinase-induced Glu-plasminogen activation. A kinetic study using the plasmin-resistant mutant pro-urokinase Ala-158-rpro-UK. *Biochemistry* 1992;31:6311.
212. Fleury V, Gurewich V, Anglés-Cano E. A study of the activation of fibrin-bound plasminogen by tissue-type plasminogen activator, single chain urokinase and sequential combinations of the activators. *Fibrinolysis* 1993;7:87.
213. Fleury V, Lijnen HR, Anglés-Cano E. Mechanism of the enhanced intrinsic activity of single-chain urokinase-type plasminogen activator during ongoing fibrinolysis. *J Biol Chem* 1993;268:18554.
214. Koie K, Ogata K, Kamiya T, et al. α_2-plasmin-inhibitor deficiency (Miyasato disease). *Lancet* 1978;2:1334.
215. Miura O, Sugahara Y, Aoki N. Hereditary α_2-plasmin inhibitor deficiency caused by a transport-deficient mutation (α_2-PI-Okinawa). Deletion of Glu137 by a trinucleotide deletion blocks intracellular transport. *J Biol Chem* 1989;264:18213.
216. Miura O, Hirosawa S, Kato A, et al. Molecular basis for congenital deficiency of α_2-plasmin inhibitor. A frameshift mutation leading to elongation of the deduced amino acid sequence. *J Clin Invest* 1989;83:1598.

217. Lijnen HR, Okada K, Matsuo O, et al. α_2-Antiplasmin gene deficiency is associated with enhanced fibrinolytic potential without overt bleeding. *Blood* 1999;93:2274.

218. Teger-Nilsson AC, Gyzander E, Myrwold H, et al. Determination of fast-acting plasmin inhibitor (α_2-antiplasmin) in plasma from patients with tendency to thrombosis and increased fibrinolysis. *Haemostasis* 1978;7:155.

219. Aoki N, Yamanaka T. The α_2-plasmin inhibitor levels in liver diseases. *Clin Chim Acta* 1978;84:99.

220. Högstorp H, Jacobsson H, Saldeen T. Effect of hepatectomy on the posttraumatic fibrinolysis inhibition and the primary fibrinolysis inhibitor in the rat. *Thromb Res* 1980;18:361.

221. Collen D, Lijnen HR. The fibrinolytic system in man. *CRC Crit Rev Oncol Hematol* 1986;4:249.

222. Collen D, Bounameaux H, De Cock F, et al. Analysis of coagulation and fibrinolysis during intravenous infusion of recombinant human tissue-type plasminogen activator in patients with acute myocardial infarction. *Circulation* 1986;73:511.

223. Kluft C, Nieuwenhuis HK, Rijken DC, et al. Alpha 2-antiplasmin Enschede: dysfunctional alpha 2-antiplasmin molecule associated with an autosomal recessive hemorrhagic disorder. *J Clin Invest* 1987;80:1391.

224. Holmes WE, Lijnen HR, Nelles L, et al. α_2-Antiplasmin Enschede: alanine insertion and abolition of plasmin inhibitory activity. *Science* 1987;238:209.

225. Loskutoff DJ. Regulation of PAI-I gene expression. *Fibrinolysis* 1991;5:197.

226. Krishnamurti C, Alving BM. Plasminogen activator inhibitor type 1: biochemistry and evidence for modulation of fibrinolysis in vivo. *Semin Thromb Hemost* 1992;18:67.

227. Ginsburg D, Zeheb R, Yang AY, et al. cDNA cloning of human plasminogen activator inhibitor from endothelial cells. *J Clin Invest* 1986;78:1673.

228. van den Berg EA, Sprengers ED, Jaye M, et al. Regulation of plasminogen activator inhibitor-1 mRNA in human endothelial cells. *Thromb Haemost* 1988;60:63.

229. Konkle BA, Kollros PR, Kelly MD. Heparin-binding growth factor-1 modulation of plasminogen activator inhibitor-1 expression. *J Biol Chem* 1990;265:21867.

230. Medcalf RL, Kruithof EK, Schleuning WD. Plasminogen activator inhibitor-1 and 2 are tumor necrosis factor/cachectin-responsive genes. *J Exp Med* 1988;168:751.

231. Medcalf RL, van den Berg E, Schleuning WD. Glucocorticoid-modulated gene expression of tissue- and urinary-type plasminogen activator and plasminogen activator inhibitor 1 and 2. *J Cell Biol* 1988;106:971.

232. Keski-Oja J, Raghow R, Sawdey M, et al. Regulation of mRNAs for type-1 plasminogen activator inhibitor, fibronectin, and type-1 procollagen by transforming growth factor-β. *J Biol Chem* 1988;263:3111.

233. Kooistra T, Bosma PJ, Töns HAM, et al. Plasminogen activator inhibitor-1: biosynthesis and mRNA level are increased by insulin in cultured human hepatocytes. *Thromb Haemost* 1989;62:723.

234. Bosma PJ, Kooistra T. Different induction of two plasminogen activator inhibitor 1 mRNA species by phorbol ester in human hepatoma cells. *J Biol Chem* 1991;266:17845.

235. Colucci M, Paramo JA, Collen D. Generation in plasma of a fast-acting inhibitor of plasminogen activator in response to endotoxin stimulation. *J Clin Invest* 1985;75:818.

236. Crutchley DJ, Conanan LB. Endotoxin induction of an inhibitor of plasminogen activator in bovine pulmonary artery endothelial cells. *J Biol Chem* 1986;261:154.

237. Medina R, Socher SH, Han JH, et al. Interleukin 1, endotoxin or tumor necrosis factor/cachectin enhance the level of plasminogen activator inhibitor messenger RNA in bovine aortic endothelial cells. *Thromb Res* 1989;54:41.

238. Emeis JJ, Kooistra T. Interleukin 1 and lipopolysaccharide induce an inhibitor of tissue-type plasminogen activator in vivo and in cultured endothelial cells. *J Exp Med* 1986;63:1260.

239. Bevilacqua MP, Schleef RR, Gimbrone MA Jr, et al. Regulation of the fibrinolytic system of cultured human vascular endothelium by interleukin 1. *J Clin Invest* 1986;78:587.

240. van Hinsbergh VW, Kooistra T, van den Berg EA, et al. Tumor necrosis factor increases the production of plasminogen activator inhibitor in human endothelial cells in vitro and in rats in vivo. *Blood* 1988;72:1467.

241. Schleef RR, Bevilacqua MP, Sawdey M, et al. Cytokine activation of vascular endothelium. Effects on tissue-type plasminogen activator and type 1 plasminogen activator inhibitor. *J Biol Chem* 1988;263:5797.

242. Saksela O, Moscatelli D, Rifkin DB. The opposing effects of basic fibroblast growth factor and transforming growth factor beta on the regulation of plasminogen activator activity in capillary endothelial cells. *J Cell Biol* 1987;105:957.

243. Santell L, Levin EC. Cyclic AMP potentiates phorbol ester stimulation of tissue plasminogen activator release and inhibits secretion of plasminogen activator inhibitor-1 from human endothelial cells. *J Biol Chem* 1988;263:16802.

244. Levin EG, Marotti KR, Santell L. Protein kinase C and the stimulation of tissue plasminogen activator release from human endothelial cells. Dependence on the elevation of messenger RNA. *J Biol Chem* 1989;264:16030.

245. Scarpati EM, Sadler JE. Regulation of endothelial cell coagulant properties. Modulation of tissue factor, plasminogen activator inhibitors, and thrombomodulin by phorbol 12-myristate 13-acetate and tumor necrosis factor. *J Biol Chem* 1989;264:20705.

246. Gelehrter TD, Sznycer-Laszuk R. Thrombin induction of plasminogen activator inhibitor in cultured human endothelial cells. *J Clin Invest* 1986;77:165.

247. Hanss M, Collen D. Secretion of tissue-type plasminogen activator and plasminogen activator inhibitor by cultured human endothelial cells: modulation by thrombin, endotoxin and histamine. *J Lab Clin Med* 1987;109:97.

248. Dichek D, Quertermous T. Thrombin regulation of mRNA levels of tissue plasminogen activator and plasminogen activator inhibitor-1 in cultured human umbilical vein endothelial cells. *Blood* 1989;74:222.

249. Stiko-Rahm A, Wiman B, Hamsten A, et al. Secretion of plasminogen activator inhibitor-1 from cultured human umbilical vein endothelial cells is induced by very low density lipoprotein. *Arteriosclerosis* 1990;10:1067.

250. Etingin OR, Hajjar DP, Hajjar KA, et al. Lipoprotein (a) regulates plasminogen activator inhibitor-1 expression in endothelial cells. A potential mechanism in thrombogenesis. *J Biol Chem* 1991;266:2459.

251. Schneider DJ, Nordt TK, Sobel BE. Stimulation by proinsulin of expression of plasminogen activator inhibitor type-1 in endothelial cells. *Diabetes* 1992;41:890.

252. Nordt TK, Klassen KJ, Schneider DJ, et al. Augmentation of synthesis of plasminogen activator inhibitor type-1 in arterial endothelial cells by glucose and its implications for local fibrinolysis. *Arterioscler Thromb* 1993;13:1822.

253. Kariko K, Rosenbaum H, Kuo A, et al. Stimulatory effect of unsaturated fatty acids on the level of plasminogen activator inhibitor-1 mRNA in cultured human endothelial cells. *FEBS Lett* 1995;361:118.

254. Nagai T, Akizawa T, Kohjiro S, et al. rHuEPO enhances the production of plasminogen activator inhibitor-1 in cultured endothelial cells. *Kidney Int* 1996;50:102.

255. Feener EP, Northrup JM, Aiello LP, et al. Angiotensin II induces plasminogen activator inhibitor-1 and -2 expression in vascular endothelial and smooth muscle cells. *J Clin Invest* 1995;95:1353.

256. Vaughan DE, Lazos SA, Tong K. Angiotensin II regulates the expression of plasminogen activator inhibitor-1 in cultured endothelial cells. A potential link between the renin-angiotensin system and thrombosis. *J Clin Invest* 1995;95:995.

257. Kerins DM, Hao Q, Vaughan DE. Angiotensin induction of PAI-1 expression in endothelial cells is mediated by the hexapeptide angiotensin IV. *J Clin Invest* 1995;96:2515.

258. Hamdan AD, Quist WC, Gagne JB, et al. Angiotensin-converting enzyme inhibition suppresses plasminogen activator inhibitor-1 expression in the neointima of balloon-injured rat aorta. *Circulation* 1996;93:1073.

259. Descheemaeker KA, Wijns S, Nelles L, et al. Interaction of AP-1-like, AP-2-like and Sp1-like proteins with two distinct sites in the upstream regulatory region of the plasminogen activator inhibitor-1 gene mediates the phorbol 12-myristate 13-acetate response. *J Biol Chem* 1992;267:15086.

260. Ding H, Descheemaeker K, Marynen P, et al. Characterization of a helicase-like transcription factor involved in the expression of the human plasminogen activator inhibitor-1 gene. *DNA Cell Biol* 1996;15;429.

261. Westerhausen DR, Hopkins WE, Billadello JJ. Multiple transforming growth factor-beta-inducible elements regulate expression of the plasminogen activator inhibitor type-1 gene in HepG2 cells. *J Biol Chem* 1991;266:1092.

262. Riccio A, Pedone P, Lund L, et al. Transforming growth factor beta-1 responsive element: closely associated binding sites for USF and CCAAT-binding transcription factor-nuclear factor I in the type 1 plasminogen activator inhibitor gene. *Mol Cell Biol* 1992;12:1846.

263. Bosma PJ, van den Berg EA, Kooistra T, et al. Human plasminogen activator inhibitor-1 gene. Promoter and structural gene nucleotide sequences. *J Biol Chem* 1988;263:9129.

264. Knudsen H, Olesen T, Riccio A, et al. A common response element mediates differential effects of phorbol esters and forskolin on type-1 plasminogen activator inhibitor gene expression in human breast carcinoma cells. *Eur J Biochem* 1994;220:63.

265. Arts J, Grimbergen J, Bosma PJ, et al. Role of c-Jun and proximal phorbol 12-myristate-13-acetate-(PMA)-responsive elements in the regulation of basal and PMA-stimulated plasminogen-activator inhibitor-1 gene expression in HepG2. *Eur J Biochem* 1996;41:393.

266. Kunz C, Pebler S, Otte J, et al. Differential regulation of plasminogen activator and inhibitor gene transcription by the tumor suppressor p53. *Nucleic Acids Res* 1995;23:3710.

267. Sawa H, Fujii S, Sobel BE. Augmented arterial wall expression of type-1 plasminogen activator inhibitor induced by thrombosis. *Arterioscler Thromb* 1992;12:1507.

268. Georg B, Riccio A, Andreasen P. Forskolin down-regulates type-1 plasminogen activator inhibitor and tissue-type plasminogen activator and their mRNAs in human fibrosarcoma cells. *Mol Cell Endocrinol* 1990;72:103.

269. Konkle BA, Ginsburg D. The addition of endothelial cell growth factor and heparin to human umbilical vein endothelial cell cultures decreases plasminogen activator inhibitor-1 expression. *J Clin Invest* 1988;82:579.

270. Fujii S, Sawa H, Sobel BE. Inhibition of endothelial cell expression of plasminogen activator inhibitor type-1 by gemfibrozil. *Thromb Haemost* 1993;70:642.

271. Krishnamurti C, Barr CF, Hassett MA, et al. Plasminogen activator inhibitor: a regulator of ancrod-induced fibrin deposition in rabbits. *Blood* 1987;69:798.

272. Levi M, Biemond BJ, van Zonneveld AJ, et al. Inhibition of plasminogen activator inhibitor-1 activity results in promotion of endogenous thrombolysis and inhibition of thrombus extension in models of experimental thrombosis. *Circulation* 1992;85:305.

273. Erickson LA, Fici GJ, Lund JE, et al. Development of venous occlusions in mice transgenic for the plasminogen activator inhibitor-1 gene. *Nature* 1990;346:74.

274. Carmeliet P, Stassen JM, Schoonjans L, et al. Plasminogen activator inhibitor-1 gene-deficient mice. II. Effects on hemostasis, thrombosis and thrombolysis. *J Clin Invest* 1993;92:2756.

275. Juhan-Vague I, Moerman B, De Cock F, et al. Plasma levels of a specific inhibitor of tissue-type plasminogen activator (and urokinase) in normal and pathological conditions. *Thromb Res* 1984;343:523.

276. Mellbring G, Dahlgren S, Wiman B, et al. Relationship between preoperative status of the fibrinolytic system and occurrence of deep vein thrombosis after major abdominal surgery. *Thromb Res* 1985;39:157.

277. Nilsson IM, Ljungner H, Tengborn L. Two different mechanisms in patients with venous thrombosis and defective fibrinolysis: low concentration of plasminogen activator or increased concentration of plasminogen activator inhibitor. *BMJ* 1985;290:1453.

278. Juhan-Vague I, Valadier J, Alessi MC, et al. Deficient t-PA release and elevated PA inhibitor levels in patients with spontaneous or recurrent deep venous thrombosis. *Thromb Haemost* 1987;57:67.

279. Landin K, Stigendal L, Eriksson E, et al. Abdominal obesity is associated with an impaired fibrinolytic activity and elevated plasminogen activator inhibitor-1. *Metabolism* 1990;39:1044.

280. Bolan CD, Krishnamurti C, Tan DB, et al. Association of protein S deficiency with thrombosis in a kindred with increased levels of plasminogen activator inhibitor-1. *Ann Intern Med* 1993;119:779.

281. Zöller B, Berntsdotter A, Garcia-de-Frutos P, et al. Resistance to activated protein C as an additional genetic risk factor in hereditary deficiency of protein S. *Blood* 1995;85:3518.

282. Dahlbäck B. New molecular insights into the genetics of thrombophilia. Resistance to activated protein C caused by Arg506 to Gln mutation in factor V as a pathogenic risk factor for venous thrombosis. *Thromb Haemost* 1995;74:139.

283. Dawson S, Hamsten A, Wiman B, et al. Genetic variation at the plasminogen activator inhibitor-1 locus is associated with altered levels of plasma plasminogen activator inhibitor-1 activity. *Arterioscler Thromb* 1991;11:183.

284. Dawson SJ, Wiman B, Hamsten A, et al. The two allele sequences of a common polymorphism in the promotor of the plasminogen activator inhibitor-1 (PAI-1) gene respond differently to interleukin-1 in HepG2 cells. *J Biol Chem* 1993;268:10739.

285. Ye S, Green FR, Scarabin PY, et al. The 4G/5G genetic polymorphism in the promotor of the plasminogen activator inhibitor-1 (PAI-1) gene is associated with differences in plasma PAI-1 activity but not with risk of myocardial infarction in the ECTIM study. *Thromb Haemost* 1995;74:837.

286. Burzotta F, Di Castelnuovo A, Amore C, et al. 4G/5G promoter PAI-1 gene polymorphism is associated with plasmatic PAI-1 activity in Italians: a model of gene-environment interaction. *Thromb Haemost* 1998;79:354.

287. Eriksson P, Kallin B, van't Hooft FM, et al. Allele-specific increase in basal transcription of the plasminogen-activator inhibitor-1 gene is associated with myocardial infarction. *Proc Natl Acad Sci U S A* 1995;92:1851.

288. Henry M, Chomiki N, Scarabin PY, et al. Five frequent polymorphisms of the PAI-1 gene: lack of association between genotypes, PAI activity, and triglyceride levels in a healthy population. *Arterioscler Thromb Vasc Biol* 1997;17:851.

289. Mansfield MW, Strickland MH, Grant PJ. Environmental and genetic factors in relation to elevated circulating levels of plasminogen activator inhibitor-1 in Caucasian patients with non-insulin-dependent diabetes mellitus. *Thromb Haemost* 1995;74:842.

290. Panahloo A, Mohamed-Ali V, Lane A, et al. Determinants of plasminogen activator inhibitor-1 activity in treated NIDDM and its relation to a polymorphism in the plasminogen activator inhibitor-1 gene. *Diabetes* 1995;44:37.

291. Henry M, Tregouet DA, Alessi MC, et al. Metabolic determinants are much more important than genetic polymorphisms in determining the PAI-1 activity and antigen plasma concentrations: a family study with part of the Stanislas cohort. *Arterioscler Thromb Vasc Biol* 1998;18:84.

292. Juhan-Vague I, Alessi MC. PAI-1, obesity, insulin resistance and risk of cardiovascular events. *Thromb Haemost* 1997;78:656.

293. Eriksson P, Nilsson L, Karpe F, et al. Very-low-density lipoprotein response element in the promoter region of the human plasminogen activator inhibitor-1 gene implicated in the impaired fibrinolysis of hypertriglyceridemia. *Arterioscler Thromb Vasc Biol* 1998;18:20.

294. Prins MH, Hirsh J. A critical review of the evidence supporting a relationship between impaired fibrinolytic activity and venous thromboembolism. *Arch Intern Med* 1991;151:1721.

295. Levi M, Lensing AWA, Buller HR, et al. Deep vein thrombosis and fibrinolysis. Defective urokinase type plasminogen activator release. *Thromb Haemost* 1991;66:426.

296. Grimaudo V, Bachmann F, Hauert J, et al. Hypofibrinolysis in patients with a history of idiopathic deep vein thrombosis and/or pulmonary embolism. *Thromb Haemost* 1992;67:397.

297. Ridker PM, Vaughan DE, Stampfer MJ, et al. Baseline fibrinolytic state and the risk of future venous thrombosis. A prospective study of endogenous tissue-type plasminogen activator and plasminogen activator inhibitor. *Circulation* 1992;85:1822.

298. Hamsten A, De Faire U, Walldius G, et al. Plasminogen activator inhibitor in plasma: risk factor for recurrent myocardial infarction. *Lancet* 1987;2:3.

299. Gram J, Jespersen J. A selective depression of tissue plasminogen activator (t-PA) activity in euglobulins characterises a risk group among survivors of acute myocardial infarction. *Thromb Haemost* 1987;57:137.

300. Cimmiello C. Tissue type plasminogen activator and risk of myocardial infarction. *Lancet* 1993;342:48.

301. Jansson JH, Nilsson TK, Johnson O. Von Willebrand factor in plasma: a novel risk factor for recurrent myocardial infarction and death. *BMJ* 1991;66:351.

302. Jansson JH, Nilsson TK, Olofsson BO. Tissue plasminogen activator and other risk factors as predictors of cardiovascular events in patients with severe angina pectoris. *Eur Heart J* 1991;12:157.

303. Jansson JH, Olofsson BO, Nilsson TK. Predictive value of tissue plasminogen activator mass concentration on long-term mortality in patients with coronary artery disease. A 7 year follow-up. *Circulation* 1993;88:2030.

304. Ridker PM, Vaughan DE, Stampfer MJ, et al. Endogenous tissue type plasminogen activator and risk of myocardial infarction. *Lancet* 1993;341:1165.

305. Salomaa V, Stinson V, Kark JD, et al. Association of fibrinolytic parameters with early atherosclerosis. The ARIC Study. *Circulation* 1995;91:284.

306. Schneiderman J, Sawdey MS, Keeton MR, et al. Increased type 1 plasminogen activator inhibitor gene expression in atherosclerotic human arteries. *Proc Natl Acad Sci U S A* 1992;89:6998.

307. Lupu F, Bergonzelli GE, Heim DA, et al. Localization and production of plasminogen activator inhibitor-1 in human healthy and atherosclerotic arteries. *Arterioscler Thromb* 1993;13:1090.

308. Chomiki N, Henry M, Alessi MC, et al. Plasminogen activator inhibitor 1 expression in human liver and healthy or atherosclerotic vessel walls. *Thromb Haemost* 1994;72:44.

309. Raghunath PN, Tomaszewski JE, Brady ST, et al. Plasminogen activator system in human coronary atherosclerosis. *Arterioscler Thromb Vasc Biol* 1995;15:1432.

310. Lupu F, Heim DA, Bachmann F, et al. Plasminogen activator expression in human atherosclerotic lesions. *Arterioscler Thromb Vasc Biol* 1995;15:1444.

311. Van de Loo JCW, Haverkate F, Thompson SG. Hemostatic factors and the risk of myocardial infarction. *N Engl J Med* 1995;332:389.

312. Thompson SG, Kienast J, Pyke SDM, et al. Hemostatic factors and the risk of myocardial infarction or sudden death in patients with angina pectoris. *N Engl J Med* 1995;332:635.

313. Prins MH, Hirsh J. A critical review of the relationship between impaired fibrinolysis and myocardial infarction. *Am Heart J* 1991;122:545.

314. Hamsten A, Eriksson P. Fibrinolysis and atherosclerosis. *Baillières Clin Haematol* 1995;8:345.

315. Juhan-Vague I, Pyke SDM, Alessi MC, et al. Fibrinolytic factors and the risk of myocardial infarction or sudden death in patients with angina pectoris. *Circulation* 1996;94:2057.

316. Juhan-Vague I, Alessi MC, Vague P. Increased plasma plasminogen activator inhibitor 1 levels. a possible link between insulin resistance and atherothrombosis. *Diabetologia* 1991;34:457.

317. Tenkanen L, Manttari M, Manninen V. Some coronary risk factors related to the insulin resistance syndrome and treatment with gemfibrozil. Experience from the Helsinki Heart Study. *Circulation* 1995;92:1779.

318. Andersen P, Smith P, Seljeflot I, et al. Effects of gemfibrozil on lipids and haemostasis after myocardial infarction. *Thromb Haemost* 1990;63:174.

319. Fujii S, Sobel BE. Direct effects of gemfibrozil on the fibrinolytic system. Diminution of synthesis of plasminogen activator inhibitor type 1. *Circulation* 1992;85:1888.

320. Andersen P, Seljeflot I, Abdelnoor M, et al. Increased insulin sensitivity and fibrinolytic capacity after dietary intervention in obese women with polycystic ovary syndrome. *Metabolism* 1995;44:611.

321. Juhan-Vague I, Thompson S, Jespersen J. Involvement of the hemostatic system in insulin resistance. A study of 1,500 patients with angina pectoris. *Arterioscler Thromb* 1993;13:1865.

322. Anfosso F, Chomiki N, Alessi MC, et al. Plasminogen activator inhibitor 1 synthesis in the human hepatoma cell line Hep G2. Metformin inhibits the stimulating effect of insulin. *J Clin Invest* 1993;91:2185.

323. Schneider DJ, Nordt TK, Sobel BE. Attenuated fibrinolysis and accelerated atherogenesis in type II diabetic patients. *Diabetes* 1993;42:1.

324. Lundgren CH, Brown NA, Nordt TK, et al. Elaboration of type 1 plasminogen activator inhibitor from adipocytes. A potential pathogenetic link between obesity and cardiovascular disease. *Circulation* 1996;93:106.

325. Samad F, Yamamoto K, Loskutoff DJ. Distribution and regulation of plasminogen activator inhibitor 1 in murine adipose tissue in vivo. *J Clin Invest* 1996;97:37.

326. Shimomura I, Funahashi T, Takahashi M, et al. Enhanced expression of PAI-1 in visceral fat: possible contributor to vascular disease in obesity. *Nat Med* 1996;2:800.

327. Samad F, Loskutoff DJ. The fat mouse: a powerful genetic model to study elevated plasminogen activator inhibitor 1 in obesity/NIDDM. *Thromb Haemost* 1997;78:652.

328. Cigolini M, Targher G, Bergamo Andreis IA, et al. Visceral fat accumulation and its relation to plasma hemostatic factors in healthy men. *Arterioscler Thromb Vasc Biol* 1996;16:368.

329. Janand-Delenne B, Chagnaud C, Raccah D, et al. Visceral fat as a main determinant of plasminogen activator inhibitor 1 level in women. *Int J Obes* 1998;22:312.

330. Alessi MC, Peiretti F, Morange P, et al. Production of plasminogen activator inhibitor 1 by human adipose tissue. *Diabetes* 1997;46:860.

331. Eriksson P, Reynisdottir S, Lönnqvist F, et al. Adipose tissue secretion of plasminogen activator inhibitor-I in non obese individuals. *Diabetologia* 1998;41:65.

332. Morange P, Aubert J, Peiretti F, et al. Glucocorticoids and insulin promote plasminogen activator inhibitor-1 production by human adipose tissue. *Diabetes* 1999;48:890.

333. Samad F, Loskutoff DJ. Tissue distribution and regulation of plasminogen activator inhibitor-1 in obese mice. *Mol Med* 1996;2:568.

334. Loskutoff DJ, Samad F. The adipocyte and hemostatic balance in obesity: studies of PAI-1. *Arterioscler Thromb Vasc Biol* 1998;18:1.
335. Hasegawa DK, Tyler BJ, Edson JR. Thrombotic disease in three families with inherited plasminogen deficiency. *Blood* 1982;60(Suppl A):213a.
336. Ten Cate JW, Peters M, Büller H. Isolated plasminogen deficiency in a patient with recurrent thromboembolic complications. *Thromb Haemost* 1983;50:59.
337. Lottenberg R, Dolly FR, Kitchens CS. Recurring thromboembolic disease and pulmonary hypertension associated with severe hypoplasminogenemia. *Am J Hematol* 1985;19:181.
338. Mannucci PM, Kluft C, Traas DW, et al. Congenital plasminogen deficiency associated with venous thromboembolism: therapeutic trial with stanozolol. *Br J Haematol* 1986;63:753.
339. Girolami A, Marafioti F, Rubertelli M, Cappellato MG. Congenital heterozygous plasminogen deficiency associated with a severe thrombotic tendency. *Acta Haematol* 1986;75:54.
340. Mingers AM, Heirriburger N, Zeitler P, et al. Homozygous type I plasminogen deficiency. *Semin Thromb Hemost* 1997;23:259.
341. Schuster V, Mingers AM, Seidenspinner S, et al. Homozygous mutations in the plasminogen gene of two unrelated girls with ligneous conjunctivitis. *Blood* 1997;90:958.
342. Schott D, Dempfle CE, Beck P, et al. Successful therapy with Lys-plasminogen in homozygous type I plasminogen deficiency. *Fibrinolysis Proteolysis* 1997;11(Suppl, 3):20.
343. Drew AF, Kaufman AH, Kombrinck KW, et al. Ligneous conjunctivitis in plasminogen-deficient mice. *Fibrinolysis Proteolysis* 1997;11(Suppl 3):21.
344. Ploplis VA, Carmeliet P, Vazirzadeh S, et al. Effects of disruption of the plasminogen gene on thrombosis, growth, and health in mice. *Circulation* 1995;92:2585.
345. Bugge TH, Flick MJ, Daugherty CC, et al. Plasminogen deficiency causes severe thrombosis but is compatible with development and reproduction. *Genes Dev* 1995;9:794.
346. Lijnen HR, Carmeliet P, Bouché A, et al. Restoration of thrombolytic potential in plasminogen-deficient mice by bolus administration of plasminogen. *Blood* 1996;88:870.
347. Carmeliet P, Schoonjans L, Kieckens L, et al. Physiological consequences of loss of plasminogen activator gene function in mice. *Nature* 1994;368:419.
348. Bugge TH, Kombrinck KW, Flick MJ, et al. Loss of fibrinogen rescues mice from the pleiotropic effects of plasminogen deficiency. *Cell* 1996;87:709.
349. Davis RD, Picoff RC. Low plasminogen levels and liver disease. *Am J Clin Pathol* 1969;59:175.
350. Kordich LC, Porterie VP, Lago O, et al. Mini-plasminogen like molecule in septic patients. *Thromb Res* 1987;47:553.
351. Jespersen J, Gram J, Bach E. A sequential study of plasma histidine-rich glycoprotein and plasminogen in patients with acute myocardial infarction and deep vein thrombosis. *Thromb Haemost* 1984;51:99.
352. Castel M, Horellou MH, Conard J, et al. Immunochemical determination of histidine-rich glycoprotein in healthy subjects and in a clinical population. In: Davidson JF, Bachmann F, Bouvier CA, Kruithof EKO, eds. *Progress in fibrinolysis*, vol. 6. Edinburgh: Churchill Livingstone, 1983:370.
353. Aoki N, Moroi M, Sakata Y, et al. Abnormal plasminogen: a hereditary molecular abnormality found in a patient with recurrent thrombosis. *J Clin Invest* 1978;61:1186.
354. Sakata Y, Aoki N. Molecular abnormality of plasminogen. *J Biol Chem* 1980; 255:5442.
355. Miyata T, Iwanaga S, Sakata Y, Aoki N. Plasminogen Tochigi: inactive plasmin resulting from replacement of alanine-600 by threonine in the active site. *Proc Natl Acad Sci U S A* 1982;79:6132.
356. Wohl RC, Summaria L, Robbins KC. Physiological activation of the human fibrinolytic system: isolation and characterization of human plasminogen variants, Chicago I and Chicago II. *J Biol Chem* 1979;254:9063.
357. Wohl RC, Summaria L, Chediak J, et al. Human plasminogen variant Chicago III. *Thromb Haemost* 1982;48:146.
358. Larsson LI, Skriver L, Nielsen LS, et al. Distribution of urokinase-type plasminogen activator immunoreactivity in the mouse. *J Cell Biol* 1984;98:894.
359. Blasi F. Surface receptors for urokinase plasminogen activator. *Fibrinolysis* 1988;2:73.
360. Fletcher AP, Alkjaersig N, Sherry S, et al. The development of urokinase as a thrombolytic agent: maintenance of a sustained thrombolytic state in man by its intravenous infusion. *J Lab Clin Med* 1965;65:713.
361. Smith D, Gilbert M, Owen WG. Tissue plasminogen activator release in vivo in response to vasoactive agents. *Blood* 1985;66:835.
362. Gelehrter TD, Snycer-Laszuk R, Zeheb R, et al. Dexamethasone inhibition of tissue-type plasminogen activator (t-PA) activity: paradoxical induction of both t-PA antigen and plasminogen activator inhibitor. *Mol Endocrinol* 1987;1:97.
363. Kooistra T, van den Berg J, Töns A, et al. Butyrate stimulates tissue-type plasminogen activator synthesis in cultured human endothelial cells. *Biochem J* 1987;247:605.
364. Moscatelli D. Urokinase-type and tissue-type plasminogen activators have different distributions in cultured bovine capillary endothelial cells. *J Cell Biochem* 1986;30:19.
365. Montesano R, Vassalli JD, Baird A, et al. Basic fibroblast growth factor induces angiogenesis in vitro. *Proc Natl Acad Sci U S A* 1986;83:7297.
366. Sakata Y, Curriden S, Lawrence D, et al. Activated protein C stimulates the fibrinolytic activity of cultured endothelial cells and decreases antiactivator activity. *Proc Natl Acad Sci U S A* 1985;82:1121.
367. Laug WE. Ethyl alcohol enhances plasminogen activator secretion by endothelial cells. *JAMA* 1983;250:772.
368. Kooistra T, Opdenberg JP, Toet K, et al. Stimulation of tissue-type plasminogen activator synthesis by retinoids in cultured human endothelial cells and rat tissues in vivo. *Thromb Haemost* 1991;65:565.
369. Bulens F, Ibanez-Tallon I, Van Acker P, et al. Retinoic acid induction of human tissue-type plasminogen activator (t-PA) gene expression via a direct repeat element (DR5) located at −7 kilobases. *J Biol Chem* 1995;270:7167.
370. Bulens F, Merchiers P, Ibanez-Tallon I, et al. Identification of a multihormone responsive enhancer far upstream from the human tissue-type plasminogen activator gene. *J Biol Chem* 1997;272:663.
371. Lansink M, Kooistra T. Stimulation of tissue-type plasminogen activator expression by retinoic acid in human endothelial cells requires retinoic acid receptor β_2-induction. *Blood* 1996;88:531.
372. Levin EG, Santell L. Stimulation and desensitization of tissue plasminogen activator release from human endothelial cells. *J Biol Chem* 1988;263:9360.
373. Levin EG, Marotti KR, Santell L. Protein kinase C and the stimulation of tissue plasminogen activator release from human endothelial cells. Dependence on the elevation of messenger RNA. *J Biol Chem* 1989;264:16030.
374. Arts J, Herr I, Lansink M, et al. Cell-type specific DNA-protein interactions at the tissue-type plasminogen activator promoter in human endothelial and HeLa cells in vivo and in vitro. *Nucleic Acids Res* 1997;25:311.
375. Shi GY, Hau JS, Wang SJ, et al. Plasmin and the regulation of tissue-type plasminogen activator biosynthesis in human endothelial cells. *J Biol Chem* 1992;267:19363.
376. Otter M, Zocková P, Kuiper J, et al. Isolation and characterization of the mannose receptor from human liver potentially involved in the plasma clearance of tissue-type plasminogen activator. *Hepatology* 1992;16:54.
377. Strickland DK, Kounnas MZ, Williams SE, et al. LDL receptor-related protein (LRP): a multiligand receptor. *Fibrinolysis* 1994;8(Suppl 1):204.
378. Stefansson S, Muhammad S, Cheng XF, et al. Plasminogen activator inhibitor-1 contains a cryptic high affinity binding site for the low density lipoprotein receptor-related protein. *J Biol Chem* 1998;13:6358.
379. Isacson S, Nilsson IM. Defective fibrinolysis in blood and vein walls in recurrent "idiopathic" venous thrombosis. *Acta Chir Scand* 1972;138:813.
380. Booth NA, Bennett B, Wijngaards G, et al. A new life-long hemorrhagic disorder due to excess plasminogen activator. *Blood* 1983;61:267.
381. Aznar J, Estellés A, Vila V, et al. Inherited fibrinolytic disorder due to an enhanced plasminogen activator level. *Thromb Haemost* 1984;52:196.
382. Schleef RR, Higgins DL, Pillemer E, et al. Bleeding diathesis due to decreased functional activity of type 1 plasminogen activator inhibitor. *J Clin Invest* 1989;83:1747.
383. Diéval J, Nguyen G, Gross S, et al. A lifelong bleeding disorder associated with a deficiency of plasminogen activator inhibitor type 1. *Blood* 1991;77:528.
384. Fay WP, Shapiro AD, Shih JL, et al. Brief report: complete deficiency of plasminogen activator inhibitor type 1 due to a frameshift mutation. *N Engl J Med* 1992;327:1729.
385. Dollery CM, McEwan JR, Henney AM. Matrix metalloproteinases and cardiovascular disease. *Circ Res* 1995;77:863.
386. Celentano DC, Frishman WH. Matrix metalloproteinases and coronary artery disease: a novel therapeutic target. *J Clin Pharmacol* 1997;150:761.
387. Newman KM, Jean Claude J, Li H, et al. Cellular localization of matrix metalloproteinase in the abdominal aortic aneurysm wall. *J Vasc Surg* 1994;20:814.
388. Galis ZS, Sukhova GK, Kranzhöfer R, et al. Macrophage foam cells from experimental atheroma constitutively produce matrix-degrading proteinases. *Proc Natl Acad Sci U S A* 1995;92:402.
389. Galis ZS, Muszynski M, Sukhova GK, et al. Cytokine-stimulated human vascular smooth muscle cells synthesize a complement of enzymes required for extracellular matrix digestion. *Circ Res* 1994;75:181.
390. Halpert I, Sires UI, Roby JD, et al. Matrilysin is expressed by lipid-laden macrophages at sites of potential rupture in atherosclerotic lesions and localizes to areas of versican deposition, a proteoglycan substrate for the enzyme. *Proc Natl Acad Sci U S A* 1996;93:9748.
391. Irizarry E, Newman KM, Gandhi RH, et al. Demonstration of interstitial collagenase in abdominal aortic aneurysm disease. *J Surg Res* 1993;54:571.
392. Sakalihasan N, Delvenne P, Nusgens BV, et al. Activated forms of MMP2 and MMP9 in abdominal aortic aneurysms. *J Vasc Surg* 1996;24:127.
393. Moons L, Shi V, Ploplis V, et al. Reduced transplant arteriosclerosis in plasminogen deficient mice. *J Clin Invest* 1998;102:1788.
394. Clowes AW, Clowes MM, Au YP, et al. Smooth muscle cells express urokinase during mitogenesis and tissue-type plasminogen activator during migration in injured rat carotid artery. *Circ Res* 1990;67:61.
395. Jackson CL, Reidy MA. The role of plasminogen activation in smooth muscle cell migration after arterial injury. *Ann N Y Acad Sci* 1992;667:141.
396. Reidy MA, Irvin C, Lindner V. Migration of arterial wall cells. Expression of plasminogen activators and inhibitors in injured rat arteries. *Circ Res* 1996;78:405.
397. Bendeck MP, Zempo N, Clowes AW, et al. Smooth muscle cell migration and matrix metalloproteinase expression after arterial injury in the rat. *Circ Res* 1994;75:539.
398. Zempo N, Kenagy RD, Au YPT, et al. Matrix metalloproteinases of vascular cells are increased in balloon-injured rat carotid artery. *J Vasc Surg* 1994;20:209.
399. Hasenstab D, Forough R, Clowes AW. Plasminogen activator inhibitor type 1 and tissue inhibitor of metalloproteinases-2 increase after arterial injury in rats. *Circ Res* 1997;80:490.

400. Zempo N, Koyama N, Kenagy RD, et al. Regulation of vascular smooth muscle cell migration and proliferation in vitro and in injured rat arteries by a synthetic matrix metalloproteinase inhibitor. *Arterioscler Thromb Vasc Biol* 1996;16:28.

401. Forough R, Koyama N, Hasenstab D, et al. Overexpression of tissue inhibitor of matrix metalloproteinase-1 inhibits vascular smooth muscle cell functions in vitro and in vivo. *Circ Res* 1996;79:812.

402. George SJ, Johnson JL, Angelini GD, et al. Adenovirus-mediated gene transfer of the human TIMP-1 gene inhibits smooth muscle cell migration and neointimal formation in human saphenous vein. *Hum Gene Ther* 1998; 9:867.

403. Kenagy RD, Hart CE, Stetler-Stevenson WG, et al. Primate smooth muscle cell migration from aortic explants is mediated by endogenous platelet-derived growth factor and basic fibroblast growth factor acting through matrix metalloproteinases 2 and 9. *Circulation* 1997;96:3555.

404. Kenagy RD, Vergel S, Mattsson E, et al. The role of plasminogen, plasminogen activators, and matrix metalloproteinases in primate arterial smooth muscle cell migration. *Arterioscler Thromb Vasc Biol* 1996;16:1373.

405. Aoyagi M, Yamamoto M, Azuma H, et al. Immunolocalization of matrix metalloproteinases in rabbit carotid arteries after balloon denudation. *Histochem Cell Biol* 1998;109:97.

406. Carmeliet P, Moons L, Stassen JM, et al. Vascular wound healing and neointima formation induced by perivascular electric injury in mice. *Am J Pathol* 1997;150:761.

407. Carmeliet P, Moons L, Ploplis V, et al. Impaired arterial neointima formation in mice with disruption of the plasminogen gene. *J Clin Invest* 1997;99:200.

408. Carmeliet P, Moons L, Herbert J-M, et al. Urokinase-type but not tissue-type plasminogen activator mediates arterial neointima formation in mice. *Circ Res* 1997;81:829.

409. Lijnen HR, Lupu F, Moons L, et al. Temporal and topographic matrix metalloproteinase expression after vascular injury in mice. *Thromb Haemost* 1999;81:799.

410. Lijnen HR, Soloway P, Collen D. Tissue inhibitor of matrix metalloproteinases-1 impairs arterial neointima formation after vascular injury in mice. *Circ Res* 1999;85:1186.

411. Schneiderman J, Bordin GM, Engelberg I, et al. Expression of fibrinolytic genes in atherosclerotic abdominal aortic aneurysm wall. A possible mechanism for aneurysm expansion. *J Clin Invest* 1995;96:639.

412. Lupu F, Heim DA, Bachmann F, et al. Plasminogen activator expression in human atherosclerotic lesions. *Arterioscler Thromb Vasc Biol* 1995;15:1444.

413. Plump AS, Smith JD, Hayek T, et al. Severe hypercholesterolemia and atherosclerosis in apolipoprotein E-deficient mice created by homologous recombination in ES cells. *Cell* 1992;71:343.

414. Carmeliet P, Moons L, Lijnen HR, et al. Urokinase-generated plasmin is a candidate activator of matrix metalloproteinases during atherosclerotic aneurysm formation. *Nat Genet* 1997:17:439.

415. Rouis M, Adamy C, Duverger N, et al. Adenovirus-mediated overexpression of tissue inhibitor of metalloproteinase-1 reduces atherosclerotic lesions in apolipoprotein E-deficient mice. *Circulation* 1999;100:533.

416. Allaire E, Forough R, Clowes M, et al. Local overexpression of TIMP-1 prevents aortic aneurysm degeneration and rupture in a rat model. *J Clin Invest* 1998;102:1413.

417. Schulman S, Wiman B. The significance of hypofibrinolysis for the risk of recurrence of venous thromboembolism. Duration of Anticoagulation (DURAC) Trial Study Group. *Thromb Haemost* 1996;75:607.

418. Malm J, Laurell M, Nilsson IM, et al. Thromboembolic disease. Critical evaluation of laboratory investigation. *Thromb Haemost* 1992;68:7.

419. Crowther MA, Roberts J, Roberts R, et al. Fibrinolytic variables in patients with recurrent venous thrombosis: a prospective cohort study. *Thromb Haemost* 2001;85:390.

420. Bauer KA. Conventional fibrinolytic assays for the evaluation of patients with venous thrombosis: don't bother. *Thromb Haemost* 2001;85:377.

421. Lijnen HR, Collen D. Impaired fibrinolysis and the risk for coronary heart disease. *Circulation* 1996;94:2052.

422. Wiman B, Anderson T, Hallqvist J, et al. Plasma levels of tissue plasminogen activator/plasminogen activator inhibitor-1 complex and von Willebrand factor are significant risk markers for recurrent myocardial infarction in the Stockholm heart epidemiology program (SHEEP) study. *Arterioscler Thromb Vasc Biol* 2000;20:2019.

423. Scarabin PY, Aillaud MF, Amoyel P, et al. Association of fibrinogen, factor VII and PAI-1 with baseline findings among 10,500 male participants in a prospective study of myocardial infarction: the PRIME Study. *Thromb Haemost* 1998;80:749.

424. Bounameaux H, Kruithof EK. On the association of elevated t-PA/PAI-1 complex and von Willebrand factor with recurrent myocardial infarction. *Arterioscler Thromb Vasc Biol* 2000;20:1857.

425. Reber G, Bounameaux H, Perrier A, et al. Performances of the fibrin monomer test for the exclusion of pulmonary embolism in symptomatic outpatients. *Thromb Haemost* 1999;81:221.

426. de Moerloose P, Michiels JJ, Bounameaux H. The place of D-dimer testing in an integrated approach of patients suspected of pulmonary embolism. *Semin Thromb Hemost* 1998;24:409.

CHAPTER 41

Disseminated Intravascular Coagulation

Marcel Levi, Erik C. M. van Gorp, and Hugo ten Cate

Disseminated intravascular coagulation (DIC) is a syndrome that may complicate a variety of diseases. Essentially, the term *DIC* comprises a clinicopathologic state in which a widespread systemic activation of coagulation occurs, leading to thrombotic obstruction of small and midsize vessels (1–4). This thrombus formation may hamper an adequate blood supply to various organs and may, therefore, contribute to multiple organ dysfunction. Due to ongoing activation of the coagulation system and other factors, such as impaired synthesis of platelets and coagulation proteins and increased degradation, exhaustion of coagulation factors, protease inhibitors, and platelets may occur (5–7). This situation may lead to a severe impairment of coagulation and may result in serious bleeding—in particular, in patients who are at risk for major blood loss, such as perioperative patients or trauma patients. In fact, bleeding may dominate the clinical picture of a patient with DIC. In this chapter, we review the current insight in the clinicopathologic presentation of DIC, secondary to various underlying conditions. Furthermore, the recently enhanced understanding of the pathogenesis of DIC is discussed and forms the basis for the review of current and novel diagnostic and therapeutic (supportive) strategies in patients with DIC.

HISTORIC ASPECTS

By the nineteenth century, some of the first clinical and pathologic observations related to DIC had been made. One of the first reports came from Dupuy in 1834, who described the effect of the intravenous injection of brain material in animals (8). The animals almost immediately died, and at autopsy there were widespread clots in the circulation, presumably due to what we would now call *tissue factor* (TF)–*dependent systemic activation of coagulation*. Thirty years later, Trousseau described the thrombotic tendency and the inclination of blood to clot in patients with advanced malignant disease (9). A more precise description of DIC and its underlying pathogenesis had to wait until 1955 when more insight in the mechanism of blood coagulation was attained and better laboratory tests had become available. Ratnoff and colleagues carefully described in two subsequent publications the hemostatic abnormalities that occurred in women with fetal death and amniotic fluid embolism (10). In 1965, MacKay, who was the first to realize that DIC was an "intermediary mechanism" in many diseases, published the first book on DIC (11). In subsequent years, the better understanding and the development of specific coagulation assays

have enabled a more precise insight into the mechanisms that play a role in DIC (12). Nevertheless, despite our increased knowledge and more refined therapy, the clinical management of patients with DIC often presents the modern clinician with major difficulties.

CLINICAL PRESENTATION AND DEFINITION OF DISSEMINATED INTRAVASCULAR COAGULATION

Patients with DIC may present with manifest thromboembolic disease or clinically less apparent microvascular thrombosis, which predominantly presents as multiple organ dysfunction (3,5). Alternatively, severe bleeding may be the leading symptom. Quite often, a patient with DIC has simultaneous thrombosis and bleeding, which does not facilitate a clinician's choice for the appropriate therapy (Fig. 41-1) (13–16). Interestingly, the clinical picture of a patient with DIC is often interpreted differently between specialists. Surgeons may primarily consider DIC as a bleeding disorder, whereas the (microvascular) thrombotic aspect is more often appreciated by hematologists and intensive care specialists. This different appraisal of DIC is also reflected in the many names that have been given to the disorder: defibrination syndrome (17,18), consumption coagulopathy (19), generalized intravascular coagulation (20), thrombohemorrhagic phenomenon and consumptive thrombohemorrhagic disorder (3), and, most recently, disseminated intravascular fibrin formation (21). In fact, both thrombosis and bleeding may occur at different locations and in varying intensities (Table 41-1). The thrombotic spectrum ranges from laboratory signs of hypercoagulability without clinical significance to vast intravascular deposition of fibrin, which may jeopardize the circulation. Similarly, the intensity of bleeding spans from mild blood loss that is only present with injury to spontaneous, massive, and life-threatening bleeding.

In the course of DIC, the fibrinolytic system may be activated concurrently with intravascular coagulation (22–24). Animal experiments have demonstrated that the activation of fibrinolysis drastically intensifies the bleeding tendency (25). The activation of fibrinolysis in the course of intravascular coagulation is a secondary phenomenon. Nevertheless, there are many indications that despite activation of the fibrinolytic system, plasmin generation is insufficiently capable of counteracting the intravascular fibrin formation (26,27). In fact, clinical and experimental studies indicate that the fibrinolytic system is essentially

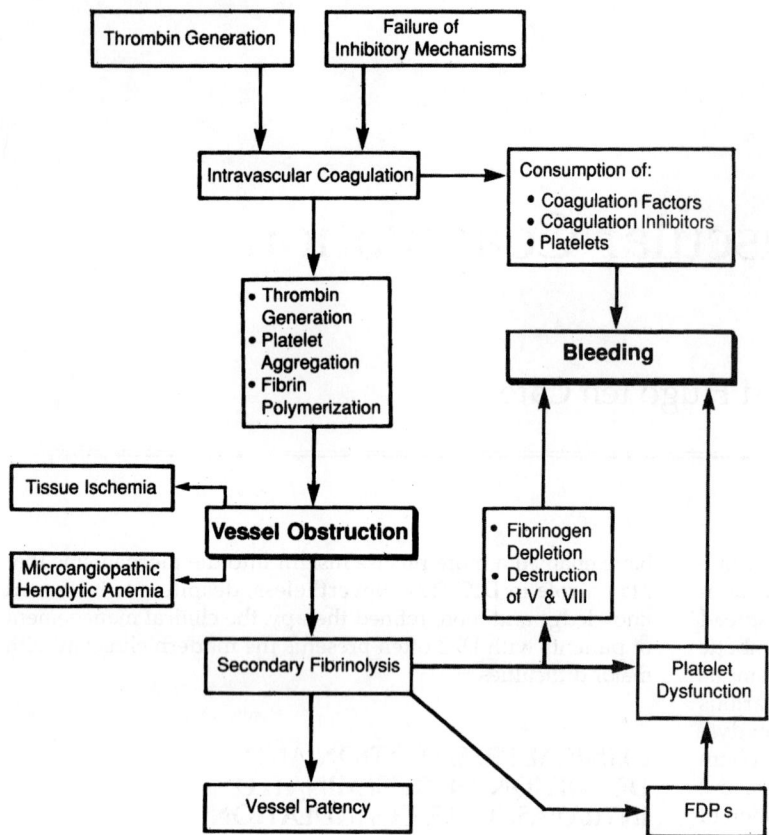

Figure 41-1. Schematic representation of the clinical picture of disseminated intravascular coagulation. FDPs, fibrin degradation products.

shut off during the initiation of DIC and may importantly contribute to the deposition of fibrin (28). An exception may be made for those rare cases of DIC, which are characterized by a severe hyperfibrinolytic state in addition to an activated coagulation system. Examples of such situations are the DIC that occurs as a complication of acute promyelocytic leukemia [acute myeloid leukemia M-3, according to the FAB (French/American/British) classification] and the DIC that may occur secondary to some forms of prostatic cancer (29,30). Although hyperfibrinolysis predominates in this situation, disseminated thrombosis is found in a considerable number of patients at

autopsy (31). Clinically, these patients suffer from severe bleeding, which (in contrast to most other forms of DIC) may benefit from therapy with antifibrinolytic agents (32).

In view of these contrasting mechanisms that occur in patients with DIC, a consensual definition of DIC has been a matter of debate for a number of years. In the 1990s, the following working definition of DIC was formulated: DIC is an acquired syndrome characterized by the activation of intravascular coagulation up to intravascular fibrin formation. The process may be accompanied by secondary fibrinolysis or inhibited fibrinolysis (21). Recently, this definition was replaced by a proposal from the subcommittee on DIC of the International Society on Thrombosis and Hemostasis, which more precisely reflects the central role of the microvascular milieu (i.e., endothelial cells, blood cells, and the plasma protease system) in the pathogenesis of DIC. This revised definition of DIC reads as follows: "DIC is an acquired syndrome characterized by the intravascular activation of coagulation without a specific localization and arising from different causes. It can originate from and cause damage to the microvasculature, which if sufficiently severe, can produce organ dysfunction" (33).

PATHOLOGIC DESCRIPTION OF DISSEMINATED INTRAVASCULAR COAGULATION

Many decades ago, disseminated microthrombi in the cerebral blood vessels of patients who presumably died from sepsis-related DIC were observed and described (34). Indeed, over the years, extensive data have been reported on postmortem findings of patients with DIC (2,11,35–41). These autopsy findings include diffuse bleeding at various sites, hemorrhagic necrosis of tissue, microthrombi in small blood vessels, and thrombi in midsize and larger arteries and veins. The observation that these

---

TABLE 41-1. Clinical Manifestations of Severe Disseminated Intravascular Coagulation

Organ	Manifestation
Skin	Purpura, bleeding from injury sites, hemorrhagic bullae, focal necrosis, acral gangrene
Cardiovascular	Shock, acidosis, myocardial infarction, cerebrovascular events, thromboembolism in all types and caliber of blood vessels
Renal	Acute renal insufficiency (acute tubular necrosis), oliguria, hematuria, renal cortical necrosis
Liver	Hepatic failure, jaundice
Lungs	Adult respiratory distress syndrome, hypoxemia, edema, hemorrhage
Gastrointestinal	Bleeding, mucosal necrosis and ulceration, intestinal ischemia
Central nervous	Coma, convulsions, focal lesions, bleeding
Adrenals	Adrenal insufficiency (hemorrhagic necrosis)

Modified from Seligsohn U. Disseminated intravascular coagulation. In: Handin RI, Lux SE, Stossel TP, eds. *Blood: principles and practice of hematology.* Philadelphia: JB Lippincott Co, 1995:1289.

TABLE 41-2. Organ Involvement by (Micro)thrombi in Patients with Disseminated Intravascular Coagulation

Organ	Mean Percentage of Patients with (Micro)thrombi at Autopsy
Kidney	70.4
Lung	70.0
Brain	41.1
Heart	40.4
Liver	39.6
Spleen	39.6
Adrenals	37.1
Pancreas	24.1
Gut	20.7

Modified from Seligsohn U. Disseminated intravascular coagulation. In: Handin RI, Lux SE, Stossel TP, eds. *Blood: principles and practice of hematology.* Philadelphia: JB Lippincott Co, 1995:1289.

findings were not present in all patients with an unambiguous clinical and laboratory picture compatible with DIC was explained by the occurrence of postmortem thrombolysis (36,40). This explanation, however, has been contested by the observation that there is no relation between the interval from death to autopsy and the apparent resolution of microthrombi (42). Furthermore, the finding of microvascular thrombosis at autopsy appeared not to be exclusively specific for the patient with DIC because this finding was occasionally also found in patients who had no apparent sign of DIC during their lives (37,38). Nevertheless, in most studies, there is a clear correlation between the presence and severity of DIC according to clinical signs, laboratory results, and the ultimate findings at autopsy. Organs most frequently involved in patients with DIC are the lungs and kidneys, followed by the brain, heart, liver, spleen, adrenals, pancreas, and intestines (Table 41-2) (35,36,39,42). Specific immunohistologic techniques and ultrastructural analysis have revealed that most thrombi consist of fibrin monomers or polymers in combination with platelets. In addition, involvement of activated mononuclear cells and other signs of inflammatory activation are frequently present. In cases of long-lasting DIC, organization and endothelialization of the microthrombi are often observed.

The relative importance of the presence of DIC in the clinical setting is not completely clear and is a subject of considerable debate. Obviously, the clinical relevance of a severe depletion of platelets and coagulation factors in patients with diffuse, widespread bleeding or in patients who need to undergo an invasive procedure is indisputable. However, it is not certain to what extent the intravascular deposition of fibrin, as a result of the systemic activation of coagulation, contributes to organ failure and mortality. Nevertheless, several lines of evidence indicate that DIC indeed contributes to multiple organ failure: First, as described above, histologic studies in patients with DIC show the presence of ischemia and necrosis due to fibrin deposition in small and midsize vessels of various organs (2,38,43). The presence of these intravascular thrombi appears to be clearly and specifically related to the clinical dysfunction of the organ. Second, experimental animal studies of DIC show fibrin deposition in various organs: Amelioration of DIC by various interventions appears to improve organ failure and, in some but not all cases, mortality (44,45). Finally, DIC has shown to be an independent predictor of mortality in patients with sepsis and severe trauma (46). Taking these data together, there appears to be sufficient evidence for a pathogenetic role of DIC in organ failure and related mortality.

PATHOGENETIC PATHWAYS IN DISSEMINATED INTRAVASCULAR COAGULATION

Initiating Factors

Traditionally, DIC was thought to be the result of activation of the combined coagulation pathways (i.e., the extrinsic and intrinsic routes) (47,48). In the classic concept of the coagulation cascade, the extrinsic route was started by a tissue-derived component, which activated plasma factor VII, leading to direct conversion of prothrombin (49). This process could proceed as long as tissue damage existed, such as during systemic infections, trauma, solutio placentae, and malignancies. Alternatively, the contact route of coagulation could be started by the contact-mediated activation of factor XII, which by the action of the cofactors kallikrein and kininogen, could convert factor XI and the further intrinsic route of coagulation (50). In the conceptual contact pathway, it has been uncertain which factors other than, perhaps, collagen and artificial surfaces would actually mediate the "contact" element. In recent years, the molecular mechanisms of both coagulation pathways have been explored and the cofactors further identified (51). In general, the current concept is that for actual thrombin and fibrin formation, the extrinsic pathway is predominant (Fig. 41-2) (52). The role, if any, of the contact system in the fibrin-forming process is currently uncertain, but several questions remain, which are addressed in the following sections.

Tissue Factor

The initiating factors comprise the molecule TF and the plasma protein factor VIIa (53). TF is a membrane-bound 4.5-kilodalton (kd) protein, which is constitutively expressed on a number of cells throughout the body (54). These cells are mostly in tissues not in direct contact with blood, such as the adventitial layer of larger blood vessels. The subcutaneous tissue also contains substantial amounts of TF, and, histologically, TF appears to be a hemostatic "envelope" (55). On expression at the cell surface, TF can interact with factor VII, either in its zymogen or activated form (56). On complexing, factor VII is activated, and the TF–factor VIIa complex catalyzes the conversion of both factors IX and X (57,58). Factors IXa and Xa enhance the activation of factors X and prothrombin, respectively (Fig 41-1). In cells that are in contact with the blood circulation, TF is induced by the action of several compounds including cytokines, C-reactive protein, and advanced glycosylated end products (55). Inducible TF is predominantly expressed by monocytes and macrophages. The expression of TF on monocytes is markedly stimulated by the presence of platelets and granulocytes in a P-selectin–dependent reaction (59). This effect may be the result of nuclear factor-κB (NF-κB) activation induced by binding of activated platelets to neutrophils and mononuclear cells. This cellular interaction also markedly enhances the production of interleukin (IL)-1B, IL-8, monocyte chemotactic protein-1, and tumor necrosis factor (TNF)-alpha (60).

Under *in vitro* conditions, different cytokines, such as TNF-α and IL-1 induce TF by vascular endothelial cells, but TF's relevance for *in vivo* coagulation is uncertain (55,61). TF's has also been localized on polymorphonuclear cells in whole blood and *ex vivo* perfusion systems, suggesting an additional pool of "bloodborne" TF (62), but it is unlikely that polymorphonuclear cells actually synthesize TF in detectable quantities (63). Finally, TF and associated procoagulant activity *in vitro* have been detected on microvesicles derived from predominantly platelets and granulocytes in patients with meningococcal sepsis (64). The localization on microvesicles may imply a highly efficient

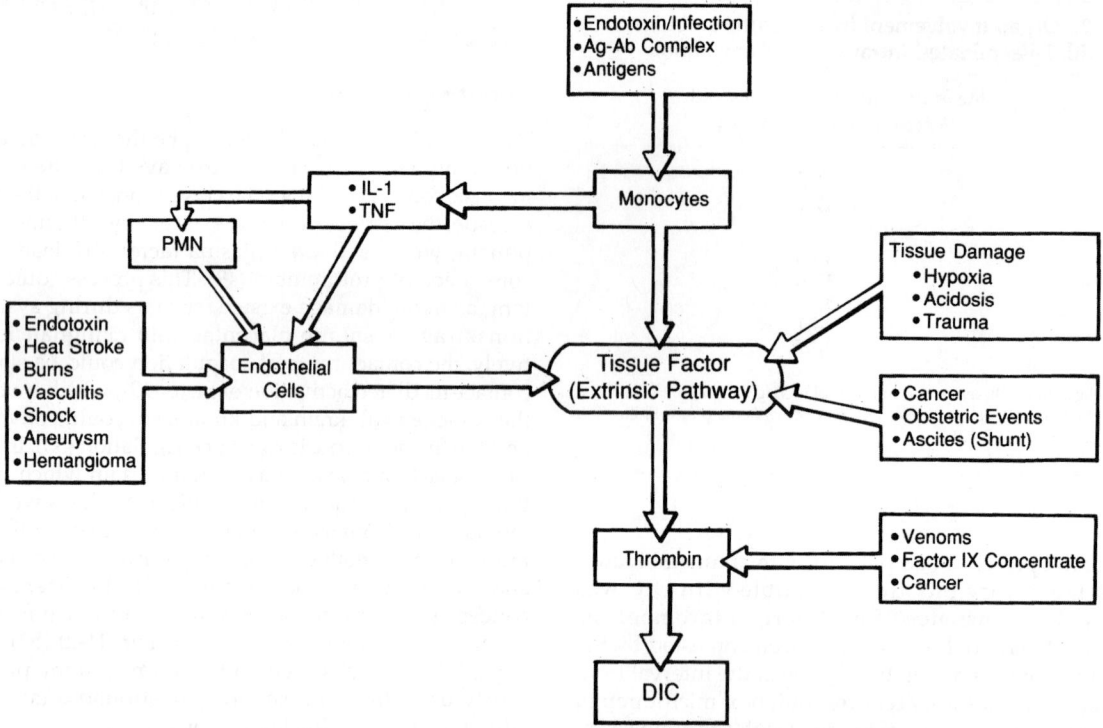

Figure 41-2. Pathogenetic pathways that may lead to disseminated intravascular coagulation (DIC). Simultaneously occurring tissue factor–driven activation of coagulation is facilitated by disruption of physiologic anticoagulant pathways, and the resulting fibrin is inadequately removed by an impaired fibrinolytic system. Ag-Ab, antigen-antibody; IL-1, interleukin-1; PMN, polymorphonuclear neutrophils; TNF, tumor necrosis factor.

pool of procoagulant material assembling not only the initiating TF–factor VIIa complex but also the phospholipid surface facilitating the development of the tenase and prothrombinase complexes. In addition, a soluble form of TF is detectable in plasma from humans, and its levels are elevated in DIC (65). The significance of soluble TF is unknown. It is likely the result of membrane cleavage by metalloproteinases produced under inflammatory conditions, and it circulates in free as well as complexed forms. Whether soluble TF is catalytically active and involved in inducing coagulation remains to be investigated.

In humans with DIC, monocytes expressing enhanced levels of TF and procoagulant activity have been demonstrated in different pathologic conditions, including sepsis (66), cancer (67), or coronary disease (68). The tissue expression of TF appears to be confined to certain organs and vascular beds, but it is uncertain whether its expression is genetically controlled in an organ-specific way. In situations of tissue trauma such as extensive surgery, brain trauma, or burns, it is likely that constitutively expressed TF at the site of injury, such as in subcutaneous tissue (69), contributes to, or is the primary source of, procoagulant stimulation of DIC, but this has not been directly demonstrated.

Contact System

Whether the contact route plays any role in humans with DIC remains unknown. Negatively charged substances including phospholipids and glycosaminoglycans are a theoretically relevant source of contact activation. Recent studies suggest that intact cell surfaces mediate the assembly of contact factor proteins that may initiate this route of activation (70). The assembly of kininogens on a multiprotein receptor leads to controlled prekallikrein (PK) activation. In the case of endothelial cells, a complex between high-molecular-weight kininogen (HMWK) and PK or factor XI binds to a multiprotein receptor on these cells. This receptor consists of cytokeratin 1, urokinase plasminogen activator receptor (uPAR), and gC1qR (70). Cytokeratin 1 was also demonstrated on platelets and granulocytes, which may allow the interaction of HMWK with these cells as well. On endothelial cells, PK activation leads to factor XII conversion, amplifying PK activation. The activation of PK causes the cleavage of HK and liberation of bradykinin. Bradykinin induces tissue plasminogen activator (TPA): This is one of the potential direct effects of the contact system on fibrinolysis (71,72).

Several lines of evidence support the important role of the contact system in activating fibrinolysis. Additional studies indicate that kininogens contain a peptide fragment that interferes with thrombin binding to platelets through preventing peptide liberation from protease-activated receptor 1 (PAR 1) by thrombin (73). Taken together, a profibrinolytic and anticoagulant function of the contact system is more likely than a procoagulant role *in vivo*.

Studies of patients suspected to have DIC have identified elevated levels of markers of activation of the contact system. Kaufmann et al. measured elevated concentrations of kininogen-a1 antitrypsin complexes (74); however, studies with similar methods for coagulation activation markers have hardly ever detected elevated levels of contact activation (75). One recent study in patients with meningococcal septicemia showed a negative correlation between plasma factor XII levels and factor XIIa–C1 inhibitor complexes (76). Although this would suggest consumption of factor XII and subsequent activation of factor XI downstream, a possible alternative explanation is a negative acute phase effect with reduced synthesis of factor XII, in conjunction with thrombin-mediated activation of factor XI (77).

Experimental studies suggested that blockade of the contact route in an *Escherichia coli* sepsis model in primates with a monoclonal antibody against factor XIIa failed to protect animals from DIC but diminished development of lethal hypotension (78). This latter study provided reasonable support for the current view that the contact activation pathway does not contribute to DIC. The contact route may play important roles in proinflammatory mechanisms related to vascular permeability, vascular proliferative processes (role of kininogen in smooth muscle cell proliferation), and stimulation of fibrinolysis (79).

Cytokines and Other Amplification Factors: Endotoxin-Induced Disseminated Intravascular Coagulation

Activation of blood coagulation requires a number of cofactors. Particularly, to develop DIC, a number of interacting surfaces from cell remnants or intact cells, inflammatory mediators, and coagulation proteins is required. The stimulus is presented by the underlying disease and can thus be diverse: a bacterial cell compound such as endotoxin; a protease induced by a malignant cell type; tissue damage exposing catalytic surfaces and constitutively expressed TF; a substance that might directly activate coagulation (fat, amniotic fluid) by unknown pathways; or others. Each of these triggers interact with other mediators: TF assembles on phospholipids; cells provide catalytic surfaces by exposure of phosphatidyl serine; and cytokines interact with receptors and induce signaling pathways that induce TF and other proinflammatory components via the NF-κB complex. To illustrate this situation, we describe in greater detail the mechanisms that lead to endotoxin-induced activation of the coagulation mechanism. This model provides the best-studied model of the complex network of interactions that involves activated coagulation in a DIC-like fashion. Endotoxin is the lipopolysaccharide compound from gram-negative bacteria inducing the sepsis syndrome and DIC. Gram-negative bacteria liberate endotoxins from their membrane, which interact with cell surfaces by different pathways. In blood, endotoxin directly binds to CD14 at monocytes and binds to endothelial cells after complexing with lipopolysaccharide binding protein (LBP) and the Toll-like receptor 4 complex (80).

By these interactions, endotoxin induces a number of signaling pathways leading to the activation of the NF-κB system, which starts the transcription of genes of proinflammatory cytokines, TF, and others. These mechanisms are further reviewed elsewhere (81).

Except for a direct positive effect of endotoxin on TF synthesis, the formation of the cytokines IL-1, TNF-α, and IL-6 stimulates TF formation (55). *Ex vivo*, this was directly demonstrated by showing that the production of TF messenger RNA was rapidly induced in blood cells after injection of endotoxin in human volunteers (82). *In vitro*, whole blood cells generate TF on incubation with endotoxin or IL-1, TNF-α, and IL-6. *In vitro*, cultured human endothelial cells also induce TF after incubation with TNF-α and IL-1, but their role in DIC remains unknown. Thus far, the only direct evidence for endothelial involvement in TF production has been the demonstration of TF's expressing circulating endothelial cells in patients with sickle cell disease (a possible DIC-associated condition) (83).

Studies in primates have revealed the molecular mechanism underlying endotoxin-induced activation of coagulation (28). After intravenous endotoxin challenge, a rapid production and liberation of proinflammatory cytokines is observed. Among these, TNF-α (84) and IL-6 (85) are important for inducing fibrinolytic and procoagulant changes in the blood. Specifically, a rapid increase in the plasma levels of TPA and the prothrombin fragment F1+2 as well as thrombin-antithrombin (AT) complexes occurs. Fibrinolytic activity indicated by plasmin-antiplasmin complexes is impaired by a subsequent rise in plasminogen activator inhibitor (PAI)-1, and a net procoagulant state results (84). Studies in baboons challenged with lethal amounts of *E. coli* (a model of gram-negative septicemia) have underscored the importance of cytokines in mediating the sepsis syndrome and have demonstrated the prolonged proinflammatory course in which the actual formation of fibrin is particularly evident at greater than 24 hours after the *E. coli* challenge (86). In fact, most fibrin appears in blood when thrombin generation is already declining, and evidence of endothelial cell activation becomes apparent, indicated by elevated levels of soluble thrombomodulin (86a). Both in the chimpanzee endotoxin model and the *E. coli* model, TF is essential for inducing coagulation activity, and inhibition of the TF pathway abolishes clotting activation (87,88). IL-6 is an important mediator of procoagulant effects, whereas TNF-α is particularly involved in the fibrinolytic response to endotoxin (89). Similarly, inhibition of TF by tissue factor pathway inhibitor (TFPI) reduced IL-6 in blood in the baboon model (44), suggesting that a more extensive crosstalk between inflammatory mediators and coagulation exists (see further). These effects may be more obvious in the sepsis model than in the endotoxin model (90); recent experiments in humans challenged with endotoxin did not reveal any effect of TFPI on IL-6 or any of the other cytokines measured in blood (91). Thus, the strength of the trigger may determine the degree of involvement of the cytokine network and its interactions with the coagulation system.

Monocytes expressing TF directly bind factor VIIa, shed TF, or become associated with the damaged vessel wall—a process probably occurring when macrophages expressing TF invade the vessel wall and play a procoagulant role in atherosclerosis (92). Circulating monocytes may trigger DIC after interacting with platelets. Microvesicles may accelerate this process, and the complex interaction between cells, membrane fragments, soluble mediators, and proteins may cause the full-blown DIC syndrome. In the endotoxin model, thrombin is an important feedback activator of the coagulation mechanism, because the thrombin-specific inhibitor hirudin reduces the procoagulant response in human volunteers (93). The extent of catalysis and exhaustion of coagulation proteins and cellular elements are primarily determined by the strength of the triggers and the potential of the inhibitory mechanisms (see below).

Coagulation Proteases Have Proinflammatory Effects: "Cross-Talk"

Coagulation activation yields proteases that interact not only with other coagulation protein zymogens but also with specific cell receptors to induce signaling pathways. Particularly, those interactions with consequences for inflammatory processes may bear importance for the development of DIC. Factor Xa, thrombin, and the factor VIIa–TF complex have each shown to elicit proinflammatory activities (94,95). In addition, fibrinogen/fibrin is of importance to the host defense mechanism, probably also by a role not directly related to clotting per se (96). Factor Xa injected into rats produced a localized inflammation, probably resulting from its interaction with endothelial protease receptor–1 (EPR-1), not mediated by thrombin (97). Exposure of cultured endothelial cells to factor Xa stimulated the production of monocyte chemotactic protein-1, IL-6, and IL-8 and up-regulated expression of adhesion proteins that mediated adhesion of polymorphonuclear leukocytes (98). Both IL-6 and IL-8 have been found to elicit TF-dependent procoagulant activity in monocytes *in vitro* (99). Furthermore, IL-6 has been identified as a critical mediator of procoagulant activity after endotoxin challenge *in vivo*, as well as a procoagulant mediator by itself (100). Thus, the stimulation of the production of these cytokines by factor Xa may have a direct impact on coagulation activity *in vivo*.

Thrombin has been shown to induce a variety of noncoagulant effects, some of which may influence DIC by influencing cytokine levels in blood. Thrombin induces production of monocyte chemotactic protein-1 (101) and IL-6 in fibroblasts, epithelial cells (102), and mononuclear cells *in vitro* (103). Stimulated whole blood produced profound IL-8 production, which had a procoagulant effect that was TF and thrombin dependent (104). Thrombin also induced IL-6 and IL-8 production in endothelial cells (103). These effects of thrombin on cell activation are probably mediated by PAR 1, 3, and 4 (105). Several studies now indicate that the factor VIIa–TF complex also activate cells by PAR binding, and it appears that, in particular, PAR 2 is involved (95). Binding of the catalytic factor VIIa–TF complex elicits a variety of inflammatory effects (106) in mononuclear cells that may influence their contribution to coagulation activity.

A direct indication of the *in vivo* relevance of these phenomena comes from a recent study showing that the infusion of recombinant factor VIIa in human volunteers caused an, albeit small, rise in plasma levels of IL-6 and IL-8 (107). Although the plasma concentrations of factor VIIa in this experiment were much higher than the endogenous factor VIIa concentrations seen in patients with sepsis, it is quite possible that the mechanism by which factor VIIa causes cytokine induction (direct or factor Xa– or thrombin-mediated) is of physiologic importance.

Taken together, a number of coagulation proteases are able to induce proinflammatory mediators that again have procoagulant effects, which may amplify the cascade that leads to DIC. The ability of the proteases to act at the cellular level is determined, among other factors, by the capacity of the coagulation inhibitors to inactivate these enzymes.

Inhibitory Mechanisms and the Balance of Proinflammatory and Procoagulant Actions

The development of DIC is counteracted by several mechanisms. First, coagulation inhibitors are present to slow down the coagulation mechanism (Fig. 41-2). Coagulation inhibitors constitute AT, protein C (PC) and protein S, and TFPI (51). AT inhibits coagulation proteases by a 1:1 complex formation, which, in the case of thrombin-antithrombin complexes, can be detected by immunoassay in plasma from patients with DIC (108,109). AT is thought to be one of the most important inhibitors of the activated coagulation system, and markedly lowered plasma levels are found in overt DIC (46,110). In the course of DIC, the function of AT may be influenced in several ways. First, a reduced absolute amount of the inhibitor may occur due to reduced protein synthesis on the one hand and clearance on the other hand. Clearance may be either in the form of protease-inhibitor complex or due to proteolytic cleavage by proteolytic enzymes including granulocyte elastase (111). Second, the function of AT may be impaired due to the possibly reduced availability of glycosaminoglycans, which may act as the physiologic heparin-like cofactor of AT (112). Under the influence of cytokines, the synthesis of glycosaminoglycans by endothelial cells may be reduced, impairing the inhibitory potential of AT (Fig. 41-3) (113). In animal models of experimental bacteremia, an AT concentrate prolonged survival and reduced the severity of DIC (45). This protective effect may have been distinct from the anticoagulant effect as such because in one of these models, an active site blocked factor Xa preparation reduced the severity of DIC but did not protect the animals from dying due to sepsis (114). The protective effect of AT may have resulted from an antiinflammatory effect. Infusion of recombinant AT at very high concentrations (approximately tenfold higher than the basal plasma concentration) markedly reduced mortality due to lethal *E. coli* infusion but also caused a significant reduction in the plasma levels of IL-6 and IL-8 (115). Despite significantly higher levels of TNF-α and lower levels of IL-10, the overall effect on DIC was apparently favorable because the reduction in fibrinogen levels was less pronounced in the AT-treated animals. An unexpected finding was that TPA levels, after an initial small rise in both groups, were markedly lower in the *E. coli*–challenged baboons that were given AT. As a result, there was no change in the levels of plasmin-antiplasmin complexes, whereas the PAI-1 levels were somewhat increased in AT-treated animals (115).

Because TNF-α is a critical mediator of fibrinolysis in primates that are given a low-dose endotoxin (84), and considering the elevated levels of TNF-α in baboons that are given AT, a marked increase in TPA and plasmin-antiplasmin complexes would have been expected in the baboon model after AT infusion. The absence of TNF-α suggests that it is not the single most important cytokine influencing fibrinolysis in sepsis. Maybe the rise of PAI-1 sufficiently blunts fibrinolysis; an alternative explanation may be a direct effect of AT at TPA release by the endothelium, which is caused by AT's binding to glycosami-

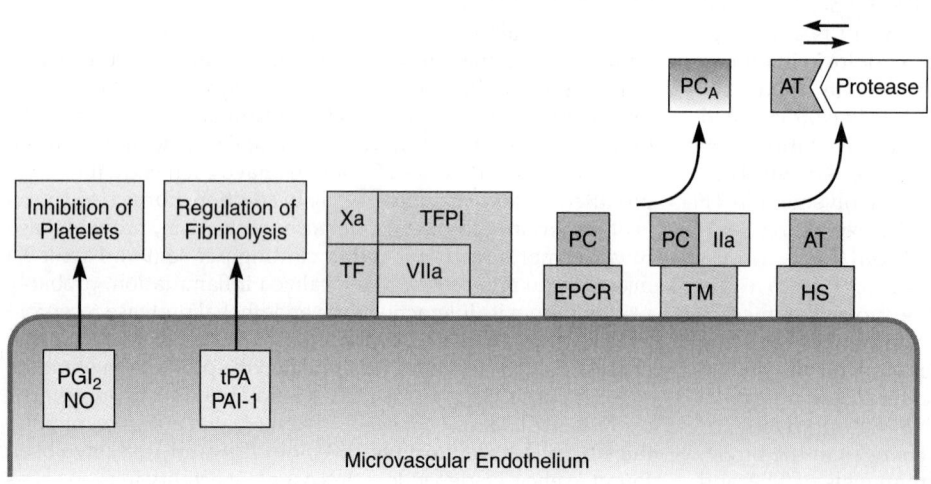

Figure 41-3. Natural endothelial cell–associated anticoagulant and regulatory mechanisms. AT, antithrombin; EPCR, endothelial protein C receptor; HS, heparan sulfate; IIa, thrombin; NO, nitrous oxide; PAI-1, plasminogen activator inhibitor-1; PC, protein C; PC$_A$, activated protein C; PGI$_2$, prostacyclin; TF, tissue factor; TFPI, tissue factor pathway inhibitor; TM, thrombomodulin; tPA, tissue plasminogen activator; VIIa, factor VIIa; Xa, factor Xa.

noglycans at the endothelial surface. Given the net negative effect on fibrinolysis and the incomplete protection achieved only at very high doses of AT, the therapeutic potential of AT may be limited.

PC and its cofactor protein S form a second line of defense. Thrombin binds to the endothelial cell membrane–associated molecule thrombomodulin, and this complex converts PC to its active form, protein Ca (PCa) (Fig. 41-3) (116). In addition, the thrombin-thrombomodulin complex accelerates the conversion of the thrombin-activatable fibrinolytic inhibitor (TAFI) (117). PCa inactivates factors Va and VIIIa by proteolytic cleavage, thus slowing down the coagulation cascade. Endothelial cells, primarily of large blood vessels, express an endothelial protein C receptor (EPCR), which augments the activation of PC at the cell surface (Fig. 41-3) (118,119). Activated PC has antiinflammatory effects on mononuclear cells and granulocytes, which may be distinct from its anticoagulant activity. Administration of PCa prevented thrombin-induced thromboembolism in mice, mainly through its antithrombotic effect (120). An antiinflammatory effect of PCa was demonstrated by Hancock et al. (121), showing reduced TNF-α production in rats challenged with endotoxin. Activated PC reduced the severity of spinal cord injury in rats, probably due to inhibition of leukocyte activity (122). In the latter model, soluble thrombomodulin had a similar antiinflammatory effect, but this was also mediated by PCa (123). In a pulmonary inflammatory model induced by endotoxin, thrombomodulin also reduced vascular permeability through a PC-dependent mechanism (124).

In contrast, defects in the PC mechanism enhance the vulnerability to inflammatory reactions and DIC. In patient studies, lowered levels of PC and protein S are associated with increased mortality. Blockade of the activity of PC by infusion of C4 binding protein turns a sublethal model of *E. coli* in baboons into a lethal model (125). Blockade of EPCR by a neutralizing monoclonal antibody also increased mortality in the *E. coli* baboon model (126). Conversely, infusion of PC in the same model protected against DIC and dying (127). Thus, it appears that the PC mechanism is of great importance in the host defense against sepsis and DIC. In situations associated with DIC and systemic inflammation, TNF-α and IL-1 may significantly down-regulate the cellular expression of thrombomodulin, as suggested by cell culture experiments (128–131). However, *in vivo* studies suggest that EPCR is not down-regulated in sepsis but up-regulated and that this effect is mediated by thrombin (132). The formation of thrombin may induce the shedding of EPCR by the endothelium due to activation of metalloproteinases by thrombin. It is presently unknown whether thrombomodulin is also cleaved by similar mechanisms.

A third inhibitory mechanism constitutes TFPI (Fig. 41-3). This molecule, which exists in several pools as either endothelial cell–associated or lipoprotein-bound in plasma, inhibits the TF–factor VIIa complex by forming a quaternary complex in which factor Xa is the fourth component (133). Clinical studies in septic patients have not provided clues as to its importance, because in the majority of patients, the levels of TFPI are not diminished as compared to normals (134). This may be explained by the lack of down-regulatory effects of inflammatory mediators on cultured endothelial cells (135). The relevance of TFPI in DIC is illustrated by two lines of experimentation. First, the depletion of TFPI sensitized rabbits to DIC that was induced with TF infusion (136). Second, TFPI infusion protected against the harmful effects of *E. coli* in primates. In this study, TFPI not only blocked DIC, but all baboons challenged with lethal amounts of *E. coli* showed a marked improvement in vital functions and survived the experiment without apparent complications (44). The benefi-

cial effects of TFPI may, in part, be due to its capacity to bind endotoxin and to interfere with its interaction with CD14 (137) and to its attenuating effect on IL-6 generation (44). A recent study in volunteers confirmed the potential of TFPI to block the procoagulant pathway triggered by endotoxin. However, in this study in healthy subjects, there was no reduction in cytokine levels, in contrast to the apparent antiinflammatory effect of TFPI in the baboon study. There are several possible explanations for this discrepancy, which all relate to the marked differences between the endotoxin and *E. coli* sepsis models in which the effects of TFPI were investigated. In the beneficial effects of TFPI on survival, antiinflammatory effects rather than antithrombotic activity may be prominent (138).

In general, the presence of intact function and normal plasma levels of inhibitors appears to be important in the defense against DIC. It should be noted, however, that there are no strong indications that individuals with congenital deficiencies of inhibitors would suffer a greater chance of developing DIC, but this issue remains to be explored. In addition, the influence of inhibitors in modifying the interaction between coagulation and inflammation deserves further attention.

Fibrinolysis

In experimental models of DIC, fibrinolysis is activated, which is demonstrated by an initial activation of fibrinolysis and followed by a marked impairment caused by the release in blood of PAI-1 (Fig. 41-2) (84,88). The latter inhibitor strongly inhibits fibrinolysis, causing a net procoagulant situation. The molecular basis is cytokine-mediated activation of vascular endothelial cells; TNF-α and IL-1 decreased TPA and increased PAI-1 production (139,140), whereas TNF-α increased urokinase-type plasminogen activator (u-PA) production in endothelial cells (141). Endotoxin and TNF-α stimulated PAI-1 production in the liver, kidney, lung, and adrenals of mice (142). The net procoagulant state is illustrated by a late rise in fibrin breakdown fragments after *E. coli* challenge of baboons. Experimental data also indicate that the fibrinolytic mechanism is active in clearing fibrin from organs and circulation. Endotoxin-induced fibrin formation in kidneys and adrenals was most dependent on a decrease in u-PA (143). PAI-1 knockout mice challenged with endotoxin did not develop thrombi in the kidney in contrast to wild-type animals (5). Endotoxin administration to mice with a functionally inactive thrombomodulin gene (TMProArg mutation) and defective PC activator cofactor function caused fibrin plugs in the pulmonary circulation, whereas wild-type animals did not develop macroscopic fibrin (144). This phenomenon proved to be temporary, with detectable thrombi at 4 hours after endotoxin and disappearance of clots at 24 hours in animals sacrificed at that time. These experiments demonstrate that fibrinolytic action is required to reduce the extent of intravascular fibrin formation.

Fibrinolytic activity is markedly regulated by PAI-1, the principal inhibitor of this system. Recent studies have shown that a functional mutation in the PAI-1 gene, the 4G/5G polymorphism, not only influenced the plasma levels of PAI-1 but also was linked to the clinical outcome of meningococcal septicemia. Patients with the 4G/4G genotype had significantly higher PAI-1 concentrations in plasma and an increased risk of death (145). Further investigations demonstrated that the PAI-1 polymorphism did not influence the risk of contracting meningitis as such but probably increased the likelihood of developing septic shock from meningococcal infection (146). These studies are the first evidence that genetically determined differences in the level of fibrinolysis influence the risk of developing complications of a gram-negative infection. In other clinical studies in cohorts of patients with DIC, high plasma levels of PAI-1 were some of the best predictors of mortality (1,22). These data suggest that DIC contributes to mortality in this situation, but as indicated earlier, owing to the fact that PAI-1 is an acute phase protein, a higher plasma concentration may also be a marker of disease rather than a causal factor.

Disseminated Intravascular Coagulation as a Systemic Complication of Disease?

The term *DIC* implies the systemic formation of fibrin in the vasculature. The terminology stems from the observation of microthrombi in the cerebral blood vessels from patients who presumably had died from sepsis-related DIC (34). Numerous subsequent studies have documented the presence of abnormalities related to DIC, including multiorgan bleeding, hemorrhagic necrosis, microthrombi in small blood vessels, and thrombi in medium and large blood vessels (11,35,147).

Several issues are involved in these observations. First, systemic activation of the coagulation mechanism is a normal phenomenon, which is quantifiable in each healthy human being, provided the test is sufficiently sensitive (148). Several factors influence coagulation activity—among these are age and disease. In a variety of disorders, systemic increased activation of coagulation can be observed in the apparent absence of thrombosis. The question of whether activated coagulation is actually DIC is a matter of definition (see diagnosis). Most definitions of DIC are based on the combination of a disease with symptoms, laboratory findings, or both that are suggestive of activated coagulation, irrespective of evidence of thrombosis (in small or large vessels) (21). Second, it is unpredictable in the individual patient whether activated coagulation actually leads to thrombosis, and this is probably dependent on several additional factors than those measured in a coagulation assay. Third, it is unclear why specific sites and organs are at greater risk of developing thrombosis; in addition, the consequences of (micro)thrombosis are still poorly understood. The occurrence of DIC may be determined by organ-specific factors that are beginning to emerge. In mice subjected to hypoxia with disturbances in fibrinolytic activity, the formation of fibrin is induced and is particularly evident in the lungs (143). Similarly, mice with a functional thrombomodulin deficiency had a marked increase in pulmonary fibrin deposition after hypoxic challenge (149). In addition, when mice with a functional defect in the thrombomodulin gene were challenged with endotoxin in sublethal amounts, fibrin formation was apparent in the lungs but not in any other organ studied. In the latter model, fibrin was only temporarily present and had disappeared after 24 hours (144). These models illustrate the assumption that fibrin formation is a localized phenomenon rather than a generalized process. Despite the limitations of the models used, it is likely that localization factors are involved. In the pulmonary circulation, granulocytes and mononuclear cells may become pooled in adherence to the endothelium after inflammatory challenge. The induction of TF on these cells in the pulmonary vasculature may cause fibrin to form. The presence of inflammatory mediators contributes to pulmonary vascular leakage and adult respiratory distress syndrome (ARDS) development when the underlying disease persists (see further) (150). Localization of coagulation activity may relate to organ- as well as cell-specific gene expression. Inflammatory mediators enhance PAI-1 gene expression in a complex and tissue-specific way (142). Recent studies have demonstrated that the von Willebrand factor promotor contains cell-specific elements, and similar response elements may be involved in protein synthesis in cells in general (151). In addition, the tissue environment may determine whether specific gene transcription occurs (152). We assume that this process is critical in determining the formation of thrombi in DIC, and this process needs further investigation.

The latter aspect is important for DIC in general: It is unknown how relevant intravascular fibrin formation is for the pathophysiology of multiorgan failure in patients with a severe underlying disease. On the basis of specific organ involvement, we consider the potential relevance of DIC for organ failure.

In a large series of autopsy examinations of patients suspected to have had DIC, the kidneys and lungs were most frequently involved by diffuse microthrombi (Table 41-2), and we focus on the association between clotting and these two organ systems in the following sections.

Disseminated Intravascular Coagulation and the Kidney

Coagulation is important in two groups of renal disorders in humans. In one group, the kidney is the major site of disease and localized thrombosis, and fibrin formation is superimposed on demonstrable immunologic and/or endothelial damage. These disorders are not discussed here. In the second group, renal lesions associated with fibrin formation are involved in a systemic disorder; in this particular group, the term *DIC* is appropriate (153). In the latter group, acute renal failure (ARF) is the usual associated renal presentation, occurring in the course of sepsis, major surgery, severe trauma, and hypovolemic and cardiogenic shock. The pathogenesis of ARF in these conditions is caused by hypoperfusion resulting in ischemia-reperfusion injury. The decrease in oxygen saturation and hormonal dysregulation causes acute tubular necrosis (154). At least in septic shock, it has been suggested that microthrombi contribute to ARF (155–157). The older literature strongly suggests that intravascular coagulation causes immediate changes that are detrimental to renal function (158). Electron-microscopic studies have shown that coagulation causes mesangial swelling and an increase in vacuoles, organelle-free ribosomes, and mitochondria (159). These changes were associated with phagocytosis of fibrin and secretion of basement membrane–like material. Within hours, increased fibrinolytic activity can be detected in glomeruli (160). The glomerular lesions occurring in the course of DIC may resemble those seen in acute glomerulonephritis, with platelets and fibrin deposits intraluminally, swollen endothelium, subendothelial deposits of fibrin cleavage fragments, and cellular proliferative effects (159). When these processes continue, complete occlusion of glomerular capillaries and hyalinization of glomeruli may follow (159,161). The pathophysiology of renal failure in shock is also thought to be influenced by vasoactive substances, and renal damage was markedly reduced by adrenergic blockade in a model of hemorrhagic shock or endotoxin shock (162,163). Catecholamine infusion in experimental animals causes shock and DIC (164). Renal cortical necrosis, as may occur late in pregnancy, can also be prevented by adrenergic blockade (163). Heparin reduces the effects of catecholamine-induced shock and endotoxin-related complications in animal models (164,165). Heparin does not abolish catecholamine-induced hemolysis (166). It thus appears that the combination of hypoperfusion-related ischemia-reperfusion injury and vasoactive reactions are of major influence on the occurrence of ARF in shock. The finding of fibrin deposits suggests that DIC contributes to organ damage, and the observed improvement under heparin treatment supports this concept. The trigger to thrombosis is probably locally induced by the ischemia-reperfusion responses of hypoxia-inducible, factor-mediated TF expression (167). In addition, systemic stimuli such as endotoxin cause the cytokine-mediated up-regulation of TF messenger RNA in the kidney, whereas local fibrinolytic defense mechanisms are also activated (u-PA and TPA, without concurrent up-regulation of PAI-1). Furthermore, experimental studies have demonstrated that specific blockade of the factor VII–TF complex reduced fibrin in the kidney (168). Infusion of hirudin caused a dose-dependent decrease in mortality and also reduced the amount of fibrin deposition in the kidney (169). It therefore appears that inhibition of coagulation also reduces the amount of fibrin in the kidney. This may imply an improvement of renal function; however, there have been no controlled trials in which the beneficial effect of anticoagulant treatment in patients with DIC and ARF was investigated. The causal association between DIC and ARF remains, in part, speculative.

Disseminated Intravascular Coagulation and the Lung

Respiratory problems occur frequently in the course of severe systemic diseases, often in association with DIC. The pulmonary syndrome occurring in the course of these disorders is referred to as *ARDS* (170). This condition is frequently associated with intraalveolar and intravascular fibrin formation (171–173). This is probably due to both systemic and local mediators of procoagulant reactions (174). It has been shown that intraalveolar fibrin formation is TF driven and may be facilitated by low concentrations of protease inhibitors (175,176). In addition, depressed intraalveolar fibrinolysis may further promote fibrin deposition (177,178). In sepsis, the liberation of endotoxin from gram-negative bacteria is known to also cause ARDS. In experimental models, these effects can be mimicked by either systemic administration of endotoxin or local infusion of endotoxin in the bronchi (178). Hemorrhagic shock may potentiate the effects of low doses of endotoxin (179), establishing a procoagulant environment in the lung mediated by reactive oxygen intermediates and TNF-α. Local production of TF, detectable in bronchoalveolar lavage fluid, may trigger the procoagulant reactions (180). Markers of DIC were markedly more elevated in patients with prolonged systemic inflammatory response syndrome and in those in whom the prevalence of ARDS was increased (181). In another study, these investigators established that all patients with ARDS had laboratory evidence of DIC (182). In addition to activated coagulation, elevated neutrophil elastase was measured in patients with ARDS, and activation of complement is probably also related to ARDS (183). The inflammatory component involved in ARDS may be distinct from the pathway that leads to fibrin formation. In a rat model of *E. coli*–induced pulmonary injury, a synthetic specific inhibitor of kallikrein prevented pulmonary vascular injury but did not inhibit DIC. In contrast, active site–blocked factor VIIa inhibited DIC but not pulmonary injury, suggesting that the inflammatory and coagulation reactions in the lungs to endotoxin are not exclusively associated (184).

CLINICAL CONDITIONS ASSOCIATED WITH DISSEMINATED INTRAVASCULAR COAGULATION

A spectrum of clinical entities has been associated with DIC (1,2,185), and the major conditions are listed in Table 41-3. The frequency of DIC in these diseases varies considerably, ranging from rare or doubtful according to current criteria for DIC to virtually obligatory (gram-negative sepsis). Here, we indicate some of the characteristic features of the listed diseases in relation to the development of DIC and indicate specific risk factors.

TABLE 41-3. Clinical Conditions That May Be Complicated by Disseminated Intravascular Coagulation

Sepsis/severe infection
Trauma
Malignancy
   Solid tumors
   Acute leukemia
Obstetric conditions
   Amniotic fluid embolism
   Abruptio placentae
   (Pre)eclampsia
Vascular abnormalities
   Kasabach-Merritt syndrome
   Other vascular malformations
   Aortic aneurysms
Severe allergic/toxic reactions
Severe immunologic reactions (e.g., transfusion reaction)
Heatstroke

Infectious Disease

Infection may result in thrombohemorrhagic syndromes such as DIC, hemolytic uremic syndrome (HUS), thrombotic thrombocytopenic purpura (TTP), or vasculitis. Symptoms and signs may be dominated by bleeding, thrombosis, or both (1,186). DIC may contribute to multiorgan failure and is associated with a high mortality (3).

Clinically overt DIC may occur in 30% to 50% of patients with gram-negative sepsis (110,187,188). Contrary to widely held belief, clinically DIC appears as commonly in patients with gram-positive sepsis as in those with gram-negative sepsis (189). Activation of the coagulation system has also been documented for nonbacterial pathogens [i.e., viruses (causing hemorrhagic fevers) (190,191), protozoa (malaria) (192,193), and fungi (194)].

Although direct interactions between the infectious agent and the coagulation system occur, cytokines are believed to be important mediators in this process, although the interactions are complicated and the effects are time dependent and transient (195).

During systemic gram-negative and gram-positive bacterial infections, activation of coagulation is mediated via the extrinsic TF pathway. Experimental studies suggest that, as a rule, coagulation and fibrinolysis occur independently of one another, and the overall result is usually a procoagulant tendency. The latter situation may result in DIC with microvascular thrombosis and multiorgan failure. Bleeding may result from consumption of platelets and clotting proteins in traumatized tissues (Fig. 41-1) (1,196).

In some cases of multiorgan failure, bleeding and (microvascular) thrombosis may be coexisting features, which make it impossible to determine the principal defect (thrombosis or bleeding). In its most severe form, this combination may present as the Waterhouse-Friderichsen syndrome, which is most commonly seen during fulminant meningococcal septicemia, although many other microorganisms may cause this clinical state (197–204). The variety and complexity of the clinical presentation of the coagulopathy syndromes confront the clinician with the difficult question of whether, when, and how to provide optimal supportive care and to combat the coagulation disorders, in addition to giving antimicrobial therapy. In making this decision, he or she is probably guided by the clinically most pronounced presenting symptom. Taking these considerations into account, the classification of clinical entities according to bleeding, thrombosis, or both is the basis for discussion, although the complexity and overlap in clinical presentation must be kept in mind.

Clinical Aspects of Hemostasis in Bacterial and Viral Infections

THROMBOSIS AND SYSTEMIC ACTIVATION OF COAGULATION

Viral and bacterial infections may result in an enhanced risk for local thromboembolic disease (i.e., deep venous thrombosis or pulmonary embolism). In a thromboembolic prevention study of low-dose subcutaneous standard heparin for hospitalized patients with infectious diseases, morbidity due to thromboembolic disease was significantly reduced in the heparin group compared to the group receiving no prophylaxis. There was, however, no beneficial effect of prophylaxis on mortality due to thromboembolic complications (205). In chronic viral diseases, such as cytomegalovirus (CMV) or human immunodeficiency virus (HIV) infection, the risk of thromboembolic complications is relatively low (206–208).

Viral hemorrhagic fever is complicated by DIC in the most severe cases (209–215). DIC is not frequently encountered in other viral infections (3) but has been reported in cases of infection with rotavirus (216,217), varicella, rubella, rubeola, and influenza (218–224).

TTP and HUS, triggered by a viral or bacterial infection (225–227), frequently lead to bleeding symptoms, as has been discussed, but also platelet and fibrin thrombi may be generated in various organs, leading to prominent symptoms with organ dysfunction.

HEMORRHAGE

Bleeding in infectious disease is most likely a multifactorial process, resulting from a combination of thrombocytopenia, consumption of clotting factors, (local) hyperfibrinolysis, and vascular damage or leakage. In addition, immunologically mediated vasculitis may contribute to bleeding in specific infections.

Hemorrhage may occur as a single clinical phenomenon or may be part of a more complex derangement of the coagulation cascade due to DIC or septic vasculitis, as in gram-negative bacterial sepsis (i.e., meningococcemia) (197–199). Severity may vary from local defects in hemostasis with oozing from arterial or venous puncture sites to more general complications such as petechiae, purpura, ecchymosis, gut bleeding, hemoptysis, or even severe adrenal bleeding (as in the Waterhouse-Friderichsen syndrome). The clinical signs are not pathogen specific and, in general, depend on the severity of infection.

In specific infections, such as viral hemorrhagic fever, bleeding complications are prominent (209–211). In other viral and bacterial infections associated with TTP or HUS, bleeding also is often the prominent and presenting symptom (Table 41-4) (225–228).

TABLE 41-4. Viral Hemorrhagic Fevers

Virus	Geographic Distribution	Source of Infection
Dengue HF	Southeast Asia, Caribbean, Middle/South America, China	Mosquito
Chikungunya	Southeast Asia	Mosquito
Ebola	Zaire, Sudan	Unknown
Marburg HF	Zimbabwe, Kenya, Uganda	Unknown
Lassa fever	West Africa	Rodent
Yellow fever	South America, Africa	Mosquito
Omsk HF	Former Soviet Union	Tick
Hantaan	Central Europe, former Soviet Union, Korea, Japan, eastern China	Rodent

HF, hemorrhagic fever.

VASCULITIS

Bacterial and viral infections may result in a vasculitis-like syndrome with either bleeding manifestations or ischemic injury (196,229,230). Vasculitis is a well-documented phenomenon in CMV infection (231,232), occurring predominantly in the vasculature of the gastrointestinal tract where it causes colitis (233,234), in the central nervous system where it causes cerebral infarction (235,236), and in the skin where it results in petechiae, purpura papules, localized ulcers, or a diffuse maculopapular eruption (237). HIV infection may be accompanied by vasculitis syndromes (e.g., polyarteritis nodosa, Henoch-Schönlein purpura, and leukocytoclastic vasculitis) (238–241). Hepatitis B and C infections may cause polyarteritis-like vasculitis (242–244). Parvovirus B19 has been suggested to be associated with vasculitis-like syndromes including Kawasaki disease, polyarteritis nodosa, and Wegener granulomatosis (245–247).

Specific Features of the Pathogenesis of Disseminated Intravascular Coagulation in Infectious Disease

Much of our knowledge on the mechanisms that play a role in DIC comes from observations in clinical and experimental infectious disease. Essentially, and as outlined in detail in the preceding paragraphs, several pathways appear to play a role, including TF-mediated generation of thrombin, impairment of physiologic anticoagulant mechanisms, and a depression of the fibrinolytic system due to elevated levels of PAI-1 (12). In addition, specific features of DIC in patients with infectious disease may be appreciated.

ENDOTHELIAL CELL ACTIVATION

Endothelial cells may turn into a procoagulant state either by stimulation of cytokines in concert with circulating blood cells, such as lymphocytes or platelets, or by direct infection (viruses) of endothelial cells. The role of endothelial cells seems to be crucial in the development of shock and activation of coagulation (248–250). Endothelial cell injury is a common feature of viral infection and can alter hemostasis in a direct or indirect manner. The endothelial cell can be directly infected by different viruses (251–253) [e.g., herpes simplex virus, adenovirus, parainfluenza virus, poliovirus, echovirus, measles virus, mumps virus (251), CMV (232), human T-cell leukemia virus type 1 (254), and HIV (255)]. The ability to infect endothelial cells has also been demonstrated in hemorrhagic fevers due to dengue virus, Marburg virus, Ebola virus, Hantaan virus, and Lassa virus (256). Such infections may result in a procoagulant state, mainly by inducing TF expression on the endothelial surface (257–259), probably mediated by cytokines such as IL-1, TNF-α, and IL-6 (257,259–267). However, not all viral infections affecting endothelial cells result in activation of coagulation, which may indicate that activation of endothelium is one factor in a multifactorial process.

The change of the endothelial cell from a resting to a procoagulant state may be associated with expression of endothelial surface adhesion molecules (264,268,269). These molecules (i.e., intercellular adhesion molecule, vascular cell adhesion molecule, E-selectin, and von Willebrand factor) play an essential role in the binding of leukocytes, resulting in a local inflammatory response, endothelial cell damage, and subsequent plasma leakage and shock (270–272). The finding of increased plasma concentrations of these endothelial surface adhesion molecules is thought to be a reflection of the level of activation and perhaps damage of the endothelial cell (273–275).

ALTERATIONS IN THE PROTEINS-C AND -S SYSTEMS

During sepsis, the PC/protein-S system is down-regulated (90,276) as described earlier. Some viruses have the ability to induce specific changes in the coagulation inhibitory system. In the course of HIV infection, the PC/protein-S system may be impaired as a result of an acquired protein-S deficiency, the pathogenesis of which is not yet clarified (277–280). In children, protein-S deficiency seems to correlate with the duration of HIV infection (277), but such a relationship has not been demonstrated in adults (278). Increased plasma concentrations of the C4b-binding protein, an acute phase protein that binds protein S, may result in decreased levels of free protein S. Antiphospholipid antibodies, which may be present in HIV patients, might interfere with the PC/protein-S complex and diminish its activity (278,281–284). In patients with dengue hemorrhagic fever, we also found decreased levels of both PC and protein-S activity (284a). As in dengue, HIV can affect the endothelial cell; hypothetically, this could lead to decreased production of protein S.

THROMBOCYTOPENIA

Thrombocytopenia is seen in the course of many viral infections but is only occasionally serious enough to lead to hemostatic impairment and bleeding complications. It is assumed that thrombocytopenia is mainly immune mediated (285). Alternative mechanisms are decreased thrombopoiesis (286), increased platelet consumption (287), or a combination of both. Direct interaction of the virus with platelets may lead to thrombocytopenia, thrombocytopathy, or both (190,288,289). Endothelial injury by the virus may lead to increased adherence and consumption of platelets (290,291).

Viral infections that have been associated with thrombocytopenia are mumps (292), rubella (293,294), rubeola (295), varicella (296,297), disseminated herpes simplex (298), CMV (299,300), infectious mononucleosis (301–303), Hantaan virus infection (304), dengue hemorrhagic fever (190,288,305), Crimean-Congo hemorrhagic fever (306), and Marburg hemorrhagic fever (212). Dengue fever is associated with thrombocytopenia even in mild and uncomplicated cases (190), and, therefore, thrombocytopenia cannot be the only explanation for the occurrence of bleeding.

Trauma

Polytrauma by physical force, due to burns, or induced by heat stroke may result in DIC due to a combination of mechanisms including hemolysis, endothelial activation, release of tissue material in the circulation (fat, phospholipids), and acidosis due to hypoperfusion. In addition, systemic infection frequently contributes to the development of DIC (185).

DIC as a consequence of trauma was first demonstrated in dogs whose femoral diaphyses were fractured (307). Shortly thereafter, clinical and laboratory signs of DIC were extensively studied in a series of patients. Several mechanisms may be responsible for the development or aggravation of DIC in patients with traumatic injuries (308–312):

- Entry of TF into the circulation, which is prominent in extensive trauma and injury of tissues rich in TF such as the brain
- Trauma-induced hemorrhage and hemorrhagic shock leading to depletion of hemostatic factors, accelerated coagulation, and impaired clearance of procoagulants
- Superimposed infections and septicemia
- Multiple transfusions of stored blood that does not contain platelets, factor V, and factor VIII, thus further diluting the concentration of these essential components

- Defense mechanisms that are impeded after direct injury to the liver or, if hepatic dysfunction follows hemorrhagic shock, from microthrombosis of hepatic vessels
- Respiratory distress syndrome, also termed *shock lung*, in which extensive damage to pulmonary vessels initiates the coagulation system
- Tissue damage inflicted by the complex mechanisms of post-ischemic reperfusion (generation of oxygen radicals, calcium overload as a consequence of severed blood vessels, or application of tourniquets)

Despite these proposed mechanisms, it has become increasingly clear that cytokines play a pivotal role in the DIC associated with trauma. In fact, systemic cytokine patterns have been shown to be virtually identical in trauma patients as compared with septic patients (313).

Fat embolism is another important factor to be considered. This syndrome, which was first described by Zenker (314) in the nineteenth century, can occur in patients within 48 hours of trauma (315–317). Fat embolism is characterized by a triad of respiratory insufficiency, neurologic dysfunction, and bleeding; in most cases, it stems from the entry into the circulation of marrow fat from injured bones. Occasionally, the syndrome follows trauma in which no involvement of bone is seen. Three types of response to fat embolism were defined (317):

1. A hyperacute fatal type in which paradoxic systemic embolization is responsible for death soon after trauma.
2. The classic type characterized by respiratory distress due to obstruction of pulmonary capillaries and arterioles with fat droplets and by interstitial pulmonary edema and slight consumption of hemostatic factors; notable in this type is the absence of extensive alveolar hemorrhage or hyaline membrane formation.
3. A third type characterized by ARDS with diffuse fat embolization of pulmonary vessels, hemorrhagic necrosis, edema, hyaline membrane formation in alveoli, and prominent laboratory evidence of DIC; the initiation of fat embolism is probably caused by damage of the endothelium of pulmonary vessels, by release of TF from ischemic pulmonary tissue or from other sites of fat embolization, and by inhibition of fibrinolysis.

The time interval between trauma and medical attention is also important. Experience with a large series of trauma cases managed during the Vietnam war proved that fast evacuation and prompt medical care reduced the risk of complications by DIC (311). This advantage probably stems from the shorter time of exposure of circulating blood to TF.

Brain tissue contains large amounts of TF. The catastrophic effects of brain extracts, which were injected intravenously into animals, were first reported by Dupuy in 1834 (8). The earliest clinical observations on DIC and bleeding after brain injury were made in 1968 (308) and thereafter were well established (318–322). The course of DIC in brain-injured patients is self-limiting, probably because of the transient exposure of blood to TF. The combination of severe injury and depleted hemostatic factors may result in significant bleeding. Transfusion of platelets and plasma components effectively arrests the bleeding (318). In fatal cases, DIC was confirmed by the presence of microthrombi in the brain, liver, lungs, kidneys, and pancreas (323). Studies of adults and children with head injuries have shown a high rate of mortality when laboratory tests were indicative of DIC (322,324,325). Moreover, a laboratory DIC score had a predictive value for prognosis of patients with head injuries, thereby supplementing the Glasgow Coma Scale (325).

Malignancy

It is quite obvious that there is a relationship between the presence of cancer and the occurrence of thrombotic disease. Less clear, however, is how much of the manifestation of clinically overt thromboembolism can be ascribed to malignancy-associated DIC. There is ample evidence for a procoagulant state in virtually all patients with advanced malignant disease; however, the incidence of overt DIC appears to be much lower (326). The exact incidence of DIC in patients with solid tumors cannot be inferred from the literature, but in patients presenting with acute leukemia, in particular acute lymphoblastic leukemia, DIC can be diagnosed in 15% to 20% (327). In patients with acute promyelocytic leukemia (acute myelogenous leukemia M-3), DIC may be diagnosed in more than 90% of patients at the time of diagnosis or after initiation of remission induction (29). As further outlined in this paragraph, the DIC that accompanies this form of leukemia has distinct features, characterized by a frank hyperfibrinolytic state, which often leads to serious bleeding. Some reports indicate that the incidence of DIC in acute leukemia patients might further increase during remission induction with chemotherapy (327).

Solid tumor cells can express different procoagulant molecules, including TF, which assembles with factor VIIa to activate factors IX and X, and a cancer procoagulant, a cysteine protease with factor X–activating properties (328). Recent studies show the occurrence of functionally active TF in vascular endothelial cells as well as tumor cells in breast cancer, whereas this does not appear in material from patients with benign fibrocystic breast disease (329,330). It should be noted that the roles of TF in pathophysiology are only partly understood as yet. Independent from its clotting cofactor function, TF appears to be involved in tumor metastasis (331) and angiogenesis (332), factors that may directly influence the course of malignancy and affect the occurrence of thrombosis.

Cellular factors presumably precipitate coagulation activation in patients with, in most cases, solid tumors. In addition, in a series of patients with malignant neoplasms, high endothelin plasma levels correlated well with progression of DIC, suggesting that this protein may influence the development of DIC in cancer (333).

In summary, the following procoagulant mechanisms have been proposed in the pathogenesis of DIC associated with malignant disease:

- TF that is found in neoplastic cells as well as in leukemic cells may initiate the activation of the coagulation cascade (330,334,335).
- TF produced by circulating monocytes in response to an interaction with tumor antigens or complexes of tumor antigens with host antibodies: A good correlation was found between the amount of TF generated *in vitro* by monocytes and markers of coagulation activation in patients with malignancies from whom these cells were obtained (67).
- A hitherto unidentified protease that activates factor X may play a role in some cases (336): This proteolytic activity has been identified in serosal fluids and in mucus, which helps to explain the predilection of DIC to patients with mucin-secreting adenocarcinomas.
- Adhesion and aggregation of platelets and extravascular fibrin deposition by malignant cells and tissues (328); these accessory mechanisms promote intravascular clotting and consumption of hemostatic components.

As mentioned before, the coagulopathy that accompanies acute promyelocytic leukemia is often seen as one of the most straightforward forms of DIC's complicating malignancy (337,338). However, this form of leukemia-associated hemostatic derangement can be considered as an exceptional type of DIC. The clinical presentation of severe bleeding associated with laboratory findings of a low fibrinogen level, very high levels of fibrin split products and fibrinogen degradation products, and massive consumption of plasminogen and α_2-antiplasmin (leading to inordinately high levels of plasmin-α_2-antiplasmin complex levels) point to a marked hyperfibrinolytic state (29,338). The precise pathogenesis of this hyperfibrinolysis has, however, not been elucidated. Plasma levels of physiologic plasminogen activators (such as u-PA and tissue-type plasminogen activator) cannot explain the massive plasminogen activation, and a role of leukocytic elastase-mediated hyperfibrinolysis is not likely. A recent report points to a potential newly described receptor for fibrinolytic proteins, annexin II, that is expressed on the surface of leukemic cells in patients with acute promyelocytic leukemia. Annexin II may facilitate plasmin generation at the surface of the cells and may thereby play a pivotal role in the development of the hyperfibrinolytic state (339). Despite the prominent role of hyperfibrinolysis in patients with acute promyelocytic leukemia, there is mounting evidence that this derangement is superimposed on a more common presentation of DIC, characterized by coagulation activation and fibrin deposition. Indeed, diffuse thrombosis is found in 15% to 25% of cases at autopsy (31,340), and recent studies have demonstrated TF-dependent activation of coagulation in this patient category. Interestingly, the current treatment with all-*trans*-retinoic acid, however, has drastically reduced the incidence of severe DIC in patients with acute promyelocytic leukemia (341).

Hepatic Disease

Although there has been considerable debate about the interpretation of clotting abnormalities in patients with liver disease, particularly liver cirrhosis, current evidence favors chronic (low-grade) DIC in this disorder (342).

Several laboratory and clinical observations support the hypothesis that DIC accompanies hepatic disorders. These observations include a shortened half-life of radiolabeled fibrinogen and prolongation of its survival by administration of heparin (343,344); failure of extensive replacement to increase significantly the levels of hemostatic factors, suggesting continuous consumption; the beneficial effects of heparin in the management of some patients with acute hepatic failure (345); and the increased blood levels of D-dimer and fibrinopeptide A indicative of thrombin generation (346,347).

Other investigators have maintained that DIC is not associated with liver disease. The observations and arguments in favor of this hypothesis include the presence of an extremely low incidence (2.2%) of microthrombosis in the tissues of patients who died of liver disease (147) and the fact that many of the hemostatic abnormalities of patients with hepatic disorders can stem from causes other than DIC or are not consistent with DIC. Examples are a prolonged thrombin time due to dysfibrinogenemia; low levels of coagulation factors and inhibitors that may be related to reduced synthesis; increased fibrin degradation product (FDP) levels that may be a consequence of primary fibrinogenolysis; increased (rather than decreased) factor VIII clotting activity; interpretation of excessive consumption of fibrinogen as loss of fibrinogen into extravascular spaces; and data showing normal decay of endogenously labeled semethionine-75 fibrinogen and plasminogen (348).

A third hypothesis maintains that patients with liver disease usually do not present with DIC but are extremely sensitive to the various triggers of DIC in view of their impeded capacity to clear procoagulants and synthesize essential components of coagulation inhibitory and fibrinolytic systems. An extreme sensitivity toward DIC has been demonstrated in patients who had primary or metastatic liver disease and who underwent a peritoneovenous shunt operation for severe ascites (see further); this is in contrast to patients who underwent the same procedure for ascites due to other causes (349).

In summary, the most important factors influencing the systemic activation of coagulation that accompanies advanced liver disease are reduced clearance in combination with reduced levels of physiologic anticoagulant proteins, due to impaired synthesis by the liver. The severity of DIC correlates with the degree of liver disease, and it is likely that the coagulopathy contributes to the hemorrhagic tendency in these patients. DIC is thus likely to be multifactorial in liver disease. Finally, but importantly, it has been shown that cirrhosis of the liver leads to enhanced circulating levels of endotoxin; this constituent of gram-negative bacteria is known to elicit a chain of events leading to enhanced coagulation activity and correlated well with coagulation activity in patients with cirrhosis (350).

Clinical and laboratory signs of DIC have been observed in some patients after a peritoneovenous shunt procedure (LeVeen shunt) for ascites associated with liver disease. The procoagulant effect of serosal fluids was already noted at the beginning of the nineteenth century (8). Subsequently, ascites fluid was found to contain the following procoagulants: TF, a factor X activator, collagen (which induces strong platelet aggregation), and endotoxin in 6 of 11 cases (351–353).

In one review of 278 patients with the LeVeen shunt, DIC was observed postoperatively in only ten patients, but other investigators have reported higher incidences (354–357). As mentioned earlier, patients with primary liver disease or with hepatic metastases are more prone to DIC after shunt than other patients are after the same procedure (349). Unsuccessful attempts have been made to control this shunt-related DIC with AT III concentrate (358).

Vascular Disorders

Vascular disorders, such as large aortic aneurysms or giant hemangiomas (Kasabach-Merritt syndrome), may result in local activation of coagulation (359–361). An association between giant hemangioma and a bleeding tendency was first described by Kasabach and Merritt in 1940 (362). They described a 2-month-old patient with purpura, thrombocytopenia, and prolonged bleeding and clotting times. All abnormalities disappeared after regression of the hemangioma by irradiation. The bleeding tendency in this patient was initially attributed to consumption of fibrinogen and platelets because of coagulation and fibrinolysis within the hemangioma. Studies using radiolabeled fibrinogen and platelets subsequently provided evidence for this hypothesis (363,364). The stimulus for the intravascular clotting and excessive fibrinolysis is apparently related to local activation of the coagulation pathway as well as to the release of large amounts of plasminogen activators by the abnormal endothelium lining the tumor vessels (365). Activated coagulation and fibrinolytic factors can ultimately "overflow" to the systemic circulation and cause DIC, but more common is the systemic depletion of coagulation factors and platelets as a result of local consumption. This may result in a clinical condition that is hardly distinguishable from DIC. Signs of DIC have also been associated with other vascular lesions such as the Klippel-Trénaunay syndrome, hemangiomas of the liver and the spleen, hemangioendotheliosarcoma, and Osler's disease (366–370). In fact, DIC may also be established in a small proportion of patients with aneurysms of large vessels, such as the aorta. In patients with giant hemangiomas, an incidence of clinically important DIC up to 25% has been

reported, but in more commonly occurring aortic aneurysms, a recent series showed an incidence of systemic activation of coagulation in only 1% of cases (361).

Obstetric Complications

(Pre)eclampsia is the most common obstetric condition associated with activation of blood coagulation, resulting in macroscopic fibrin deposits in various organs in severe cases (371,372). Thrombocytopenia is an early indicator of DIC developing in the course of the HELLP syndrome (*h*emolysis, *el*evated *l*iver enzymes, and *l*ow *p*latelets), which complicates pregnancy-induced hypertension in 5% to 10% and preeclampsia in up to 50% of cases (373). The central pathophysiologic stimuli of DIC in this syndrome appear to be microangiopathic hemolytic anemia accompanying vascular endothelial damage and platelet adhesion and activation, which may facilitate fibrin formation (see further).

Acute DIC occurs in placental abruption and amniotic fluid emboli (374). The first case of DIC complicating abruptio placentae was reported in 1901 in a 35-year-old woman in the seventh week of her pregnancy. The patient presented with acute severe pain in the abdomen, profuse vaginal bleeding, and widespread hematomas and died soon after extraction of a dead fetus and the observation of a loose placenta in the uterus. The severe hemostatic failure accompanying abruptio placentae was initially attributed to three causes: excessive consumption of fibrinogen in a retroplacental clot, loss of fibrinogen during bleeding, and diminished synthesis of fibrinogen by the liver (375). In 1947, it was shown that extracts of placenta possess thromboplastin activity, which was later related to initiation of intravascular coagulation during abruptio placentae (376). Since then, laboratory evidence of DIC and secondary fibrinolysis has repeatedly been obtained in patients with premature separation of the placenta (10,377,378). In placental abruption, the degree of placental separation appears to correlate with the extent of fibrin formation and thrombocytopenia, confirming that local factors are responsible for initiating DIC (374). In two published series, the incidence of abruptio placentae among the total number of deliveries was 0.20% and 0.37%, and 38.00% of the patients had hypofibrinogenemia (10,379). Thus, not all patients with abruptio placentae develop DIC; among those who do, different grades of severity are found with only the more severe forms resulting in shock and fetal death. It is also important to note that the DIC accompanying abruptio placentae is self-limiting and short-lasting. If no improvement is seen within 48 hours after the onset of DIC, the presence of a simultaneous other complication, such as sepsis, should be suspected.

Women surviving acute amniotic fluid emboli are at high risk (50% or more) of developing DIC within 4 hours after the insult (380). The dramatic clinical presentation of amniotic fluid embolism was initially precisely described by Steiner and Lushbaugh in 1941 (381). In old literature, the incidence of amniotic fluid embolism is approximately 1 in 8000 to 80,000 deliveries and is regarded as a significant cause of maternal death (382). Apparently, amniotic fluid is introduced into the maternal circulation through tears in the chorioamniotic membranes, rupture of the uterus, and injury of uterine veins. Amniotic fluid embolism may lead to extensive occlusion of the pulmonary vasculature by fetal debris, meconium, fat, and other elements of amniotic fluid.

Hemorrhage is particularly severe from the atonic uterus and from puncture sites, but it can also come from the gastrointestinal tract and other organs. *In vitro* data confirm that bleeding is caused by the potential of amniotic fluid to activate coagulation, involving TF (27,28), with subsequent exhaustion of coagulation factors and platelets (383–385). The mechanic obstruction of pulmonary blood vessels by the particulate matter in the amniotic fluid possibly enhances local fibrin platelet thrombi formation. Excessive fibrinogenolysis is also initiated, probably through direct activation of this system as well as indirectly by the DIC. An extremely high mortality rate (86%) in patients with amniotic fluid embolism was reported in a review of 272 cases (382).

Snake Bites

Snake bites may result in extensive hemostatic abnormalities at laboratory investigation but rarely lead to excessive bleeding or clinically manifest thromboembolic disease (386–388). The hemostatic derangement that is associated with snake bites is a result of the snake venom that may exert a powerful action on the coagulation system. In particular, snakes belonging to the Viperidae family produce venoms containing a number of hemostatic poisons. Members of the Viperidae family include the *Vipera*, *Echis* (*Echis carinatus* or *Echis coloratus*), and *Aspis* species, whereas the members of the Crotalidae family include the *Crotalus*, *Bothrops*, and *Agkistrodon* species.

The fact that blood remained fluid in animals bitten by vipers was already reported during the eighteenth century (389,390), after which the procoagulant and anticoagulant effects of venoms were described a century later (391). Subsequent analyses of Viperidae venoms showed that the active compounds in snake venom affecting coagulation are mainly enzymes or peptides with the following activities (386,387,392–396):

- Thrombinlike activity—cleaving peptide A from the αβ-chain of fibrinogen, thereby converting fibrinogen to fibrin; for example, the venom of *Agkistrodon rhodostoma*, the Malayan pit viper, has this activity.
- Activation of prothrombin in the absence of calcium ions; the component possessing this activity is found in the venom of *E. carinatus*.
- Activation of factors X and V; such a substance is present in Russell viper venom.
- Fibrinogenolytic activity (*Agkistrodon acutus* venom).
- Induction of thrombocytopenia by platelet aggregation.
- Inhibition of platelet aggregation by low-molecular-weight peptides.
- Activation of PC; in addition, snakes belonging to the Viperidae family also produce compounds that damage endothelium and other vessel wall components leading to bleeding, tissue ischemia, and edema.

Heatstroke

In the book *Travels to the City of the Caliphs* (1841), it is reported that on an extremely hot day in the Persian Gulf, the decks of one of the ships "resembled a slaughterhouse, so numerous were the bleeding patients." From the further description of the situation, it may be inferred that Wellstead here in fact described sailors that were affected by heatstroke, complicated by severe DIC (397). A few years earlier, it was already reported that in patients who had died of heatstroke, diffuse bleeding and unclottable blood was found at postmortem examination. More sophisticated clinical and experimental observations in later years indeed confirmed that heatstroke may be complicated by severe DIC, characterized by widespread fibrin deposition and hemorrhagic infarctions (398,399). Triggers for initiation of primary fibrino(geno)lysis and DIC in patients with heatstroke include endothelial cell damage and probably TF released from heat-damaged tissues (400,401). Heatstroke is caused by high environmental temperature in combination with the presence of infections, dehydration, and strenuous physical activity. Both the severity of the syndrome and the stage of its development affect the type and magnitude of hemostatic alterations (402).

Microangiopathic Hemolytic Anemias

Microangiopathic hemolytic anemia represents a spectrum of disorders encompassing TTP, HUS, chemotherapy-induced microangiopathic hemolytic anemia, malignant hypertension, and the HELLP syndrome (403). A common pathogenetic feature of these clinical entities appears to be endothelial damage, causing platelet adhesion and aggregation, thrombin formation, and an impaired fibrinolysis. In the pathogenesis of sporadic forms of TTP or HUS, infection with a verotoxin-producing *E. coli* (type HO-157) is involved (404). In patients with TTP, a deficiency of a von Willebrand factor–cleaving protease leads to ultralarge von Willebrand factor multimers in plasma, which may play an important role in the pathogenesis of this disorder (405). An acquired deficiency of this protease appears to be caused by the formation of autoantibodies, whereas familial TTP may be explained by an inherited deficiency (406,407). It has been reported that in patients with HUS a deficiency of the von Willebrand factor–cleaving protease does not occur (405).

Although some characteristics of microangiopathic hemolytic anemia and the resulting thrombotic occlusion of small and mid-size vessels leading to organ failure may mimic the clinical picture of DIC, these disorders in fact represent a distinct group of diseases that are discussed in another chapter in this book.

DIAGNOSIS OF DISSEMINATED INTRAVASCULAR COAGULATION

No single laboratory test or combination of tests is available that is sensitive or specific enough to allow a definite diagnosis. However, the diagnosis can reliably be made without ambiguity by taking into consideration the underlying disease and a combination of laboratory findings (3,5,33,408,409). Laboratory tests can be helpful in differentiating DIC from various other hemostatic disorders, such as vitamin K deficiency or liver failure. Because such conditions, however, may also occur simultaneously with DIC, this differentiation is not always simple. Laboratory tests may also be instrumental in assessing the severity of DIC and to serve as a guide for the installation of proper therapeutic or supportive interventions (410). In addition, subsequent measurements of laboratory parameters may be essential to monitor therapy. Finally, and of disputed importance, results of laboratory tests may serve as a predictor with regard to morbidity and mortality (46,411).

The abnormalities in coagulation tests are shown in Table 41-5. Because DIC encompasses a wide spectrum of hemostatic abnormalities of various severity, Müller-Berghaus has proposed to divide the stages of DIC into three phases that might be helpful in the diagnosis and the consequent therapy (185).

Phase I: Compensated Activation of the Hemostatic System

During this phase, no clinical findings are observed, but the underlying disease may arouse suspicion for the occurrence of DIC. Under these circumstances, tests should be performed for demonstrating the activation of coagulation.

TABLE 41-5. Routine Laboratory Value Abnormalities in Disseminated Intravascular Coagulation (DIC)

Test	Abnormality	Causes Other Than DIC That Contribute to Test Results
Platelet count	Decreased	Sepsis, impaired production, major blood loss, hypersplenism
Prothrombin time	Prolonged	Vitamin K deficiency, liver failure, major blood loss
Activated partial thromboplastin time	Prolonged	Liver failure, heparin treatment, major blood loss
Fibrin degradation products	Elevated	Surgery, trauma, infection, hematoma
Protease inhibitors	Decreased	Liver failure, capillary leakage

Phase II: Decompensated Activation of the Hemostatic System

In contrast to phase I, the prothrombin time as well as the activated partial thromboplastin time (aPTT) are prolonged during phase II. Under these circumstances, the thrombin time may still be normal, as the fibrinogen levels are still adequate and the level of FDP is not very high. In this phase, repeated analyses are necessary to demonstrate the dynamics of the intravascular coagulation process. The subsequent determinations demonstrate a continuous drop in platelet count as well as in fibrinogen concentration and coagulation factor activities, especially those with a short half-life (such as factor VII). Plasma levels of coagulation inhibitors, such as AT III and PC, are decreased.

Phase III: Full-Blown Disseminated Intravascular Coagulation

Full-blown DIC is characterized by an extremely prolonged or even unclottable prothrombin time as well as aPTT. Frequently, the thrombin time is pronouncedly prolonged or also unclottable. During this phase, the platelet counts are very low and the coagulation factor activities and plasma levels of physiologic anticoagulant proteins are below 50% of normal values. Tests for FDPs or other fibrin-related markers usually show high levels. If in the course of DIC hemolysis, schistocytes, or both are observed, this indicates microclot formation causing damage to the vessel wall and the red cells (microangiopathic hemolytic anemia).

Primary of dominant hyperfibrinolysis causes a specific pattern in coagulation test results (26,412). This situation is characterized by very low levels of α_2-antiplasmin and plasminogen (29). Due to the fibrinogenolytic effect of plasmin, levels of fibrinogen may be very low, causing a prolonged prothrombin time, aPTT, and thrombin time. Further analysis of coagulation factors may reveal particularly low levels of factors V and VIII, because these factors also may be degraded by plasmin. Low levels of factor VIII may be important indicators of hyperfibrinolysis, because in most normal cases of DIC, plasma levels of factor VIII are very high. Plasma levels of FDPs are extremely elevated (413,414).

Tests for Intravascular Fibrin Formation and Fibrin Degradation Products

According to the current understanding of DIC, the determination of soluble fibrin in plasma appears to be crucial for the diagnosis of DIC (415–420). Indeed, initial clinical studies indicate that

if the concentration of soluble fibrin has increased above a defined threshold, a diagnosis of DIC can be made (415,417,421–423). The only problem so far is that a reliable test is not available for quantitating soluble fibrin in plasma. The commercial semiquantitative assays can be used to support the data obtained by screening tests. Similarly, fibrin monomers can be measured and may confirm the presence of intravascular fibrin formation. Because soluble fibrin in plasma can only be generated intravascularly, this test is not influenced by extravascular fibrin formation, which, for example, may occur during local inflammation or trauma.

FDPs may be detected by specific ELISAs (enzyme-linked immunosorbent assays) or by latex agglutination assays, allowing rapid and bedside determination in emergency cases (424). None of the available assays for FDPs discriminates between degradation products of cross-linked fibrin and fibrinogen degradation, which may cause spuriously high results (425,426). The specificity of high levels of FDPs is therefore limited, and many other conditions, such as trauma, recent surgery, inflammation, or venous thromboembolism, are associated with elevated FDPs. Because FDPs are metabolized by the liver and secreted by the kidneys, FDP levels are influenced by liver and kidney function (427,428). More recently developed tests are specifically aimed at the detection of neoantigens on degraded cross-linked fibrin. One of such tests detects an epitope related to plasmin-degraded, cross-linked γ-chain, resulting in fragment D-dimer. These tests better differentiate degradation of cross-linked fibrin from fibrinogen or fibrinogen degradation products (408,421,429). D-dimer levels are high in patients with DIC but also poorly distinguish patients with DIC from patients with venous thromboembolism, recent surgery, or inflammatory conditions (346,430–432).

Markers for Thrombin Generation and Coagulation Activation

The dynamics of DIC can be judged by measuring activation markers that are released upon the conversion of a coagulation factor zymogen to an active protease. Examples of such markers are prothrombin activation fragment F1+2 and the activation peptides of factors IX and X (57,425,433,434). Indeed, these markers are markedly elevated in patients with DIC. Elevated plasma concentrations of thrombin-AT complexes may well reflect the increased generation of thrombin, and thrombin-mediated fibrinogen to fibrin conversion can be monitored by increased levels of fibrinogen activation peptide fibrinopeptide-A (108,109,435–437). All of these markers are increased in patients with DIC, and their high sensitivities may be helpful in detecting even low-grade activation of coagulation. The specificity of high levels of markers for coagulation factor activation is probably limited, because many other conditions may lead to elevated plasma levels. Another drawback may be that these assays are very much dependent on optimal venous puncture, which may be difficult in sick patients and during routine (intensive) care. The most important disadvantages of these tests may be that their use is limited to specialized coagulation laboratories and that they are not available for routine use in most clinical centers. Thus, although these tests are very relevant for research on the pathogenesis of DIC and the effect of specific interventions in the coagulation cascade of patients with DIC, their practical use in clinical medicine is very limited so far.

Platelet Count

The platelet count is a very sensitive test in the diagnosis of DIC. The platelet count in DIC is strongly correlated with markers of thrombin generation, because thrombin-induced platelet aggregation is, for a large part, responsible for platelet consumption (438,439). Because the normal platelet count varies between 150 and $450 \times 10^9/l$ l, a single determination is often not very helpful, but a continuous drop in platelet count, determined in acute DIC patients at intervals between 1 and 4 hours, indicates the generation of thrombin causing intravascular platelet aggregation. A stable platelet count suggests that thrombin formation has stopped. A low or decreasing platelet count is not very specific for DIC. Many of the underlying conditions that are associated with DIC may cause a low platelet count in the absence of DIC, such as the thrombocytopenia that may occur during severe infection or thrombocytopenia in trauma with severe bleeding. Mechanisms other than consumption, such as impaired platelet production or massive loss of platelets, may be responsible for thrombocytopenia in these situations but may also occur simultaneously.

Coagulation Factors and Inhibitors

Consumption of coagulation factors leads to low levels of coagulation factors in patients with DIC. In addition, impaired synthesis, for example, due to impaired liver function or a vitamin K deficiency, and loss of coagulation proteins due to massive bleeding may play a role in DIC as well (3,408,409). Although the accuracy of the measurement of one-stage clotting assays in DIC has been contested (due to the presence of activated coagulation factors in plasma), the level of coagulation factors appears to correlate well with the severity of the DIC. The low level of coagulation factors is reflected by prolonged coagulation screening tests, such as the prothrombin time or the aPTT. Plasma levels of factor VIII are paradoxically increased in most patients with DIC, probably due to the massive release of von Willebrand factor from the endothelium in combination with acute phase behavior of factor VIII. Measurement of fibrinogen has been widely advocated as a useful tool for the diagnosis of DIC but, in fact, is not very helpful to diagnose DIC in most cases (1). Fibrinogen acts as an acute-phase reactant, and despite ongoing consumption, plasma levels can remain well within the normal range for a long period of time. In a consecutive series of patients, the sensitivity of a low fibrinogen level for the diagnosis of DIC was only 28%, and hypofibrinogenemia was detected in very severe cases of DIC only (5).

Plasma levels of physiologic coagulation inhibitors, such as AT III or PC, are useful indicators of ongoing coagulation activation (46, 411,440). Antithrombin is the principal inhibitor of thrombin and may be readily exhausted during continuous thrombin generation. Plasma levels of AT III have been shown to be potent predictors for survival in patients with sepsis and DIC. Levels of PC may also indicate the severity of the DIC. In patients with meningococcal septicemia, very low plasma levels of PC are observed, and this may play a pivotal role in the occurrence of purpura fulminans in these patients (76,441). In fact, the plasma level of PC also may be regarded as a strong predictor for the outcome in DIC patients (110,442).

Fibrinolytic Parameters

In patients with severe DIC, enhanced fibrinolytic activity may be demonstrated by various tests. Nevertheless, as discussed in Fibrinolysis, activation of the fibrinolytic system is insufficient to counteract the ongoing systemic activation of coagulation and subsequent intravascular fibrin formation (26,28).

Plasma levels of FDPs, as discussed in the previous paragraphs, may theoretically be seen as an indicator of fibrinolytic activity but appear to correlate more strongly with fibrin formation. Fibrinolytic activation may be monitored by measurement of plasma levels of plasminogen and α_2-antiplasmin. Low levels may indicate consumption of these proteins. Due to the relatively low plasma concentration of α_2-antiplasmin, the determination of this protease inhibitor is a helpful test for judging the dynamics of fibrinolysis (440,443,444). Plasmin generation may be best judged by measurement of plasmin-α_2-antiplasmin complexes, which are indeed moderately elevated in patients with DIC (445). However, because the concentration of α_2-antiplasmin is relatively low and therefore sensitive to relatively rapid exhaustion, this test may underestimate total fibrinolytic activity. At low concentrations of α_2-antiplasmin, other protease inhibitors, such as AT, α_2-macroglobulin, α_1-antitrypsin, and C1-inhibitor, may act as plasmin inhibitors as well (446). The apparent insufficient fibrinolytic activity in patients with DIC is attributed to high levels of the inhibitor of plasminogen activation, PAI-1. Indeed, plasma levels of PAI-1 are elevated in patients with DIC and various underlying conditions and are strongly correlated with an unfavorable outcome (447–450).

The unique dominant hyperfibrinolysis that is seen in some specific situations, such as acute promyelocytic leukemia and prostatic carcinoma, has been described previously. In summary, in this situation, low levels of plasminogen, α_2-antiplasmin, and fibrinogen in combination with extremely high levels of FDPs or related markers are observed (29,338).

Diagnosis of Disseminated Intravascular Coagulation in a Routine Setting

Most of the newer, more sensitive tests described in the previous section are presently available in specialized laboratories only, and although these tests may be very helpful in clinical trials or other research, they often cannot be used in a routine setting. In these circumstances, a diagnosis of DIC may be made by a combination of platelet count, measurement of global clotting times (aPTT and PT), measurement of AT III or one or two clotting factors, and a test for FDPs (1). It should be emphasized that generally serial coagulation tests are more helpful than single laboratory results in establishing the diagnosis of DIC. A reduction in the platelet count or a clear downward trend at subsequent measurements is a sensitive (although not specific) sign of DIC. The prolongation of global clotting times may reflect the consumption and depletion of various coagulation factors, which potentially may be further substantiated by the measurement of one or two selected coagulation factors. Measurement of coagulation factors may also be helpful to detect additional hemostatic abnormalities, for example, caused by vitamin K deficiency. Measurement of AT III or PC has the additional advantage of specifically assessing the consumption of the most important inhibitor of the coagulation system. As stated earlier, measurement of fibrinogen is often not very helpful; low levels of fibrinogen are seen in the most serious cases only. Tests for FDPs (such as D-dimer) may be helpful to differentiate from other conditions that may be associated with a low platelet count and prolonged clotting times, such as chronic liver disease. However, one should realize that most of these tests are not very specific and high levels may be encountered in various clinical conditions. Nevertheless, the combination of the tests mentioned and clinical judgment enable one to establish or reject the diagnosis of DIC in most cases.

TABLE 41-6. Diagnostic Algorithm for the Diagnosis of Overt Disseminated Intravascular Coagulation (DIC)

TABLE 41-6. Diagnostic Algorithm for the Diagnosis of Overt Disseminated Intravascular Coagulation (DIC)

Presence of an underlying disorder known to be associated with DIC (Table 41-3) is a prerequisite for using this scoring system
Score global coagulation test results
    Platelet count (>100 = 0; <100 = 1; <50 = 2)
    Elevated fibrin-related marker (e.g., soluble fibrin monomers/ fibrin degradation products) (no increase = 0; moderate increase = 2; strong increase = 3)
    Prolonged prothrombin time (<3 sec = 0; >3 sec but <6 sec = 1; >6 sec = 2)
    Fibrinogen level (>1.0 g/L = 0; <1.0 g/L = 1)
Calculate score
If ≥5: Compatible with overt DIC; repeat scoring daily
If <5: Suggestive (not affirmative) for nonovert DIC; repeat next 1–2 d

Scoring System for the Diagnosis of Disseminated Intravascular Coagulation

A scoring system, using simple tests that are available in almost all hospital laboratories, is presently being developed by the subcommittee on DIC of the International Society on Thrombosis and Haemostasis. Following these objectives, the committee proposes a seven-step diagnostic algorithm to calculate a DIC score, as summarized in Table 41-6 (33). This score is partly based on a modification of the criteria for DIC, as established by the Japanese Ministry of Health and Welfare (440). In line with the previous comments, the presence of an underlying disorder known to be associated with DIC (Table 41-3) is a *conditio sine qua non* for the use of the algorithm (step 1). The result of laboratory tests contributes to a DIC score. Dependent on the type of test used, cut-off values for a "severely" or "moderately" elevated result of the test for soluble fibrin monomers or FDPs have to be established. Tentatively, and awaiting further prospective validation, a score equal to or more than 5 is compatible with DIC, whereas a score of less than 5 may be indicative (but is *not* affirmative) of nonovert DIC. It is recommended that scoring proceeds daily to characterize the severity and the course of the overt DIC.

TREATMENT OF DISSEMINATED INTRAVASCULAR COAGULATION

The proper management of patients with DIC remains controversial. The clinical picture of simultaneously occurring systemic thrombotic depositions and bleeding due to consumption does not directly indicate which specific therapy should be administered. However, adequate clinical trials on DIC treatment are hardly available, probably due to the complexity of the syndrome and its variable and unpredictable course (5). An "evidence-based" approach of the appropriate diagnosis and treatment of patients with DIC is therefore not very easy. Nevertheless, we discuss here the available and future (supportive) treatment strategies that may be used in patients with DIC and try to provide recommendations that are as much as possible based on current pathophysiologic insight and available clinical evidence.

It is well accepted that the cornerstone for the treatment of DIC is the management of the underlying disorder (3,4,409). Besides, therapeutic interventions based on our present knowledge of the pathogenesis of DIC may be appropriate. At present, these interventions may consist of replacement therapy, anticoagulant strategies or administration of physiologic coagulation

inhibitors. Future therapies may include interference in the fibrinolytic system.

Vigorous Measures to Treat Underlying Disorders and Support of Vital Functions

Aggressive medical or surgical treatment of the disorder causing the DIC is the indispensable foundation of a successful therapeutic approach. In fact, in some cases, such treatment is appropriate treatment of the underlying disorder is sufficient to eliminate the DIC, such as illustrated by the severe DIC-complicating abruptio placentae (451,452). Another example is provided by the fact that differentiating treatment of acute promyelocytic leukemia by all-*trans*-retinoic acid completely resolves the severe DIC that may be associated with this disorder (341). Vital functions are impaired both by the underlying disease and by DIC itself. Volume replacement and correction of hypotension and oxygenation improve blood flow through the microcirculation, thus restoring inhibitory functions of blood coagulation systems at the microcirculation. Although reperfusion may initially inflict further tissue injury, this is probably self-limiting.

Plasma and Platelet Transfusion

Consumption of coagulation factors and platelets during DIC can increase the risk of bleeding. Treatment with plasma or platelet concentrate is guided by the clinical condition of the patient and should not be instituted on the basis of laboratory findings alone. Replacement may be indicated in patients with active bleeding and in those requiring an invasive procedure or otherwise at risk for bleeding complications (3,5,453). On the other hand, it has been suggested that transfusion of blood components may also be harmful by further stimulating the activated coagulation system. This theory has rarely been proven to occur, and simultaneous (low-dose) heparin might be useful to prevent these complications.

The treatment with plasma is not based on evidence from controlled trials. The only randomized, controlled trial in neonates with DIC, comparing administration of fresh frozen plasma and platelets with whole blood exchange and no specific therapy, failed to show any change in outcome of DIC or survival (454). Despite the lack of evidence, most authors recommend treatment with fresh frozen plasma, at least when patients are bleeding or at increased risk for bleeding (455–458). To sufficiently correct the coagulation defect, large volumes of plasma may be needed. The use of coagulation factor concentrates may overcome this need; however, despite the fact that these concentrates usually contain only a selected number of the various clotting factors, they may be contaminated with traces of activated coagulation factors and such treatment may therefore be particularly harmful for patients with DIC. Cryoprecipitate, which contains fibrinogen as well as factor VIII, von Willebrand factor, factor XIII, and fibronectin, is also used as replacement therapy in DIC. However, its use is not supported by controlled trials. Because it is not possible to produce cryoprecipitate without risk of hepatitis C transmission, this product is not available in many countries.

Anticoagulant Strategies

HEPARIN

Heparin has been used as treatment for DIC since 1959 (459). Animal studies have shown that heparin can inhibit the activation of coagulation in experimental septicemia but does not affect mortality (460,461). Studies of heparin for treatment of DIC in humans claimed to be successful but were not controlled. Although one of these uncontrolled studies concluded in 1970 that a controlled study giving heparin to patients with gram-negative sepsis was needed (462), to date no such trial has been performed. A retrospective analysis of cases of DIC reported in the literature found similar survival for patients treated and patients not treated with heparin (463). One can conclude that there is no sound evidence in favor of the use of heparin as routine therapy in patients with DIC. An exception may be made for patients with clinical signs of extensive fibrin deposition like purpura fulminans, acral ischemia, or venous thrombosis (464). In such cases, low-dose heparin (5 to 8 U/kg/hour) is advocated, potentially in combination with plasma and, if appropriate, platelet replacement.

Low-molecular-weight heparins (LMWHs) are fractions of heparin with a molecular weight between 4000 and 8000 daltons (465). They differ from unfractionated heparins (UFHs) in their higher antifactor Xa to antifactor IIa activity ratio. This ratio varies between 2:1 and 4:1 for LMWH as compared to 1:1 for UFH. It has been postulated that these LMWHs would have a decreased bleeding risk while having at least the same antithrombotic potential as UFHs. Effective treatment of DIC with LMWH has been reported in rabbits (466). In rats, LMWH was as effective as UFH in improving the symptoms of DIC after endotoxin or thromboplastin infusion (467). Successful treatment was also reported in two small uncontrolled studies in humans (468,469). Furthermore, effects of the LMWH dalteparin as anti-DIC treatment have been studied in a multicenter, double-blind, randomized trial (470). The underlying cause of DIC in most of these patients was malignancy, and only 13% of patients suffered from infectious disease. Dalteparin was given in a dose of 75 U/kg/day, and heparin was given in a dose of 240 U/kg/day. In this study, dalteparin showed superior efficacy as compared with unfractionated heparin in improving bleeding symptoms and in improving a subjective organic symptoms score. The improvement in survival in the dalteparin group was not significant. There was no difference in laboratory parameters for DIC between the two treatment groups. Hence, based on this single study, it may be postulated that LMWH offers the benefit of decreased bleeding complications as compared with UFH in the treatment of DIC.

HIRUDIN

Hirudin is a potent and specific direct thrombin inhibitor. In contrast to heparin, its activity is not dependent on AT III (471), and therefore hirudin is capable of inhibiting clot-bound thrombin. Hirudin appeared to be effective in treating DIC in animal studies (472,473) and was shown to be able to block endotoxin-induced activation of coagulation in healthy humans (93). In one series of five patients with hematologic malignancy and DIC, hirudin treatment blocked the activation of coagulation (474). However, randomized controlled trials on the use of hirudin in patients with DIC are not available. The high risk of bleeding with hirudin treatment, as for example shown in other clinical areas, may potentially limit the use of hirudin in DIC.

TISSUE FACTOR INHIBITORS

Because TF plays a key role in the initiation of coagulation during DIC, inhibiting the actions of TF could be of value in the treatment of intravascular coagulation. In a rat model of DIC, the infusion of recombinant TFPI immediately after endotoxin administration significantly inhibited the consumption of coagulation factors and platelets (475). Furthermore, a reduced number of fibrin thrombi was formed in liver, lungs, kidney, and spleen. Similar effects were found in a rabbit model of DIC

(476). In human endotoxemia, recombinant TFPI was shown to dose-dependently reduce thrombin generation (91). Clinical trials on the use of TFPI in patients with DIC have recently been initiated, but results are not yet available. Other TF-inhibiting agents may prove to be potentially useful treatment strategies in patients with DIC.

Recently, a potent and specific inhibitor of the ternary complex between TF and factor VIIa and factor Xa has been developed (477,478). This agent (rNAPc2) is derived from the family of nematode anticoagulant proteins, which originally have been isolated from hematophagous hookworm nematodes. At present, rNAPc2 is investigated in phase II/III clinical studies, including a study in DIC patients.

Replacement of Physiologic Coagulation Inhibitors

ANTITHROMBIN III

AT III is an important physiologic inhibitor of blood coagulation, and low AT III levels are associated with increased mortality (46,411). Animal models of DIC show favorable results of AT administration, in particular normalization of hemostatic abnormalities, improvement of organ dysfunction, and better survival. Mortality due to gram-negative sepsis could be prevented by AT III infusion in baboons, but only if adequate AT III levels were achieved early in the course of sepsis (45,479). The use of AT III concentrates in patients with DIC has been studied relatively intensively. There are a number of controlled clinical trials on the use of AT concentrates in DIC patients (480–484). Most of these trials concern patients with sepsis, septic shock, or both. Blauhut et al. studied 51 patients with shock and DIC (480). They compared treatment with AT III concentrate alone to heparin treatment and to the administration of AT III concentrate plus heparin. No difference in survival was observed between the groups, but the duration of symptoms of DIC was shortened in the groups receiving AT III with or without heparin. However, the information on a number of important methodologic issues regarding this follow-up study remain unclear. A new approach was studied by Fourrier and others comparing the administration of supraphysiologic doses of AT III to placebo in patients with septic shock, DIC, or both (483). All trials show some beneficial effect in terms of improvement of a DIC score, shortening of the duration of DIC, or even improvement in organ function. Because all trials, however, used highly variable criteria for assessing these outcomes, it is hard to compare these results with one another. In the more recent clinical trials, very high doses of AT concentrate to attain supraphysiologic plasma levels were used, and the beneficial results in these trials seem to be more distinct. Some trials showed a modest reduction in mortality in AT-treated patients; however, the effect never reached statistic significance. A very large multicenter trial comparing AT administration with placebo in septic patients has recently been completed, and preliminary analyses again showed a nonsignificant trend towards reduced mortality in AT-treated patients. If one, however, performs a metaanalysis on the effect of AT III treatment on mortality in the published trials, a statistically significant reduction in mortality (from 47% to 32%) is observed (odds ratio, 0.59; 95% confidence interval, 0.39–0.87) (5). It is not clear from the literature which patients benefit most from AT III treatment in terms of clinically important outcomes (such as mortality or organ failure). In anticipation of this knowledge, it might be justified to reserve this expensive treatment for cases in which mortality attributable to DIC is expected to be high and for patients with a very active DIC, leading to substantial morbidity. An example of such a case is a patient suffering from meningococcal sepsis with purpura fulminans and acral ischemia. In such a case, the aim of the treatment should be AT concentrations of at least 100% or even higher (27). Future studies, including a large ongoing multicenter, randomized, controlled trial in patients with sepsis will probably indicate whether treatment with higher, supraphysiologic doses of AT III will result in more favorable clinical outcomes in patients with DIC.

(ACTIVATED) PROTEIN C CONCENTRATE

As mentioned above, PC levels are decreased during sepsis and clinical and experimental evidence indicates that depression of the PC/protein-S system may contribute to a fatal outcome (127,441,485). Based on these observations, suppletion of PC may be of advantage in patients with DIC. Indeed, in baboons, PC prevented the coagulopathic and lethal effects of *E. coli* infusion (127). Activated PC also appeared effective in a thromboplastin-induced DIC model in rabbits (486). There have been several reports of successful treatment with PC in sepsis in children and in adults (487–489). Clinical studies with recombinant, activated PC concentrate are ongoing and may yield promising results. One unpublished trial claims a significant reduction in mortality of septic patients who were treated with recombinant activated PC.

An alternative strategy to increase the activity of the PC system is the infusion of thrombomodulin. In several animal models of DIC, treatment with soluble thrombomodulin not only showed a beneficial effect on coagulation but also appeared to improve the pulmonary vascular injury and pulmonary accumulation of white blood cells (467,490–492). These effects were not dependent on the thrombin-binding properties of thrombomodulin but were probably mediated by the increase in activated PC. Thus far, no studies on thrombomodulin treatment in humans with DIC have been reported.

Interference in the Fibrinolytic System

Antifibrinolytic agents are effective in bleeding patients, but the use of these agents in patients with bleeding due to DIC is generally not recommended. In fact, because fibrin deposition, partly due to insufficient fibrinolysis, is an important feature of DIC, further inhibition of the fibrinolytic system seems inappropriate. An exception may be made in those rare cases in which primary or secondary hyperfibrinolysis dominates the clinical picture. This is the case in the coagulopathy associated with acute promyelocytic leukemia (acute myelogenous leukemia M-3) and in some cases of DIC secondary to malignancies (e.g., prostate carcinoma). Uncontrolled observations and one randomized controlled clinical trial have shown the beneficial effect of antifibrinolytic agents in this situation (32,493).

Because the fibrinolytic shut-down in patients with DIC appears to be due to high circulating levels of PAI-1, strategies directed against this fibrinolytic inhibitor might be useful. Anti–PAI-1 strategies have been shown to be of benefit in initial experimental studies (494); however, the effect of this treatment in clinical studies of DIC remains to be seen. An alternative strategy to enhance fibrinolysis is the administration of plasminogen activators, such as TPA or u-PA. Some case reports have been published suggesting improvement of the clinical condition of patients with meningococcemia and DIC after TPA treatment (495,496). Similarly, some initial experience with u-PA yielded interesting results. However, the risk of bleeding may be a serious drawback of this approach, and certainly controlled clinical trials should be awaited before this treatment can be advocated.

Guidelines for Therapy

First of all, treatment of DIC should consist of optimal management of the underlying disease (e.g., antibiotic therapy and abscess drainage in septicemia). As mentioned above, firm evidence for any specific therapy directed at the coagulation system for a patient with DIC is lacking. The following guidelines are based as much as possible on the available data in the literature. In case of bleeding or high risk for bleeding, plasma and platelet replacement therapy is indicated. Depending on the levels of coagulation factors and clotting times, two to three units of plasma can be given initially followed by repeated transfusion depending on PT and aPTT values. When the decision is made to give platelet transfusion, one should aim at a platelet count of 50 to 60×10^9/L. There is no evidence that treatment with heparin or LMWH is beneficial. Heparin treatment may be reserved for those cases with clinical signs of extensive fibrin deposition, such as in patients with purpura fulminans, or in cases in which DIC is likely to contribute to organ dysfunction. In those patients, heparin at a dose of 300 to 500 U/hour can be given intravenously. Finally, replacement therapy with AT III (or in the near future, activated PC) in patients with severe DIC and low levels of circulating protease inhibitors may be considered. In case of AT III administration, replacement therapy should be aimed at reaching AT III levels of greater than 100%. The optimal plasma concentration of PC during replacement therapy or the appropriate dose is not yet established and has to await further clinical trials.

CONCLUDING REMARKS

A quick literature search in the MEDLINE databases from 1966 to 2000 using the search term *disseminated intravascular coagulation* and related text words yields an impressive number of 12,371 manuscripts. Most of the published literature concerns the pathophysiology of DIC, which indeed in its main features is well understood now. However, other aspects of DIC, in particular, those related to its clinical management, remain unclear. New insights into the pathogenesis of DIC, however, are likely to yield novel supportive or therapeutic strategies for patients with DIC in the near future.

REFERENCES

1. Levi M, ten Cate H. Disseminated intravascular coagulation. *N Engl J Med* 1999;341:586–592.
2. Seligsohn U. Disseminated intravascular coagulation. In: Handin RI, Lux SE, Stossel TP, eds. *Blood: principles and practice of hematology.* Philadelphia: JB Lippincott Co, 1995:1289.
3. Marder VJ, Feinstein D, Francis C, et al. Consumptive thrombohemorrhagic disorders. In: Colman RW, Hirsh J, Marder VJ, et al., eds. *Hemostasis and thrombosis. Basic principles and clinical practice.* Philadelphia: JB Lippincott Co, 1994:1023.
4. Mammen EF, Anderson GF, Barnard MI. Disseminated intravascular coagulation in man. *Thromb Diath Haemorrh* 1969;36[Suppl]:14–21.
5. Levi M, ten Cate H, van der Poll T. Disseminated intravascular coagulation: state of the art. *Thromb Haemost* 1999;82:695–705.
6. Verstraete M, Vermylen C, Vermylen J. Excessive consumption of blood coagulation components as a cause of hemorrhagic diathesis. *Am J Med* 1965; 35:899–905.
7. Rodriguez-Erdmann F. Bleeding due to increased intravascular blood coagulation. Hemorrhagic syndromes caused by consumption of blood-clotting factors (consumption-coagulopathies). *N Engl J Med* 1965;273:1370–1378.
8. Dupuy M. Injections de matière cérébrale dans les veines. *Gaz Med Paris* 1834;2:524.
9. Trousseau A. Phlegmasia alba dolens. *Clin Med Hotel Dieu Paris* 1865;695.
10. Ratnoff OD, Pritchard JA, Colopy JE. Hemorrhagic states during pregnancy. *N Engl J Med* 1955.
11. McKay DG. *Disseminated intravascular coagulation: an intermediary mechanism of disease.* New York: Hoeber Medical Division, Harper & Row, 1965.
12. Levi M, ten Cate H, van der Poll T, et al. Pathogenesis of disseminated intravascular coagulation in sepsis. *JAMA* 1993;270:975–979.
13. Deykin D. The clinical challenge of disseminated intravascular coagulation. *N Engl J Med* 1970;283:636–644.
14. Colman RW, Robboy SJ, Minna JD. Disseminated intravascular coagulation: a reappraisal. *Annu Rev Med* 1979;30:359–374.

15. Feinstein DI. Treatment of disseminated intravascular coagulation. *Semin Thromb Hemost* 1988;14:351–362.

16. Schwartzman RJ, Hill JB. Neurologic complications of disseminated intravascular coagulation. *Neurology* 1982;32:791–797.

17. Merskey C, Johnson AJ, Kleiner GJ, et al. The defibrination syndrome: clinical features and laboratory diagnosis. *Br J Haematol* 1967;13:528–549.

18. Schneider CL. Fibrin embolism with defibrination as one of the end results during placenta abruptio. *Surg Gynecol Obstet* 1951;92:27–34.

19. Lasch HG, Heene DL, Huth K, et al. Pathophysiology, clinical manifestations and therapy of consumption-coagulopathy ("Verbrauchskoagulopathie"). *Am J Cardiol* 1967;20:381–391.

20. Müller-Berghaus G. Pathophysiologic and biochemical events in disseminated intravascular coagulation: dysregulation of procoagulant and anticoagulant pathways. *Semin Thromb Hemost* 1989;15:58–87.

21. Müller-Berghaus G, Blomback M, ten Cate JW. Attempts to define disseminated intravascular coagulation. In: Müller-Berghaus G, Madlener K, Blomback M, et al., eds. *DIC: pathogenesis, diagnosis and therapy of disseminated intravascular fibrin formation*. Amsterdam: Elsevier Science, 1993:3.

22. Brandtzaeg P, Joo GB, Brusletto B, et al. Plasminogen activator inhibitor 1 and 2, alpha-2-antiplasmin, plasminogen, and endotoxin levels in systemic meningococcal disease. *Thromb Res* 1990;57:271–278.

23. Hesselvik JF, Blomback M, Brodin B, et al. Coagulation, fibrinolysis, and kallikrein systems in sepsis: relation to outcome. *Crit Care Med* 1989;17:724–733.

24. Voss R, Matthias FR, Borkowski G, et al. Activation and inhibition of fibrinolysis in septic patients in an internal intensive care unit. *Br J Haematol* 1990;75:99–105.

25. Alkjaersig N, Fletcher AP, Sherry S. Pathogenesis of the coagulation defect developing during pathological plasma proteolytic (fibrinolytic) states. *J Clin Invest* 1962;41:917–934.

26. Levi M, van der Poll T, de Jonge E, et al. Relative insufficiency of fibrinolysis in disseminated intravascular coagulation. *Sepsis* 2000;3:103–109.

27. Vervloet MG, Thijs LG, Hack CE. Derangements of coagulation and fibrinolysis in critically ill patients with sepsis and septic shock. *Semin Thromb Hemost* 1998;24:33–44.

28. Levi M, van der Poll T, ten Cate H, et al. The cytokine-mediated imbalance between coagulant and anticoagulant mechanisms in sepsis and endotoxaemia. *Eur J Clin Invest* 1997;27:3–9.

29. Avvisati G, ten Cate JW, Sturk A, et al. Acquired alpha-2-antiplasmin deficiency in acute promyelocytic leukaemia. *Br J Haematol* 1988;70:43–48.

30. Dombret H, Scrobohaci ML, Ghorra P, et al. Coagulation disorders associated with acute promyelocytic leukemia: corrective effect of all-trans retinoic acid treatment. *Leukemia* 1993;7:2–9.

31. Albarracin NS, Haust MD. Intravascular coagulation in promyelocytic leukemia: a case study including ultrastructure. *Am J Clin Pathol* 1971;55:677–685.

32. Avvisati G, ten Cate JW, Buller HR, et al. Tranexamic acid for control of haemorrhage in acute promyelocytic leukaemia. *Lancet* 1989;2:122–124.

33. Taylor FB Jr, Toh CH, Hoots K, et al. Towards a definition, clinical and laboratory criteria, and a scoring system for disseminated intravascular coagulation. *Thromb Haemost* 2001;86(5):1327–1330.

34. Manasse P. Uber hylaine ballen und thromben in den gehirnfassen bei acuten infectionen und krankheiten. *Virchows Arch* 1882;130:217.

35. Al-Mondhiry H. Disseminated intravascular coagulation: experience in a major cancer center. *Thromb Diath Haemorrh* 1975;34:181–193.

36. Robboy SJ, Major MC, Colman RW, et al. Pathology of disseminated intravascular coagulation (DIC). Analysis of 26 cases. *Hum Pathol* 1972;3:327–343.

37. Kim HS, Suzuki M, Lie JT, et al. Clinically unsuspected disseminated intravascular coagulation (DIC): an autopsy survey. *Am J Clin Pathol* 1976;66:31–39.

38. Watanabe T, Imamura T, Nakagaki K, et al. Disseminated intravascular coagulation in autopsy cases. Its incidence and clinicopathologic significance. *Pathol Res Pract* 1979;165:311–322.

39. Shimamura K, Oka K, Nakazawa M, et al. Distribution patterns of microthrombi in disseminated intravascular coagulation. *Arch Pathol Lab Med* 1983;107:543–547.

40. Wilde JT, Roberts KM, Greaves M, et al. Association between necropsy evidence of disseminated intravascular coagulation and coagulation variables before death in patients in intensive care units. *J Clin Pathol* 1988;41:138–142.

41. Sugiura M, Hiraoka K, Ohkawa S, et al. A clinicopathological study on cardiac lesions in 64 cases of disseminated intravascular coagulation. *Jpn Heart J* 1977;18:57–69.

42. Mori K, Hizawa K. Histopathological study of disseminated intravascular coagulation. An analysis of 114 autopsy cases. *Tokushima J Exp Med* 1982;29:47–61.

43. Coalson JJ. Pathology of sepsis, septic shock, and multiple organ failure. In: *Perspective on sepsis and septic shock*. Fullerton, CA: Society of Critical Care Medicine, 1986:27.

44. Creasey AA, Chang AC, Feigen L, et al. Tissue factor pathway inhibitor reduces mortality from Escherichia coli septic shock. *J Clin Invest* 1993;91:2850–2856.

45. Kessler CM, Tang Z, Jacobs HM, et al. The suprapharmacologic dosing of antithrombin concentrate for Staphylococcus aureus-induced disseminated intravascular coagulation in guinea pigs: substantial reduction in mortality and morbidity. *Blood* 1997;89:4393–4401.

46. Fourrier F, Chopin C, Goudemand J, et al. Septic shock, multiple organ failure, and disseminated intravascular coagulation. Compared patterns of antithrombin III, protein C, and protein S deficiencies. *Chest* 1992;101:816–823.

47. Davie EW, Ratnoff OD. Waterfall sequence for intrinsic blood clotting. *Science* 1964;145:1310–1312.

48. MacFarlane RG. An enzyme cascade in the blood clotting mechanism and its function as a biochemical amplifier. *Nature* 1964;498–499.

49. Rapaport SI, Rao LV. The tissue factor pathway: how it has become a "prima ballerina." *Thromb Haemost* 1995;74:7–17.

50. Colman RW, Schmaier AH. Contact system: a vascular biology modulator with anticoagulant, profibrinolytic, antiadhesive, and proinflammatory attributes. *Blood* 1997;90:3819–3843.

51. Mann KG. Biochemistry and physiology of blood coagulation. *Thromb Haemost* 1999;82:165–174.

52. Davie EW, Fujikawa K, Kisiel W. The coagulation cascade: initiation, maintenance, and regulation. *Biochemistry* 1991;30:10363–10370.

53. Ruf W, Edgington TS. Structural biology of tissue factor, the initiator of thrombogenesis in vivo. *FASEB J* 1994;8:385–390.

54. Mann KG, van't Veer C, Cawthern K, et al. The role of the tissue factor pathway in initiation of coagulation. *Blood Coagul Fibrinolysis* 1998;9[Suppl]1:S3–S7.

55. Camerer E, Kolsto AB, Prydz H. Cell biology of tissue factor, the principal initiator of blood coagulation. *Thromb Res* 1996;81:1–41.

56. Banner DW, D'Arcy A, Chene C, et al. The crystal structure of the complex of blood coagulation factor VIIa with soluble tissue factor. *Nature* 1996;380:41–46.

57. ten Cate H, Bauer KA, Levi M, et al. The activation of factor X and prothrombin by recombinant factor VIIa in vivo is mediated by tissue factor. *J Clin Invest* 1993;92:1207–1212.

58. Bauer KA, Kass BL, ten Cate H, et al. Factor IX is activated in vivo by the tissue factor mechanism. *Blood* 1990;76:731–736.

59. Osterud B. Tissue factor expression by monocytes: regulation and pathophysiological roles. *Blood Coagul Fibrinolysis* 1998;9[Suppl]1:S9–S14.

60. Neumann FJ, Marx N, Gawaz M, et al. Induction of cytokine expression in leukocytes by binding of thrombin-stimulated platelets. *Circulation* 1997;95:2387–2394.

61. Edgington TS, Mackman N, Fan ST, et al. Cellular immune and cytokine pathways resulting in tissue factor expression and relevance to septic shock. *Nouvelle Revue Francaise d'Hematologie* 1992;34[Suppl]:S15–S27.

62. Giesen PL, Rauch U, Bohrmann B, et al. Blood-borne tissue factor: another view of thrombosis. *Proc Natl Acad Sci U S A* 1999;96:2311–2315.

63. Osterud B, Rao LV, Olsen JO. Induction of tissue factor expression in whole blood: lack of evidence for the presence of tissue factor expression on granulocytes. *Thromb Haemost* 2000;83:861–867.

64. Nieuwland R, Berckmans RJ, McGregor S, et al. Cellular origin and procoagulant properties of microparticles in meningococcal sepsis. *Blood* 2000;95:930–935.

65. Koyama T, Nishida K, Ohdama S, et al. Determination of plasma tissue factor antigen and its clinical significance. *Br J Haematol* 1994;87:343–347.

66. Osterud B, Flaegstad T. Increased tissue thromboplastin activity in monocytes of patients with meningococcal infection: related to an unfavourable prognosis. *Thromb Haemost* 1983;49:5–7.

67. Edwards RL, Rickles FR, Cronlund M. Abnormalities of blood coagulation in patients with cancer. Mononuclear cell tissue factor generation. *J Lab Clin Med* 1981;98:917–928.

68. Leatham EW, Bath PM, Tooze JA, et al. Increased monocyte tissue factor expression in coronary disease. *Br Heart J* 1995;73:10–13.

69. Weiss HJ, Turitto VT, Baumgartner HR, et al. Evidence for the presence of tissue factor activity on subendothelium. *Blood* 1989;73:968–975.

70. Schmaier AH, Rojkjaer R, Shariat-Madar Z. Activation of the plasma kallikrein/kinin system on cells: a revised hypothesis. *Thromb Haemost* 1999;82:226–233.

71. Smith D, Gilbert M, Owen WG. Tissue plasminogen activator release in vivo in response to vasoactive agents. *Blood* 1985;66:835–839.

72. Brown NJ, Nadeau JH, Vaughan DE. Selective stimulation of tissue-type plasminogen activator (t-PA) in vivo by infusion of bradykinin. *Thromb Haemost* 1997;77:522–525.

73. Hasan AA, Amenta S, Schmaier AH. Bradykinin and its metabolite, Arg-Pro-Pro-Gly-Phe, are selective inhibitors of alpha-thrombin-induced platelet activation. *Circulation* 1996;94:517–528.

74. Kaufman N, Page JD, Pixley RA, et al. Alpha 2-macroglobulin-kallikrein complexes detect contact system activation in hereditary angioedema and human sepsis. *Blood* 1991;77:2660–2667.

75. Nuijens JH, Huijbregts CC, Eerenberg-Belmer AJ, et al. Quantification of plasma factor XIIa-Cl(-)-inhibitor and kallikrein-Cl(-)-inhibitor complexes in sepsis. *Blood* 1988;72:1841–1848.

76. Wuillemin WA, Fijnvandraat K, Derkx BH, et al. Activation of the intrinsic pathway of coagulation in children with meningococcal septic shock. *Thromb Haemost* 1995;74:1436–1441.

77. Minnema MC, Pajkrt D, Wuillemin WA, et al. Activation of clotting factor XI without detectable contact activation in experimental human endotoxemia. *Blood* 1998;92:3294–3301.

78. Pixley RA, De La Cadena R, Page JD, et al. The contact system contributes to hypotension but not disseminated intravascular coagulation in lethal bacteremia. In vivo use of a monoclonal anti-factor XII antibody to block contact activation in baboons. *J Clin Invest* 1993;91:61–68.

79. Levi M. Keep in contact: the role of the contact system in infection and sepsis. *Crit Care Med* 2000;28(11):3765–3766.

80. Aderem A, Ulevitch RJ. Toll-like receptors in the induction of the innate immune response. *Nature* 2000;406:782–787.

81. Bohrer H, Qiu F, Zimmermann T, et al. Role of NFkappaB in the mortality of sepsis. *J Clin Invest* 1997;100:972–985.

82. Franco RF, de Jonge E, Dekkers PE, et al. The in vivo kinetics of tissue factor messenger RNA expression during human endotoxemia: relationship with activation of coagulation. *Blood* 2000;96:554–559.

83. Solovey A, Gui L, Key NS, et al. Tissue factor expression by endothelial cells in sickle cell anemia. *J Clin Invest* 1998;101:1899–1904.

84. Biemond BJ, Levi M, ten Cate H, et al. Plasminogen activator and plasminogen activator inhibitor I release during experimental endotoxaemia in chimpanzees: effect of interventions in the cytokine and coagulation cascades. *Clin Sci (Colch)* 1995;88:587–594.

85. van der Poll T, Levi M, Hack CE, et al. Elimination of interleukin 6 attenuates coagulation activation in experimental endotoxemia in chimpanzees. *J Exp Med* 1994;179:1253–1259.

86. Taylor FB Jr. Studies on the inflammatory-coagulant axis in the baboon response to E. coli: regulatory roles of proteins C, S, C4bBP and of inhibitors of tissue factor. *Prog Clin Biol Res* 1994;388:175–194.

86a. Wada H, Yamamurro M, Inoue A, et al. Comparison of the responses of global test of coagulation with molecular markers of neutrophil, endothelial, and hemostatic system perturbation in the baboon model of E. colisepsis—toward a distinction between uncompensated overt DIC and compensated non-overt DIC. *Thromb Haemost* 2001;86(6):1489–1494.

87. Taylor FBJ, Chang A, Ruf W, et al. Lethal E. coli septic shock is prevented by blocking tissue factor with monoclonal antibody. *Circ Shock* 1991;33:127–134.

88. Levi M, ten Cate H, Bauer KA, et al. Inhibition of endotoxin-induced activation of coagulation and fibrinolysis by pentoxifylline or by a monoclonal anti-tissue factor antibody in chimpanzees. *J Clin Invest* 1994;93:114–120.

89. van der Poll T, Levi M, van Deventer SJ, et al. Differential effects of anti-tumor necrosis factor monoclonal antibodies on systemic inflammatory responses in experimental endotoxemia in chimpanzees. *Blood* 1994;83:446–451.

90. Esmon CT. Introduction: are natural anticoagulants candidates for modulating the inflammatory response to endotoxin? *Blood* 2000;95:1113–1116.

91. de Jonge E, Dekkers PE, Creasey AA, et al. Tissue factor pathway inhibitor (TFPI) dose-dependently inhibits coagulation activation without influencing the fibrinolytic and cytokine response during human endotoxemia. *Blood* 2000;95:1124–1129.

92. Annex BH, Denning SM, Channon KM, et al. Differential expression of tissue factor protein in directional atherectomy specimens from patients with stable and unstable coronary syndromes. *Circulation* 1995;91:619–622.

93. Pernerstorfer T, Hollenstein U, Hansen JB, et al. Lepirudin blunts endotoxin-induced coagulation activation. *Blood* 2000;95:1729–1734.

94. Altieri DC. Molecular cloning of effector cell protease receptor-1, a novel cell surface receptor for the protease factor Xa. *J Biol Chem* 1994;269:3139–3142.

95. Camerer E, Huang W, Coughlin SR. Tissue factor- and factor X-dependent activation of protease-activated receptor 2 by factor VIIa. *Proc Natl Acad Sci U S A* 2000;97:5255–5260.

96. Degen JL. Hemostatic factors and inflammatory disease. *Thromb Haemost* 1999; 82:858–864.

97. Cirino G, Cicala C, Bucci M, et al. Factor Xa as an interface between coagulation and inflammation. Molecular mimicry of factor Xa association with effector cell protease receptor-1 induces acute inflammation in vivo. *J Clin Invest* 1997;99:2446–2451.

98. Senden NH, Jeunhomme TM, Heemskerk JW, et al. Factor Xa induces cytokine production and expression of adhesion molecules by human umbilical vein endothelial cells. *J Immunol* 1998;161:4318–4324.

99. Neumann FJ, Ott I, Marx N, et al. Effect of human recombinant interleukin-6 and interleukin-8 on monocyte procoagulant activity. *Arterioscler Thromb Vasc Biol* 1997;17:3399–3405.

100. Stouthard JM, Levi M, Hack CE, et al. Interleukin-6 stimulates coagulation, not fibrinolysis, in humans. *Thromb Haemost* 1996;76:738–742.

101. Grandaliano G, Valente AJ, Abboud HE. A novel biologic activity of thrombin: stimulation of monocyte chemotactic protein production. *J Exp Med* 1994;179:1737–1741.

102. Sower LE, Froelich CJ, Carney DH, et al. Thrombin induces IL-6 production in fibroblasts and epithelial cells. Evidence for the involvement of the seven-transmembrane domain (STD) receptor for alpha-thrombin. *J Immunol* 1995;155:895–901.

103. Johnson K, Choi Y, DeGroot E, et al. Potential mechanisms for a proinflammatory vascular cytokine response to coagulation activation. *J Immunol* 1998;160:5130–5135.

104. Johnson K, Aarden L, Choi Y, et al. The proinflammatory cytokine response to coagulation and endotoxin in whole blood. *Blood* 1996;87:5051–5060.

105. Kahn ML, Nakanishi-Matsui M, Shapiro MJ, et al. Protease-activated receptors 1 and 4 mediate activation of human platelets by thrombin. *J Clin Invest* 1999;103:879–887.

106. Cunningham MA, Romas P, Hutchinson P, et al. Tissue factor and factor VIIa receptor/ligand interactions induce proinflammatory effects in macrophages. *Blood* 1999;94:3413–3420.

107. de Jonge E, Friederich PW, Levi M, et al. Activation of coagulation by administration of recombinant factor VIIa elicits interleukin-6 and interleukin-8 release in healthy human subjects. 2000;(in press).

108. Kario K, Matsuo T, Kodama K, et al. Imbalance between thrombin and plasmin activity in disseminated intravascular coagulation. Assessment by the thrombin-antithrombin-III complex/plasmin-alpha-2-antiplasmin complex ratio. *Haemostasis* 1992;22:179–186.

109. Takahashi H, Wada K, Niwano H, et al. Comparison of prothrombin fragment 1 + 2 with thrombin-antithrombin III complex in plasma of patients with disseminated intravascular coagulation. *Blood Coagul Fibrinolysis* 1992;3:813–818.

110. Gando S, Kameue T, Nanzaki S, et al. Disseminated intravascular coagulation is a frequent complication of systemic inflammatory response syndrome. *Thromb Haemost* 1996;75:224–228.

111. Jochum M, Lander S, Heimburger N, et al. Effect of human granulocytic elastase on isolated human antithrombin III. *Hoppe-Seylers Zeitschrift fur Physiologische Chemie* 1981;362:103–112.

112. Bourin MC, Lindahl U. Glycosaminoglycans and the regulation of blood coagulation. *Biochem J* 1993;289:313–330.

113. Kobayashi M, Shimada K, Ozawa T. Human recombinant interleukin-1 beta- and tumor necrosis factor alpha-mediated suppression of heparin-like compounds on cultured porcine aortic endothelial cells. *J Cell Physiol* 1990;144: 383–390.

114. Taylor FBJ, Chang AC, Peer GT, et al. DEGR-factor Xa blocks disseminated intravascular coagulation initiated by *Escherichia coli* without preventing shock or organ damage. *Blood* 1991;78:364–368.

115. Minnema MC, Chang AC, Jansen PM, et al. Recombinant human antithrombin III improves survival and attenuates inflammatory responses in baboons lethally challenged with *Escherichia coli*. *Blood* 2000;95:1117–1123.

116. Esmon CT. The roles of protein C and thrombomodulin in the regulation of blood coagulation. *J Biol Chem* 1989;264:4743–4746.

117. Bouma BN, Meijers JC. Fibrinolysis and the contact system: a role for factor XI in the down-regulation of fibrinolysis. *Thromb Haemost* 1999;82:243–250.

118. Fukudome K, Esmon CT. Identification, cloning, and regulation of a novel endothelial cell protein C/activated protein C receptor. *J Biol Chem* 1994;269: 26486–26491.

119. Laszik Z, Mitro A, Taylor FBJ, et al. Human protein C receptor is present primarily on endothelium of large blood vessels: implications for the control of the protein C pathway. *Circulation* 1997;96:3633–3640.

120. Gresele P, Momi S, Berrettini M, et al. Activated human protein C prevents thrombin-induced thromboembolism in mice. Evidence that activated protein c reduces intravascular fibrin accumulation through the inhibition of additional thrombin generation. *J Clin Invest* 1998;101:667–676.

121. Hancock WW, Tsuchida A, Hau H, et al. The anticoagulants protein C and protein S display potent antiinflammatory and immunosuppressive effects relevant to transplant biology and therapy. *Transplant Proc* 1992;24:2302–2303.

122. Taoka Y, Okajima K, Uchiba M, et al. Activated protein C reduces the severity of compression-induced spinal cord injury in rats by inhibiting activation of leukocytes. *J Neurosci* 1998;18:1393–1398.

123. Taoka Y, Okajima K, Uchiba M, et al. Neuroprotection by recombinant thrombomodulin. *Thromb Haemost* 2000;83:462–468.

124. Uchiba M, Okajima K, Murakami K, et al. rhs-TM prevents ET-induced increase in pulmonary vascular permeability through protein C activation. *Am J Physiol* 1997;273:L889–L894.

125. Taylor FBJ, Dahlback B, Chang AC, et al. Role of free protein S and C4b binding protein in regulating the coagulant response to *Escherichia coli*. *Blood* 1995;86:2642–2652.

126. Taylor FBJ, Stearns-Kurosawa DJ, Kurosawa S, et al. The endothelial cell protein C receptor aids in host defense against Escherichia coli sepsis. *Blood* 2000;95:1680–1686.

127. Taylor FBJ, Chang A, Esmon CT, et al. Protein C prevents the coagulopathic and lethal effects of *Escherichia coli* infusion in the baboon. *J Clin Invest* 1987; 79:918–925.

128. Nawroth PP, Handley DA, Esmon CT, et al. Interleukin 1 induces endothelial cell procoagulant while suppressing cell-surface anticoagulant activity. *Proc Natl Acad Sci U S A* 1986;83:3460–3464.

129. Nawroth PP, Stern DM. Modulation of endothelial cell hemostatic properties by tumor necrosis factor. *J Exp Med* 1986;163:740–745.

130. Moore KL, Esmon CT, Esmon NL. Tumor necrosis factor leads to the internalization and degradation of thrombomodulin from the surface of bovine aortic endothelial cells in culture. *Blood* 1989;73:159–165.

131. Lentz SR, Tsiang M, Sadler JE. Regulation of thrombomodulin by tumor necrosis factor-alpha: comparison of transcriptional and posttranscriptional mechanisms. *Blood* 1991;77:542–550.

132. Gu JM, Katsuura Y, Ferrell GL, et al. Endotoxin and thrombin elevate rodent endothelial cell protein C receptor mRNA levels and increase receptor shedding in vivo. *Blood* 2000;95:1687–1693.

133. Broze GJ Jr. Tissue factor pathway inhibitor and the revised theory of coagulation. *Annu Rev Med* 1995;46:103–112.

134. Novotny WF, Brown SG, Miletich JP, et al. Plasma antigen levels of the lipoprotein-associated coagulation inhibitor in patient samples. *Blood* 1991;78: 387–393.

135. Ameri A, Kuppuswamy MN, Basu S, et al. Expression of tissue factor pathway inhibitor by cultured endothelial cells in response to inflammatory mediators. *Blood* 1992;79:3219–3226.

136. Sandset PM, Warn-Cramer BJ, Rao LV, et al. Depletion of extrinsic pathway inhibitor (EPI) sensitizes rabbits to disseminated intravascular coagulation induced with tissue factor: evidence supporting a physiologic role for EPI as a natural anticoagulant. *Proc Natl Acad Sci U S A* 1991;88:708–712.

137. Park CT, Creasey AA, Wright SD. Tissue factor pathway inhibitor blocks cellular effects of endotoxin by binding to endotoxin and interfering with transfer to CD14. *Blood* 1997;89:4268–4274.

138. Randolph MM, White GL, Kosanke SD, et al. Attenuation of tissue thrombosis and hemorrhage by ala-TFPI does not account for its protection against E. coli—a comparative study of treated and untreated non-surviving baboons challenged with LD100 E. coli. *Thromb Haemost* 1998;79:1048–1053.

139. Schleef RR, Bevilacqua MP, Sawdey M, et al. Cytokine activation of vascular endothelium. Effects on tissue-type plasminogen activator and type 1 plasminogen activator inhibitor. *J Biol Chem* 1988;263:5797–5803.

140. van Hinsbergh V, Kooistra T, van den Berg EA, et al. Tumor necrosis factor increases the production of plasminogen activator inhibitor in human endothelial cells in vitro and in rats in vivo. *Blood* 1988;72:1467–1473.
141. van Hinsbergh V, van den Berg EA, Fiers W, et al. Tumor necrosis factor induces the production of urokinase-type plasminogen activator by human endothelial cells. *Blood* 1990;75:1991–1998.
142. Sawdey MS, Loskutoff DJ. Regulation of murine type 1 plasminogen activator inhibitor gene expression in vivo. Tissue specificity and induction by lipopolysaccharide, tumor necrosis factor-alpha, and transforming growth factor-beta. *J Clin Invest* 1991;88:1346–1353.
143. Yamamoto K, Loskutoff DJ. Fibrin deposition in tissues from endotoxin-treated mice correlates with decreases in the expression of urokinase-type but not tissue-type plasminogen activator. *J Clin Invest* 1996;97:2440–2451.
144. ten Cate H. Pathophysiology of disseminated intravascular coagulation in sepsis. *Crit Care Med* 2000;28:S9–S11.
145. Hermans PW, Hibberd ML, Booy R, et al. 4G/5G promoter polymorphism in the plasminogen-activator-inhibitor-1 gene and outcome of meningococcal disease. Meningococcal Research Group. *Lancet* 1999;354:556–560.
146. Westendorp RG, Hottenga JJ, Slagboom PE. Variation in plasminogen-activator-inhibitor-1 gene and risk of meningococcal septic shock. *Lancet* 1999;354:561–563.
147. Oka K, Tanaka K. Intravascular coagulation in autopsy cases with liver diseases. *Thromb Haemost* 1979;42:564–570.
148. Bauer KA, Weiss LM, Sparrow D, et al. Aging-associated changes in indices of thrombin generation and protein C activation in humans. Normative Aging Study. *J Clin Invest* 1987;80:1527–1534.
149. Healy AM, Hancock WW, Christie PD, et al. Intravascular coagulation activation in a murine model of thrombomodulin deficiency: effects of lesion size, age, and hypoxia on fibrin deposition. *Blood* 1998;92:4188–4197.
150. Abraham E. Coagulation abnormalities in acute lung injury and sepsis. *Am J Respir Cell Mol Biol* 2000;22:401–404.
151. Rosenberg RD, Aird WC. Vascular-bed-specific hemostasis and hypercoagulable states. *N Engl J Med* 1999;340:1555–1564.
152. Aird WC, Edelberg JM, Weiler-Guettler H, et al. Vascular bed-specific expression of an endothelial cell gene is programmed by the tissue microenvironment. *J Cell Biol* 1997;138:1117–1124.
153. Kincaid-Smith P. Coagulation and renal disease. *Kidney Int* 1972;2:183–190.
154. Conlon PJ, Kovalik E, Schwab SJ. Percutaneous renal biopsy of ventilated intensive care unit patients. *Clin Nephrol* 1995;43:309–311.
155. Schetz MR. Coagulation disorders in acute renal failure. *Kidney Int Suppl* 1998;66:S96–S101.
156. Kanfer A. Glomerular coagulation system in renal diseases. *Ren Fail* 1992;14:407–412.
157. Davenport A. The coagulation system in the critically ill patient with acute renal failure and the effect of an extracorporeal circuit. *Am J Kidney Dis* 1997;30:S20–S27.
158. Siegal T, Seligsohn U, Aghai E, et al. Clinical and laboratory aspects of disseminated intravascular coagulation (DIC): a study of 118 cases. *Thromb Haemost* 1978;39:122–134.
159. Vassali P, Simon G, Rouiller C. Electron microscopic study of glomerular lesions resulting from intravascular fibrin formation. *Am J Pathol* 1963;43:579–617.
160. Humair L, Potter EV, Kwaan HC. The role of fibrinogen in renal disease. I. Production of experimental lesions in mice. *J Lab Clin Med* 1969;74:60–71.
161. Kincaid-Smith P. The role of coagulation in the obliteration of glomerular capillaries. In: Kincaid-Smith P, Mathew TH, Becker EL, eds. *Glomerulonephritis*. New York: John Wiley and Sons, 1972:47.
162. Grandchamp A, Ayer G, Truniger B. Pathogenesis of redistribution of intrarenal blood flow in haemorrhagic hypotension. *Eur J Clin Invest* 1971;1:271–276.
163. Müller-Berghaus G, McKay DG. Prevention of the generalized Shwartzman reaction in pregnant rats by alpha-adrenergic blocking agents. *Lab Invest* 1967;17:276–280.
164. Whitaker AN, McKay DG. Studies of catecholamine shock. I. Disseminated intravascular coagulation. *Am J Pathol* 1969;56:153–176.
165. Good RA, Thomas L. Studies on the generalized Schwartzman reaction. IV. Prevention of the local and generalized Schwartzman reaction with heparin. *J Exp Med* 1953;97:871–888.
166. McKay DG, Whitaker AN. Studies of catecholamine shock. II. An experimental model of microangiopathic hemolysis. *Am J Pathol* 1969;56:177–200.
167. O'Rourke JF, Pugh CW, Bartlett SM, et al. Identification of hypoxically inducible mRNAs in HeLa cells using differential-display PCR. Role of hypoxia-inducible factor-1. *Eur J Biochem* 1996;241:403–410.
168. Yamazaki M, Asakura H, Aoshima K, et al. Effects of DX-9065a, an orally active, newly synthesized and specific inhibitor of factor Xa, against experimental disseminated intravascular coagulation in rats. *Thromb Haemost* 1994;72:392–396.
169. Hermida J, Montes R, Paramo JA, et al. Endotoxin-induced disseminated intravascular coagulation in rabbits: effect of recombinant hirudin on hemostatic parameters, fibrin deposits, and mortality. *J Lab Clin Med* 1998;131:77–83.
170. Rinaldo JE, Rogers RM. Adult respiratory distress syndrome. *N Engl J Med* 1986;315:578–580.
171. McDonald JA. The yin and yang of fibrin in the airways. *N Engl J Med* 1990;322:929–931.
172. Idell S. Extravascular coagulation and fibrin deposition in acute lung injury. *New Horizons* 1994;2:566–574.
173. Idell S, Koenig KB, Fair DS, et al. Serial abnormalities of fibrin turnover in evolving adult respiratory distress syndrome. *Am J Physiol* 1991;261:L240–L248.
174. Chapman HA, Stahl M, Allen CL, et al. Regulation of the procoagulant activity within the bronchoalveolar compartment of normal human lung. *Am Rev Respir Dis* 1988;137:1417–1425.
175. Hasegawa N, Husari AW, Hart WT, et al. Role of the coagulation system in ARDS. *Chest* 1994;105:268–277.
176. Chapman HAJ, Bertozzi P, Reilly JJ Jr. Role of enzymes mediating thrombosis and thrombolysis in lung disease. *Chest* 1988;93:1256–1263.
177. Bertozzi P, Astedt B, Zenzius L, et al. Depressed bronchoalveolar urokinase activity in patients with adult respiratory distress syndrome. *N Engl J Med* 1990;322:890–897.
178. Levi M, van der Poll T, ten Cate H, et al. Differential effects of anti-cytokine treatment on bronchoalveolar hemostasis in endotoxemic chimpanzees. *Am J Respir Crit Care Med* 1998;158:92–98.
179. Fan J, Kapus A, Li YH, et al. Priming for enhanced alveolar fibrin deposition after hemorrhagic shock: role of tumor necrosis factor. *Am J Respir Cell Mol Biol* 2000;22:412–421.
180. Gando S, Nanzaki S, Morimoto Y, et al. Systemic activation of tissue-factor dependent coagulation pathway in evolving acute respiratory distress syndrome in patients with trauma and sepsis. *J Trauma* 1999;47:719–723.
181. Gando S, Kameue T, Nanzaki S, et al. Participation of tissue factor and thrombin in posttraumatic systemic inflammatory syndrome. *Crit Care Med* 1997;25:1820–1826.
182. Gando S, Kameue T, Nanzaki S, et al. Increased neutrophil elastase, persistent intravascular coagulation, and decreased fibrinolytic activity in patients with posttraumatic acute respiratory distress syndrome. *J Trauma* 1997;42:1068–1072.
183. Langlois PF, Gawryl MS, Zeller J, et al. Accentuated complement activation in patient plasma during the adult respiratory distress syndrome: a potential mechanism for pulmonary inflammation. *Heart Lung* 1989;18:71–84.
184. Uchiba M, Okajima K, Murakami K, et al. Effects of plasma kallikrein specific inhibitor and active-site blocked factor VIIa on the pulmonary vascular injury induced by endotoxin in rats. *Thromb Haemost* 1997;78:1209–1214.
185. Müller-Berghaus G, Levi M, ten Cate H. Disseminated intravascular coagulation. In: Verstraete M, Topol E, Fuster V, eds. *Cardiovascular thrombosis: thrombocardiology*. Philadelphia: Lippincott–Raven Publishers, 1998:781.
186. van Gorp E, Suharti C, ten Cate H, et al. Review: infectious diseases and coagulation disorders. *J Infect Dis* 1999;180:176–186.
187. Thijs LG, de Boer JP, de Groot M, et al. Coagulation disorders in septic shock. *Intensive Care Med* 1993;19[Suppl]1:S8–S15.
188. Baglin T. Disseminated intravascular coagulation: diagnosis and treatment. *BMJ* 1996;312:683–687.
189. Bone RC. Gram-positive organisms and sepsis. *Arch Intern Med* 1994;154:26–34.
190. Bhamarapravati N. Hemostatic defects in dengue hemorrhagic fever. *Rev Infect Dis* 1989;11[Suppl 4]:S826–S829.
191. Heller MV, Marta RF, Sturk A, et al. Early markers of blood coagulation and fibrinolysis activation in Argentine hemorrhagic fever. *Thromb Haemost* 1995;73:368–373.
192. Clemens R, Pramoolsinsap C, Lorenz R, et al. Activation of the coagulation cascade in severe falciparum malaria through the intrinsic pathway. *Br J Haematol* 1994;87:100–105.
193. Mohanty D, Ghosh K, Nandwani SK, et al. Fibrinolysis, inhibitors of blood coagulation, and monocyte derived coagulant activity in acute malaria. *Am J Hematol* 1997;54:23–29.
194. Fera G, Semeraro N, De Mitrio V, et al. Disseminated intravascular coagulation associated with disseminated cryptococcosis in a patient with acquired immunodeficiency syndrome. *Infection* 1993;21:171–173.
195. ten Cate JW, van der Poll T, Levi M, et al. Cytokines: triggers of clinical thrombotic disease. *Thromb Haemost* 1997;78:415–419.
196. Ackerman AB, Chongchitnant N, Sanchez J, et al. Inflammatory diseases. In: *Histologic diagnosis of inflammatory skin diseases*. Williams & Wilkins, 1997:170.
197. Ratnoff OD, Nebehay WG. Multiple coagulative defects in a patient with Waterhouse-Friderichsen syndrome. *Ann Intern Med* 1962;56:627.
198. Dennis LH, Cohen RJ, Schachner SH, et al. Consumptive coagulopathy in fulminant meningococcemia. *JAMA* 1968;205:183–185.
199. Winkelstein A, Songster CL, Caras TS, et al. Fulminant meningococcemia and disseminated intravascular coagulation. *Arch Intern Med* 1969;124:55–59.
200. Corrigan JJ Jr. Ray WL, May N. Changes in the blood coagulation system associated with septicemia. *N Engl J Med* 1968;279:851–856.
201. Robboy SJ, Minna JD, Colman RW, et al. Pulmonary hemorrhage syndrome as a manifestation of disseminated intravascular coagulation: analysis of ten cases. *Chest* 1973;63:718–721.
202. Evans RW, Glick B, Kimball F, et al. Fatal intravascular consumption coagulopathy in meningococcal sepsis. *Am J Med* 1969;46:910–918.
203. Stiehm ER, Damrosch DS. Factors in the prognosis of meningococcal infection. Review of 63 cases with emphasis on recognition and management of the severely ill patient. *J Pediatr* 1966;68:457–467.
204. Gerard P, Moriau M, Bachy A, et al. Meningococcal purpura: report of 19 patients treated with heparin. *J Pediatr* 1973;82:780–786.
205. Gardlund B. Randomised, controlled trial of low-dose heparin for prevention of fatal pulmonary embolism in patients with infectious diseases. The Heparin Prophylaxis Study Group. *Lancet* 1996;347:1357–1361.
206. Laing RB, Brettle RP, Leen CL. Venous thrombosis in HIV infection. *Int J STD AIDS* 1996;7:82–85.
207. Jenkins RE, Peters BS, Pinching AJ. Thromboembolic disease in AIDS is associated with cytomegalovirus disease. *AIDS* 1991;5:1540–1542.

208. George SL, Swindells S, Knudson R, et al. Unexplained thrombosis in HIV-infected patients receiving protease inhibitors: report of seven cases. *Am J Med* 1999;107:624–630.
209. Hayes EB, Gubler DJ. Dengue and dengue hemorrhagic fever. *Pediatr Infect Dis J* 1992;11:311–317.
210. Sumarmo, Wulur H, Jahja E, et al. Clinical observations on virologically confirmed fatal dengue infections in Jakarta, Indonesia. *Bull World Health Organ* 1983;61:693–701.
211. Kuberski T, Rosen L, Reed D, et al. Clinical and laboratory observations on patients with primary and secondary dengue type 1 infections with hemorrhagic manifestations in Fiji. *Am J Trop Med Hyg* 1977;26:775–783.
212. Egbring R, Slenczka W, Baltzer G. Clinical manifestations and mechanism of the haemorrhagic diathesis in Marburg viral disease. In: Martini GA, Siegert R, eds. *Marburg virus disease.* New York: Springer-Verlag, 1971:41.
213. Gear JS, Cassel GA, Gear AJ, et al. Outbreak of Marburg virus disease in Johannesburg. *BMJ* 1975;4:489–493.
214. WHO International Study Team. Ebola haemorrhagic fever in Sudan. *Bull World Health Organ* 1978;56:247–270.
215. International Commission. Ebola haemorrhagic fever in Zaire. *Bull World Health Organ* 1978;56:271–293.
216. Limbos MA, Lieberman JM. Disseminated intravascular coagulation associated with rotavirus gastroenteritis: report of two cases. *Clin Infect Dis* 1996; 22:834–836.
217. WHO Scientific Working Group. Rotavirus and other viral diarrheas. *Bull World Health Organ* 1980;58:183–198.
218. McKay DG, Margaretten W. Disseminated intravascular coagulation in virus diseases. *Arch Intern Med* 1967;120:129–152.
219. Linder M, Müller-Berghaus G, Lasch HG, et al. Virus infection and blood coagulation. *Thromb Diath Haemorrh* 1970;23:1–11.
220. Talley NA, Assumpcao CA. Disseminated intravascular clotting complicating viral pneumonia due to influenza. *Med J Aust* 1971;2:763–766.
221. Cumming AD, Thomson D, Davidson AM, et al. Significance of urinary C3 excretion in glomerulonephritis. *J Clin Pathol* 1976;29:601–607.
222. Whitaker AN, Bunce I, Graeme ER. Disseminated intravascular coagulation and acute renal failure in influenza A2 infection. *Med J Aust* 1974;2:196–201.
223. Settle H, Glueck HI. Disseminated intravascular coagulation associated with influenza. *Ohio State Med J* 1900;71:541–543.
224. Anderson DR, Schwartz J, Hunter NJ, et al. Varicella hepatitis: a fatal case in a previously healthy, immunocompetent adult. Report of a case, autopsy, and review of the literature. *Arch Intern Med* 1994;154:2101–2106.
225. Badesha PS, Saklayen MG. Hemolytic uremic syndrome as a presenting form of HIV infection. *Nephron* 1996;72:472–475.
226. Chu QD, Medeiros LJ, Fisher AE, et al. Thrombotic thrombocytopenic purpura and HIV infection. *South Med J* 1995;88:82–86.
227. Qadri SM, Kayali S. Enterohemorrhagic Escherichia coli. A dangerous food-borne pathogen. *Postgrad Med* 1900;103:179–180.
228. Laing RW, Teh C, Toh CH. Thrombotic thrombocytopenic purpura (TTP) complicating leptospirosis: a previously undescribed association. *J Clin Pathol* 1990;43:961–962.
229. Lie JT. Vasculitis associated with infectious agents. *Curr Opin Rheumatol* 1996; 8:26–29.
230. Guillevin L, Lhote F, Gherardi R. The spectrum and treatment of virus-associated vasculitides. *Curr Opin Rheumatol* 1997;9:31–36.
231. Golden MP, Hammer SM, Wanke CA, et al. Cytomegalovirus vasculitis. Case reports and review of the literature. *Medicine* 1994;73:246–255.
232. Ho DD, Rota TR, Andrews CA, et al. Replication of human cytomegalovirus in endothelial cells. *J Infect Dis* 1984;150:956–957.
233. Goodman MD, Porter DD. Cytomegalovirus vasculitis with fatal colonic hemorrhage. *Arch Pathol Lab Med* 1973;96:281–284.
234. Foucar E, Mukai K, Foucar K, et al. Colon ulceration in lethal cytomegalovirus infection. *Am J Clin Pathol* 1981;76:788–801.
235. Booss J, Dann PR, Winkler SR, et al. Mechanisms of injury to the central nervous system following experimental cytomegalovirus infection. *Am J Otolaryngol* 1990;11:313–317.
236. Koeppen AH, Lansing LS, Peng SK, et al. Central nervous system vasculitis in cytomegalovirus infection. *J Neurol Sci* 1981;51:395–410.
237. Lin CS, Penha PD, Krishnan MN, et al. Cytomegalic inclusion disease of the skin. *Arch Dermatol* 1981;117:282–284.
238. Libman BS, Quismorio FPJ, Stimmler MM. Polyarteritis nodosa-like vasculitis in human immunodeficiency virus infection. *J Rheumatol* 1995;22:351–355.
239. Calabrese LH. Vasculitis and infection with the human immunodeficiency virus. *Rheum Dis Clin North Am* 1991;17:131–147.
240. Gherardi R, Belec L, Mhiri C, et al. The spectrum of vasculitis in human immunodeficiency virus-infected patients. A clinicopathologic evaluation. *Arthritis Rheum* 1993;36:1164–1174.
241. Oehler R, Bierhoff E, Loos U. Vasculitis in HIV infected patients. *Medizinische Klinik* 1900;88:327–329.
242. Sergent JS, Lockshin MD, Christian CL, et al. Vasculitis with hepatitis B antigenemia: long-term observation in nine patients. *Medicine* 1976;55:1–18.
243. Carson CW, Conn DL, Czaja AJ, et al. Frequency and significance of antibodies to hepatitis C virus in polyarteritis nodosa. *J Rheumatol* 1993;20:304–309.
244. Quint L, Deny P, Guillevin L, et al. Hepatitis C virus in patients with polyarteritis nodosa. Prevalence in 38 patients. *Clin Exp Rheumatol* 1991;9:253–257.
245. Leruez-Ville M, Lauge A, Morinet F, et al. Polyarteritis nodosa and parvovirus B19. *Lancet* 1994;344:263–264.
246. Nikkari S, Mertsola J, Korvenranta H, et al. Wegener's granulomatosis and parvovirus B19 infection. *Arthritis Rheum* 1994;37:1707–1708.
247. Yoto Y, Kudoh T, Haseyama K, et al. Human parvovirus B19 infection in Kawasaki disease. *Lancet* 1994;344:58–59.
248. Cotran RS. The endothelium and inflammation: new insights. *Monogr Pathol* 1982;18–37.
249. Stemerman MB, Colton C, Morell E. Perturbations of the endothelium. *Prog Hemost Thromb* 1984;7:289–324.
250. Kaiser L, Sparks HV Jr. Endothelial cells. Not just a cellophane wrapper. *Arch Intern Med* 1987;147:569–573.
251. Friedman HM, Macarak EJ, MacGregor RR, et al. Virus infection of endothelial cells. *J Infect Dis* 1981;143:266–273.
252. Friedman HM, Wolfe J, Kefalides NA, et al. Susceptibility of endothelial cells derived from different blood vessels to common viruses. *In Vitro Cell Dev Biol* 1986;22:397–401.
253. Friedman HM. Infection of endothelial cells by common human viruses. *Rev Infect Dis* 1989;11[Suppl 4]:S700–S704.
254. Hoxie JA, Matthews DM, Cines DB. Infection of human endothelial cells by human T-cell leukemia virus type I. *Proc Natl Acad Sci U S A* 1984;81:7591–7595.
255. Wiley CA, Schrier RD, Nelson JA, et al. Cellular localization of human immunodeficiency virus infection within the brains of acquired immune deficiency syndrome patients. *Proc Natl Acad Sci U S A* 1986;83:7089–7093.
256. Butthep P, Bunyaratvej A, Bhamarapravati N. Dengue virus and endothelial cell: a related phenomenon to thrombocytopenia and granulocytopenia in dengue hemorrhagic fever. *Southeast Asian J Trop Med Public Health* 1993; 24[Suppl 1]:246–249.
257. Bevilacqua MP, Pober JS, Wheeler ME, et al. Interleukin-1 activation of vascular endothelium. Effects on procoagulant activity and leukocyte adhesion. *Am J Pathol* 1985;121:394–403.
258. Adams DH, Wyner LR, Karnovsky MJ. Experimental graft arteriosclerosis. II. Immunocytochemical analysis of lesion development. *Transplantation* 1993;56:794–799.
259. Schorer AE, Kaplan ME, Rao GH, et al. Interleukin 1 stimulates endothelial cell tissue factor production and expression by a prostaglandin-independent mechanism. *Thromb Haemost* 1986;56:256–259.
260. van Dam-Mieras MC, Bruggeman CA, Muller AD, et al. Induction of endothelial cell procoagulant activity by cytomegalovirus infection. *Thromb Res* 1987;47:69–75.
261. van Dam-Mieras MC, Muller AD, van Hinsbergh V, et al. The procoagulant response of cytomegalovirus infected endothelial cells. *Thromb Haemost* 1992;68:364–370.
262. Etingin OR, Silverstein RL, Friedman HM, et al. Viral activation of the coagulation cascade: molecular interactions at the surface of infected endothelial cells. *Cell* 1990;61:657–662.
263. Visser MR, Tracy PB, Vercellotti GM, et al. Enhanced thrombin generation and platelet binding on herpes simplex virus-infected endothelium. *Proc Natl Acad Sci U S A* 1988;85:8227–8230.
264. Etingin OR, Silverstein RL, Hajjar DP. Identification of a monocyte receptor on herpesvirus-infected endothelial cells. *Proc Natl Acad Sci U S A* 1991;88: 7200–7203.
265. Dudding L, Haskill S, Clark BD, et al. Cytomegalovirus infection stimulates expression of monocyte-associated mediator genes. *J Immunol* 1989;143: 3343–3352.
266. Smith PD, Saini SS, Raffeld M, et al. Cytomegalovirus induction of tumor necrosis factor-alpha by human monocytes and mucosal macrophages. *J Clin Invest* 1992;90:1642–1648.
267. Almeida GD, Porada CD, St Jeor S, et al. Human cytomegalovirus alters interleukin-6 production by endothelial cells. *Blood* 1994;83:370–376.
268. McEver RP. GMP-140: a receptor for neutrophils and monocytes on activated platelets and endothelium. *J Cell Biochem* 1991;45:156–161.
269. Etingin OR, Silverstein RL, Hajjar DP. von Willebrand factor mediates platelet adhesion to virally infected endothelial cells. *Proc Natl Acad Sci U S A* 1993;90:5153–5156.
270. Anderson R, Wang S, Osiowy C, et al. Activation of endothelial cells via antibody-enhanced dengue virus infection of peripheral blood monocytes. *J Virol* 1997;71:4226–4232.
271. Takahashi M, Ikeda U, Masuyama J, et al. Monocyte-endothelial cell interaction induces expression of adhesion molecules on human umbilical cord endothelial cells. *Cardiovasc Res* 1996;32:422–429.
272. Seigneur M, Constans J, Blann A, et al. Soluble adhesion molecules and endothelial cell damage in HIV infected patients. *Thromb Haemost* 1997;77:646–649.
273. Drancourt M, George F, Brouqui P, et al. Diagnosis of Mediterranean spotted fever by indirect immunofluorescence of Rickettsia conorii in circulating endothelial cells isolated with monoclonal antibody-coated immunomagnetic beads. *J Infect Dis* 1992;166:660–663.
274. George F, Brouqui P, Boffa MC, et al. Demonstration of Rickettsia conorii-induced endothelial injury in vivo by measuring circulating endothelial cells, thrombomodulin, and von Willebrand factor in patients with Mediterranean spotted fever. *Blood* 1993;82:2109–2116.
275. Solovey A, Lin Y, Browne P, et al. Circulating activated endothelial cells in sickle cell anemia. *N Engl J Med* 1997;337:1584–1590.
276. Esmon CT. The regulation of natural anticoagulant pathways. *Science* 1987;235:1348–1352.
277. Sugerman RW, Church JA, Goldsmith JC, et al. Acquired protein S deficiency in children infected with human immunodeficiency virus. *Pediatr Infect Dis J* 1996;15:106–111.

278. Stahl CP, Wideman CS, Spira TJ, et al. Protein S deficiency in men with long-term human immunodeficiency virus infection. *Blood* 1993;81:1801–1807.

279. Lafeuillade A, Alessi MC, Poizot-Martin I, et al. Endothelial cell dysfunction in HIV infection. *J Acquir Immune Defic Syndr* 1992;5:127–131.

280. Bissuel F, Berruyer M, Causse X, et al. Acquired protein S deficiency: correlation with advanced disease in HIV-1-infected patients. *J Acquir Immune Defic Syndr* 1992;5:484–489.

281. Malia RG, Kitchen S, Greaves M, et al. Inhibition of activated protein C and its cofactor protein S by antiphospholipid antibodies. *Br J Haematol* 1990;76: 101–107.

282. Lo SC, Salem HH, Howard MA, et al. Studies of natural anticoagulant proteins and anticardiolipin antibodies in patients with the lupus anticoagulant. *Br J Haematol* 1990;76:380–386.

283. Hassell KL, Kressin DC, Neumann A, et al. Correlation of antiphospholipid antibodies and protein S deficiency with thrombosis in HIV-infected men. *Blood Coagul Fibrinolysis* 1994;5:455–462.

284. Llorente MR, Carton JA, Carcaba V, et al. Antiphospholipid antibodies in human immunodeficiency virus infection. *Medicina Clinica* 1994;103:10–13.

284a. Suharti C, Van Gorp EC, Setiati TE, et al. The role of cytokines in activation of coagulation and fibrinolysis in Dengue shick syndrome. *Thromb Haemost* 2002;87(1):42–46.

285. Levin J. Bleeding with infectious disease. In: Ratnoff OD, Forbes CD, eds. *Disorders of hemostasis.* Orlando, FL: Grune & Stratton, 1984:367.

286. Nakao S, Lai CJ, Young NS. Dengue virus, a flavivirus, propagates in human bone marrow progenitors and hematopoietic cell lines. *Blood* 1989;74:1235–1240.

287. Na-Nakorn S, Suingdumrong A, Pootrakul S, et al. Bone marrow studies in Thai hemorrhagic fever. *Bull World Health Organ* 1966;35:54–55.

288. Halstead SB. Antibody, macrophages, dengue virus infection, shock, and hemorrhage: a pathogenetic cascade. *Rev Infect Dis* 1989;11[Suppl 4]:S830–S839.

289. Terada H, Baldini M, Ebbe S, et al. Interaction of influenza virus with blood platelets. *Blood* 1966;28:213–228.

290. Stemerman MB. Vascular intimal components: precursors of thrombosis. *Prog Hemost Thromb* 1974;2:1–47.

291. Curwen KD, Gimbrone MAJ, Handin RI. In vitro studies of thromboresistance: the role of prostacyclin (PGI2) in platelet adhesion to cultured normal and virally transformed human vascular endothelial cells. *Lab Invest* 1980;42:366–374.

292. Graham DY, Brown CH, Benrey J, et al. Thrombocytopenia. A complication of mumps. *JAMA* 1974;227:1162–1164.

293. Myllyla G, Vaheri A, Vesikari T, et al. Interaction between human blood platelets, viruses and antibodies. IV. Post-Rubella thrombocytopenic purpura and platelet aggregation by Rubella antigen-antibody interaction. *Clin Exp Immunol* 1969;4:323–332.

294. Morse EE, Zinkham WH, Jackson DP. Thrombocytopenic purpura following rubella infection in children and adults. *Arch Intern Med* 1966;117:573–579.

295. Charkes ND. Purpuric chickenpox: report of a case, review of the literature and classification by clinical features. *Ann Intern Med* 1961;54:745–759.

296. Tobin JDJ, Ten BR. Varicella with thrombocytopenia causing fatal intracerebral hemorrhage. *Am J Dis Child* 1972;124:577–578.

297. Brook I. Disseminated varicella with pneumonia, meningoencephalitis, thrombocytopenia, and fatal intracranial hemorrhage. *South Med J* 1979;72: 756–757.

298. Whitaker JA, Hardison JE. Severe thrombocytopenia after generalized herpes simplex-2 (HSV-2) infection. *South Med J* 1978;71:864–865.

299. Chanarin I, Walford DM. Thrombocytopenic purpura in cytomegalovirus mononucleosis. *Lancet* 1973;2:238–239.

300. Sahud MA, Bachelor MM. Cytomegalovirus-induced thrombocytopenia. An unusual case report. *Arch Intern Med* 1978;138:1573–1575.

301. Casey TP, Matthews JR. Thrombocytopenic purpura in infectious mononucleosis. *N Z Med J* 1973;77:318–320.

302. Ellman L, Carvalho A, Jacobson BM, et al. Platelet autoantibody in a case of infectious mononucleosis presenting as thrombocytopenic purpura. *Am J Med* 1973;55:723–726.

303. Mazza J, Friedenberg W. Clinical cancer. 5. Progress in acute leukemia. *Wisconsin Med J* 1986;85:26–27.

304. Lo TT, Wang SH, Hwang HF, et al. Mechanisms of bleeding and the search for treatment in epidemic hemorrhagic fever. *Chin J Infect Dis* 1986;4:716–719.

305. Suvatte V. Dengue hemorrhagic fever: hematological abnormalities and pathogenesis. *J Med Assoc Thai* 1978;61[Suppl 3]:53–58.

306. Swanepoel R, Shepherd AJ, Leman PA, et al. Epidemiologic and clinical features of Crimean-Congo hemorrhagic fever in southern Africa. *Am J Tropic Med Hyg* 1987;36:120–132.

307. Bergentz SE, Nilsson IM. Effect of trauma on coagulation and fibrinolysis in dogs. *Acta Chirurgica Scandinavica* 1961;122:21–25.

308. McGehee WG, Rapaport SI. Systemic hemostatic failure in the severely injured patient. *Surg Clin North Am* 1968;48:1247–1256.

309. McKay DG. Trauma and disseminated intravascular coagulation. *J Trauma* 1969;9:646–660.

310. Attar S, Boyd D, Layne E, et al. Alterations in coagulation and fibrinolytic mechanisms in acute trauma. *J Trauma* 1969;9:939–965.

311. Simmons RL, Collins JA, Heisterkamp CA, et al. Coagulation disorders in combat casualties. I. Acute changes after wounding. II. Effects of massive transfusion. 3. Post-resuscitative changes. *Ann Surg* 1969;169:455–482.

312. Ordog GJ, Wasserberger J, Balasubramanium S. Coagulation abnormalities in traumatic shock. *Ann Emerg Med* 1985;14:650–655.

313. Roumen RM, Hendriks T, van der Ven, et al. Cytokine patterns in patients after major vascular surgery, hemorrhagic shock, and severe blunt trauma.

Relation with subsequent adult respiratory distress syndrome and multiple organ failure. *Ann Surg* 1993;218:769–776.

314. Zenker FA. *Beitrage zur normalen und pathologischen anatomie der lungen.* Braunsdorf, Dresden, 1862.

315. Herndon JH, Riseborough EJ, Fischer JE. Fat embolism: a review of current concepts. *J Trauma* 1971;11:673–680.

316. Peltier LF. The diagnosis and treatment of fat embolism. *J Trauma* 1971;11:661–667.

317. Curtis AM, Knowles GD, Putman CE, et al. The three syndromes of fat embolism: pulmonary manifestations. *Yale J Biol Med* 1979;52:149–157.

318. Goodnight SH, Kenoyer G, Rapaport SI, et al. Defibrination after brain-tissue destruction: a serious complication of head injury. *N Engl J Med* 1974;290: 1043–1047.

319. Druskin MS, Drijansky R. Afibrinogenemia with severe head trauma. *JAMA* 1972;219:755–756.

320. Keimowitz RM, Annis BL. Disseminated intravascular coagulation associated with massive brain injury. *J Neurosurg* 1973;39:178–180.

321. Pondaag W. Disseminated intravascular coagulation related to outcome in head injury. *Acta Neurochir Suppl (Wien)* 1979;28:98–102.

322. Miner ME, Kaufman HH, Graham SH, et al. Disseminated intravascular coagulation fibrinolytic syndrome following head injury in children: frequency and prognostic implications. *J Pediatr* 1982;100:687–691.

323. Kaufman HH, Hui KS, Mattson JC, et al. Clinicopathological correlations of disseminated intravascular coagulation in patients with head injury. *Neurosurgery* 1984;15:34–42.

324. Kumura E, Sato M, Fukuda A, et al. Coagulation disorders following acute head injury. *Acta Neurochir (Wien)* 1987;85:23–28.

325. Olson JD, Kaufman HH, Moake J, et al. The incidence and significance of hemostatic abnormalities in patients with head injuries. *Neurosurgery* 1989; 24:825–832.

326. Colman RW, Rubin RN. Disseminated intravascular coagulation due to malignancy. *Semin Oncol* 1990;17:172–186.

327. Sarris AH, Kempin S, Berman E, et al. High incidence of disseminated intravascular coagulation during remission induction of adult patients with acute lymphoblastic leukemia. *Blood* 1992;79:1305–1310.

328. Donati MB. Cancer and thrombosis: from Phlegmasia alba dolens to transgenic mice. *Thromb Haemost* 1995;74:278–281.

329. Contrino J, Hair G, Kreutzer DL, et al. In situ detection of tissue factor in vascular endothelial cells: correlation with the malignant phenotype of human breast disease. *Nat Med* 1996;2:209–215.

330. Hair GA, Padula S, Zeff R, et al. Tissue factor expression in human leukemic cells. *Leuk Res* 1996;20:1–11.

331. Bromberg ME, Konigsberg WH, Madison JF, et al. Tissue factor promotes melanoma metastasis by a pathway independent of blood coagulation. *Proc Natl Acad Sci U S A* 1995;92:8205–8209.

332. Zhang Y, Deng Y, Luther T, et al. Tissue factor controls the balance of angiogenic and antiangiogenic properties of tumor cells in mice. *J Clin Invest* 1994;94:1320–1327.

333. Ishibashi M, Ito N, Fujita M, et al. Endothelin-1 as an aggravating factor of disseminated intravascular coagulation associated with malignant neoplasms. *Cancer* 1994;73:191–195.

334. Ruf W, Mueller BM. Tissue factor in cancer angiogenesis and metastasis. *Curr Opin Hematol* 1996;3:379–384.

335. Palumbo JS, Degen JL. Hemostatic factors in tumor biology. *J Pediatr Hematol Oncol* 2000;22:281–287.

336. Gordon SG, Cross BA. A factor X-activating cysteine protease from malignant tissue. *J Clin Invest* 1981;67:1665–1671.

337. Tallman MS. The thrombophilic state in acute promyelocytic leukemia. *Semin Thromb Hemost* 1999;25:209–215.

338. Rodeghiero F, Castaman G. The pathophysiology and treatment of hemorrhagic syndrome of acute promyelocytic leukemia. *Leukemia* 1994;8[Suppl 2]:S20–S26.

339. Hajjar KA, Acharya SS. Annexin II and regulation of cell surface fibrinolysis. *Ann N Y Acad Sci* 2000;902:265–271.

340. Falanga A, Consonni R, Marchetti M, et al. Cancer procoagulant and tissue factor are differently modulated by all-trans-retinoic acid in acute promyelocytic leukemia cells. *Blood* 1998;92:143–151.

341. Barbui T, Finazzi G, Falanga A. The impact of all-trans-retinoic acid on the coagulopathy of acute promyelocytic leukemia. *Blood* 1998;91:3093–3102.

342. Kelly DA, Tuddenham EG. Haemostatic problems in liver disease. *Gut* 1986;27:339–349.

343. Tytgat GN, Collen D, Verstraete M. Metabolism of fibrinogen in cirrhosis of the liver. *J Clin Invest* 1971;50:169–701.

344. Coleman M, Finlayson N, Bettigole RE, et al. Fibrinogen survival in cirrhosis: improvement by "low dose" heparin. *Ann Intern Med* 1975;83:79–81.

345. Rake MO, Flute PT, Pannell G, et al. Intravascular coagulation in acute hepatic necrosis. *Lancet* 1970;1:533–537.

346. Carr JM, McKinney M, McDonagh J. Diagnosis of disseminated intravascular coagulation. Role of D-dimer. *Am J Clin Pathol* 1989;91:280–287.

347. Coccheri S, Mannucci PM, Palareti G, et al. Significance of plasma fibrinopeptide A and high molecular weight fibrinogen in patients with liver cirrhosis. *Br J Haematol* 1982;52:503–509.

348. Straub PW. Diffuse intravascular coagulation in liver disease? *Semin Thromb Hemost* 1977;4:29–39.

349. Tempero MA, Davis RB, Reed E, et al. Thrombocytopenia and laboratory evidence of disseminated intravascular coagulation after shunts for ascites in malignant disease. *Cancer* 1985;55:2718–2721.

350. Violi F, Ferro D, Basili S, et al. Association between low-grade disseminated intravascular coagulation and endotoxemia in patients with liver cirrhosis. *Gastroenterology* 1995;109:531–539.

351. Ragni MV, Lewis JH, Spero JA. Ascites-induced LeVeen shunt coagulopathy. *Ann Surg* 1983;198:91–95.

352. Phillips LL, Rodgers JB. Procoagulant activity of ascitic fluid in hepatic cirrhosis: in vivo and in vitro. *Surgery* 1979;86:714–721.

353. Salem HH, Koutts J, Handley C, et al. The aggregation of human platelets by ascitic fluid: a possible mechanism for disseminated intravascular coagulation complicating LeVeen shunts. *Am J Hematol* 1981;11:153–157.

354. LeVeen HH, Ip M, Ahmed N, et al. Coagulopathy post peritoneovenous shunt. *Ann Surg* 1987;205:305–311.

355. Gibson PR, Dudley FJ, Jakobovits AW, et al. Disseminated intravascular coagulation following peritoneo-venous (LeVeen) shunt. *Aust N Z J Med* 1981;11:8–12.

356. Stein SF, Fulenwider JT, Ansley JD, et al. Accelerated fibrinogen and platelet destruction after peritoneovenous shunting. *Arch Intern Med* 1981;141:1149–1151.

357. Rubinstein D, McInnes I, Dudley F. Morbidity and mortality after peritoneovenous shunt surgery for refractory ascites. *Gut* 1985;26:1070–1073.

358. Buller HR, ten CJ. Antithrombin III infusion in patients undergoing peritoneovenous shunt operation: failure in the prevention of disseminated intravascular coagulation. *Thromb Haemost* 1983;49:128–131.

359. Szlachetka DM. Kasabach-Merritt syndrome: a case review. *Neonatal Netw* 1998;17:7–15.

360. Gibney EJ, Bouchier-Hayes D. Coagulopathy and abdominal aortic aneurysm. *Eur J Vasc Surg* 1990;4:557–562.

361. Aboulafia DM, Aboulafia ED. Aortic aneurysm-induced intravascular coagulation. *Ann Vasc Surg* 1996;10:396–405.

362. Kasabach HH, Merritt KK. Capillary hemangioma with extensive purpura. *Am J Dis Child* 1940;59:1063.

363. Straub PW, Kessler S, Schreiber A, et al. Chronic intravascular coagulation in Kasabach-Merritt syndrome. Preferential accumulation of fibrinogen 131 I in a giant hemangioma. *Arch Intern Med* 1972;129:475–478.

364. Warrell RPJ, Kempin SJ, Benua RS, et al. Intratumoral consumption of indium-111 labeled platelets in a patient with hemangiomatosis and intravascular coagulation (Kasabach-Merritt syndrome). *Cancer* 1983;52:2256–2260.

365. Neidhart JA, Roach RW. Successful treatment of skeletal hemangioma and Kasabach-Merritt syndrome with aminocaproic acid. Is fibrinolysis "defensive"? *Am J Med* 1982;73:434–438.

366. el-Dessouky M, Azmy AF, Raine PA, et al. Kasabach-Merritt syndrome. *J Pediatr Surg* 1988;23:109–111.

367. D'Amico JA, Hoffman GC, Dyment PG. Klippel-Trenaunay syndrome associated with chronic disseminated intravascular coagulation and massive osteolysis. *Cleve Clin Q* 1977;44:181–188.

368. Poon MC, Kloiber R, Birdsell DC. Epsilon-aminocaproic acid in the reversal of consumptive coagulopathy with platelet sequestration in a vascular malformation of Klippel-Trenaunay syndrome. *Am J Med* 1989;87:211–213.

369. Alpert LI, Benisch B. Hemangioendothelioma of the liver associated with microangiopathic hemolytic anemia. Report of four cases. *Am J Med* 1970;48:624–628.

370. Bick RL. Hereditary hemorrhagic telangiectasia and disseminated intravascular coagulation: a new clinical syndrome. *Ann N Y Acad Sci* 1981;370:851–854.

371. de Boer K, ten CJ, Sturk A, et al. Enhanced thrombin generation in normal and hypertensive pregnancy. *Am J Obstet Gynecol* 1989;160:95–100.

372. Weiner CP. Preeclampsia-eclampsia syndrome and coagulation. *Clin Perinatol* 1991;18:713–726.

373. Martin JNJ, Stedman CM. Imitators of preeclampsia and HELLP syndrome. *Obstet Gynecol Clin North Am* 1991;18:181–198.

374. Weiner CP. The obstetric patient and disseminated intravascular coagulation. *Clin Perinatol* 1986;13:705–717.

375. Dieckmann WJ. Blood chemistry and renal function in abruptio placentae. *Am J Obstet Gynecol* 1937;31:734–740.

376. Schneider CL. The active principle of placental toxin: thromboplastin; its inactivator in blood: antithromboplastin. *Am J Physiol* 1947;149:123–128.

377. Arafeh JM. Disseminated intravascular coagulation in pregnancy: an update. *J Perinat Neonat Nurs* 1997;11:30–45.

378. Lurie S, Feinstein M, Mamet Y. Disseminated intravascular coagulopathy in pregnancy: thorough comprehension of etiology and management reduces obstetricians' stress. *Arch Gynecol Obstet* 2000;263:126–130.

379. Pritchard JA, Brekken AL. Clinical and laboratory studies on severe abruptio placentae. *Am J Obstet Gynecol* 1967;97:681–700.

380. McDougall RJ, Duke GJ. Amniotic fluid embolism syndrome: case report and review. *Anaesth Intensive Care* 1995;23:735–740.

381. Steiner PE, Lushbaugh CC. Maternal pulmonary embolism by amniotic fluid as a cause of obstetric shock and unexpected death in obstetrics. *JAMA* 1941;117:1245–1250.

382. Morgan M. Amniotic fluid embolism. *Anaesthesia* 1979;34:20–32.

383. Courtney LD, Allington M. Effect of amniotic fluid on blood coagulation. *Br J Haematol* 1972;22:353–355.

384. Phillips LL, Davidson EC Jr. Procoagulant properties of amniotic fluid. *Am J Obstet Gynecol* 1972;113:911–919.

385. Weiner CP, Brandt J. A modified activated partial thromboplastin time with the use of amniotic fluid. Preliminary report of a new technique for detection of fetal lung maturity. *Am J Obstet Gynecol* 1982;144:234–240.

386. Seegers WH, Ouyang C. Snake venoms and blood coagulation. In: Chen-Yuan L, ed. *Snake venoms*. Berlin: Springer-Verlag, 1979:684.

387. Reid HA. Clinical hemostatic disorders caused by venoms. In: Ratnoff OD, Forbes CD, eds. *Disorders of hemostasis*. Orlando: Grune & Stratton, 1984.

388. Warrell DA, Pope HM, Prentice CR. Disseminated intravascular coagulation caused by the carpet viper (Echis carinatus): trial of heparin. *Br J Haematol* 1976;33:335–342.

389. Geoffroy EF, Hunauld I. *Mémoire dans lequel on examine si l'huile d'ólive est un specifique contre le morsure de vipères*. Paris, 1737.

390. Fontana F. *Treatise on the venom of the viper*. London, 1787.

391. Martin CJ. On some effects upon the blood produced by the injection of the venom of the Australian black snake. *J Physiol* 1893;15:380–391.

392. Nahas L, Denson KW, MacFarlane RG. A study of the coagulant action of eight snake venoms and proteases. *Thromb Diath Haemorrh* 1964;12:355–360.

393. Markland FS, Kettner C, Schiffman S, et al. Kallikrein-like activity of crotalase, a snake venom enzyme that clots fibrinogen. *Proc Natl Acad Sci U S A* 1982;79:1688–1692.

394. Hasiba U, Rosenbach LM, Rockwell D, et al. DiC-like syndrome after envenomation by the snake, Crotalus horridus horridus. *N Engl J Med* 1975;292:505–507.

395. Klein JD, Walker FJ. Purification of a protein C activator from the venom of the southern copperhead snake (Agkistrodon contortrix contortrix). *Biochemistry* 1986;25:4175–4179.

396. Huang TF, Holt JC, Lukasiewicz H, et al. Trigramin. A low molecular weight peptide inhibiting fibrinogen interaction with platelet receptors expressed on glycoprotein IIb-IIIa complex. *J Biol Chem* 1987;262:16157–16163.

397. Wakefield EG, Hall WW. Heat injuries: a preparatory study for experimental heat stroke. *JAMA* 1927;89:92–95.

398. Hart GR, Anderson RJ, Crumpler CP, et al. Epidemic classical heat stroke: clinical characteristics and course of 28 patients. *Medicine* 1982;61:189–197.

399. Chao TC, Sinniah R, Pakiam JE. Acute heat stroke deaths. *Pathology* 1981;13:145–156.

400. Mustafa KY, Omer O, Khogali M, et al. Blood coagulation and fibrinolysis in heat stroke. *Br J Haematol* 1985;61:517–523.

401. Meikle AW, Graybill JR. Fibrinolysis and hemorrhage in a fatal case of heat stroke. *N Engl J Med* 1967;276:911–913.

402. Perchick JS, Winkelstein A, Shadduck RK. Disseminated intravascular coagulation in heat stroke. Response to heparin therapy. *JAMA* 1975;231:480–483.

403. Ruggenenti P, Lutz J, Remuzzi G. Pathogenesis and treatment of thrombotic microangiopathy. *Kidney Int Suppl* 1997;58:S97–S101.

404. Besser RE, Griffin PM, Slutsker L. Escherichia coli O157:H7 gastroenteritis and the hemolytic uremic syndrome: an emerging infectious disease. *Annu Rev Med* 1999;50:355–367.

405. Furlan M, Robles R, Galbusera M, et al. von Willebrand factor-cleaving protease in thrombotic thrombocytopenic purpura and the hemolytic-uremic syndrome. *N Engl J Med* 1998;339:1578–1584.

406. Furlan M, Robles R, Solenthaler M, et al. Acquired deficiency of von Willebrand factor-cleaving protease in a patient with thrombotic thrombocytopenic purpura. *Blood* 1998;91:2839–2846.

407. Tsai HM, Lian EC. Antibodies to von Willebrand factor-cleaving protease in acute thrombotic thrombocytopenic purpura. *N Engl J Med* 1998;339:1585–1594.

408. Bick RL. Disseminated intravascular coagulation: objective clinical and laboratory diagnosis, treatment, and assessment of therapeutic response. *Semin Thromb Hemost* 1996;22:69–88.

409. Williams EC, Mosher DF. Disseminated intravascular coagulation. In: Hoffman R, Benz EJ Jr, Shattil SJ, eds. *Hematology. Basic principles and practice*. New York: Churchill Livingstone, 1995:1758.

410. Cembrowski GS, Griffin JH, Mosher DF. Diagnostic efficacy of six plasma proteins in evaluating consumptive coagulopathies. Use of receiver operating characteristic curves to compare antithrombin III, plasminogen, alpha 2-plasmin inhibitor, fibronectin, prothrombin, and protein C. *Arch Intern Med* 1986;146:1997–2002.

411. Mesters RM, Mannucci PM, Coppola R, et al. Factor VIIa and antithrombin III activity during severe sepsis and septic shock in neutropenic patients. *Blood* 1996;88:881–886.

412. Marx R, Meisner A. On hyperfibrinolysis and its treatment. *Angiologica* 1968;5:105–118.

413. Rodeghiero F, Castaman G. The pathophysiology and treatment of hemorrhagic syndrome of acute promyelocytic leukemia. *Leukemia* 1994;8[Suppl 2]:S20–S26.

414. Fiegl M, Weltermann A, Stindl R, et al. Massive disseminated intravascular coagulation and hyperfibrinolysis in alveolar rhabdomyosarcoma: case report and review of the literature. *Ann Hematol* 1999;78:335–338.

415. Dempfle CE, Pfitzner SA, Dollman M, et al. Comparison of immunological and functional assays for measurement of soluble fibrin. *Thromb Haemost* 1995;74:673–679.

416. Bredbacka S, Blomback M, Wiman B. Soluble fibrin: a predictor for the development and outcome of multiple organ failure. *Am J Hematol* 1994;46:289–294.

417. Okajima K, Uchiba M, Murakami K, et al. Determination of plasma soluble fibrin using a new ELISA method in patients with disseminated intravascular coagulation. *Am J Hematol* 1996;51:186–191.

418. McCarron BI, Marder VJ, Kanouse JJ, et al. A soluble fibrin standard: comparable dose-response with immunologic and functional assays. *Thromb Haemost* 1999;82:145–148.

419. Scheefers-Borchel U, Müller-Berghaus G, Fuhge P, et al. Discrimination between fibrin and fibrinogen by a monoclonal antibody against a synthetic peptide. *Proc Natl Acad Sci U S A* 1985;82:7091–7095.

420. Nieuwenhuizen W, Hoegee-De NE, Laterveer R. A rapid monoclonal antibody-based enzyme immunoassay (EIA) for the quantitative determination of soluble fibrin in plasma. *Thromb Haemost* 1992;68:273–277.

421. Shorr AF, Trotta RF, Alkins SA, et al. D-dimer assay predicts mortality in critically ill patients without disseminated intravascular coagulation or venous thromboembolic disease. *Intensive Care Med* 1999;25:207–210.

422. Bos R, Laterveer-Vreeswijk GH, Lockwood D, et al. A new enzyme immunoassay for soluble fibrin in plasma, with a high discriminating power for thrombotic disorders. *Thromb Haemost* 1999;81:54–59.

423. Dempfle CE. The use of soluble fibrin in evaluating the acute and chronic hypercoagulable state. *Thromb Haemost* 1999;82:673–683.

424. Carr ME Jr. Disseminated intravascular coagulation: pathogenesis, diagnosis, and therapy. *J Emerg Med* 1987;5:311–322.

425. Boisclair MD, Ireland H, Lane DA. Assessment of hypercoagulable states by measurement of activation fragments and peptides. *Blood Rev* 1990;4:25–40.

426. Prisco D, Paniccia R, Bonechi F, et al. Evaluation of new methods for the selective measurement of fibrin and fibrinogen degradation products. *Thromb Res* 1989;56:547–551.

427. Nakamura Y, Tomura S, Tachibana K, et al. Enhanced fibrinolytic activity during the course of hemodialysis. *Clin Nephrol* 1992;38:90–96.

428. Tomura S, Nakamura Y, Deguchi F, et al. Coagulation and fibrinolysis in patients with chronic renal failure undergoing conservative treatment. *Thromb Res* 1991;64:81–90.

429. Bick RL, Baker WF. Diagnostic efficacy of the D-dimer assay in disseminated intravascular coagulation (DIC). *Thromb Res* 1992;65:785–790.

430. Rylatt DB, Blake AS, Cottis LE, et al. An immunoassay for human D dimer using monoclonal antibodies. *Thromb Res* 1983;31:767–778.

431. Whitaker AN, Elms MJ, Masci PP, et al. Measurement of cross linked fibrin derivatives in plasma: an immunoassay using monoclonal antibodies. *J Clin Pathol* 1984;37:882–887.

432. Greenberg CS, Devine DV, McCrae KM. Measurement of plasma fibrin D-dimer levels with the use of a monoclonal antibody coupled to latex beads. *Am J Clin Pathol* 1987;87:94–100.

433. Teitel JM, Bauer KA, Lau HK, et al. Studies of the prothrombin activation pathway utilizing radioimmunoassays for the F2/F1 + 2 fragment and thrombin-antithrombin complex. *Blood* 1982;59:1086–1097.

434. Bauer KA, Kass BL, ten Cate H, et al. Detection of factor X activation in humans. *Blood* 1989;74:2007–2015.

435. Leeksma OC, Meijer-Huizinga F, Stoepman-van DE, et al. Fibrinopeptide A and the phosphate content of fibrinogen in venous thromboembolism and disseminated intravascular coagulation. *Blood* 1986;67:1460–1467.

436. Nossel HL, Yudelman I, Canfield RE, et al. Measurement of fibrinopeptide A in human blood. *J Clin Invest* 1974;54:43–53.

437. Cronlund M, Hardin J, Burton J, et al. Fibrinopeptide A in plasma of normal subjects and patients with disseminated intravascular coagulation and systemic lupus erythematosus. *J Clin Invest* 1976;58:142–151.

438. Neame PB, Kelton JG, Walker IR, et al. Thrombocytopenia in septicemia: the role of disseminated intravascular coagulation. *Blood* 1980;56:88–92.

439. Akca S, Haji-Michael P, de Mendonca A, et al. The time course of platelet counts in critically ill patients. *Crit Care Med* 2002;30:753–756.

440. Wada H, Wakita Y, Nakase T, et al. Outcome of disseminated intravascular coagulation in relation to the score when treatment was begun. Mie DIC Study Group. *Thromb Haemost* 1995;74:848–852.

441. Fijnvandraat K, Derkx B, Peters M, et al. Coagulation activation and tissue necrosis in meningococcal septic shock: severely reduced protein C levels predict a high mortality. *Thromb Haemost* 1995;73:15–20.

442. Mesters RM, Helterbrand J, Utterback BG, et al. Prognostic value of protein C concentrations in neutropenic patients at high risk of severe septic complications. *Crit Care Med* 2000;28:2209–2216.

443. Harpel PC. Alpha2-plasmin inhibitor and alpha2-macroglobulin-plasmin complexes in plasma. Quantitation by an enzyme-linked differential antibody immunosorbent assay. *J Clin Invest* 1981;68:46–55.

444. Brower MS, Harpel PC. Alpha-1-antitrypsin-human leukocyte elastase complexes in blood: quantification by an enzyme-linked differential antibody immunosorbent assay and comparison with alpha-2-plasmin inhibitor-plasmin complexes. *Blood* 1983;61:842–849.

445. Levi M, de Boer J, Roem D, et al. Plasminogen activation in vivo upon intravenous infusion of DDAVP. Quantitative assessment of plasmin-alpha 2-antiplasmin complex with a novel monoclonal antibody based radioimmunoassay. *Thromb Haemost* 1992;67:111–116.

446. Levi M, Roem D, Kamp AM, et al. Assessment of the relative contribution of different protease inhibitors to the inhibition of plasmin in vivo. *Thromb Haemost* 1993;69:141–146.

447. Mesters RM, Florke N, Ostermann H, et al. Increase of plasminogen activator inhibitor levels predicts outcome of leukocytopenic patients with sepsis. *Thromb Haemost* 1996;75:902–907.

448. Leithauser B, Matthias FR, Nicolai U, et al. Hemostatic abnormalities and the severity of illness in patients at the onset of clinically defined sepsis. Possible indication of the degree of endothelial cell activation? *Intensive Care Med* 1996;22:631–636.

449. Kidokoro A, Iba T, Fukunaga M, et al. Alterations in coagulation and fibrinolysis during sepsis. *Shock* 1996;5:223–228.

450. Gando S, Nakanishi Y, Tedo I. Cytokines and plasminogen activator inhibitor-1 in posttrauma disseminated intravascular coagulation: relationship to multiple organ dysfunction syndrome. *Crit Care Med* 1995;23:1835–1842.

451. Bonnar J. Massive obstetric haemorrhage. *Best Pract Res Clin Obstet Gynaecol* 2000;14:1–18.

452. Brandjes DP, Schenk BE, Buller HR, et al. Management of disseminated intravascular coagulation in obstetrics. *Eur J Obstet Gynecol Reprod Biol* 1991;42[Suppl]:S87–S89.

453. Rocha E, Paramo JA, Montes R, et al. Acute generalized, widespread bleeding. Diagnosis and management. *Haematologica* 1998;83:1024–1037.

454. Gross SJ, Filston HC, Anderson JC. Controlled study of treatment for disseminated intravascular coagulation in the neonate. *J Pediatr* 1982;100:445–448.

455. de Jonge E, Levi M, Stoutenbeek CP, et al. Current drug treatment strategies for disseminated intravascular coagulation. *Drugs* 1998;55:767–777.

456. Rubin RN, Colman RW. Disseminated intravascular coagulation. Approach to treatment. *Drugs* 1992;44:963–971.

457. Humphries JE. Transfusion therapy in acquired coagulopathies. *Hematol Oncol Clin North Am* 1994;8:1181–1201.

458. Spannagl M, Schramm W. Replacement of coagulation factors in liver or multiple organ dysfunction. *Thromb Res* 1999;95:S51–S56.

459. Little JR. Purpura fulminans treated successfully with anticoagulation: report of a case. *JAMA* 1959;169:36–40.

460. Gaskins RAJ, Dalldorf FG. Experimental meningococcal septicemia. Effect of heparin therapy. *Arch Pathol Lab Med* 1976;100:318–324.

461. Corrigan JJ Jr. Kiernat JF. Effect of heparin in experimental gram-negative septicemia. *J Infect Dis* 1975;131:138–143.

462. Corrigan JJ Jr. Jordan CM. Heparin therapy in septicemia with disseminated intravascular coagulation. *N Engl J Med* 1970;283:778–782.

463. Corrigan JJ Jr. Heparin therapy in bacterial septicemia. *J Pediatr* 1977;91:695–700.

464. Feinstein DI. Diagnosis and management of disseminated intravascular coagulation: the role of heparin therapy. *Blood* 1982;60:284–287.

465. Aguilar D, Goldhaber SZ. Clinical uses of low-molecular-weight heparins. *Chest* 1999;115:1418–1423.

466. Tazawa S, Ichikawa K, Misawa K, et al. Effects of low molecular weight heparin on a severely antithrombin III-decreased disseminated intravascular coagulation model in rabbits. *Thromb Res* 1995;80:391–398.

467. Takahashi Y, Hosaka Y, Imada K, et al. Human urinary soluble thrombomodulin (MR-33) improves disseminated intravascular coagulation without affecting bleeding time in rats: comparison with low molecular weight heparin. *Thromb Haemost* 1997;77:789–795.

468. Gillis S, Dann EJ, Eldor A. Low molecular weight heparin in the prophylaxis and treatment of disseminated intravascular coagulation in acute promyelocytic leukemia. *Eur J Haematol* 1995;54:59–60.

469. Audibert G, Lambert H, Toulemonde F, et al. Use of a low molecular weight heparin, CY 222, in the treatment of consumption coagulopathy. *J Maladies Vasculaires* 1987;12[Suppl B]:147–151.

470. Sakuragawa N, Hasegawa H, Maki M, et al. Clinical evaluation of low-molecular-weight heparin (FR-860) on disseminated intravascular coagulation (DIC)—a multicenter co-operative double-blind trial in comparison with heparin. *Thromb Res* 1993;72:475–500.

471. Weitz JI, Hudoba M, Massel D, et al. Clot-bound thrombin is protected from inhibition by heparin-antithrombin III but is susceptible to inactivation by antithrombin III-independent inhibitors. *J Clin Invest* 1990;86:385–391.

472. Munoz MC, Montes R, Hermida J, et al. Effect of the administration of recombinant hirudin and/or tissue-plasminogen activator (t-PA) on endotoxin-induced disseminated intravascular coagulation model in rabbits. *Br J Haematol* 1999;105:117–121.

473. Zoldhelyi P, Chesebro JH, Owen WG. Hirudin as a molecular probe for thrombin in vitro and during systemic coagulation in the pig. *Proc Natl Acad Sci U S A* 1993;90:1819–1823.

474. Saito M, Asakura H, Jokaji H, et al. Recombinant hirudin for the treatment of disseminated intravascular coagulation in patients with haematological malignancy. *Blood Coagul Fibrinolysis* 1995;6:60–64.

475. Elsayed YA, Nakagawa K, Kamikubo YI, et al. Effects of recombinant human tissue factor pathway inhibitor on thrombus formation and its in vivo distribution in a rat DIC model. *Am J Clin Pathol* 1996;106:574–583.

476. Bregengard C, Nordfang O, Wildgoose P, et al. The effect of two-domain tissue factor pathway inhibitor on endotoxin-induced disseminated intravascular coagulation in rabbits. *Blood Coagul Fibrinolysis* 1993;4:699–706.

477. Bergum PW, Cruikshank A, Maki S, et al. The potent, factor X(a)-dependent inhibition by rNAPc2 of factor VIIa/tissue factor involves the binding of its cofactor to an exosite on factor VII, followed by occupation of the active site. *Blood* 1998;92[Suppl]:669a.

478. Vlasuk GP, Bergum PW, Bradbury AE, et al. Clinical evaluation of rNAPc2, an inhibitor of the fVIIa/tissue factor coagulation complex. *Am J Cardiol* 1997;80:66S.

479. Taylor FBJ, Emerson TEJ, Jordan R, et al. Antithrombin-III prevents the lethal effects of *Escherichia coli* infusion in baboons. *Circ Shock* 1988;26:227–235.

480. Blauhut B, Kramar H, Vinazzer H, et al. Substitution of antithrombin III in shock and DIC: a randomized study. *Thromb Res* 1985;39:81–89.

481. Vinazzer H. Therapeutic use of antithrombin III in shock and disseminated intravascular coagulation. *Semin Thromb Hemost* 1989;15:347–352.

482. Baudo F, Caimi TM, de Cataldo F, et al. Antithrombin III (ATIII) replacement therapy in patients with sepsis and/or postsurgical complications: a controlled double-blind, randomized, multicenter study. *Intensive Care Med* 1998;24:336–342.

483. Fourrier F, Chopin C, Huart JJ, et al. Double-blind, placebo-controlled trial of antithrombin III concentrates in septic shock with disseminated intravascular coagulation. *Chest* 1993;104:882–888.

484. Eisele B, Lamy M, Thijs LG, et al. Antithrombin III in patients with severe sepsis. A randomized, placebo-controlled, double-blind multicenter trial plus a meta-analysis on all randomized, placebo-controlled, double-blind trials with antithrombin III in severe sepsis. *Intensive Care Med* 1998;24:663–672.

485. Hesselvik JF, Malm J, Dahlback B, et al. Protein C, protein S and C4b-binding protein in severe infection and septic shock. *Thromb Haemost* 1991;65:126–129.

486. Katsuura Y, Aoki K, Tanabe H, et al. Characteristic effects of activated human protein C on tissue thromboplastin-induced disseminated intravascular coagulation in rabbits. *Thromb Res* 1994;76:353–362.

487. Gerson WT, Dickerman JD, Bovill EG, et al. Severe acquired protein C deficiency in purpura fulminans associated with disseminated intravascular coagulation: treatment with protein C concentrate. *Pediatrics* 1993;91:418–422.

488. Dreyfus M, Magny JF, Bridey F, et al. Treatment of homozygous protein C deficiency and neonatal purpura fulminans with a purified protein C concentrate. *N Engl J Med* 1991;325:1565–1568.

489. Rintala E, Seppala O, Kotilainen P, et al. Protein C in the treatment of coagulopathy in meningococcal disease. *Lancet* 1996;347:1767.

490. Gonda Y, Hirata S, Saitoh K, et al. Antithrombotic effect of recombinant human soluble thrombomodulin on endotoxin-induced disseminated intravascular coagulation in rats. *Thromb Res* 1993;71:325–335.

491. Aoki Y, Ohishi R, Takei R, et al. Effects of recombinant human soluble thrombomodulin (rhs-TM) on a rat model of disseminated intravascular coagulation with decreased levels of plasma antithrombin III. *Thromb Haemost* 1994;71:452–455.

492. Uchiba M, Okajima K, Murakami K, et al. Effect of human urinary thrombomodulin on endotoxin-induced intravascular coagulation and pulmonary vascular injury in rats. *Am J Hematol* 1997;54:118–123.

493. Schwartz BS, Williams EC, Conlan MG, et al. Epsilon-aminocaproic acid in the treatment of patients with acute promyelocytic leukemia and acquired alpha-2-plasmin inhibitor deficiency. *Ann Intern Med* 1986;105:873–877.

494. Levi M, Biemond BJ, van Zonneveld AJ, et al. Inhibition of plasminogen activator inhibitor-1 activity results in promotion of endogenous thrombolysis and inhibition of thrombus extension in models of experimental thrombosis. *Circulation* 1992;85:305–312.

495. Aiuto LT, Barone SR, Cohen PS, et al. Recombinant tissue plasminogen activator restores perfusion in meningococcal purpura fulminans. *Crit Care Med* 1997;25:1079–1082.

496. Zenz W, Muntean W, Zobel G, et al. Treatment of fulminant meningococcemia with recombinant tissue plasminogen activator. *Thromb Haemost* 1995;74:802–803.

CHAPTER 42

Natural Anticoagulants and the Prethrombotic State

Kenneth A. Bauer and Jeffrey I. Zwicker

For many years, researchers suspected that hereditary coagulation defects underlay a large percentage of venous thromboembolic events that could not be attributed to identifiable acquired risk factors. The acquired risk factors for venous thrombosis consist of a heterogeneous group of conditions and clinical disorders with diverse and poorly understood prothrombotic mechanisms (Table 42-1). With expanding scientific knowledge of the hemostatic mechanism and the regulatory role of the natural anticoagulants, major advances have been made in identifying hereditary defects in the heparan sulfate–antithrombin and protein C pathways. This chapter reviews the biochemistry and physiology of these endogenous anticoagulant systems and the hereditary disorders associated with an increased risk of venous thromboembolism. Issues relating to the diagnosis and treatment of the hereditary thrombophilias are also discussed.

HEPARAN SULFATE–ANTITHROMBIN MECHANISM

The search for natural anticoagulants began in the early twentieth century. In 1916, while awaiting admission to medical school at Johns Hopkins, J. McLean worked for a short time in the laboratory of Dr. Howell, who was the professor of physiology at Johns Hopkins Medical School and an expert on blood coagulation. Howell asked McLean to isolate a procoagulant from the liver, which Howell had previously detected. As often happens in research, McLean isolated a powerful anticoagulant instead of a procoagulant, which was then named *heparin* because it comes from the liver (1,2). In 1973, Rosenberg and colleagues (3) suggested that the nonthrombogenic properties of blood vessels may be due, in part, to the presence of heparin-like species with anticoagulant activity on the vascular endothelium. Subsequently, the manner by which heparin expresses biologic activity and its location within vascular tissue was studied in detail (4–9). The physiologic function of the endogenous heparan sulfate–antithrombin mechanism was demonstrated using isolated rat hind-limb preparations that were free of mast cells (9). Perfusion of thrombin and antithrombin through the vascular tree accelerated enzyme-inhibitor complex formation 10- to 20-fold when compared with the calculated rate of reaction of thrombin with antithrombin alone. It is now established that heparan sulfate is associated with endothelial

cells of the vascular tree, thereby permitting a small fraction of plasma antithrombin to be activated at blood vessel wall interfaces where enzymes of the coagulation cascade are commonly generated.

Antithrombin is a plasma glycoprotein of 58 kd composed of a single chain of 432 amino acids. Antithrombin neutralizes the activity of thrombin as well as other serine proteases of the coagulation cascade, including factors Xa, IXa, XIa, and XIIa, by forming a stoichiometric complex between enzyme and antithrombin via an arginine-active center on the inhibitor and the active site serine on the enzyme (3,10–14). Complex formation between hemostatic enzymes and antithrombin occurs at a relatively slow rate in the absence of heparin (Fig. 42-1). When heparin is present, however, antithrombin dramatically accelerates the rate of complex formation (10).

The proposed mechanism for heparin-antithrombin-thrombin complex formation involves an intricate series of conformational changes and allosteric interactions. There are two major heparin-binding domains on antithrombin between residues 29 to 53 and 107 to 156 (15). Mutations of the first domain at Arg47 or Trp49 dramatically alter the kinetics of heparin binding to antithrombin (16–18), and this region of the protease inhibitor (19) is involved in a conformational transition required for heparin-dependent acceleration of complex formation. The second binding domain was confirmed by Smith et al. (15) using polyclonal antibodies directed against residues 138 to 145, which not only inhibit heparin binding but also simulate heparin activity by accelerating the inhibition of thrombin.

The heparin molecule possesses several functional domains consisting of unique sequences of sulfated and nonsulfated monosaccharide units that are responsible for accelerating interactions between antithrombin and coagulation serine proteases (20–24). At least two different domains on the heparin molecule bind to antithrombin and mediate the exposure of the Arg393-Ser394 reactive site, thereby facilitating interaction with the serine-active center of coagulation enzymes. The partial insertion of the amino-terminal region of the serine protease into the reactive site of antithrombin creates a stable tetrahedral complex between heparin-antithrombin and the serine protease (25,26). The resultant complex serves as a reservoir for the trapped serine protease until it is cleared from the circulation.

There is evidence that a third domain on longer-chain heparin oligosaccharides facilitates the neutralization of several

TABLE 42-1. Acquired Conditions and Disorders Associated with Hypercoagulable States

Disorders	Conditions
Myeloproliferative disorders	Long distance travel
Disseminated intravascular coagulation	Venous insufficiency
Thrombotic thrombocytopenic purpura	Advancing age
Nephrotic syndrome	Trauma
Antiphospholipid antibody syndrome	Immobilization
Paroxysmal nocturnal hemoglobinuria	Pregnancy
Malignancy	Oral contraception/hormone
Heparin-induced thrombocytopenia	replacement
Diabetes mellitus	
Congestive heart failure	

serine proteases. Oosta and colleagues (20) noted that cleaved heparin oligosaccharides of eight or fewer monosaccharide units accelerated factor Xa–antithrombin interactions but did not increase the rate of neutralization of other hemostatic enzymes by antithrombin (e.g., thrombin, factors IXa and XIa). However, larger oligosaccharides of approximately 16 or more monosaccharide units dramatically accelerated antithrombin-mediated factor Xa neutralization as well as the other serine

proteases including thrombin. Ultraviolet circular dichroism spectroscopy confirmed differences in binding characteristics of heparin oligosaccharides of varying lengths when complexed with antithrombin (21,27,28). This led researchers to theorize that the ability of heparin to neutralize serine proteases was due to multiple heparin-binding domains (20). A number of studies have shown that heparin can bind directly with thrombin (29,30), and Danielsson et al. (31) noted that the minimum heparin oligosaccharide chain length needed to accelerate the heparin-antithrombin-thrombin reaction corresponded to the minimum length necessary to bind both antithrombin and thrombin simultaneously. It is likely that longer-chain heparin oligosaccharides mediate thrombin inhibition through the binding of both thrombin and antithrombin independently, thus facilitating complex formation by approximating the respective binding domains (32).

PROTEIN C–THROMBOMODULIN–PROTEIN S MECHANISM

Several independent lines of evidence, obtained from animal studies and clinical observations, indicate that the protein C–

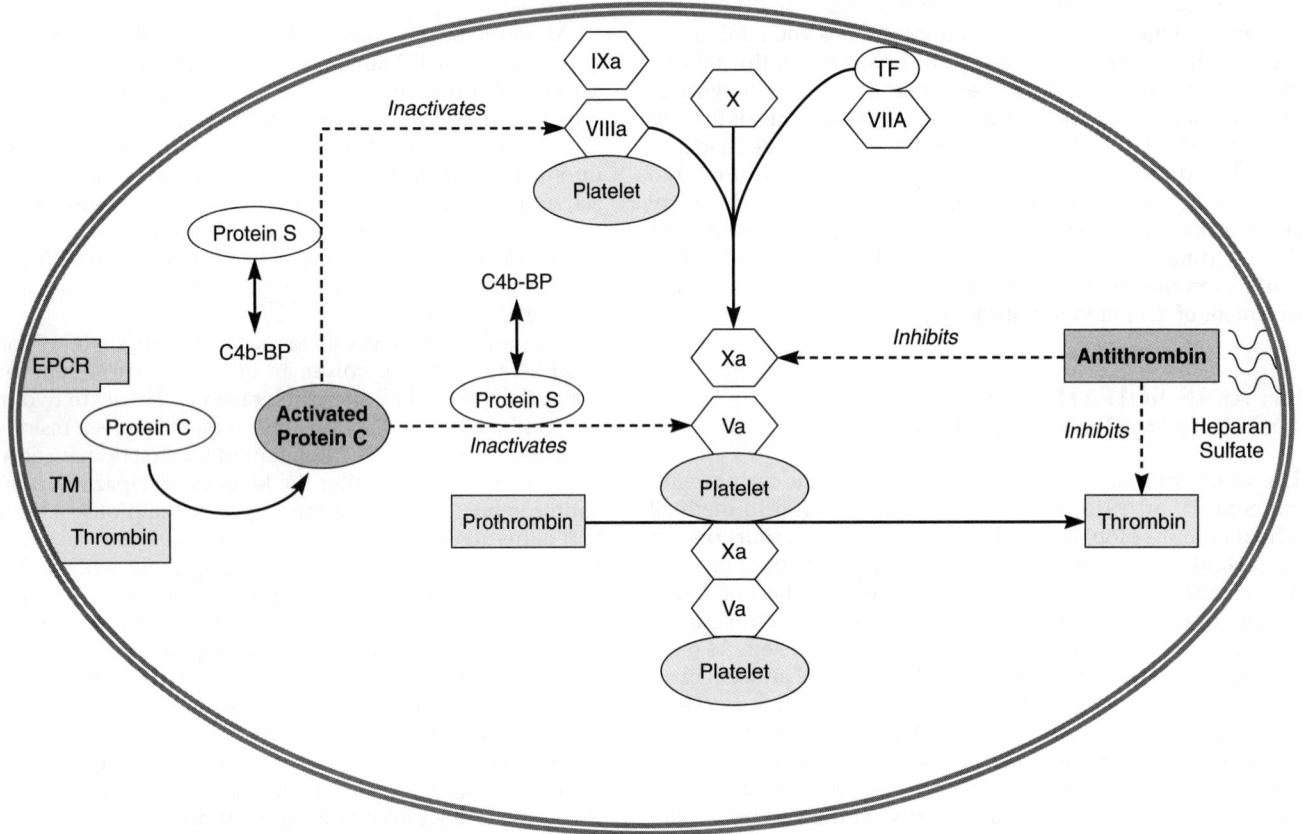

Figure 42-1. Schematic depiction of pathways that generate factor Xa, thrombin, and the natural anticoagulant mechanisms that regulate the activity of these enzymes. Factor X can be activated by the extrinsic pathway [factor VIIa–tissue factor (TF)] or the intrinsic pathway (factor IXa/VIIIa–activated cell surface complex). Factor Xa binds to factor Va on activated platelets and mediates the conversion of prothrombin to thrombin under physiologic conditions. Thrombin and factor Xa are inactivated by antithrombin bound to heparan sulfate molecules associated with the vascular endothelium. Protein C is activated by thrombin bound to thrombomodulin (TM) and endothelial cell protein C receptor (EPCR). Once evolved, activated protein C functions as a potent anticoagulant by inactivating factors VIIIa and Va. Protein S enhances the binding of activated protein C to phospholipid-containing membranes and accelerates the inactivation of factors VIIIa and Va. The complement component, C4b-binding protein (C4b-BP), forms complexes with protein S, which results in a reduction of its functional activity.

thrombomodulin mechanism functions *in vivo* to suppress thrombotic phenomena. Infusion of a small amount of thrombin into dogs induces protein C activation before there are any observable changes in the levels of factor V, fibrinogen, or platelets (33). Activated human protein C can prevent the accretion of radiolabeled fibrinogen onto preformed jugular-venous thrombi in dogs (34). Significant progress has been made in establishing the molecular basis of the protein C–thrombomodulin–protein S mechanism and defining its role as a natural anticoagulant.

Protein C is a vitamin K–dependent plasma glycoprotein of 62 kd. The amino acid sequences of the bovine and human glycoproteins were deduced from direct protein sequencing and the cloning of its cDNA, respectively (35–38). Protein C consists of a heavy chain of 41 kd and a light chain of 21 kd, which are joined by a single disulfide bridge. In human plasma, a single-chain form of the zymogen has been identified that constitutes 5% to 15% of the total protein C in the circulation (39). These observations suggest that the zymogen is initially synthesized as a single polypeptide chain and subsequently cleaved to generate a two-chain structure.

To perform its anticoagulant function, human protein C must be converted to a component with serine protease activity, which is designated *activated protein C* (APC). This process involves scission of a single Arg12–Leu13 bond at the amino-terminal end of the heavy chain of the zymogen with release of a 12–amino acid activation peptide (40). The active site serine residue is located on the heavy chain (36). Both protein C and APC possess γ-carboxyglutamic acid (Gla) residues in their light chains, which are required for the binding of the protein to calcium ions and cell membranes (35). β-Hydroxyaspartic acid, another posttranslational modification, was identified on the light chain of the protein (41). APC is slowly neutralized by several protease inhibitors in human plasma—a 57-kd protease inhibitor designated *protein C inhibitor* (PCI) (42,43), α₁-antitrypsin (44–46), and α₂-macroglobulin (47). These three inhibitors neutralize APC at a relatively slow rate, although the activity of the PCI is enhanced by high concentrations of heparin (42). Thrombin is the only physiologically relevant serine protease that can convert protein C to APC, although other activators have been described (48,49). The rate of this reaction is slow when blood is allowed to clot *in vitro*, but it is accelerated several thousand–fold by two cofactor receptors on the surface of vascular endothelium—thrombomodulin and endothelial cell protein C receptor (EPCR) (50–53).

The primary structure of thrombomodulin was deduced from the cloning of its cDNA by several groups of investigators (54–57). Thrombomodulin is a transmembrane protein of 559 amino acid residues organized in a domain structure that includes six tandem epidermal growth factor–like domains (EGF 1 to 6) joined by small interdomain peptides (56,57). Thrombin forms a 1:1 complex with thrombomodulin and rapidly activates protein C in the presence of calcium ions (58,59). Although thrombin binds initially to domains EGF5 and EGF6 (60), other EGF domains appear critical in mediating protein C activation (61).

The thrombomodulin-thrombin complex also appears to play a regulatory role in the fibrinolytic mechanism by activating thrombin-activatable fibrinolysis inhibitor (TAFI) (Fig. 42-2) (62,63). Activated TAFI regulates fibrinolysis by removing carboxy-terminal lysine and arginine residues from fibrin and limits fibrin–tissue plasminogen activator–mediated activation of plasminogen (64). Thus, the thrombin-thrombomodulin complex seemingly functions in a paradoxic manner in regulating hemostasis. On the one hand, thrombomodulin functions as an anticoagulant by activating protein C, which decreases thrombin generation and the subsequent generation of fibrin. On the

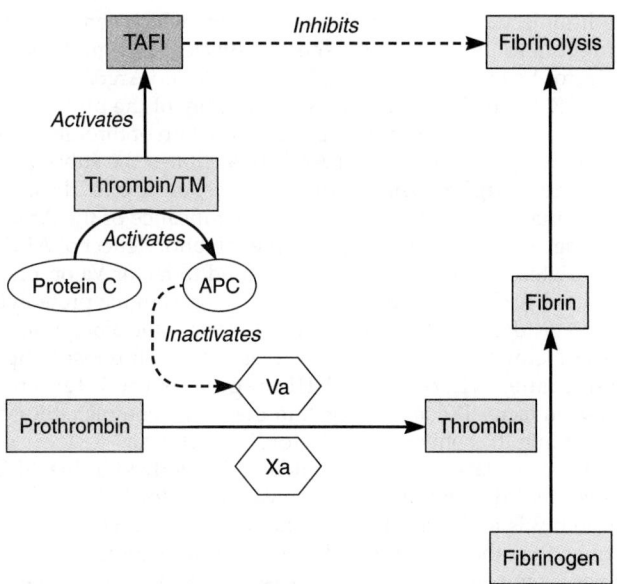

Figure 42-2. The dual role of thrombin in fibrin deposition and lysis. Thrombin promotes clot formation through the conversion of fibrinogen into fibrin. This is mediated by the release of fibrinopeptides after the cleavage of arginine-glycine bonds. The thrombin-thrombomodulin (TM) complex also regulates the fibrinolytic response by activating thrombin-activatable fibrinolysis inhibitor (TAFI). This carboxypeptidase inhibits fibrin–tissue plasminogen activator–mediated activation of plasminogen. APC, activated protein C.

other hand, TAFI activation by the thrombin-thrombomodulin complex results in diminished fibrinolysis and clot stabilization. Recent studies have suggested that this balance of clot formation and dissolution is dependent on the relative concentrations of thrombomodulin in the vasculature (65). At higher concentrations, thrombomodulin was shown to promote fibrinolysis, whereas at lower levels, there was an inhibitory effect.

Another transmembrane protein, EPCR, has recently been identified as an important regulatory component in the protein C anticoagulant pathway. EPCR is a type 1 transmembrane protein homologous in structure to the major histocompatibility complex class I family of receptors (66) and is primarily expressed on the endothelial surface of large vessels (67). EPCR binds both protein C and APC with similar affinity (68) and has been shown to augment APC formation fivefold *in vitro* by increasing the affinity of the thrombin-thrombomodulin complex for protein C (50,51). *In vitro* studies have shown that APC bound to EPCR has limited ability to inactivate factor Va, although the inhibition of APC by α₁-antitrypsin or PCI is unaffected (69). The overexpression of EPCR as well as thrombomodulin in several leukemic and breast cancer cell lines *in vitro* has been positively correlated with their ability to activate protein C (70). In animal studies, baboons treated with monoclonal antibodies, which inhibit protein C binding to EPCR, generated dramatically lower levels of APC in response to thrombin infusions than controls that were pretreated with antibody (71). It is probable that EPCR not only plays an integral role in regulating the protein C anticoagulant pathway but also is critical in regulating the inflammatory cascade seen in sepsis (see Activated Protein C and Sepsis).

Once evolved, APC functions *in vivo* as a natural anticoagulant by inactivating factor Va and factor VIIIa, which are critical cofactors in the coagulation cascade (72–74). The procofactors—factors V and VIII—are relatively resistant to the proteolytic effect of APC. APC functions on the platelet membrane surface where bound factor Va acts as a receptor for factor Xa within the multimolecular prothrombinase complex, which converts prothrombin to thrombin. APC specifically cleaves peptide bonds in factor Va in order at the Arg506, Arg306, and Arg679 residues (72,75,76), thereby preventing the assembly of the prothrombinase complex and suppressing the production of thrombin (77). The cleavage of factor Va at Arg506 facilitates the subsequent cleavage at Arg306, which is primarily responsible for the molecule's inactivation; the physiologic significance of the Arg679 cleavage site is uncertain (78,79). The inhibitory effect of APC is modulated by factor Xa, which can bind to factor Va on phospholipid surfaces and protects the cofactor from the proteolytic action of APC (80). APC also is able to destroy the biologic activity of factor VIIIa (73,74,81–83). This occurs on phospholipid membranes where factor VIIIa regulates the interaction between factor IXa and factor X in the tenase complex, thereby preventing the conversion of factor X to factor Xa.

Another plasma protein, protein S, is involved in the APC–dependent destruction of factor Va and factor VIIIa. Human protein S is a vitamin K–dependent protein of 69 kd (84,85). Unlike the other vitamin K–dependent coagulation proteins, it is not a zymogen of a serine protease. The structure of protein S was deduced from the cloning of its cDNA (86,87). It consists of a single polypeptide chain with an amino-terminal region that contains 10 Gla residues in addition to a number of β-hydroxyaspartic acid moieties (84,88). This region is homologous to other vitamin K–dependent plasma proteins, whereas the carboxy-terminal end of the molecule is similar to that of androgen-binding proteins (89).

The complement component, C4b-binding protein, complexes with protein S and is involved in regulating the function of the protein (90–93); only the free form of protein S enhances the binding of APC to cell membranes and accelerates the cleavage of factor Va and factor VIIIa by the enzyme (94–97). The inactivation of factor Va is accelerated by protein S due to a 20-fold enhancement in the rate of hydrolysis at the Arg306 cleavage site (98). Protein S also displays anticoagulant activity independent of APC by directly binding to factor Va (99,100), factor VIII (101), and factor Xa (102), although the significance of these direct interactions *in vivo* is unclear. There is also some evidence that protein S interacts with proteins outside the protein C system including tyrosine kinases (103,104) or heparin, which has been shown to limit protein S degradation *in vitro* (105).

The heparan sulfate–antithrombin and protein C–thrombomodulin anticoagulant mechanisms undoubtedly act in concert to regulate thrombin formation in circulation. The former inhibits many of the serine proteases generated by the coagulation cascade, whereas the latter acts to limit the buildup of activated cofactors. It has also been shown that heparin can enhance factor V and factor Va inactivation by APC *in vitro* (106). Heparin at a relatively high concentration *in vitro* is also able to increase the rate of APC neutralization by PCI which directly binds APC or inhibits thrombin-thrombomodulin complex activity (107,108).

Activated Protein C and Sepsis

The protein C pathway has increasingly been recognized for its role beyond that of a natural anticoagulant, especially in terms of regulating the inflammatory response seen in sepsis. Activation of the protein C pathway in severe illness can lead to significant reductions in the serum concentrations of protein C and protein S (109,110). A dramatic illustration of this effect is seen in severe meningococcemia-induced purpura fulminans. As described in later sections, purpura fulminans is characterized by an acute inflammatory response complicated by disseminated intravascular coagulation (DIC) and multiorgan failure secondary to an acquired protein C deficiency. Individuals with

this syndrome have been successfully treated with protein C concentrate (111). Taylor and colleagues have similarly highlighted the role of protein C in regulating the inflammatory cascade in animal sepsis models (112). In these studies, APC infusion before exposure to high doses of *Escherichia coli* prevented a fatal systemic inflammatory response, an effect that was reversed by the inhibition of APC (112), protein S (113), or EPCR activity (114). In fact, inhibition of the protein C pathway also magnified the adverse effects of sublethal *E. coli* infusions, transforming these lower doses into lethal exposures. *In vivo* and *in vitro* studies have shown that this antiinflammatory effect is cytokine mediated (115–119).

Recently, APC concentrates have been investigated as a therapeutic agent for patients with severe sepsis syndrome. In a randomized controlled trial of 1690 patients with sepsis, the 850 individuals who were treated with recombinant APC experienced a 6.1% absolute reduction in the 28-day mortality rate and almost a 20% reduction in the relative risk of death (118). However, this was accompanied by an increased risk of serious bleeding (3.5% vs. 2.0%, $p = .06$). These results are promising and highlight the potential role protein C in modulating inflammatory responses.

ANTITHROMBIN DEFICIENCY

In 1965, Egeberg (120) reported a Norwegian family whose members had plasma antithrombin concentrations that were 40% to 50% of normal and a history of repeated thrombotic events. Subsequently, other investigators described additional families with a similar constellation of clinical and laboratory abnormalities (121–135). Based on familial studies, original estimates of the prevalence of antithrombin deficiency were 1 in 2000 to 1 in 5000 (136,137). Subsequent screening of blood donors using a functional assay revealed a higher than expected prevalence of 1 in 600 (138); a substantial number, however, had functional abnormalities in the heparin-binding domain of the molecule, which are associated with a lower risk of thrombosis (see below).

The risk of thrombosis attributed to antithrombin deficiency depends on population selection. In familial studies, in which individuals were selected for their impressive history of thrombosis, the prevalence of thrombosis among antithrombin deficient subjects was often greater than 50% (139) with an eight- to tenfold increased risk of thrombosis as compared to noncarriers (140,141). The Leiden Thrombophilia Study investigated 474 unselected consecutive patients after an initial episode of deep vein thrombosis who were matched with an equal number of healthy controls (142). As shown in Table 42-2, the prevalence of antithrombin deficiency was only 1.1%, and the risk of thrombosis (as well as protein C and protein S deficiencies) was lower (odds ratio, 5.0) than previously seen in familial studies, although the confidence interval was relatively wide (95% confidence interval, 0.7 to 34.0) (143).

Two major types of inherited antithrombin deficiency have been delineated. The classic deficiency (type I) is a result of reduced synthesis of biologically normal protein or, less commonly, impaired secretion from hepatocytes (135,144,145). In these cases, the antigenic and biologic activity of antithrombin in plasma is reduced to the same extent. The molecular basis is either a deletion of a large segment of the gene or, more commonly, the occurrence of nonsense mutations, missense mutations, or base substitutions at splice sites (146). The second type of antithrombin deficiency (type II) is produced by a discrete molecular defect within the protein (Table 42-3). Under these circumstances, the plasma levels of antithrombin are greatly

TABLE 42-2. Prevalence of Prothrombotic Defects in the General Population and among Outpatients with Objective Deep Venous Thrombosis

Type of Prothrombotic Defect (Reference)	Prevalence in General Population (Reference)	Prevalence among Outpatients with Deep Venous Thrombosis (Reference)	Relative Risk of Thrombosis (Reference)	Confidence Intervals
Antithrombin	0.016% (138)	1.1% (143)	5.0 (143)	0.7–34.0
Protein C deficiency	0.2–0.5% (242,243)	0.5–4.0% (143,246,247)	3.8 (143)	1.3–10.0
Protein S deficiency	Unknown	1–7% (143,246,247,331)	2.4 (331)	0.8–7.9
Factor V Leiden	5–6% (369)	21% (367)	6.6 (367)	3.6–12.0
Prothrombin G20210A	2% (377)	6% (372)	2.8 (372)	1.4–5.6
Hyperhomocysteinemia (≥95th percentile)	5% (380)	10% (380)	2.5 (382)	1.8–3.5
Elevated XI (417) (≥90th percentile)	10%	19%	2.2	1.5–3.2
Elevated VIII (411) (≥90th percentile)	10%	25%	4.8	2.3–10.0

reduced as judged by biologic activity measurements relative to antigenic measurements, which are within the normal range.

The first family with a type II deficiency of antithrombin was reported by Sas and co-workers in 1974 (147). Many families with this type of deficiency have been reported, and they have been further subcategorized on the basis of two different functional assays of antithrombin activity. The first is the antithrombin–heparin cofactor assay, which measures the ability of heparin to bind to lysyl residues on antithrombin and catalyze the neutralization of coagulation enzymes such as thrombin and factor Xa. The second test is the progressive antithrombin activity assay, which quantifies the capacity of antithrombin to neutralize the enzymatic activity of thrombin in the absence of heparin. Several abnormal antithrombin molecules were identified with reductions in only heparin cofactor activity. These variants generally have mutations at a heparin-binding site at the amino-terminal end of the molecule (16,17,148–172). In one of these variants, the substitution of asparagine for isoleucine at residue 7 produces a new glycosylation site, and the resultant protein has a reduced affinity for heparin (172). Variants with decreased activity in both antithrombin activity assays generally have mutations near the Arg393-Ser394 reactive site at the carboxy-terminal end of the molecule (146,173–196). Alterations at the reactive site often impede antithrombin-protease complex formation, although some mutations result in antithrombin serving as a substrate for the protease thrombin rather than its inhibitor (194,197).

All antithrombin variants cannot be neatly characterized by this schema, however, because single amino acid substitutions can affect both functional domains of the molecule. This is perhaps best illustrated by a mutation in which arginine is replaced by histidine at residue 393 (182,198,199). This reactive site mutation markedly decreases the ability of the protein to inhibit thrombin but also leads to a conformational alteration so that the abnormal molecule has increased heparin affinity. Alternatively, single substitutions between residues 402 to 407 can result in functional defects at both the heparin-binding and reactive sites (147,170).

A review of the literature suggests that the prevalence of thrombosis is different in patients with the two types of functional antithrombin deficiency (242). On one hand, heterozygous individuals with reductions in plasma antithrombin–heparin cofactor activity to approximately 50% of normal but with normal progressive antithrombin activity have infrequent thrombotic episodes (17,152,158,200,201). Several of these cases were brought to clinical attention when young children of these heterozygous subjects developed severe venous throm-

bosis, arterial thrombosis, or both (152,158), accompanied by plasma antithrombin–heparin cofactor levels below 10%. In each instance, there was a history of parental consanguinity, and these children were homozygous for an antithrombin molecular defect. On the other hand, heterozygous type II patients with diminished progressive antithrombin activity and antithrombin–heparin cofactor activity sustain venous thromboembolism as often as type I patients.

Given the various subtypes of the familial deficiency that might be encountered, the best single screening test for the disorder is the heparin cofactor assay to measure factor Xa inhibition. The use of factor Xa in lieu of thrombin in this assay increases assay sensitivity for antithrombin deficiency due to the presence of heparin cofactor II in plasma, which is only capable of inhibiting thrombin (202,203). However, it has been observed that a factor Xa–based heparin cofactor assay failed to diagnose approximately 50% of individuals with the Cambridge II (Ala384Ser) antithrombin mutation (204).

The mean concentration of antithrombin in normal pooled plasma is approximately 140 µg/mL. In plasmas from normal individuals, the range of antithrombin concentrations, determined by immunologic or functional tests, is relatively narrow. Most laboratories report a normal range between 75% and 120% for antithrombin–heparin cofactor determinations (205) and a somewhat wider range for immunoassay results (206). Healthy newborns have approximately one-half of the normal adult concentration (207,208) and gradually reach the adult level by 6

TABLE 42-3. Type II (Functional) Deficiencies and Diagnostic Assays for Antithrombin, Protein C, and Protein S (PS)

	Type II Deficiency	Diagnostic Assay
Antithrombin	Heparin-binding site	Antithrombin-heparin cofactor assay
	Reactive site	Progressive antithrombin assay
Protein C	Catalytic site	Protac-amidolytic assay
	Other (i.e., PS-binding site)	Protac-anticoagulant assay
Protein S	PS-APC binding domains	APC anticoagulant assay with PS-depleted plasma
	PS and C4b-BP binding sites (type III)	APC anticoagulant assay; free PS antigen assay

APC, activated protein C.

TABLE 42-4. Acquired Antithrombin, Protein C, and Protein S Deficiency States

Protein C deficiency
  Warfarin
  Severe meningococcemia
Protein S deficiency
  Warfarin
  Pregnancy
  Nephrotic syndrome
  Estrogen
  Severe varicella infections
Antithrombin deficiency
  Heparin
  Preeclampsia
  Nephrotic syndrome
  Estrogen
  Cardiopulmonary bypass
  Venoocclusive disease
Common to antithrombin, protein S, and protein C deficiencies
  Liver disease
  Sepsis
  Disseminated intravascular coagulation
  Acute thrombosis
  Neonatal period
  L-Asparaginase

months of age (209). The levels may be considerably lower in infants born between 30 and 36 weeks of gestation (209).

A variety of pathophysiologic conditions can reduce the concentration of antithrombin in the blood (Table 42-4). Although acute thrombosis does not lower antithrombin levels substantially (210), DIC usually reduces the level of this inhibitor (109,211). Lowered antithrombin concentrations are known to occur in patients with liver disease (mainly cirrhosis) due to decreased protein synthesis (212) and in nephrotic syndrome as a consequence of urinary excretion (213). Furthermore, modest reductions in plasma antithrombin concentration are found in users of oral contraceptives (214,215), as well as in individuals receiving estrogens for other purposes (216). The levels of antithrombin do not change substantially during normal pregnancies (215,217) but may decrease significantly in women with pregnancy-induced hypertension, preeclampsia, or eclampsia (217). Antithrombin deficiency seen in severe sepsis is likely multifactorial, resulting from increased consumption, decreased synthesis, and vascular leak (218). Cardiopulmonary bypass is also associated with a reduction in antithrombin due to both hemodilution and consumption (219,220). Venoocclusive disease is an untoward complication of bone marrow transplantation, and low levels of antithrombin may precede clinical symptoms and directly correlate with disease severity (221,222). In addition, the administration of heparin decreases plasma antithrombin levels (223), presumably on the basis of accelerated *in vivo* clearance of the inhibitor. Evaluation of plasma samples from patients suspected of having congenital antithrombin deficiency during a period of heparinization can, therefore, potentially lead to an erroneous diagnosis of the disorder.

Because of the number of clinical disorders that can be associated with reductions in the plasma concentration of antithrombin, definitive diagnosis of the hereditary deficiency is often difficult. Although an antithrombin level in the normal range, drawn on clinical presentation, is usually sufficient to exclude the presence of the disorder, low levels should be confirmed by obtaining another sample at a subsequent time. This determination is ideally performed when the patient is no longer receiving oral anticoagulants, because these medications have occasionally been reported to raise plasma antithrombin concentrations into the normal range in individuals with the hereditary deficiency (124). In such situations, clinical assess-

ment of the individual's risk of recurrent thrombosis determines whether this approach is feasible. In most antithrombin-deficient subjects, however, this effect of oral anticoagulants is not of sufficient magnitude to obscure the diagnosis (224). Confirmation of the hereditary nature of the disorder requires the investigation of other family members. Diagnosis of other biochemically affected family members also allows for appropriate counseling regarding the need for prophylaxis against venous thrombosis.

In heterozygous antithrombin deficiency, anticoagulation therapy for acute venous thromboembolism is managed in the same manner as in other patients without this disorder. Antithrombin-deficient individuals can usually be treated successfully with intravenous unfractionated heparin or subcutaneous low-molecular-weight heparin (LMWH), although in some situations, it may be found that unusually large doses of unfractionated heparin are required to achieve adequate anticoagulation as measured by the activated partial thromboplastin time (aPTT). Indeed, the diagnosis of antithrombin deficiency is usually considered in the differential diagnosis of heparin resistance, and an occasional patient is diagnosed in this manner. Antithrombin concentrate has been used to assist in anticoagulating patients with antithrombin deficiency including patients with severe "heparin resistance." However, in patients with hereditary antithrombin deficiency receiving heparin for the treatment of acute thrombosis, the adjunctive role of antithrombin concentrate purified from human plasma is not clearly defined, because randomized, controlled trials have not been performed; retrospective studies have shown that "heparin-resistant" individuals can usually be successfully anticoagulated without the addition of antithrombin concentrate (225). It is, however, reasonable to treat asymptomatic patients with antithrombin deficiency with concentrate before major surgery or in obstetric situations in which the risks of bleeding from anticoagulation are unacceptably high.

The biologic half-life of antithrombin is approximately 48 hours in humans (145). The manufacturing processes used to prepare antithrombin concentrate from plasma result in a product that is more than 95% pure and in which the hepatitis B virus and human immunodeficiency virus I have been inactivated (226,227). The infusion of 50 units of antithrombin concentrate/kg of body weight (*1 unit* is defined as the amount of antithrombin in 1 mL of pooled normal human plasma) usually raises the plasma antithrombin level to approximately 120% in a congenitally deficient individual with a baseline level of 50% (227–229). Plasma levels should be monitored to ensure that they remain above 80%, and the administration of 60% of the initial dose at 24-hour intervals is recommended to maintain inhibitor levels in the normal range (229). A human antithrombin concentrate has also been purified from the milk of transgenic goats using recombinant DNA technology.

There are also some data for the use of antithrombin concentrates in acquired antithrombin deficiency states including sepsis, burns, and bone marrow transplantation (218,230). A metaanalysis of three small phase II trials of antithrombin therapy for septic shock revealed a nonsignificant trend towards reduction in 30-day all-cause mortality (45% vs. 35%) (231). In cases of stem cell transplantation and multiorgan failure, a randomized control trial of antithrombin versus albumin placebo showed a modest improvement in several morbidity scales without an appreciable mortality benefit (232). It can be argued, however, that the placebo arm may have been adversely affected by the use of albumin, given that its use has been associated with poor outcomes in severe illness (233). In a randomized trial of patients classified as heparin-resistant before cardiopulmonary bypass, antithrombin concentrate plus heparin was effective in achieving therapeutic activated clotting times in 42 of 44 individuals in comparison to 28 of 41 individuals treated with escalating doses of heparin alone (234). Further investigation is needed to define the potential roles of antithrombin concentrates in treating disorders associated with acquired antithrombin deficiency.

PROTEIN C DEFICIENCY

In 1981, Griffin and colleagues (235) described the first kindred in which several individuals had plasma levels of protein C antigen of approximately 50% of normal in association with a history of recurrent venous thrombotic events. Other investigators subsequently reported numerous other families with this disorder (236–239). In large cohort studies, protein C deficiency was documented in 2% to 9% of individuals with a history of venous thrombosis (237,240,241). From these cohorts, estimates placed the prevalence of protein C deficiency between 1 in 16,000 to 1 in 32,000 within the general population. These estimates were based on the assumption that protein C was an autosomal-dominant disorder with high penetrance and that at least one-half of the individuals with the deficiency would demonstrate symptomatic thrombosis (242). And yet, it was difficult to reconcile the relative infrequent history of thrombosis in parents of infants with purpura fulminans, which represents the homozygous or doubly heterozygous form of protein C deficiency. This led Miletich and others to screen healthy blood donors, and they found a much higher prevalence of heterozygosity for protein C deficiency than previously estimated, ranging from 1 in 200 to 500 (Table 42-2) (242,243).

Similar to antithrombin deficiency, the risk estimates of thrombosis attributable to protein C deficiency are subject to selection bias; in general, they are overestimated in familial studies and underestimated in healthy individuals. Among thrombophilic families, protein C deficiency is associated with an approximate sevenfold increase in risk of thrombosis (140). In asymptomatic carriers of protein C deficiency, the incidence of thrombosis is fairly low at 0.4% to 1.0% annually (141,244,245). Risk estimates more applicable to the general population were conducted in a series of case control studies of consecutive outpatients with documented deep venous thrombosis. In these studies, the prevalence of protein C deficiency ranged from 0.5% to 4.0% (143,246,247), corresponding with an approximate threefold increase in thrombotic risk (143).

Two major subtypes of heterozygous protein C deficiency can be delineated using immunologic and functional assays. The classic, or type I, deficiency is the most common form and is characterized by a reduction in both the immunologic and biologic activity of the zymogen in the blood. In families with a type II deficiency, affected individuals have normal protein C levels on immunologic examination, yet possess lowered functional levels (Table 42-3) (248–254). More than 160 different mutations in the protein C gene have been described, most commonly missense or nonsense mutations (255). Interestingly, mutations of critical domains including EGF, catalytic site, and activation sites commonly lead to type I deficiencies (256). These mutations likely interfere with the intracellular processing of the protein, thus leading to defective secretion or increased intracellular degradation. Mutations at other functional domains, including the Gla domain, typically result in type II deficiencies.

As previously noted, a clinical disorder was reported in which newborns developed purpura fulminans in association with protein C antigen levels that were less than 1% of normal (257–264). In some instances, there was a history of consanguin-

ity in the family, making it highly likely that the affected infants were homozygous for the deficiency (258,260,261). A number of case reports, however, document the existence of a form of severe protein C deficiency in which neonatal purpura fulminans is not present. These individuals generally have protein C levels of less than 20% of normal in the absence of oral anticoagulant therapy, and their clinical presentation is generally similar to that of severely affected subjects from thrombophilic kindreds with the heterozygous deficiency (265–267). The parents of these subjects have a type I deficiency, as do those of babies with purpura fulminans. In addition, two reports describe patients who are doubly heterozygous for both type I and type II alleles that were inherited separately from each of the parents (268,269). In one of these cases, a group of Japanese investigators determined that the type II defect resulted from the replacement of arginine by tryptophan at position 12 of the heavy chain. This residue is the site at which protein C is activated by the thrombin-thrombomodulin complex (269).

A variety of immunologic and functional techniques were developed to measure protein C levels in plasma samples. The most commonly used procedures for antigen determinations are electroimmunoassay (235,236), enzyme-linked immunosorbent assay (270,271), or radioimmunoassay (272,273). Functional assays use either thrombin (248,274) or the thrombin-thrombomodulin complex (249,275) to activate protein C after adsorbing the zymogen with aluminum hydroxide (248) or barium citrate (274,275). With the exception of the method of Francis and Patch (274), which measures the ability of APC to prolong the aPTT, the endpoint of these assays is the cleavage of a suitable synthetic substrate by the enzyme. The development of simpler functional assays has been facilitated by the observation that the venom from the Southern copperhead snake (*Agkistrodon contortrix*) is able to activate protein C in plasma (276–278). After activation with the venom protease (Protac), an amidolytic assay can assess the functionality of the catalytic site of protein C (277). However, several individuals have been described with a normal concentration of protein C antigen and amidolytic activity, but with substantial reductions in protein C anticoagulant activity (279). These type II variants with presumed mutations beyond the catalytic site can be diagnosed using a clotting assay based on the prolongation of the aPTT after activation of plasma protein C with venom protease. Abnormalities in this assay presumably reflect the reduced ability of APC to interact with the platelet membrane, protein S, or its substrates such as factor Va and factor VIIIa. The coagulant assay would, therefore, be expected to have greater sensitivity in screening individuals for hereditary protein C deficiency than the amidolytic assay; however, in most clinical laboratories, the latter assay is preferred for initial screening because it is technically easier to perform and has a smaller coefficient of variation than the clotting assay. "Global" coagulation assays are also being investigated as a means of screening for any major abnormality in the entire protein C pathway (e.g., protein C deficiency, protein S deficiency, or the factor V Leiden mutation) (280–283). However, the use of these assays has been limited by a poor sensitivity for protein S deficiency.

Protein C normally circulates in human plasma at an average concentration of 4 µg/mL. The levels of protein C antigen in healthy adults are log-normal distributed with 95% of the values ranging from 70% to 140% (242). There is no significant gender dependence, but mean protein C antigen concentrations increase by approximately 4% per decade and are significantly lower in newborns (284,285). Acquired protein C deficiency occurs in a number of clinical disorders (Table 42-4), including liver disease (279,286–288), DIC (279,286,287,289,290), adult respiratory distress syndrome (286), and the postoperative state

(286), and in association with L-asparaginase therapy (291) or valproic acid (292). Severe forms of acquired protein C deficiency are also seen in cases of purpura fulminans due to severe meningococcal infections (293,294). In contrast to antithrombin, the antigenic concentrations of vitamin K–dependent plasma proteins, including protein C, are often elevated in patients with the nephrotic syndrome (295).

The relatively wide normal range of protein C measurements in the general population frequently makes it difficult to identify a given individual as having heterozygous protein C deficiency. If medical and pharmacologic causes of low levels of protein C are excluded, patients with protein C values below 55% are likely to have the genetic abnormality, whereas levels of 55% to 65% are consistent with either a deficiency or the lower end of the normal distribution (242). To document this disorder, it is useful to perform repeat determinations on the individual suspected of being protein C deficient in addition to performing family studies to document the presence of an autosomal-dominant inheritance pattern.

Warfarin therapy reduces functional (248,275,279) and, to a lesser extent, immunologic measurements of protein C (235,236). This makes it difficult to diagnose individuals with heterozygous protein C deficiency in this setting. Several research laboratories have used a reduced ratio of protein C antigen or functional activity as compared by amidolytic methodology to prothrombin antigen to identify patients with a deficiency (235,236,296,297). This approach can only be used in subjects in a stable phase of oral anticoagulation, however, and the diagnostic criteria for the disorder vary with the intensity of warfarin therapy (236). Therefore, in practice, it is preferable to investigate patients suspected of having the deficiency after oral anticoagulation has been discontinued for at least 2 weeks; family studies should also be performed. If it is not possible to discontinue warfarin therapy because of the severity of the thrombotic diathesis, such individuals can be studied while receiving unfractionated or LMWH therapy, which does not alter plasma protein C levels.

Warfarin-induced skin necrosis is associated with the presence of heterozygous protein C deficiency (298–301). This syndrome typically occurs during the first several days of warfarin therapy, often in association with the administration of large loading doses of the medication. The skin lesions occur on the extremities, breasts, and trunk, as well as the penis, and marginate over a period of hours from an initial central erythematous macule. If vitamin K or a product containing protein C is not rapidly administered, the affected cutaneous areas become edematous, develop central purpuric zones, and ultimately become necrotic. Biopsies demonstrate fibrin thrombi within cutaneous vessels with interstitial hemorrhage. The dermal manifestations of warfarin-induced skin necrosis are clinically and pathologically similar to those seen in infants with purpura fulminans due to severe protein C deficiency.

The pathogenesis of warfarin-induced skin necrosis is attributable to the emergence of a transient hypercoagulable state. The initiation of the drug at standard doses leads to a decrease in protein C anticoagulant activity levels to approximately one-half of normal within a single day (279). Whereas factor VII activity measurements follow a pattern similar to that of protein C, the levels of the other vitamin K–dependent factors decline at slower rates consistent with their longer half-lives. Increased thrombin generation was documented in patients during this early phase of warfarin therapy using a sensitive immunochemical assay for fragment F_{1+2}, an index of the *in vivo* activation of prothrombin mediated by factor Xa (302). During this period, the drug's suppressive effect on protein C has a greater influence on the hemostatic mechanism than on factor VII. These effects

are likely to be augmented when loading-dose schedules are used or the patient has an underlying hereditary deficiency of protein C. However, only a third of patients with warfarin-induced skin necrosis have an inherited deficiency of protein C (300), and this complication is a rather infrequently reported event among individuals with the heterozygous deficiency state. Several case reports have also implicated other thrombophilic disorders including protein S deficiency and factor V Leiden in association with warfarin-induced skin necrosis (303–305).

Acute management of thromboembolic events in heterozygous protein C–deficient patients is similar to that of those without the disorder. It is advisable to keep the patient fully anticoagulated with unfractionated heparin or LMWH during the initiation of oral anticoagulation; large loading doses of the latter medication clearly should be avoided as has been recommended in other patient populations. Oral anticoagulants are effective in managing individuals with protein C deficiency, and the recommendations for its use in patients who have either sustained recurrent venous thrombosis or are asymptomatic are similar to those in patients with other hereditary deficiencies.

The infrequent occurrence of warfarin-induced skin necrosis and the diagnostic difficulty in making a rapid and definitive laboratory diagnosis of the deficiency are arguments against the routine measurement of plasma protein C levels in all individuals with venous thrombosis before the initiation of oral anticoagulants. If, however, one is starting oral anticoagulants in a patient who is already known or likely to be protein C deficient, it would be prudent to start the drug under the cover of full therapeutic heparinization. It would also be wise to increase the dose of warfarin gradually, starting from a relatively low level (e.g., 2 mg for the first 3 days, then increasing in increments of 2 to 3 mg until therapeutic anticoagulation is achieved). Several case reports have documented successful oral anticoagulation of a subject with heterozygous protein C deficiency and a history of warfarin-induced skin necrosis (299,306). Therapeutic doses of heparin in addition to protein C replacement in the form of fresh frozen plasma were used to prevent the development of this complication.

The management of neonatal purpura fulminans in association with severe protein C deficiency is more complicated, because heparin therapy and antiplatelet agents have not been effective (257,259,260,307–309). The administration of a source of protein C appears to be critical in the initial treatment of these patients. Fresh frozen plasma has been used successfully in these infants. The half-life of protein C in the circulation is short (6 to 16 hours) (279,310), and the administration of plasma on a frequent basis is limited by the development of hyperproteinemia, hypertension, loss of venous access, and the potential for exposure to infectious viral agents. There are also several case reports describing the successful administration of protein C concentrate (311–313), and highly purified concentrates of this protein are undergoing clinical trials for this indication. Warfarin was administered to these infants without the redevelopment of skin necrosis during the phased withdrawal of fresh frozen plasma infusions (257,261,308,314), and this medication has been used chronically to control the thrombotic diathesis.

A particularly severe form of acquired protein C deficiency is associated with purpura fulminans and DIC in individuals with severe meningococcal infections. The mortality rate seen in these cases is often in excess of 50% (315), and those who survive the acute illness often experience severe organ damage and surgical amputation. In the absence of protein C to regulate coagulation and inflammatory pathways, uncontrolled fibrin formation leads to DIC and microvascular thrombosis and, ultimately, the clinical syndrome purpura fulminans. Protein C concentrate has been used successfully in several small trials to treat meningococcus-induced purpura fulminans (111,293). In one uncontrolled, unblinded trial of 36 individuals treated with protein C concentrate, there were three deaths, and among the survivors, only four individuals underwent surgical amputation (293). These results represent an impressive benefit in both predicted morbidity and mortality rates, and thus warrant further investigation.

PROTEIN S DEFICIENCY

In 1984, members from several kindreds who exhibited reduced levels of protein S were described with a striking history of recurrent venous thrombotic disease (316,317). Subsequently, many additional families with this disorder were reported (93,318–329). Protein S deficiency is an autosomal-dominant disorder with a reported frequency of approximately 10% in families with inherited thrombophilia (140). However, the prevalence is less (between 1% and 7%) among consecutive outpatients with a deep venous thrombosis (143,246,330,331). Protein S deficiency is generally thought to confer a risk of thrombosis similar to protein C deficiency (Table 42-2) (331,332), although, as will be discussed, the association has been complicated by considerable phenotypic variability.

Three types of protein S deficiency states can be identified based on measurements of total and free antigen as well as functional activity. Type I deficiency is associated with approximately 50% of the normal total protein S antigen level (317,318) and with decrements in free protein S antigen and protein S functional activity to less than approximately 40% of normal (323). Type I deficiency is most often secondary to missense mutations, base pair insertions or deletions, and premature stop codons (333). Another type of hereditary deficiency has been described in which the APC cofactor activity of protein S is decreased but with normal total and free antigen levels (Table 42-3). Of the more than 130 different mutations documented in patients with various types of protein S deficiency, only seven different nucleotide substitutions have been identified with a type II qualitative deficiency state (333,334). The type III deficiency, most commonly due to single nucleotide substitutions, is characterized by a decreased concentration of free protein S but normal total protein S antigen levels. However, the biologic basis of the type III deficiency state remains unclear.

There appears to be a multifactorial basis for type III deficiencies. Among French individuals with the low free protein S phenotype in isolation, 82% of the genetic mutations identified were due to a single mutation thought to result in the abnormal binding of protein S to C4b-binding protein (335,336). However, a later study documented the coexistence of type I and type III deficiency in 18 protein S–deficient families. The authors concluded that the two deficiency states actually represented phenotypic variants and were not the product of distinct genetic mutations (337). In a follow-up analysis of one large family with a high prevalence of both type I and type III deficiencies, total protein S antigen but not free protein S antigen levels were shown to directly correlate with age (338). These findings were independent of gender and also seen in nondeficient family members. The researchers concluded that a single point mutation in the protein S gene was responsible for the quantitative type I deficiency, but that the type III phenotype was actually due to an age-dependent free protein S deficiency; with increasing age, the relative concentrations of free protein S to total protein S decreased.

Under normal conditions, approximately 60% of the total protein S antigen in plasma is complexed to a complement component, C4b-binding protein. Only the free 40% is functionally active as a cofactor in mediating the anticoagulant effects of APC (93). This observation led to the development of methods for measuring total (317,339,340) and free protein S antigen (323). The most reliable measurements of total protein S antigen are usually obtained using radioimmunoassay (339–341) or enzyme-linked immunosorbent assay techniques that involve dilution of plasma samples and thereby favor dissociation of the protein S–C4b-binding protein complexes. After removing protein S–C4b-binding protein complexes from plasma by polyethylene glycol precipitation (323,342), free protein S may be quantified by immunoassay of the supernatant fractions. Functional assay methods require immunodepleted protein S–deficient plasma or immobilized monoclonal antibodies to protein S (316,343–347). They are based on the ability of protein S to serve as a cofactor for the anticoagulant effect of APC. The original coagulation assays were later noted to be sensitive to the presence of the factor V Leiden mutation, which led to the development of more accurate second-generation assays (348,349).

The average concentration of total protein S antigen in normal adults is 23 µg/mL (339), but there is significant overlap between normal and heterozygous individuals. The levels also appear to increase significantly with advancing age and are lower and more variable in females than males (331,350,351), although multivariate analysis of data from the Leiden Thrombophilia Study only identified menopausal state and oral contraceptives as independent predictors of protein S levels (352). Acquired protein S deficiency occurs during pregnancy (341,342) in patients with DIC (45,46,344) and acute thromboembolic disease (344) and in association with L-asparaginase therapy (Table 42-4) (291). Several studies have noted an association with antiphospholipid antibodies and acquired protein S deficiency, especially in severe cases of varicella complicated by purpura fulminans (353–355). C4b-binding protein is an acute-phase protein, and the decline in protein S activity in inflammatory disorders is attributable to a shift of the protein to the complexed, inactive form (344). Total protein S antigen measurements are generally increased in patients with the nephrotic syndrome (295,356,357), although functional assays give reduced values. This is due, in part, to the loss of free protein S in the urine and elevations in C4b-binding protein levels. Total and free protein S antigen concentrations are moderately decreased in liver disease (340,344,356,357). Total protein S antigen values in healthy newborns at term are 15% to 30% of normal, whereas C4b-binding protein is markedly reduced to less than 20%. Thus, the free form of the protein predominates in this setting, and functional levels are only slightly reduced compared with those in normal adults (347,358,359). Finally, interpretation of protein S measurements in individuals on oral anticoagulants is complicated, because the antigenic and functional levels of the protein drop substantially in this setting. A few groups used reductions in the ratio of total protein S antigen to prothrombin antigen to infer a diagnosis of the classic type of protein S deficiency; this is accomplished by using a strategy similar to that described for protein C–deficient subjects (317,318).

The aforementioned factors confound the reliable estimation of the prevalence of heterozygous protein S deficiency in the normal population and often make it difficult to establish the diagnosis of heterozygous protein S deficiency by performing assays on a given individual at a single point in time. Therefore, resampling of patients, in addition to performing family studies, is usually required to firmly establish the diagnosis. The variability in phenotypic expression of protein S deficiency is exemplified by the disparate results of several studies that assessed the relative risk of thrombosis. Although protein S deficiency was associated with a 2.4-fold increase in risk of thrombosis in one case-control study of 327 consecutive outpatients (331), a similar study did not establish a clear causal relationship (143). Recently, genetic confirmation of a protein S gene mutation in individuals with protein S deficiency established by antigenic assays has provided further evidence that protein S deficiency is, in fact, a significant hereditary risk factor for venous thrombosis (332,360).

Recommendations for the treatment of protein S–deficient patients with anticoagulants are similar to those in individuals without this disorder. Unfractionated or LMWH therapy is generally effective for the acute treatment of thrombotic episodes, and standard warfarin schedules appear to be effective in preventing recurrent venous thromboembolism.

FACTOR V LEIDEN

Before 1993, hereditary deficiencies were infrequently identified in patients with familial thromboembolic disease. Dahlbäck et al. (361) identified a proband and family that appeared resistant to APC in an aPTT-based clotting assay. In comparison to controls, most of the family members had a blunted anticoagulant response to APC. The following year, Bertina et al. (362) identified the genotype underlying most cases of APC resistance as a single point mutation in the factor V gene leading to substitution of an arginine-506 by glutamine. This mutation at an APC cleavage site renders factor Va relatively resistant to inactivation by APC (362,363).

The description of hereditary resistance to APC led to several small clinical studies that classified APC resistance as fairly ubiquitous, with deficiencies identified in more than 30% of individuals with a first episode of venous thrombosis (364,365). The Physician's Health Study confirmed the high incidence of heterozygous factor V Leiden (366). In this nested case-control study of 14,916 healthy men older than age 40, heterozygosity for the factor V Leiden mutation was identified in 12% of men with a first episode of deep venous thrombosis or pulmonary embolism and in 6% of controls. The relative risk of venous thromboembolism was 3.5-fold in those with factor V Leiden without concomitant risk factors. Similar results were generated by the Leiden Thrombophilia Study in which 21% of patients with deep venous thrombosis were classified as having resistance to APC versus 5% of controls (odds ratio of 6.6) (367). Individuals who were homozygous for the mutation experienced an even higher risk of thromboembolism (odds ratio of 80), usually occurring at a younger age than in those heterozygous for the mutation (31 vs. 44 years old) (368). After the observation that factor V Leiden was prevalent among the general Dutch population, genetic studies confirmed the high frequency of factor V Leiden heterozygosity among European and American white populations (5% to 10%) (369,370). However, the defect was found to be extremely rare in Asian and African populations (370).

The initial observation of Dahlbäck facilitated the development of an aPTT-based assay that serves as a screening test for APC resistance. The aPTT is performed with a standardized amount of APC, and clotting times are converted to an APC ratio (aPTT with APC divided by aPTT without APC). The results can be interpreted by comparing the ratio to that of the normal range, or by normalizing it to the APC resistance ratio obtained using normal pooled plasma (APC ratio of patient divided by APC ratio of normal plasma) and comparing this to the normal range. Whereas these "first-generation" APC resistance assays were conceptually quite simple and easy to perform, they required careful standardization and determination

of the normal range in at least 50 controls. The level of APC, the aPTT reagent, and the instrumentation used for clot detection affected the performance characteristics of the assay. Some assays using this format, therefore, had inadequate sensitivity and specificity for the factor V Leiden mutation. Also, individuals receiving anticoagulants or who had an abnormal aPTT due to other coagulation defects could not be investigated with this assay, and the test was not validated in individuals with acute thrombotic events or in pregnant women.

With the finding that the factor V Leiden mutation was responsible for most cases of APC resistance, "second-generation" coagulation assays were developed by diluting an individual's plasma with factor V–deficient plasma. Consequently, the influence of the levels of other coagulation factors on clotting time determinations was minimized. With proper standardization, the modified APC resistance test can give very high sensitivity and specificity for the factor V Leiden mutation.

At present, the most cost effective approach to diagnosing individuals with the factor V Leiden mutation is to test for APC resistance using a second-generation coagulation assay. Individuals with low APC resistance ratios should then be genotyped for the mutation, although it can be argued that such confirmatory testing is unnecessary in labs that have perfect concordance between the results of their APC resistance assay and factor V Leiden genotype. Using the first-generation aPTT-based assay for APC resistance, a small number of individuals with APC resistance without the factor V Leiden mutation can be identified. Even though de Visser et al. (371) have shown that this abnormality is associated with an increased risk of venous thrombosis, this assay is not recommended as part of the routine laboratory evaluation because the commercially available APC resistance assays using undiluted plasma do not replicate the performance characteristics of the assay used in this study.

PROTHROMBIN G20210A MUTATION

A single base pair mutation in the prothrombin gene has been identified as an independent risk factor for hereditary venous thromboembolic disease and is the second most common hereditary thrombophilic defect after factor V Leiden. Originally described by Poort et al. in 1996 (372), a G to A substitution in the 3'-untranslated region at position 20210 was identified in 18% of individuals among 28 probands with a personal and familial history of venous thrombosis. Studies have shown that individuals with the prothrombin 20210A mutation have higher plasma prothrombin activity than those with a normal genotype. Linkage studies in 397 individuals from 21 Spanish families suggest that prothrombin G20210A is a functional polymorphism responsible for elevated prothrombin antigen levels and activity (373).

The prothrombin G20210A mutation has been documented at significantly higher frequency in patients with venous thrombosis than in healthy controls in numerous studies (374–376). Large population studies have shown an overall prevalence of approximately 2% in the general white population with significant geographic variation. Among southern Europeans, the prevalence was approximately 3%, but it was only very rarely identified in individuals of Asian or African descent (377). In the Leiden Thrombophilia Study, the prevalence of the prothrombin G20210A mutation was 6.2% versus 2.3% in healthy matched controls (372). This resulted in a 2.8-fold increased risk of thrombosis for carriers of the mutation, an effect that was seen in both sexes and all age groups. Similar frequencies were confirmed in a Swedish study of 99 consecutive outpatients in which 7.1% of individuals were identified with the prothrombin

G20210A allele versus 1.8% of controls, equaling a fourfold increased risk (376).

Polymerase chain reaction methods have been used to detect the prothrombin G20210A mutation in genomic DNA (372). In addition, methods are available to detect both the prothrombin G20210A mutation and factor V Leiden in the same reaction (378). Although plasma prothrombin activity and antigen levels are significantly higher in individuals with the prothrombin G20210A mutation, concentrations cannot be used to screen for the defect due to significant overlap with the normal population (372,373).

HYPERHOMOCYSTEINEMIA

Homocysteine is a sulfur-containing amino acid involved in metabolic pathways leading to the formation of other amino acids. Methionine is generated through the remethylation of homocysteine or is metabolized to cysteine via transsulfuration. Elevated levels of homocysteine are seen in a variety of disorders that affect either the concentration of substrates or the activity of enzymes involved in its metabolism (Table 42-5). Acquired hyperhomocysteinemia is most commonly seen with moderate deficiencies in folate, vitamin B_{12}, or vitamin B_6.

The association between severe hyperhomocysteinemia and premature atherosclerosis was initially described in children with homocystinuria. Homocystinuria results from several rare inborn errors of metabolism and is most frequently seen in cases of homozygous cystathionine β-synthase deficiency. Other clinical manifestations include venous thromboembolism as well as mental retardation, ectopic lenses, and skeletal abnormalities. In 1969, McCully (379) reported an infant with severe homocystinuria secondary to an inborn error of cobalamin metabolism with advanced atherosclerotic disease similar in nature to that seen with cystathionine β-synthase deficiency. The accumulation of plasma homocysteine provided the common link between these two metabolic abnormalities. Subsequent case-control and cross-sectional studies noted an association between even mild elevations in serum or plasma homocysteine and atherosclerotic or venous thromboembolic disease (380–383).

Several genetic and acquired abnormalities can lead to mild or moderate elevations in serum homocysteine concentrations. The most common genetic defects include heterozygous cystathionine β-synthase deficiency, which occurs in approximately 0.3% of the population, and homozygosity for a methylenetetrahydrofolate reductase (MTHFR) mutation, which is present in approximately 20% of Italian and U.S. Hispanic populations but less than 1% of African Americans (384). The MTHFR variant is due to an alanine for valine substitution at amino acid 677, which causes thermolability of the enzyme and a 50% reduction in its activity (385).

Mild or moderate hyperhomocysteinemia is an independent risk factor for myocardial infarction, stroke, and carotid artery disease (386–388). Data from the Framingham Heart Study showed that elderly subjects with mild hyperhomocysteinemia (>14.4 μmol/L) were twice as likely to have significant carotid artery stenosis than those with lower homocysteine levels (388). In a large cohort study, more than 5000 British men were prospectively followed for evidence of stroke or myocardial infarction. Among the 107 subjects who experienced a stroke, there was a graded increase in relative risk based on increasing homocysteine concentrations (387). There have also been numerous cross-sectional and case-control studies documenting an association between hyperhomocysteinemia and coronary disease; however, prospective studies have been less predictive, and pooled analysis of seven prospective studies found a smaller association between homocysteine levels and coronary artery disease (383).

After establishing an association between mild hyperhomocysteinemia and atherosclerotic disease, several case-control studies confirmed the role of homocysteine in venous thrombosis. The Leiden Thrombophilia Study showed that individuals with plasma homocysteine levels above the ninety-fifth percentile (>18.5 μmol/L) were 2.5 times more likely to experience an initial episode of deep venous thrombosis (380). Similarly, a metaanalysis of ten case-control studies generated a pooled estimate of the odds ratio at 2.5 (382). Curiously, although homozygosity for the thermolabile MTHFR variant or heterozygous 844ins68 mutation of the cystathionine β-synthase gene has been documented in a significant percentage of individuals with hyperhomocysteinemia, several studies have shown that the corresponding genotypes are not independent risk factors for deep venous thrombosis (389,390). This paradox may be explained by the prothrombotic effect of hyperhomocysteinemia being attributable to the interplay of environmental (such as relative vitamin deficiencies) and genetic factors.

There are several proposed mechanisms by which hyperhomocysteinemia leads to atherosclerotic or thromboembolic disease. *In vitro* studies have shown that homocysteine can induce vascular injury directly through free radical formation, impaired vasodilation due to decreased levels of nitric oxide, or its accumulation with low-density lipoprotein cholesterol in vascular macrophages (391,392). The thrombogenic effects of hyperhomocysteinemia have been attributed to the inhibition of heparan sulfate expression, tissue-type plasminogen activator binding, or factor V activation (393–395).

Hyperhomocysteinemia is usually diagnosed by measuring fasting plasma levels of homocysteine by high-pressure liquid chromatography. Normal homocysteine levels range between 5 and 15 μmol/L, and hyperhomocysteinemia has been classified as mild (15 to 30 μmol/L), moderate (30 to 100 μmol/L), or severe (>100 μmol/L). Fasting homocysteine levels have been regarded as representative of the remethylation pathway (dependent on folate, vitamin B_{12}, and MTHFR), whereas homocysteine levels 4 hours after an oral methionine load reflect the integrity of the transsulfuration pathway (dependent on vitamin B_6 and cystathionine β-synthase). Because individuals with heterozygous cystathionine β-synthase deficiency may have normal levels of fasting homocysteine, the methionine oral load has been used to diagnose these heterozygous individuals. However, recent evidence suggests that abnormal results from loading tests are not specific for heterozygous cystathionine β-synthase deficiencies (390).

Correction of hyperhomocysteinemia via vitamin supplementation is a potentially attractive means of treating a prothrombotic state. Several studies have shown that folate supplementation even in doses as low as 0.5 mg daily can lead to substantial reductions in serum homocysteine levels (382,396–398). Considering the negligible downside to folate supplementation, its use should be considered in any individ-

---

TABLE 42-5. Acquired Causes for Hyperhomocysteinemia

Smoking
Alcohol
Renal failure
Liver failure
Vitamin deficiency
    Folate, vitamin B_{12}, or vitamin B_6
Drugs
    Methotrexate, trimethoprim, cholestyramine, carbamazepine

ual with deep venous thrombosis and hyperhomocysteinemia. However, it remains to be seen if normalizing homocysteine levels results in an actual reduction in the incidence of venous or arterial thrombotic events.

HEPARIN COFACTOR II DEFICIENCY

Heparin cofactor II is a heparin-dependent glycoprotein that acts as a thrombin inhibitor. In contrast to antithrombin, this inhibitor does not inhibit factor Xa or other coagulation serine proteases. Several families have been described with quantitative deficiency of this protein, which is inherited as an autosomal-dominant trait. Heterozygous individuals have plasma heparin cofactor II concentrations that are approximately 50% of normal values.

It is uncertain whether heparin cofactor II deficiency is a risk factor for thrombosis (399). In one series of 305 patients with juvenile thromboembolic episodes, two patients had heparin cofactor II deficiency. However, each of these patients had a second defect: the factor V Leiden mutation or protein C deficiency (400).

PLASMINOGEN DEFICIENCY

Congenital plasminogen deficiency is inherited as an autosomal-dominant trait. There are both quantitative defects and functional defects. Thrombosis has been reported in young patients when the plasminogen concentration is less than 40% of control values. The development of ligneous conjunctivitis, hyperviscosity of tracheobronchial secretions, and hydrocephalus has been reported in a patient with homozygous plasminogen deficiency (401). Replacement therapy with lysine-conjugated plasminogen resulted in marked improvement.

Despite this observation, the clinical importance of plasminogen deficiency as a risk factor for thrombosis is doubtful. In a Spanish study of 2132 consecutive patients with thrombosis, plasminogen deficiency was seen in 0.75% versus 0.29% of healthy blood donors (247). Likewise, several other studies have documented no association between type I plasminogen deficiency and deep venous thrombosis (402–404).

FACTOR XII DEFICIENCY

Factor XII is the zymogen of a serine protease that initiates the contact activation reactions and intrinsic blood coagulation *in vitro*. Subjects with severe factor XII deficiency (<1% of normal) have markedly prolonged aPTTs but do not exhibit a bleeding diathesis (405); however, there have been a number of cases of venous thromboembolism or myocardial infarction in factor XII–deficient individuals (406). This thrombophilic tendency has been attributed to reduced plasma fibrinolytic activity (407). The frequency with which severe factor XII deficiency leads to thrombosis is uncertain. One review found that 8% had a history of thromboembolism (405). However, interpretation is difficult, considering that individuals with thrombotic complications are more likely to be reported than asymptomatic patients. This led to cross-sectional analyses of thromboembolic events in larger numbers of unselected families with factor XII deficiency. In a study of 14 Swiss families with factor XII deficiency, 2 of 18 homozygous or doubly heterozygous patients had sustained deep vein thrombosis; however, each episode occurred in association with predisposing thrombotic risk factors. Only 1 of the 45 heterozygotes in these families had a possible history of venous

thrombosis (408). However, other groups have found a more pronounced association with thrombosis (409,410). Thus, it remains unproven if factor XII deficiency is associated with an increased risk of thrombosis.

ELEVATED FACTORS VIII, IX, AND XI AND THROMBIN-ACTIVATABLE FIBRINOLYSIS INHIBITOR

Recently, investigators have focused on the presence of supranormal levels of clotting factors and their role in venous thrombosis. In the Leiden Thrombophilia Study, 25% of patients with a first episode of venous thrombosis and 11% of healthy controls had factor VIII coagulant (VIII:C) activity greater than 150% of normal (>150 IU/dL). Individuals with VIII:C levels greater than 150 IU/dL had a fivefold increased risk of thrombosis compared to individuals with lower VIII:C levels (<100 IU/dL) (411). Several studies confirmed this association of factor VIII activity and venous thrombosis after adjustment for other possible influences such as von Willebrand's factor and blood type. Similarly, researchers examined the possible role of VIII:C as an acute phase reactant and found that the association between elevated VIII:C levels and thrombosis was independent of immediate versus delayed testing or C-reactive protein and fibrinogen levels (411–414). An Austrian study prospectively followed 360 patients for an average of 30 months and found that among the 38 patients who developed recurrent thromboembolism, the mean VIII:C level was greater than among those without recurrence (415). Among those individuals with levels above the ninetieth percentile, the likelihood of recurrence at 2 years was 37% versus 5% with lower VIII:C levels (relative risk, 6.7) (415). Elevated antigenic levels of several other coagulation factors including factor XI, factor IX, and TAFI also confer a modest, albeit significantly increased, risk for an initial episode of deep venous thrombosis (416–418). The mechanisms for high levels of VIII:C and these other factors have yet to be elucidated, but family studies suggest that high factor VIII levels are likely to be genetically determined (419). Corroborating studies are required before recommending routine measurement of VIII:C levels in patients with a prior venous thrombotic event.

DIAGNOSIS AND MANAGEMENT OF HEREDITARY THROMBOPHILIA

The initial evaluation for an individual experiencing a thromboembolic event should be directed towards identifying acquired or potentially reversible hypercoagulable risk factors. A thorough history and physical examination should be performed with particular attention towards those disorders listed in Table 42-1. As is discussed in later sections, diagnosis of an acquired thrombophilic state has both therapeutic and diagnostic implications. Thus, only after reasonable measures have been taken to pursue such a diagnosis should testing for a hereditary thrombophilia be contemplated.

Nonetheless, screening for hereditary thrombophilias has become commonplace in the evaluation of individuals with recurrent venous thromboembolic disease and is advocated by some experts after an initial episode of deep venous thrombosis. It is estimated that more than 25,000 tests for the factor V Leiden mutation are performed each year in the United Kingdom alone (420), and it is the most commonly ordered genetic test in the United States. Even though heritable risk factors can now be identified in a substantial percentage of patients with venous thromboembolism, the practical significance of such a diagnosis has become a point of debate. At issue is whether the diagnosis of hereditary thrombophilia provides information that is beneficial in the overall management of the propositus and affected family members that adequately counterbalances the potential negative effects of establishing such a diagnosis or, in some cases, misdiagnosis. In this section, the use of testing for thrombophilia is outlined with particular attention on the clinical implications with respect to anticoagulation for thromboembolic episodes, risk of recurrent events, prophylaxis for the asymptomatic patient, and special circumstances such as surgery, oral contraception, and pregnancy.

Anticoagulation for Deep Venous Thrombosis

The initial management of acute thromboembolic disease is generally not affected by the presence of inherited risk factors for thrombosis. The usual treatment of acute venous thrombosis consists of unfractionated heparin or LMWH followed by anticoagulation with warfarin. Unfractionated heparin should be administered in adequate dosage because failure to reach a therapeutic level of anticoagulation within the first 24 hours increases the risk of recurrent thromboembolism (421). Unfractionated or LMWH should be continued for at least 5 days or until the prothrombin time reaches the desired therapeutic range, typically an international normalized ratio of 2 to 3.

Albeit infrequent, there are settings in which the diagnosis of hereditary thrombophilia can influence clinical management. In patients with hereditary antithrombin deficiency, higher doses of unfractionated heparin may be required to achieve therapeutic anticoagulation as monitored by the aPTT. In addition, antithrombin concentrate may be used in special circumstances such as recurrent thrombosis despite adequate anticoagulation, unusually severe thrombosis, or severe heparin resistance (see Antithrombin Deficiency). It is also reasonable to administer antithrombin concentrate before major surgeries or in obstetric situations when the risks of bleeding from anticoagulation are unacceptable.

Hereditary protein C deficiency is associated with warfarin-induced skin necrosis due to a transient hypercoagulable state during the initiation of warfarin. The currently recommended starting daily warfarin dose of 5 mg in warfarin-naïve patients still leads to a 50% decrease in plasma protein C anticoagulant activity from baseline within 1 day. Consequently, in patients known to have protein C deficiency, it is prudent to start treatment with warfarin only after the individual is adequately heparinized, and the dose of the drug should be increased gradually starting with a relatively low dosage (e.g., 2 mg). Individuals with a history of warfarin-induced skin necrosis can be anticoagulated after receiving a source of exogenous protein C either via fresh frozen plasma or protein C concentrate. This offers a bridge until a stable level of anticoagulation can be achieved.

Risk of Recurrence

Standard therapy for patients with deep venous thrombosis typically includes anticoagulation with warfarin for 3 to 6 months. However, after this period of anticoagulation, there is a high rate of recurrent thrombotic events of approximately 5% to 10%/year (422). A study by Kearon et al. (423) investigated 3 months versus extended therapy for an initial episode of "idiopathic" deep venous thrombosis. The study was terminated early due to a very high recurrence rate; among those receiving placebo after 3 months of warfarin, there was a 27.4% recurrence rate/year versus 1.3% in those receiving indefinite treatment. Considering the high rate of recurrent events, it would be

particularly helpful to identify those individuals who were especially prone to subsequent thrombosis.

Although uncommon in general practice, multiple studies have documented that the presence of multiple bona fide hereditary defects (e.g., doubly heterozygous or homozygous mutations) increases the likelihood of recurrent thrombosis (424,425). Conversely, the association between the most commonly encountered single hereditary thrombophilic defects, the factor V Leiden or prothrombin G20210A mutations, and recurrent thrombotic events has not been clearly established (426). On one hand, individuals in the U.S. Physician's Health Study with a first spontaneous deep venous thrombosis and heterozygosity for the factor V Leiden mutation had a significantly higher recurrence rate at 4 years (29%) than those without the mutation (11%) (427). In an Italian cohort study, Simioni et al. (428) also observed a significantly higher recurrence rate in carriers of the factor V Leiden as well as the prothrombin G20210A mutation. On the other hand, several other investigators have found that recurrence rates in individuals with heterozygosity for either of these two mutations alone were not significantly higher than those in unaffected individuals (424,429–431). Until further data are available, it is difficult to advocate testing for the hereditary thrombophilias to identify large subsets of patients at high risk for recurrent venous thromboembolic events, thus necessitating extended anticoagulation.

Long-Term Therapy

Unfortunately, controlled prospective trials to investigate the optimal duration of anticoagulant therapy in patients with hereditary thrombophilia have not been reported, and long-term treatment decisions after an initial thrombotic event must be made on an individual basis using estimates of recurrence and bleeding rates from prospective studies, which did not stratify patients with regard to the presence of the factor V Leiden or prothrombin G20210A mutation. In patients with a first thrombotic event in the setting of a transient triggering factor, anticoagulation can be discontinued after 3 to 6 months. Patients with venous thromboembolism in the absence of triggering factors should be treated for 6 months (432). Despite high recurrence rates, current evidence argues against longer warfarin therapy after a first thromboembolic episode, even in cases in which a specific hereditary thrombophilic defect can be identified.

Prolonging anticoagulation beyond 6 months after an initial episode of venous thromboembolism can be viewed in terms of mortality benefit—namely, the total number of fatal pulmonary emboli prevented versus fatal hemorrhages. Fortunately, recurrent thrombotic events are rarely fatal. In a pooled analysis of 25 prospective studies, the rate of fatal pulmonary embolism after appropriate initial therapy for deep venous thrombosis was 0.3% per year (433). This closely matches the mortality rate from bleeding seen with oral anticoagulation. In a large prospective study of 2745 patients receiving anticoagulation for varied indications, there were five fatal intracerebral hemorrhages, equaling a rate of 0.3% per year (434). Considering that the risk of recurrent thrombosis may decline 6 to 12 months after the initial event (422) and that the risk of bleeding increases with age, long-term anticoagulation at a target international normalized ratio of 2 to 3 in a population with a risk of recurrence in the range of 5% per year does not appear warranted.

This risk-benefit balance is not significantly influenced by finding the presence of heterozygosity for the factor V Leiden or prothrombin G20210A mutation, as these defects have not been clearly linked to an increased risk of recurrent venous thromboembolic events. In addition, several retrospective studies have shown that the life expectancy for individuals with hereditary thrombophilia does not differ significantly from that of the general population (435–437). Thus, it would seem doubtful that long-term anticoagulation would confer a survival benefit in cases of hereditary thrombophilia. This point was illustrated by a cohort study of individuals with the factor V Leiden mutation. The median time to recurrence after discontinuation of oral anticoagulant therapy was 9 years (438). The period was significantly shorter (3.5 years) among patients who experienced an idiopathic rather than a precipitated first event. It was estimated that, even in the latter group, death from hemorrhage would probably exceed the number of fatal pulmonary emboli prevented with chronic warfarin therapy. Decision analysis models addressed the issue for individuals with protein C, protein S, or antithrombin deficiencies as well as factor V Leiden. Although it was suggested that longer periods of anticoagulation may be warranted in certain instances, in general, anticoagulation for several years after an initial episode was not supported (439–441).

Isolated deficiencies of antithrombin, protein C, or protein S are less frequently encountered abnormalities, and there are not sufficient data regarding the risk-benefit balance of extended anticoagulation in these patients after an initial thrombotic episode. Reports of initially identified kindreds with these disorders suggest a high rate of venous thromboembolism with advancing age, but these were certainly selected for publication due to the high incidence of thrombosis among biochemically affected family members. Many experienced clinicians believe that antithrombin deficiency, particularly type I and some type II variants, is the most clinically penetrant of the hereditary thrombotic disorders; deficiencies of protein C and protein S can also be associated with a high rate of thrombosis in some families. Thus, the identification of a single thrombophilic defect in conjunction with a family history of multiple first-degree relatives with spontaneous venous thrombosis at a young age can be used as justification for extended anticoagulation after an initial episode of venous thromboembolism.

Recurrent episodes of spontaneous venous thromboembolism generally warrant indefinite anticoagulation, regardless of the presence of hereditary thrombophilia. Additional criteria for indefinite anticoagulation include the presence of more than one hereditary defect, an initial life-threatening thrombotic event or massive pulmonary embolism, or a thrombotic event in an unusual location such as cerebral, mesenteric, portal, or hepatic veins where recurrences could lead to severe morbidity or mortality.

Asymptomatic Carriers

With an increasing number of individuals identified with heterozygous thrombophilic mutations, an important consideration is the potential impact on other asymptomatic family members. These family members are at an increased risk to experience thromboembolic events and could conceivably benefit from prophylactic anticoagulation. However, prospective studies have shown that the annual incidence of a first spontaneous thrombosis in individuals with deficiencies of protein C, protein S, or antithrombin is less than 1% per year (141). Considering that less than 5% of thrombotic events typically result in fatal pulmonary emboli (422), the number of fatal hemorrhagic complications would likely exceed the benefits of prolonged anticoagulation in asymptomatic individuals. In the occasional family with hereditary thrombophilia and a very high penetrance of spontaneous venous thrombosis at an early age, the benefit of prophylactic anticoagulation in asymptomatic biochemically affected patients may be sufficiently great so that it is reasonable to consider its institution after puberty.

Transient Hypercoagulable States (Surgery, Pregnancy, and Oral Contraception)

Another potential benefit in establishing the diagnosis of hereditary thrombophilia is the possibility of prophylaxis during high-risk periods such as trauma, surgery, or pregnancy. Several retrospective studies have shown that the annual incidence of all thrombotic events in patients with hereditary thrombophilia is less than 1%, but that more than 60% occurred during periods when transient hypercoagulable risk factors were present (141,244) (Table 42-1). In fact, individuals with deficiencies of protein C, protein S, or antithrombin who were not treated with anticoagulants experienced thrombotic complications in one out of seven high-risk situations (245). Anticoagulation has been shown to be effective in preventing thrombosis in settings of trauma, immobilization, and surgery (442), and this includes patients with inherited thrombotic disorders (245,443). However, it has not yet been established if individuals with hereditary thrombophilia require more intense or longer prophylactic anticoagulation than is otherwise recommended.

The management of women with thrombophilia is especially important considering that fatal pulmonary embolism is the leading cause of maternal mortality in many developed countries (444,445). Several studies have established that the incidence of thrombotic complications during pregnancy and the postpartum period is at least eightfold higher in women with hereditary thrombophilia (244,446). Antithrombin deficiency, in particular, has been associated with an unusually high risk of thromboembolism (446,447). The treatment for women who are potentially at high risk for thrombosis depends on an individual's prior history of thromboembolism, and/or the presence of hereditary thrombophilia.

In those women who have experienced an antepartum thromboembolic episode, it is important whether the episode was in association with a reversible risk factor. In a recent prospective study of 125 pregnant women with a history of a single thromboembolic episode, there were no recurrent events among the 44 women with prior events in association with a transient hypercoagulable risk factor (448). For these women, close surveillance and postpartum anticoagulation for 4 to 6 weeks was effective. On the other hand, the rate of recurrence in women with hereditary thrombophilia was considerably higher at 20%. The appropriate management for these women has yet to be conclusively established. In general, there are two approaches to these patients—either close surveillance or prophylactic anticoagulation. In some instances, it may be reasonable to closely monitor without anticoagulation, especially in previously asymptomatic women with the factor V Leiden mutation (449,450). However, a more conservative approach is often advocated, especially for women with antithrombin deficiency. Based on an individual's perceived thrombotic risk, options for anticoagulation include prophylactic or therapeutic doses of subcutaneous unfractionated heparin or LMWH. LMWH has become an attractive, safe alternative to unfractionated heparin due to its ease of administration and lack of need for laboratory monitoring (451–453). Consideration should be given to adjusting the dosing of LMWH as the pregnancy progresses based on body weight or anti–factor Xa levels (451,452). All women with hereditary thrombophilia or history of thromboembolism should receive postpartum anticoagulation for 4 to 6 weeks (450,454).

In women who chronically take oral anticoagulants for the prevention of recurrent venous thromboembolism, it is recommended that warfarin be replaced with heparin or LMWH to

TABLE 42-6. Relative Risk of Thrombosis for Premenopausal Women with a Prothrombotic Defect Taking Oral Contraceptives

Type of Prothrombotic Defect (Reference)	Risk of Thrombosis: Odds Ratio (95% Confidence Interval)	Risk of Thrombosis: + Oral Contraceptive
Factor V Leiden (456)	3.8 (2.4–6.0)	34.7 (7.8–154.0)
Factor VIII (>150 IU/dL) (457)	4.0 (2.8–8.0)	10.3 (3.7–28.9)
Prothrombin G20210A (458)	2.7 (0.6–12.7)	16.3 (3.4–79.1)

minimize the risk of thrombotic complications as well as warfarin embryopathy. For individuals with antithrombin deficiency, replacement therapy with antithrombin concentrate until conception has infrequently been used, partly because the product needs to be administered intravenously at frequent intervals and it is costly. For women trying to conceive, some may wish to continue warfarin therapy with frequent pregnancy tests. As soon as pregnancy is diagnosed, oral anticoagulants must be discontinued and heparin therapy initiated. The risk of warfarin embryopathy appears to be small during the first 6 weeks of pregnancy (455) and is highest during the sixth to twelfth week of gestation.

Since their introduction in the 1960s, oral contraceptives have been reported to be associated with an increased risk of venous and even arterial thrombosis. The estrogen component of the pills were first identified as prothrombotic, which led to formulations with less estrogen but higher progesterone content. Yet the low-dose estrogen preparations containing older progesterones (levonorgestrel, lynestrenol, and norethisterone) still confer approximately a fourfold increase in venous thromboembolism as compared to nonusers (459). Subsequent third-generation progestins (desogesterol, gestodene, and norgestimate) were developed in an attempt to counterbalance the negative effects of estrogen on the lipid profile. Surprisingly, these agents were noted to have an even greater risk of venous thrombosis when compared to previous progestins (460,461).

The association between oral contraceptives and deep venous thrombosis is more pronounced in women with an underlying hereditary thrombophilia. Among families with deficiencies of antithrombin, protein C, or protein S, the use of oral contraceptives was associated with a sixfold increased risk of thrombosis (141). As shown in Table 42-6, case-control studies have established an impressive causal relationship between thrombophilic mutations and oral contraceptives. Consequently, there has been considerable discussion regarding the use of screening before starting such agents (462,463) due to the 30-fold increased risk of thrombosis in women with the factor V Leiden mutation (456) and the significant prevalence of factor V Leiden (5%) (369) among the U.S. white population. However, large-scale screening is unlikely to be cost effective, considering that approximately 8000 women would need to be screened in order to detect 400 women with factor V Leiden mutation and thus prevent one episode of deep venous thrombosis (462). Unfortunately, even a careful family history of thrombosis is poorly predictive of hereditary thrombophilia and is an ineffective means of screening young women before testing for hereditary thrombophilia and prescribing oral contraception (464).

Evaluation for Hereditary Thrombophilia

As outlined above, many of the issues surrounding the hereditary thrombophilias and their treatment remain unresolved. Due to this lack of consensus coupled with the high cost of performing a complete laboratory evaluation, a targeted approach to evaluate patients for the presence of hereditary thrombophilia is

warranted. Testing should be based on an understanding of the potential pros and cons of diagnosis as summarized below.

Arguments in favor of testing:

Possible diagnosis of

- Dual hereditary defects (homozygous or doubly heterozygous mutations) that are associated with an increased risk of initial thrombosis and recurrence
- Antithrombin deficiency that potentially confers a higher risk for thrombosis than the other hereditary thrombophilias
- Asymptomatic individuals that may be at higher risk of thrombosis after transient hypercoagulable states such as outpatient surgery or trauma

Better assess thrombotic risk and thereby influence management

- In older patients at risk of harboring an occult malignancy, which can later be diagnosed in more than 10% of individuals after an initial episode of deep venous thrombosis (465). In those identified to have the factor V Leiden or prothrombin G20210A mutation, the risk of an underlying malignancy is probably similar to that of the general population.
- When considering initiating oral contraception, especially in asymptomatic women with a family history of thrombosis.
- In young women with an antepartum history of deep venous thrombosis who may be at risk for recurrence during pregnancy.

Arguments against testing:

Diagnosis does not influence

- Initial choice of anticoagulant treatment for venous thromboembolism
- Duration of anticoagulation after first thrombotic event
- Risk of recurrence (except in the combined deficiency state)
- Mortality in asymptomatic carriers
- Duration of prophylaxis after surgery

Pitfalls of diagnosis

- Inaccurate or erroneous assay results, leading to deficiencies of antithrombin, protein C, or protein S being diagnosed. Other confounding factors can influence levels of these plasma proteins such as age, sex, oral contraception, liver disease, consumptive coagulopathies, thrombosis, inflammatory disease states, vitamin deficiencies, and anticoagulant therapy.
- Overaggressive prophylactic anticoagulation and increased risk of bleeding.
- Implications of assigning a genetic disorder with respect to health or life insurance.

On balance, we typically pursue a targeted approach to diagnosis for individuals after an episode of deep venous thrombosis. This involves classifying individuals as strongly or weakly thrombophilic based on three historical features: first thromboembolic event before age 50, history of recurrent thrombotic episodes, or a first-degree relative with documented venous thromboembolism before age 50. For those individuals with any of the above criteria, we perform a complete hypercoagulable evaluation, including levels of homocysteine, antithrombin, protein C, and protein S and analysis for the factor V and prothrombin G20210A mutations, as well as testing for a lupus anticoagulant and the presence of antiphospholipid antibodies. For individuals who do not meet the above criteria, deficiencies of protein C, protein S, and antithrombin are omitted due to their low prevalence in such populations (466) and the increased likelihood for assigning an erroneous diagnosis. However, such an approach should serve only as a general guideline; optimal management and evaluation of individuals with hereditary thrombophilia remains an evolving area. An appreciation of the limitations and implications of a diagnosis of hereditary thrombophilia enables the physician to pursue an evaluation that best serves the individual patient and family.

REFERENCES

1. McLean J. The thromboplastic action of cephalin. *Am J Physiol* 1916:250–257.
2. Howell WH. The nature and action of the thromboplastic (zymoplastic) substance of the tissues. *Am J Physiol* 1912;31:1–21.
3. Damus PS, Hicks M, Rosenberg RD. Anticoagulant action of heparin. *Nature* 1973;246:355–357.
4. Marcum JA, Rosenberg RD. Anticoagulantly active heparin-like molecules from vascular tissue. *Biochemistry* 1984;23:1730–1737.
5. Marcum JA, Fritze L, Galli SJ, et al. Microvascular heparin-like species with anticoagulant activity. *Am J Physiol* 1983;245:H725–H733.
6. Marcum JA, Rosenberg RD. Heparinlike molecules with anticoagulant activity are synthesized by cultured endothelial cells. *Biochem Biophys Res Commun* 1985;126:365–372.
7. Marcum JA, Atha DH, Fritze LM, et al. Cloned bovine aortic endothelial cells synthesize anticoagulantly active heparan sulfate proteoglycan. *J Biol Chem* 1986;261:7507–7517.
8. Stern D, Nawroth P, Marcum J, et al. Interaction of antithrombin III with bovine aortic segments. Role of heparin in binding and enhanced anticoagulant activity. *J Clin Invest* 1985;75:272–279.
9. Marcum JA, Conway EM, Youssoufian H, et al. Anticoagulantly active heparin-like molecules from cultured fibroblasts. *Exp Cell Res* 1986;166:253–258.
10. Rosenberg RD, Damus PS. The purification and mechanism of action of human antithrombin-heparin cofactor. *J Biol Chem* 1973;248:6490–6505.
11. Rosenberg JS, McKenna PW, Rosenberg RD. Inhibition of human factor IXa by human antithrombin. *J Biol Chem* 1975;250:8883–8888.
12. Stead N, Kaplan AP, Rosenberg RD. Inhibition of activated factor XII by antithrombin-heparin cofactor. *J Biol Chem* 1976;251:6481–6488.
13. Abildgaard U. Highly purified antithrombin 3 with heparin cofactor activity prepared by disc electrophoresis. *Scand J Clin Lab Invest* 1968;21:89–91.
14. Abildgaard U. Binding of thrombin to antithrombin III. *Scand J Clin Lab Invest* 1969;24:23–27.
15. Smith JW, Dey N, Knauer DJ. Heparin binding domain of antithrombin III: characterization using a synthetic peptide directed polyclonal antibody. *Biochemistry* 1990;29:8950–8957.
16. Owen MC, Shaw GJ, Grau E, et al. Molecular characterization of antithrombin Barcelona-2: 47 arginine to cysteine. *Thromb Res* 1989;55:451–457.
17. Borg JY, Owen MC, Soria C, et al. Proposed heparin binding site in antithrombin based on arginine 47. A new variant Rouen-II, 47 Arg to Ser. *J Clin Invest* 1988;81:1292–1296.
18. Arocas V, Bock SC, Olson ST, et al. The role of Arg46 and Arg47 of antithrombin in heparin binding. *Biochemistry* 1999;38:10196–10204.
19. Karp GI, Marcum JA, Rosenberg RD. The role of tryptophan residues in heparin-antithrombin interactions. *Arch Biochem Biophys* 1984;233:712–720.
20. Oosta GM, Gardner WT, Beeler DL, et al. Multiple functional domains of the heparin molecule. *Proc Natl Acad Sci U S A* 1981;78:829–833.
21. Stone AL, Beeler D, Oosta G, et al. Circular dichroism spectroscopy of heparin-antithrombin interactions. *Proc Natl Acad Sci U S A* 1982;79:7190–7194.
22. Rosenberg RD, Armand G, Lam L. Structure-function relationships of heparin species. *Proc Natl Acad Sci U S A* 1978;75:3065–3069.
23. Rosenberg RD, Lam L. Correlation between structure and function of heparin. *Proc Natl Acad Sci U S A* 1979;76:1218–1222.
24. Lindahl U, Backstrom G, Thunberg L, et al. Evidence for a 3-O-sulfated D-glucosamine residue in the antithrombin-binding sequence of heparin. *Proc Natl Acad Sci U S A* 1980;77:6551–6555.
25. Wright HT, Scarsdale JN. Structural basis for serpin inhibitor activity. *Proteins* 1995;22:210–225.
26. Schreuder HA, de Boer B, Dijkema R, et al. The intact and cleaved human antithrombin III complex as a model for serpin-proteinase interactions. *Nat Struct Biol* 1994;1:48–54.
27. Nordenman B, Bjork I. Binding of low-affinity and high-affinity heparin to antithrombin. Ultraviolet difference spectroscopy and circular dichroism studies. *Biochemistry* 1978;17:3339–3344.
28. Nordenman B, Danielsson A, Bjork I. The binding of low-affinity and high-affinity heparin to antithrombin. Fluorescence studies. *Eur J Biochem* 1978;90:1–6.
29. Evington JR, Feldman PA, Luscombe M, et al. Multiple complexes of thrombin and heparin. *Biochim Biophys Acta* 1986;871:85–92.
30. Jordan RE, Oosta GM, Gardner WT, et al. The binding of low molecular weight heparin to hemostatic enzymes. *J Biol Chem* 1980;255:10073–10080.
31. Danielsson A, Raub E, Lindahl U, et al. Role of ternary complexes, in which heparin binds both antithrombin and proteinase, in the acceleration of the reactions between antithrombin and thrombin or factor Xa. *J Biol Chem* 1986;261:15467–15473.
32. Olson ST, Bjork I. Regulation of thrombin activity by antithrombin and heparin. *Semin Thromb Hemost* 1994;20:373–409.
33. Comp PC, Jacocks RM, Ferrell GL, et al. Activation of protein C in vivo. *J Clin Invest* 1982;70:127–134.
34. Emerick SC, Bang NU, Yan SB, et al. Antithrombotic properties of activated protein C [abstract]. *Blood* 1985;66[Suppl 1]:349a.
35. Fernlund P, Stenflo J. Amino acid sequence of the light chain of bovine protein C. *J Biol Chem* 1982;257:12170–12179.
36. Stenflo J, Fernlund P. Amino acid sequence of the heavy chain of bovine protein C. *J Biol Chem* 1982;257:12180–12190.
37. Foster D, Davie EW. Characterization of a cDNA coding for human protein C. *Proc Natl Acad Sci U S A* 1984;81:4766–4770.
38. Beckmann RJ, Schmidt RJ, Santerre RF, et al. The structure and evolution of a 461 amino acid human protein C precursor and its messenger RNA, based upon the DNA sequence of cloned human liver cDNAs. *Nucleic Acids Res* 1985;13:5233–5247.
39. Miletich DP, Leykam JF, Broze G Jr. Detection of single chain protein C in human plasma [abstract]. *Blood* 1983;62[Suppl 1]:306a.
40. Kisiel W. Human plasma protein C: isolation, characterization, and mechanism of activation by alpha-thrombin. *J Clin Invest* 1979;64:761–769.
41. Drakenberg T, Fernlund P, Roepstorff P, et al. beta-Hydroxyaspartic acid in vitamin K-dependent protein C. *Proc Natl Acad Sci U S A* 1983;80:1802–1806.
42. Suzuki K, Nishioka J, Hashimoto S. Protein C inhibitor. Purification from human plasma and characterization. *J Biol Chem* 1983;258:163–168.
43. Suzuki K, Deyashiki Y, Nishioka J, et al. Characterization of a cDNA for human protein C inhibitor. A new member of the plasma serine protease inhibitor superfamily. *J Biol Chem* 1987;262:611–616.
44. Heeb MJ, Griffin JH. Physiologic inhibition of human activated protein C by alpha 1-antitrypsin. *J Biol Chem* 1988;263:11613–11616.
45. Heeb MJ, Espana F, Griffin JH. Inhibition and complexation of activated protein C by two major inhibitors in plasma. *Blood* 1989;73:446–454.
46. Heeb MJ, Mosher D, Griffin JH. Activation and complexation of protein C and cleavage and decrease of protein S in plasma of patients with intravascular coagulation. *Blood* 1989;73:455–461.
47. Hoogendoorn H, Nesheim ME, Giles AR. A qualitative and quantitative analysis of the activation and inactivation of protein C in vivo in a primate model. *Blood* 1990;75:2164–2171.
48. Varadi K, Philapitsch A, Santa T, et al. Activation and inactivation of human protein C by plasmin. *Thromb Haemost* 1994;71:615–621.
49. Haley PE, Doyle MF, Mann KG. The activation of bovine protein C by factor Xa. *J Biol Chem* 1989;264:16303–16310.
50. Xu J, Esmon NL, Esmon CT. Reconstitution of the human endothelial cell protein C receptor with thrombomodulin in phosphatidylcholine vesicles enhances protein C activation. *J Biol Chem* 1999;274:6704–6710.
51. Stearns-Kurosawa DJ, Kurosawa S, Mollica JS, et al. The endothelial cell protein C receptor augments protein C activation by the thrombin-thrombomodulin complex. *Proc Natl Acad Sci U S A* 1996;93:10212–10216.
52. Esmon CT, Owen WG. Identification of an endothelial cell cofactor for thrombin-catalyzed activation of protein C. *Proc Natl Acad Sci U S A* 1981;78:2249–2252.
53. Owen WG, Esmon CT. Functional properties of an endothelial cell cofactor for thrombin-catalyzed activation of protein C. *J Biol Chem* 1981;256:5532–5535.
54. Jackman RW, Beeler DL, Fritze L, et al. Human thrombomodulin gene is intron depleted: nucleic acid sequences of the cDNA and gene predict protein structure and suggest sites of regulatory control. *Proc Natl Acad Sci U S A* 1987;84:6425–6429.
55. Jackman RW, Beeler DL, VanDeWater L, et al. Characterization of a thrombomodulin cDNA reveals structural similarity to the low density lipoprotein receptor. *Proc Natl Acad Sci U S A* 1986;83:8834–8838.
56. Suzuki K, Kusumoto H, Deyashiki Y, et al. Structure and expression of human thrombomodulin, a thrombin receptor on endothelium acting as a cofactor for protein C activation. *EMBO J* 1987;6:1891–1897.
57. Wen DZ, Dittman WA, Ye RD, et al. Human thrombomodulin: complete cDNA sequence and chromosome localization of the gene. *Biochemistry* 1987;26:4350–4357.
58. Esmon NL, Owen WG, Esmon CT. Isolation of a membrane-bound cofactor for thrombin-catalyzed activation of protein C. *J Biol Chem* 1982;257:859–864.
59. Le Bonniec BF, Guinto ER, MacGillivray RT, et al. The role of thrombin's Tyr-Pro-Pro-Trp motif in the interaction with fibrinogen, thrombomodulin, protein C, antithrombin III, and the Kunitz inhibitors. *J Biol Chem* 1993;268:19055–19061.
60. Stearns DJ, Kurosawa S, Esmon CT. Microthrombomodulin. Residues 310–486 from the epidermal growth factor precursor homology domain of thrombomodulin will accelerate protein C activation. *J Biol Chem* 1989;264:3352–3356.

61. Parkinson JF, Nagashima M, Kuhn I, et al. Structure-function studies of the epidermal growth factor domains of human thrombomodulin. *Biochem Biophys Res Commun* 1992;185:567–576.

62. Molinari A, Giorgetti C, Lansen J, et al. Thrombomodulin is a cofactor for thrombin degradation of recombinant single-chain urokinase plasminogen activator "in vitro" and in a perfused rabbit heart model. *Thromb Haemost* 1992;67:226–232.

63. Bajzar L, Manuel R, Nesheim ME. Purification and characterization of TAFI, a thrombin-activable fibrinolysis inhibitor. *J Biol Chem* 1995;270:14477–14484.

64. Wang W, Boffa MB, Bajzar L, et al. A study of the mechanism of inhibition of fibrinolysis by activated thrombin-activable fibrinolysis inhibitor. *J Biol Chem* 1998;273:27176–27181.

65. Mosnier LO, Meijers JC, Bouma BN. Regulation of fibrinolysis in plasma by TAFI and protein C is dependent on the concentration of thrombomodulin. *Thromb Haemost* 2001;85:5–11.

66. Fukudome K, Kurosawa S, Stearns-Kurosawa DJ, et al. The endothelial cell protein C receptor. Cell surface expression and direct ligand binding by the soluble receptor. *J Biol Chem* 1996;271:17491–17498.

67. Laszik Z, Mitro A, Taylor FB Jr, et al. Human protein C receptor is present primarily on endothelium of large blood vessels: implications for the control of the protein C pathway. *Circulation* 1997;96:3633–3640.

68. Fukudome K, Esmon CT. Identification, cloning, and regulation of a novel endothelial cell protein C/activated protein C receptor. *J Biol Chem* 1994;269:26486–26491.

69. Regan LM, Stearns-Kurosawa DJ, Kurosawa S, et al. The endothelial cell protein C receptor. Inhibition of activated protein C anticoagulant function without modulation of reaction with proteinase inhibitors. *J Biol Chem* 1996;271:17499–17503.

70. Tsuneyoshi N, Fukudome K, Horiguchi S, et al. Expression and anticoagulant function of the endothelial cell protein C receptor (EPCR) in cancer cell lines. *Thromb Haemost* 2001;85:356–361.

71. Taylor FB Jr, Peer GT, Lockhart MS, et al. Endothelial cell protein C receptor plays an important role in protein C activation in vivo. *Blood* 2001;97:1685–1688.

72. Walker FJ, Sexton PW, Esmon CT. The inhibition of blood coagulation by activated protein C through the selective inactivation of activated factor V. *Biochim Biophys Acta* 1979;571:333–342.

73. Vehar GA, Davie EW. Preparation and properties of bovine factor VIII (antihemophilic factor). *Biochemistry* 1980;19:401–410.

74. Marlar RA, Kleiss AJ, Griffin JH. Mechanism of action of human activated protein C, a thrombin-dependent anticoagulant enzyme. *Blood* 1982;59:1067–1072.

75. Egan JO, Kalafatis M, Mann KG. The effect of Arg306→Ala and Arg506→Gln substitutions in the inactivation of recombinant human factor Va by activated protein C and protein S. *Protein Sci* 1997;6:2016–2027.

76. Kalafatis M, Rand MD, Mann KG. The mechanism of inactivation of human factor V and human factor Va by activated protein C. *J Biol Chem* 1994;269:31869–31880.

77. Dahlback B, Stenflo J. Inhibitory effect of activated protein C on activation of prothrombin by platelet-bound factor Xa. *Eur J Biochem* 1980;107:331–335.

78. Heeb MJ, Rehemtulla A, Moussalli M, et al. Importance of individual activated protein C cleavage site regions in coagulation factor V for factor Va inactivation and for factor Xa activation. *Eur J Biochem* 1999;260:64–75.

79. Gale AJ, Heeb MJ, Griffin JH. The autolysis loop of activated protein C interacts with factor Va and differentiates between the Arg506 and Arg306 cleavage sites. *Blood* 2000;96:585–593.

80. Nesheim ME, Canfield WM, Kisiel W, et al. Studies of the capacity of factor Xa to protect factor Va from inactivation by activated protein C. *J Biol Chem* 1982;257:1443–1447.

81. Kisiel W, Canfield WM, Ericsson LH, et al. Anticoagulant properties of bovine plasma protein C following activation by thrombin. *Biochemistry* 1977;16:5824–5831.

82. Fulcher CA, Gardiner JE, Griffin JH, et al. Proteolytic inactivation of human factor VIII procoagulant protein by activated human protein C and its analogy with factor V. *Blood* 1984;63:486–489.

83. Eaton D, Rodriguez H, Vehar GA. Proteolytic processing of human factor VIII. Correlation of specific cleavages by thrombin, factor Xa, and activated protein C with activation and inactivation of factor VIII coagulant activity. *Biochemistry* 1986;25:505–512.

84. DiScipio RG, Davie EW. Characterization of protein S, a gamma-carboxyglutamic acid containing protein from bovine and human plasma. *Biochemistry* 1979;18:899–904.

85. Di Scipio RG, Hermodson MA, Yates SG, et al. A comparison of human prothrombin, factor IX (Christmas factor), factor X (Stuart factor), and protein S. *Biochemistry* 1977;16:698–706.

86. Lundwall A, Dackowski W, Cohen E, et al. Isolation and sequence of the cDNA for human protein S, a regulator of blood coagulation. *Proc Natl Acad Sci U S A* 1986;83:6716–6720.

87. Hoskins J, Norman DK, Beckmann RJ, et al. Cloning and characterization of human liver cDNA encoding a protein S precursor. *Proc Natl Acad Sci U S A* 1987;84:349–353.

88. Fernlund P, Stenflo J. Beta-hydroxyaspartic acid in vitamin K-dependent proteins. *J Biol Chem* 1983;258:12509–12512.

89. Baker ME, French FS, Joseph DR. Vitamin K-dependent protein S is similar to rat androgen-binding protein. *Biochem J* 1987;243:293–296.

90. Dahlback B, Stenflo J. High molecular weight complex in human plasma between vitamin K-dependent protein S and complement component C4b-binding protein. *Proc Natl Acad Sci U S A* 1981;78:2512–2516.

91. Dahlback B. Purification of human vitamin K-dependent protein S and its limited proteolysis by thrombin. *Biochem J* 1983;209:837–846.

92. Dahlback B. Purification of human C4b-binding protein and formation of its complex with vitamin K-dependent protein S. *Biochem J* 1983;209:847–856.

93. Comp PC, Nixon RR, Cooper MR, et al. Familial protein S deficiency is associated with recurrent thrombosis. *J Clin Invest* 1984;74:2082–2088.

94. Walker FJ. Regulation of activated protein C by a new protein. A possible function for bovine protein S. *J Biol Chem* 1980;255:5521–5524.

95. Walker FJ. Regulation of activated protein C by protein S. The role of phospholipid in factor Va inactivation. *J Biol Chem* 1981;256:11128–11131.

96. Walker FJ. Regulation of bovine activated protein C by protein S: the role of the cofactor protein in species specificity. *Thromb Res* 1981;22:321–327.

97. Walker FJ, Chavin SI, Fay PJ. Inactivation of factor VIII by activated protein C and protein S. *Arch Biochem Biophys* 1987;252:322–328.

98. Rosing J, Hoekema L, Nicolaes GA, et al. Effects of protein S and factor Xa on peptide bond cleavages during inactivation of factor Va and factor VaR506Q by activated protein C. *J Biol Chem* 1995;270:27852–27858.

99. Heeb MJ, Mesters RM, Tans G, et al. Binding of protein S to factor Va associated with inhibition of prothrombinase that is independent of activated protein C. *J Biol Chem* 1993;268:2872–2877.

100. Heeb MJ, Kojima Y, Rosing J, et al. C-terminal residues 621–635 of protein S are essential for binding to factor Va. *J Biol Chem* 1999;274:36187–36192.

101. Koppelman SJ, Hackeng TM, Sixma JJ, et al. Inhibition of the intrinsic factor X activating complex by protein S: evidence for a specific binding of protein S to factor VIII. *Blood* 1995;86:1062–1071.

102. Heeb MJ, Rosing J, Bakker HM, et al. Protein S binds to and inhibits factor Xa. *Proc Natl Acad Sci U S A* 1994;91:2728–2732.

103. Stitt TN, Conn G, Gore M, et al. The anticoagulation factor protein S and its relative, Gas6, are ligands for the Tyro 3/Axl family of receptor tyrosine kinases. *Cell* 1995;80:661–670.

104. Evenas P, Dahlback B, Garcia de Frutos P. The first laminin G-type domain in the SHBG-like region of protein S contains residues essential for activation of the receptor tyrosine kinase sky. *Biol Chem* 2000;381:199–209.

105. Dougherty CS, Lowe-Krentz LJ. Heparin increases protein S levels in cultured endothelial cells by causing a block in degradation. *J Vasc Res* 1998;35:437–448.

106. Petaja J, Fernandez JA, Gruber A, et al. Anticoagulant synergism of heparin and activated protein C in vitro. Role of a novel anticoagulant mechanism of heparin, enhancement of inactivation of factor V by activated protein C. *J Clin Invest* 1997;99:2655–2663.

107. Pratt CW, Church FC. Heparin binding to protein C inhibitor. *J Biol Chem* 1992;267:8789–8794.

108. Elisen MG, von dem Borne PA, Bouma BN, et al. Protein C inhibitor acts as a procoagulant by inhibiting the thrombomodulin-induced activation of protein C in human plasma. *Blood* 1998;91:1542–1547.

109. Fourrier F, Chopin C, Goudemand J, et al. Septic shock, multiple organ failure, and disseminated intravascular coagulation. Compared patterns of antithrombin III, protein C, and protein S deficiencies. *Chest* 1992;101:816–823.

110. Vervloet MG, Thijs LG, Hack CE. Derangements of coagulation and fibrinolysis in critically ill patients with sepsis and septic shock. *Semin Thromb Hemost* 1998;24:33–44.

111. Smith OP, White B, Vaughan D, et al. Use of protein-C concentrate, heparin, and haemodiafiltration in meningococcus-induced purpura fulminans. *Lancet* 1997;350:1590–1593.

112. Taylor FB Jr, Chang A, Esmon CT, et al. Protein C prevents the coagulopathic and lethal effects of *Escherichia coli* infusion in the baboon. *J Clin Invest* 1987;79:918–925.

113. Taylor F, Chang A, Ferrell G, et al. C4b-binding protein exacerbates the host response to *Escherichia coli. Blood* 1991;78:357–363.

114. Taylor FB Jr, Stearns-Kurosawa DJ, Kurosawa S, et al. The endothelial cell protein C receptor aids in host defense against *Escherichia coli* sepsis. *Blood* 2000;95:1680–1686.

115. Murakami K, Okajima K, Uchiba M, et al. Activated protein C prevents LPS-induced pulmonary vascular injury by inhibiting cytokine production. *Am J Physiol* 1997;272:L197–202.

116. Hooper WC, Phillips DJ, Renshaw MA, et al. The up-regulation of IL-6 and IL-8 in human endothelial cells by activated protein C. *J Immunol* 1998;161:2567–2573.

117. Taylor FB Jr. Studies on the inflammatory-coagulant axis in the baboon response to *E. coli*: regulatory roles of proteins C, S, C4bBP and of inhibitors of tissue factor. *Prog Clin Biol Res* 1994;388:175–194.

118. Bernard GR, Vincent JL, Laterre PF, et al. Efficacy and safety of recombinant human activated protein C for severe sepsis. *N Engl J Med* 2001;344:699–709.

119. Grey ST, Tsuchida A, Hau H, et al. Selective inhibitory effects of the anticoagulant activated protein C on the responses of human mononuclear phagocytes to LPS, IFN-gamma, or phorbol ester. *J Immunol* 1994;153:3664–3672.

120. Egeberg O. Inherited antithrombin deficiency causing thrombophilia. *Thromb Diath Haemorrh* 1965;13:516.

121. Gruenberg JC, Smallridge RC, Rosenberg RD. Inherited antithrombin-III deficiency causing mesenteric venous infarction: a new clinical entity. *Ann Surg* 1975;181:791–794.

122. Odegard OR, Abildgaard U. Antifactor Xa activity in thrombophilia. Studies in a family with Ar-III deficiency. *Scand J Haematol* 1977;18:86–90.

123. Mackie M, Bennett B, Ogston D, et al. Familial thrombosis: inherited deficiency of antithrombin III. *BMJ* 1978;1:136–138.

124. Marciniak E, Farley CH, DeSimone PA. Familial thrombosis due to antithrombin 3 deficiency. *Blood* 1974;43:219–231.

125. Boyer C, Wolf M, Lavergne JM, et al. Thrombin generation and formation of thrombin-antithrombin III complexes in congenital antithrombin III deficiency. *Thromb Res* 1980;20:207–218.
126. van der Meer J, Stoepman-van Dalen EA, Jansen JM. Antithrombin-3 deficiency in a Dutch family. *J Clin Pathol* 1973;26:532–538.
127. Filip DJ, Eckstein JD, Veltkamp JJ. Hereditary antithrombin III deficiency and thromboembolic disease. *Am J Hematol* 1976;1:343–349.
128. Carvalho A, Ellman L. Hereditary antithrombin III deficiency. Effect of antithrombin III deficiency on platelet function. *Am J Med* 1976;61:179–183.
129. Johansson L, Hedner U, Nilsson IM. Familial antithrombin III deficiency as pathogenesis of deep venous thrombosis. *Acta Med Scand* 1978;204:491–495.
130. Gyde OH, Middleton MD, Vaughan GR, et al. Antithrombin III deficiency, hypertriglyceridaemia, and venous thromboses. *BMJ* 1978;1:621–622.
131. Matsuo T, Ohki Y, Kondo S, et al. Familial antithrombin III deficiency in a Japanese family. *Thromb Res* 1979;16:815–823.
132. Pitney WR, Manoharan A, Dean S. Antithrombin III deficiency in an Australian family. *Br J Haematol* 1980;46:147–149.
133. Beukes CA, Heyns AD. A South African family with antithrombin III deficiency. *S Afr Med J* 1980;58:528–530.
134. Ambruso DR, Jacobson LJ, Hathaway WE. Inherited antithrombin III deficiency and cerebral thrombosis in a child. *Pediatrics* 1980;65:125–131.
135. Scully MF, De Haas H, Chan P, et al. Hereditary antithrombin III deficiency in an English family. *Br J Haematol* 1981;47:235–240.
136. Rosenberg RD. Actions and interactions of antithrombin and heparin. *N Engl J Med* 1975;292:146–151.
137. Odegard OR, Abildgaard U. Antithrombin III: critical review of assay methods. Significance of variations in health and disease. *Haemostasis* 1978;7:127–134.
138. Tait RC, Walker ID, Perry DJ, et al. Prevalence of antithrombin deficiency in the healthy population. *Br J Haematol* 1994;87:106–112.
139. Demers C, Ginsberg JS, Hirsh J, et al. Thrombosis in antithrombin-III-deficient persons. Report of a large kindred and literature review. *Ann Intern Med* 1992;116:754–761.
140. Martinelli I, Mannucci PM, De Stefano V, et al. Different risks of thrombosis in four coagulation defects associated with inherited thrombophilia: a study of 150 families. *Blood* 1998;92:2353–2358.
141. Simioni P, Sanson BJ, Prandoni P, et al. Incidence of venous thromboembolism in families with inherited thrombophilia. *Thromb Haemost* 1999;81:198–202.
142. van der Meer FJ, Koster T, Vandenbroucke JP, et al. The Leiden Thrombophilia Study (LETS). *Thromb Haemost* 1997;78:631–635.
143. Koster T, Rosendaal FR, Briet E, et al. Protein C deficiency in a controlled series of unselected outpatients: an infrequent but clear risk factor for venous thrombosis (Leiden Thrombophilia Study). *Blood* 1995;85:2756–2761.
144. Fitches AC, Appleby R, Lane DA, et al. Impaired cotranslational processing as a mechanism for type I antithrombin deficiency. *Blood* 1998;92:4671–4676.
145. Ambruso DR, Leonard BD, Bies RD, et al. Antithrombin III deficiency: decreased synthesis of a biochemically normal molecule. *Blood* 1982;60:78–83.
146. Lane DA, Bayston T, Olds RJ, et al. Antithrombin mutation database: 2nd (1997) update. For the Plasma Coagulation Inhibitors Subcommittee of the Scientific and Standardization Committee of the International Society on Thrombosis and Haemostasis. *Thromb Haemost* 1997;77:197–211.
147. Sas G, Blasko G, Banhegyi D, et al. Abnormal antithrombin III (antithrombin III "Budapest") as a cause of a familial thrombophilia. *Thromb Diath Haemorrh* 1974;32:105–115.
148. Sakuragawa N, Kondo S, Katoh M, et al. Antithrombin III microheterogeneity in antithrombin III deficiency and in the antithrombin III abnormality, "antithrombin III Toyama." *Thromb Res* 1987;47:147–153.
149. Koide T, Odani S, Takahashi K, et al. Antithrombin III Toyama: replacement of arginine-47 by cysteine in hereditary abnormal antithrombin III that lacks heparin-binding ability. *Proc Natl Acad Sci U S A* 1984;81:289–293.
150. Koide T, Takahashi K, Odani S, et al. Isolation and characterization of a hereditary abnormal antithrombin III "Antithrombin III Toyama." *Thromb Res* 1983;31:319–328.
151. Duchange N, Chasse JF, Cohen GN, et al. Molecular characterization of the antithrombin III tours deficiency. *Thromb Res* 1987;45:115–121.
152. Fischer AM, Cornu P, Sternberg C, et al. Antithrombin III Alger: a new homozygous AT III variant. *Thromb Haemost* 1986;55:218–221.
153. Brunel F, Duchange N, Fischer AM, et al. Antithrombin III Alger: a new case of Arg 47→Cys mutation. *Am J Hematol* 1987;25:223–224.
154. Wolf M, Boyer C, Lavergne JM, et al. A new familial variant of antithrombin III: "antithrombin III Paris." *Br J Haematol* 1982;51:285–295.
155. Wolf M, Boyer-Neumann C, Molho-Sabatier P, et al. Familial variant of antithrombin III (AT III Bligny, 47Arg to His) associated with protein C deficiency. *Thromb Haemost* 1990;63:215–219.
156. Molho-Sabatier P, Aiach M, Gaillard I, et al. Molecular characterization of antithrombin III (ATIII) variants using polymerase chain reaction. Identification of the ATIII Charleville as an Ala 384 Pro mutation. *J Clin Invest* 1989;84:1236–1242.
157. Okajima K, Abe H, Maeda S, et al. Antithrombin III Nagasaki (Ser116-Pro): a heterozygous variant with defective heparin binding associated with thrombosis. *Blood* 1993;81:1300–1305.
158. Okajima K, Ueyama H, Hashimoto Y, et al. Homozygous variant of antithrombin III that lacks affinity for heparin, AT III Kumamoto. *Thromb Haemost* 1989;61:20–24.
159. Chowdhury V, Mille B, Olds RJ, et al. Antithrombins Southport (Leu 99 to Val) and Vienna (Gln 118 to Pro): two novel antithrombin variants with abnormal heparin binding. *Br J Haematol* 1995;89:602–609.
160. Ueyama H, Murakami T, Nishiguchi S, et al. Antithrombin III Kumamoto: identification of a point mutation and genotype analysis of the family. *Thromb Haemost* 1990;63:231–234.
161. Girolami A, Fabris F, Cappellato G, et al. Antithrombin III (AT III) Padua2: a "new" congenital abnormality with defective heparin co-factor activities but no thrombotic disease. *Blut* 1983;47:93–103.
162. Caso R, Lane DA, Thompson E, et al. Antithrombin Padua. I: Impaired heparin binding caused by an Arg47 to his (CGT to CAT) substitution. *Thromb Res* 1990;58:185–190.
163. Borg JY, Brennan SO, Carrell RW, et al. Antithrombin Rouen-IV 24 Arg→Cys. The amino-terminal contribution to heparin binding. *FEBS Lett* 1990;266:163–166.
164. de Moerloose PA, Reber G, Vernet P, et al. Antithrombin III Geneva: a hereditary abnormal AT III with defective heparin cofactor activity. *Thromb Haemost* 1987;57:154–157.
165. Gandrille S, Aiach M, Lane DA, et al. Important role of arginine 129 in heparin-binding site of antithrombin III. Identification of a novel mutation arginine 129 to glutamine. *J Biol Chem* 1990;265:18997–19001.
166. Tran TH, Bondeli C, Marbet GA, et al. Reactivity of a hereditary abnormal antithrombin III fraction in the inhibition of thrombin and factor Xa. *Thromb Haemost* 1980;44:92–95.
167. Aiach M, Francois D, Priollet P, et al. An abnormal antithrombin III (AT III) with low heparin affinity: AT III Clichy. *Br J Haematol* 1987;66:515–522.
168. Daly M, Ball R, O'Meara A, et al. Identification and characterisation of an antithrombin III mutant (AT Dublin 2) with marginally decreased heparin reactivity. *Thromb Res* 1989;56:503–513.
169. de Roux N, Chadeuf G, Molho-Sabatier P, et al. Clinical and biochemical characterization of antithrombin III Franconville, a variant with Pro 41 Leu mutation. *Br J Haematol* 1990;75:222–227.
170. Olds RJ, Lane DA, Boisclair M, et al. Antithrombin Budapest 3. An antithrombin variant with reduced heparin affinity resulting from the substitution L99F. *FEBS Lett* 1992;300:241–246.
171. Olds RJ, Lane DA, Caso R, et al. Antithrombin III Padua 2: a single base substitution in exon 2 detected with PCR and direct genomic sequencing. *Nucleic Acids Res* 1990;18:1926.
172. Brennan SO, Borg JY, George PM, et al. New carbohydrate site in mutant antithrombin (7 Ile→Asn) with decreased heparin affinity. *FEBS Lett* 1988;237:118–122.
173. Sambrano JE, Jacobson LJ, Reeve EB, et al. Abnormal antithrombin III with defective serine protease binding (antithrombin III "Denver"). *J Clin Invest* 1986;77:887–893.
174. Stephens AW, Thalley BS, Hirs CH. Antithrombin-III Denver, a reactive site variant. *J Biol Chem* 1987;262:1044–1048.
175. Olds RJ, Lane D, Caso R, et al. Antithrombin III Milano 2: a single base substitution in the thrombin binding domain detected with PCR and direct genomic sequencing. *Nucleic Acids Res* 1989;17:10511.
176. Devraj-Kizuk R, Chui DH, Prochownik EV, et al. Antithrombin-III-Hamilton: a gene with a point mutation (guanine to adenine) in codon 382 causing impaired serine protease reactivity. *Blood* 1988;72:1518–1523.
177. Perry DJ, Harper PL, Fairham S, et al. Antithrombin Cambridge, 384 Ala to Pro: a new variant identified using the polymerase chain reaction. *FEBS Lett* 1989;254:174–176.
178. Howarth DJ, Samson D, Stirling Y, et al. Antithrombin III "Northwick Park": a variant antithrombin with normal affinity for heparin but reduced heparin cofactor activity. *Thromb Haemost* 1985;53:314–319.
179. Lane DA, Flynn A, Ireland H, et al. Antithrombin III Northwick Park: demonstration of an inactive high MW complex with increased affinity for heparin. *Br J Haematol* 1987;65:451–456.
180. Wolf M, Boyer-Neumann C, Meyer D, et al. Purification and further characterization of antithrombin III Milano: lack of reactivity with thrombin. *Thromb Haemost* 1987;58:888–892.
181. Erdjument H, Lane DA, Ireland H, et al. Antithrombin Milano, single amino acid substitution at the reactive site, Arg393 to Cys. *Thromb Haemost* 1988;60:471–475.
182. Erdjument H, Lane DA, Panico M, et al. Single amino acid substitutions in the reactive site of antithrombin leading to thrombosis. Congenital substitution of arginine 393 to cysteine in antithrombin Northwick Park and to histidine in antithrombin Glasgow. *J Biol Chem* 1988;263:5589–5593.
183. Owen MC, George PM, Lane DA, et al. P1 variant antithrombins Glasgow (393 Arg to His) and Pescara (393 Arg to Pro) have increased heparin affinity and are resistant to catalytic cleavage by elastase. Implications for the heparin activation mechanism. *FEBS Lett* 1991;280:216–220.
184. Thein SL, Lane DA. Use of synthetic oligonucleotides in the characterization of antithrombin III Northwick Park (393 CGT→TGT) and antithrombin III Glasgow (393 CGT→CAT). *Blood* 1988;72:1817–1821.
185. Lane DA, Erdjument H, Flynn A, et al. Antithrombin Sheffield: amino acid substitution at the reactive site (Arg393 to His) causing thrombosis. *Br J Haematol* 1989;71:91–96.
186. Bauer KA, Ashenhurst JB, Chediak J, et al. Antithrombin "Chicago": a functionally abnormal molecule with increased heparin affinity causing familial thrombophilia. *Blood* 1983;62:1242–1250.
187. Erdjument H, Lane DA, Panico M, et al. Antithrombin Chicago, amino acid substitution of arginine 393 to histidine. *Thromb Res* 1989;54:613–619.

188. Leone G, De Stefano V, Di Donfrancesco A, et al. Antithrombin III Pescara: a defective AT III variant with no alterations of plasma crossed immunoelectrophoresis, but with an abnormal crossed immunoelectrofocusing pattern. *Br J Haematol* 1987;65:187–191.

189. Lane DA, Erdjument H, Thompson E, et al. A novel amino acid substitution in the reactive site of a congenital variant antithrombin. Antithrombin pescara, ARG393 to pro, caused by a CGT to CCT mutation. *J Biol Chem* 1989;264:10200–10204.

190. Aiach M, Nora M, Fiessinger JN, et al. A functional abnormal antithrombin III (AT III) deficiency: AT III Charleville. *Thromb Res* 1985;39:559–570.

191. Barbui T, Rodeghiero F. Hereditary dysfunctional antithrombin III (AT-III Vicenza). *Thromb Haemost* 1981;45:97.

192. Barbui T, Finazzi G, Rodeghiero F, et al. Immunoelectrophoretic evidence of a thrombin-induced abnormality in a new variant of hereditary dysfunctional antithrombin III (AT III "Vicenza"). *Br J Haematol* 1983;54:561–565.

193. Finazzi G, Tran TH, Barbui T, et al. Purification of antithrombin "Vicenza": a molecule with normal heparin affinity and impaired reactivity to thrombin. *Br J Haematol* 1985;59:259–263.

194. Caso R, Lane DA, Thompson EA, et al. Antithrombin Vicenza, Ala 384 to Pro (GCA to CCA) mutation, transforming the inhibitor into a substrate. *Br J Haematol* 1991;77:87–92.

195. Blajchman MA, Fernandez-Rachubinski F, Sheffield WP, et al. Antithrombin-III-Stockholm: a codon 392 (Gly→Asp) mutation with normal heparin binding and impaired serine protease reactivity. *Blood* 1992;79:1428–1434.

196. Picard V, Bura A, Emmerich J, et al. Molecular bases of antithrombin deficiency in French families: identification of seven novel mutations in the antithrombin gene. *Br J Haematol* 2000;110:731–734.

197. Ireland H, Lane DA, Thompson E, et al. Antithrombin Glasgow II: alanine 382 to threonine mutation in the serpin P12 position, resulting in a substrate reaction with thrombin. *Br J Haematol* 1991;79:70–74.

198. Lane DA, Lowe GD, Flynn A, et al. Antithrombin III Glasgow: a variant with increased heparin affinity and reduced ability to inactivate thrombin, associated with familial thrombosis. *Br J Haematol* 1987;66:523–527.

199. Okajima K, Abe H, Wagatsuma M, et al. Antithrombin III Kumamoto II; a single mutation at Arg393-His increased the affinity of antithrombin III for heparin. *Am J Hematol* 1995;48:12–18.

200. Chasse JF, Esnard F, Guitton JD, et al. An abnormal plasma antithrombin with no apparent affinity for heparin. *Thromb Res* 1984;34:297–302.

201. Owen MC, Borg JY, Soria C, et al. Heparin binding defect in a new antithrombin III variant: Rouen, 47 Arg to His. *Blood* 1987;69:1275–1279.

202. Demers C, Henderson P, Blajchman MA, et al. An antithrombin III assay based on factor Xa inhibition provides a more reliable test to identify congenital antithrombin III deficiency than an assay based on thrombin inhibition. *Thromb Haemost* 1993;69:231–235.

203. Beeck H, Nagel D, Pindur G, et al. Measurement of antithrombin activity by thrombin-based and by factor Xa-based chromogenic substrate assays. *Blood Coagul Fibrinolysis* 2000;11:127–135.

204. Perry DJ, Daly ME, Tait RC, et al. Antithrombin Cambridge II (Ala384Ser): clinical, functional and haplotype analysis of 18 families. *Thromb Haemost* 1998;79:249–253.

205. Odegard OR, Lie M, Abildgaard U. Heparin cofactor activity measured with an amidolytic method. *Thromb Res* 1975;6:287–294.

206. Fagerhol MK, Abildgaard U. Immunological studies on human antithrombin 3. Influence of age, sex and use of oral contraceptives on serum concentration. *Scand J Haematol* 1970;7:10–17.

207. McDonald MM, Hathaway WE, Reeve EB, et al. Biochemical and functional study of antithrombin III in newborn infants. *Thromb Haemost* 1982;47:56–58.

208. Andrew M, Paes B, Milner R, et al. Development of the human coagulation system in the full-term infant. *Blood* 1987;70:165–172.

209. Andrew M, Paes B, Milner R, et al. Development of the human coagulation system in the healthy premature infant. *Blood* 1988;72:1651–1657.

210. de Boer AC, van Riel LA, den Ottolander GJ. Measurement of antithrombin III, alpha 2-macroglobulin and alpha 1-antitrypsin in patients with deep venous thrombosis and pulmonary embolism. *Thromb Res* 1979;15:17–25.

211. Bick RL, Bick MD, Fekete LF. Antithrombin III patterns in disseminated intravascular coagulation. *Am J Clin Pathol* 1980;73:577–583.

212. Von Kaulla E, Von Kaulla KN. Antithrombin 3 and diseases. *Am J Clin Pathol* 1967;48:69–80.

213. Kauffmann RH, Veltkamp JJ, Van Tilburg NH, et al. Acquired antithrombin III deficiency and thrombosis in the nephrotic syndrome. *Am J Med* 1978;65:607–613.

214. Panicucci F, Sagripanti A, Conte B, et al. Antithrombin III, heparin cofactor and antifactor Xa in relation to age, sex and pathological condition. *Haemostasis* 1980;9:297–302.

215. Weenink GH, Kahle LH, Lamping RJ, et al. Antithrombin III in oral contraceptive users and during normotensive pregnancy. *Acta Obstet Gynecol Scand* 1984;63:57–61.

216. Thaler E, Lechner K. Antithrombin III deficiency and thromboembolism. *Clin Haematol* 1981;10:369–390.

217. Weenink GH, Treffers PE, Vijn P, et al. Antithrombin III levels in preeclampsia correlate with maternal and fetal morbidity. *Am J Obstet Gynecol* 1984;148:1092–1097.

218. White B, Perry D. Acquired antithrombin deficiency in sepsis. *Br J Haematol* 2001;112:26–31.

219. Tanaka K, Takao M, Yada I, et al. Alterations in coagulation and fibrinolysis associated with cardiopulmonary bypass during open heart surgery. *J Cardiothorac Anesth* 1989;3:181–188.

220. Hashimoto K, Yamagishi M, Sasaki T, et al. Heparin and antithrombin III levels during cardiopulmonary bypass: correlation with subclinical plasma coagulation. *Ann Thorac Surg* 1994;58:799–804; discussion 804–805.

221. Lee JH, Lee KH, Kim S, et al. Relevance of proteins C and S, antithrombin III, von Willebrand factor, and factor VIII for the development of hepatic veno-occlusive disease in patients undergoing allogeneic bone marrow transplantation: a prospective study. *Bone Marrow Transplant* 1998;22:883–888.

222. Park YD, Yasui M, Yoshimoto T, et al. Changes in hemostatic parameters in hepatic veno-occlusive disease following bone marrow transplantation. *Bone Marrow Transplant* 1997;19:915–920.

223. Marciniak E, Gockerman JP. Heparin-induced decrease in circulating antithrombin-III. *Lancet* 1977;2:581–584.

224. Kitchens CS. Amelioration of antithrombin III deficiency by coumarin administration. *Am J Med Sci* 1987;293:403.

225. Schulman S, Tengborn L. Treatment of venous thromboembolism in patients with congenital deficiency of antithrombin III. *Thromb Haemost* 1992;68:634–636.

226. Hoffman DL. Purification and large-scale preparation of antithrombin III. *Am J Med* 1989;87:23S–26S.

227. Menache D, O'Malley JP, Schorr JB, et al. Evaluation of the safety, recovery, half-life, and clinical efficacy of antithrombin III (human) in patients with hereditary antithrombin III deficiency. Cooperative Study Group. *Blood* 1990;75:33–39.

228. Mannucci PM, Boyer C, Wolf M, et al. Treatment of congenital antithrombin III deficiency with concentrates. *Br J Haematol* 1982;50:531–535.

229. Schwartz RS, Bauer KA, Rosenberg RD, et al. Clinical experience with antithrombin III concentrate in treatment of congenital and acquired deficiency of antithrombin. The Antithrombin III Study Group. *Am J Med* 1989;87:53S–60S.

230. Baudo F, Caimi TM, de Cataldo F, et al. Antithrombin III (ATIII) replacement therapy in patients with sepsis and/or postsurgical complications: a controlled double-blind, randomized, multicenter study. *Intensive Care Med* 1998;24:336–342.

231. Eisele B, Lamy M, Thijs LG, et al. Antithrombin III in patients with severe sepsis. A randomized, placebo-controlled, double-blind multicenter trial plus a meta-analysis on all randomized, placebo-controlled, double-blind trials with antithrombin III in severe sepsis. *Intensive Care Med* 1998;24:663–672.

232. Haire WD, Ruby EI, Stephens LC, et al. A prospective randomized double-blind trial of antithrombin III concentrate in the treatment of multiple-organ dysfunction syndrome during hematopoietic stem cell transplantation. *Biol Blood Marrow Transplant* 1998;4:142–150.

233. Human albumin administration in critically ill patients: systematic review of randomised controlled trials. Cochrane Injuries Group Albumin Reviewers. *BMJ* 1998;317:235–240.

234. Williams MR, D'Ambra AB, Beck JR, et al. A randomized trial of antithrombin concentrate for treatment of heparin resistance. *Ann Thorac Surg* 2000;70:873–877.

235. Griffin JH, Evatt B, Zimmerman TS, et al. Deficiency of protein C in congenital thrombotic disease. *J Clin Invest* 1981;68:1370–1373.

236. Bertina RM, Broekmans AW, van der Linden IK, et al. Protein C deficiency in a Dutch family with thrombotic disease. *Thromb Haemost* 1982;48:1–5.

237. Horellou MH, Conard J, Bertina RM, et al. Congenital protein C deficiency and thrombotic disease in nine French families. *BMJ* 1984;289:1285–1287.

238. Pabinger-Fasching I, Bertina RM, Lechner K, et al. Protein C deficiency in two Austrian families. *Thromb Haemost* 1983;50:810–813.

239. Bovill EG, Bauer KA, Dickerman JD, et al. The clinical spectrum of heterozygous protein C deficiency in a large New England kindred. *Blood* 1989;73:712–717.

240. Gladson CL, Scharrer I, Hach V, et al. The frequency of type I heterozygous protein S and protein C deficiency in 141 unrelated young patients with venous thrombosis. *Thromb Haemost* 1988;59:18–22.

241. Ben-Tal O, Zivelin A, Seligsohn U. The relative frequency of hereditary thrombotic disorders among 107 patients with thrombophilia in Israel. *Thromb Haemost* 1989;61:50–54.

242. Miletich J, Sherman L, Broze G Jr. Absence of thrombosis in subjects with heterozygous protein C deficiency. *N Engl J Med* 1987;317:991–996.

243. Tait RC, Walker ID, Reitsma PH, et al. Prevalence of protein C deficiency in the healthy population. *Thromb Haemost* 1995;73:87–93.

244. Bucciarelli P, Rosendaal FR, Tripodi A, et al. Risk of venous thromboembolism and clinical manifestations in carriers of antithrombin, protein C, protein S deficiency, or activated protein C resistance: a multicenter collaborative family study. *Arterioscler Thromb Vasc Biol* 1999;19:1026–1033.

245. Sanson BJ, Simioni P, Tormene D, et al. The incidence of venous thromboembolism in asymptomatic carriers of a deficiency of antithrombin, protein C, or protein S: a prospective cohort study. *Blood* 1999;94:3702–3706.

246. Heijboer H, Brandjes DP, Buller HR, et al. Deficiencies of coagulation-inhibiting and fibrinolytic proteins in outpatients with deep-vein thrombosis. *N Engl J Med* 1990;323:1512–1516.

247. Mateo J, Oliver A, Borrell M, et al. Laboratory evaluation and clinical characteristics of 2,132 consecutive unselected patients with venous thromboembolism—results of the Spanish Multicentric Study on Thrombophilia (EMET-Study). *Thromb Haemost* 1997;77:444–451.

248. Bertina RM, Broekmans AW, Krommenhoek-van Es C, et al. The use of a functional and immunologic assay for plasma protein C in the study of the heterogeneity of congenital protein C deficiency. *Thromb Haemost* 1984;51:1–5.

249. Comp PC, Nixon RR, Esmon CT. Determination of functional levels of protein C, an antithrombotic protein, using thrombin-thrombomodulin complex. *Blood* 1984;63:15–21.

250. Barbui T, Finazzi G, Mussoni L, et al. Hereditary dysfunctional protein C (protein C Bergamo) and thrombosis. *Lancet* 1984;2:819.

251. Sala N, Borrell M, Bauer KA, et al. Dysfunctional activated protein C (PC Cadiz) in a patient with thrombotic disease. *Thromb Haemost* 1987;57:183–186.

252. Tirindelli MC, Franchi F, Tripodi A, et al. Familial dysfunctional protein C. *Thromb Res* 1986;44:893–897.

253. Faioni EM, Esmon CT, Esmon NL, et al. Isolation of an abnormal protein C molecule from the plasma of a patient with thrombotic diathesis. *Blood* 1988;71:940–946.

254. Vasse M, Borg JY, Monconduit M. Protein C: Rouen, a new hereditary protein C abnormality with low anticoagulant but normal amidolytic activities. *Thromb Res* 1989;56:387–398.

255. Reitsma PH, Bernardi F, Doig RG, et al. Protein C deficiency: a database of mutations, 1995 update. On behalf of the Subcommittee on Plasma Coagulation Inhibitors of the Scientific and Standardization Committee of the ISTH. *Thromb Haemost* 1995;73:876–889.

256. Reitsma PH. Protein C deficiency: from gene defects to disease. *Thromb Haemost* 1997;78:344–350.

257. Branson HE, Katz J, Marble R, et al. Inherited protein C deficiency and coumarin-responsive chronic relapsing purpura fulminans in a newborn infant. *Lancet* 1983;2:1165–1168.

258. Seligsohn U, Berger A, Abend M, et al. Homozygous protein C deficiency manifested by massive venous thrombosis in the newborn. *N Engl J Med* 1984;310:559–562.

259. Sills RH, Marlar RA, Montgomery RR, et al. Severe homozygous protein C deficiency. *J Pediatr* 1984;105:409–413.

260. Marciniak E, Wilson HD, Marlar RA. Neonatal purpura fulminans: a genetic disorder related to the absence of protein C in blood. *Blood* 1985;65:15–20.

261. Peters C, Casella JF, Marlar RA, et al. Homozygous protein C deficiency: observations on the nature of the molecular abnormality and the effectiveness of warfarin therapy. *Pediatrics* 1988;81:272–276.

262. Soria JM, Brito D, Barcelo J, et al. Severe homozygous protein C deficiency: identification of a splice site missense mutation (184, Q→H) in exon 7 of the protein C gene. *Thromb Haemost* 1994;72:65–69.

263. Tarras S, Gadia C, Meister L, et al. Homozygous protein C deficiency in a newborn. Clinicopathologic correlation. *Arch Neurol* 1988;45:214–216.

264. Auletta MJ, Headington JT. Purpura fulminans. A cutaneous manifestation of severe protein C deficiency. *Arch Dermatol* 1988;124:1387–1391.

265. Manabe S, Matsuda M. Homozygous protein C deficiency combined with heterozygous dysplasminogenemia found in a 21-year-old thrombophilic male. *Thromb Res* 1985;39:333–341.

266. Sharon C, Tirindelli MC, Mannucci PM, et al. Homozygous protein C deficiency with moderately severe clinical symptoms. *Thromb Res* 1986;41:483–488.

267. Bauer KA, Broekmans AW, Bertina RM, et al. Hemostatic enzyme generation in the blood of patients with hereditary protein C deficiency. *Blood* 1988;71:1418–1426.

268. Gruppo RA, Leimer P, Francis RB, et al. Protein C deficiency resulting from possible double heterozygosity and its response to danazol. *Blood* 1988;71:370–374.

269. Matsuda M, Sugo T, Sakata Y, et al. A thrombotic state due to an abnormal protein C. *N Engl J Med* 1988;319:1265–1268.

270. Soria J, Soria C, Samama M, et al. Severe protein C deficiency in congenital thrombotic disease—description of an immunoenzymological assay for protein C determination. *Thromb Haemost* 1985;53:293–296.

271. Boyer C, Rothschild C, Wolf M, et al. A new method for the estimation of protein C by ELISA. *Thromb Res* 1984;36:579–589.

272. Bauer KA, Kass BL, Beeler DL, et al. Detection of protein C activation in humans. *J Clin Invest* 1984;74:2033–2041.

273. Epstein DJ, Bergum PW, Bajaj SP, et al. Radioimmunoassays for protein C and factor X. Plasma antigen levels in abnormal hemostatic states. *Am J Clin Pathol* 1984;82:573–581.

274. Francis RB Jr, Patch MJ. A functional assay for protein C in human plasma. *Thromb Res* 1983;32:605–613.

275. Sala N, Owen WG, Collen D. A functional assay of protein C in human plasma. *Blood* 1984;63:671–675.

276. Martinoli JL, Stocker K. Fast functional protein C assay using Protac, a novel protein C activator. *Thromb Res* 1986;43:253–264.

277. Francis RB Jr, Seyfert U. Rapid amidolytic assay of protein C in whole plasma using an activator from the venom of *Agkistrodon contortrix*. *Am J Clin Pathol* 1987;87:619–625.

278. Walker PA, Bauer KA, McDonagh J. A simple, automated functional assay for protein C. *Am J Clin Pathol* 1989;92:210–213.

279. Vigano D'Angelo S, Comp PC, Esmon CT, et al. Relationship between protein C antigen and anticoagulant activity during oral anticoagulation and in selected disease states. *J Clin Invest* 1986;77:416–425.

280. Tripodi A, Akhavan S, Asti D, et al. Laboratory screening of thrombophilia. Evaluation of the diagnostic efficacy of a global test to detect congenital deficiencies of the protein C anticoagulant pathway. *Blood Coagul Fibrinolysis* 1998;9:485–489.

281. Dati F, Hafner G, Erbes H, et al. ProC Global: the first functional screening assay for the complete protein C pathway. *Clin Chem* 1997;43:1719–1723.

282. Toulon P, Halbmeyer WM, Hafner G, et al. Screening for abnormalities of the protein C anticoagulant pathway using the ProC Global assay. Results of a European multicenter evaluation. *Blood Coagul Fibrinolysis* 2000;11:447–454.

283. Haas FJ, van Sterkenburg-Kamp BM, Scheepers HA. A protein C pathway (PCP) screening test for the detection of APC resistance and protein C or S deficiencies. *Semin Thromb Hemost* 1998;24:355–362.

284. Manco-Johnson MJ, Marlar RA, Jacobson LJ, et al. Severe protein C deficiency in newborn infants. *J Pediatr* 1988;113:359–363.

285. Karpatkin M, Mannuccio Mannucci P, Bhogal M, et al. Low protein C in the neonatal period. *Br J Haematol* 1986;62:137–142.

286. Mannucci PM, Vigano S. Deficiencies of protein C, an inhibitor of blood coagulation. *Lancet* 1982;2:463–467.

287. Griffin JH, Mosher DF, Zimmerman TS, et al. Protein C, an antithrombotic protein, is reduced in hospitalized patients with intravascular coagulation. *Blood* 1982;60:261–264.

288. Rodeghiero F, Mannucci PM, Vigano S, et al. Liver dysfunction rather than intravascular coagulation as the main cause of low protein C and antithrombin III in acute leukemia. *Blood* 1984;63:965–969.

289. Mimuro J, Sakata Y, Wakabayashi K, et al. Level of protein C determined by combined assays during disseminated intravascular coagulation and oral anticoagulation. *Blood* 1987;69:1704–1711.

290. Marlar RA, Endres-Brooks J, Miller C. Serial studies of protein C and its plasma inhibitor in patients with disseminated intravascular coagulation. *Blood* 1985;66:59–63.

291. Pui CH, Chesney CM, Bergum PW, et al. Lack of pathogenetic role of proteins C and S in thrombosis associated with asparaginase-prednisone-vincristine therapy for leukaemia. *Br J Haematol* 1986;64:283–290.

292. Gruppo R, Degrauw A, Fogelson H, et al. Protein C deficiency related to valproic acid therapy: a possible association with childhood stroke. *J Pediatr* 2000;137:714–718.

293. White B, Livingstone W, Murphy C, et al. An open-label study of the role of adjuvant hemostatic support with protein C replacement therapy in purpura fulminans-associated meningococcemia. *Blood* 2000;96:3719–3724.

294. Powars DR, Rogers ZR, Patch MJ, et al. Purpura fulminans in meningococcemia: association with acquired deficiencies of proteins C and S. *N Engl J Med* 1987;317:571–572.

295. Cosio FG, Harker C, Batard MA, et al. Plasma concentrations of the natural anticoagulants protein C and protein S in patients with proteinuria. *J Lab Clin Med* 1985;106:218–222.

296. Pabinger I, Kyrle PA, Speiser W, et al. Diagnosis of protein C deficiency in patients on oral anticoagulant treatment: comparison of three different functional protein C assays. *Thromb Haemost* 1990;63:407–412.

297. Malm J, Laurell M, Nilsson IM, et al. Thromboembolic disease—critical evaluation of laboratory investigation. *Thromb Haemost* 1992;68:7–13.

298. Samama M, Horellou MH, Soria J, et al. Successful progressive anticoagulation in a severe protein C deficiency and previous skin necrosis at the initiation of oral anticoagulant treatment. *Thromb Haemost* 1984;51:132–133.

299. Zauber NP, Stark MW. Successful warfarin anticoagulation despite protein C deficiency and a history of warfarin necrosis. *Ann Intern Med* 1986;104:659–660.

300. Broekmans AW, Bertina RM, Loeliger EA, et al. Protein C and the development of skin necrosis during anticoagulant therapy. *Thromb Haemost* 1983;49:251.

301. McGehee WG, Klotz TA, Epstein DJ, et al. Coumarin necrosis associated with hereditary protein C deficiency. *Ann Intern Med* 1984;101:59–60.

302. Conway EM, Bauer KA, Barzegar S, et al. Suppression of hemostatic system activation by oral anticoagulants in the blood of patients with thrombotic diatheses. *J Clin Invest* 1987;80:1535–1544.

303. Sallah S, Abdallah JM, Gagnon GA. Recurrent warfarin-induced skin necrosis in kindreds with protein S deficiency. *Haemostasis* 1998;28:25–30.

304. Gailani D, Reese EP Jr. Anticoagulant-induced skin necrosis in a patient with hereditary deficiency of protein S. *Am J Hematol* 1999;60:231–236.

305. Freeman BD, Schmieg RE Jr, McGrath S, et al. Factor V Leiden mutation in a patient with warfarin-associated skin necrosis. *Surgery* 2000;127:595–596.

306. Jillella AP, Lutcher CL. Reinstituting warfarin in patients who develop warfarin skin necrosis. *Am J Hematol* 1996;52:117–119.

307. Estelles A, Garcia-Plaza I, Dasi A, et al. Severe inherited "homozygous" protein C deficiency in a newborn infant. *Thromb Haemost* 1984;52:53–56.

308. Yuen P, Cheung A, Lin HJ, et al. Purpura fulminans in a Chinese boy with congenital protein C deficiency. *Pediatrics* 1986;77:670–676.

309. Rappaport ES, Speights VO, Helbert B, et al. Protein C deficiency. *South Med J* 1987;80:240–242.

310. Vigano S, Mannucci PM, Solinas S, et al. Decrease in protein C antigen and formation of an abnormal protein soon after starting oral anticoagulant therapy. *Br J Haematol* 1984;57:213–220.

311. De Stefano V, Mastrangelo S, Schwarz HP, et al. Replacement therapy with a purified protein C concentrate during initiation of oral anticoagulation in severe protein C congenital deficiency. *Thromb Haemost* 1993;70:247–249.

312. Sanz-Rodriguez C, Gil-Fernandez JJ, Zapater P, et al. Long-term management of homozygous protein C deficiency: replacement therapy with subcutaneous purified protein C concentrate. *Thromb Haemost* 1999;81:887–890.

313. Vukovich T, Auberger K, Weil J, et al. Replacement therapy for a homozygous protein C deficiency-state using a concentrate of human protein C and S. *Br J Haematol* 1988;70:435–440.

314. Hartman KR, Manco-Johnson M, Rawlings JS, et al. Homozygous protein C deficiency: early treatment with warfarin. *Am J Pediatr Hematol Oncol* 1989;11:395–401.

315. Giraud T, Dhainaut JF, Schremmer B, et al. Adult overwhelming meningococcal purpura. A study of 35 cases, 1977–1989. *Arch Intern Med* 1991;151:310–316.

316. Comp PC, Esmon CT. Recurrent venous thromboembolism in patients with a partial deficiency of protein S. *N Engl J Med* 1984;311:1525–1528.

317. Schwarz HP, Fischer M, Hopmeier P, et al. Plasma protein S deficiency in familial thrombotic disease. *Blood* 1984;64:1297–1300.

318. Broekmans AW, Bertina RM, Reinalda-Poot J, et al. Hereditary protein S deficiency and venous thrombo-embolism. A study in three Dutch families. *Thromb Haemost* 1985;53:273–277.

319. Kamiya T, Sugihara T, Ogata K, et al. Inherited deficiency of protein S in a Japanese family with recurrent venous thrombosis: a study of three generations. *Blood* 1986;67:406–410.

320. Engesser L, Broekmans AW, Briet E, et al. Hereditary protein S deficiency: clinical manifestations. *Ann Intern Med* 1987;106:677–682.

321. De Stefano V, Leone G, Ferrelli R, et al. Severe deep vein thrombosis in a 2-year-old child with protein S deficiency. *Thromb Haemost* 1987;58:1089.

322. Sas G, Blasko G, Petro I, et al. A protein S deficient family with portal vein thrombosis. *Thromb Haemost* 1985;54:724.

323. Comp PC, Doray D, Patton D, et al. An abnormal plasma distribution of protein S occurs in functional protein S deficiency. *Blood* 1986;67:504–508.

324. Mannucci PM, Tripodi A, Bertina RM. Protein S deficiency associated with "juvenile" arterial and venous thromboses. *Thromb Haemost* 1986;55:440.

325. Broekmans AW, van Rooyen W, Westerveld BD, et al. Mesenteric vein thrombosis as presenting manifestation of hereditary protein S deficiency. *Gastroenterology* 1987;92:240–242.

326. Boyer-Neumann C, Wolf M, Amiral J, et al. Familial type I protein S deficiency associated with severe venous thrombosis—a study of five cases. *Thromb Haemost* 1988;60:128.

327. Ploos van Amstel HK, Huisman MV, Reitsma PH, et al. Partial protein S gene deletion in a family with hereditary thrombophilia. *Blood* 1989;73:479–483.

328. Schwarz HP, Heeb MJ, Lottenberg R, et al. Familial protein S deficiency with a variant protein S molecule in plasma and platelets. *Blood* 1989;74:213–221.

329. Whitlock JA, Janco RL, Phillips JA III. Inherited hypercoagulable states in children. *Am J Pediatr Hematol Oncol* 1989;11:170–173.

330. Mateo J, Oliver A, Borrell M, et al. Increased risk of venous thrombosis in carriers of natural anticoagulant deficiencies. Results of the family studies of the Spanish Multicenter Study on Thrombophilia (EMET study). *Blood Coagul Fibrinolysis* 1998;9:71–78.

331. Faioni EM, Valsecchi C, Palla A, et al. Free protein S deficiency is a risk factor for venous thrombosis. *Thromb Haemost* 1997;78:1343–1346.

332. Makris M, Leach M, Beauchamp NJ, et al. Genetic analysis, phenotypic diagnosis, and risk of venous thrombosis in families with inherited deficiencies of protein S. *Blood* 2000;95:1935–1941.

333. Gandrille S, Borgel D, Sala N, et al. Protein S deficiency: a database of mutations—summary of the first update. *Thromb Haemost* 2000;84:918.

334. Gandrille S, Borgel D, Ireland H, et al. Protein S deficiency: a database of mutations. For the Plasma Coagulation Inhibitors Subcommittee of the Scientific and Standardization Committee of the International Society on Thrombosis and Haemostasis. *Thromb Haemost* 1997;77:1201–1214.

335. Borgel D, Duchemin J, Alhenc-Gelas M, et al. Molecular basis for protein S hereditary deficiency: genetic defects observed in 118 patients with type I and type IIa deficiencies. The French Network on Molecular Abnormalities Responsible for Protein C and Protein S Deficiencies. *J Lab Clin Med* 1996;128:218–227.

336. Bertina RM, Ploos van Amstel HK, van Wijngaarden A, et al. Heerlen polymorphism of protein S, an immunologic polymorphism due to dimorphism of residue 460. *Blood* 1990;76:538–548.

337. Zoller B, Garcia de Frutos P, Dahlback B. Evaluation of the relationship between protein S and C4b-binding protein isoforms in hereditary protein S deficiency demonstrating type I and type III deficiencies to be phenotypic variants of the same genetic disease. *Blood* 1995;85:3524–3531.

338. Simmonds RE, Zoller B, Ireland H, et al. Genetic and phenotypic analysis of a large (122-member) protein S-deficient kindred provides an explanation for the familial coexistence of type I and type III plasma phenotypes. *Blood* 1997;89:4364–4370.

339. Fair DS, Revak DJ. Quantitation of human protein S in the plasma of normal and warfarin-treated individuals by radioimmunoassay. *Thromb Res* 1984;36:527–535.

340. Bertina RM, van Wijngaarden A, Reinalda-Poot J, et al. Determination of plasma protein S—the protein cofactor of activated protein C. *Thromb Haemost* 1985;53:268–272.

341. Comp PC, Thurnau GR, Welsh J, et al. Functional and immunologic protein S levels are decreased during pregnancy. *Blood* 1986;68:881–885.

342. Malm J, Laurell M, Dahlback B. Changes in the plasma levels of vitamin K-dependent proteins C and S and of C4b-binding protein during pregnancy and oral contraception. *Br J Haematol* 1988;68:437–443.

343. van de Waart P, Preissner KT, Bechtold JR, et al. A functional test for protein S activity in plasma. *Thromb Res* 1987;48:427–437.

344. D'Angelo A, Vigano-D'Angelo S, Esmon CT, et al. Acquired deficiencies of protein S. Protein S activity during oral anticoagulation, in liver disease, and in disseminated intravascular coagulation. *J Clin Invest* 1988;81:1445–1454.

345. Suzuki K, Nishioka J. Plasma protein S activity measured using Protac, a snake venom derived activator of protein C. *Thromb Res* 1988;49:241–251.

346. Kobayashi I, Amemiya N, Endo T, et al. Functional activity of protein S determined with use of protein C activated by venom activator. *Clin Chem* 1989;35:1644–1648.

347. Schwarz HP, Muntean W, Watzke H, et al. Low total protein S antigen but high protein S activity due to decreased C4b-binding protein in neonates. *Blood* 1988;71:562–565.

348. Brunet D, Barthet MC, Morange PE, et al. Protein S deficiency: different biological phenotypes according to the assays used. *Thromb Haemost* 1998;79:446–447.

349. Faioni EM, Franchi F, Asti D, et al. Resistance to activated protein C in nine thrombophilic families: interference in a protein S functional assay. *Thromb Haemost* 1993;70:1067–1071.

350. Henkens CM, Bom VJ, Van der Schaaf W, et al. Plasma levels of protein S, protein C, and factor X: effects of sex, hormonal state and age. *Thromb Haemost* 1995;74:1271–1275.

351. Boerger LM, Morris PC, Thurnau GR, et al. Oral contraceptives and gender affect protein S status. *Blood* 1987;69:692–694.

352. Liberti G, Bertina RM, Rosendaal FR. Hormonal state rather than age influences cut-off values of protein S: reevaluation of the thrombotic risk associated with protein S deficiency. *Thromb Haemost* 1999;82:1093–1096.

353. Crowther MA, Johnston M, Weitz J, et al. Free protein S deficiency may be found in patients with antiphospholipid antibodies who do not have systemic lupus erythematosus. *Thromb Haemost* 1996;76:689–691.

354. Manco-Johnson MJ, Nuss R, Key N, et al. Lupus anticoagulant and protein S deficiency in children with postvaricella purpura fulminans or thrombosis. *J Pediatr* 1996;128:319–323.

355. Kurugol Z, Vardar F, Ozkinay F, et al. Lupus anticoagulant and protein S deficiency in otherwise healthy children with acute varicella infection. *Acta Paediatr* 2000;89:1186–1189.

356. Vigano-D'Angelo S, D'Angelo A, Kaufman CE Jr, et al. Protein S deficiency occurs in the nephrotic syndrome. *Ann Intern Med* 1987;107:42–47.

357. Gouault-Heilmann M, Gadelha-Parente T, Levent M, et al. Total and free protein S in nephrotic syndrome. *Thromb Res* 1988;49:37–42.

358. Melissari E, Nicolaides KH, Scully MF, et al. Protein S and C4b-binding protein in fetal and neonatal blood. *Br J Haematol* 1988;70:199–203.

359. Malm J, Bennhagen R, Holmberg L, et al. Plasma concentrations of C4b-binding protein and vitamin K-dependent protein S in term and preterm infants: low levels of protein S-C4b-binding protein complexes. *Br J Haematol* 1988;68:445–449.

360. Simmonds RE, Ireland H, Lane DA, et al. Clarification of the risk for venous thrombosis associated with hereditary protein S deficiency by investigation of a large kindred with a characterized gene defect. *Ann Intern Med* 1998;128:8–14.

361. Dahlback B, Carlsson M, Svensson PJ. Familial thrombophilia due to a previously unrecognized mechanism characterized by poor anticoagulant response to activated protein C: prediction of a cofactor to activated protein C. *Proc Natl Acad Sci U S A* 1993;90:1004–1008.

362. Bertina RM, Koeleman BP, Koster T, et al. Mutation in blood coagulation factor V associated with resistance to activated protein C. *Nature* 1994;369:64–67.

363. Kalafatis M, Bertina RM, Rand MD, et al. Characterization of the molecular defect in factor VR506Q. *J Biol Chem* 1995;270:4053–4057.

364. Svensson PJ, Dahlback B. Resistance to activated protein C as a basis for venous thrombosis. *N Engl J Med* 1994;330:517–522.

365. Griffin JH, Evatt B, Wideman C, et al. Anticoagulant protein C pathway defective in majority of thrombophilic patients. *Blood* 1993;82:1989–1993.

366. Ridker PM, Hennekens CH, Lindpaintner K, et al. Mutation in the gene coding for coagulation factor V and the risk of myocardial infarction, stroke, and venous thrombosis in apparently healthy men. *N Engl J Med* 1995;332:912–917.

367. Koster T, Rosendaal FR, de Ronde H, et al. Venous thrombosis due to poor anticoagulant response to activated protein C: Leiden Thrombophilia Study. *Lancet* 1993;342:1503–1506.

368. Rosendaal FR, Koster T, Vandenbroucke JP, et al. High risk of thrombosis in patients homozygous for factor V Leiden (activated protein C resistance). *Blood* 1995;85:1504–1508.

369. Ridker PM, Miletich JP, Hennekens CH, et al. Ethnic distribution of factor V Leiden in 4047 men and women. Implications for venous thromboembolism screening. *JAMA* 1997;277:1305–1307.

370. Rees DC, Cox M, Clegg JB. World distribution of factor V Leiden. *Lancet* 1995;346:1133–1134.

371. de Visser MC, Rosendaal FR, Bertina RM. A reduced sensitivity for activated protein C in the absence of factor V Leiden increases the risk of venous thrombosis. *Blood* 1999;93:1271–1276.

372. Poort SR, Rosendaal FR, Reitsma PH, et al. A common genetic variation in the 3'-untranslated region of the prothrombin gene is associated with elevated plasma prothrombin levels and an increase in venous thrombosis. *Blood* 1996;88:3698–3703.

373. Soria JM, Almasy L, Souto JC, et al. Linkage analysis demonstrates that the prothrombin G20210A mutation jointly influences plasma prothrombin levels and risk of thrombosis. *Blood* 2000;95:2780–2785.

374. Margaglione M, Brancaccio V, Giuliani N, et al. Increased risk for venous thrombosis in carriers of the prothrombin G→A20210 gene variant. *Ann Intern Med* 1998;129:89–93.

375. Kapur RK, Mills LA, Spitzer SG, et al. A prothrombin gene mutation is significantly associated with venous thrombosis. *Arterioscler Thromb Vasc Biol* 1997;17:2875–2879.

376. Hillarp A, Zoller B, Svensson PJ, et al. The 20210 A allele of the prothrombin gene is a common risk factor among Swedish outpatients with verified deep venous thrombosis. *Thromb Haemost* 1997;78:990–992.

377. Rosendaal FR, Doggen CJ, Zivelin A, et al. Geographic distribution of the 20210 G to A prothrombin variant. *Thromb Haemost* 1998;79:706–708.

378. Gomez E, van der Poel SC, Jansen JH, et al. Rapid simultaneous screening of factor V Leiden and G20210A prothrombin variant by multiplex polymerase chain reaction on whole blood. *Blood* 1998;91:2208–2209.

379. McCully KS. Vascular pathology of homocysteinemia: implications for the pathogenesis of arteriosclerosis. *Am J Pathol* 1969;56:111–128.

380. den Heijer M, Koster T, Blom HJ, et al. Hyperhomocysteinemia as a risk factor for deep-vein thrombosis. *N Engl J Med* 1996;334:759–762.

381. Ridker PM, Hennekens CH, Selhub J, et al. Interrelation of hyperhomocyst(e)inemia, factor V Leiden, and risk of future venous thromboembolism. *Circulation* 1997;95:1777–1782.

382. den Heijer M, Rosendaal FR, Blom HJ, et al. Hyperhomocysteinemia and venous thrombosis: a meta-analysis. *Thromb Haemost* 1998;80:874–877.

383. Christen WG, Ajani UA, Glynn RJ, et al. Blood levels of homocysteine and increased risks of cardiovascular disease: causal or casual? *Arch Intern Med* 2000;160:422–434.

384. Botto LD, Yang Q. 5,10-Methylenetetrahydrofolate reductase gene variants and congenital anomalies: a HuGE review. *Am J Epidemiol* 2000;151:862–877.

385. Frosst P, Blom HJ, Milos R, et al. A candidate genetic risk factor for vascular disease: a common mutation in methylenetetrahydrofolate reductase. *Nat Genet* 1995;10:111–113.

386. Stampfer MJ, Malinow MR, Willett WC, et al. A prospective study of plasma homocyst(e)ine and risk of myocardial infarction in US physicians. *JAMA* 1992;268:877–881.

387. Perry IJ, Refsum H, Morris RW, et al. Prospective study of serum total homocysteine concentration and risk of stroke in middle-aged British men. *Lancet* 1995;346:1395–1398.

388. Selhub J, Jacques PF, Bostom AG, et al. Association between plasma homocysteine concentrations and extracranial carotid-artery stenosis. *N Engl J Med* 1995;332:286–291.

389. de Franchis R, Fermo I, Mazzola G, et al. Contribution of the cystathionine beta-synthase gene (844ins68) polymorphism to the risk of early-onset venous and arterial occlusive disease and of fasting hyperhomocysteinemia. *Thromb Haemost* 2000;84:576–582.

390. Kluijtmans LA, den Heijer M, Reitsma PH, et al. Thermolabile methylenetetrahydrofolate reductase and factor V Leiden in the risk of deep-vein thrombosis. *Thromb Haemost* 1998;79:254–258.

391. Stamler JS, Osborne JA, Jaraki O, et al. Adverse vascular effects of homocysteine are modulated by endothelium-derived relaxing factor and related oxides of nitrogen. *J Clin Invest* 1993;91:308–318.

392. Starkebaum G, Harlan JM. Endothelial cell injury due to copper-catalyzed hydrogen peroxide generation from homocysteine. *J Clin Invest* 1986;77:1370–1376.

393. Fryer RH, Wilson BD, Gubler DB, et al. Homocysteine, a risk factor for premature vascular disease and thrombosis, induces tissue factor activity in endothelial cells. *Arterioscler Thromb* 1993;13:1327–1333.

394. Nishinaga M, Ozawa T, Shimada K. Homocysteine, a thrombogenic agent, suppresses anticoagulant heparan sulfate expression in cultured porcine aortic endothelial cells. *J Clin Invest* 1993;92:1381–1386.

395. Hajjar KA. Homocysteine-induced modulation of tissue plasminogen activator binding to its endothelial cell membrane receptor. *J Clin Invest* 1993;91:2873–2879.

396. Franken DG, Boers GH, Blom HJ, et al. Treatment of mild hyperhomocysteinemia in vascular disease patients. *Arterioscler Thromb* 1994;14:465–470.

397. Naurath HJ, Joosten E, Riezler R, et al. Effects of vitamin B12, folate, and vitamin B6 supplements in elderly people with normal serum vitamin concentrations. *Lancet* 1995;346:85–89.

398. den Heijer M, Brouwer IA, Bos GM, et al. Vitamin supplementation reduces blood homocysteine levels: a controlled trial in patients with venous thrombosis and healthy volunteers. *Arterioscler Thromb Vasc Biol* 1998;18:356–361.

399. Bertina RM, van der Linden IK, Engesser L, et al. Hereditary heparin cofactor II deficiency and the risk of development of thrombosis. *Thromb Haemost* 1987;57:196–200.

400. Bernardi F, Legnani C, Micheletti F, et al. A heparin cofactor II mutation (HCII Rimini) combined with factor V Leiden or type I protein C deficiency in two unrelated thrombophilic subjects. *Thromb Haemost* 1996;76:505–509.

401. Schott D, Dempfle CE, Beck P, et al. Therapy with a purified plasminogen concentrate in an infant with ligneous conjunctivitis and homozygous plasminogen deficiency. *N Engl J Med* 1998;339:1679–1686.

402. Shigekiyo T, Kanazuka M, Aihara K, et al. No increased risk of thrombosis in heterozygous congenital dysplasminogenemia. *Int J Hematol* 2000;72:247–252.

403. Shigekiyo T, Uno Y, Tomonari A, et al. Type I congenital plasminogen deficiency is not a risk factor for thrombosis. *Thromb Haemost* 1992;67:189–192.

404. Tait RC, Walker ID, Conkie JA, et al. Isolated familial plasminogen deficiency may not be a risk factor for thrombosis. *Thromb Haemost* 1996;76:1004–1008.

405. Saito H. Contact factors in health and disease. *Semin Thromb Hemost* 1987;13:36–49.

406. Goodnough LT, Saito H, Ratnoff OD. Thrombosis or myocardial infarction in congenital clotting factor abnormalities and chronic thrombocytopenias: a report of 21 patients and a review of 50 previously reported cases. *Medicine (Baltimore)* 1983;62:248–255.

407. Lodi S, Isa L, Pollini E, et al. Defective intrinsic fibrinolytic activity in a patient with severe factor XII-deficiency and myocardial infarction. *Scand J Haematol* 1984;33:80–82.

408. Lammle B, Wuillemin WA, Huber I, et al. Thromboembolism and bleeding tendency in congenital factor XII deficiency—a study on 74 subjects from 14 Swiss families. *Thromb Haemost* 1991;65:117–121.

409. Mannhalter C, Fischer M, Hopmeier P, et al. Factor XII activity and antigen concentrations in patients suffering from recurrent thrombosis. *Fibrinolysis* 1987;1:259–263.

410. Rodeghiero F, Castaman G, Ruggeri M, et al. Thrombosis in subjects with homozygous and heterozygous factor XII deficiency. *Thromb Haemost* 1992;67:590–591.

411. Koster T, Blann AD, Briet E, et al. Role of clotting factor VIII in effect of von Willebrand factor on occurrence of deep-vein thrombosis. *Lancet* 1995;345:152–155.

412. Kraaijenhagen RA, in't Anker PS, Koopman MM, et al. High plasma concentration of factor VIIIc is a major risk factor for venous thromboembolism. *Thromb Haemost* 2000;83:5–9.

413. Kamphuisen PW, Eikenboom JC, Vos HL, et al. Increased levels of factor VIII and fibrinogen in patients with venous thrombosis are not caused by acute phase reactions. *Thromb Haemost* 1999;81:680–683.

414. O'Donnell J, Tuddenham EG, Manning R, et al. High prevalence of elevated factor VIII levels in patients referred for thrombophilia screening: role of increased synthesis and relationship to the acute phase reaction. *Thromb Haemost* 1997;77:825–828.

415. Kyrle PA, Minar E, Hirschl M, et al. High plasma levels of factor VIII and the risk of recurrent venous thromboembolism. *N Engl J Med* 2000;343:457–462.

416. van Tilburg NH, Rosendaal FR, Bertina RM. Thrombin activatable fibrinolysis inhibitor and the risk for deep vein thrombosis. *Blood* 2000;95:2855–2859.

417. Meijers JC, Tekelenburg WL, Bouma BN, et al. High levels of coagulation factor XI as a risk factor for venous thrombosis. *N Engl J Med* 2000;342:696–701.

418. van Hylckama Vlieg A, van der Linden IK, Bertina RM, et al. High levels of factor IX increase the risk of venous thrombosis. *Blood* 2000;95:3678–3682.

419. Kamphuisen PW, Lensen R, Houwing-Duistermaat JJ, et al. Heritability of elevated factor VIII antigen levels in factor V Leiden families with thrombophilia. *Br J Haematol* 2000;109:519–522.

420. Greaves M, Baglin C, Keeling DM, et al. Workshop on screening for late onset genetic disorders. UK National Screening Committee, 2000.

421. Hull RD, Raskob GE, Hirsh J, et al. Continuous intravenous heparin compared with intermittent subcutaneous heparin in the initial treatment of proximal-vein thrombosis. *N Engl J Med* 1986;315:1109–1114.

422. Prandoni P, Lensing AW, Cogo A, et al. The long-term clinical course of acute deep venous thrombosis. *Ann Intern Med* 1996;125:1–7.

423. Kearon C, Gent M, Hirsh J, et al. A comparison of three months of anticoagulation with extended anticoagulation for a first episode of idiopathic venous thromboembolism. *N Engl J Med* 1999;340:901–907.

424. De Stefano V, Martinelli I, Mannucci PM, et al. The risk of recurrent deep venous thrombosis among heterozygous carriers of both factor V Leiden and the G20210A prothrombin mutation. *N Engl J Med* 1999;341:801–806.

425. Margaglione M, D'Andrea G, Colaizzo D, et al. Coexistence of factor V Leiden and factor II A20210 mutations and recurrent venous thromboembolism. *Thromb Haemost* 1999;82:1583–1587.

426. Lensing AW, Prins MH. Recurrent deep vein thrombosis and two coagulation factor gene mutations: quo vadis? *Thromb Haemost* 1999;82:1564–1566.

427. Ridker PM, Miletich JP, Stampfer MJ, et al. Factor V Leiden and risks of recurrent idiopathic venous thromboembolism. *Circulation* 1995;92:2800–2802.

428. Simioni P, Prandoni P, Lensing AW, et al. The risk of recurrent venous thromboembolism in patients with an Arg506 → Gln mutation in the gene for factor V (factor V Leiden). *N Engl J Med* 1997;336:399–403.

429. Eichinger S, Pabinger I, Stumpflen A, et al. The risk of recurrent venous thromboembolism in patients with and without factor V Leiden. *Thromb Haemost* 1997;77:624–628.

430. Lindmarker P, Schulman S, Sten-Linder M, et al. The risk of recurrent venous thromboembolism in carriers and non-carriers of the G1691A allele in the coagulation factor V gene and the G20210A allele in the prothrombin gene. DURAC Trial Study Group. Duration of Anticoagulation. *Thromb Haemost* 1999;81:684–689.

431. De Stefano V, Martinelli I, Mannucci PM, et al. The risk of recurrent venous thromboembolism among heterozygous carriers of the G20210A prothrombin gene mutation. *Br J Haematol* 2001;113:630–635.

432. Schulman S, Rhedin AS, Lindmarker P, et al. A comparison of six weeks with six months of oral anticoagulant therapy after a first episode of venous thromboembolism. Duration of Anticoagulation Trial Study Group. *N Engl J Med* 1995;332:1661–1665.

433. Douketis JD, Kearon C, Bates S, et al. Risk of fatal pulmonary embolism in patients with treated venous thromboembolism. *JAMA* 1998;279:458–462.

434. Palareti G, Leali N, Coccheri S, et al. Bleeding complications of oral anticoagulant treatment: an inception-cohort, prospective collaborative study (ISCOAT). Italian Study on Complications of Oral Anticoagulant Therapy. *Lancet* 1996;348:423–428.

435. van Boven HH, Vandenbroucke JP, Westendorp RG, et al. Mortality and causes of death in inherited antithrombin deficiency. *Thromb Haemost* 1997;77:452–455.

436. Hille ET, Westendorp RG, Vandenbroucke JP, et al. Mortality and causes of death in families with the factor V Leiden mutation (resistance to activated protein C). *Blood* 1997;89:1963–1967.

437. Allaart CF, Rosendaal FR, Noteboom WM, et al. Survival in families with hereditary protein C deficiency, 1820 to 1993. *BMJ* 1995;311:910–913.

438. Baglin C, Brown K, Luddington R, et al. Risk of recurrent venous thromboembolism in patients with the factor V Leiden (FVR506Q) mutation: effect of warfarin and prediction by precipitating factors. East Anglian Thrombophilia Study Group. *Br J Haematol* 1998;100:764–768.

439. van den Belt AG, Hutten BA, Prins MH, et al. Duration of oral anticoagulant treatment in patients with venous thromboembolism and a deficiency of antithrombin, protein C or protein S—a decision analysis. *Thromb Haemost* 2000;84:758–763.

440. Marchetti M, Pistorio A, Barosi G. Extended anticoagulation for prevention of recurrent venous thromboembolism in carriers of factor V Leiden—cost-effectiveness analysis. *Thromb Haemost* 2000;84:752–757.

441. Sarasin FP, Bounameaux H. Decision analysis model of prolonged oral anticoagulant treatment in factor V Leiden carriers with first episode of deep vein thrombosis. *BMJ* 1998;316:95–99.

442. Clagett GP, Anderson FA Jr, Geerts W, et al. Prevention of venous thromboembolism. *Chest* 1998;114:531S–560S.

443. Pabinger I, Kyrle PA, Heistinger M, et al. The risk of thromboembolism in asymptomatic patients with protein C and protein S deficiency: a prospective cohort study. *Thromb Haemost* 1994;71:441–445.

444. Atrash HK, Koonin LM, Lawson HW, et al. Maternal mortality in the United States, 1979–1986. *Obstet Gynecol* 1990;76:1055–1060.

445. Hogberg U, Innala E, Sandstrom A. Maternal mortality in Sweden, 1980–1988. *Obstet Gynecol* 1994;84:240–244.

446. Friederich PW, Sanson BJ, Simioni P, et al. Frequency of pregnancy-related venous thromboembolism in anticoagulant factor-deficient women: implications for prophylaxis. *Ann Intern Med* 1996;125:955–960.

447. Conard J, Horellou MH, Van Dreden P, et al. Thrombosis and pregnancy in congenital deficiencies in AT III, protein C or protein S: study of 78 women. *Thromb Haemost* 1990;63:319–320.

448. Brill-Edwards P, Ginsberg JS, Gent M, et al. Safety of withholding heparin in pregnant women with a history of venous thromboembolism. Recurrence of Clot in This Pregnancy Study Group. *N Engl J Med* 2000;343:1439–1444.

449. Conard J, Horellou M, Samama MM. Management of pregnancy in women with thrombophilia. *Haemostasis* 1999;29:98–104.

450. Ginsberg JS, Greer I, Hirsh J. Use of antithrombotic agents during pregnancy. *Chest* 2001;119:122S–131S.

451. Rey E, Rivard GE. Prophylaxis and treatment of thromboembolic diseases during pregnancy with dalteparin. *Int J Gynaecol Obstet* 2000;71:19–24.

452. Bar J, Cohen-Sacher B, Hod M, et al. Low-molecular-weight heparin for thrombophilia in pregnant women. *Int J Gynaecol Obstet* 2000;69:209–213.

453. Nelson-Piercy C, Letsky EA, de Swiet M. Low-molecular-weight heparin for obstetric thromboprophylaxis: experience of sixty-nine pregnancies in sixty-one women at high risk. *Am J Obstet Gynecol* 1997;176:1062–1068.

454. Bazzan M, Donvito V. Low-molecular-weight heparin during pregnancy. *Thromb Res* 2001;101:175–186.

455. Iturbe-Alessio I, Fonseca MC, Mutchinik O, et al. Risks of anticoagulant therapy in pregnant women with artificial heart valves. *N Engl J Med* 1986;315:1390–1393.

456. Vandenbroucke JP, Koster T, Briet E, et al. Increased risk of venous thrombosis in oral-contraceptive users who are carriers of factor V Leiden mutation. *Lancet* 1994;344:1453–1457.

457. Bloemenkamp KW, Helmerhorst FM, Rosendaal FR, et al. Venous thrombosis, oral contraceptives and high factor VIII levels. *Thromb Haemost* 1999;82:1024–1027.

458. Martinelli I, Taioli E, Bucciarelli P, et al. Interaction between the G20210A mutation of the prothrombin gene and oral contraceptive use in deep vein thrombosis. *Arterioscler Thromb Vasc Biol* 1999;19:700–703.

459. Helmerhorst FM, Bloemenkamp KW, Rosendaal FR, et al. Oral contraceptives and thrombotic disease: risk of venous thromboembolism. *Thromb Haemost* 1997;78:327–333.

460. Bloemenkamp KW, Rosendaal FR, Helmerhorst FM, et al. Enhancement by factor V Leiden mutation of risk of deep-vein thrombosis associated with oral contraceptives containing a third-generation progestagen. *Lancet* 1995;346:1593–1596.

461. Jick H, Jick SS, Gurewich V, et al. Risk of idiopathic cardiovascular death and nonfatal venous thromboembolism in women using oral contraceptives with differing progestagen components. *Lancet* 1995;346:1589–1593.

462. Vandenbroucke JP, van der Meer FJ, Helmerhorst FM, et al. Factor V Leiden: should we screen oral contraceptive users and pregnant women? *BMJ* 1996;313:1127–1130.

463. Grody WW, Griffin JH, Taylor AK, et al. American College of Medical Genetics consensus statement on factor V Leiden mutation testing. *Genet Med* 2001;3:139–148.

464. Cosmi B, Legnani C, Bernardi F, et al. Value of family history in identifying women at risk of venous thromboembolism during oral contraception: observational study. *BMJ* 2001;322:1024–1025.

465. Schulman S, Lindmarker P. Incidence of cancer after prophylaxis with warfarin against recurrent venous thromboembolism. Duration of Anticoagulation Trial. *N Engl J Med* 2000;342:1953–1958.

466. Aznar J, Vaya A, Estelles A, et al. Risk of venous thrombosis in carriers of the prothrombin G20210A variant and factor V Leiden and their interaction with oral contraceptives. *Haematologica* 2000;85:1271–1276.

CHAPTER 43

Anticoagulant Therapy

Mark A. Crowther and Jeffrey S. Ginsberg

Despite recent advances in our understanding of the coagulation system and the development of a large number of novel anticoagulants, many now entering clinical practice, heparin (and its derivatives) and coumarins continue to be the most widely used anticoagulants. This chapter focuses on the pharmacology and suggested clinical use of heparin, its derivatives, and the oral anticoagulants. In addition, we briefly review novel anticoagulants, including danaparoid, the direct thrombin inhibitors, and pentasaccharide.

HEPARIN AND LOW-MOLECULAR-WEIGHT HEPARIN

Unfractionated heparin is a sulfated, long-chain acidic glycosaminoglycan obtained by extraction from porcine intestinal mucosa. Heparin functions as a catalytic cofactor for an endogenous inhibitor of serine proteases known as *antithrombin* (AT). Although widely used and effective, heparin does have complications, including bleeding (1), heparin-induced thrombocytopenia (2), and osteoporosis (3–5).

Mechanism of Action

Heparin produces its anticoagulant effect by catalyzing the action of AT. In the presence of heparin, AT forms binary (AT–enzyme) or ternary (heparin–enzyme–AT) complexes with thrombin, factor Xa, factor IXa, and factor XIa, in order of decreasing affinity (Fig. 43-1). These enzymes are inactivated in this process (6). A specific pentasaccharide is critical for the high-affinity binding of heparin to AT and thus for heparin's anticoagulant activity (7–9). Only approximately one-third of heparin molecules contain this pentasaccharide, and these account for at least 80% of heparin's activity. A second heparin cofactor, known as *heparin cofactor II* (HCII), has been identified. When present in high concentration, heparin is able to catalyze the AT effect of HCII; however, at therapeutic heparin concentrations, HCII-mediated thrombin inhibition is not clinically important (10).

For inhibition of thrombin, heparin must bind to both the coagulation enzyme and AT, but binding to the enzyme is less important for the inhibition of factor Xa (11). Molecules of heparin with fewer than 18 saccharide units are unable to bind to thrombin and AT simultaneously and therefore do not efficiently inhibit thrombin. In contrast, very small heparin fragments that contain the high-affinity pentasaccharide sequence are able to catalyze the inhibition of factor Xa by AT (12–16). By inactivating throm-

bin, heparin not only prevents fibrin formation but also inhibits thrombin-induced activation of factor V and factor VIII (17–19).

Heparin binds to platelets *in vitro* and, depending on the experimental conditions, can either induce or inhibit platelet aggregation (20,21). The interaction of heparin with platelets (22) and endothelial cells (23) may contribute to heparin-induced bleeding by a mechanism independent of its anticoagulant effect (24). For example, binding of heparin to von Willebrand's factor results in the inhibition of von Willebrand's factor–dependent platelet function (25). In addition to its anticoagulant effects, heparin increases vessel wall permeability (23) and suppresses the proliferation of vascular smooth muscle cells (26), an effect which appears to be independent of its anticoagulant activity (27). Heparin also suppresses osteoblast formation and activates osteoclasts, effects that promote bone loss (28,29).

Clinical Use of Heparin

Intravenously administered heparin produces an immediate antithrombotic effect. The maximum effect of subcutaneous injection occurs after approximately 3 hours, and the effect lasts 12 hours or longer, depending on its dose. Heparin is cleared through a combination of a rapid saturable and a much slower first-order mechanism of clearance (30–32). The saturable phase of heparin clearance is thought to be due to heparin binding to receptors on endothelial cells (33,34) and macrophages (35), where it is internalized and depolymerized (36,37). Clearance through the slower, nonsaturable mechanism is largely renal. Because of its complex pharmacokinetics, the anticoagulant response to heparin at therapeutic doses is not linear but increases disproportionally both in its intensity and duration with increasing dose. Thus, the apparent biologic half-life of heparin increases from approximately 30 minutes with an intravenous bolus of 25 U/kg to 60 minutes with an intravenous bolus of 100 U/kg to 150 minutes with a bolus of 400 U/kg (30–32).

Heparin is usually administered by intravenous infusion or subcutaneous injection. If the subcutaneous route is selected, the initial dose must be sufficiently high to counteract the reduced bioavailability that occurs when heparin is administered by this route (38). Heparin binds to plasma proteins (39,40), a phenomenon that contributes to its reduced plasma recovery (bioavailability) at low concentrations, to the variability of the anticoagulant response to fixed doses of heparin in patients with thromboembolic disorders (38), and to the laboratory phenomenon of heparin resistance (41). Binding to plasma proteins accounts for the observation that the plasma recovery of heparin is reduced when the drug is administered by subcutaneous injection in low doses (e.g., 5000 U/12 hours) or

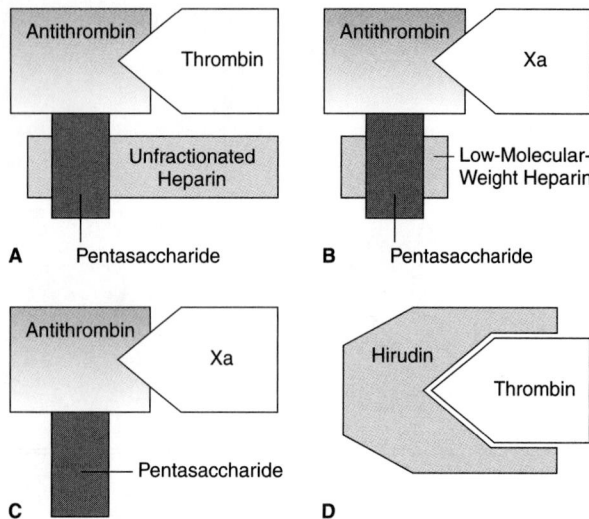

Figure 43-1. Mechanism of action of unfractionated and low-molecular-weight heparin, pentasaccharide, and hirudin. Unfractionated heparin is a template on which antithrombin (AT) and an activated clotting factor (factor IIa, Xa, IXa, or XIa) can form a complex, leading to covalent linkage of AT to the clotting factor and, thus, its inactivation. **A:** The AT–heparin interaction requires a specific five-sugar sequence known as *pentasaccharide*. Low-molecular-weight heparins are manufactured from unfractionated heparin and are unable to act as an efficient template for the interaction of factor IIa and AT. **B:** They are, however, able to catalyze the formation of an AT–factor Xa complex. The pentasaccharide sequence can be chemically manufactured and used as an anticoagulant. **C:** Its anticoagulant effect is due entirely to Xa inactivation. **D:** Hirudins and the direct thrombin inhibitors form noncovalent complexes with thrombin that are AT-independent; as a result, they are consumed in the inactivation process.

TABLE 43-1. Heparin Dosing Nomograms

Weight-based nomogram
Initial heparin dosage, 80 U/kg bolus, then 18 U/kg/h
Dosage adjustments

APTT <35 sec (<1.2 × control)	80 U/kg bolus, increase infusion 4 U/kg/h
APTT 35–45 sec (1.2–1.5 × control)	40 U/kg bolus, increase infusion 2 U/kg/h
APTT 46–70 sec (1.5–2.3 × control)	No change
APTT 71–90 sec (2.3–3.0 × control)	Decrease infusion 2 U/kg/h
APTT >90 sec (>3.0 × control)	Hold infusion for 1 h, decrease infusion 3 U/kg/h

In clinical practice, the APTT should be checked 6 to 12 h after each dosage change and at least every 24 h during continuous therapy
Nonweight-based nomogram
Initial heparin dosage, 5000 U bolus, then 1280 U/h infusion
Dosage adjustments

APTT	Intervention	Next APTT
APTT <50 sec	5000 U bolus, increase by 120 U/h	6 h
APTT 50–59 sec	Increase by 120 U/h	6 h
APTT 60–85 sec	No change	Next morning
APTT 86–95 sec	Decrease by 80 U/h	6 h
APTT 96–120 sec	Hold for 30 min, decrease by 80 U/h	6 h
APTT >120 sec	Hold for 60 min, decrease by 160 U/h	6 h

APTT, activated partial thromboplastin time.
Adapted from Cruickshank MK, Levine MN, Hirsh J, et al. A standard heparin nomogram for the management of heparin therapy. *Arch Intern Med* 1991;151:333–337; Raschke RA, Gollihare B, Peirce JC. The effectiveness of implementing the weight-based heparin nomogram as a practice guideline. *Arch Intern Med* 1996;156:1645–1649; and Raschke RA, Reilly BM, Guidry JR, et al. The weight-based heparin dosing nomogram compared with a "standard-care" nomogram: a randomized controlled trial. *Ann Intern Med* 1993;119:874–881.

moderate doses of 12,500 to 15,000 U/12 hours (38,42). However, at high therapeutic doses of subcutaneous heparin (>35,000 U/day), the plasma recovery is almost complete (43). The difference between the bioavailability of heparin when administered by subcutaneous or intravenous injection was demonstrated in a study of patients with venous thrombosis (38). In this study, patients were randomized to receive either 15,000 U/12 hours heparin by subcutaneous injection or 30,000 U heparin by continuous intravenous infusion; both regimens were preceded by an intravenous bolus dose of 5000 U. Therapeutic heparin levels and activated partial thromboplastin time (APTT) ratios were achieved at 24 hours in only 37% of patients who received subcutaneous heparin, whereas therapeutic heparin levels and APTT ratios were achieved at 24 hours in 71% given a continuous intravenous infusion.

The risk of heparin-associated bleeding is increased with increasing heparin dose (44,45) (which in turn is related to the anticoagulant response) or by the concomitant use of thrombolytics (46–49) or abciximab (50,51). The risk of bleeding is also increased by recent surgery, trauma, invasive procedures, or a generalized hemostatic abnormality (52).

Dosage and Monitoring of Heparin

The anticoagulant effect of heparin is routinely monitored using the APTT. Heparin activity levels can also be measured by protamine titration (therapeutic range of 0.2 to 0.4 U/mL) (53) or by antifactor Xa chromogenic assay (therapeutic range, 0.3 to 0.7 U/mL) (54). However, these methods are not routinely available in most clinical centers (55). On average, therapeutic anticoagulation is achieved with approximately 33,000 U heparin/day when administered by continuous intravenous infusion. Approximately 25% of patients require more than 35,000 U/day heparin (by con-

tinuous intravenous infusion) to increase their APTT into the therapeutic range, and occasional patients require more than 45,000 U/day. Heparin resistance in these patients is due, in part, to high levels of circulating heparin-binding proteins, which compete with AT for heparin binding (41,56). Heparin-resistant patients also tend to have higher levels of factor VIII than nonresistant patients, which further lowers their APTT response (54). A heparin level is useful to guide heparin dosage when APTT values have not been prolonged despite very large doses of heparin (54).

Subcutaneous injection achieves therapeutic blood levels and antithrombotic efficacy comparable with that of intravenous infusion, provided the dose is adequate (57). An insufficient initial subcutaneous heparin dose (less than approximately 35,000/day for an average-size adult) is associated with an increase in the risk of subsequent thrombotic recurrence (58); prolonged subtherapeutic APTTs probably also increase the risk of recurrence (59).

A rapid therapeutic heparin effect is achieved by starting with a loading dose of 5000 U as an intravenous bolus followed by 32,000 U/day by continuous infusion (60). If the APTT is used to monitor treatment, it should be performed approximately 6 hours after the bolus, and the heparin dose should be adjusted according to the result obtained. Alternately, the initial heparin bolus and infusion rate can be calculated using a weight-adjusted dosage regimen (61). A less intense, weight-adjusted dose is recommended after thrombolytic therapy or with abciximab treatment (51) (Tables 43-1 and 43-2).

It is also possible to achieve therapeutic heparin levels with subcutaneous injection in a dose of 35,000 U/day in two divided doses (43). However, due to interindividual variation in the response to heparin, it is recommended that patients receiving

TABLE 43-2. Recommendations for Heparin Therapy after Thrombolytic or Abciximab Therapy

After rtPA or reteplase administration
   Bolus, 75 U/kg i.v. bolus at initiation of thrombolytic therapy
   Initial maintenance, 1000–1200 U/h to maintain APTT at 1.5–2.0 × control for 48 h
   Maintenance beyond 48 h
      High-dose subcutaneous unfractionated heparin twice daily to maintain APTT at 1.5–2.0 × control 6 h injection
      OR, infusion of heparin to maintain APTT at 1.5–2.0 × control ONLY in the presence of high risk of embolism
         Anterior Q-wave myocardial infarction
         Severe left ventricular dysfunction
         Congestive heart failure
         History of embolism
         Known mural thrombus
         Atrial fibrillation
After streptokinase or anisoylated plasminogen-streptokinase activator complex administration
   Heparin should ONLY be administered in the presence of a high risk of embolism as defined above
   Initial therapy
      Measure APTT when indication emerges but NOT within 4 h of initiation of thrombolytic infusion. If APTT is 2 or more × control, do NOT start heparin, but repeat APTT as indicated clinically
      Heparin should be initiated without a bolus at an infusion rate aimed to maintain the APTT between 1.5 and 2.0 × control
   Maintenance therapy, maintain infusion as clinically indicated, or consider switching to high-dose subcutaneous therapy as outlined above
During abciximab administration
   Initial therapy, bolus of 70 U/kg (maximum)
   Maintenance therapy
      Additional boluses as needed to achieve and maintain an activated clotting time of at least 200 sec
      Discontinue heparin immediately after completion of procedure and remove vascular sheaths when activated clotting time is less than 175 sec

APTT, activated partial thromboplastin time; rtPA, recombinant tissue plasminogen activator.
From Hirsh J, Warkentin TE, Raschke R, et al. Heparin and low-molecular-weight heparin: mechanisms of action, pharmacokinetics, dosing considerations, monitoring, efficacy, and safety. *Chest* 1998;114[Suppl 5]:489S–510S; and Cairns JA, Theroux P, Lewis HDJ, et al. Antithrombotic agents in coronary artery disease. *Chest* 1998;114[Suppl 5]:611S–633S.

therapeutic doses of subcutaneous heparin be monitored with the APTT. The APTT should be drawn 6 hours after the subcutaneous injection and the dose adjusted to achieve a therapeutic APTT.

Complications of Heparin Therapy

BLEEDING

The most important side effect of heparin therapy is major bleeding. In contemporary studies, in which heparin was administered for 5 to 10 days by continuous intravenous infusion monitored by the APTT response, major or life-threatening bleeding occurred in 2% to 4% of patients (62–64). The risk of hemorrhagic complications is influenced by the dose, the method and timing of administration, and the presence of other risk factors for bleeding (e.g., thrombocytopenia, coadministration of thrombolytic therapy or antiplatelet drugs, systemic hemorrhagic tendencies, and local sources of bleeding).

The management of heparin-associated bleeding depends on the severity and site of bleeding. In all cases except the most minor, treatment should consist of immediate discontinuation of heparin and treatment of the underlying bleeding source. Surgical or endoscopic intervention may be required because bleeding can continue even after the anticoagulant effect of heparin is lost. Because of its strong positive charge, protamine sulfate binds to heparin with high affinity and neutralizes its anticoagulant effect. The effect is immediate, but rebound anticoagulation can occur because the protamine is cleared more rapidly than heparin. Patients allergic to iodine, fish, or protamine-zinc insulin should receive protamine with caution because it is derived from fish. The dose of protamine is calculated based on the estimated circulating heparin concentration. One milligram of protamine neutralizes approximately 100 U heparin. Therefore, if a patient has received a 5000-U heparin bolus followed by an infusion of 1000 U/hours for 3 hours, approximately 25 mg protamine should be administered, based on an estimated half-life of heparin of 1 hour. A sample calculation is shown in Table 43-3. The half-life of protamine is less than that of heparin; thus, repeated doses of protamine may be needed in some patients with high heparin levels, such as those who have undergone cardiopulmonary bypass or those with renal insufficiency (65).

THROMBOCYTOPENIA

Thrombocytopenia can occur as a complication of heparin therapy. An early, transient, and mild fall in the platelet count is seen in many patients after initiation of heparin. This fall is not clinically important, and its mechanism is not known. However, a fall in the platelet count 5 to 10 days after first exposure to heparin (or 1 to 3 days after reexposure) should alert the physician to the possibility of heparin-induced thrombocytopenia (HIT). HIT is due to the development of an antibody to an epitope on the heparin–platelet factor 4 complex. Platelet factor 4 is a protein released from platelets when they are activated (66,67). The heparin–platelet factor 4–antibody complex binds to platelet Fc receptors, activating the platelet (68). Platelet activation with subsequent microparticle generation causes a profound prothrombotic state (69) (Fig. 43-2). The diagnosis of HIT requires a fall in the platelet count during or soon after heparin therapy and objective confirmation of a heparin–platelet factor 4–dependent antibody. The presence of the antibody is confirmed using a serotonin release (70) or enzyme-linked immunosorbent assay (71). In a large randomized trial, HIT developed

TABLE 43-3. Calculation of Protamine Dose[a]

	Residual Heparin (Assuming Half-Life of 1 Hour)			
	End of Hour 1 (U)	End of Hour 2 (U)	End of Hour 3 (U)	Reversal (mg protamine)
Initial heparin bolus (5000 U)	2500	1250	625	6.25
Hour 1 infusion (1000 U)		500	250	2.5
Hour 2 infusion (1000 U)			500	5.0
Hour 3 infusion (1000 U)			1000	10.0

[a]Protamine doses can be calculated assuming that heparin has a half-life of 1 hour and that 1 mg protamine will inactivate 100 U heparin. To neutralize this heparin infusion, approximately 25 mg protamine should be administered.

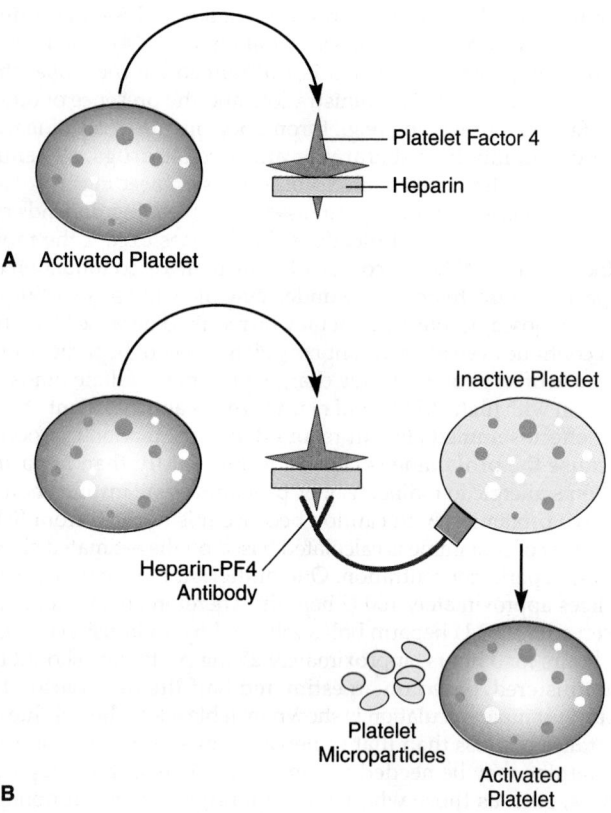

Figure 43-2. Mechanism of heparin-induced thrombocytopenia. **A:** Heparin forms a complex with platelet factor 4 (PF4), which is released during platelet activation. **B:** An autoantibody targeted to an epitope on this complex can bind to inactive platelets via their Fc receptors, resulting in activation of the platelet. Microparticle generation as a result of platelet activation produces an intensely prothrombotic state.

in 2.7% of patients undergoing elective hip surgery who received prophylactic low-dose unfractionated heparin compared with no patients who received prophylactic low-molecular-weight heparin (LMWH) (2). In this study, eight (89%) of nine patients with HIT developed thrombosis, compared with 117 (18%) of 656 patients who did not develop HIT. Patients with HIT can develop either venous or arterial thrombosis (72,73). Even with profound thrombocytopenia, hemorrhage is rare in these patients.

Patients who develop thrombosis in the setting of HIT and who require ongoing anticoagulation should not receive unfractionated heparin or LMWH, because LMWH cross-reacts with the HIT antibody. Satisfactory anticoagulation can be safely achieved with danaparoid sodium, argatroban, or hirudin (74–78). HIT antibodies can react with danaparoid, although this cross-reactivity has not been associated with worsening of thrombocytopenia or thrombosis (79). HIT antibodies do not cross-react with hirudin or the other direct thrombin inhibitors, such as argatroban. Experience with hirudin and its derivatives in the treatment of HIT is growing, and the hirudin compound known as *lepirudin* has been approved for the treatment of HIT in the United States (78). Early introduction of warfarin to a patient with active HIT or inadequate parenteral anticoagulant therapy during warfarin initiation in patients with HIT may result in worsening of thrombotic complications due to precipitous declines in the levels of protein C (72).

OSTEOPOROSIS

Osteoporosis complicates heparin therapy (4,80). Even prophylactic heparin doses are associated with a loss of bone mineral

density when administered long-term (5). Although the specific mechanism of heparin-associated osteoporosis is unknown, there is experimental evidence that heparin increases the rate of calcium resorption from bone (28). The LMWHs are likely associated with a lower risk of osteoporosis with prolonged administration (80).

No specific therapy for the prevention or treatment of heparin-associated osteoporosis has been evaluated. In the absence of clinical evidence, ensuring adequate calcium and vitamin D intake in all patients receiving long-term heparin seems appropriate.

LOW-MOLECULAR-WEIGHT HEPARINS

The development of LMWHs for clinical use has been stimulated by two main observations. Compared to heparin, LMWH has (a) a more favorable benefit to risk ratio in experimental animals (81–86) and (b) superior pharmacokinetic properties (87–92).

Synthesis and Mechanism of Action

LMWHs are derived from heparin by chemical or enzymatic depolymerization to yield fragments that are approximately one-third the size of heparin. Because these LMWHs are prepared by different methods of depolymerization and differ to some extent in their pharmacokinetic properties and anticoagulant profile, they may not be clinically interchangeable. Like heparin, LMWH preparations are heterogeneous in molecular size and anticoagulant activity. LMWHs have a mean molecular weight of 4000 to 5000, with a molecular weight distribution of 1000 to 10,000. Depolymerization of heparin produced five main changes in the properties of the resulting low-molecular-weight fragments; all are a consequence of the reduced binding of fragments to proteins or cells. Compared to heparin, LMWHs have

1. Reduced ability to catalyze the inactivation of thrombin because the smaller fragments cannot bind simultaneously to AT and thrombin. However, because bridging between AT and factor Xa is less critical for antifactor Xa activity, the smaller fragments are able to inactivate factor Xa (93–96) (Fig. 43-1)
2. Reduced nonspecific binding to plasma proteins, with a corresponding improvement in the predictability of their dose response relationship (97)
3. Reduced binding to macrophages and endothelial cells, with an associated increase in their plasma half-life (98)
4. Reduced binding to platelets (99) and PF4 (100), which may explain the lower incidence of HIT (2)
5. Reduced binding to osteoblasts, which results in less activation of osteoclasts and associated reduction in bone loss (28,29)

LMWHs are cleared principally by the renal route, and their biologic half-life is increased in patients with renal failure (101–103).

Like heparin, LMWHs produce their major anticoagulant effect by catalyzing AT. Their interaction with AT is mediated by the same unique pentasaccharide sequence found on unfractionated heparin, but these sequences are found on less than one-third of LMWH molecules. Because a minimum chain length of 18 saccharides (including the pentasaccharide sequence) is required for the formation of ternary complexes among heparin chains, AT, and thrombin, only the LMWH species above this critical chain length are able to inactivate thrombin. In contrast, all LMWH chains that contain the high-affinity pentasaccharide catalyze the inactivation of factor Xa. Consequently, commercial LMWHs have antifactor Xa to antifactor IIa ratios that vary between 4:1 and 2:1, depending on their molecular size distribution. Because virtually all heparin molecules contain at least 18 saccharide units (104,105), heparin has an antifactor Xa to antifactor IIa ratio of 1:1.

Side Effects and Their Management

The primary toxicity of the LMWH is hemorrhage. Early studies suggested that bleeding was seen less frequently in patients treated with LMWH than in similar patients treated with unfractionated heparin. However, large clinical trials comparing unfractionated and standard heparin in patients with venous thromboembolism failed to find a reduced risk of hemorrhage consistently in patients treated with LMWH. Thus, whether LMWHs are associated with a clinically important reduction in the risk of bleeding is controversial (106). The management of bleeding in patients who are anticoagulated with LMWH is problematic. Protamine sulfate will neutralize all the antifactor IIa but only approximately 75% of the antifactor Xa effect of LMWH. The remaining antifactor Xa effect is not neutralizable by protamine. In a patient anticoagulated with LMWH who develops major or life-threatening bleeding, protamine sulfate should be administered, and appropriate surgical or endoscopic evaluations should be obtained. Sequential doses of protamine might be required, particularly after subcutaneous administration of LMWH, because of its prolonged half-life. Whether long-term LMWH is associated with osteoporosis is unknown; however, preliminary data suggest that this complication is less common than that with unfractionated heparin in pregnant patients (80). As in patients receiving standard heparin, the optimal therapy to prevent the development of osteoporosis is unknown; however, ensuring adequate intake of calcium and vitamin D seems appropriate.

DANAPAROID

Pharmacokinetics and Pharmacodynamics

Danaparoid is derived from porcine and bovine mucosa and is a heterogeneous mixture of heparan sulfate, dermatan sulfate, and chondroitin sulfate, all of which are polysulfated glycosaminoglycans with structural similarities to heparin. The principal anticoagulant effect of danaparoid is due to heparan sulfate, which catalyzes AT III–mediated inactivation of thrombin and factor Xa in a manner similar to that of heparin. Approximately 10% of the anticoagulant effect of the drug is due to dermatan sulfate–mediated catalysis of thrombin by heparin cofactor II. Danaparoid has less platelet inhibitory effect than heparin, which may account for its favorable antithrombotic to hemorrhagic ratio when compared to unfractionated heparin (107). The drug is administered parenterally and is available for subcutaneous and intravenous administration. After intravenous injection, the peak anticoagulant effect of danaparoid is achieved within minutes. After subcutaneous administration, the peak anticoagulant effect is delayed, although bioavailability is nearly 100% (108). The half-life of the AT effect of danaparoid is 4.3 hours, whereas its antifactor Xa activity has a half-life of 24.5 hours (108). Renal excretion accounts for 40% to 50% of plasma clearance of the antifactor Xa activity of danaparoid (108), and its pharmacokinetics are not affected by hepatic disease (109).

Danaparoid is usually administered in a fixed dose without laboratory monitoring, although its anticoagulant activity can be measured using antifactor Xa danaparoid levels, determined using a danaparoid calibration curve. The usual prophylactic dose of danaparoid is 750 to 1000 U antifactor Xa subcutane-

ously twice daily, a dose that has been shown to reduce significantly the risk of both proximal and total deep vein thrombosis when compared with unfractionated heparin in patients with thrombotic stroke (110). For treatment of patients with acute thrombosis, danaparoid is usually administered in a dose of 1250 to 2000 U antifactor Xa subcutaneously twice daily; in one study, the latter regimen was significantly more effective than unfractionated heparin in treatment of patients with deep vein thrombosis (111). If antifactor Xa heparin levels are monitored, a therapeutic range similar to that required for the LMWHs (i.e., 0.5 to 1.0 U/mL antifactor Xa) should be targeted.

Complications of Therapy and Their Management

The principal complication of danaparoid therapy is bleeding: Danaparoid appears to cause less bleeding than unfractionated heparin in animal models in which equivalent antithrombotic doses of heparin and danaparoid are administered (107). However, studies of sufficient power to verify this finding in patients receiving danaparoid have not been performed. When administered after an intravenous bolus of danaparoid, protamine sulfate will partially reverse its antifactor IIa effect but does not affect the antifactor Xa anticoagulant effect (112). Given its prolonged anticoagulant half-life, major or life-threatening bleeding in a patient who is therapeutically anticoagulated with danaparoid is problematic. As with the LMWHs, further doses of danaparoid should be withheld until the bleeding source has been corrected, protamine sulfate should be administered, and appropriate surgical or endoscopic interventions should be undertaken. Whether long-term danaparoid therapy is associated with osteoporosis is unknown; ensuring adequate calcium and vitamin D intake in patients receiving long-term danaparoid seems appropriate.

PENTASACCHARIDE

Inhibition of factor Xa by AT requires the formation of a complex consisting of heparin, AT, and factor Xa. The interaction between AT and factor Xa is mediated by a five-sugar sequence (pentasaccharide) located on all heparin molecules that have anticoagulant activity. The pentasaccharide sequence is the smallest glycosaminoglycan able to catalyze inactivation of factor Xa by AT (113) (Fig. 43-1). Pentasaccharide is too small to act as a template on which heparin can catalyze AT-mediated inactivation of thrombin; thus, unlike heparin or the LMWHs, pentasaccharide does not inactivate thrombin to any degree. Furthermore, because of its small molecular size, pentasaccharide does not bind to platelet factor 4 and thus should not cause or potentiate HIT (114). Pentasaccharide is chemically synthesized and is currently being evaluated as a therapeutic anticoagulant (115). In early-phase clinical trials, pentasaccharide appears at least as effective as current antithrombotic agents in a variety of patient populations, including patients undergoing percutaneous coronary interventions or elective orthopedic surgery (16,116,117). Although protamine does not neutralize the antifactor Xa effect of pentasaccharide, the administration of protamine to animals anticoagulated with pentasaccharide did reduce bleeding (118).

DIRECT THROMBIN INHIBITORS

Direct thrombin inhibitors are a new class of drugs designed to inactivate thrombin via specific, high-affinity interactions with the catalytic site on the thrombin molecule (Fig. 43-1). Three types of direct thrombin inhibitors are currently in clinical trials: polypeptide congeners of the leach anticoagulant (hirudins), synthetic arginine derivatives (argatroban), and orally bioavailable compounds that block the active site of thrombin.

Hirudin is the principal anticoagulant in the saliva of the medicinal leach, *Hirudo medicinalis*. Recombinant hirudin (r-hirudin) is now being tested in various clinical settings and is approved for use in patients with HIT.

Hirudin is not absorbed after oral administration and must be administered parenterally. The direct thrombin inhibitors have predictable pharmacokinetics when compared with unfractionated heparin (119,120), presumably due to their lack of plasma and cell-surface protein binding, which allows weight-based dosing and may allow these agents to be administered with little or no monitoring of their anticoagulant effect. The lack of protein binding also suggests that direct thrombin inhibitors are not inactivated at the site of thrombus formation by locally released proteins such as platelet factor 4. These proteins, which are released in the vicinity of a thrombus by platelets, bind to and reduce the local antithrombotic effect of heparin and related compounds.

After intravenous injection, the plasma half-life of r-hirudin is 2.8 hours. Intravenous infusion of r-hirudin produces steady-state plasma concentrations proportional to the infused dose (119). Covalent linkage of hirudin with polyethylene glycol (PEG) produces a molecule with a markedly prolonged half-life that has a similar anticoagulant effect to r-hirudin. r-Hirudin is cleared mainly by the kidneys; its half-life is markedly prolonged in patients with renal failure and patients on dialysis (121).

The anticoagulant effect of hirudin is maximal within minutes of intravenous injection; the peak effect is delayed several hours after subcutaneous injection. Hirudin does not require plasma cofactors, such as AT III or heparin cofactor II, for its antithrombotic effect. Unlike heparin and related compounds, direct thrombin inhibitors are not catalysts and are therefore consumed on a mole-to-mole basis as they inhibit thrombin. Thus, to be effective, direct thrombin inhibitors must be present in sufficient quantities at the site of a thrombus to inhibit thrombin activity and must be continually delivered to the thrombus to replace the drug that is consumed when it binds to thrombin.

Plasma r-hirudin levels can be determined using a chromogenic assay (122) or one of several immunoassays (123). Hirudin produces dose-dependent prolongation of thrombin-dependent clotting tests; therefore, its anticoagulant activity can be monitored using these tests (124,125). Thrombin clotting times are sensitive to low levels of hirudin but are not useful for measuring higher levels (126).

The major side effect of r-hirudin is bleeding, and there is no specific antidote for the anticoagulant effect of this direct thrombin inhibitor. Reversal of the anticoagulant effect of r-hirudin has been attempted using protein C-depleted activated prothrombinase complex (127) or desmopressin (dDAVP) (128,129); however, neither has been adequately studied in patients receiving clinically relevant doses of r-hirudin. Hirudin can be removed by dialysis using high-flux dialysis membranes, whereas PEG hirudin binds with high affinity to polymethylmethacrylate dialysis membranes. The hemorrhagic effects of direct thrombin inhibitors are clinically relevant; excess major bleeding (in particular intracerebral hemorrhage) in patients receiving r-hirudin has been seen in three trials of the drug in patients with coronary artery disease (46,47,130) but not in others for whom lower r-hirudin doses were used (48,131). PEG-hirudin is currently in clinical trials involving patients with acute coronary syndromes and patients with end-stage renal disease. Hirudin does not cause or potentiate HIT,

nor is it known to cause osteoporosis, two well-documented complications of unfractionated heparin.

Hirudin is a protein and is therefore potentially immunogenic. Thus, patients might develop neutralizing antibodies, or antibodies that can cause allergic reactions. These antibodies would limit the number of times that patients could receive r-hirudin. To date, however, the development of clinically important antihirudin antibodies has not been reported.

Bivalirudin is a synthetic congener of hirudin that combines the catalytic site and anion binding site–blocking actions of hirudin coupled by a 10-peptide joining sequence (132). Bivalirudin has a similar mechanism of action to hirudin, although it is metabolized by thrombin to a less active metabolite, which may reduce its antithrombotic effect. Bivalirudin has been studied in the treatment of acute coronary syndromes, including administration after percutaneous interventions, after thrombolysis, and for the treatment of venous thrombosis (133–136).

Argatroban is another parenteral direct thrombin inhibitor. This small molecule blocks the active site of thrombin and is currently in clinical trials. It is approved for use in patients with HIT and has been studied in patients with unstable coronary syndromes (137).

All currently available direct thrombin inhibitors require intravenous injection. However, several direct thrombin inhibitors that can be administered orally are currently entering clinical testing (138). All these direct thrombin inhibitors are small (<1000 d) and are synthetic compounds designed to block specifically the catalytic site of thrombin. These drugs share the favorable characteristics of hirudin (predictable pharmacokinetics, lack of protein binding, and lack of inhibition by platelet factor 4) and are not antigenic. They have short half-lives (4 to 6 hours in animal models) and are thus administered in a twice-daily dosing schedule. Early results of clinical trials in patients undergoing orthopedic surgery suggest that these agents have comparable efficacy to warfarin. Phase II and III clinical trials are currently under way comparing these agents with heparin or warfarin in patients with atrial fibrillation, acute coronary syndromes, and acute venous thromboembolism, and in the setting of orthopedic surgery. As with hirudin, there are no specific antidotes to these agents. Therefore, hemorrhage should be treated symptomatically. Whether these agents are removed by dialysis is unknown.

ORAL ANTICOAGULANTS: COUMARINS

Mechanism of Action: Inhibition of Coagulation Factor Synthesis

Coumarin and its derivatives are 4-hydroxycoumarin compounds that exert their anticoagulant effect by inhibiting the hepatic synthesis of the four vitamin K–dependent coagulation proteins, prothrombin, and factors VII, IX, and X (discussed in Chapter 37). The coumarin compounds in common clinical use are warfarin, acenocoumarol, and phenprocoumon. All vitamin K antagonists have the same mechanism of action but have different pharmacokinetic characteristics. They induce their anticoagulant effect by interfering with the cyclic interconversion of vitamin K and its vitamin K epoxide (139) (Fig. 43-3). Vitamin K is a cofactor for the posttranslational carboxylation of glutamate residues to γ-carboxyglutamates (Gla) on the N-terminal regions of vitamin K–dependent proteins [factors II (prothrombin), VII, IX, and X as well as protein C and protein S] (140). The process of γ-carboxylation permits the coagulation proteins to undergo a conformational change in the presence of calcium ions, a requirement for calcium-dependent complexing of vita-

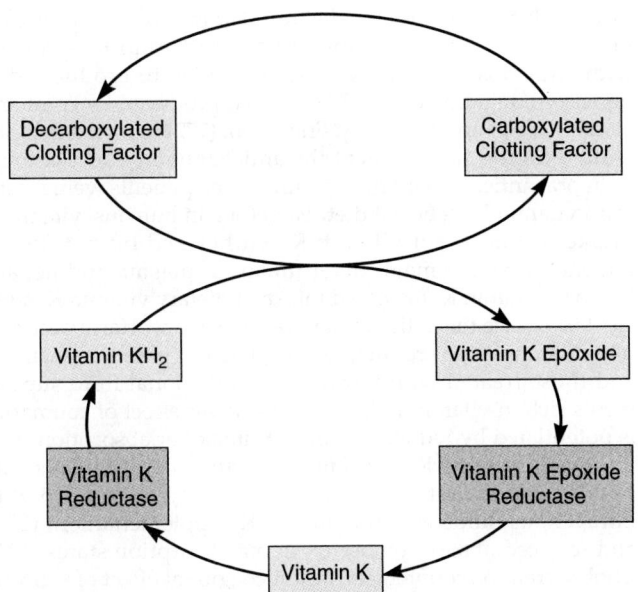

Figure 43-3. Mechanism of action of the vitamin K antagonists. γ-Carboxylation of coagulation factors II, VII, IX, and X is required for their interaction with phospholipid surfaces and thus their procoagulant effect. The formation of the γ-carboxyl residues requires reduced vitamin K; the vitamin K antagonists produce their effect by interfering with the regeneration of reduced vitamin K by competitively inhibiting two enzymes in the pathway, which regenerates reduced vitamin K (vitamin K epoxide reductase and vitamin K reductase).

min K–dependent proteins to their cofactors on phospholipid surfaces and for their biologic activity (141,142). Carboxylation of vitamin K–dependent coagulation factors is catalyzed by a carboxylase that requires the reduced form of vitamin K (vitamin KH_2), molecular oxygen, and carbon dioxide. During this reaction, vitamin KH_2 is oxidized to vitamin K epoxide, which is recycled to vitamin K by vitamin K epoxide reductase; vitamin K is, in turn, reduced to vitamin KH_2 by vitamin K (quinone) reductases (140,143). The coumarin drugs act as vitamin K antagonists by inhibiting vitamin K epoxide reductase and possibly vitamin K (quinone) reductase (144–146). This process leads to the effective intracellular depletion of vitamin KH_2 and limits γ-carboxylation of the glutamic acid residues of the vitamin K–dependent coagulant proteins (147,148). In addition, by limiting the carboxylation of protein C and protein S, the coumarins impair the function of these natural anticoagulant proteins (149). The effect of coumarins on the vitamin K–dependent clotting factors represents the basis of therapeutic anticoagulation and explains the prolongation of the prothrombin time (PT) used to monitor therapy.

Mechanism of Action:
The Antithrombotic Effect of Warfarin

The anticoagulant effect of warfarin (its ability to prolong clotting times) should be differentiated from its antithrombotic effect (its ability to reduce blood clotting). During the chronic phase of warfarin therapy, these two effects are closely correlated. However, during the initiation phase of warfarin therapy, they may be disassociated. After an initial oral warfarin dose, there is rapid (and nearly complete) absorption, but an anticoagulant effect, reflected by a rise in the international normalized ratio (INR), is delayed. This delay represents the time required for the des-carboxylated vitamin K–dependent clotting factors to replace the normal clotting factors as the latter are cleared

from the circulation. The early anticoagulant effect is caused by loss of fully carboxylated factor VII, which has a half-life of 6 hours, and their replacement with partially des-carboxylated proteins (147–150). Although the fall in factor VII occurs quickly and is associated with a rise in the INR, this reduction in the level of coagulation factor VII might not produce an antithrombotic effect. Rather, there is evidence that warfarin's antithrombotic effect requires reductions in the levels of the other three vitamin K–dependent clotting proteins (factors II, IX, and X). These clotting factors have considerably longer half-lives than factor VII (151), and therapeutic reductions in their levels require up to 60 hours. Support for the hypothesis that reductions in factor VII levels might not produce an antithrombotic effect comes from three lines of evidence. First, classic studies by Wessler and Gitel (152) demonstrated that the antithrombotic effect of vitamin K antagonists was delayed for up to 6 days irrespective of the effect of warfarin on the clotting times. Second, Zivelin et al. (153) demonstrated that reductions in the levels of factor X and II but not factor VII produced an antithrombotic effect in an animal model. Third, Patel et al. (154) demonstrated that clots formed from cord plasma, in which the prothrombin concentration is approximately 50% of control adult plasma, generated significantly less fibrinopeptide A (FPA) than clots formed from adult plasma. However, FPA generation by cord plasma clots became identical to that of adult plasma clots when the cord plasma was supplemented with adult levels of prothrombin.

The concept that the antithrombotic effect of warfarin reflects its ability to lower prothrombin levels is of potential clinical importance for the following reasons.

1. It provides a rationale for overlapping heparin with warfarin in the treatment of patients with thrombotic disease until the prothrombin level is lowered into the therapeutic range. Given that prothrombin has a half-life of approximately 60 hours, an overlap of at least 4 days is necessary to achieve this level.
2. It supports the contention of Furie et al. (155) that levels of native prothrombin antigen reflect the antithrombotic activity of warfarin more closely than the PT (INR) during warfarin therapy.
3. It supports the use of a maintenance dose of warfarin (approximately 5 mg) to initiate warfarin therapy, because based on recent studies (149,156), the rate of lowering of prothrombin levels is similar when warfarin treatment is initiated with either a 5-mg or a 10-mg dose. On the other hand, the level of the anticoagulant protein, protein C, was reduced more rapidly, producing a potential hypercoagulable state, and more patients were overanticoagulated (INR >3.0) with the 10-mg loading dose (149).

The delay in achieving an adequate antithrombotic effect, despite prolonged clotting times (e.g., the INR), has potential clinical importance because during this period, patients may have an added risk factor for thromboembolism. Thus, the natural anticoagulant protein, protein C, declines at a rate very similar to that observed with factor VII, and the resulting prothrombotic state could contribute to the observation that treatment of acute venous thromboembolism with oral anticoagulants alone (without concomitant heparin) results in an unacceptably high rate of early recurrence or extension of thrombosis (157,158).

The early decline in the levels of proteins C and S while levels of factors II and X remain near normal could also contribute to the syndrome of warfarin-induced skin necrosis. Patients with this condition present with necrotic skin lesions that develop 3 to 5 days after warfarin initiation (159). Pathologically, the condition is associated with microvascular venous thrombosis (159). Patients with hereditary forms of protein C or S deficiency are predisposed to warfarin-associated skin necrosis (160,161). The treatment of patients with warfarin-induced skin necrosis who require anticoagulant therapy for an indefinite period is problematic. Successful anticoagulation with warfarin has been reported when warfarin is reintroduced with low doses initially in combination with heparin for 10 to 14 days, during which time the warfarin dose is gradually increased (162). However, heparin treatment does not always prevent skin necrosis, and there are reports of heparin treatment failing to prevent continuing skin necrosis in patients with homozygous protein C deficiency who have very low protein C levels (163,164).

Pharmacokinetics

Warfarin is the most widely used oral anticoagulant in North America because its onset and duration of action are rapid and predictable and because it has excellent bioavailability (165). Warfarin is a racemic mixture of roughly equal amounts of two optically active isomers, the R and S forms. The isomeric composition of warfarin is important clinically, because S-warfarin is five times as potent as the R-form, and they are cleared by different pathways (166). Therefore, inhibition of the metabolic clearance of the S-isomer by drugs enhances the anticoagulant effect of warfarin much more than does the inhibition of metabolic clearance of the R-isomer. Warfarin is rapidly absorbed from the gastrointestinal tract and reaches maximal blood concentrations in healthy volunteers in 90 minutes (165,167). In healthy volunteers, warfarin has a half-life of 47 hours, with a prolonged, dose-dependent terminal phase of elimination associated with detectable levels of warfarin beyond 120 hours after a single dose (168). Warfarin rapidly accumulates in the liver, where it is metabolized into products that have little anticoagulant activity (169). The anticoagulant response to coumarins varies both within and among individuals; therefore, the dosage of coumarins must be monitored closely to prevent inappropriate dosing. The dose response to warfarin is influenced by both pharmacokinetic factors (differences in absorption or metabolic clearance of warfarin) and pharmacodynamic factors (differences in the hemostatic response to given concentrations of warfarin). Technical factors also contribute to the variability in the INR response, including inaccuracies in laboratory testing and reporting, poor patient compliance, and poor communication between patient and physician.

Alterations in Pharmacokinetics and Pharmacodynamics

The pharmacokinetics and pharmacodynamics of warfarin are influenced by vitamin K intake and absorption, by metabolic clearance of warfarin, by rates of synthesis and clearance of vitamin K–dependent clotting factors, and by drugs or disorders that impair blood coagulation or platelet function. The events leading to alterations in pharmacokinetics or pharmacodynamics occur in the gut, the plasma, and the liver, and at the site of hemostatic plug formation.

Subjects receiving coumarin therapy are sensitive to fluctuating levels of vitamin K caused by variability in dietary intake and in gut absorption of the vitamin (170). In humans, vitamin K is obtained predominantly from phylloquinones in leafy green vegetables and other plant material. Bacteria in the large bowel synthesize menaquinones (vitamin K_2) but are not an important source of vitamin K in humans. Thus, in a study of human volunteers receiving long-term warfarin therapy, treat-

ment with a vitamin K–free diet resulted in a marked prolongation of the PT, whereas suppression of vitamin K_2 synthesis with large doses of neomycin sulfate failed to produce additional prolongation of the PT over that produced by coumarin alone (171). In another study, Frick et al. (172) reported that oral antibiotics did not augment the anticoagulant effect of long-term oral anticoagulant therapy unless the patients were receiving a vitamin K–deficient diet. Therefore, in humans, vitamin K intake in food—not vitamin K synthesized by gut flora—appears to be the major determinant of plasma and hepatic levels of vitamin K. Increased intake of dietary vitamin K_1 sufficient to reduce the anticoagulant response to warfarin occurs in patients on weight reduction diets (rich in green vegetables) and those treated with intravenous nutritional fluid supplements rich in vitamin K. The anticoagulant effect of coumarins is potentiated by reduced vitamin K intake or absorption from the small intestine. Reduced intake occurs in sick patients with poor vitamin K intake (often because they are treated with intravenous fluids without vitamin K supplementation) (173), and reduced absorption occurs in malabsorption states (174). Cholestyramine counteracts the anticoagulant effect of warfarin by binding the vitamin K antagonist in the intestinal tract and reducing its absorption by increasing the excretion of the unchanged drug in the stool (175).

At therapeutic concentrations, 99% of circulating warfarin is bound to albumin, and the remaining 1% circulates unbound (165,166). The unbound fraction of warfarin binds to its receptor on hepatic cells, where it exerts its anticoagulant effect. Therefore, it might be expected that drugs that increase the concentration of the unbound warfarin by displacing it from albumin would potentiate the anticoagulant effect of warfarin. However, clear examples of the potentiation of the anticoagulant effect of warfarin by displacement from albumin have not been reported, possibly because any potential for an increased pharmacologic effect of the unbound fraction of warfarin is counteracted by its more rapid clearance (165,176).

The liver plays a central role in modulating the anticoagulant effect of vitamin K antagonists. It is the site of the pharmacologic action of coumarins; the site of synthesis of coagulation factors, including the vitamin K–dependent coagulation factors; and the site of metabolic clearance of coumarins and of coagulation proteins. As a result of these diverse actions, the liver can both potentiate and oppose the anticoagulant effect of coumarins.

Genetic factors can influence the anticoagulant response to warfarin. A recently identified common mutation in the gene coding for cytochrome P450, the hepatic enzyme responsible for oxidative metabolism of the S-isomer of warfarin (177,178), is thought to contribute to the variability in dose response to warfarin among healthy subjects (179). Hereditary resistance to warfarin has been described in rats (180) and humans (181). The affected humans require warfarin in doses 5-fold to 20-fold higher than average to achieve an anticoagulant effect. This disorder is thought to be caused by an altered affinity of the receptor for warfarin because plasma warfarin levels required to achieve an anticoagulant effect are much higher than average. More recently, a mutation in the propeptide of factor IX has been described that can cause bleeding without excessive prolongation of the INR (182,183). Patients with this disorder have factor IX activity within the normal range in the absence of coumarins, but their factor IX assay decreases precipitously to levels of 1% to 3% during anticoagulant treatment, even though the other vitamin K–dependent coagulation factors are decreased to only approximately 30% to 40%. The decline in the levels of factor IX is not reflected in an increase in the INR because the INR is not influenced by factor IX levels. Analysis of the gene for factor IX revealed two different missense mutations involv-

TABLE 43-4. Drugs That Modify Anticoagulant Effect of Coumarin Anticoagulants

Effect	Drug	Mechanism (If Known)
Potentiation	Cotrimoxazole	Reduced clearance of S enantiomer
	Erythromycin	Reduced nonstereoselective clearance
	Fluconazole	Reduced nonstereoselective clearance
	Isoniazid	—
	Metronidazole	—
	Miconazole	Reduced clearance of R and S enantiomers
	Amiodarone	Reduced nonstereoselective clearance
	Clofibrate	—
	Propafenone	—
	Propranolol	—
	Sulfinpyrazone	Reduced clearance of S enantiomer
	Phenylbutazone	Reduced nonstereoselective clearance
	Piroxicam	—
	Cimetidine	Reduced clearance of R enantiomer
	Omeprazole	Reduced clearance of R enantiomer
	Corticosteroids	—
	Mycophenolate	—
Inhibition	Griseofulvin	—
	Nafcillin	Enhanced warfarin clearance
	Rifampin	Enhanced nonstereoselective clearance
	Cholestyramine	Enhanced warfarin absorption
	Barbiturates	Enhanced nonstereoselective clearance
	Carbamazepine	Enhanced warfarin clearance
	Chlordiazepoxide	—
	Sucralfate	—

ing the propeptide coding region (183) that are expressed as a selective increase in the sensitivity of coumarin-mediated reduction of factor IX activity. The mutation is uncommon and has been estimated to occur in less than 1.5% of the population.

Many drugs have the potential to interact with coumarins or to prolong the PT when taken in combination with oral anticoagulants; however, in most of these reports, convincing evidence of a causal association is lacking (175) (Table 43-4). Nevertheless, it is prudent to monitor the INR more frequently when prescribing any new drug, changing the dose of a currently administered drug, or discontinuing a drug in patients treated with oral anticoagulants. The anticoagulant effect of warfarin is potentiated by drugs that inhibit its metabolic clearance either through stereoselective or nonselective pathways (166,184). The metabolic clearance of the more potent S-warfarin is inhibited by trimethoprim-sulfamethoxazole and sulfinpyrazone, both of which have been documented to potentiate the anticoagulant effect of coumarins (175). In contrast, drugs such as cimetidine and omeprazole, which inhibit the metabolic clearance of the less potent R-isomer, have only a moderate potentiating effect on warfarin (185,186). Amiodarone, a drug that inhibits the metabolic clearance of both the S- and R-isomers through a nonstereospecific pathway, has an important potentiating effect on warfarin's anticoagulant effect (175). Intake of 9100 mg/week or more of acetaminophen increases the risk of an INR of more than 6.0 by tenfold (95% confidence interval, 2.6 to 37.9) (187). Other drugs that potentiate the anticoagulant effect of the coumarins are listed in Table 43-4. Chronic alcohol use has the potential to increase the clearance of warfarin by hepatic enzyme induction, reducing the anticoagulant effect of coumarins (187,188). However, a study has shown that even relatively high wine consumption does not influence the PT in subjects treated with warfarin (189). Hepatic dysfunction can potentiate the response to warfarin through impaired synthesis of coagulation factors. Hypermetabolic states produced by fever, treatment with thyroxine, or hyperthyroidism potenti-

ate the effect of coumarins, probably by increasing the catabolism of vitamin K–dependent coagulation factors (190,191).

The hemorrhagic effect of coumarins is potentiated by drugs that inhibit platelet function. The most common are aspirin, ticlopidine, clopidogrel, other nonsteroidal antiinflammatory drugs (NSAIDs), high doses of penicillins, and moxalactam. Aspirin is the most important because of its widespread use and prolonged effect on hemostasis. Unlike the NSAIDs, aspirin produces an irreversible inhibition of platelet function as a result of binding to and inactivation of platelet cyclooxygenase (192,193). Aspirin can also produce gastric erosions, which increase the risk of serious upper gastrointestinal bleeding. The risk of clinically important bleeding is increased when high doses of aspirin (which increase the risk of gastric erosions) are used in combination with high-intensity warfarin therapy (INR 3.0 to 4.5) (194–196).

Aspirin and the NSAIDs produce their antiplatelet effect by blocking the activity of cyclooxygenase (COX). COX-2 inhibitors have recently become available; by selectively inhibiting COX-2, these agents should have little or no platelet inhibitory activity but should retain their antiinflammatory activity. Thus, in patients requiring an antiinflammatory medication, these agents should likely be used in preference to acetylsalicylic acid or other NSAIDs.

Adverse Effects

Bleeding is the main complication of oral anticoagulant therapy. Randomized studies have shown that the risk of bleeding is influenced by the intensity of anticoagulant therapy (Table 43-5). In these studies, the risk of clinically important bleeding is reduced by lowering the therapeutic range from 3.0 to 4.5 down to 2.0 to 3.0. Although this difference in anticoagulant intensity is produced by a reduction of the average daily dose of warfarin of only approximately 1 mg, the effect on bleeding is profound. Multivariate analysis of cohort studies also suggests that the risk of bleeding is influenced by comorbid conditions (197,198). These studies reported that the risk of major bleeding is increased by age older than 65 years, a history of stroke or gastrointestinal bleeding, and the presence of serious comorbid conditions such as renal insufficiency or anemia (199–201). Bleeding that occurs when the INR is less than 3.0 is often associated with an obvious underlying cause or an occult gastrointestinal or renal lesion (202,203). Community-based studies of the frequency of hemorrhage in patients receiving warfarin estimate that bleeding will occur in 1.6%, 3.3%, 5.3%, and 10.6% of patients after 1, 3, 12, and 24 months of therapy, respectively (204).

TABLE 43-5. Relationship between Intensity of Oral Anticoagulant Therapy and Bleeding Risk

Study	Patients (n)	Target International Normalized Ratio	Bleeding Risk (%)
Hull et al. (202)	96	3.0–4.5	22.4
		2.0–2.5	4.3
Turpie et al. (62)	210	2.5–4.0	13.9
		2.0–2.5	5.9
Saour et al. (264)	247	7.4–10.8	42.4
		1.9–3.6	21.3
Altman et al. (199)	99	3.0–4.5	24.0
		2.0–2.9	6.0

Adapted from Hirsh J, Dalen JE, Anderson DR, et al. Oral anticoagulants: mechanism of action, clinical effectiveness, and optimal therapeutic range. *Chest* 1998;114 [Suppl 5]:445S–469S.

Management of Patients with High International Normalized Ratio Values or Patients Who Bleed While Receiving Warfarin

MANAGEMENT OF ASYMPTOMATIC PROLONGATION OF THE INTERNATIONAL NORMALIZED RATIO VALUE

Patients receiving warfarin frequently have excessively prolonged INR results, which can be due to the use of concomitant medications, the presence of comorbid illnesses, or dietary changes, or they may occur for no apparent reason (175). Numerous studies have demonstrated that patients receiving warfarin frequently are found to have INR results above the therapeutic range, and that such elevations are an independent predictor for major bleeding (205), a result confirmed by other investigations (64,202,206). In a large randomized trial, Kearon et al. (63) found that 14% of the time, patients receiving warfarin with a target INR of 2.0 to 3.0 had INR values above 3.0. In this study, the annual risk of hemorrhage was 3.8%, and two of three major bleeds occurred in patients with INR values above 4.5. These findings suggest that asymptomatic prolongation of the INR value above the desired therapeutic range is a frequent and clinically important problem, and that strategies that safely and effectively reduce the INR value should be developed.

There is no generally accepted method to reduce an excessively prolonged INR in patients receiving warfarin. In some centers, warfarin is withheld and the INR allowed to fall into the therapeutic range (207). Although this method is safe in most patients, it is clear that the longer the patient has a supratherapeutic INR result and the greater the prolongation of the INR, the higher the risk of bleeding (208,209). Because of concerns about the risk of hemorrhage, vitamin K is often administered to patients with a supratherapeutic INR value. Intravenous or subcutaneous vitamin K is associated with three potential adverse experiences: (a) overreversal of the warfarin effect when high doses of vitamin K are used, resulting in long periods of warfarin resistance (210,211), (b) anaphylactoid reactions when administered by rapid intravenous injection (212–214), and (c) skin reactions when administered subcutaneously (215–226). In addition, parenteral administration is inconvenient and requires a visit to a health care provider. Oral vitamin K has the potential to avoid these complications: low doses are unlikely to overreverse the anticoagulant effect of warfarin, and anaphylactoid or skin reactions have not been reported in patients receiving oral vitamin K (227–229). Further, oral vitamin K does not require injection and, in most jurisdictions, is an over-the-counter product. Therefore, it can be administered by the patient, nurse, or pharmacist without a physician's prescription.

Patients receiving warfarin who present with an elevated INR should be screened clinically for ongoing or recent bleeding. In patients with active, major bleeding, plasma in combination with parenteral vitamin K should be administered and will quickly reduce the INR to the normal range. Because of the cost and risks of plasma therapy, it should be used only in patients with an acute indication for the immediate reversal of the anticoagulant effect of warfarin and should be administered in concert with parenteral vitamin K.

Four acceptable therapeutic strategies can be used in patients with asymptomatic prolongation of the INR who do not have an indication for immediate and complete reversal of excessive anticoagulation due to warfarin. These are (a) no treatment, allowing a spontaneous decline in the INR (207), (b) intravenous vitamin K (211,230,231), (c) subcutaneous vitamin K (210,230–232), and (d) oral vitamin K (210,211,228,229,233). The safety of no treatment has been examined in one retrospective cohort series of 48 patients (207). Intravenous vitamin K has been used in several published series. Shetty et al. (211) administered 1.0 mg or 0.5 mg of vitamin K_1 intravenously to consecutive patients presenting with excess warfarin effect. Five of ten patients receiving 1.0 mg had overreversal of anticoagulation (INR <2.0 at 24 hours), whereas two patients had persistent prolongation of INR at 24 hours. Of the 21 patients receiving 0.5 mg intravenously, seven had an INR greater than 3.0 at 24 hours, whereas none was overreversed. Two recent studies (230,231) have compared the utility of intravenous and subcutaneous vitamin K. Both of these small randomized studies demonstrated that subcutaneous vitamin K reduced the INR value more slowly than intravenous vitamin K. These findings call into question the clinical use of subcutaneous vitamin K, because intravenous vitamin K is clearly superior for rapid correction of an elevated INR value.

Oral vitamin K was evaluated in a randomized clinical trial of 92 patients performed by Crowther et al. (229). In this study, patients presenting with asymptomatic INR values of 4.5 to 10.0 were randomly allocated to 1 mg vitamin K administered orally or matching placebo. Twenty-five of 45 evaluable patients who received vitamin K and 9 of 44 who received placebo had INR values less than 3.2 on the day after study drug administration (p <.05). Similar results were reported by Pengo et al. (228). Other publications that have demonstrated the effectiveness of oral vitamin K include retrospective case series published by Weibert et al. (234), Whitling et al. (210), and Wentzien et al. (233), and two large prospective case series (235,236).

MANAGEMENT OF PATIENTS RECEIVING WARFARIN WHO BLEED

The treatment of patients who bleed while receiving oral anticoagulants must be individualized and depends on several factors, including the severity and location of the hemorrhage and the INR when bleeding occurs. For patients who have relatively minor bleeding from an accessible site, such as nose bleeding or wound bleeding, local compression with or without a reduction or discontinuation of warfarin may suffice. Patients who bleed while their INR is elevated (i.e., >3.0) may respond to a reduction of the dose of warfarin. For patients with more severe hemorrhage or hemorrhage that is intracranial or retroperitoneal, more aggressive management is necessary. Administration of vitamin K by the intravenous route in combination with either fresh frozen plasma or prothrombinase complex will result in an immediate and sustained reduction in the INR value. Doses of vitamin K as small as 1 mg used in combination with plasma or coagulation complexes are effective for this indication (211).

The long-term treatment of patients who have bled on warfarin and who require protection against systemic embolism (e.g., patients with mechanical heart valves or with atrial fibrillation and other risk factors) is problematic. If bleeding occurs when the INR is above the therapeutic range, warfarin treatment can often be started when bleeding stops and the cause (if identified) is corrected. More careful attention to warfarin control might then reduce the risk of undesired, recurrent prolongation of the INR. If bleeding occurs while the patient's INR is in the therapeutic range, treatment is more problematic. For patients with mechanical prosthetic valves (and a persisting risk of increased bleeding), it would be reasonable to aim for a less intense INR of 2.0 to 2.5 (rather than 2.5 to 3.5). For patients with atrial fibrillation (and a persisting risk of increased bleeding), the anticoagulant target range can be reduced from 2.0 to 3.0 down to 1.5 to 2.0, with the expectation that efficacy will be reduced but not abolished (237). Alternatively, aspirin can replace warfarin in patients with atrial fibrillation because it is associated with a lower risk of bleeding (but a higher risk of stroke) (238).

MANAGEMENT OF PATIENTS ON LONG-TERM WARFARIN WHO REQUIRE SURGERY

Patients frequently require temporary discontinuation of warfarin, most commonly for intervention such as surgery or dental work. The optimal management during this period is controversial. Many patients have a low risk of thrombosis during short periods of inadequate anticoagulation; these patients can be managed by simply withholding their warfarin therapy for 4 or 5 days before the procedure and restarting warfarin at their maintenance dose at the earliest possible time after the procedure. This strategy is likely to be associated with a low risk of hemorrhage and an acceptable risk of thrombosis and has been advocated in a recent review (239). In other patients, the risk of thrombosis (perceived or real) could be sufficiently high to justify the use of parenteral anticoagulants during the period of inadequate oral anticoagulation. Many such patients receive in-hospital, intravenous unfractionated heparin in the preoperative period, then heparin and warfarin begun in the immediate postoperative period, with the heparin continued until adequate oral anticoagulation had been achieved (240). This strategy is likely to be associated with a low risk of thrombosis and an increased risk of hemorrhage (compared to a strategy in which parenteral anticoagulants are not used) and is both expensive and resource-intensive. An alternative strategy is to administer full doses of LMWH for 2 to 3 days in the immediate preoperative period, followed postoperatively with warfarin and prophylactic doses of LMWH until an adequate oral anticoagulant effect is achieved.

Although evidence-based recommendations for treatment of patients receiving warfarin who require surgical intervention must await randomized trials, several approaches can be used. The first approach is to stop warfarin 4 to 5 days before surgery and administer postoperative antithrombotic prophylaxis consisting of low-dose unfractionated heparin (5000 U subcutaneously twice daily) and warfarin. The second approach is to stop warfarin 4 to 5 days before surgery, replacing the warfarin with unfractionated heparin or LMWH begun in the preoperative period. Postoperatively, low-dose heparin (unfractionated or low-molecular-weight) and warfarin are begun and the heparin is continued until the INR has returned to the therapeutic range. The third approach is to stop warfarin 4 to 5 days before surgery and replace the warfarin with therapeutic-dose heparin (unfractionated or low-molecular-weight). Heparin therapy can be administered by subcutaneous injection to an outpatient or administered as a continuous intravenous infusion when the patient is admitted to the hospital. The intravenous heparin is discontinued 6 hours before surgery with the expectation that its anticoagulant effect will cease by the time of surgery. A fourth approach is to continue warfarin at a lower than normal dose and operate on the patient when the INR is in the 1.3 to 1.5 range, an intensity that has been shown to be safe in randomized trials of gynecologic and orthopedic surgical patients. The dose of warfarin can be lowered 4 to 5 days before surgery. Warfarin can be restarted postoperatively at its usual dose, supplemented with low-dose heparin (5000 U subcutaneously) if necessary.

In addition, for many patients requiring dental or ocular surgical procedures, warfarin can be safely continued without an unacceptably high risk of hemorrhage (241–245). Alternately, tranexamic acid or ε-aminocaproic acid mouthwash can be used in patients undergoing dental procedures without interrupting anticoagulant therapy (246,247).

Discontinuation of Anticoagulant Therapy

Oral anticoagulant therapy may be discontinued temporarily or permanently. In either case, simply stopping oral anticoagulant intake should result in normal levels of coagulation factors within 4 to 7 days of the last dose. As during the initiation phase of warfarin therapy, the INR in the period immediately after warfarin is discontinued may not accurately reflect the degree of impairment of coagulation present in a patient, because the initial fall in the INR is likely due to rising levels of coagulation factor VII despite continued depression of the levels of coagulation factors II and X. The clinical importance of this phenomenon is unknown. To determine the time course of change in INR after warfarin discontinuation, White et al. (248) performed a cohort study in which patients receiving warfarin who had an average INR of 2.6 stopped their warfarin and had their INR value followed serially. The mean INR 2.7 days after warfarin was discontinued was 1.6, and 20 of 22 patients had INR values above 1.2, whereas after 4.7 days had passed, the mean INR was 1.1, with only 5 of 22 patients having INR values above 1.2. Five patients were studied in detail and demonstrated that the INR declined precipitously with a half-life of 0.5 to 1.2 days after the discontinuation of warfarin. The patient's age correlated inversely with the rate of fall of the INR. These authors concluded that normal coagulation is not achieved for a minimum of 4 days after discontinuation of warfarin, and there is substantial interindividual variation in the rate of fall of the INR.

Use of Oral Anticoagulants during Pregnancy

Oral anticoagulants cross the placenta and can produce a characteristic embryopathy if administered between 6 and 12 weeks of gestation, as well as central nervous system abnormalities or fetal bleeding at any time during the pregnancy (249). Therefore, warfarin should not be administered between 6 and 12 weeks' gestation, and, if possible, warfarin should be avoided throughout pregnancy. As a result, heparin is the anticoagulant of choice in the majority of patients who require anticoagulation during pregnancy. Reports of heparin failure in patients with mechanical heart valves (250) have led some authorities to recommend the use of warfarin in the second and early third trimester despite the risk of embryopathy and bleeding. Whether reports of valve thrombosis during pregnancy in heparin-treated patients represent true heparin failure or inadequate dosing is uncertain. However, the reports do emphasize the need for careful monitoring and appropriate dose adjustment of heparin during pregnancy. Unfractionated heparin treatment should be administered subcutaneously twice daily, starting with a dose of approximately 35,000 U/day.

Warfarin can be started immediately after delivery because there is convincing evidence that warfarin does not induce an anticoagulant effect in the breast-fed infant (251,252).

Warfarin Dosing and Monitoring

The PT is the most common method for monitoring oral anticoagulant therapy (253). The PT is responsive to depression of three of the four vitamin K–dependent procoagulant clotting factors (prothrombin and factors VII and X). These factors are reduced by warfarin at a rate proportionate to their respective half-lives. The PT assay is performed by adding a mixture of calcium and thromboplastin to citrated plasma. Thromboplastin is a recombinant or tissue-derived phospholipid–protein product that contains both tissue factor and the phospholipid necessary to promote the activation of factor X by factor VII. During induction of anticoagulant therapy, the PT reflects primarily the depression of factor VII because this factor has the shortest half-life (6 hours) of the vitamin K–dependent factors (149,150). During maintenance therapy, the test is sensitive to depression of prothrombin, factor X, and factor VII. The responsiveness of a given thromboplastin to coumarin-induced reduction in clotting factors mirrors its potential for factor X activation. A responsive or weak thromboplastin results in a greater prolongation of the PT for a given reduction in clotting factors because it is more sensitive to reduction in the plasma concentrations of these factors. Thromboplastins vary markedly in their responsiveness depending on the tissue of origin and the method of preparation; therefore, PT results reported using different reagents are not interchangeable among laboratories (254–258). To allow comparison of PT values among and within individuals when they are determined using different thromboplastins, a calibration system was developed based on the assumption that a linear relationship exists between the logarithm of the PT ratios obtained with reference and test thromboplastins. This calibration model was endorsed by the World Health Organization in 1982 and is used to standardize the reporting of the PT by converting the PT ratio observed with any local thromboplastin into an INR, which is calculated as

$$INR = observed\ PT\ ratio^C$$

where the PT ratio is patient PT divided by control PT, and C is the power value representing the international sensitivity index (ISI) for each thromboplastin. The ISI is a measure of the responsiveness of a given thromboplastin to reduction of the vitamin K–dependent coagulation factors; the lower the ISI, the more responsive the reagent and the closer the derived INR will be to the observed PT ratio. The INR is the PT ratio that would be obtained if the World Health Organization reference thromboplastin itself (ISI = 1.0) had been used to perform the PT (255,259). Suggested target INR values for various clinical conditions are presented in Table 43-6.

Initiating Warfarin: Optimal Initial Warfarin Doses and Monitoring

Before the mid-1970s, very large warfarin loading doses (up to 1 mg/kg on day 1 of therapy) were administered to patients initi-

ating warfarin. Doses of this magnitude produce rapid increases in the INR, with values of more than 2.0 frequently obtained within 24 hours of the first dose. These large initial warfarin doses are unnecessary, as demonstrated by O'Reilly and Aggeler (260). Much smaller loading doses of 10 mg on the first 2 days of warfarin therapy produce effective anticoagulation in a high proportion of patients (261). Even lower doses are effective. For example, in two randomized clinical trials that compared the effectiveness of initial 5-mg and 10-mg warfarin doses, Harrison et al. (149) and Crowther et al. (156) demonstrated that an initial warfarin dose of 10 mg did not hasten the achievement of a stable INR between 2.0 and 3.0.

Traditionally, warfarin therapy has been initiated using a fixed dose, with subsequent doses based on the INR, which is often measured daily or every other day. With the more frequent use LMWH for the outpatient treatment of deep vein thrombosis, there has been an impetus to develop warfarin dosing strategies that reduce the requirement for initial INR monitoring. Smaller initial warfarin doses reduce the need for INR monitoring because fewer patients develop INR values above 3.0 in the initial days of warfarin therapy. To date, there have been no published randomized clinical trials that examine the optimal schedule for the monitoring of warfarin therapy during the initial days of oral anticoagulation. Whether reduced monitoring of the INR during the initial days of warfarin therapy is safe and effective can be determined only by appropriately designed clinical trials. Anecdotal experience suggests that determining the INR on the day of the third and sixth doses of warfarin is adequate monitoring for the majority of patients. Few patients appear to develop clinically important overanticoagulation when their INR values are monitored only on the third and sixth days of therapy, and it is often possible to discontinue LMWH on the day of the sixth dose of warfarin if the INR is between 2.0 and 3.0. However, this strategy has not been tested in a clinical trial.

Once the INR has stabilized, the INR can be determined less frequently. Many patients with stable INR responses while taking warfarin may require INR monitoring as infrequently as once every 4 to 6 weeks. If dose adjustments are required, the cycle of more frequent monitoring is repeated until a stable dose response is again achieved. Some patients receiving long-term warfarin therapy are difficult to treat because they have unexpected fluctuations in dose response. Others have unexplained increases in dosage requirements over time. The unexpected fluctuations in dose response could be due to changes in diet, undisclosed drug use, poor compliance, surreptitious self-medication, intermittent alcohol consumption, intercurrent illness, or variability in the responsiveness of the thromboplastin used to perform the PT either among different laboratories or with different lots of PT reagents. This latter potential cause, which is often not appreciated by physicians, can occur because the ISI values reported by the manufacturer can be inaccurate.

TABLE 43-6. Target International Normalized Ratio Intensity for Selected Conditions

Condition	Recommended INR Range
Prevention of venous thromboembolism	
Hip surgery	2.0–3.0
Major gynecologic surgery	2.0–3.0
Semipermanent percutaneous catheters	1 mg warfarin daily
Patients with breast cancer receiving chemotherapy	1 mg warfarin followed by warfarin with target INR of 1.5
Treatment of venous thromboembolism	2.0–3.0
Primary prevention of myocardial ischemia	1.3–1.8 ± aspirin
Acute myocardial infarction	
Prevention of stroke and venous thromboembolism	2.0–3.0
Prevention of recurrent infarction, stroke, and death	2.5–3.5
Prosthetic heart valves	2.5–3.5 ± low-dose aspirin
Atrial fibrillation	2.0–3.0
Significant mitral valve disease in the absence of atrial fibrillation	2.0–3.0
Previous arterial embolic disease	2.0–3.0
Prevention of recurrent thrombosis in patients with antiphospholipid antibodies	2.5–3.5

INR, international normalized ratio.
Adapted from Hirsh J, Dalen JE, Anderson DR, et al. Oral anticoagulants: mechanism of action, clinical effectiveness, and optimal therapeutic range. Chest 1998;114 [Suppl 5]:445S–469S.

REFERENCES

1. Collins C, MacMahon S, Flather M, et al. Clinical effects of anticoagulant therapy in suspected acute myocardial infarction: systematic overview of randomized trials. BMJ 1996;313:652–659.
2. Warkentin TE, Levine MN, Hirsh J, et al. Heparin-induced thrombocytopenia in patients treated with low-molecular-weight heparin or unfractionated heparin. N Engl J Med 1995;332:1330–1335.
3. Dahlman T, Lindvall N, Hellgren M. Osteopenia in pregnancy during long-term heparin treatment: a radiological study post partum. Br J Obstet Gynaecol 1990;97:221–228.
4. Ginsberg JS, Kowalchuk G, Hirsh J, et al. Heparin effect on bone density. Thromb Haemost 1990;64:286–289.
5. Douketis JD, Ginsberg JS, Burrows RF, et al. The effects of long-term heparin therapy during pregnancy on bone density: a prospective matched cohort study. Thromb Haemost 1996;75:254–257.

6. Hirsh J, Warkentin TE, Raschke R, et al. Heparin and low-molecular-weight heparin: mechanisms of action, pharmacokinetics, dosing considerations, monitoring, efficacy, and safety. *Chest* 1998;114[Suppl 5]:489S–510S.

7. Rosenberg RD, Lam L. Correlation between structure and function of heparin. *Proc Natl Acad Sci U S A* 1979;76(3):1218–1222.

8. Lindahl U, Backstrom G, Hook M, et al. Structure of the antithrombin-binding site in heparin. *Proc Natl Acad Sci U S A* 1979;76:3198–3202.

9. Choay J, Petitou M, Lormeau JC, et al. Structure-activity relationship in heparin: a synthetic pentasaccharide with high affinity for antithrombin III and eliciting high anti-factor Xa activity. *Biochem Biophys Res Commun* 1983;116: 492–499.

10. Tollefsen DM, Majerus DW, Blank MK. Heparin cofactor II: purification and properties of a heparin-dependent inhibitor of thrombin in human plasma. *J Biol Chem* 1982;257:2162–2169.

11. Casu B, Oreste P, Torri G, et al. The structure of heparin oligosaccharide fragments with high anti- (factor Xa) activity containing the minimal antithrombin III-binding sequence: chemical and 13C nuclear-magnetic-resonance studies. *Biochem J* 1981;197:599–609.

12. Lindahl U, Thunberg L, Backstrom G, et al. Extension and structural variability of the antithrombin-binding sequence in heparin. *J Biol Chem* 1984; 259:12368–12376.

13. Lane DA, Denton J, Flynn AM, et al. Anticoagulant activities of heparin oligosaccharides and their neutralization by platelet factor 4. *Biochem J* 1984; 218:725–732.

14. Oosta GM, Gardner WT, Beeler DL, et al. Multiple functional domains of the heparin molecule. *Proc Natl Acad Sci U S A* 1981;78:829–833.

15. Nesheim ME. A simple rate law that describes the kinetics of the heparin-catalyzed reaction between antithrombin III and thrombin. *J Biol Chem* 1983; 258:14708–14717.

16. Vuillemenot A, Schiele F, Meneveau N, et al. Efficacy of a synthetic pentasaccharide, a pure factor Xa inhibitor, as an antithrombotic agent—a pilot study in the setting of coronary angioplasty. *Thromb Haemost* 1999;81:214–220.

17. Ofosu FA, Sie P, Modi GJ, et al. The inhibition of thrombin-dependent positive-feedback reactions is critical to the expression of the anticoagulant effect of heparin. *Biochem J* 1987;243:579–588.

18. Ofosu FA, Hirsh J, Esmon CT, et al. Unfractionated heparin inhibits thrombin-catalysed amplification reactions of coagulation more efficiently than those catalysed by factor Xa. *Biochem J* 1989;257:143–150.

19. Beguin S, Lindhout T, Hemker HC. The mode of action of heparin in plasma. *Thromb Haemost* 1988;60:457–462.

20. Eika C. Inhibition of thrombin induced aggregation of human platelets by heparin. *Scand J Haematol* 1971;8:216–222.

21. Kelton JG, Hirsh J. Bleeding associated with antithrombotic therapy. *Semin Hematol* 1980;17:259–291.

22. Fernandez F, N'Guyen P, Van Ryn J, et al. Hemorrhagic doses of heparin and other glycosaminoglycans induce a platelet defect. *Thromb Res* 1986;43:491–495.

23. Blajchman MA, Young E, Ofosu FA. Effects of unfractionated heparin, dermatan sulfate and low molecular weight heparin on vessel wall permeability in rabbits. *Ann N Y Acad Sci* 1989;556:245–254.

24. Ockelford PA, Carter CJ, Mitchell L, et al. Discordance between the anti-Xa activity and the antithrombotic activity in an ultra-low molecular weight heparin fraction. *Thromb Res* 1982;28:401–409.

25. Sobel M, McNeill PM, Carlson PL, et al. Heparin inhibition of von Willebrand factor-dependent platelet function in vitro and in vivo. *J Clin Invest* 1991;87(5):1787–1793.

26. Clowes AW, Karnowsky MJ. Suppression by heparin of smooth muscle cell proliferation in injured arteries. *Nature* 1977;265:625–626.

27. Castellot JJ Jr, Favreau LV, Karnovsky MJ, et al. Inhibition of vascular smooth muscle cell growth by endothelial cell-derived heparin: possible role of a platelet endoglycosidase. *J Biol Chem* 1982;257:11256–11260.

28. Shaughnessy SG, Young E, Deschamps P, et al. The effects of low molecular weight and standard heparin on calcium loss from fetal rat calvaria. *Blood* 1995;86:1368–1373.

29. Bhandari M, Hirsh J, Weitz JI, et al. The effects of standard and low molecular weight heparin on bone nodule formation in vitro. *Thromb Haemost* 1998;80:413–417.

30. de Swart CAM, Nijmeyer B, Roelofs JMM, et al. Kinetics of intravenously administered heparin in normal humans. *Blood* 1982;60:1251–1258.

31. Olsson P, Lagergren H, Ek S. The elimination from plasma of intravenous heparin: an experimental study on dogs and humans. *Acta Med Scand* 1963; 173:619–630.

32. Bjornsson TD, Wolfram KM, Kitchell BB. Heparin kinetics determined by three assay methods. *Clin Pharmacol Ther* 1982;31:104–113.

33. Glimelius B, Busch C, Hook M. Binding of heparin on the surface of cultured human endothelial cells. *Thromb Res* 1978;12:773–782.

34. Mahadoo J, Heibert L, Jaques LB. Vascular sequestration of heparin. *Thromb Res* 1978;12:79–90.

35. Friedman Y, Arsenis C. Studies on the heparin sulphamidase activity from rat spleen: intracellular distribution and characterization of the enzyme. *Biochem J* 1974;139:699–708.

36. Dawes J, Papper DS. Catabolism of low-dose heparin in man. *Thromb Res* 1979;14:845–860.

37. McAllister BM, Demis DJ. Heparin metabolism: isolation and characterization of uroheparin. *Nature* 1966;212:293–294.

38. Hull RD, Raskob GE, Hirsh J, et al. Continuous intravenous heparin compared with intermittent subcutaneous heparin in the initial treatment of proximal-vein thrombosis. *N Engl J Med* 1986;315:1109–1114.

39. Young E, Cosmi B, Weitz JI, et al. Comparison of the non-specific binding of unfractionated heparin and low molecular weight heparin (enoxaparin) to plasma proteins. *Thromb Haemost* 1993;70:625–630.

40. Young E, Podor TJ, Venner T, et al. Induction of the acute-phase reaction increases heparin-binding proteins in plasma. *Arterioscler Thromb Vasc Biol* 1997;17:1568–1574.

41. Young E, Prins M, Levine MN, et al. Heparin binding to plasma proteins, an important mechanism for heparin resistance. *Thromb Haemost* 1992;67:639–643.

42. Turpie AG, Robinson JG, Doyle DJ, et al. Comparison of high-dose with low-dose subcutaneous heparin to prevent left ventricular mural thrombosis in patients with acute transmural anterior myocardial infarction. *N Engl J Med* 1989;320:352–357.

43. Pini M, Pattacini C, Quintavalla R, et al. Subcutaneous vs intravenous heparin in the treatment of deep vein thrombosis—a randomized clinical trial. *Thromb Haemost* 1990;64:222–226.

44. Levine MN, Hirsh J. Heparin-induced bleeding. In: Lane DA, Lindahl U, eds. *Heparin: chemical and biological properties, clinical applications.* London: Edward Arnold, 1989:517–532.

45. Morabia A. Heparin doses and major bleedings. *Lancet* 1986;1:1278–1279.

46. Global Use of Strategies to Open Occluded Coronary Arteries (GUSTO) IIa Investigators. Randomized trial of intravenous heparin versus recombinant hirudin for acute coronary syndromes. *Circulation* 1994;90:1631–1637.

47. Antman EM, TIMI 9A Investigators. Hirudin in acute myocardial infarction: safety report from the Thrombolysis and Thrombin Inhibition in Myocardial Infarction (TIMI) 9A trial. *Circulation* 1994;90:1624–1630.

48. Global Use of Strategies to Open Occluded Coronary Arteries (GUSTO) IIb Investigators. A comparison of recombinant hirudin with heparin for the treatment of acute coronary syndromes. *N Engl J Med* 1996;335:775–782.

49. Antman EM, TIMI 9b Investigators. Hirudin in acute myocardial infarction: Thrombolysis and Thrombin Inhibition in Myocardial Infarction (TIMI) 9B trial. *Circulation* 1996;94:911–921.

50. EPIC Investigators. Use of a monoclonal antibody directed against the platelet glycoprotein IIb/IIIa receptor in high-risk coronary angioplasty. *N Engl J Med* 1994;330:956–961.

51. EPILOG investigators. Platelet glycoprotein IIb/IIIa receptor blockade and low-dose heparin during percutaneous coronary revascularization. *N Engl J Med* 1997;336:1689–1696.

52. Landefeld CS, Cook EF, Flatley M, et al. Identification and preliminary validation of predictors of major bleeding in hospitalized patients starting anticoagulant therapy. *Am J Med* 1987;82:703–713.

53. Brill-Edwards P, Ginsberg JS, Johnston M, et al. Establishing a therapeutic range for heparin therapy. *Ann Intern Med* 1993;119:104–109.

54. Levine MN, Hirsh J, Gent M, et al. A randomized trial comparing activated thromboplastin time with heparin assay in patients with acute venous thromboembolism requiring large daily doses of heparin. *Arch Intern Med* 1994;154:49–56.

55. Chiu HM, Hirsh J, Yung WL, et al. Relationship between the anticoagulant and antithrombotic effects of heparin in experimental venous thrombosis. *Blood* 1977;49:171–184.

56. Young E, Hirsh J. Contribution of red blood cells to the saturable mechanism of heparin clearance. *Thromb Haemost* 1990;64:559–563.

57. Doyle DJ, Turpie AG, Hirsh J, et al. Adjusted subcutaneous heparin or continuous intravenous heparin in patients with acute deep vein thrombosis: a randomized trial. *Ann Intern Med* 1987;107:441–445.

58. Anand S, Ginsberg JS, Kearon C, et al. The relation between the activated partial thromboplastin time response and recurrence in patients with venous thrombosis treated with continuous intravenous heparin. *Arch Intern Med* 1996;156:1677–1681.

59. Hull RD, Raskob GE, Brant RF, et al. Relation between the time to achieve the lower limit of the APTT therapeutic range and recurrent venous thromboembolism during heparin treatment for deep vein thrombosis. *Arch Intern Med* 1997;157:2562–2568.

60. Cruickshank MK, Levine MN, Hirsh J, et al. A standard heparin nomogram for the management of heparin therapy. *Arch Intern Med* 1991;151:333–337.

61. Raschke RA, Gollihare B, Peirce JC. The effectiveness of implementing the weight-based heparin nomogram as a practice guideline. *Arch Intern Med* 1996;156:1645–1649.

62. Turpie AG, Gunstensen J, Hirsh J, et al. Randomised comparison of two intensities of oral anticoagulant therapy after tissue heart valve replacement. *Lancet* 1988;1:1242–1245.

63. Kearon C, Gent M, Hirsh J, et al. A comparison of three months of anticoagulation with extended anticoagulation for a first episode of idiopathic venous thromboembolism. *N Engl J Med* 1999;340:901–907.

64. Landefeld CS, Beyth RJ. Anticoagulant-related bleeding: clinical epidemiology, prediction, and prevention. *Am J Med* 1993;95:315–328.

65. Teoh KH, Young E, Bradley CA, et al. Heparin binding proteins: contribution to heparin rebound after cardiopulmonary bypass. *Circulation* 1993;88:II420–II425.

66. Visentin GP, Ford SE, Scott JP, et al. Antibodies from patients with heparin-induced thrombocytopenia/thrombosis are specific for platelet factor 4 complexed with heparin or bound to endothelial cells. *J Clin Invest* 1994;93:81–88.

67. Greinacher A, Potzsch B, Amiral J, et al. Heparin-associated thrombocytopenia: isolation of the antibody and characterization of a multimolecular PF4-heparin complex as the major antigen. *Thromb Haemost* 1994;71:247–251.

68. Kelton JG, Smith JW, Warkentin TE, et al. Immunoglobulin G from patients with heparin-induced thrombocytopenia binds to a complex of heparin and platelet factor 4. *Blood* 1994;83:3232–3239.
69. Warkentin TE, Hayward CP, Boshkov LK, et al. Sera from patients with heparin-induced thrombocytopenia generate platelet-derived microparticles with procoagulant activity: an explanation for the thrombotic complications of heparin-induced thrombocytopenia. *Blood* 1994;84:3691–3699.
70. Fratantoni JC, Pollet R, Gralnick HR. Heparin-induced thrombocytopenia: confirmation of diagnosis with in vitro methods. *Blood* 1975;45:395–401.
71. Gruel Y, Rupin A, Darnige L, et al. Specific quantification of heparin-dependent antibodies for the diagnosis of heparin-associated thrombocytopenia using an enzyme-linked immunosorbent assay. *Thromb Res* 1991;62:377–387.
72. Warkentin TE, Elavathil LJ, Hayward CP, et al. The pathogenesis of venous limb gangrene associated with heparin-induced thrombocytopenia. *Ann Intern Med* 1997;127:804–812.
73. Warkentin TE, Chong BH, Greinacher A. Heparin-induced thrombocytopenia: towards consensus. *Thromb Haemost* 1998;79:1–7.
74. Magnani HN. Heparin-induced thrombocytopenia (HIT): an overview of 230 patients treated with orgaran (Org 10172). *Thromb Haemost* 1993;70:554–561.
75. Lewis BE, Walenga JM, Wallis DE. Anticoagulation with Novastan (argatroban) in patients with heparin-induced thrombocytopenia and heparin-induced thrombocytopenia and thrombosis syndrome. *Semin Thromb Hemost* 1997;23:197–202.
76. Greinacher A, Volpel H, Janssens U, et al. Recombinant hirudin (lepirudin) provides safe and effective anticoagulation in patients with heparin-induced thrombocytopenia: a prospective study. *Circulation* 1999;99:73–80.
77. Demers C, Ginsberg JS, Brill-Edwards P, et al. Rapid anticoagulation using ancrod for heparin-induced thrombocytopenia. *Blood* 1991;78:2194–2197.
78. Greinacher A, Janssens U, Berg G, et al. Lepirudin (recombinant hirudin) for parenteral anticoagulation in patients with heparin-induced thrombocytopenia. *Circulation* 1999;100:587–593.
79. Ramakrishna R, Manoharan A, Kwan YL, et al. Heparin-induced thrombocytopenia: cross-reactivity between standard heparin, low molecular weight heparin, dalteparin (Fragmin) and heparinoid, danaparoid (Orgaran). *Br J Haematol* 1995;91:736–738.
80. Kaaja R, Pettila P, Leinonen P, et al. Thromboprophylaxis with low molecular weight heparin (Dalteparin) compared with unfractionated heparin in pregnancy. *Blood* 1998;92[Suppl 1]:360a.
81. Carter CJ, Kelton JG, Hirsh J, et al. The relationship between the hemorrhagic and antithrombotic properties of low molecular weight heparin in rabbits. *Blood* 1982;59:1239–1245.
82. Esquivel CO, Bergqvist D, Bjorck CG, et al. Comparison between commercial heparin, low molecular weight heparin and pentosan polysulfate on hemostasis and platelets in vivo. *Thromb Res* 1982;28:389–399.
83. Cade JF, Buchanan MR, Boneu B, et al. A comparison of the antithrombotic and haemorrhagic effects of low molecular weight heparin fractions: the influence of the method of preparation. *Thromb Res* 1984;35:613–625.
84. Holmer E, Mattsson C, Nilsson S. Anticoagulant and antithrombotic effects of heparin and low molecular weight heparin fragments in rabbits. *Thromb Res* 1982;25:475–485.
85. Andriuoli G, Mastacchi R, Barbanti M, et al. Comparison of the antithrombotic and haemorrhagic effects of heparin and a new low molecular weight heparin in rats. *Haemostasis* 1985;15:324–330.
86. Bergqvist D, Nilsson B, Hedner U, et al. The effect of heparin fragments of different molecular weights on experimental thrombosis and haemostasis. *Thromb Res* 1985;38:589–601.
87. Frydman AM, Bara L, Woler M, et al. The antithrombotic activity and pharmacokinetics of enoxaparine, a low molecular weight heparin, in humans given single subcutaneous doses of 20 to 80 mg. *J Clin Pharmacol* 1988;28:609–618.
88. Briant L, Caranobe C, Saivin S, et al. Unfractionated heparin and CY 216: pharmacokinetics and bioavailabilities of the antifactor Xa and IIa effects after intravenous and subcutaneous injection in the rabbit. *Thromb Haemost* 1989;61:348–353.
89. Bratt G, Tornebohm E, Widlund L, et al. Low molecular weight heparin (KABI 2165, Fragmin): pharmacokinetics after intravenous and subcutaneous administration in human volunteers. *Thromb Res* 1986;42:613–620.
90. Matzsch T, Bergqvist D, Hedner U, et al. Effects of an enzymatically depolymerized heparin as compared with conventional heparin in healthy volunteers. *Thromb Haemost* 1987;57:97–101.
91. Bara L, Samama M. Pharmacokinetics of low molecular weight heparins. *Acta Chir Scand Suppl* 1988;543:65–72.
92. Bradbrook ID, Magnani HN, Moelker HC, et al. ORG 10172: a low molecular weight heparinoid anticoagulant with a long half-life in man. *Br J Clin Pharmacol* 1987;23:667–675.
93. Rosenberg RD, Jordan RE, Favreau LV, et al. Highly active heparin species with multiple binding sites for antithrombin. *Biochem Biophys Res Commun* 1979;86:1319–1324.
94. Danielsson A, Raub E, Lindahl U, et al. Role of ternary complexes, in which heparin binds both antithrombin and proteinase, in the acceleration of the reactions between antithrombin and thrombin or factor Xa. *J Biol Chem* 1986;261:15467–15473.
95. Andersson LO, Barrowcliffe TW, Holmer E, et al. Molecular weight dependency of the heparin potentiated inhibition of thrombin and activated factor X: effect of heparin neutralization in plasma. *Thromb Res* 1979;15:531–541.
96. Jordan RE, Favreau LV, Braswell EH, et al. Heparin with two binding sites for antithrombin or platelet factor 4. *J Biol Chem* 1982;257:400–406.
97. Young E, Wells P, Holloway S, et al. Ex-vivo and in-vitro evidence that low molecular weight heparins exhibit less binding to plasma proteins than unfractionated heparin. *Thromb Haemost* 1994;71:300–304.
98. Weitz JI. Low-molecular-weight heparins. *N Engl J Med* 1997;337:688–698.
99. Salzman EW, Rosenberg RD, Smith MH, et al. Effect of heparin and heparin fractions on platelet aggregation. *J Clin Invest* 1980;65:64–73.
100. Heparin binding and neutralizing protein. In: Lane DA, Lindahl U, eds. *Heparin: chemical and biological properties, clinical applications*. London: Edward Arnold, 1989:363–374.
101. Boneu B, Caranobe C, Cadroy Y, et al. Pharmacokinetic studies of standard and unfractionated heparins, and low molecular weight heparins in the rabbit. *Semin Thromb Hemost* 1988;14:18–27.
102. Caranobe C, Barret A, Gabaig AM, et al. Disappearance of circulating anti-Xa activity after intravenous injection of standard heparin and of a low molecular weight heparin (CY 216) in normal and nephrectomized rabbits. *Thromb Res* 1985;40:129–133.
103. Palm M, Mattsson C. Pharmacokinetics of heparin and low molecular weight heparin fragment (Fragmin) in rabbits with impaired renal or metabolic clearance. *Thromb Haemost* 1987;58:932–935.
104. Holmer E, Kurachi K, Soderstrom G. The molecular-weight dependence of the rate-enhancing effect of heparin on the inhibition of thrombin, factor Xa, factor IXa, factor XIa, factor XIIa and kallikrein by antithrombin. *Biochem J* 1981;193:395–400.
105. Holmer E, Soderberg K, Bergqvist D, et al. Heparin and its low molecular weight derivatives: anticoagulant and antithrombotic properties. *Haemostasis* 1986;16[Suppl 2]:1–7.
106. Gould MK, Dembitzer AD, Doyle RL, et al. Low-molecular-weight heparins compared with unfractionated heparin for treatment of acute deep venous thrombosis: a meta-analysis of randomized, controlled trials. *Ann Intern Med* 1999;130:800–809.
107. Meuleman DG. Orgaran (Org 10172): its pharmacological profile in experimental models. *Haemostasis* 1991;22:58–65.
108. Danhof M, de Boer A, Magnani HN, et al. Pharmacokinetic considerations on Orgaran (Org 10172) therapy. *Haemostasis* 1992;22:73–84.
109. de Boer A, Stiekema JC, Danhof M, et al. The influence of Org 10172, a low molecular weight heparinoid, on antipyrine metabolism and the effect of enzyme induction on the response to Org 10172. *Br J Clin Pharmacol* 1991;32:23–29.
110. Turpie AG, Levine MN, Hirsh J, et al. Double-blind randomised trial of Org 10172 low-molecular-weight heparinoid in prevention of deep-vein thrombosis in thrombotic stroke. *Lancet* 1987;1:523–526.
111. de Valk HW, Banga JD, Wester JW, et al. Comparing subcutaneous danaparoid with intravenous unfractionated heparin for the treatment of venous thromboembolism: a randomized controlled trial. *Ann Intern Med* 1995;123:1–9.
112. Stiekema JC, Wijnand HP, ten Cate H, et al. Partial in vivo neutralisation of plasma anticoagulant effects of Lomoparan (Org 10172) by protamine chloride. *Thromb Res* 1991;63:157–167.
113. Lormeau JC, Herault JP, Gaich C, et al. Determination of the anti-factor Xa activity of the synthetic pentasaccharide SR 90107A/ORG 31540 and of two structural analogues. *Thromb Res* 1997;85:67–75.
114. Ahmad S, Jeske WP, Walenga JM, et al. Synthetic pentasaccharides do not cause platelet activation by antiheparin-platelet factor 4 antibodies. *Clin Appl Thromb Hemost* 1999;5:259–266.
115. Herbert JM, Herault JP, Bernat A, et al. Biochemical and pharmacological properties of SANORG 34006, a potent and long-acting synthetic pentasaccharide. *Blood* 1998;91:4197–4205.
116. Lassen MR. The EPHESUS Study: comparison of the first synthetic factor Xa inhibitor with low molecular weight heparin (LMWH) for the prevention of venous thromboembolism (VTE) after elective hip replacement surgery. *Blood* 2000;96[Suppl 1]:2109(abst).
117. Eriksson BI. The PENTHIFRA Study: comparison of the first synthetic factor Xa inhibitor with low molecular weight heparin (LMWH) for the prevention of venous thromboembolism (VTE) after hip fracture surgery. *Blood* 2000;96:2110(abst).
118. Bernat A, Hoffmann P, Herbert JM. Antagonism of SR 90107A/Org 31540-induced bleeding by protamine sulfate in rats and mice. *Thromb Haemost* 1996;76:715–719.
119. Bichler J, Fichtl B, Siebeck M, et al. Pharmacokinetics and pharmacodynamics of hirudin in man after single subcutaneous and intravenous bolus administration. *Arzneimittelforschung* 1988;38:704–710.
120. Bichler J, Siebeck M, Fichtl B, et al. Pharmacokinetics, effect on clotting tests and assessment of the immunogenic potential of hirudin after a single subcutaneous or intravenous bolus administration in man. *Haemostasis* 1991;21[Suppl 1]:137–141.
121. Vanholder R, Camez A, Veys N, et al. Pharmacokinetics of recombinant hirudin in hemodialyzed end-stage renal failure patients. *Thromb Haemost* 1997;77:650–655.
122. Hafner G, Fickenscher K, Friesen HJ, et al. Evaluation of an automated chromogenic substrate assay for the rapid determination of hirudin in plasma. *Thromb Res* 1995;77:165–173.
123. Iyer L, Adam M, Amiral J, et al. Development and validation of two enzyme-linked immunosorbent assay (ELISA) methods for recombinant hirudin. *Semin Thromb Hemost* 1995;21:184–192.

124. Nurmohamed MT, Berckmans RJ, Morrien-Salomons WM, et al. Monitoring anticoagulant therapy by activated partial thromboplastin time: hirudin assessment: an evaluation of native blood and plasma assays. *Thromb Haemost* 1994;72:685–692.

125. Potzsch B, Madlener K, Seelig C, et al. Monitoring of r-hirudin anticoagulation during cardiopulmonary bypass—assessment of the whole blood ecarin clotting time. *Thromb Haemost* 1997;77:920–925.

126. Klement P, Liao P, Hirsh J, et al. Hirudin causes more bleeding than heparin in a rabbit ear bleeding model. *J Lab Clin Med* 1998;132:181–185.

127. Fareed J, Walenga JM, Pifarre R, et al. Some objective considerations for the neutralization of the anticoagulant actions of recombinant hirudin. *Haemostasis* 1991;21[Suppl 1]:64–72.

128. Amin DM, Mant TG, Walker SM, et al. Effect of a 15-minute infusion of DDAVP on the pharmacokinetics and pharmacodynamics of REVASC during a four-hour intravenous infusion in healthy male volunteers. *Thromb Haemost* 1997;77:127–132.

129. Bove CM, Casey BC, Marder VJ. DDAVP reduces bleeding during continued hirudin administration in the rabbit. *Thromb Haemost* 1996;75:471–475.

130. Neuhaus KL, von Essen R, Tebbe U, et al. Safety observations from the pilot phase of the randomized r-Hirudin for Improvement of Thrombolysis (HIT-III) study: a study of the Arbeitsgemeinschaft Leitender Kardiologischer Krankenhausarzte (ALKK). *Circulation* 1994;90:1638–1642.

131. Organisation to Assess Strategies for Ischemic Syndromes (OASIS-2) Investigators. Effects of recombinant hirudin (lepirudin) compared with heparin on death, myocardial infarction, refractory angina, and revascularisation procedures in patients with acute myocardial ischaemia without ST elevation: a randomised trial. *Lancet* 1999;353:429–438.

132. Maraganore JM. Pre-clinical and clinical studies on Hirulog: a potent and specific direct thrombin inhibitor. *Adv Exp Med Biol* 1993;340:227–236.

133. Ginsberg JS, Nurmohamed MT, Gent M, et al. Use of Hirulog in the prevention of venous thrombosis after major hip or knee surgery. *Circulation* 1994; 90:2385–2389.

134. Theroux P, Perez-Villa F, Waters D, et al. Randomized double-blind comparison of two doses of Hirulog with heparin as adjunctive therapy to streptokinase to promote early patency of the infarct-related artery in acute myocardial infarction. *Circulation* 1995;91:2132–2139.

135. Bittl JA, Strony J, Brinker JA, et al. Treatment with bivalirudin (Hirulog) as compared with heparin during coronary angioplasty for unstable or postinfarction angina. Hirulog Angioplasty Study Investigators. *N Engl J Med* 1995; 333:764–769.

136. White HD, Aylward PE, Frey MJ, et al. Randomized, double-blind comparison of Hirulog versus heparin in patients receiving streptokinase and aspirin for acute myocardial infarction (HERO). Hirulog Early Reperfusion/Occlusion (HERO) Trial Investigators. *Circulation* 1997;96:2155–2161.

137. Jang IK, Brown DF, Giugliano RP, et al. A multicenter, randomized study of argatroban versus heparin as adjunct to tissue plasminogen activator (TPA) in acute myocardial infarction: Myocardial Infarction with Novastan and TPA (MINT) Study. *J Am Coll Cardiol* 1999;33:1879–1885.

138. Mehta JL, Chen L, Nichols WW, et al. Melagatran, an oral active-site inhibitor of thrombin, prevents or delays formation of electrically induced occlusive thrombus in the canine coronary artery. *J Cardiovasc Pharmacol* 1998;31: 345–351.

139. Wallin R, Martin LF. Vitamin K-dependent carboxylation and vitamin K metabolism in liver: effects of warfarin. *J Clin Invest* 1985;76:1879–1884.

140. Furie B, Bouchard BA, Furie BC. Vitamin K-dependent biosynthesis of gamma-carboxyglutamic acid. *Blood* 1999;93:1798–1808.

141. Nelsestuen GL. Role of gamma-carboxyglutamic acid: an unusual protein transition required for the calcium-dependent binding of prothrombin to phospholipid. *J Biol Chem* 1976;251:5648–5656.

142. Borowski M, Furie BC, Bauminger S, et al. Prothrombin requires two sequential metal-dependent conformational transitions to bind phospholipid: conformation-specific antibodies directed against the phospholipid-binding site on prothrombin. *J Biol Chem* 1986;261:14969–14975.

143. Hirsh J, Dalen JE, Anderson DR, et al. Oral anticoagulants: mechanism of action, clinical effectiveness, and optimal therapeutic range. *Chest* 1998;114[Suppl 5]:445S–469S.

144. Choonara IA, Malia RG, Haynes BP, et al. The relationship between inhibition of vitamin K1 2,3-epoxide reductase and reduction of clotting factor activity with warfarin. *Br J Clin Pharmacol* 1988;25:1–7.

145. Fasco MJ, Hildebrandt EF, Suttie JW. Evidence that warfarin anticoagulant action involves two distinct reductase activities. *J Biol Chem* 1982;257:11210–11212.

146. Whitlon DS, Sadowski JA, Suttie JW. Mechanism of coumarin action: significance of vitamin K epoxide reductase inhibition. *Biochemistry* 1978;17:1371–1377.

147. Malhotra OP. Dicoumarol-induced 9-gamma-carboxyglutamic acid prothrombin: isolation and comparison with the 6-, 7-, 8-, and 10-gamma-carboxyglutamic acid isomers. *Biochem Cell Biol* 1990;68:705–715.

148. Malhotra OP. Dicoumarol-induced prothrombins containing 6, 7, and 8 gamma-carboxyglutamic acid residues: isolation and characterization. *Biochem Cell Biol* 1989;67:411–421.

149. Harrison L, Johnston M, Massicotte MP, et al. Comparison of 5-mg and 10-mg loading doses in initiation of warfarin therapy. *Ann Intern Med* 1997;126:133–136.

150. Marder VJ, Shulman NR. Clinical aspects of congenital factor VII deficiency. *Am J Med* 1964;37:182.

151. Hellemans J, Vorlat M, Verstraete M. Survival time of prothrombin and factors VII, IX, X after complete synthesis blocking doses of coumarin derivatives. *Br J Haematol* 1963;9:506–512.

152. Wessler S, Gitel SN. Warfarin: from bedside to bench. *N Engl J Med* 1984; 311:645–652.

153. Zivelin A, Rao LV, Rapaport SI. Mechanism of the anticoagulant effect of warfarin as evaluated in rabbits by selective depression of individual procoagulant vitamin K-dependent clotting factors. *J Clin Invest* 1993;92:2131–2140.

154. Patel P, Weitz J, Brooker LA, et al. Decreased thrombin activity of fibrin clots prepared in cord plasma compared with adult plasma. *Pediatr Res* 1996;39: 826–830.

155. Furie B, Diuguid CF, Jacobs M, et al. Randomized prospective trial comparing the native prothrombin antigen with the prothrombin time for monitoring oral anticoagulant therapy. *Blood* 1990;75:344–349.

156. Crowther MA, Ginsberg J, Kearon C, et al. A randomized trial comparing 5 mg and 10 mg warfarin loading doses. *Arch Intern Med* 1999;159:46–48.

157. Brandjes DP, Heijboer H, Buller HR, et al. Acenocoumarol and heparin compared with acenocoumarol alone in the initial treatment of proximal-vein thrombosis. *N Engl J Med* 1992;327:1485–1489.

158. Vigano S, Mannucci PM, Solinas S, et al. Decrease in protein C antigen and formation of an abnormal protein soon after starting oral anticoagulant therapy. *Br J Haematol* 1984;57:213–220.

159. Verhagen HJ. Local hemorrhage and necrosis of the skin and underlying tissues, during anticoagulant therapy with dicumarol or dicumacyl. *Acta Med Scand* 1954;148:453.

160. Broekmans AW, Bertina RM, Loeliger EA, et al. Protein C and the development of skin necrosis during anticoagulant therapy. *Thromb Haemost* 1983; 49:251.

161. Monagle P, Andrew M, Halton J, et al. Homozygous protein C deficiency: description of a new mutation and successful treatment with low molecular weight heparin. *Thromb Haemost* 1998;79:756–761.

162. Samama M, Horellou MH, Soria J, et al. Successful progressive anticoagulation in a severe protein C deficiency and previous skin necrosis at the initiation of oral anticoagulant treatment. *Thromb Haemost* 1984;51:132–133.

163. Pabinger-Fasching I, Deutsch E. Protein C deficiency in Austria. *Semin Thromb Hemost* 1985;11:347–351.

164. Hofmann V, Frick PG. Repeated occurrence of skin necrosis twice following coumarin intake and subsequently during decrease of vitamin K dependent coagulation factors associated with cholestasis. *Thromb Haemost* 1982;48:245–246.

165. Breckenridge A. Oral anticoagulant drugs: pharmacokinetic aspects. *Semin Hematol* 1978;15:19–26.

166. Breckenridge A, Orme M, Wesseling H, et al. Pharmacokinetics and pharmacodynamics of the enantiomers of warfarin in man. *Clin Pharmacol Ther* 1974;15:424–430.

167. Kelly JG, O'Malley K. Clinical pharmacokinetics of oral anticoagulants. *Clin Pharmacokinet* 1979;4:1–15.

168. King SY, Joslin MA, Raudibaugh K, et al. Dose-dependent pharmacokinetics of warfarin in healthy volunteers. *Pharmacol Res* 1995;12:1874–1877.

169. Sutcliffe FA, MacNicoll AD, Gibson GG. Aspects of anticoagulant action: a review of the pharmacology, metabolism and toxicology of warfarin and congeners. *Rev Drug Metab Drug Interact* 1987;5:225–272.

170. O'Reilly RA, Rytand DA. "Resistance" to warfarin due to unrecognized vitamin K supplementation. *N Engl J Med* 1980;303:160–161.

171. Udall JA. Human sources and absorption of vitamin K in relation to anticoagulation stability. *JAMA* 1965;194:127–129.

172. Frick PG, Riedler G, Brogli H. Dose response and minimal daily requirement for vitamin K in man. *J Appl Physiol* 1967;23:387–389.

173. Chakraverty R, Davidson S, Peggs K, et al. The incidence and cause of coagulopathies in an intensive care population. *Br J Haematol* 1996;93:460–463.

174. Nakamura T, Takebe K, Imamura K, et al. Fat-soluble vitamins in patients with chronic pancreatitis (pancreatic insufficiency). *Acta Gastroenterol Belg* 1996;59:10–14.

175. Wells PS, Holbrook AM, Crowther NR, et al. Interactions of warfarin with drugs and food. *Ann Intern Med* 1994;121:676–683.

176. Yacobi A, Udall JA, Levy G. Intrasubject variation of warfarin binding to protein in serum of patients with cardiovascular disease. *Clin Pharmacol Ther* 1976;20:300–303.

177. Aithal GP, Day CP, Kesteven PJ, et al. Association of polymorphisms in the cytochrome P450 CYP2C9 with warfarin dose requirement and risk of bleeding complications. *Lancet* 1999;353:717–719.

178. Mannucci PM. Genetic control of anticoagulation. *Lancet* 1999;353:688–689.

179. Harris JE. Interaction of dietary factors with oral anticoagulants: review and applications. *J Am Diet Assoc* 1995;95:580–584.

180. O'Reilly RA, Pool JG, Aggeler PM. Hereditary resistance to coumarin anticoagulant drugs in man and rat. *Ann N Y Acad Sci* 1968;151:913–931.

181. Alving BM, Strickler MP, Knight RD, et al. Hereditary warfarin resistance: investigation of a rare phenomenon. *Arch Intern Med* 1985;145:499–501.

182. Chu K, Wu SM, Stanley T, et al. A mutation in the propeptide of factor IX leads to warfarin sensitivity by a novel mechanism. *J Clin Invest* 1996;98: 1619–1625.

183. Oldenburg J, Quenzel EM, Harbrecht U, et al. Missense mutations at ALA-10 in the factor IX propeptide: an insignificant variant in normal life but a decisive cause of bleeding during oral anticoagulant therapy. *Br J Haematol* 1997;98:240–244.

184. O'Reilly RA. Studies on the optical enantiomorphs of warfarin in man. *Clin Pharmacol Ther* 1974;16:348–354.

185. Choonara IA, Cholerton S, Haynes BP, et al. Stereoselective interaction between the R enantiomer of warfarin and cimetidine. *Br J Clin Pharmacol* 1986;21:271–277.

186. Sutfin T, Balmer K, Bostrom H, et al. Stereoselective interaction of omeprazole with warfarin in healthy men. *Ther Drug Monit* 1989;11:176–184.

187. Hylek EM, Heiman H, Skates SJ, et al. Acetaminophen and other risk factors for excessive warfarin anticoagulation. *JAMA* 1998;279:657–662.

188. Kater RM, Roggin G, Tobon F, et al. Increased rate of clearance of drugs from the circulation of alcoholics. *Am J Med Sci* 1969;258:35–39.

189. O'Reilly RA. Lack of effect of fortified wine ingested during fasting and anticoagulant therapy. *Arch Intern Med* 1981;141:458–459.

190. Richards RK. Influence of fever upon the action of 3,3-methylene bis-(4-hydroxycoumarin). *Science* 1943;97:313.

191. Owens JC, Neely WB, Owen WR. Effect of sodium dextrothyroxine in patients receiving anticoagulants. *N Engl J Med* 1962;266:76.

192. Smith JB, Willis AL. Aspirin selectively inhibits prostaglandin production in human platelets. *Nat New Biol* 1971;231:235–237.

193. Vane JR. Inhibition of prostaglandin synthesis as a mechanism of action for aspirin-like drugs. *Nat New Biol* 1971;231:232–235.

194. Dale J, Myhre E, Loew D. Bleeding during acetylsalicylic acid and anticoagulant therapy in patients with reduced platelet reactivity after aortic valve replacement. *Am Heart J* 1980;99:746–752.

195. Chesebro JH, Fuster V, Elveback LR, et al. Trial of combined warfarin plus dipyridamole or aspirin therapy in prosthetic heart valve replacement: danger of aspirin compared with dipyridamole. *Am J Cardiol* 1983;51:1537–1541.

196. Turpie AG, Gent M, Laupacis A, et al. A comparison of aspirin with placebo in patients treated with warfarin after heart-valve replacement. *N Engl J Med* 1993;329:524–529.

197. Landefeld CS, Goldman L. Major bleeding in outpatients treated with warfarin: incidence and prediction by factors known at the start of outpatient therapy. *Am J Med* 1989;87:144–152.

198. Levine MN, Raskob G, Landefeld S, et al. Hemorrhagic complications of anticoagulant treatment. *Chest* 1998;114[Suppl 5]:511S–523S.

199. Altman R, Rouvier J, Gurfinkel E, et al. Comparison of two levels of anticoagulant therapy in patients with substitute heart valves. *J Thorac Cardiovasc Surg* 1991;101:427–431.

200. Petersen P, Boysen G, Godtfredsen J, et al. Placebo-controlled, randomised trial of warfarin and aspirin for prevention of thromboembolic complications in chronic atrial fibrillation: the Copenhagen AFASAK study. *Lancet* 1989;1:175–179.

201. Anonymous. Warfarin versus aspirin for prevention of thromboembolism in atrial fibrillation: Stroke Prevention in Atrial Fibrillation II Study. *Lancet* 1994;343:687–691.

202. Hull R, Hirsh J, Jay R, et al. Different intensities of oral anticoagulant therapy in the treatment of proximal-vein thrombosis. *N Engl J Med* 1982;307:1676–1681.

203. Landefeld CS, Rosenblatt MW, Goldman L. Bleeding in outpatients treated with warfarin: relation to the prothrombin time and important remediable lesions. *Am J Med* 1989;87:153–159.

204. Gitter MJ, Jaeger TM, Petterson TM, et al. Bleeding and thromboembolism during anticoagulant therapy: a population-based study in Rochester, Minnesota. *Mayo Clin Proc* 1995;70:725–733.

205. Fondu P. Heparin-associated thrombocytopenia: an update. *Acta Clin Belg* 1995;50:343–357.

206. Fihn SD, Callahan CM, Martin DC, et al. The risk for and severity of bleeding complications in elderly patients treated with warfarin. The National Consortium of Anticoagulation. *Ann Intern Med* 1996;124:970–979.

207. Glover JJ, Morrill GB. Conservative treatment of overanticoagulated patients. *Chest* 1995;108:987–990.

208. van der Meer FJM, Rosendaal FR, Vandenbroucke JP, et al. Bleeding complications in oral anticoagulant therapy: an analysis of risk factors. *Arch Intern Med* 1995;153:1557–1562.

209. Launbjerg J, Egeblad H, Heaf J, et al. Bleeding complications to oral anticoagulant therapy: multivariate analysis of 1010 treatment years in 551 outpatients. *J Intern Med* 1991;229:351–355.

210. Whitling AM, Bussey HI, Lyons RM. Comparing different routes and doses of phytonadione for reversing excessive anticoagulation. *Arch Intern Med* 1998;158:2136–2140.

211. Shetty HG, Backhouse G, Bentley DP, et al. Effective reversal of warfarin-induced excessive anticoagulation with low dose vitamin K1. *Thromb Haemost* 1992;67:13–15.

212. de la Rubia J, Grau E, Montserrat I, et al. Anaphylactic shock and vitamin K1. *Ann Intern Med* 1989;110:943.

213. Havel M, Muller M, Graninger W, et al. Tolerability of a new vitamin K1 preparation for parenteral administration to adults: one case of anaphylactoid reaction. *Clin Ther* 1987;9:373–379.

214. Martinez-Abad M, Delgado F, Palop V, et al. Vitamin K1 and anaphylactic shock. *DICP* 1991;25:871–872.

215. Joyce JP, Hood AF, Weiss MM. Persistent cutaneous reaction to intramuscular vitamin K injection. *Arch Dermatol* 1988;124:27–28.

216. Tsuboi R, Ogawa H. Skin eruption caused by fat-soluble vitamin K injection. *J Am Acad Dermatol* 1988;18:386–387.

217. Bullen AW, Miller JP, Cunliffe WJ, et al. Skin reactions caused by vitamin K in patients with liver disease. *Br J Dermatol* 1978;98:561–565.

218. Morell A, Betlloch I, Sevila A, et al. Morphea-like reaction from vitamin K1. *Int J Dermatol* 1995;34:201–202.

219. Tuppal R, Tremaine R. Cutaneous eruption from vitamin K1 injection. *J Am Acad Dermatol* 1992;27:105–106.

220. Barnes HM, Sarkany I. Adverse skin reaction from vitamin K1. *Br J Dermatol* 1976;95:653–656.

221. Finkelstein H, Champion MC, Adam JE. Cutaneous hypersensitivity to vitamin K1 injection. *J Am Acad Dermatol* 1987;16:540–545.

222. Lemlich G, Green M, Phelps R, et al. Cutaneous reactions to vitamin K1 injections. *J Am Acad Dermatol* 1993;28:345–347.

223. Guidetti MS, Vincenzi C, Papi M, et al. Sclerodermatous skin reaction after vitamin K1 injections. *Contact Dermatitis* 1994;31:45–46.

224. Bruynzeel I, Hebeda CL, Folkers E, et al. Cutaneous hypersensitivity reactions to vitamin K: 2 case reports and a review of the literature. *Contact Dermatitis* 1995;32:78–82.

225. Lee MM, Gellis S, Dover JS. Eczematous plaques in a patient with liver failure. Fat-soluble vitamin K hypersensitivity. *Arch Dermatol* 1992;128:257,260.

226. Sanders MN, Winkelmann RK. Cutaneous reactions to vitamin K. *J Am Acad Dermatol* 1988;19:699–704.

227. Harrell CC, Kline SS. Oral vitamin K1: an option to reduce warfarin's activity. *Ann Pharmacother* 1995;29:1228–1232.

228. Pengo V, Banzato A, Garelli E, et al. Reversal of excessive effect of regular anticoagulation: low oral dose of phytonadione (vitamin K1) compared with warfarin discontinuation. *Blood Coagul Fibrinolysis* 1993;4:739–741.

229. Crowther MA, Julian J, Douketis JD, et al. Treatment of warfarin-associated coagulopathy with oral vitamin K: a randomized clinical trial. *Lancet* 2000;356:1551–1553.

230. Raj G, Kumar R, McKinney WP. Time course of reversal of anticoagulant effect of warfarin by intravenous and subcutaneous phytonadione. *Arch Intern Med* 1999;159:2721–2724.

231. Nee R, Doppenschmidt D, Donovan DJ, et al. Intravenous versus subcutaneous vitamin K1 in reversing excessive oral anticoagulation. *Am J Cardiol* 1999;83:286–288.

232. Fetrow CW, Overlock T, Leff L. Antagonism of warfarin-induced hypoprothrombinemia with use of low-dose subcutaneous vitamin K1. *J Clin Pharmacol* 1997;37:751–757.

233. Wentzien TH, O'Reilly RA, Kearns PJ. Prospective evaluation of anticoagulant reversal with oral vitamin K1 while continuing warfarin therapy unchanged. *Chest* 1998;114:1546–1550.

234. Weibert RT, Le DT, Kayser SR, et al. Correction of excessive anticoagulation with low-dose oral vitamin K1. *Ann Intern Med* 1997;126:959–962.

235. Cosgriff SW. The effectiveness of an oral vitamin K1 in controlling excessive hypoprothrombinemia during anticoagulant therapy. *Ann Intern Med* 1956;45:14–22.

236. Crowther MA, Donovan D, Harrison L, et al. Low-dose oral vitamin K reliably reverses over-anticoagulation due to warfarin. *Thromb Haemost* 1998;79:1116–1118.

237. Hylek EM, Skates SJ, Sheehan MA, et al. An analysis of the lowest effective intensity of prophylactic anticoagulation for patients with nonrheumatic atrial fibrillation. *N Engl J Med* 1996;335:540–546.

238. Hart RG, Sherman DG, Easton JD, et al. Prevention of stroke in patients with nonvalvular atrial fibrillation. *Neurology* 1998;51:674–681.

239. Kearon C, Hirsh J. Management of anticoagulation before and after elective surgery. *N Engl J Med* 1997;336:1506–1511.

240. Douketis J, Crowther M, Cherian SS, et al. Physician preferences for perioperative anticoagulation in patients with a mechanical heart valve who are undergoing elective noncardiac surgery. *Chest* 1999;116:1240–1246.

241. Brickey DA, Lawlor DP. Transbronchial biopsy in the presence of profound elevation of the international normalized ratio. *Chest* 1999;115:1667–1671.

242. Wahl MJ. Dental surgery in anticoagulated patients. *Arch Intern Med* 1998;158:1610–1616.

243. Weibert RT. Oral anticoagulant therapy in patients undergoing dental surgery. *Clin Pharmacol Ther* 1992;11:857–864.

244. Saitoh AK, Saitoh A, Taniguchi H, et al. Anticoagulation therapy and ocular surgery. *Ophthal Surg Lasers* 1998;29:909–915.

245. McCormack P, Simcock PR, Tullo AB. Management of the anticoagulated patient for ophthalmic surgery. *Eye* 1993;7:749–750.

246. Ramstrom G, Sindet-Pedersen S, Hall G, et al. Prevention of postsurgical bleeding in oral surgery using tranexamic acid without dose modification of oral anticoagulants. *J Oral Maxillofac Surg* 1993;51:1211–1216.

247. Souto JC, Oliver A, Zuazu-Jausoro I, et al. Oral surgery in anticoagulated patients without reducing the dose of oral anticoagulant: a prospective randomized study. *J Oral Maxillofac Surg* 1996;54:27–32.

248. White RH, McKittrick T, Hutchinson R, et al. Temporary discontinuation of warfarin therapy: changes in the international normalized ratio. *Ann Intern Med* 1995;122:40–42.

249. Hall JG, Pauli RM, Wilson KM. Maternal and fetal sequelae of anticoagulation during pregnancy. *Am J Med* 1980;68:122–140.

250. Sbarouni E, Oakley CM. Outcome of pregnancy in women with valve prostheses. *Br Heart J* 1994;71:196–201.

251. McKenna R, Cole ER, Vasan U. Is warfarin sodium contraindicated in the lactating mother? *J Pediatr* 1983;103:325–327.

252. Lao TT, de Swiet M, Letsky SE, et al. Prophylaxis of thromboembolism in pregnancy: an alternative. *Br J Obstet Gynaecol* 1985;92:202–206.

253. Quick AJ. The prothrombin time in haemophilia and obstructive jaundice. *J Biol Chem* 1935;109:73–74.

254. Zucker S, Cathey MH, Sox PJ, et al. Standardization of laboratory tests for controlling anticoagulant therapy. *Am J Clin Pathol* 1970;53:348–354.

255. Poller L. Progress in standardization in anticoagulant control. *Hematol Rev* 1987;1:225.

256. Bailey EL, Harper TA, Pinkerton PH. The "therapeutic range" of the one-stage prothrombin time in the control of anticoagulant therapy: the effect of different thromboplastin preparations. *Can Med Assoc J* 1971;105:1041–1043.

257. Latallo ZS, Thomson JM, Poller L. An evaluation of chromogenic substrates in the control of oral anticoagulant therapy. *Br J Haematol* 1981;47:307–318.

258. Poller L, Taberner DA. Dosage and control of oral anticoagulants: an international survey. *Br J Haematol* 1982;51:479–485.

259. Kirkwood TB. Calibration of reference thromboplastins and standardisation of the prothrombin time ratio. *Thromb Haemost* 1983;49:238–244.

260. O'Reilly RA, Aggeler PM. Studies on coumarin anticoagulant drugs. Initiation of warfarin without a loading dose. *Circulation* 1968;38:169–177.

261. Kovacs M, Cruickshank M, Wells PS, et al. Randomized assessment of a warfarin nomogram for initial oral anticoagulation after venous thromboembolic disease. *Haemostasis* 1999;28:62–68.

262. Raschke RA, Reilly BM, Guidry JR, et al. The weight-based heparin dosing nomogram compared with a "standard-care" nomogram: a randomized controlled trial. *Ann Intern Med* 1993;119:874–881.

263. Cairns JA, Theroux P, Lewis HDJ, et al. Antithrombotic agents in coronary artery disease. *Chest* 1998;114[Suppl 5]:611S–633S.

264. Saour JN, Sieck JO, Mamo LA, et al. Trial of different intensities of anticoagulation in patients with prosthetic heart valves. *N Engl J Med* 1990;322:428–432.

CHAPTER **44**

Introduction to Anemias

Carlo Brugnara and Samuel E. Lux IV

The chapters that follow (Chapters 45 to 56) and some earlier chapters (Chapters 8 to 10) are devoted to specific anemias. This chapter focuses on the classification of anemias and an approach to their diagnosis.

DEFINITION OF ANEMIA

Theoretically, *anemia* refers to a reduction in red blood cell mass, but practically it refers to a decrease in the hemoglobin (Hgb) concentration or the hematocrit (packed red cell volume, or Hct). The Hgb value is more accurate because automated hematology analyzers measure it directly. The Hct used to be directly measured but now is usually calculated from the red cell count and the mean corpuscular volume (MCV). The technical limitations of this derived Hct measurement are discussed in Chapter 2. The Hgb concentration also relates more directly to physiologically important measures, like oxygen-carrying capacity. Nevertheless, old habits die hard, and for many, the Hct is easier to use.

The normal values of Hgb, Hct, and MCV for persons at different ages are presented in Table 44-1. The values shown in the neonatal period are for term infants. Premature babies have less time *in utero* to synthesize red cells and are born with lower Hgbs and Hcts (discussed in Chapter 55). The lower limits of normal in the table—2 SD below the mean for each age group—mathematically define 2.5% of the population as anemic. Other findings such as symptoms or signs of anemia, abnormal red cell indices or morphology, and coexisting leukopenia or thrombocytopenia help determine the significance of a low Hgb and Hct.

Conversely, persons who are in the upper-normal range when they are well may still be within the "normal" range when anemic. Also, patients with cardiorespiratory diseases or vascular compromise to a vital organ like the heart or brain may sometimes be functionally anemic at Hgb values that are technically normal. In both these situations, "anemia" may be recognized only after treatment.

Finally, it should be remembered that patients with hemolytic diseases can compensate for red cell destruction to a considerable degree and may have little or no anemia in their usual, steady-state condition. This situation occurs surprisingly often: Approximately half of children and adults with hereditary spherocytosis have compensated or nearly compensated hemolysis (Hgb of 12 g/dL or higher in adults) (1,2) (discussed in Chapter 51). Such patients may be recognized only when red cell indices or a reticulocyte count are obtained or when other signs or symptoms (such as splenomegaly, jaundice, or cholecystitis) reveal the hemolytic process.

CLASSIFICATION OF ANEMIAS

Anemias are usually classified according to pathophysiology (Table 44-2) or red cell size (Table 44-3). In practice, elements from both classification schemes are often used in differential diagnosis, along with information about red cell morphology (Table 44-4). The pathophysiologic classification divides anemias into four categories: (a) decreased production due to inadequate erythropoietin (such as renal disease) or bone marrow failure (such as aplasias, marrow invasion), (b) disorders of red cell nuclear or cytoplasmic maturation (such as cobalamin, folate, and iron deficiencies, and thalassemias), (c) hemolytic anemias, and (d) bleeding. The morphologic classification divides anemias into microcytic, normocytic, and macrocytic groups based on the MCV and subdivides them into hemolytic and marrow failure or dysplasia categories. Conflicts arise in each of the schemes, as might be expected.

For example, thalassemias are disorders of cytoplasmic maturation caused by poor synthesis of one globin chain, but they are also hemolytic anemias caused by membrane damage from the unpaired complementary globin chain. Red cells are macrocytic in patients with many hemolytic anemias because of the presence of reticulocytes, which have a high MCV (approximately 120 fL), and young red cells, which are also larger than average. Patients with

TABLE 44-1. Normal Values (Mean and Lower Limit of Normal [–2 SD]) for Hemoglobin, Hematocrit, and Mean Corpuscular Volume (MCV) at Various Ages[a]

Age	Hemoglobin (g/dL)		Hematocrit (%)		MCV (fL)	
	Mean	–2 SD	Mean	–2 SD	Mean	–2 SD
Cord blood	16.5	13.5	51	42	108	98
1 wk	17.5	13.5	54	42	107	88
2 wk	16.5	12.5	51	39	107	86
1 mo	14.0	10.0	43	31	104	85
2 mo	11.5	9.0	35	28	96	77
3–6 mo	11.5	9.5	35	29	91	74
0.5–2 yr	12.0	10.5	36	33	78	70
2–6 yr	12.5	11.5	37	34	81	75
6–12 yr	13.5	11.5	40	35	86	77
12–18 yr						
Female	14.0	12.0	41	36	90	78
Male	14.5	13.0	43	37	88	78
18–49 yr						
Female	14.0	12.0	41	36	90	80
Male	15.5	13.5	47	41	90	80

[a]Data were compiled from several sources, with emphasis on data obtained with electronic counters, and excluding persons likely to have iron deficiency. From Dallman PR. In: Rudolph A, ed. *Pediatrics*, 16th ed. New York: Appleton-Century-Crofts, 1977:1111, with permission.

TABLE 44-2. Pathophysiologic Classification of Anemias

Decreased production of red cells relative to degree of anemia
  Decreased erythropoietin production
    Renal disease
    Protein malnutrition
    Low-affinity hemoglobins
    Hypothyroidism
    Hypopituitarism
  Bone marrow failure
    Aplastic anemia
      Congenital
        Fanconi's anemia
        Shwachman-Diamond syndrome
        Dyskeratosis congenita
      Acquired
        Radiation
        Drugs, chemicals (including alcohol)
        Viruses: Epstein-Barr virus, hepatitis
        Autoimmune disease
        Pregnancy
        Preleukemia
        Paroxysmal nocturnal hemoglobinuria
        Protein malnutrition, anorexia nervosa
    Pure red cell aplasia
      Congenital: Diamond-Blackfan anemia
      Acquired
        Transient erythroblastopenia of childhood
        Thymoma
        Lymphoma, chronic lymphocytic leukemia, myeloma
        Other malignancies
        Autoimmune diseases
        Viruses, especially parvovirus B19
        Drugs
  Bone marrow invasion (myelophthisis)
    Leukemias, lymphomas
    Myeloma, macroglobulinemia
    Histiocytosis syndromes
    Metastatic tumors (especially breast, prostate, small cell lung, neuroblastoma, melanoma, hypernephroma, seminoma, thyroid, stomach)
    Granulomas
    Storage diseases (advanced)
    Myelofibrosis
    Osteopetrosis
Disorders of erythropoietic maturation
  Defects involving nuclear maturation (megaloblastic anemias)
    Cobalamin (vitamin B_{12}) deficiency
      Inherited disorders in absorption, transport, or cellular metabolism

      Acquired disorders
        Inadequate intrinsic factor
        Small bowel disease
        Dietary deficiencies
        Drugs (especially N_2O)
    Folic acid deficiency
      Inherited defects in absorption or metabolism
      Acquired disorders
        Dietary deficiency
        Small bowel disease
        Increased requirements (pregnancy, hemolysis)
        Drugs (methotrexate, trimethoprim, pyrimethamine)
    Other causes
      Orotic aciduria
      Myelodysplasia
      Erythroleukemia
      Thiamine-responsive anemia
      Pyridoxine-responsive anemia
      Congenital dyserythropoietic anemias I and III
  Defects involving cytoplasmic maturation
    Iron deficiency
      Nutritional deficiency
      Increased requirements (e.g., growth, pregnancy)
      Chronic blood loss (gastrointestinal, genitourinary, lungs)
      Decreased iron reuse: anemia of chronic disease
        Chronic infections (including human immunodeficiency virus)
        Connective tissue diseases
        Malignancies
    Globin deficiency
      α-Thalassemias
      β-Thalassemias
      γ-Thalassemias
      Very unstable hemoglobins
    Sideroblastic anemias
      Inherited
      Acquired
        Alcohol
        Myelodysplasia, preleukemia
        Drugs
    Congenital dyserythropoietic anemia II hereditary erythroblastic multinuclearity with positive acid serum test
    Lead poisoning
Hemolytic anemias
  Extrinsic defects
    Antibody-mediated
      Warm antibody, autoimmune

(continued)

TABLE 44-2. (*continued*)

Idiopathic
Lymphoproliferative diseases
Connective tissue diseases
Drugs
Cold antibody, autoimmune
  Idiopathic
  Infections: *Mycoplasma*, Epstein-Barr virus
  Lymphoproliferative
Paroxysmal cold hemoglobinuria
Neonatal isoimmune
  Rh(D) hemolytic disease
  ABO hemolytic disease
  Other blood group incompatibilities
Transfusion reactions
Thermal injury: severe burns
Vascular injury (fragmentation syndromes)
  Large blood vessels
    Replaced valve, prosthesis, grafts
    Aortic stenosis (severe), regurgitant jets
  Small blood vessels
    Disseminated intravascular coagulation
    Thrombotic thrombocytopenic purpura
    Hemolytic uremic syndrome
    Preeclampsia/eclampsia
    Polyarteritis
    Acute glomerulonephritis, malignant hypertension, allograft rejection
    Disseminated carcinoma
    Rickettsial diseases
  Arteriovenous malformations
    Kasabach-Merritt syndrome
    Hemangioendotheliomas
  Drugs: mitomycin C, cyclosporine
Mechanical trauma
  March hemoglobinuria
  Cardiopulmonary bypass

Osmotic hemolysis: freshwater drowning
Infections
  Erythrocyte parasites
    Malaria
    Babesia microti
    Bartonella bacilliformis
  Red cell damage from bacterial products: clostridial sepsis
Venoms, toxins: snakes, spiders
Extrinsic oxidant hemolysis
  Drugs, chemicals
  Copper: acute poisoning, Wilson's disease
Intrinsic defects
Red cell membrane
  Membrane skeleton
    Hereditary spherocytosis
    Hereditary elliptocytosis

Hereditary pyropoikilocytosis
Defective phosphoinositide-based membrane protein anchors: paroxysmal nocturnal hemoglobinuria
Blood group antigen deficiencies: Rh_{null}, McLeod's syndrome, In(Lu)
Cation permeability disorders
  Hereditary stomatocytosis
  Hereditary xerocytosis
Photooxidation: erythropoietic and hepatoerythropoietic porphyrias
Membrane lipids
  Hepatocellular disease: spur cell anemia
  Lecithin: cholesterol acyltransferase deficiency
  Vitamin E deficiency
  Abetalipoproteinemia
  Tangier disease
Other presumed membrane disorders
  Acanthocytosis with neurologic disease and normal lipoproteins
  Infantile pyknocytosis
Hemoglobin
  Structural defects
    Unstable hemoglobins (including hemoglobin E)
    Hemoglobin S
    Hemoglobins C, D
  Synthesis defects: thalassemia syndromes
Red cell metabolism
  Inherited glycolytic defects
    Hexokinase
    Glucose phosphate isomerase
    Phosphofructokinase
    Triose phosphate isomerase
    Phosphoglycerate kinase
    Pyruvate kinase
  Acquired glycolytic defects
    Malignancies, myelodysplasia
    Hypophosphatemia (severe)
  Hexose monophosphate shunt defects: glucose-6-phosphate dehydrogenase deficiency
  Glutathione metabolism defects
  Nucleotide metabolism defects
    Pyrimidine 5'-nucleotidase
    Adenylate kinase
    Adenosine deaminase overproduction
Hypersplenism
Hemophagocytic syndromes
Bleeding
  Internal
    Intracranial, especially premature infants
    Cephalohematoma
    Pulmonary cavity
    Peritoneal, retroperitoneal
  External (including gastrointestinal)

---

mild variants of the same hemolytic anemias have lower reticulocyte counts and slightly older cells and may be classified as normocytic. Similarly, patients with severe hemolytic anemias and marked reticulocytosis have normocytic red cells if the underlying disease process causes cellular dehydration, as in hereditary spherocytosis and sickle cell disease. Many other examples are possible. The point is that the classification schemes are not perfect; nevertheless, they are diagnostically useful.

EVALUATION OF ANEMIA

History, Physical Examination, and Initial Laboratory Studies

The initial diagnostic encounter includes a detailed history and physical examination and a minimum of laboratory tests. The features of the history and physical examination relevant to the differential diagnosis of anemias are covered in detail in Chapter 1. The initial laboratory tests should include determinations of the Hgb and Hct, red cell indices, reticulocyte count and indices, platelet count, white blood cell count and differential, examination of the peripheral blood smear, and additional studies of the patient or family members that derive from the history and physical examination.

BLOOD SMEAR

In evaluation of anemias, the physician should always examine the blood smear personally and not take the word of others regarding the red cell morphology. It is impossible to encompass the subtleties of the smear with terms like *anisocytosis* and *poikilocytosis*. Great care must be taken to ensure that good peripheral blood smears are obtained and that artifact-free areas of the smear are examined. This is a particular problem in very anemic or polycythemic patients (Hct <15 or >65). In these patients, it is sometimes useful to concentrate the red cells by gentle centrifugation and removal of some plasma before preparing the smear. Conversely, in polycythemic patients (or neonates), it is sometimes necessary to dilute a drop of the patient's blood with a drop of plasma (obtained from a Hct tube) to prepare a smear with optimal morphology.

TABLE 44-3. Classification of Anemias by Red Blood Cell Size

Microcytic anemias
  Microcytic-hypochromic
    Iron deficiency
    Thalassemias
    Anemia of chronic disease[a]
    Lead poisoning[a]
    Sideroblastic anemias[b]
    Very unstable hemoglobins[a]
  Microcytic-normochromic (red cell fragments)
    Hereditary pyropoikilocytosis
    Homozygous hereditary elliptocytosis
Normocytic anemias
  Hypoplastic/dysplastic bone marrow
    Aplastic anemias[b]
      Radiation, drugs, alcohol
      Viruses (Epstein-Barr, hepatitis)
      Autoimmune
      Pregnancy
      Preleukemia
      Anorexia nervosa, starvation
    Myelophthisis (bone marrow invasion) syndromes
      Leukemias, lymphomas
      Myelomas, macroglobulinemia
      Metastatic tumors
      Granulomas
      Storage diseases (advanced)
      Myelofibrosis
      Osteopetrosis
    Myelodysplastic syndromes
  Erythroid aplasia/hypoplasia
    Pure red cell aplasia
      Parvovirus B19
      Transient erythroblastopenia of childhood
      Thymoma, lymphoma, chronic lymphocytic leukemia
      Autoimmune
      Diamond-Blackfan anemia[b]
    Renal disease
    Liver disease
    Endocrine disease
      Hypothyroid
      Hypopituitary
      Hyperparathyroid
    Anemia of chronic disease
    Early iron deficiency
    Low-affinity hemoglobins
  Hemolysis with ineffective erythropoiesis: congenital dyserythropoi-
    etic anemia, type II (hereditary erythroblastic multinuclearity
    with positive acid serum test)

Hemolytic anemias
  Hemolysis with red cell dehydration
    Hereditary spherocytosis
    Sickle cell disease
    Sickle syndromes
    Hemoglobin C disease
    Hereditary xerocytosis[b]
  Hemolysis with mild red cell fragmentation
    Microangiopathic and macroangiopathic hemolytic anemias
    Hereditary elliptocytosis
  Mild variants of other hemolytic disorders
  Hypersplenism
  Hemophagocytic syndromes
Bleeding (recent)
Macrocytic anemias
  Hypoplastic bone marrow with stress erythropoiesis
    Hypoplastic anemias
      Inherited
        Fanconi's anemia
        Dyskeratosis congenita
        Shwachman-Diamond syndrome
      Acquired[a]
        Paroxysmal nocturnal hemoglobinuria[b]
    Pure red cell aplasia, especially Diamond-Blackfan anemia
  Dysplastic bone marrow
    Myelodysplastic syndromes
    Erythroleukemia
    Alcohol toxicity
    Congenital dyserythropoietic anemias I and III
  Megaloblastic bone marrow
    Cobalamin (vitamin B_{12}) deficiency
    Folic acid deficiency
    Other defects of DNA synthesis
      Inherited
      Chemotherapy
Reticulocytosis
  Hemolysis without red cell dehydration or fragmentation
    Enzyme disorders
    Immunohemolysis: warm antibody, cold agglutinin, paroxysmal cold
      hemoglobinuria
    Unstable hemoglobins
    Paroxysmal nocturnal hemoglobinuria[c]
    Hereditary stomatocytosis
  Hemolysis and apparent macrocytosis despite red cell dehydration: heredi-
    tary xerocytosis
  Bleeding (with reticulocytosis)
  Treated cobalamin (vitamin B_{12}) or folate deficiency

[a]Often normocytic, normochromic.
[b]Sometimes macrocytic.
[c]Often normocytic due to accompanying aplasia.

The blood film should first be examined under low power to assess the adequacy of staining and to find an optimal site for morphologic study. The best site is usually a few millimeters inside the feather edge of a slide smear and toward the middle of a coverslip smear. Coverslip smears prepared by an experienced technician generally provide the best morphology. Unfortunately, such experience is disappearing in our increasingly automated hematology laboratories.

In a satisfactory area, the red cells are separated from each other and central pallor is evident in most of the red cells. This is true even in blood of patients with diseases like hereditary spherocytosis in which central pallor is diminished. The red cells should not overlap significantly, or line up in "rouleaux," and they should not deform each other into polygonal shapes, as they often do at the edges of the smear. The red cells also must not be artifactually deformed by excessive water in the stain (the so-called humidity artifact) or peppered by precipitated stain. It cannot be overemphasized that it is risky and often useless to assess red cell morphology on a poorly spread or poorly stained blood smear. Another smear must be prepared.

Target cells, crenated cells, stomatocytes, and spherocytes may be produced by artifact as well as disease. Real findings should be evident in multiple areas of the smear and on multiple smears. Artifactual spherocytes are particularly common and are recognized by their complete loss of central pallor and by the fact that they are larger, not smaller, than normal red cells. It is sometimes useful, particularly with spiculated cells and stomatocytes, to dilute freshly drawn blood into phosphate-buffered saline containing 0.5% glutaraldehyde, place a drop under a coverslip, blot to remove excess liquid, and examine the wet preparation by phase microscopy (or, if necessary, under bright-field conditions with the condenser lowered). Under these conditions, the artifacts and morphologic distortions induced by drying are eliminated.

Semipermanent mounts can be prepared by sealing the coverslips with nail polish. Unfixed wet preps can also be examined, prepared by diluting the patient's blood with the patient's own plasma, but the cells must be examined immediately. They gradually change shape because of local pH changes and the so-called glass effect (3,4).

TABLE 44-4. Classification of Anemias by Predominant Morphology

Spherocytes
  Hereditary spherocytosis[a]
  Immunohemolysis with IgG-coated or C3-coated red cells[a,b]
  Acute oxidant injury (HMP shunt defects during hemolytic crisis, oxidant drugs and chemicals)[a]
  ABO incompatibility in neonates[a]
  Hemolytic transfusion reactions[a,b]
  Clostridial sepsis[a]
  Severe burns, other red cell thermal injuries[a]
  Snake venoms[a]
  Severe hypophosphatemia[a]
  Hypersplenism[a,c]
Elliptocytes
  Hereditary elliptocytosis[d]
  Thalassemias[a]
  Iron deficiency, severe
  Sideroblastic anemias
  Megaloblastic anemias
Bizarre poikilocytes
  Red cell fragmentation syndromes: microangiopathic and macroangiopathic hemolytic anemias[a]
  Acute oxidant injury[a,c]
  Hereditary elliptocytosis in some neonates[a,c]
  Hereditary pyropoikilocytosis[a]
  Homozygous hereditary elliptocytosis[a]
Stomatocytes
  Hereditary stomatocytosis[a]
  Hereditary cryohydrocytosis[a]
  Liver disease, especially acute alcoholism
  Rh$_{null}$ or Rh$_{mod}$ blood groups[a]
  Adenosine deaminase hyperactivity[a,c]
  Tangier disease[c]
  Mediterranean stomatocytosis[d]
  Duchenne's muscular dystrophy[c,d]
  Marathon runners[c,d]
Prominent basophilic stippling
  Thalassemias[a]
  Unstable hemoglobinopathies[a]
  Pyridine 5'-nucleotidase deficiency[a]
  Lead poisoning
  Sideroblastic anemias
Irreversibly sickled cells
  Sickle cell anemia[a]
  Symptomatic sickle syndromes[a]
Intraerythrocytic parasites
  Malaria[a]
  Babesiosis[a]
  Bartonellosis[a]
Spiculated or crenated red blood cells
  Acute hepatic necrosis (spur cell anemia)[a]
  Embden-Meyerhof pathway (glycolytic) defects[a,c]
  Red cell fragmentation syndromes[a,c]
  Uremia[c]
  McLeod blood group[a]
  In(Lu) blood group[d]

Abetalipoproteinemia[a]
Acanthocytosis with neurologic disease and normal lipoproteins[d]
Postsplenectomy[d]
Anorexia nervosa
Vitamin E deficiency[a,c]
Infantile pyknocytosis[a]
Heat stroke[a,c]
Transiently after massive transfusion of stored blood
Hypothyroidism
Target cells
  Hemoglobins S, C, D, E[a]
  Obstructive liver disease[d]
  Hereditary xerocytosis[a]
  Thalassemias[a]
  Iron deficiency
  Sideroblastic anemias
  Postsplenectomy[d]
  Lecithin: cholesterol acyltransferase deficiency
Teardrop erythrocytes
  Extramedullary hematopoiesis
  Myelofibrosis
  Neoplastic invasion of the bone marrow[c]
  Granulomatous diseases involving the bone marrow[c]
  Osteopetrosis
Nonspecific or normal morphology
  Anemia of chronic diseases
  Aplastic anemias
  Pure red cell aplasias
  Embden-Meyerhof pathway (glycolytic) defects[a]
  HMP shunt defects[a]
  Other red cell enzyme deficiencies[a]
  Unstable hemoglobinopathies[a]
  α-Thalassemia (heterozygous)[d]
  Warm antibody immunohemolytic anemias[a,b,c]
  Cold agglutinin disease[a,b]
  Rh hemolytic disease in neonates[a,b]
  Paroxysmal cold hemoglobinuria[a,b,c]
  Paroxysmal nocturnal hemoglobinuria[a]
  Congenital dyserythropoietic anemias[a]
  Hypothyroidism
  Hemolysis with infections[a,c]
  Erythrophagocytic disorders[a]
  Wilson's disease[a]
  Hereditary xerocytosis[a,c]
  Erythropoietic or hepatoerythropoietic porphyria[a]
  Vitamin E deficiency[a]
  Hypersplenism[a]
  Leukemias, lymphomas
  Refractory anemia, preleukemia[c]
  Myelomas, macroglobulinemia
  Metastatic tumors[c]
  Storage diseases (advanced)
  Granulomatous diseases involving the bone marrow[c]
  Bleeding

HMP, hexose monophosphate.
[a]Usually associated with increased red cell destruction.
[b]Usually associated with a positive Coombs' test.
[c]Disorder sometimes associated with this morphology.
[d]Usually no anemia.

AUTOMATED COMPLETE BLOOD CELL COUNT

Automated hematology analyzers provide values for a variety of cellular parameters, which, if properly interpreted, facilitate the diagnostic process for anemias. Values for MCV, mean corpuscular Hgb concentration (MCHC), mean corpuscular Hgb, red cell distribution width (RDW), hemoglobin concentration distribution width (HDW), absolute reticulocyte count and reticulocyte indices [mean corpuscular reticulocyte volume and reticulocyte Hgb content (CHr)] are helpful in the placement of the individual anemic patients into the major categories and in the targeted selection of the final confirmatory diagnostic tests (Fig. 44-1 and Table 44-5) (5). In addition to MCV (Fig. 44-1), values for MCHC can be indicative of hypochromia or hyperchro-

mia. The microcytic to hypochromic red blood cell (RBC) ratio is the most sensitive discriminator between iron deficiency and β-thalassemia trait (6). An increased MCHC and HDW are suggestive of SS or CC disease as well as hereditary spherocytosis or xerocytosis (7–10). The absolute reticulocyte count value is of crucial importance in distinguishing hemolytic or bone marrow expanded states from hypoproliferative anemias. A reduction in the CHr indicates a state of iron-deficient erythropoiesis well in advance of the stage at which changes in red cell parameters can be appreciated and has been shown to be useful in early detection of iron deficient erythropoietic states (11–14). Chapter 2 discusses these and other parameters provided by automated hematology analyzers.

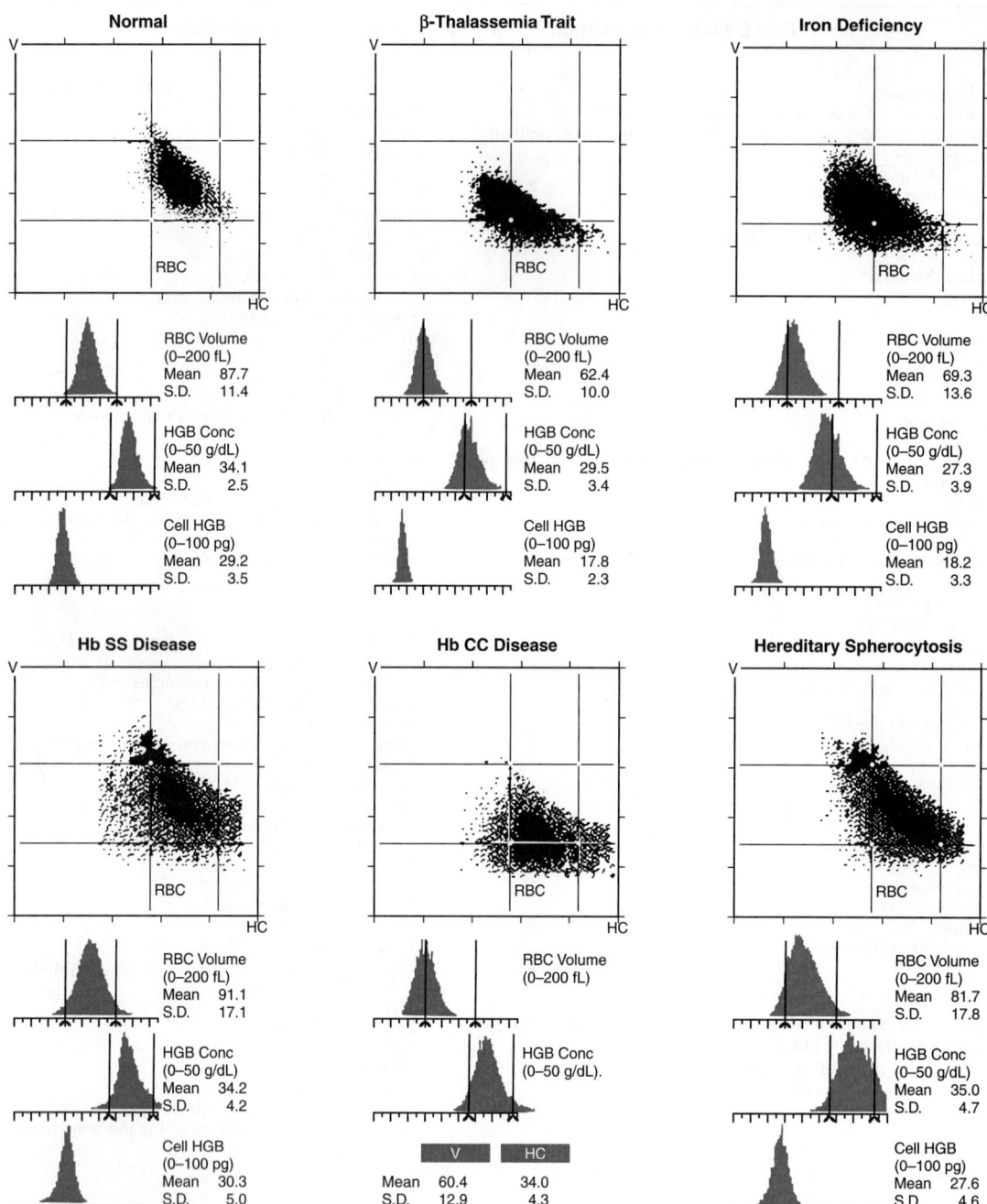

Figure 44-1. Flow cytometric characterization of mean corpuscular volume and mean corpuscular hemoglobin concentration (HGB Conc) distributions in normal blood and in selected hematologic conditions. In the top plot for each disease, the value for cellular hemoglobin concentration (HC, horizontal axis) is plotted against cell volume (V, vertical axis) for each individual erythrocyte. The plot area is divided into nine quadrants by gridlines for cell hemoglobin concentration (28 and 41 g/dL) and cell volume (60 and 120 fL). In the bottom three rows under each plot, distributions for red cell volume (goalposts at 60 and 120 μ), cell hemoglobin concentration (goalposts 60 and 120 fL), and cell hemoglobin content are presented. RBC, red blood cell.

DIAGNOSTIC APPROACH TO ANEMIA

One useful diagnostic approach to anemia is illustrated in Figure 44-2. Anemias are first divided into microcytic, normocytic, and macrocytic categories according to the MCV. It is important to remember that children have lower MCVs than adults (Table 44-1). From 1 to 6 years of age, the lower limit of normal is approximated by $MCV_{lower\ limit} = 69$ fL + (age in years); after that, the limit rises approximately 1 fL every other year until the lower adult limit (80 fL) is reached (15). The upper limit for the MCV rises linearly (0.6 fL/year) from 84 fL at 1 year to the upper limit of normal for adults (96 fL) (15). Each of these categories is subdivided into various pathophysiologic categories depending on the white cell, platelet, and reticulocyte counts and on whether the bone marrow is hypoplastic, dysplastic, or megaloblastic.

Microcytic Anemias

Microcytic anemias usually result from inadequate Hgb synthesis and are characterized by the presence of hypochromic red cells (enlarged central pallor) and target cells and in more severe cases by elliptocytes and other poikilocytes.

**TABLE 44-5. Alterations in Mean Corpuscular Volume (MCV), Mean Corpuscular Hemoglobin Concentration (MCHC),
Red Cell Distribution Width (RDW), and Hemoglobin (Hgb) Concentration Distribution Width (HDW) in Anemias**

	Low MCV	Normal MCV	High MCV
Normal RDW	Heterozygous α- and β-thalassemia	Normal Lead poisoning	Aplastic anemia
High RDW	Iron deficiency Hgb H disease Hgb H/Hgb Constant Spring Hgb S-β-thalassemia	Early stages of iron deficiency Liver disease Mixed nutritional deficiencies	Newborns Cobalamin (vitamin B$_{12}$) or folate deficiency
High RDW and high MCHC or HDW		Immune hemolysis SS and SC disease Hereditary spherocytosis Hereditary xerocytosis	Immune hemolysis

Laboratory studies typically include examination of the peripheral blood smear, a Hgb electrophoresis, and measurements of serum iron and total iron-binding capacity (TIBC)—a measure of the serum transferrin concentration. A serum ferritin and serum (circulating) transferrin receptor (sTfR) may also be useful. In young children, a blood lead should also be obtained. Although much used in the past, erythrocyte zinc protoporphyrin measurements are sensitive to a variety of biochemical interferences and are not particularly helpful in this diagnostic workup (16). In some cases, a bone marrow aspirate may also be necessary to assess iron stores and the presence or absence of ringed sideroblasts. The absolute reticulocyte count is also helpful in differentiating states of normal or increased bone marrow mass from those with reduced bone marrow mass or iron deficiency.

Iron deficiency anemia (discussed in Chapter 46) is by far the most common cause of microcytic anemias. The diagnosis is particularly common in infants from 6 months to 2 years of age and in women of reproductive age. At other ages, iron deficiency is much less common, and the physician must carefully confirm the diagnosis and establish its cause. Iron deficiency is only rarely caused by a poor diet in older children and adults who are not obviously malnourished. Chronic gastrointestinal blood loss must always be excluded in adult men and postmenopausal women, and it also must be considered in older children. Infants younger than 6 months of age should have adequate iron stores left over from intrauterine life and should not be iron deficient unless considerable bleeding or blood drawing has occurred.

Typically, the serum iron concentration is low, the TIBC is high, and the iron saturation is less than 10% in persons with iron deficiency anemia (17); these measurements are unreliable in patients who have recently taken iron supplements. The serum ferritin concentration is almost always low, regardless of the history of iron therapy (18), unless there are concomitant conditions that cause an increased ferritin, such as inflammation or infection, hyperthyroidism, liver disease (especially hepatitis C virus infection), malignancy, oral contraceptives, and alcohol consumption. Serum ferritin has been shown to provide little or no value in diagnosing iron-deficient states in infants and young children (14) and in the anemia of renal failure (19).

Because the average survival of red cells in the circulation is 4 months whereas the average survival of reticulocytes is 1 to 3 days (20), reticulocyte indices reflect changes in erythropoiesis much more quickly than do changes in the indices of the whole red cell population. The CHr is a particularly sensitive parameter of early iron deficiency. In a large study of children seen in a pediatric office setting, the CHr was more sensitive than Hgb, traditional red cell indices, zinc protoporphyrin, or any measurements of iron or ferritin in detecting iron deficiency (14,21). The probability of iron deficiency is greater than 90% when the CHr is less than 20 pg, is

50% when the CHr is 23 to 24 pg, and falls to 0% for CHr values greater than 29 pg (21). CHr also detected a response to therapy much more quickly.

Although *lead poisoning* (discussed in Chapters 46 and 47) is always included in the differential diagnosis of hypochromic-microcytic anemias, anemia is a late complication of lead intoxication and may be normocytic as well as microcytic. In many patients, the anemia of lead poisoning is actually due to concomitant iron deficiency. Both diseases occur in the same-age children, and some evidence exists that iron deficiency may exacerbate the pathophysiology of lead (22). For these reasons, all children with either disease should be tested for the other disease.

β-Thalassemia major and *β-thalassemia intermedia* (discussed in Chapter 48) are severe conditions that usually become evident between 6 and 18 months of life. The marked microcytic anemia, reticulocytosis, splenomegaly, and bony changes of β-thalassemia major or intermedia and the presence of thalassemia trait in both parents make the diagnosis relatively easy, although subsequent complications can pose many diagnostic dilemmas. One potential source of diagnostic confusion is rare Hgbs that are so unstable that they fail to assemble into Hgb tetramers and are destroyed during red cell maturation in the bone marrow. These unusual unstable Hgbs present with a thalassemic phenotype that may be dominantly inherited or may be a new mutation (discussed in Chapters 48 and 49).

β-Thalassemia trait (discussed in Chapter 49) is a common condition and must often be distinguished from other mild hypochromic-microcytic anemias, especially iron deficiency and the anemia of chronic disease. Plasma color (observed in a spun Hct tube) is frequently clear in iron deficiency but is a normal (straw) color or even abnormally yellow (due to increased bilirubin) in thalassemia trait. The blood smear also provides clues. Poikilocytosis ("animal cracker" cells) and basophilic stippling are more pronounced in thalassemia trait than iron deficiency when patients with the same degree of anemia are compared. The red cell count is increased in patients with thalassemia trait compared with those with iron deficiency, which is the basis of the Mentzer index (MCV/red cell count <13 in thalassemia trait, >13 in iron deficiency) (23) and the England and Fraser index [MCV – red cell count – (5 × Hgb) – 8.4; negative in thalassemia trait, positive in iron deficiency] (24), which attempt to differentiate the two diseases.

These classic indices have now been replaced by data provided by automated cell sizing of red cells: The microcytic to hypochromic RBC ratio is characteristically greater than 0.9 in β-thalassemia trait (reflecting the prevailing microcytosis) and lower than 0.9 in iron deficiency (reflecting the prevailing hypochromia) (6). The ratio is obtained by dividing the percentage of microcytes in a sample (obtained from a distribution of individual red cell volumes) by the percentage of hypochromic red cells (obtained from a similar

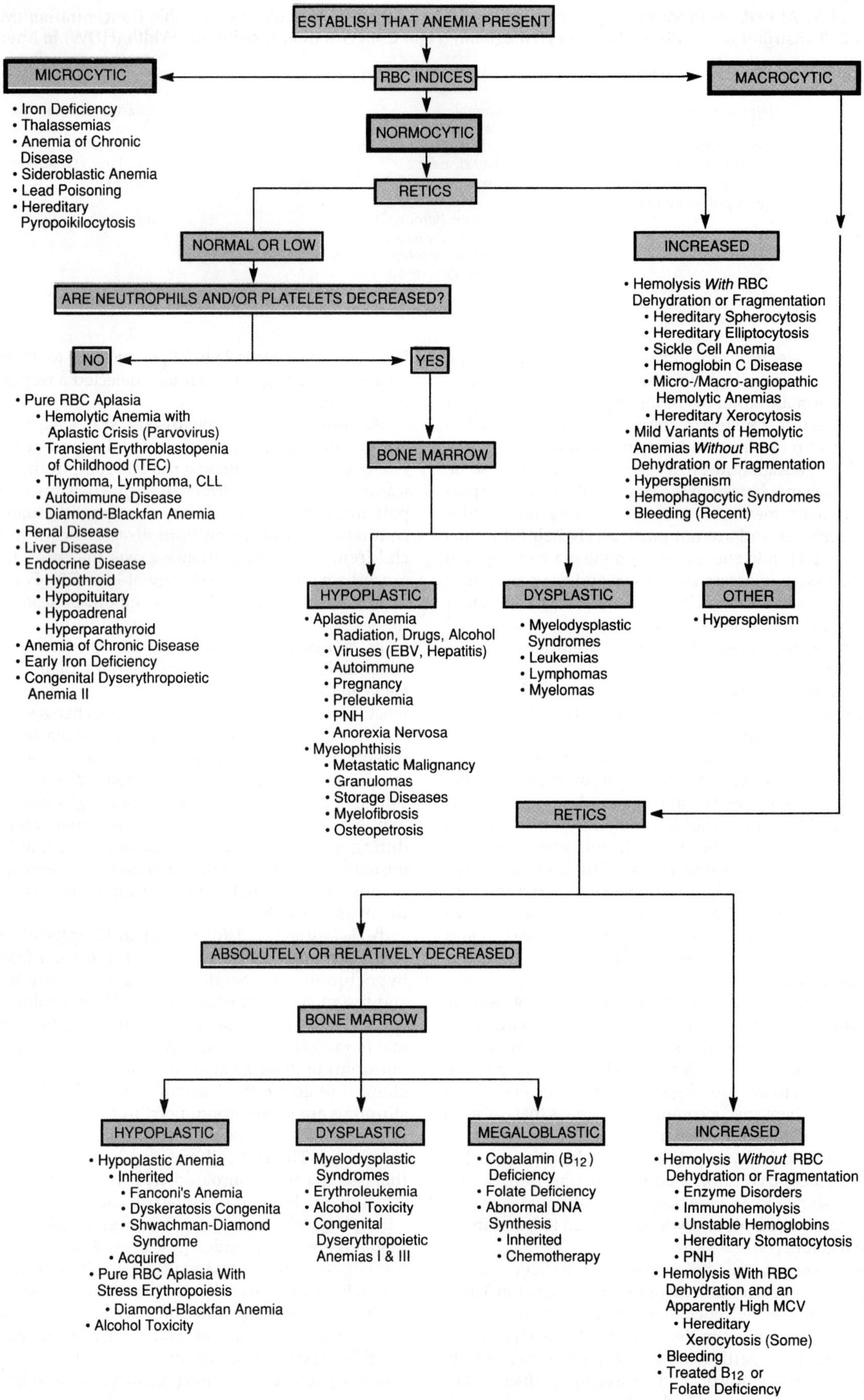

ESTABLISH THAT ANEMIA PRESENT

RBC INDICES

MICROCYTIC
- Iron Deficiency
- Thalassemias
- Anemia of Chronic Disease
- Sideroblastic Anemia
- Lead Poisoning
- Hereditary Pyropoikilocytosis

NORMOCYTIC

RETICS

MACROCYTIC

NORMAL OR LOW

ARE NEUTROPHILS AND/OR PLATELETS DECREASED?

NO
- Pure RBC Aplasia
  - Hemolytic Anemia with Aplastic Crisis (Parvovirus)
  - Transient Erythroblastopenia of Childhood (TEC)
  - Thymoma, Lymphoma, CLL
  - Autoimmune Disease
  - Diamond-Blackfan Anemia
- Renal Disease
- Liver Disease
- Endocrine Disease
  - Hypothroid
  - Hypopituitary
  - Hypoadrenal
  - Hyperparathyroid
- Anemia of Chronic Disease
- Early Iron Deficiency
- Congenital Dyserythropoietic Anemia II

YES

BONE MARROW

HYPOPLASTIC
- Aplastic Anemia
  - Radiation, Drugs, Alcohol
  - Viruses (EBV, Hepatitis)
  - Autoimmune
  - Pregnancy
  - Preleukemia
  - PNH
  - Anorexia Nervosa
- Myelophthisis
  - Metastatic Malignancy
  - Granulomas
  - Storage Diseases
  - Myelofibrosis
  - Osteopetrosis

DYSPLASTIC
- Myelodysplastic Syndromes
- Leukemias
- Lymphomas
- Myelomas

OTHER
- Hypersplenism

INCREASED
- Hemolysis *With* RBC Dehydration or Fragmentation
  - Hereditary Spherocytosis
  - Hereditary Elliptocytosis
  - Sickle Cell Anemia
  - Hemoglobin C Disease
  - Micro-/Macro-angiopathic Hemolytic Anemias
  - Hereditary Xerocytosis
- Mild Variants of Hemolytic Anemias *Without* RBC Dehydration or Fragmentation
- Hypersplenism
- Hemophagocytic Syndromes
- Bleeding (Recent)

RETICS

ABSOLUTELY OR RELATIVELY DECREASED

BONE MARROW

HYPOPLASTIC
- Hypoplastic Anemia
  - Inherited
    - Fanconi's Anemia
    - Dyskeratosis Congenita
    - Shwachman-Diamond Syndrome
  - Acquired
- Pure RBC Aplasia With Stress Erythropoiesis
  - Diamond-Blackfan Anemia
- Alcohol Toxicity

DYSPLASTIC
- Myelodysplastic Syndromes
- Erythroleukemia
- Alcohol Toxicity
- Congenital Dyserythropoietic Anemias I & III

MEGALOBLASTIC
- Cobalamin (B$_{12}$) Deficiency
- Folate Deficiency
- Abnormal DNA Synthesis
  - Inherited
  - Chemotherapy

INCREASED
- Hemolysis *Without* RBC Dehydration or Fragmentation
  - Enzyme Disorders
  - Immunohemolysis
  - Unstable Hemoglobins
  - Hereditary Stomatocytosis
  - PNH
- Hemolysis With RBC Dehydration and an Apparently High MCV
  - Hereditary Xerocytosis (Some)
- Bleeding
- Treated B$_{12}$ or Folate Deficiency

Figure 44-2. Diagnostic approach to anemias. CLL, chronic lymphocytic leukemia; EBV, Epstein-Barr virus; MCV, mean corpuscular volume; PNH, paroxysmal nocturnal hemoglobinuria; RBC, red blood cell; RETICS, reticulocyte counts.

distribution of red cell Hgb concentrations). The ratio has a high discriminant efficiency (92%) in differentiating the two disorders, better than any of the previous discriminant formulas (6).

Most patients with thalassemia trait also have an increased Hgb A_2 [and, less reliably, an increased fetal Hgb (Hgb F)], have a parent with microcytosis, and have normal or increased serum iron and ferritin values (25). It is important to remember that the elevation in Hgb A_2 is muted by iron deficiency and is not observed in forms of thalassemia that involve the δ chain (such as δβ-thalassemia). As a reflection of the slight increase in erythroid mass, the sTfR is also elevated in β-thalassemia trait (26).

Patients with α-*thalassemia trait* (discussed in Chapter 48) also have microcytosis, usually without anemia, and a normal Hgb electrophoresis. A definitive diagnosis of α-thalassemia requires DNA analysis of the α-globin loci, which is not routinely available and is rarely needed. As in β-thalassemia trait, expansion of the erythron in α-thalassemia is reflected by an increased sTfR (27).

Hgb H disease is characterized by hypochromic microcytic anemia. When Hgb Constant Spring is associated with Hgb H (H/CS), hypochromia is more pronounced and MCV values are greater than in Hgb H disease. Flow cytometric measurements of MCV, MCHC, and their respective distribution widths (RDW and HDW) have been shown to discriminate effectively between Hgb H and Hgb H/CS disease (28,29).

The *anemia of chronic disease* (discussed in Chapter 56) is often the most difficult disease to diagnose in this category. In most patients, the diagnosis can be made only by exclusion. Classically, the disorder is characterized by mild to moderate anemia, a low or low-normal serum iron concentration, a low TIBC, an iron saturation higher than 10%, and an elevated serum ferritin (30); some of these features are often missing. A very useful parameter in the differential diagnosis of this state is the sTfR. Several studies have shown that the sTfR is characteristically increased in iron-deficient states and is normal or reduced in the anemia of chronic disease (31–33). Recent work suggests that the TfR-F index [the serum transferrin receptor (mg/L) divided by the log of the serum ferritin (µg/L)] is particularly helpful in distinguishing between the anemia of chronic diseases and iron deficiency anemia (33a,33b). The bone marrow examination demonstrates adequate iron stores. The MCV is only mildly decreased in patients with anemia of chronic disease, less so than in those with iron deficiency or thalassemia trait, and it is often normocytic.

Sideroblastic anemias (discussed in Chapters 11, 46, and 47) are characterized by failure to incorporate iron into heme. The serum iron and ferritin concentrations are normal to high, and the iron-binding capacity is normal or mildly decreased (34). The inherited sideroblastic anemias present in childhood are usually X-linked and are rare. Acquired forms caused by alcohol, isoniazid, other drugs, and especially myelodysplasia, occur in adults. Some patients have the classic dimorphic blood smear (hypochromic-microcytic erythrocytes coexisting with normally hemoglobinized cells or even macrocytes), but many do not. The diagnosis of sideroblastic anemia is confirmed by demonstrating ringed sideroblasts on a Prussian blue (iron) stain of the bone marrow aspirate (35,36).

Patients with extreme red cell fragmentation may also present with microcytosis. The best examples are hereditary pyropoikilocytosis and homozygous hereditary elliptocytosis (discussed in Chapter 51), in which MCV counts in the 50s and 60s are reported, despite reticulocytosis (37,38). It is surprising that the microangiopathic hemolytic anemias that occur in disseminated intravascular coagulation, thrombotic thrombocytopenic purpura, hemolytic-uremic syndrome, and a variety of other diseases are usually not microcytic. Apparently, the percentages of fragmented cells (typically 5% to 20%) are too small to affect the MCV. However, the presence of poikilocytes and microspherocytes can result in increases of both the RDW and HDW.

Finally, anemias characterized by severe red cell dehydration, such as homozygous Hgb C disease or hereditary spherocytosis, may also have a slightly low MCV, with an increased MCHC and HDW, although generally they are classified as normocytic anemias.

Macrocytic Anemias with Normal or Low Reticulocyte Count

Macrocytic anemias are first subdivided according to the reticulocyte count. Patients with reticulocytosis and macrocytosis usually have bleeding or hemolysis and are considered in the section Hemolytic Anemias. Macrocytosis results from the relatively large size of reticulocytes, particularly stress reticulocytes, which have volumes 20% to 100% greater than erythrocytes. (The MCV of reticulocytes varies in disease, larger than normal reticulocytes in macrocytic anemias and smaller than normal in microcytic anemias.) Patients with macrocytosis and a normal to low reticulocyte count (relative to the degree of anemia) have disorders characterized by inadequate red cell production, which can be further subdivided into bone marrow failure syndromes and megaloblastic anemias. Macrocytosis in bone marrow failure syndromes is caused by stress erythropoiesis—that is, the production of red cells with characteristics of fetal erythrocytes (large size, increased Hgb F and i antigen) (39). Many classification schemes also group hypothyroidism and liver disease among the macrocytic anemias, but both diseases are more commonly associated with normocytic morphology (40–42).

Initial blood studies should include serum and red cell folate measurements, a serum cobalamin assay, and a bone marrow aspirate and biopsy. Patients who have macrocytosis and evidence of marrow failure should always have a bone marrow examination unless the diagnosis is clear from the history (e.g., chemotherapeutic agents or zidovudine) (43) or laboratory studies (e.g., folate deficiency). Additional studies will be dictated by the history, physical examination, and age of the patient and may include studies of bone marrow chromosomes; a diepoxybutane test (44); genetic and radiographic studies for Fanconi's anemia (45); tests for evidence of stress erythropoiesis (Hgb F, red cell i antigen); a test for red cell adenosine deaminase activity [increased in Diamond-Blackfan anemia (DBA)] (46); bone marrow special stains (iron, periodic acid-Schiff, and others) for evidence of sideroblastic, erythroleukemic, or other myelodysplastic features; a blood alcohol concentration; liver function tests; the Ham test; a Schilling test; tests for serum antiintrinsic factor and other autoantibodies; a gastric hydrochloric acid secretion test; or a therapeutic trial of cobalamin or folic acid.

Megaloblastic disorders such as cobalamin (vitamin B_{12}) deficiency, folic acid deficiency, and inherited disorders of DNA metabolism often leave diagnostic clues in the peripheral blood smear, particularly hypersegmented polymorphonuclear leukocytes and macroovalocytes. They damage all rapidly proliferating cells—neutrophils and megakaryocytes as well as erythrocytes—and may cause pancytopenia. Uncomplicated megaloblastic anemias are relatively easy to recognize, especially if the bone marrow is examined; however, some conditions that lead to megaloblastic hematopoiesis also cause gastrointestinal bleeding and iron deficiency (e.g., cirrhosis and alcoholism), which can mask macrocytosis and some of the megaloblastic morphology. Fortunately, the leukocyte changes (giant metamyelocytes and hypersegmented neutrophils) are not altered and serve as a marker to the underlying condition (47). In vitamin B_{12} deficiency anemia, response to therapy is characterized by the production of reticulocytes, which have a higher MCV than mature erythrocytes (48).

In addition to its effects on gastric mucosa and the liver, *alcohol* (discussed in Chapter 56) can also cause anemia through a direct toxic effect on the bone marrow, manifested by vacuolization of erythroid precursors (49) and a mild macrocytosis (50) that persists for several weeks after withdrawal of alcohol (51) or by dysplastic features (megaloblastic changes and ringed sideroblasts) (52).

In adults with macrocytic anemia, the most difficult diagnostic challenge is identification of *myelodysplastic syndromes* (discussed in Chapter 11). The typical picture is an elderly patient with macrocytosis and bicytopenia or pancytopenia combined with a normocellular or hypercellular bone marrow, dysplastic features in one or more cell lines, and, in some patients, excess myeloblasts. The dysplastic features in the erythroid series include the megaloblastic attributes, multinuclearity, nuclear budding, internuclear bridging, and ringed sideroblasts. Disordered myelopoiesis (e.g., left-shifted maturation, hypogranulation, pseudo–Pelger-Huët cells, and Auer rods) and disordered megakaryocytopoiesis (e.g., micromegakaryocytes and nuclear-cytoplasmic asynchrony) are also common (53). Clonal cytogenetic abnormalities are found in 40% to 70% of patients (54).

In children, macrocytic anemias are more often due to bone marrow failure. Megaloblastic anemias and myelodysplastic syndromes occur but are uncommon. Hypoplastic anemias may be either macrocytic or normocytic (discussed in Chapters 8 and 9). In general, they are macrocytic when the marrow insult is chronic and mild enough that a patient can produce some red cells, but less than normal. Under these conditions of stress erythropoiesis, the red cells have fetal characteristics, including macrocytosis and the presence of increased Hgb F and i antigen (39). In patients with severe aplastic anemia, virtually no erythropoiesis occurs, and the anemia is normocytic and normochromic.

Acquired aplastic anemias are often severe and normocytic, whereas congenital marrow failure syndromes are typically macrocytic. Paroxysmal nocturnal hemoglobinuria (PNH) is an exception (discussed in Chapter 10). It is an acquired disorder caused by the emergence of a complement-sensitive hematopoietic clone in persons with underlying bone marrow failure. The red cells are macrocytic because of chronic hemolysis and reticulocytosis. The diagnosis suggested by a positive Ham test and confirmed by the absence of CD59, CD55, and other glycosyl phosphatidyl inositol–linked proteins on hematopoietic cells. *Fanconi's anemia*, the most common congenital syndrome, is characterized by pancytopenia, recessive inheritance, physical anomalies (especially hyperpigmentation, café-au-lait spots, microsomy, microcephaly, thumb and radial anomalies, hypogenitalia, and renal malformations), and increased chromosomal breaks. The latter occur spontaneously but are especially common after clastogenic agents such as diepoxybutane (44). This characteristic forms the basis for a sensitive diagnostic test. The combination of immunoblot analysis and retroviral-mediated phenotypic correction of patient-derived cell lines allows a rapid method of Fanconi's anemia subtyping (45). The clinician must remember that Fanconi's anemia can present in young adults (as old as 35 years) as well as children and occurs fairly often without physical defects (approximately 25%) (55) or with subtle defects that can be detected only by an astute observer (such as loss of radial pulses or hypoplasia of the first metacarpal or of the thenar eminence).

Shwachman-Diamond syndrome (discussed in Chapter 8) begins in infancy as bicytopenia or pancytopenia combined with pancreatic insufficiency (fat malabsorption, failure to thrive), short stature, and, in some patients, metaphyseal dysostosis (56–58).

Dyskeratosis congenita (discussed in Chapter 8) is an X-linked form of ectodermal dysplasia and pancytopenia that presents from infancy to approximately 30 years. The characteristic dermatologic features are reticulated hyperpigmentation of skin, dystrophic nails, and leukoplakia (59,60).

Syndromes of pure red cell aplasia, like the aplastic anemias, are usually normocytic when acquired and macrocytic when con-

genital. DBA, an uncommon but not rare congenital disorder, classically presents in infancy (1 year or earlier) with macrocytic anemia, reticulocytopenia, selective absence of erythroid precursors beyond proerythroblasts, and sometimes (approximately 25%) physical anomalies of various types (61–63). Only approximately 30% of patients have an increased MCV at presentation, presumably because red cell production is so suppressed that even stress erythropoiesis cannot occur. As expected, almost all patients are macrocytic during recovery. For unknown reasons, adenosine deaminase activity is increased in DBA erythrocytes (46), which can be a useful point in distinguishing DBA from *transient erythroblastopenia of childhood* (discussed in Chapter 8), a more common cause of childhood red cell aplasia. Transient erythroblastopenia of childhood typically occurs in toddlers and children (1 year or older) who previously had normal Hgb levels. It is a normocytic anemia with reticulocytopenia and marrow erythroblastopenia at presentation, although macrocytosis is observed during recovery, which occurs usually within 1 to 2 months (64).

Normocytic Anemias with Normal or Low Reticulocyte Count

Normocytic anemias with an increased reticulocyte count are due to red cell destruction (hemolysis) or bleeding and are discussed in the section Hemolytic Anemias. Anemias with normal or low reticulocyte counts are due to bone marrow failure (Fig. 44-2 and Table 44-3). The differential diagnosis includes many of the disorders described in the previous sections. Under certain circumstances, particularly early in the disease, patients with iron deficiency, anemia of chronic disease, lead poisoning, acquired sideroblastic anemias, DBA, and myelodysplastic syndromes may have a normocytic anemia. Patients with combinations of disease that balance and camouflage each other, such as iron deficiency and cobalamin or folate deficiency, may also be normocytic, as may patients with mild variants of hemolytic anemias who are macrocytic when reticulocyte counts are high. Thus, knowing that red cell size is normal is not as useful diagnostically as knowing that red cells are large or small. Some conditions are typically normocytic and deserve special consideration in the workup of anemias in this category.

Patients with normocytic anemia and low reticulocyte counts should be further categorized depending on whether the granulocyte and platelet counts are normal or low. Those with bicytopenia or pancytopenia often have serious diseases and require a thorough workup, including a bone marrow aspirate and biopsy, and often, chromosome studies. Patients with isolated anemia and reticulocytopenia should also have a bone marrow examination if the condition is severe.

By definition, an empty or markedly hypoplastic bone marrow represents *aplastic anemia* (discussed in Chapter 9). Aplastic anemia has many causes (Table 44-2). In addition to drugs, radiation, toxins, and relatively obvious conditions like anorexia nervosa and postpregnancy aplasia, the physician must consider viruses [especially hepatitis viruses, Epstein-Barr virus, human immunodeficiency virus, and parvovirus B19 (which usually causes pure red cell aplasia but may cause pancytopenia)], autoimmune pancytopenia, and hypoplastic preleukemia (often clonal). In addition, in children and young adults, congenital bone marrow failure syndromes must be considered, although most patients with these syndromes have macrocytosis.

Myelophthisis is a term used to classify disorders that interfere with normal hematopoiesis due to the accumulation of malignant or reactive cells or cell products. These include malignancies of cells that are intrinsic to the marrow, such as leukemias (discussed in Chapters 15, 25, and 26), lymphomas (discussed in Chapters 27 and 28), myelomas (discussed in Chapter 29), macroglobulinemias (discussed in Chapter 29), and histiocytoses (discussed in Chapter 30) and metastatic tumors. In the last category, neuroblastomas, melanomas, seminomas, and a variety of carcinomas (breast, prostate, thyroid, stomach, renal, and small cell lung) are especially likely to involve the marrow. Myelophthisis can also be produced by granulomatous diseases, such as disseminated tuberculosis, histoplasmosis, or sarcoidosis; myelofibrosis (agnogenic myelofibrosis with myeloid metaplasia; discussed in Chapter 12); disseminated vasculitis; storage diseases in advanced stages; and osteopetrosis (discussed in Chapter 8), a rare defect of osteoclasts in which bone overgrowth occludes the marrow cavity. In addition to cytopenias, myelophthisic processes are usually accompanied by a characteristic blood smear featuring various combinations of teardrop erythrocytes, poikilocytes, nucleated erythrocytes, immature myeloid cells, and giant platelets or megakaryocyte fragments—the so-called leukoerythroblastic blood smear (65,66). Leukoerythroblastosis is also observed in patients with severe hypoxia or acidosis, especially infants; in diseases in which extramedullary hematopoiesis occurs without myelophthisis, such as thalassemia major (discussed in Chapter 48) and erythroblastosis fetalis (discussed in Chapter 55); with intrauterine infections (syphilis, cytomegalovirus, herpes simplex virus, rubella, and toxoplasmosis); with bacterial or fungal osteomyelitis (rarely); and with the transient myeloproliferative disease associated with Down's syndrome in infancy (discussed in Chapters 12 and 15).

Isolated cytopenia or pancytopenia in a patient with splenomegaly may also be due to *hypersplenism*. Usually, the spleen is large enough to be detected on physical examination; often it is massive, but ultrasound detection occasionally is required. The thrombocytopenia and neutropenia are caused by splenic pooling and are generally not severe unless the disease causing the splenomegaly also involves the bone marrow. Bone marrow examination shows normocellularity or hypercellularity of all lines, without dysplasia, unless the marrow is also affected by the underlying disease. Indium-111 platelet survival studies can aid the diagnosis by showing reduced platelet recovery and a normal platelet survival, the characteristics of platelet pooling.

Patients with normocytic anemia and reticulocytopenia who have normal neutrophil and platelet counts may have pure red cell aplasia or anemias secondary to certain systemic diseases (renal disease, liver disease, endocrine disease, or anemia of chronic disease). *Acquired pure red cell aplasia* (discussed in Chapter 9) may develop as a primary autoimmune disease, with antibody-mediated or T-cell–mediated marrow inhibition, and as a secondary condition in association with thymomas (5% to 10% of thymomas), lymphomas, leukemias (especially chronic lymphocytic leukemia), myelofibrosis, systemic lupus erythematosus, rheumatoid arthritis, and a variety of other conditions (67). Erythroblasts are almost completely lacking from the bone marrow. Other cell lines are normal. Two cases have been described of normochromic normocytic anemia due to autoantibodies against recombinant human erythropoietin (68) or native erythropoietin (69).

Transient erythroblastosis of childhood probably represents a temporary immune reaction to erythroid precursors, perhaps stimulated by childhood viral infections, although this possibility has been difficult to prove. A transient form of red cell aplasia also occurs in older children and adults from drugs (67) or viruses, especially B19 parvovirus (70). Parvovirus infections rarely produce significant anemia in normal individuals, but they can cause life-threatening aplastic crises in persons with chronic hemolytic anemias (discussed in Chapter 9).

The anemia of *renal disease* (discussed in Chapter 56) is complex. It is primarily an erythropoietin deficiency state, but bleeding, microangiopathic hemolysis, abnormal iron metabolism, and hyperparathyroidism may also be contributors (71).

Liver disease (discussed in Chapter 56) also produces a normocytic anemia, partly caused by hemodilution and hypersplenism; its complications may lead to either macrocytosis (e.g., folate deficiency, alcoholism, spur cell hemolysis) or microcytosis

(e.g., chronic gastrointestinal blood loss). Hyperbilirubinemia, increased lactate dehydrogenase (LDH), and decreased haptoglobin all may result from liver disease and not be caused by hemolysis.

Hypopituitarism, hypothyroidism, and *hyperparathyroidism* are associated with anemia (discussed in Chapter 56) that is usually normocytic, although patients with hypothyroidism may have macrocytic red cells. Whether this condition is due to accompanying pernicious anemia or is a direct effect of the lack of hormone is unclear.

HEMOLYTIC ANEMIAS

Presentation, History, and Physical Examination

Most of the signs and symptoms of anemia and hemolysis are well known to physicians and do not require detailed discussion. It is important to remember that patients with chronic hemolysis often have little or no anemia as a result of bone marrow compensation and that those who are anemic often are asymptomatic until Hgb levels fall to 8 g/dL or lower because of adjustments in the cardiovascular system and in Hgb–oxygen dissociation (72) (discussed in Chapter 49). This is particularly true in children. (73). It is also important to remember that patients with severe acute hemolysis may present with unusual symptoms such as isolated dizziness or fainting or with symptoms resembling an acute febrile illness, including headache, fever, shaking chills, vomiting, diarrhea, and abdominal or back pain. The latter symptoms are particularly likely with disorders producing acute *intravascular* hemolysis (Table 44-6) but may be seen as part of the picture of a hemolytic crisis in any chronic hemolytic anemia.

In patients with suspected hemolysis, special attention should be directed toward the family history and toward defining whether the process is acute or chronic, congenital or acquired. A history of consanguinity, anemia, jaundice, splenomegaly, splenectomy, and gallbladder disease should be sought through several generations. Unstable hemoglobins, hemolytic anemia with elevated red cell adenosine deaminase (74), and certain membrane diseases (hereditary spherocytosis, hereditary elliptocytosis, hereditary stomatocytosis, and hereditary xerocytosis) are dominantly inherited and may be discovered in abundance when fam-

---

TABLE 44-6. Hemolytic Anemias with Predominantly Intravascular Destruction and Hemoglobinuria

Immunohemolytic anemias
  Hemolytic transfusion reactions[a]
  Paroxysmal cold hemoglobinuria
  Acute onset autoimmune hemolytic anemia[a]
Acute oxidant hemolysis
  Glucose-6-phosphate dehydrogenase deficiency (after infections, drugs, favism)[a]
  Oxidant drugs, chemicals
Paroxysmal nocturnal hemoglobinuria
Red cell fragmentation syndromes
  Cardiac hemolytic anemia
  Disseminated intravascular coagulation
  March hemoglobinuria
Infections
  Clostridial sepsis
  Blackwater fever in *Plasmodium falciparum* malaria
Chemicals and toxins
  Copper toxicity[a]
  Snake venoms
  Arsine poisoning
  Water: osmotic hemolysis (freshwater drowning, infusion of hypotonic solutions)
Severe burns and other red cell thermal injuries

[a]Sometimes associated with intravascular hemolysis.

TABLE 44-7. Anemias with a Dominant or X-Linked Pattern of Inheritance

Autosomal dominant
  Membrane disorders
    Hereditary spherocytosis
    Hereditary elliptocytosis
    Hereditary stomatocytosis and cryohydrocytosis
    Hereditary xerocytosis
  Hemoglobin disorders
    Unstable hemoglobinopathies
    Heterozygous thalassemias
    Hemoglobins with diminished oxygen affinity
  Metabolic disorders
    Adenosine deaminase overproduction
    Hexokinase deficiency[a]
  Disorders of red cell production or maturation
    Diamond-Blackfan syndrome[a]
    Congenital dyserythropoietic anemia, type III
    Osteopetrosis, benign form
X-linked recessive
  Metabolic disorders
    Glucose-6-phosphate dehydrogenase deficiency
    Phosphoglycerate kinase deficiency
  Disorders of red cell production or maturation
    Congenital sideroblastic anemia[a]
    Dyskeratosis congenita
  Other diseases
    X-linked lymphoproliferative syndrome
    Hereditary elliptocytosis with mental retardation, midface hypoplasia, and Alport's syndrome
    X-linked α-thalassemia and mental retardation (ATR-X syndrome)

[a]Sometimes associated with this pattern of inheritance.

ily studies are pursued (Table 44-7). Neonatal jaundice is common in patients with congenital hemolytic anemias (it is present by history in half the patients with hereditary spherocytosis) but may be dismissed as physiologic (75). Subsequent jaundice is often mild or transiently present in association with viral illnesses and may be ignored unless it is brought out by careful questioning.

Diagnosis of Hemolysis

Hemolysis in the steady state is characterized by evidence of both increased red cell production and destruction. Many tests are available for assessing each of these processes, but few are useful.

TESTS FOR INCREASED RED CELL DESTRUCTION

The most widely used test for detecting hemolysis is the test for unconjugated (indirect) serum *bilirubin* level. In general, a level over 1 mg/dL is considered abnormal. Nonhemolytic causes of unconjugated hyperbilirubinemia are discussed in Chapter 47. With the exception of the neonatal period, unconjugated bilirubin concentrations in patients with hemolytic anemia do not exceed 4 mg/dL unless hepatic disease coexists (76). Unfortunately, the test is only moderately sensitive because the normal range for unconjugated bilirubin is so great (76). For example, 25% of patients with hereditary spherocytosis (77) and almost 50% of patients with immunohemolytic anemia (78) have normal bilirubin levels.

Gilbert syndrome (discussed in Chapter 47) is caused by the insertion of an extra TA in the TATAA element of the promoter of the UDP glycosyltransferase 1 family, polypeptide A1 (UGT1A1) gene. This gene is perhaps better known by its older name: bilirubin UDP glucuronosyltransferase 1. The gene product conjugates glucuronide to bilirubin. Homozygosity for the variant gene is common (≈ 15% of the population) and is associated with Gilbert syndrome. In hereditary spherocytosis, the reduced bilirubin conjugation due to the coexistence of Gilbert syndrome results in higher bilirubin levels (4.8 ± 1.9 mg/dL, n = 23, vs. 2.4 ± 1.3 mg/dL, n = 41) and increased risk for gallstones (80). Association of Gil-

bert syndrome with congenital dyserythropoietic anemia type II has also been shown to result in greater indirect bilirubin levels and increased risk of gallstone formation (81). Gilbert syndrome has a similar effect on the indirect bilirubin levels of acute hemolytic crises in glucose-6-phosphate dehydrogenase deficiency (82,83). It is likely that coinheritance of one or two Gilbert syndrome genes will predispose to increased indirect bilirubin levels and gallstones in all hemolytic anemias. If so, screening for the variant allele, a test that is not yet widely available, may become important in assessing the risk of gallstones or cosmetically offensive jaundice in inherited hemolytic anemias.

The most sensitive test for red cell destruction is the serum *haptoglobin* concentration (discussed in Chapter 47). In most patients, haptoglobin is absent from the plasma when the rate of red cell destruction exceeds twice normal, regardless of diagnosis (84). The haptoglobin test is very sensitive. In one large family with mild hereditary elliptocytosis and no detectable hyperbilirubinemia, 92% had low haptoglobin levels (85). The usefulness of haptoglobin determinations is complicated by the fact that the haptoglobin is an acute-phase reactant; its concentration may be normal despite hemolysis in patients with coexisting acute inflammation or malignancy or in patients taking androgens (84). This problem may be remedied if haptoglobin levels are compared with those of other acute-phase reactants (such as α₁-antitrypsin or orosomucoid), but these controls are not always available. In addition, haptoglobin is not a useful measure of hemolysis in the neonatal period because it is usually absent or diminished during the first few months of life (86). Normal adult haptoglobin concentrations are not reached until the infant is approximately 4 months old (87). Hereditary absence of haptoglobin is uncommon in white subjects but is found in approximately 4% of American blacks for unknown reasons (88).

Hemoglobinemia, hemoglobinuria, and hemosiderinuria are useful measures of hemolysis when red cell destruction is intravascular (Table 44-6). *Plasma Hgb* is readily detectable by visual observation when the concentration exceeds approximately 50 mg/dL (normal <5 mg/dL). The color may range from pink to brown, depending on the relative concentration of Hgb (red), bilirubin (yellow-green), methemoglobin (brown), and methemalbumin (brown). Hgb that passes through the glomerulus is reabsorbed by proximal tubular cells (threshold is approximately 100 to 150 mg/dL), where it is metabolized and the iron stored as ferritin and hemosiderin. Hemoglobinuria occurs if this reabsorption capacity is exceeded; it is characterized by heme-positive urine in the presence of red cells. Care must be taken to examine freshly voided specimens, because hemolysis may occur in dilute urine on standing. The color varies from pink to red to brown to almost black ("Coca-Cola urine").

Myoglobinuria produces a similar color, but it can be differentiated from hemoglobinuria by electrophoresis, gel filtration chromatography, or spectrophotometry, or by the fact that myoglobin remains in solution in fresh urine that is 80% saturated with ammonium sulfate (89). Inspection of the plasma (such as in a Hct tube) is also useful because myoglobin, with its low molecular weight (17 kd, compared with 68 kd for Hgb), is rapidly filtered by the kidneys and does not accumulate to visibly detectable levels if kidney function is normal. In addition, myoglobin does not bind to haptoglobin, so haptoglobin levels remain normal (90).

Even after intravascular hemolysis abates, iron-laden renal tubular cells continue to be sloughed, sometimes for months, and may be detected as *urine hemosiderin* (91). This is a useful test because it is simple, reliable, and sensitive, and because it permits detection of intermittent intravascular hemolysis (such as in paroxysmal nocturnal hemoglobinuria), but it may be negative in the first few days after a hemolytic episode (92). In the usual qualitative test, a smear of cells prepared from the urine sediment is stained with Prussian blue (as for bone marrow iron). Hemosiderinuria also occurs in patients with hemosiderosis or hemochromatosis.

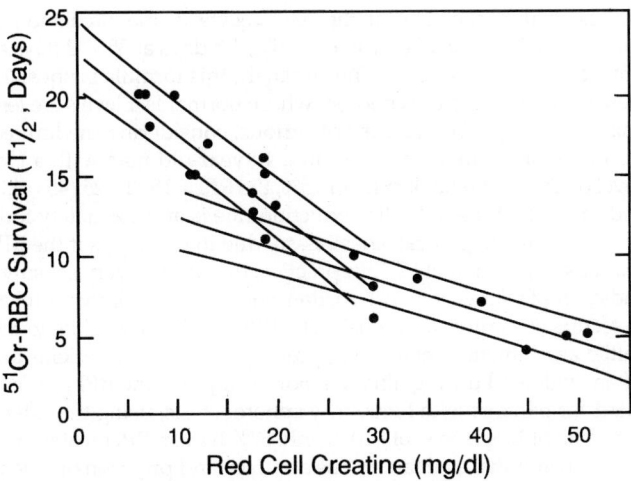

Figure 44-3. Relation of mean red cell (RBC) creatine concentration and red cell survival, measured as the half-life of chromium-51(^{51}CR)–labeled erythrocytes (normal, 25 to 31 days; regression lines ± 1 SD). (From Fehr J, Knob M. Comparison of red cell creatine level and reticulocyte count in appraising the severity of hemolytic processes. *Blood* 1979;53:966, with permission.)

The serum *LDH* level is elevated in many hemolytic anemias, especially with intravascular hemolysis or ineffective erythropoiesis, because of the release of the red cell isoenzyme (LDH-2) (93). Comparisons of the sensitivity of this readily

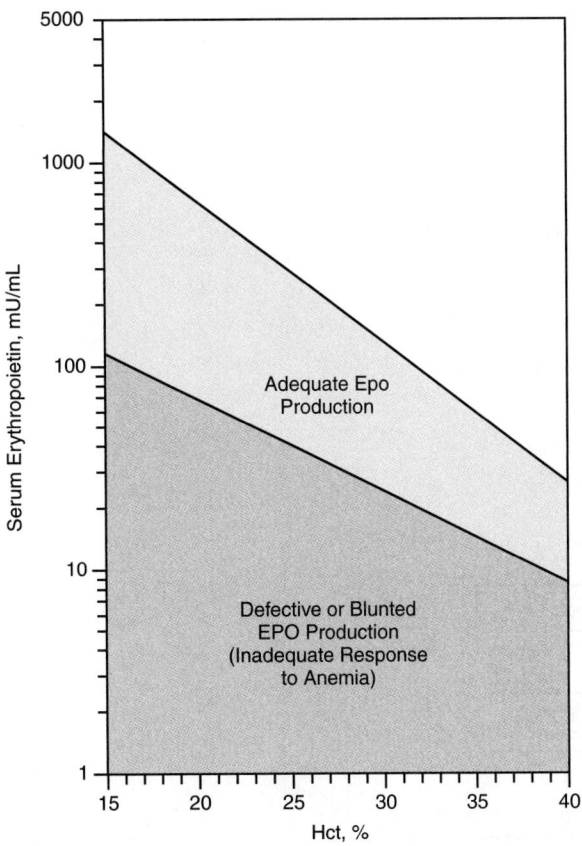

Figure 44-4. Relationship between serum erythropoietin (Epo) levels and hematocrit (Hct) in reference subjects. Area of parallel lines defines the 95% confidence limits. Values below the 95% reference range indicate a defective Epo response to anemia. Patients with aplastic or refractory anemia may show values above the reference range. (From Cazzola M, Mercuriali F, Brugnara C. Use of recombinant human erythropoietin outside the setting of uremia. *Blood* 1997;89:4248, with permission.)

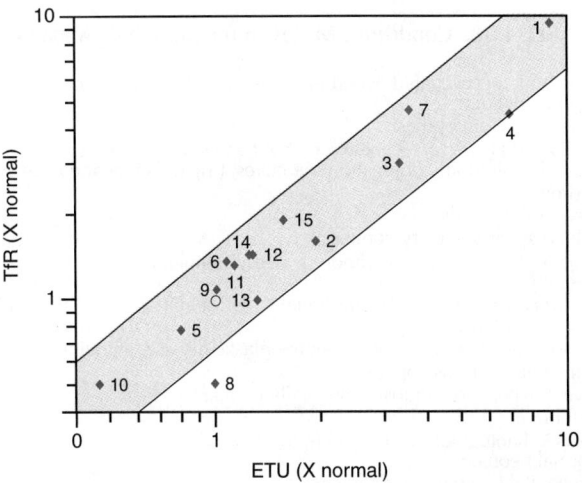

Figure 44-5. Relationship between serum transferrin receptor (TfR) and ferrokinetic measurement of the erythron transferrin uptake (ETU) shows that serum TfR is directly related to the number of erythroid precursors in the bone marrow. (*Open circle*) normal subjects; (*1*) β-Thalassemia/hemoglobin E; (*2*) angiogenic myeloid metaplasia; (*3*) autoimmune hemolytic anemia; (*4*) spherocytosis; (*5*) hypoplastic anemia; (*6*) myelodysplastic syndrome; (*7*) hemoglobin H disease; (*8*) bone marrow transplant; (*9*) myeloproliferative disorder; (*10*) renal failure; (*11*) renal failure on recombinant human erythropoietin; (*12*) secondary polycythemia; (*13*) relative polycythemia; (*14*) polycythemia of uncertain origin; (*15*) polycythemia vera. Note that ETU is overestimated in bone marrow transplant recipients because of hyperferremia. (From Beguin Y, Clemons GK, Pootrakul P, et al. Quantitative assessment of erythropoiesis and functional classification of anemia based on measurements of serum transferrin receptor and erythropoietin. *Blood* 1993;81:1067, with permission.)

available test relative to other tests of hemolysis have been made in patients with selected hemolytic anemias such as cardiac hemolysis, but its usefulness in many hemolytic anemias is unknown. One extensive study compared haptoglobin, red cell Hgb, plasma Hgb, LDH, schistocyte counts, transferrin levels, and urine hemosiderin in 1091 patients and concluded that the haptoglobin level is the most sensitive test but the serum LDH concentration value is best for quantitating intravascular hemolysis (94). Another study found haptoglobin and LDH levels to be similarly sensitive, but each was less sensitive than the chromium-51 (^{51}Cr) red cell lifespan (95).

Another useful test is that for red cell *creatine* concentration (96). Its concentration correlates closely with red cell lifespan, even in patients with mild hemolysis (Fig. 44-3). It is easily measured, the measurement requires little blood (0.1 to 0.2 mL), and the blood may be stored at 4°C for up to 1 week (97).

Other tests are available for assessing red cell destruction but are rarely needed. Tests for methemalbumin and hemopexin concentrations are insufficiently sensitive, and fecal urobilinogen levels are insufficiently practical to be useful (98,99). Carbon monoxide production tests can be precise and sensitive, but they are difficult to perform and require special apparatus (100). Carboxyhemoglobin tests are an indirect measure of carbon monoxide production but are less sensitive. ^{51}Cr-labeled red cell lifespan measurements are the gold standard. They are sensitive and can be valuable, but they are time-consuming and expensive and are rarely required.

TESTS FOR INCREASED RED CELL PRODUCTION
The most useful test for assessing red cell production and generally for detecting hemolysis is the *reticulocyte count*, especially the *absolute* reticulocyte count. When reticulocytes are expressed as a percentage of the red cell count, the normal range is approximately 0.5% to 1.5%. It is difficult to use the percentage of reticulocytes to estimate red cell production accurately in anemic patients because

TABLE 44-8. Conditions Mistaken for Hemolytic Anemia

Anemia and unconjugated hyperbilirubinemia without reticulocytosis
  Internal bleeding
  Ineffective erythropoiesis
Unconjugated hyperbilirubinemia without anemia or reticulocytosis
  Defective bilirubin conjugation: neonates, Crigler-Najjar and Arias syndromes
  Breast milk jaundice
  Gilbert syndrome (very common)
Anemia and reticulocytosis without hyperbilirubinemia
  Bleeding
  Recovery from aplastic or nutritional (iron, vitamin B_{12}, folate) anemia
Leukoerythroblastosis
  Marrow invasion (myelophthisis): neoplastic disease, granulomas, myelofibrosis, osteopetrosis
  Severe hypoxia or acidosis (especially in infants)
Myoglobinuria
Decreased haptoglobin without hemolysis
  Normal neonate
  Congenital haptoglobin deficiency

the value is increased by the fall in red cell count (the denominator) and the premature, erythropoietin-induced release of bone marrow reticulocytes (identifiable on smears by their polychromatophilia), which take longer to mature in the circulation. The reticulocyte production index (RPI) takes these factors into account and has been shown to correlate closely with ferrokinetic studies of red cell turnover (101). The usual formula for RPI corrects the Hct to a normal of 45%:

$$\text{RPI} = \% \text{ reticulocytes/reticulocyte maturation time (days)} \times \text{Hct}/45$$

The maturation time of the reticulocyte in the circulation is taken to be 1 day at a Hct value of 45%, 1.5 days at 35%, 2 days at 25%, and 2.5 days at 15%. Unfortunately, this formula is not standardized for women or children, whose normal Hct levels are less than 45% (102). The error is not serious, considering the limited accuracy of the method. Thus, in a 40-year-old man with a Hct level of 25% and reticulocytes of 15%, the RPI = $15/2 \times 25/45 = 4.2$, indicating that the red cell production rate is approximately four times normal. In general, anemias are due to hemolysis if the RPI exceeds approximately 2.5. In practice, the RPI is a very sensitive indicator of relative hypoproduction, and it is particularly useful in detecting an early aplastic crisis. The RPI may be misleading in the initial assessment of hemolysis, presumably because patients are often evaluated during illnesses. For example, if the RPI is calculated for patients with hereditary spherocytosis, using the extensive data of Emerson et al. (102), only 67% had an RPI greater than 2.5 on their initial evaluation. The accuracy and precision of reticulocyte counting with automated methods greatly exceed those of manual reticulocyte counts (103–106). Absolute reticulocyte counts (cells/µL) avoid the limitations of the percent reticulocyte count when the RBC number is outside the normal range and obviates the need for Hct corrections. If the clinical laboratory provides a normal range for absolute reticulocyte counts (typically 24,000 to 84,000 reticulocytes/µL), cases with abnormally low reticulocyte count can be quickly identified.

In patients with severe hemolysis, nucleated red cells may appear in the peripheral blood, and granulocytosis and thrombocytosis may develop; in such patients, the reticulocyte count is almost always elevated. More sophisticated measures for assessing red cell production such as the bone marrow examination or ferrokinetic studies are rarely needed.

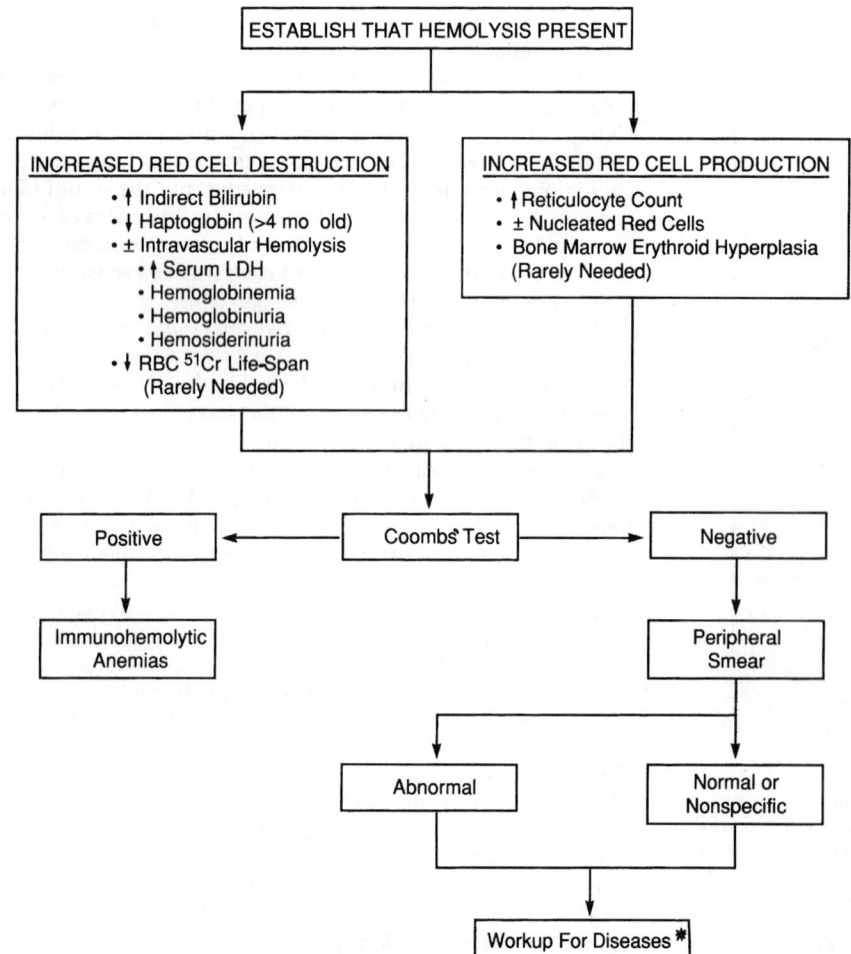

Figure 44-6. Diagnostic approach to hemolytic anemias. *Table 44-4 lists diseases included in workup based on their erythrocyte morphology. ^{51}Cr, chromium-51; LDH, lactate dehydrogenase; RBC, red blood cell.

In the assessment of difficult cases of anemia, measurements of serum erythropoietin and sTfR levels should always be obtained. The adequacy of the endogenous erythropoietin response should be evaluated with a nomogram that plots serum erythropoietin versus Hgb or Hct (Fig. 44-4), allowing identification of true erythropoietin-deficient states (107). sTfR has been shown to be an excellent indicator for the red blood cell precursor mass (108,109) (Fig. 44-5). Studies of serum erythropoietin and sTfR have shown that an inverse relationship exists between red blood cell precursor mass and serum erythropoietin—that is, for any given Hgb level, the higher the number of red cell precursors (sTfR), the lower the serum erythropoietin concentration (108,109).

DIAGNOSTIC PROBLEMS

Patients with evidence of either increased red cell destruction or increased erythropoiesis, but not both, may cause diagnostic difficulties. Conditions to consider are listed in Table 44-8.

HEMOLYSIS IN THE NEONATE

Hemolysis may be difficult to document in the first few days of life because indirect hyperbilirubinemia is common and multifaceted during this period, and serum haptoglobin levels are depressed (86). Generally, the reticulocyte count is the most useful parameter. The reticulocytosis evident in cord blood and during the first day of life (3% to 7%) normally falls to less than 3% by day 3 and to less than 1% by day 7 as a result of the termination of erythropoiesis (110). Reticulocytosis usually persists in the presence of severe hemolysis (often with nucleated red cells) but may be unimpressive in neonates with only mild to moderate hemolysis (111). Unfortunately, anoxia, infection, and acidosis also stimulate reticulocytes and nucleated red cells in neonates, and blood drawing may produce enough anemia to induce reticulocytosis and simulate hemolysis. To make matters worse, poikilocytes are common in normal neonatal blood smears (discussed in Chapter 55), particularly in premature infants, and subtle morphologic defects can easily be missed. Fortunately, time is on the side of the diagnostician. Within a few months, fetal red cells disappear, the blood smear becomes simpler to interpret, and Hgb, bilirubin, haptoglobin, and reticulocyte levels come to equilibrium.

Initial Evaluation of the Hemolytic Process

Patients with documented hemolysis are separated into a Coombs' test–positive group (immunohemolytic anemias) and a Coombs' test–negative group. The latter group is then further divided depending on whether the blood smear is characterized by predominant red cell morphology (smear abnormal in Fig. 44-6) or by normal or nonspecific red cell morphology. The anemias are classified according to their morphologic characteristics in Table 44-4. This classification is extensive but not inclusive. Occasional patients have inexplicable morphologic findings or combinations of diseases (such as hereditary spherocytosis and obstructive jaundice) that conspire to cause morphologic and diagnostic confusion.

REFERENCES

1. MacKinney AA Jr. Hereditary spherocytosis: clinical family studies. *Arch Intern Med* 1965;116:257.
2. Krueger HC, Burgert EO Jr. Hereditary spherocytosis in 100 children. *Mayo Clin Proc* 1966;41:821.
3. Furchgott RF. Disk-sphere transformation in mammalian red cells. *J Exp Biol* 1940;17:30.
4. Brecher G, Bessis M. Present status of spiculated red cells and their relationship to the discocyte-echinocyte transformation: a critical review. *Blood* 1972;40:333.
5. Brugnara C. Reticulocyte cellular indices: a new approach in the diagnosis of anemias and monitoring of erythropoietic function. *Crit Rev Clin Lab Sci* 2000;37:93–130.
6. d'Onofrio G, Zini G, Ricerca BM, et al. Automated measurement of red blood cell microcytosis and hypochromia in iron deficiency and β-thalassemia trait. *Arch Pathol Lab Med* 1992;116:84–89.
7. Mohandas N, Kim YR, Tycko DH, et al. Accurate and independent measurement of volume and hemoglobin concentration of individual red cells by laser light scattering. *Blood* 1986;68:506–513.
8. Mohandas N, Johnson A, Wyatt J, et al. Automated quantitation of cell density distribution and hyperdense cell fraction in RBC disorders. *Blood* 1989;74:442–447.
9. Gilsanz F, Ricard MP, Millan I. Diagnosis of hereditary spherocytosis with dual-angle differential light scattering. *Am J Clin Pathol* 1993;100:119–122.
10. Cynober T, Mohandas N, Tchernia G. Red cell abnormalities in hereditary spherocytosis: relevance to diagnosis and understanding of the variable expression of clinical severity. *J Lab Clin Med* 1996;128:259–269.
11. Brugnara C, Laufer MR, Friedman AJ, et al. Reticulocyte hemoglobin content (CHr): early indicator of iron deficiency and response to therapy. *Blood* 1994;83:3100.
12. Brugnara C, Colella GM, Cremins JC, et al. Effects of subcutaneous recombinant human erythropoietin in normal subjects: development of decreased reticulocyte hemoglobin content and iron-deficient erythropoiesis. *J Lab Clin Med* 1994;123:660–667.
13. Brugnara C, Zelmanovic D, Sorette M, et al. Reticulocyte hemoglobin: an integrated parameter for evaluation of erythropoietic activity. *Am J Clin Pathol* 1997;108:133–142.
14. Brugnara C, Zurakowski D, DiCanzio J, et al. Reticulocyte hemoglobin content to diagnose iron deficiency in children. *JAMA* 1999;281:2225–2230.
15. Dallman PR, Siimes MA. Percentile curves for hemoglobin and red cell volume in infancy and childhood. *J Pediatr* 1979;94:26.
16. Hastka J, Lasserre JJ, Schwarzbeck A, et al. Washing erythrocytes to remove interference in measurements of zinc protoporphyrin by front-face hematofluorometry. *Clin Chem* 1992;38:2184–2189.
17. Beutler E. Clinical evaluation of iron stores. *N Engl J Med* 1957;256:692.
18. Lipschitz DA, Cook JD, Finch CA. A clinical evaluation of serum ferritin as an index of iron stores. *N Engl J Med* 1974;290:1213.
19. Fishbane S, Galgano C, Langley RC Jr, et al. Reticulocyte hemoglobin content in the evaluation of iron status of hemodialysis patients. *Kidney Int* 1997;52:217–222.
20. Hillman RS. Characteristics of marrow production and reticulocyte maturation in normal man in response to anemia. *J Clin Invest* 1969;48:443.
21. Brugnara C. Use of reticulocyte cellular indices in the diagnosis and treatment of hematological disorders. *Int J Clin Lab Res* 1998;28:1–11.
22. Piomelli S. Lead poisoning. In: Nathan DG, Orkin FA, eds. *Hematology of infancy and childhood*. Philadelphia: WB Saunders, 1998:480–496.
23. Mentzer WC. Differentiation of iron deficiency from thalassemia trait. *Lancet* 1973;1:882.
24. England JM, Fraser PM. Differentiation of iron deficiency from thalassemia trait by routine blood count. *Lancet* 1973;1:449.
25. Johnson CS, Tegos C, Beutler E. Thalassemia minor: routine erythrocyte measurements and differentiation from iron deficiency. *Am J Clin Pathol* 1983;80:31.
26. Bianco I, Mastropiero F, D'Asero C, et al. Serum levels of erythropoietin and soluble transferrin receptor during pregnancy in non-β-thalassemic and β-thalassemic women. *Haematologica* 2000;85:902–907.
27. Rees DC, Williams TN, Maitland K, et al. Alpha thalassemia is associated with increased soluble transferrin receptor levels. *Br J Haematol* 1998;103:365–369.
28. Bunyaratvej A, Butthep P, Fucharoen S, et al. Erythrocyte volume and haemoglobin concentration in haemoglobin H disease: discrimination between the two genotypes. *Acta Haematol* 1992;87:1–5.
29. Bunyaratvej A, Fucharoen S, Greenbaum A, et al. Hydration of red cells in alpha and beta thalassemias differs: a useful approach to distinguish between these red cell phenotypes. *Am J Clin Pathol* 1994;102:217–222.
30. Lee GR. The anemia of chronic disease. *Semin Hematol* 1983;20:61.
31. Ferguson BJ, Skikne BS, Simpson KM, et al. Serum transferrin receptor distinguishes the anemia of chronic disease from iron deficiency anemia. *J Lab Clin Med* 1992;19:385–390.
32. Mast AE, Blinder MA, Gronowski AM, et al. Clinical utility of the soluble transferrin receptor and comparison with serum ferritin in several populations. *Clin Chem* 1998;44:45–51.
33a. Punnonen K, Irjala K, Rajamäki A. Serum transferrin receptor and its ratio to serum ferritin in the diagnosis of iron deficiency. *Blood* 1997;89:1052–1057.
33b. Suominen P, Möttönen T, Rajamäki A, et al. Single values of serum transferrin receptor and transferrin receptor ferritin index can be used to detect true and functional iron deficiency in rheumatoid arthritis patients with anemia. *Arthritis Rheum* 2000;43:1016–1020.
34. Hines JD, Grasso JA. The sideroblastic anemias. *Semin Hematol* 1970;7:86.
35. May A, Bishop D. The molecular biology and pyridoxine responsiveness of X-linked sideroblastic anaemia. *Haematologica* 1998;83:56–70.
36. Koc S, Harris JW. Sideroblastic anemias: variations on imprecision in diagnostic criteria, proposal for an extended classification of sideroblastic anemias. *Am J Hematol* 1998;57:1–6.
37. Silveira P, Cynober T, Dhermy D, et al. Red blood cell abnormalities in hereditary elliptocytosis and their relevance to variable clinical expression. *Am J Clin Pathol* 1997;108:391–399.
38. Palek J. Hereditary elliptocytosis and related disorders. *Clin Haematol* 1985;14:45.
39. Alter BP. Fetal erythropoiesis in stress hematopoiesis. *Exp Hematol* 1979;7:200.
40. Daughday WH, Williams RH, Daland GA. The effect of endocrinopathies on the blood. *Blood* 1948;3:1342.
41. Horton L, Coburn R, England J, et al. The haematology of hypothyroidism. *QJM* 1985;45:101.
42. Mazzaferri EL. Adult hypothyroidism: manifestations and clinical presentation. *Postgrad Med* 1986;29:64.

43. Snower DP, Weil SC. Changing etiology of macrocytosis: zidovudine as a frequent causative factor. *Am J Clin Pathol* 1993;99:57–60.

44. Auerbach AD, Wolman SR. Susceptibility of Fanconi's anemia fibroblasts to chromosome damage by carcinogens. *Nature* 1976;261:494.

45. Pulsipher M, Kupfer GM, Naf D, et al. Subtyping analysis of Fanconi anemia by immunoblotting and retroviral gene transfer. *Mol Med* 1998;4:468–479.

46. Glader BE, Backer K, Diamond LK. Elevated erythrocyte adenosine deaminase activity in congenital hypoplastic anemia. *N Engl J Med* 1983;309:1486.

47. Spivak JL. Masked megaloblastic anemia. *Arch Intern Med* 1982;142:2111.

48. d'Onofrio G, Chirillo R, Zini G, et al. Simultaneous measurement of reticulocyte and red blood cell indices in healthy subjects and patients with microcytic and macrocytic anemia. *Blood* 1995;85:818–823.

49. McCurdy P, Rath CE. Vacuolated nucleated bone marrow cells in alcoholism. *Semin Hematol* 1980;17:100.

50. Unger KW, Johnson D. Red blood cell mean corpuscular volume: a potential indicator of alcohol usage in a working population. *Am J Med Sci* 1974; 267:281.

51. Wu A, Chanarin I, Levi AJ. Macrocytosis of chronic alcoholism. *Lancet* 1974; 1:829.

52. Eichner ER, Hillman RS. The evolution of anemia in alcoholic patients. *Am J Med Sci* 1971;50:218.

53. Bennett JM. Classification of the myelodysplastic syndromes. *Clin Haematol* 1986;15:909.

54. Yunis JJ, Lobell M, Arnesen MA, et al. Refined chromosome study helps define prognostic subgroups in most patients with primary myelodysplastic syndrome and acute myelogenous leukaemia. *Br J Haematol* 1988;68:189.

55. Glanz A, Fraser FC. Spectrum of anomalies in Fanconi's anemia. *J Med Genet* 1982;19:412.

56. Shwachman HJ, Diamond LK, et al. The syndrome of pancreatic insufficiency and bone marrow dysfunction. *J Pediatr* 1964;65:645.

57. Aggett PJ, Cavanagh NPC, Matthew DJ, et al. Shwachman's syndrome: a review of 21 cases. *Arch Dis Child* 1980;55:331.

58. Dror Y, Freedman MH. Shwachman-Diamond syndrome: an inherited preleukemic bone marrow failure disorder with aberrant hematopoietic progenitors and faulty marrow microenvironment. *Blood* 1999;94:3048–3054.

59. McGrath JA. Dyskeratosis congenita: new clinical and molecular insights into ribosome function. *Lancet* 1999;353:1204–1205.

60. Coulthard S, Chase A, Pickard J, et al. Chromosomal breakage analysis in dyskeratosis congenita peripheral blood lymphocytes. *Br J Haematol* 1998; 102:1162–1164.

61. Alter BP. Childhood red cell aplasia. *Am J Pediatr Hematol Oncol* 1980;2:121.

62. Willig TN, Gazda H, Sieff CA. Diamond-Blackfan anemia. *Curr Opin Hematol* 2000;7:85–94.

63. Willig TN, Draptchinskaia N, Dianzani I, et al. Mutations in ribosomal protein S19 gene and Diamond Blackfan anemia: wide variations in phenotypic expression. *Blood* 1999;94:4294–4306.

64. Farhi DC, Luebbers EL, Rosenthal NS. Bone marrow biopsy findings in childhood anemia: prevalence of transient erythroblastopenia of childhood. *Arch Pathol Lab Med* 1998;122:638–641.

65. Weick J, Hagedorn A, Linman J. Leukoerythroblastosis: diagnostic and prognostic significance. *Mayo Clin Proc* 1974;49:110.

66. Sills RH, Hadley RAR. The significance of nucleated red blood cells in the peripheral blood of children. *Am J Pediatr Hematol Oncol* 1983;5:173.

67. Dessypris EN. *Pure red cell aplasia*. Baltimore: Johns Hopkins University Press, 1988.

68. Peces R, de la Torre M, Alcazar R, et al. Antibodies against recombinant human erythropoietin in a patient with erythropoietin-resistant anemia. *Blood* 1996;335:523–524.

69. Casadevalli N, Dupuy E, Molho-Sabatier P, et al. Autoantibodies against erythropoietin in a patient with pure red-cell aplasia. *N Engl J Med* 1996;334:630–633.

70. Young NS, Mortimer PP. Viruses and bone marrow failure. *Blood* 1984;63:7.

71. Klahr S, Slatopolsky E. Toxicity of parathyroid hormone in uremia. *Annu Rev Med* 1986;37:71.

72. Dawson AA, Ogston D, Fullerton HW. Evaluation of diagnostic significance of certain symptoms and physical signs in anaemic patients. *BMJ* 1969;3:436.

73. Cropp GJA. Cardiovascular function in children with severe anemia. *Circulation* 1969;39:775.

74. Valentine WM, Paglia DE, Tartaglia AP, et al. Hereditary hemolytic anemia with increased red cell adenosine deaminase (45- to 70-fold) and decreased adenosine triphosphate. *Science* 1977;195:783.

75. Stamey CC, Diamond LK. Congenital hemolytic anemia in the newborn. *Am J Dis Child* 1957;94:616.

76. Berk PD, Martin JF, Blaschke TF, et al. Unconjugated hyperbilirubinemia: physiologic evaluation and experimental approach to therapy. *Ann Intern Med* 1975;82:552.

77. MacKinney AAJ, Morton NE, et al. Ascertaining genetic carriers of hereditary spherocytosis by statistical analysis of multiple laboratory tests. *J Clin Invest* 1962;41:554.

78. Pirofsky B. *Autoimmunization and the autoimmune hemolytic anemias*. Baltimore: Williams & Wilkins, 1969.

79. Bosma PJ, Chowdhury JR, Bakker C, et al. The genetic basis of the reduced expression of bilirubin UDP-glucuronosyltransferase 1 in Gilbert's syndrome. *N Engl J Med* 1995;333:1171–1175.

80. del Giudice EM, Perrotta S, Nobili B, et al. Coinheritance of Gilbert syndrome increases the risk for developing gallstones in patients with hereditary spherocytosis. *Blood* 1999;94:2259–2261.

81. Perrotta S, del Giudice EM, Carbone R, et al. Gilbert's syndrome accounts for the phenotypic variability of congenital dyserythropoietic anemia type II (CDA-II). *J Pediatr* 2000;136:556–559.

82. Iolascon A, Faienza MF, Giordani L, et al. Bilirubin levels in the acute hemolytic crisis of G6PD deficiency are related to Gilbert's syndrome. *Eur J Haematol* 1999;62:307–310.

83. Iolascon A, Faienza MF, Perrotta S, et al. Gilbert's syndrome and jaundice in glucose-6-phosphate dehydrogenase deficient neonates. *Haematologica* 1999; 84:99–102.

84. Brus I, Lewis SM. The haptoglobin content of serum in haemolytic anaemia. *Br J Haematol* 1959;5:348.

85. Geerdink RA, Hellman PW, Verloop MC. Hereditary elliptocytosis and hyperhaemolysis: a comparative study of six families with 145 patients. *Acta Med Scand* 1966;179:715.

86. Bergstrand CG, Czar B, Tarukoski PH. Serum haptoglobin in infancy. *Scand J Clin Lab Invest* 1961;13:576.

87. Landaas S, Skrede S. The levels of serum enzymes, small proteins and lipids in normal infants and small children. *J Clin Chem Clin Biochem* 1981;19:1075.

88. Giblett ER. Haptoglobin types in American negroes. *Nature* 1959;183:192.

89. Blondheim SH, Margoliash E, et al. A simple test for myohemoglobinuria (myoglobinuria). *JAMA* 1958;167:453.

90. Javid J, Horowitz JI, et al. Idiopathic paroxysmal myoglobinuria: report of a case with studies on serum haptoglobin levels. *Arch Intern Med* 1959;104:628.

91. Roesser HP, Powell LW. Urinary iron excretion in valvular heart disease and after heart valve replacement. *Blood* 1970;36:785.

92. Crosby WH, Dameshek W. The significance of hemoglobinemia and associated hemosiderinuria, with particular references to various types of hemolytic anemia. *J Lab Clin Med* 1951;38:829.

93. Emerson PM, Wilkerson JH. Lactate dehydrogenase in the diagnosis and assessment of response to treatment of megaloblastic anemia. *Br J Haematol* 1966;12:678.

94. Horskotte D, Aul C, Seipl L, et al. Einfluss von Klappentyp und Klappenfunktion auf die chronische intravasale Hämolyse nach alloprothetischem Mitral-und Aortenklappenersatz. *Z Kardiol* 1983;72:119.

95. Rao KM, Learoyd PA, Rao RS, et al. Chronic haemolysis after Lillehei-Kaster valve replacement: comparison with the findings after Björk-Shiley and Starr-Edwards mitral valve replacement. *Thorax* 1980;35:290.

96. Fehr J, Knob M. Comparison of red cell creatine level and reticulocyte count in appraising the severity of hemolytic processes. *Blood* 1979;53:966.

97. Okumiya T, Jiao Y, Saibara T, et al. Sensitive enzymatic assay for erythrocyte creatine with production of methylene blue. *Clin Chem* 1998;44:1489–1496.

98. Muller-Eberhard U, Javid J, Liern HH, et al. Plasma concentrations of hemopexin, haptoglobin and heme in patients with various hemolytic diseases. *Blood* 1968;32:811.

99. Lundh B, Oski FA, Gardner FH. Plasma hemopexin and haptoglobin in hemolytic diseases of the newborn. *Acta Paediatr Scand* 1970;59:121.

100. Maisels MJ, Pathak A, Nelson NM, et al. Endogenous production of carbon monoxide in normal and erythroblastic newborn infants. *J Clin Invest* 1971;1:50.

101. Rhyner K, Ganzoni A. Erythrokinetics: evaluation of red cell production by ferrokinetics and reticulocyte counts. *Eur J Clin Invest* 1972;2:96.

102. Emerson CPJ, Shen SC, et al. Studies on the destruction of red blood cells, IX. Quantitative methods for determining the osmotic and mechanical fragility of red cells in the peripheral blood and splenic pulp: the mechanism of increased hemolysis in hereditary spherocytosis (congenital hemolytic jaundice) as related to the function of the spleen. *Arch Intern Med* 1956; 97:1.

103. Tichelli A, Gratwohl A, Driessen A, et al. Evaluation of the "Sysmex R-1000": an automated reticulocyte analyzer. *Am J Clin Pathol* 1990;93:70–78.

104. Schimenti KJ, Lacerna K, Wamble A, et al. Reticulocyte quantification by flow cytometry, image analysis and manual counting. *Cytometry* 1992;13:853–862.

105. Buttarello M, Bulian P, Venudo A, et al. Laboratory evaluation of the Miles H*3 automated reticulocyte counter: a comparative study with manual reference method and Sysmex R-1000. *Arch Pathol Lab Med* 1995;119:1141–1148.

106. Brugnara C, Hipp MJ, Irving PJ, et al. Automated reticulocyte counting and measurement of reticulocyte cellular indices: evaluation of the Miles H*3 blood analyzer. *Am J Clin Pathol* 1994;102:623–632.

107. Cazzola M, Mercuriali F, Brugnara C. Use of recombinant human erythropoietin outside the setting of uremia. *Blood* 1997;89:4248–4267.

108. Cazzola M, Guarnone R, Cerani P, et al. Red blood cell precursor mass as an independent determinant of serum erythropoietin level. *Blood* 1998;91:2139–2145.

109. Beguin Y, Clemons GK, Pootrakul P, et al. Quantitative assessment of erythropoiesis and functional classification of anemia based on measurements of serum transferrin receptor and erythropoietin. *Blood* 1993;81:1067–1076.

110. Oski FA, Naiman JL. Normal blood values in the newborn period. In: *Hematologic problems in the newborn*, vol. 1. Philadelphia: WB Saunders, 1972.

111. Trucco JI, Brown AK. Neonatal manifestations of hereditary spherocytosis. *Am J Dis Child* 1967;113:263.

112. Dallman PR. In: Rudolph A, ed. *Pediatrics*, 16th ed. New York: Appleton-Century-Crofts, 1977:1111.

CHAPTER 45

Disorders of Cobalamin and Folate Metabolism

Ralph Carmel and David S. Rosenblatt

Cobalamin and folate are essential in the metabolism of purines, pyrimidines, and amino acids. Deficiency of either of these B vitamins affects virtually all cells and has many clinical effects, the best known of which is megaloblastic anemia. Indeed, the function of these vitamins in human metabolism was discovered as a result of investigation of the hematologic defect. The history of discovery in cobalamin deficiency (especially its chief underlying clinical disorder, pernicious anemia, and its cause and treatment), folic acid, and megaloblastic anemia provides inspiring examples of clinical investigation in medicine. The stories of these discoveries are recounted in other publications (1–3).

This chapter proceeds from the details of normal function of the two vitamins to the logical sequence of thinking about their deficiency that a clinician would apply. That sequence begins with the expressions of folate and cobalamin deficiency and how to recognize and diagnose them, moves to the many specific disorders that underlie and cause deficiency and how they are recognized and diagnosed, and closes with the management of both the expressions and the causes of deficiency.

THE VITAMINS: METABOLISM AND PHYSIOLOGY

Folate

Pteroylglutamates or folates are conjugates of pterin, para-aminobenzoate, and glutamate. Pterins contain a six-member unsaturated pyrimidine ring and a pyrazole ring. The pterin is in the form of 2-amino-4-hydroxypteridine in Figure 45-1. Para-aminobenzoate binds to it through an aminomethyl group attached to position 6 of the pteridine. The C^9-N^{10} bond is labile in many of the reduced folates, and cleavage occurs readily at this point. A single glutamic acid residue can be attached (monoglutamate), or a γ-carboxy–linked chain of three or more glutamates may exist (polyglutamate).

Folic acid, which has both rings unsaturated and the pyrazole ring unreduced, is inactive unless reduced. Folate is active in reactions only as a tetrahydrofolate (THF), in which the pyrazole ring is completely reduced. Folates, especially reduced folates, are photolabile and susceptible to destruction by oxidation.

FOLATE BIOCHEMISTRY

Reduced folates bind to enzymes, for which they act as cofactors or cosubstrates (4). They acquire one-carbon units from selected reactions and transfer them to other molecules. The one-carbon units, transferred by different enzymes, are at different states of oxidation, such as those of formaldehyde, formate, or methyl. Folate-dependent enzymes are inactive without their folate cofactors (5).

The concentrations of folates within cells are much lower than the affinity constants of most of the folate-dependent enzymes for them (6,7). Intracellular metabolism would not occur if these affinities were not increased. This increase appears to be achieved by polyglutamation, because the affinity of folyl polyglutamates for most enzymes is much greater than that of folyl monoglutamates. Folyl polyglutamate synthetase, an enzyme within both cytosol and mitochondria, phosphorylates the γ-carboxyl of the folate molecule and then replaces the phosphate with another glutamate (8). Almost all intracellular folate is polyglutamated, with the predominant form usually containing five or six glutamates (6).

Many of the reactions involving folate are shown in Figure 45-2. DNA synthesis requires reaction 3, the *de novo* synthesis of thymidylate. The dihydrofolate must then be reduced to THF (reaction 1) to avoid inhibition of the many reactions requiring THF. Endogenous synthesis of purines requires reactions 8 and 9. Methionine remethylation from homocysteine is mediated by methionine synthase (5-methyl THF:homocysteine methyltransferase; reaction 5), which proceeds effectively with monoglutamated 5-methyl THF and requires methylcobalamin and S-adenosylmethionine (AdoMet) as cofactors.

The two reactions listed as reaction 6 occur on a single peptide, C1 synthase, that contains three different enzyme sites. Both enzyme sites in the two reactions listed as reaction 10 are on a single protein; the reactions appear to be restricted to hepatocytes.

Folyl polyglutamate hydrolases or conjugases are found mostly but not exclusively in lysosomes and hydrolyze polyglutamate chains to release folyl monoglutamate (9). Folyl monoglutamates cross cell membranes much better than do polyglutamates, and adequate cellular metabolism is impossible without this hydrolysis. Lysosomal conjugases have a low pH optimum and seem to function almost solely in lysosomes. Conjugases that function at neutral pH are associated with the brush border of intestinal cells. Under physiologic conditions, the relative contribution of lysosomal and neutral conjugases is unclear, but most conjugase action *in vivo* probably occurs within lysosomes.

Methionine and Homocysteine Metabolism. Dietary methionine is absorbed by an intestinal transport system shared with other neutral amino acids or dipeptides (10,11). Methionine is an essential amino acid, but the mammalian requirement for it

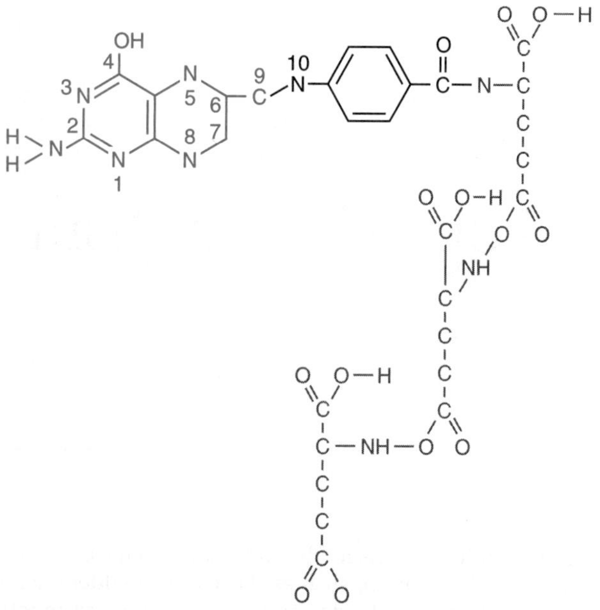

Figure 45-1. The structure of folate (tetrahydrofolyltriglutamate, in this case). Glutamates (shown in gray) are attached by ester linkage from the α amino group of the new glutamate to the γ-carboxyl of the previously added one. This produces a chain of OH-binding carbons with carboxyl groups protruding at regular intervals. The pterin (shown in blue) may vary in different folates, with attachment of one-carbon units to various nitrogen atoms. (Only the skeleton of the pterin is shown, many of the protons having been omitted for clarity.)

is decreased by two-thirds when cysteine is abundant in the diet. Plasma methionine enters cells and the cerebrospinal fluid by similar membrane transport systems.

The methionine may take several pathways in the cytoplasm: It may remain as the amino acid, it may be converted to AdoMet by adenosine triphosphate (ATP):L-methionine-S-adenosyltransferase (Fig. 45-2), or it may be incorporated into protein. AdoMet may donate its methyl group, leaving S-adenosylhomocysteine (AdoHcy). AdoHcy is toxic and is metabolized by hydrolysis to homocysteine and adenosine by AdoHcy hydrolase; however, the equilibrium favors AdoHcy synthesis, so that hydrolysis of AdoHcy requires removal of homocysteine and adenosine (10). Homocysteine can be metabolized by remethylation to methionine by methionine synthase, converted in liver only by betaine:L-homocysteine methyltransferase to form dimethylglycine and sarcosine, or converted to cystathionine by cystathionine β-synthase in the transsulfuration pathway, to be degraded subsequently by cystathionine γ-lyase to cysteine. At low concentrations of homocysteine, remethylation to methionine is favored over transsulfuration.

AdoMet is important in many transmethylation reactions in humans in addition to the remethylation of homocysteine to methionine (12). It also further regulates homocysteine metabolism by activating cystathionine β-synthase in the transsulfuration pathway, inhibiting betaine:homocysteine methyltransferase, and inhibiting methylenetetrahydrofolate reductase (MTHFR; Fig. 45-2, reaction 4), thus limiting the availability of 5-methyl THF for methionine synthesis (13).

DIETARY FOLATE INTAKE
Folate is widely distributed in the diet. Foods with high folate content include meats (especially organ meats such as liver and kidney), beans, nuts, orange juice, dairy products, grains, and cereals. As relevant to folate nutrition as the amount is the lability of folate when subjected to common storage, preservation,

and cooking procedures, such as boiling or steaming. Uncooked foods, such as fresh vegetables, retain folate activity best. Protection against oxidative damage, such as with ascorbic acid, may mitigate some of the lability of folate.

Past recommendations about intake were aimed at preventing signs of deficiency, and concerns have grown that this strategy may not maintain folate adequacy. Recommendations were revised in 1998 to indicate intakes that should maintain adequate red cell folate levels instead (Table 45-1) (14). The concept of dietary folate equivalents was also introduced to reflect that folate is not assimilated uniformly. Folic acid in supplements is viewed as having twice the availability of food folate. The availability from folic acid–fortified foods has been estimated to be 1.7 times that of food folate. A direct association with metabolic signs of folate sufficiency, such as plasma total homocysteine levels, has been shown not only for serum folate levels but also for dietary folate intake (Fig. 45-3). This association illustrates the major influence that dietary folate intake has on folate status.

Estimates of intake in Western diets have varied from 69 µg to 601 µg (15), but high-performance liquid chromatography analyses now suggest that past methods overestimated folate content (16). Folate intake has increased dramatically in North America and Europe in the past decade, in part by widespread, self-directed use of vitamin supplements. Intake in the United States has also increased with the mandated fortification of all cereal and grain products with 140 µg folic acid/g to prevent neural tube defects (17).

FOLATE ABSORPTION AND ENTEROHEPATIC RECYCLING
Folate absorption occurs predominantly in the jejunum, and the diverse processes include passive diffusion (18). There are at least two folate-binding proteins at the intestinal cell membrane. One of these, called *reduced folate carrier*, mediates low-affinity but high-capacity transport. Its membrane transport and molecular characteristics have been reviewed (19). It binds only reduced folates and is found in many tissues. The second, apparently less important binder consists of a group of proteins, *folate receptors*, with high affinity but low capacity for folate.

As mentioned, the efficiency of use of folic acid and food folate varies. Food folate, unlike folic acid supplements, is mostly polyglutamated. It must be hydrolyzed to monoglutamates within the gut lumen or brush border or in the lysosomes of enterocytes. Folyl monoglutamates are transported by a saturable transport system from the intestine into portal venous plasma. This system, which has little selectivity for monoglutamate transport, is pH-dependent (20). The folyl monoglutamates also can diffuse across the intestine by unidentified, nonsaturable processes when present in large quantities.

Folate in the intestinal lumen does not require conversion to specific folate forms for transport, although reduced folates such as 5-formyl THF tend to be rapidly converted to 5-methyl THF in the enterocyte (21). Folate appears in the portal blood within 15 minutes of entering the stomach, reaches a maximal level approximately 1 hour later, and then declines slowly over several hours.

The liver stores 7.5 to 22.5 mg folate, which decreases to approximately 1.5 mg when megaloblastic anemia appears (15). Some folate presented to the liver and some stored hepatic folate are excreted into the bile and reabsorbed. This enterohepatic recirculation of approximately 90 µg folate daily (22) provides a slow and more even absorption than would occur without it.

FOLATE TRANSPORT IN PLASMA
Plasma folate is almost all monoglutamated 5-methyl THF (23), much of it in equilibrium with newly absorbed dietary or enterohepatically recycled folate (22). Because of this equilibrium and because folate leaves the plasma to enter cells, other

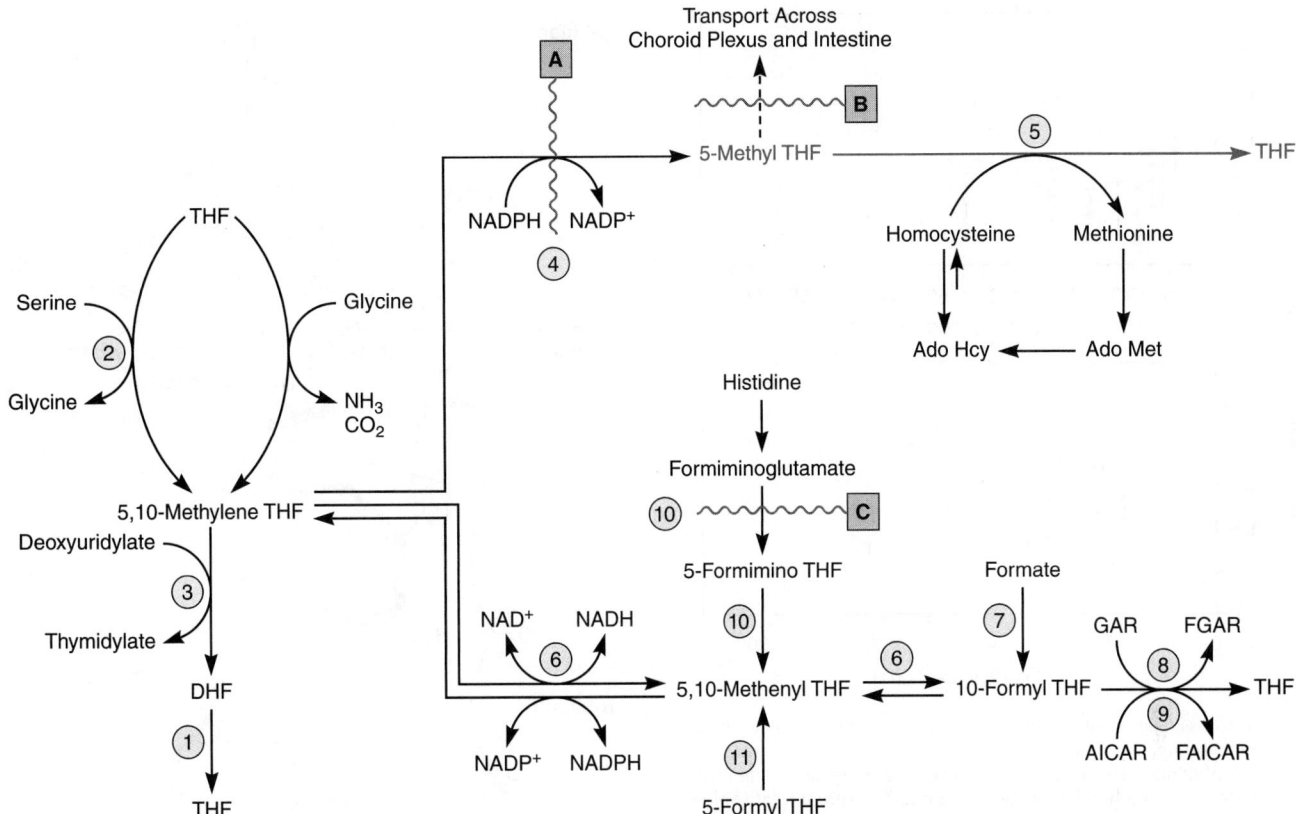

Figure 45-2. Folate metabolism, including the established hereditary blocks of metabolism and transport. The metabolic reactions numbered 1 through 11 are mediated by the following enzymes: 1, dihydrofolate reductase; 2, serine hydroxymethyltransferase; 3, thymidylate synthase; 4, methylenetetrahydrofolate reductase; 5, methionine synthase (also called *methyltetrahydrofolate:homocysteine methyltransferase*); 6, methylenetetrahydrofolate dehydrogenase and methenyltetrahydrofolate cyclohydrolase (the two enzyme activities regulating the two reactions exist on the same protein); 7, 10-formyltetrahydrofolate synthase; 8, GAR transformylase; 9, AICAR transformylase; 10, glutamate formiminotransferase and formiminotetrahydrofolate cyclodeaminase (the two enzyme activities regulating the two reactions exist on the same protein); and 11, 5,10-methenyltetrahydrofolate synthase. The sole reaction involving cobalamin in folate metabolism is reaction 5 (shown in blue). The known hereditary blocks are A, methylenetetrahydrofolate reductase deficiency; B, hereditary folate malabsorption; and C, glutamate formiminotransferase deficiency. AdoHcy, S-adenosylhomocysteine; AdoMet, S-adenosylmethionine; AICAR, 5(4)-aminoimidazole-4(5)carboxamide ribonucleotide; DHF, dihydrofolate; FAICAR, formyl-5(4)-aminoimidazole-4(5)carboxamide ribonucleotide; FGAR, formylglycinamide ribonucleotide; GAR, glycinamide ribonucleotide; THF, tetrahydrofolate.

compartments, and the kidney, plasma levels largely reflect recently absorbed folate. When intake and absorption are curtailed, plasma folate decreases rapidly over days and becomes very low within 1 to 2 weeks (24).

Most circulating folate appears to be bound only weakly and nonspecifically to plasma proteins such as albumin. Approximately one-third of circulating folate appears to be unattached. Only a tiny fraction is bound to a specific folate-binding protein, folate receptor γ/γ', which appears to be derived from folate receptors from cell membranes (25). The function of this protein, whose plasma levels increase in pregnancy, folate deficiency, renal failure, cancer, and some types of inflammation, is unclear (26).

Approximately 10% of administered folate is cleared in the kidney. Proximal convoluted tubular cells contain folate-binding protein on their brush borders and appear to reabsorb much of the filtered folate (27).

FOLATE UPTAKE BY CELLS
Folate appears to enter cells through the major transport system with affinity for reduced folates (26). The 35-kd carrier appears to exchange folate for intracellular anions, especially divalent anions; the transport system may also serve to remove organic

TABLE 45-1. Recommended Daily Allowance of Folate Proposed by the Institute of Medicine, National Academy of Sciences

Subgroup	DFE[a] (µg/d)
Infants	—
1–3 yr old	150
4–8 yr old	200
9–13 yr old	300
14–18 yr old	400
Adults	400[b]
Pregnant women	600
Lactating women	500

[a]The recommended daily allowance (RDA) is expressed in dietary folate equivalents (DFE). 1 µg DFE = 1 µg of food folate = 0.6 µg of synthetic folic acid fortifying food = 0.5 µg of synthetic folic acid supplement.
[b]For women of reproductive age, the RDA is expanded with a recommended additional intake of 400 µg of folic acid supplement or folic acid–fortified food.
From Carmel R. Folate deficiency. In: Carmel R, Jacobsen DW, eds. *Homocysteine in health and disease*. Cambridge, UK: Cambridge University Press, 2001.

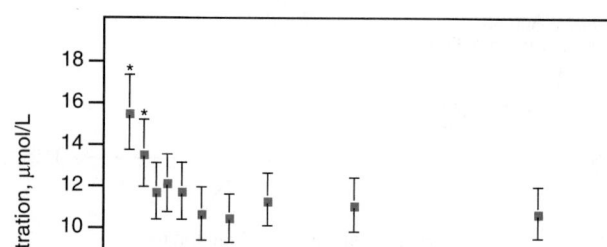
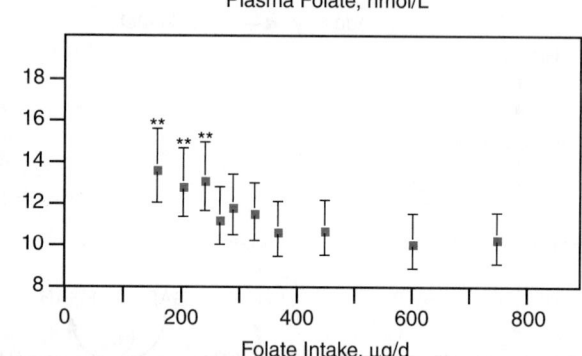

Figure 45-3. Association of serum folate levels and dietary folate intake with homocysteine levels. Mean plasma homocysteine concentrations and 95% confidence intervals are shown by deciles of serum folate levels (**top**) and deciles of daily folate intake (**bottom**). The serum folate values are expressed in nmol/L (1 nmol/L = 2.266 μg/L) and intake in μg/day. Asterisks indicate values significantly different from the mean value in the highest decile ($p < .01$). (Modified from Selhub J, Jacques PF, Wilson PW, et al. Vitamin status and intake as primary determinants of homocysteinemia in an elderly population. *JAMA* 1993;270:2693–2698.)

anions such as adenosine monophosphate and phosphate from the cell.

Several related folate-binding proteins or receptors, which vary in different tissues, are found on cell membranes (19,26,28). Two of these, folate receptors α and β, each approximately 28 kd, are anchored to glycosylphosphatidylinositol in hematopoietic cells, placenta, renal tubular cells, and other tissues (29). These receptors mediate endocytosis via clathrin-coated pits and are active at physiologic folate concentrations but vary in the folate forms they bind best. A third isoform, folate receptor γ/γ′, is truncated and thus is secreted rather than bound to the membrane. Evidence suggests that folate receptor α is also the means by which Ebola and Marburg filoviruses enter cells (30). The previously mentioned reduced folate carrier, found on most cells, including the brain, may be important where folate concentrations are high because of its high capacity (31). Some folate probably is taken up by diffusion, also.

Intracellular folate tends to be retained well if polyglutamated (32). Monoglutamates exit from cells, however. Several efflux pathways exist, one of which may be related to the multidrug resistance gene product. In red blood cells, folate retention may be enhanced by association with hemoglobin (33).

Cobalamin

Cobalamins are a subgroup of substances called *corrins*, which have structural similarity to porphyrins. The central cobalt atom of the tetrapyrrole corrin ring has linked to it, in the α axial position below the plane, 5,6-dimethylbenzimidazole, a nucleotide that also binds to one of the pyrrole rings of the corrin plate (Fig. 45-4). Linked to the central cobalt in the β axial position is any

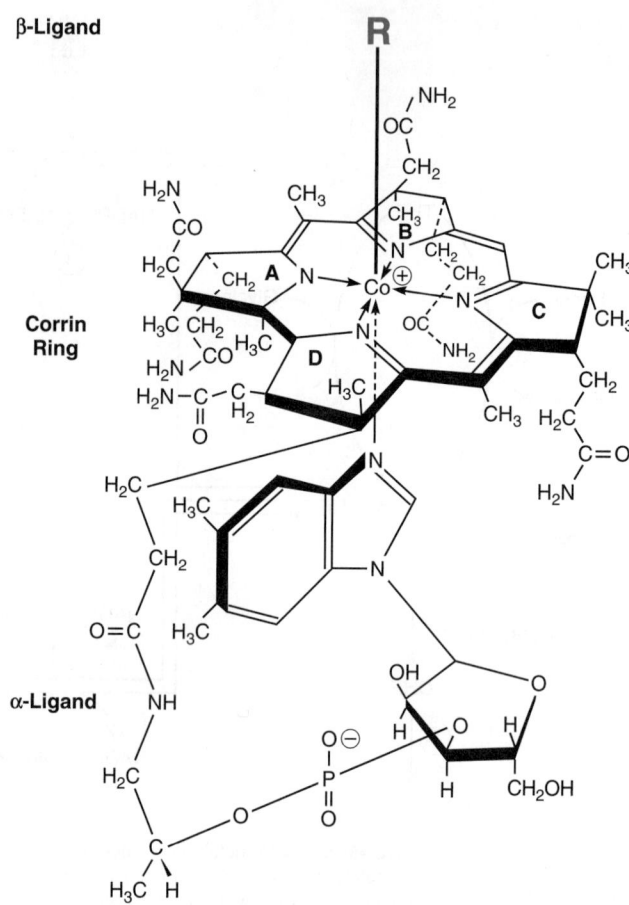

Figure 45-4. The structure of cobalamin. Different cobalamins are formed by substituting various ligands for the R (shown in blue) in the β axial plane above the tetrapyrrole plane. (From Carmel R. Cobalamin deficiency. In: Carmel R, Jacobsen DW, eds. *Homocysteine in health and disease.* Cambridge, UK: Cambridge University Press, 2001.)

one of several moieties, most often methyl (to make methylcobalamin) or 5′-deoxyadenosyl (adenosylcobalamin). The latter moieties are split from the corrin by light and are readily replaced by water (aquocobalamin), hydroxyl (hydroxocobalamin), cyanide (cyanocobalamin), or other ligands. Methylcobalamin accounts for approximately 65% of plasma cobalamin; adenosylcobalamin predominates in tissues, with hydroxocobalamin second.

The name *vitamin B$_{12}$* refers specifically to cyanocobalamin but is often used for all cobalamins active in mammalian cells, including cobalamins with the cobalt atom reduced to the divalent [cob(II)alamin] or monovalent [cob(I)alamin] states and the cobalt atom in its natural, oxidized, trivalent cob(III)alamin state.

COBALAMIN BIOCHEMISTRY

Cobalamin-Mediated Reactions. Cobalamin functions in mammalian cells as a cofactor in only two reactions: cytoplasmic synthesis of methionine from homocysteine and 5-methyl THF (34), and mitochondrial conversion of methylmalonyl-CoA to succinyl-CoA (35).

Reaction A: homocysteine + 5-methyl THF → methionine + THF

Reaction B: L-methylmalonyl–CoA → succinyl-CoA

Reaction A (also reaction 5, Fig. 45-2) is mediated by methionine synthase in the cytoplasm. Methylcobalamin is converted to cob(I)alamin and accepts a methyl group from 5-methyl THF to regenerate methylcobalamin. In reaction B, an intramolecular rearrangement converts methylmalonyl-CoA to succinyl-CoA, which is readily metabolized. The cobalamin-requiring enzyme is the mitochondrial methylmalonyl-CoA mutase (35–38).

Both reactions detoxify potentially toxic materials (homocysteine and methylmalonate). In addition, methylation of homocysteine is the major pathway for resynthesis of methionine in humans, and low levels of methionine often result when it is inactive (10). Impairment of reaction A produces hyperhomocysteinemia, and impairment of reaction B produces methylmalonic acidemia and aciduria.

Cobalamin entering a cell appears to leave if it does not either bind to methionine synthase in the cytoplasm after being reduced to cob(II)alamin [cob(III)alamin appears incapable of binding to methionine synthase] (39) or react with ATP:cob(II)alamin transferase in mitochondria (reaction C) to form adenosylcobalamin and bind to methylmalonyl-CoA mutase (40,41).

Methionine Synthesis. In the remethylation of homocysteine, if cob(I)alamin is bound to methionine synthase, it is readily methylated by 5-methyl THF to form methylcobalamin bound to the enzyme. Cob(I)alamin is readily oxidized and appears to undergo oxidation to cob(II)alamin spontaneously. The latter will not accept a methyl from 5-methyl THF. Cob(II)alamin bound to enzyme appears to be converted to methylcobalamin by donation of a methyl from AdoMet, which then permits continued acceptance of a methyl group from 5-methyl THF. The number of 5-methyl THF transfers permitted before transfer is required again from AdoMet *in vivo* is unknown, but *in vitro*, AdoMet appears to methylate the reaction every 300 to 500 methylation cycles (34,42).

In *Escherichia coli*, two flavoproteins maintain cob(I)alamin or provide other necessary reduction in the reaction (43,44). In mammalian cells, this function is provided by methionine synthase reductase, which probably represents the convergent evolution of the two genes coding for flavodoxin and flavodoxin reductase to a single human gene (45). It is methionine synthase reductase that is deficient in *cblE* patients. At least one additional protein has been postulated to play a role in the reactivation of methionine synthase (46).

Methylmalonyl-Coenzyme A Mutase. The methylmalonyl-CoA mutase pathway appears to require penetration of mitochondria by cobalamin by an unknown mechanism, reduction of cobalamin to cob(I)alamin (either before entry or in the mitochondria), and transfer of a 5'-deoxyadenosyl group from ATP.

Reaction C: ATP + cob(I)alamin → adenosylcobalamin + phosphate

The adenosylcobalamin then appears to bind to the methylmalonyl-CoA mutase enzyme to produce the active enzyme needed for reaction B. If reactions B, C, or both are impaired, levels of L-methylmalonyl–CoA, D-methylmalonyl–CoA, and propionyl-CoA increase, with subsequent hydrolysis of D-methylmalonyl–CoA to methylmalonic acid (MMA). 2-Methylcitric acid also accumulates because of the increased propionyl-CoA.

Methylfolate Trap Hypothesis. The role of cobalamin in folate-dependent methionine metabolism was discovered in the 1960s. It was proposed that cobalamin deficiency, by compromising methionine synthase activity, "trapped" folate as 5-methyl-THF, thus creating intracellular deficiency of other folates (47,48). In this way, the otherwise inexplicable megaloblastic anemia of cobalamin deficiency became understandable as the consequence of disrupted folate metabolism. Some of the predictions of this hypothesis have been challenged (49), but the interference with folate metabolism by means of slowing of the methionine synthase reaction by cobalamin deficiency is supported by many observations. The trap is amplified by the enhanced reduction of 5,10-methylene THF to 5-methyl THF as a result of decreased AdoMet end product.

DIETARY COBALAMIN INTAKE

Cobalamin is synthesized by microorganisms, which animals ingest. Bacteria also synthesize nonfunctional corrinoid analogs (50) that find their way into human plasma by an unknown process (51). Plants do not contain cobalamin, although certain algae contain cobalamin that has poor bioavailability. Consequently, the major sources of cobalamin are meat, poultry, and seafood, followed by eggs and dairy products. Cobalamin is considerably more stable in food than is folate.

Availability from the different food sources may vary. In one survey, variations in intake of dairy products and fortified cereals influenced cobalamin levels more than variations in meat consumption (52). Free, crystalline cobalamin is absorbed more efficiently than food-bound cobalamin (53,54). Most of the 0.5 to 2.0 µg cobalamin in a typical meal is absorbed as a result of intrinsic factor-mediated uptake.

Body stores of cobalamin average 2.5 µg (55). An increase in daily cobalamin intake to 2.4 µg was recommended in 1998 (56). Surveys reported mean daily intakes of 6.2 to 8.4 µg in the United States (52,57) and 5.3 µg in Dutch elderly people (58). As with folate, cobalamin supplement use has increased in recent years (52,57,59).

COBALAMIN TRANSPORT

Cobalamin crosses cell membranes poorly, and effective transmembrane transport requires mediation by a cobalamin-binding protein reacting with a receptor on the cell surface (60). This process occurs both in intestinal absorption and in cellular uptake of cobalamin by all tissues. Once within cells, released cobalamin binds to its enzymes. The three major classes of cobalamin-binding proteins in humans share several regions of structural homology (61,62), and the genes for two of them are on chromosome 11.

Intrinsic Factor. Intrinsic factor (IF), which is required for normal absorption of cobalamin, is a 48-kd glycoprotein whose gene is on chromosome 11 (63). IF is synthesized in gastric parietal cells in humans but in other cells in other species, such as chief cells in rat stomach and pancreatic cells in dogs and opossums. IF, whose concentration in stimulated gastric juice usually ranges between 10 and 50 nmol/L, binds cobalamins less tightly [dissociation constant (K_d) = 0.1 to 1.0 nmol/L] than do the transcobalamins. However, IF is highly selective and does not bind nonfunctional corrinoid analogs (51). Known activity of IF is confined to the gut, but cross-immunoreactive material has been detected in plasma and urine (64), and the kidney is rich in cubilin receptors for IF (65).

Transcobalamin II. Transcobalamin (TC) II is the transport protein crucial for cobalamin uptake via specific receptors for TC II on all cells, including brain (60,66). It is a 43-kd, single-chain polypeptide whose gene has been sequenced (61) and localized to chromosome 22 (67). TC II and IF have six conserved regions that are thought to participate in cobalamin binding, suggesting that the two proteins' genes evolved from a single gene (62); their nonconserved, receptor-binding regions, directed to separate receptors, may have evolved later. TC II binds cobalamin tightly (K_d = 5 to 18 pmol/L) and has low affinity for nonfunctional corrinoids.

TC II is synthesized by endothelial cells, by fibroblasts, and probably by ileal epithelial cells, hepatocytes, and other cells, also (68–70). Its concentration in plasma approximates 800 to 1000 pmol/L, only 10% to 20% of which is holo-TC II (i.e., TC II carrying attached cobalamin). Most of the attached cobalamin is adenosylcobalamin (71). TC II is rapidly taken up by cells and has a plasma half-life of 60 to 90 minutes (72). TC II is filtered in the kidney but is reabsorbed by tubular cells, which are rich in receptors for TC II. Semen has the highest TC II concentration of all fluids (73); cerebrospinal fluid also contains TC II.

The regulation of TC II synthesis is unknown, but a substitution polymorphism has been described that may be associated with higher TC II levels (74). TC II tends to be higher in blacks than whites (75). The tendency of serum levels to rise with active inflammatory disorders, such as collagen vascular disease and human immunodeficiency virus infection, has led to the suggestion that TC II is an acute phase reactant. High TC II levels have also been found in myeloma and Gaucher's disease.

R Binder (Haptocorrin; Transcobalamin I).

R binders are a family of 66-kd glycoproteins that are nearly identical structurally and are immunologically cross-reactive but are variably glycosylated. The gene is located on chromosome 11 and has been sequenced (76). R binder has the greatest affinity for cobalamin of all cobalamin-binding proteins (K_d = 3 to 7 pmol/L), but it also binds nonfunctional corrinoid analogs avidly (51).

R binder is synthesized and packaged in specific granules of neutrophils, with peak messenger RNA (mRNA) expression in late myeloid precursors (77), which appear to be the major source of plasma R binder. *TC I* is the name given to plasma R binder, or sometimes just to its most acidic fraction. The less sialylated fraction of R binders in plasma has sometimes been called *TC III*, but the distinction between TC I and TC III is arbitrary. Most TC III is an artifact of *in vitro* release from granulocytes, and the distinction from TC I should probably be abandoned (78).

R binder is also synthesized by exocrine glandular epithelium. It is found in virtually all secretions, such as saliva, tears, bile, breast milk, and semen, as well as in other fluids such as cerebrospinal fluid and amniotic fluid (78).

No cellular receptors for R binder are known. As a result, holo-TC I has a half-life of 6.0 to 9.3 days in plasma (79) and, in the face of the rapid clearance of holo-TC II, contains 75% or more of all circulating cobalamin (72). Most of the cobalamin in holo-TC I is methylcobalamin (71). The function of R binder is not known; clearance of nonfunctional cobalamin analogs, antimicrobial roles, and other roles have been proposed. Cross-species studies showed that desialylated R binders (i.e., TC III) are cleared rapidly but nonspecifically from the plasma by asialoglycoprotein receptors on hepatocytes (80); this clearance is thought to contribute to the enterohepatic cycle of cobalamin. R binder also serves as the intermediary carrier in the stomach for cobalamin released from food.

Mean TC I concentration in plasma approximates 300 pmol/L, most of which is holo-TC I. High plasma TC I levels occur in many disorders, have diagnostic value for some of them (such as chronic myelogenous leukemia and acute promyelocytic leukemia), and are usually accompanied by high serum cobalamin levels (78). Similarly increased levels may occur in patients with hepatoma or leukemoid reactions caused by metastatic cancer. Much less consistent elevations, with or without high cobalamin levels, occur in polycythemia vera and myelofibrosis and have no reliable diagnostic implications (81). Only plasma should be used for TC I assay, because variable and often large amounts of R binder are released artifactually by granulocytes *in vitro* after clotting.

Minor Binding Proteins.

Plasma eluted on Sephadex gel columns shows a minuscule (≈20 pmol/L) cobalamin-binding peak of approximately 800 kd (82). The nature of this binding peak, sometimes called *TC 0*, is unclear.

COBALAMIN ABSORPTION

Cobalamin absorption and transport follow the sequence of events illustrated in Figure 45-5, each event identified because of patients with defects in that step.

Cobalamin bound to proteins in food is released by gastric pepsin in the presence of acid. The released cobalamin is bound by salivary R binder preferentially over IF at the acid pH in most stomachs. In the duodenum, pancreatic secretions next provide proteases and the necessary alkalinization to digest the R binder, finally allowing cobalamin to be bound by IF (83). Biliary cobalamin is also released from biliary R binder by pancreatic secretions (84) and bound by IF for reabsorption. Nonfunctional corrinoid analogs released from R binders are not bound by IF.

Subsequent events in the luminal journey of the IF-cobalamin complex to the ileum are unknown. On reaching the ileum, the complex binds to cubilin, the specific receptor for IF. Cubilin is located on the apical brush borders of villous epithelial cells in the ileum. Cubilin derived from kidney has been characterized (65,85); it is a protein of approximately 460 kd with three structural components, one of which has epidermal growth factor–like domains and another of which has CUB domains that contain the IF-binding site. Cubilin can form trimers in the cell membrane and appears to bind other proteins, also. It is unclear whether other IF receptors exist.

Endocytosis, with separation of the cobalamin from IF in lysosomes, appears to occur in the ileal cell (60). The subsequent transport of the vitamin probably involves its specific binding to a transporter, TC II, that may be synthesized within the ileal cell (70). TC II–cobalamin exits via the basolateral membrane after several hours and enters the portal circulation (60).

When large quantities of cobalamin (e.g., 100 to 1000 µg) are fed to patients who lack IF, a tiny proportion (approximately 1%) appears to be absorbed by diffusion.

COBALAMIN TRANSPORT IN PLASMA

The essence of plasma transport has been noted in the discussion of its cobalamin-binding proteins. Absorbed cobalamin enters portal blood attached to TC II. It is not known at which point cobalamin becomes attached to TC I in plasma. Indirect data suggest that at least part of this transfer occurs after portal blood enters the liver (86). Holo-TC II is cleared rapidly via cell uptake. In the systemic circulation, therefore, cobalamin circulates largely as holo-TC I (86,87), but the proportions vary among individuals and in different diseases (86).

COBALAMIN UPTAKE BY CELLS

Holo-TC II enters cells by endocytosis after attaching to receptors for TC II (60) (Fig. 45-5). The receptor is a 62-kd glycoprotein that dimerizes in the cell membrane in a poorly understood process that depends on membrane lipids. Liver is rich in TC II receptors, with renal tubule second. Hepatic clearance transfers approximately 1.4 µg cobalamin daily to bile (84) approximately 1 µg of which is reabsorbed. The kidney also accumulates large amounts of cobalamin (88) while limiting the daily urinary loss of cobalamin to less than 1 µg. The kidney is also rich in cubilin, the function of which in this organ is unknown.

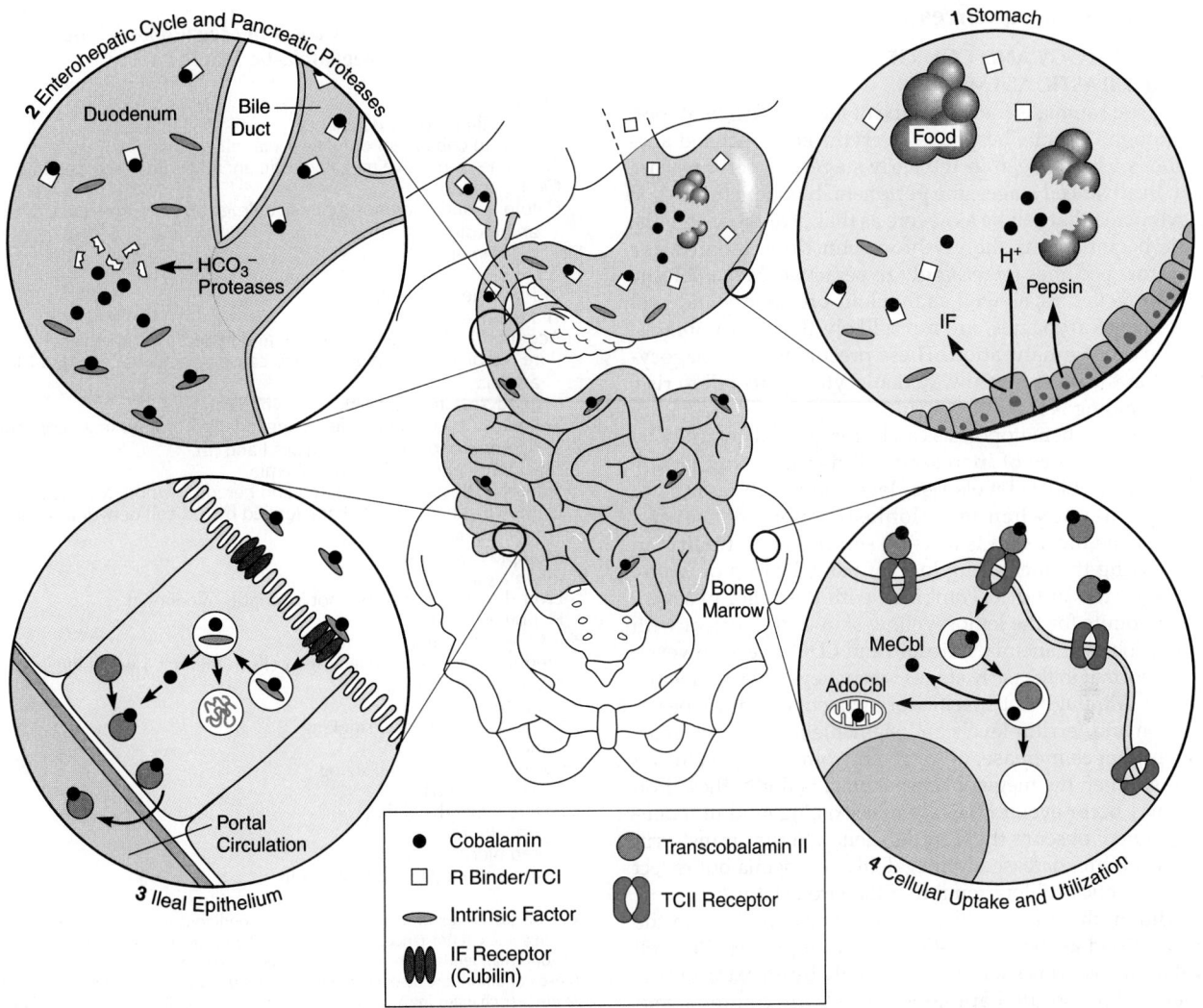

Figure 45-5. Absorption and cellular transport cycle of cobalamin in humans. 1: Secretion of gastric intrinsic factor (IF), acid, and pepsin, and release of cobalamin from food and binding to R binder. 2: Biliary and pancreatic secretion, and degradation of R binder by pancreatic enzymes. 3: Ileal cell uptake of IF-cobalamin, lysosomal processing, and transfer of transcobalamin (TC) II-cobalamin to the portal circulation. 4: Cellular uptake (e.g., in bone marrow) of TC II–cobalamin, lysosomal processing, and release of cobalamin for attachment to enzymes. AdoCbl, adenosylcobalamin; MeCbl, methylcobalamin. (Modified from Carmel R. Cobalamin deficiency. In: Carmel R, Jacobsen DW, eds. *Homocysteine in health and disease.* Cambridge, UK: Cambridge University Press, 2001.)

After cellular uptake, cobalamin enters the cytoplasm, probably after its release from TC II in lysosomes. After reduction of its cobalt, cobalamin becomes available to methionine synthase in the cytoplasm and methylmalonyl-CoA mutase in the mitochondria.

CONSEQUENCES OF VITAMIN DEFICIENCY

Many consequences and expressions of deficiency are identical in folate and cobalamin deficiency. Chief among these is megaloblastic anemia and the typical symptoms of anemia that it produces. Most of the other manifestations, even if described in deficiency of only one vitamin, probably occur in either deficiency. The chief expression that is not the same in both deficiency states is neurologic dysfunction. However, even for neurologic dysfunction, evidence of some common ground exists.

Several general characteristics of expression of deficiency should be kept in mind. The two deficiencies differ in how they usually arise. Pure folate deficiency is rare. Patients usually

become folate-deficient as part of general malnutrition or malabsorption, so that other nutrient deficiencies complicate, exacerbate, and perhaps sometimes ameliorate certain expressions. Even experimentally induced folate deficiency produced concurrent deficiencies (e.g., iron, potassium) in the study subject (24). Cobalamin deficiency, on the other hand, tends to be isolated; it is often caused by a malabsorptive defect largely limited to cobalamin.

Another major difference is that folate deficiency usually develops relatively rapidly, over a period of weeks or months, and shows a compact progression of symptoms and abnormalities (24). Cobalamin deficiency, with its minute daily turnover in relation to stores, almost always develops much more slowly, often insidiously; its symptoms and abnormalities may be more chronic, incrementally progressive ones (89,90). A third modifier is the interaction between the two vitamins, so that the expression of one deficiency may affect and be affected by the status of the other vitamin. An example is the modulation of the course and consequences of cobalamin deficiency by high intake of folate.

Hematologic Consequences

PATHOPHYSIOLOGY AND COURSE OF MEGALOBLASTIC ANEMIA

Megaloblastic anemia is the prototype of ineffective hematopoiesis. Although its name bespeaks an erythroid defect and anemia alone is usually seen in the early stages, all cell lines are affected. In advanced stages, the peripheral blood picture is one of pancytopenia that can be as severe as that of aplastic anemia.

In the beginning, as the erythropoietin drive mounts, the bone marrow becomes increasingly hyperactive. Megaloblastic erythroid precursors, as well as myeloid precursors and presumably megakaryocytes, are more likely than normoblastic cells to die during maturation. These precursors are phagocytosed within the bone marrow. Reticulocyte counts fail to rise, usually remaining below 100,000/μL.

The ineffective hematopoiesis can be recognized clinically by biochemical evidence of increased cell death. Serum lactate dehydrogenase (LDH) levels rise; levels in the thousands of units are common when megaloblastic anemia is severe. Another biochemical sign is a rising serum indirect bilirubin level, reflecting the increasing load of heme broken down by macrophages; the jaundice, combined with the pallor of severe anemia, accounts for the lemon-yellow skin of the patient with florid megaloblastic anemia. Bilirubin and LDH levels, however, tend to be normal in the early stages when megaloblastic anemia is still mild. Although not specific for ineffective erythropoiesis, plasma iron and ferritin levels and stainable iron in bone marrow macrophages increase, all derived from dying erythroid precursors. When the megaloblastic anemia is florid, these iron changes may occur even in the face of coexisting mild iron deficiency and may obscure the iron deficiency. Serum transferrin receptor levels are increased in megaloblastic anemia but reflect the erythropoietic proliferation rather than iron status (91).

In addition, there is a mild component of hemolysis in the peripheral blood as megaloblastic anemia progresses. Red cell survival in the blood is shortened randomly by an extracorpuscular defect. Low serum haptoglobin levels are common, and hemosiderinuria may occur, suggesting chronic intravascular hemolysis. The mechanism of hemolysis is unknown.

In the earliest stages, only macrocytosis may be apparent in the blood count (89). Careful attention to mean corpuscular volume (MCV) or mean corpuscular hemoglobin may identify an upward drift before the line into abnormality has been officially crossed. Many months elapse before anemia develops in cobalamin deficiency (89,92); the interval is much shorter in folate deficiency (24). A declining red cell count is discernible before hemoglobin and packed cell volume levels fall, because red cells become fewer but the overall erythroid volume and hemoglobin content are maintained by the cells' increasing size. Leukocyte and platelet counts are maintained in the early stages, but hypersegmentation of neutrophil nuclei is often apparent with careful search. Early megaloblastic changes begin to develop in the bone marrow, but a practiced eye may be needed to recognize the earliest expressions.

Megaloblastic anemia usually is macrocytic, but nonmegaloblastic causes of macrocytosis are more common than megaloblastic anemia (Table 45-2). The probability of megaloblastic anemia as the cause tends to increase with higher MCV. Nevertheless, macrocytosis is often mild in folate or cobalamin deficiency, especially in early stages, and should be suspected even when MCV is still high-normal (e.g., 95 fL).

Because macrocytosis precedes anemia, macrocytosis should always trigger attention in the nonanemic patient (89). Studies have shown that 17% to 33% of patients with diseases such as pernicious anemia have no macrocytosis, 19% to 28% have no anemia, and 14% to 28% have neither when first diagnosed (93–

TABLE 45-2. Causes of Megaloblastic and Nonmegaloblastic Macrocytosis[a]

Megaloblastic anemia
  Cobalamin or folate deficiency
  Defects in cobalamin or folate metabolism
  Thiamine-responsive megaloblastic anemia with diabetes and deafness
  Orotic aciduria
  Cytotoxic and immunosuppressive drugs (e.g., hydroxyurea, cytosine arabinoside)
Drugs and toxins
  Alcohol
  Zidovudine, acyclovir
Hematologic disorders[b]
  Acquired and congenital aplastic and hypoplastic anemias
  Pure red blood cell aplasia of any cause, including Diamond-Blackfan anemia
  Myelodysplastic syndrome, 5q- syndrome
  Refractory anemia, including congenital syndromes (e.g., congenital dyserythropoietic anemia types I and III)
  Myeloproliferative disease, leukemia
  Sideroblastic anemia, acquired and hereditary (non–X-linked)
  Hemolytic anemias not characterized by red cell dehydration or fragmentation
  Multiple myeloma
Nonhematologic diseases[b]
  Liver disease (usually, but not invariably, alcoholic)
  Hypothyroidism
Physiologic conditions[b]
  Predominance of large fetal red cells in the first 4 wk of life
Idiopathic conditions[b,c]
  Pregnancy
  Chronic lung disease, smoking
  Cancer
Artifact of electronic cell sizing
  Cold agglutinins
  Severe hyperglycemia
  Hyponatremia
  Stored blood
  Warm antibody to red blood cells

[a]Macrocytosis is not invariable in any of the conditions listed here, and is more common in some circumstances than in others. The mean corpuscular volume, even if not abnormal, tends to be higher than in the conditions' absence.
[b]These conditions are associated with nonmegaloblastic macrocytosis (i.e., without the nuclear changes in red cell precursors and white cells characteristic of folate or cobalamin deficiency). However, occasional patients (e.g., some with myelodysplasia) show nuclear atypia partially resembling megaloblastic anemia.
[c]The mechanism is unknown, and the possibility of subtle folate or cobalamin deficiency and megaloblastosis exists in some cases.

95). Of interest, cobalamin deficiency does not produce megaloblastic anemia in animals, although folate deficiency does (96).

Masked Megaloblastic Anemia. Iron deficiency, which develops at some point in half of patients with pernicious anemia (97), may hide the megaloblastic erythropoiesis (98). The MCV can be low or normal (or high, if the severity of vitamin deficiency exceeds that of iron deficiency) but will always fall if vitamin deficiency is treated first or will rise if iron deficiency is treated first. The megaloblastic morphologic changes in erythroid precursors can also be mitigated by iron deficiency, although neutrophil changes are not affected. This mitigation includes effacement of DNA synthetic abnormalities in bone marrow cells (99).

Red cell aplasia or hypoplasia has also been reported in malnourished patients with cobalamin or folate deficiency (100). The erythroid hypoplasia makes recognition of megaloblastic changes difficult, but neutrophil changes persist.

MORPHOLOGY AND CELLULAR CHANGES OF MEGALOBLASTIC ANEMIA

Erythroid Cells. The nuclei of erythroid precursors have unusually dispersed chromatin on stained smears and appear less

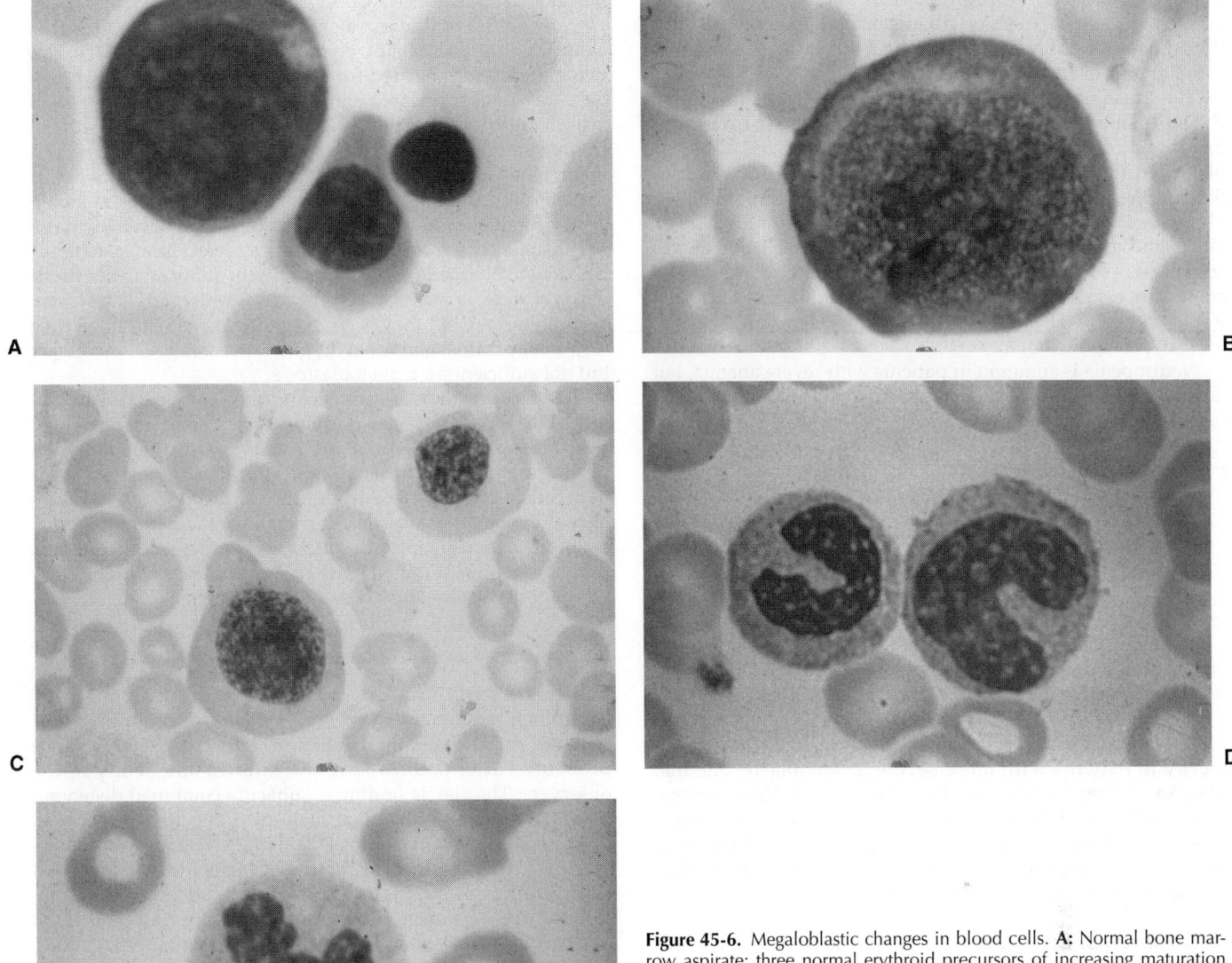

Figure 45-6. Megaloblastic changes in blood cells. **A:** Normal bone marrow aspirate: three normal erythroid precursors of increasing maturation (left to right). **B:** Megaloblastic bone marrow aspirate: a megaloblastic proerythroblast, to be compared with the normal proerythroblast in panel **A**. **C:** Megaloblastic bone marrow aspirate: two megaloblastic erythroblasts, to be compared with the normal erythroblasts in panel **A**. **D:** Megaloblastic peripheral blood: the megaloblastic, giant band cell and its smaller, normal neighbor. **E:** Megaloblastic peripheral blood: a hypersegmented neutrophil with seven or eight nuclear lobes; most of the red blood cells are large, some nearly as large as the neutrophil. (Modified from Carmel R. Folate deficiency. In: Carmel R, Jacobsen DW, eds. *Homocysteine in health and disease.* Cambridge, UK: Cambridge University Press, 2001.)

mature than the cytoplasm, producing the nuclear-cytoplasmic dissociation that characterizes the megaloblast (Fig. 45-6B and C). Typically, the mature erythrocytes in peripheral blood are not only large but have abnormal shapes and, when anemia is severe, membrane protein defects (101). Cell deformability is reduced. The shape changes include ovalocytosis and poikilocytosis. Anisocytosis with increased distribution of red cell width (RDW) is common but not invariable in the early stages. All changes become more prominent as the anemia becomes more severe. With time, nucleated red blood cells may appear in the circulation, and inclusions, such as Howell Jolly bodies and Cabot rings, may be seen.

Granulocytes. Continued DNA synthesis beyond the stage of maturation at which cell division normally occurs produces large metamyelocytes and band neutrophils (Fig. 45-6D). These

cells often have large, sometimes ribbonlike nuclei that occupy more of the cellular space than normal. Mature neutrophils may be larger than normal, but this can be hard to recognize in neutrophils. More characteristic than their size is their tendency to contain more nuclear lobes than normal (Fig. 45-6E).

The nuclear hypersegmentation has been quantified in various ways. The specific, published diagnostic cut-off numbers cannot be universalized, however, because interpretations of what constitutes a discrete lobe are highly subjective, and the quality of blood smears varies. Nuclear lobe averages per neutrophil above anywhere from 3.0 to 3.4 have been proposed by various authors to indicate hypersegmentation. Others prefer the rule that finding any neutrophil with six or more lobes indicates hypersegmentation. Alternatively, hypersegmentation may be diagnosed or at least strongly suspected if more than 3%

of neutrophils are five-lobed (meaning, in practice, that detecting any five-lobed neutrophil at all should raise suspicion, because casual observers of blood smears rarely look at more than a handful of neutrophils) or if an increased ratio of five-lobed to four-lobed neutrophils is found.

The cause of nuclear hypersegmentation is unknown, and the multilobed neutrophils do not appear to arise from giant bands and metamyelocytes. Hypersegmentation has also been observed in conditions other than megaloblastic anemia. Steroid therapy causes neutrophil hypersegmentation (102). Hypersegmentation has also been reported in iron deficiency, although the nature of the association is unclear (103), and in renal failure and myelodysplasia. A tendency to high lobe counts has also been reported in nondeficient blacks compared with whites (104). Heat stroke features nuclear changes resembling hypersegmentation.

Neutropenia is common in patients with severe anemia, but not at earlier stages when anemia is still mild. Hypersegmented neutrophils, on the other hand, appear very early and can be discerned before the MCV becomes elevated (105). However, patients with preclinical cobalamin deficiency do not have hypersegmented neutrophils (104).

Neutrophil hypersegmentation persists for more than 10 days after vitamin therapy is administered, despite the brief intravascular lifespan of neutrophils. Giant band forms and metamyelocytes persist for a similar length of time in the bone marrow.

Metabolic and bactericidal defects in leukocytes are controversial and appear variable. Neutrophil myeloperoxidase content is increased (106).

Platelets. Thrombocytopenia, like neutropenia, appears primarily in patients with more severe megaloblastic anemia. Megakaryocytes may be abundant or decreased. Thrombopoiesis is ineffective, but there are no characteristic morphologic changes. Impaired platelet function and prolonged bleeding time are often present (107,108). Platelet monoamine oxidase activity is increased in deficiency (109).

Lymphocytes. Lymphocytes, which are usually resting, nondividing cells in the peripheral blood, do not show megaloblastic changes. Metabolic evidence of deficiency has been described in cells transformed *in vitro*, but the vitamin content of the growth medium, whether normal or low, may influence the results. Lymphocyte counts in the blood have shown variable changes.

BIOCHEMISTRY OF MEGALOBLASTIC ANEMIA

When bone marrow is incubated with tritiated thymidine, cells synthesizing DNA (S phase) are labeled. These studies suggest that megaloblastic hematopoiesis is characterized by an arrest at various stages of interphase (110). In megaloblastic bone marrow, 40% to 50% of erythroid precursors are in S phase, compared with 20% to 25% in normal marrow. The erythroid abnormality is especially marked in the last dividing precursors, the early polychromatophilic megaloblasts. The giant metamyelocytes have increased DNA content compared with normal, nondividing, diploid metamyelocytes and appear to have arisen from earlier precursors slowed in S phase (111). However, studies suggest that hypersegmented neutrophils, which have a normal diploid DNA content, are derived from normal rather than giant metamyelocytes.

Flow patterns indicate two functionally distinct populations of megaloblastic precursors (112): One divides and matures normally, whereas the other matures but has stopped dividing and may be destined for intramedullary death. Apoptosis has been described in megaloblastic erythroid precursors in mice (113),

but apoptotic changes have not been found in patients with megaloblastic anemia (110,114).

How deficiency of cobalamin or folate causes the DNA changes of megaloblastic anemia is still not clear (115). The deoxynucleotides needed for DNA are synthesized *de novo*, or bases are phosphorylated and reused (salvage pathway). In *de novo* synthesis, 5,10-methylene THF is the source for methylation of deoxyuridylate to thymidylate. Insufficiency of 5,10-methylene THF, whether directly caused by folate deficiency or caused by the methylfolate trap resulting from cobalamin deficiency, limits *de novo* thymidylate synthesis. However, thymidylate insufficiency may not be the critical defect in megaloblastic cells. Monkeys made cobalamin-deficient show evidence in the deoxyuridine suppression test that *de novo* thymidylate synthesis is abnormal, but they do not develop megaloblastic anemia (96). It may be that abnormal thymidylate synthesis is necessary but not sufficient for megaloblastosis.

The accumulation of deoxyuridylate may be equally important (116–118). Uracil becomes increasingly misincorporated into the elongating DNA strand instead of thymine in megaloblastic anemia, and the ensuing high rate of excision causes both single-strand breaks and, more critically when residues opposite each other are excised, double-strand breaks.

Of incidental interest, despite the importance of folate and cobalamin in methylation reactions, hypomethylation of DNA was reportedly absent in megaloblastic anemia (119).

Neurologic Consequences

COBALAMIN DEFICIENCY

Neurologic dysfunction has been estimated to occur in 40% of patients with cobalamin deficiency (120), but the prevalence probably varies according to the interest and acuity of the observers. The classic finding is subacute combined degeneration of the spinal cord, which consists of degeneration of both posterior and lateral columns (121–124). Myelopathy is characterized by demyelination that may be secondary to axonal degeneration. The largest fibers with the thickest myelin are preferentially affected (124). The lesion begins and is most severe in the cervical spine, and its clinical manifestations commonly begin in the lower extremities (123). The cord lesion and its reversal with therapy can be documented by magnetic resonance imaging (125). Peripheral neuropathy is also common but is hard to distinguish clinically from posterior column involvement (121,126). Pathologically, the neuropathy features primarily axonal degeneration (127,128).

Signs and symptoms tend to be symmetric. Decreased vibration and position sense usually are the first objective manifestations. Pyramidal tract signs appear later but may be masked by the decreased tendon reflexes of peripheral neuropathy and sometimes become unmasked only after cobalamin treatment reverses the neuropathy. Romberg's sign may become positive. Common symptoms include numbness, paresthesias, and loss of fine sensation. As myeloneuropathy progresses, symptoms and signs in the legs ascend; the hands may also be affected. Bladder problems, impotence, bowel disturbances, ataxia, Lhermitte's sign, and other troublesome myelopathic problems may appear. Autonomic neuropathy and postural hypotension can occur (127,129). Motor difficulties are unusual, but muscle weakness and tenderness are common, fine finger movements may be impaired, and spasticity can limit mobility.

Cerebral symptoms, with patchy demyelinating lesions of the brain, can occur (121) but are unusual without other accompanying neurologic symptoms (130). In young children, especially those with inherited metabolic disorders, cerebral and developmental defects are often prominent. Common symptoms in adults are irritability, memory deficits, and difficulties with some forms of complex reasoning, but delirium and even dementia occur sometimes (94,130). Depression has also been described. Some studies of patients without overt symptoms suggest that impairment of various complex cognitive functions is more likely when cobalamin levels are only slightly diminished (131). Pseudotumor cerebri has been described in occasional patients with severe megaloblastic anemia.

Low cobalamin levels are often found in patients with Alzheimer's disease (132–134) and in some with chronic psychiatric conditions (135). However, evidence for a pathogenic role for cobalamin deficiency is infrequent in such patients, and response to cobalamin therapy is rare (136).

Electrophysiologic abnormalities are common in cobalamin deficiency (137–140). They have been reported even in asymptomatic patients by some observers (141,142) but not others (143). Electroencephalographic abnormalities, most often excess theta-wave slowing, are found in many cobalamin-deficient patients (137), including those with preclinical deficiency (136,141).

Cranial nerve involvement is not common, although disturbance of smell and taste occurs often. Optic nerve degeneration has been described, mostly in men (130). Visual acuity and color vision changes have been documented more often (130,144).

Pathogenesis. Because neurologic disease has been viewed as rare in folate deficiency, biochemical explanation of myeloneuropathy in cobalamin deficiency first focused on the folate-unrelated methylmalonyl-CoA reaction. Evidence now favors a connection with methionine metabolism instead (145,146). For example, severe neurologic problems are found in children with hereditary defects involving only methylcobalamin, methionine synthase, or MTHFR and in humans and animals exposed to nitrous oxide, which primarily oxidizes cobalamin bound to methionine synthase. Further support is provided by data in animals showing prevention of the neurologic lesion with methionine supplements. A direct role for homocysteine in cognitive dysfunction has been suggested but is far from certain and will require prospective studies (147). Special attention has been paid to the diminution of AdoMet activity and the accumulation of AdoHcy that occur in cobalamin deficiency, and to decreased AdoMet:AdoHcy ratios (148,149). The chief difficulty with the methionine pathway–related hypotheses is the paradox that folate deficiency does not cause the same frequency, severity, or form of neurologic damage that cobalamin deficiency causes.

Clinical Course. A critical clinical problem that neurologic dysfunction poses is its failure to reverse completely in some patients, especially those not treated promptly. It is impossible to predict in any patient whether neurologic symptoms will reverse. However, a longer duration of symptoms and indications of greater progression suggest the potential for irreversibility (121,122). Early diagnosis and treatment are therefore essential.

A carefully documented study showed that 28% of patients with neurologic defects, often severe, had neither anemia nor macrocytosis (94). This study confirmed a large number of older reports of this phenomenon. It is unfortunately not unusual to encounter patients with permanent neurologic dysfunction whose cobalamin deficiency was not diagnosed and treated in time because they were not anemic. The often only modestly decreased cobalamin levels in patients with predominantly neurologic involvement (130) contribute to missed diagnoses.

The neurologic and hematologic sequelae tend to be inversely related in severity to each other in cobalamin-deficient patients (130). Many patients develop one but not the other abnormality. Moreover, if relapse occurs, it tends to reproduce the predominantly hematologic or predominantly neurologic pattern seen originally (92,130,150). Various hypotheses have attempted to explain the tendency for one or the other manifestation to predominate in cobalamin-deficient patients, such as a very high folate intake (123) or high levels of nonfunctional cobalamin analogs (151) as causes of predominantly neurologic dysfunction.

Folate and the Neurologic Deficit of Cobalamin Deficiency. Folic acid given to cobalamin-deficient patients usually reverses their megaloblastic anemia, at least transiently. Neurologic disease can progress if this masking of anemia prevents or delays the diagnosis and treatment of the cobalamin deficiency. As reviewed (152), rapid neurologic deterioration was described in some patients with pernicious anemia who were treated only with high doses of folic acid (e.g., >5 mg) (153). The observations of this phenomenon, dating to the 1940s and 1950s when folic acid first became available, were uncontrolled and are hard to evaluate and impossible to repeat. The literature of that period also described occasional, transient neurologic improvement in cobalamin-deficient patients treated only with folate (152). It is worth noting, incidentally, that the glossitis of cobalamin deficiency also seemed to be unresponsive to folic acid therapy (153). It is unknown what dose of folic acid taken without cobalamin exposes patients with cobalamin deficiency to neurologic risks. This is an important question, because folate supplementation is widespread now, and the prevalence of undiagnosed, mild cobalamin deficiency is high, especially among the elderly.

FOLATE DEFICIENCY

Acquired folate deficiency only rarely causes a myelopathy or severe organic brain disorder (154–156). Mood and cognitive changes, including depression, poor judgment, and some affective disorders, occur more often (157) and may be related to a possible role of folate in neurotransmitter metabolism (158). Evidence for improvement of these changes with folate therapy has been presented (24,159), but the clinical and metabolic evidence that folate deficiency causes neurologic disorders is weaker than for cobalamin deficiency.

Neural Tube Defects. Although evidence is weak that folate deficiency causes neural tube defect births, the risk of such births is decreased by one-half or more if women take folic acid at the time of conception (160–163). The reason for the beneficial effect is unknown. One or more genetic defects involving homocysteine, folate, or cobalamin metabolism are likely explanations (164). Routine folic acid supplementation has been recommended for all women of reproductive age.

Other Consequences

Because folate and cobalamin are needed by all cells, megaloblastic changes affect many cell types. Macrocytosis and nuclear abnormality of cells of the cervix, vagina, urinary tract, nasal epithelium, buccal mucosa, and other lining tissues have been reported in patients with megaloblastic anemia. Atrophy of tongue papillae causes the smooth, sometimes beefy, red tongue of classic cobalamin deficiency (165); this condition may occur in folate deficiency, also. Aphthous stomatitis has been reported in patients with cobalamin deficiency (166). It is unknown why some patients develop oral symptoms such as soreness whereas most do not, but occasionally these symptoms predominate clinically.

Buccal cells and lymphocytes of folate-depleted volunteers show increased micronuclei (167). Decreased mitoses and shortened villi occur in ileal mucosa in untreated cobalamin or folate deficiency and reverse with vitamin therapy (168,169). Patients sometimes have gastrointestinal symptoms, the mechanisms of which are unknown. Anorexia, a sense of gastrointestinal discomfort, and, occasionally, diarrhea may occur. Reversible absorptive defects have been documented (170,171). In patients with tropical sprue, diarrhea often improves after treatment with both antibiotics and folic acid, supporting a role for folate deficiency in gut malfunction (172).

Infertility in men and women has been attributed to cobalamin deficiency in anecdotal reports. Weight loss occurs in patients with pernicious anemia (173); it averages more than 15 lb and reverses quickly with cobalamin therapy. Cholesterol and lipid levels are decreased in cobalamin or folate deficiency and respond to therapy (15).

Reversible pigment changes of skin (dark patches, especially in skin folds and knuckles), hair (lightening or reddening of dark hair), or nails (blue fingernails and toenails) may occur in cobalamin-deficient patients, especially nonwhites (174–176). Osteoblast activity appears to be impaired by cobalamin deficiency, and serum levels of alkaline phosphatase and osteocalcin are diminished (177). The risk for osteoporosis and bone fractures is increased in pernicious anemia (178,179), but the mechanism is not clear.

Hemoglobin A_2 levels vary but tend to increase slightly in cobalamin and folate deficiency and reverse with therapy (180,181). Hemoglobin S levels have changed in either direction in occasional patients with sickle cell trait who became folate-deficient (182,183). Reversible immunodeficiency has also been described (184–186).

As reviewed (187), the data supporting a contribution of chronic folate deficiency to increased cancer risk are inconclusive but appear to be most compelling for colon carcinogenesis. Folate insufficiency, perhaps by its relation to disturbed homocysteine metabolism, may also contribute to birth defects and other complications (188).

The connection between homocysteine-methionine metabolism and folate-cobalamin metabolism has been extensively reviewed (189–193). Hyperhomocysteinemia is considered an independent risk factor for vascular disease, but a direct causation awaits proof (191). Folic acid and, to a lesser extent, cobalamin supplementation are among the most effective methods of lowering mildly elevated homocysteine levels, even when evidence of deficiency is lacking.

CONSEQUENCES OF UNDERLYING DISORDERS

Patients often have signs and symptoms that arise not from the vitamin deficiency but from the underlying disorders that caused the vitamin deficiency. For example, patients may have gastrointestinal symptoms of small bowel disease, neurologic and hematologic disturbances caused by alcohol abuse, or complications of disorders that accompany pernicious anemia, such as thyroid disease.

Evolution of Deficiency

An optimal diagnostic approach requires an appreciation of the evolution of cobalamin and folate deficiency and familiarity with the types of disorders that cause the deficiencies. The early stages of deficiency have become better understood because of broader study and use of testing, the introduction of sensitive biochemical methods, the application of tests of cobalamin absorption and related phenomena, and sophisticated, multiparameter studies of asymptomatic people with early compromise of vitamin status. As a result, patients are increasingly often identified while still in the asymptomatic stage of mild preclinical deficiency.

COBALAMIN DEFICIENCY

Deficiency of cobalamin often takes several years to develop because only approximately 0.05% to 0.2% of body stores are lost per day (194). The rate of depletion is influenced by the mechanism underlying the cause of deficiency. When absorption is disrupted by loss of gastric IF or by small bowel dysfunction, both absorption of dietary cobalamin and reabsorption of enterohepatically recycled cobalamin are impaired. Presumably, the rate of depletion is slower when the malabsorption is limited to food cobalamin and the IF mechanism remains intact (90); not only is absorption not as severely compromised, but reabsorption of biliary cobalamin presumably remains unaffected. Cobalamin depletion from dietary insufficiency proceeds at least as slowly as in food cobalamin malabsorption. At the other extreme, depletion can occur in days, weeks, or a few months when the underlying disorder impairs cobalamin transport in the blood, cellular uptake, or use. The progression in any malabsorptive or dietary scenario is accelerated in patients whose stores of cobalamin are small at the outset or when a metabolic insult such as exposure to nitrous oxide or deficiency of folate becomes superimposed.

Preclinical Cobalamin Deficiency. The concept that low cobalamin levels in asymptomatic, nonanemic patients are artifactual was challenged in the 1980s (195–197). Demonstration of abnormal deoxyuridine suppression test results that reversed with cobalamin therapy (133,141,195,198,199) established the entity of mild preclinical deficiency, which is characterized by metabolic evidence of vitamin insufficiency at a still asymptomatic stage (197). Widespread metabolic testing has since made clear that mild preclinical cobalamin deficiency is present in 50% to 70% of asymptomatic patients with low cobalamin levels and is much more common than clinically overt deficiency (90,200,201). This finding is especially common in certain segments of the population, such as the elderly, as many as 10% to 15% of whom, or more, depending on the criteria that are used, may be affected (90,202–204). Such deficiency may exist even in patients with normal cobalamin levels (200), but 30% or more of patients with low cobalamin levels have no evidence of deficiency (90,200,201).

FOLATE DEFICIENCY

The evolution of folate deficiency is more rapid than that of cobalamin deficiency, as 1% to 2% of body stores turn over daily.

Preclinical Folate Deficiency. As with cobalamin deficiency, metabolic abnormalities precede clinical symptoms (198). Moreover, folate supplementation lowers homocysteine levels in many seemingly healthy people despite serum folate levels within the normal range (205). Metabolic data led to a recommendation that serum folate levels as high as 5 µg/L (11 nmol/L) be viewed as insufficient (Fig. 45-3) (206), although 2.5 µg/L (5.7 nmol/L) has generally been viewed as the low end of the reference range. A mild, preclinical folate deficiency state may persist chronically because it often remains undetected and untreated if there is no megaloblastic anemia. However, definitions in this scenario must be tempered by the nonspecificity of homocysteine changes and the lack of a gold standard for the diagnosis of folate deficiency.

Diagnosing the Deficiency

Searching for signs of megaloblastic anemia, especially neutrophil hypersegmentation, which distinguishes between megaloblastic and nonmegaloblastic macrocytosis, is important diagnostically. However, the presence of hematologic changes does not differentiate between cobalamin and folate deficiencies, is sometimes hard to recognize, and may not always occur. Specific tests must be used to define the deficiency state. Before the advent of reliable biochemical tests, the reticulocyte response to a small dose of one vitamin alone (e.g., 2 to 3 μg cobalamin or 200 μg folic acid by injection) was used to diagnose the specific vitamin deficiency (207). Although this test is now of historic interest only, evaluation of clinical response to any given therapy remains important, especially when the diagnosis is in doubt.

COBALAMIN DEFICIENCY

Serum Cobalamin Levels. Cobalamin levels fall early in the course of deficiency, usually preceding hematologic and neurologic abnormalities by months. Automated, antibody-based chemiluminescence technology is rapidly replacing radioisotope dilution assays, which replaced microbiologic assays several decades earlier. However, the newest methods have not been as thoroughly tested as the older ones, on which most existing knowledge of cobalamin levels rests (208). Questions have arisen about some of the new assay systems (209).

Serum cobalamin levels often reflect hepatic cobalamin stores, but the two occasionally diverge, and it is not always clear which is correct. Early evaluations of measurement of cobalamin in serum as a diagnostic test revealed that the level was less than 100 ng/L (78 pmol/L) in most, but not all, patients with megaloblastic anemia caused by cobalamin deficiency (208,210).

Levels that are low but above 100 ng/L are much more common than those below 100 ng/L. Although megaloblastic anemia is less frequent in patients with levels above 100 ng/L, biochemical or clinical evidence of deficiency is demonstrable in more than half of cases (90,200). In fact, clinically obvious deficiency sometimes exists in patients with cobalamin levels within the normal reference range (200,211,212). It was reported that 5.2% of cobalamin-deficient patients have normal serum cobalamin levels (211). The authors proposed that even cobalamin levels within the low part of the normal range (i.e., 250 to 350 ng/L) should be regarded as abnormal, because 20% to 30% of such levels are accompanied by abnormal metabolite levels. However, others disagree, because extending the definition of deficiency into the normal cobalamin level range will mislabel as abnormal a large number of normal people without any deficiency in order to capture a few whose deficiency is usually only preclinical (213).

Cobalamin levels always must be interpreted in context with clinical information. Although assay of cobalamin is the diagnostic mainstay, it can occasionally mislead. Serum levels can be low for reasons other than cobalamin deficiency, while falsely elevated levels occasionally mask deficiency (Table 45-3). Serum cobalamin levels usually remain normal or even rise in patients with hereditary or acquired disorders of metabolism. In addition, healthy blacks tend to have higher cobalamin levels than healthy whites (75,213).

Other Cobalamin Measurements. Assaying tissue cobalamin is theoretically preferable to serum levels but is impractical (e.g., hepatic sampling) or of limited reliability (e.g., red cell cobalamin assay). The amount of cobalamin attached to TC II (holo-TC II) is thought to fall in cobalamin deficiency even before total serum cobalamin falls (214). However, the specificity of low holo-TC II levels is unproven (215,216).

Metabolic Tests. Tests reflecting metabolic pathways are highly sensitive, although no gold standard exists at present. Homocysteine is measured in plasma as total homocysteine, of which more than 80% is protein-bound homocysteine, 10% to 15% is homocystine and homocysteine-cysteine mixed disul-

TABLE 45-3. Causes of Abnormal Serum Cobalamin Levels

Low cobalamin levels
  Cobalamin deficiency
    Overt deficiency
    Mild or preclinical deficiency[a]
      Latent pernicious anemia or other malabsorptive states, including food cobalamin malabsorption
      Old age[b]
      Vegetarianism
  Unexplained, but sometimes with compromised cobalamin status[b]
    Hydantoin therapy
    Acquired immune deficiency syndrome
  Presumed not to represent cobalamin deficit
    Pregnancy (last trimester)
    Folate deficiency[b]
    Transcobalamin I deficiency
    Multiple myeloma[b] and Waldenström's macroglobulinemia
    Aplastic anemia
    Hairy cell leukemia
    Oral contraceptive use
  Artifact
    Radioactive serum (radioassay only, after nuclear medicine procedures)
High (or inappropriately normal)[c] cobalamin levels
  Recent cobalamin injection
  Impaired cobalamin metabolism, plasma transport, or cell uptake
  Abnormalities of transcobalamin
    Elevated transcobalamin I levels
      Leukemias and myeloproliferative disorders
        Chronic myelogenous leukemia; acute promyelocytic leukemia; eosinophilic leukemia
        Some cases of polycythemia vera and myelofibrosis
      Hypereosinophilic syndrome
      Leukemoid reaction
      Cancer
        Some cases of metastatic cancer
        Some cases of hepatocellular carcinoma
    Circulating antitranscobalamin antibody
  Unknown mechanisms[d]
    Renal failure
    Liver disease[e]

[a]Only a few of the patients display clinically overt evidence of cobalamin deficiency.
[b]Some patients can have coexisting cobalamin malabsorption and either clinically overt or mild preclinical deficiency.
[c]Normal or high cobalamin levels despite coexisting cobalamin deficiency.
[d]Because of increased release of cellular cobalamin, decreased clearance of cobalamin from plasma, and other mechanisms.
[e]Most often seen with hepatic necrosis (e.g., hepatitis); seen less often with cirrhosis.

fides, and less than 2% is free homocysteine. MMA can be measured in serum or urine, although urine levels seem more readily affected by a recent meal and other variables (217). The deoxyuridine suppression test uses short-term bone marrow culture to measure the suppressive effect of preincubation with deoxyuridine on the subsequent incorporation of ^{3}H-thymidine into DNA *in vitro*. In normal cells, all but 8% (or less) of ^{3}H-thymidine incorporation is suppressed thereby, whereas folate-deficient or cobalamin-deficient cells show poor suppression (218,219). The test can be made vitamin-specific by also testing aliquots of cells to which vitamins are added *in vitro*. The precise biochemical basis of the suppression test is not fully understood (220), but the test is more sensitive than vitamin levels (221), may be slightly more sensitive than either homocysteine or MMA levels (222), and was used to provide the first documentation for subclinical cobalamin deficiency (141,195,198). The test's clinical use is limited because it is laborious and requires fresh bone marrow cells.

With the advent of accurate methods for detecting even mild elevations of total homocysteine (223) and MMA levels (224,225), wide clinical use of metabolic testing became feasible. A study of 434 patients with clinically unequivocal cobalamin deficiency showed elevated homocysteine levels in 95.9% and elevated

MMA levels in 98.4% of cases (95); levels of at least one of the metabolites were increased in 99.8% of cases. The consensus is that MMA assay, because of its greater specificity, is a more useful test for suspected cobalamin deficiency than homocysteine assay.

Metabolic tests serve other important functions. The metabolite levels do not change for several days after therapy and change only if the appropriate vitamin is used. These characteristics permit delayed diagnosis in the inadvertently or intentionally treated patient; vitamin levels are useless in this setting because they rise immediately, regardless of the appropriateness of the vitamin administered. Most important, metabolite levels and deoxyuridine suppression testing permit recognition of hereditary and acquired metabolic disorders, in which vitamin levels usually remain normal. They can also be diagnostic in the occasional patient whose acquired deficiency is not accompanied by subnormal vitamin levels. Normal metabolic test results can also help rule out the presence of vitamin deficiency. Like all tests, metabolite levels are affected by conditions other than the two vitamin deficiencies (Table 45-4).

Metabolic testing is unnecessary in patients with clear evidence of deficiency and diagnostic vitamin results, but it provides useful information in patients whose vitamin levels seem uninformative or doubtful. An oral methionine load is sometimes administered to bring out homocysteine abnormality, but this step is necessary in patients with vitamin B_6-related defects more than in cobalamin or folate deficiency.

FOLATE DEFICIENCY

Serum Folate Levels. Serum levels reflect recently absorbed folate, so that as little as 2 or 3 weeks of diminished folate intake cause levels to be low (24). For this reason, until recent years, low levels of serum folate were seen frequently in patients admitted to the hospital because of illness but were often regarded as transient phenomena rather than indicators of deficiency (15).

Ion capture and other techniques are replacing radioisotopic dilution methods, which had replaced microbiologic assays, which remain the most reliable methods. The assay of folate is not problem free. Unlike cobalamin, folate is unstable even in samples stored at $-20^\circ C$. Published reference ranges have varied, complicating the interpretation of data generated by these assays; interlaboratory variability is also high (226). Deficiency has traditionally been defined by levels below 2.5 µg/L (5.7 nmol/L), based on distinctions derived between patients with and without clinical signs of deficiency. However, because mild hyperhomocysteinemia improves by giving folic acid to people who have folate levels as high as 4.5 or 5.0 µg/L (206,227), it has been suggested that optimal folate status is misjudged by the older, lower cut-off points. Table 45-5 lists the causes of abnormal serum folate levels.

Red Blood Cell Folate. Tissue folate can be estimated in red blood cells. Folate in circulating erythrocytes reflects the mean folate that existed in plasma during maturation of the precursors. Once they mature, erythrocytes neither take up nor lose folate. Therefore, red cell folate levels do not decline in the earliest stages of insufficiency, as serum levels do.

Erythrocyte folate thus correlates better with folate status than does serum folate. However, red cell folate is also low in patients with cobalamin deficiency, whereas serum folate levels usually rise (228), presumably because 5-methyl THF accumulates in cobalamin deficiency but tends to exit from the cell into the plasma. Red cell folate levels are often normal in women with megaloblastic anemia of pregnancy, in patients with acute folate deficiency, and in patients with combined deficiency of folate and iron. Levels tend to rise with reticulocytosis and are invalid in transfused patients. Finally, technical problems are common, and results vary among laboratories (226). For all these reasons, the usefulness of red cell folate has been questioned by some (229).

TABLE 45-4. Causes of Increased Homocysteine and Methylmalonic Acid Levels

	Elevated Homocysteine	Elevated Methylmalonic Acid
Vitamin deficiency		
Folate deficiency[a]	Yes	No
Cobalamin deficiency[a]	Yes	Yes
Vitamin B_6 deficiency[a]	Yes[b]	No
Riboflavin deficiency[a]	Yes	—
Acquired disorders		
Renal failure	Yes[c]	Yes
Hypothyroidism	Yes[c]	No
Bacterial overgrowth in intestine	—	Yes?
Drugs and other agents		
Alcohol abuse	Yes	No
Lipid-lowering drugs	Yes	—
L-Dopa	Yes	No
Genetic disorders		
Cystathionine β-synthase deficiency	Yes	No
MTHFR deficiency	Yes	No
Thermolabile MTHFR	Yes[d]	No
cblE, cblG	Yes	No
cblC, cbiD, cblF	Yes	Yes
cblA, cblB, cblH	No	Yes
Methylmalonyl CoA mutase deficiency	No	Yes
Artifact		
In vitro release from cells into serum	Yes	No
Plasma volume concentration	Yes	Yes
Characteristics		
Male sex	"Yes"[e]	No
Increased muscle mass	Yes	No

CoA, coenzyme A; MTHFR, methylenetetrahydrofolate reductase; —, not studied.
[a]The metabolic changes occur regardless of the underlying cause of the deficiency (including antifols, vitamin B_6 inhibitors such as isoniazid and 6-azauridine, and nitrous oxide toxicity) or whether the deficiency is a result of an acquired or inherited disorder.
[b]Usually detectable only after an oral methionine load.
[c]Hyperhomocysteinemia may be caused by an increased creatinine level (even within the normal range) rather than failure to excrete homocysteine.
[d]May not be evident unless folate status is suboptimal.
[e]Levels are higher than in women, requiring sex-specific reference ranges.

TABLE 45-5. Causes of Abnormal Serum Folate Levels

Low serum folate levels
  Folate deficiency
  Low levels usually not reflecting overt folate deficiency
    Transiently poor dietary intake without actual folate deficiency
    Drugs (e.g., oral contraceptives, acetylsalicylic acid, alcohol)
    Idiopathic
  Artifact
    Improper handling of specimen (e.g., long storage)
    Radioactive blood[a]
    Folate-binding protein abnormality in renal failure[a]
High or falsely normal serum folate levels
  Folate therapy or supplementation
  Other disorders
    Cobalamin deficiency
  Artifact
    Hemolyzed blood sample

[a]Source of artifact in radioisotopic assay.

TABLE 45-6. Blood Test Results in the Laboratory Diagnosis of Cobalamin and Folate Deficiency

	In Deficiency of		
	Cobalamin	Folate	Cobalamin and Folate
Serum cobalamin	↓	N – ↓	↓
Serum folate	N – ↑	↓	↓
Red blood cell folate	N – ↓	↓	↓
Methylmalonic acid[a]	↑	N	↑
Homocysteine[b]	↑	↑	↑

N, normal levels; ↓, decreased levels; ↑, increased levels.
[a]Can be assayed in serum or urine.
[b]Should be assayed in ethylenediaminetetraacetic acid–anticoagulated plasma.
From Carmel R. The megaloblastic anemias. In: *Kelley's textbook of internal medicine*, 4th ed. Philadelphia: Lippincott Williams & Wilkins, 2000.

Metabolic Tests of Folate Status. The metabolic tests and their findings and applications are the same as described for cobalamin, except that folate status does not affect MMA levels. The connection between folate status and homocysteine levels has been documented extensively since the initial reports of hyperhomocysteinemia in folate deficiency (230,231), as reviewed (192) and illustrated in Figure 45-3. Table 45-6 compares the vitamin and metabolic test results found in cobalamin and folate deficiencies.

DIAGNOSTIC APPROACH

Finding a low vitamin level defines the specific deficiency in most patients who have obvious clinical manifestations. If the vitamin levels are not diagnostic, homocysteine and MMA results will often settle the issue. Metabolite levels should also be obtained immediately in any patient suspected of having a disorder of cellular metabolism or plasma transport, because vitamin levels often are not low in such patients. In patients who have an equivocal clinical picture, abnormality of vitamin levels should be accepted tentatively, and metabolic testing can be applied selectively; MMA levels are useful if cobalamin deficiency is suspected and homocysteine levels if folate deficiency is suspected. A therapeutic trial, even in the informal sense of observing response to standard monotherapy, always provides useful information.

CAUSES OF VITAMIN DEFICIENCY

Once the deficiency has been identified, attention must turn to the cause of the deficiency. Identifying the underlying disease process usually has specific implications for management and prognosis.

Causes of Cobalamin Deficiency

The disorders that cause cobalamin deficiency are presented here in the sequence of cobalamin intake, absorption, transport, and cellular use shown in Figure 45-5. The hereditary disorders are included in this sequence, but their features, summarized later in Table 45-7, often differ from those of acquired disorders. By far the most common acquired causes involve disorders of the stomach or intestine. This fact explains the lack of impact of dietary cobalamin intake on cobalamin status in population surveys (Fig. 45-7). Therefore, it is a truism that making the diagnosis of cobalamin deficiency is equivalent to saying that the patient has a gastrointestinal disorder until proven other-

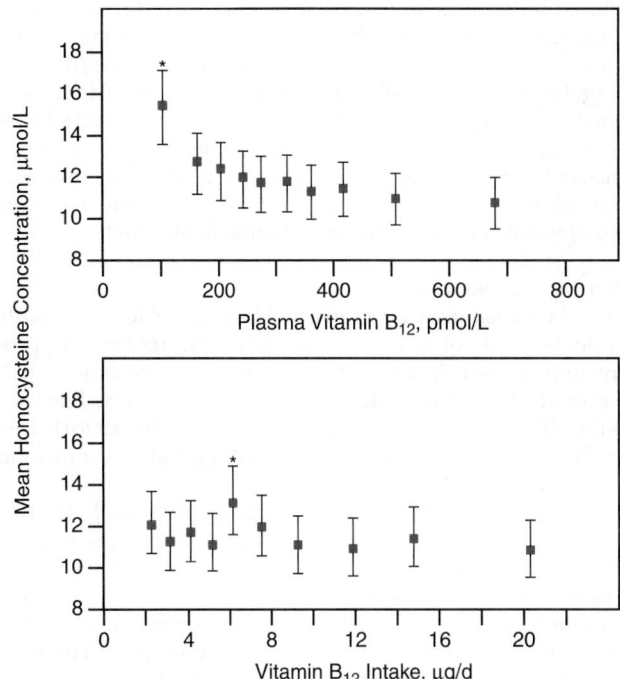

Figure 45-7. Association of serum cobalamin levels and dietary cobalamin intake with homocysteine levels. Mean plasma homocysteine concentrations and 95% confidence intervals are shown by deciles of serum cobalamin (vitamin B_{12}) levels **(top)** and deciles of daily vitamin B_{12} intake **(bottom)**. The serum vitamin B_{12} values are expressed in pmol/L (1 pmol/L = 0.738 ng/L) and intake in μg/day. Asterisks indicate values significantly different from mean in the highest decile. Note that the relationship between plasma homocysteine and cobalamin intake is not significant, unlike the significant association shown for folate intake in Figure 45-3. (Modified from Selhub J, Jacques PF, Wilson PW, et al. Vitamin status and intake as primary determinants of homocysteinemia in an elderly population. *JAMA* 1993;270:2693–2698.)

wise. However, cobalamin deficiency also takes many years to develop. A brief or transient malabsorption or dietary insufficiency usually does not, by itself, produce cobalamin deficiency.

DIETARY INSUFFICIENCY

Because cobalamin is provided only by animal-related food sources, broad malnutrition, as in alcoholics or people with anorexia, is not the usual dietary problem. Most often, the patient is a strict vegetarian or vegan (i.e., also avoids eggs and dairy products) on a religious (e.g., Hindu, Seventh Day Adventist), societal (e.g., macrobiotic community), or philosophic basis. Sometimes, the dietary restriction has a medical basis, as in phenylketonuria (232). The poor intake must be of many years' duration. Malnutrition even for several months is unlikely to cause cobalamin deficiency.

Vegetarians can show biochemical evidence of cobalamin insufficiency (233) and have slightly higher MCV than control subjects (234–236). However, megaloblastic anemia or neurologic dysfunction occurs in relatively few individuals (143,235,236). Coexisting malabsorption sometimes explains a clinically apparent cobalamin deficiency (237).

Dietary Insufficiency in Children. Those whose dietary restrictions begin in early childhood may be at greatest risk, because of both their small stores and their developmental requirements (238,239). First noted in India but increasingly reported in Western societies, babies born to and breast-fed by vegetarian mothers or mothers with unrecognized malabsorption have developed catastrophic neurologic dysfunction within the first few months of life as a result of cobalamin deficiency (240–244). The mothers have had low cobalamin levels but no symptoms or clinical signs of deficiency. As further evidence of the higher risk in children, many adolescents raised on macrobiotic diets have persistent methylmalonic acidemia despite years of taking cobalamin supplements (239).

GASTRIC DISORDERS

Food Cobalamin Malabsorption. Many people are unable to release food cobalamin adequately from its binding proteins in food (54). As a result, little cobalamin becomes available to R binder and then to IF for absorption. Because gastric IF secretion is normal, these patients absorb free cobalamin, as measured by the Schilling test, but not food cobalamin (245).

This malabsorption is mild but is also common (54). Approximately 30% to 40% of all patients with low cobalamin levels have food cobalamin malabsorption, as do approximately 10% of people with normal cobalamin levels. The frequency increases with age, and it is found in cobalamin-deficient Latin Americans and blacks more often than whites (246). The most common causes are atrophic gastritis with hypochlorhydria (that has not progressed to pernicious anemia with loss of IF), chronic suppression of gastric acid secretion (e.g., omeprazole), and partial gastrectomy or other surgical procedures affecting the stomach (245,247–251). Gastritis, hypochlorhydria, or both are frequent, but food cobalamin malabsorption can also occur without them (252). An increased frequency of *Helicobacter pylori* infection has been described (246).

Patients with food cobalamin malabsorption usually have only mild, often preclinical cobalamin deficiency (253–255). Because the malabsorption may not compromise reabsorption of biliary cobalamin and is mild, deficiency takes longer to develop than it does when the IF mechanism fails (90). However, occasional patients have severe cobalamin deficiency (237,256).

Food cobalamin malabsorption occasionally progresses to pernicious anemia when IF secretion disappears (256,257). Indeed, it seems likely that all patients with pernicious anemia go through a stage with only food cobalamin malabsorption first. Much is still unknown about food cobalamin malabsorption, its natural history, and its clinical importance. The malabsorption can be reversed with antibiotics in some patients (252,258), especially those with lesser degrees of atrophic gastritis (252); it is unclear whether the response derives from suppression of *H. pylori* or other microorganisms.

Pernicious Anemia. An apt name in the nineteenth century when the disease was fatal, the term *pernicious anemia* is misleading in many ways. The easily treated disease is no longer pernicious. Moreover, its pathophysiologic essence is gastroenterologic rather than hematologic. Although some authors continue to insist on anemia before accepting the diagnosis (259), absence of anemia is common (93,94,260,261).

The defining defect in pernicious anemia is the malabsorption of cobalamin that results from the loss of gastric IF production. The classic, acquired form occurs in the setting of a severe atrophic gastritis, in which parietal cells, which secrete both IF and acid, are lost. Atrophic gastritis itself, without the loss of IF that characterizes pernicious anemia, affects 10% or more of the population; whatever cobalamin malabsorption exists is limited to food cobalamin (54,245). Only when IF secretion is lost can pernicious anemia be said to be present. It is not known whether pernicious anemia is simply the extreme end of sever-

ity in the atrophic gastritis spectrum, destined to occur eventually in anyone with progressive atrophic gastritis, given enough time, or is a distinct disease process (262,263).

Typically, pernicious anemia occurs in the setting of type A gastritis, an antrum-sparing gastritis with severe fundic atrophy and autoimmune phenomena (264). The spared antrum often hypertrophies, and serum gastrin levels are typically very high. However, approximately 10% of patients with pernicious anemia have a pangastritis, in which autoantibodies and hypergastrinemia are not found (263). The latter, type B gastritis, is most often an end stage of *H. pylori*–induced gastritis. Patients with pernicious anemia rarely have active *H. pylori* infection (265). However, antibody to *H. pylori* is found in a few cases, suggesting that antecedent infection sometimes plays a role.

Circulating autoantibody directed against the membrane H^+,K^+-adenosine triphosphatase pump of parietal cells is typically found in 75% to 90% of patients with pernicious anemia, particularly those with underlying type A gastritis, but it is a marker for type A gastritis and not specific for pernicious anemia (266). Its prevalence declines as the patient ages (267) but also approximates only 55% to 70% in patients with onset of pernicious anemia at a younger age and in blacks (268).

Approximately 50% to 75% of patients with pernicious anemia have one or both of two circulating autoantibodies directed against different epitopes of IF. The type I (blocking) antibody is directed against the cobalamin-binding site; the target of type II antibody is unknown. The prevalence of anti-IF antibody increases as patients age (267). The anti-IF antibodies are found only infrequently in patients who do not have pernicious anemia.

A unique but uncommon setting for pernicious anemia is in the patient with agammaglobulinemia or common variable immunodeficiency (269–272). The patients have a pangastritis resembling type B atrophic gastritis, and their risk for gastric cancer is very high.

Demographic Features. Given the lengthy evolution of gastritis to pernicious anemia and the subsequent delay of several years until cobalamin deficiency develops, it is not surprising that pernicious anemia occurs most often in the sixth to eighth decades of life. A survey in 1996 found undiagnosed pernicious anemia in 1.9% of healthy subjects older than 60 years (261). Pernicious anemia can occur in young patients, also. The classic picture with type A gastritis and autoantibodies is found in adolescents, or sometimes younger children, and has been called *juvenile pernicious anemia*. However, inherited IF deficiency, sometimes called *congenital pernicious anemia*, is an unrelated hereditary disease that does not feature gastritis, and is discussed later.

Pernicious anemia is slightly more common in women. Although the highest prevalences are in Scandinavians, the disease occurs in all ethnic groups and in all parts of the world. Indeed, the prevalence in blacks in the United States is nearly as high as in whites (261). Blacks, especially black women, develop pernicious anemia disproportionately often as young adults (i.e., third to fifth decades) (273). They, and to a lesser extent affected Latin Americans, also have a higher prevalence of anti-IF antibody than whites (268,273–275); the prevalence exceeds 80% in black women with pernicious anemia. A similar picture has been observed in affected Europeans with a strong family history of pernicious anemia (276).

Immunology and Genetics. A familial link is apparent in some patients (262,276), and atrophic gastritis with or without pernicious anemia is a common familial finding.

Acquired pernicious anemia appears to be an immune disorder (266). The most compelling evidence includes the frequent autoantibodies and other signs of immune dysfunction, the frequent association with autoimmune endocrinopathy, and the amelioration of the gastric and malabsorptive abnormalities with corticosteroid therapy. An increase in CD4+ lymphocytes and lymphocytotoxic antibody, common in autoimmune disorders, has been noted (274,277). T cells may play an important role in the immune gastritis (278). Attempts to link pernicious anemia with HLA phenotypes have not shown reproducible associations (274). No pathogenic role has been reliably identified for either anti-IF or antiparietal cell antibody.

Course, Complications, and Prognosis. The symptoms arise from cobalamin deficiency and are reversible (other than the occasionally irreversible neurologic sequelae). The loss of IF is irreversible. Persistent complications unique to pernicious anemia are usually caused by disorders related to the gastric lesion and its effects. Three categories of such complications are foremost. One category is the presence of other autoimmune disorders; these may predate, accompany, or follow pernicious anemia. The most common of these immune disorders is thyroid disease, especially hypothyroidism. Evidence of thyroid abnormality, including latent disease or immune phenomena such as thyroid antibodies, is found in half of patients with pernicious anemia, and clinical disease occurs in approximately 10% (279). Other immune endocrinopathies, such as hypoadrenalism, hypoparathyroidism, and type I diabetes mellitus, also appear to be associated. Vitiligo is frequent. Other tissue-specific immune disorders such as myasthenia gravis, immune thrombocytopenia, and autoimmune hemolytic anemia are thought to coexist more often, also. Lupus erythematosus has been reported sporadically.

The second important group of complications is gastric tumors. Most studies (280–283), but not all (284,285), have found a two- to fivefold increased risk of gastric adenocarcinoma—a risk that may exist for atrophic gastritis itself (286). Early detection and excision can be curative. Gastric polyps are common and often are found to be carcinoid tumors (281–283). These tumors, attributed to the chronic hypergastrinemia of pernicious anemia, are more common than gastric cancer (281,283).

They are often benign, rarely metastasize, and sometimes regress spontaneously or after antrectomy (287).

Third, iron deficiency often complicates pernicious anemia (97). The decreased absorption of iron caused by achlorhydria may be a major factor, but a search for bleeding lesions of the stomach or colon is always indicated.

Provided cobalamin therapy is administered, the prognosis in pernicious anemia is a nearly normal life expectancy, limited primarily by the occasional development of gastric cancer or the complications of serious, irreversible neurologic dysfunction.

Inherited Intrinsic Factor Deficiency. Cobalamin malabsorption caused by absence of effective IF (Table 45-7) has been recognized as a cause of megaloblastic anemia, myelopathy, and developmental delay in at least 45 patients, mostly children. Evidence of cobalamin deficiency usually appears between the ages of 1 and 5 years, although in cases of partially defective IF, clinical deficiency has appeared as late as age 12 years (288). All patients with IF deficiency have normal gastric histology and adequate gastric acid secretion (although some may have basal hypochlorhydria) (289), and are not at increased risk for gastric cancer. In some patients, immunologically active but nonfunctional IF is produced, whereas in others, no immunologically active protein is present. An unstable IF, labile to destruction by acid and pepsin and with a low affinity for cobalamin, has also been reported (290), as has been a patient with combined deficiency of IF and R binder (291).

Human IF is coded for by a gene on chromosome 11q13, but mutations have not been described yet (63). As with the other hereditary disorders of cobalamin transport, inheritance appears to be autosomal recessive.

Gastric Surgery. Approximately 15% to 30% of patients undergoing partial gastrectomy will develop cobalamin deficiency (292,293). Because of this complication, cobalamin screening or supplementation is indicated in all patients who undergo gastric surgery. Schilling test results (see Tests of Cobalamin Absorption) are normal in more than half of patients (294), and

---

TABLE 45-7. Diagnostic Features of Inborn Errors of Cobalamin Transport and Metabolism

	Serum Cobalamin	Findings in Cultured Fibroblasts	
		Synthesis of Methylcobalamin	Synthesis of Adenosylcobalamin
Disorders of cobalamin transport[a]			
Intrinsic factor deficiency	↓	N	N
Imerslund-Gräsbeck syndrome (MGA-1)	↓	N	N
TC II deficiency	N	N	N
R binder (TC I) deficiency	↓	N?[b]	N?[b]
Cobalamin-responsive methylmalonic aciduria[c]			
cblA	N	N	↓
cblB [cob(I)alamin adenosyltransferase deficiency]	N	N	↓
cblH	N	N	↓
Combined methylmalonic aciduria and hyperhomocysteinemia[d]			
cblC	N	↓	↓
cblD	N	↓	↓
cblF	N	↓	↓
Hyperhomocysteinemia[e]			
cblE (methionine synthase reductase deficiency)	N	↓	N
cblG (methionine synthase deficiency)	N	↓	N

N, normal; TC, transcobalamin; ↓, low serum cobalamin level or deficient cobalamin synthesis.
[a]These disorders, with the exception of R binder deficiency (which does not cause identifiable cobalamin deficiency), usually include megaloblastic anemia; except in R binder deficiency, homocysteine and methylmalonic acid levels are usually high but may not be prominent.
[b]Presumably normal, but have not been determined.
[c]These three disorders are associated with acidosis and methylmalonic aciduria.
[d]Although methylmalonic aciduria is present, acidosis is not a prominent feature in these disorders. Developmental delay and megaloblastic anemia are common. A specific retinopathy is found in patients with the cblC disorder.
[e]These two disorders are associated with developmental delay, neurologic abnormalities, and megaloblastic anemia.

the cause of deficiency is often food cobalamin malabsorption (245). Bacterial overgrowth in the intestine sometimes contributes to cobalamin malabsorption. Malabsorption and deficiency of iron, folate, and other nutrients may also occur after gastrectomy (295,296). Neuropsychiatric complications thought to be caused by cobalamin deficiency often occur without anemia (297).

Gastric exclusion for obesity is often accompanied by cobalamin deficiency and iron deficiency (298–300). Food cobalamin malabsorption appears to be responsible (300). Surprisingly, response to oral cobalamin is limited unless high doses are administered (298–300).

INTRALUMINAL DISORDERS OF INTESTINAL ABSORPTION

Pancreatic Insufficiency. Because pancreatic bicarbonate and trypsin release cobalamin from R binder in the duodenum, cobalamin malabsorption occurs in one-half of patients with pancreatic insufficiency. However, cobalamin deficiency rarely develops, probably because meals ameliorate the cobalamin malabsorption (301) and because pancreatic insufficiency is unlikely to be left untreated long enough to deplete cobalamin stores.

Bacterial Contamination of the Small Intestine. Excess bacteria contaminating the small intestine, especially anaerobes, can take up cobalamin in competition with IF and prevent absorption of the cobalamin (302). This condition can occur without other clinical symptoms such as cramps and diarrhea. The bacteria also appear to synthesize inactive cobamide analogs and convert cobalamin to such analogs (50); the clinical effect of these phenomena is unknown. Conditions predisposing to bacterial overgrowth include poor motility, blind loops, large diverticula, and strictures. Gastric achlorhydria also permits bacterial growth in the upper small bowel, but its clinical relevance is unknown. Antibiotic therapy reverses the malabsorption of bacterial overgrowth quickly, but recurrence is common if the underlying cause is not corrected.

Parasitic Infestation. *Diphyllobothrium latum* takes up cobalamin, even from IF (303,304). Associated with ingestion of infected freshwater fish, infestation is rare in the United States. The risk of cobalamin deficiency has been correlated with the number of parasites and with coexistence of gastritis. Neurologic dysfunction appears to be common. An association of *Giardia lamblia* infection with cobalamin malabsorption (304) is still uncertain.

Zollinger-Ellison Syndrome. IF-cobalamin uptake by ileal cells requires a neutral pH. Cobalamin malabsorption has been reported when the intestinal pH is very low (305).

ILEAL DISORDERS

Acquired Ileal Disease. Diseases affecting the ileum are, as a group, a common cause of cobalamin deficiency. They usually cause malabsorption of other nutrients as well, including folate. However, cobalamin deficiency is sometimes the patient's sole clinical problem. Tropical sprue is a prominent example (306). Endemic to tropical regions, including the Caribbean and South Asia, the disorder may cause cobalamin deficiency long after the patient has emigrated to nonendemic regions.

Findings are more variable in other diseases. Cobalamin malabsorption in celiac disease was reported to normalize on a gluten-free diet and to be common in patients with dermatitis herpetiformis, many of whom have atrophic gastritis (307). Deficiency is variable in inflammatory bowel disease.

Cobalamin deficiency can follow surgical resection of ileum or ileal bypass, and adaptation with time does not occur (308,309). Approximately 7% of patients given a continent (Kock) ileostomy have developed cobalamin deficiency (310). The length of ileum used may be important (311). Radiation damage to the ileum after regional radiotherapy can also cause cobalamin malabsorption.

Drugs and Toxins. Several drugs, such as colchicine, neomycin, biguanides, paraaminosalicylic acid, slow-release potassium chloride, cholestyramine, and alcohol, impair absorption of cobalamin (312–314). Cobalamin deficiency results only when the drug is taken regularly for many years (e.g., metformin) (312). Deficiency is otherwise uncommon, despite abnormal tests of cobalamin absorption. The intestinal mechanisms have not been established. Sometimes, coexisting disorders rather than the drugs cause the malabsorption (314).

Cobalamin deficiency itself affects ileal epithelium and may cause an ileal defect of absorption in half of patients with pernicious anemia (168,170,171). The defect reverses after several weeks or months of cobalamin therapy.

Hereditary Cobalamin Malabsorption. Defective cobalamin transport by enterocytes (Table 45-7), also known as *Imerslund-Gräsbeck syndrome* or *Megaloblastic Anemia 1*, usually presents with clinical manifestations of cobalamin deficiency between the ages of 1 and 15 years, although the disease has appeared later (315–317). The patients have normal IF secretion, intestinal morphology, and intestinal function, aside from selective cobalamin malabsorption that is not corrected by administering IF. Some patients also have proteinuria, of the tubular type in a few cases, with all species of protein represented. Patients who excreted protein during childhood continued to do so in adulthood, but the renal lesions were not progressive (316). The literature on the renal pathology has been reviewed (318). Neurologic abnormalities such as spasticity, truncal ataxia, and cerebral atrophy may be present as a result of cobalamin deficiency. Treatment with cobalamin corrects the anemia and neurologic findings but not the proteinuria.

An apparent absence of the ileal receptor has been described (319), but other defects may exist in other cases. Imerslund-Gräsbeck syndrome is inherited as an autosomal-recessive disorder and is most commonly found in Finland, Norway, and Saudi Arabia and among North African Jews. It is not restricted to those ethnic groups, however, and more than 250 cases are known (317,318,320). The disease gene was assigned to chromosome 10p12.1 using microsatellite markers in Finnish and Norwegian families (321). Cubilin, which binds the IF-cobalamin complex, was localized to the same chromosomal region, and two mutations in the cubilin gene were found in Finnish families with this disease (322,323). Mutations in cubilin have not been found in the canine model (324,325) or in patients from Norway and the Middle East (322,326). Thus, there may be locus heterogeneity among families.

INBORN ERRORS OF COBALAMIN TRANSPORT

Diagnostic features of inborn errors of cobalamin transport are listed in Table 45-7.

Transcobalamin II Deficiency. Transcobalamin (TC) II deficiency has been reported in approximately 30 patients (327–329). The patients develop severe anemia earlier than patients with malabsorption, such as patients with Imerslund-Gräsbeck syndrome, in whom uptake of cobalamin by bone marrow cells is intact. Patients with TC II deficiency also have normal or elevated cobalamin levels, although low levels were described in two cases (330).

Patients are not clinically deficient in cobalamin at birth. Symptoms usually develop in the first few months of life and include failure to thrive, weakness, and diarrhea. The anemia is usually clearly megaloblastic; some patients have had pancytopenia or erythroid hypoplasia (331). The presence of immature white cell precursors in a marrow that is otherwise hypocellular can lead to the misdiagnosis of leukemia. Neurologic disease has appeared in patients from 6 months to 30 months after the onset of symptoms but tends to be uncommon at presentation, usually occurring in patients who have been treated with folate rather than cobalamin (328). Severely defective cellular and humoral immunity has been seen, as well as defective granulocyte function.

Homocystinuria has been tested for in only two untreated patients and was found in one of them. In 60% of untreated patients, methylmalonic aciduria was found. After discontinuation of therapy, methylmalonic aciduria may return (327,332).

In all but one patient, functional TC II, as determined by its ability to bind cobalamin, was absent. Immunologically reactive TC II was found in three patients. In one patient, TC II was able to bind cobalamin but did not mediate cobalamin uptake into cells. Cobalamin malabsorption has been found in five of seven tested patients. The two patients with normal absorption had immunoreactive TC II, suggesting that the TC II molecule may support basolateral membrane export from the ileal cell even if it cannot transport cobalamin in the circulation. The development of radioimmunoassay and enzyme-linked immunosorbent assay techniques allows the diagnosis of TC II deficiency to be made at any time (330,333), whereas assays based on cobalamin-binding capacity are unreliable if cobalamin injection was administered in the preceding 2 to 3 days.

Inheritance. Deficiency of TC II is inherited as an autosomal-recessive disease. The gene for TC II was found by linkage analysis to lie close to the P blood group system on chromosome 22q (67). As discussed in the section on TC II, the gene, complementary DNA, and amino acid sequence of TC II have been reported (61). The sequence analysis of TC II variants has also been described (334). Mutation analysis of TC II–deficient patients has revealed deletions and nonsense mutations (335,336). TC II is synthesized by cultured cells, and prenatal diagnosis is thus possible even when the mutation is not known.

Management. Serum cobalamin levels must be kept very high and titrated to the clinical response to treat TC II–deficient patients successfully. This treatment can be achieved with oral hydroxocobalamin or cyanocobalamin, 500 to 1000 μg twice weekly, or systemic hydroxocobalamin, 1000 μg weekly or more often. Folic acid or folinic acid in milligram doses has been helpful in reversing the hematologic abnormalities but should not be administered alone because of the risk of neurologic complications if cobalamin is not also administered.

R Binder (Haptocorrin) Deficiency. Absence of R binder has been described in the plasma, leukocytes, and saliva of seven people in five families (291,337–339). A subsequent prospective search identified three new cases, suggesting that the entity is not rare (R. Carmel, *unpublished data*, 2001). R binder deficiency causes low serum cobalamin levels, but evidence of tissue cobalamin deficiency has not been found because TC II–mediated delivery of cobalamin is intact. Although some patients have had neurologic dysfunction, which was severe in one case, it was most likely due to coexisting causes (337,340).

The defect in one family involved absence of lactoferrin as well as R binder (340); lactoferrin, like R binder, is synthesized both in specific granules of neutrophils and in exocrine glands (77). There was no predisposition to infection in the family. In a second family, one of the two R binder–deficient family members had coexisting inherited IF deficiency (the genes for IF and R binder are both on chromosome 11) (291).

The inheritance of R binder deficiency appears to be autosomal recessive. Presumptive heterozygotes have low but detectable levels of R binder in the blood and mildly decreased cobalamin levels but have normal R binder levels in saliva (340). A preliminary report suggested that mild R binder deficiency causes 18% of low serum cobalamin levels (341).

INBORN ERRORS OF COBALAMIN METABOLISM

Diagnostic features of inborn errors of cobalamin metabolism are listed in Table 45-7.

Methylmalonic Acidurias. The disorders causing methylmalonic aciduria are characterized by severe metabolic acidosis and accumulation of large amounts of MMA in the blood, urine, and cerebrospinal fluid (342). Megaloblastic anemia does not occur. The patients have a defect in the mitochondrial matrix enzyme methylmalonyl-CoA mutase, which requires adenosylcobalamin as a cofactor (Fig. 45-8). Classification has been based largely on studies in cultured fibroblasts in which complementation groups have been established according to whether two cell lines partially correct a defect in propionate incorporation after cell fusion.

Methylmalonyl–Coenzyme A Mutase Deficiency. Disorders of the mutase apoenzyme result in methylmalonic aciduria unresponsive to cobalamin therapy. Mature mutase purified from human liver is a homodimer of 77-kd subunits. It is coded by a nuclear gene found in the cytoplasm as a precursor with a leader sequence and processed to a mature protein in the mitochondria (36). Two classes of patients are known with mutations at the *MUT* locus. They have been characterized on the basis of studies on cultured fibroblasts. The *mut°* cell lines have no residual mutase activity, whereas the *mut⁻* cell lines show some residual activity in the presence of adenosylcobalamin. The enzyme in *mut⁻* cell lines shows decreased affinity for adenosylcobalamin. Several *mut°* cell lines synthesize no detectable protein, whereas others synthesize unstable proteins, and at least one has a mutation that interferes with transfer of the mutase to the mitochondria (343). Similarly variable levels of mRNA have been demonstrated in different *mut°* lines. Usually, no complementation between *mut°* and *mut⁻* cell lines is seen, but some cell lines have been shown to complement with most *mut⁻* and some *mut°* cell lines as a result of interallelic (intragenic) complementation (344).

Patients with mutase deficiency are clinically well at birth but may become symptomatic rapidly with protein feeding. They usually come to medical attention because of lethargy, failure to thrive, muscular hypotonia, respiratory distress, and recurrent vomiting and dehydration. Urinary excretion of MMA is usually less than 5 mg/day in normal children, whereas it is usually more than 100 mg and as much as several grams per day in mutase deficiency. In addition, these patients may have ketones and glycine in both blood and urine and metabolic acidosis with elevated levels of ammonia. Many also have hypoglycemia, leukopenia, and thrombocytopenia. One study demonstrated that mutase deficiency inhibits bone marrow stem cells in a concentration-dependent manner (345).

Follow-up of children identified by newborn screening has shown several who excrete MMA and have mutase deficiency but are clinically well and have never developed acidosis (346). It is unclear whether they are at risk for catastrophic acidosis later in life. Other children detected prospectively on newborn screening with relatively low excretion of MMA appear to have a good prognosis (347). The incidence of all forms of methylma-

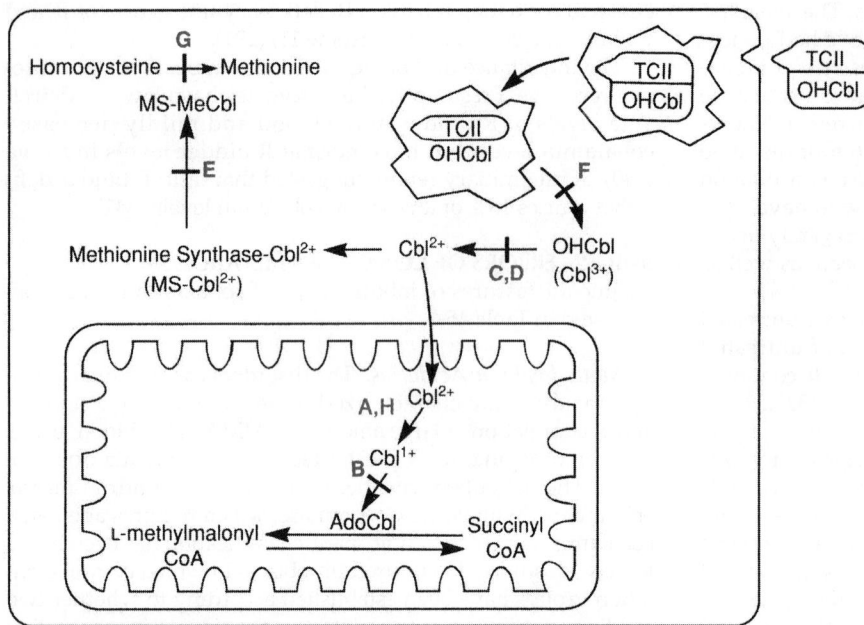

Figure 45-8. Scheme of intracellular cobalamin (Cbl) metabolism. Letters A through H represent the sites of known inherited defects (*cblA–cblH*). AdoCbl, 5'-adenosylcobalamin; $Cbl^{1+,2+,3+}$, Cbl with 1+, 2+, or 3+ oxidation states of the central cobalt; MeCbl, methylcobalamin; MS, methionine synthase; OHCbl, hydroxocobalamin; TC II, transcobalamin II.

lonic aciduria in Massachusetts is 1 in 48,000. Patients with *mut⁻* seek medical attention later than do *mut°* patients, and they tend to have a better prognosis. Neurologic sequelae may occur in patients with both types of mutase deficiency, even in the absence of a documented acidotic episode (348).

The gene for the mutase enzyme has been cloned and is located on the short arm of chromosome 6 (6p12-21.1) (37,38,349). All the methylmalonic acidurias appear to be inherited in an autosomal-recessive manner, and several mutations have been identified (344,350–354).

Mutase-deficient patients are not responsive to cobalamin. Therefore, dietary control is essential. Therapy consists of protein restriction to limit the amino acids that use the propionate pathway. Formula deficient in valine, isoleucine, methionine, and threonine is used. Maintenance of acid–base balance and therapy with carnitine have been advocated (355). Even with therapy, prognosis is guarded, with reports of brain infarcts and renal dysfunction as late complications (342). Early liver transplantation has been suggested for severe methylmalonic aciduria and has had variable results (356–359).

Adenosylcobalamin Deficiency: *cblA*, *cblB*, and *cblH*. This group of disorders results in cobalamin-responsive methylmalonic aciduria and an intracellular deficiency in adenosylcobalamin. The disorders are distinguished by complementation analysis and by the fact that patients with *cblA* and *cblH* defects are capable of adenosylcobalamin synthesis in cell extracts but not in intact cells, whereas synthesis is deficient in both systems in *cblB*. The *cblA* and *cblH* disorders are thought to reside in a reducing system, presumably mitochondrial, that converts cob(III)alamin to cob(I)alamin. Only complementation analysis can differentiate between these two disorders (360). The *cblB* defect lies in the adenosyltransferase, which is the final step in the synthesis of adenosylcobalamin (Fig. 45-8). All the patients have clinical findings virtually identical to those in patients with methylmalonyl-CoA mutase deficiency. Blood levels of cobalamin are usually within normal levels.

At least 45 *cblA* patients and 36 *cblB* patients and only one *cblH* patient are known. Both *cblA* and *cblB* are inherited in an autosomal-recessive manner; roughly equal numbers of patients of both sexes have been reported, and parents of *cblB* patients have decreased adenosyltransferase activity (361). As noted in a

classic review of methylmalonic aciduria (362), illness began in the first week of life in 5 of 12 patients with *cblA*; in six patients, it began before the end of the first year of life. Of eight patients with *cblB* disease, four presented before the age of 1 month, and one patient presented after the age of 1 year. Symptoms were similar to those reported for mutase deficiency, although usually they were less severe and were dependent on the clinical response to cobalamin therapy (362). Most *cblA* patients (90%) responded to cobalamin, and almost 70% were well at up to 14 years of age. Forty percent of *cblB* patients responded to therapy, but only 30% had a long-term survival. Therapy has been either hydroxocobalamin or cyanocobalamin injections; it is not clear if administering adenosylcobalamin offers any advantage. Prenatal cobalamin therapy has been effective (363), but it is uncertain whether therapy from birth would have been equally effective.

Combined Deficiencies of Adenosylcobalamin and Methylcobalamin: cblC, cblD, and cblF. Patients with combined deficiencies of adenosylcobalamin and methylcobalamin have a functional deficiency in both methylmalonyl–CoA mutase and methionine synthase. The precise defects are not known, but all result in a failure to synthesize both methylcobalamin and adenosylcobalamin, combined hyperhomocysteinemia and hypomethioninemia, and methylmalonic aciduria.

The defect in all three disorders occurs after the endocytosis and hydrolysis of the TC II–cobalamin complex. The *cblF* defect appears to be in the transfer of free cobalamin from the lysosome to the cytoplasm, whereas in *cblC* and *cblD*, it is presumed to be in an early cytosolic cob(III)alamin reductase needed to reduce the trivalent cobalt (Fig. 45-8). When incubated with cyanocobalamin, fibroblasts from *cblC* and *cblD* patients accumulate little intracellular cobalamin and virtually no adenosylcobalamin or methylcobalamin. In contrast, *cblF* fibroblasts accumulate excess cobalamin, but it is all free, unmetabolized, and localized to lysosomes.

Clinical Findings. We are aware of more than 100 cases of *cblC*, two patients in one sibship with *cblD*, and six unrelated patients with *cblF* disease. Most patients with *cblC* are symptomatic in the first 2 months of life, with poor feeding, failure to thrive, and lethargy. The patients usually have megaloblastic anemia, and some have thrombocytopenia. Others have a later onset, including presentation in adulthood (364): a 4-year-old boy who presented with fatigue, delirium, and spasticity (365) and a 15-year-old girl with mental deterioration and myelopathy (366). A retinal abnormality with perimacular degeneration was reported in three patients (327,365,367).

In at least two patients, diagnosis was made by neonatal screening for methylmalonic aciduria. The methylmalonic aciduria is less severe than in mutase deficiency but greater than in defects of cobalamin transport. Serum cobalamin and folate levels are never low and may be elevated. The clinical findings and outcomes in 44 early-onset and six late-onset patients have been reviewed (368). Prominent neurologic findings at diagnosis included developmental delay in 28 patients, microcephaly in nine, macrocephaly in two, hypotonia in 30, seizures in 23, dementia in four, and myelopathy in four. Major clinical and laboratory findings included feeding difficulties in 35 of the 50 patients, failure to thrive in 22, pigmentary retinopathy in 20, decreased visual acuity in 15, nystagmus in 10, hydrocephalus in eight, acidosis in nine, hematologic abnormalities in 34, and microthrombi in three.

The *cblD* sibship came to attention because of mild mental retardation and behavioral problems. Venous thrombosis was also present.

Findings in patients with *cblF* include small size for gestational age, poor feeding, growth retardation, and persistent stomatitis (369,370). One patient had glossitis, and a second had persistent skin rash; both patients also had minor facial abnormalities, and the first had dextrocardia. Only the second patient had macrocytosis and hyperhomocysteinemia (370). Although most patients present in the first year of life, one presented later in childhood (371).

Inheritance. Males and females are affected with *cblC* approximately equally. The disorder is probably inherited as an autosomal recessive. The two siblings with *cblD* are both male, so the possibility of sex linkage cannot be excluded. Male and female patients with *cblF* have been reported.

All these defects are reflected in cultured fibroblasts. Uptake of labeled cyanocobalamin is impaired in *cblC* and *cblD*, distinguishing them from all other cobalamin mutations. The incorporation of propionate and 5-methyl THF is reduced in all three disorders, as is synthesis of adenosylcobalamin and methylcobalamin. Direct measurements of total methylmalonyl-CoA mutase and methionine synthase activities in cell extracts should give low results (not measured in *cblF*). Complementation analysis between an unknown cell line and previously defined groups provides the specific diagnosis. Prenatal diagnosis has been successful in *cblC* disease using amniocytes, and the diagnosis has been ruled out using chorionic villous biopsy material and cells (371a).

Management. Therapy in *cblC* disease can be difficult, particularly in infants with early onset, many of whom have died or have severe developmental delay (361,368). Most patients have improved with parenteral hydroxocobalamin therapy (1000 μg/day), reducing their MMA and homocystine excretion. Hydroxocobalamin should be used rather than cyanocobalamin (361,368). Methylcobalamin and adenosylcobalamin have been used, but their therapeutic advantage is unclear. In a single, thorough report of therapy, parenteral hydroxocobalamin was more effective than oral therapy (372). Betaine appeared to be helpful in combination with hydroxocobalamin; neither folinic acid nor carnitine had any effect. Daily oral betaine and biweekly injections of hydroxocobalamin produced decreased MMA excretion, normal serum methionine and homocysteine

concentrations, and resolution of lethargy, irritability, and failure to thrive. The neurologic and retinal findings were not reversed, indicating that early diagnosis and treatment are essential.

Patients with *cblF* appeared to respond to hydroxocobalamin, in one case only by injection (370), and in the other first by injection and then by mouth (369). Experience is too limited to know whether parenteral therapy is essential. One patient was unable to absorb cobalamin even with added IF (371). It seems possible that *cblF* patients might store cobalamin in lysosomes to an extent that itself causes symptoms after prolonged therapy. Presence of disease has been excluded by studies on amniocytes.

Methylcobalamin Deficiency: cblE and cblG.

Functional methionine synthase deficiency is characterized by homocystinuria and hypomethioninemia without methylmalonic aciduria. Complementation analysis has identified two distinct groups, *cblE* and *cblG* (Fig. 45-8).

Clinical and Laboratory Findings. Patients usually come to medical attention in the first 2 years of life, but one patient presented at 21 years with symptoms that were mistaken for multiple sclerosis (373). There have been at least 12 patients with *cblE* and 24 with *cblG*. Both sexes are affected.

The most common findings in both disorders include megaloblastic anemia and various neurologic problems, of which developmental delay and cerebral atrophy are the most common (374). Serum cobalamin levels are within the normal range. Other findings include electroencephalographic abnormalities, nystagmus, hypotonia, hypertonia, seizures, blindness, and ataxia. Fibroblasts from both *cblE* and *cblG* patients show decreased intracellular levels of methylcobalamin but normal levels of adenosylcobalamin. Cultured *cblE* fibroblasts have normal total cyanocobalamin uptake and binding to the intracellular enzymes. In most *cblG* cells studied, cobalamin bound normally to methionine synthase, but in three cell lines, no binding was seen (375). Decreased incorporation of 5-methyl THF reflects the functional methionine synthase deficiency. Results with the standard assay for methionine synthase in *cblE* cell extracts are within the range of controls, but most *cblG* cell extracts have low enzyme activity. In *cblE* cells, a relative deficiency in enzyme activity was seen when the assay was performed under suboptimal reducing conditions, suggesting a defect in a reducing system associated with methionine synthase (376,377). The affected gene codes for methionine synthase reductase.

One patient with *cblE* disease had transient methylmalonic aciduria (378). The clinical heterogeneity is illustrated by the patient who was not diagnosed until adulthood. Her presentation was mainly neurologic, and the anemia was recognized only later.

Inheritance. Both disorders are inherited in an autosomal-recessive pattern. Decreased methylcobalamin levels have been seen in fibroblasts from obligate heterozygotes for *cblE* (379). The gene for methionine synthase has been cloned and localized to chromosome 1q43 (380–382). Both missense and nonsense mutations have been described in *cblG* patients (380,383–386). In the *cblG* cell lines that showed no binding to methionine synthase, functionally null mutations in the enzyme were found (384). The methionine synthase reductase gene has been cloned and localized to chromosome 5p15.2-15.3, and several mutations in this gene have been reported in *cblE* patients (45,387).

Management. Parenteral therapy with hydroxocobalamin, first daily, then once or twice weekly, has been used. Usually, the therapy corrects the anemia and metabolic abnormalities. The neurologic findings have been difficult to reverse, particularly in *cblG* disease. Early diagnosis and therapy are important. Prenatal diagnosis of *cblE* in amniocytes has been successful. The mother was given parenteral cobalamin from the second trimester onward, and the baby was treated from birth and has done well. It is uncertain if prenatal therapy is needed.

ACQUIRED METABOLIC DISORDERS

Exposure to Nitrous Oxide. Nitrous oxide is a commonly used inhalant in general anesthesia. Patients exposed for many consecutive hours to this gas to treat tetanus or leukemia have developed megaloblastic anemia and pancytopenia (388–390). Chronic, intermittent exposure as a result of substance abuse or leaks in operating rooms or dental offices causes myeloneuropathy typical of cobalamin deficiency, despite normal plasma concentrations of cobalamin and folate (391). In experimental animals, the neurologic dysfunction caused by chronic exposure was prevented by supplements of methionine (145,392). Hematopoietic cells in humans begin to show megaloblastic changes and changes in deoxyuridine suppression after exposure lasting 6 hours or more (393,394).

Nitrous oxide oxidatively destroys intracellular cobalamin (390,395). Cobalamin attached to methionine synthase is a primary target during turnover of the enzyme after transfer of a methyl group to form methionine, before the cobalamin is remethylated. The enzyme bound to the altered cobalamin is permanently inactivated, but in the brief exposure during routine surgery, activity is restored as new enzyme replaces the inactivated enzyme and new cobalamin attaches. During prolonged exposure, more cobalamin and enzyme are inactivated, and additional defects (e.g., methylmalonyl-CoA mutase) may occur (396).

Routine exposure during surgery raises homocysteine levels postoperatively but does not cause clinical problems related to cobalamin (397,398). However, severe problems, especially neurologic and mental dysfunction, may occur several days or weeks after prolonged surgery in patients who have concurrent but unrecognized mild cobalamin deficiency or are taking methotrexate (399–401). The neurologic problems do not always remit completely after cobalamin therapy. Concerns have been raised that administering cobalamin preoperatively may paradoxically enhance the potential for toxicity by increasing cobalamin attachment to methionine synthase just before exposure to nitrous oxide. It appears advisable to screen all patients before elective surgery and postpone it in all those with cobalamin deficiency until the deficiency has been fully treated.

MISCELLANEOUS CAUSES OF LOW COBALAMIN LEVELS

Many patients and healthy subjects fitting certain profiles have low cobalamin levels, the cause of which is not always apparent (Table 45-3). Evidence for true cobalamin deficiency is often absent.

Old Age. Approximately 10% of all elderly persons in Western countries have low serum cobalamin levels, although the reported prevalences have varied widely. The extensive literature has been reviewed (90,202–204) but includes only one longitudinal study (402,403). Most people with low cobalamin levels do not have anemia or obvious neurologic dysfunction. However, 15% to 25% of all elderly persons have elevated levels of homocysteine, MMA, or both, and metabolic evidence for cellular cobalamin insufficiency exists in 50% to 90% of the subjects with low cobalamin levels (59,200,212,213,404). Subtle neurologic or cognitive abnormalities can be demonstrated in some cases despite the lack of symptoms. These studies have formed the bulk of the evidence for the entity of mild preclinical cobalamin deficiency.

The causes of this mild deficiency state are food cobalamin malabsorption in approximately 40% and pernicious anemia and intestinal disease in approximately 10% of subjects (54,90,253,261,405,406). No explanation is apparent in the remaining 50% of subjects (90). Dietary insufficiency, often assumed to be present, is rare in the elderly (57,58,206).

Pregnancy. Cobalamin levels decline in the second half of pregnancy, and 14% to 28% of women have low cobalamin levels, sometimes below 100 ng/L, in the third trimester (15). Megaloblastic anemia is rare, and metabolic studies have not demonstrated cellular insufficiency (407,408). The cobalamin levels return to normal several days after delivery.

Folate Deficiency. Folate deficiency is a clinically important cause of low serum cobalamin levels. Cobalamin levels usually decline in folate deficiency or with use of methotrexate, sometimes falling below 100 ng/L (15). The cause is unknown, but diagnostic confusion and inappropriate cobalamin therapy can result. Measuring MMA levels, which rise only in cobalamin deficiency, may help differentiate between folate deficiency alone and combined deficiencies, as may be found in small bowel disease. Folic acid administered alone usually raises the cobalamin level within a few days in folate-deficient patients but not in cobalamin-deficient patients.

Multiple Myeloma. Low cobalamin levels were described in 29% of patients with myeloma (409). Occasional patients have coexisting pernicious anemia (410), but in most cases, no explanation for the low levels is apparent, and clinical signs of deficiency are uncommon. Evidence to support cobalamin deficiency is usually absent. A preliminary report suggested increased cobalamin uptake by bone marrow cells (411), but another study suggested that low TC I levels may be responsible (409).

Human Immunodeficiency Virus Infection. Low cobalamin levels have been found in approximately 15% of human immunodeficiency virus–infected patients (412,413). Some patients have shown evidence of deficiency of cobalamin, folate, or both, but most patients have not, and few respond to vitamin therapy. Cobalamin absorption has been normal in some studies but not in others. Low cobalamin levels may reflect low TC I levels (414) and may be associated with a poor prognosis (415).

Oral Contraceptives. Oral contraceptive use is associated with low cobalamin levels that return to normal after the contraceptives are discontinued (416). The cause is unknown.

Causes of Folate Deficiency

Acquired folate deficiency is more often multifactorial than cobalamin deficiency. Poor intake can be superimposed on all processes, the effects of drugs and alcohol may be multiple, drug effects may complicate the underlying illness for which they were used, and increased requirements sometimes potentiate the various causes of folate deficiency. The acquired and inherited disorders are presented here. The established inherited disorders of folate metabolism and transport are also summarized in Table 45-8.

DIETARY INSUFFICIENCY

Because of the relatively small ratio of body stores to daily requirements of 100:1 or less and the lability of food folate, dietary inadequacy is the most common cause of folate deficiency. Dietary insufficiency is more frequent when alcohol

TABLE 45-8. Diagnostic and Clinical Features of Known Inborn Errors of Folate Transport and Metabolism

	Serum		Clinical Findings	
	Folate	Plasma Total Homocysteine	Megaloblastic Anemia	Neurologic Abnormalities
Hereditary folate malabsorption	↓	N	Present	Present
Methylenetetrahydrofolate reductase deficiency	N or ↓	↑	Absent	Present
Glutamate formiminotransferase deficiency	N or ↓	N	Present or absent[a]	Present[b]

N, normal; ↓, low; ↑, high.
[a]Reported as present only in patients described in Japan.
[b]Neurologic abnormalities were severe in patients reported from Japan and very mild in others.

abuse is involved (although beer contains approximately 100 μg folate/L). Other persons at risk are premature babies, adolescents, and patients eating restricted diets, such as in phenylketonuria, or using unsupplemented parenteral nutrition. Blacks and Latin Americans have lower folate levels than whites (213,417,418), although the causes may not have a purely dietary explanation. Folate insufficiency has been a problem in some elderly persons, such as institutionalized ones, but no specific predisposition to folate deficiency exists in the elderly (419,420). Indeed, folate status tends to improve with age in current surveys, compared with the reverse trend for cobalamin (192,421).

There has been a dramatic change in folate status in the past decade in general in North America and Europe. Intake has improved, and the prevalence of deficiency has decreased substantially, probably because of the increased use of supplements and the introduction of food fortification.

MALABSORPTION

Gastrointestinal Causes. Achlorhydria caused by atrophic gastritis or acid-suppressive drugs can diminish folate absorption (422,423). In pernicious anemia, this effect is less noticeable because cobalamin deficiency tends to raise serum folate levels. Folate absorption is also impaired after partial gastrectomy and in giant hypertrophic gastritis (296,424).

The use of pancreatic extracts and bicarbonate may impair folate absorption in patients with pancreatic insufficiency (425). Alcohol and certain drugs can impair folate absorption but are discussed elsewhere because their effects are often multiple.

Diseases affecting the small bowel, especially its upper half, can produce folate deficiency. These include tropical sprue, in which the malabsorptive defect itself sometimes improves dramatically after folate therapy (172). Celiac disease (426), Whipple's disease, and inflammatory bowel disease can also impair folate absorption. The mechanisms producing the malabsorption have not been defined, and sometimes nonmalabsorptive causes are superimposed (427,428). Bacterial overgrowth in the small intestine does not interfere with folate absorption.

Hereditary Folate Malabsorption. Hereditary folate malabsorption (Table 45-8) is characterized by severe megaloblastic anemia, diarrhea, oral ulcers, failure to thrive, and, usually, progressive neurologic deterioration. Megaloblastic anemia in the first few months of life and low serum folate levels are the most important diagnostic features. Increased excretion of formiminoglutamic acid (FIGLU) and orotic acid may be found. All patients have a severe abnormality in the absorption of oral folic acid or reduced folates such as folinic acid and 5-methyl THF (Fig. 45-2, block B).

The disorder provides the best evidence for a specific transport system for folates across both the intestine and the choroid plexus. Except in two affected male patients (429,430), folate levels remained low in the cerebrospinal fluid even when blood levels were raised sufficiently to correct the anemia. This finding suggests that the carrier system in both intestine and brain is coded by a single gene product. The uptake of folate into other cells is probably not defective, because anemia is reversed by relatively low doses of folate, and uptake of folate into cultured cells is not abnormal.

Management. Oral folate in very high doses produces a therapeutic response in some patients, correcting the anemia. 5-Formyl THF or 5-methyl THF may be more effective in entering the cerebrospinal fluid in this disorder. Neurologic response has varied. Seizures improved with folate therapy in some patients but worsened in others (431).

Treatment must maintain high levels of folate in the blood and cerebrospinal fluid. Oral doses of folate may be increased to 100 mg or more daily, if necessary; parenteral therapy must be instituted if oral therapy is ineffective. Intrathecal folate may be needed if levels in cerebrospinal fluid cannot be normalized. Reduced folates may be more effective than folic acid.

Inheritance. The disorder has been described in fewer than 20 patients (429,430,432). Most patients have been female, but at least three male patients were reported (429,432), one of whom had atypical clinical findings. Consanguinity has been reported. The father of an affected patient had intermediate levels of folate absorption. Autosomal-recessive inheritance is likely, but the preponderance of female patients is unexplained. A complementary DNA for an intestinal transporter identical to that for the reduced folate carrier has been isolated (31). No mutations in this gene have been found yet in patients.

DRUGS AND TOXINS

Alcohol. Alcohol compromises folate balance in many ways, which, along with alcohol's folate-unrelated hematologic toxicity, has been the subject of reviews (433,434). The previously discussed dietary issues are important, yet serum folate levels fall within hours of alcohol ingestion. Studies have implicated interference with enterohepatic recycling of folate (435), although that view has been challenged. Increased folate breakdown and urinary excretion may be important (436), and acetaldehyde forms adducts with THF (437). Alcohol may also interfere with folate absorption (438). Metabolic evidence for folate deficiency has been reported in alcoholic patients without clinical signs of deficiency (439). In addition, alcohol causes red cell macrocytosis directly by unknown mechanisms unrelated to folate metabolism.

Methotrexate and Other Antifols. Methotrexate (amethopterin) binds tightly to dihydrofolate reductase (DHFR). This binding prevents binding of dihydrofolate to DHFR, even though methotrexate binds to the enzyme in a different orientation than does folate (440). Methotrexate polyglutamates also inhibit thymidylate synthase and glycinamide ribonucleotide transformylase, directly impairing thymidylate and purine synthesis.

Methotrexate was designed specifically for treatment of malignant disease. Normal hematopoietic cells appear to tolerate exposure to high concentrations for as long as 24 hours under conditions that kill many neoplastic cells and lymphocytes. High-dose methotrexate, with rescue of normal cells by leucovorin, a racemic mixture of *R* and *S*5-formyl THF, is an effective regimen. The effect of methotrexate on cell proliferation has led to its use in graft-versus-host disease, rheumatoid arthritis, psoriasis, and other diseases.

Several other folate inhibitors have been synthesized. Some have much greater affinity for prokaryotic than for mammalian DHFR and are used as antimicrobial drugs (e.g., trimethoprim and pyrimethamine). When folate status is compromised for other reasons, these drugs may produce folate deficiency in occasional patients (441). Cytopenias, especially neutropenia, have been prominent features, but their attribution to the antifol effect is not always certain.

Other Drugs. Drugs affecting folate have been reviewed (442). The postulated effect of hydantoins on folate absorption remains unclear, but folate deficiency is a common problem in patients using anticonvulsant drugs. Paraaminosalicylic acid impairs folate absorption, as does sulfasalazine, which also inhibits several folate-metabolizing enzymes and has been associated with subclinical folate deficiency (443). Trimethoprim-sulfamethoxazole and triamterene are weak DHFR inhibitors in humans. Diverse effects of oral contraceptives on folate status, including local cervical folate depletion and predisposition to cervical dysplasia in women infected with human papillomavirus, have been described but are controversial (444,445).

INCREASED FOLATE REQUIREMENTS

Physiologic settings in which folate requirements are increased include the growth-related needs of newborn infants, young children, and adolescents, and the diversion of folate that occurs in pregnant women (including their increased urinary folate loss) and lactating women (14,446–448).

Increased folate requirements have also been shown in persons with chronic hemolytic anemia and have been suggested in patients taking antiepileptic drugs and patients with certain malignant disorders such as myeloproliferative disease (449). More controversial are suggestions of increased requirements in hyperthyroidism or skin disorders with high rates of cell turnover.

The diagnosis of increased need is not easily made, because there are no clinical tests for it. Studies have relied on demonstrations of rapid clearance of folate, evidence of low folate stores in the absence of other causes, or poor clinical response of evidence of deficiency unless high doses of folic acid are used (446). Folic acid is often administered routinely to patients with conditions in which increased requirements are known to occur, but the rationale is sometimes weak, and the clinical impact is uncertain (450). The chief examples of routine supplementation are pregnancy and sickle cell anemia.

Most patients with increased requirements have a negative folate balance but do not develop clinically overt folate deficiency more often than control subjects (450). Treatable causes, such as alcoholism, poor diet, or malabsorption, should be sought whenever a patient develops megaloblastic anemia or symptomatic folate deficiency before attributing the condition to increased requirement alone.

ACUTE FOLATE DEFICIENCY

An unexplained, acute onset of megaloblastic changes has been described in catastrophically ill patients in intensive care units

(451,452). The changes, both morphologic and metabolic, are limited to the bone marrow. Although cytopenia, especially thrombocytopenia, is marked, megaloblastic changes are not found in peripheral blood. All vitamin levels are usually normal, but the deoxyuridine suppression test identifies folate deficiency in bone marrow cells. The recommendation has been made that all patients in intensive care units be given folic acid prophylactically (453). The evidence suggests a rapid superimposition of folate deficiency on patients with multiple medical problems, therapies, and interventions.

INBORN ERRORS OF FOLATE METABOLISM

Methylenetetrahydrofolate Reductase Deficiency. Methylenetetrahydrofolate reductase (MTHFR) deficiency (Table 45-8) is the most common inborn error of folate metabolism (431,454), with approximately 50 known cases. It is not associated with megaloblastic anemia because the defect impairs the conversion of 5,10-methylene THF to 5-methyl THF (Fig. 45-2, block A) but leaves intact its ability to participate in *de novo* thymidine synthesis and generate 10-formyl THF for purine metabolism. Because 5-methyl THF availability for methionine synthase diminishes, MTHFR deficiency results in elevated homocysteine levels and decreased levels of methionine. The lack of 5-methyl THF, the main circulating form of folate, also makes MTHFR deficiency one of the few inborn errors of folate metabolism that may produce low rather than high serum folate levels. A mouse model now exists for severe MTHFR deficiency (455).

Clinical Findings. Patients may become symptomatic at any age from infancy to adulthood. Most frequently, the disease appears in infancy, when its most common manifestation is developmental delay. Breathing disorders and seizures are often present, as is microcephaly. Motor and gait abnormalities and psychiatric symptoms have been reported.

Autopsy findings include dilated cerebral vessels, internal hydrocephalus, and microgyria (456–459). Perivascular changes, demyelination, macrophage infiltration, gliosis, and astrocytosis have been reported. The major factor in some deaths was thrombosis of both arteries and cerebral veins (456). The vascular changes in the brain resemble those in classic homocystinuria caused by cystathionine β-synthase deficiency. Two reports described patients with subacute combined degeneration of the cord similar to that in cobalamin deficiency (458,459). The mechanisms responsible for the neurologic dysfunction are unclear. It is important to note that, except for the absence of megaloblastic anemia, the findings in MTHFR deficiency are similar to those in *cblE* and *cblG* disease and, to a lesser extent, *cblC* disease, which also features methylmalonic aciduria.

Laboratory Investigation. Homocystinuria is seen in all patients, with a range of 15 to 667 µmol/24 hours and a mean of 130 µmol/24 hours (454). These values are much lower than those found in patients with cystathionine β-synthase deficiency. If MTHFR deficiency is suspected, more than one determination of homocystine excretion should be performed to eliminate the possibility of a false-negative value. The mentioned values are for free homocystine, which is detectable in amino acid analyses in urine. Most assays in plasma used by most clinical laboratories now measure total homocysteine.

Methionine levels have been low in plasma in severe MTHFR deficiency, with values from 0 to 18 µmol/L (mean, 12 µmol/L) (454); normal fasting plasma methionine levels are usually in the range of 23 to 35 µmol/L. Cerebrospinal fluid neurotransmitter levels have usually been low but have been measured in only a few patients (454).

The diagnosis of severe MTHFR deficiency can be confirmed by direct measurement of enzyme activity in liver, leukocytes, and cultured fibroblasts and lymphocytes. A rough correlation exists between residual enzyme activity and clinical severity (460).

Inheritance and Prenatal Recognition. Severe MTHFR deficiency is an autosomal-recessive disease. Decreased MTHFR activity has been found in the cells of obligate heterozygotes; some have levels nearly as low as those in homozygous affected patients. Prenatal diagnosis has been reported using amniocytes (461), and the enzyme is present in chorionic villi. The gene for MTHFR is on chromosome 1p36.3 (462,463); 24 mutations have been described in patients with severe deficiency (431).

Management. Early diagnosis is important because the prognosis is poor once neurologic involvement is evident. Patients are difficult to treat. A summary of the treatment protocols for some of the earliest patients with severe MTHFR deficiency has been published (454). These protocols have been highly variable and usually were unsuccessful until the introduction of betaine (464). Therapy with either methionine alone or with 5-methyl THF has not been effective. A regimen consisting of oral betaine, folinic acid, cobalamin, and vitamin B_6 has been suggested (465). Early therapy with betaine after prenatal diagnosis has produced the best outcome (466).

Glutamate Formiminotransferase Deficiency. The clinical manifestations of glutamate formiminotransferase deficiency (Table 45-8; Fig. 45-2, block C) remain unclear. Fewer than 20 patients have been described. The catabolism of histidine is associated with the transfer of a formimino group to THF followed by the release of ammonia and the formation of 5,10-methenyl THF. Two activities that share a single octomeric enzyme, found only in the liver and kidney, are involved in these reactions: glutamate formiminotransferase and formimino THF cyclodeaminase. FIGLU excretion is the one constant feature of glutamate formiminotransferase deficiency.

Two distinct phenotypes have been described, one mild and one severe. In the severe form, mental and physical retardation, an abnormal electroencephalogram, and dilation of the cerebral ventricles with cortical atrophy are seen. In the mild form, mental retardation is not found, but excretion of FIGLU is higher. It has been proposed, without direct evidence, that the mild form is caused by a defect in the formiminotransferase enzyme and the severe form by a block in the cyclodeaminase enzyme (467).

Patients with formiminotransferase deficiency range in age from 3 months to 42 years at diagnosis. Several had macrocytosis and hypersegmented neutrophils. Three had delayed speech, two had seizures, and two had mental retardation as their presenting findings. Two patients were studied because they were siblings of known patients. Mental retardation was described in most of the original patients from Japan (468), but of the remaining patients, few showed mental retardation.

Laboratory Investigation. In most cases, enzyme activity in liver has been higher than expected for a defect causing disease. The activity in five patients ranged from 14% to 54% of control values. Because the enzyme activity is expressed only in liver, it has not been possible to confirm the diagnosis using cultured cells. There is considerable debate whether the enzyme is expressed in erythrocytes (454,469).

Elevated FIGLU excretion, as well as increased FIGLU in the blood after a histidine load (Fig. 45-2), and high to normal serum folate levels have been reported. Plasma levels of amino acids, including histidine, were usually normal, but hyperhis-tidinemia and hyperhistidinuria have been found occasionally, as well as low plasma methionine levels.

Inheritance. The deficiency has been found in offspring of both sexes with unaffected parents. Autosomal-recessive inheritance is probable. Because of the lack of enzyme expression in cultured cells, definitive understanding of the inheritance awaits the cloning of the gene and localization of the molecular defect. A candidate gene for glutamate formiminotransferase deficiency has been cloned and characterized on chromosome 21q22.3 (470).

Management. Two patients in one family responded to folate therapy with decreased FIGLU excretion (471); six other patients did not (454). One of two patients responded to methionine supplementation (472,473). It is uncertain whether reducing FIGLU excretion itself has any direct clinical value.

Cellular Uptake Defects. Patients with well-characterized abnormalities of folate uptake into cells have been described, but it is unclear if any of the abnormalities represents a primary defect. In one large kindred, 34 persons had severe hematologic disease, including anemia, pancytopenia, and leukemia, resulting in the death of 18 (474). The proband had severe aplastic anemia that responded to folate therapy. The uptake of 5-methyl THF in stimulated lymphocytes was markedly reduced despite normal uptake of folic acid. One son developed the transport defect after becoming neutropenic, suggesting that it may not be the primary defect. In another family, in which the proband and three daughters had dyserythropoiesis without anemia, abnormal 5-methyl THF uptake was seen in erythrocytes and bone marrow cells but not in lymphocytes (475). No clear correlation was found between the clinical findings and the putative disorder of cellular uptake.

Enzyme Polymorphisms. A thermolabile MTHFR enzyme with slightly decreased activity was found in patients with mild hyperhomocysteinemia (476). A 677C→T polymorphism in the MTHFR gene was identified (477). Affected individuals have none of the clinical problems seen in severe MTHFR deficiency. The prevalence of homozygosity for the T allele ranges from 4% to 24% of most populations, but it is rare in blacks (478). There is a trend for homozygotes to have slightly higher homocysteine levels and lower folate levels than normal (479). The increased risk for vascular disease attributed to this common polymorphism has not been consistent. The mutation may increase the risk for neural tube defects and perhaps other obstetric complications (480). Curiously, the mutation confers a protective effect on colorectal cancer. Other MTHFR polymorphisms, such as the 1298A→C mutation, have been found. None produce the thermolability of the 677C→T mutation, and their effects on MTHFR activity and homocysteine appear to be even milder (478).

Polymorphisms that produce mildly decreased enzyme activity have been found for methionine synthase and methionine synthase reductase (478,481).

Suspect Disorders. Three patients with megaloblastic anemia were postulated to have DHFR deficiency (Fig. 45-2, reaction 1), but its existence as a true disorder is in doubt (482,483). Three patients with microcephaly, mental retardation, and abnormal electroencephalographic findings were reported to have decreased methylene-THF cyclohydrolase activity (Fig. 45-2, reaction 6) (468), but the diagnosis was retracted. Functional deficiency of methionine synthase (Fig. 45-2, reaction 5) was discussed in the section on *cblE* and *cblG* diseases. The primary defect in *cblG* is now known to be caused by mutations in methionine synthase. The diagnosis in a 6-month-old girl with megaloblastic anemia, cerebral abnormalities, and suspected decreased methionine synthase activity but no homocystinuria (484) has not been confirmed.

Megaloblastic Anemia Not Involving Cobalamin or Folate

Because of their megaloblastic anemia, these hereditary disorders can enter the differential diagnosis of cobalamin or folate disorders.

OROTIC ACIDURIA

Uridine 5'-monophosphate synthase (UMPS) is a bifunctional protein that contains activities for both orotate phosphoribosyltransferase and orotidine 5'-monophosphate decarboxylase (ODC), resulting in the *de novo* synthesis of uridine 5'-monophosphate. The protein is coded by a gene located on chromosome 3q13.

Thirteen documented patients with UMPS deficiency have been summarized (485). Most came to medical attention in the first few months of life, but two did not present until the age of 7 years. Males and females are affected. The most common findings have been megaloblastic anemia, orotic aciduria with crystalluria, and developmental delay. Clinical heterogeneity is seen, and some patients have additional clinical findings that include immune deficiencies and congenital malformations, such as cardiac malformations.

The disorder can be differentiated from other hereditary causes of megaloblastic anemia by the excretion of orotic acid. Patients with orotic aciduria excrete between 1 and 10 mmol/mmol creatinine (normal in children, <10 μmol orotic acid/mmol creatinine). The crystalluria may be sufficient to cause an obstructive uropathy. Although orotic acid excretion was also described in a patient with glutamate formiminotransferase deficiency (469), the levels were lower than in orotic aciduria.

Orotic aciduria is almost always associated with a deficiency of both orotate phosphoribosyltransferase and ODC, but one patient had decreased ODC only. The deficiency has been seen in both erythrocytes and cultured cells. When examined, mRNA of appropriate size is produced, as is immunoreactive protein. Some patients have residual enzyme activity that is more thermolabile and of different electrophoretic mobility than control enzyme (486,487). The activities are expressed in both amniocytes and chorionic villi (485). Orotic aciduria is inherited as an autosomal-recessive disorder, and heterozygotes can be detected within families by the combined study of orotic acid excretion and enzyme activity of UMPS in erythrocytes or fibroblasts. Mutations in the UMPS gene have been described in a Japanese patient (488).

Treatment with pyrimidine replacement has been successful in most patients, resulting in disappearance of megaloblastic anemia and general improvement. However, two patients died even with uridine therapy. Oral uridine in doses ranging from 100 to 200 mg/kg/day has been used. In two patients, corticosteroid therapy had some beneficial effect.

THIAMINE-RESPONSIVE MEGALOBLASTIC ANEMIA WITH DIABETES AND DEAFNESS

The triad of megaloblastic anemia, diabetes mellitus, and sensorineural deafness has been described in more than a dozen kindreds (489,490). The clinical onset has been in the first few years of life, with evidence of mild abnormalities often identifiable in retrospect. The children do not respond to cobalamin or folate, the deoxyuridine suppression test has normal results, and there is no methylmalonic aciduria. Instead, patients have responded to 25 mg thiamine daily, even though they have no signs or met-

abolic evidence of thiamine deficiency. Both the megaloblastic anemia, which includes ringed sideroblasts, and the diabetes improve, but the improvement may be partial. The first child reported had low plasma and red cell thiamine levels and poor uptake of thiamine by red blood cells *in vitro* (489). Patients have been observed for more than a decade while on thiamine maintenance. Relapse occurs if the thiamine is discontinued.

The defect appears to be recessive, and many affected patients come from consanguineous families. The affected gene, *SLC19A2*, is on chromosome 1q23.3 and codes for thiamine transporter-1, which is highly homologous to the reduced folate carrier (491–493); several mutations have been identified.

Diagnosing the Causes of Deficiency

Once it has been established that a patient has deficiency of cobalamin, folate, or both vitamins together, the task is to identify the underlying disorder responsible for the deficiency. This task seems self-evident, but there is an increasing tendency to forego this step in the diagnostic evaluation. The reasons for omission vary, but the major factors have been the ease and effectiveness of vitamin therapy, a tendency to dismiss vitamin deficiency as a minor nutritional detail rather than a sign of underlying disease, and the time and cost constraints impinging on modern medical practice. The general principles applied to acquired disorders in adults and most children are discussed here. The unique diagnostic approaches to the hereditary metabolic disorders, in which vitamin levels are often normal, have been presented in the sections discussing those disorders.

COBALAMIN DEFICIENCY

Most patients become cobalamin-deficient because of malabsorption, so the diagnostic approach must begin with a gastroenterologic orientation.

Tests of Cobalamin Absorption. Absorption is tested by administering 0.5 to 1.0 μg radiolabeled cyanocobalamin orally to a fasting patient; the dose approximates the amount in a meal but is in crystalline (free) form. Methods have varied in the means of determining how much is absorbed. The standard has become to measure urinary excretion of the absorbed isotope, the Schilling test. Tests based on stool collection, whole body counting, and plasma sampling are rarely performed now, although each has its advantages.

To allow urinary excretion to reflect absorption, the patient is given 1000 μg nonradioactive cyanocobalamin intramuscularly 1 to 2 hours after the oral dose. The injection saturates the patient's cobalamin-binding proteins, making the absorbed cobalamin readily available for urinary excretion; even with this precaution, only one-third of absorbed cobalamin is usually excreted. The radioactivity in a 24-hour urine collection is then compared against the ingested radioactivity. Impaired renal function or incomplete urine collection produces falsely abnormal (low) results; so does failure to give the injection of nonradioactive cobalamin after the oral dose or giving an injection within 48 to 72 hours before the test. A drawback of the test, besides inconvenience, is the fact that the injected cobalamin is also therapeutic and thus sometimes compromises further testing of a patient whose diagnosis was doubtful.

In most laboratories, excretion of less than 8% of the oral dose is interpreted as impaired cobalamin absorption. If the result indicates malabsorption, the test can be repeated in several days with an oral dose of IF. If the test now shows normal absorption, lack of IF (i.e., pernicious anemia) is diagnosed. If the result remains abnormal, however, the patient can be given a brief course of antibiotics and retested immediately. If the result becomes normal, malabsorption caused by bacterial overgrowth must have been present; if the result remains abnormal, an ileal defect is the diagnosis, unless one has reason to suspect pancreatic insufficiency. In case of the latter, the Schilling test can be repeated with pancreatic enzymes. If ileal malabsorption is diagnosed, disease-specific tests, up to and including biopsy, are dictated by the intestinal disease that is suspected.

A dual-isotope test that has replaced the standard Schilling test in most centers now provides the convenience of combining two tests in one procedure and one urine collection. IF-bound and unbound cobalamin, each labeled with different isotopes, are administered simultaneously in two pills. Direct comparison of the two isotopes' excretion sometimes also permits a diagnosis despite an incomplete urine collection. However, problems of isotope exchange between the IF-bound and unbound forms make the test liable to falsely normal results.

Food Cobalamin Absorption Test. None of the tests using crystalline (free) cyanocobalamin detect food cobalamin malabsorption, the inability to split cobalamin from its binders in food (245). After it was shown that food proteins labeled with radioactive cobalamin *in vitro* produced results comparable to food labeled *in vivo*, two types of *in vitro* preparations were used in most tests: eggs or egg yolks and chicken serum (54). The conditions of patient preparation, the test procedure, and the drawbacks are identical to those for the Schilling test. The test is unnecessary in patients who malabsorb free cobalamin, who by definition malabsorb food cobalamin also.

The main difficulty is the technical one of preparing and standardizing the test material, which has made the test unavailable outside research centers. The methods have not been studied as much as the high frequency of malabsorption would warrant. Important issues, such as factors affecting results and the extent of comparability among foods, remain unresolved. The low proportion of cobalamin that is normally absorbed can also be problematic. As little as 1% excretion is normal in some versions of the test. Technical issues may underlie some of the discrepancies in the literature (54). Another problem is that equivalence sometimes is automatically drawn between food cobalamin malabsorption and atrophic gastritis, leading to unwarranted substitution of surrogate findings of gastritis for direct tests of absorption. Serum gastrin levels tend to be higher and pepsinogen I levels lower in patients with food cobalamin malabsorption than in controls (246). However, the changes are usually small, and the overlap with normal results limits these tests' usefulness in individual patients.

Tests of Gastric Secretion. Analysis for IF in stimulated gastric juice usually establishes or rules out the diagnosis of pernicious anemia. Results of gastric acid analysis have only limited specificity for pernicious anemia.

Surrogate Blood Tests of Gastric Status. Gastric defects are responsible for most cobalamin deficiency. Although sensitivity and specificity of the individual blood tests are limited, the use of combinations of tests can often establish the diagnosis of pernicious anemia (but not food cobalamin malabsorption) and may obviate the need for absorption tests in some patients. For example, the patient with anti-IF antibody, especially if serum gastrin is high or pepsinogen I is low, almost certainly has pernicious anemia. Normal results in those tests makes pernicious anemia unlikely but not impossible.

Antiintrinsic Factor Antibody. The most common form of the anti-IF antibody test measures the ability of the patient's serum to inhibit binding of radiolabeled cobalamin *in vitro* by a standard IF preparation; this test detects the more common, blocking (type I) anti-IF antibody. A new enzyme-linked immunosorbent assay method measures both type I and type II anti-IF antibodies together (494). IF antibody assay has a sensitivity of approximately 60%, but its specificity exceeds 90% if the blood sample is not taken within 48 hours of the patient having received parenteral cobalamin (495). Few patients, most often those with autoimmune thyroid disease and gastritis, have the antibody without having overt or latent pernicious anemia (496,497).

Serum Gastrin. Because most patients with pernicious anemia have antral sparing, serum gastrin is elevated in more than 80% of cases (498). Levels in the thousands of units are often seen, especially in women (268,498). However, specificity is poor. Hypergastrinemia also occurs with the use of proton pump–inhibiting drugs, gastritis without pernicious anemia, and the Zollinger-Ellison syndrome.

Serum Pepsinogen I (Pepsinogen A). Derived from fundic mucosa, levels of serum pepsinogen I and pepsinogen I:II ratios are low in more than 90% of patients with pernicious anemia (498), but specificity is poor.

Antiparietal Cell Antibody. Antiparietal cell antibody is directed against the membrane H^+,K^+-adenosine triphosphatase pump in parietal cells (278). It is specific for type A gastritis, not pernicious anemia, which limits its diagnostic usefulness markedly.

FOLATE DEFICIENCY

The cause of folate deficiency can often be established with a careful history. Dietary questions should include not only how much and what a patient eats but also how the food is prepared (e.g., whether vegetables are cooked or boiled rather than eaten fresh). Inquiry must be made about alcohol use, recent pregnancy, breast feeding, symptoms that suggest gastrointestinal disease, and use of medications.

Specific tests for acquired disorders that cause folate deficiency are few. Tests of folate absorption are unreliable and not easily available. Folate malabsorption should be suspected in patients ingesting a reasonable diet in whom folate deficiency is proven. The diagnosis is usually established indirectly with standard gastroenterologic tests of intestinal function.

THERAPY AND MANAGEMENT

Treatment of the deficiency itself is usually a simple matter, except in metabolic disorders. With attention to a few basic considerations, many regimens work well. Specific schedules, doses, and routes are often more a matter of patients' preferences and physicians' habits and philosophies than of objective evidence of superiority. The most common difficulties are noncompliance by patients and inattention by physicians. The need to continue therapy for a long time, often for life, is sometimes not appreciated. Some physicians simply provide a single dose of vitamin and fail to consider the medical issues involved.

Goals of Therapy

IMMEDIATE CONSIDERATIONS

The problems that raise urgent concern most often are severe anemia and its consequences, severe neurologic dysfunction, and severe symptoms caused by the underlying or coexisting disorders (e.g., alcohol intoxication, cachexia, diarrhea). The first two problems tend to prompt immediate vitamin therapy

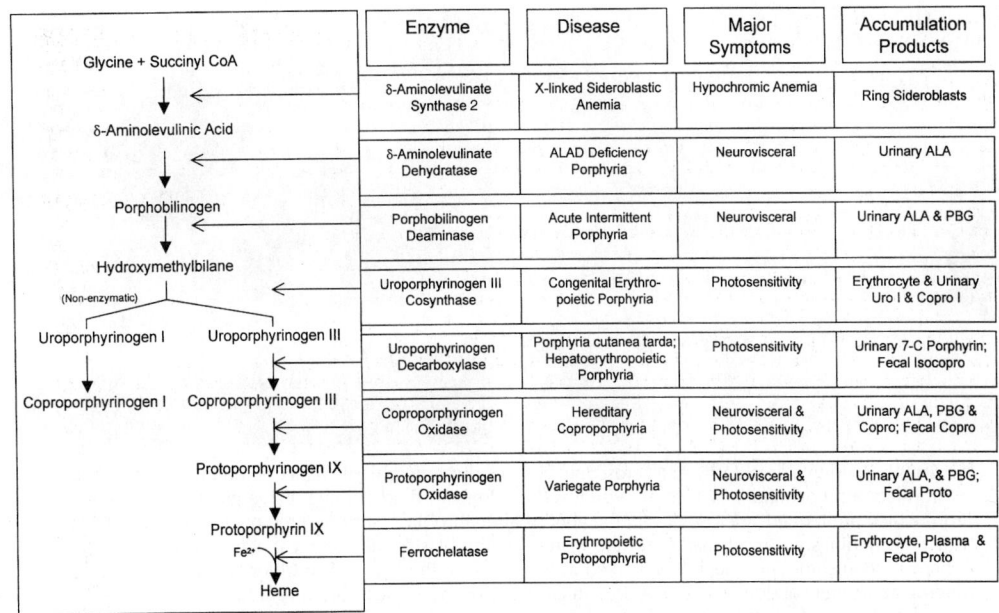

Figure 47-6. Classification and major symptoms of the porphyrias. Enzymatic defects *(Enzyme)*, associated diseases *(Disease)*, major symptoms *(Major Symptoms)*, and principal accumulation products *(Accumulation Products)* are shown. ALAS2 defect is responsible for X-linked sideroblastic anemia but is not associated with any porphyria, because the enzymatic defect blocks production of δ-aminolevulinic acid (ALA), the obligatory precursor for porphyrin synthesis. ALA dehydratase (ALAD) deficiency and porphobilinogen (PBG) deaminase deficiency are accompanied by acute hepatic porphyria but not by photocutaneous porphyria, because their enzymatic blocks result in a decrease in porphyrin synthesis. Enzymatic defects beyond uroporphyrinogen III cosynthase are all associated with photocutaneous porphyrias, because they produce excessive amounts of various porphyrins. Hereditary coproporphyria and variegate porphyria are additionally associated with acute hepatic porphyria. CoA, coenzyme A; Copro, coproporphyrin; Isocopro, isocoproporphyrin; Proto, protoporphyrin; Uro, uroporphyrin.

tryptophan and the subsequent synthesis of brain 5-hydroxytryptamine are largely determined by plasma concentrations of the amino acid (65). In turn, plasma tryptophan concentrations are largely determined by the activity of hepatic tryptophan pyrrolase, a heme-dependent enzyme that converts tryptophan to kynurenine (66). In acute attacks of AIP, deficiency of heme may lead to decreased activity of hepatic tryptophan pyrrolase, enhanced plasma levels and brain uptake of tryptophan, and, ultimately, increased 5-hydroxytryptamine synthesis. Experimental evidence for this sequence of events has been reported in a rodent model of porphyria (the 3,5-diethoxycarbonyl-1,4-dihydrocollidine-treated, phenobarbital-primed rat) (59,67). In another chemically induced model of porphyria (the AIA-treated rat), tryptophan pyrrolase activity was increased (68), which would predict a decrease in brain 5-hydroxytryptamine synthesis.

None of the previously mentioned theories can sufficiently explain the neurologic disturbances that are observed in the acute hepatic porphyrias in humans, and this issue remains unsettled.

PORPHYRIAS

Porphyrias are classified as either hepatic or erythropoietic, depending on the principal site of expression of the specific enzymatic defect in each disorder. Eight enzymes are involved in the synthesis of heme and an inherited defect has been recognized for each enzyme. Mutations of the *ALAS2* gene are associated with X-linked sideroblastic anemia (XLSA), whereas an enzymatic defect at other steps of heme synthesis is associated with each form of porphyria (Fig. 47-6). Typical values for heme pathway enzymes in human porphyrias are summarized in Table 47-3. Enzymatic defects of porphyrias can be 50% of normal for autosomal-dominant porphyrias and less than 2% of normal for recessive

porphyrias (Table 47-3). There is also derepression of ALAS1 activity during the acute attack in acute hepatic porphyrias (Table 47-3). There are also recent reviews on these subjects (69,70). In this chapter, each porphyric disorder is described according to the order of the enzymes in the heme biosynthetic sequence.

X-LINKED SIDEROBLASTIC ANEMIA

Definition

XLSA is an X-linked (Xp11.21) recessive disorder of heme biosynthesis that results from the deficient activity of erythroid-specific ALAS (ALAS-E, or ALAS2) in the mitochondria of erythroid cells. It is distinct from another XLSA, Xq13-linked sideroblastic anemia with ataxia (71), which is caused by mutations in the human *ABC7* putative mitochondrial iron transporter gene (72,73). The resultant reduction in heme synthesis in XLSA stimulates erythropoiesis, which is largely ineffective and increases erythron iron turnover. Because of ALAS2 deficiency, protoporphyrin IX formation is insufficient for ferrochelatase, which results in iron accumulation in bone marrow erythroblasts. The excess iron in the marrow is deposited as nonferritin iron in the mitochondria and produces "ring sideroblasts," a pathologic hallmark of the disease (Fig. 47-7). Most XLSA patients in whom the disease is caused by a deficiency of ALAS2 are pyridoxine-responsive, but some are refractory.

δ-Aminolevulinate Synthase

ALAS [EC 2.3.1.37], which is also known as *5-aminolevulinate synthase*, is a mitochondrial enzyme that requires pyridoxal 5'-

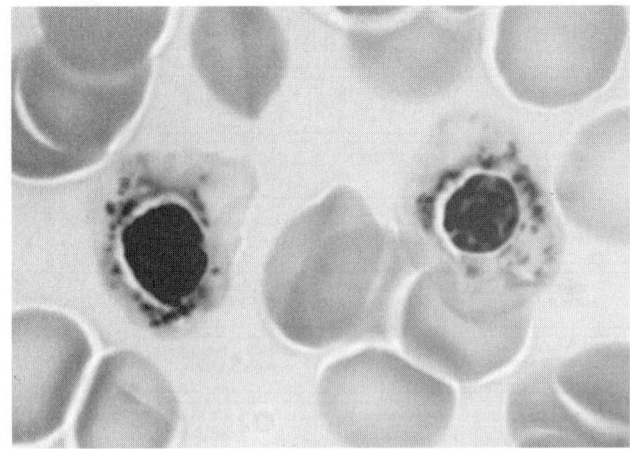
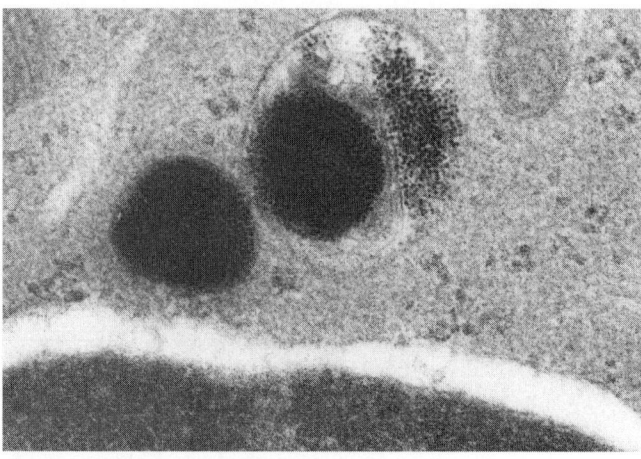

A   **B**

Figure 47-7. Ring sideroblasts. **A:** Microscopic view of ring sideroblasts. Note the perinuclear localization of iron-laden mitochondria, which are visualized by Prussian blue staining. Large granules with stainable iron, which are termed *siderosomes*, in the abnormal erythroblasts surround the nucleus of the cells like a ring. The findings are most marked in the mature erythroblasts with the most active heme biosynthesis, whereas siderosomes are much less marked in immature erythroblasts. (See Color Fig. 47-7A.) **B:** Electron micrographic view of siderosomes. Electron microscopy demonstrates that iron granules are deposited in the mitochondria and form siderosomes, which are enlarged, swollen, irregular, and show disorganized cristae. (From Yawata Y. *Atlas of blood diseases.* London: Martin Dunitz, 1996, with permission.)

phosphate (PLP) as a cofactor and catalyzes the condensation of succinyl CoA and glycine to form the aminoketone, ALA, and carbon dioxide. PLP forms a covalent Schiff base linkage with the active site lysine (Lys391) in ALAS2 (74).

Biosynthesis and Mitochondrial Import

There are unique cDNAs, *ALAS1* and *ALAS2*, for erythroid and nonerythroid *ALAS* genes, respectively (75–77). The erythroid isozyme also has been termed *ALAS-E*, and the housekeeping isozyme has been termed *ALAS-N*. The nuclear-encoded human ALAS2 precursor protein is synthesized on cytoplasmic ribosomes and is targeted to the mitochondria by signals in the polypeptide. After proteolytic processing, ALAS2 is associated with the matrix face of the inner mitochondrial membrane (78). The aminoterminal leader sequence of ALAS2 is cleaved after mitochondrial import. The predicted cleavage site in human ALAS2 is between Gln78 and Asp79 (79), which yields a mature subunit size of 56.4 kd.

The aminoterminal leader peptide of ALAS2 also contains sequence motifs that may interact with heme to block mitochondrial import. There were conserved sequences in the ALAS1 and ALAS2 leader peptides, which were termed the *heme regulatory motif* and were required for hemin-dependent inhibition of import for both proteins into isolated liver mitochondria (13,14). The heme regulatory motif consensus sequence, Cys-Pro-ϕ-X$_{12-30}$-Cys-Pro (ϕ is a hydrophobic residue, X is any amino acid) is present in all known eukaryotic ALAS leader sequences. Prevention of ALAS import into mitochondria is an effective means for down-regulation of heme biosynthesis.

It has been shown that the β-subunit of human adenosine triphosphate (ATP)–specific succinyl CoA synthetase (SCS-βA) associates with human ALAS2. An ALAS mutant, D190V, which was identified in a patient with pyridoxine-refractory XLSA, failed to associate with SCS-βA, whereas other ALAS2 mutants were able to associate with SCS-βA. When ALAS2 was transcribed, translated, and transported into mitochondria, the mature D190V mutant protein, but not its precursor protein, underwent abnormal processing, which resulted in an array of smeared bands, suggesting that appropriate association of SCS-

βA and ALAS2 is necessary for proper functioning of ALAS2 in mitochondria (80).

Purified recombinant murine ALAS2 is a homodimer (81) with a subunit molecular weight of 56,200 d (82). The active site of the mouse ALAS2 is located at the subunit interface and contains the catalytically essential residue, Lys313 (83). PLP is covalently bound via a Schiff base linkage to the first lysine residue (Lys313) that is encoded by exon 9 of the mouse *ALAS2* gene (74). Human ALAS2 also forms a homodimer, which involves a domain from amino acids 126 through 271 (84). It should be noted that four out of the five pyridoxine-refractory ALAS2 mutations in patients with XLSA occurred in this region, which suggests the critical importance of the dimer formation in ALAS function (84).

ALAS2 has a short half-life (e.g., 34 minutes for mouse ALAS2), and it is likely that mutations that result in small changes in PLP affinity or protease susceptibility, or both, can have dramatic effects on the level of mitochondrial ALAS2 and its activity.

Hemin at 10 μM inhibited the partially purified rabbit reticulocyte ALAS2 by 37% (85), but it activated rat ALAS1 by 111% (86). However, it is unlikely that heme significantly inhibits ALAS2 activity *in vivo*, because the free heme concentration in rabbit erythroblasts is estimated to be 0.7 μM (87).

Clinical Findings

Two major features in XLSA are anemia, which is due to reduced heme synthesis, and cellular toxicity, which is due to the elevated iron levels. Patients present with various signs of anemia, including pallor, shortness of breath, fatigue, weakness, or a combination of these signs (88). Clinically affected patients may present with hepatomegaly or splenomegaly, or both (88), cirrhosis, hepatocellular carcinoma, nausea and abdominal pain (88), weight loss (88), diabetes (88), skin pigmentation (88), growth delay (88), arthropathy, body hair loss, decreased libido in males, and missed menses in females. Cardiac myopathy ranges in severity from systolic murmur and tachycardia (88) to end-stage cardiac failure (88). Serum ferritin typically ranges from 400 to 14,500 μg/dL, and transferrin saturation ranges from 51% to 100%. Iron toxicity to hormone production may result in growth delay and, more frequently, in diabetes (88).

Ring sideroblasts are present in the marrow at levels generally greater than 15% (Fig. 47-7). Peripheral erythrocytes are typically microcytic and hypochromic with frequent poikilocytes, including ovalocytes, target cells, and tear-drop–, cigar-, or pencil-shaped cells, or a combination of these cell shapes.

Molecular Biology

The chromosomal localization of human *ALAS2* is at Xp11.21 (89). In contrast, the housekeeping *ALAS1* gene is present at the human chromosomal region 3p21.1 (90,91). The full-length human *ALAS2* cDNA has a 52-nucleotide (nt) 5'-untranslated region, a coding region of 587 nt encoding a predicted molecular weight of 64,689 d, and a 3'-untranslated region of 127 nt (76,92).

The human *ALAS2* gene is 22 kilobases (kb) in length and contains 11 exons. The coding region of exons 5 through 11 constitutes the catalytically competent core of the enzyme (75,93). The *ALAS2* promoter/enhancer region contains numerous erythroid-specific elements, such as a canonical CCAAT promoter element, a TATA-like promoter element, functional erythroid-specific GATA-1 enhancer elements, and a functional CACCC element (94). Although it also contains the erythroid-specific element nuclear factor erythroid 2 (NF-E2), its functionality has not been demonstrated (94). Deoxyribonuclease I hypersensitive sites have been shown to be important in transcriptional regulation (95). Although hemin inhibits transcription of the housekeeping *ALAS1* gene (96), it does not repress *ALAS2* transcription in erythroid cells (96–98).

The 5' untranslated region of the erythroid-specific *ALAS2* messenger RNA (mRNA) contains an iron-responsive element (IRE) (99–101), which acts as a binding site for the IRE binding protein 1 (IRP1) (102). This protein-mRNA complex blocks translation in iron-deficient erythroid cells (103), whereas the release of the complex from the *ALAS2* IRE in iron-replete cells allows translation to proceed.

Molecular Pathology

To date, more than 25 different mutations have been identified in more than 35 families (103–105). All have been missense mutations in the ALAS2 catalytic core that is encoded by exons 5 through 11, except for one nonsense mutation. The majority of mutations occurred in exons 5 and 9. It should be noted that exon 9 encodes lysine 391, the putative covalent binding site for PLP.

Of the 16 mutations that have been published so far, 15 were pyridoxine-responsive *in vivo* [F165L (79), R170L (105), A172T (106), Y199H (104), G291S (107), K299Q (106), T388S (108), C395Y (109), R411C (104), M426V (110), R448Q (104), R452C (104), R452H (111), I476N (112), and H524D (113)] (Fig. 47-8). Only one patient, an 18-year-old male, was pyridoxine-refractory with a D190V lesion (110). This mutant protein was PLP-responsive *in vitro*, but it was associated with abnormal processing of the precursor protein, which resulted in the loss of ALAS2 in the mitochondria of the bone marrow erythroid cells of the patient (110). The C395Y mutation was found in an elderly woman with acquired sideroblastic anemia who was heterozygous for the mutation but expressed only the mutated gene in reticulocytes (109). All women in this family showed skewed X-chromosome inactivation in leukocytes, which indicated a hereditary condition that was associated with unbalanced lyonization. Because the preferentially active X chromosome carried the C395Y mutation, acquired skewing in the elderly likely worsened the genetic condition and abolished the normal ALAS2 allele expression in the proband (109).

Excess mitochondrial iron in the marrow of XLSA patients may additionally inhibit ALAS2 activity, because high iron levels were shown to inversely correlate with pyridoxine-

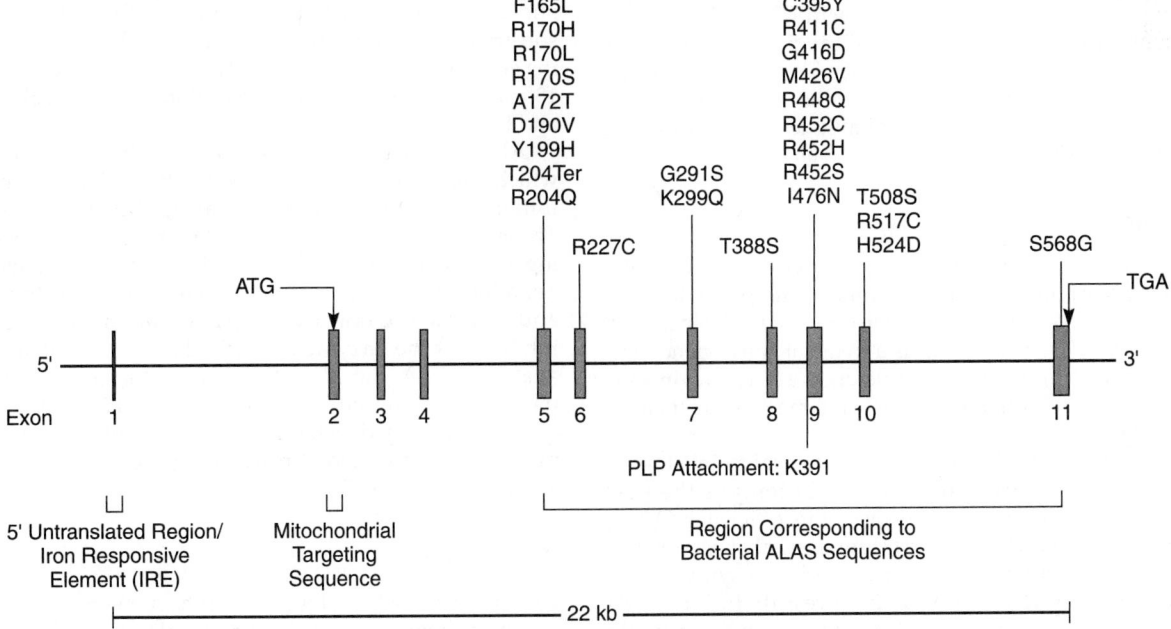

Figure 47-8. The human ALAS2 gene and the locations of mutations that are associated with X-linked sideroblastic anemia. PLP, pyridoxal 5'-phosphate. (Adapted from Anderson KE, Sassa S, Bishop DF, et al. Disorders of heme biosynthesis: X-linked sideroblastic anemia and the porphyrias. In: Scriver CR, Beaudet AL, Sly WS, et al., eds. *The metabolic and molecular bases of inherited disease.* New York: McGraw-Hill, 2001, with permission.)

responsiveness in XLSA patients (104). Chemicals that react with PLP, such as isonicotinic acid hydrazide, have also been associated with sideroblastic anemia and reduced bone marrow ALAS2 activity in patients who were treated with such chemicals (114).

Diagnosis

The presence of microcytic and hypochromic anemia, elevated iron, pyridoxine-responsiveness, and X-linked inheritance in the absence of ataxia (71) suggests the diagnosis of XLSA. The proband's erythrocyte size distribution is always microcytic, but his mother and female siblings have bimodal mean cell volumes, which consist of normal and microcytic populations. Due to the ineffective erythropoiesis, the marrow shows erythroid hyperplasia with a decreased myeloid to erythroid ratio, and ferrokinetic studies show increased erythroid iron turnover. XLSA patients generally have serum ferritin levels of greater than 200 µg/dL and a transferrin saturation of greater than 30%. Iron deficiency anemia, which also presents with microcytic, hypochromic erythrocytes, is distinguished from XLSA by the lack of excess storage iron. Bone marrow examination is diagnostic for iron deficiency anemia with the absence of hemosiderin and ringed sideroblasts.

Pyridoxine-responsiveness should always be evaluated, as most patients are pyridoxine-responsive. Some patients may respond to pyridoxine treatment only after repeated phlebotomy to remove iron (104).

Primary acquired sideroblastic anemia, which is also classified as a myelodysplastic syndrome (refractory anemia with ringed sideroblasts) is a frequent disorder in the elderly that presents with hypochromic, refractory anemia with ringed sideroblasts (see Chapter 11). The erythrocytes in this condition are, however, typically macrocytic, with a mean cell volume of greater than 100 fL, and marrow evaluation frequently demonstrates abnormal lymphocytes or granulocytes, or both.

The preferred approach in molecular diagnosis is amplification of genomic deoxyribonucleic acid (DNA) and direct sequencing of each of the 11 exons, the 5' and 3' flanking regions, and the intron-exon boundaries. Primer sets for these analyses have been published (110), and the complete genomic sequence is available online (GenBank accession numbers Z83821 and AF068624).

Treatment

Treatment of XLSA currently consists of pyridoxine and folic acid therapy to optimize heme biosynthesis and phlebotomy or chelation therapy, or both, to reverse iron overload. Splenectomy is contraindicated, as thrombosis is a frequent consequence and is often fatal (79,111). A typical pyridoxine treatment regimen is 100 to 300 mg/day initially and then 100 mg/day as maintenance therapy.

The primary cause of morbidity and mortality in XLSA is tissue damage from iron toxicity. Phlebotomy is the preferred means of iron removal because of its efficiency (0.25 g iron per unit of blood removed), low cost, absence of side effects, and stimulation of bone marrow heme synthesis. In spite of anemia, phlebotomy usually results in increased hemoglobin levels, especially if it is introduced gradually with pyridoxine therapy (115,116). Chelation therapy by continuous subcutaneous infusion of desferrioxamine is also efficient (0.2 g iron per day, removed by urinary and fecal excretion), but it is expensive and may cause optic and auditory neuropathies (117).

δ-AMINOLEVULINIC ACID DEHYDRATASE–DEFICIENCY PORPHYRIA

Definition

ALAD-deficiency porphyria (ADP) is an autosomal-recessive disorder that is due to a deficiency in ALAD, the second enzyme in the heme biosynthetic pathway. Clinical manifestations have been primarily neuropathic. The severity and the age of onset are variable. Similar to AIP, but unlike most other porphyrias, there is no cutaneous photosensitivity in this disorder. ADP is the most recently described and the rarest form of porphyria.

δ-Aminolevulinic Acid Dehydratase

ALAD (also called *5-aminolevulinic acid dehydratase* or *PBG synthase*; E.C. 4.2.1.24) catalyzes the formation of PBG from two molecules of ALA (Fig. 47-4). The substrate ALA is an amino acid that is the obligate precursor for PBG, porphyrinogens, porphyrins, heme, and other tetrapyrroles. The product PBG is a monopyrrole. In mammalian cells, this enzyme is present in vast abundance—for example, 80- to 100-fold in the liver compared to ALA synthase, the rate-limiting enzyme in heme synthesis (118). The human enzyme is a homo-octamer with a subunit size of 36,274 d (119) and is encoded by the gene localized at chromosome 9q34 (120). The enzyme requires an intact sulfhydryl group and one zinc atom (Zn^{2+}) per subunit for full activity (121). Using [$5\text{-}^{14}C$]-ALA as substrate, it was shown that, of the two molecules of ALA, it is the molecule that contributes to the propionic acid side that is initially bound to the enzyme (122). The tertiary structure of the yeast ALAD has been solved to 2.3-Å resolution, which reveals that each subunit adopts a triosephosphate isomerase barrel fold with a 39 residue N-terminal arm. Pairs of monomers then wrap their arms around each other to form compact dimers, and these associate to form a "4-2-2" symmetry (123). All eight active sites are on the surface of the octamer and possess two lysine residues (210 and 263), one of which, Lys263, forms a Schiff base link to the substrate. The two lysine side chains are close to two zinc binding sites, one of which is formed by three cysteine residues (133, 135, and 143), whereas the other binding site involves Cys234 and His142.

ALAD activity can also be deficient in other conditions in which enzyme activity is markedly inhibited. For example, lead inhibits ALAD activity by displacing Zn^{2+} from the enzyme. The enzyme activity is diminished in patients with lead poisoning, who have excess ALA in blood and urine and often develop neurologic disturbances, some of which resemble those of ADP and other acute porphyrias (124). The most potent known inhibitor of the enzyme is succinylacetone (125), a structural analog of ALA (Fig. 47-9) that is found in urine and blood of patients with hereditary tyrosinemia (126). Children with tyrosinemia may develop neurologic manifestations (approximately 40% of patients) resembling those in ADP and other acute porphyrias (127).

Prevalence

Only four cases (128–130) of ADP have been reported to date and have been confirmed by molecular analysis of the enzymatic defect. Recently reported cases, which have not yet been confirmed by these analyses, include two siblings in Chile (131) and an elderly woman in Japan (132). In addition, there was a healthy Swedish girl who had markedly decreased ALAD activity in her erythrocytes (12% of normal) in whom an F12L amino

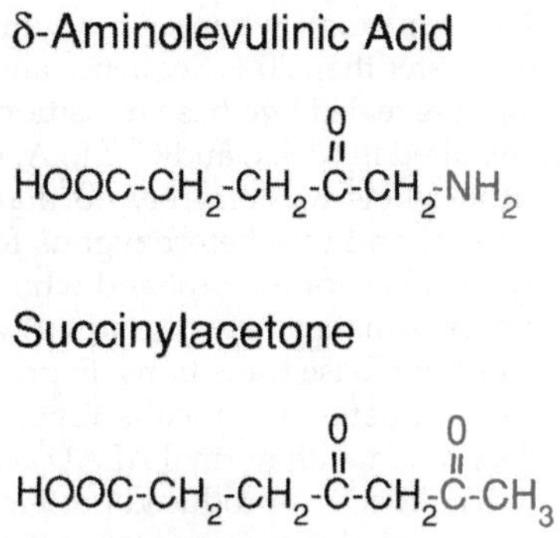

δ-Aminolevulinic Acid

$$\underset{\displaystyle HOOC\text{-}CH_2\text{-}CH_2\text{-}\overset{\displaystyle O}{\overset{\|}{C}}\text{-}CH_2\text{-}NH_2}{}$$

Succinylacetone

$$HOOC\text{-}CH_2\text{-}CH_2\text{-}\overset{O}{\overset{\|}{C}}\text{-}CH_2\overset{O}{\overset{\|}{C}}\text{-}CH_3$$

Figure 47-9. Structural formulae of δ-aminolevulinic acid (ALA) and succinylacetone. Succinylacetone (4,6-dioxoheptanoic acid) is a structural analog of ALA and a potent inhibitor of ALA dehydratase. (Adapted from Kappas A, Sassa S, Galbraith RA, et al. The porphyrias. In: Scriver CR, Beaudet AL, Sly WS, et al., eds. *The metabolic and molecular basis of inherited disease.* New York: McGraw-Hill, 1989:1305, with permission.)

acid substitution was identified in ALAD (133). This porphyria undoubtedly occurs elsewhere and is underrecognized.

The prevalence of heterozygous ALAD deficiency in Germany has been estimated to be less than 1% (134), whereas it is as high as 2% in a random normal population in Sweden (129). A potential impact of the heterozygous deficiency of ALAD on health is intriguing. Although heterozygotes usually display no clinical consequences, they may be at increased risk, if exposed, to the toxic effects of iron, lead, trichloroethylene, or styrene, which are known to potently inhibit ALAD activity (135). Indeed, it has been reported that individuals with heterozygous ALAD deficiency may show signs of subclinical lead poisoning as manifested by the marked elevation of erythrocyte zinc protoporphyrin, even if their blood lead levels are within the normal range (134).

Clinical Findings

Clinical features have differed markedly in the few patients with this disease who have been described so far. The first two German patients were male adolescents with symptoms that resembled those of AIP, including abdominal pain and neuropathy (128). The third patient was an infant who had more severe disease, including failure to thrive (129). The fourth patient was essentially healthy until 63 years of age, when he developed an acute motor polyneuropathy that was not accompanied by abdominal pain. He concurrently developed a myeloproliferative disorder (130). The fifth and sixth patients were siblings in Chile (26 and 28 years of age) who presented with similar symptoms that were typical of acute porphyria. ALAD activity in these subjects was less than 4% of normal (131); however, no molecular analysis has been made in these subjects. The disease may also be associated with hyponatremia and the syndrome of inappropriate secretion of antidiuretic hormone (ADH) (132). Heterozygotes who are identified in family studies are clinically asymptomatic and have normal amounts of ALA in urine. Subjects with partial deficiencies of ALAD do not have any clinical problems. However, as noted, they may have enhanced susceptibility to lead poisoning (134).

Biochemical Findings

The reduced erythrocyte ALAD activity in these patients is not restored to normal by the *in vitro* addition of sulfhydryl reagents, such as dithiothreitol, which is a finding that distinguishes this disease from lead poisoning. Other characteristic laboratory findings are markedly increased urinary excretion of ALA and, for

reasons yet unclear, increased urinary coproporphyrin III and increased erythrocyte protoporphyrin (complexed with zinc). Heterozygotes can be detected by demonstration of intermediate levels of erythrocyte ALAD activity in erythrocytes.

Molecular Biology

Both the mouse (136) and the human (137) *ALAD* genes contain two alternative noncoding exons, 1A and 1B, and 11 coding exons, 2 through 12. The housekeeping transcript, which includes exon 1A but not 1B, is identified in a human adult liver cDNA library, whereas an erythroid-specific transcript, which contains exon 1B but not 1A, is detected in a human K562 erythroleukemia cDNA library. The promoter region that is upstream of housekeeping exon 1A is GC-rich, and contains three potential Sp1 elements and a CCAAT box, and, further upstream, there are three potential GATA-1 binding sites and an AP1 site. The promoter region that is upstream of erythroid-specific exon 1B has several CACCC boxes and two potential GATA-1 binding sites. GATA-1 mRNA levels and exon 1B expression increase threefold during maturation of murine erythroid progenitor cells (136). These findings indicate that the mouse and the human *ALAD* genes contain two promoter regions that generate housekeeping and erythroid-specific transcripts by alternate splicing, which is analogous to the expression of the human *PBGD* gene. The novel expression of housekeeping and erythroid-specific transcripts apparently evolved to ensure sufficient heme biosynthesis for the high-level tissue-specific production of hemoglobin (136,137).

Molecular Pathology

ADP is an autosomal-recessive disorder that results from a homozygous ALAD deficiency. The first four reported cases have been studied immunochemically, and underlying mutations of the *ALAD* gene have been found. ALAD activity in erythrocytes was less than 3% of normal in these cases. Heterozygous relatives had levels of enzyme activity that were approximately one-half of normal. Because of an almost complete lack of ALAD activity, large amounts of ALA accumulate and are excreted in urine in this disease, whereas PBG is normal.

The ALAD protein in this disorder was *cross-reactive immunologic material positive* [CRIM(+)] in all four of the patients who were studied, which suggests that one or both alleles produced enzyme proteins with decreased activity. This has been confirmed by expressing mutant cDNAs in heterologous systems (Fig. 47-10) (138). In addition, a healthy Swedish girl with markedly decreased erythrocyte ALAD activity had an ALAD mutation with F12L, which resulted in aberrant premature processing of the protein (133). The disease is genetically highly heterogeneous in that there are eight distinct point mutations in these five subjects with ALAD deficiency (Fig. 47-11) (70). In other porphyrias, CRIM(–) mutations are more common than CRIM(+) mutations. Therefore, it is possible that cases of ADP with CRIM(–) mutations may be found in the future.

The first molecular analysis of the *ALAD* gene defect in ADP was made in a German patient (patient B) (139) who developed symptoms when he was 15 years of age. It was found that this patient had two distinct point mutations of the *ALAD* gene: a $G^{820} \rightarrow A$ base transition, which was termed *G1*, and $C^{718} \rightarrow T$, which was termed *G2*. G1 and G2 occurred in separate alleles and encoded ALAD with an amino acid change, A274T and R240W, respectively. The former was shown to be inherited from the father, whereas the latter was from the mother. The G1 protein had markedly decreased activity, whereas the G2 protein was highly unstable (139). The combination of the two

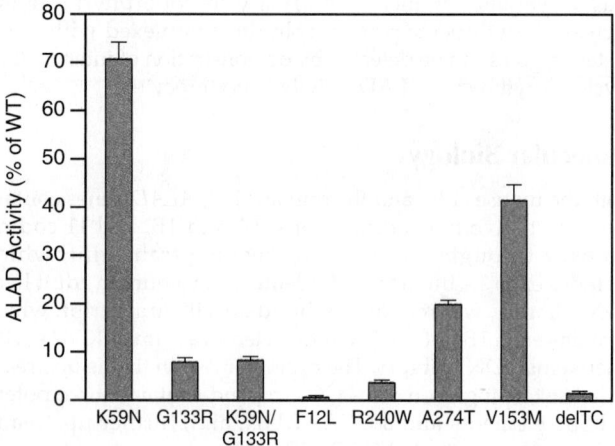

Figure 47-10. δ-Aminolevulinic acid dehydratase (ALAD) mutants and their enzyme activities. Mutant ALAD complementary deoxyribonucleic acids were expressed as glutathione-S-transferase fusion proteins in *Escherichia coli*, and expressed proteins were purified by glutathione-affinity column chromatography. ALAD activity of each mutant was assayed and expressed as the percent of the wild-type (WT) enzyme activity. [Adapted from Maruno M, Furuyama K, Akagi R, et al. Highly heterogenous nature of δ-aminolevulinate dehydratase (ALAD) deficiencies in ALAD porphyria. *Blood* 2001;97:2972, with permission.]

abnormal ALAD proteins accounted for the markedly decreased ALAD activity in the proband (<1% of normal) (139).

In the second German male patient (patient H), who also developed symptoms at 15 years of age, there were two distinct molecular defects, each occurring in separate allele. One was a G^{457}-to-A transition, which resulted in V153M, whereas the other was a deletion of T^{818} and C^{819}, which resulted in a frameshift with a premature stop codon at the amino acid position of 294 (140). Using allele-specific oligonucleotide analysis, the former was shown to be inherited from his father, whereas the latter was inherited from his mother. Expression of the former cDNA in Chinese hamster ovary cells produced an ALAD protein with little activity (approximately 10% of normal), whereas the latter produced no protein. Thus, this patient was also heteroallelic for ALAD mutations.

The third patient, a Swedish baby boy, presented from his birth on with extremely severe acute hepatic porphyria symptoms. This patient had another set of two distinct point mutations of the *ALAD* gene: a G^{823}-to-A base transition, which resulted in V275M, and a G^{397}-to-A base transition, which resulted in G133R (141). By using bacterial expression, both of these mutations were shown to encode ALAD with little activity (138).

The fourth patient was a Belgian male who was unique in that he developed ADP at 63 years of age (130). He also developed polycythemia at that time. His erythrocyte ALAD activity

was less than 1% of normal, whereas his lymphocytes had ALAD activity of greater than 20%. Sequence analysis of *ALAD* cDNA in this subject revealed two base transitions in one allele: G^{177} to C, which resulted in K59N, and G^{397} to A, which resulted in G133R. The other allele was entirely normal. This finding indicates that the proband was heterozygous for ALAD deficiency. All family members of the proband who had decreased ALAD activity (approximately 50% of normal) were shown to have the same set of two base transitions. Expression of *ALAD* cDNAs in Chinese hamster ovary cells revealed that *K59N* cDNA produced a protein with normal ALAD activity, whereas *G133R* and *K59N/G133R* cDNA produced proteins with 8% and 16% ALAD activity, respectively, compared to that expressed by the wild-type cDNA. Heterozygous ALAD deficiency, which should be clinically silent, has nevertheless produced clinical ADP in this patient, presumably because there was clonal expansion of the polycythemia clone in his erythroid cells, which carried the mutant ALAD allele (142).

The healthy asymptomatic Swedish girl was found to have markedly decreased ALAD activity (12% of normal) by neonatal ALAD screening for hereditary tyrosinemia (133). The molecular analysis of cloned *ALAD* cDNA revealed that this subject had a C^{36}-to-G base transition and a T^{168}-to-C base transition in one allele, whereas the other allele was normal. The former transition resulted in F12L amino acid substitution, whereas the latter transition was silent, which represents polymorphism. *F12L* mutant cDNA produced a protein, which underwent premature processing and resulted in no enzymatic activity (133).

In contrast to these mutations, the K59N substitution in the ALAD allele has been found to be present in approximately 10% of the population (143). Consistent with the natural abundance of this variant, modeling of the K59N mutation indicates that this mutation may not interfere with the proper folding or functioning of the human enzyme (123). In contrast, the four other mutations that were found in the German and Swedish patients with ADP are likely to have structural effects on the ALAD molecule, as judged by the yeast ALAD structure (Fig. 47-12) (123).

The fact that ADP and AIP show some similar clinical and biochemical disturbances suggests that ALA or its precursor, rather than PBG, may be a neurotoxic agent. This point is further supported by the finding that patients with hereditary tyrosinemia frequently develop symptoms that resemble acute porphyria (127,144) in association with marked inhibition of ALAD by succinylacetone (126). However, as in other acute porphyrias, the pathogenesis of the neurologic symptoms is poorly understood.

It is believed, although it has not been demonstrated directly, that acute attacks of ADP occur in association with overexpression of ALAS in the liver owing to a loss of heme-mediated repression (Fig. 47-5 and Table 47-3) (145). Therefore, this disease, like the other acute porphyrias, is often classified as one of the hepatic por-

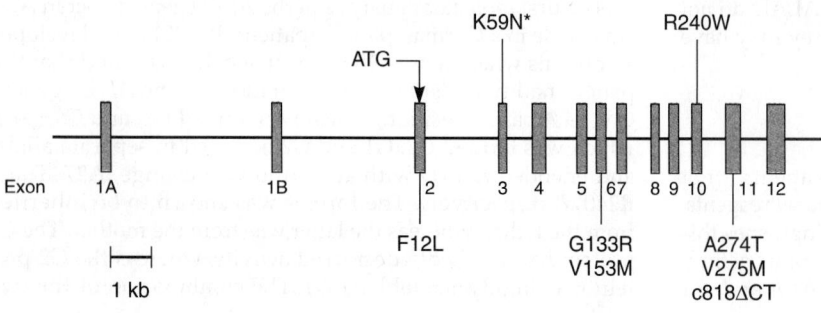

Figure 47-11. The human δ-aminolevulinic acid dehydratase gene and the mutations that are associated with δ-aminolevulinic acid dehydratase deficiency porphyria. kb, kilobase; *, common polymorphism. (Adapted from Anderson KE, Sassa S, Bishop DF, et al. Disorders of heme biosynthesis: X-linked sideroblastic anemia and the porphyrias. In: Scriver CR, Beaudet AL, Sly WS, et al., eds. *The metabolic and molecular bases of inherited disease.* New York: McGraw-Hill, 2001, with permission.)

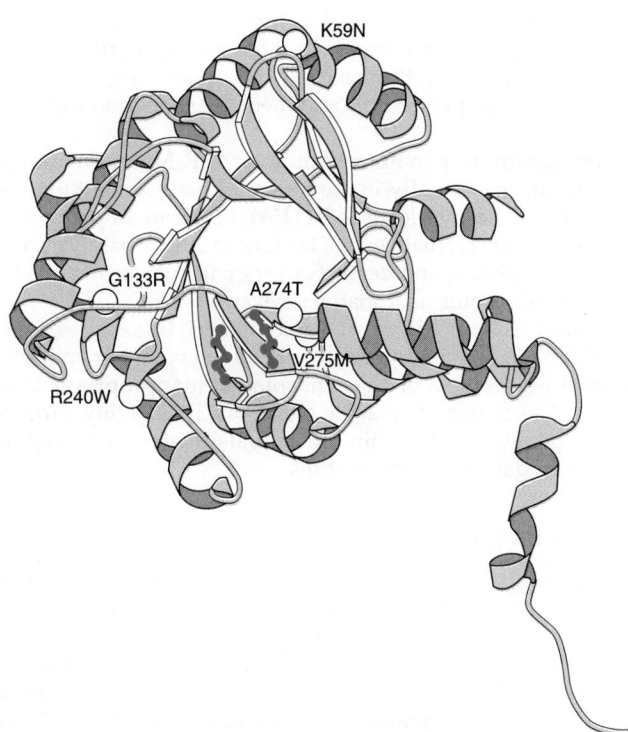

Figure 47-12. Tertiary structure of yeast δ-aminolevulinic acid dehydratase. (Adapted from Erskine PT, Senior N, Awan S, et al. X-ray structure of 5-aminolaevulinate dehydratase, a hybrid aldolase. *Nat Struct Biol* 1997;4:1025, with permission.)

phyrias. Although this may be justified, it is interesting that one patient underwent liver transplantation with only marginal clinical improvement (146). ALA and porphyrins did not decrease after transplantation in this case, which suggests that the excess intermediates originated in tissues other than the liver and, possibly, the bone marrow. The origin of excess coproporphyrin III in urine is unknown, but may be from metabolism of ALA to coproporphyrin III in a tissue other than the site of ALA overproduction. The origin of increased erythrocyte protoporphyrin also remains elusive, but may, as in all other homozygous porphyrias, be explained by accumulation of earlier pathway intermediates in bone marrow erythroid cells during hemoglobin synthesis, which is followed by their transformation to protoporphyrin.

Diagnosis

ADP should be suspected when symptoms, such as abdominal pain and peripheral neuropathy, suggest the possibility of an acute porphyria. The diagnosis is supported if urinary ALA, coproporphyrin, and erythrocyte protoporphyrin levels are increased, and erythrocyte ALAD activity is markedly reduced. The diagnosis is confirmed if other causes of this enzyme deficiency are excluded, and if both parents have activities of this enzyme that are approximately one-half of normal. ADP is differentiated from other acute porphyrias by its autosomal-recessive, rather than dominant, inheritance, by normal urinary PBG in the presence of increased ALA, and by markedly decreased ALAD activity, which is most conveniently measured in erythrocytes. This condition must be differentiated from other conditions that are associated with inhibition rather than a genetic deficiency of ALAD. Lead, styrene, and succinylacetone inhibit ALAD, thus causing increased urinary excretion of ALA and clinical manifestations that resemble those of the acute porphyrias. Lead poisoning is excluded by finding a normal blood lead level.

Treatment

There is little experience with treatment of this type of porphyria. Glucose and heme therapy was effective in some, but not in other patients with ADP (129). A Swedish ADP patient who underwent liver transplantation experienced minimal clinical improvement and urinary excretion of ALA and porphyrins (146).

ACUTE INTERMITTENT PORPHYRIA

Definition

AIP, which is also called *Swedish porphyria, pyrroloporphyria,* or *intermittent acute porphyria,* is an autosomal-dominant disorder that results from a deficiency in PBGD activity. The deficient enzyme activity is almost always approximately 50% of normal. Most (approximately 90%) persons with this genetic enzyme deficiency remain clinically normal throughout life. Clinical expression of the disease is usually linked to environmental or acquired factors, such as nutritional status, drugs, and endogenous or exogenous steroids. The cardinal pathobiology of the disease is a neurologic dysfunction that may affect the peripheral, autonomic system or the CNS.

Porphobilinogen Deaminase

PBGD (also called *HMB synthase,* or formerly called *uroporphyrinogen synthase;* E. C. 4.3.1.8) that is purified from human erythrocytes has a specific activity of approximately 2300 U/mg of protein (147). The activity of PBGD in erythroid cells is significantly lower than that of subsequent enzymes in the heme biosynthetic pathway. Molecular weights of deaminases from human and other sources are in the range of 36,000 to 40,000 d, and the enzyme functions as a monomer (147–149). PBGD is more stable when it is bound covalently to its substrate than when it is free (150).

HMB spontaneously undergoes ring closure to form uroporphyrinogen I, but, in the presence of the next enzyme in the pathway, uroporphyrinogen cosynthase, it results in the formation of uroporphyrinogen III, which has undergone flipping of the D-ring pyrrole (Fig. 47-4). PBGD activity can be measured as the amount of uroporphyrinogen that is formed from PBG, which is determined spectrophotometrically (148,151) or fluorometrically (152,153) after oxidation to uroporphyrin.

Prevalence

The highest incidence of AIP occurs in Lapland, Scandinavia, and in the United Kingdom, although it has been reported in many population groups (154). The incidence of the defective gene in the United States has been estimated at between 5 and 10 per 100,000 (155). The incidence of AIP in psychiatric populations is higher than that in the normal population (0.21%) (156). The disorder is expressed clinically after puberty almost invariably and is seen more frequently in women than in men. AIP is probably the most common of all the genetic porphyrias.

Clinical Findings

Abdominal pain is nearly always present and is often the initial symptom of an acute attack of AIP. It may be generalized or localized and, in severe cases, may mimic an acute surgical abdomen. Other gastroenterologic features are nausea, vomiting, constipation or diarrhea, abdominal distention, and ileus. Urinary incontinence, dysuria, and urinary frequency may occur, although urinary retention is probably more common. In

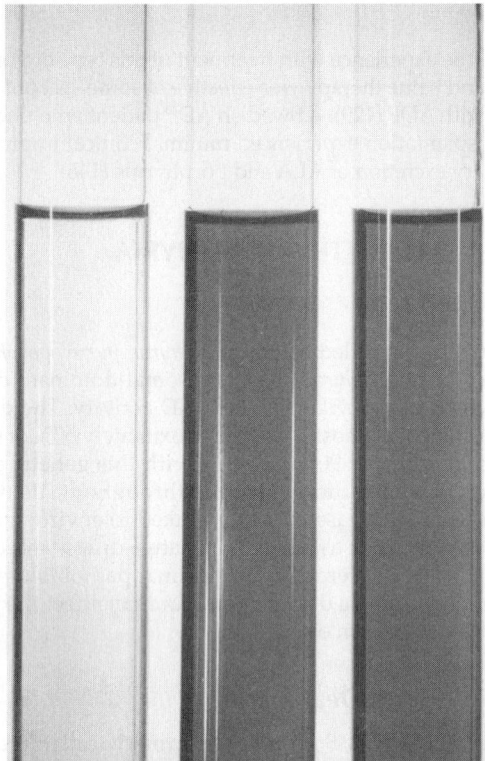

Figure 47-13. Appearance of urine samples from a healthy patient and a patient with acute intermittent porphyria. **Left:** Normal urine. **Center:** Acute intermittent porphyria urine. **Right:** Red wine that has been diluted with water. (See Color Fig. 47-13.)

severe cases of AIP, the urine may develop a port-wine color that is due to a high content of porphobilin (Fig. 47-13), an autooxidized product of PBG, and some porphyrins that are formed by nonenzymatic cyclization of PBG.

Tachycardia and hypertension, as well as, less frequently, fever, sweating, restlessness, and tremor, are also observed in patients with AIP. Catecholamine hypersecretion, when severe, has been implicated in sudden death, possibly secondary to cardiac arrhythmias (157,158). In as many as 40% of AIP patients, hypertension may become sustained between acute attacks.

Neuropathy is a common feature of AIP. Muscle weakness often begins proximally in the legs, and involvement may be symmetric, asymmetric, or focal (159). Motor neuropathy may also involve the cranial nerves, leading to bulbar paralysis, respiratory deficiency, and death. Sensory patchy neuropathy also occurs, when motor neuropathy is severe (160).

Acute attacks of AIP may be accompanied by seizures, especially in patients with hyponatremia due to vomiting, inappropriate fluid therapy, or the syndrome of inappropriate ADH release. The course of an acute attack of AIP is highly variable among patients and within individuals, with attacks lasting from a few days to several months.

Precipitating Factors

Asymptomatic heterozygotes (approximately 90% of subjects with documented PBGD deficiency) may display neither abnormal levels of heme pathway intermediates nor clinical symptoms. Persons with latent and previously clinically expressed AIP may develop an acute attack in response to endogenous or exogenous environmental factors (Fig. 47-14). There are at least five different classes of precipitating factors in this disease (154).

δ-AMINOLEVULINATE SYNTHASE 1 INDUCERS
Most precipitating factors can be related to an associated increase in the activity of ALAS1 in the liver (154). Overproduction of ALA then makes the partially deficient PBGD activity rate limiting.

ENDOCRINE FACTORS
The clinical disease is more common in women, especially at the time of menses. A subset of female patients experiences cyclical premenstrual exacerbation of the disease (161). It has been shown that C19 and C21 steroids, particularly of 5β configuration, potently induce ALAS1 activity in the liver (162,163).

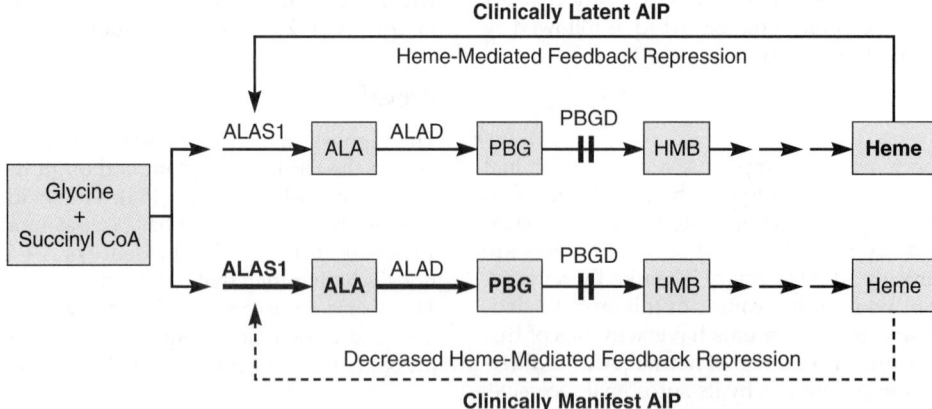

Figure 47-14. Enzymatic block in acute intermittent porphyria (AIP) and loss of heme-mediated repression of hepatic δ-aminolevulinate synthase 1 (ALAS1) (housekeeping form), when the disease is made clinically manifest by precipitating factors such as drugs, steroids, and dietary restrictions. In the presence of porphobilinogen deaminase (PBGD) deficiency, the factors that stimulate heme synthesis result in decreased availability of heme for the regulatory heme pool in hepatocytes. ALA, δ-aminolevulinic acid; ALAD, δ-aminolevulinate dehydratase; CoA, coenzyme A; HMB, hydroxymethylbilane; PBG, porphobilinogen. (Adapted from Anderson KE, Sassa S, Bishop DF, et al. Disorders of heme biosynthesis: X-linked sideroblastic anemia and the porphyrias. In: Scriver CR, Beaudet AL, Sly WS, et al., eds. *The metabolic and molecular bases of inherited disease.* New York: McGraw-Hill, 2001, with permission.)

CALORIE INTAKE

Loss of appetite or reduced calorie intake often leads to exacerbation of AIP (164). Caloric supplementation may reduce PBG excretion and may suppress clinical symptoms (165).

DRUGS AND FOREIGN CHEMICALS

Many chemicals (e.g., barbiturates, certain steroids, and other foreign substances) that exacerbate porphyria have the potential to induce cytochrome P-450 (154). The resultant enhanced demand for heme synthesis may lead to induction of hepatic ALAS1.

STRESS

Various forms of stress, including intercurrent illnesses, infections, alcoholic excess, and surgery, are known to up-regulate the heme oxygenase gene, thus leading to excessive heme catabolism and derepression of ALAS1, with clinical expression of AIP.

Biochemical Findings

Patients with clinically expressed AIP, as well as a few persons with latent AIP, excrete increased amounts of ALA and PBG in the urine between attacks. In most patients, the onset of an acute attack is accompanied by further marked to massive increases in excretion of these precursors [ALA, 25 to 100 mg/day; PBG, 50 to 200 mg/day (166)]. Acute attacks may also be associated with elevations in the plasma concentrations of ALA, PBG, and porphyrins, which are normally undetectable.

The Watson-Schwartz test is a colorimetric method that is used widely to screen for urinary PBG (167,168). More recently, a column method, which is more specific than the Watson-Schwartz test, that uses ion-exchange resin was developed by Mauzerall and Granick (169). The column method is now available as a semiquantitative resin kit (TRACE, Arlington, TX). In a direct comparison

between the resin kit and the Watson-Schwartz test, sensitivity and specificity were 95% and 99%, respectively, for the resin kit compared to 38% and 82%, respectively, for the Watson-Schwartz test (170). High-performance liquid chromatography (HPLC) method for PBG is the most recent method and is at least as sensitive and specific as the resin method (171).

Molecular Biology

The gene locus that encodes PBGD has been assigned to chromosome 11q23→11qter using somatic cell hybridization and immunologic, electrophoretic, and cytogenetic techniques (172,173). The primary sequence of the human erythroid PBGD that is deduced from its cDNA sequence indicates that the protein consists of 344 amino acid residues (174). Sequencing of the nonerythroid cDNA revealed the existence of an additional 17 amino acid residues at its N-terminus, whereas the remainder is identical to the erythroid cDNA (Fig. 47-15) (174). It was also shown that the expression of the erythroid-specific mRNA is exclusive to erythroid cells. *PBGD* cDNAs have been cloned from variety of organisms, from *Escherichia coli* to humans, and were found to have a high degree of evolutionary conservation.

Studies of the cloned human *PBGD* gene demonstrated that the gene is split into 15 exons that are spread over 10 kb of DNA (Fig. 47-15) (175). The two distinct mRNAs are produced through alternative splicing of two primary transcripts that arise from two promoters (Fig. 47-15). The upstream promoter is active in all tissues, whereas the other promoter, which is located 3 kb downstream, is active only in erythroid cells. The erythroid promoter displays some structural characteristics of other erythroid-specific promoters, including a CAAC motif, two GATA-1 sites, and one NF-E2 binding site (176). This finding suggests that some common *trans*-acting factors may co-

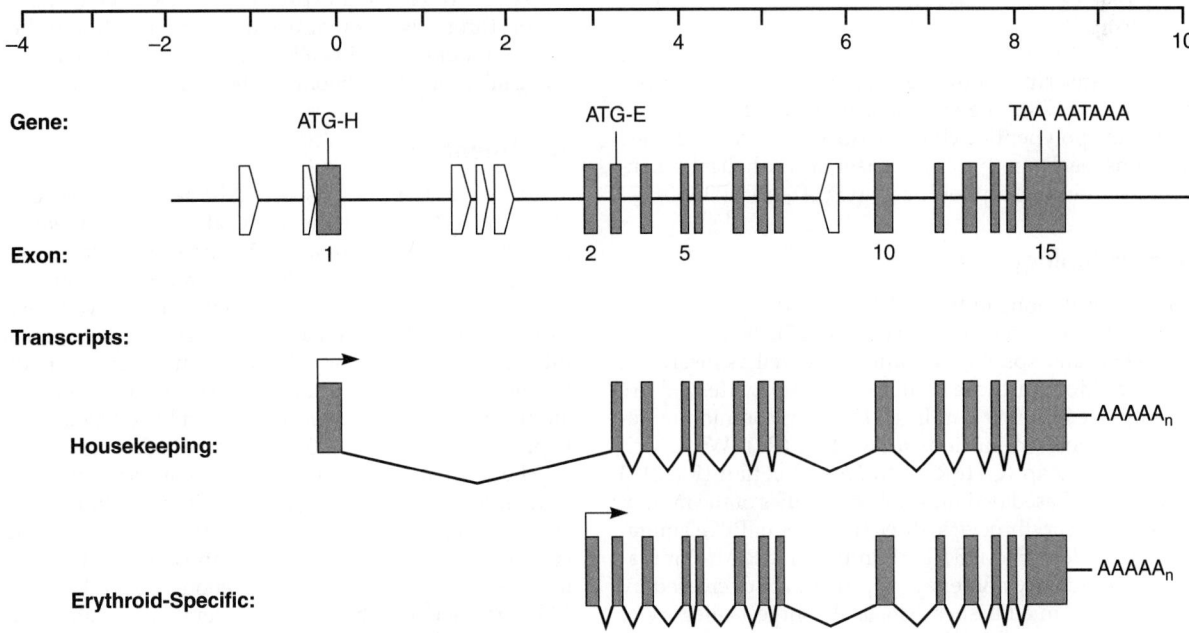

Figure 47-15. Organization of the PBGD gene and alternate splicing of the housekeeping and erythroid-specific transcripts. The 15 exons are represented as solid rectangles, and the positions and orientations of the Alu repeat elements are indicated by the pentagonal boxes. The promoter region for the housekeeping transcript is 5' to exon 1, and the promoter for the erythroid-specific transcript is immediately 5' to exon 2. Translation initiation methionines for the housekeeping and erythroid-specific enzymes are indicated (ATG-H and ATG-E, respectively). (Adapted from Anderson KE, Sassa S, Bishop DF, et al. Disorders of heme biosynthesis: X-linked sideroblastic anemia and the porphyrias. In: Scriver CR, Beaudet AL, Sly WS, et al., eds. *The metabolic and molecular bases of inherited disease.* New York: McGraw-Hill, 2001, with permission.)

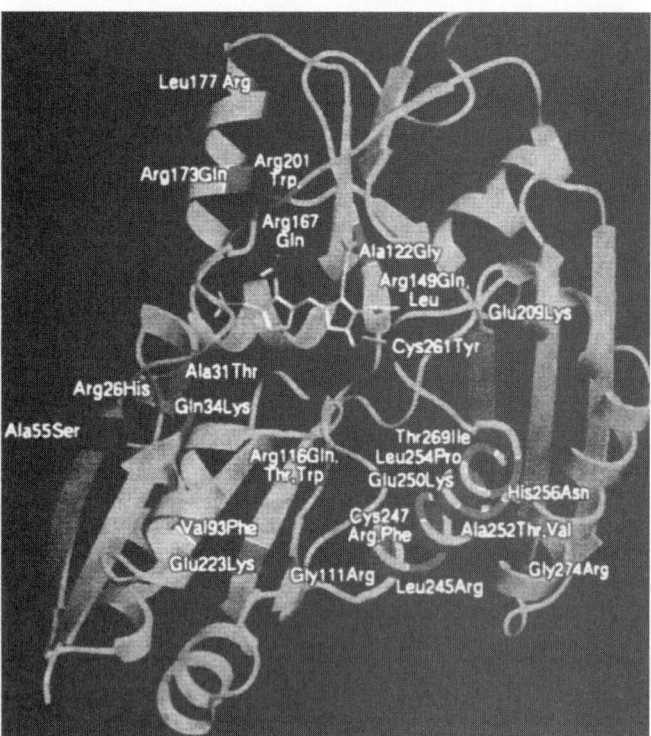

Figure 47-16. Crystal structure of *Escherichia coli* porphobilinogen deaminase (PBGD) (194). The polypeptide chain is folded into three domains, with the dipyrromethane cofactor located in the active site cavity. Suggested locations of the human PBGD mutations that cause acute intermittent porphyria are shown, as predicted by comparing the aligned amino acid sequences of *E. coli* and human PBGD. The effects of specific mutations on enzyme structure and functions can be predicted as described. (From Brownlie PD, Lambert R, Louie GV, et al. The three-dimensional structures of mutants of porphobilinogen deaminase: toward an understanding of the structural basis of acute intermittent porphyria. *Protein Sci* 1994;3:1644, with permission.)

regulate the transcription of these genes during erythroid development (177,178). The crystal structure of *E. coli* PBGD revealed that the polypeptide chain of 313 amino acids is folded into 3 domains, each comprising β-sheet and α-helical secondary structure and a hydrophobic core (Fig. 47-16) (179,180).

Molecular Pathology

More than 150 mutations in the *PBGD* gene have been identified (for a review, see reference 181) (Fig. 47-17), including missense, nonsense, and splicing mutations, as well as insertions and deletions. Most of these mutations are private and are found in only one or a few families. However, common mutations have also been identified in Swedish (R116W), Dutch (W198X), Argentinean (G116R), and Nova Scotian (R173W) patients (182–184). Based on immunologic studies of the mutant enzyme proteins in erythrocytes, three subtypes of PBGD mutations have been identified (184,185). In type I, CRIM(−) mutations, the PBGD activity and enzyme protein are decreased by approximately 50% in all tissues. This is the largest category of mutations (approximately 85%) that render the enzyme protein unstable. They include missense and nonsense mutations, small deletions and insertions, and splicing defects that cause frameshifts and early polypeptide truncation (186). Type II mutations (<5% of all AIP patients) also are CRIM(−) and include five mutations that alter the 5' splice-donor site of intron 1 and a missense mutation in the exon-1 initiation of translation codon (187–191). These mutations result in the absence of the house-keeping isozyme but normal levels of the erythroid-specific enzyme. Therefore, the erythrocyte PBGD activity in these patients is normal, whereas the activity in other tissues and cells is one-half of normal. Type III mutations are CRIM(+) and include mutations that decrease PBGD activity but do not alter the mutant enzyme's stability. Examples of type III mutations include the intron-12 point mutation IVS12^{-1} that results in abnormal splicing and skipping of exon 12, which produces an abnormal but stable polypeptide that lacks the 40 residues that are encoded by exon 12 (188), and two exon-10 missense mutations, R167Q and R173Q, that produce catalytically impaired but stable enzyme proteins (192). The R173Q mutant protein binds PBG, and stable enzyme-substrate intermediates stabilize the mutant enzyme, thereby accounting for the CRIM(+) status of this mutation (193).

As shown in Figure 47-16, modeling of the AIP lesions to the corresponding residues in the crystal structure of *E. coli* PBGD provides insight into the structure-function relationships of the human enzyme (179,193,194). For example, mutations R167Q and R173Q involve highly conserved arginines, with R167Q impairing substrate binding (194). Many other exon-10 mutations occur at conserved amino acids in the active site, whereas many exon-12 mutations alter the α-helix connecting domains 1 and 3 (193,195). Thus, with more than 150 reported mutations, there is marked molecular heterogeneity underlying AIP (181). *De novo* mutations occur in approximately 3% of cases (196).

Diagnosis

Diagnosis of AIP can be made by demonstrating decreased PBGD activity (approximately 50% of normal enzyme activity) in erythrocytes. Elevated levels of ALA (>7 mg/day) and PBG (>4 mg/day) may be seen in patients with AIP but also in patients with HCP and VP; measurement of urinary and stool porphyrins usually differentiates these conditions from AIP. The diagnosis of the subset of AIP that expresses the *PBGD* gene defect only in nonerythroid tissues requires the demonstration of PBGD deficiency in nonerythroid cells (197,198) or DNA hybridization by using allele-specific oligonucleotides (199).

Treatment

The treatment of patients with AIP, as well as those with ADP, HCP, and VP, is essentially identical. All such patients should be provided with medical alert (MedicAlert Foundation International; http://www.medicalert.org) bracelets. Treatment between attacks consists of adequate nutritional intake, avoidance of drugs that are known to exacerbate porphyria, and prompt treatment of intercurrent diseases or infections. Unresponsive patients with severe disease should be admitted to the hospital, and intravenous administration of carbohydrate should be initiated with dextrose to provide a minimum of 300 g of carbohydrate per day.

The use of intravenous hematin is generally effective in reducing ALA and PBG excretion, in curtailing acute attacks, and, perhaps, in reducing the severity of neuropathies (200–202). Hematin (Panhematin, Abbott Laboratories, Chicago, IL), as much as 4 mg/kg, is given intravenously over 30 minutes every 12 hours. Hematin therapy is frequently associated with phlebitis or thrombophlebitis (203). Coagulopathy (204–206) and hemolysis (207) have also been reported after hematin infusion. Heme arginate (Normosang, Huhtamaki Oy Pharmaceuticals, Finland) is a highly water-soluble compound and causes local phlebitis less frequently than does hematin (208).

Nasal or subcutaneous administration of long-acting agonistic analogs of luteinizing hormone-releasing hormone (Hoechst, Strasbourg, France; Salk Institute, La Jolla, CA) in dosages of

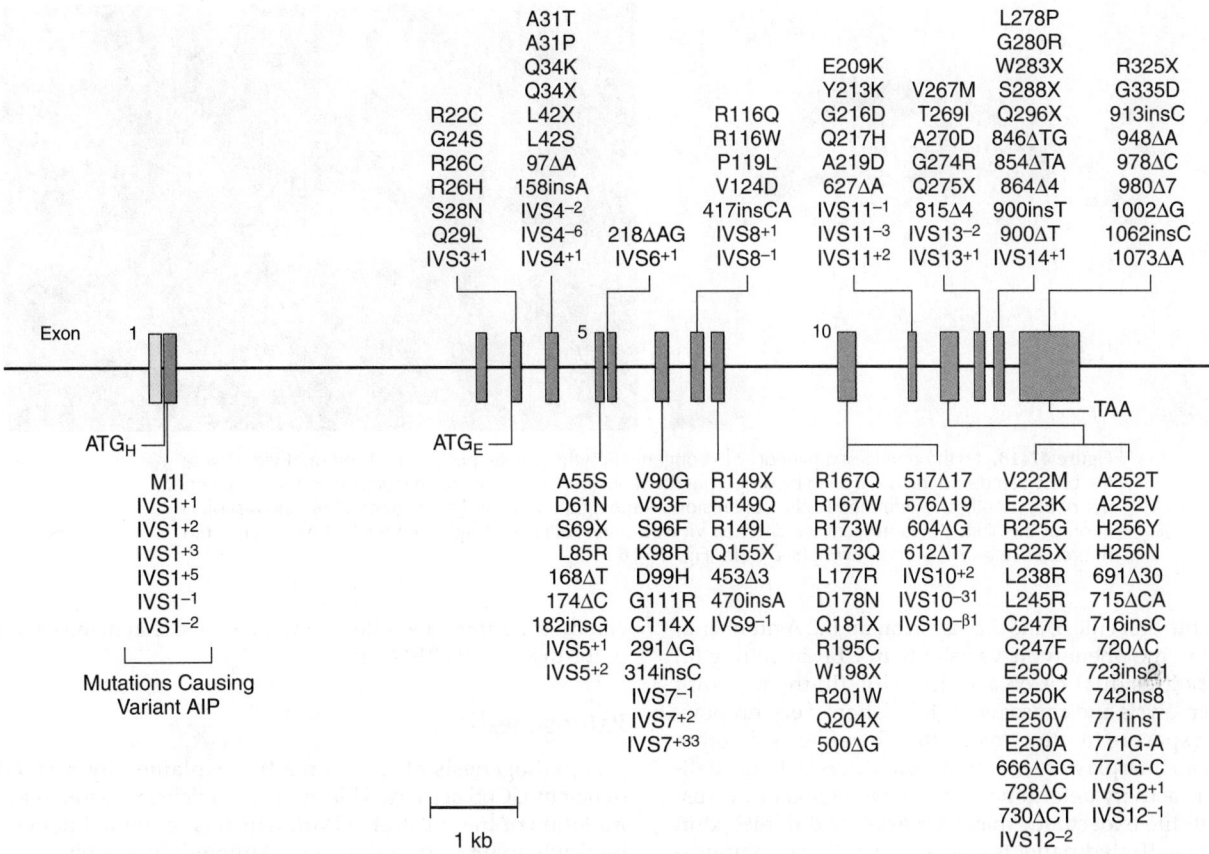

Figure 47-17. The human porphobilinogen deaminase gene, with locations of some of the many mutations that cause acute intermittent porphyria (AIP). kb, kilobase. (From Anderson KE, Sassa S, Bishop DF, et al. Disorders of heme biosynthesis: X-linked sideroblastic anemia and the porphyrias. In: Scriver CR, Beaudet AL, Sly WS, et al., eds. *The metabolic and molecular bases of inherited disease.* New York: McGraw-Hill, 2001, with permission.)

400 to 1200 µg/day has been shown to inhibit ovulation and greatly reduce the incidence of perimenstrual attacks of AIP. Synthetic heme analogs (Frontier Scientific, Logan, UT), such as tin protoporphyrin, 1 µmol/kg, and tin mesoporphyrin, 0.5 µmol/kg/day for 4 days, have also been shown to diminish the output of ALA, PBG, and porphyrins (209).

CONGENITAL ERYTHROPOIETIC PORPHYRIA

Definition

Congenital erythropoietic porphyria (CEP) is an autosomal-recessive disorder of heme biosynthesis that results from the markedly deficient activity of the cytosolic enzyme, UCoS. The enzymatic defect causes the accumulation of type I series of uroporphyrin and coproporphyrin, thus leading to the clinical manifestations of CEP. CEP has also been termed *Günther's disease, erythropoietic porphyria, congenital porphyria, congenital hematoporphyria,* and *erythropoietic uroporphyria.*

Uroporphyrinogen III Cosynthase

UCoS [HMB hydrolase (cyclizing); E. C. 4.2.1.75 (210,211)] catalyzes the cyclization of the linear tetrapyrrole, HMB, to form uroporphyrinogen III, which involves intramolecular inversion of the D-ring pyrrole in the porphyrin. Type III porphyrinogens are metabolized by subsequent enzymes to heme (Fig. 47-4)

(212). In all human cells, there is an excess of UCoS activity compared to PBGD (formerly known as *uroporphyrinogen I synthase*), thus favoring the synthesis of uroporphyrinogen III over uroporphyrinogen I under normal conditions (213).

Human UCoS has been purified to homogeneity from erythrocytes and has been shown to be a monomeric protein with an apparent molecular weight of 29.5 kd (214). The purified enzyme has a specific activity of more than 300,000 nmol/hour/mg, an isoelectric point of 5.5, and it is markedly thermolabile (the half-life at 60°C is approximately 1 minute). The enzyme's pH optimum is 7.4, and the Michaelis-Menten dissociation constant (K_m) for HMB is 5 to 20 mM. The enzyme is activated by Na^+, K^+, Mg^{2+}, and Ca^{2+} and is inhibited by Cd^{2+}, Cu^{2+}, Hg^{2+}, and Zn^{2+}.

Prevalence

CEP is rare and panethnic. As of 1997, approximately 130 cases had been reported (215).

Clinical Findings

The age at onset and clinical severity of CEP are highly variable, ranging from nonimmune hydrops fetalis due to severe hemolytic anemia *in utero* to milder, later-onset forms, which have only cutaneous lesions in adult life. In most cases, severe photosensitivity develops soon after birth. Pink or red-brown staining of diapers due to markedly increased urinary porphy-

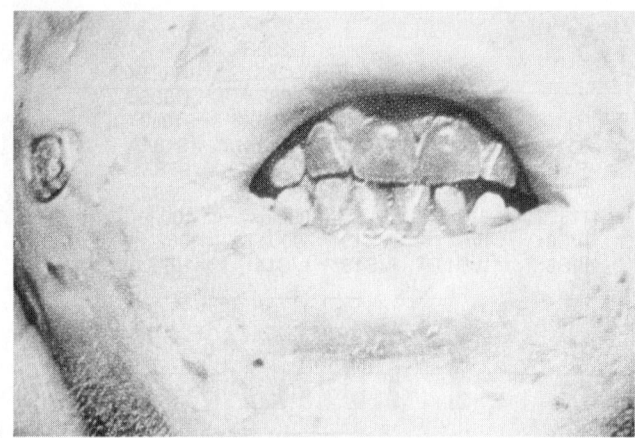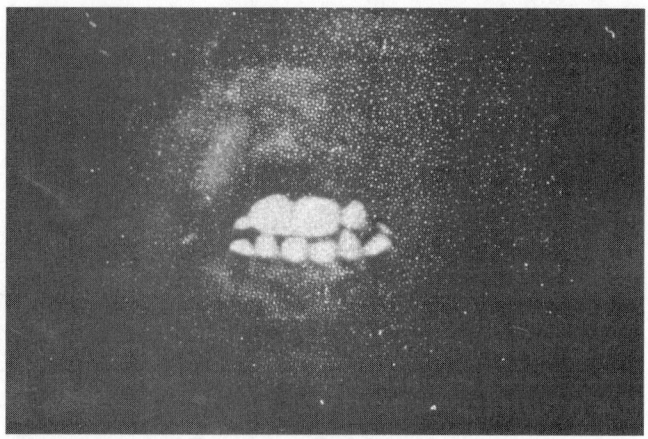

A   **B**

Figure 47-18. Erythrodontia of a patient with congenital erythropoietic porphyria. **A:** Normal view. Note the brownish discoloration of teeth by uroporphyrin deposition, the atrophic changes in the lip at the corner of the mouth, the deformed healing of erosion on the right cheek, and the pigmentation and discoloration of the skin. **B:** Fluorescent view. When viewed under ultraviolet light, the teeth show intense red fluorescence due to uroporphyrin. (See Color Fig. 47-18.)

rins may be the first clue to the disease in an infant. A number of factors lead to the phenotypic variability in CEP, including (a) the amount of residual UCoS activity (216), (b) the resultant degree of hemolysis and consequent stimulation of erythropoiesis, and (c) exposure to ultraviolet light. Therefore, as in other porphyrias, an interplay of environmental factors with the deficient enzyme activity determines clinical expression of the disease. Overall life expectancy may be markedly diminished in more severely affected patients due to hematologic complications and the increased risk of infection.

The major debilitating clinical features in patients with CEP are cutaneous photosensitivity and anemia. Mild to severe hemolysis is a feature of CEP and presumably results from the accumulated uroporphyrin I in erythrocytes. For example, two brothers, who were 5 and 1 years of age and had CEP, had a hemoglobin of 10 to 11 g/dL, a hematocrit of 30% to 36.5%, reticulocytes of 9% to 11.6%, an unconjugated bilirubin of 3 to 11.5 mg/dL (normal is 1.5 mg/dL), and a lactate dehydrogenase of 627 to 954 U/L (60–170). The serum haptoglobin level that was determined in the elder brother was 4 mg/dL (normal is 5 to 48 mg/dL), indicating that the brothers experienced intravascular hemolysis. Some erythrocytes showed red fluorescence on fluorescence microscopy, and the younger brother had 50% erythroblasts in the circulation (217). Secondary splenomegaly develops in response to the increased uptake of abnormal erythrocytes from the circulation, which may contribute to the anemia and also may result in leukopenia and thrombocytopenia.

In most cases of CEP, severe cutaneous photosensitivity usually begins in early infancy and is manifested by increased friability and blistering of the epidermis on the hands, face, and other sun-exposed areas. Bullae and vesicles contain serous fluid and are prone to rupture and infection. The skin may be thickened, with areas of hypo- and hyperpigmentation. Hypertrichosis of the face and extremities is often prominent (218). Sunlight, other sources of ultraviolet light, and minor skin trauma increase the severity of the cutaneous manifestations. Recurrent vesicles and secondary infection can lead to cutaneous scarring and deformities, as well as to loss of digits and facial features, such as the eyelids, nose, and ears. Corneal scarring can lead to blindness. Porphyrins that are deposited in the teeth produce a reddish brown color in natural light; this condition is termed *erythrodontia* (Fig. 47-18). The teeth may fluoresce on exposure to long-wavelength ultraviolet light. Later or adult-onset patients have milder

clinical symptoms and often exhibit only the skin manifestations of the disease (211,219–221).

Pathogenesis

The pathogenesis of CEP is readily explained by markedly deficient UCoS activity. This enzyme deficiency leads to accumulation of the substrate HMB, which is converted nonenzymatically to uroporphyrinogen I. Although uroporphyrinogen I can undergo decarboxylation by UROD to form hepta-, hexa-, and pentacarboxyl porphyrinogen I and, finally, coproporphyrinogen I, further metabolism cannot proceed, because the next enzyme in the pathway, CPO, is stereospecific for the III isomer. Thus, large amounts of isomer I porphyrinogens accumulate in bone marrow erythroid precursors (especially normoblasts and reticulocytes), and erythrocytes and undergo autooxidation to the corresponding porphyrins, which damage erythrocytes and cause cutaneous photosensitivity. Exposure of the skin to sunlight and other sources of long-wavelength ultraviolet light results in blistering and vesicle formation and increased friability of the skin. Hemolysis is almost always present but may not be accompanied by anemia, if erythroid hyperplasia is sufficient to compensate for the increased rate of erythrocyte destruction. Plasma iron turnover is increased in CEP (154,222).

Biochemical Findings

Urinary porphyrin excretion is markedly increased (up to 50 to 100 mg daily) and consists mostly of uroporphyrin, heptacarboxyl porphyrin, and coproporphyrin, with lesser increases in hepta-, hexa-, and pentacarboxyl porphyrins (215). Although the predominant increase is in the type I isomers, type III isomers are also increased. Urinary ALA and PBG excretion is not increased. Fecal porphyrins are markedly increased with a predominance of coproporphyrin I.

Circulating erythrocytes in most reported cases of CEP have contained large amounts of uroporphyrin I and lesser, but still excessive, amounts of coproporphyrin I. Excess plasma porphyrins, which probably originate from the bone marrow and circulating red cells, are mostly uroporphyrin and coproporphyrin. Studies of nine CEP Indian patients indicated a close relationship between the degree of porphyrin excess and the severity of disease expression (223).

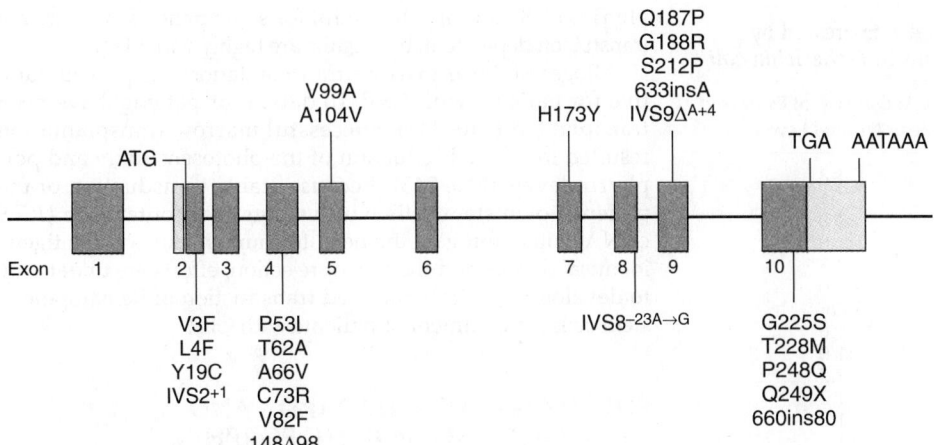

Figure 47-19. The human uroporphyrinogen III cosynthase gene, with locations of mutations that cause congenital erythropoietic porphyria. (From Anderson KE, Sassa S, Bishop DF, et al. Disorders of heme biosynthesis: X-linked sideroblastic anemia and the porphyrias. In: Scriver CR, Beaudet AL, Sly WS, et al., eds. *The metabolic and molecular bases of inherited disease.* New York: McGraw-Hill, 2001, with permission.)

Molecular Biology

The human *UCoS* cDNA consists of 1296 base pairs (bp) with 5′ and 3′ untranslated regions of 196 bp and 302 bp, respectively, and an open reading frame of 798 bp that encodes a polypeptide of 265 amino acids. The *UCoS* gene has been assigned to the chromosomal region 10q25.3→q26.3 (224,225).

Molecular Pathology

A variety of mutations that are responsible for CEP have been identified in the *UCoS* gene (Fig. 47-19). They include missense and nonsense mutations, large and small deletions and insertions, splicing defects, and intronic branch point mutations. Of the 18 single base changes, four (A66V, A104V, T228M, and G225S,) occurred at CpG dinucleotides, which are known hot spots for mutation (226–228). All but one (V82F) of the known CEP missense mutations occurred in amino acid residues that are conserved in both the mouse and human UCoS polypeptide sequences (229). V82F is a single base substitution (G to T) in the last nucleotide of exon 4, at the 5′ donor site for intron 4, which also causes a splicing defect. A branch point mutation that is 23 bp upstream from the intron-exon boundary of intron 8 has also been reported (229).

The frequencies of the *UCoS* mutations, which cause CEP, are shown in Table 47-4. Most patients were heteroallelic for the UCoS mutations. The most common mutation, C73R, was found in approximately 33% of the studied alleles. The next most common mutations were L4F and T228M (7% and 6%, respectively). Except for the previously mentioned mutations, the other mutations were private, having been detected in only one or a few CEP families. Most of the mutations were panethnic in origin.

Table 47-4 shows the UCoS activities of mutations that are expressed in *E. coli.* The mean activities ranged from essentially nondetectable activity to levels that were approximately 35% of the mean activity that was expressed in *E. coli* by the normal cDNA, with only A66V and V82F alleles having activities greater than 10% of the mean normal expressed level. However, A66V and V82F were less stable than the expressed normal enzyme, having half-lives at 37°C of 13.3, 30.5, and 49.5 minutes, respectively (229,230).

Homoallelism for the most common allele, C73R, was correlated with the most severe phenotype, nonimmune hydrops fetalis or transfusion dependency from birth, or both. Consistent with the severe phenotype of C73R/C73R homozygotes, expression of the C73R allele in *E. coli* resulted in the detection of less than 1% of the activity that was expressed by the normal

allele (Table 47-5). Of note, gene targeting of the mouse *UCoS* gene resulted in a fetal lethal (231). However, the fact that the C73R/C73R homozygotes are viable and do not die early in fetal life (i.e., fetal lethals) indicates that the mutant enzyme retains a small amount of residual activity that is sufficient to produce enough heme for the biosynthesis of hemoglobin and hemoproteins. Alternatively, if the C73R mutation produced only nonfunctional enzyme, then the fact that affected fetuses are born suggests the possibility of another gene that is responsible for UCoS activity during development. Of note, patients who were heteroallelic for C73R and a mutation that expressed little residual activity, such as P53L, also resulted in a severe or moderately severe phenotype. Patients who were heteroallelic for mutations that expressed residual activity, such as V82F

TABLE 47-4. Allele Frequency and Enzymatic Activity of Uroporphyrinogen III Cosynthase Mutations That Cause Congenital Erythropoietic Porphyria

Mutations	82 CEP Alleles (n)	82 CEP Alleles (%)	Residual Activity (% of Normal)[a]
Single base substitutions			
C73R	27	32.9	<1.0
L4F	7	8.5	1.8
T228M	6	7.3	<1.0
S212P	4	4.9	<1.0
P53L	3	3.7	<1.0
G225S	3	3.7	1.2
Q249X	2	2.4	1.1
Y19C	1	1.2	1.1
T62A	1	1.2	<1.0
A66V	1	1.2	14.5[b]
V99A	1	1.2	5.6
A104V	1	1.2	7.7
Gene rearrangements			
148del98	2	2.4	<2.0
633insA	1	1.2	1.2
660ins80	1	1.2	<2.0
Ribonucleic acid processing defects			
IVS9[A+4]	3	3.7	—
IVS2[+1]	2	2.4	—
V82F	1	1.2	35.8[b]
Unknown alleles	15	18.3	—

[a]All the mutant uroporphyrinogen III cosynthases were expressed by using the pKK223-3 vector. Results of specific activity are the mean of two to seven independent assays.
[b]Heat-inactivation experiments demonstrated the residual activities to be markedly unstable, when compared to normal activity.
Reproduced with permission from Desnick RJ, Glass IA, Xu W, et al. Molecular genetics of congenital erythropoietic porphyria. *Semin Liver Dis* 1998;18:77.

TABLE 47-5. Residual Activities That Are Expressed by Uroporphyrinogen III Cosynthase Mutants in *Escherichia coli*

Uroporphyrinogen III Cosynthase Mutations	Residual Activity (% of Expressed Mean Normal Level)
L4F	1.8
Y19C	1.1
P53L	<1.0
T62A	<1.0
A66V	14.5[a]
C73R	<1.0
V82F	35.8[a]
V99A	5.6
S212P	<1.0
A104V	7.7
633insA	1.2
G225S	1.2
T228M	<1.0
Q249X	1.1
148A98	<2.0
660ins80	<2.0

NOTE: All the mutant uroporphyrinogen III cosynthases were expressed using the pKK223-3 vector. Results of specific activity are the mean of two to seven independent assays.
[a]Heat-inactivation experiments demonstrated the residual activities to be markedly unstable, when compared to normal activity.
Reproduced with permission from Desnick RJ, Glass IA, Xu W, et al. Molecular genetics of congenital erythropoietic porphyria. *Semin Liver Dis* 1998;18:77.

(35% of normal activity), A104V (7.7% of normal activity), and A66V (14.5% of normal activity), had milder forms of CEP, even if the other allele was C73R or did not express detectable activity. For example, a teenage boy whose genotype was C73R/A66V only had mild cutaneous involvement (216).

Diagnosis

CEP should be suspected when severe photosensitivity begins in infancy or childhood, and porphyrins are markedly increased in erythrocytes and urine. In most cases, pink to dark-reddish urine or staining of the diaper, noted shortly after birth, may be the first clue to the diagnosis. In more severe cases, CEP can cause nonimmune hydrops or hemolytic anemia *in utero*.

HEP is clinically similar to CEP but is distinguishable by the predominance of protoporphyrin (complexed with zinc) in red cells and high levels of isocoproporphyrin in feces and urine.

If heterozygous parents have had a child with this disease, the disease can be detected *in utero* in future pregnancies by finding a red-brown discoloration and increased porphyrins (especially uroporphyrin I) in amniotic fluid (232), by measuring UCoS activity in cultured amniotic fluid cells (233), or by direct detection of *UCoS* gene mutations in cultured amniotic cells (234).

Treatment

Protection of the skin from sunlight and minor trauma is essential in most cases of CEP. Sunscreen lotions and β-carotene are sometimes beneficial (235). Bacterial infections that complicate cutaneous blisters require timely treatment in an effort to prevent scarring and mutilation.

Frequent blood transfusions are sometimes essential. Repeated transfusions can suppress erythropoiesis and thereby decrease porphyrin production and can greatly reduce porphyrin levels and photosensitivity (236). Treatment with hydroxyurea to reduce bone marrow porphyrin synthesis may be considered (237). Splenectomy may substantially reduce transfusion requirements in some patients (236). Oral charcoal may increase fecal loss of por-

phyrins (238) and may be useful for some patients who are not transfusion dependent, but results are highly variable (239).

Allogeneic bone marrow transplantation has proved curative for patients with CEP. To date, four patients have been transplanted (240–243). Successful marrow transplantation resulted in marked reduction of the photosensitivity and porphyrin levels (240–243). Because stable transduction of the patient's own stem cells with vectors that contain the *UCoS* cDNA would abrogate the need for human leukocyte antigen–identical donors and the risk of rejection, efforts are under way to develop retroviral-mediated transduction of hematopoietic stem cells for treatment of patients with CEP.

PORPHYRIA CUTANEA TARDA AND HEPATOERYTHROPOIETIC PORPHYRIA

Porphyria cutanea tarda (PCT) is due to a heterozygous deficiency, and hepatoerythropoietic porphyria (HEP) is due to a homozygous deficiency of UROD (E. C. 4.1.1.37).

Porphyria Cutanea Tarda

DEFINITION OF PORPHYRIA CUTANEA TARDA
PCT, also called *symptomatic porphyria*, *porphyria cutanea symptomatica*, or *idiosyncratic porphyria*, refers to a heterogeneous group of porphyric diseases that may be inherited (familial or type II) or, more commonly, acquired (sporadic or type I) (Table 47-6). Both forms display reductions in the activity of hepatic UROD; in the autosomal-dominant inherited form (type II), the enzyme is deficient in all tissues, whereas, in the acquired form, the defect is confined to the liver. Acquired PCT typically presents in adults, spontaneously or, more commonly, in conjunction with precipitating environmental factors, such as alcohol, estrogen, or polyhalogenated aromatic hydrocarbons, or in association with other disorders. Another form, which is termed *type III PCT*, has been reported, in which normal erythrocyte UROD activity and concentrations were found in more than one member in a single family, but with decreased hepatic UROD activity(244,245) (Table 47-6). The hallmark of all forms of PCT is cutaneous photosensitivity due to increased production of uroporphyrin and 7-carboxylic porphyrin.

UROPORPHYRINOGEN DECARBOXYLASE
UROD is a cytosolic enzyme that catalyzes the sequential removal of the four carboxylic groups of the acetic acid side chains in uroporphyrinogen to yield coproporphyrinogen (246) (Fig. 47-4). UROD acts only on porphyrinogen substrates, not on the corresponding porphyrins (247). The enzyme can decarboxylate all four isomers of uroporphyrinogen, but the naturally most abundant type III isomer is decarboxylated most rapidly, followed by type IV, II, and I isomers in decreasing

TABLE 47-6. Subsets of Porphyria Cutanea Tarda

Type	Familial Occurrence	Uroporphyrinogen Decarboxylase	
		Liver	Erythrocytes
I	(–)	Decreased	Normal
II	(+)	Decreased	Decreased
III	(+)	Decreased	Normal

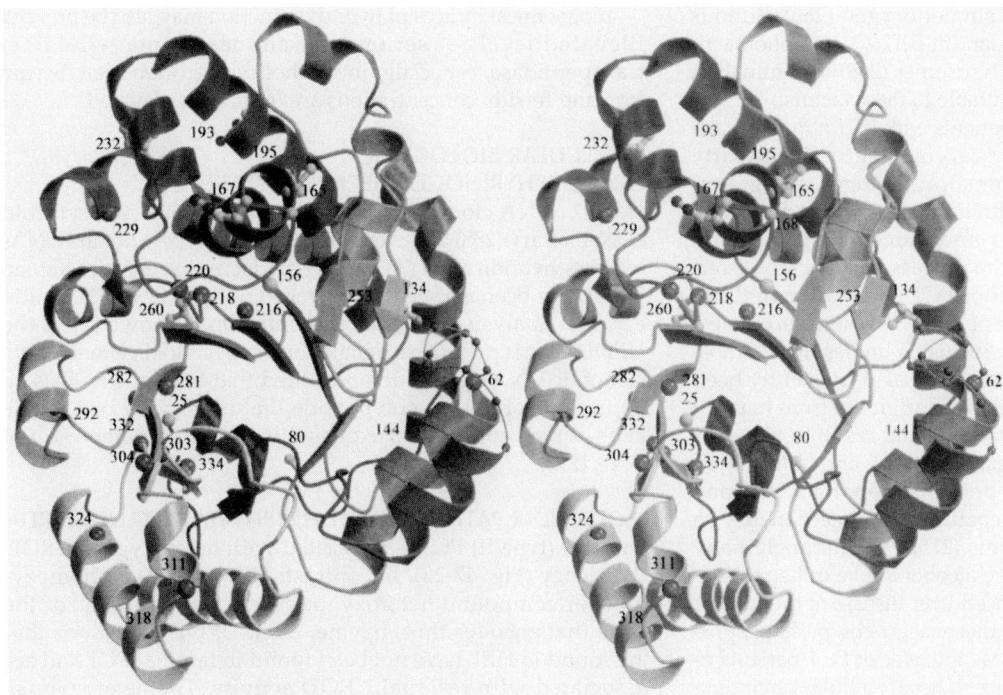

Figure 47-20. The crystal structure of human uroporphyrinogen decarboxylase (UROD), and the location of mutations in the UROD structure. Stereodiagram of the structure of a UROD monomer, from blue to green to yellow, along the amino acid sequence. The disordered loop is shown as a thin blue line with spheres on the Cα positions. Numbers indicate the positions of mutant residues. Mutated amino acids that have been identified in porphyria cutanea tarda or hepatoerythropoietic porphyria are depicted either as yellow or pink spheres. (See Color Fig. 47-20.) (From Phillips JD, Parker TL, Schubert HL, et al., *Blood* 2001;98:3179, with permission.)

order (246,248). With uroporphyrinogen III as substrate, the order of decarboxylation of acetate groups on each pyrrole ring proceeds in a clockwise fashion that starts from ring D (Fig. 47-4). Iron appears to enhance the inhibitory effect of hexachlorobenzene or polyhalogenated aromatic hydrocarbon compounds on UROD activity, although its direct effect on the enzyme activity *in vitro* remains controversial. It is also known that rats with genetic (249) or acquired siderosis (250,251) are more susceptible to hexachlorobenzene-induced porphyria than nonsiderotic rats, and experimental porphyria induced with 2,3,7,8-tetrachlorodibenzo-*p*-dioxin in mice does not occur, if animals are initially made iron deficient by phlebotomy (252).

Recombinant human UROD purified to homogeneity has been crystallized, and its crystal structure was determined at 1.60-Å resolution (253). The purified protein is a dimer with a dissociation constant of 0.1 μM (254). As shown in Figure 47-20, the 40.8-kd polypeptide forms a single domain with a distorted $(\beta/\alpha)_8$ barrel fold and a distinctive deep cleft for the enzyme's active site that is formed by loops at the C-terminal ends of the barrel strands. There is one active-site cleft per monomer, which is located adjacent to its neighbor in the dimer. This structure creates a single extended cleft that is large enough to accommodate two substrate molecules in close proximity or to allow reaction intermediates to shuttle between monomers during the four-step decarboxylation of uroporphyrinogen.

PREVALENCE OF PORPHYRIA CUTANEA TARDA

PCT is probably the most common of all the porphyrias, but its exact incidence is not clear. The disease is recognized worldwide, and no racial predilection exists except among the Bantus in South Africa (255,256), probably because of their high incidence of hemosiderosis. Sporadic PCT is generally more common than familial PCT in Europe, South Africa, and South America (257), although the trend may be less obvious or even reversed in North Americans (258). Previously, PCT was held to be more common, perhaps secondary to higher alcohol intake, in men than in women, but the incidence in women has increased of late to the level seen in men, perhaps due to increased use of contraceptive steroids, postmenopausal estrogens, and alcohol (259,260).

CLINICAL FINDINGS IN PORPHYRIA CUTANEA TARDA

Cutaneous lesions in light-exposed areas, such as the face, tip of the nose, and dorsa of hands, include skin fragility, vesicles and bullae formation (Fig. 47-21), atrophic changes, and scar formation. The lesions are often accompanied by hypopigmentation and hyperpigmentation, hypertrichosis, and pseudosclerodermoid changes. Dystrophic calcifications may occur in severely scarred tissues, forming a protrusion of calcium spicules through the epidermis and leading to chronic nonhealing ulceration as well.

PATHOGENESIS OF PORPHYRIA CUTANEA TARDA

Phototoxic porphyrins in the skin may be largely derived from the liver and, to some extent, formed locally in the skin (261). Activation of the complement system after irradiation has been demonstrated in PCT patients *in vivo* (262,263) and *in vitro* in sera (264,265) and is presumed to result from the generation of reac-

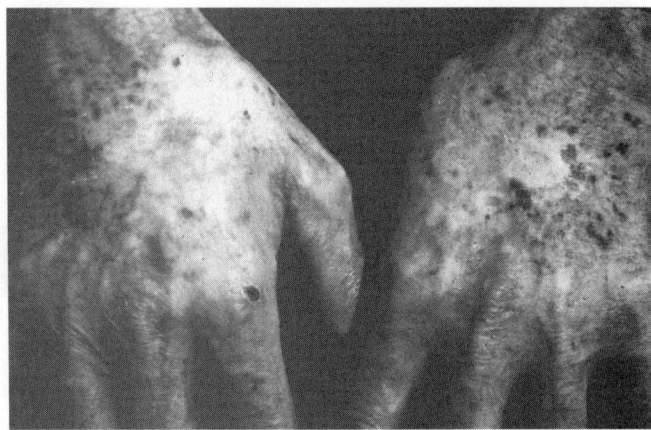

Figure 47-21. Chronic changes of a hand of a patient with porphyria cutanea tarda. Blistering and bullous eruption are seen in the acute phase of photocutaneous dermatosis. In the chronic phase, these changes are replaced with atrophic skin changes that are accompanied by (as shown in the figure) pigmentation, depigmentation, and sclerodermoid changes.

tive oxygen species, most likely singlet oxygen (266). Bullous fluid is known to contain prostaglandin E_2 (267), and photoactivation of uroporphyrin damages lysosomes (268); inflammation and autolysis may be partly attributable to these factors.

Liver biopsy specimens from patients with PCT almost invariably display siderosis of widely varying degrees, with fatty changes, necrosis, chronic inflammatory changes, and granuloma formation (269). It was also found that a significant fraction of PCT patients have associated hemochromatosis gene (HFE) mutations (270,271). Phlebotomy to decrease hepatic iron overload is effective in the treatment of PCT (272), although iron supplementation results in relapse of PCT (273). Red autofluorescence and needlelike cytoplasmic inclusion bodies, which most likely represent porphyrin crystals, have also frequently been reported (269,274). Although they may originate from hepatocytes, they accumulate in bile canaliculi and result in bile duct obstruction. Additionally, estrogens, alcohol, and chlorinated hydrocarbons, all of which are potential hepatotoxins, may aggravate PCT. The incidence of hepatitis B or C infection may be higher than normal in PCT patients (275,276). Although many patients have moderately excessive alcohol intake or hepatitis C infection, or both, few have advanced liver disease at the time of initial presentation. Any or all of these factors or, perhaps, porphyrins themselves, may predispose the liver of PCT patients to neoplastic change, and the incidence of hepatocellular carcinoma in PCT is known to be greater than in the general population (269,277–279). Rarely, primary hepatomas may secrete porphyrins and simulate PCT (280).

BIOCHEMICAL FINDINGS IN PORPHYRIA CUTANEA TARDA

Increased concentrations of uroporphyrin (mainly isomer I) and 7-carboxylic porphyrins (mainly isomer III) are found in the urine in PCT patients, with lesser increases of coproporphyrin and 5- and 6-carboxylic porphyrins (281,282). Porphyrins can be separated by thin-layer chromatography or HPLC (283). Small quantities of isocoproporphyrin may be detected in plasma or urine, but, in feces, isocoproporphyrin is often the dominant porphyrin that is excreted (284,285) and represents the most important diagnostic criterion for PCT. Coproporphyrin, 7-carboxylic porphyrin, uroporphyrin, and X-porphyrin (ether–acetic acid insoluble, extractable with urea-triton) content of stool all may be increased in patients with PCT (286). Total daily fecal porphyrin excretion exceeds total urinary porphyrin excretion. Skin porphyrins are especially increased in areas that are protected from photoactivation (287).

Biochemical indices of liver dysfunction may also be present. Elevated levels of serum transaminases and γ-glutamyl transpeptidase, especially in alcoholics, are often seen. Serum iron and ferritin concentrations are frequently elevated.

MOLECULAR BIOLOGY OF UROPORPHYRINOGEN DECARBOXYLASE

UROD cDNA clones were first isolated from a rat erythroid cDNA library (288) and were then used to isolate human cDNAs by cross-hybridization (289). The gene locus that encodes human UROD has been mapped to chromosome 1p34 (290,291). Southern blot analysis of human genomic DNA showed that the *UROD* gene is present as a single copy in a haploid genome (289). Genomic DNA studies demonstrated that human *UROD* is an approximately 41-kd polypeptide that is encoded by a single gene, which contains 10 exons within approximately 3 kb of DNA (292).

MOLECULAR PATHOLOGY OF PORPHYRIA CUTANEA TARDA

Familial (type II) PCT is associated with heterozygous UROD deficiency (Fig. 47-22). In contrast, HEP is due to a homozygous or compound heterozygous state for mutations of the gene that encodes this enzyme. Most UROD mutations that are found in HEP have not been found in familial PCT and are associated with residual UROD activity. The heterozygous UROD mutations in most cases of familial PCT appear to be more critical to the enzyme activity than those that are found in HEP. However, a few families with cases of HEP and PCT have been described. Heterozygosity for mutant UROD alleles in mice is a risk factor for the development of PCT, because heterozygous mice are much more sensitive to porphyrinogenic stimuli than wild-type animals (293). In heterozygous mice and humans that display porphyric phenotypes, hepatic UROD protein is one-half of normal, but the catalytic activity of the enzyme is reduced to approximately 20%, which suggests that there may be an inhibitor of hepatic UROD (293,294).

DIAGNOSIS OF PORPHYRIA CUTANEA TARDA

The clinical picture in patients with PCT is fairly specific but can be confused with that of other porphyric (VP) and nonporphyric (systemic lupus erythematosus) diseases. Urinary fluorescence under ultraviolet light illumination and quantitation of porphyrins and separation and identification of porphyrins by thin-layer chromatography and HPLC assist the diagnosis.

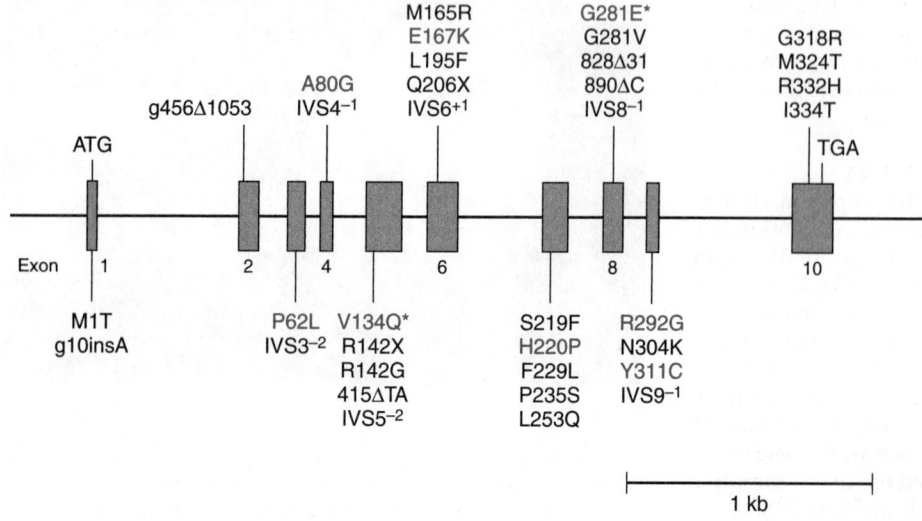

Figure 47-22. The human uroporphyrinogen decarboxylase gene, with locations of the mutations that cause familial porphyria cutanea tarda (type II) and hepatoerythropoietic porphyria (HEP). Mutations that were identified in HEP are shown in blue. The asterisk designates mutations that were identified in porphyria cutanea tarda and HEP. kb, kilobase. (From Anderson KE, Sassa S, Bishop DF, et al. Disorders of heme biosynthesis: X-linked sideroblastic anemia and the porphyrias. In: Scriver CR, Beaudet AL, Sly WS, et al., eds. *The metabolic and molecular bases of inherited disease.* New York: McGraw-Hill, 2001, with permission.)

Plasma porphyrins are elevated in patients with PCT and other photosensitizing porphyrias. Fecal porphyrins are often elevated; isocoproporphyrin (or an isocoproporphyrin to coproporphyrin ratio of 0.1 or more) is virtually diagnostic of PCT (295). The catalytic activity and the concentration of immunoreactive UROD are approximately 50% of normal in patients with type II PCT, and decreased UROD in type II PCT segregates as an autosomal-dominant trait in patients' families. In contrast, patients with type I PCT show normal erythrocyte UROD activity and concentrations and no familial occurrence of the disorder. Patients with type III PCT show familial occurrence with normal erythrocyte UROD activity.

TREATMENT OF PORPHYRIA CUTANEA TARDA

In patients with type I PCT, the identification and avoidance of precipitating factors are essential to treatment (296). The clinical response to cessation of alcohol ingestion is highly variable (297,298); nonetheless, abstinence should be recommended.

Phlebotomy is usually effective in the reduction of urinary porphyrin concentrations and the induction of clinical remissions. Strong evidence shows that the beneficial effects of phlebotomy result from a diminution in body iron stores (299–301). Replenishment of iron after remission of PCT may accelerate the onset of subsequent relapse (302), which, in the absence of supplemental iron administration, may occur from 1 to 8 years later. Reduction of porphyrin excretion usually precedes clinical improvement, which starts with an abatement of new skin lesions and may eventually progress to healing of scars and loss of skin fragility.

If phlebotomy is ineffective or contraindicated because of the presence of other diseases, such as anemia, low-dose chloroquine therapy may be effective. Efficacy of chloroquine therapy and phlebotomy is probably similar (303,304), and some reports suggest that a combined approach is useful and may diminish the incidence of side effects (305,306). The mechanism of action of chloroquine therapy is thought to be related to its ability to chelate porphyrins in a water-soluble and, hence, more easily excreted form (307).

Hepatoerythropoietic Porphyria

DEFINITION OF HEPATOERYTHROPOIETIC PORPHYRIA

HEP is a rare form of porphyria that probably results from a homozygous defect in UROD activity. Clinically, HEP is indistinguishable from CEP and is characterized by the childhood onset of severe photosensitivity and skin fragility. The term *HEP* was coined to reflect the fact that excess porphyrins are synthesized in the liver and the bone marrow. HEP is extremely rare; some 20 cases have been reported worldwide to date (308).

CLINICAL FINDINGS IN HEPATOERYTHROPOIETIC PORPHYRIA

Clinical findings in patients with HEP are similar to those that are seen in CEP. Pink urine, severe photosensitivity that leads to scarring and mutilation of sun-exposed areas of skin, sclerodermoid changes, hypertrichosis, erythrodontia, anemia (often hemolytic), and hepatosplenomegaly characterize HEP. Onset is usually in early infancy or childhood (309), but adult onset has also been described (310,311). Although photosensitivity can be similar to CEP, anemia in HEP is much milder than in CEP. For example, the first reported HEP patient, a 2-year-old boy, had a hemoglobin of 14.1 g/dL and a hematocrit of 48%, despite 95% deficiency of erythrocyte UROD activity (312). In contrast to those found in PCT patients, serum iron concentrations have usually been normal in HEP patients. Likewise, the incidence of

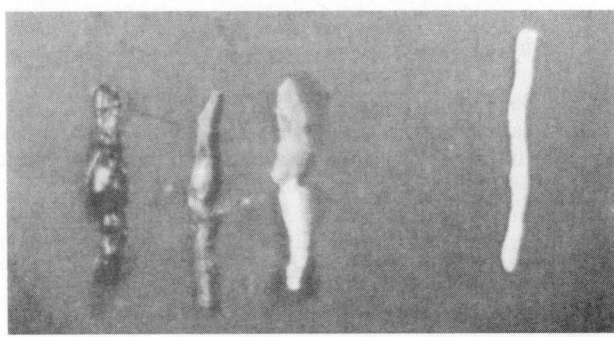

Figure 47-23. Liver biopsy sample from a patient with hepatoerythropoietic porphyria that shows various degrees of fluorescence *(far right)*, whereas samples from nonporphyric subjects do not. (See Color Fig. 47-23.)

bone marrow and liver fluorescence (Fig. 47-23), anemia, and evidence of abnormal liver function and histology have been highly variable. Skin biopsies have shown subepidermal bullae and other findings that are similar to the lesions of PCT (313).

BIOCHEMICAL FINDINGS IN HEPATOERYTHROPOIETIC PORPHYRIA

Most HEP patients have displayed elevations in urinary porphyrins, predominantly uroporphyrin I with lesser quantities of 7-carboxylic porphyrins, mainly type III. Isocoproporphyrin concentrations that are equal to or greater than coproporphyrin have also been detected in urine and feces. Elevated erythrocyte protoporphyrin (usually zinc protoporphyrin) has also been observed in HEP. Anemia and biochemical evidence of impaired hepatic function are highly variable. Serum iron is usually normal.

MOLECULAR PATHOLOGY OF HEPATOERYTHROPOIETIC PORPHYRIA

Recent availability of a human *UROD* cDNA clone (289) allowed de Verneuil et al. (314,315) to investigate the mutant gene and its expression in lymphoblastoid cell lines from a family with two cases of HEP. Southern blot analysis after digestion of genomic DNA showed the same restriction fragments in DNA that was isolated from a normal cell line and from both patients, thus excluding large deletions or rearrangements in the mutant gene. Northern and dot blot analyses demonstrated that the concentration of mRNA was similar in cell lines from controls, heterozygous parents, or homozygous patients. Synthesis, processing, and cell-free translation of the specific transcripts appear to be normal (314). Size and molecular weight of the protein were identical with those of the marker enzyme. The only explanation for the low level of UROD protein in cells (5% of control value) was provided by a study of the half-life of the enzyme (314); the half-life was 82 hours in the control cell and only 7 hours in the patients' cells. Thus, the enzyme defect appears to result from rapid degradation *in vivo* of an unstable protein.

Cloning and sequencing of a cDNA of the mutated gene in one patient from the family revealed a Gly (GGG) to Glu (GAG) change in the amino acid sequence at position 281 (314). *In vitro* experiments revealed that the cDNA with this mutation encoded a polypeptide product that was rapidly degraded when compared to the polypeptide that was encoded by the normal cDNA in the presence of cell lysate. This observation is consistent with decreased stability of the mutant protein *in vivo*. Subsequent studies showed that there are different types of mutations in this disorder, such as another homozygous mutation that involves a single base substitution within the coding region that leads to the replacement of a glutamic acid by a lysine at codon 167 (316), compound heterozygosity that involves two separate point mutations (317), or a missense mutation that is combined with a large deletion (318).

DIAGNOSIS OF HEPATOERYTHROPOIETIC PORPHYRIA

The diagnosis must be suspected in patients with severe photosensitivity and especially should be considered in the differential diagnosis of CEP. Diagnostic criteria include elevated levels of fecal or urinary isocoproporphyrin and erythrocyte zinc protoporphyrin. Included in the differential diagnosis is erythropoietic protoporphyria (EPP) in which erythrocyte protoporphyrin is also elevated, but, in contrast to HEP, urinary porphyrins are normal. EPP is also clinically milder than HEP. Measurement of erythrocyte or fibroblast UROD activities typically shows reductions from 2% to 10% of normal control values, with intermediate reductions of UROD activities in family members (309).

TREATMENT OF HEPATOERYTHROPOIETIC PORPHYRIA

Avoidance of sun exposure and use of topical sunscreens are essentially the only treatment options that can be offered to HEP patients. Because the disease is generally milder than CEP, no bone marrow or liver transplantation has been attempted. Responses to phlebotomy have not been observed, although this is perhaps not surprising, because serum iron levels, in contrast to those in PCT patients, are invariably normal (309).

HEREDITARY COPROPORPHYRIA

Definition

HCP is due to a heterozygous deficiency of CPO (E. C. 1.3.3.3) activity, which is inherited in an autosomal-dominant manner. Clinically, HCP is similar to ADP or AIP, although it is often much milder. In addition, HCP may be associated with photosensitivity. Expression of HCP is variable and influenced by the same factors that are responsible for exacerbating AIP. Rarely, homozygous deficiency of this enzyme may occur and is associated with a more severe form of the disease.

Coproporphyrinogen Oxidase

CPO utilizes coproporphyrinogen and molecular oxygen as substrates and catalyzes the oxidative decarboxylation of coproporphyrinogen to protoporphyrinogen. In contrast to UROD, which decarboxylates type I and type III uroporphyrinogens, CPO works specifically on type III coproporphyrinogen, yielding protoporphyrinogen IX (Fig. 47-4). In this process, the enzymatic conversion of two propionate side chains to two vinyl groups proceeds via a tripropionate monovinyl porphyrinogen, then to harderoporphyrinogen in a stepwise fashion.

CPO that is purified from mammalian sources is a soluble enzyme but is localized to the intermembrane space of mitochondria (319,320). The purified human CPO is a nearly globular homodimer (321) that is composed of subunits of molecular weight of approximately 39,000 d (320,321). The apparent K_m for coproporphyrinogen is 0.5 µM (321). Oxygen is an absolute requirement for the enzymatic function, and other oxidants cannot replace oxygen. Curiously, mammalian CPO does not contain redox active metals and thus is resistant to the effect of metal chelators (321,322).

Prevalence

Clinically expressed HCP is much less common than clinically expressed AIP, but, as with the latter disease, latent HCP or HCP gene carriers are being recognized more frequently since the advent of improved laboratory techniques for their detection.

Clinical Findings

Neurovisceral symptoms predominate and are essentially indistinguishable from those of ADP or AIP. Abdominal pain, vomiting, constipation, neuropathies, and psychiatric manifestations are most common in a review of 111 cases (323). In contrast to ADP or AIP, approximately 30% of cases of HCP also display cutaneous photosensitivity (323). Attacks have been precipitated by pregnancy, menses, and contraceptive steroids (324–326), but the most common precipitating factors have been drugs, notably barbiturates (327,328).

Biochemical Findings

The biochemical hallmark of HCP is hyperexcretion of coproporphyrin (predominantly type III) into the urine and feces. Fecal coproporphyrin may be chelated with copper (329), and fecal protoporphyrin may be modestly elevated. Hyperexcretion of ALA, PBG, and uroporphyrin into the urine may accompany exacerbation of the disease, but, in contrast to those seen in AIP, these findings generally normalize between attacks. CPO activity is typically reduced by approximately 50% in heterozygotes and by approximately 90% to 98% in homozygotes. Homozygotes also show elevations in urinary ALA, PBG, and uroporphyrins; in addition, patients with harderoporphyria (to be discussed in the section Harderoporphyria) have elevated erythrocyte protoporphyrin levels and higher total fecal porphyrins, of which approximately 60% is harderoporphyrin.

Molecular Biology

The human CPO gene is located on chromosome 3q12 (330). The gene spans approximately 14 kb and consists of seven exons and six introns. Its promoter is highly GC-rich and contains potential regulatory elements, such as 6 Sp1, 4 GATA, one CACCC site (331), and the CPO-gene promoter regulatory element (CPRE) (332). The CPRE binds specifically to a CPRE binding protein, which has a leucine zipperlike structure and serves as a DNA sequence-specific transcription factor that regulates gene expression (332). There is significant tissue-specific expression of CPO. For example, binding proteins to the Sp1-like element, CPRE, and GATA-1 cooperatively function in CPO gene expression in erythroid cells, whereas the CPRE binding protein by itself plays a principal role in basal expression of CPO in nonerythroid cells (333). It is also known that CPO mRNA increases during erythroid cell differentiation (334,335). Newly synthesized human CPO contains a 110–amino acid N-terminal signal peptide (331), which is removed during transport into the intermembrane space of mitochondria and yields a mature protein of 354 amino acid residues (molecular weight equals 36,842 d). A five-base insertional mutation in the middle of this presequence has been described in one patient with HCP (336).

Molecular Pathology

CPO mutations in HCP are highly heterogeneous, including missense, nonsense, and splicing mutations, as well as insertions and deletions (337). There are also three known polymorphisms, two in exon 4 and one in exon 5, in the human CPO gene (338). Except for one mutation (K404E), which occurred in two unrelated families with harderoporphyria, the CPO mutations that have been found to date are private (337). Mutations in HCP that have been identified so far are summarized in Figure 47-24. Mutations

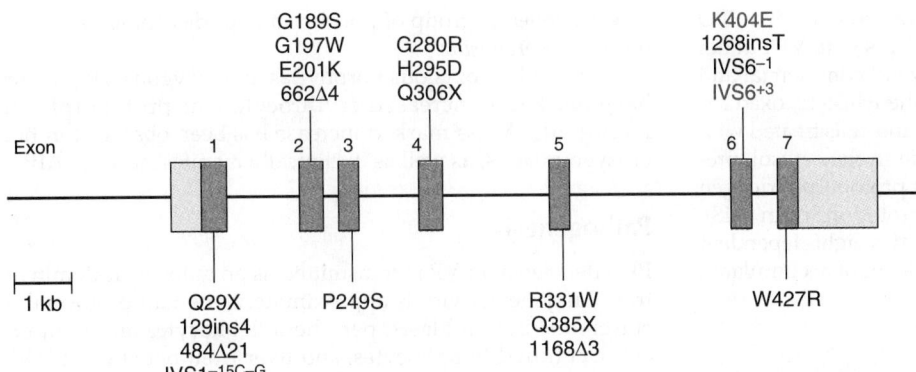

Figure 47-24. The human coproporphyrinogen oxidase gene, with locations of the mutations that cause hereditary coproporphyria. Mutations that are shown in blue were found in patients with harderoporphyria. kb, kilobase. (From Anderson KE, Sassa S, Bishop DF, et al. Disorders of heme biosynthesis: X-linked sideroblastic anemia and the porphyrias. In: Scriver CR, Beaudet AL, Sly WS, et al., eds. *The metabolic and molecular bases of inherited disease.* New York: McGraw-Hill, 2001, with permission.)

G197W, Q306X, Q385X, and W427R occur in highly conserved amino acid residues (339). K404E is located immediately after the most phylogenetically conserved region in the CPO protein, which could affect the substrate binding (340,341). Because the crystal structure of CPO is not yet available, the consequences of each mutation are conjectural.

Diagnosis

HCP should be suspected in patients with the symptoms and clinical course that are characteristic of the acute hepatic porphyrias (ADP, AIP, HCP, and VP) but in whom PBGD activity is normal. Urinary excretion of heme precursors is similar in patients with HCP and VP, but the predominant or exclusive presence of fecal coproporphyrin is more suggestive of HCP than VP, in which fecal coproporphyrin and protoporphyrin concentrations are usually approximately equal. Fecal or urinary predominance of harderoporphyrin, with greatly reduced CPO activity, indicates harderoporphyria.

Treatment

The identification and avoidance of precipitating factors are essential. Treatment of patients with acute attacks of HCP and harderoporphyria is similar to treatment of those with AIP.

HARDEROPORPHYRIA

Harderoporphyria is a variant of HCP that has been described in a white family (342). CPO catalyzes the oxidative decarboxylation of the two propionyl groups at positions 2 and 4 of coproporphyrinogen to yield the two vinyl groups of protoporphyrinogen. Harderoporphyrin, a tricarboxylate porphyrinogen, is an intermediate in this reaction. CPO activity that was determined in lymphocytes from three patients with harderoporphyria was only 10% of that of normal controls, which suggests that harderoporphyria patients were homozygous for the enzymatic defect. Enzyme kinetic studies showed that CPO in patients had an unusually high K_m (15- to 20-fold higher than the normal enzyme) and 50% of the maximum velocity of the normal enzyme. The enzyme activity in these patients was also abnormally sensitive to heat. The unique porphyrin excretion profile (harderoporphyrin predominating) and the properties of CPO in these patients are different from those of the homozygous case of HCP. It has been suggested that harderoporphyria is caused by a homozygous deficiency of a structurally altered enzyme, whereas a homozygous HCP is caused by a homozygous deficiency of the normal CPO.

VARIEGATE PORPHYRIA

Definition

VP is an autosomal-dominant hepatic porphyria and results from a partial deficiency of PPO activity. It was first described in 1937 (343). The disease was termed *variegate*, because it can present with neurologic manifestations or cutaneous photosensitivity, or both. It has also been known as *porphyria variegata*, *protocoproporphyria*, or *South African genetic porphyria*.

Prevalence

In most countries, this porphyria is less commonly recognized than AIP. VP is, however, quite common among South African whites (approximately 3 of 1000) and is known to be due to genetic drift or to a founder effect. Most VP cases in South Africa can been traced to a man or his wife who emigrated from Holland and were married in 1688 (337). As many as 20,000 South Africans may carry this gene, which is now known to be the R59W mutation of the *PPO* gene. VP has also been recognized in many countries. In Finland, the prevalence is approximately 1.3 per 100,000. VP has been termed the Royal malady, based on the suggestion that some British royalty may have had the condition (344). However, this hypothesis was based on a purely retrospective analysis of symptoms and was thought to be highly speculative (256). A more recent study, which was based on the combined use of historical records and molecular analysis of DNA samples, also suggested possible VP in the British royal lineage, but it is still far from proving this theory (345).

Protoporphyrinogen Oxidase

The penultimate step in the heme biosynthetic pathway (i.e., oxidation of protoporphyrinogen IX to protoporphyrin IX) is mediated by the mitochondrial enzyme, PPO (E. C. 1.3.3.4), which catalyzes the removal of six hydrogen atoms from the porphyrinogen nucleus (Fig. 47-4).

PPO has been purified from rat liver mitochondria and has been shown to have a molecular weight of 35,000 d, a K_m of 11 µM, a maximum velocity of 8.7 nmol/minute/mg of protein, and an absolute requirement for oxygen. The enzyme acts specifically on protoporphyrinogen and does not catalyze the oxidation of coproporphyrinogen I, coproporphyrinogen III, or uroporphyrinogen I. Low concentrations of sulfhydryl reducing agents, such as glutathione, stimulate the enzyme activity (346). Human skin fibroblasts display PPO activity [2 to 3 nmol of protoporphyrin per hour per mg of protein (346,347)], and rat liver mitochondria are known to display enzyme activity in the range of 10 to 12 nmol of protoporphyrin per hour per mg of protein (347). PPO activity is decreased in fibroblasts from patients with VP but not in those from patients with EPP (347). Several commercial and experimental herbicides such as p-nitrodiphenylesters, oxadiazoles, and cyclic imides inhibit PPO activity, and cells treated with these inhibitors accumulate protoporphyrin in the cytosol, presumably by the accumulation and export of protoporphyrinogen from mitochondria and autooxidation to protoporphyrin (348). In plants that were treated with these herbicides, light-dependent damage occurs and is correlated with the level of accumulated protoporphyrin (348).

Clinical Findings

In the past, this disease most commonly presented with neurovisceral symptoms that were identical to other acute porphyrias. In South Africa, it has been noted that acute attacks have become considerably less common and that skin manifestations are more commonly the initial presentation (349). The acute attack is identical to that seen in other acute porphyrias. Hyponatremia with evidence of sodium depletion or inappropriate ADH secretion can occur during acute attacks (350). Experience in South Africa suggests that attacks of VP are generally milder than attacks of AIP, and recurrent attacks are much less common (351).

Cutaneous photosensitivity is more common than it is in HCP. Skin manifestations generally occur apart from the neurovisceral symptoms and are usually of longer duration. They are very similar to those that are seen in PCT and HCP and include increased fragility, vesicles, bullae, erosions, milia, hyperpigmentation, and hypertrichosis of sun-exposed areas (351). Histologic changes include periodic acid-Schiff–positive thickening, immunoglobulin G deposition in the vessel walls, and reduplication of the basal lamina (352). Photosensitivity may be less commonly associated with VP in more northern countries, in which sunlight is less intense (353,354).

The same drug, steroid hormone, and nutritional factors that are detrimental in AIP can exacerbate VP (355). Restriction of calories can be detrimental, particularly near the time of menses (355,356). Women who take oral contraceptives are prone to develop cutaneous manifestations of VP.

Marked deficiencies of PPO have been reported in homozygous (or compound heterozygous) cases of VP, and clinical manifestations in such cases are likely to be more severe and to begin in childhood (357–359). In addition to photosensitivity, neurologic symptoms and developmental disturbances, including growth retardation in infancy or childhood, have been noted (357,359–362).

Biochemical Findings

Fecal protoporphyrin and coproporphyrin and urinary coproporphyrin are markedly increased when VP is clinically active. Urinary and fecal coproporphyrins are mostly type III. Urinary ALA, PBG, and uroporphyrin are increased during acute attacks but may be normal or only slightly increased during remission. Plasma porphyrins are commonly increased, particularly when photosensitivity is present. The increased plasma porphyrins in VP consist, in part, of a dicarboxyl porphyrin that is tightly bound to plasma proteins (351). It has been suggested that the risk of gallstones may be increased in VP and that the stones contain protoporphyrin (363).

The X porphyrin fraction [which is defined as ether–acetic acid–insoluble porphyrins that are extracted from feces by urea-Triton (Sigma, St. Louis, MO)] is increased in this disease more than it is in other porphyrias. In VP, this fraction contains a heterogeneous group of porphyrin-peptide conjugates that is termed X porphyrin.

As in all homozygous porphyrias, homozygous VP patients have markedly increased erythrocyte zinc protoporphyrin levels (361). A less marked increase has been observed in heterozygous cases, as well as in clinically manifest cases of AIP.

Pathogenesis

PPO deficiency in VP is transmitted as an autosomal-dominant trait. Enzyme activity is approximately one-half of normal in cultured skin fibroblasts, peripheral leukocytes and lymphocytes, cultured lymphocytes, and liver from patients with VP. Most individuals who inherit PPO deficiency remain asymptomatic. Additional influences, such as certain drugs, steroids, and nutritional alterations, many of which increase hepatic ALAS1, are important, as in other acute porphyrias. This rate-limiting enzyme is increased in liver in this disease. Therefore, as in HCP, increased ALA and PBG during acute attacks may be explained by induction of ALAS1 (364). Accumulated protoporphyrinogen IX in VP undergoes autooxidation to protoporphyrin IX before excretion in bile and feces.

Molecular Biology

Cloning of a human cDNA for PPO was achieved by complementation in vivo of a hemG mutant of E. coli (365), and, subsequently, genomic DNA fragments that contained the entire coding sequence for human PPO were cloned (366,367). The 5.5-kb gene has one noncoding and 12 coding exons, and the exon-intron boundary sequences all conform to consensus acceptor (GTn) and donor (nAG) sequences (366,367). The coding sequence of human PPO is 1431-bp long and encodes a polypeptide that is composed of 477 amino acid residues and is a protein with a molecular weight of approximately 50,800 d. The sequence data of human, mouse, and bacterial PPO indicate that there is a high degree of homology near the N-terminus of the protein. This area corresponds to a typical flavin adenine dinucleotide–binding motif. Consistent with this finding, the human PPO has been shown to contain noncovalently bound flavin adenine dinucleotide (368). The gene for human PPO has been mapped to chromosome 1q23 (369), or 1q22 (367), by fluorescence in situ hybridization.

Northern blot analyses from a variety of tissues indicate that there is a single transcript of PPO with a size of 1.8 kb in all tissues (365,368,370). Although PPO is localized to the cytosolic side of the inner mitochondrial membrane (371,372), the sequence does not indicate that PPO is synthesized with a presequence for targeting and import into mitochondria (366).

Molecular Pathology

Disease-specific PPO mutations were first reported in four patients with VP in three unrelated, French Caucasian families (373). One was a point insertion of a G at position 1022 of the PPO cDNA that produced a frameshift that resulted in a premature stop codon. In three other patients from two unrelated families, a missense mutation that led to a glycine-to-arginine substitution (G232R) was found in exon 7. Subsequently, various other mutations of the PPO gene have been reported in families from around the world who have VP (Fig. 47-25). One of the mutations (R59W) represents the founder gene that underlies the high incidence of VP in South Africa (374). Rare homozygotes for VP have been shown to be mostly heteroallelic for defects in the PPO gene, with the exception of one who was homoallelic.

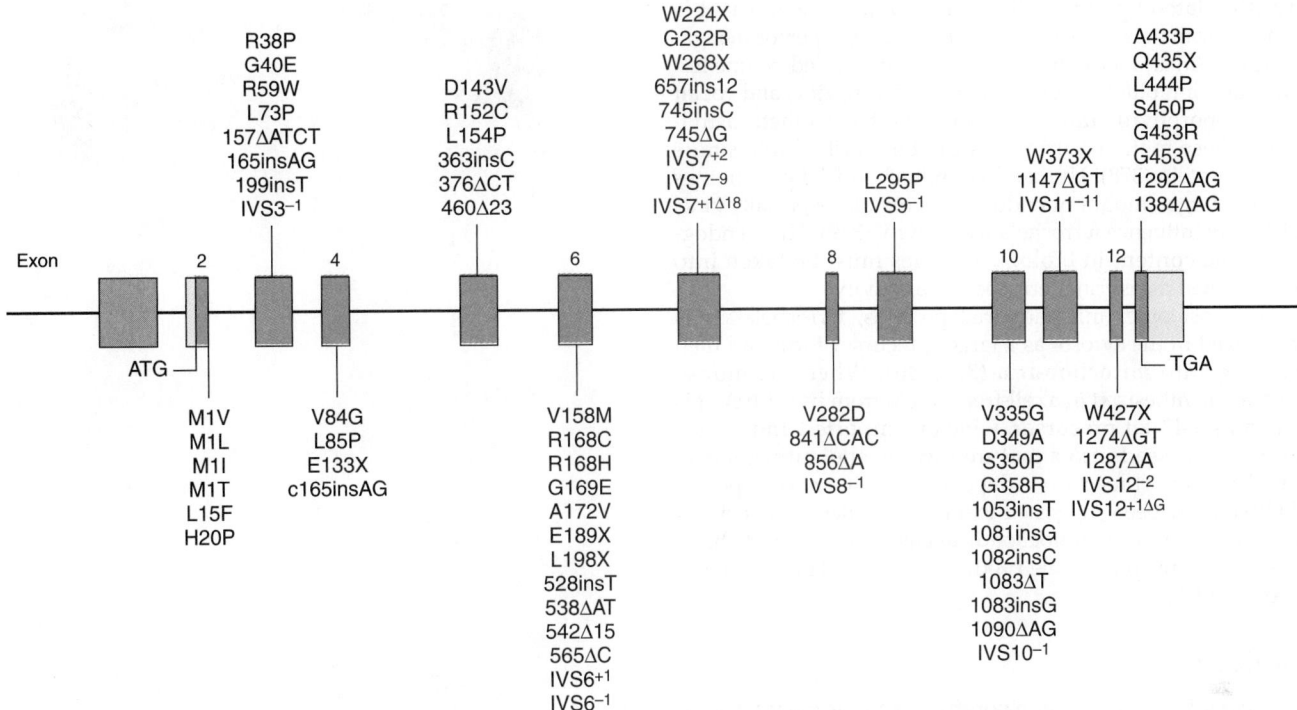

Figure 47-25. The human protoporphyrinogen oxidase gene, with the locations of the mutations that cause variegate porphyria. (From Anderson KE, Sassa S, Bishop DF, et al. Disorders of heme biosynthesis: X-linked sideroblastic anemia and the porphyrias. In: Scriver CR, Beaudet AL, Sly WS, et al., eds. *The metabolic and molecular bases of inherited disease.* New York: McGraw-Hill, 2001, with permission.)

Diagnosis

VP should be considered whenever AIP and other acute porphyrias are considered as a cause of neurovisceral symptoms. During an acute attack of VP, urinary ALA and PBG should be increased. VP can be distinguished from AIP by the finding of increased plasma porphyrins and marked increases in urinary and fecal coproporphyrin. Erythrocyte PBGD is deficient in most patients with AIP but not in those with VP. VP is differentiated from HCP by fecal and plasma porphyrin analysis. The increased plasma porphyrins in VP include a dicarboxyl porphyrin that is tightly bound to plasma proteins. Plasma porphyrin analysis provides a simple and reliable means of rapidly distinguishing VP from other cutaneous porphyrias. PPO activity can be measured in cells that contain mitochondria, such as lymphocytes, however, it has not been widely used in clinical diagnosis because of the complex nature of its assay.

Treatment

Treatment measures that are effective in AIP, such as glucose and heme therapy, are effective for acute attacks of VP but are not markedly effective for cutaneous symptoms. Protection from sunlight is highly important and may include use of protective clothing, gloves, a broad-brimmed hat, and opaque sunscreen preparations. The prognosis is usually good, once the diagnosis is established.

ERYTHROPOIETIC PROTOPORPHYRIA

Definition

EPP results from a partial deficiency of ferrochelatase, the last enzyme in the heme biosynthetic pathway. In this disorder, a large amount of protoporphyrin is synthesized and excreted from erythroid cells in the bone marrow and appears in excess amounts in plasma, circulating erythrocytes, bile, and feces. Characteristic cutaneous photosensitivity usually begins in childhood. In contrast to other cutaneous porphyrias, skin manifestations are generally mild and nonblistering. Severe liver damage occurs occasionally. Inheritance is usually autosomal dominant, but there are some pedigrees that show autosomal-recessive inheritance. EPP is also termed *protoporphyria* or *erythrohepatic protoporphyria.*

Ferrochelatase

The final step of heme biosynthesis is the insertion of iron into protoporphyrin IX, which is catalyzed by the mitochondrial enzyme, ferrochelatase (heme synthase, heme synthetase, or protoheme-ferrolyase; E. C. 4.99.1.1) (Fig. 47-4). Ferrochelatase activity in mammalian cells is localized to the inner membrane of mitochondria. Unlike other enzymatic steps, which use porphyrinogens, in the heme biosynthetic pathway, ferrochelatase uses protoporphyrin IX, the oxidized form of protoporphyrinogen IX, as a substrate. In addition to protoporphyrin IX, other synthetic 2-carboxylate porphyrins, such as deutero- and mesoporphyrin IX, also serve as good substrates for this enzyme *in vitro* (375,376). Only the reduced form of iron (Fe^{2+}), but not Fe^{3+}, is incorporated into protoporphyrin IX by the enzyme (375). Co^{2+} and Zn^{2+} are more efficient substrates than Fe^{2+} for the enzyme (375). Therefore, various rates of ferrochelatase activity can be obtained, depending on which metal and porphyrin substrates are used (375).

Ferrochelatase has been purified from rat liver mitochondria (7). The enzyme is enriched in lysine (11%) and hydrophobic amino acid residues (48%). The enzyme activity can be markedly stimulated by the addition of fatty acids, whereas it is inhibited by metals such as cobalt, zinc, lead, copper, or manganese (377). An antibody that was specific to purified bovine ferrochelatase inhibited the incorporation of iron, zinc, and cobalt into protoporphyrin, thus confirming that the synthetic activities for these metalloporphyrins can be ascribed to a single enzyme protein (378). Human liver mitochondrial membranes contain a large amount of endogenous metals, especially zinc, which may influence ferrochelatase activity (379). Thus, endogenous zinc content in biologic samples must be taken into account when measuring ferrochelatase activity.

Like most other mitochondrial proteins, ferrochelatase is synthesized in the cytosol as a larger precursor form and then imported into mitochondria (379,380). When the mouse enzyme is synthesized in a cell-free system from its mRNA, it is formed as a 43-kd precursor, which is imported and subsequently processed into a mature form in the mitochondria (381). This import reaction is dependent on membrane potential (381). It has been suggested that ferrochelatase is associated with complex I of the mitochondrial electron transport chain, and that ferrous ion may be produced on NADH oxidation in complex I (382).

Prevalence

EPP is the third most common porphyria and the most common erythropoietic porphyria. However, it was not recognized until 1961 (383), probably because the cutaneous features are usually mild, and there is no excess urinary excretion of porphyrins. As of 1976, more than 300 cases had been reported (384). It has been described mostly in whites, but it does occur in other races, including blacks and Japanese (385).

Clinical Findings

Cutaneous photosensitivity, which begins in childhood, affects sun-exposed areas and is generally worse in spring and summer. It is the major clinical feature of this disease. Common symptoms include itching, painful erythema, and swelling, which can develop within minutes of sun exposure (384). Diffuse edema of the skin in sun-exposed areas may resemble angioneurotic edema (Fig. 47-26). On occasion, burning and itching can occur without obvious skin damage. Petechiae and purpuric lesions may occur. Skin lichenification, leathery pseudovesicles, and nail changes can be pronounced (386–388). In contrast to CEP or PCT, deformities of facial features and digits do not occur. Increased fragility of the skin and hirsutism are also not characteristic of this disease. The teeth are not fluorescent, and there are no neurovisceral symptoms, except in some patients with severe hepatic complications who may develop motor neuropathy (389). Liver failure occurs in a minority of patients and is associated with a poor prognosis (390).

Mild anemia with hypochromia and microcytosis or mild anemia with reticulocytosis is sometimes present (189,384,391,392). For example, in a study in which 12 of 19 patients with EPP were classified as anemic, anemic subjects had a mean corpuscular hemoglobin concentration that ranged from 31 to 33 g/dL (normal is 32 to 36 g/dL), microcytosis, anisocytosis, and poikilocytosis (393). Depletion of iron stores may be relatively common in EPP, even in the absence of iron deficiency anemia. Iron accumulation in erythroblasts and ring sideroblasts may also occur in some EPP patients (394). Reticulocyte counts that ranged from 2% (upper limit of normal) to 9% were occasionally noted in patients with EPP (393).

Red cells from patients with EPP contain varying amounts of protoporphyrin (395). When EPP cells were analyzed by flow

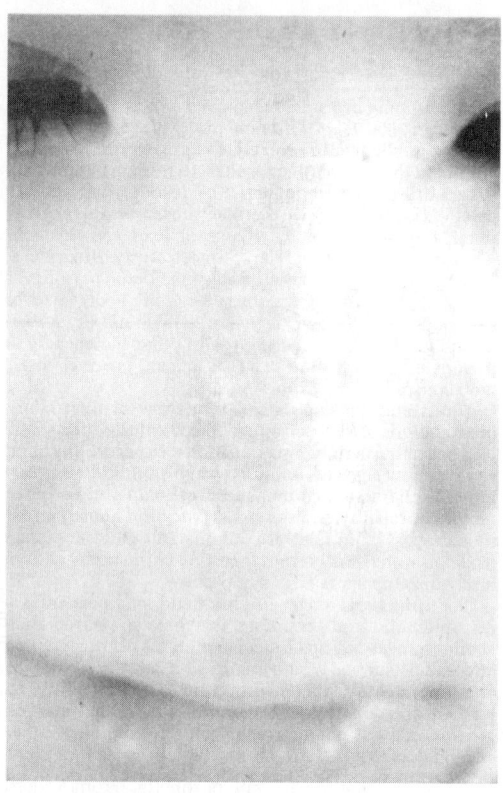

Figure 47-26. Typical shallow, elliptical scars over the nose in a child with erythropoietic protoporphyria. (See Color Fig. 47-23.) (From Poh-Fitzpatrick MB. Porphyrin-sensitized cutaneous photosensitivity: pathogenesis and treatment. *Clin Dermatol* 1985;3:41, with permission.)

cytometry, a considerable number of cells (60%) had no fluorescence, whereas the remainder showed a skewed distribution of protoporphyrin with the highest content in cells with the lowest volume. The concentration of protoporphyrin in reticulocytes was 50 to 60 times higher than the mean concentration in more mature red cells. This is because protoporphyrin leaks out of red cells with a half-life of approximately 12 to 14 days (395). There are apparently two populations of reticulocytes, with or without protoporphyrin (395). It is interesting to note that, in EPP and CEP, a heterogeneity in the cellular porphyrin content is present among reticulocytes.

Hepatobiliary complications are a feature of concern in this particular type of porphyria, but they occur only in a minority of patients. The risk of biliary stones appears to be increased, and the stones contain protoporphyrin (396). Chronic liver disease develops in a minority of patients and is associated with marked protoporphyrin accumulation in the liver, which can begin insidiously and progress rapidly to death from liver failure (397). The life-threatening hepatic complications of EPP are characteristically preceded by increasing levels of erythrocyte and plasma protoporphyrin, abnormal liver function tests, marked deposition of protoporphyrin in liver cells and bile canaliculi, and increased photosensitivity. Artificial lights, such as operating-room lights, may cause photosensitivity, with extensive burns of the skin and peritoneum, and photodamage of circulating erythrocytes (398). End-stage protoporphyric liver disease may be accompanied by a severe motor neuropathy that is similar to that seen in the acute porphyrias (389).

Bone marrow fluorescence is almost entirely in reticulocytes rather than in nucleated erythroid cells in this disease, because, during erythroid differentiation, protoporphyrin accumulation begins just before loss of cell nuclei (Fig. 47-27) (391,399). At

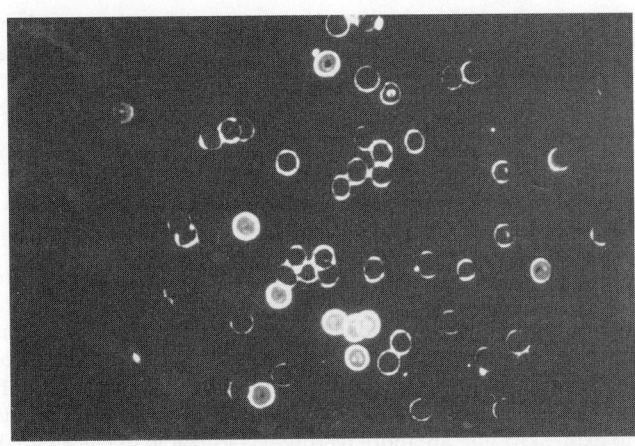 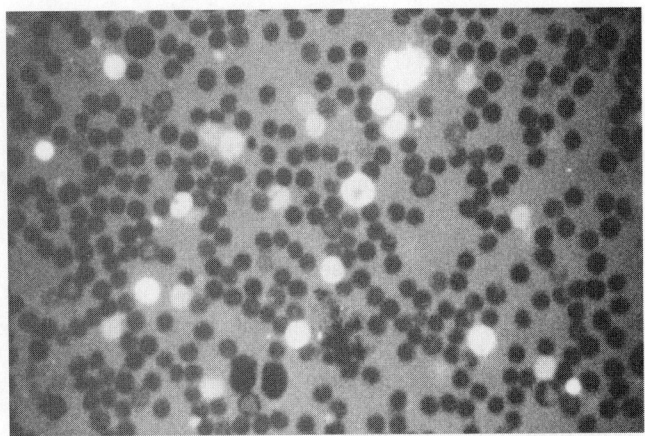

A   B

Figure 47-27. Fluorescent erythrocytes and erythroblasts in a patient with erythropoietic protoporphyria. **A:** Peripheral blood smear. Some cells contain a large amount of protoporphyrin, but others do not. **B:** Bone marrow smear. Some erythroblasts contain a large amount of protoporphyrin. Dimorphic distribution of fluorocytes in blood and of fluoroblasts in the bone marrow is characteristic of erythropoietic protoporphyria. (See Color Fig. 47-27.)

times, the liver may be an important source (391,399–402), but measuring its contribution relative to that of the erythron has not been possible (401).

Some excess protoporphyrin in EPP originates from circulating erythrocytes. Most of the excess protoporphyrin in the circulating erythrocytes in this condition is found in a small percentage of cells, and the rate of protoporphyrin leakage from these cells is proportional to their protoporphyrin content (403). Erythrocyte protoporphyrin in EPP is free and not complexed with zinc, unlike other conditions that are associated with increased erythrocyte protoporphyrin content. The content of free protoporphyrin in these cells declines much more rapidly with red-cell age than it does in conditions in which erythrocyte zinc protoporphyrin is increased (399,400). In lead poisoning and iron deficiency, the excess erythrocyte zinc protoporphyrin is bound to hemoglobin and persists in the red cell as long as it circulates, whereas free protoporphyrin in EPP binds less tightly to hemoglobin and diffuses more rapidly into the plasma. Moreover, ultraviolet light may cause free protoporphyrin to photodamage its hemoglobin binding site and thus be released from the red cell, even without disruption of the red-cell membrane. In this manner, free protoporphyrin may then diffuse into the plasma, in which it is bound to albumin (404,405). This light-mediated mechanism for the release of free protoporphyrin from hemoglobin in EPP may be important, because binding of excess free protoporphyrin to hemoglobin is usually greater than binding to plasma proteins. The capacity of the liver to take up and excrete protoporphyrin into bile may influence the flux of protoporphyrin from erythroid cells to the plasma in this disease (385). Hepatocellular uptake of protoporphyrin from plasma is favored by fatty acid–binding protein (Z protein) in hepatocytes, which binds protoporphyrin with high affinity and favors hepatocellular uptake of protoporphyrin from plasma (406).

The skin of patients with EPP is maximally sensitive to light of approximately 400 nm, which corresponds to the so-called *Soret band* (the narrow peak absorption maximum that is characteristic for all porphyrins and that photodynamically activates porphyrins) (383). Namely, when porphyrins absorb light, they enter an excited energy state, and then their energy is released as fluorescence and the formation of singlet oxygen and other oxygen radicals, thus ultimately resulting in tissue damage. This process may cause lipid peroxidation, oxidation

of amino acids, and cross-linking of proteins in cell membranes (42,266). Photoactivation of the complement system and release of histamine, kinins, and chemotactic factors may mediate skin damage (407). Damage to capillary endothelial cells in the upper dermis has been demonstrated immediately after light exposure in this disease (408).

Long-term observations of patients with EPP generally show little change in protoporphyrin levels in erythrocytes, plasma, and feces. Severe hepatic complications, when they do occur, often follow a rapid rise in protoporphyrin concentration in erythrocytes, plasma, and liver. Iron deficiency and factors that impair liver function sometimes contribute to these complications (390,409). Enterohepatic circulation of protoporphyrin may favor its return and retention in the liver, especially when liver function is impaired. Liver damage probably results, at least in part, from protoporphyrin accumulation itself, as this porphyrin is insoluble, tends to form crystalline structures in liver cells, can impair mitochondrial functions in liver cells, and can decrease hepatic bile formation and flow (397,410,411). Hepatic complications and hemolysis can be considerably improved by splenectomy (412), which suggests that the bone marrow has been the major source of excess protoporphyrin.

Biochemical Findings

Concentrations of protoporphyrin are increased in the bone marrow, circulating erythrocytes, plasma, bile, and feces. This is the only heme pathway intermediate that accumulates significantly in this disease. Erythrocyte protoporphyrin concentration can be increased in other conditions, but the increased protoporphyrin in these other conditions is less marked and is in the form of zinc protoporphyrin. Because other heme pathway intermediates do not accumulate, and protoporphyrin is excreted only in bile and feces, urinary porphyrin and porphyrin precursor concentrations are normal in EPP.

Hepatic complications of EPP are difficult to predict by laboratory tests, but they may be preceded by increased photosensitivity, increasing erythrocyte and plasma protoporphyrin levels, abnormal liver function tests, and marked deposition of protoporphyrin in liver cells and bile canaliculi. When hepatic function becomes impaired in EPP, this can contribute to further retention of protoporphyrin in the liver. An increasing ratio of erythrocyte to fecal protoporphyrin and an increasing ratio of biliary protoporphyrin to biliary bile acids also may suggest impending hepatic complications (397,413,414).

Molecular Biology

The cDNA that encodes human ferrochelatase, which has been isolated from a human placental cDNA library (415), has an open reading frame of 1269 bp that encodes a protein of 423 amino acid residues (with a molecular weight of 47,883 d). This precursor protein has a leader sequence of 54 amino acids. In contrast, the mature enzyme has only 369 amino acids (with a molecular weight of 42,168 d). Northern blot analysis for ferrochelatase showed two mRNAs of approximately 2.5 kb and approximately 1.6 kb. The variation in the length of mRNAs is due to utilization of two alternative polyadenylation signals in ferrochelatase mRNA. The human *ferrochelatase* gene contains a total of 11 exons and has a minimum size of approximately 45 kb. A major site of the transcription initiation was assigned to an adenine that was 89 bp upstream from the translation-initiating ATG. The promoter region contained a potential binding site for Sp1, NF-E2, and GATA-1 but not a typical TATA or CAAT sequence. The transcripts seemed to be identical in erythroid and nonerythroid cells.

An iron-sulfur (Fe-S) cluster, a [2Fe-2S], has been identified in the purified ferrochelatase from mouse liver and in recombinant mouse and human ferrochelatase (416–418). Comparison of amino acid sequences of ferrochelatases from humans and mice indicates that the human and the mouse enzymes contain a putative Fe-S binding site at the C-terminus. The putative binding site is a 30-residue region that contains four cysteine residues that are arranged in a sequence $(C-X_7-C-X_2-C-X_4-C)$, which is a fingerprint for a [2Fe-2S] binding motif (419). The Fe-S cluster is thought to be essential for the mammalian enzyme activity (416), but the putative binding site for the Fe-S cluster is absent from the sequences of the bacterial and yeast enzymes (417). Thus, its exact role in the enzyme reaction remains unclear.

The crystal structure of *Bacillus subtilis* ferrochelatase has been determined at 1.9-Å resolution (420). The polypeptide is folded into two similar domains, each with a four-stranded parallel β sheet that is flanked by α helices. Structural elements from both domains form a cleft, which contains several amino acid residues, including His183, that are invariant in ferroche-

latases from different organisms. This histidine residue is thought to be involved in ferrous ion binding. Based on these findings, it has been suggested that the porphyrin binds in the identified cleft, which also contains the metal binding site of the enzyme (420).

Molecular Pathology

Molecular analysis of *ferrochelatase* mutations, most of which were analyzed by cDNA sequencing, has revealed missense mutations, splicing abnormalities, intragenic deletions, and possible nonsense mutations that are associated with functional deficiency of ferrochelatase (Fig. 47-28). Among them, exon skipping was the most predominant. One possible reason for such findings is that deletions of a large fragment of DNA due to exon skipping are more readily recognizable in cDNA analysis than single nucleotide substitution.

A C→T transition at position −23 in intron 1 was first reported in a patient with EPP (421). A later study showed that the −23C→T transition was found invariably in all EPP patients, as well as in some normal controls, and there is a second and, likely, the disease-responsible mutation in patients with EPP (422). Based on these findings, it has been proposed that a mutant allele and the C→T transition in *trans* are both necessary for the expression of EPP.

Recombinant human ferrochelatase that has been engineered to have individual exon skipping that corresponds to exons 3 through 11 has been shown to lack significant enzyme activity, when it is expressed in *E. coli*. All of these mutants, with the exception of F417S, did not contain the [2Fe-2S] cluster or have enzyme activity (423).

Despite these molecular findings on the defect of the *ferrochelatase* gene, incomplete penetrance and variable clinical expression remain puzzling features of EPP. There is no strict correlation between the genetic defects and the erythrocyte protoporphyrin levels or between the abnormal ferrochelatase activity and EPP disease severity. For example, the same mutation that was found among four unrelated Swiss patients (Q59X) was associated with symptoms that ranged from mild photosensitivity to terminal liver disease (424). Clearly, the genetic background of individuals contributes to the variable expression of the disease. Gouya et al. (425) identified an EPP family in which a ferro-

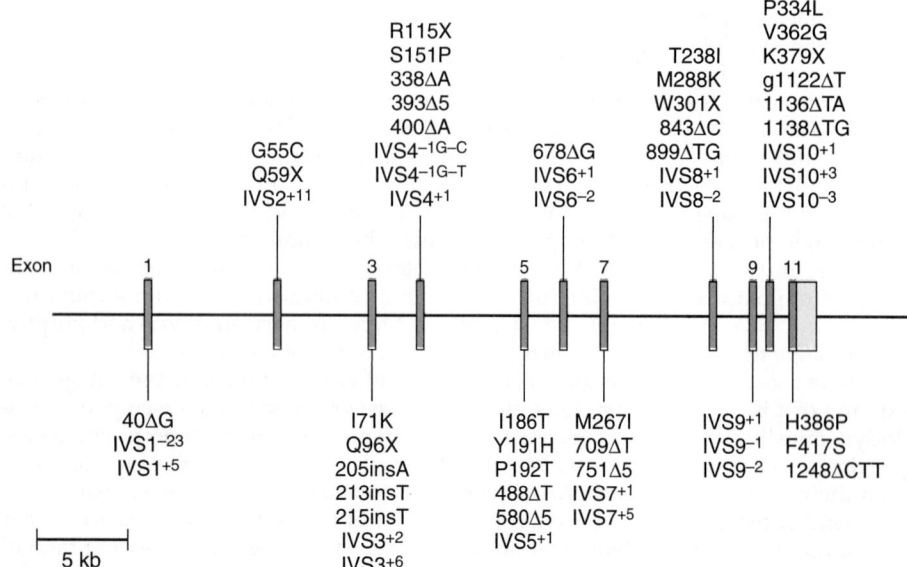

Figure 47-28. The human ferrochelatase gene, with the locations of the mutations that cause erythropoietic protoporphyria. kb, kilobase. (From Anderson KE, Sassa S, Bishop DF, et al. Disorders of heme biosynthesis: X-linked sideroblastic anemia and the porphyrias. In: Scriver CR, Beaudet AL, Sly WS, et al., eds. *The metabolic and molecular bases of inherited disease.* New York: McGraw-Hill, 2001, with permission.)

chelatase allele with a normal coding sequence was expressed at a lower than normal level. More recent studies showed five more families with EPP had a low-expression normal ferrochelatase allele, as well as a mutant allele (426). The low-expression allele, which has a particular 5' haplotype (−251A/G, IVS1-23C/T, IVS2μsatAn$_{1-10}$, 798G/C, and 1520C/T), is present in approximately 10% of the white population. Thus, inheritance of a ferrochelatase mutation in *cis* and the low expression allele in *trans* could provide an explanation for the low ferrochelatase activity and clinical expression of the disease.

Bovine EPP is an autosomal-recessive disease and probably results from a point mutation that causes only a minor to moderate change in enzyme structure (427). A potential disease-causing mutation in the bovine *ferrochelatase* gene has been associated with the bovine disease (428). A viable autosomal-recessive mutation of ferrochelatase has been described in the house mouse (429). The point mutation was the replacement of methionine by lysine at position 98 of the protein (430). Expression of the mutant *ferrochelatase* cDNA protein in *E. coli* showed a marked deficiency in enzyme activity. Similar to the human EPP, genetic background influences disease expression. This mutation (M98K) in mice has a significant effect in the BALB/c strain, with rapid development of liver failure (429), whereas it results in only mild disease in the C57Bl/6 strain (424).

Diagnosis

A markedly increased free erythrocyte protoporphyrin concentration is the hallmark of this disease. Free protoporphyrin in EPP can be differentiated from zinc protoporphyrin in other disorders by ethanol extraction or by HPLC; this differentiation is important in confirming a diagnosis of EPP.

The plasma protoporphyrin concentration is also increased in EPP and is a useful diagnostic criterion. A normal plasma porphyrin concentration in a patient with an increased erythrocyte protoporphyrin should exclude EPP, as well as other cutaneous porphyrias. Urinary porphyrin and porphyrin precursor concentrations are normal in EPP. Protoporphyrin concentrations are also increased in bile and feces in EPP. These findings help to confirm a diagnosis of EPP but should not be used in place of the measurement of porphyrins in erythrocytes and plasma.

Treatment

Oral administration of β-carotene was first reported in 1970 to be useful for treating EPP (431). Tolerance to sunlight improves in most patients who are treated with β-carotene. Improvement is usually maximal 1 to 3 months after initiation of treatment. β-Carotene dosages of 120 to 180 mg daily in adults are required to maintain serum carotene levels in the recommended range of 600 to 800 μg/dL, but dosages as large as 300 mg daily may be needed. A suntan that results from better tolerance of sunlight may lead to further protection. The mechanism of action of β-carotene may involve quenching of singlet oxygen or free radicals. The drug appears less effective in other forms of porphyria that are associated with photosensitivity, such as CEP and PCT.

Topical dihydroxyacetone and lawsone (napthoquinone) can darken the skin and have been reported to be of some benefit in EPP (384,432). Cholestyramine promotes fecal excretion of protoporphyrin and has been reported to reduce liver protoporphyrin and improve cutaneous symptoms in some EPP patients (397,433). Splenectomy may be beneficial when EPP is complicated by hemolysis and splenomegaly.

Cholestyramine and other porphyrin absorbents, such as activated charcoal, may be helpful for this situation. Other therapeutic options include red blood cell (RBC) transfusions, exchange transfusion, and intravenous hematin to suppress erythroid and hepatic protoporphyrin production (434), as well as liver transplantation (413). Although liver transplantation can be beneficial, the new liver is susceptible to protoporphyrin-induced damage (435). Unexplained increases in photosensitivity and the development of a motor neuropathy and liver failure have been observed in some EPP patients, after they are transfused with blood (436) or undergo liver transplantation (389,437).

A patient who underwent bone marrow transplantation for acute myelocytic leukemia experienced remission of EPP with marked decreases in porphyrin levels. Like other severely affected individuals with EPP, this patient had two mutations of the *ferrochelatase* gene and no normal copy of the gene. After transplant, the disease in the recipient followed the course of the donor, who, in this instance, was a sibling with one mutation and subclinical EPP.

Diagnosis of Individual Porphyrias

The porphyrias are initially diagnosed through collection of urine, plasma, or feces, or a combination of these, for analysis of porphyrin and porphyrin precursor production (Fig. 47-29).

WHEN NEUROVISCERAL SYMPTOMS ARE PRESENT

When neurovisceral symptoms that are suggestive of a hepatic porphyria are present, urinary ALA, PBG, and porphyrin concentrations should be determined in an aliquot from a 24-hour urine collection.

Urine Assays

- ALA: Normal excretion of ALA is less than 7 mg per 24 hours. During an attack of ADP, AIP, HCP, or VP, urinary ALA excretion is markedly elevated, with typical values being 3 to 10 or more times the upper limit of normal.
- PBG: Normal excretion of PBG is less than 4 mg per 24 hours. In AIP, HCP, or VP (but not ADP), increased excretion of PBG is seen, with typical values being 10 or more times the upper limit of normal.

Erythrocyte Enzyme Assay. If AIP is suspected, erythrocyte PBGD activity should be determined, because the majority of patients with AIP have approximately 50% enzyme activity compared to normal controls. In type II AIP (approximately 5% of cases), PBGD deficiency is seen only in nonerythroid cells. The decrease in enzyme activity is similar for latent gene carriers. Thus, the same test should be run in families in which a proband is identified. ALAD activity can be also determined by using erythrocytes. Moderate to low values (approximately 50% to 10% of normal levels) can be found in patients with lead poisoning, whereas extremely low values (approximately 1%) are found in patients with ADP or hereditary tyrosinemia.

All of the previously noted assays can be obtained through Quest Diagnostics, Teterboro, NJ.

WHEN PHOTOCUTANEOUS SYMPTOMS ARE PRESENT

When cutaneous or erythropoietic porphyria is suspected because of the presence of skin photosensitivity, urine and plasma porphyrin concentrations should be determined. There are always marked elevations of porphyrins, although not necessarily of ALA and PBG, in plasma and urine in these conditions, and differential diagnosis among photosensitive porphyrias is usually possible by their porphyrin excretion profiles.

Urine Porphyrin Analysis. Normal excretion of porphyrin in the urine is less than 0.3 μmol per 24 hours (<0.2 mg per 24

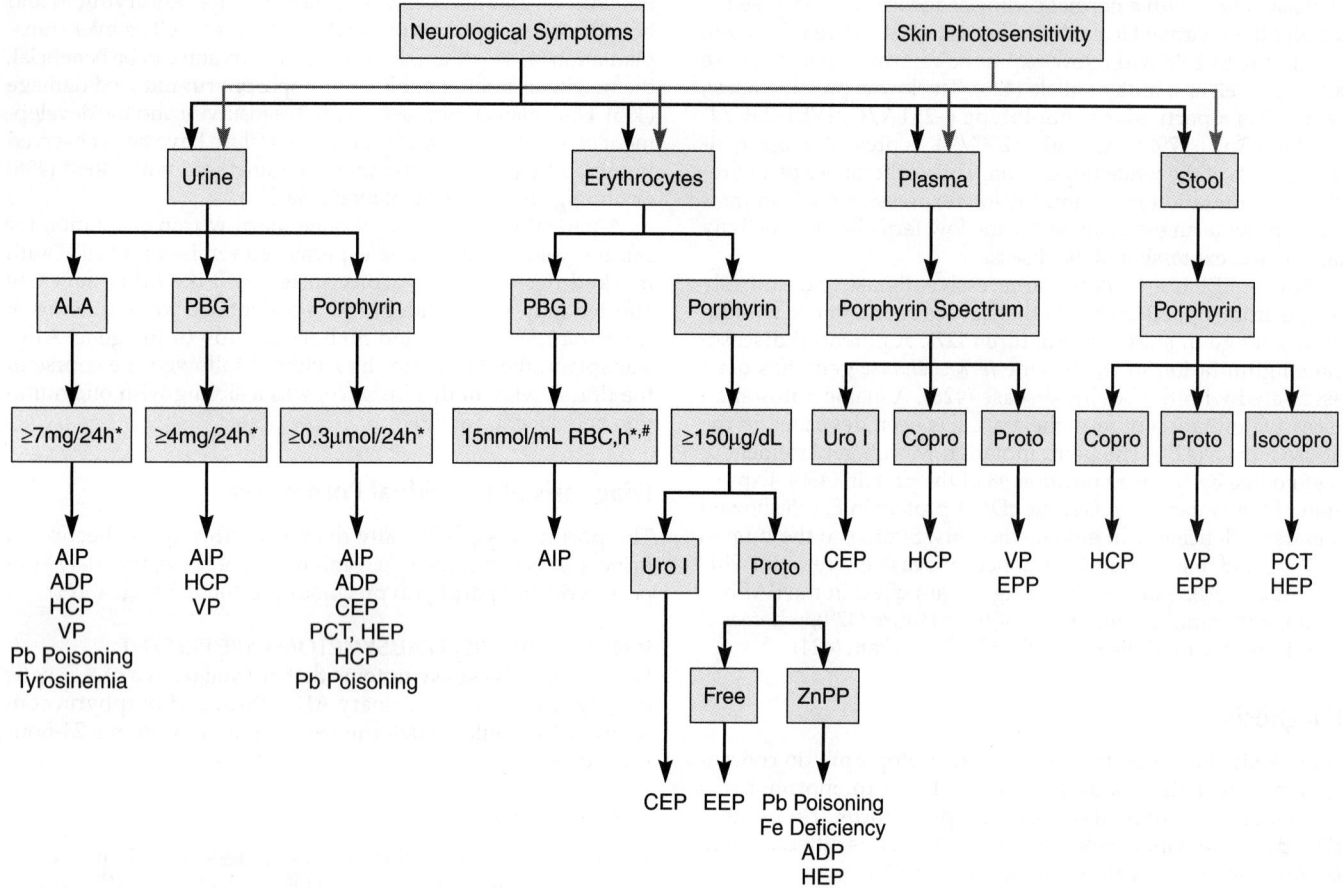

Figure 47-29. Screening strategy for porphyrias. *, values may vary, depending on the laboratory; #, 50% of normal; ADP, δ-aminolevulinic acid dehydratase–deficiency porphyria; AIP, acute intermittent porphyria; ALA, δ-aminolevulinic acid; CEP, congenital erythropoietic porphyria; Copro, coproporphyrin; EPP, erythropoietic protoporphyria; HCP, hereditary coproporphyria; HEP, hepatoerythropoietic porphyria; Isocopro, isocoproporphyrin; PBG, porphobilinogen; PBGD, porphobilinogen deaminase; PCT, porphyria cutanea tarda; Proto, protoporphyrin; RBC, red blood cell; Uro, uroporphyrin; VP, variegate porphyria. (From Sassa S. Understanding the porphyries. *Up To Date* 2001;9:2, with permission.)

hours). The presence of a large amount of porphyrin in urine (2 mg/day or more) is highly suggestive of one of the following porphyrias, which may be classified into several different types by HPLC analysis:

- If the uroporphyrin and coproporphyrin are type I isomers, this is virtually diagnostic for CEP. Type I isomers are also found in plasma and erythrocytes in these patients.
- If there is a marked increase in uroporphyrin and 7-carboxylate porphyrin that is greater than the amount of coproporphyrin in the urine, this is compatible with PCT and HEP.
- Predominant excretion of coproporphyrin or protoporphyrin favors the diagnosis of HCP, or VP and EPP, respectively.

Stool Porphyrin Analysis. Although neglected in practice, stool porphyrin analysis is extremely important in the diagnosis of porphyrias. For example:

- In PCT and HEP, but not in any other disorders, isocoproporphyrin is present, and its detection virtually establishes the diagnosis of PCT and HEP.
- HCP is characterized by a markedly elevated coproporphyrin in stool and urine (a few to many mg/day), whereas VP and EPP are associated with increases of protoporphyrin. Stool porphyrin analysis is also available at Quest Diagnostics, Teterboro, NJ.

Plasma Porphyrin Analysis. Plasma porphyrin analysis is equally as important as urinary and stool porphyrin analysis and often can replace stool porphyrin analysis because of its diagnostic value for PCT, VP, and EPP. It is also useful for finding type I uroporphyrin and coproporphyrin, which are characteristic of CEP. Unfortunately, commercial laboratories do not offer this assay.

LEAD POISONING

Adverse Effects of Lead

Lead poisoning has been recognized as a health hazard for more than 2000 years. This potentially preventable disorder is still a public health problem, despite extensive efforts to eliminate the sources of exposure. In humans, three major tissues are principally affected by lead: kidney, hematopoietic tissues, and CNS. If proper measures are taken, the renal and hematopoietic effects of lead are reversible, whereas the CNS effects are almost always irreversible, leaving clinically serious sequelae in affected persons. The major biochemical interactions of lead in the organism can be grouped into three categories: its high affinity for sulfhydryl groups, its competition with other biologically important divalent metals, and its effects on nucleic acid metabolism (124).

Adults and developing children show distinct clinical presentations of lead poisoning. Specifically, adults acquire lead poisoning mainly by occupational exposure and almost always show signs of chronic lead poisoning. This presentation is characterized by abdominal pain and peripheral motor neuropathy, such as radial palsy and house painter's wristdrop (438–440). In contrast, infants and children acquire lead poisoning mostly from ingestion of the metal and generally develop acute CNS symptoms.

The three basic stages in childhood lead poisoning are asymptomatic lead poisoning, in which measurable metabolic changes, but no clinical symptoms, occur; symptomatic lead poisoning, which manifests clinically as anorexia, vomiting, apathy, ataxia, drowsiness, or irritability; and lead encephalopathy, with cerebral edema that may progress to convulsions or coma (441,442). The sequelae of lead encephalopathy include chronic seizures, severe mental retardation, or death. Even with a less severe form of lead poisoning, minimal brain dysfunction is common, and various behavioral and functional abnormalities, such as hyperactivity, compulsive behavior, prolonged reaction time, perceptual disorders, and learning disability, may develop.

The term *critical effect* is used in lead poisoning to indicate the first definable effect of the toxic metal. The critical effect denotes the most sensitive and specific biologic change, which is beyond acceptable physiologic variation, rather than the most serious effect that is caused by metal. The critical effect occurs in the hematopoietic system, and environmental limits to prevent the irreversible effects of lead on the CNS are determined by using reversible effects in the hematopoietic system. The first metabolic effects in children become evident when the blood lead concentration exceeds 15 to 20 µg/dL. Potent inhibition of erythrocyte ALAD activity and moderate increases in erythrocyte protoporphyrin are observed at these blood lead levels (443,444). More detailed information can be found in comprehensive accounts (445–447).

Sources of Lead in the Environment

Lead occurs in nature mainly as a sulfide. Natural sources contribute little to the present daily concentrations of lead in our environment. The most useful records of natural concentrations of lead are found in chronological layers of snow strata, which are present in quiescent ice sheets in perpetually frozen polar regions (448). Annual ice layers from the interior of northern Greenland show that lead concentrations in 800 B. C. were less than 0.0005 µg/kg, whereas they were greater than 0.2 µg/kg in 1965 A. D., which is more than a 400-fold increase in 2000 years and more than a 16-fold increase after the start of the Industrial Revolution. Antarctic continental ice sheets fail to show similar changes, perhaps due to barriers to north-south tropospheric mixing that prevent the migration of the aerosol pollutants, which are mainly emitted in the Northern Hemisphere, to the Antarctic.

The relative inertness and malleability of the metal are useful features for many purposes. Lead is used widely in the electric storage battery, petroleum, and paint industries. Until the ban on the use of lead in gasoline, 98% of airborne lead could be traced to this source—the combustion of gasoline that contains lead additives. The levels of atmospheric lead in large cities are significantly higher than levels in small rural towns, because of emissions from automobiles. The number of children with blood lead levels of 60 µg/dL doubled in areas with vehicular densities that were greater than an average of 24,000 vehicles per weekday, compared to areas with vehicular densities less than 24,000 (449).

Occupational lead exposure results largely from inhalation of lead dust. In contrast, gastrointestinal absorption represents the most important route of lead absorption in children. In addition, a small amount of lead can be absorbed through the skin; this is usually of minor significance. Approximately 300 µg of lead per day is ingested naturally (450). Adults may absorb less than 10% of the daily intake of lead (399,405), whereas young children may absorb as much as 50% through the gut (451). Daily absorption of up to 40 µg/day may be tolerated for a lifetime with no apparent detrimental effects (452).

Lead in paint films is less well absorbed than dietary lead. Approximately 17% of lead in paint would be absorbed by a young child, compared to 50% absorption of dietary lead. *Pica*, the repetitive ingestion of nonfood substances, occurs in approximately 50% of children between 1 and 3 years of age. It is considered normal behavior until a child is 3 years of age; persistence of the habit beyond this age is associated with psychosocial complications or organic brain damage. Children with pica may ingest 1 to 3 g of paint chips per week (453). Children with normal blood lead levels of 20 µg/dL on a normal diet absorb lead at a rate of approximately 4.5 µg/kg/day (453). A child with pica for paint [containing the legal limit of 0.5% (weight to volume), or 5000 µg of lead per gram of paint] may absorb three to seven times more lead than a child with a normal diet. Thus, for a child with pica, 0.5% lead in paint clearly represents a hazard (453). Pica, which is often associated with iron deficiency, presents as a risk factor for lead poisoning, because lead poisoning in children is frequently found together with iron deficiency anemia. Lipids or milk in the diet may facilitate the retention of ingested lead. In addition, dietary deficiencies of calcium, copper, and iron increase the absorption of lead in experimental animals.

Hematologic Effects of Lead

One of the most evident sites of the toxic effects of lead is the hematopoietic system. Anemia and disturbances in heme biosynthesis occur in lead poisoning. Two principal enzymatic sites in the heme biosynthetic pathway are subject to inhibition by lead: ALAD and ferrochelatase (Fig. 47-30). Both enzymes are sulfhydryl dependent, and lead interferes with their activities by binding to critical sulfhydryl groups.

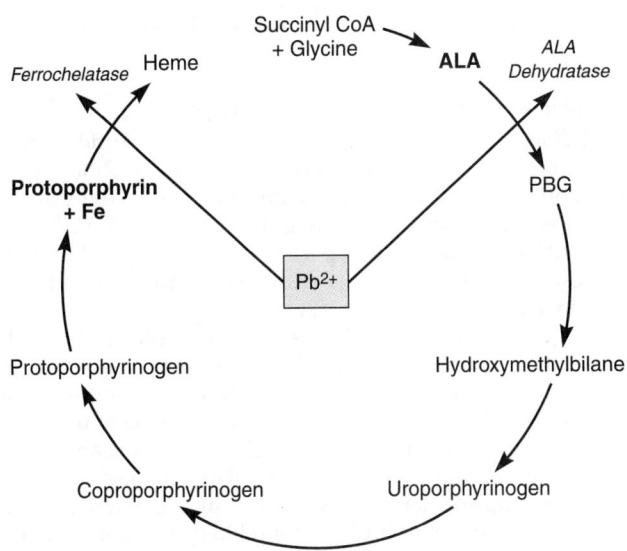

Figure 47-30. Effects of lead on heme biosynthesis. ALA, δ-aminolevulinic acid; CoA, coenzyme A; PBG, porphobilinogen.

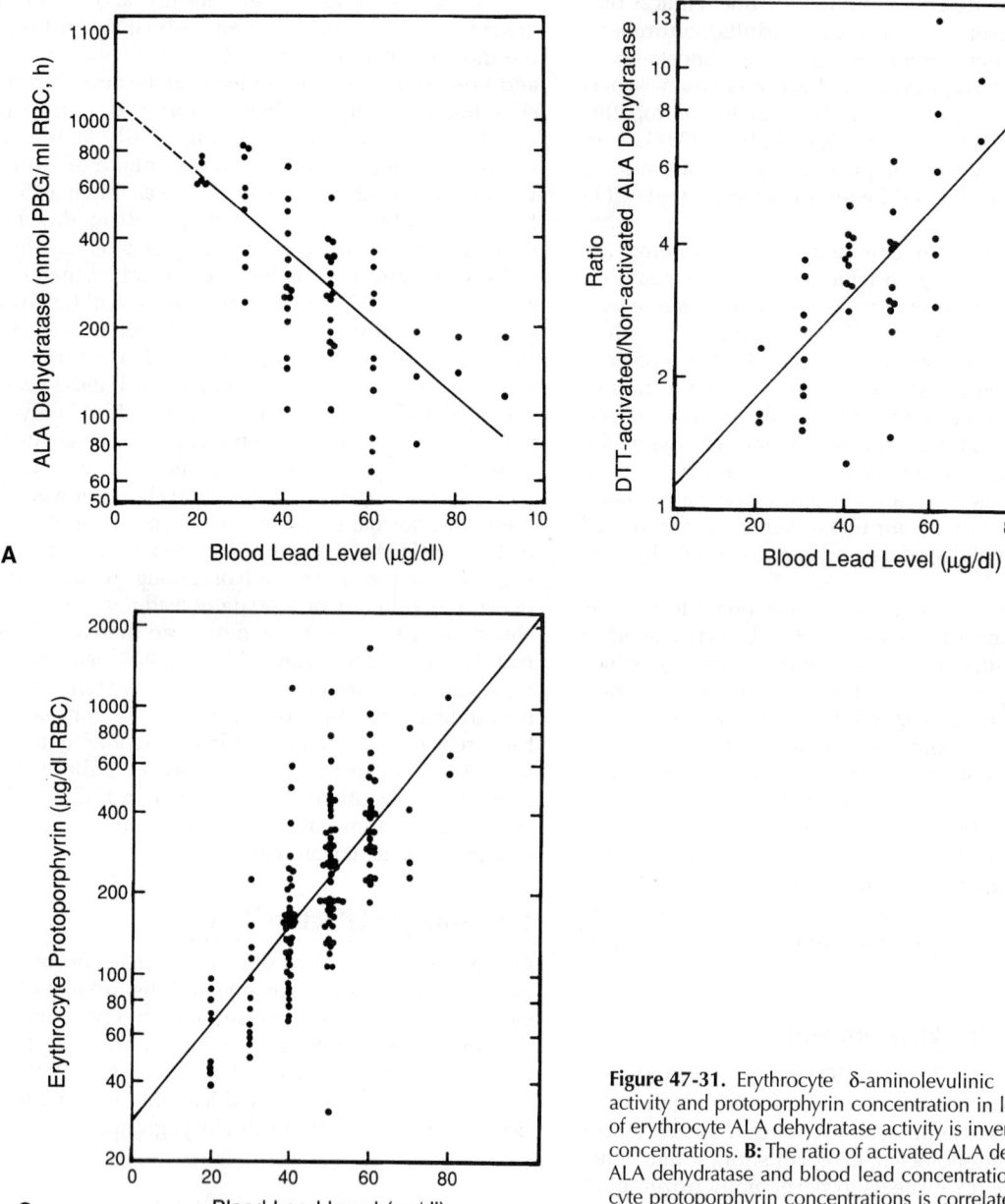

Figure 47-31. Erythrocyte δ-aminolevulinic acid (ALA) dehydratase activity and protoporphyrin concentration in lead poisoning. **A:** The log of erythrocyte ALA dehydratase activity is inversely related to blood lead concentrations. **B:** The ratio of activated ALA dehydratase to nonactivated ALA dehydratase and blood lead concentrations. **C:** The log of erythrocyte protoporphyrin concentrations is correlated with blood lead levels. DTT, dithiothreitol; PBG, porphobilinogen; RBC, red blood cell.

δ-AMINOLEVULINIC ACID DEHYDRATASE

Lead displaces the zinc atom in ALAD by mercaptide formation, thus resulting in inactivation of the enzyme. Zinc supplementation can restore the lead-inhibited enzyme activity *in vitro* (454). Lead does not interfere with the synthesis of ALAD. On the contrary, evidence in experimental animals and humans suggests that the synthesis of ALAD is stimulated in reticulocytes in lead poisoning (455–457).

The inhibition of ALAD by lead *in vivo* results in accumulation of the substrate, ALA, which is then excreted in the urine. Lead inhibition of ALAD activity in erythrocytes represents one of the most sensitive indices of the biologic effects of the metal. The log of enzyme activity is inversely related to lead concentration in blood (443) (Fig. 47-31A). The enzyme activity is decreased approximately 50%, with an increase in blood lead concentration of 20 μg/dL. Lead-inhibited ALAD activity can be completely reactivated, over a wide range of blood lead concentrations, by incubating blood samples in the presence of sulfhydryl-donating reagents, such as dithiothreitol or reduced

glutathione. Erythrocyte ALAD in normal blood is also activated twofold by dithiothreitol, which suggests that the enzyme in normal blood is present in a partially inactivated form (443).

The broad distribution of enzyme activities compared to blood lead concentrations ($r = .72$) (Fig. 47-31A) is partly due to genetic variation of enzyme activity (443). On the other hand, the ratio of dithiothreitol-activated enzyme to nonactivated enzyme activity is not influenced by genetic variation of the enzyme activity and shows a linear regression, when compared to blood lead levels with a higher correlation coefficient ($r = .8$) (Fig. 47-31B) (443). The minimum blood lead level that displays any evident effect on erythrocyte ALAD activity is approximately 15 μg/dL (443); this level can thus be considered the critical effect concentration of lead in humans.

FERROCHELATASE

Ferrochelatase, the terminal enzyme of the heme biosynthetic pathway, is also subject to marked inhibition by lead. Abnormal accumulations of iron have been reported in the mitochondria of erythroblasts from animals with experimental lead poisoning (458), presumably due to a block at the ferrochelatase step. Ferrochelatase activity in erythropoietic tissues appears to be more vulnerable to inhibition by lead than the enzyme in nonerythropoietic tissues, because the hepatic enzyme is not influenced in animals that are treated with the metal (459). Inhibition of ferrochelatase in erythropoietic tissues *in vivo* results in the accumulation of erythrocyte protoporphyrin. Because circulating erythrocytes in mammals do not contain mitochondria, the elevated erythrocyte protoporphyrin in lead-poisoned subjects must reflect the inhibition of ferrochelatase in bone marrow erythroblasts and reticulocytes.

The levels of erythrocyte protoporphyrin represent an average of the effects of bone marrow lead on erythroid ferrochelatase during the 3-month (approximate) lifespan of circulating erythrocytes (444). Erythrocyte protoporphyrin is therefore a good indicator of chronic lead exposure [see also a review (460)]. The log of erythrocyte protoporphyrin is linearly correlated with blood lead levels (Fig. 47-31C). Erythrocyte protoporphyrin has been frequently referred to as *free erythrocyte protoporphyrin*; the porphyrin is largely chelated with zinc in humans (461). Zinc cytochrome *c* has also been found in lead-poisoned animals (462). These findings suggest that zinc may be incorporated into protoporphyrin in place of iron, when iron incorporation into heme is inhibited by lead.

Effects of lead on other steps in the heme biosynthetic pathway are of lesser significance *in vivo*. Lead intoxication is known to cause coproporphyrin excretion into the urine. Studies in rabbits that were experimentally poisoned with lead indicate that decarboxylation of porphyrins that lead to production of coproporphyrin are only minimally affected by the metal (463). The source of coproporphyrin may not be erythroid but rather other tissues, such as kidney. Although lead-mediated inhibition of ALAD and ferrochelatase represents one of the most sensitive measures of the biologic effects of lead, this enzyme inhibition is rarely accompanied by severe heme deficiency in the erythropoietic system. For example, anemia of lead poisoning is almost always normochromic and normocytic in nature and is distinct from the hypochromic and microcytic anemia that is caused by iron deficiency that results in another form of ferrochelatase deficiency.

LEAD-INDUCED INCLUSION BODIES

Lead forms several inclusion bodies in the cell. Nuclear inclusion bodies in renal tubular–lining cells are characteristic signs of lead poisoning (Fig. 47-32). They occur most frequently in the proximal tubule and appear as dense bodies under light microscopy. The inclusion body is a lead-protein complex, and most of the lead in the kidney is sequestered in the complex (464). The nuclear protein has been found to be a nonhistone acidic protein that is enriched in glutamic and aspartic acid residues. Reversal of the formation of nuclear inclusion bodies, that is, extrusion of the bodies by evagination of nuclear membranes, occurs after chelation therapy. Thus, the nuclear protein complexes represent a labile and removable pool of the toxic metal (465).

A partial impairment of the respiratory and oxidative activities of kidney mitochondria has been reported in lead-poisoned rats. The adenosine diphosphate–stimulated respiration of mitochondria that are isolated from the kidneys of normal rats can be inhibited by lead *in vitro* as low as 0.15 to 0.2 μg/mg of mitochondrial protein. The maturing brain may be most vulnerable to the toxicity of lead at the critical period when rapid synthesis and increasing activity of respiratory enzymes takes place. Lead that is fed to suckling rats produces an encephalopathy that is similar to that seen in infants, and mitochondria that are isolated from brain, particularly from cerebellum, show

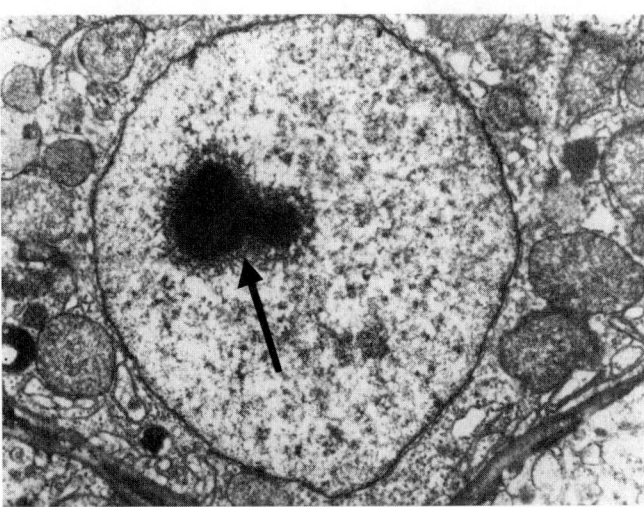

Figure 47-32. A nuclear inclusion body (*arrow*) in a proximal renal tubular lining cell of a lead-poisoned rat. (From Goyer RA, May P, Cates M, et al. Lead and protein content of isolated intranuclear inclusion bodies from kidneys of lead-poisoned rats. *Lab Invest* 1970;22:245, with permission.)

decreased nicotinamide adenine dinucleotide–linked respiration and cytochrome oxidase activity (466).

PYRIMIDINE 5'-NUCLEOTIDASE

Pyrimidine nucleotides, which result from degradation of ribosomal ribonucleic acid by ribonucleases in reticulocytes, are usually present only in minute amounts in normal erythrocytes (467). Erythrocytes that are deficient in or have inhibited pyrimidine 5'-nucleotidase activity are unable to dephosphorylate, and thus render non-diffusible, pyrimidine 5'-nucleotide monophosphates to accumulate in the cell (468). The accumulated pyrimidine nucleotides are believed to retard ribonucleic acid breakdown and result in the aggregation of undegraded and partially degraded ribosomes that are observed as basophilic stippling (468) (Fig. 47-33). Pyrimidine 5'-nucleotidase activity in normal erythrocytes can be markedly inhibited by lead or certain other heavy metals, and lead poisoning *in vivo* is associated with marked decreases in erythrocyte pyrimidine 5'-nucleotidase activity (469) (Fig. 47-34). Also, a significant correlation exists between pyrimidine 5'-nucleotidase activity and the levels of cytidine 5'-nucleotidase (CTP), as well as between erythrocyte protoporphyrin concentration and

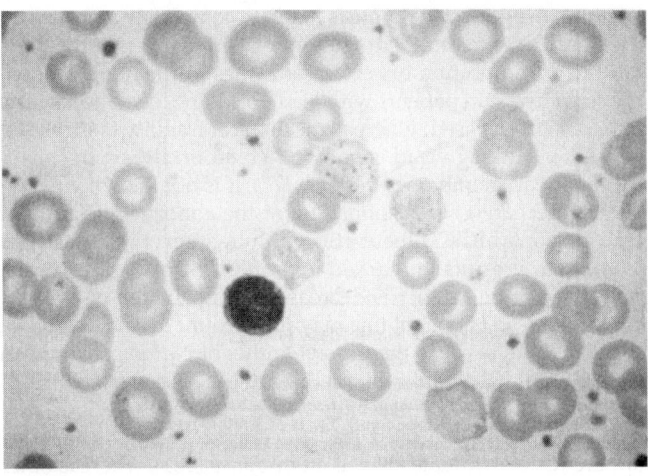

Figure 47-33. Basophilic stippling of erythrocytes in lead poisoning. (Courtesy of Dr. F. H. Bunn.)

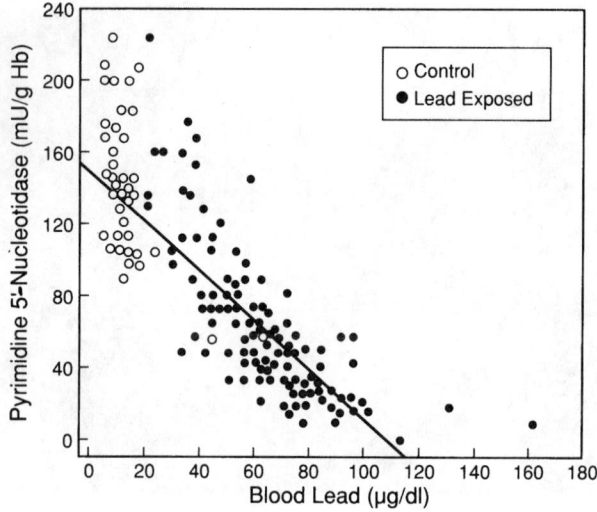

Figure 47-34. Inverse relation between blood lead and erythrocyte pyrimidine 5'-nucleotidase activity [mU/g hemoglobin (Hb); 1 U equals 1 nmol of cytidine monophosphate that is hydrolyzed per minute]. (From Angle CR, Stohs SJ, McIntire MS, et al. Lead-induced accumulation of erythrocyte pyrimidine nucleotides in the rabbit. *Toxicol Appl Pharmacol* 1980;54:161, with permission.)

CTP levels (470). The increase in CTP and uridine triphosphate antedates basophilic stippling in lead-treated animals (470). Clinically, erythrocyte pyrimidine 5'-nucleotidase activity has been shown to be a reliable and sensitive index of lead exposure (471). Decreased pyrimidine 5'-nucleotidase activity in erythrocytes reflects the chronic effects of lead on reticulocytes rather than the acute effects (472). In this respect, pyrimidine 5'-nucleotidase activity provides information that is similar to that provided by erythrocyte protoporphyrin levels. The genetic deficiency of pyrimidine 5'-nucleotidase and certain cases of lead poisoning are characterized by hemolytic anemia and basophilic stippling, and these features can be explained in part by the decreased pyrimidine 5'-nucleotidase activity that is observed in both disorders. A general discussion on hemolytic anemia and erythrocyte enzymopathies, including pyrimidine 5'-nucleotidase deficiency, can be found in a comprehensive review (473) and is discussed in detail in Chapter 53.

ANEMIA

Anemia in lead poisoning is usually normochromic and normocytic and is not associated with hypochromia. This finding suggests that sufficient heme is made to completely supplement the need for heme for hemoglobin formation, even in the presence of the inhibition of certain enzymes in the heme biosynthetic pathway. In patients with lead poisoning, osmotic fragility of RBCs is decreased, whereas mechanical fragility is increased (474,475). Although lead is known to bind firmly to phosphatidylcholine in membranes *in vitro* (476), it is not known whether such a mechanism is responsible for the abnormal fragility of lead-poisoned RBCs. Incubation of human erythrocytes with lead *in vitro* results in marked loss of K+ (477,478). Membrane [Na+,K+]ATPase activity is decreased by incubation of erythrocytes with lead (479), but this may not account for the leakage of K+ from cells, because the passive influx of Na+ is greater than the efflux of K+. Renal tubular [Na+,K+]ATPase activity is also markedly inhibited by incubation with lead (480).

Some studies that used lead tracers showed that the metal apparently accumulates in cell membranes (481), whereas other studies showed that the metal is preferentially bound to hemoglobin and some low-molecular-weight material in the cytosol

(482). At any rate, these findings suggest that anemia in lead poisoning is more likely due to a shortened lifespan of erythrocytes than to impaired heme synthesis. The extent to which the RBC lifespan is diminished also correlates most closely with the reticulocyte count (483). It should also be noted that the anemia in acute severe lead exposure is characterized by hemolysis, whereas prolonged and increased exposure leads ultimately to erythroid hypoplasia and marked morphologic changes in the bone marrow (453).

When normal erythrocytes are incubated with lead *in vitro*, suppression of pentose phosphate shunt activity is observed, together with decreased glutathione and Heinz body formation (484). This suggests that lead-poisoned erythrocytes are more sensitive to oxidant stress than normal cells and that the suppression of the pentose phosphate shunt may, in part, account for the shortened lifespan of erythrocytes in lead poisoning.

Treatment

Chelation therapy should be instituted when evidence of increased absorption or accumulation of lead in tissues is found. In addition, patients should be removed from the source of lead exposure. In the case of occupational exposure, this can be achieved by permanent isolation or, sometimes, even by rotation of workers. Physicians need to identify unusual sources of lead exposure, such as the burning of battery casings (485,486), improperly lead-glazed culinary ware (487,488), old tapestries that contain high amounts of lead (489), glass-making materials (490), artists' paint pigments (489), and lead dust in shooting galleries (491). Patients with blood lead levels that are lower than 80 μg/dL blood can be treated with chelating agents on an ambulatory basis, whereas those with higher blood lead levels should probably be treated in hospitals.

Three chelating agents are commonly used to treat lead poisoning. British antilewisite (2,3-mercaptopropanol) is given as a single injection of up to 4 mg/kg to promote excretion of lead. In adults, 3 mg/kg appears to be better tolerated (492). Although some authorities consider that British antilewisite has a place either singly or in combination therapy, this agent has been largely superseded by calcium-disodium ethylene diamine tetraacetic acid (edathamil calcium disodium, or calcium versenate) and penicillamine (492). Calcium-disodium ethylene diamine tetraacetic acid, 12.5 mg/kg, is administered intramuscularly and increases the urinary excretion of lead by 30- to 50-fold (492). D-Penicillamine can be administered orally in dosages of 150 mg twice daily for 4 to 6 weeks in children; 250 to 500 mg twice for adults increases renal lead excretion three to eight times (493), although it produces a marked zinc uresis as well (494). In addition to chelation therapy, subsequent exposure to lead should be carefully monitored, because this will ensure the most effective means of prevention of the accumulation of an increased body burden of lead. During treatment, patients should be monitored by daily total urinary lead excretion and blood lead concentrations.

HEMOGLOBIN AND HEME TRANSPORT

Senescent erythrocytes are removed and catabolized by macrophages in the reticuloendothelial system (Fig. 47-35). Free hemoglobin that is released from ruptured erythrocytes (intravascular hemolysis) is bound by haptoglobin and rapidly cleared from plasma by hepatic uptake because hemoglobin is a potent cytotoxic agent; it is especially well known as a nephrotoxin (495). Haptoglobin belongs to the members of the acute phase proteins that increase during acute inflammation or after exposure to toxic stimuli (496). Conversely, plasma haptoglobin level is decreased

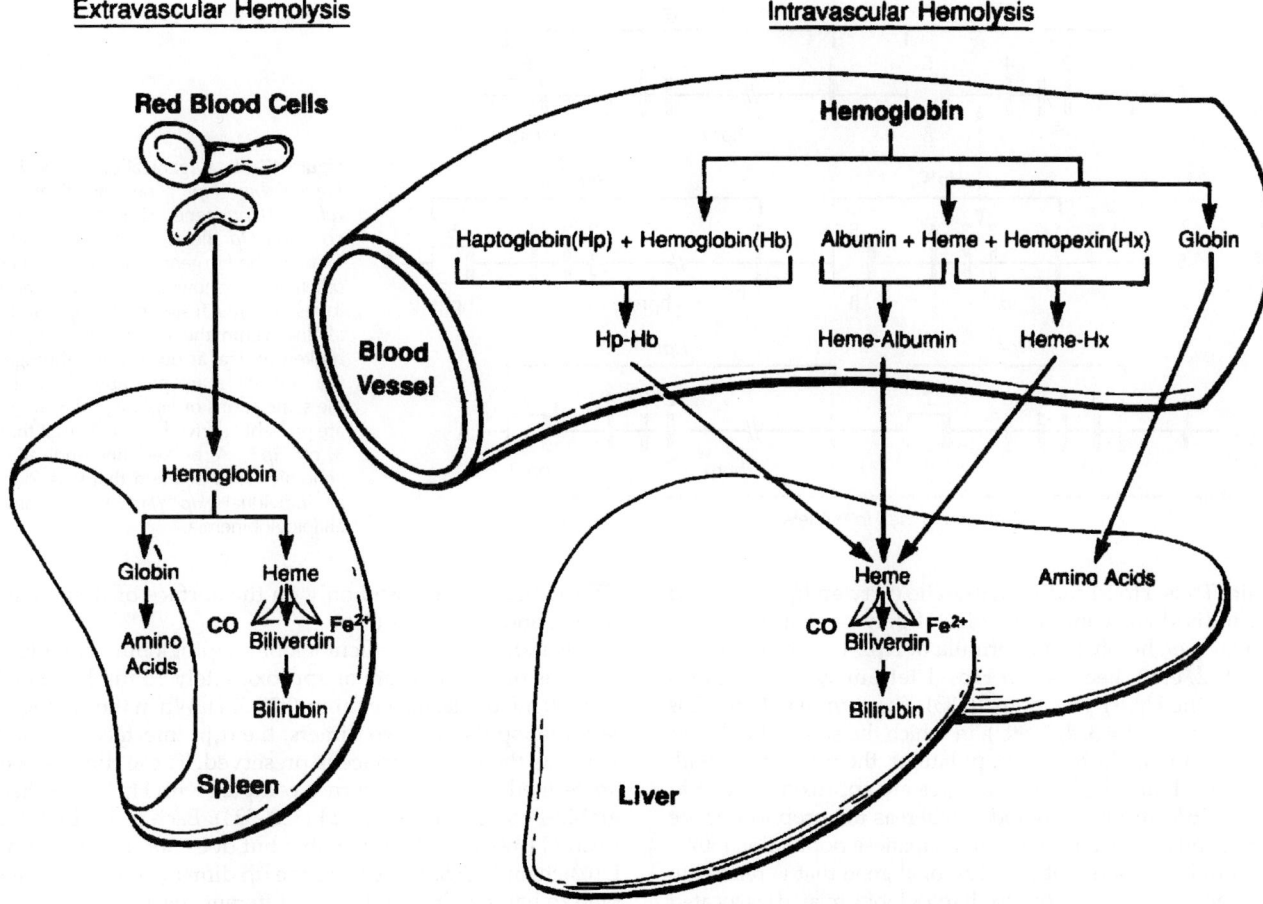

Figure 47-35. Transport and degradation of hemoglobin and heme. There are two major routes for heme disposal after hemoglobin is released from red blood cells. One is extravascular hemolysis, which occurs mainly in the spleen, and the other is intravascular hemolysis. After intravascular hemolysis, free hemoglobin forms a complex with haptoglobin, whereas heme forms a complex with albumin or hemopexin and is then transported to the liver. Heme is cleaved by heme oxygenase to release biliverdin, carbon monoxide (CO), and ferrous iron (Fe^{2+}).

in hemolytic conditions or severe hepatocellular diseases. Heme in the circulation is essentially all bound by albumin and hemopexin; thus, free heme is not usually found in plasma.

Haptoglobin

STRUCTURE AND GENETICS

Haptoglobin is a polymorphic plasma protein that belongs to the class of α_2-glycoproteins. Haptoglobin is synthesized mainly in the liver as a single chain, which is cleaved to an N-terminal α-chain and a C-terminal β-chain (497,498). The α-chain (approximately 9.5 kd) and β chain (approximately 38 kd) are also called light (L) and heavy (H) chains, respectively. Haptoglobin has been identified in all mammals and vertebrates that have been studied so far (499). Native rat haptoglobin is a heterotetramer that consists of two α-chains and two glycosylated β-chains, which are covalently attached by interchain disulfide bonds. A single disulfide bond exists between the α-chains, each of which is linked to a glycosylated β-chain by a single disulfide linkage (500). The molecular mass of the complete protein is approximately 85 kd in rats, and the protein can be symbolized as $(\alpha\beta)_2$ or H-L-L-H (501). This form of haptoglobin is equivalent to the Hp1-1 phenotype in humans.

Human haptoglobin is characterized by a molecular heterogeneity with three major phenotypes: Hp1-1, Hp2-2, and the het-

erozygous Hp2-1 (502). The polymorphism of haptoglobin is due to the presence of three common alleles on chromosome 16q22 (503), which are termed Hp^{1F}, Hp^{1S}, and Hp^2 and which code for α^{1F}, α^{1S}-, and α^2-chains, respectively (Fig. 47-36) (503,504). The symbols F and S represent *faster* and *slower*. The β-chain of 245 residues is common to the three haptoglobin α-chains. The α-chain (α^{1F} or α^{1S}) consists of 83 amino acid residues, but the α^{1F}-chain has a higher electrophoretic mobility than the α^{1S}-chain, owing to the amino acid differences at positions 53 and 54: Asp-Lys in the α^{1F}-chain and Asn-Glu in the α^{1S}-chain (504). The Hp^2 allele appears to originate from a fusion of a Hp^{1F} allele and a Hp^{1S} allele within different introns of the two alleles (Fig. 47-36). Thus, the α^2-chain consists of 142 residues, owing to a partial duplication of the α^1-chain (the fusion of exons 1 through 4 of the Hp^{1F} allele and exons 3 through 5 of the Hp^{1S} allele) (504).

Hp1-1 and Hp2-2 individuals are homozygous for the Hp^1 allele (Hp^{1F} and Hp^{1S}) and the Hp^2 allele, respectively. The Hp1-1 phenotype could come from three genotypes, Hp^{1F}/Hp^{1F}, Hp^{1F}/Hp^{1S}, and Hp^{1S}/Hp^{1S}, and the heterozygous Hp2-1 could come from two genotypes, Hp^{1F}/Hp^2 and Hp^{1S}/Hp^2. However, for simplicity, the different Hp^1 alleles are ignored in the subsequent discussion. Thus, Hp1-1 subjects contain a tetramer that consists of two α^1-chains and two β-chains that are linked by a disulfide, which is indicated as $(\alpha^1\beta)_2$. In contrast to the α^1-chain, the α^2-chain contains an additional cysteine residue that forms an intermolecular disulfide bond with the α^1-chain or the

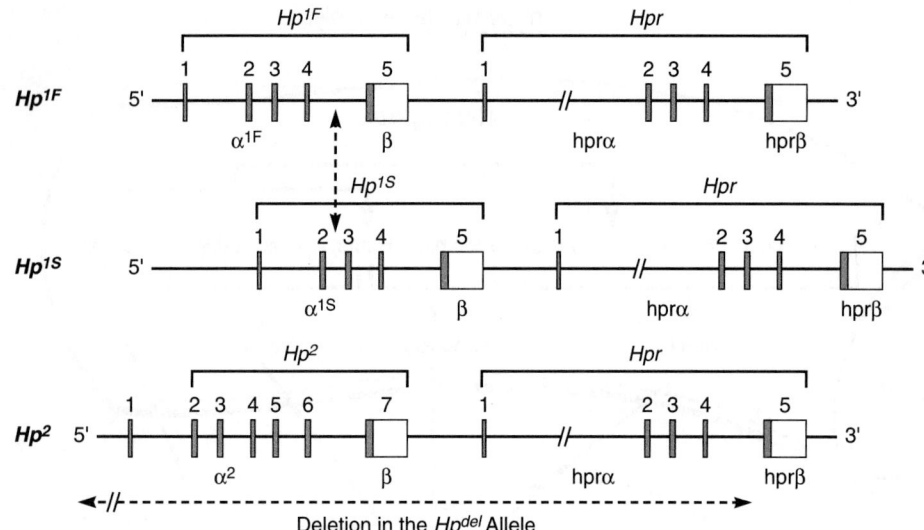

Figure 47-36. Organization of the human *haptoglobin* (*Hp*) gene and *haptoglobin-related* (*Hpr*) gene. Shown are the three common *Hp* alleles, *Hp1F*, *Hp1S*, and *Hp2*. Exons of the *Hp* genes and the *Hpr* gene are schematically shown. The *Hp2* allele appears to result from a fusion of the *Hp1F* and *Hp1S* alleles within the introns marked by the broken vertical arrow. Exons 1 through 4 of the *Hp2* allele are probably derived from the same exons of *Hp1F*. Exons 5 through 7 are probably derived from exons 3 through 5 of *Hp1S*. A broken line indicates the genomic DNA deletion that was found in an individual (*Hpdel/Hpdel*) with complete ahaptoglobinemia.

α^2-chain. Thus, Hp2-1 individuals, who carry an *Hp2* allele, and Hp2-2 individuals contain a series of polymers of increasing molecular weight (505). The formula of Hp2-1 is $(\alpha^1\beta)_2 + (\alpha^2\beta)_n$ ($n = 0, 1, 2$, etc.), because an Hp1-1 tetramer, $(\alpha^1\beta)_2$, is also present in the Hp2-1 phenotype (523). The formula of Hp2-2 is shown as $(\alpha^2\beta)_n$ ($n = 3, 4, 5$, etc.), in which the smallest polymer is a trimer. Among European populations, the proportions with Hp1-1, Hp2-1, and Hp2-2 phenotypes are approximately 16%, 48%, and 36%, respectively (506), whereas the proportions are 7%, 35%, and 58%, respectively, in a Japanese population (507).

It should be noted that an additional gene that is related to the *Hp* gene and termed *Hpr* (for haptoglobin-related) is located approximately 2.2 kb downstream from the *Hp* gene (Fig. 47-36) (508). The *Hpr* gene appears to be generated by duplication of the *Hp* gene (497). Haptoglobin-related protein (Hpr) is a serum protein that shows more than 90% identity to haptoglobin but does not bind hemoglobin (509). Hpr was suggested to be involved in the killing of trypanosomes (510–512). A more detailed discussion on the properties and genetics of haptoglobin can be found in a comprehensive review (513).

Recently, a new *Hp* allele, *Hpdel*, was identified in an individual with complete absence of serum haptoglobin. This individual was homozygous for the *Hpdel* allele. The *Hpdel* allele carries a 20-kb deletion of the *Hp* gene clusters, which includes the promoter region and the entire protein-coding exons of the *Hp1* (or *Hp2*) gene and the 5' half of the *Hpr* gene (Fig. 47-36) (514). Heterozygous carriers for the *Hpdel* allele show hypohaptoglobinemia. Thus, the *Hpdel* allele represents a cause of ahaptoglobinemia, which is also known as the *Hp0 phenotype*, and haptoglobin is not essential for human survival.

FUNCTION

Haptoglobin sequesters free hemoglobin that is released from erythrocytes as a result of hemolysis or inflammation. Haptoglobin efficiently forms a stable complex with free hemoglobin, with an association constant of greater than 10^{-15} mol/L (515), but does not bind free heme. The stable hemoglobin-haptoglobin complex is then removed from the bloodstream by the mononuclear phagocyte system through a receptor-mediated mechanism (499). The incorporated hemoglobin is degraded, and the iron atom of heme is recycled (516). In this manner, cellular injury in the kidney glomerulus by free hemoglobin is circumvented (517). Haptoglobin has also been suggested to restrict heme iron supply to pathogenic organisms (518). Recently, the scavenger receptor for the hemoglobin-haptoglobin complex was identified as

CD163 that is expressed only on the surface of tissue macrophages and monocytes (519).

Clearance of the hemoglobin-haptoglobin complex in humans occurs at a rate of approximately 15 mg hemoglobin per 100 mL of plasma per hour (520,521). When the hemoglobin tetramer splits into two dimers, the $\alpha_1\beta_2$ interface is exposed, whereas the $\alpha_1\beta_1$ interface is preserved. These dimers, which are termed $\alpha_1\beta_1$ dimers, form a complex with Hp1-1 (the haptoglobin-hemoglobin complex) (522–524). Each $\alpha_1\beta_1$ dimer binds to an H (β)-chain of haptoglobin but does not interact with the L (α)-chain (525,526). Because the $\alpha\beta$ dimers, not the tetramers, bind to haptoglobin, and many different species of hemoglobin bind to human haptoglobin, the sequence-invariant $\alpha_1\beta_2$-interdimer interface is probably the region of hemoglobin that binds to the H-chain (522). Residues 130 to 137, approximately, in the H-chain have been suggested to be the most likely sites of hemoglobin binding.

Approximately 35% homology exists between the haptoglobin structure and the structure of several serine proteases. Haptoglobin does not exhibit serine protease activity, because two of the three active-site amino acids of serine proteases have been substituted in haptoglobin (527). Various functions of haptoglobin and functional differences between haptoglobin phenotypes have been described in comprehensive reviews (528,529).

Differences in the susceptibility to malaria between haptoglobin phenotypes have been reported. The Hp1-1 phenotype was shown to be associated with susceptibility to severe *Plasmodium falciparum* malaria in Sudan (530) and in Ghana (531), whereas the Hp2-1 or Hp2-2 phenotype may confer protection against malaria. It is noteworthy that haptoglobin may function as a ligand of immune cells, thereby affecting the host defense response during *P. falciparum* infection.

A physiologically important role of haptoglobin in the protection of tissue damage from hemoglobin-driven lipid peroxidation was verified in haptoglobin deficient (−/−) mice (532). Contrary to the general view of haptoglobin, the haptoglobin (−/−) mice showed only a small reduction in postnatal viability and had normal clearance of free plasma hemoglobin. However, the renal tubular cells of the haptoglobin (−/−) mice were more susceptible to the tissue damage that was caused by hemoglobin-driven lipid peroxidation. Thus, one of the important functions of haptoglobin appears to be to inhibit hemoglobin-driven lipid peroxidation rather than to increase the clearance of free plasma hemoglobin.

NORMAL VALUES IN CHILDREN AND ADULTS

Haptoglobin concentrations can be determined by the capacity for haptoglobin to bind hemoglobin (533) or by electrophoresis of the haptoglobin-hemoglobin complex (534). In both cases, the haptoglobin-hemoglobin complex can be visualized by peroxidase activity by using benzidine. A double-decker rocket immunoelectrophoresis has also been used to determine free haptoglobin and its complex with hemoglobin (535).

Haptoglobin is undetectable in cord blood. Ahaptoglobinemia is also common in newborns (80% to 90%) or infants, and it is difficult to demonstrate haptoglobin by electrophoretic means in patients as old as 3 months of age (536). The absence of haptoglobin in the neonate is attributed to the intravascular hemolysis of fetal RBCs as well as to the immaturity of the liver.

Normal values of haptoglobin in adults vary from 40 to 180 mg/dL of plasma (537,538). The mean levels of plasma haptoglobin in subjects with Hp1-1 are generally higher than those for Hp2-2 (539,540). Individuals with the Hp1-1 phenotype seldom have ahaptoglobinemia, whereas individuals with Hp2-1 phenotype often have this condition. Despite the biologic functions of haptoglobin, there is rather a high incidence of ahaptoglobinemia among healthy Africans (approximately 30%) (541). The condition of ahaptoglobinemia is clinically silent. The area of high prevalence of ahaptoglobinemia in Africa is also closely related to the belt of malaria endemicity, and the high incidence of this condition has been suggested to be partly due to malaria infection. More recent studies, however, have revealed no association between the Hp0 phenotype (ahaptoglobinemia) and *P. falciparum* parasitemia in Ghana (531) and the Solomon Islands (542). It should be noted that an individual could be classified as ahaptoglobinemic if a serum haptoglobin level is undetectable by the method that is used for detection. Thus, so-called *ahaptoglobinemia* represents heterogeneous conditions that may be due to various environmental factors and genetic factors that may affect the *Hp* gene transcription.

Ahaptoglobinemia also exists in 4% to 10% of U.S. blacks, 2% of Micronesians, and 1% or less of Europeans and other populations (543). In addition, healthy individuals may show intermittent ahaptoglobinemia without any apparent cause (544). Sickle cell trait was implicated in increased ahaptoglobinemia among blacks, owing to possible modification of expression of Hp determinants by the genetic abnormality that is associated with the sickle cell trait (545); the tendency for ahaptoglobinemia among Greek children with HbSA was also found to be higher than in those with HbA (546).

Haptoglobin levels are decreased in females (547) during pregnancy (548) and severe malnutrition (402). Several hemolytic diseases also accompany low to undetectable levels of plasma haptoglobin. For example, low haptoglobin levels were found in paroxysmal nocturnal hemoglobinuria, hereditary spherocytosis, sickle cell disease, thalassemia major, and untreated pernicious anemia (549). On the other hand, increased levels of haptoglobin are found as a result of aging, smoking, and the occurrence of malignant lymphomas, chronic and acute leukemias, alcoholic and viral hepatitis, tuberculosis, and acute pneumonia (550). Even in some patients with hemolysis, haptoglobin levels may not be decreased during an acute phase reaction, because haptoglobin is an acute phase protein (496).

Hemopexin

The heme concentration increases in plasma after hemolysis. Free heme that is found in the circulation is largely bound to plasma proteins such as albumin, α_1-fetoprotein, and hemopexin; free heme is normally not found in plasma. Free heme can be toxic to cells by promoting peroxidation of lipids and proteins (551). The role of plasma proteins in heme binding includes prevention of potential oxidative damage of cellular constituents by heme and transport of heme to its site of metabolism. Human plasma albumin has a specific heme-binding site, with a dissociation constant of approximately 1×10^{-8} mol/L, which is distinct from the principal bilirubin-binding site (552). α-Fetoprotein, the fetal counterpart of albumin, also binds heme, but with lesser affinity than albumin (with a dissociation constant of approximately 1.5×10^{-7} mol/L) (553). Hemopexin is a 60-kd glycoprotein that is mainly synthesized by the liver. Its concentration in plasma ranges from 0.5 to 2 mg/dL (554), and it has an extremely high affinity for heme (with a dissociation constant of less than 1×10^{-13} mol/L) (555). Hemopexin binds heme in a 1:1 molar ratio by histidine-iron coordination. A review article discusses these aspects in more detail (554).

Albumin appears to be the most important protein in the delivery of heme to the liver (556). Although hemopexin is removed from the circulation after intravenous administration of large amounts of heme, its role in heme transport remains unclear (557). Hemopexin may serve to tightly bind heme, so that it can prevent heme-coupled peroxidation of other cellular constituents. Heme may also be taken up by the liver directly by a membrane heme receptor (558). A study on hemopexin deficient (−/−) mice indicates that hemopexin is not essential for survival, reproduction, or iron metabolism under physiologic conditions (559). However, hemopexin plays an important protective role in the kidney, especially to the renal tubules, after acute hemolysis. Basal plasma levels of haptoglobin are unaffected in the mutant mice, but hemopexin (−/−) mice showed delayed plasma haptoglobin turnover after hemolysis. Taken together with the phenotypic consequences of haptoglobin (−/−) mice, these studies indicate that haptoglobin is the primary defense against hemolysis, followed by hemopexin, and that the two proteins cooperate with each other in the response to hemolysis.

HEME DEGRADATION AND BILIRUBIN FORMATION

Heme Catabolism

Human erythrocytes have an average lifespan of approximately 120 days in the circulation; they are then phagocytosed by macrophages in the reticuloendothelial system. Hemoglobin is broken down intracellularly with the following results: (a) the porphyrin macrocycle is cleaved at the α-methene bridge, (b) one atom of iron is released, (c) one molecule of CO is produced, and (d) the globin moiety is ultimately hydrolyzed to its component amino acids (Fig. 47-35). The porphyrin moiety is converted to biliverdin IXα, a straight chain tetrapyrrole, which is then rapidly reduced to bilirubin IXα by cytosolic biliverdin reductase. Iron is transported to the bone marrow and reused in the formation of heme. CO is bound to hemoglobin to form carboxyhemoglobin, which is transported to the lungs and is excreted as CO in exhaled air. Amino acids that result from the hydrolysis of globin peptides are reused for protein synthesis.

In humans, 250 to 400 mg of bilirubin are formed daily, approximately 75% of which is accounted for by the degradation of hemoglobin heme (560,561). If one assumes that heme catabolism is the sole source of CO in the body, the rate of bilirubin production in humans would be 4.4 ± 0.7 (mean, plus or minus the standard error) mg/kg/day (7,562). The estimated hepatic contribution to total bilirubin production ranges from

23% to 37% (563). The turnover of hepatic heme is reflected in the so-called *early labeled bilirubin* (564), of which heme from microsomal cytochrome P-450 is the most significant (565). A high percentage of early labeled bilirubin is also derived from an erythroid source, that is, ineffective erythropoiesis, and from hepatic free heme, which serves as a precursor for hepatic heme protein synthesis and as a regulator of the synthesis of ALA synthase and of heme oxygenase (566–569). Exogenously administered hemin is quickly incorporated into the hepatic free heme pool (570), as is determined by the facts that (a) a small proportion can be incorporated into microsomal (571) or cytosolic heme proteins (572), (b) it suppresses the synthesis of ALA synthase (573), and (c) it induces heme oxygenase and is itself converted to bilirubin (574).

Heme Oxygenase

In the late 1960s, heme oxygenase was discovered by Tenhunen, Marver, and Schmid (575). They found the enzyme activity in the microsomal fraction of rat spleen, liver, and kidney that catalyzes the oxidative degradation of heme to biliverdin. Under physiologic conditions, heme oxygenase activity is higher in the tissues, such as the spleen, liver, and bone marrow, in which senescent erythrocytes are sequestered and degraded. To date, at least two isozymes of heme oxygenase, which are termed *HO-1* and *HO-2*, have been identified (576–579). The putative isozyme, HO-3, was isolated from the rat brain by cDNA cloning (580), but it lacked enzyme activity, despite sharing 90% identity with HO-2. Further studies are required to establish the identity of putative HO-3. HO-1 and HO-2 are therefore described in detail.

HO-1 can be induced in cultured cells or various tissues of many animal species by treatment with the natural substrate of the enzyme, hemin, or with a number of nonheme substances (576,581–583). In contrast, HO-2 is a constitutively expressed isozyme. HO-1 and HO-2 are encoded by separate genes; the human *HO-1* and *HO-2* genes are located on chromosomes 22q12 and 16p13.3, respectively (584,585). Human HO-1 is composed of 288 amino acids with a molecular mass of 33 kd and shares 80% amino acid sequence identity with rat HO-1 (586). HO-1 contains a hydrophobic segment of 22 amino acid residues at the carboxyl terminus (576), which may be important for the insertion of HO-1 into the endoplasmic reticulum after its synthesis on free polysomes (582). It is noteworthy that human, rat, and porcine HO-1 contain no cysteine residues, whereas one cysteine residue is present in mouse and chicken HO-1 (576,586–589). Thus, human HO-1 protein lacks a free sulfhydryl group that can be subject to an oxidative attack under various stress conditions. In contrast, human HO-2 consists of 316 amino acids, with a molecular mass of 36 kd, and contains three cysteine residues (590,591). The overall similarity in the amino acid sequences between the two isozymes is approximately 43%. HO-2 contains the extended amino terminus and a hydrophobic domain at its carboxyl terminus that is also required for membrane association (592). HO-2 has two heme-binding sites that are not involved in the heme breakdown reaction, which suggests that HO-2 may also sequester heme to reduce heme-mediated oxidative stress (593). In this context, it is interesting to note that HO-2 is expressed in hepatic parenchymal cells, whereas HO-1 expression is localized in Kupffer's cells (594).

In 1997, Poss and Tonegawa (595,596) provided direct evidence for the physiologic importance of HO-1 by generating HO-1–deficient mice. Mating between heterozygous mice showed partial prenatal lethality of the HO-1–deficient (–/–) mice, and homozygous mating pairs did not yield viable litters. The adult HO-1 (–/–) mice developed an anemia that was asso-ciated with low serum iron levels but increased serum ferritin levels. Iron accumulated in Kupffer's cells and hepatocytes and in renal proximal cortical tubules. Such iron deposits contributed to oxidative damage, tissue injury, and chronic inflammation. Moreover, adult HO-1 (–/–) mice were more vulnerable to hepatic necrosis and death, when they were challenged with endotoxin. Thus, HO-1 is required for iron reutilization, and the induction of HO-1 represents a defense mechanism to protect cells from oxidative damage. In contrast, HO-2–deficient mice showed mild phenotypes; they are fertile and survive normally for at least 1 year (597). Initially, there were no noticeable morphologic alterations in HO-2–deficient (–/–) mice, except that cerebral heme oxygenase activity was markedly reduced (597,598). Subsequent studies revealed ejaculatory abnormalities in male HO-2 (–/–) mice and increased susceptibility to hyperoxic lung damage (599,600). Thus, the function of HO-2 is not necessarily compensated by HO-1 (or vice versa).

Iron is an essential requirement for most bacteria, and *Corynebacterium diphtheriae*, a gram-positive aerobic bacterium, possesses Hmu O protein, which shares 33% identity with human HO-1 (601). This bacterium is the causative agent of diphtheria and produces a virulent diphtheria toxin, which is under the regulation of iron. Unlike mammalian HO-1, Hmu O protein lacks the hydrophobic C-terminus and functions as a soluble heme degradation enzyme (602). Heme catabolism also appears to be important for photosynthetic pigments in the plant kingdom and *Cyanobacteria* species (603,604). The *Arabidopsis thaliana* heme oxygenase isozyme shows 21% identity to human HO-1.

MECHANISM OF HEME DEGRADATION BY HEME OXYGENASE

Heme oxygenase requires the reduced form of nicotinamide-adenine dinucleotide phosphate (NADPH), molecular oxygen, and NADPH–cytochrome P-450 reductase to cleave heme (605). The HO-1 and HO-2 proteins share substrate specificity, cofactor requirements, and the ability to form biliverdin IXα (592). Heme oxygenase binds heme at an equimolar ratio and exhibits regiospecific catalytic activities by using three molecules of oxygen and at least seven electrons that are provided by NADPH–cytochrome P-450 reductase (Fig. 47-37) (605). The crystal structure of the heme-human HO-1 complex provides evidence that steric regulation is responsible for regiospecific cleavage of the α-methene bridge of heme (606). Heme catabolism by the heme oxygenase system proceeds essentially in an autocatalytic fashion on heme bound to heme oxygenase (605), in which the bound heme serves as a prosthetic group and a substrate. A review article describes this topic in more detail (607).

The initial step of heme oxygenase–dependent heme degradation is the formation of a ferric heme–heme oxygenase complex. This complex is then oxidized by a reducing equivalent that is provided by NADPH–cytochrome P-450 reductase in the presence of NADPH, yielding α-mesohydroxyheme (608–610). In the conversion of hemin to α-mesohydroxyheme, the active species of oxygen that is bound to heme on heme oxygenase attacks the α-methene bridge of heme (610–613). α-Mesohydroxyheme is further oxidized to verdoheme, consuming oxygen and another reducing equivalent (614–616). The α-methene carbon is released as CO at this step of the oxidation process. Generally, CO binds ferrous heme iron with a higher affinity than does oxygen, but the verdoheme–heme oxygenase complex has a much lower affinity for CO, thereby preventing product inhibition of the subsequent reactions by CO (617). Conversion of the ferrous verdoheme–heme oxygenase complex to the ferric iron–biliverdin complex requires oxygen and

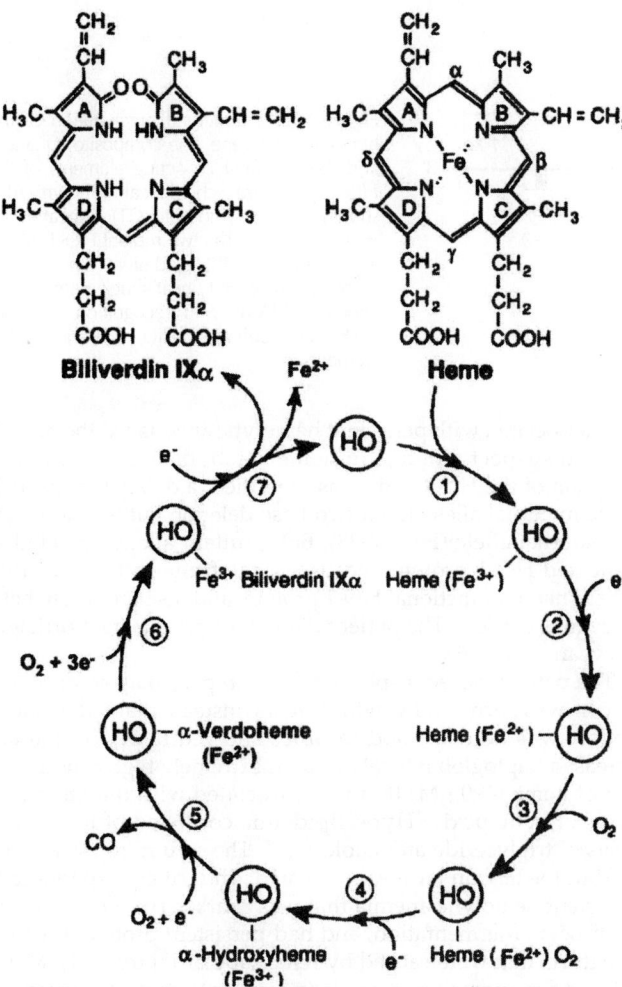

Figure 47-37. Oxidative catabolism of heme. In the series of reactions, all electrons (at least seven) are provided by nicotinamide adenine dinucleotide phosphate (NADPH)–cytochrome P-450 reductase. Heme is first bound to heme oxygenase (HO), yielding a ferric heme–HO complex (1). The subsequent heme cleavage reactions occur on the complex. Ferric heme is reduced by an electron that is provided by the NADPH–cytochrome P-450 reductase system (2). One oxygen molecule binds the ferrous heme–HO complex to form the oxygenated heme–HO complex (3). The complex receives another reducing equivalent, which is provided by NADPH–cytochrome P-450 reductase and binds the complex, and oxidative degradation of heme is initiated (4). The first oxidation product is α-hydroxyheme. Consuming another reducing equivalent, α-hydroxyheme is oxidized to verdoheme (5). The α-methene bridge carbon is released as carbon monoxide (CO) at this oxidation step. Conversion of verdoheme to the Fe^{3+}-biliverdin complex requires molecular oxygen and reducing equivalents, which presumably involves another hydroxylation reaction (6). Finally, Fe^{2+} and biliverdin IXα are released from the Fe^{3+}-biliverdin IXα complex, which consumes another reducing equivalent (7). This step is accelerated by the presence of biliverdin IXα reductase.

reducing equivalents (618). The heme oxygenase reaction is completed by the release of ferrous iron and biliverdin IXα from the ferric iron–biliverdin complex. This final step may be influenced by the presence of biliverdin reductase. In fact, biliverdin reductase appears to accelerate biliverdin release by an allosteric or direct effect (619). In this context, NADPH–cytochrome P-450 reductase, heme oxygenase, and biliverdin reductase have been shown to form a ternary complex *in vitro* in an equimolar ratio (620). This finding suggests that the cytoplasmic biliverdin reductase may interact with the binary complex of the membrane-bound NADPH–cytochrome P-450 reductase and heme oxygenase (an enzyme–enzyme interaction within

the endoplasmic reticulum). Thus, biliverdin IXα that is produced by the membrane-bound binary complex may be converted to bilirubin IXα by biliverdin reductase without leaving the enzyme complex in the membrane. The release of ferrous iron is of physiologic significance, because ferrous iron is efficiently chelated by apoferritin and stored in a ferric state within ferritin molecules or transported to the bone marrow via transferrin for recycling.

COMPETITIVE INHIBITORS OF HEME OXYGENASE

The reaction that is catalyzed by heme oxygenase can be modulated by synthetic heme analogs, in which the central iron atom of heme has been replaced by another element. These heme analogs bind more tightly to the catalytic site of the enzyme than does heme, thus resulting in various degrees of competitive inhibition of heme degradation (574,621). Such competitive inhibitors include tin, zinc, chromium, and manganese protoporphyrin and mesoporphyrin derivatives. Tin protoporphyrin and tin mesoporphyrin have been well studied and have the capacity to inhibit heme oxygenase to such an extent that they can, in small doses, significantly lower the levels of plasma bilirubin in experimental animals, normal and jaundiced adult humans, and infants with hemolytic disease of the newborn (622–626). The clinical use of these compounds is also described in the section on Prevention of Bilirubin Toxicity.

INDUCTION OF HO-1 EXPRESSION

HO-1 is characterized by its remarkable induction by hemin as well as by a number of nonheme substances, such as insulin, epinephrine, endotoxin, heavy metals, hydrogen peroxide, ultraviolet light, or sulfhydryl reagents (605,627,628). In this context, the 5'-flanking regions of the human and rat *HO-1* genes contain several potential *cis*-regulatory elements, such as heat-shock element (HSE) (Fig. 47-38) (577,628). HSE is the *cis*-acting element that is responsible for transcriptional activation of *heat-shock protein* (*HSP*) genes by heat shock. In fact, heat-shock treatment induces HO-1 in rat cells at the transcriptional level (629,630). In contrast to rat cells, heme oxygenase activity is not necessarily induced by heat shock in cultured cells that are derived from human, monkey, pig, and mouse, thus suggesting the interspecies difference in the regulation of HO-1 expression (631). In addition, there is a noticeable difference in the regulation of HO-1 expression between the cell types. For example, human HO-1 and its mRNA have been reported to be noninducible (586,632) or inducible by heat treatment (633). Thus, the HSE of the human *HO-1* gene is potentially functional (632,634), but the sequence that flanks this HSE may act as a silencer that prevents the heat-mediated activation of the *HO-1* gene under certain conditions (632). Such a silencing effect is of particular significance in the human brain, because heme degradation products possess potential toxic effects. The human *HO-1* gene has gained the silencer sequence to protect its harmful induction by heat shock. The proximal promoter region of the human *HO-1* gene also contains two copies of an interleukin-6 (IL-6)–responsive element and two functional CANNTG motifs, which is known as an *E box* (635–637). Each IL-6–responsive element overlaps the HSE or the E box. IL-6, an inducer of the acute phase reaction, increases the expression of HO-1 and haptoglobin in human hepatoma cells (635). Thus, HO-1 is a positive acute-phase reactant in hepatoma cells.

The upstream *cis*-acting element of the human *HO-1* gene, which is located at –4 kb, consists of the cadmium-responsive element and an AP-1 binding site (638,639). The AP-1 site also constitutes the NF-E2 site or Maf recognition element (640). NF-E2 is a heterodimer of an erythroid-specific subunit (p45) and a

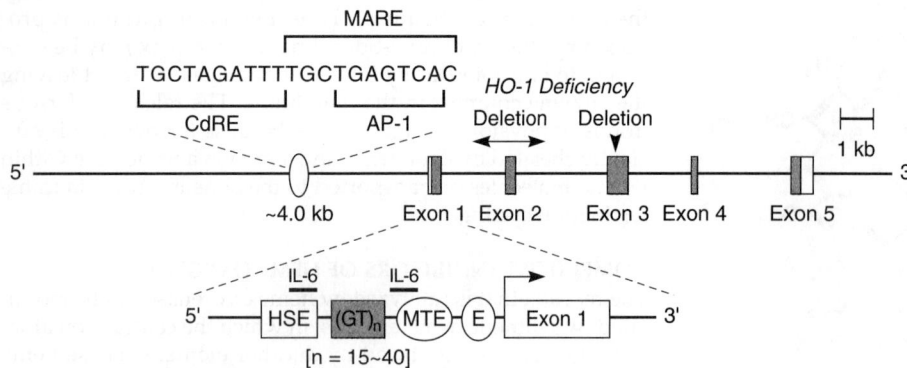

Figure 47-38. Structural organization of the human *HO-1* gene. The composite enhancer and the proximal *cis*-acting elements of the *HO-1* gene are schematically shown. Also shown is the polymorphic (GT)n repeat in the *HO-1* promoter. The two mutant HO-1 alleles are indicated. CdRE, cadmium reponse element; E, E box; HSE, heat-shock element; kb, kilobase; MARE, Maf recognition element; MTE, macrophage-specific TPA-responsive element.

member of the Maf family of transcription factors (641). Recently, a transcription repressor Bach 1 was identified as a mammalian heme-responsive transcription factor, and its repression activity was lost by heme binding, which in turn leads to transcriptional activation through the Maf recognition elements (642). Therefore, various activators and repressors, such as Bach 1, may be involved in transcriptional control of the *HO-1* gene. More detailed accounts of the induction of HO-1 can be found in review articles (631,643–645).

MICROSATELLITE POLYMORPHISM IN THE *HO-1* GENE PROMOTER

The human *HO-1* gene promoter contains a highly polymorphic (GT)n repeat that is located at –270 bp (Fig. 47-38) (646). The numbers of (GT)n repeats vary from 15 to 40 (30 to 80 bp in the Japanese population; two common repeats are 23 and 30). Because of its location at the proximal promoter, a length of (GT)n repeat may influence the basal promoter activity or the induction level of the *HO-1* gene expression under stress. It is noteworthy that polymorphic (GT)n repeats are not present at the equivalent positions in the rat and mouse *HO-1* genes. The lack of polymorphic (GT) repeats may account, in part, for the interspecies variation in the regulation of HO-1 gene expression.

The long (GT)n repeats are likely to form Z-DNA (left-handed helix), and may influence transcription from the *HO-1* gene promoter (647). In this context, longer (GT)n repeats are associated with emphysema that is caused by cigarette smoking (648). The promoter activity with a short (GT)n repeat is higher than that with a longer (GT)n repeat in cultured cells. Thus, in individuals with long (GT)n repeats (*n* >31), the degree of HO-1 induction may not be sufficient to protect the lung tissue from the damage that is caused by smoking. However, longer (GT)n repeats (n >30) might confer protection against certain pathological conditions, such as cerebral malaria, a severe complication of *Plasmodium falciparum* malaria (649). In the malaria-endemic area, the long (GT)n repeats may become fixed in a population by providing the individual with a selective advantage. Decreased production of CO, iron, or bilirubin near the site in the brain vasculature in which the parasite is sequestered may be protective against cerebral malaria. The frequency of the (GT)n repeats may vary, depending on ethnic origins or geographies, thereby modulating the expression levels of the *HO-1* gene.

HO-1 DEFICIENCY

In 1999, the first case of HO-1 deficiency was identified in Japan (650). The patient was a 26-month-old boy, who suffered from recurrent fever and severe growth retardation. His siblings and parents were healthy, except that the mother had experienced two intrauterine fetal deaths. Low serum bilirubin levels that

were associated with persistent hemolytic anemia led the physicians to suspect a defect in heme catabolism. A compound mutation of the *HO-1* gene was identified: a deletion of exon 2 in the maternal allele and a two-base deletion within exon 3 in the paternal allele (Fig. 47-38). Both mutant alleles encoded a truncated HO-1 protein because of the frameshift. Thus, the patient had no functional HO-1 protein, and his parents are heterozygous carriers. The patient died of intracranial hemorrhage at 6 years of age (651).

The patient lacked a spleen, which, in part, may account for why he was born and lived for 6 years. Instead, marked hepatomegaly was noted. Blood samples showed hyperlipidemia, increased haptoglobin levels, and an extremely high concentration of heme (490 µM) that was associated with undetectable levels of hemopexin. Hyperlipidemia consisted of increased levels of triglyceride and cholesterol. The serum iron was normal but the ferritin level was elevated. The patient experienced persistent hemolytic anemia that was characterized by marked erythrocyte fragmentation, and had persistent proteinuria and hematuria that were caused by renal tubular injury (651). Most of these symptoms are essentially similar to those observed in HO-1–deficient mice (595,596). Therefore, the essential roles for HO-1 in the host defense against oxidative stress and in iron metabolism have also been proven in humans.

Compound heterozygosity for HO-1 deficiency indicates that there are at least two inactive HO-1 alleles in the Japanese population. The one allele that lacks exon 2 may have been generated by homologous recombination that was mediated by the Alu sequence (652). This type of deletion could be relatively common in the human genome. In addition, the (GT)n repeat polymorphism generates alleles with diminished or increased transcription of the human *HO-1* gene. Because of potential cell toxicity of bilirubin, CO, and iron, the induction of HO-1 is not necessarily beneficial to the host. In fact, reports have shown that HO-1 expression is repressed in human cells by interferon-γ or hypoxia (653,654).

PATHOPHYSIOLOGIC CONDITIONS THAT ARE ASSOCIATED WITH ALTERED HO-1 EXPRESSION

Many studies show that HO-1 is involved in various human diseases and their relevant animal models. Here, only representative cases are discussed. More detailed accounts can be found in recent review articles (649,655,656).

Oxidative stress has been implicated in the pathogenesis of atherosclerosis and coronary artery disease (657,658). In the early stage of atherosclerosis, low-density lipoprotein (LDL) is oxidized in the vessel wall. Oxidized LDL is ingested by intimal macrophages, which results in the accumulation of lipid-rich foam cells. Oxidized LDL induces HO-1 expression in human endothelial and smooth muscle cell cocultures (659). In fact, HO-1 protein is expressed in atherosclerotic vessels from humans (660) and co-localizes with bilirubin IXα in foam cells of atherosclerotic lesions in cholesterol-fed rabbits, which suggests that HO-1 catalyzes heme breakdown *in situ* (661). HO-1 is also thought to be involved in the pathogenesis of various neurodegenerative disorders, including Alzheimer's disease (662–666), Parkinson's disease (667), and prion diseases (668,669). Moreover, HO-1 protein is increased in Dürck's granuloma, a typical lesion of advanced cerebral malaria (670).

Overexpression of the *HO-1* gene protects cells and hosts from the severe damage that is caused by a variety of stresses and that is of therapeutic interest (671). Protection has been reported in endothelial cells (672,673), kidney (674,675), lung (676,677), and retinal pigment epithelium (678), as well as in organ transplantation (679–681).

Carbon Monoxide

Plasma bilirubin concentrations are influenced by a number of factors and may not necessarily reflect the rate of heme degradation. In contrast, under steady-state conditions, the pulmonary CO excretion rate largely reflects the rate of heme catabolism (682). CO excretion rates have an early labeled peak, owing to the catabolism of hepatic free heme (683). The early labeled peak of CO and early labeled bilirubin are increased by treatment with phenobarbital or allylisopropylacetamide, agents that are known to increase hepatic heme turnover (682). The magnitude of the early labeled peak of CO is also increased after phlebotomy or in iron deficiency anemia and hemolysis, presumably reflecting an erythropoietic component of CO. Increased CO in exhaled air has been reported in patients with inflammatory lung diseases, such as asthma, cystic fibrosis, and upper respiratory tract infection, as well as in critically ill patients (684). Therefore, measurement of CO in exhaled air might be a good means to evaluate the degree of inflammation in patients with various disorders (685–687).

In the past decade, much attention has focused on CO as a signaling gas, similar to nitric oxide. CO has been shown to function as a neural messenger by the activation of guanylate cyclase (688–690). CO is also an endothelium-independent vasorelaxant, although it is less than one thousandth as potent as nitric oxide (691). CO reportedly inhibits platelet aggregation (692) and the proliferation of vascular smooth muscle cells (693). For example, synthetic metalloporphyrins, such as zinc- and tin-protoporphyrin, have been used to inhibit heme oxygenase activity, and results were often used to suggest the role of CO in the process. However, metalloporphyrins do not necessarily inhibit heme oxygenase activity only, thus the results may be quite complex (694).

The liver is a major site for detoxification of hemoglobin and heme. A novel role for CO has been established in the liver; CO functions as a constitutively produced modulator of hepatic sinusoidal perfusion by maintaining low hepatic vascular resistance (695,696). Moreover, CO modulates bile production and protects the liver from damage by heme overloading (697). More detailed information on this topic is available (698). CO may also have antiinflammatory effects (699) at low concentrations via the mitogen-activated protein kinase (MAPK) pathway (700).

Biliverdin Reductase

Biliverdin reductase is a cytosolic enzyme that reduces biliverdin IXα to bilirubin IXα and is present in many tissues, including the spleen and liver. A small amount of another isoform, bilirubin IXβ, is also present in the bile of newborn babies, rhesus monkeys, and dogs (701,702), as well as human adults (3% to 5% of total biliverdin) (Fig. 47-39) (703). In fact, bilirubin

IXβ is a major constituent of human fetal bile at 20 weeks of gestation, when all four possible bilirubin isomers are found [87% bilirubin IXβ, 6% bilirubin IXα, 0.6% bilirubin IXδ, and 0.5% bilirubin IXγ (704)]. Bilirubin IXβ can be excreted directly into the bile without conjugation, because bilirubin IXβ does not form internal hydrogen bonds, unlike bilirubin IXα. It is unknown how bilirubin IXβ and other isoforms are produced in the fetus.

Separate biliverdin reductases with different substrate specificities have been characterized by molecular cloning of their respective cDNAs: biliverdin IXα reductase and biliverdin IXβ reductase (705–707). The *biliverdin IXα reductase* and *biliverdin IXβ reductase* genes are localized on human chromosome 7p14→cen and 19q13.13→q13.2, respectively (708–710). Human biliverdin IXα reductase consists of 296 amino acids, with a molecular mass of 33 kd, and shows 83% amino acid sequence identity with the rat enzyme (706,710). The estimated molecular mass is consistent with that of the purified enzyme from pig spleen and rat liver (711,712), and the enzyme uses NADPH or NADH as a cofactor. Biliverdin IXα reductase shows extensive microheterogeneity that may be caused by posttranslational modification (703). Human biliverdin IXβ reductase consists of 206 amino acids with a molecular mass of 21 kd (707). It was found that biliverdin IXβ reductase is identical to NAD(P)H-linked flavin reductase (4,5). Flavin reductase is predominantly expressed in erythrocytes and may function as a methemoglobin reducing enzyme. The crystal structures of rat biliverdin IXα reductase and human biliverdin IXβ reductase suggest that the two reductases share a common reaction mechanism, despite the different amino acid sequences (713,714).

Bilirubin

CHEMISTRY

Bilirubin is lipophilic in solution *in vitro*, whereas it behaves as a relatively polar compound in circulation by binding to albumin (715). Binding of bilirubin with polar lipids may be an important factor in directing its transit through cellular membranes. Although biliverdin IXα and bilirubin IXα have two propionic acid side chains, the latter is far less soluble in aqueous solutions than the former, probably because it takes a "ridge tile" conformation by intramolecular hydrogen bonding that involves the two propionic acid side chains (716–718). As a result, rings A and B of bilirubin IXα lie in one plane, and rings C and D lie in another plane.

Bilirubin IXα in organic solvents has a strong absorption band at approximately 460 nm with a molar extinction coefficient of approximately 60,000 (719). Pure bilirubin does not fluoresce; it emits an intense fluorescence (with maxima occurring at 510 to 530 nm), when it is dissolved in a detergent, such as alkaline methanol, or albumin solution (720,721). When bilirubin in solution is exposed to light in air, it undergoes photooxidation that results in colorless products (721). These products are a mixture of maleimides and propentdyopents, and they reflect random fission of the tetrapyrrole structure by singlet oxygen. Bilirubin also undergoes geometric isomerization by light to yield more polar isomers, which are termed *photobilirubin* or *lumirubin*. Propentdyopents and photobilirubin are more polar than bilirubin, which probably explains the efficacy of phototherapy in lowering plasma bilirubin levels (722–724).

Bilirubin is toxic to a wide variety of biochemical functions in many cell types. For example, oxidative phosphorylation and ATPase activity of brain mitochondria are inhibited by bilirubin, and mitochondria swelling can be demonstrated after bilirubin treatment (725–727). Rapidly developing and irrevers-

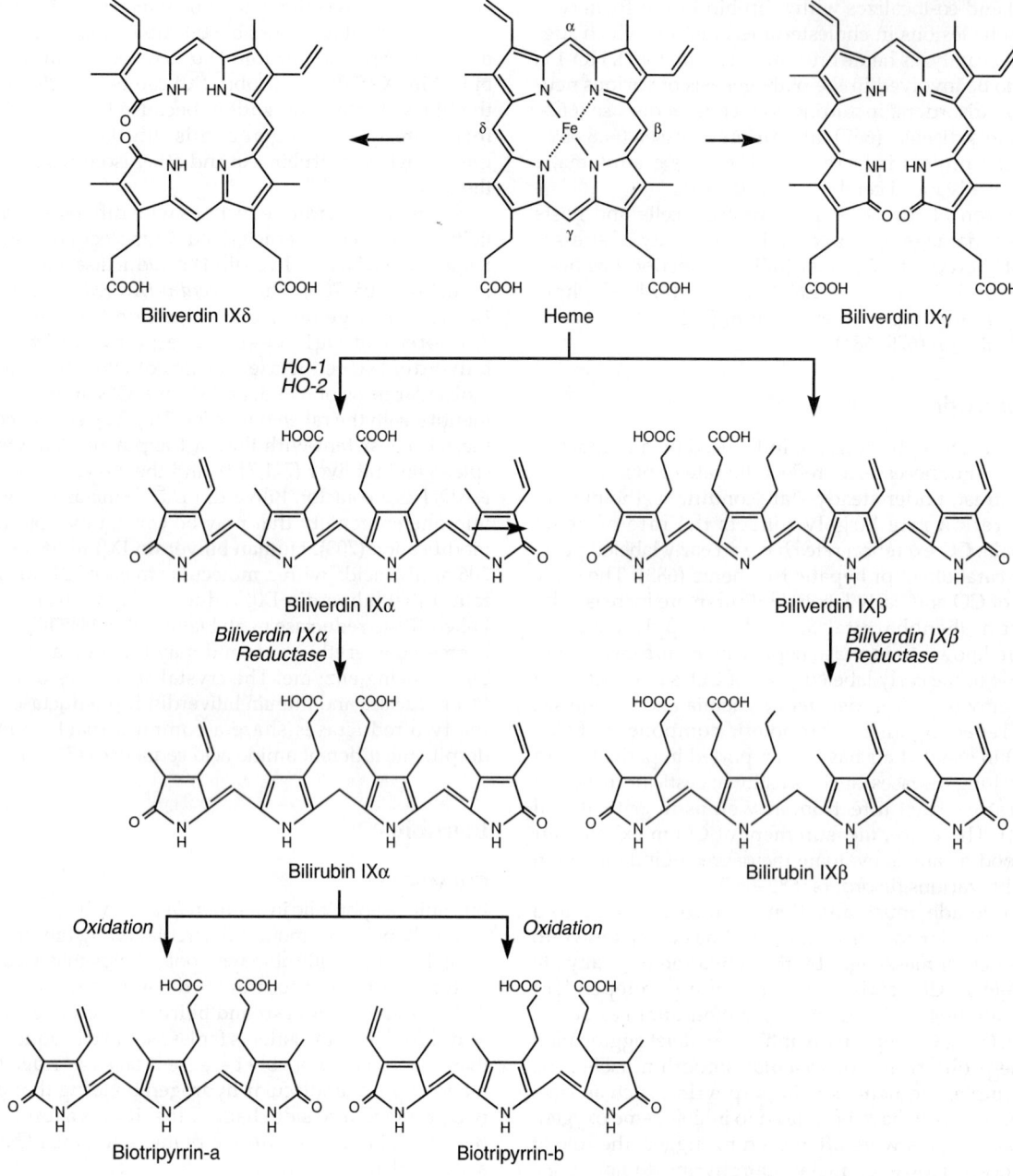

Figure 47-39. Structure of bilirubin isomers and oxidative metabolites of bilirubin IXα.

ible actions of bilirubin on CNS cells have also been described (728,729). Toxic effects of bilirubin may be decreased by albumin *in vitro* and *in vivo* (725,730). Bilirubin toxicity is discussed in the section Bilirubin Toxicity.

SERUM BILIRUBIN LEVELS

Normal serum bilirubin concentrations range from 0.3 to 1.0 mg/dL (5 to 17 μmol/L). Hyperbilirubinemia may be perceived as jaundice, when the serum bilirubin level exceeds 2 mg/dL. Serum bilirubin concentrations are influenced by age, gender, ethnic origins, and hepatic metabolism of bilirubin (uptake, conjugation, and excretion) (731). In healthy subjects, essentially all serum bilirubin (more than 90%) is in the unconjugated form. Unconjugated bilirubin (also called *indirect bilirubin*) is a nonpolar molecule and therefore circulates as a noncovalent complex with albumin. Reversible binding of unconjugated bilirubin occurs at a primary site and one or more secondary sites on albumin, and the affinity of the protein for bilirubin can be altered by other ligands, such as certain drugs and fatty acids (731). Thus, the administration of drugs, such as sulfonamides, to the newborn increases the likelihood of bilirubin toxicity, presumably by displacing bilirubin from its binding to albumin (732,733). In contrast, when bile ducts are obstructed or liver cells are diseased, conjugated bilirubin (direct or water-soluble bilirubin) refluxes into plasma, and a small portion of such conjugated bilirubin is found as an irreversible, covalent complex with albumin (734,735). The formation of the covalent albumin-bilirubin complex, which is called *delta bilirubin*, is apparently nonenzymatic and appears to occur by acyl migration of bilirubin from a bilirubin-glucuronide acid ester to a nucleophilic site on albumin (736). The protein-bound bilirubin cannot be taken up by the liver and is eliminated only when its albumin is degraded. Thus, its half-life approximates the decay of albumin (12 to 14 days).

BILIRUBIN AS AN ENDOGENOUS ANTIOXIDANT

Bilirubin and bilirubin glucuronides exhibit significant antioxidant activities *in vitro* (737,738). Unconjugated bilirubin IXα scavenges singlet oxygen (739); reacts with superoxide anion (740), peroxyl radicals (737), and lipid peroxides (741); and serves as a reducing substrate in the presence of hydrogen peroxide or organic hydroperoxides (742,743). The antioxidant activity of bilirubin appears to be due to its hydrogen-donating activity (737,744). In addition, bilirubin was shown to inhibit oxidation of LDL (741), monocyte chemotaxis that is induced by oxidized LDL (745), and adhesion of neutrophils that are elicited by ischemia reperfusion or exposure to hydrogen peroxide (746). These results suggest a role for bilirubin in the prevention of oxidative damage that is associated with cardiovascular diseases. In fact, there is an inverse relationship between plasma bilirubin levels and the risk of coronary artery disease; namely, low serum bilirubin is a risk factor for coronary artery disease (747,748).

Bilirubin oxidative metabolites have been established as direct markers for the chain-breaking antioxidative activity of bilirubin (749–751). Bilirubin reacts with reactive oxygen species to generate tripyrroles, which are termed biotripyrrin-a and biotripyrrin-b and represent a new family of bile pigments (Fig. 47-39). The bilirubin oxidative metabolites are increased in human urine after surgery (752) or psychological stress (753) and in the cerebrospinal fluid of patients with Alzheimer's disease (754).

HEPATIC METABOLISM OF BILIRUBIN

Uptake of Bilirubin. Bilirubin is rapidly removed from the circulation by the hepatocyte via diffusion (755) or active transport across the sinusoidal membrane (Fig. 47-40). In this process, bilirubin is dissociated from albumin, and albumin does not enter the liver (756). A receptorlike mechanism has been proposed for the uptake of the bilirubin-albumin complex by the liver (757). Subsequently, a family of organic anion-transporting polypeptides (OATPs) was identified by expression cloning strategies (758). OATPs are located in the hepatic sinusoidal membrane and are involved in the sodium-independent transport of several organic anions, such as bile salts and bromosulfophthalein. Especially, it was shown that OATP2 transports unconjugated bilirubin and bilirubin conjugates to hepatocytes (759,760). Other family of proteins, which are termed *organic anion transporters*, was identified in the liver, but the physiologic role of organic anion transporters in hepatic uptake of unconjugated or conjugated bilirubin is not known (758).

Bilirubin in the hepatocyte is bound to a cytosolic protein, ligandin (glutathione S-transferase B) (761,762), and is transported to the endoplasmic reticulum. Ligandin is a basic protein with a molecular mass of 47 kd, and it accounts for approximately 5% of the soluble protein in rat and human liver. Structural and immunologic studies have shown that ligandin is also identical to the protein that has been demonstrated to be an azodye carcinogen-binding protein (763), a cortisol-metabolite–binding protein (764), or glutathione S-transferase B (765). Immunochemical studies indicate that ligandin is localized in the cytosol with the highest concentration in close vicinity to the endoplasmic reticulum. Whether this finding reflects the directional movement of ligandin in the cell is not clear, and the exact role of ligandin in intracellular bilirubin transport remains conjectural (766). Intracellular movement of bilirubin may also occur by membrane–membrane transfer (767).

When bilirubin metabolism was studied by using radiolabeled precursors, such as ALA (563,768–770), heme (771), or biliverdin (772), a large proportion of bilirubin that initially was taken up by the liver refluxed into plasma (561,773). Bidirectional flux of unconjugated bilirubin was also predicted from kinetic analysis and mathematical modeling of plasma disappearance and bile excretion curves of radiolabeled bilirubin (774).

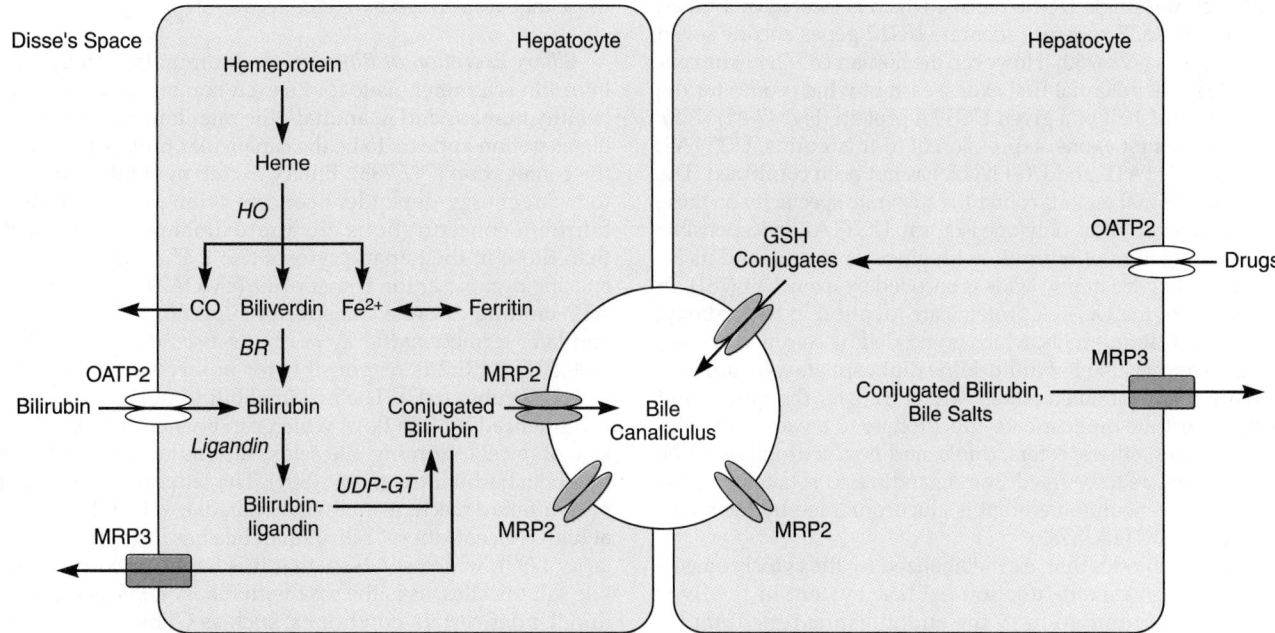

Figure 47-40. Hepatic metabolism of bilirubin. Bilirubin in circulation is largely bound by albumin, which is taken up by the liver. In hepatocytes, bilirubin is bound by bilirubin-binding proteins, such as ligandin or Z protein, the major one being ligandin. Bilirubin is conjugated with glucuronic acid by uridine diphosphate–glucuronosyltransferase (UDP-GT) before excretion into bile canaliculi. BR, biliverdin reductase; CO, carbon monoxide; GSH, glutathione; HO, heme oxygenase; MRP, multidrug resistance-associated protein; OATP2, organic anion-transporting polypeptide 2.

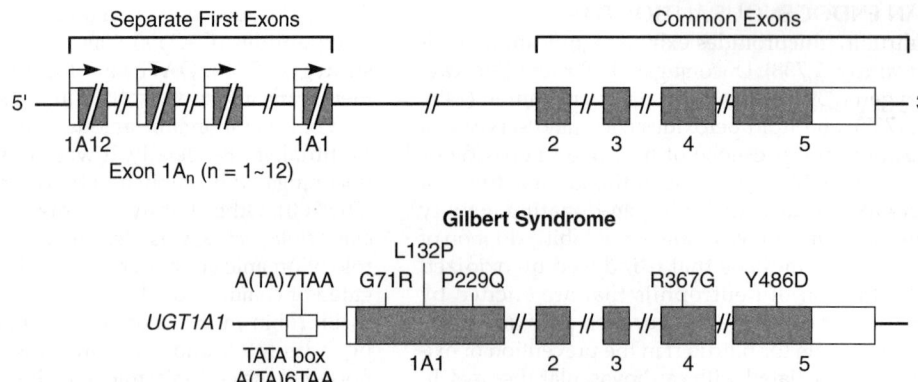

Figure 47-41. Structural organization of the human *uridine diphosphate–glucuronosyltransferase 1A (UGT1A)* gene. The *UGT1A* locus spans at least 160 kilobases and contains multiple first exons (exon 1An). Also shown is the TATA-box polymorphism that is associated frequently with Gilbert syndrome.

Bilirubin Conjugation. Under physiologic conditions, bilirubin is conjugated before excretion into bile. One or both of the two propionic acid side chains are esterified with a glucuronide moiety, yielding bilirubin monoglucuronide or bilirubin diglucuronide, respectively. Glucuronic acid is the major conjugating group, although xylosyl and glucosyl conjugates are also found to a minor degree in normal mammalian bile (775,776). Bilirubin diglucuronide constitutes a large proportion of the total bilirubin conjugates in the bile of humans, dogs, rats, and cats, whereas bilirubin monoglucuronide is the major form in bile of guinea pigs, sheep, mice, and rabbits (777).

Glucuronidation of small lipophilic compounds by uridine diphosphate–glucuronosyltransferases (UGTs) represents an important detoxification process of a large number of substrates, such as steroids, bile acids, bilirubin, dietary constituents, and various xenobiotics, including drugs and carcinogens. To date, at least 15 human UGTs have been identified and are encoded by the two loci, *UGT1A* and *UGT2* (778). Eight UGT1A proteins are encoded by the single *UGT1A* locus, which is located on human chromosome 2q37, whereas separate *UGT2* genes encode seven UGT2 proteins (778–780). However, the human *UGT1A* gene contains at least 12 potential first exons, each of which codes for the amino-terminal half of a given UGT1A protein (Fig. 47-41) (778). Among these first exons, expression of four isoforms, UGT1A2, UGT1A5, UGT1A11, and UGT1A12, has not been confirmed. The unique N-terminal regions confer the substrate specificity on these UGT1A proteins. Thus, only one isoform, UGT1A1, is responsible for the conjugation of bilirubin with glucuronic acid, and its N-terminal half of 286 amino acids is encoded by exon 1A1 (781). In contrast, all of the UGT1A proteins are identical in the carboxyl portion of 246 amino acids, which is encoded by common exons 2 through 5 and is able to bind uridine diphosphate–glucuronate. UGTs are microsomal enzymes, which transfer the glucuronyl moiety of uridine diphosphate–glucuronate to a variety of aglycones, yielding ethers, esters, thiols, and *N*-glucuronides (782). Bilirubin appears to be freed from ligandin and is taken into the endoplasmic reticulum before it is glucuronidated by the membrane-bound UGT1A1 (783).

Many xenobiotics that are metabolized by the cytochrome P-450–dependent mixed-function oxidase system in the liver undergo glucuronidation in the endoplasmic reticulum by UGTs before their excretion into bile. The enzymes that catalyze the conjugation of *p*-nitrophenol, 1-naphthol, and 3-hydroxybenzo(a)pyrene appear to be different from the enzyme that is involved in the conjugation of bilirubin and steroids (784,785).

Gunn rats that are genetically deficient in bilirubin UGT activity also have decreased activities of UGT activity for *p*-nitrophenol, *o*-aminophenol, 1-naphthol, and methyl umbelliferone (786). The reduced activities of these enzymes are due to a single base deletion in exon 4 that is common to all isoforms that are encoded by the rat *UGT1A* locus (787).

Unconjugated and conjugated bilirubin can be distinguished by the diazo reaction (788,789). Conjugated bilirubin reacts with the sulfanilic acid diazo reagent within minutes, whereas unconjugated bilirubin reacts only when an accelerator, such as methanol or caffeine, is added (788). More recently, diazotized ethyl anthranilate and *p*-iodoaniline have been used in place of sulfanilic acid, because they offer better sensitivity and greater specificity (790). The most accurate, sensitive, and quantitative determination of bile pigments is accomplished by HPLC (791–793). The irreversibly albumin-bound bilirubin can be determined by reverse-phase HPLC (794). A rapid fluorometric method for the determination of unconjugated and conjugated bilirubin and bilirubin-binding capacity has also been reported. The results that are obtained by this method are consistent with those that are verified by HPLC (795,796).

Biliary Excretion of Bilirubin. In mammals, conjugation of bilirubin is a prerequisite for its excretion into bile canaliculi. In healthy humans and in animals, the rate-limiting step for bilirubin excretion appears to be the canalicular transport rather than the conjugation (797,798). Biliary excretion of bilirubin appears to be an energy-dependent concentration process, in that bile bilirubin concentrations are approximately 100-fold greater than those in the hepatic cytosol (799). The canalicular multispecific organic anion transporter (cMOAT), a member of the ATP-binding cassette transporter superfamily, was identified and later termed *multidrug resistance-associated protein (MRP) 2* (800,801). MRP2 is responsible for biliary excretion of conjugated bilirubin (802). The maximal bilirubin excretory capacity is influenced by bile flow, which can be increased by the infusion of micelle-forming bile acids, such as taurocholate (803), or by phenobarbital treatment (804). The latter increases bile flow by a different mechanism than that mediated by bile acids. Even at high concentrations, bilirubin in bile has little effect on osmolarity (799), which suggests that it is largely incorporated into bile salt micelles, as is the case with biliary cholesterol and lecithin. Under certain conditions, such as Gilbert syndrome and chronic hemolysis, biliary excretion of bilirubin monoconjugates is increased. At the pH of bile, bilirubin monoconjugates are nonenzymatically hydrolyzed to unconjugated monohydrogenated bilirubin anions that may precipitate with calcium as calcium bilirubinate, which is the main component of pigment stones (676).

The plasma concentration of unconjugated bilirubin is known to increase linearly with increased rates of bilirubin production, if hepatic bilirubin clearance is within the normal range (805). The highest value for plasma unconjugated bilirubin that can occur as the result of sustained hemolysis in a person with normal hepatic bilirubin clearance has been estimated to be 4 mg/dL (805). When hepatic bilirubin clearance is impaired, as it is in hepatitis, obstructive disorders of bile flow, and certain metabolic disorders, bilirubin and bile salts are largely retained in the liver (cholestasis) (799). Some of these biliary components may be refluxed into plasma by MRP3, another family member of the MRPs, that is localized in the basolateral membrane of hepatocytes (677,806).

Enteric Bilirubin Absorption and Processing. Conjugated bilirubin in bile is transported to the duodenum through the biliary ducts and is excreted into the stool. In contrast to conjugated bilirubin, unconjugated bilirubin can be reabsorbed from the intestine, and the reabsorbed unconjugated bilirubin may contribute to hyperbilirubinemia in the neonate (807). A small amount of conjugated bilirubin may also undergo some nonenzymatic (alkaline hydrolysis in the duodenum or jejunum) or enzymatic deconjugation (by bacterial or intestinal mucosal β-glucuronidase) to yield unconjugated bilirubin (807). Complete lack of bile flow, such as obstruction by tumor, is associated with the absence of urobilinoids in intestinal contents.

Bilirubin in the intestinal tract is degraded by various bacteria, primarily by *Clostridium perfringens* and *E. coli,* and results in the formation of a series of products, which are termed *urobilinoids* (808). Urobilinoids include urobilin, urobilinogens, stercobilinogens, and stercobilins, in the order of their reduction steps (809,810). Urobilinogen can be reabsorbed from the small intestine and colon and enters the portal vein. Urobilinogen in the circulation is largely bound to plasma proteins (80% or more), and only a small percentage is filtered through the glomerulus. Urobilinogen excretion is influenced by a number of factors, including urinary pH (811) and diurnal rhythm (812); thus, it usually carries little clinical significance in the estimation of hepatic dysfunction. Urinary urobilinogen is increased in liver disease and in conditions that are associated with increased bilirubin production, as in hemolysis.

Renal Excretion of Bilirubin. Normally, urine contains no or only trace amounts of bilirubin, because the unconjugated bilirubin, which is bound to albumin, is not generally filtered by the renal glomeruli. In contrast, a large fraction of conjugated bilirubin, a polar molecule, is less tightly bound to albumin and is excreted into urine. Therefore, the presence of bilirubin in urine indicates conjugated hyperbilirubinemia. Because the covalent albumin–conjugated bilirubin complex is only slightly filtered through the glomerulus in the kidney (813), the resolution of jaundice generally lags behind the recovery of the hepatobiliary disease, and the plasma usually remains jaundiced longer than the urine.

DISORDERS OF BILIRUBIN METABOLISM IN THE NEONATE: NEONATAL JAUNDICE

Normal Bilirubin Metabolism and Physiologic Jaundice

DEFINITION

In normal, healthy, full-term neonates, the plasma bilirubin concentration generally rises during the first few days of life, reaching a maximum at approximately 3 days of age, then reverts to the normal range by the end of the second week of life (814). Occasionally, some infants show marked increases in plasma bilirubin during the immediate postnatal period. In a study of 4000 newborns, 16% were found to reach peak bilirubin levels that were higher than 10 mg/dL, and 5% had levels that were greater than 15 mg/dL (815). Generally, an inverse correlation exists between bilirubin levels and body weights in newborns (815,816). This type of hyperbilirubinemia, which is observed usually in the absence of documentable abnormalities, is called *physiologic jaundice* and generally is not accompanied by serious clinical consequences. Two functionally distinct periods of physiologic jaundice are seen in human newborns (817). During the first period, *phase I,* bilirubin concentrations rise to an average peak level of 6 mg/dL by the third day of life, as already noted. The duration of hyperbilirubinemia and the bilirubin concentrations are exaggerated in premature babies. In full-term infants, plasma bilirubin concentrations rapidly decline from the third day of life until the fifth day of life, when another increase in bilirubin concentration takes place. The latter increase is called *phase II.* Plasma bilirubin levels in phase II average approximately 2 mg/dL, a level that may persist until the fourteenth day of life. At that time, a return to normal concentrations of 1 mg/dL or less usually occurs. In the premature infant, the time and the magnitude of the initial peak bilirubin concentration and the duration of phase II are exaggerated.

MECHANISM

Physiologic jaundice reflects several factors, including (a) overproduction of bilirubin from the catabolism of fetal hemoglobin heme during the postnatal period; (b) insufficient activity of UGT in newborns, which is essential for the hepatic excretion of bilirubin; and (c) reabsorption in newborns of unconjugated bilirubin through the gastrointestinal tract. The erythrocyte lifespan in neonates is 70 to 90 days (818,819), which is significantly shorter than that in the adult (120 days); this results in an overload of heme with respect to the heme degrading system in the infant. The heme overload induces heme oxygenase in human newborns and may account for developmental changes in the enzyme in fetal and newborn experimental animals (820,821). Heme oxygenase induction results in a greater rate of the formation of bilirubin in the presence of excess heme substrate. Premature infants may also have an even shorter erythrocyte lifespan than full-term infants. Estimates of CO or carboxyhemoglobin production indicate that newborn infants have a several-fold higher heme turnover rate than normal adults (822,823).

UGT activity in the newborn is low and insufficient to cope with the enhanced load of bilirubin that is produced during the postnatal period (817,824,825). For example, the enzyme activity in human full-term and premature infants during the first 10 days of life is usually less than 0.1% of the normal adult value (826). This increases rapidly during the subsequent several days, ultimately reaching adult values by 6 to 14 weeks of age (827). With the rise in UGT activity, the plasma bilirubin concentration rapidly drops, an effect that is observed after 24 hours in the newborn monkey and at or after 72 hours in the human infant (817). Studies in newborn monkeys suggest that a large proportion of the bilirubin that is present in the liver cytosol is derived from intestinal reabsorption of the pigment and not from its *de novo* synthesis (828). Thus, a significant percentage of plasma bilirubin in human infants possibly originates from the enterohepatic circulation.

ETHNIC FACTORS

In full-term, healthy newborns, levels of unconjugated hyperbilirubinemia are known to be higher in infants of Asian parentage than in infants of whites and blacks (829–832). In Asian infants, hyperbilirubinemia occurs in the absence of hemolysis and appears to be due to delayed maturation of the bilirubin conjugating system, a process for which there are presumably genetic determinants. Also, reports have been made of unexplained hyperbilirubinemia in geographically localized areas (833). Several review articles deal with these aspects of bilirubin metabolism in more detail (834–836).

Neonatal Jaundice Due to Unconjugated Hyperbilirubinemia

If abnormalities of hepatic uptake, intracellular binding, or conjugation of bilirubin are present, *unconjugated* bilirubin accumulates in the plasma. In contrast, obstruction to the flow of bile into the gastrointestinal tract at any level in the canalicular-ductal system results in an increase in *conjugated* bilirubin in the plasma. Cases of diffuse hepatic injuries, such as viral hepatitis and cirrhosis, or a combined abnormality of one or more hepatic bilirubin-metabolizing systems result in a mixed type of hyperbilirubinemia. The disorders that are associated predominantly with unconjugated hyperbilirubinemia in the newborn are listed in Table 47-7. Especially, ABO blood group incompatibility and glucose-6-phosphate dehydrogenase deficiency are frequently associated with neonatal hyperbilirubinemia. Those disorders that are related to erythroblastosis fetalis and other hemolytic diseases are discussed in Chapter 56.

Hereditary Uridine Diphosphate– Glucuronosyltransferase Deficiency

CRIGLER-NAJJAR SYNDROME TYPE I AND TYPE II

Crigler-Najjar syndrome, types I and II, and Gilbert syndrome are attributable to UGT deficiencies, which result from different mutations at a single *UGT1A1* locus (allelic heterogeneity) (778). Currently, more than 50 genetic lesions have been reported (837). Homozygous or compound heterozygous mutations in the coding exons of the *UGT1A1* gene lead to Crigler-Najjar syndrome type I or type II. These conditions are recessive disorders and vary in phenotypes, depending on the nature and location of the mutations. Mutations that are associated with Crigler-Najjar syndrome type I cause a premature stop codon, a shift of the reading frame, or a single substitution of a critical amino acid (838,839). The resulting truncated or mutated protein has no enzyme activity. In contrast, Crigler-Najjar syndrome type II is always caused by a single amino acid substitution that only reduces the enzyme activity. A dominant form of Crigler-Najjar syndrome type II also occurs. In this case, the truncated enzyme, which is caused by a nonsense mutation, alters the subunit structure by forming a complex with the intact enzyme (840).

Crigler-Najjar syndrome type I (congenital nonhemolytic jaundice) is an extremely rare condition that is characterized by early onset of unconjugated hyperbilirubinemia and kernicterus (841). Affected infants usually die because of severe brain damage within 18 months of birth. Plasma bilirubin concentrations range from 25 to 45 mg/dL, and the bile of the affected children is colorless and contains no glucuronides. A few Crigler-Najjar patients survive until or past puberty (842), but thereafter they develop bilirubin encephalopathy (843,844). The reason for delayed onset of bilirubin encephalopathy is unknown, but it may be related to the combined effects of environmental factors, such as infection, and the functional consequence of the mutation. The mutation may impair the function of UGT1A1 as well as other UGT1A proteins, because many

TABLE 47-7. Disorders of the Newborn That Are Associated Predominantly with Unconjugated Hyperbilirubinemia

Transient neonatal hyperbilirubinemia
  Delayed development of hepatic uptake and conjugation system: physiologic jaundice
  Inhibitors of conjugation
    Novobiocin
    Certain breast milks (?)
  Unknown mechanisms
    Pyloric stenosis
    Upper intestinal obstruction
    Transient familial neonatal bilirubinemia
    Infants of diabetic mothers
Overproduction of bilirubin
  Isoimmune hemolysis
    Rh(D) hemolytic disease
    ABO hemolytic disease
    Other blood-group incompatibilities
  Hereditary hemolytic anemias
    Hereditary spherocytosis
    Hereditary elliptocytosis with neonatal poikilocytosis
    Hereditary stomatocytosis or xerocytosis
    Glucose-6-phosphate dehydrogenase deficiency
    Pyruvate kinase deficiency and other glycolytic defects
    Nucleotide metabolism defects
    α- or β-thalassemias or unstable hemoglobinopathies
  Acquired hemolytic anemia
    Oxidant (Heinz body) hemolytic anemias
    Vitamin E deficiency
    Infantile pyknocytosis
  Extravascular blood
    Cephalohematoma
    Occult hemorrhage
Mixed or unknown mechanism
  Sepsis
  Hypothyroidism
Inherited defects in bilirubin conjugation
  Crigler-Najjar syndrome types I and II
  Gilbert syndrome

mutations are located in the downstream exons (exons 2 through 5), which code for the common region (840). Hepatic UGT activity in typical cases of this disorder is virtually absent, and the enzyme activity in the patient's parents, who are clinically unaffected, is approximately 50% of normal (845,846). Bilirubin production in patients with Crigler-Najjar syndrome is essentially normal, whereas hepatic clearance of bilirubin and fecal excretion of urobilinoids are greatly reduced (1% or less of normal) (844,847,848). Patients with Crigler-Najjar syndrome type I require immediate orthotopic liver transplantation (849,850) or hepatocyte transplantation (851). Gene therapy is a promising treatment but is still experimental.

Crigler-Najjar syndrome type II, which was described by Arias (852), is a relatively common disorder that is characterized by substantial unconjugated hyperbilirubinemia in the newborn (8 to 20 mg/dL) and reduced hepatic UGT activity. In contrast to Crigler-Najjar syndrome type I, the clinical course of type II patients is always benign (852,853). Type II can be differentiated from type I by a reduction in plasma bilirubin concentrations after treatment with phenobarbital (845,854) and by the presence of monoglucuronidated bilirubin in bile (90% or more) (855,856). Administration of phenobarbital reduces plasma bilirubin levels to the normal range after approximately 3 days of treatment. After the immediate neonatal period, some patients with the type II syndrome have little risk of developing kernicterus.

GILBERT SYNDROME

Gilbert syndrome (constitutional hepatic dysfunction), which was described by Gilbert and Lereboullet (857) in 1901, is a

TABLE 47-8. Characteristic Symptoms of Hereditary Unconjugated Hyperbilirubinemia

	Crigler-Najjar Syndrome		
Symptoms	Type I	Type II	Gilbert Syndrome
Liver histology	Normal	Normal	Normal
Serum bilirubin	20–45 mg/dL	<20 mg/dL	<3 mg/dL
Liver function	Normal	Normal	Normal
Bromsulphalein clearance	Normal	Normal	Usually normal; occasionally enhanced
Hepatic uridine diphosphate–glucuronosyltransferase activity	Absent	Decreased	Decreased
Phenobarbital	No effect	Decreased serum bilirubin	Decreased serum bilirubin
Inheritance	Recessive	Recessive or dominant	Recessive or dominant
Prognosis	Kernicterus	Benign	Benign

common disorder that is characterized by mild, fluctuating hyperbilirubinemia, usually less than 3 mg/dL (Table 47-8). This syndrome should not be considered a disease, but rather a slow, bilirubin glucuronidation phenotype, which occurs in approximately 8% of the population (858). Gilbert syndrome has been known for a long time as a heterogeneous disorder that consists of two forms with a normal or increased bilirubin production rate, possibly due to occult hemolysis (859,860). In fact, because of the high incidence of Gilbert syndrome, it is often associated with common hemolytic disorders, such as glucose-6-phosphate dehydrogenase deficiency (861) or hereditary spherocytosis (862), which results in a severe form of neonatal hyperbilirubinemia or the early formation of pigment gallstones.

The molecular lesions of Gilbert syndrome have been identified as a homozygous promoter polymorphism or heterozygous missense mutations in the UGT1A1 gene (Fig. 47-41). Thus, Gilbert syndrome may be inherited as a recessive or dominant trait. The promoter polymorphism is the insertion of extra TA residues in the TATA box of the UGT1A1 gene, yielding the A(TA)$_7$TAA allele rather than the common A(TA)$_6$TAA (863). However, this promoter polymorphism alone is not sufficient to cause hyperbilirubinemia. Subsequently, two other alleles—five or eight repeats of (TA) at the TATA box—were identified in persons of African ancestry but not of Asian or white ancestry (863). Promoter activity decreased with increased numbers of (TA) repeats, which suggests that the promoter polymorphism may cause different levels of expression of the UGT1A1 protein. On the other hand, four heterozygous missense mutations have been identified in Japanese individuals with Gilbert syndrome (Fig. 47-41) (864,865). Each mutant protein possesses reduced enzyme activity and may function in a dominant-negative fashion. The G71R mutation, rather than the promoter polymorphism, is a common cause of Gilbert syndrome in Japanese patients. The missense mutations that are associated with Gilbert syndrome were also identified in the homozygous state in some patients with Crigler-Najjar syndrome type II (837).

Decreased hepatic UGT activity has been consistently shown in Gilbert syndrome (866,867). A male preponderance has been reported and probably relates to the known lower plasma bilirubin concentrations in women (868,869). Plasma unconjugated bilirubin concentrations in Gilbert syndrome patients increase during fasting, stress, intercurrent illness, hyperthyroidism, and menses (870). In addition, a hepatic uptake defect of bilirubin has been suggested (871,872). Despite the fact that Gilbert syndrome persists for life, patients do not develop any deleterious consequences of their hyperbilirubinemia and thus do not require treatment. However, Gilbert syndrome is a risk factor for severe neonatal hyperbilirubinemia (873–875). Several review articles deal with Gilbert syndrome in more detail (859,860,868).

Acquired Uridine Diphosphate–Glucuronosyltransferase Deficiency: Breast-Feeding Jaundice and Breast Milk Jaundice

Plasma bilirubin concentrations are increased in some newborn infants who are breast fed, compared to those who are fed formula (836,876). Two types of neonatal jaundice are known: breast-feeding jaundice and breast milk jaundice. Breast-feeding jaundice is of early onset and results from the inappropriate feeding process, such as insufficient intake of breast milk (caloric deprivation) or insufficient frequency of feeding. Breast-feeding jaundice is therefore managed by encouraging mothers to nurse as frequently as possible (at least eight times every 24 hours). In contrast, breast milk jaundice has a later onset and is more prolonged, beginning after the fifth day of birth and continuing for several weeks. Breast milk jaundice may be caused by an increased enterohepatic recirculation of bilirubin, but a causative agent in maternal milk has not been definitively identified. Gilbert syndrome may exaggerate breast milk jaundice (875). Plasma bilirubin levels in breast-fed infants may remain elevated for 3 to 16 weeks and have occasionally been reported to reach concentrations of 15 to 24 mg/dL; they slowly and steadily decline after this period. No infants with breast milk jaundice have been reported to develop kernicterus (877). Temporary interruption of nursing may help to establish the diagnosis and decrease plasma bilirubin concentration, followed by a rise in concentration when nursing is resumed. But interruption of nursing is not needed in most cases (878) and should not be required unless the plasma bilirubin concentration is near the risk level for bilirubin toxicity.

Other Disorders That Are Associated with Unconjugated Hyperbilirubinemia

Infants with pyloric stenosis and proximal small intestinal obstruction may display unconjugated hyperbilirubinemia in the absence of hemolysis. Affected infants have decreased hepatic UGT activity (879), which may account for the jaundice. The pathogenesis of the decreased bilirubin UGT activity is not clear. Novobiocin, an antibiotic that is no longer used in the United States, inhibits hepatic UGT activity (880) and can also cause unconjugated hyperbilirubinemia in treated infants.

Infants with congenital hypothyroidism occasionally develop unconjugated hyperbilirubinemia (881). Infants of diabetic mothers are also at high risk for unconjugated hyperbilirubinemia (882).

Neonatal Jaundice Due to Conjugated Hyperbilirubinemia

Marked elevations of conjugated bilirubin, which exceed 10 to 20% of total serum bilirubin, in the newborn are not physiologic

TABLE 47-9. Disorders of the Newborn That Are Associated Predominantly with Conjugated Hyperbilirubinemia

Obstruction to bile flow
  Extrahepatic
    Extrahepatic biliary atresia
    Extrahepatic stenosis and choledochal cyst
    Extrahepatic mass (tumor, stone)
    Bile plug syndrome and inspissated bile syndrome
  Intrahepatic
    Paucity of the intrahepatic ducts
    Congenital hepatic cirrhosis
    Intrahepatic biliary atresia
Hepatocellular injuries
  Infection
    Bacterial
      Syphilis
      Listeria species
      Tuberculosis
    Viral
      Hepatitis B (HBsAg+), hepatitis A (?)
      Hepatitis non-A, non-B (?)
      Rubella
      Cytomegalovirus
      Coxsackievirus B
    Protozoal: toxoplasmosis
  Toxic
    Bacterial sepsis
    Intestinal obstruction
    Diarrhea
    Intravenous alimentation
    Drugs
Metabolic disorders
  Disorders of amino acid metabolism: tyrosinemia
  Disorders of carbohydrate metabolism
    Galactosemia
    Fructosemia
    Glycogen storage disease, type IV
  Miscellaneous
    α_1-Antitrypsin deficiency
    Zellweger syndrome
Overproduction of bile pigments
  Erythroblastosis fetalis
  Hemolytic anemia due to erythrocyte enzyme deficiencies (glucose-6-phosphate dehydrogenase deficiency and others)
  Hemolytic anemia due to erythrocyte membrane structural defects (spherocytosis, elliptocytosis, pyknocytosis, and others)
  Congenital erythropoietic porphyria

and are almost always associated with hepatocellular injuries, obstructive lesions in the bile flow system, or sepsis (Table 47-9). Hepatocellular injuries result in the impaired excretion of conjugated bilirubin into the bile, whereas obstruction in the bile flow, such as biliary atresia, results in the accumulation of conjugated bilirubin in the circulation. Obstruction to bile flow can be intrahepatic (from the level of the bile canaliculi to an intrahepatic duct) or extrahepatic (the common hepatic duct). In addition, certain disorders that are discussed later in the chapter, such as Dubin-Johnson syndrome or Rotor's syndrome, are associated with specific excretory defects for bilirubin.

BILIRUBIN TOXICITY

Signs and Symptoms

Clinical findings of bilirubin toxicity range from little or no overt signs or symptoms in some affected infants to the severe expression of this toxicity, which is termed *kernicterus* and is characterized by progressive lethargy, hypotonia, muscular rigidity, opisthotonus, spasticity, high-pitched cry, fever, convulsions, and, ultimately, death (883,884). Hearing defects are probably the mildest overt neurologic expression of bilirubin toxicity (884). Aberrations of auditory brainstem responses have also

been reported in the Gunn rat, which represents an animal equivalent of the human disorder Crigler-Najjar syndrome type I (885). Infants who have survived severe bilirubin toxicity may show high-frequency deafness, sustained choreoathetosis, mental retardation, and cerebral palsy (886). Seemingly unaffected infants with unconjugated hyperbilirubinemia may also display subtle neurologic abnormalities, such as impaired motor functions, hearing loss, an aberrant cry, and psychologic dysfunction (887–890). A national collaborative survey of the relation of hyperbilirubinemia to neurodevelopmental outcome in preterm infants that was carried out in Holland indicated that the risk of an adverse neurodevelopmental outcome at 2 years of age increased by 30% for each increment of 2.9 mg/dL in maximal plasma bilirubin concentrations in the neonatal period (891).

Pathophysiology

Brains of infants with kernicterus that are examined at autopsy show characteristic yellowish staining of basal ganglia, hippocampal cortex, cerebellum, and subthalamic regions due to deposits of bilirubin (892). Conditions such as prematurity, hypoalbuminemia, hypoxia, acidosis, and hemolysis in the infant greatly enhance the risk of kernicterus. Conjugated bilirubin does not enter the CNS, whereas free bilirubin can diffuse into the brain and exert toxic effects. Unconjugated bilirubin in plasma is bound to albumin (893). Similarly, bilirubin in interstitial fluid, which represents approximately 20% of the circulating concentration, is also bound to albumin (894). Albumin-bound bilirubin is also in equilibrium with a small amount of unbound bilirubin (0.5 mg/dL or less) (894). This equilibrium can be greatly influenced by factors that compete for bilirubin binding and favor the release of free bilirubin. These factors are hypoalbuminemia, acidosis, and the presence of organic anions that bind to albumin, such as sulfonamides, salicylates, caffeine, heparin and sodium benzoate, as well as certain nonesterified fatty acids (894,895).

Free bilirubin has been shown to exert a variety of other toxic effects on cells, as was already described. Bilirubin toxicity may also be exaggerated in the presence of hypoxia, and resultant tissue acidosis may enhance this toxicity (896). Also, evidence shows that bilirubin may gain access to the CNS if the blood–brain barrier is disrupted (897,898). The blood–brain barrier also appears to be selective to bilirubin. A study using I^{125}–albumin-bound bilirubin in newborn piglets showed that the blood–brain barrier is more permeable to bilirubin than to albumin, whereas the permeability of the blood–brain barrier to bilirubin decreases with age, without alterations in the permeability to albumin (899).

Prevention of Bilirubin Toxicity

Neonatal jaundice is a frequent problem in neonatology but is generally considered to have been solved many years ago. However, the current tendency toward early hospital discharge of neonates has resulted in a reemergence of kernicterus (836,900). The two principal modes of treatment that are in current use to lower dangerously high plasma bilirubin levels are phototherapy and exchange transfusion. Experimental therapies include the use of phenobarbital to induce hepatic UGT and the use of heme oxygenase inhibitors to diminish heme degradation to bile pigments.

PHOTOTHERAPY

Products of photocatalyzed isomerization of bilirubin are more polar than the parent compound and are readily excreted in bile and urine. Phototherapy is highly effective in lowering plasma

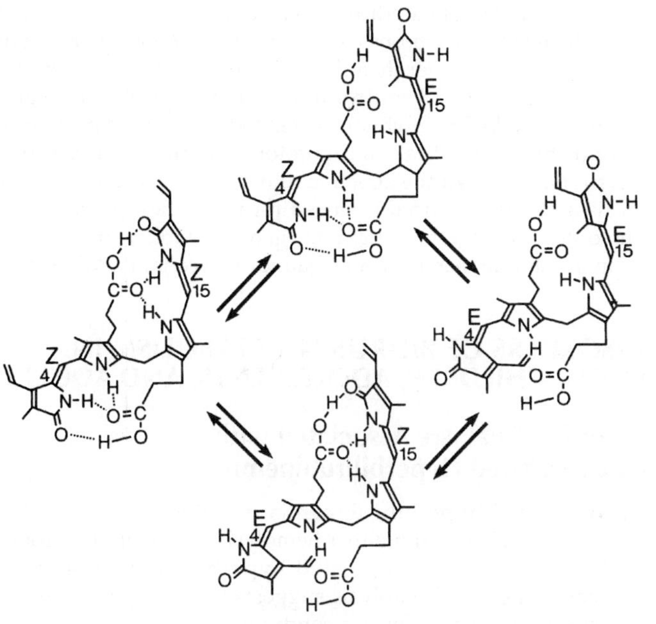

Figure 47-42. The four bilirubin configurational isomers: ZZ, ZE, EE, and EZ isomers *(from left, clockwise)*. ZZ is the stable ground-state isomer, whereas ZE, EE, and EZ are lumirubins. Lumirubin, like a bilirubin monoglucuronide, has a polar end and a nonpolar end. Like a monoglucuronide, it undergoes monoglucuronidation if the glucuronidating enzyme system in the liver is functional, and it can be excreted into bile if the glucuronidating enzyme is insufficient or inactive, as in newborns or jaundiced Gunn rats. (From Lightner DA, McDonagh AF. Molecular mechanisms of phototherapy for neonatal jaundice. *Proc Natl Acad Sci U S A* 1984;17:417, with permission.)

bilirubin concentrations in infants with unconjugated hyperbilirubinemia (901,902). Exposure of bilirubin to light in the range of 400 to 500 nm *in vitro* induces three major changes: configurational isomerization, structural isomerization, and photooxidation (903). The efficiencies of these processes are defined by the relative values of their quantum yields, that is, the number of product molecules divided by the number of photons absorbed by bilirubin.

Configurational isomerization of bilirubin that is bound to human plasma albumin has a high quantum yield, is reversible, and is completely regioselective for the 4Z, 15E isomers (904) (Fig. 47-42). This isomer appears to be excreted only slowly into bile, so that it may reach an equilibrium between the 4Z, 15E isomer and the natural 4Z, 15Z isomer during phototherapy with sufficiently bright light. Structural isomerization of bilirubin has a much lower quantum yield, but the reaction is irreversible and the primary product, lumirubin, is excreted much faster into bile and urine than in the configurational isomer. Photooxidation of bilirubin has the lowest quantum yield among the three photoprocesses and yields colorless water-soluble products—oxidized monopyrroles and dipyrroles—that are excreted rapidly into urine. Photoisomerization is a more important process than photooxidation, and lumirubin is a major contributor to the effectiveness of phototherapy (905). Lumirubin results from a "flipping-over" of one or both of the outer pyrrole rings of bilirubin IXα (Z,Z geometric isomer), which yields a mixture of geometric isomers (Z,E; E,Z; E,E) (724,906–909). Unlike the stable ground state Z,Z isomer, lumirubin cannot form intramolecular hydrogen bonds. Thus, it is more polar than the Z,Z isomer and can be excreted without glucuronidation. After excretion, it rapidly undergoes reverse isomerization to form the more stable Z,Z form. This is probably the reason why unconjugated bilirubin can be found in bile and intestine after phototherapy.

Phototherapy, first used by Cremer et al. (905) to treat infants with hyperbilirubinemia and developed as a preventive form of therapy for newborn jaundice by Lucey et al. (901), is an effective treatment modality for this common clinical problem (900). It is important to monitor plasma bilirubin concentrations before and during light treatment and to be aware of certain clinical concerns that are associated with its use, such as thermoregulatory and hydration problems (910). Otherwise, no significant long-term deleterious effects of phototherapy in newborns have been described (911).

Green light has been shown to be as effective as blue light in reducing plasma bilirubin concentrations in infants with hyperbilirubinemia (912). The reason for green light's effectiveness is not clear, but it may be related to the fact that the depth of penetration of visible light increases with increasing wavelengths (913). The use of green light may also be beneficial in the reduction of potential side effects of blue light (914).

Phototherapy is more effective than exchange transfusion in the achievement of prolonged reduction of bilirubin levels for nonhemolytic hyperbilirubinemia (915). To minimize some of the side effects of phototherapy, fiberoptic phototherapy with a blanket may be combined with conventional phototherapy (916). The fiberoptic blanket allows greater surface area to be exposed and increases convenience by eliminating the need for eye protection and incubator use. Excellent reviews of phototherapy have been published (724,916,917).

EXCHANGE TRANSFUSION

Exchange transfusion is the choice of treatment for neonates with unconjugated hyperbilirubinemia (>20 mg/dL) who have failed to respond to intensive phototherapy and other therapies. Exchange transfusion was initially used to treat infants with Rh erythroblastosis, but now it is also used in the treatment of infants with other types of unconjugated hyperbilirubinemia who are at risk for developing kernicterus (918–920). Small volumes (10 to 20 mL) of the infant's blood are replaced with equal volumes of donor blood (918). This is usually repeated until the volume of donor blood is approximately 180 mL/kg, or twice the blood volume of the infant. Approximately 90% of the RBCs can be replaced with donor RBCs by this procedure (921). A contemporary list of conditions that warrant consideration for exchange transfusion, with a summary of the various techniques for performing exchange transfusions, is available (922). Exchange transfusion physically removes bilirubin and other organic substances that may compete for binding with bilirubin to carrier proteins. The procedure also supplies albumin to help correct hypoalbuminemia, which is commonly observed in infants with Rh erythroblastosis. For example, in a study with a typical exchange of blood, it was found that plasma bilirubin concentrations decreased by 50%, and plasma bilirubin binding capacity increased by 20% for each blood replacement (923). Thus, a significant amount of albumin is extravascular and is readily exchangeable with intravascular albumin (921). Exchange transfusion can be carried out in conjunction with albumin administration to augment bilirubin binding capacity (895,924,925). In addition to complications that are common to any transfusion, complications of exchange transfusion include acidosis due to citrated blood, hyperkalemia that results from aged blood, hypocalcemia due to calcium binding by citrate, pulmonary as well as intravascular hemorrhage, and thrombosis of the portal vein with hemorrhagic infarction of the bowel (926). The mortality rate from the procedure ranges from approximately 1% (927) to 4.2% (923).

A cut-off level of 20 mg of bilirubin per 100 mL plasma for the administration of exchange transfusion has been widely used (928). In fact, it is unlikely that an otherwise-well full-term infant with a plasma bilirubin concentration of less than 25 mg/dL would develop classic kernicterus (888,928,929). On the other hand, the occurrence of kernicterus at plasma bilirubin levels lower than 20 mg/dL is also well documented in association with drug administration, hypoalbuminemia, hypoxia, and acidosis, particularly in the premature infant (930–933). The cut-off value of 20 mg/dL was determined on the basis of studies that were performed in the 1950s (934,935) and did not include sufficiently long follow-up studies (1 year or more). Thus, the value of 20 mg/dL, particularly in low-birth-weight infants, cannot be considered an absolute limit, and other factors or conditions that may complicate hepatic bilirubin metabolism must also be taken into consideration in deciding if and when to initiate exchange transfusion or phototherapy (936,937). A rate of rise in the plasma bilirubin levels greater than 1 mg/dL/hour is considered to be dangerously rapid and warrants early exchange (938). Graphs are also available, from which the risk level of bilirubin can be predicted to determine the need for exchange (834,938).

Inhibition of Bilirubin Formation

Two heme oxygenase inhibitors, tin protoporphyrin and tin mesoporphyrin, have been studied extensively at the clinical level with respect to their ability to ameliorate hyperbilirubinemia or lower normal levels of plasma bilirubin in humans (621,623,625,626,939,940). Subjects of study have included normal volunteers, patients with various forms of jaundice, a newborn infant with Crigler-Najjar syndrome type I (941,942), and a group of full-term newborns with jaundice that was associated with direct Coombs' test–positive ABO incompatibility (625). In the latter studies, incremental changes in plasma bilirubin levels were determined in control babies and inhibitor-treated infants (0.5 µmol/kg × 1, or 0.75 µmol/kg × 2 or 3) in the 96-hour period after birth; some infants were followed up for as long as 176 hours postnatally. The results indicated that inhibitor treatment diminished the incremental changes in plasma bilirubin levels at all time points that were studied after birth, with the effects being statistically significant at 48 hours and thereafter in infants who received a total of 1.5 µmol/kg (15 infants) or 2.25 µmol/kg (nine infants).

Tin protoporphyrin and tin mesoporphyrin inhibit heme oxygenase potently and rapidly (in less than 1 hour) after subcutaneous, intramuscular, and intravenous administration. Their effect is manifested by a prompt lowering of biliary bilirubin output and a decrease in respiratory CO production (943,944). A transient (approximately 6 hours) complete saturation of hepatic tryptophan pyrrolase reflects a temporary cellular accumulation of heme and the rapid excretion of unmetabolized heme into bile to an extent that quantitatively accounts for the diminution of bilirubin production that is produced by the inhibitors (943–946). The incorporation of heme oxygenase inhibitors into liposomes markedly enhances inhibition of splenic heme oxygenase. Targeting this major tissue site of heme oxygenase activity in this manner produces a profound decrease in biliary bilirubin output and a near-total inhibition of splenic heme catabolism that lasts many days after a single dose of the inhibitor-liposome preparation (947).

Extensive toxicologic examination of these compounds has shown them to be essentially innocuous; the only side effect that is noted in humans is the occurrence of transient photosensitivity, when they have been administered in doses of 1 µmol/kg (or more), and when the treated subject is then exposed to sunlight, or when newborns receive concurrent phototherapy with broad-spectrum white-light lamps. The use of high-intensity blue lamps, whose emission spectrum does not extend into the region of peak porphyrin absorbance (400 to 410 nm), has eliminated, for practical purposes, this side effect in infants.

The overall requirement for phototherapy was diminished by approximately 40% in the combined treatment groups compared to that in the control group. Inhibitor alone was sufficient to mod-erate the severity of jaundice in treated infants, because plasma bilirubin levels in newborns who receive tin protoporphyrin alone were consistently lower than those in control babies (625). In this comparison, 15 of 55 control infants required phototherapy, whereas only 1 of 35 inhibitor-treated babies required such treatment (625). Further trials of tin protoporphyrin or tin mesoporphyrin have shown the effective reduction of plasma bilirubin levels and have reduced the need for phototherapy (948,949). These studies suggest that heme oxygenase inhibitors may be useful in the clinical management of jaundice in certain newborns.

DISORDERS OF BILIRUBIN METABOLISM IN OLDER CHILDREN, ADOLESCENTS, AND ADULTS

Disorders That Are Associated with Unconjugated Hyperbilirubinemia

Unconjugated hyperbilirubinemia in older children and in adults is associated with either hemolysis or Gilbert syndrome. Prolonged, mild, unconjugated hyperbilirubinemia in the absence of signs of hemolysis suggests Gilbert syndrome. No treatment is necessary for this condition.

Disorders That Are Associated with Conjugated Hyperbilirubinemia

Conjugated hyperbilirubinemia in older children and in adults is associated with impaired hepatic excretion (intrahepatic defects) or extrahepatic biliary obstruction (Table 47-10). In acquired hepatobiliary diseases, such as hepatitis and cirrhosis, biliary excretion of conjugated bilirubin is severely impaired, thereby leading to conjugated hyperbilirubinemia. Drug-induced cholestasis is an important cause of conjugated hyperbilirubinemia. In fact, many drugs produce cholestasis or inflammation. A unique example of conjugated hyperbilirubinemia is seen in some cases of pregnancy, which are known as *cholestatic jaundice of pregnancy*. The pathogenesis of this condition is probably similar to that of cholestatic jaundice that is caused by oral contraceptive agents. In addition, the prevalence of postoperative jaundice has increased, because patients have more major surgical operations, including cardiac surgery and organ transplantation. There are various factors that contribute to postoperative jaundice, such as transfusions, anesthesia, various drugs, and infection. Here we focus on the hereditary disorders, which have provided new insights into bilirubin metabolism.

DUBIN-JOHNSON SYNDROME

Dubin-Johnson syndrome is a benign autosomal-recessive disorder that is characterized by chronic conjugated hyperbilirubinemia. Plasma bilirubin concentrations in patients with this syndrome are usually 2 to 5 mg/dL but may occasionally be elevated to as high as 17 mg/dL. The liver tissue has a dark color that is characteristic of this disorder. This is due to a lysosomal pigment (950). Plasma bilirubin is predominantly in the conjugated form, and it directly reacts with the sulfanilic acid diazo reagent (50% or more) (951,952). A major portion of plasma bilirubin in patients with Dubin-Johnson syndrome is covalently bound with albumin, a finding that is commonly observed in patients with chronic conjugated hyperbilirubinemia (735,953). In addition to conjugated hyperbilirubinemia, hepatic transport (but not uptake) of organic anions, such as sulfobromophthalein, indocyanine green, metanephrine glucuronide, and iopanoic acid, is decreased in this disorder (954). The total amount of urinary coproporphyrin in patients with Dubin-Johnson syndrome is normal, but the type I isomer of coproporphyrin is greatly

TABLE 47-10. Disorders of Adults Predominantly Associated with Conjugated Hyperbilirubinemia

Obstruction to bile flow
  Extrahepatic
    Malignancy
      Pancreatic carcinoma, lymphoma
    Inflammation
      Pancreatitis
  Intraductal and intrahepatic
    Gallstones
    Infection
      Clonorchis
      Ascaris
      Oriental cholangiohepatitis
    Malignancy
      Cholangiocarcinoma, ampullary carcinoma
    Sclerosing cholangitis
    Trauma
Impaired hepatic excretion
  Familial or hereditary disorders
    Dubin-Johnson syndrome
    Rotor syndrome
    Recurrent (benign) intrahepatic cholestasis
    Cholestatic jaundice of pregnancy (third trimester)
  Acquired hepatocellular diseases
    Cirrhosis
    Biliary cirrhosis (primary or secondary)
    Alcoholic liver disease
  Infection
    Viral hepatitis
    Bacterial hepatitis
  Toxic
    Sepsis
    Drugs
      Oral contraceptives, androgens, chlorpromazine, cyclosporin A, etc.
  Postoperative state
    Major surgical operations
    Liver transplantation

increased (more than 80%), compared to that in normal subjects (955) (20% to 25%).

Hepatobiliary excretion of conjugated bilirubin is mediated by MRP2, which is also called *cMOAT* (Fig. 47-40) (800–802). MRP2 consists of 1545 amino acids, which share 48% amino acid identity with MRP1, and is a member of the ATP-binding cassette transporter family. MRP2 is localized in the canalicular membrane of hepatocytes and mediates the efficient secretion of conjugated bilirubin and the endogenous glutathione *S*-conjugated leukotriene C_4 (677). Endotoxin reduced the expression of MRP2, which appears consistent with the impaired excretion of conjugated bilirubin into bile in sepsis. To date, 13 mutations have been reported in the *MRP2* gene of patients with Dubin-Johnson syndrome (956,957). Moreover, expression of MRP2 is not detected in patients with Dubin-Johnson syndrome, whereas MRP3, a member of the ATP-binding cassette transporter family, is overexpressed in the basolateral (sinusoidal) membrane of hepatocytes in these patients (809). MRP3 mediates secretion of conjugated bilirubin, conjugated estradiol, and sulfated bile acids into blood. Moreover, expression of MRP2 and MRP3 appears to be under an inverse regulation, thereby preventing the accumulation of conjugated chemicals in hepatocytes during cholestasis (677).

A single nucleotide deletion and a missense mutation were found in the *cMOAT* gene of TR⁻ rats and Eisai hyperbilirubinemic rats, respectively (958,959). These rats are known as models of Dubin-Johnson syndrome. A mutant strain of Corriedale sheep also has an inherited disorder that is similar to the human Dubin-Johnson syndrome (960–962). The animals have chronic conjugated hyperbilirubinemia and the characteristic lysosomal pigment of Dubin-Johnson syndrome.

ROTOR'S SYNDROME

Rotor's syndrome is a rare, benign disorder that is characterized by conjugated hyperbilirubinemia. It is inherited in an autosomal-recessive fashion (963). Plasma bilirubin concentrations rarely exceed 10 mg/dL. In contrast to that found in patients with Dubin-Johnson syndrome, no hepatocyte lysosomal pigmentation is present, and the hepatic uptake of bilirubin is diminished. Plasma disappearance curves for sulfobromosulphthalein and indocyanine green are also different from those with Dubin-Johnson syndrome. Specifically, the first slope of plasma disappearance is impaired (which suggests impaired hepatic uptake), whereas no secondary rise in plasma bilirubin occurs in those with Rotor's syndrome (964). Unlike patients with Dubin-Johnson syndrome, in whom total urinary coproporphyrin concentration is normal with a predominance of coproporphyrin I, a significant increase in total urinary coproporphyrin is found in those with Rotor's syndrome (2.5- to fivefold), with a more balanced coproporphyrin I and III excretion (965). Kinetic analyses of plasma sulfobromosulphthalein clearance suggested that this syndrome is due to a defect of hepatic storage and, to a lesser extent, of hepatic uptake (858). The unconjugated hyperbilirubinemia of Rotor's syndrome appears to have no pathologic consequences of note.

REFERENCES

1. Falk JE. *Porphyrins and metalloporphyrins*, vol 2. New York: Elsevier Science, 1964.
2. IUPAC-IUB Joint Commission on Biochemical Nomenclature (JCBN). Nomenclature of tetrapyrroles: recommendations, 1978. *Eur J Biochem* 1980;108:1.
3. Gilbert DL. Significance of oxygen on earth. In: Gilbert DL, ed. *Oxygen and living processes. An interdisciplinary approach*. New York: Springer-Verlag, 1981:73.
4. Komuro A, Tobe T, Hashimoto K, et al. Molecular cloning and expression of human liver biliverdin-IX beta reductase. *Biol Pharm Bull* 1996;19:796.
5. Shalloe F, Elliott G, Ennis O, et al. Evidence that biliverdin-IX beta reductase and flavin reductase are identical. *Biochem J* 1996;316:385.
6. Sassa S, Kappas A. Genetic, metabolic, and biochemical aspects of the porphyrias. In: Harris H, Hirschhorn K, eds. *Advances in human genetics*. New York: Plenum Publishing, 1981:121.
7. Berk PD, Rodkey FL, Blaschke TF, et al. Comparison of plasma bilirubin turnover and carbon monoxide production in man. *J Lab Clin Med* 1974;83:29.
8. Granick S, Sassa S. δ-Aminolevulinic acid synthetase and the control of heme and chlorophyll synthesis. In: Vogel HJ, ed. *Metabolic regulation*. New York: Academic Press, 1971:77.
9. Hutton JJ, Gross SR. Chemical induction of hepatic porphyria in inbred strains of mice. *Arch Biochem Biophys* 1970;141:284.
10. Tschudy DP, Marver HS, Collins A. A model for calculating messenger RNA half-life: short-lived messenger RNA in the induction of mammalian δ-aminolevulinic acid synthetase. *Biochem Biophys Res Commun* 1965;21:480.
11. Whiting MJ. Synthesis of δ-aminolevulinate synthase by isolated liver polyribosomes. *Biochem J* 1976;158:391.
12. Sassa S, Granick S. Induction of δ-aminolevulinic acid synthetase in chick embryo liver cells in culture. *Proc Natl Acad Sci U S A* 1970;67:517.
13. Lathrop JT, Timko MP. Regulation by heme of mitochondrial protein transport through a conserved amino acid motif. *Science* 1993;259:522.
14. Munakata H, Furuyama K, Norio R. The mitochondrial transfer of the nonspecific and the erythroid-specific 5-δ-aminolevulinate synthase and the heme regulatory motif. *J Biochem* 1996;68:792(abst).
15. Fujita H, Yamamoto M, Yamagami T, et al. Erythroleukemia differentiation. Distinctive responses of the erythroid-specific and the nonspecific δ-aminolevulinate synthase mRNA. *J Biol Chem* 1991;266:17494.
16. Meguro K, Igarashi K, Yamamoto M, et al. The role of the erythroid-specific delta-aminolevulinate synthase gene expression in erythroid heme synthesis. *Blood* 1995;86:940.
17. Harigae H, Suwabe N, Weinstock P, et al. Deficient heme and globin synthesis in embryonic stem cells lacking the erythroid-specific 5-aminolevulinate synthase gene. *Blood* 1998;91:798.
18. Eisen H, Keppel-Ballinet F, Georgopoulos CP, et al. Biochemical and genetic analysis of erythroid differentiation in Friend virus-transformed murine erythroleukemia cells. In: Clarkson B, Marks PA, Till J, eds. *Cold Spring Harbor Conference on differentiation of normal and neoplasmic hematopoietic cells*. Cold Spring Harbor, NY: Cold Spring Harbor Laboratory, 1978:277.
19. Sassa S, Granick JL, Eisen H, et al. Regulation of heme synthesis in mouse Friend virus-transformed cells in culture. In: Murphy MJ Jr, ed. *In vitro aspects of erythropoiesis*. New York: Springer-Verlag, 1978:135.
20. Rutherford T, Thompson GG, Moore MR. Heme biosynthesis in Friend erythroleukemia cells: control by ferrochelatase. *Proc Natl Acad Sci U S A* 1979;76:833.
21. Sassa S, Nagai T. The role of heme in gene expression. *Int J Hematol* 1996;63:167.

22. Wada O, Sassa S, Takaku F, et al. Different responses of the hepatic and erythropoietic δ-aminolevulinic acid synthetase of mice. *Biochim Biophys Acta* 1967;148:585.
23. Sassa S. Sequential induction of heme pathway enzymes during erythroid differentiation of mouse Friend leukemia virus-infected cells. *J Exp Med* 1976;143:305.
24. Sassa S. Control of heme biosynthesis in erythroid cells. In: Rossi GB, ed. *In vitro and in vivo erythropoiesis: the Friend system.* Amsterdam: Elsevier Science, 1980:219.
25. Granick JL, Sassa S. Hemin control of heme biosynthesis in mouse Friend virus-transformed erythroleukemia cells in culture. *J Biol Chem* 1978;253:5402.
26. Hoffman R, Ibrahim N, Murnane MJ, et al. Hemin control of heme biosynthesis and catabolism in a human leukemia cell line. *Blood* 1980;56:567.
27. Nagai M, Nagai T, Yamamoto M, et al. Novel regulation of delta-aminolevulinate synthase in the rat harderian gland. *Biochem Pharmacol* 1997;53:643.
28. Condie LW, Baron J, Tephly TR. Studies on adrenal δ-aminolevulinic acid synthetase. *Arch Biochem Biophys* 1976;172:123.
29. Briggs DW, Condie LW, Sedman RM, et al. δ-Aminolevulinic acid synthetase in the heart. *J Biol Chem* 1976;251:4996.
30. Tofilon PJ, Piper WN. Measurement and regulation of rat testicular δ-aminolevulinic acid synthetase activity. *Arch Biochem Biophys* 1980;201:104.
31. Wielburski A, Nelson BR. Heme a induces assembly of rat liver cytochrome c oxidase subunits I-III in isolated mitochondria. *FEBS Lett* 1984;177:291.
32. Gibson QH, Antonini E. Kinetic studies on the reaction between native globin and haem derivatives. *Biochem J* 1960;77:328.
33. Rose MY, Olson JS. The kinetic mechanism of heme binding to human apohemoglobin. *J Biol Chem* 1983;258:4298.
34. Cassoly R, Banerjee R. Structure and function of human semihemoglobins alpha and beta. *Eur J Biochem* 1971;19:514.
35. Waxman HS, Freedman ML, Rabinovitz M. Studies with ^{59}Fe-labeled hemin on the control of polyribosome formation in rabbit reticulocytes. *Biochim Biophys Acta* 1967;145:353.
36. Rabinovitz M, Freedman ML, Fisher JM, et al. Translational control in hemoglobin synthesis. *Cold Spring Harbor Symp Quant Biol* 1969;34:567.
37. Morris AJ, Liang K. Interaction of globin and heme during hemoglobin biosynthesis. *Arch Biochem Biophys* 1968;125:468.
38. Hunt T, Vanderhoff G, London IM. Control of globin synthesis. The role of hemin. *J Mol Biol* 1972;66:471.
39. Bunn HF. Subunit assembly of hemoglobin: an important determinant of hematologic phenotype. *Blood* 1987;69:1.
40. Spikes JD. Porphyrins and related compounds as photodynamic sensitizers. *Ann N Y Acad Sci* 1975;244:496.
41. Lim HW. Pathophysiology of cutaneous lesions in porphyrias. *Semin Hematol* 1989;26:114.
42. Goldstein BD, Harber LC. Erythropoietic protoporphyria: lipid peroxidation and red cell membrane damage associated with photohemolysis. *J Clin Invest* 1972;51:892.
43. Gibson SL, Goldberg A. Defects in haem synthesis in mammalian tissues in experimental lead poisoning and experimental porphyria. *Clin Sci* 1970;38:63.
44. Percy VA, Shanley BC. Studies on haem biosynthesis in rat brain. *J Neurochem* 1979;33:1267.
45. Cohn JA, Alvares AP, Kappas A. On the occurrence of cytochrome P-450 and aryl hydrocarbon hydroxylase activity in rat brain. *J Exp Med* 1977;145:1607.
46. Das M, Seth PK, Mukhtar H. NADH-dependent inducible aryl hydrocarbon hydroxylase activity in rat brain mitochondria. *Drug Metab Dispos* 1981;9:69.
47. Paterniti JR Jr, Simone JJ, Beattie DS. Detection and regulation of δ-aminolevulinic acid synthetase activity in the rat brain. *Arch Biochem Biophys* 1978;189:86.
48. Feuer G, Sosa-Lucero JC, Lund G, et al. Failure of various drugs to induce drug-metabolizing enzymes in extrahepatic tissues of the rat. *Toxicol Appl Pharmacol* 1971;19:579.
49. Nabeshima T, Fentenot J, Ho JK. Effects of chronic administration of phenobarbital or morphine on the brain microsomal cytochrome P-450 system. *Biochem Pharmacol* 1981;30:1142.
50. Sima AA, Kennedy JC, Blakeslee D, et al. Experimental porphyric neuropathy. *J Can Sci Neurol* 1981;8:105.
51. Bornstein JC, Pickett JB, Diamond I. Inhibition of the evoked release of acetylcholine by the porphyrin precursor δ-aminolevulinic acid. *Ann Neurol* 1979;5:94.
52. Dichter HN, Taddeini L, Lin S, et al. Delta aminolevulinic acid. Effect of a porphyrin precursor on an isolated neuronal preparation. *Brain Res* 1977;126:189.
53. Becker DM, Goldstuck N, Kramer S. Effect of δ-aminolevulinic acid on the resting membrane potential of frog sartorius muscle. *S Afr Med J* 1975;49:1790.
54. Durko I, Juhasz A. Porphyrin synthesis in primary nervous tissue cultures from 10-3M δ-aminolevulinic acid in the presence of metatonin and neuropeptides. *Neurochem Res* 1986;11:607.
55. Culter MG, Moore MR, Dick JM. Effects of δ-aminolevulinic acid on contractile activity of rabbit duodenum. *Eur J Pharmacol* 1980;64:221.
56. Becker DM, Viljoen D, Kramer S. The inhibition of red cell and brain ATPase by δ-aminolevulinic acid. *Biochim Biophys Acta* 1971;225:26.
57. Mueller WE, Snyder SH. δ-Aminolevulinic acid: influences on synergistic GABA receptor binding may explain CNS symptoms of porphyria. *Ann Neurol* 1977;2:340.
58. Sweeney VP, Pathak MA, Asbury AK. Acute intermittent porphyria. Increased ALA synthetase activity during an acute attack. *Brain* 1970;93:369.
59. McGillon FB, Moore MR, Goldberg A. The effect of δ-aminolevulinic acid on the spontaneous activity of mice. *Scott Med J* 1973;18:133.
60. Shanley BC, Neethling AC, Percy VA, et al. Neurochemical aspects of porphyria. Studies on the possible neurotoxicity of delta-aminolaevulinic acid. *S Afr Med J* 1975;49:576.
61. Pierach CA, Edwards PS. Neurotoxicity of δ-aminolevulinic acid and porphobilinogen. *Exp Neurol* 1978;62:810.
62. Percy VA, Shanley RC. Porphyrin precursors in blood, urine and cerebrospinal fluid in acute porphyria. *S Afr Med J* 1977;52:219.
63. Gorchein A, Webber R. δ-Aminolevulinic acid in plasma, cerebrospinal fluid, saliva and erythrocytes: studies in normal, uremic and porphyric subjects. *Clin Sci* 1987;72:103.
64. Edwards SR, Shanley BC, Reynoldson JA. Neuropharmacology of δ-aminolevulinic acid. *Neuropharmacology* 1984;23:477.
65. Green H, Greenburg SM, Erickson RW, et al. Effect of dietary phenylalanine and tryptophan upon rat brain amine levels. *J Pharmacol Exp Ther* 1962;136:174.
66. Knox WE. The regulation of tryptophan pyrrolase activity by tryptophan. *Adv Enzyme Regul* 1966;4:287.
67. Litman DA, Correia MA. Elevated brain tryptophan and enhanced 5-hydroxytryptamine turnover in acute hepatic heme deficiency: clinical implications. *J Pharmacol Exp Ther* 1985;232:337.
68. Yuwiler A, Wetterberg L, Geller E. Tryptophan pyrrolase, tryptophan and tyrosine transaminase changes during allisopropylacetamide-induced porphyria in the rat. *Biochem Pharmacol* 1970;19:189.
69. Sassa S, Kappas A. Molecular aspects of the inherited porphyrias. *J Intern Med* 2000;247:169.
70. Anderson KE, Sassa S, Bishop DF, et al. Disorders of heme biosynthesis: X-linked sideroblastic anemia and the porphyrias. In: Scriver CR, Beaudet AL, Sly WS, et al., eds. *The metabolic and molecular bases of inherited disease.* New York: McGraw-Hill, 2001:2991.
71. Raskind WH, Wijsman E, Pagon RA, et al. X-linked sideroblastic anemia and ataxia: linkage to phosphoglycerate kinase at Xq13. *Am J Hum Genet* 1991;48:335.
72. Allikmets R, Raskind WH, Hutchinson A, et al. Mutation of a putative mitochondrial iron transporter gene (ABC7) in X-linked sideroblastic anemia and ataxia (XLSA/A). *Hum Mol Genet* 1999;8:743.
73. Shimada Y, Okuno S, Kawai A, et al. Cloning and chromosomal mapping of a novel ABC transporter gene (hABC7), a candidate for X-linked sideroblastic anemia with spinocerebellar ataxia. *J Hum Genet* 1998;43:115.
74. Ferreira GC, Neame PJ, Dailey HA. Heme biosynthesis in mammalian systems: evidence of a Schiff base linkage between the pyridoxal 5'-phosphate cofactor and a lysine residue in 5-aminolevulinate synthase. *Protein Sci* 1993;2:1959.
75. Riddle RD, Yamamoto M, Engel JD. Expression of δ-aminolevulinate synthase in avian cells: separate genes encode erythroid-specific and nonspecific isozymes. *Proc Natl Acad Sci U S A* 1989;86:792.
76. Bishop DF. Two different genes encode δ-aminolevulinate synthase in humans: nucleotide sequences of cDNAs for the housekeeping and erythroid genes. *Nucleic Acids Res* 1990;18:7187.
77. Bishop DF, Henderson AS, Astrin KH. Human δ-aminolevulinate synthase: assignment of the housekeeping gene to 3p21 and the erythroid-specific gene to the X chromosome. *Genomics* 1990;7:207.
78. Aoki Y. Crystallization and characterization of a new protease in mitochondria of bone marrow cells. *J Biol Chem* 1978;253:2026.
79. Cotter PD, Rucknagel DL, Bishop DF. X-linked sideroblastic anemia: identification of the mutation in the erythroid-specific δ-aminolevulinate synthase gene (ALAS2) in the original family described by Cooley. *Blood* 1994;84:3915.
80. Furuyama K, Sassa S. Interaction between succinyl CoA synthetase and the heme-biosynthetic enzyme ALAS-E is disrupted in sideroblastic anemia. *J Clin Invest* 2000;105:757.
81. Dailey HA, Dailey TA. Expression and purification of mammalian 5-aminolevulinate synthase. *Methods Enzymol* 1997;281:336.
82. Ferreira GC, Dailey HA. Expression of mammalian 5-aminolevulinate synthase in *Escherichia coli*. Overproduction, purification, and characterization. *J Biol Chem* 1993;268:584.
83. Tan D, Ferreira GC. Active site of 5-aminolevulinate synthase resides at the subunit interface. Evidence from in vivo heterodimer formation. *Biochemistry* 1996;35:8934.
84. Furuyama K, Sassa S. Human δ-aminolevulinate synthase complexes: homodimer and heterodimer complex formation with succinyl CoA synthase. *Blood* 1999;94:190(abst).
85. Aoki Y, Wada O, Urata G, et al. Purification and some properties of δ-aminolevulinate (ALA) synthetase in rabbit reticulocytes. *Biochem Biophys Res Commun* 1971;42:568–575.
86. Woods JS, Murthy VV. δ-Aminolevulinic acid synthetase from fetal rat liver. Studies on the partially purified enzyme. *Mol Pharmacol* 1975;11:70.
87. Neuwirt J, Ponka P, Borova J. Evidence for the presence of free and protein-bound nonhemoglobin heme in rabbit reticulocytes. *Biochim Biophys Acta* 1972;264:235.
88. Bottomley SS, May BK, Cox TC, et al. Molecular defects of erythroid 5-aminolevulinate synthase in X-linked sideroblastic anemia. *J Bioenerg Biomembr* 1995;27:161.
89. Cotter PD, Willard HF, Gorski JL, et al. Assignment of human erythroid δ-aminolevulinate synthase (ALAS2) to a distal subregion of band Xp11.21 by PCR analysis of somatic cell hybrids containing X-autosome translocations. *Genomics* 1992;13:211.
90. Sutherland GR, Baker E, Callen DF, et al. 5-Aminolevulinate synthase is at 3p21 and thus not the primary defect in X-linked sideroblastic anemia. *Am J Hum Genet* 1988;43:331.

91. Cotter PD, Drabkin HA, Varkony T, et al. Assignment of the human housekeeping delta-aminolevulinate synthase gene (ALAS1) to chromosome band 3p21.1 by PCR analysis of somatic cell hybrids. *Cytogenet Cell Genet* 1995; 69:207.

92. Cox TC, Bawden MJ, Martin A, et al. Human erythroid 5-aminolevulinate synthase: promoter analysis and identification of an iron-responsive element in the mRNA. *EMBO J* 1991;10:1891.

93. Elliott WH, May BK, Bawden MJ, et al. Regulation of genes associated with drug metabolism. *Biochem Soc Symp* 1989;55:13.

94. Surinya KH, Cox TC, May BK. Transcriptional regulation of the human erythroid 5-aminolevulinate synthase gene. Identification of promoter elements and role of regulatory proteins. *J Biol Chem* 1997;272:26585.

95. Surinya KH, Cox TC, May BK. Identification and characterization of a conserved erythroid-specific enhancer located in intron 8 of the human 5-aminolevulinate synthase 2 gene. *J Biol Chem* 1998;273:16798.

96. May BK, Dogra SC, Sadlon TJ, et al. Molecular regulation of heme biosynthesis in higher vertebrates. *Prog Nucleic Acid Res Mol Biol* 1995;51:1.

97. Fujita H, Yamamoto M, Yamagami T, et al. Sequential activation of genes for heme pathway enzymes during erythroid differentiation of mouse Friend virus-transformed erythroleukemia cells. *Biochim Biophys Acta* 1991;1090:311.

98. Gardner LC, Smith SJ, Cox TM. Biosynthesis of δ-aminolevulinic acid and the regulation of heme formation by immature erythroid cells in man. *J Biol Chem* 1991;266:22010.

99. Dierks P. Molecular biology of eukaryotic 5-aminolevulinate synthase. In: Dailey HA, ed. *Biosynthesis of heme and chlorophylls*. New York: McGraw-Hill, 1990:201.

100. May BK, Bhasker CR, Bawden MJ, et al. Molecular regulation of 5-aminolevulinate synthase. Diseases related to heme biosynthesis. *Mol Biol Med* 1990; 7:405.

101. Melefors O, Goossen B, Johansson HE, et al. Translational control of 5-aminolevulinate synthase mRNA by iron-responsive elements in erythroid cells. *J Biol Chem* 1993;268:5974.

102. Ke Y, Wu J, Leibold EA, et al. Loops and bulge/loops in iron-responsive element isoforms influence iron regulatory protein binding. Fine-tuning of mRNA regulation? *J Biol Chem* 1998;273:23637.

103. May A, Bishop DF. The molecular biology and pyridoxine responsiveness of X-linked sideroblastic anaemia. *Haematologica* 1998;83:56.

104. Cotter PD, May A, Li L, et al. Four new mutations in the erythroid-specific 5-aminolevulinate synthase (ALAS2) gene causing X-linked sideroblastic anemia: increased pyridoxine responsiveness after removal of iron overload by phlebotomy and coinheritance of hereditary hemochromatosis. *Blood* 1999;93:1757.

105. Edgar AJ, Vidyatilake HM, Wickramasinghe SN. X-linked sideroblastic anaemia due to a mutation in the erythroid 5-aminolaevulinate synthase gene leading to an arginine170 to leucine substitution. *Eur J Haematol* 1998;61:55.

106. Cotter PD, May A, Fitzsimmons EJ, et al. Late-onset X-linked sideroblastic anemia. Missense mutations in the erythroid delta-aminolevulinate synthase (ALAS2) gene in two pyridoxine-responsive patients initially diagnosed with acquired refractory anemia and ringed sideroblasts. *J Clin Invest* 1995;96:2090.

107. Prades E, Chambon C, Dailey TA, et al. A new mutation of the ALAS2 gene in a large family with X-linked sideroblastic anemia. *Hum Genet* 1995;95:424.

108. Cox TC, Bottomley SS, Wiley JS, et al. X-linked pyridoxine-responsive sideroblastic anemia due to a Thr388-to-Ser substitution in erythroid 5-aminolevulinate synthase. *N Engl J Med* 1994;330:675.

109. Cazzola M, May A, Bergamaschi G, et al. Familial-skewed X-chromosome inactivation as a predisposing factor for late-onset X-linked sideroblastic anemia in carrier females. *Blood* 2000;96:4363.

110. Furuyama K, Fujita H, Nagai T, et al. Pyridoxine refractory X-linked sideroblastic anemia caused by a point mutation of the erythroid-specific 5-aminolevulinate synthase gene. *Blood* 1997;90:822.

111. Edgar AJ, Losowsky MS, Noble JS, et al. Identification of an arginine452 to histidine substitution in the erythroid 5-aminolaevulinate synthetase gene in a large pedigree with X-linked hereditary sideroblastic anaemia. *Eur J Haematol* 1997;58:1.

112. Cotter PD, Baumann M, Bishop DF. Enzymatic defect in "X-linked" sideroblastic anemia: molecular evidence for erythroid delta-aminolevulinate synthase deficiency. *Proc Natl Acad Sci U S A* 1992;89:4028.

113. Edgar AJ, Wickramasinghe SN. Hereditary sideroblastic anaemia due to a mutation in exon 10 of the erythroid 5-aminolaevulinate synthase gene. *Br J Haematol* 1998;100:389.

114. Konopka L, Hoffbrand AV. Haem synthesis in sideroblastic anaemia. *Br J Haematol* 1979;42:73.

115. Bottomley SS. Secondary iron overload disorders. *Semin Hematol* 1998;35:77.

116. Hines JD. Effect of pyridoxine plus chronic phlebotomy on the function and morphology of bone marrow and liver in pyridoxine-responsive sideroblastic anemia. *Semin Hematol* 1976;13:133.

117. Olivieri NF, Brittenham GM. Iron-chelating therapy and the treatment of thalassemia. *Blood* 1997;89:739.

118. Sassa S. δ-Aminolevulinic acid dehydratase assay. *Enzyme* 1982;28:133.

119. Wetmur JG, Bishop DF, Cantelmo C, et al. Human delta-aminolevulinate dehydratase: nucleotide sequence of a full-length cDNA clone. *Proc Natl Acad Sci U S A* 1986;83:7703.

120. Potluri VR, Astrin KH, Wetmur JG, et al. Human 5-aminolevulinate dehydratase. Chromosomal localization to 9q34 by in situ hybridization. *Hum Genet* 1987;76:236.

121. Mitchell LW, Jaffe EK. Porphobilinogen synthase from *Escherichia coli* is a Zn(II) metalloenzyme stimulated by Mg(II). *Arch Biochem Biophys* 1993;300:169.

122. Jordan PM, Seehra JS. Mechanism of action of δ-aminolevulinic acid dehydratase. Stepwise order of addition of the two molecules of delta-aminolevulinic acid in the enzyme synthesis of porphobilinogen. *J Chem Soc, Chem Commun* 1980:240–242.

123. Erskine PT, Senior N, Awan S, et al. X-ray structure of 5-aminolaevulinate dehydratase, a hybrid aldolase. *Nat Struct Biol* 1997;4:1025.

124. Granick JL, Sassa S, Kappas A. Some biochemical and clinical aspects of lead intoxication. In: Bodansky O, Latner AL, eds. *Advances in clinical chemistry*. New York: Academic Press, 1978:287.

125. Sassa S, Fujita H, Kappas A. Succinylacetone and δ-aminolevulinic acid dehydratase in hereditary tyrosinemia: immunochemical study of the enzyme. *Pediatrics* 1990;86:84.

126. Lindblad B, Lindstedt S, Steen G. On the genetic defects in hereditary tyrosinemia. *Proc Natl Acad Sci U S A* 1977;74:4641.

127. Rank JM, Pascual-Leone A, Payne W, et al. Hematin therapy for the neurologic crisis of tyrosinemia. *J Pediatr* 1991;118:136.

128. Doss M, von Tiepermann R, Schneider J, et al. New type of hepatic porphyria with porphobilinogen synthase defect and intermittent acute clinical manifestation. *Klin Wochenschr* 1979;57:1123.

129. Thunell S, Holmberg L, Lundgren J. Aminolevulinate dehydratase porphyria in infancy. A clinical and biochemical study. *J Clin Chem Clin Biochem* 1987;25:5.

130. Hassoun A, Verstraeten L, Mercelis R, et al. Biochemical diagnosis of an hereditary aminolaevulinate dehydratase deficiency in a 63-year-old man. *J Clin Chem Clin Biochem* 1989;27:781.

131. Wolff C, Piderit F, Armas-Merino R. Deficiency of porphobilinogen synthase associated with acute crisis. Diagnosis of the first two cases in Chile by laboratory methods. *Eur J Clin Chem Clin Biochem* 1992;29:313.

132. Muraoka A, Suehiro I, Fujii M, et al. Delta-aminolevulinic acid dehydratase deficiency porphyria (ADP) with syndrome of inappropriate secretion of antidiuretic hormone (SIADH) in a 69-year-old woman. *Kobe J Med Sci* 1995;41:23.

133. Akagi R, Yasui Y, Harper P, et al. A novel mutation of δ-aminolevulinate dehydratase in a healthy child with 12% erythrocyte enzyme activity. *Br J Haematol* 1999;106:931.

134. Doss M, Laubenthal F, Stoeppler M. Lead poisoning in inherited δ-aminolevulinic acid dehydratase deficiency. *Int Arch Occup Environ Health* 1984;54:55.

135. Sassa S, Fujita H, Sugita O. Genetic regulation of the heme pathway. *Ann N Y Acad Sci* 1987;514:15.

136. Bishop TR, Miller MW, Beall J, et al. Genetic regulation of delta-aminolevulinate dehydratase during erythropoiesis. *Nucleic Acids Res* 1996;24:2511.

137. Kaya AH, Plewinska M, Wong DM, et al. Human δ-aminolevulinate dehydratase (ALAD) gene: structure and alternative splicing of the erythroid and housekeeping mRNAs. *Genomics* 1994;19:242.

138. Maruno M, Furuyama K, Akagi R, et al. Highly heterogenous nature of δ-aminolevulinate dehydratase (ALAD) deficiencies in ALAD porphyria. *Blood* 2001;97:2972.

139. Ishida N, Fujita H, Fukuda Y, et al. Cloning and expression of the defective genes from a patient with δ-aminolevulinate dehydratase porphyria. *J Clin Invest* 1992;89:1431.

140. Akagi R, Shimizu R, Furuyama K, et al. Novel molecular defects of the δ-aminolevulinate dehydratase gene in a patient with inherited acute hepatic porphyria. *Hepatology* 2000;31:704.

141. Plewinska M, Thunell S, Holmberg L, et al. δ-Aminolevulinate dehydratase deficient porphyria: identification of the molecular lesions in a severely affected homozygote. *Am J Hum Genet* 1991;49:167.

142. Akagi R, Nishitani C, Harigae H, et al. Molecular analysis of δ-aminolevulinate dehydratase deficiency in a patient with an unusual late-onset porphyria. *Blood* 2000;96:3618.

143. Wetmur JG. Influence of the common human δ-aminolevulinate dehydratase polymorphism on lead body burden. *Environ Health Perspect* 1994;102:215.

144. Mitchell G, Larochelle J, Lambert M, et al. Neurologic crises in hereditary tyrosinemia. *N Engl J Med* 1990;322:432.

145. Sassa S, Kappas A. Hereditary tyrosinemia and the heme biosynthetic pathway. Profound inhibition of δ-aminolevulinic acid dehydratase activity by succinylacetone. *J Clin Invest* 1983;71:625.

146. Thunell S, Henrichson A, Floderus Y, et al. Liver transplantation in a boy with acute porphyria due to aminolaevulinate dehydratase deficiency. *Eur J Clin Chem Clin Biochem* 1992;30:599.

147. Anderson PM, Desnick RJ. Purification and properties of uroporphyrinogen-I synthase from human erythrocytes. Identification of stable enzyme-substrate intermediates. *J Biol Chem* 1980;255:1993.

148. Jordan PM, Shemin D. Purification and properties of uroporphyrinogen I synthase from *Rhodopseudomonas spheroides*. *J Biol Chem* 1973;248:1019.

149. Miyagi K, Kaneshima M, Kawakami J, et al. Uroporphyrinogen I synthase from human erythrocytes. Separation, purification, and properties of isoenzymes. *Proc Natl Acad Sci U S A* 1979;76:6172.

150. Beaumont C, Grandchamp B, Bogard M, et al. Porphobilinogen deaminase is unstable in the absence of its substrate. *Biochim Biophys Acta* 1986;882:384.

151. Grandchamp B, Phung N, Grelier M, et al. The spectrophotometric determination of uroporphyrinogen I synthetase activity. *Clin Chim Acta* 1976;70:113.

152. Strand LJ, Meyer UA, Felsher BF, et al. Decreased red cell uroporphyrinogen I synthetase activity in intermittent acute porphyria. *J Clin Invest* 1972;51:2530.

153. Sassa S, Granick S, Bickers DR, et al. A microassay for uroporphyrinogen I synthase, one of three abnormal enzyme activities in acute intermittent porphyria, and its application to the study of the genetics of this disease. *Proc Natl Acad Sci U S A* 1974;71:732.

154. Kappas A, Sassa S, Galbraith RA, et al. The porphyrias. In: Scriver CR, Beaudet AL, Sly WS, et al., eds. *The metabolic and molecular basis of inherited disease.* New York: McGraw-Hill, 1995:2103.

155. Bonkowsky HL. Porphyrin and heme metabolism and the porphyrias. In: Zakim D, Boyer TD, eds. *Hepatology.* Philadelphia: WB Saunders, 1982:351.

156. Tishler PV, Woodward B, O'Connor J, et al. High prevalence of intermittent acute porphyria in a psychiatric patient population. *Am J Psychiatry* 1985; 142:1430.

157. Stein JA, Curl FD, Valsamis M, et al. Abnormal iron and water metabolism in acute intermittent porphyria with new morphologic findings. *Am J Med* 1972;53:784.

158. Ridley A. Porphyric neuropathy. In: Dyck PJ, Thomas PK, Lambert EH, eds. *Peripheral neuropathy,* vol. 2. Philadelphia: WB Saunders, 1975:942.

159. Poser CM, Edwards K. Transient monoparesis in acute intermittent porphyria. *Arch Neurol* 1978;35:550.

160. Sorensen HW, With TK. Persistent pareses after porphyric attacks. *Acta Med Scand* 1971;190:219.

161. McColl KE, Wallace AM, Moore MR, et al. Alterations in haem biosynthesis during the human menstrual cycle. Studies in normal subjects and patients with latent and active acute intermittent porphyria. *Clin Sci (Lond)* 1982;62:183.

162. Kappas A, Song CS, Levere RD, et al. The induction of δ-aminolevulinic acid synthetase in vivo in chick embryo liver by natural steroids. *Proc Natl Acad Sci U S A* 1968;61:509.

163. Sassa S, Bradlow HL, Kappas A. Steroid induction of δ-aminolevulinic acid synthase and porphyrins in liver. Structure-activity studies and the permissive effects of hormones on the induction process. *J Biol Chem* 1979;254:10011.

164. Felsher BF, Redeker AG. Acute intermittent porphyria: effect of diet and griseofulvin. *Medicine* 1967;46:217.

165. Welland FH, Hellman ES, Gaddis EM, et al. Factors affecting the excretion of porphyrin precursors by patients with acute intermittent porphyria. I. The effects of diet. *Metabolism* 1964;13:232.

166. Granick S, van den Schreieck HG. Porphobilinogen and δ-aminolevulinic acid in acute porphyria. *Proc Soc Exp Biol Med* 1955;88:270.

167. Watson CJ, Schwartz S. A simple test for urinary porphobilinogen. *Proc Soc Exp Biol Med* 1941;47:393.

168. Watson CJ, Taddeini L, Bossermaier I. Present status of the Ehrlich aldehyde reaction for urinary porphobilinogen. *JAMA* 1964;190:501.

169. Mauzerall D, Granick S. The occurrence and determination of δ-aminolevulinic acid and porphobilinogen in urine. *J Biol Chem* 1956;219:435.

170. Deacon AC, Peters TJ. Identification of acute porphyria: evaluation of a commercial screening test for urinary porphobilinogen. *Ann Clin Biochem* 1998; 35:726.

171. Lim CK, Rideout JM, Samson DM. Determination of 5-aminolaevulinic acid and porphobilinogen by high-performance liquid chromatography. *J Chromatogr* 1979;185:605.

172. Wang AL, Arredondo-Vega FX, Giampietro PF, et al. Regional gene assignment of human porphobilinogen deaminase and esterase A4 to chromosome 11q23 leads to 11qter. *Proc Natl Acad Sci U S A* 1981;78:5734.

173. De Verneuil H, Phung N, Nordmann Y, et al. Assignment of human uroporphyrinogen-I synthase locus to region 11qter by gene dosage effect. *Hum Genet* 1982;60:212.

174. Grandchamp B, de Verneuil H, Beaumont C, et al. Tissue-specific expression of porphobilinogen deaminase. Two isoenzymes from a single gene. *Eur J Biochem* 1987;162:105.

175. Chretien S, Dubart A, Beaupain D, et al. Alternative transcription and splicing of the human porphobilinogen deaminase gene result either in tissue-specific or in housekeeping expression. *Proc Natl Acad Sci U S A* 1988; 85:6.

176. Mignotte V, Eleouet JF, Raich N, et al. Cis- and trans-acting elements involved in the regulation of the erythroid promotor of the human porphobilinogen deaminase gene. *Proc Natl Acad Sci U S A* 1989;86:6548.

177. Grandchamp B, Nordmann Y. Enzymes of the heme biosynthesis pathway: recent advances in molecular genetics. *Semin Hematol* 1988;25:303.

178. De Siervi A, Rossetti MV, Parera VE, et al. Identification and characterization of hydroxymethylbilane synthase mutations causing acute intermittent porphyria: evidence for an ancestral founder of the common G111R mutation. *Am J Med Sci* 1999;86:366.

179. Louie GV, Brownlie PD, Lambert R, et al. Structure of porphobilinogen deaminase reveals a flexible multidomain polymerase with a single catalytic site. *Nature* 1992;359:33.

180. Louie GV, Brownlie PD, Lambert R, et al. The three-dimensional structure of *Escherichia coli* porphobilinogen deaminase at 1.76-A resolution. *Proteins* 1996;25:48.

181. Grandchamp B. Acute intermittent porphyria. *Semin Liver Dis* 1998;18:17.

182. Lee JS, Anvret M. Identification of the most common mutation within the porphobilinogen deaminase gene in Swedish patients with acute intermittent porphyria. *Proc Natl Acad Sci U S A* 1991;88:10912.

183. Greene-Davis ST, Neumann PE, Mann OE, et al. Detection of a R173W mutation in the porphobilinogen deaminase gene in the Nova Scotian "foreign Protestant" population with acute intermittent porphyria: a founder effect. *Clin Biochem* 1997;30:607.

184. Gu X-F, de Rooij F, Lee JS, et al. High prevalence of a point mutation in the porphobilinogen deaminase gene in Dutch patients with acute intermittent porphyria. *Hum Genet* 1993;91:128.

185. Desnick RJ, Ostasiewicz LT, Tishler PA, et al. Acute intermittent porphyria: characterization of a novel mutation in the structural gene for porphobilino-

186. Astrin KH, Desnick RJ. Molecular basis of acute intermittent porphyria: mutations and polymorphisms in the human hydroxymethylbilane synthase gene. *Hum Mutat* 1994;4:243.

187. Grandchamp B, Picat C, Mignotte V, et al. Tissue-specific splicing mutation in acute intermittent porphyria. *Proc Natl Acad Sci U S A* 1989;86:661.

188. Grandchamp B, Picat C, Kauppinen R, et al. Molecular analysis of acute intermittent porphyria in a Finnish family with normal erythrocyte porphobilinogen deaminase. *Eur J Clin Invest* 1989;19:415.

189. Mathews-Roth MM. Anemia in erythropoietic protoporphyria [Letter]. *JAMA* 1974;230:824.

190. Puy H, Gross U, Deybach JC, et al. Exon 1 donor splice site mutations in the porphobilinogen deaminase gene in the non-erythroid variant form of acute intermittent porphyria. *Hum Genet* 1998;103:570.

191. Mustajoki S, Pihlaja H, Ahola H, et al. Three splicing defects, an insertion, and two missense mutations responsible for acute intermittent porphyria. *Hum Genet* 1998;102:541.

192. Delfau MH, Picat C, de Rooij FW, et al. Two different point G to A mutations in exon 10 of the porphobilinogen deaminase gene are responsible for acute intermittent porphyria. *J Clin Invest* 1990;86:1511.

193. Wood S, Lambert R, Jordan M. Molecular basis of acute intermittent porphyria. *Mol Med Today* 1995;5:232.

194. Brownlie PD, Lambert R, Louie GV, et al. The three-dimensional structures of mutants of porphobilinogen deaminase: toward an understanding of the structural basis of acute intermittent porphyria. *Protein Sci* 1994;3:1644.

195. Puy H, Deybach JC, Lamoril J, et al. Molecular epidemiology and diagnosis of PBG deaminase gene defects in acute intermittent porphyria. *Am J Hum Genet* 1997;60:1373.

196. Whatley SD, Roberts AG, Elder GH. De novo mutation and sporadic presentation of acute intermittent porphyria. *Lancet* 1995;346:1007.

197. Sassa S, Solish G, Levere RD, et al. Studies in porphyria. IV. Expression of the gene defect of acute intermittent porphyria in cultured human skin fibroblasts and amniotic cells: prenatal diagnosis of the porphyric trait. *J Exp Med* 1975;142:722.

198. Sassa S, Zalar GL, Kappas A. Studies in porphyria. VII. Induction of uroporphyrinogen-I synthase and expression of the gene defect of acute intermittent porphyria in mitogen-stimulated human lymphocytes. *J Clin Invest* 1978;61:499.

199. Grandchamp B, Picat C, Mignotte V, et al. Tissue-specific splicing mutation in acute intermittent porphyria. *Proc Natl Acad Sci U S A* 1989;86:661.

200. Bonkowsky HL, Tschudy DP, Collins A, et al. Repression of the overproduction of porphyria precursors in acute intermittent porphyria by intravenous infusions of hematin. *Proc Natl Acad Sci U S A* 1971;68:2725.

201. Pierach CA. Hematin therapy for the porphyric attack. *Semin Liver Dis* 1982;2:125.

202. Watson CJ, Pierach CA, Bossenmaier I, et al. Postulated deficiency of hepatic heme and repair by hematin infusions in the "inducible" hepatic porphyrias. *Proc Natl Acad Sci U S A* 1977;74:2118.

203. Lamon JM, Frykholm BC, Tschudy DP. Hematin administration to an adult with lead intoxication. *Blood* 1979;53:1007.

204. Simionatto CS, Galbraith RA, Jones R, et al. Hematin infusions impair hemostasis in normal subjects. *Clin Res* 1986;34:651A.

205. Morris DL, Dudley MD, Pearson RD. Coagulopathy associated with hematin treatment for acute intermittent porphyria. *Ann Intern Med* 1981;95:700.

206. Glueck R, Green D, Cohen I, et al. Hematin: unique effects on hemostasis. *Blood* 1983;61:243.

207. Petersen JM, Pierach CA. Hematin-induced hemolysis in acute porphyria. *Ann Intern Med* 1984;101:877.

208. Tenhunen R, Tokola O, Linden IB. Haem arginate: a new stable haem compound. *J Pharm Pharmacol* 1987;39:780.

209. Galbraith RA, Kappas A. Pharmacokinetics of tin-mesoporphyrin in man and the effects of tin-chelated porphyrins on hyperexcretion of heme pathway precursors in patients with acute inducible porphyria. *Hepatology* 1989;9:882.

210. Romeo G, Levin EY. Uroporphyrinogen 3 cosynthetase in human congenital erythropoietic porphyria. *Proc Natl Acad Sci U S A* 1969;63:856.

211. Deybach JC, de Verneuil H, Phung N, et al. Congenital erythropoietic porphyria (Gunther's disease): enzymatic studies on two cases of late onset. *J Lab Clin Med* 1981;97:551.

212. Bogorad L. The enzymatic synthesis of porphyrins from porphobilinogen. II. Uroporphyrin III. *J Biol Chem* 1958;233:510.

213. Stevens E, Frydman RB, Frydman B. Separation of porphobilinogen deaminase and uroporphyrinogen III cosynthase from human erythrocytes. *Biochim Biophys Acta* 1968;158:496.

214. Tsai SF, Bishop DF, Desnick RJ. Purification and properties of uroporphyrinogen III synthase from human erythrocytes. *J Biol Chem* 1987;262:1268.

215. Fritsch C, Bolsen K, Ruzicka T, et al. Congenital erythropoietic porphyria. *J Am Acad Dermatol* 1997;36:594.

216. Warner CA, Poh-Fitzpatrick MB, Zaider EF, et al. Congenital erythropoietic porphyria. A mild variant with low uroporphyrin I levels due to a missense mutation (A66V) encoding residual uroporphyrinogen III synthase activity. *Arch Dermatol* 1992;128:1243.

217. Saval AH, Tirado AM. Congenital erythropoietic porphyria affecting two brothers. *Br J Dermatol* 1999;141:547.

218. Poh-Fitzpatrick MB. The erythropoietic porphyrias. *Dermatol Clin* 1986;4:291.

219. Kramer S, Viljoen E, Meyer AM, et al. The anemia of erythropoietic porphyria with the first description of the disease in an elderly patient. *Br J Haematol* 1965;11:666.

220. Rank JM, Straka JG, Weimer MK, et al. Hematin therapy in late onset congenital erythropoietic porphyria. *Br J Haematol* 1990;75:617.

221. Murphy A, Gibson G, Elder GH, et al. Adult-onset congenital erythropoietic porphyria (Gunther's disease) presenting with thrombocytopenia. *J R Soc Med* 1995;88:357.

222. Schmid R, Schwartz S, Sundberg RD. Erythropoietic (congenital) porphyria: a rare abnormality of normoblasts. *Blood* 1955;10:416.

223. Freesemann AG, Bhutani LK, Jacob K, et al. Interdependence between degree of porphyrin excess and disease severity in congenital erythropoietic porphyria (Gunther's disease). *Arch Dermatol Res* 1997;289:272.

224. Astrin KH, Warner CA, Yoo HW, et al. Regional assignment of the human uroporphyrinogen III synthase (UROS) gene to chromosome 10q25.2→q26.3. *Hum Genet* 1991;87:18.

225. Xu W, Kozak CA, Desnick RJ. Uroporphyrinogen-III synthase: molecular cloning, nucleotide sequence, expression of a mouse full-length cDNA, and its localization on mouse chromosome 7. *Genomics* 1995;26:556.

226. Bensidhoum M, Ged CM, Poirier C, et al. The cDNA sequence of mouse uroporphyrinogen III synthase and assignment to mouse chromosome 7. *Mamm Genome* 1994;5:728.

227. Barker D, Schafer M, White R. Restriction sites containing CpG show a higher frequency of polymorphism in human DNA. *Cell* 1984;36:131.

228. Cooper DN, Krawczak M. The mutational spectrum of single base-pair substitutions causing human genetic disease: patterns and predictions. *Hum Genet* 1990;85:55.

229. Fontanellas A, Bensidhoum M, Enriquez DS, et al. A systematic analysis of the mutations of the uroporphyrinogen III synthase gene in congenital erythropoietic porphyria. *Eur J Hum Genet* 1996;4:274.

230. Warner CA, Yoo HW, Roberts AG, et al. Congenital erythropoietic porphyria: identification of exonic mutations in the uroporphyrinogen III synthase gene. *J Clin Invest* 1992;89:693.

231. Bensidhoum M, Audine M, Fontanellas A, et al. The disruption of mouse uroporphyrinogen III synthase (*uros*) gene is fully lethal. *Acta Haematol* 1997;98:100(abst).

232. Kaiser IH. Brown amniotic fluid in congenital erythropoietic porphyria. *Obstet Gynecol* 1980;56:383.

233. Deybach JC, Grandchamp B, Grelier M, et al. Prenatal exclusion of congenital erythropoietic porphyria (Gunther's disease) in a fetus at risk. *Hum Genet* 1980;53:217.

234. Ged C, Moreau-Gaudry F, Taine L, et al. Prenatal diagnosis in congenital erythropoietic porphyria by metabolic measurement and DNA mutation analysis. *Prenat Diagn* 1996;16:83.

235. Mathews-Roth MM. Beta-carotene in congenital porphyria. *Arch Dermatol* 1979;114:641.

236. Piomelli S, Poh-Fitzpatrick MB, Seaman C, et al. Complete suppression of the symptoms of congenital erythropoietic porphyria by long-term treatment with high-level transfusions. *N Engl J Med* 1986;314:1029.

237. Guarini L, Piomelli S, Poh-Fitzpatrick MB. Hydroxyurea in congenital erythropoietic porphyria. *N Engl J Med* 1994;330:1091.

238. Tishler PV, Winston SH. Rapid improvement in the chemical pathology of congenital erythropoietic porphyria with treatment with superactivated charcoal. *Methods Find Exp Clin Pharmacol* 1990;12:645.

239. Minder EI, Schneider-Yin X, Moll F. Lack of effect of oral charcoal in congenital erythropoietic porphyria. *N Engl J Med* 1994;330:1092.

240. Kauffman L, Evans DI, Stevens RF, et al. Bone-marrow transplantation for congenital erythropoietic porphyria. *Lancet* 1991;337:1510.

241. Tezcan I, Xu W, Gurgey A, et al. Congenital erythropoietic porphyria successfully treated by allogeneic bone marrow transplantation. *Blood* 1998; 92:4053.

242. Thomas C, Ged C, Nordmann Y, et al. Correction of congenital erythropoietic porphyria by bone marrow transplantation. *J Pediatr* 1996;129:453.

243. Zix-Kieffer I, Langer B, Eyer D, et al. Successful cord blood stem cell transplantation for congenital erythropoietic porphyria (Gunther's disease). *Bone Marrow Transplant* 1996;18:217.

244. Elder GH. Human uroporphyrinogen decarboxylase defects. In: Orfanos CS, Stadler R, Gollnick H, eds. *Dermatology in five continents.* Berlin: Springer-Verlag, 1988:857.

245. Held JL, Sassa S, Kappas A, et al. Erythrocyte uroporphyrinogen decarboxylase activity in porphyria cutanea tarda: a study of 40 consecutive patients. *J Invest Dermatol* 1989;93:332.

246. Mauzerall D, Granick S. Porphyrin biosynthesis in erythrocytes. III. Uroporphyrinogen and its decarboxylase. *J Biol Chem* 1958;232:1141.

247. Neve RA, Labbe RF, Aldrich RA. Reduced uroporphyrin III in the biosynthesis of heme. *J Am Chem Soc* 1956;78:691.

248. Smith AG, Francis JE. Decarboxylation of porphyrinogens by rat liver uroporphyrinogen decarboxylase. *Biochem J* 1979;183:455.

249. Smith AG, Francis JE. Genetic variation of iron-induced uroporphyria in mice. *Biochem J* 1993;291:29.

250. Blekkenhorst GH, Day RS, Eales L. The effect of bleeding and iron administration on the development of hexachlorobenzene-induced rat porphyria. *Int J Biochem* 1980;12:1013.

251. Louw M, Neethling AC, Percy VA, et al. Effects of hexachlorobenzene feeding and iron overload on enzymes of haem biosynthesis and cytochrome P 450 in rat liver. *Clin Sci Mol Med* 1977;53:111.

252. Sweeney GD, Jones KG, Cole FM, et al. Iron deficiency prevents liver toxicity of 2,3,7,8-tetrachlorodibenzo-p-dioxin. *Science* 1979;204:332.

253. Whitby FG, Phillips JD, Kushner JP, et al. Crystal structure of human uroporphyrinogen decarboxylase. *EMBO J* 1998;17:2463.

254. Phillips JD, Whitby FG, Kushner JP, et al. Characterization and crystallization of human uroporphyrinogen decarboxylase. *Protein Sci* 1997;6:1343.

255. Banes HD. Porphyrias in the Bantu races on the Witwatersrand. *S Afr Med J* 1955;29:781.

256. Dean G. *The porphyrias. A study of inheritance and environment.* London: Pitman Medical, 1971.

257. Elder GH. Recent advances in the identification of enzyme deficiencies in the porphyrias. *Br J Dermatol* 1983;108:729.

258. Kushner JP. The enzymatic defect in porphyria cutanea tarda. *N Engl J Med* 1982;306:799.

259. Behm AR, Unger WP. Oral contraceptives and porphyria cutanea tarda. *Can Med Assoc J* 1974;110:1052.

260. Grossman ME, Bickers DR, Poh-Fitzpatrick MB, et al. Porphyria cutanea tarda: clinical features and laboratory findings in forty patients. *Am J Med* 1979;67:277.

261. Bickers DR, Keogh L, Rifkind AB, et al. Studies in porphyria. VI. Biosynthesis of porphyrins in mammalian skin and in the skin of porphyric patients. *J Invest Dermatol* 1977;68:5.

262. Lim HW, Poh-Fitzpatrick MB, Gigli I. Activation of the complement system in patients with porphyrias after irradiation in vivo. *J Clin Invest* 1984;74: 1961.

263. Meurer M, Schulte C, Weiler A, et al. Photodynamic action of uroporphyrin on the complement system in porphyria cutanea tarda. *Arch Dermatol Res* 1985;277:293.

264. Torinuki W, Miura T, Tagami H. Activation of complement by 405-nm light in serum from porphyria cutanea tarda. *Arch Dermatol Res* 1985;277:174.

265. Pigatto PD, Polenghi MM, Altomare GF, et al. Complement cleavage products in the phototoxic reaction of porphyria cutanea tarda. *Br J Dermatol* 1986;114:567.

266. Sandberg S, Romslo I. Protoporphyrin-induced photodamage at the cellular and the subcellular level as related to the solubility of the porphyrin. *Clin Chim Acta* 1981;109:193.

267. Strandberg K, Hagermark O. Prostaglandin E2 in blister fluid of bullous diseases and experimental suction blisters. *Acta Dermatovener* 1977;57:487.

268. Sandberg S, Romslo I, Hovding G, et al. Porphyrin-induced photodamage as related to the subcellular localization of the porphyrins. *Acta Derm Venereol* 1982;100[Suppl]:75.

269. Cortes JM, Oliva H, Paradinas FJ, et al. The pathology of the liver in porphyria cutanea tarda. *Histopathology* 1980;4:471.

270. Bonkovsky HL, Poh-Fitzpatrick M, Pimstone N, et al. Porphyria cutanea tarda, hepatitis C, and HFE gene mutations in North America. *Hepatology* 1998;27:1661.

271. Bulaj ZJ, Phillips JD, Ajioka RS, et al. Hemochromatosis genes and other factors contributing to the pathogenesis of porphyria cutanea tarda. *Blood* 2000;95:1565.

272. Lundvall O. The effect of phlebotomy therapy in porphyria cutanea tarda. *Acta Med Scand* 1971;189:33.

273. Felsher BF, Jones ML, Redeker AG. Iron and hepatic uroporphyrin synthesis. *JAMA* 1973;226:663.

274. James KR, Cortes JM, Paradinas FJ. Demonstration of intracytoplasmic needle-like inclusions in hepatocytes of patients with porphyria cutanea tarda. *J Clin Pathol* 1980;33:899.

275. Uthemann H, Kotitschke R, Lissner R, et al. Serologische hepatitis-B-marker bei porphyria cutanea tarda. *Dtsch MedWochenschr* 1980;105:1718.

276. Bel A, Girard D. Porphyrie cutanee tardive avec antigene HBs of hepatite chronique agressive. *Nouv Presse Med* 1980;9:2027.

277. Pierach CA. Porphyria and hepatocellular carcinoma. *Br J Cancer* 1987;55:111.

278. Packe GE, Clarke CW. Is porphyria cutanea tarda a risk factor in the development of hepatocellular carcinoma? *Oncology* 1985;42:44.

279. Kordac V. Frequency of occurrence of hepatocellular carcinoma in patients with porphyria cutanea tarda in long-term follow-up. *Neoplasma* 1972;19:135.

280. Tio TH, Leijnse B, Jarrett A, et al. Acquired porphyria from a liver tumor. *Clin Sci Mol Med* 1959;16:517.

281. Nacht S, San Martin de Viale LC, Grinstein M. Human porphyria cutanea tarda. Isolation and properties of the urinary porphyrins. *Clin Chim Acta* 1970;27:445.

282. Smith SG, Rao KR, Jackson AH. The porphyrins of normal human urine, with a comparison of the excretion pattern in porphyria cutanea tarda. *J Biochem (Tokyo)* 1980;12:873.

283. Johansson IM, Niklasson FA. Determination of porphyrins in urine by direct injection on a liquid chromatographic column coated with tributylphosphate. *J Chromatogr* 1983;275:51.

284. Elder GH. The metabolism of porphyrins of the isocoproporphyrin series. *Enzyme* 1974;17:61.

285. Smith SG. Porphyrins found in urine of patients with symptomatic porphyria. *Biochem Soc Trans* 1977;5:1472.

286. Elder GH, Magnus IA, Handa F, et al. Faecal "X porphyrin" in the hepatic porphyrias. *Enzyme* 1973;17:29.

287. Malina L, Miller VI, Magnus IA. Skin porphyrin assay in porphyria. *Clin Chim Acta* 1978;83:55.

288. Romeo PH, Dubart A, Grandchamp B, et al. Isolation and identification of a cDNA clone coding for rat uroporphyrinogen decarboxylase. *Proc Natl Acad Sci U S A* 1984;81:3346.

289. Romeo PH, Raich N, Dubart A, et al. Molecular cloning and nucleotide sequence of a complete human uroporphyrinogen decarboxylase cDNA. *J Biol Chem* 1986;261:9825.

290. de Verneuil H, Grandchamp B, Foubert C, et al. Assignment of the gene for uroporphyrinogen decarboxylase to human chromosome 1 by somatic cell hybridization and specific enzyme immunoassay. *Hum Genet* 1984;66:202.

291. Dubart A, Mattei MG, Raich N, et al. Assignment of human uroporphyrinogen decarboxylase (URO-D) to the p34 band of chromosome 1. *Hum Genet* 1986;73:277.

292. Romeo PH, Raich N, Dubart A, et al. Molecular cloning and tissue-specific expression analysis of human porphobilinogen deaminase and uroporphyrinogen decarboxylase. In: Nordmann Y, ed. *Porphyrins and porphyrias.* London: John Libbey & Company, 1986:25.

293. Phillips JD, Jackson LK, Bunting M, et al. A mouse model of familial porphyria cutanea tarda. *Proc Natl Acad Sci U S A* 2001;98:259.

294. Elder GH, Lee GB, Tovey JA. Decreased activity of hepatic uroporphyrinogen decarboxylase in sporadic porphyria cutanea tarda. *N Engl J Med* 1978;299:274.

295. Elder GH. The differentiation of porphyria cutanea tarda symptomatica from other types of porphyria by the measurement of isocoproporphyrin in faeces. *J Clin Pathol* 1975;28:601.

296. Topi GC, Amantea A, Griso D. Recovery from porphyria cutanea tarda with no specific therapy other than avoidance of hepatic toxins. *Br J Dermatol* 1984;111:75.

297. Addy JH. Pathogenesis and natural history of porphyria cutanea tarda. *Lancet* 1974;2:213.

298. Ramsay CA, Magnus IA, Turnbull A, et al. The treatment of porphyria cutanea tarda by venesection. *QJM* 1974;169:1.

299. Ippen H. Treatment of porphyria cutanea tarda by phlebotomy. *Semin Hematol* 1977;14:253.

300. Epstein JH, Redeker AG. Porphyria cutanea tarda. A study of the effect of phlebotomy. *N Engl J Med* 1968;279:1301.

301. Sweeney GD. Porphyria cutanea tarda, or the uroporphyrinogen decarboxylase deficiency diseases. *Clin Biochem* 1986;19:3.

302. Lundvall O. Phlebotomy treatment of porphyria cutanea tarda. *Acta Derm Venereol* 1982;100[Suppl]:107.

303. Malina L, Chlumsky J, Chlumsky A. *Porphyria cutanea tarda: new facts on etiology, pathogenesis, clinical manifestations and treatment.* Czechoslovakia: Universita Karlova, 1974.

304. Malina L, Chlumsky J. A comparative study of the results of phlebotomy therapy and low-dose chloroquine treatment in porphyria cutanea tarda. *Acta Derm Venereol* 1981;61:346.

305. Swanbeck G, Wennersten G. Treatment of porphyria cutanea tarda with chloroquine and phlebotomy. *Br J Dermatol* 1977;97:77.

306. Wennersten G, Ros AM. Chloroquine in treatment of porphyria cutanea tarda. *Acta Derm Venereol* 1982;100[Suppl]:119.

307. Scholnick PL, Epstein J, Marver HS. The molecular basis of the action of chloroquine in porphyria cutanea tarda. *J Invest Dermatol* 1973;61:226.

308. Fujita H, Sassa S, Toback AC, et al. Immunochemical study of uroporphyrinogen decarboxylase in a patient with mild hepatoerythropoietic porphyria. *J Clin Invest* 1987;79:1533.

309. Toback AC, Sassa S, Poh-Fitzpatrick MB, et al. Hepatoerythropoietic porphyria: clinical, biochemical, and enzymatic studies in a three-generation family lineage. *N Engl J Med* 1987;316:645.

310. Simon N, Berko GY, Schneider I. Hepatoerythropoietic porphyria presenting as scleroderma and acrosclerosis in a sibling pair. *Br J Dermatol* 1977;96:663.

311. Pinol-Aguade J, Castells A, Indacochea A, et al. A case of biochemically unclassifiable hepatic porphyria. *Br J Dermatol* 1969;81:270.

312. Lazaro P, De Salamanca RE, Elder GH, et al. Is hepatoerythropoietic porphyria a homozygous form of porphyria cutanea tarda? Inheritance of uroporphyrinogen decarboxylase deficiency in a Spanish family. *Br J Dermatol* 1984;110:613.

313. Lim HW, Poh-Fitzpatrick MB. Hepatoerythropoietic porphyria: a variant of childhood-onset porphyria cutanea tarda. Porphyrin profiles and enzymatic studies of two cases in a family. *J Am Acad Dermatol* 1984;11:1103.

314. De Verneuil H, Grandchamp B, Romeo PH, et al. Molecular analysis of uroporphyrinogen decarboxylase in a family with two cases of hepatoerythropoietic porphyria. *J Clin Invest* 1986;77:431.

315. De Verneuil H, Beaumont C, Grandchamp B, et al. Molecular heterogeneity of uroporphyrinogen decarboxylase deficiency in hepatoerythropoietic porphyria. In: Nordmann Y, ed. *Porphyrins and porphyrias.* London: John Libbey & Company, 1986:201.

316. Romana M, Grandchamp B, Dubart A, et al. Identification of a new mutation responsible for hepatoerythropoietic porphyria. *Eur J Clin Invest* 1991;21:225.

317. Meguro K, Fujita H, Ishida N, et al. Molecular defects of uroporphyrinogen decarboxylase in a patient with mild hepatoerythropoietic porphyria. *J Invest Dermatol* 1994;102:681.

318. De Verneuil H, Bourgeois F, de Rooij F, et al. Characterization of a new mutation (R292G) and a detection at the human uroporphyrinogen decarboxylase locus in two patients with hepatoerythropoietic porphyria. *Hum Genet* 1992;89:548.

319. Elder GH, Evans JO. Evidence that the coproporphyrinogen oxidase activity of rat liver is situated in the intermembrane space of mitochondria. *Biochem J* 1978;172:345.

320. Grandchamp B, Phung N, Nordmann Y. The mitochondrial localization of coproporphyrinogen III oxidase. *Biochem J* 1978;176:97.

321. Martasek P, Camadro JM, Raman CS, et al. Human coproporphyrinogen oxidase. Biochemical characterization of recombinant normal and R231W mutated

322. Medlock AE, Dailey HA. Human coproporphyrinogen oxidase is not a metalloprotein. *J Biol Chem* 1996;271:32507.

323. Brodie MJ, Thompson GG, Moore MR, et al. Hereditary coproporphyria. Demonstration of the abnormalities in haem biosynthesis in peripheral blood. *QJM* 1977;46:229.

324. Paxton JR, Moore MR, Beattie AD, et al. Urinary excretion of 17-oxosteroids in hereditary coproporphyria. *Clin Sci Mol Med* 1975;49:441.

325. Hunter JA, Khan SA, Hope E, et al. Hereditary coproporphyria. Photosensitivity, jaundice and neuropsychiatric manifestations associated with pregnancy. *Br J Dermatol* 1971;84:301.

326. Roberts DT, Brodie MJ, Moore MR, et al. Hereditary coprophyria presenting with photosensitivity induced by the contraceptive pill. *Br J Dermatol* 1977;96:549.

327. Andrews J, Erdjument H, Nicholson DC. Hereditary coproporphyria: incidence in a large English family. *J Med Genet* 1984;21:341.

328. Houston AB, Brodie MJ, Moore MR, et al. Hereditary coproporphyria and epilepsy. *Arch Dis Child* 1977;52:646.

329. Carlson RE, Dolphin D, Bernstein M. Copper coproporphyrin: excretion in familial coproporphyria. *Clin Chem* 1978;24:2009.

330. Cacheux V, Martasek P, Fougerousse F, et al. Localization of the human coproporphyrinogen oxidase gene to chromosome band 3q12. *Hum Genet* 1994;94:557.

331. Martasek P, Camadro JM, Delfau-Larue MH, et al. Molecular cloning, sequencing, and functional expression of a cDNA encoding human coproporphyrinogen oxidase. *Proc Natl Acad Sci U S A* 1994;91:3024.

332. Takahashi S, Furuyama K, Kobayashi A, et al. Cloning of a coproporphyrinogen oxidase promoter regulatory element binding protein: differential regulation of coproporphyrinogen oxidase gene between erythroid and nonerythroid cells. *Biochem Biophys Res Commun* 2000;273:596.

333. Takahashi S, Taketani S, Akasaka J, et al. Differential regulation of mouse coproporphyrinogen oxidase gene expression in erythroid and non-erythroid cells. *Blood* 1998;92:3436.

334. Conder LH, Woodard SI, Dailey HA. Multiple mechanisms for the regulation of haem synthesis during erythroid cell differentiation. Possible role for coproporphyrinogen oxidase. *Biochem J* 1991;275:321.

335. Taketani S, Yoshinaga T, Furukawa T, et al. Induction of terminal enzymes for heme biosynthesis during differentiation of mouse erythroleukemia cells. *Eur J Biochem* 1995;230:760.

336. Lamoril J, Deybach JC, Puy H, et al. Three novel mutations in the coproporphyrinogen oxidase gene. *Hum Mutat* 1997;9:78.

337. Martasek P. Hereditary coproporphyria. *Semin Liver Dis* 1998;18:25.

338. Martasek P, Nordmann Y, Grandchamp B. Homozygous hereditary coproporphyria caused by an arginine to tryptophane substitution in coproporphyrinogen oxidase and common intragenic polymorphisms. *Hum Mol Genet* 1994;3:477.

339. Rosipal R, Lamoril J, Puy H, et al. Systematic analysis of coproporphyrinogen oxidase gene defects in hereditary coproporphyria and mutation update. *Hum Mutat* 1999;13:44.

340. Lamoril J, Martasek P, Deybach JC, et al. A molecular defect in coproporphyrinogen oxidase gene causing harderoporphyria, a variant form of hereditary coproporphyria. *Hum Mol Genet* 1995;4:275.

341. Lamoril J, Puy H, Gouya L, et al. Neonatal hemolytic anemia due to inherited harderoporphyria: clinical characteristics and molecular basis. *Blood* 1998;91:1453.

342. Nordmann Y, Grandchamp B, de Verneuil H, et al. Harderoporphyria: a variant hereditary coproporphyria. *J Clin Invest* 1983;72:1139.

343. Van der Bergh AH, Grotepass W. Ein bemerkenswerter fall von porphyrie. *Wiener Klinische Wochenschrift* 1937;50:830.

344. Macalpine I, Hunter R, Rimington C, et al. *Porphyria—a royal malady.* London: British Medical Association, 1968.

345. Röhl JC, Warren M, Hunt D. *Purple secret.* London: Bantam Press, 1998.

346. Poulson R. The enzymic conversion of protoporphyrinogen IX to protoporphyrin IX in mammalian mitochondria. *J Biol Chem* 1976;251:3730.

347. Brenner DA, Bloomer JR. A fluorometric assay for measurement of protoporphyrinogen oxidase activity in mammalian tissue. *Clin Chim Acta* 1980;100: 259.

348. Duke SO, Lydon J, Becerril JM, et al. Protoporphyrinogen oxidase-inhibiting herbicides. *Weed Sci* 1991;39:465.

349. Whatley SD, Puy H, Morgan RR, et al. Variegate porphyria in Western Europe: identification of PPOX gene mutations in 104 families, extent of allelic heterogeneity, and absence of correlation between phenotype and type of mutation. *Am J Hum Genet* 1999;65:984.

350. Eales L. Porphyrias as seen in Cape Town: a survey of 250 patients and some recent studies. *S Afr J Lab Clin Med* 1963;9:151.

351. Kirsch RE, Meissner PN, Hift RJ. Variegate porphyria. *Semin Liver Dis* 1998;18:33.

352. Timonen K, Niemi KM, Mustajoki P, et al. Skin changes in variegate porphyria. Clinical, histopathological, and ultrastructural study. *Arch Dermatol Res* 1990;282:108.

353. Muhlbauer JE, Pathak MA, Tishler PV, et al. Variegate porphyria in New England. *JAMA* 1982;247:3095.

354. Mustajoki P. Variegate porphyria. Twelve years' experience in Finland. *QJM* 1980;194:191.

355. Perloth MG, Tschudy DP, Ratner A, et al. The effect of diet in variegate porphyria. *Metabolism* 1968;17:571.

356. Quiroz-Kendall E, Wilson FA, King LE. Acute variegate porphyria following a Scarsdale gourmet diet. *J Am Acad Dermatol* 1983;8:46.

357. Murphy GM, Hawk JL, Magnus IA, et al. Homozygous variegate porphyria: two similar cases in unrelated families. *J R Soc Med* 1986;79:361.

358. Norris PG, Elder GH, Hawk JL. Homozygous variegate porphyria: a case report. *Br J Dermatol* 1990;122:253.

359. Coakley J, Hawkins R, Crinis N, et al. An unusual case of variegate porphyria with possible homozygous inheritance. *Aust N Z J Med* 1990;20:587.

360. Hift RJ, Meissner PN, Todd G, et al. Homozygous variegate porphyria: an evolving clinical syndrome. *Postgrad Med J* 1993;69:781.

361. Kordac V, Martasek P, Zeman J, et al. Increased erythrocyte protoporphyrin in homozygous variegate porphyria. *Photodermatol* 1985;2:257.

362. Mustajoki P, Tenhunen R, Niemi KM, et al. Homozygous variegate porphyria. A severe skin disease of infancy. *Clin Genet* 1987;32:300.

363. Herrick AL, Moore MR, Thompson GG, et al. Cholelithiasis in patients with variegate porphyria. *J Hepatol* 1991;12:50.

364. Elder GH, Evans JO, Thomas N, et al. The primary enzyme defect in hereditary coproporphyria. *Lancet* 1976;2:1217.

365. Nishimura K, Taketani S, Inokuchi H. Cloning of a human cDNA for protoporphyrinogen oxidase by complementation in vivo of a hemG mutant of *Escherichia coli*. *J Biol Chem* 1995;270:8076.

366. Puy H, Robreau AM, Rosipal R, et al. Protoporphyrinogen oxidase: complete genomic sequence and polymorphisms in the human gene. *Biochem Biophys Res Commun* 1996;226:226.

367. Taketani S, Inazawa J, Abe T, et al. The human protoporphyrinogen oxidase gene (PPOX): organization and location to chromosome 1. *Genomics* 1995;29:698.

368. Dailey TA, Dailey HA, Meissner P, et al. Cloning, sequence, and expression of mouse protoporphyrinogen oxidase. *Arch Biochem Biophys* 1995;324:379.

369. Roberts AG, Whatley SD, Daniels J, et al. Partial characterization and assignment of the gene for protoporphyrinogen oxidase and variegate porphyrias to human chromosome 1q23. *Hum Mol Genet* 1995;4:2387.

370. Dailey TA, Dailey HA. Human protoporphyrinogen oxidase: expression, purification, and characterization of the cloned enzyme. *Protein Sci* 1996;5:98.

371. Deybach JC, Da Silva V, Grandchamp B, et al. The mitochondrial location of protoporphyrinogen oxidase. *Eur J Biochem* 1985;149:431.

372. Ferreira GC, Andrew TL, Karr SW, et al. Organization of the terminal two enzymes of the heme biosynthetic pathway. Orientation of protoporphyrinogen oxidase and evidence for a membrane complex. *J Biol Chem* 1988;263:3835.

373. Deybach JC, Puy H, Robreau AM, et al. Mutations in the protoporphyrinogen oxidase gene in patients with variegate porphyria. *Hum Mol Genet* 1996;5:407.

374. Meissner PN, Dailey TA, Hift RJ, et al. A R59W mutation in human protoporphyrinogen oxidase results in decreased enzyme activity and is prevalent in South Africans with variegate porphyria. *Nature* 1996;13:95.

375. Johnson A, Jones OT. Enzymic formation of hemes and other metalloporphyrins. *Biochim Biophys Acta* 1964;93:171.

376. Porra RJ, Jones OT. Studies on ferrochelatase 2. An investigation of the role of ferrochelatase in the biosynthesis of various haem prosthetic groups. *Biochem J* 1963;87:186.

377. Taketani S, Tokunaga R. Rat liver ferrochelatase. Purification, properties and stimulation by fatty acids. *J Biol Chem* 1981;256:12748.

378. Taketani S, Tokunaga R. Purification and substrate specificity of bovine liver ferrochelatase. *Eur J Biochem* 1982;127:443.

379. Camadro JM, Ibrahim NG, Levere RD. Kinetics of studies of human liver ferrochelatase: role of endogenous metals. *J Biol Chem* 1984;259:5678.

380. Camadro JM, Labbe P. Purification and properties of ferrochelatase from the yeast *Saccharomyces cerevisiae*. Evidence for a precursor form of the protein. *J Biol Chem* 1988;263:11675.

381. Karr SR, Dailey HA. The synthesis of murine ferrochelatase in vitro and in vivo. *Biochem J* 1988;254:799.

382. Taketani S, Tanaka-Yoshioka A, Masaki R, et al. Association of ferrochelatase with complex I in bovine heart mitochondria. *Biochim Biophys Acta* 1986;883:277.

383. Magnus IA, Jarrett A, Prankert TA, et al. Erythropoietic protoporphyria: a new porphyria syndrome with solar urticaria due to protoporphyrinaemia. *Lancet* 1961;2:448.

384. DeLeo VA, Poh-Fitzpatrick MB, Mathews-Roth MM, et al. Erythropoietic protoporphyria. 10 years experience. *Am J Med* 1976;60:8.

385. Poh-Fitzpatrick MB. Erythropoietic porphyrias: current mechanistic, diagnostic and therapeutic considerations. *Semin Hematol* 1977;14:211.

386. Schmidt H, Snitker G, Thomsen K, et al. Erythropoietic protoporphyria. A clinical study based on 29 cases in 14 families. *Arch Dermatol* 1974;110:58.

387. Bopp C, Bakos L, da Graca B. Erythropoietic protoporphyria. *Int J Biochem* 1980;12:909.

388. Eales L. Liver involvement in erythropoietic protoporphyria (EP). *Int J Biochem* 1980;12:915.

389. Rank JM, Carithers R, Bloomer J. Evidence for neurological dysfunction in end-stage protoporphyric liver disease. *Hepatology* 1993;18:1404.

390. Bonkovsky HL, Schned AR. Fatal liver failure in protoporphyria. Synergism between ethanol excess and the genetic defect. *Gastroenterology* 1986;90:191.

391. Bottomley SS, Tanaka M, Everett MA. Diminished erythroid ferrochelatase activity in protoporphyria. *J Lab Clin Med* 1975;86:126.

392. Suurmond D. Some aspects of erythropoietic porphyria in the Netherlands. *Dermatologica* 1969;138:303.

393. Mathews-Roth MM. Anemia in erythropoietic protoporphyria [Letter]. *JAMA* 1974;230:824.

394. Rademakers LH, Koningsberger JC, Sorber CW, et al. Accumulation of iron in erythroblasts of patients with erythropoietic protoporphyria. *Eur J Clin Invest* 1993;23:130.

395. Brun A, Steen H, Sandberg S. Erythropoietic protoporphyria: two populations of reticulocytes, with and without protoporphyrin. *Eur J Clin Invest* 1996;26:270.

396. Doss MO, Frank M. Hepatobiliary implications and complications in protoporphyria, a 20-year study. *Clin Biochem* 1989;22:223.

397. Bloomer JR. The liver in protoporphyria. *Hepatology* 1988;8:402.

398. Key NS, Rank JM, Freese D, et al. Hemolytic anemia in protoporphyria: possible precipitating role of liver failure and photic stress. *Am J Hematol* 1992;39:202.

399. Piomelli S, Lamola AA, Poh-Fitzpatrick MF, et al. Erythropoietic protoporphyria and lead intoxication: the molecular basis for difference in cutaneous photosensitivity. I. Different rates of disappearance of protoporphyrin from the erythrocytes, both in vivo and in vitro. *J Clin Invest* 1975;56:1519.

400. Clark KG, Nicholson DC. Erythrocyte protoporphyrin and iron uptake in erythropoietic protoporphyria. *Clin Sci* 1971;41:363.

401. Nicholson DC, Cowger ML, Kalivas J, et al. Isotopic studies of the erythropoietic and hepatic components of congenital porphyria and 'erythropoietic' protoporphyria. *Clin Sci* 1973;44:135.

402. Scholnick P, Marver HS, Schmid R. Erythropoietic protoporphyria: evidence for multiple sites of excess protoporphyrin formation. *J Clin Invest* 1971;50:203.

403. Sassaroli M, da Costa R, Vaananen H, et al. Distribution of erythrocyte free porphyrin content in erythropoietic protoporphyria. *J Lab Clin Med* 1992; 120:614.

404. Sandberg S, Brun A. Light-induced protoporphyrin release from erythrocytes in erythropoietic protoporphyria. *J Clin Invest* 1982;70:693.

405. Sandberg S, Talstad I, Hovding G, et al. Light-induced release of protoporphyrin, but not of zinc protoporphyrin, from erythrocytes in a patient with greatly elevated erythropoietic protoporphyria. *Blood* 1983;62:846.

406. Knobler E, Poh-Fitzpatrick MB, Kravetz D, et al. Interaction of hemopexin, albumin and liver fatty acid-binding protein with protoporphyrin. *Hepatology* 1989;10:995.

407. Peterka ES, Fusaro RM, Goltz RW. Erythropoietic protoporphyria. II. Histological and histochemical studies of cutaneous lesions. *Arch Dermatol* 1965;92:357.

408. Schnait FG, Wolff K, Konrad K. Erythropoietic protoporphyria—submicroscopic events during the acute photosensitivity flare. *Br J Dermatol* 1975;92: 545.

409. Poh-Fitzpatrick MB, Whitlock RT, Leftkowitch JH. Changes in protoporphyrin distribution dynamics during liver failure and recovery in a patient with protoporphyria and Epstein-Barr viral hepatitis. *Am J Med* 1986;80:943.

410. Avner DL, Lee RG, Berenson MM. Protoporphyrin-induced cholestasis in the isolated in situ perfused rat liver. *J Clin Invest* 1981;67:385.

411. Berenson MM, Kimura R, Samowitz W, et al. Protoporphyrin overload in unrestrained rats: biochemical and histopathologic characterization of a new model of protoporphyric hepatopathy. *Int J Exp Pathol* 1992;73:665.

412. Porter S. Congenital erythropoietic protoporphyria II. An experimental study. *Blood* 1963;22:532.

413. Morton KO, Schneider F, Weimer MK, et al. Hepatic and bile porphyrins in patients with protoporphyria and liver failure. *Gastroenterology* 1988;94:1488.

414. Poh-Fitzpatrick MB. Protoporphyrin metabolic balance in human protoporphyria. *Gastroenterology* 1985;88:1239.

415. Nakahashi Y, Taketani S, Okuda M, et al. Molecular cloning and sequence analysis of cDNA encoding human ferrochelatase. *Biochem Biophys Res Commun* 1990;173:748.

416. Dailey HA, Finnegan MG, Johnson MK. Human ferrochelatase is an iron-sulfur protein. *Biochemistry* 1994;33:403.

417. Ferreira GC, Franco R, Lloyd SG, et al. Mammalian ferrochelatase, a new addition to the metalloenzyme family. *J Biol Chem* 1994;269:7062.

418. Ferreira GC. Mammalian ferrochelatase. Overexpression in *Escherichia coli* as a soluble protein, purification and characterization. *J Biol Chem* 1994;269:4396.

419. Ta DT, Vickery LE. Cloning, sequencing, and overexpression of a [2Fe-2S] ferredoxin gene from *Escherichia coli*. *J Biol Chem* 1992;267:11120.

420. Al-Karadaghi S, Hansson M, Nikonov S, et al. Crystal structure of ferrochelatase: the terminal enzyme in heme biosynthesis. *Structure* 1997;5:1501.

421. Nakahashi Y, Fujita H, Taketani S, et al. The molecular defect of ferrochelatase in a patient with erythropoietic protoporphyria. *Fourth Congress of the European Society for Photobiology* 1991:197(abst).

422. Wang X, Poh-Fitzpatrick M, Taketani S, et al. Screening for ferrochelatase mutations: molecular heterogeneity of erythropoietic protoporphyria. *Biochim Biophys Acta* 1994;1225:187.

423. Sellers VM, Dailey TA, Dailey HA. Examination of ferrochelatase mutations that cause erythropoietic protoporphyria. *Blood* 1998;91:3980.

424. Rufenacht UB, Gouya L, Schneider-Yin X, et al. Systematic analysis of molecular defects in the ferrochelatase gene from patients with erythropoietic protoporphyria. *Am J Hum Genet* 1998;62:1341.

425. Gouya L, Deybach JC, Lamoril J, et al. Modulation of the phenotype in dominant erythropoietic protoporphyria by a low expression of the normal ferrochelatase allele. *Am J Hum Genet* 1996;58:292.

426. Gouya L, Puy H, Lamoril J, et al. Inheritance in erythropoietic protoporphyria: a common wild-type ferrochelatase allelic variant with low expression accounts for clinical manifestation. *Blood* 1999;93:2105.

427. Bloomer JR, Hill HD, Morton KO, et al. The enzyme defect in bovine protoporphyria. Studies with purified ferrochelatase. *J Biol Chem* 1987;262:667.

428. Jenkins MM, LeBoeuf RD, Ruth GR, et al. A novel stop codon mutation (X417L) of the ferrochelatase gene in bovine protoporphyria, a natural animal model of the human disease. *Biochim Biophys Acta* 1998;1408:18.

429. Tutois S, Montagutelli X, Da Silva V, et al. Erythropoietic protoporphyria in the house mouse. A recessive inherited ferrochelatase deficiency with anemia, photosensitivity, and liver disease. *J Clin Invest* 1991;88:1730.

430. Boulechfar S, Lamoril J, Montagutelli X, et al. Ferrochelatase structural mutant (Fechm1Pas) in the house mouse. *Genomics* 1993;16:645.

431. Mathews-Roth MM, Pathak MA, Fitzpatrick TB, et al. Beta-carotene as a photoprotective agent in erythropoietic protoporphyria. *Trans Assoc Am Physicians* 1970;83:176.

432. Fusaro RM, Runge WJ. Erythropoietic protoporphyria. IV. Protection from sunlight. *BMJ* 1970;1:730.

433. Kniffen JC. Protoporphyrin removal in intrahepatic porphyrastasis. *Gastroenterology* 1970;58:1027.

434. Van Wijk HJ, Van Hattum J, Baart dlF, et al. Blood exchange and transfusion therapy for acute cholestasis in protoporphyria. *Dig Dis Sci* 1988;33:1621.

435. Bloomer JR, Weimer MK, Bossenmaier IC, et al. Liver transplantation in a patient with protoporphyria. *Gastroenterology* 1989;97:188.

436. Todd DJ, Callender ME, Mayne EE, et al. Erythropoietic protoporphyria, transfusion therapy and liver disease. *Br J Dermatol* 1992;127:534.

437. Nordmann Y. Erythropoietic protoporphyria and hepatic complications. *J Hepatol* 1992;16:4.

438. Campbell AM, Williams ER. Chronic lead intoxication mimicking motor neuron disease. *BMJ* 1968;4:582.

439. Lampert PW, Schochet SS Jr. Demyelination and remyelination in lead neuropathy. Electromicrographic studies. *J Neuropathol Exp Neurol* 1968;27:527.

440. Livesley B, Sissons CE. Chronic lead intoxication mimicking motor neuron disease. *BMJ* 1968;4:387.

441. Benson P. Lead poisoning in children. *Dev Med Child Neurol* 1965;7:569.

442. Perlstein MA, Attala R. Neurologic sequelae of plumbism in children. *Clin Pediatr* 1966;5:292.

443. Granick JL, Sassa S, Granick S, et al. Studies in lead poisoning. II. Correlation between the ratio of activated to inactivated δ-aminolevulinic acid dehydratase of whole blood and the blood lead level. *Biochem Med* 1973;8:149.

444. Sassa S, Granick JL, Granick S, et al. Studies in lead poisoning. I. Microanalysis of erythrocyte protoporphyrin levels by spectrophotometry in the detection of chronic lead intoxication in the subclinical range. *Biochem Med* 1973;8:135.

445. Anonymous Committee on Biologic Effects of Atmospheric Pollutants. *Lead, airborne lead in perspective.* Washington: National Academy of Sciences, 1972.

446. Grandjean P. Widening perspectives of lead toxicity. A review of health effects of lead exposure in adults. *Environ Res* 1978;17:303.

447. Moore MR. Hematological effects of lead. *Sci Total Environ* 1988;71:419.

448. Murozumi M, Chow TJ, Patterson C. Chemical concentrations of pollutant lead aerosols, terrestrial dusts, and sea salts in Greenland and Antarctic snow strata. *Geochim Cosmochim Acta* 1969;33:1247.

449. Caprio RJ, Margulis HL, Joselow MM. Lead absorption in children and its relationship to urban traffic densities. *Arch Environ Health* 1974;28:195.

450. Kehoe RA. Normal metabolism of lead. *Arch Environ Health* 1964;8:232.

451. Alexander FW, Delves HT, Clayton BE. The uptake and excretion by children of lead and other contaminants. Paper presented at: Proceedings of International Symposium on the Environmental Health Aspects of Lead; May 1973; Luxembourg.

452. Kehoe RA. Metabolism of lead under abnormal conditions. *Arch Environ Health* 1964;8:235.

453. Anonymous Committee on Toxicology of the National Research Council. *Recommendations for the prevention of lead poisoning in children.* Washington: National Academy of Sciences, 1976.

454. Tsukamoto I, Yoshinaga T, Sano S. Zinc and cysteine residues in the active site of bovine liver δ-aminolevulinic acid dehydratase. *Int J Biochem* 1980;12:751.

455. Maes J, Gerber GB. Increased ALA dehydratase activity and spleen weight in lead-intoxicated rats. A consequence of increased blood cell destruction. *Experientia* 1978;34:381.

456. Fujita H, Orii Y, Sano S. Evidence of increased synthesis of δ-aminolevulinic acid dehydratase in experimental lead-poisoned rats. *Biochim Biophys Acta* 1981;678:39.

457. Fujita H, Sato K, Sano S. Increase in the amount of erythrocyte δ-aminolevulinic acid dehydratase in workers with moderate lead exposure. *Int Arch Occup Environ Health* 1982;50:287.

458. Jensen WN, Moreno G. Les ribosomes et les ponctuations basophiles des erythrocytes dans l'intoxication par le plomb. *C R Acad Sci* 1964;258:3596.

459. Wada O, Takeo K, Yano Y, et al. δ-Aminolevulinic acid dehydratase in low level lead exposure. *Arch Environ Health* 1976;31:211.

460. Piomelli S, Seaman C, Kapoor S. Lead-induced abnormalities of porphyrin metabolism. The relationship with iron deficiency. *Ann N Y Acad Sci* 1987;514:278.

461. Lamola AA, Yamane T. Zinc protoporphyrin in the erythrocytes of patients with lead intoxication and iron deficiency anemia. *Science* 1974;186:936.

462. Vanderkooi JM, Landsberg R. In vivo synthesis of iron-free cytochrome c during lead intoxication. *FEBS Lett* 1977;73:254.

463. San Martin de Viale LC, De Calmanovici RW, Del C Rios de Molina M, et al. Studies on porphyrin biosynthesis in lead-intoxicated rabbits. *Clin Chim Acta* 1976;69:375.

464. Goyer RA, Leonard DL, Moore JF, et al. Lead dosage and the role of the intranuclear inclusion body. An experimental study. *Arch Environ Health* 1970;20:705.

465. Goyer RA. Intracellular sites of toxic metals. *Neurotoxicology* 1983;4:147.

466. Holtzman D, Hsu JS. Early effects of inorganic lead on immature rat brain mitochondrial respiration. *Pediatr Res* 1976;10:70.

467. Minakami S, Suzuki C, Saito T, et al. Studies on erythrocyte glycolysis. I. Determination of the glycolytic intermediates in human erythrocytes. *J Biochem (Tokyo)* 1965;58:543.

468. Valentine WN, Fink K, Paglia DE, et al. Hereditary hemolytic anemia with human erythrocyte pyrimidine 5'-nucleotidase deficiency. *J Clin Invest* 1974; 54:866.

469. Paglia DE, Valentine WN, Dahlgren JG. Effects of low-level lead exposure on pyrimidine 5'-nucleotidase and other erythrocyte enzymes. Possible role of pyrimidine 5'-nucleotidase in the pathogenesis of lead-induced anemia. *J Clin Invest* 1975;56:1164.

470. Angle CR, Stohs SJ, McIntire MS, et al. Lead-induced accumulation of erythrocyte pyrimidine nucleotides in the rabbit. *Toxicol Appl Pharmacol* 1980;54:161.

471. Torrance JD, Mills W, Kilroe-Smith TA, et al. Erythrocyte pyrimidine 5'-nucleotidase activity as a sensitive indicator of lead exposure. *S Afr Med J* 1985;67:850.

472. Swanson MS, Angle CR, Stohs SJ. Effect of lead chelation therapy with EDTA in children on erythrocyte pyrimidine 5'-nucleotidase and with cytidine triphosphate levels. *Int J Clin Pharmacol Toxicol* 1982;20:497.

473. Valentine WN, Tanaka KR, Paglia DE. Hemolytic anemia and erythrocyte enzymopathies. *Ann Intern Med* 1985;103:245.

474. Aub JC, Minot AS, Fairhall LT, et al. Recent investigations of absorption and excretion of lead in organism. *JAMA* 1924;83:588.

475. Aub JC, Fairhall LT, Minot AS, et al. Lead poisoning. *Medicine* 1925;4:1.

476. Hoogeveen JY, Maniloff J, Coleman JR, et al., eds. *Effects of metals on cells, subcellular elements, and macromolecules.* Springfield, IL: Thomas, 1990:207.

477. Joyce CRB, Moore H, Weatherall M. Effects of lead, mercury and gold on potassium turnover of rabbit blood cells. *Br J Pharmacol* 1954;9:463.

478. Hasan J, Hernberg S, Metsala P, et al. Enhanced potassium loss in blood cells from men exposed to lead. *Arch Environ Health* 1967;14:309.

479. Galzigna L, Corsi GC, Saia B, et al. Inhibitory effect of triethyl lead on serum cholinesterase in vitro. *Clin Chim Acta* 1969;26:391.

480. Stankovic M, Mokranjac M. *International Congress on Occupational Health, 14th Madrid International Congress, Ser.62.* Amsterdam: Excerpta Medical Foundation II, 1963.

481. Castellino N, Aloj S. Intracellular distribution of lead in the liver and kidney of the rat. *Br J Ind Med* 1969;26:139.

482. Barltrop D, Smith A. Lead binding to human haemoglobin. *Experientia* 1971;27:92.

483. Hernberg S, Nurminen M, Hasan J. Nonrandom shortening of red cell survival times in men exposed to lead. *Environ Res* 1967;1:247.

484. Lachant NA, Tomoda A, Tanaka KR. Inhibition of the pentose phosphate shunt by 2,3,-diphosphoglycerate in erythrocyte pyruvate kinase deficiency. *Blood* 1984;63:518.

485. Williams H, Schulze WH, Rothchild HB, et al. Lead poisoning from the burning of battery casings. *JAMA* 1933;100:1485.

486. Gillet JA. An outbreak of lead poisoning in the Canklow district of Rotherham. *Lancet* 1955;1:1118.

487. Harris RW, Elsea WR. Ceramic glaze as a source of lead poisoning. *JAMA* 1967;202:344.

488. Klein M, Namer R, Harpur E, et al. Earthenware containers as a source of fatal lead poisoning. Case study and public-health considerations. *N Engl J Med* 1970;283:669.

489. Fischbein A, Wallace J, Anderson KE, et al. Lead poisoning in an art conservator. *JAMA* 1982;247:2007.

490. Landrigan PJ, Tanblyn PB, Nelson M, et al. Lead exposure in stained glass workers. *Am J Ind Med* 1981;1:177.

491. Anderson KE, Fischbein A, Kestenbaum D, et al. Plumbism from airborne lead in a firing range. An unusual exposure to a toxic heavy metal. *Am J Med* 1977;63:306.

492. Chisolm JJ. The use of chelating agents in the treatment of acute and chronic lead intoxication in childhood. *J Pediatr* 1968;73:1.

493. Selander S, Cramer K, Hallberg L. Studies in lead poisoning. Oral therapy with penicillamine: relationship between lead in blood and other laboratory tests. *Br J Ind Med* 1966;23:282.

494. Rosenberg DW, Kappas A. Comparative ability of exogenously administered metals to alter tissue levels and urinary output of copper and zinc. *Pharmacology* 1989;38:159.

495. Everse J, Hsia N. The toxicities of native and modified hemoglobins. *Free Radical Biol Med* 1997;22:1075.

496. Baumann H, Held WA, Berger FG. The acute phase response of mouse liver. Genetic analysis of the major acute phase reactants. *J Biol Chem* 1984;259:566.

497. Haugen TH, Hanley JM, Heath EC. Haptoglobin: a novel mode of biosynthesis of a liver secretory glycoprotein. *J Biol Chem* 1981;256:1055.

498. Raugei G, Bensi G, Colantuoni V, et al. Sequence of human haptoglobin cDNA: evidence that the alpha and beta subunits are coded by the same mRNA. *Nucleic Acids Res* 1983;11:5811.

499. Putnam FW. *The plasma proteins—structure, function, and genetic control,* vol. 2. New York: Academic Press, 1975.

500. Kurosky A, Barnett DR, Lee T, et al. Covalent structure of human haptoglobin: a serine protease homolog. *Proc Natl Acad Sci U S A* 1980;77:3388.

501. Black JA, Dixon GH. Amino acid sequence of alpha chains of human haptoglobins. *Nature* 1968;218:736.

502. Smithies O. Zone electrophoresis in starch gels: group variations in the serum proteins of normal human adults. *Biochem J* 1955;61:629.

503. Smithies O, Walker NF. Notation for serum protein groups and the genes controlling their inheritance. *Nature* 1956;178:694.

504. Maeda N, Yang F, Barnett DR, et al. Duplication within the haptoglobin Hp2 gene. *Nature* 1984;309:131.

505. Smithies O, Connell GE. Biochemical aspects of the inherited variations in human serum haptoglobins and transferrins. In: Wolstenholme GE, O'Connor CM, eds. *Ciba Foundation Symposium on biochemistry of human genetics.* London: Churchill Livingstone, 1959.

506. Harris H. *The principles of human biochemical genetics.* New York: Elsevier Science, 1971.

507. Terano Y. Haptoglobin. *Nihon Rinsho* 1985;43:116.

508. Maeda N. Nucleotide sequence of the haptoglobin and haptoglobin-related gene pair. The haptoglobin-related gene contains a retrovirus-like element. *J Biol Chem* 1985;260:6698.

509. Muranjan M, Nussenzweig V, Tomlinson S. Characterization of the human serum trypanosome toxin, haptoglobin-related protein. *J Biol Chem* 1998;273:3884.

510. Smith AB, Esko JD, Hajduk SL. Killing of trypanosomes by the human haptoglobin-related protein. *Science* 1995;268:284.

511. Hager KM, Hajduk SL. Mechanism of resistance of African trypanosomes to cytotoxic human HDL. *Nature* 1997;385:823.

512. Smith AB, Hajduk SL. Identification of haptoglobin as a natural inhibitor of trypanocidal activity in human serum. *Proc Natl Acad Sci U S A* 1995;92:10262.

513. Maeda N, Smithies O. The evolution of multigene families: human haptoglobin genes. *Annu Rev Genet* 1986;20:81.

514. Koda Y, Soejima M, Yoshioka N, et al. The haptoglobin-gene deletion responsible for anhaptoglobinemia. *Am J Hum Genet* 1998;62:245.

515. Bowman BH, Kurosky A. Haptoglobin: the evolutionary product of duplication, unequal crossing over, and point mutation. In: Harris H, Hirschhorn K, eds. *Advances in human genetics,* vol. 12. New York: Plenum Publishing, 1982: 189.

516. Kino K, Tsunoo H, Higa Y. Hemoglobin-haptoglobin receptor in rat liver plasma membrane. *J Biol Chem* 1980;255:9616.

517. Hinton RH, Dobrota M, Mullock BM. Haptoglobin-mediated transfer of hemoglobin from serum into bile. *FEBS Lett* 1980;112:247.

518. Eaton JW, Brandt P, Mahoney JR, et al. Haptoglobin: a natural bacteriostat. *Science* 1982;215:691.

519. Kristiansen M, Graversen JH, Jacobsen C, et al. Identification of the haemoglobin scavenger receptor. *Nature* 2001;409:198.

520. Faulstick DA, Lowenstein J, Yiengst MJ. Clearance kinetics of haptoglobin-hemoglobin complex in the human. *Blood* 1962;20:65.

521. Gabrieli ER, Pyzikiewicz T. Plasma hemoglobin clearance: a clinical study. *J Reticuloendothel Soc* 1966;3:163.

522. Nagel RL, Gibson QH. The binding of hemoglobin to haptoglobin and its relation to subunit dissociation of hemoglobin. *J Biol Chem* 1971;246:69.

523. Hwang PK, Greer J. Identification of residues involved in the binding of hemoglobin alpha chains to haptoglobin. *J Biol Chem* 1979;254:2265.

524. Hwang PK, Greer J. Interaction between hemoglobin subunits in the hemoglobin-haptoglobin complex. *J Biol Chem* 1980;255:3038.

525. Valette I, Waks M, Wejamn JC, et al. Haptoglobin heavy and light chains. Structural properties, reassembly, and formation of mini complex with hemoglobin. *J Biol Chem* 1981;256:672.

526. Bernini LF, Borri-Voltattorni C. Studies on the structure of human haptoglobins. I. Spontaneous refolding after extensive reduction and dissociation. *Biochim Biophys Acta* 1970;200:203.

527. Hanley JM, Haugen TH, Heath EC. Biosynthesis and processing of rat haptoglobin. *J Biol Chem* 1983;258:7858.

528. Langlois MR, Delanghe JR. Biological and clinical significance of haptoglobin polymorphism in humans. *Clin Chem* 1996;42:1589.

529. Dobryszycka W. Biological functions of haptoglobin—new pieces to an old puzzle. *Eur J Clin Chem Clin Biochem* 1997;35:647.

530. Elagib AA, Kider AO, Akerstrom B, et al. Association of the haptoglobin phenotype (1-1) with falciparum malaria in Sudan. *Trans R Soc Trop Med Hyg* 1998;92:309.

531. Quaye IK, Ekuban FA, Goka BQ, et al. Haptoglobin 1-1 is associated with susceptibility to severe *Plasmodium falciparum* malaria. *Trans R Soc Trop Med Hyg* 2000;94:216.

532. Lim SK, Kim H, Bin AA, et al. Increased susceptibility in Hp knockout mice during acute hemolysis. *Blood* 1998;92:1870.

533. Bloomer JR, Pierach CA. Effect of hematin administration to patients with protoporphyria and liver disease. *Hepatology* 1982;2:817.

534. Javid J, Horowitz H. An improved technique for the quantitation of serum haptoglobin. *Am J Clin Pathol* 1960;34:35.

535. Brandslund I, Svehag SE. RES-saturation with accumulation of hemoglobin-haptoglobin complexes in plasma. A method for simultaneous quantitation of free haptoglobin and hemoglobin-haptoglobin complexes. *Adv Exp Med Biol* 1982;155:629.

536. Gitlin D, Biasucci A. Development of gammaG, gammaA, gammaM, betaIC/betaIA C1 esterase, hemopexin, haptoglobin, fibrinogen, plasminogen, alpha1-antitrypsin, orosomucoid, beta-lipoprotein, alpha2-macroglobulin and prealbumin in human conceptus. *J Clin Invest* 1969;48:1433.

537. Ferris TC, Easterling RE, Nelson KJ, et al. Determination of serum-hemoglobin binding capacity and haptoglobin type by acrylamide gel electrophoresis. *Am J Clin Pathol* 1966;46:385.

538. Shinton NK, Richardson RW, Williams JD. Diagnostic value of serum haptoglobins. *J Clin Pathol* 1965;18:114.

539. Nyman M. Serum haptoglobin. Methodological and clinical studies. *Scand J Clin Lab Invest* 1959;39[Suppl]:11.

540. Pintera J. The biological and clinicopathological aspects of haptoglobin. *Semin Hematol* 1971;4:12.

541. Allison AC, Blumberg BS, Rees W. Haptoglobin types in British, Spanish Basque and Nigerian African populations. *Nature* 1958;181:824.

542. Mizushima Y, Kato H, Ohmae H, et al. Relationship of haptoglobin polymorphism to malaria in the Solomon Islands. *Int Med* 1995;34:342.

543. Blumberg BS. Clinical significance of serum haptoglobins. In: Sunderman FW, Sunderman FW Jr, eds. *Hemoglobin. Its precursors and metabolites.* Philadelphia: JB Lippincott Co, 1964:318.

544. Blumberg BS, Gentile Z. Haptoglobins and transferrins in two tropical populations. *Nature* 1961;189:897.

545. Mehta SR, Jensen WR. Haptoglobins in haemoglobinopathy: a genetic and clinical study. *Br J Haematol* 1960;6:250.

546. Blumberg BS, Murray RF, Allison AC, et al. Serum protein polymorphisms in Greek populations. *Ann Hum Genet* 1964;28:189.

547. Barnicot NA, Garlick JP, Roberts DF. Haptoglobin and transferrin inheritance in northern Nigerians. *Ann Hum Genet* 1960;24:171.

548. Coryell MN, Beach EF, Robinson AR, et al. Metabolism of women during the reproductive cycle. XVII. Changes in electrophoretic pattern of plasma proteins throughout the cycle and following delivery. *J Clin Invest* 1950;29:1559.

549. Allison AC. The genetical and clinical significance of the haptoglobins. *Proc R Soc Med* 1958;51:641.

550. Swain BK, Talukder G, Sharma A. Genetic variations in serum proteins in relation to diseases. *Med Biol* 1980;58:246.

551. Vincent SH, Grady RW, Shaklai N, et al. The influence of heme-binding proteins in heme-catalyzed oxidations. *Arch Biochem Biophys* 1988;265:539.

552. Beaven GH, Chen SH, Albis AD, et al. A spectroscopic study of the haemin-human-serum-albumin system. *Eur J Biochem* 1974;41:539.

553. Zizkovsky V, Havranova M, Storp P, et al. Spectroscopic study of the hemin-human-alpha-fetoprotein system. *Ann N Y Acad Sci* 1983;417:57.

554. Muller-Eberhard U. Hemopexin. *Methods Enzymol* 1988;163:536.

555. Hrkal Z, Vodrazka Z, Kalousek I. Transfer of heme from ferrihemoglobin and ferrihemoglobin isolated chains to hemopexin. *Eur J Biochem* 1974;43:73.

556. Muller-Eberhard U, Nikkila H. Transport of tetrapyrroles by proteins. *Semin Hematol* 1989;26:86.

557. Wochner RD, Spilberg I, Lio A, et al. Hemopexin metabolism in sickle cell disease, porphyrias, and control subjects. Effects of heme injection. *N Engl J Med* 1974;290:822.

558. Galbraith RA, Sassa S, Kappas A. Heme binding to murine erythroleukemia cells. Evidence for a heme receptor. *J Biol Chem* 1985;260:12198.

559. Tolosano E, Hirsch E, Patrucco E, et al. Defective recovery and severe renal damage after acute hemolysis in hemopexin-deficient mice. *Blood* 1999;94:3906.

560. London IM, West R, Shemin D, et al. On the origin of bile pigment in normal man. *J Biol Chem* 1950;184:351.

561. Berk PD, Howe RB, Bloomer JR, et al. Studies of bilirubin kinetics in normal adults. *J Clin Invest* 1969;48:2176.

562. Landaw SA. Carbon monoxide production as a measurement of heme catabolism. In: Goresky CA, Fischer MM, eds. *Jaundice.* New York: Plenum Publishing, 1975:103.

563. Jones EA, Shrager R, Bloomer JR, et al. Quantitative studies of the delivery of hepatic synthesized bilirubin to plasma utilizing δ-aminolevulinic acid 4-^{14}C and bilirubin-^{3}H in man. *J Clin Invest* 1972;51:2450.

564. Wolkoff AW, Chowdhury JR, Arias IM. Hereditary jaundice and disorders of bilirubin metabolism. In: Stanbury JB, Wyngaarden JB, Fredrickson DS, et al., eds. *The metabolic basis of inherited disease.* New York: McGraw-Hill, 1983:1385.

565. Marver HS, Schmid R. The porphyrias. In: Stanbury JB, Wyngaarden JB, Fredrickson DS, eds. *The metabolic basis of inherited disease.* New York: McGraw-Hill, 1972:1087.

566. Granick S, Sinclair P, Sassa S, et al. Effects by heme, insulin, and serum albumin on heme and protein synthesis in chick embryo liver cells cultured in a chemically defined medium, and a spectrofluorometric assay for porphyrin composition. *J Biol Chem* 1975;250:9215.

567. Grandchamp B, Bissell DM, Licko V, et al. Formation and disposition of newly synthesized heme in adult rat hepatocytes in primary culture. *J Biol Chem* 1981;256:11677.

568. Bissell DM, Hammaker LE. Cytochrome P-450 heme and the regulation of hepatic heme oxygenase activity. *Arch Biochem Biophys* 1976;176:91.

569. Bissell DM, Hammaker LE. Effect of endotoxin on tryptophan pyrrolase and δ-aminolevulinate synthetase. Evidence for an endogenous regulatory haem fraction in rat liver. *Biochem J* 1977;166:301.

570. Farrell GC, Correia MA. Structural and functional reconstitution of hepatic cytochrome P-450 in vivo. Reversal of allylisopropylacetamide-mediated destruction of the monooxygenase by exogenous heme. *J Biol Chem* 1980;255:10128.

571. Correia MA, Farrell GC, Schmid R, et al. Incorporation of exogenous heme into hepatic cytochrome P-450 in vivo. *J Biol Chem* 1979;254:15.

572. Feigelson P, Greengaard O. A microsomal iron-porphyrin activator of rat liver tryptophan pyrrolase. *J Biol Chem* 1961;236:153.

573. Hayashi N, Yoda B, Kikuchi G. Mechanism of allylisopropylacetamide-induced increase of δ-aminolevulinate synthetase in liver mitochondria. IV. Accumulation of the enzyme in the soluble fraction of rat liver. *Arch Biochem Biophys* 1969;131:83.

574. Kappas A, Simionatto CS, Drummond GS, et al. The liver excretes large amounts of heme into bile when heme oxygenase is inhibited competitively by Sn-protoporphyrin. *Proc Natl Acad Sci U S A* 1985;82:896.

575. Tenhunen R, Marver HS, Schmid R. Microsomal heme oxygenase: characterization of the enzyme. *J Biol Chem* 1969;244:6388.

576. Shibahara S, Müller RM, Taguchi H, et al. Cloning and expression of cDNA for rat heme oxygenase. *Proc Natl Acad Sci U S A* 1985;82:7865.

577. Müller RM, Taguchi H, Shibahara S. Nucleotide sequence and organization of the rat heme oxygenase gene. *J Biol Chem* 1987;262:6795.

578. Maines MD, Trakshel GM, Kutty RK. Characterization of two constitutive forms of rat liver microsomal heme oxygenase. Only one molecular species of the enzyme is inducible. *J Biol Chem* 1986;261:411.

579. Cruse I, Maines MD. Evidence suggesting that the two forms of heme oxygenase are products of different genes. *J Biol Chem* 1988;263:3348.

580. McCoubrey WK, Huang TJ, Maines MD. Isolation and characterization of a cDNA from the rat brain that encodes hemoprotein heme oxygenase-3. *Eur J Biochem* 1997;247:725.

581. Gemsa D, Woo CH, Fudenberg HH, et al. Erythrophagocytosis by macrophages: suppression of heme oxygenase by cyclic AMP. *J Clin Invest* 1973; 52:812.

582. Shibahara S, Yoshida T, Kikuchi G. Mechanism of increase of heme oxygenase activity induced by hemin in cultured pig alveolar macrophages. *Arch Biochem Biophys* 1979;197:607.

583. Sardana MK, Sassa S, Kappas A. Hormonal regulation of heme oxygenase induction in avian hepatocyte culture. *Biochem Pharmacol* 1985;34:2937.

584. Kutty RK, Kutty G, Rodriguez IR, et al. Chromosomal localization of the human heme oxygenase genes: heme oxygenase-1 (HMOX1) maps to chromosome 22q12 and heme oxygenase-2 (HMOX2) maps to chromosome 16p13.3. *Genomics* 1994;20:513.

585. Kuwano A, Ikeda H, Takeda K, et al. Mapping of the human gene for inducible heme oxygenase to chromosome 22q12. *Tohoku J Exp Med* 1994;172:389.

586. Yoshida T, Biro P, Cohen T, et al. Human heme oxygenase cDNA and induction of its mRNA by hemin. *Eur J Biochem* 1988;171:457.

587. Kageyama H, Hiwasa T, Tokunaga K, et al. Isolation and characterization of a complementary DNA clone for a Mr 32,000 protein which is induced with tumor promoters in BALB/c 3T3 cells. *Cancer Res* 1988;48:4795.

588. Evans CO, Healey JF, Greene Y, et al. Cloning, sequencing and expression of cDNA for chick liver haem oxygenase. Comparison of avian and mammalian cDNAs and deduced proteins. *Biochem J* 1991;273:659.

589. Suzuki T, Sato M, Ishikawa K, et al. Nucleotide sequence of cDNA for porcine heme oxygenase and its expression in *Escherichia coli*. *Biochem Int* 1992;28:887.

590. McCoubrey WK, Ewing JF, Maines MD. Human heme oxygenase-2: characterization and expression of a full-length cDNA and evidence suggesting that the two HO-2 transcripts may differ by choice of polyadenylation signal. *Arch Biochem Biophys* 1992;295:13.

591. Ishikawa K, Takeuchi N, Takahashi S, et al. Heme oxygenase-2. Properties of the heme complex of the purified tryptic fragment of recombinant human heme oxygenase-2. *J Biol Chem* 1995;270:6345.

592. Maines MD. Heme oxygenase: function, multiplicity, regulatory mechanisms, and clinical applications. *FASEB J* 1988;2:2557.

593. McCoubrey WK, Huang TJ, Maines MD. Heme oxygenase-2 is a hemoprotein and binds heme through heme regulatory motifs that are not involved in heme catalysis. *J Biol Chem* 1997;272:12568.

594. Goda N, Suzuki K, Naito M, et al. Distribution of heme oxygenase isoforms in rat liver. Topographic basis for carbon monoxide-mediated microvascular relaxation. *J Clin Invest* 1998;101:604.

595. Poss KD, Tonegawa S. Heme oxygenase 1 is required for mammalian iron reutilization. *Proc Natl Acad Sci U S A* 1997;94:10919.

596. Poss KD, Tonegawa S. Reduced stress defense in heme oxygenase 1–deficient cells. *Proc Natl Acad Sci U S A* 1997;94:10925.

597. Poss KD, Thomas MJ, Ebralidze AK, et al. Hippocampal long-term potentiation is normal in heme oxygenase-2 mutant mice. *Neuron* 1995;15:867.

598. Zakhary R, Poss KD, Jaffrey SR, et al. Targeted gene deletion of heme oxygenase 2 reveals neural role for carbon monoxide. *Proc Natl Acad Sci U S A* 1997;94:14848.

599. Burnett AL, Johns DG, Kriegsfeld LJ, et al. Ejaculatory abnormalities in mice with targeted disruption of the gene for heme oxygenase-2. *Nat Med* 1998; 4:84–87.

600. Dennery PA, Spitz DR, Yang G, et al. Oxygen toxicity and iron accumulation in the lungs of mice lacking heme oxygenase-2. *J Clin Invest* 1998;101:1001.

601. Schmitt MP. Utilization of host iron sources by *Corynebacterium diphtheriae*: identification of a gene whose product is homologous to eukaryotic heme oxygenases and is required for acquisition of iron from heme and hemoglobin. *J Bacteriol* 1997;179:838.

602. Chu GC, Katakura K, Zhang X, et al. Heme degradation as catalyzed by a recombinant bacterial heme oxygenase (Hmu O) from *Corynebacterium diphtheriae*. *J Biol Chem* 1999;274:21319.

603. Muramoto T, Kohchi T, Yokota A, et al. The Arabidopsis photomorphogenic mutant hy1 is deficient in phytochrome chromophore biosynthesis as a result of a mutation in a plastid heme oxygenase. *Plant Cell* 1999;11:335.

604. Cornejo J, Willows RD, Beale SI. Phytobilin biosynthesis: cloning and expression of a gene encoding soluble ferredoxin-dependent heme oxygenase from *Synechocystis* sp. PCC 6803. *Plant J* 1998;15:99.

605. Yoshida T, Kikuchi G. Features of the reaction of heme degradation catalyzed by the reconstituted microsomal heme oxygenase system. *J Biol Chem* 1978;253:4230.

606. Schuller DJ, Wilks A, Ortiz MP, et al. Crystal structure of human heme oxygenase-1. *Nat Struct Biol*, 1999;6:860.

607. Yoshida T, Migita CT. Mechanism of heme degradation by heme oxygenase. *J Inorg Biochem* 2000;82:33.

608. Yoshida T, Noguchi M, Kikuchi G. Oxygenated form of heme: heme oxygenase complex and requirement for second electron to initiate heme degradation from the oxygenated complex. *J Biol Chem* 1980;255:4418.

609. Yoshida T, Noguchi M, Kikuchi G, et al. Degradation of mesoheme and hydroxymesoheme catalyzed by the heme oxygenase system: involvement of hydroxyheme in the sequence of heme catabolism. *J Biochem (Tokyo)* 1981;90:125.

610. Wilks A, Ortiz de Montellano PR. Rat liver heme oxygenase. High level expression of a truncated soluble form and nature of the meso-hydroxylating species. *J Biol Chem* 1993;268:22357.

611. Noguchi M, Yoshida T, Kikuchi G. Identification of the products of heme degradation catalyzed by the heme oxygenase system as biliverdin IX-alpha by reversed-phase high-performance liquid chromatography. *J Biochem (Tokyo)* 1982;91:1479.

612. Frydman RB, Awruch J, Tomaro ML, et al. Concerning the specificity of heme oxygenase: the enzymatic oxidation of synthetic hemins. *Biochem Biophys Res Commun* 1979;87:928.

613. Docherty JC, Masters BS, Firneisz GD, et al. Heme oxygenase provides alpha-specificity to physiological heme degradation. *Biochem Biophys Res Commun* 1982;105:1005.

614. Matera KM, Takahashi S, Fujii H, et al. Oxygen and one reducing equivalent are both required for the conversion of alpha-hydroxyhemin to verdoheme in heme oxygenase. *J Biol Chem* 1996;271:6618.

615. Yoshida T, Noguchi M, Kikuchi G. The step of carbon monoxide liberation in the sequence of heme degradation catalyzed by the reconstituted microsomal heme oxygenase system. *J Biol Chem* 1982;257:9345.

616. Liu Y, Moenne-Loccoz P, Loehr TM, et al. Heme oxygenase-1, intermediates in verdoheme formation and the requirement for reduction equivalents. *J Biol Chem* 1997;272:6909.

617. Migita CT, Matera KM, Ikeda-Saito M, et al. The oxygen and carbon monoxide reactions of heme oxygenase. *J Biol Chem* 1998;273:945.

618. Yoshida T, Noguchi M. Features of intermediary steps around the 688-nm substance in the heme oxygenase reaction. *J Biochem (Tokyo)* 1984;96:563.

619. Liu Y, Ortiz MP. Reaction intermediates and single turnover rate constants for the oxidation of heme by human heme oxygenase-1. *J Biol Chem* 2000;275:5297.

620. Yoshinaga T, Sassa S, Kappas A. The occurrence of molecular interactions among NADPH-cytochrome c reductase, heme oxygenase, and biliverdin reductase in heme degradation. *J Biol Chem* 1982;257:7786.

621. Kappas A, Drummond GS, Simionatto CS, et al. Control of heme oxygenase and plasma levels of bilirubin by a synthetic heme analogue, tin-protoporphyrin. *Hepatology* 1984;4:336.

622. Whitington PF, Moscioni AD, Gartner LM. The effect of tin-(IV)protoporphyrin-IX on bilirubin production and excretion in the rat. *Pediatr Res* 1987;21:487.

623. Kappas A, Drummond GS. Control of heme metabolism with synthetic metalloporphyrins. *J Clin Invest* 1986;77:335.

624. Sassa S. Inhibition of carbon monoxide production by tin-protoporphyrin. *J Pediatr Gastroenterol Nutr* 1987;6:167.

625. Kappas A, Drummond GS, Manola T, et al. Sn-protoporphyrin use in the management of hyperbilirubinemia in term newborns with direct Coombs-positive ABO incompatibility. *Pediatrics* 1988;81:485.

626. Berglund L, Angelin B, Blomstrand R, et al. Sn-protoporphyrin lowers serum bilirubin levels, decreases biliary bilirubin output, enhances biliary heme excretion and potently inhibits hepatic heme oxygenase activity in normal human subjects. *Hepatology* 1988;8:625.

627. Maines MD, Kappas A. Studies on the mechanism of induction of haem oxygenase by cobalt and other metal ions. *Biochem J* 1976;154:125.

628. Keyse SM, Tyrrell RM. Heme oxygenase is the major 32-kDa stress protein induced in human skin fibroblasts by UVA radiation, hydrogen peroxide, and sodium arsenite. *Proc Natl Acad Sci U S A* 1989;86:99.

629. Okinaga S, Shibahara S. Identification of a nuclear protein that constitutively recognizes the sequence containing a heat-shock element: its binding properties and possible function modulating heat-shock induction of the rat heme oxygenase gene. *Eur J Biochem* 1993;212:167.

630. Shibahara S, Müller RM, Taguchi H. Transcriptional control of rat heme oxygenase by heat shock. *J Biol Chem* 1987;262:12889.

631. Shibahara S. Regulation of heme oxygenase gene expression. *Semin Hematol* 1988;25:370.

632. Okinaga S, Takahashi K, Takeda K, et al. Regulation of human heme oxygenase-1 gene expression under thermal stress. *Blood* 1996;87:5074.

633. Mitani K, Fujita H, Sassa S, et al. Heat shock induction of heme oxygenase mRNA in human Hep 3B hepatoma cells. *Biochem Biophys Res Commun* 1989;165:437.

634. Mitani K, Fujita H, Sassa S, et al. A heat-inducible nuclear factor that binds to the heat-shock element of the human haem oxygenase gene. *Biochem J* 1991;277:895.

635. Mitani K, Fujita H, Kappas A, et al. Heme oxygenase is a positive acute-phase reactant in human Hep3B hepatoma cells. *Blood* 1992;79:1255.

636. Sato M, Ishizawa S, Yoshida T, et al. Interaction of upstream stimulatory factor with the human heme oxygenase gene promoter. *Eur J Biochem* 1990;188:231.

637. Muraosa Y, Shibahara S. Identification of a cis-regulatory element and putative trans-acting factors responsible for 12-O-tetradecanoylphorbol-13-acetate (TPA)-mediated induction of heme oxygenase expression in myelomonocytic cell lines. *Mol Cell Biol* 1993;13:7881.

638. Takeda K, Ishizawa S, Sato M, et al. Identification of a cis-acting element that is responsible for cadmium-mediated induction of the human heme oxygenase gene. *J Biol Chem* 1994;269:22858.

639. Alam J. Multiple elements within the 5' distal enhancer of the mouse heme oxygenase-1 gene mediate induction by heavy metals. *J Biol Chem* 1994;269:25049.

640. Igarashi K, Hoshino H, Muto A, et al. Multivalent DNA binding complex generated by small Maf and Bach1 as a possible biochemical basis for beta-globin locus control region complex. *J Biol Chem* 1998;273:11783.

641. Inamdar NM, Ahn YI, Alam J. The heme-responsive element of the mouse heme oxygenase-1 gene is an extended AP-1 binding site that resembles the recognition sequences for MAF and NF-E2 transcription factors. *Biochem Biophys Res Commun* 1996;221:570.

642. Ogawa K, Sun JY, Taketani S, et al. Heme mediates de-repression of Maf recognition element through direct binding to transcription repressor Bach1. *EMBO J* 2001;20:2835.

643. Choi AM, Alam J. Heme oxygenase-1: function, regulation, and implication of a novel stress-inducible protein in oxidant-induced lung injury. *Am J Respir Cell Mol Biol* 1996;15:9.

644. Shibahara S. Regulation of and physiological implication in heme catabolism. In: Fujita H, ed. *Regulation of heme protein synthesis*. Dayton, Ohio: AlphaMed Press, 1994:103.

645. Maines MD. The heme oxygenase system: a regulator of second messenger gases. *Ann Rev Pharmacol Toxicol* 1997;37:517.

646. Kimpara T, Takeda A, Watanabe K, et al. Microsatellite polymorphism in the human heme oxygenase-1 gene promoter and its application in association studies with Alzheimer and Parkinson disease. *Hum Genet* 1997;100:145.

647. Brahmachari SK, Meera G, Sarkar PS, et al. Simple repetitive sequences in the genome: structure and functional significance. *Electrophoresis* 1995; 16:1705.

648. Yamada N, Yamaya M, Okinaga S, et al. Microsatellite polymorphism in the heme oxygenase-1 gene promoter is associated with susceptibility to emphysema. *Am J Hum Genet* 2000;66:187.

649. Shibahara S, Kitamuro T, Takahashi K. Heme degradation and human disease: Diversity is the soul of life. *Antiox Redox Signal* 2002;4:593.

650. Yachie A, Niida Y, Wada T, et al. Oxidative stress causes enhanced endothelial cell injury in human heme oxygenase-1 deficiency. *J Clin Invest* 1999;103:129.

651. Ohta K, Yachie A, Fujimoto K, et al. Tubular injury as a cardinal pathologic feature in human heme oxygenase-1 deficiency. *Am J Kidney Dis* 2000;35:863.

652. Saikawa Y, Kaneda H, Yue L, et al. Structural evidence of genomic exon-deletion mediated by Alu-Alu recombination in a human case with heme oxygenase-1 deficiency. *Hum Mutat* 2000;16:178.

653. Takahashi K, Nakayama M, Takeda K, et al. Suppression of heme oxygenase-1 mRNA expression by interferon-gamma in human glioblastoma cells. *J Neurochem* 1999;72:2356.

654. Nakayama M, Takahashi K, Kitamuro T, et al. Repression of heme oxygenase-1 by hypoxia in vascular endothelial cells. *Biochem Biophys Res Commun* 2000;271:665.

655. Agarwal A, Nick HS. Renal response to tissue injury: lessons from heme oxygenase-1 gene ablation and expression. *J Am Soc Nephrol* 2000;11:965.

656. Otterbein LE, Choi AM. Heme oxygenase: colors of defense against cellular stress. *Am J Physiol Lung Cell Mol Physiol* 2000;279:1029.

657. Ross R. Rous-Whipple award lecture. Atherosclerosis: a defense mechanism gone awry. The pathogenesis of atherosclerosis: a perspective for the 1990s. *Am J Pathol* 1993;143:987.

658. Steinberg D. Low density lipoprotein oxidation and its pathobiological significance. *J Biol Chem* 1997;272:20963.

659. Ishikawa K, Navab M, Leitinger N, et al. Induction of heme oxygenase-1 inhibits the monocyte transmigration induced by mildly oxidized LDL. *J Clin Invest* 1997;100:1209.

660. Wang LJ, Lee TS, Lee FY, et al. Expression of heme oxygenase-1 in atherosclerotic lesions. *Am J Pathol* 1998;152:711.

661. Nakayama M, Takahashi K, Komaru T, et al. Increased expression of heme oxygenase 1 and bilirubin accumulation in foam cells of rabbit atherosclerotic lesions. *Arterioscler Thromb Vasc Biol* 2001;21:1373.

662. Smith MA, Kutty RK, Richey PL, et al. Heme oxygenase-1 is associated with the neurofibrillary pathology of Alzheimer's disease. *Am J Pathol* 1994; 145:42.

663. Schipper HM, Cisse S, Stopa EG. Expression of heme oxygenase-1 in the senescent and Alzheimer-diseased brain. *Ann Neurol* 1995;37:758.

664. Premkumar DR, Smith MA, Richey PL, et al. Induction of heme oxygenase-1 mRNA and protein in neocortex and cerebral vessels in Alzheimer's disease. *J Neurochem* 1995;65:1399.

665. Takeda A, Perry G, Abraham NG, et al. Overexpression of heme oxygenase in neuronal cells, the possible interaction with Tau. *J Biol Chem* 2000;275:5395.

666. Takahashi M, Ferris CD, Tomita T, et al. Amyloid precursor proteins inhibit heme oxygenase activity and augment neurotoxicity in Alzheimer's disease. *Neuron* 1901;28:461.

667. Schipper HM, Liberman A, Stopa EG. Neural heme oxygenase-1 expression in idiopathic Parkinson's disease. *Exp Neurol* 1998;150:60.

668. Rizzardini M, Chiesa R, Angeretti N, et al. Prion protein fragment 106-126 differentially induces heme oxygenase-1 mRNA in cultured neurons and astroglial cells. *J Neurochem* 1997;68:715.

669. Guentchev M, Voigtlander T, Haberler C, et al. Evidence for oxidative stress in experimental prion disease. *Neurobiol Dis* 2000;7:270.

670. Schluesener HJ, Kremsner PG, Meyermann R. Heme oxygenase-1 in lesions of human cerebral malaria. *Acta Neuropathol* 2001;101:65.

671. Willis D, Moore AR, Frederick R, et al. Heme oxygenase: a novel target for the modulation of the inflammatory response. *Nat Med* 1996;2:87.

672. Abraham NG, Lavrovsky Y, Schwartzman ML, et al. Transfection of the human heme oxygenase gene into rabbit coronary microvessel endothelial cells: protective effect against heme and hemoglobin toxicity. *Proc Natl Acad Sci U S A* 1995;92:6798.

673. Yang L, Quan S, Abraham NG. Retrovirus-mediated HO gene transfer into endothelial cells protects against oxidant-induced injury. *Am J Physiol* 1999; 277:127.

674. Shiraishi F, Curtis LM, Truong L, et al. Heme oxygenase-1 gene ablation or expression modulates cisplatin-induced renal tubular apoptosis. *Am J Physiol Renal Fluid Electrolyte Physiol* 2000;278:726.

675. Nath KA, Vercellotti GM, Grande JP, et al. Heme protein-induced chronic renal inflammation: suppressive effect of induced heme oxygenase-1. *Kidney Int* 2001;59:106.

676. Trotman BW. Pigment gallstone disease. *Gastroenterol Clin North Am* 1991; 20:111.

677. Keppler D, Konig J. Hepatic secretion of conjugated drugs and endogenous substances. *Semin Liver Dis* 2000;20:265.

678. Abraham NG, Da Silva JL, Dunn MW, et al. Retinal pigment epithelial cell-based gene therapy against hemoglobin toxicity. *Int J Mol Med* 1998;1:657.

679. Soares MP, Lin Y, Anrather J, et al. Expression of heme oxygenase-1 can determine cardiac xenograft survival. *Nat Med* 1998;4:1073.

680. Hancock WW, Buelow R, Sayegh MH, et al. Antibody-induced transplant arteriosclerosis is prevented by graft expression of anti-oxidant and anti-apoptotic genes. *Nat Med* 1998;4:1392.

681. Sato K, Balla J, Otterbein L. Carbon monoxide generated by heme oygenase-1 suppressed the rejection of mouse-to-rat cardiac transplant. *J Immunol* 2001;166:4185.

682. Landaw SA. Kinetic aspects of endogenous carbon monoxide production in experimental animals. *Ann N Y Acad Sci* 1970;174:32.

683. White P. Carbon monoxide production and heme catabolism. *Ann N Y Acad Sci* 1970;174:23.

684. Zayasu K, Sekizawa K, Okinaga S, et al. Increased carbon monoxide in exhaled air of asthmatic patients. *Am J Respir Crit Care Med* 1997;156:1140.

685. Yamaya M, Sekizawa K, Ishizuka S, et al. Increased carbon monoxide in exhaled air of subjects with upper respiratory tract infections. *Am J Respir Crit Care Med* 1998;158:311.

686. Paredi P, Shah PL, Montuschi P, et al. Increased carbon monoxide in exhaled air of patients with cystic fibrosis. *Thorax* 1999;54:917.

687. Scharte M, Bone HG, Van Aken H, et al. Increased carbon monoxide in exhaled air of critically ill patients. *Biochem Biophys Res Commun* 2000; 267:423.

688. Verma A, Hirsch DJ, Glatt CE, et al. Carbon monoxide: a putative neural messenger. *Science* 1993;259:381.

689. Stevens CF, Wang Y. Reversal of long-term potentiation by inhibitors of haem oxygenase. *Nature* 1993;364:147.

690. Zhuo M, Small SA, Kandel ER, et al. Nitric oxide and carbon monoxide produce activity-dependent long-term synaptic enhancement in hippocampus. *Science* 1993;260:1946.

691. Furchgott RF, Jothianandan D. Endothelium-dependent relaxation, endothelium-derived relaxing factor and photorelaxation of blood vessels. *Semin Perinatol* 1991;15:11.

692. Brune B, Ullrich V. Inhibition of platelet aggregation by carbon monoxide is mediated by activation of guanylate cyclase. *Mol Pharmacol* 1987;32:497.

693. Morita T, Perrella MA, Lee ME, et al. Smooth muscle cell-derived carbon monoxide is a regulator of vascular cGMP. *Proc Natl Acad Sci U S A* 1995; 92:1475.

694. Grundemar L, Ny L. Pitfalls using metalloporphyrins in carbon monoxide research. *Trends Pharmacol Sci* 1997;18:193.

695. Suematsu M, Kashiwagi S, Sano T, et al. Carbon monoxide as an endogenous modulator of hepatic vascular perfusion. *Biochem Biophys Res Commun* 1994;205:1333.

696. Suematsu M, Goda N, Sano T, et al. Carbon monoxide: an endogenous modulator of sinusoidal tone in the perfused rat liver. *J Clin Invest* 1995;96:2431.

697. Sano T, Shiomi M, Wakabayashi Y, et al. Endogenous carbon monoxide suppression stimulates bile acid-dependent biliary transport in perfused rat liver. *Am J Physiol* 1997;272:1268.

698. Suematsu M, Ishimura Y. The heme oxygenase-carbon monoxide system: a regulator of hepatobiliary function. *Hepatology* 2000;31:3.

699. Otterbein LE, Bach FH, Alam J, et al. Carbon monoxide has anti-inflammatory effects involving the mitogen-activated protein kinase pathway. *Nat Med* 2000;6:422.

700. Otterbein LE, Mantell LL, Choi AM. Carbon monoxide provides protection against hyperoxic lung injury. *Am J Physiol* 1999;276:688.

701. Blumenthal SG, Taggart DB, Ikeda RM, et al. Conjugated and unconjugated bilirubins in bile of humans and rhesus monkeys. Structural identity of adult human and rhesus monkey bilirubins. *Biochem J* 1977;167:535.

702. Blumenthal SG, Taggart DB, Rasmussen RD, et al. Conjugated and unconjugated bilirubins in humans and rhesus monkeys. Structural identity of bilirubins from biles and meconium of newborn humans and rhesus monkeys. *Biochem J* 1979;179:537.

703. Yamaguchi T, Komoda Y, Nakajima H. Biliverdin-IXα reductase and biliverdin-IXβ reductase from human liver: purification and characterization. *J Biol Chem* 1994;269:24343.

704. Yamaguchi T, Nakajima H. Changes in the composition of bilirubin-IX isomers during human prenatal development. *Eur J Biochem* 1995;233:467.

705. Komuro A, Tobe T, Nakano Y, et al. Cloning and characterization of the cDNA encoding human biliverdin-IX alpha reductase. Molecular cloning and expression of human liver biliverdin-IX beta reductase. *Biochim Biophys Acta* 1996;1309:89.

706. Fakhrai H, Maines MD. Expression and characterization of a cDNA for rat kidney biliverdin reductase. Evidence suggesting the liver and kidney enzymes are the same transcript product. *J Biol Chem* 1992;267:4023.

707. Yamaguchi T, Komuro A, Nakano Y, et al. Complete amino acid sequence of biliverdin-IX beta reductase from human liver. *Biochem Biophys Res Commun* 1993;197:1518.

708. Meera-Khan P, Wijnen LM, Wijnen JT, et al. Electrophoretic characterization and genetics of human biliverdin reductase (BLVR; EC 1.3.1.24); assignment of BLVR to the p14 leads to cen region of human chromosome 7 in mouse-human somatic cell hybrids. *Biochem Genet* 1983;21:123.

709. Parkar M, Jeremiah SJ, Povey S, et al. Confirmation of the assignment of human biliverdin reductase to chromosome 7. *Ann Hum Genet* 1984;48:57.

710. Saito F, Yamaguchi T, Komuro A, et al. Mapping of the newly identified biliverdin-IX beta reductase gene (BLVRB) to human chromosome 19q13.13→q13.2 by fluorescence in situ hybridization. *Cytogenet Cell Genet* 1995;71:179.

711. Noguchi M, Yoshida T, Kikuchi G. Purification and properties of biliverdin reductase from pig spleen and rat liver. *J Biochem (Tokyo)* 1979;86:833.

712. Kutty RK, Maines MD. Purification and characterization of biliverdin reductase from rat liver. *J Biol Chem* 1981;256:3956.

713. Kikuchi A, Park SY, Miyatake H, et al. Crystal structure of rat biliverdin reductase. *Nat Struct Biol* 2001;8:221.

714. Pereira PJ, Macedo-Ribeiro S, Parraga A, et al. Structure of human biliverdin IXβ reductase, an early fetal bilirubin IXb producing enzyme. *Nat Struct Biol* 2001;8:215.

715. McDonagh AF. Bile pigments, bilatrienes and 5,15-biladienes. In: Dolphin D, ed. *The porphyrins*, vol. 6. New York: Academic Press, 1979.

716. Fog J, Jellum E. Structure of bilirubin. *Nature* 1963;198:88.

717. Kuenzle CC, Weibel MH, Pelloni RR. A proposed novel structure for the metal chelates of bilirubin. *Biochem J* 1973;130:1147.

718. Kuenzle CC, Weibel MH, Pelloni RR. The reaction of bilirubin with diazomethane. *Biochem J* 1973;133:357.

719. Kuenzle CC. Bilirubin conjugates of human bile. Nuclear magnetic resonance, infrared and optical spectra of model compounds. *Biochem J* 1970;119:395.

720. Cu A, Bellah GG, Lightner DA. On the fluorescence of bilirubin. *J Am Chem Soc* 1975;97:2579.

721. McDonagh AF, Palma LA. Mechanism of bilirubin photodegradation: role of singlet oxygen. In: Berk PD, Berlin NI, eds. *Chemistry and physiology of bile pigments*. Washington: US Government Printing Office, 1977:81; DHEW Publ. No. (NIH) 77-1100.

722. McDonagh AF. Phototherapy of neonatal jaundice. *Biochem Soc Trans* 1976;4:219.

723. McDonagh AF. Light effects on transport and excretion of bilirubin in newborns. *Ann N Y Acad Sci* 1985;453:65.

724. Ennever JF. Phototherapy for neonatal jaundice. *Photochem Photobiol* 1988;47:871.

725. Mustafa MG, Cowger ML, King TW. Effects of bilirubin on mitochondrial reaction. *J Biol Chem* 1969;244:6403.

726. Diamond I, Schmid R. Oxidative phosphorylation in experimental bilirubin encephalopathy. *Science* 1967;155:1288.

727. Menken M, Waggoner JG, Berlin NI. The influence of bilirubin on oxidative phosphorylation and related reactions in brain and liver mitochondria. Effects of protein binding. *J Neurochem* 1966;13:1241.

728. Amit Y, Chan G, Fedunec S, et al. Bilirubin toxicity in a neuroblastoma cell line N-115: I. Effects on Na$^+$K$^+$ ATPase, [3H]-Thymidine uptake, L-[35S]-Methionine incorporation, and mitochondrial function. *Pediatr Res* 1989;25:364.

729. Amit Y, Poznansky MJ, Schiff D. Bilirubin toxicity in a neuroblastoma cell line N-115: II. Delayed effects and recovery. *Pediatr Res* 1989;25:369.

730. Odell GB. Influence of binding on the toxicity of bilirubin. *Ann N Y Acad Sci* 1973;226:225.

731. Chowdhury JR, Wolkoff AW, Arias IM. Hereditary jaundice and disorders of bilirubin metabolism. In: Scriver CR, Beaudet AL, Sly WS, et al., eds. *The metabolic basis of inherited disease*. New York: McGraw-Hill, 1989.

732. Silverman WA, Anderson DH, Bland DA, et al. A difference in mortality rate and incidence of kernicterus among premature infants allotted to prophylactic antibacterial regimens. *Pediatrics* 1956;18:614.

733. Odell GB. The dissociation of bilirubin from albumin and its clinical implications. *J Pediatr* 1959;55:268.

734. Blankaert N, D'Argenio G. Presence of bilirubins linked covalently to albumin in serum of patients with cholestasis. *Gastroenterology* 1982;82:1222.

735. Weiss JS, Gautam A, Lauff JJ, et al. The clinical importance of a protein-bound fraction of serum bilirubin in patients with hyperbilirubinemia. *N Engl J Med* 1983;309:147.

736. McDonagh AF, Palma LA, Lauff JJ, et al. Origin of mammalian biliprotein and rearrangement of bilirubin glucuronides in vivo in the rat. *J Clin Invest* 1984;74:763.

737. Stocker R, Yamamoto Y, McDonagh AF, et al. Bilirubin is an antioxidant of possible physiological significance. *Science* 1987;235:1043.

738. Stocker R, Ames BN. Potential role of conjugated bilirubin and copper in the metabolism of lipid peroxides in bile. *Proc Natl Acad Sci U S A* 1987;84:8130.

739. Stevens B, Small RD Jr. The photoperoxidation of unsaturated organic molecules—XV. O$_2$^{1} Delta g quenching by bilirubin and biliverdin. *Photochem Photobiol* 1976;23:33.

740. Kaul R, Kaul HK, Murti CR. An alternate pathway for bilirubin catabolism. *FEBS Lett* 1980;111:240.

741. Neuzil J, Stocker R. Free and albumin-bound bilirubin are efficient co-antioxidants for alpha-tocopherol, inhibiting plasma and low density lipoprotein lipid peroxidation. *J Biol Chem* 1994;269:16712.

742. Brodersen R, Bartels P. Enzymatic oxidation of bilirubin. *Eur J Biochem* 1969;10:468.

743. Jacobsen J, Fedders O. Determination of non-albumin-bound bilirubin in human serum. *Scand J Clin Lab Invest* 1970;26:237.

744. Stocker R, Glazer AN, Ames BN. Antioxidant activity of albumin-bound bilirubin. *Proc Natl Acad Sci U S A* 1987;84:5918.

745. Otterbein LE, Kolls JK, Mantell LL, et al. Exogenous administration of heme oxygenase-1 by gene transfer provides protection against hyperoxia-induced lung injury. *J Clin Invest* 1999;103:1047.

746. Hayashi S, Takamiya R, Yamaguchi T, et al. Induction of heme oxygenase-1 suppresses venular leukocyte adhesion elicited by oxidative stress: role of bilirubin generated by the enzyme. *Circ Res* 1999;85:663.

747. Schwertner HA, Jackson WG, Tolan G. Association of low serum concentration of bilirubin with increased risk of coronary artery disease. *Clin Chem* 1994;40:18.

748. Hopkins PN, Hunt SC, Wu LL, et al. Hypertension, dyslipidemia, and insulin resistance: links in a chain or spokes on a wheel? *Curr Opin Lipidol* 1996;7:241.

749. Yamaguchi T, Shioji I, Sugimoto A, et al. Chemical structure of a new family of bile pigments from human urine. *J Biochem (Tokyo)* 1994;116:298.

750. Yamaguchi T, Horio F, Hashizume T, et al. Bilirubin is oxidized in rats treated with endotoxin and acts as a physiological antioxidant synergistically with ascorbic acid in vivo. *Biochem Biophys Res Commun* 1995;214:11.

751. Yamaguchi T, Hashizume T, Tanaka M, et al. Bilirubin oxidation provoked by endotoxin treatment is suppressed by feeding ascorbic acid in a rat mutant unable to synthesize ascorbic acid. *Eur J Biochem* 1997;245:233.

752. Tsujinaka T, Fujita J, Morimoto T, et al. Increased urinary excretion of bilirubin metabolites in association with hyperbilirubinemia after esophagectomy. *Surg Today* 1998;28:1119.

753. Yamaguchi T, Shioji I, Sugimoto A, et al. Psychological stress increases bilirubin metabolites in human urine. *Biochem Biophys Res Commun* 2002;293:517–520.

754. Kimpara T, Takeda A, Yamaguchi T, et al. Increased bilirubins and their derivatives in cerebrospinal fluid in Alzheimer's disease. *Neurobiol Aging* 2000;21:551.

755. Zucker SD, Goessling W, Hoppin AG. Unconjugated bilirubin exhibits spontaneous diffusion through model lipid bilayers and native hepatocyte membranes. *J Biol Chem* 1999;274:10852.

756. Bloomer JR, Berk PD, Bergalla J, et al. Influence of albumin on the hepatic uptake of unconjugated bilirubin. *Clin Sci Mol Med* 1973;45:505.

757. Weisiger RA. Dissociation from albumin. A potential rate-limiting step in the clearance of substances by the liver. *Proc Natl Acad Sci U S A* 1985;82:1563.

758. Kamisako T, Kobayashi Y, Takeuchi K, et al. Recent advances in bilirubin metabolism research: the molecular mechanism of hepatocyte bilirubin transport and its clinical relevance. *J Gastroenterol* 2000;35:659.

759. Konig J, Cui Y, Nies AT, et al. A novel human organic anion transporting polypeptide localized to the basolateral hepatocyte membrane. *Am J Physiol Gastrointest Liver Physiol* 2000;278:156.

760. Cui Y, Konig J, Leier I, et al. Hepatic uptake of bilirubin and its conjugates by the human organic anion transporter SLC21A6. *J Biol Chem* 2001;276:9626.

761. Kaplowitz N. Physiological significance of glutathione S-transferases. *Am J Physiol* 1980;239:439.

762. Bhargava MM, Arias IM. Ligandin. *Trends Biochem Sci* 1981;6:131.

763. Ketterer B, Ross-Mansell P, Whitehead JK. The isolation of carcinogen-binding protein from livers of rats given 4-dimethylaminoazobenzene. *Biochem J* 1967;103:316.

764. Morley KS, Litwack G. Isolation and properties of cortisol metabolite binding proteins of rat liver cytosol. *Biochemistry* 1969;8:4813.

765. Habig WH, Pabst MJ, Fleischner G, et al. The identity of glutathione S-transferase B with ligandin, a major binding protein of liver. *Proc Natl Acad Sci U S A* 1974;10:3879.

766. Wolkoff AW, Goresky CA, Sellin J, et al. Role of ligandin in transfer of bilirubin from plasma into liver. *Am J Physiol* 1978;236:638.

767. Gollan JL, Schmid R. Bilirubin update: formation, transport, and metabolism. *Prog Liver Dis* 1982;7:261.

768. Kirshenbaum G, Shames DM, Schmid R. An expanded model of bilirubin kinetics: effect of feeding, fasting and phenobarbital in Gilbert's syndrome. *J Pharmacokinet Biopharm* 1976;4:115.

769. Jones EA, Bloomer JR, Berk PD, et al. Quantitation of hepatic bilirubin synthesis in man. In: Berk PD, Berlin NI, eds. *The chemistry and physiology of bile pigments*. Washington: US Government Printing Office, 1977:189; DHEW Publ. No. (NIH) 77-1100.

770. Anwer MS, Gronwall R. A compartmental model for bilirubin kinetics in isolated perfused rat liver. *Can J Physiol Pharmacol* 1976;54:277–286.

771. Farrell GC, Gollan JL, Schmid R. Efflux into plasma following hepatic degradation of exogenous heme. *Proc Soc Exp Biol Med* 1980;163:504.

772. Gollan JL, McDonagh AF, Schmid R. Biliverdin IXalpha: a new probe of hepatic bilirubin metabolism. *Gastroenterology* 1977;72:1186(abst).

773. Gollan JL, Hammaker L, Licko V, et al. Bilirubin kinetics in intact rats and isolated perfused liver. Evidence for hepatic deconjugation of bilirubin glucuronides. *J Clin Invest* 1981;67:1016.

774. Carson ER, Jones EA. Use of kinetic analysis and mathematical modeling in the study of metabolic pathways in vivo: applications to hepatic organic anion metabolism. *N Engl J Med* 1979;300:1016.

775. Heirwegh KP, van Hees GP, Leroy P, et al. Heterogeneity of bile pigment conjugates as revealed by chromatography of their ethyl anthranilate azopigments. *Biochem J* 1970;120:877.

776. Fevery J, van Damme B, Michiels R, et al. Bilirubin conjugates in bile of man and rat in the normal state and in liver disease. *J Clin Invest* 1972;51:2482.

777. Fevery J, van de Vijver M, Michiels R, et al. Comparison in different species of biliary bilirubin-IXalpha conjugates with the activities of hepatic and renal bilirubin-IXalpha-uridine diphosphate glycosyltransferases. *Biochem J* 1977; 164: 737.

778. Tukey RH, Strassburg CP. Human UDP-glucuronosyltransferases: metabolism, expression, and disease. *Annu Rev Pharmacol Toxicol* 2000;40:581.

779. Moghrabi N, Sutherland L, Wooster R, et al. Chromosomal assignment of human phenol and bilirubin UDP-glucuronosyltransferase genes (UGT1A-subfamily). *Ann Hum Genet* 1992;56:81.

780. Van Es HH, Bout A, Liu J, et al. Assignment of the human UDP-glucurono-syltransferase gene (UGT1A1) to chromosome region 2q37. *Cytogenet Cell Genet* 1993;63:114.

781. Ritter JK, Chen F, Sheen YY, et al. A novel complex locus UGT1 encodes human bilirubin, phenol, and other UDP-glucuronosyltransferase isozymes with identical carboxyl termini. *J Biol Chem* 1992;267:3257.

782. Tephly T, Green M, Puig J, et al. Endogenous substrates for UDP-glucurono-syltransferases. *Xenobiotica* 1988;26:975.

783. Whitmer DL, Russell PE, Ziurys JC, et al. Hepatic microsomal glucuronida-tion of bilirubin is modulated by the lipid microenvironment of membrane-bound substrate. *J Biol Chem* 1986;261:7170.

784. Tomlison GA, Yaffe SJ. The formation of bilirubin and p-nitrophenol glucu-ronides by rabbit liver. *Biochem J* 1964;99:507.

785. Halac E, Reff A. Studies on bilirubin UDP–glucuronyl transferase. *Biochim Biophys Acta* 1967;139:328.

786. Nakata D, Zakim D, Vassey DA. Defective function of a microsomal UDP–glucuronyl transferase in Gunn rats. *Proc Natl Acad Sci U S A* 1976;73:289.

787. Iyanagi T, Watanabe T, Uchiyama Y. The 3-methylcholanthrene-inducible UDP-glucuronosyltransferase deficiency in the hyperbilirubinemic rat (Gunn rat) is caused by a −1 frameshift mutation. *J Biol Chem* 1989;264:21302.

788. Van den Bergh AA, Muller P. Uber eine direkte und eine indirekte diazoreak-tion aus bilirubin. *Biochem Z* 1916;77:90.

789. Hutchinson DW, Johnson B, Knell AJ. The reaction between bilirubin and aromatic diazo compounds. *Biochem J* 1972;127:907.

790. Heirwegh KP, Fevery JB, Meuwissen JA, et al. Recent advances in the separa-tion and analysis of diazo-positive bile pigments. *Methods Biochem Anal* 1974;22:205.

791. Blankaert N, Kabra PM, Farina FA, et al. Measurement of bilirubin and its mono- and di-conjugates in human serum by alkaline methanolysis and high performance liquid chromatography. *J Lab Clin Med* 1980;96:198.

792. Onishi S, Itho S, Kawade N, et al. An accurate and sensitive analysis by high pressure liquid chromatography of conjugated and unconjugated bilirubin IX and in various biological fluids. *Biochem J* 1980;185:281.

793. Chowdhury JR, Arias IM. Dismutation of bilirubin. *Methods Enzymol* 1981;77:192.

794. Lauff JJ, Kasper ME, Ambros RT. Quantitative liquid chromatography esti-mation of bilirubin species in pathological serum. *Clin Chem* 1983;29:800.

795. Dappen GM, Smedberg MW, Wu TW, et al. A diazo-based dry film for deter-mination of total bilirubin in serum. *Clin Chem* 1983;29:37.

796. Brown AK, Eisinger J, Blumberg WE, et al. A rapid fluorometric method for determining bilirubin levels and binding in the blood of neonates: compari-son with other methods. *Pediatrics* 1980;65:762.

797. Jansen PL, Roy Chowdhury J, Fischberg EB, et al. Enzymatic conversion of bilirubin monoglucuronide to diglucuronide by rat liver plasma mem-branes. *J Biol Chem* 1977;252:2710.

798. Chowdhury JR, Fischberg EB, Daniller A, et al. Hepatic conversion of biliru-bin monoglucuronide to bilirubin diglucuronide in uridine diphosphate glu-curonyl transferase deficient in man and rat by bilirubin glucuronyl transferase. *J Clin Invest* 1978;62:191.

799. Gartner LM, Lane DL, Cornelius CE. Bilirubin transport by liver in adult *Macaca mulatta*. *Am J Physiol* 1971;220:1528.

800. Paulusma CC, Kothe MJ, Bakker CT, et al. Zonal down-regulation and redis-tribution of the multidrug resistance protein 2 during bile duct ligation in rat liver. *Hepatology* 2000;31:684.

801. Taniguchi K, Wada M, Kohno K, et al. A human canalicular multispecific organic anion transporter (cMOAT) gene is overexpressed in cisplatin-resis-tant human cancer cell lines with decreased drug accumulation. *Cancer Res* 1996;56:4124.

802. Kamisako T, Leier I, Cui Y, et al. Transport of monoglucuronosyl and bisglu-curonosyl bilirubin by recombinant human and rat multidrug resistance pro-tein 2. *Hepatology* 1999;30:485.

803. Upson DW, Gronwall RR, Cornelius CE. Maximal hepatic excretion of biliru-bin in sheep. *Proc Soc Exp Biol Med* 1970;134:9.

804. Klaassen CD, Plaa GL. Studies on the mechanism of phenobarbital-enhanced sulfobromophthalein disappearance. *J Pharmacol Exp Ther* 1968;161:361.

805. Berk PD, Martin JF, Blaschke TF, et al. NIH conference: unconjugated hyper-bilirubinemia. Physiologic evaluation and experimental approaches to ther-apy. *Ann Intern Med* 1975;82:552.

806. König J, Rost D, Cui Y, et al. Characterization of the human multidrug resis-tance protein isoform MRP3 localized to the basolateral hepatocyte mem-brane. *Hepatology* 1999;29:1156.

807. Brodersen R, Herman LS. Intestinal reabsorption of unconjugated bilirubin: a possible contributing factor in neonatal jaundice. *Lancet* 1963;1:1242.

808. Schmid R, McDonagh AF. The enzymatic formation of bilirubin. *Ann N Y Acad Sci* 1975;244:533.

809. Watson CJ. The urobilinoids. Milestones in their history and some recent devel-opments. In: Berk PD, Berlin NI, eds. *The chemistry and physiology of bile pigments.* Washington: US Government Printing Office, 1977:469; USDEW, NIH.

810. Stoll MS, Lim CK, Gray CH. Chemical variants of the urobilins. In: Berk PD, Berlin NI, eds. *The chemistry and physiology of bile pigments.* Washington: US Government Printing Office; 1977:483; USDEW, NIH.

811. Levy M, Lester R, Levinsky NG. Renal excretion of urobilinogen in the dog. *J Clin Invest* 1968;47:2117.

812. Watson CJ. Recent studies of the urobilin problem. *J Clin Pathol* 1963;16:1.

813. Gollan JL, Dallinger KJ, Billing BH. Excretion of conjugated bilirubin in the isolated perfused rat kidney. *Clin Sci Mol Med* 1978;54:381.

814. Davidson LT, Merritt KK, Weech AA. Hyperbilirubinemia in the newborn. *Am J Dis Child* 1941;61:958.

815. Hardy JB, Peeples MO. Serum bilirubin levels in newborn infants. Distribu-tions and associations with neurological abnormalities during the first year of life. *Johns Hopkins Med J* 1971;128:265.

816. Lang FC, Stroder J, Alao M. Die Korrelation zwischen hyperbilirubinaemie und korpergewicht bei reifen neugeborenen. *Z Kinderh* 1968;104:161.

817. Gartner LM, Lee KS, Vaisman S, et al. Development of bilirubin transport and metabolism in the newborn rhesus monkey. *J Pediatr* 1977;90:513.

818. Pearson H. Life-span of the fetal red blood cell. *J Pediatr* 1967;70:166.

819. Vest MF, Grieder AR. Erythrocyte survival in newborn infants as measured by chromium 51 and its relation to postnatal serum bilirubin level. *J Pediatr* 1961;54:194.

820. Fallstrom SP. On the endogenous formation of carbon monoxide in full-term newborn infants. *Acta Paediatr Scand* 1969;189[Suppl]:1.

821. Maines MD, Kappas A. Study of the developmental pattern of heme catabo-lism in liver and the effects of cobalt on cytochrome P-450 and the rate of heme oxidation during the neonatal period. *J Exp Med* 1975;141:1400.

822. Maisels MJ, Pathak A, Nelson NM, et al. Endogenous production of carbon monoxide in normal and erythroblastotic newborn infants. *J Clin Invest* 1971;50:1.

823. Bartoletti AL, Stevenson DK, Ostrander CR, et al. Pulmonary excretion of carbon monoxide in the human infant as an index of bilirubin production. I. Effects of gestational and postnatal age and some common neonatal abnor-malities. *J Pediatr* 1979;94:952.

824. Brown AK, Zuelzer WW. Studies on the neonatal development of the glucu-ronide conjugating system. *J Clin Invest* 1958;37:332.

825. Lathe GH, Walker MJ. The synthesis of bilirubin glucuronide in animal and human liver. *Biochem J* 1958;70:705.

826. Maisels MJ. Neonatal jaundice. *Semin Liver Dis* 1988;8:148.

827. Onishi S, Kawade N, Itoh S, et al. Postnatal development of uridine diphos-phate glucuronyl transferase activity towards bilirubin and 2-aminophenol in human liver. *Biochem J* 1979;184:705.

828. Gartner LM. Disorders of bilirubin metabolism. In: Nathan DG, Oski FA, eds. *Hematologic disorders of the fetus and newborn.* Philadelphia: WB Saun-ders, 1981:86.

829. Brown WR, Boon WH. Ethnic group differences in plasma bilirubin levels of full-term healthy Singapore newborns. *Pediatrics* 1965;36:745.

830. Horiguchi T, Bauer C. Ethnic differences in neonatal jaundice: comparison of Japanese and Caucasian newborn infants. *Am J Obstet Gynecol* 1975;121:71.

831. Lu TC, Wei H, Blackwell RQ. Increased incidence of severe hyperbilirubin-emia among newborn Chinese infants with G-6-PD deficiency. *Pediatrics* 1966;37:994.

832. Ose T, Tsuruhara T. Follow-up study of exchanges transfusion for hyperbili-rubinemia in infants in Japan. *Pediatrics* 1976;40:196.

833. Valaes T, Petmezaki S, Doxiadis SA. Effect on neonatal hyperbilirubinemia of phenobarbital during pregnancy or after birth. Practical value of the treat-ment in a population with high risk of unexplained severe neonatal jaundice. *Birth Defects* 1970;6:46.

834. Lee KS, Gartner LM. Management of unconjugated hyperbilirubinemia in the newborn. *Semin Liver Dis* 1983;3:52.

835. Levine RL. Neonatal jaundice. *Acta Paediatr Scand* 1988;77:177.

836. Rubaltelli FF. Current drug treatment options in neonatal hyperbilirubi-naemia and the prevention of kernicterus. *Drugs* 1998;56:23.

837. Kadakol A, Ghosh SS, Sappal BS, et al. Genetic lesions of bilirubin uridine-diphosphoglucuronate glucuronosyltransferase (UGT1A1) causing Crigler-Najjar and Gilbert syndromes: correlation of genotype to phenotype. *Hum Mutat* 2000;16:297.

838. Ritter JK, Yeatman MT, Ferreira P, et al. Identification of a genetic alteration in the code for bilirubin UDP-glucuronosyltransferase in the UGT1 gene complex of a Crigler-Najjar type I patient. *J Clin Invest* 1992;90:150.

839. Bosma PJ, Chowdhury NR, Goldhoorn BG, et al. Sequence of exons and the flanking regions of human bilirubin-UDP–glucuronyl transferase gene com-plex and identification of a genetic mutation in a patient with Crigler-Najjar syndrome, type I. *Hepatology* 1992;15:941.

840. Koiwai O, Aono S, Adachi Y, et al. Crigler-Najjar syndrome type II is inher-ited both as a dominant and as a recessive trait. *Hum Mol Genet* 1996;5:645.

841. Crigler JF, Najjar VA. Congenital familial nonhemolytic jaundice with ker-nicterus. *Pediatrics* 1952;10:169.

842. Blumenschein SD, Kallen RJ, Storey B, et al. Familial nonhemolytic jaundice with late onset of neurological damage. *Pediatrics* 1968;42:786.

843. Berk PD, Martin JF, Blaschke TF, et al. Unconjugated hyperbilirubinemia. Physiologic evaluation and experimental approaches to therapy. *Ann Intern Med* 1975;82:552.

844. Blaschke TF, Berk PD, Scharschmidt BF, et al. Crigler-Najjar syndrome: an unusual course with development of neurologic damage at age eighteen. *Pediatr Res* 1974;8:573.

845. Arias IM, Gartner LM, Cohen M, et al. Chronic non-hemolytic unconjugated hyperbilirubinemia with glucuronyl transferase deficiency: clinical, biochemical, pharmacologic, and genetic evidence for heterogeneity. *Am J Med* 1969;47:395.

846. Axelrod J, Schmid R, Hammaker L. A biochemical lesion in congenital, non-obstructive, non-hemolytic jaundice. *Nature* 1957;180:1426.

847. Berk PD, Blaschke TF, Scharschmidt BF, et al. A new approach to quantita-tion of the various sources of bilirubin in man. *J Lab Clin Med* 1976;87:767.

848. Schmid R, Hammaker L. Metabolism and disposition of C14 bilirubin in congenital nonhemolytic jaundice. *J Clin Invest* 1963;42:1720.
849. Kaufman SS, Wood RP, Shaw BW, et al. Orthotopic liver transplantation for type I Crigler-Najjar syndrome. *Hepatology* 1986;6:1259.
850. Fox IJ, Chowdhury JR, Kaufman SS, et al. Treatment of the Crigler-Najjar syndrome type I with hepatocyte transplantation. *N Engl J Med* 1998;338:1422.
851. Gupta S, Gorla GR, Irani AN. Hepatocyte transplantation: emerging insights into mechanisms of liver repopulation and their relevance to potential therapies. *J Hepatol* 1999;30:162.
852. Arias IM. Chronic unconjugated hyperbilirubinemia without overt signs of hemolysis in adolescents and adults. *J Clin Invest* 1962;41:2233.
853. Berk PD, Wolkoff AW, Berlin NI. Inborn errors of bilirubin metabolism. *Med Clin North Am* 1975;59:803.
854. Arias IM, Gartner LM, Furman M, et al. Studies of the effect of several drugs on hepatic glucuronide formation in newborn rats and humans. *Ann N Y Acad Sci* 1963;111:274.
855. Gordon EF, Shaffer EA, Sass-Kortsaka A. Bilirubin secretion and conjugation in the Crigler-Najjar syndrome type II. *Gastroenterology* 1976;70:761.
856. Fevery J, Blankaert N, Heirwegh KP, et al. Unconjugated bilirubin and an increased proportion of bilirubin monoconjugates in the bile of patients with Gilbert's syndrome and Crigler-Najjar syndrome. *J Clin Invest* 1977;60:970.
857. Gilbert A, Lereboullet P. La cholemie simple familiale. *Sem Med* 1901;21:241.
858. Jansen PL, Elferink RP. Hereditary hyperbilirubinemias: a molecular and mechanistic approach. *Semin Liver Dis* 1988;8:168.
859. Watson KJ, Gollan JL. Gilbert's syndrome. *Baillieres Clin Gastroenterol* 1989;3:337.
860. Schmid R. Gilbert's syndrome—a legitimate genetic anomaly? *N Engl J Med* 1995;333:1217.
861. Kaplan M, Renbaum P, Levy-Lahad E, et al. Gilbert syndrome and glucose-6-phosphate dehydrogenase deficiency: a dose-dependent genetic interaction crucial to neonatal hyperbilirubinemia. *Proc Natl Acad Sci U S A* 1997;94:12128.
862. Del Giudice EM, Perrotta S, Nobili B, et al. Coinheritance of Gilbert syndrome increases the risk for developing gallstones in patients with hereditary spherocytosis. *Blood* 1999;94:2259.
863. Beutler E, Gelbart T, Demina A. Racial variability in the UDP-glucuronosyltransferase 1 (UGT1A1) promoter: a balanced polymorphism for regulation of bilirubin metabolism? *Proc Natl Acad Sci U S A* 1998;95:8170.
864. Koiwai O, Nishizawa M, Hasada K, et al. Gilbert's syndrome is caused by a heterozygous missense mutation in the gene for bilirubin UDP-glucuronosyltransferase. *Hum Mol Genet* 1995;4:1183.
865. Aono S, Adachi Y, Uyama E, et al. Analysis of genes for bilirubin UDP-glucuronosyltransferase in Gilbert's syndrome. *Lancet* 1995;345:958.
866. Black M, Billing BH. Hepatic bilirubin UDP–glucuronyl transferase activity in liver disease and Gilbert's syndrome. *N Engl J Med* 1969;280:1266.
867. Felsher BF, Craig JR, Carpio N. Hepatic bilirubin glucuronidation in Gilbert's syndrome. *J Lab Clin Med* 1973;81:829.
868. Powell LW, Hemingway EH, Billing BH, et al. Idiopathic unconjugated hyperbilirubinemia (Gilbert's syndrome): a study of 42 families. *N Engl J Med* 1967;217:1108.
869. Owens D, Evans J. Population studies on Gilbert's syndrome. *J Med Genet* 1975;12:152.
870. Foulk WT, Butt HR, Owen CA, et al. Constitutional hepatic dysfunction (Gilbert's disease): its natural history and related syndrome. *Medicine* 1959;38:25.
871. Berk PD, Bloomer JR, Howe RB, et al. Constitutional hepatic dysfunction (Gilbert's syndrome): a new definition based on kinetic studies with unconjugated radiobilirubin. *Am J Med* 1970;49:296.
872. Okolicsanyi L, Ghidini O, Orlando, et al. An evaluation of bilirubin kinetics with respect to the diagnosis of Gilbert's syndrome. *Clin Sci Mol Med* 1978;54:539.
873. Bancroft JD, Kreamer B, Gourley GR. Gilbert syndrome accelerates development of neonatal jaundice. *J Pediatr* 1998;132:656.
874. Maruo Y, Sato H, Yamano T, et al. Gilbert syndrome caused by a homozygous missense mutation (Tyr486Asp) of bilirubin UDP-glucuronosyltransferase gene. *J Pediatr* 1998;132:1045.
875. Monaghan G, McLellan A, McGeehan A, et al. Gilbert's syndrome is a contributory factor in prolonged unconjugated hyperbilirubinemia of the newborn. *J Pediatr* 1999;134:441.
876. Arthur LJH, Beva BR, Holton JB. Neonatal hyperbilirubinemia and breast feeding. *Dev Med Child Neurol* 1966;8:279.
877. Arias IM, Gartner LM, Seifter S, et al. Prolonged neonatal unconjugated hyperbilirubinemia associated with breast feeding and a steroid, pregnane-3-alpha, 20-beta-diol, in maternal milk that inhibits glucuronide formation in vitro. *J Clin Invest* 1964;43:2037.
878. Maisels MJ, Gifford K. Normal serum bilirubin levels in the newborn and the effect of breast-feeding. *Pediatrics* 1986;78:839.
879. Woolley MM, Felsher BF, Asch J, et al. Jaundice, hypertrophic pyrrolic stenosis and hepatic glucuronyl transferase. *J Pediatr Surg* 1974;9:359.
880. Lokietz H, Dowben RM, Hsia DY. Studies on the effect of novobiocin on glucuronyl transferase. *Pediatrics* 1963;32:47.
881. Akerren Y. Prolonged jaundice in the newborn associated with congenital myxedema. *Acta Paediatr* 1954;43:411.
882. Taylor PM, Wolfson JH, Bright NH, et al. Hyperbilirubinemia in infants of diabetic mothers. *Biol Neonate* 1963;5:289.
883. Van Praagh R. Diagnosis of kernicterus in the neonatal period. *Pediatrics* 1961;28:870.
884. Perlstein MA. The late clinical syndrome of post-icteric encephalopathy. *Pediatr Clin North Am* 1960;7:665.
885. Shapiro SM, Hecox KE. Brain stem auditory evoked potentials in jaundiced Gunn rats. *Ann Otol Rhinol Laryngol* 1989;98:308.
886. Hyman CB, Keaster J, Hanson V, et al. CNS abnormalities after neonatal hemolytic disease or hyperbilirubinemia. *Arch Dis Child* 1969;117:395.
887. Johnson L, Boggs TR. Bilirubin-dependent brain damage. Incidence and indications for treatment. In: Odell GB, Schaffer R, Simopoulos AP, eds. *Phototherapy in the newborn: an overview.* Washington: National Academy of Sciences, 1974:122.
888. Johnston WH, Angara V, Baumal R, et al. Erythroblastosis fetalis and hyperbilirubinemia. A five-year follow-up with neurological, psychological and audiological evaluation. *Pediatrics* 1967;39:88.
889. Scheidt PC, Mellits ED, Hardy JB, et al. Toxicity to bilirubin in neonates: infant development during first year in relation to maximal neonatal serum bilirubin concentration. *J Pediatr* 1977;91:292.
890. Corwin MJ, Golub HL. Spectral analysis of a cry is abnormal in infants who have moderate hyperbilirubinemia. *Pediatr Res* 1984;18:102A.
891. Van de Bor M, van Aeben-van der Aa TM, Verloove-Vanhorick SP, et al. Hyperbilirubinemia in preterm infants and neurodevelopmental outcome at 2 years of age: results of a national collaborative survey. *Pediatrics* 1989; 83:915.
892. Rose AL, Johnson A. Bilirubin encephalopathy: neurological and histochemical studies in the Gunn rat model. *Neurology* 1972;22:420.
893. Odell GB. Studies in kernicterus. The protein binding of albumin. *J Clin Invest* 1959;38:823.
894. Odell GB. The distribution and toxicity of bilirubin. *Pediatrics* 1970;46:16.
895. Odell GB. Neonatal jaundice. In: Popper H, Schaffner F, eds. *Progress in liver disease*, V. New York: Grune & Stratton, 1977:457.
896. Brodersen R. Prevention of kernicterus, based on recent progress in bilirubin chemistry. *Acta Paediatr Scand* 1977;66:625.
897. Levine RL, Fredericks WR, Rapoport SI. Entry of bilirubin into the brain due to opening of the blood-brain barrier. *Pediatrics* 1982;69:255.
898. Hansen TW, Bratlid D. Bilirubin and brain toxicity. *Acta Paediatr Scand* 1986;75:513.
899. Lee C, Oh W, Stonestreet BS, et al. Permeability of the blood brain barrier of 125I-albumin-bound bilirubin in newborn piglets. *Pediatr Res* 1989;25:452.
900. Schwoebel A, Sakraida S. Hyperbilirubinemia: new approaches to an old problem. *J Perinat Neonat Nurs* 1997;11:78.
901. Lucey JF, Ferreiro M, Hewitt J. Prevention of hyperbilirubinemia of prematurity by phototherapy. *Pediatrics* 1968;41:1047.
902. Hodgman JE, Schwartz A. Phototherapy and hyperbilirubinemia of the premature. *Am J Dis Child* 1963;119:473.
903. McDonagh AF, Agati G, Fusi F, et al. First observation of the wavelength-dependent photoproduction of the 4E,15Z configurational isomer of bilirubin bound to human serum albumin. *Soc Photo Opt Instr Engin* 1987;701:367.
904. Lightner DA, McDonagh AF. Molecular mechanisms of phototherapy for neonatal jaundice. *Proc Natl Acad Sci U S A* 1984;17:417.
905. Cremer RJ, Perryman PW, Richards DW. Influences of light on the hyperbilirubinemia of infants. *Lancet* 1958;1:1094.
906. Lightner DA, Wooldridge TA, McDonagh AF. Photobilirubin: an early bilirubin photoproduct detected by absorbance difference spectroscopy. *Proc Natl Acad Sci U S A* 1979;76:29.
907. Lightner DA, Wooldridge TA, McDonagh AF. Configuration isomerization of bilirubin and mechanism of jaundice phototherapy. *Biochem Biophys Res Commun* 1979;86:235.
908. Stoll MS, Zenone FA, Ostrow JD, et al. Preparation and properties of bilirubin photoisomers. *Biochem J* 1979;183:139.
909. Cohen AN, Ostrow JD. New concepts in phototherapy: photoisomerization of bilirubin IXalpha and potential toxic effects of light. *Pediatrics* 1980; 65:740.
910. Sisson TR, Voge TP. Phototherapy of hyperbilirubinemia. In: Regan JD, Parrish JA, eds. *The science of photomedicine.* New York: Plenum Publishing, 1982:477.
911. National Institutes of Child Health and Human Development. Randomized controlled trial of phototherapy for neonatal hyperbilirubinemia. *Pediatrics* 1985;75[Suppl]:385.
912. Vecchi C, Donzelli GP, Migliorini MG, et al. Green light in phototherapy. *Pediatr Res* 1983;17:461.
913. Anderson RR, Parrish JA. The optics of human skin. *J Invest Dermatol* 1981;77:13.
914. Donzelli GP. Green light phototherapy: towards new trends. *J Photochem Photobiol B* 1989;4:126.
915. Tan KL. Comparison of the effectiveness of phototherapy and exchange transfusion in the management of nonhemolytic neonatal hyperbilirubinemia. *J Pediatr* 1975;87:609.
916. American Academy of Pediatrics. Provisional Committee for Quality Improvement and Subcommittee on Hyperbilirubinemia. Practice parameter: management of hyperbilirubinemia in the healthy term newborn. *Pediatrics* 1994;94:558.
917. McDonagh AF, Lightner DA. Phototherapy and the photobiology of bilirubin. *Semin Liver Dis* 1988;8:272.
918. Allen FH Jr, Diamond LK. Erythroblastosis fetalis including exchange transfusion technique. *N Engl J Med* 1957;257:659.
919. Allen FH Jr, Diamond LK, Vaughan VC III. Erythroblastosis fetalis. VI. Prevention of kernicterus. *Am J Dis Child* 1950;80:779.
920. Diamond LK. Replacement transfusion as a treatment for erythroblastosis. *Pediatrics* 1948;2:520.
921. Valaes T. Bilirubin distribution and dynamics of bilirubin removal by exchange transfusion. *Acta Paediatr Scand* 1962;52[Suppl]:1.

922. Baumgart S, Kim HC. Exchange transfusion in the neonate. In: Stockman JA III, Pochedly C, eds. *Developmental neonatal hematology.* New York: Raven Press, 1988:199.

923. Keenan WJ, Novak KK, Sutherland JM, et al. Morbidity and mortality associated with exchange transfusion. *Pediatrics* 1985;75:417.

924. Odell GB. Administration of albumin in the management of hyperbilirubinemia by exchange transfusion. *Pediatrics* 1962;30:613.

925. Waters WJ, Porter E. Indications for exchange transfusion based upon the role of albumin in the treatment of hemolytic disease of the newborn. *Pediatrics* 1964;33:749.

926. Oski FA, Naiman JL. *Hematologic problems in the newborn.* Philadelphia: WB Saunders, 1972.

927. Boggs TR Jr, Westphal MD Jr. Mortality of exchange transfusion. *Pediatrics* 1960;26:745.

928. Culley P, Powell J, Waterhouse J, et al. Sequelae of jaundice. *BMJ* 1970;3:383.

929. Rubin RA, Balow B, Fisch RO. Neonatal serum bilirubin levels related to cognitive development at ages 4 through 7 years. *J Pediatr* 1979;94:601.

930. Gartner IM, Snyder RN, Chabon RS, et al. High incidence in premature infants with low serum bilirubin concentrations. *Pediatrics* 1970;45:906.

931. Keenan WJ, Perlstein PH, Light IJ, et al. Kernicterus in small sick premature infants receiving phototherapy. *Pediatrics* 1972;49:652.

932. Odell GB, Storey GN, Rosenberg LA, et al. Studies in kernicterus. III. The saturation of serum proteins with bilirubin during neonatal life and its relationship to brain damage at five years. *J Pediatr* 1970;76:12.

933. Stern L, Denton RL. Kernicterus in small premature infants. *Pediatrics* 1965;35:483.

934. Hsia D-Y, Allen FH, Gellis SS, et al. Erythroblastosis fetalis: studies of serum bilirubin in relation to kernicterus. *N Engl J Med* 1952;247:668.

935. Mollison PL, Cutbush M. Haemolytic disease of the newborn. In: Gardiner D, ed. *Recent advances in pediatrics.* New York: P Blakiston & Sons, 1954:110.

936. Lucey JF. Bilirubin and brain damage—a real mess. *Pediatrics* 1982;69:381.

937. Watchko JF, Oski FA. Bilirubin 20 mg/dl = vigintiphobia. *Pediatrics* 1983; 71:660.

938. Phipps RH. Hemolytic anemias. Hemolytic diseases of the newborn (erythroblastosis fetalis). In: Rudolph AM, Hoffman JI, eds. *Pediatrics.* Norwalk, CT: Appleton-Century-Crofts, 1982:1057.

939. Galbraith RA, Kappas A. Pharmacokinetics of tin-mesoporphyrin in man and the effects of tin-chelated porphyrins on hyperexcretion of heme pathway precursors in patients with acute inducible porphyria. *Hepatology* 1989; 9:882.

940. Anderson KE, Simionatto CS, Drummond GS, et al. Disposition of tin-protoporphyrin and suppression of hyperbilirubinemia in humans. *Clin Pharmacol Ther* 1986;39:510.

941. Rubaltelli FF, Guerrini P, Reddi E, et al. Tin-protoporphyrin in the management of Crigler-Najjar Disease. *Pediatrics* 1989;84:728.

942. Galbraith RA, Drummond GS, Kappas A. Suppression of bilirubin production in the Crigler-Najjar type I syndrome: studies with the heme oxygenase inhibitor, Sn-mesoporphyrin. *Pediatrics* 1992;89:175.

943. Milleville GS, Levitt MD, Engel RR. Tin protoporphyrin inhibits carbon monoxide production in adult mice. *Pediatr Res* 1985;19:94.

944. Landaw SA, Sassa S, Drummond GS, et al. Proof that Sn-protoporphyrin inhibits the enzymatic catabolism of heme in vivo. Suppression of 14CO generation from radiolabeled endogenous and exogenous heme sources. *J Exp Med* 1987;165:1195.

945. Simionatto CS, Anderson KE, Drummond GS, et al. Studies on the mechanism of Sn-protoporphyrin suppression of hyperbilirubinemia. Inhibition of heme oxidation and bilirubin production. *J Clin Invest* 1985;75:513.

946. Kappas A, Drummond GS, Sardana MK. Sn-protoporphyrin rapidly and markedly enhances the heme saturation of hepatic tryptophan pyrrolase. Evidence that this synthetic metalloporphyrin increases the functional content of heme in the liver. *J Clin Invest* 1985;75:302.

947. Landaw SA, Drummond GS, Kappas A. Targeting of heme oxygenase inhibitors to the spleen markedly increases their ability to diminish bilirubin production. *Pediatrics* 1989;84:1091.

948. Kappas A, Drummond GS, Henschke C, et al. Direct comparison of Sn-mesoporphyrin, an inhibitor of bilirubin production, and phototherapy in controlling hyperbilirubinemia in term and near-term newborns. *Pediatrics* 1995; 95:468.

949. Martinez JC, Garcia HO, Otheguy LE, et al. Control of severe hyperbilirubinemia in full-term newborns with the inhibitor of bilirubin production Sn-mesoporphyrin. *Pediatrics* 1999;103:1.

950. Seymour CA, Neale G, Peters TJ. Lysosomal changes in liver tissue from patients with Dubin-Johnson-Sprinz syndrome. *Clin Sci Mol Med* 1977; 52:241.

951. Cohen L, Lewis C, Arias IM. Pregnancy, oral contraceptives, and chronic hyperbilirubinemia (Dubin-Johnson syndrome). *Gastroenterology* 1972;62: 1182.

952. Kondo T, Kuchiba K, Ohtsuka Y, et al. Clinical and genetic studies on Dubin-Johnson syndrome in a clustered area in Japan. *Jinrui Idengaku Zasshi* 1974; 18:378.

953. Jansen PL, Peters WH, Janssens AR. Clinical value of serum bilirubin subfractionation by high-performance liquid chromatography and conventional methods in patients with primary biliary cirrhosis. *J Hepatol* 1986;2:485.

954. Schoenfield LJ, McGill DB, Hutton DB, et al. Studies of chronic idiopathic jaundice (Dubin-Johnson syndrome). I. Demonstration of hepatic excretory defect. *Gastroenterology* 1963;44:101.

955. Kaplowitz N, Javitt N, Kappas A. Coproporphyrin I and 3 excretion in bile and urine. *J Clin Invest* 1972;51:2895.

956. Paulusma CC, Kool M, Bosma PJ, et al. A mutation in the human canalicular multispecific organic anion transporter gene causes the Dubin-Johnson syndrome. *Hepatology* 1997;25:1539.

957. Wada M, Toh S, Taniguchi K, et al. Mutations in the canalicular multispecific organic anion transporter (cMOAT) gene, a novel ABC transporter, in patients with hyperbilirubinemia II/Dubin-Johnson syndrome. *Hum Mol Genet* 1998;7:203.

958. Paulusma CC, Bosma PJ, Zaman GJ, et al. Congenital jaundice in rats with a mutation in a multidrug resistance-associated protein gene. *Science* 1996; 271:1126.

959. Ito K, Suzuki H, Hirohashi T, et al. Molecular cloning of canalicular multispecific organic anion transporter defective in EHBR. *Am J Physiol* 1997; 272:16.

960. Cornelius CE, Arias IM, Osburn BI. Hepatic pigmentation with photosensitivity: a syndrome in Corriedale sheep resembling Dubin-Johnson syndrome in man. *J Am Vet Med Assoc* 1965;146:709.

961. Cornelius CE, Osburn BI, Gronwall RR, et al. Dubin-Johnson syndrome in immature sheep. *Am J Dig Dis* 1968;13:1072.

962. Mia AS, Gronwall RR, Cornelius CE. Unconjugated bilirubin transport in normal and mutant Corriedale sheep with Dubin-Johnson syndrome. *Proc Soc Exp Biol Med* 1970;135:33.

963. Rotor AB, Manahan L, Florentin A. Familial non-hemolytic jaundice with direct Van den Bergh reaction. *Acta Med Phillipp* 1948;5:37.

964. Wolpert E, Pascasio FM, Wolkoff AW, et al. Abnormal sulfobromophthalein metabolism in Rotor's syndrome and obligate heterozygotes. *N Engl J Med* 1977;296:1091.

965. Wolkoff AW, Wolpert E, Pascasio FN, et al. Rotor's syndrome, a distinct inheritable pathophysiologic entity. *Am J Med* 1976;60:173.

966. Poh-Fitzpatrick MB. Porphyrin-sensitized cutaneous photosensitivity: pathogenesis and treatment. *Clin Dermatol* 1985;3:41.

967. Goyer RA, May P, Cates M, et al. Lead and protein content of isolated intranuclear inclusion bodies from kidneys of lead-poisoned rats. *Lab Invest* 1970;22:245.

CHAPTER 48

Hemoglobin Synthesis and the Thalassemias

Bernard G. Forget and Nancy F. Olivieri

HEMOGLOBIN SYNTHESIS

Normal Human Hemoglobins and Their Genes

Many different normal human hemoglobins exist, as well as numerous abnormal hemoglobins. Before precise knowledge of globin gene organization by gene mapping and gene cloning procedures was gained, a general picture of the number and arrangement of the normal human globin genes emerged from the genetic analysis of normal and abnormal hemoglobins and their pattern of inheritance. The number and subunit composition of different normal human hemoglobins (Fig. 48-1) indicated that there must be at least one different globin gene for each of the different globin chains: α, β, γ, δ, ε, and ζ. Evidence then accumulated from the study of hemoglobin variants and the analysis of the biochemical heterogeneity of the chains in fetal hemoglobin (Hb F) that the α-globin and γ-globin genes were duplicated. Persons were identified whose red blood cells (RBCs) contained more than two structurally different α-globin chains that could be best explained by duplication of the α-globin gene locus, and the characterization of the structurally different $^G\gamma$-globin and $^A\gamma$-globin chains of Hb F imposed a requirement for duplication of the γ-globin gene locus.

From the study of the pattern of inheritance of Hb variants from persons carrying both an α-chain and a β-chain variant, it became clear that the α-globin and β-globin genes must be on different chromosomes, or at least widely separated if on the same chromosome; α-chain and β-chain Hb variants were always observed to segregate independently in offspring of doubly affected parents (1). Linkage of the various β-like globin genes to one another was established from the study of interesting Hb variants, which contained fused globin chains presumably resulting from nonhomologous crossover among different β-like globin gene loci. The characterization of Hb Lepore (2), with its $\delta\beta$ fusion chain, established that the δ-globin gene was linked to and located on the 5' (or N-terminal) side of the β-globin gene, whereas the analysis of Hb Kenya (3), with its $^A\gamma\beta$ fusion chain, provided evidence for linkage of the $^A\gamma$ gene, and presumably the $^G\gamma$ gene as well, to the 5' side of the δ-globin and β-globin genes. Thus, the general concept of the arrangement of the globin genes that emerged from these various genetic analyses can be represented as illustrated in Figure 48-1. It was also assumed, but unsupported by genetic evidence, that the embryonic α-like (ζ) and β-like ε-globin genes were likely to be linked to the loci for their adult counterparts.

Chromosomal Localization of Globin Genes

By the use of rodent–human somatic hybrid cells containing only one or a limited number of human chromosomes, Deisseroth et al. (4,5) clearly established that the human α-globin and β-globin genes resided on different chromosomes, and that the α genes were located on chromosome 16, whereas the β genes were located on chromosome 11. The latter results were obtained by solution hybridization assays of total cellular DNA from the various somatic hybrid cells hybridized to radioactive complementary DNAs synthesized from α-globin and β-globin messenger RNAs (mRNAs) by use of the enzyme reverse transcriptase. These results were later confirmed and extended by various groups using the gene mapping procedure of Southern blot analysis with DNA from various hybrid cell lines containing different translocations or deletions of the involved chromosomes.

These studies led to the regional localization of the globin gene loci on their respective chromosomes: the β-globin gene cluster to the short arm of chromosome 11 and the α-globin gene cluster to the short arm of chromosome 16. These chromosomal assignments were further confirmed and refined by *in situ* hybridization of radioactive cloned globin gene probes to metaphase chromosomes as well as by fluorescence *in situ* hybridization. Thus, the β-globin gene cluster was assigned to 11p15.5 and the α-globin gene cluster to 16p13.3.

Detailed Chromosomal Organization of Human Globin Genes

A precise picture of the chromosomal organization of the α-like and β-like human globin gene clusters, with respect to the number of structural loci and intergene distances, was obtained by the technique of restriction endonuclease mapping using the gel blotting procedure of Southern as well as actual isolation, gene cloning technology, and characterization of large fragments of human DNA containing the various globin genes (6–8). Sets of overlapping genomic DNA fragments spanning the entire α-globin and β-globin gene clusters have been obtained by gene cloning, initially in bacteriophage l as well as larger fragments in cosmid vectors. Detailed analysis of these recombinant DNA clones has led to the determination of the gene organization illustrated in Figure 48-2. Some of the results were expected, such as the finding of single δ- and β-globin gene loci and duplication of the α-globin and γ-globin gene loci. In addition, single loci for the embryonic ζ-globin and ε-globin chains were found to be linked to the α-globin and β-globin gene clusters, respectively.

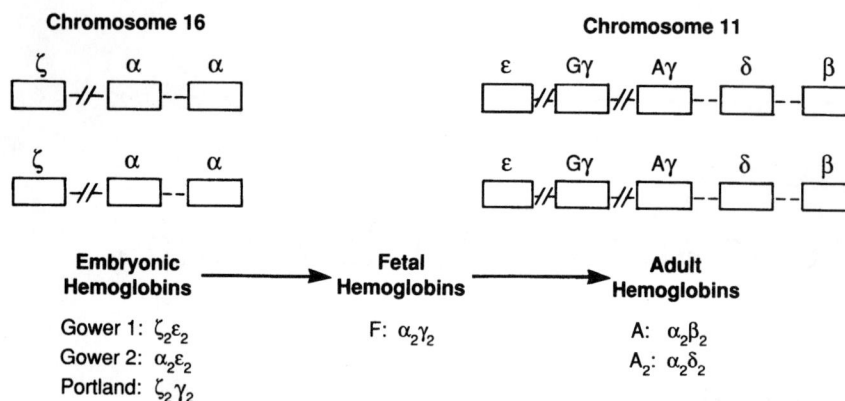

Figure 48-1. Model of the human globin gene system based on genetic information available before the actual cloning of the genes. The various hemoglobins expressed at different stages of development are indicated below the model.

An unexpected finding was the presence in the globin gene clusters of additional genelike structures with structural homology to the authentic globin genes: one in the β gene cluster between the γ-globin and δ-globin genes and three in the α gene cluster, between the ζ- and authentic α-globin genes. These structures have been called *pseudogenes*. They are characterized by the presence of one or more mutations that render them incapable of encoding a functional globin chain. These pseudogenes appear to have arisen by gene duplication events within the globin gene clusters followed by mutation and inactivation of the duplicated gene and subsequent accumulation of additional mutations through loss of selective pressure.

Another α-like globin gene has been identified and characterized in the α-globin gene cluster: the θ gene located toward the 3' or C-terminal side of the duplicated α-globin genes (9). This gene is evolutionarily related to and coexpressed with the α-globin genes (10,11). mRNA transcripts are only at very low levels (less than 1% of α), and no Hb containing the θ-globin chains has been identified. Furthermore, the predicted structure (translated amino acid sequence) of the θ-globin chain suggests that it is unlikely to function normally as a Hb subunit (12).

Globin Gene Structure

INTERVENING SEQUENCES OR INTRONS
The coding region of the globin genes of humans and other animals is interrupted at two positions by considerable stretches of noncoding DNA called *intervening sequences* or *introns* (6–8). In the β-like globin genes, the intervening sequences interrupt the

sequence between codons 30 and 31 and between codons 104 and 105; in the α-globin gene family, the intervening sequences interrupt the coding sequence between codons 31 and 32 and between codons 99 and 100 (Fig. 48-3). Although the precise codon position numbers at which the interruption occurs differ between the α-like and β-like globin genes, the introns occur at precisely the same position with regard to the regions of the primary structure of the α-globin and β-globin chains that are homologous and can be aligned if one assumes that the α-globin and β-globin gene families originally evolved from a single ancestral globin gene. The first intervening sequence (IVS-1) is shorter than the second intervening sequence (IVS-2) in both α-globin and β-globin genes, but IVS-2 of the human β-globin gene is considerably larger than that of the α-globin gene.

As illustrated in Figure 48-2, the pattern of intron sizes of the ζ-like globin genes is different from that of the other α-like globin genes; whereas the introns in the α and ψα genes are small (fewer than 150 base pairs [bp]), those of the ζ and ψζ genes are considerably larger. Furthermore, IVS-1 is much larger than IVS-2 and is 8 to 10 times larger than the IVS-1 of any other globin gene.

The presence of intervening sequences that interrupt the coding sequences of structural genes imposes a requirement for some cellular process to prevent the occurrence of these sequences in the mature mRNA. Intervening sequences have been found to be transcribed into globin (and other) precursor mRNA molecules but subsequently excised and the proper ends of the coding sequences relegated to yield the mature mRNA. This posttranscriptional processing of mRNA precursors has been termed *splicing* and is illustrated schematically in Figure 48-4A.

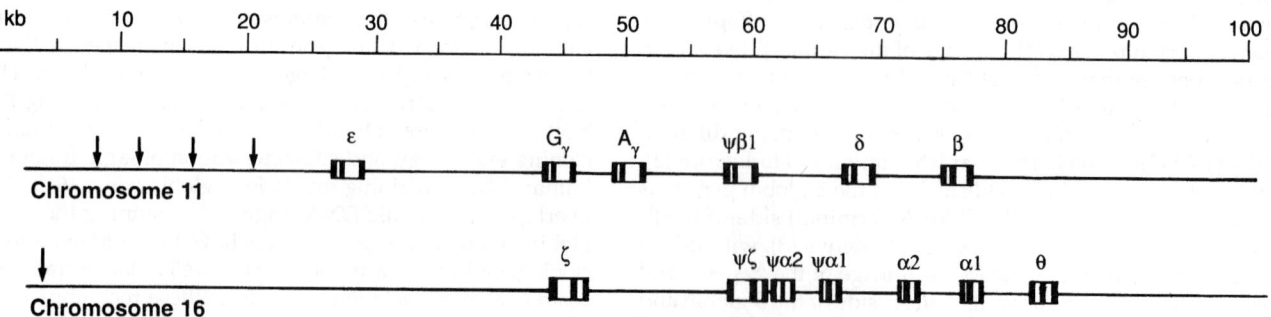

Figure 48-2. Structure of the human α-globin and β-globin gene loci based on information obtained by gene cloning and DNA sequence analysis. The vertical arrows indicate the positions of developmentally stable, erythroid-specific DNase I–hypersensitive sites that, in the β locus, constitute the 5' locus control region, and in the α locus, the HS-40 enhancer. The fine structure of the genes (exon–intron organization) is shown in Figure 48-3. (From Bunn HF, Forget BG. *Hemoglobin: molecular, genetic and clinical aspects.* Philadelphia: WB Saunders, 1986, with permission.)

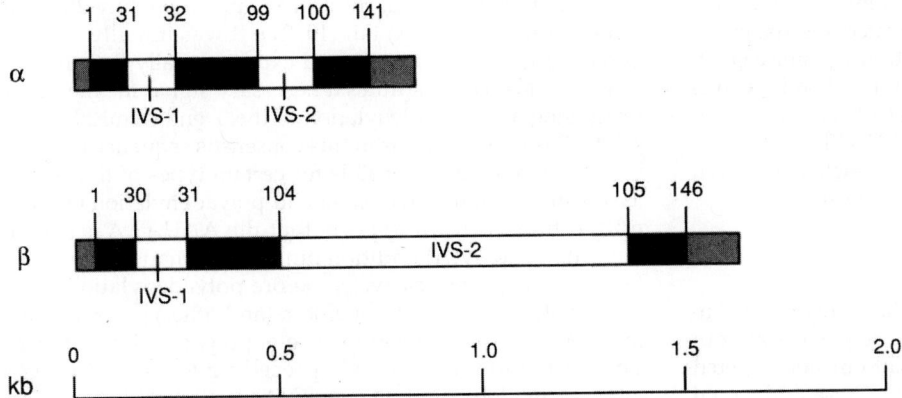

Figure 48-3. Fine structure of the human α-globin and β-globin genes. The black blocks represent the coding regions of the gene; the gray blocks at either end represent the 5' and 3' untranslated sequences; IVS-1 and IVS-2 are the intervening sequences (introns) that interrupt the coding sequences of the genes. The numbers above the diagram indicate the amino acid codon positions of the coding sequence. (From Bunn HF, Forget BG. *Hemoglobin: molecular, genetic and clinical aspects*. Philadelphia, WB Saunders, 1986, with permission.)

A crucial prerequisite for the proper splicing of globin (and other) precursor mRNA molecules is the presence of specific nucleotide sequences at the junctions between coding sequences (exons) and intervening sequences (introns). Comparison of these sequences in many different genes has permitted the derivation of two different "consensus" sequences, which are universally found at the 5' and 3' ends, respectively, of introns (13,14). The consensus sequences thus derived are the following:

donor splice site   acceptor splice site

$(5')(C/A) AG \quad \underline{GT} (A/G) AGT \ldots (T/C)_nN(C/T)\underline{AG} \quad G(3')$

where N = any nucleotide and n = a variable number of pyrimidine nucleotides, equal to or greater than 11. The 5' sequence is sometimes called the *donor splice site* and the 3' sequence, the *acceptor splice site*. The underlined dinucleotides GT and AG, located at the 5' and 3' ends, respectively, of the intron, are

essentially invariant and are thought to be required for proper splicing—the so-called GT-AG rule. Rare examples have been described in which GC instead of GT is found at the donor splice site junction. The importance or significance of these consensus sequences is underscored by the fact that mutations that alter these normal consensus sequences, or mutations that create consensus sequences at new sites in a globin gene, lead to abnormal processing of globin mRNA precursors and constitute the molecular basis for many types of thalassemia.

The mechanism by which introns are excised from pre-mRNAs involves a cellular organelle called the *spliceosome* (15–17). The spliceosome is a large macromolecular complex consisting of five RNA species (called *small nuclear RNAs*: U1, U2, U4, U5, and U6) and a large number of different proteins. In the presplicing complex, U1 RNA binds to the 5' end of the intronic sequence, whereas U2 RNA binds to a sequence called the *branch site* near the 3' end of the intronic sequence. The excision is a two-step adenosine triphosphate–independent process involving two trans-esterification reactions. As a result of the first reaction, the 5'

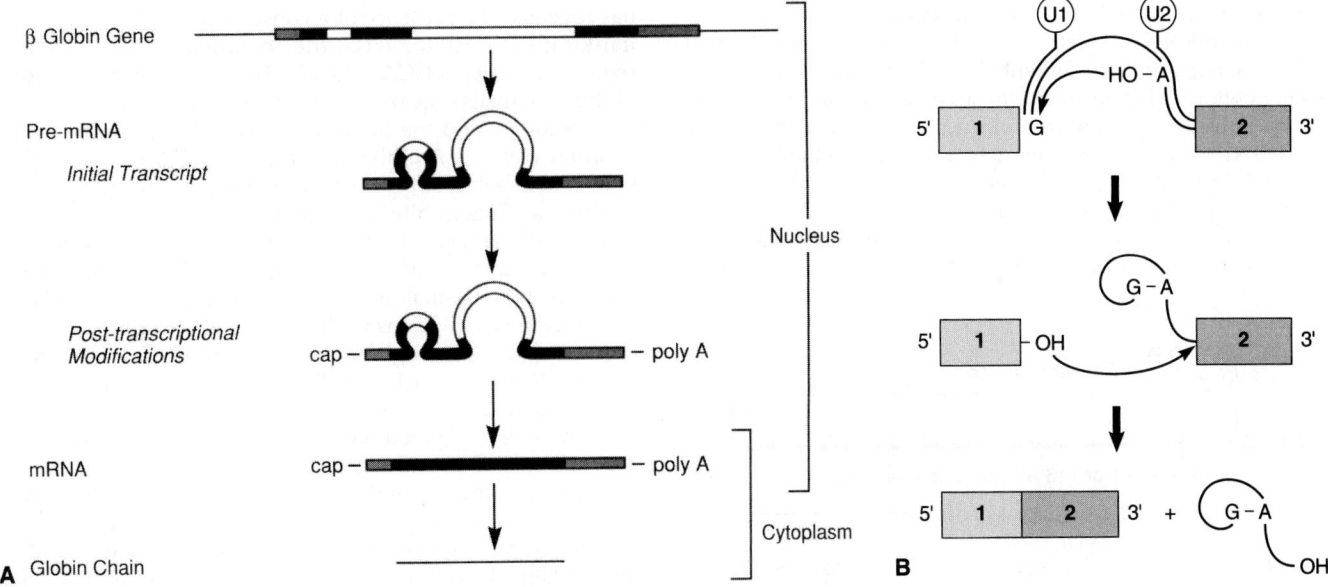

Figure 48-4. Schematic representation of the process of β-globin gene expression. **A:** Overall process, including gene transcription, posttranscriptional processing of the messenger RNA (mRNA), transport of mRNA from nucleus to cytoplasm, and mRNA translation. (From Bunn HF, Forget BG. *Hemoglobin: molecular, genetic and clinical aspects*. Philadelphia: WB Saunders, 1986, with permission.) **B:** Steps involved in the excision of an intron. (From Forget BG. Molecular genetics of the human globin genes. In: Steinberg MH, Forget BG, Higgs DR, et al., eds. *Disorders of hemoglobin*. New York: Cambridge University Press, 2001:117, with permission.)

end of the intronic sequence forms a covalent bond with the region of the intron called the *branch site*, located approximately 18 to 37 nucleotides from the 3' end of the intron, forming a lariat-like or branched RNA structure (Fig. 48-4B). This bond involves the G of the GU dinucleotide of the 5' donor site and the A residue in the branch site recognition sequence ACT(TT/CC) or ATC (TT/CC). After the second transesterification reaction, the lariat is released and the two adjacent exons joined (Fig. 48-4B).

CONSERVED FUNCTIONAL SEQUENCES OF MATURE GLOBIN MESSENGER RNA

The transcript of the human globin genes that is represented in mature globin mRNA contains additional sequences at both extremities of the mRNA in addition to the information required to encode the globin polypeptide chains. These additional untranslated nucleotides account for approximately 30% of the total length of globin mRNA. The 3' (C-terminal) untranslated sequences are two to three times the length of the 5' (N-terminal) untranslated sequences. The lengths of these sequences in the major human globin mRNAs are illustrated in Figure 48-5. In addition to the nucleotides that are transcribed from the globin gene, the globin mRNA contains nucleotides that are added to it within the cell nucleus after transcription: a methylated guanylic acid (m^7G) cap structure at the 5' end of the mRNA and a number of adenylic acid residues forming a poly(A) tail at the 3' end of the mRNA. The precise functions of these untranslated sequences in globin and other mRNAs are not completely known. The 5'-methylated cap structure appears to be important for the initiation of polypeptide chain synthesis through its interaction with specific initiation factors. The poly(A) tail of mRNAs appears to contribute to the stability of the mRNA (6–8).

Two general consensus sequences are at or near the extremities of these untranslated sequences and are important for the efficient processing of mRNA transcripts. The cap site in globin (and most eukaryotic) mRNAs is usually located at an A residue that is preceded in genomic DNA by a C. The DNA sequence to either side of the CA is generally rich in pyrimidines. The cap site consensus sequence appears to be important not only for accurate initiation of transcription and 5' processing of the mRNA but also for service as a promoter element called the *initiator* (Inr) element (18), which is capable of influencing both the efficiency and the accuracy of transcription initiation. This is especially true in the case of certain genes that lack a TATA box in their promoters (discussed in the following section). At least one β-thalassemia mutation involves a base substitution in the cap site consensus sequence.

The one common feature of the 3' noncoding sequence of globin and other mRNAs is the presence of the hexanucleotide

AAUAAA (AATAAA in the DNA) approximately 20 nucleotides from the poly(A) tail (19–21). It was initially assumed and subsequently demonstrated experimentally that this consensus sequence constitutes a necessary signal for the proper processing and polyadenylation of the 3' end of mRNA transcripts. Base substitutions in this consensus sequence have also been shown to be responsible for certain types of thalassemia as a result of faulty processing and polyadenylation of globin mRNA transcripts. It appears that the AAUAAA is a signal not only for poly(A) addition but also (perhaps more important) for the proper cleavage, before polyadenylation, of the primary RNA transcripts of globin (and other) genes that normally extend well beyond the site of polyadenylation (19–21). The nucleotide immediately preceding the site of poly(A) addition in globin and other mRNAs is almost always C, and GC is the most common, although not invariant, dinucleotide at this site.

Translation of globin (and other eukaryotic) mRNAs starts at the initiator codon ATG, which is generally the first ATG encountered in any reading frame of the mature mRNA. The initiator ATG, like ATG codons elsewhere in the mRNA, encodes the amino acid methionine, which is present at the N-terminal of all nascent polypeptide chains. During the process of peptide chain elongation, the N-terminal methionine is cleaved from nascent globin chains and is thus absent from the full-length chains. The nature of the first two amino acids encoded immediately after the initiator methionine is important in determining whether the N-terminal methionine is cleaved from a nascent peptide chain. Generally, if the second amino acid is also a methionine or is a charged residue or if the third amino acid is a proline, the N-terminal methionine is retained (22). A number of human β-globin chain variants in which such amino acid replacements have occurred at codon positions 2 or 3 have retained the initiator methionine at the N-terminal of the full-length mutant globin chain.

The sequence surrounding the initiator ATG is important for the efficiency of peptide chain initiation. Comparison of the nucleotide sequence of a large number of eukaryotic mRNAs has revealed the presence of a conserved consensus sequence flanking the initiator ATG, the so-called Kozak consensus sequence: CC(**A/G**)CC**ATGG** (23). The most important features of this consensus sequence are the presence of a purine (A or G) at position –3 and the presence of a G at position +4 (where position +1 is the A of the initiator ATG). These positions are indicated in boldface type. The consensus sequence presumably facilitates efficient binding of the mRNA to ribosomes. One form of α-thalassemia is caused by a base substitution changing the purine to a pyrimidine at position –3 of the consensus sequence. Other α-thalassemia and β-thalassemia mutations are due to base substitutions in the ATG itself, resulting in a complete block to normal globin chain initiation (discussed in the sections Molecular Basis of α-Thalassemia and Molecular Basis of β-Thalassemia).

Termination of globin chain synthesis occurs when one of the three possible chain termination codons (UAA, UAG, or UGA) is encountered in the mRNA sequence. Point mutations in the termination codon result in the insertion of a novel amino acid residue at that position and translation of the normally untranslated 3' portion of the mRNA into an abnormally elongated peptide chain until a new in-phase termination codon is encountered. A number of different termination codon mutations are the cause of Hb variants associated with α-thalassemia (discussed in the section Hemoglobin H Disease Due to Interactions with Hemoglobin Constant Spring).

The synthesis of normal globin chains requires that the triplet codons of the mRNA encoding each amino acid of the pep-

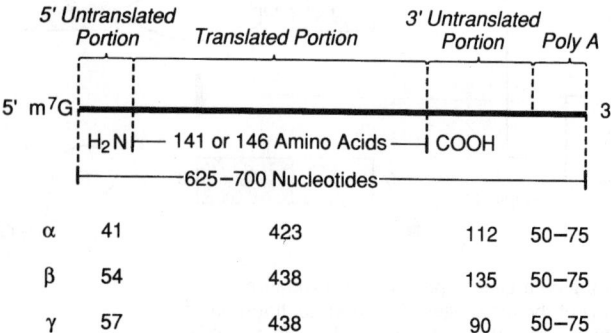

Figure 48-5. Diagram of the relative sizes of translated and untranslated regions of the major human globin messenger RNAs. (From Forget BG. Molecular genetics of human hemoglobin synthesis. *Ann Intern Med* 1979;91:605, with permission.)

tide chain be arrayed in the proper uninterrupted alignment. Nucleotide insertions or deletions other than those in multiples of three will lead to a shift in the reading frame (frameshift) of mRNA translation and the synthesis of a novel peptide sequence until a new in-phase termination codon is encountered, which usually occurs within a relatively short distance. The mutant globin chain thus encoded usually accumulates in markedly reduced amounts because either the mutant globin chain itself or its mRNA is unstable, resulting in a-thalassemia phenotype. A large number of different forms of α-thalassemia and β-thalassemia are the result of such frameshift mutations. Point mutations (nonsense mutations) can also change a normal amino acid codon to a chain termination codon, resulting in the synthesis of a truncated, unstable globin chain and α-thalassemia phenotype. A number of such nonsense mutations have also been documented as causes of α-thalassemia and β-thalassemia (discussed in the sections Molecular Basis of α-Thalassemia and Molecular Basis of β-Thalassemia).

CONSERVED SEQUENCES AND TRANSCRIPTION FACTOR BINDING SITES IN 5' FLANKING DNA OF GLOBIN GENES

The DNA flanking the 5' extremity of the globin genes contains a number of sequences (Fig. 48-6) that are common to all of these genes and are situated at relatively similar distances from the site of initiation of transcription of the genes (cap site) (6–8). The first preserved sequence is ATA, situated approximately 30 nucleotides from the cap site. A second preserved sequence is CCAAT, situated approximately 70 to 80 nucleotides from the cap site. In the case of the human δ-globin gene, there are three CCAAT-like sequences, but none has the perfect canonical sequence; the closest is CCAAC. In the case of both γ-globin genes, the CCAAT sequence is duplicated. A third preserved 5' flanking sequence is slightly more variable in location and is found 80 to 140 nucleotides from the cap site. It has the general structure CACCC or the inverted form GGGTG and is duplicated in the 5' flanking DNA of the β gene. In the case of the δ-globin gene, the proximal CACCC sequence is missing. The abnormalities of CCAAT and CACCC sequences of the δ-globin gene are thought to be responsible in great part for its normally low level of transcription: Correction by site-directed mutagenesis of the CCAAT sequence and insertion of a β-like CACCC sequence

into the promoter confer a high level of expression to the δ gene (24,25).

Site-directed mutagenesis or deletion of these preserved sequences, followed by testing of the modified genes in various cell-free and tissue culture cell systems capable of transcribing cloned genes, have demonstrated the importance of these sequences for the efficiency and accuracy of gene transcription. Their importance for normal globin gene expression is also underscored by the fact that decreased expression of the β-globin genes in certain forms of β-thalassemia has been found to be due to base substitutions in these sequences, specifically in and around the ATA box and the proximal as well as distal CACCC box of the β-globin gene (discussed in the section Molecular Basis of β-Thalassemia).

The promoter sequences described are common to a large number of other nonglobin eukaryotic genes and constitute binding sites for the general transcription apparatus of the cell: RNA polymerase II and its associated accessory transcription factors that are ubiquitously expressed (26,27). In addition, the 5' flanking DNA of the globin genes contains one or more copies of a consensus sequence having the motif (A/T)GATA(A/G), which has been shown to be the binding site of a hematopoietic-specific transcription factor called *GATA-1* (28–35).

GATA-1 sites are also present in globin gene enhancers and locus control regions (LCRs) (discussed in following section). The importance of GATA-1 for gene expression in erythroid cells is underscored by the fact that chimeric mice that developed from male embryonic stem (ES) cells with a disruption of their single X-linked GATA-1 gene failed to produce erythroid cells of the ES cell lineage (36). Normal definitive erythropoiesis was totally absent in hemizygous mice derived from these mutated ES cells, resulting in an embryonic lethal phenotype (37). Using *in vitro* tissue culture systems for hematopoietic differentiation of ES cells, or of yolk sac progenitors of GATA-1⁻ embryos or both, it has been shown that GATA-1⁻ ES cells or erythroid progenitor cells can differentiate to the proerythroblast stage of erythroid cell maturation (38–40), but the cells then fail to differentiate terminally, and they undergo apoptosis (41). The ability of the mutant ES cell line to undergo normal erythroid differentiation *in vitro* was restored after transfer of a functional GATA-1 gene to the cells (38,42,43).

Using various mutants of GATA-1 to rescue erythroid differentiation of GATA-1⁻ ES cells, it was subsequently demonstrated that the N-terminal (non-DNA binding) zinc finger of GATA-1 was essential for the effect, suggesting that it might be the binding site for a second *trans*-acting factor essential for erythroid differentiation. This factor was subsequently isolated and named *Friend of GATA-1* (FOG) (44). Homozygous disruption of the FOG-1 gene leads to an embryonic lethal phenotype very similar to that of the GATA-1 gene disruption, with severe anemia, partial block of terminal erythroid differentiation and, in addition, failure of megakaryocytopoiesis (45). There is also evidence that GATA-1 forms a number of different multimeric protein complexes with other transcription factors—CBP/p300 (46) and erythroid Kruppel-like factor (EKLF) and Sp1 (47,48)—and a pentameric complex with SCL/tal1, Rbtn2/Lmo2, the LIM-binding protein Ldb-1/NL1, and helix-loop-helix proteins such as the E2A proteins, E12 and E47 (49). The pentameric complex binds to a DNA element consisting of one or two GATA sites flanking an E box motif, the general consensus site for basic helix-loop-helix proteins (49,50).

In the γ-globin gene promoters, two GATA-1 binding sites flank the octameric consensus sequence ATTTGCAT for a ubiquitous octamer binding transcription factor (OCT-1) which is

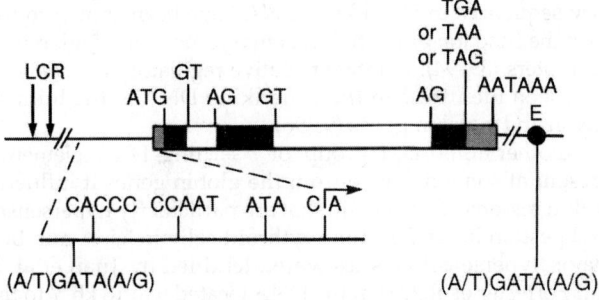

Figure 48-6. Model of the structure of a typical globin gene showing specific sequences and *cis*-acting elements that are important for the regulation of gene expression. The same conventions are used as in Figure 48-3. The following elements and consensus sequences are shown: LCR, locus control region; CACCC, CCAAT, ATA, consensus sequences of the promoter; CA, cap site; ATG, initiator codon; 5' GT . . . AG 3', consensus dinucleotides at exon–intron junctions; TGA, TAA, or TAG, termination codons; AATAAA, polyadenylation signal; E, enhancer element. The bottom line shows the consensus binding sequences for the erythroid-specific factor GATA-1, found within the LCR, promoter, and enhancer.

related to the lymphoid-specific octamer binding transcription factor (OCT-2) that is involved in immunoglobulin gene regulation (26). A base substitution involving one of the GATA-1 consensus sequences of the γ gene promoter is associated with a form of nondeletion hereditary persistence of Hb F (HPFH) (discussed in the section Nondeletion Forms of δβ-Thalassemia and Hereditary Persistence of Fetal Hemoglobin).

Andrews et al. (51) have also characterized a hematopoietic-specific *trans*-acting factor, called *NF-E2*, that binds to the LCR of the β-globin gene cluster and a related sequence in the α cluster called *HS-40* (discussed in the following section). The NF-E2 binding site of the DNase I hypersensitive site 2 (HS2) of the β cluster LCR has been shown to be very important for the functional ability of the LCR to enhance globin gene expression (52–54). The promoter of the gene encoding the heme synthetic enzyme porphobilinogen deaminase also contains a consensus binding site for NF-E2 (55). NF-E2 is a heterodimer consisting of an erythroid/megakaryocytic-specific subunit of 45 kd (p45) and a ubiquitously expressed subunit of 18 kd (p18) (56), both of which are members of the basic region-leucine zipper family of transcription factors. The ubiquitously expressed p18 subunit is a member of the Maf family of transcription factors, and the binding site for the complex is referred to as a *maf-recognition element* (MARE), which is used by proteins related to AP1. Disruption of the p45 gene in mice results in a major defect of megakaryocytopoiesis, but only a minor defect in erythropoiesis resulting in a mild hypochromic anemia (57). One possible explanation for the lack of a more dramatic effect of p45 deficiency on globin gene expression is the finding of other genes encoding p45-related proteins such as LCRF1/Nrf1, Nrf2/ECH, Bach 1, and Bach 2, which may compensate for the absence of p45 NF-E2 gene expression (58–63).

The extended proximal CACCC sequence of the β-globin gene promoter is a binding site for yet another erythroid-specific transcription factor, EKLF (64). This transcription factor is a member of the large family of zinc finger transcription factors that includes the ubiquitous factor Sp1 (20) that is capable of binding CACCC motifs in addition to its more usual G+C rich consensus sequence. EKLF binds preferentially to the β-globin gene promoter compared to its binding activity to other globin gene promoters, and β-thalassemic point mutations of the proximal CACCC/EKLF binding sequence result in markedly decreased binding of EKLF in gel mobility shift assays (65). Disruption of the EKLF gene in mice results in a β-thalassemic phenotype (66,67), but does not cause a generalized defect in erythropoiesis, as does disruption of the GATA-1 gene. Thus, EKLF appears to be a quasi–β-globin gene-specific transcription factor, and it has been referred to by some as a *hemoglobin switching factor* (68). However, although EKLF is necessary for full activity of the β-globin gene, it is not sufficient to cause the γ-globin to β-globin gene switch, because it is present and fully functional in embryonic erythroid tissues before switching occurs (69). Therefore, the γ-globin to β-globin gene switch is regulated by mechanisms other than differential expression or function of EKLF during development. More recently, Asano and Stamatoyannopoulos (70) have identified two other EKLF-like factors, called *FKLF-1* and *FKLF-2*. FKLF-1 is preferentially expressed in fetal erythroid cells and appears to activate selectively the transcription of embryonic and fetal β-like globin genes (71).

Additional transcription factors have been identified that appear to have preferential activity on the expression of one or another globin gene. The –50 region of the γ-globin gene promoter contains a G+C rich region called the *stage selector element*, which fosters preferential activity of the γ gene promoter over the β gene promoter in competitive reporter gene assays (72). A heteromeric protein complex called the *stage selector protein* (SSP) binds to this sequence and contains the ubiquitous transcription factor CP2 (73) as well as an erythroid-specific component that has been called *NF-E4* (74) by analogy to the related factor involved in embryonic to definitive globin gene switching in the chicken (75) (discussed in the sections Ontogeny of Globin Gene Expression and Molecular Mechanisms and Models). Another multimeric protein complex, called the *PYR complex*, containing proteins of the SWI/SNF family of chromatin-modifying factors, binds to a polypyrimidine region 5' to the δ-globin gene and appears to influence the timing of human γ-globin to β-globin gene switching in a transgenic mouse model (76).

ENHANCERS AND OTHER *cis*-ACTING SEQUENCES THAT INFLUENCE GLOBIN GENE EXPRESSION

Enhancer elements are *cis*-acting DNA sequences in the vicinity of a gene that confer to the gene a high level of expression, frequently in a tissue-specific or developmentally specific manner. Originally described in viral genomes, enhancer elements were subsequently discovered in many chromosomal genes, either in 5' or 3' flanking DNA or in introns (77). Typically, enhancers are functional in a position-independent and orientation-independent fashion when tested in various gene transfer–expression systems. The mechanisms of action of enhancers are not completely understood. Enhancers are known to bind various ubiquitous as well as tissue-specific *trans*-acting protein factors with resulting alterations in the configuration of the local chromatin, such as the creation of sites that are hypersensitive to various nucleases—DNase I, for example (78). Such perturbations in the structure or configuration of chromatin are probably associated with activation of transcription of the adjacent gene through various protein–protein interactions (79,80).

A well-defined tissue-specific and developmental stage-specific enhancer element has been identified and characterized in the 3' flanking DNA of the β-globin gene in humans (81–85) as well as other animal species, particularly the chicken. This element confers a high level of gene expression specifically in adult erythroid cells and contains multiple binding sites for the erythroid-specific transcription factor GATA-1 (86). A less well-defined enhancer element has also been identified in the 3' flanking DNA of the human ^{A}γ-globin gene (87). Thus far, no analogous enhancer elements have been identified in proximity to the human α-globin genes, although an enhancer has been found in the 3' flanking DNA of the chicken α-globin gene (88). In contrast to such positive regulatory sequences, which are found adjacent to adult and fetal globin genes, negative regulatory sequences in 5' flanking DNA have been shown to influence the function of the human embryonic ε- and ζ-globin gene promoters (89–94). Putative negative regulatory elements have also been identified in the 5' flanking DNA of the human β-globin and γ-globin genes (95,96).

Another important group of *cis*-acting DNA elements is present at some distance from the globin genes it influences, within regions of chromatin that are particularly hypersensitive to digestion by DNase I in erythroid cell nuclei. A number of major hypersensitive sites were identified by Tuan et al. (97) and Forrester et al. (98) in the DNA located 6 to 18 kb 5' to the ε-globin gene, and an additional site was found in the DNA approximately 20 kb 3' to the β-globin gene. In contrast to hypersensitive sites located in promoter regions of the individual globin genes that are usually present only at developmental stages, when the particular globin gene is expressed, these remote HS sites were found to be present in erythroid cells at all developmental stages. The human β-globin gene locus contains four 5' erythroid-specific, developmentally stable DNase I HS sites (5' HS1, HS2, HS3, and HS4). A fifth site (5' HS5) is not erythroid-specific and is thought to act as an insulator element

(99), as does HS4 in the chicken β-globin gene cluster (100–102). More recently, two additional HS sites (5' HS6 and HS7) have been identified (103).

The presence and sequences of these DNase I HSs at the 5' end of the β gene locus are conserved in all mammalian animal species examined to date, but not in the chicken, in which the 3' β enhancer sequence appears to be the evolutionarily and functionally corresponding sequence.

The functional significance of the 5' HSs of the human β locus in vivo was initially suggested by the fact that naturally occurring deletions of these sites (discussed in the section Deletions Associated with γδβ-Thalassemia) are associated with total silencing of any remaining downstream structurally intact β-like globin genes, and these globin genes remain in a DNase I-resistant chromatin configuration in erythroid cells (104). The smallest deletion with this phenotype (Hispanic γδβ-thalassemia) encompasses 35 kb, including 5' HS2 through HS5.

The suspected functional significance of the DNA encompassing these DNase I hypersensitive sites was then demonstrated by Grosveld et al. (105) and subsequently by other investigators in experiments involving transfer of human globin genes into transgenic mice and mouse erythroleukemia (MEL) cells (106).

When DNA containing the DNase I hypersensitive sequences normally located 5' to the ε gene is linked to a human β-globin gene that is used to produce transgenic mice, the level of expression of the transferred β-globin gene is virtually equivalent, on a per copy basis, to that of the endogenous murine β-globin gene and does not vary significantly with the site of integration of the transgene (i.e., there is a position-independent high level of gene expression) (105). Similar results were also obtained in MEL cells. Previous gene transfer–expression studies in transgenic mice and MEL cells using human β-globin genes without these sequences resulted in low levels of expression of the transferred gene. The expression level on the average was less than 10% of that of the endogenous murine β-globin gene and frequently varied depending on the site of integration of the transferred gene. Because of its functional properties, this region of DNA was initially called the *locus activating region* (107) or the *dominant control region* (108), but was subsequently renamed the *locus control region*, or *LCR* (30).

A similar region (HS-40) has also been identified in the α-globin gene cluster, in the DNA located between 28 kb and 65 kb 5' to the ζ-globin gene, and was found to be essential for obtaining high levels of human α-globin gene expression in transgenic mice (109). Naturally occurring deletions involving this region of DNA were also found to be associated with various forms of α-thalassemia in which the α-globin genes themselves were structurally intact (discussed in the section on α-thalassemia). The critical region was subsequently narrowed down to a 0.35-kb segment of DNA located 40 kb upstream of the ζ-globin gene (HS-40) (110). The α HS-40 and β 5' HS2 share many features, such as conservation of many sequence motifs and the ability to serve as strong enhancers of globin gene expression in transient and stable transfection assays as well as in transgenic mice. However, there are several differences between HS-40 and the β cluster LCR [reviewed by Higgs et al. (111)]: (a) the HS-40 consists of a single element, in contrast to the multiple elements in the β LCR complex; (b) the HS-40 does not confer a copy number-dependent level of expression to transgenes; (c) the level of expression of HS-40/α-globin transgenes is not equivalent to that of the endogenous murine genes; (d) deletion of HS-40 has no effect on long-range chromatin structure in the α-globin gene cluster; and (e) deletion of HS-40 has no effect on the timing of replication of the α gene cluster during the cell cycle.

The conserved sequence motifs in α HS-40, β 5' HS2, and the other β 5' HSs consist of consensus sequences and functional *in vitro* binding sites in gel mobility shift assays for a number of

ubiquitous as well as hematopoietic-specific transcription factors, such as GATA-1, EKLF (and other CACCC binding proteins), Sp1, AP-1, and NF-E2 (112–116). These factor binding sites have been shown by *in vivo* footprinting experiments to be protected or "occupied" in the chromatin of erythroid cell nuclei, strongly suggesting that transcription factors are actually bound to these sites in erythroid cells *in vivo* (117–119). The ubiquitous factor AP-1 and the erythroid-specific factor NF-E2 share a very similar DNA binding consensus sequence; evidence shows that competitive binding of these two factors occurs at a duplicated MARE consensus sequence in HS2 of the β cluster LCR, which is critical for the activity of the β LCR (52–52,122). A duplicated MARE in α HS-40 also serves as a binding site for NF-E2 (110,117) and has been shown to be important for the function of HS-40 (119).

Each of the β LCR HS sequences can individually influence the expression of β-like globin genes in transgenic mice. HS2 and HS3 have a particularly strong positive regulatory effect on globin gene expression. HS2 acts as a strong enhancer in transient transfection assays, and this effect is mediated by a core element that contains a duplicated MARE that serves as a binding site for NF-E2 (120,121). HS3 is particularly effective in rendering surrounding chromatin DNase I sensitive or "open." Although initial experiments suggested some selectivity of different HS sites for regulatory effects on the γ- versus the β-globin gene during development (123), the current consensus is that the entire LCR, with its bound *trans*-acting factors, acts as a holocomplex in mediating its effects on globin gene expression (124–127).

When transgenic mice are generated that carry the β LCR linked to a globin gene, the DNA region containing the transgene becomes DNase I–sensitive in erythroid cells, and the globin gene is expressed at high levels. Thus, the β LCR has long been considered not only to function as a traditional enhancer element but also to possess chromatin opening (or activating) properties. However, recent LCR deletion experiments using homologous recombination in an erythroid cell line as well as in β LCR knockout mice *in vivo* have demonstrated that the negative effect of LCR loss on globin gene expression can occur without the loss of DNase I-sensitive, open chromatin in the β cluster (128). Thus, other regions of the β cluster outside the LCR region may be sufficient for maintaining an open chromatin configuration (129).

The general molecular processes or mechanisms by which the LCRs carry out their effects on globin gene expression from their remote locations are not known. The prevailing opinion is that of the "looping" model in which the LCR holocomplex, including its bound *trans*-acting protein factors, form a loop and interact in a combinatorial manner through protein–protein interactions with the promoter or enhancer regions or both of the target globin genes and their bound transcription factor complexes, thus facilitating high levels of expression of the globin genes in contact with the LCR holocomplex at a particular time in development: the ε-globin and ζ-globin genes in yolk sac–derived erythroid cells, the α-globin and γ-globin genes during fetal development, and the α-globin and β-globin genes in adult erythroid cells (30,34,106). A modification of the looping model is the "linking" model, in which there is a continuous complex of *trans*-acting factors extending from the LCR to the globin gene promoters (134,135). An alternative hypothesis is the "tracking" model, in which RNA transcripts originating from the LCR extend to and include globin gene transcripts and form very long pre-mRNA molecules (137,138).

Ontogeny of Globin Gene Expression

The pattern of human globin gene expression during development is illustrated in Figure 48-7. Two switches in globin gene expression are observed in development (139,140): an embry-

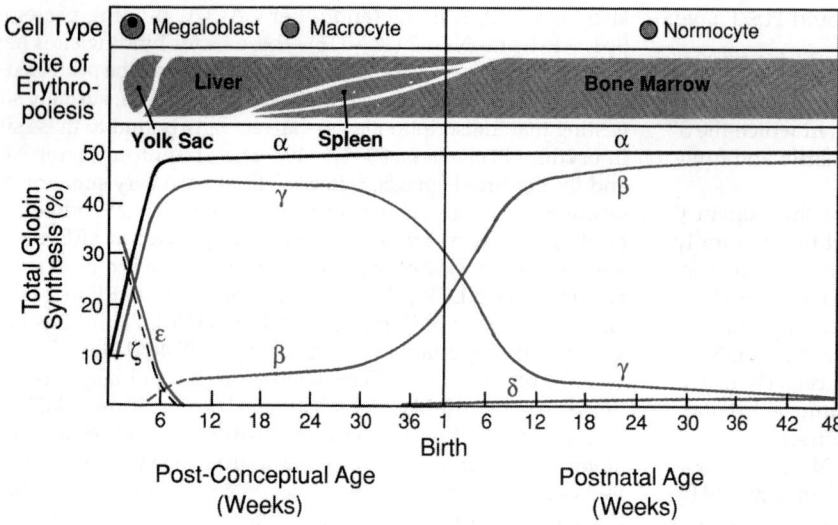

Figure 48-7. Schematic representation of the pattern of synthesis of the different globin chains at various stages of development, showing the sites of erythropoiesis as well as the morphologic features of the red cells at the different developmental stages. (From Weatherall DJ, Clegg JB. *The thalassemia syndromes*, 3rd ed. Oxford: Blackwell Science, 1981, with permission.)

onic to fetal switch, which occurs in the early weeks of gestation, during which α-chain and γ-chain synthesis replaces ζ-chain and ϵ-chain synthesis; and a perinatal fetal to adult switch, during which β-chain synthesis replaces γ synthesis. The α-like globin genes switch only once at the time of the $\zeta \rightarrow \alpha$ switch, whereas the β-like globin genes switch twice: $\epsilon \rightarrow \gamma \rightarrow \beta$. The embryonic to fetal switch coincides with the shift of erythropoiesis from yolk sac to fetal liver and is associated with a dramatic change in the morphology of circulating erythroid cells from nucleated megaloblastic cells to anucleated macrocytic cells. It was long assumed that this embryonic to fetal switch represented the replacement of one population or lineage of erythropoietic stem cells by another. Evidence suggests that a population of yolk sac–derived erythroid cells synthesizes α-chains and γ-chains (141). Therefore, the embryonic to fetal globin gene switch may not be strictly regulated at the level of cell lineage; it is feasible that the definitive lineage of erythroid cells may derive from seeding of the liver by yolk sac–derived hematopoietic stem cells. In the absence of separate stem cell lineages, the basis for the dramatic change in gene expression program and phenotype in fetal versus embryonic erythroid cells remains essentially unexplained.

The mechanism by which erythroid cells switch from the synthesis of Hb F ($\alpha_2\gamma_2$) to that of Hb A ($\alpha_2\beta_2$) during the perinatal period has been the subject of much study and speculation. The issue has generated a great deal of interest because it constitutes an excellent model system for study of the developmental regulation of gene expression and also because of the practical consideration that reactivation, or prevention of suppression, of γ-globin gene expression potentially constitutes a form of gene therapy for serious β-chain hemoglobinopathies such as sickle cell anemia and β-thalassemia. Despite a large body of work on this topic, the precise mechanisms that regulate the normal switch from γ-globin to β-globin gene expression remain essentially unknown.

DEVELOPMENTAL CLOCK

The switch seems to be regulated more by a developmental clock and by gestational age than by intrauterine or extrauterine environmental factors, as evidenced by the fact that prematurity has little effect on the process (142,143,160–162). The apparent developmental programming of fetal versus adult globin gene expression, independent of environmental factors, is also illustrated by a number of transplantation experiments between fetal and adult

donor–recipient pairs in sheep as well as in humans. When fetal liver cells were transplanted into lethally irradiated adult sheep, the pattern of Hb synthesis in reconstituted animals was essentially the same as that observed with fetal liver erythroid cells of a fetal lamb of the same gestational age as the donor; substantial synthesis of Hb F was found, with only slightly more than expected Hb A synthesis for the age of the donor cells (144,145). Analogous results were obtained when human fetal liver (instead of adult bone marrow) was transplanted into children after marrow ablation for therapy of acute leukemia; the pattern of Hb synthesis after engraftment was similar to that expected for the donor cells (146,147).

The reverse experiment was also performed, in which adult bone marrow cells were transplanted into fetal lambs *in utero* at midgestation, a time when they synthesized only Hb F. The transplanted cells were derived from animals that were homozygous for the adult variant Hb B, whereas the recipient animals were homozygous for adult Hb A. Repeated sampling of the blood of the transplanted fetuses revealed the appearance of substantial amounts of β^B-globin chains at a time before the appearance of β^A-globin chains resulting from the fetal to adult switch in the recipient's endogenous erythroid cells (148). Similar results were obtained in analogous midgestational transplantation experiments in mice (149). These results were consistent with the lack of influence of the fetal environment on the pattern of globin gene expression by the transplanted adult erythroid cells.

Together, these various transplantation experiments provide convincing evidence for a predetermined program of γ-globin and β-globin gene expression that is intrinsic to erythroid precursor cells derived from different developmental stages or ages and that cannot be significantly altered by transferring the cells into a different developmental environment.

The intrinsic programming of the β-globin gene cluster during the period of the fetal to adult switch is also illustrated by experiments using hybrid tissue culture cell lines, established by fusion between human fetal erythroid cells and MEL cells, which were selected for retention of human chromosome 11 bearing the human β-globin gene cluster (150). MEL cells express adult mouse globin genes after induction of erythroid differentiation by various chemical agents and are considered to provide an adult erythroid environment for globin gene expression. After induction, the hybrid cell lines initially produced both human γ-globin and β-globin chains, but with a marked predominance of cells expressing γ-globin. The cell lines were maintained in culture for longer periods of time before induction, and the proportion of cells expressing human β-globin progressively increased in a manner similar to the pattern of Hb switching usually observed *in vivo* during the same period of time.

Nevertheless, there is some evidence for plasticity in the developmental program of globin gene expression of hematopoietic stem cells. In a study by Geiger et al. (151), it was shown that stem cells from an adult mouse injected into blastocysts give rise in the resulting mouse embryos to erythroid cell progeny that express embryonic/fetal globin genes. Conversely, it was shown that when embryonic and fetal stem/progenitor cells derived from transgenic mice carrying the human β-globin gene cluster are transplanted into irradiated adult mice, the human adult globin transgene is expressed in the hematopoietic splenic colonies that subsequently develop (151). Thus, it appears that the developmental stage of the marrow microenvironment can regulate the developmental program of globin gene expression in the erythroid progeny of transplanted stem/progenitor cells. The apparent discrepancy between those results and those of the earlier studies described may be related to the higher degree of immaturity or primitiveness (and therefore plasticity) of the stem/progenitor cells used in this more recent study. It is also possible that in order for adult erythroid progenitors to revert to an embryonic/fetal program of globin gene expression, they need to be exposed to the very early embryonic hematopoietic microenvironment, and then, exposure to the midgestational fetal microenvironment alone is not capable of mediating the transition.

CLONAL MODEL

Another issue related to the mechanisms of Hb switching is whether fetal and adult erythroid cells derive from the same family or lineage of erythroid progenitor or stem cells. One hypothetic model (clonal model) for the mechanism of the fetal switch would be the progressive replacement of cells derived from a fetal stem cell or progenitor cell lineage by cells derived from an adult cell lineage. The apparent correlation between the switch in the sites of erythropoiesis from liver and spleen to bone marrow associated with the switch in type of Hb synthesized from Hb F to Hb A initially suggested the possibility of different, organ-specific, erythroid cell populations with different programs of Hb synthesis. However, despite a limited number of studies demonstrating some qualitative differences in functional properties of fetal versus adult erythroid progenitors (152,153), the prevailing model is that a single ancestral lineage of stem/progenitor cells progressively migrates to and colonizes the fetal liver, fetal spleen, and bone marrow.

Throughout fetal development, the ratio of γ-globin to β-globin chain synthesis is the same in erythroid cells isolated from different sites of erythropoiesis, indicating the presence of a common progenitor cell population in the fetal liver, spleen, and bone marrow (154,155). Furthermore, during the perinatal switching period, virtually all of the RBCs contain both Hb F and Hb A in variable amounts, consistent with a gradual and progressive change in the program of globin gene expression in cells derived from a single lineage of progenitor cells. If the switch were due to the differential proliferation or output of two totally distinct progenitor cell pools (one strictly fetal and the other strictly adult), one would expect to find variable admixtures of two different RBC populations during the perinatal switch: one containing exclusively (or predominantly) Hb F and the other containing Hb A. Such a phenomenon is not observed, and the postnatal decline in Hb F synthesis is generally smooth and gradual (142,143). In addition, studies of globin chain synthesis in individual erythroid colonies derived from

neonatal progenitor cells revealed a continuous distribution of γ:β synthesis ratios consistent with a range of globin gene expression programs in different progenitors, rather than a biphasic distribution, as would be expected with two different progenitor cell populations (139).

Additional evidence against the clonal model is provided by the following observations, described in more detail by Stamatoyannopoulos and Grosveld (139): the presence of both embryonic and adult Hbs in single erythrocytes of various animals during the switch from embryonic to definitive erythropoiesis; the presence of both ε and γ or of both γ and β globins in erythroid colonies derived from single progenitors of embryonic, fetal, or adult origin (156–159); and, as described in the section Developmental Clock, the phenomenon of Hb switching in individual clones of MEL X human fetal erythroid cell hybrids (150).

HUMORAL INFLUENCES

Considerable speculation has focused on the possibility that some hormonal or humoral factors may normally regulate Hb switching, but little evidence supports this contention. A number of ablation experiments of endocrine organs in fetal sheep have been performed to study this possibility. In one study, hypophysectomy *in utero* did not affect the time of onset of the fetal to adult Hb switch, but it did result in a moderate slowing of the rate at which switching occurred, concomitant with an overall delay in the development of the animals (155,165). In another study, adrenalectomy *in utero* did not affect the initiation of the switch but was associated with a significant delay in its completion, which could be reversed by replacement therapy with cortisol (166). In humans, a number of observations have suggested the possible influence of humoral or hormonal factors on Hb switching (1,6). These include increased maternal synthesis of Hb F during pregnancy shortly after the time of peak secretion of human chorionic gonadotropin by the placenta; increased Hb F production in patients with human chorionic gonadotropin-producing tumors or with thyrotoxicosis; and an apparent delay in the switch in infants of insulin-dependent diabetic mothers (167,168). It has been suggested that butyrate, a metabolite that is elevated in diabetic mothers and their infants, may mediate this effect. In fact, butyrate has been shown to be capable of increasing the level of expression of embryonic or fetal globin genes in a number of animal and cell culture model systems (169–174), as well as in humans (175,176).

In most circumstances in which there is increased synthesis of Hb F in adults, usually some accelerated production of erythroid cells (erythropoietic stress) is found in association with the presence of substantial amounts of Hb F in some of the circulating erythrocytes. This subpopulation of Hb F–containing cells is referred to as *F cells* (discussed in the section Stress Erythropoiesis and Increased F-Cell Production). The increased production of F cells in the face of erythropoietic stress is usually associated with increased erythropoietin levels, but no evidence exists that the physiologic neonatal fetal to adult switch is induced by changes in the amount or type of erythropoietin produced.

STRESS ERYTHROPOIESIS AND INCREASED F-CELL PRODUCTION

The normal level of Hb F in adults is rarely above 1%, and it is distributed within a subset of only 1% to 7% of the total RBCs called *F cells* (177,178). F cells contain both Hb A and Hb F (in a ratio of approximately 2:1) and have membrane antigens as well as other characteristics of adult rather than fetal erythrocytes. A model for the origin of normal F cells and their increase in conditions of erythropoietic stress has been proposed by

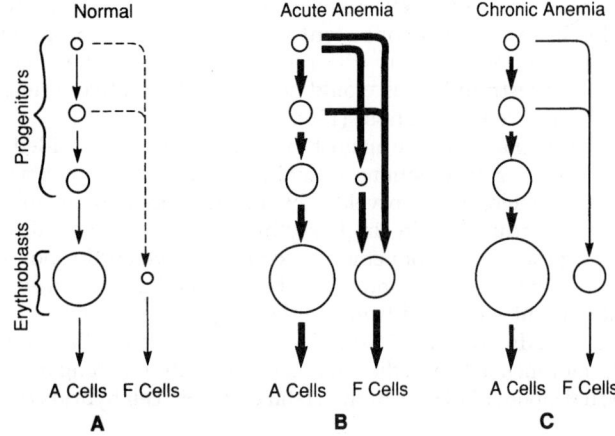

Figure 48-8. Model of F-cell formation **(A)** in a normal situation, **(B)** in acute anemia or sudden erythroid regeneration, and **(C)** in chronic anemia with expanded erythropoiesis. (From Stamatoyannopoulos G, Veith R, Al-Khatti A, et al. Induction of fetal hemoglobin by cell-cycle–specific drugs and recombinant erythropoietin. *Am J Pediatr Hematol Oncol* 1990;12:21, with permission.)

Stamatoyannopoulos and Grosveld (139) and is illustrated in Figure 48-8. Erythroid progenitor cells at the early or burst-forming unit–erythroid (BFU-E) stage of committed erythroid progenitor cell maturation are thought to have the potential to express both Hb F and Hb A. Nevertheless, during the progressive maturation of these progenitor cells from BFU-Es to colony-forming units–erythroid, most of the progenitors lose their potential for γ-globin gene expression, and their progeny become predominantly A cells, with relatively few progenitors giving rise to F cells (which should be more accurately designated *A + F cells*).

A hypothetic corollary of the model shown in Figure 48-8 is that normal F cells may derive directly from BFU-E progenitor cells that short-circuit the normal pathway of maturation through the colony-forming unit–erythroid stage and give rise slightly prematurely to differentiated erythroid cell progeny that manifest the early potential of their immediate progenitors and contain both Hb F and Hb A (Fig. 48-8A). This model is attractive because it reconciles the results of *in vitro* culture experiments and the *in vivo* observations of increased F-cell production in conditions associated with erythropoietic stress. The model proposes that under conditions of erythropoietic stress, the short-circuit pathway of progenitor cell maturation becomes favored and quantitatively more significant, resulting in the production of increased numbers of erythroid cells containing Hb F (Fig. 48-8B and C). This model also potentially explains, at least partially, how the administration of some chemotherapeutic agents such as 5-azacytidine, cytosine arabinoside, and hydroxyurea can result in increased Hb F and F-cell production (139,140) (discussed in the section Gene Therapy and Manipulation of Gene Expression).

MOLECULAR MECHANISMS AND MODELS
Studies of DNA methylation and chromatin structure by nuclease sensitivity have demonstrated that hypomethylation and DNase I hypersensitivity of the 5' flanking DNA of the γ-globin genes are associated with activity of these genes, and that hypermethylation and loss of DNase I hypersensitivity are associated with lack of gene activity (139). These phenomena are probably secondary to other regulatory events that are not well understood.

It was hoped that further insights into the mechanisms of the Hb switch would be provided by elucidation of the molecular

basis of the HPFH syndromes in which Hb F expression persists at a high level and in a pancellular fashion in adult erythroid cells. In the deletion types of HPFH, it was once thought that the basis of the marked increase in γ-globin gene expression might be the loss of regulatory sequences located in the intergene DNA between the ${}^{A}γ$-globin and δ-globin genes, which would be preserved in other deletion syndromes such as δβ-thalassemia, in which Hb F is produced at a lower level and in a heterocellular fashion (179). Comparison of the 5' deletion endpoints in HPFH with those in a large number of δβ-thalassemia syndromes does not allow construction of a comprehensive model for the regulation of γ-globin gene expression by putative control sequences in the intergene DNA between the ${}^{A}γ$-globin and δ-globin genes (discussed in the sections Deletions Associated with δβ-Thalassemia, and Deletions Associated with Hb Kenya and Hereditary Persistence of Fetal Hemoglobin).

In nondeletion forms of HPFH, a number of point mutations have been identified in the promoter region of the affected γ-globin genes (discussed in the section Nondeletion Forms of δβ-Thalassemia and Hereditary Persistence of Fetal Hemoglobin). These mutations are thought to interfere with the normal pattern of binding of various transcriptional regulatory protein factors to the affected γ-gene promoter and thereby prevent the normal postnatal suppression of γ-gene expression. Even though a number of human erythroid-specific *trans*-acting factors have been described (discussed in the section on transcription factor binding sites), their role in the regulation of Hb switching remains to be determined. In particular, the mRNA for the erythroid-specific factor GATA-1 is present in erythroid cells of all developmental stages (29,181,182). Therefore, if GATA-1 plays a role in Hb switching, it is not by its *de novo* appearance or disappearance during development. Nonetheless, subtle quantitative differences in the level of GATA-1 or its posttranslational modification (resulting in activation or inactivation) could play roles in the human Hb switching process. Furthermore, in the mouse, the levels of GATA-1 mRNA in fetal liver erythroid cells are markedly higher than those of yolk sac–derived cells; this finding suggests a role for GATA-1 in the embryonic to definitive Hb switch (183). Differences in levels of various transcription factors, including GATA-1, have also been observed during the embryonic to definitive Hb switch in the chicken (184).

In addition, GATA-1 binding to the γ promoter is essential for the increased promoter activity of one type of nondeletion HPFH with a point mutation at position –175 of the promoter, because mutations that abolish GATA-1 binding to this promoter also abolish its overexpression (28,185).

The erythroid-specific transcription factor EKLF that selectively activates β-globin gene expression was discussed in the section on transcription factor binding sites. Although it has been referred to as a *hemoglobin switching factor* (68) and it is necessary for full activity of the β-globin gene, it is not sufficient to cause the γ-globin to β-globin gene expression switch, because it is present and fully functional in embryonic erythroid tissues before switching occurs.

The most convincing evidence for the role of a *trans*-acting factor in Hb switching is found in the embryonic to adult Hb switch in the chicken, in which the onset of adult β-globin chain synthesis coincides with the appearance of an erythroid-specific *trans*-acting factor (NF-E4) (75). This factor appears to promote, in a looping model, the competitive interaction between the 3' β enhancer and β promoter at the expense of the interaction between the 3' β enhancer and the downstream chicken embryonic ε-globin gene promoter (75,186). The human analog of this factor has been characterized and is called the *SSP*; it binds to the stage selector element of the γ-globin gene promoter (see

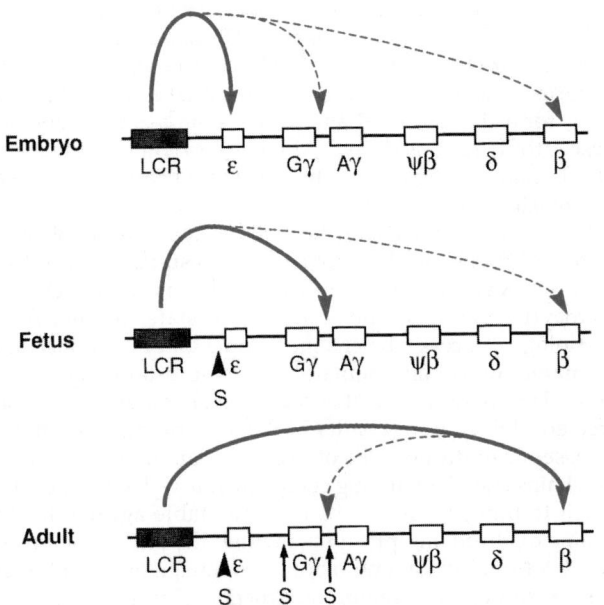

Figure 48-9. Model of the regulation of human globin gene switching. Arrows illustrate the competition between genes for interaction with the locus control region. *S* denotes silencing sequences; the arrowhead indicates a proven silencer, and the thin arrows indicate postulated silencing sequences. LCR, locus control region. (From Stamatoyannopoulos G. Human hemoglobin switching. *Science* 1991;252:383, with permission.)

previous section on transcription factor binding sites) (72,186). SSP is a heteromeric protein complex that contains a ubiquitously expressed transcription factor called *CP2* and an erythroid-specific component that has been called *NF-E4* (72,73). Developmental stage-specific factors that are capable of binding to the γ gene promoters and the ^Aγ gene enhancer element have been identified in fetal erythroid cells of humans and nonhuman primates (187–190).

As discussed in the section Enhancers and Other *cis*-Acting Sequences That Influence Globin Gene Expression, a major advance in the field has been the demonstration of the functional importance of the region of DNA, located 6 to 20 kb 5' to the ε-globin gene, which contains a number of erythroid-specific but developmentally stable DNase I hypersensitive sites and has been called the *LCR*. It has been proposed that the LCR plays a role in Hb switching (30,106,130–140). When linked to an isolated human ε-globin gene, the LCR allows proper developmental control of the gene, which is expressed in yolk sac erythroid cells of transgenic mice but not at later stages (191). On the other hand, when linked to isolated γ-globin or β-globin genes, the LCR appears to disrupt the normal developmental pattern of globin gene expression by conferring activity to the γ genes in adult erythroid cells and to β genes in embryonic erythroid cells of transgenic mice (192–194). However, in another study (195), the LCR γ gene was expressed in a developmentally appropriate manner; this finding suggests that the expression of the γ gene, like that of the ε gene, can be appropriately regulated in the absence of a linked β gene, most likely due to the binding of *trans*-acting factors to silencer elements near the genes (89,190,191,195). When the LCR is linked to larger DNA fragments containing both γ-globin and β-globin genes, or when the entire β gene cluster is used as a transgene, proper developmental regulation is observed (193–197). A looping model has been proposed in which the fetal to adult switch may be associated with differential competition between the β-globin and γ-globin gene promoter or enhancer elements for the influence of the LCR (30,106,130–140,193,194), as

illustrated schematically in Figure 48-9. This is possibly mediated by the presence or absence of developmentally specific *trans*-acting factors.

INTRODUCTION TO THE THALASSEMIAS

Definition

The thalassemia syndromes are a group of hereditary disorders in which a defect in the synthesis of one or more of the globin polypeptide chains of Hb is present (1). This defect causes absent or decreased synthesis of the affected globin chain. As a result, the erythrocytes are characterized by decreased intracellular Hb content (hypochromia) and small size (microcytosis). In addition, the continued normal synthesis of the unaffected globin chain leads to the accumulation of unstable aggregates of these unmatched globin chains. These unstable aggregates precipitate within the erythroid cell, leading to oxidative membrane damage and premature destruction of erythroid cells in the peripheral circulation as well as at earlier stages of maturation in the bone marrow. In α-thalassemia, synthesis of the α-chain of Hb A ($\alpha_2\beta_2$) is impaired, whereas in β-thalassemia, the synthesis of β-chains is reduced or absent.

Prevalence, Geographic Distribution, and Influence of Malaria

Thalassemia affects primarily people of Mediterranean, African, and Asian ancestry. Sporadic cases have been reported in many varied ethnic groups. Malaria is believed to have exerted selective pressure for the increased prevalence of the thalassemia genes in certain populations, although the precise scientific basis for the probable protection of the thalassemia heterozygote against malaria is unknown (2). It has been proposed that in β-thalassemia heterozygotes, the main protection may be against cerebral malaria in the first 1 to 1 $1/2$ years of life because of a slower than normal decline of neonatal Hb F levels and growth retardation of malarial parasites in RBCs containing Hb F (1,198). An alternative explanation proposes that the RBC membrane in heterozygous thalassemia is particularly susceptible to damage by oxidation and that infection with the malaria parasite gives rise to sufficient oxidative stress to perturb intracellular metabolism in a manner that leads to premature death of the parasite (199–201). This latter hypothesis provides a unifying theory for the selective survival of heterozygotes for α-thalassemia as well as β-thalassemia, glucose-6-phosphate dehydrogenase deficiency, and sickle Hb (Hb S).

The prevalence of thalassemia in various populations has been estimated in a number of surveys (1). In Southern Italian, Sicilian, and Greek populations, approximately 10% are heterozygotes for β-thalassemia. In certain Greek islands and some villages of Sardinia, the incidence reaches 20% to 30%. In Southeast Asian populations, the incidence of heterozygous β-thalassemia is approximately 5%, although a higher incidence is encountered in certain regions. In African and American blacks, the percentage of heterozygous β-thalassemia is approximately 1.5%.

The highest incidence of heterozygous α-thalassemia occurs in blacks and Southeast Asians. As discussed in detail in the section Molecular Basis of α-Thalassemia, phenotypically apparent α-thalassemia trait with hypochromic and microcytic RBCs is almost always associated with the deletion or malfunction of two of the four α-globin genes. This condition is referred to as α-*thalassemia-1*. When only one of the four α genes is deleted or dysfunctional, the RBCs are usually phenotypically normal (without apparent hypochromia and microcytosis), and the condition is referred to as α-*thalassemia-2* or the *silent carrier state*. Approximately 3% of blacks have phenotypically apparent α-thalassemia trait (α-thalassemia-1 phenotype); this phenotype results from homozygosity for the α-thalassemia-2 genotype, with the deletion of a single α-globin gene on each chromosome—that is, there is the deletion of two α-globin genes in *trans*.

Thus, to account for the 3% incidence of the α-thalassemia-1 phenotype due to homozygosity for α-thalassemia-2, approximately 25% to 30% of blacks must be heterozygous for the α-thalassemia-2 gene deletion; this fact has been confirmed experimentally (202). The cause of this extraordinarily high gene frequency is poorly understood. It is difficult to explain a selective advantage against malaria when the RBCs in heterozygous α-thalassemia-2 are difficult to distinguish hematologically from normal RBCs.

In Thailand, where the α-thalassemia-1 phenotype is due to the deletion of two α-globin genes on the same chromosome (in *cis*), the prevalence of this form of heterozygous thalassemia is approximately 10%. An additional 10% or so of Thais are heterozygous for α-thalassemia-2. Thus, the combined prevalence of heterozygous α-thalassemia in Thailand is approximately 20%, although in northern Thailand it is higher, approaching 30%. In certain regions of New Guinea, the combined prevalence of heterozygous and homozygous α-thalassemia-2 is greater than 80% (203). In other Southeast Asian populations, the evidence of heterozygous α-thalassemia is approximately 5%. In Mediterranean populations, α-thalassemia is less common than β-thalassemia, with an incidence of approximately 5% in Sardinia and Greece and a slightly higher incidence of approximately 10% in Cyprus.

Pathophysiology of the Anemia

As stated, the primary biochemical abnormality in thalassemia is a quantitative defect in the synthesis or accumulation of one or more of the polypeptide chains of Hb. As a result of the deficient production of the affected globin chain, an overall deficit of Hb A occurs in thalassemic erythrocytes. As a consequence, these cells are microcytic and hypochromic in both the heterozygous and homozygous states.

The imbalance of globin chain synthesis that is characteristic of thalassemia can be directly demonstrated by a technique that consists of incubating peripheral blood reticulocytes for 1 to 2 hours in the presence of a radioactive amino acid precursor, usually leucine, followed by separation of the individual globin chains by column chromatography and quantitation of incorporated radioactivity into the different peaks (1,6). The results are usually expressed as the ratio of β-globin to α-globin chain radioactivity (β:α synthetic ratio), which in normal cells is equal to 1.

When applied to the study of thalassemic reticulocytes, a decrease in β-chain synthesis relative to α-chain synthesis can be demonstrated in β-thalassemia, and a decrease in α-chain synthesis relative to β-chain synthesis can be demonstrated in α-thalassemia. In the usual heterozygotes for β-thalassemia, approximately half as much radioactivity is incorporated into β-chains as into α-chains. In homozygotes for β-thalassemia, either a total absence of β-chain radioactivity (β⁰-thalassemia) or a marked decrease in β-chain radioactivity (β⁺-thalassemia) with β:α ratios of 0.1:0.3 is observed.

When globin chain synthesis is studied in reticulocytes of α-thalassemia heterozygotes, the observed imbalance in globin chain synthesis is less striking than in β-thalassemia heterozygotes. In the phenotypically apparent form of heterozygous α-thalassemia (α-thalassemia-1), the α:β ratio is 0.7 to 0.8, whereas in the mild form of heterozygous α-thalassemia (silent carrier

state or α-thalassemia-2 trait), it is 0.8 to 0.95. In homozygous α-thalassemia-1 (hydrops fetalis with Hb Bart's), there is a total absence of α-chain synthesis. In Hb H disease, which is a less severe α-thalassemia syndrome usually due to double heterozygosity for α-thalassemia-1 and α-thalassemia-2, the globin synthesis profile reveals decreased incorporation of radioactivity into α-chains compared with that into β chains, with an α:β ratio of 0.3 to 0.6.

It is easy to understand how reduced synthesis of one or another of the globin chains of Hb A can result in an overall deficit of Hb A accumulation in RBCs and cause a hypochromic, microcytic anemia. In the homozygous state, another pathophysiologic process worsens the anemia and is responsible for the major clinical and hematologic manifestations of thalassemia. The continued synthesis in normal amounts of the non-affected globin chain results in the accumulation within the thalassemic erythroid cells of excessive amounts of these normal chains (1,6). Not finding complementary globin chains with which to bind, these chains form unstable aggregates that become oxidized and precipitate within the cell. These precipitates lead to physical and oxidative damage of the cell membrane, resulting in premature destruction of erythroid cells.

In β-thalassemia, the resulting α-chain aggregates are called *inclusion bodies* or, perhaps improperly, *Heinz bodies*. In contrast to true Heinz bodies, which are made up of total precipitated Hb ($\alpha_2\beta_2$), the β-thalassemic inclusions consist of only α-globin chains, which have some attached heme in the form of hemichromes. The process of inclusion body formation occurs extensively in the erythroid precursor cells of the marrow and is responsible for the marked ineffective erythropoiesis that characterizes homozygous β-thalassemia.

In α-thalassemia, the resulting β_4 tetramers constitute Hb H, which is more soluble than α-chain aggregates. In the neonatal and fetal periods, γ_4 tetramers are formed and constitute Hb Bart's.

In β-thalassemia, the role of thalassemic inclusions in the pathophysiology of the hemolytic anemia provides an explanation for the genesis of the heterogeneous RBC population found in this disorder. The peripheral blood of patients with homozygous β-thalassemia usually contains increased amounts of Hb F. The Hb F is heterogeneously distributed among such β-thalassemic RBCs, consistent with a relative increase in the normal number of circulating F cells (discussed in the section Ontogeny of Globin Gene Expression). The cells with the most Hb F are those that have the least relative excess of α chains, because the γ chains can combine with α chains to form Hb F. It has been demonstrated in β-thalassemia that Hb A has a more rapid turnover (shorter half-life) than Hb F. This finding is consistent with the presence of at least two different populations of RBCs; those containing mainly Hb A are short-lived, and those containing much more Hb F (F cells) have a longer survival.

Differential centrifugation of RBCs in β-thalassemia reveals that the older, more rapidly sedimenting RBCs contain much Hb F and have relatively few α-chain inclusions, whereas the younger, more slowly sedimenting cells are relatively deficient in Hb F and contain many α-chain inclusions. These results are consistent with selective survival of F cells in homozygous β-thalassemia; this selective survival of F cells, combined with some increase in F-cell production due to stress erythropoiesis, is the major cause of the increased Hb F levels observed in this condition. The severity of the disease in homozygous β-thalassemia correlates well with the size of the free α-chain pool and the degree of α-chain to non–α-chain imbalance. Furthermore, coinheritance of α-thalassemia together with homozygous β-thalassemia reduces the degree of α-globin to non–α-globin chain imbalance and leads to a milder clinical course.

Finally, persons with high Hb F levels and therefore less α-chain/non-α-chain imbalance due to higher α-globin:(β+γ)-globin chain synthetic ratios also generally have a milder clinical course. These findings indicate that a relation exists between α-chain inclusion body formation and processes of peripheral hemolysis and intramedullary ineffective erythropoiesis. They also illustrate the beneficial role of γ-chain synthesis in decreasing the imbalance of globin chain synthesis, decreasing the formation of α-chain inclusions, and thus increasing the effective production of RBCs and prolonging their survival in the circulation.

In homozygous β-thalassemia, the α-chain inclusions are found in large quantities in the maturing bone marrow erythroid precursor cells, a phenomenon that is thought to be the cause of the marked ineffective erythropoiesis or intramedullary destruction of erythroid cells observed in this condition. Before splenectomy, these inclusion bodies are practically never seen in peripheral RBCs, but after splenectomy, they appear in large numbers. This observation correlates well with the demonstrated role of the spleen (and reticuloendothelial system) in removing inclusion bodies of the Heinz body type from RBCs, thereby damaging or destroying these cells.

One cause of RBC injury and destruction in homozygous β-thalassemia may be direct physical trauma due to the presence of the rigid α-chain inclusions and the mechanical injury resulting from the interactions between the abnormal erythroid cells and the reticuloendothelial cells. In addition, other abnormalities of RBC metabolism occur that further damage the erythroid cell membrane and contribute to the premature destruction of the cell (1,204,205). These abnormalities include oxidant damage to the membrane (lipid peroxidation and protein oxidation or cross-linking) resulting from increased superoxide generation and hemichrome formation due to excessive oxidation of the unstable globin chain aggregates. Such oxidant effects may be further enhanced by vitamin E deficiency and iron overload resulting from transfusions. β-Thalassemic RBCs exhibit markedly reduced cellular deformability. Their membranes, to which are associated large amounts of α-globin chains, are characterized by increased rigidity as well as decreased mechanical stability (206). These changes are consistent with damage to the RBC membrane skeleton. In fact, a number of abnormalities of the membrane and membrane skeleton proteins have been identified in β-thalassemic RBCs (206–213), including a specific acquired abnormality in the ability of protein 4.1 molecules to bind normal spectrin (207).

In addition, cross-linking of protein 3 molecules by hemichromes may occur and result in the formation of an external antigenic site for the binding of a specific antibody, which leads to premature destruction of the RBCs in the reticuloendothelial system (205,213).

In the α-thalassemia syndrome of Hb H disease, the resulting β_4 tetramers (Hb H) are more stable than α-chain aggregates and precipitate more slowly. Therefore, one does not observe the marked ineffective erythropoiesis and intramedullary destruction of erythroid precursor cells that is characteristic of homozygous β-thalassemia, although some Hb H inclusions are occasionally seen in marrow normoblasts. The precipitation of β_4 tetramers (Hb H) to form inclusion bodies proceeds more gradually and occurs mainly in mature RBCs rather than in nucleated erythroid precursor cells. The spleen removes these inclusion bodies and thus damages the RBCs, resulting in their premature destruction. Before splenectomy, no preformed Hb H inclusion bodies are seen in the peripheral RBCs, although soluble Hb H is present and can be induced to precipitate in the form of small, stippled inclusions after *in vitro* incubation of the blood with the oxidant compound brilliant cresyl blue. After splenectomy, large, usually single, round preformed inclusion

bodies are seen in the RBCs after staining with supravital stains, by phase and electron microscopy, and occasionally on routine blood smears. The membrane lesion that develops in Hb H disease erythrocytes is different from that observed in homozygous β-thalassemia. The RBCs in both disorders display increased membrane rigidity and viscosity (123). The mechanical stability of the RBC membrane is normal or slightly increased in Hb H disease, whereas it is markedly decreased in homozygous β-thalassemia (208).

Analysis of membrane skeleton protein interactions has also revealed a different defect in Hb H disease compared with that in homozygous β-thalassemia: a qualitative defect in the binding of normal spectrin to inside-out vesicles, suggesting either oxidative damage to the protein ankyrin or interference of spectrin binding to ankyrin due to steric hindrance by Hb H that is bound to the membrane (207).

In addition to the primary pathophysiologic processes operative in thalassemia, a number of secondary abnormalities occur that can worsen the anemia or its consequences on the affected patient. In patients with β-thalassemia intermedia with no transfusion or in patients on low transfusion programs, the anemia may be aggravated by folic acid deficiency. This condition can easily develop because of the high folic acid requirement resulting from the massive marrow erythroid hyperplasia and cellular turnover. Such patients may also experience sudden worsening of their anemia during aplastic crises induced by various bacterial or viral infections, including that caused by parvovirus B19, as also occurs in patients with sickle cell anemia and other chronic hemolytic anemias. The splenomegaly invariably associated with homozygous β-thalassemia also contributes to the anemia either by simply acting as a third space, increasing intravascular volume and causing hemodilution, or by causing true hypersplenic destruction of RBCs. After splenectomy, the liver may act in a similar fashion but less effectively. Finally, because RBCs containing Hb F have a high oxygen affinity, actual tissue hypoxia may exist at Hb levels that would otherwise be adequate to provide proper tissue oxygenation if the Hb were all normal adult Hb A. In fact, thalassemic RBCs appear to adapt poorly to anemia, as reflected by inappropriately low levels of RBC 2,3-diphosphoglycerate (2,3-DPG) and relatively increased oxygen affinity (1).

A schematic outline of the interactions between the various pathophysiologic processes in severe β-thalassemia is illustrated in Figure 48-10. More detailed discussions of the pathophysiologic processes in α-thalassemia and β-thalassemia have recently been published (214,215).

Classification of the Thalassemia Syndromes

The thalassemia syndromes are usually classified according to the type of globin chain that is absent or present in decreased amounts. The clinical types of thalassemia syndromes are listed in Table 48-1. The two major categories are α-thalassemia and β-thalassemia, each of which can be subdivided into a number of different subtypes that may be inherited in the heterozygous state, in the homozygous state, or in various doubly heterozygous states to generate a large number of diverse clinical and hematologic syndromes.

In the α-thalassemia syndromes, heterozygous α-thalassemia can occur in two forms: a phenotypically apparent form, referred to as *α-thalassemia-1*, and a mild defect, with minimal or no hematologic abnormalities, called *α-thalassemia-2* or the *silent carrier state*. The α-thalassemia-1 phenotype can also result from homozygosity for α-thalassemia-2. The heterozygous state for the structurally abnormal hemoglobin Hb Con-

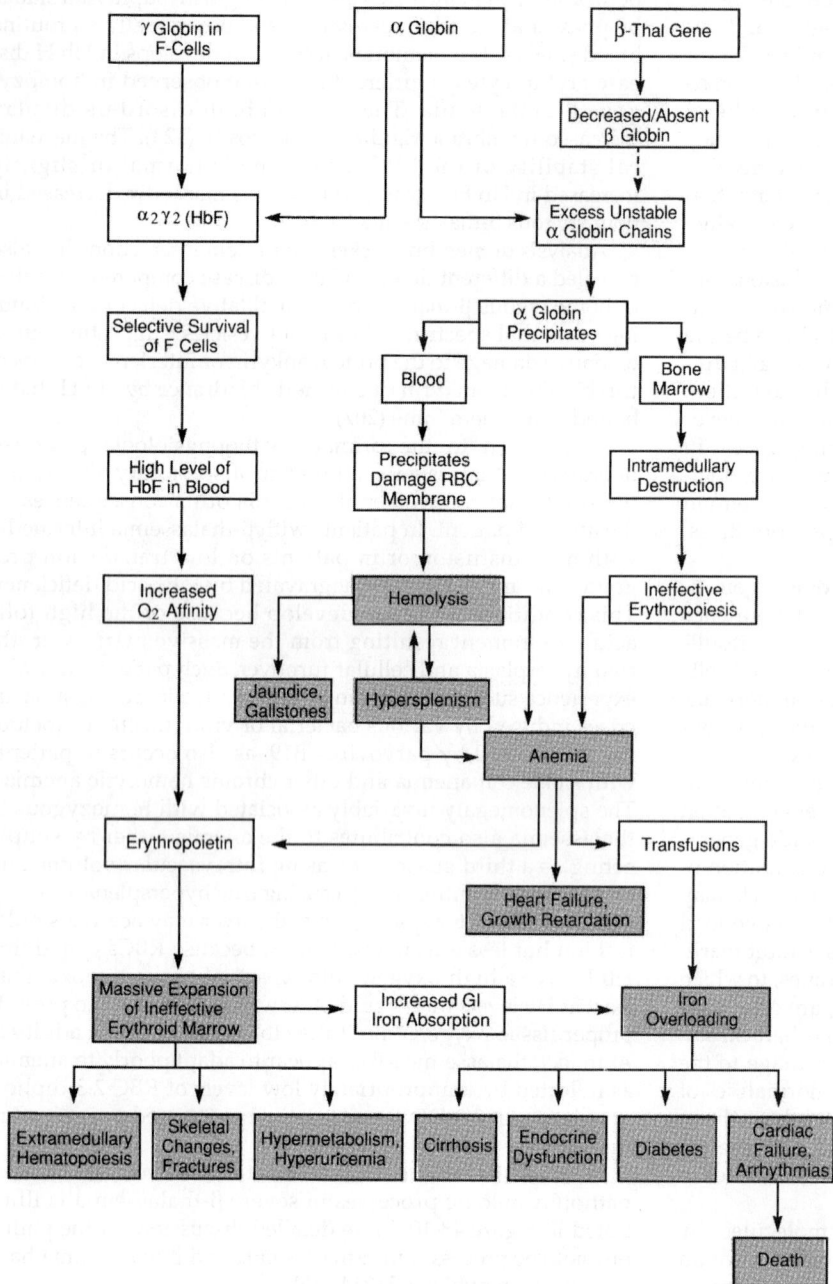

Figure 48-10. Pathophysiology of severe β-thalassemia. The colored boxes indicate clinical consequences. GI, gastrointestinal; HbF, fetal hemoglobin; RBC, red blood cell. (From Weatherall DJ, Clegg JB. *The thalassemia syndromes*, 3rd ed. Oxford: Blackwell Science, 1981, with permission.)

stant Spring is phenotypically similar to α-thalassemia-2, except that small amounts (1% to 2%) of the abnormal Hb are detectable. The homozygous state for α-thalassemia-1 is the syndrome of hydrops fetalis with Hb Bart's. The doubly heterozygous state for α-thalassemia-1 and α-thalassemia-2 (or Hb Constant Spring) results in the less severe syndrome of Hb H disease.

In the β-thalassemia syndromes, the heterozygous state for β-thalassemia (β-thalassemia minor or β-thalassemia trait) is heterogeneous, as indicated by the variations in the amounts of the minor components of Hb present in RBCs of affected persons. The various heterozygous states include (a) β-thalassemia with elevated Hb A_2; (b) δβ-thalassemia or F thalassemia, characterized by normal Hb A_2 but elevated Hb F; (c) β-thalassemia trait with normal levels of Hb F and Hb A_2; and (d) Hb Lepore trait, a condition that is phenotypically similar to heterozygous β-thalassemia but characterized by normal

levels of Hb A_2, the presence of small amounts (10% to 15%) of the structurally abnormal Hb (Hb Lepore), and usually some elevation of Hb F. β-Thalassemia major or Cooley's anemia may result from the combination of any two of these genes.

Occasionally, a person inherits a combination of thalassemic genes that result in a syndrome that is clinically less severe than the typical cases of homozygous β-thalassemia. Typically, such a condition is not associated with a chronic transfusion requirement and is referred to as β-*thalassemia intermedia*. A number of different genotypes can be associated with β-thalassemia intermedia, including a form of unusually severe heterozygous β-thalassemia associated with inclusion body formation (discussed in the section Molecular Basis of β-Thalassemia).

Thalassemia can also be classified according to the nature of the molecular defect. In the sections that follow, the various

TABLE 48-1. Clinical and Hematologic Classification of the Thalassemias and Thalassemia-Like Syndromes

α-Thalassemia syndromes
  Heterozygous α-thalassemia-2 or silent carrier state
  Heterozygous α-thalassemia-1 or α-thalassemia trait
  Hb H disease: double heterozygosity for α-thalassemia-1 and α-thalassemia-2
  Hydrops fetalis with Hb Bart's: homozygous α-thalassemia-1
    Hb Constant Spring syndromes
    α + β-Thalassemia
    Hb S or Hb SS/α-thalassemia
β-Thalassemia syndromes
  Heterozygous β-thalassemia, β-thalassemia trait, or β-thalassemia minor
    With elevated Hb A$_2$, with or without elevated Hb F
    With normal Hb A$_2$ and elevated Hb F: δβ-thalassemia, or F thalassemia
      $^{G}\gamma^{A}\gamma(\delta\beta)^{0}$ Thalassemia
      $^{G}\gamma(^{A}\gamma\delta\beta)^{0}$ Thalassemia
    With normal Hb A$_2$ and Hb F
      Silent carrier, including Hb Knossos
      Concomitant δ + β-thalassemia, in *cis* or in *trans*
      γδβ-Thalassemia
      Other: atypical δβ-thalassemia, concomitant iron deficiency
    Hb Lepore trait
  Homozygous β-thalassemia, Cooley's anemia, or β-thalassemia major
    True homozygosity for one β-thalassemia gene
    Double heterozygosity for any two different β-thalassemia genes
    β-Thalassemia intermedia
Rare forms of thalassemia
  γ-Thalassemia
  δ-Thalassemia
  γδβ-Thalassemia
Interacting thalassemia
  α-Thalassemia + α-chain variant
    Hb Q/α-thalassemia
    Hb G/α-thalassemia
  β-Thalassemia + β-chain variant
    Sickle/β-thalassemia
    Hb C/β-thalassemia
    Hb E/β-thalassemia
Hereditary persistence of fetal hemoglobin
  Pancellular
    $^{G}\gamma^{A}\gamma(\delta\beta)^{0}$ HPFH
    Hb Kenya ($^{G}\gamma$ HPFH)
    Black $^{G}\gamma\beta^{+}$ HPFH with high Hb F
    Greek $^{A}\gamma$ HPFH
    Chinese $^{A}\gamma$ HPFH
  Heterocellular
    Swiss type $^{G}\gamma^{A}\gamma$ HPFH
    British type $^{A}\gamma$ HPFH
    Other: Seattle type $^{G}\gamma^{A}\gamma$ HPFH; Atlanta type—black $^{G}\gamma\beta^{+}$ HPFH with low Hb F; Saudi high Hb F determinant

Hb, hemoglobin; HPFH, hereditary persistence of fetal hemoglobin.

molecular lesions associated with α-thalassemia and β-thalassemia and their related syndromes are discussed.

MOLECULAR PATHOPHYSIOLOGY

Despite having a relatively limited range of clinical, hematologic, and biochemical phenotypes, the thalassemias have been shown to be due to a surprisingly large number of different genetic defects. The reviews of normal gene structure and function presented at the beginning of this chapter and in Chapter 4 illustrate the many steps of gene expression at which a mutation can result in the absent or markedly decreased production or accumulation of a normal gene product such as α-globin or β-globin. The α-thalassemias are generally due to deletions in the α-globin gene cluster, whereas the β-thalassemias are generally due to point mutations in the β-globin gene. Nondeletion forms of α-thalassemia and deletion forms of β-thalassemia have also been identified. In the following sections, we describe

the different genetic lesions that result in α-thalassemia and β-thalassemia.

Molecular Basis of β-Thalassemia

Most mutations that cause β-thalassemia are point mutations in functionally important regions of the β-globin gene. More than 175 different point mutations have thus far been identified as causes of β-thalassemia, although a relatively small number of mutations account for the majority of cases in a given racial group (discussed in the section Prenatal Diagnosis). These point mutations can be classified according to the type or category of defect in gene expression that they cause (Table 48-2). These mutations have been cataloged by Huisman et al. (216), and the updated listing is accessible electronically through the Globin Gene Server Web site (http://globin.cse.psu.edu) (217,218).

PROMOTER MUTATIONS

As discussed at the beginning of this chapter, a number of conserved sequence motifs in the 5' flanking DNA of globin (and other) genes constitute important functional elements of the gene promoter and are therefore important for efficient transcription of the gene. Three of these consensus sequences are found in the promoter regions of all globin genes: the CACCC box, the CCAAT box, and the ATAA (or TATA) box. Mutations in two of these three conserved sequence motifs have been identified in different patients with β-thalassemia—that is, in the CACCC and ATAA boxes. No mutations of the CCAAT box have been identified as causes of β-thalassemia, although mutations in this motif are associated with certain cases of HPFH (discussed in the section Nondeletion Forms of δβ-Thalassemia and Hereditary Persistence of Fetal Hemoglobin).

In general, the degree of diminished β-chain synthesis associated with mutations of the β-globin gene promoter is relatively minor. Patients have β^{+}-thalassemias which, in the homozygous or doubly heterozygous form, are relatively mild and frequently associated with the clinical phenotype of β-thalassemia intermedia. This finding is consistent with studies of transcription of the mutant genes in gene transfer–expression studies in tissue culture cells, which reveal only a mild to moderate decrease in transcriptional activity of these genes (219–222).

As shown in Table 48-2, there are a number of mutations at five different positions of the ATAA box (nucleotides –28 to –32 from the cap site) and at five different positions of the proximal CACCC box (nucleotides –86, –87, –88, and –92 from the cap site). One mutation has been identified at position –101 within a second (distal) CACCC element of the β-globin gene promoter. This mutation is extremely mild and is associated in heterozygotes with the silent carrier phenotype characterized by little or no hypochromia and microcytosis of the RBCs. The ATAA box mutations at position –28 (A → G) and –29 (A → G) are relatively common causes of β-thalassemia in Chinese and black populations, respectively. Although the –29 mutation results in a relatively mild disorder in blacks (220), the same mutation is associated with severe transfusion-dependent thalassemia in a homozygous Chinese patient (223). The cause of this striking difference in phenotype is not known but may be related to different levels of γ-gene expression associated with the different chromosomal backgrounds on which these apparently identical mutations occurred in the two different racial groups (223–225).

As discussed, the cap site or transcription initiation site is part of a conserved sequence motif which, in the case of genes lacking a TATA box, serves as a promoter element (Inr element) (15). It is not known if the Inr element plays a significant role in transcription of the globin genes that do contain a

TABLE 48-2. Mutations Causing β-Thalassemia (Reported through May 1993)[a]

Mutation	Phenotype β⁰ or β⁺	Racial Group	References
Promoter mutations			
ATA box			
−28 (A → G)	+	Chinese	219
−28 (A → C)	+	Kurdish	1486
−29 (A → G)	+	American black, Chinese	220,223
−30 (T → C)	+	Chinese	1487
−30 (T → A)	+	Eastern Mediterranean	1488
−31 (A → G)	+	Japanese	221
−32 (C → A)	+	Taiwanese	1489
CACCC box			
−86 (C → G)	+	Lebanese	224,296
−86 (C → A)	+	Italian	1490
−87 (C → G)	+	Mediterranean	301
−87 (C → T)	+	German, Italian	1491
−87 (C → A)	+	Yugoslavian	1492
		American black	1493
−88 (C → A)	+	Kurdish	1494
−88 (C → T)	+	American black, Asian Indian	222
−90 (C → T)	+	Portuguese	1495
		Ashkenazi Jewish	1496
−92 (C → T)	+	Mediterranean	224,296
−101 (C → T)	+	Italian, Eastern Mediterranean	598
Cap site			
+1 (A → C)	+	Asian Indian	225
Cleavage and polyadenylation mutations			
AATAAA → AACAAA	+	American black	227
AATAAA → AATAAG	+	Kurdish	1494
AATAAA → AATAGA	+	Malaysian	1497
AATAAA → AATGAA	+	Mediterranean	1497
AATAAA → A(−AATAA)	+	Arab	1498
AATAAA → AAAA(−AT)	+	French	1499
Splicing mutations			
Splice site junction mutations			
IVS-1 position 1 (G → A)	0	Mediterranean	301
IVS-1 position 1 (G → T)	0	Asian Indian, Chinese	253
IVS-1 position 2 (T → G)	0	Tunisian	1500
IVS-1 position 2 (T → C)	0	American black	1501
		Algerian	1502
IVS-1 position 2 (T → A)	0	Algerian	1503
IVS-1 5' end (−44 bp)	0	Mediterranean	261
IVS-1 position 130 (G → A)	0	Egyptian	1504
IVS-1 position 130 (G → C)	0	Italian	224,296
		Turkish	1505
		Japanese	1506
IVS-1 3' end (−17 bp)	0	Kuwaiti	261
IVS-1 3' end (−25 bp)	0	Asian Indian	1507
IVS-2 position 1 (G → A)	0	Mediterranean	228
		Tunisian	1500
		American black	1508
		Japanese	1509
IVS-2 position 1 (G → C)	0	Iranian	1510
IVS-2 position 849 (A → G)	0	American black	220,229
IVS-2 position 849 (A → C)	0	American black	1511
IVS-2 position 850 (G → C)	0	Yugoslavian	1512
IVS-2 position 850 (−G)	0	Italian	1513
Consensus sequence mutations			
IVS-1 position −3 (C → T) (codon 29)	?	Lebanese	1514
IVS-1 position −1 (G → C) (codon 30) (Hb Kairoran or Monroe)	+	Tunisian, American black	1500,1515,1516
IVS-1 position −1 (G → A) (codon 30)	?	Bulgarian	1517
IVS-1 position 5 (G → C)	+	Asian Indian	253
		Chinese	230
		Melanesian	1518
IVS-1 position 5 (G → T)	+	Mediterranean	232
		American black	1519
IVS-1 position 5 (G → A)	+	Greek[b]	375,376
		Algerian	1520
IVS-1 position 6 (T → C)	+	Mediterranean	301
IVS-1 position 128 (T → G)	+	Saudi Arabian	1521
		Chinese	1522
IVS-2 positions 4–5 (−AG)	0	Portuguese	1495
IVS-2 position 848 (C → A)	+	Mediterranean, Iranian, Egyptian, American black	376,1521,1523
IVS-2 position 848 (C → G)	+	Japanese	1509
IVS-2 position 844 (C → G)	+	Italian	1524

(continued)

TABLE 48-2. Continued

Mutation	Phenotype β^0 or β^+	Racial Group	References
IVS-2 position 843 (T → G)	+	Algerian	1525
IVS-2 position 837 (T → G)	?	Asian Indian	1526
Mutations creating alternative splice sites			
In introns			
IVS-1 position 110 (G → A)	+	Mediterranean	1527,1528
IVS-1 position 116 (T → G)	0	Mediterranean	238
IVS-2 position 654 (C → T)	0	Chinese	230
IVS-2 position 705 (T → G)	0	Mediterranean	239
IVS-2 position 745 (C → G)	+	Mediterranean	301
In exons			
Codon 19 (A → G) Hb Malay	+	Malaysian	1529
Codon 24 (T → A)	+	American black	239
		Japanese	1530
Codon 26 (G → A) Hb E	+	Southeast Asian	233
Codon 27 (G → T) Hb Knossos	+	Mediterranean	235
Mutations producing nonfunctional messenger RNAs			
Nonsense mutations			
Codon 15 (TGG → TAG)	0	Asian Indian	253
Codon 15 (TGG → TGA)	0	Portuguese	1531
Codon 17 (A → T)	0	Chinese	1532
Codon 22 (G → T)	0	Reunion Islander	296,1499
Codon 26 (G → T)	0	Thai	1533
Codon 35 (C → A)	0	Thai	1534
Codon 37 (G → A)	0	Saudi Arabian	1535
Codon 39 (C → T)	0	Mediterranean, European	1536–1542
Codon 43 (G → T)	0	Chinese	1543
Codon 61 (A → T)	0	American black	1523
Codon 90 (G → T)	0	Japanese	1509,1544
Codon 112 (T → A)	0	Czechoslovakian	1545
Codon 121 (G → T) truncated β-chain variant	(+)	Polish, Swiss, British, Japanese	257,1506,1546,1547
Codon 127 (C → T)	0	English	1548
Frameshift mutations			
Codon 1 (–G)	0	Mediterranean	1549
Codon 5 (–CT)	0	Mediterranean	1550
Codon 6 (–A)	0	Mediterranean, American black	1523,1551,1552
Codon 8 (–AA)	0	Turkish	1538
Codons 8/9 (+G)	0	Asian Indian	253
		Mediterranean	376
Codon 11 (–T)	0	Mexican	1553
Codons 14/15 (+G)	0	Chinese	1554
Codon 15 (–T)	0	Asian Indian, Thai	1499
Codon 16 (–C)	0	Asian Indian	253
Codons 20/21 (+G)	0	Ashkenazi Jewish	1496
Codon 24 (–G, +CAC)	0	Egyptian	1555
Codons 25/26 (+T)	0	Tunisian	1556
Codons 27/28 (+C)	0	Chinese	1557
Codon 35 (–C)	0	Malaysian	1529
Codons 36/37 (–T)	0	Kurdish (Iranian)	1494
Codons 37–39 (–GACCCAG)	0	Turkish	1558
Codons 38/39 (–C)	0	Czechoslovakian	1559
Codon 41 (–C)	0	Thai	1560
Codons 41/42 (–TTCT)	0	Asian Indian	253
		Chinese	254
Codon 44 (–C)	0	Kurdish	1561
Codon 47 (+A)	0	Surinamese black	1562
Codon 54 (+G)	0	Japanese	1544
Codon 64 (–G)	0	Swiss	1563
Codon 71 (+T)	0	Chinese	1564
Codons 71/72 (+A)	0	Chinese	230
Codons 74/75 (–C)	0	Turkish	1565
Codon 76 (–C)	0	Italian	1566
Codons 82/83 (–G)	0	Azerbaijani	1567
		Czechoslovakian	1568
Codon 88 (+T)	0	Asian Indian	1526
Codon 94 (+TG) β Agnana	(+)	Italian	1569
Codon 95 (+A)	0	Thai	1499
Codons 106/107 (+G)	0	American black	225
Codons 109/110 (–G) β Manhattan	(+)	Lithuanian	252
+1 codon 114 (–CT, +G) β Geneva	(+)	French	1570
Codon 123 (–A) β Makabe	(+)	Japanese	1571
Codons 123–125 (–ACCCCACC) β Khon Kaen	0	Thai	1572
Codon 126 (–T) β Vercelli	(+)	Italian	1524
Codons 127/128 (–AGG) β Gunma	(+)	Japanese	1532,1573

(continued)

TABLE 48-2. Continued

Mutation	Phenotype β^0 or β^+	Racial Group	References
Codons 128/129 (–4, +5) (–GCTG, +CCACA) and codons 132–135 (–11) (–AAAGTGGTGGC)	(+)	Irish	1547
Codons 134–137 (–10, +4) (–TGGCTGGTGT, +GCAC)	0	Portuguese	1574
Initiation codon mutations			
ATG → AGG	0	Korean	1499
		Chinese	1575
		Japanese	1576
ATG → ACG	0	Yugoslavian	1577
		Swiss	1578
ATG → GTG	0	Japanese	1579
ATG → ATT	0	White	1580
Other			
5' Untranslated sequence			
+22 G → A	+	Eastern Mediterranean	1581
		Italian	1582
+43 → +40 (–AAAC)	+	Chinese	1583
3' Untranslated sequence			
Cap site + 1570 (T → C)^c	+	Irish	1582,1584
Termination codon +6 (C → G)	+	Greek	1585
Unstable globin chains with thalassemic phenotype due to missense mutations^d			
Codon 28 (Leu → Arg) β Chesterfield	+	English	1586
Codon 60 (Val → Glu)	+	Italian	1587
Codon 106 (Leu → Arg) β Terre Haute, formerly β Indianapolis	+	European	259
Codon 110 (Leu → Pro) β Showa-Yakushiji	+	Japanese	1588
Codon 114 (Leu → Pro) β Durham N.C.	+	Irish	1589
Codon 127 (Gln → Pro) β Houston	+	British	252
Codon 127 (CAG → CGG)	+	French	1491

Hb, hemoglobin; IVS, intervening sequence.
^{a}Additional mutations have subsequently been reported (http://globin.cse.psu.edu) (216,218).
^{b}Combined with 7.2-kb deletion of δ-globin gene (Corfu δβ-thalassemia) (375).
^{c}This base change has subsequently been determined to be a polymorphism linked to the IVS-2 position 654 mutation (1584).
^{d}See also frameshift mutations for additional unstable β chains or variants associated with inclusion bodies, indicated by (+). A number of additional, usually unstable, β-chain variants are also associated with a mild β-thalassemia phenotype (260,1499).

TATA box. Nevertheless, one mutation of the cap site (+1 A → C) has been found to be associated with a mild form of β-thalassemia similar to the silent carrier state (226). It is not known whether this mutation causes β-thalassemia by decreasing β-globin gene transcription or by decreasing the efficiency of capping (posttranscriptional addition of m^{7}G) and mRNA translation.

MUTATIONS CAUSING ABNORMAL POSTTRANSCRIPTIONAL MODIFICATION

As discussed earlier in this chapter, the nascent precursor globin mRNA molecule is modified at both of its ends: A methylated (m^{7}G) cap structure is added at the 5' end, and a poly(A) tail is added at the 3' end of the mRNA. One mutation of the cap site has been described, although it is not known whether the principal effect of the mutation is on transcription or on the capping modification. On the other hand, a number of different β-thalassemias have been associated with defective polyadenylation due to mutations involving the consensus sequence AATAAA required for the cleavage–polyadenylation reaction: four base substitutions at different positions of the consensus sequence and two short deletions (2 and 5 bp; Table 48-2). These mutations markedly decrease the efficiency of the cleavage–polyadenylation process but do not abolish it completely. Therefore, the associated phenotype is that of β$^+$-thalassemia of typical severity, because only approximately 10% of the β mRNA is properly modified. The remainder of the transcripts extend far beyond the normal polyadenylation site and are probably cleaved and polyadenylated after the next AATAAA consensus sequences, which occur approximately 0.9 to 3.0 kb downstream (227). These elongated transcripts are presumably

unstable because they constitute only a minor portion of the β mRNA in affected erythroid cells.

MUTATIONS CAUSING ABNORMAL PRECURSOR MESSENGER RNA SPLICING

The precursor globin mRNA must be processed posttranscriptionally to remove sequences corresponding to the introns of the gene. The complex, multistep process is referred to as *splicing*, and the consensus sequences required for efficient and accurate splicing were discussed at the beginning of this chapter. Defects in splicing can be either complete or partial, resulting in β^0-thalassemia or β$^+$-thalassemia, respectively. These defects are described individually in the sections that follow.

Mutations of the Splice Site Junction That Totally Abolish Normal Splicing. The dinucleotides GT and AG are nearly always present at the 5' (donor) and 3' (acceptor) splice junctions, respectively, forming the boundaries of the intronic sequence. Base substitutions that change one or the other of these invariant dinucleotides, or short deletions that remove them, are associated with total absence of normal pre-mRNA splicing. Therefore, the phenotype is that of β^0-thalassemia. A number of base substitutions or short deletions involving the invariant dinucleotides of the β-globin gene introns have been identified (Table 48-2). In some cases, the mutated intron is totally retained within the mutant mRNA. In other cases, the mutation appears to activate (or facilitate the use of) cryptic splice sites present elsewhere in the intron or, in the case of mutations of the IVS-1 5' splice junctions, in the adjacent exon, resulting in partial splicing of the mutant intron or removal of the intron together with a portion of the 5' flanking exon (220,228–231). The partially or abnormally spliced mRNA species can sometimes be detected in small amounts in affected erythroid cells. They are presumably unstable or poorly transported from nucleus to cytoplasm to account for their low abundance, and they are nonfunctional because translation of the abnormally spliced or frameshifted mRNAs would usually stop prematurely because of the presence of chain termination (nonsense) codons (discussed in the section Mutations That Produce Nonfunctional β-Globin Messenger RNAs).

Mutations of Splice Site Consensus Sequence That Partially Block Normal Splicing. The invariant dinucleotides GT at AG, which are present at the 5' and 3' splice junctions, respectively, are necessary but not sufficient to ensure efficient and accurate splicing. They are normally part of a larger consensus sequence that contains a number of other conserved sequence features, as previously discussed in this chapter. Mutations of certain residues in this consensus sequence result in a partial block of normal mRNA splicing, the severity of which varies with the site of the mutation within the consensus sequence. As a group, these mutations are generally associated with a phenotype of β+-thalassemia. The mutation at position +6 of the IVS-1 5' (donor) consensus sequence is particularly mild and is usually associated with β-thalassemia intermedia because of a relatively high level of normal mRNA splicing. In contrast, three different mutations at position +5 of the same consensus sequence result in a severe form of β-thalassemia with a markedly reduced amount of normally spliced β-globin mRNA. Other positions of the donor consensus sequences affected by mutations include positions –1 and –3 from the GT (Table 48-2). The 3' consensus mutations affect nucleotides at different positions of the polypyrimidine tract upstream from the acceptor AG.

The pattern of splicing that occurs with mutations of the 5' consensus sequence of IVS-1 is complex. Mutations at this site result in the activation or use of three neighboring alternative or cryptic splice sites, two of which are present in adjacent exon 1 and one of which is located downstream in IVS-1 (231,232) (Fig. 48-11). The alternative splice site that is preferentially used over all others is located within exon 1 at codon positions 24 to 27. This cryptic splice site, GTG<u>GT</u>-GAGG, consists of a good, although imperfect, match with the generic or canonical consensus sequence (A/C)AG<u>GT</u>(A/G)AGT. Preferential use of this same alternative or cryptic splice site also occurs in the case of Hb E (233), as well as two other Hb variants with base substitutions in the same region of the β mRNA (234,235), and is presumably responsible for the β-thalassemia phenotype associated with these disorders (discussed in the section Mutations That Create New Alternative Splice Sites in Exons). The resulting abnormally spliced mRNA species have been characterized after gene transfer and expression in tissue culture cells. They are presumably highly unstable *in vivo* because they are not present in easily detectable amounts in erythroid cells of affected patients. Even if these abnormally spliced β-globin mRNAs did accumulate within the cell, the two main species would be nonfunctional because of premature termination due to frameshift (discussed in the section Mutations That Produce Nonfunctional β-Globin Messenger RNAs).

Mutations That Create New Alternative Splice Sites in Introns. A third category of splicing mutation is due to base substitutions in introns that generate new splicing signals preferentially used instead of the normal splice sites. Five such mutations have been identified in the β-globin gene: two in IVS-1 and three in IVS-2 (Table 48-2). The associated phenotype may

be either β+-thalassemia or β0-thalassemia, depending on the site and nature of the mutation.

The first base substitution identified in a β-thalassemia gene was at position 110 of IVS-1. This mutation has subsequently been shown to be the most common form of β-thalassemia in the Mediterranean population. The mutation is a substitution of G to A that creates an acceptor AG in a favorable consensus sequence environment, 19 bp 5' to the normal acceptor AG of IVS-1 (Fig. 48-12A). Gene transfer and expression studies in tissue culture cells have demonstrated that this newly created alternative splice site is preferentially used in 80% to 90% of the transcripts, whereas the normal splice site is used in only 10% to 20% of the transcripts (236,237), thus giving the phenotype of β+-thalassemia (Fig. 48-12B). The mutant mRNA is presumably unstable or poorly transported from nucleus to cytoplasm because it is not detected in significant quantity in affected erythroid cells. Even if it were to accumulate, it would be nonfunctional because the 19-bp segment of retained intronic sequence contains an in-phase termination codon; thus, a truncated β-globin peptide would be synthesized.

Another mutation was later identified in a different Mediterranean family, 6 bp farther 3' in IVS-1 at position 116 (238). This mutation (T → G) also creates a new acceptor AG in a good consensus sequence, but in this case the phenotype is that of β0-thalassemia. The normal acceptor sequence, although intact, is not used, presumably because the new AG occurs at a position that is too proximal to the normal AG and thus totally interferes with its recognition and use as a splice site (238). In a survey of normal acceptor sites, a second AG was virtually never found at positions –5 to –15 from the normal acceptor AG (14); the new AG in the IVS-1 position 116 mutation occurs at positions –13 and –14.

In IVS-2, a mutation at position 654 (C → T) has been identified as a relatively common cause of β0-thalassemia in Chinese persons (230). The mutation creates a new donor GT splice site within IVS-2. Gene transfer and expression studies revealed that IVS-2 sequences of the mutant precursor β mRNA are partially spliced out in two steps: from the normal 5' donor GT to a cryptic acceptor at position 579, then from the mutant donor site at position 654 to the normal 3' acceptor (230). As a result, a 75-bp segment of IVS-2 sequence is retained in the abnormally processed mRNA (Fig. 48-13). It is surprising that although the normal splice sites of IVS-2 are intact and located at a considerable distance from the mutation, no normal splicing is observed. A similar phenomenon occurs in the case of the mutation of IVS-2 at position 705 (T → G). There is an apparent absence of normal splicing, and two-step partial excision of IVS-2 occurs (1) from the normal 5' GT to the naturally occurring cryptic acceptor at position 579 and (2) from the cryptic donor site created by the mutation at position 705 to the normal 3' acceptor AG (239,240).

In contrast, another mutation of IVS-2 at position 745 also creates a new alternative donor splice site and is associated with a similar two-step excision of IVS-2 with use of the cryptic acceptor at position 654 (231). Some normal splicing of IVS-2 does occur (231); therefore, this mutation results in β+-thalassemia rather than β0-thalassemia (231). The β0 versus β+ phenotype associated with these different mutations must be related to different affinities of the enzymatic splicing complex for a given mutant splice site versus the normal splice sites.

Mutations That Create New Alternative Splice Sites in Exons. Four mutations have been identified in exon 1 that are associated with activation of cryptic or alternative splice sites within exon 1 in a manner analogous to the mutations of the normal

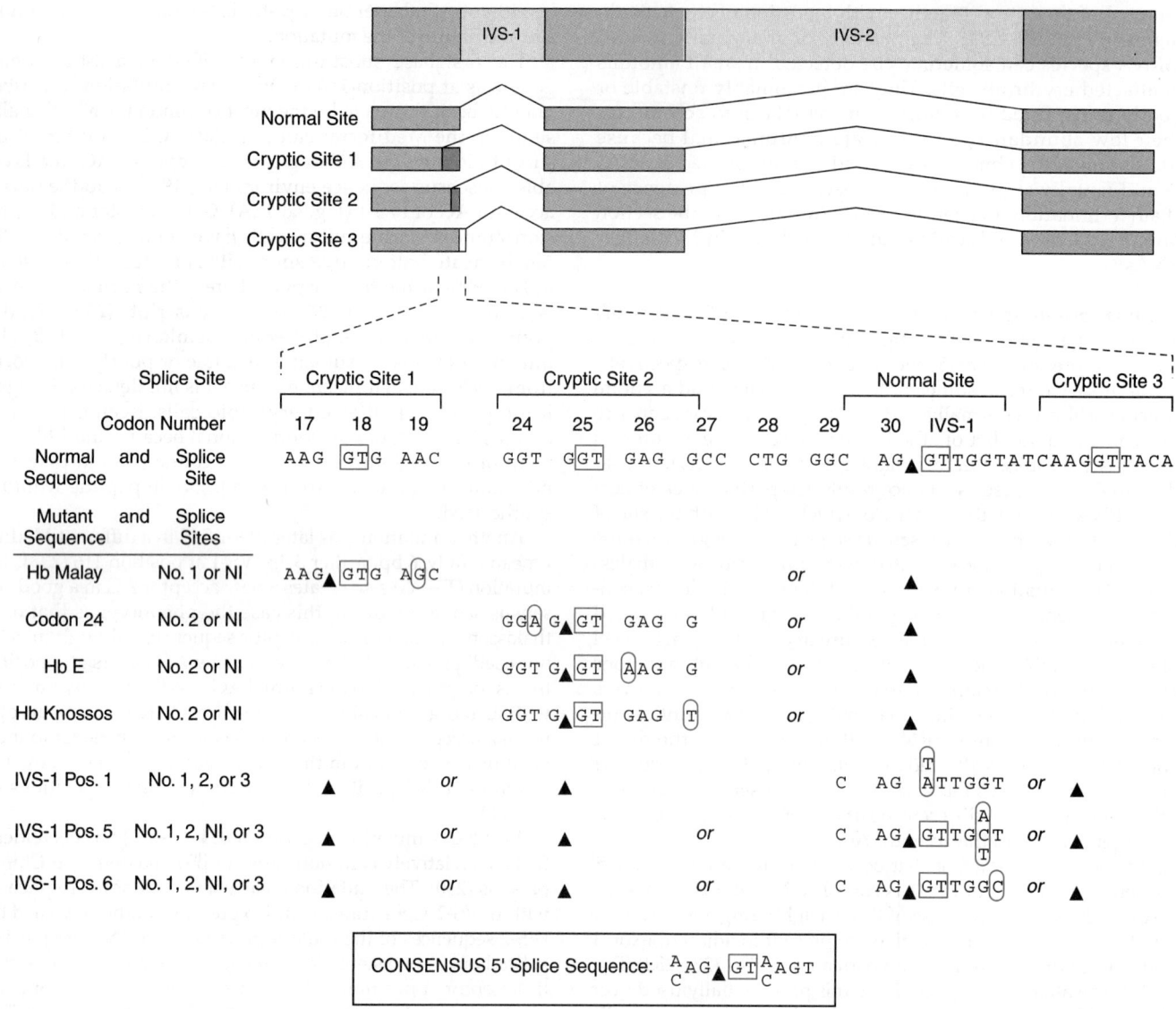

Figure 48-11. Splicing patterns associated with different thalassemic mutations in exon 1 and the first intervening sequence (IVS-1) of the β-globin gene. The normal and abnormal 5' (donor) splice sites are indicated by arrowheads. The GT dinucleotide sequences required for the splicing events are indicated by the boxes. The nucleotide base substitutions resulting from the mutations are indicated by circled bold letters. The cross-hatched boxes indicate the portions of exon 1 that are removed from the processed messenger RNA (mRNA) by alternative splicing; the open box represents the portion of IVS-1 retained in the processed mRNA. Hb, hemoglobin; IVS-2, second intervening sequence.

IVS-1 5' consensus sequence (discussed in the section Mutations of Splice Site Consensus Sequence That Partially Block Normal Splicing). In contrast to the latter group of mutations that activate three cryptic splice sites, the exon mutations activate only the one cryptic splice site that they modify. Three of these mutations are located in codons 24 to 27 (Table 48-2) and activate the cryptic donor site that has a preexisting GT derived from codon 25. The mutations involve the nucleotides at positions –2, +3, and +6 of the consensus sequence (Fig. 48-11). These mutations presumably increase the affinity of the preexisting cryptic splice site for the enzymatic splicing complex so that it is more readily recognized and used. The mutation at codon 24 is silent and does not change the encoded amino acid in the normally spliced β mRNA (234).

The mutations at codon positions 26 and 27 do result in the encoding of amino acid replacements by the normally spliced β mRNA and the synthesis of structurally abnormal variant Hbs:

Hb E (233) and *Hb Knossos* (235), respectively. The phenotype associated with these mutations is that of β⁺-thalassemia, because the normal 5' splice site of IVS-1 is intact and variably used instead of the cryptic site at codon positions 24 to 27. The mutation at codon 24 is associated with a β⁺-thalassemia phenotype of typical severity (234). In contrast, Hb E and Hb Knossos are associated with relatively mild forms of β⁺-thalassemia. In fact, Hb Knossos is usually associated with the silent carrier state for β-thalassemia (241,242). Hb E, which is a common Hb variant in Southeast Asia, was long known to be associated with the phenotype of mild β-thalassemia with hypochromia, microcytosis, and interaction with typical β-thalassemia resulting in a more severe clinical syndrome. The basis for the thalassemic phenotype did not become clear until gene cloning and expression studies (233).

A mutation at codon 19 also results in a Hb variant, *Hb Malay*, which is associated with a mild β⁺-thalassemia pheno-

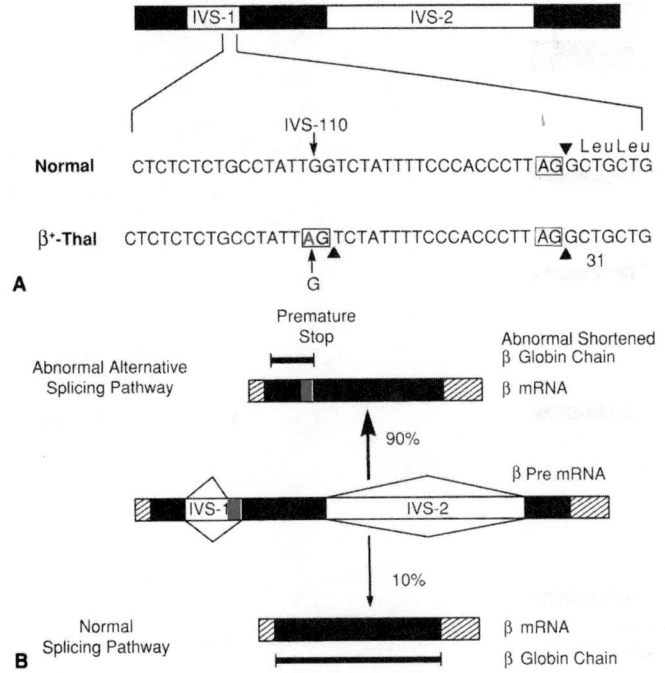

Figure 48-12. Alternative splicing of precursor β-globin messenger RNA (mRNA) resulting in β⁺-thalassemia associated with the mutation at first intervening sequence (IVS-1) position 110. **A:** Diagram of the β-globin gene showing the DNA sequence at the 3' end of IVS-1 and the G to A base substitution at position 110, creating an AG dinucleotide within a potential consensus 3' (acceptor) splice site in the β⁺-thalassemic gene. The arrowheads indicate potential splice sites. **B:** Schematic representation of alternative splicing pathways caused by the mutation. The colored area in IVS-1 indicates the portion of IVS-1 that is abnormally spliced into the β mRNA. IVS-2, second intervening sequence. (From Bunn HF, Forget BG. *Hemoglobin: molecular, genetic and clinical aspects.* Philadelphia: WB Saunders, 1986, with permission.)

type (243). The mutation involves the nucleotide at position +5 of the consensus sequence of a preexisting cryptic donor site at codon positions 17 to 19 of exon 1 (Fig. 48-11). This same cryptic site is also used in the case of mutations of the normal IVS-1 donor consensus sequence (discussed in the section Mutations of Splice Site Consensus Sequence That Partially Block Normal Splicing). Gene expression studies have demonstrated that approximately 25% of the mRNA from the β Malay gene is abnormally spliced at the alternative splice site (244).

MUTATIONS THAT PRODUCE NONFUNCTIONAL β-GLOBIN MESSENGER RNAS

Nonsense Mutations. Nonsense mutations result from single base substitutions that change a codon for a given amino acid to a chain termination codon and cause premature cessation of mRNA translation. Three mRNA chain termination codons are possible: UAA, UAG, and UGA; their corresponding DNA codons are TAA, TAG, and TGA.

Truncated globin chains should be produced as a result of such mutations, but they are not usually detected, presumably because they are unstable and rapidly degraded. The phenotype is that of β⁰-thalassemia, with total absence of normal β-chain synthesis from the affected gene.

One of the first nonsense mutations to be characterized and extensively studied is the mutation at codon 39 (CAG to TAG), which is the second most common cause of β-thalassemia in the

Mediterranean population. An interesting and poorly understood feature of this and other nonsense mutations is the finding of very low levels of the mutant β-globin mRNA in affected erythroid cells. Initial studies of this phenomenon revealed that the gene was transcribed normally, but there appeared to be defective mRNA stability in the nucleus or defective processing, transport, or both of the mRNA from nucleus to cytoplasm; mRNA stability in the cytoplasm appears to be normal (245–248).

Based on a large number of subsequent experimental studies, it now appears that the deficiency of globin mRNA in association with nonsense mutations is due to both posttranscriptional processing and translational mechanisms. The splicing out of intronic sequences from the pre-mRNA apparently marks the mature mRNA in such a manner that if the translational machinery of the cell encounters a nonsense mutation before nucleotides upstream of the last (3'-most) exon–exon splice junction, degradation of the mRNA occurs (249–251). This process, called *nonsense-mediated decay*, may be a mechanism by which the cell protects itself from the potential noxious effects of dominant negative proteins resulting from the translation of abnormal mRNAs. However, when the nonsense mutations occur in the terminal exon of a gene (such as exon 3 of the globin gene), the protective process does not occur, and the abnormal mRNA can accumulate and be translated to produce the abnormal protein (discussed in the section Mutations Resulting in Unstable Globin Chains: Dominant β-Thalassemia).

In addition to the β 39 codon mutation, a number of other nonsense mutations have subsequently been described, ranging in location from codon 15 to codon 127 of the β-globin gene (Table 48-2). In general, the resulting β⁰-thalassemia has a phenotype similar to that associated with the β 39 codon mutation: β⁰-thalassemia with little or no detectable β-globin mRNA. However, the nonsense mutations that occur in exon 3 (β gene codons 112, 121, and 127) are associated with an unusually severe phenotype in the heterozygous state, with hemolytic anemia and, in some cases, the formation of inclusion bodies, so-called *dominant β-thalassemia* (discussed in the section Mutations Resulting in Unstable Globin Chains: Dominant β-Thalassemia) (252). In these cases, there is sufficient accumulation of the abnormal mRNA (due to absence of nonsense-mediated decay) to result in the synthesis of a highly unstable truncated β globin chain responsible for the hemolysis. Nevertheless, some carriers of the β 112, β 121, and β 127 nonsense mutations have the phenotype of typical β-thalassemia trait without hemolysis, perhaps because of enhanced proteolytic capacity of their erythroid cells.

Frameshift Mutations. Frameshift mutations result from the deletion or insertion of one or more nucleotides (other than multiples of three) in the protein-encoding region of the gene. This deletion or insertion causes a change in the normal reading frame of the encoded mRNA at the site of the mutation. Such mutations usually allow the continued translation of the mRNA for some distance, yielding a novel abnormal amino acid sequence until a chain termination codon is encountered in the new reading frame. Chain termination usually occurs at a position well before the normal termination codon and results in the synthesis of a truncated unstable mutant globin chain that is presumably rapidly degraded. The frameshift due to a 4-bp deletion at codon positions 41 and 42 is a particularly common mutation in persons of Chinese and Asian Indian ancestry (253,254). The frameshift due to a single base deletion at codon 44 in Kurdish Jewish persons is associated with an unusually short β-globin mRNA half-life of 30 minutes (255). This marked mRNA instability appears to be restricted to erythroid cells, because the abnormal β-globin mRNA is stable after gene transfer and expression in HeLa cells (256). The basis for the mRNA

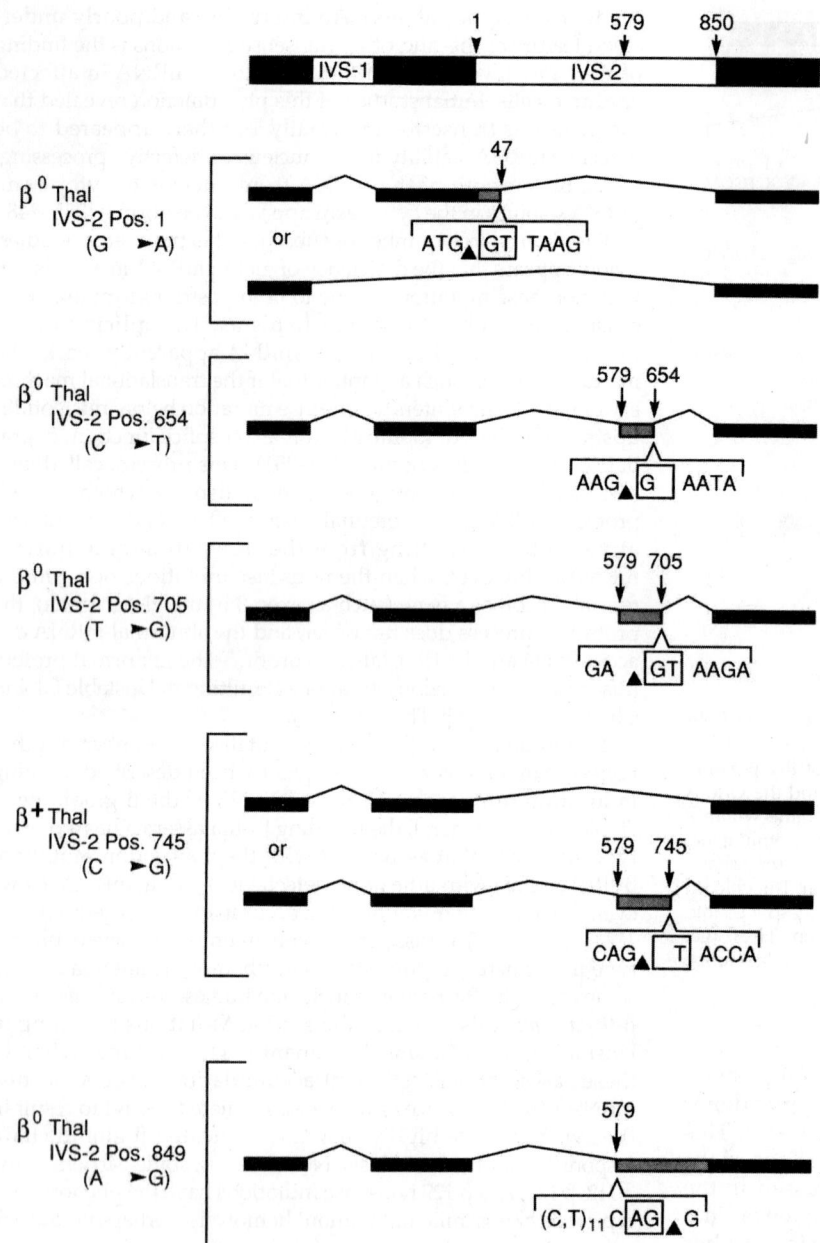

Figure 48-13. Splicing patterns associated with different thalassemic mutations in the second intervening sequence (IVS-2) of the β-globin gene. The nucleotide sequences at the cryptic or alternative splicing sites are indicated, with the same conventions as in Figure 48-11. The same cryptic acceptor site at IVS-2 position 579 is used in many of the mutations. The portions of IVS-2 retained in the processed messenger RNAs are indicated by the gray boxes. (From Bunn HF, Forget BG. *Hemoglobin: molecular, genetic and clinical aspects.* Philadelphia: WB Saunders, 1986, with permission.)

instability is probably the process of nonsense-mediated mRNA decay described in the section Nonsense Mutations. A large number of other frameshift mutations have been identified, some of which are listed in Table 48-2.

Although most frameshift mutations are associated with β⁰-thalassemia, those that occur relatively far into the coding sequence (in exon 3) can result in the synthesis of detectable amounts of mutant β-globin chains and are therefore classified as β(+)-thalassemia (Table 48-2). In such cases, heterozygotes are more severely affected than persons with typical forms of heterozygous β+-thalassemia or β⁰-thalassemia and manifest moderately severe anemia, splenomegaly, and inclusion body formation. The nonsense mutation at codon 121 of exon 3 is also associated with such a phenotype. The striking difference in phenotype between these cases and the more common forms of heterozygous β-thalassemia is probably due to the length and stability of the mutant β-globin chain, together with its ability to bind heme and produce aggregates that are relatively resistant to proteolytic degradation (257,258).

Initiation Codon Mutations. As discussed earlier in this chapter, translation of globin mRNAs begins at the initiation codon AUG (or ATG in DNA), which encodes methionine. The initiator ATG is usually located within a consensus sequence (Kozak consensus) that probably constitutes part of the ribosome binding site of the mRNA (19). A number of different point mutations of the initiator ATG have been identified as causes of β⁰-thalassemia (Table 48-2). It is theoretically possible for the mutant mRNAs to be initiated at the next downstream ATG. In β-globin mRNA, the next ATG occurs in a different reading frame at codon positions 21 and 22, and the abnormal translation product would terminate approximately 40 codons further downstream, giving a short missense peptide unrelated to β-globin. In addition, this ATG is not located within a good Kozak consensus sequence. The only other in-frame ATG in β-globin mRNA is at codon 55, and it is part of a better Kozak consensus sequence. Even if it were used, a nonfunctional and possibly unstable N-terminal truncated globin chain would be produced.

MUTATIONS RESULTING IN UNSTABLE GLOBIN CHAINS: DOMINANT β-THALASSEMIA

Many base substitutions result in amino replacements at residues that are crucial for globin chain stability. The globin chain that is synthesized is so unstable that little or no soluble mutant Hb is detectable. In certain cases, such as in *Hb Terre Haute* (formerly called *Hb Indianapolis*) (259), the phenotype may be similar to that previously described for nonsense and frameshift mutations involving exon 3: so-called dominant β-thalassemia with hypochromia, microcytosis, and hemolytic anemia in heterozygotes, presumably due to membrane damage caused by precipitation and association of the mutant globin chain aggregates with the erythrocyte membrane (258). In other cases, simply hypochromia and microcytosis without inclusion body formation or hemolysis are present, presumably because of more rapid and efficient proteolysis of the mutant globin chain. A number of such mutations have been identified in the β-globin gene (Table 48-2; Chapter 49). A mild degree of hypochromia can also be associated with a number of additional unstable Hbs caused by the progressive loss of intracellular Hb from precipitation and degradation (260). In these cases, the β-globin chain that is initially synthesized is stable and assembled into Hb tetramers that become progressively unstable. Variants of this type are not included in Table 48-2 but are discussed in Chapter 49.

DELETIONS OF THE β-GLOBIN GENE RESULTING IN β⁰-THALASSEMIA

Although most cases of β-thalassemia are due to point mutations, a few cases occur in which the cause is a partial or total deletion of the β-globin gene (Fig. 48-14). These deletions involve only the β-globin gene and its flanking DNA without affecting any of the other neighboring β-like globin genes (261–285). In contrast, δβ-thalassemia and HPFH are associated with deletions, which encompass multiple genes in the cluster (discussed in the sections Deletions Associated with δβ-Thalassemia, Deletions Associated with γδβ-Thalassemia, and Deletions Associated with Hemoblobin Kenya and Hereditary Persistence of Fetal Hemoglobin). The β-thalassemic deletions vary in size between 105 bp and approximately 67 kb, excluding the smaller intragenic dele-

tions of 17, 25, and 44 bp listed in Table 48-2 under splice site junction mutations. The phenotype associated with these deletions is that of β⁰-thalassemia.

The 0.6-kb deletion involving the 3' of the β-globin gene is a relatively common cause of β⁰-thalassemia in Asian Indians and accounts for approximately one-third of cases of β-thalassemia in this population (253,269,272). The other β-gene deletions are relatively rare. Most of these deletions have an interesting phenotype with unusually high levels of Hb A₂ in heterozygotes (263–265,268,275). A common feature of these mutations is the deletion of the promoter region of the β-globin gene. It has been proposed that the unusually high level of Hb A₂ may be due to the lack of competition between δ-globin and β-globin gene promoters for transcription factors, thus allowing more efficient expression of the δ-globin gene (268). In this regard, the β-gene promoter mutation at position –88, and possibly that at position –29, are also associated with unexpectedly high levels of Hb A₂ (286).

UNKNOWN, POSSIBLY DISTANT, MUTATIONS CAUSING β-THALASSEMIA

A small number of β-thalassemic patients carry β-globin genes that are entirely normal in structure. The cause of β-thalassemia in these cases is presumably a more remote mutation either within the β-globin gene cluster (perhaps in the LCR) or in another gene such as one for a specific transcription factor. The first family of this type to be studied was an Albanian family in which two children had β-thalassemia of intermediate severity (β-thalassemia intermedia). The mother had typical β-thalassemia trait, whereas the father apparently had the silent carrier trait (287). One of the cloned β-globin genes from one of the affected children had a normal DNA sequence except for some sequence variation (–T, +ATA) at position –530 from the cap site (288). This region of DNA is characterized by the presence of variable numbers of repeated AT and T residues in different persons that is suggestive of a polymorphism (289–291) (see the following section). Analysis of other β-globin cluster polymorphisms in this family initially indicated that the two affected children had inherited different β-globin gene clusters from

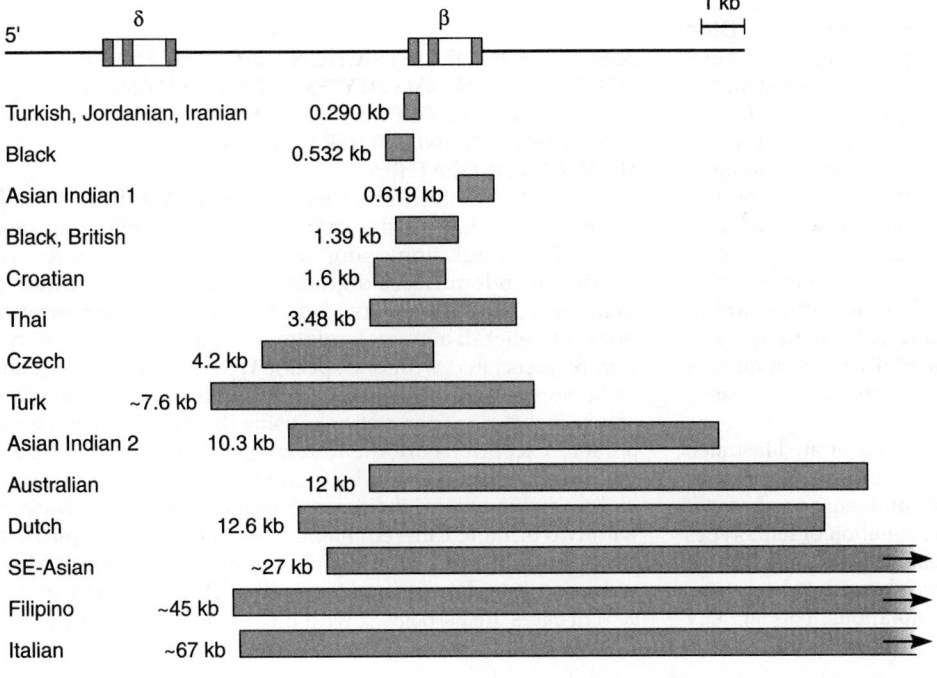

Figure 48-14. Deletions of the β-globin gene and flanking DNA associated with β⁰-thalassemia. (From Forget BG. Molecular mechanisms of β-thalassemia. In: Steinberg MH, Forget BG, Higgs DR, et. al., eds. *Disorders of hemoglobin.* New York: Cambridge University Press, 2001:252, with permission.)

their father. This finding suggests that the β-thalassemia determinant in the father did not reside nearby on chromosome 11 and could even be located on a different chromosome (288).

Subsequent analysis revealed that both of the affected children had inherited the same sequence variation at –530, and the difference in the polymorphisms was attributed to a first-generation crossover between the two paternal alleles (292). It has been proposed that the base changes found in the –530 region of the β gene in this family may be responsible for the β-thalassemia phenotype because of the increased binding of a putative negative regulatory *trans*-acting factor (293). The same changes were also found in three siblings (of a Southern Italian family) who had β-thalassemia intermedia and an otherwise normal β gene (294), further suggesting that the sequence variation point –530 might be functionally significant.

In another Italian family, two brothers with β-thalassemia intermedia also had the complex rearrangement at –530 (with an otherwise normal β-globin gene) in *trans* to the β 39 nonsense mutation (295); one of the affected brothers had a child with β-thalassemia major who inherited the father's β 39 nonsense mutation (without the –530 rearrangement) and a structurally normal β-globin gene from an apparently normal mother.

In a study of 100 β-thalassemia genes, Kazazian et al. (222,296) identified nine persons in whom the β-globin gene had a normal DNA sequence from a point 600 nucleotides 5' to the cap site to a point 200 nucleotides 3' to the end of the gene, as well as a normal DNA sequence of the 400-bp enhancer region located approximately 0.7 kb 3' to the gene. These cases appear to represent truly unknown mutations. Other similar cases have also been reported (215,297).

POLYMORPHISMS OF THE GLOBIN GENE CLUSTERS

In contrast to the DNA of exons that shows little or no sequence variability among individuals, the DNA between genes and that of introns can vary significantly in its nucleotide sequence from one person to another; an estimated 1 of every 200 to 400 nucleotides of extragenic DNA may be different in any two persons. Such sequence variability has proved to be informative in a number of genetic studies because it provides a marker or fingerprint for a person's genome.

Sequence variability is most frequently detected by restriction endonuclease digestion and Southern gel blotting of total cellular DNA, followed by hybridization to a labeled DNA probe from the gene region of interest. The generation of DNA fragments of different sizes in different persons provides evidence for sequence variability in the region of DNA tested; this is called *restriction fragment length polymorphism* (RFLP). A large number of such polymorphisms have been identified in the β-globin gene cluster. They are found in intergene as well as intervening sequence DNA, and one polymorphism is even present in the coding sequence of the β-globin gene, but without causing a change in amino acid sequence. Most of these polymorphisms are common and widely distributed among different racial groups. The location and nature of some of these RFLPs are illustrated in Figure 48-15. These different polymorphisms are not associated with one another in a totally random manner but tend to occur in certain groupings or subsets called *haplotypes* (298–300).

The nine major haplotypes of the β-gene cluster are illustrated in Figure 48-15. Orkin et al. (301) first demonstrated that, in Mediterraneans, different specific β-thalassemia mutations were associated with different haplotypes. The determination of haplotypes by gene mapping therefore provided a relatively simple screening test to identify the most probable mutation in an affected person or to help identify the persons with novel mutations. This strategy was successfully applied to a systematic survey of β-thalassemia

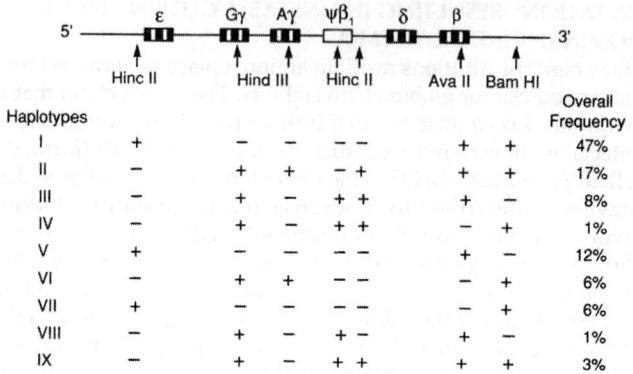

Haplotypes	Hinc II	Hind III	Hind III	Hinc II	Hinc II	Ava II	Bam HI	Overall Frequency
I	+	–	–	–	–	+	+	47%
II	–	+	+	–	+	+	+	17%
III	–	+	–	+	+	+	–	8%
IV	–	+	–	+	+	–	+	1%
V	+	–	–	–	–	+	–	12%
VI	–	+	+	–	–	–	+	6%
VII	+	–	–	–	–	–	+	6%
VIII	–	+	–	+	–	+	–	1%
IX	–	+	–	+	+	+	+	3%

Figure 48-15. Different haplotypes of restriction site polymorphisms in the β gene cluster and their frequency in Mediterranean individuals with β-thalassemia. A plus sign indicates the presence and a minus sign the absence of the particular restriction endonuclease cleavage site. (From Orkin SH, Kazazian HH Jr, Antonarakis SE, et al. Linkage of β-thalassemic mutations and β-globin gene polymorphisms with DNA polymorphisms in the human β-globin gene cluster. *Nature* 1982;296:627, with permission.)

mutations in different population groups such as Asian Indians, Chinese, and American blacks (299,300). Haplotype analysis was also a useful procedure in prenatal diagnosis of β-thalassemia by analysis of DNA from amniocentesis samples or chorionic villus biopsies before the availability of direct DNA-based prenatal diagnosis (discussed in the section Use of Restriction Fragment Length Polymorphisms).

RFLPs have also been identified in the α-globin gene cluster, and a number of different α cluster haplotypes have been defined (302–305). As in the β-globin gene cluster, many of these RFLPs are due to single base changes that abolish or create a restriction endonuclease site. A second type of RFLP is also present that is due to the presence of variable numbers of short, tandemly repeated DNA sequences. Such clusters of variable DNA, called *hypervariable regions*, have been identified at the 3' end of the cluster, within the introns of the ζ and ψζ genes, between the ψζ and ζ genes, and at a site approximately 70 kb 5' of the ζ gene (303). These polymorphisms have proved useful in the study of the population genetics of α-thalassemia mutations.

ASSOCIATION OF RESTRICTION FRAGMENT LENGTH POLYMORPHISM HAPLOTYPES WITH β-THALASSEMIA MUTATIONS AND POPULATION GENETICS OF β-THALASSEMIA AND OTHER β-CHAIN HEMOGLOBINOPATHIES

The prevalence of different haplotypes in Mediterranean β-thalassemic patients is shown in Figure 48-15. Follow-up studies of this population using synthetic oligonucleotides (or restriction endonuclease digestion) for direct identification of thalassemic mutations have led to some interesting observations. In general, a given haplotype within this population is usually associated with one specific type of thalassemia. Thus, by haplotype analysis, one can predict with approximately 90% accuracy the specific mutation causing β-thalassemia in a given person. Exceptions are the following: More than one type of thalassemia mutation can be found within a given haplotype, and a specific type of thalassemia mutation may be associated with two or more different haplotypes in the same population. In haplotype I, which is the most common haplotype in Mediterranean β-thalassemic patients (Fig. 48-15), approximately 90% of cases are associated with the mutation at IVS-1 position 110 (306).

Other β-thalassemia mutations are also associated with haplotype I in Mediterraneans: the frameshift mutation at codon 6, Hb Knossos, and even the β codon 39 nonsense mutation. Thus, it cannot be assumed that all Mediterranean β-thalassemic persons with haplotype I have the IVS-1 position 110 mutation. This result is not totally surprising; multiple different independent mutations might be expected to occur on the same chromosomal background if the background is particularly common in a given normal population, as is haplotype I.

Although a number of examples have been found of the association of a given specific β-thalassemia mutation with more than one different haplotype, the most interesting cases consist of the β-codon 39 nonsense and β^E-globin genes. The β-codon 39 nonsense mutation was shown to be associated with at least nine different chromosomes (307). In seven of these chromosomes, RFLPs within (or close to) the β-globin gene itself were identical. Thus, one could explain the observation of a single mutation in an ancestral β-globin gene that then spread to other chromosomes by recombination, with the crossover site located between the 5' side of the β-globin gene and the 3' side of the polymorphic *HincII* sites around the ψβ1 gene (Fig. 48-15). It has been proposed that this region of DNA contains a hot spot for recombination (298,308).

The β-codon 39 nonsense mutation has also been identified in β-globin genes with different intragenic polymorphic sites or, in the terminology of Orkin and Kazazian (299,300), in different β-globin gene "frameworks." There are three (or four) basic β-globin gene frameworks that differ by two to five intragenic nucleotide base substitutions (305,306). The occurrence of the same mutation in two different β-gene frameworks, especially in two frameworks differing by five nucleotides (one in exon 1 and four in IVS-2), implies that the identical mutation must have arisen spontaneously at least twice, once in each framework.

Alternatively, if one holds to the theory of a single ancestral mutation, the findings can be explained only by a rare localized interchromosomal recombination event called *gene conversion*. Such short discrete recombination or gene conversion events appear to have occurred in the γ-globin genes (in IVS-2) as well as in the histocompatibility and immunoglobulin genes. The Hb E mutation in Asian populations has been identified in two different β-globin gene frameworks, differing by four nucleotides (309). This finding must also be explained by the occurrence of independent identical mutations or short gene conversion events. A similar phenomenon has also been observed with the Hb S mutation.

The comparison of haplotypes and β-thalassemic mutations in different populations has provided the interesting finding that the same haplotype is generally associated with different forms of β-thalassemia in different populations. In fact, a given β-thalassemia mutation generally appears to be restricted to a particular population, because the same mutation is not usually found in two different racial groups. Of the more than 100 mutations listed in Table 48-2, only 11 have been described in more than one racial group (224). In such instances, the chromosomal background (haplotype or β-globin gene framework or both) is almost always different in the separate racial groups, indicating that the mutations most likely had independent origins in the different populations (224).

Molecular Basis of α-Thalassemia

In contrast to β-thalassemia, with most cases due to point mutations, the major cause of α-thalassemia is deletions that remove one or both α-globin genes from the affected chromosome 16. Nevertheless, a number of nondeletion cases of α-thalassemia have been characterized, and these are generally due to types of point mutations similar to those that cause β-thalassemia.

α-Thalassemia was first intensively studied in Asian populations, in which it occurs at a very high incidence. Four main

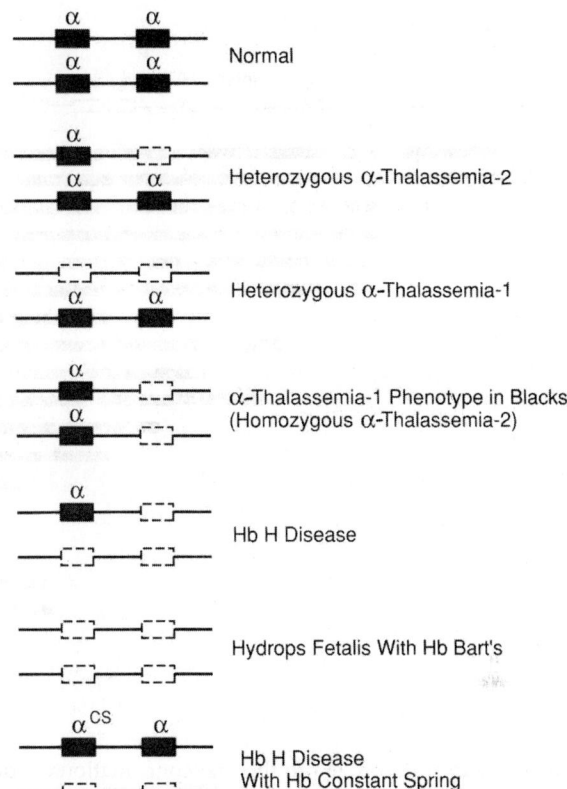

Figure 48-16. Model of α-globin gene deletions as the molecular basis for the various α-thalassemia syndromes. Gene deletions are represented by the dashed blocks. Hb, hemoglobin. (From Bunn HF, Forget BG. *Hemoglobin: molecular, genetic and clinical aspects.* Philadelphia: WB Saunders, 1986, with permission.)

clinical types of α-thalassemia syndromes of progressively increasing severity were defined in this population and were thought to be caused by deletion or inactivating mutation of one, two, three, or four of the α-globin gene loci (Fig. 48-16). The four syndromes were called (a) α-*thalassemia-2* or *silent carrier state* (one inactive α-globin gene); (b) α-*thalassemia-1* (two inactive α-globin genes); (c) *Hb H disease* (three inactive α-globin genes), due to double heterozygosity for α-thalassemia-2 plus α-thalassemia-1; and (d) *hydrops fetalis with Hb Bart's* (four inactive α-globin genes), due to homozygosity for α-thalassemia-1. An additional common type of α-thalassemia syndrome identified in Asians is associated with the inheritance of Hb Constant Spring, a Hb variant with an elongated α-globin chain due to an α-chain termination mutation (discussed in the section Nondeletion Forms of α-Thalassemia), which interacts with α-thalassemia-1 in the same manner as does α-thalassemia-2 to cause Hb H disease. The hematologic and clinical characteristics of these different conditions are discussed later in this chapter.

On the other hand, the results of genetic analyses in blacks with α-thalassemia did not fit the model proposed for the inheritance of α-thalassemia in Asians. Although the incidence of apparent heterozygous α-thalassemia (α-thalassemia-1 phenotype) was high in blacks, hydrops fetalis was never observed, and Hb H disease was rare. It was therefore proposed that the α-thalassemia-1 phenotype in blacks might be associated with the deletion or inactivation of two α-globin genes, but on opposite chromosomes (in *trans*) rather than on the same chromosome (in *cis*), as in Asians (Fig. 48-16).

The availability of molecular hybridization assays, in particular gene quantitation by DNA–complementary DNA hybrid-

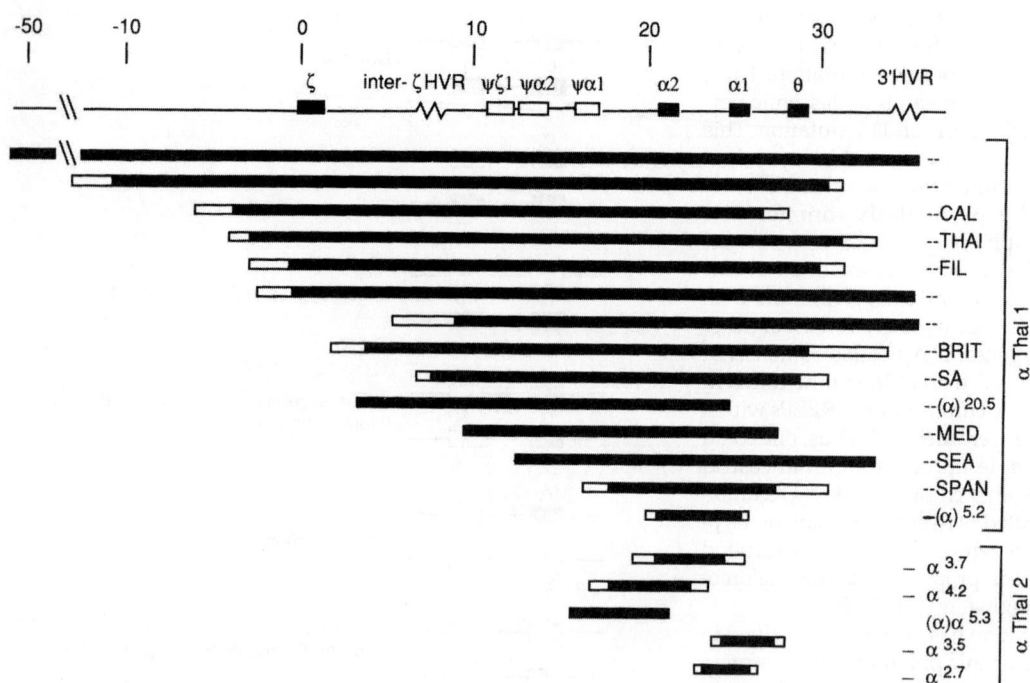

Figure 48-17. Extent of various deletions in the α-globin gene cluster associated with α-thalassemia. Reference citations for the individual mutations can be found in the text and elsewhere (303). Additional deletions have been reported (328). BRIT, British; CAL, Calabrian; FIL, Filipino; HVR, hypervariable region; MED, Mediterranean; SA, South African; SEA, Southeast Asian; SPAN, Spanish. (From Higgs DR, Vickers MA, Wilkie AOM, et al. A review of the molecular genetics of the human α-globin gene cluster. *Blood* 1989;73:1081, with permission.)

ization assays in solution, led to the first confirmation of some of the genetic theories on the molecular basis of α-thalassemia by demonstrating the actual absence or deletion of the predicted number of α-globin genes in the different α-thalassemia syndromes (310). The refinement of gene mapping technology (Southern gel blotting) provided additional confirmation of α-globin gene deletions as a cause of α-thalassemia and permitted the characterization of the location and extent of these deletions within the affected α-globin gene cluster. More than 20 different deletions have been identified in the α-globin gene cluster, most of which are illustrated in Figure 48-17. Most result in deletion or inactivation of both α-globin genes on the same chromosome, whereas some are associated with the deletion of only one α-globin gene per chromosome (303–305).

DELETION OF A SINGLE α-GLOBIN GENE CAUSING α-THALASSEMIA-2, OR α⁺-THALASSEMIA, DESIGNATED –α

The heterozygous state for the deletion of a single α-globin gene or silent carrier state can be easily detected by the technique of Southern gel blotting. Normal DNA with two α-globin genes per haploid genome after digestion with the restriction endonuclease *Bam*HI and hybridization to an α gene probe yields a single band of approximately 14 kb. DNA from persons who are obligate carriers for α-thalassemia-2 yields a second shorter band of approximately 10.5 kb in addition to the normal band.

Detailed restriction endonuclease mapping of the shorter abnormal α-globin gene DNA fragment found in α-thalassemia-2 has established that it contains only one of the two α-globin genes. By using various restriction endonucleases, five different types of (–α) deletions have been defined (224,303–305) (Fig. 48-17):

1. A deletion of approximately 3.7 kb (by far the most common) found in Asians, Mediterraneans, and blacks, consistent with a deletion created by nonhomologous crossing over between two α-globin loci, which has been called the *rightward deletion* and designated –α³·⁷ (311). There are three distinct subtypes of this deletion—designated types I, II, and III—because of the different sites of crossover between the two α loci.

2. A deletion of approximately 4.2 kb, found in Southeast Asians and rarely in blacks, consistent with deletion of the 5' or α2-globin gene, which has been called the *leftward deletion* and designated α⁴·² (311).

3. A rare deletion of approximately 3.5 kb, identified in two Asian Indians, consistent with deletions of the 3' or α1-globin gene and designated –α³·⁵ (312).

4. A rare deletion of approximately 2.7 kb in a Chinese family, designated –α²·⁷ (313).

5. A rare deletion of 5.3 kb in an Italian family, designated (α)α⁵·³ (314).

MECHANISMS OF α-GLOBIN GENE DELETION

Structural analysis of the α-globin gene cluster has revealed the presence of homologous stretches of flanking or intergene DNA sequences, which form α-globin gene duplication units of approximately 4 kb and could serve as foci for nonhomologous crossover or recombination. These homologous duplicated segments are indicated by the boxes labeled X, Y, and Z in Figure 48-18. The two common forms of α-thalassemia-2, –α³·⁷ and –α⁴·², are thought to result from recombination events involving different segments of this duplication unit. Thus, the common rightward –α³·⁷ deletion would result from mispairing and recombination between the duplicated homologous sequences located in segment Z. The leftward –α⁴·² deletion would result from mispairing and recombination between the homologous sequences located in segment X (Fig. 48-18). When recombinant DNA bacteriophages containing the cloned normal human α-globin gene cluster are grown in culture, recombination frequently occurs, generating deletions of a similar nature to those observed in the naturally occurring –α³·⁷- and –α⁴·²-thalassemias. As noted, the –α³·⁷ deletion is itself heterogeneous, and three different forms have been described—designated –α³·⁷ᴵ, –α³·⁷ᴵᴵ, and –α³·⁷ᴵᴵᴵ—because of crossovers occurring at different points within segment Z.

The unequal crossover mechanism described predicts the occurrence in some persons of the reciprocal product of such a recombination event—that is, a chromosome bearing three α-

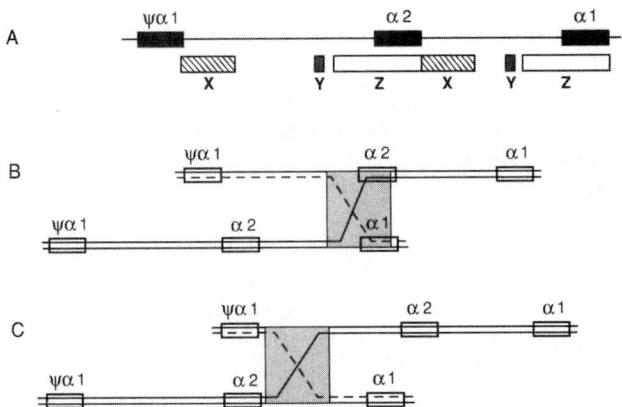

Figure 48-18. Model of unequal crossover events in the α-globin gene cluster resulting in α-thalassemia-2 deletions and reciprocal triple α gene clusters. **A:** The X, Y, and Z homology blocks in the region of the α-globin genes are shown. **B:** Mispairings and crossing over in the Z homology block produce the $-\alpha^{3.7}$ chromosome containing a 3.7-kb deletion (*dashed line*). The reciprocal of this event (*solid line*) is a triple α chromosome. **C:** Mispairing and crossing over in the X homology block produces a single chromosome with a 4.2-kb deletion (*dashed line*). The reciprocal of this event (*solid line*) is also a triple α chromosome. (From Kazazian HH Jr. The thalassemia syndromes: molecular basis and prenatal diagnosis in 1990. *Semin Hematol* 1990;27:209, with permission.)

globin gene loci. Such is the case, and both possible reciprocal chromosomes, $\alpha\alpha\alpha^{anti-3.7}$ and $\alpha\alpha\alpha^{anti-4.2}$, have been found (303–305). Occasional chromosomes with quadruplicated α-globin genes, $\alpha\alpha\alpha\alpha^{anti-3.7}$ and $\alpha\alpha\alpha\alpha^{anti-4.2}$, have also been observed, presumably resulting from subsequent recombination events involving a triplicated locus with a normal locus (303). The frequency of the $\alpha\alpha\alpha$ chromosome is unexpectedly high, ranging from 0.01 to 0.08; it has been found in most populations that have been studied, including those in which α-thalassemia is rare (303).

The possible role of malaria and other selective pressures in causing the high frequency of the $\alpha\alpha\alpha$ chromosome is unknown. Another interesting feature of the $\alpha\alpha\alpha$ locus is that affected homozygotes are hematologically normal even with an excess of α-globin mRNA and α-globin chain synthesis in their erythroid cells (315). The possibility exists that in some circumstances, a mild β-thalassemia phenotype may be conferred by the excess α-globin chain synthesis as a result of the $\alpha\alpha\alpha$ cluster, resulting in a more severe than expected phenotype when one or two $\alpha\alpha\alpha$ chromosomes are coinherited with heterozygous β-thalassemia (315–317).

The two linked α-globin genes are known to be expressed at different levels: The 5' or α2-globin gene is expressed at a level approximately threefold higher than that of the 3' or α1-globin gene (318,319). Therefore, the clinical phenotype of α-thalassemia would be expected to be more severe with deletion or inactivity of the α2 gene. This is generally the case in the nondeletion forms of α-thalassemia (discussed in the section Nondeletion Forms of α-Thalassemia). In deletions causing α-thalassemia-2, the situation is more complex, and compensatory mechanisms appear to modify the expected result. Thus, homozygotes for the leftward deletion, who lack both α2 genes, express more α-globin than the expected 25% of normal, and homozygotes for the rightward deletion, who have two hybrid α2/α1 genes, express less α-globin than the expected 75% of normal (320). Nevertheless, the clinical phenotype associated with homozygosity for the $-\alpha^{4.2}$ deletion is more severe than that associated with homozygosity for the $-\alpha^{3.7}$ deletion (320). It has been estimated that the level of

expression of the $-\alpha^{3.7}$ hybrid gene is intermediate between that of a normal α2 and α1 gene (321), even though the promoter and 5' flanking DNA of the $-\alpha^{3.7}$ gene are those of the α2 gene and would be expected to direct the synthesis or accumulation of more α-globin mRNA than is actually observed. The precise mechanisms responsible for this phenomenon are unknown.

HOMOZYGOSITY FOR α-THALASSEMIA-2 (–α) AS A CAUSE OF THE α-THALASSEMIA-1 PHENOTYPE

When Southern gel blotting was carried out using DNA from blacks with the α-thalassemia-1 phenotype (hematologically apparent α-thalassemia trait), the results were consistent with the genotype –α /–α (202,322). This observation confirmed earlier theories that black persons with the α-thalassemia-1 phenotype were likely to carry deletions of two α-globin genes *in trans*, –α /–α (homozygosity for α-thalassemia-2), rather than *in cis*, – – / αα, as is the case in Asian subjects heterozygous for α-thalassemia-1 (Fig. 48-16; discussed in the following section). These findings, therefore, provided a definitive explanation for the lack of hydrops fetalis and the rarity of Hb H disease in blacks. Because the α-thalassemia chromosome prevalent in the black population almost always carries one normal α-globin gene (–α), it is virtually impossible for blacks to inherit the genotype found in Asian infants with hydrops fetalis, who lack all four globin genes. The rare cases of Hb H disease in blacks result from inheritance of the prevalent α-thalassemic chromosome together with a much rarer α-thalassemic chromosome in which both α-globin genes are deleted or inactive (discussed in the next section).

Another corollary of these findings is that the heterozygous state for α-thalassemia-2 must be extremely prevalent in the black population. If the prevalence of the α-thalassemia-1 phenotype (homozygous α-thalassemia-2) is 1% to 2% in the black population, then heterozygosity for α-thalassemia-2 must approach 30%. In fact, a survey of a large number of black Americans revealed that 27.5% were heterozygous for the α-thalassemia genotype (–α/αα) and 1.9% were homozygous (–α/–α); the overall frequency of the single α-globin locus was calculated to be 0.16 in this population (117).

DELETION CAUSING LACK OF EXPRESSION OF BOTH α-GLOBIN GENES ON ONE CHROMOSOME: α-THALASSEMIA-1 OR α⁰-THALASSEMIA

A large number of different deletions have been characterized that inactivate both α-globin genes on the same chromosome (in *cis*) and result in the phenotype of α-thalassemia-1 in heterozygotes. Most of these deletions completely remove both α genes and are designated as – –; two deletions retain portions of one α-globin gene and are designated $-(\alpha)^{5.2}$ and $-(\alpha)^{20.5}$, respectively, according to the total size of the deletion (303,304,323) (Fig. 48-17). Another interesting set of deletions, designated $(\alpha\alpha)^{RA}$, $(\alpha\alpha)^{MM}$, $(\alpha\alpha)^{TI}$, and $(\alpha\alpha)^{IJ}$ (Fig. 48-19), leave both α-globin genes intact but involve varying amounts of DNA located 5' to the α cluster. In $(\alpha\alpha)^{RA}$, the approximately 62-kb deletion includes the ζ-globin gene and approximately 50 kb of upstream DNA (323,324). In $(\alpha\alpha)^{MM}$, the deletion begins approximately 7 kb 5' to the ζ gene and extends in the 5' for at least 105 kb, without involving the telomere (325). In $(\alpha\alpha)^{TI}$, the deletion begins approximately 30 kb 5' to the gene and extends to and includes the telomere (tip) of the short arm of chromosome 16 (326). In $(\alpha\alpha)^{IJ}$, the deletion involves approximately 35 kb of DNA 5' to the ζ gene, starting at a point 28 kb 5' to the gene (327). The clinical phenotype associated with these unusual deletions is that of α-thalassemia-1, and it is thought that the α-globin genes on the

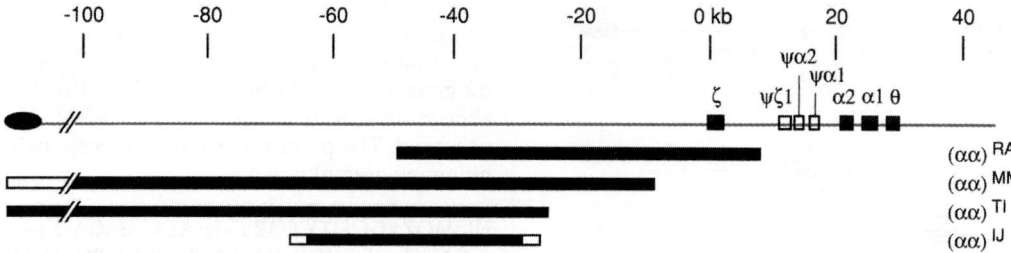

Figure 48-19. α-Thalassemia-1 deletions involving the upstream regulatory sequences of the α-globin gene cluster. The α-globin genes are intact but inactive. The telomere of the short arm of chromosome 16 is indicated by the oval at the far left of the α gene cluster. Additional deletions have been reported (328). (From Higgs DR. α-Thalassemia. *Baillieres Clin Haematol* 1993;6:117, with permission.)

affected chromosomes are totally (or partially) inactive because of the absence in the upstream DNA of an important *cis*-acting element analogous to the β-gene cluster LCR (discussed in the section Enhancers and Other *cis*-Acting Sequences That Influence Globin Gene Expression and the section γδβ-Thalassemia). Functional studies in transgenic mice and in MEL cells after gene transfer, as well as *in vivo* footprinting studies of erythroleukemia cell lines, have confirmed the existence of an LCR-like sequence in the 5' flanking DNA of the α cluster, called *HS-40*, which is deleted in the (αα)-thalassemia syndromes (109–111,117). In addition to the four deletions shown in Figure 48-19, a number of similar deletions associated with the same phenotype have been subsequently identified (328).

The most frequently encountered α-thalassemia-1 mutations are the – –[EA] deletion found in Southeast Asians, the – –[MED] deletion found in Mediterranean persons, and the – –[FIL] deletion found in Filipinos (Fig. 48-17). The – –[FIL] deletion, which accounts for approximately 30% of α-thalassemia genes in Filipinos, involves the entire α-globin gene cluster including the functional ζ-globin gene. Homozygosity for this and other deletions involving the ζ gene would not be expected to allow development of the embryo beyond the earliest stages of pregnancy because of total absence of functional embryonic Hb. In contrast, heterozygotes develop normally. The common – –[SEA] deletion, which reaches a gene frequency of 0.1 to 0.2 in certain regions of Southeast Asia, encompasses the θ-globin gene located 3' to the α1-globin gene. Homozygosity for this deletion clearly allows development beyond the early stages of gestation, and there is at least one child with hydrops fetalis due to this deletion who has survived through treatment with blood transfusions and who has apparently developed normally (329,330). These observations indicate that the presence (or function) of the θ-globin gene is not essential for normal development. Heterozygotes for this and other deletions that preserve the ζ gene express low levels of ζ-globin (less than 1% of total globin) in adult life (331).

The infrequent cases of Hb H disease in blacks are associated with the inheritance of the following α-thalassemia-1 mutations: – –[BRIT] (303,332) (Fig. 48-17), an incompletely characterized deletion involving the entire α cluster (333), an approximately 8.5 kb deletion including the α2-globin, α1-globin, and θ1-globin genes (334) and mutations, including an initiation codon mutation (335), a framework mutation in codon 31 (336), and the Hb Evanston missense mutation (337), affecting the remaining α gene on an $-\alpha^{3.7}$ α-thalassemia-2 allele.

The mechanism that gave rise to most of the α^0-thalassemia deletions is different from that described for the α^+-thalassemia deletions and usually consists of illegitimate recombination events between nonhomologous segments of DNA (323). In the human genome, a number of different types of repetitive DNA sequences exist and are primarily located in the intergene DNA

and sometimes in introns. One of these families of repetitive DNA sequences is called the *Alu*I family because of the usual presence of the recognition site for that particular restriction endonuclease within the repetitive sequence. *Alu*I repetitive sequences are approximately 300 bp in length, occur approximately 300,000 times within the human genome, and share approximately 80% homology with one another (338,339). A number of copies of *Alu*I repetitive sequences are found in both the α-globin and β-globin gene clusters. In some gene systems, recombination between homologous *Alu*I repetitive sequences has resulted in gene deletion events. The $(\alpha\alpha)^{RA}$ α-thalassemia deletion appears to have resulted from such a recombination event between two *Alu*I repetitive sequences located 62 kb apart (323).

In other α^0-thalassemia deletions, *Alu*I repetitive DNA sequences are frequently found at or near one of the breakpoints, but the significance of this finding is unclear. The 3' breakpoints of many of the α-thalassemia deletions tend to cluster in a 6-kb to 8-kb region of DNA between the α-globin gene and a hypervariable region of DNA (3' HVR in Fig. 48-17) located approximately 10 kb downstream. Analysis of polymorphisms (RFLPs) in the 5' flanking DNA of the common – –[MED] and – –[SEA] α^0-thalassemia deletions indicates that these mutations probably arose only once during evolution. Therefore, their high frequency must be attributed to positive selection due to malaria (303).

NONDELETION FORMS OF α-THALASSEMIA

Although rare, a number of different point mutations have been identified as causes of α-thalassemia (Table 48-3). In general, these mutations fall into the same categories or classes of point mutations that have been identified and discussed as causes of β-thalassemia (in the section Molecular Basis of β-Thalassemia): nonfunctional mRNA due to initiation codon mutations, nonsense mutations or frameshifts, splicing defects, polyadenylation signal defects, and unstable globin chains. In fact, nondeletion forms of α-thalassemia provided the first examples of initiator codon (340) and polyadenylation signal (341) mutations. The unstable $\alpha^{\text{Quong Sze}}$ globin chain is the prototypical example of an extremely unstable globin chain associated in heterozygotes with a phenotype of typical thalassemia trait without detectable hemolysis or abnormal globin chains, except as a radioactive product in short (5 to 20 minutes) pulse-labeling experiments (342). One unusual initiator codon mutation involves the adjacent Kozak consensus sequence (deletion of nucleotides –2 and –3) rather than the ATG itself: CCC<u>ACC</u>ATG → CCCCATG (343). This mutation illustrates the importance for proper chain initiation of the nucleotides flanking the ATG, particularly the requirement for a purine (usually A) in position –3 (19).

An especially novel form of nondeletion α-thalassemia consists of the chain termination mutants *Hb Constant Spring*

TABLE 48-3. Nondeletion Forms of α-Thalassemia[a]

Mutation	Racial Group	Affected Gene	References
Cleavage/polyadenylation mutations			
AATAAA → AATAAG	Arab	α2	341,1590
AATAAA → AATGAA	Turkish	α2	1591
Splicing mutation			
IVS-1 donor site, 5-bp deletion	Mediterranean	α2	1592,1593
Mutations producing nonfunctional messenger RNAs			
Nonsense mutation			
Codon 116 (G → T)	Black	α2	1594
Frameshift mutation			
–2 codon 31 (–AG)	Black	$-\alpha^{3.7}$	336
Initiator codon mutations			
ATG → ACG	Mediterranean	α2	340
ATG → GTG	Mediterranean	α1	353
	Black	$-\alpha^{3.7}$	335
CCACCATG → CC—CATG	North African	$-\alpha^{3.7}$	343
	Mediterranean	$-\alpha^{3.7}$	1595
Chain termination mutations			
Hb Constant Spring (TAA → CAA)	Southeast Asian	α2	344,345
Hb Icaria (TAA → AAA)	Mediterranean	α2	346
Hb Koya Dora (TAA → TCA)	Asian Indian	α2	347
Hb Seal Rock (TAA → GAA)	Black	α2	348
Missense mutations producing unstable globins			
Codon 14 (Trp → Arg), Hb Evanston	Black	$-\alpha^{3.7}$	337
Codon 109 (Leu → Arg), Hb Suan Dok	Southeast Asian	α2	1596
Codon 110 (Ala → Asp), Hb Petah Tikvah	Middle Eastern	α	1597
Codon 125 (Leu → Pro) Hb Quong Sze	Southeast Asian	α2	342

Hb, hemoglobin; IVS, intervening sequence.
[a]Additional mutations have been reported (http://globin.cse.psu.edu) (216,328).

(found not uncommonly in Southeast Asians), *Hb Koya Dora*, *Hb Icaria*, and *Hb Seal Rock* (344–348). These mutants are due to four different base substitutions in the normal α-chain termination codon, changing it to a codon for one of four different amino acids and allowing read-through of the 3' untranslated sequence of the α mRNA until a new in-phase termination codon is encountered 31 codons later. The striking feature of these four elongated α-chain variants is that they are present in only very low amounts in RBCs of heterozygotes (1% to 2% of the total Hb)—hence the α-thalassemia phenotype.

The precise molecular basis for the uniformly very low level of expression of these chain termination mutants is not completely understood. However, it is clear that the low level of Hb Constant Spring is not due primarily to instability of the mutant globin chain itself, because biosynthetic studies reveal that the variant globin chain does not have a high specific activity and is therefore not rapidly turning over in reticulocytes or marrow cells. The rate of globin chain elongation, or translation time, was also measured and found to be the same for α^{CS}-globin chains as for normal α^{A}-globin chains. The mutant α-globin chain is synthesized almost exclusively in bone marrow erythroid cells rather than in peripheral blood, and α^{CS}-globin mRNA is virtually absent in reticulocyte mRNA of affected persons, suggesting the possibility of instability of α^{CS} mRNA as a basis for the low level of synthesis of the mutant globin chain (319,349). It has been demonstrated that read-through of the α mRNA results in disruption of an RNA/protein complex within the usually untranslated (3' UTR) region of the mRNA, a complex that is normally required for increased stability of the α mRNA (350–352).

Most of the nondeletion α-thalassemia mutations affect the more strongly expressed α2-globin gene. In contrast to the $-\alpha^{4.2}$ deletion of the α2 gene, no compensatory increase occurs in the expression of the linked α1 gene. Therefore, the clinical pheno-

type associated with these nondeletion mutants is more severe than that of the common –α determinants and more closely resembles that of α-thalassemia-1 than α-thalassemia-2. The initiator codon mutation that affects the α1-globin gene is associated with a mild clinical phenotype (353).

ACQUIRED α-THALASSEMIA

Two distinct α-thalassemia syndromes are due to acquired or *de novo* mutations of the α-globin genes: Hb H disease associated with myeloproliferative or myelodysplastic disorders, and Hb H disease associated with mental retardation.

Acquired Hemoglobin H Disease Associated with Myeloproliferative Disorders.
Hb H disease has occasionally been observed to develop during the course of erythroleukemia or other myeloproliferative disorders, including preleukemic syndromes, such as myelofibrosis and refractory anemia, which eventually progress to acute nonlymphocytic leukemia (303,305,354). The disorder usually affects elderly men older than 60 years and is characterized by a dimorphic blood smear containing both normal RBCs and hypochromic RBCs from the leukemic clone that show numerous inclusion bodies of Hb H after incubation with brilliant cresyl blue. As the disease progresses, the abnormal clone becomes increasingly predominant. The degree of imbalance of globin chain synthesis and of α-globin mRNA deficiency is greater than that observed in the hereditary type of Hb H disease. It is even conceivable that cells of the abnormal leukemic clone synthesize no α-globin chains at all, but this phenomenon is difficult to document in total blood as long as some normal erythroid cells are being produced.

The molecular basis of this fascinating disorder remains obscure. It is clear that the marked deficiency of α-globin chain synthesis is not due to a major deletion or rearrangement in the α-globin gene cluster (354–356). The defect probably involves the suppression or silencing of all four α-globin genes in affected cells (355,356). The results of various studies, including chromosome transfer experiments, suggest that the defect responsible for this disorder may involve the abnormal expression of a *trans*-acting factor—either the absence of a positive regulatory factor required for normal α-globin gene expression, or the presence of a negative regulatory factor capable of suppressing α-gene expression (356,357).

Hemoglobin H Disease in Association with Mental Retardation.

A second syndrome that is associated with Hb H as a *de novo* abnormality is the disorder of mental retardation with Hb H disease, α-thalassemia and mental retardation (ATR) (358–362). In this disorder, those affected have mental retardation (with IQs of 50 to 70), dysmorphic features, and Hb H disease that is inherited in a nontraditional manner. Although one parent may have α-thalassemia-2 by various criteria, the other parent is usually completely normal. Two distinct syndromes have been identified. In some cases, there is the *de novo* appearance of large (2000 kb or so) deletions involving the entire α-globin gene cluster and adjacent DNA of the top of chromosome 16, the so-called *ATR-16 syndrome*. In some of these persons, the deletion produces detectable cytogenetic abnormalities of chromosome 16, indicating that a very large segment of the chromosome is deleted, sometimes because of unbalanced chromosomal translocations involving the telomeres of the affected chromosomes (259,363,364). In the second syndrome, without detectable deletions of the α-globin gene complex (360), the molecular basis of the disorder consists of mutations of a gene on the X chromosome (365–369), the so-called ATR-X syndrome. The affected gene encodes a *trans*-acting factor called *XH2* that is thought to influence the expression of the α-globin genes as well as other genes (361,362).

δβ-Thalassemia, γδβ-Thalassemia, Hereditary Persistence of Fetal Hemoglobin, Hemoglobin Lepore, and Related Disorders

A group of β-thalassemia-like disorders is distinguished from the more typical forms of β-thalassemia by the presence of a substantial elevation of Hb F in heterozygotes as well as in homozygotes and compound heterozygotes. These disorders are usually due to deletions of different sizes involving the β-globin gene cluster, but nondeletion types of disorders have also been identified (370–374).

Although δβ-thalassemia and HPFH are generally described or referred to as distinct disorders with different phenotypes, they should probably not be considered as unambiguously separate entities but as a group of disorders with a variety of partially overlapping phenotypes that sometimes defy classification as one syndrome or the other. The following are working definitions generally applied to the classification of these disorders. δβ-*Thalassemia* usually refers to a group of disorders associated with a mild but definite thalassemia phenotype of hypochromia and microcytosis together with a modest elevation of Hb F, which, in heterozygotes, is heterogeneously distributed among RBCs. In contrast, *HPFH* refers to a group of disorders with substantially higher levels of Hb F, in which there is usually no associated phenotype of hypochromia and microcytosis. In addition, the increased Hb F in heterozygotes with the typical forms of HPFH is distributed in a relatively uniform (pancellular) fashion among all the RBCs rather than being distributed in a heterogeneous (heterocellular) fashion among a subpopulation of so-called F cells, as in δβ-thalassemia.

Homozygotes for both conditions totally lack Hb A and Hb A₂, indicating absence of δ- and β-globin gene expression in *cis* to the δβ-thalassemia and HPFH determinants. Although the apparent striking qualitative difference in cellular distribution of Hb F between HPFH and β-thalassemia may be due in great part to the quantitative differences in Hb F per cell and the sensitivity of the methods used to detect Hb F cytologically, it appears that the increased amount of Hb F in HPFH is caused by a genetically determined failure to suppress γ-globin gene activity postnatally in all erythroid cells, rather than by selective survival of the normally occurring subpopulation of F cells as occurs in sickle cell anemia, β⁺-thalassemia, and β⁰-thalassemia. In the final analysis, some overlap definitely exists between the two sets of syndromes at the level of their clinical and hematologic phenotypes as well as at the level of their molecular basis.

DELETIONS ASSOCIATED WITH δβ-THALASSEMIA

A large number of different deletions of the β-globin gene cluster have been identified as causes of δβ-thalassemia (Fig. 48-20). In almost all patients, partial or total deletions of both the δ- and β-globin genes are the bases for absent δ- and β-globin chain synthesis. The one exception is the so-called Corfu δβ-thalassemia, in which the deletion involves only the δ gene, with the defect in β-gene expression due to a point mutation (G → A) at position 5 of IVS-1 of the linked β-globin gene (376,377). The δβ-thalassemias can be classified into two general categories: $^{G}\gamma^{A}\gamma(\delta\beta)^{0}$-thalassemia, in which both γ genes are intact, and $^{G}\gamma(^{A}\gamma\delta\beta)^{0}$-thalassemia, in which the deletion also involves part or all of the $^{A}\gamma$ gene and results in increased Hb F that is all of the $^{G}\gamma$ type. In general, the δβ-thalassemia deletions are relatively circumscribed and do not extend far beyond the β-gene cluster. Three δβ-thalassemia mutations (Chinese, Spanish, and Japanese deletions) encompass a considerable region of DNA with 3' endpoints approximately 75 kb, 100 kb, and more than 100 kb, respectively, to the 3' side of the β-globin gene. A particularly interesting DNA rearrangement is that causing the Indian $^{G}\gamma(^{A}\gamma\delta\beta)^{0}$-thalassemia, in which there are two deletions involving portions of the $^{A}\gamma$, δ, and β genes and an inversion of the intergene DNA between the $^{A}\gamma$ and δ genes.

As indicated by their names, these deletions are usually limited in their geographic distribution. In those cases in which the endpoints have been sequenced, the deletions appear to have arisen by illegitimate recombination events between nonhomologous segments of DNA (discussed in section Molecular Mechanisms Associated with the Generation of Deletions in the β-Globin Gene Cluster).

The cause of the increased Hb F production in δβ-thalassemia is poorly understood, and a number of theories have been advanced. One theory proposes that the deletions may lead to disruption of the normal adult chromatin configuration between the fetal and adult domains of the β cluster and thereby allow the γ genes to escape normal repression and be expressed in a subpopulation of adult erythroid cells (377). Based on observations of possible competition between γ and β promoters for various *cis*-acting and *trans*-acting factors, such as the LCR (30,130–139) (discussed in the section Molecular Mechanisms and Models), another theory proposes that deletion of the δ and β gene promoters allows the γ gene promoters to compete more successfully for the influence of the LCR or other *cis*-acting and *trans*-acting factors. Finally, as proposed in the case of deletion type HPFH (discussed in the section Deletions Associated with Hemoglobin Kenya and Hereditary Persistence of Fetal Hemoglobin), the DNA sequences at the 3' breakpoint of certain deletions may contain enhancer-like sequences that activate the γ genes when translocated into their vicinity by the recombination–deletion event.

For example, certain δβ-thalassemia deletions, such as the black $^{G}\gamma(^{A}\gamma\delta\beta)^{0}$ and Indian $^{G}\gamma(^{A}\gamma\delta\beta)^{0}$ deletions, leave the 3' β

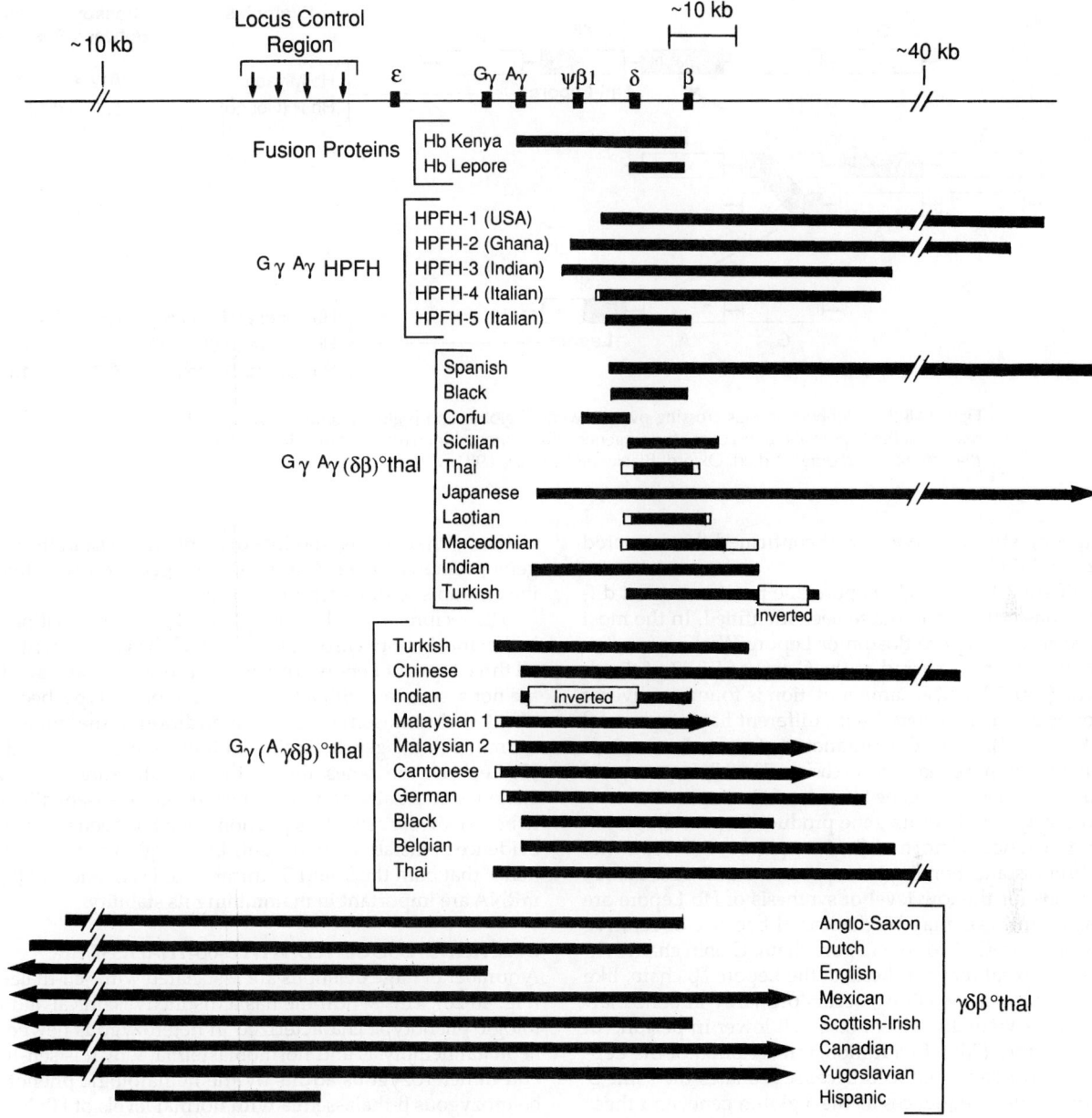

Figure 48-20. Deletions involving multiple genes or the locus control region of the β-globin gene cluster associated with fusion proteins, hereditary persistence of fetal hemoglobin (HPFH), δβ-thalassemia, or γδβ-thalassemia. The extents of the deletions are indicated by the closed bars, with open bars representing regions where the precise endpoints of the deletions are indeterminate. The open bars in the Indian $^{G}\gamma(^{A}\gamma\delta\beta)^{0}$-thalassemia and Turkish $^{G}\gamma^{A}\gamma(\delta\beta)^{0}$-thalassemia indicate a DNA inversion. The reference citations for the individual mutations are listed elsewhere (370). Additional deletions have been reported (373). Hb, hemoglobin. (From Bollekens JA, Forget BG. δβ-Thalassemia and hereditary persistence of fetal hemoglobin. *Hematol Oncol Clin North Am* 1991;5:399, with permission.)

gene enhancer intact and result in its translocation closer to the γ gene promoters. The Chinese, German, and black $^{G}\gamma(^{A}\gamma\delta\beta)^{0}$-thalassemia deletions have 3' breakpoints similar to those of certain types of deletional $^{G}\gamma^{A}\gamma$-HPFH but are presumably associated with a δβ-thalassemia rather than an HPFH phenotype because only one γ gene remains functional, whereas in the HPFH deletions, both γ genes are functional.

HEMOGLOBIN LEPORE SYNDROMES
The Hb Lepore syndromes can be considered related to the δβ-thalassemia syndromes because they are associated with a β-thalassemia phenotype, absence of normal δ- and β-globin

gene expression in *cis*, and usually a modest elevation of Hb F. The increase in Hb F is not as striking as that seen in typical cases of δβ-thalassemia. Hb Lepore is a structurally abnormal Hb in which the abnormal globin chain is a hybrid or fused globin chain, having the N-terminal amino acid sequence of the normal δ-chain and the C-terminal amino acid sequence of the normal β-chain (2). The Lepore gene is almost certainly the result of an unequal crossover event or recombination between the homologous (but nonidentical) δ-globin and β-globin genes, with the resulting deletion of the 5' end of the β gene, the 3' end of the δ gene, and approximately 7 kb of intergene DNA between the δ and β genes (Figs. 48-20 and 48-21).

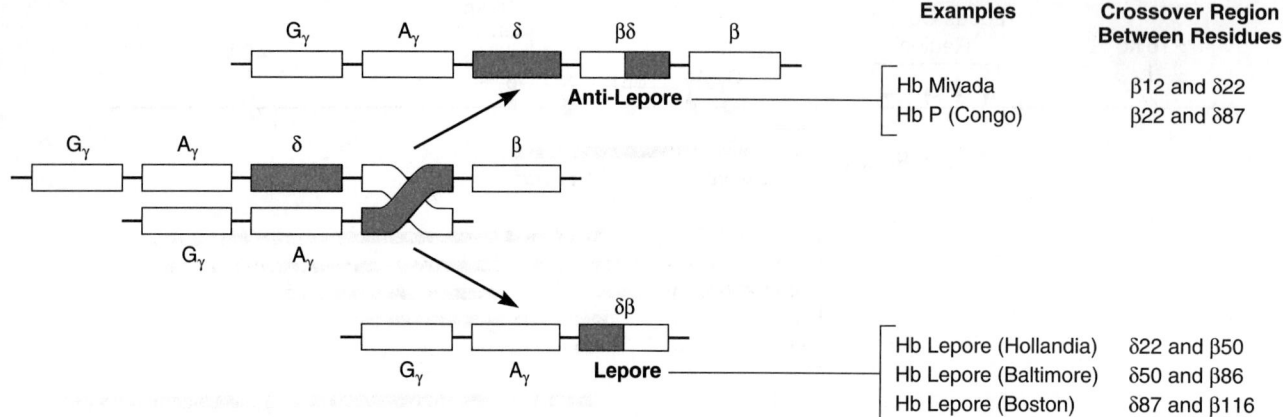

Figure 48-21. Nonhomologous crossing over between δ-globin and β-globin genes resulting in the formation of the Lepore and anti-Lepore fusion genes. Hb, hemoglobin. (From Weatherall DJ, Clegg JB. *The thalassemia syndromes*, 3rd ed. Oxford: Blackwell Science, 1981, with permission.)

Gene mapping studies have in fact confirmed the expected gene deletion (378,379).

Three different types of Hb Lepore due to crossovers at different positions of the genes have been identified. In the most common form, Hb Lepore Boston or Lepore Washington, the recombination event occurred at the 5' end of IVS-2 of the β-globin gene (380–382). The same mutation is found in diverse racial groups and is associated with different haplotypes of β cluster RFLPs (383). Thus, the mutation appears to have arisen independently on more than one occasion. The Hb Lepore gene behaves as a β-thalassemic gene because of the presence of only a low level of synthesis of its gene product (Lepore δβ-globin chain) and absence of normal β-chain production from the affected chromosome; homozygotes produce no Hb A or Hb A_2.

The reasons for the low level of synthesis of Hb Lepore are not known. Synthesis may be decreased because of relative instability of the mRNA for the Lepore chain. Globin chain synthetic studies reveal that synthesis of the Lepore δβ chain, like that of the δ chain of the Hb A_2, occurs primarily in bone marrow cells and is virtually absent or much lower in peripheral blood reticulocytes (384). In addition, transcription of the Lepore δβ gene is probably reduced because it shares the same 5' flanking (promoter) sequences as the δ-globin gene, and these sequences, which differ from the corresponding sequences of the β gene, are likely responsible (at least partly) for the normally low level of δ-globin gene expression (discussed in the section Conserved Sequences and Transcription Factor Binding Sites in 5' Flanking DNA of Globin Genes).

Whatever the relative contributions of mRNA instability and decreased gene transcription, Hb Lepore accumulates to a level of approximately 10% to 15% of the total Hb, whereas Hb A_2 is rarely increased to levels much greater than 5%. The 5' flanking DNA adjacent to the δ gene cannot be the only factor influencing the level of expression of the Lepore δβ gene; otherwise, Hb Lepore would be expected to accumulate only to a level similar to that of Hb A_2. It is possible that the enhancer elements in IVS-2, exon 3, and the 3' flanking DNA of the β-globin gene, now in proximity to the δ promoter because of the recombination event, increase the activity of the δ promoter in the Lepore δβ-fusion gene (discussed in the section Enhancers and Other *cis*-Acting Sequences That Influence Globin Gene Expression). Other possible mechanisms to explain the differences between steady-state amounts of Hb Lepore and Hb A_2 are stabilization of the δβ mRNA by 3' untranslated sequences from the β gene, different affinities of the δ-globin and δβ-globin chains for asso-

ciation with α-chains, and loss of competition from the β-globin gene promoter (deleted in the Lepore gene) for possibly limiting amounts of transcription factors.

The reciprocal product of Lepore-type recombination events is the anti-Lepore chromosome, which has been identified for all three types of Lepore crossovers. The anti-Lepore syndromes are not associated with a β-thalassemia phenotype, because the affected chromosome carries, in addition to the mutant gene, normal β and δ genes. Similar to the situation observed in the Hb Lepore syndromes, the synthesis of the anti-Lepore globin chain is almost absent in reticulocytes and is essentially limited to bone marrow cells. This phenomenon has been interpreted as evidence of instability of the anti-Lepore globin mRNA and evidence that both the 5' and 3' untranslated sequences of β-globin mRNA are important in maintaining its stability.

DELETIONS ASSOCIATED WITH γδβ-THALASSEMIA
A number of large deletions are associated with γδβ-thalassemia (Fig. 48-20). This syndrome has a distinctive clinical and hematologic phenotype characterized in heterozygous newborns by neonatal hemolysis and normoblastemia, which is self-limited, and in heterozygous adults by the hematologic phenotype of heterozygous β-thalassemia with normal levels of Hb F and Hb A_2. Because of the associated absence of γ gene expression, homozygosity for this disorder is expected to be lethal early in gestation.

The location and extent of the deletions associated with γδβ-thalassemia are illustrated in Figure 48-20 (385–394). Both endpoints of the deletions have been mapped in the Anglo-Saxon and Dutch deletions, and in these, the total size of the deletion is approximately 100 kb, with the breakpoints staggered by only 3 to 5 kb (386). Gene mapping studies suggest that in many of the other deletions, the total extent of the deletion probably encompasses even more DNA. For instance, the 5' breakpoints of five of the deletions are located at an unknown distance 5' to the breakpoints of the Dutch and the Anglo-Saxon deletions.

The basis for the total absence of γ-globin, δ-globin, and β-globin chain synthesis in *cis* to these mutations is clearly understandable in the case of five of the eight deletions shown in Figure 48-20, because the involved genes are either totally or partially deleted. In the case of the three other deletions, the β-globin gene or one or both of the γ-globin genes on the affected chromosome are intact but inactive. This surprising finding was initially studied in some detail in the Dutch deletion, in which the β-globin gene with 2.5 kb of its 5' flanking DNA is intact but appears to be totally inactive. The cloned β-globin gene from this chromosome was shown to be structurally normal and to function normally in gene transfer–expression studies. In fetal liver erythroid cells of an affected fetus, the β-globin gene from the deletion chromosome was found to be hypermethylated, whereas the β gene from the normal chromosome in *trans* was hypomethylated, as is usually found in actively transcribing genes (395).

The cause of the inactivity and hypermethylation of the β-globin gene on the deletion chromosome was initially poorly understood. Proposed explanations included disruption of chromatin structure preventing normal expression of the β gene, or juxtaposition of negative regulatory sequences from the upstream DNA brought into the vicinity of the β gene as a result of the deletion–recombination event. Subsequently, two other families were described in which the 3' breakpoint of the deletion was found to be located substantially farther 5' in the β cluster, leaving considerable amounts of normal β cluster DNA situated 5' to the silent β-globin gene. These include the English deletion, in which the 3' breakpoint is located between the $^G\gamma$-globin and $^A\gamma$-globin genes (389), and the Hispanic deletion, in which the entire β cluster is intact and the 3' breakpoint of the deletion is located approximately 10 kb 5' to the ε-globin gene (393). An explanation for this puzzling inactivity of the structurally normal γ-globin, δ-globin, and β-globin genes on these various deletion chromosomes came to light with the discovery of important regulatory sequences located 5' to the ε-globin gene, the LCR associated with the presence of DNase I hypersensitive or superhypersensitive sites in erythroid cells (discussed in the section Enhancers and Other *cis*-Acting Sequences That Influence Globin Gene Expression).

The most plausible explanation for the inactivity of the β-globin gene (and other nondeleted globin genes) in the Dutch, English, and Hispanic γδβ-thalassemias is the deletion of the LCR region 5' to the ε gene, which is required for normal activity of the globin genes in the β cluster. The Hispanic γδβ deletion spares hypersensitive site 1 while deleting the other 5' sites together with approximately 30 kb of 5' DNA. These findings suggest that the presence of site 1 alone is not sufficient to allow high levels of activity of the β gene cluster. In fact, a short deletion involving only site 1 is not associated with a clinical phenotype of γδβ-thalassemia (396). Studies in transgenic mice and MEL cells suggest that the 5' hypersensitive sites 2 and 3, which are effectively deleted in the Hispanic γδβ-thalassemia, contain most of the sequences responsible for conferring high levels of globin gene expression (182,397,398).

DELETIONS ASSOCIATED WITH HEMOGLOBIN KENYA AND HEREDITARY PERSISTENCE OF FETAL HEMOGLOBIN

Hb Kenya is a structurally abnormal Hb that, like Hb Lepore, contains a fused β-like globin chain resulting from a nonhomologous crossover event between two globin genes in the β cluster. Whereas the Lepore crossover occurred between the δ-globin and β-globin genes, the Kenya gene resulted from crossover between the $^A\gamma$-globin and β-globin genes (3) (Fig. 48-20). The crossover occurred in the second exons of the $^A\gamma$ and β genes between the codons for amino acids 80 to 87 and resulted in deletion of approximately 24 kb of DNA from the $^A\gamma$ to the β gene (399). Unlike Hb Lepore, which is associated with a β-thalassemic phenotype, Hb Kenya is associated with a phenotype of pancellular $^G\gamma$-HPFH. Erythrocytes of affected heterozygotes have normal RBC indices and contain 7% to 23% Hb Kenya as well as approximately 10% Hb F, all of which is of the $^G\gamma$ type and is relatively uniformly distributed among the RBCs.

The finding of Hb Kenya was initially thought to add support to an early theory that proposed the existence of control elements in the $^A\gamma$ to δ intergene DNA, deletion of which in HPFH (and Hb Kenya) but not in δβ-thalassemia resulted in incomplete postnatal suppression of γ gene activity in all erythroid cells (179). The most likely explanation for the HPFH phenotype associated with Hb Kenya is the influence on the $^G\gamma$ and Kenya gene promoters of the 3' β-globin gene enhancer translocated into closer proximity of the γ-globin gene promoters by the crossover–deletion event (discussed in the section Enhancers and Other *cis*-Acting Sequences That Influence Globin Gene Expression).

A number of deletions have been described in the β-globin gene cluster that are associated with a phenotype of pancellular $^G\gamma^A\gamma$-HPFH (377,388,400–410) (Fig. 48-20). One of these deletions, HPFH-5, identified in an Italian family, is relatively short and extends from a point approximately 3 kb 5' to the δ gene to a point 0.7 kb 3' to the β gene, within the proximal portion of its 3' enhancer (410). The molecular basis of the HPFH phenotype associated with this deletion is presumably the influence of the translocated 3' β gene enhancer on the γ gene promoters in a manner analogous to that proposed for the basis of the HPFH phenotype of the Hb Kenya syndrome. The other four deletions are considerably more extensive and fall into two different size classes. HPFH-1 and HPFH-2, found in blacks, are the result of extensive deletions of nearly identical sizes, involving approximately 105 kb of DNA, with breakpoints staggered by only 5 to 6 kb (377,388,400–405) (Fig. 48-20). The deletions associated with HPFH-3 (in Asian Indians) and HPFH-4 (in Southern Italians) are less extensive, encompassing approximately 50 kb and 40 kb, respectively. The 3' breakpoints of these two deletions are separated by only approximately 2 kb and are located approximately 30 kb 3' to the site of the β-globin gene, or approximately 50 to 60 kb more proximal than the 3' breakpoints of HPFH-1 and HPFH-2 (406–410).

The 5' breakpoints of all five HPFH deletions are located between the ψβ and δ genes. The clustering of the 3' breakpoints of the four largest deletions in two discrete regions has focused attention on the nature of the DNA sequences at these sites and their possible role in the generation of the HPFH phenotype. The DNA sequences at the 3' breakpoint of HPFH-1 and HPFH-2 have a number of interesting properties: They have gene enhancer activity in various assay systems; they are specifically hypomethylated and contain a DNase I hypersensitive site in erythroid cells (401,411); and they contain a large open reading frame that encodes a protein homologous to members of the superfamily of G protein-coupled receptors, and in particular to members of the family of olfactory receptors (401,412). All these properties suggest the presence in this DNA of a gene that is active in erythroid cells. The Spanish type of $^G\gamma^A\gamma$ (δβ)^0-thalassemia has a 5' breakpoint close to that of HPFH-1 (413) (Fig. 48-20) but extends for an additional 6 to 7 kb in the 3' direction (401,414). Thus, the deletion of the additional DNA containing the interesting sequences at the 3' breakpoint of the HPFH-1 and HPFH-2 deletions is associated with a δβ-thalassemia rather than a HPFH phenotype, suggesting a role for these sequences in the generation of the HPFH phenotype in HPFH-1 and HPFH-2. In fact, when a DNA fragment with a structure very similar to that of HPFH-2 (and containing the HPFH-1 3' breakpoint DNA) is used to generate transgenic mice, the mice express the γ-globin transgene at a high level and in a virtually pancellular fashion in adult erythroid cells (415). The 3' breakpoints of HPFH-3 and HPFH-4 are located within a complex array of repetitive DNA sequences (406), but these DNA sequences have been shown to possess enhancer-like properties in different assay systems, including transgenic mice (416).

The unifying theory that emerges from the study of the four largest HPFH deletions is that the DNA sequences at the 3' deletion breakpoints become juxtaposed to the γ genes as a result of the deletion events and may influence γ gene expression in a manner analogous to the presumed influence of the 3' β gene enhancer on γ gene expression in Hb Kenya and HPFH-5. Mechanisms by which this could occur include the presence of enhancer sequences in the translocated 3' breakpoint DNA or the presence in this DNA of an active chromatin configuration, which could have a spreading and activating effect on the expression of the neighboring γ-globin genes.

A number of $^Gγ(^Aγδβ)^0$-thalassemia deletions have 3' breakpoints located near those of the HPFH deletions. These include the Chinese (417) and Thai deletions (418), with 3' breakpoints near that of HPFH-2, and the German (419) and Belgian (420) deletions, with 3' breakpoints near those of HPFH-3 and HPFH-4 (Fig. 48-20). The Thai deletion is associated with a high level and pancellular distribution of Hb F and has been reclassified by some authors as HPFH-6 (421). The DNA at the 3' breakpoint of this deletion has enhancer-like activity and an open reading frame that appears to encode an olfactory receptor pseudogene with approximately 55% sequence identity to that of the olfactory receptor gene at the 3' breakpoint of the HPFH-1 and HPFH-2 deletions (422).

MOLECULAR MECHANISMS ASSOCIATED WITH THE GENERATION OF DELETIONS IN THE β-GLOBIN GENE CLUSTER

Considerable discussion in the literature has addressed the molecular mechanisms responsible for generating the various deletions observed in the β-globin gene cluster (409). With the exceptions of Hb Lepore and Hb Kenya, all the deletions in the β gene cluster are the result of "illegitimate" recombination events in which no significant DNA sequence homology is present at the deletion breakpoints. Sometimes, a simple rejoining of the normal DNA sequences flanking the breakpoints occurs; other times, short segments of foreign DNA are inserted between the breakpoints. In some cases, one of the breakpoints involves a repetitive DNA sequence, either of the AluI family or of the L1 family, and some speculation has occurred concerning whether such repetitive DNA sequences serve as hot spots for recombination. Although examples of recombination events between two repetitive DNA sequences of the AluI family are found in the α-globin gene cluster and in other gene systems, these are not found in the β-globin gene cluster. It is likely that the finding of repetitive DNA sequences at one or the other breakpoint of a deletion event often occurs by chance alone, given the abundance of such sequences in the β cluster, as in the human genome in general.

A striking feature of the deletions in the β-globin gene locus is the clustering of sets of deletions of approximately the same size. To explain this phenomenon, Vanin et al. (388) proposed a model in which recombination may occur during DNA replication between sequences located at the attachment points of DNA or chromatin to the structure in the cell nucleus (called the *nuclear matrix*), resulting in loss of an entire chromatin loop. Because chromatin loops are thought to move through the nuclear matrix attachment points during DNA replication like a cable through a reel, different deletions of approximately the same size, but with different breakpoints, could result from random breakage and joining of DNA at different points in time as they travel through the nuclear matrix.

NONDELETION FORMS OF δβ-THALASSEMIA AND HEREDITARY PERSISTENCE OF FETAL HEMOGLOBIN

δβ-*Thalassemia.* Although most cases of δβ-thalassemia are due to deletions in the β-globin gene cluster, two distinct syndromes occur in which a δβ-thalassemia phenotype is not asso-

ciated with a deletion. In these cases, two separate mutations have been found: a point mutation causing β-thalassemia, and a second mutation causing increased Hb F production. The form of δβ-thalassemia found in Sardinia is characterized by the synthesis of predominantly $^Aγ$-globin chains of Hb F (423). The β-globin gene on the affected chromosome carries the common nonsense mutation at codon 39 as the cause of the β-thalassemia phenotype (424,425), whereas the $^Aγ$-globin gene carries a C → T base substitution at position −196 of the $^Aγ$ gene promoter (426), which is associated with one form of nondeletion HPFH (see the following section).

A Chinese family has also been described in which a δβ-thalassemia phenotype with increased levels of both $^Gγ$-chains and $^Aγ$-chains of Hb F is not associated with a deletion in the β-globin gene cluster (427). The β-globin gene on the affected chromosome was found to contain an A → G substitution at position −29 of the β-gene promoter as the cause of the β-thalassemia phenotype (428), but the mutation responsible for the increased production of Hb F remains unknown.

Hereditary Persistence of Fetal Hemoglobin. In contrast to the deletional HPFH syndromes in which both linked $^Gγ$ and $^Aγ$ genes are overexpressed, only one or the other γ gene is usually overexpressed in the best characterized nondeletional types of HPFH, although less well-characterized nondeletion forms of $^Gγ^Aγ$-HPFH also exist. Because of the restricted pattern of γ-globin gene expression in the $^Gγ$ and $^Aγ$ forms of nondeletion HPFH, it was assumed that the mutations in these syndromes must be located near the affected gene, and molecular studies focused initially on the DNA sequence analysis of the overexpressed γ genes in these disorders.

The results of these structural analyses revealed a number of different point mutations in the promoter region of the overexpressed γ gene in persons with different types of nondeletion HPFH (Table 48-4 and Fig. 48-22). These point mutations have clustered in three distinct regions of the 5' flanking DNA of the affected γ genes. Five different mutations have been identified in the region located approximately 200 bp from the cap site or site of transcription initiation of the γ genes, specifically at position −202 (C → G) of the $^Gγ$ gene and positions −202 (C → T), −198 (T → C), −196 (C → T), and −195 (C → G) of the $^Aγ$ gene (429–434) (Fig. 48-22). This region of DNA, which had not previously been suspected of playing a role in the regulation of γ gene expression, is very G+C rich, and its sequence bears homology to that of known control elements of other genes, such as the 21-bp repeat of the SV40 virus promoter and the distal element of the thymidine kinase gene of herpes simplex virus.

The G+C rich sequence of the latter genes is known to be the binding site of a ubiquitous *trans*-acting protein factor called *Sp1*. Subsequent studies of the γ gene promoters have demonstrated that the −200 region is also a binding site for Sp1 and at least one other ubiquitous DNA-binding protein (190,435–438). The −202 (G → C) and −196 mutations are associated with high levels of Hb F (15% to 20%), expressed in a pancellular fashion, whereas the −202 (C → T), −198, and −195 mutations are associated with lower levels of Hb F (3% to 10%), expressed in a heterocellular fashion (1,370,372) (Table 48-4).

The second region containing a mutation associated with nondeletion HPFH is located at position −175 (Fig. 48-22). A point mutation (T → C) at this position of either the $^Gγ$ or $^Aγ$ gene is associated with a phenotype of pancellular HPFH with high levels of Hb F (15% to 25%) (439–441). This region of DNA is noteworthy because it contains an octanucleotide sequence that is present in the promoter region of a number of genes and is the binding site of another ubiquitous *trans*-acting factor called *OCT-1*. In addition, the octamer consensus sequence of

**TABLE 48-4. Nondeletion Forms of Hereditary Persistence
of Fetal Hemoglobin (HPFH) and δβ-Thalassemia**[a]

Type and Racial Group	Mutation in Globin Gene	Percentage of Hb F in Heterozygotes	References
Pancellular ^Gγ HPFH			
Black	^Gγ: −202 (C → G)	15–25	429
Black	^Gγ: −175 (T → C)	20–30	439
Sardinian	^Gγ: −175 (T → C)	17–21	440
Japanese	^Gγ: −114 (C → T)	11–14	445
Pancellular ^Aγ HPFH			
Southern Italian	^Aγ: −196 (C → T)	12–16	432
Chinese	^Aγ: −196 (C → T)	14–21	433
Black	^Aγ: −175 (T → C)	36–41[b]	441
Greek	^Aγ: −117 (G → A)	10–20	442,443
Sardinian	^Aγ: −117 (G → A)	12–16	1598
Black	^Aγ: −117 (G → A)	11–16	1599
Black	^Aγ: −114 to −102 deleted	30–32	444
Pancellular ^Gγ^Aγ HPFH			
Chinese	Unknown	20–25	1600
Heterocellular ^Gγ HPFH			
Black (Atlanta)	^Gγ^Gγ: −158 (C → T)	2.3–3.8	465,469
Heterocellular ^Aγ HPFH			
Black	^Aγ: −202 (C → T)	1.6–3.9	430
British	^Aγ: −198 (T → C)	3.5–10	431
Brazilian	^Aγ: −195 (C → G)	4.5–7	434
Black (Georgia)	^Aγ: −114 (C → T)	2.6–6	1598
Heterocellular ^Gγ^Aγ HPFH			
Swiss	Unknown	1–4	1
Black (Seattle)	Normal γ-gene promoters	3–8	464,465
^Aγ-δβ-Thalassemia			
Sardinian	^Aγ: −196 (C → T)	10–20	423,425
	β: codon 39 (CAG → TAG)		424
^Gγ^Aγ-δβ-Thalassemia			
Chinese	Normal γ-gene promoters	22.3	427,428
	β: −29 (A → G)		

Hb, hemoglobin.

[a]Additional mutations have been reported (http://globin.cse.psu.edu) (216,373).

[b]The one patient studied was doubly heterozygous for Hb A and Hb C. Approximately 20% of the Hb F (or 8% of the total Hb) was of the ^Gγ type, and the ^Gγ gene in *cis* to the −175 ^Aγ mutation carried the −158 C → T change.

---

the γ gene promoters is flanked on either side by a consensus sequence for the erythroid-specific factor GATA-1 (28,31,180–185). The point mutation at position −175 affects the one nucleotide that is present in the partially overlapping binding sites of both OCT-1 and GATA-1.

The third region affected by a point mutation in nondeletion HPFH is the area of a well-known regulatory element of globin and other genes: the CCAAT box sequence. In the γ genes, the CCAAT box is duplicated, and the mutation associated with the Greek (^Aγ) type of nondeletion HPFH is a G → A substitution at position −117, two bases upstream of the distal CCAAT box of the ^Aγ-globin gene promoter (442,443). The base change disrupts a pentanucleotide sequence, YYTTGA (Y, pyrimidine), which is highly conserved immediately upstream of the CCAAT sequence in all animal fetal and embryonic genes (442). Another mutation with a similar phenotype involves the deletion of 13 bp of DNA, from positions −102 to −114, encompassing the distal CCAAT box and adjacent 3' DNA of the ^Aγ-globin gene (444) (Fig. 48-22). The CCAAT box region is known to be the binding site of a number of *trans*-acting factors, including the ubiquitous factors CCAAT-binding protein (CP1) and CCAAT displacement factor (CDP), as well as an erythroid-specific factor, NF-E3. A third mutation has also been identified that consists of a C → T base substitution at position −114 of the ^Gγ-globin or ^Aγ-globin gene, within the distal CCAAT consensus sequence (445,446).

The unifying model by which these various mutations are thought to affect Hb switching proposes that these base changes alter the binding of a number of different *trans*-acting factors to

critical regions of the γ gene promoters and thereby prevent the normal postnatal suppression of γ gene expression (372). The mutations could prevent the binding of negative regulatory factors or enhance the binding of positive regulatory factors. Either mechanism could be operative with one mutation or the other.

The following abnormalities of protein–DNA interactions have been observed when nondeletion HPFH γ-globin gene promoter sequences have been compared with normal γ gene promoter sequences.

The point mutation at position −198 clearly results in increased binding affinity of the ubiquitous *trans*-acting factor, Sp1, whereas the mutations at positions −202 (C → T) and −196 result in either no change or reduced Sp1 binding (435–438). The C → G mutation at position −202 gives variable results: increased Sp1 binding in some studies (435,436) but not in others (437,438). At least one other ubiquitous activity has been identified, the binding of which is decreased by the −202 C → G and −198 mutations (190,435–438). Finally, the −202 C → G mutation leads to the binding of yet another activity, called −50γ, that usually binds to the −50 region of the γ promoter and may be important for selective γ-globin over β-globin gene expression during the fetal stage of development (189,190,438).

The T → G mutation at position −175 results in markedly decreased binding of the ubiquitous factor OCT-1 (28,447–449), whereas the binding of the erythroid-specific factor GATA-1 is either unaffected (28,447) or slightly enhanced (448) in different studies. The mutation does alter the DNase I "footprint" pattern of the GATA-1–DNA complex (28), and the increased functional activity of the mutant promoter in gene transfer–expression

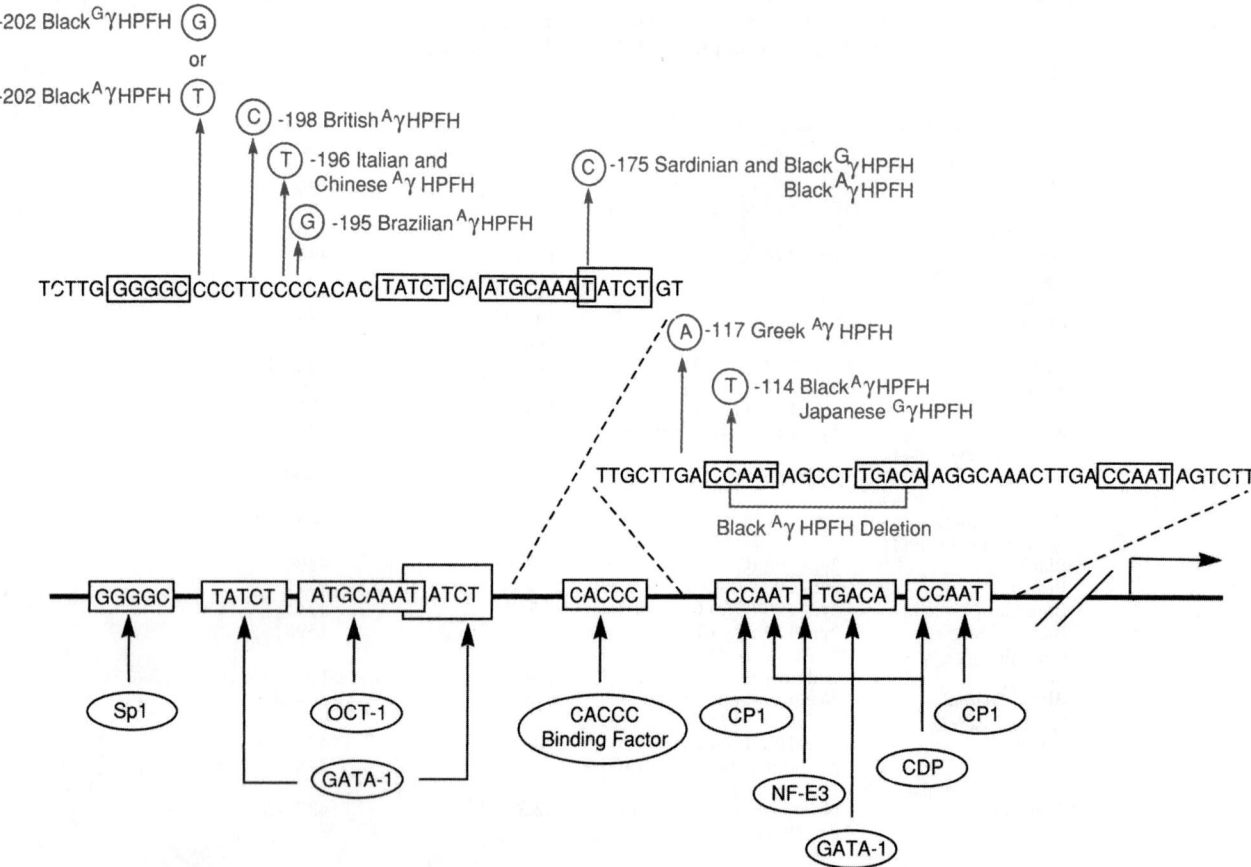

Figure 48-22. *Cis*-acting and *trans*-acting elements of the human γ-globin gene promoters and mutations associated with nondeletion forms of hereditary persistence of fetal hemoglobin (HPFH). (From Bollekens JA, Forget BG. δβ-Thalassemia and hereditary persistence of fetal hemoglobin. *Hematol Oncol Clin North Am* 1991;5:399, with permission.)

studies is dependent on the presence and ability of GATA-1 to bind to the promoter, because additional mutations that abolish GATA-1 binding to the HPFH promoter also abolish its overexpression (28,185).

The G → A mutation at position −117 results in reduced binding of the erythroid-specific factors GATA-1 and NF-E3 and enhanced binding of the ubiquitous factors CP1 and CDP (447,448,450,451). The 13-bp deletion involving the distal CCAAT box and adjacent 3' DNA results in the loss of binding of NF-E3, CP1, and CDP, but it leaves GATA-1 binding intact (451). The C → T mutation at position −114 abolishes binding of CP1 to the distal CCAAT box without affecting the binding of GATA-1 (445).

Studies of nondeletion HPFH mutations in transgenic mice have given variable results. The HPFH phenotype can be reproduced in mice with some, but not all, transgenes (452–457).

In addition to the nondeletion forms of HPFH associated with point mutations of the Gγ or Aγ promoters, there exists another group of related disorders, the molecular basis of which is less well characterized. These disorders include the Swiss, Seattle, and German types of heterocellular HPFH, in which the increased Hb F is of both the Gγ and the Aγ types; the Atlanta type of heterocellular HPFH, in which the elevated Hb F is all of the Gγ type; and the Saudi and other related high Hb F determinants, with predominance of Gγ gene expression.

The Swiss type of the heterocellular HPFH consists of a heterogeneous group of disorders associated with only a slight elevation of Hb F (2% to 3%) in simple heterozygotes but with

substantially higher than usual levels of Hb F when coinherited with homozygous sickle cell anemia, homozygous β-thalassemia, or Hb S/β-thalassemia (1). In some families, the disorder appears to be linked to the β gene cluster on chromosome 11, but the finding of a small number of crossover events suggests that the locus may be at some distance from the β cluster (458). In other families, the locus is clearly not linked to the β-gene cluster (373). In some of these families, an X-chromosome–linked pattern of inheritance of the high Hb F determinant is seen (459–461), whereas in another family, there is evidence for linkage to a locus on chromosome 6 (462,463).

Heterozygotes with the Seattle type of HPFH have slightly higher levels of Hb F (3% to 8%) than heterozygotes with the Swiss type HPFH (464). The promoters of the overexpressed Gγ and Aγ genes have a normal DNA sequence (465). A cluster of three base substitutions was identified in the 3' Aγ gene enhancer of affected persons (465), but this was later shown to be a polymorphism also found in persons without HPFH (466).

The German type of heterocellular HPFH (5% to 8% Hb F) was described in a family in which the mother and daughter were found to have a balanced cyclic translocation involving four chromosomes: 46,XX,t(6;9;11;20), including the portion of chromosome 11 containing the β gene cluster (467). The breakpoint of the translocation did not appear to occur within the β cluster itself.

The Atlanta type of Gγ-HPFH (2.5% to 4% Hb F) (468) is associated with a β locus that contains two Gγ genes, perhaps as the result of a gene conversion event (469). Both Gγ genes have a

C → T base substitution at position –158 of the $^{G}\gamma$ promoter. The possible significance of the –158 C → T base change is discussed in relation to the high Hb F determinants associated with sickle cell anemia in certain Saudi Arabians and in Africans.

In eastern Saudi Arabia, many patients with homozygous sickle cell anemia or Hb S/β^0-thalassemia have an unusually mild clinical course, associated with consistently high levels of Hb F—in the range of 25% to 40%—and with predominance of $^{G}\gamma$ chains (470,471). A similar syndrome has also been described in certain Asian Indians with sickle cell anemia (472,473). In contrast to the situation in blacks of African ancestry with sickle cell anemia and high levels of Hb F, one cannot usually identify in the Saudi or Indian families a parent with slight elevation of Hb F or F-cell numbers consistent with the Swiss type of heterocellular HPFH. The high Hb F genetic determinant appears to be inherited in *cis* to the sickle gene but seems to be expressed only in the presence of erythropoietic stress induced by hemolysis due to the homozygosity for the β^S gene or double heterozygosity for one β^S gene and a β^0-thalassemia gene.

The molecular basis of high Hb F expression in Saudis with sickle cell anemia is poorly understood. Analysis of the cloned genes of affected persons has revealed the presence of the C → T base change at position –158 of the $^{G}\gamma$ gene promoter and one other probably polymorphic base change (A → G) 29 bp upstream of the initiator codon in the 5' untranslated sequence of the $^{A}\gamma$ gene (474). The C → T base change at position –158 is also found in the $^{G}\gamma$ gene promoter of African β^S chromosomes bearing the so-called Senegal haplotype of β cluster RFLPs (475). Sickle cell anemia patients with the Senegal haplotype have a predominance of Hb F of the $^{G}\gamma$ type, but the total elevation of Hb F, although generally higher than that in sickle cell anemia patients with other haplotypes, is not nearly as great as that observed in the Saudi. As in the case of Saudi heterozygotes, heterozygotes for the Senegal haplotype have normal levels of Hb F. The Saudi and Senegal β^S-haplotypes, although similar, differ at the polymorphic *Hinc*II site 5' to the ε gene. Thus, the β cluster chromosomal background is not identical in the two populations.

The significance of the –158 C → T base change is not entirely clear. It creates a polymorphism for the enzyme *Xmn*I (469), which is commonly found in the general population and is associated with high $^{G}\gamma$:$^{A}\gamma$ ratios of Hb F in normal adults. Simple heterozygotes for the –158 C → T base change do not have significantly elevated levels of Hb F and therefore are not classified as having HPFH. When the –158 base change is coinherited with conditions that cause erythroid stress, such as sickle cell anemia, Hb S/β-thalassemia, or homozygous β-thalassemia, usually a significantly higher than usual synthesis of Hb F occurs, which is predominantly of the $^{G}\gamma$ type.

The precise role of the –158 base change in the phenomenon of high total levels of Hb F in the presence of erythroid stress remains to be determined. It is conceivable that the base change itself is not directly responsible for the high level of Hb F production but is simply a polymorphism that marks chromosomes with high Hb F genetic determinants, the nature of which is still unknown. Another base change has been identified in the same region of the $^{G}\gamma$ gene promoter (–161 G → A) in a black family with low levels of Hb F (1% to 2%) and marked predominance of $^{G}\gamma$ chains (476).

ISOLATED δ-THALASSEMIA AND γ-THALASSEMIA

δ-*Thalassemia.* Isolated thalassemia affecting the δ-globin gene has been identified in persons who totally lack Hb A$_2$ and are either homozygous for δ^0-thalassemia or doubly heterozygous for δ^0-thalassemia and (δβ)^0-thalassemia. A form of δ$^+$-thalassemia has also been described in Sardinians in whom partial rather than

total suppression of δ-chain synthesis occurs. The clinical significance of heterozygous δ-thalassemia is that if it is coinherited with heterozygous β-thalassemia, the affected person will have a normal level of Hb A$_2$; thus, the diagnosis of β-thalassemia trait may be missed. In such cases, the δ-thalassemia gene is usually coinherited in *trans* to the β-thalassemia gene. There are two syndromes in which a δ-thalassemia gene is coinherited as a second independent mutation in *cis* to a β-thalassemia gene: δ^0-thalassemia in *cis* to the structurally abnormal β^{Knossos} gene (in Mediterraneans, but not blacks of the French West Indies) (477), and δ-thalassemia in *cis* to the β$^+$-thalassemia caused by a point mutation (C → G) at position 745 of IVS-2 (478).

With one exception [the 7.2-kb Corfu δβ-thalassemia deletion without associated β-thalassemia (479)], gene mapping studies have failed to reveal any deletion or rearrangement of the affected δ-globin gene in cases of isolated δ thalassemia. Gene cloning or polymerase chain reaction (PCR) analysis and DNA sequence analysis have identified a number of different point mutations in the δ-globin genes of affected persons (216), some of which are listed in Table 48-5.

Many of the molecular defects causing δ thalassemia are similar in type to those that cause β-thalassemia: premature chain termination due to frameshifts, splicing defects, unstable globin chains, and so on. Two defects are novel and noteworthy because they are associated with point mutations in GATA-1 consensus sequences in either the promoter region (480,481) or 3' flanking DNA of the δ gene (482) with resulting abnormal binding of the transcription factor GATA-1. The promoter mutation at position –77 is associated with decreased GATA-1 binding (481), whereas the point mutation 69 bp 3' to the poly(A) addition site is associated with increased binding affinity of GATA-1 (482).

δ^0-Thalassemia also occurs in nonhuman primates such as the Old World monkeys, which do not synthesize Hb A$_2$ despite the presence of δ-globin genes in their DNA. A number of different mutations have been identified by cloning and DNA sequence analysis of δ-globin genes from various nonhuman primates, including a frameshift mutation associated with a 1-base insertion at codon 55 in rhesus monkeys and baboons and a 20-bp deletion at the cap site in colobus monkeys (483,484). It has been postulated that these mutations may be secondary events that occurred by evolutionary drift after a different δ-gene silencing event such as a promoter mutation (483). The cloned δ-globin genes of colobus and rhesus monkeys have been shown to be transcribed inefficiently, compared with the human δ-globin gene, in a cell-free transcription system. Although the 20-bp deletion could account in part for decreased transcription of the colobus δ gene, the frameshift mutation by itself should not cause decreased transcription of the rhesus δ gene.

The only differences in the promoter sequences of these different δ-globin genes consist of three base substitutions at positions –92, –52, and –23 from the cap site; the base change at position –52 was not found in the baboon (483). Thus, it has been proposed that one (or both) of the other differences between the human and monkey sequences may be the primary cause of the silencing of the δ gene in all of the Old World monkeys by markedly decreasing the transcriptional activity of the gene (483).

In an evolutionarily more distant prosimian, the brown lemur, a δ pseudogene has resulted from a crossover between the ψβ1 gene and the δ gene, leading to the formation of a Leporelike fusion gene having the 5' end of the nonfunctional ψβ1 gene and the 3' end (including IVS-2) of the δ-globin gene (485).

γ-*Thalassemia.* Isolated thalassemia affecting the γ-globin gene has been identified during the course of cord blood screen-

TABLE 48-5. Molecular Defects Causing δ-Thalassemia[a]

Mutation	Phenotype δ⁰ or δ⁺	Racial Group	References
Gene deletion			
7.2 kb	0	Sardinian	479
Frameshift mutations			
Codon 59 (–A)	0	Greek	1601
		Egyptian	1602
Codon 91 (+T)	0	Belgian	1603
Splicing defects			
IVS-1, position 1 (T → C)	0	Italian	1604
IVS-2, 3' end (AG → GG)	0	Greek Cypriot	1605
? Codon 30 (G → C)	0	Southern Italian	1606
Amino acid substitutions			
Codon 27 (G → T) (Ala → Ser)	+	Sardinian	1604
		Greek Cypriot	1605
Codon 30 (G → C) (Arg → Thr) (? consensus splice site mutation)	0	Southern Italian	1606
Codon 116 (C → T) (Arg → Cys)	+	Greek	1605,1607
Codon 141 (T → C) (Leu → Pro)	+	Greek Cypriot	1605
GATA-1 consensus site			
–77 (T → C)	0	Japanese	480,481
Poly(A) addition site +69 (G → A)	+	Sardinian	482

IVS, intervening sequence.
[a]Additional mutations have been reported (http://globin.cse.psu.edu) (216).

ing surveys in infants with unusually high levels of the ᴬγ type of Hb F. Gene mapping studies revealed a deletion of 5 kb consistent with a nonhomologous crossover between ᴳγ-globin and ᴬγ-globin genes, creating a single fused γ-globin gene having the 5' end of the ᴳγ gene and the 3' end of the ᴬγ (486). Because the homozygous Indian child originally studied synthesized Hb F containing only ᴬγ^T chains with threonine instead of the usual isoleucine at position 75, the crossover in that family must have occurred 5' to codon 75 in the ᴬγ-globin gene, as the γ^T polymorphism has been identified only in ᴬγ-globin chains.

The (–γ) thalassemia deletion is analogous to the (–α) deletion causing α-thalassemia-2 and is the reciprocal product of the recombination event leading to chromosomes with triplicated γ-globin genes. Both single and triple γ-gene chromosomes are found in a number of different populations, especially Asian populations (487–489). The homozygous state for the (–γ) deletion is essentially asymptomatic and is characterized by a lower than normal percentage of Hb F in cord blood, all of which is of the ᴬγ type, and by a rapid decrease in the amount of Hb F in the first 2 to 3 months of life. Heterozygotes have an increased proportion of ᴬγ chains in cord blood Hb F; a similar phenotype can result from the inheritance of a chromosome with two ᴬγ genes (490).

A different deletion has been described that involves 2.5 kb of DNA encompassing the 5' end of the ᴬγ gene and constitutes a form of isolated ᴬγ⁰-thalassemia (491). Cord blood of affected children should have Hb F with disproportionately high levels of ᴳγ chains in heterozygotes and total absence of ᴬγ chains in homozygotes. A similar phenotype can result from inheritance of chromosomes with two ᴳγ genes (490), as observed in the Atlanta type of nondeletion HPFH (469) (discussed in the section Nondeletion Forms of δβ-Thalassemia and Hereditary Persistence of Fetal Hemoglobin).

A 4-bp deletion at positions –222 to –225 of the ᴬγ-globin gene promoter was found to be associated with unusually low levels of ᴬγ-chains in a black family (492) and in certain Sardinian β⁰-thalassemia (codon 39) patients (493), and may be the cause of a form of ᴬγ⁺-thalassemia. Other studies suggest that this small deletion is a common polymorphism that does not affect ᴬγ-globin gene expression (494).

IMPLICATIONS OF MOLECULAR FINDINGS FOR PRENATAL DIAGNOSIS AND GENE THERAPY

Prenatal Diagnosis

An important step in the prevention of cases of severe homozygous α- or β-thalassemia is the detection of the heterozygous state in adults of reproductive age. Physicians should be aware of the possibility of thalassemia trait occurring in persons with hypochromic anemias that are refractory to iron therapy, and they should perform the necessary diagnostic studies to confirm the diagnosis. In areas where a high incidence of thalassemia trait is present, general population screening is often available. Once identified, affected persons can be educated and counseled about the disease process and its genetics. Two affected heterozygotes contemplating marriage and planning to have a family should be aware of the one in four chance of having a severely affected homozygous child. Identification of such couples provides the opportunity for their counseling and education regarding the option of prenatal diagnosis. Nevertheless, such information rarely alters the reproductive behavior of couples at risk.

Prenatal diagnosis for hemoglobinopathies has gone through many changes during the past decade because of rapid advances in our understanding of the molecular basis of the thalassemias. Much of this new knowledge has been applied to prenatal diagnosis of thalassemia at the DNA level (224,296,495).

FETAL BLOOD SAMPLING

Before the availability of DNA-based diagnosis, prenatal diagnosis of thalassemia required fetal blood sampling at 18 to 20 weeks of gestation and analysis of globin chain synthesis by isotopic labeling and separation of globin chains to identify the quantitative defect in globin chain synthesis (496). Although fetal blood sampling has been successfully accomplished by various techniques in many medical centers, the procedure cannot be considered totally safe. In a few cases, fetal loss has occurred because of infection, hemorrhage, premature labor, or undetermined causes. It is estimated from large surveys of the worldwide experience with this procedure that even in the best of hands, there exists a risk of death or serious injury to the fetus in the order of approximately 5% (496), which is a much higher risk than that associated with amniocentesis.

With the availability of DNA-based prenatal diagnosis, the demand for prenatal diagnosis by fetal blood sampling and analysis of globin chain synthesis has decreased markedly. Fetal blood sampling is usually limited to cases in which DNA diagnosis is not possible, either because of lack of knowledge of the genotype of the parents or lack of sufficient information concerning linkage of RFLPs, or because the case presents itself too late in the course of the pregnancy to obtain the necessary baseline DNA information from parents and other family members. Such situations are becoming increasingly rare because of the speed and efficiency of DNA-based prenatal diagnosis using PCR.

DNA-BASED PRENATAL DIAGNOSIS

The characterization of thalassemia mutations at the DNA level has led to the application of various molecular techniques for the prenatal detection of thalassemia (224,296). The source of DNA may be amniotic fluid cells obtained by amniocentesis between 14 and 20 weeks of gestation or chorionic villi obtained by ultrasound-guided transcervical or transabdominal sampling (aspiration biopsy) between 8 and 10 weeks of gestation. The latter procedure is increasingly preferred because it allows much earlier diagnosis, counseling, and decision-making. Both procedures are considerably safer than fetal blood sampling.

DETECTION OF GLOBIN GENE DELETIONS

The earliest applications of molecular biology to prenatal detection of thalassemia consisted of molecular hybridization assays in solution or Southern gel blotting assays to detect thalassemia syndromes due to gene deletions, such as the common forms of α-thalassemia and $\delta\beta$-thalassemia. Theoretically, any thalassemia defect associated with an abnormal globin gene pattern on Southern gel blotting can be detected in this way. However, most of the demand for prenatal diagnosis involves pregnancies at risk for homozygous β-thalassemia, in which the molecular defects are mostly the result of point mutations rather than gene deletions.

USE OF RESTRICTION FRAGMENT LENGTH POLYMORPHISMS

A widely applied procedure for the prenatal diagnosis of thalassemia in the absence of gene deletion or of a direct assay for the gene mutation was developed after the characterization of RFLPs in the β-globin gene cluster (discussed in the section Polymorphisms of the Globin Gene Clusters). Thus, it is possible by Southern gel blotting to identify and track, in a given family, linkage of one or more polymorphisms to a β-thalassemic gene that is coinherited with the marker polymorphisms in the family.

Use of this technique for prenatal diagnosis of β-thalassemia is facilitated by the fact that polymorphisms occur at a high frequency at multiple different sites in the β-globin gene cluster and are associated with one another in a nonrandom fashion, forming haplotypes (Fig. 48-15) that are associated in a given population group with specific molecular forms of thalassemia. Thus, haplotype analysis of RFLPs in fetal DNA became a widely used and precise method to achieve prenatal diagnosis of β-thalassemia (497).

Although accurate, haplotype analysis remains a labor-intensive procedure requiring analysis of DNA from many family members using a number of different enzymes. With standard Southern gel blotting, this technique may also require substantial amounts of fetal DNA, which may not always be available. Finally, the test does not provide a definitive answer

in approximately 10% to 15% of cases because of lack of heterozygosity of RFLPs in key family members or lack of sufficient numbers or types of informative family members. For these various reasons, a procedure with 100% applicability would be preferred that can directly rather than indirectly identify mutations in a single assay requiring a small amount of DNA. Such procedures have been devised and are discussed in the following section.

DIRECT DEMONSTRATION OF POINT MUTATIONS IN DNA

Polymerase Chain Reaction. Point mutations causing β-thalassemia can be detected by Southern gel blotting of total cellular DNA followed by hybridization to allele-specific oligonucleotide (ASO) probes (498–500) (discussed in the section Direct Identification of Single Base Substitutions by the Use of Synthetic Oligonucleotide Probes). The introduction of the PCR has greatly facilitated the process of mutation detection (501,502). The PCR technique uses synthetic oligonucleotides corresponding to sequences flanking a DNA region of interest as primers for the amplification of this DNA segment. This is done in repeated cycles of DNA synthesis *in vitro*, using a DNA polymerase. The reaction is carried out in an automated apparatus that subjects the sample to repeated cycles of heating to denature the DNA, followed by lowering of the temperature to allow annealing of the primers to the denatured DNA and synthesis of DNA between the two primers by primer extension. A thermostable DNA polymerase is used, which is resistant to inactivation during the heating cycles. After 30 or more cycles, the target sequence is amplified approximately 1 million-fold over its starting concentration and can be seen as a discrete band after gel electrophoresis. Thus, starting with 1 µg total cellular DNA in which the β-globin gene is less than 1 part per million, the PCR technique can yield 1 µg of β-globin gene fragment.

The amplified DNA can then be subjected to various analyses, which are discussed in detail in sections that follow: (a) restriction endonuclease digestion and gel electrophoresis to visualize the digestion pattern, and (b) blotting of the DNA to filters (dot blots or slot blots) followed by hybridization with normal and mutant ASO probes. The PCR approach is much quicker and simpler than previously used techniques, such as Southern gel blotting of total cellular DNA followed by ASO hybridization. An added advantage is that only tiny amounts of DNA are required; thus, the size of the fetal tissue sample is almost never a limiting factor.

Although ^{32}P-labeled oligonucleotide probes are most frequently used, the procedure has been adapted to nonisotopic techniques, increasing its access to geographic areas where use of isotopes is not feasible or inconvenient (503,504). A longer shelf-life of probes can also be achieved by use of ^{35}S-labeled rather than ^{32}P-labeled adenosine triphosphate for end labeling of the oligonucleotide probes (505). Other modifications of the technique include the use of fluorescence-based color complementation assays (506), use of specific primers to amplify selectively only a normal or mutant allele (507), use of immobilized sequence-specific probes in nonisotopic detection assays (508), and PCR-based mutagenesis to create a restriction endonuclease cleavage site difference between a normal and a mutant allele (509,510). The PCR technique can also be used to detect RFLPs either singly (511) or in groups using multiplex reactions containing multiple sets of matched primer pairs. Thus, it is possible to perform haplotyping of β gene cluster RFLPs using one or two PCR reactions and direct visualization of the PCR products after enzyme digestion and gel electrophoresis, circumventing the need for multiple Southern gel blots and hybridization to multiple different ^{32}P-labeled probes (512).

TABLE 48-6. Common β-Thalassemia Mutations in Different Racial Groups

Mediterranean
    IVS-1 position 110 (G → A)
    Codon 39, nonsense
    IVS-1 position 1 (G → A)
    IVS-2 position 745 (C → G)
    IVS-1 position 6 (T → C)
    IVS-2 position 1 (G → A)
Black
    −29 (A → G)
    −88 (C → T)
    Poly(A), (AATAAA → AACAAA)
Southeast Asian
    Codons 41/42, frameshift
    IVS-2 position 654 (C → T)
    Codon 17, nonsense
    −28 (A → G)
Asian Indian
    IVS-1 position 5 (G → C)
    619-bp deletion
    Codons 8/9, frameshift
    Codons 41/42, frameshift
    IVS-1 position 1 (G → T)

IVS, intervening sequence.
Data from Kazazian HH Jr, Boehm CD. Molecular basis and prenatal diagnosis of β-thalassemia. *Blood* 1988;72:1107.

Identification of the Mutations in the Couple at Risk. Prenatal diagnosis of β-thalassemia by direct detection of point mutations using PCR or traditional approaches requires previous demonstration of the specific mutations present in the family at risk. In view of the multiplicity of β-thalassemic mutations (Table 48-2), this demonstration may appear a daunting task. However, a given mutation usually occurs within only one racial group, and within a given racial group, five or six specific mutations usually account for approximately 90% of all cases of β-thalassemia (224,296,495) (Table 48-6). In addition, a given mutation within a given racial group is usually associated with only one particular haplotype of β gene cluster RFLPs. Thus, when a couple who are at risk present for the first time for prenatal diagnosis of β-thalassemia, it should be relatively easy to establish the nature of the β-thalassemic mutation in each parent (and in any affected offspring) by using PCR-based technology to carry out haplotype analysis and screening for the most likely mutations, based on knowledge of the racial origin and haplotypes of the affected persons. In those cases in which a common mutation is not detected in this initial screening procedure, PCR can be used to amplify and directly sequence the β-globin genes of the undiagnosed parent to identify the nature of the mutation (225,513).

Another screening procedure to identify the general location of a point mutation is the technique of *denaturing gradient gel electrophoresis* (514). By initially determining the approximate location of a point mutation in the β-globin gene, the process of specific mutation identification by DNA sequence analysis can be achieved more quickly and efficiently. The technique consists of fractionating DNA fragments, usually PCR products, in a specialized acrylamide gel electrophoresis system that subjects the migrating DNA fragments to a gradient of denaturing forces. Thus, DNA fragments that are identical except for the presence of a single base substitution will denature and acquire altered mobility at different positions in the gel, because different DNA sequences usually require different conditions of denaturation for the two strands to separate or "melt." The differential mobility between mutant and normal fragments can be further enhanced by mixing them together and then subjecting them to denatur-

ation and renaturation, thus allowing the formation of heteroduplexes or hybrid DNA fragments in which one strand is normal and the complementary strand contains the base substitution.

The heteroduplexes are substantially more unstable than the parent molecules and thus are more widely separated from the parent molecules after gel electrophoresis. This technique, which was initially applied to the study of cloned globin genes, has also been used successfully to detect single base substitution in thalassemic globin genes by analysis of total cellular DNA digested with appropriate restriction enzymes (515) and, more recently, to identify β-thalassemic mutations efficiently in PCR-generated fragments derived from genomic DNA (516,517). Computer programs have been derived to facilitate the selection of the location and sequence of PCR primers that are most likely to provide the most efficient detection of mutations by this procedure (514). This technique constitutes another screening procedure for the identification of those carrying novel or specific mutations in a given region of a globin (or other) gene.

Direct Identification of Mutations by Differences in Restriction Endonuclease Cleavage Pattern Due to the Mutation Itself. A number of the base substitutions (or other subtle mutations) causing α-thalassemia or β-thalassemia abolish or create cleavage sites for different restriction endonucleases at the precise point of the mutation (495). They are therefore directly detectable by Southern gel blotting of total cellular DNA or enzymatic digestion and gel electrophoresis of appropriate PCR products. This approach was first used for the successful prenatal diagnosis of Hb O^{Arab} (β$^{121\ Glu}$→^{Lys}), in which the base substitution abolishes the intragenic *Eco*RI site of the β-globin gene (518). Widespread use of this approach occurred with the identification of restriction enzymes, such as *Mst*II, having recognition sites encompassing β-globin gene codon 6, which are abolished by the base substitution causing sickle cell Hb (β$^{6\ Glu}$→^{Val}). Direct detection of the β^S mutation using PCR followed by digestion of the PCR product with *Mst*II (or other enzymes with similar specificity) constitutes the method of choice for prenatal diagnosis of sickle cell anemia (519,520).

In β-thalassemia, approximately 30% to 40% of the mutations, including five of seven common Mediterranean mutations, are directly detectable by restriction endonuclease digestion of DNA (224,296,495). In some cases, the size of the affected DNA fragments is small, making detection difficult or impossible by traditional Southern gel blotting but not by analysis of PCR products. Nevertheless, some common forms of β-thalassemia, such as the IVS-1 position 110 mutation, do not directly affect restriction endonuclease sites and are therefore not normally detectable by enzymatic digestion and gel analysis. A different strategy was initially devised for the direct DNA diagnosis of these thalassemic mutations, as described in the following section.

Direct Identification of Single Base Substitutions by the Use of Synthetic Oligonucleotide Probes. The precedent-setting work of Wallace and colleagues (521,522) established the feasibility of direct detection of single nucleotide base substitutions in globin gene DNA by the use of labeled synthetic oligonucleotide probes approximately 19 nucleotides long, in which the central nucleotide is either identical with or different from that of the target DNA sequence being analyzed. Hybridization conditions were established that would allow annealing of the synthetic probe to its target only if all 19 nucleotides were perfectly complementary. If the one central nucleotide was different, no hybridization was observed. Thus, it was possible to distinguish with such oligonucleotide probes DNA containing the β^A-globin gene from that containing the β^S-globin gene, initially in cloned DNA samples, then in total cellular DNA. This ability established the basis for using this procedure in the prenatal detection of β-thalassemic point mutations in fetal DNA samples.

The general strategy for this approach consists of using two ASO probes: one complementary to the normal sequence, the other complementary to the mutant sequence with a single nucleotide substitution. By using the different probes in parallel or sequential hybridization assays, the presence or absence of the normal or the mutant sequence can be detected in the test sample, allowing the detection of heterozygotes as well as homozygotes for the target sequences. Before the introduction of PCR, this procedure was applied to the study of total cellular DNA. Because total cellular DNA contains multiple regions that can hybridize to a given 19-base oligonucleotide, it was not possible to carry out the analysis directly on dots or spots of total unfractionated DNA. If the DNA was first digested with a restriction endonuclease and fractionated by agarose gel electrophoresis, it became possible to separate the specific target DNA fragment containing the β-globin gene away from the nonspecifically hybridizing fragments located elsewhere in the genome (522).

*Bam*HI is a convenient enzyme for detecting β-thalassemic mutations (498–500). It yields a 1.8-kb fragment containing the 5' end of the β-globin gene, which is well separated from higher molecular weight fragments that hybridize to oligonucleotide probes corresponding to sequences in exon 1, exon 2, or IVS-1 of the β-globin gene, the sites of common point mutations causing β-thalassemia.

With the introduction and availability of PCR, use of ASO hybridization has been made much simpler and quicker. Because of the tremendous amplification of the target sequence, the background hybridization to nonspecific DNA sequences is negligible relative to the authentic hybridization signal. Thus, it is not necessary to fractionate the sample; it can be directly applied to filters and hybridized to the probes. Nevertheless, the specificity of the hybridization and washing conditions must be established for each probe set to ensure accuracy of the assay. Conditions for specificity may vary between different probe sets because of differences in the G+C content of the probes and the nature of the single base-pair mismatch that disrupts hybridization; that is, G to T mismatches are more stable than A to C mismatches.

As stated, it is possible to use nonisotopically tagged probes, which have the advantage of a long shelf-life, providing more flexibility to the assay (503,504). Such probes usually consist of oligonucleotides tagged with horseradish peroxidase or with biotin (or other haptens) and are detected by histochemical assay or enzyme-linked immunosorbent assay. A variation on the nonisotopic detection assay uses reverse dot hybridization, in which the unmodified oligonucleotide probe is immobilized on a filter and the target DNA is amplified using biotinylated primers (508).

Allele-specific oligonucleotide probes are commonly used in the detection of those thalassemia mutations for which there is no detection assay using naturally occurring restriction enzyme sites. Nevertheless, in such cases, it is frequently possible to generate by PCR-based mutagenesis restriction enzyme sites, which distinguish the mutant from the normal allele (509,510), or to use allele-specific primers for the PCR reaction, which allow the amplification of only the normal or mutant allele (507). This latter approach is called *amplification refractory mutation system* (ARMS) and has been widely used for the prenatal diagnosis of β-thalassemia (522–525). This technique relies on the ability of properly designed normal and mutation-specific primers to allow the exclusive amplification of DNA containing the normal or the mutant allele, respectively. ARMS-PCR is rapid and inexpensive, making it the preferred technique for prenatal diagnosis of β-chain hemoglobinopathies in developing countries.

Finally, approaches have been developed to isolate fetal nucleated RBCs from the maternal circulation as a source of DNA for PCR-based prenatal diagnosis of hemoglobinopathies (526).

A detailed description of DNA-based approaches to the diagnosis of hemoglobinopathies has recently been published (527).

SUMMARY AND CONCLUSIONS

Safe, rapid, and accurate procedures are available for the prenatal diagnosis of thalassemia. The method of choice consists of chorionic villus biopsy performed between 8 and 10 weeks of gestation. DNA extracted from the sample is then amplified by using PCR or ARMS-PCR and the amplified DNA analyzed by gel electrophoresis or by hybridization of slot–dot blots with ASOs. Systematic programs to educate the public and provide comprehensive testing and counseling services in countries and regions where the prevalence of thalassemia is high have resulted in a dramatic decrease in the incidence of new cases of the disease in recent years (520–522). Information regarding laboratories providing DNA-based diagnosis of thalassemia mutations can be obtained from the Web site http://www.genetests.com.

Gene Therapy and Manipulation of Gene Expression

GENE TRANSFER APPROACHES

It is clear from the heterogeneity and nature of the molecular defects that cause thalassemia that any practical attempts at gene therapy for thalassemia should be directed at substituting, by various gene transfer technologies, normal globin genes for the defective thalassemic genes, rather than directly correcting the specific defect associated with the mutant gene. Nevertheless, a number of targeted, mutation-specific approaches have been proposed. One such approach is the potential for correcting the effect of nonsense mutations in thalassemic globin mRNAs by the transfer of suppressor transfer RNA genes into hematopoietic stem cells, thus providing erythroid cells with a means of translating the mutant globin mRNA into a full-length, functional globin chain. The mutant β-globin mRNA associated with the nonsense mutation at β-globin codon 17 has been successfully translated into normal β-globin chains in frog oocytes after transfer into these cells of genes for an amber suppressor transfer RNA capable of inserting a lysine at the position of a UAG chain termination codon (528).

Although attractive on a theoretical level, this approach is not being actively pursued as a possible modality of human gene therapy.

Other approaches to targeted correction of disorders of globin gene expression include (a) correction of alternative splicing due to thalassemic mutations by antisense oligonucleotides capable of modifying pre-mRNA splicing (529,530); (b) use of triplex-forming (or other) oligonucleotides to carry out site-directed mutagenesis of single nucleotides, thereby correcting single base changes that cause β-thalassemia or sickle cell disease (531–533); and (c) ribozyme-mediated *trans*-splicing techniques to repair mutant globin mRNAs (534). The applicability in practice of such technologies in actual future therapy of thalassemia remains unclear.

With regard to gene therapy by transfer of normal globin genes into hematopoietic stem cells, a number of obstacles must be overcome: those related to the level of expression of globin genes after transfer into a foreign chromosomal environment, and those related to the cell biology of hematopoietic stem cells and the difficulty of introducing genes into the self-renewing or reconstituting hematopoietic stem cell. Great progress has been made in the technical ability to transfer globin gene DNA into a variety of tissue culture cells as well as into primary hematopoietic cells of the bone marrow (535–538). It has become apparent during the course of these experiments that the transferred globin genes are not usually expressed at high levels in their new chromosomal environment and that the marrow cells successfully transfected are not predominantly self-renewing.

RETROVIRAL VECTORS

The most efficient method of transferring genes into cells is by the use of retroviral vectors (535–538). The gene of interest is inserted into a DNA copy of the virus from which most of the viral genes and control elements have been removed. The DNA is then transfected into a viral packaging cell line that produces all of the necessary components to package RNA copies of the modified retroviral genome into infectious viral particles. After entry of these particles into a target cell, a DNA copy of the viral genome (produced by the reverse transcription of the viral RNA) is integrated randomly into the chromosomal DNA of the host cell. Because the modified retroviral genome lacks essential genes, such as those for viral envelope proteins, no further cycles of viral production can occur. Nevertheless, the integrated viral genome can be transcribed and can produce mRNA copies of the gene inserted into it for the purpose of gene therapy. In globin gene transfers, the retrovirus is constructed in such a way that the globin gene is transcribed from its own promoter in an opposite direction from that of viral gene transcription, which occurs from the promoter of the viral long terminal repeat sequence.

One of the earliest successful globin gene transfer experiments in a long-term living animal model system was performed by Dzierzak et al. (539). This experiment illustrated some of the practical difficulties of the approach that must be overcome before future applications in humans. The human β-globin gene was successfully transferred by means of a retrovirus into self-renewing hematopoietic stem cells of mice; this was evidenced by the fact that DNA of the transferred globin retrovirus was still detectable in blood cells of the mice 4 to 9 months after transplantation of the virally transduced bone marrow cells. The extent of donor marrow cell engraftment varied between 40% and 98%, whereas the efficiency of infection of the engrafted donor marrow cells ranged between 2% and 100%. The transferred human globin gene was expressed in virtually a tissue-specific manner, with globin mRNA detected in significant amounts essentially only in erythroid cells, although trace amounts were observed in lymphoid cells and macrophages of some of the animals (539). A disappointing result was the very low level of β-globin mRNA expression that was estimated to correspond to only 0.4% to 4.0% of the level of the endogenous murine β-globin mRNA when considered on a single copy per genome basis. Another disappointing observation was that the human β-globin genes were expressed in only 17% of the transplanted animals. This low efficiency of transduction was attributed to low viral titers and suboptimal transduction conditions. Nonetheless, these experiments demonstrated the feasibility of long-term expression of a transduced β-globin gene in erythroid cells *in vivo*, albeit at a level that is not sufficient to ameliorate the clinical manifestations of human Hb disorders. These findings were also confirmed independently by other groups (540,541). The transduction of the pluripotent hematopoietic stem cell in those studies was demonstrated by serial marrow reconstitution in secondary recipients (541,542).

An important feature of the normal chromosomal environment that confers a high level of expression to globin genes is the LCR (106,129,132–136) (discussed in the section Enhancers and Other *cis*-Acting Sequences That Influence Globin Gene Expression). It was therefore thought that incorporation of LCR sequences into the retroviral vectors would overcome the problem of low expression levels. Unfortunately, initial attempts to include LCR sequences in gene transfer vectors had unexpected deleterious effects on the ability to obtain retroviral stocks of sufficiently high titer to be efficient vehicles for gene transfer into bone marrow hematopoietic stem cells (543). Nevertheless, the use of LCR-containing retroviral vectors for human β-globin gene transfers into MEL tissue culture cells did result in enhanced levels of expression of the transferred gene (544–547), which, in some cell lines, was equal to or higher than that of the endogenous murine β-globin gene (544,545). Mice were also successfully engrafted with LCR/β-globin retrovirus-transduced hematopoietic stem cells and expressed significantly higher levels of human β-globin than in previous studies (547).

More recently, a number of different groups have described the production of genetically stable retroviral vectors that can give rise to high level expression of transferred globin genes in transduced erythroid cells. Previous studies by Miller et al. (543) had suggested that sequences within IVS-2 may be responsible for the genetic instability of retroviruses that carry the β-globin gene. When Leboulch et al. (548) deleted a 372-bp fragment from IVS-2 of the β-globin gene, the titer of the corresponding retroviruses increased approximately tenfold with some improvement in genetic stability in the presence of simple β LCR cassettes (548). They also performed extensive site-directed mutagenesis of the human β-globin gene to remove all potential splice sites and polyadenylation sites that could interfere with the stable propagation of these retroviruses. Although these additional modifications did not increase the titers further, they appeared to improve stability in the presence of complex β LCR cassettes. The viral titers ranged from 10^4 to 10^5 colony-forming units/mL, and the expression of the β-globin gene in transduced MEL cells ranged between 54% and 108% of the mouse β^{maj}-globin gene (548). When bone marrow cells were transduced with a retrovirus of this type and transplanted into lethally irradiated mice, long-term expression of human β-globin mRNA, at variable but generally low levels, was observed in only a small percentage of the mice that survived more than 4 months (549).

Sadelain et al. (550) used a similar strategy in which a portion of IVS-2 was deleted from the β-globin gene in retroviral vectors that carried multiple core hypersensitive sites from the β LCR in different configurations (550). They examined a large number of such recombinant retroviruses and were able to identify only one genetically stable retrovirus that contained the modified β-globin gene linked to the core elements of HS2, HS3, and HS4. Although stocks of this retroviral vector had titers greater than 10^6 colony-forming units/mL, the expression of the integrated β-globin gene in transduced erythroid cells was clearly not position independent. The level of expression of the transduced human β-globin gene in cultured MEL cells ranged from 4% to 146% of the murine β-globin gene. They concluded that even though their β LCR cassette demonstrated significant enhancer activity, it clearly did not satisfy the criteria of position independence that defines LCR function (550). Primary murine bone marrow cells were efficiently transduced by this retrovirus, but after transplantation, human β-globin mRNA expression decreased from a level of 5 ± 5% at 10 weeks posttransplantation to undetectable levels at 4 months (537).

Ren et al. (551) used a totally different approach in an attempt to solve the problems of genetic instability and low level expression of globin genes in transduced erythroid cells (551). They incorporated the human γ-globin gene instead of the β-globin gene in their retroviral vectors. They also replaced the β LCR element with the much simpler α LCR-like enhancer (i.e., HS-40) to stimulate the expression of the target globin gene in an erythroid-specific manner. These two modifications allowed the generation of retroviral vectors whose titers exceeded 7 × 10^6 colony-forming units/mL. These retroviruses were capable of expressing the transferred γ-globin gene at a high level in a position-independent manner in cultured MEL cells (551). Unfortunately, transduction of bone marrow cells with this type of retrovirus followed by transplantation into mice did not result in the expression of human γ-globin mRNA *in vivo* (552).

Subsequently, Sadelain et al. (553) inserted their β-globin gene cassette, as well as another cassette containing larger fragments of the β LCR HSs, into a lentiviral vector derived from human immunodeficiency virus type-1 (HIV-1). Such vectors have the ability to regulate packaging of unspliced viral genomes, thereby avoiding splicing and other alterations such as rearrangements that can affect stability and transduction efficiency of the recombinant genomes. Long-term engraftment of unselected transduced murine bone marrow cells was achieved, with expression and accumulation of human β-globin chains at a level up to 13% of the total β-chains. When marrow cells from heterozygous β-thalassemic mice were similarly transduced and transplanted, the levels of human β-globin chains ranged between 17% and 24% (553). Such expression levels could potentially be of therapeutic benefit if they could be achieved after transduction of human thalassemic bone marrow cells.

A more detailed discussion of approaches to gene therapy for Hb disorders, including the use of alternative vector systems, has recently been published by Sorrentino and Nienhuis (538).

Potential safety problems associated with the use of retroviral vectors as gene transfer vehicles include the following (554): insertional mutagenesis due to the random nature of the DNA integration event, resulting either in inactivation of an essential gene or inappropriate activation of a nearby latent, potentially harmful gene such as a protooncogene; and inadvertent infection of the marrow and therefore the patient with oncogenic wild-type retrovirus, which may contaminate the gene transfer virus stock because of recombination with the viral genome in the packaging cell line. Although these are definite risks, they occur very infrequently. In particular, the use of more recently developed disabled viruses and newer generations of packaging cell lines has greatly reduced the risk of contaminating wild-type retroviruses.

GENE TARGETING APPROACH

An alternative approach to the problem of low expression levels of transferred globin genes is to attempt targeted insertion by homologous recombination. Although targeted transfer of globin and other genes has been successfully accomplished in tissue culture cells as well as in mouse embryonic stem cells, such homologous recombination events occur at a very low frequency (555–557). To be useful in practical terms for gene therapy, this targeting approach requires the ability to carry out selection and subsequent *in vitro* expansion of the rare cell in which the event has taken place. Unfortunately, *in vitro* techniques for selection and expansion of self-renewing hematopoietic stem cells are not readily available. Recently, however, Kyba and his colleagues have devised a method for converting ES cells to hematopoietic stem cells, using the HoxB4 gene product (557a). This technique was combined with nuclear transfer (cloning) and homologous recombination to correct a genetic defect of the lymphoid system in a proof-of-principle experiment in mice (557b). In theory, it should be possible to make customized, genetically corrected human hematopoietic stem cells by similar approaches, although much preliminary work must first be done. Further progress along these lines can be anticipated in the near future.

STEM CELL BIOLOGY

For gene therapy to be effective, the gene must be transferred into the self-renewing hematopoietic stem cell. If the gene is transferred only into the more differentiated, nonself-renewing progenitor or precursor cells, the cell lineage containing the transferred gene will persist only transiently. Unfortunately, the efficiency of gene transfer into hematopoietic stem cells is generally much lower than the efficiency of transfer into committed progenitors, which may be in part a result of the presence of very low levels of amphotropic retrovirus receptors in murine and human hematopoietic stem cells (558). In addition, gene transfer with chromosomal integration using retroviral vectors requires cell division. The majority of the self-renewing stem cells in the bone marrow are usually in the nondividing (G_0) phase of the cell cycle and are therefore relatively refractory to successful gene transfer. Although transfer of globin (and other) genes into the self-renewing hematopoietic stem cell of the mouse has been successfully accomplished (539), experiments in larger animal species have been generally disappointing, and suggest that gene transfer into self-renewing hematopoietic stem cells of these species occurs at too low a level to achieve any practical therapeutic impact. One approach to this problem is the exposure of the bone marrow to various combinations of hematopoietic growth factors—before or during infection with the retroviral vector—to stimulate the self-renewing cell to enter into the cell cycle and divide.

Experiments in the murine model system indicate that a higher proportion of reconstituting or self-renewing stem cells can be infected after prestimulation of the marrow *in vitro* with hematopoietic growth factors such as interleukin (IL)-3 and IL-6 (542,559). The addition of stem cell factor (kit ligand) to IL-3 and IL-6 may also be beneficial (560,561). Such prestimulation approaches, combined with the use of high-titer viral producer cell lines, have resulted in the successful transfer of a retroviral vector into self-renewing stem cells of the rhesus monkey, but at a very low frequency of approximately 1% of the reconstituting stem cells (562–565). More recently, the efficiency of transfer into rhesus monkey hematopoietic stem cells was shown to be enhanced significantly by priming with stem cell factor and granulocyte colony-stimulating factor *in vivo*. More than 5% of the circulating cells in these monkeys contained the retroviral genome up to 1 year after transplantation (566).

In conclusion, much progress in the successful transfer of globin (and other) genes into hematopoietic cells has been achieved, but more progress is required before gene therapy by globin gene transfer is a reality for the management of thalassemia. If advances in this field continue to occur with the same explosive rapidity as they have, numerous breakthroughs can be anticipated, and perhaps the realization of what has been for many the impossible dream. In fact, successful gene therapy for severe combined immunodeficiency –X1 disease by retroviral transduction of bone marrow CD34+ cells has been reported (567).

CLINICAL ASPECTS OF THE THALASSEMIAS

Thalassemia Syndromes

The primary biochemical abnormality in the thalassemias is a quantitative defect in the synthesis or accumulation of one or more of the polypeptide chains of Hb (568). Reduced synthesis of one or another of the globin chains of adult Hb, Hb A ($\alpha_2\beta_2$) results in an overall deficit of Hb accumulation in red cells, and hypochromic-microcytic anemia in the heterozygous and homozygous states. In the homozygous state, the continued synthesis in normal amounts of the nonaffected globin chain results in the accumulation within the thalassemic erythroid cells of excessive amounts of normal chains (569). These chains form unstable aggregates that become oxidized and precipitate within the cell, causing physical and oxidative damage of its membrane and premature destruction of the red cell.

The thalassemia syndromes are usually classified according to the type of globin chain that is absent, or present in decreased amounts. The two major categories are the α-thalassemias and β-thalassemias, each of which can be subdivided into a number of different subtypes that may be inherited in the heterozygous state, in the homozygous state, or in various doubly heterozygous states to generate a large number of diverse clinical and hematologic syndromes.

World Distribution and Population Genetics

The thalassemia syndromes are widespread throughout the Mediterranean region, Africa, the Middle East, the Indian subcontinent and Burma, Southeast Asia, southern China, the Malay peninsula, and Indonesia (570,571). Although an inhomogeneous distribution of the disease precludes accurate gene frequencies in many populations, estimates vary between 3% and 10% in these areas. A high frequency of this disorder arising independently in different regions points to the action of a local selective agent (572). As proposed over 50 years ago (573,574), the high frequency of the α-thalassemias (575,576) and almost certainly of the β-thalassemias (572,577) is a reflection of heterozygote advantage against *Plasmodium falciparum* malaria (578). α-Thalassemia appears to enhance the susceptibility of children to infection with *Plasmodium vivax* and, to a lesser extent, to *P. falciparum* at a time when maternal immunity and other factors may still confer some protection against these infections (575). Thus, early increased exposure to *P. vivax* may act as a natural vaccine, inducing cross-species protection later in life against the more dangerous *P. falciparum* (576,578). Varying susceptibility to malaria may also be reflected by polymorphisms at other loci (578–582).

β-Thalassemias

The majority of the β-thalassemias are caused by mutations at the β-globin gene loci that result in either no output of β-globin chains, or β^0-thalassemia; or a reduced output, or β^+-thalassemia. Hence, compound heterozygotes may be heterozygous for both β^+- and β^0-thalassemia, or for two different forms of either β^0- or β^+-thalassemia. The term β^{++}-*thalassemia* is sometimes used to describe β-thalassemia with a particularly mild reduction in β-chain synthesis (583,584). Within each population at risk for β-thalassemia are found a small number of common mutations as well as some rarer ones; each mutation exists in strong linkage dysequilibrium with specific arrangements of RFLPs, or haplotypes, within the β-globin cluster. A limited number of haplotypes is found in each population at risk, such that 80% of β-thalassemia mutations appear to arise in only 20 different haplotypes (585). This observation has proven of considerable value in evolutionary studies of the β-globin genes and has helped demonstrate the independent origin of β-thalassemia in several populations (586).

The β-thalassemias have extremely diverse phenotypes (569). At the severe end of the spectrum are homozygous and compound heterozygous states, which are characterized by profound anemia. They present to medical attention in the first year of life, and subsequently require regular transfusions for survival (587)—the condition known as β-*thalassemia major*. Many patients with inheritance of two mutant β alleles have a milder illness, with a broad range of severity—from only slightly less severe than thalassemia major to an asymptomatic state. This group of patients with varying severity who present later or remain largely transfusion-free are said to have *thalassemia intermedia*. The terms *thalassemia major* and *intermedia* have no specific molecular correlate and encompass a wide spectrum of clinical and laboratory abnormalities (588). A period of observation and folate repletion after diagnosis may be useful in sorting out the phenotypes of thalassemia intermedia. These may include patients in whom early growth and development is normal, and whose well-compensated anemia may be exacerbated only by infection, folate deficiency, or increasing hypersplenism (587–590), but who, with advancing age, may develop osteopenia,

tissue iron loading, or ectopic marrow expansion. The classic changes of untreated thalassemia major are now regularly observed only in countries without resources to support long-term transfusion programs (570).

Even individuals with the heterozygous (carrier) state for β-thalassemia exhibit wide phenotypic diversity. Although usually associated with mild asymptomatic anemia, the effect of inheritance of a single thalassemic allele may vary from no definable hematologic abnormalities to a phenotype as severe as the major forms of the disease, known as *dominantly inherited β-thalassemia* (578,591–595).

GENOTYPE/PHENOTYPE RELATIONSHIPS

Although it is relatively easy to define the most severe and mildest phenotypes of β-thalassemia, many forms in between are difficult to categorize. Further, the phenotype of β-thalassemia is often not static but may vary with age, progressive splenomegaly, recurrent infections, and other factors, and some complications of the disease are unrelated to the levels of steady-state Hb. The remarkable variability in clinical severity of the β-thalassemias reflects both genetic and environmental factors. The genetic modifiers may be classified as *primary*, including the different mutations that underlie β-thalassemia; *secondary*, or loci involved in globin synthesis; and *tertiary*, those factors not involved in globin synthesis that modify disease complications in other ways (578) (Fig. 48-23).

Primary Modifiers of Clinical Severity. More than 200 different mutations have been identified as causing β-thalassemia (596). Some of these are β^0 mutations, which are usually but not always associated with a severe phenotype, and β^+ mutations or β^{++} mutations, which are diverse in their effects on β-chain output. A few rare β-thalassemia mutations are completely silent, with no demonstrable effect in carriers (597–599); certain alleles are associated with minor disease in heterozygotes and intermediate disease in homozygotes; and several mutations may cause severe disease in the heterozygous state (600,601).

Secondary Modifiers of Clinical Severity. Anything that modifies the magnitude of the surfeit of α-chain should have an important effect on the severity of β-thalassemia. Two such modifiers include the coinheritance of α-thalassemia and increased synthesis of Hb F. Coinheritance of α-thalassemia can ameliorate the severity of β-thalassemia (569,602). Although red cells with individuals with both α-thalassemia and β-thalassemia are grossly underhemoglobinized, the anemia is less severe because of the overall reduction in imbalance of globin chains (578,603).

Several determinants within the β-globin cluster are involved in determining the level of Hb F in β-thalassemia (604,605). Deletions involving the cluster or point mutations in the promoters of one of the γ-globin genes result in persistent synthesis of high levels of Hb F in adults (569,570,606,607). A common polymorphism at position −158 in the Gγ gene in homozygous individuals is associated with increased synthesis of Hb F (585,608–611). There are also genetic determinants that are not encoded by the β-globin gene cluster that increase the output of Hb F in some patients (590,612–615). Many different interactions with structural Hb variants may also result in a complex series of clinical phenotypes. The interactions of β-thalassemia with different structural Hb variants have been reviewed recently (569). Only two, Hb S and Hb E, are of global importance. The laboratory and clinical manifestations of Hb E are described in a later section. Hb S is discussed in Chapter 50.

Tertiary Modifiers of Clinical Severity. Finally, a number of acquired and environmental factors (616), including progressive splenomegaly, exposure to infections, social conditions and the

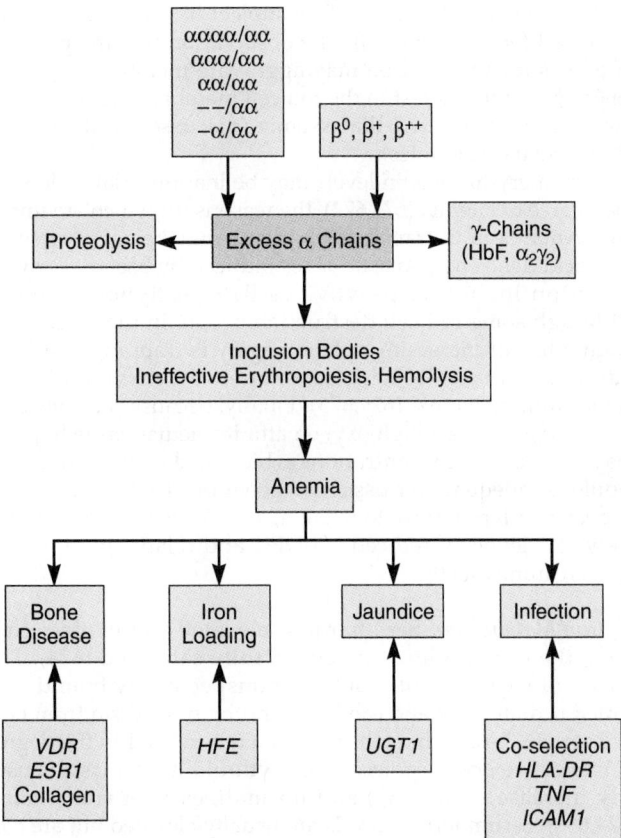

Figure 48-23. Summary of genetic mechanisms that contribute to the phenotypic diversity of β-thalassemia. The secondary modifiers—that is, the α-globin and γ-globin genes—are shown at the top of the figure, as they affect the magnitude of the excess of α-chains. The tertiary modifiers are shown at the bottom of the figure: VDR, vitamin D receptor; ESR1, estrogen receptor; collagen, several genes determined in collagen synthesis; HbF, fetal hemoglobin; HFE, the locus for hereditary hemochromatosis; HLA-DR, major histocompatibility complex locus; ICAM1, intercellular adhesion molecule 1; TNF, tumor necrosis factor-α; UGT1, UGT glucuronosyltransferase involved in bilirubin glucuronidation. (From Weatherall DJ. Phenotype-genotype relationships in monogenic disease: lessons from the thalassaemias. *Nat Rev Genet* 2001;2:245–255, with permission.)

availability of medical care, may also modify the phenotype of β-thalassemia. As well, polymorphisms affecting bilirubin metabolism (617,618), iron metabolism (619–621), bone disease (622,624), and susceptibility to infections, especially malaria (575,576,578–582), may influence the phenotype of β-thalassemia (Fig. 48-23).

In the following section, the main laboratory features of severe β-thalassemia are described.

HOMOZYGOUS β-THALASSEMIA

Peripheral Blood and Bone Marrow. Homozygous β-thalassemia is characterized by severe hypochromic and microcytic anemia and marked abnormalities of red cell morphology, including anisocytosis, poikilocytosis, misshapen microcytes, occasional macrocytes, target cells, and erythroblasts (Fig. 48-24) (625). Before and after splenectomy, ragged inclusion bodies in the cytoplasm of nucleated red cells and reticulocytes consisting of precipitated α-chains are evident after incubation with methyl violet (626). In well transfused patients, the blood picture may appear virtually normal, reflecting almost total suppression of endogenous erythropoiesis. The total white cell and platelet counts are normal or slightly elevated; neutropenia and thrombo-

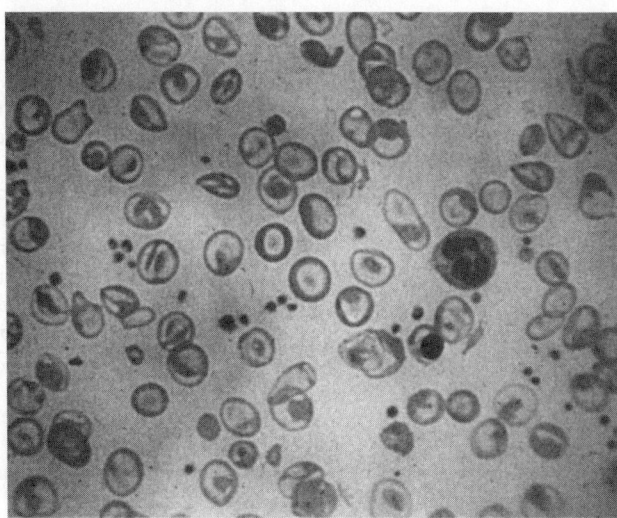

Figure 48-24. Peripheral blood of thalassemia major. Marked hypochromia anisocytosis and poikilocytosis and nucleated red blood cells are notable. Many of the red blood cells contain dense masses of precipitated α-globin chains (inclusion bodies) not visible in the Wright stain.

cytopenia may reflect hypersplenism or folate deficiency. There is a variable degree of anemia. In some of the dominantly inherited forms of β-thalassemia, hypochromia is less marked, and poikilocytosis is the main feature (578,592–595).

In the peripheral blood, red cell survival is reduced, with values ranging from 7 to 22 days (627–629), and is not directly related to the level of Hb F or severity of anemia (630). Red cell survival studies in milder genotypes may be slightly longer, varying from 10 to 16 days (631,632). The osmotic fragility is markedly decreased. Levels of glucose-6-phosphate dehydrogenase are elevated, reflecting the young age of the red cells (578).

The bone marrow in untransfused patients is characterized by intense erythroid hyperplasia, reflected in an alteration in the myeloid to erythroid ratio from the normal 3 or 4 to 0.1 or less. If the marrow is incubated with methyl violet, Fessas bodies will be found in large numbers within erythroid precursors, in which they result in intramedullary hemolysis and ineffective erythropoiesis (632). Extensive findings characteristic of the thalassemic marrow have been recently reviewed (578).

Ferrokinetics and Erythrokinetics. There is gross ineffective erythropoiesis (628,633). Plasma iron turnover is higher than in any other disease, up to ten times greater than normal; red cell iron turnover is only slightly elevated (634), representing a massive breakdown of developing red cells in the bone marrow. Marked suppression of erythropoiesis after blood transfusion has been demonstrated (635).

Other Changes. Hemolysis may be reflected by a mild elevation of unconjugated bilirubin, low or absent haptoglobin and hemopexin (636,637), and increased plasma Hb (638) and methemalbumin (639). There is increased urobilinogen in the feces (640), increased level of urates in the urine, and elevated serum uric acid. There is a postnatal persistence of i antigen, possibly related to the marrow transit time, and a decrease of the red cell enzyme carbonic anhydrase (641,642).

Hemoglobin Constitution. The red cells in severe forms of β-thalassemia contain increased amounts of Hb F, the main diagnostic feature of the disorder (569). Homozygous β⁰-thalassemics have only Hb F and A₂; Hb A is absent. The level of Hb F in β⁺-thalassemia homozygotes is variable and is always elevated after the first few months of life (643,644), although insufficiently to compensate for reduced β-chain synthesis and relative α-chain excess. The production of Hb F in β-thalassemia reflects marked erythroid expansion, which may favor γ-chain synthesis in the postnatal period, together with selective survival of red cell precursors and mature red cells that have relatively higher levels of γ-chain production and hence less severe globin–chain imbalance (645,646). These mechanisms together account for synthesis of between 2 and 4 g/dL Hb F; greater synthesis is associated with specific β-thalassemia alleles or other genetic determinants within, or linked to, the β-globin complex. At least two other determinants that may affect Hb F synthesis appear to be unlinked to the β-globin gene cluster: one on chromosome 6 (647) and the other on the X chromosome (613,648).

There is heterogeneity in the amount of Hb F in the red cell (649–651), with no evidence that Hb F synthesis is localized to a single clone of red cells. The Gγ:Aγ ratios of Hb F show a broad scatter of values (652).

Hemoglobin A_2 levels in the homozygous or compound heterozygous states may be subnormal, normal, or elevated, and hence are of no diagnostic value. Occasionally, levels exceeding 10% are encountered, usually in association with deletions removing the 5' end of the β gene and its associated promoter regions, or in homozygotes or compound heterozygotes for β-thalassemia who also have inherited the genotype associated with Hb H disease. Hb A synthesis varies from 5% to 10% of normal in the case of severe alleles to a modest reduction in the case of the extremely mild or silent alleles. There seems to be a reciprocal relationship between Hb A and F synthesis (653). The only other abnormal finding on Hb electrophoresis is the occasional presence of free α-chains.

In Vitro Hemoglobin Synthesis. In nonthalassemic reticulocytes, α-chain and β-chain synthesis is nearly synchronous. If reticulocytes or bone marrow cells from patients with thalassemia are incubated with radioactive amino acids for a few minutes to several hours, a decrease in β-chain synthesis relative to α-chain synthesis in β-thalassemia, and a decrease in α-chain synthesis relative to β-chain synthesis in α-thalassemia, can be demonstrated (568,654–667). In severe β-thalassemia, the ratio of α/(β + γ) radioactivity varies considerably, with a published range of 1.5 to 30. The measurement of globin synthesis does not offer information about the absolute rates of synthesis of individual chains, but gives some indication of the overall severity of the defect in β-globin synthesis such that in less severe forms of β-thalassemia, the degree of imbalance of globin chain synthesis is less (631,658).

Mechanisms of Anemia. Imbalanced globin synthesis leads to a substantial amount of free α-chains in the red cells and their precursors (659). Ineffective erythropoiesis, the hallmark of β-thalassemia, is a result of the myriad deleterious effects of relative excess of α-chains (625). In severe untreated β-thalassemia, erythropoiesis may be increased up to tenfold, of which 5% or less may be effective. The relative excess of α-chains interferes with most stages of normal erythroid maturation: Both intramedullary death of red cell precursors through arrest in the G_1 phase of the cell cycle, and accelerated intramedullary apoptosis of late erythroblasts have been demonstrated (660–663). Accumulation of excess α-chains and their degradation products within the membrane and its skeleton also results in abnormalities in the spectrin to band 3 ratio and in the function of band 4.1 (662–667). Cross-linking of protein 3 molecules by hemichromes may occur and result in the formation of an external antigenic site for the binding of a specific antibody, which leads to premature destruction of the red cells in the reticuloendothelial system (668,669). This subject has been thoroughly reviewed (569,663,665,670). The observation that the presence of excess membrane iron may aggravate membrane changes (666) has led to interest in the red cell membrane as a potential therapeutic target in β-thalassemia (discussed in the section Experimental Therapies).

Serum erythropoietin levels may be inappropriately low for the degree of anemia (671,672), the reasons for which are uncertain. Anemia in untransfused patients may be aggravated by folic acid deficiency, aplastic crises induced by bacterial or viral infection including parvovirus B19, or hypersplenism. Although some red cell destruction occurs in the spleen, the main effect of increasing splenomegaly is trapping of a large number of red cells with consequent hypervolemia and hemodilution anemia (629,673). Finally, because red cells containing Hb F have a high oxygen affinity, actual tissue hypoxia may exist at Hb concentrations which, if the Hb were Hb A, would be adequate for tissue oxygenation. Thalassemic RBCs appear to adapt poorly to anemia, as reflected by inappropriately low levels of red cell 2,3-DPG and relatively increased oxygen affinity (569).

Iron Metabolism. Serum iron is elevated and in older children, the iron-binding capacity is fully saturated (674). The serum of such patients contains nonspecifically bound iron which is dialyzable and can be bound by transferrin from normal sera (675–679). Iron absorption likely related to the degree of ineffective erythropoiesis and erythroid hyperplasia is usually increased (680–682) and normalizes after transfusion (674,683). Serum ferritin levels are usually elevated but are correlated imprecisely with concentrations of tissue iron (discussed in the section Management).

A schematic outline of the interactions between the various pathophysiologic processes in severe β-thalassemia is illustrated in Figure 48-10.

CLINICAL FINDINGS IN SEVERE β-THALASSEMIA

Severe Transfusion-Dependent β-Thalassemia (Cooley's Anemia). The early descriptions of severe thalassemia by Cooley and Lee (684) and others (685,686) [reviewed in (569)] present a picture of the disease as it was, and still is, seen in children who have either not been transfused or have received inadequate transfusion. If children are adequately transfused, many of the "typical" features of thalassemia do not appear in early childhood, during which growth and development is usually normal. Most of the clinical problems in transfused patients develop as a result of iron accumulation after the first decade.

In the inadequately treated child and the child who has been transfused adequately, the disease phenotype is very different.

Age and Symptoms at Presentation. β-Thalassemia usually becomes manifest during the first year of life, as β-chain synthesis replaces γ-chain synthesis. The mean age at presentation may vary from 2 to 36 months (597,687). Although a later mean age at presentation has been observed in patients with nontransfusion-dependent β-thalassemia (569), many infants who eventually will be diagnosed with thalassemia major come to clinical attention well after the first year of life.

Diagnostic Difficulties at Presentation. Many infants may present with an acute infection and severe anemia and may be assumed to have a transfusion-dependent phenotype. Observation in the steady state may identify potential milder, intermediate forms of the disease possibly exacerbated by an intercurrent illness. In developing countries, difficulties may arise in an undiagnosed infant during coinfection with malaria and severe anemia and splenomegaly; reassessment after antimalarial treatment should confirm the diagnosis. Other diagnoses that may superficially resemble β-thalassemia may include severe iron deficiency, juvenile chronic myeloid leukemia, and congenital dyserythropoietic anemia (569), although usually, the clinical and laboratory findings differ markedly from those of β-thalassemia (569,688).

Course throughout Childhood in Inadequately Transfused Patients. Growth retardation, pallor, icterus, and the dirty gray-brown pigmentation first described (684) are observed. Failure to thrive and features of a hypermetabolic state are characteristic. Severe ineffective erythropoiesis, an increased plasma volume as a result of shunting through expanded marrow, and progressive hepatosplenomegaly exacerbate anemia. Increased erythropoietin synthesis may stimulate formation of extramedullary erythropoietic tissue, primarily in the thorax and paraspinal region. Marrow expansion results not only in characteristic deformities of the skull and face, with bossing of the skull, maxillary hypertrophy, and prominent malar eminences with depression of the bridge of the nose (Fig. 48-25), but also in osteopenia and focal defects in bone mineralization (623,689–691). Marrow hyperplasia leads to increased iron absorption, and ultimately to progressive tissue iron deposition. The characteristic radiologic changes include dilatation of the diploic space of the skull, with subperiosteal bone growth in a series of radiating striations and the typical "hair-on-end" appearance (Fig. 48-26). There may be cortical thinning and porous rarefaction of the long bones and of those of the hands and feet (692–695), and pathologic fractures (696).

Throughout early childhood, progressive bone deformity, folate deficiency, increasing hypersplenism, gallstones, recurrent ulceration of the legs, recurrent infections associated with worsening of the anemia, and tumor masses resulting from extramedullary hemopoiesis often complicate the clinical

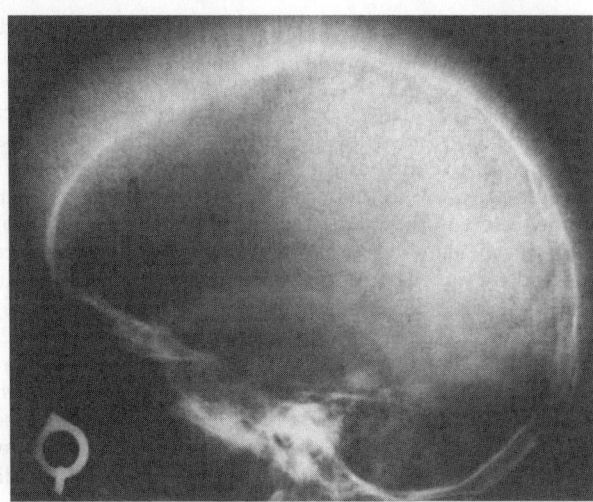

Figure 48-26. Lateral roentgenogram of the skull of a patient with thalassemia major. There is marked widening of the diploe of the skull, producing a "hair-on-end" appearance.

course (569,688). If they survive to puberty, these children may develop complications similar to those experienced by adequately transfused children. By contrast, in well transfused thalassemic children who usually remain asymptomatic until the second decade of life, morbidity and mortality are influenced by the adequacy of control of body iron burden (697,698).

MAJOR COMPLICATIONS OF SEVERE β-THALASSEMIA

Hypersplenism and Plasma-Volume Expansion. Progressive splenomegaly with shortening of the red cell survival, a marked expansion of the total blood volume, and trapping of up to 40% of the total red cell mass may be observed (629,673,699–701). These features are less frequently observed in adequately transfused children (698,702). Splenic enlargement may cause physical discomfort and may constitute a mass of ineffective hemopoietic tissue that increases the metabolic demands of the growing child.

Iron Overload. If not prevented or adequately treated, tissue iron overload is fatal in both transfused and untransfused patients (698). After approximately 1 year of transfusions, iron is deposited in parenchymal tissues (704), where it may cause significant toxicity, as compared to that within reticuloendothelial cells (676,705). As iron loading progresses, the capacity of serum transferrin, the main transport protein of iron, to bind and detoxify iron may be exceeded, and a "nontransferrin-bound" fraction of plasma iron may promote the generation of free hydroxyl radicals, propagators of oxygen-related damage (675,676,706). Although the body maintains a number of antioxidant mechanisms against free radical damage, in heavily iron-loaded patients, these may be inadequate to prevent oxidative damage.

In untransfused patients, abnormally regulated iron absorption results in increases in body iron burden which, depending on the severity of erythroid expansion, may vary between 2 and 5 g per year (707,708). Regular transfusions may double this rate of iron accumulation. Although most clinical manifestations of iron loading do not appear until the second decade of life even in inadequately chelated individuals, in many chronically transfused patients, iron-related tissue damage may occur as early as 8 years of age (709–713) and is common after age 11 years (703,714–719). During transfusion of the initial 50 to 100 units of blood, a steep rise in ferritin levels is observed, followed by a less marked rate of increase (720); the correlation between transfusion load

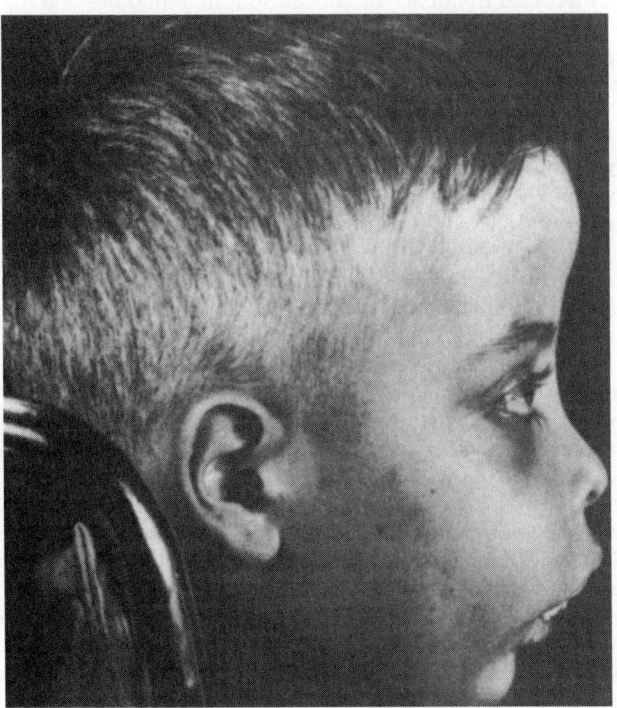

Figure 48-25. Profile of a 12-year-old boy with thalassemia major treated by a low transfusion regimen. He demonstrates a classic mongoloid facies. The skull is enlarged, and there is expansion of the maxilla with severe overbite.

and serum ferritin concentration is not clear (721), as described in the section Iron Chelating Therapy.

Cardiac Complications. Cardiac disease may reflect several pathologic processes, including chronic anemia, iron overload, pulmonary disease, myocarditis, and pericarditis. In irregularly transfused children, adaptive changes to hypoxia may include enhanced left ventricular contractility, elevated cardiac output, and left ventricular hypertrophy and dilatation; ultimately, profound anemia may induce congestive cardiac failure. Recently, observations of impaired relaxation patterns suggest a state of asymptomatic cardiac anoxia even in transfused patients (722). High transfusion regimens rescued many younger children from clinical cardiac failure due to anemia but, until effective iron chelating therapy was developed, merely deferred death to the second or third decade of life (723,724). Ventricular hypertrophy and conduction disturbances were frequently observed by late childhood, and ventricular arrhythmias and refractory congestive failure often developed by the mid-teens (724). The duration of life after the onset of cardiac failure was less than 3 months in over half the patients; one-third died within a month of onset. In addition to the effects of anemia and iron loading, myocarditis (158) and right heart strain due to chronic pulmonary hypertension (726) resulting in right heart failure (723,727,728) may also complicate the clinical course. Attacks of transient idiopathic pericarditis, once common (700,724,729–732), have been reported less frequently in recent years.

In adequately transfused patients in the present era, the magnitude of the body iron burden is the primary determinant of cardiac disease (698). Patients with body iron burdens corresponding to hepatic iron concentrations exceeding 15 mg/g liver, dry weight, have been shown to be at heightened risk of cardiac disease and premature death (733). Often there are no abnormalities until the rapid onset of overt cardiac failure (734). Effective use of deferoxamine results in long-term survival and the prevention of clinically apparent cardiac disease in most patients.

Cardiac Pathology and Pathophysiology. Autopsy studies reported diffuse rust-brown staining of the heart, right and left ventricular hypertrophy (711) and dilatation (723,724), a greatly increased cardiac weight, and pericarditis of unknown etiology (711,723,724,735). Iron content may be elevated up to 20 times normal with heterogeneous deposition of iron, maximally concentrated in the left ventricular epicardium (711,723,724,736,737). Preferential iron deposition in the epicardium, only later involving the transmural wall thickness, may explain the preservation of systolic ventricular function early in the course of disease. Although iron concentrations correlate reasonably well with the degree of dysfunction, in many patients who died of cardiac arrhythmias, iron deposition within the conduction system appears to be relatively mild (736,737). Fibrosis varied from minimal (711) to variable (723,724,736) to extensive (723,724,738), and may be unrelated to myocardial iron content (711,723,724,735,739–741).

Very low levels of myocardial iron may interfere directly with diastolic function (742). This interference may resemble the effect of hypercalcemia and is characterized by inadequate relaxation, spontaneous early depolarization, and subsequent failure of contractility (743). In a Mongolian gerbil model of human iron overload, the arrhythmogenesis of iron-induced cardiac disease may be caused by abnormal excitability and heterogeneous cardiac iron deposition (744). Decreased antioxidant activity of apolipoprotein E, related to the frequency of the apolipoprotein E4 allele, has been proposed as a genetic risk for left ventricular failure in thalassemia (745). Genetically defined immune mechanisms may also play a role in the pathogenesis of heart failure in β-thalassemia (746).

Lung Disease. Several different pathologic processes may provoke pulmonary hypertension and right ventricular strain, dilatation, and failure (747). Small airway obstruction, hyperinflation, hypoxemia (726,748–750), and a restrictive pattern of lung disease (726,751–754) have been described. Studies of total lung capacity have provided inconsistent results, as with the effects of transfusion on pulmonary function (750,752,755). Massive accumulation of hemosiderin in alveolar phagocytes in the perivascular and supporting framework (711,751), fibrosis, sclerotic vascular lesions, and thromboemboli (756) are observed on autopsy. Iron-induced tissue damage, abnormalities of the alveolar capillary membrane, alveolitis (757), or abnormal development of the alveolus secondary to intrinsic disease or frequent transfusions (758) may account for this pathology. Pulmonary hypertension, which has been described in nonthalassemic patients who have undergone splenectomy (759), may be related to iron overload or recurrent pulmonary emboli (760). An acute pulmonary syndrome has also been described in patients receiving excessive doses of deferoxamine (761).

Thromboembolic Disease. In older transfused and nontransfused patients, incidence rates approximating 5% per patient are reported for thromboembolic disease, including stroke, pulmonary embolism, mesenteric or portal thrombosis, and deep venous thrombosis (728,762–764). An increased risk for thromboembolic events has been associated with cardiac disease, diabetes, nonspecific liver-function abnormalities, and hypothyroidism, age older than 20 years, previous splenectomy, high platelet counts, and reduced plasma protein C and plasminogen levels (763,764). Other reports have observed that evidence of a chronic hypercoagulable state associated with increased platelet activation and enhanced thrombin generation exists in children as well as adults (765). Other genetic and acquired factors may contribute to an increased likelihood of thromboembolic disease [reviewed in (569)]; for example, patients with heart failure who carry the apolipoprotein E4 allele (745), or those with an increased frequency of anticardiolipin antibodies and lupus anticoagulant associated with hepatitis C infection (766), may have an increased risk of thromboembolic events.

Liver Disease. In young adults, liver disease remains a common cause of morbidity and mortality (728). Iron produces cellular injury with progression to fibrosis and cirrhosis through the promotion of free radical-mediated lipid peroxidation and mitochondrial dysfunction (666,676,767,768). Iron accumulation also promotes excess collagen deposition (769) and may potentiate further iron loading through up-regulation of the transport of nontransferrin bound plasma iron (770), and may also potentiate the effects of viral hepatitis.

Severe hepatic fibrosis and siderosis are regular findings at autopsy even in irregularly transfused patients (710,711,738,771), including those as young as 2 years (714,772–774). In most patients, fibrosis progressed to frank cirrhosis during the second decade of life (709–711,713,717,771–779). In transfused patients, age, liver iron content, and the presence of viral hepatitis all play a role in the rate of development of significant fibrosis and cirrhosis (777,780). Fibrosis is observed in approximately 50% of transfused, irregularly chelated patients younger than 6 years and in 90% of those older than 5 years (718,719). Early studies observed that fibrosis was observed only in patients in whom hepatic iron exceeded 7.6 mg/g liver, dry weight (711). Later studies reported chronic persistent or active hepatitis and severe fibrosis only in patients with hepatic irons exceeding 10 to 12 mg/g liver, dry weight (781), although mild to moderate fibrosis was observed in the presence of lower concentrations (778). In patients with hereditary hemochromatosis, liver iron concentrations exceeding 7 mg/

g liver, dry weight, appear to place patients at risk for hepatic fibrosis. Screening tests of liver function were of limited clinical value in these studies, and there were frequently no observed biochemical changes in the presence of substantial liver damage.

Clearly, though, the toxic manifestations of iron overload do not depend only on the severity of tissue iron loading, but are modified by the rate of iron accumulation; the duration of exposure to increased iron; ascorbate status, which influences the partition of the iron load (between relatively harmless sites in macrophages and more hazardous deposits in parenchymal cells); and noniron-related factors, including viral hepatitis (698). For example, in patients with hepatitis C infection, both liver damage and the response to therapy may be considerably modified by the presence of excess iron (782–784).

Endocrine Disease. Iron loading of the tissues has a particular predilection for the endocrine organs (710,785–787). Over a wide range of ages, populations, and body iron burdens, the most common endocrine abnormalities in the present era are hypogonadotropic hypogonadism, growth hormone deficiency, and diabetes mellitus (788–809). Lower frequencies of hypothyroidism, hypoparathyroidism, and adrenal insufficiency are reported (810).

Retarded Growth. In inadequately transfused patients, growth retardation is extremely common and may be related to hypoxia (785,811,812). Bone age is frequently delayed after age 6 to 7 years (785), when growth retardation becomes evident. Growth disturbances associated with low-transfusion regimens are characterized by lack of weight gain, reduced muscle mass, and delayed development (687) and are usually correctable by adequate transfusion (687,703,813,814). Growth rates and final heights may be related to the Hb levels maintained throughout early life (814).

In well transfused but inadequately chelated patients, iron-mediated damage to the hypothalamic/pituitary axis represents the main factor affecting growth; the first observable change may be failure or reduction of the pubertal growth spurt, associated with delayed sexual maturation (687). For reasons that are not entirely understood, even adequately chelated patients may show some degree of delayed pubertal growth (687,800,810). This finding has been attributed to iron-induced selective central hypogonadism (798,799,815,816) or interference by iron with the production of insulin-like growth factor (IGF)-1 (817–819). Other proposed mechanisms include impaired growth hormone response to growth hormone–releasing hormone (820), abnormalities in growth hormone secretion (821), or, as growth hormone reserves are often normal (822,823), a defect in the growth hormone receptor. In some adequately transfused, chelated patients, reduced growth hormone reserve and reduced levels of IGF-1 and IGF-BP3 (the growth hormone–dependent, IGF-1–binding protein that prolongs the serum half-life of IGF peptides) do not correlate with reduction in height or delay in bone age (824). Even if stimulated growth hormone secretion is normal, *spontaneous* nocturnal growth hormone secretion may be abnormal in patients with severe iron-induced pituitary gonadotrophin insufficiency (825). A state of partial growth hormone insensitivity due to a postreceptor defect in growth hormone action, which can be overcome with supraphysiologic doses of exogenous growth hormone (826,827), may also be present. Other factors possibly related to growth failure include a reduced level of secretion of adrenal androgen (795,828), zinc deficiency (829), and free Hb-induced inhibition of cartilage growth (830). Excessive deferoxamine may have a damaging effect on spinal cartilage (814,831,832) and may be associated with reduction in sitting height (814,831,832) (Figs. 48-27 and 48-28). Sitting height may also be more proportionally

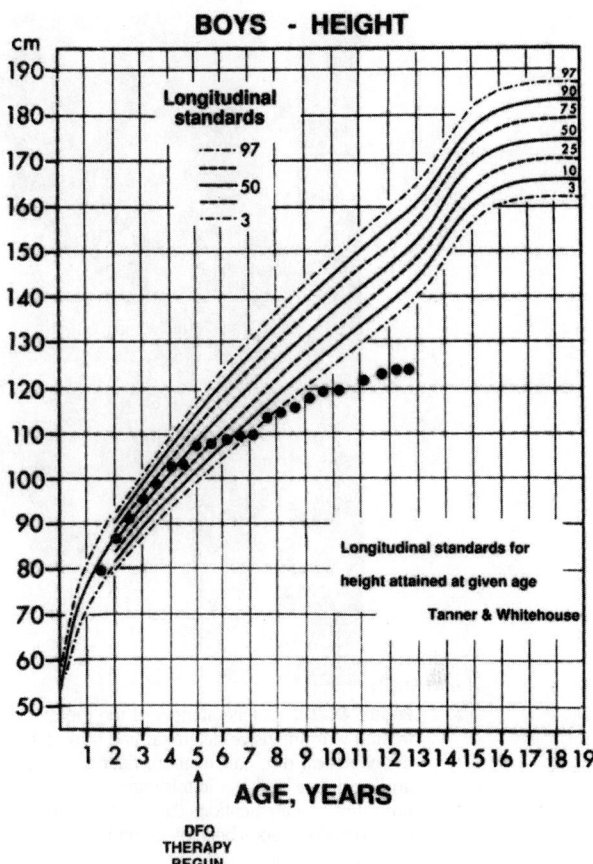

Figure 48-27. Decline in height percentile observed in a child with thalassemia major. The patient began therapy at age 4 years, 11 months (*arrow*) with nightly subcutaneous deferoxamine (initial dose, 11 mg deferoxamine/kg/day; mean dose over the first 3 years of therapy, 55 ± 17 mg/kg/day). This patient had normal radiographs before the start of deferoxamine but subsequently developed marked growth failure with a dramatic decline in height percentile, from the thirty-seventh percentile for age, 6 months before initiation of deferoxamine, to less than the third percentile 36 months later. (From Olivieri NF, Koren G, Harris J, et al. Growth failure and bony changes induced by deferoxamine. *Am J Ped Hematol Oncol* 1992;14:48, with permission.)

compromised in girls with hypogonadotropic hypogonadism than in those with spontaneous puberty, because estrogens are essential for normal pubertal skeletal growth in girls (834).

Delayed Puberty and Defective Function of the Hypothalamic/Pituitary Axis. Hypogonadism may be a reflection of chronic anemia, deficiency of IGF-1 secondary to liver dysfunction, cirrhosis, diabetes, low adrenal-androgen production, or a combination of any of these factors. In generally adequately treated patients, failure of sexual maturation is caused by selective central hypogonadism (779,799,815) as a result of the vulnerability of the hypothalamic/pituitary axis to the effects of iron loading. There may be selective deposition in pituitary gonadotropes (837) and radiologic evidence of loss of anterior pituitary volume (838). Testicular and ovarian iron loading (791) and defective ovarian function (839) are unusual.

Arrest or failure of puberty is observed in approximately 50% of males and females in the modern era, and secondary amenorrhea develops in nearly one-fourth of females by the mid-twenties (806), presumably reflecting reduced secretion of gonadotropin-releasing hormone (GnRH) from the hypothalamus (835,836). In developing countries, where adequate transfusion and chelation programs are not widely available, these complications may be

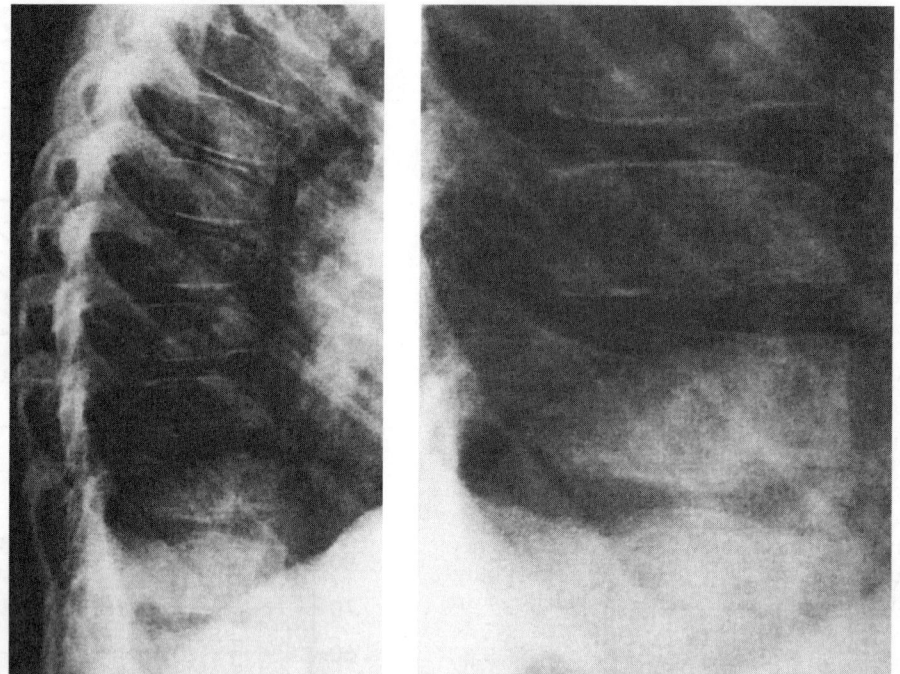

Figure 48-28. A: Lateral view of the thoracic spine in a girl 11 years, 9 months old with thalassemia major treated with intensive deferoxamine throughout childhood. The spine shows decreased vertebral height with intervertebral disc calcification; flattening, lengthening, and anterior tapering of the vertebrae; and wedging and moderate kyphosis in this region. **B:** Detail shows a bone-within-bone appearance, demarcating a zone of pronounced calcification. (From Hartkamp MJ, Babyn PS, Olivieri F. Spinal deformities in deferoxamine-treated homozygous beta thalassemia major patients. *Pediatr Radiol* 1993;23:525–528, with permission.)

even more prevalent (840). A residual gonadotrophin response to pulsatile GnRH infusions may identify patients as having potentially reversible hypogonadism (841). Although there is debate regarding the effects of deferoxamine therapy on sexual maturation, most recent studies have observed an improvement in the prevalence of attainment of normal puberty (806,808,842) compared to historical studies (800). In parallel, over the past decade, a number of reports have reported successful and safe pregnancies in women with thalassemia (discussed in the section Management) (843–850).

Diabetes Mellitus. Diabetes and insulin resistance (710,793,797,806,851–858) are observed in the present era in up to 6% of transfused and chelated patients. Early, progressive loss of β-cell mass is manifested by decreased insulin release in response in secretagogues before the development of clinically significant insulin resistance or diabetes (859,860). Diabetes has been attributed to impaired secretion of insulin secondary to chronic pancreatic iron overload due to exhaustion of β cells, decreased insulin sensitivity, and, as iron-related liver dysfunction progresses, reduced hepatic insulin extraction. There appears to be a reduction in the frequency of diabetes in adequately chelated patients (733).

Exocrine Pancreatic Dysfunction. Markedly increased echogenicity and decreased size of the pancreas and reductions in serum trypsin and lipase concentrations have all been correlated with age and duration of transfusion (861,862). The clinical significance of these findings is not clear.

Hypothyroidism. Abnormalities of thyroid function described in the previous era (792,794) are less common in patients treated by transfusion and chelation in the modern era (802,805,863,864), but a correlation between (estimates of) body iron burden and thyroid dysfunction has been reported (808). An underlying defect in thyroid function may be present without clinical hypothyroidism (865) and may also be induced by treatment with amiodarone (866).

Hypoparathyroidism. Defective parathyroid function (794,798,867,868) and florid, clinical hypoparathyroidism (794,795,869,870) have been reported. In a recent study of transfusion-dependent patients, 12.4% showed evidence of subclinical hypoparathyroidism (871). The full clinical syndrome of acute irritability, memory impairment, lethargy, and convulsions is rarely observed.

Adrenal Insufficiency. Measurable abnormalities of adrenal function (792,828) are rarely associated with overt adrenal failure (789,791,795,802). A decreased adrenocorticotropic hormone response to surgical stress may suggest decreased adrenal reserve in some patients (872). In developing countries, adrenal hypofunction may be more common, and patients have reportedly benefited from steroid replacement (840).

Bone Disease. In poorly transfused patients, expansion of the bone marrow mass leads to gross skeletal deformities, pathologic fractures (873,874), poor dentition (875), and attacks of recurrent sinusitis due to inadequate drainage (876). High transfusion regimens prevent these complications (877,878). In well transfused patients, the etiology of osteoporosis, exceeding frequencies of 50% in some studies, is less well understood (623,879). Although bone formation may not be impaired, bone resorption may be greatly increased (880). Hypogonadotropic-hypogonadism and diabetes are likely significant risk factors (881–883); males may be more commonly and severely affected (883). Many patients are symptomatic with varying degrees of bone pain. This complication may be modified by polymorphisms at loci involved in bone metabolism, including the genes for the vitamin D receptor, collagen, the estrogen receptor, and transforming growth factor β1 gene (616,622–624,883,884), but these relationships require further study.

Infection. In children maintained at variable Hb levels, the most serious reported infections include pneumonia, pericarditis, meningitis, peritonitis, osteomyelitis, and sequelae of streptococcal infections (687). Pneumonia and septicemia are significantly associated with splenectomy and a low-transfusion regimen, whereas meningitis, peritonitis, and osteomyelitis are seen only in splenectomized patients and have no obvious relationship to anemia. These observations were in keeping with the earlier studies of the dangers of infection in splenectomized children (885,886), including those with thalassemia (887,888). Widespread use of prophylactic penicillin and appropriate immunization have reduced the frequency of severe infections with *Streptococcus pneumoniae, Haemophilus influenzae,* and *Neisseria meningitidis.* Infections with *Yersinia* genus, which normally have a low pathogenicity and an unusually high requirement for iron, may become pathogenic in the presence of iron (889) and cause substantial morbidity in patients with thalassemia (890,891).

Hepatitis Viruses. Transfusion-dependent children are at risk for *hepatitis B virus,* primarily a bloodborne infection, depending on its prevalence in their community and the effectiveness of donor screening programs. By contrast to previous studies [summarized in (687,892)], in which the frequency of antibody positivity ranged from 30% to 90% in Europe, the application of adequate screening and vaccination programs has decreased greatly the frequency of infection (893). Hepatitis B virus–related hepatitis is still seen frequently in the absence of these programs; it is estimated that approximately 350 million individuals worldwide are persistent carriers of hepatitis B. Approximately 25% of patients with chronic hepatitis progress to cirrhosis, and approximately 20% of these may develop hepatocellular carcinoma.

In the modern era, infection with *hepatitis C virus* is a more widespread risk. Its prevalence in thalassemia patients varies worldwide, from approximately 12% in Turkish Cypriots, through 30% in Malaysians and Chinese, to nearly 75% in Italians (894–900). Approximately 50% of patients develop persistent viremia with hepatitis C after an initial infection, and approximately 20% of these will develop cirrhosis and increased risk of hepatocellular carcinoma.

Human Immunodeficiency Viruses. Infections with HIV-1 and HIV-2, which may give rise to the acquired immunodeficiency syndrome (AIDS) and can be transmitted by blood transfusion, has become a major concern for patients with thalassemia (901,902). Early prevalence figures from Italy and Greece ranged from 2% to 11% (903–905); those in the United States were reported to be approximately 12% (906). Further data collected after establishment of screening (907) revealed a sharp decrease in the number of HIV-positive patients, although there is a small risk of transmission from blood from seronegative donors (340). In countries where screening started later or is not established, current prevalences of infection of approximately 9% are reported (569,908–910). In patients becoming HIV-positive, the risk of progression to AIDS appears to be approximately 9% at 5 years (911); progression does not appear to be influenced by splenectomy, age, or gender.

Malaria. Thalassemic children from emerging countries are at risk because of the high frequency of chronic malaria in blood

donors in endemic regions (569). In one study, 6.4% of children showed evidence of malaria immediately after a transfusion (912). Chronic malaria may aggravate splenomegaly and exacerbate anemia (913).

Vitamin and Trace Metal Deficiencies. In inadequately transfused patients, folate deficiency is relatively common (914–916). In many patients, leukocyte and serum ascorbic acid concentrations may be reduced (917–921) (discussed in the section on therapy). Serum vitamin E levels may also be reduced, reflecting consumption of this vitamin in the continual process of peroxidation of thalassemic red cell membranes (918,922,923). The significance of observations of increased concentrations of serum copper and decreased concentrations of magnesium and zinc (924–927) is unclear. Trace metal deficiency may be exacerbated by excessive treatment with deferoxamine.

Other. Because of the rapid turnover of red cells, gallstone formation is common in undertransfused patients (928); hyperuricemia, secondary gout, and gouty arthropathy have also been reported (639,929).

Neuromuscular Abnormalities. In inadequately transfused patients, walking may be delayed beyond 18 months, and a syndrome of proximal weakness has been reported, mainly in the lower extremities, associated with a myopathic electromyographic pattern (841). Focal neurologic episodes suggesting cerebral ischemia have been described (841,930). Neurosensory deafness, involvement of the optic nerve, and compression of other nerves by hemopoietic cell tumor masses resulting from massive expansion of the bone marrow (876,931) are all described. Finally, administration of excessive deferoxamine may cause neurologic and sensory complications (932).

Intelligence and Behavioral Patterns. Intelligence testing has revealed no difference from normal children of similar age and social group (933). Abnormalities of behavior and character and abnormal emotional responses, including depression and anxiety, were similar to those in any group of children with chronic disease.

Pregnancy. A number of reports have appeared over recent years of successful pregnancies in transfusion-dependent patients. Spontaneous pregnancies, twin pregnancies, and pregnancies after ovulation induction with and without subsequent *in vitro* fertilization have been reported (843–845). Pregnancies in patients with thalassemia are high-risk and require careful monitoring (846,847) (discussed in the section on therapy).

β-THALASSEMIA INTERMEDIA

Thalassemia intermedia, a descriptive title with no clear genetic meaning, can result from the interaction of many different thalassemia alleles (569). Its molecular pathology and pathophysiology (934,935), its molecular basis in certain populations (588–590,611,936–938), and its clinical features (569,588,939,940) have been reviewed thoroughly. Any thalassemic patient with a Hb level persistently between 6 and 9 g/dL, particularly if there are associated other abnormalities, falls into the intermediate class of β-thalassemias. Some children classified in early life as having thalassemia intermedia do not thrive or develop normally and probably should be classified as having thalassemia major. By contrast, some children with Hbs between 6 and 9 g/dL are fully active and thriving, and their clinical course is usually one of chronic well compensated anemia that may be exacerbated by infection, folate deficiency, or increasing hypersplenism. Clearly, the diagnosis of thalassemia intermedia can be made only after a considerable period of observation, and often requires revision.

Complications of Thalassemia Intermedia. Iron Overload.
Iron overload becomes a problem in adolescence or young adulthood, because gastrointestinal iron loading is increased up to four times normal (707,939,941–943), resulting in positive iron balances of 3 to 9 mg iron per day. There are few reports of iron-induced cardiac disease (787,944); nonspecific symptoms and signs consistent with cardiac disease have been reported (939), but similar changes have been ascribed to anemia (940). By the third or fourth decade, a significant incidence of diabetes mellitus and other endocrine deficiencies is observed (787,795,854,939). The coinheritance of mutations for hereditary hemochromatosis on iron overload may adversely increase iron loading in thalassemia intermedia (945,946), although not in patients with thalassemia major (947–949).

Complications of Anemia and Ineffective Erythropoiesis.
Increasing splenomegaly leading to hypersplenism is a relatively common complication. Bone marrow expansion resulting in severe skeletal deformities, acetabular protrusion, and pathologic fractures may occur in older patients. A painful periarticular syndrome of thalassemic osteoarthropathy is characterized histologically by microfractures and osteomalacia (950). Tumor masses composed of extramedullary erythropoietic tissue, most commonly located in the paraspinal region, can be identified by conventional radiography and are evident in up to 65% of patients evaluated with computed tomography (951–954). Usually asymptomatic, these masses may cause spinal cord compression (955,956), cauda equina lesions (957), and hemorrhage resulting in hemothorax (958). After transfusion, these lesions may regress or undergo fatty transformation (569,959), and they may regress after a course of hydroxyurea treatment (960,961).

Other Complications.
The pattern of infection appears to be similar to that outlined for transfusion-dependent patients. Leg ulcers, possibly related to abnormal rheologic properties of the red cells, are common (588,687,942,962). A hypercoagulable state associated with platelet activation may be related to abnormal red cell phospholipid exposure [reviewed in (763,764,963)] and may be more common after splenectomy (964,965). Pulmonary hypertension and right heart failure, as well as recurrent priapism, possibly related to recurrent thrombosis, have also been reported after splenectomy (966,967). Gallstones developing as a result of both ineffective erythropoiesis and hemolysis (218,373,401,968), folate deficiency (687,785,787), and hyperuricemia are also described (950).

HETEROZYGOUS FORMS OF β-THALASSEMIA
True heterozygous states for the common forms of β-thalassemia are usually symptom-free and associated with only a mild degree of anemia. The most common varieties are associated with an elevated level of Hb A_2 and a normal or slightly elevated level of Hb F. Rarer variants have unusually high levels of Hb A_2 or F. Another heterogeneous group is characterized by normal levels of Hb A_2. Finally, a much rarer group is characterized by more severe hematologic abnormalities that may result from coinheritance of a single β-thalassemia allele with chromosomes containing extra α-globin genes, or may reflect the action of a genuinely dominant β-thalassemia allele (569).

Laboratory Findings.
Completely normal hematologic findings in heterozygous β-thalassemia are unusual and usually occur in individuals who have coinherited forms of α-thalassemia (569). In the usual forms, red cell indices and Hb do not differ significantly from normal in newborns, but by the age of 3 months, clear differences emerge. After 6 months, carrier screening by determination of mean cell volume or mean cell Hb is feasible. Most individuals have mild anemia (969); in blacks, compared to individuals from the Mediterranean region (970–972), anemia is less marked. The anemia is the result of ineffective erythropoiesis secondary to imbalanced globin chain synthesis, with precipitation of excess α-chains. There are a relatively high red cell count, microcytosis and hypochromia, target cells, and basophilic stippling (687,973–977); reticulocytes are elevated to approximately twice normal. Red cell survival is usually normal (627) or nearly normal (978–981). Elevations in serum bilirubin may be correlated with the degree of anemia (974). Serum iron, ferritin, and iron-binding capacity are usually close to normal (973,982–985). Reports of patients with heterozygosity for β-thalassemia and evidence of increased body iron burden (983,986–991) may reflect previous inappropriate iron administration, more severe forms of β-thalassemia, or coinheritance of an allele for hereditary hemochromatosis. A microcytic anemia that does not respond to iron therapy should suggest the possibility of β-thalassemia trait.

The cardinal finding in the common forms is an elevated level of Hb A_2 (992,993), averaging approximately 5% [reviewed in (569)]. Diagnostically elevated levels are established by 4 to 6 months of age. In the presence of severe iron deficiency anemia, Hb A_2 may be normal (994) or, more usually, may remain slightly elevated (982,995); Hb A_2 should be determined after a course of iron replacement, if necessary. Hb F is slightly but significantly elevated in approximately 50% of cases (970,996,997), probably due to preferential survival of F cells. Hb F is distributed heterogeneously within the red cells (651,998) and is not modified by coexisting iron deficiency (982). The rate of decline of Hb F is retarded and does not seem to reach adult levels until well into childhood. 2,3-DPG levels are elevated appropriately to the degree of anemia, but the expected increase in p50 (reduction in oxygen affinity) is not observed (999,1000). A variety of metabolic abnormalities of the red cell are described and include a decrease in osmotic fragility (1001), elevated free red cell protoporphyrin (1002–1004), and normal or slightly elevated plasma ferritin (984,1005).

Clinical Findings.
The great majority of individuals are asymptomatic; reported symptoms, including fatigue and lassitude (974,1006,1007), are difficult to evaluate, and may reflect another diagnosis (569). Many patients are treated with iron for years due to an erroneous diagnosis of iron deficiency anemia. In the majority of individuals, there are no abnormal physical signs. Although palpable splenomegaly has been reported in 10% to 50% of cases in the older literature (974,1007,1008), if splenomegaly is found in what otherwise appears to be true heterozygosity for β-thalassemia, another diagnosis should be sought (569).

Complications.
The vast majority of patients heterozygous for β-thalassemia go through life without any manifestations that can be ascribed to the disease. Anemia may worsen during pregnancy because pregnant thalassemic women are unable to increase red cell mass to the same degree as normal women (1009). Although anemia is usually mild, placental hypertrophy and fetal distress may be observed (1010). Any pregnant β-thalassemia carrier with Hb concentrations less than 8 to 9 g/dL should be investigated for iron or folic acid deficiency (1011). Because of the unreliability of serum iron and iron-binding capacity determinations in pregnancy, it is important to assess iron status using the serum ferritin concentration. Transfusions have been administered during the last trimester in some patients.

Iron overload is not a feature of β-thalassemia trait. Some of the variability in iron loading reported in β-thalassemia trait may be related to coinheritance of an allele for hereditary hemochromatosis. As discussed in Chapter 46, the H63D mutation at the locus for hereditary hemochromatosis (1012,1013) is dispersed in parts of the world where thalassemia is common (619).

Folic acid deficiency in nonpregnant persons is extremely rare (1014,1015). Although lifespan is reported as normal (1016), in males, a significant degree of protection against myocardial infarction and an advanced age at which myocardial infarction occurred have also been reported (1017), observations that require further investigation.

***Variant Forms of Heterozygous β-Thalassemia.* Normal Hemoglobin A$_2$ β-Thalassemia.** The more important variant forms of heterozygous β-thalassemia are the normal Hb A$_2$ β-thalassemias. Based on the hematologic findings, it is useful to divide these into *type 1*, in which there are minimal red cell abnormalities and in which the thalassemia allele is clinically "silent"; and *type 2*, in which the hematologic changes are indistinguishable from those of heterozygous β-thalassemia with an elevated level of Hb A$_2$ (1018).

"Silent" β-Thalassemia. The importance of the "silent" β-thalassemias are that they may interact with more severe alleles to produce thalassemia intermedia (597). There are no significant hematologic abnormalities. On globin chain synthesis analysis, there is mild imbalance, with α/β-chain synthesis ratios in the 1.2 to 1.3:1 range.

Type 2 Normal Hemoglobin A$_2$ β-Thalassemia. The causes of this heterogeneous condition include compound heterozygous inheritance of both δ thalassemia and β-thalassemia (1019), forms of εγδβ-thalassemia involving long deletions of the β-globin gene complex, and the Corfu form of δβ-thalassemia, in which a 7.2-kb deletion involves the δ gene but leaves the γ-thalassemic genes in *cis* to this deletion intact. Some forms of normal Hb A$_2$ β-thalassemia, which are associated with only very slightly elevated levels of Hb A$_2$ include carriers for the −101 C-T mutation associated with "silent" β-thalassemia, another mild (IVS1-6 T-C) allele, compound heterozygosity for δ thalassemia and β-thalassemia, triplicated α-globin genes, and single α-globin gene deletions (1020). Many of these may interact with β-thalassemia to produce severe phenotypes (discussed in the section on screening).

Heterozygous β-Thalassemia with Unusually High Levels of Hemoglobin A$_2$ or F. Levels of Hb A$_2$ in excess of 5% to 6% result from deletions removing the 5' promoter region of the β-globin gene, including the promoter boxes (reviewed in [1021]). Hb A$_2$ levels may be as high as 8% to 9%. These deletions are also associated with unusually high Hb F levels in heterozygotes (1022).

Isolated Elevated Hemoglobin A$_2$ Levels; Heterozygous β-Thalassemia with α-Thalassemia and Related Conditions. During population screening or family studies, occasionally individuals with elevated Hb A$_2$ levels are found, in the absence of the usual hematologic findings of heterozygous β-thalassemia. Many of these individuals may reflect the coinheritance of α$^+$- or α^0-thalassemia with β-thalassemia, which may result in normalization of the red cell indices and balanced globin chain synthesis (1023,1024). In some, detailed analyses of the α-, β-, and δ-globin genes reveal no abnormalities (1025).

Heterozygous β-Thalassemia with an Unusually Severe Clinical Course. There are two main mechanisms whereby heterozygous thalassemia may run a more severe course. First,

there is the coinheritance of a chromosome containing additional α-globin genes, either ααα or αααα. Second, there are the dominant β-thalassemias, which result from mutations that give rise to products that are able to form inclusion bodies (Heinz bodies) in the red cell precursors (600,601). This form of β-thalassemia arises from a heterogeneous series of mutations, most within the third exon of the β-globin gene, that lead to the synthesis of unstable β-chains (591–594,1026,1027) (discussed in Chapter 49). These unstable chains act in a dominant-negative fashion and damage red cell precursors. A wide range of phenotypes result, from typical thalassemia disorders, through conditions in which there is defective erythropoiesis and severe hemolysis, to pure hemolytic anemia (578).

β-Thalassemia Unlinked to the β-Globin Gene Complex or of Unknown Cause. A form of phenotypically characteristic heterozygous β-thalassemia appears to segregate independently from the β-globin gene complex (1028–1031). This may involve the action of a mutant *trans*-acting factor involved in β-globin gene regulation. The red cell indices, Hb A$_2$ levels, and globin chain synthesis findings are indistinguishable from β-thalassemia trait associated with mutations in the β-globin genes. In some families with the phenotype of β-thalassemia, no abnormality has been found (1032); these families may reflect the type of unlinked forms of β-thalassemia described.

AVOIDANCE AND POPULATION CONTROL

Mass screening programs, when combined with prenatal diagnosis, have significantly decreased the incidence of new cases of β-thalassemia major in many areas of the world (1033–1036). The finding of reduced mean cell volume or mean cell Hb (MCH) values in the vast majority of heterozygous β thalassemics has been used for population screening for these disorders (1037–1039). Cut-off values for the mean cell volume and MCH of 80 fl and 27 pg, respectively, in adults detect 95% or more of β-thalassemia heterozygotes (1039), although these values would still miss some carriers of unusually mild alleles. Although similar red cell changes are sometimes found in iron deficiency anemia, several formulas have been established that relate the mean cell volume, red cell count, and Hb as an approach to discriminating between iron deficiency and thalassemia. Some forms of β-thalassemia associated with normal Hb A$_2$ can interact with other forms to produce severe phenotypes; hence, in any screening program, such patients should be investigated carefully. Mass screening may be fraught with similar difficulties and should be undertaken only with expert professional and laboratory backup. It is essential to ensure voluntary informed participation, confidentiality of results, and well-informed counseling (570).

MANAGEMENT

Over the last three decades, profound changes in the treatment of patients with severe β-thalassemia have resulted in one of the most dramatic alterations in morbidity and mortality associated with a genetic disease. This interesting history is described in detail elsewhere (569,1040). On the other hand, effective treatment of these disorders is costly (1041). Treatment poses a major drain on health care resources in emerging countries, where improvements in public health measures have dramatically reduced the number of deaths in affected infants who are surviving to require long-term treatment (569).

For most patients, the mainstays of therapy are adequate transfusions (475) and iron chelation therapy (698,1040,1042–1046). For patients with appropriate donors in countries where the facilities exist, bone marrow transplantation now offers the possibility of curing thalassemia (569,688,1043).

Transfusions. **Decision to Transfuse.** The decision to initiate regular transfusions is a complex one and should ideally be based on the presence and severity of the symptoms and signs of anemia, failure of growth and development, deterioration in appetite or activity level, or the presence of disfiguring skeletal changes. If possible, it is often useful to assess the patient for at least a few months after diagnosis before making this decision. Many patients with intermediate forms of thalassemia embark on a life of unnecessary regular transfusion if, for example, they present with an unusually low Hb during an intercurrent illness. Before the start of transfusions, most centers establish the DNA mutations causing thalassemia and obtain a full red cell phenotype (Table 48-7).

Transfusion Regimens. Avoidance or reduction of the frequency of transfusions in an effort to ameliorate iron loading does not prevent this complication. When erythropoiesis is increased more than fivefold, as in severe thalassemia, the amount of iron absorbed surpasses iron loss, resulting in increases in body iron (708). The goals of transfusion, therefore, include not only correction of the anemia but also suppression of erythropoiesis and inhibition of increased gastrointestinal absorption of iron (878). Both *hypertransfusion* and *supertransfusion* regimens, in which pretransfusion Hbs are maintained above 10 and 12 g/dL, respectively, prevent most complications of anemia and ineffective erythropoiesis (687,1047), but the substantial additional iron loading associated with supertransfusion has limited application of this regimen (569,688). Pretransfusion

Hb concentrations should be maintained at approximately 9.5 g/dL; this moderate transfusion regimen reduces transfusion requirements, adequately suppresses marrow activity, and has been reported in early studies to be associated with a lower incidence of endocrine and cardiac complications (1048). A typical transfusion schedule involves administration of approximately 15 mL packed red cells/kg body weight every 28 to 35 days. There is no proven benefit of transfusions administered at 2-week intervals, although some centers have used this regimen to ameliorate volume overload (569,688). One center has achieved preliminary promising results in a program of home transfusions for patients with thalassemia (1049).

Clinical Effects of Different Transfusion Regimens. In patients with Hb concentrations exceeding 8 g/dL, a reduction in the incidence of pathologic fractures (873), reduced endosteal resorption, increased periosteal deposition, and greater thickness of cortical bone were observed (877). Maintenance of steady-state Hb exceeding 9 g/dL reduces the incidence of bone malformations and causes regression of bone changes in some patients (878,1048). There is no direct evidence with respect to improved impact of supertransfusion on bone metabolism. Linear growth is improved on hypertransfusion programs in most studies (813,873,878,1050), particularly in patients in whom a long period of hypersplenism is avoided (687). Many adequately chelated patients show linear growth equal to midparental height if pubertal maturation is normal (842,1040), but growth delay and failure are still observed (see above). There is no evidence that supertransfusion is associated with linear growth superior to that of other regimens. After the adoption of hypertransfusion programs, the incidence of splenectomy has decreased (687,1051). No data exist to suggest that supertransfusion has an added favorable effect on hypersplenism.

Procurement of Donors. Blood shortages are not uncommon in many countries throughout Europe and Asia. The principles of recruitment of the lowest-risk donors, including the use of products from repeat donors, the evaluation of risk behavior of donors, and careful screening for infectious agents, has been emphasized (1042,1052).

Type of Red Cell Concentrates. All patients should receive leukocyte-reduced red cell preparations. The most convenient and cost-effective procedure for preparing this product depends on the financial resources of the center (1042,1052). Current generation filters, although practical and effective in reducing white cell numbers and the frequency of nonhemolytic febrile transfusion reactions, are expensive (1052,1053). Early clinical experience with *neocytes*, young RBCs separated from older cells by density centrifugation (1054), suggested that their use is associated with modest extensions of transfusion intervals and reduction in annual transfusional iron load of 10% to 25% (1055–1059). Because these potential benefits are offset by major increases in preparation expenses and donor exposure over those of standard concentrates (1058), neocytes have had a minor impact on the long-term management of patients with thalassemia. This is also true of the use of exchange transfusions (erythrocytapheresis) (1060), which, when combined with administration of neocytes in one study (1061), was associated with an approximately 30% reduction in red cell consumption, but also with greatly increased costs and donor exposure.

Complications of Blood Transfusions

ALLOIMMUNIZATION. A variable frequency of red cell alloimmunization is reported, which is higher in patients in whom blood transfusion was begun after the age of 1 to 2 years and in

---

TABLE 48-7. Evaluation of the Patient with Thalassemia

Initial	Clinical assessment	
	Hematologic evaluation (CBC, hemoglobin electrophoresis)	
	α:non–α-globin chain synthesis ratio	
	Red cell phenotype	
	Serum iron, total iron-binding capacity	
	Serum ferritin concentration	
	Red blood cells and serum folate	
	Total and direct bilirubin	
	Serum ALT, albumin, PT, partial thromboplastin time	
	Hepatitis screen	
	Initiation of hepatitis B vaccine series	
	Parental counseling and education	
Monthly	History and physical examination	
	CBC	
	Parental counseling	
	If receiving iron chelation therapy, compliance review	
Q6 mo	Serum ALT, ferritin	
Yearly		
Age <10 yr	Liver	Biopsy
		Hepatitis screen
		Serum ALT, albumin, PT
	Endocrine	Serum Ca^{2+}, PO$_4$, Mg^{2+}, Zn^{2+}, PTH, TSH
	Monitoring of deferoxamine toxicity	
Age >10 yr	Liver	Biopsy
		Hepatitis screen
		Serum ALT, albumin, PT
	Heart	Cardiology consultation
		Radionuclide angiography
		If indicated, 48-h Holter monitoring
	Endocrine	Endocrinology consultation
		Fasting blood glucose
		Serum Ca^{2+}, PO$_4$, Mg^{2+}, Zn^{2+}
		Serum PTH, TSH
		GnRH stimulation test
	Monitoring of deferoxamine toxicity	

ALT, alanine aminotransferase; CBC, complete blood count; GnRH, gonadotropin-releasing hormone; PT, prothrombin time; PTH, parathyroid hormone; TSH, thyroid-stimulating hormone.

those who have received the highest number of transfusions (1042,1062–1064). Overall, the incidence of alloimmunization in Mediterranean patients appears lower (between approximately 3% and 10%) than in Asian individuals (estimated at approximately 21%); this finding is attributed to the differences in antigenic distribution between these patients and the largely (in the United States) white donor population (1065). Most antibodies are to antigens of the Rh or Kell systems (1042,1064,1065), and lower rates of alloimmunization are reported in patients who have received ABO, Rh, and Kell antigen-matched blood from their first transfusion (1063,1065). Hence, if possible, patients with thalassemia—particularly those in whom transfusions are begun after the age of 12 months—should receive blood matched for ABO, CcDdEe, and Kell antigens (1063,1065). *Autoantibody* formation in thalassemia may be more common in splenectomized patients (1062,1065); treatment has included steroids, splenectomy (1066), and high-dose immunoglobulins (1067).

OTHER COMPLICATIONS. Hepatitis B and hepatitis C virus, HIV, human T-cell lymphoma virus, and cytomegalovirus are transmitted by blood transfusion and cause significant morbidity and mortality in humans (1042,1052). The relevance to the transfused patient of Epstein-Barr virus, parvovirus B19, and human herpesvirus 6, also transmittable through blood, is uncertain (1068). *Yersinia enterocolitica* contamination of blood, because of its frequency (1069) and because its growth is enhanced in iron-rich environments (322), poses a risk to thalassemia patients (891), as does transfusion-acquired malaria (912). The use of kits to detect the presence of malarial antigen may reduce the incidence of this complication.

Alterations in circulating B lymphocytes, natural killer cell activity, HLA-DR–expressing cells, and T-helper/suppressor cell ratios (903,1070–1072) may be related to repeated exposure to transfusions, but the long-term consequences of these abnormalities are not clear (1073). The cause of a syndrome of hypertension, convulsions, and cerebral hemorrhage in thalassemia patients after blood transfusion (1074,1075) is unknown. To prevent this complication, transfusions should gradually increase Hb concentrations, and blood pressure should be monitored carefully.

Iron overload is discussed above, and in the section Iron Chelating Therapy.

Splenectomy. In the past, an increase in transfusion requirements due to hypersplenism was frequently observed at approximately 10 years of age (687). When annual transfusion requirements exceed 200 to 250 mL packed cells/kg body weight, splenectomy significantly reduces these requirements (687,1076–1078). In the modern era, with improved transfusion practices, hypersplenism is reduced, and many patients do not require splenectomy (698,1051).

Concerns that splenectomy may be associated with acceleration of iron loading in other organs (711,1079–1081) remain unproven (777); the spleen does not appear to be a significant repository of transfused iron (1082). Partial splenectomy (1083,1084) has been used to preserve splenic function, but early reductions in transfusion requirements observed after this procedure have been followed by recurrence of hypersplenism. Splenic embolization (1085) and partial vascular disconnection of the spleen (1086) have been proposed but are not used widely. The biliary tract should always be carefully assessed at surgery, but in the absence of disease, there seems little place for prophylactic cholecystectomy.

Infection. The major complication of splenectomy is severe, sometimes overwhelming infection (699,701,732,886–888,1076,1087–1092). Although likely more severe in the early years of life (1093), the ages at which postsplenectomy infec-

tion occurs in thalassemic children show a broad scatter (687,1076,1092). Overall, the pattern of postsplenectomy infection appears similar in different populations [reviewed in (687)] and is most often associated with *S. pneumoniae*, *H. influenzae*, and *N. meningitidis*. There are no published data on the risks to splenectomized children in countries where malaria is still endemic. When absolutely necessary, splenectomy should be delayed until the age of at least 5 years. At least 1 month before splenectomy, patients should receive pneumococcal, *H. influenzae* type B, and meningococcal vaccines, although the effectiveness of these vaccines in thalassemia has not been studied prospectively. After surgery, daily prophylactic penicillin should be administered, at least during childhood and probably indefinitely; erythromycin is usually substituted for patients allergic to penicillin.

Other Complications. When followed by maintenance of low steady-state Hbs, splenectomy may be complicated by progressive hepatic enlargement (687,1092). This may reflect more intensive extramedullary hematopoiesis as a response to continued anemia, with trapping of abnormal cells in an enlarged hepatic pool (687). Except for the problem of pulmonary thrombotic complications in patients with thalassemia intermedia, there is limited evidence for an increased risk of thrombotic disease after splenectomy, as outlined above.

Iron Chelating Therapy. Iron overload may be treated or prevented with a chelating agent capable of complexing with iron and promoting its excretion. The only iron chelating agent approved for first-line therapy is deferoxamine B, a trihydroxamic acid produced by *Streptomyces pilosus* with relative specificity for ferric iron. Deferoxamine, which is poorly absorbed from the gastrointestinal tract and rapidly metabolized in the plasma, is usually given by prolonged, parenteral infusion (1094). The sources of iron chelatable by deferoxamine have been reviewed (1094). Several studies have permitted the design of regimens of nightly subcutaneous deferoxamine infusions using portable ambulatory pumps [reviewed in (698,1094)]. Iron chelation is also discussed in Chapter 46.

Evidence of the Clinical Effectiveness of Deferoxamine. The appropriate use of deferoxamine has led to survival curves for patients with thalassemia that approximate those of normal individuals (569,697,698,733,1040,1041–1046,1095). A recent survey of survival of patients in the United Kingdom, which reported a mortality rate of approximately 50% before the age of 35 years, should be interpreted with caution: Included in this analysis were patients born more than 20 years before the implementation of deferoxamine (1096), whereas many more had not received adequate deferoxamine before adulthood. The survival of this study's most recent birth cohort, now age 17 to 25 years (Fig. 48-29) (1096), is markedly superior and is consistent with reports from other centers (569,697,698,733,1044–1046,1095). Misunderstanding arising from similar analyses should not permit rationalization of the implementation of alternative therapies of uncertain efficacy and safety.

It may be possible to reverse some, although not all, complications of iron overload with regular use of deferoxamine (697,698). Even in patients unable or unwilling to administer regular subcutaneous infusions, protocols for alternate means of administration have been developed, and because of the rarity of genuine allergic reactions to the drug, few patients exist who cannot tolerate some modified regimen. The observation that even low doses of deferoxamine arrest progression of hepatic fibrosis at doses which stabilize but do not reduce body iron burden (1097) justifies attempts to provide even low doses of deferoxamine to patients.

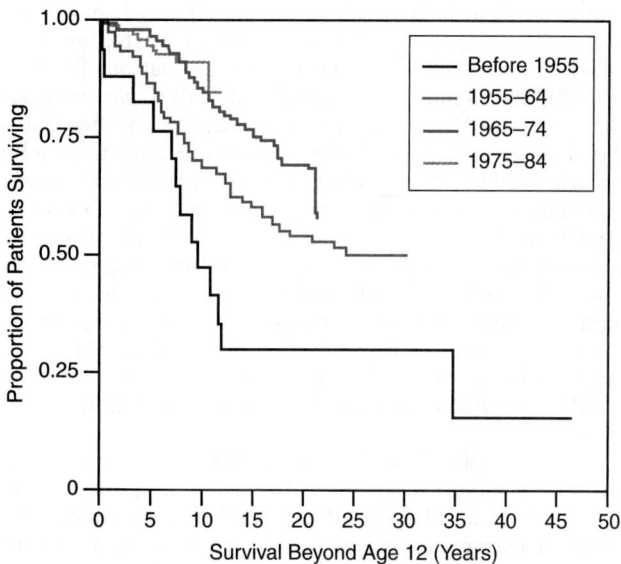

Figure 48-29. Survival beyond 12 years of age by 10-year birth cohort.

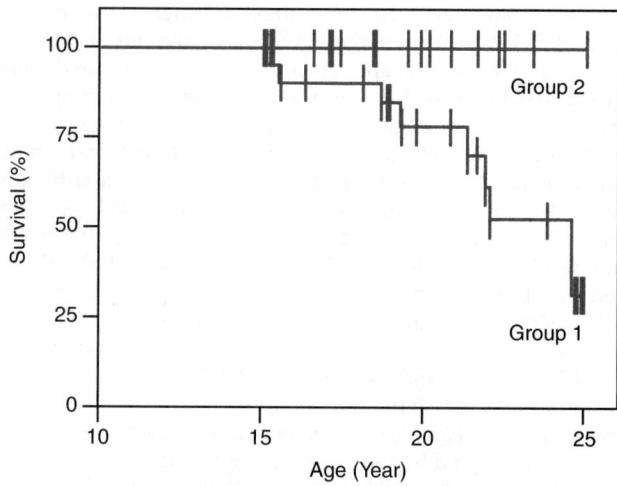

Figure 48-30. Survival of noneffectively (group 1) and effectively (group 2) chelated patients. Age-adjusted survival analysis indicated that the cumulative probability of survival to at least the age of 25 years was 32% (95% confidence interval, 4–60%) in group 1. A comparison of the survival distributions in the two groups over the 10 years of the study showed that survival was significantly better in group 2 (L = 10.04, p = .0015 by log-rank test). (From Brittenham GM, Griffith PM, Nienhuis AW, et al. Efficacy of deferoxamine in preventing complications of iron overload in patients with thalassemia major. *N Engl J Med* 1994;331:567–573, with permission.)

The beneficial effects of deferoxamine on the complication of iron overload in patients with β-thalassemia have been reviewed (569,697,698) and are outlined briefly here.

Heart. Iron-induced cardiac disease is the leading cause of death in thalassemia major (728). The early observation that adequate deferoxamine may be associated with survival free of the cardiac complications of iron overload (1098) has been confirmed in larger studies in which the primary determinant of survival was the magnitude of the body iron burden (733,1095). Patients in whom most serum ferritin concentrations are maintained at less than 2500 μg/L appear to have an estimated cardiac disease-free survival of 91% after 15 years (1095). Similarly, patients with hepatic storage irons less than 15 mg iron/g liver, dry weight, appear to be protected from cardiac disease, if not other complications of iron overload (Fig. 48-30) (733). In a cohort of patients who had received deferoxamine from an early age, the prevalence of heart disease by age 15 years was 2% (1044).

Liver. The beneficial effects of deferoxamine on the liver include reduction in iron concentration, improvement in liver function, and arrest of fibrosis (778,1097,1099), even in patients with massively elevated hepatic iron concentrations (1100).

Endocrine Function. The impact of chelation therapy on endocrine function is still under evaluation. Many studies have reported only short periods of observation in treated patients, or have been complicated by a relatively advanced age at the start of deferoxamine or inadequate compliance with therapy (779,800,807,825,828,831). Overall, long-term deferoxamine appears to have some beneficial effect on growth, sexual maturation, and other endocrine complications (805,806,808,842,1101). Normal pubertal development, for which the age of commencing chelation therapy may be an important factor (842), has been reported in approximately 50% to 70% of patients (697,806,1044).

Diabetes Mellitus. Adequate chelation therapy appears to reduce the likelihood of the development of diabetes mellitus (733).

Reversal of Iron-Induced Organ Dysfunction. Established iron-induced dysfunction of the heart and liver may improve

during intensive deferoxamine therapy (1102–1105). In patients with true end-stage iron-related disease, both cardiac transplantation (1106–1108) and combined cardiac and liver transplantation (1109) have been successful in extending survival in patients with thalassemia major. There have been no reports of improvement in gonadal function after reduction of iron load in thalassemia major, as has been described in hereditary hemochromatosis (1110,1111), but a potential therapeutic benefit to pulsatile subcutaneous gonadotrophin-releasing hormone infusions has been reported in males with evidence of mild hypogonadism (841).

Optimal Body Iron Concentrations in Patients with Thalassemia Major. The optimal body iron should minimize both the risk of adverse effects from iron chelating therapy and the risk of complications from iron overload. With stable transfusion requirements and in the absence of other confounding factors, the lower the level of body iron desired, the higher the dose of iron chelator needed. The risk of many adverse reactions is increased with administration of excessive doses of deferoxamine. Therapy to maintain normal body iron stores, corresponding to a hepatic iron of approximately 0.2 to 1.6 mg iron/g liver, dry weight, greatly increases the probability of dose-related drug toxicity (1112). Maintenance of hepatic iron concentrations exceeding 15 mg iron/g liver, dry weight, is associated with a heightened risk of cardiac disease and early death (733). Slightly lower iron burdens, corresponding to hepatic irons between 7 and 15 mg iron/g liver, dry weight, are associated with an increased risk of other complications of iron overload, including hepatic fibrosis, in individuals with hereditary hemochromatosis (1113,1114) and thalassemia (1115,1116). By contrast, minor iron loading develops in approximately one quarter of those *heterozygous* for hereditary hemochromatosis, but body iron stores in these individuals do not seem to increase beyond approximately two to four times the upper limit of normal, corresponding to hepatic irons between 3.2 and 7 mg iron/g liver, dry weight. This body iron burden is associated with no morbidity and a normal life expectancy (1117). These data suggest

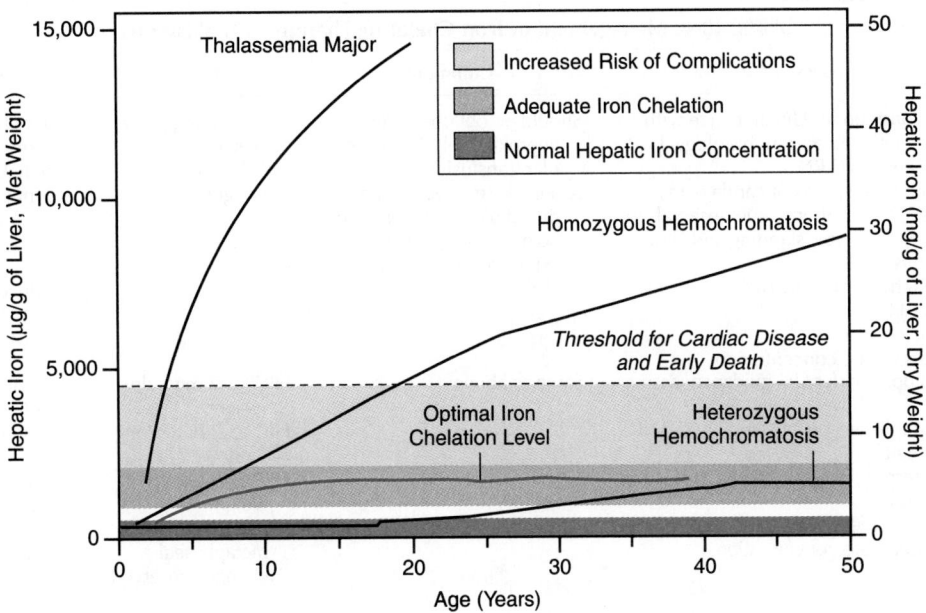

Figure 48-31. Hepatic iron burden over time and the effect of various hepatic iron concentrations in patients with thalassemia major, homozygous hemochromatosis, and heterozygous hemochromatosis. Because efforts to maintain normal hepatic iron concentrations in patients with thalassemia major are frequently associated with adverse reactions to deferoxamine, an optimal range within which hepatic iron may be safely maintained, derived in part from clinical experience with the iron-loading disorder hereditary hemochromatosis, has been proposed. In a proportion of patients who are heterozygous for hemochromatosis, moderate iron loading corresponding to concentrations of approximately 3.2 to 7.0 mg iron/g liver, dry weight (indicated in medium blue), is associated with normal survival without complications of iron overload (117). In patients who are homozygous for this disorder, concentrations exceeding this range, up to approximately 15 mg iron/g liver, dry weight (indicated in light blue), are associated with an increased risk of complications of overload (114), whereas maintenance of levels exceeding 15 mg iron/g liver, dry weight, greatly increases the risk of cardiac disease and early death in patients with thalassemia major (733). In patients with thalassemia major who receive regular transfusions, the rate of iron loading is much more accelerated, and death usually occurs before the third decade of life. The goal of treatment is the maintenance of a body iron burden corresponding to a hepatic iron concentration of approximately 3.2 to 7.0 mg iron/g liver, dry weight, achievable with regular deferoxamine therapy (698). The serum ferritin concentrations corresponding to these ranges of hepatic iron are not clearly defined.

that a conservative goal for iron chelation therapy in thalassemia is maintenance of a body iron burden corresponding to hepatic storage iron of approximately 3.2 to 7 mg iron/g liver, dry weight. The risks of deferoxamine toxicity associated with regimens to maintain body iron within this range are probably minor. Patients with higher body iron burdens, up to approximately 15 mg iron/g liver, dry weight, are at increased risk of hepatic fibrosis and other complications (1113,1114,1118). Patients with higher iron burdens have an increased risk of cardiac disease and early death (733) and are candidates for continuous intravenous ambulatory deferoxamine (698,1119). These ranges are shown graphically in Figure 48-31, and suggestions for management are summarized in Table 48-8.

Serum ferritin concentrations are a more commonly used, but less reliable, method to *estimate* body iron (Fig. 48-32). The serum ferritin concentrations corresponding to the ranges of hepatic iron shown in Figure 48-31 are not defined. Although serum ferritin concentrations of approximately 2500 μg/L, when maintained over a period of 15 years, may identify *retrospectively* patients who develop cardiac disease (1095), further evidence is emerging that the level of body iron truly protective with respect to the development of complications of iron overload is lower than is estimated by this level (1116,1120).

Initiation of Chelating Therapy. Uncertainties exist regarding the optimal age to start chelation therapy. There are reports of abnormal linear growth and metaphyseal dysplasia in chil-

dren treated with intensive regimens of deferoxamine before the age of 3 years (831,1121–1123). On the other hand, there is some urgency to beginning therapy, because transfused children often develop variable iron loading associated with hepatic fibrosis before this age, which is not always evident by determinations of serum ferritin or liver function (718,1115). Early chelating therapy probably reduces the frequency of failure of growth and sexual maturation (842). Hepatic iron concentrations should, ideally, be measured after approximately 1 year of regular transfusion (698); the value that should prompt therapy is approximately 6 mg iron/g liver, dry weight. If a liver biopsy is not possible at the start of therapy, subcutaneous deferoxamine not exceeding 25 to 35 mg/kg body weight/24 hours should be initiated approximately 1 year after the start of regular transfusions.

Usually, patients and parents administer deferoxamine by means of an overnight subcutaneous infusion over 8 to 12 hours through a needle inserted into the abdomen, thigh, or upper arm. Net negative iron balance is usually maintained with 50 mg/kg body weight/night, 5 nights each week.

Rescue of Patients with Intravenous Deferoxamine. Reduction of body iron is most rapidly implemented by regimens of intravenous deferoxamine administered through implantable venous ports (1100,1119,1124). Such regimens eliminate the irritation associated with subcutaneous infusions, and those that overcome the disadvantages of drug preparation and self-

TABLE 48-8. Management of Iron Chelating Therapy in Thalassemia

Time Point	Assessment	Comment	Results	Treatment Recommendations
At start of therapy	Liver biopsy under U/S guidance with quantitative liver iron, histology, PCR for hepatitis C RNA Baseline radiographs of cartilage in wrists, knees, thoracolumbosacral spine; bone age; standing and sitting heights Serum ferritin, Fe, and TIBC Serum ALT Hepatitis screen WBC ascorbate concentration	Should be obtained after approximately 1 yr of regular transfusion Should be reviewed by pediatric radiologist and endocrinologist with previous experience in toxicity of DFO	HIC <3.2 mg/g dry weight HIC ≥3.2 mg/g dry weight	Defer chelation; reassess HIC in 6 mo Initiate DFO at 25 mg/kg/night × 5 nights/wk If reduced, administer vitamin C PO 100 mg/night during DFO infusion
Yearly, before age 5 yr	Liver biopsy under U/S guidance; assessments as above Radiographs as above; standing and sitting heights Serum ferritin; serum iron and TIBC Serum ALT Hepatitis screen WBC ascorbate concentration	Same as above	HIC <3.2 mg/g dry weight HIC ≥3.2 but <7 mg/g dry weight HIC ≥7 mg/g dry weight Severe spinal or metaphyseal changes observed	Discontinue DFO; reassess HIC in 6 mo Continue DFO at 25 mg/kg/night × 5 nights/wk Increase DFO to 35 mg/kg/night × 6 nights/wk Reduce DFO to 25 mg/kg/night × 4 nights/wk even if HIC ≥7 mg/g dry weight; reassess HIC in 12 mo If reduced, administer vitamin C PO 100 mg/night during DFO infusion
Q18 mo, from age 5–10 yr	Liver biopsy under U/S guidance with quantitative HIC, histology, PCR for hepatitis C RNA Radiographs as above; standing and sitting heights Serum ferritin, Fe, and TIBC Serum ALT Hepatitis screen WBC ascorbate concentration	Same as above	HIC <3.2 mg/g dry weight HIC ≥3.2 but <7 mg/g dry weight HIC ≥7 but <15 mg/g dry weight HIC ≥15 mg/g dry weight Severe spinal or metaphyseal changes observed WBC ascorbate concentration low	Discontinue DFO; reassess HIC in 6 mo Maintain DFO at 40 mg/kg/night × 5 nights/wk Increase DFO to 50 mg/kg/night × 6 nights/wk Increase DFO to 50 mg/kg/night × 7 nights/wk Reduce DFO to 25 mg/kg/night × 4 nights/wk even if HIC ≥7 mg/g dry weight; reassess HIC in 12 mo Administer vitamin C PO 100 mg/night during DFO infusion
Q18 mo, after age 10 yr	Liver biopsy under U/S guidance; assessments as above Radiographs as above; standing and sitting heights Serum ferritin, Fe, and TIBC Serum ALT Hepatitis screen WBC ascorbate concentration	Same as above	HIC <3.2 mg/g dry weight HIC ≥3.2 but <7 mg/g dry weight HIC ≥7 but <15 mg/g dry weight HIC ≥15 mg/g dry weight but <18 mg/g dry weight HIC ≥18 mg/g dry weight Severe spinal or metaphyseal changes observed	Discontinue DFO; reassess HIC in 6 mo Maintain DFO at 40 mg/kg/night × 5 nights/wk Increase DFO to 50 mg/kg/night × 6 nights/wk Increase DFO to 50 mg/kg/night × 7 nights/wk Consider continuous IV DFO 50 mg/kg/24 h through implantable port Reduce DFO to 25 mg/kg/night × 4 nights/wk even if HIC ≥7 mg/g dry weight; reassess HIC in 12 mo If reduced, administer vitamin C PO 100 mg/night during DFO infusion

ALT, alanine aminotransferase; DFO, deferoxamine; HIC, hepatic iron concentration; PCR, polymerase chain reaction; TIBC, total iron-binding capacity; U/S, ultrasound; WBC, white blood cell.

administration improve compliance greatly (1119,1124). Except in exceptional circumstances, *doses of deferoxamine should not exceed 50 mg/kg body weight/day.* Although requiring scrupulous attention to the care of access sites and regular visits for surveillance by experienced medical personnel (1119,1124), long-term intravenous deferoxamine is associated with improvement in clinical cardiac disease and cardiac function and an acceptably low incidence of line infections, thrombosis, and deferoxamine toxicity (1119).

Assessment of Body Iron Burden. Both direct and indirect means for the assessment of body iron are available, and no single indicator or combination of indicators is ideal for the evaluation of iron status in all clinical circumstances (Table 48-9).

INDIRECT ASSESSMENT. The measurement of plasma or serum ferritin is the most commonly used indirect estimate of body iron stores (1125). Normally, ferritin concentrations decrease with depletion of storage iron and increase with storage iron accumulation. Interpretation of ferritin values may be complicated by condi-

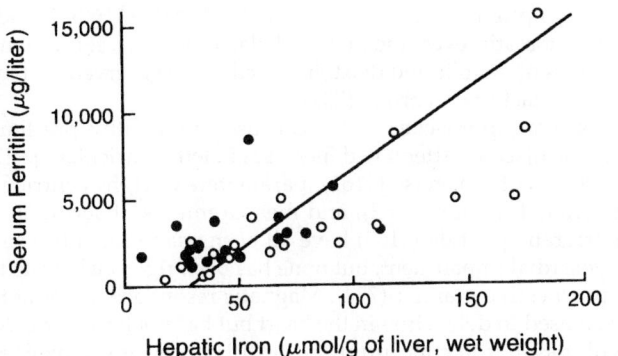

Figure 48-32. Comparison of hepatic iron and serum ferritin concentrations in patients with thalassemia major. Indirect estimation of body iron load, based on serum ferritin concentrations, is compared with the reference method, direct measurement of hepatic iron concentrations (by chemical analysis or magnetic-susceptibility studies) in patients with thalassemia major treated with deferiprone therapy. Open circles denote the values determined before deferiprone therapy and solid circles those at the time of final analysis after 1 to 5 years of treatment. The diagonal line denotes the simple linear least-squares regression between the two variables. (From Olivieri NF, Brittenham GM, Matsui D, et al. Iron-chelation therapy with oral deferiprone in patients with thalassemia major. *N Engl J Med* 1995;332:918–922, with permission.)

tions that alter concentrations independently of changes in body iron burden, including ascorbate deficiency, fever, infection and inflammation, acute and chronic hepatic damage, hemolysis, and ineffective erythropoiesis, all of which are common in thalassemia major. The 95% prediction intervals for hepatic iron concentration, given the plasma ferritin, are too broad to make the latter a useful predictor of body iron stores (1126). As a consequence, the serum ferritin is an imperfect index of iron overload, and reliance on this modality alone usually leads to inaccurate assessment of iron burden in individual patients (Fig. 48-32). Similarly, of serum iron, transferrin, transferrin saturation, transferrin receptor concentration, and urinary iron excretion after an infusion of deferoxamine, none evaluates body iron quantitatively. The usefulness of determining the iron content of serum ferritin is unclear (1127–1130). The availability of a simple assay for monitoring nontransferrin-bound plasma iron could provide a useful measurement of iron status but has not been applied widely (677–679,1131).

Tissue iron has been imaged with many methods, including computed tomography (1132–1134), nuclear resonance scattering (1135), and magnetic resonance imaging (1136–1140) [summarized in (1125)]. The most widely used of these is magnetic resonance imaging, which can identify the presence of iron in the liver, heart, and pituitary. Studies of the correlation obtained between hepatic irons determined at biopsy and by magnetic resonance imaging have shown that present magnetic resonance imaging techniques do not distinguish patients with dangerous levels of body iron from those who require regular approaches to chelating therapy (1141), or provide an accurate measurement of hepatic iron in patients with concentrations exceeding 20 mg/g or fibrosis (1142). Although the potential utility of other magnetic resonance imaging techniques in the evaluation of tissue iron deposition (1143) should be confirmed, current applications of this modality do not provide measurements of tissue iron that are quantitatively equivalent to those determined at biopsy. The utility of measurement of skin iron with x-ray fluorescence has been examined in animals (1144).

DIRECT ASSESSMENT. Measurement of hepatic iron stores is the most quantitative, specific, and sensitive means of assessing body iron burden (1145). In thalassemia, hepatic iron concentrations are correlated closely with total body iron burden (1146). Data accumulated over the past 10 years permit a quantitative

TABLE 48-9. Assessment of Body Iron Burden in Thalassemia

Test	Comments
Indirect	
Serum/plasma ferritin concentration	Noninvasive
	Lacks sensitivity and specificity
	Poorly correlated with hepatic iron concentration in individual patients
Serum transferrin saturation	Poorly correlated with hepatic iron concentration in individual patients
Tests of 24-h deferoxamine-induced urinary iron excretion	Less than half of outpatient aliquots collected correctly
	Ratio of stool:urine iron variable; poorly correlated with hepatic iron concentration
Imaging of tissue iron	
Computed tomography: liver	Variable correlation with hepatic iron concentration reported
Magnetic resonance Liver	Variable correlations with hepatic iron concentration reported; cannot distinguish acceptable and dangerous ranges; imprecise if hepatic iron >20 mg/g, or if fibrosis present
Heart Anterior pituitary	Only modality available to image cardiac or pituitary iron stores; correlations with tissue iron not demonstrated
Evaluation of organ function	Most tests lack sensitivity and specificity; may provide limited information regarding functional status
Direct	
Cardiac iron quantitation Biopsy	Imprecise because of inhomogeneous distribution of cardiac iron
Hepatic iron quantitation Biopsy	Reference method; provides precise assessment of body iron burden; information on fibrotic and inflammatory changes
	Safe when performed under ultrasound guidance
Superconducting susceptometry (SQUID)	Noninvasive; excellent correlation with biopsy-determined hepatic iron

SQUID, superconducting *quantum interference device.*

approach to the management of iron overload and provide guidelines for the control of body iron burden in individual patients treated with chelating therapy, including maintenance of balance between the effectiveness and toxicity of deferoxamine (698). Biopsies of adequate weight permit a chemical measurement of the nonheme storage iron concentration, the pattern of iron accumulation, and evaluation of the extent of inflammation, fibrosis, and cirrhosis (1147).

The observation that quantitation of liver iron from a single liver biopsy has limited value in long-term monitoring of body storage iron (1116) highlights the importance of regular monitoring in patients with thalassemia who require life-long control of body iron. Resistance of many thalassemia centers to monitor body iron burden using regular liver biopsies is usually related to the perceived dangers and discomforts of liver biopsy. The frequency of complications appears to be lower in children, in whom a 0.5% rate of major complications and no fatalities were reported (718), compared to that in adults (1148). Overall, large numbers of liver biopsies have been undertaken safely using ultrasound guidance over the past decade (1115), and this procedure, in expert hands, is safe and cost-effective.

Although some investigators have proposed that iron determined in hepatic biopsies is not representative of total body

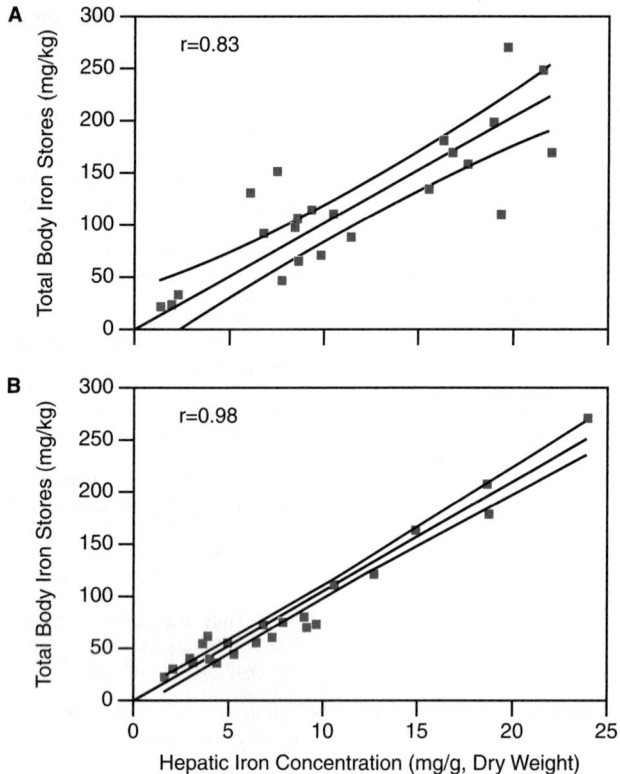

Figure 48-33. Correlation between hepatic iron concentration and total body iron stores in 48 patients without cirrhosis. The correlation is shown for two groups of patients: **(A)** 23 patients with liver samples that had a dry weight of less than 1.0 mg, and **(B)** 25 with samples that had a dry weight of 1.0 mg or more. The regression line (*middle line*) and 95% confidence limits (*upper and lower lines*) are shown.

iron burden (1149–1151), recent elegant studies have shown unequivocally that hepatic iron is indeed a reliable indicator of total body iron stores in noncirrhotic thalassemia patients in whom adequate amounts of tissue are obtained (Fig. 48-33) (1146). The variability in hepatic irons determined in needle biopsy specimens that has been reported in some (1152), but not all (1153), studies may be related to evaluation of hepatic iron in cirrhotic specimens or those of inadequate size.

Magnetic susceptometry using a *s*uperconducting *qu*antum *i*nterference *d*evice (SQUID) magnetometer provides a direct measure of hepatic storage iron that is quantitatively equivalent to that determined at biopsy (1125,1154–1156). Magnetic susceptometry has been useful in clinical investigation of iron overload but is not generally available, in part because only two sites, one in the United States (1125,1154) and one in Germany (1155,1156), have the specialized equipment needed for measurements of hepatic magnetic susceptibility. The correlations between hepatic iron concentration determined by SQUID and from biopsy specimens do not appear to be equivalent in these two centers (1125,1154–1156). The development of high transition temperature superconductors that can operate at liquid nitrogen temperatures promise to make SQUID susceptometers widely available at low cost (1125).

Assessment of Organ Function. CARDIAC FUNCTION. Diagnosis of asymptomatic cardiac disease may be difficult. Because cardiac iron distribution is not uniform (1157), endomyocardial biopsy may not reflect iron deposition accurately. Electrocardiographic and echocardiographic findings are nonspecific (734) and systolic function is usually normal until there are unequiv-

ocal symptoms of cardiac failure (725,742,1158–1160). In older, asymptomatic, even adequately chelated patients, subtle abnormalities of systolic and diastolic function are observed that may be multifactorial in origin (734).

Several approaches have been used to identify preclinical cardiac disease. Attenuated increases in left ventricular ejection fraction with exercise (1161), parameters of right ventricular diastolic function (1162), and measurements of serum atrial natriuretic peptide (1163) have all been used to identify early myocardial impairment, but none has been rigorously tested in a prospective manner (734). Magnetic resonance imaging has been used to detect iron in the heart but has not been correlated with tissue iron concentrations (698,1164), whereas magnetic susceptometry has not yet been applied to the evaluation of cardiac iron (1125). To date, information on the number of transfusions, details of their adherence to a chelation regimen, and, primarily, hepatic iron concentration appear to provide as much predictive power as any noninvasive test (734).

Tests of liver function do not regularly identify patients with fibrosis or cirrhosis. Hence, these tests are of limited value in identification of patients with severe histologic abnormalities.

ANTERIOR PITUITARY FUNCTION AND RESERVE. Measurement of gonadotrophin response to pulsatile infusions of GnRH may identify patients with potentially reversible hypogonadism (841). Correlations between measurements of iron in the anterior pituitary by magnetic resonance imaging and serum ferritin concentration (1165) as well as the identification of magnetic resonance parameters that may predict anterior pituitary failure (1166) will require confirmation.

Balance between Effectiveness and Toxicity of Deferoxamine. Most serious toxic effects of deferoxamine are observed in only modestly iron-loaded patients who are receiving excessive doses of deferoxamine relative to body iron burden (932,1121). Attempts to maintain normal hepatic iron concentrations with deferoxamine may be associated with increased toxicity, whereas titration of hepatic iron to the levels described above usually avoids most potential adverse effects (932).

ACUTE DEFEROXAMINE TOXICITY. Local cutaneous reactions with itching, pain, and weal formation are by far the most commonly observed adverse effects associated with deferoxamine. Although hypertonicity of the solution may increase the frequency of such reactions, these effects are observed even with adequate dilution of deferoxamine and may be related to unidentified contaminants in different drug batches or to poor injection technique. Very rarely, patients experience more severe, generalized hypersensitivity reactions to deferoxamine (687) with acute inflammation and edema at the site of infusion, sometimes associated with wheezing, tachypnea, tachycardia, hypotension, and coma. Although these reactions suggest an allergic mechanism, evidence is lacking. Immunoglobulin E–independent activation of dermal mast cells by deferoxamine has been demonstrated (1167). A total of 20 or fewer such reactions is reported in the literature (569,687); these are almost always managed effectively using rapid intravenous desensitization similar to protocols recommended for penicillin allergy (1168–1170).

CHRONIC DEFEROXAMINE TOXICITY. Cataracts reported during deferoxamine therapy (1171–1173) usually improve after its temporary withdrawal and are not usually associated with visual loss. Once symptomatic recovery is complete, the drug can be safely restarted at a lower dose (932). Retinal damage, characterized by impaired peripheral and night vision not always reversible with drug withdrawal, and optic atrophy are also reported (1173–1175). When such symptoms are detected, quantitative assessment of body iron burden—*not* substitution of experimental drugs—is indicated. If symptomless electrophysiologic changes are observed, deferoxamine may be continued with careful regular follow-up if the severity of body iron loading mandates continued chelating therapy (365). Ototoxicity, reported in patients receiving high doses of deferoxamine (1175–1179), is managed by assessment of body iron burden and appropriate alterations in the dose, or temporary withdrawal, of deferoxamine. Impaired linear growth in young children, associated with evidence of cartilaginous dysplasia of the long bones and spine (831–833,1122,1123,1180–1186), appears to be preventable with management protocols that maintain hepatic iron within the ranges (3.2 to 7 mg/g liver, dry weight) described above (698). Up to 30% of patients will show *radiologic* abnormalities presumed secondary to deferoxamine treatment in cartilage (Fig. 48-28). *Histologic* examination may show abnormal chondrocytes, irregularities in columnar cartilage and in bone mineralization, and microfractures, even in patients without radiographic signs of lesions (1185).

Less common side effects ascribed to deferoxamine include loss of consciousness (1186), acute aphasia with visual loss (1187), and acute pulmonary syndrome during administration of high doses (761,1188,1189). There may be an increased susceptibility to infection with *Yersinia* species (891), and possibly *Pneumocystis carinii* and mucormycosis (invasive zygomycosis) (1190). By contrast, the progression of HIV infection may be slower in patients receiving 40 mg or more deferoxamine per kilogram per day (911). Other, rarer adverse effects, including zinc and copper deficiency, thrombocytopenia, nausea and vomiting, and renal toxicity, have been reported (932).

Prevention of Deferoxamine Toxicity. Deferoxamine-induced toxicity can be avoided by regular, direct assessment of body storage iron burden with evaluation of hepatic iron concentration. If the hepatic iron concentration is not regularly assessed, a toxicity index [the mean daily dose of deferoxamine (in milligrams per kilogram body weight) divided by the serum ferritin concentration] should be calculated regularly for each patient, and should not exceed 0.025 (932). Except in exceptional circumstances, doses should not exceed 50 mg/kg/24 hours. Attempts to rescue patients with organ failure using higher doses have been associated with permanent hearing loss and fatal pulmonary toxicity (932). Annual screening for deferoxamine toxicity, including regular assessments of height and weight, expert examination of vision and hearing, and radiologic examination of bones (Table 48-10), is strongly recommended. With these efforts, it is possible to administer deferoxamine with minimal likelihood of side effects.

Ascorbate Supplementation. Low ascorbic acid levels have been demonstrated in iron-loaded thalassemic patients. Ascorbate supplementation may result in a marked improvement in deferoxamine-induced iron excretion through expansion of the chelatable iron pool to which deferoxamine has access. In parallel, ascorbate-induced expansion of this pool may aggravate the toxicity of iron *in vivo* [reviewed in (698)]. Although routine ascorbate supplementation has therefore been discouraged in patients with iron overload, evidence of diminishing efficacy of deferoxamine should prompt determination of tissue ascorbate concentrations. If supplementation is required, 100 mg ascorbic acid should be administered approximately 30 to 60 minutes after initiation of an infusion of deferoxamine, only on days during which deferoxamine is administered.

The most common difficulty associated with long-term subcutaneous deferoxamine is erratic compliance with therapy, which may decline as supervision of this regimen becomes increasingly the responsibility of the patient. Compliance with deferoxamine may be improved with intensive social and psychological support (1191,1192).

Other Indications for Chelating Therapy. DEFEROXAMINE IN PREGNANCY. Because of unproven concerns about the teratogenicity of deferoxamine, whenever possible, the drug should be avoided in pregnancy. If transfusion throughout pregnancy is required and iron levels exceed thresholds of risk, deferoxamine can be used with caution after the first trimester (1193).

THALASSEMIA INTERMEDIA. Iron loading secondary to increased gastrointestinal iron absorption in patients with thalassemia intermedia is less accelerated than that in transfused patients (707,942). Direct determination of body iron burden is indicated in any patient with thalassemia intermedia and an elevated serum ferritin concentration, and therapy should be initiated if the hepatic iron exceeds 6 to 7 mg/g liver, dry weight.

DEFEROXAMINE THERAPY AFTER BONE MARROW TRANSPLANTATION. Successful allogeneic bone marrow transplantation in thalassemia liberates patients from chronic transfusions but does not eliminate the necessity for iron chelating therapy in all patients. Timely reduction of hepatic iron concentration is observed only in younger patients with low pretransplantation

---

TABLE 48-10. Monitoring of Deferoxamine-Related Toxicity

Toxicity	Investigations	Frequency	Alteration in Therapy
High frequency sensorineural hearing loss	Audiogram	Yearly; if patient symptomatic, immediate reassessment	Interrupt DFO immediately; directly assess body iron burden; discontinue DFO × 6 mo if HIC ≤3 mg/g dry weight tissue; repeat audiogram at 3-mo intervals until normal or stable; adjust DFO to HIC
Retinal abnormalities	Retinal examination	Yearly; if patient symptomatic, immediate reassessment	Interrupt DFO immediately; directly assess body iron burden; discontinue DFO × 6 mo if HIC ≤3 mg/g dry weight tissue; review at 3-mo intervals until normal or stable; adjust DFO to HIC
Metaphyseal and spinal abnormalities	X-rays of wrists, knees, thoraco-lumbar-sacral spine; bone age of wrist	Yearly	Reduce DFO to 25 mg/kg/d; directly assess body iron burden; discontinue DFO × 6 mo if HIC ≤3 mg/g dry weight tissue; reassess HIC and radiographs after 6 mo; adjust DFO to HIC
Decline in height velocity, sitting height, or both	Determination of sitting and standing heights	Twice yearly	Reduce DFO to 25 mg/kg/d; directly assess body iron burden; discontinue DFO × 6 mo if HIC ≤3 mg/g dry weight tissue; reassess HIC and radiographs after 6 mo; adjust DFO to HIC; regular (6-mo) assessment by pediatric endocrinologist

DFO, deferoxamine; HIC, hepatic iron concentration.

body iron burdens; by contrast, parenchymal hepatic iron overload persists for up to 6 years after marrow transplantation in most patients who do not receive posttransplant deferoxamine treatment (1194), resulting in hepatic fibrosis and cirrhosis (1195). In formerly thalassemic patients who cannot be phlebotomized safely (1196,1197), deferoxamine appears to be safe and effective in the reduction of tissue iron (1043,1198,1199). Therapy should be initiated after successful marrow transplantation if hepatic iron exceeds 7 mg/g dry weight liver tissue (1198). A recent study has suggested that deferoxamine may be started as early as 3 months after transplantation (1200).

Other Aspects of Symptomatic Treatment. ABNORMAL GROWTH AND PUBERTAL DEVELOPMENT. Evaluation and treatment should be undertaken in collaboration with endocrinologists expert in the management of thalassemic children and adults. Patients should be investigated thoroughly to rule out nonendocrine causes of poor growth, including the toxic effects of deferoxamine. In patients with genuine growth hormone insufficiency, daily recombinant growth hormone, self-administered subcutaneously, is associated with variable increments in growth velocity (623). In children with short stature, subnormal height velocity, and normal growth hormone response to conventional stimulation tests, supraphysiologic doses of recombinant growth hormone caused a significant improvement in short-term growth and in serum insulin-like growth factor-1 levels (623,825,827,1201,1202). No studies have yet determined whether administration of growth hormone increases final height in thalassemic children.

In patients with delayed sexual maturation, androgen or estrogen replacement is usually implemented (802). Initiation of estrogen therapy has been recommended before a bone age of 12 years in an effort to obtain better truncal growth in girls with thalassemia major (834). More physiologic approaches to hormone replacement include pulsatile GnRH infusions to induce puberty (1203,1204). Some gonadotrophin (luteinizing hormone and follicle-stimulating hormone) response to pulsatile GnRH infusion may identify patients with potentially reversible hypogonadism, at least in males, suggesting a potential therapeutic benefit to pulsatile subcutaneous GnRH infusions (841).

The management of diabetes mellitus and thyroid and parathyroid deficiency involves standard replacement therapy.

CARDIAC DISEASE. Intensive intravenous deferoxamine therapy should be implemented if possible (1102–1105). The judicious use of diuretics, digoxin, inotropes and, most recently, an angiotensin-converting enzyme inhibitor (1205) may result in improvement in both systolic and diastolic function. As noted, cardiac transplantation (1106–1108) and combined heart and liver transplantation (1109) have been successful in patients with advanced disease.

BONE DISEASE. All thalassemic patients should undergo regular assessment of bone densitometry with dual-energy x-ray absorptiometry or *in vivo* neutron activation (623,688,689). As noted, even well transfused, properly chelated patients with normal gonadal function may have bone densities below normal (688), and the risk is increased by low transfusion schemes and hypogonadism (1206). Inadequately transfused patients should be placed on an adequate transfusion regimen. If indicated, patients should also receive hormone-replacement therapy. If osteopenic, patients should be supplemented with oral calcium and vitamin D and advised to exercise and not to smoke. Investigational treatments including bisphosphonates, calcitonin, and fluoride are under evaluation (623,1207).

VITAMIN SUPPLEMENTATION. Patients maintained at low Hb levels should be maintained on folate supplements; transfused patients may require folate supplementation in times of increased bone marrow activity and, in particular, pregnancy.

As noted, patients with severe β-thalassemia may also be vitamin E–depleted (918,920,923), but, overall, studies that have attempted to improve red cell survival with vitamin E supplementation have proven disappointing (1208).

INFECTION. In addition to the life-threatening infections related to previous splenectomy (discussed above), patients infected with *Yersinia* species may present with severe abdominal pain and diarrhea, vomiting, fever, and sore throat. In any iron-loaded patient who presents with this clinical picture, deferoxamine (if administered) should be discontinued and stools cultured for *Yersinia* species, and empirical treatment should commence immediately with either an aminoglycoside or cotrimoxazole (891). In 40% of thalassemia patients infected with hepatitis C, a complete response to treatment with interferon-α, defined as both sustained normalization of serum ALT and clearance of hepatitis C virus RNA from serum, was observed over a mean follow-up period of 3 years (1209). The rate of relapse was lower (18%) than in nonthalassemic individuals (50%). This finding suggests that in most patients with thalassemia, interferon-α should not be stopped after 3 to 6 months but should be continued at least until the serum alanine aminotransferase level declines to normal. Iron loading may influence the response to interferon-α therapy (782,1210). The results of coadministration of ribavirin with interferon-α (1211,1212) and of therapy with pegylated interferon (1213,1214) remain to be evaluated.

Bone Marrow Transplantation. Bone marrow transplantation from HLA-identical donors has been successfully performed in over 1000 patients with severe β-thalassemia worldwide (1199,1215). Survival and disease-free survival appear to be influenced significantly by three characteristics before transplantation: hepatomegaly (greater than 2 cm below the costal margin), portal fibrosis, and a history of effective chelating therapy. Patients in class I have none of these characteristics, patients in class II have one or two, and patients in class III have all three (1216). In class III children younger than 16 years, survival and disease-free survival 3 years after transplantation are 62% and 51%, respectively. Increasingly better outcomes are observed after transplantation of class II patients (86% and 82%, respectively), whereas excellent outcomes are observed in class I patients (90% and 93%, respectively). Transplantation of thalassemic adults older than 16 years achieves results approximately equivalent to those observed in class III patients (1217,1218). Survival and disease-free survival rates vary considerably among centers (1219–1222). Posttransplantation management involves complications related directly to the transplantation procedure itself, including acute and chronic graft-versus-host disease and mixed chimerism, the persistence of host hematopoietic cells. After transplantation for thalassemia, the probability of development of moderate chronic graft-versus-host disease is approximately 8%, whereas that of severe chronic graft-versus-host disease is approximately 2% (1223). Mixed chimerism has been described in approximately one-fourth of patients and is a risk factor for graft failure. Also observed are complications unique to the posttransplant, formerly thalassemic patient as a result of the primary disease or previous treatment, including management of hepatic iron loading using either deferoxamine (1198,1215) or phlebotomy (1196), and improvement of iron-induced cardiac disease (1224–1226), endocrine dysfunction (1227), and viral hepatitis (1228).

Experimental approaches to marrow replacement in thalassemia include cord blood transplantation (1229), the use of unrelated phenotypically matched marrow donors (1230) and mismatched donors (949,1231), *in utero* transplantation (1232,1233), and transplantation with both umbilical cord blood and bone marrow (1234).

***Experimental Therapies.* Hydroxyethyl Starch Deferoxamine.**
Attachment of deferoxamine to a hydroxyethyl starch polymer
creates a high-molecular-weight chelator with affinity for iron
identical to, but with a vascular half-life 10 to 30 times longer
than, that of standard deferoxamine. Pilot studies of this agent
have been promising (1235).

Bolus Injections of Subcutaneous Deferoxamine. Preliminary
studies suggest that twice-daily subcutaneous injections of
deferoxamine may induce urinary iron excretion equal to that
induced by prolonged subcutaneous infusion of the same dose
(1236,1237). Long-term regimens have reduced serum ferritin
concentrations, particularly in patients who are not regularly
transfused (1238). If confirmed, such regimen could offer an
alternative to prolonged deferoxamine infusions.

Therapy Directed at the Thalassemic Red Cell Membrane.
The observation that excess red cell membrane iron may aggravate membrane changes (666) has led to interest in the cell
membrane as a potential therapeutic target in β-thalassemia. In
a mouse model, increased cellular rigidity and decreased stability associated with membrane-associated α-chains (664) have
reportedly been ameliorated during exposure to agents that
bind membrane iron (1239,1240). Further understanding of
these processes may guide future therapies.

Orally Active Iron Chelators. The expense and inconvenience of deferoxamine have led to a continued search for iron
chelators that are effective when administered orally. The only
such agent to reach extended clinical trials is 1,2-dimethyl-3-
hydroxypyridin-4-one (deferiprone; L1) (1241), evaluated in
several short-term and long-term studies over the last decade
(1242–1257). Most trials have estimated changes in body iron
burden using serum ferritin concentration. The largest such
study to evaluate serial changes in serum ferritin, a toxicity trial
overseen by consultants and employees of a pharmaceutical
company (Apotex) in patients "unwilling or unable" to use
deferoxamine, was characterized by a high (31%) dropout rate
in which nearly half the dropouts discontinued deferiprone
because of "increasing iron stores" (1258). Changing incidences
of parameters of efficacy and toxicity have been reported in
triplicate publications of this trial (1258–1260); in the most
recent, a unusual *post hoc* analysis observed "positive slopes" of
serum ferritin in 49% to 55% of patients (1258).

Only a few studies of deferiprone have evaluated tissue iron
stores (1138,1248–1252,1255–1257). The poor correlation between
the serum ferritin and hepatic iron concentrations in these studies emphasizes the importance of quantitative determinations of
body storage iron in the evaluation of this, and any, new chelating agent. Support for two Canadian studies that obtained serial
determinations of hepatic iron in all deferiprone patients was terminated prematurely by Apotex in 1996 under circumstances
that have recently been exposed (1261–1268). Nonetheless,
follow-up of data in these and other studies have provided useful information about the long-term effectiveness of deferiprone.
As recently reviewed (1269), deferiprone therapy has been
acknowledged to be inadequately effective in a substantial proportion of patients in all peer-reviewed articles to have quantitated body storage iron (1138,1248–1252,1255,1256). In all of these
studies, hepatic iron concentrations have exceeded the threshold
for cardiac disease and premature death (733) in between 18%
and 65% of patients after extended therapy; hepatic irons in
approximately 70% have exceeded 7 mg iron/g liver, dry weight,
the threshold of increased risk of other iron-related complications. Nonetheless, all reports published in non–peer-reviewed
conference proceedings by consultants and employees of Apotex

remain emphatically supportive of the effectiveness and safety of
deferiprone [summarized in (1270)].

Although the only randomized trial to compare the effectiveness of deferiprone and deferoxamine using prospective measurements of hepatic iron was terminated prematurely by
Apotex, 90% of patients underwent a follow-up assessment of
hepatic iron during the therapy to which each had been randomized (1271). The proportion of deferiprone-treated patients
in whom final hepatic iron exceeded the threshold for cardiac
disease and premature death increased nearly fivefold over 2
years; in most patients randomized to deferoxamine, hepatic
iron remained within optimal range. These findings confirm
those of previous iron balance studies, which observed markedly less short-term efficacy of standard-dose deferiprone relative to that of deferoxamine (1245,1272), results confirmed more
recently by Apotex-supported investigators (1273).

Recent short-term studies have attempted to achieve iron
balance by combining deferiprone with intermittent deferoxamine (1274,1275). In one study, deferoxamine was administered
in full doses (1274), somewhat undermining the logic of combination therapy. Without full supplemental doses of deferoxamine, deferiprone does not appear sufficiently effective in most
patients (1277). Until this combination is evaluated in controlled clinical trials in which body iron burden is quantitated
rather than estimated, patients should not be exposed to the
combined risks of both drugs without the assurance of benefits
surpassing those of deferoxamine as a single agent.

TOXICITY OF DEFERIPRONE. During limited toxicity studies in
rodents, adrenal hypertrophy, gonadal and thymic atrophy,
bone marrow atrophy and pancytopenia, growth retardation,
and embryotoxicity were observed [summarized in
(1277,1278)]. In humans, the major previously recognized
adverse effects include embryotoxicity, teratogenicity, neutropenia, and agranulocytosis (1278,1279). Different incidences of
neutropenia and agranulocytosis have been reported in duplicate publications of the study designed originally to evaluate
this complication (1258–1260).

Later concerns that hydroxypyridinones might *exacerbate*
iron-related tissue damage were first raised on theoretic
grounds (1280–1282). Deferiprone is a bidentate chelator, three
molecules of which are needed to occupy the six coordination
sites of a single atom of iron. At low deferiprone concentrations
relative to available iron, partially liganded (bound to only one
or two molecules of deferiprone) forms of iron appear; the
unoccupied coordination sites remain reactive, able to catalyze
the formation of hydroxyl radical or other reactive oxygen species (1281), implicated in the pathogenesis of hepatic fibrosis.
Recently, the potential for deferiprone to produce cellular toxicity has been confirmed experimentally in studies of hepatocytes
(1283) and myocyte cultures (1284). By contrast to deferiprone,
one molecule of deferoxamine binds a single atom of iron, and
the chelate (ferrioxamine) is virtually inert biologically.

In gerbils, chronic coadministration of iron and 1,2-diethyl-3-
hydroxypyridin-4-one, a hydroxypyridinone closely related to
deferiprone, results in increased iron accumulation in the liver
and heart, worsening of hepatic fibrosis, and development of cardiac fibrosis (1285); similar studies with deferiprone itself in gerbils (1286) and in guinea pigs (1287) have observed similar
changes. These findings were paralleled in the only human trial
to obtain serial systematic liver biopsies over 6 years, in which
deferiprone-treated patients but not a group treated with deferoxamine showed accelerated progression of hepatic fibrosis over a
median period of 3.2 years (1249). Similarly, at a different center,
nearly 30% of deferiprone-treated patients demonstrated significant progression of hepatic fibrosis, more than three times the rate
in deferoxamine-treated patients over 2 to 3 years (1256). In the

group of patients studied by Apotex consultants (1259), a significant increase in serum alanine aminotransferase was observed, evidence of hepatotoxicity that was not reported in earlier analyses of the same trial (1259,1260). Liver histology, determined in less than 20% of patients, reportedly showed no acceleration of fibrosis (1288). This delayed appearance of hepatocellular dysfunction appears consistent with the observation that the time to progression of deferiprone-associated fibrosis may exceed 3 years (1249). Together, a pattern of findings based on theoretic grounds, *in vitro* studies, animal testing, and human trials lends biologic plausibility to a relationship between deferiprone and accelerated hepatic fibrosis, for which no other established cause has been identified. The prolonged period, exceeding 3 years, over which progression of fibrosis has developed in humans indicates that extended observation of adequate numbers of patients will be required to permit meaningful assessment of this risk (1289).

Deaths from cardiac disease in several patients during deferiprone therapy (1250) and development of fulminant cardiac failure associated with cardiac fibrosis at body iron burdens not usually associated with the development of heart disease (1290) parallel findings in animals in which deferiprone treatment was associated with cardiac fibrosis. These findings indicate, as suggested early in this drug's development (1282), that deferiprone's impact on this complication must be evaluated thoroughly.

In summary, before deferiprone can be considered for clinical use, evaluation of its long-term toxicity in controlled clinical trials in which hepatic iron and histology are evaluated prospectively is mandatory. This step is particularly important in view of the grave prognostic implications of the progression of liver and cardiac disease in iron-loaded patients (1289). The decision in 1999 to permit licensing of deferiprone in Europe is under legal challenge (1289a).

Augmentation of Fetal Hemoglobin Production. Standard treatment for severe β-thalassemia is effective if used under ideal circumstances but is expensive and inconvenient; definitive therapy to reduce the globin chain imbalance that is the hallmark of this disorder remains elusive. Since the discovery of Hb F ($\alpha_2\gamma_2$), augmentation of its synthesis has been proposed as a therapeutic goal in patients with β-thalassemia. Although the switch from Hb F to adult Hb ($\alpha_2\beta_2$) observed in humans around the time of birth usually proceeds on schedule in thalassemia, the γ-globin genes remain intact and functional. Increasing their output would be expected to ameliorate the severity of the disease (645) because of the mild phenotype of individuals with coinheritance of homozygous β-thalassemia and heterocellular HPFH and of patients with homozygous β⁰-thalassemia who synthesize no adult Hb, but in whom reduced requirements for transfusions are observed in the presence of unusually high levels of Hb F production (1291).

The therapeutic approaches to date, and the possible mechanisms for the way in which different agents might stimulate Hb F synthesis, have been reviewed recently (1292,1293). Clinical trials aimed at augmentation of Hb F synthesis in β-thalassemia have included administration of cell cycle–specific agents, hematopoietic growth factors, and short-chain fatty acids, all of which stimulate γ-globin synthesis by different mechanisms (1294). Presently, the compounds of most interest are hydroxyurea and the butyric acid analogs.

Hydroxyurea. The results of treatment with hydroxyurea have been reported in only approximately 100 thalassemia patients worldwide. Although in one patient in whom baseline values were not determined, the requirement for transfusions was eliminated (1295), hydroxyurea has generally been ineffective with only modest increases in Hb level or Hb F production

(1296–1303). In one patient with Hb Lepore and β⁰-thalassemia, increases in fetal and total Hb exceeding 4 g/dL were observed during hydroxyurea therapy (1304). As outlined above, administration of hydroxyurea may result in regression of extramedullary erythropoietic tissue (960,961).

Butyrate Analogs. Interest in the butyric acid compounds, derivatives of natural short-chain fatty acids, as potential therapy for β-thalassemia arose from observations that elevated plasma concentrations of amino-*N*-butyric acid in infants of diabetic mothers delay the switch from γ-globin to β-globin synthesis around the time of birth (1305). Arginine butyrate, the first butyric acid compound to be administered in humans with thalassemia, induced a 5 g/dL increase in Hb concentration over 7 weeks in a homozygote for Hb Lepore (1306). Unfortunately, extended treatment with arginine butyrate in more common forms of thalassemia resulted in virtually no change in Hb concentration (1307). Further evidence supporting the utility of pulse doses of arginine butyrate in thalassemia (1308) is awaited.

SODIUM PHENYLBUTYRATE. The observation that sodium phenylacetate and its prodrug, sodium-4-phenylbutyrate, increased Hb F production in patients with sickle cell disease (1309,1310), stimulating a pilot trial of sodium phenylbutyrate in thalassemia (1311). Sustained increases exceeding 1 g/dL in Hb concentration were noted in selected thalassemia intermedia patients, generally those with the highest pretherapy Hb F and the most marked degree of erythroid expansion. These observations support those of studies suggesting that acute erythroid expansion is associated with increased Hb F synthesis after bone marrow transplantation (1312), treatment for leukemia (1313), or hemolysis (1314).

ISOBUTYRAMIDE. Treatment with 1 month of oral isobutyramide was associated with few hematologic changes, although, curiously, a progressive increase of Hb F was observed in some patients up to 1 month after cessation of therapy (1315). One year of treatment with higher doses induced increases in Hb F in several patients (1316), an effect that appeared greatest in patients with high pretreatment Hb F and evidence of marked marrow expansion (1316). These findings require confirmation in larger studies.

Recombinant Human Erythropoietin. Hb F may be induced during rapid erythroid regeneration and recruitment of erythroid progenitor cells with an active Hb F program (1317); recombinant human erythropoietin induces red cell formation by stimulating proliferation, downstream differentiation, and maturation of erythroid progenitors. These effects stimulated interest in administration of high pulsed doses of erythropoietin to patients with thalassemia. Early studies of administration of erythropoietin, alone or with hydroxyurea, to baboons demonstrated that the combination accelerates erythroid regeneration beyond the level achieved by either agent alone (1318,1319). Administration of erythropoietin to a β-thalassemic mouse increased Hb and hematocrit, reduced globin chain imbalance, and was associated with improvement in erythrocyte membrane defects (1320). In the first studies of erythropoietin in thalassemia (1321), no consistent changes in Hb F or red cell indices were observed. Subsequent trials in both transfused and untransfused patients reported modest increases in peripheral Hb concentrations (1322–1324); in only one study was a consistent effect on Hb F synthesis, possibly secondary to coadministration of hydroxyurea, observed (1324).

The mechanism of the observed effects of erythropoietin in patients with thalassemia is still undefined, as are the usefulness of combination therapy with hydroxyurea or other agents, the effect of erythropoietin dose and dosing regimen, and the range of adverse effects. Bone pain has been reported during erythropoietin therapy (1322), and erythropoietin-induced marrow expansion poses at least a theoretic risk that may be reduced with coadministration of hydroxyurea. Gastrointestinal absorption of iron is also increased by erythropoietin-induced increase in hematopoiesis and may aggravate tissue iron overload in thalassemia.

Cytosine Arabinoside. Studies of cytosine arabinoside in anemic baboons (1325), and in two patients (1326) in whom substantial increases in Hb F were reported during short-term treatment, confirmed that cell cycle agents, by inhibiting proliferation of rapidly dividing erythroid cells, may lead to premature commitment of early progenitors having an active Hb F program (1327).

5-Azacytidine. The β minor Hb of the thalassemic mouse has been shown to increase in response to cytotoxic agents such as 5-azacytidine (1328). Intravenous 5-azacytidine has been shown to be associated with increased γ-globin mRNA synthesis, normalization of globin chain imbalance, and increases in total Hb concentration exceeding 2 g/dL in a few patients (1296,1329). Although these studies were of great interest, the potential adverse effects of 5-azacytidine shifted further interest to less toxic chemotherapeutic agents to stimulate Hb F.

Combination Therapy. There have been a few reports of combinations of therapies to augment Hb F in patients with β-thalassemia. Administration of sodium phenylbutyrate with 5-azacytidine produced a synergistic effect on Hb F synthesis in baboons (1330). Sodium phenylbutyrate added to daily hydroxyurea in anemic rhesus monkeys produced substantial augmentation in production of reticulocytes containing Hb F; superpharmacologic doses of recombinant erythropoietin added to hydroxyurea produced a similar effect (1331). These findings support those of earlier primate studies, which observed that hydroxyurea and erythropoietin accelerated erythroid regeneration beyond the level achieved by each agent alone (1318,1319). Studies in patients with thalassemia in which short-term (but not chronic) coadministration of erythropoietin with hydroxyurea was associated with increases in Hb F (1324) also suggest that erythropoietin might be usefully combined with agents that exert their effects, in part, by cytoreduction and regeneration from the progenitor pool.

COMBINATION OF THERAPIES. Combination therapy with butyrate and hydroxyurea in a patient homozygous for Hb Lepore has resulted in long-term steady-state Hb concentrations exceeding 10 g/dL, an increase of approximately 6 g/dL over untreated values; a similar response has been observed in an affected sibling (1332,1333). The marked elevation of Hb F in these siblings, and a response of almost equal magnitude in a compound heterozygote for Hb Lepore and β-thalassemia (1304), raise the question of whether the molecular pathology that underlies Hb Lepore may be related in some way to these unusual pharmacologic responses.

Although these attempts to increase the synthesis of Hb F in β-thalassemia have, with a few exceptions, been disappointing, the handful of successes offer some encouragement for the future. Therefore, it is important that attempts are made to determine the reasons for the marked variability of response, particularly whether this variability relates to the underlying mutations, the kinetics of erythropoiesis, or the particular dosages and regimens of the drugs that have been used (1292). Although it may not be possible to raise the level of Hb F sufficiently to treat patients with transfusion-dependent forms of thalassemia, this level may be achievable in β-thalassemia intermedia, including some patients with Hb E/β-thalassemia who might benefit very considerably by a modest elevation of their Hb levels.

MECHANISMS OF ACTION OF SWITCHING AGENTS. The *methylation status* of DNA sequences near the globin genes correlates with their activity in particular tissues (1334). Increased Hb F observed during administration of 5-azacytidine is associated with hypomethylation of DNA in the region of the γ-globin genes (1335). Early observations of transient increases in Hb F after marrow transplantation (1312), treatment for leukemia, and phlebotomy suggest that *acute erythroid expansion* might be associated with increased Hb F synthesis (1312,1313,1335). Perturbation of erythroid division and maturation by hydroxyurea and cytosine arabinoside may induce an alteration in cell kinetics of erythroid progenitors, leading to a premature commitment to maturation with an increased likelihood of Hb F production. These deductions are confirmed by *in vitro* studies (1336,1337). Although the butyric acid compounds may act directly on 5' flanking sequences in the chicken (1338) and through the γ-globin promoter in humans, it was not recognized until recently that responses to butyrate and other agents may require activated globin genes (1339).

α-Thalassemias

Because of the restricted distribution of their more severe forms, the α-thalassemias pose a less serious global health problem than the β-thalassemias. The severity of the α-thalassemias is largely related to the degree of imbalanced globin production: A spectrum of different clinical disorders reflects gene dosage effects, from the normal complement of four genes, αα/αα, to the loss of all four genes, --/--.

The α-globin genes are duplicated and lie near each other on chromosome 16. There are two major classes of α-thalassemia, α^0- and α^+-thalassemia. In α^0-thalassemia, both α-globin genes are inactivated (--/αα), whereas in α^+-thalassemia, only one of the pair is defective, due to either a deletion (-α) or another form of mutation ($\alpha^T\alpha$ or $\alpha\alpha^T$). α-Thalassemia may also be classified as α-thalassemia-2 trait or silent carrier (-α/αα) and α-thalassemia-1 or classic trait (αα/-- or -α/-α). The inactivation of two α genes from the same chromosome in *cis* (--/αα) is common in Asia, whereas the inactivation of one α gene on each chromosome in *trans* (-α/-α) is common in black populations. The excess γ-chains and β-chains produced in the α-thalassemias form γ_4 or β_4 tetramers, Hb Bart's and H, respectively. In Hb H disease, three genes are deleted (--/-α). Hydrops fetalis is associated with deletion of all four genes (--/--). Because deletions in *cis* are rare in black individuals, hydrops fetalis and Hb H disease are rarely encountered, and are found predominantly in the Mediterranean region and Southeast Asia.

GLOBIN CHAIN IMBALANCE

When globin chain synthesis is studied in reticulocytes of α-thalassemia heterozygotes, the observed imbalance in globin chain synthesis is less striking than in β-thalassemia heterozygotes. In the mild form of heterozygous α-thalassemia (-α/αα), the α:β ratio is 0.8 to 0.95, whereas in the phenotypically apparent forms of heterozygous α-thalassemia (--/αα or -α/-α), it is 0.7 to 0.8. Patients with Hb H disease (--/-α) usually have α:β ratios of 0.3 to 0.6. In hydrops fetalis with Hb Bart's (--/--), there is a total absence of α-chain synthesis.

STRUCTURALLY ABNORMAL HEMOGLOBINS ASSOCIATED WITH α-THALASSEMIA

Hb *Quong Sze* ($\alpha^{125\ Leu\rightarrow Pro}_2\beta_2$) has a labile α-chain that is destroyed so rapidly after its synthesis on ribosomes that no Hb tetramers can be formed. *Hb Constant Spring* results from a single base mutation in the termination codon that normally signals the cessation of mRNA translation. Translation thus continues 31 additional amino acids beyond the normal stop, into the usually untranslated regions of the α mRNA, resulting in an elongated α-chain. Four other Hbs convert the α-chain stop codon to another amino acid, which results in a similar elongation [*Hb Icaria* (Ter→Lys), *Hb Koya Dora* (Ser), *Hb Seal Rock* (Glu), and *Hb Paksé* (Tyr)].

HEMOGLOBIN BART'S AND HYDROPS FETALIS

Because α-globin chains are normally produced throughout development, contributing to embryonic ($\alpha_2\varepsilon_2$), fetal ($\alpha_2\gamma_2$), and adult ($\alpha_2\beta_2$) Hbs, infants who inherit no functional α genes (––/––) from their parents suffer from severe anemia *in utero*, which causes hypoxia, heart failure, and, consequently, hydrops fetalis. These infants produce large amounts of Hb Bart's (γ_4), which binds oxygen very tightly and is useless for oxygen transport. They also synthesize small amounts of the embryonic Hb, Portland ($\zeta_2\gamma_2$), which may allow sufficient tissue oxygenation for them to survive until the third trimester of pregnancy. After a gestation of 23 to 43 weeks, infants with the Hb Bart's hydrops fetalis syndrome usually die *in utero*, during delivery, or within an hour or two of birth (1340–1344). Occasionally, even without specific treatment, they survive for a few days (1345). There are a few long-term survivors (1344). Typically, affected infants are pale, slightly jaundiced, growth retarded, and edematous (1344). Ascites, cardiomegaly, and hepatomegaly (more marked than splenomegaly) (1346) are usually observed, along with retarded development of the lungs, thymus, adrenals, and kidneys (1342,1347,1348). A progressive decrease in brain weight relative to that expected for gestational age is noted from approximately 8 weeks of gestation.

This condition is characterized by severe anemia with a mean Hb level of 6.5 g/dL (1342), a very high proportion of Hb Bart's (1349–1352), a variable amount of Hb Portland, and small amounts of Hb H and Portland II ($\zeta_2\beta_2$) are also observed. The condition can be identified toward the end of the first trimester by chorion villus sampling, and later by amniotic fluid DNA analysis or fetal blood sampling. Ultrasound findings of a fetal cardiothoracic ratio greater than 0.05 may identify fetuses by 13 to 14 weeks of gestation (1353).

As neonatal care has improved, several individuals with Hb Bart's hydrops fetalis have survived. Nine babies, usually delivered prematurely by cesarean section and transfused *in utero* from approximately 25 weeks onward, or soon after birth, are reported (Table 48-11) (569). Subsequent development has been abnormal in many children, and all have required regular blood transfusions and chelation therapy. Developmental abnormalities (1341,1343,1354), including hydrocephaly (1341), microcephaly (1341), abnormal limb development (1341,1355–1358) possibly due to occlusion of small blood vessels (1358), pulmonary hypoplasia (1342), and cardiac defects (1341,1342) are reported in up to 17% of cases. Urogenital abnormalities are common and include undescended testes, hypospadias, ambiguous genitalia, and male pseudohermaphroditism (1341,1344,1347,1348,1357,1359).

MATERNAL COMPLICATIONS

An increased incidence of serious maternal complications has been reported in pregnancies complicated by hydrops fetalis (569,1344), including anemia, preeclampsia, polyhydramnios, oligohydramnios, antepartum hemorrhage, and premature labor (1341–1343,1354). Although it has been suggested that, without medical care, up to 50% of women would die as a direct result of these pregnancies (1342), this estimate is unconfirmed.

HEMOGLOBIN H DISEASE

Hb H disease is usually a moderately severe, but variable, anemia resulting from the interaction of α-thalassemia-2 with α-

thalassemia-1 (––/–α), Hb Constant Spring (––/αα^{CS}), or nondeletional forms of α-thalassemia (––/α^{T}α). Hb H disease can also occur in homozygotes for some nondeletional forms of α$^+$-thalassemia (α^{T}α/α^{T}α) in Southeast Asia and the Mediterranean. The disorder spans a wide range of clinical phenotypes, but the majority of affected individuals are healthy, and the term *disease* may be inappropriate (569). Some have thalassemia intermedia, whereas the most severe forms may be lethal late in gestation or in the perinatal period. There have been relatively few systematic studies of the natural history of Hb H disease or of the relationship between its genotype and phenotype (1347,1348,1360–1367).

At birth, infants have near normal Hb levels and no hepatosplenomegaly. The clinical features evolve slowly over the first year of life. The age at presentation is widely variable, from birth to 74 years (1348). Patients most frequently come to medical attention because of a hypochromic-microcytic anemia. Common physical findings include mild pallor, scleral icterus, and hepatosplenomegaly (1348). Gallstones (1368), leg ulcers (1369), an increased frequency of infection (1291,1348,1370), and significant reductions in serum and red cell folate (916), but not clinical folate deficiency, are also described.

Anemia in Hb H disease results from a shortened red cell survival due to the damaging effects of the interaction between precipitated β-chains and the red cell membrane. This condition is aggravated by the fact that Hb H shows no heme–heme interaction or Bohr effect and is useless as an oxygen carrier. The marked ineffective erythropoiesis and intramedullary destruction of erythroid precursor cells in β-thalassemia are not observed. The mechanical stability of the RBC membrane is normal or slightly increased, compared to homozygous β-thalassemia, in which it is markedly decreased (663,1371). Analysis of membrane skeleton protein interactions has revealed a qualitative defect in the binding of normal spectrin to inside-out vesicles, suggesting either oxidative damage to the protein ankyrin or interference of spectrin binding to ankyrin due to steric hindrance by Hb H that is bound to the membrane (663,1371).

There is a very broad scatter in Hb levels; the reported mean is approximately 7.5 g/dL (1370,1372,1373). The blood film shows hypochromia and polychromasia. In Hb H disease resulting from interaction with Hb Constant Spring trait, the slowly migrating Hb Constant Spring band is noted on electrophoresis. Before splenectomy, soluble Hb H is present and can be induced to precipitate in the form of small, stippled inclusions after *in vitro* incubation of the blood with the oxidant brilliant cresyl blue. After splenectomy, large, usually single, round preformed inclusion bodies (H bodies) are seen in red cells by phase and electron microscopy after staining with supravital stains, and occasionally on routine blood films. Hb H levels may fall in association with iron deficiency and rise again after iron therapy (1374).

It is unusual for patients with Hb H disease to require regular blood transfusions. When profound anemia is observed, it is usually complicated by iron or folic acid deficiency. Hypersplenism occurs in approximately 10% of patients (1348). After splenectomy, a sometimes fatal combination of superficial migrating thrombophlebitis, deep venous disease, and major pulmonary emboli has been described (1375).

Older patients may accumulate considerable amounts of iron through increased gastrointestinal absorption. The clinical manifestations of iron overload frequently encountered in patients with severe β-thalassemia are rarely seen (1360,1361,1376,1377). Coexistence with the common form of hereditary hemochromatosis (1012) may explain more severe iron overload in occasional patients (1365,1378).

TABLE 48-11. Summary of Clinical and Hematologic Data of Living Infants with Hemoglobin Bart's Hydrops Fetalis Syndrome

Case	Sex	Delivery (Wk of Gestation)	Method	First Transfusion	Neonatal Problems	Hb at Birth, g/dL	Weight at Birth, g	Hb Portland, %	Subsequent Development	References
1	M	34	CS	Intrauterine at 25 wk	Missing one-third of foot, syndactyly, hand defects, hypospadias, incompletely descended right testicle	Transfused	2100	Transfused	Psychological testing at 21 mo showed developmental delay, 16 mo; motor delay at 21 mo; growth below the third percentile at 21 mo	1355,1357
2	M	32	CS	At birth	Cardiopulmonary convulsions, PDA, hypospadias, cholestatic jaundice, subarachnoid hemorrhage	9.7	2300	20	At 14 mo, 6–9 mo; at 6 yr, delay in speech and hearing; height at tenth percentile, weight at fifth percentile	329, Jackson et al. (1990a)
3	F	28	CS	At birth	Respiratory distress, jaundice	(Hct 29.1%)	1080	19	At 5 yr, normal development; 50% height, 25% weight	330,323, Jackson et al. (1990a)
4	NR	28	PV (breech)	At birth	NR	NR	NR	7	Gross motor delay 10 mo, 5% height, 5% weight	Jackson et al. (1990a)
5	F	31	CS	At birth	Jaundice, PDA, heart failure	7.9	1600	NR	At 27 mo, growth retarded (less than third percentile), spastic quadriplegia, and profound developmental delay	1353
6	M	33	CS	At birth	Jaundice, metabolic instability, cortical infarcts on CT scan, right inguinal hernia	9.7	1850	17[a]	Spastic diplegia at 20 mo; mild global development delay	S. Howarth, *personal communication,* 1996, and C. Cole, *personal communication,* 1998
7	F	32	PV	At birth	PDA, cardiopulmonary "blueberry muffin" rash	~7.0	1623	10	Severe growth retardation, asymmetry in hand size; limited neuropsychiatric assessment appears normal at 5 yr	D.K. Bowden, *unpublished data,* 1992
8	M	35	PV	At birth	Penoscrotal hypospadias	(Hct 30%)	1900	22	At 6 mo, weight at tenth percentile, length at third percentile	C.K. Li, *personal communication*
9	NR	37	CS	Intrauterine at 26 wk	Cardiopulmonary, thrombocytopenia left portal vein obstruction	NR	NR	NR	Neurologically normal at 3 yr	Naqvi et al. (1997)

CS, cesarean section; CT, computed tomography; Hb, hemoglobin; Hct, hematocrit; NR, not recorded; PDA, patent ductus arteriosus; PV, *per vaginam.*
[a]Not confirmed as Hb Portland.
Modified from The α thalassemias and their interactions with structural hemoglobin varients. In: Weatherall DJ, Clegg JB, eds. The thalassemia syndromes. Oxford: Blackwell Science, 2001:489.

Hemoglobin H Disease Due to Interactions with Hemoglobin Constant Spring. Hb H disease due to interactions with the nondeletional forms of α-thalassemia, notably that associated with Hb Constant Spring, may have a more severe phenotype than the more common disorder described above. Individuals with Hb H disease associated with Hb Constant Spring are more likely to have splenomegaly or to have undergone splenectomy, to have received transfusions (1366), and to have a significantly lower Hb level and red cell counts, a significantly higher level of Hb H, and higher numbers of red cells containing Hb H inclusions (1366,1379). The membranes of the red cells containing Hb Constant Spring are even more rigid and hyperstable than in other forms of α-thalassemia, related to both the accumulation of excess β-chains and the attachment of partially oxidized α^{CS}-chains to the red cell membrane and its skeleton. More recent insights into the pathophysiology of the red cell changes associated with Hb Constant Spring have been reviewed (663,1371).

Homozygotes for Hb Constant Spring have a mild hemolytic anemia, whereas heterozygotes have no hematologic abnormality other than the 1% Hb Constant Spring demonstrated by electrophoresis.

Although most patients with Hb H disease survive into adult life, there have been no long-term studies analyzing longevity compared with normal individuals in the same population.

MILDER α-THALASSEMIA PHENOTYPES
The milder α-thalassemia phenotypes include the heterozygous and homozygous states for the deletion forms of α^+-thalassemia (−α/αα and −α/−α), the heterozygous state for α-thalassemia (−−/αα), the equivalent states for nondeletional forms of α-thalassemia (−α^Tα/αα) or (α^Tα/α^Tα), and the various compound heterozygous states for the deletion and nondeletion forms of α-thalassemia (−α/α^Tα). There is an overlapping continuum of hematologic findings and Hb constitutions across interactions of α-thalassemia.

SILENT CARRIER (−α/αα)
The heterozygous state for α-thalassemia, or α-thalassemia-2 trait, resulting from deletion of one α gene, is usually hematologically silent. The red cells are not microcytic; Hb A_2 and F are normal. A mild decrease in α-chain synthesis occurs, with β-globin:α-globin synthesis ratios slightly exceeding 1. In the newborn period, small amounts (1% to 3%) of Hb Bart's may be seen in Asian populations, but they have not been regularly seen in black or Mediterranean peoples (1380).

α-THALASSEMIA TRAIT
Patients usually have lower levels of total Hb, mean cell Hb concentration, mean cell volume, and mean corpuscular Hb than normal, but higher RBC counts. Adequate Hb levels are maintained, within approximately 1.0 to 1.5 g/dL of normal, at all stages of development (1380,1381). As a group, these patients have slightly lower levels of Hb A_2. It is possible to generate Hb H inclusions in a few red cells in α-thalassemia carriers (−−/αα), but rarely in heterozygotes or homozygotes for α-thalassemia.

NONDELETIONAL FORMS OF α-THALASSEMIA
(α^Tα/αα) OR (α^Tα/α^Tα)
The heterozygous states for the nondeletional forms of α-thalassemia (α^Tα/αα) show slightly more marked hematologic changes than the deletion forms. The homozygous states for the nondeletional forms of α-thalassemia (α^Tα/α^Tα) have very similar hematologic findings to those of patients with Hb H disease. Using standard Hb H preparation, inclusions are usually found in those with the genotypes α^Tα/αα and −α/α^Tα (1382).

The α-thalassemias pose particular difficulties in certain settings: (a) with an unexplained mild hypochromic anemia on routine blood testing, (b) with a mild hypochromic anemia with normal Hb A_2 level in a parent whose partner has a typical β-thalassemia trait as part of prenatal counseling, (c) during studies of the relatives of patients with Hb H disease, and (d) as part of a screening program for thalassemia in newborn infants. In all these situations, the finding of a microcytic, hypochromic anemia in an individual who is iron-replete and in whom the Hb A_2 level is normal should always raise the possibility of α-thalassemia. A hypochromic-microcytic picture in individuals of African origin, in whom α-thalassemia trait (−−/αα) is extremely uncommon, nearly always reflects the homozygous state for α-thalassemia of the deletional variety (−α/−α). On the other hand, in persons of Mediterranean or Southeast Asian descent, in whom both α-thalassemia and β-thalassemia are common, it is not safe to make this distinction without globin gene analysis.

α-THALASSEMIA WITH MENTAL RETARDATION OR MYELODYSPLASIA
There are other forms of α-thalassemia not inherited in the usual Mendelian way and which do not have any particular geographic pattern of occurrence, including two conditions in which mild forms of α-thalassemia are associated with *mental retardation*. Studies of these disorders have provided valuable information about the regulation of the α-globin genes. Another unusual form of α-thalassemia is associated with *myelodysplasia*. This form also has important implications for our further understanding of the regulation of the α-globin genes and insights into the etiology of the myelodysplasias. In these conditions, the α-globin genes, as "innocent bystanders," have been caught up in a pathologic process that leads to a completely different disorder (569).

α-THALASSEMIA AND MENTAL RETARDATION
The combination of ATR, together with associated developmental abnormalities, was first described in three children of North European origin, in which α-thalassemia is uncommon (1383). It has subsequently emerged that there are two distinct syndromes (1384,1385). The first, ATR-16, is characterized by large (1 to 2 Mb) chromosomal rearrangements that delete many genes from the short arm of chromosome 16: It is therefore an example of a contiguous gene syndrome. In the second, ATR-X, a complex phenotype, including α-thalassemia, results from mutations in an X-encoded factor that is a putative regulator of gene expression. Mutations within this gene down-regulate α gene expression and also perturb the expression of other, as yet unidentified, genes (1386).

ATR-16 Syndrome. Worldwide, fewer than 20 individuals who have α-thalassemia/mental retardation (ATR-16) syndrome are known (569). In all cases, the patients did not inherit the entire α-globin cluster from one or other of the parents. The clinical features, including the degree of mental retardation, are extremely diverse (2). At least three types of chromosomal rearrangements, inherited or *de novo* translocations, inversion/deletions, and truncations, as well as other less well characterized chromosomal abnormalities, have now been found in patients with ATR-16.

ATR-X Syndrome. In some patients with α-thalassemia and mental retardation, no structural abnormalities of the α cluster on chromosome 16p can be found. By contrast to the ATR-16 syndrome, patients in this nondeletional group are phenotypically uniform: They are male and have severe mental retardation with a similar facial appearance (1384,1387,1388). Ultimately, it was shown that this syndrome results from an X-linked abnormality, a condition now referred to as the *ATR-X syndrome* (1389,1390). Over 100 cases from more than 70 families have been characterized. The majority of children have profound and global developmental delay, which may vary within families (1391); marked hypotonia as neonates and in early childhood; and delayed development. The facial features are distinctive (569), and there is a wide spectrum of associated abnormalities affecting many systems, including striking genital abnormalities (1392–1394). There is generalized gut dysmotility, and aspiration is implicated as a cause of death in early childhood. The Hb and MCH are not as severely affected as in the common forms of α-thalassemia (1395). Female carriers have a normal appearance and intellect, although approximately one in four have subtle signs of α-thalassemia, with very rare cells containing Hb H inclusions (1390).

The ATR-X gene (1386) spans approximately 300 kb of genomic DNA, and is more fully described under molecular mechanisms responsible for α-thalassemia earlier in the chapter (1396–1398). ATR-X mutations appear to down-regulate expression of the α-globin genes, and the gene presumably plays an important part in the development of the central nervous system. To date, 33 different mutations have been documented. Patients with identical mutations may have very different degrees of α-thalassemia, suggesting that the effect of ATR-X protein on α-globin expression may be modified by other genetic factors. Further analysis of the ATR-16 syndrome is important to identify the target genes that are regulated by ATR-X. These genes will provide some answers for how chromosomal imbalance may give rise to developmental abnormalities.

α-Thalassemia with Myelodysplasia. Rarely, patients with myelodysplasia develop an unusual form of Hb H disease with a severe hypochromic-microcytic anemia, Hb H inclusions, and detectable levels of Hb H in the peripheral blood. Most are of North European origin, and in all cases for which archival data are available, there is no evidence of preexisting α-thalassemia. This condition is referred to as the *α-thalassemia/myelodysplasia syndrome* (ATMDS) (1399). Patients are predominantly older males. The predominant clinical features, which are those associated with myelodysplasia, include symptoms and signs of anemia and thrombocytopenia, and increased infections. Patients have hypochromic-microcytic red cells, marked anisopoikilocytosis, variable amounts of Hb H in the peripheral blood, and in some, trace amounts of Hb Bart's (1400). The α-globin:β-globin synthesis ratio is reduced (1400,1401), and in the most severely affected individuals, α-chain synthesis is almost abolished (1401). Most patients eventually develop acute myeloid leukemia or refractory cytopenias, as expected in a group of patients with myelodysplasia.

It is likely that in this disorder, the α genes are down-regulated by a *trans*-acting mutation, in a gene for a factor that either controls α gene expression or exerts a dominant-negative effect. It is also possible that the very low levels of α mRNA and α-chain synthesis may be the product of a small number of normal or myelodysplastic clones that are unaffected by the α-thalassemia mutation. Clonal evolution would explain the variations in Hb H and α-globin/β-globin synthesis observed during the course of the disease. Alternatively, the ATMDS mutation might cause variable down-regulation of α-globin expression in all cells within a single myelodysplasia clone. Localization and identification of a putative acquired *trans*-acting abnormality in ATMDS might be of great importance to understanding α gene regulation and the molecular pathway to clonal evolution in myelodysplasia (569,1402,1403).

Clinical Aspects of Hereditary Persistence of Fetal Hemoglobin

HPFH is characterized by high levels of Hb F within the red cells that persist after infancy. The genetic mechanisms responsible for HPFH were reviewed earlier in the chapter. In heterozygotes with the deletional form of HPFH, no anemia or microcytosis is observed, and levels of 20% to 30% Hb F are present in otherwise normal red cells. The distribution of Hb F is pancellular in the Kleihauer-Betke acid elution test. Homozygotes have slightly microcytic-hypochromic red cells containing 100% Hb F. There is a left shift of the oxygen dissociation curve. Because of the high oxygen affinity of Hb F-containing RBCs, a slight increase in the total Hb level occurs (1404).

The levels of Hb F in heterozygotes for nondeletional HPFH are variable, ranging from 3% to 30%. The distribution of Hb F may be pancellular or heterocellular (645,1404).

Hemoglobin E Thalassemia

Globally, Hb E/β-thalassemia is one of the most important varieties of thalassemia (570). From the gene frequencies of Hb E and β-thalassemia (1347), it is estimated there are approximately 49,000 patients in Thailand. The disease is also widespread in Vietnam (1405), Malaysia (1406,1407), Indonesia (1408–1410), Burma (1411,1412), parts of the Indian subcontinent, (1413–1415), Thailand (1416), and Sri Lanka (1417,1418).

The base substitution at codon 26, GAG → AAG, that gives rise to Hb E, β26 Glu → Lys, also activates a cryptic splice site that causes abnormal mRNA processing. Because the usual donor site has to compete with this new site, the level of normally spliced β^E mRNA is reduced (1419). The abnormally spliced mRNA is nonfunctional, because part of exon 1 is missing and a new stop codon is generated. Thus, the β^E chain is produced in reduced amounts, resulting in a β-thalassemic phenotype.

Although Hb E appears mildly unstable *in vitro* (1420), there is no evidence that this is the case *in vivo* in either the heterozygous or homozygous states (1421). Heterozygotes for Hb E have a mild microcytosis; homozygotes have red cell changes and indices similar to those of heterozygous β-thalassemia: mild anemia, normal red cell survival, and little or no elevation of Hb F (1421–1423). Homozygotes have imbalanced globin synthesis, with α-chain:β-chain synthesis ratios very similar to those of heterozygous β-thalassemia (1421,1423–1425). Hence, inheritance of Hb E produces the phenotype of a mild form of β-thalassemia.

The majority of the β-thalassemia alleles commonly associated with Hb E are of the β^0 or of the severe β^+ variety; mild β-thalassemia alleles are relatively uncommon in the Southeast Asian populations in which Hb E occurs.

There is marked clinical heterogeneity in the disorder (1368,1426–1430). Coinheritance of different α-thalassemia alleles or increased levels of Hb F production, at least as evidenced by the presence or absence of the *Xmn*1 polymorphism –158 to the $^G\gamma$-globin gene, may play a minor role in modifying the phenotype (1431). With the possible exception of the interaction of the rare mild forms of β^+-thalassemia with Hb E, there seems to be very little relationship between the remarkable phenotypic variation of this disease and the particular β-thalassemia allele that has been inherited (1415).

HEMATOLOGIC FINDINGS
There is a variable and sometimes severe degree of anemia from early life (1347,1370,1432,1433), with most patients' Hbs in the 5 to 7 g/dL range. The red cell indices (865) and bone marrow findings (1434) are similar to those of homozygous β-thalas-

semia. Red cell survival is considerably shortened (1435,1436), and intravascular hemolysis results in elevations in serum bilirubin and plasma Hb levels (1437).

HEMOGLOBIN ANALYSIS

The usual finding in families is Hb E trait in one parent and β-thalassemia trait in the other (1438). Most cases of Hb E/β-thalassemia in Southeast Asia and India are due to the interaction of $β^0$ or severe types of $β^+$-thalassemia with Hb E. Hence, the Hb is a mixture of E, F, and A_2; Hb A is absent, or present in low amounts. Hb F in the peripheral blood varies widely, from 5% to nearly 90% (1409,1432,1437,1439) (mean, 48%) (1347), and is heterogeneously distributed in the red cell (1439). The degree of globin chain imbalance is usually comparable to that in homozygous β-thalassemia (659,1429,1436,1440).

CLINICAL FEATURES

Many of these children develop clinical features of severe homozygous or compound heterozygous thalassemia as they age (1405,1415,1432,1437,1441). However, in every population, some patients do not require chronic transfusions and have relatively normal growth and development (848,1429), similar to the clinical course of β-thalassemia intermedia.

COURSE AND COMPLICATIONS

Although few data are available, the average age of presentation is later than in other forms of β-thalassemia. In 120 patients studied in Sri Lanka, patients presented from 1 to 54 years of age. Even the severely affected children tended to present later than homozygotes or compound heterozygotes for β-thalassemia (*unpublished data*, 2001).

Growth. Retardation of growth and development is noted in early descriptions of Hb E/β-thalassemia (1405,1432,1442,1443). Reduction in height is related to the Hb level. Preliminary studies from Sri Lanka suggest that much more needs to be learned about the relationship between the steady-state Hb level, and growth and sexual maturation in this disease.

Infection. Children with Hb E/β-thalassemia are prone to infection, which is probably the most common cause of death in all age groups (1347,1432,1444–1448). Apart from the effects of splenectomy and of neutropenia associated with hypersplenism, there are no explanations for such a high rate of infection in this form of thalassemia.

Hypersplenism. Massive enlargement of the spleen occurs (1347,1432,1437), and patients may improve after splenectomy (1347,1437). Although hepatomegaly is reported to occur after splenectomy (1432), this finding is not well documented. Liver biopsies after splenectomy suggest that extramedullary erythropoiesis, inflammatory change, and early evidence of hepatic fibrosis all contribute to the development of hepatomegaly.

Other Changes. Temporary aplasia of the bone marrow with worsening anemia has been well documented (1437). Serum and red cell folate levels are reduced in a substantial proportion of patients in Thailand (916), and megaloblastic anemia may complicate the clinical course (1437).

As in all forms of severe thalassemia intermedia, tumor masses caused by extension of bone marrow due to massive erythroid hyperplasia may simulate a mediastinal mass on chest x-ray (1449). Large bone marrow masses may form an intracranial mass (1450) or compress the spinal cord or other structures and cause severe paraplegia (1451,1452) or obstructive uropathy (1453).

Iron Overload. Severe iron loading may occur in Hb E/β-thalassemia due to increased gastrointestinal iron absorption (1454). A consistent relationship is noted between the degree of erythropoiesis and the rate of absorption of radioactive iron occurs (708). Even in nontransfused patients, serum ferritin (1455) and nontransferrin-bound plasma iron (1456) increase significantly with age. Elevated hepatic iron concentrations associated with varying degrees of fibrosis (1457,1458) are observed even in untransfused patients (1459). Pathologic data show extensive iron loading of liver, spleen, lymph nodes, pancreas, adrenals, kidneys, alimentary tract, and heart (1460–1463).

Cardiopulmonary Dysfunction. Although the cardiac complications in heavily transfused patients are similar to those in transfusion-dependent β-thalassemia (1368), specific cardiopulmonary manifestations differ from those of other forms of β-thalassemia. Pulmonary arterial obstruction, pulmonary hypertension, chronic hypoxemia, and right heart failure occur in patients with Hb E/β-thalassemia, particularly after splenectomy, and are partially reversed by the administration of aspirin (1464–1467). These findings may reflect chronic right ventricular strain and hypoxia, possibly resulting from postsplenectomy thrombocytosis and platelet aggregation in the pulmonary arterial vessels. Autopsy studies show obliterative changes in the pulmonary arterioles and, in some cases, large pulmonary emboli (1462,1468). Restrictive and obstructive defects, arterial hypoxemia, and abnormalities of platelet function are reported (1469,1470).

Coagulation Abnormalities. As in other thalassemias, abnormalities of platelet numbers and function, or of clotting factors and their antagonists, are reported in Hb E/β-thalassemia; however, no clear pattern has emerged. These abnormalities include increases in spontaneous platelet aggregation (1471,1472), a variety of abnormalities of platelet aggregation and function (1473), reduced levels of proteins C and S (1474), changes in platelet factor III availability (1475), and an acquired abnormality of von Willebrand's factor (1476). These coagulation abnormalities may have important implications for the management of this disease, particularly in splenectomized patients.

Endocrine Dysfunction. Endocrine dysfunction secondary to iron loading has been reported in a few studies (1370,1477,1478). Its full clinical spectrum remains to be determined.

Other Complications. There is progressive reduction in bone density as patients age, which may be associated with an increasing tendency for spontaneous fractures (1368,1479). Chronic ulceration of the lower legs and ankles is common in some populations (1347). Gallstones are reported in up to 50% of patients (1480).

An unexplained syndrome of posttransfusion hypertension, convulsions, and cerebral hemorrhage after multiple blood transfusions has been described in patients with Hb E/β-thalassemia (507,1481–1483). At autopsy, the brains were edematous and congested, with visible cerebral hemorrhages. Microscopically, small focal or perivascular hemorrhages were detected, but there were no lesions characteristic of hypertensive cerebral damage or underlying vascular disease.

Hb E/β-thalassemia has a variable prognosis. In some populations, the disorder is associated with a considerable mortality in childhood. It is not clear how many patients survive to adult life or the extent to which the poor socioeconomic conditions of many children in Southeast Asia and India contribute to early mortality. Infection is a major factor (1432,1460), particularly in splenectomized patients (1370,1484). Posttransfusion cerebral hemorrhage and a curious syndrome of progressive wasting, severe weakness, weight loss, and general malaise in young patients (1416) are other causes of death. Apart from congestive cardiac failure associated with severe anemia, cardiac deaths of the type observed in well transfused, poorly chelated patients with β-thalassemia are rare (1485). It is becoming clear that some patients go through childhood and adolescence relatively symptom-free. Thus, although the disease may kill in infancy or adolescence, there is no doubt that it is compatible with survival into adult life.

REFERENCES

1. Weatherall DJ, Clegg JB. *The thalassemia syndromes*, 3rd ed. Oxford: Blackwell Science, 1981.
2. Baglioni C. The fusion of two peptide chains in hemoglobin Lepore and its interpretation as a genetic deletion. *Proc Natl Acad Sci U S A* 1962;48:1880.
3. Kendall AG, Ojwang PJ, Schroeder WA, et al. Hemoglobin Kenya, the product of a γ-β fusion gene: studies of the family. *Am J Hum Genet* 1973;25:548.
4. Deisseroth A, Nienhuis A, Turner P, et al. Localization of the human α-globin structural gene to chromosome 16 in somatic cell hybrids by molecular hybridization assay. *Cell* 1977;12:205.
5. Deisseroth A, Nienhuis A, Lawrence J, et al. Chromosomal localization of human β-globin gene on human chromosome 11 in somatic cell hybrids. *Proc Natl Acad Sci U S A* 1978;75:1456.
6. Bunn HF, Forget BG. *Hemoglobin: molecular, genetic and clinical aspects*. Philadelphia: WB Saunders, 1986.
7. Collins FS, Weissman SM. The molecular genetics of human hemoglobin. *Prog Nucleic Acid Res Mol Biol* 1984;31:315.
8. Nienhuis AW, Maniatis T. Structure and expression of globin genes in erythroid cells. In: Stamatoyannopoulos G, Nienhuis AW, Leder P, et al., eds. *The molecular basis of blood diseases*. Philadelphia: WB Saunders, 1987:28.
9. Hsu S-L, Marks J, Shaw J-P, et al. Structure and expression of the human θ globin gene. *Nature* 1988;331:44.
10. Ley TJ, Maloney KA, Gordon JI, et al. Globin gene expression in erythroid human fetal liver cells. *J Clin Invest* 1988;83:1032.
11. Albitar M, Peschle C, Liebhaber SA. Theta, zeta, and epsilon globin messenger RNAs are expressed in adults. *Blood* 1989;74:629.
12. Clegg JB. Can the product of the θ-gene be a real globin? *Nature* 1987;329:465.
13. Padgett RA, Grabowski PJ, Konaroka MM, et al. Splicing of messenger RNA precursors. *Annu Rev Biochem* 1986;55:1119.
14. Mount SM. A catalogue of splice junction sequences. *Nucleic Acids Res* 1982; 10:459.
15. Madhani HD, Guthrie C. Dynamic RNA-RNA interactions in the spliceosome. *Annu Rev Genet* 1994;28:1.
16. Nilsen TW. RNA-RNA interactions in the spliceosome: unraveling the ties that bind. *Cell* 1994;78:1.
17. Staley JP, Guthrie C. Mechanical devices of the spliceosome: motors, clocks, springs, and things. *Cell* 1998;92:315.
18. Smale ST, Baltimore D. The "initiator" as a transcription control element. *Cell* 1989;57:103.
19. Wickens M. How the messenger got its tail: addition of poly(A) in the nucleus. *Trends Biochem Sci* 1990;15:277.
20. Wahle E, Keller W. The biochemistry of 3'-end cleavage and polyadenylation of messenger RNA precursors. *Annu Rev Biochem* 1992;61:419.
21. Proudfoot N. Ending the message is not so simple. *Cell* 1996;87:779–781.
22. Boissel J-P, Kasper TJ, Shah SC, et al. Amino-terminal processing of proteins: hemoglobin South Florida, a variant with retention of initiator methionine and Nα-acetylation. *Proc Natl Acad Sci U S A* 1985;82:8448.
23. Kozak M. The scanning model for translation: an update. *J Cell Biol* 1989;108:229.
24. Donze D, Jeancake P, Townes T. Activation of delta-globin gene expression by erythroid Krupple-like factor: a potential approach for gene therapy of sickle cell disease. *Blood* 1996;88:4051.
25. Tang DC, Ebb D, Hardison RC, et al. Restoration of the CCAAT box and insertion of the CACCC motif activate δ-globin gene expression. *Blood* 1997;90:421.
26. Lewin B. Commitment and activation at Pol II promoters: a tail of protein-protein interactions. *Cell* 1990;61:1161.
27. Kadonaga J. Eukaryotic transcription: an interlaced network of transcription factors and chromatin-modifying machines. *Cell* 1998;92:307.
28. Martin D, Tsai S, Orkin S. Increased γ-globin expression in a non-deletion HPFH is mediated by an erythroid-specific DNA-binding factor. *Nature* 1989;338:435.
29. Tsai S, Martin D, Zon L, et al. Cloning of the cDNA for the major DNA-binding protein of the erythroid lineage through expression in mammalian cells. *Nature* 1989;339:446.
30. Orkin SH. Globin gene regulation and switching: circa 1990. *Cell* 1990;63:665.
31. Orkin SH. GATA-binding transcription factors in hematopoietic cells. *Blood* 1992;80:575.
32. Engel JD, George KM, Ko LJ, et al. Transcription factor regulation of hematopoietic lineage cells. *Semin Hematol* 1991;28:158.
33. Orkin SH. Transcription factors and hematopoietic development. *J Biol Chem* 1995;270:4955.

34. Orkin SH. Regulation of globin gene expression in erythroid cells. *Eur J Biochem* 1995;231:271.
35. Weiss MJ, Orkin SH. GATA transcription factors: key regulators of hematopoiesis. *Exp Hematol* 1995;23:99.
36. Pevny L, Simon MC, Robertson E, et al. Erythroid differentiation in chimaeric mice blocked by a targeted mutation in the gene for transcription factor GATA-1. *Nature* 1991;349:257.
37. Fujiwara Y, Browne CP, Cunniff K, et al. Arrested development of embryonic red cell precursors in mouse embryos lacking transcription factor GATA-1. *Proc Natl Acad Sci U S A* 1996;93:12355.
38. Simon MC, Pevny L, Wiles MV, et al. Rescue of erythroid development in gene targeted GATA-1 mouse embryonic stem cells. *Nat Genet* 1992;1:92.
39. Pevny L, Lin CS, D'Agati V, et al. Development of hematopoietic cells lacking transcription factor GATA-1. *Development* 1995;121:13.
40. Weiss MJ, Keller G, Orkin SH. Novel insights into erythroid development revealed through *in vitro* differentiation of GATA-1 embryonic stem cells. *Genes Dev* 1994;8:1184.
41. Weiss MJ, Orkin SH. Transcription factor GATA-1 permits survival and maturation of erythroid precursors by preventing apoptosis. *Proc Natl Acad Sci U S A* 1995;92:9623.
42. Blobel GA, Simon MC, Orkin SH. Rescue of GATA-1-deficient embryonic stem cells by heterologous GATA-binding proteins. *Mol Cell Biol* 1995;15:626.
43. Weiss MJ, Yu C, Orkin SH. Erythroid-cell-specific properties of transcription factor GATA-1 revealed by phenotypic rescue of a gene-targeted cell line. *Mol Cell Biol* 1997;17:1642.
44. Tsang AP, Visvader JE, Turner CA, et al. FOG, a multitype zinc finger protein, acts as a cofactor for transcription factor GATA-1 in erythroid and megakaryocytic differentiation. *Cell* 1997;90:109.
45. Tsang AP, Fujiwara Y, Hom DB, et al. Failure of megakaryopoiesis and arrested erythropoiesis in mice lacking the GATA-1 transcriptional cofactor FOG. *Genes Dev* 1998;12:1176.
46. Blobel GA, Nakajima T, Eckner R, et al. CREB-binding protein cooperates with transcription factor GATA-1 and is required for erythroid differentiation. *Proc Natl Acad Sci U S A* 1998;95:2061.
47. Merika M, Orkin SH. Functional synergy and physical interactions of the erythroid transcription factor GATA-1 with the Kruppel family proteins Sp1 and EKLF. *Mol Cell Biol* 1995;15:2437.
48. Gregory RC, Taxman DJ, Seshasayee D, et al. Functional interaction of GATA1 with erythroid Kruppel-like factor and Sp1 at defined erythroid promoters. *Blood* 1996;87:173.
49. Wadman IA, Osada H, Grutz GG, et al. The LIM-only protein Lmo2 is a bridging molecule assembling an erythroid, DNA-binding complex which includes the TAL1, E47, GATA-1 and Ldb1/NLI proteins. *EMBO J* 1997;16:3145.
50. Anderson, KP, Crable SC, Lingrel JB. Multiple proteins binding to a GATA-E box-GATA motif in the erythroid Kruppel-like factor (EKLF) gene. *J Biol Chem* 1998;273:14347.
51. Andrews NC, Erdjument-Bromage H, Davidson MB, et al. Erythroid transcription factor NF-E2 is a haematopoietic-specific basic-leucine zipper protein. *Nature* 1993;363:722.
52. Ney PA, Sorrentino BP, McDonagh KT, et al. Tandem AP-1-binding sites within the human β-globin dominant control region function as an inducible enhancer in erythroid cells. *Genes Dev* 1990;4:993.
53. Ney PA, Sorrentino BP, Lowrey CH, et al. Inducibility of the HS II enhancer depends on binding of an erythroid specific nuclear protein. *Nucleic Acids Res* 1990;18:6011.
54. Talbot D, Grosveld F. The 5' HS2 of the globin locus control region enhances transcription through the interaction of a multimeric complex binding at two functionally distinct NF-E2 binding sites. *EMBO J* 1991;10:1391.
55. Mignotte V, Wall L, deBoer E, et al. Two tissue-specific factors bind the erythroid promoter of the human porphobilinogen deaminase gene. *Nucleic Acids Res* 1989;17:37.
56. Andrews NC, Kotkow KJ, Ney PA, et al. The ubiquitous subunit of erythroid transcription factor NF-E2 is a small basic-leucine zipper protein related to the v-maf oncogene. *Proc Natl Acad Sci U S A* 1993;90:11488.
57. Shivdasani RA, Orkin SH. Erythropoiesis and globin gene expression in mice lacking the transcription factor NF-E2. *Proc Natl Acad Sci U S A* 1995;92:8690.
58. Chan JY, Han X-L, Kan YW. Cloning of Nrf1, an NF-E2-related transcription factor, by genetic selection in yeast. *Proc Natl Acad Sci U S A* 1993;90:11371.
59. Caterina JJ, Donze D, Sun C-W, et al. Cloning and functional characterization of LCR-F1: a bZIP transcription factor that activates erythroid-specific, human globin gene expression. *Nucleic Acids Res* 1994;22:2383.
60. Moi P, Chan K, Asunis I, et al. Isolation of NF-E2 like basic leucine zipper transcriptional activator that binds to the tandem NF-E2/AP1 repeat of the β-globin locus control region. *Proc Natl Acad Sci U S A* 1994;91:9926.
61. Chui DHK, Tang W, Orkin SH. cDNA cloning of murine Nrf2 gene, coding for a p45 NF-E2 related transcription factor. *Biochem Biophys Res Commun* 1995;209:40.
62. Oyake T, Itoh K, Motohashi H, et al. Bach proteins belong to a novel family of BTB-basic leucine zipper transcription factors that interact with MafK and regulate transcription through the NF-E2 site. *Mol Cell Biol* 1996;16:6083–6095.
63. Itoh K, Igarashi K, Hayashi N, et al. Cloning and characterization of a novel erythroid cell-derived CNC family transcription factor heterodimerizing with the small Maf family proteins. *Mol Cell Biol* 1995;15:4184.
64. Miller U, Bieker JJ. A novel, erythroid cell-specific murine transcription factor that binds to the CACCC element and is related to the Kruppel family of nuclear proteins. *Mol Cell Biol* 1993;13:2776.

65. Feng WC, Southwood CM, Bieker JJ. Analyses of β-thalassemia mutant DNA interactions with erythroid Kruppel-like factor (EKLF), an erythroid cell-specific transcription factor. *J Biol Chem* 1994;269:1493.

66. Nuez B, Michalovich D, Bygrave A, et al. Defective hematopoiesis in fetal liver resulting from inactivation of the EKLF gene. *Nature* 1995;375:316–318.

67. Perkins AC, Sharpe AH, Orkin SH. Lethal β-thalassemia in mice lacking the erythroid CACCC-transcription factor EKLF. *Nature* 1995;375:318.

68. Donze D, Townes TM, Bieker JJ. Role of erythroid Kruppel-like factor in human γ- to β-globin gene switching. *J Biol Chem* 1995;270:1955.

69. Guy L-G, Mei Q, Perkins AC, et al. Erythroid Kruppel-like factor is essential for β-globin gene expression even in absence of gene competition, but is not sufficient to induce the switch from γ-globin to β-globin gene expression. *Blood* 1998;91:2259.

70. Asano H, Stamatoyannopoulos G. Activation of β-globin promoter by erythroid Kruppel-like factor. *Mol Cell Biol* 1998;118:102.

71. Asano H, Li XS, Stamatoyannopoulos G. FKLF-2: a novel Kruppel-like transcriptional factor that activates globin and other erythroid lineage genes. *Blood* 2000;95:3578.

72. Jane SM, Ney PA, Vanin EF, et al. Identification of a stage selector element in the human γ-globin gene promoter that fosters preferential interaction with the 5' HS2 enhancer when in competition with the β-promoter. *EMBO J* 1992;11:2961.

73. Jane SM, Nienhuis AW, Cunningham JM Hemoglobin switching in man and chicken is mediated by a heteromeric complex between the ubiquitous transcription factor CP2 and a developmentally specific protein. *EMBO J* 1995;14:97–105.

74. Zhou W, Clouston DR, Wang X, et al. Induction of human fetal globin gene expression by a novel erythroid factor, NF-E4. *Mol Cell Biol* 2000;20:7662.

75. Gallarda JL, Foley KP, Yang ZY, et al. The beta-globin stage selector element factor is erythroid-specific promoter/enhancer binding protein NF-E4. *Genes Dev* 1989;3:1845.

76. O'Neill D, Yang J, Erdjument-Bromage H, et al. Tissue-specific and developmental stage-specific DNA binding by a mammalian SWI/SNF complex associated with human fetal-to-adult globin gene switching. *Proc Natl Acad Sci U S A* 1999;96:349.

77. Khoury G, Gruss P. Enhancer elements. *Cell* 1983;33:313.

78. Svaren J, Chalkley R. The structure and assembly of active chromatin. *Trends Genet* 1990;6:52.

79. Lewin B. Commitment and activation at Pol II promoters: a tale of protein-protein interactions. *Cell* 1990;61:1161.

80. Ptashne M, Gann AAF. Activators and targets. *Nature* 1990;346:329.

81. Kollias G, Hurst J, DeBoer E, et al. The human β-globin gene contains a downstream developmental specific enhancer. *Nucleic Acids Res* 1987;15:5739.

82. Trudel M, Magram J, Bruckner L, et al. Upstream G δ-globin and downstream β-globin sequences required for stage-specific expression in transgenic mice. *Mol Cell Biol* 1987;7:4024.

83. Behringer RR, Hammer RE, Brinster RL, et al. Two 3' sequences direct adult erythroid-specific expression of human β-globin genes in transgenic mice. *Proc Natl Acad Sci U S A* 1987;84:7056.

84. Trudel M, Costantini F. A 3' enhancer contributes to the stage-specific expression of the human β-globin gene. *Genes Dev* 1987;1:954.

85. Antoniou M, deBoer E, Habets G, et al. The human β-globin gene contains multiple regulatory regions: identification of one promoter and two downstream enhancers. *EMBO J* 1988;7:377.

86. Wall L, deBoer E, Grosveld F. The human β-globin gene 3' enhancer contains multiple binding sites for an erythroid-specific protein. *Genes Dev* 1988;2:1089.

87. Bodine DM, Ley TJ. An enhancer element lies 3' to the human ᴬγ-globin gene. *EMBO J* 1987;6:2997.

88. Knezetic JA, Felsenfeld G. Identification and characterization of a chicken α-globin enhancer. *Mol Cell Biol* 1989;9:893.

89. Cao SX, Gitman PD, Dave HPG, et al. Identification of a transcriptional silencer in the 5'-flanking region of the human ε-globin gene. *Proc Natl Acad Sci U S A* 1989;86:5306.

90. Watt P, Lamb P, Proudfoot NJ. Distinct negative regulation of the human embryonic globin genes zeta and epsilon. *Gene Expr* 1993;3:61–75.

91. Liebhaber SA, Wang Z, Cash FE, et al. Developmental silencing of the embryonic ζ-globin gene: concerted action of the promoter and the 3'-flanking region combined with stage-specific silencing by the transcribed segment. *Mol Cell Biol* 1996;16:2637.

92. Li Q, Blau CA, Clegg CH, et al. Multiple ε-promoter elements participate in the developmental control of ε-globin genes in transgenic mice. *J Biol Chem* 1998;273:17361.

93. Li J, Noguchi CT, Miller W, et al. Multiple regulatory elements in the 5'-flanking sequence of the human ε-globin gene. *J Biol Chem* 1998;273:10202.

94. Wang Z, Liebhaber SA. A 3'-flanking NK-κB site mediates developmental silencing of the human ζ-globin gene. *EMBO J* 1999;18:2218–2228.

95. Berg PE, Williams DM, Quian RL, et al. A common protein binds to two silencers 5' to the human β-globin gene. *Nucleic Acids Res* 1989;17:8833.

96. Stamatoyannopoulos G, Josephson B, Zhang J-W, et al. Developmental regulation of human γ-globin genes in transgenic mice. *Mol Cell Biol* 1993;13:7636.

97. Tuan D, Solomon W, Li Q, et al. The "β-like-globin" gene domain in human erythroid cells. *Proc Natl Acad Sci U S A* 1985;82:6384.

98. Forrester WC, Thompson C, Elder JT, et al. A developmentally stable chromatin structure in the human β-globin gene cluster. *Proc Natl Acad Sci U S A* 1986;83:1359.

99. Li Q, Stamatoyannopoulos G. Hypersensitive site 5 of the human β locus control region functions as a chromatin insulator. *Blood* 1994;84:1399.

100. Chung JH, Whiteley M, Felsenfeld G. A 5'element of the chicken beta-globin domain serves as an insulator in human erythroid cells and protects against position effect in *Drosophila*. *Cell* 1993;74:505.

101. Chung JH, Bell AC, Felsenfeld G. Characterization of the chicken beta-globin insulator. *Proc Natl Acad Sci U S A* 1997;94:575.

102. Receillas-Targa F, Bell AC, Felsenfeld G. Positional enhancer-blocking activity of the chicken beta-globin insulator in transiently transfected cells. *Proc Natl Acad Sci U S A* 1999;96:14354.

103. Bulger M, Hikke von Doorninck J, Saitoh N, et al. Conservation of sequence and structure flanking the mouse and human β-globin loci: the β-globin genes are embedded within an array of odorant receptor genes. *Proc Natl Acad Sci U S A* 1999;96:5129.

104. Forrester WC, Epner E, Driscoll MC, et al. A deletion of the human β-globin gene locus activation region causes a major alteration in chromatin structure and replication across the entire β-globin locus. *Genes Dev* 1990;4:1637.

105. Grosveld F, Blom van Assendelft G, Greaves DR, et al. Position-independent, high-level expression of the human β-globin gene in transgenic mice. *Cell* 1987;51:975.

106. Townes TM, Behringer RR. Human globin locus activation region (LAR): role in temporal control. *Trends Genet* 1990;6:219.

107. Forrester WC, Takegawa S, Papayanopoulou T, et al. Evidence for a locus activating region: the formation of developmentally stable hypersensitive sites in globin-expressing hybrids. *Nucleic Acids Res* 1987;15:10159.

108. Talbot D, Collis P, Antoniou M, et al. A dominant control region from the human β-globin locus conferring integration site-independent gene expression. *Nature* 1989;338:352.

109. Higgs DR, Wood WG, Jarman AP, et al. A major positive regulatory region located far upstream of the human α-globin gene locus. *Genes Dev* 1990;4:1588.

110. Jarman AP, Wood WG, Sharpe JA, et al. Characterization of the major regulatory element upstream of the human alpha-globin gene cluster. *Mol Cell Biol* 1991;11:4679.

111. Higgs DR, Sharpe JA, Wood WG. Understanding α globin gene expression: a step towards effective gene therapy. *Semin Hematol* 1998;35:93.

112. Moi P, Kan YW. Synergistic enhancement of globin gene expression by activator protein-1-like proteins. *Proc Natl Acad Sci U S A* 1990;87:9000.

113. Philipsen S, Talbot D, Fraser P, et al. The β-globin dominant control region: hypersensitive site 2. *EMBO J* 1990;9:2159.

114. Philipsen S, Talbot D, Fraser P, et al. Detailed analysis of the site 3 region of the human β-globin dominant control region. *EMBO J* 1990;9:2169.

115. Ikuta T, Kan YW. In vivo protein-DNA interactions at the β-globin gene locus. *Proc Natl Acad Sci U S A* 1991;88:10188.

116. Strauss EC, Orkin SH. In vivo protein-DNA interactions at hypersensitive site 3 of the human β-globin locus control region. *Proc Natl Acad Sci U S A* 1992;89:5809.

117. Strauss EC, Andrews NC, Higgs DR, et al. *In vivo* footprinting of the human α-globin locus upstream regulatory element by guanine and adenine ligation-mediated polymerase chain reaction. *Mol Cell Biol* 1992;12:2135.

118. Reddy PMS, Stamatoyannopoulos G, Papayannopoulou T, et al. Genomic footprinting and sequencing of human β-globin locus: tissue specificity and cell line artifact. *J Biol Chem* 1994;269:8287.

119. Zhang Q, Reddy PM, Yu CY, et al. Transcriptional activation of human zeta 2 globin promoter by the alpha globin regulatory element (HS-40): functional role of specific nuclear factor-DNA complexes. *Mol Cell Biol* 1998;13:2298.

120. Ney PA, Sorrentino BP, McDonagh KT, et al. Tandem AP-1 binding sites within the human β-globin dominant control region. *Genes Dev* 1990;4:993.

121. Talbot D, Grosveld F. The 5'HS2 of the globin locus control region enhances transcription through the interaction of a multimeric complex binding at two functionally distinct NF-E2 binding sites. *EMBO J* 1991;10:1391.

122. Liu D, Chang JC, Moi P, et al. Dissection of the enhancer activity of β-globin 5' DNaseI-hypersensitive site 2 in transgenic mice. *Proc Natl Acad Sci U S A* 1992;89:3899.

123. Engel JD. Developmental regulation of human β-globin gene transcription: a switch of loyalties? *Trends Genet* 1993;9:304.

124. Fraser P, Pruzina S, Antoniou M, et al. Each hypersensitive site of the human β-globin locus control region confers a different developmental pattern of expression on the globin genes. *Genes Dev* 1993;7:106.

125. Ellis J, Tan-Un KC, Harper A, et al. A dominant chromatin-opening activity in 5' hypersensitive site 3 of the human beta-globin locus control region. *EMBO J* 1996;15:562.

126. Wijgerde M, Grosveld F, Fraser P. Transcription complex stability and chromatin dynamics in vivo. *Nature* 1995;377:209.

127. Milot E, Strouboulis J, Trimborn T, et al. Heterochromatin effects on the frequency and duration of LCR-mediated gene transcription. *Cell* 1996;87:105.

128. Reik A, Telling A, Zitnik G, et al. The locus control region is necessary for gene expression in the human β-globin locus but not the maintenance of an open chromatin structure in erythroid cells. *Mol Cell Biol* 1998;18:5992.

129. Higgs DR. Do LCRs open chromatin domains? *Cell* 1998;95:299.

130. Stamatoyannopoulos G. Human hemoglobin switching. *Science* 1991;252:383.

131. Grosveld F, Antoniou M, Berry M, et al. The regulation of human globin gene switching. *Philos Trans R Soc Lond B Biol Sci* 1993;339:183.

132. Hardison R, Slightom JL, Gumucio DL, et al. Locus control regions of mammalian β-globin gene clusters: combining phylogenetic analyses and experimental results to gain functional insights. *Gene* 1997;205:73.

133. Grosveld F. Activation by locus control regions? *Curr Opin Genet Dev* 1999; 9:152.
134. Bulger M, Groudine M. Looping versus linking: toward a model for long-distance gene activation. *Genes Dev* 1999;13:2465.
135. Engel JD, Tanimoto K. Looping, linking, and chromatin activity: new insights into beta-globin locus regulation. *Cell* 2000;100:499.
136. Li Q, Harju S, Peterson KR. Locus control regions: coming of age at a decade plus. *Trends Genet* 1999;15:403.
137. Tuan D, Kong S, Hu K. Transcription of the hypersensitive site HS2 enhancer in erythroid cells. *Proc Natl Acad Sci U S A* 1992;89:11219.
138. Kong S, Bohl D, Li C, et al. Transcription of the HS2 enhancer toward a cis-linked gene is independent of the orientation, position, and distance of the enhancer relative to the gene. *Mol Cell Biol* 1997;17:3955.
139. Stamatoyannopoulos G, Grosveld F. Hemoglobin switching. In: Stamatoyannopoulos G, Majerus PW, Perlmutter RM, et al., eds. *The molecular basis of blood diseases*, 3rd ed. Philadelphia: WB Saunders, 2001:135.
140. Ley TJ. The pharmacology of hemoglobin switching: of mice and men. *Blood* 1991;77:6.
141. Peschle C, Mavilio F, Carè A, et al. Haemoglobin switching in human embryos: asynchrony of ζ → α and ε → γ-globin switches in primitive and definitive erythropoietic lineage. *Nature* 1985;313:235.
142. Bard H. Postnatal fetal and adult hemoglobin synthesis in early preterm newborn infants. *J Clin Invest* 1973;52:1789.
143. Bard H, Prosmanne J. Postnatal fetal and adult hemoglobin synthesis in preterm infants whose birth weight was less than 1,000 grams. *J Clin Invest* 1982;70:50.
144. Bunch C, Wood WG, Weatherall DJ, et al. Haemoglobin synthesis by foetal erythroid cells in an adult environment. *Br J Haematol* 1981;49:325.
145. Wood WG, Bunch C, Kelly S, et al. Control of haemoglobin switching by a developmental clock? *Nature* 1985;313:320.
146. Delfini C, Saglio G, Mazzo, U, et al. Fetal haemoglobin synthesis following fetal liver transplantation in man. *Br J Haematol* 1983;55:609.
147. Papayannopoulou T, Nakamoto B, Agostinelli, F, et al. Fetal to adult hemopoietic cell transplantation in man: insights into hemoglobin switching. *Blood* 1986;67:99.
148. Zanjani ED, Lim G, McGlave PB, et al. Adult haematopoietic cells transplanted to sheep fetuses continue to produce adult globins. *Nature* 1982;295:244.
149. Blanchet JP, Fleischman RA, Mintz B. Murine adult hematopoietic cells produce adult erythrocytes in fetal recipients. *Dev Genet* 1982;3:197.
150. Papayannopoulou T, Brice M, Stamatoyannopoulos G. Analysis of human globin switching in MEL X human fetal erythroid cell hybrids. *Cell* 1986;46:469.
151. Geiger H, Sick S, Bonifer C, et al. Globin gene expression is reprogrammed in chimeras generated by injecting adult hematopoietic stem cells into mouse blastocysts. *Cell* 1998;93:1055.
152. Weinberg RS, Goldberg JD, Schofield JM, et al. Switch from fetal to adult hemoglobin is associated with change in progenitor cell population. *J Clin Invest* 1983;71:785.
153. Alter BP, Jackson BT, Lipton JM, et al. Control of the simian fetal hemoglobin switch at the progenitor cell level. *J Clin Invest* 1981;67:458.
154. Wood WG, Weatherall DJ. Haemoglobin synthesis during human foetal development. *Nature* 1973;244:162.
155. Wood WG, Nash J, Weatherall DJ, et al. The sheep as an animal model for the switch from fetal to adult hemoglobins. In: Stamatoyannopoulos G, Nienhuis AW, eds. *Cellular and molecular regulation of hemoglobin switching*. New York: Grune & Stratton, 1979:153.
156. Peschle C, Migliaccio AR, Migliaccio G, et al. Embryonic to fetal Hb switch in humans: studies on erythroid bursts generated by embryonic progenitors from yolk sac and liver. *Proc Natl Acad Sci U S A* 1984;81:2416.
157. Stamatoyannopoulos G, Constantoulakis P, Brice M, et al. Coexpression of embryonic, fetal, and adult globins in erythroid cells of human embryos: relevance to the cell-lineage models of globin switching. *Dev Biol* 1987;123:191.
158. Kidoguchi K, Ogawa M, Karam JD, et al. Hemoglobin biosynthesis in individual bursts in culture: studies of human umbilical cord blood. *Blood* 1979;53:519.
159. Papayannopoulou TH, Brice M, Stamatoyannopoulos G. Hemoglobin F synthesis in vitro: evidence for control at the level of primitive erythroid stem cells. *Proc Natl Acad Sci U S A* 1977;74:2923.
160. Colombo B, Kim B, Perez Atencio R, et al. The pattern of fetal haemoglobin disappearance after birth. *Br J Haematol* 1976;32:79.
161. Terrenato L, Bertilaccio C, Spinelli P, et al. The switch from Haemoglobin F and A: the time course of qualitative and quantitative variations of haemoglobins after birth. *Br J Haematol* 1981;47:31.
162. Shepart MK, Weatherall DJ, Conley CL. Semi-quantitative estimation of the distribution of fetal hemoglobin in red cell populations. *Bull Johns Hopkins Hosp* 1962;110:293.
163. Weinberg RS, Goldberg JD, Schofield JM, et al. Switch from fetal to adult hemoglobin is associated with a change in progenitor cell population. *J Clin Invest* 1983;71:785.
164. Alter BP, Jackson BT, Lipton JM, et al. Control of the simian fetal hemoglobin switch at the progenitor cell level. *J Clin Invest* 1981;67:458.
165. Wood WG, Pearce K, Clegg JB, et al. Switch from foetal to adult haemoglobin synthesis in normal and hypophysectomised sheep. *Nature* 1977;264:799.
166. Wintour EM, Smith MB, Bell RJ, et al. The role of fetal adrenal hormones in the switch from fetal to adult globin synthesis in the sheep. *J Endocrinol* 1985;104:165.
167. Perrine SP, Greene MF, Faller DV. Delay in the fetal globin switch in infants of diabetic mothers. *N Engl J Med* 1985;312:334.
168. Bard H, Prosmanne J. Relative rates of fetal hemoglobin and adult hemoglobin synthesis in cord blood of infants of insulin-dependent diabetic mothers. *Pediatrics* 1985;75:1143.
169. Perrine SP, Rudolph A, Faller DV, et al. Butyrate infusions in the ovine fetus delay the biologic clock for globin gene switching. *Proc Natl Acad Sci U S A* 1988;85:8540.
170. Burns LJ, Glauber JG, Ginder GD. Butyrate induces selective transcriptional activation of a hypomethylated embryonic globin gene in adult erythroid cells. *Blood* 1988;72:1536.
171. Constantoulakis P, Papayannopoulou TH, Stamatoyannopoulos G. α-Amino-N-butyric acid stimulates fetal hemoglobin in the adult. *Blood* 1988;72:1961.
172. Constantoulakis P, Knitter G, Stamatoyannopoulos G. On the induction of fetal hemoglobin by butyrates: in vivo and in vitro studies with sodium butyrate and comparison of combination treatments with 5-AzaC and AraC. *Blood* 1989;74:1963.
173. Perrine SP, Miller BA, Faller DV, et al. Sodium butyrate enhances fetal globin gene expression in erythroid progenitors of patients with Hb SS and β thalassemia. *Blood* 1989;74:454.
174. Blau AC, Constantoulakis P, Shaw CM, et al. Fetal hemoglobin induction with butyric acid: efficacy and toxicity. *Blood* 1993;81:529.
175. Dover GJ, Brusilow S, Samid D. Increased fetal hemoglobin in patients receiving sodium 4-phenylbutyrate. *N Engl J Med* 1992;327:569.
176. Perrine SP, Ginder GD, Faller DV, et al. A short-term trial of butyrate to stimulate fetal-globin-gene expression in the β-globin disorders. *N Engl J Med* 1993;328:81.
177. Boyer SH, Belding TK, Margolet L, et al. Fetal hemoglobin restriction to a few erythrocytes (F cells) in normal human adults. *Science* 1975;188:361.
178. Wood WG, Stamatoyannopoulos G, Lim G, et al. F-cells in the adult: normal values and levels in individuals with hereditary and acquired elevations of Hb F. *Blood* 1975;46:671.
179. Huisman THJ, Schroeder WA, Efremov GD, et al. The present status of the heterogeneity of fetal hemoglobin in β-thalassemia: an attempt to unify some observations on thalassemia and related conditions. *Ann N Y Acad Sci* 1974;232:107.
180. Evans T, Felsenfeld G. The erythroid-specific transcription factor Eryf1: a new finger protein. *Cell* 1989;58:877.
181. Zon LI, Tsai S-F, Burgess S, et al. The major human erythroid DNA-binding protein (GF-1): primary sequence and localization of the gene to the X chromosome. *Proc Natl Acad Sci U S A* 1990;87:668.
182. Trainor CD, Evans T, Felsenfeld G, et al. Structure and evolution of a human erythroid transcription factor. *Nature* 1990;343:92.
183. Whitelaw E, Tsai S-F, Hogben P, et al. Regulated expression of globin chains and the erythroid transcription factor GATA-1 during erythropoiesis in the developing mouse. *Mol Cell Biol* 1990;10:6596.
184. Minie ME, Kimura T, Felsenfeld G. The developmental switch in embryonic rho-globin expression is correlated with erythroid lineage-specific differences in transcription factor levels. *Development* 1992;115:1149.
185. Nicolis S, Ronchi A, Malgaretti N, et al. Increased erythroid-specific expression of a mutated HPFH γ-globin promoter requires the erythroid factor NFE-1. *Nucleic Acids Res* 1989;17:5509.
186. Foley KP, Engel JD. Individual stage selector element mutations lead to reciprocal changes in β- versus ε-globin gene transcription: genetic confirmation of promoter competition during globin gene switching. *Genes Dev* 1992;6:730.
187. Purucker M, Bodine D, Lin H, et al. Structure and function of the enhancer 3' to the human ^Aγ-globin gene. *Nucleic Acids Res* 1990;18:7408.
188. Lavelle D, Ducksworth J, Eves E, et al. A homeodomain protein binds to γ-globin gene regulatory sequences. *Proc Natl Acad Sci U S A* 1991;88:7318.
189. Jane SM, Ney PA, Vanin EF, et al. Identification of a stage selector element in the human γ-globin gene promoter that fosters preferential interaction with the 5' HS2 enhancer when in competition with the β-promoter. *EMBO J* 1992;11:2961.
190. Gumucio DL, Heilstedt-Williamson H, Gray TA, et al. Phylogenetic footprinting reveals a nuclear protein which binds to silencer sequences in the human γ and ε globin genes. *Mol Cell Biol* 1992;12:4919.
191. Raich N, Enver T, Nakamoto B, et al. Autonomous developmental control of human embryonic globin gene switching in transgenic mice. *Science* 1990;250:1147.
192. Enver T, Ebens AJ, Forrester WC, et al. The human β-globin locus activation region alters the developmental fate of a human fetal globin gene in transgenic mice. *Proc Natl Acad Sci U S A* 1989;86:7033.
193. Behringer RR, Ryan TM, Palmiter RD, et al. Human γ- to β-globin gene switching in transgenic mice. *Genes Dev* 1990;4:380.
194. Enver T, Raich N, Ebens AJ, et al. Developmental regulation of human fetal-to-adult globin gene switching in transgenic mice. *Nature* 1990;344:309.
195. Dillon N, Grosveld F. Human γ-globin genes silenced independently of other genes in the β-globin locus. *Nature* 1991;350:252.
196. Strouboulis J, Dillon N, Grosveld F. Developmental regulation of a complete 70-kb human β-globin locus in transgenic mice. *Genes Dev* 1992;6:1857.
197. Peterson KR, Clegg CH, Josephson BM, et al. Transgenic mice containing a 248 Kb human β locus YAC display proper developmental control of human globin genes. *Clin Res* 1993;41:258a(abst).
198. Pasvol G, Weatherall DJ, Wilson RJM. Effects of foetal haemoglobin on susceptibility of red cells to *Plasmodium falciparum*. *Nature* 1977;270:171.
199. Friedman MJ, Traeger W. The biochemistry of resistance to malaria. *Sci Am* 1981;244:154.
200. Nagel RL, Roth EF Jr. Malaria and red cell genetic defects. *Blood* 1989;74:1213.
201. Nagel RL. Malaria and hemoglobinopathies. In: Steinberg MH, Forget BG, Higgs DR, et al., eds. *Disorders of hemoglobin*. New York: Cambridge University Press, 2001:832.

202. Dozy AM, Kan YW, Embury SH, et al. α-Globin gene organization in blacks precludes the severe form of α-thalassemia. *Nature* 1979;280:605.
203. Oppenheimer SJ, Higgs DR, Weatherall DJ, et al. α-Thalassemia in Papua New Guinea. *Lancet* 1984;2:424.
204. Rachmilewitz EA, Shinar E, Shalev O, et al. Erythrocyte membrane alterations in beta-thalassemia. *Clin Hematol* 1985;14:163.
205. Shinar E, Rachmilewitz EA. Oxidative denaturation of red blood cells in thalassemia. *Semin Hematol* 1990;27:70.
206. Shinar E, Shalev O, Rachmilewitz EA, et al. Erythrocyte membrane skeleton abnormalities in severe beta thalassemia. *Blood* 1987;70:158.
207. Shinar E, Rachmilewitz EA, Lux SE. Differing erythrocyte membrane skeletal protein defects in alpha and beta thalassemia. *J Clin Invest* 1989;83:404.
208. Schrier SL, Rachmilewitz E, Mohandas N. Cellular and membrane properties of alpha and beta thalassemic erythrocytes are different: implication for differences in clinical manifestations. *Blood* 1989;74:2194.
209. Rouyer-Fessard P, Garel M-C, Domenget C, et al. A study of membrane protein defects and α-hemoglobin chains of red blood cells in human β thalassemia. *J Biol Chem* 1989;264:19092.
210. Sorensen S, Rubin E, Polster H, et al. The role of membrane skeletal-associated α-globin in the pathophysiology of β-thalassemia. *Blood* 1990;75:1333.
211. Adavani R, Sorenson S, Shinar E, et al. Characterization and comparison of the red blood cell membrane damage in severe human α- and β-thalassemia. *Blood* 1992;79:1058.
212. Scott MD, Rouyer-Fessard P, Ba MS, et al. α- and β-Haemoglobin chain induced changes in normal erythrocyte deformability: comparison to β thalassemia intermedia and Hb H disease. *Br J Haematol* 1992;80:519.
213. Yuan J, Kannan R, Shinar E, et al. Isolation, characterization, and immunoprecipitation studies of immune complexes from membranes of β-thalassemic erythrocytes. *Blood* 1992;79:3007.
214. Rachmilewitz EA, Schrier SL. Pathophysiology of β thalassemia. In: Steinberg MH, Forget BG, Higgs DR, et al., eds. *Disorders of hemoglobin*. New York: Cambridge University Press, 2001:233.
215. Leibhaber SA, Schrier SL. Pathophysiology of β thalassemia. In: Steinberg MH, Forget BG, Higgs DR, et al., eds. *Disorders of hemoglobin*. New York: Cambridge University Press, 2001:391.
216. Huisman THJ, Carver MFH, Baysal E. A syllabus of thalassemia mutations. The Sickle Cell Anemia Foundation. Augusta, GA, USA (http://globin.cse.psu.edu).
217. Hardison R, Riemer C, Chui DH, et al. Electronic access to sequence alignments, experimental results and human mutations as an aid to studying globin gene regulation. *Genomics* 47:429–437.
218. Forget BG. Molecular mechanisms of β-thalassemia. In: Steinberg MH, Forget BG, Higgs DR, et al., eds. *Disorders of hemoglobin*. New York: Cambridge University Press, 2001:252.
219. Orkin SH, Sexton JP, Cheng T-C, et al. ATA box transcription mutation in β-thalassemia. *Nucleic Acids Res* 1983;11:4727.
220. Antonarakis SE, Orkin SH, Cheng T-C, et al. β-Thalassemia in American blacks: novel mutations in the TATA box and IVS-2 acceptor splice site. *Proc Natl Acad Sci U S A* 1984;81:1154.
221. Takihara Y, Nakamura T, Yamada H, et al. A novel mutation in the TATA box in a Japanese patient with β⁺-thalassemia. *Blood* 1986;67:547.
222. Orkin SH, Antonarakis SE, Kazazian HH Jr. Base substitution at position −88 in a β-thalassemic globin gene: further evidence for the role of distal promoter element ACACCC. *J Biol Chem* 1984;259:8679.
223. Huang S-Z, Wong C, Antonarakis SE, et al. The same TATA box β-thalassemia mutation in Chinese and US blacks: another example of independent origins of mutation. *Hum Genet* 1986;74:152.
224. Kazazian HH Jr. The thalassemia syndromes: molecular basis and prenatal diagnosis in 1990. *Semin Hematol* 1990;27:209.
225. Wong C, Dowling CE, Saiki RK, et al. Characterization of β-thalassemic mutations using direct genomic sequencing of amplified single copy DNA. *Nature* 1987;330:384.
226. Wong C, Dowling CE, Saiki RK, et al. Characterization of β-thalassaemia mutation using direct genomic sequencing of amplified single copy DNA. *Nature* 1987;330:384.
227. Orkin SH, Cheng T-C, Antonarakis SE, et al. Thalassemia due to a mutation in the cleavage-polyadenylation signal of the human β-globin gene. *EMBO J* 1985;4:453.
228. Treisman R, Proudfoot NJ, Shander M, et al. A single base change at a splice site in a β⁰-thalassemic gene causes abnormal RNA splicing. *Cell* 1982;29:903.
229. Atweh GF, Anagnou NP, Forget BG, et al. β-Thalassemia resulting from a single nucleotide substitution in an acceptor splice site. *Nucleic Acids Res* 1985;13:777.
230. Cheng T-C, Orkin SH, Antonarakis SE, et al. β-Thalassemia in Chinese: use of in vivo RNA analysis and oligonucleotide hybridization in systematic characterization of molecular defects. *Proc Natl Acad Sci U S A* 1984;81:2821.
231. Treisman R, Orkin SH, Maniatis T. Specific transcription and RNA splicing defects in five cloned β-thalassaemia genes. *Nature* 1983;302:591.
232. Atweh GF, Wong C, Reed R, et al. A new mutation in IVS-1 of the human β globin gene causing β-thalassemia due to abnormal splicing. *Blood* 1987;70:147.
233. Orkin SH, Kazazian HH Jr, Antonarakis SE, et al. Abnormal RNA processing due to the exon mutation of the βᴱ-globin gene. *Nature* 1982;300:768.
234. Goldsmith ME, Humphries RK, Ley T, et al. Silent substitution in β⁺-thalassemia gene activating a cryptic splice site in β-globin RNA coding sequence. *Proc Natl Acad Sci U S A* 1983;80:2318.
235. Orkin SH, Antonarakis SE, Loukopoulos D. Abnormal processing of βᴷⁿᵒˢˢᵒˢ RNA. *Blood* 1984;64:311.

236. Busslinger M, Moschonas N, Flavell RA. β⁺-Thalassemia: aberrant splicing results from a single point mutation in an intron. *Cell* 1981;27:289.
237. Fukumaki Y, Ghosh PK, Benz EJ Jr, et al. Abnormally spliced messenger RNA in erythroid cells from patients with β⁺-thalassemia and monkey cells expressing a cloned β⁺-thalassemia gene. *Cell* 1982;28:585.
238. Metherall JE, Collins FS, Pan J, et al. β⁰-Thalassemia caused by a base substitution that creates an alternative splice acceptor site in an intron. *EMBO J* 1986;5:2551.
239. Dobkin C, Pergolizzi RG, Bahre P, et al. Abnormal splice in a mutant β-globin gene not at the site of a mutation. *Proc Natl Acad Sci U S A* 1983;80:1184.
240. Dobkin C, Bank A. Reversibility of IVS 2 missplicing in a mutant human β-globin gene. *J Biol Chem* 1985;260:16332.
241. Fessas P, Loukopoulos D, Loutradi-Anagnostou A, et al. "Silent" β-thalassaemia caused by a "silent" β-chain mutant: the pathogenesis of a syndrome of thalassaemia intermedia. *Br J Haematol* 1982;51:577.
242. Rouabhi F, Chardin P, Boissel JP, et al. Silent β-thalassaemia associated with Hb Knossos β27 (B9) Ala→Ser in Algeria. *Hemoglobin* 1983;7:555.
243. Yang KG, Kutlar F, George E, et al. Molecular characterization of β-globin gene mutations in 243 Malay patients with Hb E-β-thalassaemia and thalassaemia major. *Br J Haematol* 1989;72:73.
244. Gonzalez-Redondo JM, Brickner HE, Atweh GF. Abnormal processing of β-Malay globin RNA. *Biochem Biophys Res Commun* 1989;163:8.
245. Takeshita K, Forget BG, Scarpa A, et al. Intranuclear defect in β globin mRNA accumulation due to a premature translation termination codon. *Blood* 1984;64:13.
246. Humphries RK, Ley TJ, Anagnou NP, et al. β⁰-Thalassemia gene: a premature termination codon causes β mRNA deficiency without changing cytoplasmic β mRNA stability. *Blood* 1984;64:23.
247. Baserga SJ, Benz EJ Jr. Nonsense mutations in the human β-globin gene affect mRNA metabolism. *Proc Natl Acad Sci U S A* 1988;85:2056.
248. Baserga SJ, Benz EJ Jr. β-Globin nonsense mutation: deficient accumulation of mRNA occurs despite normal cytoplasmic stability. *Proc Natl Acad Sci U S A* 1992;89:2935.
249. Nagy E, Maquat LE. A rule for termination-codon position within intron-containing genes: when nonsense affects RNA abundance. *Trends Biochem Sci* 1998;23:198.
250. Thermann R, Neu-Yilik G, Deters A, et al. Binary specification of nonsense codons by splicing and cytoplasmic translation. *EMBO J* 1998;17:3484.
251. Hentze MW, Kulozik AE. A perfect message: RNA surveillance and nonsense-mediated decay. *Cell* 96:307–310.
252. Kazazian HH Jr, Dowling CE, Hurwitz RL, et al. Dominant thalassemia-like phenotypes associated with mutations in exon 3 of the β-globin gene. *Blood* 1992;79:3014.
253. Kazazian HH Jr, Orkin SH, Antonarakis SE, et al. Molecular characterization of seven β-thalassemia mutations in Asian Indians. *EMBO J* 1984;3:593.
254. Kimura A, Matsunaga E, Takihara Y, et al. Structural analysis of a β-thalassemia gene found in Taiwan. *J Biol Chem* 1983;258:2748.
255. Maquat LE, Kinninberg AJ, Rachmilewitz EA, et al. Unstable β-globin mRNA in mRNA-deficient β⁰-thalassemia. *Cell* 1981;27:543.
256. Maquat LE, Kinninburgh AJ. A β⁰-thalassemic β-globin RNA that is labile in bone marrow cells is relatively stable in HeLa cells. *Nucleic Acids Res* 1985;13:2855.
257. Thein SL, Hesketh C, Taylor P, et al. Molecular basis for dominantly inherited inclusion body β-thalassemia. *Proc Natl Acad Sci U S A* 1990;87:3924.
258. Thein SL. Dominant β thalassemia: molecular basis and pathophysiology. *Br J Haematol* 1992;80:273.
259. Coleman MB, Steinberg MH, Adams JG III. Hemoglobin Terre Haute arginine β¹⁰⁶: a posthumous correction to the original structure of hemoglobin Indianapolis. *J Biol Chem* 1991;266:5798.
260. Adams JG, Coleman MB. Structural hemoglobin variants that produce the phenotype of thalassemia. *Semin Hematol* 1990;27:229.
261. Gonzalez-Redondo JM, Kattamis C, Huisman THJ. Characterization of three types of β⁰ thalassemia resulting from a partial deletion of the β-globin gene. *Hemoglobin* 1989;13:377.
262. Padanilam BJ, Felice AE, Huisman THJ. Partial deletions of the 5' β-globin gene region causes β⁰-thalassemia in members of an American black family. *Blood* 1984;4:941.
263. Anand R, Boehm CD, Kazazian HH, et al. Molecular characterization of a β⁰-thalassemia resulting from a 1.4 kilobase deletion. *Blood* 1988;72:636.
264. Thein SL, Hesketh C, Brown JM, et al. Molecular characterization of a high A₂β thalassemia by direct sequencing of single strand enriched amplified genomic DNA. *Blood* 1989;73:924.
265. Diaz-Chico JC, Yang KG, Kutlar A, et al. An approximately 300 bp deletion involving part of the 5' β-globin gene region is observed in members of a Turkish family with β-thalassemia. *Blood* 1987;70:583.
266. Spiegelberg R, Aulehla-Scholz C, Erlich H, et al. A β-thalassemia gene caused by a 290-base pair deletion: analysis by direct sequencing of enzymatically amplified DNA. *Blood* 1989;73:1695.
267. Gilman J. The 12.6 kilobase DNA deletion in Dutch β-thalassemia. *Br J Haematol* 1987;67:369.
268. Popovich BW, Rosenblatt DS, Kendall AG, et al. Molecular characterization of an atypical β-thalassemia caused by a large deletion in the 5' β-globin gene region. *Am J Hum Genet* 1986;39:797.
269. Spritz R, Orkin SH. Duplication followed by deletion accounts for the structure of an Indian deletion β⁰-thalassemia gene. *Nucleic Acids Res* 1982;10:8025.

270. Sanguansermsri T, Pape M, Laig M, et al. β-Thalassemia in a Thai family is caused by a 3.4 kb deletion including the entire β-globin gene. *Hemoglobin* 1990;14:157.

271. Wayne JS, Cai SP, Eng B, et al. High hemoglobin A^{2B}_0-thalassemia due to a 532-basepair deletion of the 5' β-globin gene region. *Blood* 1991;77:1100.

272. Thein SL, Old JM, Wainscoat JS, et al. Population and genetic studies suggest a single origin for the Indian deletion $β^0$ thalassemia. *Br J Haematol* 1984;57:271.

273. Spritz R, Orkin SH. Duplication followed by deletion accounts for the structure of an Indian deletion $β^0$-thalassemia gene. *Nucleic Acids Res* 1982;10:8025.

274. Motum PI, Lindeman R, Hamilton TJ, et al. Australian $β^0$-thalassaemia due to a 12 kb deletion commencing 5' to the β-globin gene. *Br J Haematol* 1992;82:107.

275. Craig JE, Kelly SJ, Barnetson R, et al. Molecular characterization of a novel 10.3 kb deletion causing β-thalassaemia with unusually high Hb A_2. *Br J Haematol* 1992;82:735.

276. Motum PI, Kearney A, Hamilton TJ, et al. Filipino $β^0$ thalassaemia: a high Hb $A^2β_0$ thalassaemia resulting from a large deletion of the 5' β globin gene region. *J Med Genet* 1993;30:240.

277. Lynch JR, Brown JM, Best S, et al. Characterization of the breakpoint of a 3.5-kb deletion of the beta-globin gene. *Genomics* 1991;10:509–511.

278. Dimovski AJ, Efremov DG, Jankovic L, et al. A $β^0$-thalassaemia due to a 1605 bp deletion of the 5' beta-globin gene region. *Br J Haematol* 1993;85:143.

279. Dimovski AJ, Divoky V, Adekile AD, et al. A novel deletion of approximately 27 kb including the beta-globin gene and the locus control region 3'HS-1 regulatory sequence: beta zero-thalassemia or hereditary persistence of fetal hemoglobin? *Blood* 1994;83:822–827.

280. Dimovski AJ, Baysal E, Efremov DG, et al. A large beta-thalassemia deletion in a family of Indonesian-Malay descent. *Hemoglobin* 1996;20:277–392.

281. Gilman J. The 12.6 kilobase DNA deletion in Dutch β-thalassemia. *Br J Haematol* 1987;67:369.

282. Spiegelberg R, Aulehla-Scholz C, Erlich H, et al. A β-thalassemia gene caused by a 290-base pair deletion: analysis by direct sequencing of enzymatically amplified DNA. *Blood* 1989;73:1695.

283. Öner C, Öner R, Gurgey A, et al. A new Turkish type of beta-thalassemia major with homozygosity for two non-consecutive 7.6 kb deletions of the psi beta and beta genes and an intact delta gene. *Br J Haematol* 1995;89:306–312.

284. Nopparatana C, Panich V, Saechan V, et al. The spectrum of beta-thalassemia mutations in southern Thailand. *Southeast Asian J Trop Med Public Health* 1995;26[Suppl 1]:229–234.

285. Lacerra G, DeAngioletti M, Sabato V, et al. South-Italy beta⁰-thalassemia: a novel deletion, with 3' breakpoint in a hsRTVL-H element, associated with beta⁰-thalassemia and HPFH. In: *6th International Conference on Thalassemia and the Haemoglobinopathies, Malta, 1997*(abst 152).

286. Codrington JF, Li HW, Kutlar F, et al. Observations on the level of Hb A_2 in patients with different β-thalassemia mutations and a chain variant. *Blood* 1990;76:1246.

287. Schwartz E. The silent carrier of β-thalassemia. *N Engl J Med* 281:1327.

288. Semenza GL, Delgrosso K, Poncz M, et al. The silent carrier allele: β thalassemia without a mutation in the β-globin gene or its immediate flanking regions. *Cell* 1984;39:123.

289. Chebloune Y, Pagnier J, Trabuchet G, et al. Structural analysis of the 5' flanking region of the β-globin gene in African sickle cell anemia patients: further evidence for three origins of the sickle cell mutation in Africa. *Proc Natl Acad Sci U S A* 1988;85:4431.

290. Wong SC, Stoming TA, Efremov GD, et al. High frequencies of a rearrangement (+ATA; -T) at -530 to the β-globin gene in different populations indicate the absence of a correlation with a silent β-thalassemia determinant. *Hemoglobin* 1989;13:1.

291. Balanello R, Meloni A, Gasperini D, et al. The repeated sequence $(AT)_x(T)_y$ upstream to the β-globin gene is a simple polymorphism. *Blood* 1993;81:1974.

292. Schwartz E, Cohen A, Surrey S. Overview of the β-thalassemias: genetic and clinical aspects. *Hemoglobin* 1988;12:551.

293. Berg PE, Mittelman M, Elion J, et al. Increased protein binding to a -530 mutation of the human β-globin gene associated with decreased β-globin synthesis. *Am J Hematol* 1991;36:42.

294. Murru S, Loudianos G, Cao A, et al. A β-thalassemia carrier with normal sequence within the β-globin gene. *Blood* 1990;76:2164.

295. Murru S, Loudianos G, Porcu S, et al. A β-thalassemia phenotype not linked to the β-globin cluster in an Italian family. *Br J Haematol* 1992;81:283.

296. Kazazian HH Jr, Dowling CE, Boehm CD, et al. Gene defects in β-thalassemia and their prenatal diagnosis. *Ann N Y Acad Sci* 1990;612:1.

297. Thein SL, Wood WG, Wickramasinghe SN, et al. β-Thalassemia unlinked to the β-globin gene in an English family. *Blood* 1993;82:961–967.

298. Antonarakis SE, Boehm CD, Giardina PJ, et al. Nonrandom association of polymorphic restriction sites in the β-globin gene cluster. *Proc Natl Acad Sci U S A* 1982;79:137.

299. Antonarakis SE, Kazazian HH Jr, Orkin SH. DNA polymorphism and molecular pathology of the human globin gene clusters. *Hum Genet* 1985;69:1.

300. Orkin SH, Kazazian HH Jr. The mutation and polymorphism of the human β-globin gene and its surrounding DNA. *Annu Rev Genet* 1984;18:131.

301. Orkin SH, Kazazian HH Jr, Antonarakis SE, et al. Linkage of β-thalassemia mutations and β-globin gene polymorphisms with DNA polymorphisms in the human β-globin gene cluster. *Nature* 1982;296:627.

302. Higgs DR, Wainscoat JS, Flint J, et al. Analysis of the human α-globin gene cluster reveals a highly informative genetic locus. *Proc Natl Acad Sci U S A* 1986;83:5165.

303. Higgs DR, Vickers MA, Wilkie AOM, et al. A review of the molecular genetics of the human α-globin gene cluster. *Blood* 1989;73:1081.

304. Higgs DR. The molecular genetics of the α-globin gene family. *Eur J Clin Invest* 1990;20:340.

305. Lienhaber SA. α-Thalassaemia. *Hemoglobin* 1989;13:685.

306. Kazazian HH Jr, Orkin SH, Markham AF, et al. Quantification of the close association between DNA haplotypes and specific β-thalassaemia mutations in Mediterraneans. *Nature* 1984;310:152.

307. Pirastu M, Galanello R, Doherty MA, et al. The same β-globin gene mutation is present on nine different β-thalassemia chromosomes in a Sardinian population. *Proc Natl Acad Sci U S A* 1987;84:2882.

308. Chakravarti A, Buetow KH, Antonarakis SE, et al. Nonuniform recombination within the human β-globin gene cluster. *Am J Hum Genet* 1984;36:1239.

309. Antonarakis SE, Orkin SH, Kazazian HH Jr, et al. Evidence for multiple origins of the $β^E$- globin gene in Southeast Asia. *Proc Natl Acad Sci U S A* 1982;79:6608.

310. Kan YW, Dozy AM, Varmus HE, et al. Deletion of α-globin genes in haemoglobin H disease demonstrates multiple α-globin structural loci. *Nature* 1975;255:255.

311. Embury SH, Miller JA, Dozy AM, et al. Two different molecular organizations account for the single α-globin gene of the α-thalassemia-2 genotype. *J Clin Invest* 1980;66:1319.

312. Kulozik AE, Kar BC, Serjeant GR, et al. The molecular basis of α-thalassemia in India: its interactions with the sickle cell gene. *Blood* 1988;71:467.

313. Zhao J-B, Zhao L, Fei Y-J, et al. A novel α-thalassemia-2 (-2.7 kb) observed in a Chinese patient with Hb H disease. *Am J Hematol* 1991;38:248.

314. Lacerra G, Fioretti G, De Angioletti M, et al. (α) $α^{5.3}$: a novel $α^+$ thalassemia deletion with the breakpoints in the α2-globin gene and in close proximity to an *Alu* family repeat between the ψα2- and ψα1-globin genes. *Blood* 1991;78:2740.

315. Camaschella C, Bertero MT, Serra A, et al. A benign form of thalassaemia intermedia may be determined by the interaction of triplicated α locus and heterozygous β-thalassaemia. *Br J Haematol* 1987;66:103.

316. Galanello R, Ruggeri R, Paglietti E, et al. A family with segregating triplicated alpha globin loci and beta thalassemia. *Blood* 1983;62:1035.

317. Kulozik AE, Thein SL, Wainscoat JS, et al. Thalassaemia intermedia: interaction of the triple α-globin gene arrangement and heterozygous β-thalassaemia. *Br J Haematol* 1987;66:109.

318. Orkin SH, Goff SC. The duplicated human α-globin genes: their relative expression as measured by RNA analysis. *Cell* 1981;24:345.

319. Liebhaber SA, Kan YW. Differentiation of the mRNA transcripts originating from the α1- and α2-globin loci in normals and α-thalassemics. *J Clin Invest* 1981;68:439.

320. Bowden DK, Hill AVS, Higgs DR, et al. Different hematologic phenotypes are associated with leftward ($-α^{4.2}$) and rightward ($-α^{3.7}$) $α^+$-thalassemia deletions. *J Clin Invest* 1987;79:39.

321. Liebhaber SA, Cash FE, Main DM. Compensatory increase in α1-globin gene expression in individual heterozygous for the α thalassemia-2 deletion. *J Clin Invest* 1985;76:1057.

322. Higgs DR, Old JM, Clegg JB, et al. Negro α-thalassemia is caused by deletion of a single α-globin gene. *Lancet* 1979;2:272.

323. Nicholls RD, Fischel-Ghodsian N, Higgs DR. Recombination at the human α-globin gene cluster: sequence features and topological constraints. *Cell* 1987;49:369.

324. Hatton CSR, Wilkie AOM, Drysdale HC, et al. α-Thalassemia caused by a large (62 kb) deletion upstream of the human α-globin gene cluster. *Blood* 1990;76:221.

325. Romao L, Osorio-Almeida L, Higgs DR, et al. α-Thalassemia resulting from deletion of regulatory sequences far upstream of the α-globin structural genes. *Blood* 1991;78:1589.

326. Wilkie AOM, Lamb J, Harris PC, et al. A truncated human chromosome 16 associated with α-thalassaemia is stabilized by addition of telomeric repeat (TTAGGG). *Nature* 1990;346:868.

327. Liebhaber SA, Griese E-U, Weiss I, et al. Inactivation of human α-globin gene expression by a de novo deletion located upstream of the α-globin gene cluster. *Proc Natl Acad Sci U S A* 1990;87:9431.

328. Higgs DR. Molecular mechanisms of α thalassemia. In: Steinberg, MH, Forget BG, Higgs DR, et al., eds. *Disorders of hemoglobin*. New York: Cambridge University Press, 2001:405.

329. Beaudry MA, Ferguson DJ, Pearse K, et al. Survival of a hydropic infant with homozygous α-thalassemia-1. *J Pediatr* 1986;108:713.

330. Bianchi DW, Beyer EC, Stark AR, et al. Normal long-term survival with α-thalassemia. *J Pediatr* 1986;108:716.

331. Chui DHK, Wong SC, Chung S-W, et al. Embryonic ζ-globin chains in adults: a marker for α-thalassemia-1 haplotype due to a >17.5 kb deletion. *N Engl J Med* 1986;314:76.

332. Steinberg MH, Coleman MB, Adams JH III, et al. A new gene deletion in the α-like globin gene cluster as the molecular basis for the rare α-thalassemia-1 (—/αα) in blacks: Hb disease in sickle cell trait. *Blood* 1986;67:469.

333. Felice AE, Cleek MP, McKie K, et al. The rare α-thalassemia-1 of blacks is a ζα-thalassemia-1 associated with deletion of all α- and ζ-globin genes. *Blood* 1984;63:1253.

334. Fei YJ, Liu JC, Walker ELD III, et al. A new gene deletion involving the α2-, α1-, and ξ-globin genes in a black family with Hb H disease. *Am J Hematol* 1992;39:299.

335. Olivieri NF, Chang LS, Poon AO, et al. An α-globin gene initiation codon mutation in a black family with Hb H disease. *Blood* 1987;70:729.

336. Safaya S, Rieder RF. Dysfunctional α-globin gene in hemoglobin H disease in blacks. *J Biol Chem* 1988;263:4328.
337. Honig GR, Shamsuddin M, Vida LN, et al. Hemoglobin Evanston (α14 Trp →Arg): an unstable α-chain variant expressed as α-thalassemia. *J Clin Invest* 1984;73:1740.
338. Schmid CW, Jelinek WR. The *Alu* family of dispersed repetitive sequences. *Science* 1982;216:1065.
339. Jelinek WR, Schmid CW. Repetitive sequences in eukaryotic DNA and their expression. *Annu Rev Biochem* 1982;51:813.
340. Pirastu M, Saglio G, Chang JC, et al. Initiation codon mutation as a cause of α-thalassemia. *J Biol Chem* 1984;259:12315.
341. Higgs DR, Goodbourn SEY, Lamb J, et al. α-Thalassaemia caused by a poly-adenylation signal mutation. *Nature* 1983;306:398.
342. Goosens M, Lee KY, Liebhaber SA, et al. Globin structural mutant α$^{125Leu\to Pro}$ is a novel cause of α-thalassaemia. *Nature* 1982;296:864.
343. Morle F, Lopez B, Henni T, et al. α-Thalassaemia associated with the deletion of two nucleotides at position -2 and -3 preceding the AUG codon. *EMBO J* 1985;44:1245.
344. Milner PF, Clegg JB, Weatherall DJ. Haemoglobin H disease due to a unique haemoglobin variant with an elongated α-chain. *Lancet* 1971;1:729.
345. Clegg JB, Weatherall DJ, Milner PG. Haemoglobin Constant Spring: a chain termination mutant? *Nature* 1971;234:337.
346. Clegg JB, Weatherall DJ, Contopoulos-Griva I, et al. Haemoglobin Icaria, a new chain termination mutant which causes α-thalassaemia. *Nature* 1974;251:245.
347. De Jong WW, Khan PM, Bernini LF. Hemoglobin Koya Dora: high frequency of a chain termination mutant. *Am J Hum Genet* 1975;27:81.
348. Bradley TB, Wohl RC, Smith GJ. Elongation of the α-globin chain in a black family: interaction with Hb G Philadelphia. *Clin Res* 1975;23:1314(abst).
349. Hunt DM, Higgs DR, Winichagoon P, et al. Haemoglobin Constant Spring has an unstable α-chain messenger RNA. *Br J Haematol* 1982;51:405.
350. Weiss IM, Liebhaber SA. Erythroid-cell specific determinants of α-globin mRNA stability. *Mol Cell Biol* 1994;14:8123.
351. Wang X, Kiledjian I, Weiss M, et al. Detection and characterization of a 3' untranslated region ribonucleoprotein complex associated with human α-globin mRNA stability. *Mol Cell Biol* 1995;15:1769.
352. Liebhaber SA, Russell JE. Expression and developmental control of the human α-globin gene cluster. *Ann N Y Acad Sci* 1998;850:54.
353. Moi P, Cash FE, Liebhaber SA, et al. An initiation codon mutation (AUG → GUG) of the human α1-globin gene: structural characterization and evidence for a mild thalassemic phenotype. *J Clin Invest* 1987;80:1416.
354. Higgs DR, Wood WG, Barton C, et al. Clinical features and molecular analysis of acquired Hb H disease. *Am J Med* 1983;75:181.
355. Anagnou NP, Ley TJ, Chesbro B, et al. Acquired α-thalassemia in preleukemia is due to decreased expression of all four α-globin genes. *Proc Natl Acad Sci U S A* 1983;80:6051.
356. Higgs DR, Bowden DK. Clinical and laboratory features of the α-thalassemia syndromes. In: Steinberg MH, Forget BG, Higgs DR, et al., eds. *Disorders of hemoglobin.* New York: Cambridge University Press, 2001:431.
357. Helder J, Deisseroth A. S1 nuclease analysis of α-globin gene expression in preleukemic patients with acquired hemoglobin H disease after transfer to mouse erythroleukemia cells. *Proc Natl Acad Sci U S A* 1987;84:2387.
358. Weatherall DJ, Higgs DR, Bunch C, et al. Hemoglobin H disease and mental retardation. *N Engl J Med* 1981;305:607.
359. Wilkie AOM, Buckle VJ, Harris PC, et al. Clinical features and molecular analysis of the α-thalassemia/mental retardation syndromes, I: cases due to deletions involving chromosome band 16p13.3. *Am J Hum Genet* 1990;46:1112.
360. Wilkie AOM, Zeitlin HC, Lindenbaum RH, et al. Clinical features and molecular analysis of the α thalassemia/mental retardation syndromes, II: cases without detectable abnormality of the α-globin complex. *Am J Hum Genet* 1990;46:1127.
361. Gibbons RJ, Higgs DR. The alpha-thalassemia/mental retardation syndromes. *Medicine* 1996;75:45.
362. Gibbons RJ, Higgs DR. The alpha thalassemia/mental retardation syndromes. In: Steinberg MH, Forget BG, Higgs DR, et al., eds. *Disorders of hemoglobin.* New York: Cambridge University Press, 2001:470.
363. Lamb J, Harris PC, Lindenbaum RH, et al. Detection of breakpoints in submicroscopic chromosomal translocation, illustrating an important mechanism for genetic disease. *Lancet* 1989;2:819.
364. Lamb J, Harris PC, Wilkie AOM, et al. *De novo* truncation of chromosome 16p and healing with (TTAGGG)$_n$ in the α-thalassemia/mental retardation syndrome (ATR-16). *Am J Hum Genet* 1993;52:668.
365. Wilkie AOM, Pembrey ME, Gibbons RJ, et al. The non-deletion type of alpha thalassemia/mental retardation: a recognizable dysmorphic syndrome with X-linked inheritance. *J Med Genet* 1991;28:724.
366. Gibbons RJ, Suthers GK, Wilkie AOM, et al. X-linked alpha thalassemia/mental retardation (ATR-X) syndrome: localization to Xq12-21:31 by X-inactivation and linkage analysis. *Am J Hum Genet* 1992;51:1136.
367. Lefort G, Taib J, Toutain A, et al. X-linked alpha-thalassemia/mental retardation (ATR-X) syndrome: report of three male patients in a large French family. *Ann Genet* 1993;36:200.
368. Gibbons RJ, Brueton I, Buckle VJ, et al. The clinical and hematological features of the X-linked alpha thalassemia/mental retardation syndrome (ATR-X). *Am J Med Genet* 1995;55:288.
369. Gibbons RJ, Picketts DJ, Villard L, et al. Mutations in a putative global transcriptional regulator cause X-linked mental retardation with alpha-thalassemia (ATR-X syndrome). *Cell* 1995;80:837.
370. Bollekens JA, Forget BG. δβ Thalassemia and hereditary persistence of fetal hemoglobin. *Hematol Oncol Clin North Am* 1991;5:399.
371. Poncz M, Henthorn P, Stoeckert C, et al. Globin gene expression in hereditary persistence of fetal hemoglobin and (δβ)^0 thalassemia. In: MacLean N, ed. *Oxford surveys on eukaryotic genes,* 5th vol. Oxford: Oxford University Press, 1988:163.
372. Ottolenghi S, Mantovani R, Nicolis S, et al. DNA sequences regulating human globin gene transcription in nondeletional hereditary persistence of fetal hemoglobin. *Hemoglobin* 1989;13:523.
373. Wood WG. Hereditary persistence of fetal hemoglobin and δ/β thalassemia. In: Steinberg MH, Forget BG, Higgs DR, et al., eds. *Disorders of hemoglobin.* New York: Cambridge University Press, 2001:356.
374. Forget BG. Molecular basis of hereditary persistence of fetal hemoglobin. *Ann N Y Acad Sci* 1998;850:38.
375. Kulozik AE, Yarwood N, Jones RW. The Corfu δβ^0 thalassemia: a small deletion acts at a distance to selectively abolish β globin gene expression. *Blood* 1988;71:457.
376. Kattamis C, Hu H, Cheng G, et al. Molecular characterization of β-thalassaemia in 174 Greek patients with thalassaemia major. *Br J Haematol* 1990;74:342.
377. Bernards R, Flavell RA. Physical mapping of the globin gene deletion in hereditary persistence of foetal haemoglobin (HPFH). *Nucleic Acids Res* 1980;8:1521.
378. Flavell RA, Kooter JM, deBoer E, et al. Analysis of the βδ-globin gene loci in normal and Hb Lepore DNA: direct determination of gene linkage and intergene distance. *Cell* 1978;15:25.
379. Mears JG, Ramirez F, Leibowitz D, et al. Organization of human δ and β-globin genes in cellular DNA and the presence of intragenic inserts. *Cell* 1978;15:15.
380. Baird M, Schreiner H, Driscoll C, et al. Localization of the site of recombination in formation of the Lepore Boston globin gene. *J Clin Invest* 1981;68:560.
381. Mavilio F, Giampaolo A, Care A, et al. The δβ crossover region in Lepore Boston hemoglobinopathy is restricted to a 59 base pairs region around the 5' splice junction of the large globin gene intervening sequence. *Blood* 1983;62:230.
382. Chebloune Y, Verdier G. The delta-beta-crossing-over site in the fusion gene of the Lepore-Boston disease might be localized in a preferential recombination region. *Acta Haematol* 1983;69:294.
383. Lanclos KD, Patterson J, Efremov GD, et al. Characterization of chromosomes with hybrid genes for Hb Lepore-Washington, Hb Lepore-Baltimore, Hb P-Nilotic, and Hb Kenya. *Hum Genet* 1987;77:40.
384. Wood WG, Old JM, Roberts AVS, et al. Human globin gene expression: control of β, δ and δβ chain production. *Cell* 1978;15:437.
385. Orkin SH, Goff SC, Nathan DG. Heterogeneity of DNA deletion in γδβ thalassemia. *J Clin Invest* 1981;67:878.
386. Taramelli R, Kioussis D, Vanin E, et al. γδβ-Thalassemias 1 and 2 are the result of a 100 kbp deletion in the human β-globin cluster. *Nucleic Acids Res* 1986;14:7017.
387. Van der Ploeg LHT, Konings A, Oort M, et al. γ β-Thalassemia studies showing that deletion of the γ and δ influences β-globin gene expression in man. *Nature* 1980;283:637.
388. Vanin EF, Henthorn PS, Kioussis D, et al. Unexpected relationships between four large deletions in the human β-globin gene cluster. *Cell* 1983;35:701.
389. Curtin P, Pirastu M, Kan YW, et al. A distant gene deletion affects β-globin gene function in an atypical γδβ-thalassemia. *J Clin Invest* 1985;76:1554.
390. Fearon ER, Kazazian HH, Waber PG, et al. The entire globin cluster is deleted in a form of γδβ-thalassemia. *Blood* 1983;61:1273.
391. Pirastu M, Kan YW, Lin CC, et al. Hemolytic disease of the newborn caused by a new deletion of the entire β-globin cluster. *J Clin Invest* 1983;72:602.
392. Trent RJ, Williams BG, Kearney A, et al. Molecular and hematologic characterization of Scottish-Irish type (εγδβ)^0 thalassemia. *Blood* 1990;76:2132.
393. Driscoll MC, Dobkin CS, Alter BP. γδβ-Thalassemia due to a de novo mutation deleting the 5' β-globin gene activating-region hypersensitive sites. *Proc Natl Acad Sci U S A* 1989;86:7470.
394. Diaz-Chico JC, Huang HJ, Juricic D, et al. Two new large deletions resulting in εγδβ thalassemia. *Acta Haematol* 1988;80:79.
395. Kioussis D, Vanin E, deLange T, et al. β-Globin gene inactivation by DNA translocation in γ β-thalassemia. *Nature* 1983;306:662.
396. Kulozik AE, Bail S, Bellan-Koch A, et al. The proximal element of the β globin locus control region is not functionally required in vivo. *J Clin Invest* 1990;87:2142.
397. Collis P, Antoniou M, Grosveld F. Definition of the minimal requirements within the human β-globin gene and the dominant control region for high level expression. *EMBO J* 1990;9:223.
398. Ryan TM, Townes TM, Reilly MP, et al. A single erythroid-specific DNAse I superhypersensitive site activates high levels of human β-globin gene expression in transgenic mice. *Genes Dev* 1989;3:314.
399. Ojwang PJ, Nakatsuji T, Gardiner MB, et al. Gene deletion as the molecular basis for the Kenya-^{G}γ-HPFH condition. *Hemoglobin* 1983;7:115.
400. Collins FS, Cole JL, Lockwood WK, et al. The deletion in both common types of hereditary persistence of fetal hemoglobin is approximately 105 kilobases. *Blood* 1987;70:1797.
401. Feingold EA, Forget BG. The breakpoint of a large deletion causing hereditary persistence of fetal hemoglobin occurs within an erythroid DNA domain remote from the β-globin gene cluster. *Blood* 1989;74:2178.
402. Fritsch EF, Lawn RM, Maniatis T. Characterization of deletions which affect the expression of fetal globin genes in man. *Nature* 1979;279:598.
403. Tuan D, Feingold E, Newman M, et al. Different 3'-end points of deletions causing δβ-thalassemia and hereditary persistence of fetal hemoglobin:

implications for the control of γ-globin gene expression in man. *Proc Natl Acad Sci U S A* 1983;80:6937.

404. Tuan D, Murnane MJ, de Riel JK, et al. Heterogeneity in the molecular basis of hereditary persistence of fetal hemoglobin. *Nature* 1980;285:335.

405. Henthorn PS, Smithies O, Mager DL. Molecular analysis of deletions in the human β-globin cluster: deletion junctions and locations of breakpoints. *Genomics* 1990;6:226.

406. Henthorn PS, Mager DL, Huisman THJ, et al. A gene deletion ending with a complex array of repeated sequences 3' to the human β-globin gene cluster. *Proc Natl Acad Sci U S A* 1986;83:5194.

407. Kutlar A, Gardiner MB, Headlee MG, et al. Heterogeneity in the molecular basis of three types of hereditary persistence of fetal hemoglobin and the relative synthesis of the $^Gγ$ and $^Aγ$ types of γ chain. *Biochem Genet* 1984;22:21.

408. Wainscoat JS, Old JM, Wood WG, et al. Characterization of an Indian (δβ)^0 thalassemia. *Br J Haematol* 1984;58:353.

409. Saglio G, Camaschella C, Serra A, et al. Italian type of deletional hereditary persistence of fetal hemoglobin. *Blood* 1986;68:646.

410. Camaschella C, Serra A, Gottardi E, et al. A new hereditary persistence of fetal hemoglobin deletion has a breakpoint within the 3' β-globin gene enhancer. *Blood* 1990;75:1000.

411. Elder JT, Forrester WC, Thompson C, et al. Translocation of an erythroid-specific hypersensitive site in deletion-type hereditary persistence of fetal hemoglobin. *Mol Cell Biol* 1990;10:1382.

412. Feingold EA, Penny LA, Nienhuis AW, et al. An olfactory receptor gene is located in the extended human β-globin gene cluster and is expressed in erythroid cells. *Genomics* 1999;61:15.

413. Ottolenghi S, Giglioni B. The deletion in a type of β thalassemia begins in an inverted Alu I repeat. *Nature* 1982;300:770.

414. Camaschella C, Serra A, Saglio G, et al. The 3' end of the deletions of Spanish (β)^0-thalassemia and Black HPFH 1 and 2 lie within 17 kilobases. *Blood* 1987;70:593.

415. Arcasoy M, Romana M, Fabry ME, et al. High levels of human γ-globin gene expression in adult mice carrying a transgene of deletion-type hereditary persistence of fetal hemoglobin. *Mol Cell Biol* 1997;17:2076.

416. Anagnou NP, Perez-Stable C, Gelinas R, et al. Sequences located 3' to the breakpoint of HPFH-3 exhibit enhancer activity and can modify the developmental expression of the $^Aγ$ globin gene in transgenic mice. *J Biol Chem* 1995; 270:10256.

417. Mager DL, Henthorn PS, Smithies O. A Chinese $^Gγ^+(^Aγδβ)^0$ thalassemia deletion: comparison to other deletions in the human β-globin gene cluster and sequence analysis of the breakpoints. *Nucleic Acids Res* 1985;13:6559.

418. Winichagoon S, Fucharoen S, Thonglairoam V, et al. Thai $^Gγ^+(^Aγδβ)^0$ thalassemia and its interaction with a single γ-globin gene on a chromosome carrying β^0 thalassemia. *Hemoglobin* 1990;14:185.

419. Anagnou NP, Papayannopoulou T, Nienhuis AW, et al. Molecular characterization of a novel form of ($^Aγδβ)^0$-thalassemia deletion with a 3' breakpoint close to those of HPFH-3 and HPFH-4: insights into a common regulatory mechanism. *Nucleic Acids Res* 1988;16:6057.

420. Fodde R, Losekoot M, Casula L, et al. Nucleotide sequence of the Belgian $^Gγ^+(^Aγβ)^0$-thalassemia deletion breakpoint suggests a common mechanism for a number of such recombination events. *Genomics* 1990;8:732.

421. Kosteas T, Palena A, Anagnou NP. Molecular cloning of the breakpoints of the hereditary persistence of fetal hemoglobin type-6 (HPFH-6) deletion and sequence analysis of the novel juxtaposed region from the 3' end of the β-globin gene cluster. *Hum Genet* 1997;100:441.

422. Kosteas T, Pavlou A, Palena A, et al. Complete sequencing and functional analysis of the HPFH-6 enhancer detection of multiple motifs for transcription factors and identification of an opening reading frame. *Blood* 1996;88 [Suppl 1]:150a.

423. Cao A, Melis MA, Galanello T, et al. δβ(F)-Thalassemia in Sardinia. *J Med Genet* 1982;19:184.

424. Guida S, Giglioni B, Comi P, et al. The β-globin gene in Sardinian δβ^0-thalassemia carries a C → T nonsense mutation at codon 39. *EMBO J* 1984;3:785.

425. Pirastu M, Kan YW, Galanello R, et al. Multiple mutations produce δβ^0 thalassemia in Sardinia. *Science* 1983;223:929.

426. Ottolenghi S, Giglioni B, Pulazzini A, et al. Sardinian β-thalassemia: a further example of a C to T substitution at position -196 of the $^Aγ$ globin gene promoter. *Blood* 1987;69:1058.

427. Atweh GF, Zhu D-E, Forget BG. A novel basis for β-thalassemia in a Chinese family. *Blood* 1986;68:1108.

428. Atweh GF, Zhu X-X, Brickner HE, et al. The δβ-globin gene on the Chinese β-thalassemic chromosome carries a promoter mutation. *Blood* 1988;70:1470.

429. Collins FS, Stoeckert CJ Jr, Serjeant GR, et al. $^Gγβ^+$ Hereditary persistence of fetal hemoglobin: cosmid cloning and identification of a specific mutation 5' to the $^Gγ$ gene. *Proc Natl Acad Sci U S A* 1984;81:4894.

430. Gilman JG, Mishima N, Wen XJ, et al. Upstream promoter mutation associated with modest elevation of fetal hemoglobin expression in human adults. *Blood* 1988;72:78.

431. Tate VE, Wood WG, Weatherall DJ. The British form of hereditary persistence of fetal hemoglobin results from a single base pair mutation adjacent to an S1 hypersensitive site 5' to the $^Aγ$ globin gene. *Blood* 1986;68:1389.

432. Giglioni B, Casini C, Mantovani R, et al. A molecular study of a family with Greek hereditary persistence of fetal hemoglobin and β-thalassemia. *EMBO J* 1984;3:2641.

433. Gelinas R, Bender M, Lotshaw C, et al. Chinese $^Aγ$ fetal hemoglobin: C to T substitution at position -196 of the $^Aγ$ gene promoter. *Blood* 1986;67:1777.

434. Costa FF, Zago MA, Cheng G, et al. The Brazilian type of nondeletional $^Aγ$-fetal hemoglobin has a C to G substitution at nucleotide-195 of the $^Aγ$-globin gene. *Blood* 1990;76:1896.

435. Sykes K, Kaufman R. A naturally occurring gamma globin gene mutation enhances SP1 binding activity. *Mol Cell Biol* 1989;10:95.

436. Ronchi A, Nicolis S, Santoro C, et al. Increased Sp1 binding mediates erythroid-specific overexpression of a mutated (HPFH) γ-globin promoter. *Nucleic Acids Res* 1989;24:10231.

437. Fischer K-D, Nowock J. The T to C substitution at -198 of the $^Aγ$-globin gene associated with the British form of HPFH generates overlapping recognition sites for two DNA-binding proteins. *Nucleic Acids Res* 1990;18:5685.

438. Gumucio D, Rood KL, Blanchard-McQuate KL, et al. Interaction of Sp1 with the human γ globin promoter: binding and transactivation of normal and mutant promoters. *Blood* 1991;78:1853.

439. Surrey S, Delgrosso K, Malladi P, et al. A single base change at position -175 in the 5'-flanking region of the $^Gγ$-globin gene from a black with $^Gγβ^+$-HPFH. *Blood* 1988;71:807.

440. Ottolenghi S, Nicolis S, Taramelli R, et al. Sardinian $^Gγ$-HPFH: a T → C substitution in a conserved "octamer" sequence in the $^Gγ$-globin promoter. *Blood* 1988;71:815.

441. Stoming TA, Stoming GS, Lanclos KD, et al. An $^Aγ$ type of nondeletional hereditary persistence of fetal hemoglobin with a T → C mutation at position -175 to the cap site of the $^Aγ$ globin gene. *Blood* 1989;73:329.

442. Collins FS, Metherall JE, Yamakawa M, et al. A point mutation in the $^Aγ$-globin gene promoter in Greek hereditary persistence of fetal haemoglobin. *Nature* 1985;313:325.

443. Gelinas R, Endlich B, Pfeiffer C, et al. G to A substitution in the distal CCAAT box of the $^Aγ$-globin gene in Greek hereditary persistence of fetal haemoglobin. *Nature* 1985;313:323.

444. Gilman JF, Mishima N, Wen XJ, et al. Distal CCAAT box deletion in the $^Aγ$ globin gene of two black adolescents with elevated fetal $^Aγ$ globin. *Nucleic Acids Res* 1988;16:10635.

445. Fucharoen S, Shimizu K, Fukumaki Y. A novel C-T transition within the distal CCAAT motif of the G γ-globin gene in the Japanese HPFH: implication of factor binding in elevated fetal globin expression. *Nucleic Acids Res* 1990;18:5245.

446. Oner R, Kutlar F, Gu L-H, et al. The Georgia type of nondeletional hereditary persistence of fetal hemoglobin has a C → T mutation at nucleotide -114 of the $^Aγ$-globin gene. *Blood* 1991;77:1124.

447. Gumucio DL, Rood KL, Gray TA, et al. Nuclear proteins that bind to the human γ-globin gene promoter: alterations in binding produced by point mutation associated with hereditary persistence of fetal hemoglobin. *Mol Cell Biol* 1988;8:5310.

448. Mantovani R, Malgaretti N, Nicolis S, et al. The effects of HPFH mutations in the human γ-globin promoter on binding of ubiquitous and erythroid-specific nuclear factors. *Nucleic Acids Res* 1988;16:7783.

449. Lloyd JA, Lee RF, Lingrel JB. Mutation in two regions upstream of the $^Aγ$ globin gene canonical promoter affect gene expression. *Nucleic Acids Res* 1989;17:4339.

450. Superti-Furga G, Barberis A, Schaffner G, et al. The -117 mutation in Greek HPFH affects the binding of three nuclear factors to the CCAAT region of the γ-globin gene. *EMBO J* 1988;7:3099.

451. Mantovani R, Superti-Furga G, Gilman J, et al. The deletion of the distal CCAAT-box region of the $^Aγ$-globin gene in black HPFH abolishes the binding of the erythroid specific protein NFE3 and of the CCAAT displacement protein. *Nucleic Acids Res* 1989;17:6681.

452. Berry M, Grosveld F, Dillon N. A single point mutation is the cause of the Greek form of hereditary persistence of fetal hemoglobin. *Nature* 1992;358:499.

453. Peterson KR, Li Q, Clegg CH, et al. Use of yeast artificial chromosomes (YACs) in studies of mammalian development: production of β-globin locus YAC mice carrying human globin developmental mutants. *Proc Natl Acad Sci U S A* 1995;92:5655.

454. Ronchi A, Berry M, Raguz S, et al. Role of the duplicated CCAAT box region in γ-globin gene regulation and hereditary persistence of fetal hemoglobin. *EMBO J* 1996;45:143.

455. Morley BJ, Abbott CA, Sharpe JA, et al. A single β-globin locus control region element (5' hypersensitive site 2) is sufficient for developmental regulation of human globin genes in transgenic mice. *Mol Cell Biol* 1992;12:2057.

456. Starck J, Sarkar R, Romana M, et al. Developmental regulation of human γ- and β-globin genes in the absence of the locus control region. *Blood* 1994;84:1656.

457. Li Q, Duan ZJ, Stamatoyannopoulos G. Analysis of the mechanism of action of non-deletion hereditary persistence of fetal hemoglobin mutants in transgenic mice. *EMBO J* 2001;20:157.

458. Old JM, Ayyub H, Wood WG, et al. Linkage analysis of non-deletion hereditary persistence of fetal hemoglobin. *Science* 1982;215:981.

459. Miyoshi K, Kaneto Y, Kawai H, et al. X-linked dominant control of F-cells in normal adult life. *Blood* 1988;72:1854.

460. Dover GJ, Smith KD, Chang YC, et al. Fetal hemoglobin levels in sickle cell disease and normal individuals are partially controlled by an X-linked gene located at Xp22.2. *Blood* 1992;80:816.

461. Chang YC, Smith KD, Moore RD, et al. An analysis of fetal hemoglobin variation in sickle cell disease: the relative contributions of the X-linked factor, β-globin haplotypes, α-globin gene number, gender and age. *Blood* 1995;85:1111.

462. Thein SI, Sampietro M, Rohde K, et al. Detection of a major gene for heterocellular hereditary persistence of fetal hemoglobin after accounting for genetic modifiers. *Am J Hum Genet* 1994;54:214.

463. Craig JE, Rochette J, Fischer CA, et al. Dissecting the loci controlling fetal hemoglobin production on chromosomes 11p and 6q by the regressive approach. *Nat Genet* 1996;12:58.

464. Stamatoyannopoulos G, Wood WF, Papayanopoulou T, et al. A new form of hereditary persistence of fetal hemoglobin in blacks and its association with sickle cell trait. *Blood* 1975;46:683.

465. Gelinas RE, Rixon M, Magis W, et al. γ-Gene promoter and enhancer structure in Seattle variant of hereditary persistence of fetal hemoglobin. *Blood* 1988;71:1108.

466. Bouhassira EE, Rajagopal K, Ragusa A, et al. The enhancer-like sequence 3' to the ᴬγ gene is polymorphic in human populations. *Blood* 1989;73:1050.

467. Jensen M, Wirtz A, Walther J-U, et al. Hereditary persistence of fetal haemoglobin (HPFH) in conjunction with a chromosomal translocation involving the haemoglobin β locus. *Br J Haematol* 1984;56:87.

468. Altay C, Huisman TH, Schroeder WA. Another form of hereditary persistence of fetal hemoglobin (the Atlanta type)? *Hemoglobin* 1977;1:125.

469. Gilman JG, Huisman THJ. DNA sequence variation associated with elevated fetal ᴳγ globin production. *Blood* 1985;66:783.

470. Pembrey ME, Wood WG, Weatherall DJ, et al. Fetal haemoglobin production and the sickle gene in the oases of eastern Saudi Arabia. *Br J Haematol* 1978;40:415.

471. Perrine RP, Pembrey ME, John P, et al. Natural history of sickle cell anaemia in Saudi Arabs: a study of 270 subjects. *Ann Intern Med* 1978;88:1.

472. Kar BC, Satapathy RK, Kulozik RK, et al. Sickle cell disease in Orissa state, India. *Lancet* 1986;2:1198.

473. Kulozik AE, Kar BC, Satapathy RK, et al. Fetal hemoglobin levels and βˢ globin haplotypes in an Indian population with sickle cell disease. *Blood* 1987;69:1742.

474. Miller BA, Olivieri N, Salameh M, et al. Molecular analysis of the high-hemoglobin-F phenotype in Saudi Arabian sickle cell anemia. *N Engl J Med* 1987;316:244.

475. Nagel RL, Fabry ME, Pagnier J, et al. Hematologically and genetically distinct forms of sickle cell anemia in Africa: the Senegal type and the Benin type. *N Engl J Med* 1985;312:880.

476. Gilman JG, Kutlar F, Johnson ME, et al. A G to A nucleotide substitution 161 base pairs 5' of the ᴳγ globin gene cap site (-161) in a high ᴳγ non-anemic person. In: Stamatoyannoupoulos G, Nienhuis AW, eds. *Developmental control of globin gene expression*. New York: Alan R. Liss, 1987:383.

477. Galacteros F, Garin DJ, Monplaisir N, et al. Two new cases of heterozygosity for hemoglobin Knossos α₂β₂ 27 Ala → Ser detected in the French West Indies and Algeria. *Hemoglobin* 1984;8:215.

478. Oggiano L, Pirastu M, Moi P, et al. Molecular characterization of a normal Hb A₂β-thalassaemia determinant in a Sardinian family. *Br J Haematol* 1987;67:225.

479. Galanello R, Melis MA, Podda A, et al. Deletion δ-thalassemia: the 7.2 Kb deletion of Corfu δβ-thalassemia in a non-β-thalassemia chromosome. *Blood* 1990;75:1747.

480. Nakamura T, Takihara Y, Ohta Y, et al. A δ globin gene derived from patients with homozygous δ⁰-thalassemia functions normally on transient expression in heterologous cells. *Blood* 1987;70:809.

481. Matsuda M, Sakamoto N, Fukumaki Y. δ Thalassemia caused by disruption of the site for an erythroid-specific transcription factor, GATA-1, in the δ-globin gene promoter. *Blood* 1992;80:1347.

482. Moi P, Loudianos G, Lavinha J, et al. δ-Thalassemia due to a mutation in an erythroid-specific binding protein sequence 3' to the δ-globin gene. *Blood* 1992;79:512.

483. Martin SL, Vincent KA, Wilson AC. Rise and fall of the delta globin gene. *J Mol Biol* 1983;164:513.

484. Kimura A, Takagi Y. A frameshift addition causes silencing of the δ-globin gene in an old world monkey, an anubis. *Nucleic Acids Res* 1985;11:2541.

485. Jeffreys AJ, Barrie PA, Harris S, et al. Isolation and sequence analysis of a hybrid δ-globin pseudogene from the brown lemur. *J Mol Biol* 1982;156:487.

486. Nakatsuji T, Gardiner MB, Reese AI, et al. Gamma thalassemia resulting from the deletion of a γ-globin gene. *Nucleic Acids Res* 1983;11:4635.

487. Shimasaki S, Iuchi I. Diversity of human γ-globin gene loci including a quadruplicated arrangement. *Blood* 1986;67:784.

488. Hill AVS, Bowden DK, Weatherall DJ, et al. Chromosomes with one, two, three, and four fetal globin genes: molecular and hematologic analysis. *Blood* 1986;67:1611.

489. Liu JZ, Gilman JG, Cao Q, et al. Four categories of γ-globin gene triplications: DNA sequence comparison of low ᴳγ and high ᴳγ triplications. *Blood* 1988;72:480.

490. Powers PA, Altay C, Huisman THJ, et al. Two novel arrangements of the human fetal globin genes: ᴳγ-ᴳγ and ᴬγ-ᴬγ. *Nucleic Acids Res* 1984;12:7023.

491. Tate VE, Hill AVS, Bowden DK, et al. A silent deletion in the β-globin gene cluster. *Nucleic Acids Res* 1986;14:4743.

492. Gilman JG, Johnson ME, Mishima N. Four base-pair DNA deletion in human ᴬγ globin-gene promoter associated with low ᴬγ expression in adults. *Br J Haematol* 1988;68:455.

493. Manca L, Cocco E, Gallisai D, et al. Diminished ᴬγᵀ fetal globin levels in Sardinian haplotype II β⁰-thalassaemia patients are associated with a four base pair deletion in the ᴬγᵀ. *Br J Haematol* 1991;78:105.

494. Coleman MB, Steinberg MN, Adams JG III. A four-base deletion 5' to the ᴬγ globin gene is a common polymorphism. *Blood* 1991;78:2473.

495. Kazazian HH Jr, Boehm CD. Molecular basis and prenatal diagnosis of β-thalassemia. *Blood* 1988;72:1107.

496. Alter BP. Antenatal diagnosis. *Ann N Y Acad Sci* 1990;612:237.

497. Boehm CD, Antonarakis SE, Phillips JA III, et al. Prenatal diagnosis using DNA polymorphisms: report on 95 pregnancies at risk for sickle-cell disease or β-thalassemia. *N Engl J Med* 1983;308:1054.

498. Orkin S, Markham AF, Kazazian HH. Direct detection of the common Mediterranean β-thalassemia gene with synthetic DNA probes. *J Clin Invest* 1983;71:775.

499. Pirastu M, Kan YW, Cao A, et al. Prenatal diagnosis of β-thalassemia: detection of a single nucleotide mutation in DNA. *N Engl J Med* 1983;309:284.

500. Rosatelli C, Falchi AM, Tuveri T, et al. Prenatal diagnosis of beta-thalassaemia with the synthetic-oligomer technique. *Lancet* 1985;1:241.

501. Eisenstein BI. The polymerase chain reaction: a new method of using molecular genetics for medical diagnosis. *N Engl J Med* 1990;322:178.

502. Mullis KB. The unusual origin of the polymerase chain reaction. *Sci Am* 1990;263:56.

503. Saiki RK, Chang C-A, Levenson CH, et al. Diagnosis of sickle cell anemia and β-thalassemia with enzymatically amplified DNA and nonradioactive allele-specific oligonucleotide probes. *N Engl J Med* 1988;319:537.

504. Cai S-P, Chang CA, Zhang JZ, et al. Rapid prenatal diagnosis of β thalassemia using DNA amplification and nonradioactive probes. *Blood* 1989;73:372.

505. Cai S-P, Zhang J-Z, Huang D-H, et al. A simple approach to prenatal diagnosis of β-thalassemia in a geographic area where multiple mutations occur. *Blood* 1988;71:1357.

506. Chehab FF, Kan YW. Detection of specific DNA sequences by fluorescence amplification: a color complementation assay. *Proc Natl Acad Sci U S A* 1989;86:9178.

507. Wu DY, Ugozzoli L, Pal BK, et al. Allele-specific enzymatic amplification of β-globin genomic DNA for diagnosis of sickle cell anemia. *Proc Natl Acad Sci U S A* 1989;86:2757.

508. Saiki RK, Walsh SP, Levenson CH, et al. Genetic analysis of amplified DNA with immobilized sequence-specific oligonucleotide probes. *Proc Natl Acad Sci U S A* 1989;86:6230.

509. Lindeman R, Hu SP, Volpato F, et al. Polymerase chain reaction (PCR) mutagenesis enabling rapid non-radioactive detection of common β-thalassaemia mutations in Mediterraneans. *Br J Haematol* 1991;78:100.

510. Change J-G, Chen P-H, Chiou S-S, et al. Rapid diagnosis of β-thalassemia mutation in Chinese by naturally and amplified created restriction sites. *Blood* 1992;80:2092.

511. Sutton M, Bouhassira EE, Nagel RL. Polymerase chain reaction amplification applied to the determination of β-like globin gene cluster haplotypes. *Am J Hematol* 1989;32:66.

512. Sallee D, Kazazian HH Jr. Multiplex analysis of β-globin restriction site polymorphisms by PCR: a method for rapid haplotyping and identity exclusion. *Am J Hum Genet* 1989;45:A216(abst).

513. Engelke DR, Hoener PA, Collins FS. Direct sequencing of enzymatically amplified human genomic DNA. *Proc Natl Acad Sci U S A* 1988;85:544.

514. Myers RM, Maniatis T, Lerman LS. Detection and localization of single base changes by denaturing gradient gel electrophoresis. *Methods Enzymol* 1987;155:501

515. Myers RM, Lumelsky N, Lerman LS, et al. Detection of single base substitutions in total genomic DNA. *Nature* 1985;313:495.

516. Cai S-P, Kan YW. Identification of the multiple β-thalassemia mutations by denaturing gradient gel electrophoresis. *J Clin Invest* 1990;85:550.

517. Losekoot M, Fodde R, Harteveld CL, et al. Denaturing gradient gel electrophoresis and direct sequencing of PCR amplified genomic DNA: a rapid and reliable diagnostic approach to beta thalassaemia. *Br J Haematol* 1990;76:269.

518. Phillips JA III, Scott AF, Kazazian HH, et al. Prenatal diagnosis of hemoglobinopathies by restriction endonuclease analysis: pregnancies at risk for sickle cell anemia and S-Oᴬʳᵃᵇ disease. *Johns Hopkins Med J* 1979;145:57.

519. Embury SH, Scharf SJ, Saiki RK, et al. Rapid prenatal diagnosis of sickle cell anemia by a new method of DNA analysis. *N Engl J Med* 1987;316:656.

520. Chehab FF, Doherty M, Cai S, et al. Detection of sickle cell anaemia and thalassaemias. *Nature* 1987;329:293.

521. Wallace RB, Schold M, Johnson MJ, et al. Oligonucleotide directed mutagenesis of the human β-globin gene: a general method for producing specific point mutations in cloned DNA. *Nucleic Acids Res* 1981;9:3647.

522. Conner BJ, Reys AA, Morin C, et al. Detection of sickle cell βˢ-globin allele by hybridization with synthetic oligonucleotides. *Proc Natl Acad Sci U S A* 1983;80:278.

523. Old JM, Varawalla NY, Weatherall DJ. The rapid detection and prenatal diagnosis of β thalassemia in the Asian Indian and Cypriot populations in the UK. *Lancet* 1990;336:834–837.

524. Old J. Haemoglobinopathies. *Prenat Diagn* 1996;16:1181–1186.

525. Saxena R, Jain PK, Thomas E, et al. Prenatal diagnosis of β-thalassaemia: experience in a developing country. *Prenat Diagn* 1998;18:1–7.

526. Cheung MC, Goldberg JD, Kan YW. Prenatal diagnosis of sickle cell anaemia and thalassemia by analysis of fetal cells in maternal blood. *Nat Genet* 1996;14:264–268.

527. Old JM. DNA-based diagnosis of the hemoglobin disorders. In: Steinberg MH, Forget BG, Higgs DR, et al., eds. *Disorders of hemoglobin*. New York: Cambridge University Press, 2001:941.

528. Temple GF, Dozy AM, Roy KL, et al. Construction of a functional human suppressor tRNA gene: an approach to gene therapy for β-thalassaemia. *Nature* 1982;296:537.

529. Sierakowska H, Sambade MJ, Agrawal S, et al. Repair of thalassemic human β-globin mRNA in mammalian cells by antisense oligonucleotides. *Proc Natl Acad Sci U S A* 1996;93:12840.

530. Lacerra G, Sierakowska H, Carestia C, et al. Restoration of hemoglobin A synthesis in erythroid cells from peripheral blood of thalassemic patients. *Proc Natl Acad Sci U S A* 2000;97:9591.

531. Chan PP, Glazer PM. Triplex DNA: fundamentals, advances, and potential applications for gene therapy. *J Mol Med* 1997;75:267.

532. Broitman S, Amosova O, Dolinnaya NG, et al. Repairing the sickle cell mutation, I: specific covalent binding of a photoreactive third strand to the mutated base pair. *J Biol Chem* 1999;274:21763.

533. Cole-Strauss A, Yoon K, Xiang Y, et al. Correction of the mutation responsible for sickle cell anemia by an RNA-DNA oligonucleotide. *Science* 1996;273:1386.

534. Lan H, Howrey RP, Lee SW, et al. Ribozyme-mediated repair of sickle beta-globin mRNAs in erythrocyte precursors. *Science* 1998;280:1593.

535. Sadelain M. Genetic treatment of the haemoglobinopathies: recombinations and new combinations. *Br J Haematol* 1997;98:247–253.

536. Atweh GH, Forget BG. Clinical applications of gene therapy: animals. In: Quesenberry PJ, Stein GS, Forget BG, et al., eds. *Stem cell biology and gene therapy*. New York: Wiley-Liss, 1998:411.

537. Rivella S, Sadelain M. Genetic treatment of severe hemoglobinopathies: the combat against transgene variegation and transgene silencing. *Semin Hematol* 1998;35:112–125.

538. Sorrentino BP, Nienhuis AW. Prospects for gene therapy of sickle cell disease and thalassemia. In: Steinberg MH, Forget BG, Higgs DR, et al., eds. *Disorders of hemoglobin*. New York: Cambridge University Press, 2001:1118.

539. Dzierzak EA, Papayannopoulou T, Mulligan RC. Lineage-specific expression of a human β-globin gene in murine bone marrow transplant recipients reconstituted with retrovirus-transduced stem cells. *Nature* 1988;331:35.

540. Karlsson S, Bodine DM, Perry L, et al. Expression of the human β-globin gene following retroviral-mediated transfer into multipotential hematopoietic progenitors of mice. *Proc Natl Acad Sci U S A* 1987;84:2411.

541. Bender MA, Gelinas RE, Miller AD. A majority of mice show long-term expression of a human β-globin gene after retrovirus transfer into hematopoietic stem cells. *Mol Cell Biol* 1989;9:1426.

542. Bodine DM, Karlsson S, Nienhuis AW. Combination of interleukins 3 and 6 preserves stem cell function in culture and enhances retrovirus-mediated gene transfer into hematopoietic stem cells. *Proc Natl Acad Sci U S A* 1989;86:8897.

543. Miller AD, Bender MA, Harris EAS, et al. Design of retrovirus vectors for transfer and expression of the human β-globin gene. *J Virol* 1988;62:4337–4345.

544. Gelinas R, Novak U. Retroviral vectors for the β-globin gene that demonstrate improved titer and expression. *Ann N Y Acad Sci* 1990;612:427.

545. Novak U, Harris EAS, Forrester W, et al. High level β-globin expression after retroviral transfer of locus activation region-containing human β-globin gene derivatives into murine erythroleukemia cells. *Proc Natl Acad Sci U S A* 1990;87:3386.

546. Chang JC, Liu D, Kan YW. A 36-base-pair core sequence of the locus control region enhances retrovirally transferred β-globin gene expression. *Proc Natl Acad Sci U S A* 1992;89:3107.

547. Plavec I, Papayannopoulou T, Maury C, et al. A human β-globin gene fused to the human β-globin locus control region is expressed at high levels in erythroid cells of mice engrafted with retrovirus-transduced hematopoietic stem cells. *Blood* 1993;81:1384.

548. Leboulch P, Huang GMS, Humphries RK, et al. Mutagenesis of retroviral vectors transducing human beta-globin gene and beta-globin locus control region derivatives results in stable transmission of an active transcriptional structure. *EMBO J* 1994;13:3065.

549. Raftopoulos H, Ward M, Leboulch P, et al. Long-term transfer and expression of the human beta-globin gene in a mouse transplant model. *Blood* 1997;90:3414.

550. Sadelain M, Wang CH, Antoniou M, et al. Generation of a high-titer retroviral vector capable of expressing high levels of the human beta-globin gene. *Proc Natl Acad Sci U S A* 1995;92:6728.

551. Ren S, Wong BY, Li J, et al. Production of genetically stable high-titer retroviral vectors that carry a human γ-globin gene under the control of the α-globin locus control region. *Blood* 1996;87:2518.

552. Lung H-Y, Meeus IS, Atweh GF. In vivo silencing of the human γ-globin gene in murine erythroid cells following retroviral transduction. *Blood Cells Mol Dis* 2000;26:613–619.

553. May C, Rivella S, Callegari J, et al. Therapeutic haemoglobin synthesis in β-thalassaemic mice expressing lentivirus-encoded human β-globin. *Nature* 2000;406:82–86.

554. Cornetta K. Safety aspects of gene therapy. *Br J Haematol* 1992;80:421.

555. Smithies O, Gregg RG, Boggs SS, et al. Insertion of DNA sequences into the human chromosomal β-globin locus by homologous recombination. *Nature* 1985;317:230.

556. Nandi AK, Roginski RS, Gregg RG, et al. Regulated expression of genes inserted at the human chromosomal β-globin locus by homologous recombination. *Proc Natl Acad Sci U S A* 1988;85:3845.

557. Popovich BW, Kim H-S, Shesely EG, et al. Correction of the human sickle cell gene using targeted gene replacement. In: Stamatoyannopoulos G, Nienhuis AW, eds. *The regulation of hemoglobin switching*. Baltimore: Johns Hopkins University Press, 1991:526.

557a. Kyba M, Perlingeiro RC, Daley GQ. HoxB4 confers definitive lymphoid-myeloid engraftment potential on embryonic stem cell and yolk sac hematopoietic progenitors. *Cell* 2002;109:29–37.

557b. Rideout WM III, Hochedlinger K, Kyba M, et al. Correction of a genetic defect by nuclear transplantation and combined cell and gene therapy. *Cell* 2002;109:17–27.

558. Orlic D, Girard LJ, Jordan CT, et al. The level of mRNA encoding the amphotropic retrovirus receptor in mouse and human hematopoietic stem cells is low and correlates with the efficiency of retrovirus transduction. *Proc Natl Acad Sci U S A* 1996;93:11097.

559. Bodine DM, Crosier PS, Clark SC. Effects of hematopoietic growth factors on the survival of primitive stem cells in liquid suspension culture. *Blood* 1991;78:914.

560. Bodine DM, Orlic D, Birkett NC, et al. Stem cell factor increases CFU-S number *in vitro* in synergy with interleukin-6, and *in vivo* as a single factor. *Blood* 1992;79:913.

561. Toksoz D, Zsebo KM, Smith KA, et al. Support of human hematopoiesis in long-term bone marrow cultures by murine stromal cells selectively expressing the membrane-bound and secreted forms of the human homolog of the steel gene product, stem cell factor. *Proc Natl Acad Sci U S A* 1992;89:7350.

562. Bodine DM, McDonagh KT, Brandt SJ, et al. Development of a high-titer retrovirus producer cell line capable of gene transfer into rhesus monkey hematopoietic stem cells. *Proc Natl Acad Sci U S A* 1990;87:3738.

563. Bodine DM, McDonagh KT, Seidel NE, et al. Retrovirus mediated gene transfer to pluripotent hematopoietic stem cells. In: Stamatoyannopoulos G, Nienhuis AW, eds. *The regulation of hemoglobin switching*. Baltimore: Johns Hopkins University Press, 1991:505.

564. van Beusechem VW, Kukler A, Heidt PJ, et al. Long-term expression of human adenosine deaminase in rhesus monkeys transplanted with retrovirus-infected bone-marrow cells. *Proc Natl Acad Sci U S A* 1992;89:7640.

565. Bodine DM, Moritz T, Donahue RE, et al. Long-term in vivo expression of a murine adenosine deaminase gene in rhesus monkey hematopoietic cells of multiple lineages after retroviral mediated gene transfer into CD34+ bone marrow cells. *Blood* 1993;82:1975.

566. Dunbar CE, Seidel NE, Doren S, et al. Improved retroviral gene transfer into murine and Rhesus peripheral blood or bone marrow repopulating cells primed in vivo with stem cell factor and granulocyte colony-stimulating factor. *Proc Natl Acad Sci U S A* 1996;93:11871.

567. Cavazzana-Calvo M, Hacein-Bey S, de Saint Basile G, et al. Gene therapy of human severe combined immunodeficiency (SCID)-XI disease. *Science* 2000;288:669.

568. Weatherall DJ, Clegg JB, Naughton MA. Globin synthesis in thalassemia: an in vitro study. *Nature* 1965;208:1061–1065.

569. Weatherall DJ, Clegg JB. *The thalassaemia syndromes*. Oxford: Blackwell Science, 2001.

570. Weatherall DJ, Clegg JB. Thalassaemia: a global public health problem. *Nat Med* 1996;2:847–849.

571. Weatherall DJ, Clegg JB, Higgs DR, et al. The hemoglobinopathies. In: Scriver CR, Beaudet AL, Sly WS, et al., eds. *The metabolic and molecular bases of inherited disease*, 8th vol. New York: McGraw-Hill, 2000.

572. Clegg JB, Weatherall DJ. Thalassemia and malaria: new insights into an old problem. *Proc Assoc Am Physicians* 1999;111:278–282.

573. Haldane JBS. The rate of mutation of human genes. *Proc VIII Int Cong Genet Hereditas* 1949;35:267–273.

574. Silvestroni E, Bianco I, Montalenti G. On genetics and geographical distribution of a human blood disease. *Proc VIII Int Cong Genet Hereditas* 1949;35:662.

575. Williams TN, Maitland K, Bennett S, et al. High incidence of malaria in α-thalassaemic children. *Nature* 1996;383:522–525.

576. Allen SJ, O'Donnell A, Alexander ND, et al. alpha+-Thalassaemia protects children against disease caused by other infections as well as malaria. *Proc Natl Acad Sci U S A* 1997;94:14736–14741.

577. Weatherall DJ, Clegg JB, Kwiatkowski D. The role of genomics in studying genetic susceptibility to infectious disease. *Genome Res* 1997;7:967–973.

578. Weatherall DJ. Phenotype-genotype relationships in monogenic disease: lessons from the thalassaemias. *Nat Rev Genet* 2001;2:245–255.

579. Hill AVS, Allsop CEM, Kwiatkowski D. Common west African HLA antigens are associated with protection from severe malaria. *Nature* 1991;352:595–600.

580. McGuire W, Hill AV, Allsopp CE, et al. Variation in the TNF-alpha promoter region associated with susceptibility to cerebral malaria. *Nature* 1994;371:508–510.

581. Weatherall D, Clegg J, Kwiatkowski D. The role of genomics in studying genetic susceptibility to infectious disease. *Genome Res* 1997;7:967–973.

582. Fernandez-Reyes D, Craig AG, Kyes SA, et al. A high frequency African coding polymorphism in the N-terminal domain of ICAM-1 predisposing to cerebral malaria in Kenya. *Hum Mol Genet* 1997;6:1357–1360.

583. Weatherall DJ, Wainscoat JS, Thein SL, et al. Genetic and molecular analysis of mild forms of homozygous β-thalassemia. *Ann N Y Acad Sci* 1985;445:68–80.

584. Weatherall DJ, Clegg JB. Genetic disorders of hemoglobin. *Semin Hematol* 1999;36:24.

585. Weatherall DJ. Pathophysiology of thalassaemia. *Baillieres Clin Haematol* 1998;11:127–146.

586. Flint J, Harding RM, Boyce AJ, et al. The population genetics of the haemoglobinopathies. In: Higgs DR, Weatherall DJ, eds. *Baillière's Clinical Haematology*, vol 11, *Haemoglobinopathies*. London: Baillière Tindall and WB Saunders, 1998:1–51.

587. Cao A. Diagnosis of β-thalassemia intermedia at presentation. *Birth Defects: Original Articles Series* 1988;23:219–226.

588. Camaschella C, Cappellini MD. Thalassemia intermedia. *Haematologica* 1995; 80:58–68.

589. Rund D, Oron-Karni V, Filon D, et al. Genetic analysis of β-thalassemia intermedia in Israel: diversity of mechanisms and unpredictability of phenotype. *Am J Hematol* 1997;54:16–22.

590. Ho PJ, Hall GW, Luo LY, et al. Beta thalassaemia intermedia: is it possible to predict phenotype from genotype? *Br J Haematol* 1998;100:70–78.

591. Kazazian HH, Dowling CE, Hurwitz RL, et al. Thalassemia mutations in exon 3 of the β-globin gene often cause a dominant form of thalassemia and show no predilection for malarial-endemic regions of the world. *Am J Hum Genet* 1989;45:A242.

592. Thein SL, Hesketh C, Taylor P, et al. Molecular basis for dominantly inherited inclusion body beta-thalassemia. *Proc Natl Acad Sci U S A* 1990;87:3924–3928.

593. Thein SL. Dominant beta thalassaemia: molecular basis and pathophysiology. *Br J Haematol* 1992;80:273–277.

594. Ho PJ, Wickramasinghe SN, Rees DC, et al. Erythroblastic inclusions in dominantly inherited β thalassaemias. *Blood* 1997;89:322–328.

595. Thein SL. Is it dominantly inherited β thalassaemia or just a β-chain variant that is highly unstable? *Br J Haematol* 1999;107:12–21.

596. Huisman TH, Carver MFH, Baysal E. *A syllabus of thalassemia mutations.* Augusta: The Sickle Cell Anemia Foundation, 1997.

597. Schwartz E. The silent carrier of beta thalassemia. *N Engl J Med* 1969; 281:1327–1333.

598. Gonzalez-Redondo JM, Stoming TA, Kutlar A, et al. A C→T substitution at nt–101 in a conserved DNA sequence of the promotor region of the beta-globin gene is associated with "silent" beta-thalassemia. *Blood* 1989;73:1705–1711.

599. Bianco I, Cappabianca MP, Foglietta E, et al. Silent thalassemias: genotypes and phenotypes. *Haematologica* 1997;82:269–280.

600. Weatherall DJ, Clegg JB, Knox-Macaulay HH, et al. A genetically determined disorder with features both of thalassaemia and congenital dyserythropoietic anaemia. *Br J Haematol* 1973;24:681–702.

601. Stamatoyannopoulos G, Woodson R, Papayannopoulou T, et al. Inclusion-body β-thalassemia trait: a form of β thalassemia producing clinical manifestations in simple heterozygotes. *N Engl J Med* 1974;290:939–943.

602. Kan YW, Nathan DG. Mild thalassemia: the result of interactions of alpha and beta thalassemia genes. *J Clin Invest* 1970;49:635–642.

603. Knox-Macaulay HHM, Weatherall DJ, Clegg JB, et al. Clinical and biosynthetic characterization of αβ-thalassemia. *Br J Haematol* 1972;22:497–512.

604. Craig JE, Rochette J, Fisher CA, et al. Dissecting the loci controlling fetal haemoglobin production on chromosomes 11p and 6q by the regressive approach. *Nat Genet* 1996;12:58–64.

605. Garner C, Tatu T, Reittie JE, et al. Genetic influences on F cells and other hematologic variables: a twin heritability study. *Blood* 2000;95:342–346.

606. Weatherall DJ, Clegg JB, Higgs DR, et al. In: Scriver CR, ed. *The metabolic and molecular bases of inherited disease.* New York: McGraw Hill, 2001:4571–4636.

607. Stamatoyannopoulos G, Grosveld F. In: Stamatoyannopoulos G, Majerus PW, Perlmutter RM, et al., eds. *The molecular basis of blood disease.* New York: Saunders, 2001.

608. Gilman JG, Huisman TH. DNA sequence variation associated with elevated fetal G gamma globin production. *Blood* 1985;66:783–787.

609. Labie D, Pagnier J, Lapoumeroulie C, et al. Common haplotype dependency of high ᴳγ-globin gene expression and high Hb F levels in β-thalassemia and sickle cell anemia patients. *Proc Natl Acad Sci U S A* 1985;82:2111–2114.

610. Thein SL, Sampietro M, Old JM, et al. Association of thalassemia intermedia with a beta-globin gene haplotype. *Br J Haematol* 1987;65:370–373.

611. Galanello R, Dessi E, Melis MA, et al. Molecular analysis of beta zero-thalassemia intermedia in Sardinia. *Blood* 1989;74:823–827.

612. Thein SL, Weatherall DJ. In: Stamatoyannopoulos G, Niehuis AW, eds. *Hemoglobin switching, B: cellular and molecular mechanisms.* New York: Alan R. Liss, 1989:97–112.

613. Dover GJ, Smith KD, Chang YC, et al. Fetal hemoglobin levels in sickle cell disease and normal individuals are partially controlled by an X-linked gene located at Xp22.2. *Blood* 1992;80:816–824.

614. Craig JE, Rochette J, Fisher CA, et al. Haemoglobin switch: dissecting the loci controlling fetal haemoglobin production on chromosomes 11p and 6q by the regressive approach. *Nat Genet* 1996;12:58–64.

615. Craig JE, Rochette J, Sampietro M, et al. Genetic heterogeneity in heterocellular hereditary persistence of fetal hemoglobin. *Blood* 1997;90:428–434.

616. Dresner Pollack R, Rachmilewitz E, Blumenfeld A, et al. Bone mineral metabolism in adults with beta thalassemia major and intermedia. *Br J Haematol* 2000;111:902–907.

617. Galanello R, Perseu L, Melis MA, et al. Hyperbilirubinaemia in heterozygous beta-thalassaemia is related to co-inherited Gilbert's syndrome. *Br J Haematol* 1997;99:433–436.

618. Sampietro M, Lupica L, Perrero L, et al. The expression of uridine diphosphate glucuronosyltransferase gene is a major determinant of bilirubin level in heterozygous β-thalassaemia and in glucose-6-phosphate dehydrogenase deficiency. *Br J Haematol* 1997;99:437–439.

619. Merryweather-Clarke AT, Pointon JJ, Shearman JD, et al. Global prevalence of putative haemochromatosis mutations. *J Med Genet* 1997;34:275–278.

620. Rees DC, Singh BM, Luo LY, et al. Nontransfusional iron overload in thalassemia: association with hereditary hemochromatosis. *Ann N Y Acad Sci* 1998;850:490–494.

621. Andrews NC. Iron homeostasis: insights from genetics and animal models. *Nat Rev Genet* 2000;1:208–217.

622. Rees DC, et al. Genetic influences on bone disease in thalassemia. *Blood* 1998;2:S532a.

623. Wonke B. Annotation: bone disease in β-thalassaemia major. *Br J Haematol* 1998;103:897–901.

624. Perrotta S, Cappellini MD, Bertoldo F, et al. Osteoporosis in beta-thalassaemia major patients: analysis of the genetic background. *Br J Haematol* 2000;111:461–466.

625. Nathan DG, Gunn RB. Thalassemia: the consequences of unbalanced hemoglobin synthesis. *Am J Med* 1966;41:815–830.

626. Fessa P. Inclusions of hemoglobin in erythroblasts and erythrocytes of thalassemia. *Blood* 1963;21:21.

627. Kaplan E, Zuelzer WW. Erythrocyte survival studies in childhood, II: studies in Mediterranean anemia. *J Lab Clin Med* 1950;36:517–523.

628. Sturgeon P, Finch CA. Erythrokinetics in Cooley's anemia. *Blood* 1957;12:64–73.

629. Blendis LM, Modell CB, Bowdler AJ, et al. Some effects of splenectomy in thalassaemia major. *Br J Haematol* 1974;28:77–87.

630. Erlandson ME, Schulman I, Stern G, et al. Studies of congenital hemolytic syndromes, I: rates of destruction and production of erythrocytes in thalassemia. *Pediatrics* 1958;22:910–922.

631. Gallo E, Massaro P, Miniero R, et al. The importance of the genetic picture and globin synthesis in determining the clinical and haematological features of thalassaemia intermedia. *Br J Haematol* 1979;41:211–221.

632. Nathan DG, Stossel TB, Gunn RB, et al. Influence of hemoglobin precipitation on erythrocyte metabolism in alpha and beta thalassemia. *J Clin Invest* 1969;48:33–41.

633. Crosby WH, Akeroyd JH. The limit of hemoglobin synthesis in hereditary hemolytic anemia. *Am J Med* 1952;13:273.

634. Finch CA, Deubelbeiss K, Cook JD, et al. Ferrokinetics in man. *Medicine (Baltimore)* 1970;49:17–53.

635. Cavill I, Ricketts C, Jacobs A, et al. Erythropoiesis and the effect of transfusion in homozygous beta-thalassemia. *N Engl J Med* 1978;298:776–778.

636. Yamak B, Ozsoylu S. Haptoglobin in thalassemia. *Acta Haematol* 1969;42:176.

637. Cutillo S, Meloni T. Serum concentrations of haptoglobin and hemopexin in favism and thalassemia. *Acta Haematol* 1974;52:65.

638. Crosby WH, Dameshek W. The significance of hemoglobinuria and associated hemosiderinuria, with particular reference to various types of hemolytic anemia. *J Lab Clin Med* 1951;38:829.

639. Fessas P, Loukopoulos D. The β thalassaemias. *Clin Haematol* 1974;3:411–435.

640. Sturgeon P, Chen LPL, Bergren WR. Free erythrocyte porphyrins in thalassemia: preliminary observation. In: *6th International Congress of the International Society of Hematology.* New York: Grune & Stratton, 1958.

641. Giblett ER, Crookston MC. Agglutinability of red cells by anti-i in patients with thalassemia major and other haematological disorders. *Nature* 1964;201:1138.

642. Hillman RS, Giblett ER. Red cell membrane alteration associated with marrow stress. *J Clin Invest* 1965;10:1730.

643. Vecchio F. Sulla resistenza della emoglobina alla denaturazione alcalina in alcune sindromi emopatiche. *Pediatria* 1946;54:545.

644. Weatherall DJ, Clegg JB, Na-Nakorn S, et al. The pattern of disordered haemoglobin synthesis in homozygous and heterozygous β-thalassaemia. *Br J Haematol* 1969;16:251–267.

645. Wood WG. Increased HbF in adult life. *Baillieres Clin Haematol* 1993;6:177–213.

646. Stamatoyannopoulos G, Perlmutter RM, Marjerus PW, et al. *Molecular basis of blood diseases.* Philadelphia: WB Saunders, 1999.

647. Thein SL, Sampietro M, Rohde K, et al. Detection of a major gene for heterocellular HPFH after accounting for genetic modifiers. *Am J Hum Genet* 1994;54:214–228.

648. Chang YC, Smith KD, Moore RD, et al. An analysis of fetal hemoglobin variation in sickle cell disease: the relative contributions of the X-linked factor, β-globin haplotypes, α-globin gene number, gender and age. *Blood* 1995;85:1111–1117.

649. Kattamis C, Ladis V, Metaxatou-Mavromati A. Hemoglobins F and A₂ in Greek patients with homozygous β and β/δβ thalassemia. In: Schmidt RM, ed. *Abnormal haemoglobins and thalassaemia: diagnostic aspects.* New York: Academic Press, 1975:209–228.

650. Mitchiner JW, Thompson RB, Huisman THJ. Foetal haemoglobin synthesis in some haemoglobinopathies. *Lancet* 1961;i:1169.

651. Shepard MK, Weatherall DJ, Conley CL. Semi-quantitative estimation of the distribution of fetal hemoglobin in red cell populations. *Bull Johns Hopkins Hosp* 1962;110:293.

652. Huisman TH, Schroeder WA, Efremov GD, et al. The present status of the heterogeneity of fetal hemoglobin in beta-thalassemia: an attempt to unify some observations in thalassemia and related conditions. *Ann N Y Acad Sci* 1974;232:107–124.

653. Steinberg MH, Adams JG III. Hemoglobin A₂: origin, evolution and aftermath. *Blood* 1991;78:2165–2177.

654. Heywood JD, Karon M, Weissman S. Asymmetrical incorporation of amino acids into the alpha and beta chains of hemoglobin synthesized in thalassemia reticulocytes. *J Lab Clin Med* 1965;66:476.

655. Bank A, Marks PA. Excess α chain synthesis relative to β chain synthesis in thalassaemia major and minor. *Nature* 1966;212:1198–1200.

656. Bargellesi A, Pontremoli S, Conconi F. Absence of beta globin synthesis and excess alpha globin synthesis in homozygous β thalassemia. *Eur J Biochem* 1967;1:73–79.

657. Modell CB, Latter A, Steadman JH, et al. Haemoglobin synthesis in beta-thalassaemia. *Br J Haematol* 1969;17:485–501.

658. Bianco I, Graziani B, Carboni C. Genetic patterns in thalassemia intermedia (constitutional microcytic anemia): familial, hematologic and biosynthetic studies. *Hum Hered* 1977;27:257.

659. Weatherall DJ, Clegg JB. Disorders globin synthesis in thalassemia. *Ann N Y Acad Sci* 1969;165:242–252.

660. Wickramasinghe SN. The morphology and kinetics of erythropoiesis in homozygous β-thalassaemia. *Congenital disorders of erythropoiesis.* North Holland, Amsterdam: Ciba Foundation Symposium, 1976:221–237.

661. Yuan J, Angelucci E, Lucarelli G, et al. Accelerated programmed cell death (apoptosis) in erythroid precursors of patients with severe beta-thalassemia (Cooley's anemia). *Blood* 1993;82:374–377.

662. Schrier SL. Thalassemia: pathophysiology of red cell changes. *Annu Rev Med* 1994;45:211–218.

663. Schrier SL. Pathobiology of thalassemic erythrocytes. *Curr Opin Hematol* 1997;4:75–78.

664. Sorensen S, Rubin E, Polster H, et al. The role of membrane skeletal-associated alpha-globin in the pathophysiology of beta-thalassemia. *Blood* 1990;75:1333–1336.

665. Shinar E, Rachmilewitz EA. Haemoglobinopathies and red cell membrane function. *Clin Haematol* 1993;6:357–369.

666. Grinberg LN, Rachmilewitz EA. Oxidative stress in beta-thalassemic red blood cells and potential use of antioxidants. In: *Sickle cell disease and thalassemia: new trends in therapy.* Colloque INSERN/John Libby Eurotext Ltd., 1995:519–524.

667. Shalev O, Shinar E, Lux SE. Isolated beta-globin chains reproduce, in normal red cell membranes, the defective binding of spectrin to alpha-thalassaemic membranes. *Br J Haematol* 1996;94:273–278.

668. Shinar E, Shalev O, Rachmilewitz EA, et al. Erythrocyte membrane skeleton abnormalities in severe beta-thalassemia. *Blood* 1987;70:158–164.

669. Shinar E, Rachmilewitz EA. Oxidative denaturation of red blood cells in thalassemia. *Semin Hematol* 1990;27:70–82.

670. Lux SE, Palek J. Disorders of red cell membrane. In: Handin RI, Lux SE, Stossel TP, eds. *Blood: principles and practice of hematology.* Philadelphia: JB Lippincott, 1995:1701–1818.

671. Dore F, Bonfigli S, Gaviano E, et al. Serum erythropoietin levels in thalassemia intermedia. *Ann Hematol* 1993;67:183–186.

672. Camaschella C, Gonella S, Calabrese R, et al. Serum erythropoietin and circulating transferrin receptor in thalassemia intermedia patients with heterogeneous genotypes. *Haematologica* 1996;81:397–403.

673. Prankerd TAJ. The spleen and anaemia. *BMJ* 1963;ii:517–524.

674. Smith CH, Sisson TRC, Floyd WHJ, et al. Serum iron and iron binding capacity of the serum in children with severe Mediterranean (Cooley's) anemia. *Pediatrics* 1950;5:799.

675. Hershko C, Graham G, Bates CW, et al. Non-specific serum iron in thalassemia: an abnormal serum iron fraction of potential toxicity. *Br J Haematol* 1978;40:255–263.

676. Hershko C, Link G, Cabantchik I. Pathophysiology of iron overload. *Ann N Y Acad Sci* 1998;850:191–201.

677. Breuer W, Ermers MJ, Pootrakul P, et al. Desferrioxamine-chelatable iron (DCI), a component of serum non-transferrin-bound iron (NTBI) used for assessing iron chelation therapy. *Transfus Sci* 2000;23:241–242.

678. Breuer W, Hershko C, Cabantchik ZI. The importance of non-transferrin bound iron in disorders of iron metabolism. *Transfus Sci* 2000;23:185–192.

679. Breuer W, Ermers MJ, Pootrakul P, et al. Desferrioxamine-chelatable iron, a component of serum non-transferrin-bound iron, used for assessing chelation therapy. *Blood* 2001;97:792–798.

680. Bannerman RM. Iron absorption in thalassaemia. *Br J Haematol* 1964;10:490.

681. Shahid MJ, Abu Haydar N. Absorption of inorganic iron in thalassaemia. *Br J Haematol* 1967;13:713.

682. Necheles TF, Allen DM, Finkel HE. *Clinical disorders of hemoglobin structure and synthesis.* New York: Appleton Century Crofts, 1969.

683. Erlandson ME, Walden B, Stern G, et al. Studies on congenital hemolytic syndromes, IV: gastrointestinal absorption of iron. *Blood* 1962;19:359.

684. Cooley TB, Lee P. A series of cases of splenomegaly in children with anemia and peculiar bone changes. *Trans Am Pediatr Soc* 1925;37:29.

685. Rietti F. Ittero emolitico primitivo. *Atti Acad Sci Med Nar Ferrara* 1925;2:14.

686. Micheli F, Penati F, Momigliano LG. Ulteriori richerche sulla anemia ipocromica splenomegalica con poichilocitosi. *Haematologica* 1935;16[Suppl]:10.

687. Modell B, Bedoukas V. *The clinical approach to thalassemia.* Orlando: Grune & Stratton, 1984.

688. Olivieri NF. The beta-thalassemias. *N Engl J Med* 1999;341:99–109.

689. Rioja L, Girot R, Garabedian M, et al. Bone disease in children with homozygous beta-thalassemia. *Bone Miner* 1990;8:69–86.

690. Orvieto R, Leichter I, Rachmilewitz EA, et al. Bone density, mineral content, and cortical index in patients with thalassemia major and the correlation to their bone fractures, blood transfusions, and treatment with desferrioxamine. *Calcif Tissue Int* 1992;50:397–399.

691. Vichinsky EP. The morbidity of bone disease in thalassemia. *Ann N Y Acad Sci* 1998;850:344–348.

692. Voght EC, Diamond LK. Congenital anemias, roentgenologically considered. *Am J Roentgenol* 1930;23:625.

693. Baker DH. Roentgen manifestations of Cooley's anemia. *Ann N Y Acad Sci* 1964;119:641–661.

694. Middlemis JH, Raper AB. Skeletal changes in the haemoglobinopathies. *J Bone Joint Surg* 1966;48:693.

695. Cammisa M, Sabella G. Clinico-radiological considerations on the pathogenesis of bone changes in thalassemia major. *Nunt Radiol* 1967;33:77–101.

696. Michelson J, Cohen A. Incidence and treatment of fractures in thalassemia. *J Orthop Trauma* 1988;2:29–32.

697. Gabutti V, Piga A. Results of long-term iron-chelating therapy. *Acta Haematol* 1996;95:26–36.

698. Olivieri NF, Brittenham GM. Iron-chelating therapy and the treatment of thalassemia. *Blood* 1997;89:739–761.

699. Lichtman HC, Watson RJ, Feldman F, et al. Studies on thalassemia, I: an extracorpuscular defect in thalassemia major; II: the effects of splenectomy in thalassemia major with an associated acquired hemolytic anemia. *J Clin Invest* 1953;32:1229–1235.

700. Smith CH, Schulman I, Ando RE, et al. Studies in Mediterranean (Cooley's) anemia, I: clinical and hematologic aspects of splenectomy with special reference to fetal hemoglobin synthesis. *Blood* 1955;10:582–599.

701. Reemsta K, Elliot RH. Splenectomy in Mediterranean anemia: an evaluation of long-term results. *Ann Surg* 1956;144:999–1007.

702. O'Brien RT, Pearson HA, Spencer RP. Transfusion-induced decrease in spleen size in thalassemia major: documentation by radioisotopic scan. *J Pediatr* 1972;81:105–107.

703. Modell B. Management of thalassaemia major. *Br Med Bull* 1976;32:270–276.

704. Risdon RA, Flynn DM, Barry M. The relation between liver iron concentration and liver damage in transfusional iron overload in thalassaemia and the effect of chelation therapy. *Gut* 1973;14:421.

705. Hershko C, Weatherall DJ. Iron-chelating therapy. *Crit Rev Clin Lab Sci* 1988;26:303–345.

706. Link G, Tirosh R, Pinson A, et al. Role of iron in the potentiation of anthracycline toxicity: identification of heart cell mitochondria as the site of iron-anthracycline interaction. *J Lab Clin Med* 1996;127:272–278.

707. Pippard MJ, Callender ST, Warner GT, et al. Iron absorption and loading in beta-thalassaemia intermedia. *Lancet* 1979;2:819–821.

708. Pootrakul P, Kitcharoen K, Yansukon P, et al. The effect of erythroid hyperplasia on iron balance. *Blood* 1988;71:1124–1129.

709. Whipple GH, Bradford WL. Mediterranean disease—thalassemia (erythroblastic anemia of Cooley). *J Pediatr* 1936;9:279–311.

710. Ellis JT, Schulman I, Smith CH. Generalized siderosis with fibrosis of liver and pancreas in Cooley's (Mediterranean) anemia. *Am J Pathol* 1954;30:287–309.

711. Witzleben CL, Wyatt JP. The effect of long survival on the pathology of thalassaemia major. *J Pathol Bacteriol* 1961;82:1–12.

712. Masera G, Jean G, Gazzola G, et al. Role of chronic hepatitis in development of thalassaemic liver disease. *Arch Dis Child* 1976;51:680–685.

713. Iancu TC, Landing BH, Neustein HB. Pathogenetic mechanisms in hepatic cirrhosis of thalassemia major: light and electron microscopic studies. *Pathol Annu* 1977;12:171–200.

714. Iancu TC, Neustein HB, Landing BH. The liver in thalassaemia major: ultrastructural observations. *Ciba Found Symp* 1977;51:293–307.

715. Masera G, Jean G, Conter V, et al. Sequential study of liver biopsy in thalassaemia. *Arch Dis Child* 1980;55:800–802.

716. De Virgiliis S, Cossu P, Sanna G, et al. Iron chelation in transfusion-dependent thalassemia with chronic hepatitis. *Acta Haematol* 1982;67:49–56.

717. Jean G, Terzoli S, Mauri R, et al. Cirrhosis associated with multiple transfusions in thalassaemia. *Arch Dis Child* 1984;59:67–70.

718. Angelucci E, Baronciani D, Lucarelli G, et al. Needle liver biopsy in thalassaemia: analyses of diagnostic accuracy and safety in 1184 consecutive biopsies. *Br J Haematol* 1995;89:757–761.

719. Thakerngpol K, Fucharoen S, Boonyaphipat P, et al. Liver injury due to iron overload in thalassemia: histopathologic and ultrastructural studies. *Biometals* 1996;9:177–183.

720. Letsky EA, Miller F, Worwood M, et al. Serum ferritin in children with thalassaemia regularly transfused. *J Clin Pathol* 1974;27:652–655.

721. Pippard MJ, Callender ST, Letsky EA, et al. Prevention of iron loading in transfusion-dependent thalassaemia. *Lancet* 1978;i:1178–1180.

722. Fiorillo A, Farina V, D'Amore R, et al. Longitudinal assessment of cardiac status by echocardiographic evaluation of left ventricular diastolic function in thalassaemic children. *Acta Paediatr* 2000;89:436–441.

723. Engle MA. Cardiac involvement in Cooley's anemia. *Ann N Y Acad Sci* 1964;119:694–702.

724. Engle MA, Erlandson M, Smith CH. Late cardiac complications of chronic severe refractory anaemia with haemochromatosis. *Circulation* 1964;30:698.

725. Kremastinos DT, Tiniakos G, Theodorakis GN, et al. Myocarditis in beta-thalassemia major: a cause of heart failure. *Circulation* 1996;91:66–71.

726. Grisaru D, Rachmilewitz EA, Mosseri M, et al. Cardiopulmonary assessment in beta-thalassemia major. *Chest* 1990;98:1138–1142.

727. Ehlers KH, Levin AR, Markenson AL, et al. Longitudinal study of cardiac function in thalassemia major. *Ann N Y Acad Sci* 1980;344:397–404.

728. Zurlo MF, De Stefano P, Borgna-Pignatti C, et al. Survival and causes of death in thalassaemia major. *Lancet* 1989;ii:27–30.

729. Smith CH, Erlandson ME, Stern G, et al. The role of splenectomy in the management of thalassemia. *Blood* 1960;15:197–211.

730. Orsini A, Louchet E, Raybaud C, et al. Les pericardites de la maladie de Cooley. *Pediatrie* 1970;15:831–842.

731. Orsini A, Louchet E, Raybaud C, et al. [Pericarditis in Cooley's disease]. *Pediatrie* 1970;25:831–842.

732. Wasi P. Adverse effects of splenectomy. *J Med Assoc Thai* 1972;55:1.

733. Brittenham GM, Griffith PM, Nienhuis AW, et al. Efficacy of deferoxamine in preventing complications of iron overload in patients with thalassemia major. *N Engl J Med* 1994;331:567–573.

734. Jessup M, Manno CS. Diagnosis and management of iron-induced heart disease in Cooley's anemia. *Ann N Y Acad Sci* 1998;850:242–250.

735. Arnett EN, Nienhuis AW, Henry WL, et al. Massive myocardial hemosiderosis: a structure-function conference at the National Heart and Lung Institute. *Am Heart J* 1975;90:777–787.

736. Schellhammer PF, Engle MA, Hagstrom JW. Histochemical studies of the myocardium and conduction system in acquired iron-storage disease. *Circulation* 1967;35:631–637.

737. Buja LM, Roberts WC. Iron in the heart: etiology and clinical significance. *Am J Med* 1971;51:209–221.

738. Howell J, Wyatt JP. Development of pigmentary cirrhosis in Cooley's anaemia. *Arch Pathol* 1953;55:423–431.

739. Short EM, Winkle RA, Billingham ME. Myocardial involvement in idio-

pathic hemochromatosis: morphologic and clinical improvement following venisection. *Am J Med* 1981;70:1275–1279.

740. Lombardo T, Tamburino C, Bartoloni G, et al. Cardiac iron overload in thalassemic patients: an endomyocardial biopsy study. *Ann Hematol* 1995;71:135–141.

741. Kyriacou K, Al Quobaili F, Pavlou E, et al. Molecular characterization of beta-thalassemia in Syria. *Hemoglobin* 2000;24:1–13.

742. Spirito P, Lupi G, Melevendi C, et al. Restrictive diastolic abnormalities identified by Doppler echocardiography in patients with thalassemia major. *Circulation* 1990;82:88–94.

743. Liu P, Olivieri N. Iron overload cardiomyopathies: new insights into an old disease. *Cardiovasc Drugs Ther* 1994;8:101–110.

744. Kuryshev YA, Brittenham GM, Fujioka H, et al. Decreased sodium and increased transient outward potassium currents in iron-loaded cardiac myocytes: implications for the arrhythmogenesis of human siderotic heart disease. *Circulation* 1999;100:675–683.

745. Economou-Petersen E, Aessopos A, Kladi A, et al. Apolipoprotein E epsilon4 allele as a genetic risk factor for left ventricular failure in homozygous beta-thalassemia. *Blood* 1998;92:3455–3459.

746. Kremastinos DT, Flevari P, Spyropoulou M, et al. Association of heart failure in homozygous beta-thalassemia with the major histocompatibility complex. *Circulation* 1999;100:2074–2078.

747. Koren A, Garty I, Antonelli D, et al. Right ventricular cardiac dysfunction in β-thalassemia major. *Am J Dis Child* 1987;141:93–96.

748. Keens TG, O'Neal MH, Ortega JA, et al. Pulmonary function abnormalities in thalassemia patients on a hypertransfusion program. *Pediatrics* 1980;65:1013–1017.

749. Hoyt RW, Scarpa N, Wilmott RW, et al. Pulmonary function abnormalities in homozygous β-thalassemia. *J Pediatr* 1986;109:452–455.

750. Santamaria F, Villa MP, Werner B, et al. The effect of transfusion on pulmonary function in patients with thalassemia major. *Pediatr Pulmonol* 1994;18:139–143.

751. Cooper DM, Mansell AL, Weiner MA, et al. Low lung capacity and hypoxemia in children with thalassemia. *Am Rev Respir Dis* 1980;121:639–646.

752. Grant GP, Graziano JH, Seaman C, et al. Cardiorespiratory response to exercise in patients with thalassemia major. *Am Rev Respir Dis* 1987;136:92–97.

753. Bacalo A, Kivity S, Heno N, et al. Blood transfusion and lung function in children with thalassemia major. *Chest* 1992;101:362–370.

754. Factor JM, Pottipati SR, Rappaport I, et al. Pulmonary function abnormalities in thalassemia major and the role of iron overload. *Am J Respir Crit Care Med* 1994;149:1570–1574.

755. Kanj N, Shamseddine A, Gharzeddine W, et al. Relation of ferritin levels to pulmonary function in patients with thalassemia major and the acute effects of transfusion. *Eur J Haematol* 2000;64:396–400.

756. Sonakul D, Pacharee P, Thakerngpol K. Pathologic findings in 76 autopsy cases of thalassemia. *Birth Defects: Original Articles Series* 1988;23:157–176.

757. Filosa A, Esposito V, Meoli I, et al. Evidence of lymphocyte alveolitis by bronchoalveolar lavage in thalassemic patients with pulmonary dysfunction. *Acta Haematol* 2000;103:90–95.

758. Tai DY, Wang YT, Lou J, et al. Lungs in thalassaemia major patients receiving regular transfusion. *Eur Respir J* 1996;9:1389–1394.

759. Hoeper MM, Niedermeyer J, Hoffmeyer F, et al. Pulmonary hypertension after splenectomy. *Ann Intern Med* 1999;130:506–509.

760. Wasi P, Fucharoen S, Youngchaiyud P, et al. Hypoxemia in thalassemia. *Birth Defects: Original Articles Series* 1982;18:213–217.

761. Freedman MH, Grisaru D, Olivieri N, et al. Pulmonary syndrome in patients with thalassemia major receiving intravenous deferoxamine infusions. *Am J Dis Child* 1990;144:565–569.

762. Michaeli J, Mittelman M, Grisaru D, et al. Thromboembolic complications in beta thalassemia major. *Acta Haematol* 1992;87:71–74.

763. Borgna Pignatti C, Carnelli V, Caruso V, et al. Thromboembolic events in beta thalassemia major: an Italian multicenter study. *Acta Haematol* 1998;99:76–79.

764. Moratelli S, De Sanctis V, Gemmati D, et al. Thrombotic risk in thalassemic patients. *J Pediatr Endocrinol Metab* 1998;11:915–921.

765. Eldor A, Durst R, Hy-Am E, et al. A chronic hypercoagulable state in patients with β-thalassaemia major is already present in childhood. *Br J Haematol* 1999;107:739–746.

766. Giordano P, Galli M, Del Vecchio GC, et al. Lupus anticoagulant, anticardiolipin antibodies and hepatitis C virus infection in thalassaemia. *Br J Haematol* 1998;102:903–906.

767. Gutteridge JM, Halliwell B. Iron toxicity and oxygen radicals. *Baillieres Clin Haematol* 1989;2:195–256.

768. Tsukamoto H, Horne W, Kamimura S, et al. Experimental liver cirrhosis induced by alcohol and iron. *J Clin Invest* 1995;96:620–630.

769. Iancu TC, Neustein HB. Ferritin in human liver cells of homozygous beta-thalassaemia: ultrastructural observations. *Br J Haematol* 1977;37:527–535.

770. Parkes JG, Randell EW, Olivieri NF, et al. Modulation by iron loading and chelation of the uptake of non-transferrin-bound iron by human liver cells. *Biochim Biophys Acta* 1995;1243:373–380.

771. Frumin AM, Miller EE. Exogenous hemochromatosis in sickle cell anemia. *Am J Pathol* 1952;24:130–132.

772. Wollstein M, Kreidel KV. Familial hemolytic anemia of childhood—von Jaksch. *Am J Dis Child* 1930;39:115–130.

773. Koch LA, Shapiro B. Erythroblastic anemia, review of cases reported showing roentgenographic changes in bones and five additional cases. *Am J Dis Child* 1932;44:318–335.

774. Panizon F, Vullo C. Sulla envoluzione della siderosi e fibrosi epatica nella malattia di Cooley: studio bioptico su 20 casi. *Acta Paediat Lat* 1952;10:71.

775. Cooley TB, Witer ER, Lee P. Anemia in children with splenomegaly and peculiar changes in bones: report of cases. *Am J Dis Child* 1927;34:347.

776. Baty JM, Blackfan KD, Diamond LK. Blood studies in infants and in children, I: erythroblastic anemia; a clinical and pathologic study. *Am J Dis Child* 1932;43:667–704.

777. Risdon AR, Barry M, Fynn DM. Transfusional iron overload: the relationship between tissue iron concentration and hepatic fibrosis in thalassaemia. *J Pathol* 1975;116:83–95.

778. Aldouri MA, Wonke B, Hoffbrand AV, et al. Iron state and hepatic disease in patients with thalassaemia major, treated with long term subcutaneous desferrioxamine. *J Clin Pathol* 1987;40:1353–1359.

779. Maurer HS, Lloyd-Still JD, Ingrisano C, et al. A prospective evaluation of iron chelation therapy in children with severe β-thalassemia: a six-year study. *Am J Dis Child* 1988;142:287–292.

780. Barry M. Iron and the liver. *Gut* 1974;15:324–334.

781. De Virgiliis S, Fiorelli G, Fargion S, et al. Chronic liver disease in transfusion-dependent thalassaemia: hepatitis B virus marker studies. *J Clin Pathol* 1980;33:949–953.

782. Clemente MG, Congia M, Lai ME, et al. Effect of iron overload on the response to recombinant interferon-alfa treatment in transfusion-dependent patients with thalassemia major and chronic hepatitis C. *J Pediatr* 1994;125:123–128.

783. Olynyk JK, Bacon BR. Hepatitis C: recent advances in understanding and management. *Postgrad Med J* 1995;98:79–81.

784. Rubin RB, Barton AL, Banner BF, et al. Iron and chronic viral hepatitis: emerging evidence for an important interaction. *Dig Dis* 1995;13:223–238.

785. Erlandson M, Brilliant R, Smith CH. Comparison of sixty-six patients with thalassemia major and thirteen patients with thalassemia intermedia: including evaluations of growth, development, maturation, and prognosis. *Ann N Y Acad Sci* 1964;119:727–735.

786. Fink H. Transfusion hemachromatosis in Cooley's anemia. *Ann N Y Acad Sci* 1964;119:680.

787. Bannerman RM, Keusch G, Kreimer-Birnbaum M, et al. Thalassemia intermedia, with iron overload, cardiac failure, diabetes mellitus, hypopituitarism and porphyrinuria. *Am J Med* 1967;42:476–486.

788. Kuo B, Zaino E, Roginsky MS. Endocrine function in thalassemia. *J Clin Endocrinol Metab* 1968;28:805–808.

789. Toccafondi R, Maioli M, Meloni T. Plasma insulin response to oral carbohydrate in Cooley's anemia. *Riv Clin Med* 1970;70:96–101.

790. Toccafondi R, Maioli M, Meloni T. The plasma HGH and 11-OHCS response to insulin induced hypoglycaemia in children affected by thalassaemia major. *Riv Clin Med* 1970;70:102–109.

791. Canale VC, Steinherz P, New M, et al. Endocrine function in thalassemia major. *Ann N Y Acad Sci* 1974;232:333–345.

792. Lassman MN, O'Brien RT, Pearson HA, et al. Endocrine evaluation in thalassemia major. *Ann N Y Acad Sci* 1974;232:226–237.

793. Lassman MN, Genel M, Wise JK, et al. Carbohydrate homeostasis and pancreatic islet cell function in thalassemia. *Blood* 1974;80:65–69.

794. Flynn DM, Fairney A, Jackson D, et al. Hormonal changes in thalassemia major. *Arch Dis Child* 1976;51:828–836.

795. McIntosh N. Endocrinopathy in thalassaemia major. *Arch Dis Child* 1976;51:195–201.

796. Anoussakis C, Alexiou D, Abatxis D, et al. Endocrinological investigation of pituitary gonadal axis in thalassaemia major. *Acta Paediatr Scand* 1977;66:49–51.

797. Costin G, Kogut MD, Hyman C, et al. Carbohydrate metabolism and pancreatic islet-cell function in thalassemia major. *Diabetes* 1977;26:230–240.

798. Costin G, Kogut MD, Hyman CB, et al. Endocrine abnormalities in thalassemia major. *Am J Dis Child* 1979;133:497–502.

799. Kletsky OA, Costin G, Marrs RP, et al. Gonadotrophin insufficiency in patients with thalassemia major. *J Clin Endocrinol Metab* 1979;48:901–905.

800. Borgna-Pignatti C, De Stefano P, Zonta L, et al. Growth and sexual maturation in thalassemia major. *J Pediatr* 1985;106:150–155.

801. De Sanctis V, Vullo C, Katz M, et al. Endocrine complications in thalassaemia major. *Prog Clin Biol Res* 1989;309:77–83.

802. Vullo C, De Sanctis V, Katz M, et al. Endocrine abnormalities in thalassemia. *Ann N Y Acad Sci* 1990;612:293–310.

803. Perignon F, Brauner R, Souberbielle JC, et al. Growth and endocrine function in thalassemia major. *Arch Fr Pediatr* 1993;50:657–663.

804. El-Hazmi MA, Warsy AS, Al Fawaz I. Iron-endocrine pattern in patients with beta-thalassaemia. *J Trop Pediatr* 1994;40:219–224.

805. Grundy RG, Woods KA, Savage MO, et al. Relationship of endocrinopathy to iron chelation status in young patients with thalassaemia major. *Arch Dis Child* 1994;71:128–132.

806. Italian Working Group on Endocrine Complications in Non-endocrine Diseases. Multicentre study on prevalence of endocrine complications in thalassaemia major. *Clin Endocrinol (Oxf)* 1995;42:581–586.

807. Kwan EY, Lee AC, Li AM, et al. A cross-sectional study of growth, puberty and endocrine function in patients with thalassaemia major in Hong Kong. *J Paediatr Child Health* 1995;31:83–87.

808. Jensen CE, Tuck SM, Old J, et al. Incidence of endocrine complications and clinical disease severity related to genotype analysis and iron overload in patients with β-thalassaemia. *Eur J Haematol* 1997;59:76–81.

809. Low LC. Growth, puberty and endocrine function in β-thalassaemia major. *J Pediatr Endocrinol Metab* 1997;10:175–184.

810. Kattamis C, Liakopoulou T, Kattamis A. Growth and development in children with thalassemia major. *Acta Paediatr Scand* 1990;366:111.
811. Logothetis J, Constantoulakis M, Economidou J, et al. Thalassemia major (homozygous beta-thalassemia): a survey of 138 cases with emphasis on neurologic and muscular aspects. *Neurology* 1972;22:294–304.
812. Constantoulakis M, Panagopoulos G, Augoustaki O. Stature and longitudinal growth in thalassemia major: a study of 229 Greek patients. *Clin Pediatr* 1975;14:355–362.
813. Beard ME, Necheles TF, Allen DM. Clinical experience with intensive transfusion therapy in Cooley's anemia. *Ann N Y Acad Sci* 1969;165:415–422.
814. De Sanctis V, Katz M, Vullo C, et al. Effect of different treatment regimes on linear growth and final height in β-thalassaemia major. *Clin Endocrinol (Oxf)* 1994;40:791–798.
815. Wang C, Tso SC, Todd D. Hypogonadotropic hypogonadism in severe beta-thalassemia: effect of chelation and pulsatile gonadotropin-releasing hormone therapy. *J Clin Endocrinol Metab* 1989;68:511–516.
816. Landau H, Matoth I, Landau-Cordova Z, et al. Cross-sectional and longitudinal study of the pituitary-thyroid axis in patients with thalassaemia major. *Clin Endocrinol (Oxf)* 1993;38:55–61.
817. Saenger P, Schwartz E, Markenson AL, et al. Depressed serum somatomedin activity in beta-thalassemia. *J Pediatr* 1980;96:214–218.
818. Herington AC, Werthe GA, Matthews RN, et al. Studies on the possible mechanism for deficiency of nonsuppressible insulin-like activity in thalassemia major. *J Clin Endocrinol Metab* 1981;52:393–398.
819. Werther GA, Matthews RN, Burger HG, et al. Lack of response of nonsuppressible insulin-like activity to short term administration of human growth hormone in thalassemia major. *J Clin Endocrinol Metab* 1981;53:806–809.
820. Pintor C, Cella SG, Manso P, et al. Impaired growth hormone (GH) response to GH-releasing hormone in thalassemia major. *J Clin Endocrinol Metab* 1986;62:263–267.
821. Shehadeh N, Hazani A, Rudolf MC, et al. Neurosecretory dysfunction of growth hormone secretion in thalassemia major. *Acta Paediatr Scand* 1990;79:790–795.
822. Masala A, Meloni T, Gallisai D, et al. Endocrine functioning in multitransfused prepubertal patients with homozygous beta-thalassemia. *J Clin Endocrinol Metab* 1984;58:667–670.
823. Leger J, Girot R, Crosnier H, et al. Normal growth hormone (GH) response to GH-releasing hormone in children with thalassemia major before puberty: a possible age-related effect. *J Clin Endocrinol Metab* 1989;69:453–456.
824. Cavallo L, Gurrado R, Gallo F, et al. Growth deficiency in polytransfused beta-thalassaemia patients is not growth hormone dependent. *Clin Endocrinol (Oxf)* 1997;46:701–706.
825. Roth C, Pekrun A, Bartz M, et al. Short stature and failure of pubertal development in thalassaemia major: evidence for hypothalamic neurosecretory dysfunction of growth hormone secretion and defective pituitary gonadotropin secretion. *Eur J Pediatr* 1997;156:777–783.
826. Scacchi M, Damesi L, De Martin M, et al. Treatment with biosynthetic growth hormone of short thalassaemic patients with impaired growth hormone secretion. *Clin Endocrinol (Oxf)* 1991;35:335–339.
827. Low LC, Kwan EY, Lim YJ, et al. Growth hormone treatment of short Chinese children with beta-thalassaemia major without GH deficiency. *Clin Endocrinol (Oxf)* 1995;42:359–363.
828. Sklar CA, Lew LQ, Yoon DJ, et al. Adrenal function in thalassemia major following long-term treatment with multiple transfusions and chelation therapy: evidence for dissociation of cortisol and adrenal androgen secretion. *Am J Dis Child* 1987;141:327–330.
829. Arcasoy A, Cavdar A, Cin S, et al. Effects of zinc supplementation on linear growth in beta thalassemia (a new approach). *Am J Hematol* 1987;24:127–136.
830. Vassilopoulou-Sellin R, Oyedeji CO, Foster PL, et al. Haemoglobin as a direct inhibitor of cartilage growth *in vitro*. *Horm Metab Res* 1989;21:11.
831. Rodda CP, Reid ED, Johnson S, et al. Short stature in homozygous β-thalassaemia is due to disproportionate truncal shortening. *Clin Endocrinol (Oxf)* 1995;42:587–592.
832. Hatori M, Sparkman J, Teixeira CC, et al. Effects of deferoximine on chondrocyte alkaline phosphatase activity: proxidant role of deferoximine in thalassemia. *Calcif Tissue Int* 1995;57:229–236.
833. Olivieri NF, Basran RK, Talbot AL, et al. Abnormal growth in thalassemia major associated with deferoxamine-induced destruction of spinal cartilage and compromise of sitting height. *Blood* 1995;86:482a.
834. Filosa A, Di Maio S, Lamba M, et al. Bone age progression during five years of substitutive therapy for the induction of puberty in thalassemic girls: effects on height and sitting height. *J Pediatr Endocrinol Metab* 1999;12:525–530.
835. De Sanctis V, Vullo C, Katz M, et al. Hypothalamic-pituitary-gonadal axis in thalassemic patients with secondary amenorrhea. *Obstet Gynecol* 1988;72:643–647.
836. Chatterjee R, Katz M, Cox TF, et al. A prospective study of the hypothalamic-pituitary axis in thalassaemic patients who developed secondary amenorrhoea. *Clin Endocrinol (Oxf)* 1993;39:287–296.
837. Bergeron C, Kovacs K. Pituitary siderosis: a histologic, immunocytologic, and ultrastructural study. *Am J Pathol* 1978;93:295–309.
838. Chatterjee R, Katz M, Oatridge A, et al. Selective loss of anterior pituitary volume with severe pituitary-gonadal insufficiency in poorly compliant male thalassemic patients with pubertal arrest. *Ann N Y Acad Sci* 1998;850:479–482.
839. De Sanctis V, Vullo C, Katz M, et al. Gonadal function in patients with beta thalassaemia major. *J Clin Pathol* 1988;41:133–137.
840. Gulati R, Bhatia V, Agarwal SS. Early onset of endocrine abnormalities in beta-thalassemia major in a developing country. *J Pediatr Endocrinol Metab* 2000;13:651–656.
841. Chatterjee R, Katz M. Reversible hypogonadotrophic hypogonadism in sexually infantile male thalassaemic patients with transfusional iron overload. *Clin Endocrinol (Oxf)* 2000;53:33–42.
842. Bronspeigel-Weintrob N, Olivieri NF, Tyler NF, et al. Effect of age at the start of iron chelation therapy on gonadal function in β-thalassemia major. *N Engl J Med* 1990;323:713.
843. Seracchioli R, Porcu E, Colombi C, et al. Transfusion-dependent homozygous β-thalassaemia major: successful twin pregnancy following *in vitro* fertilization and tubal embryo transfer. *Hum Reprod* 1994;9:1964–1965.
844. Tampakoudis P, Tsatalas C, Mamopoulos M, et al. Transfusion-dependent homozygous beta-thalassaemia major: successful pregnancy in five cases. *Eur J Obstet Gynecol Reprod Biol* 1997;74:127–131.
845. Skordis N, Christou S, Koliou M, et al. Fertility in female patients with thalassemia. *J Pediatr Endocrinol Metab* 1998;11:935–943.
846. Tuck SM, Jensen CE, Wonke B, et al. Pregnancy management and outcomes in women with thalassemia major. *J Pediatr Endocrinol Metab* 1998;11:923–928.
847. Protonotariou AA, Tolis GJ. Reproductive health in female patients with beta-thalassemia major. *Ann N Y Acad Sci* 2000;900:119–124.
848. Pafumi C, Farina M, Pernicone G, et al. At term pregnancies in transfusion-dependent beta-thalassemic women. *Clin Exp Obstet Gynecol* 2000;27:185–187.
849. Pafumi C, Zizza G, Caruso S, et al. Pregnancy outcome of a transfusion-dependent thalassemic woman. *Ann Hematol* 2000;79:571–573.
850. Perniola R, Magliari F, Rosatelli MC, et al. High-risk pregnancy in beta-thalassemia major women: report of three cases. *Gynecol Obstet Invest* 2000;49:137–139.
851. Saudek CD, Hemm RM, Peterson CM. Abnormal glucose tolerance in beta-thalassemia major. *Metabolism* 1977;26:43–52.
852. Zuppinger K, Molinari B, Hirt A, et al. Increased risk of diabetes mellitus in beta-thalassemia major. *Hel Paediatr Acta* 1979;4:197–207.
853. Dandona P, Hussain MA, Varghese Z, et al. Insulin resistance and iron overload. *Ann Clin Biochem* 1983;20:77–79.
854. De Sanctis V, D'Ascola G, Wonke B. The development of diabetes mellitus and chronic liver disease in long term chelated β-thalassaemic patients. *Postgrad Med J* 1986;62:831–836.
855. De Sanctis V, Zurlo MG, Senesi E, et al. Insulin dependent diabetes in thalassaemia. *Arch Dis Child* 1988;63:58–62.
856. Merkel PA, Simonson DC, Amiel SA, et al. Insulin resistance and hyperinsulinemia in patients with thalassemia major treated by hypertransfusion. *N Engl J Med* 1988;318:809–814.
857. Dmochowski K, Finegood DT, Francombe W, et al. Factors determining glucose tolerance in patients with thalassemia major. *J Clin Endocrinol Metab* 1993;77:478–483.
858. Cavallo-Perin P, Pacini G, Cerutti F, et al. Insulin resistance and hyperinsulinemia in homozygous beta-thalassemia. *Metabolism* 1995;44:281–286.
859. Karahanyan E, Stoyaniva A, Moumdzhiev I, et al. Secondary diabetes in children with thalassaemia major (homozygous thalassemia). *Folia Med (Plovdiv)* 1994;35:29–34.
860. Soliman AT, el Banna N, alSalmi I, et al. Insulin and glucagon responses to provocation with glucose and arginine in prepubertal children with thalassemia major before and after long-term blood transfusion. *J Trop Pediatr* 1996;42:291–296.
861. Gullo L, Corcioni E, Brancati C, et al. Morphologic and functional evaluation of the exocrine pancreas in beta-thalassemia. *Pancreas* 1993;8:176–180.
862. Theochari M, Ioannidou D, Nounopoulos H, et al. Ultrasonography of the pancreas, as a function index, in children with beta-thalassemia. *J Pediatr Endocrinol Metab* 2000;13:303–306.
863. Sabato A, De Sanctis V, Atti G, et al. Primary hypothyroidism and the low T$_3$ syndrome in thalassemia major. *Arch Dis Child* 1983;58:120–127.
864. Magro S, Puzzonia P, Consarino C, et al. Hypothyroidism in patients with thalassemia syndromes. *Acta Haematol* 1990;84:72–76.
865. Alexandrides T, Georgopoulos N, Yarmenitis S, et al. Increased sensitivity to the inhibitory effect of excess iodide on thyroid function in patients with beta-thalassemia major and iron overload and the subsequent development of hypothyroidism. *Eur J Endocrinol* 2000;143:319–325.
866. Mariotti S, Loviselli A, Murenu S, et al. High prevalence of thyroid dysfunction in adult patients with beta-thalassemia major submitted to amiodarone treatment. *J Endocrinol Invest* 1999;22:55–63.
867. Gertner JM, Broadus AE, Anast CS, et al. Impaired parathyroid response to induced hypocalcemia in thalassemia major. *J Pediatr* 1979;95:210–213.
868. De Sanctis V, Vullo C, Bagni B, et al. Hypoparathyroidism in β-thalassemia major: clinical and laboratory observations in 24 patients. *Acta Haematol* 1992;88:105–108.
869. Gabriele OF. Hypoparathyroidism associate with thalassemia. *South Med J* 1971;64:115–116.
870. Oberklaid F, Seshadri R. Hypoparathyroidism and other endocrine dysfunction complicating thalassaemia major. *Med J Aust* 1975;1:304–306.
871. Pratico G, Di Gregorio F, Caltabiano L, et al. Calcium phosphate metabolism in thalassemia. *Pediatr Med Chir* 1998;20:265–268.
872. Banani SA, Omrani GH. Cortisol and adrenocorticotropic hormone response to surgical stress (splenectomy) in thalassemic patients. *Pediatr Surg Int* 2000;16:400–403.

873. Wolman IJ. Transfusion therapy in Cooley's anemia: growth and health as related to long-range hemoglobin levels, a progress report. *Ann N Y Acad Sci* 1964;119:736–747.

874. Herrick RT, Davis GL. Thalassemia major and non-union of pathologic fractures. *J La State Med Soc* 1975;127:341–347.

875. Tas I, Smith P, Cohen T. Metric and morphologic characteristics of the dentition in beta thalassaemia major in man. *Arch Oral Biol* 1976;21:583–586.

876. Hazell JW, Modell CB. E.N.T. complications in thalassaemia major. *J Laryngol Otol* 1976;90:877–881.

877. Johnston FE, Roseman JM. The effects of more frequent transfusions upon bone loss in thalassemia major. *Pediatr Res* 1967;1:479–483.

878. Piomelli S, Danoff SJ, Becker MH, et al. Prevention of bone malformations and cardiomegaly in Cooley's anemia by early hypertransfusion regimen. *Ann N Y Acad Sci* 1969;165:427–436.

879. Jensen CE, Tuck SM, Agnew JE, et al. High prevalence of low bone mass in thalassaemia major. *Br J Haematol* 1998;103:911–915.

880. Voskaridou E, Kyrtsonis MC, Terpos E, et al. Bone resorption is increased in young adults with thalassaemia major. *Br J Haematol* 2001;112:36–41.

881. Fabbri G, Petraglia F, Segre A, et al. Reduced spinal bone density in young women with amenorrhoea. *Eur J Obstet Gynecol Reprod Biol* 1991;41:117–122.

882. Anapliotou ML, Kastanias IT, Psara P, et al. The contribution of hypogonadism to the development of osteoporosis in thalassaemia major: new therapeutic approaches. *Clin Endocrinol (Oxf)* 1995;42:279–287.

883. Jensen CE, Tuck SM, Agnew JE, et al. High prevalence of low bone mass in thalassaemia major. *Br J Haematol* 1998;103:911–915.

884. Hanslip JI, Prescott E, Lalloz M, et al. The role of the Sp1 polymorphism in the development of osteoporosis in patients with thalassaemia major. *Br J Haematol* 1998;101:26.

885. Eraklis AJ, Kevy SV, Diamond LK, et al. Hazard of overwhelming infection after splenectomy in childhood. *N Engl J Med* 1967;276:1225–1229.

886. Erikson WD, Burgert EO, Lynn HB. The hazard of infection following splenectomy in children. *Am J Dis Child* 1968;116:1–12.

887. Smith CH, Erlandson ME, Stern G, et al. Postsplenectomy infection in Cooley's anemia. *Ann N Y Acad Sci* 1964;119:748–757.

888. Smith CH, Erlandson ME, Stern G, et al. Postsplenectomy infection in Cooley's anemia: an appraisal of the problem in this and other blood disorders, with consideration of prophylaxis. *N Engl J Med* 1962;266:737–743.

889. Green NS. Yersinia infections in patients with homozygous beta-thalassemia associated with iron overload and its treatment. *Pediatr Hematol Oncol* 1992;9:247–254.

890. Mazzoleni G, de Sa D, Gately J, et al. *Yersinia enterocolitica* infection with ileal perforation associated with iron overload and deferoxamine therapy. *Dig Dis Sci* 1991;36:1154–1160.

891. Adamkiewicz TV, Berkovitch M, Krishnan C, et al. *Yersinia enterocolitica* and beta thalassemia: a report of 15 years' experience. *Clin Infect Dis* 1998;27:1367–1368.

892. Schanfield MS, Scalise G, Economidou I, et al. Immunogenetic factors in thalassemia and hepatitis B infection: a multicentre study. *Dev Biol Stand* 1975;30:257–269.

893. Politis C. Complications of blood transfusion in thalassemia. In: Buckner CD, Gale RP, Lucarelli G, eds. *Advances and controversies in thalassemia therapy: bone marrow transplantation and other approaches*, 309th vol. New York: Alan R. Liss, 1989:67–76.

894. Wonke B, Hoffbrand AV, Brown D, et al. Antibody to hepatitis C virus in multiply transfused patients with thalassaemia major. *J Clin Pathol* 1990;43:638–640.

895. Bozkurt G, Dikengil T, Alimoglu O, et al. Hepatitis C among Turkish Cypriot thalassemic patients. Fifth International Conference on Thalassemias and Hemaglobinopathies. Nicosia, Cyprus, 1993.

896. Cancado RD, Guerra LGM, Rosenfeld MOJA, et al. Prevalence of hepatitis C virus antibody in beta thalassemic patients. Fifth International Conference on Thalassemia and Hemoglobinopathies, Nicosia, Cyprus, 1993.

897. Lau YL, Chow CB, Lee AC, et al. Hepatitis C virus antibody in multiply transfused Chinese with thalassaemia. *Bone Marrow Transplant* 1993;12:26–28.

898. Kaur P, Kaur B. Thalassemia in Penang. First Asian Congress on Thalassemia, Penang, Malaysia, 1995.

899. Cao A, Galanello R, Rosatelli MC, et al. Clinical experience of management of thalassemia: the Sardinian experience. *Semin Hematol* 1996;33:66–75.

900. Wonke B, Hoffbrand AV, Bouloux P, et al. New approaches to the management of hepatitis and endocrine disorders in Cooley's anemia. *Ann N Y Acad Sci* 1998;850:232–241.

901. Girot R, Lefrere JJ, Schettini F, et al. HIV infections and AIDS in thalassemia. 5th Annual Meeting of the COOLEYCARE Group, Athens, 1991.

902. Manconi PE, Dessi C, Sanna G, et al. Human immunodeficiency virus infection in multi-transfused patients with thalassemia major. *Eur J Pediatr* 1998;147:304–307.

903. De Martino M, Quarta G, Melpignano A, et al. Antibodies to HTLV III and the lymphadenopathy syndrome in multi-transfused beta-thalassemia patients. *Vox Sang* 1985;41:230–233.

904. Politis C, Roumeliotou A, Germenis A, et al. Risk of acquired immune deficiency syndrome in multi-transfused patients with thalassemia major. *Plasma Ther Transfus Technol* 1986;7:41–43.

905. Zanella A, Mozzi F, Ferroni A, et al. Anti-HTLV III screening in multi-transfused thalassaemia patients. *Vox Sang* 1986;50:192.

906. Robert-Guroff M, Giardina PJ, Robey WG, et al. HTLV III neutralizing antibody development in transfusion-dependent seropositive patients with β-thalassemia. *J Immunol* 1987;138:3731–3736.

907. Jullien AM, Courouce AM, Richard D, et al. Transmission of HIV blood from seronegative donors. *Lancet* 1988;2:1248–1249.

908. Sen S, Mishra NM, Giri T, et al. Acquired immunodeficiency syndrome (AIDS) in multitransfused children with thalassemia. *Indian Pediatr* 1993;30:455–460.

909. Kumar RM, Uduman S, Hamo IM, et al. Incidence and clinical manifestations of HIV-1 infection in multitransfused thalassaemia Indian children. *Trop Geogr Med* 1994;46:163–166.

910. Kumar RM, Khuranna A. Pregnancy outcome in women with beta-thalassemia major and HIV infection. *Eur J Obstet Gynecol Reprod Biol* 1998;77:163–169.

911. Costagliola DG, Girot R, Rebulla P, et al. Incidence of AIDS in HIV-1 infected thalassaemia patients. *Br J Haematol* 1992;81:109–112.

912. Choudhury NJ, Dubey ML, Jolly JG, et al. Post-transfusion malaria in thalassaemia patients. *Blut* 1990;61:314–316.

913. Looareesuwan S, Suntharasamai P, Webster HK, et al. Malaria in splenectomized patients: report of four cases and review. *Clin Infect Dis* 1993;16:361–366.

914. Jandl JH, Greenberg MS. Bone marrow failure due to relative nutritional deficiency in Cooley's hemolytic anemia. *N Engl J Med* 1959;266:461–468.

915. Luhby AL, Cooperman JM, Feldman R, et al. Folic acid deficiency as a limiting factor in the anemias of thalassemia major. *Blood* 1961;18:786.

916. Vatanavicharn S, Avunatankulchai M, Na-nakorn S, et al. Serum and erythrocyte folate levels in thalassemia patients. *J Med Assoc Thai* 1978;61:56.

917. Wapnick AA, Lynch SR, Charlton RW, et al. The effect of ascorbic acid deficiency on desferrioxamine-induced iron excretion. *Br J Haematol* 1969;17:563–568.

918. Modell CB, Beck J. Long-term desferrioxamine therapy in thalassemia. *Ann N Y Acad Sci* 1974;232:201–210.

919. O'Brien RT. Ascorbic acid enhancement of desferrioxamine-induced urinary iron excretion in thalassemia major. *Ann N Y Acad Sci* 1974;232:221–225.

920. Cohen A, Cohen IJ, Schwartz E. Scurvy and altered iron stores in thalassemia major. *N Engl J Med* 1981;304:158–160.

921. Chapman RWG, Hussein MAM, Gorman A, et al. Effect of ascorbic acid deficiency on serum ferritin concentrations in patients with β-thalassaemia major and iron overload. *J Clin Pathol* 1982;35:487–491.

922. Hyman CB, Landing B, Alfin-Slater R, et al. Dl-alpha-tocopherol, iron, and lipofuscin in thalassemia. *Ann N Y Acad Sci* 1974;232:211–220.

923. Rachmilewitz EA. The role of intracellular hemoglobin precipitation, low MCHC and iron overload on red blood cell membrane peroxidation in thalassemia. In: Bergsma D, Cerami A, Peterson CM, et al., eds. *Birth Defects: Original Articles Series*. New York: Alan R. Liss, 1976:123.

924. Erlandson M, Golubow J, Smith CH. Bivalent cations in homozygous thalassemia. *J Pediatr* 1965;66:637–648.

925. Prasad AS, Diwany M, Gabr M, et al. Biochemical studies in thalassemia. *Ann Intern Med* 1965;62:87–96.

926. Hyman CB, Ortega JA, Costin G, et al. The clinical significance of magnesium depletion in thalassaemia. *Ann N Y Acad Sci* 1980;344:436.

927. Silprasert A, Laokuldilok T, Kulapongs P. Zinc deficiency in β-thalassemic children. *Birth Defects: Original Articles Series* 1998;23:473–476.

928. Dewey KW, Grossman H, Canale VC. Cholelithiasis in thalassemia major. *Radiology* 1970;96:385–388.

929. Paik CH, Alavi I, Dunea G, et al. Thalassemia and gouty arthritis. *JAMA* 1970;213:296–297.

930. Sinniah D, Vegnaendra V, Kammaruddin A. Neurological complications of beta-thalassaemia major. *Arch Dis Child* 1977;52:977–979.

931. McIntosh N. Beneficial effects of transfusing a patient with non-transfusion-dependent thalassemia major. *Arch Dis Child* 1976;51:471–472.

932. Porter JB, Huehns ER. The toxic effects of desferrioxamine. *Baillieres Clin Haematol* 1989;2:459–474.

933. Logothetis J, Haritos-Fatouros M, Constantoulakis M, et al. Intelligence and behavioral patterns in patients with Cooley's anemia (homozygous beta-thalassemia); a study based on 138 consecutive cases. *Pediatrics* 1971;48:740–744.

934. Wainscoat JS, Thein SL, Weatherall DJ. Thalassaemia intermedia. *Blood Rev* 1987;1:273–279.

935. Cao A, Galanello R, Rosatelli MC. Molecular pathology of thalassemia intermedia. *Eur J Intern Med* 1990;1:227–236.

936. Antonarakis SE, Kang J, Lam VM, et al. Molecular characterization of beta-globin gene mutations in patients with beta-thalassaemia intermedia in south China. *Br J Haematol* 1988;70:357–361.

937. Thein SL, Hesketh C, Wallace RB, et al. The molecular basis of thalassaemia major and thalassaemia intermedia in Asian Indians: application to prenatal diagnosis. *Br J Haematol* 1988;70:225–231.

938. Kanavakis E, Traeger-Synodinos J, Tzetis M, et al. Molecular characterization of homozygous (high Hb A_2) β-thalassaemia intermedia in Greece. *Pediatr Hematol Oncol* 1995;12:37–45.

939. Pippard MJ, Rajagopalan B, Callender ST, et al. Iron loading, chronic anaemia, and erythroid hyperplasia as determinants of the clinical features of β-thalassaemia intermedia. In: Weatherall DJ, Fiorelli G, Gorini S, eds. *Advances in red blood cell biology*. New York: Raven Press, 1982:103–113.

940. Fiorelli G, Sampietro M, Romano M, et al. Clinical features of thalassemia intermedia in Italy. *Birth Defects: Original Articles Series* 1988;23:287–295.

941. Heinrich HC, Gabbe EE, Oppitz KH, et al. Absorption of inorganic and food iron in children with heterozygous and homozygous beta-thalassemia. *Z Kinderheilkd* 1973;115:1–22.

942. Cossu P, Toccafondi C, Vardeu F, et al. Iron overload and desferrioxamine chelation therapy in beta-thalassemia intermedia. *Eur J Pediatr* 1981;137:267–271.

943. Pippard MJ, Weatherall DJ. Iron absorption in non-transfused iron loading anaemias: prediction of risk for iron loading, and response to iron chelation

treatment, in beta thalassaemia intermedia and congenital sideroblastic anaemias. *Haematologia* 1984;17:17–24.

944. Mancuso L, Iacona MA, Marchi S, et al. Severe cardiomyopathy in a woman with intermediate beta-thalassemia: regression of cardiac failure with desferrioxamine. *G Ital Cardiol* 1985;15:916–920.

945. Rees DC, Luo LY, Thein SL, et al. Nontransfusional iron overload in thalassemia: association with hereditary hemochromatosis. *Blood* 1997;90:3234–3236.

946. Cappellini MD, Fargion SR, Sampietro M, et al. Nontransfusional iron overload in thalassemia intermedia: role of the hemochromatosis allele. *Blood* 1998;92:4479–4480.

947. Borgna-Pignatti C, Solinas A, Bombieri C, et al. The haemochromatosis mutations do not modify the clinical picture of thalassaemia major in patients regularly transfused and chelated. *Br J Haematol* 1998;103:813–816.

948. Longo F, Zecchina G, Sbaiz L, et al. The influence of hemochromatosis mutations on iron overload of thalassemia major. *Haematologica* 1999;84:799–803.

949. Konstantopoulos K, Theocharis S, Karagiorga M, et al. Iron stores in multitransfused thalassaemic patients seem not to be influenced by the HLA system. *Haematologica* 2000;30:319–323.

950. Gratwick GM, Bullough PG, Bohne WH, et al. Thalassemic osteoarthropathy. *Ann Intern Med* 1978;88:494–501.

951. Ben-Bassat I, Hertz M, Selzer G, et al. Extramedullary hematopoiesis with multiple tumor-simulating mediastinal masses in a patient with β-thalassemia intermedia. *Isr J Med Sci* 1977;13:1206–1210.

952. Papavasiliou C, Gouliamos A, Vlahos L, et al. CT and MRI of symptomatic spinal involvement by extramedullary haemopoiesis. *Clin Radiol* 1990;42:91–92.

953. Yu YC, Kao EL, Chou SH, et al. Intrathoracic extramedullary hematopoiesis simulating posterior mediastinal mass: report of a case in patient with beta-thalassemia intermedia. *Gaoxiong Yi Xue Ke Xue Za Zhi* 1991;7:43–48.

954. Alam R, Padmanabhan K, Rao H. Paravertebral mass in a patient with thalassemia intermedia. *Chest* 1997;112:265–267.

955. David CV, Balasubramaniam P. Paraplegia with thalassaemia. *Aust N Z J Surg* 1983;53:283–284.

956. Cardia E, Toscano S, La Rosa G, et al. Spinal cord compression in homozygous β-thalassemia intermedia. *Pediatr Neurosurg* 1994;20:186–189.

957. Mancuso P, Zingale A, Basile L, et al. Cauda equina compression syndrome in a patient affected by thalassemia intermedia: complete regression with blood transfusion therapy. *Childs Nerv Sys* 1993;9:440–441.

958. Smith PR, Manjoney DL, Teitcher JB, et al. Massive hemothorax due to intrathoracic extramedullary hematopoiesis in a patient with thalassemia intermedia. *Chest* 1988;94:658–660.

959. Martin J, Palacio A, Petit J, et al. Fatty transformation of thoracic extramedullary hematopoiesis following splenectomy: CT features. *J Comput Assist Tomogr* 1990;14:477–478.

960. Saxon BR, Rees D, Olivieri NF. Regression of extramedullary haemopoiesis and augmentation of fetal haemoglobin concentration during hydroxyurea therapy in beta thalassaemia. *Br J Haematol* 1998;101:416–419.

961. Cianciulli P, di Toritto TC, Sorrentino F, et al. Hydroxyurea therapy in paraparesis and cauda equina syndrome due to extramedullary haematopoiesis in thalassaemia: improvement of clinical and haematological parameters. *Eur J Haematol* 2000;64:426–429.

962. Gimmon Z, Wexler MR, Rachmilewitz EA. Juvenile leg ulceration in beta-thalassemia major and intermedia. *Plast Reconstr Surg* 1982;69:320–325.

963. Ruf A, Pick M, Deutsch V, et al. *In vivo* platelet activation correlates with red cell anionic phospholipid exposure in patients with β-thalassaemia major. *Br J Haematol* 1997;98:51–56.

964. Skarsgard E, Doski J, Jaksic T, et al. Thrombosis of the portal venous system after splenectomy for pediatric hematologic disease. *J Pediatr Surg* 1993;28:1109–1112.

965. Cappellini MD, Robbiolo L, Bottasso BM, et al. Venous thromboembolism and hypercoagulability in splenectomized patients with thalassemia intermedia. *Br J Haematol* 2000;111:467–473.

966. Dore F, Bonfigli S, Pardini S, et al. Priapism in thalassemia intermedia. *Haematologica* 1991;76:523.

967. Aessopos A, Stamatelos G, Skoumas V, et al. Pulmonary hypertension and right heart failure in patients with β-thalassemia intermedia. *Chest* 1995;107:50–53.

968. Goldfarb A, Grisaru D, Gimmon Z, et al. High incidence of cholelithiasis in older patients with homozygous beta-thalassemia. *Acta Haematol* 1990;83:120–122.

969. Castaldi G, Zavagli G. Anaemia in thalassaemia. *Lancet* 1972;ii:1254–1255.

970. Weatherall DJ. Biochemical phenotypes of thalassemia in the American Negro populations. *Ann N Y Acad Sci* 1964;119:450–462.

971. Charache S, Conley CL, Doeblin TD, et al. Thalassemia in black Americans. *Ann N Y Acad Sci* 1974;232:125–134.

972. Millard DP, Mason K, Serjeant BE, et al. Comparison of haematological features of the β⁰ and β⁺ thalassaemia traits in Jamaican Negroes. *Br J Haematol* 1977;36:161–170.

973. Pootrakul P, Wasi P, Na-Nakorn S. Haematological data in 312 cases of β thalassaemia trait in Thailand. *Br J Haematol* 1973;24:703–712.

974. Mazza U, Saglio G, Cappio FC, et al. Clinical and haematological data in 254 cases of beta-thalassaemia trait in Italy. *Br J Haematol* 1976;33:91–99.

975. Knox-Macaulay HH, Weatherall DJ. Studies of red-cell membrane function in heterozygous beta thalassaemia and other hypochromic anaemias. *Br J Haematol* 1974;28:277–297.

976. Pearson HA, McPhedran P, O'Brien RT, et al. Comprehensive testing for thalassemia trait. *Ann N Y Acad Sci* 1974;232:135–144.

977. Tatsumi N, Tsuda I, Funahara Y, et al. Size distribution curves of blood cells in thalassemias and hemoglobin H. *Southeast Asian J Trop Med Public Health* 1992;23:79–85.

978. Pearson HA, McFarland W, King ER. Erythrokinetic studies in thalassemia trait. *J Lab Clin Med* 1960;56:866–873.

979. Malamos B, Belcher EH, Gyftaki E, et al. Simultaneous studies with Fe⁵⁹ and Cr⁵¹ in congenital haemolytic anaemias. *Nucl Med (Stuttgart)* 1961;2:1–20.

980. Gallo E, Pich P, Ricco G, et al. The relationship between anemia, fecal stercobilinogen, erythrocyte survival, and globin synthesis in heterozygotes for beta-thalassemia. *Blood* 1975;46:693–698.

981. Pippard MJ, Wainscoat JS. Erythrokinetics and iron status in heterozygous beta thalassaemia, and the effect of interaction with alpha thalassaemia. *Br J Haematol* 1987;66:123–127.

982. Kattamis C, Lagos P, Metaxatou-Mavromati A, et al. Serum iron and unsaturated iron-binding capacity in the β-thalassaemia trait: their relation to the levels of haemoglobins A, A₂ and F. *J Med Genet* 1972;9:154–159.

983. Knox-Macaulay HH, Weatherall DJ, Clegg JB, et al. Thalassaemia in the British. *BMJ* 1973;3:150–155.

984. Hussein S, Hoffbrand AV, Laulicht M, et al. Serum ferritin levels in beta-thalassaemia trait. *BMJ* 1976;2:920.

985. Economidou J, Augustaki O, Georgiopoulou V, et al. Assessment of iron stores in subjects heterozygous for β-thalassaemia based on serum ferritin levels. *Acta Haematol* 1980;64:205–208.

986. Bowdler AJ, Huehns ER. Thalassaemia major complicated by excessive iron storage. *Br J Haematol* 1963;9:13–24.

987. Williams CE, Siemsen AW. Hemosiderosis in association with thalassaemia minor. *Arch Intern Med* 1968;121:356–360.

988. Tolot F, Bocquet B, Baron M. Hemochromatosis and pigmentary cirrhosis in minor thalassemia in adults. *J Med Lyon* 1970;51:655–660.

989. Parfrey PS, Squier M. Thalassaemia minor, iron overload and hepatoma. *BMJ* 1978;i:416.

990. Fargion S, Piperno A, Panaiotopoulos N, et al. Iron overload in subjects with β-thalassaemia trait: role of idiopathic haemochromatosis gene. *Br J Haematol* 1985;61:487–490.

991. Van der Weyden MB, Fong H, Hallam LJ, et al. Red cell ferritin and iron overload in heterozygous β-thalassemia. *Am J Hematol* 1989;30:201–205.

992. Kunkel HG, Wallenius G. New hemoglobin in normal adult blood. *Science* 1955;122:288.

993. Kunkel HG, Ceppellini R, Müller-Eberhard U, et al. Observations on the minor basic hemoglobin component in blood of normal individuals and patients with thalassemia. *J Clin Invest* 1957;36:1615–1625.

994. Wasi P, Disthasongchan P, Na-Nakorn S. The effect of iron deficiency on the levels of hemoglobins A2 and E. *J Lab Clin Med* 1968;71:85–91.

995. Steinberg MH. Case report: effects of iron deficiency and the -88 C→T mutation on Hb A₂ levels in β-thalassemia. *Am J Med Sci* 1993;305:312–313.

996. Fessas P, Mastrokalos N. Demonstration of small components in red cell haemolysates by starch-gel electrophoresis. *Nature* 1959;183:30.

997. Beaven GH, Ellis MJ, White JC. Studies in human foetal haemoglobin, III: the hereditary haemoglobinopathies and thalassaemia. *Br J Haematol* 1961;7:169–186.

998. Wood WG, Stamatoyannopoulos G, Lim G, et al. F-cells in the adult: normal values and levels in individuals with hereditary and acquired elevations of Hb F. *Blood* 1975;46:671–682.

999. Schettini F, Mautone A, de Lucia I. 2,3-Diphosphoglycerate content of erythrocytes in the thalassaemic trait. *Boll Soc Ital Biol Sper* 1974;50:215.

1000. Pearson HA, Motoyama E, Genel M, et al. Intraerythrocytic adaptation (2,3 DPG, P50) in thalassemia minor. *Blood* 1977;49:463.

1001. Selwyn JG, Dacie JV. Autohemolysis and other changes resulting from the incubation in vitro of red cells from patients with congenital hemolytic anemia. *Blood* 1954;9:414–438.

1002. Ziegler G, Marti HR. Protoporphyrin and coproporphyrin of erythrocytes in heterozygotic thalassemia. *Schweiz Med Wschr* 1966;96:1272–1273.

1003. Lyberatos C, Chalevelakis G, Platis A, et al. Erythrocyte content of free protoporphyrin in thalassaemic syndromes. *Acta Haematol* 1972;47:164–167.

1004. Hinchliffe RF, Lilleyman JS, Steel GJ, et al. Usefulness of red cell zinc protoporphyrin concentration in the investigation of microcytosis in children. *Pediatr Hematol Oncol* 1995;12:455–462.

1005. Loria A, Konijn AM, Hershko C. Serum ferritin in β thalassaemia trait. *Isr J Med Sci* 1978;14:1127–1131.

1006. Bannerman RM, Callender ST. Thalassaemia in Britain. *BMJ* 1961;ii:1288.

1007. Gardikas C. Modes of presentation of thalassaemia minor. *Acta Haematol* 1968;40:34–36.

1008. Fessas P. Thalassaemia and the alterations of the haemoglobin pattern. In: Jonxis JHP, Delafresnaye JF, eds. *Abnormal haemoglobins*. Oxford: Blackwell Science, 1959:134–155.

1009. Schuman JE, Tanser CL, Peloquin R, et al. The erythropoietic response to pregnancy in β thalassaemia minor. *Br J Haematol* 1973;25:249–260.

1010. Fleming AF. Maternal anemia and fetal outcome in pregnancies complicated by thalassaemia minor and "stomatocytosis." *Am J Obstet Gynecol* 1973;116:309–319.

1011. Landman H. *Haemoglobinopathies and pregnancy*. Groningen: Van Denderen Printing, 1988.

1012. Feder JN, Gnirke A, Thomas W, et al. A novel MHC class I-like gene is mutated in patients with hereditary haemochromatosis. *Nat Genet* 1996;13:399–408.

1013. Feder JN, Penny DM, Irrinki A, et al. The hemochromatosis gene product complexes with the transferrin receptor and lowers its affinity for ligand binding. *Proc Natl Acad Sci U S A* 1998;95:1472–1477.

1014. Chanarin I, Dacie JV, Mollin DL. Folic-acid deficiency in haemolytic anaemia. *Br J Haematol* 1959;5:245–256.

1015. Silva AE, Varella-Garcia M. Plasma folate and vitamin B_{12} levels in β-thalassemia heterozygotes. *Braz J Med Biol Res* 1989;22:1225–1226.

1016. Gallerani M, Cicognani I, Ballardini P, et al. Average life expectancy of heterozygous beta thalassemic subjects. *Haematologica* 1990;75:224–227.

1017. Gallerani M, Scapoli C, Cicognani I, et al. Thalassaemia trait and myocardial infarction: low infarction incidence in male subjects confirmed. *J Intern Med* 1991;230:109–111.

1018. Kattamis C, Metaxatou-Mavromati A, Wood WG, et al. The heterogeneity of normal Hb A_2-β thalassaemia in Greece. *Br J Haematol* 1979;42:109–123.

1019. Silvestroni E, Bianco I, Graziani B, et al. First premarital screening of thalassaemia carriers in intermediate schools in Latium. *J Med Genet* 1978;15:202–207.

1020. Galanello R, Barella S, Ideo A, et al. Genotype of subjects with borderline hemoglobin A2 levels: implication for beta-thalassemia carrier screening. *Am J Hematol* 1994;46:79–81.

1021. Thein SL. β-Thalassaemia. In: Higgs DR, Weatherall DJ, eds. *Baillière's Clinical Haematology*. International Practice and Research: The Haemoglobinopathies. London: Baillière Tindall, 1993:151–176.

1022. Schokker RC, Went LN, Bok J. A new genetic variant of beta-thalassaemia. *Nature* 1966;209:44–46.

1023. Kanavakis E, Wainscoat JS, Wood WG, et al. The interaction of α thalassaemia with heterozygous β thalassaemia. *Br J Haematol* 1982;52:465–473.

1024. Melis MA, Pirastu M, Galanello R, et al. Phenotypic effect of heterozygous α and $β^0$-thalassaemia interaction. *Blood* 1983;62:226–229.

1025. Gasperini D, Cao A, Paderi L, et al. Normal individuals with high Hb A2 levels. *Br J Haematol* 1993;84:166–168.

1026. Thein SL. Is it dominantly inherited beta thalassemia or just a beta chain variant that is highly unstable? *Br J Haematol* 1999;107:12–21.

1027. Vetter B, Neu-Yilik G, Kohne E, et al. Dominant beta-thalassaemia: a highly unstable haemoglobin is caused by a novel 6 bp deletion of the beta-globin gene. *Br J Haematol* 2000;108:176–181.

1028. Semenza GL, Delgrosso K, Poncz M, et al. The silent carrier allele: beta thalassemia without a mutation in the beta-globin gene or its immediate flanking regions. *Cell* 1984;39:123–128.

1029. Schwartz E, Cohen A, Surrey S. Overview of the beta thalassemias: genetic and clinical aspects. *Hemoglobin* 1988;12:551–564.

1030. Murru S, Loudianos G, Porcu S, et al. A beta-thalassaemia phenotype not linked to the beta-globin cluster in an Italian family. *Br J Haematol* 1992;81:283–287.

1031. Thein SL, Wood WG, Wickramasinghe SN, et al. Beta-thalassaemia unlinked to the beta-globin gene in an English family. *Blood* 1993;82:961–967.

1032. Kazazian HH Jr. The thalassemia syndromes: molecular basis and prenatal diagnosis in 1990. *Semin Hematol* 1990;27:209–228.

1033. Pearson HA, Guiliotis DK, Rink L, et al. Patient age distribution in thalassemia major: changes from 1973 to 1985. *Pediatrics* 1987;80:53–57.

1034. Cao A, Rosatelli MC. Screening and prenatal diagnosis of the haemoglobinopathies. *Clin Haematol* 1993;6:263–286.

1035. Angastiniotis M, Modell B, Englezos P, et al. Prevention and control of haemoglobinopathies. *Bull World Health Organ* 1995;73:375–386.

1036. Modell B, Petrou M, Layton M, et al. Audit of prenatal diagnosis for haemoglobin disorders in the United Kingdom: the first 20 years. *BMJ* 1997;315:779–784.

1037. Pearson HA, O'Brien RT, McIntosh S. Screening for thalassemia trait by electronic measurement of mean corpuscular volume. *N Engl J Med* 1973;288:351–353.

1038. Klee GG. Role of morphology, and erythrocyte indices in screening and diagnosis, A: the automated hematology group (CBC) as a screen for thalassemias and hemoglobinopathies. In: Fairbanks VF, ed. *Hemoglobinopathies and thalassemias: laboratory methods and clinical cases*. New York: Decker, 1980:38.

1039. Letsky EA, Weatherall DJ. Acquired haematological disorders. In: Wald N, ed. *Antenatal and neonatal screening*, 2nd vol. Oxford: Oxford University Press, 1998.

1040. Rund D, Rachmilewitz E. New trends in the treatment of beta-thalassemia. *Crit Rev Oncol Hematol* 2000;33:105–118.

1041. Karnon J, Zeuner D, Brown J, et al. Lifetime treatment costs of beta-thalassaemia major. *Clin Lab Haematol* 1999;21:377–385.

1042. Prati D. Benefits and complications of regular blood transfusion in patients with beta-thalassaemia major. *Vox Sang* 2000;79:129–137.

1043. Giardini C. Treatment of beta-thalassemia. *Curr Opin Hematol* 1997;4:79–87.

1044. Borgna-Pignatti C, Rugolotto S, De Stefano P, et al. Survival and disease complications in thalassemia major. *Ann N Y Acad Sci* 1998;850:227–231.

1045. Cario H, Stahnke K, Sander S, et al. Epidemiological situation and treatment of patients with thalassemia major in Germany: results of the German multicenter beta-thalassemia study. *Ann Hematol* 2000;79:7–12.

1046. Ladis V, Berdousi H, Palamidou F, et al. Morbidity and mortality of iron intoxication in adult patients with thalassemia major, and effectiveness of chelation. *Transfus Sci* 2000;23:255–256.

1047. Fosburg MT, Nathan DG. Treatment of Cooley's anemia. *Blood* 1990;76:435–444.

1048. Cazzola M, Borgna-Pignatti C, Locatelli F, et al. A moderate transfusion regimen may reduce iron loading in beta-thalassemia major without producing excessive expansion of erythropoiesis. *Transfusion* 1997;37:135–140.

1049. Madgwick KV, Yardumian A. A home blood transfusion programme for beta-thalassaemia patients. *Transfus Med* 1999;9:135–138.

1050. Necheles TF, Chung S, Sabbah R, et al. Intensive transfusion therapy in thalassemia major: an eight-year follow-up. *Ann N Y Acad Sci* 1974;232:179–185.

1051. Viens AM, Sharma S, Olivieri NF. Re-assessment of the value of splenectomy in thalassemia major (TM). *Blood* 1998;92:533a.

1052. Rebulla P. Blood transfusion in beta thalassaemia major. *Transfus Med* 1995;5:247–258.

1053. Lane TA. Leukocyte reduction of cellular blood components: effectiveness, benefits, quality control, and costs. *Arch Pathol Lab Med* 1994;118:392–404.

1054. Piomelli S, Seaman C, Reibman J, et al. Separation of younger red cells with improved survival *in vivo*: an approach to chronic transfusion therapy. *Proc Natl Acad Sci U S A* 1978;75:3474–3478.

1055. Cohen AR, Schmidt JM, Martin MB, et al. Clinical trial of young red cell transfusions. *J Pediatr* 1984;104:865–868.

1056. Kevy SV, Jacobson MS, Fosburg M, et al. A new approach to neocyte transfusion: preliminary report. *J Clin Apheresis* 1988;4:194–197.

1057. Simon TL, Sohmer P, Nelson EF. Extended survival of neocytes produced by a new system. *Transfusion* 1989;29:221–225.

1058. Collins AF, Dias GC, Haddad S, et al. Evaluation of a new neocyte transfusion preparation vs. washed cell transfusion in patients with homozygous beta thalassemia. *Transfusion* 1994;34:51520.

1059. Spanos T, Ladis V, Palamidou F, et al. The impact of neocyte transfusion in the management of thalassaemia. *Vox Sang* 1996;70:217–223.

1060. Valbonesi M, Bruni R. Clinical application of therapeutic erythrocytapheresis (TEA). *Transfus Sci* 2000;22:183–194.

1061. Berdoukas VA, Kwan YL, Sansotta ML. A study on the value of red cell exchange transfusion in transfusion dependent anaemias. *Clin Lab Haematol* 1986;8:209–220.

1062. Sirchia G, Zanella A, Parravicini A, et al. Red cell alloantibodies in thalassemia major: results of an Italian cooperative study. *Transfusion* 1985;25:110–112.

1063. Spanos T, Karageorga M, Ladis V, et al. Red cell alloantibodies in patients with thalassemia. *Vox Sang* 1990;58:50–55.

1064. Rebulla P, Modell B. Transfusion requirements and effects in patients with thalassaemia major. Cooleycare Programme. *Lancet* 1991;337:277–280.

1065. Singer ST, Wu V, Mignacca R, et al. Alloimmunization and erythrocyte autoimmunization in transfusion-dependent thalassemia patients of predominantly Asian descent. *Blood* 2000;96:3369–3373.

1066. Kruatrachue M, Sirisinha S, Pacharee P, et al. An association between thalassaemia and autoimmune haemolytic anaemia (AIHA). *Scand J Haematol* 1980;25:259–263.

1067. Argiolu F, Diana G, Arnone M, et al. High-dose intravenous immunoglobulin in the management of autoimmune hemolytic anemia complicating thalassemia major. *Acta Haematol* 1990;83:65–68.

1068. Sayers MH. Transfusion-transmitted viral infections other than hepatitis and human immunodeficiency virus infection: cytomegalovirus, Epstein-Barr virus, human herpesvirus 6, and human parvovirus B19. *Arch Pathol Lab Med* 1994;118:346–349.

1069. Sazama K. Bacteria in blood for transfusion: a review. *Arch Pathol Lab Med* 1994;118:350–365.

1070. Guglielmo P, Cunsolo F, Lombardo T, et al. T-subset abnormalities in thalassaemia intermedia: possible evidence for a thymus functional deficiency. *Acta Haematol* 1984;72:361–367.

1071. Li Q, Clegg C, Peterson K, et al. Binary transgenic mouse model for studying the trans control of globin gene switching: evidence that GATA-1 is an *in vivo* repressor of human ε gene expression. *Proc Natl Acad Sci U S A* 1997;94:2444–2448.

1072. Walker EM Jr, Walker SM. Effects of iron overload on the immune system. *Ann Clin Lab Sci* 2000;30:354–365.

1073. Cunningham-Rundles S, Giardina PJ, Grady RW, et al. Effect of transfusional iron overload on immune response. *J Infect Dis* 2000;182[Suppl 1]:S115–S121.

1074. Wasi P, Na-Nakorn S, Pootrakul P, et al. A syndrome of hypertension, convulsions, and cerebral haemorrhage in thalassaemic patients after multiple blood transfusions. *Lancet* 1978;ii:602.

1075. Constantopoulos A, Matsaniotis N. Hypertension, convulsion, and cerebral haemorrhage in thalassaemic patients after multiple blood transfusions. *Helv Paediatr Acta* 1980;35:269–271.

1076. Modell B. Total management of thalassaemia major. *Arch Dis Child* 1977;52:489–500.

1077. Graziano JH, Piomelli S, Hilgartner M, et al. Chelation therapy in beta-thalassemia major, III: the role of splenectomy in achieving iron balance. *J Pediatr* 1981;99:695–699.

1078. Cohen A, Gayer E, Mizanin J. Long-term effect of splenectomy on transfusion requirements in thalassemia major. *Am J Hematol* 1989;30:254–256.

1079. Berry CL, Marshall WC. Iron distribution in the liver of patients with thalassaemia major. *Lancet* 1967;1:1031–1033.

1080. Okon E, Levij IS, Rachmilewitz EA. Splenectomy, iron overload and liver cirrhosis in beta-thalassemia major. *Acta Haematol* 1976;56:142–150.

1081. Pootrakul P, Rugkiatsakul R, Wasi P. Increased transferrin iron saturation in splenectomized thalassaemia patients. *Br J Haematol* 1980;46:143–145.

1082. Borgna-Pignatti C, de Stefano P, Bongo IG, et al. Spleen iron content is low in thalassemia. *Am J Pediatr Hematol Oncol* 1984;6:340–343.

1083. Kheradpir MH, Albouyeh M. Partial splenectomy in the treatment of thalassaemia major. *Kinderchirurgie* 1985;40:195–198.

1084. de Montalembert M, Girot R, Revillon Y, et al. Partial splenectomy in homozygous beta thalassaemia. *Arch Dis Child* 1990;65:304–307.

1085. Politis C, Spigos DG, Georgiopoulou P, et al. Partial splenic embolisation for hypersplenism of thalassaemia major: five year follow-up. *BMJ* 1987;294:665–667.

1086. Revillon Y, Girot R. Désartérialisation partielle de la rate et splénectomie partielle chez l'enfant. *Presse Med* 1985;14:423–425.

1087. Penberthy GC, Cooley TB. Results of splenectomy in childhood. *Ann Surg* 1935;102:645.

1088. Clement DH, Taffel M. Splenectomy in Mediterranean anemia. *Pediatrics* 1955;16:353.

1089. Smith CH, Erlandson ME, Schulman I, et al. Hazard of severe infections in splenectomized infants and children. *Am J Med* 1957;22:390.

1090. Mainzer RA, O'Connor WJ. Evaluation of splenectomy in the treatment of Cooley's anemia. *Ann Surg* 1958;148:44.

1091. Wolff JA, Sitarz AL, VonHofe FH. Effect of splenectomy on thalassemia. *Pediatrics* 1960;26:674.

1092. Engelhard D, Cividalli G, Rachmilewitz EA. Splenectomy in homozygous beta thalassaemia: a retrospective study of 30 patients. *Br J Haematol* 1975;31:39.

1093. Wahidijat I, Markum AH, Adang ZK. Early splenectomy in the management of thalassemic children in Djakarta. *Acta Haematol* 1972;48:28.

1094. Hershko C, Konijn AM, Link G. Iron chelators for thalassaemia. *Br J Haematol* 1998;101:399–406.

1095. Olivieri NF, Nathan DG, MacMillan JH, et al. Survival in medically treated patients with homozygous beta-thalassemia. *N Engl J Med* 1994;331:574–578.

1096. Modell B, Khan M, Darlison M. Survival in beta-thalassaemia major in the UK: data from the UK Thalassaemia Register. *Lancet* 2000;355:2051–2052.

1097. Barry M, Flynn DM, Letsky EA, et al. Long-term chelation therapy in thalassaemia major: effect on liver iron concentration, liver histology, and clinical progress. *BMJ* 1974;2:16–20.

1098. Wolfe L, Olivieri N, Sallan D, et al. Prevention of cardiac disease by subcutaneous deferoxamine in patients with thalassemia major. *N Engl J Med* 1985; 312:1600–1603.

1099. Cohen A, Martin M, Schwartz E. Depletion of excessive liver iron stores with desferrioxamine. *Br J Haematol* 1984;58:369–373.

1100. Cohen AR, Mizanin J, Schwartz E. Rapid removal of excessive iron with daily, high-dose intravenous chelation therapy. *J Pediatr* 1989;115:151–155.

1101. Papadimas J, Mandala E, Pados G, et al. Pituitary-testicular axis in men with β-thalassaemia major. *Hum Reprod* 1996;11:1900–1904.

1102. Freeman AP, Giles RW, Berdoukas VA, et al. Early left ventricular dysfunction and chelation therapy in thalassemia major. *Ann Intern Med* 1983;99:450–454.

1103. Marcus RE, Davies SC, Bantock HM, et al. Desferrioxamine to improve cardiac function in iron-overloaded patients with thalassaemia major. *Lancet* 1984;1:373.

1104. Rahko PS, Salerni R, Uretsky BF. Successful reversal by chelation therapy of congestive cardiomyopathy due to iron overload. *J Am Coll Cardiol* 1986;8:426.

1105. Aldouri MA, Wonke B, Hoffbrand AV, et al. High incidence of cardiomyopathy in beta-thalassaemia patients receiving regular transfusion and iron chelation: reversal by intensified chelation. *Acta Haematol* 1990;84:113.

1106. Perrimond H, Michel G, Orsini A, et al. First report of a cardiac transplantation in a patient with thalassaemia major. *Br J Haematol* 1991;78:467.

1107. Koerner MM, Tenderich G, Minami K, et al. Heart transplantation for end-stage heart failure caused by iron overload. *Br J Haematol* 1997;97:293–296.

1108. Detry O, Defechereux T, Honore P, et al. [Combined liver and heart transplantation in a patient with thalassaemia major]. *Rev Med Liege* 1997;52:532–534.

1109. Olivieri NF, Liu PP, Sher GD, et al. Successful combined cardiac and liver transplantation in an adult with homozygous beta-thalassemia. *N Engl J Med* 1994;330:1125–1127.

1110. Kelly TM, Edwards CQ, Meikle AW, et al. Hypogonadism in hemochromatosis: reversal with iron depletion. *Ann Intern Med* 1984;101:629–632.

1111. Siemons LJ, Mahler CH. Hypogonadotropic hypogonadism in hemochromatosis: recovery of reproductive function after iron depletion. *J Clin Endocrinol Metab* 1987;65:585–587.

1112. Porter JB, Jaswon MS, Huehns ER, et al. Desferrioxamine ototoxicity: evaluation of risk factors in thalassaemia patients and guidelines for safe dosage. *Br J Haematol* 1989;73:403–409.

1113. Loreal O, Deugnier Y, Moirand R, et al. Liver fibrosis in genetic hemochromatosis: respective roles of iron and non-iron-related factors in 127 homozygous patients. *J Hepatol* 1992;16:122–127.

1114. Niederau C, Fischer R, Purschel A, et al. Long-term survival in patients with hereditary hemochromatosis. *Gastroenterology* 1996;110:1107–1119.

1115. Saxon BR, Brittenham GM, Nisbet-Brown E, et al. Liver biopsy is safe and provides quantitative guidelines for initiation of chelating therapy in children with thalassaemia major. *Blood* 1997;90[Suppl 1]:130a.

1116. Telfer PT, Prestcott E, Holden S, et al. Hepatic iron concentration combined with long-term monitoring of serum ferritin to predict complications of iron overload in thalassaemia major. *Br J Haematol* 2000;110:971–977.

1117. Cartwright GE, Edwards CQ, Kravitz K, et al. Hereditary hemochromatosis: phenotypic expression of the disease. *N Engl J Med* 1979;301:175–179.

1118. Telfer P, De la Salle B, Ridler C. Antenatal testing for haemoglobinopathies. *Br J Haematol* 2000;110:1003–1004.

1119. Davis BA, Porter JB. Long-term outcome of continuous 24-hour deferoxamine infusion via indwelling intravenous catheters in high-risk beta-thalassemia. *Blood* 2000;95:1229–1236.

1120. Lai E, Belluzzo N, Muraca MF, et al. The prognosis for adults with thalassemia major: Sardinia. *Blood* 1995;86:251a.

1121. De Virgiliis S, Congia M, Frau F, et al. Deferoxamine-induced growth retardation in patients with thalassemia major. *J Pediatr* 1988;113:661–669.

1122. Piga A, Luzzatto L, Capalbo P, et al. High-dose desferrioxamine as a cause of growth failure in thalassaemia patients. *Eur J Haematol* 1988;40:380.

1123. Olivieri NF, Koren G, Harris J, et al. Growth failure and bony changes induced by deferoxamine. *Am J Pediatr Hematol Oncol* 1992;14:48–56.

1124. Olivieri NF, Berriman AM, Tyler BJ, et al. Reduction in tissue iron stores with a new regimen of continuous ambulatory intravenous deferoxamine. *Am J Hematol* 1992;41:61–63.

1125. Brittenham GM, Sheth S, Allen CJ, et al. Noninvasive methods for quantitative assessment of transfusional iron overload in sickle cell disease. *Semin Hematol* 2001;38:37–56.

1126. Brittenham GM, Cohen AR, McLaren C, et al. Hepatic iron stores and plasma ferritin concentration in patients with sickle cell anemia and thalassemia. *Am J Hematol* 1993;42:81–85.

1127. Herbert V, Shaw S, Jayatilleke E. High serum ferritin protein does not distinguish iron overload from inflammation, but a new assay, high serum-ferritin-iron does. *Am J Clin Nutr* 1995;61:911.

1128. Herbert V, Shaw S, Jayatilleke E. Serum ferritin-iron (holoferritin): the first reliable (not confounded by inflammation) serum measurement of body iron stores. *J Invest Med* 1995;43[Suppl 1]:198a.

1129. Herbert V, Jayatilleke E, Shaw S, et al. Serum ferritin iron, a new test, measures human body iron stores unconfounded by inflammation. *Stem Cells* 1997;15:291–296.

1130. Nielsen P, Gunther U, Durken M, et al. Serum ferritin iron in iron overload and liver damage: correlation to body iron stores and diagnostic relevance. *J Lab Clin Med* 2000;135:413–418.

1131. Breuer W, Ronson A, Slotki IN, et al. The assessment of serum nontransferrin-bound iron in chelation therapy and iron supplementation. *Blood* 2000;95:2975–2982.

1132. Houang MTW, Arozena X, Skalicka A, et al. Correlation between computed tomographic values and liver iron content in thalassaemia major with iron overload. *Lancet* 1979;1:1322–1323.

1133. Long JAJ, Doppman JL, Nienhuis AW, et al. Computed tomographic analysis of beta-thalassemic syndromes with hemochromatosis: pathological findings with clinical and laboratory correlations. *J Comput Assist Tomogr* 1980;4:159.

1134. Olivieri NF, Grisaru D, Daneman A, et al. Computed tomography scanning of the liver to determine efficacy of iron chelation therapy in thalassemia major. *J Pediatr* 1989;114:427–430.

1135. Wielopolski L, Zaino EC. Noninvasive *in-vivo* measurement of hepatic and cardiac iron. *J Nucl Med* 1992;33:1278–1282.

1136. Stark DD, Moseley ME, Bacon BR, et al. Magnetic resonance imaging and spectroscopy of hepatic iron overload. *Radiology* 1985;154:137–142.

1137. Gomori JM, Horev G, Tamary H, et al. Hepatic iron overload: quantitative MR imaging. *Radiology* 1991;179:367–369.

1138. Olivieri NF, Koren G, Matsui D, et al. Reduction of tissue iron stores and normalization of serum ferritin during treatment with the oral iron chelator L1 in thalassemia intermedia. *Blood* 1992;79:2741–2748.

1139. Villari N, Caramella D, Lippi A, et al. Assessment of liver iron overload in thalassemic patients by MR imaging. *Acta Radiol* 1992;4:347.

1140. Lui P, Henkelman M, Joshi J, et al. Quantitation of cardiac and tissue iron by nuclear magnetic resonance in a novel murine thalassemia-cardiac iron overload model. *Can J Cardiol* 1996;12:155–164.

1141. Bonkovsky HL, Rubin RB, Cable EE, et al. Hepatic iron concentration: noninvasive estimation by means of MR imaging techniques. *Radiology* 1999;212:227–234.

1142. Angelucci E, Giovagnoni A, Valeri G, et al. Limitations of magnetic resonance imaging in measurement of hepatic iron. *Blood* 1997;90:4736–4742.

1143. Papanikolaou N, Ghiatas A, Kattamis A, et al. Non-invasive myocardial iron assessment in thalassaemic patients: T2 relaxometry and magnetization transfer ratio measurements. *Acta Radiol* 2000;41:348–351.

1144. Farquharson MJ, Bagshaw AP, Porter JB, et al. The use of skin Fe levels as a surrogate marker for organ Fe levels, to monitor treatment in cases of iron overload. *Phys Med Biol* 2000;45:1387–1396.

1145. Pippard MJ. Measurement of iron status. *Prog Clin Biol Res* 1989;309:85–92.

1146. Angelucci E, Brittenham GM, McLaren CE, et al. Hepatic iron concentration and total body iron stores in thalassemia major. *N Engl J Med* 2000;343:327–331.

1147. Crisponi G, Ambu R, Cristiani F, et al. Does iron concentration in a liver needle biopsy accurately reflect hepatic iron burden in beta-thalassemia? *Clin Chem* 2000;46:1185–1188.

1148. Sherlock S, Dick R, van-Leeuwen DJ. Liver biopsy today: the Royal Free Hospital experience. *J Hepatol* 1985;1:75–85.

1149. Faa G, Sciot R, Farci AM, et al. Iron concentration and distribution in the newborn liver. *Liver* 1994;14:193–199.

1150. Ambu R, Crisponi G, Sciot R, et al. Uneven hepatic iron and phosphorus distribution in beta-thalassemia. *J Hepatol* 1995;23:544–549.

1151. Aragoni MC, Crisponi G, Nurchi VM, et al. Chemometric methods applied to an ICP-AES study of chemical element distributions in autopsy livers from subjects affected by Wilson and beta-thalassemia. *J Trace Elem Med Biol* 1995;9:215–221.

1152. Villeneuve JP, Bilodeau M, Lepage R, et al. Variability in hepatic iron concentration measurement from needle-biopsy specimens. *J Hepatol* 1996;25:172–177.

1153. Overmoyer BA, McLaren CE, Brittenham GM. Uniformity of liver density and nonheme (storage) iron distribution. *Arch Pathol Lab Med* 1987;111:549–554.

1154. Brittenham GM, Farrell DE, Harris JW, et al. Magnetic-susceptibility measurement of human iron stores. *N Engl J Med* 1982;307:1671–1675.

1155. Fischer R, Tiemann CD, Engelhardt R, et al. Assessment of iron stores in children with transfusion siderosis by biomagnetic liver susceptometry. *Am J Hematol* 1999;60:289–299.

1156. Nielsen P, Engelhardt R, Duerken M, et al. Using SQUID biomagnetic liver susceptometry in the treatment of thalassemia and other iron loading diseases. *Transfus Sci* 2000;23:257–258.

1157. Fitchett DH, Coltart DJ, Littler WA, et al. Cardiac involvement in secondary haemochromatosis: a catheter biopsy study and analysis of myocardium. *Cardiovasc Res* 1980;14:719–724.

1158. Henry WL, Nienhuis AW, Wiener M, et al. Echocardiographic abnormalities in patients with transfusion-dependent anemia and secondary myocardial iron deposition. *Am J Med* 1978;64:547–555.

1159. Bahl VK, Malhotra OP, Kumar D, et al. Noninvasive assessment of systolic and diastolic left ventricular function in patients with chronic severe anemia: a combined M-mode, two-dimensional, and Doppler echocardiographic study. *Am Heart J* 1992;124:1516–1523.

1160. Lattanzi F, Bellotti P, Picano E, et al. Quantitative ultrasonic analysis of myocardium in patients with thalassemia major and iron overload. *Circulation* 1993;87:748–754.

1161. Leon MB, Borer JS, Bacharach SL, et al. Detection of early cardiac dysfunction in patients with severe beta-thalassemia and chronic iron overload. *N Engl J Med* 1979;301:1143–1148.

1162. Hahalis G, Manolis AS, Gerasimidou I, et al. Right ventricular diastolic function in beta-thalassemia major: echocardiographic and clinical correlates. *Am Heart J* 2001;141:428–434.

1163. Derchi G, Bellone P, Forni GL, et al. Cardiac involvement in thalassaemia major: altered atrial natriuretic peptide levels in asymptomatic patients. *Eur Heart J* 1992;13:1368–1372.

1164. Liu P, Henkelman M, Joshi J, et al. Quantification of cardiac and tissue iron by nuclear magnetic resonance relaxometry in a novel murine thalassemia-cardiac iron overload model. *Can J Cardiol* 1996;12:155–164.

1165. Argyropoulou MI, Metafratzi Z, Kiortsis DN, et al. T2 relaxation rate as an index of pituitary iron overload in patients with beta-thalassemia major. *AJR Am J Roentgenol* 2000;175:1567–1569.

1166. Sparacia G, Iaia A, Banco A, et al. Transfusional hemochromatosis: quantitative relation of MR imaging pituitary signal intensity reduction to hypogonadotropic hypogonadism. *Radiology* 2000;215:818–823.

1167. Shalit M, Tedeschi A, Miadonna A, et al. Desferal (desferrioxamine): a novel activator of connective tissue-type mast cells. *J Allergy Clin Immunol* 1991;6:854–860.

1168. Miller KB, Rosenwasser LJ, Bessette JA, et al. Rapid desensitisation for desferrioxamine anaphylactic reaction. *Lancet* 1981;i:1059.

1169. Bousquet J, Navarro M, Robert G, et al. Rapid desensitization for desferrioxamine anaphylactoid reactions. *Lancet* 1983;ii:859–860.

1170. Lombardo T, Ferro G, Frontini V, et al. High-dose intravenous desferrioxamine (DFO) delivery in four thalassemic patients allergic to subcutaneous DFO administration. *Am J Hematol* 1996;51:90–92.

1171. Waxman HS, Brown EB. Clinical usefulness of iron chelating agents. *Prog Hematol* 1969;6:338–373.

1172. Modell B. Advances in the use of iron-chelating agents for the treatment of iron overload. *Prog Hematol* 1979;11:267–312.

1173. Davies SC, Marcus RE, Hungerford JL, et al. Ocular toxicity of high dose intravenous desferrioxamine. *Lancet* 1983;ii:181–184.

1174. Borgna-Pignatti C, De Stefano P, Broglia AM. Visual loss in patient on high-dose subcutaneous desferrioxamine. *Lancet* 1984;i:681.

1175. Olivieri NF, Buncic JR, Chew E, et al. Visual and auditory neurotoxicity in patients receiving subcutaneous deferoxamine infusions. *N Engl J Med* 1986;314:869–873.

1176. Marsh MN, Holbrook IB, Clark C, et al. Tinnitus in a patient with beta-thalassaemia intermedia on long term treatment with desferrioxamine. *Postgrad Med J* 1981;57:582–584.

1177. Guerin A, London G, Marchais S, et al. Acute deafness and desferrioxamine. *Lancet* 1985;ii:39–40.

1178. Porter JB, East CA, Jaswon MS, et al. Audiometric abnormalities in thalassaemia: risk factor associated with the use of desferrioxamine. *Br J Haematol* 1988;69:88.

1179. Wonke B, Hoffbrand AV, Aldouri M, et al. Reversal of desferrioxamine induced auditory neurotoxicity during treatment with G-DTPA. *Arch Dis Child* 1989;6:77–82.

1180. Brill PW, Winchester P, Giardina PJ, et al. Desferrioxamine-induced bone dysplasia in patients with thalassemia major. *AJR Am J Roentgenol* 1991;156:561.

1181. Orxincolo C, Scutellari PN, Castaldi G. Growth plate injury of the long bones in treated β-thalassaemia. *Skeletal Radiol* 1992;21:39.

1182. Hartkamp MJ, Babyn PS, Olivieri NF. Spinal deformities in deferoxamine-treated beta-thalassemia major patients. *Pediatr Radiol* 1993;23:525.

1183. Sher GD, Belluzzo N, Babyn P, et al. Improvement in deferoxamine-induced bony abnormalities in transfusion-dependent patients following withdrawal or reduction of deferoxamine and initiation of the oral chelator. *Blood* 1993;82:360a.

1184. Chan YL, Li CK, Pang LM, et al. Desferrioxamine-induced long bone changes in thalassaemic patients: radiographic features, prevalence and relations with growth. *Clin Radiol* 2000;55:610–614.

1185. de Sanctis V, Stea S, Savarino L, et al. Osteochondrodystrophic lesions in chelated thalassemic patients: an histological analysis. *Calcif Tissue Int* 2000;67:134–140.

1186. Blake DR, Winyard P, Lunec J, et al. Cerebral and ocular toxicity induced by desferrioxamine. *QJM* 1985;56:345–355.

1187. Dickerhoff R. Acute aphasia and loss of vision with desferrioxamine overdose. *Am J Pediatr Hematol Oncol* 1987;9:287–288.

1188. Castriota Scanderbeg A, Izzi GC, Butturini A, et al. Pulmonary syndrome and intravenous high-dose desferrioxamine. *Lancet* 1990;336:1511.

1189. Tenenbein M, Kowalski S, Sienko A, et al. Pulmonary toxic effects of continuous desferrioxamine administration in acute iron poisoning. *Lancet* 1992;339:699.

1190. Boelaert JR, Vergauwe PL, Vandepitte JM. Mucormycosis infections in dialysis patients. *Ann Intern Med* 1987;107:782–783.

1191. Piga A, Magliano M, Bianco L, et al. Compliance with chelation therapy in Torino. Thalassaemia Today: Second Mediterranean Meeting on Thalassaemia, Milano, Italy, Policlinico di Malano, 1987.

1192. Zani B, Di Palma A, Vullo C. Psychosocial aspects of chronic illness in adolescents with thalassaemia major. *J Adolesc* 1995;18:387.

1193. Singer ST, Vichinsky EP. Deferoxamine treatment during pregnancy: is it harmful? *Am J Hematol* 1999;60:24–26.

1194. Muretto P, Del Fiasco S, Angelucci E, et al. Bone marrow transplantation in thalassemia: modifications of hepatic iron overload and associated lesions after long-term engrafting. *Liver* 1994;14:14–24.

1195. Lucarelli G, Angelucci E, Giardini C, et al. Fate of iron stores in thalassaemia after bone marrow transplantation. *Lancet* 1993;342:1388–1391.

1196. Angelucci E, Muretto P, Lucarelli G, et al. Phlebotomy to reduce iron overload in patients cured of thalassemia by bone marrow transplant. Italian Cooperative Group for Phlebotomy Treatment of Transplanted Thalassemia Patients. *Blood* 1997;90:994–998.

1197. Angelucci E, Muretto P, Lucarelli G, et al. Treatment of iron overload in the "ex-thalassemic": report from the phlebotomy program. *Ann N Y Acad Sci* 1998;850:288–293.

1198. Giardini C, Galimberti M, Lucarelli G, et al. Desferrioxamine therapy accelerates clearance of iron deposits after bone marrow transplantation for thalassaemia. *Br J Haematol* 1995;89:868–873.

1199. Giardini C, Lucarelli G. Bone marrow transplantation for beta-thalassemia. *Hematol Oncol Clin North Am* 1999;13:1059–1064.

1200. Li CK, Lai DH, Shing MM, et al. Early iron reduction programme for thalassaemia patients after bone marrow transplantation. *Bone Marrow Transplant* 2000;25:653–656.

1201. Katzos G, Papakostantinou-Athanasiadou E, Athanasiou-Metaxa M, et al. Growth hormone treatment in short children with beta-thalassemia major. *J Pediatr Endocrinol Metab* 2000;13:163–170.

1202. Kwan EY, Tam SC, Cheung PT, et al. The effect of 3 years of recombinant growth hormone therapy on glucose metabolism in short Chinese children with beta-thalassemia major. *J Pediatr Endocrinol Metab* 2000;13:545–552.

1203. Chatterjee R, Katz M, Wonke B, et al. Induction of puberty in patients with beta-thalassemia major. *Birth Defects: Original Articles Series* 1988;23:453–458.

1204. Chatterjee R, Katz M, Cox T, et al. Evaluation of growth hormone in thalassaemic boys with failed puberty: spontaneous versus provocative test. *Eur J Pediatr* 1993;152:721–726.

1205. Karvounis HI, Zaglavara TA, Parharidis GE, et al. An angiotensin-converting enzyme inhibitor improves left ventricular systolic and diastolic function in transfusion-dependent patients with beta-thalassemia major. *Am Heart J* 2001;141:281.

1206. Collins AF, Belluzzo N, Lewis N, et al. Osteopenia in young adults with homozygous beta thalassemia: persistence of an old problem. *Blood* 1993;82:358a.

1207. Canatan D, Akar N, Arcasoy A. Effects of calcitonin therapy on osteoporosis in patients with thalassemia. *Acta Haematol* 1995;93:20–24.

1208. Rachmilewitz EA, Shifter A, Kahane I. Vitamin E deficiency in β-thalassemia major: changes in hematological and biochemical parameters after a therapeutic trial with α-tocopherol. *Am J Clin Nutr* 1979;32:1850–1858.

1209. Di Marco V, Lo Iacono O, Almasio P, et al. Long-term efficacy of α-interferon in β-thalassemics with chronic hepatitis C. *Blood* 1997;90:2207–2212.

1210. Donohue SM, Wonke B, Hoffbrand AV, et al. Alpha interferon in the treatment of chronic hepatitis C infection in thalassaemia major. *Br J Haematol* 1993;83:491–497.

1211. Sherlock S. Antiviral therapy for chronic hepatitis C viral infection. *J Hepatol* 1995;23:3–7.

1212. Preston H, Wright TL. Interferon therapy for hepatitis C. *Lancet* 1996;348:973–974.

1213. Zeuzem S, Feinman SV, Rasenack J, et al. Peginterferon alfa-2a in patients with chronic hepatitis C. *N Engl J Med* 2000;343:1666–1672.

1214. Heathcote EJ, Shiffman ML, Cooksley WG, et al. Peginterferon alfa-2a in patients with chronic hepatitis C and cirrhosis. *N Engl J Med* 2000;343:1673–1680.

1215. Giardini C. Ethical issue of bone marrow transplantation for thalassemia. *Bone Marrow Transplant* 1995;15:657–658.

1216. Lucarelli G, Galimberti M, Polchi P, et al. Bone marrow transplantation in patients with thalassemia. *N Engl J Med* 1990;322:417–421.

1217. Lucarelli G, Giardini C, Baronciani D. Bone marrow transplantation in β-thalassemia. *Semin Hematol* 1995;32:297–303.

1218. Lucarelli G, Clift RA, Galimberti M, et al. Marrow transplantation for patients with thalassemia: results in class 3 patients. *Blood* 1996;87:2082–2088.

1219. Vellodi A, Picton S, Downie CJ, et al. Bone marrow transplantation for thalassaemia: experience of two British centres. *Bone Marrow Transplant* 1994;13:559–562.

1220. Walters MC, Sullivan KM, O'Reilly RJ, et al. Bone marrow transplantation for thalassemia: the USA experience. *Am J Pediatr Hematol Oncol* 1994;16:11–17.

1221. Clift RA, Johnson FL. Marrow transplants for thalassemia: the USA experience. *Bone Marrow Transplant* 1997;19[Suppl 2]:57–59.

1222. Roberts IAG, Darbyshire PJ, Will AM. B.M.T. for children with β-thalassemia major in the U.K. *Bone Marrow Transplant* 1997;19[Suppl 2]:60–61.

1223. Gaziev D, Polchi P, Galimberti M, et al. Graft-versus-host disease after bone marrow transplantation for thalassemia: an analysis of incidence and risk factors. *Transplantation* 1997;63:854–860.

1224. Mariotti E, Agostini A, Angelucci E, et al. Echocardiographic study in ex-thalassemic patients with iron overload, preliminary observations during phlebotomy therapy. *Bone Marrow Transplant* 1993;12:106–107.

1225. Mariotti E, Agostini A, Angelucci E, et al. Reversal of the initial cardiac damage in thalassemic patients treated with bone marrow transplantation and phlebotomy. *Bone Marrow Transplant* 1997;19[Suppl 2]:139–141.

1226. Mariotti E, Angelucci E, Agostini A, et al. Evaluation of cardiac status in iron-loaded thalassaemia patients following bone marrow transplantation:

improvement in cardiac function during reduction in body iron burden. *Br J Haematol* 1998;103:916–921.

1227. Kattamis AC, Antoniadis M, Manoli I, et al. Endocrine problems in ex-thalassemic patients. *Transfus Sci* 2000;23:251–252.

1228. Giardini C, Galimberti M, Lucarelli G, et al. Alpha-interferon treatment of chronic hepatitis C after bone marrow transplantation for homozygous beta-thalassemia. *Bone Marrow Transplant* 1997;20:767–772.

1229. Issaragrisil S, Visuthisakchai S, Suvatte V, et al. Brief report: transplantation of cord-blood stem cells into a patient with severe thalassemia. *N Engl J Med* 1995;332:367–369.

1230. Contu L, La Nasa G, Arras M, et al. Successful unrelated bone marrow transplantation in beta-thalassaemia. *Bone Marrow Transplant* 1994;13:329–331.

1231. Kottaridis PD, Peggs K, Lawrence A, et al. One antigen mismatched related donor bone marrow transplant in a patient with acute lymphoblastic leukaemia and beta-thalassaemia major: potential cure of both marrow disorders. *Bone Marrow Transplant* 2000;25:677–678.

1232. Westgren M, Ringden O, Eik-Nes S, et al. Lack of evidence of permanent engraftment after in utero fetal stem cell transplantation in congenital hemoglobinopathies. *Transplantation* 1996;61:1176–1179.

1233. Cowan MJ, Chou SH, Tarantal AF. Tolerance induction post in utero stem cell transplantation. *Ernst Schering Res Found Workshop* 2001;33:145–171.

1234. Goussetis E, Peristeri J, Kitra V, et al. Combined umbilical cord blood and bone marrow transplantation in the treatment of beta-thalassemia major. *Pediatr Hematol Oncol* 2000;17:307–314.

1235. Dragsten PR, Hallaway PE, Hanson GJ, et al. First human studies with a high-molecular-weight iron chelator. *J Lab Clin Med* 2000;135:57–65.

1236. Jensen PD, Jensen FT, Christensen T, et al. Evaluation of transfusional iron overload before and during iron chelation by magnetic resonance imaging of the liver and determination of serum ferritin in adult non-thalassaemic patients. *Br J Haematol* 1995;89:880–889.

1237. Borgna-Pignatti C, Cohen AR. An alternative method of subcutaneous deferoxamine administration. *Blood* 1996;86:483a.

1238. Franchini M, Gandini G, de Gironcoli M, et al. Safety and efficacy of subcutaneous bolus injection of deferoxamine in adult patients with iron overload. *Blood* 2000;95:2776–2779.

1239. Shalev O, Repka T, Goldfarb A, et al. Deferiprone (L1) chelates pathologic iron deposits from membranes of intact thalassemic and sickle red blood cells both in vitro and in vivo. *Blood* 1995;86:2008–2013.

1240. de Franceschi L, Shalev O, Piga A, et al. Deferiprone therapy in homozygous human beta-thalassemia removes erythrocyte membrane free iron and reduces KCl cotransport activity. *J Lab Clin Med* 1999;133:64–69.

1241. Hider RC, Kontoghiorghes GJ, Silver J. United Kingdom patent GB-2118176. 1982.

1242. Kontoghiorghes GJ, Bartlett AN, Hoffbrand AV, et al. Long-term trial with the oral iron chelator 1,2-dimethyl-3-hydroxypyrid-4-one (L1), I: iron chelation and metabolic studies. *Br J Haematol* 1990;76:295–300.

1243. Tondury P, Kontoghiorghes GJ, Ridolfi-Luthy AR, et al. L1 (1,2-dimethyl-3-hydroxypyrid-4-one) for oral iron chelation in patients with beta-thalassaemia major. *Br J Haematol* 1990;76:550–553.

1244. Olivieri NF, Koren G, Hermann C. Comparison of oral iron chelator L1 and desferrioxamine in iron-loaded patients. *Lancet* 1990;336:1275–1279.

1245. al-Refaie FN, Wonke B, Hoffbrand AV, et al. Efficacy and possible adverse effects of the oral iron chelator 1,2-dimethyl-3-hydroxypyrid-4-one (L1) in thalassemia major. *Blood* 1992;80:593–599.

1246. Agarwal MB, Gupte SS, Viswanathan C, et al. Long-term assessment of efficacy and safety of L1, an oral iron chelator, in transfusion-dependent thalassaemia: Indian trial. *Br J Haematol* 1992;82:460–466.

1247. al-Refaie FN, Hershko C, Hoffbrand AV, et al. Results of long-term deferiprone (L1) therapy: a report by the International Study Group on Oral Iron Chelators. *Br J Haematol* 1995;91:224–229.

1248. Olivieri NF, Brittenham GM, Matsui D, et al. Iron-chelation therapy with oral deferiprone in patients with thalassemia major. *N Engl J Med* 1995;332:918–922.

1249. Olivieri NF, Brittenham GM, McLaren CE, et al. Long-term safety and effectiveness of iron chelation therapy with deferiprone for thalassemia major. *N Engl J Med* 1998;339:417–423.

1250. Hoffbrand AV, al-Refaie F, Davis B, et al. Long-term trial of deferiprone in 51 transfusion-dependent iron overloaded patients. *Blood* 1998;91:295–300.

1251. Mazza P, Anurri B, Lazzari G, et al. Oral iron chelating therapy: a single center interim report on deferiprone (L1) in thalassemia. *Haematologica* 1998;83:496–501.

1252. Tondury P, Zimmermann A, Nielsen P, et al. Liver iron and fibrosis during long-term treatment with deferiprone in Swiss thalassaemic patients. *Br J Haematol* 1998;101:413–415.

1253. Taher A, Chamoun FM, Koussa S, et al. Efficacy and side effects of deferiprone (L1) in thalassemia patients not compliant with desferrioxamine. *Acta Haematol* 1999;101:173–177.

1254. Lucas GN, Perera BJ, Fonseka EA, et al. A trial of deferiprone in transfusion-dependent iron overloaded children. *Ceylon Med J* 2000;45:71–74.

1255. Del Vecchio GC, Crollo E, Schettini F, et al. Factors influencing effectiveness of deferiprone in a thalassaemia major clinical setting. *Acta Haematol* 2000;104:99–102.

1256. Berdoukas V, Bohane T, Eagle C, et al. The Sydney Children's Hospital experience with the oral iron chelator deferiprone (L1). *Transfus Sci* 2000;23:239–240.

1257. Rombos Y, Tzanetea R, Konstantopoulos K, et al. Chelation therapy in patients with thalassemia using the orally active iron chelator deferiprone (L1). *Haematologica* 2000;85:115–117.

1258. Cohen AR, Galanello R, Piga A, et al. Long-term safety of the oral iron chelator deferiprone. *Blood* 2000;96:443a.

1259. Cohen A, Galanello R, Piga A, et al. A multi-center safety trial of the oral iron chelator deferiprone. In: Cohen AR, ed. *Cooley's Anemia Seventh Symposium*, 850th vol. New York: New York Academy of Sciences, 1998:223–226.

1260. Cohen AR, Galanello R, Piga A, et al. Safety profile of the oral iron chelator deferiprone: a multicentre study. *Br J Haematol* 2000;108:305–312.

1261. Bonetta L. Inquiry into clinical trial scandal at Canadian research hospital. *Nat Med* 1998;4:1095.

1262. Birmingham K. Controversial HSC clinical trials report made public. Hospital for Sick Children. *Nat Med* 1999;5:7.

1263. Bonetta L. Canadian fight over thalassemia drug worsens. *Nat Med* 1999;5:1223.

1264. Nathan DG, Weatherall DJ. Academia and industry: lessons from the unfortunate events in Toronto. *Lancet* 1999;353:771–772.

1265. Birmingham K. Second HSC researcher sends anonymous "Olivieri" note. Hospital for Sick Children. *Nat Med* 2000;6:485.

1266. Birmingham K. No dismissal for hate-mail author. *Nat Med* 2000;6:609–610.

1267. Bonetta L. Hate-mail author trapped by DNA. *Nat Med* 2000;6:364.

1268. Bonetta L. Olivieri to testify against Apotex in Europe. *Nat Med* 2001;7:644.

1269. Pippard MJ, Weatherall DJ. Oral iron chelation therapy for thalassaemia: an uncertain scene. *Br J Haematol* 2000;111:2–5.

1270. Addis A, Loebstein R, Koren G, et al. Meta-analytic review of the clinical effectiveness of oral deferiprone (L1). *Eur J Clin Pharmacol* 1999;55:1–6.

1271. Olivieri NF, Brittenham GM. Final results of the randomized trial of deferiprone (L1) and deferoxamine (DFO). *Blood* 1997;90:264a.

1272. Collins AF, Fassos FF, Stobie S, et al. Iron-balance and dose-response studies of the oral iron chelator 1,2-dimethyl-3-hydroxypyrid-4-one (L1) in iron-loaded patients with sickle cell disease. *Blood* 1994;83:2329–2333.

1273. Grady RW, Berdoukas VA, Rachmilewitz EA, et al. Optimizing chelation therapy: combining deferiprone and desferroxamine. *Blood* 2000;96:604a.

1274. Wonke B, Wright C, Hoffbrand AV. Combined therapy with deferiprone and desferrioxamine. *Br J Haematol* 1998;103:361–364.

1275. Balveer K, Pyar K, Wonke B. Combined oral and parenteral iron chelation in beta thalassaemia major. *Med J Malaysia* 2000;55:493–497.

1276. Aydinok Y, Nisli G, Kavakli K, et al. Sequential use of deferiprone and desferrioxamine in primary school children with thalassaemia major in Turkey. *Acta Haematol* 1999;102:17–21.

1277. Brittenham GM. Development of iron-chelating agents for clinical use. *Blood* 1992;80:569–574.

1278. Porter JB. A risk-benefit assessment of iron-chelation therapy. *Drug Saf* 1997;17:407–421.

1279. Hoffbrand AV. Oral iron chelation. *Semin Hematol* 1996;33:1–8.

1280. Halliwell B. Drug antioxidant effects: a basis for drug selection? *Drugs* 1991;42:569–605.

1281. Motekitis RJ, Martell AE. Stabilization of the iron (III) chelates of 1,2-dimethyl-3-hydroxypyrid-4-ones and related ligands. *Inorg Chim Acta* 1991;183:71–80.

1282. Nathan DG. An orally active iron chelator. *N Engl J Med* 1995;332:953–954.

1283. Cragg L, Hebbel RP, Miller W, et al. The iron chelator L1 potentiates oxidative DNA damage in iron-loaded liver cells. *Blood* 1998;92:632–638.

1284. Hershko C, Link G, Pinson A, et al. Deferiprone fails to mobilize iron and promotes iron cardiotoxicity at suboptimal L1/iron concentrations. *Blood* 1997;90:11a.

1285. Carthew P, Smith AG, Hider RC, et al. Potentiation of iron accumulation in cardiac myocytes during the treatment of iron overload with the hydroxypyridinine iron chelator CP94. *Biometals* 1994;7:267–271.

1286. Hershko C, Link G, Konjin AM. Ability of deferiprone to protect tissues from non-transferrin-bound iron (NTBI) toxicity. 9th International Conference on Oral Chelation in the Treatment of Thalassemia and Other Diseases, Hamburg, 1999.

1287. Wong A, Alder V, Robertson D, et al. Liver iron depletion and toxicity of the iron chelator deferiprone (L1, CP20) in the guinea pig. *Biometals* 1997;10:247–256.

1288. Wanless IR, Sweeney G, Dhillon AP, et al. Absence of deferiprone-induced hepatic fibrosis: a multi-center study. *Blood* 2000;96:606a.

1289. Pippard MJ, Weatherall DJ. Deferiprone for thalassaemia. *Lancet* 2000;356:1444–1445.

1289a. Bonetta L. Olivieri to testify against Apotex in Europe. *Nat Med* 2001;7:644.

1290. Olivieri NF, Butany J, Templeton DM, et al. Cardiac failure and myocardial fibrosis in a patient with thalassemia major (TM) treated with long-term deferiprone. *Blood* 1998;92:532a.

1291. Cao A, Rosatelli C, Pirastu M, et al. Thalassemias in Sardinia: molecular pathology, phenotype-genotype correlation and prevention. *Am J Pediatr Hematol Oncol* 1991;13:179–188.

1292. Olivieri NF, Weatherall DJ. The therapeutic reactivation of fetal haemoglobin. *Hum Mol Genet* 1998;7:1655–1658.

1293. Swank RA, Stamatoyannopoulos G. Fetal gene reactivation. *Curr Opin Genet Dev* 1998;8:366–370.

1294. Olivieri NF. Reactivation of fetal hemoglobin in patients with β thalassemia. *Semin Hematol* 1996;33:24–42.

1295. Arruda VR, Lima CS, Saad ST, et al. Successful use of hydroxyurea in beta-thalassemia major. *N Engl J Med* 1997;336:964.

1296. Nienhuis AW, Ley TJ, Humphries RK, et al. Pharmacological manipulation of fetal hemoglobin synthesis in patients with severe beta thalassemia. *Ann N Y Acad Sci* 1985;445:198–211.

1297. McDonagh KT, Orringer EP, Dover GJ, et al. Hydroxyurea improves erythropoiesis in a patient with homozygous beta thalassemia. *Clin Res* 1990;38:346A.

1298. Hajjar FM, Pearson HA. Pharmacologic treatment of thalassemia intermedia with hydroxyurea. *J Pediatr* 1994;125:490–492.

1299. Huang SZ, Ren ZR, Chen MJ, et al. Treatment of beta-thalassemia with hydroxyurea (HU)—effects of HU on globin gene expression. *Sci China B* 1994;37:1350–1359.

1300. Cohen AR, Martin MB, Schwartz E. Hydroxyurea therapy in thalassemia intermedia. In: Beuzard Y, Lubin B, Rosa J, eds. *Sickle cell disease and thalassemia: new trends in therapy*, 234th vol. Colloque INSERM, 1995:193–194.

1301. Bachir D, Drame M, Lee K, et al. Clinical effects of hydroxyurea in thalassemia intermedia patients. In: Beuzard Y, Lubin B, Rosa J, eds. *Sickle cell disease and thalassemia: new trends in therapy*, 234th vol. Colloque INSERM, 1995:195.

1302. Zeng YT, Huang SZ, Ren ZR, et al. Hydroxyurea therapy in β-thalassaemia intermedia: improvement in haematological parameters due to enhanced β-globin synthesis. *Br J Haematol* 1995;90:557–563.

1303. Fucharoen S, Siritanaratkul N, Winichagoon P, et al. Hydroxyurea increases hemoglobin F levels and improves the effectiveness of erythropoiesis in beta-thalassemia/hemoglobin E disease. *Blood* 1996;87:887–892.

1304. Rigano P, Manfre L, La Galla R, et al. Clinical and hematological response to hydroxyurea in a patient with Hb Lepore/beta-thalassemia. *Hemoglobin* 1997;21:219–226.

1305. Perrine SP, Greene MF, Faller DV. Delay in the fetal globin switch in infants of diabetic mothers. *N Engl J Med* 1985;312:334–338.

1306. Perrine SP, Ginder GD, Faller DV, et al. A short-term trial of butyrate to stimulate fetal-globin-gene expression in the β-globin disorders. *N Engl J Med* 1993;328:81–86.

1307. Sher GD, Ginder G, Little JA, et al. Extended therapy with arginine butyrate in patients with thalassemia and sickle cell disease. *N Engl J Med* 1995;332:106–110.

1308. Atweh GF, Dover GJ, Faller G, et al. Sustained hematologic response to pulse butyrate therapy in beta globin disorders. *Blood* 1996;88[Suppl]:652a.

1309. Dover GJ, Charache SC, Brusilow SW. Sodium phenylbutyrate increases fetal hemoglobin production in patients with sickle cell disease. *Blood* 1992;80[Suppl 1]:73A(abst).

1310. Dover GJ, Brusilow S, Charache S. Induction of fetal hemoglobin production in subjects with sickle cell anemia by oral sodium phenylbutyrate. *Blood* 1994;84:339–343.

1311. Collins AF, Pearson HA, Giardina P, et al. Oral sodium phenylbutyrate therapy in homozygous beta thalassemia: a clinical trial. *Blood* 1995;85:43–49.

1312. Alter BP, Rappeport JM, Huisman THJ, et al. Fetal erythropoiesis following bone marrow transplantation. *Blood* 1976;48:843.

1313. Sheridan BL, Weatherall DJ, Clegg JB, et al. The patterns of fetal haemoglobin production in leukaemia. *Br J Haematol* 1976;32:487.

1314. De Simone J, Biel SI, Heller P. Stimulation of fetal hemoglobin synthesis in baboons by hemolysis and hypoxia. *Proc Natl Acad Sci U S A* 1978;75:2937–2940.

1315. Cappellini MD, Graziadei G, Ciceri L, et al. Butyrate trials. *Ann N Y Acad Sci* 1998;850:110–119.

1316. Reich S, Buhrer C, Henze G, et al. Oral isobutyramide reduces transfusion requirements in some patients with homozygous beta-thalassemia [in process citation]. *Blood* 2000;96:3357–3363.

1317. Papayannopoulou T, Brice M, Stamatoyannopoulos G. Hemoglobin F synthesis in vitro: evidence for control at the level of primitive erythroid stem cells. *Proc Natl Acad Sci U S A* 1977;74:2923–2927.

1318. Al-Khatti A, Veith RA, Papayannopoulou T, et al. Stimulation of fetal hemoglobin synthesis by erythropoietin in baboons. *N Engl J Med* 1987;317:415–420.

1319. Al-Khatti A, Papayannopoulou T, Knitter G, et al. Cooperative enhancement of F-cell formation in baboons treated with erythropoietin and hydroxyurea. *Blood* 1988;72:817–819.

1320. Leroy-Viard K, Rouyer-Fessard P, Beuzard Y. Improvement of mouse beta-thalassemia by recombinant human erythropoietin. *Blood* 1991;78:1596–1602.

1321. Rachmilewitz EA, Goldfarb A, Dover G. Administration of erythropoietin to patients with β-thalassemia intermedia: a preliminary trial. *Blood* 1991;78:1145–1147.

1322. Olivieri NF, Freedman M, Perrine S, et al. Trial of recombinant human erythropoietin in thalassemia intermedia. *Blood* 1992;80:3258–3260.

1323. Aker M, Kapelushnik J, Pugatsch T, et al. Donor lymphocyte infusions to displace residual host hematopoietic cells after allogeneic bone marrow transplantation for beta-thalassemia major. *J Pediatr Hematol Oncol* 1998;20:145–148.

1324. Loukopoulos D, Voskaridou E, Stamoulakatou A. Clinical trials with hydroxyurea and recombinant human erythropoietin. In: Stamatoyannopoulos G, ed. *Hemoglobin switching*. New York: Alan R. Liss, 1995:365–372.

1325. Papayannopoulou T, Torrealba-de-Ron A, Veith R, et al. Arabinosylcytosine induces fetal hemoglobin in baboons by perturbing erythroid cell differentiation kinetics. *Science* 1984;224:617–619.

1326. Veith R, Galanello R, Papayannopoulou T, et al. Stimulation of F-cell production in patients with sickle-cell anemia treated with cytarabine or hydroxyurea. *N Engl J Med* 1985;313:1571–1575.

1327. Torrealba-de Ron AT, Papayannopoulou T, Knapp MS, et al. Perturbations in the erythroid marrow progenitor cell pools may play a role in the augmentation of HbF by 5-azacytidine. *Blood* 1984;63:201–210.

1328. Ley TJ, DeSimone J, Noguchi CT, et al. 5-Azacytidine increases gamma-globin synthesis and reduces the proportion of dense cells in patients with sickle cell anemia. *Blood* 1983;62:370–380.

1329. Ley TJ, DeSimone J, Anagnou NP, et al. 5-Azacytidine selectively increases gamma-globin synthesis in a patient with beta+ thalassemia. *N Engl J Med* 1982;307:1469–1475.

1330. Constantoulakis P, Knitter G, Stamatoyannopoulos G. On the induction of fetal hemoglobin by butyrates: in vivo and in vitro studies with sodium butyrate and comparison of combination treatments with 5-AzaC and AraC. *Blood* 1989;74:1963–1971.

1331. McDonagh KT, Dover GJ, Donahue RE, et al. Hydroxyurea-induced HbF production in anemic primates: augmentation by erythropoietin, hematopoietic growth factors, and sodium butyrate. *Exp Hematol* 1992;20:1156–1164.

1332. Olivieri NF, Rees DC, Ginder GD, et al. Treatment of thalassaemia major with phenylbutyrate and hydroxyurea. *Lancet* 1997;350:491–492.

1333. Olivieri NF, Rees DC, Ginder GD, et al. Elimination of transfusions through induction of fetal hemoglobin synthesis in Cooley's anemia. *Ann N Y Acad Sci* 1998;850:100–109.

1334. Van der Ploeg LH, Konings A, Oort M, et al. gamma-beta-Thalassaemia studies showing that deletion of the gamma- and delta-genes influences beta-globin gene expression in man. *Nature* 1980;283:637–642.

1335. DeSimone J, Heller P, Hall L, et al. 5-Azacytidine stimulates fetal hemoglobin synthesis in anemic baboons. *Proc Natl Acad Sci U S A* 1982;79:4428–4431.

1336. Humphries RK, Dover G, Young NS, et al. 5-Azacytidine acts directly on both erythroid precursors and progenitors to increase production of fetal hemoglobin. *J Clin Invest* 1985;75:547–557.

1337. Galanello R, Stamatoyannopoulos G, Papayannopoulou T. Mechanism of Hb F stimulation by S-stage compounds: in vitro studies with bone marrow cells exposed to 5-azacytidine, Ara-C, or hydroxyurea. *J Clin Invest* 1988;81:1209–1216.

1338. Ginder GD, Whitters MJ, Pohlman JK. Activation of a chicken embryonic globin gene in adult erythroid cells by 5-azacytidine and sodium butyrate. *Proc Natl Acad Sci U S A* 1984;81:3954–3958.

1339. Pace B, Li Q, Peterson K, et al. alpha-Amino butyric acid cannot reactivate the silenced gamma gene of the beta locus YAC transgenic mouse. *Blood* 1994;84:4344–4353.

1340. Thumasathit B, Nondasuta A, Silpisornkosol S, et al. Hydrops fetalis associated with Bart's hemoglobin in northern Thailand. *J Pediatr* 1968;73:132–138.

1341. Liang ST, Wong VCW, So WWK, et al. Homozygous α-thalassaemia: clinical presentation, diagnosis and management: a review of 46 cases. *Br J Obstet Gynaecol* 1985;92:680–684.

1342. Vaeusorn O, Fucharoen S, Ruangpiroj T, et al. Fetal pathology and maternal morbidity in hemoglobin Bart's hydrops fetalis: an analysis of 65 cases. International Conference on Thalassemia, Bangkok, Thailand, 1985.

1343. Nakayama R, Yamada D, Steinmiller V, et al. Hydrops fetalis secondary to Bart hemoglobinopathy. *Obstet Gynecol* 1986;67:176–180.

1344. Chui DHK, Waye JS. Hydrops fetalis caused by α-thalassemia: an emerging health care problem. *Blood* 1998;91:2213–2222.

1345. Israngkura P, Siripoonya P, Fucharoen S, et al. Hemoglobin Barts disease without hydrops manifestation. *Birth Defects: Original Articles Series* 1987;23:333–342.

1346. Wong HB. Haemoglobinopathies in Singapore: the first Haridas Memorial Lecture. Singapore: Stamford College Press, 1966.

1347. Wasi P, Na-Nakorn S, Pootrakul S, et al. Alpha- and beta-thalassemia in Thailand. *Ann N Y Acad Sci* 1969;165:60.

1348. Wasi P, Na-Nakorn S. The alpha thalassemia. *Clin Haematol (Oxf)* 1974;3:383.

1349. Lie-Injo LE, Jo BH. Hydrops foetalis with a fast-moving haemoglobin. *BMJ* 1960;ii:1649.

1350. Lie-Injo LE, Jo BH. A fast moving haemoglobin in hydrops foetalis. *Nature* 1960;185:698.

1351. Weatherall DJ, Clegg JB, Boon WH. The haemoglobin constitution of infants with the haemoglobin Bart's hydrops foetalis syndrome. *Br J Haematol* 1970;18:357–367.

1352. Todd D, Lai MCS, Beaven GH, et al. The abnormal haemoglobins in homozygous α-thalassaemia. *Br J Haematol* 1970;19:27–31.

1353. Lam YH, Tang MHY. Prenatal diagnosis of haemoglobin Bart's disease by cordocentesis at 12-14 weeks' gestation. *Prenat Diagn* 1997;17:501–504.

1354. Guy G, Coady DJ, Jansen V, et al. α-Thalassemia hydrops fetalis: clinical and ultrasonographic considerations. *Am J Obstet Gynecol* 1985;153:500–504.

1355. Carr S, Rubin L, Dixon D, et al. Intrauterine therapy for homozygous α-thalassemia. *Obstet Gynecol* 1995;85:876–879.

1356. Harmon JV, Osathanondh R, Holmes LB. Symmetrical terminal transverse limb defects: report of twenty-week fetus. *Teratology* 1995;51:237–242.

1357. Abuelo DN, Forman EN, Rubin LP. Limb defects and congenital anomalies of the genitalia in an infant with homozygous α-thalassemia. *Am J Med Genet* 1997;68:158–161.

1358. Chitayat D, Silver MM, O'Brien K, et al. Limb defects in homozygous α-thalassemia: report of three cases. *Am J Med Genet* 1997;68:162–167.

1359. Ongsangkoon T, Vawesorn O, Pootakul S-N. Pathology of hemoglobin Bart's hydrops fetalis, I: gross autopsy findings. *J Med Assoc Thai* 1978;61:71.

1360. Weatherall DJ, Clegg JB. *The thalassaemia syndromes*. Oxford: Blackwell Science, 1981.

1361. Wasi P. Hemoglobinopathies in Southeast Asia. In: Bowman JE, ed. *Distribution and evolution of the hemoglobin and globin loci*. New York: Elsevier, 1983: 179–209.

1362. Wong HB. Thalassemias in Singapore. *J Singapore Paediatr Soc* 1984;26:1–14.

1363. Kattamis C, Tzotzos S, Kanavakis E, et al. Correlation of clinical phenotype to genotype in haemoglobin H disease. *Lancet* 1988;i:442–444.

1364. George E, Ferguson V, Yakas J, et al. A molecular marker associated with mild hemoglobin H disease. *Pathology* 1989;21:27–30.

1365. Galanello R, Aru B, Dessi C, et al. HbH disease in Sardinia: molecular, hematological and clinical aspects. *Acta Haematol* 1992;88:1–6.

1366. Styles L, Foote DH, Kleman KM, et al. Hemoglobin H-Constant Spring disease: an under recognized, severe form of α thalassemia. *Int J Pediatr Hematol Oncol* 1997;4:69–74.

1367. Chen FE, Ooi C, Ha SY, et al. Genetic and clinical features of hemoglobin H disease in Chinese patients. *N Engl J Med* 2000;343:544–550.

1368. Fucharoen S, Winichagoon P. Hemoglobinopathies in Southeast Asia: molecular biology and clinical medicine. *Hemoglobin* 1997;21:299–319.

1369. Daneshmend TK, Peachey RD. Leg ulcers in α thalassaemia (haemoglobin H disease). *Br J Dermatol* 1978;98:233.

1370. Piankijagum A, Palungwachira P, Lohkoomgunpai A. Beta thalassemia, hemoglobin E and hemoglobin H disease: clinical analysis 1964-1966. *J Med Assoc Thai* 1978;61:50.

1371. Schrier SL, Bunyaratvej A, Khuhapinant A, et al. The unusual pathobiology of hemoglobin Constant Spring red blood cells. *Blood* 1997;89:1762–1769.

1372. Wasi P, Pravatmuang P, Winichagoon P. Immunologic diagnosis of α-thalassemia traits. *Hemoglobin* 1979;3:21–31.

1373. Kanavakis E, Papassotiriou I, Karagiorga M, et al. Phenotypic and molecular diversity of haemoglobin H disease: a Greek experience. *Br J Haematol* 2000;111:915–923.

1374. O'Brien RT. The effect of iron deficiency on the expression of hemoglobin H. *Blood* 1973;41:853–856.

1375. Tso SC, Chan TK, Todd D. Venous thrombosis in haemoglobin H disease after splenectomy. *Aust N Z J Med* 1982;12:635–638.

1376. Tso SC, Loh TT, Todd D. Iron overload in patients with haemoglobin H disease. *Scand J Haematol* 1984;32:391–394.

1377. Chim CS, Chan V, Todd D. Hemosiderosis with diabetes mellitus in untransfused hemoglobin H disease. *Am J Hematol* 1998;57:160–163.

1378. Lin CK, Peng HW, Ho CH, et al. Iron overload in untransfused patients with hemoglobin H disease. *Acta Haematol (Basel)* 1990;83:137–139.

1379. Winichagoon P, Adirojnanon P, Wasi P. Levels of haemoglobin H and proportions of red cells with inclusion bodies in the two types of haemoglobin H disease. *Br J Haematol* 1980;46:507–509.

1380. Higgs DR. α-Thalassaemia. *Bailliere's Clin Haematol* 1993;6:117.

1381. Higgs DR, Vickers MA, Wilkie AO, et al. A review of the molecular genetics of the human alpha-globin gene cluster. *Blood* 1989;73:1081–1104.

1382. Higgs DR, Pressley L, Aldridge B, et al. Genetic and molecular diversity in nondeletion HbH disease. *Proc Natl Acad Sci U S A* 1981;78:5833–5837.

1383. Weatherall DJ, Higgs DR, Bunch C, et al. Hemoglobin H disease and mental retardation: a new syndrome or a remarkable coincidence? *N Engl J Med* 1981;305:607–612.

1384. Wilkie AO, Zeitlin HC, Lindenbaum RH, et al. Clinical features and molecular analysis of the alpha thalassemia/mental retardation syndromes, II: cases without detectable abnormality of the alpha globin complex. *Am J Hum Genet* 1990;46:1127–1140.

1385. Wilkie AOM, Zeitlin HC, Lindenbaum RH, et al. Clinical features and molecular analysis of the α thalassemia/mental retardation syndromes, II: cases without detectable abnormality of the α globin complex. *Am J Hum Genet* 1990;46:1127–1140.

1386. Gibbons RJ, Picketts DJ, Villard L, et al. Mutations in a putative global transcriptional regulator cause X-linked mental retardation with alpha-thalassemia (ATR-X syndrome). *Cell* 1995;80:837–845.

1387. Gibbons RJ, Wilkie AO, Weatherall DJ, et al. A newly defined X linked mental retardation syndrome associated with alpha thalassaemia. *J Med Genet* 1991;28:729–733.

1388. Wilkie AOM, Pembrey ME, Gibbons RJ, et al. The non-deletion type of α thalassaemia/mental retardation: a recognisable dysmorphic syndrome with X-linked inheritance. *J Med Genet* 1991;28:724.

1389. Donnai D, Clayton-Smith J, Gibbons RJ, et al. α Thalassaemia/Mental retardation syndrome (non-deletion type): report of a family supporting X linked inheritance. *J Med Genet* 1991;28:734–737.

1390. Gibbons RJ, Suthers GK, Wilkie AO, et al. X-linked alpha-thalassaemia/mental retardation (ATR-X) syndrome: localization to Xq12-q21.31 by X inactivation and linkage analysis. *Am J Hum Genet* 1992;51:1136–1149.

1391. Guerrini R, Shanahan JL, Carrozzo R, et al. A nonsense mutation of the *ATRX* gene causing mild mental retardation and epilepsy. *Ann Neurol* 2000;47:117.

1392. Gibbons RJ, Picketts DJ, Higgs DR. Syndromal mental retardation due to mutations in a regulator of gene expression. *Hum Mol Genet* 1995;4:1705–1709.

1393. Gibbons RJ, Brueton L, Buckle VJ, et al. Clinical and hematologic aspects of the X-linked alpha-thalassemia/mental retardation syndrome (ATR-X). *Am J Med Genet* 1995;55:288–299.

1394. McPherson E, Clemens M, Gibbons RJ, et al. X-linked alpha thalassemia/mental retardation (ATR-X) syndrome: a new kindred with severe genital anomalies and mild hematologic expression. *Am J Med Genet* 1995;55:302–306.

1395. Lefort G, Taib J, Toutain A, et al. X-linked α-thalassemia/mental retardation (ATR-X) syndrome: report of three male patients in a large French family. *Ann Genet* 1993;36:200–205.

1396. Aasland R, Gibson TJ, Stewart AF. The PHD finger: implications for chromatin-mediated transcriptional regulation. *Trends Biol Sci* 1995;20:56–59.

1397. Picketts DJ, Higgs DR, Bachoo S, et al. *ATRX* encodes a novel member of the SNF2 family of proteins: mutations point to a common mechanism underlying the ATR-X syndrome. *Hum Mol Genet* 1996;5:1899–1907.

1398. Gibbons RJ, Bachoo S, Picketts DJ, et al. Mutations in transcriptional regulator ATRX establish the functional significance of a PHD-like domain. *Nat Genet* 1997;17:146–148.

1399. Craddock CF. Normal and abnormal regulation of human α globin expression. Oxford: University of Oxford, 1994.

1400. Weatherall DJ, Old J, Longley J, et al. Acquired haemoglobin H disease in leukaemia: pathophysiology and molecular basis. *Br J Haematol* 1978;38:305–322.

1401. Higgs DR, Wood WG, Barton C, et al. Clinical features and molecular analysis of acquired hemoglobin H disease. *Am J Med* 1983;75:181–191.

1402. Higgs DR, Weatherall DJ. The haemoglobinopathies. *Clin Haematol (Oxf)* 1993;6:1–331.

1403. Higgs DR, Sharpe JA, Wood WG. Understanding α globin gene expression: a step towards effective gene therapy. *Semin Hematol* 1998;35:93–104.

1404. Wood WG, Weatherall DJ, Clegg JB. Interaction of heterocellular hereditary persistence of foetal haemoglobin with β thalassaemia and sickle cell anaemia. *Nature* 1976;264:247–249.

1405. Khanh NC, Thu LT, Truc DB, et al. Beta-thalassemia/haemoglobin E disease in Vietnam. *J Trop Pediatr* 1990;36:43–45.

1406. Vella F. The incidence of abnormal haemoglobin variants in Singapore and Malays. *Indian J Child Health* 1958;7:804–808.

1407. Bolton JM, Eng L-IL. Hb E-beta thalassaemia in the West Malaysian Oran Asli (aborigines). *Med J Malaysia* 1969;24:36–40.

1408. Punt K, Van Gool J. Thalassaemia-haemoglobin E disease in two Indo-European boys. *Acta Haematol* 1957;17:305.

1409. Lie-Injo LE. Haemoglobin of newborn infants in Indonesia. *Nature* 1959;183:1125–1126.

1410. Oman H, Wiradisuria S. Thalassemia and Hb E thalassemia in Bandung. *Paediatr Indones* 1969;9:269.

1411. Lehmann H, Story P, Thein H. Hemoglobin E in Burmese. *BMJ* 1956;i:544.

1412. Aung-Than-Batu, Hla-Pe U. Haemoglobinopathies in Burma, I: the incidence of haemoglobin E. *Trop Geogr Med* 1971;23:15–19.

1413. Chatterjea JB. Haemoglobinopathies, glucose-6-phosphate dehydrogenase deficiency and allied problems in the Indian sub-continent. *Bull World Health Organ* 1966;35:837–856.

1414. Saha N, Banerjee B. Haemoglobinopathies in the Indian sub-continent. *Acta Genet Med Gemellol (Roma)* 1973;22:117–138.

1415. Agarwal S, Gulati R, Singh K. Hemoglobin E-beta thalassemia in Uttar Pradesh. *Indian Pediatr* 1997;34:287–292.

1416. Fucharoen S, Winichagoon P. Clinical and hematologic aspects of hemoglobin E beta-thalassemia. *Curr Opin Hematol* 2000;7:106–112.

1417. de Silva S, Fisher CA, Premawardhena A, et al. Thalassaemia in Sri Lanka: implications for the future health burden of Asian populations. Sri Lanka Thalassaemia Study Group. *Lancet* 2000;355:786–791.

1418. de Silva S, Fisher CA, Premawardhena A, et al. Thalassaemia in Sri Lanka: implications for the future health burden of Asian populations. *Lancet* 2000;355:786–791.

1419. Orkin SH, Kazazian HH Jr, Antonarakis SE, et al. Abnormal RNA processing due to the exon mutation of beta E-globin gene. *Nature* 1982;300:768–769.

1420. Yuthavong Y, Ruenwongsa P, Benyajati C, et al. Studies on the structural stability of haemoglobin E. *J Med Assoc Thai* 1975;58:351.

1421. Fairbanks VF, Oliveros R, Brandabur JH, et al. Homozygous hemoglobin E mimics β-thalassemia minor without anemia or hemolysis: hematologic, functional, and biosynthetic studies of first North American cases. *Am J Hematol* 1980;8:109–121.

1422. Fairbanks VF, Gilchrist GS, Brimhall B, et al. Hemoglobin E trait reexamined: a cause of microcytosis and erythrocytosis. *Blood* 1979;53:109–115.

1423. Wong SC, Ali MAM. Hemoglobin E diseases: hematological, analytical, and biosynthetic studies in homozygotes and double heterozygotes for α-thalassemia. *Am J Hematol* 1982;13:15–21.

1424. Pagnier J, Wajcman H, Labie D. Defect in hemoglobin synthesis possibly due to a disturbed association. *FEBS Lett* 1974;45:252.

1425. Traeger J, Wood WG, Clegg JB, et al. Defective synthesis of Hb E is due to reduced levels of βE mRNA. *Nature* 1980;288:497–499.

1426. Wasi P, Pootrakul P, Fucharoen S, et al. Thalassemia in Southeast Asia: determination of different degrees of severity of anemia in thalassemia^α. *Ann N Y Acad Sci* 1985;445:119–126.

1427. Winichagoon P, Thonglairoam V, Fucharoen S, et al. Severity differences in β-thalassaemia haemoglobin E syndromes: implication of genetic factors. *Br J Haematol* 1993;83:633–639.

1428. Kalpravidh RW, Komolvanich S, Wilairat P, et al. Globin chain turnover in reticulocytes from patients with β⁰-thalassaemia/Hb E disease. *Eur J Haematol* 1995;55:322–326.

1429. Rees DC, Styles J, Vichinsky EP, et al. The hemoglobin E syndromes. *Ann N Y Acad Sci* 1998;850:334–343.

1430. Fucharoen S, Ketvichit P, Pootrakul P, et al. Clinical manifestation of beta-thalassemia/hemoglobin E disease. *J Pediatr Hematol Oncol* 2000;22:552–557.

1431. Fucharoen S, Winichagoon P, Pootrakul P, et al. Determination for different severity of anemia in thalassemia: concordance and discordance among sib pairs. *Am J Med Genet* 1984;19:39–44.

1432. Chernoff AI, Minnich V, Na-Nakorn S, et al. Studies on hemoglobin E, I: the clinical, hematologic, and genetic characteristics of the hemoglobin E syndromes. *J Lab Clin Med* 1956;47:455–498.

1433. Fucharoen S, Winichagoon P, Thonglairuam V, et al. EF Bart's disease: interaction of the abnormal alpha- and beta-globin genes. *Eur J Haematol* 1988;40:75–78.

1434. Wickramasinghe SN, Lee MJ. Observations on the relationship between γ-globin chain content and globin chain precipitation in thalassaemic erythroblasts and on the composition of erythroblastic inclusions in Hb E/β-thalassaemia. *Eur J Haematol* 1997;59:305–309.

1435. Swarup S, Chatterjea JB, Ghosh SK, et al. Observations on erythropoiesis in Hb E-thalassaemia disease: a study with Cr[51] and Fe[59]. *Indian J Pathol Bacteriol* 1961;4:1.
1436. Feldman R, Rieder RF. The interaction of hemoglobin E with beta thalassemias: a study of hemoglobin synthesis in a family of mixed Burmese and Iranian origin. *Blood* 1973;42:783.
1437. Chatterjea JB. Haemoglobinopathy in India. In: Jonxis JHP, Delafresnaye JF, eds. *Abnormal haemoglobins*. Oxford: Blackwell Science, 1959:322–339.
1438. Weatherall DJ. Hemoglobin E β-thalassemia: an increasingly common disease with some diagnostic pitfalls. *J Pediatr* 1998;132:765–767.
1439. Rakshit MM, Chatterjea JB, Mitra SS. Observations on the intraerythrocytic distribution of foetal haemoglobin in Hb E-thalassaemia disease. *Indian J Pathol Bacteriol* 1973;16:41.
1440. Testa U, Dubart A, Hinard N, et al. Beta⁰-thalassaemia/Hb E association: hemoglobin synthesis in blood reticulocytes and bone marrow cells fractionated by density gradient and in blood erythroid colonies in culture. *Acta Haematol* 1980;64:42–52.
1441. De Silva CC, Jonxis JHP, Wickramasinghe RL. Haemoglobinopathies in Ceylon. In: Jonxis JHP, Delafresnaye JF, eds. *Abnormal haemoglobins*. Oxford: Blackwell Science, 1959:340.
1442. Israngkura P, Hathirat P, Sanaskul W, et al. The relationship of growth rate and hemoglobin level in thalassemia. *J Med Assoc Thai* 1978;61:51.
1443. Israngkura P, Khemapiratana T, Tuchinda P. Bone age and bone changes in thalassemia. *J Med Assoc Thai* 1978;61:53.
1444. Tanphaichitr V, Suvatte V, Mahasandana C, et al. Host defense in thalassemias and the effects of splenectomy, I: incidence of mild and severe infections. *J Med Assoc Thai* 1978;61:66.
1445. Aswapokee N, Aswapokee P, Fucharoen S, et al. A study of infective episodes in patients with β-thalassemia/Hb E disease in Thailand. *Birth Defects: Original Articles Series* 1988;23:513–520.
1446. Aswapokee P, Aswapokee N, Fucharoen S, et al. Severe infection in thalassemia: a prospective study. *Birth Defects: Original Articles Series* 1988;23:521–526.
1447. Issaragrisil S, Wanachinwanawin W, Bhuripanyo K, et al. Infection in thalassemia: a retrospective study of 1,018 patients with β-thalassemia/Hb E disease. *Birth Defects: Original Articles Series* 1988;23:505–511.
1448. Wasi C, Kuntang R, Louisirirotchananakul S, et al. Viral infections in β-thalassemia/hemoglobin E patients. *Birth Defects: Original Articles Series* 1988;23:547–555.
1449. De Costa JL, Loh YS, Hanam E. Extramedullary hemopoiesis with multiple tumor-stimulating mediastinal masses in hemoglobin E-thalassemia. *Chest* 1974;65:210.
1450. Fucharoen S, Suthipongchai S, Poungvarin N, et al. Intracranial extramedullary hematopoiesis inducing epilepsy in a patient with beta-thalassemia—hemoglobin E. *Arch Intern Med* 1985;145:739–742.
1451. Mihindukulasuriya JC, Chanmugam D, Machado V, et al. A case of paraparesis due to extramedullary haemopoiesis in Hb E thalassaemia. *Postgrad Med J* 1977;53:393.
1452. Fucharoen S, Tunthanavatana C, Sonakul D, et al. Intracranial extramedullary hematopoiesis in beta-thalassemia/hemoglobin E disease. *Am J Hematol* 1981;10:75–78.
1453. Intragumtornchai T, Arjhansiri K, Posayachinda M, et al. Obstructive uropathy due to extramedullary haematopoiesis in β thalassaemia/haemoglobin E. *Postgrad Med J* 1993;69:75–77.
1454. Vatanavicharn S, Anuwatanakulchai M, Tuntawiroon M, et al. Iron absorption in patients with β-thalassaemia/haemoglobin E disease and the effect of splenectomy. *Acta Haematol* 1983;69:414–416.
1455. Fouladi M, Macmillan ML, Nisbet-Brown E, et al. Hemoglobin E/beta thalassemia: the Canadian experience. *Ann N Y Acad Sci* 1998;850:410–411.
1456. Anuwatanakulchia M, Pootrakul P, Thuvasethakul P, et al. Non-transferrin plasma iron in β-thalassaemia/Hb E and haemoglobin H diseases. *Scand J Haematol* 1984;32:153.
1457. Thakerngpol K, Fucharoen S, Sumiyoshi A, et al. Liver tissue injury secondary to iron overload in beta-thalassemia/hemoglobin E disease. *Southeast Asian J Trop Med Public Health* 1992;23:110–115.
1458. Mitra R, Sarkar S, Ganguli S, et al. Haemochromatosis in a case of thalassaemia haemoglobin E disease. *J Indian Med Assoc* 1996;94:29–30.
1459. Olivieri NF, De Silva S, Premawardena A, et al. Iron overload and iron-chelating therapy in hemoglobin E-beta thalassemia. *J Pediatr Hematol Oncol* 2000;22:593–597.
1460. Bhamapravati N, Na-Nakorn S, Wasi P, et al. Pathology of abnormal hemoglobin diseases seen in Thailand, I: pathology of beta-thalassemia hemoglobin E disease. *Am J Clin Pathol* 1967;47:745–758.
1461. Sonakul D, Sook-aneak M, Pacharee P. Pathology of thalassemic diseases in Thailand. *J Med Assoc Thai* 1978;61:72.
1462. Sonakul D, Pacharee P, Wasi P, et al. Cardiac pathology in 47 patients with beta thalassaemia/haemoglobin E. *Southeast Asian J Trop Med Public Health* 1984;15:554–563.
1463. Sonakul D. *Pathology of thalassemic diseases*. Thailand: Amarin Printing Group, 1989.
1464. Sonakul D, Pacharee P, Laohapand T, et al. Pulmonary artery obstruction in thalassaemia. *Southeast Asian J Trop Med Public Health* 1980;11:516–523.
1465. Fucharoen S, Youngchaiyud P, Wasi P. Hypoxaemia and the effect of aspirin in thalassaemia. *Southeast Asian J Trop Med Public Health* 1981;12:90–93.
1466. Winichagoon P, Fucharoen S, Wasi P. Increased circulating platelet aggregates in thalassaemia. *Southeast Asian J Trop Med Public Health* 1981;12:556–560.
1467. Jootar P, Fucharoen S. Cardiac involvement in β-thalassemia/hemoglobin E disease: clinical and hemodynamic findings. *Southeast Asian J Trop Med Public Health* 1990;21:269–273.
1468. Sonakul D, Suwananagool P, Sirivaidyapong P, et al. Distribution of pulmonary thromboembolic lesions in thalassemic patients. *Birth Defects: Original Articles Series* 1988;23:375–384.
1469. Youngchaiyud P, Suthamsmai T, Fucharoen S, et al. Lung function tests in splenectomized β-thalassemia/Hb E patients. *Birth Defects: Original Articles Series* 1988;23:361–370.
1470. Israngkura P, Chantarojanasiri T, Sudhas Na Ayuthya P, et al. Studies of cardiopulmonary and platelet function in thalassemic children. *Birth Defects: Original Articles Series* 1988;23:385–393.
1471. Laosombat V, Fucharoen S-P, Panich V, et al. Molecular basis of beta thalassemia in the South of Thailand. *Am J Hematol* 1992;41:194–198.
1472. Opartkiattikul N, Funahara Y, Fucharoen S, et al. Increase in spontaneous platelet aggregation in β-thalassemia/haemoglobin E disease: a consequence of splenectomy. *Southeast Asian J Trop Med Public Health* 1992;23:36–41.
1473. Visuphiphan S, Ketsa-Ard K, Tumliang S, et al. Significance of blood coagulation and platelet profiles in relation to pulmonary thrombosis in β-thalassemia/Hb E. *Southeast Asian J Trop Med Public Health* 1994;25.
1474. Shirahata A, Funahara Y, Opartkiattikul N, et al. Protein C and S deficiency in thalassaemic patients. *Southeast Asian J Trop Med Public Health* 1992;23:65–73.
1475. Opartkiattikul N, Funahara Y, Hijikata-Okunomiya A, et al. Detection of PF3 availability in whole blood from volunteers and β-thalassemia/Hb E patients: a promising method for prediction of thrombotic tendency. *Southeast Asian J Trop Med Public Health* 1992;23:52–59.
1476. Benson PJ, Peterson LC, Hasegawa DK, et al. Abnormality of von Willebrand factor in patients with hemoglobin E-β⁰ thalassemia. *Am J Clin Pathol* 1990;93:395–399.
1477. Tuchinda C, Punnakanta L, Angsusinga K. Endocrine disturbances in thalassemia children. *J Med Assoc Thai* 1978;61:55–56.
1478. Vannassaeng S, Ploybutr S, Visutakul P, et al. Endocrine functions in thalassemia patients. *J Med Assoc Thai* 1978;61:54.
1479. Pootrakul P, Hungsprenges S, Fucharoen S, et al. Relation between erythropoiesis and bone metabolism in thalassemia. *N Engl J Med* 1981;304:1470–1473.
1480. Chandcharoensin-Wilde C, Chairoongruang S, Jitnuson P, et al. *Birth Defects: Original Articles Series* 1988;23:263.
1481. Chuansumrit A, Isarangkura P, Hathirat P, et al. A syndrome of post-transfusion hypertension, convulsion and cerebral hemorrhage in β-thalassemia Hb E disease: a case report with high plasma renin activity. *J Med Assoc Thai* 1986;69:1–5.
1482. Thirawarapan SS, Snongchart N, Fucharoen S, et al. Study of mechanisms of post-transfusion hypertension in thalassaemic patients. *Southeast Asian J Trop Med Public Health* 1989;20:471–478.
1483. Sonakul D, Fucharoen S. Brain pathology in 6 fatal cases of post-transfusion hypertension, convulsion and cerebral hemorrhage syndrome. *Southeast Asian J Trop Med Public Health* 1992;23:116–119.
1484. Wanachiwanawin W. Infections in E-beta thalassemia. *J Pediatr Hematol Oncol* 2000;22:581–587.
1485. Yipintsoi T, Haraphongse M, Wasi P, et al. Cardiological examinations in hemoglobin E and thalassemia diseases. *J Med Assoc Thai* 1968;51:131.
1486. Poncz M, Ballantine M, Solowiejczyk D, et al. β-Thalassemia in a Kurdish Jew. *J Biol Chem* 1983;257:5994.
1487. Cai SP, Zhang JZ, Doherty M, et al. A new TATA box mutation detected in prenatal diagnosis. *Am J Hum Genet* 1989;45:112.
1488. Fei YJ, Stoming TA, Efremov GD, et al. β-Thalassemia due to a T→A mutation within the ATA box. *Biochem Biophys Res Commun* 1988;153:741.
1489. Lin L-I, Lin K-S, Lin K-H, et al. A novel -32 (C→A) mutant identified in amplified genomic DNA of a Chinese β-thalassemic patient. *Am J Hum Genet* 1992;50:237.
1490. Meloni A, Rosatelli MC, Faa V, et al. Promoter mutations producing mild β-thalassemia in the Italian population. *Br J Haematol* 1992;80:222.
1491. Kulozik AE, Bellan-Koch A, Bail S, et al. Thalassemia intermedia: moderate reduction of β-globin gene transcriptional activity by a novel mutation of the proximal CACCC promoter element. *Blood* 1991;77:2054.
1492. Efremov DG, Dimovski AJ, Efremov GD. Detection of β-thalassemia mutations by ASO hybridization of PCR amplified DNA with digoxigenin ddUTP labeled oligonucleotides. *Hemoglobin* 1991;15:525.
1493. Coleman MB, Steinberg MH, Harrell AH, et al. The -87 (C→A) β⁺-thalassemia mutation in a black family. *Hemoglobin* 1992;16:399.
1494. Rund D, Cohen T, Filon D, et al. Evolution of a genetic disease in an ethnic isolate: β-thalassemia in the Jews of Kurdistan. *Proc Natl Acad Sci U S A* 1991;88:310.
1495. Faustino P, Osorio-Almeida L, Barbot J, et al. Novel promoter and splice junction defects add to the genetic, clinical or geographical heterogeneity of β-thalassemia in the Portuguese population. *Hum Genet* 1992;89:573.
1496. Oron V, Filon D, Fearon C, et al. Two novel β-thalassemia mutations in Ashkenazi Jews. *Blood* 1992;80[Suppl 1]:5a(abst).
1497. Jankovic L, Efremov GD, Petkov G, et al. Two novel polyadenylation mutations leading to β⁺-thalassemia. *Br J Haematol* 1990;75:122.
1498. Rund D, Dowling C, Najjar K, et al. Two mutations in the β-globin polyadenylylation signal reveal extended transcripts and new RNA polyadenylylation sites. *Proc Natl Acad Sci U S A* 1992;89:4324.
1499. Huisman THJ. The β- and δ-thalassemia repository. *Hemoglobin* 1992;16:237.
1500. Chibani J, Vidaud M, Duquesnoy P, et al. The peculiar spectrum of β-thalassemia genes in Tunisia. *Hum Genet* 1988;78:190.

1501. Gonzalez-Redondo JM, Stoming TA, Kutlar F, et al. Severe Hb S-β⁰-thalas-saemia with a T→C substitution in the donor splice site of the first intron of the β-globin gene. *Br J Haematol* 1989;71:113.

1502. Lossi AM, Milland M, Berge-Lefranc JL. A further case of β-thalassemia with an homozygous T→C substitution at the donor splice site of the first inter-vening sequence of the β-globin gene. *Hemoglobin* 1989;13:619.

1503. Bouhass R, Aguercif M, Trabuchet G, et al. A new mutation at IVS1 nt 2(T→A), in β-thalassemia from Algeria. *Blood* 1990;76:1054.

1504. Deidda G, Novelletto A, Hafez M, et al. A new β-thalassemia mutation pro-duced by a single nucleotide substitution in the conserved dinucleotide sequence of the IVS-1 consensus acceptor site (AG→AA). *Hemoglobin* 1990;14:431.

1505. Oner R, Altay C, Gurgey A, et al. β-Thalassemia in Turkey. *Hemoglobin* 1990;14:1.

1506. Yamamoto Ku, Yamamoto Ki, Hattori Y, et al. Two β-thalassemia mutations in Japan: codon 121 (GAA→TAA) and IVS-I-130 (G→C). *Hemoglobin* 1992;16:295.

1507. Orkin SH, Sexton JP, Goff SC, et al. Inactivation of an acceptor RNA splice site by a short deletion in β-thalassemia. *J Biol Chem* 1983;258:7249.

1508. Wong C, Antonarakis SE, Goff SC, et al. On the origin and spread of β-thalas-semia: recurrent observation of four mutations in different ethnic groups. *Proc Natl Acad Sci U S A* 1986;83:6529.

1509. Hattori Y, Yamamoto K, Yamashiro Y, et al. Three β-thalassemia mutations in the Japanese: IVS-II-1 (G → A), IVS-II-848 (C → G), and codon 90 (GAC → TAG). *Hemoglobin* 1992;16:93.

1510. Nozari G, Rahbar S, Rahmanzadeh S, et al. Splice junction [IVS-II-1 (G→C)] thalassemia: a new mutation detected in an Iranian patient. *Hemoglobin* 1993;17:279.

1511. Padanilam BJ, Huisman THJ. The β⁰-thalassemia in an American black fam-ily is due to a single nucleotide substitution in the acceptor splice junction of the second intervening sequence. *Am J Hematol* 1986;22:259.

1512. Jankovic L, Dimovski AJ, Sukarova E, et al. A new mutation in the β-globin gene (IVS II-850 G → C) found in a Yugoslavian β-thalassemia heterozygote. *Haematologica* 1992;77:119.

1513. Rosatelli MC, Tuveri T, Scalas MT, et al. Molecular screening and fetal diag-nosis of β-thalassemia in the Italian population. *Hum Genet* 1992;89:585.

1514. Chehab FF, Der Kaloustian V, Khouri FP, et al. The molecular basis of β-thalas-semia in Lebanon: application to prenatal diagnosis. *Blood* 1987;69:1141.

1515. Vidaud M, Gattoni R, Stevenin J, et al. A 5' splice-region G → C mutation in exon 1 of the human β-globin gene inhibits pre-mRNA splicing: a mecha-nism for β⁺-thalassemia. *Proc Natl Acad Sci U S A* 1989;86:1041.

1516. Gonzalez-Redondo JM, Stoming TA, Kutlar F, et al. Hb Monroe or α₂β₂30(B12)Arg → Thr, a variant associated with β-thalassemia due to a G → C substitution adjacent to the donor splice site of the first intron. *Hemoglobin* 1989;13:67.

1517. Kalaydjieva L, Eigel A, Argiris A, et al. The molecular basis of thalassemia in Bulgaria. Third International Conference on Thalassemia and the Hemoglo-binopathies, Sardinia, April 1989;43(abst).

1518. Hill AVS, Bowden DK, O'Shaughnessy DF, et al. β-Thalassemia in Melanesia: association with malaria and characterization of a common variant (IVS-1 nt 5 G → C). *Blood* 1988;72:9.

1519. Gonzalez-Redondo JM, Kutlar A, Kutlar F, et al. Molecular characterization of Hb S(C) β-thalassemia in American blacks. *Am J Hematol* 1991;38:9.

1520. Lapoumeroulie C, Pagnier J, Bank A, et al. β-Thalassemia due to a novel mutation in IVS-1 sequence donor site consensus sequence creating a restric-tion site. *Biochem Biophys Res Commun* 1986;139:709.

1521. Wong C, Antonarakis SE, Goff SC, et al. β-Thalassemia due to two novel nucleotide substitutions in consensus acceptor site sequences of the β-globin gene. *Blood* 1989;73:914.

1522. Chiou SS, Chang TT, Chen PH, et al. Molecular basis and haematological characterization of β-thalassaemia major in Taiwan, with a mutation of IVS-1 3' end TAG → GAG in a Chinese patient. *Br J Haematol* 1993;83:112.

1523. Gonzalez-Redondo JH, Stoming TA, Lanclos KD, et al. Clinical and genetic/heterogeneity in black patients with homozygous β-thalassemia from the southeastern United States. *Blood* 1988;72:1007.

1524. Murru S, Loudianos G, Deiana M, et al. Molecular characterization of β-thalassemia intermedia in patients of Italian descent and identification of three novel β-thalassemia mutations. *Blood* 1991;77:1342.

1525. Beldjord C, Lapoumeroulie C, Pagnier J, et al. A novel β-thalassemia gene with a single base mutation in the conserved polypyrimidine sequence at the 3' end of IVS-II. *Nucleic Acids Res* 1988;16:4927.

1526. Varawalla NY, Old JM, Weatherall DJ. Rare β-thalassemia mutations in Asian Indians. *Br J Haematol* 1991;79:640.

1527. Spritz RA, Jagadeeswaran P, Choudary PV, et al. Base substitution in an intervening sequence of a β⁺-thalassemic human globin gene. *Proc Natl Acad Sci U S A* 1981;78:2455.

1528. Westaway D, Williamson R. An intron nucleotide sequence variant in a cloned β⁺-thalassemia globin gene. *Nucleic Acids Res* 1981;9:1777.

1529. Yang KG, Kutlar F, George E, et al. Molecular characterization of β-globin gene mutations in Malay patients with Hb E-β-thalassaemia and thalas-saemia major. *Br J Haematol* 1989;72:73.

1530. Hattori Y, Yamane A, Yamashiro Y, et al. Gene analysis of β-thalassemia among Japanese. *Hemoglobin* 1989;13:657.

1531. Ribeiro MLS, Baysal E, Kutlar F, et al. A novel β⁰-thalassaemia mutation (codon 15, TGG → TGA) is prevalent in a population of central Portugal. *Br J Haematol* 1992;80:567.

1532. Chang JC, Kan YW. β⁰-Thalassemia: a nonsense mutation in man. *Proc Natl Acad Sci U S A* 1979;76:2886.

1533. Fucharoen G, Fucharoen S, Jetsrisuparb A, et al. Molecular basis of HbE-β-thalassemia and the origin of HbE in northeast Thailand: identification of one novel mutation using amplified DNA from buffy coat specimens. *Bio-chem Biophys Res Commun* 1990;170:698.

1534. Fucharoen S, Fucharoen G, Fucharoen P, et al. A novel ochre mutation in the β-thalassemia gene of a Thai. *J Biol Chem* 1989;264:7780.

1535. Boehm CD, Dowling CD, Waber PG, et al. Use of oligonucleotide hybridiza-tion in the characterization of a β⁰-thalassemia gene (β³⁷ᵀᴳᴳ→ᵀᴳᴬ) in a Saudi Arabian family. *Blood* 1986;67:1185.

1536. Trecartin RF, Liebhaber SA, Chang JC, et al. β⁰-Thalassemia in Sardinia is caused by a nonsense mutation. *J Clin Invest* 1981;68:1012.

1537. Moschonas N, deBoer E, Grosveld FG, et al. Structure and expression of a cloned β⁰-thalassemic globin gene. *Nucleic Acids Res* 1981;9:4391.

1538. Orkin SH, Goff SC. Nonsense and frameshift mutations in β⁰-thalassemia detected in cloned β globin genes. *J Biol Chem* 1981;256:9782.

1539. Pergolizzi R, Spritz RA, Spence S, et al. Two cloned β-thalassemia genes are associated with amber mutations at codon 39. *Nucleic Acids Res* 1981;9:7065.

1540. Jackson IJ, Freund RM, Wasylyk B, et al. The isolation, mapping and trans-cription in vitro of a β⁰-thalassemia globin gene. *Eur J Biochem* 1981;121:27.

1541. Gorski J, Fiori M, Mach B. A new nonsense mutation as the molecular basis for β⁰-thalassemia. *J Mol Biol* 1982;154:537.

1542. Chehab FF, Honig GR, Kan YW. Spontaneous mutation in β-thalassemia pro-ducing the same nucleotide substitution as that in a common hereditary form. *Lancet* 1986;1:3.

1543. Atweh GF, Brickner HE, Zhu XX, et al. A new amber mutation in a β-thalas-semia gene with non-measurable levels of mutant mRNA in vivo. *J Clin Invest* 1988;82:557.

1544. Fucharoen S, Katsube T, Fucharoen G, et al. Molecular heterogeneity of β-thalassaemia in the Japanese: identification of two novel mutations. *Br J Hae-matol* 1990;74:101.

1545. Divoky V, Gu L-H, Indrak K, et al. A new β⁰-thalassaemia nonsense mutation (codon 112, T → A) not associated with a dominant type of thalassaemia in the heterozygote. *Br J Haematol* 1993;83:523.

1546. Kazazian HH Jr, Orkin SH, Boehm CD, et al. Characterization of a spontane-ous mutation to a β-thalassemia allele. *Am J Hum Genet* 1986;38:860.

1547. Fei YJ, Stoming TA, Kutlar A, et al. One form of inclusion body β-thalassemia is due to a GAA → TAA mutation at codon 121 of the β chain. *Blood* 1989;73:1075.

1548. Hall GW, Franklin IM, Sura T, et al. A novel mutation (nonsense β127) in exon 3 of the β globin gene produces a variable thalassaemia phenotype. *Br J Haematol* 1991;79:342.

1549. Rosatelli MC, Dozy A, Faa V, et al. Molecular characterization of β-thalas-semia in the Sardinian population. *Am J Hum Genet* 1992;50:422.

1550. Kollia P, Gonzalez-Redondo JM, Stoming TA, et al. Frameshift codon 5 [FSC-5 (-CT)] thalassemia: a novel mutation detected in a Greek patient. *Hemoglo-bin* 1989;13:597.

1551. Kazazian HH Jr, Orkin SH, Boehm CD, et al. β-Thalassemia due to deletion of the nucleotide which is substituted in sickle cell anemia. *Am J Hum Genet* 1983;35:1028.

1552. Chang JC, Alberti A, Kan YW. A β-thalassemia lesion abolishes the same *Mst*II site as the sickle mutation. *Nucleic Acids Res* 1983;11:7789.

1553. Economou EP, Antonarakis SE, Dowling CC, et al. Molecular heterogeneity of β-thalassaemia in Mestizo Mexicans. *Genomics* 1991;11:474.

1554. Chan V, Chan TK, Kan YW, et al. A novel β-thalassemia frameshift mutation (codon 14/15) detectable by direct visualization of abnormal restriction frag-ment in amplified genomic DNA. *Blood* 1988;72:1420.

1555. Deidda G, Novelletto A, Hafez M, et al. A new β-thalassaemia frameshift mutation detected by PCR after selective hybridization to immobilized oli-gonucleotides. *Br J Haematol* 1991;79:90.

1556. Fattoum S, Guemira F, Öner C, et al. β-Thalassemia, Hb S-β-thalassemia, and sickle cell anemia among Tunisians. *Hemoglobin* 1991;15:11.

1557. Lin L-I, Lin K-S, Lin K-H, et al. The spectrum of β-thalassemia mutations in Tai-wan: identification of a novel frameshift mutation. *Am J Hum Genet* 1991;48:809.

1558. Schnee J, Griese EV, Eigel A, et al. β-Thalassemia gene analysis in a Turkish family reveals a 7 bp deletion in the coding region. *Blood* 1989;73:3224.

1559. Indrak K, Indrakova J, Kutlar F, et al. Compound heterozygosity for a β⁰-thalassemia (frameshift codons 38/39;-C) and a non-deletional Swiss type of HPFH (A → C at nt -110, ᴳγ) in a Czechoslovakian family. *Ann Hematol* 1991;63:111.

1560. Fucharoen S, Fucharoen G, Laosombat V, et al. Double heterozygosity of the β-Malay and a novel β-thalassemia gene in a Thai patient. *Am J Hematol* 1991;38:142.

1561. Kinniburgh AJ, Maquat LE, Schedl T, et al. mRNA-deficient β⁰-thalassemia results from a single nucleotide deletion. *Nucleic Acids Res* 1982;10:5421.

1562. Losekoot M, Fodde R, van Heeren H, et al. A novel frameshift mutation [FSC 47 (A+)] causing β-thalassemia in a Surinam patient. *Hemoglobin* 1990;14:467.

1563. Chehab FF, Winterhalter KH, Kan YW. Characterization of a spontaneous mutation in β-thalassemia associated with advanced paternal age. *Blood* 1989;74:852.

1564. Chan V, Chan TK, Todd D. A new codon 71 (+T) mutant resulting in β⁰-thalassemia. *Blood* 1989;74:2304.

1565. Basak AN, Özer A, Özcelik H, et al. A novel frameshift mutation: deletion of C in codons 74/75 of the β-globin gene causes β⁰-thalassemia in a Turkish patient. *Hemoglobin* 1992;16:309.

1566. DiMarzo R, Dowling CE, Wong C, et al. The spectrum of β-thalassemia mutations in Sicily. *Br J Haematol* 1988;69:393.

1567. Schwartz E, Goltsov AA, Kaboaev OK, et al. A novel frameshift mutation causing β-thalassemia in Azerbaijan. *Nucleic Acids Res* 1989;17:3997.

1568. Indrak K, Brabec V, Indrakova J, et al. Molecular characterization of β-thalassemia in Czechoslovakia. *Hum Genet* 1992;88:399.

1569. Ristaldi MS, Pirastu M, Murru S, et al. A spontaneous mutation produced a novel elongated β-globin chain structural variant (Hb Agnana) with a thalassemia-like phenotype. *Blood* 1990;75:1378.

1570. Beris PH, Miescher PA, Diaz-Chico JC, et al. Inclusion-body β-thalassemia trait in a Swiss family is caused by an abnormal hemoglobin (Geneva) with an altered and extended β chain carboxy-terminus due to a modification in codon β114. *Blood* 1988;72:801.

1571. Fucharoen S, Kobayashi Y, Gucharoen G, et al. A single nucleotide deletion in codon 123 of the β-globin gene causes an inclusion body β-thalassemia trait: a novel elongated globin chain β^{Makabe}. *Br J Haematol* 1990;75:393.

1572. Fucharoen S, Fucharoen S, Jetsrisuparb A, et al. Eight-base deletion in exon 3 of the β-globin gene produced a novel variant (β Khon Kaen) with an inclusion body thalassemia trait. *Blood* 1991;78:537.

1573. Fucharoen S, Fucharoen G, Fukumaki Y, et al. Three-base deletion in exon 3 of the β-globin gene produced a novel variant (β^{Gunma}) with a thalassemia-like phenotype. *Blood* 1990;76:1894.

1574. Öner R, Öner C, Wilson JB, et al. Dominant β-thalassemia trait in a Portuguese family is caused by a deletion of (G)TGGCTGGTGT(G) and an insertion of (G)GCAG(G) in codons 134, 135, 136, and 137 of the β-globin gene. *Br J Haematol* 1991;79:306.

1575. Lam VMS, Xie SS, Tam JWO, et al. A new single nucleotide change at the initiation codon (ATG → AGG) identified in amplified genomic DNA of a Chinese β-thalassemic patient. *Blood* 1990;75:1207.

1576. Koo MS, Kim SI, Cho HI, et al. A β-thalassemia mutation found in Korea. *Hemoglobin* 1992;16:313.

1577. Jankovic L, Efremov GD, Josifovska O, et al. An initiation codon mutation as a cause of a β-thalassemia. *Hemoglobin* 1990;14:169.

1578. Beris P, Darbellay R, Speiser D, et al. *De novo* initiation codon mutation (ATG → ACG) of the β-globin gene causing β-thalassemia in a Swiss family. *Am J Hematol* 1993;42:248.

1579. Hattori Y, Yamashiro Y, Ohba Y, et al. A new β-thalassemia mutation (initiation codon ATG → GTG) found in the Japanese population. *Hemoglobin* 1991;15:317.

1580. Rahbar S, Nozari G. A novel β-thalassemia mutation (initiation codon ATG → ATT) with a β-thalassemia intermedia phenotype. *Blood* 1992;80[Suppl 1]:5a(abst).

1581. Öner R, Agarwal S, Dimovski AJ, et al. The G → A mutation at position +22 3' to the cap site of the β-globin gene as a possible cause for a β-thalassemia. *Hemoglobin* 1991;15:67.

1582. Cai S-P, Eng B, Francombe WH, et al. Two novel β-thalassemia mutations in the 5' and 3' noncoding regions of the β-globin gene. *Blood* 1992;79:1342.

1583. Huang S-Z, Xu Y-H, Zeng F-Y, et al. A novel β-thalassaemia mutation: deletion of 4 bp (-AAAC) in the 5' transcriptional sequence. *Br J Haematol* 1991;78:125.

1584. Eng B, Waye JS, Chui DHK. The T → C substitution at nucleotide +1570 of the β-globin gene is a polymorphism. *Blood* 1992;80:1365.

1585. Jankovic L, Dimovski AJ, Kollia P, et al. A C → G mutation at nt position 6 3' to the terminating codon may be the cause of a silent β-thalassemia. *Int J Hematol* 1991;54:289.

1586. Thein SL, Best S, Sharpe J. Hemoglobin Chesterfield (β28 Leu → Arg) produces the phenotype of inclusion body β thalassemia. *Blood* 1991;77:2791.

1587. Podda A, Galanello R, Maccioni L, et al. A new unstable hemoglobin variant producing a β-thalassemia-like phenotype. Third International Conference on Thalassemia and the Hemoglobinopathies, Sardinia, 1989; 51(abst).

1588. Kobayashi Y, Fukumaki Y, Komatsu N, et al. A novel globin structural mutant, Showa-Yakushiji (β110 Leu-Pro) causing a β-thalassemia phenotype. *Blood* 1987;70:1688.

1589. de Castro CM, Lee M, Fleenor DE, et al. A novel β-globin mutation, β Durham-N.C. [β(114) Leu → Pro], detected by SSCP, produces a dominant thalassemia-like phenotype. *Blood* 1992;80[Suppl 1]:6a(abst).

1590. Thein SL, Wallace RB, Pressley L, et al. The polyadenylation site mutation in the α-globin gene cluster. *Blood* 1988;71:313.

1591. Yüregir GT, Aksoy K, Cürük MA, et al. Hb H disease in a Turkish family resulting from the interaction of a deletional α-thalassaemia-1 and a newly discovered poly A mutation. *Br J Haematol* 1992;80:527.

1592. Orkin SH, Goff SC, Hechtman RL. Mutation in an intervening sequence splice junction in man. *Proc Natl Acad Sci U S A* 1981;78:5041.

1593. Felber BK, Orkin SH, Hamer DH. Abnormal RNA splicing causes one form of α-thalassemia. *Cell* 1982;29:895.

1594. Liebhaber SA, Coleman MB, Adams JG III, et al. Molecular basis for non-deletion α-thalassemia in American blacks α2$^{116GAG→UAG}$. *J Clin Invest* 1987;80:154.

1595. Morle F, Starck J, Godet J. α-Thalassemia due to the deletion of nucleotides -2 and -3 preceding the AUG initiation codon affects translation efficiency both in vitro and in vivo. *Nucleic Acids Res* 1986;14:3279.

1596. Sanguansermsri T, Matragoon S, Changloah L, et al. Hemoglobin Suan-Dok (α$^{109(G16)LEU→ARG}_2$β$_2$): an unstable variant associated with α-thalassemia. *Hemoglobin* 1979;3:161.

1597. Honig GR, Shamsuddin M, Zaizov R, et al. Hemoglobin Petah Tikvah (α110 Ala → Asp): a new unstable variant with α-thalassemia-like expression. *Blood* 1981;57:705.

1598. Ottolenghi S, Camaschella C, Comi P, et al. A frequent ^{A}γ-hereditary persistence of fetal hemoglobin in Northern Sardinia: its molecular basis and haematological phenotype in heterozygotes with β thalassemia. *Hum Genet* 1988;79:13.

1599. Huang HJ, Stoming TA, Harris HF, et al. The Greek ^{A}γβ-HPFH observed in a large black family. *Am J Hematol* 1987;25:401.

1600. Zeng Y-T, Huang S-Z, Chen B, et al. Hereditary persistence of fetal hemoglobin or (δβ)^0-thalassemia: three types observed in South Chinese families. *Blood* 1985;66:1430.

1601. Loudianos G, Cao A, Pirastu M, et al. Molecular basis of the δ thalassemia in *cis* to hemoglobin Knossos variant. *Blood* 1991;77:2087.

1602. Olds RJ, Sura T, Jackson B, et al. A novel δ^0 mutation in *cis* with Hb Knossos: a study of different genetic interactions in three Egyptian families. *Br J Haematol* 1991;78:430.

1603. Losekoot M, Fodde R, Giordano PC, et al. A novel δ^0-thalassemia arising from a frameshift insertion, detected by direct sequencing of enzymatically amplified DNA. *Hum Genet* 1989;83:75.

1604. Moi P, Paglietti E, Sanna A, et al. Delineation of the molecular basis of δ- and normal HbA$_2$β-thalassemia. *Blood* 1988;72:530.

1605. Trifillis P, Ioannou P, Schwartz E, et al. Identification of four novel δ-globin gene mutations in Greek Cypriots using polymerase chain reaction and automated fluorescence-based DNA sequence analysis. *Blood* 1991;78:3298.

1606. Loudianos G, Murru S, Ristaldi MS, et al. A novel δ-thalassemia mutation A G → C substitution at codon 30 of the δ-globin gene in a person of southern Italian origin. *Hum Mutat* 1992;1:169.

1607. Loudianos G, Murru S, Kanavakis E, et al. A new δ chain variant hemoglobin A2-Corfu or α$_2$δ$_2$ 116 Arg → Cys (G18), detected by δ-globin gene analysis in a Greek family. *Hum Genet* 1991;87:237.

CHAPTER 49

Disorders of Hemoglobin Function and Stability

Ronald L. Nagel

This chapter deals with disorders stemming from structural abnormalities (mutations of the coding sequence) that lead to clinical manifestations secondary to alterations of the function (oxygen affinity, electronic state of the heme iron) or stability of the hemoglobin molecule. Not included are disorders resulting from the presence of hemoglobin (Hb) S or related conditions or the thalassemias.

At last count (mid 2002), 854 human hemoglobin mutations had been cataloged: 214 involving the $\alpha 1$ gene, 254 the $\alpha 2$ gene, 650 the β gene, 56 the δ gene, 44 the $^A\gamma$ gene, and 54 the $^G\gamma$ gene. Of these, 83 have high affinity for oxygen and are stable, 66 have low affinity for oxygen and are stable, and 125 are unstable. [A list of the mutants can be found in the Globin Gene Server (http://globin.cse.psu.edu), a Web site founded by Ross Hardison and initially based on Titus Huisman's database. The site has recently been expanded and updated significantly and is user friendly.]

Hemoglobin disorders can be classified according to the genetic mechanisms involved, the functional abnormalities they engender, or the clinical syndrome with which they are associated. Table 49-1 depicts the classification of these disorders according to the functional abnormality and the clinical syndrome they generate.

NORMAL HEMOGLOBIN STRUCTURE AND FUNCTION

Overall Hemoglobin Structure: Myoglobin Fold

The adult major hemoglobin molecule is a tetramer because it is formed by four polypeptide chains: two α-chains (141 amino acids long) and two β-chains (146 amino acids long). The primary structure (amino acid sequence) is illustrated in Table 49-2. Each of these chains is attached to a prosthetic group called *heme*, formed by protoporphyrin IX complexed with an iron molecule. To understand the secondary and tertiary structure—that is, the three-dimensional shape—of each of the globin polypeptide chains forming the tetramer, we need to consider (a) the "myoglobin fold," the overall architectural strategy that nature has devised for constructing all globin-based oxygen carriers; (b) the peculiarities of the α-chains and β-chains that form the major adult human hemoglobin; and (c) the heme and its relation to the protein moiety.

The myoglobin fold is a time-proven structural solution to the secondary and tertiary structure of globin chains. In effect, it has been found to be the structural blueprint of all myoglobin analyzed by x-crystallography, but also of the individual chains of all globin chains so far examined, including vertebrate and mollusk hemoglobins (two dissimilar hemoglobin constructs). Even hemoglobin present in the root nodules of legumes has the same myoglobin fold. This structure clearly was the best solution for heme–globin complexes early in evolution.

Myoglobin, the oxygen-carrying pigment in muscle, is a single polypeptide chain of 153 amino acids and was the first protein in which secondary and tertiary structures were elucidated by x-ray crystallography. John C. Kendrew from Cambridge, England, was awarded a Nobel Prize for his pioneering contribution on this subject (1) (Fig. 49-1).

Myoglobin is a globular and well-packed molecule in which most of the 153 amino acids are arranged in eight (labeled A to H) predominantly α-helical structures. The amide (–CO–NH–) backbone forms a helical structure with 3.6 residues per turn, stabilized by hydrogen bonds between a –C=O with the NH four residues further down the chain (Fig. 49-2).

All the α helices are right-handed and vary in length between four amino acids (minimum number required to construct an α helix) and 28 amino acids. Nevertheless, the terminal portions of the α helices are anomalous because they fit either a 3_{10} helix (four residues per turn) or a π helix (five residues per turn). The remaining amino acids (23 of 153 total) are not arranged in helices but are participants in two other types of molecular structures: (a) the elbows, hairpin corners of different degrees of sharpness that connect α helices and allow the sequence to wrap itself around the heme; and (b) terminal portions of the sequence (C-terminal and N-terminal portions of the polypeptide chain).

Not all elbows contain residues in nonhelical configuration; the sharp turns between helices A and B, B and C, and D and E do not leave room for them. When there is room for amino acids in the elbows, they are mostly amino acid residues that are not helix makers. For example, the side chain of proline (Pro) introduces strains to the amide plane; when present in the midst of an α helix, it results in either bending (as in helix E) or interruption (as in C and G helices) of the helix. Other residues, such as glycine (Gly), are also α-helix busters.

Another cardinal feature of the myoglobin fold is that different types of amino acid residues tend to occupy the surface of the molecule and the interior portions. The charged amino acids [aspartic acid (Asp), glutamic acid (Glu), lysine (Lys), arginine (Arg), and histidine (His)] all are present almost exclusively in the exterior of the molecule, in direct contact with the solvent. Also, the uncharged but polar asparagine (Asn) and glutamine

TABLE 49-1. Classification of Structural Nonsickle Hemoglobinopathies

Functional Abnormalities	Clinical Syndrome
High-affinity hemoglobins	Erythrocytosis
Low-affinity hemoglobins	Cyanosis
Ferric-heme hemoglobins	Pseudocyanosis
Unstable hemoglobins	Heinz body hemolytic anemia
Hemoglobins with abnormal assembly	Dominant thalassemia

(Gln) tend to be in the exterior of the molecule. The true hydrophobic residues [phenylalanine (Phe), leucine (Leu), isoleucine (Ile), methionine (Met), and valine (Val)] are mostly present pointing toward the interior of the molecule, away from the solvent, and they stabilize the packing arrangement. Finally, some residues are not strong in either polarity or hydrophobicity because their side chains are too short and have an –OH group or a ring structure [Pro, threonine (Thr), serine (Ser), cysteine (Cys), alanine (Ala), Gly, tyrosine (Tyr), tryptophan (Trp)].

These are trump card amino acids; they can be located in the interior or exterior of the molecule. Nevertheless, they play critical roles in the secondary structure, because some of these amino acids can interrupt α helices and others can form structurally and functionally critical hydrogen bonds.

Violations of any of these myoglobin fold rules make the protein unstable in solution, change its functional properties, or both, resulting in pathologic states.

The myoglobin fold has been conserved by nature for several millions of years in all globin-based oxygen carriers. The central achievement of this structure is that it solves two fundamental problems: It makes heme water soluble, and it helps maintain the heme iron in the ferrous state. These two physical properties are central and indispensable for the oxygen-carrying capacity of myoglobin and hemoglobin.

Heme

The myoglobin fold is wrapped around the heme, the combination of a porphyrin ring and an iron molecule. The porphy-

TABLE 49-2. Primary Structure of Human Globin Subunits[a]

Helix	α	ζ	Helix	β	δ	γ	ε
NA1	1Val	Ser	NA1	1Val	Val	Gly	Val
—	—	—	NA2	2His	His	His	His
NA2	2Leu	Leu	NA3	3Leu	Leu	Phe	Phe
A1	3Ser	Thr	A1	4Thr	Thr	Thr	Thr
A2	4Pro	Lys	A2	5Pro	Pro	Glu	Ala
A3	5Ala	Thr	A3	6Glu	Glu	Glu	Glu
A4	6Asp	Glu	A4	7Glu	Glu	Asp	Glu
A5	7Lys	Arg	A5	8Lys	Lys	Lys	Lys
A6	8Thr	Thr	A6	9Ser	Thr	Ala	Ala
A7	9Asn	Ile	A7	10Ala	Ala	Thr	Ala
A8	10Val	Ile	A8	11Val	Val	Ile	Val
A9	11Lys	Val	A9	12Thr	Asn	Thr	Thr
A10	12Ala	Ser	A10	13Ala	Ala	Ser	Ser
A11	13Ala	Met	A11	14Leu	Leu	Leu	Leu
A12	14Trp	Trp	A12	15Trp	Trp	Trp	Trp
A13	15Gly	Ala	A13	16Gly	Gly	Gly	Ser
A14	16Lys	Lys	A14	17Lys	Lys	Lys	Lys
A15	17Val	Ile	A15	18Val	Val	Val	Met
A16	18Gly	Ser	—	—	—	—	—
AB1	19Ala	Thr	—	—	—	—	—
B1	20His	Gln	B1	19Asn	Asn	Asn	Asn
B2	21Ala	Ala	B2	20Val	Val	Val	Val
B3	22Gly	Asp	B3	21Asp	Asp	Glu	Glu
B4	23Glu	Thr	B4	22Glu	Ala	Asp	Glu
B5	24Tyr	Ile	B5	23Val	Val	Ala	Ala
B6	25Gly	Gly	B6	24Gly	Gly	Gly	Gly
B7	26Ala	Thr	B7	25Gly	Gly	Gly	Gly
B8	27Glu	Glu	B8	26Glu	Glu	Glu	Glu
B9	28Ala	Thr	B9	27Ala	Ala	Thr	Ala
B10	29Leu	Leu	B10	28Leu	Leu	Leu	Leu
B11	30Glu	Glu	B11	29Gly	Gly	Gly	Gly
B12	31Arg	Arg	B12	30Arg	Arg	Arg	Arg
B13	32Met	Leu	B13	31Leu	Leu	Leu	Leu
B14	33Phe	Phe	B14	32Leu	Leu	Leu	Leu
B15	34Leu	Leu	B15	33Val	Val	Val	Val
B16	35Ser	Ser	B16	34Val	Val	Val	Val
C1	36Phe	His	C1	35Tyr	Tyr	Tyr	Tyr
C2	37Pro	Pro	C2	36Pro	Pro	Pro	Pro
C3	38Thr	Gln	C3	37Trp	Trp	Trp	Trp
C4	39Thr	Thr	C4	38Thr	Thr	Thr	Thr
C5	40Lys	Lys	C5	39Gln	Gln	Gln	Gln
C6	41Thr	Thr	C6	40Arg	Arg	Arg	Arg
C7	42Tyr	Tyr	C7	41Phe	Phe	Phe	Phe
CE1	43Phe	Phe	CD1	42Phe	Phe	Phe	Phe
CE2	44Pro	Pro	CD2	43Glu	Glu	Asp	Asp
CE3	45His	His	CD3	44Ser	Ser	Ser	Ser
CE4	46Phe	Phe	CD4	45Phe	Phe	Phe	Phe
—	—	—	CD5	46Gly	Gly	Gly	Gly

(continued)

TABLE 49-2. (*continued*)

Helix	α	ζ	Helix	β	δ	γ	ε
CE5	47Asp	Asp	CD6	47Asp	Asp	Asn	Asn
CE6	48Leu	Leu	CD7	48Leu	Leu	Leu	Leu
CE7	49Ser	His	CD8	49Ser	Ser	Ser	Ser
CE8	50His	Pro	D1	50Thr	Ser	Ser	Ser
—	—	—	D2	51Pro	Pro	Ala	Pro
—	—	—	D3	52Asp	Asp	Ser	Ser
—	—	—	D4	53Ala	Ala	Ala	Ala
—	—	—	D5	54Val	Val	Ile	Ile
—	—	—	D6	55Met	Met	Met	Leu
CE9	51Gly	Gly	D7	56Gly	Gly	Gly	Gly
E1	52Ser	Ser	E1	57Asn	Asn	Asn	Asn
E2	53Ala	Ala	E2	58Pro	Pro	Pro	Pro
E3	54Gln	Gln	E3	59Lys	Lys	Lys	Lys
E4	55Val	Leu	E4	60Val	Val	Val	Val
E5	56Lys	Arg	E5	61Lys	Lys	Lys	Lys
E6	57Gly	Ala	E6	62Ala	Ala	Ala	Ala
E7	58His	His	E7	63His	His	His	His
E8	59Gly	Gly	E8	64Gly	Gly	Gly	Gly
E9	60Lys	Ser	E9	65Lys	Lys	Lys	Lys
E10	61Lys	Lys	E10	66Lys	Lys	Lys	Lys
E11	62Val	Val	E11	67Val	Val	Val	Val
E12	63Ala	Val	E12	68Leu	Leu	Leu	Leu
E13	64Asp	Ser	E13	69Gly	Gly	Thr	Thr
E14	65Ala	Ala	E14	70Ala	Ala	Ser	Ser
E15	66Leu	Val	E15	71Phe	Phe	Leu	Phe
E16	67Thr	Gly	E16	72Ser	Ser	Gly	Gly
E17	68Asn	Asp	E17	73Asp	Asp	Asp	Asp
E18	69Ala	Ala	E18	74Gly	Gly	Ala	Ala
E19	70Val	Val	E19	75Leu	Leu	Ile, Thr	Ile
E20	71Ala	Lys	E20	76Ala	Ala	Lys	Lys
EF1	72His	Ser	EF1	77His	His	His	Asn
EF2	73Val	Ile	EF2	78Leu	Leu	Leu	Met
EF3	74Asp	Asp	EF3	79Asp	Asp	Asp	Asp
EF4	75Asp	Asp	EF4	80Asn	Asn	Asp	Asn
EF5	76Met	Ile	EF5	81Leu	Leu	Leu	Leu
EF6	77Pro	Gly	EF6	82Lys	Lys	Lys	Lys
EF7	78Asn	Gly	EF7	83Gly	Gly	Gly	Pro
EF8	79Ala	Ala	EF8	84Thr	Thr	Thr	Ala
F1	80Leu	Leu	F1	85Phe	Phe	Phe	Phe
F2	81Ser	Ser	F2	86Ala	Ser	Ala	Ala
F3	82Ala	Lys	F3	87Thr	Gln	Gln	Lys
F4	83Leu	Leu	F4	88Leu	Leu	Leu	Leu
F5	84Ser	Ser	F5	89Ser	Ser	Ser	Ser
F6	85Asp	Glu	F6	90Glu	Glu	Glu	Glu
F7	86Leu	Leu	F7	91Leu	Leu	Leu	Leu
F8	87His	His	F8	92His	His	His	His
F9	88Ala	Ala	F9	93Cys	Cys	Cys	Cys
FG1	89His	Tyr	FG1	94Asp	Asp	Asp	Asp
FG2	90Lys	Ile	FG2	95Lys	Lys	Lys	Lys
FG3	91Leu	Leu	FG3	96Leu	Leu	Leu	Leu
FG4	92Arg	Arg	FG4	97His	His	His	His
FG5	93Val	Val	FG5	98Val	Val	Val	Val
G1	94Asp	Asp	G1	99Asp	Asp	Asp	Asp
G2	95Pro	Pro	G2	100Pro	Pro	Pro	Pro
G3	96Val	Val	G3	101Glu	Glu	Glu	Glu
G4	97Asn	Asn	G4	102Asn	Asn	Asn	Asn
G5	98Phe	Phe	G5	103Phe	Phe	Phe	Phe
G6	99Lys	Lys	G6	104Arg	Arg	Lys	Lys
G7	100Leu	Leu	G7	105Leu	Leu	Leu	Leu
G8	101Leu	Leu	G8	106Leu	Leu	Leu	Leu
G9	102Ser	Ser	G9	107Gly	Gly	Gly	Gly
G10	103His	His	G10	108Asn	Asn	Asn	Asn
G11	104Cys	Cys	G11	109Val	Val	Val	Val
G12	105Leu	Leu	G12	110Leu	Leu	Leu	Met
G13	106Leu	Leu	G13	111Val	Val	Val	Val
G14	107Val	Val	G14	112Cys	Cys	Thr	Ile
G15	108Thr	Thr	G15	113Val	Val	Val	Ile
G16	109Leu	Leu	G16	114Leu	Leu	Leu	Leu
G17	110Ala	Ala	G17	115Ala	Ala	Ala	Ala
G18	111Ala	Ala	G18	116His	Arg	Ile	Thr
G19	112His	Arg	G19	117His	Asn	His	His
GH1	113Leu	Phe	GH1	118Phe	Phe	Phe	Phe
GH2	114Pro	Pro	GH2	119Gly	Gly	Gly	Gly
GH3	115Ala	Ala	GH3	120Lys	Lys	Lys	Lys
GH4	116Glu	Asp	GH4	121Glu	Glu	Glu	Glu
GH5	117Phe	Phe	GH5	122Phe	Phe	Phe	Phe

(*continued*)

TABLE 49-2. (*continued*)

Helix	α	ζ	Helix	β	δ	γ	ε
H1	118Thr	Thr	H1	123Thr	Thr	Thr	Thr
H2	119Pro	Ala	H2	124Pro	Pro	Pro	Pro
H3	120Ala	Glu	H3	125Pro	Gln	Glu	Glu
H4	121Val	Ala	H4	126Val	Met	Val	Val
H5	122His	His	H5	127Gln	Gln	Gln	Gln
H6	123Ala	Ala	H6	128Ala	Ala	Ala	Ala
H7	124Ser	Ala	H7	129Ala	Ala	Ser	Ala
H8	125Leu	Trp	H8	130Tyr	Tyr	Trp	Trp
H9	126Asp	Asp	H9	131Gln	Gln	Gln	Gln
H10	127Lys	Lys	H10	132Lys	Lys	Lys	Lys
H11	128Phe	Phe	H11	133Val	Val	Met	Leu
H12	129Leu	Leu	H12	134Val	Val	Val	Val
H13	130Ala	Ser	H13	135Ala	Ala	Thr	Ser
H14	131Ser	Val	H14	136Gly	Gly	Gly, Ala	Ala
H15	132Val	Val	H15	137Val	Val	Val	Val
H16	133Ser	Ser	H16	138Ala	Ala	Ala	Ala
H17	134Thr	Ser	H17	139Asn	Asn	Ser	Ile
H18	135Val	Val	H18	140Ala	Ala	Ala	Ala
H19	136Leu	Leu	H19	141Leu	Leu	Leu	Leu
H20	137Thr	Thr	H20	142Ala	Ala	Ser	Ala
H21	138Ser	Glu	H21	143His	His	Ser	His
HC1	139Lys	Lys	HC1	144Lys	Lys	Arg	Lys
HC2	140Tyr	Tyr	HC2	145Tyr	Tyr	Tyr	Tyr
HC3	141Arg	Arg	HC3	146His	His	His	His

*a*The α and α-related (δ) subunits are shown at the left. The β and β-related (δ, γ, and ε) chains are at the right. The amino acids' relationship to the eight globin helices (A to H) is also shown. Thus, A16 is the sixteenth amino acid in the A helix. *Interhelical elbows* are named for the two adjacent helices (e.g., AB1 is the first amino acid between helices A and B). The N-terminal and C-terminal residues are labeled NA and HC, respectively. The residues are aligned to maximize the homology between subunits, which causes some gaps. Modified from Bunn HF, Forget BG. *Hemoglobin: molecular, genetic, and clinical aspects.* Philadelphia: WB Saunders, 1986.

rin, in turn, is composed of four pyrrole rings tied together by methenyl (=CH–) bridges. The porphyrin ring in heme is protoporphyrin IX, defined by the type of substitutions found in the carbons not involved in methenyl bridging (Fig. 49-3). All the structural components of heme are arranged in a single plane, resulting in a waferlike structure, hence representing the heme as a flat plate in the myoglobin model. The centerpiece of the structure is a tetracoordinated iron atom in which the bonds with pyrrole rings 4 and 2 are identical, as well as the bonds between the iron and pyrrole rings 1 and 3. This structure, weighing 616 Da, contains a large number of alternating double-bond rings and consequently delocalized π electrons.

HOW DOES THE HEME INTERACT WITH THE GLOBIN PORTION OF MYOGLOBIN?

The heme fits snugly in the heme pocket formed by the F and E helices, to which it is tied. It is surrounded by the H, G, and B helices on one side and the C and D helices on the other.

WHY IS THE HEME SEMIBURIED IN THE GLOBIN HEME POCKET?

Model compound studies suggest that hydrophobic environments are best for the maintenance of the ferrous state of the iron, and the heme pocket is highly hydrophobic and narrow (2). The heme leaves only the charged propionic side chains significantly exposed to the solvent at the entrance of the niche.

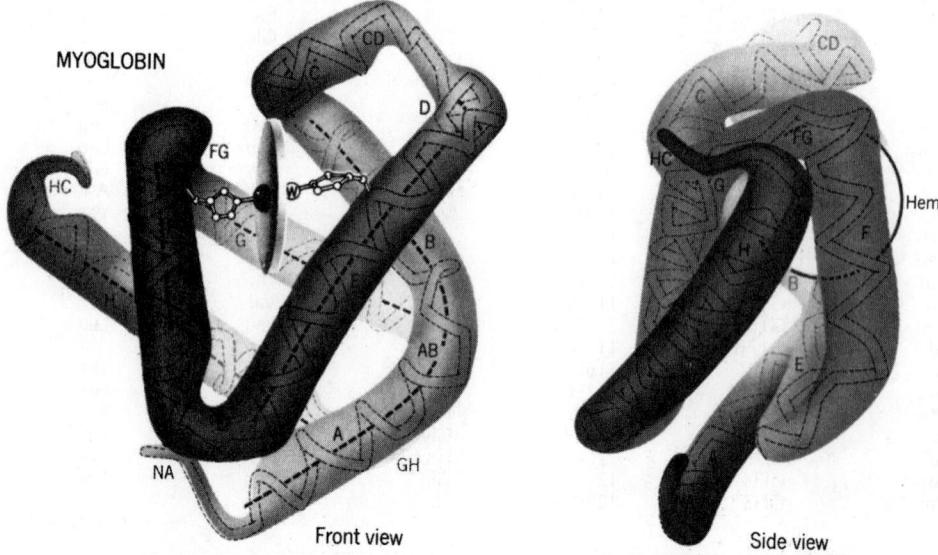

MYOGLOBIN

Front view

Side view

Figure 49-1. The myoglobin fold. The myoglobin molecule consists of eight stretches of helix that surround the heme group, forming a pocket. Single letters signify a helix; double letters, a corner or bend (nonhelical regions). The heme pocket is formed by helices E and F. Helices B, G, and H are at the bottom, and the CD corner closes the open end. Histidine side chains interact with the heme from both sides. W depicts the place occupied by the oxygen molecule when it binds to the iron. (From Dickerson RE, Geis I. *Hemoglobin: structure, function, evolution, and pathology.* Menlo Park, CA: Benjamin/Cummings, 1983, with permission.)

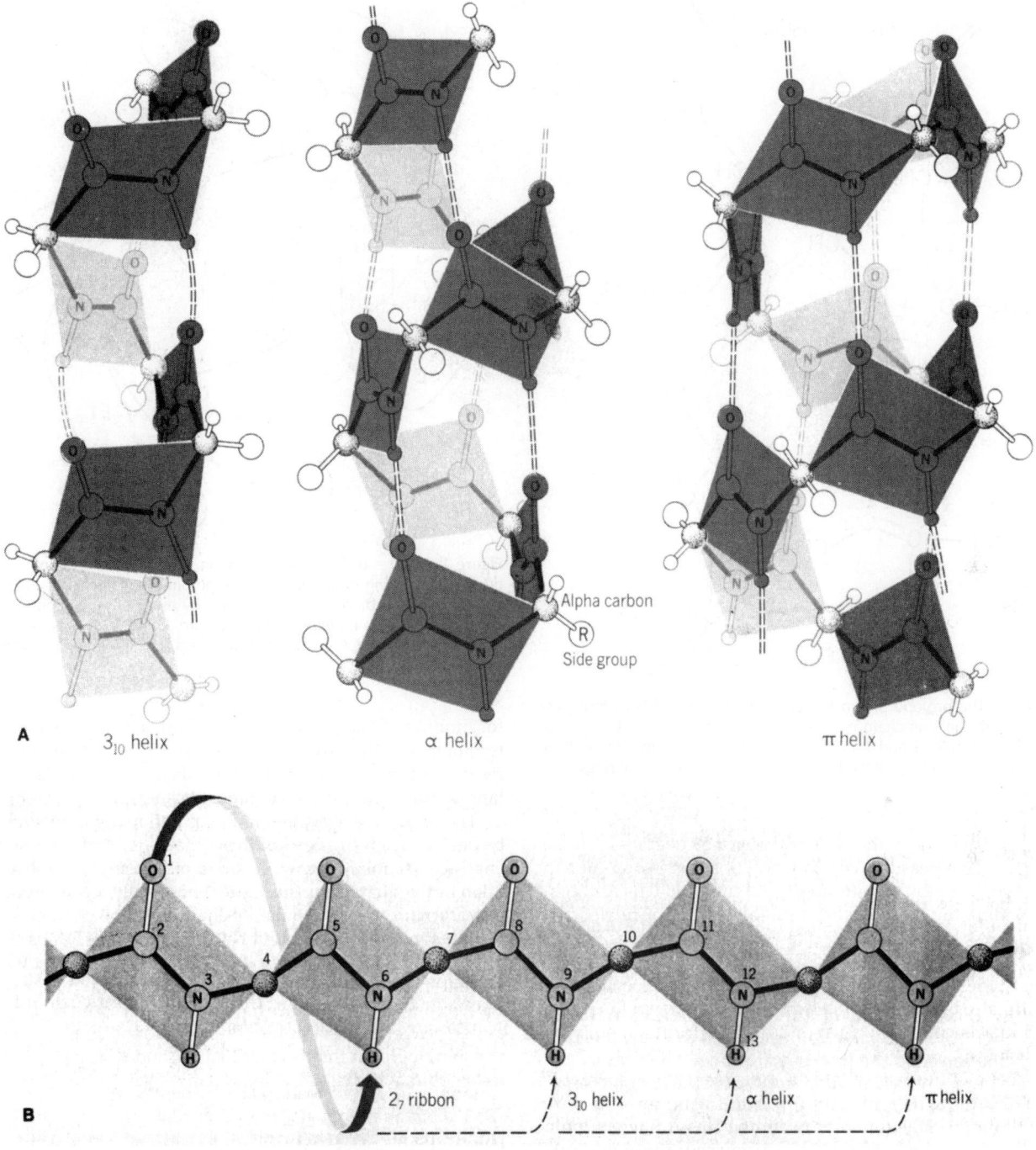

Figure 49-2. Coiling of polypeptide chains into helices. **A:** The 3_{10}, α, and π helices differ in their patterns of hydrogen bonding, shown in **(B)**. Hydrogen bonds in the helix are particularly unstrained, making the helix especially stable. The carbons are stippled, with small attached spheres for hydrogens and larger spheres for side chains. **B:** Hydrogen-bonding pattern from one turn of the helix to the next turn for four related helices. Only the helix is found extensively in proteins; the others are found only occasionally for very short stretches, usually winding down or unwinding the last turn of an helix. (From Dickerson RE, Geis I. *Hemoglobin: structure, function, evolution, and pathology.* Menlo Park, CA: Benjamin/Cummings, 1983, with permission.)

The niche is large enough for oxygen to penetrate, although with slight difficulty, as judged by micropath kinetic measurements. Ligands (molecules capable of binding to the iron) that are significantly larger than oxygen, such as those in the family of isocyanates, have progressive difficulty in reaching the iron in direct proportion to their bulk.

HOW DOES THE IRON OF THE HEME INTERACT WITH THE GLOBIN?

Four valences are consumed by coordination with the four pyrrole rings. The fifth coordination occurs with a His residue in the eighth position of the F helix (His F8), the proximal His. The sixth coordination is potentially occupied by an oxygen mole-

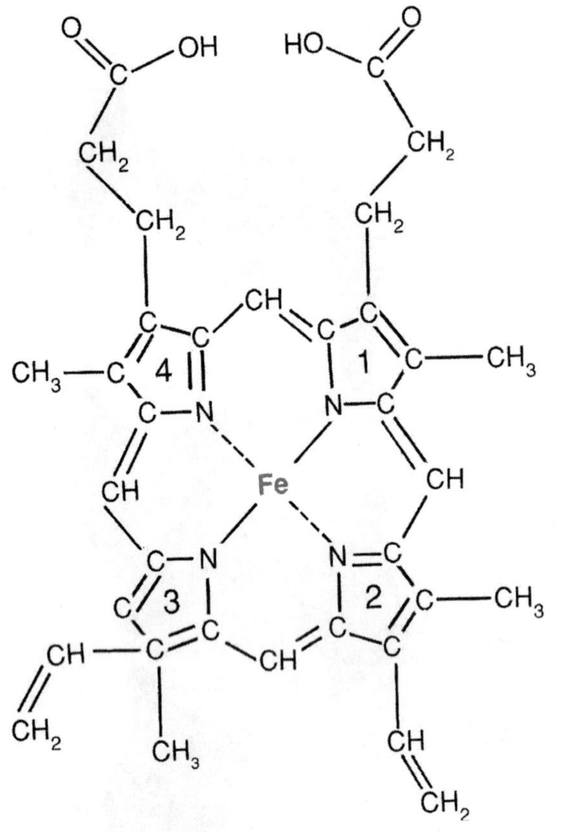

Figure 49-3. The protoporphyrin IX heme structure consists of four pyrrole rings with the side-chain replacements: two methyl and two propionic acids in pyrroles 1 and 4, and two methyl and two vinyls in pyrroles 2 and 3. Iron is tetracoordinated by the nitrogens of the pyrrole rings.

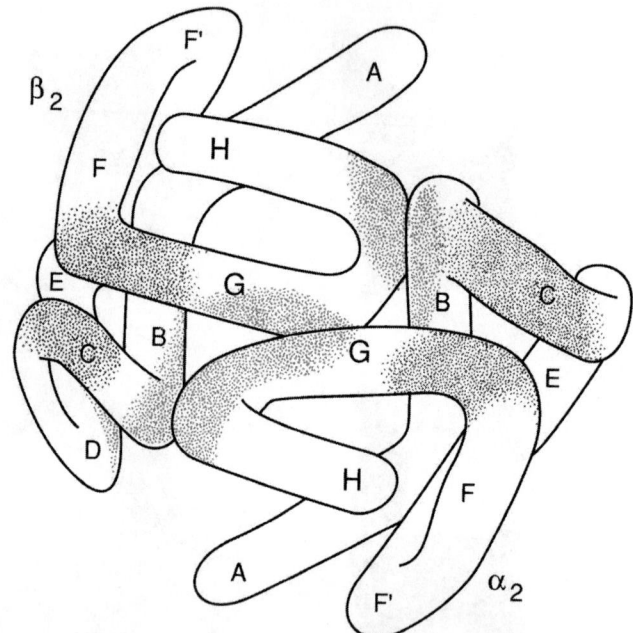

Figure 49-4. The $\alpha_2\beta_2$ dimer is seen in a side view. The colored areas depict the packing contacts that hold the dimer together. The sliding contacts with the $\alpha_1\beta_1$ dimer are depicted by areas of gray stippling. (From Dickerson RE, Geis I. *Hemoglobin: structure, function, evolution, and pathology.* Menlo Park, CA: Benjamin/Cummings, 1983, with permission.)

cule: In oxymyoglobin, the –O–O– axis is at 59 degrees from the heme plane, whereas this coordination position is occupied in deoxymyoglobin by a water molecule instead. This arrangement renders the favored structure for ferrous or ferric iron, octahedral coordination. Nevertheless, this structure is further complicated by the presence of an interacting His, the E7 or distal His, on the far site of the oxygen. This residue is too far away to coordinate directly with the iron, but the nitrogen in its side chain interacts with the oxygen or the water, further modifying ligand binding.

The fact that the heme–globin arrangement is indispensable for retaining the oxygen-binding iron in the ferrous state becomes abundantly apparent when the class of hemoglobin mutants called *M hemoglobins* are discussed; these variants result from mutations of the proximal and distal His.

α-Chains of Hemoglobin

The α-chains have the general architecture of the myoglobin fold, but they are shorter chains, involving 141 amino acids rather than 153. This difference comes from the absence of the five residues that form the myoglobin D helix and six residues from the C-terminal portion (two are the last members of the H helix and four are from the nonhelical tail of myoglobin; Fig. 49-4).

The deletion of the D helix in the α-chains has no explanation. The disappearance of the nonhelical C-terminal residues could be related to the important bond between Argα141 and Tyrα140 and the appropriate receptor, which are important to the conformational changes involved in the oxy to deoxy transformation (discussed in the section Structure–Function Relations

for Binding of Oxygen by Hemoglobin), a central feature of the tetramer structural–functional relation. The N-terminal–added residues in myoglobin might strain these critical molecular distances and make the conformational change impossible.

The differences between α-chains and myoglobin could also be derived from the need of the α-chains to bind several different β-like chains (γ, δ, ε) with varied requirements for the generation of the quaternary structure. Specifically, the generation of a quaternary structure implies changes in the character of the residues involved in subunit contact. That is, residues that are polar in myoglobin (because they are in direct contact with the solvent) might be buried in an intersubunit contact in several of the hemoglobins and hence have to be replaced by hydrophobic amino acids. Two examples of this are found in residue B15, a Lys in myoglobin that becomes a Leu, and residue C1, a His in myoglobin, which is a Phe in human α-chains (3).

β-Chains of Hemoglobin

The human β-chains are also shorter than myoglobin, but longer than α-chains, containing 146 residues. The general architecture of the chain, its secondary and tertiary structure, complies closely with the myoglobin fold (4–6).

Two small structural differences with myoglobin are apparent: the disappearance of two residues from the junction of A and B helices, making the AB elbow sharper, and six residues missing from the C-terminal sequence (as in the α-chains). The reason for the change in the AB elbow is not understood. The critical bonds involving His β142 and Tyr β145 might be incompatible with the presence of the nonhelical terminal residues found in myoglobin. In the β-chains, changes of charged residues to hydrophobic ones can also be observed in the areas of the sequence involved in subunit interaction.

The main secondary and tertiary structural differences between α-chains and β-chains are in the D helix, which are

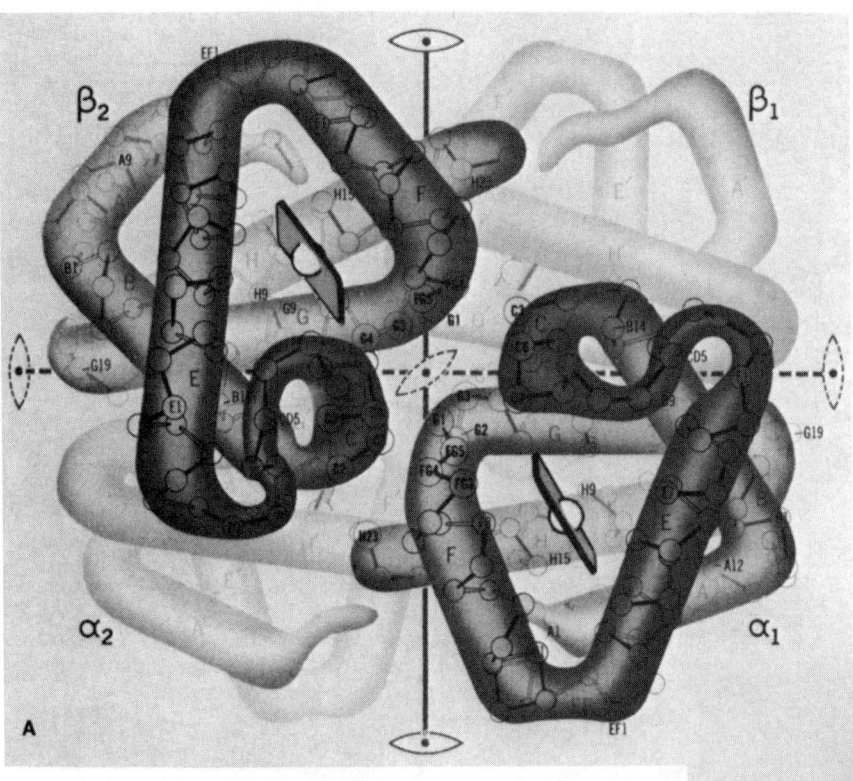

Figure 49-5. The four chains of methemoglobin. **A:** Front view: $\alpha_1\beta_2$ contacts (the $\alpha_2\beta_1$ contacts are identical on the back side of the molecule). **B:** Right side view: $\alpha_1\beta_1$ contacts (the $\alpha_2\beta_2$ contacts are identical). The two perpendicular pseudoaxes are indicated in **(A)** by dashes. Only the carbons of the main chains are shown. Those side chains involved in contacts between subunits are given boldface numbers in large circles. (From Dickerson RE, Geis I. *Hemoglobin: structure, function, evolution, and pathology.* Menlo Park, CA: Benjamin/Cummings, 1983, with permission.)

absent in the former and present in the latter. The reason for this difference is also not known.

Tetramer (Quaternary Structure)

The hemoglobin molecule is a tetramer formed by two α-chains and two β-chains, with a total molecular weight of 64.5 kd.

HOW DO THE TWO PAIRS OF CHAINS ARRANGE THEMSELVES IN SPACE TO GENERATE A TETRAMER (QUATERNARY STRUCTURE)?

The arrangement of the two types of chains in the tetramer complies with a 2-2-2 symmetry. This designation means that the structure can be characterized by three twofold axes of symmetry, perpendicular to each other, as illustrated in Figure 49-5. To understand this symmetry, consider the upper half (the dark

pair of chains) in the vertical axis. If you rotate these two chains by 180 degrees, they will coincide perfectly with the light-colored pair of chains: This is called a *twofold* or *diad axis of symmetry,* hence the 3 twos. Of course, α-chains are not identical to β-chains. Therefore, in a real hemoglobin molecule, this symmetry is only approximate. The homotetramer of β-chains (β_4 or Hb H), observed in a severe form of α-thalassemia, exhibits the perfect 2-2-2 symmetry in the oxygenated tetramer because all chains are truly identical.

HOW DO THE FOUR CHAINS INTERACT WITH EACH OTHER?

The tetramer $\alpha_2\beta_2$ exhibits several types of subunit interactions. First, little contact occurs between identical chains, that is, in the $\alpha_1\alpha_2$ or $\beta_1\beta_2$ interfaces. Most of the strong interactions between subunits are in the contacts between the dissimilar pair of chains, that is, in the interface $\alpha_1\beta_1$ and or the equivalent $\alpha_2\beta_2$.

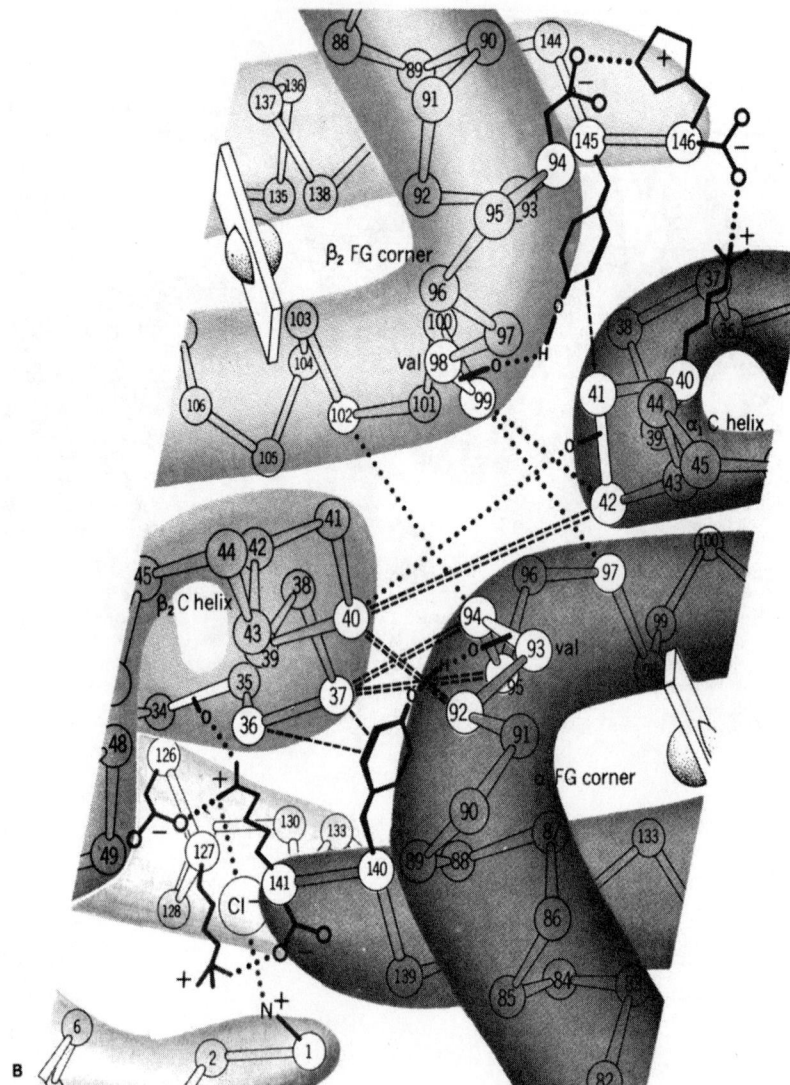

Deoxyhemoglobin:

····· H bonds or salt bridges

----- Nonbonded packing contacts

Oxyhemoglobin:

····· H bonds or salt bridges

----- Nonbonded packing contacts

Figure 49-6. Front view of hemoglobin shows extensive subunit interactions between FG corners and C helices in the $\alpha_1\beta_2$ contacts. The area in **(A)** is enlarged in **(B)**. Important interaction regions from top to bottom are the β-chain carboxy terminal, the switch region, the flexible joint, and the α-chain terminal. (From Dickerson RE, Geis I. *Hemoglobin: structure, function, evolution, and pathology.* Menlo Park, CA: Benjamin/Cummings, 1983, with permission.)

The next level of complexity is the contact between these two pairs of unlike chains. The contact occurs in two areas in the surfaces of these dimers: the $\alpha_1\beta_2$ contact (Fig. 49-6) and the equivalent $\alpha_2\beta_1$, called the *sliding contact*. Conversely, the $\alpha_1\beta_2$ dimer has areas of interaction between the α-chain and β-chain called *packing contacts*. The packing contacts are strong and can be disrupted only with very high urea concentrations and certain salts, and they remain intact through all the conformational changes of hemoglobin. The sliding contact, on the other hand, is weaker and has strategically located hydrogen bonds and salt bridges that can be broken and reformed elsewhere, allowing the mobility of the two surfaces indispensable for conformational changes (discussed in the section Structure–Function Relations for Binding of Oxygen by Hemoglobin). The interactions between like chains are weak, whereas the interactions between unlike chains are strong; hence, when the tetramer dissociates, $\alpha_1\beta_2$ dimers are generated.

Chothia et al. (7) have shown that approximately 20% of the surface area of the subunits is consumed in subunit–subunit interaction, of which 60% is involved in packing contacts and 35% in sliding contacts.

Structure–Function Relations for Binding of Oxygen by Hemoglobin

The primary task of hemoglobin is to carry oxygen from the lungs to the capillaries and carbon dioxide (CO_2) in the reverse direction. In addition, in mammals, hemoglobin must be able to adapt to sudden changes in oxygenation requirements; therefore, the modulation of its oxygen carrying capacity must be available. The functions of hemoglobin are summarized as follows:

1. It binds CO_2 when it is delivering oxygen and releases CO_2 when it is binding oxygen.
2. It binds H^+ efficiently in a low pH environment and releases it when it encounters high pH (Bohr effect).
3. Oxygen affinity is modulated by allosteric effectors—that is, 2,3-diphosphoglyceric acid (DPG), chloride (Cl^-), H^+, and CO_2.

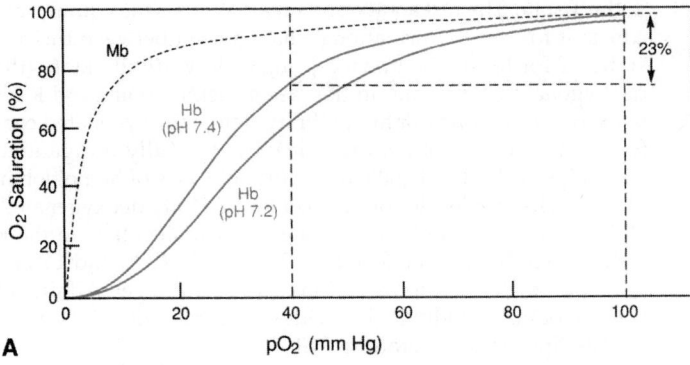

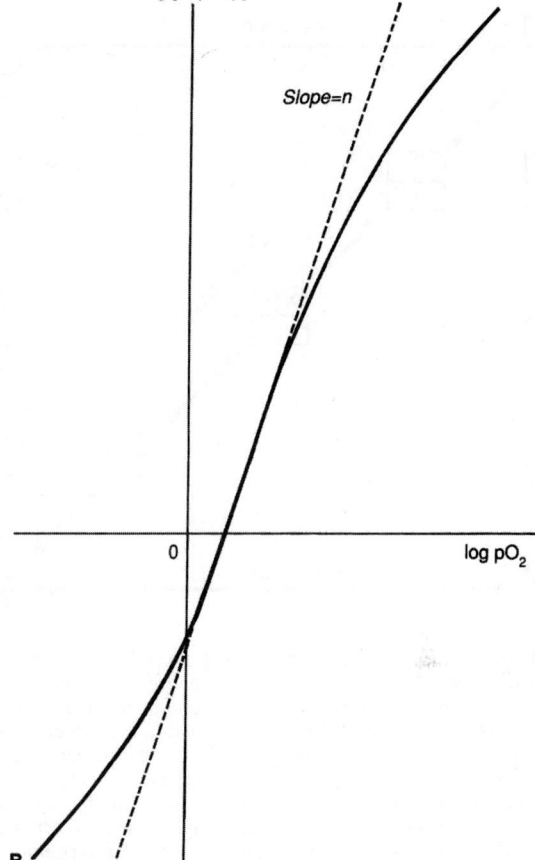

Figure 49-7. A: Oxygen equilibrium curves of sperm whale myoglobin (Mb) and hemoglobin (Hb) in human red cells. At pH 7.4 and 37°C, the oxygen saturation of the red cells is 98% at the arterial blood partial pressure of oxygen (pO$_2$) (100 mm Hg) and 75% at the mixed venous blood pO$_2$ (40 mm Hg) so that oxygen corresponding to 23% saturation difference is transported by circulating red blood cells. **B:** Logarithmic (Hill) plot of oxygen equilibrium curve of human hemoglobin. n, Hill coefficient; Y, fractional saturation of hemoglobin with oxygen. (From Imai K. *Allosteric effects in haemoglobin.* Cambridge: Cambridge University Press, 1982, with permission.)

These properties and their molecular mechanisms are described in the following sections.

HEMOGLOBIN BINDS OXYGEN ALLOSTERICALLY

The myoglobin molecule, a monomer with one heme, binds oxygen as predicted by mass law: A plot of partial pressure of oxygen (pO$_2$) versus oxygen saturation can be described by a hyperbole. On the other hand, the hemoglobin tetramer with four hemes, binds oxygen with a sigmoidal curve (Fig. 49-7). Myoglobin binding of oxygen can be described at equilibrium by the simple relation

$$y = K_a\, pO_2 / 1 + K_a\, pO_2$$

where y is the fractional saturation of the myoglobin molecule with oxygen and K_a is the association constant. For the hemoglobin molecule, the binding of oxygen is different, and at equilibrium this reaction can be described by the formula

$$y = K_a\, pO_2^{\,n} / 1 + K_a\, pO_2^{\,n}$$

The difference is the power of n to which pO$_2$ is elevated: *n* is the Hill coefficient, an empiric number that is an index of the sigmoidicity of the curve and a feature of the function that is related to the extent of cooperativity. The Hill coefficient is 2.8 for hemoglobin, whereas it is 1 for myoglobin.

What Is Cooperativity? Cooperativity is the reason for the sigmoid shape of the oxygen equilibrium curve of hemoglobin. The initial portion of the curve has a very low slope, reflecting a low affinity for oxygen by hemoglobin at the beginning of the loading process. That is, when hemoglobin is totally deoxygenated, it has a rather poor avidity for oxygen (Fig. 49-7). As the

loading proceeds and as the molecule binds more oxygen molecules, the slope of the reaction begins to change rapidly and becomes steep, meaning that the affinity for oxygen has become much higher despite the sluggish beginnings. In other words, the initial molecules of oxygen that bind a deoxyhemoglobin tetramer change the protein's avidity for oxygen. This property, called *cooperativity*, ensures that the hemoglobin tetramer, after it begins to accept oxygen, is fully oxygenated promptly. Thus, if we could measure the distribution of oxygen in all the hemoglobin molecules in a solution that contains enough oxygen to oxygenate only half of the hemes available, most molecules would not be oxygenated at all or would be entirely oxygenated, with a small compartment of partially oxygenated hemoglobins.

How Can Cooperativity Be Explained at the Molecular Level? Formally, there are two overall models for cooperativity. The *sequential*, or Koshland-Nemethy-Filmer (KNF), model (8) (Fig. 49-8) involves the change of conformation of each subunit after binding oxygen, combined with a slight modification of the conformation of their neighbors and, as a consequence, progressive increase in their affinity for oxygen. This model predicts a family of conformations between fully deoxygenated and totally oxygenated molecules, each one exhibiting slightly higher overall affinity for the ligand.

The *two-state* (or *concerted*) model of Monod, Wyman, and Changeaux (9) (MWC model) contains two fundamentally different conformations, one for oxygenated hemoglobin, another for the deoxygenated molecule. In its strictest form, this model does not accept meaningful intermediate conformations, only two extreme ones. It predicts that the molecule of hemoglobin

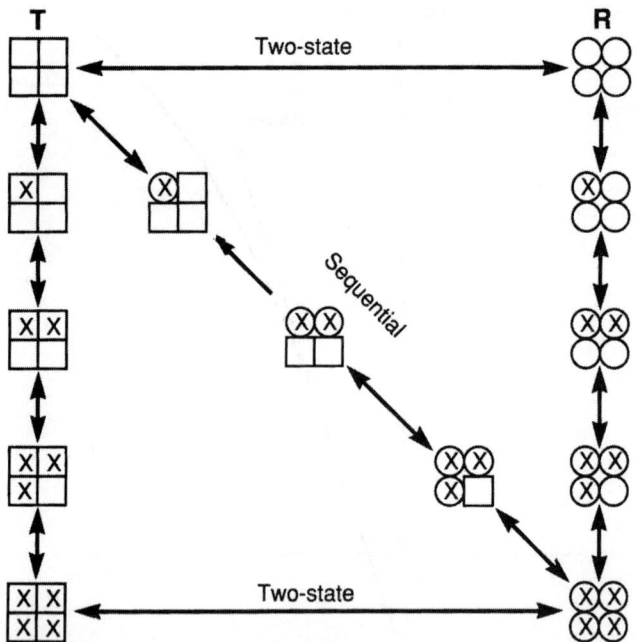

Figure 49-8. Contrasting ways of generating cooperativity according to the two-state (Monod-Wyman-Changeaux) and sequential (Koshland-Nemethy-Filmer) models. Each subunit has two distinct tertiary conformations, one with higher ligand affinity for ligand X. In the two-state model, the oligomeric molecule is postulated to exist in only two global conformations, T and R. In quaternary T, all subunits have the low-affinity tertiary conformation t (*squares*); in quaternary R, they all have the high-affinity conformation r (*circles*). The fully unligated oligomer favors T, whereas the R form predominates in fully ligated molecules. Changes in conformation of individual subunits occur in a concerted or all-or-none fashion so that the oligomer is always symmetric. The sequential model is indicated by the diagonal, where species proceed through a sequence of intermediate conformations. Ligand binding induces a change to the high-affinity conformation (r) in each ligated subunit, whereas the unligated subunits retain their low-affinity conformations (t). Altered pairwise contacts of each ligated subunit with its neighbors influence the neighboring subunit's tendency to bind the next ligand and to switch to the high-affinity form. The sequential model can account for both positive and negative cooperativity (binding a ligand diminishes the affinity for subsequent binding), whereas the two-state model can accommodate only positive cooperativity. (From Komiyama N, Shih DT, Looker D, et al. Was the loss of the D helix in alpha globin a functional neutral mutation? *Nature* 1991;352:349, with permission.)

will bind two or three molecules of oxygen at low affinity (deoxy conformation); then, suddenly, the molecule will flip to the oxygenated conformation, drastically increasing the oxygen affinity of the molecule as a whole. Perutz et al. (14a) have applied this model with great success to hemoglobin.

The two-state model was originally developed to explain the function of enzymes, particularly the role of effectors; these effectors, although not binding at the active site, were able to modify the activity of protein. The conceptual breakthrough came with the realization that the effector induces a change in conformation of the molecule as a whole, producing, from a distance, a significant change in the conformation and function of the active site. This process was called *allostery* or produced *allosteric changes*, meaning different shapes.

Formally, the two-state model can be defined by two quantities. The first, c, represents the difference in activity between the two enzyme states, but in the special case of hemoglobin, corresponds to the ratio in oxygen affinity constants between the two conformation states (K_a oxy/K_a deoxy = c). The second quantity, the allosteric constant L, is the fraction of hemoglobin molecules

in the T state. The rest are R structures. L defines the equilibrium constant for the conformational change itself between the two states: T for tense, the nonaccepting or low-affinity state (the deoxygenated conformer in the case of hemoglobin) and R for relaxed, the accepting or high-affinity state (the oxygenated conformer in the case of hemoglobin). For the fully unliganded state, $(T_o)/(R_o)$ = L = 10,000 for *in vitro* solutions of hemoglobin. That is, when molecules of hemoglobin are fully deoxygenated, 10,000 molecules are in the T state and 1 molecule is in the R state. The influence of effectors (2,3-DPG, H^+, CO_2, and Cl^-) on these parameters is discussed in the section Oxygen Affinity of Hemoglobin Is Modulated by Other Allosteric Effectors, Such As 2,3-Diphosphoglycerate and Cl^-.

As soon as the first molecule of oxygen is added, the ratio of the two conformers will be defined by $(T_1)/(R_1)$ = Lc. In a study by Baldwin and Chothia (10), the number for c is approximately 0.01; therefore, the ratio will be 10 to 1. When two molecules of oxygen are added, the ratio will be $(T_2)/(R_2)$ = Lc_2 = 1; hence, the same number of T molecules and R molecules will be present. When three molecules are bound, the ratio becomes $(T_3)/(R_3)$ = Lc_3 = –100, which means that 100 molecules are in the R form and 1 is in the T form. Finally, when all four sites are saturated, $(T_4)/(R_4)$ = Lc_4 = –10,000. There are 10,000 molecules in the R form for every T hemoglobin molecule. Thus, the significant switch of conformation must occur in hemoglobin somewhere between the binding of two and three molecules of oxygen. In physiologic conditions of pH, in the presence of effectors and osmolarity, at full saturation, only 1 out of 3 million hemoglobin molecules has the T structure.

Why is the hemoglobin tetramer of higher organisms allosteric? Allosterism makes hemoglobin a molecule with lower affinity for oxygen than myoglobins or the isolated hemoglobin chains. Allosteric effectors such as 2,3-DPG, chloride, hydrogen ions, and so forth, modulate the reduced affinity by lowering K_T (the association constant for the T state) and raising the L constant. The K_R (association constant of the R state) and L at oxygen saturation are not modified (11).

In contrast, the sequential (KNF) model has progressive subunit conformation changes that are stepwise but not necessarily equal. The first subunit oxygenated will change conformation from t_1 to r_1 and so progressively, until $t_4 \rightarrow R_4$. This reaction produces stepwise but nonequal increments in affinity for the successive subunits liganded.

The question is which of these two models better explains the data available on hemoglobin ligand binding. Crystallography has defined two extreme conformations of hemoglobin, one oxy and one deoxy, both of which are different, but this result does not decide the issue, because the two models proposed have different initial and final conformers. The present evidence suggests that, in general, the two-state model explains most of the experimental data accumulated for the functional properties of the hemoglobin molecule. The broad categories of evidence are the following:

1. In the cyanomethemoglobin–oxyhemoglobin hybrids of the type of $\alpha_2\beta_2$CMet and α_2CMetβ_2 (12), two hemes are frozen in the liganded oxygenated-like state (cyanomethemoglobin), and they can be interrogated [by nuclear magnetic resonance (NMR) spectroscopy] as to their R or T state when the other two hemes are deoxygenated or oxygenated. The experiment demonstrates that the cyanomet hemes do not change when the ferrous hemes are either oxygenated or deoxygenated. In other words, they are fixed in the R (oxy) conformer. Nevertheless, if the R conformer is forced into the T state by a powerful allosteric inhibitor (such as inositol hexaphosphate), the spectrum of the cyanomet hemes

changes to the T state. Therefore, the environment of the hemes is sensitive to protein conformational changes and not to the individual state of the subunits.

2. Hybrid hemoglobin molecules constructed with nitrous oxide-bound hemoglobins have been examined by spectral methods (13,14b,14c). They can also be driven to the deoxy conformer, even when fully liganded, by the superallosteric inhibitor, inositol hexaphosphate. Iron–His interactions can be observed to go from the R to the T state in spite of the liganded state of the molecule. Again, these results are a strong argument for the two-state model.

3. The properties of hemoglobin mutants are largely concordant with the two-state model (15,19).

Nevertheless, detailed thermodynamic descriptions of the hemoglobin molecule by Gary Ackers et al. (16) and other data by Ho and Russu (15) indicate that the two-state model must be relaxed to accept some amount of stepwise conformational change. Miura et al. (17) find NMR evidence of tertiary conformational changes that are incompatible with the strict two-state model system. Ackers et al. (16) find thermodynamic evidence of a third allosteric structure. Perella et al. (18), using low temperature isoelectric focusing techniques, find that the distribution of intermediate ligand states is compatible with a third allosteric structure, which in effect brings features of the KNF sequential model to the MWC two-state model.

Nevertheless, the extent of departure from the MWC model is well settled: The use of mixed-state hybrids for defining some of the evidence overstates the KNF feature of heme–heme interaction. In other words, the big picture remains the overall T to R transition of the whole hemoglobin molecule (two-state model), but the small (but significant) picture is the T to R transitions in each subunit. Eaton's (19,20) analysis argues convincingly that the two-state model of Perutz defines the fundamental function of hemoglobin and, in addition, casts doubt on the interpretation of some of the experiments by Acker et al.

An important area that has not been fully defined is subunit specificity. Does oxygen (or other ligands) bind differently to α-chains and β-chains? Are the two chains equally likely to bind the first molecule of ligand? Are the pathways that lead to conformational changes identical if the first ligand bound attaches to the α-chains or the β-chains? Some of these questions have been answered for bulky ligands that fit differently in the heme slits of the α-chains and β-chains, but they have not been conclusively answered for smaller, physiologically relevant ligands such as oxygen and carbon monoxide.

What Are the Precise Structural Events Underlying Cooperativity? We will examine the conformational restraints characterizing the T and R states, the triggering mechanism at the heme, and the micropath that leads from the iron to the switching of conformers.

The critical differences between R and T conformers are confined to the areas of contact between the $\alpha_1\beta_2$ and $\alpha_2\beta_1$ dimers. The $\alpha_1\beta_1$ and $\alpha_2\beta_2$ areas of contact are essentially immobile during the conformational change, because these dimers move as a unit. These events are depicted in Figure 49-9.

Three regions of the molecule sustain the major changes during the R to T conformational change, which is a 15-degree rotation of the $\alpha_1\beta_1$ dimer with respect to the $\alpha_2\beta_1$ dimer around a pivot passing through the terminal portions of the H helix in both chains. The asymmetry of the pivot results in great changes (7-Å translation) in the way the two β-chains are deployed with respect to each other and in considerably smaller changes between the two α-chains. The movements involve exclusively the residues that touch each other in the $\alpha_1\beta_2$ areas of contact. These are of two types: one between the FG corner of the β-chains and the C helix of the α-chains, and the other involving the FG corner of the α-chains contacting the C helix of the β-chains. In the pivotal sliding of the two dimers with respect to each other, the contact involving the β FG corner is farther away from the pivotal axis; therefore, the translation is farther. Baldwin and Chothia (10) have called this contact point the *switch region* (Fig. 49-6A). The other contact is less affected

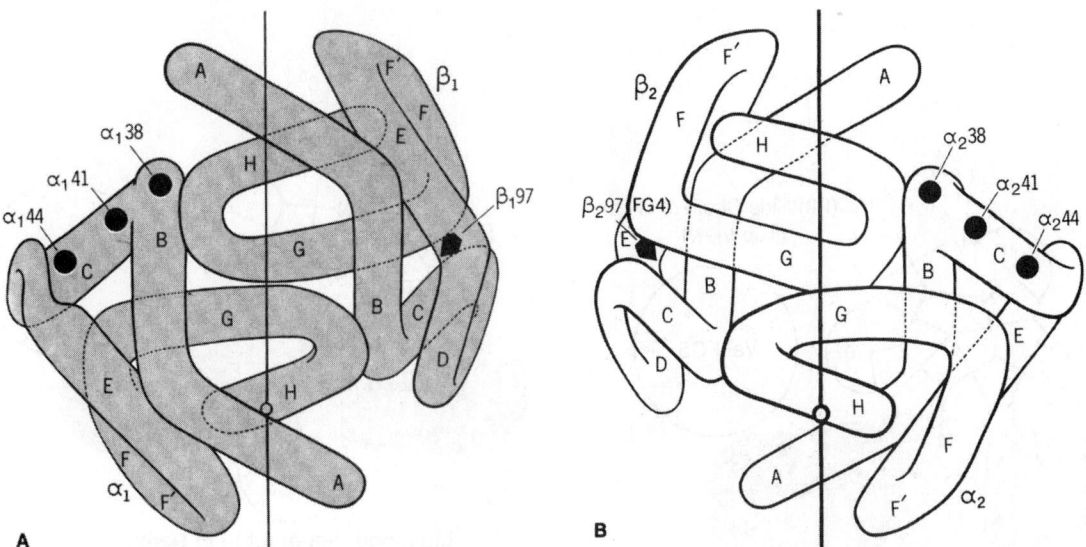

Figure 49-9. Subunit motion in hemoglobin. Side views of the separated $\alpha_1\beta_1$ and $\alpha_2\beta_2$ dimers and their combination into deoxyhemoglobin and oxyhemoglobin. **A:** The $\alpha_1\beta_1$ dimer is seen from outside the molecule, and the four critical residues appear on the undersides of the helices. **B:** The $\alpha_2\beta_2$ dimer is seen from inside the molecule. These two dimers are superimposed in (**C**) and (**D**). Critical-chain residues in the switch region are noted. (*continued*)

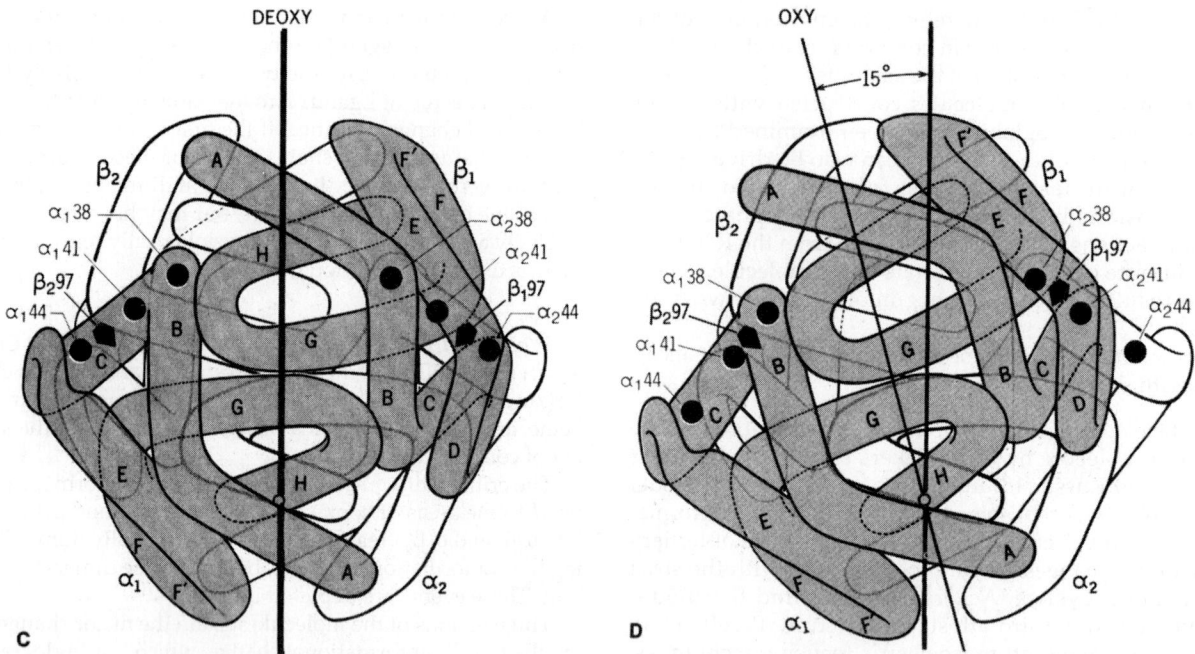

Figure 49-9. (*continued*) **C:** The complete tetramer is shown in its deoxyhemoglobin conformation. Note the position of β97 relative to 41 and 44. **D:** In oxyhemoglobin, the $\alpha_1\beta_1$ is rotated 15 degrees relative to $\alpha_2\beta_2$. The new position of β97 is between 41 and 38. (From Dickerson RE, Geis I. *Hemoglobin: structure, function, evolution, and pathology.* Menlo Park, CA: Benjamin/Cummings, 1983, with permission.)

because the α FG corner is much closer to the pivotal axis. The same authors have called this area the *flexible joint*. The third important change is in the set of salt bridges between the H helix (C-terminal portion of the β-chain) and the C helix of the α-chain and between the C-terminal portion of the α-chains and the C helix of the β-chain. These contact points have no particular name, but they are referred to here as the *C-terminal changes*. Detailed residue interactions are depicted in Figure 49-9.

All these H bonds and salt bridges are broken in the oxy conformer, providing one of the most important sources of the difference in free energy between the T and R states in hemoglobin.

What Is the Triggering Mechanism at the Level of the Heme for the Conformational Change? The iron in deoxyhemoglobin is slightly out of the plane of the heme (domed configuration) because the pyrrole rings are also slightly pyramidal (Fig. 49-10). The angle between the heme plane and the iron is 8 degrees in the α heme and 7 degrees in the β heme. The His F8 axis is 8 degrees off center (Fig. 49-11), and the Val FG5 is in contact with the vinyl side chain of pyrrole 3 (Fig. 49-10B). When the ligand binds the sixth coordinating position of the iron, significant steric stresses are introduced, particularly between the heme and the proximal His, the ligand and the heme, and the heme and the Val FG5. To

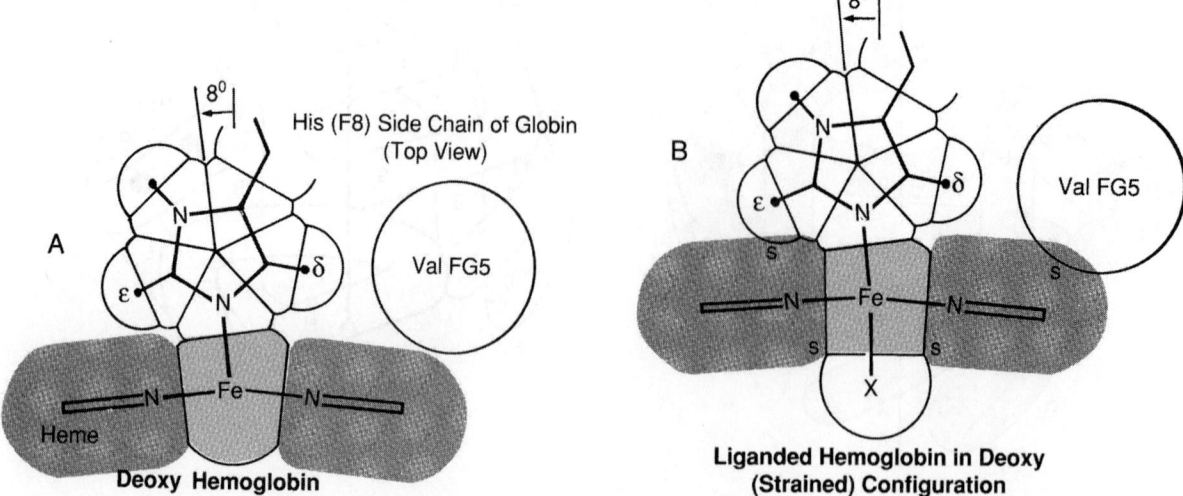

Figure 49-10. Ligation and strain in the heme environment. **A:** Unliganded heme in deoxyhemoglobin, with the histidine tilted, the iron out of plane, and the heme in contact with the Val FG5 side chain. **B:** Liganded heme held in its deoxy configuration before the T to R subunit transition. Steric strain (s) among heme, histidine, ligand (X), and Val can be relieved only after this transition. (*continued*)

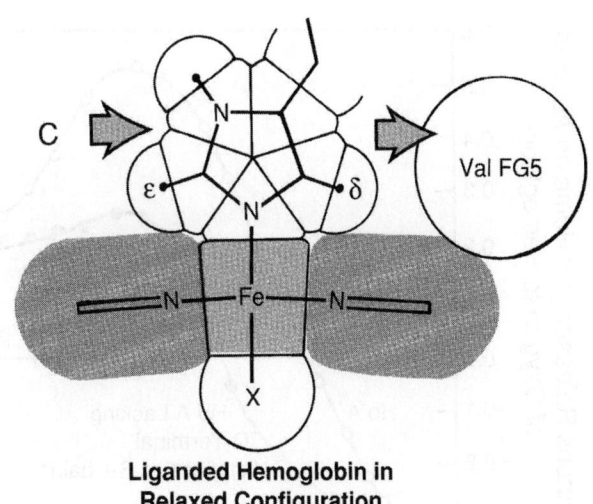

**Liganded Hemoglobin in
Relaxed Configuration**

Figure 49-10. *(continued)* **C:** Relaxed, unstrained liganded heme after the T to R shift. Both His F8 and Val FG5 have shifted to the right, and the histidine now is perpendicular to the heme plane. The heme is largely undomed. (From Dickerson RE, Geis I. *Hemoglobin: structure, function, evolution, and pathology*. Menlo Park, CA: Benjamin/Cummings, 1983, with permission.)

relieve this strain, the His moves 8 degrees to become perpendicular to the heme (Fig. 49-10C), significantly decreasing the doming of the iron (the angle between iron and the heme falls to 4 degrees). Also, displacement of FG5 is present in the direction of His F8. The configuration around the heme has now changed to the oxygenated or R state, and a chain of events follows involving the critical interactions in the $\alpha_1\beta_2$ area of contact.

What Is the Micropath Followed by Conformational Change Extending from the Heme to the Globin?

The best interpretation of the available data is the following. In the α-chain, the displacement of the His F8 to straighten up its 8-degree tilt in the liganded heme requires that the F helix (Fig. 49-11) move with it. This displacement of the F helix along its axis is accompanied by a shift downward, which moves closer to the heme. The heme shifts toward the interior of the heme pocket. The changes in the F helix are propagated along the E and G helices but leave the rest of the α-chain unchanged. In the β-subunit, the changes are similar, except that the heme also tilts around a pyrrole 2–4 axis. In both heme niches, the Val FG5 moves closer to the vinyl side chains; this Van der Waals contact breaks the critical H bonds between Val98 and Tyr145 in the β-chain and between Val98 and Tyr140 in the α-chain. The rest of the H bonds and salt bridges described for the C-terminals become weakened to the point of

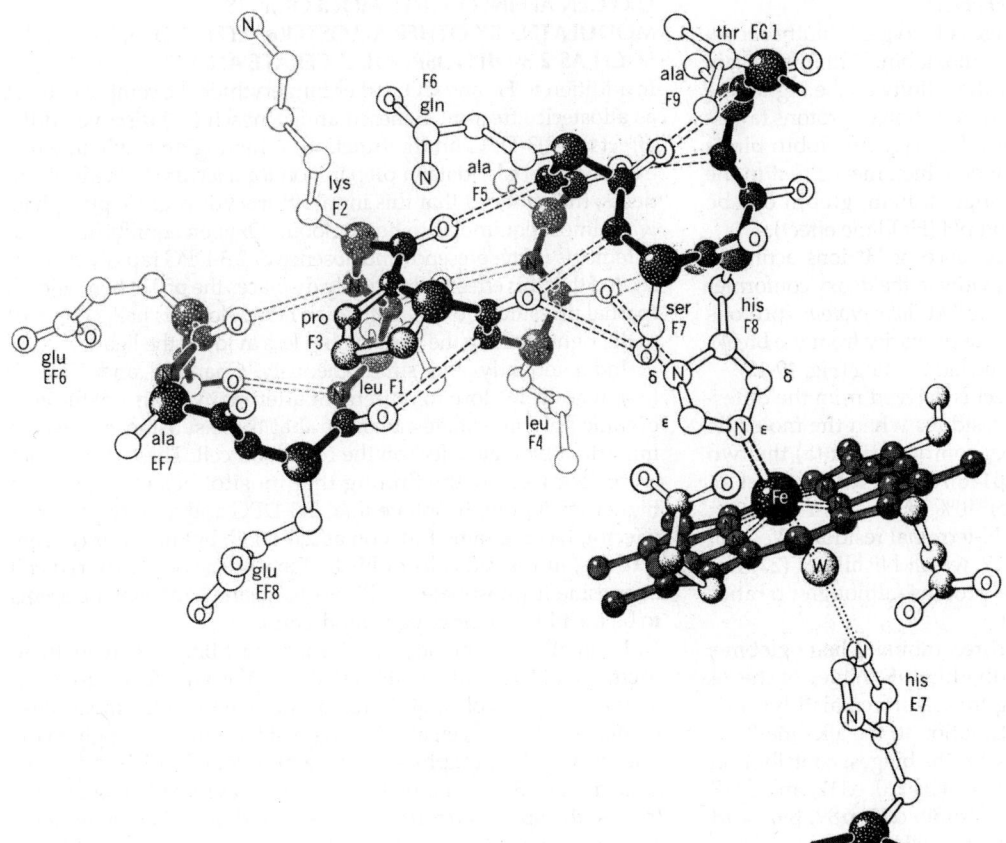

Figure 49-11. The F helix. Pro in position F3 interrupts the hydrogen bonding of the F helix. Because Pro lacks a free NH, it can appear at the beginning of helices but not in the middle or at the end. Pro frequently introduces bends into the polypeptide chain. In the heme environment, octahedral coordination about the iron atom is completed in metmyoglobin by a water molecule at (W). In deoxymyoglobin, the water molecule is gone, and in oxymyoglobin, it is replaced by oxygen. The hydrogen bond between N of the histidine and CO of F4 helps to hold the histidine ring rigidly in place. (From Dickerson RE, Geis I. *Hemoglobin: structure, function, evolution, and pathology*. Menlo Park, CA: Benjamin/Cummings, 1983, with permission.)

breakage, releasing the molecule from the T state (closed and low affinity) to the R state (open and high affinity).

The general features of this micropath for the conformational changes of hemoglobin were proposed early with insufficient evidence (21). Significant proof had to wait for high-resolution x-ray crystallography, extended x-ray absorption fine structure, and the experiments of Perutz et al. (14a–c).

HEMOGLOBIN BINDS CARBON DIOXIDE WHEN IT IS DELIVERING OXYGEN AND RELEASES CARBON DIOXIDE WHEN IT IS BINDING OXYGEN

The hemoglobin molecule is designed to bind CO_2 after delivering oxygen to the tissues, helping to dissipate the increase in concentration of CO_2 in the tissues and conveniently delivering this metabolic end product to the alveoli of the lungs. It accomplishes this task with ease because CO_2 is an allosteric inhibitor of hemoglobin, decreasing the oxygen affinity of the molecule.

Carbon dioxide binds hemoglobin by forming carbamates with the α-amino groups of the α-chains. Through this new negative charge, CO_2 can bind Arg141 in the absence of Cl^- ions. This bond stabilizes the T conformer and decreases the oxygen affinity of the molecule (25,26). The basic reaction is

$$Hb\text{–}NH_2 + CO_2 \rightarrow Hb\text{–}NH\text{–}COO^- + H^+$$

Although CO_2 also binds the α-amino groups of the β-chains, helping to transport more of this metabolic end product, the reaction does not contribute to the allosteric effect. The β-chain carbamate reaction favors the deoxy conformer by the production of H^+, but this effect is counteracted by the reduction of positive charges in the central cavity, an event that favors the R state. Nothing gained, nothing lost.

HEMOGLOBIN BINDS H^+ EFFICIENTLY IN A LOW pH ENVIRONMENT AND RELEASES PROTONS WHEN IT ENCOUNTERS HIGH pH (BOHR EFFECT)

The Bohr effect describes the changes of oxygen affinity secondary to pH changes exhibited by hemoglobin. Within a certain range, the lower the pH, the lower the affinity or the higher the p50 (27,28). That is, an increased concentration of protons favors a low-affinity state in hemoglobin. Deoxyhemoglobin binds more protons than the oxy conformer, which means that in the absence of a buffer, a ligand change in hemoglobin can be recorded by a change in the solution pH (Haldane effect).

All these features are the consequence of H^+ ions acting as allosteric inhibitors: H^+ binds more avidly to the deoxy conformer (T state) than the oxy state. The so-called *Bohr protons* (protons released during oxygenation) originate primarily from the breakage of the C-terminal bonds during ligand binding (Fig. 49-12).

Seventy percent of the Bohr effect is derived from the differences in the pK of the following residues when the molecule changes from the oxy to the deoxy conformation: (a) the two terminal His of the β-chains (Hisβ146), which Kilmartin et al. (26) have determined account for 40% of the Bohr protons; (b) the α-amino groups of the two N-terminal residues (Val1) of the α-chains (25%); and (c) Hisα122, which Nishikura (27) has found contributes 10% of the Bohr protons (although no rationale for this effect has been found).

Using proton NMR spectra and recombinant hemoglobins, Fang et al. (29) have measured individual pK values of the 24 histidyl residues of Hb A. Among those surface histidyl residues, Hisβ146 has the biggest contribution to the alkaline Bohr effect (63% at pH 7.4), and β143 His has the biggest contribution to the acid Bohr effect (71% at pH 5.1). Hisα20, α112, and β117 have essentially no contribution; Hisα50, α72, α89, β97, and β116 have moderate positive contributions; Hisβ2 and β77 have a moderate negative contribution to the Bohr effect. The sum of

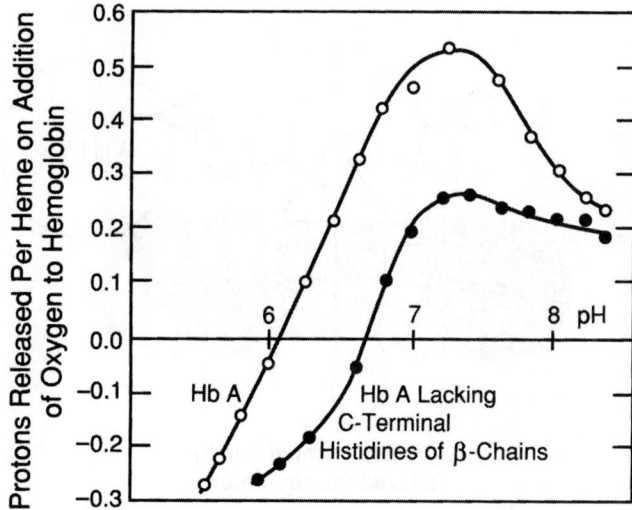

Figure 49-12. Discharge of protons on uptake of oxygen (Bohr effect) by normal human hemoglobin (Hb) A and hemoglobin from which the C-terminal histidines of the β-chains have been cleaved with carboxypeptidase B (des Hisβ146 hemoglobin). Note the reversal of the alkaline Bohr effect at pH 6.0 in Hb A and at the pH 6.7 in des His hemoglobin and the halving of the alkaline Bohr effect in the latter. (From Kilmartin JV, Wootton JF. Inhibition of Bohr effect after removal of C-terminal histidines from haemoglobin β chains. *Nature* 1970;228:766, with permission.)

the contributions from 24 surface histidyl residues accounted for 86% of the alkaline Bohr effect at pH 7.4 and approximately 55% of the acid Bohr effect at pH 5.1. The present study argues in favor of a global electrostatic network in regulating the Bohr effect of the hemoglobin molecule.

OXYGEN AFFINITY OF HEMOGLOBIN IS MODULATED BY OTHER ALLOSTERIC EFFECTORS, SUCH AS 2,3-DIPHOSPHOGLYCERATE AND Cl^-

In addition to H^+ and CO_2, other intraerythrocytic components act as allosteric effectors. Benesch and Benesch (30) discovered the effects of 2,3-DPG on the function of hemoglobin when, while examining tabular data in preparation for a lecture to medical students, they noticed that this intraerythrocytic organic phosphate was almost equimolar to hemoglobin. Oxygen equilibrium measurements in the presence and absence of 2,3-DPG rapidly demonstrated that this effector drastically displaces the p50 of hemoglobin (partial pressure of oxygen at which hemoglobin is half saturated) to the right, making the hemoglobin less avid for the ligand.

Independently and simultaneously, Chanutin and Cumish (31), who were close to retirement after many years of studying organic polyphosphates, realized that these substances have an important biologic effect on the red blood cell. These discoveries were followed by the finding that inositol hexaphosphate, a higher-level polyphosphate than 2,3-DPG and a more powerful effector, has the same function as 2,3-DPG, but at lower concentrations, in the red cells of birds. Finally, in some fish, red cell adenosine triphosphate (ATP) or guanosine triphosphate seems to be the physiologic oxygen modulator.

In an allosteric model, the effector must bind differentially to each one of the conformational states. For an effector to be an inhibitor (a molecule that decreases the activity of the molecule—in this case, the oxygen affinity), it must bind more strongly to the T form. Crystallographic evidence by Arnone (32) has demonstrated that 2,3-DPG binds to the central cavity of hemoglobin—that is, the space surrounding the true diad axis of symmetry between the two β-chains (Fig. 49-13). The displacement of the β-chains away from each other by 7 Å in deoxyhemoglobin makes

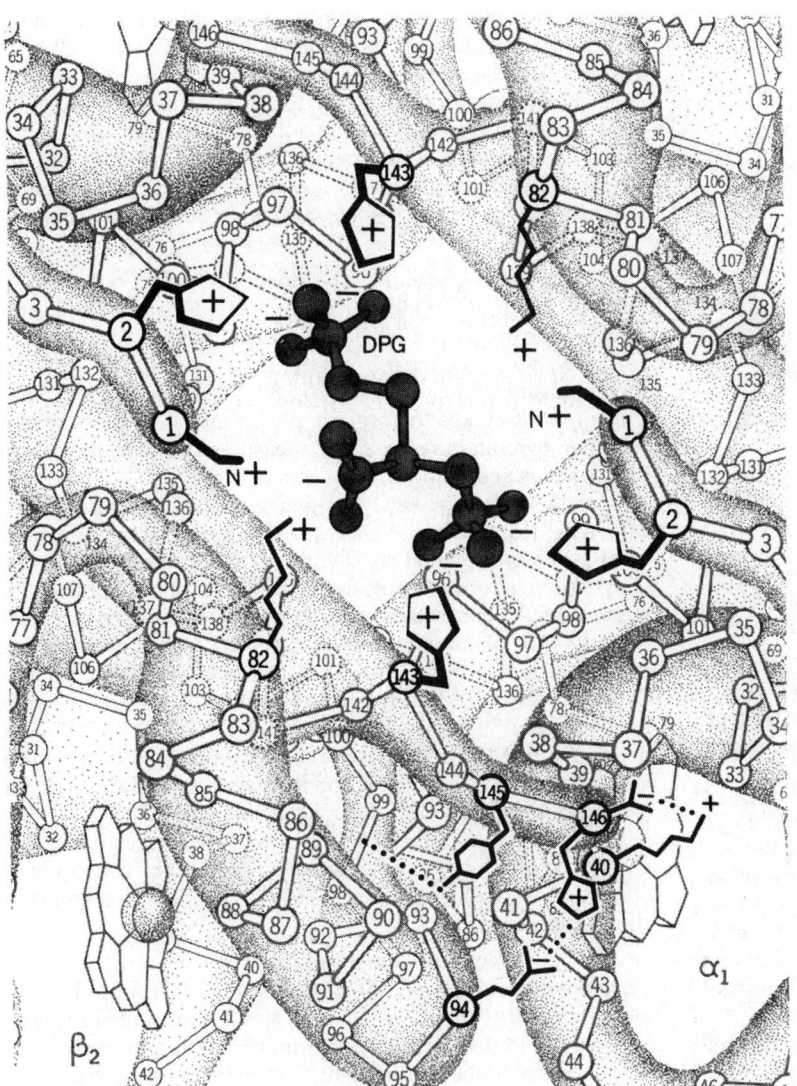

Figure 49-13. Amino acid side chains around the 2,3-diphosphoglycerate (DPG) binding site. This top view of the central cavity in human deoxyhemoglobin shows the positive charges lining the DPG site: two each from the amino terminal (Valβ1), Hisβ2, Lysβ82, and Hisβ143. The DPG molecule with its five negative charges sits in the middle of this ring of positive charges. The fetal γ chain loses two of its eight positive charges by substituting Ser for His at β143, decreasing the affinity for DPG. Also shown are the salt bridges and the hydrogen-bonding pattern around the carboxyl terminus of the β chain (*lower part of figure*), which emphasizes their contribution to the Bohr effect. (From Dickerson RE, Geis I. Hemoglobin: structure, function, evolution, and pathology. Menlo Park, CA: Benjamin/Cummings, 1983, with permission.)

this single site in the tetramer capable of accommodating the highly negatively charged 2,3-DPG molecule, whereas the tighter β–β interaction in oxyhemoglobin does not allow the effector to penetrate the central cavity. The five negative charges of 2,3-DPG find proper positive charges to form salt bridges just under the edge of the central cavity between the β-chains. The globin residues involved in the binding are the two amino terminals of the α-chains and β-chains, the two Hisβ143, and one of the two Lysβ82.

This site in the central cavity is the only binding site for 2,3-DPG in hemoglobin; therefore, one 2,3-DPG molecule binds per tetramer of hemoglobin. This is unusual, because in hemoglobin, because of its 2-2-2 symmetry, most binding sites have an equivalent counterpart on the other side of the molecule. The central cavity is the exception, reinforcing that this molecule does not have perfect 2-2-2 symmetry due to the nonidentity of the α-chains and β-chains. The other end of the central cavity, surrounded by α-chains, does not move apart much during deoxygenation, as previously discussed, and does not form a proper binding site for 2,3-DPG.

The purpose of this effector is to modulate the oxygen equilibrium curve according to physiologic requirements. For example, in anemia, the synthesis of 2,3-DPG increases, favoring the release of oxygen and partially coping with the decrease in the number of oxygen carriers.

Chloride is another allosteric inhibitor of hemoglobin. It also decreases the oxygen affinity of the molecule. Two mechanisms are involved. Cl^- binds preferentially to the deoxy conformer, the classic mechanism by which allosteric inhibitors work in hemoglobin. As noted earlier, Argα141, among its many interactions, forms a salt bridge with the amino terminals of the opposite α-chain across the $\alpha_1\beta_1$ area of contact through a Cl^- ion (Fig. 49-14). These bonds are broken in the oxy conformer, and the binding of Cl^- is no longer possible. The other type of Cl^- binding to hemoglobin is less clear. Bonaventura et al. (33) have found that anions, including Cl^-, in the absence of 2,3-DPG can bind the positive charges available in the central cavity. This binding might not affect the oxygen affinity of hemoglobin through the T to R conversion because the same effect is observed in isolated chains. The physical basis of this effect remains unresolved.

Oxygen Transport by the Red Cell

OXYGEN-BINDING PROPERTIES OF THE RED CELL

The oxygen equilibrium of red cells depends on (a) the intrinsic oxygen affinity of the hemoglobin molecule (determined in solutions stripped of phosphate), (b) intraerythrocytic pH, (c) the intraerythrocytic concentration of 2,3-DPG, (d) temperature, and (e) partial pressure of carbon dioxide.

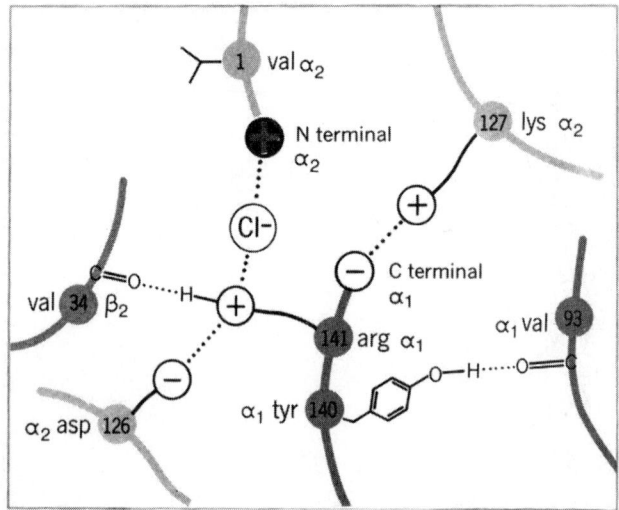

Figure 49-14. Salt bridges and hydrogen bonds (the distinction is often unclear from radiographic analyses) between other groups and the N-terminal and C-terminal residues in the chains of deoxyhemoglobin. All these bonds are ruptured in oxyhemoglobin. A shift to the oxy configuration brings the carboxy terminals closer together. The side chain of $Arg_1 141(HC3)$ is squeezed out, rupturing all the bonds shown. One of the two groups that contribute to the Bohr effect by becoming partially deprotonated in the oxy configuration is shown by a black-encircled plus sign. (From Dickerson RE, Geis I. *Hemoglobin: structure, function, evolution, and pathology.* Menlo Park, CA: Benjamin/Cummings, 1983, with permission.)

Intraerythrocytic pH. The Bohr effect of whole blood is remarkably similar to hemoglobin in solution. For normal blood (37°C and 40 mm Hg CO_2), the log p50/pH is close to 0.5. Intracellular pH is 0.2 units below the extracellular pH, determined by the concentration of permeant ions H^+, OH^-, Cl^-, and bicarbonate, the major impermeant ions, hemoglobin itself, and 2,3-DPG.

The concentrations of solutes inside and outside the red cell follow the Gibbs-Donnan relation that requires electroneutrality and due consideration to activity coefficient differences in the two compartments. As hemoglobin and 2,3-DPG, which are negatively charged at pH 7.4, are trapped inside the red cell, erythrocyte Cl^- concentration has to be decreased, thus the ratio of 0.7 between intracellular and extracellular Cl^-. Calculation of the Gibbs-Donnan equilibrium predicts the observed 0.2 pH unit difference between the inside and outside of the red cell, suggesting that no significant participant is missing in this phenomenon.

2,3-Diphosphoglycerate. The normal level of red cell 2,3-DPG is 12.8 (μmol/g Hb) for males and 13.8 (μmol/g Hb) for females for the Sigma kit based on the method of Rose (34). Children younger than 5 years and elderly patients have increased and decreased levels of 2,3-DPG, respectively (35,36). This amount makes the organic phosphate almost equimolar with hemoglobin in red cells, whereas in other cells, it exists in very small concentrations.

Metabolically, 2,3-DPG is generated by the Rapoport-Luebering shunt from 1,3-DPG by DPG synthase or mutase. Its level depends on the rates of synthesis and hydrolysis. The rate of synthesis is complex and depends on the amount of the substrate 1,3-DPG generated by glycolysis, which in turn increases directly with pH, and on the amount of 1,3-DPG entering the Rapoport-Luebering shunt. The alternative pathway for 1,3-DPG, and the most energetic, is to be converted into 3-phosphoglycerate and generate an ATP molecule. This alternative is probably greatly affected by the activity of the synthase, which is stimulated in direct proportion to the red cell pH and is under end product inhibition by the concentration of 2,3-DPG.

Hypoxia has a tremendous impact on these relations, and Duhm has put together a scheme that clarifies the consequence of acidosis and alkalosis (Fig. 49-15), an event with significant clinical implications.

Temperature. The p50 of blood is almost doubled by an increase of 10°C (between 20° and 30°C). This reaction seems appropriate to deal with hypothermia and hyperthermia. Cold decreases metabolic requirements and reduces the need for oxy-

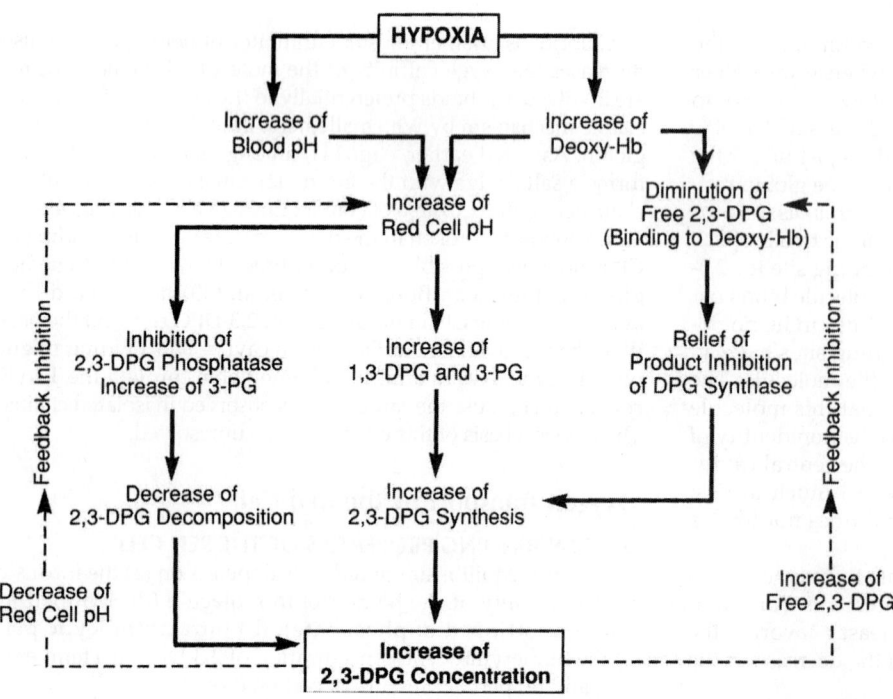

Figure 49-15. Effect of hypoxia on red cell pH and 2,3-diphosphoglycerate (DPG). (From Bunn HF, Forget BG. *Hemoglobin: molecular, genetic, and clinical aspects.* Philadelphia: WB Saunders, 1986, with permission.)

gen. During fever, metabolism is increased dramatically, and an increase in the delivery of oxygen is required. The basis for this phenomenon is primarily the temperature-induced changes on the hemoglobin molecule.

Oxygen Transport to the Tissues

The fundamental relation that describes the delivery of oxygen to the tissues is the Fick equation:

$$Vo_2 = 0.139(Q)(Hb)(Sao_2 - Svo_2)$$

The equation indicates that the amount of oxygen delivered to the tissues (Vo_2) in liters per minute is the product of three independent variables: (a) the blood flow (Q); (b) the amount of O_2 carried by that flow, which is the product of 0.139 and the grams of hemoglobin (1.39 is the amount of oxygen, in millimeters of mercury, that a fully saturated gram of hemoglobin is capable of carrying); and (c) the extraction of oxygen at the level of the tissues, which is the difference between the saturations of the arterial blood and the mixed venous blood.

The consequence of this analysis is that when regulation of oxygen release is desired, it is best performed in the following areas.

BLOOD FLOW
Blood flow is in turn affected by cardiac output and by microcirculatory size and distribution.

HEMOGLOBIN CONCENTRATION
For hemoglobin concentration (Hb), the red cell mass is the balance between erythropoiesis and red cell destruction and is actively regulated by erythropoietin. This hormone responds to hypoxia detected in the postarterial side of the renal circulation by a detection system that uses a prolyl hydroxylase (the likely oxygen detector), the von Hippel-Lindau tumor suppressor, and the hypoxia-inducing factor (see Chapters 7 and 56).

OXYGEN EXTRACTION BY THE TISSUES
The parameter oxygen extraction by the tissues ($Sao_2 - Svo_2$) depends on the shape of the oxygen equilibrium curve, as discussed in the section Hemoglobin Binds Oxygen Allosterically, and on tissue po_2. The determinants of tissue po_2 and its regulation are poorly understood.

Nitric Oxide Binding to Hemoglobin

PHYSIOLOGY AND CHEMISTRY
Nitric oxide (NO) is the product of the action of endothelial synthases and macrophage synthase (mNOS)—on L-Arg (Table 49-3).

They are differentially stimulated by Ca^{2+}-dependent calmodulin, tumor necrosis factor, and other cytokines. In addition, the NO synthases are cell-specific (37), including endothelium, macrophages, neutrophils, adrenal tissue, cerebellum, and others.

Nitric oxide action is mediated by the activation of a soluble guanylyl cyclase to produce cyclic guanosine monophosphate. This second messenger is involved in many cellular functions. The NO formed diffuses out of the originating cells and affects only nearby target cells (because NO has a short half-life), binding the heme group of cytosolic guanylate cyclase and activating this enzyme by breaking the iron–proximal His bond. A similar mechanism occurs when NO binds to the heme of hemoglobin (discussed in the section Toxicity and Pathophysiology of Nitric Oxide). Nevertheless, most NO activity may involve direct cell-to-cell interactions and may not be mediated by blood NO.

The steady-state level of blood NO is balanced between the production of NO by NOSs and the binding or scavenging of NO by hemoglobin (bound at the heme level). One of the main functions of NO is the maintenance of an appropriate vascular tone.

The affinity of NO for hemoglobin is 100 times higher than CO and 20,000 times higher than oxygen, which explains the reputation of NO as an extremely toxic compound without physiological or therapeutic importance.

The chemistry of NO is complex; an attempt to demystify it is shown in Fig. 49-16.

Head et al. (38) observed that pharmacologic concentrations of NO shift the oxygen equilibrium binding curve of sickle blood to the left but do not affect the oxygen equilibrium of normal blood. However, others have failed to reproduce these data (39). This shift can be induced by methemoglobin, which is formed at toxic levels of NO. When NO dissolved in buffer is used, the p50 of hemoglobin correlates with the amount of methemoglobin generated (39).

Gow and Stamler (40) propose that another physiologic function of red blood cell NO is related to the formation of S-nitrosohemoglobin (S-NO-Hb), which is generated by the binding of NO to the Cysβ93 of hemoglobin. They suggest that S-NO-Hb is generated in the lungs, where hemoglobin is in the R or oxygenated state, and that NO is released in the microcirculation, where the transition of the R→T conformation induced by deoxygenation liberates NO from the Cys93 site to relax subendothelial muscle and increase blood flow.

Gladwin et al. (39) find that less than 1% of hemoglobin has S-NO in patients breathing NO at several concentrations, which makes the physiologic or pathophysiologic role of S-NO-Hb controversial. In addition, in the hypothesis by Gow and Stamler (40), the deoxy form of Hb releases NO from S-NO-Hb. Recent data by Patel et al. (42) show that S-NO-Hb has a higher affinity for oxygen than native Hb, implying that NO transfer from S-NO-Hb *in vivo*

TABLE 49-3. Nitric Oxide Synthases

	NOS1	NOS2	NOS3
Synonyms	Type 1 NOS, (n)eural NOS, (b)rain NOS	Type 2 NOS, (mac)rophage NOS, (i)nducible NOS	Type 3 NOS, (e)ndothelial NOS
Localization	Cytosol and attached to membrane	Cytosol and vesicles	Plasmalemmal caveolae
Synthesis	Constitutive	Cytokine induced	Constitutive
C^{2+} dependence	Yes	No	Yes
Regulation by cytokines	Weak	Strong	Weak
NO production	Low	High	Low
Some cell types	Neurons, skeletal muscle	Microphages, microglia, hepatocytes	Endothelium, some epithelium
Key functions	Neurotransmission, neuroprotection	Antimicrobial, immunoregulation, tissue damage	Inhibition of platelet aggregation, vasodilation, hypotension

Modified from Bogdan C. Nitric oxide and the regulation of gene expression. *Trends Cell Biol* 2001;11:66.

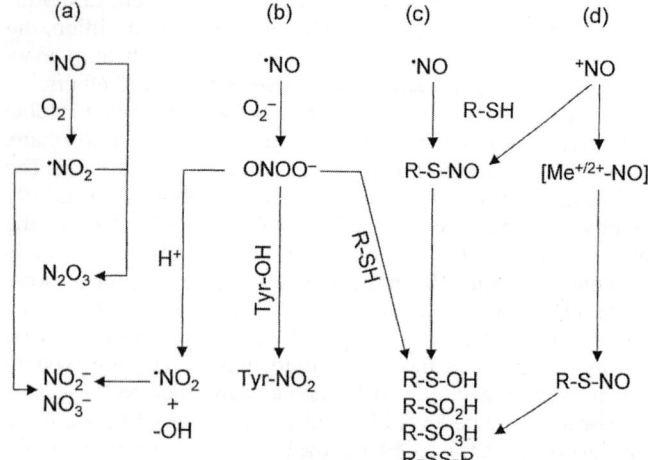

Figure 49-16. Fate of nitric oxide (NO) and NO radicals (·NO) by nitric oxide synthase (NOS) or NO donors. **A:** Oxygen oxidizes ·NO to ·NO$_2$; in turn ·NO oxidizes ·NO to N$_2$O$_3$. **B:** In the presence of superoxide (O$_2^-$), ·NO can form ONOO$^-$ (peroxynitrite), which in turn results in the formation of ·NO$_2$ and the hydroxyl radical (·OH), in nitration of tyrosines, and in oxidation of thiols. **C:** ·NO can nitrosylate thiol groups of protein cysteines to intramolecular disulfide bonds (–S–S–), sulfenic acids (R–S–OH), sulfinic acids (R–SO$_2$H), or sulfonic acids (R–SO$_3$H). **D:** NO$^+$ (nitrosonium ions) in the presence of trace metals (Fe, Zn, or Cu) form metal-nitrosyl complexes and nitrosylate thiol groups, also resulting in sulfenic, sulfinic, and sulfonic acids and disulfides. (Adapted from Bogdan C. Nitric oxide and the regulation of gene expression. *Trends Cell Biol* 2001;11:66–75.)

would be limited to regions of extremely low oxygen tension. Furthermore, the kinetics of the transnitrosation reactions between glutathione (GSH) and S-NO-Hb (NO bound to –SH groups in Hb), another potentially physiologically important reaction also proposed by Gow and Stamler (40), are relatively slow, according to Patel et al. (42), making transfer of NO$^+$ from S-NO-Hb to GSH less likely as a mechanism to elicit vessel relaxation. These data suggest that oxygen-dependent S-nitrosation of GSH from S-NO-Hb involves biochemical mechanisms that are not intrinsic to the hemoglobin molecule and are not well understood.

Yonetani (43) does not find evidence that NO is liberated from the Cys93 site as hemoglobin turns into the T state. Also, the nitroso compounds do not liberate NO but NO$^+$, which needs to be deprotonated before it is active. The mechanisms involved in deprotonation are not fully known nor necessarily available in red cells. Finally, the process of exporting of NO$^+$ from the red cell needs further elucidation. Overall, the physiologic and potential pathophysiologic significance of NO binding to Cysβ92 requires further research.

TOXICITY AND PATHOPHYSIOLOGY OF NITRIC OXIDE
Nitric oxide was long thought highly toxic, until physicians began using low concentrations of the gas, generally 5 to 10 ppm, to manage the acute pulmonary hypertension seen in adult respiratory distress syndrome. The use of NO is still considered dangerous in the presence of sepsis because production of NO is increased in this situation (44).

Animal studies show that concentrations of 10 to 40 ppm of NO inhaled for 6 months have no ill effects and do not produce hypotension. The common explanation is that rapid binding of NO by hemoglobin mops up this dangerous vasodilator. However, the binding of NO to the heme in hemoglobin results in a low affinity for oxygen, so an explanation for the lack of effects of this alteration is needed.

Yonetani (43) offers the following scheme: NO binds preferentially to the hemes of the α-chains, inducing a conformational

change of hemoglobin to a super-T state due to the breakage of the bond between the iron and the proximal His. The hemes that bind NO exclude oxygen; hence, the two remaining hemes have a particularly low oxygen affinity, or a super-T state. This unique T form delivers oxygen to the tissues more effectively than the normal T state. Hence, in spite of the fact that the NO-Hb tetramer has only two ligand-carrying oxygenated hemes, it delivers oxygen almost as well as the normal hemoglobin tetramer.

The tetramers with hemes containing NO will, in approximately half an hour, be converted to methemoglobins, lose their NO, and be reduced by the methemoglobin reductase system of the red cell to normal hemoglobin molecules. This is the reason why NO, within limits, is not as toxic as initially feared.

What is the mechanism of methemoglobin formation in the NO-bound heme? Eich et al. (45) found that NO-dependent hemoglobin oxidation to methemoglobin varies linearly with NO concentration but not with oxygen concentration. Nonreversible NO binding and NO-induced oxidation occur in two steps: (a) bimolecular entry of NO into the distal portion of the heme pocket, and (b) rapid reaction of noncovalently bound NO with iron to produce Fe^{2+}–N=O or with Fe^{2+}–O-O to produce Fe^{3+}–OH$_2$ and nitrate.

A related issue in NO metabolism is the formation of peroxynitrate (ONOO$^-$) when L-Arg becomes rate-limiting. Peroxynitrate forms nitrotyrosine and modifies proteins with functional consequences. In addition, it promotes apoptosis. In hemoglobinopathies, the kidneys of α^{H}β^S[β^{MDD}] mice express NOS strongly in the tubular endothelium (46–49).

Mercaptoethylguanidine, a compound that selectively inhibits iNOS and scavenges ONOO$^-$, virtually eliminates renal immunostaining of iNOS and nitrotyrosine and prevents DNA strand breakage when administered to sickle mice intraperitoneally (50). In addition, PARP, a nuclear DNA-repairing enzyme that is activated by DNA strand breakage, is cleaved in hypoxic sickle mice but is partially protected by mercaptoethylguanidine. Apoptosis was also markedly reduced, suggesting that NO, ONOO$^-$, or both are responsible for initiating cell damage that leads to apoptosis in sickle cell mouse kidneys.

More recently, to define the relative contributions of endothelial and intravascular NO in the regulation of human blood flow, Gladwin et al. (51) simultaneously measured forearm blood flow, arterial and venous plasma nitrite, low-molecular-weight and high-molecular-weight S-NO, and red cell S-nitrosohemoglobin (S-NO-Hb). Measurements were made at rest and during regional inhibition of NO synthesis, followed by forearm exercise. They found significant circulating arterial-venous (AV) plasma nitrite gradients, suggesting a novel delivery source for intravascular NO. Further supporting the notion that circulating nitrite is bioactive, the consumption of nitrite increased significantly with exercise when regional endothelial synthesis of NO was inhibited. The role of circulating S-nitrosothiols and S-NO-Hb in the regulation of basal vascular tone is less certain in these experiments. Low-molecular-weight S-nitrosothiols were undetectable, and S-nitroso-albumin levels were two logs lower than previously reported. S-nitroso-albumin primarily formed in the venous circulation, even during NOS inhibition. S-NO-Hb was measurable in the human circulation, but AV gradients were not significant, and the delivery of NO from S-NO-Hb was minimal. The authors draw the following conclusions: (a) circulating nitrite is bioactive and provides a delivery gradient of intravascular NO, (b) S-nitroso-albumin does not deliver NO from the lungs to the tissue but forms in the peripheral circulation, and (c) S-NO-Hb and S-nitrosothiols play a minimal role in the regulation of basal vascular tone, even during exercise stress. Some of these conclusions are based on the notion that AV gradients are informative, but that assumption requires that very low levels of S-NO-Hb are physiologically insignificant.

Gladwin et al. (52) have also measured NO-Hb reaction products in normals with and without NO inhalation. NO inhalation markedly raised total NO-Hb, with a significant AV gradient, supporting a role for hemoglobin in the transport and delivery of NO. The predominant species accounting for this gradient is nitrosyl(heme)-Hb. NO inhalation increased S-nitrosylation of hemoglobin β-chain Cys92, but only to a fraction of the level of nitrosyl(heme)-Hb, and without an AV gradient. A strong correlation between methemoglobin and plasma nitrate formation was observed, suggesting that NO metabolism is a primary physiologic cause of hemoglobin oxidation. The authors draw the following conclusions: (a) NO binding to heme groups is rapidly reversible, and (b) S-nitrosohemoglobin formation is probably not a primary transport mechanism for NO but may facilitate NO release from heme.

Finally, although both O_2 and NO diffuse into red blood cells, only O_2 diffuses out. For dilatation of blood vessels to take place by red blood cell–mediated events, export of NO-related vasoactivity is indispensable. Pabloski et al. (53) have recently shown

that hemoglobin-derived S-nitrosothiol (S-NO-Hb), generated from NO, associates predominantly with the red blood cell membrane and principally with Cys residues in the hemoglobin-binding cytoplasmic domain of band 3 (also called *AE1*). The authors postulate that the interaction with band 3 promotes the deoxygenated structure in S-NO-Hb, which facilitates NO transfer to the membrane. Furthermore, they show that vasodilatory activity is released from the red cell membrane with the help of deoxygenation. If confirmed, this model would overcome the criticisms of the original postulate.

HIGH LIGAND AFFINITY HEMOGLOBINS: ERYTHROCYTOSIS

Structural Defects

Mutations resulting in changes in the primary structure of the α-chains or β-chains can lead to changes in the affinity toward ligand of these hemoglobin variants (Table 49-4). Increases in the oxygen affinity of hemoglobin can come about by various

TABLE 49-4. High-Affinity Hemoglobins

	Mutation	Name	Hb Level and Additional Properties
α-Chain sites			
α2 (NA2)	Leu→Arg	Chongqing	UN
α6 (A4)	Asp→Ala	Sawara	
	Asp→Asn	Dunn	
	Asp→Val	Ferndown	
	Asp→Tyr	Woodville	
	Asp→Gly	Swan River	
α14 (A12)	Trp→Arg	Evanston	
α16 (A14)	Lys→Met	Harbin	UN
α40 (C5)	Lys→Glu	Kariya	UN
	Lys→Met	Kanagawa	
α44 (CE2)	Pro→Leu	Milledgeville	
	Pro→Arg	Kawachi	
α45 (CE3)	His→Arg	Fort de France	
α84 (F5)	Ser→Arg	Etobioke	
α85 (F6)	Asp→Asn	G-Norfolk	
	Asp→Tyr	Atago	
	Asp→Val	Inksten	
α88 (F9)	Ala→Ser	Loire	
	Ala→Val	Columbia-Missouri	
α90 (FG2)	Lys→Met	Handa Munakate	
α92 (FG5)	Arg→Gln	J Capetown	
	Arg→Ser	Chesapeake	
α95 (G2)	Pro→Ala	Denmark Hill	
	Pro→Ser	Rampa	
	Pro→Arg	St. Lukes	
	Pro→Leu	G-Georgia	
α97 (G4)	Asn→His	Dallas	
α126 (H9)	Asp→His	Sassai	
	Asp→Asn	Tarrant	
	Asp→Val	Fukitomi	Hb: 15–19
	Asp→Tyr	Montefiore	
α138 (H21)	Ser→Pro	Attleboro	
α139 (HCl)	Lys→Thr	Tokoname	
	Lys→Glu	Hanamaki	
α140–α141	(Tyr-Arg)→O	Natal	
α141 (HC3)	Arg→His	Suresnes	Hb: 15–19
	Arg→Cys	Nunobiki	
	Arg→Leu	Legnano	Hb: 16–20
β-Chain sites			
β2 (NA2)	His→Arg	Deer Lodge	
	His→Gln	Okayama	
β9 (A6)	Ser→Cys	Porto Alegre	Polymerization
β17–18	(Lys-Val)→O	Lyon	
β20 (B2)	Val→Met	Olympia	
β23 (B5)	Val→O	Freiburg	

(continued)

TABLE 49-4. (continued)

	Mutation	Name	Hb Level and Additional Properties
	Val→Asp	Strasbourg	
	Val→Phe	Palmerston North	
β27 (B9)	Ala→Val	Grange Blanche	
β34 (B16)	Val→Phe	Pitie-Salpetriere	Hb: 17–20
β36 (C2)z	Pro→Ser	North Chicago	
β37 (C3)	Trp→Ser	Hirose	Dissoc
β40 (C6)	Arg→Lys	Athens-Ga, Waco	Dissoc
	Arg→Ser	Austin	
β51 (D2)	Pro→Arg	Williamette	UN
β68 (E12)	Leu→His	Brisbane, Great Lakes	Hb: 15–20; UN
β79 (EF3)	Asp→Gly	G-Hsi-Tsou	
β82 (EF6)	Lys→Thr	Rahere	Hb: 19
	Lys→Met	Helsinki	Hb: 14–17
β86 (F2)	Ala→Asp	Olomouc	
β87 (F3)	Thr→O	Tours	
β89 (F5)	Ser→Asn	Creteil	
	Ser→Arg	Vanderbilt	Hb: 19–22
β90 (F6)	Gly→Asp	Pierre Benite	
β93 (F9)	Cys→Arg	Okazaki	
β94 (FG1)	Asp→His	Barcelona	Hb: 18
	Asp→Asn	Bunbury	
β96 (FG3)	Leu→Val	Regina	
β97 (FG4)	His→Gln	Malmo	Hb: 17–21
	His→Leu	Wood	Hbhb: 17–22
	His→Pro	Nagoya	UN
β99 (G1)	Asp→Asn	Kempsey	Hb: 17–20
	Asp→His	Yakima	Hb: 16–18
	Asp→Ala	Radcliffe	Hb: 17–19
	Asp→Tyr	Ypsilanti	Hb: 15–19
	Asp→Gly	Hotel-Dieu	Hb: 20–24
	Asp→Val	Chemilly	Hb: 19
	Asp→Glu	Cormora	
β100 (G2)	Pro→Leu	Brigham	Hb: 16–18
β101 (G3)	Glu→Lys	British	Hb: 17
	Glu→Gly	Columbia Alberta	Hb: 20
	Glu→Asp	Potomac	Hb: 17–19
β103 (G5)	Phe→Leu	Heathrow	Hb: 16–21
β105 (G7)	Leu→Phe	South Milwaukee	
β109 (G11)	Val→Met	San Diego	Hb: 16–18
	Val→Leu	Johnston	
β124 (H2)	Pro→Gln	Ty Gard	Hb: 19
β140 (HC2)	(Tyr-Arg)→O	Natal	
β141 (HC3)			
β140 (H18)	Ala→Thr	Saint Jacques	Hb: 19
β142 (H20)	Ala→Asp	Ohio	Hb: 19–20
β143 (H21)	His→Arg	Abruzzo	
	His→Gln	Little Rock	Hb: 20–13
	His→Pro	Syracuse	Hb: 19–24
	His→Asp	Rancho Mirage	
β144 (HC1)	Lys→Asn	Andrew-Minneapolis	Hb: 20
	Lys→Glu	Mito	
β145 (HC2)	Tyr→His	Bethesda	Hb: 16–21
	Tyr→Cys	Rainier	Hb: 17–21; alkaline resistance
	Tyr→Asp	Fort Gordon	Hb: 17–23
	Tyr→Term	Osler, Nancy McKees Rocks	Hb: 18–21
β146 (HC3)	His→Asp	Hiroshima	Hb: 15–17
	His→Pro	York	
	His→Leu	Cowtown	Hb: 18–19
	His→Gln	Kodaira	

Insertions

After β144(HC1): Ser-Ile-Thr-Lys-Leu-   Cranston
   Ala-Phe-Leu-Leu-Ser-Asn-Phe-Thr-
   COOH

Dissoc, tendency to increased dissociation; Hb, hemoglobin in g/dL; UN, unstable.

mechanisms. In most instances, the changes in oxygen affinity are in concordance with our understanding of the structure–function relations of hemoglobin. In a few instances, the known alterations of the primary structure are not sufficient to explain the observed effect, given the state of our knowledge.

The mutations that generate high-affinity hemoglobins can arise from single-point substitutions, double-point substitutions (although some of these could be crossover events between two mutated chains), deletions, additions, frameshift mutations, and fusion genes.

The molecular mechanisms of ligand high-affinity hemoglobin mutants are summarized here and described in the following sections (for some high-affinity hemoglobins, there is no explanation for their functional behavior).

- Alteration of the switch region, the flexible joint, or the C-terminals in the $\alpha_1\beta_2$ area of contact that favor the R (or oxy) state, either by stabilizing this conformer or by destabilizing the T (or deoxy) state
- Alteration of the $\alpha_1\beta_1$ area of contact with disruption of the overall architecture of hemoglobin that favors the R state
- Mutations that decrease the affinity of hemoglobin for 2,3-DPG
- Reduction of heme interaction by restraining the quaternary conformation due to a tendency to aggregate or polymerize
- Elongation of the globin chains, disrupting the quaternary structure

ALTERATIONS OF THE SWITCH REGION, FLEXIBLE JOINT, OR C-TERMINALS IN THE $\alpha_1\beta_2$ AREA OF CONTACT

Alterations of the switch region, flexible joint, or C-terminals in the $\alpha_1\beta_2$ area of contact favor the R state either by stabilizing this conformer or by destabilizing the T state.

α-Chain Abnormalities. Hb Chesapeake [α92 (FG4) Arg→Leu] (54–56) was the first high-affinity mutant described in a classic paper by Charache et al. (54). At pH 8.61, it is a fast-moving electrophoretic variant, representing approximately 20% of the hemolysate. It has a moderately high oxygen affinity (whole blood p50: 19 mm Hg) and normal Bohr and 2,3-DPG effects, and it produces moderate erythrocytosis. It involves a substitution of an invariant residue (a residue in most α-chains analyzed regardless of species). The molecular mechanism is the stabilization of the R state at the level of the $\alpha_1\beta_2$ area of contact.

Hb J Capetown [α92 (FG4) Arg→Gln] occurs at the same site as Hb Chesapeake and has similar characteristics, although the stabilization of the R state is probably less significant. The initial report that this abnormal hemoglobin had a very low n value proved to be incorrect (57). The observation was based on total hemolysate data that corresponded to the addition of two curves with a very displaced p50 but a not so different n value (58). The copresence of two hemoglobins (the patient was a heterozygote)—Hb A and Hb Capetown—generates a flattened oxygen equilibrium curve because Hb Capetown begins loading oxygen first because of its high affinity. From this combination curve, a reliable n value cannot be calculated for each individual hemoglobin.

Hb Nunobiki [α141 (HC3) Arg→Cys] is one of four mutations at the same site, all of which exhibit a high affinity for oxygen, significantly decreased heterotropic interactions (effect of H⁺, Cl⁻, and 2,3-DPG), and moderate to mild erythrocytosis (59). The mutation affects an invariant residue. Hb Nunobiki merits special mention. At pH 8.6, it is an electrophoretically fast-moving abnormal hemoglobin expressed at a low level (13%). Most α-chain abnormalities represent 20% to 25% of the hemolysate because they are produced by one of four α-genes.

The consequences of the presence of the Cys residue in position α141 are varied. First, during storage, the hemoglobin changes mobility (becomes faster), presumably through the oxidation of the Cys residue to a negatively charged sulfoxide ($-SO^-$) or sulfitic acid ($-SOO^-$). Second, Hb Nunobiki is more resistant to autoxidation, probably because of two circumstances: the protection toward oxidants rendered by its high-affinity status, and the addition of a new site (Cys residue) for the consumption of the oxidants. Third, the low percentage of the α mutant is explained by the fact that it is a mutant of the α_1-gene (closest to the 3' region of the α-globin gene cluster), which Orkin has

shown to be expressed one-third to two-thirds less than the α_2-gene. Finally, as with other mutations of the N-terminal end of the α-chains, Hb Nunobiki produces little erythrocytosis in spite of its high affinity because of the low percentage present in the red cells. The high ligand affinity is due to the breaking of the C-terminal to C-terminal salt bridge indispensable for the stabilization of the T state. Hence, the R state is greatly favored.

β-Chain Abnormalities. Hb Howick [β37 (C3) Trp→Gly] (60) is one of three mutations at codon β37. Hb Howick and Hb Hirose (Trp→Ser) have increased oxygen affinity, whereas Hb Rothschild (Trp→Gly) has low oxygen affinity (see below). Hb Howick comprises 29% of the hemolysate and migrates electrophoretically with Hb D at alkaline pH and with Hb F on citrate agar electrophoresis. The red cell p50 of the heterozygote carrier was 20 mm Hg (normal, 26 mm Hg), and the Bohr effect was reduced. Oxygen affinity was very high at low pH. β37 sits in the $\alpha_1\beta_2$ area of contact, and the absence of Trp is expected to alter the bonds between the two dimers critical in the R→T transition, destabilizing the T conformer. There is also evidence (60) that purified Hb Howick is nearly totally dimerized in the R state (associated equilibrium constant = 35 mM), whereas the T form is highly tetrameric (associated equilibrium constant = 3 μM). These vastly different values are due to the large increase in the dissociation rate of oxy Hb Howick. Simulation of the protein concentration dependence of O_2 binding fits well with experimental data and is also consistent with the free-energy change associated with the change of the Gly residue from a hydrophilic to a hydrophobic environment during dimerization.

The pivotal role of β37 has stimulated studies of recombinant hemoglobins at this site (61,62). The high resolution crystal structure of four recombinant mutants, β37 Trp→Tyr, β37 Trp→Ala, β37 Trp→Glu, and β37 Trp→Gly (Hb Howick), has been determined. None of these mutations altered tertiary structure at the mutation site. However, they altered the $\alpha_1\beta_2$ interface, caused distal tertiary structural change involving Aspα94 and Proα95, produced distal tertiary changes involving Aspβ99 and Asnβ102, increased the mobility of the α-globin subunit C-terminal dipeptide, and shortened the Fe-His bond in both chains in the Tyrβ37 and Gluβ37 mutants. Overall, the magnitude of the structural changes increased in the order Trpβ37→Tyr > Trpβ37→Ala > Trpβ37→Glu and Trpβ37→Gly (Hb Howick) and paralleled the disruption of function detected in these recombinant mutants.

Hb Poissy [β56 (D7) Gly→Arg and 86 (F2) Ala→Pro] (63) is a double-site mutation; one mutation (Arg at the β56 site) had been described previously as *Hb Hamadan*, exhibiting no functional abnormalities. When a second case was found in 1982 in France, the patient had erythrocytosis and red cells with a high affinity for oxygen. A discrepancy that needed explanation was apparent. Recent reexamination of the structure of the mutant hemoglobin by high-performance liquid chromatography (HPLC) revealed that the French propositus carries a β-chain with two mutations, one identical to Hb Hamadan, the other an electrophoretically silent mutation in the same β-chain but at position 86, in which an Ala has been substituted by a Pro. This new hemoglobin has a threefold increase in oxygen affinity, with a low n (Hill) coefficient and a diminished Bohr effect. It also shows a biphasic curve in the autooxidation rate, suggesting a great inequivalency in the propensity for methemoglobin formation (conversion of heme iron from ferrous to ferric) of the α and β hemes. NMR studies in this mutant suggest that the helix-breaking Pro residue displaces the F helix toward the heme, destabilizing this helix toward the critical FG corner. This change interferes with the $\alpha_1\beta_2$ contact area, favors the R state, and modifies the environment of the hemes.

There are six known mutations of the β99 [Gl] site: *Hb Kempsey* (Asp→Asn) (64), *Hb Yakima* (Asp→His) (65), *Hb Radcliffe* (Asp→Ala) (66), *Hb Ypsilanti* (Asp→Tyr) (67), *Hb Hotel-Dieu* (Asp→Gly) (68), and *Hb Chemilly* (Asp→Val) (69). These six electrophoretically apparent mutations constitute approximately 40% to 50% of the hemolysate, exhibit moderately high oxygen affinity, show a 25% to 60% decrease in the Bohr effect, exhibit clinically apparent erythrocytosis, and are the molecular consequence of disturbances in the $\alpha_1\beta_2$ area of contact. In Hb Yakima, as determined by x-ray crystallography of the deoxy form, the intersubunit deoxy bonds between β99 [Gl] and αC7 and αG4 are broken, a situation that favors the R or oxy conformation. More recently, crystallography of CO Hb Ypsilanti, another mutation of β99, has disclosed an important characteristic of this mutant. At a 3-Å resolution, it appears that CO Hb Ypsilanti has a feature never before observed in abnormal hemoglobins: a different and stable quaternary structure along the $\alpha_1\beta_1$ area of contact. The two stable dimers in the liganded form of carboxyhemoglobin (CO-Hb) Ypsilanti rotate beyond the limit observed in the R/T difference. The consequence of this rotation is that many of the salt bridges stabilizing the R structure are lost, but the H bonding between Aspβ94 and β102 is retained, and new bonds are formed by the mutated Tyrβ99 with Asnα97 and Thrα38. This new quaternary conformation, baptized as Y by the authors to differentiate it from the R and T conformers, could be a transient conformation attained during the normal RT transition that is stabilized by the mutation.

The response to 2,3-DPG is moderately decreased in Kempsey and Hb Radcliffe and is slightly decreased in Hb Hotel Dieu. In other mutations, it has not been measured. It is interesting that Hb Ypsilanti and Hb Radcliffe form stable hybrids in the hemolysates in which the abnormal β-chains coexist with normal β-chains.

Hb Puttelange [β140 (H18) Ala→Val] (70) was found as an apparent *de novo* mutation in a French family in which affected members had erythrocytosis. On isoelectric focusing, Hb Puttelange migrated slightly cathodically to Hb A. Although high oxygen affinity was present, more interesting was that β-globin gene DNA analysis strongly suggested that the mutation was not *de novo* but rather an example of paternal germ line mosaicism, leading to a recurrent risk of transmission.

Four mutations are described for site β146 [HC3]: *Hb Hiroshima* (His→Asp) (71,72), *Hb York* (His→Pro), *Hb Cowtown* (His→Leu), and *Hb Cochin-Port Royal* (His→Arg) (73,74). These hemoglobins are detectable by electrophoresis. They have moderately increased oxygen affinity and a Bohr effect that is half-normal (Fig. 49-17). In addition, Hb Cowtown has a decreased 2,3-DPG effect. All of these mutants disrupt a T state salt bridge and eliminate the residue originating 50% of the Bohr protons. The decrease of the 2,3-DPG binding might be secondary to the reduction of positive charges in the central cavity or to the destabilization of the T state. Hb Cochin-Port Royal exhibits normal oxygen affinity and a very reduced Bohr effect. All these mutants disrupt a salt bridge that stabilizes the T state, and the absence of the Hisβ146 reduces by half the Bohr protons. Reduced 2,3-DPG binding might be secondary to the reduction of positive charges in the central cavity, the destabilization of the T state, or both.

ALTERATION OF THE $\alpha_1\beta_1$ AREA OF CONTACT WITH DISRUPTION OF THE OVERALL ARCHITECTURE OF HEMOGLOBIN THAT FAVORS THE R STATE

Hb San Diego [β109 (Gll) Val→Met] is an electrophoretically silent mutation with moderately high oxygen affinity, a normal Bohr effect, and clinically apparent erythrocytosis (75). The molecular mechanism probably involves a steric hindrance,

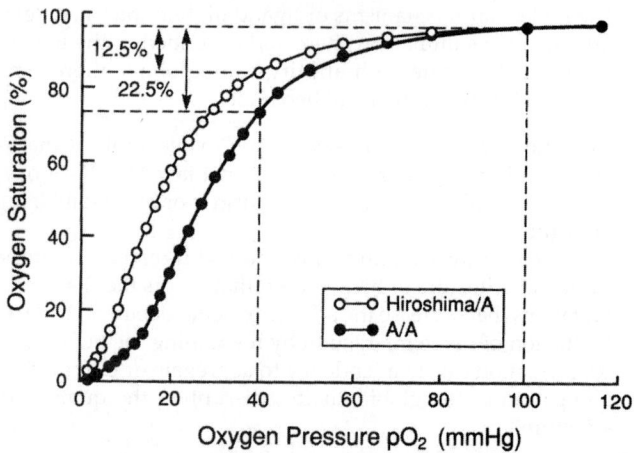

Figure 49-17. Oxygen equilibrium curves of red cells from a healthy person (*A/A*) and from a hemoglobin Hiroshima heterozygote (*Hiroshima/A*). Oxygen pressure is plotted against oxygen saturation. Vertical dotted lines mark the typical pO_2 of the lungs (100 mm Hg) and of the tissues (40 mm Hg). Horizontal dotted lines mark the oxygen extraction (lungs, tissues) for normal red cells (22.5%) and the reduction observed for the high-affinity red cells (15%).

induced by the larger bulk of Met compared with Val in the $\alpha_1\beta_1$ contact, particularly in the deoxy configuration. This biases the molecule toward the R state.

Hb Crete [β129 (H7) Ala→Pro] (76) presented with a unexpected combination of erythrocytosis, hemolysis, splenomegaly, abnormal red cell morphology, and marked erythroid hyperplasia. The propositus was a combined heterozygote for Hb Crete and δβ thalassemia, with 67% Hb Crete and 30% Hb F. The red cell p50 was 11.3, whereas isolated Hb Crete had a p50 of 2.2 mm Hg at pH 7.3 compared with 5.4 for Hb A, moderately decreased cooperativity, and a normal Bohr effect. Hb Crete was also mildly unstable. Pro is not well accommodated in the α-helix structure and disturbs H helix while also having a longer-range effect on nearby residues in the $\alpha_1\beta_1$ interface, perturbing this area of subunit contact.

This case is instructive for several reasons. Splenomegaly is not usually associated with erythrocytosis caused by high oxygen affinity hemoglobins and is reminiscent of polycythemia vera. However, in this instance, it was caused by δβ thalassemia. The high affinity of Hb Crete may have complex origins. Another family member who was heterozygous for Hb Crete alone had only 38% of this variant and a hematocrit of 50%. In the propositus, the magnitude of the erythrocytosis is greater because the level of Hb Crete is much higher, and the situation is compounded by the presence of high levels of the high ligand affinity Hb F.

MUTATIONS THAT DECREASE THE AFFINITY OF HEMOGLOBIN FOR 2,3-DIPHOSPHOGLYCERATE

Three mutations of β82 [EF6] have been described: *Hb Rahere* (Lys→Thr) (77), *Hb Helsinki* (Lys→Met) (78), and *Hb Providence* (Lys→Asn→Asp) (79). All these mutants have moderately high oxygen affinity and moderate erythrocytosis. Hb Helsinki, in addition, has a mild decrease in the Bohr effect. In Hb Providence, the new Asn suffers deamidation *in vivo*, generating an Asp (electrophoretically detectable). All these mutants have drastically reduced 2,3-DPG binding due to the elimination of one of the normal binding sites for this allosteric effect. This position in the β-chains involves an invariant residue, suggesting the importance that nature places on the binding of polyphosphates.

Hb Old Dominion/Burton-upon-Trent [β143 (H21) His→Tyr] (80), found among Scotch-Irish people, has a mild increase in oxygen affinity and no clinical abnormalities. This hemoglobin elutes before Hb A by reverse-phase HPLC and forms 50% of the hemolysate. Of interest, the mutation disrupts the 2,3-DPG binding site in the central cavity. Hb Old Dominion/Burton-upon-Trent coelutes with Hb A_{1C} on ion exchange chromatography and may therefore lead to the erroneous diagnosis of diabetes or to mismanagement of a diabetic patient with this variant.

REDUCTION OF HEME INTERACTION BY RESTRAINING THE QUATERNARY CONFORMATION DUE TO A TENDENCY TO AGGREGATE OR POLYMERIZE

Hb Porto Alegre [β9 (A6) Ser→Cys] is an extremely interesting mutant with higher than normal oxygen affinity and a tendency to aggregate (80,81). No erythrocytosis is apparent in the carriers. The polymerization of Hb Porto Alegre is based on the formation of –S–S– bonds in oxygenated samples and thus is different from Hb S. The polymerization of this mutant diminishes heme–heme interaction and increases the oxygen affinity (82). This is a unique molecular mechanism.

Hb Olympia [β20 (B2) Val→Met] is a silent mutation that is hard to detect (not detectable by isoelectric focusing) and that produces moderate erythrocytosis because of a moderately increased oxygen affinity with a normal Bohr effect (83,84). Difficulties in isolation impaired the study of this mutation. The mutation is particularly intriguing because it affects an exterior residue that is not involved in any of the areas of contact associated with quaternary conformational changes. However, the mystery has been solved. Using a case of β thalassemia associated with Hb Olympia (thus, an almost pure solution of Hb Olympia hemolysate), Edelstein et al. (84) confirmed its high affinity, low n value, and normal heterotropic interactions with 2,3-DPG and Cl⁻. In addition, detailed analysis of the oxygen equilibrium curve showed a pH dependency of the n value, suggesting that the tetramer molecules aggregate in the deoxy state at a high pH. This possibility was confirmed with centrifugation studies in the liganded and unliganded states. Small-angle diffraction studies need to be performed to determine the actual size of the aggregate (84).

ELONGATION OF THE GLOBIN CHAINS DISRUPTING THE QUATERNARY STRUCTURE

In *Hb Tak* insertion of the dinucleotide CA into codon 146 [CAC→CA(CA)C] abolishes the normal stop codon at position 147. This insertion causes a frameshift, which results in elongation of the β-chains by 11 residues (157 residues total), probably due to unequal crossing over (85–87). The abnormal hemoglobin constitutes 40% of the hemolysate and has a high oxygen affinity with no cooperativity (n = 0) and no allosteric effects with pH or 2,3-DPG. This finding is not surprising, because the C-terminus of the β-chain is actively involved in the conformational changes of the hemoglobin molecule by stabilizing the T state. Hence, by having these stabilizing interactions disrupted, Hb Tak is totally frozen in the R state. It is also slightly unstable. In spite of these severe functional abnormalities, the heterozygous patient exhibited no erythrocytosis. This puzzling situation could be explained by the extraordinarily biphasic oxygen affinity curve observed with mixtures of Hb Tak and Hb A, suggesting that no hybrid formation is present. The top portion of the oxygen equilibrium curve of the mixture is normal and begins to be abnormal only below 40% saturation. As physiologic oxygen exchange occurs (most frequently above that level of saturation), the tissues might not be aware of the presence of the abnormal hemoglobin.

Hb Saverne corresponds to an elongation of the β-chains due to a frameshift mutation involving a deletion of the second base of the triplet coding for His143 (88,89). New residues are added, for a total of 156. This abnormal hemoglobin is 30% of the hemolysate, has a slightly faster electrophoretic mobility than Hb A, has a high oxygen affinity, lacks cooperativity, and has a low Bohr effect. Again, the disruption of the C-terminals due to the excess residues also disrupts the stabilization of the T conformer, favoring the R state. The patient has a compensated hemolytic anemia that could be the consequence of the conflicting effects of high affinity and instability.

Another extended chain, *Hb Thionville* (90) (αNH₂-terminal Val→Glu), has intrinsically high affinity due to changes in the $\alpha_1\beta_1$ contact surface, but because it is an α-chain abnormality, it is expressed only at a 21% level and does not reach functional importance or cause clinical consequences. Nevertheless, this abnormality illuminates another feature of hemoglobin synthesis. In humans, globin translation is initiated by a Met residue that is cleaved after the chain has reached approximately 30 amino acids by the enzyme Met aminopeptidase. If a charged amino acid is introduced, as in α Thionville, the cleavage does not take place, and there is one amino acid extension at the N-terminal. In the β-chain, this same phenomenon has been described in *Hb Doha* (91). In another case, the β_1 Val is replaced by Met (*Hb South Florida*) (92). The posttranslation modification continues because a globin chain with an N-terminal Met is acetylated when the chain reaches approximately 50 residues in length. As discussed below, N-terminal Val strongly inhibits acetylation, as demonstrated in normal α-chains and β-chains, whereas the Met–Glu dimer is a particularly good acceptor for complete acetylation. This is the case not only for globin but also for other proteins (such as band 3 protein in the red cell membrane). In *Hb Long Island–Marseille* (93), the Met is not acetylated because the second position in the β-chain (β2) is Val instead of Glu.

Finally, Hb Thionville is interesting for two other reasons. Because it is an α-chain abnormality, it identifies the allosteric interactions in which α-chains participate. It shows a reduced Bohr effect and reduced Cl⁻ binding, whereas 2,3-DPG binding, which is mainly due to an allosteric interaction of the β-chains, is normal. It also illustrates how acetylation of the N-terminal interferes with the R→T transition. This demonstrates the need to keep the N-terminal nonacetylated—that is, without Met—for the conformational changes of hemoglobin to take place.

SOME HIGH-AFFINITY HEMOGLOBINS THAT LACK AN EXPLANATION FOR THEIR FUNCTIONAL BEHAVIOR

Hb Heathrow [β103 (G5) Phe→Leu] is an intriguing, electrophoretically silent mutation with moderately high oxygen affinity and clinically apparent erythrocytosis (94). This mutation affects an invariant residue that guards the entrance of the heme pocket. The molecular mechanism is not known. The smaller side chain at the bottom of the heme pocket might alter ligand micropaths or the electronic environment of the prosthetic group, but this is speculation. We might not know why this mutant has a high oxygen affinity, but nature surely does, because the mutated residue is invariant.

Diagnosis of High Oxygen Affinity Hemoglobins

In 1966, Samuel Charache et al. (54) described an 81-year-old patient who presented with erythrocytosis, was found to have an abnormal band in his hemoglobin electrophoresis, had an increased oxygen affinity of red cells, and complained of mild angina.

The abnormal hemoglobin proved to be a substitution of Leu for Arg in residue 92 of the α-chains. The discovery of the first carrier of Hb Chesapeake opened a new chapter in the study of hemoglobinopathies, because it demonstrated that a variant of this molecule could generate another clinical syndrome. The discovery of this abnormal hemoglobin and others has been useful in the elucidation of the molecular mechanisms underlying the function of normal hemoglobin.

Because the propositus of the Hb Chesapeake pedigree presented with mild angina, it is legitimate to ask whether this is a characteristic of the carriers of high-affinity hemoglobins. The study of other members of the same pedigree and a large number of carriers of high-affinity hemoglobins have convinced most observers that the presence of these variants is largely without clinical consequences, except for inappropriate iatrogenic interventions when the diagnosis has been ignored or the patients have been confused with having polycythemia vera.

High-affinity hemoglobin patients do not have increased white cell and platelet counts and do not have splenomegaly (except for patients with concomitant β thalassemia). They sometimes have a family history of "thick blood," but a significant number of high-affinity hemoglobins are new mutations—that is, no abnormal hemoglobin is found among parents or siblings.

The differential diagnosis of erythrocytosis is outlined in Table 49-5. Erythrocytosis should not be confused with polycythemia, in which there is also elevation of white cells and platelets and usually splenomegaly. The diagnosis of the entities in Table 49-5 requires different methodologic approaches. For example, an increase in erythropoietin can be suspected in the appropriate clinical environment but can be certified only by measuring blood erythropoietin levels. For this purpose, the best method available is radioimmunoassay (95). This method is available in commercial kits, and the test is also available from commercial laboratories and some academic institutions. Hypoxia of pulmonary or cardiovascular origin can be excluded on the basis of arterial blood gases. Affected patients characteristically have a low p50 and low O_2 saturations. Patients with red cells that have an altered capacity to transport O_2 have a normal pO_2.

Among the patients with abnormal red cells, the different subtypes can be distinguished by a strategy based on comparing the oxygen affinity of hemolysates (those that contain only hemoglobin at defined conditions of pH and salt) with the oxygen equilibrium of the red cells. The hemolysates identify intrinsic defects in the hemoglobin molecule; study of intact red cells identifies other red cell factors (such as 2,3-DPG) that alter the oxygen affinity of an otherwise normal hemoglobin. Specifically, abnormal hemoglobins have red cells with a high oxygen affinity, a high oxygen affinity hemolysate, and a near-normal 2,3-DPG concentration. The enzymatic defects of 2,3-DPG mutase are characterized by high oxygen affinity red cells, normal oxygen affinity of the red cell hemolysate, and a very low 2,3-DPG (96). All of these have a normal absorption spectrum of their hemolysates.

Methemoglobin (e.g., congenital methemoglobinemia) can be identified by the presence of an abnormal peak at 620 nm, and carboxyhemoglobin (e.g., carbon monoxide poisoning) (97) can be assayed by a three-wavelength measurement, because the spectra of carbon monoxy Hb and oxy Hb differ significantly. Several gas-measuring apparatuses available in hospitals (IL CO-oximeter) (Instrumentation Laboratory) can give an accurate reading of methemoglobinemia and carboxyhemoglobinemia in whole blood.

Finally, patients with familial erythrocytosis have a normal oxygen affinity, whether red cells or hemolysate is used. The disease has a recessive inheritance pattern and is sometimes associated with clubbing (98). Two interesting groups of patients have been identified with erythrocytosis that is not related to hemoglobin variants or enzyme abnormalities.

ERYTHROPOIETIN RECEPTOR MUTATIONS

Several patients have been identified in whom erythrocytosis is associated with truncation of the cytosolic portion of the erythropoietin (Epo) receptor, eliminating the negative regulatory domain of the receptor. The truncation does not allow the physiologically appropriate shut-off of the signaling cascade induced by Epo binding and receptor dimerization. This change leads to inappropriate Epo signaling, increased red cell formation relative to the plasma levels of Epo, and higher plasma hemoglobin levels than would be expected for the patients' blood oxygenation.

CHUVASHIAN ERYTHROCYTOSIS

Familial and congenital erythrocytosis not due to hemoglobin or red cell enzyme mutations is common in the Chuvash population of the Chuvashia Autonomous Republic of Russian Federation, located in the European portion of Russia, southeast from Moscow (99). Hundreds of individuals appear to be affected in an autosomal-recessive and severe form of the disease, with hemoglobins of approximately 22 g/dL. In addition, the phenotype has features of polycythemia vera, with a high incidence of thrombosis, stroke, and occasionally, splenomegaly. However, platelet and white blood cell counts are normal. Analysis of the BglII and minisatellite polymorphisms of the erythropoietin gene showed no evidence of linkage. This finding was confirmed by Vasserman et al. (100) by microsatellite linkage analysis, which placed the disease locus on chromosome 11q23 between the markers D11S4142 and D11S1356, with a maximal lod score of 6.61. The Chuvash erythrocytosis represents a distinct disease involving an unknown gene that has the potential of increasing our understanding of the regulation of red cell production.

In terms of the diagnosis of high-affinity hemoglobin variants, the following points should be remembered:

1. Routine hemoglobin electrophoresis is capable of detecting only a fraction of high-affinity mutants. More sophisticated methods, such as agar electrophoresis or isoelectric focusing, can improve detection, but a group of abnormal hemoglobins with high affinity and neutral substitutions cannot be detected by any electrophoretic methods. Some of these cases apparently can be detected by HPLC. Nevertheless, a normal electrophoresis does not exclude the diagnosis of a high-affinity hemoglobin.

2. A p50 value useful for the diagnosis of a high-affinity hemoglobin cannot be a calculated p50 from pO_2 data. One has to be able to measure directly the saturation of hemoglobin and the pO_2 to obtain a useful p50. Types of apparatus like the Hem-o-Scan are perfectly adequate for this purpose, but the state of the art equipment is the Imai cell as an attachment to a good recording spectrophotometer.

TABLE 49-5. Differential Diagnosis of Erythrocytosis (Isolated Increase in Hematocrit and Hemoglobin)

Relative erythrocytosis (normal red cell mass) due to decreased plasma volume
Absolute erythrocytosis (increased red cell mass)
  Idiopathic familial erythrocytosis
  Primary (physiologically inappropriate increase in erythropoietin)
    Neoplasms that secrete erythropoietin
    Renal lesions that produce erythropoietin
    Abnormality in erythropoietin receptor
  Secondary (physiologically appropriate increase in erythropoietin)
    Arterial hypoxemia
      High altitude
      Chronic pulmonary disease
      Right-to-left cardiac shunts
      Massive obesity (pickwickian syndrome)
    Hypoxemia secondary to intrinsic red cell changes
      High-affinity hemoglobin variants
      Decreased or absence of 2,3-diphosphoglyceric acid mutase
      Congenital or acquired methemoglobinemia
      Chronic carbon monoxide poisoning (including heavy smoking)

PATHOPHYSIOLOGIC AND CLINICAL ASPECTS OF HIGH-AFFINITY HEMOGLOBINS

Most patients with high-affinity hemoglobins and erythrocytosis have a benign clinical course and no apparent complications. Although the first case of a high-affinity hemoglobin was identified in the course of a workup for angina, this circumstance was probably fortuitous.

Patients with *Hb Malmo* [β97(FG-4)His→Gln] (100a) have been reported to be symptomatic and have benefited from phlebotomy and the transfusion of normal blood, but this course is the exception and not the rule (101). A significant number of these patients are diagnosed in the course of a routine hematologic examination or when the pedigree of a propositus is examined. There are generally no physical findings, except occasionally a ruddy complexion. The hemoglobin and hematocrit levels are only moderately increased.

The most pressing reason to diagnose these high-affinity hemoglobins early and accurately is to avoid submitting the patient to unnecessary invasive diagnostic procedures and inappropriate and often dangerous therapeutic interventions. Many of these patients have undergone expensive and unnecessary cardiac catheterization. Others have suffered several courses of radioactive phosphorus (^{32}P) treatment based on a mistaken diagnosis of polycythemia vera. As a rule of thumb, any patient with polycythemia vera about to undergo a serious therapeutic intervention should have a whole blood oxygen equilibrium measurement.

The main pending issues that concern students of this subject follow.

DO THE CARRIERS OF HIGH-AFFINITY HEMOGLOBINS HAVE PROBLEMS IN THE DELIVERY OF OXYGEN TO THE TISSUES?

Patients carrying a physiologically significant high-affinity hemoglobin all their lives are probably reasonably compensated. The reduced delivery of oxygen to the tissues is compensated primarily by increases in erythropoietin-induced red cell mass, and probably compensated by increases in blood flow and changes in perfusion patterns in selected regions (Fig. 49-18).

The best evidence of an erythropoietin-mediated increase in red cell mass, responding to hypoxic stimuli, comes from Adamson and Finch (102,104) and Adamson and Hayashi (103). These authors determined that patients with several high-affinity hemoglobins with erythrocytosis had normal urinary erythropoietin levels that dramatically increased when they were phlebotomized to a normal red cell mass. This effect was not observed among patients with idiopathic familial erythrocytosis. Charache et al. (105) have determined that patients with high-affinity hemoglobins have normal oxygen consumption, normal arterial pO_2, slightly reduced mixed venous pO_2 in some cases, and slightly decreased resting cardiac output. More important, these numbers change significantly on phlebotomy or measured exercise, with marked increases in cardiac output and lowering of the mixed venous pO_2. The compensatory mechanisms might include increased perfusion efficiency. For example, patients with Hb Malmo have been shown to have increased myocardial blood flow, and patients with Hb Yakima have increased cerebral flow.

Charache et al. (106) have also addressed the issue of the risk involved in pregnancy for mothers with high-affinity hemoglobins. No increase in morbidity or mortality in the infant or mother is observed, suggesting that compensatory mechanisms other than the differences in oxygen affinity between Hb F and Hb A (the former has a lower affinity) must operate in pregnancies in which the mother's hemoglobin has a higher oxygen affinity than Hb F.

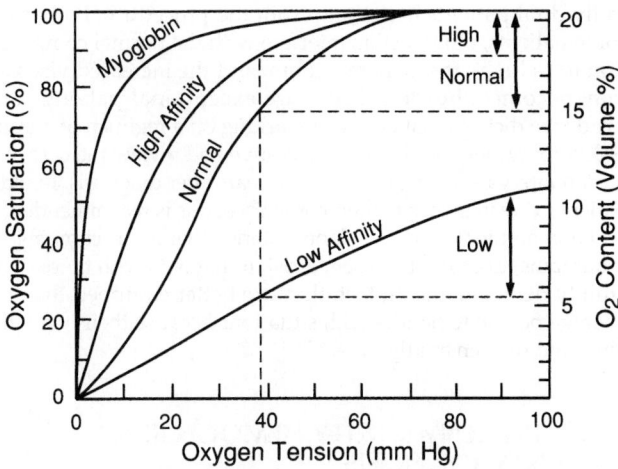

Figure 49-18. Oxygen equilibrium curves of myoglobin (no heme–heme interaction, hence n = 1) and of normal hemoglobin red cells, flanked by curves of high-affinity hemoglobin red cells and low-affinity hemoglobin-containing red cells. Oxygen tension (pO_2) is plotted against percentage of oxygen saturation and oxygen content in volume percentage. Oxygen content takes into account the amount of hemoglobin present. The oxygen extraction is the difference in oxygen content of red cells at a pO_2 of 100 mm Hg in the lungs and a pO_2 of 40 mm Hg in the tissues. That subtraction renders approximately 5 volumes of oxygen for normal hemoglobin. The high-affinity hemoglobin renders 2.5 volumes and causes tissue hypoxia. The very low oxygen affinity hemoglobin (p50 of 85 mm Hg as in hemoglobin Beth Israel) results in an extraction of a little over 5 volumes, essentially normal. Nevertheless, any curve between this and the normal will have an increased oxygen extraction, and it is possible that the tissues will respond to this increased oxygen delivery with a decrease in the release of erythropoietin and anemia.

WHAT IS THE BASIS OF THE DIFFERENCES IN LEVELS OF HEMOGLOBIN AMONG CARRIERS OF THE SAME HIGH-AFFINITY HEMOGLOBIN?

Charache et al. (106) observed that carriers of *Hb Osler* had the same oxygen affinity as patients with *Hb McKees Rocks*, but hemoglobin levels were significantly higher (by more than 4 g/dL) in male carriers of the former. When oxygen transport was assessed in these two groups, only a small decrease in mixed venous pO_2 was observed. This finding could be the consequence of better oxygen extraction by carriers of Hb McKees Rocks, who therefore may require a smaller increase in red cell mass than carriers of Hb Osler.

These results imply that epistatic genetic effects might be operating, making the level of increase in red cell mass variable according to a person's genetic makeup. Charache et al. (106) have pointed out that adaptation to hypoxia at high altitude is also different in different ethnic groups. Among Sherpas of Nepal, a lower hematocrit, no chronic mountain sickness, and a normal oxygen equilibrium curve are found, whereas in the populations adapted to the Andes (Quechuas and Aymaras), a higher hematocrit, chronic mountain sickness, and right-shifted oxygen equilibrium curves are observed. These findings suggest that adaptation might involve choosing among several possible strategies (with potential differences in success) according to the different genetic background.

SHOULD CARRIERS OF HIGH-AFFINITY HEMOGLOBINS UNDERGO PHLEBOTOMY?

The preceding discussion suggests that patients with high-affinity hemoglobins have reached a reasonable compensation of their abnormality with correction of the delivery of oxygen to the tissues in spite of increases in blood viscosity, and therefore, no intervention is needed. Butler et al. (107) have performed exercise studies before and after phlebotomy in patients with Hb Osler and have found no need for phlebotomy. Nevertheless, there are reports of individual patients benefiting from the procedure. Perhaps in some patients, other factors interfere with the normal compensation for a high-affinity hemoglobin, and the increased viscosity may become a burden. These are exceptional patients, and prudence dictates that before embarking on a regimen of chronic phlebotomy, one should be conservative and review the case at 6-month intervals during the first few years after diagnosis. In older patients, due vigilance to their coronary status is recommended.

Low ambient pO_2 (airplane cabins, living or climbing in mountains) does not represent a risk to patients with these high-affinity hemoglobins. In fact, they are better equipped than the average person to handle such situations because their hemoglobins bind oxygen avidly.

LOW OXYGEN AFFINITY HEMOGLOBIN MUTANTS: CYANOSIS

Carriers of some low ligand affinity hemoglobin variants are characterized by a slate gray color of the skin and other teguments secondary to cyanosis. Cyanosis can be present from birth in the α-chain abnormalities and from the middle to the end of the first year of life in the β-chain mutants. This pattern results because α-chains are expressed from the second trimester of fetal life, whereas β-chains begin to be synthesized in the perinatal period and reach a significant concentration after approximately 6 months of age. This congenital noncardiopulmonary cyanotic syndrome, secondary to abnormal hemoglobins, must be distinguished from other causes of cyanosis.

Description and Clinical Features of Low-Affinity Hemoglobins

Many fewer low-affinity hemoglobins are described than high-affinity hemoglobins (Table 49-6). They can be classified as resulting from these three conditions discussed at length in the following section:

- Alteration of the switch region, the flexible joint, or the C-terminals of the $\alpha_1\beta_2$ area of contact that favor the T state, either by stabilizing this conformer or by destabilizing the R state
- Steric hindrance to the heme, resulting in decreased affinity for ligands
- Alteration of the $\alpha_1\beta_1$ area of contact with disruption of the overall architecture of the hemoglobin that favors the T state

ALTERATION OF THE SWITCH REGION, FLEXIBLE JOINT, OR C-TERMINAL IN THE $\alpha_1\beta_2$ AREA OF CONTACT THAT FAVORS THE T STATE, EITHER BY STABILIZING THIS CONFORMER OR BY DESTABILIZING THE R STATE

Hb Bruxelles [β42 (CD1) Phe→0] (108,109) is a deletion of the most phylogenetically conserved amino acid residue of hemoglobin. Phe residues at β41 and β42 are conserved in all normal mammalian non–α-globin chains and are indispensable for the structural integrity and oxygen-binding functions of the molecule. Sequence analysis was insufficient to differentiate between Pheβ41 or β42 as the site of the Hb Bruxelles deletion. DNA analysis showed that the missing codon was the TTT of β42.

From age 4 years, the propositus for Hb Bruxelles had severe hemolytic anemia and cyanosis, requiring blood transfusion on one occasion. Later in life, her hemoglobin concentration stabilized at approximately 10 g/dL. The reasons for this switch of phenotype is unknown. A discussion follows of other mutations of β41 and β42, which are predominately unstable hemoglobins.

The striking feature of the oxygen equilibrium curve of Hb Bruxelles is that unlike the normal curve, which is roughly symmetric with maximum cooperativity at half saturation, Hb Bruxelles has almost nonexistent cooperativity and a shift of the allosteric equilibrium almost entirely to the T or deoxy state. Confirming the latter, CO rebinding kinetics showed, even at low photolysis levels, the T conformation; hence, the switch between R and T occurs after the third heme is liganded, not after second heme ligation, as in normal hemoglobin. Hb Bruxelles provides a fine example of the separation of ligand affinity and allosteric effects. The shift to T state is so large (allosteric effect) that the

TABLE 49-6. Stable Low-Affinity Hemoglobins

	Mutation	Name	Cyanosis	Other Properties
α-Chain sites				
α94 (G1)	Asp→Asn	Titusville	(−)	↑ Dimer
α130 (H13)	Ala→Asp	Yuda	(−)	
β-Chain sites				
β1 (NA1)	Val→AcAla	Raleigh	(−)	↓ Dimer
β11 (A8)	Val→Phe	Washtenaw	(−)	
β21 (B3)	Asp→Gly	Connecticut	(−)	
β37 (C3)	Trp→Arg	Rothschild	(−)	
β41 (C7)	Phe→Ser	Denver	(+)	
β61 (E7)	Lys→Met	Bologna	(−)	
β65 (E9)	Lys→Glu	J Cairo	(−)	↑ Met
β66 (E10)	Lys→Thr	Chico	(−)	
β73 (E17)	Asp→Tyr	Vancouver	(−)	
	Asp→Asn	Korle Bu, G Accra	(−)	
	Asp→Val	Mobile	(−)	
	Asp→Gly	Tilburg	(−)	
β76 (E20)	Ala→Pro	Calais	(−)	↑ Met
β82 (EF6)	Lys→Asn→Asp	Providence	(−)	
β83 (EF7)	Gly→Asp	Pyrgos, Mizunami	(−)	
β90 (F6)	Glu→Lys	Agenogi	(−)	
β102 (G4)	Asn→Thr	Kansas	(+)	↑ Dimer
	Asn→Ser	Beth Israel	(+)	
	Asn→Tyr	Saint Mandé	(+)	
β108 (G11)	Asn→Asp	Yoshisuka	(−)	
	Asn→Lys	Presbyterian	(−)	
β121 (GH4)	Glu→Gln	D Los Angeles, D Punjab	(−)	

Dimer, dissociation into dimers; Met, methemoglobin formation.

oxygen equilibrium/CO kinetics show essentially T state properties. Because cooperativity is minimal in the absence of effectors, the shift in p50 observed with 2,3-DPG is exclusively a ligand affinity effect. The molecule is already nearly totally in the T state. In Hb A, the contributions of allosteric effects and ligand affinity contribute equally to the 2,3-DPG shift in oxygen affinity.

Hb Titusville [α94 (G1) Asp→Asn] (110) is the only α-chain mutation described with low oxygen affinity. This mutant has an abnormal electrophoretic mobility in cellulose acetate and makes up 35% of the hemolysate. The propositus had a hemoglobin level of 12.5 g/dL. The mutant hemoglobin has a low oxygen affinity combined with a reduction of the Bohr effect by over 60% and a clear tendency of the molecule to dimerize. Nevertheless, the patient has no apparent cyanosis. The molecular defect involves the $\alpha_1\beta_2$ area of contact, and the substitution favors the T state of the molecule.

Other examples are the three mutations described for the β102 [G4] site: *Hb Kansas* (Asn→Thr) (111,112), *Hb Beth Israel* (Asn→Ser) (113), and *Hb St. Mandé* (Asn→Tyr) (114). These three abnormal hemoglobins all have low oxygen affinity and produce clinically apparent cyanosis.

Hb Kansas (the first low-affinity hemoglobin described and the most extensively studied) has a very high p50 (approximately 70 mm Hg for whole blood in a heterozygous person compared with 26 mm Hg for a normal person), decreased cooperativity, and a normal Bohr effect. The Asn residue at this site is invariant for the β-chains; this finding is not surprising because the only hydrogen bond across the $\alpha_1\beta_2$ interface in oxyhemoglobin is formed between this Asn and Asp94. This bond is broken when the molecule assumes the T state. Examination of deoxy Hb Kansas by difference Fourier x-ray diffraction analysis at 5.5-Å resolution has shown that the new Thr residue is incapable of forming this bond (115). Thus, the low oxygen affinity results from destabilization of the oxy (R) conformer. In addition, other structural changes occur at the $\alpha_1\beta_2$ interface, which accounts for the increased tendency of Hb Kansas to dissociate into αβ dimers.

Replacement of the same Asn residue by Lys in *Hb Richmond* has not been reported to produce abnormal oxygen-binding properties (116). With this mutant, Greer (115) has shown that the introduced Lys residue is capable of bridging the $\alpha_1\beta_2$ region by forming a salt bridge with Asp94 that replaces the original hydrogen bond. Because there are some abnormalities in the $\alpha_1\beta_2$ region on the difference Fourier maps, Greer (115) suggests that detailed analyses of oxygen equilibrium curve might be useful.

Hb Beth Israel was found in a person of Italian descent, but the abnormal hemoglobin was not detected in his parents. The propositus exhibited clinically apparent cyanosis involving fingers, lips, and nailbeds (113). He had been severely disciplined in the past for constantly having "dirty hands," and the abnormal skin color was not noticeable to him or his parents. The cyanosis was detected by a surgeon about to perform a herniorrhaphy. The whole blood p50 was 88 mm Hg (normal, 26), and the arterial blood was only 63% saturated despite a normal pO$_2$ of 97 mm Hg. The red cell 2,3-DPG was mildly elevated. The hemolysate showed a low oxygen affinity and a normal Bohr effect. The molecular mechanism involved here is the same as in Hb Kansas, although the defect might be more disruptive locally because Ser is shorter than Thr.

Hb St. Mandé is a mutant making up 38% of the hemolysate that migrates electrophoretically as Hb F. It was found in a person who exhibited labial cyanosis and moderate anemia (hemoglobin, 9.6 g/dL). The p50 was 52 mm Hg (normal in that laboratory was 28), and the 2,3-DPG concentration was normal. The measured oxygen saturation of arterial blood was 81%. Recent one-dimensional and two-dimensional NMR spectros-

copy demonstrated that the quaternary structure of liganded Hb St. Mandé is different from the R state but also different from the T state (117). This special ligand quaternary structure also differs from Hb Kansas, which has an NMR spectrum similar to the T state in the liganded molecule. The tertiary conformation around the heme of both chains is altered, suggesting that the β-chain mutation propagates its modification to the α-subunit: and one of them, involving Leuβ141, is a long-range interaction as detected by NMR.

The intensity of the cyanosis and the extent of the decrease in oxygen affinity are inversely proportional to the length of the substituted side chain at β102. It is maximal when Ser is present, less when Thr is present, and least in Tyr-substituted hemoglobins.

Hb Rothschild (β37 [C3] Trp→Arg) (71,118) is a remarkably interesting abnormal hemoglobin that Sharma et al. (86) have characterized as alternatively exhibiting low and high affinity, depending on conditions. The overall oxygen affinity curve of this mutant exhibits low affinity (119). Nevertheless, the situation is far more complicated (120). This mutant extensively dissociates into dimers in the liganded state. This feature, in turn, explains the low affinity of this hemoglobin, because fully liganded dimers have lower affinity than partially unsaturated dimers, and they predominate overwhelmingly in this abnormal hemoglobin.

On the other hand, the fully deoxy state of Hb Rothschild has a higher affinity for ligands than the T state of Hb A. This feature explains that this mutant simultaneously has low and high ligand affinity: The introduction of a positively charged Arg at position 37 brings this residue in direct conflict with another Arg at position 92 [FG4]. This clash of positive charges destabilizes the $\alpha_1\beta_2$ subunit contacts and explains the extensive dissociation into αβ dimers, a situation not present in normal hemoglobin T state (the normal T tetramer dissociates into dimers with much difficulty). In Hb Rothschild addition, the destabilization of the $\alpha_1\beta_2$ contact makes the T state less constrained (explaining the decrease in low affinity of the tetramer and, hence, the higher affinity of the deoxy form). To make matters worse, the monoliganded tetramers (which should retain the T state conformation) have increased dissociation in Hb Rothschild, again conspiring against a true T state behavior. Hb Rothschild has considerable alterations in the intradimer stability and in its capacity to refold (120). These findings predict small but potentially significant changes in the areas of the molecule distal to the substitution.

Hb Aalborg [β74 (E18) Gly→Arg] (121), comprising 21 percent of the hemolysate, has decreased oxygen affinity, has increased affinity for 2,3-DPG, and is moderately unstable. Clinically, it is associated with mild anemia. Electrophoretically, it moves between Hb F and Hb S. Crystallographic analysis (122) and comparison with *Hb Shepherds Bush* [β74 (E18) Gly→Asp], an unstable high oxygen affinity mutant, shed light on this mutation. Hb Shepherds Bush has an opposite charge substitution and exhibits increased ligand affinity, diminished affinity for phosphate, and instability. Fermi et al. (122) superimposed the B, G, and H helices of Hb A, known not to be affected by ligand binding, on those of Hb Aalborg. This analysis revealed a shift of the F helix of deoxy Hb Aalborg toward the EF corner, a movement opposite the normal change with ligand binding. On transition to the R state, this shift is linked to an increased tilt of the proximal His away from the heme axis, accounting for the bias toward the T state and the low oxygen affinity. The opposite effects of 2,3-DPG binding between Hb Aalborg and Shepherds Bush are the consequence of the opposite charges of the introduced residues.

STERIC HINDRANCE TO THE HEME RESULTING IN DECREASED AFFINITY FOR LIGANDS

Hb Connecticut [β21 (B3) Asp→Gly] might be an example of this steric hindrance to the heme (123). It is an electrophoretically apparent mutation that makes up 39% of the hemolysate. It shows a slightly elevated p50 (whole blood p50, 28.5 mm Hg; normal, 26), a normal Bohr effect, and normal 2,3-DPG interactions. Cyanosis is not apparent clinically, and patients with this mutation are not anemic. Hb Connecticut is of theoretic interest because it involves a residue that lies outside the areas critical for ligand-dependent conformational changes. Moo-Penn et al. (123) have suggested, on the basis of preliminary radiographic data, that the molecular abnormality probably involves the disruption of the salt bridges between Asp21 and Lys residues 61 and 65. This event might allow the E helix to come closer to the heme plate, inducing potential steric hindrance to the binding of ligands.

Hb Bologna [β61 (E5) Lys→Met] has an abnormal electrophoretic mobility and accounts for 48% of the hemolysate (124). The propositus was not anemic or cyanotic. This mutation has also been found in conjunction with $β^0$ thalassemia, in which the abnormal hemoglobin makes up 90% of the hemolysate. Remarkably, affected patients had no apparent cyanosis in spite of a whole blood p50 of 37.6 mm Hg (normal, 26) in the compound heterozygotes and 31 in the simple heterozygotes.

Lysβ61 is an external residue close to the distal heme-linked E7 His and forms a salt bridge with Asp21 of the same β-chain. It is also in contact with β25 of the B helix and two residues in the D helix (β55 and β56). The disruption of any or all of these contacts is likely to alter the oxygen-binding properties of the β heme. Note that the compensatory erythrocytosis observed commonly in thalassemia traits is abolished in the compound heterozygote for $β^0$ thalassemia and Hb Bologna, demonstrating the increased oxygen delivery secondary to the right shift of the oxygen equilibrium curve.

Hb Chico is a mutation of β66 [E10], in which the normal Lys is replaced by Thr. The interesting feature of this variant is the low affinity (p50 approximately 50% of normal) (125). This feature is not limited to the tetramer but it is also present in the isolated β Chico chain, suggesting that the mutation creates conditions of decreased affinity for ligands by changes in the heme environment unrelated to the R→T transition. The most facile interpretation is that this effect is a consequence of the rupture of the salt bridge that Lys66 forms with one of the propionate side chains of the β heme. Crystallography shows hydrogen bonding of the introduced Thrβ66 to the distal β63 [E7] His. Nevertheless, although distal His are important in ligand binding in α-chains, site-directed mutagenesis shows they are not significant in β-chains (124–126). Hence, the low affinity of Hb Chico must be secondary to direct steric hindrance.

ALTERATION OF THE $α_1β_1$ AREA OF CONTACT WITH DISRUPTION OF THE OVERALL ARCHITECTURE OF HEMOGLOBIN THAT FAVORS THE T STATE

Two mutant hemoglobins have been described for site β108 [G10]: *Hb Yoshisuka* (Asn→Asp) (127) and *Hb Presbyterian* (Asn→Lys) (128). Hb Yoshisuka is electrophoretically distinct, amounts to 51% of the hemolysate, and has significantly low oxygen affinity and a decreased Bohr effect (by 30%). Affected carriers usually have mild anemia and no cyanosis. Asn108 lies in the central cavity and is hydrogen-bonded to His 103, a residue located in the $α_1β_1$ area of contact. In addition, this residue is linked extensively through hydrogen bonding (by water molecules) to other residues in both the α-chains and β-chains. The introduction of the carbonyl group of the Asp residue disrupts this contact severely and changes the electrostatic properties of the central cavity, resulting in destabilization of the oxy conformation.

Hb Presbyterian, in which the mutation introduces a residue with opposite charge from Yoshisuka (Lys instead of Asp), amounts to 40% of the hemolysate, is an electrophoretically fast

component, exhibits significantly low oxygen affinity, and has an abnormally high Bohr effect (increased by 30%) and normal interactions with 2,3-DPG. Heterozygotes are mildly anemic. The molecular mechanism involved here is probably similar to that of Hb Yoshisuka. This hemoglobin does not dissociate normally in the R state, suggesting that it is abnormally biased toward the T state (93).

These two hemoglobins teach us that any charge (positive or negative) disrupts drastically the $α_1β_1$ area of contact. The difference in Bohr effects can be resolved only after high-resolution crystallography of these hemoglobins.

The three mutations at β73 [E17]: *Hb Vancouver* (Asp→Tyr) (129), *Hb Korle Bu* (Asp→Asn) (130), and *Hb Mobile* (Asn→Val) (131) belong in the same category as the preceding two hemoglobins. These three mutants are similar and account for close to 40% of the hemolysate. Affected patients have no evident cyanosis. Hb Vancouver has a p50 of 29.5 mm Hg for whole blood, but this variant (as well as Hb Mobile) has an increased Bohr effect (approximately 20% higher than normal). The isolated mutants are in the following order of increasing p50: Vancouver > Mobile > Korle Bu > A (132). The molecular mechanism of these effects is not obvious. Residue β73 is on the surface, and one of its well-known properties is its capacity to interfere with the polymerization of Hb S, as demonstrated by Bookchin and Nagel (133) and confirmed in the crystallographic studies of Wishner et al. (134). The possibility that bulkier side changes could interfere with the entrance of ligands to the heme and alter the oxygen affinity by steric hindrance has been suggested (129). Because the size of asparaginyl and aspartyl residues is almost identical, Wajcman and Jones (132) have argued that this theory does not explain the differences in p50 observed. These authors note that the increase in p50 is proportional to the hydrophobicity of the newly introduced residue. Hence, it is likely that the effect is the result of the formation of a hydrophobic bond of increasing strength that perturbs the conformation. A good candidate for the receptor of this interaction is Thr84, located in the EF segment.

Pathophysiologic Considerations

Low-affinity hemoglobins deliver more oxygen to the tissues. Figure 49-18 depicts the amount of oxygen extracted from a curve situated to the right of the normal oxygen equilibrium curve. The oxygen binding at 100 mm Hg (lungs) and 40 mm Hg (tissues) in a low-affinity curve can be as high as double the difference of a normal oxygen equilibrium curve. Nevertheless, the increase in extraction is not monotonic with the increase in p50. This analysis predicts that patients with moderately right-shifted red cell oxygen equilibrium curves (p50 between 35 and 55 mm Hg) could be anemic, but that no anemia should be expected in patients with severely right-shifted curves (p50 approximately 80 mm Hg). The clinical picture observed in patients with Hb Kansas, Hb Beth Israel, Hb Titusville, and Hb Seattle confirms this analysis. Clinically apparent cyanosis is observed only in carriers whose red cells have significantly right-shifted curves—that is, a p50 over 50 mm Hg.

The effect of the right-shifted curve on the level of 2,3-DPG is of interest. In erythrocytes, approximately 20% of the conversion of 1,3-DPG to 3-phosphoglycerate occurs indirectly through the formation of 2,3-DPG. The level of red cell 2,3-DPG is known to rise in many conditions associated with hypoxia, as previously discussed (Fig. 49-15). This effect is probably related to the decrease in oxygen saturation of red cells and is independent of the presence of hypoxia per se; therefore, it applies to the low-affinity hemoglobins despite the absence of tissue hypoxia.

Desaturation increases intraerythrocytic pH as a result of deoxyhemoglobin binding more protons than oxyhemoglobin

(Bohr effect). This slight intraerythrocytic alkalosis, in turn, stimulates two enzymes involved in 2,3-DPG synthesis: phosphofructokinase, which controls the overall glycolytic rate, and DPG mutase, which directly controls the rate of 2,3-DPG synthesis. In addition, high pH inhibits 2,3-DPG phosphatase. Hence, high pH simultaneously increases the synthesis of 2,3-DPG and decreases its destruction. Finally, release of end product inhibition may also be involved. Red cells with low-affinity hemoglobin have an increased proportion of deoxyhemoglobin and will bind more 2,3-DPG, decreasing the free 2,3-DPG and thus inhibiting DPG mutase (34). Figure 49-19 depicts the oxygen affinity effect of the increased 2,3-DPG in Hb Beth Israel–containing red cells.

Diagnosis of Low-Affinity Hemoglobin Variants

The diagnosis of a low-affinity hemoglobin should always be considered in patients with cyanosis, particularly when cardiopulmonary causes can be ruled out. In patients with cyanosis of unknown origin, it is probably advisable to obtain a hemoglobin electrophoresis and a whole blood p50 before undertaking expensive or risky invasive diagnostic procedures. The search for low-affinity hemoglobins as the explanation for anemia is less compelling, because the yield is probably very low and the tests are not cost-effective. Nevertheless, if other investigations prove fruitless, unexplained normocytic anemias deserve to be explored with a hemoglobin electrophoresis and a whole blood p50.

A simple test (even bedside) to distinguish low-affinity hemoglobins and cardiopulmonary cyanosis from methemoglobinemia, Hb M, and sulfhemoglobinemia involves exposing blood from the patient to pure oxygen. This exposure will turn the purple-greenish blood of healthy persons and that of patients with low-affinity hemoglobins to the bright red color of fully oxygenated blood. In contrast, the blood of patients with methemoglobinemia, sulfhemoglobinemias, or Hb M retains its abnormal color in spite of the exposure to pure oxygen.

M HEMOGLOBINS: PSEUDOCYANOSIS

Description and Pathophysiologic Features of the M Hemoglobins

The German physicians Horlein and Weber (135) described a family with congenital cyanosis due to abnormal red cells 1 year before Pauling's discovery of Hb S. These authors determined that the defect was autosomal dominant and was produced by red cells with an abnormal pigment similar to methemoglobin. They showed that the genetic defect resided in the globin and not in the heme. This last finding was based on recombination experiments in which the patients' globin was bound to normal heme and the patients' heme to normal globin. The amino acid substitutions characterizing three of these types of Hb M were reported by Gerald and Efron (136). At approximately the same time, Shibata et al. (137) in Japan solved the problem of hereditary nigremia (kuroko or "black child"), which had been observed by clinicians in the Shiden village of the Iwate prefecture for over 160 years. They found a brownish-colored hemoglobin in the hemolysate of a patient of this type, which was later characterized as Hb Iwate.

In the types of Hb M, each mutated globin chain (α or β) creates an abnormal microenvironment for the heme iron, displacing the equilibrium toward the oxidized or ferric state. The combination of the Fe^{3+} and its abnormal coordination with the substituted amino acid generates an abnormal visible spectrum that resembles but is clearly different from methemoglobin (oxidized heme iron in a normal globin chain). The strength by which the abnormal hemes are locked into this situation differs from one Hb M to another. Figure 49-20 is a diagram of the Hb M mutations.

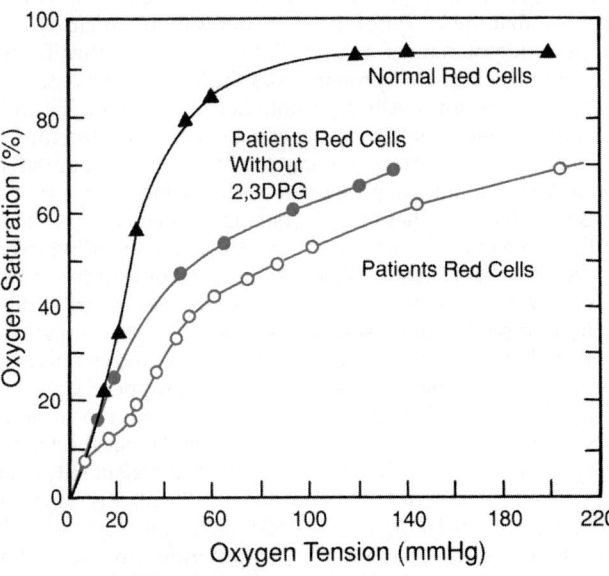

Figure 49-19. Oxygen equilibrium curves of normal red cells (*triangles*) and red cells from a patient heterozygous for hemoglobin Beth Israel before (*open circles*) and after (*closed circles*) depletion of 2,3-diphosphoglycerate (DPG). The p50 for hemoglobin Beth Israel–containing cells was 88 mm Hg (normal, 27 mm Hg). Patient's cells depleted of 2,3-DPG had a p50 of 55 mm Hg. Normal red cells subjected to the same procedure had a p50 of 16 mm Hg. The heterozygous patient's red cells have a biphasic or triphasic curve composed of the oxygen affinity curves of normal hemoglobin (*particularly the bottom portion of the composite patient curve*), the abnormal hemoglobin Beth Israel (*top of the composite curve*), and probably hybrid molecules containing one β Beth Israel chain and one normal β chain (*intermediate portion of the curve*). (From Nagel RL, Joshua L, Johnson J, et al. Hemoglobin Beth Israel: a mutant causing clinically apparent cyanosis. *N Engl J Med* 1976;295:125, with permission.)

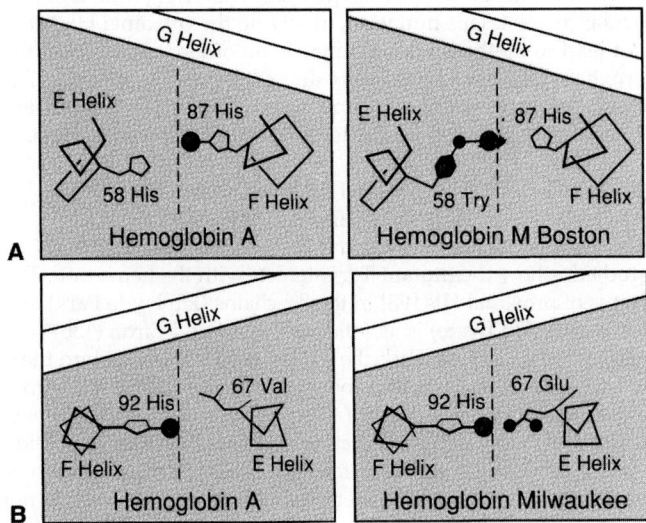

Figure 49-20. Schematic depiction of the crystallographic findings in **(A)** hemoglobin M Boston [α58 (E7) His→Tyr] and **(B)** hemoglobin M Milwaukee-1 [β67 (E11) Val→Glu] compared with normal. The heme iron is represented by the shaded circle in the center. [**(A)** From Pulsinelli PD, Perutz MF, Nagel RL. Structure of hemoglobin M Boston, a variant with a five-coordinated ferric heme. *Proc Natl Acad Sci U S A* 1973;70:3870, with permission; **(B)** from Perutz MF, Pulsinelli PD, Ranney HM. Structure and subunit interaction of haemoglobin M Milwaukee. *Nature* 1972;237:259, with permission.]

TABLE 49-7. Human M Hemoglobins

	Hb M Milwaukee	Hb M Boston	Hb M Iwate	Hb M Saskatoon	Hb M Hyde Park	Normal Values
Substitution	β67 (E11) Val→Glu	α58 (E7) His→Tyr	α87 (F8) His→Tyr	β63 (E7) His→Tyr	β92 (F8) His→Tyr	E7: distal histidine F8: proximal histidine
Percentage of total Hb	50	—	19	35	—	—
Hb, g/dL	14–15	—	17	13–16	10–125	13–16
Reticulocytes, %	1–2	—	—	0.8–3.2	4–6	1–2
Rate of reduction of Fe^{3+} by dithionite, $T_{1/2}$	23	260	—	15	55	Too fast to measure
Rate of autooxidation of abnormal chains	13	—	—	26	—	1440 min
p50	Decreased	Decreased	Decreased	Normal	Normal	—
Value in Hill equation	n = 1.2	n = 1.2	n = 1.1	n = 1.2	n = 1.3	n value for Hb A = 2.7
Bohr effect	Present	Decreased	Decreased	Present	Present	—
Conversion of abnormal subunits to cyanmet with potassium cyanide	Fast	Slow	Very slow	Fast	Slow	Very fast

Hb, hemoglobin.

As shown in Table 49-7, in four of the five known types of Hb M, the distal or proximal His that interacts with the heme iron is replaced by Tyr either in the α-chains or in the β-chains. In the fifth, *Hb Milwaukee*, Valβ67 [E11] is replaced by a Glu, which has longer side chains that can reach and perturb the heme iron.

Several molecular abnormalities are associated with Hb M. They can be classified as follows.

WEAK HEME ATTACHMENT

The x-ray crystallographic studies of deoxy *Hb M Hyde Park* [β92 (F8) His→Tyr] showed a loss of 20% to 30% of the heme (138). Others detected a minor component (5%) in the hemolysate of these patients that migrated between Hb A$_2$ and Hb A Hyde Park (139). The α-chains of the abnormal component were normal, but only one of the two β^{HP}-chains contained heme.

In this context, *Hb Auckland* [α97 (F8) His→Asn] (140) is of particular interest. This mutation, involving the proximal His, does not lead to methemoglobinemia, as do other mutations of the proximal His, but to instability and accelerated heme loss. The clinical picture is of a mild compensated hemolytic anemia and not methemoglobinemia, due to the absence of the ferric heme.

BINDING OF THE IRON TO THE REMAINING HISTIDINE AND TO THE NEWLY INTRODUCED TYROSINE

The question that has intrigued investigators since Hb M was first studied is how the mutant Tyr interacts with the heme iron. The status of proximal His [F8] in the β^M-chains (Hb Hyde Park) and α^M-chains (Hb Iwate) is as follows: Gerald and Efron (136) suggested that in *Hb Hyde Park*, the β heme would move toward the E helix, allowing the iron to be bound by the distal His, accommodating the bulkier side chain of the new Tyr, and generating a phenolic bond to the sixth coordinating position of the iron; this action would stabilize it in the ferric form. Crystallographic studies contradicted this interpretation, demonstrating that the heme was not displaced toward the E helix (138). Therefore, the Tyr must be accommodated by movements of the F helix, which appears largely destabilized. Independent confirmation was provided by the application of electron nuclear double-resonance spectroscopy (141). Examination of the N^{14} interactions in Hb M Hyde Park show none of the high-frequency peaks assigned to the normal proximal His, indicating that the distal His does not take over the role of the proximal His. It is likely that that the Tyr in Hb Hyde Park binds the heme iron through a phenolic anion.

The findings in *Hb Iwate* (α87 [F8] His→Tyr) are the opposite. Here, crystallographic studies (138) show that the E helix of the α-chains is displaced toward the heme plate by approximately 2 Å, which is the distortion expected if the distal His [α58 (E7)] moves to bind the fifth coordinating position in the heme iron (136). To complicate matters, NMR studies indicate that when the abnormal heme is reduced and bound to a ligand, the iron binds the distal His (142–144).

Ultraviolet (UV) resonance Raman and visible resonance Raman spectroscopy have been used by Nagai et al. (141) to establish that the F8 Tyr of the abnormal subunit in Hb M Iwate adopts a deprotonated form. UV Raman bands of other Tyr residues indicated that the protein takes the T-quaternary structure even in the met form. Although both hemes of α-subunits and β-subunits in met Hb take a six-coordinate high-spin structure, the resonance Raman spectrum of met Hb M Iwate indicates that the abnormal α-subunit adopts a five-coordinate high-spin structure. These results show that F8-tyrosinate is covalently bound to the Fe(III) heme in the α-subunit of Hb M Iwate, pretending to be a His residue. As a result, peripheral groups of porphyrin ring, especially the vinyl and the propionate side chains, are strongly influenced so that the resonance Raman spectrum is distinctly abnormal. When Hb M Iwate is fully reduced, the characteristic UV resonance Raman bands of tyrosinate disappear. Coordination of distal His [E7] to the Fe(II) heme in the reduced α-subunit of Hb M Iwate was proven by the resonance Raman spectrum.

The interactions of the distal His [E7] that are substituted by Tyr in the β^M-chain of *Hb M Saskatoon* [β63 (E7) His→Tyr] and the α^M-chain in *Hb M Boston* [α58 (E7) His→Tyr] are also known. The data for Hb M Boston are more precise and are illustrated in Figure 49-20. Pulsinelli et al. (145) demonstrated by x-ray crystallography that the new residue Tyr58 [E7] surprisingly fills the fifth coordinating position of the heme iron in spite of the presence of a normal proximal His. This bond moves the plane of the heme sufficiently to make the interaction between the proximal His and the heme iron impossible. This interpretation has been confirmed by NMR data (143). No crystallographic data are available for Hb M Saskatoon.

Finally, *Hb M Milwaukee* occupies a particular place in the constellation of Hb M because it is not a mutation of the proximal or distal His but of a residue nearby [Val67 (E11)]. When substituted by a residue with an appropriate side chain (such as Glu), it perturbs the heme iron and generates a Hb M (defined as a variant having an abnormal methemoglobin-like spectrum). Other mutations of that site, such as Hb Bristol (Asp) or Hb Sydney (Ala), are unstable or have low affinity but do not generate an abnormal ferric state for the heme iron. Perutz et al. (146) found by x-ray crystallography that the carboxylic group of the new glutamate occupies the sixth coordinating position of the iron and that the proximal His maintains its role as the tenant of the fifth coordinating position. This situation, of course, stabilizes the abnormal ferric state of Hb Milwaukee (Fig. 49-19).

OXYGEN-BINDING PROPERTIES AND R→T TRANSITION OF M HEMOGLOBINS

Hb M Milwaukee, Hb M Hyde Park, and Hb M Boston all adopt deoxy or deoxylike conformation on the deoxygenation of the two normal chains (in spite of the fact that the abnormal chains cannot deoxygenate). This finding helps in understanding the function of normal hemoglobin. It affirms that after two hemes become deoxygenated, the molecule as a whole adopts a deoxy conformation (T state). The finding is based on crystallography, electron paramagnetic resonance spectroscopy, NMR spectroscopy (147), binding of 2,3-DPG (147), and studies of copolymerization of deoxy Hb C Harlem (148).

The presence of the Bohr effect and a normal p50 strongly suggests that in Hb M Milwaukee, Hb M Saskatoon, and Hb M Hyde Park, the molecule adopts the R state when the two normal chains are oxygenated. NMR studies on Hb M Milwaukee by Lindstrom et al. (149) support the theory that the conformational changes take place when the normal hemes are oxygenated. On the other hand, Hb M Iwate is in the crystallographic T-configuration state when the normal hemes are in the ferric state, explaining its decreased affinity. The molecule does not shift to the R state when the normal hemes are liganded and remains in the low-affinity T state. A similar situation probably exists in Hb M Boston, because the habit of the deoxyhemoglobin crystal remains intact after oxygenation, suggesting that no conformational change has occurred that would necessitate a different crystal structure (145).

The reason Hb M Saskatoon and Hb M Boston have different properties (despite their common substitution of the distal His) is that the former does not change conformation when oxygenated and the latter does. Why β-chains differ from α-chains when their distal His is substituted has not been resolved.

IRON OXIDATION AND SPECTRAL CHARACTERISTICS

The fundamental characteristic of the types of Hb M is that their hemes are stabilized in the abnormal ferric state. Hence, they exhibit an abnormal visible spectrum that can be easily distinguished from regular methemoglobins (Figs. 49-21 and 49-22). This characteristic separates these variants from hemoglobin mutants that have a tendency to form normal methemoglobin, such as Hb St. Louis (150), Hb Bicetre (151), Hb I Toulouse (152), and Hb Seattle (153), all of which are unstable (see text that follows).

The iron atoms in the abnormal subunits of the types of Hb M exhibit an abnormally low redox potential. Hence, they are oxidized much more rapidly than normal by molecular oxygen (154) and are variably resistant to reduction by dithionite. Nagai et al. (155) have examined the rate of reduction of the five types of Hb M with various reductases, including the enzyme active in the normal erythrocyte, nicotinamide adenine dinucleotide (NADH)-cytochrome b_5 reductase. The surprise is that Hb M Iwate, Hb M Hyde Park, and Hb M Boston are not reduced at all, but Hb M Milwaukee is reduced slowly and Hb M Saskatoon is reduced normally by this reductase. These findings suggest the possibility that *in vivo* the latter two types of Hb M might be less oxidized than expected. Full ferric conversion might occur only *in vitro* due to the high autooxidation rate of

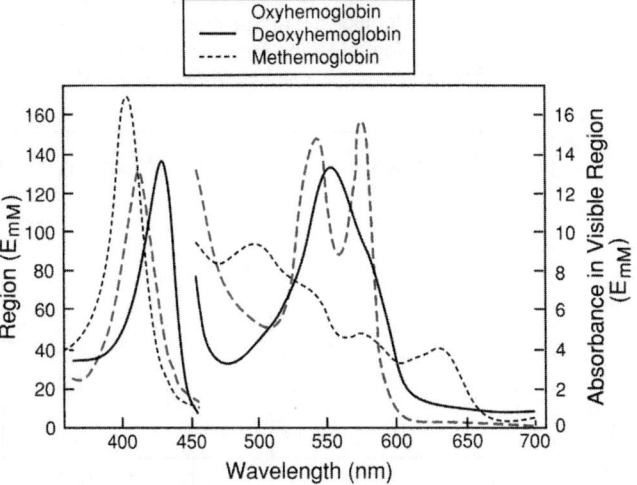

Figure 49-21. Light absorption spectra of oxyhemoglobin, deoxyhemoglobin, and methemoglobin in the visible and near ultraviolet regions. E_{mM} is the millimolar extinction coefficient in 0.1 mol/L potassium phosphate buffer (pH 7.4). (From Imai K. *Allosteric effects in haemoglobin.* Cambridge: Cambridge University Press, 1982, with permission.)

these abnormal hemoglobins. Older red cells might nevertheless have fully oxidized abnormal chains, in keeping with the presence of clinically apparent cyanosis.

Column chromatography, which separates the types of Hb M from Hb A, dramatically demonstrates the differences in the state of the iron in the two hemoglobins.

CLINICAL ASPECTS AND DIAGNOSIS

The predominant clinical feature associated with Hb M carriers is a condition similar to cyanosis that can be called *pseudocyanosis* (156–166). The skin and mucosal membranes may be brownish or slate-colored, more like those seen in methemoglobinemia, but not as blue-purple as in true cyanosis. The distinction is subtle and might not be apparent without contrasting the two conditions directly. The reason for the difference is that the color of the skin is induced by hemoglobin molecules that have an abnormal methemoglobin state, whereas cyanosis is caused by the presence of more than 5 g/dL deoxyhemoglobin. The cyanosis is present from birth in α-chain abnormalities and from the middle of the first year in the β-chain mutants. In addition, a mixture of the abnormal pigment and true cyanosis due to hemoglobin desaturation (of the normal chains) is observed in the types of low-affinity Hb M (Hb M Boston and Hb M Iwate).

Pseudocyanosis is not associated with dyspnea or clubbing, and affected persons apparently have a normal life expectancy. A mild hemolytic anemia (with increased reticulocyte count) has been observed in Hb M Hyde Park and can be explained by the instability of the hemoglobin induced by partial loss of the hemes.

The possibility of Hb M should be considered in all patients with abnormal homogeneous coloration of the skin and mucosa, particularly when pulmonary and cardiac function is normal. The diagnosis can be reinforced by observing an abnormal brown coloration of the blood in a tube. To distinguish this coloration from methemoglobin, the addition of potassium cyanide to the hemolysate is useful. Hemolysates containing methemoglobin turn red; those containing Hb M often change color more slowly. The rate of color conversion varies among the types of Hb M. A recording spectrophotometer is required for the next step in the diagnosis, although any spectrophotometer can be used for the overall technique recommended for the differential diagnosis of

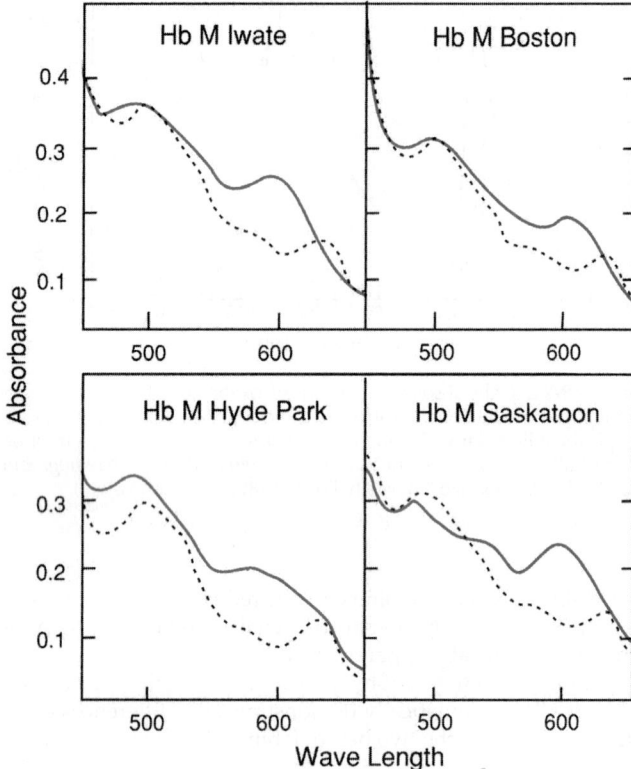

Figure 49-22. Spectra between 450 and 650 μm of the oxidized form of four M hemoglobins are compared in each case with the normal methemoglobin spectra. In these spectra, the normal chains are methemoglobin, and the abnormal chains have their own particular spectral properties. (From Shibata S, Miyaji T, Iuchi I. Methemoglobin M's of the Japanese. *Bull Yamaguchi Med Sch* 1967;14:141, with permission.)

cyanotic syndromes [discussed in the section Differential Diagnosis of Red Cell-Induced Cyanosis (Low-Affinity Hemoglobins) and Pseudocyanosis (M Hemoglobins) from Methemoglobinemia and Sulfhemoglobinemia]. Figure 49-22 illustrates the differences in the spectra observed with the types of Hb M, but all clearly differ from the normal methemoglobin spectrum with its maximum at 620 nm.

Electrophoresis is of limited value because the oxy forms are not separable from normal hemoglobin by cellulose acetate. Agar electrophoresis is a little better. Ion exchange chromatography (Biorex 70 equilibrated and developed with 0.196 M Na$_2$PO$_4$, pH 6.42) can separate the brown hemoglobin from the normal hemoglobin, rendering the diagnosis. Hemoglobin chains can be prepared by blocking the Cys thiols with *p*-chloromercuribenzoate and separating the chains electrophoretically or chromatographically. This procedure allows determination of which chain has an abnormal color.

Perhaps the greatest hazard for carriers of Hb M is misdiagnosis and the risk of expensive and hazardous workups. I am aware of one instance in which a 1-week-old infant was misdiagnosed as having a pseudotruncus arteriosus and underwent surgery with a procedure (Blalock) that did not allow the surgeons to realize the error. When the family study was completed many years later, the father was identified as a carrier of Hb M Boston and the child was also recognized as a carrier of this abnormal hemoglobin.

Differential Diagnosis of Red Cell–Induced Cyanosis (Low-Affinity Hemoglobins) and Pseudocyanosis (M Hemoglobins) from Methemoglobinemia and Sulfhemoglobinemia

In this section, a more general problem is analyzed: the pathophysiologic and diagnostic aspects of the patient with cyanosis not of cardiopulmonary origin.

Although the cardiac and pulmonary systems are major targets in the evaluation of a patient with apparent cyanosis, the differential diagnosis of this clinical sign includes two classes of hemoglobinopathies. First, the presence of an abnormal hemoglobin with a normal visible spectrum but a markedly right-shifted p50 results in significant arterial desaturation (167,168). Second, in sulfhemoglobin, methemoglobin, and Hb M, the altered visible spectrum of the abnormal pigments is responsible for the gray skin. The comparative spectral properties of sulfhemoglobin with those of methemoglobin are such that less of the former is needed to produce cyanosis. A patient can be markedly cyanotic with only 12% (1.6 g/dL) sulfhemoglobin (169,170).

The respiratory status of persons with cyanosis resulting from an abnormal hemoglobin varies with the entity. There is general agreement that clinically apparent dyspnea is not associated with the mutant hemoglobins with right-shifted p50s (167,168) or with the types of Hb M (154,171) but can be associated with even relatively mild degrees of methemoglobinemia (172). For sulfhemoglobinemia, there is no agreement. Most case reports indicate that dyspnea is not a feature, but others state that the symptoms associated with methemoglobinemia and sulfhemoglobinemia are identical (172).

Because the altered hemes in Hb M, sulfhemoglobin, and methemoglobin do not transport oxygen, affected persons with all three entities may have normal hemoglobin levels but suffer the physiologic effects of an anemia simply because insufficient functional hemes remain. This effect in isolation would be clinically significant only in extreme cases of methemoglobinemia and sulfhemoglobinemia or in cases in which the overall hemoglobin level was low. Severe cases of both sulfhemoglobinemia (173) and methemoglobinemia (174) have been reported in which the abundance of nonfunctional hemes was the major concern. In contrast, with Hb M, the proportion of normal to abnormal hemes is genetically determined as greater than 75% (because the carriers are heterozygotes and there are two genetically different chains), so that the decrease of oxygen-binding capacity is a problem only when superimposed on underlying anemia.

The clinical effects of nonfunctional hemes need not be limited to their inability to transport oxygen. Small amounts of nonfunctional hemes can have clinical significance beyond that of comparable degrees of anemia if their presence in partially modified tetramers produces a physiologically dysfunctional shift in the oxygenation curve of neighboring unmodified subunits. This explanation is the molecular basis of the left-shifted oxygenation curve, the impaired oxygen delivery to the periphery, and the resulting respiratory distress seen in relatively mild degrees of methemoglobinemia. This phenomenon, called the *Darling-Roughton effect*, occurs because the oxidized subunits in partially oxidized tetramers are held in an R-like (or liganded) conformation, increasing the oxygen affinity of the remaining subunits in those tetramers (175). Although mixed venous blood is unusually saturated, the abnormal spectrum of the methemoglobin outweighs this effect, and the person appears cyanotic. An analogous left shift in the oxygenation curve occurs to a more pronounced degree in carbon monoxide poisoning, and here, too, the impaired oxygen delivery is thought to exacerbate dyspnea.

In the types of Hb M, the presence of the abnormal nonfunctional hemes in the affected tetramers results in a marked flattening of the oxygen affinity curve. The curve is also right-shifted, especially in the most physiologically relevant pO$_2$ range (154,175). This shift leads to normal or even enhanced ability to deliver oxygen to the periphery, which is consistent with the absence of respiratory insufficiency in these syndromes.

The following system has been suggested by Park et al. (167) for evaluating the blood of persons with pseudocyanosis with exposure to drugs or chemicals associated with methemoglobinemia or sulfhemoglobinemia.

- Procedure: if the visible spectrum of the hemolysate reveals a peak in the 610 to 640 nm range, the following sequence of spectra should be obtained:
  - The air-equilibrated sample with and without potassium cyanide
  - The sample with dithionite
  - The sample with carbon monoxide

- Interpretation: if only methemoglobin is present, the abnormal peak will disappear immediately after the addition of dithionite or cyanide. For Hb M, the peak disappears more slowly and can require hours. For sulfhemoglobin, the peak undergoes a very slow decrease as a result of instability.
- Differentiation: to distinguish sulfhemoglobin from Hb M, compare the spectra of the air-equilibrated and CO-equilibrated samples. If CO results in an augmentation and downfield shift of the peak, the sample contains sulfhemoglobin.

UNSTABLE HEMOGLOBIN VARIANTS: CONGENITAL HEINZ BODY HEMOLYTIC SYNDROME

Some hemoglobin mutants have substitutions that alter the solubility of the molecule in the red cell (Table 49-8). The

TABLE 49-8. Unstable Hemoglobins

	Mutation	Name	Molecular Mechanism[a]	Reticulocytes and Additional Abnormalities
α-Chain site				
α6 (A3)	Asp→O	Boyle Heights		HA
α24 (B5)	Tyr→His	Luxembourg	4	Low
α26 (B7)	Ala→Glu	Shenyang		
α27 (B8)	Glu→Lys	Shuangfeng		Medium
α31 (B12)	Arg→Ser	Prato		
α43 (CE1)	Phe→Val	Torino	1	Medium, LA
	Phe→Leu	Hirosaki		
α47 (CE5)	Asp→Gly	Kokura, Umi, Beilinson	2	Medium, HA
	Asp→His	Hasharon, Sealy, L-Ferrara		Low
	Asp→Asn	Arya		Low
	Asp→Ala	Cordele		Low
α50 (CE8)	His→Arg	Aichi		
α53 (E2)	Ala→Asp	J-Rovigo		Low
α59 (E8)	Gly→Val	Tettori		Medium
α62 (E11)	Val→Met	Evans	1	High
α63 (E12)	Ala→Asp	Pontoise		
α80 (F1)	Leu→Arg	Ann Arbor	2	Medium
α86 (F7)	Leu→Arg	Moabit	1	Medium, LA
α87 (F8)	His→Arg	Iwata		Low, Met
α91 (FG3)	Leu→Pro	Port Philip	2	Low
α103 (G10)	His→Arg	Contaldo		Medium
α109 (G16)	Leu→Arg	Suan-Dok	2	
α110 (G17)	Ala→Asp	Petah Tikva		Low
α112 (G19)	His→Asp	Hopkins II	2	Low, HA
α130 (H13)	Ala→Pro	Sun Prairie	2	High, Hypo
α131 (H14)	Ser→Pro	Questembert		
α136 (H19)	Leu→Pro	Bibba	2	Medium
	Leu→Arg	Toyama		
β-Chain mutations				
β6 or 7 (A3)	Glu→O	Leiden	3b	Low
β7 (A4)	Glu→Gly	G-San Jose		
β11 (A8)	Val→Asp	Windsor	1	Low, HA
β14 (A11)	Leu→Arg	Sogn		
	Leu→Pro	Saki	2	Low
β15 (A12)	Trp→Arg	Belfast	2	Low, LA
	Trp→Gly	Radwick	3	Low
β22 (B4)	Glu→Lys	E-Saskatoon	3	
β23 (B5)	Val→Gly	Miyashiro		Low, HA
β24 (B6)	Gly→Arg	Riverdale-Bronx	3	Medium, HA
	Gly→Val	Savannah	3	High, HA
	Gly→Asp	Moscva	3	
β26 (B8)	Glu→Lys	E		
	Glu→Val	Mondor		
β27 (B9)	Ala→Asp	Volga, Drenthe	3a	H
β28 (B10)	Leu→Gln	St. Louis	1	HA
	Leu→Arg	Chesterfield		Thal
	Leu→Pro	Genova, Hyogo	2	HA
β29 (B11)	Gly→Asp	Lufkin		Medium
β30 (B12)	Arg→Ser	Tacoma	2	Low
β31 (B13)	Leu→Pro	Yokohama	2	Medium

(continued)

TABLE 49-8. (continued)

	Mutation	Name	Molecular Mechanism[a]	Reticulocytes and Additional Abnormalities
β32 (B14)	Leu→Pro	Perth, Lincoln	2	High
	Leu→Arg	Kobe	3a	High
	Leu→Val	Castilla Muscat		
β33 (B15) or β34 (B16)	Val→O	Korea		
β35 (C1)	Tyr→Phe	Philly	4	Low, HA
β36 (C2)	Pro→Thr	Linkoping		
β38 (C4)	Thr→Pro	Hazebrouck	2	Medium
β39 (C5)	Gln→Glu	Vassa		Low
β41 (C7)/β42 (CD1)	Phe→O	Bruxelles		
β42 (CD1)	Phe→Ser	Hammersmith		High, LA
	Phe→Leu	Chiba		Medium, LA
	Phe→Val	Louisville, Bucaresti, Sendagi, Warsaw		LA
β43 (CD2)	(Phe-Glu-Ser)→O or (Glu-Ser-Phe)→O	Niteroi		LA
β45 (CD4)	Phe→Ser	Cheverly		Low, LA
β48 (CD7)	Leu→Arg	Okaloosa	3a	Low, LA
β49 (CD8)	Phe→Val	Las Palmas		Low
β54 (D5)	Sen→Pro	Jacksonville	3a, 4	High, HA
β55 (D6)	Met→Lys	Matera		
β56 (D7)	(Gly-Asn-Pro-Lys)→O	Tochigi		
β57 (E1)	Asn→Lys	G-Ferrara	2	
β60 (E4)	Val→Ala	Collingwood		
	Val→Glu	Cagliari		High, Thal
β62 (E6)	Ala→Pro	Duarte	2	Medium, HA
β63 (E7)	His→Pro	Bicetre	2	Medium, Met
	His→Arg	Zurich		
β64 (E8)	Gly→Asp	J-Calabria, J Bari		Low, HA
β66 (E10)	Lys→Glu	I-Toulouse	1	Low, Met
β67 (E11)	Val→Asp	Bristol	1	High, LA
	Val→Ala	Sydney	1	Medium
β68 (E12)	Leu→Pro	Mizuho	2	
β70 (E14)	Ala→Asp	Seattle	1	Low
β71 (E15)	Phe→Ser	Christchurch	3c	Medium
β74 (E18)	Gly→Val	Bushwick		Low
	Gly→Arg	Aalborg	3a	Low
	Gly→Asp	Shepherds Bush	3	Medium, HA
β74–β75	(Gly-Leu)→O	St. Antoine	3b	Medium
β75 (E19)	Leu→Pro	Atlanta	2	
	Leu→Arg	Pasadena		HA
β81 (EF5)	Leu→Arg	Baylor	3a	Low, HA
β83 (EF7)	Gly→Cys	Ta-Li		Polym
β85 (F1)	Phe→Ser	Buenos Aires, Bryn Mawr	1	Medium, HA
β87 (F3)	Thr→O	Tours	2	Medium
β88 (F4)	Leu→Arg	Borås	1	
	Leu→Pro	Santa Ana	2	High
β91 (F7)	Leu→Pro	Sabrine	2	High
	Leu→Arg	Caribbean	1	Low, LA
β91–β95 (F7–FG1)	(Leu-His-Cys-Asp-Lys)→O	Gun Hill	3b	Medium
β92 (F8)	His→Gln	St. Etienne, Istanbul	1	Low, HA
	His→Asp	J-Altgeld Gardens		Low
	His→Pro	Newcastle	2	Medium, HA
	His→Arg	Mozhaisk		Medium
	His→Asn→Asp	Redondo, Ishehara	1	
β97 (FG4)	His→Pro	Nagoya		
β98 (FG5)	Val→Met	Koln, San Francisco, Ube I	1, 4	Medium, HA
	Val→Gly	Nottingham	1, 3c	High, HA
	Val→Ala	Djelfa	1, 3c	
β101 (G3)	Glu→Gln	Rush		Low
β106 (G8)	Leu→Pro	Southampton, Casper	2	High, HA
	Leu→Gln	Tubingen	1, 3a	High, HA
	Leu→Arg	Terre Haute		
β107 (G9)	Gly→Arg	Burke		Medium, LA
β111 (G13)	Val→Phe	Peterborough	3, 4	Low, LA
	Val→Ala	Stanmore		LA
β112 (G14)	Cys→Arg	Indianapolis	3a, 4	High
β113 (G15)	Val→Glu	New York, Kaohsiung		LA
β115 (G17)	Ala→Pro	Madrid	2	High
β117 (G19)	His→Pro	Saitama	2	High
β119 (GH2)	Gly→Asp	Fannin-Lubbock		
	Gly→Val	Bougardirey-Mali		
β124 (H2)	Pro→Arg	Khartoum	4	
β126 (H4)	Val→Glu	Hofu		
	Val→Gly	Dhonburi, Neapolis	2	M, Thal

(continued)

TABLE 49-8. (continued)

	Mutation	Name	Molecular Mechanism[a]	Reticulocytes and Additional Abnormalities
β127 (H5)	Gln→Lys	Brest	4	High
β128 (H6)	Ala→Asp	J-Guantanamo	4	Low
β129 (H7)	Ala→Pro	Crete		
	Ala→Val	LaDesirade		LA
β130 (H8)	Tyr→Asp	Wien	3a	High
β131 (H9)	Gln→Lys	Shelby	2	
	Gln→Pro	Shanghai		
	Gln→Arg	Sarrebourg		
β134 (H12)	Val→Glu	North Shore	3	Low
β135 (H13)	Ala→Pro	Altdorf	2	Medium
	Ala→Glu	Beckman		
β136 (H14)	Gly→Asp	Hope		
β138 (H16)	Ala→Pro	Brockton	2	Medium
β139 (H17)	Asn→Asp	Geelong		
β140 (H18)	Ala→Asp	Himeji		LA
β141 (H19)	Leu→Arg	Olmsted	3	Low
	Leu→O	Coventry	3b	Medium
β142 (H20)	Ala→Pro	Toyoake	2	Low
δ Chain				
δ98 (FG5)	Val→Met	A₂ Wrens		
δ121 (GH4)	Glu→Val	A₂ Manzanares		
Gγ Chain				
γ130 (H8)	Trp→Gly	F-Poole		
AγT Chain				
AγT25 (B7)	Gly→Arg	F-Xin Jiang		
Extension (frameshift)				
144 (β)		Cranston	3	Medium
Lys-Ser-Ile-Thr-150				
Lys-Leu-Ala-Phe-Leu-L				
eu-Ser-Asn-155				
Phe-Tyr-COOH				

HA, high affinity; high, 15% reticulocytes; Hypo, hypochromia; LA, low affinity; low, <5% reticulocytes; medium, 5% to 15% reticulocytes; Met, tendency to methemoglobin formation; Polym, tendency to polymerize; Thal, thalassemia.

[a]1, heme environment; 2, secondary structure; 3, tertiary structure; 3a, change residue in interior; 3b, deletion; 3c, steric hindrance; 4, α₁β₁ contact.

intraerythrocytic precipitated material derived from the unstable abnormal hemoglobin is detectable by a supravital stain as dark globular aggregates called *Heinz bodies*. These intracellular inclusions reduce the life expectancy of the red cell and generate a hemolytic syndrome of varied severity called the *Heinz body hemolytic syndrome*. The word *syndrome* is advisable because this clinical picture is not exclusive to unstable hemoglobins but can also be generated by congenital enzyme deficiencies.

Cathie (173) in 1952 was the first to describe and publish data on a patient with a congenital Heinz body hemolytic anemia. The baby was diagnosed at 10 months of age when it presented with jaundice, splenomegaly, and pigmenturia. Because this syndrome did not respond to splenectomy, the authors concluded that it was not familial spherocytosis. Eighteen years later, it was identified as a case of Hb Bristol, an unstable variant. In the intervening years, a number of unstable hemoglobins were described and an easy diagnostic test was devised: the heat stability test.

Structural Abnormalities Involved in Unstable Hemoglobins

Substitutions in the primary sequence can lead to alterations in the tertiary or quaternary structure and result in a globin polypeptide chain or a hemoglobin tetramer that is relatively unstable and tends to precipitate inside the red cell. The structural alterations leading to this event can be classified as follows.

MUTATIONS THAT WEAKEN OR MODIFY THE HEME–GLOBIN INTERACTIONS

The binding of the heme to the globin is important not only for the oxygen-binding properties of the molecule but also for its stability and solubility. Figure 49-23 depicts several of the mutations involving residues with defined interactions with the heme group. These mutations include the following:

- Substitutions that introduce a charged side chain into the heme pocket where a nonpolar side chain existed previously; examples are Hb Borås, Hb Bristol, Hb Olsted, Hb Himeji, and others
- Deletions involving residues that directly interact with the heme, such as Hb Gun Hill
- The nontyrosine substitutions of the proximal His [F8] such as Hb St. Etienne (also known as *Hb Istanbul*), Hb J-Altgeld Gardens, Hb Mozhaisk, Hb Newcastle, Hb Iwata, and Hb Redondo (also known as *Hb Ishehara*)
- Nontyrosine substitutions of the distal His [E7], such as Hb Zurich and Hb Bicetre

Hb Zurich [β63 (E7) His→Arg] is an interesting mutation that deserves special mention. Caughey's group (174–181) have dissected the molecular pathology associated with this hemoglobin variant. The substitution of an Arg for the distal His in the β-chains makes the space available for ligand binding around the iron much larger, fundamentally changing some of its interactions with ligands.

Although the extra space in the heme pocket has little effect on the oxygen molecule that binds iron at an angle, a significant

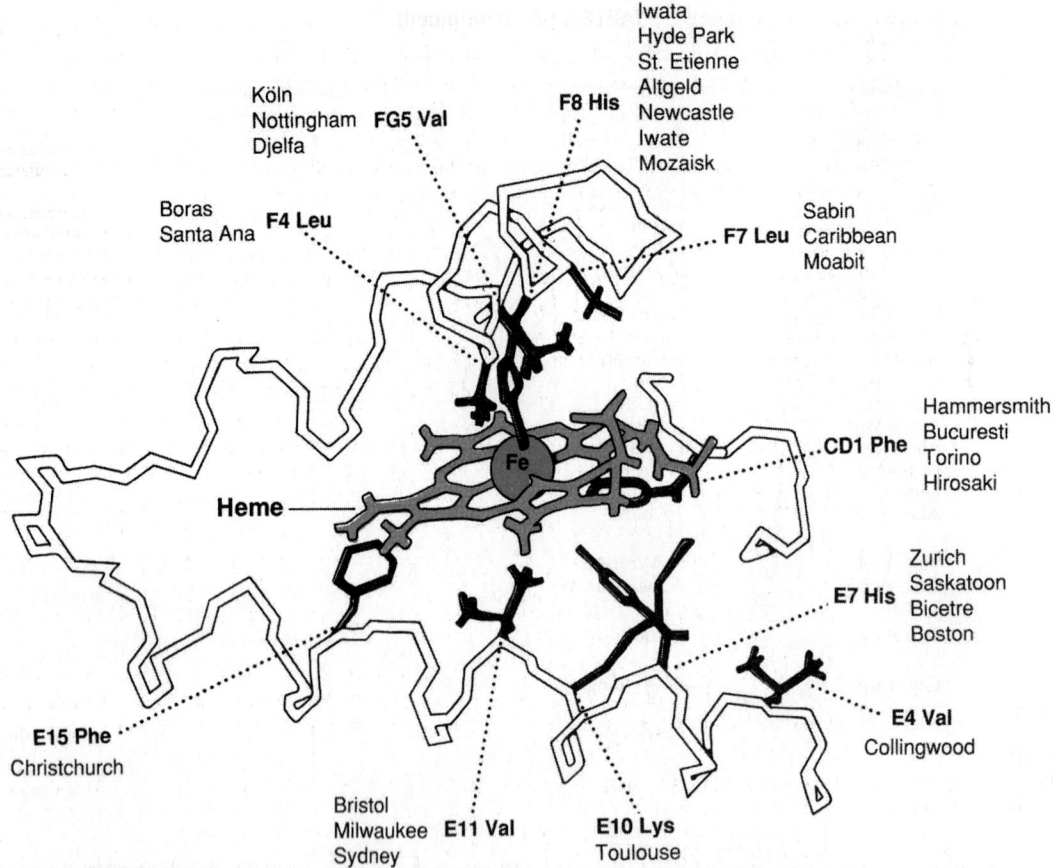

Figure 49-23. Diagram of the heme pocket, showing the replacement site of several of the unstable hemoglobins. Val E4 is at the corner of the pocket, and its side chain does not make contact with the heme but does affect the placement of adjacent amino acid side chains. [From Williamson D, Brennan SO, Muir H, et al. Hemoglobin Collingwood beta 60 (E4) Val replaced by Ala: a new unstable hemoglobin. *Hemoglobin* 1983;7:511, with permission.]

difference for carbon monoxide becomes apparent. The biatomic carbon monoxide binds perpendicular to the heme, and because of steric constraints present in the normal heme pocket, its binding to iron is reduced with respect to oxygen. This reduction of the binding constant is a normal adaptation to the endogenous generation of CO (one CO molecule evolves from each heme catabolized) and protects us from excessive accumulation of carboxy hemoglobin (CO Hb). The toxicity of CO stems from the significant reduction in the dissociation constant compared with oxygen, making CO Hb a particularly stable ligand species.

Carriers of Hb Zurich exhibit an increased affinity for CO due to the increase in the binding constant. This molecular pathology is a protective mechanism of sorts. It does not allow the abnormal β-chain to become ferric, which would increase its instability. Smokers with Hb Zurich have high levels of CO Hb, but nonsmoking carriers also have abnormal CO Hb levels. Because of the partially protective effect of CO Hb Zurich, Heinz bodies are less common among smokers than nonsmokers with this abnormal hemoglobin (175).

Hb Zurich carriers have a special susceptibility to hemolytic crises induced by sulfanilamide. The increased aperture of the heme pocket also explains this phenomenon: Sulfanilamide is now capable of binding to the heme and producing methemoglobin directly. Again, CO is protective.

Substitutions involving the proximal β-chain His [F8] are also interesting. If the substituting residue is Tyr, a Hb M is the result, but if it is another residue, the consequences vary. For example, *Hb Redondo* (176) results from substitution of this residue by Asn

[β92 (F8) His→Asn]. The phenotype includes compensated hemolytic anemia, macrocytosis [mean corpuscular volume (MCV) = 111 fL], and the presence of two abnormal hemoglobin bands on electrophoresis (at pH 8.6). The major band migrates in the position of Hb A_2 (10% of total hemoglobin). The minor component (6%) migrates close to the position of Hb S. Both bands lack heme in their β-globin subunits and hence are semihemoglobins. A phenotypic consequence of this phenomenon is that mean corpuscular hemoglobin, mean corpuscular hemoglobin concentration (MCHC), and total hemoglobin are artifactually low because these parameters are determined by spectrophotometric methods that depend on heme absorption.

The slower electrophoretic band increases during storage, suggesting a posttranslational modification. Adding heme to the hemolysate dramatically decreases the slow-moving band. Amino acid analysis demonstrates that this band has Asp instead of Asn in position β92. Hence, deamidation is the posttranslation event generating the second band. Other hemoglobins in which deamidation takes place in Asn residues that have been introduced by mutation are *Hb Providence* (β82 Lys→Asn) and *Hb Wayne* (frameshift mutation introduces an Asn at position α139). All these mutations comply with the requirements of Robinson (177) that Asn residues that lose their side-chain amide are usually in α-helix/interhelix interface regions, which increases their flexibility and chances of interaction. In addition, they are usually preceded by Thr, Ser, or Cys and followed by a charged residue. Another interesting hemoglobin is the unstable *Hb La Roche sur Yon* (β81 Leu→His). This substitution makes the neighboring Asn at β80 labile because it becomes partially deamidated. His might have to be added to the list of residues that promote deamidation when they precede an Asn residue (assuming the rest of these requirements are met, as in this case).

The two Phe residues at β41 and β42 are conserved in all mammalian globins. Hb Bruxelles, in which β42 is deleted, has high oxygen affinity (discussed in the section Alteration of the Switch Region, Flexible Joint, or C-Terminal in the $\alpha_1\beta_2$ Area of Contact That Favors the T State, Either by Stabilizing This Conformer or by Destabilizing the R State). Hb Bucaresti [β42 (CD1) Phe→Leu] (182) patients have anemia, reticulocytosis, Heinz bodies, splenomegaly, and a heat-unstable hemolysate. Hb Hammersmith [β42 (CD1) Phe→Ser] (183) was discovered in a patient with very similar characteristics. Hb Warsaw/Sendagi [β42 (CD1) Phe→Val] (184) was found in an individual with moderate hemolytic anemia and thermoinstability of the hemolysate. The purified variant had low oxygen affinity and a normal response to 2,3-DPG. Five to six percent of the hemolysate consisted of partially heme-depleted tetramers. A heme-intact fraction of Hb Warsaw had a high oxygen affinity, decreased cooperativity and 2,3-DPG interaction, and a very low Bohr effect. A heme-depleted fraction consisted mainly of dimers. Hb Mequon [β41 (C7) Phe→Tyr] (185) presented with episodic hemolytic anemia, Heinz bodies, and instability of the hemolysate. Hb Denver [β41 (C7) Phe→Ser] (186) was present in an individual with chronic cyanosis, moderate reticulocytosis, and mild anemia. Although this hemoglobin did not separate from Hb A by standard electrophoretic means, it was separated by isoelectric focusing and HPLC. A hemolysate was heat-unstable, and the isolated variant had low oxygen affinity.

Another interesting posttranslational modification is illustrated by Hb Atlanta-Coventry (178). In the first report of this hemoglobin, the propositus had a chronic hemolytic anemia and the products of three β-globin genes: 66% of the hemolysate was normal Hb A, 23% was Hb Atlanta (β75 Leu→Pro), and 11% was the β Atlanta mutation plus a deletion previously identified in Hb Coventry (β141 Leu→O). Elaborate theories were advanced to explain this occurrence, including a β-gene rearrangement generating three β-genes due to a Lepore-type unequal crossover (discussed in the section δ-Gene) involving the β Atlanta gene and the normal neighboring δ-genes. Nevertheless, when the genome was examined, no β-gene rearrangement was found and, even more striking, the β141 deletion was not found in the sequence, because the codon for Leu was intact. The authors rechecked the protein to see if they had missed a posttranslational modification, and they found by mass spectrometry a 129-Da amino acid in the β141 position. The only common amino acid with this weight is Glu, which was impossible, given the charge of the peptide. The likely explanation is the presence in position 141 of hydroxyleucine, which fits the weight and other properties of the peptide. The failure to detect this modification by amino acid analysis is probably related to the formation of lactones.

The story does not end here. The Hb Atlanta (β75 Leu→Pro) mutation affects the heme-linked E helix, decreasing the strength of the heme–globin bond. Hb Sydney (β67 Val→Ala) is another unstable hemoglobin with the same mechanism. Hb Coventry was first described in a patient who was also heterozygous for Hb Sydney. Because the peptide mapping of Hb Coventry and Hb Sydney was performed from the hemolysate, the authors could not exclude the possibility that the two defects were located in the same chain. The possibility that Hb Sydney could be posttranslationally modified at Leu 141 should be contemplated, particularly because Brennan et al. (179) have identified a mutation in the same site as Hb Sydney, β67 Val→Gly, and found that 5% of the chains had the same 129-Da residue in position 141.

The question is, therefore, what is it about β141 and mutations in the E helix that makes this residue susceptible to

hydroxylation? Could Hb Vicksburg, which is expressed at an 8% level and is considered a deletion (β75 Leu→O), be another case of hydroxyleucine?

MUTATIONS THAT INTERFERE WITH THE SECONDARY STRUCTURE OF THE SUBUNITS

As previously mentioned, hemoglobin is over 75% α-helical, and any disruption of this secondary structure reduces the solubility of the subunit. Unstable hemoglobin mutants can result from the introduction of Pro in the helical structure or the substitution of Gly by a mutation in invariant positions in the bands. Twenty-one of the 139 mutations depicted in Table 49-8 correspond to the introduction of a Pro residue.

Hb Brockton [β138 (H16) Ala→Pro] (187) is associated with moderate anemia. It cannot be separated from Hb A by standard electrophoretic procedures. Crystallography showed that the tertiary structure was disrupted in the vicinity of the mutated residue. Molecular instability is probably the result of the breakage of a buried H bond normally tying β138 Ala with β134 Val, a task that the Pro side chain cannot accomplish.

One special case does not constitute an exception. Hb Singapore (α141 Arg→Pro) is an abnormal hemoglobin in which the introduction of a Pro is not accompanied by instability. The reason is simple. The substituted residue is the last amino acid of the α-chain, Arg 141, and no disruption of an α helix takes place.

MUTATIONS THAT INTERFERE WITH THE TERTIARY STRUCTURE OF THE SUBUNITS

Hemoglobin is a globular protein, quite tightly bound, which means that the α-helical regions must be folded into a solid sphere. This design introduces enormous constraints to the architecture. Substitutions of the sequence can occur with no change in solubility as long as (a) no charged residues (hydrophilic) are allowed to point inward, (b) no bulky side chains are allowed to substitute for less bulky residues inside the molecule, and (c) the loss of critical nonpolar residues from the surface of the subunit is avoided. A special case is what Fermi and Perutz called the loss of a nonpolar plug, a reference to hydrophobic residues that are located on the surface and serve to prevent water from invading the interior of the molecule. This loss is a common cause of instability for hemoglobin, and approximately half of the cases correspond to substitution of an Arg for a Leu.

Hb J Biskra is the result of an eight-residue deletion between either α50-57 or α52-59; clearly altering the tertiary structure by amino acid reduction. This is the longest described amino acid deletion of the hemoglobin molecule (188). Although the deletion includes the distal His and neighboring residues, the hemoglobin is only mildly unstable in vitro, hemolysis is absent, and the concentration of this variant is approximately that expected for a variant of the α_1-globin gene. This mutation might appear to defy the rules, but it does not: Hb J Biskra involves the removal of a string of amino acids, and it does not add inappropriate side chains to the interior of the molecule. It gets away with a major deletion because it does not break the rules.

MUTATIONS THAT AFFECT SUBUNIT INTERACTIONS: INTERFERENCE WITH QUATERNARY STRUCTURE

These mutations involve the introduction of charged residues in the interior or the loss of intersubunit contact hydrogen bonds or salt bridges in the $\alpha_1\beta_1$ contact. This contact is critical for stability because it does not dissociate normally, unlike the $\alpha_1\beta_2$ area of contact, which dissociates under conditions found in the red cell, yielding hemoglobin dimers. Because dimerization is a first-order reaction (concentration-independent) and tetramerization is a second-order reaction (concentration-dependent), the proportion of dimers in the concentrated hemoglobin milieu of the red cell is small. Nevertheless, dissociation is possible and is constantly occurring.

In contrast, the breakdown of $\alpha_1\beta_1$ dimers normally occurs to a very small extent but is a great threat to the molecule because it generates methemoglobin and consequent instability. Dissociation of $\alpha_1\beta_1$ dimers generates monomeric α-chains and β-chains that uncoil, loosening their heme–globin interaction and favoring methemoglobin formation. Several unstable hemoglobin mutations involve residues located in the $\alpha_1\beta_1$ area of contact: Hb Philly (189), Hb Peterborough (190), Hb Stanmore (191), Hb J Guantanamo (192), and Hb Khartoum (193).

MUTATIONS THAT INTERFERE WITH HEME BINDING TO GLOBIN

Hb Auckland is a newly described unstable hemoglobin with a mutation of α97 [F8] His$\rightarrow$Asn (194). This substitution involving the proximal His does not lead to methemoglobinemia but to instability, accelerated heme loss, and low oxygen saturation. Usual oxygen saturation was 92%. The clinical picture is a mild compensated hemolytic anemia. The isopropanol stability test (discussed in the section Heat Stability Test) was positive. The abnormal hemoglobin was further studied by electrospray ionization mass spectrometry of the total lysate: 14% of the α-chains had a mass of 15,103.4 Da, which is 23 Da less than normal and is due to the Asn substitution.

HYPERUNSTABLE HEMOGLOBINS

Hyperunstable hemoglobin is a term coined by Ohba (195) to characterize unstable hemoglobins that are either barely detectable or undetectable in hemolysates. These hemoglobins are presumably synthesized normally but are rapidly destroyed in the bone marrow, creating a phenotype closer to thalassemia than to the hemolytic anemia normally associated with unstable hemoglobins.

Hb Hirosaki [α43 (CE1) Phe$\rightarrow$Leu] accounts for 1% of the hemolysate and is clinically silent in some carriers and expressed as a hemolytic anemia in others (196).

Hb Quong Sze [α125 (H8) Leu$\rightarrow$Pro] is undetectable in red cells by electrophoresis, chromatography, or biosynthetic studies (197). It was discovered by sequencing the α_2-gene and confirmed by biosynthesis in a cell-free system.

Hb Toyama [α136 (H19) Leu$\rightarrow$Arg] (198) corresponds to less than 1% of the hemolysate and is detectable only in biosynthetic studies. Although some of the carriers have severe normocytic hemolytic anemias, others are not anemic but have microcytic red cells.

Presumably, the disappearance of these chains in the cytosol is the consequence of proteases that are particularly effective in digesting the mutated chains. The interesting variability in phenotype strongly suggests the phenomenon of epistasis (the effect of other genes besides the one affected—*epistatic genes* or *modifier genes*—in defining the phenotype). It is possible that persons differ in the level or type of proteases expressed in the red cell cytosol. Carriers have microcytosis and hypochromia if they express effective proteases and have hemolytic anemia if they do not.

Clinical Characteristics of the Congenital Heinz Body Hemolytic Anemias

Anemia is the centerpiece of the syndrome, but its intensity varies widely among patients, depending on the hemoglobin variant.

Unstable hemoglobins are uncommon mutational events generally limited to a single pedigree. The exception is *Hb Köln* [β98 (FG5) Val$\rightarrow$Met], which has been detected in several different pedigrees and geographic locations. The time when anemia appears depends on the chain affected. One of the α-chain mutants, *Hb Hasharon* [α47 (CE5) Asp$\rightarrow$His], which is found predominantly among Ashkenazi Jews, produces significant hemolysis in newborns but is milder in adults (199,200). In some carriers, it produces a mild anemia, whereas no hemolysis is observed in other carriers of the same pedigree. Epistatic effects of other nonlinked genes are probably involved here.

Unstable γ-chain variants such as *Hb Poole* have been associated with significant hemolysis in the first semester of life (201). The condition disappears with the emergence of the β-chains as the predominant hemoglobin chain at the end of the first year.

Patients with unstable hemoglobin may have hemolytic crises (abrupt increases in hemolysis over the levels usually found during the steady state) in association with bacterial or viral infections or with exposure to chemical oxidants. The mechanism of the infection-mediated hemolysis is not clear, but pyrexia and transient acidosis contribute to the phenomenon. Both are capable of increasing hemoglobin denaturation. Drugs such as sulfonamides have been directly implicated in the hemolytic crisis of Hb Zurich, as discussed in the section Mutations That Weaken or Modify the Heme–Globin Interactions, as well as Hb Hasharon, Hb Shepherds Bush, Hb Peterborough, and others. The crises are generally self-limited, and stopping all drugs is the prudent course. These patients, like all patients with chronic hemolysis, are susceptible to parvovirus B19–induced aplastic crises.

Patients with unstable hemoglobins can have characteristically dark urine or pigmenturia. The color change is due not to bilirubin but to the presence of dipyrrole methylenes of the mesobilifuscin group (202). The origin of these fluorescent compounds is not clear. Their structure—two pyrrole rings still bound to each other by a methenyl bridge—suggests the malfunctioning of the methenyl oxygenase, the enzyme involved in the breaking of the –CH= bridges. Apparently, fluorescent dipyrroles are also present in Heinz bodies (203).

The absence of pigmenturia does not exclude the diagnosis of unstable hemoglobin because not all unstable mutants exhibit pigmenturia and the severity of hemolysis is unrelated to pigmenturia. For example, Hb Köln (which induces a severe hemolytic anemia) has in common with Hb Zurich (very little hemolysis) significant pigmenturia.

Congenital Heinz body hemolytic anemias secondary to unstable hemoglobins are generally mild and do not require therapy except for supportive and preventive measures, including administration of folic acid to ensure that the overworked marrow does not become deficient in this nutrient, prevention and prompt treatment of infections, avoidance of pyrexia with aspirin, and avoidance of oxidant drugs, including acetaminophen.

The question of splenectomy arises in the more severe hemolytic cases. No doubt the spleen plays an important pathophysiologic role in the destruction of Heinz body–containing red cells. This fact must be balanced with the role of the spleen in the susceptibility to pneumococcal infections early in life and the need to use antipneumococcal vaccines when splenectomy occurs during childhood (discussed in Chapters 21 and 55). According to Koler et al. (204), splenectomy is beneficial, in balance, for the most severe cases of unstable hemoglobinopathies, and partial correction of the anemia has been achieved in some instances. Nevertheless, the patient should be informed that the success of the splenectomy cannot be ensured.

DIAGNOSIS

The elements for the differential diagnosis of unstable hemoglobins are the following:

- Heinz bodies, spontaneously present in the blood (less frequent) or induced by 24-hour incubation of a sterile sample on sterile saline and stained by supravital pigments

- Hemoglobin electrophoresis, only when positive (sometimes a smeared band is observed); negative results are not diagnostically useful
- Positive heat stability test

All these tests are useful and should be pursued because any one of them could be negative. The heat stability test is the least likely to result in a false-negative outcome.

The differential diagnosis of an unstable hemoglobinopathy in the adult is listed with the other causes of congenital Heinz body hemolytic syndrome (G6PD deficiency is discussed in Chapter 55) and acquired forms of Heinz body hemolytic anemias (acquired methemoglobinemia, chemical and drug oxidants, and other conditions). In rare cases, several of these entities interact with each other to the detriment of the patient (205).

Because the spleen removes Heinz bodies efficiently, many patients with unstable hemoglobins lack Heinz bodies before splenectomy, and the differential diagnosis is with autoimmune hemolytic anemias (see Chapter 52) and other disorders with nonspecific red cell morphology, such as glycolytic and other red cell enzyme defects (see Chapters 53 and 54), Wilson disease (see Chapter 51), paroxysmal nocturnal hemoglobinuria (see Chapter 10), hereditary xerocytosis (see Chapter 51), and (very rarely) erythropoietic porphyria (discussed in Chapter 47).

SMEAR AND HEINZ BODY PREPARATION
The blood smear is not specific. It reveals anisocytosis, sometimes hypochromia, and often *prominent basophilic stippling*. The last is frequently the most useful clue to the diagnosis because prominent basophilic stippling is uncommon in other hemolytic anemias, except for the rare pyridine-5'-nucleotidase deficiency (discussed in Chapter 53). Howell-Jolly bodies, normoblasts, and some microspherocytes may also be observed in the peripheral blood.

Heinz body detection requires the use of methyl blue or crystal violet supravital stains. Heinz bodies appear as irregular pale purple inclusions, 2 μm in diameter or less, singly or a few, and frequently have the appearance of being attached to the membrane. In some cases, Heinz bodies are apparent in fresh blood, but in most cases, sterile incubation of the blood for 24 hours in the absence of glucose is required to elicit them. A normal sample should always be run simultaneously as a control. After splenectomy, red cells containing Heinz bodies become much more frequent and easier to detect. Indeed, in some patients, Heinz bodies can be detected only after splenectomy.

ELECTROPHORESIS
Hemoglobin electrophoresis can demonstrate an abnormal component, but many times, the unstable hemoglobin appears as a diffuse band. This alteration is probably secondary to the partial denaturation of hemoglobin molecules during electrophoresis (because of the heat generated) or during the preelectrophoresis manipulations of the hemolysate. Occasionally, only precipitated material at the origin is observed. Many unstable hemoglobins are not detectable by electrophoresis.

HEAT STABILITY TEST
The heat denaturation test, consisting of the incubation of a hemolysate for 1 or 2 hours at 50°C, is a simple and reliable procedure described by Grimes and Meisler (206) and Grimes et al. (207) almost 40 years ago. Normal hemolysates are stable under these conditions, and the presence of an unstable hemoglobin is signaled by the appearance of a visible precipitate. Some abnormal hemoglobins, such as Hb Hasharon, precipitate at higher temperatures than 50°C, but if higher temperatures are used, controls are indispensable, because normal hemoglobin begins to precipitate at approximately 55°C.

Other similar laboratory procedures are available. For example, the isopropanol test of Carrell and Kay (208) is used by many laboratories, but it gives false-positive results when the sample contains over 5% Hb F. Zinc acetate precipitation is free from interference with Hb F (209). The mechanical agitation procedure of Asakura et al. (210) has also been shown useful in the diagnosis of unstable hemoglobins in several cases (211).

Pathophysiology of the Heinz Body Hemolytic Syndrome Produced by Unstable Hemoglobins

THERMOSTABILITY OF HEMOGLOBINS
When heat-unstable hemoglobins were related to the presence of a Heinz body hemolytic anemia by Grimes and Meisler (206) and Grimes et al. (207), the conceptual framework for the understanding of this syndrome was generated. Homeothermic mammals and birds have relatively thermostable hemoglobins. If a hemolysate is incubated for 1 or 2 hours at 50°C, little protein precipitate occurs. This property is observed even among the reptile hemoglobins, although to a lesser degree. Among amphibians and fish, the thermostability of hemoglobin decreases substantially.

At first approximation, these differences may be connected with the environmental mean temperature. Thus, the hemoglobins of heterothermic animals (exposed to low mean temperatures) must have evolved to the hemoglobins of homeothermic animals (exposed to higher mean temperatures) by accumulating mutations in their globin genes (and other genes) that provide thermostable (instead of thermolabile) gene products (212,213).

The molecular basis of thermostability is not clear. Perutz (214) has suggested that thermostability of some proteins, including hemoglobin, can be attributed to electrostatic interactions and salt bridge formations, whereas Bigelow (215) contends that hydrophobic interactions are critical. Others claim that both electrostatic and hydrophobic interactions are contributory (216). Most of this evidence comes from the structural analysis of homologous proteins obtained from thermophilic and mesophilic bacteria (217) or from comparison of amino acid sequences in hemoglobins of organisms that prefer different temperatures (218).

Borgese et al. (213) have studied several fish hemoglobins and found that they can be classified into four categories: those stable at all levels of pH (for example, skate hemoglobins); those stable at acid but unstable at alkaline pH (like the *Mustelus canis*, or dogfish, hemoglobins); those unstable at acid but stable at alkaline pH (such as the toadfish hemoglobins); and those unstable at all levels of pH (most fish hemoglobins). Furthermore, the effect of salt (which interferes with electrostatic interactions) and alkylureas (which interfere with hydrophobic interactions) are revealing: Electrostatic interactions are not consistently related to thermostability, whereas all hemoglobins demonstrate increased thermoinstability in the presence of alkylureas. In this model system, hydrophobic interactions are at the heart of the thermostability properties of hemoglobins.

Other contributions to the thermostability come from the strength of the heme–globin bonds. Bunn and Jandl (219) demonstrated that heme exchange between hemoglobin and albumin and between hemoglobins decreases considerably when the methemoglobin heme is ligated with cyanide. Presumably, cyanomethemoglobin has a stronger heme–globin attachment than methemoglobin and is more similar to liganded hemoglobin. Deoxyhemoglobin has the tighter bond.

AUTOOXIDATION OF HEMOGLOBIN
An old observation is that the generation of methemoglobin decreases the thermostability of hemoglobin. Thus, the pathways

and events accompanying the conversion of Fe^{2+} to Fe^{3+} in hemoglobin are important in understanding unstable hemoglobins.

When a hemoglobin solution is left on the counter at room temperature, it turns into a brown material that is predominantly methemoglobin. This process occurs even more rapidly at 37°C. The chemical basis of autooxidation is probably the generation of superoxide anion (oxygen). This is an infrequent event because most of the time, oxyhemoglobin gives up dimolecular oxygen and converts itself partially into deoxyhemoglobin. The generation of superoxide anion comes from the transfer of a d electron from the heme iron to the unoccupied $\Pi2$ orbital. The loss of this electron converts iron into the low spin ferric state. This reaction is catalyzed by H^+, Cl^-, the superoxide anion itself, and probably the T state of hemoglobin (generated by 2,3-DPG and other polyphosphates, T-stabilizing mutations, and partial deoxygenation). All of these conditions favor autooxidation. Totally deoxygenated hemoglobin, although in the T state, has no oxygen to contribute to the reaction. Hence, it is more stable with respect to autooxidation (220).

The decrease in the autooxidation of hemolysates in the presence of ethylenediaminetetraacetic acid suggests that bivalent cations could play a catalytic role in this process. The best-known effect is that of copper. Long known to bind hemoproteins (221), Cu^{2+} binds specifically to the β-chains (and converts the β-hemes into methemoglobin) with two high-affinity sites (222,223). Later work (224,225) confirmed these findings and determined that Cu^{2+} reacts with Cysβ93. The mechanism by which the bound Cu^{2+} oxidizes the β-hemes is not known.

In contrast, the α-chains are a preferred site for autooxidation (226). Isoelectric focusing is an excellent tool to separate and quantitate the different forms of the autooxidation process.

From the previous discussion, we conclude that the autooxidation of hemoglobin is favored by increased temperature, 2,3-DPG, trace metals, and low pH.

DENATURATION OF HEMOGLOBIN AND HEMICHROME FORMATION

Heinz bodies, one of the hallmarks of the hemolytic syndrome generated by unstable hemoglobins, are the product of hemoglobin denaturation. Initial suggestions were that Heinz bodies are composed by heme-depleted globin chains (227,228). The pioneering work of Rachmilewitz et al. (229–232) allowed the identification of the precipitated material as hemichromes. These are derivatives of the low-spin forms of ferric hemoglobin that have the sixth coordinating position occupied by a ligand provided by the globin: a hydroxyl group (–OH) or unprotonated histidyl (reversible hemichromes) or a protonated histidyl (irreversible hemichrome) (233) (Fig. 49-24).

Another type of irreversible hemichrome can be generated by having the fifth coordinating position of Fe occupied by a Cys and the sixth by an aliphatic amine. All these compounds can be resolved by electron paramagnetic resonance spectroscopy but not by absorption spectroscopy, because their visible spectra are similar. Hemichromes are generated when the heme is dissociated from the heme pocket and rebinds elsewhere in the globin after the α-chains or β-chains have suffered some form of uncoiling or denaturation. Irreversible hemichromes seem to be an indispensable stage in the formation of Heinz bodies. Winterbourne and Carrell (234) have found both α-chains and β-chains in Heinz bodies. In addition, these authors have worked out a general scheme for the process involved in the generation of Heinz bodies (235) (Fig. 49-25).

From the preceding discussion, it is understandable that any weakening of the heme–globin bond will accelerate hemoglobin denaturation.

ANEMIA IN THE UNSTABLE HEMOGLOBINS GENERATING HEINZ BODIES HEMOLYTIC SYNDROME

The primary cause of the anemia resides in the reduced lifespan of the red cells that contain Heinz bodies. Evidence indicates that Heinz bodies, at least in part, adhere to the cytosolic side of the membrane (236,237) by hydrophobic interactions and not through covalent bonds, as previously suggested (238,239).

The anion exchanger (AE-1 or band 3: 103 kdkd) is the most common transmembrane protein in the mature red cell. It spans the membrane with a glycosylated portion on the surface of the red cell, a hydrophobic portion across the lipid bilayer, and a cytosolic domain of approximately 43 kd (discussed in Chapter 52). The most N-terminal portion of the cytosolic domain is highly negatively charged and ends in an acetylated N-terminus. The enzymes phosphofructokinase, glyceraldehyde-3-phosphate dehydrogenase, and aldolase bind to this region of band 3 (discussed in Chapter 51). In addition, this is the portion of the molecule to which hemoglobin and hemichromes bind (240,241).

The negatively charged band 3 sequence threads itself into the positively charged central cavity of hemoglobin, so that it binds deoxyhemoglobin preferentially and in a reversible way; the higher the positive charge, the higher the affinity. This is why Hb A_2 and Hb C (particularly the latter) attach tenaciously to the membrane. Hb S is intermediate in affinity. Hb C also exhibits reversible binding, and Hb S has an irreversible component that may be due to hemichrome binding to band 3. Hemichromes bind at the same site as hemoglobin, but the binding seems to be irreversible and causes band 3 molecules (and associated membrane proteins) to aggregate (240–247).

Unstable hemoglobins generate considerable amounts of hemichromes, and some of these bind to band 3. It is not surpris-

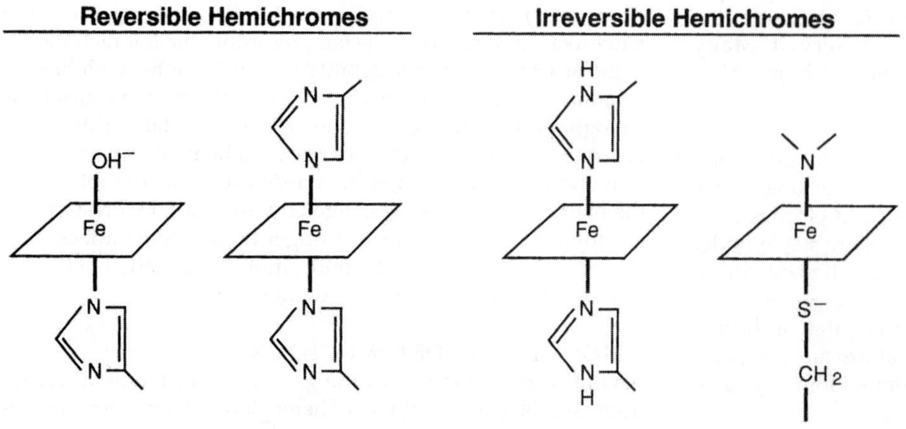

Reversible Hemichromes   **Irreversible Hemichromes**

Figure 49-24. Diagrammatic structure of hemichromes, showing proximal histidine below the plane of the heme and distal histidine above the plane. One or both of the histidines can be substituted. (From Peisach J, Blumberg WE, Rachmilewitz EA. The demonstration of ferrihemochrome intermediates in Heinz body formation after the reduction of oxyhemoglobin A by acetylphenylhydrazine. *Biochem Biophys Acta* 1975;393:404, with permission.)

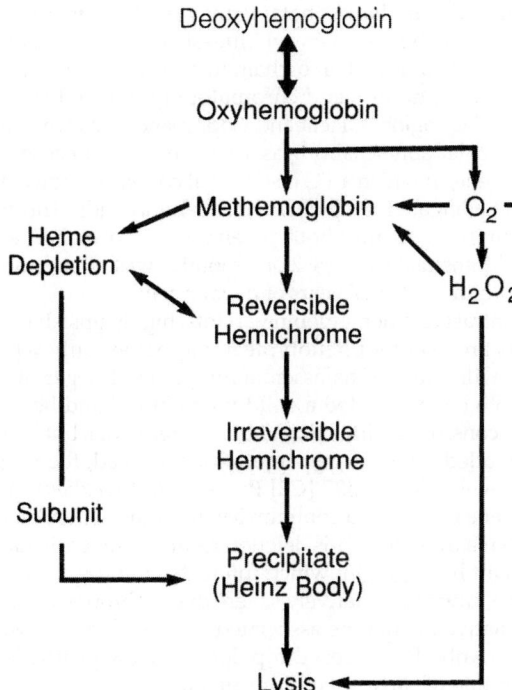

Figure 49-25. Scheme of the intraerythrocyte denaturation of unstable hemoglobins as proposed by Winterbourne and Carrell. (From Winterbourne CC, Carrell DW. Studies of hemoglobin denaturation and Heinz body formation in the unstable hemoglobins. *J Clin Invest* 1974;54:678, with permission.)

ing that these red cells exhibit decreased deformability, a characteristic that will condemn them to be preferentially trapped in the red cell quality control organ, the spleen (248,249). It is possible that Heinz body–containing red cells are pitted initially. The term *pitting* refers to the mechanism by which Heinz bodies and a portion of the overlying plasma membrane are excised from the cell during their passage through the spleen. This manipulation converts red cells progressively into spherocytes through membrane loss, producing a rigid remnant that will be eliminated eventually from the circulation.

Other potential sources of membrane damage come from peroxidation and cross-linking of membrane proteins. These sources are probably secondary to the presence of free heme and iron and to free radicals generated during methemoglobin formation and hemoglobin denaturation (250–252). Other evidence of membrane alteration is the presence of abnormal K^+ efflux in some of these cells (249,253).

Another determinant of the anemia in patients with unstable hemoglobins is the oxygen equilibrium curve. The level of 2,3-DPG is generally normal (254), but some of the unstable variants have a high or low oxygen affinity. For the reasons discussed, the high-affinity unstable hemoglobins tend to have less anemia, and the low-affinity unstable hemoglobins are characterized by more anemia. Nevertheless, there is considerable overlapping of these abnormal properties.

Unstable hemoglobins with abnormal oxygen affinity include the following:

- High oxygen affinity: the β-chain mutant Hb Etobioke and the β-chain mutants (in increasing order of sequence number) St. Louis, Genova, Tacoma Philly, Duarte, Zurich, Bicetre, Shepherds Bush, Baylor, Buenos Aires, Borås, Gun Hill, Istanbul, Mozhaisk, Köln, Nottingham, Southampton, Tubingen, Altdorf, Toyoake, and Cranston

- Low oxygen affinity: the α-chain mutant Torino and the β-chain mutants Leiden, Hazebrouck, Hammersmith, Louisville, Cheverly, Okaloosa, Bristol, Seattle, Christchurch, Caribbean, and Burke

The question of alterations in the synthesis or catabolism of the unstable hemoglobins is also of interest. The extreme case is that in which the hemoglobin is so unstable that none can be detected in the red cell. This is the case for *Hb Quong Sze*, an α-chain mutant that can be identified only by DNA sequencing. Adams et al. (256,257) have demonstrated that *Hb Terre Haute* (β106 Leu→Arg), originally incorrectly identified as Hb Indianapolis (β112 Cys→Arg), is an extremely unstable hemoglobin and is expressed as a dominant thalassemic syndrome (see next section), with an α-globin to β-globin synthesis ratio of 0.4:1 (normal, 1:1). In Hb Quong Sze, the abnormal chain is so unstable that it does not have the opportunity to form dimers or tetramers, and it is destroyed by proteolysis. In Hb Terre Haute, the synthesis of the abnormal hemoglobin is reduced drastically. Other, less dramatic instances are represented by unstable hemoglobins with lower than normal synthesis: *Hb Borås, Hb Abraham Lincoln*, and *Hb Riverdale-Bronx*. An increase in free heme in erythroblasts (which has been found in unstable hemoglobins with weak heme–globin interactions) may inhibit heme synthesis and significantly reduce δ-aminolevulinic synthetase levels (258).

Many unstable hemoglobins have a normal rate of synthesis, sometimes unexpectedly, as in *Hb Gun Hill* (260), which contains a five-residue deletion. With this hemoglobin, Rieder (259) demonstrated that the unstable α-chains can exchange with stable α-chains from the small surplus pool. Hence, paradoxically, very unstable hemoglobins tend to have more abnormal hemoglobin, more Heinz bodies, and more severe hemolysis. In contrast, naturally, patients with unstable chains that are incapable of assembly will have less abnormal hemoglobin, less hemolysis, and fewer Heinz bodies.

Finally, several unstable hemoglobins coexist in the genome with α or β thalassemia: the α-chain mutants *Hb Suan-Dok* and *Hb Petah Tikva* coexist in *cis* with α thalassemia, and the β-chain mutant *Hb Leiden* coexists in *cis* with a β thalassemia mutation.

Hemoglobin Structural Mutations with Abnormal Assembly: Dominant Thalassemia Syndrome

The dominant thalassemia syndrome includes mutations of the coding region of the globin genes that lead to a significant deficit in synthesis and that present clinically as autosomal-dominant thalassemia. This definition does not include structural mutations associated with phenotypes resembling β thalassemia trait. For example, not considered in this group are the δβ fusion genes (Lepore and anti-Lepore hemoglobins) or mutations affecting the translation termination codon (Hb Constant Spring, Hb Icaria, Hb Koya Dora, and Hb Seal Rock). We also exclude α or β structural mutations that are linked in *cis* with α or β thalassemia, respectively. Finally, neither Hb North Shore-Caracas nor Hb K Woolrich, both of which have a thalassemia syndrome of unknown origin, nor the abnormal messenger RNA splicing observed in Hb E, Hb Knossos, and Hb Monroe, nor proteolytically hypersusceptible Hb Mississippi qualify for this group because the clinical presentation of the heterozygotes is mild.

CLINICAL PICTURE AND DIAGNOSIS
The dominant thalassemia syndrome is characterized by significant anemia, often transfusion-dependent, by splenomegaly, and by a blood smear with prominent hypochromia, microcytosis, and basophilic stippling. The reticulocyte count is often high. Inclusion bodies are frequently observed in erythrocyte precursors with

supravital staining, which is why some authors call this syndrome *inclusion body thalassemia*. The bone marrow exhibits considerable erythroid hyperplasia, and evidence of ineffective erythropoiesis can be obtained. Finally, the full-fledged thalassemic syndrome is found in members of different generations in the same pedigree, frequently in one of the parents or progeny of the propositus. Although the syndrome is similar to thalassemia intermedia, an astute clinician can exclude this diagnosis when the intensity of the disease in the parents or descendants is equal to that seen in the propositus. Thalassemia intermedia usually results from homozygosity or double heterozygosity for much milder defects; hence, the parents or progeny have a much milder disease. Nevertheless, lack of parental involvement does not exclude the diagnosis, because the mutation can be *de novo*. A thalassemia picture in a patient with an ethnic origin not associated with β thalassemia should also increase suspicion for this syndrome.

An important point to keep in mind is that electrophoresis might not reveal an abnormal band because the abnormal hemoglobin is synthesized at an extremely low level, catabolized rapidly, or both. Specific examples of dominant thalassemia syndrome follow.

Hb Sowa-Yakushiji (β110 Leu→Pro) (261) was found in a Japanese family (β thalassemia is uncommon in the Japanese). The three affected adults had hemoglobin of 7.6 to 9.0 g/dL, MCV of approximately 60, low MCHC, reticulocytes of 2.4 to 4.1, Hb F of 1.2% to 2.0%, Hb A_2 of 5%, hypochromia, a normal hemoglobin electrophoresis (no abnormal bands), and negative heat denaturation and isopropanol tests. Sequence of the β-genes and Southern blotting demonstrated a nucleotide mutation affecting codon 110 (CTG→CCG) in all three affected members of the pedigree. HPLC was incapable of detecting the synthesis of the abnormal β-chain. The α–chain to β-chain synthesis ratio was 0.7 to 0.8.

Hb Terre Haute (β106 Leu→Arg) (262) was observed in a person of Irish descent. It was originally described as Hb Indianapolis and was incorrectly identified as β112 Cys→Arg. The proband and father had intense anemia [hemoglobin 4.7 to 5.7, MCV 72 to 75, low MCHC, 14% to 15% reticulocytes (some of which could have been inclusion bodies in red cells), hypochromia, nucleated red cells, and basophilic stippling]. Hemoglobin electrophoresis was normal, Hb A_2 was normal, and Hb F was 10% to 12%. Labeled amino acids allowed the detection of the β-chain of Hb Terre Haute by HPLC. The synthesis ratio of β Terre Haute to β normal was 0.8:1 at 1.25 minutes of incubation during the *in vitro* synthesis study, but at 20 minutes it had dropped to 0.46:1. Undoubtedly, Hb Terre Haute was rapidly precipitating with subsequent proteolysis.

Most of the residues involved in the packing contact ($\alpha_1\beta_1$ area of contact) correspond to amino acids coded by exon 3, which starts at G6 (β104 and α99) and includes the β106 residue. The pathophysiologic differences with a β thalassemia trait are the celerity of the precipitation of the abnormal chains and the potential that this process will overwhelm the antifree radical-protecting mechanisms of the red cell and cause oxidative damage.

Hb Manhattan (β109→0) (263) is a frameshift mutation produced by a single nucleotide deletion in codon 109 in a 78-year-old Lithuanian Jew with chronic hemolytic anemia and thalassemic features. Labs revealed a hemoglobin of 8.5, a MCV of 67, marked anisocytosis with hypochromia, marked basophilic stippling, reticulocyte count of 1.2%, and no spontaneous or incubated Heinz bodies. It leads to an abnormal globin (β Manhattan) that is elongated to 156 amino acids. This mutation was discovered in a Lithuanian Jew with life-long hemolytic anemia. Synthetic studies did not reveal the abnormal chain, and the α to β ratio was 0.5:1.

Hb Agnana [β94 (+TG)→extension to 156aa] (264) is another frameshift mutation first observed in a Southern Italian child who had a hemoglobin level of 6.6 g/dL at the age of 3 years, hepato-

splenomegaly, moderate thalassemia type bone manifestations, large inclusion bodies in cresyl blue–stained smears, normal Hb A_2, 10% level Hb F, and an α-chain to non–α-chain synthetic ratio of 5:1. Electrophoresis and chromatography failed to detect an abnormal hemoglobin. Heat and isopropanol tests were negative. The molecular abnormality was ascertained by direct sequencing of the β-gene, in which a TG insertion at codon 94 created a frameshift that elongated the β-chain by 10 amino acids. This was a *de novo* mutation, because both parents were normal. The patient required transfusions every 2 or 3 months, was splenectomized at 14 years, and died at 27 years of hepatic coma.

In contrast to β-hemoglobin variants, highly unstable α-globin variants are usually phenotypically apparent only when they interact with other α thalassemia mutations. Traeger-Synodinos et al. (265) have reported a child with clinical and hematologic features consistent with β thalassemia intermedia, but DNA analysis excluded β-globin gene mutations. Instead, the propositus had a novel deletion β37 [C2] Pro→0 (*Hb Heraklion*) in the α_1-globin gene in *trans* to a common Mediterranean nondeletional α thalassemia mutation. This deletion results in severe instability of the variant hemoglobin, which interacts with the α thalassemia mutation, causing a relatively severe dyserythropoietic anemia—an alternative phenotype associated with the highly unstable α-chain variants. The dyserythropoietic marrow picture is due to the alteration of early red cell precursors.

PATHOPHYSIOLOGY

The molecular basis of the dominant thalassemia syndrome is generally of two types: (a) single-point mutations (substitutions or deletions) affecting particularly, but not exclusively, exon 3; and (b) chain-length abnormalities secondary to either a shorter chain (premature termination) or an elongated chain (frameshift mutation leading to an altered stop codon). These mutations also affect exon 3.

The central question of this syndrome is why the phenotype is significantly more severe than β^0 thalassemia trait, in which a similar deficit in the α-globin to β-globin synthetic ratio exists. The answer lies in the notion that in dominant thalassemia, the abnormal chain is probably synthesized at a close to normal rate but is rapidly destroyed because it cannot assemble into tetramers. This phenomenon creates inclusions and generates large amounts of free radicals (because of conversion of the heme groups to metheme). The reason for the lack of assembly is that all these mutations affect the residues coded in exon 3 and involved in the $\alpha_1\beta_1$ area of contact, the contact that stabilizes the $\alpha_1\beta_1$ dimer. Without this contact, a tetramer cannot be built. The mutations found in dominant thalassemia affect the $\alpha_1\beta_1$ area of contact, either directly, as in most cases, or indirectly, as in *Hb Chesterfield* (β28 Leu→Arg) or *Hb Cagliari* (β60 Val→Glu), in which an internal amino acid is replaced by a bulky, charged amino acid, or *Hb Korea* (β33 or β34 Val→0), in which a deletion completely destroys the tertiary structure.

Oxidative damage to the red cell membrane has not been studied in these syndromes but is probably severe and may even be the primary basis for the hemolysis.

DYSHEMOGLOBINS: SULFHEMOGLOBINEMIA AND METHEMOGLOBINEMIA

Dyshemoglobins are hemoglobins with abnormal ligands that generate disease.

Sulfhemoglobinemia

The discussion that follows is largely based on the work of Constance M. Park in collaboration with the author (166,167).

Sulfhemoglobin, a green-pigmented molecule with a sulfur atom incorporated into the porphyrin, is associated with drug abuse (266–271), with direct occupational exposure to sulfur compounds (272), and with environmental exposure to polluted air (273). Although sulfurated hemoglobin was not separated from unmodified hemoglobin until recently (169), it is known that the modified hemes have a drastically right-shifted oxygenation curve that renders them ineffective for oxygen transport (274). In addition, the fully sulfurated tetramer seems to have no heme–heme interaction (n close to 1) (170). The oxygenation curve shows a right shift in the physiologically relevant pO_2. Full saturation of unaltered hemes in the lungs and enhanced oxygen unloading at the tissues would be expected. Because this right shift would ameliorate any decrease in functional hemoglobin mass, sulfuration of hemes may have little physiologic significance as long as sufficient unmodified hemoglobin remains.

For equivalent amounts of abnormal pigment, the patient with sulfhemoglobinemia would be expected to have a bluer appearance than the patient with methemoglobinemia as a result of spectral differences between the pigments, but the patient with sulfhemoglobinemia would be less symptomatic as a result of the differences in p50—a fortunate difference, because no known treatment is analogous to methemoglobin reduction for reconverting sulfhemoglobin to functional hemoglobin.

An understanding of the molecular basis of the right-shifted oxygenation curve emerges from isoelectric focusing data. In a clinical sample that contains only 12% modified hemes, the distribution of these hemes among partially sulfurated tetramers results in a larger percentage of the abnormal tetramers (169). Between 24% and 48% of the hemoglobin tetramers in a clinical sample are abnormal and may contribute to the shift of the oxygenation curve (170). The actual effect of partially modified molecules on the oxygenation curve depends on their conformation. Because the half-sulfurated, half-liganded tetramers have an isoelectric point between deoxy and oxyhemoglobin and bind 2,3-DPG under conditions when oxyhemoglobin does not, their conformation must be closer to the T state than that of oxyhemoglobin.

Whereas in methemoglobinemia some tetramers have subunits frozen in an oxidized R-like state (Darling-Roughton effect), in sulfhemoglobinemia, some tetramers have subunits frozen in a T-like state because they remain unliganded at physiologic pO_2 (175). In the former, a left-shifted oxygenation curve and impaired oxygen delivery results; in the latter, a right-shifted curve and enhanced oxygen delivery occur. The slightly high 2,3-DPG in the blood of patients with sulfhemoglobinemia probably reflects increased binding to the T-like sulfurated tetramers rather than an actual increase in free 2,3-DPG (169).

Sulfhemoglobin and methemoglobin have been reported as coexisting in a number of patients with drug-induced hemoglobinopathy (173,266–272), and the lists of chemicals and drugs reported to produce these syndromes are overlapping. Acetanilid, usually in the form of Bromo-Seltzer, and phenacetin were the main offenders in 62 cases of sulfhemoglobinemia seen at the Mayo Clinic (267). The aryl hydroxylamine metabolites of these drugs can serve as reducing agents in a cyclic process capable of generating both sulfhemoglobin (272) and methemoglobin (275). The origin of the sulfur atom in the former remains unclear, but H_2S generated by both intestinal flora (276) and GSH (277) have been suggested. It has been noted that laboratory documentation is often inadequate to distinguish between the various hemoglobin entities, and it is likely that sulfhemoglobin is underdiagnosed (279). Although acetanilid was removed from Bromo-Seltzer a number of years ago and the Food and Drug Administration removed phenacetin from the

U.S. market, sulfhemoglobinemia is not likely to vanish. Sulfonamides, dapsone, and sulfur-containing ointments are reported offenders (272,280,281) and are still widely used. Some drugs reported to produce methemoglobin, including acetaminophen, may also be found to produce sulfhemoglobin when more careful analysis is performed.

Furthermore, accidents involving occupational exposure to H_2S are expected to increase (282), and exposure of red cells to H_2S produces sulfhemoglobin within minutes (283). Although sulfhemoglobin is seldom sought in this setting, it has been reported, and interest has increased with more attention to occupational and environmental pollutants. Screening of populations at risk may reveal many more subclinical cases (273,274).

Sulfhemoglobinemia is probably a relatively nontoxic syndrome in persons with Hb A, but it may prove surprisingly toxic in those with Hb S, especially compared with methemoglobinemia, which would be expected to ameliorate sickling (284). The presence of sulfurated subunits shifts the conformation of Hb S tetramers toward the unliganded, polymerizing T form, even in the presence of high pO_2. Microvascular occlusion could be exacerbated by the fact that these tetramers remain in the polymerizing conformation in both the arterial and the venous circulation. We have shown that a solution of Hb S that is half sulfurated gels at atmospheric pO_2 in concentrations found in red cells.

In summary, the features to remember about sulfhemoglobin are the following. It is a green-pigmented protein that can be accurately identified by spectrophotometric and isoelectric focusing methods (Fig. 49-26). At low concentrations, sulfurated tetramers are shifted toward the deoxy or T form, producing a right shift of the oxygen equilibrium curve. For this reason, dyspnea is absent unless the levels of sulfhemoglobin are extraordinarily high. Mild cases that now go undiagnosed may be revealed in screening studies looking for toxic effects of drugs and environmental pollutants. Even small amounts of sulfhemoglobin may exacerbate sickling disorders. Awareness of this entity and a proper diagnostic approach will allow assessment of its true incidence.

Methemoglobinemia

Methemoglobinemia is the consequence of the oxidation of the iron (from ferrous to ferric) in the center of the protoporphyrin IX ring that forms the prosthetic group (heme) of hemoglobin. The term *methemoglobinemia* is a misnomer, as Jaffe (286) has noted, because it is not oxidized hemoglobin circulating in plasma but oxidized hemoglobin inside the red cells. The more precise name, *methemoglobincythemia*, is too cumbersome. Potentially, methemoglobinemia can induce problems because it renders hemoglobin incapable of binding oxygen (an exclusive property of ferrous heme).

The clinical consequences of methemoglobinemia are generally (but not always) benign, but the change in skin color may be dramatic. Methemoglobinemia belongs in the differential diagnosis of cyanosis. It may be the consequence of genetic abnormalities of the mechanisms involved in maintaining the hemoglobin in the ferrous state and may be capable of binding oxygen (hereditary methemoglobinemia), or it may be due to exogenous oxidizing agents that gain access to the interior of red cells (acquired methemoglobinemia).

HEREDITARY METHEMOGLOBINEMIA DUE TO ENZYME MUTATIONS

History and Background. The discovery of methemoglobin takes us back 50 years to a town near Belfast called Banbridge. As Quentin H. Gibson (285) recalls, the event can be traced to the practice of Dr. Deeny. This country doctor had tried Albert Szent-Görgyi's great discovery (ascorbic acid) in a few patients with

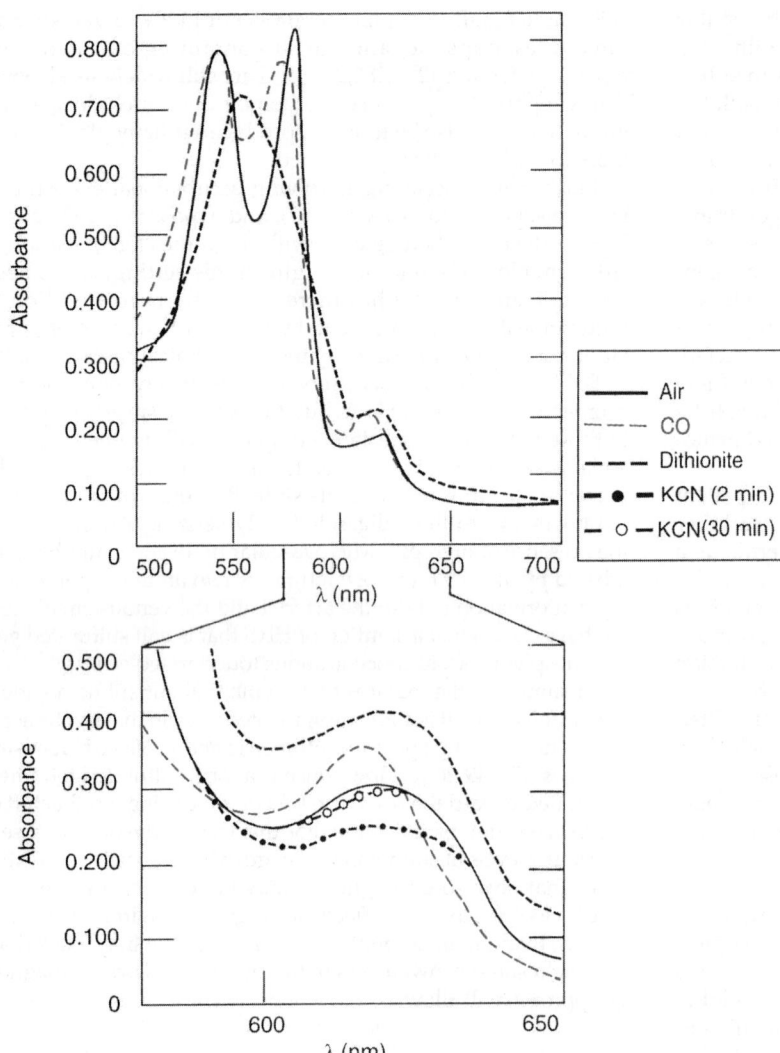

Figure 49-26. Visible spectra of the hemolysate of a patient with sulfhemoglobinemia. **A:** The spectrum of the air-equilibrated sample, the sample after equilibration with carbon monoxide, and the sample treated with the reducing agent dithionite. **B:** The abnormal peak in the air-equilibrated sample at 2 and 30 minutes after the addition of potassium cyanide (KCN). The augmentation and shift of the peak toward lower wavelength with the addition of carbon monoxide provide the basis for the diagnostic procedure for sulfhemoglobinemia. (From Park CM, Nagel RL. Sulfhemoglobin: clinical and molecular aspects. *N Engl J Med* 1984;310:1579, with permission.)

congestive heart failure and was convinced of its efficacy, although his colleagues were reluctant. It is understandable that when, in the streets of Banbridge, he encountered two brothers—Fred and Russell—who were blue (cyanotic in aspect), he jumped at the opportunity to try ascorbic acid again. He treated one brother and used the other as a control. Sure enough, the treated patient saw his cyanosis disappear quickly and dramatically. The untreated brother remained blue. Deeny's skeptical cardiologist colleagues rapidly poked a hole in Deeny's proof: The hearts of Fred and Russell were in excellent and normal condition. One brother was even a member of a field hockey team. Fortunately for all concerned and for hematology, the patients were next studied at the Physiology Laboratory at Belfast, where it was established that their blood contained methemoglobin. The calculated amount of hemoglobin based on gasometry (which depended on the binding of oxygen) was lower than the calculated amount based on colorimetry (which depended on the amount of visible light absorbed by the heme). The diagnosis was clinched by the "observation of the band at 630 nm made with a pocket spectroscope" (285).

Gibson's work in Belfast included using gas manometers to study gas exchange in solutions. Armed with the knowledge that methylene blue speeded methemoglobin reduction (conversion of ferric to ferrous iron in the heme), he obtained Fred's blood, exposed it to the dye, and observed a burst of oxygen uptake, indicating the reduction of methemoglobin. In addition, by observing that glycolysis was normal in Fred and Russell's red cells and that

neither lactate nor glucose, which were known to serve as substrates for the reduction of methemoglobin, were effective in reducing the brothers' methemoglobin, Gibson concluded that the defect had to be in coenzyme factor I (diaphorase I). He tested this hypothesis using an enzymatic assay in which fructose diphosphate was converted to triosephosphate by aldolase. This exercise is an example of how an enlightened analysis of a genetic defect can produce powerful insights, even when the only clinical material available is two affected members of a pedigree.

Although mutations of relevant enzymes were the first methemoglobinemias described, we now know that there are two kinds of hereditary methemoglobinemia: enzyme mutations and abnormal hemoglobins.

Clinical Aspects. The principal symptom of methemoglobinemia is cyanosis, but the critical question is how much methemoglobin is needed to make cyanosis apparent on examination of the skin and mucosa. Jaffe (286) has calculated that the degree of cyanosis produced by 5 g/dL deoxyhemoglobin (in the ferrous state) is equivalent to 1.5 g/dL of methemoglobin (in the ferric state) or 0.5 g/dL of sulfhemoglobin.

According to Jaffe (286), hereditary methemoglobinopathies that are the product of an enzyme deficiency (excluding carriers of Hb M) can be classified into the four following categories.

Type I. Patients affected with this group of methemoglobinopathies are more cyanotic than sick. They have no symptoms

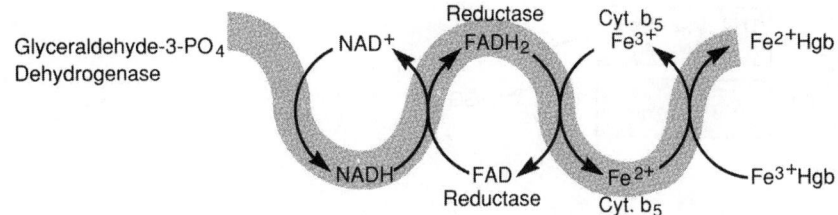

Figure 49-27. The absence of methemoglobin-reducing reaction in hemolysates of human erythrocytes suggests the need for a biochemical carrier between red cell–reduced nicotinamide adenine dinucleotide (NADH) and methemoglobin. Because intact erythrocytes contain cytochrome (Cyt.) b_5 and a flavin-containing cytochrome b_5 reductase that is capable of reducing methemoglobin, the sequence shown has been postulated. Hgb, hemoglobin.

except for some fatigue with strenuous exercise in the worst cases. The patients have a normal survival and normal pregnancies. Levels of methemoglobin vary from between 20% and 40% of the total hemoglobin. Despite the mild course, affected patients can develop toxic levels of methemoglobin on exposure to methemoglobin-inducing drugs or chemicals.

Gibson's original patients belonged in this category. The original article describing type I disease contained the solution: The defect was a diaphorase deficiency. Later, Scott (287) confirmed Gibson's findings by demonstrating decreased activity of the red cell-reduced NADH-dependent methemoglobin reductase system in Eskimos and American Indians with hereditary methemoglobinemia. NADH was formerly called *DNPH* or *coenzyme I*. *Methemoglobin reductase* is the new name for diaphorase I. Passon and Hultquist (288) made the next major contribution by demonstrating that NADH-methemoglobin reductase works in conjunction with cytochrome b_5 to reduce methemoglobin. It is interesting that NADH-methemoglobin (cytochrome b_5) reductase turns out to have a totally different function in red cell progenitors; it serves as a protease and clips the hydrophobic C-terminal portion of microsomal cytochrome b_5 (288).

Methylene blue works in methemoglobin reductase deficiency because it reduces methemoglobin through a different pathway, using an NADH-phosphate (NADPH)–dependent methemoglobin reductase (diaphorase II), as Gibson had already predicted.

Type II. Hereditary methemoglobinemia type II affects approximately 10% to 15% of patients. It is a severe and lethal disease with a strong neurologic component. Although the methemoglobinemia can be treated, the neurologic syndrome is refractory. As Beauvais and Kaplan (289) and Kaplan et al. (290,291) have demonstrated, the disease is secondary to a defective NADH-methemoglobin reductase (cytochrome b_5 reductase) in all tissues. The mutation apparently affects the whole molecule.

The defect is autosomal-recessive because only the homozygote is affected. The elucidation of this genetic disease involved the finding of Leroux et al. (292) that there are two NADH-methemoglobin reductases in the red cell. One is attached to the membrane, and the other is a soluble form that has been modified by proteolysis so that it no longer assembles itself on the membrane. Because both enzymes are deficient in type II methemoglobinemia patients, Leroux et al. (292) concluded that the primary defect affects the original gene in a way that makes both enzyme forms deficient; hence, the symptomatology affects other organs.

Prenatal diagnosis is available for hereditary methemoglobinemia type II, but it is generally useful only after the propositus is ascertained because the disease is recessive.

Type III. Only a few families have been described with type III methemoglobinemia, which is intermediate in severity between types I and II but closer to type I symptomatically

(293,294). The deficiency of NADH-methemoglobin (cytochrome b_5) reductase is expressed in some nonerythroid cells, including leukocytes, lymphocytes, and platelets. The methemoglobin level is approximately 25%. The existence of type III methemoglobinemia forces us to be cautious in the use of leukocyte enzyme analyses in the diagnosis of type II.

Type IV. The patient who generated the type IV category of methemoglobinopathy presented with congenital deficiency of cytochrome b_5 (the cofactor, not the enzyme) with a reduction of 23% of the normal level and methemoglobinemia of 12% to 19% (295). This disorder has no neurologic symptoms and definitely establishes the importance of cytochrome b_5 in the reduction of methemoglobin. The NADH methemoglobin (cytochrome b_5) reductase level is normal in red cells.

Pathophysiology. **Reduction of Methemoglobin.** If normal red cell hemolysates are analyzed for the presence of methemoglobin, less than 0.5% is usually found. Much more is produced, but the red cell has an elaborate mechanism by which the ferric hemes are constantly reduced to the ferrous form (Figs. 49-27 and 49-28). Autooxidation of hemoglobin is discussed in the section Description and Pathophysiologic Features of the M Hemoglobins.

Mechanisms capable of reducing methemoglobin include the cytochrome b_5 reductase system, the NADPH reductase system, ascorbic acid, and reduced GSH.

Cytochrome b_5 Reductase System. This system contains several components.

NICOTINAMIDE ADENINE DINUCLEOTIDE–DEPENDENT ENZYME: CYTOCHROME B_5 REDUCTASE. Cytochrome b_5 reductase was purified by Yubisui and Takeshita (296) in 1980. It exists in two forms in erythroid cells. It is also known as *diaphorase I, NADH-methemoglobin reductase*, and *NADH-dehydrogenase*. It is a soluble enzyme that reduces methemoglobin and has a molecular weight of approximately 31,000 Da without flavin adenine dinucleotide. It contains 275 amino acids, and its N-terminal amino acid is a Phe. The membrane-bound cytochrome b_5 reductase is found in erythroblasts and is probably similar or identical to the liver microsomal enzyme (297). It contains 300 amino acids, including a membrane-binding domain at the N-terminal end. A 14-carbon fatty acid, myristic acid, is attached to the N-terminal Gly and anchors the enzyme to the membrane. The soluble erythrocyte form is derived from the membrane-bound form by proteolysis of the membrane-binding domain during erythroid maturation. The functions of the membrane-bound enzyme in somatic cells are drug metabolism and desaturation and elongation of fatty acids in cholesterol biosynthesis.

The human gene for this enzyme has been cloned (298) (Fig. 49-29) and consists of nine exons and eight introns (30 kb). Some of the exons and introns are short. For example, the first

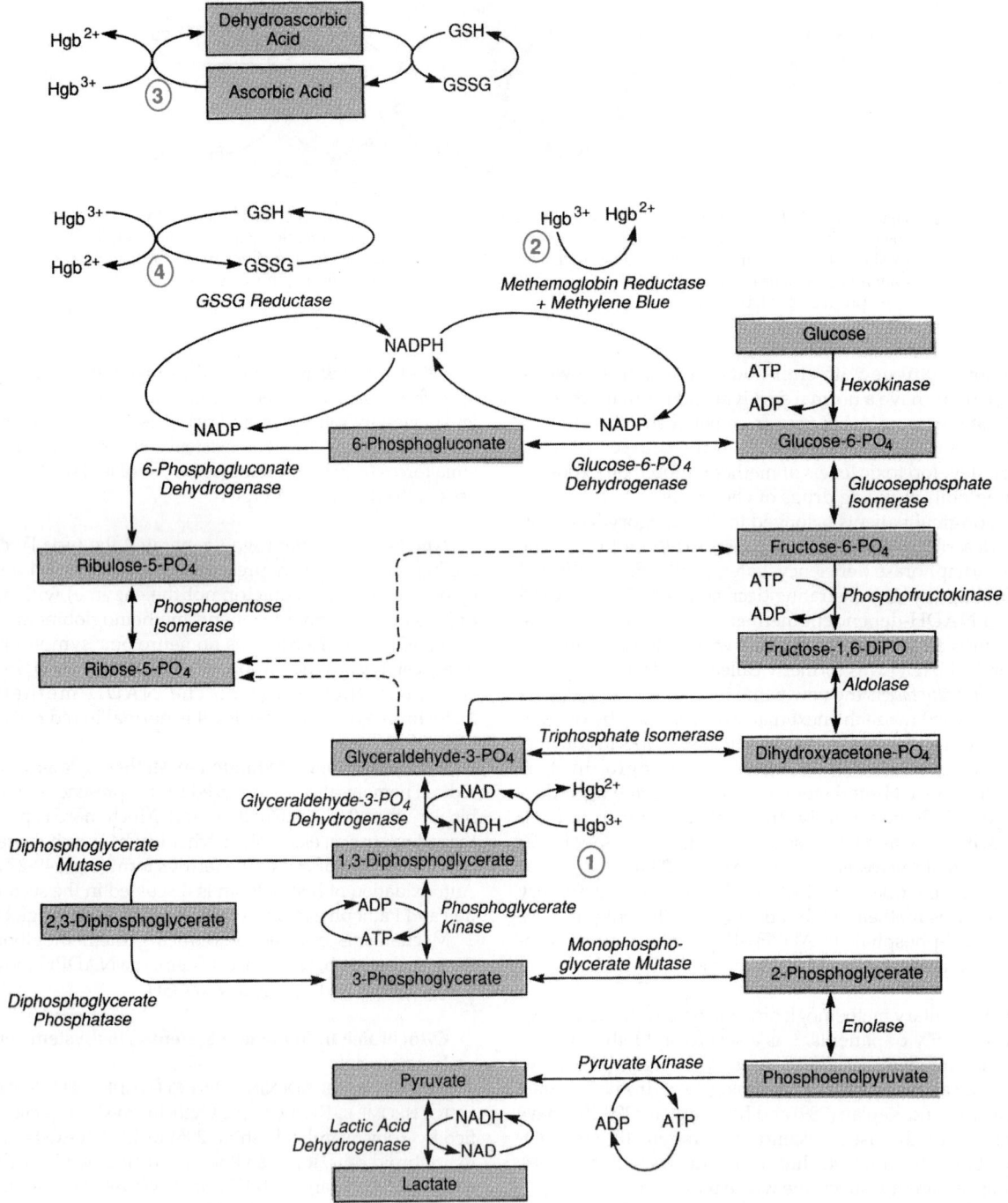

Figure 49-28. Pathway for the reduction of methemoglobin. ADP, adenosine diphosphate; ATP, adenosine triphosphate; GSH, glutathione; GSSG, oxidized glutathione; Hgb, hemoglobin; NAD, nicotinamide adenine dinucleotide; NADH, red cell–reduced nicotinamide adenine dinucleotide; NADPH, red cell–reduced nicotinamide adenine dinucleotide phosphate.

exon encodes only seven amino acids. The first encoded amino acid is Met. As Met is removed, the underlying Gly is spontaneously modified by myristic acid. The cleavage site of the membrane-binding domain lies in the center of the second exon, making it unlikely that the soluble form is generated by alternative splicing. The promoter is of the housekeeping gene type, with no TATA box or CAAT box but several GC boxes.

Some of the mutations that generate NADP-dependent cytochrome b_5 reductase deficiency have been elucidated (Fig. 49-30). Type I hereditary methemoglobinemia can be the result of a point mutation involving a G→A change in codon 57 of the cytochrome b_5 reductase gene (b_5R-*Toyoake*). This codon corresponds to residue 32 in the protein. It is normally an Arg and is substituted by a Gln in the mutated protein (299). This residue is constant in all enzymes sequenced. The mutation is probably located between an α helix and a β-pleated sheet and might disrupt the conformation of the enzyme (296,297,300,301).

Type II hereditary methemoglobinemia is also the result of a single-base mutation in position 102 (b_5R-*Hiroshima*) in which a Ser is replaced by a Pro. The substitution is in a region likely to be α-helical. The introduction of a Pro in an α helix tends to disrupt the secondary structure and has high probability of inducing signifi-

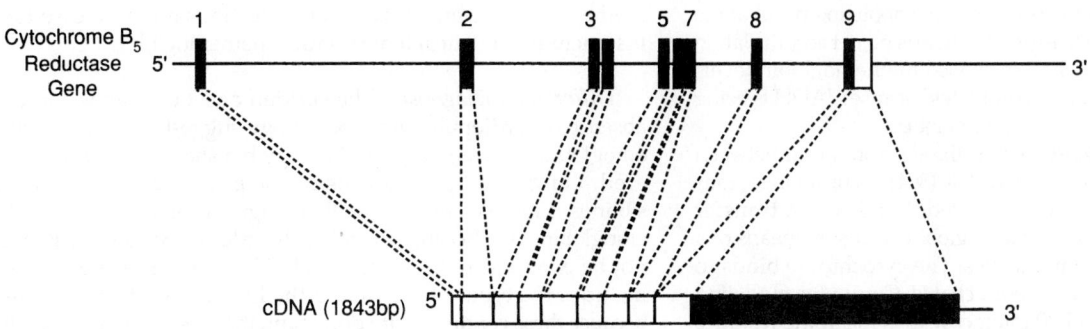

Figure 49-29. Organization of the cytochrome b_5 reductase gene and complementary DNA (cDNA).

cant conformational changes. The mutation is located in exon 5. A mutation associated with type III hereditary methemoglobinemia is located 21 amino acids downstream at position 123: Leu→Pro (b_5R-$Kurobe$) (302). Again, the introduction of the Pro should be disruptive. Why type II is so severe and generalized and why type III is generalized but not severe remain to be elucidated. These mutations, unlike type II, are likely to disrupt the function of the membrane form of the enzyme, particularly its participation in the metabolism of lipids. Fatty acid composition might be altered in patients with type II hereditary methemoglobinemia (303). Of

course, all persons of the same type are unlikely to have the same mutation; it is more likely within one ethnic group but less likely as patients from other ethnic backgrounds are examined.

NICOTINAMIDE ADENINE DINUCLEOTIDE. Nicotinamide adenine dinucleotide is an indispensable cofactor for cytochrome b_5 reductase. It is generated (reaction 1 in Fig. 49-27) by glyceraldehyde-3-phosphate dehydrogenase, which reduces NAD to NADH in the process of converting glyceraldehyde-3-phosphate to 1,3-diphosphoglycerate in the glycolytic pathway. Lactic acid dehydrogenase, another enzyme of the glycolytic pathway, converts

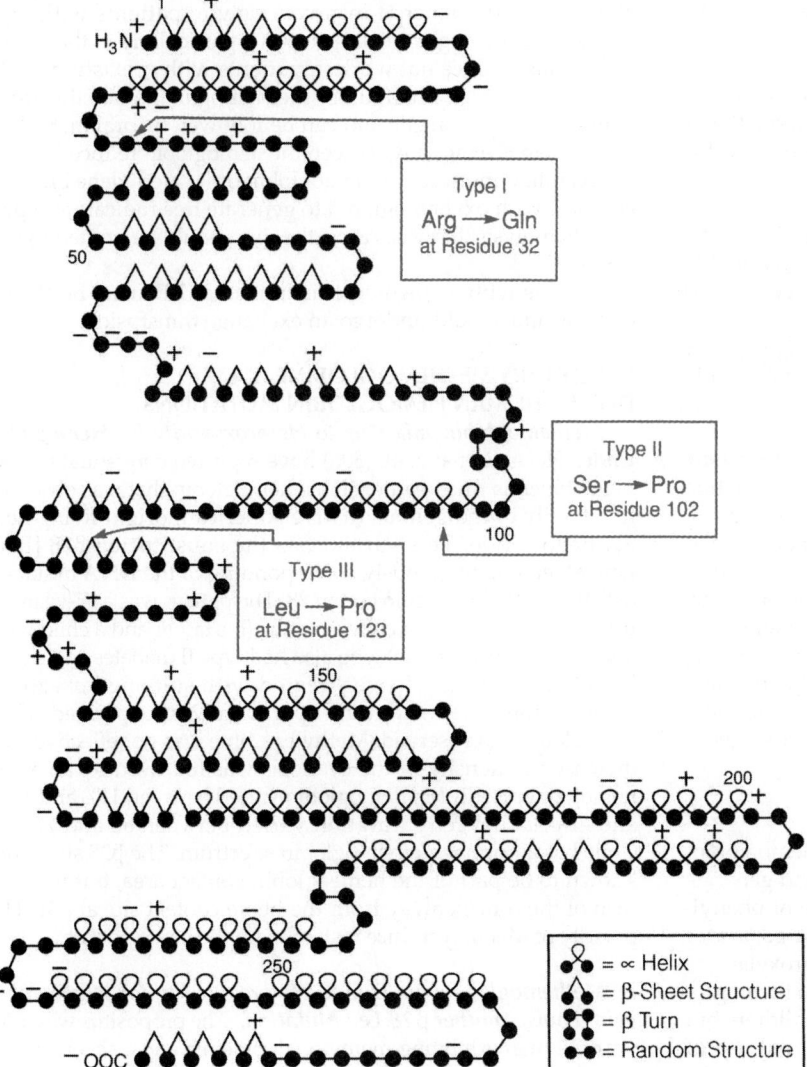

Figure 49-30. Location of a few of the amino acid substitutions found in cytochrome b_5 reductase (b5R) of homozygotes for hereditary methemoglobinemia types I to III. The secondary structure of the soluble type (erythrocyte type) of b5R is shown. Residue 1 of the soluble type of b5R corresponds to residue 26 of the membrane-bound type. Each substitution is indicated by an arrow. Plus signs indicate positively charged residues, and minus signs indicate negatively charged residues. The variant with Arg-Gln at residue 32 is named *b5R Toyoake*, that with Ser-Pro at residue 1023 is *b5R Hiroshima*, and the variant with Leu-Pro at residue 123 is *b5R Kurobe*. (From Kobayashi Y, Fukumaki Y, Yubisui T, et al. Ser-Pro replacement at residue 127 of NADH-cytochrome b5 reductase causes hereditary methemoglobinemia, generalized type. *Blood* 1990;75:1408, with permission.)

NADH back into NAD in the process of metabolizing pyruvate to lactic acid. Hence, during steady state, there is no net accumulation of NADH. Nevertheless, when increased methemoglobin levels need to be reduced, pyruvate accumulates because NADH is being consumed in the reduction of methemoglobin.

CYTOCHROME B_5. Cytochrome b_5 is the electron carrier between NADH and methemoglobin. Gacon et al. (304), using an ingenious isoelectric focusing technique, showed that electron transfer between cytochrome b_5 and methemoglobin occurs by means of a complex between the two molecules. The cytochrome binds to four Lys in the heme pocket in both chains. Computer modeling predicts that Lys 56, 60, and 90 interact with cytochrome residues 43 (Glu), 44 (Glu), and 60 (Asp). In addition, an H bond between Lys61 of the cytochrome acts as a bridge between the two heme propionic side chains of both heme proteins, serving as the micropath for electron transfer. An almost identical interaction occurs in the β-chains (305).

The whole cytochrome b_5 reductase system and the reactions in which this enzyme and its cofactors are involved are depicted in Figure 49-27.

Nicotinamide Adenine Dinucleotide Phosphate Reductase System.
The NADH system reaction (reaction 2 in Fig. 49-28) is probably nonphysiologic because patients with glucose-6-phosphate dehydrogenase (G6PD) deficiency do not have methemoglobinemia. Nevertheless, in the presence of nonphysiologic electron carriers such as methylene blue, this system becomes active. It is the basis for use of methylene blue in the treatment of hereditary methemoglobinemia.

Ascorbic Acid. Ascorbic acid can reduce methemoglobin at a low rate in red cells (reaction 3 in Fig. 49-28). The reduction is combined with oxidation of ascorbic acid to dehydroascorbic acid, which occurs without the help of an enzyme.

Reduced Glutathione System. Glutathione can reduce methemoglobin directly, without enzyme assistance (reaction 4 in Fig. 49-28). The resulting oxidized GSH (GSSG) is recycled by GSH reductase.

These four metabolic systems generate a reducing capacity 250 times greater than that required to reduce physiologically generated red cell methemoglobin (286).

Protective Mechanisms to Avoid Methemoglobin Formation.
Several metabolic processes protect hemoglobin from oxidation to methemoglobin. For example, superoxide dismutase mops up the toxic superoxide ion, generating hydrogen peroxide. H_2O_2 is also toxic but can be removed by GSH peroxidase and, less effectively, by the low-affinity enzyme catalase, which intervenes only when peroxides reach an excess. This situation explains why patients with acatalasemia do not have any methemoglobinemia, whereas patients with an inherited deficiency of GSH peroxidase have low levels of methemoglobin. GSH peroxidase is deficient in the red cells of newborns, which might explain their susceptibility to acquired methemoglobinemia (286).

ACQUIRED METHEMOGLOBINEMIA
Several chemical agents and drugs can induce methemoglobinemia. Dyes and anilines reduce molecular oxygen and generate methemoglobin, sometimes in cycles, as in the case of phenylhydroxylamine. After reducing oxyhemoglobin, it generates nitrobenzene, which is reduced again to phenylhydroxylamine by red cell enzymes and in turn generates more methemoglobin. Nitrites are common offenders, particularly in children, but the mechanism is less well understood. Recreational use of amyl, butyl, or isobutyl nitrites is another cause of acquired methemoglobinemia. In addition, infections might release toxins (including nitrites) that produce methemoglobin.

Differential Diagnosis. The sudden onset of cyanosis in the absence of cardiopulmonary pathology suggests acquired methemoglobinemia, although sulfhemoglobin should also be considered. Long-standing cyanosis or the presence of cyanosis in siblings is more compatible with a diagnosis of hereditary methemoglobinemia. Because the latter disorder is recessive, it should not be expected in the parents. The differential diagnosis also includes the types of Hb M and the low-affinity hemoglobins; because these conditions are dominant, the presence of cyanosis in a parent is diagnostically useful (details of the laboratory differential diagnosis are covered in previous sections). Enzymatic assays or spot tests are available for the methemoglobin reductases, and genetic ascertainment is available for the known mutations. Prenatal diagnosis is available for type II hereditary methemoglobinemia. The efficacy of methylene blue is also diagnostic.

An unusually high incidence of hereditary methemoglobinemia is found among Alaskan Eskimos and Northwest Indians, Navajo Indians, and natives of Yakutsk, Siberia, all of whom may be ethnically connected. The disease has also been observed among Puerto Ricans and in Mediterranean populations.

TREATMENT OF METHEMOGLOBINEMIA
Acquired methemoglobin is treated first by stopping the offending agent, if it can be identified. Methylene blue, 1 or 2 mg/kg, should be administered intravenously in patients with high levels of methemoglobin (40% to 60%), particularly in those with symptoms. It does not work in patients with coexisting G6PD deficiency. In type I hereditary methemoglobinemia, this intervention is only cosmetic and can be followed by oral methylene blue, 100 to 300 mg/day, to keep the hemoglobin reduced.

In aniline-induced methemoglobinemia, methylene blue can combine with oxyhemoglobin to generate free radicals and produce hemolysis. In these cases, the dye should be limited to two doses.

Patients with methemoglobinemia over 70% may be at serious risk and should undergo an exchange transfusion.

HEREDITARY METHEMOGLOBINEMIA DUE TO HUMAN HEMOGLOBIN MUTATIONS
Methemoglobinemia Due to Heterozygosity for Hemoglobin Chile. Hojas-Bernal et al. (306) have reported congenital methemoglobinemia due to an unstable hemoglobin that was observed in a family of indigenous (native American) origin living near Santiago, Chile. This variant has the substitution β28 [B10] Leu→Met, unambiguously corresponding to the DNA mutation of CTG→ATG in β-globin codon 28. The patient was a 57-year-old man known to be chronically cyanotic (his father and a child were also chronically cyanotic) who also had type II diabetes and a pyeloureteral stenosis. He was treated with sulfamethoxazole 2 weeks before surgery, but the operation was suspended when dark blood was observed. Methylene blue was not effective. The increase in intensity of the cyanosis was followed by an acute hemolytic episode. Methemoglobin varied between 11% and 18%, and arterial oxygen saturation varied between 88 and 79. Hb Chile has a normal methemoglobin spectrum. The β28 site is not known to be part of the heme–globin contact area, but it is one turn of the α helix away from the heme contact site at β31. The polarity of Met may induce instability in the heme pocket.

Methemoglobinemia Due to Heterozygosity for Hemoglobin Saint Louis, Another β28 Leu Mutation. The propositus was a 20-year-old man exhibiting methemoglobinemia and a severe Heinz body hemolytic anemia due to Hb St. Louis (β28 [B10] Leu→Gln).

This unstable hemoglobin represented 30% of the total and was isolated by starch block electrophoresis at pH 8.6. Electrophoretic and spectral studies showed Hb St. Louis to be a valency hybrid, $\alpha_2\beta^+_2$. The presence of hemichrome in this hemoglobin was detected by electron paramagnetic resonance spectroscopy. Purified Hb St. Louis had a high oxygen affinity and a markedly reduced cooperativity. The Bohr effect was normal, but the interaction of the hemoglobin with 2,3-DPG was decreased. The oxidation rate of Hb St. Louis was normal. The ferric form was completely reduced by dithionite and ferrous citrate, and the functional properties of the reduced form were normal. In contrast, Hb St. Louis was only partially reduced by methemoglobin reductase.

Thillet et al. (307) have proposed that the mechanism of the oxidation of Hb St. Louis involves a stable bond between β28 Gln and the distal His, β63, with intercalation of a water molecule of the form: Glnβ28–HOH–Hisβ-His63. This bond would disrupt the normal stereochemistry of Hisβ63 and the heme iron, accelerating the oxidation of Fe^{2+} to Fe^{3+}, without major disruption of the B helix. A similar mechanism could be involved in Hb Chile: Metβ28–HOH–Hisβ-His63. Diaphorase could fail to reduce the ferric iron because of steric hindrance induced by the anomalous bond, a severely shifted equilibrium toward Fe^{3+}, or both.

OTHER NORMAL HEMOGLOBINS AND THEIR MUTATIONS

Hemoglobin F

In 1966, Korber (308) discovered that the red cells of newborns are resistant to alkaline denaturation, which was the first suggestion that these cells contain a hemoglobin different from normal adult hemoglobin. Another easily measurable property is found in the ultraviolet spectrum of Hb F ($\alpha_2\gamma_2$), which contains a *tryptophan notch* at 252 nm as the result of an extra Trp at position 130, compared with the β-chains (309).

The γ-chains are different from the β-chains in 39 to 40 positions in the sequence (310). γ-Chains are the product of two genes placed in tandem between the ε-genes and pseudo–β-genes in the β-like globin cluster on chromosome 11. The only difference between the two gene products is the presence of Gly in position γ136 in the ^{G}γ-gene, the left gene, and Ala in the same position in the ^{A}γ-gene, to the right. A common polymorphism occurs in the ^{A}γ-gene in which Thr γ^{A}γ^T) replaces Ile γ^{A}γ^I) (311). The striking similarities in the protein sequence are reflected at the nucleotide level, where the homology between the two genes is high. Slightom et al. (312) were the first to point out that this homology is a consequence of gene conversion, a mutational event in which the sequences upstream replace sequences downstream, particularly in tandem genes, homogenizing them in the process.

That this process is ongoing in this portion of the genome was demonstrated by Bouhassira et al. (313) in the Bantu haplotype linked to the β^S-gene. They found a subgroup of this haplotype that had undergone an even more recent gene conversion, eliminating several of the few differences in sequence between the two γ-genes. One interpretation of this phenomenon is that considerable selective value is placed on the sequence of γ-chains and on the structure of Hb F. This possibility is not surprising, because Hb F is present throughout most of fetal life (although mostly during the last three trimesters), and abnormalities could easily be fatal.

There are functionally important differences between γ-chains and β-chains.

SEQUENCE DIFFERENCES

The 39 differences occur mostly on the surface of the molecule, exactly 22 of them. Four critical substitutions occur in the $\alpha_1\beta_1$

area of contact (the packing contact). This is the strong contact that dissociates only under extreme conditions (very high butyl urea concentration, iodine salts, extreme pH). Nevertheless, two of these substitutions (Thr112 and Try130) in the $\alpha_1\gamma_1$ contact could be involved in providing the molecule (Hb F) with its alkaline resistance as well as its decreased dissociation to monomers. In the β-chains, position β112 is a Cys, and β130 is a Tyr. Both of these residues ionize at alkaline pH, which could promote dissociation of the dimer into monomers. Thr and Trp are polar but not ionizable. No sequence changes affect the $\alpha_1\beta_2$ area of contact (sliding contact), which is the center of ligand-dependent conformational changes. Other critical sequence differences are discussed with the anomalous functional properties.

PROTEIN CONFORMATION

Crystallographic studies of Hb F at 2.5 Å resolution show almost entire isomorphism between Hb A and Hb F (314). The only difference occurs in the N-terminal portion. This change increases the distance of 2,3-DPG inserted in the central cavity to Hisγ2, which may contribute to the reduction in the effect of 2,3-DPG on Hb F.

LIGAND BINDING

Red cells of newborns (containing mostly Hb F) have a higher oxygen affinity than adult red cells (p50 = 29 mm Hg compared with 26 mm Hg in adults), but the oxygen affinities of neonatal and adult red cell hemolysates are indistinguishable (315). This finding suggests that the Hb F and Hb A molecules have identical oxygen-binding properties, but the red cells contain effectors that interact abnormally with Hb F.

2,3-DPG has decreased binding to Hb F (316). The primary structural basis of this effect is the replacement of Hisβ143 (phosphate-binding site in the central cavity) with a Ser residue at γ143, abolishing an important binding site. Secondary effects come from displacement of the N-terminal portion of the γ-chains, which inhibits the binding of phosphates with Hisγ2. Finally, Hb F molecules that are acetylated at the γ-chain N-terminal are incapable of binding 2,3-DPG (317).

The effect of Cl⁻ is also impaired (318). This anion binds in the 2,3-DPG site in the central cavity. At low NaCl concentrations (up to 0.05 mol/L), Hb F has a lower affinity for oxygen than does Hb A. At higher Cl⁻ concentrations, the differences disappear. This effect is not well understood but might have to do with the diminution of positive charges in the central cavity; therefore, the binding affinity for anions and the destabilizing effect on the T state are reduced. The increased stability of the T state induced by the absence of anion-neutralizing positive charges would favor low ligand affinity.

The binding of CO_2 to Hb F is drastically decreased (319). Fewer carbamates are formed at the N-terminus over a wide range of partial pressure of carbon dioxide. The γ-chain N-terminal amino acid has a pKa of 8.1, which is considerably higher than the pKa of β-chains (pKa 6.6). Under physiologic conditions, 90% of the γ sites are protonated and unable to bind CO_2.

Cerebral fractional oxygen extraction (FOE) represents the balance between cerebral oxygen delivery and consumption and has been studied in preterm infants during hypotension, during moderate anemia, and with changes in CO_2 (320). There was a significant negative correlation between cerebral FOE and pace within individuals, but there was no correlation between individuals. Cerebral FOE was not significantly altered in neonates with either mild anemia or hypotension. Cerebral FOE decreased after blood transfusion and increased with decreasing partial arterial pressure of CO_2. These properties of Hb F–containing cells need further investigation.

The alkaline Bohr effect (relation between high pH and ligand affinity) is increased by 20% in Hb F–containing red cells

(321). This seems to be a Cl⁻ effect, because in isolated Hb F at low anion concentrations, Hb A and F have an identical Bohr effect, and the Bohr effect of Hb F increases *pari passu* with the Cl⁻ concentration. A plausible explanation is that the binding of Cl⁻ at low pH to β143 His stabilizes the R state. The absence of this Cl⁻ site in γ-chains would lower the low pH Bohr effect because it is a situation that favors the T state. As a consequence, the alkaline Bohr effect is favored in Hb F.

PHYSIOLOGY OF HEMOGLOBIN F–CONTAINING RED CELLS

The central question is how the modified properties of Hb F benefit the fetus and the newborn. Perhaps the main feature of fetal circulation, in terms of its differences with postnatal life, is that the oxygen loading occurs under more difficult circumstances in the fetus (liquid–liquid interface) than in the neonate (gas–liquid interface). On the plus side, the tissues of the fetus have a high metabolic rate. Therefore, the limitation may be on loading sufficient oxygen rather than on delivery of oxygen, because a significant difference between the pO_2 of blood and that of tissue is likely to exist in the fetus.

This analysis explains why the oxygen affinity of Hb F–containing red cells is increased, a situation that favors uptake of oxygen in the placenta. It also explains why modulation of delivery of oxygen is less needed, because modulation generally consists in the decrease of the affinity of Hb A for oxygen. Therefore, no 2,3-DPG response is found in Hb F. Moreover, the analysis explains why the Bohr effect is increased, because fetal blood increases its pH when it passes through the intravillous spaces because of release of CO_2. The Bohr effect accounts for 40% of the normal fetal gas exchange (321). In addition, by having an increased Bohr effect, the fetus can modulate delivery of oxygen to tissues if it is really needed, even in the absence of 2,3-DPG. Approximately 50% of the delivery to tissues is accounted for by the increased Bohr effect. Finally, the increased Bohr effect could also explain the paradox observed by Charache et al. (106) in which mothers with high-affinity hemoglobin variants did not have pregnancy complications or fetal morbidity. The advantage of Hb F is not limited to the p50 difference with Hb A; if the affinity difference is erased, as in the patients of Charache et al. (106), the enhanced Bohr effect can make up at least some of the difference.

GENETIC HETEROGENEITY

As noted earlier, γ-chains are synthesized by two sequence-identifiable genes. This genetic heterogeneity is unique among globins. Additional heterogeneity comes from the fact that approximately 10% to 15% of newborns have a posttranslation modification of the N-terminal Gly of the γ-chains. Acetylation is common in proteins that have N-terminal Ala, Ser, and, to a lesser extent, Gly residues. Hemoglobin needs to have its N-terminus free for functional reasons; therefore, it is not surprising that acetylation has been excluded largely by selection. In the case of Hb F, it contributes to the decrease in 2,3-DPG binding, apparently a welcome feature. Acetylation occurs after synthesis, probably early in the process, and involves catalytic transfer of the acetyl moiety from acetyl-CoA to the protein by acetyltransferase. *Hb Raleigh*, which involves the replacement of Valβ1 by an acetylatable Ala, is 100% acetylated. Cat hemoglobin, in which the β1 residue is Ser, is also 100% acetylated (and does not bind 2,3-DPG well).

GENDER-RELATED AND *TRANS*-ACTING MODULATION OF HEMOGLOBIN F LEVELS

Miyoshi et al. (322) found that in normal, healthy Japanese adults, the ranges of Hb F (0.17% to 2.28%) and Hb F–containing erythrocytes or *F cells* (0.3% to 16.0%) were affected by gender. Family studies with high Hb F levels and F cells suggested a dominant X-linked pattern of inheritance. In another study in patients with

sickle cell anemia, there were higher Hb F levels among females (323), complementing the findings of others (324,325).

These results suggest but do not prove that a factor linked to the X chromosome may influence the level of Hb F in normal individuals and patients with sickle cell anemia. Boyer et al. (326) and Chang et al. (327) reported that F cells are increased in females with sickle cell anemia and sickle cell trait and postulated that there are two genes and three alleles (LL, HL, and HH) linked to the F-cell production locus on the X chromosomes. A restriction fragment length polymorphism detected by anonymous probes seems to locate this locus to the end of the short arm of the X chromosome. In one study, this locus accounted for approximately 40% of Hb F variability in sickle cell anemia (327). Nevertheless, the interpretation of these results is heavily dependent on the still unproven accuracy of the postulated locus structure. We need to wait for the cloning, localization, and structure of the locus before this result can be properly evaluated.

Variation of Hb F levels and F cells has also been linked to chromosome 6q22.3-23.2 in an Asian Indian family (328). Linkage analysis using microsatellite markers showed that this *quantitative trait locus* was located in the 1.5 Mb region between markers D6S270 and D6S1626. Several candidate genes within this locus are being studied further (329). Evidence for another *trans*-acting quantitative trait locus unlinked to chromosome 6 or the X chromosome has been found in an English family (330). In studies of monozygotic and dizygotic twins, 15% of the variability of F-cell levels could be ascribed to the Xmn I restriction site polymorphism 5' to the ᴳγ-globin gene, leaving over 70% to be explained by other genetic modulators (329,330).

The description of a major human erythroid DNA binding protein (GF-1) capable of binding a locus in the X chromosome (Xp21-11) (332) opens the possibility that this is the determinant related to the excess Hb F expression in females.

LABORATORY DIAGNOSIS OF HEMOGLOBIN F

The best methods for determining the level of Hb F in the hemolysate depend on its concentration. For normal levels, between 0.1% and 1.5% of the total hemoglobin, the immunologic assays are best. Between 1.5% and 40%, alkaline denaturation is accurate. Over 40%, HPLC is probably the best method, although it can also be used at lower concentrations. A method of enriching the Hb F by chromatography or isoelectric focusing followed by HPLC allows this technique to be applied to all concentrations of fetal hemoglobins. Disposable columns for the determination of Hb F in hemolysates that contain no Hb A (such as red cells from Hb SS or Hb CC disease patients) are also available and are accurate.

Hemoglobin F is unevenly distributed among red cells in normals and in those with most medical conditions, except for some forms of hereditary persistence of fetal hemoglobin (333). Immunologic techniques that allow the identification of red cells containing Hb F (F cells and F reticulocytes) and measurement of the average amount of Hb F per cell have become powerful tools for the study of Hb F expression (334–336). Approximately 0.5% to 7.0% of red cells are F cells in normal adults.

Agar electrophoresis at pH 6.4 (available as a kit) offers an interesting method to isolate or identify Hb F. Hemoglobins are subjected to a combination of chromatography and electrophoresis in agar. The agar matrix interacts with the central cavity of hemoglobins (337), and hemoglobins with abnormalities in that region (such as Hb F) tend to migrate faster (or slower) than their electrophoretic mobility would predict at pH 6.4. Therefore, when a hemoglobin is found in which the electrophoretic mobility in agar is anomalous compared with the mobility under standard conditions (cellulose acetate, pH 8.6), a mutation of the central cavity should be suspected. *Hb Hope* is an example of this phenomenon.

MEDICAL CONDITIONS OUTSIDE OF HEMOGLOBINOPATHIES ASSOCIATED WITH HIGH FETAL HEMOGLOBIN EXPRESSION IN INFANTS AND ADULTS

Newborns have between 65% and 95% Hb F. This amount decreases progressively during the first year of life. The normal adult level is approached by 1 year of age and is achieved by 5 years. Normal subjects have a gender-determining dispersion of their Hb F levels. As noted earlier, Miyoshi et al. (322) have detected an excess of high normal values in women and have presented evidence that this finding is inherited as an X-linked characteristic. Identification of an X-linked modulator of Hb F expression is being actively pursued.

Pregnancy is associated with a modest increase in Hb F in the second trimester. Hydatidiform moles are associated with particularly high values. Although maternal pregnancy hormones have been implicated, the mechanism of this elevation is not clear (323).

Some conditions (besides hemoglobinopathies) retard the down-regulation of Hb F in the first 5 years of life. Affected are premature infants and infants of diabetic mothers (324). Acceleration of the fall in Hb F is observed in patients with Down's syndrome and those with C/D translocations.

Hemolytic anemias, acute bleeding, and treatment with hydroxyurea or Ara-C all can be associated with higher than normal values of Hb F, a phenomenon that has been interpreted to mean that under these conditions, early progenitors are rushed through development while retaining their fetal hemoglobin program, because the reduction in cell divisions precluded their down-regulation.

Invariably, juvenile chronic myeloid leukemia and Fanconi's anemia are accompanied by significant elevations of Hb F. Erythroleukemia, paroxysmal nocturnal hemoglobinuria, kala-azar, preleukemia, and recovery from marrow aplasia are also accompanied by variable elevations of Hb F. The highest levels are found in erythroleukemia (DiGuglielmo's disease). Many other conditions, including solid tumors, exhibit occasionally increased levels of Hb F (325,326,338).

MUTATIONS IN THE $^G\gamma$-GENES

Variants of the $^G\gamma$-Gene. Thirty-three variants with a single amino acid substitution in the $^G\gamma$-gene have been described. Of these, two are unstable: *Hb Poole* [$^G\gamma$130 (H8) Trp→Gly], which is significantly unstable, and *Hb F Xin Jin* [$^G\gamma$119 (GH2) Gly→Arg] (201). A mutation of the same site but not the same amino acid as Hb Poole has also been identified in β-chains [*Hb Wein* (β130 Tyr→Asp)].

Also found in Hb F is the equivalent of Hb M in the β-chains: *Hb F-M Fort Ripley,* which has a cyanotic phenotype in the newborn and corresponds to the substitution of the proximal Hisγ92 [F8] His→Tyr. It is the perfect equivalent to Hb Hyde Park. The other mutation, *Hb F-M Osaka* (341), involves the distal His, γ63 [E7] His→Tyr, and is equivalent to Hb M Saskatoon. Newborns with α-chain substitutions of the proximal or distal His have the same cyanotic phenotype as adults, with the cyanosis appearing early in the neonatal period (339,340).

Finally, one high-affinity variant has been described: *Hb F Onoda* [$^G\gamma$146 (HC3) His→Tyr] (342).

Variants of the $^A\gamma$-Gene and the Common Variant $^A\gamma^T$ (Hemoglobin F Sardinia). Twenty variants of the $^A\gamma$-gene have been described, but none have functional abnormalities. Six variants of the common $^A\gamma^T$ variant have been described (343), but only *Hb F Xin Jiang* [$^A\gamma$25 (B7) Gly→Arg] is unstable.

Note that Hb F Texas, Hb F Alexandria, and Hb F Ube have not been assigned to the corresponding γ-gene.

Hemoglobin A$_2$

Hemoglobin A$_2$ is the product of the combination of α-chains with δ-chains ($\alpha_2\delta_2$). The δ-chains are the product of the δ-gene, which transcribes δ message at a low level. Hb A$_2$ represents approximately 2.4% of the hemoglobins present in normal hemolysates. The δ-gene resides in the cluster of β-like genes between the pseudo–β-gene and the β-gene.

δ-GENE

The δ-gene arose from a duplication of the β-gene approximately 40 million years ago (although one cannot exclude the possibility that gene conversion could have erased differences of an older gene). The δ-gene also exists and is expressed at low levels in the new-world primates (1% to 6%). In some old-world primates, the δ-gene is present but not expressed. The δ-gene is absent in other mammals. In any case, the distribution among animals suggests that this was the last globin gene to emerge in the β-like gene cluster. Its relatively recent appearance (or recent gene conversion) explains why the δ-chain exhibits only ten sequence differences from the β-gene.

The low level of transcription might be the consequence of changes in the 5' flanking region. Of the three CCAAT boxlike sequences, none are perfectly conserved. Instability of the δ-messenger RNA may also contribute to the poor expression of the δ-gene.

FUNCTIONAL AND STRUCTURAL ASPECTS

Hemoglobin A and Hb A$_2$ have similar ligand binding curves, although the latter has slightly higher oxygen affinity. The Bohr effect, the cooperativity of ligand binding, and the response to 2,3-DPG are identical.

Among the differences, Hb A$_2$ is more thermostable because of a change at δ116, in which there is an Arg instead of the Proβ114. This Arg forms a salt bridge with Proα114, increasing even further the stability of the $\alpha_1\beta_1$ packing contact. Another difference is that Hb A$_2$ binds to the red cell membrane better than does Hb A (344).

The low levels of Hb A$_2$ and the multiple functionally abnormal mutations found in primate δ-like genes have been quoted as reasons for the lack of functional importance for this minor component. According to this view, the δ-gene is condemned to the biologic heap of history as a pseudogene. This possibility presupposes that the only functional role of any hemoglobin is to carry oxygen. If so, Hb A$_2$ is clearly useless. Alternatively, the increased binding of Hb A$_2$ to the membrane could indicate another role for this hemoglobin. It is necessary to know what proteins in addition to band 3 are capable of binding this hemoglobin and whether such binding has any functional role. The finding of Hb A$_2$ at polymorphic frequencies in the Dogon (see following text) stimulates this type of thinking.

MUTATIONAL EVENTS INVOLVING THE δ-GENE

Twenty-three single amino acid substitutions, all due to single base changes, have been described in Hb A$_2$. This number might be the tip of the iceberg, because these substitutions are more difficult to detect. Two mutations, *Hb A$_2$ Wrens* [γ98 (FG5) Val→Met] (345) and *Hb A$_2$ Manzanares* [γ121 (GH4) Glu→Val] (346), are unstable. *Hb A$_2$ Canada* (γ99 Asp→Asn) (347) has very high affinity for oxygen, but no erythrocytosis is present.

A common mutation found mostly among African-Americans and Africans is *Hb A'$_2$*, also called *Hb B$_2$*. In Africa, it has been described in samples from different geographic locations including Ghana. Hb A'$_2$ has been found at polymorphic frequencies in one of the castes in the Dogon region of the Republic of Mali. Haplotype analysis of the Mali β-like gene cluster demonstrates that all unrelated persons carrying this mutation have the same haplotype. Samples from unrelated African Americans with this mutation also demonstrate haplotype homogeneity. Hence, it is possible that Hb A'$_2$ arose in Africa unicentrally and distributed itself to other regions of Africa by gene flow.

An interesting set of mutational events involves the unequal crossover between the δ-gene and the β-gene. This crossover generates hemoglobins with portions of δ-chains and portions of β-chains. They are termed *Lepore-type hemoglobins* after the first family described. The first three examples of this type of event were characterized in heterozygotes by low levels of the Lepore-type hemoglobin (approximately 20%), electrophoretic migration similar to Hb S, and a thalassemic phenotype (microcytosis, hypochromia, hemolytic anemia). In homozygotes for this condition, severity varies from transfusion dependency to moderate anemia. Populations at risk are principally Italians, Greeks, and Yugoslavians (the last having the highest risk), but examples have been found in Turkish Cypriots, inhabitants of Papua New Guinea, African-Americans, Indians, and Romanians.

Hb Lepore Hollandia, Hb Lepore Baltimore, and Hb Lepore Washington-Boston (the first described) (348–350) have different lengths of the δ-sequence in the N-terminal portion of the hybrid chain and complementary portions of the β-chains at the C-terminal end. All have a total of 146 amino acids. The more recently described Lepore-type hemoglobin, Hb Parchman, is a patchwork in which a segment of the β-sequence is located in the center of the chain. The location of the crossover is uncertain because, with only 10 amino acid differences between the δ-chains and β-chains, there are too few informative sites.

If a Lepore-type unequal crossover occurs, an anti-Lepore hemoglobin molecule is also generated, but finding it depends on its prevalence and on luck. Hb P Nilotic is the anti-Lepore of Lepore Hollandia. Hb Lincoln Park is probably the same with an added deletion at position δ137. The hemoglobins Miyada and P Congo could be anti-Lepores of Lepore hemoglobins that are yet to be found. Electrophoretically, hemoglobins P Congo, P Nilotic, and Lincoln Park migrate like Hb S, whereas Hb Miyada and Hb Parchman migrate like Hb C.

VARIATION OF HEMOGLOBIN A$_2$ LEVELS WITH OTHER CLINICAL CONDITIONS

The levels of Hb A$_2$ are elevated in a number of conditions; in some instances, this feature is of diagnostic value. The most common clinical instance is β thalassemia. Hb A$_2$ is also elevated in sickle trait; in SS blood, particularly SS with α thalassemia; and in acquired conditions such as megaloblastic anemias and hyperthyroidism. Controversial evidence exists that Hb A$_2$ is elevated in malaria patients. Elevation of Hb A$_2$ is not due to an increase in the synthesis of δ-chains but is a consequence of the preferential assemblage of δ-chains with α-chains, particularly if α-chains are in short supply. Decreases of the levels of Hb A$_2$ are found in iron deficiency, α thalassemia, δβ thalassemia, δ thalassemia, and hereditary persistence of fetal hemoglobin, either because the δ-gene is not present (deletions) or because the α-chains are more avid for γ-chains or β-chains than for δ-chains.

Embryonic Hemoglobins

At 4 to 14 weeks of gestation, the human embryo synthesizes three distinct hemoglobins in yolk sac–derived primitive nucleated erythroid cells: ζ$_2$ε$_2$ (*Hb Gower I*), ζ$_2$γ$_2$ (*Hb Portland*), and α$_2$ε$_2$ (*Hb Gower II*) (351). ζ-Globin and ε-globin chains are expressed before the γ-globin and α-globin chains. After the establishment of the placenta, at 14 days of development, embryonic hemoglobins are replaced by Hb F, but ζ-globin and ε-globin chains can be found in definitive fetal erythrocytes (352). At 15 to 22 weeks of

gestation, 53% of fetal cells contained ζ-globin chains, and 5% had ε-globin chains. At term, cord blood contained 34% ζ-globin and 0.6% ε-globin chain–positive cells. Erythrocytes from normal adults do not contain embryonic globins.

Developmental timing of the synthesis of embryonic hemoglobins has been studied in erythroid cells of embryos 35 to 56 days old (353). Embryonic, fetal, and adult globins are synthesized *in vivo* and in cultures of erythroid burst-forming units in the yolk sac (where primitive erythropoiesis occurs) and in liver cells (the site of definitive erythropoiesis). Similarly, the adult α-globin gene and the corresponding embryonic α-like chains (ζ-globin gene) are coexpressed in the earliest murine erythrocyte progenitors (354). Because of these studies and the recent finding of embryonic hemoglobin in cord blood, it appears that embryonic globin is expressed in both primitive and definitive erythroblasts, although in vastly different quantities. These results are compatible with the notion that the switch from embryonic to fetal globin synthesis represents a time-dependent change in programs of progenitor cells rather than a change in hemopoietic cell lineages.

Hoffman et al. (355) analyzed embryonic hemoglobins obtained from an *in vitro* expression system and found that in the absence of any effector of hemoglobin function, including Cl⁻, they all have oxygen affinities and ligand-binding rates similar to Hb A. In the presence of organic phosphates, the oxygen affinities of ζ$_2$ε$_2$ and α$_2$ε$_2$ are lowered, in the case of Gower II, to a lesser extent than normal Hb A. This finding demonstrates that the ζ-globin and ε-globin chains do bind 2,3-DPG, but different than Hb A, which requires explanation (see below). Hb Portland does not bind organic phosphates well, which is not surprising, because its central cavity is formed by γ-globin chains.

The rates of oxygen dissociation from the embryonic hemoglobins have been measured by Hoffmann and Brittain (356) and appear to be responsible for the high oxygen-binding affinity of the embryonic proteins. The pH dependence of the oxygen dissociation rate constants also accounts for the rather unusual Bohr effects characteristic of embryonic hemoglobins.

Bonaventura et al. (356a), studying Hb A and Hb Hinsdale (Asnβ139→Lys), were among the first to realize that it is indispensable to reduce the destabilizing effect of an excess of positive charges in the central cavity. Cl⁻ binding to oxyhemoglobin accomplishes that task and preserves the physiologic oxygen affinity of hemoglobin. Perutz et al. (357) proposed that Cl⁻ binding in embryonic hemoglobins differed from that of Hb A. The Cl⁻ interactions with embryonic hemoglobins are particularly interesting (358).

Hb Portland is completely insensitive to Cl⁻, whereas Hb Gower I has a small effect and Hb Gower II a chloride effect approaching that of Hb A. Chloride binding and the Bohr effect of these hemoglobins are in accordance with the allosteric model proposed by Perutz et al. (357).

For α$_2$ε$_2$ (Hb Gower II), crystallographic data on the CO form are available (358) (Fig. 49-27). Compared to Hb A and Hb F, the tertiary structure of the α-globin chain is unchanged. The ε-globin chain has a structure very similar to the β-globin chain, with small differences in the N-terminus and A helix. The Cl⁻ binding sites involve the polar residues within the central cavities (anionic α94, α126, and β101 and the cationic α1, α99, α103, β1, β2, β82, β104, and β143). Of these residues, only Argβ104 is changed to a Lys in the ε-globin chain. The ε-globin Lys residue might be involved in an ionic interaction with Gluε101, but whether the pK of Lys is low enough to be nonionized in physiologic conditions and whether this sequence change can explain the decrease in Cl⁻ binding is uncertain. Other candidate residues that may influence Cl⁻ binding are the sequence changes Hisβ77→Asnε77, Hisβ116→Thrε116, and Proβ125→Glyε125. A better understanding of the consequence of these changes will require knowledge of the T crystal structure of Hb Gower II. It is possible that the decrease of the Cl⁻ effect is the sum of small aggregated changes and not the result of a single amino acid substitution.

The most distinct change in Hb Gower II compared to Hb A is a shift of the N-terminus and the A helix similar to that seen in Hb F. The α-helix moves into the central cavity as a consequence of a complex disruption of the N-terminal region due to sequence changes at Leuβ3→Pheϵ3, Leuβ78→Metϵ78, Proβ5→Alaϵ5, and Tyrβ130→Trpϵ130. To establish definitively the mechanism of the decrease in 2,3-DPG binding, it is necessary to know the T crystal structure of Gower II, but the A helix shift remains a likely candidate.

The embryonic ϵ-globin chain has a Lys residue at position 87, compared to a Thr residue in the β-globin chain. Is there a microconformational change at this site? Any change would have to be only solution-active, because crystallography does not support this interpretation.

Hoffmann et al. (355) have studied the effect of CO_2, ATP, and lactate ions on the oxygen affinity of the three human embryonic hemoglobins. CO_2 and ATP lower the affinity of both the adult and embryonic hemoglobins for oxygen. Lactate ions have no effect on the oxygen equilibrium process over the concentration range studied. The three embryonic hemoglobins have reduced values of CO binding compared to previously reported mammalian fetal or adult hemoglobin (360). It is possible that this feature is a mechanism to protect the embryo from CO poisoning.

The three embryonic hemoglobins exhibit lower oxidation rates than the adult protein (361) and are significantly less susceptible to anion-induced oxidation. The heme groups are more tightly bound, similar to Hb F (see above).

Finally, embryonic ζ-globin and ϵ-globin subunits assemble with each other and with adult α-globin and β-globin subunits into hemoglobin heterotetramers in both primitive and definitive erythrocytes. A complex transgenic knock-out mouse that expresses these hemoglobins at high levels has allowed functional characterization of these hybrids (362). The exchange of ζ-chains for α-chains increases the p50 and decreases the Bohr effect, increasing oxygen transport capacity. By comparison, the ϵ-chain for β-chain exchange has little impact on these parameters. Hb Gower-1, assembled entirely from embryonic subunits, displays an elevated p50, a reduced Bohr effect, and increased 2,3-DPG binding compared to Hb A. The data support the hypothesis that Hb Gower-2, assembled from reactivated ϵ-globin in individuals with hemoglobinopathies and thalassemias, would serve as a physiologically acceptable substitute for deficient or dysfunctional Hb A. In addition, the unexpected properties of Hb Gower-1 call into question its primary role in embryonic development.

MUTATIONS AFFECTING EMBRYONIC HEMOGLOBINS

The most common mutation producing lethal hydrops fetalis is the Southeast Asian (–/SEA) double α-globin gene deletion (363). Erythrocytes from adults heterozygous for the (–/SEA) deletion have minute amounts of embryonic ζ-globin chains detectable by anti-ζ-globin monoclonal antibodies. The majority of subjects are of Filipino, Chinese, or Laotian ancestry. The (–/SEA) double α-deletion was the only abnormality in two-thirds of these patients. In the others, it was combined with α-globin or β-globin mutations or coincidental iron deficiency. Four other samples from (–/SEA) heterozygotes were negative by this immunologic assay. Anti-ζ-negative samples included deletions of the total α-globin region (–/Tot), single α-globin deletions, and a variety of β-globin mutations; normocytic samples with normal α-genes were also negative. Benign triplicated ζ-globin genes were also detected. Anti-ζ immunobinding testing provides rapid, simple, and reliable screening for the (–/SEA) double α-globin deletion, although it does not detect the (–/Tot) total α-deletions.

REFERENCES

1. Kendrew JC, Dickerson RE, Strandberg BE, et al. Structure of myoglobin: a three-dimensional Fourier synthesis at 2 Å resolution. *Nature* 1960;185:422.
2. Tetreau C, Lavalette D, Momenteau M, et al. Energy barriers in the binding of CO and O_2 bindings to heme model compounds. *Proc Natl Acad Sci U S A* 1987;84:2267.
3. Komiyama NH, Shih DT, Looker D, et al. Was the loss of the D helix in α-globin a functionally neutral mutation? *Nature* 1991;352:349.
4. Perutz MF, Rossman MG, Cullis AF, et al. Structure of haemoglobin: a three-dimensional Fourier synthesis at 5.5 Å resolution, obtained by X-ray analysis. *Nature* 1960;185:416.
5. Baldwin JM. The structure of human carbonmonoxy haemoglobin at 2.7 Å resolution. *J Mol Biol* 1980;136:103.
6. Fermi G, Perutz MF, Shaanan B, et al. The crystal structure of human deoxyhaemoglobin at 1.7 Å resolution. *J Mol Biol* 1984;175:159.
7. Chothia C, Wodak S, Janin J. Role of subunit interfaces in the allosteric mechanism of hemoglobin. *Proc Natl Acad Sci U S A* 1976;73:3793.
8. Koshland DE Jr, Nemethy G, Filmer D. Comparison of experimental binding data and theoretical model in proteins containing subunits. *Biochemistry* 1966;5:365.
9. Monod J, Wyman J, Changeaux JP. On the nature of allosteric transition: a plausible model. *J Mol Biol* 1967;12:88.
10. Baldwin J, Chothia C. Haemoglobin: the structural changes related to ligand binding and its allosteric mechanism. *J Mol Biol* 1979;129:175.
11. Perutz MF, Sanders JKM, Chenery DH, et al. Interactions between the quaternary structure of the globin and the spin state of the heme in ferric mixed spin derivatives of hemoglobin. *Biochemistry* 1978;17:3640.
12. Perutz MF, Kilmartin JV, Nagai K, et al. Influence of globin structures on the state of the heme: ferrous low spin derivatives. *Biochemistry* 1976;15:378.
13. Maxwell JC, Caughey WS. An infrared study of NO bonding to heme B and hemoglobin A: evidence for inositol hexaphosphate induced cleavage of proximal histidine to iron bonds. *Biochemistry* 1976;15:388.
14a. Perutz MF. Stereochemistry of the cooperative effects in haemoglobin. *Nature* 1970;288:726.
14b. Perutz MF, Gronenbom AM, Clore GM, et al. The pKa values of two histidine residues in human haemoglobin, the Bohr effect, and the dipole moments of α-helices. *J Mol Biol* 1985;183:491.
14c. Perutz MF. Molecular anatomy and physiology of hemoglobin. In: MH Steinberg, BG Forget, DR Higgs, et al., eds. *Disorders of hemoglobin: genetics, pathophysiology, clinical management.* Cambridge: Cambridge University Press, 2000.
15. Ho C, Russu IM. Proton nuclear magnetic resonance studies of sickle cell hemoglobin. In: Caughey WS, ed. *Biochemical and clinical aspects of hemoglobin abnormalities.* New York: Academic Press, 1978:179.
16. Ackers GK, Doyle ML, Myers D, et al. Molecular code for cooperativity in hemoglobin. *Science* 1992;255:54.
17. Miura S, Ikeda-Saito T, Yonetani T, et al. Oxygen equilibrium studies of cross-linked asymmetrical cyanomet valency hybrid hemoglobins: models for partially oxygenated species. *Biochemistry* 1987;26:2149.
18. Perrella M, Colosimo A, Benazzi L, et al. What the intermediate compounds in ligand binding to hemoglobin tell about the mechanism of cooperativity. *Biophys Chem* 1990;37:211.
19. Eaton WA, Henry ER, Hofrichter J, et al. Is cooperative oxygen binding by hemoglobin really understood? *Nat Struct Biol* 1999;6:351–358.
20. Henry ER, Jones CM, Hofrichter J, et al. Can a two-state MWC allosteric model explain hemoglobin kinetics? *Biochemistry* 1997;3:6511–6518.
21. Nagel RL, Ranney HM, Kucinskies LL. Tyrosine ionization in human CO and deoxyhemoglobin. *Biochemistry* 1966;5:1934.
22. Ishimor K, Hashimoto M, Imai K, et al. Site-directed mutagenesis in haemoglobin: functional and structural role of the penultimate tyrosine in the alpha subunit. *Biochemistry* 1994;33:2546.
23. Ackers GK, Hazzard JH. Transduction of binding energy into hemoglobin cooperativity. *Trends Biochem Sci* 1993;18:385.
24. Perrella M, Bresciani D, Rossi-Bemardi L. The binding of CO_2 to human hemoglobin. *J Biol Chem* 1975;250:5413.
25. Perrella M, Kilmartin JV, Fogg J, et al. Identification of the high and low affinity CO_2 binding sites of human haemoglobin. *Nature* 1975;256:759.
26. Kilmartin JV, Fogg JH, Perutz MF. Role of C-terminal histidine in the alkaline Bohr effect of human hemoglobin. *Biochemistry* 1980;19:3189.
27. Nishikura K. Identification of histidine-122 in human haemoglobin as one of the unknown alkaline Bohr groups by hydrogen-tritium exchange. *Biochem J* 1978;173:651.
28. Russu IM, Ho NT, Ho C. Role of the β146 histidyl residue in the alkaline Bohr effect of hemoglobin. *Biochemistry* 1980;19:1043.
29. Fang TY, Zou M, Simplaceanu V, et al. Assessment of roles of surface histidyl residues in the molecular basis of the Bohr effect and of β143 histidine in the binding of 2,3-bisphosphoglycerate in human normal adult hemoglobin. *Biochemistry* 1999;38:13423–13432.
30. Benesch R, Benesch RE. The effect of organic phosphates from the human erythrocyte on the allosteric properties of hemoglobin. *Biochem Biophys Res Commun* 1967;26:162.
31. Chanutin A, Cumish RR. Effect of organic and inorganic phosphates on the oxygen equilibrium of human erythrocytes. *Arch Biochem Biophys* 1967;121:96.
32. Arnone A. X-ray diffraction study of binding of 2,3-diphosphoglycerate to human deoxyhaemoglobin. *Nature* 1972;237:146.

33. Bonaventura J, Bonaventura C, Amiconi G, et al. Allosteric interactions in non-chains isolated from normal human hemoglobin, fetal hemoglobin, and hemoglobin Abruzzo [β143 (H21) His→Arg]. *J Biol Chem* 1975;250:6278.

34. Rose ZB. The enzymology of 2,3-bisphosphoglycerate. *Adv Enzymol* 1980;51:211.

35. Card R, Brain M. The "anemia" of childhood. *N Engl J Med* 1973;288:388.

36. Purcell Y, Brozovic B. Red cell 2,3-diphosphoglycerate concentration in man decreases with age. *Nature* 1974;251:511.

37. Ignarro LJ. A novel signal transduction mechanism for transcellular communication. *Hypertension* 1990;16:477–483.

38. Head CA, Brugnara C, Martinez-Ruiz R, et al. Low concentrations of nitric oxide increase oxygen affinity of sickle erythrocytes in vitro and in vivo. *J Clin Invest* 1997;100:1193–1198.

39. Gladwin MT, Schechter AN, Shelhamer JH, et al. Inhaled nitric oxide transport on sickle cell hemoglobin without affecting oxygen affinity. *J Clin Invest* 1999;104:937–945.

40. Gow AJ, Stamler JS. Reactions between nitric oxide and haemoglobin under physiological conditions. *Nature* 1998; 391:169–173.

41. Hrinczenko BW, Alayash AI, Wink DA, et al. Effect of nitric oxide and nitric oxide donors on red blood cell oxygen transport. *Br J Haematol* 2000;110:412–419.

42. Patel RP, Hogg N, Spencer NY, et al. Biochemical characterization of human S-nitrosohemoglobin: effects on oxygen binding and transnitrosation. *J Biol Chem* 1999;274:15487–15492.

43. Yonetani T. Nitric oxide and hemoglobin. *Nippon Yakurigaku Zasshi* 1998;112:155–160.

44. Holzmann A. Nitric oxide and sepsis. *Respir Care Clin North Am* 1997;3:537–550.

45. Eich RF, Li T, Lemon DD, et al. Mechanism of NO-induced oxidation of myoglobin and hemoglobin. *Biochemistry* 1996;35:976–983.

46. Bank N, Kiroycheva M, Singhal PC, et al. Inhibition of nitric oxide synthase ameliorates cellular injury in sickle cell mouse kidneys. *Kidney Int* 2000; 58:82–89.

47. Kiroycheva M, Ahmed F, Anthony GM, et al. Mitogen-activated protein kinase phosphorylation in kidneys of β^S sickle cell mice. *J Am Soc Nephrol* 2000;11:1026–1032.

48. Bank N, Kiroycheva M, Ahmed F, et al. Peroxynitrite formation and apoptosis in transgenic sickle cell mouse kidneys. *Kidney Int* 1998;54:1520–1528.

49. Bank N, Aynedjian HS, Qiu JH, et al. Renal nitric oxide synthases in transgenic sickle cell mice. *Kidney Int* 1996;50:184–189.

50. Bank N, Kiroycheva M, Singhal PC, et al. Inhibition of nitric oxide synthase ameliorates cellular injury in sickle cell mouse kidneys. *Kidney Int* 2000;58: 82–89.

51. Gladwin MT, Shelhamer JH, Schechter AN, et al. Role of circulating nitrite and S-nitrosohemoglobin in the regulation of regional blood flow in humans. *Proc Natl Acad Sci U S A* 2000;97:11482–11487.

52. Gladwin MT, Ognibene FP, Pannell LK, et al. Relative role of heme nitrosylation and P-cysteine 93 nitrosation in the transport and metabolism of nitric oxide by hemoglobin in the human circulation. *Proc Natl Acad Sci U S A* 2000; 97:9943–9948.

53. Pabloski JR, Hess DT, Stamler JS. Export by red blood cells of nitric oxide bioactivity. *Nature* 2001;409:622–626.

54. Charache S, Weatherall DJ, Clegg JB. Polycythemia associated with a hemoglobinopathy. *J Clin Invest* 1966;45:813.

55. Clegg JB, Naughton MA, Weatherall DJ. Abnormal human haemoglobins: separation and characterization of the α and β chains by chromatography, and the determination of two new variants, Hb Chesapeake and Hb J (Bangkok). *J Mol Biol* 1966;19:91.

56. Nagel RL, Gibson QH, Charache S. Relation between structure and function in hemoglobin Chesapeake. *Biochemistry* 1967;6:2395.

57. Lines JG, McIntosh R. Oxygen binding by haemoglobin J Capetown (α₂92 Arg→Gln). *Nature* 1967;215:297.

58. Nagel RL, Gibson OH, Jenkins T. Ligand binding in the Hb J Capetown. *J Mol Biol* 1971;58:643.

59. Shimasaki S. A new hemoglobin variant, hemoglobin Nunobiki [α141 (HC3) Arg→Cys]: notable influence of the carboxy-terminal cysteine upon various physico-chemical characteristics of hemoglobin. *J Clin Invest* 1985;75:695.

60. Owen MC, Ockelford PA, Wells RM. Hb Howick [β37(C3)Trp→Gly]: a new high oxygen affinity variant of the α₁β₂ contact. *Hemoglobin* 1993;17:513.

61. Moo-Perm WF, Swan DC, Hine TK, et al. Hb Catonsville (glutamic acid inserted between Pro37(C2)alpha and Thr38(C3)alpha): nonallelic gene conversion in the globin system? *J Biol Chem* 1989;264:21454.

62. Kavanaugh JS, Weydert JA, Rogers PH, et al. High-resolution crystal structures of human hemoglobin with mutations at tryptophan 37beta: structural basis for a high-affinity T-state. *Biochemistry* 1998;37:4358–4373.

63. Lacombe C, Craescu CT, Blouquit Y, et al. Structural and functional studies of hemoglobin Poissy α₂β₂56 (D7) Gly→Arg and 86 (F2) Ala→Pro. *Eur J Biochem* 1985;153:655.

64. Reed CS, Hampson R, Gordon S, et al. Erythrocytosis secondary to increased oxygen affinity of a mutant hemoglobin, hemoglobin Kempsey. *Blood* 1968; 31:623.

65. Jones RT, Osgood EE, Brimhall B, et al. Hemoglobin Yakima, I. Clinical and biochemical studies. *J Clin Invest* 1967;46:1840.

66. Weatherall DJ, Clegg JB, Callender ST, et al. Haemoglobin Radcliffe (α₂β₂ 99(G1)Ala): a high oxygen-affinity variant causing familial polycythaemia. *Br J Haematol* 1977;35:177.

67. Rucknagel DL, Glynn KP, Smith JR. Hemoglobin Ypsilanti characterized by increased oxygen affinity, abnormal polymerization and erythremia. *Clin Res* 1967;15:270.

68. Blouquit Y, Braconnier F, Galacteros F, et al. Hemoglobin Hotel-Dieu β99 Asp→Gly (G1): a new abnormal hemoglobin with high oxygen affinity. *Hemoglobin* 1981;5:19.

69. Rochette J, Poyart C, Varet B, et al. A new hemoglobin variant altering the α₁β₂ contact: Hb Chemilly α₂β₂ 99 (G1) Asp→Val. *FEBS Lett* 1984;166:8.

70. Wajcman H, Girodon E, Prome D, et al. Germline mosaicism for an alanine to valine substitution at residue β140 in hemoglobin Puttelange, a new variant with high oxygen affinity. *Hum Genet* 1995;96:711.

71. Imai K. Oxygen-equilibrium characteristics of abnormal hemoglobin Hiroshima (α₂β₂ 143 Asp). *Arch Biochem Biophys* 1968;127:543.

72. Nagel RL, Gibson OH, Hamilton HB. Ligand kinetics in hemoglobin Hiroshima. *J Clin Invest* 1971;50:1772.

73. Wajcman H, Kilmartin JV, Najman A, et al. Hemoglobin Cochin-Port-Royal: consequences of the replacement of the beta chain C-terminal by an arginine. *Biochim Biophys Acta* 1975;400:354

74. Russu IM, Ho C. Assessment of role of beta 146-histidyl and other histidyl residues in the Bohr effect of human normal adult hemoglobin. *Biochemistry* 1986;25:1706.

75. Nute PE, Stamatoyannopoulos G, Hermodson MA, et al. Hemoglobinopathic erythrocytosis due to a new electrophoretically silent variant, hemoglobin San Diego (β109 [G11] Val→Met). *J Clin Invest* 1974;53:320.

76. Maniatis A, Bousios T, Nagel RL, et al. Hemoglobin Crete (β129 Ala→Pro): a new high-affinity variant interacting with β°- and δβ°-thalassemia. *Blood* 1979;54:54.

77. Lorkin PA, Stephens AD, Beard ME, et al. Haemoglobin Rahere (β82 Lys→Thr): a new high affinity haemoglobin associated with decreased 2,3 diphosphoglycerate binding and relative polycythaemia. *BMJ* 1975;4:200.

78. Ikkala E, Koskela J, Pikkarainen P, et al. Hb Helsinki: a variant with a high oxygen affinity and a substitution at a 2,3-DPG binding site (β82 [EF6] Lys→Met). *Acta Haematol* 1976;56:257.

79. Bonaventura J, Bonaventura C, Sullivan B, et al. Hemoglobin Providence: functional consequences of the two alterations of the 2,3-diphosphoglycerate binding site at position β82. *J Biol Chem* 1976;251:7563.

80. Elder GE, Lappin TR, Horne AB, et al. Hemoglobin Old Dominion/Burton-upon-Trent, β143 (H21) His→Tyr, codon 143 CAC→TAC—a variant with altered oxygen affinity that compromises measurement of glycated hemoglobin in diabetes mellitus: structure, function, and DNA sequence. *Mayo Clin Proc* 1998;73:321–328.

81. Tondo CV, Bonaventura J, Bonaventura C, et al. Functional properties of hemoglobin Porto Alegre (α₂β₂ 9 Ser→Cys) and the reactivity of its extra cysteinyl residue. *Biochim Biophys Acta* 1974;342:15.

82. Bonaventura J, Riggs A. Polymerization of hemoglobins of mouse and man: structural basis. *Science* 1967;158:800.

83. Stamatoyannopoulos G, Nute PE, Adamson JW, et al. Hemoglobin Olympia (β20 valine→methionine): an electrophoretically silent variant associated with high oxygen affinity and erythrocytosis. *J Clin Invest* 1973;52:342.

84. Edelstein SJ, Poyart C, Blouquit Y, et al. Self-association of haemoglobin Olympia (α₂β₂ 20 (B2) Val→Met): a human haemoglobin bearing a substitution at the surface of the molecule. *J Mol Biol* 1986;187:277.

85. Flatz G, Kinderlerer JL, Kilmartin JV, et al. Haemoglobin Tak: a variant with additional residues at the end of the β-chains. *Lancet* 1971;10:732.

86. Imai K, Lehmann H. The oxygen affinity of haemoglobin Tak, a variant with elongated β-chain. *Biochim Biophys Acta* 1975;412:288.

87. Lehmann H, Casey R, Lang A, et al. Haemoglobin Tak: a β-chain elongation. *Br J Haematol* 1975;31:119.

88. Delano J, North ML, Arous N, et al. Hb Saverne: a new variant having an elongated β-chain. *Blood* 1984;64[Suppl 1]:56a(abst).

89. Delanoe-Garin J, Blouquit Y, Arous N, et al. Hemoglobin Saverne: a new variant with elongated β chains: structural and functional properties. *Hemoglobin* 1988;12:337.

90. Vasseur C, Blouquit Y, Kister J, et al. Hemoglobin Thionville: an alpha-chain variant with a substitution of a glutamate for valine at NA-1 and having an acetylated methionine NH₂ terminus. *J Biol Chem* 1992;267:12682–12691.

91. Kamel K, el-Najjar A, Webber BB, et al. Hb Doha or α2β2[X-N-Met-1(NA1)Val→Glu]; a new beta-chain abnormal hemoglobin observed in a Qatari female. *Biochim Biophys Acta* 1985;831:257–260.

92. Boissel JP, Kasper TJ, Shah SC, et al. Amino-terminal processing of proteins: hemoglobin South Florida, a variant with retention of initiator methionine and N-alpha-acetylation. *Proc Natl Acad Sci U S A* 1985;82:8448–8452.

93. Prchal JT, Cashman DP, Kan YW. Hemoglobin Long Island is caused by a single mutation (adenine to cytosine) resulting in a failure to cleave amino-terminal methionine. *Proc Natl Acad Sci U S A* 1986;83:24–27.

94. White JM, Szur L, Gillies IDS, et al. Familial polycythaemia caused by a new haemoglobin variant: Hb Heathrow: Hb β103 (G5) phenylalanine→leucine. *BMJ* 1973;3:665.

95. Sherwood JB, Goldwasser E. A radioimmunoassay for erythropoietin. *Blood* 1979;54:885.

96. Rosa R, Prehu MO, Beuzard Y, et al. The first case of a complete deficiency of diphosphoglycerate mutase in human erythrocytes. *J Clin Invest* 1978; 62:907.

97. Kales SN. Carbon monoxide intoxication. *Am Fam Physician* 1993;48:1100.

98. Adamson JW. Familial polycythemia. *Semin Hematol* 1975;12:383.

99. Sergeyeva A, Gordeuk VR, Tokarev YN, et al. Congenital polycythemia in Chuvashia. *Blood* 1997;89:2148–2154.

100. Vasserman NN, Karzakova LM, Tverskaya SM, et al. Localization of the gene responsible for familial benign polycythemia to chromosome 11q23. *Hum Hered* 1999;49:129–132.

100a. Giordano PC, Harteveld CL, Brand A, et al. Hb Malmo [β97(FG4)His→Gln] leading to polycythemia in a Dutch family. *Ann Hematol* 1996;73:183–188.

101. Grace RJ, Gover PA, Treacher DF, et al. Venesection in haemoglobin Yakima, a high oxygen affinity haemoglobin. *Clin Lab Haematol* 1992;14:1995.

102. Adamson JW, Finch CA. Erythropoietin and the polycythemias. *Ann N Y Acad Sci* 1968;149:560.

103. Adamson JW, Hayashi A, Stamatoyannopoulos G, et al. Erythrocyte function and marrow regulation in hemoglobin Bethesda (β145 Histidine). *J Clin Invest* 1972;51:2883.

104. Adamson JW, Finch CA. Hemoglobin function, oxygen affinity and erythropoietin. *Annu Rev Physiol* 1975;37:351.

105. Charache S, Achuff S, Winslow R, et al. Variability of the homeostatic response to altered P(50). *Blood* 1978;52:1156.

106. Charache S, Catalano P, Bums S, et al. Pregnancy in carriers of high-affinity hemoglobins. *Blood* 1985;65:713.

107. Butler WM, Spratling L, Kark JA, et al. Hemoglobin Osier: report of a new family with exercise studies before and after phlebotomy. *Am J Hematol* 1982; 13:293.

108. Blouquit Y, Bardakdjian J, Lena-Russo D, et al. Hb Bruxelles: α₂β₂ 41 or 42(C7 or CDI) Phe deleted. *Hemoglobin* 1989;13:465.

109. Griffon N, Badens C, Lena-Russo D, et al. Hb Bruxelles, deletion of Phe β42, shows a low oxygen affinity and low cooperativity of ligand binding. *J Biol Chem* 1996;271:25916.

110. Schneider RG, Atkins RJ, Hosty TS, et al. Haemoglobin Titusville: α94 Asp→Asn, a new haemoglobin with a lowered affinity for oxygen. *Biochem Biophys Acta* 1975;400:365.

111. Bonaventura J, Riggs A. Hemoglobin Kansas: a human hemoglobin with a neutral amino acid substitution and an abnormal oxygen equilibrium. *J Biol Chem* 1968;243:980.

112. Reismann KR, Ruth WE, Nomura T. A human hemoglobin with lowered oxygen affinity and impaired heme-heme interactions. *J Clin Invest* 1961; 40:182.

113. Nagel RL, Lynfield J, Johnson J, et al. Hemoglobin Beth Israel: a mutant causing clinically apparent cyanosis. *N Engl J Med* 1976;295:125.

114. Arous N, Braconnier F, Thillet J, et al. Hemoglobin Saint Mande β102 (G4) Asn→Tyr: a new low oxygen affinity variant. *FEBS Lett* 1981;126:114.

115. Greer J. Three dimensional structure of abnormal haemoglobins Kansas and Richmond. *J Mol Biol* 1971;59:99.

116. Efremov GD, Huisman THJ, Smith LL, et al. Hemoglobin Richmond: a human hemoglobin which forms asymmetric hybrids with other hemoglobins. *J Biol Chem* 1969;244:6105.

117. Andersen L. Structures of deoxy and carbonmonoxy haemoglobin Kansas in the deoxy quaternary conformation. *J Mol Biol* 1975;94:33.

118. Gacon G, Belkhodja O, Wajcman H, et al. Structural and functional studies of Hb Rothschild β37(C3) Trp→Arg: a new variant of the α₁β₂ contact. *FEBS Lett* 1977;82:243.

119. Sharma VS, Newton GL, Ranney HM, et al. Hemoglobin Rothschild (β37(C3) Trp→Arg): a high/low affinity haemoglobin variant. *J Mol Biol* 1980;144:267.

120. Craik CS, Vallette I, Beychok A, et al. Refolding defects in hemoglobin Rothschild. *J Biol Chem* 1980;255:6219.

121. Williamson D, Nutkins J, Rosthoj S, et al. Characterization of Hb Aalborg, a new unstable hemoglobin variant, by fast atom bombardment mass spectrometry. *Hemoglobin* 1990;14:137.

122. Fermi G, Perutz MF, Williamson D, et al. Structure-function relationships in the low-affinity mutant haemoglobin Aalborg (Gly74 (E18)β→Arg). *J Mol Biol* 1992;226:883.

123. Moo-Penn WF, McPhedran P, Bobrow S, et al. Hemoglobin Connecticut (β21 (B3) Asp→Gly): a hemoglobin variant with low oxygen affinity. *Am J Hematol* 1981;11:137.

124. Marinucci M, Giuliani A, Maffi D, et al. Hemoglobin Bologna (α₂β₂ 61(E5) Lys→Met), an abnormal human hemoglobin with low oxygen affinity. *Biochim Biophys Acta* 1981;668:209.

125. Bonaventura C, Cashon R, Bonaventura J, et al. Involvement of the distal histidine in the low affinity exhibited by Hb Chico (Lys β66→Thr) and its isolated β chains. *J Biol Chem* 1991;266:23033–23040.

126. Olson JS, Mathews AJ, Rohlfs RJ, et al. The role of the distal histidine in myoglobin and hemoglobin. *Nature* 1988;336:265–266.

127. Imamura T, Fujita S, Ohta Y, et al. Hemoglobin Yoshizuka (G10 (108) β asparagine→aspartic acid): a new variant with a reduced oxygen affinity from a Japanese family. *J Clin Invest* 1969;48:2341.

128. Moo-Penn WF, Wolff JA, Simon A, et al. Hemoglobin Presbyterian: βl08 (G10) asparagine→lysine. A hemoglobin variant with low oxygen affinity. *FEBS Lett* 1978;92:53.

129. Jones RT, Brimhall B, Pootrakul S, et al. Hemoglobin Vancouver [α₂β₂ 73 (E17) Asp→Tyr]: its structure and function. *J Mol Evol* 1976;9:37.

130. Konotey-Ahulu FID, Gallo E, Lehmann H, et al. Haemoglobin Korle-Bu (73 aspartic acid→asparagine) showing one of the two amino acid substitutions of haemoglobin C, Harlem. *J Med Genet* 1968;5:107.

131. Schneider RG, Hosty TS, Tomlin G, et al. Hb Mobile (α₂β₂ 73 (E17) Asp→Val): a new variant. *Biochem Genet* 1975;13:411.

132. Wajcman H, Jones RT. Propriétés fonctionelles des hemoglobines humaines mutees en position 73. *INSERM* 1977;70:269.

133. Bookchin RM, Nagel RL. Molecular interactions of sickling hemoglobin. In: Abramson H, Bertles JF, Wethers DC, eds. *Sickle cell disease*. St. Louis: CV Mosby, 1973;140.

134. Wishner BC, Ward KB, Lattman EE, et al. Crystal structure of sickle-cell deoxyhemoglobin at 5 Å resolution. *J Mol Biol* 1975;98:179.

135. Horlein H, Weber G. Uber chronisch familiare Methamoglobinanue und eine neue Modifikation des Methamoglobins. *Dtsch Med Wochenschr* 1948;73:476.

136. Gerald DS, Efron ML. Chemical studies of several varieties of Hb M. *Proc Natl Acad Sci U S A* 1961;47:1758.

137. Shibata S, Tanuira A, Iuchi I. Hemoglobin M₁ demonstration of a new abnormal hemoglobin in hereditary nigremia. *Acta Haematol Jpn* 1960;23:96.

138. Greer J. Three dimension studies of abnormal human hemoglobins M Hyde Park and M Iwate. *J Mol Biol* 1971;59:107.

139. Ranney HM, Nagel RL, Heller P, et al. Oxygen equilibrium of hemoglobin M-Hyde Park. *Bichim Biophys Acta* 1968;160:112–115.

140. Brennan SO, Matthews JR. Hb Auckland [β87(F8) His→Asn]: a new mutation of the proximal histidine identified by electrospray mass spectrometry. *Hemoglobin* 1997;21:393–403.

141. Nagai M, Aki M, Li R, et al. Heme structure of hemoglobin M Iwate [α87(F8) His→Tyr]: a UV and visible resonance Raman study. *Biochemistry* 2000; 39:13093.

142. Feher G, Isaacson RA, Scholes CP. Endor studies on normal and abnormal hemoglobins. *Ann N Y Acad Sci* 1973;222:86.

143. Peisach J, Gersonde K. Binding of CO to mutant chains of HbM Iwate: evidence for distal imidazole ligation. *Biochemistry* 1977;16:2539.

144. LaMar GR, Nagai K, Jue T, et al. Assignment of proximal histidyl imidazole exchangeable proton NMR resonances to individual subunits in HbA, Boston, Iwate and Milwaukee. *Biochem Biophys Res Commun* 1980;96:1177.

145. Pulsinelli PD, Perutz MF, Nagel RL. Structure of hemoglobin M Boston, a variant with a five-coordinated ferric heme. *Proc Natl Acad Sci U S A* 1973; 70:3870.

146. Perutz MF, Pulsinelli PD, Ranney HM. Structure and subunit interaction of haemoglobin M Milwaukee. *Nature* 1972;237:259.

147. Raftery MA, Huestis WH. Molecular conformation and cooperativity in hemoglobin. *Ann N Y Acad Sci* 1973;222:40.

148. Caldwell PRB, Nagel RL. The binding of 2,3 diphosphoglycerate as a conformational probe of human hemoglobins. *J Mol Biol* 1973;74:605.

149. Lindstrom TR, Ho C, Pisciotta AV. Nuclear magnetic resonance studies of haemoglobin M Milwaukee. *Nature* 1972;237:263.

150. Thillet J, Cohen-Solal M, Seligmann M, et al. Functional and physiochemical studies of hemoglobin St. Louis β28 (B10) Leu→Gln. *J Clin Invest* 1976; 58:1098.

151. Wajcman H, Krishnamoorthy R, Gacon G, et al. A new hemoglobin variant involving the distal histidine: Hb Bicetre (β63 (E7) His→Pro). *J Mol Med* 1976;1:187.

152. Rosa J, Labie D, Wajcman H, et al. Haemoglobin I Toulouse: β66 (E10) Lys→ Glu: a new abnormal haemoglobin with a mutation localized on the E10 porphyrin surrounding zones. *Nature* 1969;223:190.

153. Kurachi S, Hermodson M, Hornung S, et al. Structure of haemoglobin Seattle. *Nature* 1973;243:275.

154. Bunn HF, Forget BG. *Hemoglobin: molecular, genetic and clinical aspects*. Philadelphia: WB Saunders, 1986.

155. Nagai M, Yubisui T, Yoneyama Y. Enzymatic reduction of hemoglobin M Milwaukee I and M Saskatoon by NADH: cytochrome b₅ reductase and NADPH flavin reductase purified from human erythrocytes. *J Biol Chem* 1980;255:4599.

156. Shibata S, Mijaji T, Iuchi I. Methemoglobin M's of the Japanese. *Bull Yamaguchi Med Sch* 1967;14:141.

157. Shibata S. Hemoglobinopathies in Japan. *Hemoglobin* 1981;5:509.

158. Hayashi A, Suzuki T, Shimizu A, et al. Properties of hemoglobin M: unequivalent nature of the alpha and beta subunits in the hemoglobin molecule. *Biochim Biophys Acta* 1968;168:262.

159. Ranney HM, Nagel RL, Heller P, et al. Oxygen equilibrium of hemoglobin M (Hyde Park). *Biochim Biophys Acta* 1968;160:112.

160. Suzuki T, Hayashi A, Shimizu A, et al. The oxygen equilibrium of hemoglobin M Saskatoon. *Biochim Biophys Acta* 1966;127:280.

161. Suzuki T, Hayashi A, Yamamura Y, et al. Functional abnormality of hemoglobin M. *Biochim Biophys Res Commun* 1965;19:691.

162. Udem L, Ranney HM, Bunn HF, et al. Some observations on the properties of hemoglobin M$_{Milwaukee}$. *J Mol Biol* 1970;48:489.

163. Hayashi A, Suzuki T, Imai K, et al. Properties of hemoglobin M Milwaukee I variant and its unique characteristics. *Biochem Biophys Acta* 1969;194:6.

164. Nagel RL, Bookchin RM. Human hemoglobin mutants with abnormal oxygen binding. *Semin Hematol* 1974;11:385.

165. Moo-Penn WF, Bechtel KC, Schmidt RM, et al. Hemoglobin Raleigh (β1 valine→acetylamine). *Biochemistry* 1977;16:4872.

166. Park CM, Nagel RL. Sulfhemoglobin: clinical and molecular aspects. *N Engl J Med* 1984;310:1579.

167. Park CM, Nagel RL, Blumberg WE, et al. Sulfhemoglobin: properties of partially sulfurated tetramers. *J Biol Chem* 1986;261:8805.

168. Beutler E. Hemoglobinopathies producing cyanosis. In: Williams J, Beutler E, Erslev AJ, et al., eds. *Hematology*. New York: McGraw-Hill, 1983.

169. Finch CA. Methemoglobinemia and sulfhemoglobinemia. *N Engl J Med* 1948; 239:470.

170. Pinkas J, Pjaldetti M, Joshua H, et al. Sulfhemoglobinemia and acute hemolytic anemia with Heinz bodies following contact with a fungicide-zinc ethylanol bisthiocarbamate in a subject with glucose-6-phosphate dehydrogenase deficiency and hypocatalasemia. *Blood* 1963;21:484.

171. Greenberg HB. Syncope and shock due to methemoglobinemia. *Arch Environ Health* 1964;9:762.

172. Darling RC, Roughton FJW. The effect of methemoglobin on the equilibrium between oxygen and hemoglobin. *Am J Physiol* 1942;137:56.

173. Cathie AB. Apparent idiopathic Heinz body anemia. *Great Ormond St J* 1952;3:3.
174. Asakura T, Adachi K, Shapiro M, et al. Mechanical precipitation of hemoglobin Koln. *Biochim Biophys Acta* 1975;412:197.
175. Roth EF Jr, Elbaum D, Bookchin RM, et al. The conformational requirements for the mechanical precipitation of hemoglobin S and other mutants. *Blood* 1976;48:265.
176. Wajcman H, Vasseur C, Blouquit Y, et al. Hemoglobin Redondo [β92(F8)His→Asn]: an unstable hemoglobin variant associated with heme loss which occurs in two forms. *Am J Hematol* 1991;38:194.
177. Robinson AB. Evolution and the distribution of glutamyl and asparaginyl residues in proteins. *Proc Natl Acad Sci U S A* 1974;71:885.
178. George PM, Myles Y, Williamson D, et al. A family with haemolytic anaemia and three beta-globins: the deletion in haemoglobin Atlanta-Coventry (β 75 Leu→Pro, 141 Leu deleted) is not present at the nucleotide level. *Br J Haematol* 1992;81:93.
179. Brennan SO, Shaw J, Allen J, et al. Beta 141 Leu is not deleted in the unstable haemoglobin Atlanta-Coventry but is replaced by a novel amino acid of mass 129 daltons. *Br J Haematol* 1992;81:99.
180. Tucker PW, Phillips SEV, Perutz MF, et al. Structure of hemoglobins Zurich [His E7(63) β→Arg] and Sydney [Val E11(67)→Ala] and role of the distal residues in ligand binding. *Proc Natl Acad Sci U S A* 1978;75:1076.
181. Virshup DM, Zinkham WH, Sirota RL, et al. Unique sensitivity of Hb Zurich to oxidative injury by phenazopyridine: reversal of the effects by elevating carboxyhemoglobin in vivo and in vitro. *Am J Hematol* 1983;14:315.
182. Bratu V, Lorkin PA, Lehmann H, et al. Haemoglobin Buccuresti 42(CD1) Phe→Leu, a cause of unstable haemoglobin haemolytic anaemia. *Biochim Biophys Acta* 1971;251:1.
183. Wajcman H, Leroux A, Labie D. Functional properties of hemoglobin Hammersmith. *Biochimie* 1973;55:119.
184. Honig GR, Vida LN, Rosenblum BB, et al. Hemoglobin Warsaw (Phe beta 42(CD1)→Val), an unstable variant with decreased oxygen affinity: characterization of its synthesis, functional properties, and structure. *J Biol Chem* 1990;265:126.
185. Burkert LB, Sharma VS, Pisciotta AV, et al. Hemoglobin Mequon beta 41 (C7) phenylalanine leads to tyrosine. *Blood* 1976;48:645.
186. Stabler SP, Jones RT, Head C, et al. Hemoglobin Denver [alpha 2 beta 2(41) (C7) Phe→Ser]: a low-O2-affinity variant associated with chronic cyanosis and anemia. *Mayo Clin Proc* 1994;69:237–243.
187. Moo-Penn WF, Jue DL, Johnson MH, et al. Hemoglobin Brockton [beta 138 (H16) Ala→Pro]: an unstable variant near the C-terminus of the beta-subunits with normal oxygen-binding properties. *Biochemistry* 1988;27:7614.
188. Wajcman H, Dahmane M, Prehu C, et al. Haemoglobin J-Biskra: a new mildly unstable alpha1 gene variant with a deletion of eight residues (alpha50-57, alpha51-58 or alpha52-59) including the distal histidine. *Br J Haematol* 1998;100:401–406.
189. Reider RF, Oski FA, Clegg JB. Hemoglobin Philly (β35 tyrosine→phenylalanine): studies in the molecular pathology of hemoglobin. *J Clin Invest* 1969;48:1627.
190. King MAR, Wiltshire BG, Lehmann H, et al. An unstable haemoglobin with reduced oxygen affinity: haemoglobin Peterborough, β111 (G13) valine→phenylalanine, its interaction with normal haemoglobin and with haemoglobin Lepore. *Br J Haematol* 1972;22:125.
191. Como PF, Wylie BR, Trent RJ, et al. A new unstable and low oxygen affinity hemoglobin variant: Hb Stanmore [111(G13)→βAla]. *Hemoglobin* 1991;15:53.
192. Martinez G, Lima F, Colombo B. Haemoglobin J Guantanamo (α₂β₂ 128 (H6) Ala→Asp). A new fast unstable haemoglobin found in a Cuban family. *Biochim Biophys Acta* 1977;491:1.
193. Clegg JB, Weatherall DJ, Boon WH, et al. Two new haemoglobin variants involving proline substitutions. *Nature* 1969;22:379.
194. Brennan SO, Matthews JR. Hb Auckland [alpha 87(F8) His→Asn]: a new mutation of the proximal histidine identified by electrospray mass spectrometry. *Hemoglobin* 1997;21:393–403.
195. Ohba Y. Unstable hemoglobins. *Hemoglobin* 1990;14:353.
196. Ohba Y, Miyaji T, Matsouka M, et al. Hemoglobin Hirosaki [x43(CE1) Phe→Leu]: a new unstable variant. *Biochim Biophys Acta* 1975;405:155.
197. Goosens M, Lee KY, Liebhaber SA, et al. Globin structural mutant α125 Leu→Pro is a novel cause of α-thalassemia. *Nature* 1982;296:864.
198. Ohba Y, Yamamoto K, Hattori Y, et al. Hyperunstable hemoglobin Toyama α₂136 (H19) Leu→Arg β₂: detection and identification by in vitro biosynthesis with radioactive amino acids. *Hemoglobin* 1987;11:539.
199. Tatsis B, Dosik H, Rieder R, et al. Hemoblogin Hasharon: severe hemolytic anemia and hypersplenism associated with a mildly unstable hemoglobin. *Birth Defects* 1972;8:25.
200. Levine RL, Lincoln DR, Buchholz WM, et al. Hemoglobin Hasharon in a premature infant with hemolytic anemia. *Pediatr Res* 1975;9:7.
201. Lee-Potter JP, Deacon-Smith RA, Simpkiss MJ, et al. A new cause of haemolytic anemia in the newborn: a description of an unstable fetal haemoglobin—F Poole ᴳγ 130 Tryptophan→glycine. *J Clin Pathol* 1975;28:317.
202. Schmid R, Brecher G, Clemens T. Familial hemolytic anemia with erythrocyte inclusion bodies and a defect in pigment metabolism. *Blood* 1959;14:991.
203. Eisinger J, Flores J, Tyson JA, et al. Fluorescent cytoplasm and Heinz bodies of Koln erythrocytes: evidence for intracellular heme catabolism. *Blood* 1985;65:886.
204. Koler RD, Jones RT, Bigley RH, et al. Hemoglobin Casper: β106 (G8) Leu→Pro, a contemporary mutation. *Am J Med* 1973;55:549.
205. Nagel RL, Ranney HM. Drug-induced oxidative denaturation of hemoglobin. *Semin Hematol* 1973;10:269.

206. Grimes AJ, Meisler A. Possible cause of Heinz bodies in congenital Heinz body anaemia. *Nature* 1962;194:190.
207. Grimes AJ, Meisler A, Dacie JV. Congenital Heinz-body anaemia: further evidence on the cause of Heinz-body production in red cells. *Br J Haematol* 1964;10:281.
208. Carrell RW, Kay R. A simple method for the detection of unstable hemoglobins. *Br J Haematol* 1972;23:615.
209. Ohba Y, Hattori Y, Yoshinaka H, et al. Urea polyacrylamide gel electrophoresis of PCMB precipitate as a sensitive test for the detection of the unstable hemoglobin subunit. *Clin Chim Acta* 1982;119:179–188.
210. Asakura T, Adachi K, Shapiro M, et al. Mechanical precipitation of hemoglobin Koln. *Biochim Biophys Acta* 1975;412:197.
211. Roth EF Jr, Elbaum D, Bookchin RM, et al. The conformational requirements for the mechanical precipitation of hemoglobin S and other mutants. *Blood* 1976;48:265.
212. Tondo CV, Mendez HM, Reischl E. Thermostability of hemoglobins in homeothermic and non-homeothermic vertebrates. *Comp Biochem Physiol* 1980;66B:151.
213. Borgese TA, Harrington J, Borgese JM, et al. Thermostability of fish hemoglobins. *Comp Biochem Physiol* 1982;72B:7.
214. Perutz MF. Electrostatic effects in proteins. *Science* 1978;201:1187.
215. Bigelow C. On the average hydrophobicity of proteins and the relation between it and protein structure. *J Theor Biol* 1967;16:187.
216. Kauzmann W. Some factors in the interpretation of protein denaturation. *Adv Protein Chem* 1959;14:1.
217. Argos P, Rossman MG, Grau UM, et al. Thermal stability and protein structure. *Biochemistry* 1979;18:5698.
218. Perutz MF, Raidt H. Stereochemical bases of heat stability in bacterial ferredoxins and in hemoglobin A₂. *Nature* 1975;255:256.
219. Bunn FH, Jandl JH. Exchange of heme among hemoglobins and between hemoglobin and albumin. *J Biol Chem* 1968;243:465.
220. Brooks J. The oxidation of haemoglobin to methaemoglobin by oxygen, II. The relation between the rate of oxidation and the partial pressure of oxygen. *Proc R Soc Lond B Biol Sci* 1935;118:560.
221. Gurd FRN, Falk KE, Malstrom BG, et al. The conformational transition of sperm whale ferrimyoglobin in the presence of several equivalents of cupric ion. *J Biol Chem* 1967;242:5731.
222. Bemski G, Arends T, Blanc G. Electron spin resonance of Cu (II) in copper hemoglobin complexes. *Biochem Biophys Res Commun* 1969;35:599.
223. Nagel RL, Bemski G, Pincus P. Some aspects of the binding of Cu (II) to human hemoglobin and its subunits. *Arch Biochem Biophys* 1970;137:428.
224. Rifkind J. Copper and the autoxidation of hemoglobin. *Biochemistry* 1974;13:2475.
225. Winterbourne CC, Carrell RW. Oxidation of human hemoglobin by copper. *Biochem J* 1977;165:141.
226. Mansouri A, Winterhalter KH. Nonequivalence of chains in hemoglobin oxidation. *Biochemistry* 1973;12:4946.
227. Jacob HS, Winterhalter KH. The role of hemoglobin heme loss in Heinz body formation: studies with a partially heme-deficient hemoglobin and with genetically unstable hemoglobin. *J Clin Invest* 1970;49:2008.
228. Jacob HS, Winterhalter KH. Unstable hemoglobins: the role of heme loss in Heinz body formation. *Proc Natl Acad Sci U S A* 1970;65:697.
229. Rachmilewitz EA, Peisach J, Blumberg WE. Studies on the stability of oxyhemoglobin A and its constituent chains and their derivatives. *J Biol Chem* 1971;246:3356.
230. Rachmilewitz EA, Harari E. Intermediate hemichrome formation after oxidation of three unstable hemoglobins (Freiburg, Riverdale-Bronx and Koln). *Haematol Bluttransfus* 1972;10:241.
231. Rachmilewitz EA, White JM. Haemichrome formation during the in vitro oxidation of haemoglobin Koln. *Nature* 1973;241:115.
232. Rachmilewitz EA. Denaturation of the normal and abnormal hemoglobin molecule. *Semin Hematol* 1974;11:441.
233. Peisach J, Blumberg WE, Rachmilewitz EA. The demonstration of ferrihemochrome intermediates in Heinz body formation following the reduction of oxyhemoglobin A by acetylphenylhydrazine. *Biochem Biophys Acta* 1975;393:404.
234. Winterbourne CC, Carrell RW. Studies of hemoglobin denaturation and Heinz body formation in the unstable hemoglobins. *J Clin Invest* 1974;54:678.
235. Winterbourne CC, McGrath BM, Carrell RW. Reactions involving superoxide and normal and unstable haemoglobins. *Biochem J* 1976;155:503.
236. Rifkind RA. Heinz body anemia: an ultrastructural study, II. Red cell sequestration and destruction. *Blood* 1965;26:433.
237. Schnitzer B, Rucknagel DL, Spencer HH, et al. Erythrocytes: pits and vacuoles as seen with transmission and scanning electron microscopy. *Science* 1971;173:251.
238. Winterbourne CC, Carrell RW. Characterization of Heinz bodies in unstable haemoglobin haemolytic anaemia. *Nature* 1972;240:150.
239. Chan E, Desforges J. Role of disulfide bonds in Heinz body attachment to membranes. *Blood* 1974;44:921.
240. Low P. Interaction of native and denatured hemoglobins with band 3: consequences for erythrocyte structure and function. In: Agre P, Parker JC, eds. *Red blood cell membranes*. New York: Marcel Dekker, 1989.
241. Low PS, Westfall MA, Allen DP, et al. Characterization of the reversible conformational equilibrium of the cytoplasmic domain of erythrocyte membrane band 3. *J Biol Chem* 1984;259:13070.
242. Waugh SM, Low PS. Hemichrome binding to band 3: nucleation of Heinz bodies on the erythrocyte membrane. *Biochemistry* 1985;24:34.

243. Cho N, Song S, Asher SA. UV resonance Raman and excited-state relaxation rate studies of hemoglobin. *Biochemistry* 1994;33:5932.

244. Fisher S, Nagel RL, Bookchin RM, et al. The binding of hemoglobin to membranes of normal and sickle erythrocytes. *Biochim Biophys Acta* 1975;375:422.

245. Shaklai N, Sharma VS, Ranney HM. Interaction of sickle cell hemoglobin with erythrocyte membrane. *Proc Natl Acad Sci U S A* 1981;78:65.

246. Reiss GH, Ranney HM, Shaklai N. Association of Hb C with erythrocyte ghosts. *J Clin Invest* 1982;70:946.

247. Walder JA, Chatterjee R, Steck T, et al. The interaction of hemoglobin with the cytoplasmic domain of band 3 of the human erythrocyte membrane. *J Biol Chem* 1984;259:10238.

248. Jandl JH, Simmons RL, Castle WB. Red cell filtration and the pathogenesis of certain hemolytic anemias. *Blood* 1961;18:133.

249. Miller DR, Weed RI, Stamatoyannopoulos G, et al. Hemoglobin Koln disease occurring as a fresh mutation: erythrocyte metabolism and survival. *Blood* 1971;38:715.

250. Chou AC, Fitch CD. Mechanism of hemolysis induced by ferriprotoporphyrin IX. *J Clin Invest* 1981;68:672.

251. Allen DW, Burgoyne CF, Groat JD, et al. Comparison of hemoglobin Koln erythrocyte membranes with malondialdehyde-reacted normal erythrocyte membranes. *Blood* 1984;64:1263.

252. Flynn TP, Allen DW, Johnson GJ, et al. Oxidant damage of the lipids and proteins of the erythrocyte membranes in unstable hemoglobin disease: evidence for the role of lipid peroxidation. *J Clin Invest* 1983;71:1215.

253. Jacob HS, Brain MK, Dacie JV. Altered sulfhydryl reactivity of hemoglobins and red blood cell membranes in congenital Heinz body hemolytic anemia. *J Clin Invest* 1968;47:2664.

254. DeFuria FG, Miller DR. Oxygen affinity in hemoglobin Koln disease. *Blood* 1972;39:398.

255. Goosens M, Lee KY, Liebhaber SA, et al. Globin structural mutant α125 Leu→Pro is a novel cause of α-thalassemia. *Nature* 1982;296:864.

256. Adams JG III, Boxer LA, Baehner RL, et al. Hemoglobin Indianapolis (β112[G14]→arginine): an unstable β-chain variant producing the phenotype of severe β-thalassemia. *Nature* 1982;296:864.

257. Adams JG, Steinberg MH, Boxer LA, et al. The structure of hemoglobin Indianapolis (β 112 [G14]→arginine): an unstable variant detectable only by isotopic labeling. *J Biol Chem* 1979;254.

258. Kolski GB, Miller DR. Heme synthesis in hereditary hemolytic anemias: decreased–amino-levulinic acid synthetase in hemoglobin Koln disease. *Pediatr Res* 1976;10:702.

259. Rieder RF. Synthesis of hemoglobin Gun Hill: increased synthesis of the heme-free β^{GH} globin chain and subunit exchange with a free alpha chain pool. *J Clin Invest* 1971;50:388.

260. Bradley TB, Wohl RC, Rieder RF. Hemoglobin Gun Hill: deletion of five amino acid residues and impaired heme-globin binding. *Science* 1967;157:1581.

261. Kobayashi Y, Fukumaki Y, Komatsu N, et al. A novel globin structural mutant, Showa-Yakushiji (beta 110 Leu-Pro) causing a beta-thalessemia phenotype. *Blood* 1987;70:1688–1691.

262. Coleman MB, Steinberg MH, Adams JG III. Hemoglobin Terre Haute arginine beta 106: a posthumous correction to the original structure of hemoglobin Indianapolis. *J Biol Chem* 1991;266:5798–5800.

263. Kazazian HH Jr, Dowling CE, Hurwitz RL, et al. Dominant thalassemia-like phenotypes associated with mutations in exon 3 of the beta-globin gene. *Blood* 1992;79:3014–3018.

264. Ristaldi MS, Pirastu M, Murru S, et al. A spontaneous mutation produced a novel elongated beta-globin chain structural variant (Hb Agnana) with a thalassemia-like phenotype. *Blood* 1990;75:1378–1379.

265. Traeger-Synodinos J, Papassotiriou I, Metaxotou-Mavrommati A, et al. Distinct phenotypic expression associated with a new hyperunstable alpha globin variant (Hb Heraklion, alpha1cd37(C2)Pro→0): comparison to other alpha-thalassemic hemoglobinopathies. *Blood Cells Mol Dis* 2000;26:276.

266. Kneezel LD, Kitchens CS. Phenacetin-induced sulfhemoglobinemia: report of a case and review of the literature. *Johns Hopkins Med J* 1967;139:175.

267. Brandenburg RO, Smith HL. Sulfhemoglobinemia: a study of 62 clinical cases. *Am Heart J* 1951;42:582.

268. Cumming RLC, Pollock A. Drug-induced sulfhaemoglobinemia and Heinz body anemia in pregnancy with involvement of the foetus. *Scott Med J* 1967;12:320.

269. Reynolds TB, Ware AG. Sulfhemoglobinemia following habitual use of acetanilid. *JAMA* 1952;149:1538.

270. Evans AS, Enzer N, Eder HA, et al. Hemolytic anemia with paroxysmal methemoglobinemia and sulfhemoglobinemia. *Arch Intern Med* 1950;86:22.

271. Lambert M, Sonnet J, Mahien P, et al. Delayed sulfhemoglobinemia after acute dapsone intoxication. *Clin Toxicol* 1982;19:45.

272. Ford R, Shkov J, Akman WV, et al. Deaths from asphyxia among fishermen. *MMWR Morb Mortal Wkly Rep* 1978;27:309.

273. Medeiros M, Bechara EJ, Naoum PC, et al. Oxygen toxicity and hemoglobinemia in subjects from a highly polluted town. *Arch Environ Health* 1983;38:11.

274. Carrico RJ, Blumberg WE, Peisach J. The reversible binding of oxygen to sulfhemoglobin. *J Biol Chem* 1978;253:7212.

275. Nichol AW, Hendry I, Movell DB, et al. Mechanism of formation of sulfhemoglobin. *Biochim Biophys Acta* 1968;156:97.

276. Kiese M. The biochemical production of ferrihemoglobin-forming derivatives from aromatic amines and mechanisms of ferrihemoglobin formation. *Pharmacol Rev* 1966;18:1091.

277. Gibson GA, Douglas CC. Microbic cyanosis. *Lancet* 1906;2:72.

278. McCutcheon AD. Sulfhaemoglobinaemia and glutathione. *Lancet* 1960;2:290.

279. Suzuki T, Hayshi A, Shimizu A, et al. The oxygen equilibrium of hemoglobin M Saskatoon. *Biochim Biophys Acta* 1966;127:280.

280. Basch F. On hydrogen sulfide poisoning from external application of elementary sulfur as an ointment. *Arch Exp Pathol Pharmacol* 1926;111:126.

281. Glud TK. Complete recovery from acquired met- and sulfhemoglobinemia following treatment with neomycin and bacitracin. *Ugeskr Laeger* 1979;141:1410.

282. Burnett E, King EG, Grace M, et al. Hydrogen sulfide poisoning: review of 5 years' experience. *Can Med Assoc J* 1977;117:1277.

283. Baker CH, Sutton ET, Davis DL. Microvessel mean transit time and blood flow velocity of sulfhemoglobin-RBC. *Am J Physiol* 1980;238:745.

284. Beutler E, Milcus BJ. The effect of methemoglobin formation in sickle cell disease. *J Clin Invest* 1961;40:1856.

285. Gibson QH. The reduction of methaemoglobinaemia in red blood cells and studies on the cause of idiopathic methaemoglobinaemia. *Biochem J* 1948; 42:13–23.

286. Jaffe ER. Methemoglobinemia in the differential diagnosis of cyanosis. *Hosp Pract* 1985;20:92.

287. Scott EM. The relation of diaphorase of human erythrocytes to inheritance of methemoglobinemia. *J Clin Invest* 1960;39:1176.

288. Passon PG, Hultquist DE. Soluble cytochrome b5 reductase from human erythrocytes. *Biochim Biophys Acta* 1972;275:62.

289. Beauvais P, Kaplan JC. La methemoglobinemie congenitale recessive: etude de huit cas avec encephalopathie—nouvelle conception nosologique. *J Pediatr* 1978;10:145.

290. Kaplan JC, Leroux A, Beauvais P. Formes cliniques et biologiques de déficit en cytochrome b5 réductase. *C R Seances Soc Biol* 1979;173:368.

291. Kaplan JC, Leroux A, Bakouri S, et al. La lésion enzymatique dans la méthémoglobinemie congénital récessive avec encephalopathie. *Nouv Rev Fr Hematol* 1974;14:755.

292. Leroux A, Junien C, Kaplan JC, et al. Generalised deficiency of cytochrome b5 reductase in congenital methaemoglobinaemia with mental retardation. *Nature* 1975;258:619.

293. Arnold H, Botcher HW, Hufnagel D, et al. Hereditary methemoglobinemia due to methemoglobin reductase deficiency in erythrocytes and leukocytes without neurological symptoms. In: *Abstracts of the XVII Congress of the International Society of Hematology, Paris, 1978* (abst 752).

294. Tanishima K, Tanimoto K, Tomoda A, et al. Hereditary methemoglobinemia due to cytochrome b5 reductase deficiency in blood cells without associated neurologic and mental disorders. *Blood* 1985;66:1288.

295. Hegesh E, Avron M. The enzymatic reduction of ferrihemoglobin. II. Purification of a ferrihemoglobin reductase from human erythrocytes. *Biochim Biophys Acta* 1967;146:397.

296. Yubisui T, Takeshita M. Characterization of the purified NAH-cytochrome b5 reductase of human erythrocytes as a FAD-containing enzyme. *J Biol Chem* 1980;255:2454.

297. Ozols J, Korza G, Heinemann FS, et al. Complete amino acid sequence of steer liver microsomal NADH-cytochrome b$_5$ reductase. *J Biol Chem* 1985;260:11953.

298. Tomatsu S, Kobayashi Y, Fukumaki Y, et al. The organization and the complete nucleotide sequence of the human NADH-cytochrome b5 reductase gene. *Gene* 1989;80:353.

299. Katsube T, Sakamoto N, Kobayashi Y, et al. Exonic point mutations in NADH-cytochrome B$_5$ reductase genes of homozygotes for hereditary methemoglobinemia, types I and III: putative mechanisms of tissue-dependent enzyme deficiency. *Am J Hum Genet* 1991;48:799.

300. Yubisui T, Murakami K, Shirabe K, et al. Structural analysis of NADH-cytochrome B$_5$ reductase in relation to hereditary methemoglobinemia. In: Brewer GJ, ed. *The red cell.* New York: Alan R Liss, 1989;107.

301. Zenno S, Hattori M, Misumi Y, et al. Molecular cloning of a cDNA inducting rat NADH cytochrome B$_5$ reductase and the corresponding gene. *Biochem J (Tokyo)* 1990;107:810.

302. Kobayashi Y, Fukumaki Y, Yubuisi T, et al. Serine-proline replacement at residue 127 of NADH-cytochrome B$_5$ reductase causes hereditary methemoglobinemia, generalized type. *Blood* 1990;75:1408.

303. Hiono H. Lipids of myelin, white matter and gray matter in a case of generalized deficiency of cytochrome B$_5$ reductase in congenital methemoglobinemia with mental retardation. *Lipids* 1980;15:272.

304. Gacon G, Lostanlen D, Labie D, et al. Interaction between cytochrome B$_5$ and hemoglobin: involvement of β66(E10) and β95(FG2) lysyl residues of hemoglobin. *Proc Natl Acad Sci U S A* 1980;77:1917.

305. Poulos TL, Mauk AG. Models of the complexes formed between cytochrome b$_5$ and the subunits of methemoglobin. *J Biol Chem* 1983;258:7369.

306. Hojas-Bernal R, McNab-Martin P, Fairbanks VF, et al. Hb Chile [beta28(B10)Leu→Met]: an unstable hemoglobin associated with chronic methemoglobinemia and sulfonamide or methylene blue-induced hemolytic anemia. *Hemoglobin* 1999;23:125–134.

307. Thillet J, Cohen-Solal M, Seligmann M, et al. Functional and physicochemical studies of hemoglobin St. Louis beta 28 (B10) Leu replaced by Gln: a variant with ferric beta heme iron. *J Clin Invest* 1976;58:1098–1106.

308. Korber E. Inaugural dissertation: Uber differenzen Blutfarbstoffes: Dorpat, 1866. In: Bischoff H, ed. *Z Exp Med* 1926;48:472.

309. Jope EM. The ultra-violet spectral absorption of haemoglobin inside and outside the red blood cell. In: Roughton FJW, Kendrew JC, eds. *Haemoglobin.* London: Butterworths, 1949:205.

310. Schroeder WA, Shelton JR, Shelton JB, et al. The amino acid sequence of the α-chain of human fetal hemoglobin. *Biochemistry* 1963;2:992.

311. Schroeder WA, Huisman THJ, Efremov GD, et al. Further studies on the frequency and significance of the $^T\alpha$ chain of human fetal hemoglobin. *J Clin Invest* 1979;63:268.

312. Slightom JL, Blechl AE, Smithies O. Human fetal $^G\gamma$- and $^A\gamma$-globin genes: complete nucleotide sequences suggest that DNA can be exchanged between these duplicated genes. *Cell* 1980;21:627.

313. Bouhassira EE, Lachman H, Krishnamoorthy R, et al. A gene conversion located 5' to the A gamma gene is in linkage disequilibrium with the Bantu haplotype in sickle cell anemia. *J Clin Invest* 1989;83:2070.

314. Frier JA, Perutz M. Structure of human foetal deoxyhemoglobin. *J Mol Biol* 1977;112:97.

315. Allen DW, Wyman J, Smith CA. The oxygen equilibrium of foetal and adult human hemoglobin. *J Biol Chem* 1953;203:81.

316. Tyuma I, Shimizu K. Different response to organic phosphates of human fetal and adult hemoglobins. *Arch Biochem Biophys* 1969;129:404.

317. Schroeder WA, Cua JT, Matsuda G, et al. Hemoglobin F_1, an acetyl-containing hemoglobin. *Biochim Biophys Acta* 1962;63:532.

318. Poyart C, Bursaux E, Guesnon P, et al. Chloride binding and Bohr effect of human fetal erythrocytes and HbF_{II} solutions. *Pfluegers Arch* 1978;37:169.

319. Gros G, Bauer C. High pK value of the N-terminal amino group of the γ chains causes low CO_2 binding of human fetal hemoglobin. *Biochem Biophys Res Commun* 1978;80:56.

320. Wardle SP, Yoxall CW, Weindling AM. Determinants of cerebral fractional oxygen extraction using near infrared spectroscopy in preterm neonates. *J Cereb Blood Flow Metab* 2000;20:272–279.

321. Bursaux E, Poyart C, Guesnon P, et al. Comparative effects of CO_2 on the affinity for O_2 of fetal and adult hemoglobins. *Pfluegers Arch* 1979;378:197.

322. Miyoshi K, Kaneto Y, Kawai H, et al. X-linked dominant control of F-cells in normal adult life: characterization of the Swiss type as hereditary persistence of fetal hemoglobin regulated dominantly by gene(s) on X chromosome. *Blood* 1988;72:1854.

323. Pembrey ME, Weatherall DJ, Clegg JB. Maternal synthesis of haemoglobin F in pregnancy. *Lancet* 1973;16:1351.

324. Huehns ER, Hecht F, Keil JV, et al. Developmental hemoglobin anomalies in a chromosomal triplication: D_1 trisomy syndrome. *Proc Natl Acad Sci U S A* 1964;51:89.

325. Wood WG, Stamatoyannopoulos G, Lim G, et al. F-cells in the adult: normal values and levels in individuals with hereditary and acquired elevations of Hb F. *Blood* 1975;46:671.

326. Boyer SH, Belding TK, Margolet L, et al. Variations in the frequency of fetal hemoglobin-bearing erythrocytes (F-cells) in well adults, pregnant women, and adult leukemics. *Johns Hopkins Med J* 1975;137:105.

327. Chang YC, Smith KD, Moore RD, et al. An analysis of fetal hemoglobin variation in sickle cell disease: the relative contributions of the X-linked factor, β-globin haplotypes, β-globin gene number, gender, and age. *Blood* 1995;85:1111–1117.

328. Thein SL, Sampietro M, Rohde K, et al. Detection of a major gene for heterocellular hereditary persistence of fetal hemoglobin after accounting for genetic modifiers. *Am J Hum Genet* 1994;54:214–228.

329. Thein SL, Craig JE. Genetics of Hb F/F cell variance in adults and heterocellular hereditary persistence of fetal hemoglobin. *Hemoglobin* 1998;22:401–414.

330. Craig JE, Rochette J, Sampietro M, et al. Genetic heterogeneity in heterocellular hereditary persistence of fetal hemoglobin. *Blood* 1997;90:428–434.

331. Garner C, Tatu T, Reittie J, et al. Twins en route to QTL mapping for heterocellular HPFH. *Blood* 1998;92:694a.

332. Zon LI, Tsai SF, Burgess S, et al. The major human erythroid DNA-binding protein (GF-1): primary sequence and localization of the gene to the X chromosome. *Proc Natl Acad Sci U S A* 1990;87:668–672.

333. Kleinhauer E, Braun H, Betke K. Demonstration von fetalem Hamoglobin in den Erythrozyten eines Blutausstrichs. *Klin Wochenschr* 1957;35:637.

334. Dover GJ, Boyer SH, Bell WR. Microscopic method for assaying F cell production: illustrative changes during infancy and in aplastic anemia. *Blood* 1978;52:664.

335. Dover GJ, Boyer SH, Pembrey ME. F cell production in sickle cell anemia: regulation by genes linked to β-hemoglobin locus. *Science* 1981;211:1441.

336. Dover GJ, Boyer SH, Charache S, et al. Individual variation in the production and survival of F-cells in sickle cell disease. *N Engl J Med* 1978;299:1428.

337. Winters WP, Seale WR, Yodh J. Interaction of hemoglobin S with anionic polysaccharides. *Am J Pediatr Hematol Oncol* 1984;6:77.

338. Newman DR, Pierre RV, Linman JW. Studies on the diagnostic significance of hemoglobin F levels. *Mayo Clin Proc* 1973;48:199.

339. Priest JR, Watterson J, Jones RT, et al. Mutant fetal hemoglobin causing cyanosis in a newborn. *Pediatrics* 1989;83:734.

340. Glader BE. Hemoglobin FM-Fort Ripley: another lesson from the neonate. *Pediatrics* 1989;83:792.

341. Hayashi A, Fujita T, Fujimura M, et al. A new fetal hemoglobin, HbF M Osaka ($\alpha_2\gamma_2$ 63 His→Leu): a mutant with high oxygen affinity and erythrocytosis. *Am J Clin Pathol* 1979;72:1028.

342. Harano T, Harano K, Doi K, et al. HbF-Onoda or $\alpha_2\gamma_2$146(HC3)His→Tyr, a newly discovered fetal hemoglobin variant in a Japanese newborn. *Hemoglobin* 1990;14:217.

343. Huisman THJ. The human fetal hemoglobins. *Texas Rep Biol Med* 1980–1981;40:29–42.

344. Fischer S, Nagel RL, Bookchin RM, et al. The binding of hemoglobin to membranes of normal and sickle erythrocytes. *Biochim Biophys Acta* 1975;375:422.

345. Codrington JF, Kutlar F, Harris HF, et al. Hb A_2-Wrens or $\alpha_2\gamma_2$^{G} 98(FG5) Val→Met, an unstable chain variant identified by sequence analysis of amplified DNA. *Biochim Biophys Acta* 1989;1009:87.

346. Garcia CR, Navarro JL, Lam H, et al. Hb A_2-Manzanares or $\alpha_2\gamma_2$^{G} 121(GH4) Glu→Val, an unstable chain variant observed in a Spanish family. *Hemoglobin* 1983;7:435.

347. Salkie ML, Gordon PA, Rigal WM, et al. Hb A_2-Canada or $\alpha_2\gamma_2$^{G} 99(G1) Asp→Asn: a newly discovered chain variant with increased oxygen affinity occurring in cis to β-thalassemia. *Hemoglobin* 1982;6:223.

348. Baglioni C. The fusion of two peptide chains in hemoglobin Lepore and its interpretation as a genetic deletion. *Proc Natl Acad Sci U S A* 1962;48:1880–1886.

349. Flavell RA, Kooter JM, De Boer E, et al. Analysis of the beta-delta-globin gene loci in normal and Hb Lepore DNA: direct determination of gene linkage and intergene distance. *Cell* 1978;15:25–41.

350. Mears JG, Ramirez F, Leibowitz D, et al. Organization of human delta- and beta-globin genes in cellular DNA and the presence of intragenic inserts. *Cell* 1978;15:15–23.

351. Huehns ER, Dance N, Beaven GH, et al. Human embryonic hemoglobins. *Cold Spring Harb Symp Quant Biol* 1964a;19:327–331.

352. Luo HY, Liang XL, Frye C, et al. Embryonic hemoglobins are expressed in definitive cells. *Blood* 1999;94:359–361.

353. Stamatoyannopoulos G, Constantoulakis P, Brice M, et al. Coexpression of embryonic, fetal, and adult globins in erythroid cells of human embryos: relevance to the cell-lineage models of globin switching. *Dev Biol* 1987;123:191–197.

354. Leder A, Kuo A, Shen MM, et al. In situ hybridization reveals co-expression of embryonic and adult alpha globin genes in the earliest murine erythrocyte progenitors. *Development* 1992;116:1041–1049.

355. Hoffmann OM, Brittain T, Wells RM. The control of oxygen affinity in the three human embryonic haemoglobins by respiration linked metabolites. *Biochem Mol Biol Int* 1997;42:553–566.

356. Hoffmann OM, Brittain T. Ligand binding kinetics and dissociation of the human embryonic haemoglobins. *Biochem J* 1996;315:65–70.

356a. Bonaventura C, Arumugam M, Cashon R, et al. Chloride masks effects of opposing positive charges in Hb A and Hb Hinsdale (beta 139 Asn→Lys) that can modulate cooperativity as well as oxygen affinity. *J Mol Biol* 1994;239:561–568.

357. Perutz M, Fermi G, Poyart C, et al. A novel allosteric mechanism in haemoglobin: structure of bovine deoxy-haemoglobin, absence of specific chloride-binding sites and origin of the chloride-linked Bohr effect in bovine and human haemoglobin. *J Mol Biol* 1993;233:536–545.

358. Hoffman O, Currucan G, Robson N, et al. The chloride effect in the human embryonic haemoglobins. *Biochem J* 1995;309:959–962.

359. Sutherland-Smith AJ, Baker HM, Hoffmann OM, et al. Crystal structure of human embryonic haemoglobin: the carbon monoxide for Gower II (alpha2epsilon2) haemoglobin at 2.9 Å resolution. *J Mol Biol* 1998;280:475–484.

360. Hoffmann OM, Brittain T. Partitioning of oxygen and carbon monoxide in the three human embryonic hemoglobins. *Hemoglobin* 1998;22:313–319.

361. Robson N, Brittain T. Heme stability in the human embryonic hemoglobins. *J Inorg Biochem* 1996;64:137–147.

362. He Z, Russell JE. Expression, purification, and characterization of human hemoglobins Gower-1 (zeta(2)epsilon(2)), Gower-2 (alpha(2)epsilon(2)), and Portland-2 (zeta(2)beta(2)) assembled in complex transgenic-knockout mice. *Blood* 2001;97:1099–1105.

363. Ireland JH, Luo HY, Chui DH, et al. Detection of the (-SEA) double alpha-globin gene deletion by a simple immunologic assay for embryonic zeta-globin chains. *Am J Hematol* 1993;44:22–28.

364. Dickerson RE, Geis I. *Hemoglobin: structure, function, evolution, and pathology.* Menlo Park, CA: Benjamin/Cummings, 1983.

365. Imai K. *Allosteric effects in haemoglobin.* Cambridge: Cambridge University Press, 1982.

366. Kilmartin JV, Wootton JF. Inhibition of Bohr effect after removal of C-terminal histidines from haemoglobin β chains. *Nature* 1970;228:766.

367. Williamson D, Brennan SO, Muir H, et al. Hemoglobin Collingwood beta 60 (E4) Val replaced by Ala: a new unstable hemoglobin. *Hemoglobin* 1983;7:511.

CHAPTER 50

Sickle Syndromes

Orah S. Platt

The sickle mutation is a single base change (A to T) in the middle of the triplet that codes for glutamic acid as the sixth amino acid of the hemoglobin β-chain (Fig. 50-1). This mutation substitutes valine (Val) for glutamic acid (Glu) and is common among people whose origins are in areas where malaria has been endemic (Fig. 50-2). Nagel and Flemming reviewed the worldwide distribution of the sickle gene and the influence of malaria, spontaneous mutation, and migration (most often forced by slave trade) (1). In the various populations of equatorial Africa, the gene frequency ranges from 5% to more than 14%; it is approximately 4% among Caribbean people, Europeans, and North and South Americans of African descent. The sickle gene is also indigenous to Sicily (2–4), Greece (5,6), India (7–13), Saudi Arabia (14,15), Israel (16), Turkey (17), and Iran (18).

Studies of β-gene cluster polymorphisms from different populations suggest that the sickle mutation arose at least five times, each in the context of a different ancient β haplotype (Fig. 50-2). In Africa, there are three major sickle haplotypes, each associated with a particular geographic region: Senegal (Atlantic west Africa), Benin (central west Africa), and Bantu [also called CAR (Central African Republic)] (19). The relative geographic isolation and certain structural features of the 5'-flanking region of these β genes support the hypothesis that they are independent mutations and not recombination events (20). The Benin type is the most widely dispersed, found not only in Benin but also in Ibadan (21), Algeria (19,22), Sicily (23–25), Turkey (26), Greece (5), Yemen, and southwest Saudi Arabia (21). A fourth haplotype is described in a small population found in the Cameroon (27). Among Jamaican and American sickle cell patients of African heritage, approximately 50% to 70% of chromosomes are Benin, 15% to 30% are Bantu-CAR, and 5% to 15% are Senegal. In Africa, the geographic isolation is strong, and virtually all patients are homozygous for a given haplotype. Nagel and co-workers (28,29) document that different homozygotes have different hematologic characteristics. The Bantu-CAR and Senegalese patients have higher levels of fetal hemoglobin and fewer dense cells compared with Beninians. The Senegalese have a high proportion of γ^G fetal hemoglobin; the Bantu-CAR and Beninians do not. In contrast to what is found among Africans living in Africa, African Americans are mainly heterozygotes. In Los Angeles, 38% of patients are Benin homozygotes (Benin/Benin); 25% are Benin/Bantu-CAR; 13% are Benin/Senegal; 5% are Bantu-CAR homozygotes; and 3% are Bantu-CAR/Senegal (30). There is some evidence to suggest that these haplotypes influence overall clinical severity, with the Bantu-

CAR being the most and the Senegalese being the least severely affected (31).

A fifth haplotype is found in India and parts of Saudi Arabia (21). In Riyadh, Saudi Arabia, all patients with sickle cell anemia are from southwest Saudi Arabia and Yemen and are homozygous Benin. In the eastern oases of Saudi Arabia, the African haplotypes are not seen; an Arab-Indian haplotype is the only one associated with the sickle mutation. This haplotype is also seen in patients from Orissa, India (whether they are of tribal origin or not) and Poona, India. Patients from these regions have long been recognized as having mild disease and elevated levels of fetal hemoglobin (32–40). The Arab-Indian and Senegalese haplotypes are both associated with elevated fetal hemoglobin and, as seen in Figure 50-2, are structurally similar in the regions near and in the γ genes.

MALARIA AND SICKLING

Nagel and Roth (41) and Weatherall (42) have reviewed the impact of malaria on the prevalence of genetic red cell disorders and the impact of those disorders on the malaria parasite. Two observations on the epidemiology of malaria in Africa support the concept of balanced polymorphism: (a) children with the sickle cell trait are less likely to die from Plasmodium falciparum than children without the trait (43), and (b) the prevalence of the trait increases with age (44). Balanced polymorphism correctly predicts that because those with the sickle trait have a selective advantage, the prevalence of the trait rises in endemic areas until it is offset by the early death of patients with homozygous disease. It is important to emphasize that this selective advantage translates into a lower death rate for individuals with the trait—it does not mean that individuals with the sickle trait are less likely to develop malaria in the first place. It also does not mean that individuals with sickle cell anemia have an advantage when it comes to malaria: As with other overwhelming infections, patients with sickle cell anemia have a high death rate from malaria.

In humans, P. falciparum has exoerythrocytic and intraerythrocytic phases. It is presumably the intraerythrocytic phase that is affected by sickle hemoglobin. Deoxygenated sickle trait red cells containing P. falciparum are more likely to sickle than unparasitized cells (45,46). Sickling probably accelerates removal of these cells and their parasites from the circulation. In addition, the loss of potassium, water, or both that accompanies sickling may provide an inhospitable environment for the parasite (47). In culture, oxygenated trait cells support the growth of P. falciparum,

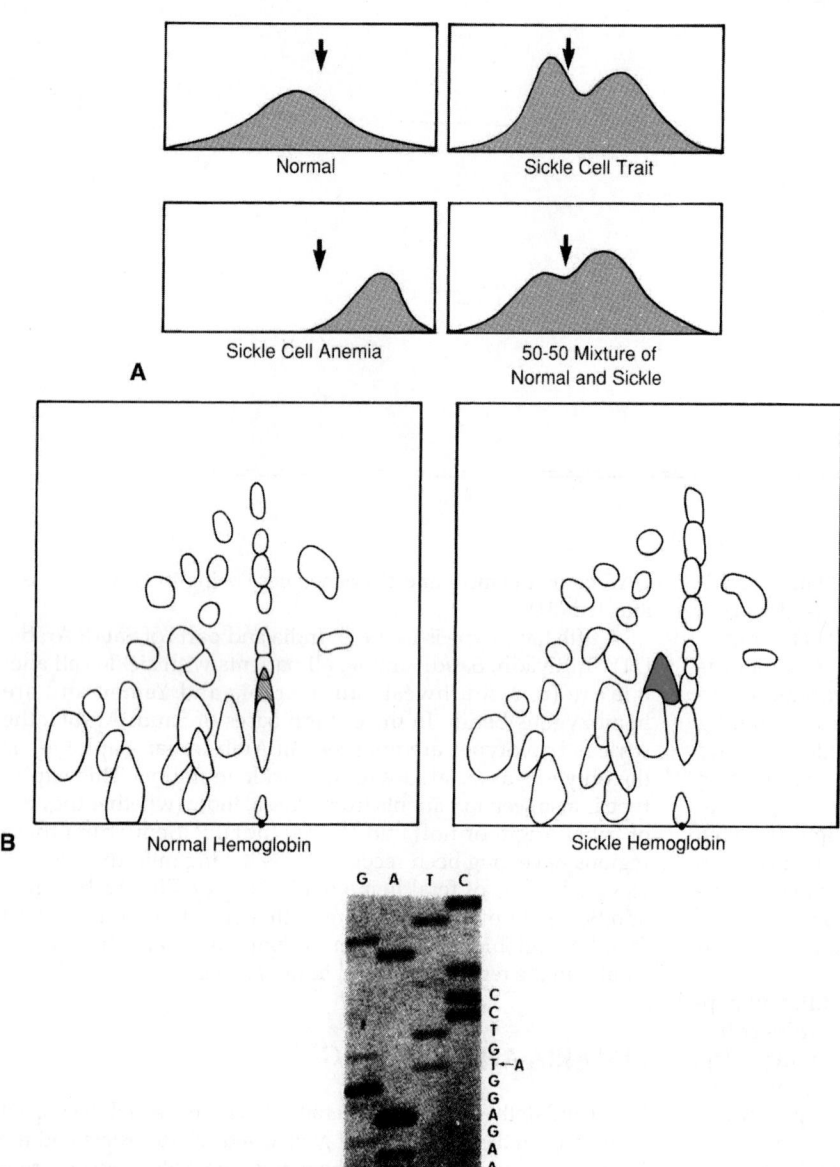

Figure 50-1. History of the investigation of the sickle mutation. **A:** Hemoglobin electrophoresis: the first demonstration of the abnormal electrophoretic mobility of sickle hemoglobin. **B:** Hemoglobin fingerprinting: the classic globin "fingerprint," demonstrating the specific peptide abnormality (*shaded peptide*) of sickle hemoglobin. **C:** β-Globin sequencing gel of sickle β-globin DNA. [**(A)** from Pauling L, Itano HA, Singer SJ, et al. Sickle cell anemia: a molecular disease. *Science* 1949;110:543; and **(B)** from Ingram VM. A specific chemical difference between globins of normal human and sickle cell anaemia hemoglobin. *Nature* 1956;178:792, with permission.]

whereas deoxygenated trait cells do not (48,49). The parasites may die because they are unable to metabolize polymerized hemoglobin (50) or because they get skewered by it (51). Many of the ambiguities regarding the precise mechanism by which sickle hemoglobin protects against malaria are related to the logistics of studying malaria *in vitro*. The recent observations that transgenic mice expressing human sickle hemoglobin are partially protected from malaria will allow these obstacles to be overcome (52,53).

SICKLE HEMOGLOBIN POLYMER

The critical early work of Hahn and Gillespie (54), Ham and Castle (55), and Harris (56) contributed to our knowing that deoxygenation causes sickle hemoglobin to polymerize. This fundamental fact remains at the center of our concept of the pathophysiology of the disease. The fascinating history of the early clinical and scientific discoveries in the field are beautifully described by Conley (57). The basic unit of sickle hemoglobin polymerization is the fiber, which is responsible for the viscosity and shape changes characteristic of sickle red cells.

Understanding the fine structure of the fiber and the factors that influence its formation is central to understanding the clinical manifestations of the disease and to designing rational therapy.

Structure of the Sickle Hemoglobin Fiber

ELECTRON MICROSCOPY

Electron microscopy has proved to be one of the most powerful tools in dissecting the anatomy of the sickle hemoglobin fiber. Electron micrographs of deoxygenated sickle red cells display slender cables of hemoglobin fibers running along their long axes (58–62) (Fig. 50-3). Detailed examination of high-resolution micrographs provides a consistent depiction of the geometry of the fiber (63–69). It is approximately 21 nm in diameter and is composed of 14 strands. Cross-sectional analysis shows that the 14 strands are arranged as seven staggered, twisted pairs with a repeat of approximately 300 nm, as shown in Figure 50-4. The double strands are not symmetric because they are staggered by half a tetramer, and each tetramer is tilted slightly off the *x*-axis of the fiber, creating a relative polarity.

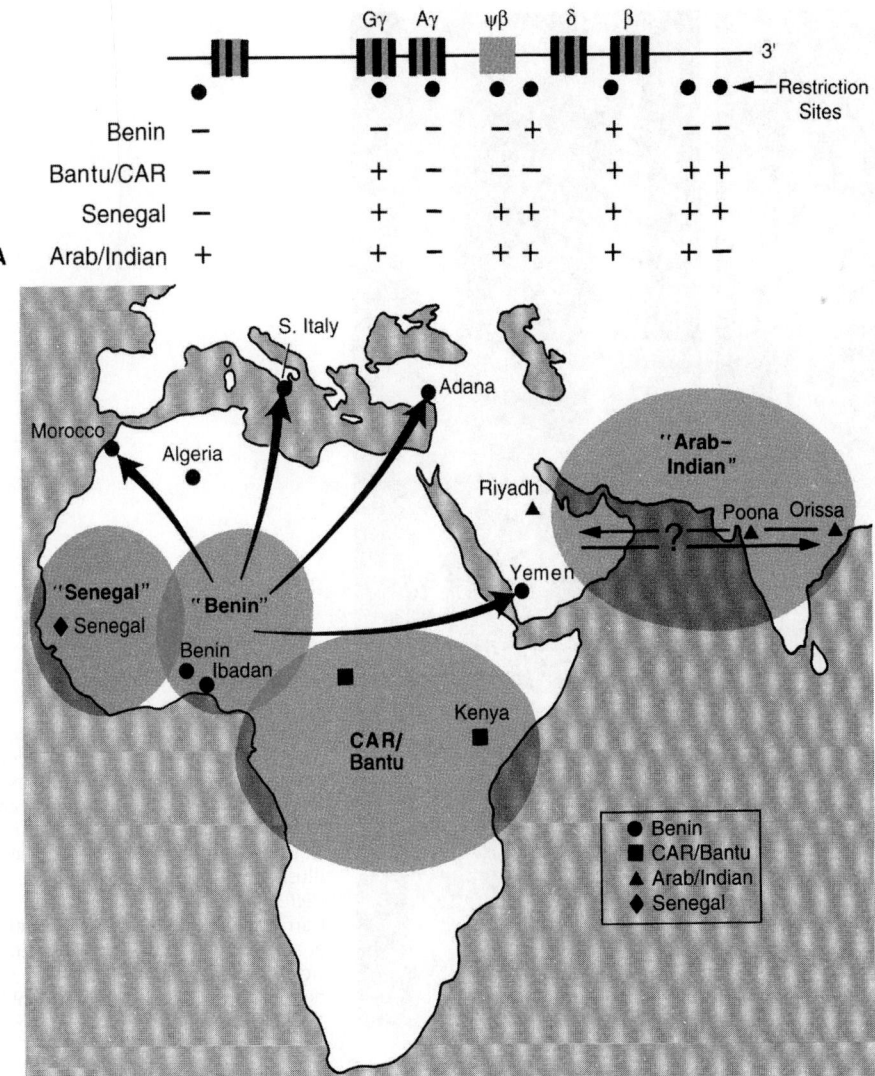

		Gγ	Aγ	ψβ		δ	β		
Benin	−		−	−	−	+	+	−	−
Bantu/CAR	−		+	−	−	−	+	+	+
Senegal	−		+	−	+	+	+	+	+
A Arab/Indian	+		+	−	+	+	+	+	−

● Benin
■ CAR/Bantu
▲ Arab/Indian
◆ Senegal

Figure 50-2. Worldwide distribution of the sickle haplotypes. **A:** Each haplotype shown is distinguished by different patterns of restriction enzyme polymorphisms within the β-globin gene cluster on chromosome 11. β^S is associated with each of the different haplotypes shown, indicating it arose independently several times during evolution. **B:** The distribution and spread of the major sickle haplotypes. CAR, Central African Republic. (From Ragusa A, Lombardo M, Sortino G, et al. Beta S gene in Sicily is in linkage disequilibrium with the Benin haplotype: implications for gene flow. *Am J Hematol* 1988;27:139, with permission.)

X-RAY CRYSTALLOGRAPHY

Although electron micrographs provide tremendous insight into the arrangement and orientation of tetramers in sickle hemoglobin fibers, details at the molecular level are available only by x-ray crystallography. This technique requires the use of large crystals of sickle hemoglobin grown in polyethylene glycol. Fortunately, even though the structures of the crystal and the fiber are not identical, many of the important molecular interactions are maintained. In fact, with time (70) or stirring (71), naturally occurring fibers convert spontaneously to crystals. By x-ray diffraction, the crystal and the fiber are both composed of the same basic structural unit: the double strand (69,70). The major difference between the fiber and the crystal is that the crystal does not have the twisted, 14-stranded arrangement shown in Figure 50-5; instead, it has a larger array of evenly matched straight parallel and antiparallel double strands.

The crystal structure was first described at the resolution of 5 Å by Wishner and colleagues (72) and is commonly known as the *Wishner-Love double strand*. Padlan and Love refined the resolution to 3 Å (73,74); most recently, Harrington and colleagues resolved the structure to 2 Å (Fig. 50-6) (75). Most of the atomic pair interactions are of the van der Waals type, with only rare potential hydrogen bonds and even rarer ionic interactions. Several of these important interactions are shown in Figure 50-6.

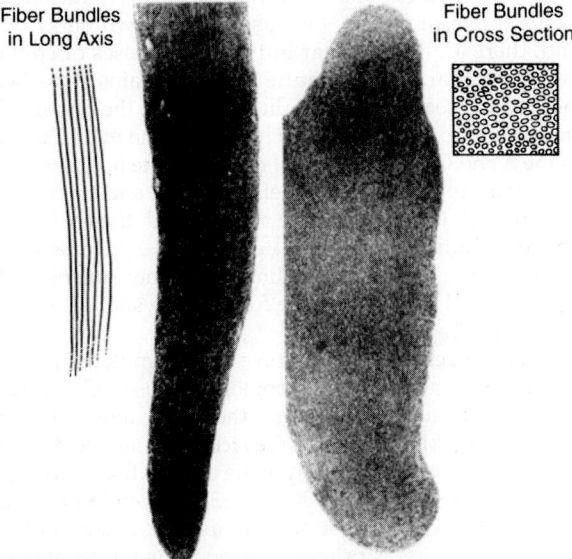

Fiber Bundles in Long Axis

Fiber Bundles in Cross Section

Figure 50-3. Electron micrograph of deoxygenated sickle erythrocyte, demonstrating deoxyhemoglobin S fibers. (From Bertles JF, Dobler J. Reversible and irreversible sickling: a distinction by electron microscopy. *Blood* 1969;33:884, with permission.)

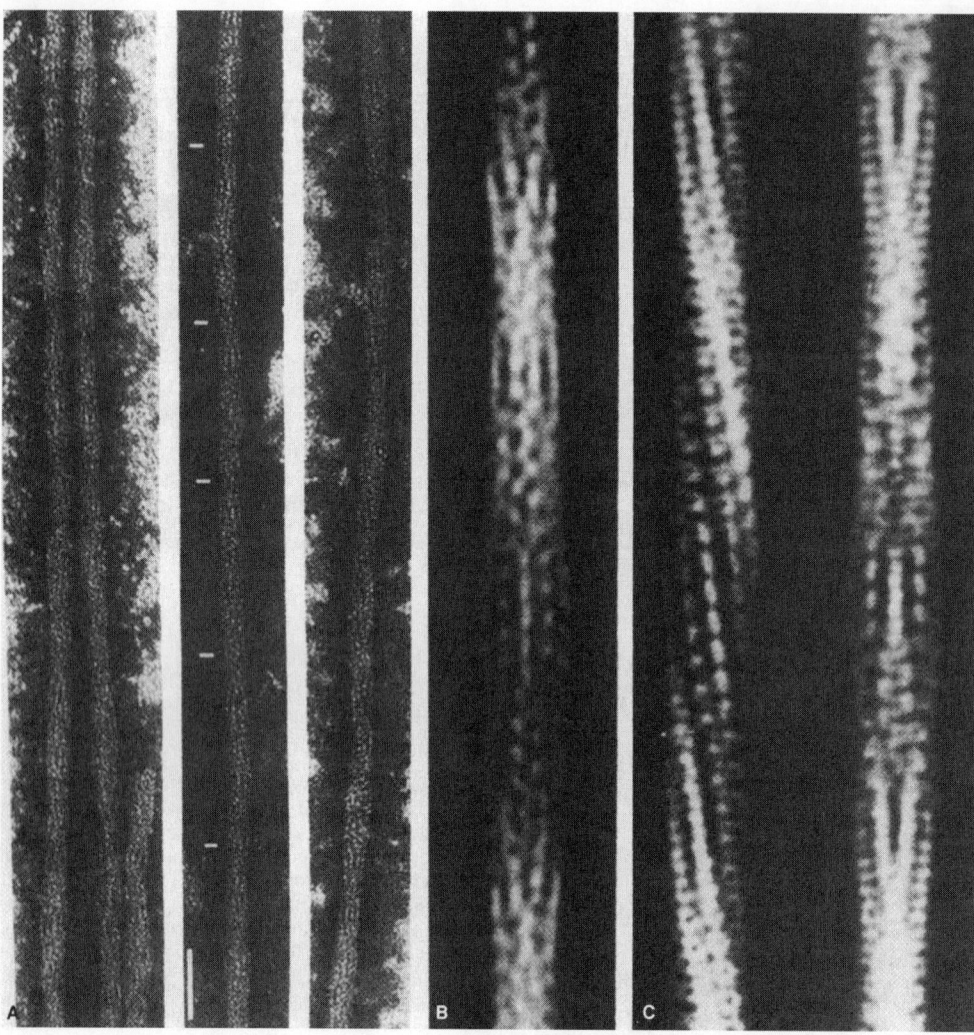

Figure 50-4. Structure of the sickle hemoglobin fiber. **A:** Electron micrographs of negatively stained fibers of deoxyhemoglobin S. **B:** Fourier transform of the electron microscopic data. **C:** Electron density models of the fiber, illustrating both the helical projection (*left*) and the surface map (*right*). (From Carragher B, Bluemke DA, Gabriel B, et al. Structural analysis of polymers of sickle cell hemoglobin. I. Sickle cell hemoglobin fibers. *J Mol Biol* 1988; 199:315, with permission.)

In each double strand, there are axial and lateral contacts. Axial contacts consist of interactions between the α_1- and β_1-chains of one tetramer and the α_2- and β_2-chains of the tetramer directly above or below. Because of the asymmetry of the strand, there are two similar but distinct classes of contacts. Using the standard nomenclature for the domains of the hemoglobin chains (see Chapter 49), in one strand, the dimer below contributes residues from the GH region of the α_1 and residues from the A and G helices and GH regions of the β_1. The tetramer above contributes from the G helix of the β_2 and from the GH regions of both α_2 and β_2. In the other strand, there is an additional contribution from the A helix of the α_2. None of these interactions involves the β-6 valine, so it is not surprising that almost identical interactions are found in crystals of hemoglobins A, F, and C.

Lateral contacts strongly involve the β-6 mutation. Because this mutation is not seen in hemoglobins A, F, or C, crystals of these hemoglobins do not contain the strong interactions that stabilize the double strands. In the sickle crystal, the β-6 valine of the β_2-chain interacts strongly, lying deep within a hydrophobic pocket lined with the Ala 70, Phe 85, and Leu 88 of the adjacent β_1. This key contact is shown in three dimensions in Figure 50-6. This interaction is primarily responsible for the abnormal solubility of deoxy sickle hemoglobin.

The interactions between double strands largely involve residues from the α-chains. Antiparallel pairs are loosely held, interacting with only a few residues of the α_1-chains. Parallel pairs interact more extensively than antiparallel pairs, with α residues reacting with adjacent β residues.

Interaction of Sickle with Other Hemoglobins

There is a long scientific tradition of studying the properties of mixtures of sickle and nonsickle hemoglobins. Although the methods have changed over the years, these studies continue to provide insight into the structure of the sickle hemoglobin fiber, the clinical behavior of patients with various hemoglobin combinations, and the manipulation of hemoglobin as a therapeutic tactic. A summary of the important hemoglobins that affect sickle hemoglobin polymerization is shown in Table 50-1.

BEHAVIOR OF HEMOGLOBIN MIXTURES IN SOLUTION

In solution, hemoglobin tetramers continuously dissociate into dimers and reassociate. In the process, tetramers exchange dimers. Consider preparing a solution of equal parts hemoglobin A and hemoglobin S. Initially, there are two types of tetramer, $\alpha_2\beta_2^S$ (hemoglobin S) and $\alpha_2\beta_2^A$ (hemoglobin A). As the dissociation to dimer and reassociation to tetramer proceeds, hybrid tetramers $\alpha_2\beta^A\beta^S$ are formed. At equilibrium, approximately one-half of the tetramers are hybrids, and one-fourth are of pure starting material. Experimentally, the tetramers can be frozen so no hybrid forms. This can be performed either by deoxygenating (deoxyhemoglobin does not dissociate) or by

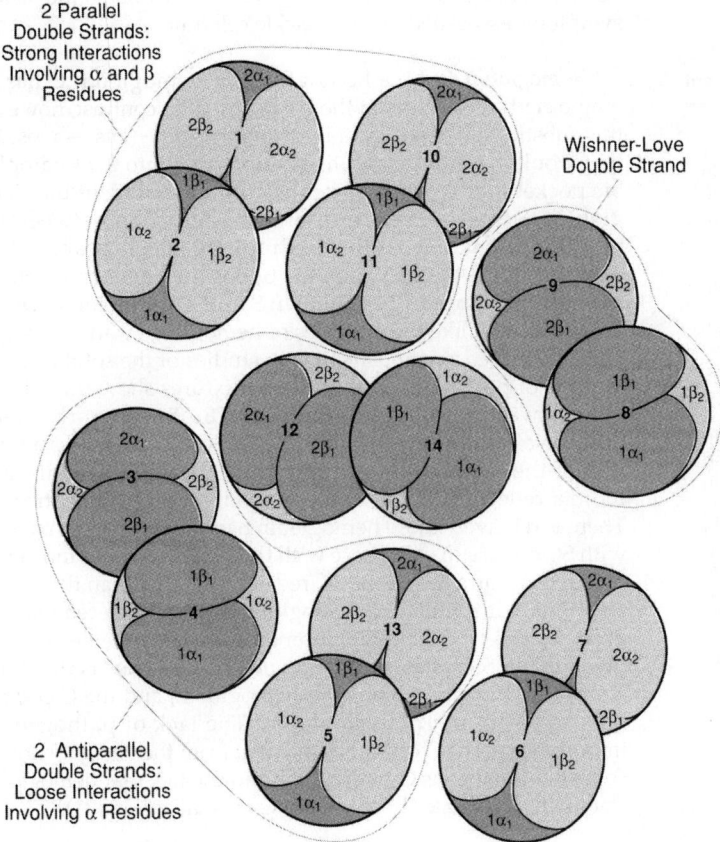

Figure 50-5. Model indicating the arrangement of the double strands to form a fiber, using the conventional numbering system. (From Dickerson RE, Geis I. *Hemoglobin: structure, function, evolution, and pathology.* Menlo Park, CA: Benjamin/Cummings Pub. Co., 1983, with permission.)

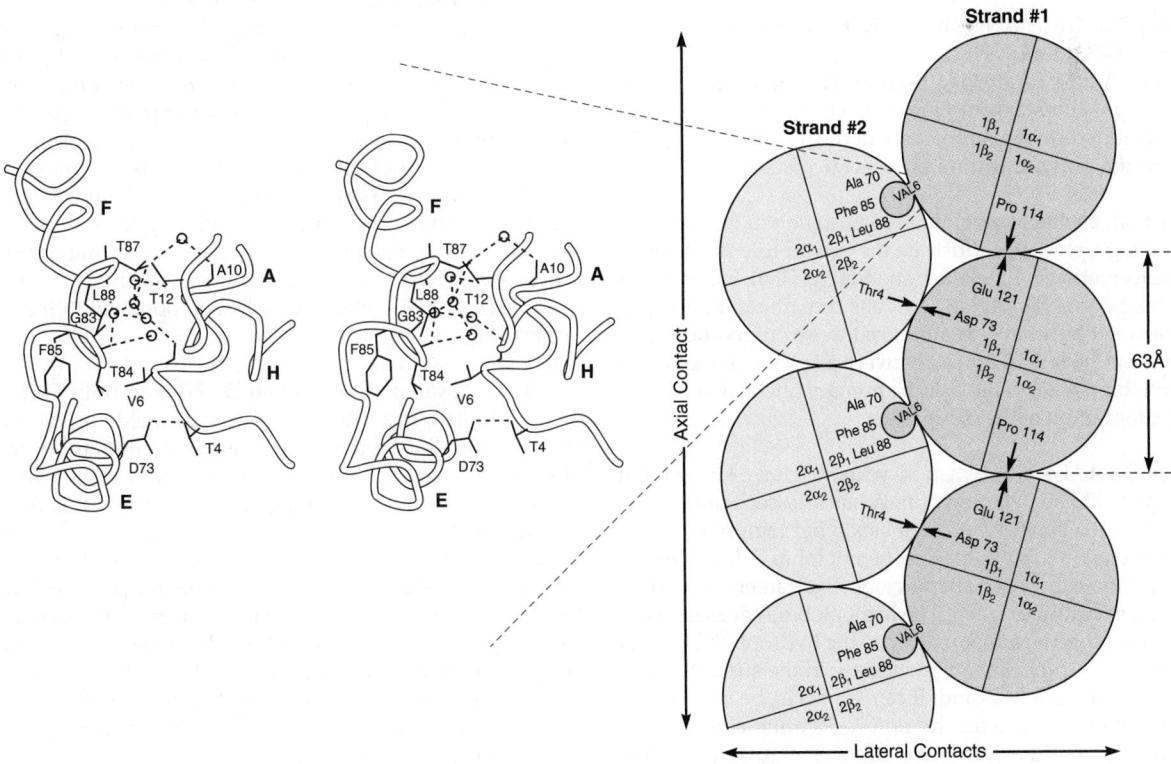

Figure 50-6. The Wishner-Love double strand, indicating a number of the key contact residues. The stereo drawing in the inset shows the key contact points surrounding the mutant valine (Val6) at 3 Å resolution. (From Wishner BC, Ward KB, Lattman EE, et al. Crystal structure of sickle-cell deoxyhemoglobin at 5 Å resolution. *J Mol Biol* 1975;98:179; and Harrington DJ, Adachi K, Royer WE Jr. The high resolution crystal structure of deoxyhemoglobin S. *J Mol Biol* 1997;272:398–407, with permission.)

TABLE 50-1. Variant Hemoglobins with Effects on Sickle Hemoglobin Polymerization

Name	Residue	Normal	Mutant
α-Chain variants			
Sawara	α6	Asp	Ala
Anantharaj	α11	Lys	Glu
I	α16	Lys	Glu
Le Lamentin	α20	His	Gln
Memphis	α23	Glu	Gln
Sealy	α47	Asp	His
J-Mexico	α54	Gln	Glu
G-Philadelphia	α69	Asn	Lys
Winnipeg	α75	Asp	Tyr
Stanleyville	α78	Asn	Lys
O-Indonesia	α116	Glu	Lys
β-Chain variants			
C	β6	Glu	Lys
Machida	β6	Glu	Gln
J-Baltimore	β16	Gly	Asp
J-Amiens	β17	Lys	Gln
D-Ouled Rabah	β19	Asn	Lys
I-Toulouse	β66	Lys	Glu
Korle Bu	β73	Asp	Asn
G-Szunu	β80	Asn	Lys
Pyrgos	β83	Gly	Asp
D-Ibadan	β87	Thr	Lys
Detroit	β95	Lys	Asn
N-Baltimore	β95	Lys	Glu
O-Arab	β121	Glu	Lys
D-Los Angeles	β121	Glu	Gln

chemically cross-linking the hemoglobin before mixing. Hybrid formation also takes place in cells. Routine hemoglobin electrophoresis does not reveal the presence of hybrids because electrophoresis conditions favor the formation of dimer.

SICKLE HEMOGLOBIN AND HEMOGLOBINS WITH NONSICKLE β-CHAINS

Hemoglobin A and numerous β-chain variants affect sickle hemoglobin polymerization (Table 50-1). In this section, the variants that illustrate the importance of the β-6, β-73, and β-121 positions on the polymerization process are discussed.

β-6 Position. Sickle hemoglobin is a mutation in the β-6 position. Crystallographic data illustrate the critical role this residue plays in the formation of the double strand (Fig. 50-6). Experiments that examine polymerization in solutions containing mixtures of different hemoglobins have strengthened these observations and established that the lateral contact between the Val-6 of the β_2 and the hydrophobic pocket of the β_1 is the primary interaction responsible for the formation of the sickle fiber.

Hemoglobin A. For more than 30 years, we have known that a mixture of sickle and hemoglobin A has a lesser tendency to polymerize than a pure solution of sickle hemoglobin (76,77). This mixture contains three species: hemoglobin S, hemoglobin A, and the hybrid $\alpha_2\beta^A\beta^S$. The hemoglobin S tetramer can participate in polymerization as usual. The hemoglobin A does not contain the β-6 valine, so it cannot reach into the hydrophobic pocket of the neighboring β-chain and participate in the strengthening and growth of the double strand. It can, however, be *incorporated* into the polymer because all the non–β-6 valine contacts are maintained. The hybrid exists in two forms. In one, the β-6 valine is in the correct position to enter the hydrophobic pocket (the β_2-chain) and behaves exactly like hemoglobin S in all its contacts. In the other, the β-6 valine is in the chain that provides the pocket (the β_1-chain). This hybrid behaves exactly like hemoglobin A. The effect of hemoglobin A on the kinetics of polymerization of

hemoglobin S is shown in Figure 50-7 and explains the lack of symptoms associated with the sickle cell trait.

Hemoglobin C. Like hemoglobin S, hemoglobin C has an amino acid substitution at the β-6 position. In contrast, however, this substitution codes for a hydrophilic lysine (Lys)—a residue that would have difficulty insinuating itself into the hydrophobic pocket that accommodates the mutant valine of the sickle globin. Because the critical lateral interaction between the hydrophobic valine and its hydrophobic pocket cannot take place when the β^C-chain is in the β_2 position, one would anticipate that mixtures of hemoglobin S and hemoglobin C would behave exactly like the mixtures of hemoglobin S and hemoglobin A described previously. In fact, studies of the solubility and kinetics of polymerization of these mixtures show little difference between S plus A and S plus C (78,79). The stark clinical difference between the sickle trait and SC disease is less a function of the physical interaction of the two hemoglobins and more a reflection of their cellular content and concentration. There is relatively more hemoglobin S in the red cells of patients with SC disease than in those with the sickle trait, and the hemoglobin concentration of the SC red cell is higher than the AS red cell (78,80). Interestingly, hemoglobin C also has a tendency to crystallize *in vivo*. The key difference between the behavior of hemoglobin S crystals and hemoglobin C crystals is that the S crystals are formed from *deoxy* hemoglobin, and the C crystals are formed from *oxy* hemoglobin. The lack of pathogenetic importance of the C crystals is evident from the benign, clinical-course homozygous C individuals and the fact that hemoglobin S actually accelerates hemoglobin C crystallization (81).

β-73 Position. **Hemoglobins C-Harlem and Korle Bu.** Hemoglobin C-Harlem is a mutant hemoglobin with two amino acid substitutions: β-6 Glu → Val (as in hemoglobin S) and β-73 Asp → Asn. This hemoglobin should theoretically polymerize as well as hemoglobin S because it has the critical β-6 valine in every β-chain, but it does not (82,83). Deoxyhemoglobin C-Harlem is three times more soluble than deoxyhemoglobin S, illustrating the importance of having asparagine (Asn) in position 73. Additional studies using the mutant hemoglobin Korle Bu (β-73 Asp → Asn) indicate that this hemoglobin is more effective than hemoglobin A in inhibiting the polymerization of hemoglobin S—convincing evidence that the impact of the β-73 residue is in the *trans* (β_1) position. This contact is found in the crystal (Fig. 50-6), where it hydrogen-bonds with the β-4 threonine (Thr).

β-121 Position. **Hemoglobin D.** Hemoglobin D (Los Angeles or Punjab) is a mutant with amino acid substitution β-121 Glu → Gln. This hemoglobin is less efficient than hemoglobin A in reducing the polymerization of hemoglobin S in mixtures (84), and patients heterozygous for S and D-Los Angeles are symptomatic (85–87). This suggests that the β-121 residue is important in the formation of the fiber and that a glutamine (Gln) in this position is more favorable for polymerization than glutamic acid (Glu). The crystal structure suggests that this residue is part of an axial contact in which the Glu-121 contacts the α-114 Pro of the tetramer above (Fig. 50-6). Because this is already a favorable interaction, it is possible that the Gln-121 interacts even more strongly with another residue and enhances the axial contact.

Hemoglobin O-Arab. Hemoglobin O-Arab is another mutation at the β-121 position, a substitution of a lysine for glutamic acid. In a minimal gelling capacity assay at high ionic strength, this hemoglobin actually enhanced the polymerization of

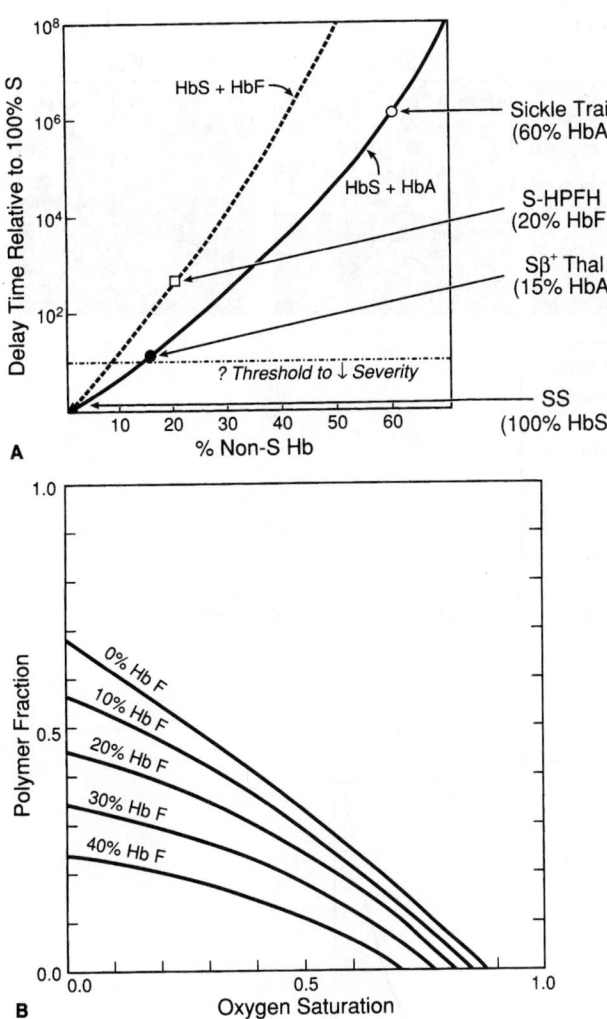

Figure 50-7. Effect of nonsickle hemoglobin (non-S Hb) on sickle Hb (HbS) polymerization. **A:** Effect of hemoglobins A and F (HbA; HbF) on the kinetics of polymerization. The locations of four common sickle syndromes and their relative severity are shown. **B:** Effect of different percentages of HbF on the fraction of sickle polymer at equilibrium. S-HPFH, hemoglobin S-hereditary persistence of fetal hemoglobin. [(**A**) from Sunshine HR, Hofrichter J, Eaton WA. Requirements for therapeutic inhibition of sickle hemoglobin gelation. *Nature* 1978;275:238; (**B**) from Schechter AN, Noguchi CT, Rodgers GP. Sickle cell disease. In: Stamatoyannopoulos G, Neinhuis AW, Leder P, et al., eds. *Molecular basis of blood diseases.* Philadelphia: WB Saunders, 1987, with permission.]

hemoglobin S (88). The observation confirms the importance of the β-121 in the formation of the polymer and accurately predicts that patients doubly heterozygous for S and O-Arab are clinically severe (89).

SICKLE AND HEMOGLOBINS WITHOUT β-CHAINS

Hemoglobin F. In mixing experiments, hemoglobin F is the most efficient hemoglobin for solubilizing hemoglobin S (90–92) (Fig. 50-7). The effect of hemoglobin F is mediated through the formation of hybrid tetramers—$\alpha_2\beta^S\gamma$. This hybrid interferes with polymerization in the solution phase. Unlike the hybrids formed with hemoglobin A, almost no γ-chains are incorporated into the polymer until the amount of hemoglobin F exceeds 30%. The γ loci that are critical in interfering with hemoglobin S polymerization are the γ-80 Asp and γ-87 Gln (93). In the crystal, the β-87 Thr is an important lateral contact site (75), as shown in the three-dimensional section of Figure 50-6.

Hemoglobin A₂. Hemoglobin A_2 is comparable to hemoglobin F in its ability to interfere with the polymerization of hemoglobin S (93,94). The critical contact residues are the δ-87 Gln and the δ-22 Ala (93).

SICKLE HEMOGLOBIN AND α-CHAIN VARIANTS

Numerous α-chain variants influence hemoglobin S polymerization (95–100). As can be seen in Table 50-1, effective α mutants generally represent axial or inter–double-strand contacts.

Polymerization of Sickle Hemoglobin

Excellent reviews and views of the polymerization of hemoglobin S present different emphases on the relative importance of equilibrium, kinetic, and structural issues in the pathophysiology of disease (101–103). An overview of the relevant data and some of the areas of controversy are considered in this section.

POLYMERIZATION IN SOLUTION

Studies at Equilibrium. As seen in Figure 50-8, a sickle hemoglobin gel is a two-phase system with polymer coexisting in equilibrium with tetramers in solution (104–106). The solubility of sickle hemoglobin can be determined by measuring the concentration of hemoglobin in the supernatant (105–108). The solubility depends on temperature (105–107), pH (90,109), and 2,3-diphosphoglycerate concentration (110,111). The most dramatic environmental influence on the solubility of sickle hemoglobin is oxygen. Complete saturation with oxygen prevents polymer formation, whereas removal of oxygen promotes polymerization. Between the extremes of a pO_2 of 100 and one of 0, the degree of polymerization of the gel depends on the relative oxygen affinities of the hemoglobin in the polymer phase and the hemoglobin in solution.

As a respiratory pigment, soluble sickle hemoglobin behaves exactly like hemoglobin A. The *solution* oxygen-binding curve (Fig. 50-9) is normal (112); in contrast, the *polymer*-binding curve is far from normal, exhibiting low affinity and no cooperativity (113–116) (Fig. 50-9A). Knowledge of the solubility as a function of oxy-

O₂ Saturation

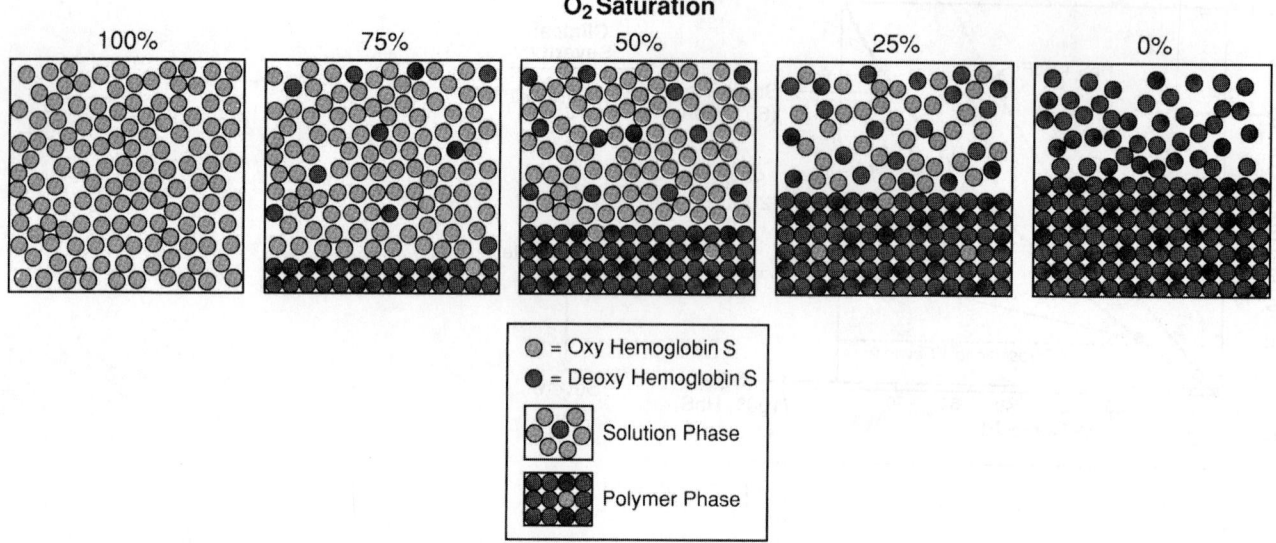

Figure 50-8. Sickle hemoglobin at equilibrium at various oxygen saturations. (From Noguchi CT, Schechter AN. Intracellular polymerization of sickle hemoglobin and its relevance to sickle cell disease. *Blood* 1981;58:1057, with permission.)

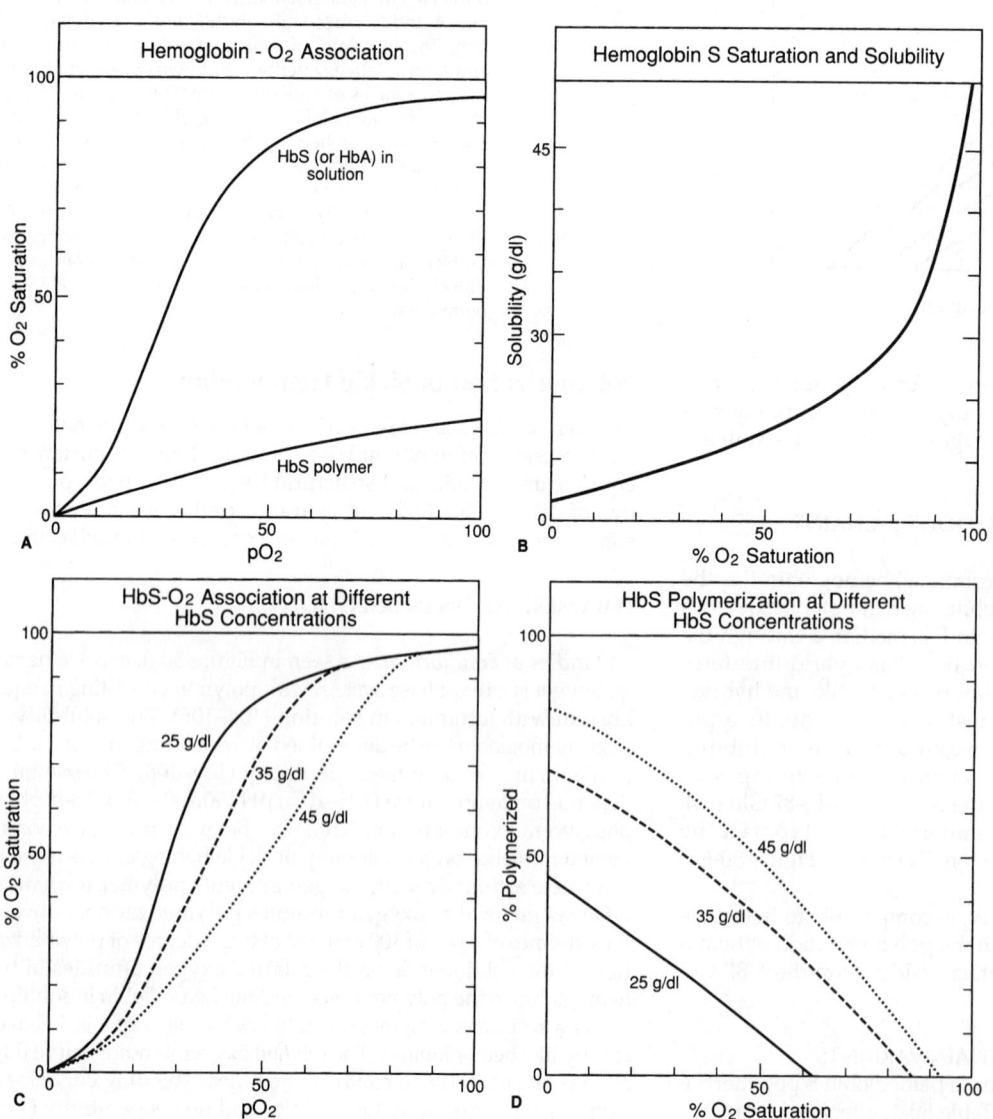

Figure 50-9. Relationship between sickle hemoglobin (Hbs) and oxygen (O₂). [(**A** to **E**) from Eaton WA, Hofrichter J. Hemoglobin S gelation and sickle cell disease. *Blood* 1987;70:1245, with permission.] (*continued*)

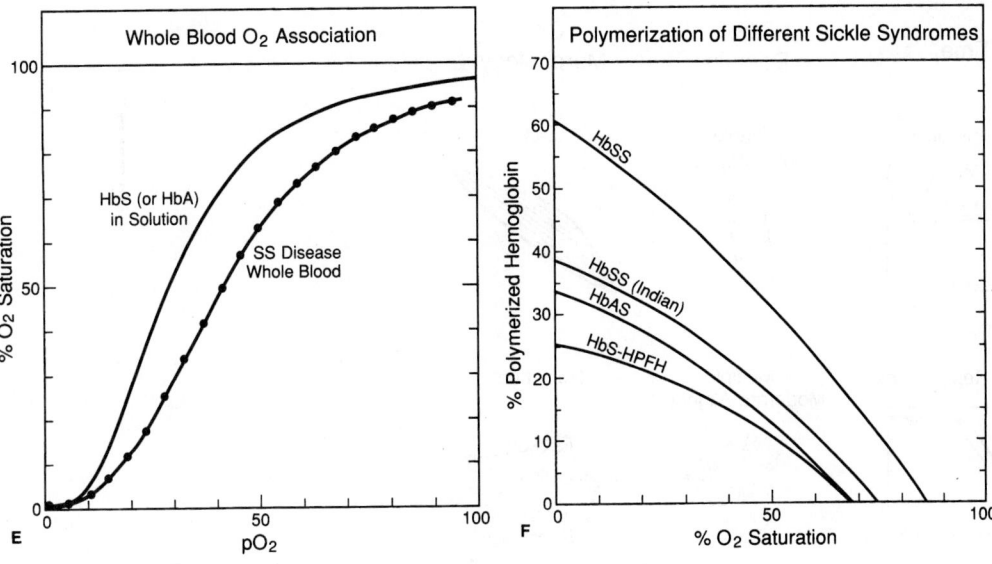

Figure 50-9. (*continued*) HPFH, hereditary persistence of fetal hemoglobin. (**F** from Brittenham GM, Schechter AN, Noguchi CT. Hemoglobin S polymerization: primary determinant of the hemolytic and clinical severity of the sickling syndromes. *Blood* 1985;65:183, with permission.)

gen saturation (114) (Fig. 50-9B) combined with the data on the oxygen binding of solution and polymer phases can be used to construct binding curves and polymerization curves of gels at different hemoglobin concentrations (Fig. 50-9C and D). The more concentrated the solution, the more likely there is to be polymer at a given pO_2, and the more the binding curve deviates from normal and toward the polymer-binding curve. As discussed later, this phenomenon, combined with the increased 2,3-diphosphoglycerate, results in the right-shifted oxygen dissociation curve found in patients with sickle cell disease (Fig. 50-9E). After controlling for 2,3-diphosphoglycerate content and the presence of other hemoglobins (Fig. 50-9F), these curves accurately predict the behavior of cells with different concentrations of hemoglobin S.

Studies of Kinetics. The binding curves presented in Figure 50-9 are the result of experiments in which hemoglobin solutions were exposed to specific oxygen tensions for relatively long periods of time, allowing polymers to form and reach equilibrium before being analyzed. Understanding the process of polymer assembly required an experimental set-up that allowed rapid induction of polymer in a polymer-free solution while continuously monitoring polymer accumulation. Polymer could be induced by temperature jump, and the amount of polymer formed could be monitored by birefringence (117–119), viscometry (120–125), turbidity (108,113,118,126,127), or nuclear magnetic resonance (NMR) (128–131). Regardless of the detection system used, the results were the same. After the temperature jump, there was a quiet delay period during which there was no apparent polymerization. After the delay, there was a characteristic precipitous and rapid appearance of polymer. These studies illustrated the unprecedented sensitive dependence of the delay on the concentration of sickle hemoglobin. Although most reactions depend on the first or second power of the concentration, this reaction is sensitive to the thirtieth to fiftieth power of the hemoglobin S concentration (132). As discussed later, this has important therapeutic implications because small changes in hemoglobin S concentration translate into profound changes in the delay time. The temperature jump experiments were informative regarding the kinetics of polymerization for solutions with delay times longer than 100 seconds. To study the process at more realistic physiologic time and hemoglobin concentrations, a technique that could deoxygenate hemoglobin S in milliseconds was devised (133–135). In these experiments, 10^{-11} mL of solution was saturated with carbon monoxide [carboxyhemoglobin S is soluble at concentrations greater

than 45 g/dL (136)] and then rapidly dissociated from the carbon monoxide ligand by laser photolysis. The effect of hemoglobin concentration (up to 40 g/dL) on the delay time (down to milliseconds) is shown in Figure 50-10. The reproducibility of delay

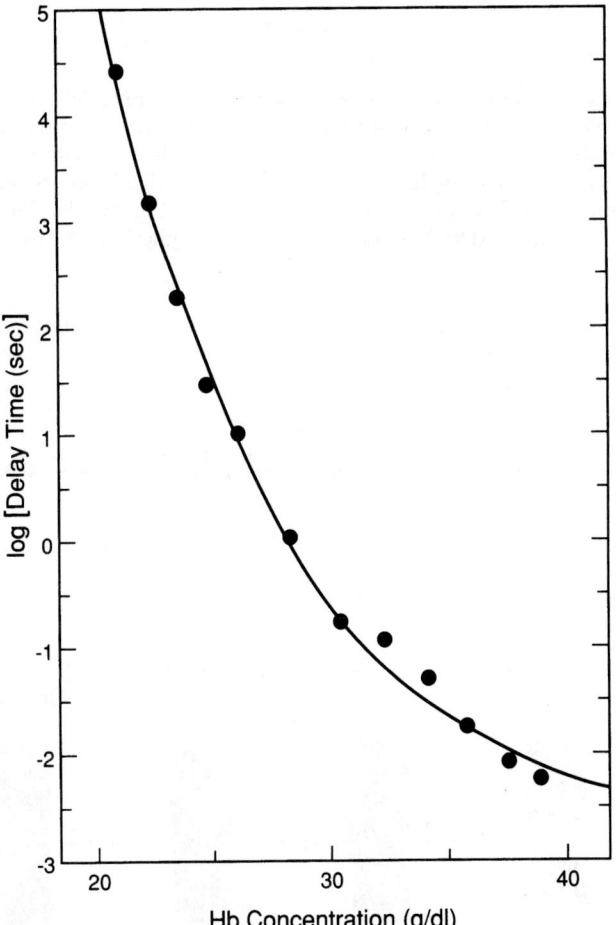

Figure 50-10. Effect of hemoglobin (Hb) concentration on the delay time of polymerization. (From Ferrone FA, Hofrichter J, Eaton WA. Kinetics of sickle hemoglobin polymerization. I. Studies using temperature-jump and laser photolysis techniques. *J Mol Biol* 1985;183:591, with permission.)

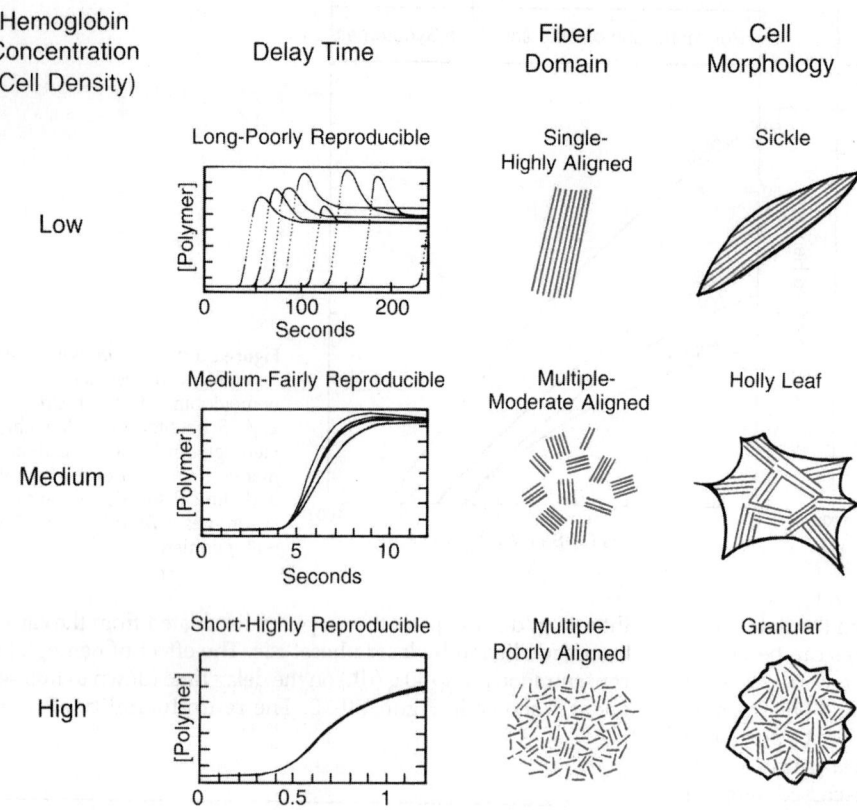

Hemoglobin Concentration (Cell Density) | Delay Time | Fiber Domain | Cell Morphology

Low — Long-Poorly Reproducible — Single-Highly Aligned — Sickle

Medium — Medium-Fairly Reproducible — Multiple-Moderate Aligned — Holly Leaf

High — Short-Highly Reproducible — Multiple-Poorly Aligned — Granular

Figure 50-11. Illustration of the dependence of delay time, fiber domain, and cell morphology on cell hemoglobin concentration (a measure of cell density). (From Eaton WA, Hofrichter J. Hemoglobin S gelation and sickle cell disease. *Blood* 1987;70:1245, with permission.)

curves is shown in Figure 50-11. Solutions with long delay times exhibit poor reproducibility and, microscopically, a highly aligned single domain of polymer. In contrast, the solutions with short delay times have highly reproducible curves and, microscopically, multiple small domains of short polymers (Fig. 50-11). These observations led to the double-nucleation hypothesis for the mech-

anism of hemoglobin S polymerization (137) (Fig. 50-12). This model suggests that two related processes take place in a polymerizing solution: (a) a homogeneous nucleation that occurs free in solution, and (b) a heterogeneous nucleation that occurs on the surface of polymer. Homogeneous nucleation starts the process. The initial aggregation of monomers in

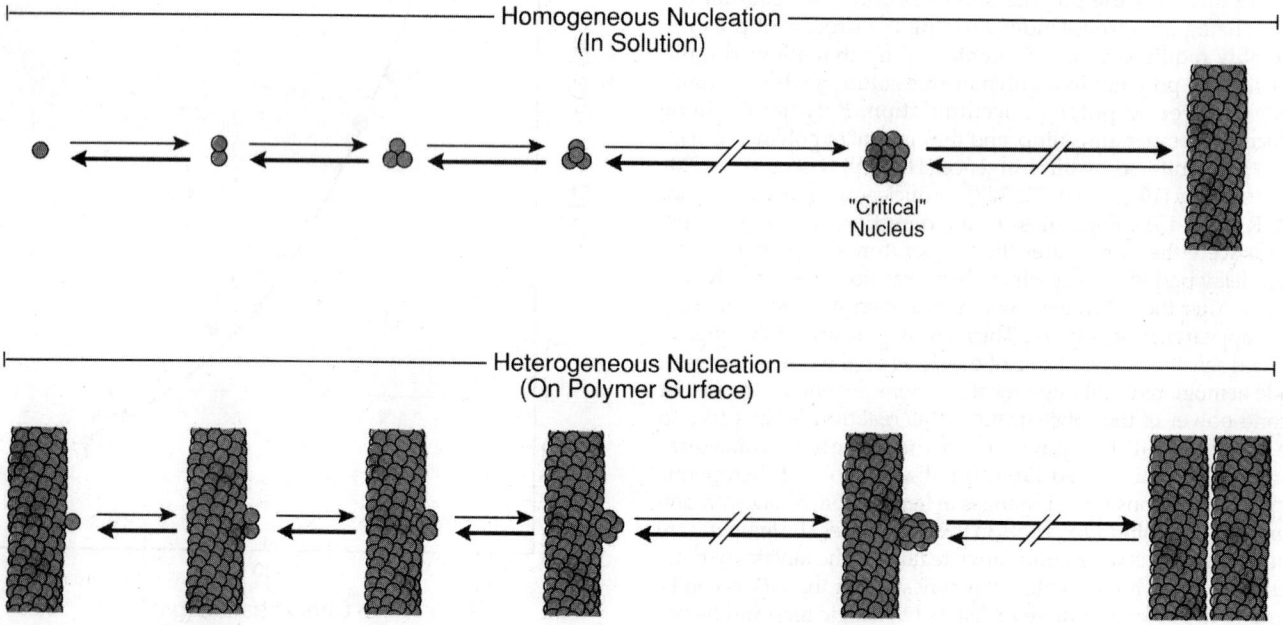

Homogeneous Nucleation (In Solution)

"Critical" Nucleus

Heterogeneous Nucleation (On Polymer Surface)

Figure 50-12. The double nucleation mechanism of hemoglobin S polymerization hypothesized by Ferrone and colleagues. Gray circles represent molecules of deoxyhemoglobin S. (From Ferrone FA, Hofrichter J, Eaton WA. Kinetics of sickle hemoglobin polymerization. II. A double nucleation mechanism. *J Mol Biol* 1985;183:611, with permission.)

solution is relatively unfavorable until the size of the critical nucleus is reached. At this point, entropy is overcome, and the deposition of more monomers becomes favorable. Heterogeneous nucleation can now proceed on the surface of the already formed polymer—an autocatalytic process because the surface area available for aggregation is constantly increasing. In slowly polymerizing solutions, homogeneous nucleation is relatively slow and random and is followed by the rapid heterogeneous nucleation and polymerization of a single, highly ordered domain. In contrast, rapidly polymerizing solutions contain multiple homogeneous nuclei that ultimately provide polymer surface for the production of multiple small polymer domains by heterogeneous nucleation. What results is a dynamic network of growing and crosslinking fibers (138).

POLYMERIZATION IN CELLS

Several independent pieces of evidence suggest that polymerization data derived from hemoglobin S solutions apply equally well to intact cells.

¹³C Nuclear Magnetic Resonance Studies at Equilibrium.

Natural abundance ¹³C NMR spectroscopy has been used to quantitate polymer as a function of oxygen saturation at equilibrium in intact cells in a number of different sickle syndromes and density-separated cells (139–142). As seen in Figure 50-13, sickle cells of different density (and therefore different hemoglobin concentration) have different polymerization curves. The experimental data are close to theoretical expectations, supporting the hypothesis that hemoglobin S in the cell behaves much like hemoglobin S in a cuvette. The ¹³C NMR data in Figure 50-13 demonstrate the presence of small amounts of polymer in dense cells even at the relatively high oxygen tensions that are encountered in the arterial circulation of some patients with sickle cell disease (143). This point has been stressed by Noguchi and Schechter and their colleagues (101,144–148) as being of prime importance in understanding the pathophysiology of sickle cell anemia. Two factors powerfully influence the presence of polymer in cells at high oxygen tension: the nonideal behavior of concentrated hemoglobin solutions and the heterogeneous distribution of cell density. Nonideality results from the molecular crowding that takes place in concentrated hemoglobin solutions and roughly translates into the observation that "hemoglobin in the red cell behaves chemically as if it

were almost 100 times more concentrated than it actually is" (144). Heterogeneous distribution of cell density is a hallmark of the sickle syndromes and results from a complex interplay between sickling and membrane permeability changes. Sickle syndromes with a large number of dense cells have more cells with polymer at high oxygen saturations and are generally more severe (Fig. 50-9F). The presence of cells with small amounts of polymer on the arterial side of the circulation focuses interest on a part of the vascular tree that, because of its high oxygen tension, has received little attention. Although it remains to be determined which, and to what extent, arteriolar beds are affected in sickle cell disease, these beds are potentially pharmacologically manipulable (149).

Laser Photolysis Studies of Kinetics.

The laser photolysis technique that was used to study the kinetics of polymerization of hemoglobin S solutions has been used to study individual red cells (150). These experiments underscore the concordance between the behavior of hemoglobin S in the test tube and its behavior in the cell. In cells, the distribution of delay times observed correlates with the expected distribution based on cell heterogeneity. In addition, as in solution, the reproducibility of delay time in cells is best for rapidly polymerizing cells and worst for slowly polymerizing cells. The double-nucleation mechanism (Fig. 50-12) appears to apply to cells and predicts that dense cells with short delays have multiple small domains of polymer and that light cells have long delays and large single domains (Fig. 50-11). This view is supported by morphologic studies (151) and may have clinical implications because domains with long fibers are more likely to be rigid and to stretch and potentially damage the membrane than domains with small fibers (103).

To answer some basic questions as to where, if, and how cells polymerize or sickle in the circulation, a second laser was added to the basic photolysis experiment, allowing cells to be studied at partial desaturation (152). Eaton and Hofrichter (102) emphasized the importance of polymerization kinetics in the pathophysiology of sickle cell disease. The relevant time frame for cells in the circulation is approximately 1 second in the alveoli, 3 seconds on the arterial side, 1 second in the capillaries, and 10 seconds in the venous return (152). Cells with delay times longer than 1 second pass through the microcirculation without sickling. At equilibrium, approximately 5% of cells would be

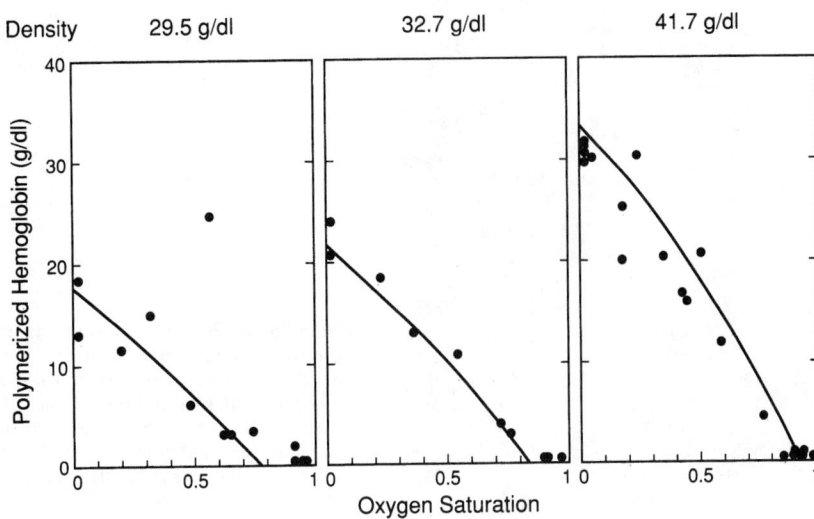

Figure 50-13. Relationship between the concentration of polymerized hemoglobin S and oxygen saturation for cells of different density. Density is measured as the mean corpuscular hemoglobin concentration. (A fractional oxygen saturation of 1 represents 100% saturation.) (From Noguchi CT, Torchia DA, Schechter AN. Intracellular polymerization of sickle cell hemoglobin: effects of cell heterogeneity. *J Clin Invest* 1983;72:846, with permission.)

sickled at arterial oxygen tensions and 85% at venous tensions. In contrast, the kinetic experiment predicts only approximately 5% sickled at venous tensions. This implies that under steady-state conditions, the delay time is sufficiently long that approximately 80% of cells are prevented from sickling in the capillaries. This is close to the figure of 10% sickled cells in the arteries and 20% in the veins, compiled from a number of morphologic studies (143,153–155) by Eaton and Hofrichter (102). Vasoocclusion is favored by factors that either shorten the delay time or increase the transit time.

POLYMERIZATION, RED CELLS, AND THE CIRCULATION

Membrane Damage in Sickle Red Cells

The pathophysiology of sickle cell disease starts with the abnormal gene and its unstable hemoglobin product that polymerizes when deoxygenated. The clinical manifestation is a secondary phenomenon: tissue damage caused by the hemoglobin. Because hemoglobin is packaged as a highly concentrated solution encased by the red cell membrane, the membrane is an important modulator of clinical expression. It is the tissue in most intimate contact with the abnormal gene product and is precariously exposed to its noxious by-products and subject to gross physical distortion. The membrane also influences the degree of concentration of the hemoglobin and is the surface that is recognized by proteins and cells in the plasma, by the vascular endothelium, and by reticuloendothelial cells. In this section, the evidence for membrane damage is presented, its cause is considered, and its clinical implications are discussed.

Irreversibly Sickled Cells

Irreversibly sickled cells are the long, slender, pointed cells that persist in well-oxygenated peripheral smears of patients with hemoglobin SS disease (Fig. 50-14). These dense, hemoglobin F–poor cells contain virtually no polymerized hemoglobin when they are fully oxygenated and survive for only a few days

(156,157). Their number correlates well with hemolytic rate (158) and spleen size (159) but not with vasoocclusive severity. Experimentally, irreversibly sickled cells can be produced from reversibly sickled cells using a variety of deoxy incubation strategies, including adenosine triphosphate depletion (160), calcium accumulation (161), adenosine triphosphate maintenance (162), and oxy-deoxy cycling (163–166). They provide the most graphic evidence of membrane damage in SS disease. As seen in Figure 50-15, the abnormal shape of an irreversibly sickled cell is maintained by the membrane ghost. Furthermore, when the cell ghost is exposed to a detergent that removes the membrane lipid and integral proteins, the abnormal shape survives in the residual protein skeleton (167). In normal red cells, the skeleton influences cell shape, permeability, lipid organization, deformability, and movement of intramembranous particles. There are abnormalities other than shape in irreversibly sickled cells and other abnormalities in cells with normal shape.

Membrane Control of the Internal Environment

As discussed previously, the red cells in sickle cell anemia are extremely heterogeneous with respect to their hemoglobin concentration. The proportion of dehydrated cells (including irreversibly sickled cells) directly influences the amount of polymer present at a given pO_2. Extreme dehydration, which in itself may cause membrane damage (168), is a reflection of the abnormal permeability of sickle membranes. Three transport pathways contribute in varying degrees under varying conditions to pathologic dehydration.

NA$^+$-K$^+$ PUMP

Almost 40 years ago, Tosteson and colleagues (169–171) demonstrated that sickle cells have the unique tendency to lose K$^+$ and gain Na$^+$ when deoxygenated. Physical deformation of the membrane is closely associated with the increased permeability (172,173), and the leak is relatively insensitive to charge but restrictive in size (174). Because the K$^+$ lost is balanced by the Na$^+$ gained, there is no net water movement and no dehydration (161,175). When the internal Na$^+$ becomes sufficiently high, however, the Na$^+$-K$^+$ pump is stimulated, and the excess Na$^+$ is

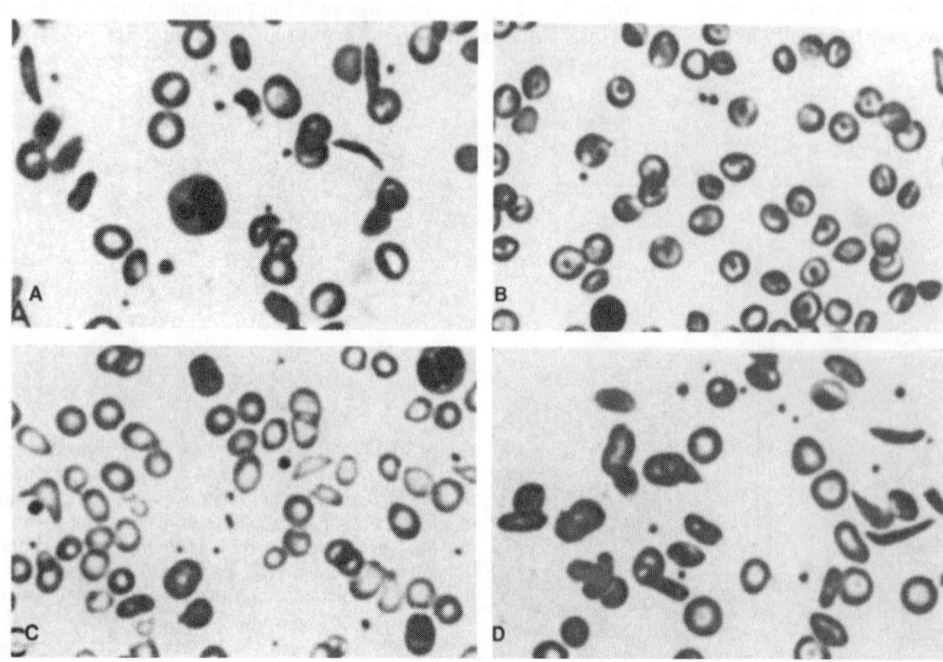

Figure 50-14. Peripheral blood smears from persons with sickle cell (SC) anemia **(A)**, hemoglobin SC disease **(B)**, Sβ-thalassemia **(C)**, and hemoglobin SD disease **(D)**. (From Platt OS, et al. Hematology of infancy and childhood. In: Nathan DG, Oski FA, eds. *Hematology of infancy and childhood*. WB Saunders, 1993, with permission.)

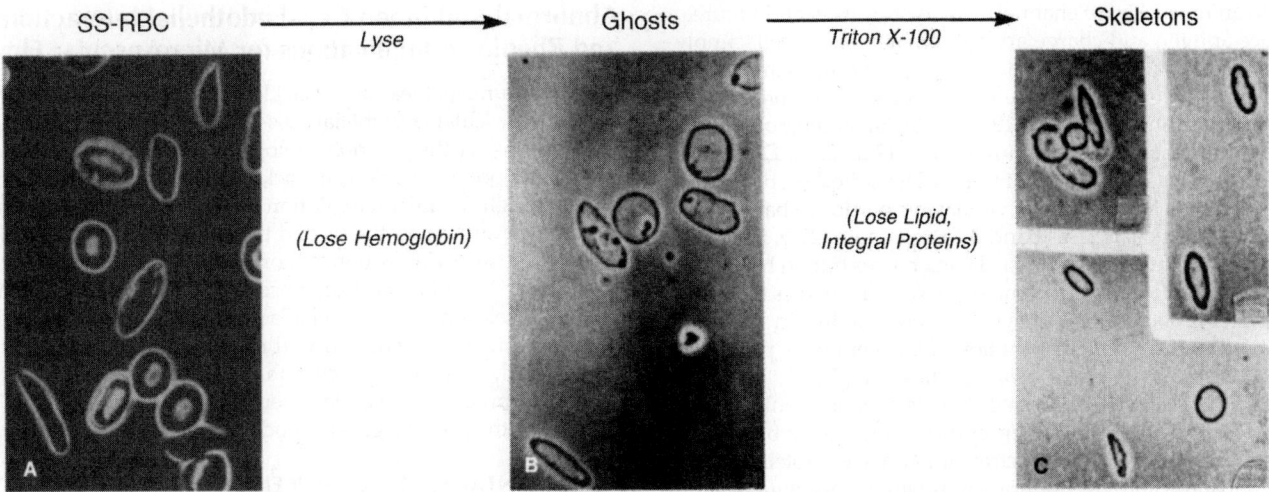

SS-RBC → *Lyse* → Ghosts → *Triton X-100* → Skeletons

(Lose Hemoglobin)

(Lose Lipid, Integral Proteins)

Figure 50-15. Demonstration that membrane ghosts and membrane protein skeletons of irreversibly sickled red blood cells (SS-RBCs) maintain the sickle shape. (From Lux SE, John KM, Karnovsky MJ. Irreversible deformation of the spectrin-actin lattice in irreversibly sickled cells. *J Clin Invest* 1976;58:955, with permission.)

expelled. The stoichiometry of the pump is such that for every three Na$^+$ that are extruded, only two K$^+$ are imported. This imbalance creates a situation in which the stimulated pump can cause net cation loss and cell dehydration (176–179).

CA^{2+}-ACTIVATED K$^+$ CHANNEL

As discussed previously, morphologic sickling is associated with a transient increase in both Na$^+$ and K$^+$ permeability. Similarly, Ca^{2+} permeability is increased during sickling, allowing the red cell to accumulate large amounts of calcium (180,181). Normally, red cells contain 2 to 8 μmol calcium/L of red cells (182). In contrast, unfractionated sickle cells contain 40 to 60 μmol calcium, and irreversibly sickled cells contain as much as 200 μmol calcium/L of red cells (183,184). In 1956, Gardos (185) showed that red cells with elevated levels of calcium undergo selective K$^+$ and water loss if they become adenosine triphosphate depleted. The *Gardos phenomenon* is an attractive hypothesis to explain dehydration in calcium-loaded sickle cells (160,161,163,164,186). However, the excessive Ca^{2+} that is needed to provoke the Gardos phenomenon is not free in the cytosol (187) but is safely sequestered—it is actively pumped into endocytic vesicles (188). Compartmentalization may explain why there is no easily measurable Ca^{2+}-dependent K$^+$ loss in sickle red cells (189,190) but does not exclude the possibility that brief dehydrating pulses of increased cytosolic Ca^{2+} develop during polymerization. Brugnara has shown the importance of this channel in producing cellular dehydration in sickle red cells *in vitro* by blocking its activity with clotrimazole and demonstrating the prevention of cellular dehydration (191). *In vivo*, he has shown that clotrimazole reduces dehydration in a mouse model of sickle cell disease (192) as well as in patients with sickle cell anemia (193). This strategy is now being explored therapeutically.

KCL COTRANSPORT SYSTEM

The KCl cotransport system is probably the most important dehydrating transport pathway in sickle red blood cells (RBCs) and does not require deoxygenation, polymerization, or sickling for its activation (194–196). This system is found in normal reticulocytes (197,198), which partially explains its enhanced activity in sickle cell anemia. Its high activity in cells from patients with hemoglobin C trait (199) and homozygous C disease who do not have elevated reticulocyte counts (200) supports the hypothesis that an interaction between the positively

charged hemoglobin and the membrane activates the system. KCl cotransport activity results in a net loss of water and KCl and may explain why cells with hemoglobin C tend to be dehydrated. The pathway is chloride dependent and is stimulated by acid pH (<7.4), cell swelling, and sulfhydryl modification (201,202). Incubation of sickle red cells at low pH suggests that this pathway can lead to cellular dehydration (196). It is inhibited by magnesium *in vitro* (195,203), *in vivo* in a mouse model of sickle cell disease (204), and in patients with sickle cell anemia (205,206). Blockade of this transport channel is an emerging therapeutic strategy that is undergoing clinical trial.

Membrane and Outside Surface of the Cell

ABNORMAL LIPID ORIENTATION

The phospholipids of the red cell bilayer are constantly flipping between the inner and outer leaflets (see Chapter 51). Despite this rapid continuous movement, a degree of asymmetry is maintained, with the amino phospholipids (phosphatidylserine and phosphatidylethanolamine) spending relatively more time in the inner leaflet and the choline-phospholipids (phosphatidylcholine and sphingomyelin) on the external surface. This asymmetry is poorly maintained in sickle cells. Phosphatidylserine and phosphatidylethanolamine partition normally in oxygenated reversibly sickled cells, are more exposed on the surface of deoxygenated reversibly sickled cells, and are permanently externalized in irreversibly sickled cells (207–212). This anomalous partitioning, which, in part, is related to the deposition of denatured hemoglobin on the inner surface of the membrane (213), results in abnormal cell-surface characteristics and reactions. Phosphatidylserine is capable of promoting coagulation, and its exposure on the surface of sickle cells is associated with increased procoagulant activity (210). It is not known whether such enhanced clotting influences microvascular occlusion. The abnormal surface lipids are also associated with the increased tendency of sickle cells to bind and fuse with lipid vesicles (214), dehydrate (215), and adhere to macrophages (216).

ABNORMAL SURFACE TOPOGRAPHY AND MEMBRANE PROTEINS

Surface charge and antigens of red cells are largely carried on the transmembrane proteins glycophorin and band 3 (the erythrocyte anion exchange channel). The distribution and nature of surface antigen and charge are abnormal in sickle cells, implying an abnormality in the protein structure of the membrane.

Hemoglobin A binds to the membrane (217,218) on the cytoplasmic portion of band 3 (219–221). Sickle hemoglobin binds even more readily than hemoglobin A (222–225). Denatured hemoglobin, the major constituent of Heinz bodies, binds with extremely high affinity to the cytoplasmic portion of band 3 (226) and, in intact cells, causes band 3 to aggregate (227). Sickle red cells do not contain large classic Heinz bodies but do have small inclusions made of hemichrome—micro-Heinz bodies (228–231). These Heinz bodies are visible in the ghosts shown in Figure 50-15. There is a marked redistribution of the membrane proteins of sickle cells near the micro-Heinz bodies. Membrane-associated Heinz bodies underlie abnormal clusters of band 3, ankyrin, and glycophorins (232), and even cytoplasmic Heinz bodies are coated with a film of lipid spectrin, ankyrin, and proteins 4.1 and 3 (213). Band 3 and glycophorin are progressively aggregated in increasingly dehydrated sickle and normal red cells (233), and clustered or clusterable band 3 and glycophorins may be responsible for the electron microscopic appearance of uneven clumps of negative charge on the surface of sickle red cells (234).

The skeletal proteins, which interact with and provide structural support for band 3 and the glycophorins, are also affected in sickle cell disease. Long polymers of sickle hemoglobin can physically dissociate the membrane lipid and its associated band 3 from the underlying skeleton (235). This causes the release of spectrin-free vesicles (236,237). Chemically, there is good evidence that the thiol redox status of spectrin, ankyrin, and protein 4.1 is abnormal (238). Functionally, both ankyrin and protein 3 have abnormal binding characteristics in sickle red cells (239–241), similar to what is found in other cells with Heinz bodies, such as erythrocytes containing unstable hemoglobins (242). The pathogenesis of the membrane abnormalities is not known precisely but is likely to be some combination of hemoglobin interaction and oxidation.

Several convincing convergent lines of evidence implicate oxidation as the major contributor to the membrane abnormalities of sickle cells; these are reviewed in detail by Hebbel (243). Sickle red cells generate twice the normal amount of the potent oxidants, superoxide, peroxide, and hydroxyl radical (244). The inherent tendency of oxyhemoglobin S to autooxidize and form methemoglobin results in the generation of superoxide and the loss of free heme (245). The liberated heme is capable of damaging the membrane by oxidizing proteins or lipids and also by acting as a structure-perturbing detergent (246,247). Even circulating low-density lipoprotein is susceptible to oxidation in patients with sickle cell disease, generating potentially endothelial-toxic by-products (248). Various components of the sickle membrane contain excessive amounts of free or globin-bound heme, which may cause site-specific damage (249). For example, free heme may target membrane lipids, whereas denatured globin-bound heme (hemichrome) may target band 3 and its neighbors, such as ankyrin. Nonheme iron is also found in sickle cells and is enriched in dense cells (250). Because phospholipase D can liberate free iron from membranes, it is likely that the iron is associated with and can potentially specifically damage amino phospholipids (250). Many of the abnormal membrane properties of sickle membranes can be circumstantially linked to oxidation. Oxidation of normal cells can result in abnormal cation homeostasis (251,252), membrane deformability (253), interaction with phagocytes (254), lipid asymmetry (255), tendency to form vesicles (256), abnormal binding function of ankyrin (242), and increased binding of anti–band 3 surface immunoglobulin (Ig) G (257). Antioxidant therapy has potential benefit in sickle cell disease, although there are currently no supportive clinical data.

Abnormal Red Blood Cell–Endothelial Interactions and Rheology: Implications for Microvascular Flow

One of the unusual features of sickle red cells is their tendency to adhere to vascular endothelial cells—a tendency that has obvious implications for the pathophysiology of occlusion. As discussed previously, polymerization and sickling takes time (117), and passage through the microcirculation also takes time. Under most physiologic situations, the second that it takes a sickle red cell to traverse the microcirculation is shorter than the time it takes for it to sickle (152), and no occlusion occurs. The more the movement of cells is held up by endothelial adherence, the more likely it is that sickling and occlusion will occur. One of the attractive aspects of the adherence/occlusion hypothesis is that it provides another approach to designing therapeutic interventions and for examining the possible genetic modifiers of clinical severity.

EXPERIMENTAL EVIDENCE FOR ENDOTHELIAL ADHERENCE

The first observations that sickle RBCs adhere to endothelial cells were made using static assays incubating sickle RBCs on monolayers of cultured endothelial cells from calf aorta (258) or human umbilical vein (234). These pioneering experiments were met with initial skepticism but were bolstered by the observation that endothelial adherence correlated with clinical severity (259). Since then, hundreds of experiments have demonstrated increased adherence of sickle RBCs to endothelial cells (Fig. 50-16), but the full impact of adhesion on the pathophysiology of occlusion is still not known. The experimental systems for studying the interactions between RBCs and endothelial cells are primitive. Measurements of adherence are extremely variable and depend not only on inter- and intrapatient differences but also on experimental design. These assays can be performed under static and flow conditions (with a variety of shear rates and turbulence conditions), with and without plasma, *in vitro* and *in vivo*, and using endothelial cells and cell lines of humans and animals and a variety of tissue sources. Each system is optimized to answer specific questions, but each has pitfalls, and the comparison of results across experimental systems can be misleading. Despite these methodologic issues, it appears that sickle RBCs can develop multiple attachment sites to endothelial cells (260) that are at least strong enough to withstand the detaching forces found in low-shear vascular beds *in vivo* (261,262).

INFLUENCE OF RED BLOOD CELL CHARACTERISTICS ON ENDOTHELIAL CELL ADHERENCE
See Figure 50-17.

Red Cell Youth. The extreme heterogeneity of circulating RBCs in sickle cell disease reflects the competing forces of increased production and release of very young cells and premature aging. The characteristics of the very young and the prematurely aged cells are quite different and translate into different behavior with respect to endothelial cell adherence.

As normal reticulocytes mature, they shed surface receptors that are no longer necessary to bring iron into the cell or to enhance the cell's affinity for the matrix of the bone marrow. Circulating stress reticulocytes briefly retain these surface receptors, which can serve as useful markers but may also constitute receptors directly involved in adhesion. In part, these developmental receptors explain the consistent observation that reticulocytes are the most adhesive cells in the blood. The best examples of age-related receptors that mediate endothelial cell adherence are VLA4 ($\alpha_4\beta_1$ integrin) and CD36 (glycoprotein IV) (263).

Sickle reticulocyte VLA4 binds to VCAM-1 (vascular cell adhesion molecule–1) on endothelial cells (264) and VCAM-1–transfected COS cells (265). Increased adherence during infec-

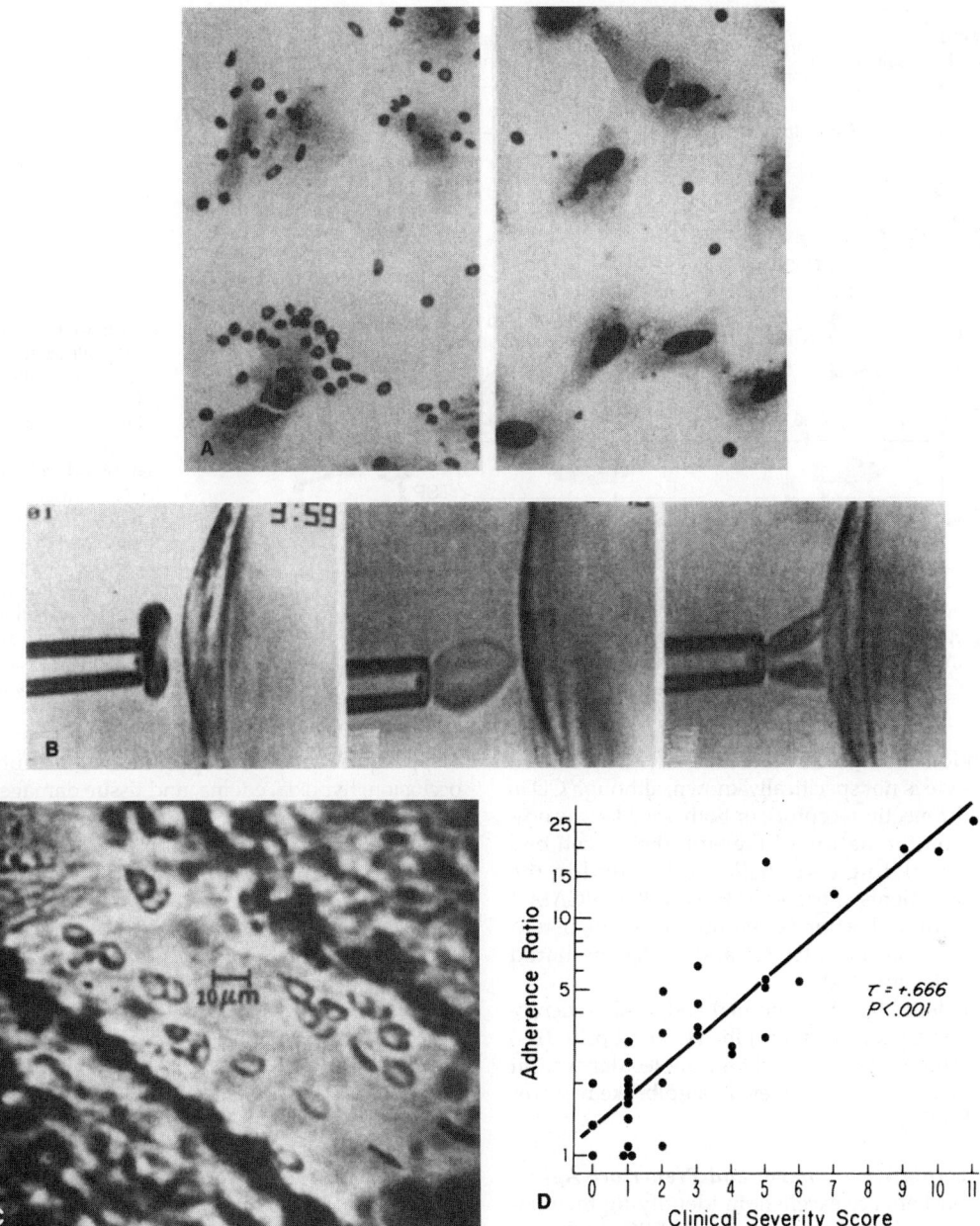

Figure 50-16. Sickle erythrocytes and endothelial adherence. Three measures of adherence are shown. **A:** Increased adherence of sickle (*left*) compared to normal (*right*) red cells to cultured endothelial cells. The small dark sickle red cells rosette around the much larger endothelial cells (*left*), whereas none of the normal red cells is close to an endothelial cell. **B:** Increased force of adherence of individual erythrocytes to cultured cells: nonadherent normal cell (*left*), sickle cell with one attachment site (*center*), and sickle cell with multiple attachment sites (*right*). **C:** Increased adherence of sickle erythrocytes in a flow system (small blood vessels in the rat mesocecum) that mimics *in vivo* conditions. Transfused sickle cells are adherent to the wall of the blood vessel in the center of the photomicrograph. **D:** Positive correlation between clinical severity and increased adherence of sickle cells to cultured human venous endothelial cells. (**A** from Hebbel RP, Yamada O, Moldow CF, et al. Abnormal adherence of sickle erythrocytes to cultured vascular endothelium: possible mechanism for microvascular occlusion in sickle cell disease. *J Clin Invest* 1980;65:154; **B** from Mohandas N, Evans E. Sickle erythrocyte adherence to vascular endothelium. *J Clin Invest* 1985;76:1605; **C** from Kaul DK, Fabry ME, Nagel RL. Microvascular sites and characteristics of sickle cell adhesion to vascular endothelium in shear flow conditions: pathophysiological implications. *Proc Natl Acad Sci U S A* 1989;86:3356; and **D** from Hebbel RP, Boogaerts MAB, Eaton JW, et al. Erythrocyte adherence to endothelium in sickle-cell anemia: a possible determinant of disease severity. *N Engl J Med* 1980;302:992, with permission.)

tion (266), hypoxia (267), or exposure to inflammatory cytokines (264) may be mediated through this interaction by up-regulating VCAM-1 expression on endothelial cells. The decreased adherence found in patients receiving hydroxyurea (268) may relate to the decrease in VLA4 (and/or CD36) on those RBCs (269).

RBC VLA4 can also be activated by exposure to phorbol ester or interleukin (IL)-8 to bind fibronectin and adhere to endothelial cells independent of VCAM-1 (270).

CD36 found on sickle stress reticulocytes mediates binding to endothelial cells via a thrombospondin bridge (271,272). The

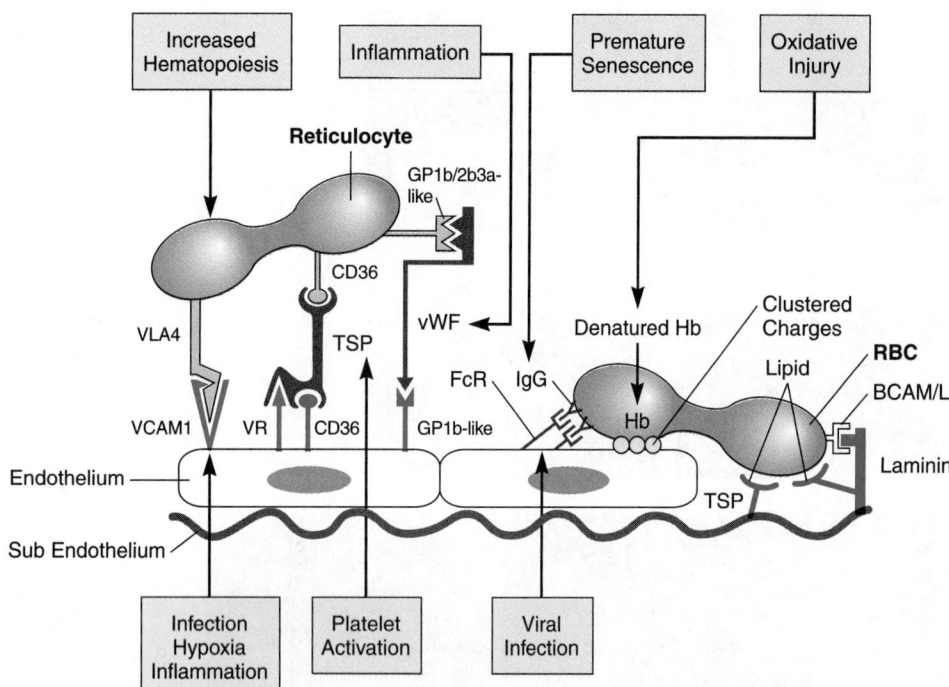

Figure 50-17. Summary of key interactions between sickle red cells and endothelial cells. BCAM/Lu, basal cell adhesion molecule/Lutheran; FcR, Fc receptor; GP, glycoprotein; Hb, hemoglobin; IgG, immunoglobulin G; RBC, red blood cell; TSP, thrombospondin; VCAM, vascular cell adhesion molecule; VR, vitronectin receptor ($\alpha_v\beta_3$-integrin); vWF, von Willebrand's factor. (Modified from Nagel RL, Platt OS. General pathophysiology of sickle cell anemia. In: Steinberg MH, Forget BG, Higgs DR, et al., eds. *Disorders of hemoglobin.* Cambridge: Cambridge University Press, 2001:494–527.)

receptor on the endothelial cell that binds the thrombospondin-decorated reticulocyte is not specifically known, although CD36 or $\alpha_v\beta_3$ integrin (vitronectin receptor), or both, are likely candidates, depending on the nature of the endothelial cell bed involved (272). Circulating endothelial cells found in the peripheral blood of patients express CD36 as well as VCAM-1 and other markers of activation/inflammation—consistent with the hypothesis that both CD36- and VLA4-mediated adherence may be relevant (272).

There is also evidence that both normal and sickle reticulocytes express platelet glycoprotein (gp) Ib–like and gpIIb/IIIa-like receptors that allow them to bind high-molecular-weight von Willebrand's factor and then adhere to a gpIb-like receptor on endothelial cells (273).

Cell Density, Oxidative Damage, and Premature Aging. Whereas surface markers are excellent in identifying the relatively homogeneous population of the youngest RBCs in the circulation, the remaining prematurely aging cells are very heterogeneous. One of the hallmarks of this heterogeneity is the wide distribution of cell density. The low density of reticulocytes, the relationship between density and deformability, and the unusual and dense irreversibly sickled cell population complicate understanding the effects of cell density on adherence. *In vitro*, the adherence of sickle RBCs can be increased by exposing the cells to oxidizing conditions that cause the cells to become dehydrated (274). As discussed earlier in this chapter, these are conditions that alter the external surface of the cell and may enhance adherence by increasing the binding of denatured hemoglobin to the inner surface of the membrane and clustering integral membrane proteins, thereby clustering charges at the cell surface. In contrast, experiments designed to examine the adhesion and flow of sickle RBCs in living vascular beds reveal a complex interplay between cells of different density, deformability, and shape, which are influenced by plasma proteins and the geometry of the vessels they encounter. Synthesizing the results of these experiments performed in rats and mice suggests a picture as follows: high-molecular-weight von Willebrand's factor → adherence of low-density cells in postcapillary venules →

trapping denser cells (especially irreversibly sickled cells) → occlusion, hypoxia, edema, and tissue damage (275–279).

The modulation of adherence by high-molecular-weight von Willebrand's factor multimers is an example of how intercurrent infection or inflammation, or both, may influence vasoocclusion. Another example results from the pathologic accumulation of IgG on the surface of sickle RBCs—a marker of their premature senescence. These cells become increasingly adherent to virus-infected endothelial cells that display Fc receptor on their surface (280).

INFLUENCE OF ENDOTHELIAL CELL CHARACTERISTICS ON ENDOTHELIAL CELL ADHERENCE
See Figure 50-17.

Source of Endothelial Cells. Endothelial cells from different vascular beds differ in surface receptors and behavior in response to external signals. The impact of the relationship between the heterogeneity of endothelial cells and the heterogeneity of sickle RBCs is far from being understood. For example, although most of the *in vitro* work performed on sickle red cell–endothelial cell adherence used human umbilical vein endothelial cells, these cells do not express CD36, which is a theoretically important receptor for thrombospondin-coated sickle reticulocytes (281). In contrast, endothelial cells isolated from the blood of patients with sickle cell disease do express CD36, suggesting a microvascular source (282). The complexity of these systems is illustrated by the observation that plasma and von Willebrand's factor multimers have differential effects on red cell adherence that depend on whether the experimental endothelial cells are of large vessel or microvascular origin (283).

Inflammation, Infection, and Hypoxia. Endothelial cells can also modulate their surface receptors in response to external stimuli. Infection itself can cause changes in endothelial cells by at least two different mechanisms. Herpes simplex virus type 1 can infect endothelial cells and cause them to display an Fc receptor on their surface. This receptor can increase adherence of sickle red cells by binding to the IgG pathologically found on the surface of sickle red cells (280). Endothelial cells exposed to parainfluenza 1 or virus-mimicking double-stranded RNA demonstrated increased adherence mediated by and up-regulated by the VCAM-1–VLA4 mechanism (266).

Like parainfluenza 1, tumor necrosis factor-α, a proinflammatory cytokine, induced increased adhesion of sickle RBCs (284) through the VCAM-1–VLA4 interaction (264). A more complex reaction to another cytokine, IL-1β, was demonstrated when the adherence phenomenon was examined after endothelial cells were exposed to the cytokine for up to 24 hours. In this series of experiments, adherence was increased 16-fold over baseline, and, at different times, different endothelial cell receptors were critical: first, vitronectin receptor, then E-selectin, and, finally, VCAM-1 (285).

Hypoxia can induce endothelial cells to become more adhesive to $CD36^+/VLA4^+$ sickle reticulocytes. Hypoxic endothelial cells have increased expression of VCAM-1 and intracellular adhesion molecule–1, although VCAM-1 appears to be the key receptor involved in the increased adherence (267). In contrast, exposing endothelial cells to hydroxyurea decreases RBC adherence and changes endothelial cell morphology and cation transport (286).

Endothelial Cell Alteration by Sickle Red Blood Cells. The adhesion process can alter endothelial cells. Endothelial cells culled from the peripheral blood of patients with sickle cell disease demonstrate an activated phenotype, displaying intracellular adhesion molecule–1, VCAM-1, E-selectin, P-selectin, and tissue factor (282,287). In the IL-1β experiments described above, morphologic evidence of damage was found after the stimulated endothelial cells were exposed to sickle RBCs, and the morphologic changes correlated with the degree of adherence (285). Biochemically, change in endothelial cell function after exposure to sickle red cells can be demonstrated generally by decreased DNA synthesis (288) and specifically by increased expression of endothelin-1 (289). Similarly, arachidonate metabolites generated by endothelial cells are implicated in increasing adherence and appear to be stimulated by adherence of sickle red cells (290–292).

Subendothelium. The presence of circulating endothelial cells in patients with sickle cell disease (282,287) suggests that these cells have lost their mooring and that areas of exposed subendothelium may be present along the vasculature. Three subendothelial matrix proteins, laminin, thrombospondin, and fibronectin, are adhesive to sickle RBCs.

Two classes of binding sites for laminin have been identified on normal and sickle RBCs. An acidic lipid that binds both laminin and thrombospondin has been isolated (293). The membrane protein BCAM/LU (basal cell adhesion molecule/Lutheran) has been identified as the receptor for laminin (294). The epitope on laminin that binds to red cells appears to lie within the α_5-chain of the protein (295).

Thrombospondin behaves differently depending on whether it is in solution or immobilized (as it would be in the subendothelium). In contrast to soluble thrombospondin, immobilized thrombospondin binds sickle red cells by an interaction that does *not* appear to involve red cell CD36 (296). This interaction is inhibited by von Willebrand's factor, even at concentrations found normally in plasma (297).

Sickle reticulocytes appear to bind to fibronectin (298,299), although such binding is not consistently demonstrated in all assay systems (296). Interestingly, neutrophils from patients with sickle cell disease are particularly adhesive to fibronectin—an interaction that correlates with plasma levels of IL-6 (298).

INFLUENCE OF PLASMA PROTEINS, PLATELETS, AND WHITE CELLS ON ENDOTHELIAL CELL ADHERENCE

Soluble thrombospondin plays an important role in modulating endothelial adherence. Thrombospondin in the supernatant from activated platelets enhances the adherence of sickle red cells to microvascular endothelium (300) (Fig. 50-17) and may explain the observation that platelet-rich plasma promotes adherence (301). A strong pathophysiologic link comes from the observation that thrombospondin levels are increased in the plasma of patients with acute sickle crisis to the levels that are demonstrated to increase adherence *in vitro* (302).

Another key plasma protein that modulates endothelial adherence is von Willebrand's factor. Ultra–high-molecular-weight von Willebrand's factor multimers promote adhesion of sickle red cells (303). Reticulocytes bind these multimers through a gpIb- and gpIIa/IIIb-like receptor and bind to a gpIb-like receptor on endothelial cells (273) (Fig. 50-17). The importance of von Willebrand's factor in enhancing adherence is most dramatically shown in *in vivo* experiments in which desmopressin (DDAVP) stimulation causes a marked increase in the adhesion of light sickle red cells (275,279).

Polymorphonuclear leukocytes (PMNs) from patients with sickle cell disease are more adherent to endothelial cells (304) as well as subendothelium (298). Sickle red cells are also adherent to PMNs—a process that activates the PMNs, much as red cell adherence activates endothelial cells (305). This type of interaction between sickle red cells and PMNs increases oxidative damage to the red cells (306).

SICKLE RED CELLS IN THE CIRCULATION

A variety of rheologic techniques demonstrates that even fully oxygenated sickle red cells are less deformable than normal (307–310). When these cells are fractionated by density and studied, it becomes clear that the major rheologic impairment comes from the very dense cells with high intracellular viscosity (311–313). When rehydrated to a normal hemoglobin concentration, the rheology of these cells improves but does not normalize. This partial correction implies that there may be a residual abnormal membrane component—perhaps one described previously or one related to the formation of a complex between spectrin and sickle hemoglobin (314). Sickle hemoglobin can be experimentally packaged in normal membranes, creating a hybrid cell with an abnormal shear modulus. Packaging of hemoglobin A in sickle membranes normalizes the shear modulus (315). This observation suggests that the interaction of sickle hemoglobin with the membrane causes the abnormal cellular characteristics. In the same series of experiments, however, the abnormal plastic behavior of the very dense sickle cells could not be normalized by exchanging the sickle hemoglobin for hemoglobin A.

If oxygenated sickle cells have difficulty traversing the microvasculature, the situation drastically deteriorates when the cells become deoxygenated. As oxygen tension is reduced, so is the deformability of sickle cells (316–318). The filterability of sickle red cells declines with oxygen tension, and the densest cells appear to be the most sensitive to deoxygenation (319). Very dense cells become less filterable, even in oxygen tensions found on the arterial side of the circulation (320). The observation that the rheologic properties of minimally desaturated dense cells correlate with clinical parameters stresses the potential pathophysiologic importance of polymer in the arterial circulation (321). Ironically, ektacytometric measurements of cell deformability suggest that the cells with the highest hemoglobin concentration require the greatest amount of polymer to be present before deformability is impaired (322).

Hebbel has articulated a view of flow in the microvascular circulation that emphasizes the role of the reticulocyte in the pathogenesis of occlusion and illustrates the potential to exploit the blockade of endothelial adherence as a strategy for therapy (323).

STRATEGIES FOR THERAPY

Replace Defective Marrow

Expression of the sickle gene is limited to the erythroid cells of the bone marrow—a tissue that can be transplanted. Although the first bone marrow transplants in patients with sickle cell anemia were performed for other indications [acute myeloblastic leukemia (324), Morquio's syndrome (325)], transplantation has now been performed on more than 150 patients with the intent to cure sickle cell disease (326–330). In most cases, transplant criteria have included some indication of increased severity including combinations of stroke, high rates of pain episodes or acute chest syndrome, and evidence of lung or kidney damage. Overall, approximately 80% to 85% of patients were reported alive and free of sickle cell disease; approximately 6% to 8% died; and approximately 9% to 14% had graft failure. Evidence of spleen regeneration has been observed after transplant (331,332), a phenomenon that has also been described after transfusion (333) and hydroxyurea treatment (334,335). Most of this experience reflects treatment that was modeled after regimens designed to treat thalassemia including myeloablation and immunosuppression. Early experience with these myeloablative regimens also revealed a particular vulnerability of sickle cell anemia patients to thrombocytopenia-related intracranial hemorrhage and other neurologic complications (336) and led to improved transplant protocols, including a higher threshold platelet count for platelet transfusion and prophylactic antiseizure therapy. With these aggressive preparative regimens, gonadal dysfunction and secondary malignancy have been observed. Newer nonmyeloablative regimens hold promise for reducing transplant morbidity and mortality. In addition to designing safer transplant regimens, one of the major challenges in the field includes overcoming the practical barrier of having so few HLA-identical sibling donors (337). In one study, only 14% of patients meeting entry criteria for transplant had an HLA-identical sibling (338).

More specific gene therapy, repairing the sickle gene defect by inserting a normal β gene (339) or "correcting" the product of the abnormal gene (340,341), is still years from clinical trial.

Stimulate Fetal Hemoglobin Production

Because fetal hemoglobin has such a profound inhibitory effect on sickle hemoglobin polymerization, there has been substantial interest in trying to stimulate the dormant γ-globin genes. The first evidence that the chemotherapeutic agent 5-azacytidine could enhance fetal hemoglobin production in anemic primates (342) led to encouraging proof-of-principle trials in patients with thalassemia and sickle cell disease (343,344). The increased production of fetal hemoglobin was thought to be related to the ability of 5-azacytidine to directly reduce methylation and therefore restore transcription of fetal genes. Subsequent trials with other cytotoxic drugs that do not influence DNA methylation, such as cytosine arabinoside (345) and hydroxyurea (346), revealed that "safer" drugs than 5-azacytidine can also stimulate fetal hemoglobin production. Complete understanding of the precise mechanism of this effect continues to be elusive, but it is, in part, related to drawing more erythroid production from primitive precursor cells that have a propensity for producing F cells. Short-chain fatty acids such as butyrate and acetate

enhance fetal hemoglobin synthesis in sickle red cell progenitors (347–351) and in vivo (352–359). The mechanism for this effect is also not precisely known, although it is probably associated with inhibition of histone deacetylase and its effect on chromatin structure. The observation that hydroxyurea and fatty acid compounds appear to work by two independent mechanisms implies that their use may be additive.

Hydroxyurea has been tested extensively in several clinical settings, including a prospective, randomized, placebo-controlled efficacy trial that ultimately resulted in its approval by the U.S. Food and Drug Administration for the treatment of sickle cell anemia (360). The clinical use of hydroxyurea is discussed in the section Use of Hydroxyurea.

Decrease the Concentration of Hemoglobin S

The polymerization of sickle hemoglobin is exquisitely concentration dependent. Any therapy that reduced the mean corpuscular hemoglobin concentration of sickle cells would drastically reduce polymerization. Two approaches to decrease hemoglobin concentration have been tried: (a) lowering plasma osmolarity, and (b) blocking the pathologic cation channels that dehydrate sickle red cells. The first approach uses DDAVP and severe dietary salt restriction to decrease the serum sodium to 120 mEq/L. This treatment causes cell swelling, lower mean corpuscular hemoglobin concentration, and fewer painful episodes (361). Although theoretically promising as a strategy, this regimen has ultimately proven to be too difficult to maintain, neurologically toxic, and ineffective (362,363).

As discussed previously, the two major dehydrating channels of the sickle red cell are inhibitable in vivo. The Gardos channel is inhibited by the imidazole antifungal agent clotrimazole (193,364), and magnesium blocks K-Cl cotransport (195). Both agents have been shown to be effective physiologically in a mouse model of disease (192,204) and in small-scale studies in patients (193,205,206). These promising agents act independently and are amenable to being added into regimens including hydroxyurea (365). New Gardos blockers without the potentially dose-limiting imidazole toxicities associated with clotrimazole have been identified (366) and are in the early phases of human testing. It is likely that combination therapy including mixtures of channel blockers and hydroxyurea will undergo clinical efficacy studies within the next few years.

Inhibit the Polymerization of Hemoglobin S

Despite the detailed knowledge of the structure of the sickle polymer and the effort that excellent laboratories have expended in designing and demonstrating antisickling compounds, none is used to treat patients. Pragmatic issues of toxicity and red cell membrane permeability are serious problems that may take years to solve. The potentially useful antisickling agents are generally classified as either noncovalent or covalent modifiers of hemoglobin and have a variety of effects on hemoglobin solubility, oxygen affinity, and cell sickling (367). Urea is the classic noncovalent reagent that disrupts hydrophobic interactions. It is an antisickling agent at molar concentrations in vitro (368) but is ineffective in concentrations that can be achieved clinically (369). A more specific approach to noncovalent disruption of polymerization is exemplified by the use of p-aminobenzoylpolyglutamates with hydrophobic end groups (370). These relatively potent compounds are designed to interfere with the interaction of the β-6 valine of one strand and the hydrophobic pocket on the adjacent strand.

The covalent modifiers were reviewed by Ueno and colleagues (371). A variety of effective antisickling agents target a variety of residues. For example, nitrogen mustard reacts with histidine (372); glyceraldehyde (373) and aspirins (374) react with lysine and cystamine (375); and glutathione (376) reacts with cysteine. The only agent of this class that has undergone clinical trial is cyanate, a chemical that carbamylates the amino-terminal groups of the α- and β-chains (377,378). Despite some initial encouraging clinical experience, serious neurotoxicity (379) and cataract stimulation (380) preclude its use.

Increase the Flow in Small Vessels or Decreasing Sickle Cell Interactions with Endothelial Cells

As shown in Figure 50-17, a variety of factors conspire to impede the flow of sickle red cells as they come in contact with the endothelium. As knowledge of and interest in the roles of coagulation, inflammation, oxidation, reperfusion (381), and endothelial pathophysiology grow, it is likely that new classes of agents or a combination of agents will be tested in clinical trials in sickle cell disease.

CLINICAL FEATURES

Nomenclature

In this chapter, the term *sickle cell disease* includes all the symptomatic sickle syndromes (e.g., SS disease, S-thalassemias, SC disease) and specifically excludes the asymptomatic carrier state—sickle trait. Table 50-2 lists the shorthand notation for the different sickle syndromes.

Diagnosis

PRENATAL DIAGNOSIS
Old (382) has reviewed the history of the development of technology for performing prenatal diagnosis and the U.K. experience to date. Interesting innovations include preimplantation prenatal diagnosis (383) and avoiding chorionic villus sampling by isolating fetal cells from the maternal peripheral blood (384).

NEWBORN SCREENING
One of the most important therapeutic trials in sickle cell disease literature is the trial by Gaston and co-workers (385) that demonstrated the efficacy of prophylactic penicillin in the prevention of pneumococcal sepsis in young children (Fig. 50-18). This study established that early identification and intervention can have an impact on mortality. As a result, most of the United States has developed procedures to screen newborns for sickle cell disease (386). The benefit of screening *all* newborns is illustrated by the experience of the state of California, in which 58 non-black infants with sickle cell disease were identified in a 4-year period (387).

In newborn samples, an FA electrophoretic or chromatographic pattern is normal; FAS is sickle trait [or, rarely, Sβ+-thalassemia or a transfused baby (388)]; FS is sickle cell anemia (or, rarely, sickle hereditary persistence of fetal hemoglobin or Sβ0-thalassemia); FSC is SC disease; FAC is C trait; and the presence of Bart's hemoglobin indicates α-thalassemia. The sickle preparation and solubility tests are inaccurate in this age group (389).

DIAGNOSING SICKLE SYNDROMES IN THE OLDER CHILD AND ADULT
Such a wide variation exists in the clinical severity of the sickle syndromes that it is not uncommon to be faced with making a new diagnosis in a relatively asymptomatic adult. This is particularly true for the syndromes that tend to be milder, such as SC disease or Sβ+-thalassemia. As shown in Table 50-2, a reliable diagnosis of the major sickle syndromes can be made on the basis of a complete blood count, reticulocyte count, peripheral smear, sickle solubility test, and hemoglobin electrophoresis or chromatography. For prenatal counseling or research situations, a more specific genetic diagnosis can be assigned at the DNA level, determining α-gene number and β-globin haplotype.

Anemia of Sickle Cell Disease

CHRONIC ANEMIA
After the first few months of life, the level of fetal hemoglobin declines (Table 50-3), the production of hemoglobin S dominates, and the typical chronic hemolytic pattern of SS disease develops (390,391). As seen in Figure 50-15, in SS disease, the peripheral blood has some normal-looking red cells as well as targets, Howell-Jolly bodies, nucleated red cells, fragments, spherocytes, and irreversibly sickled cells. This is a hemolytic anemia with a red cell survival of 10 to 30 days (normal, 120 days) and a rate of heme catabolism (endogenous carbon monoxide production) that is six times normal (392). The degree of hemolysis is relatively constant for a given patient (393) and is essentially unchanged during uncomplicated vasoocclusive events. The degree of anemia inversely correlates with the irreversibly sickled cell count (158,394), the reticulocyte count, and the mean corpuscular volume (MCV) (395).

Theoretically, the expanded bone marrow should be able to compensate for the hemolytic rate of this disease and produce a normal hematocrit (Hct). There are several possible explanations for the apparent lack of complete compensation: (a) The amount of erythropoietin is lower than seen in other comparable anemias (396), possibly due to an altered renal response or the right-shifted O_2 dissociation curve; (b) the plasma volume is expanded to a greater extent than in other anemias (394), making the Hct appear lower than it really is; and (c) there is some degree of ineffective erythropoiesis because polymerization and phagocytosis can occur in and to red cell precursors in the marrow (397,398) (Fig. 50-19).

Anemia is probably more of a help than a hindrance in this disease because the increased blood viscosity that accompanies a higher Hct may augment sludging and vasoocclusion. This may explain why patients with SS disease and coexisting α-thalassemia—who have fewer dense cells, less intracellular polymer, and less hemolysis—typically have considerable symptoms, with acute pain episodes (399) and avascular necrosis of bones (400,401). It also explains why patients with higher Hcts have a tendency toward more pain crises (399) and episodes of acute chest syndrome (402). This apparent paradox suggests that phlebotomy might be useful in the treatment of some patients with high Hcts and high rates of vasoocclusive events.

EXACERBATIONS OF STEADY-STATE ANEMIA

Iron Deficiency. Florid iron deficiency that causes anemia to worsen is relatively rare in SS disease, although mild deficiency certainly occurs (403–406), and the resultant microcytosis can contribute to misdiagnosing Sβ0-thalassemia (404). Because of the decreased hemoglobin concentration, iron deficiency may result in less hemolysis and fewer painful episodes (407–409), but inducing iron deficiency is not recommended as treatment.

Folic Acid Deficiency. As in all patients with chronic hemolysis, patients with SS disease have increased folic acid requirements. Patients with poor dietary intake of folate may develop a

TABLE 50-2. Clinical Features of Sickle Cell Syndromes: Typical Findings

Syndrome	Abbreviation	Complete Blood Cell Count			Morphology		Hemoglobin Electrophoresis					Percentage with Splenomegaly (%)	Vasoocclusive Severity (Range)
		Hemoglobin (g/dL)	Mean Corpuscular Volume (fL)	Reticulocytes (%)	Irreversibly Sickled Cells	Targets	S	A	F	A$_2$	Other		
Sickle cell trait	AS (αα/αα)	N	80–90	N	0	0	35–40	50–60	<2	<3.5	—	0	0
Sickle trait (+ α-thalassemia silent carrier)	AS (-α/αα)	13–14	75–85	—	—	—	30–35	55–65	—	—	—	—	—
Sickle trait (+ α-thalassemia trait)	AS (-α/-α)	12–13	70–75	—	—	—	25–30	60–75	—	—	—	—	—
Sickle trait (+ hemoglobin H disease)	AS (--/-α)	7–10	50–55	—	—	—	17–25	65–80	—	—	—	—	—
Sickle cell anemia	SS (αα/αα)	8	95	>10	4+	3+	80–99	0	2–20	2.8	—	80 in children; ~10 in adults	4+ (1+ to 4+)
SS (+ α-thalassemia silent carrier)	SS (-α/αα)	8.5	85	~10	3+	3+	80–99	0	2–20	3.3	—	—	—
SS (+ α-thalassemia trait)	SS (-α/-α)	9	75	<10	2+	3+	80–90	0	2–20	3.8	—	—	—
Sickle C disease	SC	11	80	<10	1+	4+	50	0	<2	<3.5	50% C	60	2+ (1+ to 4+)
Sickle β+-thalassemia	Sβ+ thal	10	75	<5	2+	4+	75	15	5	>3.5	—	60	2+ (1+ to 4+)
Sickle β0-thalassemia	Sβ0 thal	8	70	~10	3+	4+	90	0	5	>3.5	—	60	4+ (1+ to 4+)

N, normal.

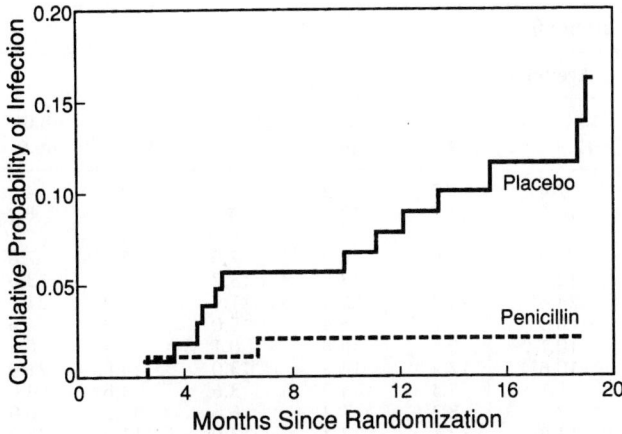

Figure 50-18. Effect of prophylactic penicillin on the probability of bacterial sepsis in children with sickle cell anemia younger than 5 years of age. (From Gaston MH, Verter JI. Prophylaxis with oral penicillin in children with sickle cell anemia: a randomized trial. *N Engl J Med* 1986;314:1593, with permission.)

superimposed megaloblastic anemia, particularly if they are not supplemented during pregnancy or a period of rapid growth. Mild chemical folate deficiency without megaloblastosis is relatively common (410). It has become general clinical practice to provide prophylactic folate supplementation (1 mg/day), although a controlled trial of placebo versus folate showed a

difference of only 4 fL in MCV and no difference in Hct or growth in children (411,412). There is no evidence to suggest that mild folate deficiency causes increased levels of homocysteine in children with sickle cell disease, a concern because of the endothelial damage and vascular compromise that hyperhomocysteinemia might cause (413).

Renal Failure. When patients with SS disease develop renal failure, erythropoietin levels fall, and anemia worsens (414). Many of these patients develop chronic congestive heart failure, become transfusion dependent, and, like other patients with renal failure, may benefit from high-dose exogenous erythropoietin (396,415,416).

Acute Splenic Sequestration. Acute splenic sequestration crisis has a peak incidence of 5 to 6 episodes/100 patient-years in the 0.5- to 3.0-year age group (Table 50-4) (417). It remains one of the leading causes of death in children with SS disease (417–423). These young children frequently present in hypovolumic shock, having trapped a considerable portion of intravascular volume in a rapidly enlarging spleen. There is often history of dyspnea, left-sided abdominal pain, vomiting, and abdominal distention blossoming over a period of hours. The hemoglobin is at least 2 g/dL lower than usual, with increased reticulocytes, erythroblastosis, and mild to moderate thrombocytopenia. For those who survive the initial episode, approximately one-half have a recurrence (418,420,421), usually within 6 months (420,421). In the Jamaican series (421), the mortality

TABLE 50-3. Hematologic Findings in SS, SC, and Sβ⁺-Thalassemia

		Age (mo)										
	Percentile	2.0–3.9	4.0–5.9	6.0–8.9	9.0–11.9	12.0–14.9	15.0–17.9	18.0–23.9	24.0–29.9	30.0–35.9	36.0–47.9	48.0–60.0
Hemoglobin (g/dL)												
SS	5th	7.0	7.0	7.1	7.2	7.2	7.2	7.1	6.9	6.7	6.4	6.6
	50th	9.3	9.2	9.2	9.2	9.1	9.0	8.9	8.6	8.3	8.1	8.3
	95th	11.4	11.3	11.4	11.5	11.5	11.5	11.3	11.1	10.9	10.5	10.4
SC	5th	8.0	8.2	8.6	8.9	9.2	9.3	9.5	9.5	9.4	9.3	9.6
	50th	9.7	9.8	10.1	10.3	10.5	10.6	10.7	10.8	10.7	10.6	10.6
	95th	11.6	11.5	11.7	11.8	12.0	12.0	12.1	12.2	12.2	12.1	11.9
Sβ⁺-thal	5th	9.2	9.4	9.1	8.5	9.1	9.1	9.9	10.0	9.8	9.3	10.0
	50th	10.8	10.9	11.0	10.8	10.6	11.2	10.9	11.0	10.7	10.6	10.8
	95th	12.4	12.7	13.5	11.8	14.1	12.0	12.0	13.0	11.3	11.6	11.2
Mean corpuscular volume (fL)												
SS	5th	72	69	68	67	67	67	67	68	69	71	72
	50th	84	81	81	82	82	83	84	85	86	88	90
	95th	96	94	94	95	95	96	96	97	97	98	100
SC	5th	68	65	64	63	63	63	63	63	64	66	69
	50th	81	78	77	75	74	74	74	74	76	77	77
	95th	91	88	86	85	84	84	84	84	86	88	87
Sβ⁺-thal	5th	70	64	61	61	63	62	63	61	66	64	66
	50th	80	73	72	69	72	70	70	70	72	76	68
	95th	88	83	84	75	84	77	77	79	76	76	76
Reticulocyte (%)												
SS	5th	1.0	1.1	1.2	1.3	1.4	1.6	1.9	2.3	2.6	2.7	1.8
	50th	4.0	5.1	5.9	6.7	7.4	8.0	8.7	9.3	9.8	10.4	11.8
	95th	15.5	17.9	19.4	20.7	21.8	22.5	23.2	23.5	23.6	23.6	25.8
SC	5th	0.8	0.8	0.8	0.7	0.7	0.7	0.7	0.7	0.7	0.7	0.9
	50th	2.8	2.8	2.7	2.6	2.5	2.5	2.5	2.6	2.7	2.9	2.8
	95th	8.2	8.8	8.9	9.0	8.9	8.7	8.4	8.0	7.9	8.8	13.4
Sβ⁺-thal	5th	1.1	0.0	1.1	0.9	0.8	0.9	0.7	1.5	1.2	1.0	3.0
	50th	2.6	1.8	2.5	2.5	3.0	2.5	2.4	2.2	3.4	2.2	4.1
	95th	8.5	6.4	2.5	4.6	5.9	7.4	5.1	6.2	7.4	7.6	5.7
Hemoglobin F (%)												
SS	5th	14.6	12.3	10.8	9.1	7.8	6.7	5.6	4.8	4.5	4.4	3.3
	50th	43.5	34.1	29.1	24.3	20.6	17.7	14.8	12.8	12.4	12.4	9.0
	95th	68.5	59.0	53.0	47.3	42.7	39.1	35.3	32.5	31.2	29.6	21.9
SC	5th	13.6	2.9	2.9	3.1	3.1	2.9	2.4	1.4	0.5	0.0	2.0

(continued)

TABLE 50-3. (continued)

	Percentile	Age (mo)										
		2.0–3.9	4.0–5.9	6.0–8.9	9.0–11.9	12.0–14.9	15.0–17.9	18.0–23.9	24.0–29.9	30.0–35.9	36.0–47.9	48.0–60.0
	50th	31.6	17.9	14.5	11.6	9.3	7.4	5.5	4.2	3.9	4.4	4.2
	95th	54.0	39.1	32.1	25.7	20.9	17.6	14.7	13.8	14.7	15.9	8.3
White blood cell count (×10³/µL)												
SS	5th	6.0	6.0	6.3	6.6	6.9	6.9	6.9	6.8	7.0	7.8	7.8
	50th	9.5	9.4	10.2	11.3	12.2	12.9	13.4	13.7	13.7	13.5	13.6
	95th	15.7	15.8	18.6	22.1	24.1	24.8	24.4	22.4	21.9	23.9	21.2
SC	5th	6.2	6.1	6.3	6.5	6.5	6.3	6.0	5.4	5.0	4.9	4.6
	50th	9.5	9.3	9.7	10.2	10.3	10.1	9.6	8.6	8.1	8.4	8.2
	95th	15.1	13.6	15.0	17.5	18.6	18.6	17.2	14.5	13.0	14.8	21.0
Sβ⁺-thal	5th	6.3	5.0	4.3	6.9	5.1	5.1	5.3	4.9	3.6	3.8	4.8
	50th	8.7	7.9	8.3	9.5	8.2	8.6	8.2	7.2	6.6	7.2	8.0
	95th	13.4	15.0	22.5	14.6	14.5	13.6	12.1	12.2	13.9	11.5	23.0
Platelets (×10³/µL)												
SS	5th	224	216	207	199	192	186	182	181	182	187	198
	50th	419	405	390	376	366	361	361	374	387	405	423
	95th	683	649	615	586	572	571	596	667	719	743	674
SC	5th	192	191	191	190	189	188	187	185	188	203	242
	50th	424	423	420	414	405	395	375	342	317	298	309
	95th	704	681	655	624	595	567	530	487	462	463	533

from recurrences reached 14%, although such devastating outcomes are not found in contemporary American series (424). As used here, the phrase *acute splenic sequestration* refers to a rapidly evolving dramatic event, typically with the spleen palpable below the umbilicus, an Hct 40% to 70% of baseline, and fewer than 150,000 platelets. Some patients, who, between routine visits, may superficially appear to have acute sequestration and whose Hcts are falling, reticulocytes are increasing, and spleens are enlarging, are in fact going through the typical hematologic changes of infancy (Table 50-3). Some patients develop mild hypersplenism in association with viral illness, with a larger than usual spleen and a 20% to 25% drop in Hct. At initial presentation, these patients may resemble an early sequestration and should be examined frequently to assess the tempo of the process. It is not known whether these children with a tendency for transient hypersplenism are at high risk for developing fulminant sequestration, but they should be seen frequently, and their parents should be alerted to the possibility.

The acute management of sequestration is straightforward and noncontroversial: immediately restore intravascular volume and oxygen-carrying capacity by transfusion of packed red cells. Once a normal cardiovascular status is restored, the patient usually improves rapidly, and the spleen size and platelet count normalize over days. There is no role for emergency splenectomy.

Chronic management is less straightforward and more controversial. The obvious approach to preventing the recurrence of splenic sequestration is to remove the spleen (425). There is understandable reluctance, however, to remove what may be a functional spleen in a very young child, and some have suggested that a maintenance transfusion program (426) or partial splenectomy (427) be used to prevent recurrence. A review of 23 cases of splenic sequestration from Duke University illustrates the problems of transfusion as prevention (424). In this series, 4 patients underwent prompt splenectomy, 7 were observed carefully without transfusion, and 12 received transfusions (6 to 12 months) and were maintained with a hemoglobin S less than 30%. Of the seven observed patients, four experienced recurrences 3 to 11 months after the initial episode. Of the 12 patients who received transfusions, 2 are still receiving transfusions and are well. Of the remaining ten, three experienced recurrences while on transfusion (3 to 9 months after the initial episode), and four had recurrences within 3 months

of the last transfusion. Only three of the patients remained well 11.0 months to 3.9 years off transfusion therapy. In this series, 14% of children developed red cell antibodies, and one child developed non-A, non-B hepatitis. Eventually, 14 of the 23 patients came to splenectomy. All were immunized against pneumococcus and were prescribed prophylactic penicillin. None has experienced a life-threatening infection in a total follow-up period of 65.6 patient-years. Several important lessons can be learned from this series: (a) Sequestration can occur while on a transfusion program, (b) sequestration can recur soon after stopping a transfusion program, (c) transfusions are not without risk, (d) children who are immunized and treated with prophylactic penicillin can tolerate splenectomy, and (e) sequestration need not be a fatal complication if families are alerted to early signs. In one series of 35 patients treated with partial splenectomy, one developed overwhelming pneumococcal sepsis (428). Routine care of children should include teaching parents to palpate the child's spleen and to be alert to a rapid increase in size.

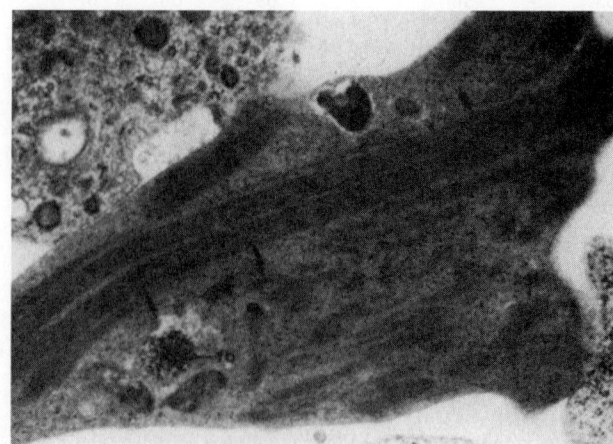

Figure 50-19. Sickle hemoglobin polymer (*arrows*) in a bone marrow reticulocyte. (From Grasso JA, Sullivan AL, Sullivan LW. Ultrastructural studies of the bone marrow in sickle cell anemia. I. The structure of sickled erythrocytes and reticulocytes and their phagocytic destruction. *Br J Haematol* 1975;31:135, with permission.)

TABLE 50-4. Incidence of Acute Events (Per 100 Patient-Years) by Age and Genotype in a Cohort of Patients Followed Prospectively, Starting Before 6 Months of Age

Event	Genotype	<6 mo	6–12 mo	1 yr	2 yr	3 yr	4 yr	5 yr	6 yr	7 yr	8–10 yr
Pain episode	SS	2.9	9.5	24.0	38.3	42.4	49.6	40.8	39.2	41.6	37.9
	SC	0	3.8	8.5	15.3	28.5	23.3	33.6	29.1	40.3	23.0
Acute chest syndrome	SS	6.8	16.4	26.8	26.3	34.2	25.5	22.5	28.9	20.8	15.2
	SC	3.5	18.2	10.6	10.4	13.1	9.7	5.2	1.8	5.8	3.3
Bacteremia	SS	1.9	9.9	6.5	8.7	4.7	2.0	0	4.1	1.5	0
	SC	0	7.7	5.8	1.2	0	0	0	1.8	0	0
Splenic sequestration	SS	1.0	5.5	6.2	5.3	2.0	1.5	1.4	1.0	0	0
	SC	0	0	0.5	0	1.5	2.9	1.3	1.8	0	0
Hand-foot	SS	14.6	31.3	20.0	11.0	3.5	2.0	0	0	0	0
	SC	0	1.0	3.2	1.2	0	0	0	0	0	0
Cerebrovascular accident	SS	0	0	0.3	1.3	0.4	1.5	0.7	2.1	1.5	0
	SC	0	0	0	0	0	0	0	0	0	0

Splenic sequestration is primarily a disease of young children with SS disease, and it had been documented to occur as early as 8 weeks of age (429). Occasionally, it occurs in older patients with SC disease and Sβ-thalassemia (430–433). In adults with these syndromes, acute splenic sequestration is usually not a life-threatening complication (434) and behaves more like a transient episode of hypersplenism, often in the setting of an acute viral illness. One patient with SC disease and hereditary spherocytosis is described who experienced five episodes of sequestration (435).

Acute Liver Sequestration. Sequestration may also take place in the liver, but because the liver is not as distensible as the spleen, there is rarely associated cardiovascular collapse. These patients experience worsening anemia, an enlarged tender liver, right upper quadrant pain, extreme hyperbilirubinemia (unconjugated bilirubin >50 mg/dL), elevated transaminases, and increased reticulocytosis (436). These patients usually recover spontaneously within a week but may be indistinguishable at presentation from those rare patients who go on to die of fulminant hepatic failure (437,438).

Aplastic Episode. Patients with SS disease are vulnerable to the same life-threatening, parvovirus-induced transient cessation of erythropoiesis as patients with other chronic hemolytic anemias (439). In Jamaica, approximately 40% of SS and AA children developed parvovirus-specific IgG by age 15 years, although approximately 20% of these children did not develop aplasia (440). Typical patients with aplastic crises present with various combinations of increased fatigue, headache, gastrointestinal symptoms, pallor, thrombocytopenia, and arthralgia—but not the typical rash of fifth disease (441,442). The short-lived, hemoglobin F–poor cells disappear first from the circulation, causing an apparent increase in the percentage of hemoglobin F during these episodes (443). The Hct falls 10% to 15%/day without compensatory reticulocytosis (444). The virus is highly transmissible to medical personnel as well as other close contacts. If one patient in a household becomes aplastic, others are almost certain to follow within a few days (445). Spontaneous recovery is usually preceded by a sharp increase in peripheral nucleated red cells and then a brisk reticulocytosis, an increase in serum transferrin receptor (446), and, often, hyperbilirubinemia. This recovery phase is probably responsible for many of the cases referred to as *hyperhemolytic episodes.* Spontaneous recovery may not occur before cardiovascular compromise occurs. In the Jamaican experience, 87% of patients required transfusion to tide them over until marrow activity

resumed (441). In one series of aplastic crisis, approximately 70% of cases were associated with positive diagnostic tests for parvovirus (447). Recurrence is generally not seen.

Glucose-6-Phosphate Dehydrogenase Deficiency. Glucose-6-phosphate dehydrogenase (G6PD) deficiency is a common genetic variant among people of African heritage. An unexpectedly high prevalence of G6PD deficiency among patients with SS disease originally suggested that the enzyme deficiency confers a protective effect (448,449), but subsequent studies suggest that there is no increased prevalence (450). In a study of 801 males with SS disease from the Cooperative Study of Sickle Cell Disease (CSSCD), 4% were G6PD deficient (451) and demonstrated no difference in degree of anemia, MCV, reticulocyte count, bilirubin, serum glutamic-oxaloacetic transaminase, or incidence of painful or acute anemic episodes. Because the sickle red cell is young and the A– variant of G6PD deficiency typically maintains normal activity in young cells, hemolysates from enzyme-deficient SS red cells have normal activity, whereas those from enzyme-sufficient SS red cells have elevated activity. Episodes of accelerated hemolysis in patients with both SS disease and G6PD deficiency have been described (452). It appears that such accelerated "hyperhemolysis" would be more likely when the average age of the circulating cells is higher, as it is during an aplastic episode.

Growth and Development

Infants with SS disease have normal birthweight (453,454) but may exhibit growth delay and delayed bone age during childhood (455–458). In the CSSCD, the 2115 patients studied had normal height and weight until 7 years of age (459). At this age, growth was delayed compared with healthy black patients, the controls in the study (Fig. 50-20). Weight was more affected than height. Patients with SS disease or Sβ0-thalassemia were more delayed than patients with SC disease or Sβ+-thalassemia. In general, by late adolescence, patients caught up with the normal population and attained normal adult height, although weight continued to be low. Similar findings have been reported from Jamaica (460).

Sexual development is also delayed in sickle cell disease (459,461) (Table 50-5). The pattern of sexual delay is similar to that found for growth delay: SS disease and Sβ0-thalassemia patients are more delayed than the SC disease and Sβ+-thalassemia patients. Although there is a delay in sexual maturity, males and females eventually mature, suggesting that there is no permanent underlying endocrinopathy. This was supported by the careful study of female fertility in Jamaica, which revealed no

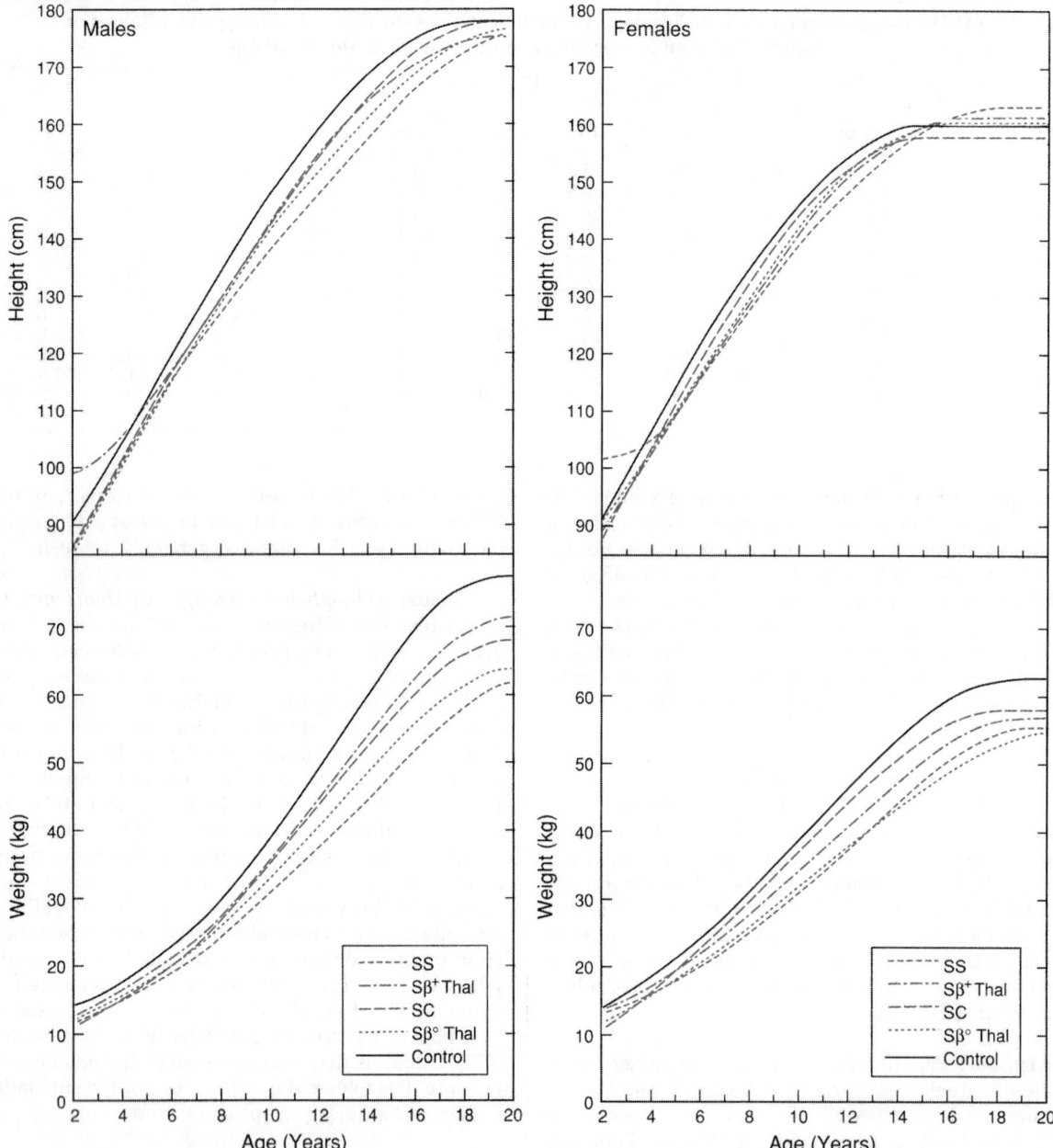

Figure 50-20. Height and weight growth curves for patients with sickle cell syndromes. (From Platt OS, Rosenstock W, Espeland MA. Influence of sickle hemoglobinopathies on growth and development. *N Engl J Med* 1984;311:7, with permission.)

difference in the interval between sexual exposure and pregnancy between patients and normal controls (462). Normal thyroid function (461) and hypothalamic-pituitary axis (461,463) have been shown, although some men are infertile and have decreased sperm motility and number (464). Primary hypogonadism (465,466) and hypothalamic hypogonadism responsive to clomiphene (467) have also been described.

The cause of delayed growth and development among patients with sickle cell disease is not known. The fact that growth is more delayed in SS disease and Sβ⁰-thalassemia than in SC disease and Sβ⁺-thalassemia suggests that the degree of anemia or clinical severity may be relevant. Analyses from the CSSCD showed that growth and maturation delays are inversely correlated with Hct (468) and do not correlate with the incidence of painful episodes (M. Espeland, unpublished data). Perhaps the hematopoietic and cardiovascular compensation for anemia

causes the increased metabolic needs (469–471) that impair growth if unmet. This is supported by the finding that supplemental nasogastric feeding improves the growth of children with SS disease (472), although major nutritional deficiencies in patients with delayed growth are not readily demonstrable (473). In one series, zinc deficiency was also a factor in growth retardation (474).

Susceptibility to Infection

Although sickle cell disease is a disorder of hemoglobin, the single most common cause of death in children is not polymerization but infection (417,418,423,475). The organisms encountered are generally not unusual pathogens, but the infections they cause are more frequent and severe. Characteristically, the infections of children are fulminant, without focus, often fatal, and

TABLE 50-5. Estimated Median Age at Attainment of Tanner Stages, According to Hemoglobinopathy

Tanner Stage		SS	SC	Sβ⁺	Sβ⁰
			Median Age (yr)		

Females
Breasts 2   11.8   9.8 10.6 11.8
3   13.5 11.9 12.6 12.8
4   15.0 13.9 13.8 14.8
5   17.3 16.0 16.5 17.2
Pubic hair 2 12.0 10.1 10.0 11.5
3 13.5 11.8 11.2 12.8
4 15.2 14.0 13.8 14.2
5 19.2 17.0 17.0 20.8
Males
Penis 2 12.0 10.4 11.9 12.4
3 14.2 13.0 13.0 13.2
4 16.0 14.1 13.5 15.5
5 17.6 16.6 16.6 18.8
Pubic hair 2 13.2 11.5 12.0 13.2
3 14.8 13.2 13.0 13.9
4 16.2 14.2 13.9 16.2
5 17.9 16.6 17.1 18.5

From Platt OS, Rosenstock W, Espeland MA. Influence of sickle hemoglobinopathies on growth and development. *N Engl J Med* 1984;311:7, with permission.

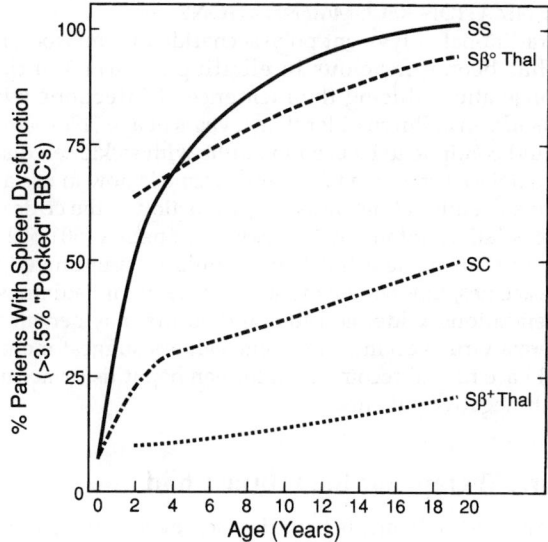

Figure 50-21. Splenic function (as measured by peripheral blood "pocked" erythrocytes) by age in the various sickle syndromes. RBC, red blood cell. (From Pearson HA, Gallagher D, Chilcote R, et al. Developmental pattern of splenic dysfunction in sickle cell disorders. *Pediatrics* 1985;76:392, with permission.)

typically caused by the encapsulated *Streptococcus pneumoniae* and, to a much lesser degree, *Haemophilus influenzae*. In adults, death from sepsis is less common (476), urinary tract and bone foci are more frequent, and *Escherichia coli*, *Salmonella* spp., and *Staphylococcus aureus* are prominent pathogens (477).

Functional Asplenia and Bacterial Sepsis

The function of the spleen is invariably destroyed in sickle cell disease. During the first year of life, most patients with SS disease lose the spleen's ability to clear particulate matter from the blood, referred to as *functional asplenia* (478,479). This dysfunction is heralded by the appearance of Howell-Jolly bodies and irregular "pocking" of the red cell surface (which can only be seen using a microscope equipped with interference or Nomarski optics). Despite their palpable splenomegaly, these children have no uptake of technetium 99m sulfur colloid and are susceptible to the most virulent complication of asplenia: *S. pneumoniae* sepsis. Chronic transfusion may temporarily restore splenic function (333,480,481), even in adults (482). Similar restoration of splenic function has been documented in some patients after bone marrow transplantation (331,332) and during hydroxyurea treatment (334,335).

The timing of the development and the ultimate prevalence of splenic dysfunction varies by genotype (483) (Fig. 50-21). Patients with Sβ⁰-thalassemia have a spleen pattern virtually identical to that of SS disease; Sβ⁺-thalassemia has little dysfunction; and SC disease is intermediate. In one series, the risk of a child with SS disease younger than 5 years of age acquiring *S. pneumoniae* sepsis or meningitis was greater than 15%; the associated mortality was approximately 30% (484). It appears that children with SC disease may be at somewhat less risk of bacterial sepsis overall (485–487). The CSSCD experience showed that the children with SC disease who were younger than 2 years of age had a rate of sepsis indistinguishable from that of the SS disease group (417,477) but had a lower mortality rate.

Clinically, the most worrisome organism is *S. pneumoniae*. There may be as high as a 400-fold increase in the incidence of *S. pneumoniae* sepsis in children with SS disease who are younger than 5 years of age (488). The course is fulminant and often fatal. In contrast, *H. influenzae* sepsis is only two to four times more common in SS disease than in the general population (which is extremely rare given the success of infant immunization programs) and typically follows a several-day prodrome with low-grade fever, symptoms of upper respiratory tract infection, or otitis media (488).

PROPHYLACTIC PENICILLIN

Prophylactic penicillin prevents 80% of *S. pneumoniae* sepsis in children with SS disease who are younger than 3 years of age (385) (Fig. 50-18), and given the low incidence of disease after age 5, it has not been shown to be effective in children older than 5 years of age (489). Discontinuation after age 5 is becoming increasingly important as penicillin-resistant organisms are becoming more prevalent (490–494). The impact of prophylaxis is tremendous, and newborn screening programs are in place in most of the United States so that infants with sickle cell disease can be identified early and begun on penicillin. Our approach is as follows:

- Give prophylaxis to all newborns with sickle cell disease (SS, SC, Sβ-thalassemia). (Note that some clinicians do not recommend penicillin to newborns with SC disease or Sβ⁺-thalassemia.)
- Start as early as possible, optimally by 2 to 3 months of age.
- Prescribe penicillin, 125 mg orally twice daily, until 3 years of age; then, increase to 250 mg orally twice daily.
- Prescribe erythromycin for penicillin-allergic children.
- Do not use ampicillin prophylactically—efficacy is unproved, side effects are common, and resistant organisms are likely to emerge.
- Develop an educational program to encourage compliance and recognition of early signs of infection.
- Discontinue penicillin after age 5.

This program does not—and is not intended to—eradicate nasopharyngeal carriage of *S. pneumoniae* (495). The goal is to prevent mortality from bacteremia. The appearance of this organism in the pharynx of a patient does not necessarily indicate poor compliance.

IMMUNIZATION RECOMMENDATIONS

The traditional polyvalent polysaccharide pneumococcal vaccine has been efficacious in eliciting a normal antibody response and reducing the incidence of infections with *S. pneumoniae* in children older than 2 years of age (496–500), and it should continue to be used in adults with sickle cell disease. Fortunately, a conjugated 7-valent vaccine is now in use and is effective in stimulating antibody production in the critical target population: infants with sickle cell anemia (501,502). All children with sickle cell disease should be immunized with both vaccines, following American Academy of Pediatrics recommendations. Older children and adults may benefit from influenza virus vaccine, and some centers suggest meningococcal vaccine and recombinant human hepatitis B vaccine for HbsAb-negative patients.

Empiric Therapy for the Febrile Child

For the child with sickle cell disease, fever may be the only indication of a potentially fatal infection. As a rule, the higher the temperature (503) and the higher the erythrocyte sedimentation rate, leukocyte count, and band count (504), the more likely there will be a serious bacterial infection. Unfortunately, however, there is no absolutely safe set of numbers that clearly separate febrile children into bacteremic or nonbacteremic groups. This issue is further complicated because the baseline leukocyte count is typically elevated (Table 50-3) and the sedimentation rate may be lower (because of the anemia and poikilocytosis that disfavor rouleaux formation). The following are guidelines for empiric therapy of febrile children younger than 12 years of age without an obvious source (505):

- Basic laboratory investigation includes complete blood count, urine analysis, chest radiograph, and cultures of the blood, urine, and throat.
- Toxic children, or those with temperatures greater than 39.9°C, should be treated with parenteral antibiotics promptly before radiographs are taken or laboratory results are available. These children should be admitted to the hospital.
- Lumbar puncture should be performed on toxic children and those with any signs of meningitis.
- Nontoxic children with temperatures lower than 39.9°C, but with an infiltrate on chest radiograph or a white blood cell (WBC) count greater than 30,000/μL or less than 5000/μL, should be treated parenterally and admitted to the hospital.
- Nontoxic children with temperatures lower than 39.9°C, normal chest radiograph, normal leukocyte count, and caretakers who can recognize problems and bring the child in quickly can be treated with a long-acting antibiotic (such as ceftriaxone), observed over a period of hours, and discharged, with follow-up evaluation and repeated antibiotic dosing the next day.
- Antibiotics should be selected based on their ability to kill *S. pneumoniae* and *H. influenzae* (Table 50-6) and to enter the central nervous system. In areas where β-lactamase–producing *H. influenzae* are regularly encountered, β-lactamase–resistant antibiotics should be used. Where resistant *S. pneumoniae* is common, antibiotics should be chosen on the basis of the local susceptibility profiles.
- If children do well and cultures remain negative after 72 hours, antibiotics can be discontinued.
- Documented sepsis should be treated parenterally for a minimum of 7 days.
- Bacterial meningitis should be treated for a minimum of 10 days parenterally or for at least 7 days after cerebrospinal fluid sterilization.

TABLE 50-6. Selection Criteria for Antibiotic Use

Empiric Therapy for	Should Include Coverage for	Consider Broadening to Include
Fever without source (rule out sepsis)	*Streptococcus pneumoniae*	*Salmonella*
	Haemophilus influenzae	Gram-negative enterics
Meningitis	*S. pneumoniae* *H. influenzae*	*Neisseria meningitidis*
Chest syndrome	*S. pneumoniae* *Mycoplasma pneumoniae* *Chlamydia pneumoniae*	*Legionella* Respiratory syncytial virus
Osteomyelitis/septic arthritis	*Salmonella* *Staphylococcus aureus* *S. pneumoniae*	
Urinary tract infection	*Escherichia coli* Other gram-negative enterics	

Organ System Involvement

MUSCULOSKELETAL

Acute Painful Episodes. Acute episodes of bone pain (or *pain crises*) are such a prominent clinical feature that African tribal names for sickle cell disease are onomatopoetic repetitive descriptions of pain: *chwechweechwa* (Ga tribe), *nwiinii* (Fante tribe), *nucdudui* (Ewe tribe), and *ahotutuo* (Twi tribe). Roughly translated, these names mean *beaten up, body biting,* and *body chewing* (506). The variation in incidence by age is shown in Figure 50-22 and Table 50-4. The rate increases over the first 3 decades and then declines. The decline does not reflect an improvement with age but rather the early mortality of adults with high rates of pain (399). There is also tremendous variation in pain rate between individuals, even in those of a given genotype (Fig. 50-23). In SS, those with the highest rate of pain had a higher baseline Hct and a lower level of fetal hemoglobin (Fig. 50-24) (399).

The patient experiences a deep, gnawing, throbbing pain, usually with few physical findings. The underlying event appears to be ischemia or infarction of the marrow (507). In one study, marrow was aspirated serially from a patient with acute sternal pain. The aspirates revealed a pattern that evolved from frank necrosis to purulent neutrophil infiltration and, over a

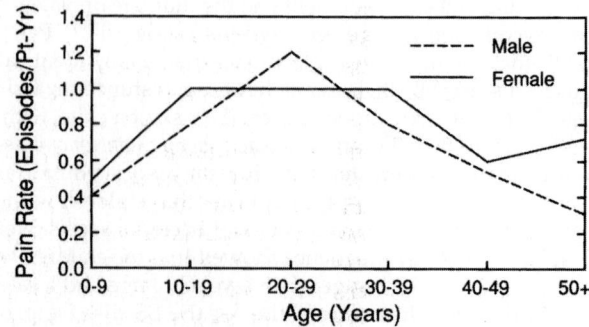

Figure 50-22. Pain rate [episodes requiring medical attention/patient-year (Pt-Yr)] by age among patients with sickle cell anemia. (From Platt OS, Thorington BD, Brambilla DJ, et al. Pain in sickle cell disease. Rates and risk factors. *N Engl J Med* 1991;325:11–16, with permission.)

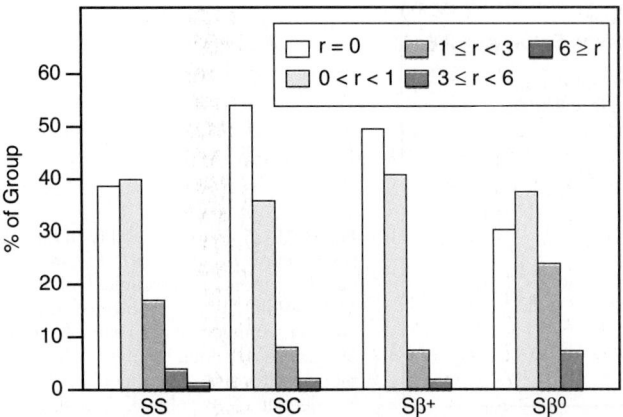

Figure 50-23. Variability in clinical manifestations: distribution of pain rates (r) among patients with different sickle hemoglobinopathies. (Modified from Platt OS, Thorington BD, Brambilla DJ, et al. Pain in sickle cell disease. Rates and risk factors. *N Engl J Med* 1991;325:11–16.)

period of weeks, to restored normal marrow (508). It is difficult to distinguish these infarctive changes from bone infection because both processes produce similar physical findings and similar purulent infiltrate, fever, leukocytosis, and acute-phase response. Even with systemic and local signs, the diagnosis of infarction is statistically more likely. The results of one study suggest that acute long-bone infarction is at least 50 times more common than osteomyelitis (509). Forty-one acute long-bone infarcts were examined (38%, humerus; 23%, tibia; 19%, femur). All patients had local tenderness, with swelling in 85%, joint findings in 68%, and localized warmth in 65%. Fourteen percent of patients appeared toxic, and 21% had a temperature above 39°C. The total leukocyte count varied between 7200 and 43,000/μL (mean, 17,000/μL); absolute band counts ranged from 0 to 2940/μL (mean, 442/μL). Although most of the patients did not have impressive systemic signs of inflammation, some clearly had classic findings of osteomyelitis. Various radionuclide scans have been reported to be helpful in making the distinction between infarction and infection (510–513); in

this study, however, they did not eliminate osteomyelitis as a possibility.

Most often, patients with acute painful episodes have no local physical findings and only a modest elevation in temperature, heart rate, blood pressure, and leukocyte count. Numerous laboratory changes have been observed in patients experiencing painful episodes, including decreased platelets (514,515), abnormal platelet function (516–518), normal platelet function (519,520), increased fibrin turnover (514,521–524), elevated myoglobin (525), elevated α-hydroxybutyrate (356,525), and a decreased proportion of dense red cells (526). These findings are interesting from a pathophysiologic point of view, but none is a sufficiently definitive marker of vasoocclusion to warrant its use to identify malingerers. Infections (524), changes in climate (527–529), and psychologic factors have been suggested as possible precipitating events, although in most cases, no such factors can be identified.

The most frequently involved areas are the knee, lumbosacral spine, elbow, and femur. Less often, the ribs, sternum, clavicles, calcaneus, iliac crest, zygoma, mandible, and maxilla are affected (524). Involvement of facial bones may result in impressive facial swelling (394), and rib infarction is commonly associated with the acute chest syndrome (530). When the knees or elbows are involved, joint effusions (usually noninflammatory) are common. They should be tapped only if the clinical course is strongly suggestive of infection. Sterile purulent effusions can be encountered (531), so the diagnosis of infection necessarily relies on culture results.

In children younger than 5 years of age, the small bones of the hands and feet may become involved in dactylitis, the so-called *hand-foot syndrome* (532). This is often the first clinical manifestation of the disease (533). As shown in Table 50-4, the peak incidence is 20 to 30 episodes/100 patient-years in the 0.5- to 3.0-year age group. Children who experience an episode before age 1 are unusual and are at an increased risk of having a severe clinical course by the time they are 10 years of age (Fig. 50-25) (534). The young patient experiences severe discomfort, refuses to use the extremity, and has hot, tender, swollen hands or feet. As in other patients experiencing acute bone involvement, the child may be febrile and have a leukocyte count as

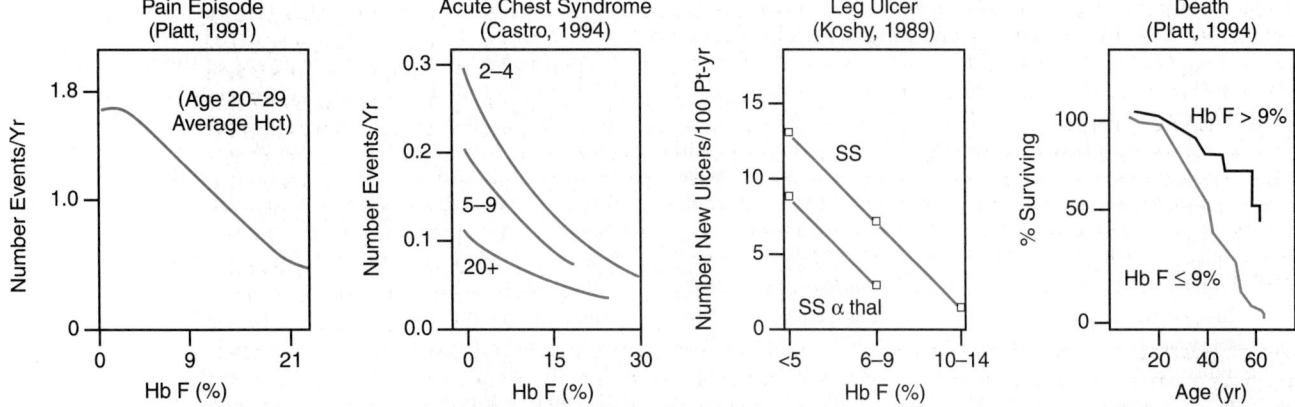

Figure 50-24. High levels of fetal hemoglobin (Hb F) are associated with decreased pain rate, decreased acute chest syndrome rate, number of new leg ulcers, and increased life expectancy in patients with sickle cell anemia. Hct, hematocrit; Pt-yr, patient-year. (Modified from Platt OS, Thorington BD, Brambilla DJ, et al. Pain in sickle cell disease. Rates and risk factors. *N Engl J Med* 1991;325:11–16; Castro O, Brambilla DJ, Thorington B, et al. The acute chest syndrome in sickle cell disease: incidence and risk factors. The Cooperative Study of Sickle Cell Disease. *Blood* 1994;84:643–649; Koshy M, Entsuah R, Koranda A, et al. Leg ulcers in patients with sickle cell disease. *Blood* 1989;74:1403–1408; and Platt OS, Brambilla DJ, Rosse WF, et al. Mortality in sickle cell disease. Life expectancy and risk factors for early death. *N Engl J Med* 1994;330:1639–1644.)

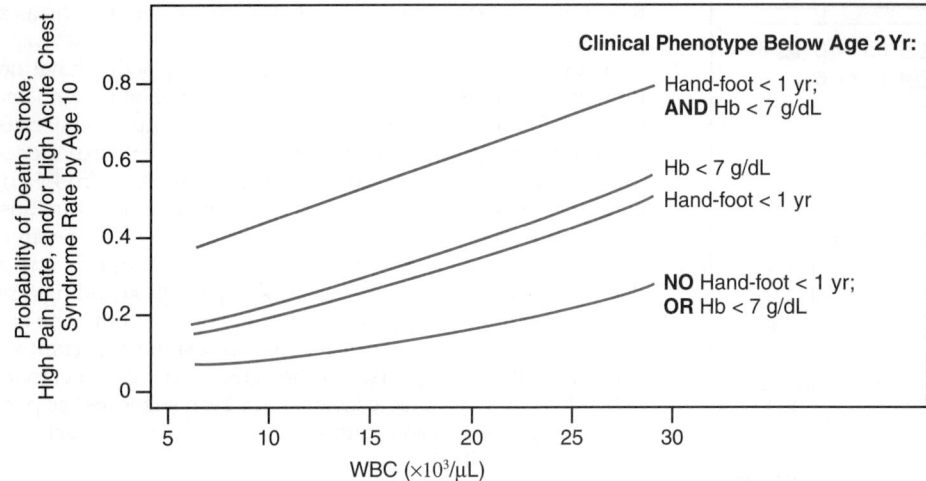

Figure 50-25. The probability of having a severe clinical course by 10 years of age can be predicted by clinical phenotype and baseline white blood cell count in children younger than 2 years of age with SS disease. Hb, hemoglobin; WBC, white blood cell count. (Modified from Miller ST, Sleeper LA, Pegelow CH, et al. Prediction of adverse outcomes in children with sickle cell disease. *N Engl J Med* 2000;342:83–89.)

high as 60,000/μL. At the onset of soft-tissue swelling, bony changes are not usually seen on radiograph. One to 2 weeks later, films demonstrate subperiosteal new bone, irregular areas of radiolucency, and cortical thinning. These bone changes generally resolve spontaneously over a period of 4 to 8 months. Rarely, permanent shortening of the digits is seen (535).

No specific treatment is directed toward the underlying ischemia of the painful episode. Treatment is supportive. The goals are to alleviate pain and to treat aggravating problems such as infection, hypoxia, acidosis, or dehydration. Patients in pain should always be evaluated for possible infection—fever should not be assumed to be simply part of the vasoocclusive process. Hypoxia is a serious problem for patients because of the relation between deoxygenation and polymerization. Oxygen therapy is important for hypoxemic patients but does little besides causing bone marrow suppression (536) for those who are not. Even hyperbaric oxygen is not beneficial in painful crises (537). Dehydrated patients, particularly those with concurrent gastrointestinal fluid losses, need careful restoration of normal volume status. Overhydration (managing fluids at 1.5 or 2.0 times normal maintenance) must be done with caution because these patients handle rapid infusions poorly and easily develop acute chest syndrome and pulmonary edema—especially when being "run wet" and treated with narcotics at the same time (538,539). Careful monitoring of weight, electrolytes, and fluid balance is essential.

The careful, consistent, and compassionate use of analgesics in the context of an experienced multidisciplinary team is key to the management of painful episodes (540). The choice, route, and dosage of narcotic agents is a highly charged subject that is unfortunately contaminated by the misimpression that the iatrogenic addiction rate is high among sickle cell disease patients (541). Other subtle misconceptions interfere with providing appropriate pain relief. In one study, standardized patients presenting with a chief complaint of pain who gave histories of frequent pain crises were given less narcotic by nurses than the identical patients whose scripts included a history of infrequent pain episodes (542). Our approach emphasizes empirically determining a fixed dose and rate schedule (not as-needed dosing) that is clinically effective for the particular patient. This requires an expert application of the knowledge of analgesic pharmacokinetics and equianalgesic dosing and the careful monitoring and documentation of the effectiveness of the pain relief. This subject is reviewed in detail in an important chapter by Benjamin (543).

Transfusion (even exchange transfusion) rarely works acutely, and it is not recommended for the treatment of uncomplicated pain episodes. Hydroxyurea is effective in lowering the pain rate in individuals with frequent pain episodes, but it has no role in the acute setting.

Osteomyelitis. Definitive diagnosis and appropriate therapy of osteomyelitis require the identification of a specific pathogen. Although blood (and stool in the case of *Salmonella* sp.) cultures may be positive, needle aspiration and culturing of suspicious bone lesions are critical. Careful culturing before starting antibiotics is essential to avoid unnecessary or inappropriate protracted intravenous therapy. The predominant pathogen is *Salmonella* sp. Pending culture results, empiric antibiotic treatment should cover *Salmonella* and *Staphylococcus* spp. (Table 50-6). Fortunately, osteomyelitis is a relatively rare disease. In one study, the New York City Department of Health reviewed its cases of *Salmonella* osteomyelitis between 1964 and 1978 (544); 37 cases were reported, and 14 were in patients with sickle cell disease. Only four patients developed chronic osteomyelitis, and *all* of these patients had been treated parenterally for less than 1 week. The perfusion of these lesions is severely compromised, and clearing these infections requires a more aggressive approach than is generally required in the normal population. A minimum of 6 weeks of treatment with documented efficacious blood levels of antibiotics is recommended.

Aseptic Necrosis. Aseptic necrosis of the femoral head is a serious and often debilitating complication that occurs in young adults with sickle cell disease. This is one of the few complications that is a prominent feature of SC disease, although the incidence is slightly higher among patients with SS disease and is highest among those with SS and α-thalassemia (401). In the CSSCD, in which patients were screened for the presence of hip disease, 3% of those younger than 15 years of age had osteonecrosis (all had SS disease, Sβ⁰-thalassemia, or SC disease). Among those patients older than 45 years of age, 35% with SS disease, 25% with Sβ⁰-thalassemia, 29% with SC disease, and 40% with Sβ⁺-thalassemia had osteonecrosis of the hip. Bilateral disease developed in approximately one-half of the patients with hip disease, usually by 25 years of age. Approximately one-half of the patients had no signs or symptoms at the time of diagnosis, but 21% had signs or symptoms at a later date. The typical radiographic findings (545) of aseptic necrosis are generally not present when the patient first becomes symptomatic, but magnetic resonance imaging (MRI) is useful in documenting subtle early disease (546). Treatment of these lesions is not satisfying. Proscription of weightbearing for long periods (months) may be helpful in the early stages. For patients who have progressed to severe disease, total hip replacement may be the only way to provide relief of pain and improve mobility. Because the underlying bone is generally of poor quality, hip replacement surgery carries a high complication rate, and early revisions are common (547,548). The CSSCD experience with hip prosthesis suggests a failure of approximately 10%/year. Experience at the Medical College of Georgia suggests that a relatively simple procedure in which the increased pressure found in the necrotic femoral head is decompressed by removing a small portion of ischemic cancellous bone—core decompression (549)—may be a beneficial technique in early lesions (550). In the CSSCD, aseptic necrosis of the humeral head followed a genetic pattern similar to that of necrosis of the femoral head (400). In fact, approximately 75% of SS and SC patients with shoulder disease also had hip disease, although only 20% had shoulder symptoms.

Other Chronic Bone Findings. Chronic hemolytic anemia results in an expanded marrow cavity that can be easily seen in radiographs of the skull, which typically show a widened diploic space. Overgrowth of the anterior maxilla may lead to orthodontic problems. Vertebrae are usually flattened, with a characteristic biconcave codfishlike shape on radiograph. Older patients may develop chronic back pain as a result of vertebral collapse.

PULMONARY

Acute Chest Syndrome. Episodes of acute lung injury with radiographic evidence of infiltrate are usually accompanied by hypoxia, chest pain, fever, cough, and tachypnea and are referred to as the *acute chest syndrome*. The vague terminology *chest syndrome* used to be an admission that the etiology was largely unknown. Now that recent studies have clarified the etiologies, the imprecise terminology emphasizes the fact that in individual patients, knowing the specific etiology is less important than accurately assessing the magnitude and pace of lung injury.

The critical pathophysiologic points are that only deoxygenated sickle hemoglobin polymerizes and that reoxygenation abolishes the polymer. The lung is the critical depolymerizing organ that protects the arterial side of the circulation from the sludge of sickle polymers. When the lung is injured, underventilated, and inflamed—regardless of the cause, the protection is incomplete, and downstream tissues, including the injured lung itself, become increasingly vulnerable to sickling and impaired blood flow. In fact, the restoration of that flow may cause reperfusion injury, as suggested in the study by Kaul and Hebbel using a sickle mouse model. They found that cycles of oxygenation/deoxygenation caused the classic P-selectin–inhibitable efflux of white cells to tissue (381).

It is no surprise that the acute chest syndrome is a leading cause of morbidity and mortality. It represents the second most common complication (pain episode is the first), with a rate of 12.8 cases/100 patient-years (402), and it is the most common condition at the time of death (476). The highest incidence is in children 2 to 4 years of age (Table 50-4), and the lowest incidence is in adults (8.8/100 patient-years in SS) (402). Patients with lower rates of acute chest syndrome have a longer life expectancy (402), and those with a higher level of fetal hemoglobin have a lower attack rate (Fig. 50-24). Hydroxyurea therapy lowers the attack rate in adults by 50%, as would be predicted on the basis of the associated increase in fetal hemoglobin (360).

Vichinsky and colleagues studied 671 episodes (551). The most common etiologies were fat embolus (some from bone marrow) and infection with chlamydia, *Mycoplasma*, or virus. In contrast to patients with infection, patients with bone marrow embolus were more likely to have an associated episode of bone pain, chest pain, abnormal neurologic symptoms, and fall in platelet count (552). Classically, fat embolization is associated with thrombocytopenia, hypocalcemia, hyperuricemia, lipemia, retinalis, and lipid droplets in the sputum or urine (553), although these are rarely found in patients with acute chest syndrome.

Bacterial pneumonia was rare overall but more common in children than adults, in whom it was associated with bacteremia in 58% of cases of *S. pneumoniae* and 18% of cases of *H. influenzae* (554). Regardless of etiology, virtually every case of acute chest syndrome is associated with some degree of localized sickling and lung ischemia; in 16% of cases, no precipitating embolus or pathogen was identified. Overall, the prognosis is poor. Thirteen percent of patients required mechanical ventilation, 11% developed new abnormal neurologic findings, and 9% of the patients aged 20 years or older died. In general, the death rate from acute chest syndrome is four times higher in adults than children (554).

Several important therapeutic principles emerged from the Vichinsky study: (a) Bronchodilator therapy was remarkably effective in 20% of the patients with wheezing or pulmonary function tests that indicated obstruction at the time of presentation (61% of all patients). This is not surprising because measurable airway hyperactivity has been documented in as many as 73% of children with SS, even without any history of asthma (555). (b) Red cell transfusion improved oxygenation. Simple transfusion was used in 68% of patients and appeared to be as effective as exchange transfusion—although the study was not designed to test this hypothesis. It may be that the efficacy of simple transfusion is related to the fact that acute chest syndrome is typically associated with a 0.5- to 1.0-g/dL decrease in hemoglobin at presentation. (c) The prominence of chlamydia and *Mycoplasma* underscores the importance of including macrolide antibiotics in the initial empiric therapy (Table 50-6).

Although some patients, particularly adults, initially present with the full-blown picture of chest pain, hypoxia, and abnormal x-ray findings, the diagnosis often becomes clear only days into an event that starts as a fever without source, abdominal pain, or extremity pain. This diagnosis can be very difficult to make. Children younger than 4 years of age often had few signs at presentation: 35% to 40% had a normal lung examination; 30 to 40% had no tachypnea; and 30% to 50% had no tachycardia (554). The x-ray examination is notoriously slow in turning positive; only 36% of patients had an abnormal x-ray on presentation, although all eventually developed abnormal radiographic findings (556).

There was considerable change in blood counts at the time of presentation in patients with acute chest syndrome. The hemoglobin dropped an average of 0.7 g/dL, and white blood counts increased an average of 69%. The mean pO_2 was 71 mm Hg, with one-fifth of the patients presenting with a pO_2 less than 60 mm Hg. Because the hemoglobin-oxygen dissociation curve varies among patients and the shallow portion of the curve is between a pO_2 of 50 and 100 mm Hg, transcutaneous oxygen saturation measurements are not sufficient unless there are enough simultaneous direct measurements of arterial pO_2 to detect trends (557). In one study, all children with SS disease and acute chest syndrome had transcutaneous saturation measurements below 96% or only three points below their steady-state values (558). Given that it is not unusual for a transcutaneous measurement to vary as much as three points with slight differences in the positioning of the probe, it is inappropriate to place too much reliance on this single measurement in isolation. Unfortunately, there are no clinical findings that are reliably predictive of the degree of hypoxia (554).

Although most patients with acute chest syndrome recover uneventfully, the course is unpredictable, and rapid unexpected deterioration is common. Most series of acute chest syndrome include a section on autopsy findings. Pulmonary postmortem findings typically include areas of alveolar wall necrosis and focal parenchymal scars (559). In one autopsy finding, multiple large infarcts but no accompanying occluded vessels were found, suggesting that severe vasospasm may play a role in some cases (560).

All patients with chest syndrome must be managed in the hospital, a setting where they can have frequent monitoring of vital signs and arterial blood gases. A pO_2 of less than 75 mm Hg (or a decrease of 25% from baseline, if the patient is chronically hypoxic) carries a poor prognosis (561). Oxygen therapy is of critical importance, and mechanical ventilation is sometimes required. Preliminary evidence suggests that inhaled nitric oxide may be of benefit in severe cases (562). Antibiotics should be used empirically after careful culturing, keeping in mind the prevalence of chlamydia, *Mycoplasma*, *S. pneumoniae*, and *H. influenzae*. Bronchodilator therapy should be tried, especially in patients with a history of obstructive lung disease or who have wheezing on presentation. Transfusion is critical for persistently hypoxic patients (pO_2 <75 mm Hg, or a decrease of 25% from baseline). Exchange transfusion is indicated if the Hct is high, if the patient is hypoxic, if the patient is deteriorating rapidly, or if the patient continues to deteriorate after simple red cell transfusion. In one series, intravenous dexamethasone was effective in reducing the length of stay (563).

Chronic Pulmonary Disease. In one survey, the lung volumes of asymptomatic adolescents with SS disease were normal compared with those of a black control population (564). In these patients, resting arterial pO_2 was 65 to 85 mm Hg (normal is >87 mm Hg). Large alveolar-arterial oxygen pO_2 differences were found in room air (27 to 42 mm Hg; normal is <16 mm Hg) and on 100% O_2 (186 to 246 mm Hg; normal is <86 mm Hg). These values are consistent with increased pulmonary shunting of 12% to 16% (normal is <7%). Progressive deterioration in pulmonary function is discussed in detail in a comprehensive review by Powars and colleagues (565). They identified a group of patients with increasing hypoxia, decreasing lung volumes and flow rates, increasing chest pain, increasing right ventricular dysfunction, and increasing pulmonary artery pressure. These patients had a high mortality rate compared with their matched controls. One-half of the identified patients died; some died suddenly, with postmortem evidence of myocardial infarction without coronary artery disease and with cor pulmonale. Risk factors for developing chronic lung disease include

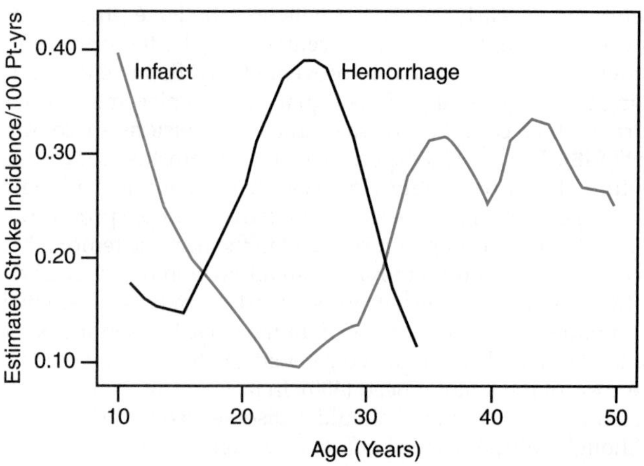

Figure 50-26. Incidence of hemorrhagic and infarctive stroke in patients with SS disease. Pt-yrs, patient-years. (Modified from Ohene-Frempong K, Weiner SJ, Sleeper LA, et al. Cerebrovascular accidents in sickle cell disease: rates and risk factors. *Blood* 1998;91:288–294.)

increased incidence of acute chest syndrome and painful episodes associated with chest pain.

Central Nervous System

In patients with sickle cell disease, the risk of stroke is higher than in the general population. In the CSSCD, the overall incidence of clinical stroke in patients without a prior episode was 0.46/100 patient-years (566). The rates in children are included in Table 50-4. In patients with SS, the chance of having a first stroke by age 20 is 11%, by age 30 is 15%, and by age 45 is 24%. In patients with SC, the incidence of stroke is much lower, reaching only 10% by age 45 (566). As shown in Figure 50-26, the strokes were either infarctive or hemorrhagic, with the peak age for infarctive stroke in the first decade and the peak for hemorrhagic stroke in the second decade. In this series, no deaths occurred within 14 days after the 62 infarctive strokes that occurred during the study. In contrast, there was a 24% mortality rate in the 2 weeks after the 35 hemorrhagic strokes that were observed during the study. Risk factors for infarctive stroke included history of transient ischemic attack, low steady-state hemoglobin level, an episode of acute chest syndrome in the prior 2 weeks, a high acute chest syndrome rate, and high systolic blood pressure (Table 50-7). Risk factors for hemorrhagic stroke were low steady-state hemoglobin and high steady-state WBC count. In contrast to what has been observed regarding risk factors for high pain rate and acute chest syndrome, a high level of fetal hemoglobin was not protective against stroke. Individuals with α-thalassemia had a marginally lower rate of stroke, which mul-

TABLE 50-7. Blood Pressure in Patients with Sickle Cell Anemia

			Age (yr)										
		Percentile	2–3	4–5	6–7	8–9	10–11	12–13	14–15	16–17	18–24	25–34	35–44
Female	Systolic	50th	90	95	96	96	104	106	110	110	110	110	110
		90th	100	110	110	110	110	118	120	122	122	125	130
	Diastolic	50th	52	60	60	60	60	62	70	70	64	68	70
		90th	62	70	70	70	74	74	80	78	80	80	84
Male	Systolic	50th	90	95	100	100	100	110	108	112	112	114	110
		90th	104	110	108	116	112	120	120	128	130	130	132
	Diastolic	50th	54	60	60	60	60	64	64	70	68	70	70
		90th	66	68	68	70	70	72	78	80	80	80	84

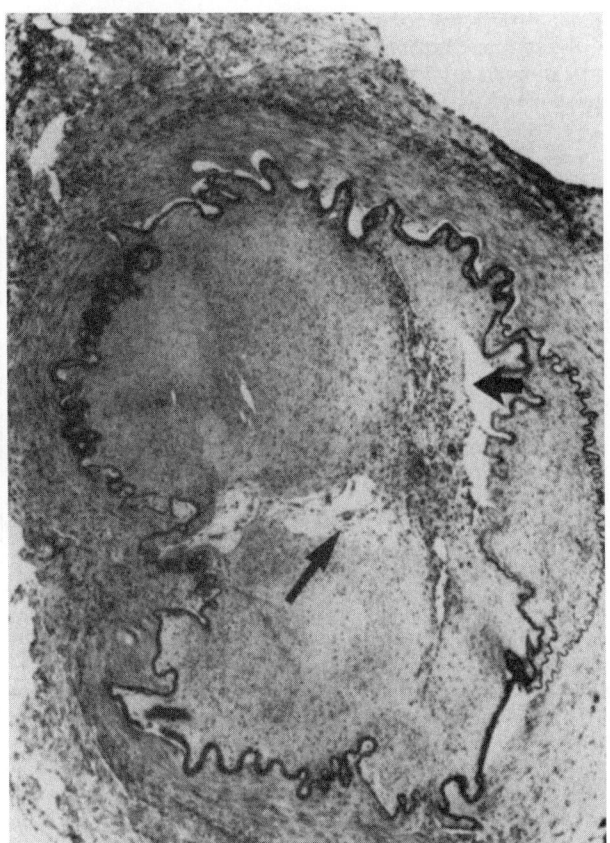

Figure 50-27. Cerebral blood vessel pathology in sickle cell anemia patient. Narrowed vessel lumen (*thick arrow*) and marked intimal hyperplasia (*thin arrow*) are visible. [From Koshy M, Thomas C, Goodwon J. Vascular lesions in the central nervous system in sickle cell disease (neuropathology). *J Assoc Acad Minor Phys* 1990;1:71, with permission.]

tivariate analysis suggested was related to their higher steady-state hemoglobin. As discussed later in this section, the most highly predictive risk factor for stroke is an abnormal transcranial Doppler study.

Stroke is a potential disaster that usually occurs spontaneously and without warning, but it also notably occurs during episodes of acute chest syndrome, aplasia, viral illness, pain, priapism, hyperventilation, and dehydration (567–570). In infarctive strokes, hemiplegia, seizures, speech defects, coma, and visual disturbances are the most common features. With modern management (see below), the abnormal signs and symptoms typically improve dramatically with treatment, although some may remain constant (571,572). In untreated patients, acute mortality approaches 20%, and approximately 70% recur within 3 years. Angiographic and postmortem examinations usually reveal more vessel involvement than anticipated on clinical grounds. Typically, there are multiple stenoses of internal carotid and anterior and middle cerebral arteries that appear to originate at sites of bifurcations; less frequently, single or no lesions are found (567,573–575). This is not simple *in situ* sickling but a definite vasculopathy with intimal, fibroblast, and smooth muscle proliferation (576,577) (Fig. 50-27). Associated HLA genotypes (578) and increased levels of homocysteine (579) are preliminary hints that a variety of vascular pathologies may be in play.

Hemorrhagic strokes are usually subarachnoid and present as a severe sudden headache, frequently with vomiting, signs of meningismus, and photophobia. They progress rapidly, and the overall mortality rate approaches 50% in some series (571),

although others report a more favorable outcome (580,581). Not all patients with arteriographically demonstrated bleeds have diagnostic cerebrospinal fluid or computed tomography (CT) findings (580). Bleeding aneurysms probably balloon from damaged intima and fragile collaterals [often resembling moyamoya disease (576)] formed during childhood. This sequence of events is suggested in a series of patients with hemorrhage 4 to 20 or more years after ischemia (582), although a history of stroke is not invariable (580). As more is learned about the pathogenesis of vascular lesions in sickle cell disease as well as other disorders, it is not surprising that certain markers of inflammation, such as baseline WBC count, are risk factors for hemorrhagic and silent infarcts in sickle cell disease.

The ability to image watershed infarcts by MRI has highlighted the vulnerability of these areas of the brain that are supplied by the distal arteries and that are susceptible to changes in cerebral perfusion (583). The sensitivity of this technique also creates important clinical conundrums, as exemplified by the finding of unexpected infarcts in 11% of patients without history of central nervous system symptoms (584). A prospective MRI examination of 312 children enrolled in the CSSCD demonstrated infarction/ischemia in 13% of children without history of stroke (585). These "silent" lesions were typically confined to the deep white matter, whereas the ischemic lesions in those who had experienced a clinical stroke characteristically involved both the cortex and the deep white matter. Emerging evidence suggests that silent infarcts are associated with subtle neuropsychologic defects in the realms of verbal, mathematic, and visual motor performance (586). These lesions indicate a propensity toward clinical stroke. In the CSSCD cohort, stroke occurred in 8% of children with silent infarct and in less than 1% of those without silent infarct. Risk factors for silent infarcts include a low rate of pain episodes, a history of seizures, and an elevated steady-state WBC count (587). Whether silent or not, 78% of abnormal MRI lesions were in the frontal lobe, 51% were in the parietal lobe, and 15% were in the temporal lobe. Lesions were also common in the basal ganglia or thalamus but rare in the occipital lobe cerebellum and brainstem. Among those individuals with demonstrable lesions, 60% had them in both hemispheres, and the rest were evenly divided between the right and left hemispheres (585).

CT scanning, MRI, and/or magnetic resonance angiography is essential in the acute setting to rule out potentially treatable disorders such as subdural hematoma, berry aneurysm, or tuberculous granuloma—all of which have been described in patients with sickle cell disease (567,588). CT scans are more likely to demonstrate middle cerebral infarcts several days after an acute event and are less sensitive than MRI in demonstrating deep white matter infarcts in patients with transient ischemic attacks or seizures (584). Positron emission tomography (PET) has been systematically evaluated in 49 patients with SS who also had MRI scans and appears to have increased sensitivity (589). The use of this technology is likely to grow in the next few years.

Acute treatment for stroke includes exchange transfusion. Following up with maintenance transfusion therapy has had a profound influence on the prognosis of patients with stroke (567,574,590–592). A regular transfusion program designed to keep the hemoglobin S level below 30% lowers the recurrence rate to 10%, although 30% of patients may continue to have residual motor impairment, and 10% develop intelligence quotient levels below 70. Transient ischemic attacks can occur in patients who are still on transfusion (567,593–595). In three such patients (592), the hemoglobin S levels were 17% to 35%. In patients undergoing transfusion, repeated arteriograms generally show stabilization and smoothing of intimal lesions, whereas patients not receiving transfusions demonstrate progressive vessel damage (567). Even after improvement of arteriograms, however, patients continue to be at risk of recurrence, as demonstrated by two patients whose arteriograms improved after 1 year of transfusion but who had recurrences after cessation of therapy (567).

A study of 12 children in Memphis who had been on transfusion therapy for 1 to 2 years revealed a 70% recurrence rate within 5 weeks to 11 months of stopping transfusion (574). The St. Jude's and LeBonheur Children's group reported its updated results on patients who received transfusions for 5.0 to 12.5 years before discontinuation (596). All ten patients had abnormal arteriograms and evidence of encephalomalacia by MRI at the time transfusions were stopped. Five patients had recurrent strokes, and one died suddenly and without explanation (no new stroke at postmortem) 2.5 to 12.0 months after discontinuation. A study of adult patients who had their long-term transfusion therapy discontinued was more optimistic, with no recurrent episodes in nine patients (597). Although theoretically beneficial, a lifetime of maintenance transfusion carries risks of infection, red cell antigen sensitization, and iron overload. Despite these hazards, life-long therapy may be the only way to prevent recurrent strokes. The study of a group of children from the Children's Hospital of Philadelphia, who had undergone 4 years of a transfusion program designed to keep the pretransfusion hemoglobin S level below 30%, suggests an alternative strategy: The target hemoglobin S level can be safely increased to 50% (598). Hydroxyurea has also been used to prevent the recurrence of stroke in patients who, for a variety of reasons, could not continue on maintenance transfusion (599). Although these patients had a good response with respect to increasing their levels of fetal hemoglobin, there was a 19% stroke recurrence rate. Given the data, hydroxyurea does not appear to be effective in this setting, but it is a reasonable approach for those who cannot be transfused. Bone marrow transplantation has been used in patients on maintenance transfusion after stroke. Although the experience is not large, with careful attention to preventing posttransplant bleeding and seizures and the use of prophylactic platelet transfusions and anticonvulsants, bone marrow transplant may prove to be the ideal treatment.

Because the clinical experience with hemorrhage is limited and the mortality is high, there are not enough data on survivors to be dogmatic about long-term management. One reasonable approach is to use chronic maintenance transfusion for those who are found to have abnormal vascular anatomy (600), although three patients are known to have bled while on a transfusion program that maintained their hemoglobin S level lower than 20% (582).

One of the most exciting new developments in the treatment of children with sickle cell disease has been the discovery that an abnormal transcranial Doppler study can identify a child at high risk of infarctive stroke, and that a maintenance transfusion program can reduce the subsequent incidence of stroke (601). In this study, 130 children with an abnormal mean blood flow velocity in the internal carotid or middle cerebral artery of 200 cm/second or higher were randomized to receive maintenance transfusions or standard care (Fig. 50-28). The standard care group experienced ten infarctive strokes and one intracerebral hematoma. There was only one infarctive stroke in the transfusion group—a 92% difference in the risk of stroke. Because of the potential impact of this important clinical observation, the trial was terminated early. This noninvasive technique that measures blood flow velocity through intracranial vessels can easily be performed as part of a routine screening evaluation. Special training of the ultrasonographer is important to assure that the results obtained are valid in this clinical setting. Many clinical centers are now routinely screening all

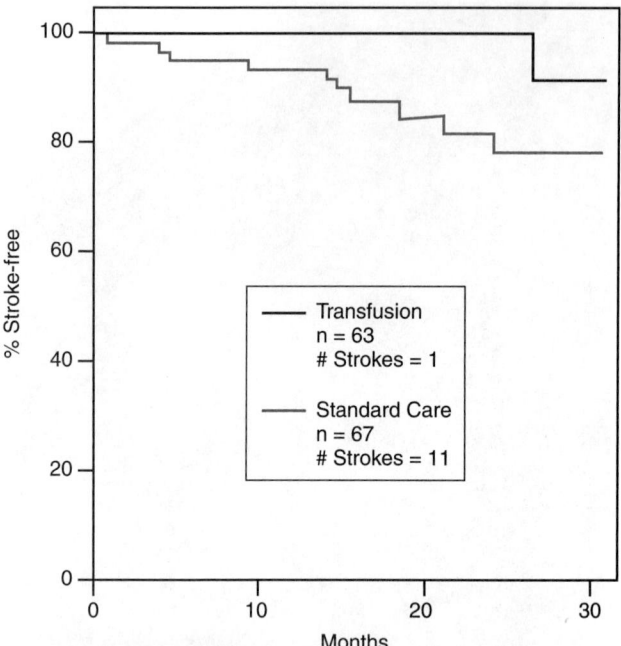

Figure 50-28. Impact of prophylactic maintenance transfusion therapy on the prevention of stroke in children with abnormal transcranial Doppler screening. n, number. (Modified from Adams RJ, McKie VC, Brambilla D, et al. Stroke prevention trial in sickle cell anemia. *Control Clin Trials* 1998;19:110–129.)

children using the laser Doppler technique and offering chronic transfusion to those children who have a rate of 200 cm/second or higher. The ideal age range for the studies and the frequency of screening have not been rigorously evaluated yet.

Cardiovascular

The chronic anemia of sickle cell disease causes a compensatory increase in cardiac output (602), with a normal heart rate (603). As a result, most patients have abnormal cardiac findings (604–610). On examination, the most common signs are cardiomegaly, systolic ejection murmur, third heart sound, suprasternal notch thrill, split first heart sound, and diastolic murmur (609).

Discrete episodes of acute myocardial infarction are relatively rare, although this is a disease marked by vasoocclusion and tissue infarction (610,611). In one review of the postmortem literature, only four classic infarcts were reported among 153 hearts (611), although 20% of another series of 72 cases had lesions that could be interpreted as ischemic (612). Despite the high oxygen extraction in the coronary circulation, blood in the coronary sinus has no more sickling than blood in the general circulation (154), presumably because of the rapid transit time (602). Atherosclerosis is virtually absent in this population—appearing in none of the 100 hearts of patients between 16 and 47 years of age (611). This is in marked contrast to the findings among those who died on the battlefields of Vietnam, of whom 45% had atherosclerosis (613). When injected at autopsy, hearts from patients with SS disease had larger than normal caliber vessels (614).

The most comprehensive prospective examination of cardiac function in an unselected population of patients with sickle cell anemia was performed as part of the CSSCD, a study that has proven to be critical in understanding the impact of the disease on cardiac function (603). One hundred ninety-one steady-state patients, 13 years of age or older, underwent echocardiography; all of the measurements were performed centrally by an investi-

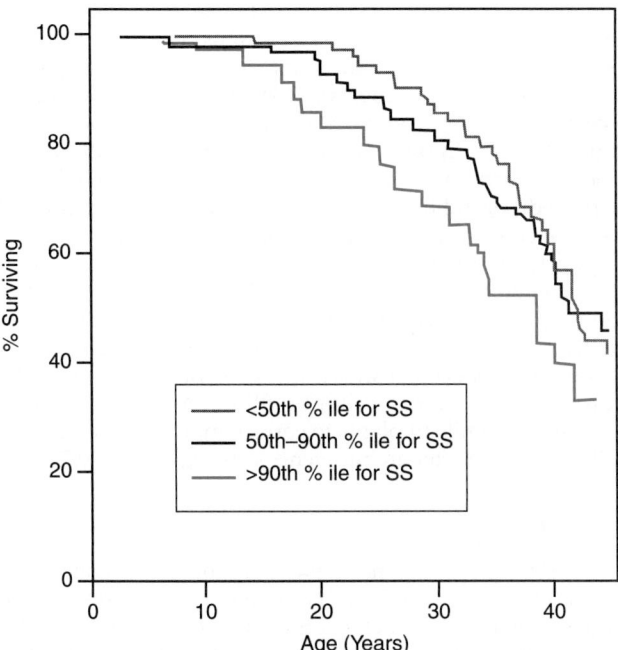

Figure 50-29. Impact of blood pressure on overall mortality in patients with SS disease. Percentiles for blood pressure are detailed in Table 50-7. % ile, percentile. (Modified from Pegelow CH, Colangelo L, Steinberg M, et al. Natural history of blood pressure in sickle cell disease: risks for stroke and death associated with relative hypertension in sickle cell anemia. *Am J Med* 1997;102:171–177.)

gator without access to other patient data. After appropriately adjusting for body surface area, the left and right ventricles, the aortic root, and the left atrium were found to be larger than normal. Significant wall thickening was found only in the septum. The left ventricular dilatation correlated with hemoglobin and age, suggesting that the major cardiac findings are indeed related to the years of increased stroke volume in compensation for anemia and abnormal rheology. The finding of normal left and right ventricular function suggests that if a specific "sickle myocardiopathy" exists, it is rare. Pulmonary hypertension and right ventricular dysfunction are also rare, except in those with acute or chronic pulmonary disease (615,616). As discussed in the section Chronic Pulmonary Disease, patients with cor pulmonale and right ventricular dysfunction have a high mortality rate.

Arrhythmia appears to be common during painful episodes. In one study, 80% of patients experienced arrhythmia during the first hour of treatment for pain (617); 67% were atrial, 60% were ventricular, and none was thought to be clinically significant.

The blood pressure in steady-state patients with sickle cell anemia (and, to a lesser extent, SC disease) from the CSSCD is lower than in a race-, gender-, and age-matched normal population (618). The reason for this difference is not known, but the authors speculate that it might be related to the defect in urine-concentrating ability and the tendency to lose sodium in the urine. Most important, this study demonstrates that high blood pressure is a risk factor for stroke and early mortality (Fig. 50-29), and that the diagnosis of high blood pressure depends on knowing the "normal values" for this population (Table 50-7). Blood pressures above the 90% percentile in the sickle cell anemia population overlap with the normal range in a normal population. It is not known whether, or to what extent, the treatment of hypertension would benefit this population, but a steady-state blood pressure of 140/90 is an ominous risk factor, and patients with such measurements should be considered appropriate candidates for antihypertensive therapy.

Genitourinary

HYPOSTHENURIA AND TUBULAR DEFECTS

Hyposthenuria (619–621) develops during the first 10 years of life and, as with functional asplenia, may be temporarily reversed with transfusion (622,623). The hypertonic environment of the renal medulla enhances sickling (624), thereby reducing medullary blood flow and disturbing the countercurrent multiplier system. The abnormal countercurrent multiplier may be the cause of the hyposthenuria, or it may result from the diversion of blood flow away from nephrons with long Henle loops and toward those with short loops (625). The obligatory water loss results in a tendency toward dehydration and invalidates the use of urine flow or specific gravity as an indicator of the patient's state of hydration. Nocturia and enuresis are common complaints of patients who excrete large volumes of dilute urine (626). Urinary sodium is rarely high enough to cause hyponatremia (627). A defect in renal tubular acidification (628,629), as well as hyporeninemic hypoaldosteronism (630) and impaired potassium excretion (631,632), has been identified and may result in hyperkalemic acidosis (633). Mild hyperuricemia is found in patients with impaired secretion of uric acid in the distal tubule (634). This may rarely lead to urate stones or clinical gout.

HEMATURIA

Approximately one-fourth of patients with SS disease and renal papillary necrosis do not have hematuria (635); nevertheless, this pathologic entity is thought to be responsible for most of the occasional episodes of hematuria (636) that occur in all the sickle syndromes, including sickle trait. Hematuria is usually mild but can be severe enough to cause significant blood loss (637,638). Maintenance transfusion may allow bleeding lesions to heal. ε-Aminocaproic acid can be used for refractory bleeding (639–641), but this must be done cautiously. Patients should be kept on bed rest in the hospital, and a high urine flow should be maintained because of the risk of clotting and obstruction of the ureter or renal pelvis. In patients with long-standing hematuria, iron supplements may be necessary.

NEPHROTIC SYNDROME AND RENAL FAILURE

Proteinuria and nephrotic syndrome occur mainly in adults with SS disease (642). Despite the well-described histology (643,644), the cause of the glomerular lesion is not known. It may represent a response to iron (645) or immune complex (646,647) deposition. Results from the series of patients observed at Chapel Hill suggest that proteinuria is caused by glomerular capillary hypertension and that it can be reduced by therapy with the inhibition of angiotensin-converting enzyme (648). In one series, a group of patients randomized to take captopril (25 mg/day) had a 37% reduction in microalbuminuria, whereas those randomized to placebo had a 17% increase in microalbuminuria (649). Bakir and colleagues (650) reviewed the Chicago experience and reported that 4% of adult SS patients developed nephrotic syndrome; two-thirds of these patients developed renal failure, and one-half of these patients died within 2 years. In the Jamaican experience, 6 of 25 patients older than 40 years of age had diminished creatinine clearance (651). In Los Angeles, chronic renal failure was found in approximately 4% of SS patients (median age at onset, 25 years) and in approximately 2% of SC patients (median age at onset, 50 years). Chronic renal failure contributed little to mortality in patients younger than 10 years of age but accounted for approximately 15% of deaths in those older than 10 years of age (31). Sickle cell patients with chronic renal failure can be managed remarkably well with peritoneal dialysis, hemodialysis, or transplantation (652–654).

PRIAPISM

Priapism is a distressing problem that occurs in males of all ages. In a Jamaican questionnaire study of 104 males between 10 and 62 years of age, 42% reported at least one episode of priapism, with a median age of onset of 21 years (655). The experience in Los Angeles indicated that approximately 7% of SS males and approximately 2% of SC males develop priapism, with a median age of onset of approximately 22 years (31). A questionnaire survey administered to 98 patients younger than 20 years of age in Dallas found the mean age at the initial episode to be 12 years, with an average number of episodes per patient of 15.7 and an average duration of 125 minutes (656). Priapism most commonly occurred around 4:00 a.m.—during sleep or soon after waking. There was a surprisingly high prevalence of priapism in this age group, with an 89% actuarial probability of experiencing priapism by age 20. Because early intervention and treatment may prevent irreversible penile fibrosis and impotence, patients and parents should be educated about this complication in advance of its occurrence.

Four clinical entities are described: stuttering priapism, with short (<2 to 3 hours), often multiple episodes; acute prolonged priapism (>24 hours), which can persist for weeks; chronic priapism, a painless induration that may last for years; and acute-on-chronic priapism, acute painful episodes complicating chronic induration. Sexual dysfunction was reported by 46% of patients with a history of priapism (655). In general, young patients with brief episodes restricted to the corpora cavernosa ("bicorporal priapism") are less likely to become dysfunctional (657,658), whereas adults with involvement of the corpora cavernosa and corpus spongiosa ("tricorporal priapism") tend to have prolonged episodes and a greater than 50% chance of becoming impotent (659). Urinary retention requiring catheterization may complicate such acute episodes (660). Patients with tricorporal involvement are also particularly susceptible to acute severe neurologic complications and overall increased morbidity—even those treated with exchange transfusion (570,659). They should be monitored closely for early neurologic symptoms, especially headache.

Diagnostic studies such as technetium scans, MRI, Doppler flow studies, and measurements of corporal pressures, hemoglobin electrophoresis, and blood gases are currently being used in a variety of settings to help define the anatomy and potential prognostic features of priapism. As yet, they have not had an impact on clinical decision making in individual patients (661–663).

The approach to treatment of priapism is not entirely uniform; there are no controlled clinical trials to guide therapy. Short episodes of acute priapism usually occur on awakening and can be managed at home. Patients should be instructed to urinate frequently, do some vigorous exercise, increase fluid intake, and soak in a warm tub. If the episode does not resolve within a few hours, the patient should appear for medical treatment. In a small series of pediatric patients in Dallas, corporal aspiration and irrigation with dilute epinephrine were used successfully in an outpatient setting (664). In general, treatment of acute priapism that has lasted more than a few hours should include analgesics, and preparation for possible transfusion should be made. Priapism may respond to simple red cell transfusion (657), and this may be a reasonable temporizing measure in the first 6 to 8 hours. Some patients begin to improve within hours of exchange transfusion (665,666), although most do not show signs of detumescence for 24 to 48 hours, and some do not respond at all (667). Use of intracorporal and oral α-adrenergic agents has been tried successfully in a small experimental group in Paris in both acute and chronic settings (668); in one group of patients with stuttering priapism in Jamaica, stilbestrol was helpful in preventing recurrences (669).

Surgical shunting procedures should be considered for patients who have not shown any signs of detumescence 24 hours after exchange transfusion or corporal irrigation, particularly if they are postpubertal. Historically, these procedures have carried a high complication rate with subsequent penile deformities and impotence. In fairness, it is difficult to determine how many of the observed adverse effects are related to the procedure, and how many are related to the priapism itself. The most conservative shunt is Winter's procedure or one of its modifications, whereby a needle or scalpel is inserted through the glans into one of the corpora, and the viscous blood is aspirated. This temporarily allows for drainage of cavernous blood into the systemic circulation and has been successfully used in SS disease patients (670). Intermittent compression with a blood pressure cuff is critical to limit refilling. Anecdotal evidence suggests that penile implants to correct impotence may be more easily done soon after an impotence-causing episode (671,672).

Hepatobiliary

Liver and biliary tract abnormalities are common among SS disease patients (673,674). Liver pathology typically results from various combinations of cholelithiasis, iron overload, drug toxicity, viral hepatitis, alcohol toxicity, and hepatic ischemia (675). Most asymptomatic patients have chronic hyperbilirubinemia [average bilirubin, 3 mg/dL (674)], mild to moderate hepatomegaly, and moderately elevated transaminases (676). Chronically elevated levels of alkaline phosphatase are usually of bone origin (677).

GALLSTONES

Bilirubin stones are common (678,679). In one informative series, 226 patients with SS disease had routine sonograms of the gallbladder (680). Among patients 2 to 4 years of age, the prevalence of stones was 12%. With increasing age, the prevalence increased, reaching 42% in those 15 to 18 years of age. Fourteen patients were noted to have sludge in the gallbladder. They were reexamined up to 2 years later; four had developed stones, six still had sludge, and the sludge had disappeared in four patients. The patients with stones had an average, steady-state, total bilirubin (3.8 ± 0.3 mg/dL) that was higher than that of the patients without stones (2.6 ± 0.12 mg/dL). Total hemoglobin and reticulocyte counts did not differ significantly between the two groups. Acute cholecystitis presents in these patients with the same signs and symptoms as in other populations, but it is not known what proportion of patients with bilirubin stones eventually develop cholecystitis.

Common bile duct stones can be difficult to diagnose solely on the basis of routine laboratory tests and ultrasonography and may require direct examination of the duct (681). Convincing evidence suggests that children tolerate *elective* cholecystectomy with little morbidity (682,683), whereas operating in the setting of acute cholecystitis carries a significant risk of serious complication (684). Laparoscopic cholecystectomy has been particularly effective in reducing the postoperative hospital stay in children with sickle cell disease (685).

INTRAHEPATIC SICKLING AND HEPATITIS

All episodes of right upper quadrant pain are not cholecystitis (437). Pain, worsening jaundice, elevations in transaminases, nausea, and low-grade fever are also features of intrahepatic sickling (436,686) and viral hepatitis (687). Schubert (686) recalls the second reported case of sickle cell disease, described by Washburn in 1911 (688). Although 107 gallstones were removed at cholecystectomy, the patient continued to have episodes of right upper quadrant pain postoperatively. Acute intrahepatic sickling usually resolves fairly abruptly, in days to weeks (686). In contrast, in viral hepatitis, the resolution is more gradual and takes longer (686). Fulminant hepatic failure with massive cholestasis and rapid progression to hepatic encephalopathy and shock is a rare, often fatal complication that may be amenable to emergency exchange transfusion (689,690).

A review of postmortem liver pathology among 70 patients from Johns Hopkins Hospital (438) revealed unexpected hepatic injury. Necrosis, portal fibrosis, regenerative nodules, and cirrhosis were common features thought to be a result of recurrent ischemia and repair.

Skin

Leg ulcers have been described in a number of different anemias, including hereditary spherocytosis, thalassemia, elliptocytosis, and pyruvate kinase deficiency (691); their presence in sickle cell anemia should, therefore, not necessarily imply that they represent vasoocclusion. Ulceration may result from increased venous pressure in the legs caused by the expanded blood volume in the hypertrophied bone marrow (692). Koshy and colleagues reviewed the CSSCD experience (693) and revealed that there were no ulcers found among 1700 patients younger than 10 years of age, and that there was an inverse relationship between fetal hemoglobin level and the appearance of new ulcers (Fig. 50-24). Among older patients with SS disease, the incidence/100 person-years was as follows: ages 10 to 20, 3; ages 20 to 30, 15; ages 30 to 40, 17; ages 40 to 50, 18; older than age 50, 19. For every age group, the presence of α-thalassemia resulted in a lower incidence—for example, 9% in the 20- to 30-year-old group (Fig. 50-24). There were also fewer ulcers among the $S\beta^0$-thalassemia patients, and no ulcers were found in either $S\beta^+$-thalassemia or SC patients. In tropical areas where shoes are not always worn and insect bites are common, leg ulcers are more frequent (694–696). In Jamaica, leg ulcers typically start in the 10- to 20-year-old group and eventually appear in 75% of adults. Chronic lesions become a major source of morbidity and have a profound negative impact on educational achievement and employment (697).

Ulcers are usually present over the medial surface of the lower tibia or just posterior to the medial malleolus. They begin as a small depression with central necrosis and, if unattended, may widen to encircle the entire lower leg. In one case, ulcers resulted in chronic osteomyelitis requiring amputation (693). Initially, the surrounding skin appears healthy; however, as the ulcer becomes chronic, the skin becomes darker, the follicles and subcutaneous fat are lost, and chronic cellulitis and local adenitis can be severely painful. These ulcers can persist for years.

Treatment of ulcers is a long-term and relatively frustrating process. In the CSSCD, the recurrence rate was high (25% to 52%) regardless of the treatment program (693). The National Institutes of Health management and therapy guide (698) suggests an escalating regimen that starts with local cleaning (several weeks of wet-to-dry dressings every 3 hours) and moves to protection (3 to 4 weeks of weekly changing of Unna boot), transfusion (6 months of maintenance), and, eventually, skin grafting (split thickness, with continued postoperative maintenance transfusion) for ulcers that have not healed. Logic suggests that early intervention should be beneficial. Patients should be advised to be particularly careful about leg injuries and to seek early care for any skin lesions on the legs that do not heal promptly.

Ocular

The review by Cohen and colleagues (699–703) illustrates the often subtle and always complex nature of the ocular manifesta-

tions of sickle cell disease. Before describing the common complications, three important clinical points need to be stressed:

1. Proliferative retinopathy can cause blindness and can be diagnosed reliably only by an ophthalmologist.
2. Eye trauma resulting in blood in the anterior chamber (hyphema) can cause blindness even in patients with sickle cell trait.
3. Retinal surgery should not be performed without preoperative transfusion treatment.

Some of the most dramatic and exotic ocular lesions of sickle cell disease are not associated with blindness. Saccular comma-shaped dilatations of conjunctival vessels occur in virtually all patients with SS disease, more than one-half of patients with SC disease, and no patients with sickle trait (704). These benign lesions curiously disappear with the administration of oxygen, with transfusion, or under the heat of the slit lamp (705–707); they appear more prominently with vasoconstricting eyedrops; and they are correlated with the number of circulating irreversibly sickled cells (708).

Retinopathy is conveniently classified as either proliferative or nonproliferative (709). Nonproliferative retinopathy generally does not cause blindness and marks localized areas of hemorrhage. Depending on the age, layer, and extent of the bleed, the lesion appears as a salmon patch, schisis cavity, iridescent spot, black sunburst, or mottled brown area (710,711). In contrast, proliferative retinopathy can ultimately cause blindness by vitreous hemorrhage or retinal detachment. These lesions occur peripherally—out of the view of nonophthalmologists. The initial insult appears to be cessation of blood flow at the end or bifurcation of an arteriole. Endothelial damage at the site of occlusion is inferred by the abnormal angiographic pattern (699–703). Goldberg (712) defined five stages of proliferative retinopathy that progress from discrete peripheral occlusions, through the development of characteristic "sea-fan" neovascularization, and, ultimately, to retinal hemorrhage and detachment (Fig. 50-30). Although 20% to 60% of patients with sea-fans may cure their own lesions by autoinfarction (713,714), in well-selected patients with stage III retinopathy, blindness can be prevented by photocoagulation (715). Surgically amenable lesions typically occur in patients older than 15 years of age and are more common among patients with SC disease. It is reasonable, therefore, that regular yearly ophthalmologic examinations begin in the teenage years, particularly in patients with SC disease. Unfortunately, surgery carries the risk of potentially blinding complications (716,717) and should be undertaken only by retinal specialists.

Rarely, acute painless loss of vision results from central retinal artery occlusion. Although spontaneous restoration of sight may occur, exchange transfusion has been recommended when bilateral disease occurs (718).

The aqueous humor is an ascorbate-rich fluid that promotes sickling (699–703). With even minimal amounts of hyphema, intraocular pressure can be elevated by outflow obstruction. As reviewed by Cohen and colleagues (699–703), optimal intraocular pressure for sickle cell patients is less than 25 mm Hg. Higher pressure may result in retinal infarction or central retinal artery occlusion. Pressure reduction therapy is complicated because most antiglaucoma medications, at least theoretically, enhance sickling or vasoconstriction (mannitol, acetazolamide, epinephrine). Timolol maleate has been well tolerated in some patients, although if this therapy fails, repeated paracentesis may be required. Hyphema is an ophthalmologic emergency, even in patients with sickle trait.

Auditory

In patients with SS disease, sensorineural hearing loss can be found at both ends of the auditory spectrum (719,720). In one

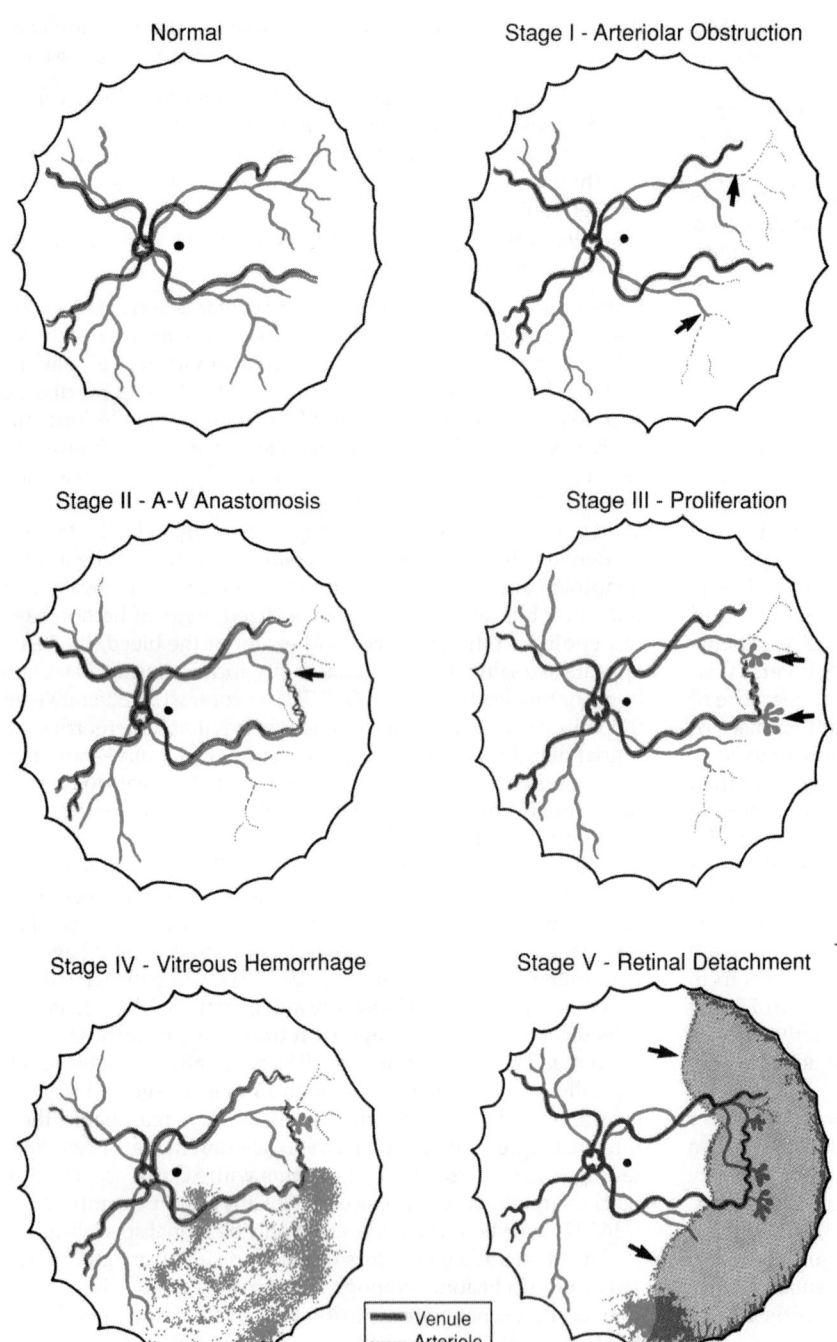

Figure 50-30. Goldberg classification of sickle cell retinopathy. (From Goldberg MF. Retinal vaso-occlusion in sickling hemoglobinopathies. *Birth Defects* 1976;12:475, with permission.)

study, 12% of children had deficiencies in the high-frequency range (721). Although there was no excess of meningitis or otitis media in the affected group, five of the six children with central nervous system disease had abnormal hearing. The underlying pathology appears to be sickling in the cochlear vasculature and loss of hair cells (722).

PROGNOSIS AND LIFE EXPECTANCY IN SICKLE CELL DISEASE

As shown in Figure 50-31, the median age at death for patients with sickle cell anemia is 42 years for men and 48 years for women. In those with SC disease, the median age at death is 60 years for men and 68 years for women (476). The rate and cause of death

vary with age. In children, the peak mortality is in the 1- to 3-year-old group, with pneumococcal sepsis, stroke, and splenic sequestration being the most often defined causes of death (418,419,423). Older patients die during acute chest syndrome, painful episodes, cerebral vascular accidents, and chronic renal or lung failure (31,422,476,723). Approximately 85% of SS and 95% of SC patients survive to age 20 (423). It is encouraging that the widespread use of prophylactic penicillin in young children, aggressive treatment of pulmonary disease and infection, careful selection of patients for transfusion therapy, and thoughtful comprehensive care has coincided with an improvement in survival (Fig. 50-32) (724).

Much is known about the risk factors for early mortality in patients with sickle cell anemia. As shown in Figure 50-24, those with a higher level of fetal hemoglobin have a longer life expectancy (476). The same is true for patients with low baseline

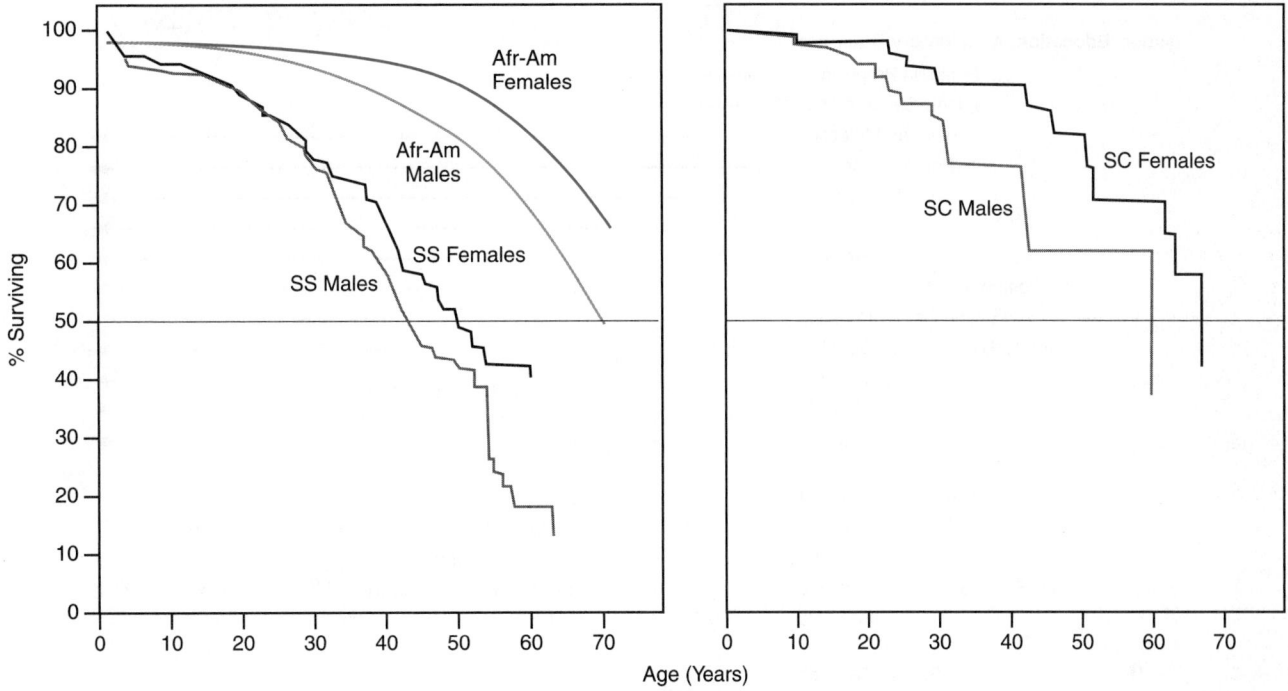

Figure 50-31. Life expectancy among male and female African American (Afr-Am) individuals in the general population and patients with SS and SC disease. (Modified from Platt OS, Brambilla DJ, Rosse WF, et al. Mortality in sickle cell disease. Life expectancy and risk factors for early death. *N Engl J Med* 1994;330:1639–1644.)

WBC counts (476), low rate of pain crisis (476), low rate of acute chest syndrome (402), no hand-foot crisis before 1 year of age (534) (Fig. 50-25), no severe anemia before 2 years of age (Fig. 50-25) (534), and relatively low blood pressure (Fig. 50-29) (618).

MANAGEMENT OF PATIENTS WITH SICKLE CELL DISEASE

Routine Health Maintenance

Patients with sickle cell anemia should be followed on a routine basis by a multidisciplinary team of caregivers familiar with the prevention and treatment of the various complications of the disease. The emphasis of the routine visit should be on patient education and anticipation of problems. Patients should be encouraged to participate in self-help groups that are ideally organized and run by patients outside the medical bureaucracy. Routine dental care is critical in avoiding serious oral infections that may lead to osteomyelitis (725). Regular visits with routine laboratory studies when the patient is well establish the patient's steady-state normal values and baseline physical findings. These baseline data are extremely helpful in sorting out the problems when the patient is ill. The issues and data of importance differ with age. Figure 50-33 briefly highlights some of the issues and studies that should be considered at each routine visit. This figure is not meant to be exhaustive and deals with neither normal routine care nor the management of a patient with a specific chronic problem.

Use and Abuse of Transfusions

Patients with sickle cell disease tolerate (and ironically may benefit from) their anemia. They require transfusion only under unusual situations: acute splenic sequestration, aplastic crisis, central nervous system infarction, acute chest syndrome with hypoxia, pro-

longed priapism, preparation for some surgery, chronic heart failure (especially with the anemia of renal failure), and complicated pregnancy. Specifically, there is no role for transfusion in managing uncomplicated painful episodes, and transfusion is not indicated to simply improve the baseline Hct of otherwise well patients.

CHOICE OF RED CELL PRODUCT

In studies of sickle cell disease patients who received blood cross-matched by standard techniques, the rate of sensitization varied

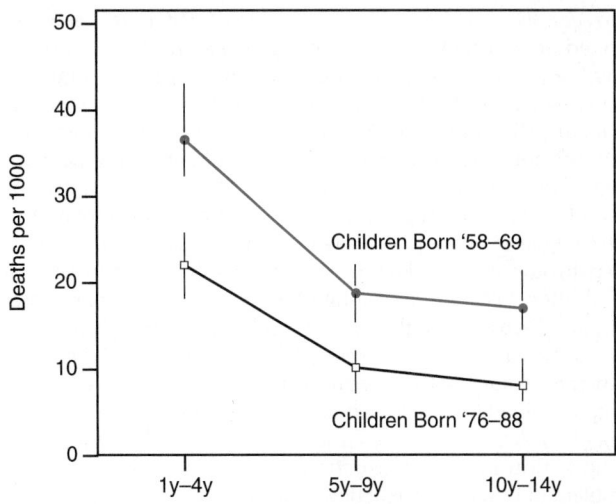

Figure 50-32. Improvement in the death rate in children with SS disease born from 1976 to 1988 compared to those born from 1958 to 1969. (Data from Davis H, Schoendorf KC, Gergen PJ, et al. National trends in the mortality of children with sickle cell disease, 1968 through 1992. *Am J Public Health* 1997;87:1317–1322.)

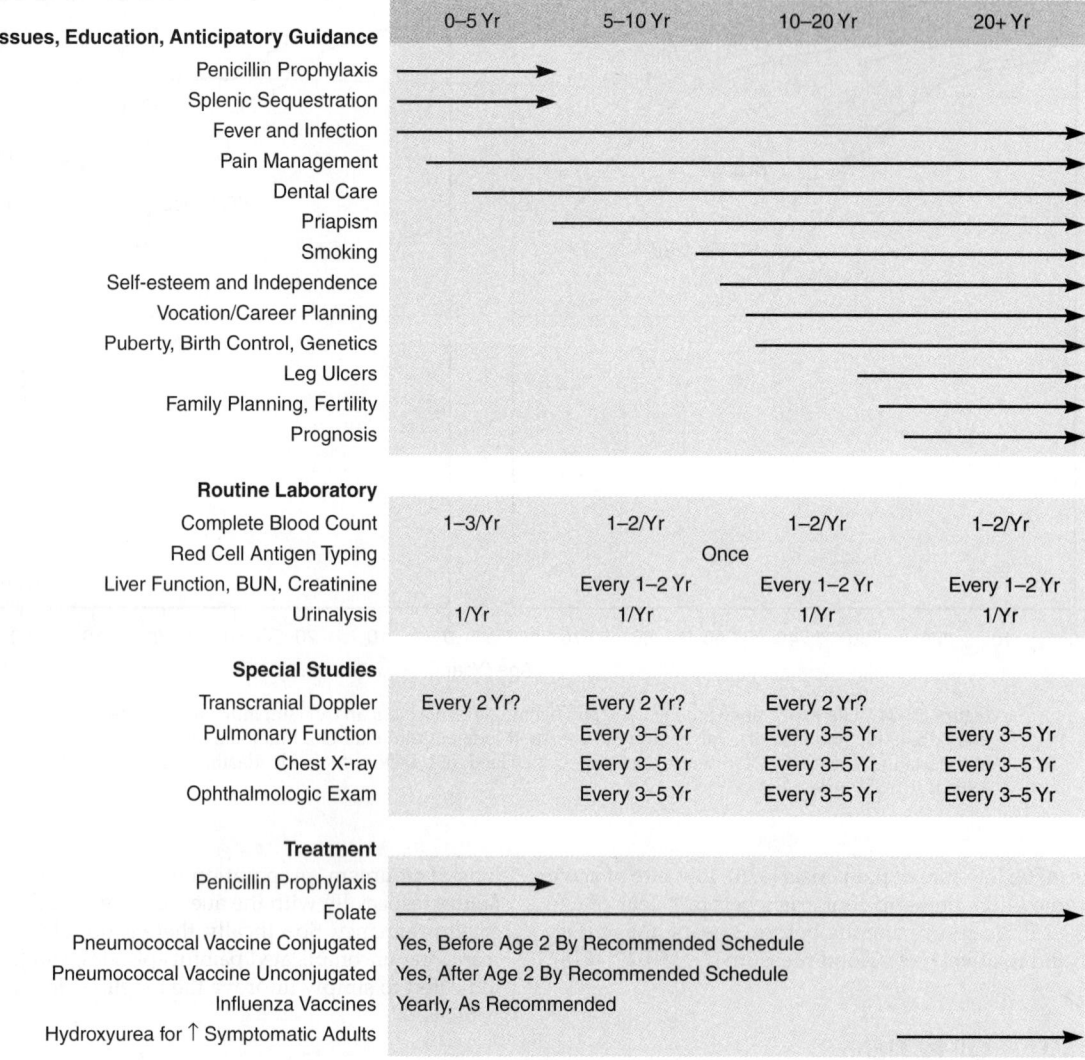

Issues, Education, Anticipatory Guidance	0–5 Yr	5–10 Yr	10–20 Yr	20+ Yr
Penicillin Prophylaxis	⟶			
Splenic Sequestration	⟶			
Fever and Infection	⟶			⟶
Pain Management	⟶			⟶
Dental Care	⟶			⟶
Priapism		⟶		⟶
Smoking		⟶		⟶
Self-esteem and Independence			⟶	⟶
Vocation/Career Planning			⟶	⟶
Puberty, Birth Control, Genetics			⟶	⟶
Leg Ulcers			⟶	⟶
Family Planning, Fertility			⟶	⟶
Prognosis			⟶	⟶

Routine Laboratory				
Complete Blood Count	1–3/Yr	1–2/Yr	1–2/Yr	1–2/Yr
Red Cell Antigen Typing		Once		
Liver Function, BUN, Creatinine		Every 1–2 Yr	Every 1–2 Yr	Every 1–2 Yr
Urinalysis	1/Yr	1/Yr	1/Yr	1/Yr

Special Studies				
Transcranial Doppler	Every 2 Yr?	Every 2 Yr?	Every 2 Yr?	
Pulmonary Function		Every 3–5 Yr	Every 3–5 Yr	Every 3–5 Yr
Chest X-ray		Every 3–5 Yr	Every 3–5 Yr	Every 3–5 Yr
Ophthalmologic Exam		Every 3–5 Yr	Every 3–5 Yr	Every 3–5 Yr

Treatment				
Penicillin Prophylaxis	⟶			
Folate	⟶			⟶
Pneumococcal Vaccine Conjugated	Yes, Before Age 2 By Recommended Schedule			
Pneumococcal Vaccine Unconjugated	Yes, After Age 2 By Recommended Schedule			
Influenza Vaccines	Yearly, As Recommended			
Hydroxyurea for ↑ Symptomatic Adults			⟶	⟶

Figure 50-33. General recommendations for routine health care maintenance in patients with sickle cell disease. BUN, blood urea nitrogen.

between 8% and 50% (726–732). In the CSSCD series, which looked at 1814 patients receiving transfusions, the overall rate was 18.6%—a rate that increased with the increasing number of transfusions (733). The following antibodies are the most common: anti-E, anti-C, anti-K, anti-Le[a], anti-Fy[a], anti-D, anti-Le[b], anti-Jk[b], anti-S, anti-M, anti-Fy[b], anti-e, and anti-c. It is likely that these antibodies arise as a result of the difference in the distribution of antigens between the largely white donor pool and the predominantly black patients (734). Sensitization (especially multisensitization) can make transfusion difficult or even impossible. In addition, because these antibodies may be transient and therefore not discovered at the time of a subsequent transfusion, they can cause serious delayed transfusion reactions (735). Sensitization can be successfully reduced by transfusing antigenically matched blood (730), a worthwhile strategy despite the increased cost (727). An alternative solution is to increase the pool of black donors. Routine leukoreduction of blood products avoids the problem of transfusion reactions related to infused white cells.

SIMPLE AND EXCHANGE RED CELL TRANSFUSIONS
During episodes of acute splenic sequestration or erythroid aplasia, a standard simple red cell transfusion is the most effective way to restore the abnormally low red cell mass. When the

patient is not excessively anemic (Hct >25%), however, simple transfusion increases the viscosity of the blood and can potentially lead to decreased oxygen delivery (736). For patients who are not severely anemic, some form of exchange transfusion is recommended to decrease the number of circulating sickle cells while increasing the Hct. Partial red cell exchange can be performed manually, as described by Charache (737). A 50-kg adult with an Hct of 20% to 27% can have 500 mL of blood removed through a 14- or 16-gauge needle, followed immediately by the infusion of 500 mL of saline. Another 500 mL of blood is removed, and five units of packed cells are then infused. Vital signs and Hct must be monitored closely during the procedure. The most rapid and efficient way to perform red cell exchange is by using automated cytapheresis (738–742).

MAINTENANCE TRANSFUSION
Maintenance transfusion programs are designed to suppress erythropoiesis by consistently transfusing to an Hct level that is in the 30% to 35% range. The goal is to keep the level of hemoglobin S below 30% or, in some cases, below 50%. First, a partial exchange is done; then, the patient receives a simple transfusion every 3 to 5 weeks. Hemoglobin electrophoresis is monitored at the time of each transfusion to ensure that the transfusion

the transmembrane domain results in homodimerization into a right-handed pair of α helices (306,307). Nuclear magnetic resonance spectroscopy showed that I^{76}, V^{80}, and V^{84} on the α helix of one monomer interface with L^{75}, G^{79}, G^{83}, and T^{87} on the second monomer (308). This dimeric interaction is strong enough to resist dissociation by detergents. Recent evidence suggests that a sequence in the transmembrane domain of GPA is important for horizontal interactions with band 3 (236) and that GPA may function as a chaperone for membrane targeting of band 3 (239) (see section Membrane Domain). Finally, a specific role for the cytoplasmic domain of GPA (amino acids 96 to 131) has not been defined. Interestingly, the treatment of red cells with antibodies (or monovalent Fab fragments) to GPA induces cellular rigidity as measured by ektacytometry, and the quantity of GPA that becomes associated with the membrane skeleton in experimental systems increases (309). Both of these changes are dependent on the presence of the cytoplasmic tail of GPA, suggesting that the cytoplasmic domain binds to the membrane skeleton in response to a transmembrane signal initiated by antibody treatment (310). Hypothetically, cellular rigidity induced by the adherence of pathogens to glycophorins may serve the beneficial role of heightening reticuloendothelial clearance of infected cells (310). GPA has been used as a specific marker for the erythroid lineage due to its early detection in proerythroblasts (311). In addition, assays to gauge radiation exposure and consequent somatic mutation have been developed based on measuring the frequencies of variant GPA phenotypes in red cells (312,313).

GLYCOPHORIN B

The gene for GPB (glycophorin B) lies just downstream of GPA on chromosome 4 and is believed to have arisen by gene duplication (314,315). The first 26 amino acids of the extracellular N-terminal domain are almost identical to the N blood group form of GPA, except that GPB lacks the N-linked complex oligosaccharide (267) (Fig. 51-9B). In addition to N blood group reactivity, GPB carries the S, s, and U blood group antigens, with the S and s antigens differing by substitutions at residue 29 (S = Met; s = Thr) (316). Distally, GPB lacks a portion of the extracellular domain that corresponds to exon 3 of GPA and almost all of the cytoplasmic domain. Because GPB is expressed exclusively in erythrocytes, the GPB promoter has been the subject of transcriptional regulation studies. Repression of the GPB promoter in nonerythroid cells is accomplished by the binding of a ubiquitous factor that recognizes a GATA motif centered at position −75 of the promoter (317); recent evidence suggests that the Ku70 protein may function as the GPB repressor (318). Erythroid-specific derepression of the GPB promoter is accomplished by the erythroid transcription factor GATA-1 (317).

GLYCOPHORINS C AND D

GPC and glycophorin D (GPD) have a general domain structure similar to that of GPA and GPB (Fig. 51-9C), but they are encoded by a distinct gene located on chromosome 2 (2q14-2q21) (319,320). GPD is generated from the same mRNA as GPC by means of an alternate initiation codon (163). GPC is a 32-kd protein bearing one N-linked oligosaccharide and approximately 12 O-linked oligosaccharides in the N-terminal extracellular domain. The desialylated form of GPC is exposed on the surface of early erythroid progenitors [erythroid blast-forming units (BFU-E)] and is a useful marker of early normal or leukemic erythroid differentiation (321). Normally, glycosylated GPC first appears in the erythroid colony-forming unit (CFU-E) cells (322). Amino acids 41 to 50 of the extracellular domain contain the Gerbich blood group antigens. Like GPA and GPB, the transmembrane domain passes through the lipid bilayer as a single α helix. The cytoplasmic domain of GPC forms a ternary complex with protein 4.1 and p55, and it is a major site of attachment of the spectrin-actin–based skeleton to the plasma membrane. The 30-kd membrane binding domain (MBD) of protein 4.1 interacts with amino acids 82 to 98 of GPC and the corresponding residues 61 to 77 of GPD (323). p55 is a member of the membrane-associated guanylate kinase (MAGUK) family of proteins and contains a single PDZ domain, which binds to GPC at residues 112 to 128 and to GPD at the corresponding amino acids 91 to 107 (323,324). The ternary complex of GPC/GPD, protein 4.1, and p55 (Fig. 51-5) is believed to be important in maintaining and perhaps regulating red cell membrane deformability and mechanical stability. Unlike GPA and GPB, GPC and GPD are expressed in a variety of tissues (although at lower levels than in erythroid cells and with different glycosylation patterns) (325,326), and they may have analogous functions in the membrane mechanics of nonerythroid cells.

GLYCOPHORIN E

The gene for glycophorin E (GPE) lies just downstream of GPB on chromosome 4 and encodes a 78–amino acid protein with structural similarities to GPB (327) (Fig. 51-9B). The extracellular domain of GPE corresponds to exon 2 of GPB, but the amino acid sequence specifies blood group M rather than N (327). The transmembrane domain is encoded by exon 5 and contains an 8–amino acid insertion. Like GPB, GPE has a markedly truncated cytoplasmic domain. GPE is believed to have arisen by gene duplication of GPB, which, in turn, derived from the ancestral duplication of GPA (315). Thus, GPA, GPB, and GPE define an erythroid-specific family of integral membrane sialoglycoproteins. The level of expression of GPE and its specific functional role have not been determined.

GLYCOPHORIN MUTATIONS

Defects in Glycophorin A, Glycophorin B, and Glycophorin E Give Rise to Approximately 40 Variant Phenotypes of the MNS Blood Group System. These are reviewed in reference 328. Complete loss of GPA, GPB, or both, often by gene deletion from the unequal recombination of the neighboring loci, gives rise to En(a–), (S–s–), and M^kM^k red cells, respectively (Table 51-3) (Fig. 51-10). En(a–) red cells, for example, are completely deficient in GPA and have weak MN blood group antigens (272,275). The affected red cells compensate for a potential 60% loss of surface charge by increasing the glycosylation of band 3, so that the overall surface charge is only reduced by approximately 20% (276). Given the proximity and homology of GPA, GPB, and GPE genes, hybrid glycophorin molecules may be generated by recombination events during meiosis. In the MiV variant, for example, Lepore-like recombination yields a fusion gene containing the N-terminus of GPA and C-terminus of GPB (294). In the St^a variant, anti-Lepore recombination produces the reverse hybrid (N-terminal GPB with C-terminal GPA), which is inserted between the normal GPA and GPB genes—neither of which is lost (294). Interestingly, none of the GPA and GPB variants produces detectable changes in erythropoiesis or in the shape, function, or lifespan of the affected red cells. Rarely, individuals with complete absence of GPA and GPB apparently exhibit no erythrocyte abnormalities (279). Thus, either GPA, GPB, and GPE do not serve any critical basal functions in red cells or such functions are assumed by other protein(s), such as GPC or band 3, when GPA/GPB/GPE are deficient.

Variations in Glycophorin C and Glycophorin D Affect the Gerbich Antigen System. Mutations in exons 1, 2, and most of 3 modify the N-terminal extracellular domain of GPC and GPD;

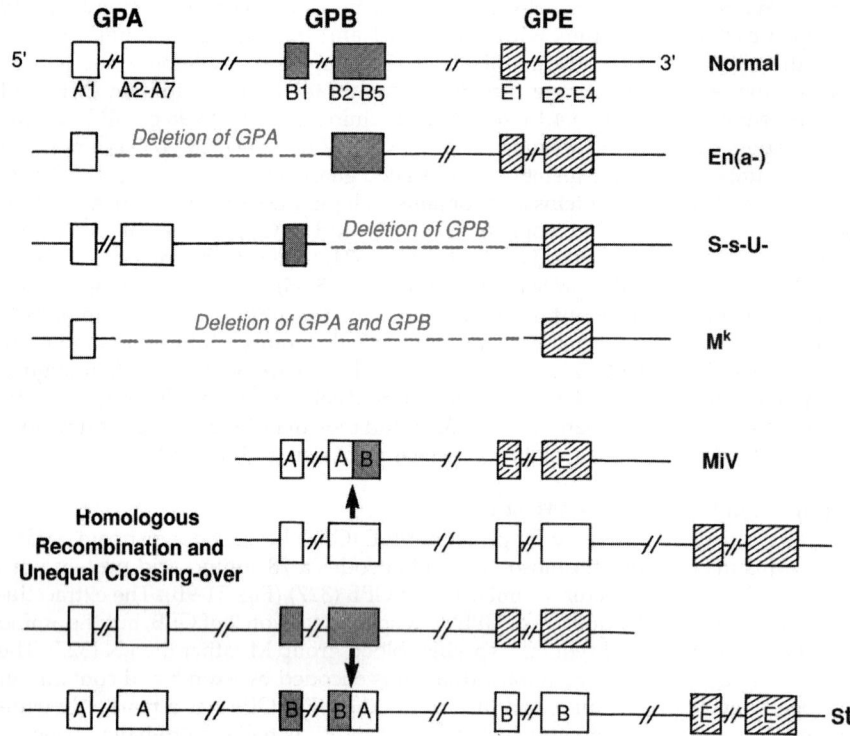

Figure 51-10. Glycophorin variants. Organization of the glycophorin A (GPA), glycophorin B (GPB), and glycophorin E (GPE) genes on chromosome 4 and probable deletions in the En(a-), S-s-U-, M^k, Miltenburger type V (MiV), and Stones (St^a) variants. The MiV and St^a variants arise from unequal crossing over, analogous to the Lepore hemoglobins. In MiV red cells, the normal GPB gene is replaced by a fusion gene (Lepore-type recombination). In St^a erythrocytes, the product of the reciprocal exchange is inserted between the GPA and GPB loci, but no normal genes are lost (anti–Lepore-type recombination). (Adapted from Vignal A, London J, Rahuel C, et al. Promoter sequence and chromosomal organization of the genes encoding glycophorins A, B, and E. *Gene* 1990;5:289.)

thus, they alter the antigenicity of red cells but do not affect cellular mechanical properties (326,329). Examples include Gerbich-type cells, which lack exon 2; Yus-type cells, which lack exon 3; and Webb-type cells, which have a missense mutation of GPC that converts Asn at position 8 to Ser, thereby precluding N-glycosylation at this site (330,331). In contrast, in the Leach phenotype, there is a complete loss of GPC and GPD secondary to the deletion of exons 3 and 4 (332,333) or to a frameshift mutation (333); affected individuals do not have significant hemolysis, but their red cells are elliptocytic (334,335) and exhibit decreased membrane deformability and mechanical stability (329,336,337). GPC-deficient cells also demonstrate partial deficiencies of protein 4.1 and p55 (338); thus, the disturbance in membrane mechanical properties exhibited by Leach cells likely derives from a deficiency of the GPC/protein 4.1/p55 ternary complex. Individuals with homozygous protein 4.1 deficiency likewise exhibit a deficiency of GPC (~70%) in their elliptocytic red cells (339,340), underscoring that the cellular content of each component of the ternary complex depends on the expression level of the others. Interestingly, the absence of the *Drosophila* protein neurexin IV, which contains a cytoplasmic domain homologous to that of GPC, results in the mislocalization of coracle (the *Drosophila* homolog of protein 4.1) at septate junctions, with attendant defects in the formation of septate-junction septa and intercellular barriers (such as the blood–nerve barrier) (341).

GLYCOPHORINS AS RECEPTORS FOR MALARIAL INVASION

Experiments by Perkins published in 1981 identified GPA as a likely red cell surface attachment site for *P. falciparum* on merozoite invasion (342). Subsequently, erythrocytes deficient in GPA were shown to resist malarial invasion presumably by lacking the requisite attachment site for parasitic invasion (343). It has since been learned that there are alternative pathways for the malarial invasion of red cells that depend on the strain of *P. falciparum* and the ability of the parasite to switch its invasion requirements (344). For example, sialic acid–dependent invasion results from the binding of merozoite protein EBA-175 to the ter-

minal sialic acid-galactose moiety on the O-linked tetrasaccharides of GPA (345). Another sialic acid–dependent, but EBA-175–independent, pathway is believed to involve merozoite binding to GPB (346). The identification of specific *P. falciparum* strains that invade neuraminidase-treated red cells (i.e., desialylated cells) (344,347) and GPA/GPB-deficient M^{k}M^k cells (348) highlighted the existence of a sialic-acid–independent mechanism for malarial invasion. One such mechanism may involve merozoite adhesion to band 3 (349). Protein 4.1–deficient red cells (which exhibit partial GPC deficiency) and GPC/GPD-deficient Leach-type cells both demonstrate significant resistance to malarial invasion *in vitro* (350), suggesting that GPC/GPD may also function as an extracellular attachment site for *P. falciparum*.

Stomatin

Stomatin, or band 7.2b, is of particular interest because it is missing in the classic type of hereditary stomatocytosis: a severe hemolytic anemia characterized by red cell membranes that are extremely leaky to Na$^+$ and K$^+$ ions. The disease is discussed in the later section Inherited Disorders of Red Cell Cation Permeability and Volume. Recent data make it clear that hereditary stomatocytosis is not caused by the absence of stomatin, and its role in the pathophysiology of the disease is one of the biggest mysteries in the red cell membrane field.

STOMATIN IS A SMALL INTEGRAL MEMBRANE PROTEIN THAT MAY REGULATE A NA$^+$ CHANNEL

The 31.5-kd stomatin protein (~28-kd on SDS gels) has been isolated (351,352) and cloned (352–354). It is a positively charged, homooligomeric (n = 9 to 12), phosphorylated [cyclic adenosine 3',5'-monophosphate (cAMP)-dependent kinase], palmitoylated integral membrane protein with a single transmembrane helix, a small external segment, and a relatively large cytoplasmic domain (351,353–356). As noted earlier, it is located, in part, in membrane lipid rafts (109,110). Stomatin is a member of a protein superfamily—the PID superfamily, which stands for *prolif-*

eration, *ion*, and *death*. Red cells contain other members of this family, such as SLP-2 (357) and STORP (stomatin-related protein) (358), but nothing is known about their functions or interactions. The stomatin gene (EPB72) is located on chromosome 9 at 9q34.1 (359).

Stomatin is expressed in all of the tissues and in the red cells of all tested species, from human to frog (354), and stomatin-like proteins, of which there are at least 50, are found throughout evolution—even in very primitive organisms such as *Rhizobium* (360). A homolog of stomatin, MEC-2, has been cloned from *Caenorhabditis elegans* (361–364). It is involved in touch sensation and is linked to an Na^+ channel called the *DEG/ENaC channel*. The channel is believed to be mechanically gated by linkage to the extracellular matrix and membrane skeleton or cytoskeleton. Displacement of the membrane (e.g., by touch) pulls the channel open. MEC-2 greatly increases the activity of the Na^+ channel. By analogy, human stomatin may localize, structurally support, activate, or regulate an Na^+ channel—perhaps one that is sensitive to shear stress.

STOMATIN INTERACTS WITH PEROXIREDOXIN-2, A GLUCOSE TRANSPORTER, AND ADDUCIN

Stomatin also interacts with peroxiredoxin-2 (see the section Peroxiredoxin-2) (365), binds and represses Glut1, the erythrocyte glucose transporter (366,367), and may bind to adducin (368). The relationship of stomatin to peroxiredoxin-2 is interesting because this peroxide-reducing protein binds Ca^{2+} and translocates to the membrane (365,369,370), where it seems to be involved with the activation of a K^+ egress channel (the Gárdos channel) (371). Excess K^+ is a major feature of hereditary stomatocytosis membranes. The interaction with the glucose transporter reinforces the emerging concept that stomatin and its paralogs somehow regulate transporters. Stomatin-adducin binding has only been reported in preliminary form (368). If confirmed, it implies that stomatin is attached to the junctional complex of the membrane skeleton.

Other Integral Membrane Proteins

Although band 3 and the glycophorins are the major integral membrane constituents of the red cell membrane, a large number of other integral membrane proteins with specific functions have also been identified and characterized (372).

AQUAPORIN

Aquaporin-1, a 28-kd channel-forming protein (CHIP28), is the major water channel in red cells (373). The human aquaporin-1 gene is located on chromosome 7p14 and encodes a 269–amino acid polypeptide with six membrane-spanning domains. Aquaporin-1 is expressed in red cells, as well as in the kidney and the endothelial cells in the lung. There are approximately 200,000 copies of aquaporin-1/cell, and the protein carries the antigens of the Colton blood group. It exists as a tetramer in the red cell membrane, and the crystal structure of the protein has recently been determined (374). Human red cells lacking aquaporin-1 exhibit markedly reduced osmotic water permeability. Recent studies have shown defective urinary-concentrating ability as well as decreased pulmonary vascular permeability in humans with complete deficiency of aquaporin-1 (375,376). Aquaporin-1 knock-out mice appear normal but become severely dehydrated and lethargic compared to control mice after water deprivation for 36 hours (377).

RH PROTEINS (RHD, RHCE, AND RHAG)

The Rh blood group system is comprised of at least 40 independent antigens carried by two nonglycosylated, palmitoylated proteins that are encoded by two homologous genes, RHD and RHCE, located on chromosome 1 (378,379). RHCE encodes the CcEe set of antigens, and RHD encodes the D antigen. Rh antigen expression at the red cell surface requires the presence of the Rh-associated glycoprotein (RhAG), which exhibits 36% sequence identity with RH proteins and is encoded by a gene located on chromosome 6. All three Rh proteins are predicted to have 12 membrane-spanning domains. There are approximately 10,000 to 30,000 copies of RhD and RhCE proteins and 100,000 to 200,000 copies of RhAG protein/cell. The interaction between RhAG and Rh proteins in the membrane appears to be stabilized by *N*-terminal domain and C-terminal domain (CTD) interactions. In addition to the interaction between the three Rh subunits, the Rh core complex also appears to contain several other proteins: LW glycoprotein (intracellular adhesion molecule-4), integrin-associated protein (IAP, CD47), GPB, protein 4.2, and, possibly, Duffy protein. Recent evidence suggests that the Rh complex also interacts with band 3 and its associated proteins (379a).

Although the function of the Rh protein complex in the normal red cell has yet to be defined, it is postulated to act as an ammonium transporter based on a weak homology to the Mep/Ant family of proteins and a single complementation study in yeast (380). Others speculate that the Rh proteins facilitate the diffusion of CO_2 gas (381). It should be noted, however, that there is not yet definitive evidence regarding the transport function of the Rh protein complex in the red cell membrane. The importance of the Rh complex in regulating red cell membrane structure is revealed by the altered phenotype of Rh_{null} red cells, which exhibit stomatocytic morphology with loss of membrane surface area, cell dehydration, cation permeability abnormalities, and shortened red cell survival, leading to a mild compensated hemolytic anemia (382).

KIDD GLYCOPROTEIN

The Kidd glycoprotein is the urea transporter in the red cell membrane (383). The human Kidd glycoprotein gene is located on chromosome 18q11-q12 and encodes a 391–amino acid polypeptide with ten membrane-spanning domains. There are 14,000 copies of Kidd glycoprotein/cell, and the protein carries the antigens of the Kidd blood group system (384). The urea transporter in red cells functions by rapidly transporting urea into and out of red cells as they pass through the high urea concentration in the renal medulla and thereby prevents red cell dehydration (385). Urea transport across $Kidd_{null}$ red cell membranes is approximately 1000 times slower than across normal membranes (386). However, no phenotypic changes in either red cell shape or red cell survival have been noted in association with the absence of Kidd glycoprotein.

XK PROTEIN

Xk protein, a 37-kd protein (444 amino acids) with ten membrane-spanning domains, is encoded by a gene on the short arm of the X chromosome (387). Although the Xk protein has structural but not sequence similarity with a family of proteins involved in the transport of neurotransmitters, its transport substrates have not been defined. The Xk protein carries the Kx blood group antigen. In the red cell membrane, the Xk protein is covalently linked to the Kell glycoprotein by a disulfide bond (388). Lack of the Xk protein in McLeod syndrome results in acanthocytic red cells, compensated hemolytic anemia, and, in later life, muscle wasting and choreiform movements.

KELL GLYCOPROTEIN

The Kell glycoprotein is a 93-kd (732–amino acid) single-pass type II membrane protein encoded by a gene on chromosome 7q33 (389). It has sequence homology with a family of neutral endopeptidases and has been shown to be an endothelin-3 converting enzyme (390). In addition to cleaving the precursor of endothelin-3, Kell glycoprotein can cleave the precursors of endothelin-1 and endothelin-2—but much less effectively. As endothelins are potent vasoactive peptides, it is thought that the Kell glycoprotein may be involved in the regulation of vascular tone. The Kell glycoprotein carries the antigens of the Kell blood group system. In contrast to the red cell pathology seen in the Xk-deficient red cells, Kell glycoprotein deficiency does not result in red cell alterations (391).

DUFFY GLYCOPROTEIN

The Duffy glycoprotein is a promiscuous chemokine receptor present in the red cell membrane (392). It binds a variety of proinflammatory cytokines of both the C-X-C class (acute inflammation) and the C-C class (chronic inflammation), including interleukin-8, MGSA (melanoma growth stimulatory activity), monocyte chemotactic protein-1, and RANTES (regulated on activation, normal T-expressed and secreted). The Duffy glycoprotein gene is located on chromosome 1q22-23 and encodes a 333–amino acid polypeptide with seven membrane-spanning domains (393). There are 6000 to 13,000 copies of Duffy glycoprotein/cell, and the protein carries the antigens of the Duffy blood group system. The Duffy glycoprotein is the receptor for the malarial parasite *Plasmodium vivax*, and Duffy glycoprotein–deficient red cells are refractory to invasion by *P. vivax* (394). The function of Duffy glycoprotein in normal red cell physiology remains to be defined.

LUTHERAN GLYCOPROTEIN

The Lutheran blood group glycoprotein (Lu gp) belongs to the Ig superfamily and is the receptor on erythroid cells for the extracellular matrix protein, laminin (395). The glycoprotein consists of five disulfide-bonded extracellular Ig superfamily domains, a single hydrophobic transmembrane domain, and a cytoplasmic tail. Two isoforms of this membrane protein (85-kd and 78-kd isoforms) are expressed by alternative splicing of a single gene located on human chromosome 19q13.2. Both isoforms bind laminin. The two isoforms are distinguished by differences in their cytoplasmic domains: The 78-kd isoform has a truncated cytoplasmic tail. There are approximately 1500 to 4000 copies of Lu gp on the mature red cell. Although the function of the Lu gp in normal red cells remains to be defined, it has been shown to mediate adhesion of sickle red cells to laminin (396). As Lu gp is expressed late during erythroid differentiation, it has been suggested that it may play a functional role in mediating erythroblast–extracellular matrix interactions in the bone marrow that regulate egress of reticulocytes from the bone marrow into the circulation.

LW GLYCOPROTEIN

The LW glycoprotein (also termed *intracellular adhesion molecule-4*) present on the red cell membrane also belongs to the Ig superfamily (397). The glycoprotein consists of two extracellular Ig-like domains, which show strong sequence homology with the protein superfamily known as *intracellular adhesion molecules*. The 40- to 42-kd LW glycoprotein is encoded by a gene on chromosome 19. There are approximately 4000 copies of LW glycoprotein on the mature red cell. Preliminary evidence suggests that extracellular domains of LW glycoprotein can interact with the integrin LFA1 (CD11/CD18) (398) and α4β1 and αV integrins (399). In contrast to Lu gp, which is expressed late during erythroid development, LW glycoprotein is expressed early during erythropoiesis. Based on this expression pattern, it has been suggested that LW glycoprotein may play a role in erythroblast-macrophage interactions that are critical for erythropoiesis.

MEMBRANE SKELETON PROTEINS

Spectrin

Erythroid spectrin is the major constituent of the red cell skeleton, accounting for 50% to 75% of the membrane skeletal mass (400,401). The spectrin-based skeleton is anchored to the plasma membrane by an ankyrin-mediated linkage to band 3 (402) and a protein 4.1–mediated attachment to GPC (403). As a result of these vertical attachments, spectrin represents approximately 25% of the membrane-associated mass of the red cell. Spectrin is composed of two large polypeptide chains that associate side-by-side in an antiparallel arrangement (404); the 280-kd α-chain and the 246-kd β-chain are structurally similar but functionally distinct (405–407) (Fig. 51-11). Electron micrographs of spectrin reveal a slender, twisted, wormlike molecule that is 100 nm in length (408) (Fig. 51-12). Spectrin is a highly flexible protein that assumes a variety of conformational and oligomerization states; in concert with its associated membrane skeletal proteins, spectrin generates a deformable juxtamembranous meshwork that affords stability and flexibility to the circulating red cell.

FAMILY OF SPECTRIN PROTEINS IN HUMANS ENCODED BY AT LEAST SEVEN DISTINCT GENES

Two genes encoding for α-spectrin and five genes encoding for β-spectrin have been characterized (409,410). The αI- (or α_R-) spectrin gene (*SPTA*) is located on chromosome 1q22-q23 adjacent to the Duffy blood group (411) and encodes the erythroid-specific α-chain (412). The αII- (or α_G-) spectrin (also called *α-fodrin*) gene (*SPTAN1*) has been mapped to chromosome 9q34.1 and encodes an α-spectrin homolog found in nearly all cells except mature red cells (413). The βI- (or β_R-) spectrin gene (*SPTB*) is located on chromosome 14q23-q24.2 and encodes the β subunit of the erythroid-specific spectrin, designated βIΣ1 (414,415). The βI gene promoter region contains specific GATA-1 and CACCC-related protein-binding sites that account for specific, high-level expression in erythroid cells (416). Differential 3' processing of the βI-spectrin pre-mRNA generates an alternative βI-spectrin subunit, which is found in brain (predominantly cerebellum) and muscle and is designated βIΣ2 (417).

The βII- (or β_G-) spectrin (also called *β-fodrin*) gene (*SPTBN1*) has been mapped to chromosome 2p21 and encodes the generally expressed β subunit of spectrin, which shares 60% amino acid identity with βI-spectrin (418). Thus, erythrocyte spectrin (or spectrin$_R$) is composed of αI- and βIΣ1-chains, and the widely expressed spectrin (called *fodrin, tissue spectrin, brain spectrin*, or *spectrin$_G$*) contains αII and βII subunits. Muscle spectrin is believed to contain predominantly αII and βIΣ2 subunits. Alternative splicing of spectrin genes, in addition to the interchangeability of α- and β-chain isoforms in heterodimer formation, gives rise to a rich diversity of spectrin proteins that likely have distinct localizations and functions.

The most recently cloned spectrin subunits, designated βIII, βIV, and βV, have been localized to chromosomes 11q13, 19q13.13, and 15q21, respectively (419–422). βIII-spectrin is associated with Golgi membranes and intracellular vesicles rather than the plasma membrane. βIV-spectrin associates with the electrogenic Na+ channel in the axon initial segments and the nodes of Ranvier in neurons, presumably through ankyrin$_G$ (see below) (420). Mice lacking this βIV-spectrin have the quivering (qv) mutation, characterized by progressive ataxia with hind limb paralysis, deafness, and tremor (423). A truncated isoform of βIV-spectrin is associated with a subnuclear structure (promyelocytic leukemia bodies) and may be part of a nuclear scaffold (421). βV-spectrin is detected prominently in the outer segments of photoreceptor rods and cones and in the

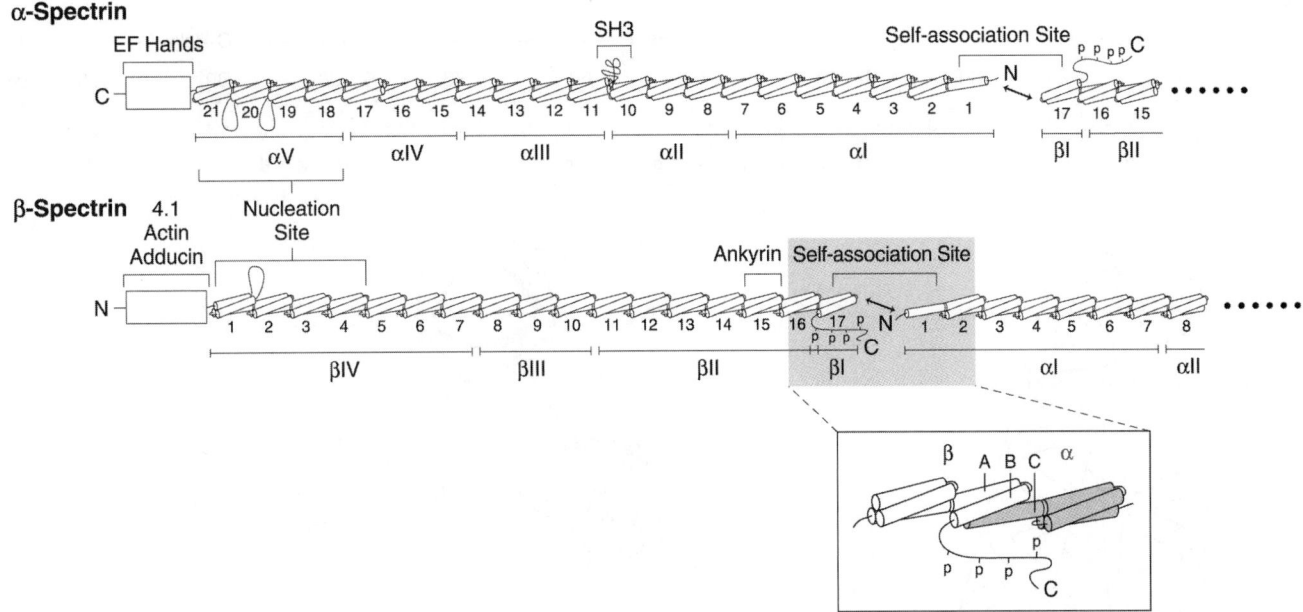

Figure 51-11. Spectrin structure. The α- and β-chains are aligned antiparallel with respect to their *N-* and *C*-terminal ends. The ~106–amino acid "spectrin repeats" are numbered from the N-terminus of each chain. Each repeat is composed of three α-helices (A, B, and C) (407). Note that the spectrin self-association site is formed **(blue shaded area and inset)** by joining parts of a repeat that are leftover at the "head" ends of the two chains. The α-chain contributes helix C; the β-chain contributes helices A and B. Some repeats are specialized, such as β15, which forms the ankyrin binding site, and the parts of the first four repeats at the "tail" of each chain, which nucleate interchain interactions. Rectangles denote peptide segments that differ from the repeats. They include the actin–protein 4.1–adducin binding sites, a potential Ca²⁺ binding region (EF Hands), and an SH3 domain. Each chain can be further divided into large structural domains by gentle proteolysis with trypsin. These are marked below each chain. In patients with hereditary elliptocytosis or pyropoikilocytosis, which are usually due to spectrin defects, the defects lie in the α-I (80-kd), α-II, and βI domains.

basolateral membrane and cytosol of gastric epithelial cells (422). Presumably, these homologs of β-spectrin perform a specialized function related to their association with intracellular and nuclear compartments.

SPECTRINS CONSIST MOSTLY OF TANDEM 106–AMINO ACID REPEATS

Each spectrin chain is composed of a series of 106–amino acid repeats and folds into three helices that self-associate to

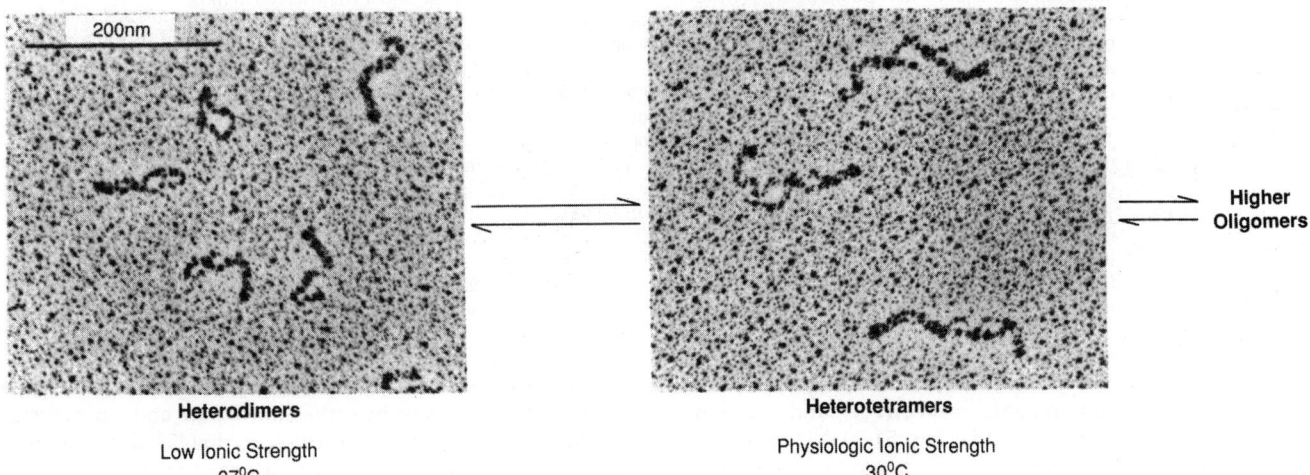

Figure 51-12. Electron micrographs (rotary shadowed) of spectrin heterodimers and heterotetramers. Note that the α- and β-chains of heterodimers are flexible and twisted about each other and that heterotetramers are made by end-to-end association of dimers. The chains sometimes separate, suggesting they are loosely attached, but this is probably an artifact. The scale marker indicates 200 nm (2000 Å). Factors that favor the dimer or tetramer-oligomer state are listed under the photographs. The dimer-tetramer-oligomer equilibrium is kinetically frozen at 0°C. Spectrin extracted and maintained at 0°C retains the distribution of dimers and tetramers that exists on the membrane.

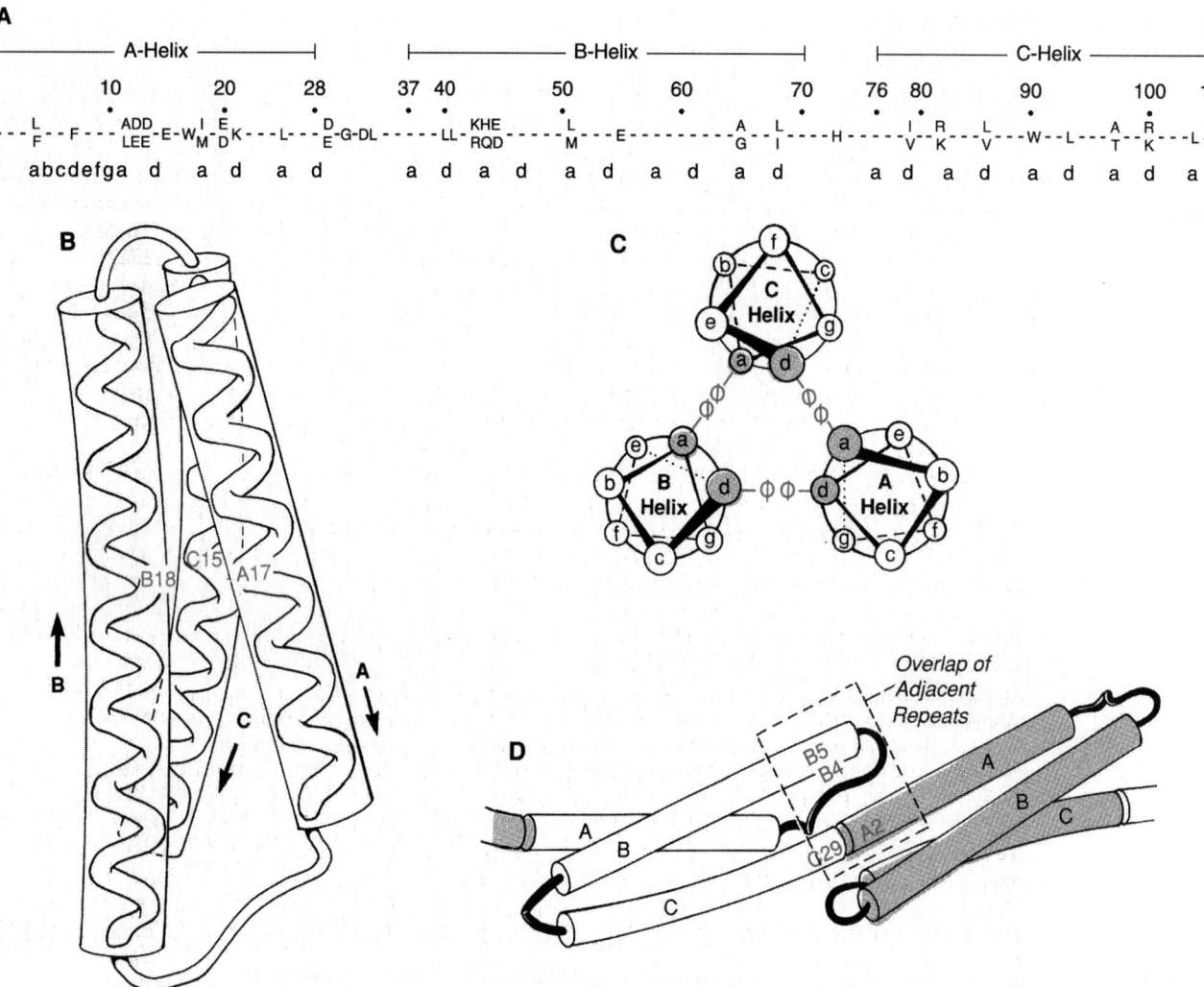

Figure 51-13. Structure of spectrin repeats. **A:** Consensus sequence of a typical 106–amino acid, human erythrocyte spectrin repeat phased according to crystallographic data (424), which identifies three α helices per repeat. Less conserved amino acids are marked with a dash. The amino acids in the repeat are designated a through g. The distance from one a to the next corresponds to two turns of the α-helix. Residues a and d are the major contact points between helices. They tend to be hydrophobic and are conserved in most spectrins. **B:** Model of a single repeat based on the crystal structure of *Drosophila* αII-spectrin (424). The positions of the nearly invariant tryptophans at A17 (amino acid 17 of the repeat) and C15 (repeat amino acid 90) are shown. They interact with surrounding residues, including B18 (repeat amino acid 54), at the central junction where the A helix crosses over from B to C. **C:** Cross-section of a typical repeat. Note that the A, B, and C helices are in a triangular array and that the a and d residues lie on one face of each helix. The side chains of these amino acids are usually hydrophobic (Φ) and interact with each other to stabilize the triple helical configuration. Salt bonds between the typically polar amino acids at positions e and g also help attach the BC and AC pairs of helices to each other. **D:** Interconnection of two adjacent repeats. The A and C helices are colinear, forming one long helix. The distal repeat of each pair is rotated 60 degrees (right-handed). Note that the B helix of the proximal repeat (*white*) overlaps the A helix of the following repeat (*blue*). Interactions in the overlap region among conserved hydrophobic residues, such as C29, B4, and B5 (repeat amino acids 104, 40, and 41, respectively), and the mostly hydrophobic residues at A2 (repeat amino acid 2) probably stabilize the connection and limit mobility at the repeat junction.

form a triple-helical bundle (424,425). α- and β-spectrins contain 20 and 16 complete repeats, respectively, and each contains one partial repeat (412,415) (Fig. 51-11). The primary sequence of each repeat exhibits extensive heptad (seven-residue) symmetry, with conserved hydrophobic residues situated in the first and fourth positions of each heptad motif (designated as positions *a* and *d* in Fig. 51-13A) (407,424). Each spectrin repeat forms a triple-helical structure that is approximately 5 nm long, 2 nm wide, and is rotated 60 degrees (right-handed) relative to the neighboring repeats (424) (Fig. 51-13B).

The prototypical three-dimensional structure of the spectrin repeats was determined by expression studies and x-ray crystallographic analysis of *Drosophila* αII-spectrin (424,425). The first 28 amino acids of αII-spectrin forms a straight α helix designated helix A. The polypeptide chain then reverses itself and forms a second 34–amino-acid-long, straight α helix designated helix B. After another reverse turn, a third α helix is formed and is comprised of 31 amino acids with a bend in the middle of the structure. The three helices are arranged in a triangular array held together by hydrophobic interactions between the hydrophobic faces of the helices and by electrostatic interactions, particularly between heli-

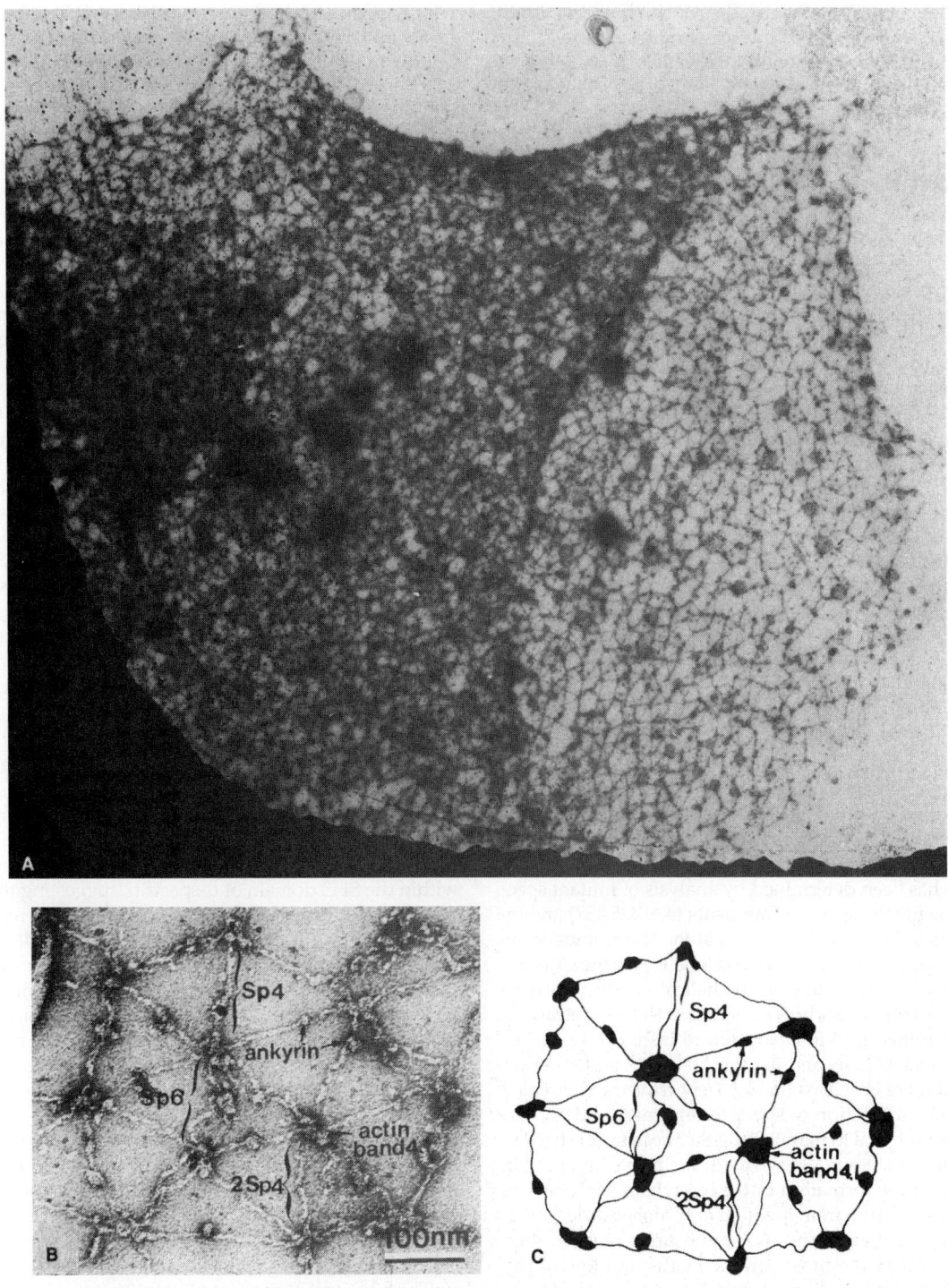

Figure 51-14. Electron microscopy of red cell membrane skeletons. The negative-stained skeletons have been stretched during preparation to reveal details of their structure. **A:** Low magnification to emphasize the ordered, netlike structure. **B,C:** High-magnification view and schematic showing the predominantly hexagonal organization of the skeleton. The location of various skeletal elements is shown in **(C)**. Sp4, spectrin tetramer; Sp6, spectrin hexamer. (Reprinted from Palek J, Sahr KE. Mutations of the red blood cell membrane proteins: from clinical evaluation to detection of the underlying genetic defect. *Blood* 1992;80:308, with permission.)

ces A to C and B to C, in which mostly polar amino acids are found in positions e and g of the helices (Fig. 51-13C).

Interestingly, the three helices of αII are tilted away from each other by 10 to 20 degrees so that the C-terminal end of each repeat is wider than the N-terminal end (Fig. 51-14B). This tilted structure enables the subsequent repeat to attach without any adjustment in the architecture of the preceding repeats. Thus, the C helix of one

triple-helical bundle connects to the A helix of the subsequent triple-helical bundle, forming one long α helix (Fig. 51-13D). The tight connection between repeats causes the B helix of a proximal repeat to overlap the A helix of the distal repeat; the resultant interactions between the two helices restrict movement at the junction between repeats, thereby limiting the overall range of motion of αII-chains. Recent analysis of four related crystal structures of two connected repeats of chicken brain αII-spectrin, however, highlights that flexibility in the spectrin structure may be preserved by conformational rearrangement within the repeat (causing movement in the position of an interhelical loop, for example) and by various degrees of bending at the linker region (426).

SIDE-TO-SIDE INTERACTIONS BETWEEN α- AND β-CHAINS RESULT IN ZIPPERLIKE DIMERIZATION

Nucleation sites located at repeats 18 to 21 of the α-chain and 1 to 4 of the β-chain are implicated in triggering the zipping up of α- and β-chains (427) (Fig. 51-11). Eight residue insertions in two of the α repeats and one of the β repeats may help nucleate the interchain dimerization (427–429). After the initial tight association of the complementary nucleation sites, a conformational change is propagated, causing the remainder of the α- and β-chains to pair together, forming a supercoiled ropelike structure (329). A common polymorphism of the α-spectrin allele, α^{LELY}, encodes α-chains that lack one of the nucleation sites and therefore do not form stable heterodimers (430–432). This clinically relevant allele is discussed further in the section Common Hereditary Elliptocytosis.

SPECTRIN TETRAMERIZATION OCCURS IN HEAD-TO-HEAD FASHION BY ASSOCIATION OF INCOMPLETE REPEATS AT THE ENDS OF THE α- AND β-CHAINS

The "self-association" sequences required for tetramerization are located at the N-terminus of the α-spectrin chain and the C-terminus of the β-spectrin chain (i.e., at the opposite end of the chain from where the nucleation site is found) (408,433,434) (Fig. 51-11). For spectrin dimers to associate into tetramers, the dimer bonds located at the opposite end of the chains from the nucleation sites must reversibly open to allow the formation of two new αβ attachments. Thus, opening of the αβ contact, whether present as the internal bond of heterodimers or the αβ attachment site for tetramers, is the rate-limiting step in dimer-tetramer interconversion (435). The specific structure of the spectrin self-association site has been determined by analysis of mutant spectrins (436) and synthetic spectrin fragments (429,435,437) and by proteolytic studies (438). The free C helix at the N-terminus of the α-spectrin associates with the free A and B helices at the C-terminus of β-spectrin to form a stable triple-helical bundle repeat; in this manner, spectrin heterodimers associate to form tetramers and higher-order oligomers in head-to-head fashion (Fig. 51-11). The isolated α-chain C helix and the free β-chain A and B helices only associate if there is at least one adjacent triple-helical repeat present (437). The formation of spectrin tetramers and higher-order oligomers is critical to maintaining the mechanical strength of the membrane skeleton (439). Mutations in α- or β-spectrin that interfere with the formation of the interchain triple-helical bundle prevent spectrin tetramerization and higher-order oligomerization, thereby weakening the membrane skeleton; such defects in spectrin are the most common causes of hereditary elliptocytosis (HE) and hereditary pyropoikilocytosis (HPP).

SPECTRIN EXISTS PREDOMINANTLY AS TETRAMERS *IN VIVO*

The association constant for the formation of tetramers is substantially higher than that for larger oligomers (441). Whereas physiologic ionic strength and lower temperatures (25°C) favor tetramer formation, low ionic strength and physiologic temperatures favor dissociation to dimers (433,442). At 4°C, the dimer-tetramer equilibrium is virtually kinetically frozen due to the high activation energy (434). The oligomerization state of spectrin can be studied directly by extracting spectrin from red cell membranes at various temperatures and by manipulating *in vitro* conditions to alter the degree of oligomerization (433,434,438,439). In red cell ghosts, driving the equilibrium toward dimerization produces exceedingly fragile structures, underscoring the importance of spectrin

tetramerization in membrane skeletal stability (439). Quantitation of spectrin eluted from normal ghosts at 4°C indicates that approximately 5% of the spectrin is in the dimer form, 50% exists as a tetramer, and the remainder is divided between higher-order oligomers and very-high-molecular-weight complexes of spectrin, actin, protein 4.1, and dematin (440,443).

SPECTRIN HAS SPRINGLIKE PROPERTIES

In vivo, spectrin is believed to have springlike properties, with the 200-nm tetramers intermittently coiled up to achieve a 76-nm end-to-end distance (444). Spectrin molecules condense by twisting the α and β subunits around a common axis. The degree to which the chains condense is regulated by varying the pitch and diameter of the twisted double strand; native spectrin has approximately 10 turns, with a pitch of 7.0 nm and a diameter of 5.9 nm (445,446). Thus, the coiled spectrin tetramers can condense and extend reversibly within the 76- to 200-nm contour length parameter, enabling the red cell to exhibit the properties of deformability and flexibility required during circulation. There is also evidence that individual spectrin repeats are elastic and can partially unfold, extending the molecule (446a).

SPECTRIN CONTAINS IMPORTANT FUNCTIONAL DOMAINS INVOLVED IN PROTEIN-PROTEIN INTERACTIONS

In addition to the critical sequences involved in spectrin nucleation and self-association, the α- and β-chains interface with other proteins via defined structural domains (Fig. 51-11). The tenth repeat of α-spectrin encodes a *src* homology (SH3) domain. SH3 domains generally function as sites of protein-protein attachment at cell membranes. Although the target of the α-spectrin SH3 domain is not definitively known, a recent candidate belongs to a family of tyrosine kinase binding proteins, suggesting a mechanism for association of tyrosine kinases to the spectrin-based membrane skeleton (447). Interestingly, plasmepsin II, the aspartic protease of *P. falciparum*, has been shown to cleave spectrin mainly within the SH3 domain of α-spectrin, suggesting that specific targeting of the SH3 domain by *P. falciparum* may represent a strategy to dismantle the membrane skeleton (448). In polarized epithelial cells, the SH3 domain of α-spectrin interacts with a unique proline-rich sequence within the C-terminal region of the amiloride-sensitive Na⁺ channel (alpha ENaC) and is believed to specifically target the Na⁺ channel to the apical membrane (449). This interaction exemplifies an important function of the spectrin-based skeleton in organizing integral membrane proteins in specialized domains of the plasma membrane.

The C-terminus of α-spectrin shares homology with the actin-binding protein α-actinin and contains two or three EF hands, which are structures that bind and mediate the regulatory effects of calcium (450,451). Whereas calcium binding to EF hands regulates the functions of αIIβII-spectrin and α-actinin (450,452–454), there is no such evidence for αIβI-spectrin.

The β subunit of spectrin contains structural domains that interact with multiple membrane skeletal proteins, including ankyrin, protein 4.1, actin, and adducin (455) (Fig. 51-5). The fifteenth repeat and the last third of the fourteenth repeat of β-spectrin (I1768→Q1898) form the minimal binding site for ankyrin (456). Spectrin's strongest link to the erythrocyte plasma membrane is achieved by the interaction of β-spectrin with ankyrin, which, in turn, binds to the integral membrane protein band 3 (402,457). In nonerythroid cells, ankyrin homologs mediate the linkage of spectrin to other proteins of the plasma membrane, including Na⁺,K⁺-ATPase (458), and voltage-dependent sodium channels (459). The N-terminal 272 amino acids of β-spectrin contain the binding site for protein 4.1 (460,461), which provides an additional link between the spectrin-based skeleton and the red cell membrane through vertical interactions with GPC (323).

The *N*-terminal region of β-spectrin also binds actin (461–463) and shares sequence homology with several actin-binding proteins, including α-actinin, dystrophin, filamin, gelation factor (ABP 120), adducin, and fimbrin. A 27–amino acid peptide within the conserved actin-binding domain of gelation factor has specifically been shown to account for actin binding (464). The interaction of spectrin with actin is enhanced by protein 4.1 binding (465–468). The tail ends of spectrin tetramers and oligomers bind to short, double-helical protofilaments of F-actin with the aid of protein 4.1. Approximately six spectrins can be accommodated on each actin protofilament, leading to the characteristic hexagonal network that forms the basic framework of the membrane skeleton (Fig. 51-14). The actin–protein 4.1 complexes, which reside at the nodal junctions of the network, are associated with multiple other proteins, including adducin, dematin, tropomyosin, tropomodulin, and p55. Assembly of the spectrin-actin skeleton is further enhanced by adducin, a heteromeric calmodulin-binding phosphoprotein, which recruits spectrin to fast-growing ends of actin filaments in addition to binding, bundling, and barbed-end–capping actin (469–472). The *N*-terminal domain and first two β-spectrin repeats participate in forming the spectrin-adducin-actin complex (473).

Isoforms of β-spectrin with *C*-terminal extensions, such as βIΣ2- and βIII-spectrin, contain pleckstrin homology (PH) domains (419,474). The specialized 100-residue PH domain has been identified in proteins involved in signal transduction [e.g., protein kinases and their substrates, phospholipase C isoforms, guanosine triphosphatases (GTPases), GTPase-activating proteins, and GTPase-exchange factors]. The domain also contributes to membrane skeletal organization (e.g., dynamin, β-spectrin) and is believed to mediate membrane targeting of proteins (474,475). The PH domain of βIΣ2 is targeted to the plasma membrane *in vivo* (476) and has been shown to bind with equal affinity to PI-4,5-bisphosphate and PI-3,4,5-trisphosphate (477,478). The association of βIII-spectrin with Golgi membranes (419) is enhanced by adenosine 5'-diphosphate ribosylation factor (ARF)–induced elevations of PI-4,5-bisphosphate (PI-4,5-P_2) in Golgi membranes. PI-4,5-P_2 recruits βIII-spectrin by binding to its PH domain (479).

Finally, the *C*-terminal region of βI-spectrin contains a 52–amino acid extension that is phosphorylated just beyond the site of self-association by a membrane-associated casein kinase-I (480,481). *In vitro* phosphorylation of βI-spectrin has no effect on spectrin self-association (434,482–484). However, increased phosphorylation of βI-spectrin *in vivo* has been shown to decrease membrane mechanical stability, whereas decreased phosphorylation strengthens the mechanical properties of the red cell membrane (485).

The tryptic domains of spectrin have important historical, structural, and clinical significance. Gentle proteolysis of spectrin generates nine structural domains, each composed of several 106–amino acid repeats (404,486). Thus, spectrin was initially demonstrated to contain a series of proteolytically resistant domains joined by protease-sensitive regions. Five tryptic fragments represent the α-chain and include the αI (80 kd), αII (46 kd), αIII (52 kd), αIV (52 kd), and αV (41 kd) domains; the β-chain is digested into four domains, including βI (17 kd), βII (65 kd), βIII (33 kd), and βIV (74 kd) (Fig. 51-11). Many of the molecular defects in HE have been identified as abnormalities in spectrin domain maps after proteolytic digestion (see section Common Hereditary Elliptocytosis).

SPECTRIN IS SYNTHESIZED EARLY IN ERYTHROID DEVELOPMENT

Spectrin is abundant in pronormoblasts (487) and is detectable in undifferentiated erythroleukemia cells (488) and, possibly, in immature committed erythroid stem cells, BFU-Es, and CFU-Es (489). α-Spectrin is synthesized in at least threefold excess compared to β-spectrin (490–492) and has a distinctly slower degradative pathway (493). The limited synthesis and more rapid degradation of β-spectrin suggest that its association with the membrane is the rate-limiting step in spectrin assembly (492,493). The difference in the rate of α- and β-spectrin production is relevant to the molecular pathophysiology that underlies spectrin-related red cell membrane disorders (see sections Common Hereditary Elliptocytosis and Hereditary Spherocytosis).

SPECTRIN DEGRADATION IS A MARKER FOR CELL REMODELING, CELL INJURY, AND CELL DEATH

Calpain I is a calcium-activated thiol-protease, which cleaves αII- and βII-spectrin into characteristic fragments during regulated or pathologic calcium influx (494,495). This cleavage leads to the disassembly of the spectrin-actin network from cell membranes and the perturbation of cellular architecture. Excitatory stimulation of specific neurons during early postnatal development, for example, activates calpain I and generates spectrin breakdown products in a distribution corresponding to regions of synapse formation and neuronal remodeling (496). Thus, regulated transient elevations in intracellular calcium may serve to modify the membrane skeleton to achieve a change in cellular state. Monitoring calpain-mediated proteolysis of spectrin has become a useful tool in studying neurodegeneration and apoptosis. Apoptosis, which occurs after ischemic cellular injury, for example, is accompanied by rapid dissolution of the spectrin-based skeleton. Calpain inhibitors have been shown to prevent the extent of cellular injury after a cellular insult that activates calcium entry. In erythrocytes, cell aging correlates with a decrease in α-spectrin ubiquitination at domains αIII and αV (497,498). The progressive decline in spectrin ubiquitination with aging is believed by some to alter the stability and deformability of the red cell membrane.

MUTATIONS IN ERYTHROID SPECTRIN AFFECT THE INTEGRITY OF THE RED CELL AND LEAD TO CLINICAL DISEASE

Spectrin defects are the major cause of HE and are also important in the pathogenesis of HS (see sections Common Hereditary Elliptocytosis and Hereditary Spherocytosis).

Actin

The red cell contains β-type actin, which is the actin subtype found in a variety of nonmuscle cells (499). Whereas red cell actin shares structural and functional similarities with β-type actin found in nonerythroid cells (500,501), the assembly of protofilaments or short, double-helical F-actin filaments comprised of 12 to 18 monomers is a characteristic feature of red cell actin (502). Actin protofilaments are stabilized by (a) interactions with spectrin, protein 4.1, and tropomyosin; (b) capping of the pointed or slow-growing end by tropomodulin (503); and (c) capping of the barbed or fast-growing end by adducin (504). Another unique feature of the membrane-associated actin filaments in red cells is that actin filaments are capped by adducin instead of CapZ, the ubiquitous barbed-end–capping protein of nonerythroid cells (505). Interestingly, this occurs even though red cells contain CapZ (505).

Actin protofilaments function within the red cell skeleton meshwork as junctional centers intertriangulated by spectrin (Fig. 51-14). Recent data further demonstrate that the protofilaments are oriented tangent to the lipid bilayer and are specifically localized within 20 degrees of the membrane tangent plane (506). This suggests that the protofilaments additionally function as points of reinforcement between the membrane skeleton and the lipid bilayer. Spectrin dimers bind to the side of actin filaments at a site near the tail of the spectrin molecule (Fig. 51-11) (462). Spectrin tetramers are bivalent and, therefore, cross-link actin filaments, although binding is weak (Kd ~10^{-3} M) and ineffectual in the absence of protein 4.1 (507). Spectrin-actin interactions are specifically enhanced by protein 4.1 and adducin [see sections Protein 4.1 (4.1R) and Adducin].

Protein 4.1 (4.1R)

Red cell protein 4.1 (4.1R) is a major component of the erythrocyte membrane skeleton, with approximately 200,000 copies present in each red cell. 4.1R confers stability and flexibility to circulating red cells by potentiating the interaction of spectrin tetramers with F-actin (508) and by linking this membrane skeletal scaffold to the plasma membrane through vertical interactions with GPC (403). In the mature red cell, 4.1R exists as a globular protein that is 4.7 nm in diameter and has a molecular weight of 66 kd, although it runs as an 80-kd protein on SDS gels. Two forms of the protein are resolved on high-resolution SDS gels: an 80-kd protein designated *4.1Ra* and a 78-kd protein designated *4.1Rb*. 4.1Ra derives from 4.1Rb by progressive deamidation of Asn502 during the lifespan of the red cell; thus, 4.1Ra is more prominent in senescent red cells (509). Proteolysis of 4.1R generates four structural domains, including the N-terminal 30-kd MBD [also called the *FERM domain* (510)], a 16-kd linker domain, the 8- to 10-kd spectrin-actin binding domain (SABD), and the 22- to 24-kd CTD (511) (Fig. 51-15). Two posttranslational modifications of the CTD include the previously mentioned deamidation of Asn502 coincident with red cell aging (509) and O-linked glycosidation of cytosolic 4.1R with *N*-acetylglucosamine (512). The functional significance of these modifications is unclear. 4.1R is phosphorylated *in vitro* and *in vivo* by protein kinase A (PKA), protein kinase C (PKC), and casein kinase II; in each case, 4.1R phosphorylation leads to a marked decrease in its ability to bind spectrin and promote the spectrin-actin interaction (513). PKC phosphorylation of 4.1R inhibits its binding to membranes by blocking its interaction with band 3 (514).

SPECTRIN-ACTIN BINDING DOMAIN

4.1R Significantly Enhances the Interaction of Spectrin with Actin. In physiologic solvent conditions, spectrin tetramers bind weakly to F-actin (Kd ~10^{-4} M), whereas the addition of 4.1R generates a high-affinity ternary complex (Kd ~10^{-12} M^2) (468). The 10-kd domain of 4.1R specifically facilitates spectrin-actin interactions (508) and is encoded by alternatively spliced exon 16 and constitutive exon 17 (515,516). The 21–amino acid peptide (encoded by exon 16) and amino acids 27 to 43 (encoded by the constitutive exon 17) form the spectrin binding site (515,516,516a). The F-actin binding site (517) is located in the first 26 amino acids of exon 17. An 8-amino acid motif (LKKNFMES) within that region is critical for actin binding (516a). Thus, the actin site is straddled by the bipartite spectrin binding site (516a,518). The stoichiometry of 4.1R-actin binding is 1:1, and the interaction is highly cooperative, so that the binding of one 4.1R molecule induces a conformational change in the actin protofilament that promotes further 4.1R binding (517,518). Thus, the available data suggest that 4.1R facilitates spectrin-actin binding by bridging spectrin and actin in a strong ternary complex.

The interactions of spectrin, actin, and 4.1R within the red cell membrane skeleton are dynamic, enabling red cell membranes to be stable yet deformable as the cells course through the circulation. 4.1R phosphorylation by PKA, which labels Ser331 in the 16-kd domain and Ser467 in the 10-kd domain, inhibits 4.1R binding to spectrin-actin (519). The interaction is also inhibited by tyrosine phosphorylation at Tyr418, which is located in the 10-kd domain (520). Formation of the ternary complex is further regulated by Ca^{2+} and calmodulin (521), with attendant consequences in red cell membrane stability (522). The critical role of 4.1R in maintaining red cell membrane stability is underscored by the erythrocyte membrane fragility and resultant hemolysis observed in patients who lack 4.1R (see section Common Hereditary Elliptocytosis). Interestingly, normal membrane stability is completely restored when patient red cell ghosts are reconstituted with a 64–amino acid fusion protein containing the spectrin-actin binding site (i.e., the 21 amino acids encoded by exon 16 and the first 43 amino acids encoded by exon 17) (518). This finding highlights the critical functional role of the 10-kd domain of 4.1R in red cell function.

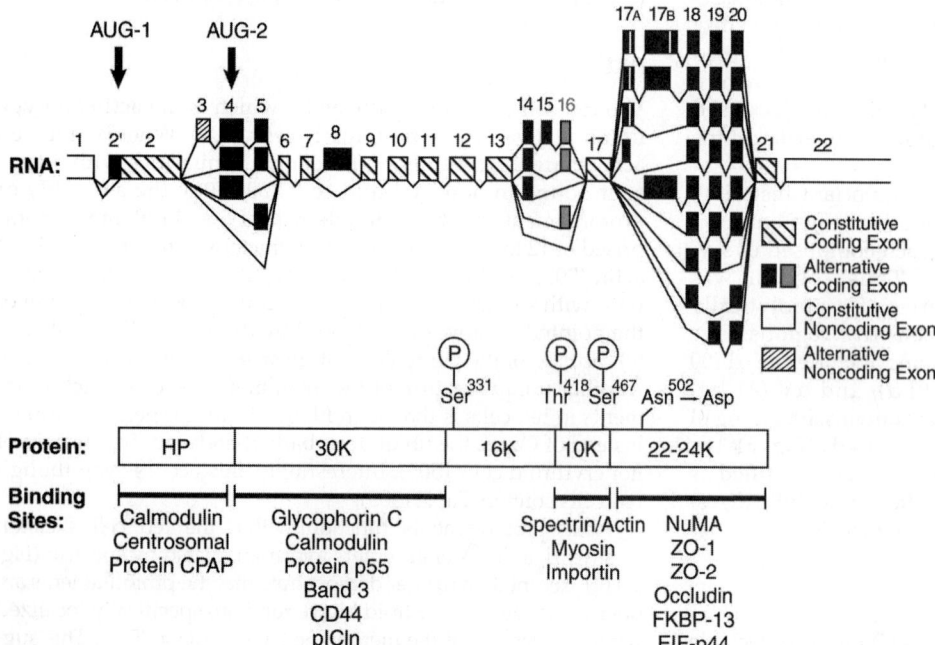

Figure 51-15. Protein 4.1. **Top:** Alternative splicing map of protein 4.1 messenger RNA. Erythrocyte 4.1 is translated from AUG-2 and includes a 63–base pair (21 amino acid) erythroid-specific sequence (*blue*) that is critical for spectrin-actin interactions. The nonerythroid protein that begins at AUG-1 contains an additional headpiece (HP) domain. Many combinations of exons are expressed, particularly in the C-terminal domain, although many of these are only observed in nonerythroid tissues. **Bottom:** Domain map of protein 4.1 indicating binding sites, phosphorylation sites, and the location of a C-terminal asparagine that is deamidated in old red cells. The deamidation reaction accounts for the variability in the apparent molecular weight of the C-terminal domain. (Adapted from Conboy JG. Structure, function, and molecular genetics of erythroid membrane skeletal protein 4.1 in normal and abnormal red blood cells. *Semin Hematol* 1993;30:58.)

Spectrin-Actin Binding Domain Also Interacts with Myosin.

4.1R binds to heavy meromyosin with a 1:1 stoichiometry and partially inhibits the actin-activated Mg^{2+}-ATPase activity of myosin (523). This interaction may be relevant in modulating the Mg^{2+}-ATPase–dependent function in erythroid cells (523).

MEMBRANE BINDING DOMAIN

Thirty-kd Membrane Binding Domain of 4.1R Conserved among Entire Family of Proteins Known as Ezrin-Radixin-Moesin Proteins.

The ERM family is composed of a diverse and interesting group of proteins, including ezrin, radixin, moesin, merlin (or schwannomin), talin, coracle, and several tyrosine phosphatases (e.g., PTPH1, PTPMEG). Merlin, for example, is a tumor-suppressor protein that binds to the C-terminal end of βII- (or β_G-) spectrin (525) and regulates cell growth and organization of the actin-based cytoskeleton (526). The merlin gene is defective in neurofibromatosis type 2 and is absent in virtually all schwannomas and many meningiomas and ependymomas. Despite the diverse functions of ERM proteins, they each use the conserved 30-kd MBD to facilitate interactions with cellular membranes (524).

4.1R Links the Membrane Skeleton to the Plasma Membrane through Interactions with the Integral Membrane Protein Glycophorin C/D.

The majority of membrane-associated 4.1R is bound to the carboxy terminus of glycophorin C/D (GPC/D) via the 30-kd MBD (403) (Fig. 51-15). Although 4.1R also associates with GPA *in vitro*, there is considerable evidence indicating that the physiologically relevant interaction is the association of 4.1R with GPC/D; for example, (a) 4.1R-deficient red cells also lack GPC/D but not GPA (403); (b) any residual GPC/D in 4.1R-deficient red cells is only loosely bound to the membrane skeleton and becomes tightly bound if the cells are reconstituted with 4.1R (403); (c) stripped, inside-out membrane vesicles from normal red cells bind five times more 4.1R than vesicles prepared from red cells lacking GPC/D (150); (d) treatment of membrane vesicles with antibodies that block the 4.1R-binding sites on GPC/D reduces the ability of 4.1R to promote spectrin-actin binding to the vesicles by 85% (527); and (e) GPC/D-deficient red cells, like 4.1R-deficient cells, are elliptocytic and mechanically unstable, whereas GPA-deficient cells are morphologically and structurally normal (322).

4.1R and GPC/D can occur as a ternary complex with p55, a MAGUK protein. The residues Tyr94 to Arg166 of the 30-kd MBD of 4.1R interact with a positively charged peptide in the cytoplasmic domain of GPC localized to residues 82 to 98 (150,528,529). The residues Tyr214 to Glu246 of the 4.1R MBD bind to p55 at a positively charged, 39–amino acid segment found between the SH3 domain and the guanylate kinase domain (528); in turn, p55 binds via its PDZ domain to C-terminal amino acids 112 to 128 of GPC (323,530).

4.1R Membrane Binding Domain Also Interacts with Other Integral Membrane Proteins of the Red Cell, Including Band 3 and CD44.

Binding sites for the 4.1R MBD include the two positively charged motifs LRRRY and IRRRY, located near the beginning of the band 3 transmembrane domain (531). Approximately 20% or less of 4.1R in red cells is believed to associate with band 3 (532), and 4.1R–band 3 interactions do not appear to link the spectrin-actin–based skeleton to the plasma membrane (205). Instead, the 4.1R–band 3 interaction may function to modulate the association of band 3 with ankyrin. *In vitro*, 4.1R competes with ankyrin for binding to band 3. Displacement of 4.1R from band 3 decreases membrane deformability and increases membrane mechanical stability, presumably due to the resultant increase in band 3–ankyrin interactions (204). Whether 4.1R regulates band 3–ankyrin binding

in vivo remains to be demonstrated. One recent experiment implies that it may. Zebrafish lacking red cell band 3 have a nearly bloodless phenotype, which can be rescued by injecting normal mouse band 3 cRNA into the early band 3 (–/–) fish embryos (533). Rescue is markedly reduced if mouse band 3 containing a mutation in either the LRRRY or IRRRY site is used, and it is nearly abolished if both sites are mutated (Paw BH, personal communication, 2001).

The MBD also binds to CD44, a transmembrane glycoprotein present in erythroid and nonerythroid cells; the binding sites on CD44 are the positively charged motifs SRRRC and QKKKL, which are homologous to the interacting peptides found in band 3 (535). Analogous to band 3, 4.1R competes with ankyrin for CD44 binding and may thus regulate CD44-ankyrin interactions (535). Ca^{2+}-dependent and -independent calmodulin binding sites have been located within the MBD (536), and MBD interactions with transmembrane proteins are subject to regulation by Ca^{2+}-calmodulin. For example, Ca^{2+}-calmodulin specifically reduces the affinity of the 4.1R-CD44 interaction (535) as well as 4.1R interactions with band 3, GPC, and p55. Thus, the intracellular concentration of Ca^{2+} is an important influence on the dynamic nature of 4.1R MBD–integral membrane protein associations. The crystal structure of the MBD domain of 4.1R has recently been solved and provides a mechanistic understanding of the binding of 4.1R to various membrane proteins and the regulation of these interactions by Ca^{2+}-calmodulin (537).

4.1R Also Interacts with the Plasma Membrane through Direct Associations with Negatively Charged Phospholipids.

Specifically, 4.1R binds to phosphatidyl serine (538) and phosphatidylinositol (539). The interaction with negatively charged phospholipids may account for some of the low-affinity binding of 4.1R to membranes, suggesting that the membrane may directly serve as a depot for 4.1R that is temporarily unbound from its protein targets. A recent study showed that 4.1R binding to phosphatidylserine is a two-step process in which 4.1R first interacts with serine head groups through the positively charged amino acids YKRS in the MBD domain and, subsequently, forms a tight hydrophobic interaction with the fatty acid moieties (540). Importantly, it was shown that acyl-chain interactions with 4.1R impaired its ability to interact with band 3, GPC, and calmodulin.

C-TERMINAL DOMAIN

Whereas the functional roles of the SABD and the MBD have been well known for years, the 16-kd domain and CTD of 4.1R are poorly understood. Several human mutations in the 4.1R CTD have recently been identified (541). Rather than affect the primary structure and assembly of 4.1R within the membrane skeleton, the CTD mutations depress the accumulation of 4.1R mRNA and reduce the amount of functional protein in the red cell (541). The 4.1R CTD also contains a consensus sequence for binding to FKBP13, an immunophilin found to be enriched in red cell membranes (542). The physiologic role of this interaction is unclear.

ALTERNATIVE SPLICING

The 4.1R gene undergoes complex alternative pre-mRNA splicing. The human 4.1R gene, designated EPB4.1, maps to human chromosome 1p36.1 (543), whereas the mouse 4.1 gene (Epb4.1) localizes to the syntenic region on mouse chromosome 4 (154). The 4.1R gene is more than 200 kb in length and contains at least 24 exons, 13 of which are alternatively spliced (155–159) (Fig. 51-15). Thus, complex arrays of 4.1R isoforms composed of distinct peptide cassettes are found in erythroid and nonerythroid cells. Whereas complex alternative splicing of the 4.1R gene was previously believed to account for the diversity of isoforms observed by immunologic methods across a range of tissues (544–546), the molecular cloning of three new 4.1 genes

(542,547–549) has specifically clarified which 4.1 gene products are expressed in each tissue. Interestingly, this work revealed that 4.1R expression is relatively limited and predominantly localized to hematopoietic tissues and specific cell populations in the brain, kidney, heart, and stomach (550–551).

The two major isoforms of 4.1R derive from the alternate use of two distinct translation-initiation codons. The 17-bp motif at the 5' end of exon 2 encodes an inframe ATG start site used by early erythroid cells and most nonerythroid cells to produce a 135-kd 4.1R isoform that contains a 209–amino acid N-terminal extension. The upstream translation initiation sequence is spliced out late in erythroid differentiation, and a downstream ATG is used instead, producing the prototypical 80-kd isoform of 4.1R found in mature red cells (552,553). The selective incorporation of exon 16 late in erythroid differentiation inserts a 21–amino acid sequence into the 10-kd domain of 4.1R, generating the domain essential for spectrin-actin binding. In nucleated cells, the incorporation of exon 5 and exon 16 into the 4.1R transcript yields a gene product capable of importin-mediated nuclear import (554). The selective exclusion of exon 17b from the CTD of 4.1R occurs in cultured mammary epithelial cells that are induced to divide, whereas nondividing cells in suspension uniformly include this exon; thus, the incorporation of a specific exon correlates dramatically with changes in cell morphology induced by altering cell culture conditions (155). Understanding the functional significance of each of the many 4.1R spliceoforms continues to be an active area of research.

4.1R MUTATIONS

Mutations in the human 4.1R gene cause HE, a disease characterized by red cells with (a) elliptical rather than biconcave morphology, (b) decreased membrane stability, and (c) decreased circulatory half-life, leading to varying degrees of hemolytic anemia (555,556) (see section Common Hereditary Elliptocytosis). The targeted deletion of 4.1R in mice produces an analogous phenotype of moderate hemolytic anemia, with decreased hematocrit and increased reticulocyte count (557). The erythrocytes of 4.1R knock-out mice have an abnormal spherocytic morphology, decreased membrane stability, and reduced expression of 4.1R-interacting proteins, including spectrin, p55, and GPC (557). Interestingly, the knock-out mice exhibit specific neurobehavioral deficits in movement, coordination, balance, and learning that correspond with the selective localization of 4.1R in granule cells of the cerebellum and dentate gyrus (551). Thus, the data generated by the 4.1R knock-out mice underscore the relevance of 4.1R to the cellular physiology of both erythroid *and* nonerythroid cells.

NONERYTHROID PROTEIN 4.1

4.1R Is Expressed in Selected Nonerythroid Cells, in Which New Roles for 4.1R Are Being Elucidated. The 4.1R MBD has recently been shown to interact with pICln, an actin-binding protein thought to play a role in cell volume regulation (558). It is hypothesized that pICln may join the 4.1R-linked membrane skeleton to a volume-sensitive membrane channel (558). 4.1R has been localized to the tight junctions of epithelial cells, where the 4.1R CTD specifically interacts with ZO-2, a tight-junction MAGUK protein (559). The 4.1R CTD also associates with NuMA (560), a nuclear protein involved in organizing the spindle apparatus during mitosis and in reassembling the nucleus at the end of mitosis (561). Depletion of 4.1R or addition of the spectrin-actin binding domain or CTD to nuclear reconstitution assays interferes with normal nuclear assembly (561a). As previously mentioned, specific spliceoforms of 4.1R contain defined residues that enable importin-mediated nuclear import (554);

these 4.1R spliceoforms are associated with the nuclear matrix and colocalize with several proteins involved in mRNA splicing (562,563). In resting cells, 4.1R associates with centrosomes (564); in dividing cells, 4.1R colocalizes with the mitotic spindle and the midbody at defined times during the cell cycle (563). The specific functions of 4.1R at these novel sites are unknown.

4.1G, Closest Homolog to 4.1R, Is General, Widely Expressed Version of Protein 4.1. 4.1G was the second 4.1 gene to be discovered, and comparison of 4.1R and 4.1G expression patterns revealed that 4.1G was indeed the ubiquitous 4.1 protein found in almost all body tissues (542,547). The human 4.1G gene (EPB41L2) has been mapped to human chromosome 6q22-23, and the mouse homolog (*Epb4.1l2*) is found at the syntenic region on mouse chromosome 10 (154). The mouse 4.1G cDNA encodes a 988–amino acid protein with a predicted molecular weight of 110 kd (542). Mouse 4.1G is 53% identical to mouse 4.1R at the amino acid level, with 70%, 68%, and 64% amino acid identities in the MBD, SABD, and CTD, respectively. As previously indicated, 4.1G is expressed in a variety of tissues, including the central nervous system, olfactory epithelium, skeletal muscle, thymus, thyroid, spleen, bone marrow, liver, lung, intestine, adrenal, and testis (542). In each of these locations, 4.1G co-localizes with the immunophilin FKBP13, which binds to the 4.1G CTD (542). 4.1G exhibits a cytoplasmic filamentous distribution in transfected cells (554), consistent with its likely general function as a component of the membrane skeleton.

4.1N, a Neuronal Homolog of 4.1R, Expressed in Almost All Central and Peripheral Neurons of the Body. The human 4.1N gene (EPB41L1) maps to human chromosome 20q11.2-13.1 (565), and the mouse homolog (*Epb4.1l1*) is found at the syntenic region on mouse chromosome 2 (154). The mouse 4.1N gene encodes an 879–amino acid protein, which shares 70%, 36%, and 46% amino acid identities with mouse 4.1R in the MBD, SABD, and CTD, respectively (548) (Fig. 51-15). Like 4.1R, 4.1N has multiple spliceoforms, with a predominant 135-kd form found in the brain and a smaller 100-kd isoform enriched in peripheral tissues (548). Immunohistochemical studies reveal several patterns of neuronal staining, with localizations in the neuronal cell body, dendrites, and axons (548). A distinct punctate-staining pattern is observed in certain neuronal locations, consistent with a synaptic localization; in neuronal cultures, 4.1N co-localizes with the postsynaptic density protein of 95 kd (PSD95), a postsynaptic marker, and with glutamate receptor type 1 (GluR1), an excitatory postsynaptic marker, confirming that 4.1N is a component of the synapse (548). By analogy to the role of 4.1R in red cells, 4.1N may function to confer stability and plasticity to the neuronal membrane via interactions with multiple binding partners, including the neuronal cytoskeleton, integral membrane channels and receptors, and MAGUK proteins. Like the 4.1R CTD, the 4.1N CTD has recently been shown to interact with NuMA (566). PC12 cells stimulated to differentiate with nerve growth factor exhibit translocation of 4.1N into the nucleus concomitant with cell cycle arrest at the G_1 phase (566). Thus, nuclear 4.1N may mediate the antiproliferative effect of nerve growth factor by antagonizing the role of NuMA in mitosis. Interestingly, 4.1N expression is detected in embryonal neurons at the earliest stage of postmitotic differentiation (548).

4.1B, Another Neuronal Homolog of 4.1R, Is Focally Expressed in Brain and in Selected Other Tissues, Including Adrenal Gland, Kidney, Testis, and Heart. Human 4.1B (EPB41L3) maps to human chromosome 18p11.32, and the mouse 4.1B gene (*Epb4.1l3*) is found at the syntenic region on mouse chromosome 17 (154). The mouse 4.1B gene encodes a 951–amino acid protein with a predicted molecular weight of 103 kd. Like 4.1G and 4.1N, 4.1B exhibits a domain organization similar to that of 4.1R (Fig. 51-15). Both the 4.1B MBD and CTD are 70% to 80% identical to the corresponding domains of 4.1R. Alternative splicing produces a brain isoform that lacks the 21–amino acid peptide important in spectrin-actin binding and a skeletal and heart muscle isoform that incorporates this sequence into the SABD (549). Even the 4.1B isoforms that have a complete SABD do not promote gelation of a hematopoietic spectrin-actin mixture as efficiently as the 4.1R SABD (549), suggesting that the 4.1B SABD may bind neuronal cytoskeletal targets more effectively. Interestingly, 4.1B is highly expressed in certain neuronal populations of the brain that do not contain 4.1N, namely Purkinje cells of the cerebellum and thalamic nuclei. This finding demonstrates the selective and complementary nature of 4.1 gene expression. Immunofluorescence studies with cultured PC12 cells demonstrate that 4.1B is enriched at sites of cell–cell contact (549).

Diversity of 4.1 Gene Products and Their Spliceoforms Participate in Generating an Array of Tissue-Specific and Subcellular Compartment-Specific Membrane Skeleton Scaffolds. Current research efforts are focused on identifying the specific protein targets of the MBDs, SABDs, and CTDs of the various 4.1 proteins, as well as elucidating the functional roles of the novel interactions. Furthermore, each 4.1 gene encodes unique domains that may have new, heretofore unappreciated functions. Recent discoveries, such as the association of 4.1R and 4.1N with NuMA and the localization of 4.1N to synapses, underscore the possibility that, in addition to functioning as structural proteins, 4.1 gene products may indeed participate in diverse cellular functions, including cell cycle dynamics and signal transduction.

p55

p55 is a MAGUK homolog found in the red cell membrane as part of a ternary complex with GPC and 4.1R (567). The p55 gene has been localized to Xq28 and is situated just distal to the factor VIII locus (568). The protein is heavily palmitoylated, which contributes to its tight association with the plasma membrane (569). The structure of p55 is composed of five domains, including an N-terminal PDZ domain, an SH3 domain, a central 4.1R-binding (HOOK) region, a tyrosine phosphorylation zone, and a C-terminal guanylate kinase domain (570) (Fig. 51-16). The single PDZ domain of p55 interacts with C-terminal residues 112 to 128 of GPC (323,324). The PDZ domain binding specificity of p55 is distinct from that of the *Drosophila* tumor-suppressor protein Dlg, for example, but is similar to the PDZ domains of LIN-2 and Tiam-1, which preferentially bind to targets containing hydrophobic or aromatic amino acids at the three C-terminal amino acid positions (571). The central 39–amino acid, positively charged HOOK-motif binds to the 30-kd domain of 4.1R. Interestingly, this 4.1-binding domain is conserved in other MAGUK proteins (572). It is not known whether p55 shares functional characteristics with other MAGUKs, which participate, for example, in ion channel clustering, signal transduction, and regulation of cell proliferation and tumor suppression. It is clear, however, that p55 forms a tight complex with GPC and 4.1R (573), so that red cells lacking either 4.1R or GPC are also deficient in p55 (338). There are 80,000 copies of p55/red cell (569)—a number less than the available binding sites for p55 on GPC and 4.1R. Thus, it remains to be determined whether there are functional differences between GPC-4.1R complexes that contain p55 and those that do not.

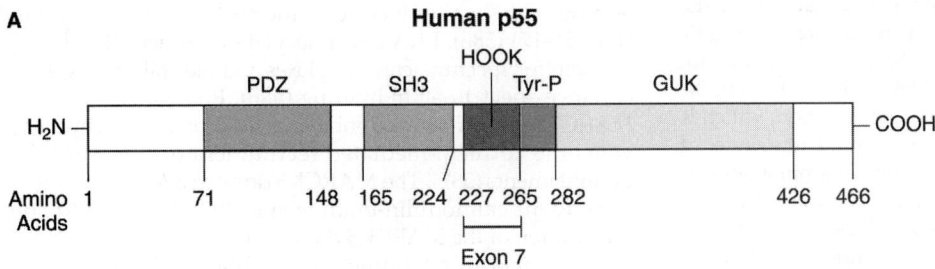

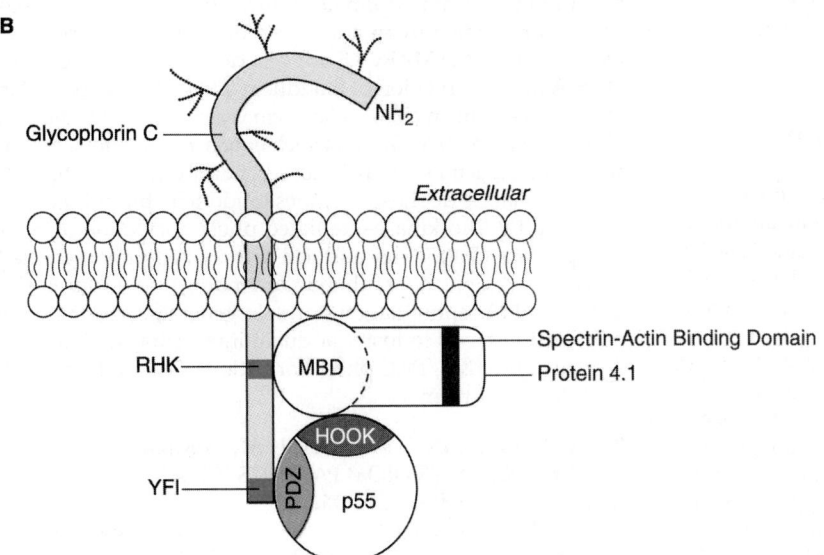

Figure 51-16. Model of p55 and its interactions. **A:** Domain structure of p55. Protein p55 belongs to the membrane-associated guanylate kinase protein family. **B:** Ternary interactions between glycophorin C, protein 4.1, and p55. Note that p55 and glycophorin C (GPC) bind at two distinct sites on the 30K membrane binding domain of protein 4.1R (the GPC site resides in exon 8, the p55 site in exon 10). Although p55 is shown as distant from the lipid bilayer, it is probably adjacent, as it is heavily palmitoylated. GUK, guanylate kinase domain; HOOK, protein 4.1-binding site; MBD, membrane binding domain; PDZ, PSD-95/discs large/ZO-1 domain; SH3, Src homology 3 domain; Tyr-P, site of tyrosine phosphorylation. (Adapted from Chishti AH. Function of p55 and its nonerythroid homologues. *Curr Opin Hematol* 1998;5:116.)

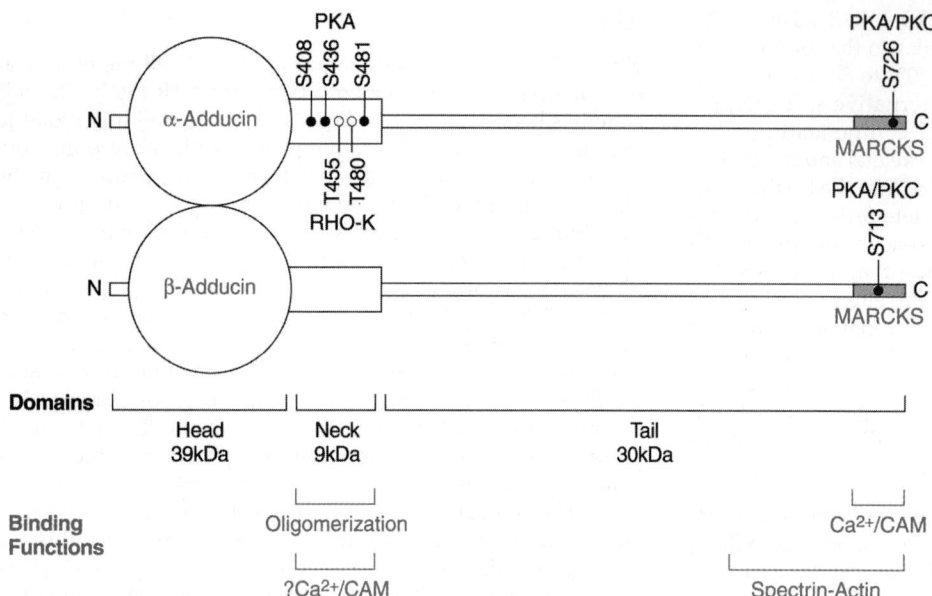

Figure 51-17. Domain organization of adducin. Model for the structure of the αβ-adducin heterodimer showing the three structural domains, the phosphorylation sites, and the identified binding regions. Although the dimer is shown for simplicity, the $\alpha_2\beta_2$ heterotetramer is probably the physiologic form. Binding functions include αβ oligomerization, spectrin-actin binding, and Ca^{2+}-dependent calmodulin (Ca^{2+}/CAM) binding. PKA, protein kinase A; PKC, protein kinase C; RHO-K, Rho kinase. (Adapted from Matsuoka Y, Hughes CA, Bennett V. Adducin regulation. Definition of the calmodulin-binding domain and sites of phosphorylation by protein kinases A and C. *J Biol Chem* 1996;271:25157.)

Adducin

Adducin is a heteromeric membrane skeleton protein that functions in the regulated assembly of the spectrin-actin network. Adducin is composed of an 81-kd α subunit associated with either an 80-kd β subunit or a 70-kd γ subunit (469,574,575). The predominant form of adducin in red cells is the $\alpha_2\beta_2$ heterotetramer. The human genes for adducins α (ADD1), β (ADD2), and γ (ADD3) have been mapped to human chromosomes 4p16.3 (576,577), 2p13-p14 (578), and 10q24.2-q24.3 (575), respectively. Whereas α and γ subunits are widely expressed throughout the body, β-adducin is selectively expressed in brain and hematopoietic tissues (574,575,579). The subunits of adducin are approximately 50% identical to each other at the amino acid level (574,575) and are composed of three distinct domains (574,580) (Fig. 51-17). The N-terminal 39-kd domain forms the globular head region, which is protease resistant and generally more basic than the remainder of the protein (581). A 9-kd neck region links the N-terminal domain to the 30-kd carboxy tail. The carboxy tail is protease sensitive, composed almost entirely of hydrophilic residues, and contains a highly basic 22-residue C-terminal motif that is homologous to the myristoylated alanine-rich C kinase substrate (MARCKS) protein (Fig. 51-17) (574). There are multiple alternative spliceoforms of adducin subunits, many of which generate truncated isoforms that may subserve tissue-specific functions (582–585).

ADDUCIN BINDS, BUNDLES, AND CAPS ACTIN, IN ADDITION TO ENHANCING THE ASSOCIATION OF SPECTRIN WITH ACTIN

In solution, adducin exists as a mixture of heterodimers and tetramers, with the 39-kd head domains contacting one another to form a globular core (580). An important oligomerization site has been localized within the 9-kd neck domain (471). The adducin tails, which extend from the head and neck domains, interact directly with the fast-growing ends of actin filaments and together recruit spectrin to the membrane skeletal complex (471). The N-terminal domain and first two α-helical repeats of β-spectrin are involved in complex formation (473). Adducin-actin interactions require both the C-terminal MARCKS domain and the oligomerization site present in the neck domain (471). In red cells, adducin also functions as the barbed-end–capping protein, stabilizing actin network assemblies by preventing elongation and depolymerization at the barbed ends of actin filaments (470).

CapZ, the major barbed-end–capping protein found in most cells, is also present in red cells, but it is confined to the cytoplasm and binds to the membrane only if adducin is removed (505). Of note, the entire adducin protein is required for capping activity, consistent with the presence of stoichiometric amounts of adducin and actin protofilaments in the red cell membrane skeleton (470).

ADDUCIN ACTIVITY REGULATED BY PHOSPHORYLATION AND CA²⁺-CALMODULIN

The C-terminal MARCKS domain contains a serine phosphorylation site targeted by PKA and PKC (586). There are also three additional PKA sites located in the neck domain of α-adducin (Fig. 51-17) (586). PKA phosphorylation reduces the affinity of adducin for spectrin-actin complexes and the ability of adducin to enhance spectrin-actin binding (586). Phosphorylation of the MARCKS domain by PKC inhibits actin-capping activity and prevents the adducin-mediated recruitment of spectrin to actin protofilaments (587). The MARCKS domain also contains a Ca^{2+}-dependent calmodulin-binding site (493). PKA or PKC phosphorylation of the MARCKS domain inhibits calmodulin binding (586). Calmodulin binding reduces both adducin-actin binding and adducin-mediated enhancement of spectrin-actin binding (472). Calmodulin also blocks the binding of a second spectrin molecule to an adducin-actin-spectrin complex (469). Once bound to the MARCKS domain, calmodulin reduces the rate of PKA phosphorylation of β-adducin and PKC phosphorylation of α- and β-adducin (586). α-Adducin is also subject to Rho-kinase phosphorylation (Fig. 51-17), which enhances the interaction of α-adducin with actin filaments and, secondarily, with spectrin. Myosin phosphatase dephosphorylates α-adducin, but this activity is inhibited by Rho-kinase–mediated phosphorylation of myosin phosphatase (588). Thus, adducin activity is tightly regulated *in vivo* by Ca^{2+}-dependent calmodulin binding and a complexity of differential phosphorylation states. In general, Rho-kinase phosphorylation tends to foster adducin interaction with actin and spectrin, and PKA/PKC phosphorylation or calmodulin binding tends to inhibit them.

RED CELLS LACKING β-ADDUCIN ARE SIMILAR TO ERYTHROCYTES FROM PATIENTS WITH HEREDITARY SPHEROCYTOSIS

Mice with targeted deletion of β-adducin have osmotically fragile, spherocytic, and dehydrated red cells (579). The incorporation of α-adducin into the membrane skeleton is decreased by 30%, perhaps due to decreased α subunit stability in the absence of its heteromeric partner (579). Interestingly, there is a compensatory fivefold increase in the amount of γ-adducin associated with the red cell membrane skeleton (579). The defective red cell phenotype and resultant hemolytic anemia produced by β-adducin deficiency underscore a role of β-adducin in stabilizing the red cell membrane skeletal network.

ADDUCIN ENRICHED AT SITES OF CELL–CELL CONTACT IN NONERYTHROID CELLS

α- and γ-Adducin are the predominant adducin subunits found in nonerythroid cells (574,575), with β-adducin expression mostly limited to hematopoietic and neural tissues (579). In cultured epithelial cells, adducin promptly localizes to sites of intercellular contact in response to the addition of calcium (0.3 mM) to the medium (589,590). Treatment with nanomolar concentrations of phorbol esters, which stimulate PKC phosphorylation of adducin, redistributes adducin away from the cell–cell contact sites (589). Transfection of MDCK cells with a mutated, unphosphorylatable form of adducin results in a dramatic change in intracellular localization from the usual intercellular contact sites to a diffuse, punctate cytoplasmic distribution. These data indicate that focal cytoskeletal assembly and stability are regulated by calcium and PKC-induced modulation of adducin function. Interestingly, phosphoadducin-specific antibodies localize the phosphorylated form of adducin in hippocampal neurons to postsynaptic sites, the specialized regions of neuronal membranes that undergo dynamic morphologic changes and membrane skeletal rearrangement in response to extracellular signals (587). Immunohistochemical techniques were also used to demonstrate increased PKC phosphorylation of adducin during the progression of renal carcinoma, with changes in adducin expression level and phosphorylation state and intracellular localization correlating with tumor growth potential and degree of dedifferentiation (591).

POLYMORPHISMS IN ADDUCIN GENES GENETICALLY LINKED TO CERTAIN FORMS OF ESSENTIAL HYPERTENSION

In rat models, a single point mutation in the α-adducin gene accounts for 50% of hypertension cases, with the mechanism of action related to changes in actin polymerization and increased Na^+,K^+-ATPase activity, resulting in elevated renal tubular salt reabsorption (592–594). A G460W polymorphism in α-adducin is associated with a salt-sensitive form of essential hypertension in certain human populations (595) but not in others (596–599).

Dematin (Protein 4.9)

Dematin is an actin-binding protein that bundles actin filaments into cables within the red cell membrane skeleton (600). The dematin gene has been mapped to human chromosome 8p21.1 (160) and is widely expressed throughout the body. Red cells contain both a 48-kd gene product and a 52-kd spliceoform that incorporates a 22–amino acid insertion (160,601); additional alternative spliceoforms have been identified in the brain (602). The protein is comprised of two domains, a rod-shaped N-terminal tail and a C-terminal actin-binding headpiece that shares homology with villin, an actin-bundling protein localized to the epithelial brush border (601). The 22–amino acid insertion contains an ATP-binding site within a conserved 11–amino acid motif also found in protein 4.2 (161). The native protein exists as a trimer composed of two 48-kd subunits and one 52-kd subunit held together by disulfide bonds (160). Dematin is phosphorylated by PKA and PKC (603), with cAMP-dependent phosphorylation completely abolishing its actin-bundling

capability (604). Like villin, which participates in the assembly of epithelial microvilli, dematin functions as an important structural protein that organizes and stabilizes actin within the membrane skeletal network. Interestingly, the dematin gene maps to a genetic locus frequently deleted in certain cancers. Overexpression of dematin in a prostate adenocarcinoma cell line restored a more polarized epithelial phenotype, highlighting dematin's role in regulating cell shape (605). A knock-out mouse, in which the exons that encode the carboxy-terminal domain of dematin involved in actin binding were deleted, was recently generated (606). The red cells are very mildly spherocytic and osmotically fragile. *In vitro* membrane mechanical stability measurements show that membrane stability of the mutant red cells are slightly decreased compared to normal membranes. These findings suggest that dematin may contribute modestly to regulating red cell membrane stability.

Tropomyosin

Tropomyosin is a heterodimeric protein that functions in red cells to stabilize F-actin protofilaments in uniform segments measuring 33 to 37 nm in length (162,607). The α-helical 27- and 29-kd subunits of tropomyosin form a rodlike coiled coil *in vivo* and migrate in the region of band 7 when subjected to SDS gel electrophoresis (608) (Fig. 51-4). The two major human tropomyosin isoforms found in red cells are designated hTM5 and hTM5b and derive from the γ- and α-TM genes, respectively (162). hTM5 and hTM5b are each composed of 248 amino acid residues, measure 33 to 35 nm in length, and have high affinities for F-actin and tropomodulin. Each actin protofilament is composed of 12 to 18 actin monomers and is associated with two tropomyosin molecules, so that one tropomyosin molecule binds to each of the two grooves of the double helical protofilament (608). Thus, all actin protofilaments within the red cell membrane skeleton are coated with tropomyosin, which strengthens the filamentous network. The corresponding lengths of tropomyosin and actin protofilaments has led to the hypothesis that tropomyosin participates, with actin-capping proteins, in dictating the length of the actin protofilaments. The N-terminus of tropomyosin binds with high affinity to tropomodulin, the capping protein for the pointed or slow-growing end of actin. This interaction limits the cooperativity of actin-tropomyosin associations, thereby restricting the length of actin filaments to the length of tropomyosin itself (609). The binding of tropomyosin to actin is unaffected by spectrin, but spectrin-actin interactions are inhibited by saturating concentrations of tropomyosin (610). This finding suggests that actin-tropomyosin interactions may dictate the site specificity or the extent, or both, of spectrin binding along the actin filament.

Caldesmon

Caldesmon is a 71-kd protein identified in red cells in 1:1 stoichiometry with tropomyosin. In conjunction with tropomyosin, actin-bound caldesmon has been shown to modify actin-activated myosin ATPase activity (611). It has been speculated that caldesmon may function as the inhibitory component of an incompletely characterized contractile system that may be present within the red cell.

Tropomodulin

Tropomodulin is a 41-kd protein that functions as an actin-capping protein at the pointed or slow-growing end of actin filaments. The C-terminal end of tropomodulin has pointed end actin-capping activity, whereas the N-terminal portion binds with high affinity to tropomyosin, which results in further strengthening of actin capping (612). Among tropomyosin homologs, tropomodulin binds with highest affinity to the erythrocyte isoforms (hTM5 and hTM5b) (162,609,613). The interaction of tropomodulin with tropomyosin inhibits the head-to-tail associations of tropomyosin molecules along actin filaments, thereby restricting the lengths of tropomyosin-stabilized actin filaments (614). Tropomodulin remains attached to the red cell membrane even after removal of spectrin, actin, and tropomyosin. The membrane binding site for tropomodulin and the significance of this membrane interaction are unknown.

Myosin

Red cells contain a nonmuscle myosin composed of two light chains (19 kd and 25 kd) and one heavy chain (200 kd) (611,616). The protein has two globular heads, a rodlike tail that self-associates to form bipolar filaments, and the characteristic actin-activated Mg^{2+}-ATPase activity (616). There are approximately 80 actin monomers for every myosin molecule in the red cell, yielding an actin to myosin ratio comparable to other nonmuscle cells (617). Interestingly, neonatal red cells have 2.5 times the myosin of adult cells, perhaps accounting for the enhanced motility of neonatal reticulocytes (618). The SABD of protein 4.1R binds to myosin and partially inhibits its actin-activated Mg^{2+}-ATPase activity (523). Thus, 4.1R binding may function as a means of regulating myosin activity in erythroid cells.

Ankyrin

Erythrocyte ankyrin (ankyrin-1 or ankyrin$_R$) is a 206-kd protein (619,620) that links spectrin to band 3 and thus forms the basis of the skeleton membrane attachment that is so critical to the mechanical and viscoelastic properties of the red cell. Ankyrin$_R$ is encoded by the ANK1 gene, which has been localized to the short arm of chromosome 8 near the centromere (8p11.2) (621). The protein is comprised of three domains, including an 89-kd membrane domain (amino acids 2 to 827) that interacts with band 3 (and other integral membrane proteins in nonerythroid cells), a 62-kd spectrin-binding domain (amino acids 828 to 1382), and a 55-kd CTD (amino acids 1383 to 1881) that modulates ankyrin$_R$'s interactions with spectrin and band 3 (Fig. 51-18). Alternative splicing, particularly in the CTD, generates several ankyrin species in the red cell and accounts for the presence of ankyrin bands 2.1, 2.2, 2.3, and 2.6 on SDS gel electrophoresis (Fig. 51-4) (619). Disruption of the ankyrin–band 3 interaction by exposing intact red cells to alkaline pH causes marked membrane instability, thereby emphasizing the importance of the ankyrin linkage to red cell physiology (623). Indeed, defects in ankyrin$_R$ are the most common cause of HS (194) (see section Hereditary Spherocytosis).

MEMBRANE DOMAIN

The 89-kd N-Terminal Domain of Ankyrin Contains 24 Consecutive 33–Amino Acid Repeats. The ankyrin repeats (619,620) are organized functionally into four subdomains of six repeats each (624), and contain two distinct and cooperative binding sites for band 3 (625). One band 3 binding site occurs at repeats 7 to 12 (subdomain 2), and the other occurs at repeats 13 to 24 (subdomains 3 and 4) (Fig. 51-18). The presence of two binding sites on ankyrin$_R$ for dimeric band 3 facilitates the tetramerization of band 3 on ankyrin binding (201). High-affinity binding interfaces for ankyrin$_R$ on the cytoplasmic domain of band 3 (Kd $\sim10^{-7}$ to 10^{-8} M) have been localized to the N-terminus (193,626) and in the middle of the cytoplasmic domain (627,628) in a region corresponding to an external loop in the crystal structure (Fig. 51-7).

These two regions are close to each other in the crystal structure (Fig. 51-7) and probably form a single site (198).

Ankyrin Repeats Are Found in a Variety of Proteins in All Phyla and Are One of the Most Common Protein Sequence Motifs. The ankyrin repeat motif functions as a site of protein–protein interaction in a range of proteins involved in development, cell cycle control, and oncogenesis (619,629–633). In several crystallized proteins, the ankyrin repeats form a novel L-shaped structure consisting of a β hairpin (bottom of the L) followed by two α helices that pack side-to-side in an antiparallel fashion (stem of the L) (622,634–638) (Fig. 51-18). In ankyrin$_R$, the repeats correspond to individual exons (639). They start at the tip of the β hairpin and line up side-to-side like overlapping Ls, with the hairpins forming a β sheet that is perpendicular to the plane of the α helices. The concave and convex surfaces of the connected repeats provide an ideal interface for protein–protein interactions, making the ankyrin repeat a versatile binding partner. Because the crystallized proteins only contain four to six ankyrin repeats, it is not definitively known how the 24 repeats of ankyrin$_R$ pack. However, it is likely that they maintain the same structure that they have in the crystallized proteins and form a linear domain that is shaped like a twisted piano keyboard, on which each key represents a repeat.

SPECTRIN DOMAIN

The central 62-kd domain of ankyrin$_R$ binds to βI-spectrin and attaches the spectrin-actin–based skeleton to the plasma membrane. Ankyrin-spectrin interactions are cooperative, so that ankyrin binding promotes spectrin tetramer and oligomer formation (640,1564). The spectrin binding interface involves regions at the beginning and middle of the domain (641,642) (Fig. 51-18). The site in the middle of the spectrin domain is highly conserved among erythroid and nonerythroid ankyrins and likely represents a critical point of spectrin attachment; the amino acid sequence at the beginning of the domain is less well conserved among ankyrins and may account for selective interactions with distinct β-spectrin homologs (642). The minimal binding site on spectrin is formed by the last third (helix C) of β-spectrin repeat 14 and all of repeat 15 (456) (Fig. 51-11). β-Spectrin repeat 15 is distinguished by the lack of a conserved tryptophan at position 17 of the repeat (amino acid 1812 of βI-spectrin) and by a nonhomologous 43-residue segment in the middle third of the repeat (helix B). The last 28 residues of repeat 14 are highly conserved among erythroid and nonerythroid β-spectrins and are believed to be critical for ankyrin binding (456).

C-TERMINAL (REGULATORY) DOMAIN

The 55-kd CTD contains sequences that regulate ankyrin interactions (643,644) and has been dubbed the "regulatory domain" (619). Alternative splicing within the CTD yields at least 15 ankyrin isoforms, which differ in size and, presumably, function (639) (Fig. 51-18). For example, one isoform of ankyrin, represented by band 2.2, lacks an acidic 162–amino acid peptide present in full-sized ankyrin (band 2.1). Omission of this sequence generates an activated ankyrin, which exhibits enhanced binding to band 3 and spectrin (644), and facilitates the binding of ankyrin to additional distinct targets in nonerythroid membranes (645). The identification of a membrane-associated protease that cleaves ankyrin$_R$ suggests that cleavage of a repressor region within the CTD may activate ankyrin (645). The CTD also contains a region homologous to the "death domain" of proteins implicated in apoptosis (646), suggesting that ankyrins may additionally play a role in this signaling pathway. There is a reasonable possibility that the C-terminus of ankyrin also contains other functional domains because the most C-terminal amino acids are also conserved.

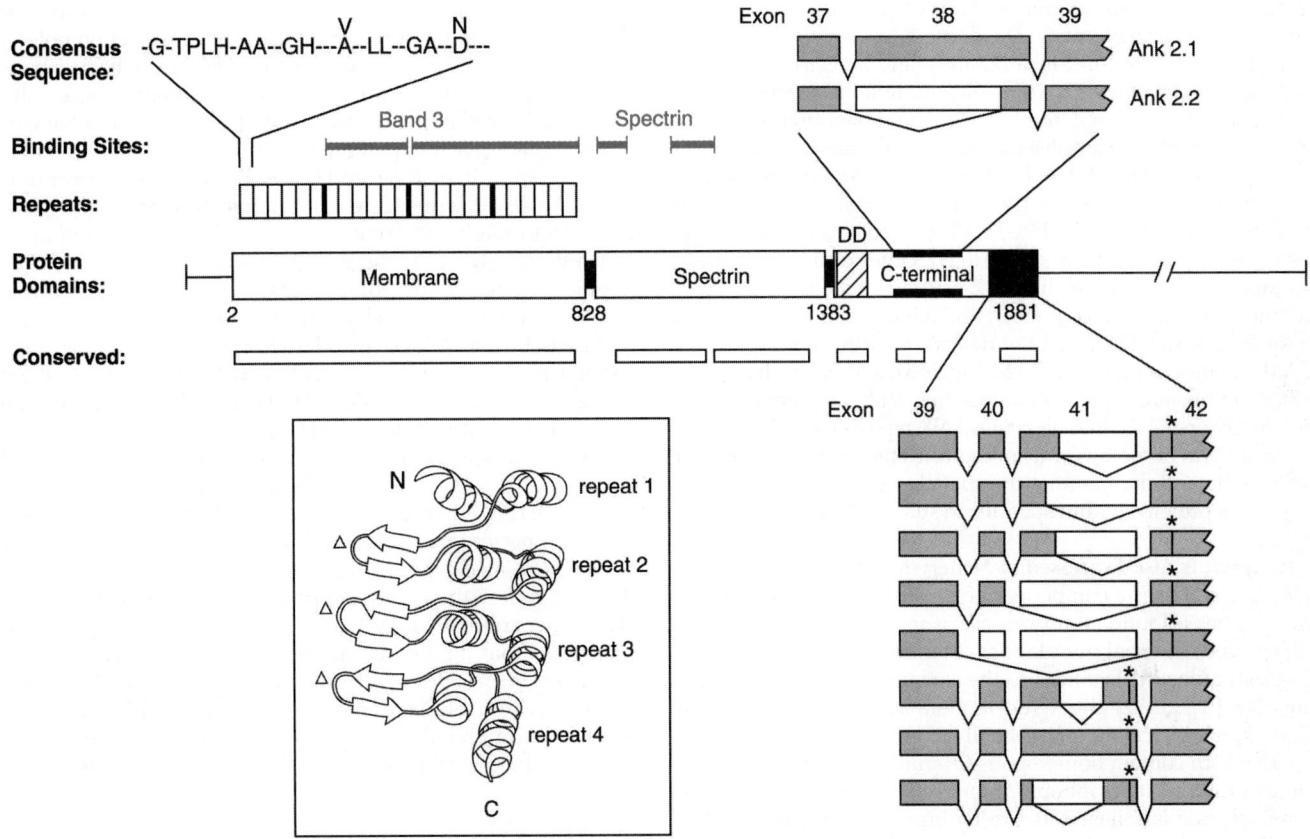

Figure 51-18. Model of erythroid ankyrin (Ank1 or AnkR) structure. The membrane domain (89 kd) contains 24 "Ank" repeats (33 amino acids each) grouped functionally into subdomains of six repeats. Their consensus sequence is shown at the top left in single-letter amino acid code. Dashes indicate less conserved residues. There are two binding sites for band 3, one involving repeats 7 to 12 and one involving repeats 13 to 24. The spectrin domain (62 kd) contains the binding site(s) for spectrin. These two domains are the most conserved. The C-terminal (regulatory) domain (55 kd) is thought to modulate the binding functions of the other two domains. A conserved death domain (DD) resides at the beginning of this domain. It is similar to DDs in proteins involved in apoptosis, but its function in ankyrins is unknown. In the middle of the domain, a highly acidic inhibitory region in exon 38 is spliced out of full length Ank 2.1 to make Ank 2.2. At least eight isoforms of the last three exons exist. In addition, isoforms lacking exons 38 and 39, 36 through 39, and 36 through 41 have been detected. The asterisk and vertical line under it indicate the location of the translation terminator codon. The inset shows the structure of four consecutive ankyrin repeats (622). Each repeat forms an L-shaped structure. A β hairpin loop (arrows) makes up the bottom of the L, and two antiparallel α helical coils form the vertical stem. The hairpin loops of neighboring repeats interact to create an antiparallel β sheet, and the α helices interact to form helical bundles. The small triangles in the inset indicate the junction between adjacent repeats.

PHOSPHORYLATION

Phosphorylation of ankyrin regulates its interactions with spectrin and band 3. *In vitro*, up to seven phosphates are added to ankyrin by casein kinase I (647), and three to four phosphates are contributed by casein kinase II (648). Unphosphorylated ankyrin preferentially binds to spectrin tetramers and oligomers rather than spectrin dimers (640,647,649). This preference is abolished by phosphorylation, which also reduces the capacity of ankyrin binding to band 3 (650).

ANKYRIN$_R$ MUTATIONS

Mice with Normoblastosis (nb/nb) Produce Defective Ankyrin, Which Causes Severe Hemolytic Anemia.
Red cells from nb/nb mice contain no full length ankyrin and, as a result, are also moderately spectrin deficient despite normal spectrin synthesis (491,651). The resultant red cells exhibit severe OF and shortened lifespan due to a defective membrane skeleton. Interestingly, mature nb/nb mice also develop ataxia secondary to a

drop out of Purkinje cells in the cerebellum (652). Ankyrin$_R$ is highly expressed in cerebellar Purkinje cells of normal mice; the observed reduction of ankyrin$_R$ in Purkinje cells of nb/nb mice may cause cell fragility and contribute to their degeneration.

ANK-1 Mutations Are the Most Common Cause of Hereditary Spherocytosis in Humans.
Ankyrin$_R$ mutations lead to combined deficiencies of ankyrin and spectrin. The defective cells produce a variable clinical presentation ranging from mild hemolysis to severe transfusion-dependent anemia (194) (see section Hereditary Spherocytosis).

NONERYTHROID ANKYRINS

The Three Known Ankyrin Genes ANK1, ANK2, and ANK3.
The corresponding proteins ankyrin$_R$ (ankyrin-1), ankyrin$_B$ (ankyrin-2), and ankyrin$_G$ (ankyrin-3) exhibit distinct patterns of expression in the body and have multiple spliceoforms. Whereas ankyrin$_B$ and ankyrin$_G$ both contain membrane and spectrin

domains highly homologous to those of ankyrin$_R$, distinctions arise from heterogeneous CTDs, domain insertions, differential cellular and intracellular localizations, and an eclectic array of binding partners. Nonerythroid ankyrins link the spectrin-actin–based skeleton to a large number of integral membrane proteins other than band 3. Examples include transporters such as anion exchanger 2 (AE2) (653); Na$^+$,K$^+$-ATPase (458,654,655); the electrogenic and amiloride-sensitive Na$^+$ channels (459,656); the Na$^+$,Ca^{2+} exchanger (657); H$^+$,K$^+$-ATPase (658); and the hepatic system A amino acid transporter (659). Other examples include receptors, such as the inositol 1,4,5-trisphosphate receptor (660) and the ryanodine receptor (661), and adhesive proteins, such as CD44 (662,663), CD45, and the neural cell adhesion molecules (CAMs) neurofascin, L1, NrCAM, NgCAM, and neuroglian (664–667). Ankyrins are capable of associating with a variety of target proteins as a result of their versatile ANK repeats (666). The diversity of ankyrin homologs and spliceoforms has been implicated in establishing and maintaining the spatial organization of integral membrane proteins within specialized subcellular compartments.

Ankyrin$_R$ Is Also Expressed in Nonerythroid Cells. In addition to its critical role as a component of the red cell membrane skeleton, ankyrin$_R$ is found in muscle cells, macrophages, endothelium, and specific neuronal populations. In muscle cells, for example, full-sized ankyrin$_R$ localizes to the sarcolemma and nuclei and functions to stabilize the myocyte membrane skeleton (668). In addition, muscle cells express small ankyrin$_R$ spliceoforms (20 to 26 kd), which contain homologous *C*-terminal sequences in addition to a unique, hydrophobic *N*-terminal extension. The hydrophobic peptide is believed to directly insert into the sarcoplasmic reticulum membrane, functioning to stabilize the sarcoplasmic reticulum through an ankyrin-based linkage to the contractile apparatus (668). In the brain, ankyrin$_R$ isoforms are first expressed during the postmitotic phase of neuronal development (669) and, ultimately, localize to the cell bodies and dendrites of selective neuronal populations, with particularly robust expression in the Purkinje and granule cells of the cerebellum (670).

Ankyrin$_B$ Is the Major Ankyrin Homolog Expressed in the Brain. The ANK2 gene is localized to chromosome 4 (4q25-q27) (671) and encodes both 220-kd and 440-kd isoforms of ankyrin$_B$ (672). The 220-kd isoform is the predominant ankyrin isoform expressed in the adult brain and localizes to neuronal cell bodies and dendrites and glial membranes (673). The 440-kd spliceoform contains a large, extended, hydrophilic, filamentous tail domain inserted between the spectrin domain and CTD (674). The 440-kd ankyrin$_B$ is specifically associated with the plasma membranes of unmyelinated and premyelinated axons and, accordingly, is the predominant ankyrin found in the neonatal brain (675). The inserted domain targets the protein to unmyelinated and premyelinated sites, and expression is subsequently down-regulated on axonal myelination (674). Ankyrin$_B$ knock-out mice exhibit hypoplasia of the corpus callosum and pyramidal tracts, ventriculomegaly, optic nerve degeneration, and death by postnatal day 21 (676). This phenotype shares similarities to mice and humans with deficiencies of L1, a member of the L1 CAM family of cell adhesion molecules. These data suggest that 440-kd ankyrin$_B$, in conjunction with L1, plays an essential role in the maintenance of premyelinated axons during development.

Ankyrin$_G$ Generally Expressed Throughout the Body, with Spliceoforms Localized to Specialized Membrane Domains. The 200-kd isoform of ankyrin$_G$, which has a typical three-domain ankyrin structure, is expressed in the plasma membranes of many cells—particularly epithelial and muscle cells—throughout the body (677). The 480- and 270-kd spliceoforms of ankyrin$_G$ localize to axon initial segments and the nodes of Ranvier, an axonal membrane site where ion fluxes propagate neuronal action potentials (678). Mice that do not express ankyrin$_G$ in the cerebellum become ataxic due to the loss of Purkinje neurons, cannot localize voltage-gated sodium channels to axon initial segments, and have difficulty initiating action potentials (679). In addition to membrane binding, spectrin binding, and CTDs, the neural spliceoforms contain (a) a 46-kd serine/threonine-rich region that is glycosylated with *N*-acetylglucosamine residues and shares homology with mucins and glycoproteins; and (b) a large, extended, rodlike tail region. The neural spliceoforms of ankyrin$_G$ co-localize with voltage-dependent sodium channels and the cell adhesion proteins neurofascin and NrCAM at nodal axon segments, and they may be responsible for targeting and anchoring these proteins to the specialized membrane sites (678,680,681). In addition, neuronal ankyrin$_G$ interacts with βIV-spectrin (423).

A 119-kd isoform of ankyrin$_G$, which was first identified in the human kidney, co-localizes with βI-spectrin in the endoplasmic reticulum (ER), Golgi apparatus, and early endosomes. Thus, this ankyrin species is not associated with the plasma membrane. The Golgi-associated cytoskeletal network may serve to organize protein microdomains critical to polarized vesicle transport (682). Two other approximately 120-kd isoforms of ankyrin$_G$ have been identified that do not interact with plasma membranes: One is localized in an unknown cytoplasmic structure (677); the other associates with late lysosomes (683). Ankyrin$_G$ also interacts with clathrin through ankyrin repeat domain 4, and it plays a role in the budding of clathrin-coated pits during endocytosis (684).

Protein 4.2

PROTEIN 4.2 PARTICIPATES IN STABILIZING THE RED CELL MEMBRANE SKELETON THROUGH INTERACTIONS WITH BAND 3 AND THE LIPID BILAYER

Protein 4.2, an 80-kd peripheral membrane protein (685), has been mapped to human chromosome 15q15 (686) and shares homology with transglutaminases but lacks transglutaminase activity (687). Protein 4.2 is first detected in late erythroblasts; there are at least seven spliceoforms that arise from alternative splicing of 90-bp and 234-bp exons in the *N*-terminal region of the protein (688). The synthesis, stability, and membrane localization of protein 4.2 and band 3 are interrelated. The band 3 binding site has been mapped to a sequence, 64RRGQPFTIILYF, near the beginning of protein 4.2 (206). A second site (689) has been localized to amino acids 187 to 211. The protein is palmitoylated on Cys203; palmitoylation enhances band 3 binding (689). Mutant mice that lack band 3 also lack protein 4.2, despite normal protein 4.2 synthesis (689). Human cells that are partially deficient in band 3 are proportionally deficient in protein 4.2. Conversely, band 3 is partially deficient in mice that lack protein 4.2 (209). Interactions between protein 4.2 and band 3 stabilize the proteins within the membrane skeleton. For example, protein 4.2–deficient red cells exhibit increased band 3 rotational mobility and a weaker interaction between band 3 and the membrane skeleton (208,690). Protein 4.2 may also interact with ankyrin and spectrin because nb/nb mice that lack ankyrin$_R$ and patients with one ANK1 deletion have decreased red cell protein 4.2, and a spectrin binding site is located between Gly470 and Asn492 (690a). An ATP binding site is also present (Gly346-Gly351) (690b), but its function, if any, is unknown. Finally, protein 4.2 is both myristylated (691,692) and palmitoylated (693), which suggests a direct means for protein 4.2 to target and interact with lipid bilayers.

Protein 4.2 Deficiency Is a Cause of Hereditary Spherocytosis and Ovalostomatocytosis. Mutations in the human protein 4.2 gene are associated with the production of dysmorphic and osmotically fragile red cells, resulting in hemolytic anemia (197,694–696). Protein 4.2–null mice exhibit mild HS (209). The defective red cells demonstrate a loss of membrane surface area and defective cation transport, with cell shrinkage associated with increased Na$^+$ permeability (209). Whereas the spectrin and ankyrin content of the 4.2-null red cells is normal, there is decreased band 3 protein and a corresponding decline in anion transport activity (209).

Peroxiredoxin-2

Peroxiredoxin-2, also known as *thioredoxin peroxidase B, calpromotin, thiol-specific antioxidant protein, protector protein, natural killer–enhancing factor B, acidic peroxidoxin, torin,* and *band 8,* is 198 residues in length (~22 kd) and the third most abundant protein in the red cell. It is a soluble cytoplasmic protein that translocates to the membrane in the presence of Ca^{2+}. There are approximately 14 million copies/cell (369,371,697), but only approximately 200,000 molecules appear to be associated with the membrane in normal red cells, judging from the intensity of band 8 on SDS gels. The accumulation of peroxiredoxin-2 is maximal in early erythroid development, before the start of Hb synthesis (698). Like the glutathione peroxidases, peroxiredoxins are able to reduce hydrogen peroxide and lipid hydroperoxides to water or the corresponding alcohol, respectively. The activity of peroxiredoxin-2 depends on a pair of highly conserved cysteine residues that catalyze the peroxide reduction step. Thioredoxin is the hydrogen donor. Peroxiredoxin-2 is especially abundant in adrenal glands, brain, and lung, as well as blood. There are four other mammalian peroxiredoxins. These proteins are widely distributed and conserved in evolution. They protect cells from insult by reactive oxygen species and regulate signal transduction pathways that influence cell growth and apoptosis (699).

In the red cell, peroxiredoxin-2 activates the Gárdos channel, a charybdotoxin-sensitive, Ca^{2+}-dependent, K$^+$ channel, which leads to the loss of K$^+$ and water (371). This activation is associated with increased Ca^{2+}-dependent binding of dimeric calpromotin to the red cell membrane as a pentamer of the dimers (365,369,370). Peroxiredoxin-2 is especially abundant on the red cell membranes of sickle cells, particularly the dense, dehydrated fraction of sickle cells (700). Interestingly, peroxiredoxin-2 binds stomatin (365), a protein that is absent in hereditary stomatocytosis, a severe hemolytic anemia associated with markedly increased Na$^+$ and K$^+$ permeability (see Hereditary Stomatocytosis).

ORGANIZATION OF THE MEMBRANE SKELETON

By analogy, the skeleton is sometimes compared to a sweater, which reveals its nodes and individual filaments when stretched but not when collapsed. When viewed by high-resolution, negative-stain electron microscopy, stretched skeletons reveal complexes of F-actin (the nodes) cross-linked by molecular filaments of spectrin (502,701,702) (Fig. 51-14). Dematin, adducin, and protein 4.1 co-localize with these complexes on immunoelectron microscopy (701) (Fig. 51-19). Most of the complexes are connected by spectrin tetramers (85%) and three-armed hexamers (10%) (702) (Fig. 51-14). Ankyrin and band-3–containing globular complexes attach to spectrin approximately 80 nm from its distal end, near the site of self-association (Fig. 51-14). The average thickness of the skeletal protein layer has been estimated to be 3 to 6 nm from x-ray diffraction data (703) and 7 to 10 nm from electron micrographs (704). These dimensions suggest that the skeleton is only one or two molecules thick on average, which means that it must cover approximately 25% to 50% of the inner membrane surface area (like a

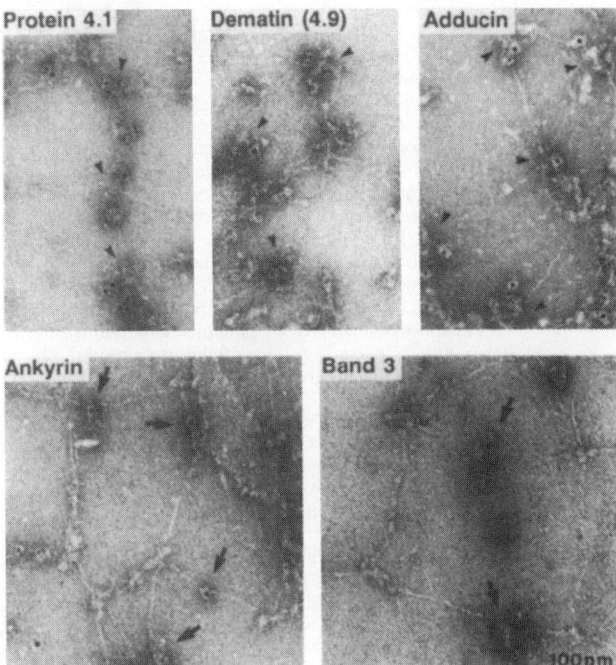

Figure 51-19. Immunogold labeling of proteins in red cell membrane skeletons. Expanded membrane skeletons were incubated with affinity-purified antibodies to the membrane skeletal proteins indicated and then washed and stained with 5-nm gold-labeled anti–immunoglobulin G. Note that protein 4.1, dematin, and adducin are located in junctional complexes (*arrowheads*), whereas band 3 and ankyrin reside in globular structures (*arrows*) on spectrin filaments midway between junctional complexes. (Reprinted from Liu S-C, Derick LH. Molecular anatomy of the red blood cell membrane skeleton: structure-function relationships. *Semin Hematol* 1992;29:231, with permission.)

loose-knit sweater). This corresponds reasonably to micrographs of unspread skeletons, in which the contracted, collapsed spectrin filaments appear to cover most, but not all, of the inner membrane surface.

A model of the membrane skeleton based on this and other evidence is shown in Figure 51-5. Similar models have existed, with gradual refinement since 1979 (705). Spectrin dimers are depicted as twisted, flexible polymers joined head to head to form tetramers and higher-order oligomers. Self-association occurs between the N-terminal end of the spectrin α-chain and the C-terminal end of the β-chain (Fig. 51-11), as described in detail in the earlier section Spectrin. Spectrin molecules are linked into a two-dimensional network by interactions with a complex of actin protofilaments, protein 4.1, dematin, adducin, and tropomyosin (Fig. 51-19). These associations occur at the tail ends of the bifunctional spectrin tetramer. The predicted complexes are morphologically similar to isolated spectrin-actin-4.1 complexes and to structures observed *in situ* in normal ghosts (Figs. 51-14 and 51-19). They appear to serve as a branch point or "molecular junction" in skeletal construction. On average, six spectrin molecules emanate from each complex, although there is some variation. This is evident in the hexagonal arrangement of spectrin in spread skeletons (Fig. 51-14). In unperturbed skeletons, most spectrin molecules probably fold up to approximately one-third their length and do not extensively overlap or intertwine (706,707).

Individual spectrin tetramers and oligomers are attached to the overlying lipid bilayer through high-affinity interactions with ankyrin and band 3, probably with the assistance of protein 4.2. Current evidence suggests that band 3 is a mixture of dimers and tetramers in the membrane (201) and that the tetramer prob-

TABLE 51-4. Posttranslational Modifications of the Major Red Cell Membrane Proteins

Protein	Modification	Functional Effect/Comment
α-Spectrin	Phosphorylation: PKA	Unknown.
β-Spectrin	Phosphorylation: CK-I	No effects detected *in vitro*. In intact erythrocytes, increased phosphorylation of β-spectrin decreases membrane mechanical stability, whereas decreased phosphorylation strengthens the membrane.
	Phosphorylation: PKA	Unknown.
Ankyrin	Phosphorylation: CK-I and CK-II	Decreased affinity for spectrin tetramers and oligomers and decreased affinity of ankyrin for band 3.
	Phosphorylation: PKA	Unknown.
Adducin	Phosphorylation: PKA	Reduces affinity of adducin for spectrin-actin complexes, reduces adducin enhancement of spectrin-actin binding, and inhibits calmodulin binding.
	Phosphorylation: PKC	Inhibits barbed-end actin capping activity, reduces adducin enhancement of spectrin-actin binding, and inhibits calmodulin binding.
	Phosphorylation: Rho kinase	Enhances binding to F-actin.
Band 3	Phosphorylation: CK[a]	Unknown.
	Phosphorylation: TK (Tyr 8)[b]	Inhibits binding of glycolytic enzymes, increased glycolysis, may be activated by oxidants.
	Glycosylation (Asn 642)	No effects detected.
	Palmitoylation (Cys 843)	Unknown.
	Methylation	Unknown (low stoichiometry).
Protein 4.1	Phosphorylation: PKA (Ser 331, Ser 467)	Inhibits 4.1-spectrin binding and spectrin-actin-4.1 complex formation.
	Phosphorylation: PKC	Inhibits 4.1-spectrin binding, spectrin-actin-4.1 complex formation, and 4.1–band 3 binding.
	Phosphorylation: CK-II	Inhibits 4.1-spectrin binding and binding of 4.1 to membrane.
	Phosphorylation: TK (Tyr 418)[c]	Inhibits spectrin-actin-4.1 complex formation.
	Deamidation (Asn 502)	Unknown (converts SDS gel band 4.1b to 4.1a).
	Glycosylation	Unknown (only 20% to 40% of protein modified).
Protein 4.2	N-myristoylation (Gly 1)	Unknown.
Protein p55	Palmitoylation	Unknown, possibly membrane attachment.
Dematin (4.9)	Phosphorylation: PKA	Inhibits actin-filament bundling.
	Phosphorylation: PKC	No effects detected.
	Phosphorylation: CK	Unknown.

CK, casein kinase; PKA, protein kinase A; PKC, protein kinase C; SDS, sodium dodecyl sulfate; TK, tyrosine kinase.
[a]Several amino acids in the N-terminal region are partially phosphorylated (total incorporated PO_4 ~1 mol/mol): Ser 29, Thr 39, Thr 42, Thr 48, Thr 49, Ser 50, and Thr 54.
[b]Also some phosphorylation of Tyr 21, Tyr 359, and Tyr 904.
[c]May only occur in nonerythroid cells.
Adapted from Cohen CM, Gascard P. Regulation and post-translational modification of the erythrocyte membrane and membrane-skeletal proteins. *Semin Hematol* 1992;29:244–292.

ably binds only one molecule of ankyrin (708,709). If so, approximately 40% of the band 3 molecules are involved in anchoring the membrane skeleton. Although the spectrin tetramer contains two ankyrin-binding sites, there is only enough ankyrin to fill one, and, on average, only one is filled *in situ* (Fig. 51-14). Interactions between protein 4.1, protein p55, and GPC or between protein 4.1 and band 3 provide secondary sites of attachment.

Modulation of Membrane Skeletal Structure

Red cell membrane proteins are subject to a large number of posttranslational modifications or other regulatory effects: phosphorylation, fatty acid acylation, methylation, glycosylation, deamidation, calpain cleavage, polyphosphoinositide and calmodulin regulation, oxidation, and modification by polyanions (Tables 51-4 and 51-5). Detailed discussion of all these pathways is beyond the scope of this chapter. Fortunately, they have been thoroughly reviewed (125).

PHOSPHORYLATION

Almost all of the membrane skeletal proteins are phosphorylated by one or more protein kinases (Table 51-4). These include casein kinases (spectrin, ankyrin, band 3, protein 4.1, and dematin); PKA (spectrin, ankyrin, adducin, protein 4.1, and dematin); PKC (adducin, protein 4.1, and dematin); and tyrosine kinases (band 3 and protein 4.1) (125).

In all cases studied so far, phosphorylation inhibits membrane protein interactions: (a) Ankyrin phosphorylation (casein

kinase) abolishes the preference of ankyrin for spectrin tetramer (710,711) and decreases binding to band 3 (712); (b) phosphorylation of protein 4.1 (several kinases) diminishes its binding to spectrin and its ability to promote spectrin-actin binding (713–715) and decreases its attachment to the membrane (716); (c) phosphorylation by PKC inhibits binding of protein 4.1 to band 3 (717); (d) phosphorylation of protein 4.9 by PKA prevents actin bundling (718); and (e) phosphorylation of Tyr8 at the N-terminus of band 3 blocks the binding of glycolytic enzymes (719) and, presumably, Hb and results in increased glycolysis (1). In contrast, despite extensive study (434,482,720,721), no functional effect of spectrin phosphorylation on *in vitro* protein–protein interactions has yet been identified. However, increased phosphorylation of β-spectrin *in vivo* has been shown to decrease membrane mechanical stability, whereas decreased phosphorylation strengthens the mechanical properties of the red cell membrane (722).

POLYANIONS
Physiologic concentrations of organic polyanions such as 2,3-diphosphoglycerate (2,3-DPG) and ATP weaken and dissociate the membrane skeleton (723,724) and increase the lateral mobility of band 3 in ghosts (725). Although some studies suggest that even supraphysiologic concentrations of 2,3-DPG have little or no effect on intact erythrocytes (726,727) in terms of membrane *deformability*, there is convincing evidence that increased 2,3-DPG levels decrease membrane mechanical *stability* (724). It has been suggested that the developmental switch

TABLE 51-5. Red Cell Membrane Regulatory Pathways

Pathway	Effect	Activation
Ca^{2+}/calmodulin	Regulates membrane mechanical properties by effects on the spectrin-actin-4.1 complex and/or by effects on adducin.	Increased intracellular Ca^{2+}.
	Regulates interaction of 4.1 with CD44, band 3 glycophorin C and p55.	
Calpain-mediated proteolysis	Degradation of spectrin, ankyrin, band 3, and protein 4.1.	Increased intracellular Ca^{2+}.
Deamidation	See Table 51-4.	
2,3-Diphosphoglycerate (2,3-DPG)	Decreases membrane mechanical stability, disrupts spectrin-actin-4.1 complexes, inhibits membrane casein kinases.	Increased oxygenation or hemoglobin F increase free 2,3-DPG because 2,3-DPG does not bind to deoxyhemoglobin A or hemoglobin F.
Glycosylation	See Table 51-4.	—
Methylation	See Table 51-4.	—
Phosphoinositides	Regulate binding of protein 4.1 to membrane sites (probably glycophorins). May affect casein kinase activity, cation homeostasis, and/or cell shape.	Increased intracellular Ca^{2+} (via activation of phosphoinositidase C), metabolic depletion, PKC activation.
Phosphorylation	See Table 51-4.	—
Sulfhydryl oxidation	Formation of cross-linked complexes of membrane proteins. Some specific effects of SH oxidation on protein interactions: Spectrin: decreased 4.1 binding and decreased self-association. Ankyrin: decreased spectrin binding. Band 3: decreased ankyrin binding.	Oxidative stress, G6PD deficiency, sickle cell disease, unstable hemoglobinopathies, thalassemias.

G6PD, glucose-6-phosphate dehydrogenase; PKC, protein kinase C.
Adapted from Cohen CM, Gascard P. Regulation and post-translational modification of the erythrocyte membrane and membrane-skeletal proteins. *Semin Hematol* 1992;29:244–292.

from fetal to adult Hb, by diminishing available free 2,3-DPG (which does not bind to fetal Hb), may explain the abatement of cell fragmentation and hemolytic anemia that accompanies maturation of infants with HE (724).

CALCIUM AND CALMODULIN

There is strong evidence that calmodulin modifies the membrane properties of the red cell (728). Physiologic concentrations of calmodulin, sealed in red cell ghosts, destabilize membranes in the presence, but not in the absence, of micromolar concentrations of Ca^{2+}. Recent studies suggest that the effect may result from interactions of calmodulin with protein 4.1 (729). Submicromolar concentrations of calmodulin—even lower than those that exist in the red cell (~3 to 6 µM)—block the protein 4.1–induced gelation of actin in the presence of spectrin (729). The effect is Ca^{2+} dependent. It begins at a Ca^{2+} concentration of 10^{-6} to 10^{-7} M, which is relatively low but still higher than the free Ca^{2+} concentration in the erythrocyte (20 to 40 nM). Surprisingly, Ca^{2+}-calmodulin does not block spectrin-actin-4.1 complex formation under these conditions (729); it blocks only the extensive cross-linking needed to cause gelation. Calmodulin also binds to the spectrin β-chain in a Ca^{2+}-dependent manner (730); however, the affinity of spectrin for calmodulin is not great, and it is unclear whether this effect occurs at the concentrations of calmodulin that exist in erythrocytes.

β-Adducin also binds calmodulin (Kd = 2.3×10^{-7} M) (731). Adducin that is bound to spectrin and actin fosters the attachment of a second, neighboring spectrin. This reaction is blocked by calmodulin in the presence of Ca^{2+} (>10^{-7} M) (469,732). The physiologic consequences of this effect are unclear.

Several other Ca^{2+}-dependent events do not require the presence of calmodulin. One is membrane protein cross-linking, which is catalyzed by a Ca^{2+}-dependent transglutaminase (733). This cross-linking acts as an endogenous fixative that stabilizes red cell shape (734,735). However, the Ca^{2+} concentration required by this reaction is more than 100-fold greater than the normal red cell Ca^{2+} concentration, making it unlikely that transglutaminase permanently stabilizes red cell shape *in vivo* (734).

A second calmodulin-independent effect of Ca^{2+} is the so-called Gárdos phenomenon (736) (described later in this chap-

ter), a unidirectional K$^+$ and water loss producing cellular dehydration. In contrast to transamidative cross-linking, the Ca^{2+} concentration required to trigger the Gárdos channel is low (in the micromolar range) and, thus, physiologically significant. As discussed elsewhere in this textbook (see Chapter 50), this pathway contributes to cellular dehydration of sickle red cells.

A third calmodulin-independent Ca^{2+} effect involves calpain, one of a family of Ca^{2+}-stimulated neutral proteases, which are present in a variety of tissues including red cells (125). Susceptible membrane substrates include adducin, ankyrin, protein 4.1, and, to a lesser extent, spectrin and band 3.

Finally, Ca^{2+} also induces phospholipid scrambling, as discussed earlier in the section Calcium Induces Rapid Phospholipid Scrambling. Thus, increases in intracellular calcium produce a range of deleterious effects. Although these phenomena are well studied *in vitro*, their role in erythrocyte pathology, particularly in acquired disorders associated with abnormal red cell shape, is not well understood.

Biogenesis of the Membrane Skeleton

SYNTHESIS OF BAND 3 INITIATES ASSEMBLY OF STABLE MEMBRANE SKELETON

Spectrin and ankyrin synthesis is detectable at very early stages of erythroid development in avian and mammalian erythroid cells (reviewed in 737–739). However, these proteins turn over rapidly, and they do not assemble into a permanent network. Synthesis of band 3 (the anion exchange protein) and protein 4.1 begins at the proerythroblast stage and increases throughout terminal erythroid maturation up to the late erythroblast stage. During this time, the mRNA levels and the synthesis of spectrin and ankyrin decline. Even so, the proportion (and actual amounts) of newly assembled spectrin and ankyrin on the membrane progressively increase, and these proteins become more stable, as indicated by their slower turnover. This increased recruitment and stabilization of spectrin and ankyrin, despite declining synthesis, is thought to be related to the progressive increase in the synthesis of band 3 and protein 4.1 because these proteins are the principal sites for the attachment of the skeleton to the membrane (737).

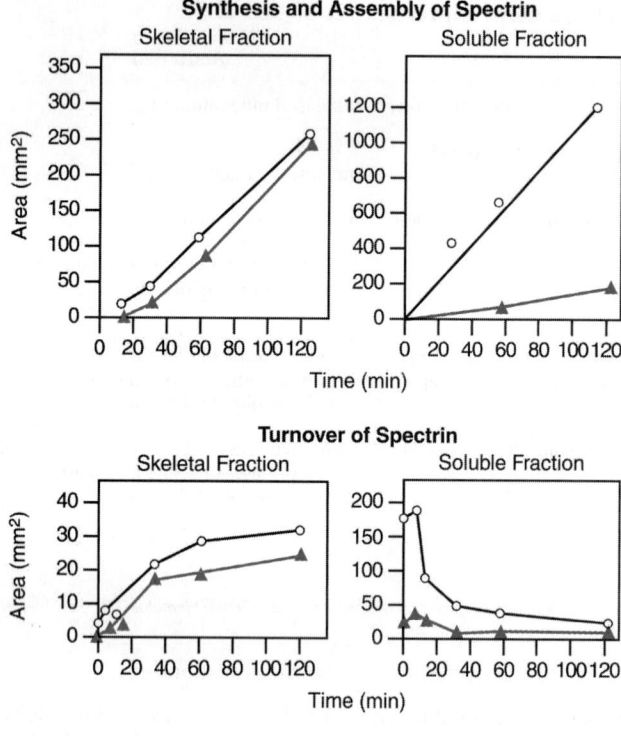

Figure 51-20. Synthesis, assembly, and turnover of spectrin in erythroblasts. **Top:** Synthesis and assembly of α- and β-spectrin. Membrane skeletons and soluble (cytoplasmic) proteins from red cell precursors labeled with a radioactive amino acid were immunoprecipitated with an antispectrin antibody, and the proteins were separated on a sodium dodecyl sulfate gel and autoradiographed. The areas of the scanned autoradiogram peaks are plotted with time. Note that α-spectrin is synthesized in excess of β-spectrin **(top right)**, but both subunits assemble in equivalent amounts on the membrane **(top left)**. **Bottom:** Turnover of spectrin. After a brief period of labeling ("pulse"), erythroblasts were incubated with nonradioactive amino acids ("chase"), and the amounts of α- and β-spectrin were followed with time. Note that the newly synthesized spectrins are stable if they are incorporated into the membrane skeleton **(bottom left)** but are rapidly degraded if they remain in the cytoplasm **(bottom right)**. (Adapted from Palek J, Lambert S. Genetics of the red cell membrane skeleton. *Semin Hematol* 1990;27:290.)

SKELETAL PROTEINS ARE SYNTHESIZED IN EXCESS

The synthesis of membrane skeletal proteins is wasteful. Only a fraction of newly synthesized spectrin, ankyrin, and protein 4.1 is assembled into the permanent skeletal network (Fig. 51-20). The excess proteins are rapidly catabolized (738,740,741). Furthermore, skeletal protein synthesis is highly asymmetric. This is most striking in the case of spectrin, in which three- to four-fold more α-spectrin is produced than β-spectrin (Fig. 51-20). Even so, the two chains are assembled into the membrane skeleton in equimolar amounts as mixed heterodimers. Because of this high α-spectrin to β-spectrin synthetic ratio, heterozygotes for a deleted or synthetically inactive α-spectrin allele are asymptomatic, because sufficient α-spectrin is still made to pair with all of the β-spectrin.

RATE-LIMITING STEPS OF MEMBRANE SKELETAL ASSEMBLY

As discussed above, the principal rate-limiting step in membrane skeletal assembly *in vitro* is the synthesis of band 3, which contains a high-affinity ankyrin-binding site that recruits and stabilizes spectrin and ankyrin on the membrane (742,743). This

view, however, has to be reconciled with the observation that some patients with dominantly inherited HS and partial band 3 deficiency do not have a proportional decrease in the amounts of spectrin and ankyrin in their membranes (744,745). The explanation that has been offered is that band 3 is synthesized in excess. Approximately fivefold more band 3 is made than spectrin or ankyrin, but only the tetrameric fraction of band 3 binds ankyrin with high affinity (201,709,744). Excess dimeric band 3 is selectively lost in band 3–deficient spherocytes (744). However, mouse red cells with *complete* deficiency of band 3 also assemble a functional spectrin-based membrane skeleton (255). This means that *in vivo* there must be other means of attaching spectrin or spectrin-ankyrin complexes to the membrane of developing erythroblasts, allowing the skeleton to assemble. How this is done remains a mystery.

The second rate-limiting step is the availability of ankyrin, which provides the high-affinity binding sites for β-spectrin. This is best illustrated by studies of membrane skeletal synthesis in nb/nb spherocytic mice (491) and in a severe form of human HS associated with a combined deficiency of spectrin and ankyrin (490). In both disorders, ankyrin synthesis is markedly reduced, which leads to the decreased assembly of spectrin and ankyrin on the membrane, despite normal spectrin synthesis.

The third rate-limiting step involves the synthesis of β-spectrin. Because α- and β-spectrin polypeptides are assembled on the membrane in equimolar amounts, and because β-spectrin binds to ankyrin with high affinity, the availability of β-spectrin seems to regulate the amounts of membrane-assembled α/β-spectrin heterodimers. This regulatory role of β-spectrin is illustrated by the effects of erythropoietin on membrane protein assembly. Erythropoietin stimulates the synthesis of β-spectrin and increases assembly of α/β-spectrin heterodimers on the membrane (746). In contrast, α-spectrin, which is made in excess, does not seem to have a limiting role in the skeletal assembly. α-Spectrin becomes rate limiting only when its synthesis is markedly reduced, as it is in some patients with recessive HS or HPP.

MEMBRANE REMODELING DURING ENUCLEATION AND RETICULOCYTE MATURATION

At the orthochromatic erythroblast stage when membrane biogenesis is nearly complete, the cell membrane undergoes a series of critical remodeling steps. The cell nucleus is surrounded by an actin ring, which likely participates in the expulsion of the nucleus from the erythroblast. At the same time, the spectrin skeleton segregates into the incipient reticulocyte, while some surface receptors cluster in the membrane surrounding the soon-to-be-extruded nucleus (487,747). Further membrane remodeling takes place as the young multilobular reticulocyte attains the biconcave shape (748–751). This involves a loss of lipids and certain surface proteins, including receptors for transferrin and fibronectin. Autophagocytosis plays an important role in removing cytoplasmic organelles and some membrane receptors (745,747) and in initiating the changes in shape and volume that characterize the transition from reticulocyte to mature erythrocyte. Cholesterol-loaded reticulocytes from mice that lack the high-density lipoprotein (HDL) receptor and are cholesterol fed or from hypercholesterolemic mice that lack the receptors for both HDL and apolipoprotein E, are anemic and contain targeted, macrocytic red cells with large abnormal autophagolysosomes (751). The cholesterol-loaded reticulocytes also retain ribosomes and transferrin receptor. Removal of cholesterol, incubation in normolipemic serum, or transfusion into normal recipients leads to the expulsion of autophagolysosomes and the reinitiation of reticulocyte maturation (751). How cholesterol accumulation inhibits reticulocyte maturation remains to be determined.

RED CELL MEMBRANE DEFORMABILITY AND STABILITY

Material Properties

The material properties of the membrane reflect the properties of both the lipid bilayer and the skeleton. During deformation of the red cell membrane, bending is restricted by the incompressibility of the lipid bilayer and is facilitated by rapid translocation of cholesterol from the inner to the outer half of the bilayer (121). The lipid bilayer cannot expand its surface area more than 3% to 4%. Consequently, when red cells are suspended in hypotonic solutions (such as during OF testing), they swell to a spherical shape and then rupture, discharging their Hb into the supernatant (752).

The membrane skeleton determines the solid and semisolid properties of the membrane (753). The solid properties are exemplified by an elastic extension of cells, which completely restore their normal shape after the applied force has been removed. An example is a cell that has been deformed when passing through fenestrations of the splenic sinus wall. This elastic recovery of the biconcave shape is facilitated by the unique molecular anatomy of the skeletal lattice. In normal red cells, individual spectrin molecules are arranged in a hexagonal array and are folded in a compact configuration. The junctional complexes are close to each other and are linked by shortened spectrin tetramers, thus allowing large unidirectional extensions without disruption of the lattice (Fig. 51-21). The skeletal connections are generally assumed to be unperturbed during such deformations. However, recent evidence shows that the spectrin dimer-tetramer link is continuously breaking and reforming ("breathing") *in vivo* (753a). This process is greatly accentuated by shear stresses well below those in the circulation. Whether the rate is rapid enough to allow membrane reorganization during normal blood flow requires further investigation. It almost certainly plays a role in the reorganization

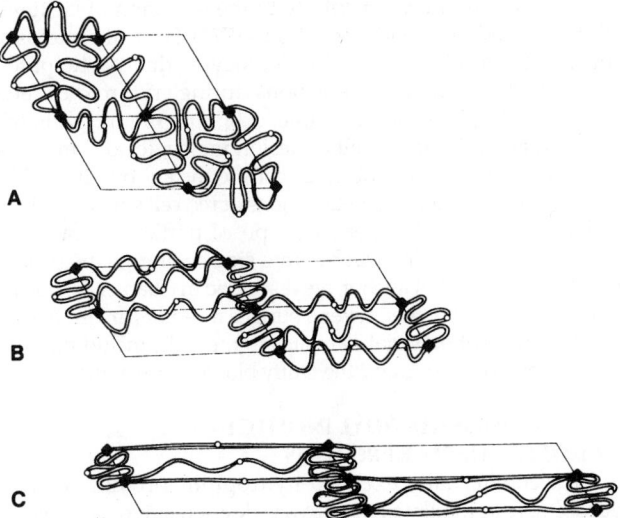

Figure 51-21. Model of the effects of deformation on the membrane skeleton. The red cell membrane cannot expand its area. When a force is applied to a section of nondeformed membrane **(A)** extending the lipid bilayer and its attached spectrin molecules **(B)**, the bilayer and spectrin molecules in the nonstressed dimension must shrink to maintain a constant area. Eventually, spectrins reach the limit of their length **(C)**. Further extension disrupts membrane skeleton interconnections and leads to membrane fragmentation. Spectrin-actin-4.1 junctions (*solid diamonds*) and sites of spectrin-spectrin association (*open circles*) are shown. (Reprinted from Mohandas N, Chasis JA. Red cell deformability, membrane material properties, and shape: regulation by transmembrane, skeletal, and cytosolic proteins and lipids. *Semin Hematol* 1993;30:171, with permission.)

of the skeleton that occurs when large or prolonged forces are applied to the membrane. This produces a permanent "plastic" deformation (see below). When the force is excessive, membrane fragmentation ensues. An example is the poikilocytosis produced in microangiopathic blood vessels in which red cells may adhere to damaged endothelium and be stretched by the vascular torrent or may be clotheslined by fibrin strands (754). After release, many of the cells are either permanently deformed or fragmented.

Cellular and Molecular Determinants of Red Cell Deformability

The need to undergo large deformations is best exemplified in the wall of the splenic sinus where red cells have to "squeeze" through narrow slits between the endothelial cells that line the splenic sinus wall (see Chapter 21 and the later section Spherocytes Are Detained at the Cordal-Sinus Junction in this chapter). This whole cell deformability is determined by three factors: (a) cell geometry (i.e., a large cell surface to volume ratio, which allows cells to undergo large deformations at a constant volume); (b) viscosity of the cell contents, which is principally determined by the properties and the concentration of Hb in the cells; and (c) intrinsic viscoelastic properties of the red cell membrane (753). Among these factors, the contribution of the surface to volume ratio is the most important, as exemplified by the cellular lesion of hereditary spherocytes, discussed later in this chapter. On the other hand, the intrinsic deformability of the red cell membrane has a relatively small effect on red cell survival. This is best illustrated by the red cell membrane properties of Southeast Asian ovalocytes, which carry a mutant band 3 protein. As will be discussed, both the intact SAO red cells and their membranes are extremely rigid, yet the SAO red cells have normal survival *in vivo*.

Several molecular alterations increase membrane rigidity. One is the accretion of denatured Hb, which may contribute to the membrane rigidity of Heinz body–containing red cells (755). Others are transamidative or oxidative cross-linking, which rigidify the membrane *in vitro* (733–735). Oxidative cross-linking may also be important *in vivo*, as evidenced by aggregates of oxidant cross-linked proteins in red cells containing unstable Hbs (756). On the other hand, transamidative cross-linking is probably not physiologically significant because the high Ca^{2+} concentrations needed for the reaction are unlikely to be attained *in vivo* (734).

Recent studies emphasize the role of integral proteins in regulating membrane deformability. For example, the treatment of red cells by antibodies against GPA, including their Fab fragments, leads to reduced deformability via transmembrane signaling. This is exemplified by red cells that lack the cytoplasmic domain of GPA (e.g., Miltenberger V red cells), which are not influenced by such treatment (238,757). Another important factor is the aggregation state of band 3. Membrane rigidity is increased when band 3 molecules are cross-linked with antibodies (758) or, as in SAO (see the section Southeast Asian Ovalocytosis), when mutant band 3s spontaneously stack into linear aggregates (759,760). This finding presumably also explains the marked restriction of band 3 mobility in SAO red cells. Because aggregates of SAO band 3 contain ankyrin, which attaches the skeleton to the membrane, the decreased mobility of SAO band 3 may impede skeletal deformation when red cells deform, resulting in a rigid erythrocyte.

MEMBRANE STRUCTURAL INTEGRITY AND FRAGMENTATION

The skeleton is also the principal determinant of membrane stability. As noted earlier, it is possible to manipulate the proportion of spectrin dimers and tetramers *in situ* by exposing ghosts to temperatures and salt concentrations that favor or discourage self-association. Ghosts enriched in spectrin dimers are strikingly

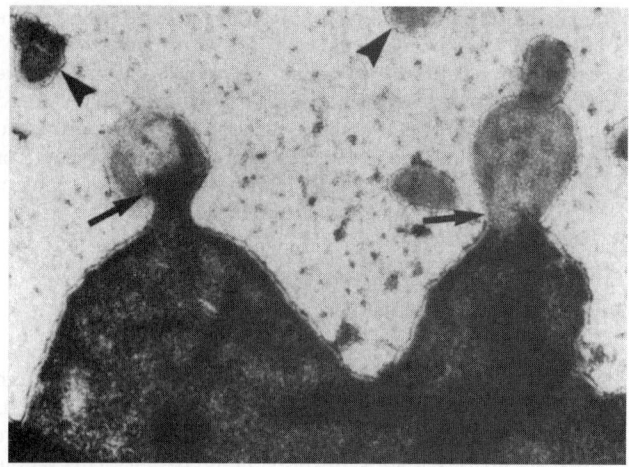

Figure 51-22. Microvesiculation. Red cell ghosts treated with hypertonic saline develop spicules. At the end of the spicules, the lipid bilayer often separates from the underlying membrane skeleton. The arrows point to the boundary between the skeleton (dark material, *below*) and the unsupported lipids (light material, *above*), which are unstable and tend to be released as vesicles (*arrowheads*). A similar process is thought to occur in a variety of disorders associated with spiculation, such as spur cell anemia and hereditary spherocytosis. (Adapted from Liu S-C, Derick LH. Molecular anatomy of the red blood cell membrane skeleton: structure-function relationships. *Semin Hematol* 1992;29:231–243.)

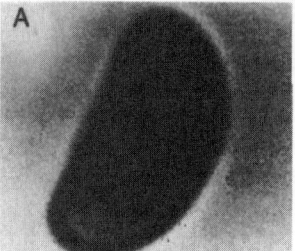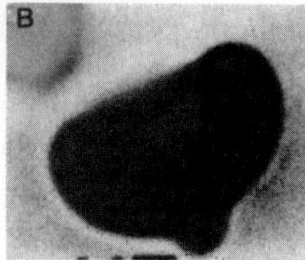

Figure 51-23. Plastic deformation. **A:** Discocytic shape of a red cell at rest in solution. If a nipple of membrane from such a cell is aspirated into a micropipette and immediately released, it snaps back to its original position. However, if the aspirated membrane is deformed for some time, a permanent nipple forms **(B)** due to reorganization of the membrane skeleton in the stressed portion of the membrane. This semisolid behavior is called *plastic deformation* and is believed to be responsible for the irregular shape of poikilocytes, especially in diseases such as hereditary pyropoikilocytosis, in which skeletal reorganization is fostered by genetically weakened skeletal interconnections. (Reprinted from Mohandas N, Chasis JA. Red cell deformability, membrane material properties, and shape: regulation by transmembrane, skeletal, and cytosolic proteins and lipids. *Semin Hematol* 1993;30:171, with permission.)

fragile (761). Similarly, HE and pyropoikilocytosis are often due to α- or β-spectrin mutations that weaken spectrin self-association. In such cells, the hexagonal skeletal lattice is disrupted (762), usually in association with red cell fragmentation and poikilocytosis.

LIPID BILAYER LOSS AND MICROVESICULATION

The fluid lipid bilayer is stabilized by the underlying membrane skeleton and the transmembrane proteins. *In vitro*, the bilayer can be uncoupled from the skeleton at the tips of spiculated red cells by force or by various treatments (763,764) (Fig. 51-22). The lipids are released in the form of microvesicles, which contain integral proteins but lack skeletal components (764). Such loss of membrane material may underlie the surface area deficiency of red cells subjected to prolonged storage (765,766) or of ATP-depleted red cells (767). Aggregation of the band 3–containing intramembrane particles (IMPs) in the membrane also destabilizes the lipid bilayer (768). In ghosts, such aggregation can be induced by treatment with Ca^{2+}, Mg^{2+}, polylysine, or basic proteins (768). The particle-free regions bleb and release lipid microvesicles. As discussed later, all these pathways may contribute to the surface deficiency of hereditary spherocytes.

PLASTIC DEFORMATION OF RED CELLS

The role of the membrane skeleton in red cell shape is best illustrated by irreversibly sickled cells (ISCs) or hereditary elliptocytes, in which the abnormal shape is retained in the ghosts and membrane skeletons (769,770). This process is probably an example of "plastic deformation"—the result of the prolonged exposure of red cells to deforming forces, when the proteins of the deformed skeleton undergo active rearrangement that permanently stabilizes the cells in the deformed shape (Fig. 51-23) (753). Existing protein–protein contacts disconnect and new associations form. In HE, shape transformations may be facilitated by the weakened skeletal protein interactions. *In vitro*, plastic deformation occurs more rapidly in normal red cells with skeletons weakened by exposure to urea (771).

In addition, both normal and abnormal red cell shapes can be stabilized by intermolecular cross-linking of membrane proteins, either by the formation of intermolecular disulfide bridges induced by oxidants (734) or by transamidative protein cross-linking catalyzed by a Ca^{2+}-activated cytosolic transglutaminase (734). These protein modifications are like endogenous fixatives and permanently stabilize cell shape *in vitro*.

Red Cell Surface

The red cell surface is rich in sialic acid residues accounting for the negative surface charge. Ninety percent of these residues reside on GPA; the remainder are shared by other glycophorins, the anion exchange protein, and glycolipids. Alterations in surface charge distribution are deleterious. For example, surface charge clustering may contribute to the adhesion of sickle red cells to the surface of endothelial cells (772). Several proteins are removed from the surface of reticulocytes that participate in cell–cell and cell–matrix interactions during erythroid differentiation (747,750,773). One example, $\alpha_4\beta_1$ integrin, interacts with VCAM-1, an endothelial cell adhesion molecule, and may contribute to the attachment of sickle cells to the endothelium (773).

The structure and the genetic origins of red cell surface antigens, residing on glycolipids, externally exposed portions of transmembrane proteins or their carbohydrate side chains, or the proteins linked via a glycosyl PI anchor, are discussed in Chapter 57. Furthermore, as discussed earlier, several surface receptors are involved in the attachment of malarial parasites to the cells, including glycophorins, band 3 protein, and the Duffy blood group antigen.

GLYCOSYL PHOSPHATIDYL INOSITOL–ANCHORED SURFACE PROTEINS

To connect externally exposed hydrophilic proteins with the hydrophobic lipid bilayer, nature has devised a hydrophobic glycosyl phosphatidyl inositol (GPI) anchor, which is embedded in the outer leaflet of the bilayer. Among the large number of GPI-linked surface proteins, a group of complement-regulatory proteins are clinically the most important (774). Defective biosynthesis of the GPI anchor precludes the attachment of these proteins to the membrane, causing increased susceptibility to hemolysis by complement, as clinically manifest by paroxysmal nocturnal hemoglobinuria (Chapter 10). Because this glycolipid anchor is embedded only in the outer leaflet of the bilayer, GPI-anchored surface proteins, such as CD59, are not restricted by the membrane skeleton, in contrast to most transmembrane proteins, and are much more laterally mobile (774,775). This high mobility may be important in recruiting complement regulatory proteins to sites of complement activation. These regulatory proteins are preferentially enriched in the lipid vesicles that are released from abnormal red cells (776), such as vesicles derived from spicules of deoxygenated sickle cells. Consequently, GPI-linked proteins are diminished in the densest fraction of sickle cells, rendering them more susceptible to complement-mediated injury (776).

LATERAL MOBILITY OF TRANSMEMBRANE AND SURFACE PROTEINS

The mobilities of membrane surface molecules influence the interaction of red cells with the outside environment. For example, cell agglutination requires rapid lateral movements of surface antigens. Their immobilization (e.g., by glutaraldehyde) inhibits agglutination (777).

The lateral mobility of proteins that are anchored exclusively in the outer leaflet of the bilayer (e.g., GPI-linked proteins) is very fast (see above). Conversely, transmembrane proteins, such as band 3, are much less mobile. In the case of band 3, this occurs because of (a) specific binding to ankyrin and the skeleton; (b) steric hindrance by spectrin strands, which entangle the internal portions of band 3; (c) self-association of band 3 into tetramers and higher oligomers; and (d) interaction of band 3 with other transmembrane proteins, such as the glycophorins (778).

MEMBRANE PERMEABILITY

Normally, the red cell membrane is nearly impermeable to monovalent and divalent cations, thereby maintaining a high potassium, low sodium, and very low calcium content. In contrast, the red cell is highly permeable to water and anions, which are readily exchanged by the water channel and the anion transport protein, respectively. Glucose is taken up by the glucose transporter (779), whereas larger charged molecules, such as ATP and related compounds, do not cross the normal red cell membrane.

The transport pathways for cations and anions in the human red cell membrane can be divided into five categories (Fig. 51-24).

- Exchangers, such as the Na^+,H^+ exchanger and anion exchanger discussed earlier.
- Cotransporters, in which the transmembrane movements of more than one solute are coupled in the same direction (e.g., the K^+,Cl^- cotransporter and the $Na^+,K^+,2Cl^-$ cotransporter).
- The Ca^{2+}-activated K^+ channel (Gárdos channel), discussed below.
- The cation "leak" pathways, which allow Na^+ and K^+ to move in the direction of their concentration gradients.
- Membrane pumps, such as the ouabain-inhibitable Na^+,K^+ pump and the Ca^{2+} pump, respectively.

A detailed review of these pathways is beyond the scope of this chapter. The interested reader is referred to several excellent reviews that discuss them in the pathophysiology of sickle cell disease (780,781).

An important feature of the normal red cell is its ability to maintain a constant volume. One of the very intriguing yet unanswered questions is how cells "sense" changes in cell volume and activate appropriate volume regulatory pathways. One possibility is that they sense mechanical events, such as membrane stretching (782). Such a mechanism is unlikely to operate in red cells, which, by virtue of their large surface area, can undergo a substantial volume increase without stretching. Another possibility is that cell volume is controlled by the crowding of cytoplasmic macromolecules (782). According to this theory, cell shrinkage stimulates and swelling inhibits a putative protein kinase, which, in turn, changes the activity of a volume regulatory cation transporter, such as the K^+,Cl^- cotransporter (782).

Water Permeability

Water permeability of many cell types is similar to the permeability of pure lipid bilayer membranes, in which water is postulated to enter through small "cavities" in the bilayer (783). When phospholipids are in the liquid crystalline state, these cavities are thought to be caused by a noncooperative rotation and kinking around the C-C bonds (783). In addition, water permeability may be facilitated by lipids with large polar head

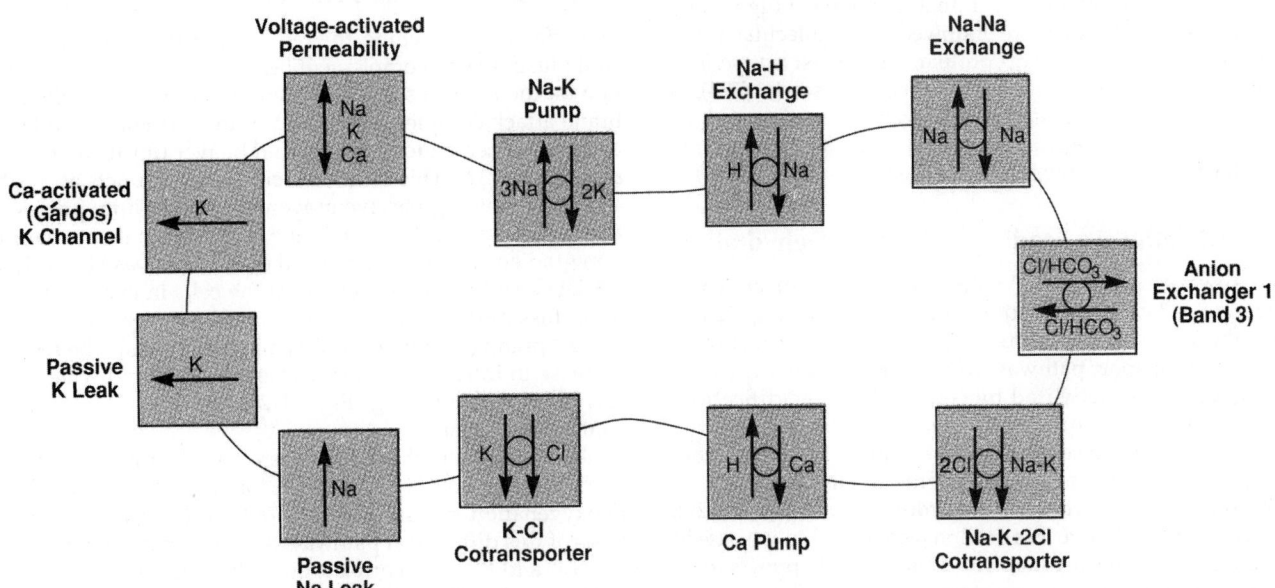

Figure 51-24. Red cell membrane ion transport channels, ion exchange channels, and passive permeability pathways.

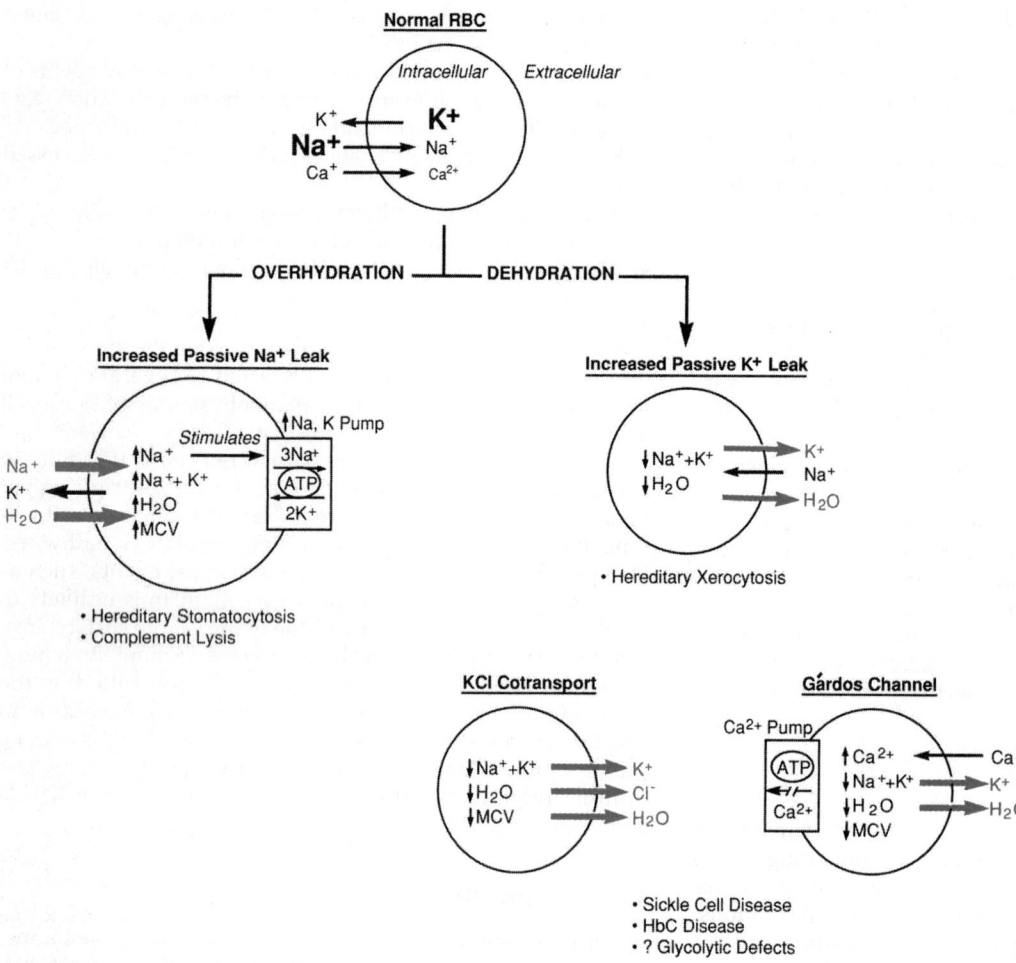

Figure 51-25. Cation changes leading to dehydration or overhydration of red cells. **Left:** Overhydration is caused by a massive, unbalanced influx of Na^+ that overwhelms the Na^+,K^+-pump and leads to an increase in total monovalent cations ($Na^+ + K^+$) and cell water. **Right:** Dehydration is caused by excess, unbalanced K^+ leakage or by activation of K^+-losing channels such as the K^+Cl^- cotransport channel or the Ca^{2+}-activated Gárdos pathway. Dehydration is associated with a decline in total monovalent cations ($Na^+ + K^+$) and cell water. ATP, adenosine triphosphate; HbC, hemoglobin C; MCV, mean cell volume; RBC, red blood cell.

groups, such as gangliosides and lysophospholipids, which, when dispersed in water, prefer a micellar rather than bilayer configuration. Additionally, integral proteins are likely to enhance water diffusion by producing localized discontinuities in the lipid bilayer (783).

Membranes of red cells and some kidney tubules differ from membranes of most other cells in that they have a high water permeability because they are endowed by a molecular water channel protein (784,785). This protein, designated *aquaporin-1*, has been cloned (373), and its structure has been solved (374), as has previously been discussed. The suggested function of aquaporin-1 is to facilitate rehydration of red cells after their shrinkage in the hypertonic environment of the renal medulla (786).

Transport Pathways Leading to Cellular Dehydration

Two pathways exert a critical volume regulatory effect, which can lead to red cell dehydration and destruction (Fig. 51-25). One is the K^+,Cl^- cotransporter (Fig. 51-24), a typical carrier-mediated cotransport pathway, which is particularly active in reticulocytes. It is activated by cell swelling, acidification, depletion of intracellular Mg^{2+}, and thiol oxidation. It is increased in sickle red cells and HbC erythrocytes, accounting, in part, for the cellular dehydration of these cells (787–789).

The second transporter is the Gárdos channel (Fig. 51-24), which causes the selective loss of K^+ in response to an increase in intracellular ionized calcium (736). This channel appears to be regulated by a cytoplasmic protein called *peroxiredoxin-2* or *calpromotin* and by cAMP. The channel is inhibited by insect toxins, such as charybdotoxin, and by the Ca^{2+}-channel blockers

nitrendipine and nifedipine. In sickle cells, the combination of the Gárdos pathway and the K^+,Cl^- cotransporter accounts for the net loss of K^+ and water, leading to cellular dehydration (788).

Disruption of the Permeability Barrier in Abnormal Red Cells

The effects of breaching the red cell permeability barrier are well illustrated by complement hemolysis. Complement activation on the red cell surface leads to the formation of the membrane attack complex, composed of the terminal complement components embedded in the lipid bilayer (for further details, see Chapter 22). This multimolecular complex acts as a cation channel, allowing passive movements of sodium, potassium, and calcium across the membrane according to their concentration gradients. Attracted by fixed anions, such as Hb, ATP, and 2,3-DPG, sodium accumulates in the cells in excess of potassium loss and in excess of the compensatory efforts of the Na^+,K^+ pump (see the section Membrane Pumps). The resulting increase in intracellular monovalent cations and water is followed by cell swelling (Fig. 51-25) and, ultimately, colloid osmotic hemolysis.

Another leak pathway has been described in sickle cells. It involves an influx of Na^+ and Ca^{2+} and an efflux of K^+ during deoxygenation and sickling (787,788). Although the molecular basis of this diffusional pathway is unknown, the magnitude of the Na^+ and K^+ leaks correlates with the degree of morphologic sickling and with lipid bilayer–skeleton uncoupling, suggesting that it is caused by mechanical events (788). This conclusion is further supported by the observation that Ca^{2+} permeability is increased by mechanical stress (790). Such permeability pathways may be related to stretch-activated channels, described in various tissues, including endothelial, epithelial, and muscle cells (for references see 791). The mechanism of activation of these channels is unknown, but one of the possibilities involves the deformation of the submembrane skeleton.

Membrane Pumps

To maintain low intracellular concentrations of sodium and calcium and a high potassium concentration, the membrane is endowed with two cation pumps, both using intracellular ATP as an energy source. The ouabain-inhibitable Na^+,K^+ pump extrudes sodium and takes up potassium, with a stoichiometry of three Na^+ pumped outward for two K^+ pumped inward. This exactly balances the normal passive leaks (Na^+ influx = 1.0 to 2.0 mEq/liter RBCs (LRBC)/hour; K^+ efflux = 0.8 to 1.5 mEq/LRBC/hour). The enzyme is activated by intracellular Na^+ (Km = 25 mM) and extracellular K^+ (Km = 2.5 mM) (792). Because plasma K^+ is high enough to saturate the extracellular K^+ site, Na^+ and K^+ transport is primarily regulated by increases in red cell Na^+ concentration, and cell K^+ losses are rectified only if there is a concomitant Na^+ gain to stimulate active transport. Even then, the ratio between the inward Na^+ leak and outward K^+ leak must not be less than the physiologic ratio of 3:2. At lower ratios, the Na^+,K^+ pump, driven by the Na^+ leak and internal Na^+ concentration, does not balance the leaks and actually exacerbates K^+ loss (793,794). Consequently, conditions in which K^+ loss approaches or exceeds Na^+ gain, as in the disease hereditary xerocytosis, lead to irreversible K^+ depletion and cell dehydration.

The calmodulin-activated, Mg^{2+}-dependent Ca^{2+} pump extrudes Ca^{2+} and maintains a very low intracellular free Ca^{2+} concentration (~20 to 40 nM). It protects red cells from the multiple deleterious effects of Ca^{2+} (echinocytosis, membrane vesiculation, calpain activation, membrane proteolysis, and cell dehydration) described earlier in the chapter.

RED CELL MEMBRANE ALTERATIONS OF SENESCENT RED CELLS

Pleiotropic Effects of Red Cell Aging

The removal of senescent red cells from the circulation is a subject of a long-standing interest. As discussed in a comprehensive review of the literature published before 1988 (795), the concept of red cell senescence is based on results of radioactive labeling of a cohort of reticulocytes and bone marrow erythroblasts. In many species, including humans, the fraction of labeled cells remains constant for a defined time period, followed by a rapid decline of radioactivity, suggesting that the red cells are removed from the circulation in an age-dependent manner. Many techniques have been used to isolate senescent red cells, including methods based on differences in cell density, OF, and cell size (reviewed in 795). Density separation is most widely used, but the results obtained by this technique must be interpreted with caution. Although red cells exhibit a progressive increase in density as they age *in vivo*, not all dense red cells are senescent (795–797).

In addition to *in vitro* separation techniques, various *in vivo* animal models have been used to study red cell aging (795). For example, red cells can be labeled with biotin and then removed at defined times with avidin, which complexes tightly to biotin (798,799). The senescent cells defined by these techniques exhibit numerous membrane abnormalities (795,796,799). Of particular note is the loss of potassium and water, leading to cell

dehydration and increased cell density, and the loss of surface area, presumably due to the gradual release of membrane microvesicles (795,800). The latter phenomenon is probably caused by constant exposure of red cells to the shearing forces of the microcirculation. In addition, red cell membrane proteins and lipids experience oxidative damage, as evidenced by high-molecular-weight aggregates containing Hb, spectrin, and band 3 (801,802) and by adducts of proteins and malonyldialdehyde, a product of lipid peroxidation (802).

Early results suggested that the loss of red cell surface charge (803), due to the *in vivo* loss of sialic acid residues, and the exposure of the penultimate β-galactose residues (804) of the carbohydrate side chains were important factors in the recognition and removal of aged erythrocytes. However, other studies reveal that the mild surface charge loss can be entirely explained by the loss of cell-surface area (805) and that the surface charge density and the number of sialic acid residues/sialoglycoprotein in senescent red cells is normal (806,807).

In addition to red cell membrane abnormalities, red cell aging is associated with the decline of many red cell enzyme activities (808). However, red cell ATP concentration is normal (795). Likewise, no major abnormalities have been detected in Ca^{2+} transport, and there is no compelling evidence that Ca^{2+} accumulates in senescent cells (reviewed in 795).

Autologous Immunoglobulin G Targets Senescent Red Cells for Destruction by Macrophages

Although some of the above alterations may compromise red cell microcirculatory flow, none is likely to destroy old cells. In a creative series of studies begun almost three decades ago, Kay and colleagues have shown that senescent red cells have small amounts (a few hundred molecules/cell) of autologous IgG on their surface that target the cells for destruction by macrophages (809). The nature of the "senescent antigen" has been a source of some dispute. Possibilities include band 3 molecules (810–812) and exposed α-galactosyl residues on membrane glycoproteins (813,814). The contribution of the latter modification is probably minimal because the removal of antibodies to α-galactosyl residues by extensive washing does not affect phagocytosis of senescent erythrocytes (815). On the other hand, there is considerable evidence that antibodies are bound to band 3 in aged and pathologic red cells (799,810–812,816–820).

It is not clear why. The most popular view is that antibodies to senescent antigen bind to aggregated or oligomerized band 3 (799,811,817,819,820). There is evidence that the epitope resides on the band 3 carbohydrate (821,822). Band 3 clusters have been visualized by immunofluorescence microscopy and detected by biochemical methods in aged red cells (811,817). Aggregation probably results from cumulative oxidative damage because similar damage, including the binding of autologous IgG, takes place on oxidized red cells or red cells containing Heinz bodies, a product of oxidative denaturation of Hb (76,811,817,823,824). The senescent antigen is also exposed on red cells infected with *P. falciparum* (825,826).

It should be noted, however, that IMPs, which are half band 3, are not reproducibly clustered in cells that bear senescent IgG (827). This suggests that other band 3 modifications account for increased binding of autologous IgG. For example, band 3 could be structurally modified by proteolysis, oxidation, or other posttranslational modification, or band 3 molecules could be vertically displaced, exposing new antigenic sites or rendering existing sites more accessible to antibodies.

In addition to targeting senescent red cells for macrophage destruction, band 3 antibodies also trigger complement deposition on senescent cells (828). As noted earlier, this process may be facilitated by loss of GPI-linked complement regulatory proteins from old cells through microvesiculation.

Although the role of autologous IgG in the destruction of senescent erythrocytes is widely accepted, two observations suggest that other mechanisms must be considered. First, the blockade of the Fc portion of autologous "senescent" IgG with protein G fails to inhibit red cell phagocytosis (829). Second, red cell survival is the same in agammaglobulinemic mice as in controls (829). However, the latter data may not be applicable to humans, because the removal of mouse red cells from the circulation is random (795).

Altered phospholipid asymmetry might also contribute to the removal of senescent erythrocytes. This could occur from damage to the aminophospholipid translocase by products of lipid peroxidation (830). Disordered phospholipid asymmetry reportedly activates the alternate complement pathway (831) and targets apoptotic red cells for destruction by the CD36 receptor on macrophages (86–91,832,833). Although there is no convincing evidence that senescent red cells expose phosphatidyl serine on their surface, this hypothesis is favored by some (834), presumably because it is a proven mechanism for removing other types of damaged cells (89–91).

Other alterations of possible pathologic significance include postsynthetic modification of red cell proteins by nonenzymatic glycosylation (835) or carboxymethylation (836,837). Glycosylation of membrane proteins, like Hb (to form HbA_{1c}), occurs gradually over the life of the cell and is proportional to the glucose concentration. Methylation of membrane proteins occurs primarily in older red cells. Ankyrin and protein 4.1 are the principal substrates.

Transamidation of membrane proteins may also play a role in aging. Aged red cells from mice lacking transglutaminase-2 are more osmotically resistant than aged normal red cells (838), suggesting that the knock-out red cells lose less membrane surface as they age. Transglutaminase-2 catalyzes the formation of peptide bonds between ε-amino groups on lysine side chains and side chain carboxyls on aspartic and glutamic acids in the presence of Ca^{2+}.

HEREDITARY SPHEROCYTOSIS

HS is a common, inherited hemolytic anemia in which defects of spectrin or the proteins that attach spectrin to the membrane (ankyrin, protein 4.2, band 3) lead to spheroidal, osmotically fragile cells that are selectively trapped in the spleen and that survive almost normally after splenectomy.

History

In 1871, two Belgian physicians, Vanlair and Masius, described the story of a young woman who experienced recurrent abdominal pains over her enlarged spleen, associated with prostration, vomiting, jaundice, anemia, aphonia, and marked muscular weakness, in a lengthy report in the Bulletin of the Royal Academy of Medicine of Belgium (839). The authors noted that during the attack (presumably a hemolytic crisis) most of the woman's red cells were spherical and smaller than normal, averaging only 4 μm in diameter. The authors named the disease *microcythemia* and depicted the patient's unstained cells, which they called *microcytes*, in a beautiful lithograph drawn and tinted by Vanlair (Fig. 51-26). The drawing shows numerous spherocytes and some elliptocytes (19% of the evaluable cells), which suggests that iron deficiency or thalassemia may have contributed to the anemia and cell size. The patient's red cells remained abnormal after her recovery, and her splenomegaly persisted. Vanlair and Masius thought that the microcytes were senile red cells ("*globules atrophiques*") and that the spleen assisted in their aging. They argued that when red cells are sequestered in the splenic pulp, they lose volume and become dense, spherical, and microcytic. They reasoned that an enlarged spleen might produce even more of such cells than a normal spleen, and that the liver might complete the work of the spleen by destroying microcytes it received via the splenic vein. They suggested that the large number of microcytes in their patient was due to a combination of splenic enlargement and liver atrophy. Finally, they noted that the patient's sister had experienced an identical illness and died during a crisis, and that her mother was also subject to jaundice.

In retrospect, the paper is remarkably prescient. The authors not only described the first example of a hereditary hemolytic anemia well before the microscope was in general use in the analysis of blood diseases, but their deductions concerning the pathophysiology of HS, particularly the role of the spleen, predated Ham and Castle's concept of erythrostasis (840) by more than two-thirds of a century. Their paper is placed in perspective by the fact that five to seven decades later respected hematologists were still ascribing HS to causes such as hereditary syphilis (841) and splenic hemolysins (842).

However, Vanlair and Masius's report went unnoticed, as did subsequent descriptions of HS in the 1890s by the British physicians Wilson and Stanley (843,844), who clearly recognized the hereditary nature of the disease and were the first to describe the characteristic pathology of the spleen engorged with red cells. However, a report by Minkowski in 1900 in the German literature (845) received wide attention, and many

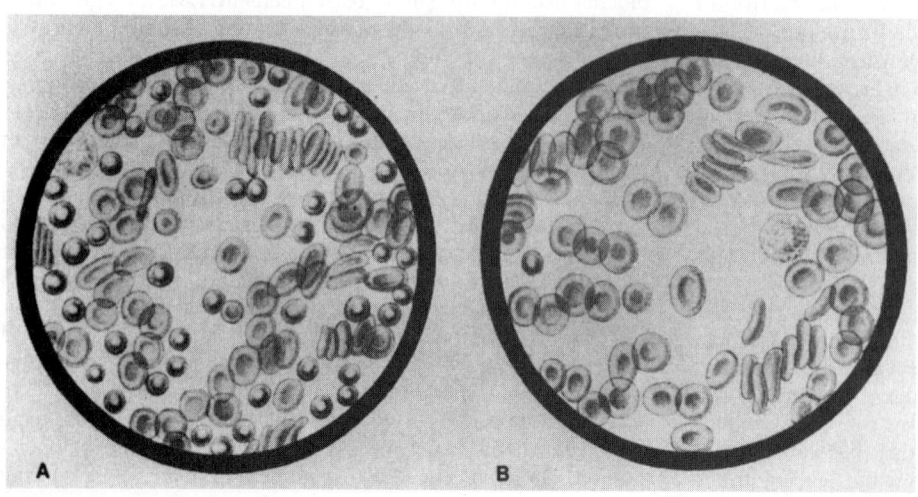

Figure 51-26. Lithograph of normal blood cells **(B)** and cells from a patient **(A)** with "microcythemia" (now *hereditary spherocytosis*) described by Vanlair and Masius in 1871. (Reprinted from De la microcythémie. *Bull R Acad Med Belg* 1871;5:515, with permission.)

additional papers soon appeared (846,847), including Chauf-fard's classic description of OF (848) and reticulocytosis (849) as hallmarks of the disease. During this time, Widal (850) defined an acquired form of the disease, which we now recognize as warm-antibody immunohemolytic anemia. Because Hayem had previously reported similar cases (851), the congenital and acquired diseases were soon accorded the Minkowski-Chauf-fard and Hayem-Widal eponyms.

The use of splenectomy was soon advocated, and in 1911 Micheli (852) removed the spleen from a patient with acquired hemolytic jaundice. The favorable result, combined with the subsequent success of splenectomy in congenital disease (853), led rapidly to widespread acceptance of the procedure. Actually, the first successful splenectomy for HS was unintentionally per-formed by Wells in England in 1887 (854)—3 years before Wil-son's description of HS in that country! While operating on a jaundiced woman for a supposed uterine fibroid, he instead encountered and removed an enormous spleen. The patient recovered and her jaundice disappeared. The events were recon-structed 40 years later by Dawson (854), who found the charac-teristic OF during an examination of the woman and her son.

Thus, almost all the major clinical features of HS were defined by the time of Tileston's (855) and Gänsslen's (856) reviews in 1922. The spleen was thought to be involved in red cell destruction, and splenectomy was known to be curative. Nevertheless, except for Vanlair and Masius's farsighted (and still unrecognized) deductions, nothing significant was known about the pathogenesis of the disease.

Readers interested in more details about these and other aspects of the history of HS should consult the delightful chap-ters by Dacie, Crosby, and Wintrobe in *Blood, Pure and Eloquent*, a captivating account of the history of hematology (857).

Prevalence and Genetics

HS occurs in all racial and ethnic groups. It is particularly com-mon in Northern European peoples, where it affects approxi-mately one person in 5000 (858). In fact, this is probably an underestimate of the prevalence. Surveys of red cell OF that use sensitive assays suggest that very mild forms of the disease may be four or five times as common (859,860). There are no good esti-mates of the prevalence in other populations, but clinical experi-ence suggests it is less common in blacks and Southeast Asians.

HS exhibits both dominant and recessive phenotypes. Approximately 75% of families have the autosomal-dominant disease (858,861,862). Homozygotes for dominant HS are very rare; from the frequency of the disease, one would estimate that they should occur approximately once in 100 million births. Only two well documented cases are reported: a baby who was homo-zygous for band 3 Coimbra (Y488M) (862) and another who was homozygous for band 3 Neapolis (16+2T>C), in which a splicing defect impedes initiation of translation (864). Band 3 Coimbra is a conservative mutation and produced only mild HS in the par-ents, but the infant was extremely anemic and hydropic at birth and has remained transfusion dependent. Homozygous band 3 Neapolis is a splicing mutation and, therefore, may not abolish all synthesis of the normal protein. It also caused a life-threaten-ing anemia. These patients suggest that homozygosity for more typical dominant HS, due to null mutations, is incompatible with life. A report of near lethal HS (severe intrauterine hydrops feta-lis, marked spherocytosis, and extreme spectrin deficiency) in a family in which one parent has moderate dominant HS and the other has clinically silent disease, with only a slightly abnormal OF test, supports this supposition (865). Three other reports of less severe "homozygous" HS have appeared (866–868), but in none of these was homozygosity proved.

In approximately 20% to 25% of HS cases, both parents are clinically normal. Some of these patients have an autosomal-recessive form of the disease (164,861,869). In these families, careful measurements may detect subtle laboratory abnormali-ties in the parents that suggest a carrier state (861,869), but clin-ically they are well and do not manifest hemolysis, anemia, or spherocytosis. However, recent evidence shows that one-half or more of the HS patients with normal parents have new muta-tions of the type seen in dominant HS (870–873). These muta-tions tend to occur at CpG dinucleotides and are associated with small insertions or deletions. Parental mosaicism also occurs and must be considered in genetic counseling (874). Patients with recessive disease are often more severely affected (164,875), but there is considerable clinical variability.

The first clue that pointed to a genetic locus for congenital spherocytosis was the identification of two unrelated HS fami-lies with balanced translocations involving the short arm of chromosome 8 (876,877). Chilcote and his colleagues then iden-tified two sisters with moderate to severe splenectomy-responsive anemia, spherocytosis, dysmorphic features, micrognathia, nys-tagmus, psychomotor retardation, and deletion of chromosome bands 8p11.1-p21.2 (878); subsequently, similar deletions (879–882) and a pericentric inversion (883) have been discovered in other HS patients. Together, these and other (884) observations provide evidence for a genetic locus for congenital spherocyto-sis in the proximal part of 8p (8p11.1-p11.2). The nature of this HS locus was clarified when it was shown that the gene for ankyrin resides in this region and that the individuals reported by Chilcote and another unrelated patient with a similar condi-tion lacked the ankyrin gene on the abnormal chromosome (Fig. 51-27) (621). This conclusion was supported by genetic analysis of a large kindred with typical autosomal-dominant HS and no chromosome deletion. Spherocytosis was linked to a restriction fragment length polymorphism in the ankyrin gene, whereas linkage to other candidate genes (α-spectrin, β-spectrin, or pro-tein 4.1 genes) was excluded (885).

In an analysis of 15 other families with HS, Kimberly et al. observed a weak association of HS with the IgGm type (886), which is located on 14q34. This observation suggested that the cause of HS is heterogeneous and that there is at least one other genetic locus. This turns out to be true. The chromosome 14 locus is probably the β-spectrin gene, which was later mapped to 14q23-q24.2 (887). As will be shown, other loci involve the genes for band 3, protein 4.2, α-spectrin, and, possibly, β-adducin and dematin.

Clinical Presentation

TYPICAL HEREDITARY SPHEROCYTOSIS

The typical clinical picture of HS combines evidence of hemoly-sis (anemia, jaundice, reticulocytosis, gallstones, and spleno-megaly) with spherocytosis [positive OF or acidified glycerol lysis tests (AGLTs), or both] and a positive family history (Table 51-6). Mild, moderate, and severe forms of HS have been defined according to differences in the Hb and bilirubin concen-trations and the reticulocyte count (Table 51-7) (667,888).

HS typically presents in infancy or childhood, but it may present at any age (889). In children, anemia is the most fre-quent presenting complaint (50%), followed by splenomegaly, jaundice, or a positive family history (all 10% to 15%) (890). No comparable data exist for adults.

The majority of HS patients (~60% to 75%) have incom-pletely compensated hemolysis and mild to moderate anemia. The anemia is often asymptomatic except for fatigue and mild pallor or, with children, nonspecific parental complaints such as "crabbiness."

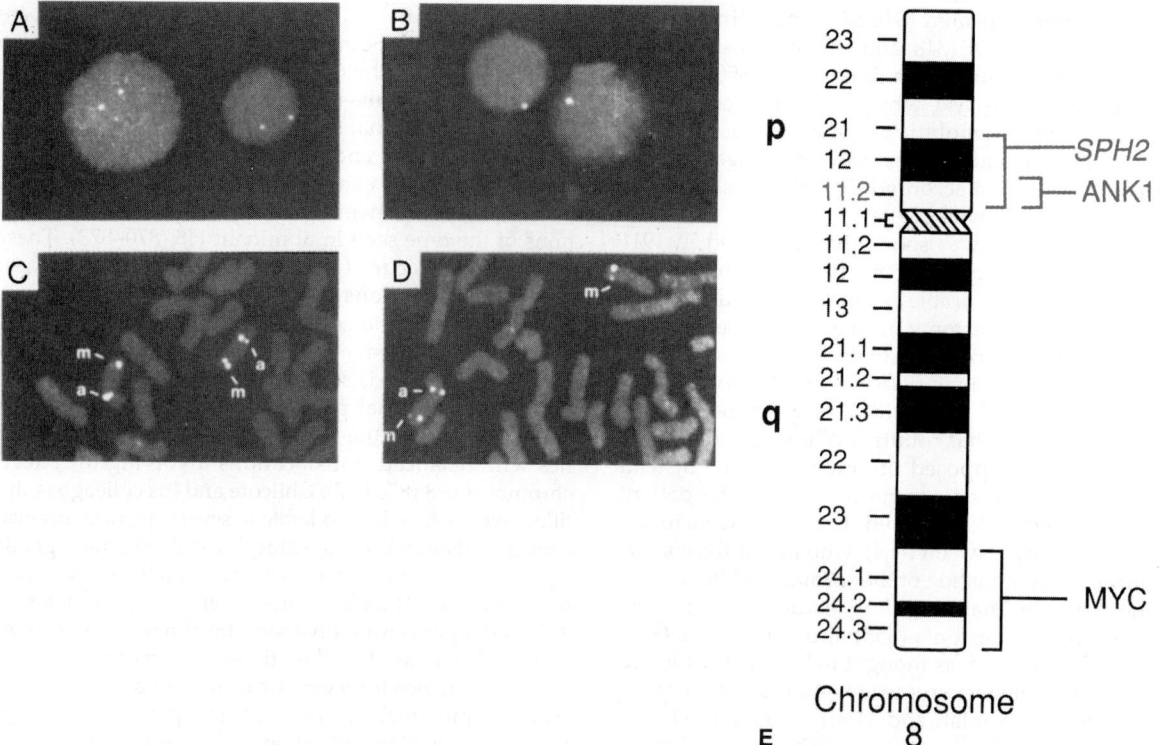

Figure 51-27. Demonstration of ANK1 (erythrocyte ankyrin) gene deletion in hereditary spherocytosis by fluorescence *in situ* hybridization. **A,B:** Interphase nuclei from a control (*left*) and a patient with hereditary spherocytosis and a small, heterozygous deletion (8p11.1–p21.1) of part of the short arm of chromosome 8 that defines the spherocytosis 2 (SPH2) locus (*right*). Two fluorescent spots represent the two normal ankyrin genes in the control, but only a single spot is seen in the nuclei of the patient. **C,D:** Metaphase spreads of control (*left*) and patient (*right*) cells hybridized with ANK1 *a* and MYC *m* genomic probes. The MYC gene is located at 8q24, near the end of the long arm of chromosome 8. Both normal chromosomes 8 are labeled by both probes, whereas both hereditary spherocytosis chromosomes 8 contain MYC signals, but the one at the top of (**D**) does not react with the ankyrin probe. **E:** Map of human chromosome 8 indicating the location of the ANK1 and MYC genes and the SPH2 locus. (Adapted from Lux SE, Tse WT, Menninger JC, et al. Hereditary spherocytosis associated with deletion of the human erythrocyte ankyrin gene on chromosome 8. *Nature* 1990;345:736.)

Jaundice is seen at some time in approximately one-half of patients, usually in association with viral infections. When present, it is acholuric [i.e., characterized by unconjugated (indirect) hyperbilirubinemia and the absence of bilirubinuria].

The incidence of palpable splenomegaly varies from approximately 50% in young children to 75% to 95% in older children and adults (890–892). Typically, the spleen is modestly enlarged (2 to 6 cm), but it may be massive (854,855,893,894). There is no proven correlation between the size of the spleen and the severity of HS, although, given the pathophysiology (see below) and the response of the disease to splenectomy, such a correlation probably exists.

SILENT CARRIER STATE
The parents of patients with "nondominant" HS are clinically asymptomatic and do not have anemia, splenomegaly, hyperbilirubinemia, or spherocytosis on peripheral blood smears (861,869). However, many have subtle laboratory signs of HS (861,869) including slight reticulocytosis (average, 2.1% ± 0.8%), diminished haptoglobin levels, elevated OF, shortened acidified glycerol lysis time (860), or elevated autohemolysis (Table 51-7). These tests are described in detail below. The incubated OF test is probably the most sensitive measure of this condition, particularly the 100% lysis point, which is significantly elevated in carriers (0.43 ± 0.05 g NaCl/dL) compared to normals (0.23 ± 0.07) (861). However, no single test is sufficient. Carriers can

only be detected reliably by considering the results of a battery of tests.

From the estimated prevalence of recessive HS [1 in 40,000 (i.e., ~12.5% of all HS, which is 1 in 5000 in the United States [858])], one can estimate that approximately 1% of the population should be silent carriers. Interestingly, screens of normal Norwegian (859) or German (860) blood donors with OF or AGLTs show a 0.9% to 1.1% incidence of previously unsuspected "very mild" HS.

MILD HEREDITARY SPHEROCYTOSIS

Patients with Mild Hereditary Spherocytosis Have Compensated Hemolysis. Red cell production and destruction are balanced or nearly balanced in approximately 20% to 30% of HS patients (891,895). They are said to have "compensated hemolysis." Such patients are not anemic and are usually asymptomatic. In some cases, diagnosis may be difficult because hemolysis, splenomegaly, and spherocytosis are unusually mild. For example, reticulocyte counts are generally less than 6%, and only 60% have significant spherocytosis on peripheral blood smears (861) (Table 51-7).

Pregnancy, Exercise, and Splenic Enlargement May Exacerbate Mild Hereditary Spherocytosis. Hemolysis may become severe with illnesses that cause splenomegaly, such as infectious mono-

TABLE 51-6. Characteristics of Hereditary Spherocytosis

Clinical manifestations
  Anemia
  Splenomegaly
  Intermittent jaundice
    From hemolysis
    From biliary obstruction
  Aplastic crises
  Inheritance
    Dominant—75%
    Nondominant—25%
  Rare manifestations
    Leg ulcers
    Extramedullary hematopoietic tumors
    Spinocerebellar ataxia
    Myocardiopathy
  Excellent response to splenectomy
Laboratory features
  Reticulocytosis
  Spherocytosis
  Elevated mean corpuscular hemoglobin concentration
  Increased osmotic fragility (especially the incubated osmotic fragility test)
  Normal Coombs' test
  Decreased red cell spectrin, or spectrin and ankyrin, or protein 3, or
    protein 4.2

nucleosis (896). Hemolysis may also be exacerbated by pregnancy (893,894) or exercise (899) to the point at which it may impair athletic performance in endurance sports, even in patients with mild disease. Many of these patients are diagnosed during family studies or discovered as adults when splenomegaly or gallstones appear. Although mild HS is usually familial, it develops sporadically in families with more severe disease (891). Presumably, this is due to the coinheritance of modifying genes, such as those affecting splenic function or the synthesis or function of membrane skeletal proteins.

How Is "Compensated Hemolysis" Achieved? One of the interesting aspects of HS is why patients with compensated hemolysis continue to have erythroid hyperplasia when their Hb levels are normal. It is difficult to reconcile this phenomenon with the generally accepted theory that erythropoiesis is regulated by tissue hypoxia. One possibility is the concentration of 2,3-DPG, which reportedly is low in hereditary spherocytes before splenectomy (900,901) [although the P_{50} of HS blood is normal (901)]. Another possibility is that the dehydrated HS red

cells are rheologically impaired and do not perfuse the peritubular renal cells (where erythropoietin is made) normally, even when the hematocrit is normal. This hypothesis fits with recent observations that the level of serum erythropoietin is inappropriately high in HS patients with compensated hemolysis and maintains bone marrow hyperplasia (902). If this is true, then erythropoietin production at any Hb level should correlate inversely with red cell deformability, and compensated hemolysis should mostly occur in disorders with dehydrated erythrocytes (e.g., HS, sickle cell disease, Hb CC disease, and hereditary xerocytosis).

MODERATELY SEVERE AND SEVERE HEREDITARY SPHEROCYTOSIS

A small fraction of HS patients (~5% to 10%) have moderately severe to severe anemia (164,861,865,878,903–906). Patients with "moderately severe" disease typically have an Hb of 6 to 8 g/dL, reticulocytes of at least 10%, and a bilirubin of 2 to 3 mg/dL (Table 51-7). This category includes patients with both dominant and recessive HS and a variety of molecular defects (see below).

Patients with "severe" disease, by definition, have life-threatening anemia and are transfusion dependent (Table 51-7). They almost always have recessive HS. In addition to the risks of recurrent transfusions, these patients are particularly prone to aplastic crises and occasionally develop growth retardation (164,893,894; Lux SE, *unpublished observations*), delayed sexual maturation (893), or aspects of thalassemic facies (893; Lux SE, *unpublished observations*).

HEREDITARY SPHEROCYTOSIS IN PREGNANCY

In general, unsplenectomized patients with HS have no significant complications during pregnancy except for anemia, which worsens due to plasma volume expansion (908) and sometimes due to increased hemolysis (897,898). Folic acid deficiency is also a risk (909,910). One group reported that transfusions were required in 20% of HS pregnancies (898), but, in our experience, few pregnant HS patients need to be transfused.

HEREDITARY SPHEROCYTOSIS IN THE NEONATE

HS frequently presents as jaundice in the first few days of life (911–913). Perhaps as many as one-half of all HS patients have a history of neonatal jaundice (914), and 91% of infants discovered to have HS in the first week of life are jaundiced (bilirubin >10 mg/dL) (912). Recent evidence shows that neonatal hyper-

TABLE 51-7. Clinical Classification of Hereditary Spherocytosis

	Trait	Mild Spherocytosis	Moderate Spherocytosis	Moderately Severe[a] Spherocytosis	Severe Spherocytosis[a,c]
Hemoglobin (g/dL)	Normal	11–15	8–12	6–8	<6
Reticulocytes (%)	1–3	3–8	≥8	≥10	≥10
Bilirubin (mg/dL)	0–1	1–2	≥2	2–3	≥3
Spectrin content (% of normal)[b]	100	80–100	50–80	40–80	20–50
Peripheral smear	Normal	Mild spherocytosis	Spherocytosis	Spherocytosis	Spherocytosis and poikilocytosis
Osmotic fragility					
Fresh blood	Normal	Normal or slightly increased	Distinctly increased	Distinctly increased	Distinctly increased
Incubated blood	Slightly increased	Distinctly increased	Distinctly increased	Distinctly increased	Markedly increased

[a]Values in untransfused patients.
[b]Spectrin content varies. Is only relevant for patients with spectrin or ankyrin defects. Hereditary spherocytosis patients who lack band 3 or protein 4.2 have mild to moderate spherocytosis, with normal or near normal amounts of spectrin and ankyrin. Normal spectrin content = 245 ± 27 (SD) × 10^5 spectrin dimers per erythrocyte.
[c]By definition in references 861–888, patients with severe spherocytosis are transfusion dependent.
Adapted from references 861–888.

bilirubinemia in HS (915) and other hemolytic diseases (916–918), in breast-fed infants (915), and maybe even in normals (920) is more frequent in infants with the TATA box polymorphism in the bilirubin uridine diphosphate glucuronosyltransferase gene (UGT1A1) (921) that causes Gilbert syndrome. A similar relationship is seen in Japanese neonates, in whom a G71R polymorphism in UGT1A1 is a frequent cause of Gilbert syndrome (922).

Hyperbilirubinemia usually appears in the first 2 days of life (911,913,914) and may rise rapidly, driven by the combination of hemolysis and the reduced capacity of the neonatal liver to conjugate bilirubin, particularly in Gilbert syndrome. Because neonates are discharged from the nursery earlier than in the past, physicians and parents must be alert for this delayed jaundice. Kernicterus is a risk (911,923), so exchange transfusions are sometimes necessary, but, in most cases, the jaundice can be controlled with phototherapy.

Only 43% of neonates with HS are anemic (Hb ≤15 g/dL) (912), and severe anemia is rare. Hydrops fetalis has been reported, but it probably only occurs in infants with homozygous dominant HS (863,864) or the most severe forms of recessive HS (865). Such infants may require intrauterine transfusions.

DIAGNOSIS OF HEREDITARY SPHEROCYTOSIS CAN BE DIFFICULT IN NEONATES

The diagnosis of HS is often more difficult in the neonatal period than later in life. Splenomegaly is uncommon—at most, the spleen tip is palpable (913,914)—and reticulocytosis is variable and usually not severe. Only 35% of affected neonates have a reticulocyte count of at least 10% (912). In addition, the haptoglobin level is not a reliable indicator of hemolysis during the first few months of life (924). An even greater problem is that 33% of neonates with HS do not have significant numbers of spherocytes on their peripheral blood smears (912). Moreover, because fetal red cells are more osmotically resistant than adult cells when fresh and more osmotically sensitive after incubation at 37°C for 24 hours (912,925), the OF test may theoretically give false-positive (incubated OF) or false-negative (unincubated OF) results unless fetal controls are used. Fortunately, these have been published (912), and they appear to reliably discriminate neonates with HS, particularly when the incubated OF test is used (912–915). In more than 30 years of pediatric practice, we have not seen an infant for whom the diagnosis of HS was missed because of a false-negative OF test. Preliminary reports indicate that neonates with HS, like older children and adults with HS, have a fraction of hyperdense cells in the blood that can be detected by cell counters that measure the mean corpuscular hemoglobin count (MCHC) directly (see the section Red Cell Indices) (926). This simple and reliable measurement can be very helpful diagnostically.

HS can also be hard to differentiate from ABO incompatibility in the neonatal period because microspherocytosis is prominent in both, and the Coombs' test is sometimes negative in ABO disease. Fortunately, a negative Coombs' test is rare in symptomatic infants with ABO incompatibility (those with anemia and spherocytosis), and even then anti-A (or -B) antibodies can usually be eluted from the red cells, and free anti-A (or -B) IgG antibodies can be detected in the infant's serum. However, ABO incompatibility is much more common than HS. In a recent report (926), 1% of full-term icteric newborns had HS, which is 25 to 50 times more common than the incidence in the population generally; however, ABO incompatibility and symptomatic ABO disease were 25 times and 4 to 5 times as common as HS, respectively. The patients with ABO disease had hyperdense red cells, like HS patients, but they also had positive Coombs' tests.

MANY NEONATES WITH HEREDITARY SPHEROCYTOSIS HAVE TRANSIENT SLUGGISH ERYTHROPOIESIS

There is no evidence that patients with HS who are symptomatic as neonates have a more severe form of the disease, but many develop severe disease transiently. As noted above, the majority of infants with HS are not anemic at birth, but Hb values typically decrease sharply during the subsequent 20 days, which leads in many cases to a transient and severe anemia (927). The inordinate anemia is due to the inability to mount an appropriate erythropoietic response, as the reticulocyte count is relatively low for the degree of anemia. Postnatal improvement in splenic function may also play a role. The anemia is severe enough to warrant blood transfusions in a large number of infants. In a recent series, 24% of HS infants required no transfusion; 34% needed a single transfusion, usually before 2 months; 24% required multiple transfusions and up to 9 months to reach transfusion independence; and 18% had severe HS and required chronic transfusions (927). In our experience, a larger number of infants require no transfusions or only one, a smaller number require multiple transfusions, and less than 5% are indefinitely transfusion dependent. If the child is otherwise well, we allow the Hb to fall to approximately 5.5 to 6.5 g/dL before transfusing to try and stimulate the marrow, and we only raise the Hb to 9 to 11 g/dL after transfusion to avoid suppressing the desired marrow response. Sluggish erythropoiesis also occurs late in the course of hemolytic disease of the newborn, and, in a few tested patients, it was associated with relatively low erythropoietin levels (928), but this was not confirmed in other studies (929). In four preliminary studies, the anemia responded to recombinant human erythropoietin (926,930–932). It is not known if erythropoietin treatment averts transfusions in the late anemia of HS, but this possibility should be formally tested.

These findings indicate that it is important to carefully monitor Hb levels and reticulocyte counts in infants with HS during the first 6 months of life to detect and treat late anemia.

Etiology: Membrane Protein Defects

The primary molecular defects in HS reside in membrane skeletal proteins, particularly the proteins whose "vertical interactions" connect the membrane skeleton to the lipid bilayer: spectrin, ankyrin, protein 4.2, and band 3 (AE1).

SPECTRIN DEFECTS
See Table 51-8.

Spectrin Deficiency Common in Hereditary Spherocytosis. Red cells from HS patients with defects in spectrin or ankyrin are spectrin deficient (861,869,903,953). The degree of deficiency correlates well with the spheroidicity of HS erythrocytes (869,903,954), the severity of hemolysis (672,869,903), and the response of patients to splenectomy (869). The spectrin deficiency is evident microscopically (Fig. 51-28). The HS red cells show fewer spectrin filaments interconnecting spectrin-actin-4.1 junctional complexes (955), but overall skeletal architecture is preserved, except in the most severe forms of HS. The mechanical properties of the cells, particularly their ability to withstand shear stress, also correlate with their spectrin content (954,956) (Fig. 51-29).

α-Spectrin: Association with Recessive Hereditary Spherocytosis. The characteristics of HS due to α-spectrin defects are listed in Table 51-9. In general, HS caused by α-spectrin defects is a recessive trait, and HS due to β-spectrin mutations is a dominant trait. This is probably because in several species, including humans (957), α-spectrin exceeds β-spectrin synthesis by approximately three or four to one. Heterozygotes for α-spectrin

TABLE 51-8. Spectrin Defects in Hereditary Spherocytosis (HS)

Name of Variant	Location/Domain	Exon	Codon	Nucleotide Change	Amino Acid Change	Systemic Name[a]	Type of Mutation	Inheritance	No. of Kindreds	Clinical Severity[b]	Comment	Selected References
α-Spectrin												
LEPRA	Repeat	99 nt before exon 31	—	C→T	PCT	4339-99 C>T	Splicing	AR	12	Severe	Common; allele frequency ~3% to 4%; linked to αSp Bughill (A970D) polymorphism that is found in ~70% of severe recessive HS; αSp^LEPRA exaggerates a normal alternate splice of intron 30 that leads to PCT; only approximately 20% of normal α-spectrin production; frequently seen in cis to presumed severe α-spectrin defects in severe recessive HS.	936–940
Prague	Repeat	2 nt before exon 37	—	A→G	PCT	5187-2A>G	Splicing	AR	1	Severe	Compound heterozygote with αSp^LEPRA.	937
β-Spectrin												
Promissão	Actin-4.1	2	1	ATG→GTG	Met→Val	M1V	Missense	AD	1	Mild-moderate	Mutation interferes with translation initiation; some acanthocytes.	941
Guemene-Penfao	Actin-4.1	3	100	CTG→CTC	Silent mutation alters splicing→PCT	300G>C	Splicing	AD	1	?Mild	Silent mutation in last base of exon 3 interferes with splicing (only 4% of RNA normally spliced); some acanthocytes.	942
Atlanta	Actin-4.1	5	182	TGG→GGG	Trp→Gly	W182G	Missense	AD	1	Mild	Trp182 is highly conserved in actin binding proteins. Some acanthocytes.	943
Unnamed	Actin-4.1	5	189	GGC→GAC	Gly→Ala	G189A	Missense; ?splicing	AD	1	?	Mutation is at last base of exon 5; may affect splicing; some acanthocytes.	944
Kissimmee	Actin-4.1	6	202	TGG→CGG	Trp→Arg	W202R	Missense	AD	1	Mod-moderately severe	Mutant protein (40% of spectrin) unstable, oxidizes easily and binds 4.1 weakly causing spectrin loss; some acanthocytes.	945–948
Ostrava	Actin-4.1	6	202	TGG→GG	PCT	604delT	Frameshift	AD	1	Mild-moderate	—	943
Oakland	Actin-4.1	7	220	ATC→GTC	Ile→Val	I220V	Missense	AD	1	Moderate	This residue is Val in spectrin βIV; reason for hemolysis unclear; some acanthocytes.	943
Bicêtre	Repeat	11	444-446	GCCTCGTGGCC→GCC	PCT	1331-1338del8	Frameshift	AD	1	?	Some acanthocytes.	944
Alger	Repeat	12	514	CAG→TAG	Gln→Ter	Q514X	Nonsense	AD	1	?	Some acanthocytes.	944
Philadelphia	Repeat	13	589	GAA→GAAA	PCT	1767-1768insA	Frameshift	AD	1	Mild-moderate	—	943
Santa Barbara	Repeat	14	638	CGA→GA	PCT	1912delC	Frameshift	S	1	Mild	—	949,950
Bergen	Repeat	14	783-784	AAAAG→AAAAAG	PCT	2351-2352insA	Frameshift	AD	1	Mild-moderate	Very large family; some acanthocytes.	943
Baltimore	Repeat	14	845	CAG→TAG	Gln→Ter	Q845X	Nonsense	AD	1	Moderate	—	943

(continued)

TABLE 51-8. Continued

Name of Variant	Location/Domain	Exon	Codon	Nucleotide Change	Amino Acid Change	Systemic Name[a]	Type of Mutation	Inheritance	No. of Kindreds	Clinical Severity[b]	Comment	Selected References
Houston	Repeat	15	926	AAG→AG	PCT	2777delA	Frameshift	AD	1	Mild-moderate	—	943
Winston-Salem	Repeat	1 nt after exon 17	936-1255	G→A	Deletion of W936-R1255 (320 AA)	3764 + 1G>A	Splicing	S	1	Mild-moderate	Mutant protein truncated (~200 kd band between 2.1 and 2.2; 12% of spectrin) due to skipping exons 16 and 17; it is synthesized poorly and is unstable; some acanthocytes.	951
Columbus	Repeat	17	1227	CCT→TCT	Pro→Ser	P1227S	Missense	AD	1	Mild-moderate	Pro1227 not conserved in β-spectrins.	943
Durham	Repeat	22-23	1492-1614	4.6-kb deletion from intron 21 to intron 23	Deletion of L1492-K1614 (123 AA)	L1492-K1614del	Deletion	S	1	Mild-moderate	Mutant protein truncated (205 kd; 10% of spectrin) due to in-frame deletion of exons 22 and 23. It is synthesized and stable but weak ankyrin binding →poor membrane incorporation; some acanthocytes.	952
Birmingham	Repeat	25	1684	CGC→TGC	Arg→Cys	R1684C	Missense	AR	1	Severe	Assumed to have second mutation in trans; Arg1684 not conserved in β-spectrins.	943
Sao Paulo	Repeat	27	1884	GCG→GTG	Ala→Val	A1884V	Missense	S	1	Mild	Spherocytic elliptocytosis; Ala1884 not conserved in β-spectrins.	949
Tabor	Repeat	28	1946	CAG→TAG	Gln→Ter	Q1946X	Missense	AD	1	Moderate	—	943

AD, autosomal dominant; AR, autosomal recessive; LEPRA, low-expression Prague allele; nt, nucleotide; PCT, premature chain termination; Repeat, spectrin repeats region; S, sporadic mutation; SDS, sodium dodecyl sulfate; Ter, terminator codon.

[a]Mutations are abbreviated according to a described convention (933). Note that nucleotide numbers refer to the first nucleotide in the translation start ATG codon, which is numbered 1. The preceding codon is numbered –1 (there is no zero). This system conforms to the convention noted (933) but contrasts with that used by many previous authors (194,873,934), who numbered nucleotides from the beginning of a reported cDNA. Because more than one complete cDNA is available for many proteins, and the cDNAs often begin at different places in the 5'UTR, numbering from the beginning of the cDNA can be variable and confusing.

[b]Clinical severity was estimated using reported hematologic values presplenectomy and the criteria of Eber et al. (861) as modified by Eber and Lux (935).

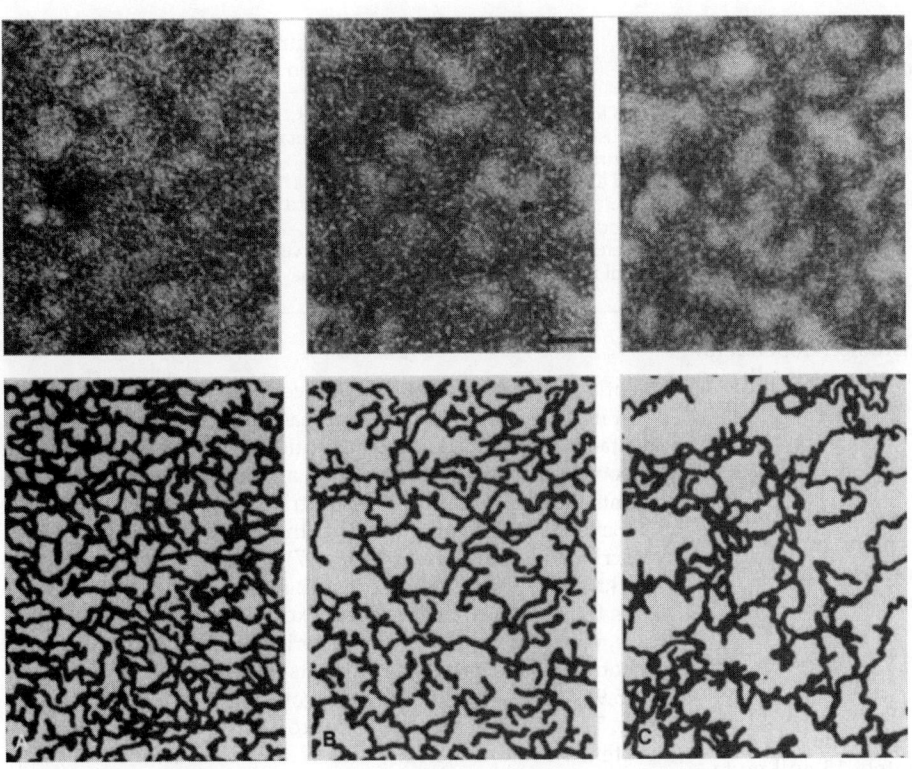

Figure 51-28. Density of spectrin on the membrane. Spectrin *in situ* was visualized by negative-stain electron microscopy **(top row)** in normal ghosts **(A)**, 50% spectrin-deficient ghosts **(B)**, and 70% spectrin-deficient ghosts **(C)**. Tracings of the skeletal network **(bottom row)** indicate the relative change in spectrin density. (Bar = 100 nm.) (Reprinted from Liu S-C, Derick LH, Agre PA, et al. Alteration of the erythrocyte membrane skeletal ultrastructure in hereditary spherocytosis, hereditary elliptocytosis and pyropoikilocytosis. *Blood* 1990;76:198–205, with permission.)

synthetic defects should still produce enough normal α subunits to pair with all or nearly all of the β-chains that are made, so spectrin deficiency would only be evident in the homozygous state.

This fits with the limited amount of data available. Defects in α-spectrin have been implicated in a subset of patients with a life-threatening form of nondominant HS associated with marked spectrin deficiency (25% to 50% of normal) (953). Many, but not all, of these families carry a variant α-spectrin peptide, designated αIIa- or α-spectrin Bughill (936). It bears the amino acid substitution alanine to asparagine at residue 309 of the α-spectrin chain (936). Peptide analysis of the α-spectrin peptides from the affected HS patients shows only the αIIa variant, but genomic DNA analysis reveals both an allele with the αIIa/α-spectrin Bughill mutation and one without, indicating that the second α-spectrin allele in these patients may be functionally silent (936). A candidate gene for this silent mutation was discovered in a family with severe, nondominant HS (938). One of the alleles, designated α-spectrin Prague, had a mutation in the penultimate position of intron 36, leading to the skipping of exon 37 and the premature termination of the α-spectrin peptide (Fig. 51-30). The other α-spectrin allele had a partial splicing abnormality in intron 30 and produced only approximately one-sixth of the normal amount of α-spectrin. This low-expression allele, named α-*spectrin*^LEPRA (low-expression allele Prague), is linked to the αIIa/α-spectrin Bughill variant in this patient and several other patients with severe, nondominant HS (937). Recently, another family with severe HS has been discovered in which the affected children inherited α-spectrin^LEPRA and α-spectrin Bughill from one parent and a proven but undefined null mutation of α-spectrin from the other (939). The families are not likely to be related because the first is Czech, and the second is Norwegian. Five other patients with severe HS are known who carry the α-spectrin^LEPRA allele on one chromosome and are presumed to have a second α-spectrin mutation in transit (940). This suggests that the combination of α-spectrin^LEPRA and an α-spectrin allele encoding a nonfunctional peptide may

be a frequent cause of severe nondominant HS. Homozygosity for α-spectrin^LEPRA alone does not appear to cause disease.

Patients with recessive HS and α-spectrin mutations are rare—probably less than 5% of HS. They have all had moder-

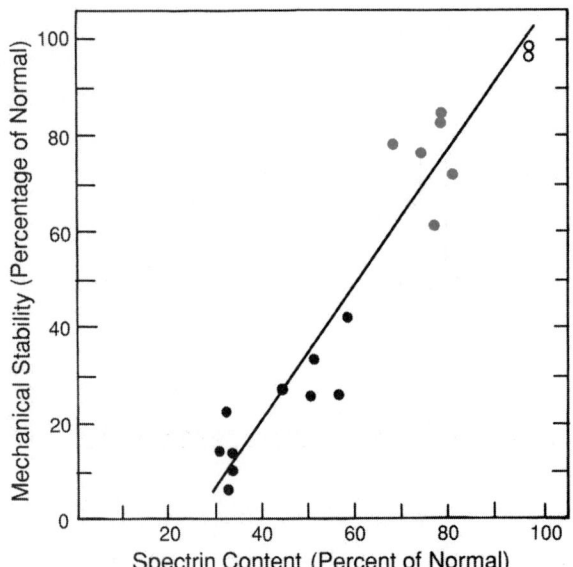

Figure 51-29. Relationship between membrane mechanical stability, measured with the ektacytometer, and spectrin content in red cells from patients with heterozygous dominant hereditary spherocytosis (*solid blue circles*), homozygous recessive hereditary spherocytosis (*solid black circles*), and heterozygous recessive hereditary spherocytosis (*open circles*). Membranes from dominant and recessive hereditary spherocytosis patients fall on the same curve, suggesting that similar mechanisms may be responsible for membrane fragility in the two conditions. (Adapted from Chasis JA, Agre PA, Mohandas N. Decreased membrane mechanical stability and in vivo loss of surface area reflect spectrin deficiencies in hereditary spherocytosis. *J Clin Invest* 1988;82:617.)

TABLE 51-9. Hereditary Spherocytosis Due to α-Spectrin Mutations

<5% of hereditary spherocytosis.
Autosomal recessive.
α-Spectrin LEPRA, a common, low expression splicing defect, is often paired with a second, presumably null allele.
Severe hemolysis and anemia, often transfusion dependent.
50% to 75% spectrin deficiency.
Red cell morphology not well defined.

TABLE 51-10. Hereditary Spherocytosis Due to β-Spectrin Mutations

15% to 30% of hereditary spherocytosis.
Almost all individual, dominant null mutations. No common mutations.
Spectrin content decreased 15% to 40%.
Mild to moderate hemolysis and anemia.
Spherocytosis *plus* 5% to 10% spiculated red cells (acanthocytes or echinocytes).
Spherocytosis *plus* elliptocytosis is observed in some patients with C-terminal mutations. They are classified as having spherocytic elliptocytosis.

ately severe to severe HS, sometimes transfusion dependent (869,903,938–940,953). Blood smears contain numerous spherocytes and microspherocytes. Patients with very severe spectrin deficiency may also have misshapen spherocytes, spiculated red cells, and bizarre poikilocytes (869,903,953).

β-Spectrin: Association with Dominant Hereditary Spherocytosis. Deficiency of the scarce β-spectrin chains, on the other hand, should limit the formation of spectrin heterodimers and be expressed as a dominant defect; in general, this seems to be the case (Table 51-10). Twenty mutations have been described so far (Fig. 51-31; Table 51-8), of which 19 are dominant. Each is found in a single family.

Monoallelic expression of β-spectrin occurs frequently in HS patients with spectrin deficiency (871,872), suggesting that null mutations are common defects. Approximately 15 null mutations have been described in patients with dominant HS. The defects include initiation codon disruption (941), frameshift and nonsense mutations (943,951), gene deletions (952), and splicing defects (942,944,951) (Fig. 51-31). A 4.6-kb genomic deletion in spectrin Durham results in a truncated peptide that is ineffi-

ciently incorporated into the red cell (952). A splice site mutation in spectrin Winston-Salem leads to exon skipping and an unstable truncated β-spectrin peptide (951). A similar defect in spectrin Guemene-Penfao causes an intron to be retained and blunts the accumulation of β-spectrin transcripts (942).

Several missense mutations in the β-spectrin gene have been described in dominant HS (943,947). In most of these cases, it is not known if the mutation causes a functional defect or destabilizes the mRNA or protein. One exception is β-spectrin Kissimmee, which has been well characterized on the protein level and is both unstable and defective in its capacity to bind protein 4.1 (945,947,948). Affected heterozygotes have two types of spectrin. The abnormal fraction, approximately 40%, cannot bind protein 4.1 and therefore binds weakly to actin (945,959) (Fig. 51-32). Peptide mapping shows that the defect resides near the N-terminus of the β-spectrin chain (947,948), near the site where protein 4.1 binds (959,960). The mutant spectrin is unstable and susceptible to thiol oxidation (947). This either causes or exacerbates the defect in binding to protein 4.1, because chemical reduction almost completely restores normal binding activity (947). Interestingly, very mild oxidation of normal spectrin (946) or storage of normal cells under aerobic conditions in the blood bank (961) produces similar defects in spectrin-4.1 interactions. Patients with the spectrin-4.1 binding defect have only 80% of normal red cell spectrin (947), which may be the real explanation why they have spherocytosis. Presumably, the defective spectrin detaches from the membrane more easily than normal and falls prey to proteases that specifically degrade unbound or oxidized spectrin chains (962). Loss of the abnormal spectrin explains why the ratio of normal to abnormal spectrin is 60:40 instead of the expected 50:50.

Molecular analysis shows a Trp→Arg substitution at position 202 of the β-spectrin Kissimmee cDNA (948) but not in the other two described kindreds with a similar functional defect (958). The mutation inserts a positively charged amino acid in a highly conserved region of largely hydrophobic amino acid sequence, and it could thus disrupt a region that is critical for protein 4.1 binding. Two other mutations, spectrins Atlanta and Oakland, have missense mutations at positions 182 and 220 of the β-spectrin cDNA, flanking the position of the spectrin Kissimmee mutation. These mutations may potentially also cause defective protein 4.1 binding, but this hypothesis has not been tested.

A mutation in β-spectrin has only been identified in one case of presumed recessive HS. A point mutation in position 1684 of the β-chain in spectrin Birmingham changes an arginine to cystine (943). There presumably is another mutation in the second allele to account for the recessive nature of the disease, but it has not been found.

Overall, β-spectrin defects account for approximately 15% to 30% of HS in Northern European populations. Patients with β-spectrin deficiency typically have mild to moderately severe HS. Where described, their blood smears have contained some (8% to 20%) spiculated red cells (echinocytes and acanthocytes)

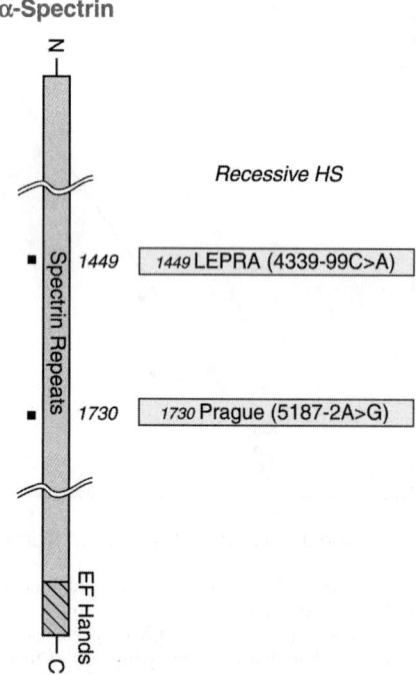

Figure 51-30. Two α-spectrin mutations associated with recessive hereditary spherocytosis (HS) are shown next to a schematic representation of the α-spectrin peptide. (Adapted from Tse WT, Lux SE. Hereditary spherocytosis and hereditary elliptocytosis. In: Scriver CR, Beaudet AL, Sly WS, Valle D, eds. *The metabolic and molecular bases of inherited disease,* 8th ed. New York: McGraw-Hill, 2001:4665.)

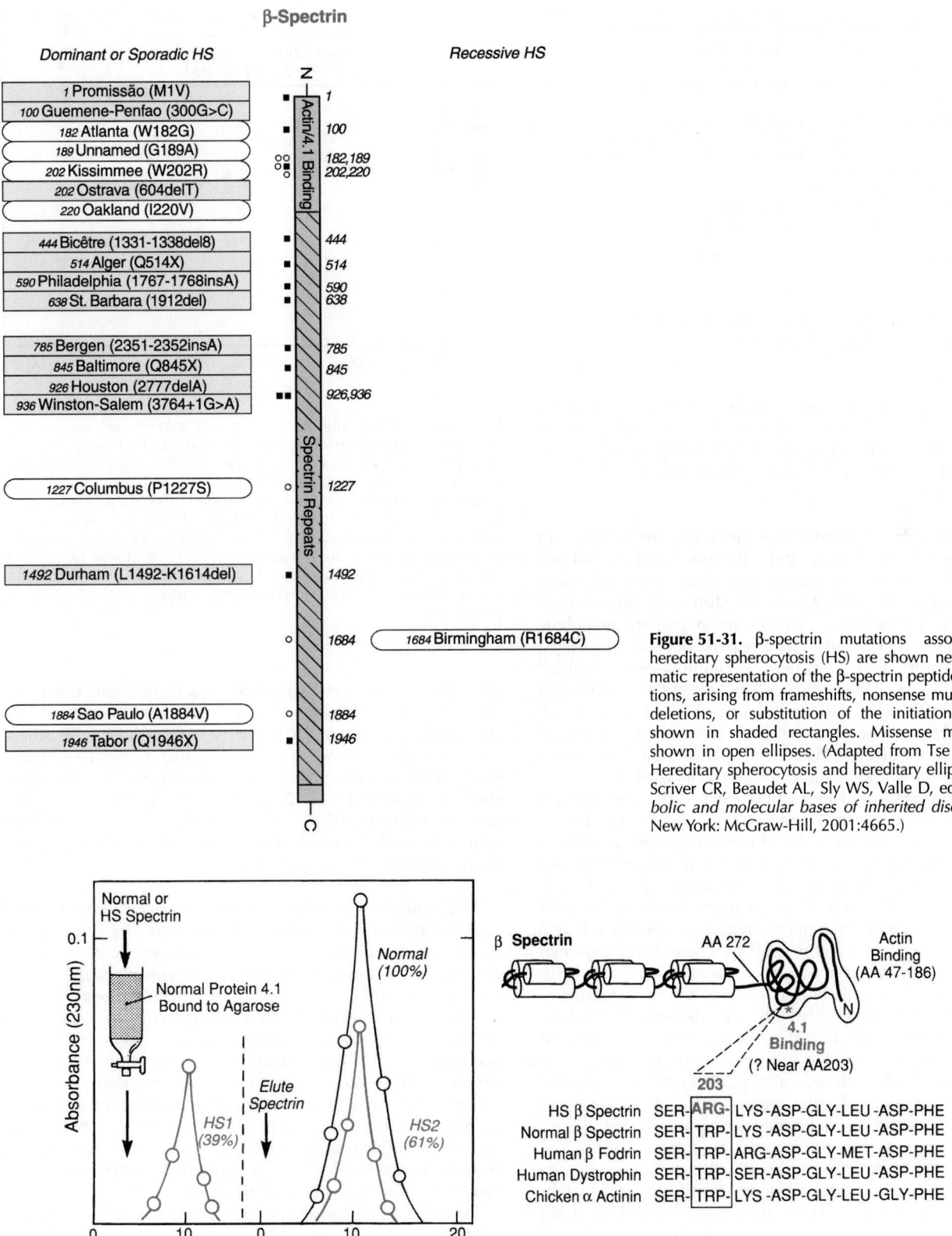

β-Spectrin

Dominant or Sporadic HS   *Recessive HS*

1 Promissão (M1V)
100 Guemene-Penfao (300G>C)
182 Atlanta (W182G)
189 Unnamed (G189A)
202 Kissimmee (W202R)
202 Ostrava (604delT)
220 Oakland (I220V)

444 Bicêtre (1331-1338del8)
514 Alger (Q514X)
590 Philadelphia (1767-1768insA)
638 St. Barbara (1912del)

785 Bergen (2351-2352insA)
845 Baltimore (Q845X)
926 Houston (2777delA)
936 Winston-Salem (3764+1G>A)

1227 Columbus (P1227S)

1492 Durham (L1492-K1614del)

1684 Birmingham (R1684C)

1884 Sao Paulo (A1884V)
1946 Tabor (Q1946X)

N
Actin/4.1 Binding
1
100
182,189
202,220
444
514
590
638
785
845
926,936
Spectrin Repeats
1227
1492
1684
1884
1946
C

Figure 51-31. β-spectrin mutations associated with hereditary spherocytosis (HS) are shown next to a schematic representation of the β-spectrin peptide. Null mutations, arising from frameshifts, nonsense mutations, large deletions, or substitution of the initiation codon, are shown in shaded rectangles. Missense mutations are shown in open ellipses. (Adapted from Tse WT, Lux SE. Hereditary spherocytosis and hereditary elliptocytosis. In: Scriver CR, Beaudet AL, Sly WS, Valle D, eds. *The metabolic and molecular bases of inherited disease,* 8th ed. New York: McGraw-Hill, 2001:4665.)

Normal or HS Spectrin

Normal Protein 4.1 Bound to Agarose

0.1

Normal (100%)

Elute Spectrin

HS1 (39%)

HS2 (61%)

Absorbance (230nm)

0   10   0   10   20
Fraction Number

β **Spectrin**   AA 272   Actin Binding (AA 47-186)

N

4.1 Binding (? Near AA203)

203

HS β Spectrin	SER-	ARG-	LYS -ASP-GLY-LEU -ASP-PHE
Normal β Spectrin	SER-	TRP-	LYS -ASP-GLY-LEU -ASP-PHE
Human β Fodrin	SER-	TRP-	ARG-ASP-GLY-MET-ASP-PHE
Human Dystrophin	SER-	TRP-	SER-ASP-GLY-LEU -ASP-PHE
Chicken α Actinin	SER-	TRP-	LYS -ASP-GLY-LEU -GLY-PHE

Figure 51-32. Defect in binding site for protein 4.1 in β-spectrin Kissimmee. Spectrin from a normal individual or from a patient with β-spectrin Kissimmee was passed over a column containing immobilized normal protein 4.1. All normal spectrin and 61% of the hereditary spherocytosis (HS) spectrin bound and could be eluted under conditions unfavorable for spectrin-4.1 interactions. However, 39% of the HS spectrin failed to bind to the column, and, in a separate assay, this fraction (Sp Kissimmee) lacked the ability to bind protein 4.1 (945). Subsequent studies have localized the defect to β-spectrin (947) and defined a mutation in amino acid (AA) 202 (Trp→Arg) (948). The mutation is in a conserved region in the N-terminal end of β-spectrin, just beyond the actin binding domain (AA 47-186). The region is a likely location for the 4.1 binding site.

TABLE 51-11. Hereditary Spherocytosis Due to Ankyrin Mutations

30% to 60% of hereditary spherocytosis in the Unites States and Europe; 5% to 10% in Japan.
Autosomal dominant and autosomal recessive.
Dominant mutations individual, null mutations. No common defects.
Recessive mutations missense and promoter defects. −108 T→C promoter mutation relatively common.
Both spectrin and ankyrin equally deficient: 15% to 50%.
Mild to moderately severe hemolysis and anemia.
Spherocytosis without other abnormal morphology.

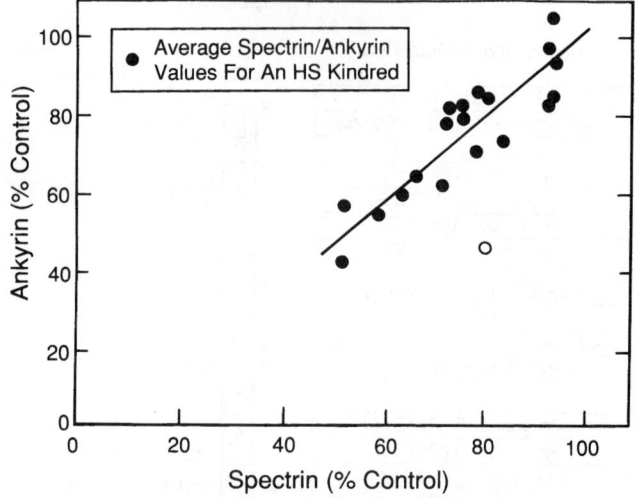

Figure 51-33. Correlation of spectrin and ankyrin deficiencies in 20 dominant hereditary spherocytosis (HS) kindreds. Each point, expressed as a percentage of the control, taken as 100%, represents the mean value for a kindred for both red cell spectrin and ankyrin levels. Note that, within experimental error, the degree of spectrin and ankyrin deficiencies is essentially identical in these families with one exception (*open circle*), an otherwise typical family in which red cells are primarily ankyrin deficient. (Reprinted from Savvides P, Shalev O, John KM, Lux SE. Combined spectrin and ankyrin deficiency is common in autosomal dominant hereditary spherocytosis. *Blood* 1993;82:2953, with permission.)

(942–945,949,950) as well as spherocytes. It seems this may be a fairly reliable differentiating feature.

ANKYRIN DEFECTS

See Table 51-11. Because spectrin heterodimers are only stable when bound to the membrane (978) and ankyrin, the high-affinity binding site is normally present in limiting amounts, and deficiency of ankyrin should lead to loss of both proteins. This is, in fact, observed.

Many Hereditary Spherocytosis Red Cells Are Deficient in Spectrin and Ankyrin. Coetzer and colleagues first described two patients with an atypical, severe form of spherocytosis who were deficient in spectrin and ankyrin. The clinical picture of these patients was characterized by transfusion-dependent hemolytic anemia, marked spherocytosis, bizarre poikilocytosis, and only a partial response to splenectomy (904). The authors showed that red cell membranes from the patients were deficient in spectrin and ankyrin. Each was reduced to approximately 50% to 60% of normal. They studied the synthesis, assembly, and turnover of spectrin and ankyrin in the reticulocytes in one of the patients and found that a defect in ankyrin synthesis was the primary abnormality.

Other studies showed that combined spectrin and ankyrin deficiency is not limited to these atypical patients but is common in patients with typical HS (149,888). Savvides and co-workers used a radioimmunoassay (RIA) to measure the spectrin and ankyrin content in 20 kindreds with dominant HS (149). The values ranged from 40% to 100% of the normal cellular levels of 242,000 ± 20,500 spectrin heterodimers and 124,500 ± 11,000 ankyrins. Spectrin and ankyrin levels were less than the normal range in 75% and 80% of the kindreds, respectively, and, with one exception, the degree of deficiency of the two proteins in each kindred correlated strictly with each other (Fig. 51-33). Pekrun and co-workers used an enzyme-linked immunosorbent assay (ELISA) to measure the ankyrin and spectrin contents in the erythrocytes of 45 patients with typical HS (888). They found concomitant deficiency of both proteins in all of the patients and showed that the degree of deficiency is proportional to the clinical severity.

Several surveys have used SDS gel electrophoresis to estimate the relative frequencies of different membrane protein deficiencies in HS (979–983). They show that 30% to 45% of HS patients have combined ankyrin and spectrin deficiency, and approximately 30% have isolated spectrin deficiency. The reasons for the difference between SDS polyacrylamide gel electrophoresis (SDS-PAGE) and RIA measurements are unknown but seem to be methodologic because different groups have reported similar results with each technique. SDS-PAGE should be less accurate because ankyrin runs so close to β-spectrin on SDS gels that it is hard to quantitate. A high reticulocyte count may also mask the detection of ankyrin deficiency (984). However, patients defined as solely spectrin deficient on SDS gels have

often proved to have β-spectrin defects, whereas those with combined spectrin and ankyrin deficiency have usually had ankyrin mutations. For unknown reasons, patients with isolated spectrin deficiency were not detected in either RIA/ELISA study, which seems improbable given the number of patients studied (approximately 80) and the estimated frequency of β-spectrin mutations (15% to 30%) (149,888). Also, the SDS-PAGE method is much easier to set up for most laboratories and seems likely to become the method of choice.

Different Types of Ankyrin Mutations Are Prevalent in Dominant and Recessive Hereditary Spherocytosis. As discussed above, genetic linkage analyses and cytogenetic evidence first showed that a defect in ankyrin is the primary cause of HS in some families (621,885). Using a dinucleotide repeat polymorphism in the ankyrin cDNA as a marker to distinguish between the two ankyrin alleles, Jarolim and co-workers showed that one ankyrin allele has reduced expression in one-third of HS patients with combined spectrin and ankyrin deficiency (985). This may be caused by either the reduced transcription of one of the ankyrin alleles or the instability of its mRNA. By the same method, it has been shown that *de novo* mutations leading to the decreased expression of one ankyrin allele are frequent in HS patients without a positive family history (870).

Eber et al. examined 46 kindreds with dominant and recessive spherocytosis and identified 12 different ankyrin mutations in 13 kindreds (194). Considering the inaccuracies in the technique used to detect mutations, they concluded that ankyrin defects account for 45% to 65% of HS in European populations. Other investigators have reported additional mutations (966,967,971,972,977) (Table 51-12). Most of these are family specific, private mutations. Null mutations (frameshift and nonsense mutations) that result in either unstable ankyrin transcripts or truncated peptides predominate in dominant HS. They are located throughout the ankyrin peptide (Fig. 51-34). One of the

TABLE 51-12. Ankyrin Defects in Hereditary Spherocytosis

Name of Variant	Location/ Domain	Exon	Codon	Nucleotide Change	Amino Acid Change	Systemic Name[a]	Type of Mutation	Inheritance	No. of Kindreds	Clinical Severity[b]	Comment	Selected References
Unnamed	Promoter	—	204 nt before codon 1	TGCGG→TGGGG	—	-204C>T	Promoter	AD	1	Moderate	—	194
Campinas	Promoter	—	153 nt before codon 1	G→A	—	-153G>A	Promoter	AR	1	Moderately severe	Linked to -108T>C.	963
Unnamed	Promoter	—	108 nt before codon 1	CCTGG→CCCGG	—	-108T>C	Promoter	AR	6	Mild to severe	Compound heterozygote with second mutation or presumed second mutation.	194
Unnamed	Promoter	—	-72/-73 nt before codon 1	GGTGAGG→GGAGG	—	-72/-73delTG	Promoter	AR	2	?	Disrupts promoter function in transgenic mice.	964,965
Chiba II	Memb	1	2-4	del 10 (CCCT TATCTG)	PCT	4-13del10	Frameshift	AD	1	?	—	873
Nara II	Memb	5 nt after exon 1	—	G→C	Deletion and/or PCT	27 + 5G>C	Splicing?	AD	1	?	—	873
Saitama	Memb	5	112	TTT→TT	PCT	334delT	Frameshift	S	1	?	—	873
Shiga	Memb	3-4 nt after exon 5	—	GTAAGT→GTAAAGT	PCT	427 + 3-4insA	Frameshift	S	1	?	—	873
Bugey	Memb	6	146	ACG→AG	PCT	437delC	Frameshift	S	1	Mild-moderate	—	966
Osterholz	Memb	6	174	del 20 (CTCC ... TCGC)	PCT	520-539del20	Frameshift	S	1	Mild-moderate	—	194
Tokyo II	Memb	6	187-190	del 10 (CACG GCTGCG)	PCT	561-570del10	Frameshift	S	1	?	—	873
Limeira	Memb	9	277	CAC→CGC	His→Arg	H277R	Missense	AD	1	Mild-moderate	—	962
Stuttgart	Memb	10	329	GCA→A	PCT	985-986delGC	Frameshift	AD	1	Mild-moderate	—	194
Bari	Memb	12	426-428	$(G)_6 \rightarrow (G)_5$	PCT	1282delG	Frameshift	S	1	Mild-moderate	—	967
Walsrode	Memb	14	463	GTC→ATC	Val→Ile	V463I	Missense	AR	1	Severe	Compound heterozygote with -108T>C; defect in binding band 3.	194,968
Florianopolis	Memb	14	505-507	$(C)_6 \rightarrow (C)_7$	PCT	1519insC	Frameshift	AD	3	Moderately severe-severe	—	969
Laguna	Memb	15	535	AAA→AA	PCT	1605delA	Frameshift	?	1	?	—	970
Tokyo III	Memb	16	571-573	$(C)_6 \rightarrow (C)_5$	PCT	1717delC	Frameshift	S	1	?	—	873
Einbeck	Memb	16	571-573	$(C)_6 \rightarrow (C)_7$	PCT	1717-1718insC	Frameshift	AD	1	Mild	—	194
Napoli I	Memb	16	573	CTG→CG	PCT	1717-1718delT	Frameshift	S	1	Moderate	—	971

(continued)

TABLE 51-12. Continued

Name of Variant	Location/Domain	Exon	Codon	Nucleotide Change	Amino Acid Change	Systemic Name[a]	Type of Mutation	Inheritance	No. of Kindreds	Clinical Severity[b]	Comment	Selected References
Munster	Memb	16	596	CAC→CA	PCT	1788delC	Frameshift	AD	1	?	Parental mosaicism.	874
Duisberg	Memb	18 nt before exon 17	—	C→A	PCT	1801-18C>A	Splicing	AD	1	Mild-moderate	Parental mosaicism.	194,874
Osaka II	Memb	17	612	CAG→TAG	Gln→Ter	Q612X	Nonsense	S	1	?	—	873
Votice	Memb	17	631	GAG→TAG	Glu→Ter	E631X	Nonsense	AD	1	Mild	—	972,973
Osaka I	Memb	17	637	ACG→ACCG	PCT	1909-1911insC	Frameshift	S	1	?	—	873
Olomouc	Memb	20	765	TCG→TAG	Ser→Ter	S765X	Nonsense	AD	1	Mild	—	972,973
Horovice	Memb	2 nt before exon 21	—	A→T	Deletion and/or PCT	2296-2A>T	Splicing	AD	1	Moderate	—	972,973
Marburg	Memb	22	797-798	TTAGTC→TC	PCT	2389-2392del4	Frameshift	AD	1	Severe	—	194
Kagoshima (or Yamanishi)	Memb	22	798-799	GTCAGT→GT	PCT	2394-2397del4	Frameshift	S	2	?	—	873
Yamagata	Memb	1 nt after exon 22	—	G→C	Deletion and/or PCT	2461+1G>C	Splicing	S	1	?	—	873
Tabor	Spectrin	25	907	AGC→AC	PCT	2720delG	Frameshift	AD	1	Moderate	—	972,973
Napoli II	Spectrin	26	933-934	GGCCTG→GGCTG	PCT	2800delC	Frameshift	S	1	Moderate	—	967
Benesov	Spectrin	26	941	ACG→ACCGGACG	PCT	2825-2826ins5	Frameshift	AD	1	Mild	—	973
Mie	Spectrin	26	951-953	TGCCGCCTG→TTCTGG	PCT	2852del7 ins4(TCTG)	Frameshift	S	1	?	—	873
Anzio	Spectrin	26	983	GCA→G	PCT	2948-2949delCA	Frameshift	S	1	Moderate	—	966
Nara I / Melnik	Spectrin	28 / 28	1046 / 1053	CTA→CCA / CGA→TGA	Leu→Pro / Arg→Ter	L1046P / R1053X	Missense / Nonsense	? / AD	1 / 1	? / Mild	— / —	873 / 972,973
Jaguariúna / Tubarao / Chiba I	Spectrin / Spectrin / 1 nt after exon 28	28 / 28 / —	1054 / 1075 / —	ATC→ACC / ATC→ACC / G→C	Ile→Thr / Ile→Thr / Deletion and/or PCT	I1054T / I1075T / 3327+1G>C	Missense / Missense / Splicing	AD / ? / S	1 / ? / 1	Moderate / ? / ?	— / — / —	963 / 970 / 873
Porta Westfalica	Spectrin	29	1127	ACA→AA	PCT	3380delC	Frameshift	S	1	Moderately severe	—	194
Unnamed	Spectrin	30	1185	TGG→CGG or AGG	Trp→Arg	W1185R	Missense	?	?	?	—	974
Chiba III	Spectrin	31	1230	TAC→TAG	Tyr→Ter	Y1230X	Nonsense	S	1	?	—	873

Name	Domain	Location	Codon	Nucleotide change	Amino acid effect	Mutation	Type	AD/AR	No.[a]	Severity[b]	Comments	Ref.
Tokyo I	Spectrin	31	1252	CGA→TGA	Arg→Ter	R1252X	Nonsense	AD	1	?	—	873
Kalrupy	Spectrin	34	1382	CTG→CG	PCT	4145delT	Frameshift	AD	1	Mild-moderate	Extra 150 kd band on SDS gels.	973
Bovenden	CTD	36	1436	CGA→TGA	Arg→Ter	R1436X	Nonsense	AD	1	Mild-moderate	—	194
Karlov	CTD	37	1488	CGA→TGA	Arg→Ter	R1488X	Nonsense	AD	1	Mild-moderate	—	973
Prague	CTD	37	1512	Insert 201 nt	Insert 67 amino acids	4537-4538ins201	Splicing?	?	1	?	Insertion occurs between exons 37 and 38; deficiency of band 2.1 on SDS gels; new band at 174 kd.	975
Düsseldorf	CTD	38	1592	GAC→AAC	Asp→Asn	D1592N	Missense	AR	1	Moderately severe	Presumed second mutation in trans	194
Toyama	CTD	38	1640	CAG→TAG	Gln→Ter	Q1640X	Nonsense	AD	1	?	—	873
Rakovnik	CTD	38	1669	GAA→TAA	Glu→Ter	E1699X	Nonsense	AD	1	Mild	Decreased band 2.1 on SDS gels; normal 2.2.	976
Unnamed	CTD	34 nt before exon 39	—	C→T	Deletion and/or PCT	5097-34C>T	Splicing?	AD	1	Moderate	—	194
St. Etienne I	CTD	39	1721	TGG→TGA	Trp→Ter	W1721X	Nonsense	AD	1	Mild-moderate	Additional band between 2.1 and 2.2 on SDS gels.	977
St. Etienne II	CTD	40	1833	CGA→TGA	Arg→Ter	R1833X	Nonsense	AD	1	Mild-moderate	Two additional bands between 2.1 and 2.2 on SDS gels.	977
Bocholt	CTD	16 nt after exon 41	—	C→T	Deletion or PCT	5619+16C>T	Splicing?	AR	1	Mild-moderate	Compound heterozygote with −108C>T mutation.	194

AD, autosomal dominant; AR, autosomal recessive; CTD, c-terminal (or regulatory) domain; del, delete; ins, insert; Memb, membrane domain; nt, nucleotide; PCT, premature chain termination; S, sporadic mutation; SDS, sodium dodecyl sulfate; Ter, terminator codon.

[a] Mutations are abbreviated according to a described convention (933). Note that nucleotide numbers refer to the first nucleotide in the translation start ATG codon, which is numbered 1. The preceding codon is numbered −1 (there is no zero). This system conforms with the convention noted (933) but contrasts with that used by many previous authors (194,873,934), who numbered nucleotides from the beginning of a reported comDNA. Because more than one complete cDNA is available for many proteins, and the cDNAs often begin at different places in the 5′UTR, numbering from the beginning of the cDNA can be variable and confusing.

[b] Clinical severity was estimated using reported hematologic values presplenectomy and the criteria of Eber et al. (861) as modified by Eber and Lux (935).

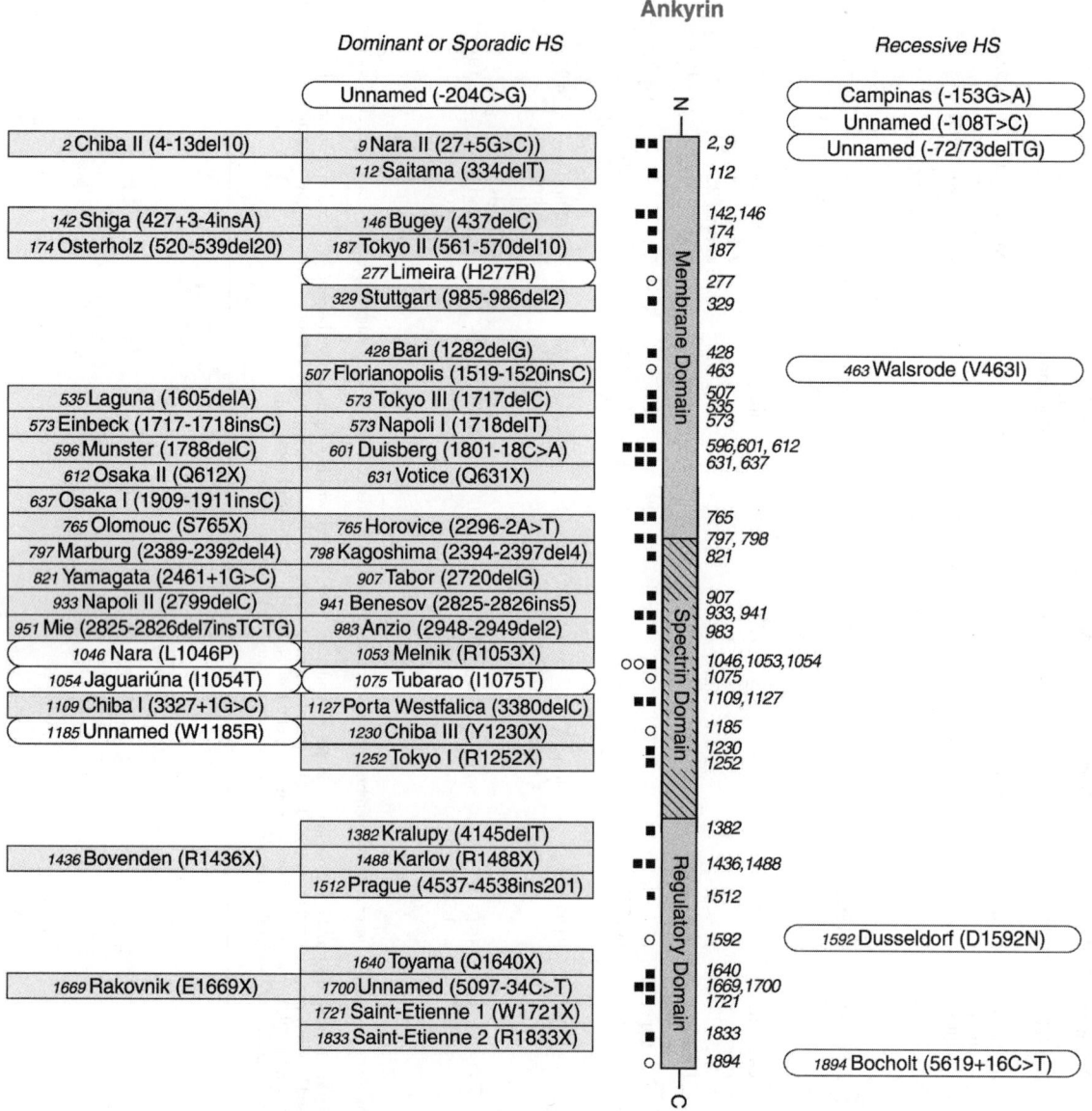

Figure 51-34. Ankyrin mutations associated with hereditary spherocytosis (HS). Null mutations, arising from frameshifts or nonsense mutations, are shown in shaded rectangles. Missense and putative promoter mutations are shown in open ellipses. (Adapted from Tse WT, Lux SE. Hereditary spherocytosis and hereditary elliptocytosis. In: Scriver CR, Beaudet AL, Sly WS, Valle D, eds. *The metabolic and molecular bases of inherited disease,* 8th ed. New York: McGraw-Hill, 2001:4665.)

more interesting is ankyrin Rakovnik, a nonsense mutation within the CTD that leads to selective deficiency of the major ankyrin isoform, band 2.1, but preserves the minor isoform, band 2.2 (986).

All of the ankyrin defects lead to combined and equivalent deficiencies of ankyrin and spectrin. Most of the null mutations are not detectable in reticulocyte mRNA, suggesting instability of the mutant transcript. The clinical manifestations are quite variable and range from mild hemolysis to severe transfusion-dependent anemia (194). This variability may be explained by different degrees of compensation for the null mutation, from either overproduction of the normal ankyrin allele or diminished ankyrin degradation, or it may be due to modifying genes involving other proteins. An example of such a modifying gene is described later in the section Animal and Fish Models of Hereditary Spherocytosis.

Several ankyrin defects have been identified in patients with recessive HS (194). These are mostly missense or promoter muta-

tions. A point mutation in the ankyrin promoter, $-108T \rightarrow C$, is particularly common and was found in four of seven families with recessive HS. In transgenic animals, the mutation reduces ankyrin expression, confirming that the mutation is significant (987). In two of four families, a second mutation was identified on the other allele: ankyrins Walsrode and Bocholt. Ankyrin Walsrode contains a missense mutation (V463I) in the band 3 binding domain and has a decreased affinity for band 3 (968). It is present in a patient whose red cells are more deficient in band 3 than in spectrin or ankyrin, which is opposite the trend in other ankyrin defects. Ankyrin Bocholt bears a missense mutation in a rare alternative splice product that may result in aberrant splicing.

Overall, ankyrin defects are estimated to account for 30% to 60% of HS in Northern European populations (194,979–983), but they account for much less (5% to 10%) in Japan (988). HS patients with ankyrin defects have prominent spherocytosis without other morphologic defects. Hemolysis and anemia vary

TABLE 51-13. Hereditary Spherocytosis Due to Band 3 Mutations

20% to 30% of hereditary spherocytosis.
Individual, dominant, functionally null mutations. No common defects.
15% to 40% decrease in band 3 and similar decrease in protein 4.2.
Mild to moderate hemolysis and anemia.
Spherocytosis with a small number of characteristic mushroom-shaped or "pincered" cells.

from mild to moderately severe (194,966,967,971,977). In general, patients with dominant defects are less affected than those with recessive mutations; however, there is considerable overlap.

BAND 3 (ANION EXCHANGE PROTEIN 1) DEFECTS

The characteristics of HS due to band 3 deficiency are listed in Table 51-13. Molecular defects have been described in many of these patients (Fig. 51-35; Table 51-14). Conserved arginine residues in band 3 are frequent sites of mutations. Examples include arginines 490, 518, 760, 808, and 870 (194,242,981). These highly conserved residues are positioned at the internal boundaries of transmembrane segments, and substitution probably interferes with cotranslational insertion of band 3 into the membranes of the ER during synthesis of the protein. In one case, mRNAs for both

alleles were present, but the mutant band 3 protein was not detected in the membrane, demonstrating either a functional defect in the incorporation of the protein into the membrane or an instability of the mutant protein (242). Missense mutations or short inframe deletions affecting other residues in the transmembrane domain of band 3 have been identified and, presumably, also impair insertion of the mutant band 3 into the membrane (194,979,991,998,1001,1003). This has recently been proved for a number of the mutations (1004). A ten-nucleotide duplication near the C-terminal end of band 3 Prague leads to a shift in the reading frame and an altered C-terminus after amino acid 821. This mutation affects the last transmembrane helix and may eliminate the carbonic anhydrase II binding site on band 3 (1005). It may also impair insertion of band 3 into the membrane and abolish anion transport function (1000).

Mutations in the cytoplasmic domain of band 3 can interfere with its binding to other membrane skeleton proteins, resulting in a functional defect. An amino acid substitution (Gly→Arg) at residue 130 in the cytoplasmic domain in band 3 Fukuoka affects protein 4.2 binding (1003). Patients with band 3 Montefiore and Tuscaloosa also have spherocytic hemolytic anemia with protein 4.2 deficiency and missense mutations in the cytoplasmic domain of band 3 at residues 40 and 327, respectively

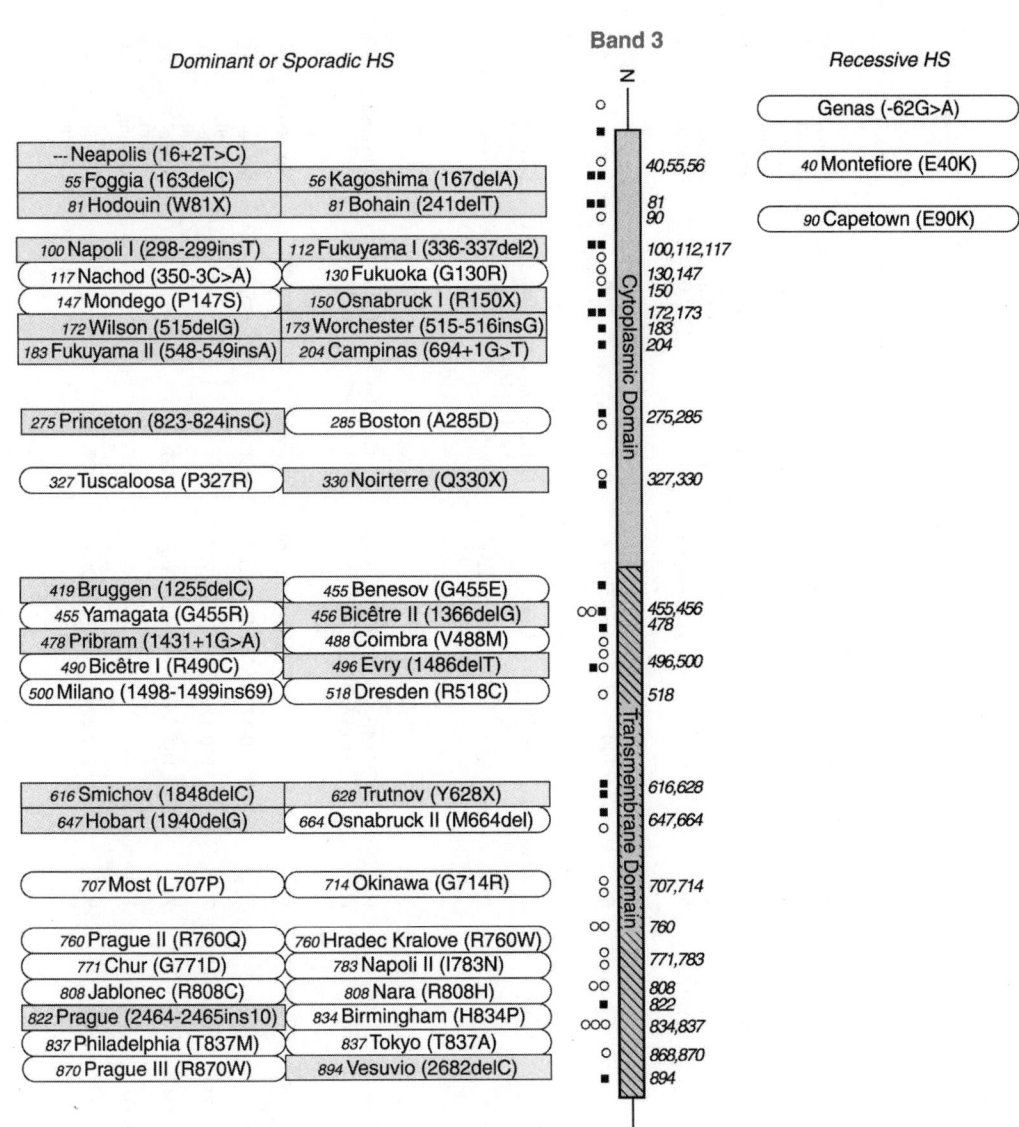

Figure 51-35. Band 3 mutations associated with hereditary spherocytosis (HS). Null mutations arising from either frameshift or nonsense mutations are shown in shaded rectangles, as is a mutation associated with loss of the translation start site (band 3 Neapolis). Missense mutations or short in-frame deletions or insertions are shown in open ellipses. (Adapted from Tse WT, Lux SE. Hereditary spherocytosis and hereditary elliptocytosis. In: Scriver CR, Beaudet AL, Sly WS, Valle D, eds. *The metabolic and molecular bases of inherited disease,* 8th ed. New York: McGraw-Hill, 2001:4665.)

TABLE 51-14. Band 3 (AE1) Defects in Hereditary Spherocytosis

Name of Variant	Location/Domain	Exon	Codon	Nucleotide Change	Amino Acid Change	Systemic Name[a]	Type of Mutation	Inheritance	No. of Kindreds	Clinical Severity[b]	Comment	Selected References
Genas	5'UTR	2	62 nt before codon 1	G→A	—	-62G>A	Promoter	?AR	1	Silent	Aggravates Bd 3 defects in trans (e.g., Bd 3 Lyon).	989
Neapolis	Cyto	2 nt after exon 2	—	T→C	(1) Loss of ATG, (2) PCT	15+2T>C	Splicing	AD	1	Mild	Two transcripts: (1) exon 2 skipped → abolishes initiation and (2) intron 2 retained → PCT; homozygote = very severe but no renal tubular acidosis.	864
Montefiore	Cyto	4	40	GAG→AAG	Glu→Lys	E40K	Missense	?AR	Many	None	E40K identified in patient with a partial deficiency of protein 4.2, but not clear the mutation alters 4.2 binding. May be a polymorphism, but Bd 3 Mondego (E40K plus P147S) worsens HS due to Bd 3 Coimbra in trans.	197, 990
Foggia	Cyto	4	55	ACCCAC→ACCAC	PCT	163delC	Frameshift	AD	1	Mild-moderate	—	991
Kagoshima	Cyto	4	56	AAG→AG	PCT	167delA	Frameshift	S	1	Mild	—	988
Bohain	Cyto	4	81	GCTGGG→GCGGG	PCT	241delT	Frameshift	AD	1	Mild	—	981
Hodouin	Cyto	5	81	TGG→TGA	Trp→Ter	W81X	Nonsense	?AR	1	?		979
Capetown	Cyto	5	90	GAG→AAG	Glu→Lys	E90K	Missense				E80 conserved in vertebrate AEs. Compound heterozygote with B3 Prague III is severe.	992
Napoli I	Cyto	5	100	TCTCT→TCTTCT	PCT	298-299ins1	Frameshift	AD	1	Mild-moderate	—	981
Fukuyama I	Cyto	5	112-113	AGAGTC→AGTC	PCT	336-337del2	Frameshift	AD	1	Mild	—	988
Nachod	Cyto	3 nt before exon 6	117-121	C→A	Del Gly-Thr-Val-Leu-Leu	349-3C>A	Splicing	AD	1	?	Conserved sequence.	979
Fukuoka	Cyto	6	130	GGA→AGA	Gly→Arg	G130R	Missense	AR	2	Silent	Binds 4.2 poorly. Homozygous Bd 3 Fukuoka shows mild HS with 91% Bd 3 and only 45% 4.2 (see also Bd 3 Okinawa).	993, 994
Mondego	Cyto	(1) 4 (2) 6	(1) 40 (2) 147	(1) GAG→AAG (2) CCT→ICT	(1) Glu→Lys (2) Pro→Ser	(1) E40K (2) E147S	Missense	AD	1	Silent	By itself, Bd 3 Modego is silent, but it aggravates other Bd 3 mutations in trans.	990
Osnabrück I (or Lyon)	Cyto	6	150	CGA→TGA	Arg→Ter	R150X	Nonsense	AD	2	Mild	Moderate severity when Bd 3 Genas in trans.	194, 989
Wilson	Cyto	7	170-172	$(G)_6 \to (G)_5$	PCT	515delG	Frameshift	AD	1	Mild	Original case of Bd 3 deficiency.	907,995
Worchester	Cyto	7	170-172	$(G)_6 \to (G)_7$	PCT	515-516insG	Frameshift	AD	1	?		979
Fukuyama II	Cyto	7	183	GAT→GAAT	PCT	548-549insA	Frameshift	AD	1	Mild		988
Campinas	Cyto	1 nt after exon 8	—	G→T	Del exon 8 and PCT	694+1G>T	Splicing	AD	1	Mild	Mild distal renal tubular acidosis.	996
Princeton	Cyto	9	273-275	$(C)_6 \to (C)_7$	PCT	823-824insC	Frameshift	S	1	?		979

Boston	Cyto	9	285	Ala→Asp	GCT→GAT	A285D	Missense	AD	1	?	Conserved in AE1s since birds.	979
Tuscaloosa	Cyto	10	327	Pro→Arg	CCC→CGC	P327R	Missense	?	1	?	P327 is conserved in all AE1s but not other AEs.	195
Noirterre	Cyto	10	330	Gln→Stop	CAG→TAG	Q330X	Nonsense	AD	1	Mild-moderate	—	997
Brüggen	Memb	11	418-419	PCT	CACCCG→CACCG	1257delC	Frameshift	AD	1	Mild	—	194
Benesov	Memb	12	455	Gly→Glu	GGG→GAG	G455E	Missense	AD	1	?	G455 highly conserved; introduction of charged residues in second TM segment. Bd 3 Benesov present in cis with duplication of 3'UTR nt 2785-2821 of unknown consequence.	979
Yamagata	Memb	12	455	Gly→Arg	GGG→AGG	G455R	Missense	S	1	Mild-moderate	—	988
Bicêtre II	Memb	12	456	PCT	CTGGGGCT→CTGGGGCT	1366 delG	Frameshift	AD	1	Mild	—	981
Pribram	Memb	1 nt after exon 12	—	PCT	G→A	1431+1 G>A	Splicing	AD	1	?	—	979
Coimbra	Memb	13	488	Val→Met	GTG→ATG	V488M	Missense	AD	1	Mild	Homozygote hydropic and transfusion-dependent, with spherocytes and bizarre poikilocytes, distal RTA, and nephrocalcinosis.	863,970
Bicêtre I	Memb	13	490	Arg→Cys	CGC→TGC	R490C	Missense	AD	3	Mild	—	981
Evry	Memb	13	496	PCT	TTCTGG→TTCGG	1486 delT	Frameshift	AD	1	Mild	—	981
Milano	Memb	13	499	New Gln + duplicate of 478-499	Duplicate 69 nt: from 1432 to 1500	1497-1498 ins69	Insertion	AD	1	Mild	Anti-Lepore type variant. Mutant protein not incorporated in membrane.	998
Dresden	Memb	13	518	Arg→Cys	CGC→TGC	R518C	Missense	AD	1	Moderate	R518 highly conserved in TM 4-5 internal loop.	194
Smichov	Memb	15	616	PCT	ATC→AT	1848delC	Frameshift	AD	1	?	—	979
Trutnov	Memb	15	628	Tyr→Ter	TAC→TAA	Y628X	Nonsense	AD	1	?	—	979
Hobart	Memb	16	646-647	PCT	CCGGGGC→CGGGC	1940delG	Frameshift	S	1	?	—	979
Osnabrück II	Memb	16	663-664	del Met	ATGATG→ATG	delM664	Deletion	AD	1	Mild	Met664 conserved in TM8 in all anion exchangers.	194
Tochigi II	Memb	5 nt before start of 17	—	Splicing with PCT?	del A	2058-5 delA	Splicing?	S	1	Mild	—	988
Most	Memb	17	707	Leu→Pro	CTG→CCG	L707P	Missense	AD	1	?	L707 highly conserved.	979
Okinawa	Memb	17	714	Gly→Arg	GGG→AGG	G714R	Missense	AD	1	Mild-moderate	G714 is a perfectly conserved TM residue. In cis to Bd 3 Okinawa are the Memphis I (K56E) and Memphis II (P854L) polymorphisms. This allele combined with Bd 3 Fukuoka in trans → severe hemolysis with 66% band 3 and no 4.2.	993
Prague II (or Kumamoto)	Memb	17	760	Arg→Gln	CGG→CAG	R760Q	Missense	AD	2	?	R760 at cytoplasmic side of TM11; highly conserved.	242,988
Hradec Kralove (or Tochigi I)	Memb	17	760	Arg→Trp	CGG→TGG	R760W	Missense	AD	2	Mild	—	242,988

(continued)

TABLE 51-14. Continued

Name of Variant	Location/ Domain	Exon	Codon	Nucleotide Change	Amino Acid Change	Systemic Name[a]	Type of Mutation	Inheritance	No. of Kindreds	Clinical Severity[b]	Comment	Selected References
Chur	Memb	18	771	GGC→GAC	Gly→Asp	G771D	Missense	AD	1	Mild	G771 highly conserved.	999
Napoli II	Memb	18	783	ATC→AAC	Ile→Asn	I783N	Missense	AD	1	Mild-moderate	Propositus has severe anemia in neonatal period for unexplained reasons.	991
Jablonec	Memb	18	808	CGC→TGC	Arg→Cys	R808C	Missense	AD	1	?	R808 perfectly conserved in all AEs since worms.	242
Nara	Memb	18	808	CGC→CAC	Arg→His	R808H	Missense	S	1	Mild	—	988
Prague I	Memb	18	822	TGTG→TG (10nt)TG	PCT	2464-2465 ins 10	Frame-shift	AD	1	Mild	—	1000
Birmingham	Memb	19	834	CAC→CCC	His→Pro	H834P	Missense	AD	1	?	H834 highly conserved.	979
Philadelphia	Memb	19	837	ACG→ATG	Thr→Met	T837M	Missense	AD	3	?	T837 highly conserved.	979
Tokyo	Memb	19	837	ACG→GCG	Thr→Ala	T837A	Missense	S		Mild	T837 perfectly conserved in all AEs since worms.	1001
Nagoya	Memb	19	837	ACG→AGG	Thr→Arg	T837R	Missense	AD	1	Mild-moderate	—	988
Prague III	C-ter	19	870	CGG→TGG	Arg→Trp	R870W	Missense	AD	1	?	R870 conserved in AE1 since birds.	242
Vesuvio	C-ter	20	894	ACC→AC	Elongated C-ter (terminates at AA 1026 instead of 911)	2681delC	Frame-shift	AD	6	Moderate	Frameshift → elongated C-terminus; mutant expressed but not incorporated in membrane; potentially unable to bind carbonic anhydrase.	1002

AA, amino acid; AD, autosomal dominant; AE, anion exchanger; AR, autosomal recessive; Bd, band; Cyto, cytoplasmic domain; del, delete; HS, hereditary spherocytosis; ins, insert; Memb, membrane domain; nt, nucleotide; PCT, premature chain termination; RTA, renal tubular acidosis; S, sporadic mutation; Ter, terminator codon; TM, transmembrane.

[a]Mutations are abbreviated according to a described convention (933). Note that nucleotide numbers refer to the first nucleotide in the translation start ATG codon, which is numbered 1. The preceding codon is numbered −1 (there is no zero). This system conforms to the convention noted (933) but contrasts with that used by many previous authors in references 194,873,934, who numbered nucleotides from the beginning of a reported cDNA. Because more than one complete cDNA is available for many proteins, and the cDNAs often begin at different places in the 5′UTR, numbering from the beginning of the cDNA can be variable and confusing.

[b]Clinical severity was estimated using reported hematologic values presplenectomy and the criteria of Eber et al. (861) as modified by Eber and Lux in reference 935.

(195,197), although the mild decrement in protein 4.2 in patients with band 3 Tuscaloosa suggests that it may simply reflect the loss of band 3, rather than damage to the 4.2 binding site, as originally proposed. All patients with band 3 deficiency have a proportional decrease in protein 4.2.

Null mutations in the band 3 gene also occur. They include nonsense mutations, single nucleotide insertions or deletions, and splicing defects (194,864,979,981,989,991,996,997). These mutations presumably lead to mRNA instability and protein deficiency (997).

Clinically, band 3 mutations account for approximately 20% to 30% of HS in European and Japanese populations (194,979–983,988). The amount of band 3 is decreased by 15% to 40% in patient red cells, and there is a variable decrease in protein 4.2. Band 3 HS is somewhat milder, on average, than HS caused by ankyrin or spectrin defects, although the diseases overlap. Interestingly, many patients have a small number of mushroom-shaped cells in blood smears. These are sometimes called "pincered" cells, as though they had been pinched by tweezers. It would be interesting to know how this unique morphology forms, and whether it accurately predicts a band 3 abnormality.

DISTAL RENAL TUBULAR ACIDOSIS

Because band 3 functions as an anion exchanger and is expressed in the acid-secreting intercalated cells of the kidney cortical collecting ducts, patients with HS and band 3 deficiency have been tested for a defect in acid-base homeostasis. Two HS patients with band 3 Pribram have incomplete dRTA (1006), as does a patient with homozygous band 3 Coimbra (863), but most other HS patients with band 3 deficiency have no evidence of metabolic acidosis (1006,1007). The patient with homozygous band 3 Coimbra, however, has chronic hyperchloremic metabolic acidosis (plasma HCO_3 = 15 mEq/L), a borderline low serum K^+ (3.5 mEq/L), nephrocalcinosis, and evidence of a distal urinary acidification defect (863). She has no detectable band 3 and is chronically transfused for life-threatening hemolysis and anemia.

In HS patients with band 3 Campinas, there is increased basal urinary bicarbonate excretion but efficient urinary acidification (996). A bovine model of band 3 deficiency exhibits only mild acidosis (1008), and there are no obvious metabolic disturbances in mice that have a targeted deletion of band 3 that eliminates both the red cell and kidney isoform (255). Band 3 missense mutations have been found in patients with dominant dRTA, but these patients have no red cell abnormality, and the mutations identified are different from those associated with HS (1007,1009–1011). Mutations affecting Arg589 are particularly common in dRTA (8 of 11 families). The mechanism by which these mutations produce RTA is a mystery. The disease does not correlate with the anion transport activity of the band 3 mutants (1007,1009), and the one tested mutant (R589H) does not have a dominant negative effect when coexpressed with normal band 3 (1007). The best possibility is that the mutant proteins may impair the trafficking of band 3 (1011).

PROTEIN 4.2 DEFECTS

The characteristics of HS due to protein 4.2 deficiency are summarized in Table 51-15. The molecular etiology of protein 4.2 deficiency has been defined in several cases. The most common mutation is protein 4.2 Nippon (Ala142→Thr) (Fig. 51-36; Table 51-16) (539,1018). It affects the processing of 4.2 mRNA, so that red cells contain only traces of the 72-/74-kd isoforms of protein 4.2 instead of the usual abundant 72-kd species. This mutation is common in Japanese HS patients. It is homozygous in some patients (1018) or compound heterozygous with a second mutant allele such as protein 4.2 Fukuoka, Notame, or Shiga (696,1013,1016).

TABLE 51-15. Hereditary Spherocytosis Due to Protein 4.2 Mutations

<5% of hereditary spherocytosis in the United States and Europe. Much more common in Japan (45% to 50%).
Autosomal recessive.
95% to 100% deficiency of protein 4.2.
4.2 Nippon common in Japan.
Variable red cell morphology: spherocytes, acanthocytes, ovalostomatocytes, normal discocytes.

Band 4.2 Komatsu contains an amino acid substitution in codon 175 that causes a moderate hemolytic anemia with ovalostomatocytosis and an increased OF in the homozygous state (809).

The only three protein 4.2 mutations reported outside the Japanese population are protein 4.2 Tozeur, protein 4.2 Lisboa, and protein 4.2 Nancy, which were found in homozygous form in Tunisian, Portuguese, and French patients, respectively (694,1014,1017). In protein 4.2 Tozeur (1014,1015), the propositus and her sister had a chronic hemolytic anemia and no protein 4.2 in their red cells. Molecular analysis showed a missense mutation in codon 310, in a region that is conserved in protein 4.2 and other members of the transglutaminase family. A recombinant protein bearing the mutation was abnormally sensitive to proteolysis, which may explain the absence of protein 4.2 in the patients' erythrocytes. In protein 4.2 Lisboa (694), a single nucleotide deletion at nucleotide 265 of the cDNA causes a frameshift mutation and premature termination of the peptide. The heterozygous parents are clinically asymptomatic. The proband presented with a hemolytic anemia and splenomegaly at the age of 20. Peripheral blood films showed only a few spherocytes. Her symptoms improved markedly after splenomegaly.

Finally, as noted above, erythrocyte protein 4.2 deficiency is sometimes secondary to mutations in the cytoplasmic domain of band 3 that affect 4.2 binding—such as band 3 Montefiore (Glu40→Lys) (203).

Protein 4.2 Nippon–deficient membranes lose 70% of their ankyrin with low ionic strength extraction (988,1019), and the

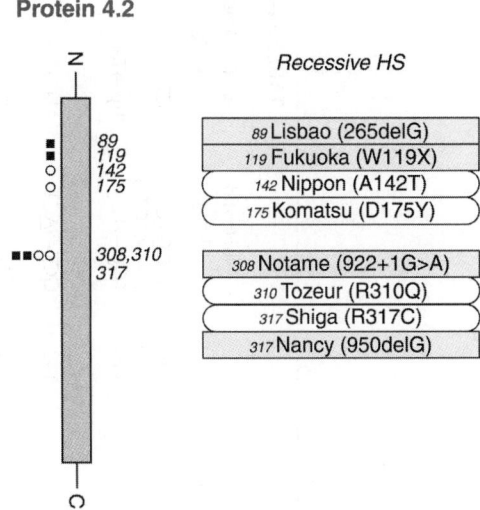

Figure 51-36. Protein 4.2 mutations associated with recessive hereditary spherocytosis (HS). Null mutations, arising from frameshifts or nonsense mutations are shown in shaded rectangles. Missense mutations are shown in open ellipses. (Adapted from Tse WT, Lux SE. Hereditary spherocytosis and hereditary elliptocytosis. In: Scriver CR, Beaudet AL, Sly WS, Valle D, eds. *The metabolic and molecular bases of inherited disease,* 8th ed. New York: McGraw-Hill, 2001:4665.)

TABLE 51-16. Protein 4.2 Defects in Hereditary Spherocytosis

Name of Variant	Exon	Codon	Nucleotide Change	Amino Acid Change	Systemic Name[a]	Type of Mutation	Inheritance	No. of Kindreds	Clinical Severity[b]	Comment	Selected References
Lisbao	2	89	AAGGTG →AAGTG	PCT	265 delG	Frameshift	AR	1	Mild	—	694
Fukuoka	3	119	TCG→TGA	Trp→Ter	W119X	Nonsense	AR	1	Mild	Compound heterozygote with Bd 4.2 Nippon	695,994
Nippon	3	142	GCT→ACT	Ala→Thr	A142T	Missense	AR	>20	Mild	Ovalostomatocytosis	539
Komatsu	4	175	GAT→TAT	Asp→Tyr	D175Y	Missense	AR	1	Moderate	Ovalostomatocytosis	1012
Notame	First base after exon 6	—	GT→AT	Ex 6 spliced out→PCT	922+1G>A	Frameshift; splicing	AR	1	Mild	Compound heterozygote with Bd 4.2 Nippon	1013
Tozeur	7	310	CGA→CAA	Arg→Gln	R310Q	Missense	AR	1	Mild	Normal red cell morphology	1014,1015
Shiga	7	317	CGC→TGC	Arg→Cys	R317C	Missense	AR	1	Mild	Spherocytosis; compound heterozygote with Bd 4.2 Nippon	1016
Nancy	7	317	CGC→CC	PCT	950 delG	Frameshift	AR	1	Mild	—	1017

AR, autosomal recessive; Bd, band; del, delete; Memb, membrane domain; PCT, premature chain termination; S, sporadic mutation; Ter, terminator codon.

[a]Mutations are abbreviated according to a described conventions in reference 933. Note that nucleotide numbers refer to the first nucleotide in the translation start ATG codon, which is numbered 1. The preceding codon is numbered −1 (there is no zero). This system conforms to the convention noted (933) but contrasts with that used by many previous authors (191,194,844,873,905,934), who numbered nucleotides from the beginning of a reported cDNA. Because more than one complete cDNA is available for many proteins, and the cDNAs often begin at different places in the 5'UTR, numbering from the beginning of the cDNA can be variable and confusing.

[b]Clinical severity was estimated using reported hematologic values presplenectomy and the criteria of Eber et al. (861) as modified by Eber and Lux (935).

ankyrin loss is blocked by preincubation of the membranes with purified protein 4.2, which suggests that 4.2 stabilizes ankyrin on the membrane. This hypothesis is supported by the observations that protein 4.2 content is low in ankyrin-deficient *nb/nb* mice (see section Animal and Fish Models of Hereditary Spherocytosis) and in HS patients who lack one ankyrin gene (621). In addition, red cells from patients homozygous for 4.2 Nippon are fragile and exhibit heat-sensitive skeletons, clumped intramembranous particles (probably band 3 molecules), and increased lateral mobility of band 3 (988,1020). However, ankyrin lability is not evident in other patients with protein 4.2 deficiency (1015,1021).

Clinically, only a small fraction of HS is due to mutations in protein 4.2 in Europeans (probably <5%), but the proportion is much higher in Japanese (45% to 50%) (988). HS due to 4.2 deficiency is usually mild and is not always uniformly spherocytic. Some patients have normal morphology (1015), some have typical microspherocytosis (1016), but most have ovalostomatocytosis (988,1022). Whether the variation is due to the specific molecular defect in protein 4.2 or to other modifier genes is unclear. The latter possibility seems more likely because affected patients have, at most, only traces of the mutant protein in their red blood cells. Red cells lacking 4.2 also show increased Na⁺ influx, a disrupted membrane skeleton when viewed in the electron microscope, and a curious heat sensitivity, in which the cells become relatively indeformable at temperatures at which normal red cells show no change (988). The molecular explanations for these phenomena are unknown.

SECONDARY DEFECTS
A large number of presumably secondary abnormalities have been identified over the years. These are catalogued and discussed in detail in earlier reviews (1023,1024).

Tight Binding of Spectrin to the Membrane. Inextractable spectrin was first observed many years ago in 2 of 12 HS patients in whom spectrin did not elute from the membrane after exposure to low ionic strength for 72 hours (1025). These are conditions that generally produce greater than 90% spectrin extraction. A second patient was subsequently discovered (1026). The molecular basis of this phenomenon has not been investigated, although the possibility that it might be secondary to a defect in ankyrin or β-spectrin seems obvious. In addition, some tightly bound spectrin is palmitoylated (1027), and this fraction might be increased. Alternatively, the muscle isoform of erythrocyte spectrin, which contains a PH domain (409) that binds to phosphoinositides, could be expressed in red cells in these patients.

Increased Membrane Hemoglobin. HS membranes contain increased amounts of Hb and catalase (1028). This is a relatively nonspecific finding that is observed in a number of hemolytic anemias. Its molecular basis is not understood.

Enolase Deficiency. Two reports of apparent HS combined with partial enolase deficiency (~50%) have appeared (1029,1030). In the first patient, a French woman, red cell OF and autohemolysis tests were typical of HS, although spherocytes were not apparent on the blood smear (1029). Dominant inheritance was suggested by history but could not be established, as the affected father was deceased. However, dominant inheritance of both HS and partial enolase deficiency was clearly evident in the second family, in which both diseases could be traced through four generations (1030). In this kindred, the enolase-deficient spherocytes resisted lysis in the AGLT—another characteristic of typical HS (see the section Acidified Glycerol Lysis Test and Pink Test). The similarity of these two cases suggests that they may represent a unique sub-

group of HS. In particular, the combination of dominant inheritance and half-normal levels of enolase raises the possibility that the primary defect could lie in an enolase-binding membrane protein, assuming such a protein exists. Conceivably, this could be one of the known HS target proteins, such as band 3 or protein 4.2. Enolase (1p36.2-36.3) and protein 4.1 (1p36.1) are only 38.2 million base pairs apart on chromosome 1, which raises the possibility of a contiguous gene deletion, but this seems unlikely given the large number of intervening genes and the lack of other stigmata.

Diminished Membrane Protein Phosphorylation. The discovery that red cell membrane proteins are phosphorylated was followed in the late 1970s and early 1980s by numerous reports that phosphorylation was defective in HS. These reports are summarized and analyzed in previous reviews (1023,1024). In short, the effects were variable from lab to lab, and they generally were only demonstrable in ghosts incubated in low ionic strength buffers for relatively long periods. Initial rates of phosphorylation in HS ghosts were normal (1031–1033), as was membrane protein phosphorylation of intact spherocytes from splenectomized individuals (1033). It now appears that the phosphorylation defects were secondary effects.

Phosphorylation-Induced Gelation of Membrane Skeletons Is Defective in Hereditary Spherocytosis. Homogenized suspensions of membrane skeletons from hereditary spherocytes gel poorly or not at all when treated with spectrin kinase, whereas normal skeletons gel firmly under the same conditions (1034). The phenomenon is not understood on a molecular level, but it is specific and reproducibly abnormal in HS (1034,1035).

Membrane Lipids. The principal lipid abnormality of hereditary spherocytes is a symmetric loss of membrane lipids as part of the overall loss of membrane surface, which is the hallmark of HS pathobiology. The relative proportions of cholesterol and the various phospholipids are normal (1036), and the phospholipids show the usual transmembrane asymmetry, even in severe cases (69). It has been reported that very-long-chain fatty acids are missing from certain classes of phospholipids in HS (1037), but this has not been confirmed (1038). It is unclear whether this difference is due to technical factors or to genetic heterogeneity of the disease. Even if real, however, it seems likely that the changes in fatty acid composition would be secondary to underlying membrane protein defects.

Cations and Transport. It has been known for many years that HS red cells are intrinsically more leaky to sodium and potassium ions than normal cells (1039,1040). Interestingly, a similar defect exists in spectrin-deficient mice (1041). The excessive sodium influx activates Na⁺,K⁺-ATPase and the monovalent cation pump, and the accelerated pumping, in turn, increases ATP turnover and glycolysis. At one time, it was believed that this modest sodium leak was responsible for the hemolysis of hereditary spherocytes (1040), particularly those cells trapped in the unfavorable metabolic environment of the spleen, but it now is clear that this is incorrect, because the magnitude of the sodium flux does not correlate with the extent of hemolysis in HS (1042). In addition, patients with hereditary stomatocytosis (to be discussed) and a much greater defect in sodium permeability do not develop microspherocytes and, sometimes, have very little hemolysis (1043). As discussed later in this chapter, the leak of sodium into red cells in hereditary stomatocytosis is accompanied by the entry of water and cell swelling—a finding that contrasts with the well-established dehydration of hereditary spherocytes.

The dehydration of HS red cells is likely to be inflicted, in part, by the adverse environment of the spleen, because spherocytes from surgically removed spleens are the most dehydrated (1044). The pathways causing HS red cell dehydration have not been clearly defined. One likely candidate is increased K^+,Cl^- cotransport, which is activated by acid pH (789). HS red cells, particularly from unsplenectomized subjects, have a low intracellular pH (1045), reflecting the low pH of the splenic environment. The K^+,Cl^- cotransport pathway is also activated by oxidation (1046), which is likely to be inflicted by splenic macrophages. The Ca^{2+}-activated, K^+ efflux (Gárdos) channel pathway is probably not involved because Ca^{2+} concentrations are not elevated in HS red cells. Finally, hyperactivity of the Na^+,K^+ pump, triggered by increased intracellular Na^+, can dehydrate red cells directly, because three Na^+ ions are extruded in exchange for only two K^+ ions (793,794). The loss of monovalent cations is accompanied by water.

Alternatively, spherocyte dehydration could be related to surface area loss. Normal cells become dehydrated during aging, with attendant surface area loss, and the red cells that lose the most surface area in patients with autoimmune hemolytic anemias or with HS are the most dehydrated. How surface area and dehydration are related is not clear. Perhaps compensatory transport channels are preferentially lost when surface area is lost.

Glycolysis. In general, glycolysis is mildly accelerated in HS red cells (1040,1047,1048), mostly to support increased cation pumping (1040), and 2,3-DPG concentrations are slightly depressed (900,901,1049), probably due to the activation of 2,3-DPG phosphatase by the acidic intracellular pH of the cell (1049). The latter abnormalities are partly due to splenic detention, because the acidosis and DPG deficiency both improve after splenectomy (900,901).

Phosphoenolpyruvate Transport. An apparently specific decrease in carrier-mediated transport of phosphoenolpyruvate has been noted in the red cells of some patients with HS (1050).

However, only nonsplenectomized patients were studied, so it is possible that the defect is secondary to the metabolic derangements these cells acquire during their detention in the spleen (to be discussed). More likely, it is caused by diminished anion exchange. Band 3 transports pyruvate, and, probably, phosphoenolpyruvate. If so, reduced phosphoenolpyruvate transport would be expected in HS patients with band 3 deficiency. Diminished phosphoenolpyruvate transport has only been reported in Japanese patients with HS, a population in which band 3 deficiency is particularly common.

ANIMAL AND FISH MODELS OF HEREDITARY SPHEROCYTOSIS

The availability of several well-characterized mouse and zebrafish models has contributed to our understanding of the pathophysiology of HS. Four types of hereditary spherocytic or elliptocytic hemolytic anemia have been identified in the common house mouse *Mus musculus* (1051): *ja/ja* (jaundice); *sph/sph* (spherocytosis) and its alleles [*sph^J^/sph^J^* (hemolytic anemia), *sph^2BC^/sph^2BC^*, and *sph^Dem^/sph^Dem^*]; *nb/nb* (normoblastosis); and *wan/wan* (Fig. 51-37). The nomenclature indicates that anemia is observed only in the homozygous state and that the mutants represent four loci: *ja*, *sph*, *nb*, and *wan*. All of the mutants have severe hemolysis, with marked spherocytosis, jaundice, bilirubin gallstones, and massive hepatosplenomegaly except the *sph^Dem^/sph^Dem^* mice, which have hereditary elliptocytosis. The defects are autosomal recessive, and the homozygotes have drastically impaired viability (491,1051,1052). There is a similar but much milder condition, designated *sp/sp*, in the deer mouse *Peromyscus maniculatus* (1053). The deer mice have mild (~20%) spectrin deficiency (Falcone JC, Lux SE, *unpublished observations*) and a phenotype that resembles typical human HS.

Spectrin Mutants. The *ja/ja* mutant has no detectable spectrin. The mice carry a nonsense mutation in the β-spectrin gene (R1160X) (1055) and lack the ability to produce stable β-chains (491).

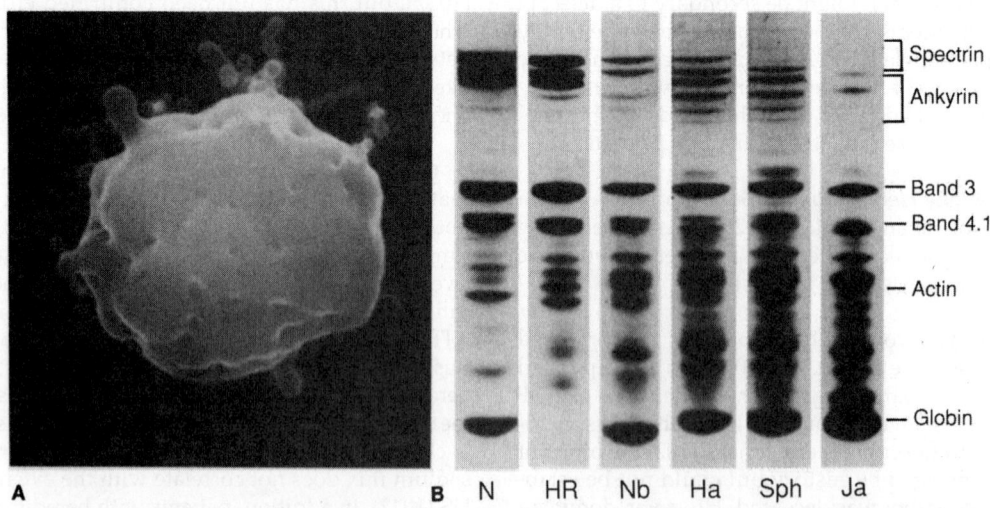

Figure 51-37. Hereditary spherocytosis mutants in mice (*Mus musculus*). **A:** Scanning electron micrograph of *sph^J^/sph^J^* ("hemolytic anemia" mutation) red cell. The marked membrane instability and spontaneous vesiculation are evident. **B:** Sodium dodecyl sulfate gels of red cell membrane proteins from normal (N) and high reticulocyte control (HR) mice and from four *Mus* mutants: *nb/nb* (Nb), *sph^J^/sph^J^* (Ha), *sph/sph* (Sph), and *ja/ja* (Ja). The *ja/ja* and *sph/sph* mutations are defects in β- and α-spectrin synthesis, respectively. Mice with the *sph^J^/sph^J^* mutation synthesize an unstable α-spectrin. The *nb/nb* mice lack ankyrin. (Reprinted from Lux SE. Spectrin-actin membrane skeleton of normal and abnormal red blood cells. *Semin Hematol* 1979;16:21, with permission.)

The *sph/sph* variants lack α-spectrin but have small amounts of β-spectrin. They have defects in α-spectrin synthesis, function, and stability (491). The *sph* and *sph²ᴮᶜ* alleles are frameshift mutations and null alleles (1056,1057). *sphʲ/sphʲ* mice, in contrast, synthesize normal amounts of spectrin mRNA and protein; however, the protein is not stably incorporated into the membrane skeleton. Surprisingly, the *sphʲ* allele contains a nonsense mutation near the C-terminus that deletes the last 13 amino acids from the protein (1057a). Apparently, these amino acids, in the EF hand region at the spectrin tail (Fig. 51-11), are functionally important in attaching spectrin to actin. The *sph⁻ᴰᵉᵐ/sphᴰᵉᵐ* mutation arose spontaneously in the CeS3/Dem strain and is missing exon 11 and 46 amino acids from spectrin repeat 5. The mice have spherocytes, elliptocytes, and some poikilocytes, and they are a cross between HS and HPP (see Hereditary Pyropoikilocytosis) (1058).

Cardiac thrombi, fibrotic lesions, and renal hemochromatosis are found in *ja/ja* and *sph/sph* mice in adulthood (1059). Transplantation of hematopoietic cells from *sph/sph* mice is sufficient to induce thrombotic events in the recipients (1060). One possibility is that the membrane vesicles released from the very unstable mouse red cells expose PS on their outer surface, which would be very thrombogenic (85). However, the amount of exposed PS is not predictive of thrombotic risk in *sphʰᵃ/sphʰᵃ* mice (1061), which suggests that it is not the critical factor.

Reisling is an induced mutation in zebrafish that results in a nearly bloodless phenotype. It is caused by a null mutation of β-spectrin (1062). Fish that are homozygous for the *reisling* defect have severe anemia and congestive heart failure. Their blood cells are spherical instead of elliptical, which is the normal shape of fish red blood cells. Scanning electron micrographs show marked membrane loss, as in other severe forms of HS. One of the interesting things about red cell β-spectrin in zebrafish is that it contains a C-terminal PH domain. This domain is spliced out of mammalian red cell spectrins (409). PH domains localize signaling components such as inositol polyphosphates and certain G-proteins within membranes, but their functions in spectrins are unknown. The fact that fish red cells are elliptical and mammalian red cells are not raises the possibility that the PH domain helps determine red cell shape.

Ankyrin Mutants. The *nb/nb* mice have 50% to 70% of the normal quantity of spectrin and no ankyrin (491,1051,1052). They have normal spectrin synthesis (491) but are moderately spectrin deficient because their ankyrin is very unstable. This contrasts with human ankyrin deficiency in which ankyrin and spectrin levels are comparably depressed. The *nb* mutation causes premature termination of the ankyrin protein in exon 36 at the beginning of the CTD (1063). A small amount of the 157-kd remnant is found in mature *nb/nb* red cells (1063,1064) and, along with some expression of an Ank-2 (or Ankᴳ)–related peptide, may explain why fetal *nb/nb* mice have normal reticulocyte counts and no anemia at birth (1064,1065) and, perhaps, why the red cell membranes are not more spectrin deficient. Humans may also be protected *in utero*, at least partially, because hydrops fetalis has not been reported in patients with ankyrin defects or probable ankyrin defects (i.e., combined spectrin-ankyrin deficiency)—even in patients who become transfusion dependent after birth.

The *nb/nb* mice develop ataxia when they reach maturity due to the loss of cerebellar Purkinje cells (652). Ank-1 (or Ankᴿ) protein is markedly reduced in the Purkinje cells, which may explain their fragility. Spinocerebellar degeneration and related syndromes have also been reported in a few adults with HS, although it is not yet known whether ankyrin is affected.

Band 3. New mouse mutants with defects in membrane skeleton proteins have been generated by targeted mutagenesis in embryonic stem cells. Mice completely deficient in band 3 survive gestation but tend to die in the neonatal period (255), often from thrombotic complications (254). Those that survive have a severe spherocytic hemolytic anemia that closely resembles severe HS in humans. The mice have undetectable amounts of protein 4.2 and GPA (241,255) but normal amounts of spectrin, actin, and protein 4.1 in their red cell membrane skeletons, and they have normal membrane skeleton architecture by electron microscopy (255). Despite their normal skeletons, the band 3–deficient red cells shed astonishing amounts of membrane surface in small vesicles and long tubules (Fig. 51-38). These observations indicate that band 3 is, surprisingly, not required for membrane skeleton assembly, but it has a critical function in

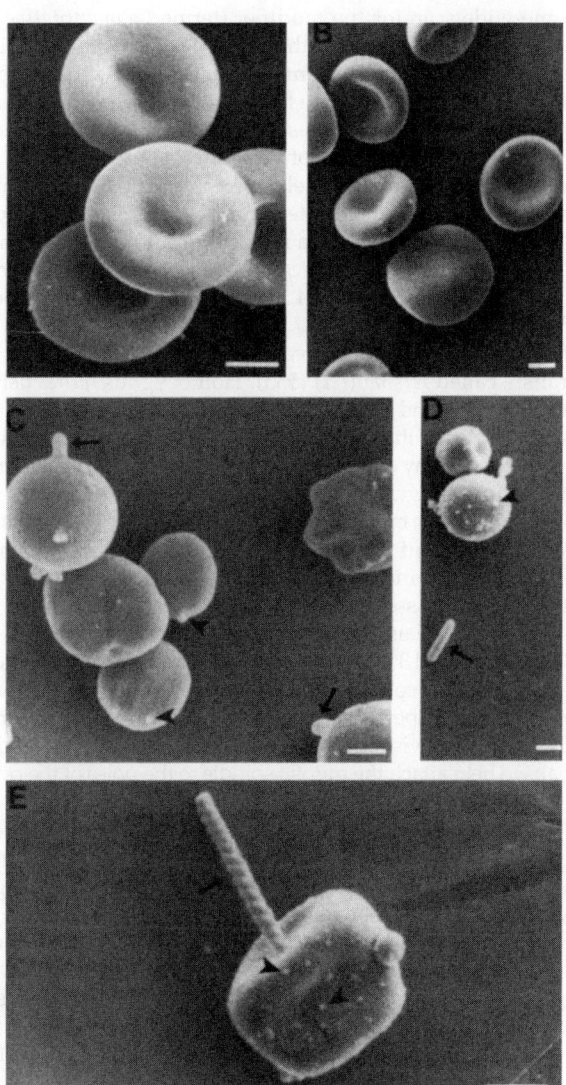

Figure 51-38. Marked membrane fragility of mice lacking band 3. Scanning electron micrographs of red cells from wild-type (**A**), heterozygous (**B**), and homozygous band 3–deficient (**C–E**) mice. Note the markedly spherocytic shape of the band 3⁻/⁻ red blood cells. Many are shedding multiple tiny membrane vesicles (*arrowheads*). Others extrude rodlike membrane extensions (*arrows*), which are frequently detached (**D**, *arrow*). The membrane extensions often reach considerable length and are highly coiled (**E**). (Bar = 1 μm.) [Adapted from Peters LL, Shivdasani RA, Liu SC, et al. Anion exchanger 1 (band 3) is required to prevent erythrocyte membrane surface loss but not to form the membrane skeleton. *Cell* 1996;86:917.]

stabilizing membrane lipids. Loss of this function may be critical to the pathogenesis of HS.

These mice also provide an unexpected clue about the genetic control of anemia in band 3–deficient HS. Approximately 15% of the band 3 knock-out mice, in a C57BL/6J and 129/Sv (B6/129) hybrid genetic background, survived beyond weaning; however, later generations of the mice, inbred on a C57BL/6 background, show a striking decrease in survival; all die in the neonatal period.

A newly discovered mouse mutant (*wan*) in a C3H/HeJ background that has a null defect in the band 3 gene (1066) has an equally severe anemia (100% lethal in neonatal period). But when the *wan/wan* mice are crossed to wild-type *Mus castaneus* mice, the F$_2$ generation shows a wide variation in severity, from lethal anemia to normal hematologic values [Hb, hematocrit, mean corpuscular volume (MCV)]. These observations show that a strong genetic modifier is segregating in the *M. castaneus* background. A genome-wide scan for the modifier (termed a *quantitative trait locus*, or QTL), using MCV as the variable trait, identified a single QTL on chromosome 12 centered over the β-spectrin gene (1067)—an obvious candidate for a modifier gene. *M. castaneus*- and *M. musculus*-C3H/HeJ β-spectrins differ by 3 amino acids, but it is not yet known if one of these affects function.

In addition to mouse models, there is a recessive form of HS in cattle with mild to moderate hemolytic anemia and complete deficiency of band 3, due to a nonsense mutation at codon 646 (1008). The cattle, like band 3–deficient mice, have defective anion transport, lack protein 4.2, and have a reduced number of IMPs by electron microscopy.

There is also an informative induced mutation in band 3 in zebrafish, called *retsina* (*ret*) (533). Homozygous *ret/ret* fish are almost bloodless and have a lethal anemia. The rare *ret/ret* red cells are spherical rather than elliptical and shed a large number of membrane vesicles. Many of the red cells are binucleate, as are late erythroblasts. Interestingly, band 3–*wan/wan* and band 3 knock-out mice also contain excess binucleate erythroblasts, which suggests that the absence of band 3 is associated with a defect in cytokinesis. Indeed, mitotic spindles in *ret/ret* erythroblasts are grossly disrupted, and the masses of DNA separate poorly and interfere with cell cleavage, explaining the high frequency of binucleate cells (533). Because band 3 is only expressed in erythroblasts and one cell type in the kidney collecting duct, the data imply that vertebrates have developed a special kind of cytokinesis for the last one or two erythroblast cell divisions: a cytokinesis that depends on band 3— perhaps to help attach the mitotic spindle to the poles of the cell.

Protein 4.2. The absence of protein 4.2 is not responsible for the severe phenotype observed in band 3 knock-out mice, because mice with a targeted deletion of the protein 4.2 gene survive normally and have only a mild spherocytic hemolytic anemia (209). Interestingly, the 4.2-deficient mouse red cells have *dramatic* increases in several cation transport pathways, suggesting that protein 4.2 directly or indirectly regulates the associated transporters. This totally unexpected finding illustrates the value of gene knock-outs for uncovering new biology.

Protein 4.1. Mice lacking erythrocyte protein 4.1 (protein 4.1R) have also been generated by gene targeting (557). Homozygotes have moderate hemolysis with increased fragmentation and decreased red cell membrane stability. In addition to the total absence of protein 4.1, the mice lack protein p55 and have reduced levels of GPC. There is also partial deficiency of ankyrin and spectrin, suggesting that loss of protein 4.1 compromises membrane skeleton assembly. Erythrocyte morphology shows spherocytosis instead of elliptocytosis; this is probably related to the spectrin deficiency. Interestingly, these

mice also have neurologic deficits in movement, coordination, and learning, presumably because neuronal isoforms of erythroid protein 4.1 are also disrupted (551).

Two zebrafish mutants, *merlot* (*mot*) and *chablis* (*cha*), also lack protein 4.1 and have a very severe hemolytic anemia characterized by marked membrane loss, microshperocytosis, osmotic fragility, and disruption of the marginal band of microtubules found in fish RBCs (1067a).

β-Adducin. Due to a targeted gene deletion, mice deficient in β-adducin have recently been described (575). The mice have a mild hemolytic anemia characterized by spherocytes, spherostomatocytes, and rounded elliptocytes; a partial deficiency of α-adducin; and a compensatory increase in γ-adducin, which, like β-adducin, pairs with α-adducin. The phenotype indicates that β-adducin is needed for the maintenance of normal red cell surface area. This is an original observation, because no human patient deficient in adducin has yet been described.

Dematin. Mice lacking the headpiece of dematin (band 4.9), which contains the actin-binding and -bundling functions of the protein, have less actin associated with the skeleton and more extractable spectrin and actin than normal (1068). They also exhibit a very mild spherocytic hemolytic anemia. The data support a model in which the headpiece of one dematin molecule interacts with the tail of a neighbor to form the dematin trimer.

Pathophysiology

LOSS OF MEMBRANE SURFACE BY VESICULATION

The primary membrane lesions described above, almost all involving "vertical interactions" between the skeleton and the bilayer, fit the prevailing theory that HS is caused by the local disconnection of the skeleton and bilayer, followed by the vesiculation of the unsupported surface components. This, in turn, leads to progressive reduction in membrane surface area and to a shape called a *spherocyte*, although it usually ranges between a thickened discocyte and a spherostomatocyte (1069). The phospholipid and cholesterol contents of isolated spherocytes are decreased by 15% to 20%, which is consistent with the loss of surface area (1070,1071).

The evidence supporting the vesiculation theory is substantial. Careful biomechanical measurements show that HS membranes are fragile. The force required to fragment the membrane is diminished and is proportional to the density of spectrin on the membrane (Figs. 51-28 and 51-29) (954,956). Membrane elasticity and bending stiffness are also reduced and proportional to spectrin density (956). In addition, HS red cells lose membrane more readily than normal when metabolically deprived (1072–1074) or when their ghosts are subjected to conditions facilitating vesiculation. This has not been shown to occur in metabolically healthy spherocytes in typical autosomal-dominant HS, perhaps because it occurs slowly (~1% to 2%/day) under such conditions. However, massive vesiculation is evident in mice or fish with extremely severe spherocytic hemolytic anemias, such as the homozygous band 3 knock-out or band 3-*wan/wan* mice or homozygous *reisling*, *retsina*, or *merlot/chablis* zebrafish (255,533,1062,1066).

Because budding red cells are rarely observed in typical HS blood smears, even when many cells are examined, membrane loss probably involves microscopic vesicles and may occur preferentially in bywaters of the circulation such as the reticuloendothelial system. When membrane vesicles are induced in normal red cells, they originate at the tips of spicules, where the lipid bilayer uncouples from the underlying skeleton (Fig. 51-22) (763). The vesicles are small (approximately 100 nm) and devoid of Hb and skeletal proteins, so they are invisible during a conventional examination of stained blood films. Tiny (50 to 80 nm) bumps on the surface of HS

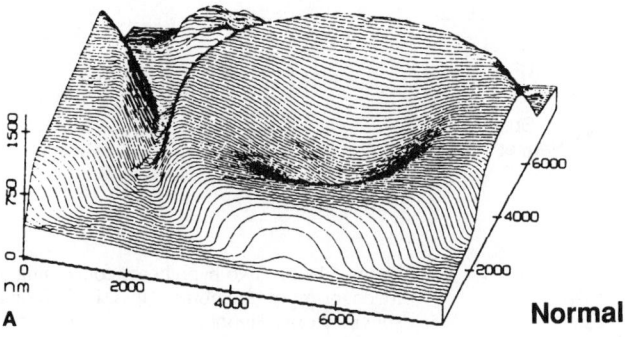

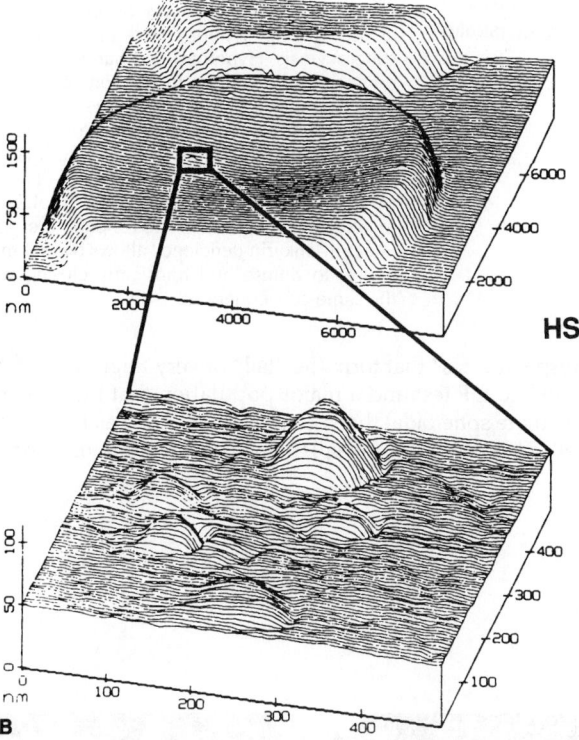

Figure 51-39. Comparison of the surface of a normal red cell (**A**) and a hereditary spherocyte (HS) (presplenectomy) (**B**) by atomic force microscopy. Note that at high magnification, 50- to 80-nm pseudopodia are evident on the surface of the spherocyte, which may represent membrane microvesicles (bottom of **B**). These were not observed postsplenectomy. (Reprinted from Zachèe P, Boogaerts MA, Hellemans L, Snauwaert J. Adverse role of the spleen in hereditary spherocytosis: evidence by the use of the atomic force microscope. *Br J Haematol* 1992;80:264, with permission.)

red cells obtained from patients who are actively hemolyzing have been detected in studies with an atomic force microscope (1075) (Fig. 51-39). The bumps are probably microvesicles, although this needs to be proven using more conventional microscopic techniques. They are approximately the length of a spectrin molecule (100 nm) and are not present on red cells from splenectomized patients—consistent with the slower rate of surface loss and much longer lifespan of HS red cells postsplenectomy.

Is Hereditary Spherocytosis Caused by Spectrin Deficiency or a Lack of Lipid–Band 3 Interactions? The observation that spectrin or spectrin-ankyrin deficiencies are common in HS has led to the suggestion that they are the primary cause of spherocytosis. According to this hypothesis (Fig. 51-40; hypothesis 1), interactions of spectrin with bilayer lipids or proteins are

required to stabilize the membrane. Spectrin-deficient areas would tend to bud off, leading to spherocytosis. However, this conjecture does not explain how spherocytes develop in patients whose red cells are deficient in band 3 or protein 4.2 but have normal amounts of spectrin (745,1019,1076).

The alternate hypothesis (Fig. 51-40; hypothesis 2) argues that the bilayer is stabilized by interactions between lipids and the abundant band 3 molecules. Each band 3 contains approximately 14 hydrophobic transmembrane helices, many of which must interact with lipids. Such interactions presumably spread beyond the first layer of lipids and influence the mobility of lipids in successive layers. In deficient red cells, the area between band 3 molecules would increase, on average, and the stabilizing effect would diminish. Transient fluctuations in the local density of band 3 could aggravate this situation and allow unsupported lipids to be lost, resulting in spherocytosis. Such a hypothesis is supported by early microscopic studies of the aggregation of IMPs, which leads to IMP-free domains (768). These domains are unstable, giving rise to surface blebs that are subsequently released from the cells as vesicles.

Spectrin- and ankyrin-deficient red cells could become spherocytic by a similar mechanism. Because spectrin filaments corral band 3 molecules and limit their lateral movement (1077), a decrease in spectrin would allow band 3s to diffuse and transiently cluster, fostering vesiculation. However, it is more likely that both mechanisms operate to different degrees in different diseases—hypothesis 1 dominating in spectrin and ankyrin defects, and hypothesis 2 controlling in band 3 and protein 4.2 disorders.

LOSS OF CELLULAR DEFORMABILITY

Hereditary spherocytes hemolyze because of the rheologic consequences of their decreased surface to volume ratio. The red cell membrane is very flexible, but it can only expand its surface area approximately 3% before rupturing (1078). Hence, the cell becomes less and less deformable as surface area is lost. For HS red cells, poor deformability is only a hindrance in the spleen, because the cells have a nearly normal lifespan after splenectomy (1079,1080).

SEQUESTRATION OF HEREDITARY SPHEROCYTES IN THE SPLEEN

Spherocytes Are Detained at the Cordal-Sinus Junction. In the spleen, most of the arterial blood empties directly into the splenic cords—a tortuous maze of interconnecting narrow passages formed by reticular cells and lined with phagocytes (1081–1086). Histologically, this is an "open" circulation, but, apparently, most of the blood that enters the cords normally travels by fairly direct (i.e., functionally closed) pathways (1085,1086). If passage through these channels is impeded, red cells are diverted deeper into the labyrinthine portions of the cords where blood flow is slow, and the cells may be detained for minutes to hours. Whichever route is taken, the circulation red cells must squeeze through spaces between the endothelial cells that form the walls of the venous sinuses to reenter. Even when maximally distended, these narrow slits are always much smaller than red cells (Fig. 51-41), which are greatly distorted during their passage (1083,1085).

Experiments show that spherocytes are selectively sequestered at this juncture (1087). As a consequence, spleens from HS patients have massively congested cords and relatively empty sinuses (1081,1088–1090). In electron micrographs, few spherocytes are seen in transit through the sinus wall (1081,1089,1091) in contrast to normal spleens in which transiting cells are readily found (1085).

Hypothesis 1:

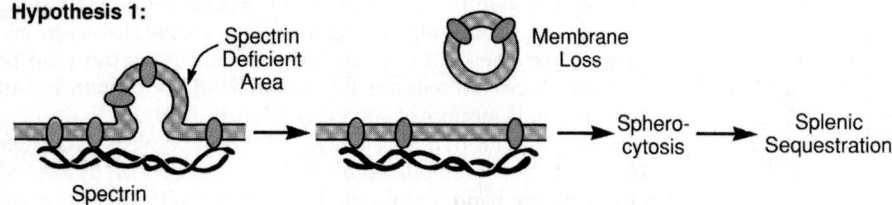

Hypothesis 2:

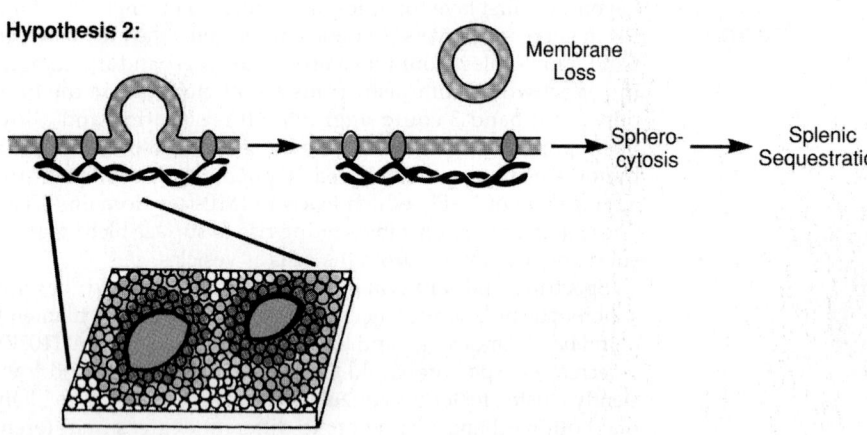

Figure 51-40. Two hypotheses concerning the mechanism of membrane loss in hereditary spherocytosis. Hypothesis 1 assumes that the "membrane" (i.e., the lipid bilayer and integral membrane proteins) is directly stabilized by interactions with spectrin or other elements of the membrane skeleton. Spectrin-deficient areas, lacking support, bud off, leading to spherocytosis. Hypothesis 2 assumes the membrane is stabilized by interactions of band 3 with neighboring lipids. The influence of band 3 extends into the lipid milieu because the first layer of immobilized lipids slows the lipids in the next layer and so on. In band 3–deficient cells, the area between lipid molecules increases, and unsupported lipids are lost. Spectrin-ankyrin deficiency allows band 3 molecules to diffuse and transiently cluster, with the same consequences.

Spherocytes Are "Conditioned" in the Spleen. There is also abundant evidence that HS red cells suffer during detention in the spleen. In unsplenectomized HS patients, two populations of spherocytes are detectable: a minor population of hyperchromic "microspherocytes" that form the "tail" of very fragile cells in the unincubated OF test and a major population that may be only slightly more spheroidal than normal. By 1913, it was known that red cells obtained from the splenic vein were more osmotically

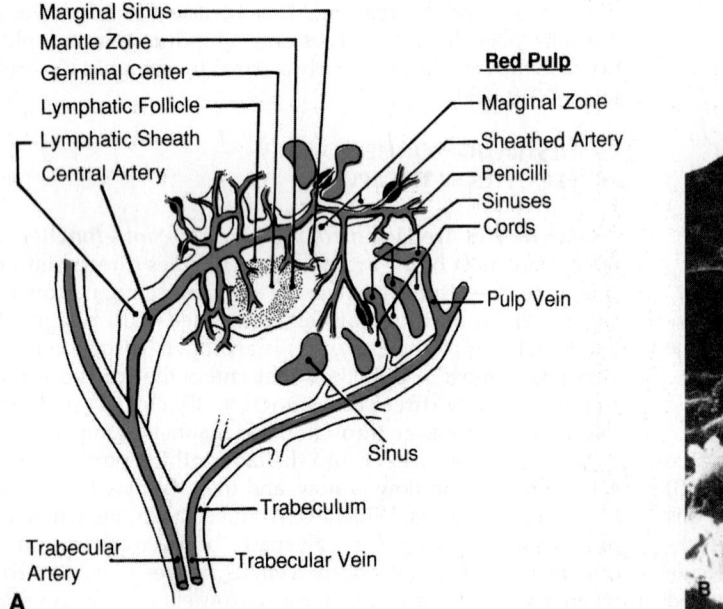

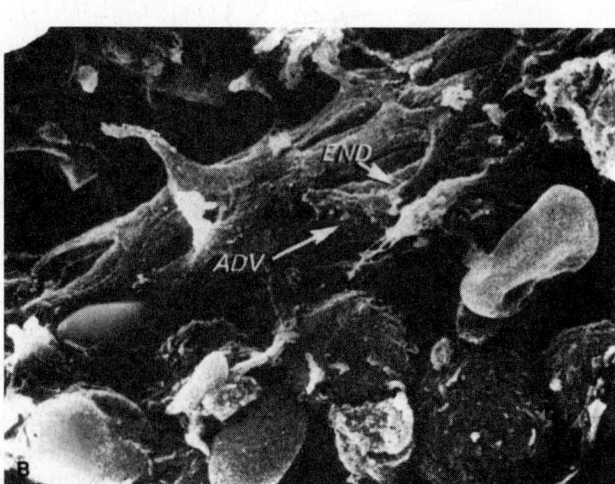

Figure 51-41. Splenic anatomy. **A:** Schematic illustration of the anatomy of the spleen. Note that blood entering the splenic cords must pass through the walls of the splenic sinuses to reenter the venous circulation. **B:** Scanning electron micrograph of a splenic sinus viewed from within the splenic cords. The narrow transmural slits between the endothelial cells (END) and adventitial cells (ADV) of the sinus are evident. The edges of these slits probably touch each other in the normal spleen, so the openings are potential structures rather than fixed pores. They are revealed here because of a drying artifact. Note that the adjacent erythrocytes are considerably larger than the slits and, hence, must be flexible to pass into the splenic sinuses and return to the venous circulation. (Electron micrograph reprinted from Weiss L. A scanning electron microscopic study of the spleen. *Blood* 1974;43:665, with permission.)

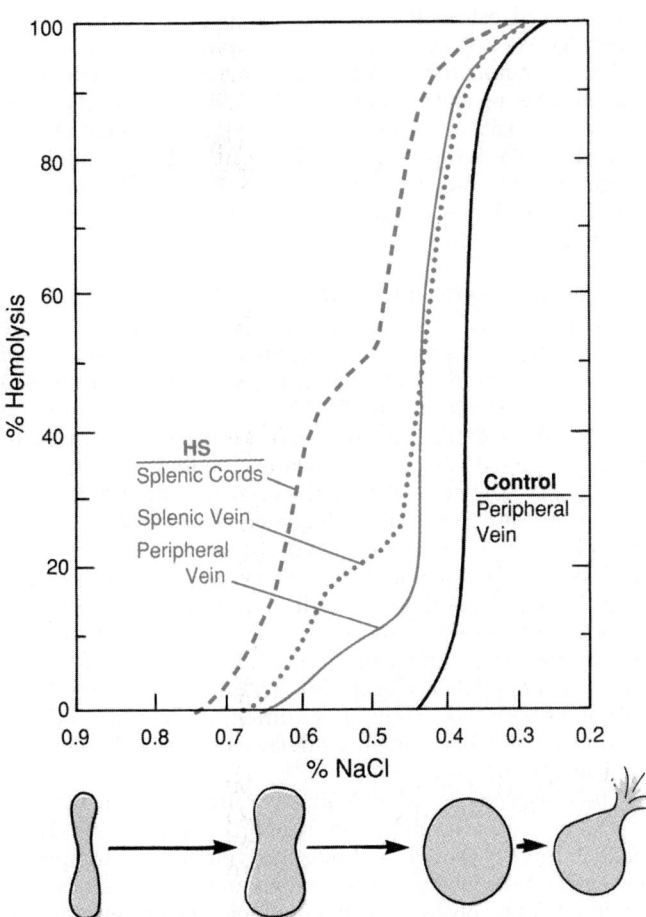

Figure 51-42. Osmotic fragility in hereditary spherocytosis (HS). In the osmotic fragility test, red cells are suspended in salt solutions of varying tonicities between isotonic saline (0.9% NaCl) (*left*) and distilled water (*right*). Normal red cells swell in hypotonic media and eventually reach a limiting spheric shape, beyond which they hemolyze (*bottom*). Spherocytes, which begin with a lower than normal surface to volume ratio, can swell less before they reach their limiting volume; hence, their osmotic fragility curve is shifted to the left (higher salt concentrations). They are said to be *osmotically fragile*. Before splenectomy, a small proportion of the red cells are extra fragile and produce a "tail" on the osmotic fragility curve. The cells have been "conditioned" by the spleen as shown by their higher concentration in the splenic vein and especially in the splenic cords.

fragile than those in the peripheral circulation (1092), and this fact was confirmed by other hematologists of the time (854,855,1093); however, its significance was not clear until the classic studies of Emerson (1094) and Young (1087) in the early 1950s. These investigators showed that osmotically fragile microspherocytes are concentrated in and emanate from the splenic pulp (Fig. 51-42). After splenectomy, spherocytosis persists, but the tail of hyperfragile red cells is no longer evident (1087,1094,1095). These and other data led to the conclusion that the spleen detains and "conditions" circulating HS red cells in a way that increases their spheroidicity and hastens their demise (1087,1094,1096). The kinetics of this process were beautifully illustrated *in vivo* by Griggs (1096), who found that a cohort of ^{59}Fe-labeled HS red cells gradually shifted from the major, less fragile population to the more fragile, conditioned population 7 to 11 days after their release into the circulation. Although most conditioned HS red cells that escape the spleen are probably recaptured and destroyed, the damage incurred is sufficient to permit extrasplenic recognition and removal, because conditioned spherocytes, isolated from the spleen and reinfused postoperatively, are rapidly eliminated (1096,1097).

Splenic Cords Are Metabolically Inhospitable. The mechanism of splenic conditioning is less certain. It is difficult to obtain accurate information about the cordal environment, but the existing data suggest that it is metabolically inhospitable (1094,1098,1099), although perhaps less so than originally believed (1086). Crowded red cells must compete for limited supplies of glucose (1099) in acidic surroundings (pH ~6.8 to 7.2) (1086,1094,1098) in which glycolysis is inhibited (1100,1101). The acidic environment induces chloride and water entry and cell swelling (1102), but it also stimulates the K^+,Cl^- cotransporter, which produces a net loss of potassium and water from the cells. The adverse effects of the cordal environment are further compounded by the oxidant-producing macrophages. Hence, the spherocyte, detained in the splenic cords because of its surface deficiency, is stressed by erythrostasis in a metabolically threatening environment.

ERYTHROSTASIS

As Ham and Castle (840) and Dacie (1103) first recognized, the HS red cell is particularly vulnerable to erythrostasis. This is the basis of the well-known autohemolysis test. During prolonged sterile incubation in the absence of supplemental glucose, red cells undergo a series of changes that culminate in hemolysis (1024). The sequence of the changes is the same for HS and normal erythrocytes; however, because HS cells are abnormally leaky and bear unstable membranes, their degeneration is accelerated.

HS red cells are initially jeopardized because their membrane permeability to Na^+ is mildly increased (1039,1040). Their propensity to accumulate Na^+ and water is normally balanced by increased Na^+ pumping; however, the increased dependence on glycolysis is detrimental in erythrostasis in which substrate is limited (1040). HS red cells exhaust serum glucose and become ATP depleted more rapidly than normal red cells. As ATP levels fall, ATP-dependent Na^+,K^+ and Ca^{2+} pumps fail, and the cells gain Na^+ and water and swell. Later, when the Ca^{2+}-dependent K^+ (Gárdos) pathway is activated, K^+ loss predominates, and the cells lose water and shrink. The Na^+ gain is accelerated in HS red cells but is insufficient by itself to induce hemolysis. However, HS red cells are doubly jeopardized. As noted earlier, they are inherently unstable and fragment excessively during metabolic depletion (1072–1074). Membrane lipids (and probably integral membrane proteins) are lost at more than twice the normal rate (1073). At first, this surface loss is balanced by cell dehydration, but eventually (30 to 48 hours) membrane loss predominates, the cells exceed their critical hemolytic volume, and autohemolysis ensues (1024).

CONSEQUENCES OF SPLENIC TRAPPING

Calculations (1024) indicate that the average normal red cell passes through the splenic cords approximately 14,000 times during its lifetime and has an average transit time of 30 to 40 seconds—surprisingly close to measured transient times in normal human spleens *in vivo* (1104). The calculated residence time of the average HS red cell in the splenic cords is much longer—perhaps as long as 15 to 150 minutes (1024)—but is still far short of the time required for metabolic depletion to occur.

This conclusion is supported by direct analysis of splenic red cells. As shown in Table 51-17, HS red cells obtained from the splenic pulp and containing 80% to 100% conditioned cells are moderately cation depleted and show changes in ADP and 2,3-DPG concentrations consistent with metabolism in an acidic environment, but their ATP levels are normal (1044). Others have reported similar findings (1105,1106).

Oxidants May Exacerbate Membrane and Water Loss in Hereditary Spherocytosis Red Cells. The data suggest that splenic conditioning is caused by mechanisms other than ATP

TABLE 51-17. Comparison of Splenic Cordal and Circulating Red Blood Cells in Hereditary Spherocytosis

	Peripheral RBCs (30% Conditioned)[a]	Splenic Cordal RBCs (90% Conditioned)[a]
Na$^+$ (mEq/L RBC)	10 ± 2	17 ± 3
K$^+$ (mEq/L RBC)	78 ± 7	58 ± 12
Na$^+$ + K$^+$ (mEq/L RBC)	89 ± 9	75 ± 13
ATP (mmol/L RBC)	1.48 ± 0.16	1.46 ± 0.18
ADP (mmol/L RBC)	0.40 ± 0.08	0.85 ± 0.14
2,3-DPG (mmol/L RBC)	4.72 ± 0.35	3.02 ± 0.57
ATP turnover (relative specific activity)	102 ± 9	93 ± 7

ADP, adenosine diphosphate; ATP, adenosine triphosphate; DPG, diphosphoglycerate; RBC, red blood cell.
[a]As measured by osmotic fragility tests.
Data from Mayman D, Zipursky A. Hereditary spherocytosis: the metabolism of erythrocytes in the peripheral blood and in the splenic pulp. *Br J Haematol* 1974;27:201–217.

depletion. For example, potassium loss and membrane instability may be exacerbated by the high concentrations of acids and oxidants that must exist in a spleen filled with activated macrophages lunching on trapped HS red cells. *In vitro*, oxidants from activated phagocytes can diffuse across the membranes of bystander red cells and damage intracellular proteins within minutes. Red cells moving through the rapid transit pathways in the spleen might escape damage, but those trapped in cordal traffic would be vulnerable. Oxidants, even in relatively low concentrations, cause selective K$^+$ loss by a variety of mechanisms (1107–1109) and also damage membrane skeletal proteins (75,801,823,824,945,961,1110,1111). Finally, there is preliminary evidence that HS red cells may be abnormally sensitive to oxidants (1112). When exposed to peroxides, they undergo remarkable blebbing (and presumably vesiculation) (1113) due to skeletal damage (1114). If a similar process occurs in the spleen, it could be responsible for the excessive surface loss observed in conditioned cells.

Splenic Residence May Activate Membrane Proteases.
Residence in the spleen may also activate proteolytic enzymes in the red cell membrane. Membrane proteins of HS red cells from patients with splenomegaly are excessively digested during *in vitro* incubations, and the degree of proteolysis correlates with splenic size (1115). Oxidatively damaged membrane proteins are also subject to proteolysis *in vitro* (962). Whether this occurs *in vivo* is uncertain, but, if so, it could contribute to skeletal weakness and membrane loss.

Macrophages May Directly Condition Hereditary Spherocytes. The possibility that macrophages may directly condition HS red cells must also be considered. It is well known that spherocytosis often results from the interaction of IgG-coated red cells with macrophages, but HS red cells do not have abnormal levels of surface IgG (1116). Macrophages also bear receptors for oxidized lipids (scavenger receptor) and PS, but there is no evidence at present that HS red cells expose the relevant ligands. The involvement of macrophages is supported by the careful, but frequently ignored, observations of Coleman and Finch (1117), who found that large doses of cortisone markedly ameliorated HS in nonsplenectomized patients. The effects were similar to those produced by splenectomy. Hb production, reticulocytosis, and fecal urobilinogen declined; red cell lifespan doubled; and hyperspheroidal, conditioned red cells disappeared from the circulation. This has subsequently been confirmed in HS patients treated with prednisone (1118). It is well known that similar

doses of corticosteroids inhibit splenic processing and destruction of IgG- or C3b-coated red cells in patients with immunohemolytic anemias, probably by suppressing macrophage-induced red cell sphering and phagocytosis (1119,1120). Electron microscopy shows that splenic erythrophagocytosis is common in HS, particularly in the splenic cords (1089,1091,1121). In addition, phagocytes expressed from the cords of HS patients contain bits of ghostlike "debris" (1122), presumably resulting from membrane fragmentation.

SUMMARY OF PATHOPHYSIOLOGY

It is clear that HS red cells are selectively detained by the spleen and that this custody is detrimental, leading to a loss of membrane surface that fosters further splenic trapping and eventual destruction (Fig. 51-43). The primary membrane defects involve deficiencies of spectrin, ankyrin, protein 4.2, or band 3, but much remains to be learned about how this causes surface loss. The current speculation is that the HS skeleton (including band 3) may not adequately support all regions of the lipid bilayer, leading to loss of small areas of untethered lipids and integral membrane proteins. As discussed earlier, it is not clear whether this is due directly to a deficiency of spectrin and ankyrin or to a spectrin-ankyrin deficiency that operates indirectly by increasing the lateral mobility of band 3 molecules and decreasing their stabilization of the lipid bilayer, or both (Fig. 51-40). In addition, the loss of band 3 in HS due to band 3 or protein 4.2 defects may directly diminish lipid anchoring.

The mechanisms of splenic conditioning and red cell destruction are also uncertain. Kinetic considerations (1024) make it unlikely that HS red cells are continuously trapped in the cords for the long periods required to induce passive sphering and autohemolysis by metabolic depletion; however, repetitious accrual of metabolic damage remains a possibility. A special susceptibility of the HS red cell to the acidic, oxidant-rich environment of the spleen and to the active intervention of macrophages in the processing of damaged spherocytes must also be considered.

Laboratory Features

Many of the laboratory features of HS are common to all hemolytic processes. These include reticulocytosis, erythroid hyperplasia of the bone marrow, unconjugated (indirect) hyperbilirubinemia, and increased fecal urobilinogens (890,891).

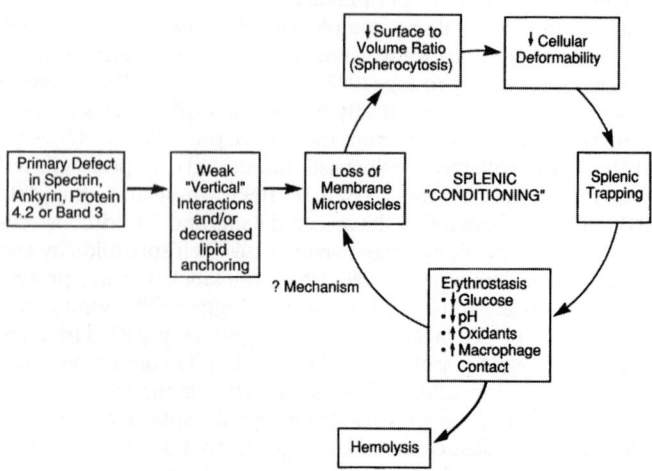

Figure 51-43. Pathophysiology of the splenic conditioning and destruction of hereditary spherocytes.

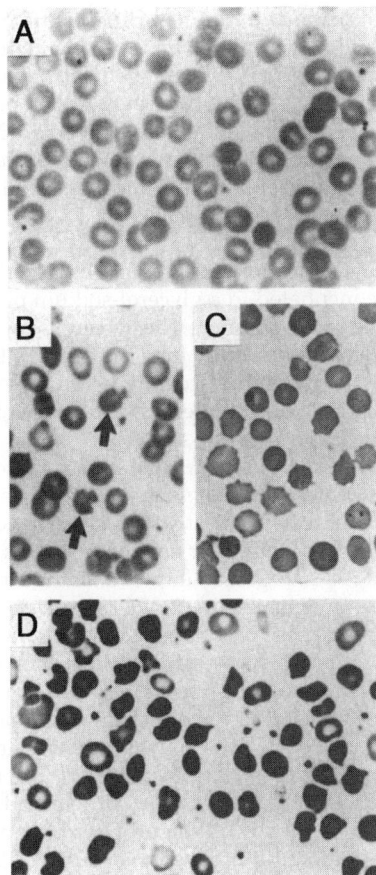

Figure 51-44. Red cell morphology in hereditary spherocytosis (HS). **A:** HS due to an ankyrin defect. Microspherocytes are evident among red cells with some central pallor. **B:** Band 3–deficient HS. Mushroom-shaped ("pincered") red cells (*arrows*) are found in approximately 80% of patients with this form of HS (1124). **C:** HS due to a β-spectrin mutation. Echinocytes and acanthocytes (5% to 15%) are usually observed in addition to typical spherocytes. **D:** Severe HS with spherocytes and bizarre poikilocytes (490,906). (Reprinted from Palek J, Lambert S. Genetics of the red cell membrane. *Semin Hematol* 1990;27:290, with permission.)

Plasma Hb is normal, and haptoglobin is only variably reduced (1123), because most of the Hb that is released when hereditary spherocytes are destroyed is catabolized at the site of destruction ("extravascular hemolysis"). Besides the spherocytic morphology, the laboratory tests that distinguish HS from other causes of hemolysis usually measure the biophysical properties of the affected red cells, among which the OF test is the standard test. Biochemical analysis and DNA analysis of the membrane skeleton proteins, which are performed only in a few research laboratories, allow determination of the primary molecular defects underlying HS.

RED CELL MORPHOLOGY
Spherocytes are the hallmark of HS and are reliably present (97%) (861) in patients with moderate or moderately severe disease. However, approximately 25% to 35% of mild HS patients lack the characteristic microspherocytes (861,890,891). Although hereditary spherocytes appear spheroidal in conventional dried smears, most are actually thickened diskocytes, stomatocytes, or spherostomatocytes when examined in the scanning electron microscope (1069).

The various subtypes of HS, discussed above, have subtle differences in red cell morphology (1123a). Patients with ankyrin defects and combined spectrin and ankyrin deficiency (the most

common subtype) (194,888) have typical round spherocytes and microspherocytes (Fig. 51-44; panel A). Combinations of spiculated red cells (acanthocytes) and spherocytes are observed in HS due to defects in β-spectrin (panel C) (941–945,1125). Patients with more severe spectrin deficiency, such as those who are homozygotes or compound heterozygotes for α-spectrin defects or who have severe spectrin and ankyrin deficiency, have proportionally more misshapen spherocytes, spiculated red cells, and bizarre poikilocytes, which may dominate the blood smear in the most severe cases (904,953) (panel D). Most patients with band 3 deficiency have rare (0.2% to 2.3%) mushroom-shaped (or "pincered") red cells in their peripheral blood smears (979,1126) (panel B). Red cell morphology is variable in protein 4.2 deficiency and may even be normal (1015). Most patients appear to have mild spherocytosis or ovalostomatocytosis, but acanthocytes and poikilocytes are sometimes observed (1012). Spherocytes combined with elliptocytes suggest spherocytic HE, which is most often associated with truncated β-spectrin chains (see Spherocytic Hereditary Elliptocytosis).

Recent work indicates that HS red cells lose most of their surface area in the bone marrow before their emergence as reticulocytes (1127). Once in the circulation, they lose surface at the same rate as normal erythrocytes. This contrasts with the spherocytes observed in autoimmune hemolytic anemia, in which most of the cells' surface area is lost in the circulation (1127).

Nucleated red cells are uncommon in HS blood smears (890) except in the most severe forms (953). Howell-Jolly bodies are also uncommon before splenectomy (only 4% of patients) (890) and suggest reticuloendothelial blockade (906).

RED CELL INDICES
The MCHC of HS red cells is increased due to cellular dehydration. Spherocyte Na^+ concentrations are normal or slightly increased, but K^+ concentration and water content are low (1044,1128), particularly in cells harvested from the splenic pulp. The nature of the permeability defect has not been thoroughly investigated with modern techniques. The average MCHC exceeds the upper limit of normal (36%) in approximately one-half of HS patients (891), but all patients have some dehydrated cells.

The mean corpuscular hemoglobin (MCH) and MCV fall within the normal range in HS (891), except in severe HS, in which the MCV may be slightly low (953). However, the MCV is relatively low for the age of the cells (reticulocytes have a high MCV) in all HS patients, reflecting the dehydrated state of HS red cells. In addition, the reticulocyte MCV is also low, which contrasts with the spherocytosis of autoimmune hemolytic anemia, in which reticulocyte indices are normal and total cellular MCV is increased (1127).

The profile of the volume and Hb concentration of individual red cells can now be measured with automated blood counters using dual angle laser light scattering [Bayer (Technicon/Advia) analyzers] (1129). In HS blood samples, there is almost always a right shift of the Hb concentration histogram, with a population of hyperdense cells (MCHC >40 g/dL) due to red cell dehydration, and a broadening of the volume curve, due to the mixture of small microspherocytes and large young erythrocytes (1130,1131). In our and others' experience (1132,1133), this is sufficient to identify all, or nearly all, HS patients (Fig. 51-45). We find this simple method is one of the easiest and most accurate ways to diagnose HS. It is particularly useful when one member of a family is already known to have HS and an inexpensive method of screening other family members is needed.

Similar diagnostic information can be obtained from the data generated by aperture impedance (Coulter) analyzers (1134). The combination of a high MCHC, a widened red cell distribu-

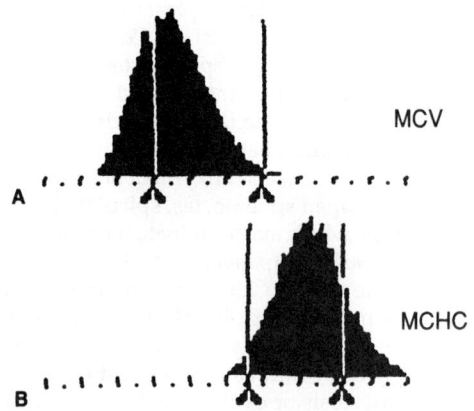

Figure 51-45. Histograms of the distribution of mean cell volume (MCV) **(A)** and mean cell hemoglobin concentration (MCHC) **(B)** in red cells of a patient with hereditary spherocytosis before splenectomy. The vertical lines mark the normal limits of the distributions. For the volume distribution, they separate microcytic (less than 60 fL) and macrocytic (greater than 120 fL) cells from normocytic red cells (60 to 120 fL). For the hemoglobin concentration distribution, they separate hypochromic (less than 28 g/dL) and hyperdense (greater than 41 g/dL) cells from normochromic red cells (28 to 41 g/dL). The data were collected with a Technicon H1 laser scattering blood counter. Note that the hereditary spherocytosis patient has subpopulations of microcytes (low MCV) and dehydrated cells (high MCHC). All patients in this study (n = 21) (1133) had similar subpopulations. (Reprinted from Pati AR, Patton WN, Harris RI. The use of the Technicon H1 in the diagnosis of hereditary spherocytosis. *Clin Lab Haematol* 1989;11:27, with permission.)

tion width, and shifts in distribution curves is often enough to suggest a diagnosis of HS (1134). Studies also show that in nonsplenectomized HS patients, the percentage of microcytes best reflects the severity of the disease, whereas the percentage of hyperdense cells best discriminates HS patients from normal individuals (1131). The presence of hyperdense cells is, however, not specific to HS, as it is also seen in other disorders such as Hb SC and Hb CC disease, hereditary xerocytosis, and autoimmune hemolytic anemia.

FRAGILITY AND AUTOHEMOLYSIS TESTS

Osmotic Fragility Test. The OF test is performed by suspending red cells in buffered solutions containing various concentrations of sodium chloride (1094,1135). In hypotonic solutions, red cells swell until they become spherical and then burst (Fig. 51-42). Cells that begin with a decreased surface to volume ratio, like spherocytes or stomatocytes, reach the spherical limit at a lower salt concentration than normal cells and are termed *osmotically fragile*. The method of Parpart (1135) is recommended with the modified buffers introduced by Godal (1136).

The OF test, particularly the incubated OF, is the most useful test available for HS. This is surprising because OF reflects a secondary property of HS red cells (the loss of surface area) instead of the primary molecular defect. However, in our experience, direct quantitation of membrane proteins rarely, if ever, detects patients missed by the incubated OF test and is *much* more difficult and expensive to perform.

The unincubated OF test provides useful information on the proportion of "conditioned" red cells—data that are lost in the incubated test (1087,1094,1095). However, 20% to 25% of HS patients have a normal unincubated OF, particularly patients with mild HS (who are the most difficult to diagnose) (892,1137).

The incubated OF test is more sensitive than the unincubated OF test (1137) and is almost always positive. The test is performed the same way, but the whole blood sample is first

incubated for 24 hours at 37°C. During this time, HS red cells become metabolically depleted and lose membrane fragments more rapidly than normal, which accentuates their spheroidicity and enhances the sensitivity of the test. HS patients with a normal incubated OF have been described (1138), and such patients may be even more common than reported (1131), but the incubated OF test remains the gold standard in the diagnosis of HS.

Acidified Glycerol Lysis Test and Pink Test. In this test, red blood cells are incubated in a glycerol-sodium phosphate–buffered hypotonic saline solution. The glycerol slows the entry of water into the cells, so that the time for the cells to lyse is prolonged and can be measured accurately. The glycerol lysis time is shortened for hereditary spherocytes because of the reduced surface to volume ratio.

The original test (1139) lacked the necessary sensitivity and specificity (1140). An acidified version (AGLT) was more sensitive (1141), although insufficiently so in some hands (1142), and was not completely specific. For unknown reasons, the accuracy of the standard AGLT is greatly improved if the samples are preincubated at room temperature for 24 hours (incubated AGLT) (1143–1145). Under these conditions, the sensitivity and specificity of the test approach 100%—similar to the incubated OF test.

Eber (860) reinvestigated the buffers used in the test and found that simply increasing the sodium phosphate concentration from 5.3 to 9.3 mM gives 100% sensitivity and specificity without the need for the preincubation step. The modified test is easy to perform and requires very little blood. Ethylenediaminetetraacetic acid (EDTA) blood (20 µL) is diluted into a solution of 9.3 mM sodium phosphate–buffered 2 M glycerol-saline with a pH of 6.9, and the fall in absorbance at 625 nm (largely turbidity) is measured as the red cells hemolyze. The $T_{1/2}$ for AGLT lysis is more than 30 minutes for normals and less than 5 minutes for HS samples (860). The simplicity and sensitivity of this test make it an excellent test for rapid screening of a large number of microblood samples.

Another adaptation of the original glycerol lysis test, called the *Pink test*, is more reproducible and accurate than the original test (1146), but it also profits from a 1-day preincubation (1147). The test has been adapted for fingerstick blood samples (1147,1148); however, direct comparisons suggest it is less specific than the OF or incubated AGLT tests (1143,1148).

Hypertonic Cryohemolysis Test. This relatively new method (1149) is based on the fact that HS red cells are particularly sensitive to cooling at 0°C in hypertonic conditions, which causes them to lyse and release their Hb. Hypertonic cryohemolysis is said to be more sensitive than other tests, especially in mild cases of HS and asymptomatic carriers (1150); however, although some find it is specific (1151), others find it is positive in some patients with elliptocytosis and other hemolytic anemias and in some forms of congenital dyserythropoietic anemia (1152). The advantages of the test include its simplicity, its high sensitivity, and the ability to use EDTA-preserved blood samples obtained for routine hematologic studies. However, the hypertonic cryohemolysis test is still new, and its limitations are not yet fully understood.

Autohemolysis Test. The autohemolysis of HS red cells, incubated in their own plasma in the absence of added glucose, is increased at 48 hours (892,1103,1153). In most HS patients, less autohemolysis occurs if supplemental glucose is added (892,1153,1154). This is not always true in more severe HS (1155), which can cause diagnostic confusion because autohemolysis that is unresponsive to glucose is a feature of some

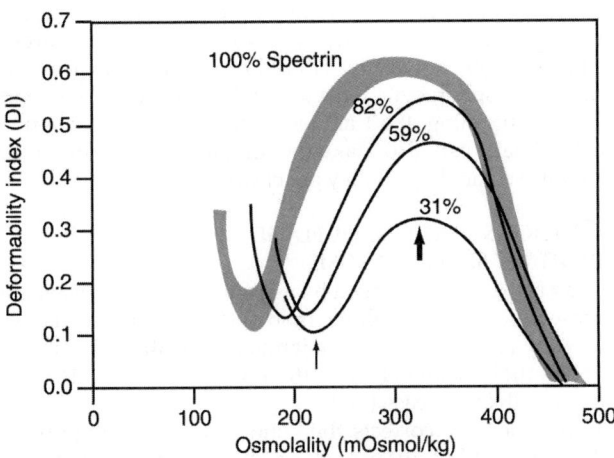

Figure 51-46. Osmotic gradient ektacytometry of red blood cells with varying degrees of spectrin deficiency. In the spectrin-deficient cells, the minimum deformability index observed in the hypotonic region (*thin arrow*) is shifted to the right of the control (*shaded area*), indicating a decrease in the cell surface area to volume ratio. The maximum deformability index (DI_{max}) associated with the spectrin-deficient cells (*thick arrow*) is less than that of control cells, implying reduced surface area. The more pronounced the spectrin deficiency, the greater is the loss of surface area and the lower is the DI_{max}. The osmolality in the hyperosmolar region at which the DI reaches half its maximum value is a measure of the hydration state of the red cells. It is decreased in the patient with the lowest spectrin content, indicating cellular dehydration. (Adapted from Tse WT, Lux SE. Hereditary spherocytosis and hereditary elliptocytosis. In: Scriver CR, Beaudet AL, Sly WS, Valle D, eds. *The metabolic and molecular bases of inherited disease*, 8th ed. New York: McGraw-Hill, 2001:4665.)

other hemolytic anemias (1153). In general, the autohemolysis test lacks specificity but is relatively sensitive, and it is occasionally useful in confirming the diagnosis of mild or sporadic cases of HS.

EKTACYTOMETRY
Ektacytometry is a very useful method for measuring the biophysical properties of intact erythrocytes (1156). The ektacytometer is described in the section Hereditary Elliptocytosis and Pyropoikilocytosis. "Osmotic gradient ektacytometry," a modification of the original technique, is particularly useful in the diagnosis of HS. In this method, the deformability index of the red cell sample is measured as a function of the osmolarity of the suspending medium, which is continuously varied (Fig. 51-46). The osmolality of the suspending medium at which the red cell deformability index reaches a minimum is the same as the osmolarity at which 50% of the red cells hemolyze in an OF test (954,1157). This value indirectly measures the surface area to volume ratio of the red cells. The maximum deformability index of the curve quantitatively reflects the surface area of the red cells (1131). In patients with HS, there is a shift of the curve to the right, demonstrating the reduced surface area to volume ratio of the cells, and a decline in the height of the curve, reflecting a decrease of the absolute surface area. Even though this technique is only available in a small number of laboratories at present, it provides useful diagnostic information that cannot be obtained otherwise and deserves greater availability. Cynober and co-workers, for instance, showed that increased OF is only detected in 66% of nonsplenectomized HS patients, whereas decreased membrane surface area can be demonstrated in all the patients by osmotic gradient ektacytometry (1131).

MEMBRANE PROTEIN, RNA, AND DNA MEASUREMENTS
Membrane protein concentrations are most easily assessed using SDS gels. Individual stained bands are quantified by densitometry

or by eluting the dye from an excised band and measuring its concentration spectrophotometrically (149). This technique is satisfactory for detecting spectrin deficiency (expressed as a spectrin to band 3 ratio) (1158), although it is not as accurate as an RIA (149,164) or ELISA immunoassay (888), in part because band 3 is lost with other surface components as spherocytes circulate. This is even truer for ankyrin, which is present in smaller amounts and migrates close to β-spectrin on gels. SDS gels do not give reliable results even with a gel system that optimizes the spectrin-ankyrin separation (164) (Fig. 51-4). The popular Laemmli SDS gels are completely unsatisfactory because ankyrin migrates between the spectrin bands in this system. SDS gels are satisfactory for detecting band 3 deficiency (elevated spectrin to band 3 ratio) or protein 4.2 deficiency, and they are useful in combination with antibody staining (Western blots) for detecting mutant proteins of altered size.

However, SDS gels do not always identify the abnormal protein in HS, partly because deficiencies as small as 10% can cause disease, and partly because missense mutations may cause functional rather than quantitative defects. Several approaches have been used to define specific molecular defects.

1. In families with multiple affected members, lack of genetic linkage between HS and polymorphic markers for α- or β-spectrin, ankyrin, band 3, or protein 4.2 can be used to *exclude* specific proteins from consideration.

2. Frameshift and nonsense mutations are common in HS and are often accompanied by absence of the mutant mRNA as well as protein due to nonsense-mediated mRNA decay (1159–1162). This can be detected by loss of heterozygosity of a polymorphic reticulocyte cDNA marker of one of the five candidate HS genes compared to the same marker in genomic DNA (985). This method has also been used to detect *de novo* dominant mutations in HS patients without a positive family history (870).

3. Finally, suspect proteins can be sequenced using genomic DNA and polymerase chain reaction (PCR) primers to amplify each exon (194). However, most of the proteins that cause HS are large and contain many exons, so this approach is arduous.

At present, there are no laboratories that identify the molecular defects in HS membrane proteins commercially. Analyses are limited to research studies. Because most of the mutations are one-of-a-kind defects restricted to a specific family, and because the nature of the mutation does not predict the severity or complications of the disease or the response to splenectomy, this is not a serious limitation. The few common mutations, such as α-spectrin[LEPRA] or protein 4.2 Nippon can be detected by PCR, if needed.

Diagnosis

The diagnosis of HS is usually easy if there are typical laboratory findings of spherocytosis, Coombs'-negative hemolysis, increased OF, and a positive family history. There are several situations in which the diagnosis can be more difficult. Other causes of spherocytosis are listed in Table 51-18.

ABO INCOMPATIBILITY
In the neonatal period, it may be hard to differentiate HS from ABO incompatibility because microspherocytosis is prominent in both and the Coombs' test is occasionally negative in ABO disease that is severe enough to produce spherocytosis (1163). In most affected infants with ABO incompatibility, anti-A (or anti-B) antibodies can be eluted from the red cells, and free anti-A or anti-B IgG antibodies can be detected in the infants' serum.

IMMUNOHEMOLYTIC ANEMIAS
Occasionally, older patients with immunohemolytic anemias and spherocytosis have so few antibody molecules attached to

TABLE 51-18. Diseases in Which Spherocytosis Is the Predominant Morphology

Common
  Hereditary spherocytosis
  Immunohemolytic anemias (warm antibody type)
  ABO incompatibility in neonates
Uncommon to rare
  Clostridial sepsis
  Hemolytic transfusion reactions
  Severe burns and other red cell thermal injuries
  Spider, bee, and snake venoms
  Severe hypophosphatemia
  Acute red cell oxidant injury (glucose-6-phosphate dehydrogenase deficiency during hemolytic crisis or favism, oxidant drugs, and chemicals)[a]
  Hawkinsinuria

[a]Acute red cell oxidant injury is common, but spherocytosis is only rarely the predominant morphology.

their red cells that the Coombs' test is negative, and the differentiation of the disease from HS is possible only with the use of radioactive antiglobulin reagents, the so-called super-Coombs' test (1164).

HEINZ BODY HEMOLYTIC ANEMIAS
Spherocytosis is also seen in Heinz body hemolytic anemias during an acute hemolytic crisis (see Chapter 49). The diagnosis is suggested by the presence of bite cells and blister cells on peripheral blood films and by detecting Heinz bodies in red cells stained with methyl violet.

APLASTIC CRISES
As discussed below, diagnostic difficulties also arise in patients who present during an aplastic crisis. Early in the crisis, the acute nature of the symptoms may suggest an acquired process, and the absence of reticulocytes may divert the physician from

a diagnosis of hemolytic anemia. Later, as marrow function returns, physicians may occasionally be misled by the properties of the emerging young HS red cells, which acquire their typical microspherocytic form only with age and reticuloendothelial conditioning. If a transfusion has been given, the transfused red cells can also make the diagnosis of the underlying HS disease difficult until they are cleared.

CONDITIONS THAT CAMOUFLAGE HEREDITARY SPHEROCYTOSIS
HS may also be camouflaged by association with disorders that increase the surface to volume ratio of the red cells, such as iron deficiency (1165), obstructive jaundice (1070), β-thalassemia (1166), α-thalassemia (1167), vitamin B_{12} or folate (1168) deficiency, or Hb SC disease (1169).

Iron deficiency corrects the abnormal shape, fragility, and high MCHC of hereditary spherocytes but does not improve their lifespan (1165), whereas obstructive jaundice improves both shape and survival (1070). For example (Fig. 51-47), we have seen a young girl who developed jaundice and symptoms of biliary obstruction at 6 years of age. She had a palpable spleen tip, evidence of mild compensated hemolysis (Hb = 14 g/dL; reticulocytes = 3.3%) and a normal peripheral blood smear and OF test (fresh and incubated). Abdominal x-ray studies showed calcified stones in the gallbladder and common bile duct. After cholecystectomy and relief of the partial biliary obstruction, the child's hemolysis worsened (reticulocytes = 10.8%), and she developed anemia (Hb = 10.2 g/dL), spherocytosis, and a definitely abnormal incubated OF test. She subsequently responded to splenectomy.

The variability of HS in a large French family in which HS and the β-thalassemia trait are independently segregating (1166) strongly suggests that β-thalassemia ameliorates and partially masks HS. Patients with both traits have signs of both diseases: small, HbA₂-rich, osmotically fragile cells and some spherocytes on peripheral blood smears.

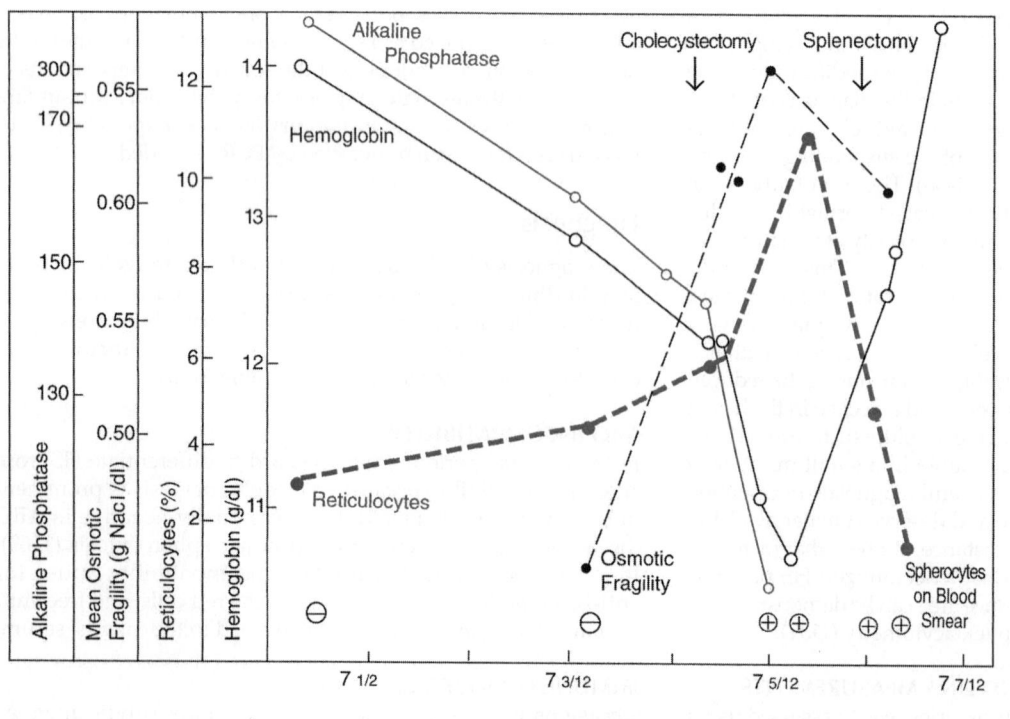

Figure 51-47. Hereditary spherocytosis camouflaged by obstructive jaundice. Patient CD presented at 7 years, 1 month of age with a history of recurrent abdominal pain, vomiting, jaundice, and evidence of biliary obstruction (four gallstones in the common duct). She had a normal hemoglobin, a normal osmotic fragility test, a near normal reticulocyte count, and normal red cell morphology. After cholecystectomy and relief of her obstruction (note fall in alkaline phosphatase), she developed florid hereditary spherocytosis (increased osmotic fragility, reticulocytosis, anemia, and spherocytosis), which improved, as expected, after splenectomy. CD's course clearly shows that loss of red cell surface area is responsible for hemolysis in hereditary spherocytosis and that conditions that increase red cell surface area, such as biliary obstruction (1070), can camouflage hereditary spherocytosis.

TABLE 51-19. Classification of Crises

Type	Anemia	Reticulocytes	Jaundice	Cause	Comment
Hemolytic	Increased	Increased	Increased	Viral infections → splenomegaly	Frequent, usually mild.
Aplastic	Increased	Decreased	Decreased	Parvovirus B19	Occurs once, severe, risk to pregnant contacts.
Megaloblastic	Increased	No change or decreased	No change or increased	Relative folic acid deficiency	Rare, preventable. Particularly likely during pregnancy.

α-Thalassemia also modifies HS (1167). The hemolytic rate is diminished by the increased osmotic resistance of the α-thalassaemia trait in the patients with both disorders. Coexistence of Hb H disease and HS results in an asymptomatic state.

Megaloblastic anemia can also mask HS (1168)—at least the morphologic characteristics of the disease. OF is also improved. The masking effect is observed in both vitamin B_{12} (Lux SE, *unpublished observations*) and folate (1168) deficiencies and is rapidly reversed after correction of the nutritional deficit.

Coinheritance of HS and Hb SC disease may exacerbate the hemoglobinopathy. A 14-year-old boy with both diseases was much more anemic than his SC siblings and had five splenic sequestration crises (1169). However, the two diseases may also disguise each other, at least partially. Only a few spherocytes or target cells were evident on the boy's blood smear, and the surface area to volume ratio of his red cells (and probably their OF) was normal. Presumably, this is due to the balancing effects of HS (loss of surface area) and Hb SC (loss of cell volume) on red cells. Even sickle trait may be worsened by HS. Yang et al. (1170) recently reported two patients with the combination who experienced multiple splenic sequestration crises. On the other hand, spontaneous regression of HS, presumably due to the development of a hyposplenic state, has been observed in two family members who had HS and the sickle cell trait (1171).

In these unusual cases, special tools may be needed to confirm the diagnosis of HS, such as immunoassays for red cell membrane proteins (149,888,953) or osmotic gradient ektacytometry (Fig. 51-46), which independently measures surface area and volume (1156,1157).

ATYPICAL HEREDITARY SPHEROCYTOSIS

Zail and co-workers have described a family with a dominantly inherited disorder characterized by spherocytosis and mild compensated hemolysis in which fresh red cells had a normal or decreased OF, and ^{51}Cr-labeled red cells lacked the characteristic pattern of splenic sequestration that is typical of HS (1172).

HEREDITARY SPHEROCYTOSIS WITH INVOLVEMENT OF NONERYTHROID TISSUES

Two adults with HS and a poorly defined, slowly progressive spinocerebellar degenerative syndrome have been described (1173). The existence of similar cases in the older European literature (1174–1180) and the subsequent discoveries that erythrocyte ankyrin (652,678) and β-spectrin (409) are expressed in the cerebellum and spinal cord and that mice with an inherited lack of ankyrin develop delayed cerebellar ataxia due to slow loss of Purkinje cells (652) suggests that these patients might have unique spectrin or ankyrin defects.

Similarly, the recent reports of hypertrophic cardiomyopathy segregating with HS in three generations of a Russian family (1181) and of spherocytosis with a movement disorder and myopathy in two brothers (1182) are of interest because erythroid spectrin and ankyrin are also known to be expressed in muscle (409,1183–1185).

Complications

CRISES

Patients with HS, like patients with other hemolytic diseases, are subject to crises (Table 51-19).

Hemolytic Crises. Hemolytic crises are probably the most frequent, particularly mild hemolytic crises, which usually occur with viral syndromes, particularly in children. They are characterized by a mild transient increase in jaundice, splenomegaly, anemia, and reticulocytosis. Severe hemolytic crises occur, but they are rare. Characteristic features include jaundice, anemia, vomiting, abdominal pain, and tender splenomegaly. Hemolysis can also be aggravated during pregnancy (1186,1187). For most patients with a hemolytic crisis, supportive care is all that is needed; red cell transfusions are rarely required. Corticosteroids can be beneficial during severe episodes of acute hemolysis (1118) but are generally not indicated.

Aplastic Crises. Aplastic crises are less frequent but more serious. Severe anemia and death (854,893) can result. The sequence of events is best described in the classic article of Owren (1188) and is illustrated in Figure 51-48. During the aplastic phase, the hematocrit level and reticulocyte count fall, marrow erythroblasts disappear, and unused iron accumulates in the serum (1188). As production of new red cells declines, the cells that remain age, and microspherocytosis and OF increase. However, bilirubin levels may decrease as the number of abnormal red cells that can be destroyed declines. The return of marrow function is heralded by a fall in the serum iron concentration and the emergence of granulocytes, platelets, and, finally, reticulocytes (Fig. 51-48). The serum phosphorus can fall to very low levels (0.5 to 1.0 mg/dL) during this recovery.

It is now clear that aplastic crises are usually caused by parvovirus B19 (1189,1190) [see Chapter 9 or recent reviews (1191,1192)]. Parvovirus B19 typically causes erythema infectiosum or fifth disease in small children and fever, rash, and polyarthropathy in older children and adults. In children with HS, the viral infection often presents with fever, vomiting, and abdominal pain, along with pallor, extreme lassitude, and other symptoms of anemia (1193,1194).

The virus infects and kills early erythroid precursors (1195–1197) and drastically impairs red cell production, resulting in aplastic crises in patients who have erythrocytes with a shortened lifespan, like HS patients. Sometimes, multiple family members are affected simultaneously (1193,1198). Parvovirus infections are often associated with mild neutro-

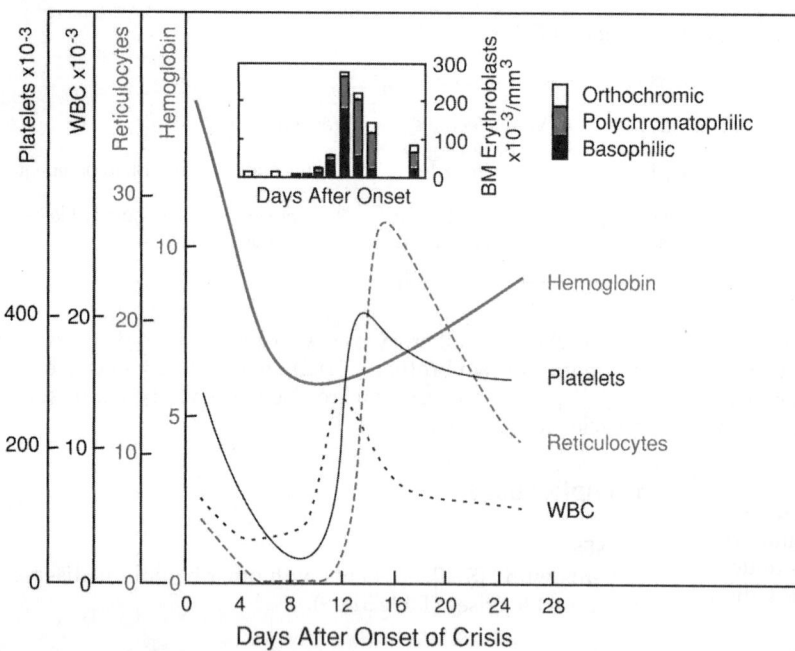

Figure 51-48. The temporal sequence of a severe aplastic crisis in a patient with hereditary spherocytosis. Note the marked reticulocytopenia and the mild-moderate leukopenia and thrombocytopenia during the aplastic phase (in this case, the leukopenia and thrombocytopenia are more severe than usual). Note also that reticulocytosis and recovery are heralded by a rise in peripheral blood granulocytes and platelets and by reappearance of bone marrow (BM) normoblasts. WBC, white blood cell. (Adapted from Owren PA. Congenital hemolytic jaundice. The pathogenesis of the hemolytic crisis. *Blood* 1948;3:231.)

penia (~20%) or thrombocytopenia (~40%) (1199), and isolated cases of transient pancytopenia (1200–1202), hemophagocytosis (1203–1205), and myelodysplasia (1206,1207) are reported in HS patients and others. Rarely, glomerulonephritis, Henoch-Schönlein purpura, meningitis, and other rheumatic manifestations (including Raynaud's phenomenon, lupuslike diseases, antiphospholipid antibodies, and microangiopathic vasculitic syndromes) have also been associated with parvovirus B19.

The virus is a particular danger to pregnant women because it can cause fetal death due to anemia and nonimmune hydrops fetalis (1208–1210). Fortunately, the risk of hydrops for women who become infected during pregnancy is low (1209,1211,1212). For example, in one recent study, none of the 52 fetuses of infected woman developed hydrops (1212). Nevertheless, because the virus is highly contagious and is easily transmitted to patients and staff (1213,1214), and because nearly 50% of the pregnant population does not have protective antibodies (1212,1215), all patients who have or are suspected of having an aplastic crisis should be placed on precautions while hospitalized, and IgG-negative contacts who are pregnant should be tested for evidence of seroconversion. Hydrops can be detected by ultrasound and has been successfully treated with intrauterine transfusions (1216–1219).

The infection is diagnosed by immunologic tests or by PCR (1220). Examination of the bone marrow shows loss of erythroblasts beyond the pronormoblast stage and, in some cases, characteristic giant pronormoblasts with cytoplasmic vacuoles.

It is important to realize that an aplastic crisis may be first evidence of HS in a patient with compensated hemolysis (mild HS) (1221–1223) and that the lack of reticulocytes should not eliminate hemolytic anemias from diagnostic consideration. Diagnostic confusion may also arise during reemergence of marrow function when the physician may mistake an aplastic crisis for a hemolytic one.

Because aplastic crises usually last 10 to 14 days (1188) (approximately one-half the lifespan of HS red cells) (1104,1224), the Hb value typically falls to approximately one-half its usual level before recovery occurs. For this reason, aplastic crises are a serious threat to young children with HS,

particularly children with more severe forms of the disease, and require careful observation.

Treatment is supportive until the aplastic episode is over. Red cell transfusions may be necessary if the anemia is severe. Intravenous Ig helps clear persistent parvovirus infection in immunocompromised patients but is not necessary for most HS patients. Persons with erythema infectiosum are infectious before the onset of illness and not infectious once the rash appears, but patients in aplastic crisis are contagious from before the onset of symptoms to at least 1 week afterward (1225). HS patients should avoid exposure to other family members with HS during this period. Droplets and contact precautions to prevent spread of parvovirus through respiratory secretions are necessary (1225). A parvovirus vaccine is currently undergoing phase I trials and may be available in the future for patients with HS.

Megaloblastic Crises. Megaloblastic crises are rare. They occur when the dietary intake of folic acid is inadequate for the increased needs of the erythroid HS bone marrow. This need is particularly acute during pregnancy (909,910) and during recovery from an aplastic crisis. Even though megaloblastic crises are rare, recent evidence suggests that folic acid intake in normal individuals may be inadequate to minimize plasma homocysteine (1226), a known atherogenic risk factor. Presumably, the risk of folate deficiency is even greater in HS patients. Accordingly, we recommend that all patients with HS (or other hemolytic anemias) routinely receive folic acid supplements (~1 mg/day) to prevent megaloblastic crises and to optimize homocysteine metabolism.

GALLSTONES

Pigment gallstones have been detected in young children with HS (1227) but are most common in adolescents and adults. In a retrospective study of 152 consecutive cases of HS conducted before the development of ultrasonography, Bates and Brown (1228) only found gallstones in 5% of children younger than 10 years of age who were adequately examined, but the incidence rose to 40% to 50% in the second to fifth decades and 55% to 75% thereafter (Fig. 51-49). The rise in the incidence of gallstones after 30 years of age paralleled the incidence in the general population (1229), which suggests that cholelithiasis due to HS is primarily manifest in the second and third decades.

The incidence of gallstones in HS patients is apparently related to the ability of the liver to metabolize bilirubin. A very common mutation in the promoter of the uridine diphosphate–glucuronyl transferase gene (*UGT-1A*) has recently been shown to be associated with reduced uridine diphosphate–glucuronyl transferase activity in heterozygotes and to cause Gilbert syndrome in homozygotes (920). A preliminary study of the frequency of gallstones in 103 HS children showed that the rate of gallstone formation in patients homozygous for the mutated *UGT-1A* allele is 2.1 times that of heterozygous patients and 4.5 times that of normals (1230). If this result is confirmed, analysis of this allele should be useful in predicting the risk of gallstones in HS.

The pigment stones typical of HS and other hemolytic anemias are easily detected by ultrasonography. All HS patients should have ultrasound examinations approximately every 5 years and before splenectomy. The high incidence of cholelithiasis and the risks of its complications are the major impetus for splenectomy in many HS patients. However, it is not clear how often patients with pigment gallstones develop symptomatic gallbladder disease or biliary obstruction. Anecdotal reports in the old HS literature suggest that 40% to 50% of HS patients with cholelithiasis have symptoms and that a high proportion of stone-containing gallbladders have histologic evidence of cholecystitis (1231). However, studies that include large numbers of patients with mild HS show a much lower incidence of symptomatic gallbladder disease (1232). Clearly, more accurate data about the long-term complications of pigment stone disease are needed to assess the risk to benefit ratio of splenectomy in HS and the need for cholecystectomy in the asymptomatic patient with stones.

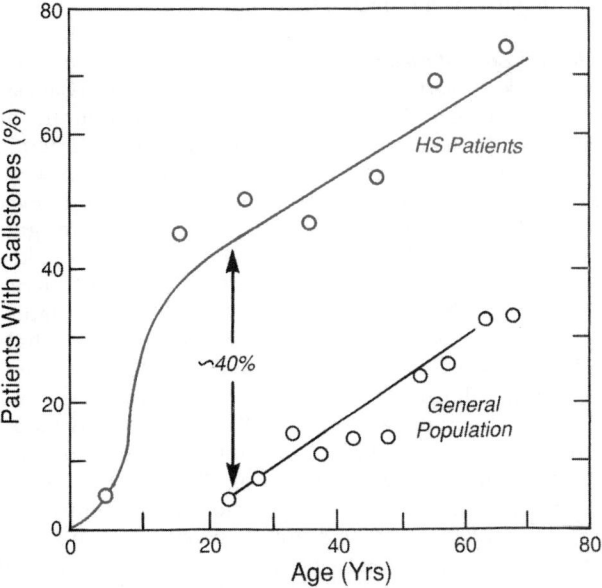

Figure 51-49. Proportion of normal and hereditary spherocytosis (HS) patients with gallstones as a function of age. Data are from a study (1228) of gallbladder disease in 152 consecutive patients seen at The Cleveland Clinic before 1952. Only patients whose gallbladders were examined at surgery or by cholecystography are included. Data for the general population are from an autopsy series of patients who did not have hemolytic anemia (1229). Note that the prevalence of gallstones rises sharply between the ages of 10 and 30 years and parallels the general population after age 30 years.

The treatment of gallbladder disease in HS is debatable, especially in patients with mild hemolytic disease or asymptomatic gallstones. An initial period of observation is advisable (1233). Surgery may be necessary if there are recurrent symptoms or complications such as cholecystitis or biliary obstruction. Laparoscopic cholecystectomy is the procedure of choice among most surgeons and the general public (1234). If a patient needs splenectomy for ongoing hemolysis or its complications, gallbladder ultrasound should be performed first and concomitant cholecystectomy considered if gallstones are present (1235). Splenectomy solely as a prophylaxis for gallstone development is probably not indicated, nor is prophylactic cholecystectomy. For patients with mild HS who do not receive a splenectomy in childhood, and subsequently develop gallstones, a recent Markov analysis (1236) suggests that splenectomy and cholecystectomy should be performed if the patient is younger than 39 years of age and has no gallbladder symptoms. If the patient has occasional biliary colic, both operations are recommended up to 52 years of age. Cholecystectomy alone is the preferred strategy in older patients with biliary colic.

OTHER COMPLICATIONS

Gout and Leg Ulcers. Rarely, adults with HS develop gout (855,1236), indolent leg ulcers (1234,1235), or a chronic erythematous dermatitis on the legs (1239). All three problems are corrected by splenectomy.

Extramedullary Hematopoietic Tumors. Adults with HS may also develop extramedullary masses of hematopoietic tissue, particularly along the posterior thoracic or lumbar spine (855,1237,1241–1245) or in the hila of the kidneys (854). Surprisingly, the tumors often arise in patients with mild HS, perhaps because they frequently escape splenectomy. The masses gradually enlarge and may be mistaken for neoplasms (1237). Biopsy can lead to extensive bleeding (1237). These bone marrow tumors can be diagnosed by magnetic resonance imaging (1245), which may make biopsies unnecessary, but, if necessary, an open biopsy should be performed. The masses stop growing and undergo fatty metamorphosis after splenectomy (1241,1243), but they do not shrink in size.

Malignancy. Four HS patients have developed multiple myeloma (1246–1248), and ten patients have developed myeloproliferative diseases (1249), leading to the suggestion that chronic reticuloendothelial stimulation may predispose HS patients, especially unsplenectomized patients, to these neoplasms. Splenic clearance of abnormal red cells induces proliferation of macrophages, lymphocytes, and plasma cells (1250). HS patients have a mild, polyclonal hypergammaglobulinemia (1246,1251), and there is evidence favoring the association of myeloma and chronic gallbladder disease (1246,1252); however, it is not clear if the proposed association of HS with myeloma and myeloproliferative disease is a real phenomenon or a chance relationship.

Hemochromatosis. Untreated HS may also exacerbate hemochromatosis in patients who are heterozygous for the hereditary disease (1253–1256). Several patients subsequently died of liver failure or hepatoma.

Congestive Heart Disease. Of course, untreated HS may also aggravate underlying heart disease and precipitate heart failure. Occasionally, this may be the presenting complaint (1257).

Angioid Streaks. Angioid streaks, brownish or gray streaks resembling veins in the optic fundus, have been reported in adult members of several kindreds with HS (1258,1259). The frequency of this association is unknown. Angioid streaks are relatively common in some other hematologic disorders, notably sickle cell disease and thalassemia (1260), and may be complicated by retinal vascular proliferation requiring photocoagulation (1261).

Pseudohyperkalemia. Because HS red cells leak K^+ ions more rapidly than normal cells, pseudohyperkalemia may be reported if the samples are allowed to sit for a long time at low temperatures before plasma electrolytes are analyzed (1262).

Splenic Rupture. Even though splenomegaly is often seen in patients with HS, traumatic rupture of the enlarged spleen in HS patients is very rare (1263). This contrasts with the higher frequency of splenic rupture in patients with Epstein-Barr virus infection and may reflect the different pathophysiology of splenic enlargement in the two conditions. We do not restrict normal activities in children with HS and splenomegaly, but if the spleen extends below the rib cage, we recommend that older children and adults avoid activities that could inflict a violent blow directly to the unprotected spleen.

Splenectomy

Splenectomy cures almost all patients with HS by eliminating anemia and reducing the reticulocyte count to near normal levels (1% to 3%). Patients with the most severe forms of the disease may not achieve a complete remission (869,953) but still benefit greatly from the procedure. The major issues today are who should have a splenectomy, what kind of operation should be performed, and how the patients should be treated postoperatively.

Before splenectomy, HS patients, like patients with other hemolytic disorders, should take folic acid (1 mg/day p.o.) to prevent folate deficiency.

RISKS OF SPLENECTOMY

Immediate Postsplenectomy Complications. Immediate postoperative complications include bleeding and subphrenic abscess. Hemorrhage usually comes from peritoneal and diaphragmatic surfaces of the splenic bed rather than from identifiable blood vessels. Subphrenic abscess is more likely to occur when adjacent organs are injured during the surgery. Acute pancreatitis can also occur in the postoperative period (1264).

Postsplenectomy Sepsis. Overwhelming postsplenectomy sepsis is one of the most serious complications of splenectomy. The risk is particularly high for encapsulated organisms, such as *Streptococcus pneumoniae*, *Neisseria meningitidis*, and *Haemophilus influenzae*. Postsplenectomy sepsis can be extremely rapid and potentially fatal; although it is most common in the first few years after surgery, it can occur years or decades later (1265). It is difficult to estimate the true incidence. King and Shumacker first drew attention to the high risk of fulminant sepsis in splenectomized infants with HS in 1952 (1266), and numerous reports of postsplenectomy sepsis have since been published. The results are summarized in a number of reviews (1267–1271). In adults, the incidence of overwhelming postsplenectomy infection is estimated to be 0.2 to 0.5/100 person-years of follow-up, with a death rate of 0.1/100 person-years (1272,1273). In addition, other serious bacterial infections (e.g., pneumonia, meningitis, peritonitis, bacteremia) are much more common (4.5/100 person-years) than normal, particularly in the first few years after the operation. The incidence is much higher in children, particularly younger children (1274–1276).

However, the majority of studies of postsplenectomy sepsis in children have serious methodologic problems (1270,1277). Most are retrospective studies or case reports, which have an inherent bias towards reporting the more serious cases. The duration of observation is often poorly documented, so it is impossible to establish risk as a function of time. In some studies, a large fraction of patients are not followed up. In others, splenectomized infants and young children are included. Many patients did not receive pneumococcal vaccine or antibiotic prophylaxis. The underlying diseases of the patients and the reasons for splenectomy are highly heterogeneous.

In our experience, overwhelming postsplenectomy sepsis is a serious or even devastating problem, but it is relatively uncommon in HS patients compared to patients with underlying immunologic dysfunction, such as Hodgkin's disease, or with portal hypertension or continuing extravascular hemolysis (e.g., thalassemia) (1264,1267,1275,1278). A recent 30-year follow-up of more than 200 splenectomized adult HS patients found that four patients had died from overwhelming sepsis, making the mortality rate from postsplenectomy sepsis 0.073/100 person-years (1279). Three of the four deaths occurred 18 years or more after the operation, and none of the patients who died had received pneumococcal vaccine or antibiotic prophylaxis. There is evidence of a dramatic decrease in the incidence of postsplenectomy sepsis in children who are given pneumococcal vaccine(s) and prophylactic antibiotics (1280,1281) (see Vaccination and Antibiotic Prophylaxis). This suggests that the incidence of postsplenectomy sepsis may continue to decline, even though preventive measures still may not be completely successful (1282). Continued research is needed to quantitate the true risk of overwhelming postsplenectomy sepsis in HS patients treated according to current practice guidelines (1265).

Babesiosis and Malaria. After splenectomy, HS patients are also at risk for serious parasitic infections, such as babesiosis and malaria. Babesiosis is a tick-transmitted zoonotic infection by an intraerythrocytic protozoan that is endemic in Europe and in the northeastern, north central, and western United States (1283). The causative agents include *Babesia microti*, *Babesia divergens*, and a related organism designated WA1. In healthy individuals, the infection is usually mild and often asymptomatic, but in patients without a functional spleen, it can be rapidly progressive and life threatening (1284). Patients may have malaise, headache, fever, shaking chills, profuse sweating, jaundice, and dark urine. There may be intravascular hemolysis and, occasionally, pancytopenia (1285) and hemophagocytosis (1286). Diagnosis is made by finding the parasites in blood smears or by serologic tests or amplification of parasitic DNA using PCR. Current treatment of symptomatic cases is with quinine plus clindamycin, but unsuccessful treatments have been reported in asplenic patients. Splenectomized HS patients, when traveling in endemic areas, should take measures to avoid tick bites by, for instance, wearing long pants and using tick repellents. The nymphal ticks that cause the disease are only 1 to 2 mm in size and are difficult to detect.

Animal experiments have shown that the spleen is essential for limiting malaria parasitemia in the acute stage of infection (1287,1288), but, surprisingly, other than anecdotal reports (1289–1291), there are no studies that definitively demonstrate an increased risk of severe malaria in asplenic individuals. It is, nevertheless, prudent for postsplenectomy HS patients to adhere strictly to malaria chemoprophylaxis protocols when traveling to endemic areas and to take measures to reduce exposure to malaria parasites.

THROMBOSIS AND ATHEROSCLEROSIS

There are occasional reports of thromboembolic events occurring many years after splenectomy for HS (1292,1293) and other diseases (1294–1296). A systematic study of long-term causes of death in Swedish patients after splenectomy also showed a slightly increased incidence of thromboembolism (1297). However, a causal relationship between splenectomy and thrombotic disease has not been convincingly demonstrated, except for patients with hereditary stomatocytosis and hereditary xerocytosis, in whom the risk of thrombotic complications after splenectomy approaches 100% (1298).

There is also some evidence that the incidence of atherosclerosis is elevated after splenectomy. A carefully controlled, long-term follow-up of splenectomy in 740 World War II servicemen after battlefield injuries showed excess mortality from pneumonia and atherosclerotic heart disease (1.9 times relative risk) in the splenectomized patients (1299). The authors suggest that the chronically elevated platelet counts that occur after splenectomy may have contributed to vascular disease. Circulating membrane fragments released from HS red cells may also be a contributing factor because such fragments are highly thrombogenic if PS is exposed (1300,1301). A more recent study found that the cumulative incidence of atherosclerosis after the age of 40 is six times higher in patients who have had a splenectomy compared to those who have not had the procedure (1302). Although these results need to be confirmed by other studies, they support a conservative approach to splenectomy.

INDICATIONS FOR SPLENECTOMY

In view of the potential risks, splenectomy should be performed only if there are clear indications. We believe the procedure is clearly warranted for the rare patients with severe HS who require transfusions or who have serious complications, such as growth failure or thalassemic facies. It is probably also indicated for patients with moderate or moderately severe disease who are symptomatic with chronic fatigue, decreased physical stamina, or, later in life, leg ulcers, extramedullary hematopoietic tumors, or reduced perfusion of vital organs. Whether patients with moderate HS and asymptomatic anemia

should have a splenectomy is controversial. Subtotal splenectomy may have a particular role in these patients. Splenectomy can be deferred, probably indefinitely, in patients with mild HS and compensated hemolysis. The presence of gallbladder disease may influence the decision, as discussed above. In young children, splenectomy, if indicated, should be delayed until at least 3 years of age and, if possible, until 7 to 9 years of age—after the peak incidence of fevers and common viral infections. There is probably no additional benefit in postponing splenectomy beyond 10 years of age, because the risk of gallstone development rises sharply after that. In some patients, splenectomy may not be needed until old age, when complications such as leg ulcers and extramedullary hematopoietic tumors develop.

SURGICAL PROCEDURES

Splenectomy. Laparoscopic splenectomy, sometimes with concomitant laparoscopic cholecystectomy, has now become a viable alternative to open splenectomy (1303–1305). The benefits of this approach are its minimal invasiveness, shortened hospital stay, lower need for narcotic pain control, and more appealing cosmetic result. The liabilities include the longer operation time, the potential difficulty in control of bleeding, capsular fracture with subsequent splenosis, and the chance of missing an accessory spleen. Experience with the procedure has accumulated tremendously in the past few years, although there are few multicenter, controlled trials comparing it with the traditional open surgical approach (1306–1308). The current consensus is that if the surgical staff is experienced with the procedure and the spleen is not very large, laparoscopic splenectomy is the method of choice.

Subtotal (Partial) Splenectomy. Because of the risk of postsplenectomy sepsis, subtotal splenectomy (or partial splenectomy) has been advocated as an alternative to total splenectomy for HS (1309,1310). In this procedure, approximately 80% to 90% of the enlarged spleen is removed, leaving behind a remnant with approximately 25% of the volume of a normal spleen (Fig. 51-50). Subtotal splenectomy is usually performed as an open operation, although a laparoscopic procedure has been reported. It is more time consuming than complete splenectomy, and recovery is longer (4 to 7 days of hospitalization) (1310), but the procedure is safe and decreases the rate of hemolysis (1309,1310). After partial

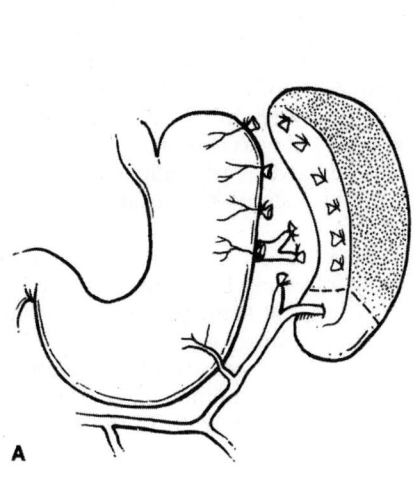

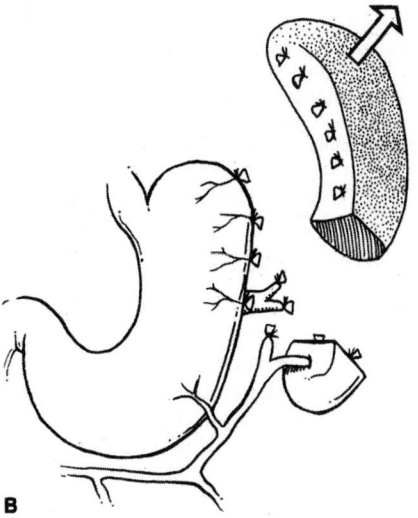

A   **B**

Figure 51-50. Surgical technique used for subtotal (partial, ~80%) splenectomy. **A:** All vascular pedicles supplying the spleen are divided except those arising from the left gastroepiploic vessels. **B:** The upper pole of the spleen is removed at the boundary between the well-perfused and poorly perfused tissue. (Reprinted from Tchernia G, Gauthier F, Mielot F, et al. Initial assessment of the beneficial effect of partial splenectomy in hereditary spherocytosis. *Blood* 1993;81:2014, with permission.)

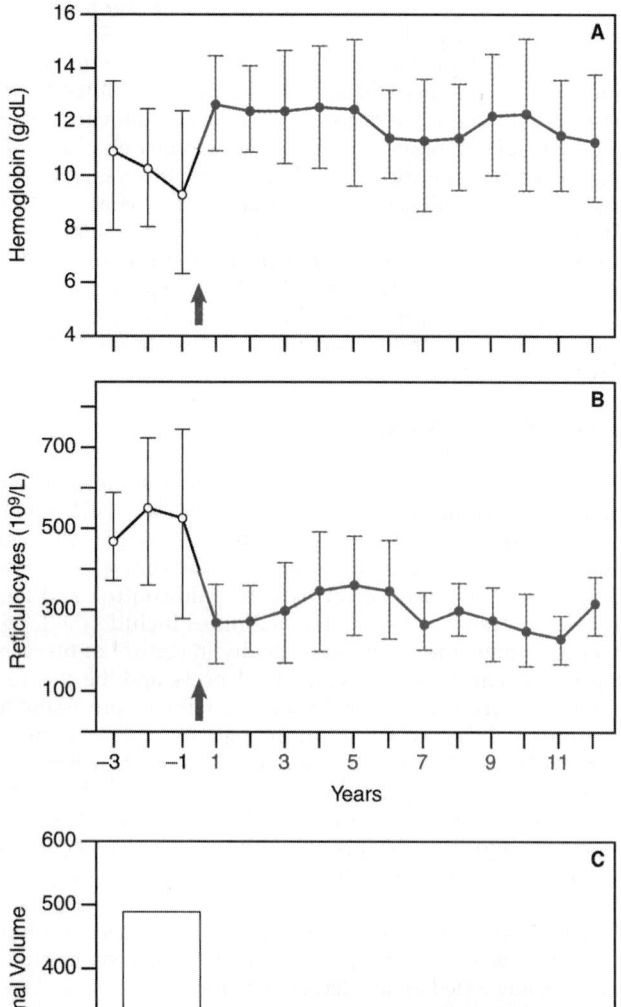

Figure 51-51. Long-term follow-up of subtotal splenectomy in hereditary spherocytosis. The data are the results of 12 years of experience with the procedure in 40 patients (1 to 25 years of age). **A,B:** Change in hemoglobin and reticulocyte count with time before and after the subtotal splenectomy (*arrow*). The mean and standard deviations are shown. Both the rise in hemoglobin and fall in reticulocytes have been sustained for more than a decade. **C:** The size of the spleen during the same period. There is some regrowth of the splenic remnant, especially in the first few years. It remains to be seen whether the remnant will reach a stable size or continue to regrow slowly. (Adapted from Bader-Meunier B, Gauthier F, et al. Long-term evaluation of the beneficial effect of subtotal splenectomy for management of hereditary spherocytosis. *Blood* 2001;97:399.)

splenectomy, the mean Hb in a group of 40 HS patients increased from 9.2 to 12.7 g/dL, and the absolute reticulocyte count decreased from 523 to 267×10^9 cells/L (Fig. 51-51) (1310). In the children with at least 10 years of follow-up, no significant differences were noted between the 1- and 10-year postoperative Hb values and reticulocyte counts. Significant regrowth of the splenic remnant was noted during the first year after surgery

(Fig. 51-51); however, after this initial spurt, the rate of growth was reduced and appeared either to reach a plateau value or to show only a modest increase over the years. Some of the phagocytic function of the spleen was preserved. Howell-Jolly bodies appeared transiently in the first week after surgery but then disappeared in almost all patients (1310). The percentage of pitted erythrocytes also remained normal in all patients during up to 14 years of follow-up. The uptake of ^{99}Tc-labeled heat-damaged red cells was also normal in 97% of patients. Presumably, the risk of postsplenectomy sepsis is also decreased, although this may be impossible to prove. There was improved quality of life in 92% and gain in physical growth in all patients studied. However, the reduction in hemolytic rate was not as great as that observed after total splenectomy, and partial splenectomy did not prevent the development of gallstones completely (4 of 18 patients whose gallbladder was not removed) (1310). Total splenectomy was subsequently required in 8% of patients. It is not clear if these "failures" occurred primarily in patients with severe HS, but, in the study discussed above, 12 of the 40 patients required repeated transfusions (1310). In our view, the procedure is more suited for patients with mild to moderate HS, in whom splenectomy is often not performed. It is likely that a second operation will rarely be needed in these patients. However, given the relatively high rate of gallstone formation after subtotal splenectomy, it may be necessary to do a prophylactic cholecystectomy with the procedure.

Partial splenic artery embolization has been performed as an alternative to splenectomy in patients with hypersplenism and has been performed in a child with HS (1311). The experience with this procedure in HS is limited, and it cannot be recommended as a routine procedure.

VACCINATION AND ANTIBIOTIC PROPHYLAXIS

All HS patients undergoing splenectomy should receive vaccines against encapsulated bacteria. The 23-valent polysaccharide pneumococcal vaccine (Pneumovax) is highly effective (1280) after 2 years of age and should be given at least 2 weeks before splenectomy (1312). A conjugated heptavalent pneumococcal vaccine (Prevnar), effective before 2 years of age, has recently been released. It is safe and effective (1313–1315) and is now recommended for all infants (<2 years of age) by the Advisory Committee on Immunization Practices and may be given to children up to 5 years of age (1316). Prevnar has not been studied sufficiently among older children or adults for the Committee to recommend its use at the present time. The 23-valent polysaccharide vaccine (Pneumovax) is still recommended before splenectomy for patients older than 2 years of age, followed by boosters every 5 years.

The conjugated *H. influenzae* type b vaccine is now given to all children and should also be given to splenectomized adult HS patients (1317). The *N. meningitidis* vaccine is currently effective against only serogroup A and C strains, not the common serogroup B, but it probably should still be given to patients undergoing splenectomy (1317). Revaccination with meningococcal vaccine in 2 years is advised. Yearly influenza vaccination may help reduce the chance of secondary bacterial infection.

Prophylactic antibiotics against *S. pneumoniae* should be given to HS patients after splenectomy. Penicillin V (125 to 250 mg twice/day) is usually used, but some physicians recommend amoxicillin because of its improved absorption (1317). Patients who are allergic to penicillin may be offered erythromycin (1318). Antibiotic prophylaxis should be given to splenectomized patients throughout their childhood or, for teenagers and adults, in the first 2 to 5 years after splenectomy when the risk of overwhelming infection is highest. Some authorities recommend life-long antibiotic prophylaxis (1318), which is also our recommendation, but there are concerns of poor patient compliance and emergence of resistant organisms (1319). Patients not on prophylaxis should have a supply of oral antibiotics at hand, which they should take immediately if fever or other symptoms of infection develop. They should then seek medical attention right away (see Chapter 21 for advice regarding the workup and antibiotic treatment of splenectomized patients presenting with fever).

The risk of infection must be decreased in immunized patients because 50% to 70% of postsplenectomy sepsis is due to *S. pneumoniae*, and 80% of pneumococcal disease is due to strains contained in the 23-valent vaccine. Further risk reductions would be anticipated from the chronic use of prophylactic penicillin. Nevertheless, the risk cannot be reduced to zero. Postsplenectomy infections occur occasionally in successfully immunized patients (1320–1323), and compliance regarding prophylactic medications is a problem, particularly in teenagers (1324).

Penicillin-resistant pneumococci are increasing very rapidly all over the world. In some countries, more than one-half of all isolates are resistant (1325). In the United States, the prevalence is closer to 5% to 10% (1326,1327), but it is rising. Although most of the strains show some sensitivity to penicillin, some are highly resistant, and others are multiply resistant (1327). The emergence of these strains will greatly complicate the use of antibiotics for pneumococcal prophylaxis during the next decades.

POSTSPLENECTOMY CHANGES

After splenectomy, spherocytosis persists, but conditioned microspherocytes disappear, and changes typical of the postsplenectomy state, including Howell-Jolly bodies, target cells, siderocytes, and acanthocytes, become evident in the peripheral blood smear. On average, the MCV and mean red cell surface area increase, and the MCHC and OF decrease, but the effects are modest (5% to 10%) (1328). In typical dominant HS, reticulocyte counts fall to normal or near normal levels (869), although the red cell lifespan, if carefully measured, remains slightly shortened (96 ± 13 days) (1080). In all except the most severe cases, anemia and jaundice remit and do not recur.

SPLENECTOMY FAILURE

The rare splenectomy failure (i.e., recurrence of hemolysis) is usually caused by an accessory spleen that was missed during surgery (1329,1330) or by another red cell disorder, such as pyruvate kinase deficiency (1331,1332). Accessory spleens occur in 15% to 40% of patients (1231,1267,1333) and must always be sought at the time of splenectomy. Recurrence of hemolytic anemia years (1330) or even decades (1329) after splenectomy should raise suspicion of an accessory spleen, particularly if Howell-Jolly bodies are no longer evident on peripheral blood smears. The absence of "pitted" red cells with craterlike surface indentations (readily seen by interference contrast microscopy) is also a sensitive measure of recrudescent splenic function (1334,1335). The ectopic splenic tissue can be confirmed by a radiocolloid liver/spleen scan or a scan using ^{51}Cr- or ^{99}Tc-labeled, heated red cells (1329,1336).

HEREDITARY ELLIPTOCYTOSIS AND PYROPOIKILOCYTOSIS

HE is a relatively common, clinically and genetically heterogeneous disorder characterized by the presence of a large number of elliptically shaped red cells in the peripheral blood. Oval or elliptical erythrocytes are normally found in fish, reptiles, birds, camels, and South American Camelids (llamas, alpacas, guana-cos, and vicunas); however, in humans, elliptocytosis indicates a defect in the erythrocyte membrane skeleton. In the more severe forms of the disease, spherocytes or bizarre poikilocytes are also present, and, sometimes, these shapes predominate. HPP is an example of the latter situation. Although HPP was once considered to be a separate entity, biochemical and genetic information clearly indicates that it is related to HE, and the two disorders are considered together here.

History

According to Lambrecht (1337), elliptocytosis was first observed in 1860 by Goltz in Königsburg, Germany, but no written report of this observation is known. The disease was first reported in 1904 by Dresbach, a physiologist at Ohio State University, in one of his histology students during a laboratory exercise in which the students were examining their own blood (1338). His brief report elicited some controversy, as the student died soon thereafter, leading the prominent American physician Austin Flint to suggest that he actually had incipient pernicious anemia (1339). Dresbach replied that the student died of acute rheumatic carditis and took his slides to Germany, where famous pathologists such as Ewing, Ehrlich, and Arneth supported his view that the red cell disorder was primary (1340). This was substantiated during the next two decades by the reports of Bishop (1341), Sydenstricker (1342), and Huck and Bigelow (1343). Hunter's demonstration of elliptocytosis in three generations of one family firmly established the hereditary nature of the disease (1344,1345).

In the 1930s and early 1940s, there was considerable debate about whether HE was a disease or simply a morphologic curiosity. In retrospect, it is surprising because a number of individuals with hemolytic HE were described during this interval (1337,1346–1350), and some authors had clearly differentiated hemolytic and nonhemolytic forms (1337,1346,1349). In fact, as early as 1928 van den Bergh even reported that anemia and jaundice cleared after splenectomy in one patient (1350). Early on, some confusion also existed in differentiating HE from sickle cell anemia and thalassemia and, later, in differentiating hemolytic HE from HS (1351). These reports illustrate a point that is emphasized later—namely, that HE, particularly its hemolytic variants, can sometimes be morphologically deceptive.

For the reader interested in the historical aspects of HE, the reports of Wyandt and co-workers (1351), Wolman and Ozge (1352), and Dacie (1353,1354) are particularly recommended.

The recognition of HPP as a clinical entity came more recently. Zarkowsky and co-workers first described children with congenital hemolytic anemia who had fragmented and irregularly shaped erythrocytes that resembled red cells seen in patients with severe cutaneous burns (1355). They showed that these red cells were thermally unstable and called them *pyropoikilocytes*. Other reports described patients who presented with a similar clinical picture, but the thermal properties of their erythrocytes were not examined (1356). In a follow-up study, Zarkowsky noted that neonates with elliptocytosis and hemolysis also have heat-induced fragmentation of their red cells, prompting the author to suggest that elliptocytosis and pyropoikilocytosis may be caused by a similar defect in the red cell membrane (1357). This predication turned out to be true when the molecular defects of the two disorders were later elucidated.

Prevalence and Genetics

The prevalence of all forms of HE in the United States has been estimated to be between 1 in 2000 to 1 in 4000 (1351,1358), but the true incidence is unknown because the disease is heterogeneous and often asymptomatic. HE is observed in all racial and ethnic groups but is more prevalent in Africans, with an incidence as high as 1% in some groups (1359–1361). The high frequency of the gene in these populations suggests the disease may confer some protection against malaria. There is some preliminary evidence supporting this idea (1362), but it has not been adequately tested. SAO is a distinct and homogeneous subgroup of elliptocytosis that is very prevalent in some parts of Asia and is discussed separately (1363).

HE is generally inherited as an autosomal-dominant trait. It is clinically variable in severity, reflecting genetic heterogeneity at the molecular level. Patients who are homozygous or compound heterozygous for HE usually have a more severe phenotype with significant hemolysis and splenomegaly. The clinical picture may be indistinguishable from HPP.

Genetic studies show that one of the elliptocytosis genes (El1) is closely linked to the Rh locus on the short arm of chromosome 1 (1p36→p34) (1364–1366). This is the location of the protein 4.1 gene (158). Another gene (El2) is located on the long arm of chromosome 1 near the Duffy blood group locus (1q22→q23) (1367) in the region where the spectrin α-chain gene is located (1q21) (411). The identification of numerous mutations in both of these proteins in HE confirms the linkage studies. There may also be an X-linked elliptocytosis locus (1368).

HPP is a much rarer disorder than HE. It usually occurs sporadically, but, not infrequently, one of the parents or siblings of the proband can be shown to have common HE

(1355,1369,1370). The pattern of inheritance of HPP in most cases cannot be explained by the transmission of a single genetic determinant, but it can often be explained by the cosegregation of two genetic determinants—one of which may be silent in the carrier state. Recent research suggests that the HPP phenotype is produced by homozygosity for certain HE genes, compound heterozygosity for two different HE alleles, or coinheritance of an HE gene and a modifying gene, such as the α^{LELY} allele (see below) (346).

Clinical Syndromes

Most of the reported cases of HE can be classified into one of four clinical categories: heterozygous common HE, homozygous common HE or HPP, spherocytic HE, and SAO (Table 51-20). With the exception of the latter disorder, which is homogeneous in molecular genetic terms, these appellations denote clinical phenotypes and not specific molecular etiologies, although correlations between the two exist. Numerous molecular defects in the membrane proteins of HE have been identified in recent years, and HE can also be classified based on these defects.

Common Hereditary Elliptocytosis

Common HE is, by far, the most prevalent form of HE. It is observed in all populations but is particularly common in Afri-

---

TABLE 51-20. Clinical Subtypes of Hereditary Elliptocytosis (HE)

Clinical Manifestations	Laboratory Features
Heterozygous common HE	
Asymptomatic	Blood smear: elliptocytes, rod forms, few or no poikilocytes
Dominant inheritance: one parent with HE	No anemia, little or no hemolysis (reticulocytes = 1% to 3%)
No splenomegaly	Normal osmotic fragility
Variants	Usually there is a defect in α- or β-spectrin → decreased spectrin self-association
Some neonates with moderately severe hemolytic anemia and hereditary pyropoikilocytosis (HPP)-like smear; converts to typical common HE by ~1 yr	Sometimes common HE is caused by a partial deficiency or dysfunction of protein 4.1
Some patients with mild-moderate chronic hemolysis, due either to coinheritance of the low expression α-spectrin variant α^{LELY}, or to coexistence of a chronic disease-producing splenomegaly, or unknown factors	
Homozygous common HE or HPP	
Moderate to severe hemolytic anemia	Blood smear: bizarre poikilocytes, fragments, ± spherocytes, ± elliptocytes
Splenomegaly	Reticulocytosis
Intermittent jaundice	Decreased mean cell volume due to red cell fragmentation
Aplastic crises	Increased osmotic fragility
Recessive inheritance: typically one parent with HE and one with α^{LELY} or both parents with HE	α-Spectrin defects in most patients
Good improvement after splenectomy	Decreased red cell heat stability
	Marked defect in spectrin self-association
	In most severe variants, partial spectrin deficiency (indicated by more spherocytes on the blood smear)
Spherocytic HE	
Mild-moderate hemolytic anemia	Blood smear: rounded elliptocytes, ± spherocytes; may see variable morphology within a kindred
Splenomegaly	Reticulocytosis
Intermittent jaundice	Increased osmotic fragility
Aplastic crises	Glucose-responsive autohemolysis
Dominant inheritance pattern	Variable molecular defects: C-terminal truncations of β-spectrin; protein 4.2 deficiency (some patients) → ovalostomatocytosis, which resembles spherocytic HE; glycophorin C deficiency (rare)
Excellent response to splenectomy	
Southeast Asian ovalocytosis	
Asymptomatic	Blood smear: rounded elliptocytes, some with a transverse bar that divides the central clear space
Dominant inheritance (homozygous state lethal)	Little or no hemolysis or anemia
Lowland aboriginal tribes, especially in Melanesia and Malaysia	Normal osmotic fragility
Very rigid red cells	Mutant band 3 that lacks anion exchange function and shows increased interactions with membrane skeleton → rigid membrane
Decreased susceptibility to malaria	

cans. In West Africa, the prevalence of some variants is 0.4% to 3.0% (1371,1372). Almost all of the African mutations involve α-spectrin. Common HE is at least 15 to 25 times less common in Western populations, in which, in some laboratories, approximately 60% to 80% of the cases of HE are due to α-spectrin defects, and approximately 20% to 40% are due to defects in protein 4.1 (1373). Occasionally, patients with common HE lack GPC or have mutations in β-spectrin that affect the structure of the α-chain. The truncated β-spectrins, which are usually included among mutations causing common HE, are discussed in the section Spherocytic Hereditary Elliptocytosis later in the chapter. The fact that mutations in different membrane proteins result in a similar clinical phenotype suggests that they disrupt red cell membrane integrity by a common mechanism.

HETEROZYGOUS COMMON HEREDITARY ELLIPTOCYTOSIS
The clinical picture of the common HE trait varies enormously—from the silent carrier state to moderately severe hemolytic HE. Several clinical patterns can be defined. However, it is important to emphasize that different members of the same family may exhibit different clinical patterns. The clinical patterns are probably more useful for illustrating the spectrum of common HE than for classifying the disease into genetic or molecular phenotypes.

Silent Carrier State. This condition was identified by analyzing asymptomatic members of kindreds with HE or HPP. The affected persons have normal red cell shape and no evidence of hemolysis, but careful measurements show a subtle defect in their membrane skeletons, with decreased red cell thermal stability, decreased mechanical stability of isolated skeletons, an increased fraction of spectrin dimers in 0°C spectrin extracts, abnormal tryptic peptide maps of spectrin, and various combinations of these defects (1374–1381). (These tests are discussed in more detail in the section Etiology.) It is notable that some patients classified as "silent carriers" have the same molecular defect as patients with common HE (1378–1381). This underscores the natural variability of these mutations.

More commonly, the silent carrier state is associated with the low-expression α-spectrin allele α^{LELY} (1382,1383). This very common allele is described in detail in the section Spectrin α^{LELY} Polymorphism. It contains a mutation within a nucleation site of α-spectrin that diminishes the propensity of α^{LELY}-spectrin to associate, side by side, with β-spectrin. When present in *trans* with an α-spectrin mutant that causes HE, incorporation of the HE α-chain into spectrin αβ heterodimers is favored, leading to an increased proportion of the elliptocytogenic spectrin in the cells and, consequently, more severe hemolytic disease. The α^{LELY} locus is clinically silent by itself, even when homozygous, but it greatly augments the effects of the *trans* allele and plays a major role in the clinical expression of HE.

Common Hereditary Elliptocytosis. Common hereditary elliptocytosis (also called *mild hereditary elliptocytosis* or *mild common hereditary elliptocytosis*) is the most prevalent clinical form of HE (1351,1384–1400). It is typically dominantly inherited. Patients are asymptomatic and are often discovered by accident when a blood smear is examined. They have no anemia and no splenomegaly, except for an occasional "spleen tip" (Table 51-20). Red cell survival may be normal (1399), but, more often, there is very mild, compensated hemolysis with a slight reticulocytosis and a decreased haptoglobin level (1351,1389,1392,1397,1398,1401). In these patients, HE is hardly more than a morphologic curiosity.

The peripheral blood smear shows prominent elliptocytosis with little red cell budding or fragmentation and without spherocytosis. Elliptocytes exceed 10% of the red cells by definition and

usually exceed 30% (Fig. 51-52A) (1351,1380,1381,1395,1397,1401). In some patients, they approach 100%. In contrast, normal individuals have no more than 2% to 5% elliptocytes (1380,1381,1401). Somewhat higher proportions are seen in patients with anemia, particularly megaloblastic anemias, hypochromic-microcytic anemias, myelodysplastic syndromes or refractory anemia (1402–1404), and myelofibrosis; however, even in these individuals, elliptocytes usually do not exceed 35% (1395).

Hence, the morphologic diagnosis of common HE is rarely difficult. This may not be true in the neonatal period. Early investigators noted that elliptocytes are infrequent in the cord blood of infants with common HE and become more prominent with time (1345,1351). For example, Wyandt and co-workers detected only 11% elliptocytes at birth in one infant, whereas by 4 months of age, 80% of the cells were elliptical (1351). These observations, although few, suggest that the disease may be expressed differently in fetal red cells.

Common Hereditary Elliptocytosis with Chronic Hemolysis. More severe variants of common HE occur frequently, even within a kindred (1376,1389,1391,1405,1406). In general, the hemolysis is accompanied by evidence of membrane instability on the peripheral blood smear: budding red cells, fragments, and other bizarre poikilocytes.

In patients with α-spectrin mutations, significant hemolysis is usually due to coinheritance of the α^{LELY} allele and one of the more deleterious HE alleles (1382,1407–1410). Of the common mutations (discussed below), $\alpha^{I/74}$-spectrin is more severe than $\alpha^{I/46}$-spectrin and much more severe than $\alpha^{I/65}$-spectrin (1373,1411). Patients with $\alpha^{LELY}/\alpha^{I/74}$ have marked hemolysis and elliptopoikilocytosis compared to their $\alpha/\alpha^{I/74}$ siblings, whereas patients with $\alpha^{LELY}/\alpha^{I/65}$ have more elliptocytes than their $\alpha/\alpha^{I/65}$ siblings but no significant hemolysis (1382).

Less often, hemolysis is caused by the inheritance of a mutant spectrin that is grossly dysfunctional (1405). This is indicated by the dominant transmission of the hemolytic syndrome and by an unusually high fraction of spectrin dimers in 0°C spectrin extracts.

Common Hereditary Elliptocytosis with Sporadic Hemolysis. Patients with common HE may also develop uncompensated hemolysis in response to stimuli that cause hyperplasia of the reticuloendothelial system, particularly if the spleen is involved. Examples include viral hepatitis (1412), cirrhosis (1413), infectious mononucleosis (1398), cytomegalovirus (1414), bacterial infections (1398), and malaria (1415,1416). Hemolysis has also been observed with thrombotic thrombocytopenic purpura (1417) and during a renal transplant rejection complicated by disseminated intravascular coagulation (1417), which suggests that elliptocytes may be especially susceptible to microangiopathic damage. For unknown reasons, pregnancy (1398,1418) and cobalamin (vitamin B_{12}) deficiency (1419) may also transiently aggravate the disease.

Finally, acquired elliptocytosis is sometimes observed in myelodysplastic syndromes (1403,1404) and leukemias (1420). In one recent study, nearly 50% of children with leukemia (both acute lymphocytic leukemia and chronic myelogenous leukemia) had elliptocytosis and poikilocytosis at diagnosis (1420). This was associated with an increase of spectrin dimers (42% ± 16%) and slightly enhanced phosphorylation of β-spectrin. These alterations disappeared during remission of the leukemia.

Common Hereditary Elliptocytosis with Infantile Poikilocytosis. Some infants with common HE begin life with moderately severe hemolytic anemia, characterized by marked red cell budding, fragmentation, and poikilocytosis (Table 51-20) and by

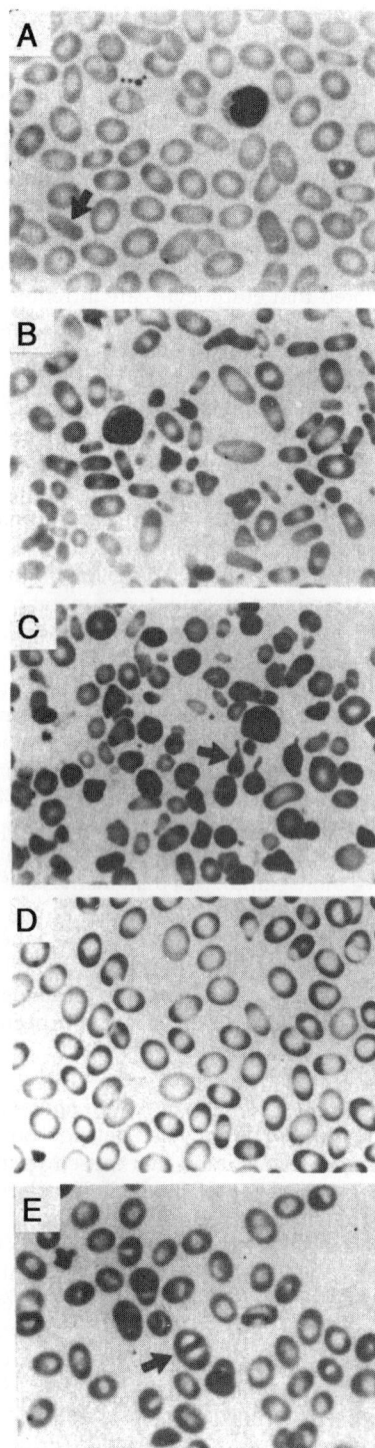

Figure 51-52. Blood films of patients with hereditary elliptocytosis or hereditary pyropoikilocytosis. **A:** Heterozygous common hereditary elliptocytosis. Elliptocytosis predominates with some rod-shaped cells (*arrow*) and virtual absence of poikilocytes. **B:** Homozygous common hereditary elliptocytosis. There are many elliptocytes as well as numerous fragments and poikilocytes. **C:** Hereditary pyropoikilocytosis with prominent microspherocytosis, micropoikilocytosis, and fragmentation. Only a few elliptocytes are present. Some poikilocytes are in the process of budding (*arrow*). **D:** Spherocytic elliptocytosis. Rounded elliptocytes are visible. **E:** Southeast Asian ovalocytosis. The majority of cells are rounded elliptocytes, some of them containing either a longitudinal slit or transverse ridge (*arrow*). (Reprinted from Palek J, Lambert S. Genetics of the red cell membrane skeleton. *Semin Hematol* 1990;27:290, with permission.)

neonatal jaundice, which may require an exchange transfusion (724,1387,1391,1401,1406,1421–1425). In most cases, enough elliptocytes are present to suggest the diagnosis, but, sometimes, this is not so, and the disorder is mistaken for sepsis, infantile pyknocytosis, or a microangiopathic or oxidant-induced hemolytic anemia (1421,1422). Neonatal HE can easily be distinguished from these conditions if the parents' smears are examined, because one will have common HE—typically due to a defect in α- or β-spectrin that affects spectrin self-association. However, it is more difficult to distinguish HE with neonatal poikilocytosis from HPP.

Most α-spectrin variants have been associated with the neonatal poikilocytosis syndrome; however, not all neonates are affected (1406,1425). The factors that determine susceptibility are unknown. With time, fragmentation and hemolysis decline, and the clinical picture of common HE emerges. This transition requires from 4 months to 2 years. Subsequently, the disease is clinically indistinguishable from typical common HE. The prevalence is unknown, but, in our experience, it is not rare.

The fragmenting neonatal red cells are very sensitive to heat like hereditary pyropoikilocytes, but unlike pyropoikilocytes, this sensitivity lessens as the patients mature (1424). During the conversion, the poikilocytic red cells are dense and rich in HbF, whereas the smooth elliptocytes are light and enriched in HbA (Lux SE, John KM, *unpublished observations*). This suggests the change in the disease corresponds to the change from fetal to adult erythropoiesis. No variations in the primary α-spectrin defect or in its functional effects on spectrin self-association occur during the conversion (1401), so other skeletal interactions must differ in fetal and adult red cells. Mentzer has made the interesting suggestion that 2,3-DPG is the critical agent (724). Free 2,3-DPG is elevated in fetal red cells because it is not bound by HbF. The free anion is known to weaken spectrin-actin-4.1 interactions (723,725), to interfere with 4.1 binding to GPC (1427), to inhibit ankyrin binding to band 3 (1427). It also increases the fragility of isolated ghosts at physiologic concentrations (724), although it is controversial whether it does so in intact red cells (726,727). If so, this would certainly aggravate the underlying defect in spectrin self-association (to be discussed).

HOMOZYGOUS AND COMPOUND HETEROZYGOUS COMMON HEREDITARY ELLIPTOCYTOSIS

A number of patients who are homozygotes or compound heterozygotes for common HE have been reported (334,1351,1385,1401,1411,1428–1441). Some have had a very severe or even fatal (1440) transfusion-dependent hemolytic anemia (Hb = 2 to 6 g/dL) with marked fragmentation, poikilocytosis, spherocytosis, and elliptocytosis (Table 51-20; Fig. 51-52B). In others, hemolysis was less rampant (Hb = 7 to 11 g/dL). It appears that these differences reflect variations in the severity of the many α-spectrin mutations that produce common HE (1401,1411,1412). In one interesting case, a proband with moderate HE inherited an α-spectrin self-association site mutation from his mother and a β-spectrin self-association site mutation from his father (1453). Clinically homozygous HE resembles HPP (1401,1430), except for the mildest forms. All treated patients have responded dramatically to splenectomy.

HEREDITARY PYROPOIKILOCYTOSIS

HPP is an interesting, rare, recessive disease that presents in infancy or early childhood as a severe hemolytic anemia (Hb = 4 to 8 g/dL) (1401) characterized by extreme poikilocytosis with budding red cells, fragments, spherocytes, triangulocytes, and other bizarre-shaped cells (1378,1444–1446) (Fig. 51-52C; Table 51-20) and, in some cases, with few or no elliptocytes. The morphology somewhat resembles the fragmented and irregularly

TABLE 51-21. Molecular Defects in Hereditary Elliptocytosis (HE) and Hereditary Pyropoikilocytosis (HPP)

Name of Variant	Codon	Amino Acid Change	Systemic Name[a]	Type of Mutation	Mechanism	Peptide Designation (Repeat)[b]	Comments[c]	Selected References
α-Spectrin								
Lograno	24	Ile→Ser	I24S	Missense	—	—		1467
Corbeil	28	Arg→His	R28H	Missense	—	αI/74 (R1)	Arg 28 mutations are relatively common; found in whites, blacks, Arabs, and Melanesians; severe defect.	1405–1407
Unnamed	28	Arg→Cys	R28C	Missense	—	αI/74 (R1)	—	1405,1443,1468
Unnamed	28	Arg→Leu	R28L	Missense	—	αI/74 (R1)	—	1405,1469
Unnamed	28	Arg→Ser	R28S	Missense	—	αI/74 (R1)	—	1405,1469
Marseille	31	Val→Ala	V31A	Missense	—	αI/74 (R1)	—	1470
Genova	34	Arg→Trp	R34W	Missense	—	αI/74 (R1)	Especially in North Africa; severe defect.	1467,1471
Tunis	41	Arg→Trp	R41W	Missense	—	αI/78 (R1)		1386,1472
Clichy	45	Arg→Ser	R45S	Missense	—	αI/78 (R1)	—	1387
Anastasia	45	Arg→Thr	R45T	Missense	—	αI/74 (R1)	—	1473
Culoz	46	Gly→Val	G46V	Missense	—	αI/74 (R1)	—	1474
Unnamed	48	Lys→Arg	K48R	Missense	—	αI/74 (R1)	—	1469
Lyon	49	Leu→Phe	L49F	Missense	—	αI/74 (R1)	—	1474
Unnamed	128	Arg→Ser	R128S	Missense	—	αI/65 (R2-R3 linker)	—	1475
Ponte de Sôr	151	Gly→Asp	G151D	Missense	—	αI/65 (R2-R3 linker)	—	1476
Unnamed	154	Leu→LeuLeu	L154-155ins	1-aa insertion	—		Common in blacks; incidence = 0.4% in Benin; mild defect.	1361,1389– 1391,1401,1408,1429, 1442,1477–1481
Dayton	178	Glu178→ Glu226del	E178-E226del	49-aa deletion	Splicing (exon 5 skipped, mobile element insertion)	αI/50a (R3)	—	1482
Saint Louis	207	Leu→Pro	L207P	Missense	—	αI/50a (R3)	Common in blacks; incidence = 0.5% in Benin; mild defect.	1361,1478,1483,1484
Nigerian	260	Leu→Pro	L260P	Missense	—	αI/50a (R3-R4 linker)	—	1478
Unnamed	261	Ser→Pro	S261P	Missense	—	αI/50a (R3-R4 linker)	—	1478
Sfax	363	Tyr363→ Trp371del	1086A>G	9-aa deletion	Splicing	αI/36 (R4-R5 linker)	Mild defect.	1409
Alexandria	469	His del	H469del	1-aa deletion	Cryptic splice site	αI/50b (R5-R6 linker)	Moderate to marked poikilocytosis.	1485
Barcelona	469	His→Pro	H469P	Missense	—	αI/50b (R5-R6 linker)	Asymptomatic unless combined with α^LELY, then moderately severe.	1410
Unnamed	469	His→Arg	H469R	Missense	—	αI/50b (R5-R6 linker)	—	1483,1486
Unnamed	471	Gln→Pro	Q471P	Missense	—	αI/50b (R5-R6 linker)	—	1478,1483
Jendouba	791	Asp→Glu	D791E	Missense	—	αII/31 (R8-R9 linker)	Mild defect; relatively few, roundish elliptocytes; only slight defect in spectrin self-association.	1487
Oran	822	822→862 del	2465-1G>A	41-aa deletion	Splicing (exon 18 skipped)	αII/21 (R9)	Heterozygotes silent; homozygotes mild-moderate HE.	1431,1432
St. Claude	936	936→966 del	2806-13T>G	31-aa deletion	Splicing → two messenger RNAs: one has 12-nt of intron 20 → PCT. The other skips exon 20 → truncated α-spectrin.	αII/47 (R10); truncated: 277 kd	Heterozygotes: asymptomatic; homozygotes: severe poikilocytic anemia; common in blacks; incidence = 3% in Benin, Africa.	1372,1433

(continued)

TABLE 51-21. Continued

Name of Variant	Codon	Amino Acid Change	Systemic Name[a]	Type of Mutation	Mechanism	Peptide Designation (Repeat)[b]	Comments[c]	Selected References
LELY	2177	2177 → 2182 del (AYFLDG)	6528-12C>T	6-aa deletion (exon 46)	Splicing → two mRNAs: one (50%) deletes exon 46; the other is normal.	αV/41 due to linked L1847V mutation	Heterozygote and homozygote asymptomatic; gene frequency 20% to 30%; exacerbates severity of HE mutations in *trans*.	1383
β-Spectrin								
Yamagata	Unknown	Unknown	Unknown	Unknown	Unknown	Truncated: ~210 kd on SDS gels	Unknown.	1488
Prague	Intron 29 (within codon 2008)	PCT	6023-1G>C	Frameshift	Splicing	Truncated: ~214 kd on SDS gels	Spherocytic elliptocytosis; ↑OF; ↓synthesis of β-spectrin; moderate spectrin deficiency.	1466
Kuwaitino	2018	Ala→Asp	A2018D	Missense	—	—	Heterozygote asymptomatic with very slight reticulocytosis; no elliptocytes and no spectrin deficiency; moderately severe HE/HPP when coinherited with αSp R28C and αSp^LELY	1443
Cagliari	2018	Ala→Gly	A2018G	Missense	—	αI/74	Heterozygote: mild HE; homozygotes: severe anemia with hydrops fetalis.	1489
Providence	2019	Ser→Pro	S2019P	Missense	—	αI/74	Heterozygote: mild HE, nl OF; homozygote: severe anemia with hydrops fetalis.	1490
Paris	2023	Ala→Val	A2023V	Missense	—	—	Highly conserved residue; heterozygote: very mild HE with a few rounded elliptocytes and low MCV; nl OF; homozygote: hydrops fetalis or near fatal anemia with marked spherocytosis, few elliptocytes.	1467
Linguere	2024	Trp→Arg	W2024R	Missense	—	—		1467
Buffalo	2025	Leu→Arg	L2025R	Missense	—	—		1491
Tandil	2042	PCT	6124-6130del7	Frameshift	7-nt deletion	Truncated: ~216 kd on SDS gels	Moderate spherocytic HE; GOE = HS pattern; rounded elliptocytes.	1460
Nice	2046	PCT	6136-6137insGA	Frameshift	2-nt insertion	Truncated: ~216 kd on SDS gels	Moderate spherocytic HE; GOE = HS pattern; hemolytic crises.	1458,1459
Kayes (Mali)	2053	Ala→Pro	A2053P	Missense	—	αI/74		1374
Napoli	2053	PCT	6160-6167del8	Frameshift	8-nt deletion	Truncated: ~216 kd on SDS gels		1492
Tokyo	2059	PCT	6177delC	Frameshift	1-nt deletion	Truncated: ~216 kd on SDS gels		1493
Cotonou	2061	Trp→Arg	W2061R	Missense	—	αI/74		1361
Cosenza	2064	Arg→Pro	R2064P	Missense	—	—		1494
Nagoya	2069	Glu→Ter	E2069X	Nonsense	—	—		1495
Campinas	Intron 30 (after codon 2073)	PCT	6219+1G>A	Frameshift	Splicing	Truncated: ~200 kd on SDS gels, plus αI/74		1496
Göttingen	Intron 30 (after codon 2073)	PCT	6219+2T>A	Frameshift	Splicing	Truncated: ~214 kd on SDS gels	Moderately severe spherocytic HE; MCV 70–90, ↑OF, hemolytic crises.	1461,1462

Name	Location[a]	Amino acid change	Nucleotide/mutation[a]	Type	Effect	Protein[b]	Clinical features[c]	References
LePuy	Intron 30 after codon 2073	PCT	6219+4A>G	Frameshift	Splicing	Truncated: ~214 kd on SDS gels	Elliptocytes and poikilocytes; OF normal.	1463,1464
Rouen	Intron 31 in codon 2090	PCT	6269+3G>T	Frameshift	Splicing	Truncated: ~218 kd on SDS gels	Moderate spherocytic HE; GOE = HS pattern; hemolytic crises.	1456,1457
Protein 4.1 Algeria	1	—	—	318-nt deletion	Abolition of initiation codon	—	Heterozygote: mild HE, 50% 4.1; homozygote: severe HE; 0% 4.1 and 9% glycophorin C.	1385,1497–1500
Annecy	1	—	—	70-kd deletion	Abolition of initiation codon	—	—	1501
Lille	1	Met→Thr	M1T	Missense	Substitution of initiation codon	—	—	1502
Madrid	1	Met→Arg	M1R	Missense	Substitution of initiation codon	—	Heterozygote: silent; homozygote: severe HE.	1434
Unnamed	407	Lys407-Gly486 deletion	K407-G486 deletion	Deletion	80-aa deletion (2 exons)	65- and 68-kd 4.1 isoforms on SDS gels	Heterozygote: mild HE; deletion removes spectrin-actin binding domain; membranes mechanically unstable.	1394,1503–1505
Hurdle-Mills	407	Lys407-Gln529 duplication	K407-Q529 duplication	Duplication	123-aa duplication	95 kd 4.1 isoform on SDS gels	Heterozygote: mild HE; duplication of spectrin-actin binding domain; normal membrane stability.	1394,1403,1405
Aravis	447	Lys deletion	K447 deletion	Deletion	1-aa deletion	—	—	1506
Glycophorin C Leach	—	Deletion of exons 3 and 4	—	—	—	—	Rare; Leach phenotype of Gerbich-negative blood group; heterozygote = silent carrier, 50% GPC; homozygote = mild HE, 0% GPC and 30% protein 4.1.	1384,1507–1515
Unnamed	44–45	—	PCT	—	2-nt deletion	—	Leach phenotype.	1509

GOE, gradient osmotic ektacytometry; GPC, glycophorin C; MCHC, mean corpuscular hemoglobin concentration; MCV, mean cellular volume; nl, normal; nt, nucleotide; OF, osmotic fragility; PCT, premature chain termination; Repeat, spectrin repeats region; SDS, sodium dodecyl sulfate; Ter, terminator codon.

[a]Mutations are abbreviated according to a described convention (933). Note that nucleotide numbers refer to the first nucleotide in the translation start ATG codon, which is numbered 1. The preceding codon is numbered −1 (there is no zero). This system conforms to the convention noted (933) but contrasts with that used by many previous authors (194,873,934), who numbered nucleotides from the beginning of a reported cDNA. Because more than one complete cDNA is available for many proteins, and the cDNAs often begin at different places in the 5′UTR, numbering from the beginning of the cDNA can be variable and confusing.

[b]This column indicates the α-spectrin domain that is altered on tryptic peptide maps (αI to αV; see Fig. 51-11) and the size of the largest tryptic peptide that is generated from the mutant domain. Thus, Sp αI/65 indicates that the αI domain is affected and that a 65-kd peptide is generated by tryptic cleavage instead of the usual 80-kd peptide. The number in parentheses indicates which spectrin repeat contains the defect. The nomenclature for β-spectrin truncation mutations reflects the size of the abnormal peptide. Finally, note that some point mutations of β-spectrin cause abnormal tryptic cleavage of the α-spectrin chain and are therefore included in the αI/74 group, the phenotype of their tryptic cleavage.

[c]Clinical severity was estimated using reported hematologic values presplenectomy and the criteria of Eber et al. (861) as modified by Eber and Lux (935).

shaped erythrocytes seen when red cells are heated (*pyro-*, fire; *poikilo-*, variegated), which explains the peculiar name. Similar red cell shapes are observed in homozygous common HE and common HE with infantile poikilocytosis.

Patients typically present with hyperbilirubinemia in the neonatal period or with anemia in the first few months of life (1447). The anemia is characterized by splenomegaly, red cell fragmentation, and erythroblastosis (1447). Complications of severe anemia, including growth retardation, frontal bossing, and early gallbladder disease, are reported (1445,1446). OF tests are very abnormal, particularly after incubation (1429,1444–1446). The MCV is very low (25 to 75 μ^3) because of the large number of fragmented red cells (1379–1381,1401,1444,1445). Another characteristic feature of these cells is their remarkable thermal sensitivity. Hereditary pyropoikilocytes fragment at 45°C to 46°C (normal = 49°C) after heating for 10 to 15 minutes (1446). After splenectomy, hemolysis is greatly lessened but not eliminated (1445,1446). Typically, the Hb after splenectomy is 10 to 14 g/dL with 3% to 10% reticulocytes (1401).

Although HPP was initially considered as a separate disease, there is convincing evidence that it is related to HE. As noted above, HPP is clinically and morphologically similar to the more severe forms of hemolytic elliptocytosis. In addition, in many cases, one of the parents or siblings has typical common HE, and in some of these kindreds, an identical molecular defect is observed in siblings with phenotypically different diseases (i.e., HPP and common HE). In other families, all of the first-degree relatives are phenotypically normal.

HPP red cells, but not hereditary elliptocytes, are partially deficient in spectrin (742,1401,1448). Typically, one parent of the HPP offspring carries an α-spectrin mutation, and the other parent is fully asymptomatic and has no detectable biochemical abnormality. Studies of spectrin synthesis and mRNA levels reveal that such asymptomatic parents carry α^{LELY} or another silent "thalassemia-like" defect of spectrin synthesis (742). When coinherited with the elliptocytogenic spectrin mutation in the HPP offspring, this thalassemia-like defect enhances the expression of the mutant spectrin in the cells and leads to a superimposed spectrin deficiency. The spectrin deficiency is thought to be responsible for the large number of spherocytes and relative paucity of elliptocytes in some HPP blood smears (Fig. 51-52C).

Spherocytic Hereditary Elliptocytosis

This dominant disorder is a phenotypic hybrid of common HE and HS. Its prevalence is unknown, but, judging from the number of published reports (1398,1449–1453) and our own experience, it is relatively rare, probably accounting for no more than 5% to 10% of HE in patients of European ancestry. Unlike common HE, almost all of the affected patients have some hemolysis. This is usually mild to moderate and is often incompletely compensated. The elliptocytes are fewer and plumper than in common HE, and some spherocytes, microspherocytes, and microelliptocytes are usually present. Poikilocytes and red cell fragments are uncommon, which distinguishes this disorder from common HE with hemolysis. Red cell morphology may vary, even within the same family. Some family members may have relatively prominent spherocytes and as few as 10% to 20% elliptocytes, whereas in others, elliptocytes predominate, and spherocytes are rare (Lux SE, *unpublished observations*;1346,1450). This may cause diagnostic confusion initially, particularly if the propositus has few elliptocytes. Family studies almost always reveal some members with obvious elliptocytosis.

Like HS red cells, spherocytic elliptocytes are osmotically fragile, particularly after incubation (Lux SE, *unpublished observations*;1450,1452,1453). Excessive mechanical fragility and

increased autohemolysis that responds to glucose are also characteristic (1450,1452,1453). Gallbladder disease is common (1450,1452), and aplastic crises are a risk. The splenic pathology also mimics HS (1450,1451). Splenic sequestration is evident, red cells are conditioned during splenic passage, and hemolysis abates after splenectomy (1450,1452,1453,1455).

It appears that spherocytic HE has several molecular etiologies. C-terminal truncations of β-spectrin are one of the most common causes (1456–1466). Ten such truncations have been identified (Table 51-21). The affected patients typically have moderate hemolysis and anemia punctuated by recurrent, severe hemolytic crises (1457,1458,1461,1496). Blood smears show plump elliptocytes (1457,1458,1460,1465,1466,1496), which are usually smooth, although in three cases, poikilocytosis was prominent (1461,1463,1496). In all but one instance (1457) when tested, the HE red cells were mildly heat sensitive. All patients had a positive OF test or an osmotic gradient ektacytometry pattern that resembled the pattern in HS, and one patient also had a positive AGLT (1458).

Synthesis of the truncated spectrin was decreased in one tested patient with spectrin Prague and was associated with a moderate to marked decrease in spectrin content of the red cells (1466), indicating that the synthetic defect was not adequately compensated by the normal allele. This is likely to be the cause of the spherocytic part of the phenotype, because deficiency of β-spectrin is a major cause of HS (see earlier section Hereditary Spherocytosis). Presumably, the other truncated β-spectrins that cause spherocytic HE are also associated with spectrin deficiency.

In one tested patient (1496), tryptic digestion gave an α$^{I/74}$ pattern. This supports the idea that the extra helix in the partial repeat at the N-terminal end of the α-chain is unstable when it is not associated with the β-chain, and it is more susceptible to tryptic cleavage to the 74-kd fragment (1511).

Like HS, the spleen is enlarged and selectively destroys labeled elliptocytes (1463) (T$_{1/2}$ = 11 days; normal = 24 to 34 days), and splenectomy is effective (1496).

Patients who lack GPC also have positive OF tests and rounded, smooth elliptocytes (1510–1512). They should probably also be classified as a recessive (and unusually mild) variant of spherocytic HE.

Many patients who lack protein 4.2 (another recessive condition) display features of spherocytic HE, such as ovalostomatocytosis (988,1022,1512), whereas others have spherocytes and are classified as HS. Because protein 4.2 is part of the spectrin-ankyrin-band 3 complex that attaches the membrane skeleton to the lipid bilayer, and because deficiencies of the other proteins in the complex cause HS, 4.2 deficiency is better classified as a variant of that disorder.

Mice with a knock-out of the β-adducin gene also have the phenotype of spherocytic elliptocytosis (see Animal and Fish Models of Hereditary Spherocytosis) (575). Whether β-adducin deficiency is also a cause of spherocytic HE in humans has not been tested.

Rarely, patients appear to be compound heterozygotes for HS and HE. One Turkish girl (1513) is a particularly good candidate. Her mother and father had mild HS and common HE (probably), respectively, whereas she experienced a moderately severe hemolytic anemia (Hb = 8.4; reticulocytes = 24.0%; bilirubin 1.6 mg/dL) with frontal bossing, osteoporosis, splenomegaly (10 cm), and a mixture of microspherocytes and rounded elliptocytes.

Hereditary Elliptocytosis with Dyserythropoiesis

In a small number of families with HE, the sporadic occurrence of hemolysis and anemia is at least partially due to the development of dysplastic and ineffective erythropoiesis. All reported patients with this rare syndrome (1514,1515) are from Italy, have somewhat less elongated red cells than is typical for common HE, and show the characteristic findings of ineffective erythropoiesis (relatively low retic counts, indirect hyperbilirubinemia, high serum iron and ferritin, and rapid clearance of ^{59}Fe combined with poor incorporation of ^{59}Fe into new erythrocytes). Some patients are macrocytic. The patients' bone marrows are hyperplastic, with decreased late erythroblasts and dysplastic features (asynchrony of nuclear-cytoplasmic maturation, binuclearity, internuclear bridges, and a small number of ringed sideroblasts) (1514,1515). Anemia and, presumably, erythroid dysplasia usually commence during adolescence or early adult life and advance gradually over years. Because dysplasia persists after splenectomy, response to the operation is incomplete. The available data suggest that dysplasia and elliptocytosis cosegregate because no individuals with dysplasia have been observed who did not have elliptocytosis (1514,1515). If so, these families must represent a unique subtype of common HE. This is supported by the fact that none of the typical HE protein defects (see Etiology) was observed in one well-studied family (1515). Spectrin self-association, spectrin peptide maps, and the concentration of protein 4.1 and other major membrane proteins were normal.

Southeast Asian Ovalocytosis

This fascinating condition, also known as *hereditary ovalocytosis, Melanesian elliptocytosis,* or *stomatocytic elliptocytosis,* is inherited in an autosomal-dominant pattern (1516–1520). Homozygosity is probably lethal (1521,1522). It is observed in the aboriginal populations of Melanesia and Malaysia and in portions of Indonesia, Madagascar, and the Philippines (1517,1518,1523–1526a). The disease occurs but is rare in Western populations (1527,1528). It is very common in Melanesia (1517,1520,1526,1529).

RESISTANCE TO MALARIA

Malaria is endemic in the lowland tribes in which SAO is common (1516,1520,1526,1529). In these tribes, 5% to 25% of the natives are affected. *In vivo,* there is evidence that SAO provides some protection against all forms of malaria (1516,1517,1520,1526,1529,1530), particularly against heavy infections (1189), but protection is incomplete. Nevertheless, the prevalence of SAO increases with age in populations challenged by malaria, suggesting that ovalocytic individuals have a survival advantage (1530). Recent work indicates that the SAO band 3 variant prevents cerebral malaria but exacerbates malaria anemia (1531,1532). *In vitro,* SAO red cells are resistant to invasion by malarial parasites (1533–1535), apparently because the membrane is 10 to 20 times more rigid than normal (1536–1539) (Fig. 51-53A). Other membrane characteristics reflect this property. For example, the cells are unusually heat resistant. They easily withstand heating to 49°C, at which temperature normal red cells disintegrate (1534); they do not undergo endocytosis in response to drugs that produce dramatic endocytosis in normal cells (1538); and they strongly resist crenation (1538), even after several days of storage in plasma or buffered salt solutions (Fig. 51-53B). The latter property, combined with the distinctive red cell morphology provides a simple means of diagnosing the disease.

HEMATOLOGY

In the typical patient, more than 20% of the cells are rounded elliptocytes, a few of which are traversed by one or two transverse bars that divide the central clear space (1519,1523–1526) (Fig. 51-52D). These "elliptical knizocytes" or "stomatocytic elliptocytes" are not seen in any other condition. Stomatocytes or red cells (or both) with multiple linear or nonlinear ("S," "C," or bizarre-shaped) pale regions are present in all patients,

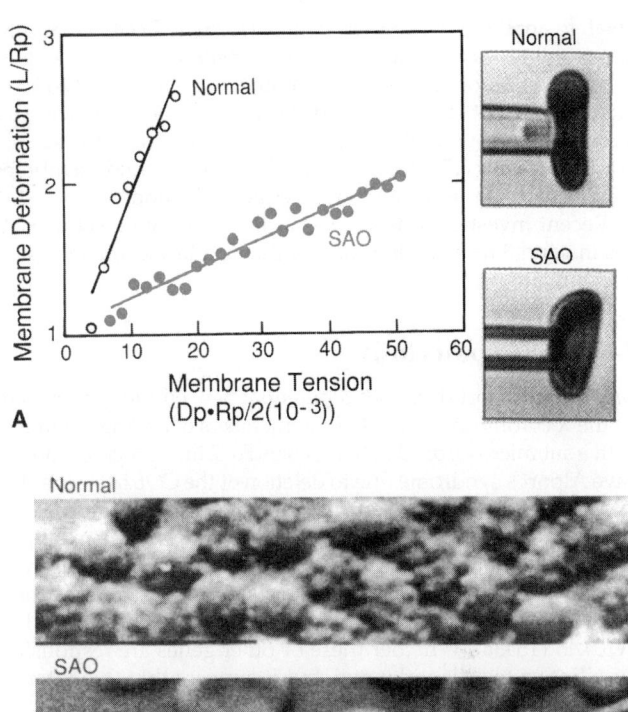

Figure 51-53. Membrane stiffness of Southeast Asian ovalocytosis (SAO) red cells as measured by micropipette (**A**), and lack of crenation (**B**). Membrane rigidity of normal and SAO red cells. **Top right:** Videomicrographs of pipette aspirations of normal and SAO red cells. Note that the SAO cell forms a much smaller tongue of membrane than the normal cell at the same aspiration pressure. **Top left:** Plots of membrane tension, where D_p = aspiration pressure versus tongue length (L), both normalized by the pipette radius (Rp). A much higher tension is required to aspirate an equal length of SAO membrane into the pipette (*solid blue circles*) than normal membrane (*open black circles*). **Bottom:** Failure of SAO red cells to crenate, compared to normal cells, when diluted in saline. This is one of the simplest methods for demonstrating the rigidity of SAO membranes. [Adapted from Mohandas N, Chasis JA. Red cell deformability, membrane material properties, and shape: regulation by transmembrane, skeletal, and cytosolic proteins and lipids. *Semin Hematol* 1993;30:171 (**A**); and Saul A, Lamont G, Sawyer WH, Kidson C. Decreased membrane deformability in Melanesian ovalocytes from Papua New Guinea. *J Cell Biol* 1984;98:1348 (**B**).]

including patients who have the characteristic molecular lesion (see Protein 3 Mutations: Southeast Asian Ovalocytosis) but lack elliptocytes (25% of patients in one series) (1531). The latter cells look like stomatocytes with curved "stoma." These are also quite characteristic, although similar cells are seen in cryohydrocytosis (see section Cryohydrocytosis). A large subpopulation of hyperdense red cells was observed on MCHC histograms in two white patients with SAO (1540). These may be an artifact of cold storage because recent studies show that cation permeability is greatly increased at 4°C (1541). If not, there should be an easy way to screen for the disease.

Hemolysis is mild or absent (1517,1523–1525,1531,1539,1542). For example, one patient had compensated hemolysis (no anemia), with mild splenomegaly, an absolute reticulocyte count of 150 to 300 × 10³ (normal = 40 to 80 × 10³), mild hyperbilirubinemia, and gallstones (1542). However, most patients seem to have no more anemia than control children when well, but they are more anemic when infected with malaria (1531). This indicates that membrane rigidity is not a major determinant of red cell survival. In another well-studied patient (1525), red cell Na^+ and K^+ permeability was increased, glucose consumption was elevated to compensate for increased cation pumping, autohemolysis was increased, and the cells were osmotically resistant. Curiously, many blood group antigens are poorly expressed on the surface of SAO red cells (1526), conceivably because the rigid membrane inhibits their clustering and impedes agglutination.

Recent investigations show that the primary defect in SAO lies in band 3 near the interface of the membrane and cytoplasmic domains.

X-Linked Elliptocytosis

One recent report describes a potential new elliptocytosis locus on the X chromosome (1543). Four members of an English family with a submicroscopic deletion of band q22 in the X chromosome have Alport's syndrome due to deletion of the COL4A5 gene. The two affected male members also have mental retardation, dysmorphic facies with midface hypoplasia, and prominent elliptocytosis but no anemia, reticulocytosis, or red cell membrane fragility. These individuals have a contiguous gene syndrome that includes the FACL4 and AMMECR1 genes as well as COL4A5 (1543a). Whether these or other genes are responsible for elliptocytosis is unknown, but it appears that this interval contains a previously unknown elliptocytosis locus.

Etiology

METHODS TO DEFINE ABNORMAL SPECTRIN STRUCTURE AND FUNCTION IN HEREDITARY ELLIPTOCYTOSIS

Thermal Sensitivity of Red Cells and Spectrin. Red cells heated to temperatures approaching 50°C for short periods become unstable and fragment spontaneously (1544–1546), probably due to the denaturation of spectrin (1547). Normal spectrin denatures at 49°C (10 minutes of exposure) (766,1547), and normal red cells fragment at the same temperature (766,1446,1538). As noted earlier, all patients with HPP (by definition) and some patients with other forms of HE have thermally sensitive red cells. Hereditary pyropoikilocytes and red cells from infants with common HE and neonatal poikilocytosis fragment after 10 minutes at 44°C to 46°C (1424,1446). Red cells from some, but not all, patients with common HE fragment at 47°C to 48°C (766,1446). As expected, purified spectrin from these red cells is also heat sensitive (766,1547). This test is limited because we do not understand, in molecular terms, why specific mutations are thermally sensitive. However, it remains one of the simplest tests available for assessing HPP in laboratories that do not specialize in membrane protein analysis.

Abnormal Spectrin Oligomerization. Many patients with HE and all patients with HPP are unable to properly convert spectrin dimers to tetramers and higher oligomers *in vitro* or on the membrane (Fig. 51-54). This important functional property is easily assessed in low-temperature spectrin extracts. At 0°C, the equilibrium between spectrin dimer and tetramer is greatly slowed—virtually frozen (434). If spectrin is extracted from the membrane at 0°C and carefully protected from warming during the separation of dimers, tetramers, and oligomers (usually on nondenaturing polyacrylamide gels), the proportion of each spectrin species reflects its relative proportion on the membrane (1548). Patients with defects in spectrin self-association have abnormally high proportions of spectrin dimer in 0°C spectrin extracts (i.e., >10% of total spectrin dimers and tetramers) (1376,1549,1550). The fraction of spectrin dimers is an important functional assessment in patients with α-spectrin defects. It cor-

relates well with clinical severity (1411) and accurately predicts unusually severe mutations (1405). Conversely, discordance between the degree of hemolysis and fraction of spectrin dimers may alert the physician to an underlying, secondary complication (see earlier section Common Hereditary Elliptocytosis with Sporadic Hemolysis).

Ektacytometry. The ektacytometer can be used to assess red cell membrane deformability and stability in patients with hemolytic disorders (1551,1552). Isolated red cell ghosts are subjected to a high shear stress in a laser diffraction viscometer, and the "deformability index" (a measure of the average elongation of the sheared ghosts) is recorded as a function of time. Fragile ghosts fragment more quickly than normal, causing their "deformability" to fall (Fig. 51-55). The technique is a useful screening test because membrane stability is reduced in almost all membrane skeletal diseases, particularly HE and HPP.

In addition, the ektacytometer can be modified to measure cellular deformability at different osmolalities, a technique termed *osmotic gradient ektacytometry* (1553). This was discussed in detail in the section Hereditary Spherocytosis (Fig. 51-46). The resulting curves are dependent on both membrane surface area and cell volume and are a sensitive measure of the surface loss that characterizes many skeletal defects.

Two-Dimensional Spectrin Domain Maps. In the past, spectrin structure was analyzed by "domain mapping" (1554,1555)—limited tryptic digestion, performed at 0°C, followed by one-dimensional (SDS-PAGE) or two-dimensional (isoelectric focusing, then SDS-PAGE) separation of the resulting trypsin-resistant domains into characteristic, reproducible maps. The relationship of these domains to spectrin structure is depicted in Fig. 51-11. A two-dimensional separation of normal spectrin domains is shown in Figure 51-56. Among these peptides, the 80-kd αI domain peptide, which contains the self-association site of normal α-spectrin, is the most prominent. Almost all α- or β-spectrin HE and HPP mutations are associated with tryptic peptides of abnormal size and mobility that are generated instead of the normal 80-kd peptide (Fig. 51-57). The cleavage sites of the most common abnormal tryptic peptides are located near the end of the or in the adjoining "linker" region between repeats third helix (helix C) of the triple-helical spectrin repeats (1556). The reported mutations reside in the vicinity of these cleavage sites either in the same helix or, less commonly, at neighboring sites in helices one or two (1556). Consequently, tryptic peptide mapping is a powerful tool to map the approximate sites of the underlying spectrin mutations; the mutations can subsequently be defined by PCR amplification and sequencing of the respective region of the cDNA or genomic DNA.

In this era of high throughput DNA sequencing, two-dimensional spectrin peptide mapping is used less than it once was, but it is important to understand the technique because the old literature on spectrin defects in HE is so dependent on the technology.

Molecular Analysis. There are two general approaches used to identify mutations in membrane proteins. One is to analyze the cDNA made from the patient's mRNA. Reticulocyte mRNA is isolated, reverse transcribed, and amplified using the PCR. The cDNA product is subjected to nucleic acid sequencing or other forms of analysis. For heterozygotes, several independent subclones must be sequenced because, on average, only one-half have the mutant allele. The major problem with this approach is that the mutant mRNA is often destroyed by the process of "nonsense-mediated mRNA decay" (1557,1558) when a nonsense or frameshift mutation is present. Such mutations are common in HS and occur in HE, although missense mutations are more common in HE.

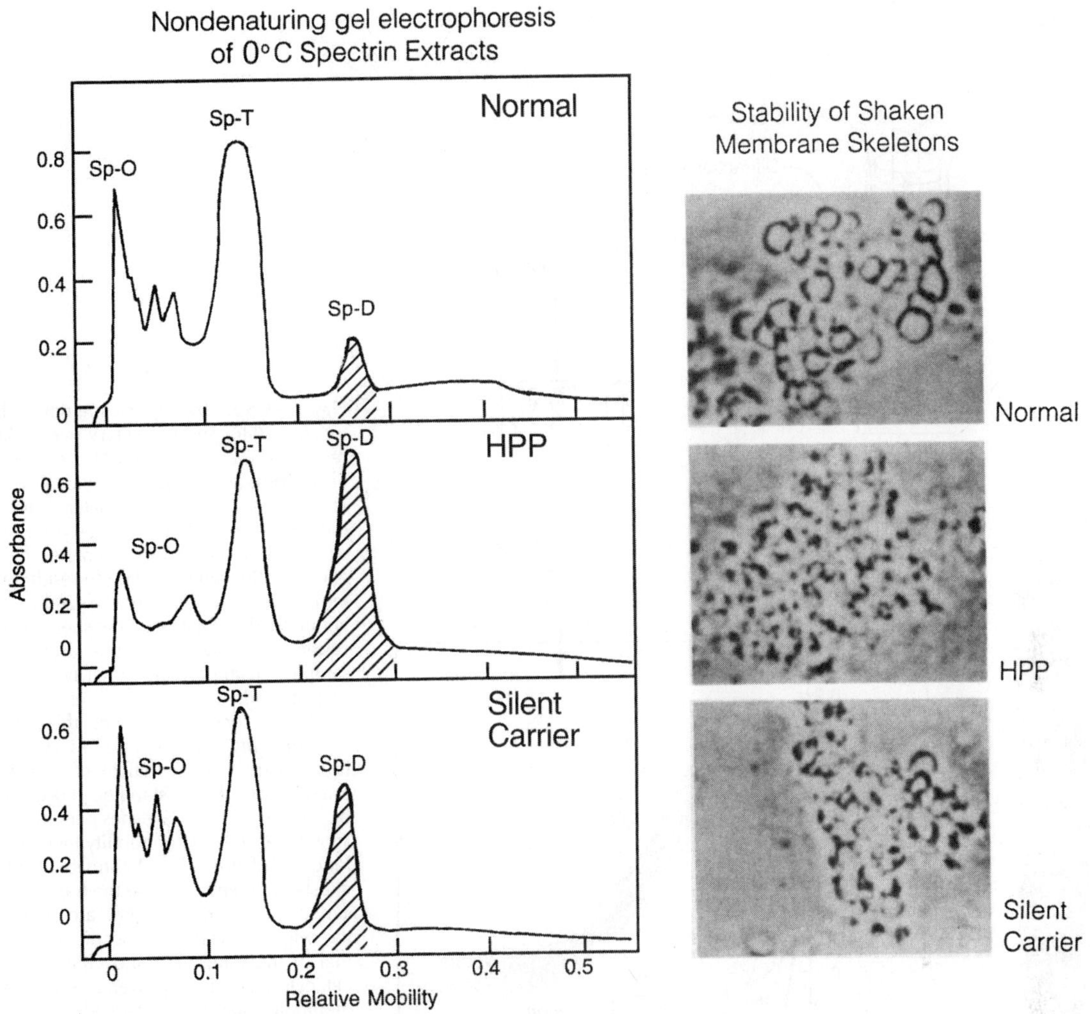

Figure 51-54. Increased spectrin dimers (Sp-D) and membrane fragility in hereditary elliptocytosis and hereditary pyropoikilocytosis (HPP). **Left:** Analysis of Sp-D, tetramers (Sp-T), and oligomers (Sp-O) by nondenaturing gel electrophoresis in a normal individual, a patient with HPP, and his mother, a silent carrier. The densitometric tracing of the scanned gel is shown. **Right:** Membrane skeletons from each of the three persons were shaken for 1 hour and examined microscopically. Note the increased fraction of Sp-D in the HPP patient (~50%) and his asymptomatic mother (~30%) compared to normal (8 ± 3%). Note also that the membrane skeletons of the patient, and to a lesser extent his mother, are fragile and disintegrate with shaking, whereas normal skeletons remain intact. (Reprinted from Liu S-C, Palek J, Prchal J, Castlebury RP. Altered spectrin dimer-dimer association and instability of erythrocyte membrane skeletons in hereditary pyropoikilocytosis. *J Clin Invest* 1981;68:597, with permission.)

Alternatively, genomic DNA can be substituted for mRNA if intron-exon boundaries are known, and the PCR-amplified exons can be sequenced directly or first screened for mutations. Screening is particularly advantageous for large proteins with dozens of exons, such as spectrin or ankyrin. The SSCP (single-strand conformation polymorphism) method (1559,1560) is a simple, sensitive, and appropriately popular example of such a screening test. It detects approximately 70% to 90% of mutations. In some regions where common elliptocytogenic mutations have been identified, multiplex PCR techniques or simple restriction endonuclease digestion of amplified genomic DNA have been developed to screen rapidly for these mutations.

α-SPECTRIN DEFECTS: GENERAL CONCEPTS*

Defects in the αI or αII Domains Impair Spectrin Self-Association. Defects of spectrin self-association are found in many patients with common HE and in all patients with HPP. Most of the defects lie in the 80-kd αI domain at the N-terminal

end of the α-spectrin chain (Fig. 51-11). Nine tryptic cleavage defects of the αI domain have been identified by peptide mapping (Table 51-21; Figs. 51-58 and 51-59). These are characterized by the loss of the normal 80-kd αI peptide and the appearance of one of the following:

A new 78-kd peptide ($\alpha^{I/78}$) (1386,1387,1472)
A new 74-kd peptide ($\alpha^{I/74}$) (1375,1376,1388,1401,1405–1407,1428,1442,1469,1474,1561)
A new 65- or 68-kd peptide ($\alpha^{I/65}$ or $\alpha^{I/68}$) (1389–1391,1401,1408,1429,1442,1477–1481,1483,1562)
A new 61-kd peptide ($\alpha^{I/61}$) (1430)
A new 46-kd peptide ($\alpha^{I/46}$) (1482)

---

*The nomenclature for α-spectrin defects in HE includes an abbreviation for spectrin (Sp) followed by a superscript designation of the α-spectrin domain that is altered on tryptic peptide maps (αI to αV) and the size of the largest tryptic peptide that is generated from the mutant domain (1379). Thus, Sp $\alpha^{I/65}$ indicates that the αI domain (80 kd) is affected and that a 65-kd peptide is generated by tryptic cleavage instead of the usual 80-kd peptide.

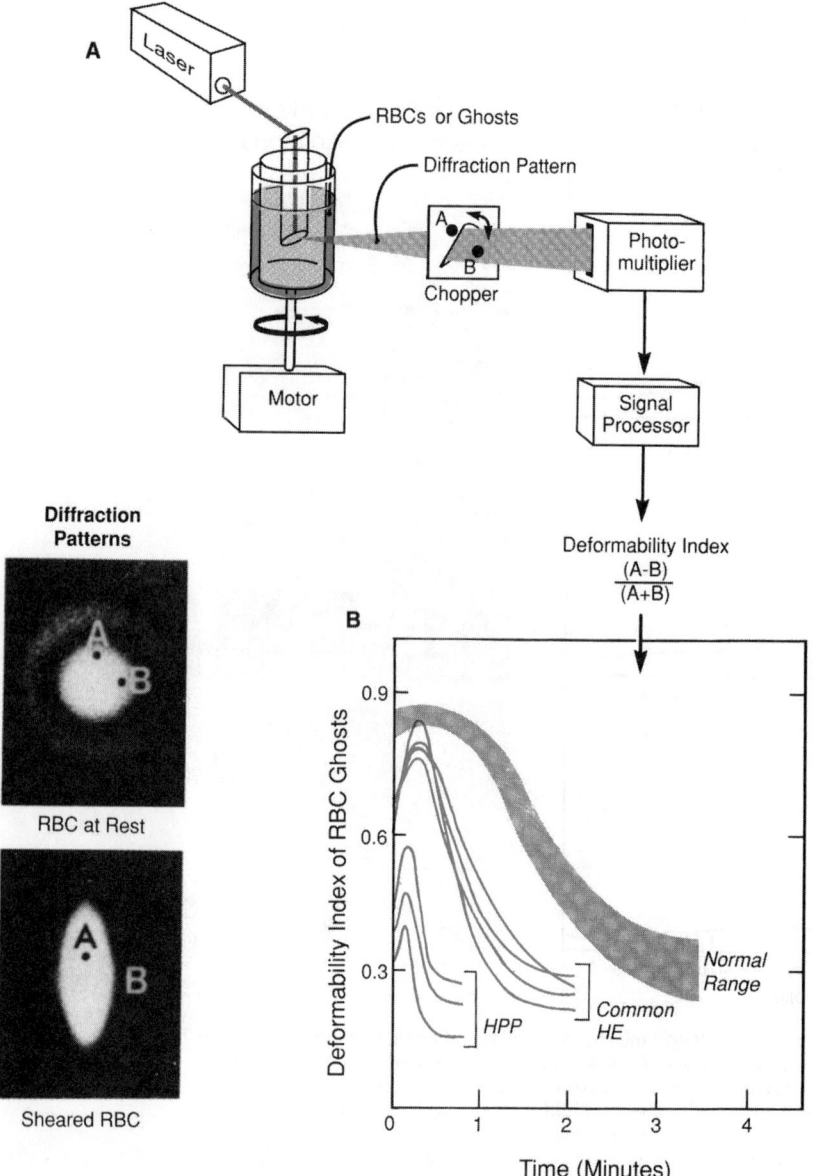

Diffraction Patterns

RBC at Rest

Sheared RBC

Figure 51-55. Membrane fragility of hereditary elliptocytosis (HE) and hereditary pyropoikilocytosis (HPP) red cells measured with the ektacytometer. **A:** The ektacytometer combines a concentric cylinder viscometer with a laser diffractometer. The outer cylinder of the viscometer is spun to produce a uniform shear stress. The laser beam is diffracted by the red cells or ghosts in the sample, and the resulting diffraction patterns (photos at left) are analyzed to give information about the deformation of the sheared cells. In the usual system, the intensity of the laser light is alternately sampled, using a chopper, at two points (A,B), which lie just inside the edge of the resting diffraction pattern. A signal processor converts this information into a *deformability index*, defined as (A − B)/(A + B), which is a measure of the ellipticity of the sheared cells. **B:** To measure membrane stability, ghosts are subjected to a high shear stress (575 dynes per cm^2 in the experiment shown), and the deformability index is determined as a function of time. The deformability index falls as the ghosts fragment, because the fragments have a smaller surface to volume ratio (i.e., are more spheroidal) than the original ghosts. This occurs more rapidly than normal in the fragile HE and HPP red cells. In general, ektacytometry is a powerful screening test because membrane stability is reduced in almost all membrane skeletal disorders. (Adapted from Mohandas N, Clark MR, Health BO, et al. A technique to detect reduced mechanical stability of red cell membranes: relevance to elliptocytic disorders. *Blood* 1982;59:768; and Mohandas N, Clark MR, Jacobs MS, Shohet SB. Analysis of factors regulating erythrocyte deformability. *J Clin Invest* 1980;66:563.)

A new 50-kd (or 46-kd) peptide ($\alpha^{I/50a}$ or $\alpha^{I/46-50a}$) (673,685,688,692,709,710,716,1174,1175)

A new 50-kd peptide with a more basic isoelectric point than $\alpha^{I/50a}$ ($\alpha^{I/50b}$) (1410,1478,1483,1485,1486)

Two new peptides of 43- and 42-kd ($\alpha^{I/43}$) (1563)

Two new peptides of 36- and 33-kd ($\alpha^{I/36}$) (1409)

All of these defects produce a similar functional deficit: diminished spectrin self-association, reflected in the increased proportion of spectrin dimers in 0°C low ionic strength extracts of spectrin (Fig. 51-54) and the decreased conversion of spectrin dimers to tetramers in solution, in ghosts, and on inside-out vesicles. In addition, all patients show decreased red cell thermal stability. The fragile spectrin-spectrin links weaken the membrane skeleton and diminish the resistance of the isolated membrane or skeleton to shear stresses (749,1378,1552) (Fig. 51-55).

Morrow and colleagues have recently shown that spectrin self-association, the binding of spectrin to ankyrin, and the binding of ankyrin to the cytoplasmic domain of band 3 are all coupled in a positively cooperative way (1564). This important observation may explain why spectrin mutations distal to the self-association sites that do not directly destabilize self-association

or ankyrin binding can cause hemolysis. Three classes of mutations appear to disrupt cooperative coupling between self-association and ankyrin binding (1564).

Many α-spectrin mutations that cause HE occur at the C-terminal end of helix C of the spectrin repeat, in the linker region connecting one repeat with the next (Fig. 51-59; Table 51-21). Examples include α-spectrin Ponte de Sôr, the Leu154 duplication, and α-spectrins Nigerian, Sfax, and Barcelona. Presumably, such mutations block the repeat-to-repeat transfer of conformational information and prevent the cooperative linkage of the various binding interactions.

Mutations in α-spectrin repeats 5 to 7 presumably disrupt the ability of this region to transregulate ankyrin binding by the adjacent β-spectrin repeats 14 to 15. Examples include α-spectrins Alexandria and Barcelona (Table 51-21). The unnamed spectrin αGln471→Pro, in particular, lies immediately adjacent to the ankyrin-binding site in β-spectrin.

Distal exon-skipping mutations shorten α-spectrin and force repeats 5 to 7 to fall out of register with the ankyrin-binding motif in β-spectrin. Presumably, these also interfere with the transregulation of ankyrin binding. Examples

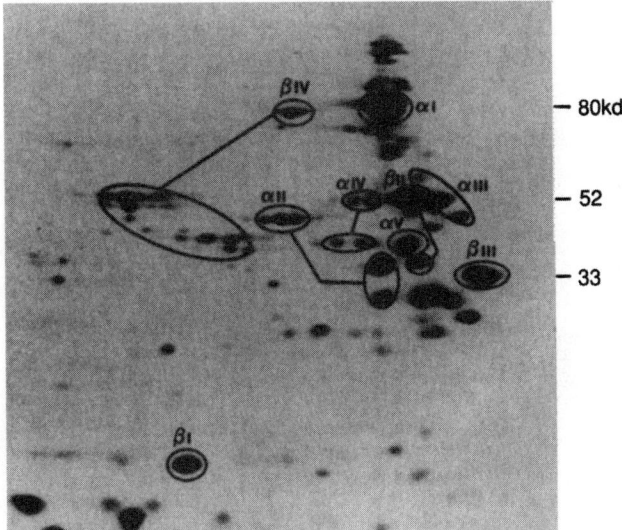

Figure 51-56. Tryptic domains of spectrin. The partial tryptic digest is separated by isoelectric focusing, pH 6.5 to 4.5 (*left to right*), followed by sodium dodecyl sulfate gel electrophoresis (*top to bottom*). The major α- and β-chain domain peptides are labeled. (Reprinted from Gallagher PG, Forget BG. Spectrin genes in health and disease. *Semin Hematol* 1993;30:4, with permission.)

include spectrins Oran ($\alpha^{II/21}$) and St Claude ($\alpha^{II/47}$) (Table 51-21). These defects are relatively mild and are only clinically evident in the homozygous or compound heterozygous state. This is also true for another distal defect, spectrin Jendouba ($\alpha^{II/31}$).

Severity Depends on the Amount of Mutant Spectrin and Its Effect on Self-Association. In general, patients with spectrin defects in the αI or αII domains have common HE (or HPP). The severity of a particular mutation correlates especially with the degree of impairment of spectrin self-association and with the degree of structural disruption, as measured by the deviation of the predicted backbone structure of the mutant spectrin

from the crystal structure of a normal spectrin repeat (1565). Electron micrographs of negatively stained red cell membrane skeletons from patients with various α-spectrin mutations corroborate this association (697,758,1401) (Fig. 51-60). Severity is also affected by the amount of the mutant spectrin, which is strongly influenced by the spectrin α^{LELY} polymorphism.

SPECTRIN α^{LELY} (OR $\alpha^{V/41}$) POLYMORPHISM

Differences in clinical expression are at least partially due to the presence or absence of the α^{LELY} (*low expression allele from Lyon*, France) polymorphism on the "normal" spectrin allele (i.e., in *trans* to α-spectrin mutations that cause HE) (1382). This polymorphism is very common, affecting approximately 30% of the α-spectrin alleles of European whites and 20% of the alleles of Japanese and African blacks (1382). This means that approximately 42% of the European white population are heterozygous for Sp α^{LELY}, and 9% are homozygous. (The comparable figures in Japan and Africa are 32% and 4%, respectively.) The exceptional frequency of the polymorphism suggests that it may be experiencing genetic selection. If so, its advantage is presently unclear.

Sp α^{LELY} is actually a combination of two linked mutations: one in exon 40 and one in intron 45 (1383). The effect of each is shown in Figure 51-61. Exon 40 contributes a point mutation in helix B of α-spectrin repeat 19 that converts Leu1857→Val. When folded according to the crystallographic model (Fig. 51-11), this valine lies next to the tryptic site (Lys1920) that is cleaved to generate the αIV and αV domains. This results in more rapid cleavage of the αIV-αV junction and an increased concentration of the 41-kd αV domain, the so-called $\alpha^{V/41}$ polymorphism (Fig. 51-61).

The linked defect is responsible for low expression. It is a C→T substitution at position –12 in the 3' ("acceptor") splice site of intron 45, and it interferes with the splicing of the neighboring exon 46, so that half of the resulting RNAs and proteins contain exon 46, and half do not (1383,1568) (Fig. 51-61). Exon 46 is very small—only six amino acids (1569)—so its absence is not evident on SDS gels. However, it lies in the middle of the site that nucleates the assembly of the spectrin α and β subunits (1566). The α-chains that lack exon 46 do not assemble into stable spectrin dimers and are rapidly degraded (1567).

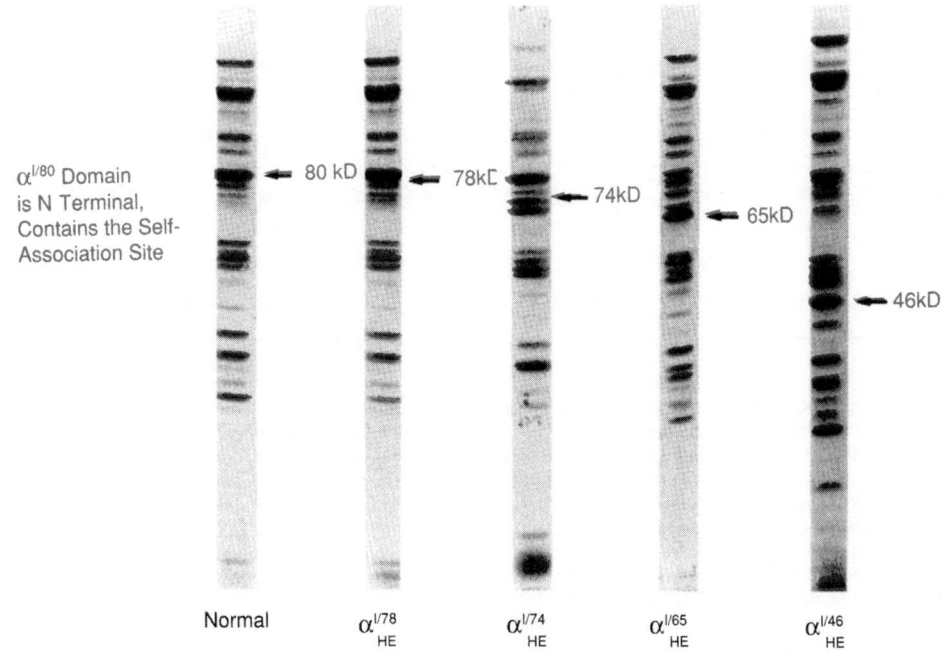

$\alpha^{I/80}$ Domain is N Terminal, Contains the Self-Association Site

Normal $\alpha^{I/78}_{HE}$ $\alpha^{I/74}_{HE}$ $\alpha^{I/65}_{HE}$ $\alpha^{I/46}_{HE}$

Figure 51-57. Spectrin domains in hereditary elliptocytosis (HE). One-dimensional peptide maps of partial tryptic digests of normal spectrin (*left*). The tryptic digestion releases an 80-kd peptide from the N-terminus of the normal α chain. In the $\alpha^{I/78}$, $\alpha^{I/74}$, $\alpha^{I/65}$, and $\alpha^{I/46}$ mutant α-spectrins the 80-kd domain is degraded to smaller peptides (*arrows*) by trypsin, due to local conformational changes produced by the mutations. (Adapted from Delaunay J, Dhermy D. Mutations involving the spectrin heterodimer contact site: clinical expression and alterations in specific function. *Semin Hematol* 1993;30:21.)

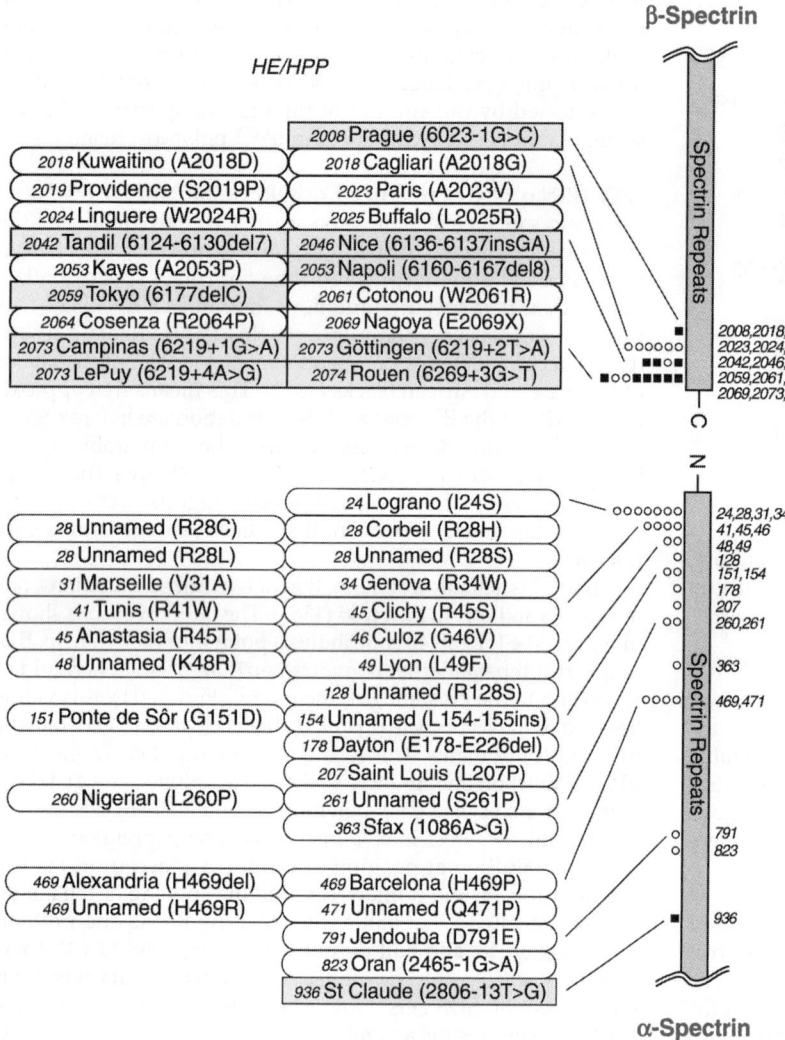

Figure 51-58. Spectrin mutations associated with hereditary elliptocytosis (HE) and hereditary pyropoikilocytosis (HPP) are shown alongside a schematic representation of the N-terminus of α-spectrin and the C-terminus of β-spectrin. On the left, missense mutations are shown in open ellipses, and mutations causing peptide truncation are shown in shaded rectangles. The nucleotide numbers of the mutations are relative to the first nucleotide of the ATG initiation codon and may differ from the numbering in some published reports. (Adapted from Tse WT, Lux SE. Hereditary spherocytosis and hereditary elliptocytosis. In: Scriver CR, Beaudet AL, Sly WS, Valle D, eds. *The metabolic and molecular bases of inherited disease*, 8th ed. New York: McGraw-Hill, 2001:4665.)

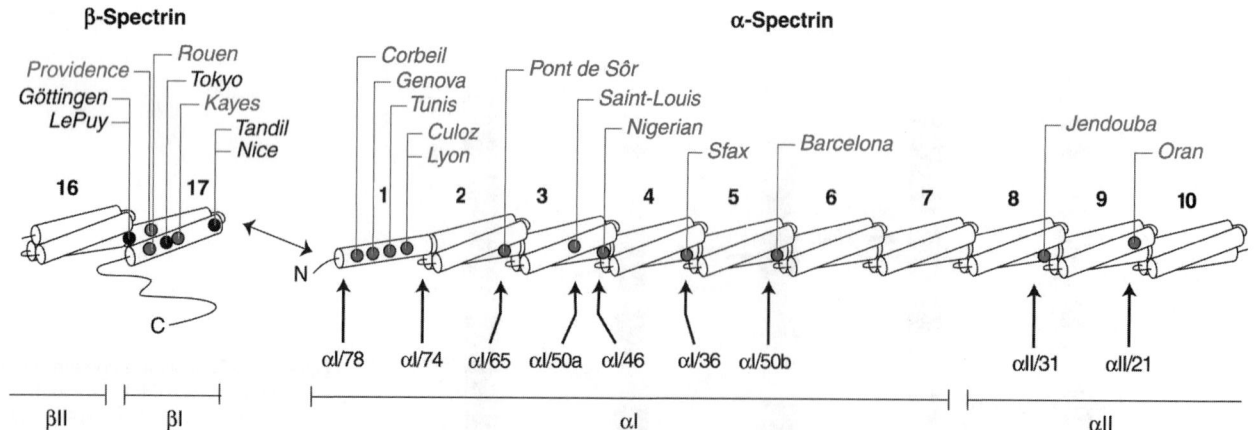

Figure 51-59. Location of some of the spectrin defects in hereditary elliptocytosis and hereditary pyropoikilocytosis on the triple helical model of spectrin structure. The tryptic cleavage sites observed in α-spectrin defects are also indicated. Note that the majority of defects are close to the site of spectrin self-association. Nearly all the α-spectrin mutations are missense mutations or in-frame deletions or insertions (*blue circles*). Many of the more distal mutations are in helix C near the junction between one spectrin repeat and the next and are thought to interfere with cooperative effects linking spectrin self-association to spectrin-ankyrin and ankyrin–band 3 interactions. Most β-chain defects are C-terminal truncations (*black circles*) or missense mutations directly affecting spectrin self-association (*blue circles*). The truncations also impair synthesis of the mutant spectrin and lead to a spherocytic hereditary elliptocytosis phenotype. (Adapted from Tse WT, Lux SE. Hereditary spherocytosis and hereditary elliptocytosis. In: Scriver CR, Beaudet AL, Sly WS, Valle D, eds. *The metabolic and molecular bases of inherited disease*, 8th ed. New York: McGraw-Hill, 2001:4665.)

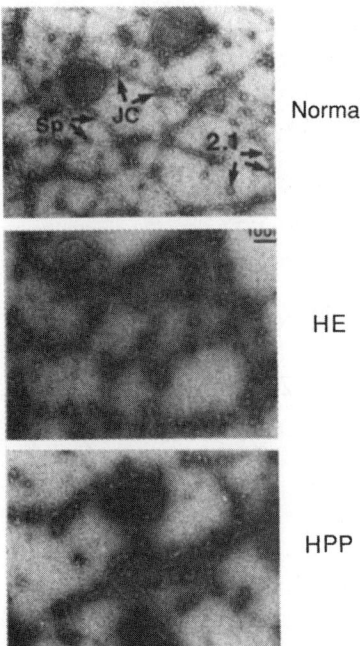

Normal

HE

HPP

Figure 51-60. Electron micrographs of negative-stained membrane skeletons from normal hereditary elliptocytosis (HE) and hereditary pyropoikilocytosis (HPP) red cells. Note that the regular structure of the normal skeleton is moderately disrupted in the HE skeleton and severely damaged in HPP. JC, junctional complexes; Sp, spectrin tetramers; 2.1, ankyrin molecules. (Reprinted from Liu S-C, Derick LH. Molecular anatomy of the red blood cell membrane skeleton: structure-function relationships. *Semin Hematol* 1992;29:231, with permission.)

The polymorphism is completely silent by itself, even when homozygous, probably because α-spectrin is normally synthesized in a three- or fourfold excess (736). However, when Sp α^{LELY} is inherited in *trans* to an α-spectrin mutation, it has the effect of increasing the concentration of the mutant spectrin and the severity of the associated disease (1382) (Fig. 51-62). The effect can be quite dramatic. For example, in one family, a patient who was heterozygous for the $\alpha^{I/74}$ mutation ($\alpha^{I/74}/\alpha$) had mild disease and almost no morphologic abnormality, whereas a relative who had also inherited the α^{LELY} allele ($\alpha^{I/74}/\alpha^{LELY}$) had severe elliptocytosis (1382). Similarly, in another family, the α^{LELY} allele increased the proportion of Sp $\alpha^{I/65}$ in heterozygotes from 45% to 65% of the total spectrin (1382,1570). This was associated with an increase in the proportion of elliptocytes from none or only a few to nearly 100%. A similar effect (1571) is observed with Sp $\alpha^{I/50}$. All α-spectrin mutations seem to be similarly affected (1382). Conversely, when the α^{LELY} allele is on the same chromosome as an α-spectrin mutation, it mutes the elliptocytic phenotype (1377) (Fig. 51-62).

Sp α^{LELY} should be distinguished from other thalassemia-like defects of α-spectrin synthesis that, when coinherited with some of the α-spectrin mutations, produce a phenotype of HPP (see section Hereditary Pyropoikilocytosis). The defect is characterized by reduced α-spectrin mRNA levels and diminished α-spectrin synthesis (738). Deletion of the α-spectrin gene, although not yet reported, would produce a similar effect. In contrast, α-spectrin mRNA levels are normal in Sp α^{LELY}.

α-SPECTRIN DEFECTS: SPECIFIC MUTATIONS

Spectrin $\alpha^{I/74}$. The $\alpha^{I/74}$ defect is heterogeneous and is caused by mutations in codons 24, 28, 31, 34, 46, 48, or 49 (1405–1407,1467–1471,1474) (Table 51-21). Codon 28, containing a CpG dinucleotide,

may be a mutation "hot spot" and is associated with four different mutations. The defects result in enhanced tryptic cleavage following Arg45 or Lys48 in repeat 1, an extra helical segment (helix C) that juts out from the N-terminal end of the α-spectrin chain. This is the end that participates in spectrin self-association (Fig. 51-11). The corresponding (C-terminal) end of the β-chain also contains extra helices (helices A and B) in repeat 17, followed by a phosphorylated segment (Fig. 51-11). These three helices pair, as they do all along the spectrin chain, and form the bond responsible for spectrin self-association (1374,1511,1572).

Because the Sp $\alpha^{I/74}$ mutations disrupt one of the three interacting terminal helices, they should markedly disrupt spectrin self-association. Curiously, the mutations arising in codon 45 or 48 result in severe HPP, whereas those arising in codons 41, 46, or 49 result in a milder HE condition. The severe $\alpha^{I/74}$ mutations are generally considered to be the most severe of the common α-spectrin mutations that cause HE. Rarely, patients who are homozygous for the severe forms of $\alpha^{I/74}$ usually have life-threatening hemolysis and an HPP-like syndrome (1401,1411). Patients who are compound heterozygotes for $\alpha^{I/74}$ and $\alpha^{I/46}$ or $\alpha^{I/61}$ also have severe hemolysis. Both groups of patients have partial (~30%) spectrin deficiency (1448) similar to HS (148,888,903). These $\alpha^{I/74}$ patients also have marked microspherocytosis on their blood smears and sometimes have so many bizarre poikilocytes and so few elliptocytes that the diagnosis of HE is not considered until the parents' smears are examined.

In most cases, the primary defect in Sp $\alpha^{I/74}$ lies near the site of enhanced tryptic cleavage in the α-chain. However, in some instructive families, the primary defects occur in helices A or B of repeat 17 of β-spectrin (1361,1374,1389–1391). Examples include spectrins Campinas, Cagliari, Providence, Kayes, and Cotonou (Table 51-21). These two helices are adjacent to the $\alpha^{I/74}$ cleavage site in helix C at the N-terminus of the α-chain. Presumably, the β-spectrin mutation exposes the N-terminus of the α-spectrin peptide to increased tryptic digestion because of the abnormal spectrin self-association caused by the β-spectrin mutation.

Spectrin $\alpha^{I/78}$. The $\alpha^{I/78}$ defect arises due to substitutions in codons 41 or 45 of the α-spectrin peptide (1386,1387,1472). It has been observed mostly in North Africans to date. Symptoms are quite variable, ranging from asymptomatic to moderately severe hemolysis, perhaps related to the coinheritance of Sp α^{LELY}, which is common in this population (1382). Primary mutations occur amid those that cause Sp $\alpha^{I/74}$ defects (1387,1472) (Table 51-21); however, for unknown reasons, these mutations induce tryptic cleavage at a more proximal site (Lys16).

Spectrin $\alpha^{I/65}$. This common mutation arises from the duplication of a leucine residue in codon 154 (1361,1389–1391,1401,1408,1429,1442,1477–1481) or from a missense mutation in codon 151 (spectrin Ponte de Sôr) (1476). It is quite mild. It causes common HE in blacks and is even milder in North Africans, who sometimes have little or no elliptocytosis (i.e., are silent carriers). Even homozygotes have only mild to moderate hemolysis.

The disorder is widely distributed in blacks in West Africa [where the prevalence of HE is 1.6% to 3.0% or more (1361,1372)], in blacks in Central Africa (1573), and in their descendants in the West Indies and North America. It is also seen in Arab populations and is the most common cause of HE in North Africa. The high frequency of $\alpha^{I/65}$ and its homogeneous expression strongly suggest that it has experienced genetic selection, and that it may provide some protection from malaria or other tropical bloodborne parasites. This has not yet been systematically tested, although there is preliminary evidence that the growth of *P. falciparum* is inhibited in $\alpha^{I/65}$ erythrocytes (1574).

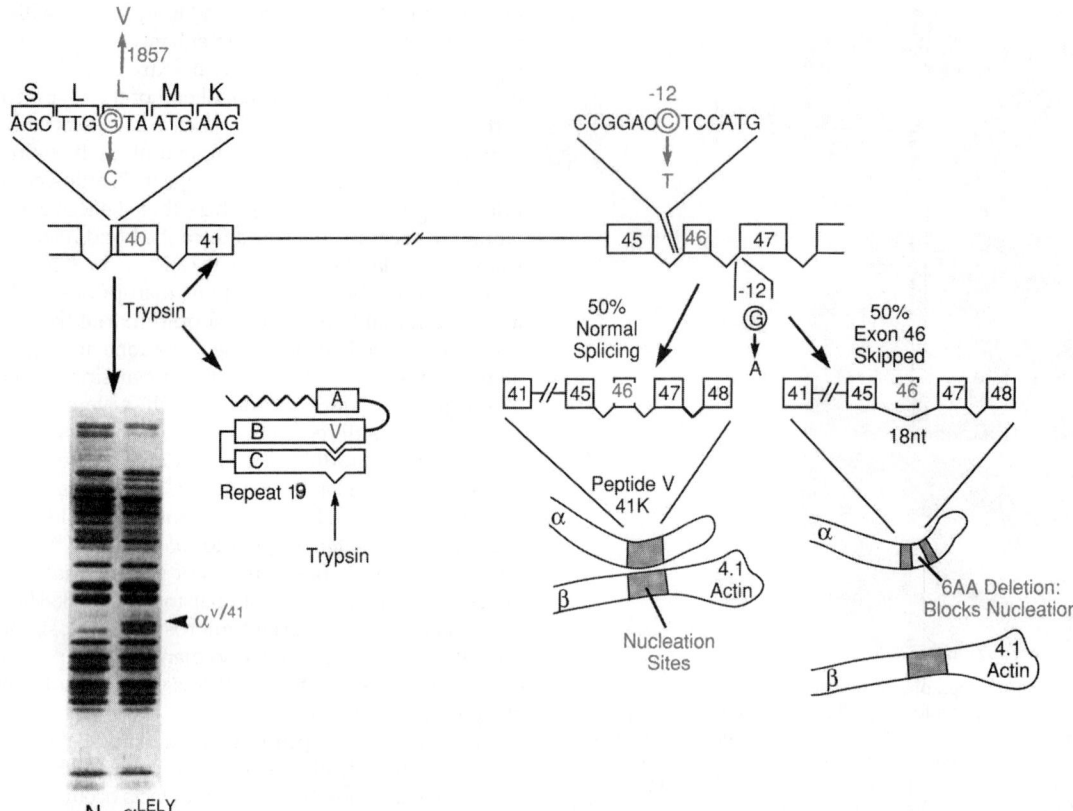

Figure 51-61. Nature of the low-expression α^{LELY} allele. The allele contains two linked mutations (1383): a marker mutation, the $\alpha^{V/41}$ defect, and a splicing mutation, the α^{LELY} defect. **Left:** The $\alpha^{V/41}$ defect is caused by a GC substitution at the beginning of exon 40, which changes Leu1857$\rightarrow$Val in helix B of spectrin repeat 19. The valine impinges on the neighboring helix C of the repeat and makes it more trypsin sensitive, leading to a more rapid release of the $\alpha^{V/41}$ peptide from trypsin-treated spectrin derived from the α^{LELY} allele. Sodium dodecyl sulfate gels of trypsin-treated normal and α^{LELY}-containing spectrin are shown at the bottom left. The $\alpha^{V/41}$ peptide is marked. **Right:** The linked splicing mutation is a C$\rightarrow$T substitution at position –12 in the acceptor splice site of intron 45 (a second linked mutation, G$\rightarrow$A, at position –12 of intron 46 may also contribute). This causes exon 46 to be skipped in 50% of α^{LELY} spectrin molecules (far right). Exon 46 is very small, only 6 amino acids, but it lies in the center of the nucleation site required for side-to-side association of the spectrin α and β chains (1566,1567). The half of α^{LELY} spectrin that lacks exon 46 cannot form spectrin heterodimers and is destroyed. Note that the other 50% of α^{LELY} spectrin contains exon 46 and will be functionally normal (though marked by the $\alpha^{V/41}$ tryptic peptide).

Spectrin $\alpha^{I/50a}$ (or $\alpha^{I/46}$). The $\alpha^{I/50a}$ defect often results from the substitution of a proline, which is an amino acid known to disrupt helix formation (Table 51-21) (1361,1478,1483,1484). Spectrin Dayton, which has a 48-residue deletion in codons 178 to 226, also gives rise to an $\alpha^{I/50a}$ phenotype (1482). This disorder is variable in severity (1376,1391,1401,1442,1478,1482,1484,1575), but, generally, it is less severe than Sp $\alpha^{I/74}$ and more severe than Sp $\alpha^{I/65}$ (1411). It is particularly common in black populations.

Other α-Spectrin Mutations. The mutation responsible for the $\alpha^{I/61}$ defect has not yet been defined. The $\alpha^{I/50b}$ defect originates either by proline substitutions (1410,1478,1483) or by a single residue deletion in codon 469 (1484). The $\alpha^{I/36}$ mutation (spectrin Sfax) derives from the deletion of codons 363 to 371 due to the activation of a cryptic splice site (1409). The $\alpha^{II/31}$ mutation (spectrin Jendouba) is caused by a point mutation in codon 791 (1487), whereas the $\alpha^{II/21}$ defect (spectrin Oran) is produced by a deletion of amino acids 822 to 862, from a mutation in the acceptor splice site for exon 18, resulting in the skipping of exon 18 (1432).

Unlike mutations associated with β-spectrin, which often result in premature chain termination, very few truncated α-spectrin peptides have been described in patients with HE/HPP. They would presumably have impaired actin binding, because there is evidence that the C-terminus of α-spectrin is needed for actin binding (1576). The spectrin dimer nucleation site might also be affected. Either way, the truncated α-spectrin would not be incorporated into the membrane skeleton. But, because α-spectrin synthesis exceeds β-spectrin synthesis by three- to fourfold, enough α-spectrin chains would be still be produced by the single normal α-spectrin allele to bind all of the β-spectrin chains and form a complete membrane skeleton.

Homozygous C-terminal truncations of α-spectrin would be expected to produce a phenotype, and do in the sph^J/sph^J mouse, where the last 13 amino acids of α-spectrin are lost and the resulting spectrin binds poorly to the membrane skeleton (1057a). However, the phenotype is HS rather than HE.

DEFECTS OF SPECTRIN SELF-ASSOCIATION INVOLVING THE β-CHAIN

At least 20 mutations in β-spectrin associated with HE/HPP have been described (Table 51-21). They all cluster near the C-terminus of β-spectrin, where the spectrin dimer self-association site is situated (Fig. 51-59). The abnormalities identified include truncations that delete various amounts of the C-terminus as well as missense mutations (Fig. 51-58; Table 51-21). Both kinds of mutations presumably alter spectrin self-association by dis-

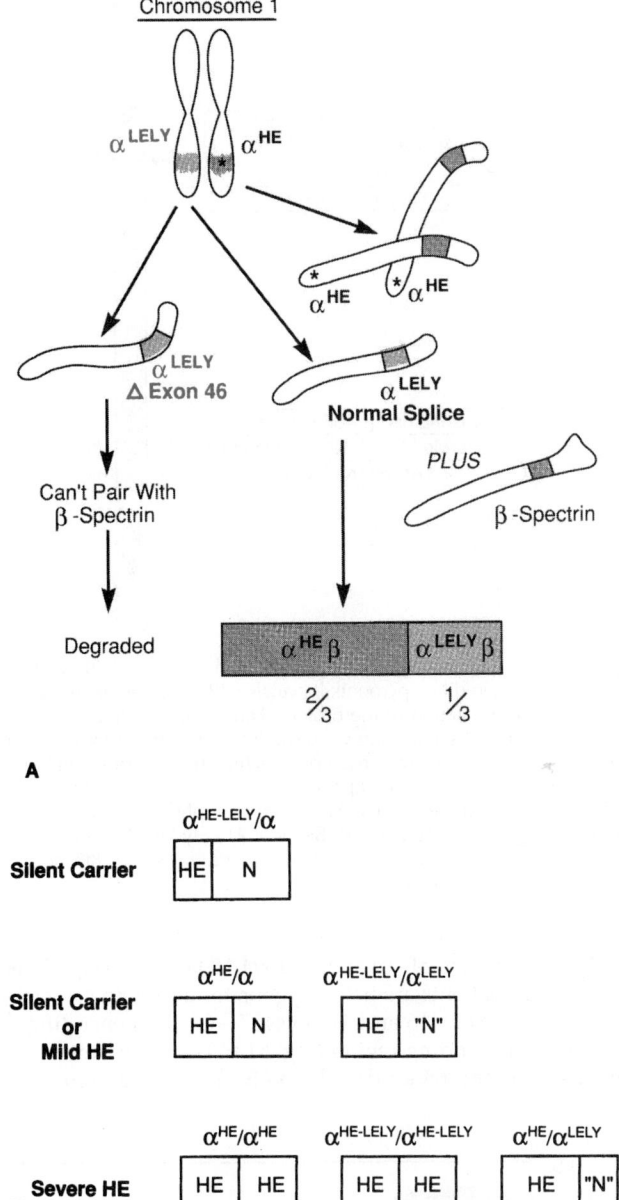

A

B

Figure 51-62. Effect of α^{LELY} on the proportion of spectrins containing normal and hereditary elliptocytosis (HE) α chains. **A:** When an α^{LELY} allele (*blue*) pairs with an α allele bearing an HE mutation (*asterisk*), the abnormal splicing associated with the α^{LELY} polymorphism decreases the concentration of normal α chains and results in an increased proportion of spectrin containing the HE α chain. **B:** The consequences of different combinations of normal α chains (α), low-expression α chains (α^{LELY}), HE α chains (α^{HE}), and HE mutations developing on an α chain carrying the common α^{LELY} polymorphism ($\alpha^{HE-LELY}$). The proportions of normal (N) and HE spectrins and the resulting phenotypes are illustrated. (Adapted from Delaunay J, Dhermy D. Mutations involving the spectrin heterodimer contact site: clinical expression and alterations in specific function. *Semin Hematol* 1993;30:21.)

rupting the coiled-coil triple-helical structure that forms the spectrin dimer self-association site. For example, for one of the β-spectrin truncated variants, β216, where approximately 4 kd are lost from the C-terminus of normal (220-kd) β-spectrin, low-temperature spectrin extracts contain increased spectrin dimer (~50% of the dimer-tetramer pool as compared with the normal 5% to 10%), and nearly all of the abnormal β216 spectrin is found in the dimer fraction (1461,1463,1465), indicating that the

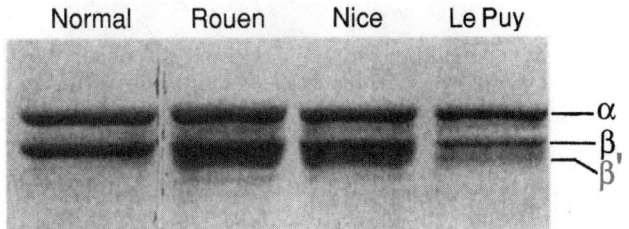

Figure 51-63. Sodium dodecyl sulfate gel electrophoretic patterns of the α- and β-spectrin subunits and some shortened β' chains due to C-terminal truncations. Normal, Sp Rouen ($\beta^{220/218}$), Sp Nice ($\beta^{220/216}$), and Sp Le Puy ($\beta^{220/214}$) are shown. (Reprinted from Delaunay J, Dhermy D. Mutations involving the spectrin heterodimer contact site: clinical expression and alterations in specific function. *Semin Hematol* 1993;30:21, with permission.)

inability of the β216 peptide to oligomerize is responsible for the functional defect.

Several molecular defects causing truncated β-spectrin chains have been characterized (Fig. 51-63). They include frameshift mutations, exon skipping, and a nonsense mutation (Table 51-21). Defective β-spectrins with missense mutations in the partial repeat that forms the spectrin dimer association site (repeat 17) have also been identified (Table 51-21). Several of these missense mutations result in the substitution of a proline residue in the mutant peptide. Because proline is known to disrupt α helices, this fact underscores the importance of the triple-helical conformation of spectrin in maintaining its structural stability. In many of these β-spectrin mutations, an associated α-spectrin abnormality, $\alpha^{I/74}$, can also be seen on tryptic maps (1458). As noted earlier, this is a secondary effect, a result of the exposure of the N-terminus of the α-spectrin peptide to increased tryptic digestion because of the abnormal spectrin self-association caused by the β-spectrin mutation (1374,1400,1577).

Clinically, HE patients with β-spectrin missense mutations have common HE. In contrast, patients with truncated β-spectrins typically have spherocytic HE, with mild to moderate hemolysis, rounded elliptocytes, and, sometimes, spherocytes or fragmented red cells. Where measured, OF is increased. It appears that synthesis of the truncated β-spectrin and the concentration of spectrin on the membrane is decreased (1466), which probably accounts for the spherocytic aspect of the phenotype. Thermal stability is unusual; the red cells become echinocytic at 47°C (normal = 49°C) but do not fragment. In the occasional patients who are homozygous for β-spectrin mutations, a clinical picture of HPP with severe neonatal hemolysis, or even lethal hydrops fetalis, has been described (1374,1490,1491).

DEFICIENCY OF PROTEIN 4.1

Tchernia (1385) and Féo (1578) and their colleagues first described the association between HE and protein 4.1R deficiency in a consanguineous Algerian family (Fig. 51-64). Subsequent investigators showed that this is a relatively common cause of HE in some Arab and European populations (~40%) (1373,1392–1394,1442,1579). It is not observed in blacks (1361,1372).

In one well-studied Algerian patient (1385), the 4.1(–) mRNA is not translated (1499), owing to a 318-bp deletion that encompasses the "downstream" translational start site that is used by the 80-kd erythroid isoform of protein 4.1 (1580) (Fig. 51-65). Two families have point mutations in the same initiation codon (4.1R Madrid and 4.1R Lille), with the same consequences (1434,1502). A large 70-kb deletion of the gene causes the deficiency seen in protein 4.1R Annery (1501), and a deletion of a single residue in the spectrin-binding domain in protein 4.1 Aravis abolishes its capacity to bind spectrin (1506).

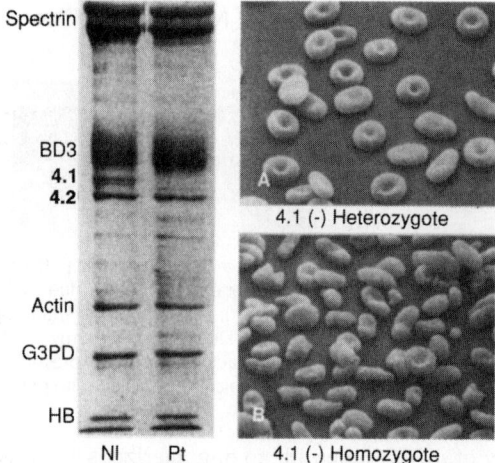

Figure 51-64. Deficiency of protein 4.1 in hereditary elliptocytosis. **Left:** Sodium dodecyl sulfate gels of red cell membrane proteins from a normal individual (NI) and a patient with homozygous hereditary elliptocytosis who lacks protein 4.1 (Pt). **Right:** Scanning electron micrographs of red blood cells in 4.1-deficient patients. **A:** Elliptocytes in a patient with heterozygous hereditary elliptocytosis and 50% protein 4.1. **B:** Elliptocytes, poikilocytes, and fragmented red cells in a patient with homozygous hereditary elliptocytosis and no 4.1. BD, band 3; G3PD, glyceraldehyde-3-phosphate dehydrogenase. (Reprinted from Tchernia G, Mohandas N, Shohet SB. Deficiency of cytoskeletal membrane protein band 4.1 in homozygous hereditary elliptocytosis: implications for erythrocyte membrane stability. *J Clin Invest* 1981;68:454, with permission.)

In addition to 4.1R deficiency, homozygotes have only approximately 30% of the normal content of GPC and GPD (1434,1511,1581,1582) and lack protein p55 (1434,1583). This and other evidence (1581,1584) argue persuasively that GPC is one of the membrane attachment sites of protein 4.1R, probably with the aid of p55 (1583,1585). Completely 4.1R-deficient red cells also manifest other defects. Membrane phospholipid asymmetry is disturbed (1586), and protein 4.9 appears to be missing from isolated membrane skeletons, although not from intact red cell membranes (1385).

Clinically, heterozygotes have "classic" common HE with a high proportion of elongated, smooth elliptocytes and little or no hemolysis. They have approximately 50% of the normal amount of protein 4.1.

No protein 4.1 is detectable in homozygotes (Fig. 51-64). Consequently, they have a severe, transfusion-dependent hemolytic anemia with marked OF, normal thermal stability, fragmenting elliptocytes (Fig. 51-64), and a very good response to splenectomy (1385,1434,1587). The homozygous red cells fragment much more rapidly than normal at moderate shear stresses (Fig. 51-66)—an indication of their intrinsic instability (1552). Cells from heterozygotes show intermediate stability similar to those of other patients with common HE. Membrane mechanical stability can be completely restored by reconstituting the deficient red cells with normal protein 4.1 (1497) (Fig. 51-66) or even with a fusion protein containing only 62 amino acids (the 21–amino acid spectrin-actin binding site plus the next 41 amino acids) (1588).

STRUCTURAL AND FUNCTIONAL DEFECTS OF PROTEIN 4.1
Two structural defects of protein 4.1 have been identified in patients with HE.

Shortened Protein 4.1 (4.1⁶⁵/⁶⁸) with Defective Spectrin-Actin Binding.
This disorder was discovered in an Italian family with a mild form of common HE (no anemia or reticulocytosis) and

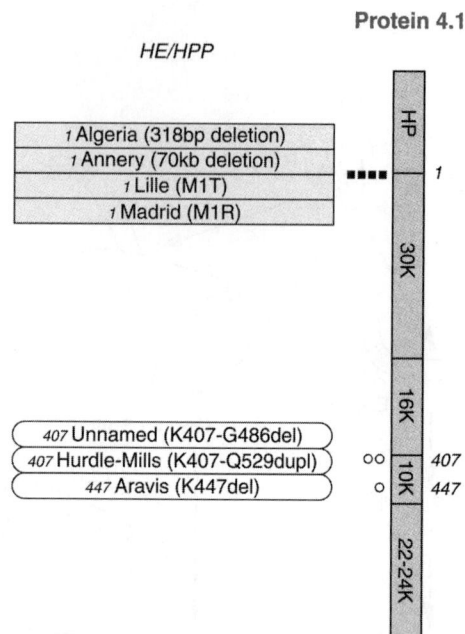

Figure 51-65. Protein 4.1 mutations associated with hereditary elliptocytosis (HE) and hereditary pyropoikilocytosis (HPP) are shown alongside a schematic representation of the protein. **Left:** Four mutations abolishing the translation start site are shown in shaded rectangles. A large in-frame deletion and a large in-frame insertion affecting the spectrin-actin binding domain are shown as open ellipses, as is a missense mutation at codon 447. (Adapted from Tse WT, Lux SE. Hereditary spherocytosis and hereditary elliptocytosis. In: Scriver CR, Beaudet AL, Sly WS, Valle D, editors, *The metabolic and molecular bases of inherited disease*, 8th ed. New York: McGraw-Hill, 2001:4665.)

mechanically unstable red cells (1394,1503–1505) (Fig. 51-66). The affected patients are heterozygous for a protein 4.1 variant that has lost exons 16 and 17 (Lys407→Gly486) encoding the spectrin-actin binding region (Fig. 51-65). The mutant protein runs as a 65- and 68-kd doublet on SDS gels and seems to be

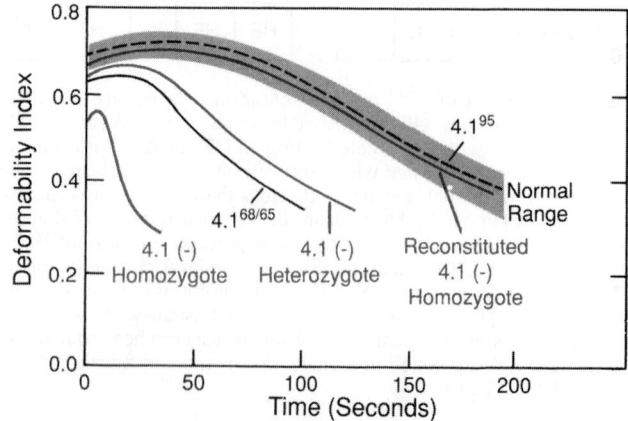

Figure 51-66. Red cell membrane stability in defects of protein 4.1. Red cell membranes were subjected to high shear stress in an ektacytometer, and their deformability was measured as a function of time. A fall in deformability occurred as the membranes fragmented. Note that the patient lacking protein 4.1 [4.1 (–) homozygote] has very fragile membranes and that normal fragility can be restored by reconstituting the membranes with normal 4.1. (Adapted from Mohandas N, Chasis JA. Red cell deformability, membrane material properties, and shape: regulation by transmembrane, skeletal, and cytosolic proteins and lipids. *Semin Hematol* 1993;30:171.)

present in nearly normal amounts (1394). It is presumed—but not proven—to be functionally inept.

High-Molecular-Weight Protein 4.1 (4.1[95] or 4.1 Hurdle Mills). This variant was discovered in a family of Scotch-Irish ancestry with very common HE (1394). The patients are heterozygous for a 95-kd form of protein 4.1 that results from the duplication of exons 16 to 18, encoding the sequences between Lys407 and Gln529 (1503,1505) (Fig. 51-65). This leads to the duplication of the spectrin-actin binding region; however, function appears to be preserved because 4.1[95] red cell membranes have normal mechanical stability (Fig. 51-66) (1580). It is not clear why this functionally normal variant causes HE.

DEFICIENCY OF GLYCOPHORINS C AND D
Deficiency of these two closely related minor sialoglycoproteins occurs in homozygous 4.1 deficiency, as described earlier, and in patients with the rare Leach phenotype of Gerbich-negative (Ge–) red cells. The Gerbich antigen system is carried on both GPC and GPD. Patients with the Leach phenotype of Ge– lack both of these glycophorins (1384,1507,1509–1515). These patients have a mild form of HE (1384,1507,1510,1512) with increased OF (i.e., a mild form of spherocytic HE). In one patient, transient GPC deficiency and elliptocytosis were associated with the development of an autoantibody to GPC (1513). Patients who lack some but not all Ge antigens (so-called Yus and Ge phenotypes) have normal amounts of red cell 4.1 and do not have HE. Their red cells contain a hybrid and, apparently, functionally active glycophorin with features of both GPC and GPD (1589,1590).

Red cells that lack GPC also lack protein p55 (1583), which binds to GPC and protein 4.1 (1585). The levels of protein 4.1 are reduced, reflecting a weakened interaction with the membrane. This and other information, discussed earlier, suggest that GPC and protein p55 may create a membrane binding site for protein 4.1.

In contrast to GPC, patients lacking GPA or GPB, or both, are entirely asymptomatic and have normal red cell morphology and mechanical stability.

ABNORMAL BAND 3 IN SOUTHEAST ASIAN OVALOCYTOSIS
The finding of tight linkage between an abnormal proteolytic digest of band 3 protein and the SAO phenotype led to the detection of the underlying molecular defect (1519). All carriers of the SAO phenotype are heterozygotes. One band 3 allele is normal, and the other contains two mutations in *cis*: a deletion of nine codons encoding amino acids 400 to 408, located at the boundary of the cytoplasmic and membrane domains, and the replacement of Lys56 by Glu (1537,1591,1592). The Lys56→Glu substitution is an asymptomatic polymorphism known as *band 3 Memphis* (1593–1595). The inframe deletion of amino acids 400 to 408 is found in all or almost all patients with the morphology of SAO (1596) and is thought to be entirely responsible for the phenotype—although this has not been proven.

SAO band 3 is made and inserted in the plasma membrane, but it appears to be misfolded and is functionally inept. It cannot transport anions (1597,1598). It is subject to increased tyrosine phosphorylation (1599). It forms linear aggregates within the lipid bilayer (755). Presumably, as a consequence, it has markedly restricted lateral and rotational mobility in the membrane (755,1519,1537) and binds more tightly than normal to ankyrin (755,1519). Other studies show that the wild-type and SAO band 3 interact to form heterodimers, but the mutant subunit alters the conformation of its wild-type partner (1600). Whether it also impairs the function of the wild-type protein is uncertain.

Because SAO is caused by the deletion of 27 bases from the band 3 gene, amplification of the deleted region in genomic DNA or reticulocyte cDNA is the most specific diagnostic test. This produces a single band in control red cells and a doublet, with the second band shorter by 27 base pairs, in SAO cells (1537,1591,1592).

Molecular Basis of Membrane Rigidity and Malaria Resistance in Southeast Asian Ovalocytosis. SAO red cells are unique among axially deformed cells because they are rigid and hyperstable rather than unstable (1536) (Fig. 51-53). The SAO band 3 mutation is the first example of a defect of an integral membrane protein leading to red cell membrane rigidity, a property that had previously been attributed to the membrane skeleton (reviewed in 1601).

The molecular mechanism underlying SAO red cell membrane rigidity is not clear. Tanner and colleagues have recently examined the structure of a band 3 by nuclear magnetic resonance from Arg389 to Lys430, a fragment that encompasses the SAO deletion. The wild-type peptide begins with an α helix (Pro391-Ala400) that presumably lies in the cytoplasm, followed by a sharp bend at Pro403 and a second helix that presumably represent the first transmembrane domain (1602). The SAO deletion would remove this bend and leave a stable helix from Pro391 to Ala416. A peptide containing this deletion would not insert stably into microsomal membranes when translated, unlike the normal peptide (1602). The results suggest that in SAO band 3, the region of the first membrane span of normal band 3 does not integrate properly into the membrane because it lacks a sufficiently long hydrophobic segment, and the deletion also disrupts a conserved structural subdomain at the membrane surface.

One hypothesis proposes that the long stiff SAO band 3 α helix observed in the studies above, protrudes rigidly into the membrane skeleton and precludes lateral movement (extension) of the skeletal network during deformation (749,1537,1539). A second possibility is that SAO band 3 binds abnormally tightly to ankyrin and, thus, to the underlying skeleton (1519). Or, SAO band 3 may adhere to the skeleton nonspecifically, possibly due to denaturation of the membrane-spanning domain (1603). Finally, the increased propensity of SAO band 3 to aggregate into higher oligomers may be important because the oligomers can strengthen band 3 attachment to ankyrin (755,756). All of these ideas are attractive and have some experimental support. It may be that the true answer is some combination of the possibilities.

The resistance of SAO red cells to malaria is presumably related to the altered properties of SAO band 3. The invasion and multiplication of *P. falciparum* parasites are decreased in the mutant red cells (1604). Band 3 serves as one of the malaria receptors, as evidenced by the inhibition of *in vitro* invasion by band 3–containing liposomes (1605). In normal red cells, parasite invasion is associated with marked membrane remodeling and redistribution of band 3–containing IMPs (1606). IMPs cluster at the site of parasite invasion, forming a ring around the orifice through which the parasite enters the cell. The invaginated red cell membrane, which surrounds the invading parasite, is free of IMPs. The reduced lateral mobility of band 3 protein in SAO red cells (1519,1537) may preclude band 3 receptor clustering and thus prevent attachment or entry of the parasites.

Resistance to malaria has also been attributed to diminished anion exchange due to the inability of SAO band 3 to transport anions (1596,1597). In addition, SAO red cells consume ATP at a higher rate than normal cells; the ensuing partial depletion of ATP levels in ovalocytes has been proposed to account, in part, for the resistance of these cells to malaria invasion *in vitro* (1535). However, diminished anion transport and ATP depletion do not appear to play a critical role in malaria resistance of SAO erythrocytes *in vivo*. This is evidenced by the fact that band 3–deficient HS red cells are considerably less resistant to malaria invasion than SAO red cells (although both cell types have a similar decrease of anion transport) and by the fact that malaria resistance of SAO red cells is detected *in vitro* even when red cell ATP levels are maintained.

It is important to reemphasize that SAO red cells are much more leaky to sodium and potassium than normal red cells when stored in the cold (1541). Many of the defects in SAO red cells were detected in cells that were stored in the cold. These defects need to be reevaluated using never-chilled SAO red cells. For example, fresh SAO cells are invaded by the parasites but become resistant to invasion on storage, presumably because intracellular ATP is depleted more rapidly than normal.

Patients with SAO sometimes have dRTA, but this is due to compound heterozygosity for a missense mutation of band 3, G701D—not to the 9–amino acid deletion of band 3 that causes SAO (1540).

Pathophysiology of Hereditary Elliptocytosis and Hereditary Pyropoikilocytosis

SPECTRIN MUTATIONS
The principal functional consequence of the elliptocytogenic spectrin mutations is a weakening, or even a disruption, of the spectrin dimer-tetramer contact and, consequently, the two-dimensional integrity of the membrane skeleton (697). These "horizontal defects" are readily detected by ultrastructural examination of membrane skeletons, which reveals the disruption of the normally uniform hexagonal lattice (758). Consequently, membrane skeletons, cell membranes, and the red cells are mechanically unstable (reviewed in 697,749). In patients carrying severely dysfunctional spectrin mutations or in subjects who are homozygous or compound heterozygous for milder mutations, this membrane instability is sufficient to cause hemolytic anemia with red cell fragmentation.

How elliptocytes are formed is less clear. In common HE, red cell precursors are round, and the scant data available suggest that the cells become progressively more elliptical as they age *in vivo* (1351,1607). Red cells distorted by shear stress *in vitro* or flowing through the microcirculation *in vivo* have elliptical or parachute-like shapes, respectively (749,1608). Even normal spectrin dimer-tetramer interactions are loosened by shear stress (753a). Perhaps elliptocytes and poikilocytes are permanently stabilized in their abnormal shape because the weakened skeletal interactions facilitate skeletal reorganization after prolonged or repetitive cellular deformation. Skeletal reorganization is likely to involve breakage of the unidirectionally stretched protein connections and formation of new contacts that reduce stress on the skeleton and stabilize the deformed shape (reviewed in 749). This hypothesis, first proposed in 1978 (1609), has been shown to account for the permanent deformation of irreversibly sickle cells (1609,1610).

As noted above, HPP red cells have two abnormalities: They contain a mutant spectrin that disrupts spectrin self-association, and they are partially deficient in spectrin (738,1448). This is due either to an elliptocytogenic α-spectrin mutation and a defect involving reduced α-spectrin synthesis or to two elliptocytogenic spectrin alleles. In the latter situation, spectrin deficiency might be a consequence of spectrin instability, which would reduce the amount of spectrin available for membrane assembly. In red cells carrying a lot of unassembled spectrin dimers, the fact that one ankyrin is bound/one spectrin tet-

ramer (i.e., two spectrin heterodimers) may also contribute to spectrin deficiency. At best, only approximately one-half of the spectrin dimers could succeed in attaching to the available ankyrin-binding sites. In fact, it would be substantially less because ankyrin binds spectrin dimers approximately ten times less avidly than spectrin tetramers (706,707,1564).

The phenotype of HPP, characterized by the presence of fragments and elliptocytes, together with evidence of red cell surface area deficiency (i.e., microspherocytes) suggests that the membrane dysfunction involves both vertical interactions (a consequence of the spectrin deficiency) and horizontal interactions (a consequence of the elliptocytogenic spectrin mutations).

PROTEIN 4.1 MUTATIONS
Hereditary elliptocytes that are deficient in protein 4.1 are similar in shape and membrane instability to elliptocytes that result from spectrin mutations (749). This suggests that 4.1 deficiency principally affects the spectrin-actin contact (i.e., a horizontal interaction) rather than the skeletal attachment to GPC (a vertical interaction).

PROTEIN 3 MUTATIONS: SOUTHEAST ASIAN OVALOCYTOSIS
The genesis of the ovalocytosis (actually, elliptocytosis—the cells are not egg shaped) in SAO is a mystery. As noted above, SAO red cells are more rigid than normal and are believed to have more firm attachment between ankyrin and spectrin. Because ankyrin-spectrin interactions are linked to the nearby spectrin-spectrin interactions in a positively cooperative way (1564), spectrin self-association should be stronger than normal in SAO, which is the opposite of what is expected in elliptocytosis. Even if this is incorrect, it seems clear that the membrane skeleton is more rigid than normal in SAO red cells, which does not fit with the idea above that elliptocytes form by progressive plastic deformation of the skeleton. It is also not clear why homozygosity for SAO is lethal (1521,1522). It was once thought this was due to the absence of anion transport, but rare children are living with severe HS and homozygous band 3 deficiency, although their growth is stunted as a consequence of chronic metabolic acidosis (863,864).

PERMEABILITY OF HEREDITARY ELLIPTOCYTOSIS RED CELLS
HE red cells consume more ATP and 2,3-DPG than normal erythrocytes (1611), probably due to increased transmembrane sodium movements (1612). As a result of the underlying skeletal defect, HE and HPP red cells are abnormally permeable to Na^+, K^+, and Ca^{2+} ions (1445,1612). The excessive Ca^{2+} leak was originally thought to be the primary molecular lesion in a patient with a severe microcytic hemolytic anemia and red cell thermal instability (1445), who was subsequently shown to have a spectrin mutation and, probably, HPP (1575).

Common Hereditary Elliptocytosis and Malaria
Epidemiologic studies of the elliptocytogenic mutations of spectrin in central Western Africa, including Benin, suggest that their prevalence is considerably greater than would be expected for sporadic mutations. The prevalence of certain α-spectrin mutations in that area ranges from 0.4% to 5.0% (1361). The unnamed Leu154→LeuLeu (0.4% in Benin), Leu207Pro (0.5% in Benin), and spectrin St Claude (3.0% in Benin) are particular examples (1361,1372). The 154LeuLeu mutation is always linked to a series of α-spectrin polymorphisms (701R, 809I, and 853T), indicating that the mutation has a single origin (1361). These data are of considerable interest in light of *in vitro* studies demonstrating diminished malarial parasite entry or growth (or

both) in red cells that contain some of the elliptocytogenic spectrin mutants or are deficient in protein 4.1 (1574,1613).

OTHER CAUSES OF MEMBRANE INJURY LEADING TO SPHEROCYTOSIS

Relatively few conditions cause "spherocytosis," meaning that spherocytes predominate and are the only significant red cell shape on the peripheral blood smear (Table 51-18). The definition excludes diseases like HPP, in which spherocytes are common but are clearly only one of many morphologic elements.

Other than HS, immunohemolytic anemias are the most common cause of spherocytosis: AB(H)-related hemolysis in newborns and warm antibody-type (IgG-mediated) autoimmune or drug-related hemolytic anemias in older children and adults. These are discussed in Chapters 55 and 52, respectively. Severe hemolytic transfusion reactions (see Chapter 57) are also a form of immunohemolysis and are often marked by spherocytosis, but they are relatively uncommon.

Patients with acute red cell oxidant injury may also develop spherocytes, although they are rarely the principal morphology. Usually, bite cells, blister cells, and dense, irregular, contracted cells predominate. Oxidant injury occurs during acute hemolytic episodes in patients with glucose-6-phosphate dehydrogenase (G6PD) deficiency (see Chapter 54) and in normal individuals exposed to toxic concentrations of oxidant drugs or chemicals. Powerful reducing agents, such as arsine (AsH_3), may also cause a spherocytic hemolytic anemia after toxic exposure. Little is known about the specific nature of the membrane injury in any of these conditions.

Other acquired causes of membrane damage and spherocytosis are discussed in the sections that follow.

Thermal Injury

Almost 140 years ago, Schultze observed that red cells fragment and sphere when heated to temperatures approaching 50°C for short periods (1614). This phenomenon was further defined by the careful studies of Ham and co-workers (1544,1545) and others (1546) and is now believed to be due to heat denaturation of spectrin or other membrane proteins (1587). Essentially identical changes are observed acutely in patients with major cutaneous burns—presumably due to heat exposure of red cells in the skin and subcutaneous tissues. Intravascular hemolysis develops, with red cell fragmentation and spherocytosis, during the first 24 to 48 hours after the burn (1615,1616). The severity of the reaction is related to the extent and degree of the burn. Hemolysis is usually evident in patients with third-degree burns involving 15% to 20% or more of the skin (1615,1617). In severely burned patients, up to 30% of the red cell mass may be destroyed. Acute hemolysis is usually complete by the third postburn day and is followed by the anemia of chronic disease (1618,1619), which often does not respond to erythropoietin (1620) and may require transfusions. A rare variant of this disorder has been reported after infusion of red cells that were inadvertently overheated in a blood warmer (1621,1622).

Hypophosphatemia

In patients with severe hypophosphatemia (serum phosphorus level ≤0.1 to 0.3 mg/dL), red cell glucose metabolism is compromised, ATP and 2,3-DPG levels decline, and Hb oxygen affinity increases (1623,1624). If red cell ATP falls to very low levels (approximately 10% to 20% of normal), a severe hemolytic anemia characterized by marked microspherocytosis or sphero-

acanthocytosis results (1623,1624). Rhabdomyolysis may also occur (1624). Hemolysis remits after phosphate repletion and ATP regeneration (1623,1624).

Toxins and Venoms

CLOSTRIDIAL SEPSIS

Patients with Clostridial Sepsis May Have Spherocytosis and Massive Intravascular Hemolysis. *Clostridium perfringens* septicemia occurs in a variety of clinical situations, but it must particularly be considered in immunosuppressed patients with gastrointestinal or hematologic malignancies (1625), in infants with necrotizing enterocolitis (1626–1629), and in patients with penetrating wounds, septic abortions (1630), peritonitis after a perforated viscus, and cholecystitis or cholangitis (1625,1631–1636). Severe, rapidly progressive intravascular hemolysis and marked microspherocytosis occur in approximately 10% of patients with *C. perfringens* sepsis (1625,1634), often in association with shock, disseminated intravascular coagulation, acute renal failure, and a fatal outcome. Hemolysis of the entire red cell mass has been reported (1630,1636–1638) and, remarkably, is compatible with good tissue oxygenation and survival for hours (1638) despite ineffective transfusion therapy. *Clostridium sordellii* can produce similar hemolysis (1639).

The mechanism of red cell damage is disputed and may not be the same for all patients. The bacteria produce several hemolytic toxins, of which α-toxin and θ-toxin are the best characterized. α-Toxin is a 43-kd protein that has an *N*-terminal, zinc-binding domain with phospholipase C and sphingomyelinase activities and a *C*-terminal, calcium-dependent domain (1640). It appears that both domains are needed for hemolysis (1641–1644). The protein is secreted as an inactive 46-kd protoxin. It is activated by the protease furin, which cleaves near the C-terminus. The proteolyzed toxin oligomerizes and forms pores on the plasma membrane, resulting in colloid osmotic lysis (1645). θ-Toxin is a 54-kd, thiol-sensitive, cholesterol-binding protein (1646,1647) that also aggregates and forms membrane pores (1647,1648), leading to colloid osmotic hemolysis.

In addition, *C. perfringens* contains a neuraminidase that cleaves terminal sialic acids from red cell membrane glycoproteins in some [but not all (1649)] infected patients. The underlying galactose residues form the so-called Thomsen-Friedenreich cryptantigen or red cell T antigen. The antigen is easily detected because the affected red cells are agglutinated by peanut lectin (1632). Because anti-T antibodies are present in most adult plasma, T activation can cause hemolysis. In septic infants and children who lack T antibodies, hemolysis may follow transfusions (1626,1627,1629). On the other hand, T activation may precede frank intravascular hemolysis and, for the savvy clinician, permit early detection of clostridial sepsis and life-saving therapeutic intervention (1632). Aggressive treatments with antibiotics, exchange transfusions, hemodialysis, and hyperbaric oxygen are sometimes successful in treating clostridial infections (1628,1632,1633,1650–1652).

VENOMS

The venoms of cobras and certain vipers and rattlesnakes may produce severe hemolysis and spherocytosis (1653–1656). Occasionally, the anemia is Coombs'-positive (1656). Spherocytic hemolytic anemia may also be seen in persons bitten by the common brown spiders (*Loxosceles reclusa*, *Loxosceles laeta*, and *Loxosceles intermedia*) of the central and southern United States and South America (1657–1660) and in individuals afflicted by massive numbers of honeybee (1661,1662), wasp (1662–1665), or yellow jacket (1666) stings. Hemolysis has also been reported in a child stung by a Portuguese man-of-war jellyfish (1667).

A full description of the numerous toxins in these venoms and their mechanisms of action is beyond the scope of this chapter. In general, the mechanisms of hemolysis after envenomation are not fully understood. The venoms of snakes and insects often contain phospholipases (particularly phospholipase A_2) and protein toxins that enhance their action. Examples of the latter are the mastoparans of wasp and hornet venoms (1668–1670) and melittin, a polypeptide contained in honeybee (*Apis mellifera*) venom that immobilizes and clusters erythrocyte band 3 (1671–1673), exposing protein-free areas of lipid bilayer to phospholipase attack (1674).

Brown Spider Bites Sometimes Cause Coombs'-Positive Hemolytic Anemia. Hemolysis after brown spider bites is characteristically delayed from 1 to 5 days (1658) and is caused by a different mechanism. Affected patients develop a transient, spherocytic, Coombs'-positive hemolytic anemia (1675–1677) with intravascular hemolysis, erythrophagocytosis, and deposition of IgG (1676) and C3 (1675) on the red cell surface. *In vitro*, venom components, including a sphingomyelinase (1678), bind to the red cell membrane (1679) and induce IgG attachment (1676) and activation of complement by the alternative pathway (1680). The purified sphingomyelinase is sufficient to induce hemolysis and dermonecrosis in experimental models (1678). The hemolysis usually subsides within a week, but it may be fatal (1658,1681,1682). The role of complement seems to be critical because C'-deficient guinea pigs are resistant to the venom (1683).

With the exception of spider bites, which may initially be clinically deceptive (1658), the potential for a hemolytic catastrophe should be clear in patients who have been bitten or stung. Sometimes, the impending hemolysis is signaled by a rapid rise in the serum potassium level, due to a prelytic leak of this ion from damaged red cells. Once hemolysis is established, therapies other than transfusions are usually of little use. In snake bites, localization or drainage of the venom and prompt administration of antivenom can be life-saving.

Hawkinsinuria

Hawkinsinuria is a rare, autosomal-dominant disorder associated with urinary excretion of hawkinsin, (2-L-cystein-S-yl-1,4-dihydroxycyclohex-5-en-1-yl)-acetic acid, a toxic amino acid

by-product of a defect in tyrosine metabolism. The disorder presents with failure to thrive and persistent acidosis in infancy that responds to phenylalanine and tyrosine restriction. In one well-studied family, hemolytic anemia with anisocytosis and spherocytosis was also observed (1684).

ECHINOCYTES AND ACANTHOCYTES

There are two basic types of spiculated red cells: echinocytes and acanthocytes (Fig. 51-67). Echinocytes have a serrated outline with small, uniform projections evenly spread over the circumference of the cell. Acanthocytes have fewer spicules that vary in size and project irregularly from the red cell surface. These differences are easily appreciated in scanning electron micrographs (Fig. 51-67) and can usually be discerned in wet preparations, but they are sometimes hard to distinguish in dried smears. In general, echinocytes have relatively uniform scalloped edges in smears (i.e., appear crenated), whereas acanthocytes are contracted, dense, and irregular (Fig. 51-67). However, the distinction is not critical. Although echinocytes can appear on their own, acanthocytes are almost always accompanied by echinocytes. From a diagnostic point of view, it is usually best to consider all spiculated red cells as a group and not attempt to include or exclude diseases based on this fine morphologic distinction.

However, it is important to realize that echinocytes in peripheral blood smears are often artifactual. They are readily produced *in vitro* by washing red cells in buffers or diluting them in saline (1685), by contact between red cells and glass surfaces (1685,1686), and by amphipathic molecules that partition into and expand the outer half of the lipid bilayer (see section Bilayer Couple Hypothesis). High pH values, ATP depletion, and Ca^{2+} accumulation also cause echinocytosis (1687–1690).

It is important to be sure that spiculated red cells are consistently present in different parts of a blood smear and on different smears, and it is often useful to examine "wet preps" or red cells fixed with glutaraldehyde (0.5% in phosphate buffered saline). Wet preps are easily made by diluting a small drop of blood with the plasma from the top of a hematocrit tube and covering the mixture with a coverslip. The cells should be viewed with phase contrast optics or, if necessary, under brightfield conditions with the microscope condenser lowered.

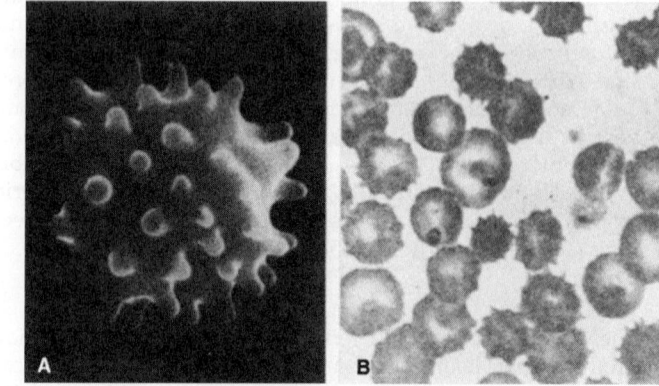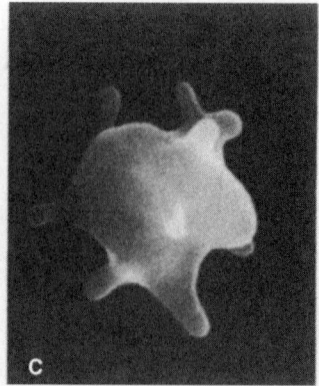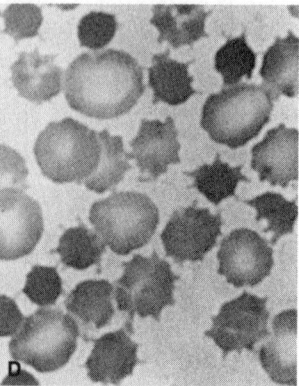

Figure 51-67. Morphology of echinocytes and acanthocytes. **A:** Scanning electron micrograph of a spheric echinocyte. **B:** Peripheral blood smear of echinocytes in a splenectomized patient with pyruvate kinase deficiency. **C:** Scanning electron micrograph of an acanthocyte. **D:** Peripheral smear of acanthocytes in a patient with hepatitis and spur cell anemia. (Reprinted from Becker PS, Lux SE. Disorders of the red cell membrane. In: Nathan DG, Oski FA, eds. *Hematology of infancy and childhood*, 4th ed. Philadelphia: WB Saunders, 1993:529, with permission.)

TABLE 51-22. Conditions Associated with Echinocytosis, Acanthocytosis, or Target Cells

Echinocytes or acanthocytes (spiculated red cells)
  Echinocytes
    Premature infants[a,b]
    Embden-Meyerhof pathway (glycolytic) defects[a,b]
    Uremia[a]
    Red cell fragmentation syndromes[a]
    Transiently after massive transfusion of stored blood
    Divers after decompression[a]
    Heat stroke[a]
    Snake envenomation (low dose)
    Bee venom
    Hemodialysis (during procedure)
    Ionizing radiation
    Oxidative damage
  Acanthocytes and echinocytes
    Abetalipoproteinemia
    Acute hepatic necrosis (spur cell anemia)
    Acanthocytosis with neurologic disease and normal lipoproteins
      Choreoacanthocytosis
      Hallervorden-Spatz syndrome
    McLeod blood group
    In(Lu) blood group
    Vitamin E deficiency[a,b]
    Infantile pyknocytosis
    Anorexia nervosa[a,b]
    Hypothyroidism[a,b]
    Postsplenectomy[a,b]
Target cells
  Obstructive liver disease
  Hypochromic-microcytic anemias
    Iron deficiency[a]
    Hemoglobins S, C, D, and E[a]
    Thalassemias
    Sideroblastic anemias[a,b]
  Hereditary xerocytosis[a,b]
  Lecithin:cholesterol acyltransferase deficiency
  Fish-eye disease
  Postsplenectomy[a,b]

[a]Disorder sometimes associated with this morphology.
[b]Indicated morphology usually only affects a small proportion of the red cells.

According to Dacie, normal adults may have up to 3% spiculated red cells in their peripheral blood (1691); however, in our experience, the limit is less than 1% and probably closer to 0.5%. This is increased in states of functional or actual splenectomy and after the ingestion of certain drugs (e.g., salicylates, ethanol, furosemide, and indomethacin) (1692). Postsplenectomy, the median number of acanthocytes is 1.7%, with a range of 0.0% to 8.5% (1685). In term infants, the median number of spiculated red cells is 2% (range, 0% to 6%), whereas in premature babies, it is 5.5% (range, 1% to 25%) (1693,1694).

Echinocytes are found in patients with advanced uremia (1695,1696); in patients with defects of glycolytic metabolism (1697), especially after splenectomy; in some patients with microangiopathic hemolytic anemias (1698); and in divers after decompression from pressures of more than 3 to 4 bar (1699) (Table 51-22). They are seen transiently after transfusions with large amounts of stored blood, because red cells become echinocytic after a few days of storage. They are also seen after exposure to various venoms in concentrations too low to cause spherocytosis (1700,1701), after exposure to ionizing radiation (1602), and during hemodialysis (1603,1704).

Acanthocytes and echinocytes are common in patients with severe hepatocellular damage (1705), abetalipoproteinemia (1706), infantile pyknocytosis (1707), and the McLeod (1708) and In(Lu) (1709) blood groups (Table 51-22). Occasionally, they are a predominant morphologic feature (5% to 10% of red cells) in patients with myelodysplasia (1710,1711). Small numbers of

acanthocytes are present in many patients with hypothyroidism (1712) and anorexia nervosa (1713,1714).

Uremia

Red cell survival is reduced in patients with advanced renal failure (1715,1716). An extracorporeal factor is involved, because red cells from uremic patients survive normally when infused into normal persons, whereas normal red cells survive poorly in uremic patients (1716). The factor is nondialyzable, and some studies suggest it is parathyroid hormone (PTH) (1717–1719). PTH is elevated in renal failure due to hyperphosphatemia and secondary hyperparathyroidism; PTH levels correlate closely with red cell survival in chronic renal failure patients on dialysis (1719), and parathyroidectomy abolishes hemolysis in dogs with uremia (1717). *In vitro*, relevant levels of PTH or its bioactive N-terminal peptide augment Ca^{2+} entry into red cells via a cAMP-independent pathway and cause the cells to develop filamentous extensions and to lose membrane surface (presumably by vesiculation) (1718). These effects are largely blocked by the calcium channel blocker verapamil (1718). It is possible that they are responsible for the increased numbers of echinocytes observed in some uremic patients, because increased intracellular Ca^{2+} is markedly echinocytogenic (1720); however, this remains to be tested.

Hepatocellular Damage (Spur Cell Anemia)

Anemia in liver disease is complex. Common causes include blood loss, hypersplenism, iron deficiency, folic acid deficiency, and marrow suppression from alcohol, hepatitis virus, and other poorly understood factors (1721,1722) (see Chapter 56). In addition, in some patients, acquired abnormalities of the red cell membrane may contribute to anemia. Two morphologic syndromes are recognized. In one, target cells predominate. In the other, a syndrome of brisk hemolysis develops in association with acanthocytes or "spur" cells—so-called "spur cell anemia" (1705,1723–1733).

Typically, target cells are associated with obstructive liver disease, and acanthocytes are associated with hepatocellular disease. In practice, the situation is more complex. It is not uncommon for both morphologies to coexist, and some experimental data suggest they are different stages of the same process. For example, when the bile duct is ligated in a rat, acanthocytes appear within 8 hours, but they convert to target cells if the obstruction persists for 7 days or more (1734). Nevertheless, acanthocytes (spur cells) and target cells differ in many important respects, and we consider them separately in this chapter.

CLINICAL FEATURES

Spur cell anemia is most often observed in patients with alcoholic cirrhosis (1705,1725–1727,1731,1732). However, it is also reported with cardiac cirrhosis (1727), metastatic liver disease (1730), hemochromatosis (1729), neonatal hepatitis (1735), cholestasis (1723,1724,1733), Wilson disease (Lux SE, *unpublished observations*), and fulminant hepatitis (Lux SE, *unpublished observations*). It probably can occur in any disease in which damage to hepatocytes is severe.

Typically, patients have moderately severe hemolysis (hematocrits of 20% to 30%), marked indirect hyperbilirubinemia, splenomegaly, and clinical and laboratory evidence of severe hepatic dysfunction. By definition, greater than 20% acanthocytes are evident in multiple areas on several peripheral blood smears. Morphologically, the acanthocytes of spur cell anemia are indistinguishable from those seen in patients with abetalipoproteinemia. Echinocytes and target cells are also present in

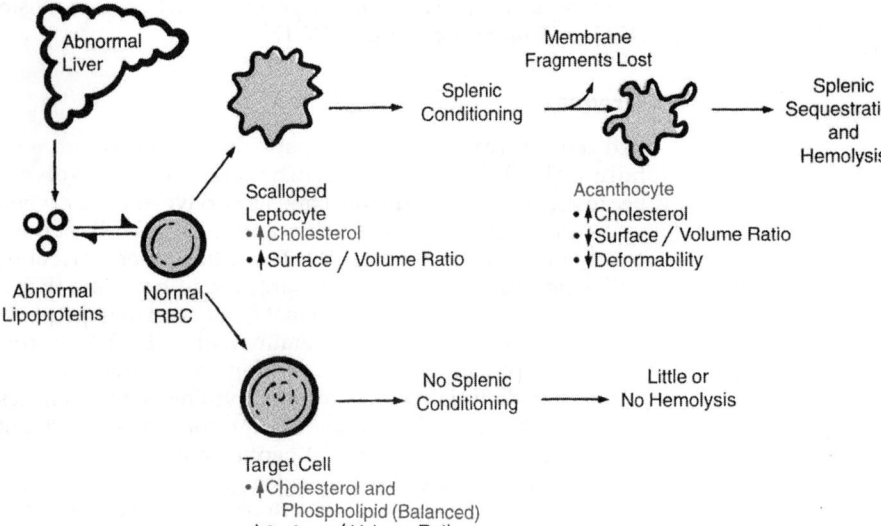

Figure 51-68. Pathophysiology of acanthocyte (spur cell) and target cell formation in liver disease. RBC, red blood cell. (Adapted from Becker PS, Lux SE. Disorders of the red cell membrane. In: Nathan DG, Oski FA, eds. *Hematology of infancy and childhood*, 4th ed. Philadelphia: WB Saunders, 1993:529.)

some patients, and spherocytes may develop, presumably from vesiculation (Fig. 51-22). Occasionally, this may be confusing. In our experience, however, many of these "spherocytes" have fine spicules on close examination (i.e., are spheroechinocytes), which distinguishes them from true microspherocytes.

The red cell lifespan of spur cells is shortened by splenic sequestration (1705,1726,1731,1736) and improves after splenectomy (1736); however, spur cell anemia has developed in a splenectomized patient (1728). Because splenectomy is a dangerous and often fatal procedure (1736) in these very sick patients, it is not generally recommended. Some success has been reported in treating patients with either phospholipid infusions (1737) of flunarizine (1738), or, recently, with a combination of flunarizine, pentoxifylline, and cholestyramine (1739); however, these approaches, although promising, are still experimental, and their efficacy has not been confirmed in controlled studies.

ETIOLOGY AND PATHOGENESIS

It appears that the clinical syndrome of spur cell anemia can be produced by at least two different pathogenic mechanisms. In one group, typically patients with alcoholic cirrhosis (1705,1727,1732,1736), the disorder is due to an acquired abnormality of red cell lipids. The pathophysiology of spurring in these patients has been defined and reviewed by Cooper and associates in a classic series of investigations (17,131,1705,1736,1740–1742) and is illustrated in Figure 51-68. It occurs in two stages: cholesterol loading and splenic remodeling. In the first stage, abnormal, cholesterol-laden, apolipoprotein A-II–deficient lipoproteins, produced by the spur cell patient's diseased liver, transfer their excess cholesterol to circulating erythrocytes and increase erythrocyte membrane cholesterol concentration, the cholesterol to phospholipid ratio, and membrane surface area (Figs. 51-68 and 51-69) (1740,1743). This is an acquired process and can be mimicked *in vitro* by incubating normal red cells in spur cell plasma (Fig. 51-70) (1705,1736) or in artificial media containing cholesterol-phospholipid dispersions with a cholesterol to phospholipid ratio greater than 1.0 (1741). It can be reproduced *in vivo* in dogs (1742) and rabbits (1743a) fed a high-cholesterol diet. In scanning electron micrographs, these cholesterol-laden cells are flattened and often folded, with an undulating periphery (1741). They appear scalloped or crenated on dried smears (Fig. 51-70) (1705,1736).

In vivo, the scalloped cells are converted into spur cells by a process involving "splenic conditioning." Over a period of 1 to 7

days (1705), membrane lipids and surface area are lost, cellular rigidity increases (presumably because of a decline in the surface to volume ratio), and the cells become acanthocytes (Fig. 51-67) (1705,1736). Splenectomy blocks the formation of spur cells and retards their premature destruction (1736), but, as noted earlier, it is a high-risk procedure and is seldom indicated.

Cholesterol-laden incipient spur cells are presumably detained and conditioned by the spleen because they are less deformable than normal. It is not known how this occurs at a molecular level, but, presumably, it must involve effects of the excess cholesterol on the membrane skeleton or on interconnections between the skeleton and integral membrane proteins. There is evidence that cholesterol interacts directly with band 3 (1744) and, possibly, with membrane skeleton proteins (1745) and that a slight increase in the cholesterol to phospholipid ratio above normal markedly alters cholesterol organization in the membrane (as measured by accessibility to cholesterol oxidase) (1746) and increases the helical content of one or more of the major membrane proteins (1747). There is also evidence that membrane proteolytic activity is increased in

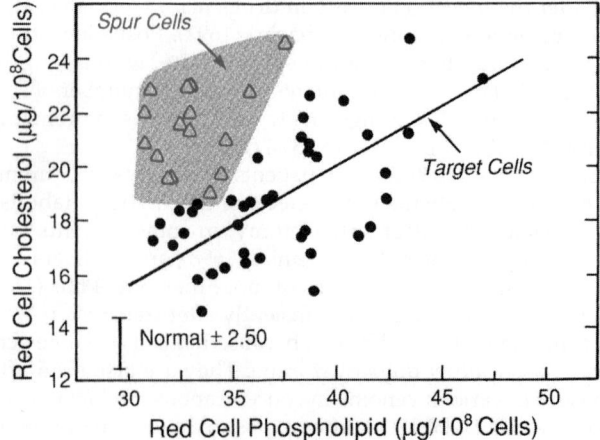

Figure 51-69. The cholesterol and phospholipid content of target and spur cells. Note that target cells (*solid circles*) tend to have a balanced increase in cholesterol and phospholipid, whereas spur cells (*open triangles*) are selectively enriched in cholesterol. (Adapted from Cooper RA, Diloy Puray M, et al. An analysis of lipoproteins, bile acids, and red cell membranes associated with target cells and spur cells in patients with liver disease. *J Clin Invest* 1972;31:3182.)

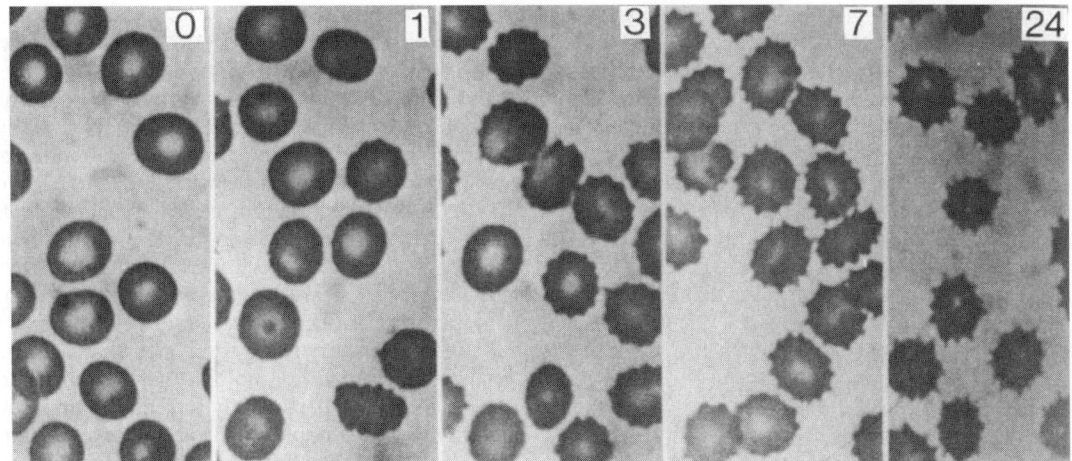

Figure 51-70. Production of spur cells *in vitro* by incubation of normal red cells in heated serum from a patient with spur cell anemia. The hours of incubation are shown in the upper right corner of each panel. (Reprinted from Cooper RA. Anemia with spur cells: a red cell defect acquired in serum and modified in the circulation. *J Clin Invest* 1969;48:1820, with permission.)

spur cells and that spur cell plasma can stimulate membrane protein degradation in normal red cells (1748). Spur cells and cholesterol-laden normal cells also have decreased fatty acid acylation of phospholipids—a mechanism for repair of oxidized phospholipids (1749,1750). Finally, RBC membrane lipid "rafts" are cholesterol-rich microdomains within the lipid bilayer that contain unique proteins (109, 110). When red cell Ca^{2+} is increased, some of the lipid rafts are shed in vesicles (see section *cis* Asymmetry) (111). Addition of excess cholesterol may enhance this process. Overall, these observations are interesting, but more specific information is obviously needed.

The second group of patients with liver disease and spur cell anemia differs because red cell membrane lipids are normal, and incubation of normal red cells in the patients' plasma does not induce spurring (1726,1730,1731). The pathophysiology of this condition is unknown and largely unstudied. It has been reported in patients with alcoholic cirrhosis (1726,1733) and metastatic liver disease (1730), and we have observed it in some children with spur cell anemia.

Both of these forms of spur cell anemia appear to differ from Zieve syndrome, a poorly defined syndrome of hyperlipoproteinemia, jaundice, and spherocytic hemolytic anemia that is occasionally observed in patients with alcoholic liver disease (1751).

Abetalipoproteinemia

Abetalipoproteinemia [Bassen-Kornzweig syndrome (1706,1752)] is the paradigm of disorders associated with acanthocytosis. Progressive ataxic neurologic disease, retinitis pigmentosa, fat malabsorption, and the absence of chylomicrons, very-low-density lipoproteins (VLDL; preβ-lipoproteins), and low-density lipoproteins (LDL; β-lipoproteins) are the other major features of this rare autosomal-recessive disorder. The disease is caused by failure to synthesize or secrete lipoproteins containing products of the apolipoprotein B (apoB) gene (1753) due to lack of the *microsomal triglyceride transfer protein* (1754,1755), which catalyzes the transport of triglyceride, cholesteryl ester, and phospholipid between phospholipid surfaces. It is located in the lumen of the ER in liver and intestinal epithelial cells, the sites of lipoprotein synthesis, and is required for transferring triglycerides into the ER for the assembly of apoB-containing lipoproteins (1756). Microsomal triglyceride transfer protein is a heterodimer of a multifunctional protein called *disulfide isomerase* and a unique 97-kd subunit. The 97-kd subunit is missing in abetalipoproteinemia (1755), and homozygous mutations have been demonstrated in the p97 cDNA in all tested patients (1754,1757,1758). A liver-specific knock-out of the microsomal triglyceride transfer protein gene reproduces the lipoprotein defects of the disease (1756). apoB is synthesized (1759) but cannot be secreted without its lipid coat.

Related entities such as hypobetalipoproteinemia, normotriglyceridemic abetalipoproteinemia, and chylomicron retention disease (Anderson's disease) are associated with the partial production of apoB-containing lipoproteins or with the secretion of lipoproteins containing truncated forms of apoB (1753,1760,1761). Patients with these diseases may also manifest acanthocytosis and neurologic disease, depending on the severity of the lipoprotein defect. Even patients with heterozygous hypobetalipoproteinemia may have acanthocytosis (1762), although often they do not.

In abetalipoproteinemia, typically 50% to 90% of the red cells are acanthocytes (1753,1763). The shape defect is not evident in nucleated red cells or reticulocytes and worsens as the erythrocytes age (1753,1763). Membrane protein composition is normal, but membrane lipids are not. PC concentration is decreased by approximately 20%, and SM is correspondingly increased. The cholesterol to phospholipid ratio is normal or mildly elevated (131,1763–1765). These changes reflect abnormalities in the distribution of plasma phospholipids and a decrease in LCAT activity (1766). The elevated cholesterol and SM decrease lipid fluidity (131,1764), particularly in the outer half of the bilayer (1767), and, presumably, contribute to the acanthocytic shape. They probably do so by expanding the outer bilayer relative to the inner bilayer, because drugs that selectively intercalate into the inner bilayer convert acanthocytes to biconcave disks (1768). However, this is almost impossible to prove because the difference in the surface areas of the outer bilayers of an echinocyte or acanthocyte compared to a discocyte is less than 1% (111).

Because of the fat malabsorption and the absence of LDL [which transports vitamin E (1769)], the red cells of these patients are markedly deficient in vitamin E (1770). Lipid-soluble oxidants such as hydrogen peroxide generate lipid peroxides; damage phospholipids rich in unsaturated fatty acids, such as PE and PS; oxidize membrane proteins; and cause hemolysis (1770). Oxidant sensitivity can be blocked by treatment with a water-soluble form of vitamin E (e.g., d-α-tocopherol polyethylene glycol succinate) (1770). It is widely believed that vitamin E deficiency is the primary stimulus for secondary manifestations of the disease, such as neuropathy (1753), because a similar neuropathy is observed (rarely) in patients with chronic cholestasis (1771–1773), selective malabsorption of vitamin E, or deficiency of α-tocopherol transfer protein (1774–1776). In these latter defects (1777) and, probably, in abetalipoproteinemia (1753,1778), the neurologic symptoms can be delayed or prevented by chronic vitamin E administration.

Surprisingly, despite the increased lipid viscosity and vitamin E deficiency, hemolysis is mild (1753,1763). This contrasts with spur cell anemia, in which hemolysis of similarly shaped cells is often quite severe. Several authors have attributed the difference to the spleen, which is normal in abetalipoproteinemia but is enlarged and congested by portal hypertension (131) in spur cell anemia. Whether this is a sufficient explanation is unknown.

Vitamin E Deficiency

Premature infants (<36 weeks' gestation or weighing <2000 g) and children or adults with steatorrhea are susceptible to vitamin E deficiency because of the decreased absorption of the vitamin (1779, reviewed in 1780). The diagnosis has largely disappeared in modern nurseries, partly from increased breastfeeding and adjustments to the composition of infant formulas, and partly from the realization that the disease was overdiagnosed (1781) and that overdoses of parenteral vitamin E can be toxic. However, experience with disorders of fat malabsorption, such as abetalipoproteinemia (see previous section Abetalipoproteinemia), and with rare infants with cystic fibrosis who present with hemolysis and edema (1782–1784) that respond to vitamin E, suggest that vitamin E deficiency can be deleterious. Moreover, isolated chronic vitamin E deficiency (e.g., due to congenital lack of tocopherol transfer protein) is associated with spinocerebellar dysfunction and ataxia (1774–1776).

Hemolysis and thrombocytosis are hallmarks of classic vitamin E deficiency (1785–1787); generalized firm edema is seen occasionally in severely affected infants (1782–1784,1786,1787). Peripheral blood smears are usually normal but sometimes show variable numbers of irregularly contracted, spiculated cells (acanthocytes or pyknocytes) and small numbers of spherocytes and fragmented red cells (1783,1786). The mechanism of hemolysis is uncertain. Vitamin E is a lipid-soluble antioxidant, and in its absence, lipid peroxidation occurs with damage to the double bonds of unsaturated fatty acids. Phospholipids rich in unsaturated acyl chains, such as PE, are particularly susceptible (1765,1770,1788); however, there is some evidence that damage to membrane protein sulfhydryls may also contribute to hemolysis (1789).

Vitamin E–deficient rat erythrocytes have many of the characteristics of aged normal red cells (1790), especially exposure of the so-called senescent antigen (809,810) (see section Red Cell Membrane Alterations of Senescent Red Cells). This cryptic antigen is exposed by incompletely defined modifications of band 3. It is recognized by an IgG autoantibody that initiates removal of the cells by macrophages (809). Autoantibody attachment is blocked by vitamin E and reversed by thiol-reducing agents in experimental situations (823), which suggests that membrane lipid oxidation occurs first and leads to the oxidation of band 3 thiols. Presumably, similar processes accelerate red cell destruction *in vivo* in vitamin E deficiency.

Acanthocytosis with Neurologic Disease and Normal Lipoproteins

CHOREA-ACANTHOCYTOSIS

Chorea-acanthocytosis (amyotrophic chorea-acanthocytosis, Levine-Critchley syndrome) was first described by Estes, Levine, and co-workers in 1967 (1791) and 1968 (1792). Since then, a number of reports have appeared (1692,1793–1804) (reviewed in 1692 and 1805). More than 30 patients have been described in the Western literature, and more than 50 patients have been described in Japan. The disorder is characterized by acanthocytosis, normolipoproteinemia, and progressive neurologic disease beginning in adolescence or adult life (8 to 62 years of age) and having a variety of manifestations, including orofacial dyskinesia, vocalizations, lip and tongue biting, limb chorea, dysarthria, dysphagia, axonal sensorimotor polyneuropathy, decreased or absent tendon reflexes, muscle hypotonia, distal muscle wasting, and increased creatine phosphokinase. Antibodies to ganglioside GM1 have also been observed in one patient (1806). Magnetic resonance imaging and pathologic examinations show atrophy of the basal ganglia, particularly the caudate and putamen. Mental deterioration is variable (1348), and little or no hemolysis occurs.

In some patients, acanthocytosis precedes neurologic symptoms (1799); in others, it is delayed (1807). Sometimes, spiculation is not evident in peripheral blood smears but can be induced *in vitro* more easily than normal by echinocytogenic stimuli (e.g., saline, contact with glass, etc.) (1808). The acanthocytic red cells are dense due to excessive K⁺ loss (1795) and may (1795) or may not (1803) have an increased proportion of sphingomyelin.

It is likely that more than one disorder is represented by these reports, because both dominant (1792,1793,1799) and recessive (1793,1798,1802,1807) inheritance is recorded. In addition, variant syndromes with chorea-acanthocytosis and myopathy (1809) or cardiomyopathy (1797) and with chorea-acanthocytosis, spherocytosis, and hemolysis (1810) have been observed. The recessive disease is caused by defects in a previously unknown protein called *chorein*, located on chromosome 9q21 (1811,1812). The protein is conserved and postulated to play a role in protein sorting (1811).

OTHER NEUROLOGIC SYNDROMES

Acanthocytosis is also associated with five other unusual neurologic syndromes. One features acanthocytosis and parkinsonism and is sometimes associated with motor neuron disease (1813) or diurnal dystonia (1814).

The second combines acanthocytosis, mitochondrial myopathy, encephalopathy, lactic acidosis, and a strokelike syndrome (1815).

The third couples acanthocytosis and a Hallervorden-Spatz disease, which is also called *pantothenate kinase–associated neurodegeneration* (progressive dementia, dystonia, spasticity, pallidal degeneration, and, often, retinitis pigmentosa or retinal degeneration) (1358–1360). The pallidal degeneration is characterized by iron deposition, gliosis, and axonal enlargements consisting of mitochondria, dense bodies, vesicles, and amorphous material. Magnetic resonance imaging shows a characteristic "tiger's eye" appearance of the globus pallidus.

The fourth unites acanthocytosis, abnormal lipoproteins, and a Hallervorden-Spatz–like disorder called *HARP syndrome* [*h*ypoprebetalipoproteinemia (decreased VLDL), *a*canthocytosis, *r*etinitis pigmentosa, and *p*allidal degeneration with iron deposition] (1361). Recent investigations show that this syndrome, like Hallervorden-Spatz disease, is caused by a defect in pantothenate kinase (1361a).

Finally, a specific molecular defect near the C-terminus of band 3, Pro868→Leu, has been identified (1816) in one kindred with chorea-acanthocytosis and mild hemolytic anemia (hematocrit ~34%; retics ~5%) (1817,1818). The affected siblings have 20% to 25% acanthocytes, a slight increase in the apparent molecular weight of band 3 on SDS gels (97 to 99 kd instead of 95 kd), a modest increase in anion transport, and a decrease in ankyrin-binding sites (1817). It is possible that this is only a polymorphism or an unrelated defect. It is difficult to understand how a band 3 mutation could cause chorea because band 3 is not expressed in the brain. It will be interesting to learn whether similar defects are found in other chorea-acanthocytosis kindreds.

MCLEOD SYNDROME

The McLeod syndrome is an X-linked anomaly of the Kell blood group system in which red cells or white cells, or both, react poorly with Kell antisera but behave normally in other blood group reactions (reviewed in 1819,1820). The affected cells lack XK, a 51-kd membrane protein that is disulfide cross-linked (1821) to Kell, a 93-kd zinc endopeptidase that carries the Kell antigens (1822–1825). The XK protein resembles a transport channel, but its transport function (1823), if any, is unknown.

XK is highly expressed in brain and muscle, which fits with the phenotype of its deficiency. A variety of null mutations are found in affected patients (1825a). The resemblance of McLeod syndrome to Huntington's disease and autosomal-recessive chorea-acanthocytosis suggests that the affected proteins—XK, huntingtin, and chorein—may belong to a common pathway, the dysfunction of which causes degeneration of the basal ganglia.

The XK gene is located on the X chromosome and is referred to as the *XK locus* (1826). Male hemizygotes who lack Kx on their red cells have variable echinocytosis or acanthocytosis (8% to 85%) and mild, compensated hemolysis (3% to 7% reticulocytes) (1708,1827,1828). Some teardrop erythrocytes and bizarre poikilocytes are also present. Female heterozygotes have occasional acanthocytes (as expected by chromosome X in activation) and very mild hemolysis (1708,1827). The abnormal shape is apparently due to a lack of lipid or protein in the inner bilayer, because it can be corrected by substances such as chlorpromazine, which accumulate between inner bilayer lipids (1829).

Patients with McLeod syndrome also have a myopathy or neuropathy, or both (1692,1825,1830–1836). This is first manifest as areflexia and an elevated serum creatine phosphokinase (1830) but may become severe (1835,1836). Later, in adult life, a cardiomyopathy (cardiomegaly) or slowly progressive neuropathy (dystonic or choreiform movements, with or without peripheral neuropathy, psychiatric disturbances, and seizures) may appear. Imaging studies then show caudate atrophy and decreased dopamine D2 receptors (1825,1832,1834). At this stage, the disease is sometimes confused with chorea-acanthocytosis (1833). The skeletal muscle myopathy is usually not evident clinically, although myopathic changes may be seen in biopsy specimens (1692,1831,1835,1836).

The cause of the red cell membrane defect is unknown. The XK protein is present in very small amounts (~500 copies/red cell). Membrane protein and lipid composition is normal (1837,1838), but the density of IMPs is increased (1837). This suggests that band 3, the major IMP protein, may be more dissociated in McLeod red cells than in normal red cells, in which it exists primarily as dimers and tetramers (201). There is also increased phosphorylation of some lipids and membrane proteins, notably band 3, spectrin, phosphatidic acid, and polyphosphoinositides (1838). The meaning of these changes is unknown.

The XK gene is less than 500 kilobases distal to the chronic granulomatous disease locus on the short arm of the X chromosome (Xp21.1) (1839,1840). As a consequence, some males have both chronic granulomatous disease and McLeod syndrome due to deletions that encompass both loci. It is important to recognize chronic granulomatous disease patients with McLeod syndrome (i.e., XK-deficient red cells) because, if transfused, they may produce antibodies that are only compatible with McLeod red cells (1841,1842).

In(Lu) Gene

The major antigens of the Lutheran blood group system are Lu^a and Lu^b. They are located on two low-abundance glycoproteins of 85 and 78 kd (1843). Approximately 1 person in 3000 to 5000 (1709,1844) inherits a dominantly acting inhibitor, called In(Lu), located on chromosome 11p, which greatly suppresses the expression of Lu^a and Lu^b to the extent that they are not detectable by routine agglutination tests. This is the most common cause of the null Lutheran phenotype Lu(a–b–). It is of interest for three reasons. First, the In(Lu) gene product has broad regulatory powers. It inhibits the expression of CD44 (an adhesive protein), MER2 (a common red cell antigen), CR1 (the C3b/C4b complement receptor), AnWj (the erythroid *H. influenzae* receptor), and the glycolipid antigens P_1 and i, as well as the Lutheran antigens (1845). The Lutheran glycoproteins (Lu; also called *B-cell adhesion molecules*) are the erythrocyte receptors for lamin (1846–1848). Second, although some of these proteins are widely expressed (e.g., CD44), the action of In(Lu) is limited to erythroid cells (1849). Third, patients with the In(Lu) Lu(a–b–) phenotype have abnormally shaped red cells (1709). The morphology varies from normal or mild poikilocytosis (bumpy, irregular cells) to marked acanthocytosis (1709). No hemolysis or anemia is evident. OF of fresh In(Lu) Lu(a–b–) red cells is normal, but, during *in vitro* incubations, the cells lose K^+ and become osmotically resistant (1709). The molecular mechanisms responsible for this cation loss and for the regulatory effects of the In(Lu) protein are not known, mostly because the In(Lu) gene has not yet been cloned, but they should be of considerable interest.

Anorexia Nervosa

Acanthocytosis or echinocytosis is conspicuous in many, but not all, patients with severe anorexia nervosa (1713,1714). The reason is unknown. Patients with undetectable LDL and VLDL have been reported (1850), but plasma lipids and LDL are usually normal or mildly decreased (1714). In contrast, patients who are heterozygous for congenital hypobetalipoproteinemia typically have normal red cell morphology even when LDL levels are only 10% to 20% of normal (1763). Severe starvation or malnutrition due to causes other than anorexia nervosa can also produce acanthocytosis (1851–1853) or target cells (1854) and hypobetalipoproteinemia.

Despite the morphologic defect, only a small proportion (~7%) of anorexia patients are anemic. However, mild to moderate leukopenia/neutropenia is fairly common (~38%), and mild thrombocytopenia is not rare (1713,1714,1855–1857). The various cytopenias are due to bone marrow hypoplasia (1714,1855), and their severity correlates with body weight (1855). The number of colony-forming units granulocyte-monocyte was only one-third of normal in one study, and granulocyte-macrophage colony-stimulating factor levels were low (1857). The hypoplastic marrow is also deficient in fat, which is replaced by a gelatinous, amorphous ground substance that is, possibly, acid mucopolysaccharide (1714,1858).

Infantile Pyknocytosis

In 1959, Tuffy and colleagues described a syndrome of neonatal jaundice and hemolysis associated with variable numbers of distorted, hyperchromic, irregularly contracted, spiculated cells, which they called *pyknocytes* (1707). Morphologically, these cells are very similar (and possibly identical) to acanthocytes. Normal full-term infants have 0.3% to 1.9% pyknocytes on peripheral blood smears. In premature infants, the normal range is 0.3% to 5.6% (1707). The affected infants typically present with jaundice and slight hepatosplenomegaly in the first few days of life, although intrauterine hemolysis is reported (1859). Pyknocytosis and hemolytic anemia peak at 3 to 4 weeks of age and then decline spontaneously. Clinical severity is variable; however, some infants are severely affected (Hb = 4 to 6 g/dL, 15% to 20% reticulocytes, and 25% to 50% pyknocytes), and some require exchange transfusions (1707,1859). Transfused erythrocytes become pyknocytic (1707,1860,1861) and survive poorly (1861), indicating an extracorpuscular defect. The syndrome is seen in both premature and term infants. The only consistent chemical abnormality is a mild elevation in serum glutamic-oxaloacetic transaminase (50 to 250 IU). Parents and siblings are normal (1861).

The etiology of this syndrome has not been clearly defined, and, for unknown reasons, the diagnosis is seldom made today. Infants with severe G6PD deficiency (1862), neonatal Heinz body hemolytic anemias (1707,1863), vitamin E deficiency (1792,1795), glycolytic enzyme deficiencies (1697), neonatal hepatitis (1734), HE with neonatal poikilocytosis (1421,1422), HPP, and microangiopathic hemolytic anemias may present with hemolysis and pyknocytes (or cells resembling pyknocytes) and are sometimes misdiagnosed as having infantile pyknocytosis. However, in most of the original case reports, there is sufficient evidence to exclude those disorders. The transient nature, onset after the first week of life, mild transaminase elevation, morphology, and extracorpuscular etiology are a reasonably distinctive combination and imply that infantile pyknocytosis may be a valid entity. The morphology and timing suggest oxidant damage; however, other hypotheses are tenable.

Hypothyroidism

Patients with hypothyroidism frequently (20% to 65%) have a small number (0.5% to 2.0%) of acanthocytes in their peripheral blood smears (1685,1712,1864,1865). Given the high frequency of hypothyroidism relative to other diseases associated with echinocytosis or acanthocytosis (Table 51-22), the presence of acanthocytes should prompt physicians to consider testing thyroid function, particularly in adults. Sometimes, this uncovers unsuspected cases of hypothyroidism (1866).

TARGET CELLS

Red cells increase their surface area by an increase in membrane lipids. In dried smears, the excess surface accumulates and bulges outward in the red cell's central clearing, producing the characteristic target cell morphology. In wet preps, they are bowl shaped. Target cells also occur when red cell volume is diminished due to decreased Hb synthesis (e.g., thalassemia, iron deficiency), abnormal Hb charge or aggregation, or decreased cell cations and water (e.g., HbS, HbC, and HbE). In these cases, there is a relative increase in the surface to volume ratio. With the exception of dehydrated red cells, an increase in membrane surface, whether relative or absolute, has little effect on red cell deformability or lifespan and, hence, is usually innocuous.

Obstructive Liver Disease

Target cells are particularly characteristic of biliary obstruction (1867,1868) but also occur in other forms of liver disease. Like spur cells, they form when red cells accumulate excess lipids from abnormal lipoproteins (Fig. 51-68) (1740,1868). However, unlike spur cells, target cells are characterized by a balanced increase in both free cholesterol and phospholipids (Fig. 51-69) (1740,1869,1870). The phospholipid increase is confined to PC (1740).

PATHOGENESIS OF TARGET CELLS: ROLE OF LP-X

The pathogenesis of lipid accumulation in target cells is relatively clear. The process is extracorpuscular and reversible and is due to an abnormal serum component. Normal cells acquire target cell

surface area, morphologic characteristics, and osmotic resistance when they are transfused into patients with obstructive jaundice or are incubated in their serum, whereas target cells from such patients lose their excess lipids and revert to biconcave discs in normal persons or their sera (1868). Cooper and co-workers found a close relation between the cholesterol to phospholipid ratios of target cells and serum lipoproteins, particularly LDL (1740). It is known that in obstructive jaundice and LCAT deficiency (see section Familial Lecithin-Cholesterol Acyltransferase Deficiency), a unique, abnormal lipoprotein called *lipoprotein X* (Lp-X) accumulates in the LDL density class (1871–1873). Lp-X is a lipid vesicle that contains approximately 30% unesterified cholesterol and 60% PC, plus small amounts of apolipoproteins C and E, albumin, cholesterol esters, triglycerides, and lithocholic acid (1872–1874). It appears to arise from bile lipids and requires the Mdr2 P-glycoprotein, which translocates lipids across the bile canalicular membrane (1875). Lp-X is a substrate for LCAT in the presence of apolipoprotein A-I (1874), so a deficiency of LCAT or apolipoprotein A-I may also be needed to produce Lp-X. Normal red cells rapidly acquire excess cholesterol, PC, and surface area when incubated with Lp-X *in vitro* (1870), and it is almost certainly the source of lipids for membrane expansion and targeting *in vivo*.

Interestingly, membrane proteins may also be abnormal in these cells. Iida and co-workers (1876) found that protein 4.2 was diminished or absent in 11 of 11 Japanese patients with obstructive jaundice and typical lipid-laden target cells. Red cell morphology, membrane lipids, and protein 4.2 content returned to normal in one patient after surgical relief of the biliary obstruction (1876). To date, this curious observation has never been confirmed or denied, and its relevance to the pathophysiology of targeting, if any, remains obscure.

Familial Lecithin-Cholesterol Acyltransferase Deficiency

Familial LCAT deficiency is a rare autosomal-recessive disorder characterized by anemia, corneal opacities, hyperlipemia, proteinuria, chronic nephritis, and premature atherosclerosis. An excellent review of the disease has been published (1878). LCAT deficiency is relatively asymptomatic during childhood. Proteinuria and corneal opacities are among the earliest manifestations. The latter consist of minute grayish dots that concentrate near the edge of the cornea, resembling arcus senilis (1878). Almost all of the reported patients have had a moderate normochromic anemia (Hb = 8 to 11 g/dL) characterized by prominent target cell formation and decreased OF (1878–1881). Hematologic studies suggest that the anemia is due to a combination of moderate hemolysis and decreased erythropoietic compensation, but interpretation of the evidence is complicated by the coexisting renal disease. Other studies have shown that the red cells are abnormally susceptible to peroxidative threat and have mechanically fragile membranes (1880). There is no obvious explanation for these changes, but it is possible that they contribute to the shortened red cell lifespan.

The disease is caused by a variety of mutations of the LCAT gene (1878). As expected from the absence of LCAT activity, there is a pronounced decrease in cholesteryl esters and an increase in free cholesterol and PC in plasma lipoproteins (1878). Because LCAT is required for normal lipoprotein formation and catabolism, nascent lipoproteins and abnormal lipoprotein remnants accumulate in the plasma (1878). One of the latter is Lp-X (1875,1878,1882). As discussed in the previous section, this lipoprotein is believed to be responsible for target cell formation in patients with the acquired LCAT deficiency of obstructive liver disease (1870) and presumably plays the same role in the familial disease. Unesterified cholesterol and PC levels are markedly elevated in the red cell membranes of LCAT-deficient patients (1883); however, total red cell phospholipid levels are normal because the increase in PC is balanced by a decrease in PE and SM (1883). As in liver disease, red cell targeting and lipid abnormalities can be induced by incubation of normal red cells in LCAT-deficient serum and reversed by incubation in normal serum (1882). Other plasma membranes are probably also affected by the abnormal LCAT-deficient lipoproteins. For example, accumulations of lipid from Lp-X may stimulate the proliferation of mesangial cells and lead to nephritic complications (1884). In addition, phagocytosis of abnormal lipoproteins by reticuloendothelial cells generates foam cells (1879) and sea-blue histiocytes (1885) in the bone marrow, spleen, and other organs. Serum and red cell lipids are improved *in vivo* when LCAT is supplied by infusions of normal plasma (1878); however, the short half-life of this protein (approximately 4 to 5 days) and the large amount of plasma required make chronic replacement therapy impractical. Therapy with recombinant human LCAT remains a hope.

FISH-EYE DISEASE
Fish-eye disease is caused by a partial deficiency of LCAT. It is characterized by corneal opacities (which give the disease its name), hypertriglyceridemia, and very low levels of HDL (1878). One report notes increased target cells and decreased OF (1886).

Postsplenectomy

In the first several weeks after splenectomy, target cells gradually increase in number (1867,1887–1889), eventually (in otherwise normal persons) reaching levels of 2% to 10% (1889). This change is associated with an increase in osmotic resistance (1867), membrane lipid content (1070), and mean surface area relative to volume (1887), indicating expansion of the red cell membrane surface (1887). By deduction, the spleen must normally remove surplus membrane from such cells—a process referred to as *surface remodeling*. Experimental studies clearly document that the stress reticulocytes induced by acute blood loss or hemolysis undergo extensive surface remodeling (1890,1891) and suggest that normal reticulocytes are remodeled to a lesser degree. In addition to membrane lipids, transferrin receptors (745), fibronectin receptors (746), and a high-molecular-weight membrane protein complex (1892) are removed during the remodeling process. Nuclei and internal organelles with their membranes are also removed. Autophagocytosis and expulsion of phagolysosomes are believed to be the major mechanisms for this remodeling (1893). Interestingly, plasma lipoproteins are involved in this process, perhaps functioning as the "garbage trucks" that remove the detritus. Hypercholesterolemic mice lacking the HDL receptor develop large, irregular erythrocytes packed with autophagolysosomes. These are expelled when the immature red cells are transfused into normal hosts or incubated with normolipidemic serum (1893).

Postsplenectomy blood smears also show increased numbers of acanthocytes (1685,1894), poikilocytes, and red cells burdened with useless or potentially harmful inclusions (e.g., Heinz bodies, Howell-Jolly bodies, siderotic granules, and endocytic vesicles) (1895–1897). The presence of these inclusions attests to the "culling" and "pitting" functions of the spleen (1895). These and other aspects of splenic function are discussed more fully in Chapter 21.

INHERITED DISORDERS OF RED CELL CATION PERMEABILITY AND VOLUME

Red cell hydration is determined, in part, by the intracellular concentration of monovalent cations (1898). A net increase in

$[Na^+ + K^+]$ causes water to enter, forming *stomatocytes*, or *hydrocytes*, whereas a net loss of monovalent cations produces dehydrated red cells, or *xerocytes*.*

In the last 34 years, numerous descriptions of congenital or familial hemolytic anemias associated with abnormal cation permeability and, in some cases, disturbed red cell hydration have appeared (1525,1899–1942). These span the range from severe stomatocytosis (1930) to severe xerocytosis (1905) and are clinically very heterogeneous. They can be divided into six provisional categories based on differences of severity, morphology, cation content, lipid and protein composition, genetics, and response to splenectomy (Table 51-23); however, it is not certain that these categories are unique entities. Indeed, none of these apparent disorders is precisely defined in either clinical or molecular terms.

Reviews of these disorders are available (1950,1957,1957a).

Hereditary Stomatocytosis

Stomatocytes are erythrocytes with a mouth-shaped (stoma) area of central pallor on peripheral blood smears (Fig. 51-71A). Classic hereditary stomatocytosis is a rare syndrome characterized by extraordinary monovalent cation leaks, relative Na^+,K^+ pump failure, and stomatocytic red cell morphology. Stomatocyte membranes are remarkably permeable to Na^+ and K^+ ions, particularly Na^+ ions. Intracellular Na^+ is increased, and K^+ is decreased, but the total monovalent cation content ($Na^+ + K^+$) is high, which leads to an increase in cell water and cell volume. Consequently, the cells are sometimes called *hydrocytes* or *overhydrated stomatocytes*. The clinical severity of hereditary stomatocytosis is variable: Some patients have hemolysis and anemia, whereas others are asymptomatic (reviewed in 1460,1461). Ten definite families with the classic phenotype have been described (353,1902,1904,1913,1915,1919,1920,1923,1924,1930).

PATHOPHYSIOLOGY

Hereditary Stomatocytes Have a Huge Passive Sodium Leak. The major detectable defect in hereditary stomatocytosis is a marked asymmetric increase in passive Na^+ and K^+ permeability ($Na^+_{in} > K^+_{out}$). Permeabilities as great as 15 to 40 times normal are observed (353,1923,1930). Because the influx of Na^+ exceeds the loss of K^+, stomatocytic red cells progressively gain cations and water and swell. As a consequence, their average density is less than normal (Fig. 51-72), and the swollen stomatocytes are osmotically fragile. Unlike normal cells, aged stomatocytes are less dense and more stomatocytic than stomatocytic reticulocytes (1043,1902).

Monovalent cation transporters are stimulated by the influx of Na^+, particularly the Na^+,K^+ pump and K^+,Cl^- cotransporter (1919), but are unable to keep up with the exaggerated cation leaks and are overwhelmed. There is no convincing evidence that Na^+,K^+ pumping is defective: Pump kinetics are normal (1043), and the number of pumps is increased several-fold (1930,1954)—even after correcting for red cell age (1958). Some authors have observed that Na^+ and K^+ are not transported in the usual ratio (3 Na^+:2 K^+) (1043,1920) and have argued that the Na^+,K^+ pump is "decoupled" (1920); however, other work suggests that this is, at least partly, an artifact of the methods used to measure cation permeability (1959).

Remarkably, bifunctional imidoesters, which cross-link proteins, reverse the abnormal shape and permeability of hereditary stomatocytes, and normalize stomatocyte survival in the

---

*These cells have also been dubbed *desiccytes*; however, this term, a Latin-Greek chimera, is less desirable.

TABLE 51-23. Features of Hereditary Stomatocytosis-Xerocytosis Syndromes

	Stomatocytosis (Overhydrated Stomatocytosis)		Intermediate Syndromes			
	Severe Hemolysis[a]	Mild Hemolysis[b]	Cryohydrocytosis[c]	Stomatocytic Xerocytosis[d]	Pseudo-Hyperkalemia[e]	Xerocytosis[f,g] (Dehydrated Stomatocytosis)
Hemolysis	Severe	Mild-moderate	Mild-moderate	Mild	Mild or none	Moderate
Anemia	Severe	Mild-moderate	Mild-moderate	None	None	Mild-moderate
Blood smear	Stomatocytes	Stomatocytes	Stomatocytes or normal	Stomatocytes	Targets, few stomatocytes	Targets; occasional echinocytes, stomatocytes
MCV (80–100 µ³)[h]	110–150	95–130	90–105	91–98	82–104	84–122
MCHC (32–36g/dL)	24–30	26–29	34–38	33–39	33–39	34–38
Unincubated osmotic fragility	Very increased	Increased	Normal-slt. increased	Slt. decreased	Slt. decreased	Very decreased
RBC Na+ (5–12 mEq/L)	60–100	30–60	15–50	10–20	10–25	10–30
RBC K+ (90–103 mEq/L)	20–55	40–85	55–65	75–85	75–100	60–90
RBC Na+ + K+ (95–110 mEq/L)	110–140	115–145	75–105	87–109	87–109	75–99
RBC passive membrane leak[i]	20–40	~3–10	1–6	?	1–2	2–4
Cold autohemolysis	No	No	Yes	No	No	± No
Pseudohyperkalemia	?Yes	?Yes	Yes	?	Yes	Sometimes
Perinatal ascites	No	?	No	?	No	Sometimes
Stomatin absent	Yes	?	± No[j]	?	?	?No
Phosphatidylcholine content	Normal	± Increased	Normal	Normal	Normal	Increased
Effect of splenectomy	Good	Good	Fair-none	?	?	Poor
Thromboembolism postsplenectomy	Yes	?	No	?	?	Yes
Genetics	AD	AD	AD	AD	AD 16q23-q24	AD 16q23-q24

AD, autosomal dominant; MCHC, mean cell hemoglobin concentration; MCV, mean cellular volume; RBC, red blood cell; slt., slightly.
[a]Data from references 1902,1904,1909,1911–1913,1916,1919,1923,1924,1930.
[b]Data from references 1043,1920,1943.
[c]Data from references 1908,1917,1932,1934,1937,1944,1945.
[d]Data from reference 1918.
[e]Data from references 1932,1935,1936,1938,1941,1946–1953.
[f]Data from references 1900,1903,1905,1910,1914,1921,1922,1925,1926,1928,1929,1931,1933,1936,1941–1943,1948,1949,1954–1956.
[g]Hereditary xerocytosis is identical (1931) to dehydrated hereditary stomatocytosis and to high phosphatidyl choline hemolytic anemia.
[h]Normal values are given in parentheses.
[i]Defined as the ouabain- and bumetanide-resistant (86) Rb+ influx at 37°C and expressed as the ratio of patient to normal residual leak (normal = 0.06 – 0.10 mmol/L RBC/h).
[j]One patient reported with cryohydrocytosis and absence of stomatin (1909), but this patient may have typical (overhydrated) hereditary stomatocytosis.

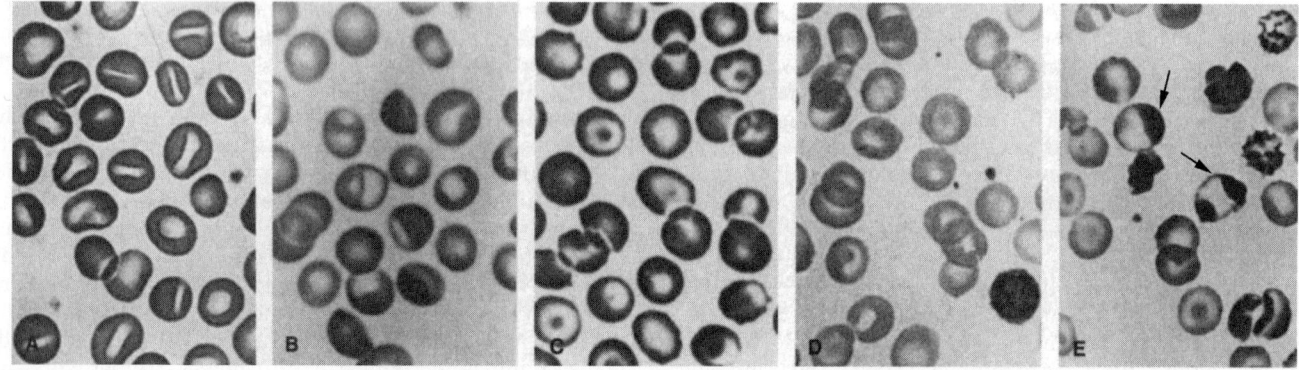

Figure 51-71. Peripheral blood morphology in hereditary stomatocytosis and hereditary xerocytosis. **A:** Stomatocytosis. Many stomatocytes and occasional spherocytes are seen (1927). **B:** Cryohydrocytosis. Some of the stomatocytes are bowl shaped, some have curvilinear slits, and some have a transverse bar dividing the central clearing (1917). **C:** Stomatocytic xerocytosis. Moderate numbers of target cells and some crenated cells are present (1928). **D:** Xerocytosis (mild). Some target cells are evident, but most red cells are morphologically unremarkable (1948). **E:** Xerocytosis (severe). Target cells, echinocytes, and dense crenated cells predominate. In occasional cells (*arrows*), the hemoglobin appears to be puddled in one portion of the cell (1905).

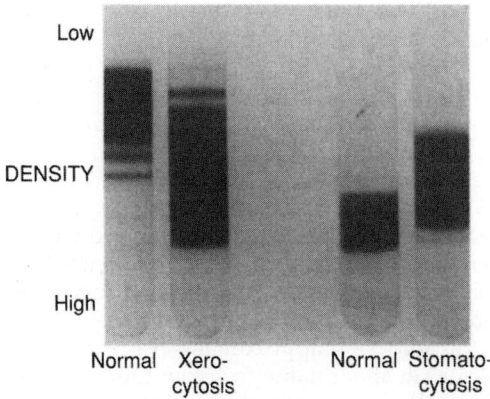

Figure 51-72. Separation of hydrocytes and xerocytes by density. **Left:** Normal and hereditary xerocytosis samples. The cells were separated on Stractan density gradients. The xerocytes extend to higher densities than normal red cells. **Right:** Normal and hereditary stomatocytosis samples. Many of the stomatocytes are lighter than the normal red cells. (Reprinted from Lande WM, Mentzer WC. Haemolytic anaemia associated with increased cation permeability. *Clin Haematol* 1985;14:89, with permission.)

circulation (1960). The critical proteins have not been identified because many red cell membrane proteins are cross-linked at the concentrations required to achieve this effect.

Stomatocytes are relatively rigid (1916) and expend extraordinary amounts of ATP to pump Na⁺ and K⁺, attempting to defend the threat of osmotic rupture. They should be uniquely vulnerable to splenic sequestration, and, predictably, splenectomy has been uniformly beneficial in patients with severe hemolysis (1902,1903,1919,1920,1924,1930)—but not without serious risk (see section Treatment) (1961).

STOMATIN

Many Patients with Hereditary Stomatocytosis Lack Stomatin (Protein 7.2b). The excess cation permeability is often (353,1894,1909,1919,1923) but not always (1906,1907) associated with the absence of stomatin, a membrane protein that migrates in the band 7 region on SDS gels (Fig. 51-73). Lande and Mentzer first observed that stomatin (they called it *protein 7.2b*) was absent in the red cell membranes of a patient with classic hereditary stomatocytosis (1909). Subsequently, the same defect has been found in all eight patients tested from seven other typical stomatocytosis kindreds (353,1904,1919,1923) and from a patient said to have cryohydrocytosis (1909) (see following section), who probably should be reclassified as having hereditary stomatocytosis.

Stomatin Deficiency Is Not the Cause of Hereditary Stomatocytosis. If stomatin deficiency is the cause of hereditary stomatocytosis, one must explain why stomatin is completely absent in patients with autosomal-dominant stomatocytosis. One would expect a 50:50 mixture of normal and mutant proteins. One possibility is that stomatin behaves as a dominant-negative mutation. If the protein forms higher-order oligomers, then the introduction of even one mutant protomer might destabilize the structure or interfere with its membrane assembly. However, four groups have cloned and sequenced cDNAs from stomatocytosis patients with stomatin deficiency (1962–1964; John KM, Lux SE, *unpublished observations*, 1996), including the most severe patient yet reported (1930). All four find that the coding sequence of stomatin is normal, which is not compatible with a dominant-negative mutation.

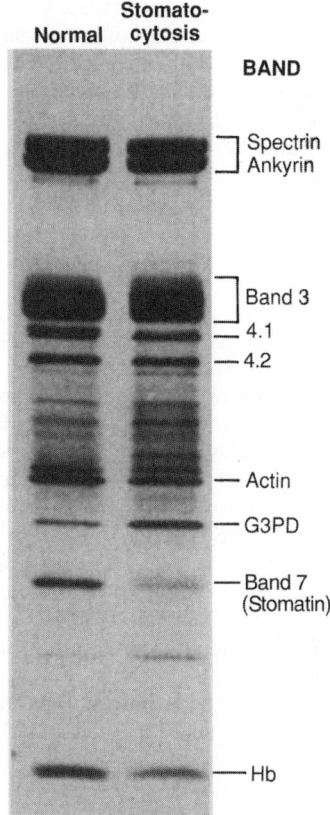

Figure 51-73. Stomatin deficiency in hereditary stomatocytosis. Sodium dodecyl sulfate gels of normal and stomatocytosis red cells show that the principal (28-kd) band in the band 7 region (stomatin) is missing. A similar picture is observed in most patients with severe hereditary stomatocytosis. Immunoblots confirm that stomatin is absent in these cells. G3PD, glyceraldehyde-3-phosphate dehydrogenase; Hb, hemoglobin. (Reprinted from Rix M, Bjerrum PJ, Wieth JO, Frandsen B. Congenital stomatocytosis with hemolytic anemia—with abnormal cation permeability and defective membrane proteins. *Ugeskrift for Laeger* 1991;153:724, with permission.)

In addition, mice with targeted disruption of stomatin are clinically and hematologically normal (1966). Thus, it seems more likely that the defect resides in a protein that interacts with stomatin and causes its destruction secondarily. For example, the defect could lie in a chaperone that brings stomatin to the membrane. Or, it could activate a protein that modifies stomatin (e.g., a kinase, a phosphatase, or a ubiquitinating enzyme) so that it is recognized and destroyed; that destroys stomatin directly (e.g., a protease); or that directs stomatin to be lost with other proteins and organelles during reticulocyte maturation.

Also, stomatin and other red cell lipid raft proteins are lost when raft cholesterol is depleted (109), but there is no discernible effect on red cell deformability or membrane transport to the extent tested. Monovalent cation transport was not directly measured; however, marked leakiness of the type observed in severe hereditary stomatocytosis should have decreased cellular deformability.

Finally, stomatin-deficient patients apparently do not experience any nonhematologic symptoms (1962), which suggests that either the deficiency is confined to erythrocytes or stomatin is not essential for the function of other tissues.

Hereditary Stomatocytosis Is Heterogeneous. Some patients with severe permeability defects have little or no hemolysis (1043). In addition, studies of 44 Japanese patients with stomatocytosis (1907) show that the proportion of stomatocytes and the degree of Na^+ influx do not correlate with each other, and neither correlates with the amount of hemolysis or anemia. Furthermore, stomatin (protein 7.2b) deficiency was not observed in Japanese patients with the most severe permeability defects and was only present, to a mild degree, in five of nine patients with more moderate Na^+ leaks. This suggests that hereditary stomatocytosis is either a complex mixture of diseases or that factors other than Na^+ leak and stomatin content are critical to the demise of the stomatocyte.

CLINICAL FEATURES

The diagnostic features of typical, stomatin-deficient hereditary stomatocytosis include the unique red cell morphology (5% to 50% stomatocytes) (Fig. 51-71A), macrocytosis, greatly elevated erythrocyte Na^+ concentration, greatly reduced K^+ concentration, and increased total ($Na^+ + K^+$) content (Table 51-23). The excess cations elevate cell water (Fig. 51-25), producing osmotically fragile cells (Table 51-23) and severe hemolytic anemia. In many patients, hereditary stomatocytes are also moderately deficient in 2,3-DPG (1916,1930,1954). Perhaps a portion of the 1,3-DPG normally used for 2,3-DPG synthesis is diverted through phosphoglycerate kinase to provide extra ATP for cation transport (1954). The 2,3-DPG deficiency mildly enhances oxygen affinity (1954) and causes additional water entry and cell swelling. Some patients (1912,1918) and dogs (1967,1968) with hereditary stomatocytosis have an unexplained decrease in red cell glutathione; however, it is unlikely that this is pathophysiologically significant.

TREATMENT

Splenectomy reduces the hemolytic rate of patients with severe hereditary stomatocytosis (1902,1919,1920,1924,1930), presumably because the swollen, poorly deformable stomatocytes are filtered by the spleen. The acidic, hypoxic, metabolic splenic environment compromises red cell metabolism, which is fatal for cells that are dependent on maximal activity of the ATP-driven Na^+,K^+ pump to survive (1916). However, although splenectomy is beneficial from the red cell's point of view, it is very dangerous in these patients. A high proportion have experienced thrombotic or thromboembolic complications, sometimes with fatal results (1961). Venous thrombi predominate and sometimes give rise to portal hypertension or embolism and pulmonary hypertension. The reasons why hereditary stomatocytosis patients are hypercoagulable and why thrombosis is only observed after splenectomy are unknown. One possibility is that phospholipid asymmetry is altered, exposing PS, which is highly thrombogenic (83–85) (see section Asymmetric Organization of Phospholipids in the Bilayer at the beginning of this chapter). This has not been tested to our knowledge. Red cells with exposed PS are cleared by macrophages (27,86–89), and this function would presumably be impaired by splenectomy. A second possibility is that hereditary stomatocytes are more adherent to the endothelium. This has been observed in a splenectomized patient with hereditary xerocytosis (1969) (see following section) but has not been examined in classic hereditary stomatocytosis.

Hereditary Xerocytosis (Dehydrated Hereditary Stomatocytosis, High Phosphatidyl Choline Hemolytic Anemia)

This disorder is the most common, and perhaps the most subtle, of the cation permeability defects. It is often called *dehydrated stomatocytosis*, although stomatocytes are rarely prominent as they are in classic hereditary stomatocytosis ("overhydrated stomatocytosis"). Unfortunately, early articles often confused

the two conditions and called the disease *stomatocytosis* or focused on membrane lipid changes with the term *high phosphatidyl choline hemolytic anemia* (HPCHA) (1931). We prefer *hereditary xerocytosis*, which is the name given by Glader, who described the first case (1905), and a name that emphasizes the hallmark of the disease: cellular dehydration.

K+ AND WATER EFFLUX INCREASED

Since the first report, other families with hereditary xerocytosis have been described (Table 51-23). Physiologically, the major red cell abnormality in these patients is a change in the relative membrane permeability to potassium. K^+ efflux is increased (two- to fourfold) and approximates Na^+ influx. There is no metabolic or Hb abnormality to account for this permeability lesion, and red cell Ca^{2+} content is not increased. The nature of the permeability defect (i.e., the pathways involved) has not been well studied. Monovalent cation pump activity is increased appropriately for the slightly elevated Na^+ content, but the Na^+,K^+ pump cannot compensate for K^+ losses in excess of Na^+ gain. In fact, the action of the pump significantly exacerbates the rate of K^+ loss because three Na^+ ions are pumped out for every two K^+ ions returned (793,794). As a consequence, xerocytes gradually become cation depleted and lose water in response to decreased intracellular osmolality. This is easily detected by centrifugation on Stractan gradients (Fig. 51-72).

HEREDITARY XEROCYTOSIS MAPS TO CHROMOSOME 16Q23-Q24

Little is known about the molecular pathology of the disease. The disease maps to a 9-cM interval on chromosome 16q23-q24 (1945,1970), but the specific molecular defect has not been identified. There are no obvious candidate genes in the immediate genomic neighborhood; however, we note that the gene for the red cell KCl cotransporter (SLP12A4 or KCC1) lies suspiciously nearby at 16q22.1 (1971). Although xerocytosis is usually considered to be a defect in the passive permeability of the membrane, overactivity or leakiness of the KCl cotransporter could account for the K^+ loss and should be investigated.

XEROCYTE MEMBRANES CONTAIN DISPROPORTIONATE AMOUNTS OF PHOSPHATIDYL CHOLINE

When measured, the proportion of red cell membrane PC is increased in xerocytes (12 to 20 fmol/cell; nl = 10 to 12) (1931). As noted above, the combination of hereditary xerocytosis and high PC is sometimes given the name *high phosphatidyl choline hemolytic anemia* (1910,1925,1929,1931,1948), but there appears to be little reason to distinguish HPCHA from hereditary xerocytosis (1931). Early studies suggested the excess PC was due to diminished transfer of PC fatty acids to PE (1924), a pathway that is normally stimulated by cellular dehydration (1972). It is not clear why this pathway is inhibited in hereditary xerocytosis or how it relates to the underlying membrane leakiness and hemolysis.

XEROCYTE MEMBRANES ARE OXIDANT SENSITIVE

Red cells in hereditary xerocytosis are also shear sensitive (1922) and are exceptionally prone to membrane fragmentation in response to metabolic stress (1900). This suggests a membrane skeletal defect, but no systematic studies of xerocytic membrane skeletons have been conducted to date. Conventional analyses of red cell membrane proteins have been normal (1901,1936), except for an increase in the proportion of membrane-associated G3PD in one family (1973). Quantitatively, all membrane components are increased because, for unknown reasons, xerocytes have 15% to 25% more surface area than normal (1974). Xerocytes are relatively rigid cells (1903) and probably develop a dehydration-induced membrane injury (1919). This poorly defined lesion is also found in ISCs (1975) and presumably is important in the pathophysiology of hemolysis. Hereditary xerocytes are also unusually sensitive to oxidants (1976–1978). Exposure of xerocytes to concentrations of hydrogen peroxide that do not affect normal cells causes a rapid loss of intracellular K^+, conversion of Hb to methemoglobin, and cross-linking of Hb to spectrin (1977,1978). Similar sensitivity occurs in dehydrated normal red cells. Conversely, rehydrated xerocytes exhibit a normal reaction to hydrogen peroxide. Native xerocytes contain the abnormal spectrin-globin complex, and the amount correlates with the extent of dehydration in various cellular fractions and with membrane rigidity (1979). Finally, oxidation of normal erythrocytes with peroxide generates the spectrin-globin complex and rigid membranes (1980). Complex formation is blocked by carbon monoxide, which prevents Hb oxidation, but is not blocked by lipid antioxidants (1980). This implies a direct role for Hb in cross-linking spectrin. However, the relevance of these interesting findings to the pathophysiology of hereditary xerocytosis remains a complete mystery.

CLINICAL AND LABORATORY FEATURES

Xerocytes Are Uniquely Dehydrated But Macrocytic. Hereditary xerocytosis is inherited as an autosomal-dominant trait. The characteristic biochemical abnormality is a reduced concentration of red cell K^+ and total monovalent cations [i.e., $(Na^+ + K^+)$] (Table 51-23). In older erythrocytes, K^+ approaches half-normal levels (1931). Most patients have well-compensated hemolysis with little or no anemia by laboratory evaluation. Diagnostic laboratory features include an increased MCHC, an increased MCV, and a decreased OF (i.e., resistance to osmotic lysis) (Table 51-23) (1936). The combination of a high MCHC and a high MCV is unique and should suggest the diagnosis. Surprisingly, the fraction of hyperdense cells is not a reliable marker (1936), in contrast to HS (Fig. 51-46). Osmotic gradient ektacytometry shows a leftward shift (1157,1936)—the opposite of HS. The leftward shift of the minimum (O_{min}) in the deformability index at low osmolarities in the ektacytometer (see *thin arrow* in Fig. 51-46) is the most reliable diagnostic parameter (1936). This point corresponds to the 50% hemolysis point in the unincubated OF curve. In the absence of ektacytometry, an increase in the osmotic resistance measured on *fresh* blood appears to be the best diagnostic test (1936).

The large size of hereditary xerocytes is probably partly an artifact of cellular stiffness. In Coulter-type electronic counters, the conversion of pulse height (from the resistance of a cell passing through an electric field) to a cellular volume is dependent on cell shape. Xerocytes do not deform to the same degree as normal cells, which causes the electronically measured MCV to be approximately 10% too high (1972). However, after correction for this, the cells are still too large.

Autohemolysis is increased and responds to glucose (1900,1913,1928,1948)—similar to the pattern in HS.

Red Cell Morphology Is Relatively Normal. In the most severely affected patients (1905), blood smears contain contracted and spiculated red cells and red cells in which the Hb appears to be "puddled" or "gelled" on one side of the cell (Fig. 51-71E). Most patients, however, have nearly normal erythrocyte morphology, with a small number of target cells or stomatocytes and an occasional echinocyte (Fig. 51-71D). Despite the name *dehydrated stomatocytosis*, stomatocytes are *not* a prominent feature of the disease ($\leq 10\%$) in most patients. However, there are exceptions (1933).

Xerocytes Are 2,3-Diphosphoglycerate Deficient. Red cell 2,3-DPG concentrations are moderately decreased in hereditary xerocytosis (1900,1901,1905,1913,1921), as well as in hereditary stomatocytosis. The reasons for this deficiency are unknown. Because loss of the polyvalent 2,3-DPG is compensated by an influx of monovalent chloride ions and water, patients with xerocytosis and unusually low 2,3-DPG levels have fewer dehydrated red cells than expected for the degree of cation loss and, in rare cases, have almost no dehydration (1901). Patients with low 2,3-DPG also have *increased* whole blood oxygen affinity and, consequently, often have little apparent anemia (1901). It should be noted, however, that such patients have relative polycythemia and are *physiologically* more anemic than their Hb levels suggest. This is even more so if the hematocrit is used to judge anemia, because cellular stiffness may artifactually elevate the hematocrit value on certain electronic counters.

Some Patients with Hereditary Xerocytosis Have Pseudohyperkalemia or Perinatal Edema. It has recently become clear that hereditary xerocytosis is a pleiotropic syndrome. In addition to the familiar presentation as a well-compensated hemolytic anemia, patients also present with pseudohyperkalemia (see section Familial Pseudohyperkalemia) and perinatal edema (1933,1936,1942,1956). Various combinations of these features occur in different families—and even within the same family (1936). The term *perinatal edema* encompasses a variety of fluid collections, including ascites, hydrothorax, pericardial effusion, and subcutaneous edema. It may occur *in utero* or in the neonatal period. Hydrops fetalis (a combination of at least two of the manifestations above) is also observed. It is notable that the edema is *not* caused by the anemia, which, as noted above, is mild. The mechanism is unknown. However, the fluid collections are transient and resolve spontaneously within weeks to months after birth (1936) and, possibly, even *in utero* (1942). It is not clear if treatment is necessary or what treatment should be given. Intrauterine transfusions were tried in one instance and were ineffective (1956), but repeated intrauterine administration of red cells and albumin was judged effective in another instance (1942). The effectiveness of any treatment is hard to judge because of the spontaneous remissions.

Splenectomy Is Not Beneficial and Is Associated with High Risk of Thrombosis. In contrast to hereditary stomatocytosis, in which splenectomy is beneficial, the limited experience available to date suggests that removing the spleen does not significantly reduce hemolysis in patients with hereditary xerocytosis (1429,1434). Presumably, xerocytes are so functionally compromised that they are easily detected and eliminated in other areas of the reticuloendothelial system. Moreover, there is such a remarkably high risk of venous thrombosis and thromboembolism—and even death—after splenectomy (1910,1936,1961,1981) that, in our judgment, *splenectomy is absolutely contraindicated in this disease.* The reason why patients are so hypercoagulable is not known. As noted in the section on hereditary stomatocytosis, which also carries a risk of thromboembolism, the possibilities of PS exposure and enhanced endothelial adherence of the defective cells must be considered. There is evidence for the latter possibility (1969). Fortunately, almost all patients are able to maintain an Hb level of at least 9 g/dL (1936) so that splenectomy is not an issue.

Intermediate Syndromes

Hereditary stomatocytosis and hereditary xerocytosis represent the extremes of a spectrum of red cell permeability defects. A number of families with features of both conditions have been reported. The reported cases seem to fall into three groups whose red cells differ principally in morphology, OF, and sensitivity to cold (Table 51-23).

CRYOHYDROCYTOSIS

Seven unrelated families have been reported with this disease (1908,1917,1930,1932,1934,1937), and we have seen an eighth (Lux SE, Lanzkowsky P, et al., *unpublished observations*). The inheritance is autosomal dominant. The patients have a mild congenital hemolytic anemia characterized by marked autohemolysis that is greater at 4°C than at 37°C (1908,1917,1930,1932,1937,1945). Fresh erythrocytes are Na^+ loaded and K^+ depleted (Table 51-23). The total concentration of $Na^+ + K^+$ is normal (1908; Lux SE, Lanzkowsky P, et al., *unpublished observations*) or low (1934,1937), but the measurements are complicated by the ion shifts that occur in storage, especially in the cold (1934). In the cold, Na^+ and K^+ passive permeabilities are markedly increased; however, because Na^+ entry greatly predominates, the red cells rapidly swell and lyse. Nevertheless, K^+ leak is high enough that pseudohyperkalemia has been noted (1934,1937). Perinatal edema has not been reported. Curiously, this cold autohemolysis is sensitive to the method of anticoagulation. It is increased in the cold in heparin, EDTA, and defibrinated plasma but not in acid citrate dextrose (1908,1917).

The primary molecular lesion of this interesting disorder is unknown. Membrane lipids are quantitatively normal (1908) except for an increase in ether lipids (1932,1937), and, with the exception of a mild decrease in red cell glutathione (1908,1917), no defects in metabolism have been detected. Na^+,K^+ pumping and $Na^+,K^+,2Cl^-$ cotransport activities are appropriately high (1934), and red cell membrane protein content is normal (1937; Lux SE, Lanzkowsky P, et al., *unpublished observations*). One patient was reported to be missing stomatin (1909), but it is likely this patient actually has classic stomatocytosis. Recent studies show that the abnormal cold permeability of cryohydrocytes can be mimicked by suspending normal cells in media in which either Na^+ or Cl^- has been replaced by an organic cation or anion, respectively (1937). This suggests that the membrane element responsible for the abnormal permeability is responsive to the local ordering of water molecules.

Blood smears show stomatocytes, some of which have an eccentric or curvilinear slit or a transverse bar bisecting the area of central pallor (1917,1934; Lux SE, Lanzkowsky P, et al., *unpublished observations*) (Fig. 51-71B). The MCV and MCHC are normal or increased, but, again, the measurements are difficult because the MCV rapidly rises, and the MCHC dramatically falls during storage (1934,1937). *In this disease, red cell measurements need to be performed immediately on freshly drawn blood that is not allowed to cool.* The Pink test (a variant of the glycerol lysis test) is positive (1937), and the unincubated OF test shows a crossover pattern, with some fragile cells (1934). These results, combined with the dominant inheritance and the positive autohemolysis (which corrects with glucose) (1937), may easily lead to the mistaken diagnosis of atypical HS (1934). Splenectomy seems to provide no benefit and so far has not been associated with thromboembolic complications (1934,1937).

FAMILIAL PSEUDOHYPERKALEMIA

A number of families with pseudohyperkalemia have been described (1932,1935,1936,1938,1941,1947,1949,1951–1953) since the original description (1946). The dominantly inherited disorder is characterized by erythrocyte K^+ loss that is relatively greater just below ambient temperature or in the cold (1932,1935,1946,1947,1982). Electrolyte analyses of plasma obtained from blood samples stored for only a few hours at room temperature or below may falsely suggest that affected individuals are hyperkalemic. The disorder resembles cryohydrocytosis except that K^+ loss and dehydration predominate instead of Na^+ gain and cryohemolysis. Fortunately, there is little K^+ loss at physiologic temperatures, so patients have only mildly dehydrated red cells and little or no hemolysis and anemia. The disorder maps to 16q23-q24, the same locus as hereditary xerocytosis (1983), and probably is just a subset of the manifestations of that disease (1936), as discussed above. However, pseudohyperkalemia is also observed in cryohydrocytosis (1934,1937) and has been reported in HS (1984,1985). In addition, at least one family with pseudohyperkalemia has been described (1939) that does *not* map to chromosome 16 (1938), indicating genetic heterogeneity. Nonfamilial pseudohyperkalemia occurs in patients with very high platelet (1986–1988) or leukocyte (1989–1991) counts, either reactive or malignant, if precautions are not taken to draw the blood gently and analyze electrolyte levels immediately in plasma. Pseudohyperkalemia is also reported in Akita dogs (1992). This has not been well studied but might be a useful model system.

STOMATOCYTIC XEROCYTOSIS

In 1971, Miller and colleagues reported 54 patients with dominantly inherited stomatocytosis in a large Swiss-German family (1918). Apparent heterozygotes (51 of 54 patients) had mild hemolysis, 1% to 25% stomatocytes, moderate numbers of target cells, some crenated cells on their peripheral blood smears (Fig. 51-71C), and no anemia. Intracellular potassium and total monovalent cations were mildly decreased, and fresh red cells were osmotically resistant (Table 51-23). Three probable homozygotes from a consanguineous mating had mild anemia, moderately severe hemolysis, marked stomatocytosis (20% to 35%), and greater cation permeability (1918,1959); however, because net sodium and potassium levels were relatively balanced, cell hydration was not seriously deranged. It is not clear that this syndrome is unique. It may only be an example of hereditary xerocytosis with an unusual proportion of stomatocytes. Genetic mapping could resolve the issue.

CLASSIFICATION BASED ON THE TEMPERATURE DEPENDENCE OF CATION LEAKS

Gordon Stewart and his colleagues have pioneered a classification system of the stomatocytosis-xerocytosis syndromes based on the effects of temperature on passive cation permeability (1932,1934–1937,1982,1983). They measure the residual influx of $^{86}Rb^+$ (a convenient radioactive substitute for K^+) across the red cell membrane in the presence of ouabain (to inhibit the Na^+,K^+ pump) and bumetanide (to inhibit the $Na^+,K^+,2Cl^-$ cotransporter). This measurement is often taken as a measure of the passive permeability of monovalent cations, although it does not exclude contributions of the Gárdos channel and the K^+Cl^- cotransporter. This is not a significant problem in normal red cells but that may not always be true in pathologic erythrocytes. Nevertheless, this estimate of monovalent cation "leak" is useful in understanding the pathophysiology of these permeability disorders.

The temperature profile of the passive leak varies in each disorder (Fig. 51-74). Normal red cells have a low leak that falls with temperature, reaching a minimum at approximately 10°C (Figs. 51-74 and 51-75). The reason for this minimum is unknown. The capacity of the Na^+,K^+ pump far exceeds the normal leak rate at physiologic temperatures, but pump activity falls sharply below room temperature and approximates the normal leak at 0°C (Fig. 51-75; normal curves). In classic, severe stomatin-deficient stomatocytosis, however, the leak rate, particularly the Na^+ leak, is extremely high at body temperatures

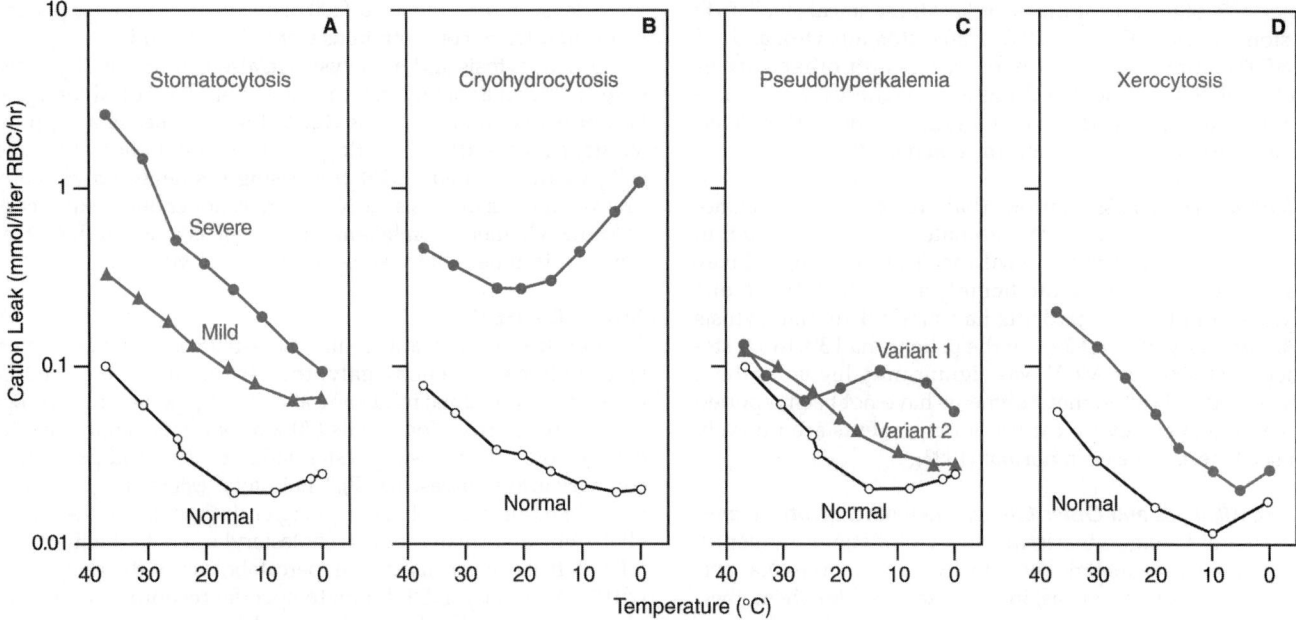

Figure 51-74. Passive permeability of monovalent cations as a function of temperature in the hereditary stomatocytosis-xerocytosis disorders (*solid blue circles* and *triangles*) compared to normals (*open black circles*). Stomatocytosis (1943,1982) (**A**), cryohydrocytosis (1937) (**B**), pseudohyperkalemia (1935,1982) (**C**), and xerocytosis (1936) (**D**) are shown. *Passive permeability* is defined as the uptake of $^{86}Rb^+$ in the presence of ouabain (to inhibit the Na^+,K^+-pump) and bumetanide (to inhibit the $Na^+,K^+,2Cl^-$ cotransporter). RBC, red blood cell.

and exceeds the capacity of the Na^+,K^+ pump, which leads to cell swelling and hemolysis. Stomatocytosis patients with a milder leak (1943) are better compensated and have much milder disease (Fig. 51-74A). Patients with cryohydrocytosis have a similar mild to moderate cation leak at body temperatures and mild to moderate hemolysis, but their leak increases dramatically at below-ambient temperatures. It exceeds the capacity of the Na^+,K^+ pump below 10°C to 15°C (Fig. 51-75), which explains why these red cells lyse in the cold.

The temperature profile of monovalent cation leaks in hereditary xerocytosis parallels the normal, but the leak is three- to fourfold greater (Fig. 51-74D). Although this is a relatively small leak, it favors K^+. This is a problem because the Na^+,K^+ pump extrudes three Na^+ ions for every two K^+ ions returned. Hence, the red cell cannot compensate for leaks of K^+_{out} to Na^+_{in} that exceed the normal 2:3 ratio. In fact, the pump exacerbates the loss of intracellular cations and water and probably contributes to the dehydration of xerocytes (794).

Individuals with pseudohyperkalemia typically have a nearly normal cation leak at physiologic temperatures and therefore little or no hemolysis, but the slope of the leak is flatter than normal and sometimes even bulges at below-ambient temperatures (Fig. 51-74C), so that K^+ loss occurs during storage at room temperature or below.

Other Stomatocytic Disorders

ACQUIRED STOMATOCYTOSIS

In normal people, 3% or less of the red cells on peripheral blood smears are stomatocytic (1993–1995), although more stomatocytic forms are evident (up to 10%) if sensitive techniques such as scanning electron microscopy are used (1996). Because stomatocytes may occasionally occur as a drying artifact in limited areas of the smear, care must be taken to examine multiple areas on several smears before diagnosing stomatocytosis. In wet preparations, stomatocytes are bowl shaped (uniconcave). Such

preparations are useful in excluding artifactual stomatocytes, but the presence of bowl-shaped cells cannot be used as proof of stomatocytes because target cells are also bowl shaped in solution (1867).

In a prospective study of 4291 peripheral blood smears, Davidson and co-workers found increased numbers of stomato-

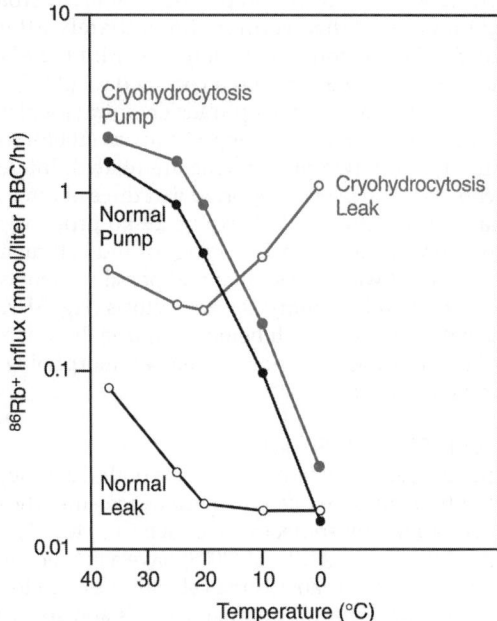

Figure 51-75. Comparison of passive monovalent cation permeabilities (*open circles*) and the capacity of the Na^+,K^+-pump (*solid circles*) in hereditary cryohydrocytosis (*blue circles*) and normals (*black circles*) (1937). Note that the rate of cation leak exceeds the pump rate in cryohydrocytes at low temperatures, causing the cells to swell and hemolyze. RBC, red blood cell.

cytes in 2.3% of the preparations (59% of these smears had 5% to 20% stomatocytes, 35% had 20% to 50% stomatocytes, and 6% had >50% stomatocytes) (1995). In this and other studies (1911,1917,1997), a variety of drugs and diagnoses were associated with stomatocytosis. Further studies are needed to determine which associations are specific and repeatable.

Alcoholism. Two associations that are specific are alcohol and vinca alkaloids. Acquired stomatocytosis is common in alcoholics, particularly in those with acute alcoholism, and may be associated with moderate hemolysis (1993,1994). In one study, 15% of alcoholic patients had marked stomatocytosis (≥10% stomatocytes), and 29% of the patients had 3% to 9% stomatocytes (1998). The MCV was significantly higher in these patients. Red cell cation measurements have not been reported to date; however, severe cation derangements are unlikely because OF tests have been normal (1993).

Vinca Alkaloids and Other Cancer Chemotherapeutic Agents.
Vinca alkaloids (e.g., vincristine and vinblastine) frequently induce hemolysis, sometimes with increased membrane Na^+ permeability and stomatocytosis, in the doses used for chemotherapy of leukemias and lymphomas (1999). Stomatocytosis is also reported in association with cytosine arabinoside and thioguanine therapy (2000) and with ifosfamide (2001). This is a particular problem in the rare instances in which these drugs must be given to patients with cancer who also have HS. We have seen two such patients, and, in both cases, very severe hemolysis occurred. Presumably, the explanation is that spherocytes and stomatocytes both have a decreased surface to volume ratio. Imposing a stomatocytic stress on HS red cells makes them even more spheroidal and hastens their demise.

Occasionally, patients with myelodysplasia (2002) or dyserythropoiesis (2003) develop stomatocytosis, which may even be the presenting symptom (2002).

Long Distance Runners. Stomatocytes have also been observed transiently on wet preparations of blood from marathon or longer distance runners immediately after a race (2004,2005). The morphologic change is mild (12.8% ± 1.8% after the race vs. 4.3% ± 1.8% on a control day) (2005). Because some marathon runners develop transient intravascular hemolysis after running (march hemoglobinuria) (2006), there is a possibility that the two phenomena are related. Interestingly, some years ago, Banga et al. reported that three of three patients with march hemoglobinuria lacked a 29-kd protein (presumably stomatin) in the band 7.2 region of red cell membranes (2007). The defect was very similar and possibly identical to the defect observed in hereditary stomatocytosis (Fig. 51-73); however, the patients with march hemoglobinuria did not have any significant hemolysis or abnormal red cell morphology under basal conditions (2007).

RH_{NULL} AND RH_{MOD} DISEASES

The Rh(D) antigen and the other antigens of the Rh group (cCeE) are part of two minor red cell membrane proteins whose structures have recently been deciphered (see Chapter 57). Patients who lack all Rh antigens (Rh$_{null}$) (2008) have a moderately severe hemolytic anemia (^{51}Cr-labeled red cell half-life of 10 to 14 days) (2009–2012) characterized by stomatocytosis and spherocytosis. OF is only mildly increased (2000,2012), but ektacytometry shows a significant loss of membrane surface, particularly in denser (and presumably older) cells (2009). Red cell membrane K^+ or Rb^+ (a K^+ analog) permeability is approximately twice normal, which is compatible with a mild xerocytosis syndrome (2009,2013). Indeed, in one patient, a majority of the Rh$_{null}$ cells

were dense and K^+ depleted (2009); however, in another patient, cation and water concentrations were normal (2013).

Stomatocytosis and hemolysis are also features of Rh$_{mod}$ disease, a related anomaly in which the expression of Rh antigens is suppressed but not absent, due to the influence of a suppressor gene (2014–2016). Like Rh$_{null}$, reduced OF indicates the red cells are dehydrated (2016). Surprisingly, splenectomy greatly improved the hemolysis (2016). There is not enough experience to know whether thromboembolic disease is a risk in this situation as it is in hereditary xerocytosis (1936,1961,1981).

TANGIER DISEASE

Tangier disease is an autosomal-recessive condition characterized by hepatosplenomegaly; the virtual absence of HDLs; hypertriglyceridemia; mild corneal clouding; peripheral neuropathy; bone marrow foam cells (70% of patients); characteristic orange-colored, cholesteryl ester–laden tonsils; and premature coronary artery disease (2017). Cholesteryl esters are greatly elevated in tissue macrophages in Tangier disease due to the lack of HDL, which normally returns cholesteryl esters to the liver. The HDL deficiency is caused by hypercatabolism of the lipoprotein (2018). Normally, HDL binds to specific receptors on macrophages, is internalized to load up on cholesteryl esters, and then recycles to the membrane surface. In Tangier disease, the protein is misrouted to macrophage lysosomes and destroyed (2018). Recently, three groups independently discovered that the primary defect is in a gene in the ABC transporter superfamily called ABCA1 (originally ABC1) (2019–2021). This protein mediates the first step in the reverse transport of cholesterol from cells to the liver: the transfer of cellular cholesterol and phospholipids to lipid-poor nascent apolipoproteins, particularly to apolipoprotein A-I, the major protein of HDL. Recent evidence suggests ABCA1 is involved in vesicular budding and transfer of vesicles between the Golgi and the plasma membrane (2022) and promotes transbilayer redistribution of PS to the outer surface of the bilayer and microvesiculation (2023). From the bilayer couple hypothesis (Fig. 51-2), the loss of this activity in Tangier cells should lead to the accumulation of excess PS in the inner leaflet of the bilayer and a tendency for endocytosis and stomatocytosis.

As predicated, Tangier fibroblasts have more than a 50% increase in receptor-mediated endocytosis (2024), and careful hematologic examination of one patient disclosed stomatocytosis, hemolysis (Hb = 8.5 g/dL; reticulocytes = 6% to 9%), and osmotically sensitive red cells with a decreased surface to volume ratio (2025). Membrane cholesterol was low, the cholesterol to phospholipid ratio was decreased, and phospholipid analysis showed high PC and low SM (2025). Red cell monovalent cation fluxes were normal. The low content of cholesterol and SM suggests that membrane lipid raft formation may be disturbed, but this was not examined. Because hematologic data have rarely been reported in Tangier disease, it is difficult to be certain that this patient is not exceptional. However, previous reports of unexplained hemolysis in three patients (2026–2028) suggest that he is not.

MEDITERRANEAN STOMATOCYTOSIS

Over 30 years ago, several groups independently observed that stomatocytosis was remarkably common among Mediterranean immigrants to Australia (1997,2029–2032). Norman and Jackson and Knight (2029,2030) recorded 41 patients within one small private practice, and Ducrou and Kimber (1997) added an additional 20 patients. The typical stomatocytic morphology was associated with mild-moderate hemolytic anemia, normal red cell cations, and normal OF (1997,2030). Many patients also had macrothrombocytopenia (40,000 to 150,000 platelets, 3 μ^3 to 120 μ^3 in size) and slight splenomegaly.

A study of healthy Mediterranean immigrants confirmed the increased incidence of stomatocytosis (36% with more than 5% stomatocytes); however, affected individuals were not anemic (2032). Splenomegaly and macrothrombocytopenia were also common, but they segregated independently of the red cell defect.

The cause of this phenomenon remains a mystery. Indeed, it is not even clear if it still exists, as no further reports have appeared in the past quarter century. There is a general impression that stomatocytosis is not unusually prevalent in Mediterranean countries or in Mediterranean immigrants in other parts of the world, which suggests an environmental influence; however, accurate data concerning the prevalence of stomatocytosis are lacking.

FAMILIAL STOMATOCYTOSIS-HYPERTROPHIC GASTRITIS
Dogs of the Drentse patrijshond breed are reported (2033,2034) with an autosomal-recessive syndrome featuring hemolytic anemia with osmotically fragile, stomatocytic red cells, ataxia, polyneuropathy, progressive liver disease, and hypertrophic gastritis resembling Ménétrier's disease in humans. Studies of membrane cation permeability and stomatin have not been reported but would be of interest.

Other Diseases Associated with Stomatocytosis

Stomatocytosis is also observed in at least some patients with the hemolytic anemia that results from adenosine deaminase overproduction (2035). A curious report of pseudohomozygous hypercholesterolemia in a young girl with marked (50% to 80%) stomatocytosis and megathrombocythemia but no defect in red cell membrane lipids, proteins, or cation transport has also appeared (2036).

Other Causes of Xerocytosis

ADENOSINE TRIPHOSPHATE DEPLETION
When red cell ATP concentrations fall below 5% to 15% of normal, the cells leak cations and become rigid and echinocytic (2037). In plasma or other Ca^{2+}-containing media, a specific K^+ permeability lesion (the Gárdos channel) (732) is superimposed on the unchecked normal leak of Na^+ and K^+ and leads to cation depletion and dehydration. Coincidentally, poorly defined changes occur in membrane skeletal structure (2038,2039).

Presumably, these phenomena are involved in the hemolysis that occurs in inherited defects of glycolysis such as pyruvate kinase deficiency (see Chapter 53). Studies by Nathan (2040), Mentzer (2041), Glader (2042), and their co-workers show that pyruvate kinase–deficient red cells rapidly lose ATP and K^+ and become dehydrated, spiculated, and viscous when incubated *in vitro*, particularly under conditions in which residual mitochondrial production of ATP is curtailed. In splenectomized patients, contracted, crenated red cells are more numerous (1697,2043). These "deflated echinocytes" (2043) are more rigid than normal (2044) and are relatively scarce in unsplenectomized patients (1697,2043), which implies that they are premorbid cells given temporary reprieve by removal of the spleen.

Little is known about the status of membrane proteins in red cells with compromised ATP production. Small amounts of disulfide-linked spectrin complexes and marked diminution of spectrin extractability were detected in a patient with glucose phosphate isomerase deficiency (2045), which suggests that membrane protein damage may be pathologically relevant in these disorders; however, further experience is required to assess this point accurately.

IRREVERSIBLY SICKLED CELLS
ISCs are circulating erythrocytes from patients with sickle cell anemia that retain a sickled shape when oxygenated because of an acquired defect in the membrane skeleton (765). Biochemically, ISCs are deficient in total monovalent cations and water (2046,2047). The mechanism of their formation and the nature of the acquired membrane defects responsible for their abnormal shape, cation content, and surface topography are detailed in Chapter 50.

OTHER MEMBRANE DISORDERS

Oxidant Hemolysis

Oxidant damage is incurred by the red cell membrane in a variety of inherited disorders involving abnormal Hbs or defects in the cell's endogenous system for the detoxification of oxidants. These include sickle cell disease (Chapter 50), thalassemias (Chapter 48), unstable hemoglobinopathies (Chapter 49), G6PD deficiency (Chapter 54), and disorders of glutathione metabolism (Chapter 54). A complete description of the membrane lesions associated with these diseases is beyond the scope of this chapter and, in most instances, is covered in the chapters indicated.

Membrane oxidant damage may also result from encounters with exogenous oxidants, one of the most important of these being copper, as discussed in the following section.

Copper Toxicity and Wilson Disease

ACUTE INTOXICATION
Acute copper-induced hemolysis has been reported in humans after accidental or suicidal ingestion, copper sulfate therapy of burns, and copper contamination of hemodialysis units (2048–2052). It is characterized by flushing, chills, nausea and vomiting, diarrhea, abdominal pain, a metallic taste in the mouth, excessive salivation, headache, weakness, and acute intravascular hemolysis.

WILSON DISEASE
Wilson disease (hepatolenticular degeneration) is an autosomal-recessive disorder of copper metabolism characterized by defective biliary excretion of copper, low plasma ceruloplasmin, and toxic accumulation of copper in liver, erythrocytes, kidneys, corneas, and brain (2053). The toxic consequences include liver disease, varying from cirrhosis to fulminant hepatitis and hepatic failure; hemolysis (2054–2074); Fanconi's renal tubular syndrome; corneal Kayser-Fleischer rings; and a progressive neurologic syndrome (psychiatric symptoms, loss of coordination, dystonic posturing, involuntary movements, and dysarthria).

Primary Defect Is in ATP7B, a Protein Involved in Copper Secretion. The Wilson disease gene (ATP7B) is located on chromosome 13q14.3 and encodes an integral membrane P-type ATPase (2075–2082). More than 100 mutations have been identified, including some in which functional protein is made but is misrouted in the cell (2079,2080). The protein is expressed in hepatocytes where it is located in the *trans*-Golgi network. It transports copper into the post-Golgi secretory pathway for incorporation into ceruloplasmin (see Chapter 46) and excretion into the bile (2081–2083) (reviewed in 2084). This is the only physiologic pathway for copper excretion, so when the protein is missing, copper accumulates in the liver, eventually reaching toxic levels. Hepatocyte death follows, with the release of copper into the plasma, where it accumulates in red cells, causing hemolysis, or in the brain, causing neuropsychiatric symptoms.

Depending on the rate of hepatic damage, the liver disease may range from chronic hepatitis to cirrhosis to fulminant hepatic failure. Often, the liver disease has a metabolic phenotype, in which failure of protein synthesis is out of proportion to other signs of liver disease. The liver disease tends to occur in childhood, and the neuropsychiatric disease tends to occur in adolescents and young adults, but there are many exceptions. The disease has been reported from 3 to 58 years of age (2085,2086).

Hemolytic Anemia Is Common and May Be the Presenting Manifestation. It is important to remember that hemolysis is an early feature of Wilson disease. It is seen in 20% to 50% of patients who present with liver disease (2054,2087) and is the first manifestation in approximately 5% (2055–2059,2066,2067,2073,2086,2088,2088a). Because the disease is treatable and because hemolysis may presage fulminant liver disease by days to years (2057), *the clinician must always consider Wilson disease in children and young to middle-aged adults with Coombs'-negative hemolytic anemia who do not have another clear diagnosis.* Typically, these previously well individuals have chemical evidence of acute hepatocyte damage, mild hepatosplenomegaly, and chemical signs of Wilson disease (low ceruloplasmin concentration, increased erythrocyte and hepatic copper levels, and increased urinary copper excretion) (2053). However, 15% to 20% of patients have a normal ceruloplasmin or a normal urine copper concentration, or both. For unknown reasons, a low serum alkaline phosphatase is often present and can provide a clue to the diagnosis (2070). Kayser-Fleischer rings are diagnostic, if present, but may only be seen on slit lamp examination. Elevated hepatic copper is the gold standard, but the risk of a diagnostic liver biopsy in a patient with severe liver disease and a coagulopathy is often deemed too great.

Hematologic Picture. Jaundice is frequent in patients with Wilson disease and hemolysis and may be extreme. Hemolysis is usually at least partially intravascular, and Hb or hemosiderin may be detected on urine analysis, but gross hemoglobinuria is uncommon. Hemolysis may be acute and fulminant or chronic and may be episodic. Patients with G6PD deficiency are especially susceptible (2067,2089), and the combination may account for some episodes of particularly severe hemolysis. Peripheral blood smears *usually show nonspecific changes in red cell morphology*, but a picture of oxidant hemolysis sometimes occurs. Crenated and contracted cells, spherocytes, schistocytes, and Heinz bodies have all been reported (2068,2088). One patient was even misdiagnosed as thrombotic thrombocytopenic purpura for a time (2066). In patients with concomitant liver disease, spur cells and target cells may also be prominent.

Free Copper Is a Potent Oxidant. As noted above, it is believed that copper accumulates in the liver in Wilson disease until it reaches a toxic level. The resulting hepatocellular necrosis releases stored copper into the bloodstream (2059) where it is rapidly taken up by red cells (2090). "Free" copper (unbound to ceruloplasmin) is detectable in untreated patients with Wilson disease (2091). Serum copper is particularly high in those with hemolysis (2059), and, because ceruloplasmin is usually low, much of the copper must be free. Free copper, like free iron, is capable of generating free radicals and activated forms of oxygen. Hemolysis occurs as a consequence of oxidative damage. The oxidative effects of copper are manifold. *In vitro*, copper inactivates numerous red cell glycolytic and hexose monophosphate shunt enzymes; directly oxidizes nicotinamide adenine dinucleotide phosphate and glutathione; oxidizes and denatures Hb; damages membrane ATPases, fatty acid acylase, and

probably other membrane enzymes; generates lipid peroxides; and cross-links membrane skeletal proteins into disulfide-bonded high-molecular-weight complexes, increasing membrane permeability and rigidity (2056,2092). It should be noted, however, that most of these effects have not been demonstrated at concentrations of copper observed in hemolyzing erythrocytes (150 to 400 µg/100 mL red cells = 2.4×10^{-5} to 6.3×10^{-5} M) (2060,2064). So far, it has not been possible to determine the exact cause of the red cells' demise.

Final Lesson. Hematologists must always keep Wilson disease in mind, particularly in patients with the combination of liver disease (even subtle liver disease) and hemolysis, because life-saving therapy is available and the liver disease can rapidly progress to a fulminant stage if the diagnosis is delayed, with a lethal outcome or, at best, a liver transplant.

REFERENCES

1. Harrison ML, Rathinavelu P, Arese P, et al. Role of band 3 tyrosine phosphorylation in the regulation of erythrocyte glycolysis. *J Biol Chem* 1991;266:4106–4111.
2. Wieth JO, Andersen OS, Brahm J, et al. Chloride-bicarbonate exchange in red blood cells: physiology of transport and chemical modification of binding sites. *Philos Trans R Soc Lond B Biol Sci* 1982;299:383–399.
3. Danielli JF, Davson HA. A contribution to the theory of the permeability of thin films. *J Cell Comp Physiol* 1936;9:89.
4. Singer SJ, Nicolson GL. The fluid mosaic model of the structure of cell membranes. *Science* 1972;175:720–731.
5. Dodge JT, Mitchell C, et al. The preparation and chemical characteristics of hemoglobin free ghosts of human erythrocytes. *Arch Biochem Biophys* 1963;100:119–130.
6. Kant JA, Steck TL. Cation-impermeable inside-out and right-side-out vesicles from human erythrocyte membranes. *Nat New Biol* 1972;240:26–28.
7. Fairbanks G, Steck TL, Wallach DF. Electrophoretic analysis of the major polypeptides of the human erythrocyte membrane. *Biochemistry* 1971;10:2606–2617.
8. Shapiro AL, Vinuela E, Maizel JV. Molecular weight estimation of polypeptide chains by electrophoresis in SDS polyacrylamide gels. *Biochem Biophys Res Commun* 1967;28:815–820.
9. Marchesi VT, Steers E Jr. Selective solubilization of a protein component of the red cell membrane. *Science* 1968;159:203–204.
10. Marchesi VT, Tillack TW, Jackson RL, et al. Chemical characterization and surface orientation of the major glycoprotein of the human erythrocyte membrane. *Proc Natl Acad Sci U S A* 1972;69:1445–1449.
11. Blair L, Bittman R. Cholesterol distribution between the two halves of the lipid bilayer of human erythrocyte ghost membranes. *J Biol Chem* 1978;253:8366-8368.
12. Low MG, Finean JB. Modification of erythrocyte membranes by a purified phosphatidylinositol-specific phospholipase C (Staphylococcus aureus). *Biochem J* 1977;162:235–240.
13. Verkleij AJ, Zwaal RF, Roelofsen B, et al. The asymmetric distribution of phospholipids in the human red cell membrane: a combined study using phospholipase and freeze-etch electron microscopy. *Biochim Biophys Acta* 1973;323:178–193.
14. Ferrell JE Jr, Huestis WH. Phosphoinositide metabolism and the morphology of human erythrocytes. *J Cell Biol* 1984;98:1992–1998.
15. Van Deenen LLM, De Gier J. Lipids of the red blood cell membrane. In: Surgenor DM, ed. *The red blood cell*, 2nd ed. New York: Academic Press, 1974:148.
16. Sweeley CC, Dawson G. Lipids of the erythrocyte. In: Jamieson GA, Greenwalt TJ, eds. *Red cell membrane structure and function*. Philadelphia: JB Lippincott Co, 1969:172.
17. Cooper RA. Lipids of human red cell membranes: normal composition and variability in disease. *Semin Hematol* 1970;7:296–332.
18. Turner JD, Rouser G. Precise quantitative determination of human blood lipids by thin layer and triethylaminoethyl cellulose column chromatography. *Anal Biochem* 1970;38:437–445.
19. Ways P, Hanahan DJ. Characterization and quantification of red cell lipids in normal man. *J Lipid Res* 1964;5:318.
20. Weinstein RS. The morphology of adult red cells. In: Surgenor DM, ed. *The red blood cell*, 2nd ed, vol. 1. New York: Academic Press, 1974:214–269.
21. Cullis PR, Hope MJ. Effects of fusogenic agents on membrane structure of erythrocyte ghosts and the mechanism of membrane fusion. *Nature* 1978;271:672–674.
22. Bergelson LD, Barsukov LI. Topological asymmetry of phospholipids in membranes. *Science* 1977;197:224–230.
23. Etemadi AH. Membrane asymmetry: a survey and critical appraisal of the methodology. Methods for assessing the unequal distribution of lipids. *Biochim Biophys Acta* 1980;604:423–475.
24. Op den Kamp JAF. Lipid asymmetry in membranes. *Annu Rev Biochem* 1979;48:47–71.

25. Devaux PF. Protein involvement in transmembrane lipid asymmetry. *Annu Rev Biophys Biomol Struct* 1992;21:417–439.

26. Devaux PF. Lipid transmembrane asymmetry and flip-flop in biological membranes and in lipid bilayers. *Curr Opin Struct Biol* 1993;3:489–494.

27. Kuypers FA. Phospholipid asymmetry in health and disease. *Curr Opin Hematol* 1998;5:122–131.

28. Bevers EM, Comfurius P, Dekkers DW, et al. Lipid translocation across the plasma membrane of mammalian cells. *Biochim Biophys Acta* 1999;1439:317–330.

29. Daleke DL, Lyles JV. Identification and purification of aminophospholipid flippases. *Biochim Biophys Acta* 2000;1486:108–127.

30. Morrot G, Hervè P, Zachowski A, et al. Aminophospholipid translocase of human erythrocytes: phospholipid substrate specificity and effect of cholesterol. *Biochemistry* 1989;28:3456–3462.

31. Connor J, Schroit AJ. Transbilayer movement of phosphatidylserine in non-human erythrocytes: evidence that the aminophospholipid transporter is a ubiquitous membrane protein. *Biochemistry* 1989;28:9680–9685.

32. Zachowski A, Henry JP, Devaux PF. Control of transmembrane lipid asymmetry in chromaffin granules by an ATP-dependent protein. *Nature* 1989;340:75–76.

33. Connor J, Schroit AJ. Transbilayer movement of phosphatidylserine in erythrocytes: inhibition of transport and preferential labeling of a 31,000-dalton protein by sulfhydryl reactive reagents. *Biochemistry* 1988;27:848–851.

34. Zachowski A, Favre E, Cribier S, et al. Outside-inside translocation of aminophospholipids in the human erythrocyte membrane is mediated by a specific enzyme. *Biochemistry* 1986;25:2585–2590.

35. Williamson P, Kulick A, Zachowski A, et al. Ca2+ induces transbilayer redistribution of all major phospholipids in human erythrocytes. *Biochemistry* 1992;31:6355–6360.

36. Auland ME, Roufogalis BD, Devaux PF, et al. Reconstitution of ATP-dependent aminophospholipid translocation in proteoliposomes. *Proc Natl Acad Sci U S A* 1994;91:10938–10942.

37. Tang X, Halleck MS, Schlegel RA, et al. A novel subfamily of P-type ATPases with aminophospholipid transporting activity. *Science* 1996;272:1495–1497.

38. Siegmund A, Grant A, Angeletti C, et al. Loss of Drs2p does not abolish transfer of fluorescence-labeled phospholipids across the plasma membrane of *Saccharomyces cerevisiae*. *J Biol Chem* 1998;273:34399–34405.

39. Schroit AJ, Madsen J, Ruoho AE. Radioiodinated, photoactivatable phosphatidylcholine and phosphatidylserine transfer properties and differential photoreactive interaction with human erythrocyte membrane proteins. *Biochemistry* 1987;26:1812–1819.

40. Schroit AJ, Bloy C, Connor J, et al. Involvement of Rh blood group polypeptides in the maintenance of aminophospholipid asymmetry. *Biochemistry* 1990;29:10303–10306.

41. Chèrif-Zahar B, Bloy C, Le Van Kim C, et al. Molecular cloning and protein structure of a human blood group Rh polypeptide. *Proc Natl Acad Sci U S A* 1990;87:6243–6247.

42. Walker JE, Saraste M, Runswick J, et al. Distantly related sequences in the alpha and beta subunits of ATP synthase, myosin, kinases, and other ATP-requiring enzymes and a common nucleotide binding fold. *EMBO J* 1982;8:945–951.

43. Dekkers DWC, Comfurius P, Schroit AJ, et al. Transbilayer movement of NBD-labeled phospholipids in red blood cell membranes: outward-directed transport by the multidrug resistance protein 1 (MRP1). *Biochemistry* 1998;37:14833–14837.

44. Kamp D, Haest CWM. Evidence for a role of the multi-drug resistance protein (MRP) in the outward translocation of NBD-phospholipids in the erythrocyte membrane. *Biochim Biophys Acta* 1998;1372:91–101.

45. Connor J, Pak CH, Zwaal RFA, et al. Bidirectional transbilayer movement of phospholipid analogs in human red blood cells. *J Biol Chem* 1992;267:19412–19417.

46. Bitbol M, Devaux PF. Measurement of outward translocation of phospholipids across human erythrocyte membrane. *Proc Natl Acad Sci U S A* 1998;85:6783–6787.

47. Connor J, Gillum K, Schroit AJ. Maintenance of membrane lipid asymmetry in red blood cells and ghosts: effect of divalent cations and serum albumin on the transbilayer distribution of endogenous and NBD-labeled phosphatidylserine. *Biochim Biophys Acta* 1990;1025:82–86.

48. Dekkers DWC, Comfurius P, Schroit AJ, et al. Transbilayer movement of NBD-labeled phospholipids in red blood cell membranes: outward-directed transport by the multidrug resistance protein 1 (MRP1). *Biochemistry* 1998;37:14833–14837.

49. Higgins CF, Gottesman MM. Is the multidrug transporter a flippase? *Trends Biochem Sci* 1992;17:18–21.

50. Smit JJ, Schinkel AH, Oude Elferink RP, et al. Homozygous disruption of the murine mdr2 P-glycoprotein gene leads to a complete absence of phospholipid from bile and to liver disease. *Cell* 1993;75:451–462.

51. Smith AJ, Timmermans-Hereijgers JLPM, Roelofsen B, et al. The human MDR3 P-glycoprotein promotes translocation of phosphatidylcholine through the plasma membrane of fibroblasts from transgenic mice. *FEBS Lett* 1994;354:263–266.

52. van Helvoort A, Smith AJ, Sprong H, et al. MDR1 P-glycoprotein is a lipid translocase of broad specificity, while MDR3 P-glycoprotein specifically translocates phosphatidylcholine. *Cell* 1996;87:507–517.

53. Bezombes C, Maestre N, Laurent G, et al. Restoration of TNFα-induced ceramide generation and apoptosis in resistant human leukemia KG1a cells by the P-glycoprotein blocker PSC833. *FASEB J* 1998;12:101–109.

54. Basse F, Stout JG, Sims PJ, et al. Isolation of an erythrocyte membrane protein that mediates Ca2+-dependent transbilayer movement of phospholipid. *J Biol Chem* 1996;271:17205–17210.

55. Zhou QS, Zhao J, Stout JG, et al. Molecular cloning of human plasma membrane phospholipid scramblase: a protein mediating transbilayer movement of membrane phospholipids. *J Biol Chem* 1997;272:18240–18244.

56. Wiedmer T, Zhou Q, Kwoh DY, et al. Identification of three new members of the phospholipid scramblase gene family. *Biochim Biophys Acta* 2000;1467:244–253.

57. Zhou QS, Sims PJ, Wiedmer T. Identity of a conserved motif in phospholipid scramblase that is required for Ca2+-accelerated transbilayer movement of membrane phospholipids. *Biochemistry* 1998;37:2356–2360.

58. Zhao J, Zhou QS, Wiedmer T, et al. Palmitoylation of phospholipid scramblase is required for normal function in promoting Ca2+-activated transbilayer movement of membrane phospholipids. *Biochemistry* 1998;37:6361–6366.

59. Kasukabe T, Kobayashi H, Kaneko Y, et al. Identity of human normal counterpart (MmTRA1b) of mouse leukemogenesis-associated gene (MmTRA1a) product as plasma membrane scramblase and chromosome mapping of the human MmTRA1b/phospholipid scramblase gene. *Biochem Biophys Res Commun* 1998;249:449–455.

60. Bonnet D, Begard E. Interaction of anilinonaphthyl labeled spectrin with fatty acids and phospholipids: fluorescence study. *Biochem Biophys Res Commun* 1984;120:344–350.

61. Cohen AM, Liu SC, Derick LH, et al. Ultrastructural studies of the interaction of spectrin with phosphatidylserine liposomes. *Blood* 1986;68:920–926.

62. Maksymiw R, Sui SF, Gaub H, et al. Electrostatic coupling of spectrin dimers to phosphatidylserine containing lipid lamellae. *Biochemistry* 1987;26:2983–2990.

63. Mombers C, De Gier J, Demel RA, et al. Spectrin-phospholipid interaction. A monolayer study. *Biochim Biophys Acta* 1980;603:52–62.

64. Bergmann WL, Dressler V, Haest CW, et al. Crosslinking of SH groups in the membrane enhances transbilayer orientation of phospholipids. Evidence for a limited access of phospholipids to the reorientation sites. *Biochim Biophys Acta* 1984;769:390–398.

65. Dressler V, Haest CWM, Plasa G, et al. Stabilizing factors of phospholipid asymmetry in the erythrocyte membrane. *Biochim Biophys Acta* 1984;775:189–196.

66. Franck PFH, Roelofsen B, Op den Kamp JAF. Complete exchange of phosphatidylcholine from intact erythrocytes after protein crosslinking. *Biochim Biophys Acta* 1982;687:105–108.

67. Haest CWM, Plasa G, Kamp D, et al. Spectrin as a stabilizer of the phospholipid asymmetry in the human erythrocyte membrane. *Biochim Biophys Acta* 1978;509:21–32.

68. Calvez JY, Zachowski A, Herrmann A, et al. Asymmetric distribution of phospholipids in spectrin-poor erythrocyte vesicles. *Biochemistry* 1988;27:5666–5670.

69. Kuypers FA, Lubin BH, Yee M, et al. The distribution of erythrocyte phospholipids in hereditary spherocytosis demonstrates a minimal role for erythrocyte spectrin on phospholipid diffusion and asymmetry. *Blood* 1993;81:1051–1057.

70. de Jong K, Larkin SK, Styles L, et al. Characterization of the phosphatidylserine-exposing subpopulation of sickle cells. *Blood* 2001;98:860–867.

71. Blumenfeld N, Zachowski A, Galacteros F, et al. Transmembrane mobility of phospholipids in sickle erythrocytes: effect of deoxygenation on diffusion and asymmetry. *Blood* 1991;77:849–854.

72. Franck PF, Chiu DT, Op den Kamp JAF, et al. Accelerated transbilayer movement of phosphatidylcholine in sickled erythrocytes: a reversible process. *J Biol Chem* 1983;258:8436–8442.

73. Lubin B, Chiu D, Bastacky J, et al. Abnormalities in membrane phospholipid organization in sickled erythrocytes. *J Clin Invest* 1981;67:1643–1649.

74. Platt OS, Falcone JF, Lux SE. Molecular defect in the sickle erythrocyte skeleton. Abnormal spectrin binding to sickle inside-out vesicles. *J Clin Invest* 1985;75:266–271.

75. Schwartz RS, Rybicki AC, Heath RH, et al. Protein 4.1 in sickle erythrocytes. Evidence for oxidative damage. *J Biol Chem* 1987;62:15666–15672.

76. Waugh SM, Willardson BM, Kannan R, et al. Heinz bodies induce clustering of band 3, glycophorin, and ankyrin in sickle cell erythrocytes. *J Clin Invest* 1986;78:1155–1160.

77. Liu SC, Derick LH, Zhai S, et al. Uncoupling of the spectrin based skeleton from the lipid bilayer in sickled red cells. *Science* 1991;252:574–576.

78. Kuypers FA, Yuan J, Lewis RA, et al. Membrane phospholipid asymmetry in human thalassemia. *Blood* 1998;91:3044–3051.

79. Wautier JL, Paton RC, Wautier MP, et al. Increased adhesion of erythrocytes to endothelial cells in diabetes mellitus and its relationship to vascular complications. *N Engl J Med* 1981;305:237–242.

80. Hebbel RP, Yamada O, Moldow CF, et al. Abnormal adherence of sickle erythrocytes to cultured vascular endothelium. Possible mechanism for microvascular occlusion in sickle cell disease. *J Clin Invest* 1980;65:154–160.

81. Hebbel RP, Boogaerts MA, Eaton JW, et al. Erythrocyte adherence to endothelium in sickle-cell anemia. A possible determinant of disease severity. *N Engl J Med* 1980;302:992–995.

82. Mohandas N, Evans E. Adherence of sickle erythrocytes to vascular endothelial cells: requirement for both cell membrane changes and plasma factors. *Blood* 1984;64:282.

83. Bevers EM, Comfurius P, van Rijn JL, et al. Generation of prothrombin-converting activity and the exposure of phosphatidylserine at the outer surface of platelets. *Eur J Biochem* 1982;122:429–436.

84. Chiu D, Lubin B, Roelofsen B, et al. Sickled erythrocytes accelerate clotting in vitro: an effect of abnormal membrane lipid asymmetry. *Blood* 1981;58:398–401.

85. Zwaal RFA, Comfurius P, van Deenen LL, et al. Membrane asymmetry and blood coagulation. *Nature* 1977;268:358–360.

86. Allen TM, Williamson P, Schlegel RA. Phosphatidylserine as a determinant of reticuloendothelial recognition of liposome models of the erythrocyte surface. *Proc Natl Acad Sci U S A* 1988;85:8067–8071.

87. McEvoy L, Williamson P, Schlegel RA. Membrane phospholipid asymmetry as a determinant of erythrocyte recognition by macrophages. *Proc Natl Acad Sci U S A* 1986;83:3311–3315.

88. Tanaka Y, Schroit AJ. Insertion of fluorescent phosphatidylserine into the plasma membrane of red blood cells: recognition by autologous macrophages. *J Biol Chem* 1983;258:11335–11343.

89. Fadok VA, Voelker DR, Campbell PA, et al. Exposure of phosphatidylserine on the surface of apoptotic lymphocytes triggers specific recognition and removal by macrophages. *J Immunol* 1992;148:2207–2216.

90. Verhoven B, Schlegel RA, Williamson P. Mechanisms of phosphatidylserine exposure, a phagocyte recognition signal, on apoptotic T lymphocytes. *J Exp Med* 1995;182:1597–1601.

91. Bratton DL, Fadok VA, Richter DA, et al. Appearance of phosphatidylserine on apoptotic cells requires calcium-mediated nonspecific flip-flop and is enhanced by loss of the aminophospholipid translocase. *J Biol Chem* 1997;272:26159–26165.

92. Devaux PF. Static and dynamic lipid asymmetry in cell membranes. *Biochemistry* 1991;30:1163–1173.

93. Toti F, Satta N, Fressinaud E, et al. Scott syndrome, characterized by impaired transmembrane migration of procoagulant phosphatidylserine and hemorrhagic complications, is an inherited disorder. *Blood* 1996;87:1409–1415.

94. Weiss HJ, Lages B. Family studies in Scott syndrome. *Blood* 1997;90:475–476.

95. Weiss HJ. Scott syndrome: a disorder of platelet coagulant activity. *Semin Hematol* 1994;31:312–319.

96. Zhou Q, Sims PJ, Wiedmer T. Expression of proteins controlling transbilayer movement of plasma membrane phospholipids in the B-lymphocytes from a patient with Scott syndrome. *Blood* 1998;92:1707–1712.

97. Rodgers W, Glaser M. Characterization of lipid domains in erythrocyte membranes. *Proc Natl Acad Sci U S A* 1991;88:1364–1368.

98. Jost PC, Nadakavukaren KK, Griffith OH. Phosphatidyl choline exchange between the boundary lipid and bilayer domains in cytochrome oxidase containing membranes. *Biochemistry* 1977;16:3110–3114.

99. Smith RL, Oldfield E. Dynamic structure of membranes by deuterium NMR. *Science* 1984;225:280–288.

100. Armitage IM, Shapiro DL, Furthmayr H, et al. 31P nuclear magnetic resonance evidence for polyphosphoinositide associated with the hydrophobic segment of glycophorin A. *Biochemistry* 1977;16:1317–1320.

101. Mendelsohn R, Dluhy RA, Crawford T, et al. Interaction of glycophorin with phosphatidylserine: a Fourier transform infrared investigation. *Biochemistry* 1984;23:1498–1504.

102. Ong RL. 31P and 19F NMR studies of glycophorin-reconstituted membranes: preferential interaction of glycophorin with phosphatidylserine. *J Membr Biol* 1984;78:1–7.

103. Yeagle PL, Kelsey D. Phosphorus nuclear magnetic resonance studies of lipid-protein interactions: human erythrocyte glycophorin and phospholipids. *Biochemistry* 1989;28:2210–2215.

104. Boyd D, Beckwith J. The role of charged amino acids in the localization of secreted and membrane proteins. *Cell* 1990;62:1031–1033.

105. Parks GD, Lamb RA. Topology of eukaryotic type II membrane proteins: importance of N-terminal positively charged residues flanking the hydrophobic domain. *Cell* 1991;64:777–787.

106. Yamane K, Akiyama Y, Ito K, et al. A positively charged region is a determinant of the orientation of cytoplasmic membrane proteins in *Escherichia coli*. *J Biol Chem* 1990;265:21166–21171.

107. Simons K, Ikonen E. Functional rafts in cell membranes. *Nature* 1997;387:569–572.

108. Brown DA, London E. Functions of lipid rafts in biological membranes. *Annu Rev Cell Dev Biol* 1998;14:111–136.

109. Samuel BU, Mohandas N, Harrison T, et al. The role of cholesterol and glycosylphosphatidylinositol-anchored proteins of erythrocyte rafts in regulating raft protein content and malaria infection. *J Biol Chem* 2001;276:29319–29329.

110. Salzer U, Prohaska R. Stomatin, flotillin-1, and flotillin-2 are major integral proteins of erythrocyte lipid rafts. *Blood* 2001;97:1141–1143.

111. Salzer U, Hinterdorfer P, Hunger U, et al. Ca⁺⁺-dependent vesicle release from erythrocytes involves stomatin-specific lipid rafts, synexin (annexin VII) and sorcin. *Blood* 2002;99:2569–2577.

112. Lauer S, VanWye J, Harrison T, et al. Vacuolar uptake of host components, and a role for cholesterol and sphingomyelin in malarial infection. *EMBO J* 2000;19:3556–3564.

113. Beck JS. Relations between membrane monolayers in some red cell shape transformations. *J Theor Biol* 1978;75:487–501.

114. Ferrell JE Jr, Lee KJ, Huestis WH. Membrane bilayer balance and erythrocyte shape: a quantitative assessment. *Biochemistry* 1985;24:2849–2857.

115. Sheetz MP, Singer SJ. Biological membranes as bilayer couples: a molecular mechanism of drug erythrocyte interactions. *Proc Natl Acad Sci U S A* 1974;71:4457–4461.

116. Christiansson A, Kuypers FA, Roelofsen B, et al. Lipid molecular shape affects erythrocyte morphology: a study involving replacement of native phosphatidylcholine with different species followed by treatment of cells with sphingomyelinase C or phospholipase A. *J Cell Biol* 1985;101:1455–1462.

117. Isomaa B, Hagerstrand H, Paatero G. Shape transformation induced by amphiphiles in erythrocytes. *Biochim Biophys Acta* 1987;899:93–103.

118. Sheetz MP, Painter RG, Singer SJ, et al. Biological membranes as bilayer couples. III. Compensatory shape changes induced in membranes. *J Cell Biol* 1986;70:193–203.

119. Lange Y, Steck TL. Mechanism of red blood cell acanthocytosis and echinocytosis in vivo. *J Membr Biol* 1984;77:153–159.

120. Brown K, Anderson SM, Young NS. Erythrocyte P antigen: cellular receptor for B19 parvovirus. *Science* 1993;262:114–117.

121. Lange Y, Dolde J, Steck TL. The rate of transmembrane movement of cholesterol in the human erythrocyte. *J Biol Chem* 1981;256:5321–5323.

122. Lange Y, Slayton JM. Interaction of cholesterol and lysophosphatidylcholine in determining red cell shape. *J Lipid Res* 1982;23:1121–1127.

123. Huang CH. A structural model for the cholesterol phosphatidyl choline complexes in bilayer membranes. *Lipids* 1977;12:348–356.

124. Berridge MJ. Inositol trisphosphate and calcium signalling. *Nature* 1993;361:315–325.

125. Cohen CM, Gascard P. Regulation and post-translational modification of the erythrocyte membrane and membrane-skeletal proteins. *Semin Hematol* 1992;29:244–292.

126. Levine YK, Birdsall NJM, Lee AG, et al. ¹³C nuclear magnetic resonance relaxation measurements of synthetic lecithins and the effect of spin labeled lipids. *Biochemistry* 1972;11:1416–1421.

127. McConnell HM, McFarland BG. The flexibility gradient in biological membranes. *Ann N Y Acad Sci* 1972;195:207–217.

128. Barton PG, Gunstone FD. Hydrocarbon chain packing and molecular motion in phospholipid bilayers formed from unsaturated lecithins. *J Biol Chem* 1975;250:4470–4476.

129. Seelig A, Seelig J. Effect of a single cis double bond on the structure of a phospholipid bilayer. *Biochemistry* 1977;16:45–50.

130. Oldfield E, Chapman D. Effects of cholesterol and cholesterol derivatives on hydrocarbon chain mobility in lipids. *Biochem Biophys Res Commun* 1971;43:610.

131. Lee AG, Birdsall NJM, Metcalfe JC, et al. Measurement of fast lateral diffusion of lipids in vesicles and in biological membranes by 3H nuclear magnetic resonance. *Biochemistry* 1973;12:1650–1659.

132. Seigneuret M, Devaux PF. ATP dependent asymmetric distribution of spin labeled phospholipids in the erythrocyte membrane: relation to shape changes. *Proc Natl Acad Sci U S A* 1984;81:3751–3755.

133. Cooper RA, Durocher JR, Leslie MH. Decreased fluidity of red cell membrane lipid in abetalipoproteinemia. *J Clin Invest* 1977;60:115–121.

134. Cooper RA. Abnormalities of cell membrane fluidity in the pathogenesis of disease. *N Engl J Med* 1977;297:371–377.

135. Vanderkooi J, Fischkoff S, Chance B, et al. Fluorescent probe analysis of the lipid architecture of natural and experimental cholesterol rich membranes. *Biochemistry* 1974;13:1589–1595.

136. Devaux P, McConnell HM. Lateral diffusion in spin labeled phosphatidyl choline multilayers. *J Am Chem Soc* 1972;94:4475.

137. Wu ES, Jacobson K, Papahadjopoulos D, et al. Lateral diffusion in phospholipid multilayers measured by fluorescence recovery after photobleaching. *Biochemistry* 1977;16:3836–3841.

138. Koppel DE, Sheetz MP, Schindler M, et al. Matrix control of protein diffusion in biological membranes. *Proc Natl Acad Sci U S A* 1981;78:3576.

139. Reed CF. Incorporation of orthophosphate ³²P into erythrocyte phospholipids in normal subjects and in patients with hereditary spherocytosis. *J Clin Invest* 1968;47:2630–2638.

140. Renooij W, Van Golde LMG. The transposition of molecular classes of phosphatidyl choline across the rat erythrocyte membrane and their exchange between the red cell membrane and plasma lipoproteins. *Biochim Biophys Acta* 1977;470:465–474.

141. Shohet SB. Release of phospholipid fatty acid from human erythrocytes. *J Clin Invest* 1970;49:1668–1678.

142. Norum KR, Gjone E, Glomset JA. Familial lecithin: cholesterol acyltransferase deficiency, including fish eye disease. In: Scriver CS, Beaudet AL, Sly WS, et al., eds. *The metabolic basis of inherited disease*, 6th ed. New York: McGraw-Hill, 1989:1181–1194.

143. Mulder E, Van Deenen LLM. Metabolism of red cell lipids. I. Incorporation in vitro of fatty acids into phospholipids from mature erythrocytes. *Biochim Biophys Acta* 1965;106:106.

144. Oliveria MM, Vaughan M. Incorporation of fatty acids into phospholipids of erythrocyte membranes. *J Lipid Res* 1964;5:156.

145. Shohet SB, Nathan DG, et al. Stages in the incorporation of fatty acids into red blood cells. *J Clin Invest* 1968;47:1096–1108.

146. Renooij W, Van Golde LMG, Zwaal RF, et al. Preferential incorporation of fatty acids at the inside of human erythrocyte membranes. *Biochim Biophys Acta* 1974;363:287–292.

147. Farquhar JW, Ahrens EH Jr. Effects of dietary fats on human erythrocyte fatty acid patterns. *J Clin Invest* 1963;42:675–685.

148. Rubin RW, Milikowski C. Over two hundred polypeptides resolved from the human erythrocyte membrane. *Biochim Biophys Acta* 1978;988:107.

148a. Low TY, Seow TK, Chung MCM. Separation of human erythrocyte membrane associated proteins with one-dimensional and two-dimensional gel electrophoresis followed by identification with matrix-assisted laser desorption/ionization-time of flight mass spectrometry. *Proteomics* 2002;2:1229–1239.

149. Savvides P, Shalev O, John KM, et al. Combined spectrin and ankyrin deficiency is common in autosomal dominant hereditary spherocytosis. *Blood* 1993;82:2953–2960.

150. Hemming NJ, Anstee DJ, Mawby WJ, et al. Localization of the protein 4.1-binding site on human erythrocyte glycophorins C and D. *Biochem J* 1994;299:191–196.

151. Fukuda M. Molecular genetics of the glycophorin A gene cluster. *Semin Hematol* 1993;30:138–151.

152. Pinder JC, Gratzer WB. Structural and dynamic states of actin in the erythrocyte. *J Cell Biol* 1983;96:768–775.

153. Inaba M, Guptka KC, Kuwabara M, et al. Deamidation of human erythrocyte membrane protein 4.1: possible role in aging. *Blood* 1992;79:3355–3361.

154. Peters LL, Weier HU, Walensky LD, et al. Four paralogous protein 4.1 genes map to distinct chromosomes in mouse and human. *Genomics* 1998;54:348–350.

155. Schischmanoff PO, Yaswen P, Parra MK, et al. Cell shape-dependent regulation of protein 4.1 alternative pre-mRNA splicing in mammary epithelial cells. *J Biol Chem* 1997;272:10254–10259.

156. Baklouti F, Huang SC, Vulliamy TJ, et al. Organization of the human protein 4.1 genomic locus: new insights into the tissue-specific alternative splicing of the pre-mRNA. *Genomics* 1997;39:289–302.

157. Huang JP, Tang CJ, Kou GH, et al. Genomic structure of the locus encoding protein 4.1. Structural basis for complex combinational tissue-specific alternative RNA splicing. *J Biol Chem* 1993;268:3758–3766.

158. Conboy JG. Structure, function, and molecular genetics of erythroid membrane skeletal protein 4.1 in normal and abnormal red blood cells. *Semin Hematol* 1993;30:58–73.

159. Gascard P, Lee G, Coulombel L, et al. Characterization of multiple isoforms of protein 4.1R expressed during erythroid terminal differentiation. *Blood* 1998;92:4404.

160. Azim AC, Knoll JH, Beggs AH, et al. Isoform cloning, actin binding, and chromosomal localization of human erythroid dematin, a member of the villin superfamily. *J Biol Chem* 1995;270:17407–17413.

161. Azim AC, Marfatia SM, Korsgren C, et al. Human erythrocyte dematin and protein 4.2 (pallidin) are ATP binding proteins. *Biochemistry* 1996;35:3001–3006.

162. Sung LA, Gao KM, Yee LJ, et al. Tropomyosin isoform 5b is expressed in human erythrocytes: implications of tropomodulin-TM5 or tropomodulin-TM5b complexes in the protofilament and hexagonal organization of membrane skeletons. *Blood* 2000;95:1473–1480.

163. Cartron JP, Le Van Kim C, Colin Y. Glycophorin C and related glycoproteins: structure, function, and regulation. *Semin Hematol* 1993;30:152–168.

164. Agre P, Orringer EP, Bennett V. Deficient red-cell spectrin in severe, recessively inherited spherocytosis. *N Engl J Med* 1982;306:1155–1161.

165. Dodge JT, Mitchell C, et al. The preparation and chemical characteristics of hemoglobin-free ghosts of human erythrocytes. *Arch Biochem Biophys* 1963; 100:119.

166. Sheetz MP. Integral membrane protein interaction with Triton cytoskeletons of erythrocytes. *Biochim Biophys Acta* 1979;557:122.

167. Yu J, Fischman DA, Steck TL. Selective solubilization of proteins and phospholipids from red blood cell membranes by nonionic detergents. *J Supramol Struct* 1973;1:233.

168. Showe LC, Ballantine M, Huebner K. Localization of the gene for the erythroid anion exchange protein, band 3 (EMPB3), to human chromosome 17. *Genomics* 1987;1:71–76.

169. Lux SE, John KM, Kopito RR, et al. Cloning and characterization of band 3, the human erythrocyte anion-exchange protein (AE1). *Proc Natl Acad Sci U S A* 1989;86:9089–9093.

170. Tanner MJ, Martin PG, High S. The complete amino acid sequence of the human erythrocyte membrane anion-transport protein deduced from the cDNA sequence. *Biochem J* 1988;256:703–712.

171. Landolt-Marticorena C, Charuk JH, Reithmeier RA. Two glycoprotein populations of band 3 dimers are present in human erythrocytes. *Mol Membr Biol* 1998;15:153–158.

171a. Sterling D, Alvarez BV, Casey JR. The extracellular component of a transport metabolon. Extracellular loop 4 of the human AE1 Cl⁻/HCO₃⁻ exchanger binds carbonic anhydrase IV. *J Biol Chem* 2002;277:25239–25246.

172. Vince JW, Reithmeier RA. Carbonic anhydrase II binds to the carboxyl terminus of human band 3, the erythrocyte C1⁻/HCO3⁻exchanger. *J Biol Chem* 1998;273:28430–28437.

172a. Scozzafava A, Supuran CT. Carbonic anhydrase activators: human isozyme II is strongly activated by oligopeptides incorporating the carboxyterminal sequence of the bicarbonate anion exchanger AE1. *Bioorg Med Chem Lett* 2002;12:1177–1180.

173. Bennett V, Stenbuck PJ. Association between ankyrin and the cytoplasmic domain of band 3 isolated from the human erythrocyte membrane. *J Biol Chem* 1980;255:6424–6432.

174. Low PS. Structure and function of the cytoplasmic domain of band 3: center of erythrocyte membrane-peripheral protein interactions. *Biochim Biophys Acta* 1986;864:145–167.

175. Kliman HJ, Steck TL. Association of glyceraldehyde-3-phosphate dehydrogenase with the human red cell membrane. A kinetic analysis. *J Biol Chem* 1980;255:6314–6321.

176. De B, Kirtley M. Interaction of phosphoglycerate kinase with human erythrocyte membranes. *J Biol Chem* 1977;252:6715.

177. Strapazon E, Steck T. Interaction of aldolase and the membrane of human erythrocytes. *Biochemistry* 1977;16:2966.

178. Murthy SN, Liu T, Kaul RK, et al. The aldolase-binding site of the human erythrocyte membrane is at the NH2 terminus of band 3. *J Biol Chem* 1981; 256:11203–11208.

179. Jenkins J, Madden D, Steck T. Association of phosphofructokinase and aldolase with the membrane of the intact erythrocyte. *J Biol Chem* 1984;259:9374.

180. Tsai IH, Murthy SN, Steck TL. Effect of red cell membrane binding on the catalytic activity of glyceraldehyde-3-phosphate dehydrogenase. *J Biol Chem* 1982;257:1438–1442.

181. Low PS, Allen DP, Zioncheck TF, et al. Tyrosine phosphorylation of band 3 inhibits peripheral protein binding. *J Biol Chem* 1987;262:4592–4596.

182. Low PS, Rathinavelu P, Harrison ML. Regulation of glycolysis via reversible

183. enzyme binding to the membrane protein, band 3. *J Biol Chem* 1993; 268:14627–14631.

183. Chetrite G, Cassoly R. Affinity of hemoglobin for the cytoplasmic fragment of human erythrocyte membrane band 3. Equilibrium measurements at physiological pH using matrix-bound proteins: the effects of ionic strength, deoxygenation and of 2,3-diphosphoglycerate. *J Mol Biol* 1985;185:639–644.

184. Walder JA, Chatterjee R, Steck TL, et al. The interaction of hemoglobin with the cytoplasmic domain of band 3 of the human erythrocyte membrane. *J Biol Chem* 1984;259:10238–10246.

185. Waugh SM, Low PS. Hemichrome binding to band 3: nucleation of Heinz bodies on the erythrocyte membrane. *Biochemistry* 1985;24:34–39.

186. Waugh SM, Walder JA, Low PS. Partial characterization of the copolymerization reaction of erythrocyte membrane band 3 with hemichromes. *Biochemistry* 1987;26:1777–1783.

187. Kannan R, Labotka R, Low PS. Isolation and characterization of the hemichrome-stabilized membrane protein aggregates from sickle erythrocytes. Major site of autologous antibody binding. *J Biol Chem* 1988;263:13766–13773.

188. McPherson RA, Sawyer WH, Tilley L. Rotational diffusion of the erythrocyte integral membrane protein band 3: effect of hemichrome binding. *Biochemistry* 1992;31:512–518.

189. Rettig MP, Low PS, Gimm JA, et al. Evaluation of biochemical changes during in vivo erythrocyte senescence in the dog. *Blood* 1999;93:376–384.

190. Beppu M, Ando K, Kikugawa K. Poly-N-acetyllactosaminyl saccharide chains of band 3 as determinants for anti-band 3 autoantibody binding to senescent and oxidized erythrocytes. *Cell Mol Biol (Noisy-le-grand)* 1996;42:1007–1024.

191. Thevenin BJ, Willardson BM, Low PS. The redox state of cysteines 201 and 317 of the erythrocyte anion exchanger is critical for ankyrin binding. *J Biol Chem* 1989;264:15886–15892.

192. Davis L, Lux S, Bennett V. Mapping the ankyrin-binding site of ankyrin with band 3 in erythrocyte membranes and in lipid vesicles. *J Biol Chem* 1989;264:9665.

193. Willardson BM, Thevenin BJ, Harrison ML, et al. Localization of the ankyrin-binding site on erythrocyte membrane protein, band 3. *J Biol Chem* 1989; 264:15893–15899.

194. Eber SW, Gonzalez JM, Lux ML, et al. Ankyrin-1 mutations are a major cause of dominant and recessive hereditary spherocytosis. *Nat Genet* 1996;13:214–218.

195. Jarolim P, Palek J, Rubin HL, et al. Band 3 Tuscaloosa: Pro327→Arg327 substitution in the cytoplasmic domain of erythrocyte band 3 protein associated with spherocytic hemolytic anemia and partial deficiency of protein 4.2. *Blood* 1992;80:523–529.

196. Jarolim P, Murray JL, Rubin HL, et al. Characterization of 13 novel band 3 gene defects in hereditary spherocytosis with band 3 deficiency. *Blood* 1996;88:4366–4374.

197. Rybicki AC, Qiu JJ, Musto S, et al. Human erythrocyte protein 4.2 deficiency associated with hemolytic anemia and a homozygous 40glutamic acid→lysine substitution in the cytoplasmic domain of band 3 (band 3Montefiore). *Blood* 1993;81:2155–2165.

198. Zhang D, Kiyatkin A, Bolin J, et al. Crystallographic structure and functional interpretation of the cytoplasmic domain of erythrocyte membrane band 3. *Blood* 2000;96:2925–2933.

199. Van Dort HM, Moriyama R, Low PS. Effect of band 3 subunit equilibrium on the kinetics and affinity of ankyrin binding to erythrocyte membrane vesicles. *J Biol Chem* 1998;273:14819–14826.

200. Yi SJ, Liu SC, Derick LH, et al. Red cell membranes of ankyrin-deficient nb/nb mice lack band 3 tetramers but contain normal membrane skeletons. *Biochemistry* 1997;36:9596–9604.

201. Casey JR, Reithmeier RA. Analysis of the oligomeric state of band 3, the anion transport protein of the human erythrocyte membrane, by size exclusion high performance liquid chromatography. Oligomeric stability and origin of heterogeneity. *J Biol Chem* 1991;266:15726–15737.

202. Pasternack GR, Anderson RA, Leto TL, et al. Interactions between protein 4.1 and band 3. An alternative binding site for an element of the membrane skeleton. *J Biol Chem* 1985;260:3676–3683.

203. Lombardo CR, Willardson BM, Low PS. Localization of the protein 4.1-binding site on the cytoplasmic domain of erythrocyte membrane band 3. *J Biol Chem* 1992;267:9540–9546.

204. An XL, Takakuwa Y, Nunomura W, et al. Modulation of band 3-ankyrin interaction by protein 4.1. Functional implications in regulation of erythrocyte membrane mechanical properties. *J Biol Chem* 1996;271:33187–33191.

205. Workman RF, Low PS. Biochemical analysis of potential sites for protein 4.1-mediated anchoring of the spectrin-actin skeleton to the erythrocyte membrane. *J Biol Chem* 1998;273:6171–6176.

206. Rybicki AC, Musto S, Schwartz RS. Identification of a band-3 binding site near the N-terminus of erythrocyte membrane protein 4.2. *Biochem J* 1995;309:677–681.

207. Rybicki AC, Schwartz RS, Qiu JJ, et al. Molecular cloning of mouse erythrocyte protein 4.2: a membrane protein with strong homology with the transglutaminase supergene family. *Mamm Genome* 1994;5:438–445.

208. Rybicki AC, Schwartz RS, Hustedt EJ, et al. Increased rotational mobility and extractability of band 3 from protein 4.2-deficient erythrocyte membranes: evidence of a role for protein 4.2 in strengthening the band 3-cytoskeleton linkage. *Blood* 1996;88:2745–2753.

209. Peters LL, Jindel HK, Gwynn B, et al. Mild spherocytosis and altered red cell ion transport in protein 4.2-null mice. *J Clin Invest* 1999;103:1527–1537.

210. Wieth JO, Anderson OS, Brahm J, et al. Chloride—bicarbonate exchange in red blood cells: physiology of transport and chemical modification of binding sites. *Philos Trans R Soc Lond B Biol Sci* 1982;299:383–399.

211. Fujinaga J, Tang XB, Casey JR. Topology of the membrane domain of human erythrocyte anion exchange protein, AE1. *J Biol Chem* 1999;274:6626–6633.

212. Jennings ML, Smith JS. Anion-proton cotransport through the human red blood cell band 3 protein. Role of glutamate 681. *J Biol Chem* 1992;267:13964–13971.

213. Chernova MN, Jiang L, Crest M, et al. Electrogenic sulfate/chloride exchange in Xenopus oocytes mediated by murine AE1 E699Q. *J Gen Physiol* 1997;109:345–360.

214. Milanick MA, Gunn RB. Proton-sulfate cotransport: external proton activation of sulfate influx into human red blood cells. *Am J Physiol* 1984;247:C247–259.

215. Tang XB, Fujinaga J, Kopito R, et al. Topology of the region surrounding Glu681 of human AE1 protein, the erythrocyte anion exchanger. *J Biol Chem* 1998;273:22545–22553.

216. Tang XB, Kovacs M, Sterling D, et al. Identification of residues lining the translocation pore of human AE1, plasma membrane anion exchange protein. *J Biol Chem* 1999;274:3557–3564.

217. Tanner MJ. Molecular and cellular biology of the erythrocyte anion exchanger (AE1). *Semin Hematol* 1993;30:34.

218. Lindenthal S, Schubert D. Monomeric erythrocyte band 3 protein transports anions. *Proc Natl Acad Sci U S A* 1991;88:6540–6544.

219. Wang DN, Kuhlbrandt W, Sarabia VE, et al. Two-dimensional structure of the membrane domain of human band 3, the anion transport protein of the erythrocyte membrane. *EMBO J* 1993;12:2233–2239.

220. Salhany JM, Schopfer LM. Interactions between mutant and wild-type band 3 subunits in hereditary Southeast Asian ovalocytic red blood cell membranes. *Biochemistry* 1996;35:251–257.

221. Salhany JM. Allosteric effects in stilbenedisulfonate binding to band 3 protein (AE1). *Cell Mol Biol (Noisy-le-grand)* 1996;42:1065–1096.

222. Jennings ML. Structure and function of the red blood cell anion transport protein. *Annu Rev Biophys Biophys Chem* 1989;18:397–430.

223. Fukuda M, Dell A, Oates JE, et al. Structure of branched lactosaminoglycan, the carbohydrate moiety of band 3 isolated from adult human erythrocytes. *J Biol Chem* 1984;259:8260–8273.

224. Fukuda M, Dell A, Fukuda MN. Structure of fetal lactosaminoglycan. The carbohydrate moiety of band 3 isolated from human umbilical cord erythrocytes. *J Biol Chem* 1984;259:4782–4791.

225. Jay DG. Glycosylation site of band 3, the human erythrocyte anion-exchange protein. *Biochemistry* 1986;25:554–556.

226. Fukuda M, Fukuda MN, et al. Developmental change and genetic defect in the carbohydrate structure of band 3 glycoprotein of human erythrocyte membrane. *J Biol Chem* 1979;254:3700–3703.

227. Bruce LJ, Tanner MJ. Structure-function relationships of band 3 variants. *Cell Mol Biol (Noisy-le-grand)* 1996;42:953–973.

228. Jarolim P, Murray JL, Rubin HL, et al. Blood group antigens Rb(a), Tr(a), and Wd(a) are located in the third ectoplasmic loop of erythroid band 3. *Transfusion* 1997;37:607–615.

229. Jarolim P, Murray JL, Rubin HL, et al. A Thr552→Ile substitution in erythroid band 3 gives rise to the Warrior blood group antigen. *Transfusion* 1997;37:398–405.

230. Zelinski T, Punter F, McManus K, et al. The ELO blood group polymorphism is located in the putative first extracellular loop of human erythrocyte band 3. *Vox Sang* 1998;75:63–65.

231. Zelinski T, McManus K, Punter F, et al. A Gly565→Ala substitution in human band 3 accounts for the Wu blood group polymorphism. *Transfusion* 1998;38:745–748.

232. Zelinski T. Erythrocyte band 3 antigens and the Diego Blood Group System. *Transfus Med Rev* 1998;12:36–45.

233. Jarolim P, Rubin HL, Zakova D, et al. Characterization of seven low incidence blood group antigens carried by erythrocyte band 3 protein. *Blood* 1998;92:4836–4843.

234. Huang CH, Reid ME, Xie SS, et al. Human red blood cell Wright antigens: a genetic and evolutionary perspective on glycophorin A-band 3 interaction. *Blood* 1996;87:3942–3947.

235. Bruce LJ, Ring SM, Anstee DJ, et al. Changes in the blood group Wright antigens are associated with a mutation at amino acid 658 in human erythrocyte band 3: a site of interaction between band 3 and glycophorin A under certain conditions. *Blood* 1995;85:541–547.

236. Poole J, Banks J, Bruce LJ, et al. Glycophorin A mutation Ala65→Pro gives rise to a novel pair of MNS alleles ENEP (MNS39) and HAG (MNS41) and altered Wrb expression: direct evidence for GPA/band 3 interaction necessary for normal Wrb expression. *Transfus Med* 1999;9:167–174.

237. Telen MJ, Chasis JA. Relationship of the human erythrocyte Wrb antigen to an interaction between glycophorin A and band 3. *Blood* 1990;76:842–848.

238. Knowles DW, Chasis JA, Evans EA, et al. Cooperative action between band 3 and glycophorin A in human erythrocytes: immobilization of band 3 induced by antibodies to glycophorin A. *Biophys J* 1994;66:1726–1732.

239. Groves JD, Tanner MJ. Glycophorin A facilitates the expression of human band 3-mediated anion transport in Xenopus oocytes. *J Biol Chem* 1992;267:22163–22170.

240. Tanphaichitr VS, Sumboonnanonda A, Ideguchi H, et al. Novel AE1 mutations in recessive distal renal tubular acidosis. Loss-of-function is rescued by glycophorin A. *J Clin Invest* 1998;102:2173–2179.

241. Hassoun H, Hanada T, Lutchman M, et al. Complete deficiency of glycophorin A in red blood cells from mice with targeted inactivation of the band 3 (AE1) gene. *Blood* 1998;91:2146–2151.

242. Jarolim P, Rubin HL, Brabec V, et al. Mutations of conserved arginines in the membrane domain of erythroid band 3 lead to a decrease in membrane-associated band 3 and to the phenotype of hereditary spherocytosis. *Blood* 1995;85:634–640.

243. Liu SC, Zhai S, Palek J, et al. Molecular defect of the band 3 protein in southeast Asian ovalocytosis. *N Engl J Med* 1990;323:1530–1538.

244. Jarolim P, Palek J, Amato D, et al. Deletion in erythrocyte band 3 gene in malaria-resistant Southeast Asian ovalocytosis. *Proc Natl Acad Sci U S A* 1991;88:11022–11026.

245. Mohandas N, Winardi R, Knowles D, et al. Molecular basis for membrane rigidity of hereditary ovalocytosis. A novel mechanism involving the cytoplasmic domain of band 3. *J Clin Invest* 1992;89:686–692.

246. Karet F, Gainza F, Gyory A, et al. Mutations in the chloride-bicarbonate exchanger gene AE1 cause autosomal dominant but not autosomal recessive distal renal tubular acidosis. *Proc Natl Acad Sci U S A* 1998;96:6337–6342.

247. Jarolim P, Shayakul C, Prabakaran D, et al. Autosomal dominant distal renal tubular acidosis is associated in three families with heterozygosity for the R589H mutation in the AE1 (band 3) Cl$^-$/HCO$_3$$^-$ exchanger. *J Biol Chem* 1998;273:6380–6388.

248. Bruce LJ, Cope DL, Jones GK, et al. Familial distal renal tubular acidosis is associated with mutations in the red cell anion exchanger (Band 3, AE1) gene. *J Clin Invest* 1997;100:1693–1707.

249. Bruce LJ, Tanner MJA. Erythroid band 3 variants and disease. *Baillieres Clin Haematol* 1999;12:637–654.

250. Bruce LJ, Unwin RJ, Wrong O, et al. The association between familial distal renal tubular acidosis and mutations in the red cell anion exchanger (band 3, AE1) gene. *Biochem Cell Biol* 1998;76:723–728.

251. De Franceschi L, Turrini F, del Giudice EM, et al. Decreased band 3 anion transport activity and band 3 clusterization in congenital dyserythropoietic anemia type II. *Exp Hematol* 1998;26:869–873.

252. Iolascon A, D'Agostaro G, Perrotta S, et al. Congenital dyserythropoietic anemia type II: molecular basis and clinical aspects. *Haematologica* 1996;81:543–559.

253. Bruce LJ, Kay MM, Lawrence C, et al. Band 3 HT, a human red-cell variant associated with acanthocytosis and increased anion transport, carries the mutation Pro868→Leu in the membrane domain of band 3. *Biochem J* 1993;293:317–320.

254. Hassoun H, Wang Y, Vassiliadis J, et al. Targeted inactivation of murine band 3 (AE1) gene produces a hypercoagulable state causing widespread thrombosis in vivo. *Blood* 1996;87:1785–1792.

255. Peters LL, Shivdasani RA, Liu SC, et al. Anion exchanger 1 (band 3) is required to prevent erythrocyte membrane surface loss but not to form the membrane skeleton. *Cell* 1996;86:917–927.

256. Demuth DR, Showe LC, Ballantine M, et al. Cloning and structural characterization of a human non-erythroid band 3-like protein. *EMBO J* 1986;5:1205–1214.

257. Alper SL, Kopito RR, Libresco SM, et al. Cloning and characterization of a murine band 3-related cDNA from kidney and from a lymphoid cell line. *J Biol Chem* 1988;263:17092–17099.

258. Kopito RR, Lee BS, Simmons DM, et al. Regulation of intracellular pH by a neuronal homolog of the erythrocyte anion exchanger. *Cell* 1989;59:927–937.

259. Brosius FC, Alper SL, Garcia AM, et al. The major kidney band 3 gene transcript predicts an amino-terminal truncated band 3 polypeptide. *J Biol Chem* 1989;264:7784–7787.

260. Richards SM, Jaconi ME, Vassort G, et al. A spliced variant of AE1 gene encodes a truncated form of band 3 in heart: the predominant anion exchanger in ventricular myocytes. *J Cell Sci* 1999;112:1519–1528.

261. Zhang Y, Chernova MN, Stuart-Tilley AK, et al. The cytoplasmic and transmembrane domains of AE2 both contribute to regulation of anion exchange by pH. *J Biol Chem* 1996;271:5741–5749.

262. Rahuel C, London J, d'Auriol L, et al. Characterization of cDNA clones for human glycophorin A. Use for gene localization and for analysis of normal of glycophorin-A-deficient (Finnish type) genomic DNA. *Eur J Biochem* 1988;172:147–153.

263. Kudo S, Fukuda M. Structural organization of glycophorin A and B genes: glycophorin B gene evolved by homologous recombination at Alu repeat sequences. *Proc Natl Acad Sci U S A* 1989;86:4619–4623.

264. Irimura T, Tsuji T, Tagami S, et al. Structure of a complex-type sugar chain of human glycophorin A. *Biochemistry* 1981;20:560–566.

265. Gahmberg CG, Andersson LC. Role of sialic acid in the mobility of membrane proteins containing O-linked oligosaccharides on polyacrylamide gel electrophoresis in sodium dodecyl sulfate. *Eur J Biochem* 1982;122:581–586.

266. Morrow B, Rubin CS. Biogenesis of glycophorin A in K562 human erythroleukemia cells. *J Biol Chem* 1987;262:13812–13820.

267. Furthmayr H. Structural comparison of glycophorins and immunochemical analysis of genetic variants. *Nature* 1978;271:519–524.

268. Dahr W, Gielen W, et al. Structure of the Ss blood group antigens. I. Isolation of Ss active glycopeptides and differentiation of the antigens by modification of methionine. *Hoppe Seylers Z Physiol Chem* 1980;361:145.

269. Dahr W, Kordowicz M, et al. The amino acid sequence of the Mc-specific major red cell membrane sialoglycoprotein: an intermediate of the blood group M and N active molecules. *Hoppe Seylers Z Physiol Chem* 1981;362:363.

270. Dahr W, Beyreuther K, et al. Amino acid sequence of the blood group M9-specific major human erythrocyte membrane sialoglycoprotein. *Hoppe Seylers Z Physiol Chem* 1981;362:81.

271. Dahr W, Kordowicz M, et al. Structural analysis of the Ss sialoglycoprotein specific for Henshaw blood group from human erythrocyte membranes. *Eur J Biochem* 1984;141:51.

272. Tanner M, Anstee D. The membrane change in En(a-) human erythrocytes. *Biochem J* 1976;153:271.
273. Tanner MJA, Jenkins RE, et al. Abnormal carbohydrate composition of the major penetrating membrane protein of En(a-) human erythrocytes. *Biochem J* 1976;155:701.
274. Gahmberg CG, Myllyla G, Leikola J, et al. Absence of the major sialoglycoprotein in the membrane of human En(a-) erythrocytes and increased glycosylation of band 3. *J Biol Chem* 1976;251:6108–6116.
275. Dahr W, Uhlenbruck G, et al. Studies on the membrane glycoprotein defect of En(a-) erythrocytes, I. Biochemical aspects. *J Immunogenet* 1976;3:329.
276. Tanner MJA, Anstee DJ. A carbohydrate deficient membrane glycoprotein in human erythrocytes of phenotype S-s-. *Biochem J* 1977;165:151.
277. Dahr W, Uhlenbruck G, et al. SDS polyacrylamide gel electrophoretic analysis of the membrane glycoproteins from S-s-U-erythrocytes. *J Immunogenet* 1975;2:249.
278. Huang CH, Johe K, Moulds JJ, et al. δ glycophorin (glycophorin B) gene deletion in two individuals homozygous for the S-s-U-blood group phenotype. *Blood* 1987;70:1830–1835.
279. Tokunaga E, Sasakawa S, et al. Two apparently healthy Japanese individuals of type MkMk have erythrocytes which lack both blood group MN and Ss-active sialoglycoproteins. *J Immunogenet* 1979;6:383.
280. Anstee DJ. The blood group MNSs active sialoglycoproteins. *Semin Hematol* 1981;15:13.
281. Blanchard D, Asseraf A, et al. Miltenberger class I and II erythrocytes carry a variant of glycophorin A. *Biochem J* 1983;213:399.
282. Dahr W, Newman RA, Contreras M, et al. Structures of Miltenberger class I and II specific major human erythrocyte membrane sialoglycoproteins. *Eur J Biochem* 1984;138:259.
283. Dahr W, Beyreuther K, Moulds JJ. Structural analysis of the major human erythrocyte membrane sialoglycoproteins from Miltenberger class VII cells. *Eur J Biochem* 1987;166:27.
284. Dahr W, Vengelen-Tyler V, Dybkjaer E, et al. Structural analysis of glycophorin A from Miltenberger class VIII erythrocytes. *Biol Chem Hoppe Seyler* 1989;370:855.
285. Johe KK, Smith AJ, Blumenfeld OO. Amino acid sequence of MiIII glycophorin: demonstration of δ-α and α-δ junction regions and expression of δ pseudoexon by direct protein sequencing. *J Biol Chem* 1991;266:7256.
286. Johe KK, Vengelen-Tyler V, Leger R, et al. Synthetic peptides homologous to human glycophorins of the Miltenberger complex of variants of MNSs blood group system specify the epitopes for Hil, S JL, Hop, and Mur antisera. *Blood* 1991;78:2456–2461.
287. Mawby WJ, Anstee DJ, et al. Immunochemical evidence for hybrid sialoglycoproteins of human erythrocytes *Nature* 1981;291:161.
288. Tanner MJ, Anstee DJ, et al. A new human erythrocyte variant (Ph) containing an abnormal membrane sialoglycoprotein. *Biochem J* 1980;187:493.
289. Johe KK, Smith AJ, Vengelen-Tyler V, et al. Amino acid sequence of an α-δ glycophorin hybrid: a structure reciprocal to Sta δ-α glycophorin hybrid. *J Biol Chem* 1989;264:17486–17492.
290. Anstee DJ, Mawby WJ, et al. Abnormal blood group Ss active sialoglycoproteins in the membrane of Miltenberger class III, IV, and V erythrocytes. *Biochem J* 1979;183:19.
291. Huang CH, Guizzo ML, Kikuchi M, et al. Molecular genetic analysis of a hybrid gene encoding Sta glycophorin of the human erythrocyte membrane. *Blood* 1989;74:836–843.
292. Blumenfeld OO, Smith AJ, Moulds JJ. Membrane glycophorins of Dantu blood group erythrocytes. *J Biol Chem* 1987;262:11864–11870.
293. Blanchard D, Cartron JP, et al. Pj variant, a new, hybrid MNSs glycoprotein of the human red cell membrane. *Biochem J* 1982;203:419.
294. Huang CH, Blumenfeld OO. Identification of recombination events resulting in three hybrid genes encoding human MiV, MiV(J.L.), and Sta glycophorins. *Blood* 1991;77:1813–1820.
295. Huang CH, Blumenfeld OO. Molecular genetics of human erythrocyte MiIII and MiVI glycophorins. Use of a pseudoexon in construction of two δ-α-δ hybrid genes resulting in antigenic diversification. *J Biol Chem* 1991;266:7248–7255.
296. Huang CH, Blumenfeld OO. Multiple origins of the human glycophorin Sta gene. Identification of hot spots for independent unequal homologous recombinations. *J Biol Chem* 1991;266:23306–23314.
297. Huang CH, Kikuchi M, McCreary J, et al. Gene conversion confined to a direct repeat of the acceptor splice site generates allelic diversity at human glycophorin (GYP) locus. *J Biol Chem* 1992;267:3336–3342.
298. Huang CH, Skov F, Daniels G, et al. Molecular analysis of human glycophorin MiIX gene shows a silent segment transfer and untemplated mutation resulting from gene conversion via sequence repeats. *Blood* 1992;80:2379–2387.
299. Huang CH, Blumenfeld OO. Characterization of a genomic hybrid specifying the human erythrocyte antigen Dantu: dantu gene is duplicated and linked to a δ glycophorin gene deletion. *Proc Natl Acad Sci U S A* 1988;85:9640–9644.
300. Kudo S, Fukuda M. Structural organization of glycophorin A and B genes: glycophorin B gene evolved by homologous recombination at Alu repeat sequences. *Proc Natl Acad Sci U S A* 1989;86:4619–4623.
301. Cartron JP, Blanchard D. Association of human erythrocyte membrane glycoproteins with blood group Cad specificity. *Biochem J* 1982;207:497.
302. Blanchard D, Cartron JP, et al. Primary structure of the oligosaccharide determinant of blood group Cad specificity. *J Biol Chem* 1983;258:7691.
303. Herkt F, Parente JP, et al. Structure determination of oligosaccharides isolated from Cad erythrocyte membranes by permethylation analysis and 500 MHz ¹H NMR spectroscopy. *Eur J Biochem* 1985;146:125.
304. Armitage IM, Shapiro DL, Furthmayr H, et al. ³¹P nuclear magnetic resonance evidence for polyphosphoinositide associated with the hydrophobic segment of glycophorin A. *Biochemistry* 1977;16:1317–1320.
305. Mendelsohn R, Dluhy RA, Crawford T, et al. Interaction of glycophorin with phosphatidylserine: a Fourier transform infrared investigation. *Biochemistry* 1984;23:1498–1504.
306. Smith SO, Bormann BJ. Determination of helix-helix interactions in membranes by rotational resonance NMR. *Proc Natl Acad Sci U S A* 1995;92:488–491.
307. Brosig B, Langosch D. The dimerization motif of the glycophorin A transmembrane segment in membranes: importance of glycine residues. *Protein Sci* 1998;7:1052–1056.
308. MacKenzie KR, Prestegard JH, Engelman DM. A transmembrane helix dimer: structure and implications. *Science* 1997;276:131–133.
309. Chasis JA, Mohandas N, Shohet SB. Erythrocyte membrane rigidity induced by glycophorin A-ligand interaction. Evidence for a ligand-induced association between glycophorin A and skeletal proteins. *J Clin Invest* 1985;75:1919–1926.
310. Chasis JA, Reid ME, Jensen RH, et al. Signal transduction by glycophorin A: role of extracellular and cytoplasmic domains in a modulatable process. *J Cell Biol* 1988;107:1351–1357.
311. Andersson LC, Gahmberg CG, Teerenhovi L, et al. Glycophorin A as a cell surface marker of early erythroid differentiation in acute leukemia. *Int J Cancer* 1979;24:717–720.
312. Langlois RG, Bigbee WL, Kyoizumi S, et al. Evidence for increased somatic cell mutations at the glycophorin A locus in atomic bomb survivors. *Science* 1987;236:445–448.
313. Kyoizumi S, Nakamura N, Hakoda M, et al. Detection of somatic mutations at the glycophorin A locus in erythrocytes of atomic bomb survivors using a single beam flow sorter. *Cancer Res* 1989;49:581–588.
314. Siebert PD, Fukuda M. Molecular cloning of a human glycophorin B cDNA: nucleotide sequence and genomic relationship to glycophorin A. *Proc Natl Acad Sci U S A* 1987;84:6735–6739.
315. Rearden A, Magnet A, Kudo S, et al. Glycophorin B and glycophorin E genes arose from the glycophorin A ancestral gene via two duplications during primate evolution. *J Biol Chem* 1993;268:2260–2267.
316. Dahr W, Beyreuther K, Steinbach H, et al. Structure of the Ss blood group antigens, II: a methionine/threonine polymorphism within the N-terminal sequence of the Ss glycoprotein. *Hoppe Seylers Z Physiol Chem* 1980;361:895–906.
317. Rahuel C, Vinit MA, Lemarchandel V, et al. Erythroid-specific activity of the glycophorin B promoter requires GATA-1 mediated displacement of a repressor. *EMBO J* 1992;11:4095–4102.
318. Camara-Clayette V, Thomas D, Rahuel C, et al. The repressor which binds the -75 GATA motif of the GPB promoter contains Ku70 as the DNA binding subunit. *Nucleic Acids Res* 1999;27:1656–1663.
319. Colin Y, Rahuel C, London J, et al. Isolation of cDNA clones and complete amino acid sequence of human erythrocyte glycophorin C. *J Biol Chem* 1986;261:229–233.
320. Mattei MG, Colin Y, Le Van Kim C, et al. Localization of the gene for human erythrocyte glycophorin C to chromosome 2, q14-q21. *Hum Genet* 1986;74:420–422.
321. Villeval JL, Le Van Kim C, Bettaieb A, et al. Early expression of glycophorin C during normal and leukemic human erythroid differentiation. *Cancer Res* 1989;49:2626–2632.
322. Chasis J, Mohandas N. Red blood cell glycophorins. *Blood* 1992;8:1869.
323. Hemming NJ, Anstee DJ, Staricoff MA, et al. Identification of the membrane attachment sites for protein 4.1 in the human erythrocyte. *J Biol Chem* 1995;270:5360–5366.
324. Marfatia SM, Morais-Cabral JH, Kim AC, et al. The PDZ domain of human erythrocyte p55 mediates its binding to the cytoplasmic carboxyl terminus of glycophorin C. Analysis of the binding interface by in vitro mutagenesis. *J Biol Chem* 1997;272:24191–24197.
325. Le Van Kim C, Colin Y, Mitjavila MT, et al. Structure of the promoter region and tissue specificity of the human glycophorin C gene. *J Biol Chem* 1989;264:20407–20414.
326. Colin Y. Gerbich blood groups and minor glycophorins of human erythrocytes. *Transfus Clin Biol* 1995;2:259–268.
327. Kudo S, Fukuda M. Identification of a novel human glycophorin, glycophorin E, by isolation of genomic clones and complementary DNA clones utilizing polymerase chain reaction. *J Biol Chem* 1990;265:1102–1110.
328. Blumenfeld OO, Huang CH. Molecular genetics of glycophorin MNS variants. *Transfus Clin Biol* 1997;4:357–365.
329. Reid ME, Anstee DJ, Jensen RH, et al. Normal membrane function of abnormal β–related erythrocyte sialoglycoproteins. *Br J Haematol* 1987;67:467–472.
330. Chang S, Reid ME, Conboy J, et al. Molecular characterization of erythrocyte glycophorin C variants. *Blood* 1991;77:644–648.
331. Telen MJ, Le Van Kim C, Guizzo ML, et al. Erythrocyte Webb-type glycophorin C variant lacks N-glycosylation due to an asparagine to serine substitution. *Am J Hematol* 1991;37:51–52.
332. Anstee D, Ridgewell K, Tanner M, et al. Individuals lacking the Gerbich blood-group antigens have alterations in the human erythrocyte membrane sialoglycoproteins β and γ. *Biochem J* 1984;221:97.

333. Telen MJ, Le Van Kim C, Chung A, et al. Molecular basis for elliptocytosis associated with glycophorin C and D deficiency in the Leach phenotype. *Blood* 1991;78:1603–1606.

334. Anstee D, Parsons S, Ridgewell K, et al. Two individuals with elliptocytic red cells apparently lack three minor sialoglycoproteins. *Biochem J* 1984;218:615.

335. Daniels G, Shaw MA, Judson P, et al. A family demonstrating inheritance of the Leach phenotype, a Gerbich-negative phenotype associated with elliptocytosis. *Vox Sang* 1986;50:117.

336. Nash GB, Palmer J, Reid ME. Effects of deficiencies of glycophorins C and D on the physical properties of the red cell. *Br J Haematol* 1990;76:282–287.

337. Reid ME, Chasis JA, Mohandas N. Identification of a functional role for human erythrocyte sialoglycoproteins β and γ (C and D). *Blood* 1987;69:1068–1072.

338. Alloisio N, Dalla Venezia N, Rana A, et al. Evidence that red blood cell protein p55 may participate in the skeleton-membrane linkage that involves protein 4.1 and glycophorin C. *Blood* 1993;82:1323–1327.

339. Dhermy D, Garbarz M, Lecomte MC, et al. Hereditary elliptocytosis: clinical, morphological and biochemical studies of 38 cases. *Nouv Rev Fr Hematol* 1986;28:129–140.

340. Dalla Venezia N, Gilsanz F, Alloisio N, et al. Homozygous 4.1(−) hereditary elliptocytosis associated with a point mutation in the downstream initiation codon of protein 4.1 gene. *J Clin Invest* 1992;90:1713–1717.

341. Baumgartner S, Littleton JT, Broadie K, et al. A Drosophila neurexin is required for septate junction and blood-nerve barrier formation and function. *Cell* 1996;87:1059–1068.

342. Perkins M. Inhibitory effects of erythrocyte membrane proteins on the in vitro invasion of the human malarial parasite (*Plasmodium falciparum*) into its host cell. *J Cell Biol* 1981;90:563–567.

343. Pasvol G, Wainscoat JS, Weatherall DJ. Erythrocytes deficiency in glycophorin resist invasion by the malarial parasite *Plasmodium falciparum*. *Nature* 1982;297:64–66.

344. Dolan SA, Miller LH, Wellems TE. Evidence for a switching mechanism in the invasion of erythrocytes by *Plasmodium falciparum*. *J Clin Invest* 1990;86:618–624.

345. Orlandi PA, Klotz FW, Haynes JD. A malaria invasion receptor, the 175–kilodalton erythrocyte binding antigen of *Plasmodium falciparum* recognizes the terminal Neu5Ac(alpha 2-3)Gal-sequences of glycophorin A. *J Cell Biol* 1992;116:901–909.

346. Dolan SA, Proctor JL, Alling DW, et al. Glycophorin B as an EBA-175 independent *Plasmodium falciparum* receptor of human erythrocytes. *Mol Biochem Parasitol* 1994;64:55–63.

347. Sharma A, Mishra NC, Biswas S. Receptor heterogeneity and invasion on erythrocytes by *Plasmodium falciparum* merozoites in Indian isolates. *Indian J Exp Biol* 1994;32:486–488.

348. Hadley TJ, Klotz FW, Pasvol G, et al. *Falciparum* malaria parasites invade erythrocytes that lack glycophorin A and B (MkMk). Strain differences indicate receptor heterogeneity and two pathways for invasion. *J Clin Invest* 1987;80:1190–1193.

349. Okoye VC, Bennett V. *Plasmodium falciparum* malaria: band 3 as a possible receptor during invasion of human erythrocytes. *Science* 1985;227:169–171.

350. Chishti AH, Palek J, Fisher D, et al. Reduced invasion and growth of *Plasmodium falciparum* into elliptocytic red blood cells with a combined deficiency of protein 4.1, glycophorin C, and p55. *Blood* 1996;87:3462–3469.

351. Wang D, Mentzer WC, Cameron T, et al. Purification of band 7.2b, a 31-kDa integral membrane phosphoprotein absent in hereditary stomatocytosis. *J Biol Chem* 1991;266:17826–17831.

352. Hiebl-Dirschmied CM, Adolf GR, Prohaska R. Isolation and partial characterization of the human erythrocyte band 7 integral membrane protein. *Biochim Biophys Acta* 1991;1065:195–202.

353. Stewart GW, Hepworth-Jones BE, Keen JN, et al. Isolation of cDNA coding for an ubiquitous membrane protein deficient in high Na+, low K+ stomatocytic erythrocytes. *Blood* 1992;79:1593–1601.

354. Hiebl Dirschmied C, Entler B, et al. Cloning and nucleotide sequence of cDNA encoding human erythrocyte band 7 integral membrane protein. *Biochim Biophys Acta* 1991;1090:123.

355. Snyers L, Umlauf E, Prohaska R. Oligomeric nature of the integral membrane protein stomatin. *J Biol Chem* 1998;273:17221–17226.

356. Snyers L, Umlauf E, Prohaska R. Cysteine 29 is the major palmitoylation site on stomatin. *FEBS Lett* 1999;449:101–104.

357. Wang Y, Morrow JS. Identification and characterization of human SLP-2, a novel homologue of stomatin (band 7.2b) present in erythrocytes and other tissues. *J Biol Chem* 2000;275:8062–8071.

358. Gilles F, Glenn M, Goy A, et al. A novel gene STORP (STOmatin-Related Protein) is localized 2 kb upstream of the promyelocytic gene on chromosome 15q22. *Eur J Haematol* 2000;64:104–113.

359. Westberg JA, Entler B, Prohaska R, et al. The gene coding for erythrocyte protein band 7.2b (EPB72) is located in band q34.1 of human chromosome 9. *Cytogenet Cell Genet* 1993;63:241–243.

360. You Z, Gao X, Ho MM, et al. A stomatin-like protein encoded by the slp gene of Rhizobium etli is required for nodulation competitiveness on the common bean. *Microbiology* 1998;144:2619–2627.

361. Huang M, Gu G, Ferguson EL, et al. A stomatin-like protein necessary for mechanosensation in *C. elegans*. *Nature* 1995;378:292–295.

362. Mannsfeldt AG, Carroll P, Stucky CL, et al. Stomatin, a MEC-2 like protein, is expressed by mammalian sensory neurons. *Mol Cell Neurosci* 1999;13:391–404.

363. Sedensky MM, Siefker JM, Morgan PG. Model organisms: new insights into ion channel and transporter function. Stomatin homologues interact in *Caenorhabditis elegans*. *Am J Physiol Cell Physiol* 2001;280:C1340.

364. Goodman MB, Ernstrom GG, Chelur DS, et al. MEC-2 regulates *C. elegans* DEG/ENaC channels needed for mechanosensation. *Nature* 415:1039–1042.

365. Moore RB, Shriver SK. Protein 7.2b of human erythrocyte membranes binds to calpromotin. *Biochem Biophys Res Commun* 1997;232:294–297.

366. Zhang JZ, Hayashi H, Ebina Y, et al. Association of stomatin (band 7.2b) with Glut1 glucose transporter. *Arch Biochem Biophys* 1999;372:173–178.

367. Zhang JZ, Abbud W, Prohaska R, et al. Overexpression of stomatin depresses GLUT-1 glucose transporter activity. *Am J Physiol Cell Physiol* 2001;280:C1277–C1283.

368. Sinard JH, Stewart GW, et al. Stomatin binding to adducin: a novel link between transmembrane transport and the cytoskeleton. *Mol Cell Biol* 1994;5:421a (abst).

369. Schroder E, Littlechild JA, Lebedev AA, et al. Crystal structure of decameric 2-Cys peroxiredoxin from human erythrocytes at 1.7 A resolution. *Structure Fold Des* 2000;8:605–615.

370. Plishker GA, Chevalier D, Seinsoth L, et al. Calcium-activated potassium transport and high molecular weight forms of calpromotin. *J Biol Chem* 1992;267:21839–21843.

371. Moore RB, Mankad MV, Shriver SK, et al. Reconstitution of Ca²⁺-dependent K+ transport in erythrocyte membrane vesicles requires a cytoplasmic protein. *J Biol Chem* 1991;266:18964–18968.

372. Reid ME, Yahalom V. Blood groups and their function. *Baillieres Clin Haematol* 2000;13:485–509.

373. Preston GM, Carroll TP, Guggino WB, et al. Appearance of water channels in *Xenopus* oocytes expressing red cell CHIP28 protein. *Science* 1992;256:385–387.

374. Sui H, Han BG, Lee JK, et al. Structural basis of water specific transport through the AQP1 water channel. *Nature* 2001;414:872–878.

375. King LS, Choi M, Fernandez PC, et al. Defective urinary-concentrating ability due to a complete deficiency of aquaporin-1. *N Engl J Med* 2001;345:175–179.

376. King LS, Nielsen S, Agre P, et al. Decreased pulmonary vascular permeability in aquaporin-1-null humans. *Proc Natl Acad Sci U S A* 2002;99:1059–1063.

377. Ma T, Yang B, Gillespie A, et al. Severely impaired urinary concentrating ability in transgenic mice lacking aquaporin-1 water channels. *J Biol Chem* 1998;273:4296–4299.

378. Avent ND, Reid ME. The Rh blood group system: a review. *Blood* 2000;95:375–387.

379a. Bruce LJ, Ghosh S, King MJ, et al. Absence of CD47 in protein 4.2–deficient hereditary spherocytosis in man: an interaction between the Rh complex and the band 3 complex. *Blood* 2002;100:1878–1885.

379. Haung CH, Liu PZ, Cheng JG. Molecular biology and genetics of Rh blood group system. *Semin Hematol* 2000;37:150–165.

380. Marini AM, Matassi G, Raynal V, et al. The human Rhesus-associated RhAG protein and a kidney homologue promote ammonium transport in yeast. *Nat Genet* 2000;26:341–344.

381. Soupene E, Ramirez RM, Kustu S. Evidence that fungal MEP proteins mediate diffusion of the uncharged species NH3 across the cytoplasmic membrane. *Mol Cell Biol* 2001;21:5733–5741.

382. Ballas SK, Clark MR, Mohandas N, et al. Red cell membrane and cation deficiency in Rh null syndrome. *Blood* 1984;63:1046–1055.

383. Olives B, Neau P, Bailly P, et al. Cloning and functional expression of a urea transporter from human bone marrow cells. *J Biol Chem* 1994;269:31649–31652.

384. Olives B, Mattei MG, Huet M, et al. Kidd blood group and urea transport function of human erythrocytes are carried by the same protein. *J Biol Chem* 1995;270:15607–15610.

385. Macey RI, Yousef LW. Osmotic stability of red cells in renal circulation requires rapid urea transport. *Am J Physiol* 1988;254:C669–C674.

386. Frohlich O, Macey RI, Edwards-Moulds J, et al. Urea transport deficiency in Jk (a-b-) erythrocytes. *Am J Physiol* 1991;260:C778–C783.

387. Ho M, Chelly J, Carter N, et al. Isolation of a gene for McLeod syndrome encodes a novel membrane transport protein. *Cell* 1994;77:869–880.

388. Russo D, Redman C, Lee S. Association of Xk and Kell blood group proteins. *J Biol Chem* 1998;273:13950–13956.

389. Lee S, Zambas E, Green ED, et al. Organization of the gene encoding the human Kell blood group protein. *Blood* 1995;85:1364–1370.

390. Lee S, Lin M, Mele A, et al. Proteolytic processing of big endothelin-3 by the Kell blood group protein. *Blood* 1999;94:1440–1450.

391. Lee S, Russo D, Redman CM. The Kell blood group system: Kell and XK membrane proteins. *Semin Hematol* 2000;37:113–121.

392. Pogo O, Chaudhuri A. The Duffy protein: a malarial and chemokine receptor. *Semin Hematol* 2000;37:122–129.

393. Chaudhuri A, Polyakova J, Zbrzezna V, et al. Cloning of glycoprotein D cDNA, which encodes the major subunit of the Duffy blood group system and the receptor for the Plasmodium vivax malaria parasite. *Proc Natl Acad Sci U S A* 1993;90:10793–10797.

394. Hadley TJ, Peiper SC. From malaria to chemokine receptor: the emerging physiologic role of the Duffy blood group antigen. *Blood* 1997;89:3077–3091.

395. Parsons SF, Mallinson G, Holmes CH, et al. The Lutheran blood group glycoprotein, another member of the immunoglobulin superfamily, is widely expressed in human tissues and is developmentally regulated in human liver. *Proc Natl Acad Sci U S A* 1995;92:5496–5500.

396. Udani M, Zen Q, Cottman M, et al. Basal cell adhesion molecule/Lutheran protein. The receptor critical for sickle cell adhesion to laminin. *J Clin Invest* 1998;101:2550–2558.

397. Bailly P, Hermand P, Callebault I, et al. The LW blood group glycoprotein is homologous to intracellular adhesion molecules. *Proc Natl Acad Sci U S A* 1994;91:5306–5310.

398. Bailly P, Tontti E, Hermand P, et al. The red cell LW blood group glycoprotein is an intracellular adhesion molecule (ICAM-4) which binds to CD11/CD18 leukocyte integrin. *Eur J Immunol* 1995;25:3316–3320.

399. Spring FA, Parsons SF, Ortlepp S, et al. Intracellular adhesion molecule-4 binds α4 β1 and αV integrins through novel integrin-binding mechanisms. *Blood* 2001;98:458–466.

400. Yu J, Fischman D, Steck T. Selective solubilization of proteins and phospholipids from red blood cell membranes by nonionic detergents. *J Supramol Struct* 1973;1:233.

401. Sheetz MP. Integral membrane protein interaction with Triton cytoskeletons of erythrocytes. *Biochim Biophys Acta* 1979;557:122–134.

402. Bennett V, Stenbuck PJ. The membrane attachment protein for spectrin is associated with band 3 in human erythrocyte membranes. *Nature* 1979;280:468–473.

403. Reid ME, Takakuwa Y, Conboy J, et al. Glycophorin C content of human erythrocyte membrane is regulated by protein 4.1. *Blood* 1990;75:2229–2234.

404. Speicher DW, Morrow JS, Knowles WJ, et al. A structural model of human erythrocyte spectrin. Alignment of chemical and functional domains. *J Biol Chem* 1982;257:9093–9101.

405. Dunn MJ, Kemp RB, Maddy AH. The similarity of the two high-molecular-weight polypeptides of erythrocyte spectrin. *Biochem J* 1978;173:197–205.

406. Anderson JM. Structural studies on human spectrin. Comparison of subunits and fragmentation of native spectrin. *J Biol Chem* 1979;254:939–944.

407. Speicher DW, Marchesi VT. Erythrocyte spectrin is comprised of many homologous triple helical segments. *Nature* 1984;311:177–180.

408. Shotton DM, Burke BE, Branton D. The molecular structure of human erythrocyte spectrin. Biophysical and electron microscopic studies. *J Mol Biol* 1979;131:303–329.

409. Winkelmann JC, Forget BG. Erythroid and nonerythroid spectrins. *Blood* 1993;81:3173–3185.

410. Bennett V, Baines AJ. Spectrin and ankyrin based pathways: metazoan inventions for integrating cells into tissues. *Physiol Rev* 2001;81:1353–1392.

411. Huebner K, Palumbo AP, Isobe M, et al. The alpha-spectrin gene is on chromosome 1 in mouse and man. *Proc Natl Acad Sci U S A* 1985;82:3790–3793.

412. Sahr KE, Laurila P, Kotula L, et al. The complete cDNA and polypeptide sequences of human erythroid alpha-spectrin. *J Biol Chem* 1990;265:4434–4443.

413. Leto TL, Fortugno-Erikson D, Barton D, et al. Comparison of nonerythroid alpha-spectrin genes reveals strict homology among diverse species. *Mol Cell Biol* 1988;8:1–9.

414. Winkelmann JC, Leto TL, Watkins PC, et al. Molecular cloning of the cDNA for human erythrocyte beta-spectrin. *Blood* 1988;72:328–334.

415. Winkelmann JC, Chang JG, Tse WT, et al. Full-length sequence of the cDNA for human erythroid beta-spectrin. *J Biol Chem* 1990;265:11827–11832.

416. Gallagher PG, Sabatino DE, Romana M, et al. A human beta-spectrin gene promoter directs high level expression in erythroid but not muscle or neural cells. *J Biol Chem* 1999;274:6062–6073.

417. Winkelmann JC, Costa FF, Linzie BL, et al. Beta spectrin in human skeletal muscle. Tissue-specific differential processing of 3' beta spectrin pre-mRNA generates a beta spectrin isoform with a unique carboxyl terminus. *J Biol Chem* 1990;265:20449–20454.

418. Hu RJ, Watanabe M, Bennett V. Characterization of human brain cDNA encoding the general isoform of beta-spectrin. *J Biol Chem* 1992;267:18715–18722.

419. Stankewich MC, Tse WT, Peters LL, et al. A widely expressed βIII spectrin associated with Golgi and cytoplasmic vesicles. *Proc Natl Acad Sci U S A* 1998;95:14158–14163.

420. Berghs S, Aggujaro D, Dirkx R Jr, et al. βIV spectrin, a new spectrin localized at axon initial segments and nodes of Ranvier in the central and peripheral nervous system. *J Cell Biol* 2000;151:985–1001.

421. Tse WT, Tang J, Jin O, et al. A new spectrin, βIV, has a major truncated isoform that associates with promyelocytic leukemia protein nuclear bodies and nuclear matrix. *J Biol Chem* 2001;276:23974–23985.

422. Stabach PR, Morrow JS. Identification and characterization of βV spectrin, a mammalian ortholog of Drosophila βH spectrin. *J Biol Chem* 2000;275:21385–21395.

423. Parkinson NJ, Olsson CL, Hallows JL, et al. Mutant β-spectrin 4 causes auditory and motor neuropathies in quivering mice. *Nat Genet* 2001;29:61–65.

424. Yan Y, Winograd E, Viel A, et al. Crystal structure of the repetitive segments of spectrin. *Science* 1993;262:2027–2030.

425. Winograd E, Hume D, Branton D. Phasing the conformational unit of spectrin. *Proc Natl Acad Sci U S A* 1991;88:10788–10791.

426. Grum VL, Li D, MacDonald RI, et al. Structures of two repeats of spectrin suggest models of flexibility. *Cell* 1999;98:523–535.

427. Speicher DW, Weglarz L, DeSilva TM. Properties of human red cell spectrin heterodimer (side-to-side) assembly and identification of an essential nucleation site. *J Biol Chem* 1992;267:14775–14782.

428. Viel A, Branton D. Interchain binding at the tail end of the *Drosophila* spectrin molecule. *Proc Natl Acad Sci U S A* 1994;91:10839–10843.

429. Ursitti JA, Kotula L, DeSilva TM, et al. Mapping the human erythrocyte beta-spectrin dimer initiation site using recombinant peptides and correlation of its phasing with the alpha-actinin dimer site. *J Biol Chem* 1996;271:6636–6644.

430. Wilmotte R, Harper SL, Ursitti JA, et al. The exon 46-encoded sequence is essential for stability of human erythroid alpha-spectrin and heterodimer formation. *Blood* 1997;90:4188–4196.

431. Alloisio N, Morle L, Marechal J, et al. Sp alpha V/41: a common spectrin polymorphism at the alpha IV-alpha V domain junction. Relevance to the expression level of hereditary elliptocytosis due to alpha-spectrin variants located in trans. *J Clin Invest* 1991;87:2169–2177.

432. Wilmotte R, Marechal J, Morle L, et al. Low expression allele alpha LELY of red cell spectrin is associated with mutations in exon 40 (alpha V/41 polymorphism) and intron 45 and with partial skipping of exon 46. *J Clin Invest* 1993;91:2091–2096.

433. Morrow JS, Marchesi VT. Self-assembly of spectrin oligomers in vitro: a basis for a dynamic cytoskeleton. *J Cell Biol* 1981;88:463–468.

434. Ungewickell E, Gratzer W. Self-association of human spectrin. A thermodynamic and kinetic study. *Eur J Biochem* 1978;88:379–385.

435. DeSilva TM, Peng KC, Speicher KD, et al. Analysis of human red cell spectrin tetramer (head-to-head) assembly using complementary univalent peptides. *Biochemistry* 1992;31:10872–10878.

436. Tse WT, Lecomte MC, Costa FF, et al. Point mutation in the beta-spectrin gene associated with alpha I/74 hereditary elliptocytosis. Implications for the mechanism of spectrin dimer self-association. *J Clin Invest* 1990;86:909–916.

437. Nicolas G, Pedroni S, Fournier C, et al. Spectrin self-association site: characterization and study of beta-spectrin mutations associated with hereditary elliptocytosis. *Biochem J* 1998;332:81–89.

438. Speicher DW, DeSilva TM, Speicher KD, et al. Location of the human red cell spectrin tetramer binding site and detection of a related "closed" hairpin loop dimer using proteolytic footprinting. *J Biol Chem* 1993;268:4227–4235.

439. Liu SC, Palek J. Spectrin tetramer-dimer equilibrium and the stability of erythrocyte membrane skeletons. *Nature* 1980;285:586–588.

440. Liu SC, Windisch P, Kim S, et al. Oligomeric states of spectrin in normal erythrocyte membranes: biochemical and electron microscopic studies. *Cell* 1984;37:587–594.

441. Ralston G, Dunbar J, White M. The temperature-dependent dissociation of spectrin. *Biochim Biophys Acta* 1977;491:345–348.

442. Ralston GB, Dunbar JC. Salt and temperature-dependent conformation changes in spectrin from human erythrocyte membranes. *Biochim Biophys Acta* 1979;579:20–30.

443. Beaven GH, Jean-Baptiste L, Ungewickell E, et al. An examination of the soluble oligomeric complexes extracted from the red cell membrane and their relation to the membrane cytoskeleton. *Eur J Cell Biol* 1985;36:299–306.

444. Vertessy BG, Steck TL. Elasticity of the human red cell membrane skeleton. Effects of temperature and denaturants. *Biophys J* 1989;55:255–262.

445. McGough AM, Josephs R. On the structure of erythrocyte spectrin in partially expanded membrane skeletons. *Proc Natl Acad Sci U S A* 1990;87:5208–5212.

446. Ursitti JA, Pumplin DW, Wade JB, et al. Ultrastructure of the human erythrocyte cytoskeleton and its attachment to the membrane. *Cell Motil Cytoskeleton* 1991;19:227–243.

446a. Altmann SM, Grünberg RG, Lenne P-F, et al. Pathways and intermediates in forced unfolding of spectrin repeats. *Structure* 2002;10:1085–1096.

447. Ziemnicka-Kotula D, Xu J, Gu H, et al. Identification of a candidate human spectrin Src homology 3 domain-binding protein suggests a general mechanism of association of tyrosine kinases with the spectrin-based membrane skeleton. *J Biol Chem* 1998;273:13681–13692.

448. Le Bonniec S, Deregnaucourt C, Redeker V, et al. Plasmepsin II, an acidic hemoglobinase from the *Plasmodium falciparum* food vacuole, is active at neutral pH on the host erythrocyte membrane skeleton. *J Biol Chem* 1999;274:14218–14223.

449. Rotin D, Bar-Sagi D, O'Brodovich H, et al. An SH3 binding region in the epithelial Na+ channel (alpha rENaC) mediates its localization at the apical membrane. *EMBO J* 1994;13:4440–4450.

450. Wallis CJ, Wenegieme EF, Babitch JA. Characterization of calcium binding to brain spectrin. *J Biol Chem* 1992;267:4333–4337.

451. Dubreuil RR, Brandin E, Reisberg JH, et al. Structure, calmodulin-binding, and calcium-binding properties of recombinant alpha spectrin polypeptides. *J Biol Chem* 1991;266:7189–7193.

452. Noegel A, Witke W, Schleicher M. Calcium-sensitive non-muscle α-actinin contains EF-hand structures and highly conserved regions. *FEBS Lett* 1987;221:391.

453. Waites G, Graham I, Jackson P, et al. Mutually exclusive splicing of calcium-binding domain exons in chick α-actinin. *J Biol Chem* 1992;267:6263.

454. Fishkind DJ, Bonder EM, Begg DA. Isolation and characterization of sea urchin egg spectrin: calcium modulation of the spectrin-actin interaction. *Cell Motil Cytoskeleton* 1987;7:304–314.

455. Coleman TR, Fishkind DJ, Mooseker MS, et al. Functional diversity among spectrin isoforms. *Cell Motil Cytoskeleton* 1989;12:225–247.

456. Kennedy SP, Warren SL, Forget BG, et al. Ankyrin binds to the 15th repetitive unit of erythroid and nonerythroid beta-spectrin. *J Cell Biol* 1991;115:267–277.

457. Bennett V, Stenbuck PJ. Identification and partial purification of ankyrin, the high affinity membrane attachment site for human erythrocyte spectrin. *J Biol Chem* 1979;254:2533–2541.

458. Devarajan P, Scaramuzzino DA, Morrow JS. Ankyrin binds to two distinct cytoplasmic domains of Na,K-ATPase alpha subunit. *Proc Natl Acad Sci U S A* 1994;91:2965–2969.

459. Srinivasan Y, Elmer L, Davis J, et al. Ankyrin and spectrin associate with voltage-dependent sodium channels in brain. *Nature* 1988;333:177–180.

460. Becker PS, Tse WT, Lux SE, et al. Beta spectrin Kissimmee: a spectrin variant associated with autosomal dominant hereditary spherocytosis and defective binding to protein 4.1. *J Clin Invest* 1993;92:612–616.

461. Becker PS, Schwartz MA, Morrow JS, et al. Radiolabel-transfer cross-linking demonstrates that protein 4.1 binds to the N-terminal region of beta spectrin and to actin in binary interactions. *Eur J Biochem* 1990;193:827–836.

462. Cohen CM, Tyler JM, Branton D. Spectrin-actin associations studied by electron microscopy of shadowed preparations. *Cell* 1980;21:875–883.

463. Karinch AM, Zimmer WE, Goodman SR. The identification and sequence of the actin-binding domain of human red blood cell beta-spectrin. *J Biol Chem* 1990;265:11833–11840.

464. Bresnick AR, Warren V, Condeelis J. Identification of a short sequence essential for actin binding by Dictyostelium ABP-120. *J Biol Chem* 1990;265:9236–9240.

465. Ungewickell E, Bennett PM, Calvert R, et al. In vitro formation of a complex between cytoskeletal proteins of the human erythrocyte. *Nature* 1979;280:811–814.

466. Cohen CM, Korsgren C. Band 4.1 causes spectrin-actin gels to become thixiotropic. *Biochem Biophys Res Commun* 1980;97:1429–1435.

467. Fowler V, Taylor DL. Spectrin plus band 4.1 cross-link actin. Regulation by micromolar calcium. *J Cell Biol* 1980;85:361–376.

468. Ohanian V, Wolfe LC, John KM, et al. Analysis of the ternary interaction of the red cell membrane skeletal proteins spectrin, actin, and 4.1. *Biochemistry* 1984;23:4416–4420.

469. Gardner K, Bennett V. Modulation of spectrin-actin assembly by erythrocyte adducin. *Nature* 1987;328:359–362.

470. Kuhlman PA, Hughes CA, Bennett V, et al. A new function for adducin. Calcium/calmodulin-regulated capping of the barbed ends of actin filaments. *J Biol Chem* 1996;271:7986–7991.

471. Li X, Matsuoka Y, Bennett V. Adducin preferentially recruits spectrin to the fast growing ends of actin filaments in a complex requiring the MARCKS-related domain and a newly defined oligomerization domain. *J Biol Chem* 1998;273:19329–19338.

472. Mische SM, Mooseker MS, Morrow JS. Erythrocyte adducin: a calmodulin-regulated actin-bundling protein that stimulates spectrin-actin binding. *J Cell Biol* 1987;105:2837–2845.

473. Li X, Bennett V. Identification of the spectrin subunit and domains required for formation of spectrin/adducin/actin complexes. *J Biol Chem* 1996;271:15695–15702.

474. Macias MJ, Musacchio A, Ponstingl H, et al. Structure of the pleckstrin homology domain from beta-spectrin. *Nature* 1994;369:675–677.

475. Ingley E, Hemmings BA. Pleckstrin homology (PH) domains in signal transduction. *J Cell Biochem* 1994;56:436–443.

476. Wang DS, Miller R, Shaw R, et al. The pleckstrin homology domain of human beta I sigma II spectrin is targeted to the plasma membrane in vivo. *Biochem Biophys Res Commun* 1996;225:420–426.

477. Wang DS, Shaw G. The association of the C-terminal region of beta I sigma II spectrin to brain membranes is mediated by a PH domain, does not require membrane proteins, and coincides with a inositol-1,4,5 triphosphate binding site. *Biochem Biophys Res Commun* 1995;217:608–615.

478. Rameh LE, Arvidsson A, Carraway KL, et al. A comparative analysis of the phosphoinositide binding specificity of pleckstrin homology domains. *J Biol Chem* 1997;272:22059–22066.

479. Godi A, Santone I, Pertile P, et al. ADP ribosylation factor regulates spectrin binding to the Golgi complex. *Proc Natl Acad Sci U S A* 1998;95:8607–8612.

480. Tao M, Conway R, Cheta S. Purification and characterization of a membrane-bound protein kinase from human erythrocytes. *J Biol Chem* 1980;255:2563.

481. Harris HW Jr, Lux SE. Structural characterization of the phosphorylation sites of human erythrocyte spectrin. *J Biol Chem* 1980;255:11512–11520.

482. Shahbakhti F, Gratzer WB. Analysis of the self-association of human red cell spectrin. *Biochemistry* 1986;25:5969–5975.

483. Harris HW Jr, Levin N, Lux SE. Comparison of the phosphorylation of human erythrocyte spectrin in the intact red cell and in various cell-free systems. *J Biol Chem* 1980;255:11521–11525.

484. Anderson JM, Tyler JM. State of spectrin phosphorylation does not affect erythrocyte shape or spectrin binding to erythrocyte membranes. *J Biol Chem* 1980;255:1259–1265.

485. Manno S, Takakuwa Y, Nagao K, et al. Modulation of erythrocyte membrane mechanical function by beta-spectrin phosphorylation and dephosphorylation. *J Biol Chem* 1995;270:5659–5665.

486. Speicher DW, Morrow JS, Knowles WJ, et al. Identification of proteolytically resistant domains of human erythrocyte spectrin. *Proc Natl Acad Sci U S A* 1980;77:5673–5677.

487. Geiduschek JB, Singer SJ. Molecular changes in the membranes of mouse erythroid cells accompanying differentiation. *Cell* 1979;16:149–163.

488. Eisen H, Bach R, Emery R. Induction of spectrin in erythroleukemic cells transformed by Friend virus. *Proc Natl Acad Sci U S A* 1977;74:3898–3902.

489. Hasthorpe S. Quantification of spectrin-containing erythroid precursor cells in normal and perturbed erythropoiesis. *Exp Hematol* 1980;8:1001–1008.

490. Hanspal M, Yoon SH, Yu H, et al. Molecular basis of spectrin and ankyrin deficiencies in severe hereditary spherocytosis: evidence implicating a primary defect of ankyrin. *Blood* 1991;77:165–173.

491. Bodine DM, Birkenmeier CS, Barker JE. Spectrin deficient inherited hemolytic anemias in the mouse: characterization by spectrin synthesis and mRNA activity in reticulocytes. *Cell* 1984;37:721–729.

492. Moon RT, Lazarides E. Beta-spectrin limits alpha-spectrin assembly on membranes following synthesis in a chicken erythroid cell lysate. *Nature* 1983;305:62–65.

493. Woods CM, Lazarides E. Degradation of unassembled alpha- and beta-spectrin by distinct intracellular pathways: regulation of spectrin topogenesis by beta-spectrin degradation. *Cell* 1985;40:959–969.

494. Siman R, Baudry M, Lynch G. Brain fodrin: substrate for calpain I, an endogenous calcium-activated protease. *Proc Natl Acad Sci U S A* 1984;81:3572–3576.

495. Hu RJ, Bennett V. In vitro proteolysis of brain spectrin by calpain I inhibits association of spectrin with ankyrin-independent membrane binding site(s). *J Biol Chem* 1991;266:18200–18205.

496. Bi X, Chen J, Baudry M. Developmental changes in calpain activity, GluR1 receptors and in the effect of kainic acid treatment in rat brain. *Neuroscience* 1997;81:1123–1135.

497. Corsi D, Galluzzi L, Lecomte MC, et al. Identification of alpha-spectrin domains susceptible to ubiquitination. *J Biol Chem* 1997;272:2977–2983.

498. Corsi D, Paiardini M, Crinelli R, et al. Alteration of alpha-spectrin ubiquitination due to age-dependent changes in the erythrocyte membrane. *Eur J Biochem* 1999;261:775–783.

499. Pinder J, Gratzer W. Structural and dynamic states of actin in the erythrocyte. *J Cell Biol* 1983;96:768.

500. Puszkin S, Puszkin E, Maimon J, et al. α-Actinin and tropomyosin interactions with a hybrid complex of erythrocyte-actin and muscle-myosin. *J Biol Chem* 1977;252:5529.

501. Tilney LG, Detmers P. Actin in erythrocyte ghosts and its association with spectrin. Evidence for a nonfilamentous form of these two molecules in situ. *J Cell Biol* 1975;66:508–520.

502. Byers T, Branton D. Visualization of the protein associations in the erythrocyte membrane skeleton. *Proc Natl Acad Sci U S A* 1985;82:6153.

503. Fowler V, Sussman M, Miller P, et al. Tropomodulin is associated with the free (pointed) ends of the thin filaments in rat skeletal muscle. *J Cell Biol* 1993;120:411.

504. Kuhlman P, Hughes C, Bennett V, et al. A new function for adducin: calcium/calmodulin-regulated capping of the barbed ends of actin filaments. *J Biol Chem* 1996;271:7986.

505. Kuhlman PA, Fowler VM. Purification and characterization of an α1β2 isoform of CapZ from human erythrocytes: cytosolic location and inability to bind to Mg2+ ghosts suggest that erythrocyte actin filaments are capped by adducin. *Biochemistry* 1997;36:13461–13472.

506. Picart C, Discher DE. Actin protofilament orientation at the erythrocyte membrane. *Biophys J* 1999;77:865–878.

507. Ohanian V, Gratzer W. Preparation of red-cell-membrane cytoskeletal constituents and characterisation of protein 4.1. *Eur J Biochem* 1984;144:375–379.

508. Correas I, Leto TL, Speicher DW, et al. Identification of the functional site of erythrocyte protein 4.1 involved in spectrin-actin associations. *J Biol Chem* 1986;261:3310–3315.

509. Inaba M, Gupta KC, Kuwabara M, et al. Deamidation of human erythrocyte protein 4.1: possible role in aging. *Blood* 1992;79:3355–3361.

510. Chishti A, Kim A, Marfatia S, et al. The FERM domain: a unique module involved in the linkage of cytoplasmic proteins to the membrane. *Trends Biochem Sci* 1998;23:281.

511. Leto TL, Marchesi VT. A structural model of human erythrocyte protein 4.1. *J Biol Chem* 1984;259:4603–4608.

512. Holt GD, Haltiwanger RS, Torres CR, et al. Erythrocytes contain cytoplasmic glycoproteins: O-linked GlcNAc on band 4.1. *J Biol Chem* 1987;262:14847.

513. Cohen CM, Gascard P. Regulation and post-translational modification of erythrocyte membrane and membrane-skeletal proteins. *Semin Hematol* 1992;29:244–292.

514. Danilov YN, Fennell R, Ling E, et al. Selective modulation of band 4.1 binding to erythrocyte membranes by protein kinase C. *J Biol Chem* 1990;265:2556–2562.

515. Schischmanoff PO, Winardi R, Discher DE, et al. Defining of the minimal domain of protein 4.1 involved in spectrin-actin binding. *J Biol Chem* 1995;270:21243–21250.

516. Discher DE, Winardi R, Schischmanoff PO, et al. Mechanochemistry of protein 4.1's spectrin-actin-binding domain: ternary complex interactions, membrane binding, network integration, structural strengthening. *J Cell Biol* 1995;130:897–907.

516a. Gimm JA, An X, Nunomura W, et al. Functional characterization of spectrin-actin-binding domains in 4.1 family of proteins. *Biochemistry* 2002;41:7275–7282.

517. Morris MB, Lux SE. Characterization of the binary interaction between human erythrocyte protein 4.1 and actin. *Eur J Biochem* 1995;231:644–650.

518. Discher DE, Winardi R, Schischmanoff PO, et al. Mechanochemistry of protein 4.1's spectrin-actin-binding domain: ternary complex interactions, membrane binding, network integration, structural strengthening. *J Cell Biol* 1995;130:897–907.

519. Horne WC, Prinz WC, Tang EK. Identification of two cAMP-dependent phosphorylation sites on erythrocyte protein 4.1. *Biochim Biophys Acta* 1990;1055:87–92.

520. Subrahmanyam G, Bertics PJ, Anderson RA. Phosphorylation of protein 4.1 on tyrosine-418 modulates its function in vitro. *Proc Natl Acad Sci U S A* 1991;88:5222–5226.

521. Tanaka T, Kadowaki K, Lazarides E, et al. Ca2(+)-dependent regulation of the spectrin/actin interaction by calmodulin and protein 4.1. *J Biol Chem* 1991;266:1134–1140.

522. Takakuwa Y, Mohandas N. Modulation of erythrocyte membrane material properties by Ca2+ and calmodulin. Implications for their role in regulation of skeletal protein interactions. *J Clin Invest* 1988;82:394–400.

523. Pasternack GR, Racusen RH. Erythrocyte protein 4.1 binds and regulates myosin. *Proc Natl Acad Sci U S A* 1989;86:9712–9716.

524. Tsukita S, Yoneumura S. ERM proteins: head-to-tail regulation of actin-plasma membrane interaction. *Trends Biochem Sci* 1997;22:53.

525. Scoles DR, Huynh DP, Morcos PA, et al. Neurofibromatosis 2 tumour suppressor schwannomin interacts with beta II-spectrin. *Nat Genet* 1998;18:354–359.

526. La Jeunesse DR, McCartney BM, Fehon RG. Structural analysis of *Drosophila* merlin reveals functional domains important for growth control and subcellular localization. *J Cell Biol* 1998;141:1589.

527. Workman RF, Low PS. Biochemical analysis of potential sites for protein 4.1-mediated anchoring of the spectrin-actin skeleton to the erythrocyte membrane. *J Biol Chem* 1998;11:6171.

528. Marfatia SM, Leu RA, Branton D, et al. Identification of the protein 4.1 binding interface on glycophorin C and p55, a homologue of the Drosophila discs—large tumor suppressor protein. *J Biol Chem* 1995;270:715–719.

529. Nunomura W, Takakuwa Y, Parra M, et al. Regulation of protein 4.1R, p55, and glycophorin C ternary complex in human erythrocyte membrane. *J Biol Chem* 2000;275:24540–24546.

530. Marfatia SM, Cabral JHM, Kim AC, et al. The PDZ domain of human erythrocyte p55 mediates its binding to the cytoplasmic carboxyl terminus of glycophorin C: analysis of binding interface by in vitro mutagenesis. *J Biol Chem* 1997;272:24191–24197.

531. Jons T, Drenckhahn D. Identification of the binding interface involved in linkage of cytoskeletal protein 4.1 to the erythrocyte anion exchanger. *EMBO J* 1992;11:2863–2867.

532. Hemming NJ, Anstee DJ, Staricoff MA, et al. Identification of the membrane attachment sites for protein 4.1 in the human erythrocyte. *J Biol Chem* 1995;270:5360–5366.

533. Paw BH, Zhou Y, Li R, et al. Cloning of the zebrafish *retsina* blood mutation: mutations in erythroid band 3 result in dyserythropoiesis and cytokinesis defects. *Blood* 2000;96[Suppl 1]:440a (abst).

534. Reference deleted.

535. Nunomura W, Takakuwa Y, Tokimitsu R, et al. Regulation of CD44-protein 4.1 interaction by Ca2+ and calmodulin. Implications for modulation of CD44-ankyrin interaction. *J Biol Chem* 1997;272:30322–30328.

536. Nunomura W, Takakuwa Y, Parra M, et al. Ca2+-dependent and Ca2+-independent calmodulin binding sites in erythrocyte protein 4.1. Implications for regulation of protein 4.1 interaction with transmembrane proteins. *J Biol Chem* 2000;275:6360–6367.

537. Han BG, Nunomura W, Takakuwa Y, et al. Protein 4.1R core domain structure and insights into regulation of cytoskeletal organization. *Nat Struct Biol* 2000;7:871–875.

538. Rybicki AC, Heath R, Lubin B, et al. Human erythrocyte protein 4.1 is a phosphatidylserine binding protein. *J Clin Invest* 1988;81:255–260.

539. Gascard P, Cohen CM. Absence of high-affinity band 4.1 binding sites from membranes of glycophorin C- and D-deficient (Leach phenotype) erythrocytes. *Blood* 1994;83:1102–1108.

540. An XL, Takakuwa Y, Manno S, et al. Structure and functional characterization of protein 4.1R-phosphatidylserine interaction. *J Biol Chem* 2001;276:35778–35785.

541. Moriniere M, Ribeiro L, Dalla Venezia N, et al. Elliptocytosis in patients with C-terminal domain mutations of protein 4.1 correlates with encoded messenger RNA levels rather than with alterations in primary protein structure. *Blood* 2000;95:1834–1841.

542. Walensky LD, Gascard P, Fields ME, et al. The 13-kD FK506 binding protein, FKBP13, interacts with a novel homologue of the erythrocyte membrane cytoskeletal protein 4.1. *J Cell Biol* 1998;141:143–153.

543. Huang S, Lichtenauer UD, Pack S, et al. Reassignment of the EPB4.1 gene to 1p36 and assessment of its involvement in neuroblastomas. *Eur J Clin Invest* 2001;31:907–914.

544. Constantinescu E, Heltianu C, Simionescu M. Immunological detection of an analogue of the erythroid protein 4.1 in endothelial cells. *Cell Biol Int Rep* 1986;10:861–868.

545. Davies GE, Cohen CM. Platelets contain proteins immunologically related to red cell spectrin and protein 4.1. *Blood* 1985;65:52–59.

546. Goodman SR, Casoria LA, Coleman DB, et al. Identification and location of brain protein 4.1. *Science* 1984;224:1433–1436.

547. Parra M, Gascard P, Walensky LD, et al. Cloning and characterization of 4.1G (EPB41L2), a new member of the skeletal protein 4.1 (EPB41) gene family. *Genomics* 1998;49:298–306.

548. Walensky LD, Blackshaw S, Liao D, et al. A novel neuron-enriched homolog of the erythrocyte membrane cytoskeletal protein 4.1. *J Neurosci* 1999;19:6457–6467.

549. Parra M, Gascard P, Walensky LD, et al. Molecular and functional characterization of protein 4.1B, a novel member of the protein 4.1 family with high level, focal expression in brain. *J Biol Chem* 2000;275:3247–3255.

550. Shi ZT, Afzal V, Coller B, et al. Protein 4.1R-deficient mice are viable but have erythroid membrane skeleton abnormalities. *J Clin Invest* 1999;103:331–340.

551. Walensky LD, Shi ZT, Blackshaw S, et al. Neurobehavioral deficits in mice lacking the erythrocyte membrane cytoskeletal protein 4.1. *Curr Biol* 1998;8:1269–1272.

552. Baklouti F, Huang SC, Tang TK, et al. Asynchronous regulation of splicing events within protein 4.1 pre-mRNA during erythroid differentiation. *Blood* 1996;87:3934–3941.

553. Chasis JA, Coulombel L, Conboy J, et al. Differentiation-associated switches in protein 4.1 expression. Synthesis of multiple structural isoforms during normal human erythropoiesis. *J Clin Invest* 1993;91:329–338.

554. Gascard P, Nunomura W, Lee G, et al. Deciphering the nuclear import pathway for the cytoskeletal red cell protein 4.1R. *Mol Biol Cell* 1999;10:1783–1798.

555. Conboy J, Mohandas N, Tchernia G, et al. Molecular basis of hereditary elliptocytosis due to protein 4.1 deficiency. *N Engl J Med* 1986;315:680–685.

556. Palek J, Lux SE. Red cell membrane skeletal defects in hereditary and acquired hemolytic anemias. *Semin Hematol* 1983;20:189.

557. Shi ZT, Afzal V, Coller B, et al. Protein 4.1R-deficient mice are viable but have erythroid membrane skeletal abnormalities. *J Clin Invest* 1999;103:331.

558. Tang CJ, Tang TK. The 30-kD domain of protein 4.1 mediates its binding to the carboxyl terminus of pICln, a protein involved in cellular volume regulation. *Blood* 1998;92:1442–1447.

559. Mattagajasingh SN, Huang SC, Hartenstein JS, et al. Characterization of the interaction between protein 4.1R and Z0-2. A possible link between the tight junction and the actin cytoskeleton. *J Biol Chem* 2000;275:30573–30585.

560. Mattagajasingh SN, Huang SC, Hartenstein JS, et al. A nonerythroid isoform of protein 4.1R interacts with the nuclear mitotic apparatus (NuMA) protein. *J Cell Biol* 1999;145:29–43.

561. Compton DA, Cleveland DW. NuMA, a nuclear protein involved in mitosis and nuclear reformation. *Curr Opin Cell Biol* 1994;6:343.

561a. Krauss SW, Heald R, Lee G, et al. Two distinct domains of protein 4.1 critical for assembly of functional nuclei *in vitro*. *J Biol Chem* 2002 (in press).

562. De Carcer G, Lallena MJ, Correas I. Protein 4.1 is a component of the nuclear matrix of mammalian cells. *Biochem J* 1995;312:871–877.

563. Krauss SW, Larabell CA, Lockett S, et al. Structural protein 4.1 in the nucleus of human cells: dynamic rearrangements during cell division. *J Cell Biol* 1997;137:275–289.

564. Krauss SW, Chasis JA, Rogers C, et al. Structural protein 4.1 is located in mammalian centrosomes. *Proc Natl Acad Sci U S A* 1997;94:7297–7302.

565. Kim AC, Van Huffel C, Lutchman M, et al. Radiation hybrid mapping of EPB41L1, a novel protein 4.1 homologue, to human chromosome 20q11.2-q12. *Genomics* 1998;49:165–166.

566. Ye K, Compton DA, Lai MM, et al. Protein 4.1N binding to nuclear mitotic apparatus protein in PC12 cells mediates the antiproliferative actions of nerve growth factor. *J Neurosci* 1999;19:10747.

567. Chishti AH. Function of p55 and its nonerythroid homologues. *Curr Opin Hematol* 1998;5:116–121.

568. Metzenberg AB, Gitschier J. The gene encoding the palmitoylated erythrocyte membrane protein, p55, originates at the CpG island 3' to the factor VIII gene. *Hum Mol Genet* 1992;1:97–101.

569. Ruff P, Speicher DW, Husain-Chishti A. Molecular identification of a major palmitoylated erythrocyte membrane protein containing the src homology 3 motif. *Proc Natl Acad Sci U S A* 1991;88:6595–6599.

570. Kim AC, Metzenberg AB, Sahr KE, et al. Complete genomic organization of the human erythroid p55 gene (MPP1), a membrane-associated guanylate kinase homologue. *Genomics* 1996;31:223–229.

571. Songyang Z, Fanning AS, Fu C, et al. Recognition of unique carboxyl-terminal motifs by distinct PDZ domains. *Science* 1997;275:73–77.

572. Marfatia SM, Leu RA, Branton D, et al. Identification of the protein 4.1 binding interface on glycophorin C and p55, a homologue of the *Drosophila* discs—large tumor suppressor protein. *J Biol Chem* 1995;270:715–719.

573. Marfatia SM, Lue RA, Branton D, et al. In vitro binding studies suggest a membrane-associated complex between erythroid p55, protein 4.1, and glycophorin C. *J Biol Chem* 1994;269:8631–8634.

574. Joshi R, Gilligan DM, Otto E, et al. Primary structure and domain organization of human alpha and beta adducin. *J Cell Biol* 1991;115:665–675.

575. Katagiri T, Ozaki K, Fujiwara T, et al. Cloning, expression and chromosome mapping of adducin-like 70 (ADDL), a human cDNA highly homologous to human erythrocyte adducin. *Cytogenet Cell Genet* 1996;74:90–95.

576. Taylor SA, Snell RG, Buckler A, et al. Cloning of the alpha-adducin gene from the Huntington's disease candidate region of chromosome 4 by exon amplification. *Nat Genet* 1992;2:223–227.

577. Goldberg YP, Lin BY, Andrew SE, et al. Cloning and mapping of the alpha-adducin gene close to D4S95 and assessment of its relationship to Huntington disease. *Hum Mol Genet* 1992;1:669–675.

578. Gilligan DM, Lieman J, Bennett V. Assignment of the human beta-adducin gene (ADD2) to 2p13-p14 by in situ hybridization. *Genomics* 1995;28:610–612.

579. Gilligan DM, Lozovatsky L, Gwynn B, et al. Targeted disruption of the beta adducin gene (Add2) causes red blood cell spherocytosis in mice. *Proc Natl Acad Sci U S A* 1999;96:10717–10722.

580. Hughes CA, Bennett V. Adducin: a physical model with implications for function in assembly of spectrin-actin complexes. *J Biol Chem* 1995;270:18990–18996.

581. Joshi R, Bennett V. Mapping the domain structure of human erythrocyte adducin. *J Biol Chem* 1990;265:13130–13136.

582. Suriyapperuma SP, Lozovatsky L, Ciciotte SL, et al. The mouse adducin gene family: alternative splicing and chromosomal localization. *Mamm Genome* 2000;11:16–23.

583. Lin B, Nasir J, McDonald H, et al. Genomic organization of the human alpha-adducin gene and its alternately spliced isoforms. *Genomics* 1995;25:93–99.

584. Sinard JH, Stewart GW, Stabach PR, et al. Utilization of an 86 bp exon generates a novel adducin isoform (beta 4) lacking the MARCKS homology domain. *Biochim Biophys Acta* 1998;1396:57–66.

585. Gilligan DM, Lozovatsky L, Silberfein A. Organization of the human beta-adducin gene (ADD2). *Genomics* 1997;43:141–148.

586. Matsuoka Y, Hughes CA, Bennett V. Adducin regulation. Definition of the calmodulin-binding domain and sites of phosphorylation by protein kinases A and C. *J Biol Chem* 1996;271:25157–25166.

587. Matsuoka Y, Li X, Bennett V. Adducin is an in vivo substrate for protein kinase C: phosphorylation in the MARCKS-related domain inhibits activity in promoting spectrin-actin complexes and occurs in many cells, including dendritic spines of neurons. *J Cell Biol* 1998;142:485–497.

588. Kimura K, Fukata Y, Matsuoka Y, et al. Regulation of the association of addu-

cin with actin filaments by Rho-associated kinase (Rho-kinase) and myosin phosphatase. *J Biol Chem* 1998;273:5542–5548.

589. Kaiser HW, O'Keefe E, Bennett V. Adducin: Ca⁺⁺-dependent association with sites of cell-cell contact. *J Cell Biol* 1989;109:557–569.

590. Kaiser HW, Ness W, O'Keefe E, et al. Localization of adducin in epidermis. *J Invest Dermatol* 1993;101:783–788.

591. Fowler L, Everitt J, Stevens JL, et al. Redistribution and enhanced protein kinase C-mediated phosphorylation of alpha- and gamma-adducin during renal tumor progression. *Cell Growth Differ* 1998;9:405–413.

592. Bianchi G, Tripodi G, Casari G, et al. Two point mutations within the adducin genes are involved in blood pressure variation. *Proc Natl Acad Sci U S A* 1994;91:3999–4003.

593. Tripodi G, Szpirer C, Reina C, et al. Polymorphism of gamma-adducin gene in genetic hypertension and mapping of the gene to rat chromosome 1q55. *Biochem Biophys Res Commun* 1997;237:685–689.

594. Manunta P, Cusi D, Barlassina C, et al. Alpha-adducin polymorphisms and renal sodium handling in essential hypertensive patients. *Kidney Int* 1998;53:1471–1478.

595. Cusi D, Barlassina C, Azzani T, et al. Polymorphisms of alpha-adducin and salt sensitivity in patients with essential hypertension. *Lancet* 1997;349:1353–1357.

596. Alam S, Liyou N, Davis D, et al. The 460Trp polymorphism of the human alpha-adducin gene is not associated with isolated systolic hypertension in elderly Australian Caucasians. *J Hum Hypertens* 2000;14:199–203.

597. Busch CP, Harris SB, Hanley AJ, et al. The ADD1 G460W polymorphism is not associated with variation in blood pressure in Canadian Oji-Cree. *J Hum Genet* 1999;44:225–229.

598. Wang WY, Adams DJ, Glenn CL, et al. The Gly460Trp variant of alpha-adducin is not associated with hypertension in white Anglo-Australians. *Am J Hypertens* 1999;12:632–636.

599. Ishikawa K, Katsuya T, Sato N, et al. No association between alpha-adducin 460 polymorphism and essential hypertension in a Japanese population. *Am J Hypertens* 1998;11:502–506.

600. Siegel DL, Branton D. Partial purification and characterization of an actin-bundling protein, band 4.9, from human erythrocytes. *J Cell Biol* 1985;100:775.

601. Rana AP, Ruff P, Maalouf GJ, et al. Cloning of human erythroid dematin reveals another member of the villin family. *Proc Natl Acad Sci U S A* 1993;90:6651–6655.

602. Kim AC, Azim AC, Chishti AH. Alternative splicing and structure of the human erythroid dematin gene. *Biochim Biophys Acta* 1998;1398:382–386.

603. Horne WC, Leto TL, Marchesi VT. Differential phosphorylation of multiple sites in protein 4.1 and protein 4.9 by phorbol ester-activated and cyclic AMP-dependent protein kinases. *J Biol Chem* 1985;260:9073–9076.

604. Husain-Chishti A, Levin A, Branton D. Abolition of actin-bundling by phosphorylation of human erythrocyte protein 4.9. *Nature* 1988;334:718–721.

605. Lutchman M, Pack S, Kim AC, et al. Loss of heterozygosity on 8p in prostate cancer implicates a role for dematin in tumor progression. *Cancer Genet Cytogenet* 1999;115:65–69.

606. Khanna R, Chang SH, Andrabi S, et al. Headpiece domain of dematin is required for the stability of the erythrocyte membrane. *Proc Natl Acad Sci U S A* 2002;99:6637–6642.

607. Fowler VM. Regulation of actin filament length in erythrocytes and striated muscle. *Curr Opin Cell Biol* 1996;8:86–96.

608. Fowler VM, Bennett V. Erythrocyte membrane tropomyosin. Purification and properties. *J Biol Chem* 1984;259:5978–5989.

609. Sung LA, Lin JJ. Erythrocyte tropomodulin binds to the N-terminus of hTM5, a tropomyosin isoform encoded by the gamma-tropomyosin gene. *Biochem Biophys Res Commun* 1994;201:627–634.

610. Mak AS, Roseborough G, Baker H. Tropomyosin from human erythrocyte membrane polymerizes poorly but binds F-actin effectively in the presence and absence of spectrin. *Biochim Biophys Acta* 1987;912:157–166.

611. der Terrossian E, Deprette C, Lebbar I, et al. Purification and characterization of erythrocyte caldesmon. Hypothesis for an actin-linked regulation of a contractile activity in the red blood cell membrane. *Eur J Biochem* 1994;219:503–511.

612. Fowler VM. Capping actin filament growth: tropomodulin in muscle and nonmuscle cells. *Soc Gen Physiol Ser* 1997;52:79–89.

613. Sussman MA, Fowler VM. Tropomodulin binding to tropomyosins. Isoform-specific differences in affinity and stoichiometry. *Eur J Biochem* 1992;205:355–362.

614. Sung LA, Fowler VM, Lambert K, et al. Molecular cloning and characterization of human fetal liver tropomodulin. A tropomyosin-binding protein. *J Biol Chem* 1992;267:2616–2621.

615. Wong AJ, Kiehart DP, Pollard TD. Myosin from human erythrocytes. *J Biol Chem* 1985;260:46–49.

616. Fowler VM, Davis JQ, Bennett V. Human erythrocyte myosin: identification and purification. *J Cell Biol* 1985;100:47–55.

617. Matovcik LM, Groschel-Stewart U, Schrier SL. Myosin in adult and neonatal human erythrocyte membranes. *Blood* 1986;67:1668–1674.

618. Colin FC, Schrier SL. Myosin content and distribution in human neonatal erythrocytes are different from adult erythrocytes. *Blood* 1991;78:3052.

619. Lux SE, John KM, Bennett V. Analysis of cDNA for human erythrocyte ankyrin indicates a repeated structure with homology to tissue-differentiation and cell-cycle control proteins. *Nature* 1990;344:36–43.

620. Lambert S, Yu H, Prchal JT, et al. cDNA sequence for human erythrocyte ankyrin. *Proc Natl Acad Sci U S A* 1990;87:1730–1734.

621. Lux SE, Tse WT, Menninger JC, et al. Hereditary spherocytosis associated with deletion of human erythrocyte ankyrin gene on chromosome 8. *Nature* 1990;345:736–739.

622. Gorina S, Pavletich NP. Structure of the p53 tumor suppressor bound to the ankyrin and SH3 domains of 53BP2. *Science* 1996;274:1001–1005.

623. Low PS, Willardson BM, Mohandas N, et al. Contribution of the band 3-ankyrin interaction to erythrocyte membrane mechanical stability. *Blood* 1991;77:1581–1586.

624. Michaely P, Bennett V. The membrane-binding domain of ankyrin contains four independently folded subdomains, each comprised of six ankyrin repeats. *J Biol Chem* 1993;268:22703–22709.

625. Michaely P, Bennett V. The ANK repeats of erythrocyte ankyrin form two distinct but cooperative binding sites for the erythrocyte anion exchanger. *J Biol Chem* 1995;270:22050–22057.

626. Ding Y, Casey JR, Kopito RR. The major kidney AE1 isoform does not bind ankyrin (Ank1) in vitro. An essential role for the 79 NH2-terminal amino acid residues of band 3. *J Biol Chem* 1994;269:32201–32208.

627. Davis L, Lux SE, Bennett V. Mapping the ankyrin-binding site of the human erythrocyte anion exchanger. *J Biol Chem* 1989;264:9665–9672.

628. Ding Y, Kobayashi S, Kopito R. Mapping of ankyrin binding determinants on the erythroid anion exchanger, AE1. *J Biol Chem* 1996;271:22494–22498.

629. Bennett V. Ankyrins: adaptors between diverse plasma membrane proteins and the cytoplasm. *J Biol Chem* 1992;267:8703.

630. Sedgwick SG, Smerdon SJ. The ankyrin repeat: a diversity of interactions on a common structural framework. *Trends Biochem Sci* 1999;24:311–316.

631. Albert S, Despres B, Guilleminot J, et al. The EMB 506 gene encodes a novel ankyrin repeat containing protein that is essential for the normal development of Arabidopsis embryos. *Plant J* 1999;17:169–179.

632. Hamada Y, Kadokawa Y, Okabe M, et al. Mutation in ankyrin repeats of the mouse Notch2 gene induces early embryonic lethality. *Development* 1999;126:3415–3424.

633. Dumont E, Fuchs KP, Bommer G, et al. Neoplastic transformation by Notch is independent of transcriptional activation by RBP-J signalling. *Oncogene* 2000;19:556–561.

634. Shiohara M, Spirin K, Said JW, et al. Alterations of the cyclin-dependent kinase inhibitor p19 (INK4D) is rare in hematopoietic malignancies. *Leukemia* 1996;10:1897–1900.

635. Venkataramani R, Swaminathan K, Marmorstein R. Crystal structure of the CDK4/6 inhibitory protein p18INK4c provides insights into ankyrin-like repeat structure/function and tumor-derived p16INK4 mutations. *Nat Struct Biol* 1998;5:74–81.

636. Baumgartner R, Fernandez-Catalan C, Winoto A, et al. Structure of human cyclin-dependent kinase inhibitor p19INK4d: comparison to known ankyrin-repeat-containing structures and implications for the dysfunction of tumor suppressor p16INK4a. *Structure* 1998;6:1279–1290.

637. Jacobs MD, Harrison SC. Structure of an IκBα/NF-κB complex. *Cell* 1998;95:749–758.

638. Yang Y, Nanduri S, Sen S, et al. The structural basis of ankyrin-like repeat function as revealed by the solution structure of myotrophin. *Structure* 1998;6:619–626.

639. Gallagher PG, Tse WT, Scarpa AL, et al. Structure and organization of the human ankyrin-1 gene. Basis for complexity of pre-mRNA processing. *J Biol Chem* 1997;272:19220–19228.

640. Cianci CD, Giorgi M, Morrow JS. Phosphorylation of ankyrin down-regulates its cooperative interaction with spectrin and protein 3. *J Cell Biochem* 1988;37:301–315.

641. Davis LH, Bennett V. Mapping the binding sites of human erythrocyte ankyrin for the anion exchanger and spectrin. *J Biol Chem* 1990;265:10589–10596.

642. Platt OS, Lux SE, Falcone JF. A highly conserved region of human erythrocyte ankyrin contains the capacity to bind spectrin. *J Biol Chem* 1993;268:24421–24426.

643. Hall TG, Bennett V. Regulatory domains of erythrocyte ankyrin. *J Biol Chem* 1987;262:10537–10545.

644. Davis LH, Davis JQ, Bennett V. Ankyrin regulation: an alternatively spliced segment of the regulatory domain functions as an intramolecular modulator. *J Biol Chem* 1992;267:18966–18972.

645. Davis J, Davis L, Bennett V. Diversity in membrane binding sites of ankyrins. Brain ankyrin, erythrocyte ankyrin, and processed erythrocyte ankyrin associate with distinct sites in kidney microsomes. *J Biol Chem* 1989;264:6417–6426.

646. Cleveland JL, Ihle JN. Contenders in FasL/TNF death signaling. *Cell* 1995;81:479.

647. Lu PW, Soong CJ, Tao M. Phosphorylation of ankyrin decreases its affinity for spectrin tetramer. *J Biol Chem* 1985;260:14958–14964.

648. Wei T, Tao M. Human erythrocyte casein kinase II: characterization and phosphorylation of membrane cytoskeletal proteins. *Arch Biochem Biophys* 1993;307:206–216.

649. Weaver DC, Pasternack GR, Marchesi VT. The structural basis of ankyrin function. II. Identification of two functional domains. *J Biol Chem* 1984;259:6170–6175.

650. Soong CJ, Lu PW, Tao M. Analysis of band 3 cytoplasmic domain phosphorylation and association with ankyrin. *Arch Biochem Biophys* 1987;254:509–517.

651. White RA, Birkenmeier CS, Lux SE, et al. Ankyrin and the hemolytic anemia mutation, *nb*, map to mouse chromosome 8: presence of the nb allele is associated with a truncated erythrocyte ankyrin. *Proc Natl Acad Sci U S A* 1990;87:3117–3121.

652. Peters LL, Birkenmeier CS, Bronson RT, et al. Purkinje cell degeneration associated with erythroid ankyrin deficiency in *nb/nb* mice. *J Cell Biol* 1991;114:1233–1241.

653. Jons T, Drenckhahn D. Anion exchanger 2 (AE2) binds to erythrocyte ankyrin and is colocalized with ankyrin along the basolateral plasma membrane of human gastric parietal cells. *Eur J Cell Biol* 1998;75:232–236.

654. Zhang Z, Devarajan P, Dorfman AL, et al. Structure of the ankyrin-binding domain of alpha-Na,K-ATPase. *J Biol Chem* 1998;273:18681–18684.

655. Jordan C, Puschel B, Koob R, et al. Identification of a binding motif for ankyrin on the alpha-subunit of Na⁺,K⁺-ATPase. *J Biol Chem* 1995;270:29971–29975.

656. Smith PR, Saccomani G, Joe EH, et al. Amiloride-sensitive sodium channel is linked to the cytoskeleton in renal epithelial cells. *Proc Natl Acad Sci U S A* 1991;88:6971–6975.

657. Li ZP, Burke EP, Frank JS, et al. The cardiac Na⁺-Ca²⁺ exchanger binds to the cytoskeletal protein ankyrin. *J Biol Chem* 1993;268:11489–11491.

658. Smith PR, Bradford AL, Joe EH, et al. Gastric parietal cell H(+)-K(+)-ATPase microsomes are associated with isoforms of ankyrin and spectrin. *Am J Physiol* 1993;264:C63–70.

659. Handlogten ME, Dudenhausen EE, Yang W, et al. Association of hepatic system A amino acid transporter with the membrane-cytoskeletal proteins ankyrin and fodrin. *Biochim Biophys Acta* 1996;1282:107–114.

660. Bourguignon LY, Jin H. Identification of the ankyrin-binding domain of the mouse T-lymphoma cell inositol 1,4,5-trisphosphate (IP3) receptor and its role in the regulation of IP3-mediated internal Ca2+ release. *J Biol Chem* 1995;270:7257–7260.

661. Bourguignon LY, Chu A, Jin H, et al. Ryanodine receptor-ankyrin interaction regulates internal Ca2+ release in mouse T-lymphoma cells. *J Biol Chem* 1995;270:17917–17922.

662. Zhu D, Bourguignon LY. The ankyrin-binding domain of CD44s is involved in regulating hyaluronic acid-mediated functions and prostate tumor cell transformation. *Cell Motil Cytoskeleton* 1998;39:209–222.

663. Lokeshwar VB, Fregien N, Bourguignon LY. Ankyrin-binding domain of CD44(GP85) is required for the expression of hyaluronic acid-mediated adhesion function. *J Cell Biol* 1994;126:1099–1109.

664. Tuvia S, Garver TD, Bennett V. The phosphorylation state of the FIGQY tyrosine of neurofascin determines ankyrin-binding activity and patterns of cell segregation. *Proc Natl Acad Sci U S A* 1997;94:12957–12962.

665. Dubreuil RR, MacVicar G, Dissanayake S, et al. Neuroglian-mediated cell adhesion induces assembly of the membrane skeleton at cell contact sites. *J Cell Biol* 1996;133:647–655.

666. Michaely P, Bennett V. Mechanism for binding site diversity on ankyrin. Comparison of binding sites on ankyrin for neurofascin and the Cl⁻/HCO₃⁻ anion exchanger. *J Biol Chem* 1995;270:31298–31302.

667. Davis JQ, Bennett V. Ankyrin binding activity shared by the neurofascin/L1/NrCAM family of nervous system cell adhesion molecules. *J Biol Chem* 1994;269:27163–27166.

668. Zhou D, Birkenmeier CS, Williams MW, et al. Small, membrane-bound, alternatively spliced forms of ankyrin 1 associated with the sarcoplasmic reticulum of mammalian skeletal muscle. *J Cell Biol* 1997;136:621–631.

669. Lambert S, Bennett V. Postmitotic expression of ankyrinR and beta R-spectrin in discrete neuronal populations of the rat brain. *J Neurosci* 1993;13:3725–3735.

670. Kordeli E, Bennett V. Distinct ankyrin isoforms at neuron cell bodies and nodes of Ranvier resolved using erythrocyte ankyrin-deficient mice. *J Cell Biol* 1991;114:1243–1259.

671. Tse WT, Menninger JC, Yang-Feng TL, et al. Isolation and chromosomal localization of a novel nonerythroid ankyrin gene. *Genomics* 1991;10:858–866.

672. Otto E, Kunimoto M, McLaughlin T, et al. Isolation and characterization of cDNAs encoding human brain ankyrins reveal a family of alternatively spliced genes. *J Cell Biol* 1991;114:241–253.

673. Kunimoto M. A neuron-specific isoform of brain ankyrin, 440-kD ankyrinB, is targeted to the axons of rat cerebellar neurons. *J Cell Biol* 1995;131:1821–1829.

674. Chan W, Kordeli E, Bennett V. 440-kD AnkyrinB: structure of the major developmentally regulated domain and selective localization in unmyelinated axons. *J Cell Biol* 1993;123:1463–1473.

675. Kunimoto M, Otto E, Bennett V. A new 440-kD isoform is the major ankyrin in neonatal rat brain. *J Cell Biol* 1991;115:1319–1331.

676. Scotland P, Zhou D, Benveniste H, et al. Nervous system defects of AnkyrinB (-/-) mice suggest functional overlap between the cell adhesion molecule L1 and 440-kD AnkyrinB in premyelinated axons. *J Cell Biol* 1998;143:1305–1315.

677. Peters LL, John KM, Lu FM, et al. Ank3 (epithelial ankyrin), a widely distributed new member of the ankyrin gene family and the major ankyrin in kidney, is expressed in alternatively spliced forms, including forms that lack the repeat domain. *J Cell Biol* 1995;130:313–330.

678. Kordeli E, Lambert S, Bennett V. AnkyrinG A new ankyrin gene with neural-specific isoforms localized at the axonal initial segment and node of Ranvier. *J Biol Chem* 1995;270:2352–2359.

679. Zhou D, Lambert S, Malen PL, et al. AnkyrinG is required for clustering of voltage-gated Na channels at axon initial segments and for normal action potential firing. *J Cell Biol* 1998;143:1295–1304.

680. Davis JQ, Lambert S, Bennett V. Molecular composition of the node of Ranvier: identification of ankyrin-binding cell adhesion molecules neurofascin (mucin+/third FNIII domain-) and NrCAM at nodal axon segments. *J Cell Biol* 1996;135:1355–1367.

681. Zhang, X, Bennett, V. Restriction of 480/270-kd ankyrinG to axon proximal segments requires multiple ankyrinG-specific domains. *J Cell Biol* 1998;142:1571–1581.

682. Devarajan P, Stabach PR, Mann AS, et al. Identification of a small cytoplasmic ankyrin (AnkG119) in the kidney and muscle that binds BIΣ* spectrin and associates with the Golgi apparatus. *J Cell Biol* 1996;133:819–830.

683. Hoock TC, Peters LL, Lux SE. An isoform of ankyrin 3 that lack the N-terminal repeat domain associate with mouse macrophage lysosomes. *J Cell Biol* 1997;136:1059–1070.

684. Michaely P, Kamal A, Anderson RGW, et al. A requirement for ankyrin binding to clathrin during coated pit budding. *J Biol Chem* 1999;50:35908–35913.

685. Sung LA, Chien S, Chang LS, et al. Molecular cloning of human protein 4.2: a major component of the erythrocyte membrane. *Proc Natl Acad Sci U S A* 1990;87:955–959.

686. Najfeld V, Ballard SG, Menninger J, et al. The gene for human erythrocyte protein 4.2 maps to chromosome 15q15. *Am J Hum Genet* 1992;50:71–75.

687. Korsgren C, Lawler J, Lambert S, et al. Complete amino acid sequence and homologies of human erythrocyte membrane protein band 4.2. *Proc Natl Acad Sci U S A* 1990;87:613.

688. Wada H, Kanzaki A, Yawata A, et al. Late expression of red cell membrane protein 4.2 in normal human erythroid maturation with seven isoforms of the protein 4.2 gene. *Exp Hematol* 1999;27:54–62.

689. Bhattacharyya R, Das AK, Moitra PK, et al. Mapping of a palmitoylatable band 3-binding domain of human erythrocyte membrane protein 4.2. *Biochem J* 1999;340:505–512.

690. Golan DE, Corbett JD, Korsgren C, et al. Control of band 3 lateral and rotational mobility by band 4.2 in intact erythrocytes: release of band 3 oligomers from low-affinity binding sites. *Biophys J* 1996;70:1534.

690a. Mandal D, Moitra PK, Basu J. Mapping of a spectrin-binding domain of human erythrocyte membrane protein 4.2. *Biochem J* 2002;364:841–847.

690b. Azim AC, Marfatia SM, Korsgren C, et al. Human erythrocyte dematin and protein 4.2 (pallidin) are ATP-binding proteins. *Biochemistry* 1996;35:3001–3006.

691. Risinger MA, Korsgren C, Cohen CM. Role of N-myristylation in targeting of band 4.2 (pallidin) in nonerythroid cells. *Exp Cell Res* 1996;229:421–431.

692. Risinger MA, Dotimas EM, Cohen CM. Human erythrocyte protein 4.2, a high copy number membrane protein, is N-myristylated. *J Biol Chem* 1992;267:5680–5685.

693. Das AK, Bhattacharya R, Kundu M, et al. Human erythrocyte membrane protein 4.2 is palmitoylated. *Eur J Biochem* 1994;224:575–580.

694. Hayette S, Dhermy D, dos Santos ME, et al. A deletional frameshift mutation in protein 4.2 gene (allele 4.2 Lisboa) associated with hereditary hemolytic anemia. *Blood* 1995;85:250–256.

695. Takaoka Y, Ideguchi H, Matsuda M, et al. A novel mutation in the erythrocyte protein 4.2 gene of Japanese patients with hereditary spherocytosis (protein 4.2 Fukuoka). *Br J Haematol* 1994;88:527–533.

696. Gallagher PG, Forget BG. Hematologically important mutations: band 3 and protein 4.2 variants in hereditary spherocytosis. *Blood Cells Mol Dis* 1997;23:417–421.

697. Shau H, Butterfield LH, Chiu R, et al. Cloning and sequence analysis of candidate human natural killer enhancing factor genes. *Immunogenetics* 1994;40: 129–134.

698. Rabilloud T, Berthier R, Vincon M, et al. Early events in erythroid differentiation: accumulation of the acidic peroxidoxin (PRP/TSA/NKEF-B). *Biochem J* 1995;312:699–705.

699. Butterfield LH, Merino A, Golub SH, et al. From cytoprotection to tumor suppression: the multifactorial role of peroxiredoxins. *Antioxid Redox Signal* 1999;1:385–402.

700. Moore RB, Shriver SK, Jenkins LD, et al. Calpromotin, a cytoplasmic protein, is associated with the formation of dense cells in sickle cell anemia. *Am J Hematol* 1997;56:100–106.

701. Liu SC, Derick LH. Molecular anatomy of the red blood cell membrane skeleton: structure-function relationships. *Semin Hematol* 1992;29:231–243.

702. Liu SC, Derick LH, Palek J. Visualization of the hexagonal lattice in the erythrocyte membrane skeleton. *J Cell Biol* 1987;104:527–536.

703. McCaughan L, Krimm S. X-ray and neutron scattering density profiles of the intact human red blood cell membrane. *Science* 1980;207:1481–1483.

704. Tsukita S, Tsukita S, Ishikawa H. Cytoskeletal network underlying the human erythrocyte membrane. Thin-section electron microscopy. *J Cell Biol* 1980;85:567–576.

705. Lux SE. Dissecting the red cell membrane skeleton. *Nature* 1979;281:426–429.

706. McGough AM, Josephs R. On the structure of erythrocyte spectrin in partially expanded membrane skeletons. *Proc Natl Acad Sci U S A* 1990;87:5208–5212.

707. Ursitti JA, Pumplin DW, Wade JB, et al. Ultrastructure of the human erythrocyte cytoskeleton and its attachment to the membrane. *Cell Motil Cytoskeleton* 1991;19:227–243.

708. Hargreaves WR, Giedd KN, Verkleij A, et al. Reassociation of ankyrin with band 3 in erythrocyte membranes and in lipid vesicles. *J Biol Chem* 1980; 255:11965–11972.

709. Thevenin BJM, Low PS. Kinetics and regulation of the ankyrin-band 3 interaction of the human red blood cell membrane. *J Biol Chem* 1990;265:16166–16172.

710. Cianci CD, Giorgi M, Morrow JS. Phosphorylation of ankyrin down-regulates its cooperative interaction with spectrin and protein 3. *J Cell Biochem* 1988;37:301–315.

711. Lu PW, Soong CJ, Tao M. Phosphorylation of ankyrin decreases its affinity for spectrin tetramer. *J Biol Chem* 1985;260:14958–14964.

712. Soong CJ, Lu PW, Tao M. Analysis of band 3 cytoplasmic domain phosphorylation and association with ankyrin. *Arch Biochem Biophys* 1987;254: 509–517.

713. Ling E, Danilov YN, Cohen CM. Modulation of red cell band 4.1 function by cAMP-dependent kinase and protein kinase C phosphorylation. *J Biol Chem* 1988;263:2209–2216.

714. Subrahmanyam G, Bertics PJ, Anderson RA. Phosphorylation of protein 4.1 on tyrosine-418 modulates its function in vitro. *Proc Natl Acad Sci U S A* 1991;88:5222–5226.

715. Eder PS, Soong CJ, Tao M. Phosphorylation reduces the affinity of protein 4.1 for spectrin. *Biochemistry* 1986;25:1764–1770.

716. Chao TS, Tao M. Modulation of protein 4.1 binding to inside-out membrane vesicles by phosphorylation. *Biochemistry* 1991;30:10529–10535.

717. Danilov YN, Fennell R, Ling E, et al. Selective modulation of band 4.1 binding to erythrocyte membranes by protein kinase C. *J Biol Chem* 1990;265:2556–2562.

718. Husain-Chishti A, Faquin W, Wu CC, et al. Purification of erythrocyte dematin (protein 4.9) reveals an endogenous protein kinase that modulates actin-bundling activity. *J Biol Chem* 1989;264:8985–8991.

719. Low PS, Allen DP, Zioncheck TF, et al. Tyrosine phosphorylation of band 3 inhibits peripheral protein binding. *J Biol Chem* 1987;262:4592–4596.

720. Anderson JM, Tyler JM. State of spectrin phosphorylation does not affect erythrocyte shape or spectrin binding to erythrocyte membranes. *J Biol Chem* 1980;255:1259–1265.

721. Harris HW Jr, Levin N, Lux SE. Comparison of the phosphorylation of human erythrocyte spectrin in the intact red cell and in various cell-free systems. *J Biol Chem* 1980;255:11521–11525.

722. Manno S, Takakuwa Y, Nagoa K, et al. Modulation of erythrocyte membrane mechanical function by beta-spectrin phosphorylation and dephosphorylation. *J Biol Chem* 1995;270:5969–5975.

723. Sheetz MP, Casaly J. 2,3-Diphosphoglycerate and ATP dissociate erythrocyte membrane skeletons. *J Biol Chem* 1980;255:9955–9960.

724. Mentzer WC Jr, Iarocci TA, Mohandas N, et al. Modulation of erythrocyte membrane mechanical fragility by 2,3-diphosphoglycerate in the neonatal poikilocytosis/elliptocytosis syndrome. *J Clin Invest* 1987;79:943–949.

725. Schindler M, Koppel D, Sheetz MP. Modulation of membrane protein lateral mobility by polyphosphates and polyamines. *Proc Natl Acad Sci U S A* 1980; 77:1457–1461.

726. Suzuki Y, Nakajima T, Shiga T, et al. Influence of 2,3-diphosphoglycerate on the deformability of human erythrocytes. *Biochim Biophys Acta* 1990;1029:85–90.

727. Waugh RE. Effects of 2,3-diphosphoglycerate on the mechanical properties of erythrocyte membrane. *Blood* 1986;68:231–238.

728. Takakuwa Y, Mohandas N. Modulation of erythrocyte membrane material properties by Ca²⁺ and calmodulin. Implications for their role in regulation of skeletal protein interactions. *J Clin Invest* 1988;78:80–85.

729. Tanaka T, Kadowaki K, Lazarides E, et al. Ca²⁺-dependent regulation of the spectrin/actin interaction by calmodulin and protein 4.1. *J Biol Chem* 1991; 266:1134–1140.

730. Anderson JP, Morrow JS. The interaction of calmodulin with erythrocyte spectrin. Inhibition of protein 4.1-stimulated actin binding. *J Biol Chem* 1987;262:6365–6372.

731. Gardner K, Bennett V. A new erythrocyte membrane-associated protein with calmodulin binding activity. Identification and purification. *J Biol Chem* 1986;261:1339–1348.

732. Mische SM, Mooseker MS, Morrow JS. Erythrocyte adducin: a calmodulin-regulated actin-bundling protein that stimulates spectrin-actin binding. *J Cell Biol* 1987;105:2837–2845.

733. Lorand L, Siefring GE Jr, Lowe Krentz L. Enzymatic basis of membrane stiffening in human erythrocytes. *Semin Hematol* 1979;16:65–74.

734. Palek J, Liu PA, Liu SC. Polymerisation of red cell membrane protein contributes to spheroechinocyte shape irreversibility. *Nature* 1978;274:505–507.

735. Smith BD, La Celle PL, Siefring J, et al. Effects of the calcium mediated enzymatic cross linking of membrane proteins on cellular deformability. *J Membr Biol* 1981;61:75–80.

736. Gárdos G. The role of calcium in the potassium permeability of human erythrocytes. *Acta Physiol Acad Sci Hung* 1959;15:121–125.

737. Hanspal M, Palek J. Biogenesis of normal and abnormal red blood cell membrane skeletons. *Semin Hematol* 1992;29:305–319.

738. Lazarides E. From genes to structural morphogenesis: the genesis and epigenesis of a red blood cell. *Cell* 1987;51:345–356.

739. Lazarides E, Woods C. Biogenesis of the red blood cell membrane skeleton and the control of erythroid morphogenesis. *Annu Rev Cell Biol* 1989;5:427–452.

740. Hanspal M, Palek J. Synthesis and assembly of membrane skeletal proteins in mammalian red cell precursors. *J Cell Biol* 1987;105:1417–1424.

741. Hanspal M, Hanspal J, Kalraiya R. Asynchronous synthesis of membrane skeletal proteins during terminal maturation of murine erythroblasts. *Blood* 1992;80:530–539.

742. Hanspal M, Hanspal JS, Sahr KE, et al. Molecular basis of spectrin deficiency in hereditary pyropoikilocytosis. *Blood* 1993;82:1652–1660.

743. Woods CM, Boyer B, Vogt PK, et al. Control of erythroid differentiation: asynchronous expression of the anion transporter and the peripheral components of the membrane skeleton in AEV- and S13-transformed cells. *J Cell Biol* 1986;103:1789–1798.

744. Jarolim P, Rubin HL, Liu SC, et al. Duplication of 10 nucleotides in the erythroid band 3 (AE1) gene is a kindred with hereditary spherocytosis and band 3 protein deficiency (Band 3 PRAGUE). *J Clin Invest* 1994;93:121–130.

745. Lux S, Bedrosian C, Shalev O, et al. Deficiency of band 3 in dominant hereditary spherocytosis with normal spectrin content. *Clin Res* 1990;38:300a (abst).

746. Hanspal M, Kalraiya R, Hanspal J. Erythropoietin enhances the assembly of α β spectrin heterodimers on the murine erythroblast membranes by increasing β spectrin synthesis. *J Biol Chem* 1991;266:15626–15630.

747. Patel VP, Lodish HF. A fibronectin matrix is required for differentiation of murine erythroleukemia cells into reticulocytes. *J Cell Biol* 1987;105:3105–3112.

748. Chasis JA, Prenant M, Leung A, et al. Membrane assembly and remodeling during reticulocyte maturation. *Blood* 1989;74:1112–1120.

749. Johnstone RM. The transferrin receptor. In: Agre P, Parker JC, eds. *Red blood cell membranes: structure, function, and clinical implications.* New York: Marcel Dekker Inc., 1989:325–366.

750. Patel VP, Lodish HF. The fibronectin receptor on mammalian erythroid precursor cells: characterization and developmental regulation. *J Cell Biol* 1986;102:449–456.

751. Holm TM, Braun A, Trigatti BL, et al. Failure of red blood cell maturation in mice with defects in the high-density lipoprotein receptor SR-BI. *Blood* 2002;99:1817–1824.

752. Rand RP, Burton AC. Area and volume changes in hemolysis of single erythrocytes. *J Cell Comp Physiol* 1963;61:245–253.

753. Mohandas N, Chasis JA. Red cell deformability, membrane material properties, and shape: regulation by transmembrane, skeletal, and cytosolic proteins and lipids. *Semin Hematol* 1993;30:171–192.

753a. An X, Lecomte MC, Chasis JA, et al. Shear-response of the spectrin dimer-tetramer equilibrium in the red blood cell membrane. *J Biol Chem* 2002;277:31796–31800.

754. Bull BS, Kuhn IN. The production of schistocytes by fibrin strands (a scanning electron microscope study). *Blood* 1970;35:104.

755. Reinhart WH, Sung LA, Chien S. Quantitative relationship between Heinz body formation and red blood cell deformability. *Blood* 1986;68:1376–1383.

756. Flynn TP, Allen DW, Johnson GJ, et al. Oxidant damage of the lipids and proteins of the erythrocyte membranes in unstable hemoglobin disease. Evidence for the role of lipid peroxidation. *J Clin Invest* 1983;71:1215–1223.

757. Chasis JA, Reid ME, Jensen RH, et al. Signal transduction by glycophorin A: role of extracellular and cytoplasmic domains in a modulatable process. *J Cell Biol* 1988;107:1351–1357.

758. Chasis JA, McGee S, Anstee D, et al. Different transmembrane signalling mechanisms mediated by band 3 and glycophorin A. *Blood* 1993;82[Suppl 1]:174a (abst).

759. Liu SC, Palek J, Yi SJ, et al. Molecular basis of altered red blood cell membrane properties in Southeast Asian ovalocytosis: role of the mutant band 3 protein in band 3 oligomerization and retention by the membrane skeleton. *Blood* 1995;86:349–358.

760. Che A, Cherry RJ, Bannister LH, et al. Aggregation of band 3 in hereditary ovalocytic red blood cell membranes. Electron microscopy and protein rotational diffusion studies. *J Cell Sci* 1993;105:655–660.

761. Liu SC, Palek J. Spectrin tetramer-dimer equilibrium and the stability of erythrocyte membrane skeletons. *Nature* 1980;285:586–588.

762. Liu SC, Derick LH, Agre P, et al. Alteration of the erythrocyte membrane skeletal ultrastructure in hereditary spherocytosis, hereditary elliptocytosis, and pyropoikilocytosis. *Blood* 1990;76:198–205.

763. Liu SC, Derick LH, Duquette MA, et al. Separation of the lipid bilayer from the membrane skeleton during discocyte-echinocyte transformation of human erythrocyte ghosts. *Eur J Cell Biol* 1989;49:358–365.

764. Knowles DW, Tilley L, Mohandas N, et al. Erythrocyte membrane vesiculation: model for the molecular mechanism of protein sorting. *Proc Natl Acad Sci U S A* 1997;94:12969–12974.

765. Wagner GM, Chiu DT, Qju JH, et al. Spectrin oxidation correlates with membrane vesiculation in stored RBC's. *Blood* 1987;69:1777–1781.

766. Wolfe LC. The membrane and the lesions of storage in preserved red cells. *Transfusion* 1985;25:185–203.

767. Lutz HU, Liu SC, Palek J. Release of spectrin-free vesicles from human erythrocytes during ATP depletion. Characterization of spectrin free vesicles. *J Cell Biol* 1977;73:548–560.

768. Elgsaeter A, Shotton DM, Branton D. Intramembrane particle aggregation in erythrocyte ghosts II. The influence of spectrin aggregation. *Biochim Biophys Acta* 1996;426:101–122.

769. Lux SE, John KM, Karnovsky MJ. Irreversible deformation of the spectrin actin lattice in irreversibly sickled cells. *J Clin Invest* 1976;58:955–963.

770. Tomaselli MB, John KM, Lux SE. Elliptical erythrocyte membrane skeletons and heat-sensitive spectrin in hereditary elliptocytosis. *Proc Natl Acad Sci U S A* 1981;78:1911–1915.

771. Khodadad JK, Waugh RE, Podolski JL, et al. Remodeling the shape of the skeleton in the intact red cell. *Biophys J* 1996;70:1036–1044.

772. Hebbel RP. Beyond hemoglobin polymerization: the red blood cell membrane and sickle cell disease pathophysiology. *Blood* 1991;77:214–237.

773. Swerlick RA, Eckman JR, Kumar A, et al. α4β1-Integrin expression on sickle reticulocytes: vascular cell adhesion molecule-1-dependent binding to endothelium. *Blood* 1993;82:1891–1899.

774. Rosse WF. The glycolipid anchor of membrane surface proteins. *Semin Hematol* 1993;30:219–231.

775. Discher DE, Mohandas N, Evans EA. Molecular maps of red cell deformation: hidden elasticity and in situ connectivity. *Science* 1994;266:1032–1035.

776. Test ST, Butikofer P, Yee MC, et al. Characterization of the complement sensitivity of calcium-loaded human erythrocytes. *Blood* 1991;78:3056–3065.

777. Victoria EJ, Muchmore EA, Sudora EJ, et al. The role of antigen mobility in anti Rh(D) induced agglutination. *J Clin Invest* 1975;56:292–301.

778. Golan DE. Red blood cell membrane protein and lipid diffusion. In: Agre P, Parker JC, eds. *Red blood cell membranes: structure, function, and clinical implications.* New York: Marcel Dekker, Inc., 1989:367–400.

779. Mueckler MM, Caruso C, Baldwin SA, et al. Sequence and structure of a human glucose transporter. *Science* 1985;229:941–945.

780. Brugnara C. Erythrocyte dehydration in pathophysiology and treatment of sickle cell disease. *Curr Opin Hematol* 1995;2:132–138.

781. Bookchin RM, Lew VL. Sickle red cell dehydration; mechanisms and interventions. *Curr Opin Hematol* 2002;9:107–110.

782. Parker JC. In defense of cell volume? *Am J Physiol* 1993;265:1191–1200.
783. De Gier J. Permeability barriers formed by membrane lipids. *Bioelectrochem Bioenerg* 1992;27:1–10.
784. Nielsen SB, Smith L, Christensen EI, et al. CHIP28 water channels are localized in constitutively water permeable segments of the nephron. *J Cell Biol* 1993;120:371–383.
785. Zeidel ML, Ambudkar SV, Smith BL, et al. Reconstitution of functional water channels in liposomes containing purified red cell CHIP28 protein. *Biochemistry* 1992;31:7436–7440.
786. Smith BL, Baumgarten R, Nielsen S, et al. Concurrent expression of erythroid and renal aquaporin CHIP and appearance of water channel activity in perinatal rats. *J Clin Invest* 1993;92:2035–2041.
787. Brugnara C. Membrane transport of Na and K and cell dehydration in sickle erythrocytes. *Experientia* 1993;49:100–109.
788. Joiner CH. Cation transport and volume regulation in sickle red blood cells. *Am J Physiol* 1993;264:C251–C270.
789. Lauf PK, Bauer J, Adragna NC, et al. Erythrocyte K-Cl cotransport: properties and regulation. *Am J Physiol* 1992;263:C917–C932.
790. Johnson RM, Gannon SA. Erythrocyte cation permeability induced by mechanical stress: a model for sickle cell cation loss. *Am J Physiol* 1990;259:C746–C751.
791. Kim YK, Dirksen ER, Sanderson MJ. Stretch activated channels in airway epithelial cells. *Am J Physiol* 1993;265:1306–1318.
792. Garrahan PJ, Glynn IM. Factors affecting the relative magnitude of the sodium:potassium and sodium:sodium exchanges catalyzed by the sodium pump. *J Physiol* 1967;192:189.
793. Clark MR, Guatelli JC, White AT, et al. Study of dehydrating effect of the red cell Na$^+$/K$^+$ pump in nystatin treated cells with varying Na$^+$ and water content. *Biochim Biophys Acta* 1981;646:422–432.
794. Joiner CH, Platt OS, Lux SE. Cation depletion by the sodium pump in red cells with pathologic cation leaks. *J Clin Invest* 1986;78:1487–1496.
795. Clark MR. Senescence of red blood cells: progress and problems. *Physiol Rev* 1988;68:503–554.
796. Beutler E. Isolation of the aged. *Blood Cells* 1988;14:1–5.
797. Dale GL, Norenberg SL. Density fractionation of erythrocytes by Percoll/Hypaque results in only a slight enrichment for aged cells. *Biochim Biophys Acta* 1990;1036:183–187.
798. Suzuki T, Dale GL. Senescent erythrocytes: isolation of in vivo aged cells and their biochemical characteristics. *Proc Natl Acad Sci U S A* 1988;85:1647–1651.
799. Rettig MP, Low PS, Gimm JA, et al. Evaluation of biochemical changes during in vivo erythrocyte senescence in the dog. *Blood* 1999;93:376–384.
800. Waugh RE, Mohandas N, Jackson CW, et al. Rheologic properties of senescent erythrocytes: loss of surface area and volume with red blood cell age. *Blood* 1992;79:1351–1358.
801. Snyder LM, Fortier NL, Trainor J, et al. Effect of hydrogen peroxide exposure on normal human erythrocyte deformability, morphology, surface characteristics and spectrin hemoglobin crosslinking. *J Clin Invest* 1985;76:1971–1977.
802. Jain SK. Evidence for membrane lipid peroxidation during the in vivo aging of human erythrocytes. *Biochim Biophys Acta* 1988;937:205–210.
803. Danon D, Marikovsky Y. The aging of the red blood cell. A multifactor process. *Blood Cells* 1988;14:7–15.
804. Aminoff D, Ghalambor MA, Henrich CJ. GOST, galactose oxidase and sialyl transferase, substrate and receptor sites in erythrocyte senescence. In: Eaton JW, ed. *Erythrocyte membranes. 2: Recent clinical and experimental advances.* New York: Alan R. Liss, 1981:269–278.
805. Gattegno L, Bladier D, Garnier M, et al. Changes in carbohydrate content of surface membranes of human erythrocytes during ageing. *Carbohydr Res* 1976;52:197–208.
806. Lutz HU, Fehr J. Total sialic acid content of glycophorins during senescence of human red blood cells. *J Biol Chem* 1979;254:11177–11180.
807. Seaman GVF, Korok FJ, Nordt FJ. Red cell aging. I. Surface charge density and sialic acid content of density fractionated human erythrocytes. *Blood* 1977;50:1001–1011.
808. Beutler E. Biphasic loss of red cell enzyme activity during in vivo aging. *Prog Clin Biol Res* 1985;95:317–325.
809. Kay MMB. Mechanism of removal senescent cells by human macrophages in situ. *Proc Natl Acad Sci U S A* 1975;72:3521–3525.
810. Kay MMB. Localization of senescent cell antigen on band 3. *Proc Natl Acad Sci U S A* 1984;81:5753–5757.
811. Schlüter K, Drenckhahn D. Co-clustering of denatured hemoglobin with band 3: its role in binding of autoantibodies against band 3 to abnormal and aged erythrocytes. *Proc Natl Acad Sci U S A* 1986;83:6137–6141.
812. Lutz HU, Stringaro-Wipf G. Senescent red cell bound IgG is attached to band 3 protein. *Biomed Biochim Acta* 1983;42:117–121.
813. Galili U, Macher BA, Buehler J, et al. Human natural anti-α-galactosyl IgG. II. The specific recognition of (113) linked galactose residues. *J Exp Med* 1985;162:573–582.
814. Galili U, Flechner I, Knyszynski A, et al. The natural anti-α-galactosyl IgG on human normal senescent red blood cells. *Br J Haematol* 1986;62:317–324.
815. Kay MMB, Bosman GJCGM. Naturally occurring human "antigalactosyl" IgG antibodies are heterophile antibodies recognizing blood group related substances. *Exp Hematol* 1985;13:1103–1112.
816. Kay MMB, Marchalonis JJ, Hughes J, et al. Definition of a physiologic aging autoantigen by using synthetic peptides of membrane protein band 3: localization of the active antigenic sites. *Proc Natl Acad Sci U S A* 1990;87:5734–5738.
817. Kannan R, Labotka R, Low PS. Isolation and characterization of the hemichrome-stabilized membrane protein aggregates from sickle erythrocytes. Major site of autologous antibody binding. *J Biol Chem* 1988;263:13766–13773.
818. Kay MMB, Marchalonis JJ, Schluter SF, et al. Human erythrocyte aging: cellular and molecular biology. *Transfus Med Rev* 1991;5:173–195.
819. Turrini F, Mannu F, Arese P, et al. Characterization of the autologous antibodies that opsonize erythrocytes with clustered integral membrane proteins. *Blood* 1993;81:3146–3152.
820. Hornig R, Lutz HU. Band 3 protein clustering on human erythrocytes promotes binding of naturally occurring anti-band 3 and anti-spectrin antibodies. *Exp Gerontol* 2000;35:1025–1044.
821. Ando K, Kikugawa K, Beppu M. Involvement of sialylated poly-N-acetyllactosaminyl sugar chains of band 3 glycoprotein on senescent erythrocytes in anti-band 3 autoantibody binding. *J Biol Chem* 1994;269:19394–19398.
822. Ando K, Kikugawa K, Beppu M. Induction of band 3 aggregation in erythrocytes results in anti-band 3 autoantibody binding to the carbohydrate epitopes of band 3. *Arch Biochem Biophys* 1997;339:250–257.
823. Beppu M, Mizukami A, Nagoya M, et al. Binding of anti-band 3 autoantibody to oxidatively damaged erythrocytes. Formation of senescent antigen on erythrocyte surface by an oxidative mechanism. *J Biol Chem* 1990;265:3226–3233.
824. Lutz HU, Bussolino F, Flepp R, et al. Naturally occurring anti-band-3 antibodies and complement together mediate phagocytosis of oxidatively stressed human erythrocytes. *Proc Natl Acad Sci U S A* 1987;84:7368–7372.
825. Winograd E, Greenan JRT, Sherman IW. Expression of senescent antigen on erythrocytes infected with a knobby variant of the human malaria parasite *Plasmodium falciparum. Proc Natl Acad Sci U S A* 1987;84:1931–1935.
826. Giribaldi G, Ulliers D, Mannu F, et al. Growth of *Plasmodium falciparum* induces stage-dependent haemichrome formation, oxidative aggregation of band 3, membrane deposition of complement and antibodies, and phagocytosis of parasitized erythrocytes. *Br J Haematol* 2001;113:492–499.
827. Lelkes G, Fodor I, Lelkes G, et al. The distribution and aggregatability of intramembrane particles in phenylhydrazine-treated human erythrocytes. *Biochim Biophys Acta* 1988;945:105–110.
828. Lutz HU. Erythrocyte clearance. In: Harris JR, ed. *Blood cell biochemistry, volume 1, erythroid cells.* New York: Plenum Publishing, 1990:81–120.
829. Gershon H. Is the sequestration of aged erythrocytes mediated by natural autoantibodies? *Isr J Med Sci* 1992;28:818–828.
830. Herrmann A, Devaux PF. Alteration of the aminophospholipid translocase activity during in vivo and artificial aging of human erythrocytes. *Biochim Biophys Acta* 1990;1027:41–46.
831. Wang RH, Phillips G Jr, Medof ME, et al. Activation of the alternative complement pathway by exposure of phosphatidylethanolamine and phosphatidylserine on erythrocytes from sickle cell disease patients. *J Clin Invest* 1993;92:1326–1335.
832. Schroit AJ, Madsen JW, Tanaka Y. In vivo recognition and clearance of red blood cells containing phosphatidylserine in their plasma membranes. *J Biol Chem* 1985;260:5131–5138.
833. Tait JF, Smith C. Phosphatidylserine receptors: role of CD36 in binding of anionic phospholipid vesicles to monocytic cells. *J Biol Chem* 1999;274:3048–3054.
834. Kiefer CR, Snyder LM. Oxidation and erythrocyte senescence. *Curr Opin Hematol* 2000;7:113–116.
835. Vlassara H, Valinsky J, Brownlee M, et al. Advanced glycosylation end products on erythrocyte cell surface induce receptor mediated phagocytosis by macrophages. A model for turnover of aging cells. *J Exp Med* 1987;166:539–549.
836. Barber JR, Clarke S. Membrane protein carboxyl methylation increases with human erythrocyte age. *J Biol Chem* 1983;258:1189–1196.
837. Galletti P, Ingrosso D, Nappi A, et al. Increased methyl esterification of membrane proteins in aged red-blood cells. Preferential esterification of ankyrin and band-4.1 cytoskeletal proteins. *Eur J Biochem* 1983;135:25–31.
838. Bernassola F, Boumis G, Corazzari M, et al. Osmotic resistance of high-density erythrocytes in transglutaminase 2-deficient mice. *Biochem Biophys Res Commun* 2002; 291:1123–1127.
839. Vanlair CF, Masius JB. De la microcythémie. *Bull Acad R Med Belg* 1871;5:515–613.
840. Ham TH, Castle WB. Studies on destruction of red blood cells. Relation of increased hypotonic fragility and erythrostasis to the mechanism of hemolysis in certain anemias. *Proc Am Philos Soc* 1940;82:411–419.
841. Chauffard MA. Pathogénie de l'ictère hémolytique congénitale. *Ann Méd* 1914;1:3–17.
842. Dameshek W, Schwartz SO. Hemolysins as the cause of clinical and experimental hemolytic anemias. With particular reference to the nature of spherocytosis and increased fragility. *Am J Med Sci* 1938;196:769–792.
843. Wilson C. Some cases showing hereditary enlargement of the spleen. *Trans Clin Soc (London)* 1890;23:162.
844. Wilson C, Stanley D. A sequel to some cases showing hereditary enlargement of the spleen. *Trans Clin Soc (London)* 1893;26:163.
845. Minkowski O. Über eine hereditäre, unter dem Bilde eines chronischen Ikterus mit Urobilinurie, Splenomegalie und Nierensiderosis verlaufende Affektion. *Verh Dtsch Kongr Med* 1900;18:316.
846. Gilbert A, Castaigne J, Lereboullet P. De l'ictère familial. Contribution Ö l'étude de la diathäse biliaire. *Bull Mem Soc Med Hop Paris* 1900;17:948–959.
847. Barlow T, Shaw HB. Inheritance of recurrent attacks of jaundice and of abdominal crises with hepatosplenomegaly. *Trans Clin Soc (London)* 1902; 35:155.

848. Chauffard MA. Pathogénie de l'ictère congénital de l'adulte. *Semaine Méd (Paris)* 1907;27:25–29.
849. Chauffard MA. Les ictères hémolytiques. *Semaine Méd (Paris)* 1908;28:49–53.
850. Widal F, Abrami P, Brulè M. Differentiation de plusieurs types d'ictères hémolytiques par le procédédes hématies déplasmatisées. *Presse Med* 1907;15:641.
851. Hayem G. Sur une variété particuliàre d'ictère chronique. Ictäre infectieux chronique splénomégalique. *Presse Med* 1898;6:121–125.
852. Micheli F. Unmittelbare Effekte der Splenektomie bei einem Fall von erworbenem hämolytischen splenomegalischen Ikterus Typus-Hayem-Widal (Splenohämolytischer Ikterus). *Wien Klin Wochenschr* 1911;24:1269.
853. Giffin HZ. Haemolytic jaundice: a review of 17 cases. *Surg Gynecol Obstet* 1917;25:152–161.
854. Dawson of Penn. The Hume Lectures on haemolytic icterus. *BMJ* 1931;1:921–928 and 1931;1:963–966.
855. Tileston W. Hemolytic jaundice. *Medicine* 1922;1:355.
856. Gänsslen M. Über hämolytischen Ikterus. *Dtsch Arch Klin Med* 1922;140:210.
857. Wintrobe MM. *Blood, pure and eloquent.* New York: McGraw-Hill, 1980.
858. Morton NE, MacKinney AA, Kosower N, et al. Genetics of spherocytosis. *Am J Hum Genet* 1962;14:170.
859. Godal HC, Heist H. High prevalence of increased osmotic fragility of red blood cells among Norwegian donors. *Scand J Haematol* 1981;27:30–34.
860. Eber SW, Pekrun A, Neufeldt A, et al. Prevalence of increased osmotic fragility of erythrocytes in German blood donors: screening using a modified glycerol lysis test. *Ann Hematol* 1992;64:88–92.
861. Eber SW, Armbrust R, Schröter W. Variable clinical severity of hereditary spherocytosis: relation to erythrocytic spectrin concentration, osmotic fragility and autohemolysis. *J Pediatr* 1990;177:409–416.
862. Race RR. On the inheritance and linkage relations of acholuric jaundice. *Ann Eugen* 1942;11:365–384.
863. Ribeiro ML, Alloisio N, Almeida H, et al. Severe hereditary spherocytosis and distal renal tubular acidosis associated with the total absence of band 3. *Blood* 2000;96:1602–1604.
864. Perrotta S, Nigro V, Iolascon A, et al. Dominant hereditary spherocytosis due to band 3 Neapolis produces a life-threatening anemia at the homozygous state. *Blood* 1998;92:9a (abst).
865. Whitfield CF, Follweiler JB, Lopresti-Morrow L, et al. Deficiency of α-spectrin synthesis in burst-forming units-erythroid in lethal hereditary spherocytosis. *Blood* 1991;78:3043–3051.
866. Olim G, Marques S, Saldanha C, et al. Red cell abnormalities in a kindred with an uncommon form of hereditary spherocytosis. *Acta Med Port* 1984;6:137–141.
867. Bernard J, Boiron M, Estager J. Une grand famille hémolytique. Trieze cas de maladie de Minkowski-Chauffard observés dans la màme fratrie. *Semaine Hop Paris* 1952;28:3741–3744.
868. Duru F, Gürgey A, Öztürk G, et al. Homozygosity for dominant form of hereditary spherocytosis. *Br J Haematol* 1992;82:596–600.
869. Agre P, Asimos A, Casella JF, et al. Inheritance pattern and clinical response to splenectomy as a reflection of erythrocyte spectrin deficiency in hereditary spherocytosis. *N Engl J Med* 1986;315:1579–1583.
870. Miraglia del Giudice E, Francese M, Nobili B, et al. High frequency of de novo mutations in ankyrin gene (ANK1) in children with hereditary spherocytosis. *J Pediatr* 1998;132:117–120.
871. Miraglia del Giudice E, Lombardi C, Francese M, et al. Frequent de novo monoallelic expression of beta-spectrin gene (SPTB) in children with hereditary spherocytosis and isolated spectrin deficiency. *Br J Haematol* 1998;101:251–254.
872. Miraglia del Giudice E, Nobili B, Francese M, et al. Clinical and molecular evaluation of non-dominant hereditary spherocytosis. *Br J Haematol* 1991;112:42–47.
873. Nakanishi H, Kanzaki A, Yawata A, et al. Ankyrin gene mutations in Japanese patients with hereditary spherocytosis. *Int J Hematol* 2001;73:54–63.
874. Özcan R, Kugler W, Feuring-Buske M, et al. Parental mosaicism for ankyrin-1 mutations in two families with hereditary spherocytosis. *Blood* 1997;90[Suppl 1]:4a (abst).
875. Wichterle H, Hanspal M, Palek J, et al. Combination of two mutant α spectrin alleles underlies a severe spherocytic hemolytic anemia. *J Clin Invest* 1996;98:2300–2307.
876. Bass EB, Smith SW Jr, Stevenson RE, et al. Further evidence for localization of the spherocytosis gene on chromosome 8. *Ann Intern Med* 1983;99:192–193.
877. Kimberling WJ, Fulbeck T, Dixon L, et al. Localization of spherocytosis to chromosome 8 or 12 and report of a family with spherocytosis and a reciprocal translocation. *Am J Hum Genet* 1975;27:586–594.
878. Chilcote RR, Le Beau MM, Dampier C, et al. Association of red cell spherocytosis with deletion of the short arm of chromosome 8. *Blood* 1987;69:156–159.
879. Cohen H, Walker H, Delhanty JDA, et al. Congenital spherocytosis, B19 parvovirus infection and inherited deletion of the short arm of chromosome 8. *Br J Haematol* 1991;78:251–257.
880. Kitatani M, Chiyo H, Ozaki M, et al. Localization of the spherocytosis gene to chromosome segment 8p11.22–8p21.1. *Hum Genet* 1988;78:94–95.
881. Cohen H, Walker H, Delhanty JDA, et al. Congenital spherocytosis, B19 parvovirus infection and inherited deletion of the short arm of chromosome 8. *Br J Haematol* 1991;78:251–257.
882. Okamoto N, Wada Y, Nakamura Y, et al. Hereditary spherocytic anemia with deletion of the short arm of chromosome 8. *Am J Med Genet* 1995;58:225–229.
883. Ganguly BB, Dalvi R, Mehta AV. Pericentric inversion in human chromosome 8 and spherocytosis. *Cytobios* 2000;102:119–126.

884. Stratton RF, Crudo DF, Varela M, et al. Deletion of the proximal short arm of chromosome 8. *Am J Med Genet* 1992;42:15–18.
885. Costa FF, Agre P, Watkins PC, et al. Linkage of dominant hereditary spherocytosis to the gene for the erythrocyte membrane-skeleton protein ankyrin. *N Engl J Med* 1990;323:1046–1050.
886. Kimberling WJ, Taylor RA, Chapman RG, et al. Linkage and gene localization of hereditary spherocytosis (HS). *Blood* 1978;52:859–867.
887. Fukushima Y, Byers MG, Watkins PC, et al. Assignment of the gene for β spectrin (SPTB) to chromosome 14q23-q24.2 by in situ hybridization. *Cytogenet Cell Genet* 1990;53:232–233.
888. Pekrun A, Eber SW, Kuhlmey A, et al. Combined ankyrin and spectrin deficiency in hereditary spherocytosis. *Ann Hematol* 1993;67:89–93.
889. Friedman EW, Williams JC, Van Hook L. Hereditary spherocytosis in the elderly. *Am J Med* 1988;84:513–516.
890. Krueger HC, Burgert EO Jr. Hereditary spherocytosis in 100 children. *Mayo Clin Proc* 1966;41:821–830.
891. MacKinney AA Jr, Morton NE, Kosower NS, et al. Ascertaining genetic carriers of hereditary spherocytosis by statistical analysis of multiple laboratory tests. *J Clin Invest* 1962;41:554–567.
892. Young LE, Izzo MJ, Platzer RF. Hereditary spherocytosis. I. Clinical, hematologic and genetic features in 28 cases, with particular reference to the osmotic and mechanical fragility of incubated erythrocytes. *Blood* 1951;6:1073–1096.
893. Debre R, Lamy M, See G, et al. Congenital and familial hemolytic disease in children. *Am J Dis Child* 1938;56:1189–1214.
894. Diamond LK. Indications for splenectomy in childhood. Results in fifty-two operated cases. *Am J Surg (NS)* 1938;39:400–421.
895. Jensson O, Jonasson JL, et al. Studies on hereditary spherocytosis in Iceland. *Acta Med Scand* 1977;201:187.
896. Gehlbach SH, Cooper BA. Haemolytic anaemia in infectious mononucleosis due to inapparent congenital spherocytosis. *Scand J Haematol* 1970;7:141–144.
897. Ho-Yan DO. Hereditary spherocytosis presenting in pregnancy. *Acta Haematol* 1984;72:29–33.
898. Pajor A, Lehoczky D, Szakacs Z. Pregnancy and hereditary spherocytosis. Report of 8 patients and a review. *Arch Gynecol Obstet* 1993;253:37–42.
899. Godal HC, Refsum HE. Haemolysis in athletes due to hereditary spherocytosis. *Scand J Haematol* 1979;22:83–86.
900. Palek J, Mirevova L, Brabec V. 2,3-Diphosphoglycerate metabolism in hereditary spherocytosis. *Br J Haematol* 1969;17:59.
901. Fernandez LA, Erslev AJ. Oxygen affinity and compensated hemolysis in hereditary spherocytosis. *J Lab Clin Med* 1972;80:780–785.
902. Guarnone R, Centenara E, Zappa M, et al. Erythropoietin production and erythropoiesis in compensated and anaemic states of hereditary spherocytosis. *Br J Haematol* 1996;92:150–154.
903. Agre P, Casella JF, Zinkham WH, et al. Partial deficiency of erythrocyte spectrin in hereditary spherocytosis. *Nature* 1985;314:380–383.
904. Coetzer TL, Lawler J, Liu SC, et al. Partial ankyrin and spectrin deficiency in severe, atypical hereditary spherocytosis. *N Engl J Med* 1988;318:230–234.
905. Garwicz S. Atypical spherocytosis, a disease of spleen as well as of red blood cells. *Lancet* 1975;1:956–957.
906. Wiley JS, Firkin BG. An unusual variant of hereditary spherocytosis. *Am J Med* 1970;48:63.
907. Reference deleted.
908. Maberry MC, Mason RA, Cunningham FG, et al. Pregnancy complicated by hereditary spherocytosis. *Obstet Gynecol* 1992;79:735–738.
909. Delamore IW, Richmond J, Davies SH. Megaloblastic anaemia in congenital spherocytosis. *BMJ* 1961;1:543–545.
910. Kohler HG, Meynell MJ, Cooke WT. Spherocytic anaemia, complicated by megaloblastic anaemia of pregnancy. *BMJ* 1960;1:779–781.
911. Burman D. Congenital spherocytosis in infancy. *Arch Dis Child* 1958;33:335–341.
912. Schröter W, Kahsnitz E. Diagnosis of hereditary spherocytosis in newborn infants. *J Pediatr* 1983;103:460–463.
913. Trucco JI, Brown AK. Neonatal manifestations of hereditary spherocytosis. *Am J Dis Child* 1967;113:263–270.
914. Stamey CC, Diamond LK. Congenital hemolytic anemia in the newborn. *Am J Dis Child* 1957;94:616–622.
915. Kaplan M, Renbaum P, Levy-Lahad E, et al. Gilbert syndrome and glucose-6-phosphate dehydrogenase deficiency: a dose-dependent genetic interaction crucial to neonatal hyperbilirubinemia. *Proc Natl Acad Sci U S A* 1997;94:12128–12132.
916. Iolascon A, Faienza MF, Giordani L, et al. Bilirubin levels in the acute hemolytic crisis of G6PD deficiency are related to Gilbert's syndrome. *Eur J Haematol* 1999;62:307–310.
917. Galanello R, Cipollina MD, Dessì C, et al. Co-inherited Gilbert's syndrome: a factor determining hyperbilirubinemia in homozygous beta-thalassemia. *Haematologica* 1999;84:103–105.
918. Monaghan G, McLellan A, McGeehan A, et al. Gilbert's syndrome is a contributory factor in prolonged unconjugated hyperbilirubinemia of the newborn. *J Pediatr* 1999;134:441–446.
919. Bancroft JD, Kreamer B, Gourley GR. Gilbert syndrome accelerates development of neonatal jaundice. *J Pediatr* 1998;132:656–660.
920. Bosma PJ, Chowdhury JR, Bakker C, et al. The genetic basis of the reduced expression of bilirubin UDP-glucuronosyltransferase 1 in Gilbert's syndrome. *N Engl J Med* 1995;333:1171–1175.
921. Akaba K, Kimura T, Sasaki A, et al. Neonatal hyperbilirubinemia and a common mutation of the bilirubin uridine diphosphate-glucuronosyltransferase gene in Japanese. *J Hum Genet* 1999;44:22–25.

922. Iolascon A, Faienza MF, Moretti A, et al. UGT1 promoter polymorphism accounts for increased neonatal appearance of hereditary spherocytosis. *Blood* 1998;91:1093.

923. Ebbesen F. Recurrence of kernicterus in term and near-term infants in Denmark. *Acta Paediatr* 2000;89:1213–1217.

924. Bergstrand CG, Czar B, et al. Serum haptoglobin in infancy. *J Lab Clin Invest* 1961;13:576.

925. Erlandson ME, Hilgartner M. Hemolytic disease in the neonatal period and early infancy. *J Pediatr* 1959;54:566.

926. Saada V, Da Costa L, Brossard Y, et al. Screening for hereditary spherocytosis in icteric neonates. *Blood* 2000;96[Suppl 1]:539a (abst).

927. Delhommeau F, Cynober T, Schischmanoff PO, et al. Natural history of hereditary spherocytosis during the first year of life. *Blood* 2000;95:393–397.

928. Dallacasa P, Ancora G, Miniero R, et al. Erythropoietin course in newborns with Rh hemolytic disease transfused and not transfused in utero. *Pediatr Res* 1996;40:357–360.

929. al-Alaiyan S, al Omran A. Late hyporegenerative anemia in neonates with rhesus hemolytic disease. *J Perinat Med* 1999;27:112–115.

930. Scaradavou A, Inglis S, Peterson P, et al. Suppression of erythropoiesis by intrauterine transfusions in hemolytic disease of the newborn: use of erythropoietin to treat the late anemia. *J Pediatr* 1993;123:279–284.

931. Ovali F, Samanci N, Dagoglu T. Management of late anemia in Rhesus hemolytic disease: use of recombinant human erythropoietin [a pilot study]. *Pediatr Res* 1996;39:831–834.

932. Dhodapkar KM, Blei F. Treatment of hemolytic disease of the newborn caused by anti-Kell antibody with recombinant erythropoietin. *J Pediatr Hematol Oncol* 2001;23:69–70.

933. Antonarakis SE. Recommendations for a nomenclature system for human gene mutations. *Hum Mutat* 1998;11:1.

934. Gallagher PG, Forget BG. Hematologically important mutations: spectrin and ankyrin variants in hereditary spherocytosis. *Blood Cells Mol Dis* 1998;24:539–543.

935. Eber SW, Lux SE. Genetic disorders of the red-cell membrane. In: Weatherall D, Ledingham JGG, Warrell DA, eds. *Oxford textbook of medicine,* 3rd ed. Oxford: Oxford University Press, 1995:3527–3533.

936. Tse WT, Gallagher PG, Jenkins PB, et al. Amino-acid substitution in α-spectrin commonly coinherited with nondominant hereditary spherocytosis. *Am J Hematol* 1997;54:233.

937. Jarolim P, Wichterle H, Palek J, et al. The low expression α spectrin LEPRA is frequently associated with autosomal recessive/nondominant hereditary spherocytosis. *Blood* 1996;88[Suppl 1]:4a (abst).

938. Wichterle H, Hanspal M, Palek J, et al. Combination of two mutant α spectrin alleles underlies a severe spherocytic hemolytic anemia. *J Clin Invest* 1996;98:2300–2307.

939. Dhermy D, Steen-Johnsen J, Bournier O, et al. Coinheritance of two alpha-spectrin gene defects in a recessive spherocytosis family. *Clin Lab Haematol* 2000;22:329–336.

940. Miraglia del Giudice E, Nobili B, Francese M, et al. Clinical and molecular evaluation of non-dominant hereditary spherocytosis. *Br J Haematol* 2001;112:42–47.

941. Bassères DS, Vicentim DL, Costa FF, et al. β-spectrin Promissão: a translation initiation codon mutation of the β-spectrin gene (ATG→GTG) associated with hereditary spherocytosis and spectrin deficiency in a Brazilian family. *Blood* 1998;91:368–369.

942. Garbarz M, Galand C, Bibas D, et al. A 5′ splice region G→C mutation in exon 3 of the human β-spectrin gene leads to decreased levels of β-spectrin mRNA and is responsible for dominant hereditary spherocytosis (spectrin Guemene-Penfao). *Br J Haematol* 1998;100:90–98.

943. Hassoun H, Vassiliadis JN, Murray J, et al. Characterization of the underlying molecular defect in hereditary spherocytosis associated with spectrin deficiency. *Blood* 1997;90:398–406.

944. Dhermy D, Galand C, Bournier O, et al. Hereditary spherocytosis with spectrin deficiency related to null mutations of the β-spectrin gene. *Blood Cells Mol Dis* 1998;24:251–261.

945. Wolfe LC, John KM, Falcone JC, et al. A genetic defect in the binding of protein 4.1 to spectrin in a kindred with hereditary spherocytosis. *N Engl J Med* 1982;307:1367–1374.

946. Becker PS, Cohen CM, Lux SE. The effect of mild diamide oxidation on the structure and function of human erythrocyte spectrin. *J Biol Chem* 1986;261:4620–4628.

947. Becker PS, Morrow JS, Lux SE. Abnormal oxidant sensitivity and beta-chain structure of spectrin in hereditary spherocytosis associated with defective spectrin-protein 4.1 binding. *J Clin Invest* 1987;80:557–565.

948. Becker PS, Tse WT, Lux SE, et al. β Spectrin Kissimmee: a spectrin variant associated with autosomal dominant hereditary spherocytosis and defective spherocytosis and defective binding to protein 4.1. *J Clin Invest* 1993;92:612–616.

949. Bassères DS, Tavares AC, Bordin S. Novel β-spectrin variants associated with hereditary spherocytosis. *Blood* 1997;90[Suppl 1]:4b(abst).

950. Bassères DS, Duarte AS, Hassoun H, et al. β Spectrin S(ta) Barbara: a novel frameshift mutation in hereditary spherocytosis associated with detectable levels of mRNA and a germ cell line mosaicism. *Br J Haematol* 2001;115:347–353.

951. Hassoun H, Vassiliadis JN, Murray J, et al. Hereditary spherocytosis with spectrin deficiency due to an unstable truncated β spectrin. *Blood* 1996;87:2538–2545.

952. Hassoun H, Vassiliadis JN, Murray J, et al. Molecular basis of spectrin deficiency in β spectrin Durham: a deletion within β spectrin adjacent to the ankyrin-binding site precludes spectrin attachment to the membrane in hereditary spherocytosis. *J Clin Invest* 1995;96:2623–2629.

953. Agre P, Orringer EP, Bennett V. Deficient red-cell spectrin in severe, recessively inherited spherocytosis. *N Engl J Med* 1982;306:1155–1161.

954. Chasis JA, Agre PA, Mohandas N. Decreased membrane mechanical stability and in vivo loss of surface area reflect spectrin deficiencies in hereditary spherocytosis. *J Clin Invest* 1988;82:617–623.

955. Liu SC, Derick LH, Agre P, et al. Alteration of the erythrocyte membrane skeletal ultrastructure in hereditary spherocytosis, hereditary elliptocytosis, and pyropoikilocytosis. *Blood* 1990;76:198–205.

956. Waugh RE, Agre P. Reductions of erythrocyte membrane viscoelastic coefficients reflect spectrin deficiencies in hereditary spherocytosis. *J Clin Invest* 1988;81:133–141.

957. Hanspal M, Yoon SH, Yu H, et al. Molecular basis of spectrin and ankyrin deficiencies in severe hereditary spherocytosis: evidence implicating a primary defect of ankyrin. *Blood* 1991;77:165–173.

958. Goodman SR, Shiffer KA, Casoria LA, et al. Identification of the molecular defect in the erythrocyte membrane skeleton of some kindreds with hereditary spherocytosis. *Blood* 1982;60:772–784.

959. Cohen CM, Tyler JM, Branton D. Spectrin-actin associations studied by electron microscopy of shadowed preparations. *Cell* 1980;21:875–883.

960. Becker PS, Schwartz MA, Morrow JS, et al. Radiolabel-transfer crosslinking demonstrates that protein 4.1 binds to the N-terminal region of beta spectrin and to actin in binary interactions. *Eur J Biochem* 1990;193:827–836.

961. Wolfe LC, Byrne AM, Lux SE. Molecular defect in the membrane skeleton of blood bank-stored red cells. Abnormal spectrin-protein 4.1-actin complex formation. *J Clin Invest* 1986;78:1681–1686.

962. Fujino T, Ishikawa T, Inoue M, et al. Characterization of membrane-bound serine protease related to degradation of oxidatively damaged erythrocyte membrane proteins. *Biochim Biophys Acta* 1998;1374:47–55.

963. Leite RC, Bassères DS, Ferreira JS, et al. Low frequency of ankyrin mutations in hereditary spherocytosis: identification of three novel mutations. *Hum Mutat* 2000;16:529.

964. Eber SW, Lux ML, Gonzalez JM, et al. Discovery of 8 ankyrin mutations in hereditary spherocytosis (HS) indicates that ankyrin defects are a major cause of dominant and recessive HS. *Blood* 1993;82[Suppl 1]:308a (abst).

965. Nilson DG, Wong C, et al. A dinucleotide deletion in the downstream promoter element of the ankyrin gene associated with hereditary spherocytosis disrupts promoter function in transgenic mice. *Blood* 2001;98[Suppl 1]:8a (abst).

966. Morlé L, Bozon M, Alloisio N, et al. Ankyrin Bugey: a de novo deletional frameshift variant in exon 6 of the ankyrin gene associated with spherocytosis. *Am J Hematol* 1997;54:242.

967. Randon J, Miraglia del Giudice E, Bozon M, et al. Frequent de novo mutations of the ANK1 gene mimic a recessive mode of transmission in hereditary spherocytosis: three new ANK1 variants: ankyrins Bari, Napoli II and Anzio. *Br J Haematol* 1997;96:500–506.

968. Eber SW, Pekrun A, Reinhardt D, et al. Hereditary spherocytosis with ankyrin Walsrode, a variant ankyrin with decreased affinity for band 3. *Blood* 1994;84[Suppl 1]:362a (abst).

969. Gallagher PG, Ferreira JD, Costa FF, et al. A recurrent frameshift mutation of the ankyrin gene associated with severe hereditary spherocytosis. *Br J Haematol* 2000;111:1190–1193.

970. Gallagher PG, Ferreira JD, Costa FF, et al. A recurrent frameshift mutation of the ankyrin gene associated with severe hereditary spherocytosis. *Br J Haematol* 2000;111:1190–1193.

971. Miraglia del Giudice E, Hayette S, Bozon M, et al. Ankyrin Napoli: a de novo deletional frameshift mutation in exon 16 of ankyrin gene (ANK1) associated with spherocytosis. *Br J Haematol* 1996;93:828–834.

972. Özcan R, Jarolim P, Brabec V, et al. High frequency of frameshift/nonsense mutations of ankyrin-1 in Czech patients with dominant hereditary spherocytosis. *Blood* 1996;88[Suppl 1]:5a (abst).

973. Reference deleted.

974. Reference deleted.

975. Jarolim P, Brabec V, Lambert S, et al. Ankyrin Prague: A dominantly inherited mutation of the regulatory domain of ankyrin associated with hereditary spherocytosis. *Blood* 1990;76[Suppl 1]:37a (abst).

976. Jarolim P, Rubin HL, Brabec V, et al. Abnormal alternative splicing of erythroid ankyrin mRNA in two kindred with hereditary spherocytosis (Ankyrin Prague and Ankyrin Rakovnik). *Blood* 1993;82[Suppl 1]:5a (abst).

977. Hayette S, Carre G, Bozon M, et al. Two distinct truncated variants of ankyrin associated with hereditary spherocytosis. *Am J Hematol* 1998;58:36–41.

978. Woods CM, Lazarides E. Spectrin assembly in avian erythroid development is determined by competing reactions of subunit homo- and hetero-oligomerization. *Nature* 1986;321:85–89.

979. Jarolim P, Murray JL, Rubin HL, et al. Characterization of 13 novel band 3 gene defects in hereditary spherocytosis with band 3 deficiency. *Blood* 1996;88:4366–4374.

980. Miraglia del Giudice E, Iolascon A, Pinto L, et al. Erythrocyte membrane protein alterations underlying clinical heterogeneity in hereditary spherocytosis. *Br J Haematol* 1994;88:52–55.

981. Dhermy D, Galand C, Bournier O, et al. Heterogenous band 3 deficiency in hereditary spherocytosis related to different band 3 gene defects. *Br J Haematol* 1997;98:32–40.

982. Lanciotti M, Perutelli P, Valetto A, et al. Ankyrin deficiency is the most common defect in dominant and non dominant hereditary spherocytosis. *Haematologica* 1997;82:460.

983. Saad ST, Costa FF, Vicentim DL, et al. Red cell membrane protein abnormalities in hereditary spherocytosis in Brazil. *Br J Haematol* 1994;88:295.

984. Miraglia del Giudice E, Francese M, Polito R, et al. Apparently normal ankyrin content in unsplenectomized hereditary spherocytosis patients with the inactivation of one ankyrin (ANK1) allele. *Haematologica* 1997;82:332–333.

985. Jarolim P, Rubin HL, Brabec V, et al. Comparison of the ankyrin (AC)n microsatellites in genomic DNA and mRNA reveals absence of one ankyrin mRNA allele in 20% of patients with hereditary spherocytosis. *Blood* 1995;85:3278–3282.

986. Jarolim P, Rubin HL, Brabec V, et al. A nonsense mutation 1669Glu→Ter within the regulatory domain of human erythroid ankyrin leads to a selective deficiency of the major ankyrin isoform (band 2.1) and a phenotype of autosomal dominant hereditary spherocytosis. *J Clin Invest* 1995;95:941–947.

987. Gallagher PG, Sabatino DE, Basseres DS, et al. Erythrocyte ankyrin promoter mutations associated with recessive hereditary spherocytosis cause significant abnormalities in ankyrin expression. *J Biol Chem* 2001;276:41683–41689.

988. Yawata Y, Kanzaki A, Yawata A, et al. Characteristic features of the genotype and phenotype of hereditary spherocytosis in the Japanese population. *Int J Hematol* 2000;71:118–135.

989. Alloisio N, Maillet P, Carre G, et al. Hereditary spherocytosis with band 3 deficiency. Association with a nonsense mutation of the band 3 gene (allele Lyon), and aggravation by a low-expression allele occurring in trans (allele Genas). *Blood* 1996;88:1062–1069.

990. Alloisio N, Texier P, Vallier A, et al. Modulation of clinical expression and band 3 deficiency in hereditary spherocytosis. *Blood* 1997;90:414–420.

991. Miraglia del Giudice E, Vallier A, Maillet P, et al. Novel band 3 variants (bands 3 Foggia, Napoli I and Napoli II) associated with hereditary spherocytosis and band 3 deficiency: status of the D38A polymorphism within the EPB3 locus. *Br J Haematol* 1997;96:70–76.

992. Bracher NA, Lyons CA, Wessels G, et al. Band 3 Cape Town (E90K) causes severe hereditary spherocytosis in combination with band 3 Prague III. *Br J Haematol* 2001;113:689–693.

993. Kanzaki A, Takezono M, Kaku M. Molecular and genetic characteristics in Japanese patients with hereditary spherocytosis: frequent band 3 mutations and rarer ankyrin mutations. *Blood* 1997;90[Suppl 1]:6b (abst).

994. Inoue T, Kanzaki A, Kaku M, et al. Homozygous missense mutation (band 3 Fukuoka: G130R): a mild form of hereditary spherocytosis with near-normal band 3 content and minimal changes of membrane ultrastructure despite moderate protein 4.2 deficiency. *Br J Haematol* 1998;102:932–939.

995. Lux S, Bedrosian C, Shalev O, et al. Deficiency of band 3 in dominant hereditary spherocytosis with normal spectrin content. *Clin Res* 1990;38:300a (abst).

996. Lima PR, Gontijo JA, Lopes de Faria JB, et al. Band 3 Campinas: a novel splicing mutation in the band 3 gene (AE1) associated with hereditary spherocytosis, hyperactivity of Na$^+$/Li$^+$ countertransport and an abnormal renal bicarbonate handling. *Blood* 1997;90:2810–2818.

997. Jenkins PB, Abou-Alfa GK, Dhermy D, et al. A nonsense mutation in the erythrocyte band 3 gene associated with decreased mRNA accumulation in a kindred with dominant hereditary spherocytosis. *J Clin Invest* 1996;97:373–380.

998. Bianchi P, Zanella A, Alloisio N, et al. A variant of the EPB3 gene of the anti-Lepore type in hereditary spherocytosis. *Br J Haematol* 1997;98:283–288.

999. Maillet P, Vallier A, Reinhart WH, et al. Band 3 Chur: a variant associated with band 3-deficient hereditary spherocytosis and substitution in a highly conserved position of transmembrane segment 11. *Br J Haematol* 1995;91:804–810.

1000. Jarolim P, Rubin HL, Liu SC, et al. Duplication of 10 nucleotides in the erythroid band 3 (AE1) gene in a kindred with hereditary spherocytosis and band 3 protein deficiency (Band 3 PRAGUE). *J Clin Invest* 1994;93:121–130.

1001. Iwase S, Ideguchi H, Takao M, et al. Band 3 Tokyo: Thr837→Ala837 substitution in erythrocyte band 3 protein associated with spherocytic hemolysis. *Acta Haematol* 1999;100:200–203.

1002. Perrotta S, Polito F, Cone ML, et al. Hereditary spherocytosis due to a novel frameshift mutation in AE1 cytoplasmic COOH terminal tail: band 3 Vesuvio. *Blood* 1999;93:2131–2132.

1003. Kanzaki A, Hayette S, Morlé L, et al. Total absence of protein 4.2 and partial deficiency of band 3 in hereditary spherocytosis. *Br J Haematol* 1997;99:522.

1004. Quilty JA, Reithmeier RA. Trafficking and folding defects in hereditary spherocytosis mutants of the human red cell anion exchanger. *Traffic* 2000;1:987–998.

1005. Vince JW, Reithmeier RA. Carbonic anhydrase II binds to the carboxyl terminus of human band 3, the erythrocyte C1$^-$/HCO$_3^-$ exchanger. *J Biol Chem* 1998;273:28430.

1006. Rysava R, Tesar V, Jirsa M Jr, et al. Incomplete distal renal tubular acidosis coinherited with a mutation in the band 3 (AE1) gene. *Nephrol Dial Transplant* 1997;12:1869.

1007. Jarolim P, Shayakul C, Prabakaran D, et al. Autosomal dominant distal renal tubular acidosis is associated in three families with heterozygosity for the R589H mutation in the AE1 (band 3) Cl$^-$/HCO$_3^-$exchanger. *J Biol Chem* 1998;273:6380.

1008. Inaba M, Yawata A, Koshino I, et al. Defective anion transport and marked spherocytosis with membrane instability caused by hereditary total deficiency of red cell band 3 in cattle due to a nonsense mutation. *J Clin Invest* 1996;97:1804.

1009. Bruce LJ, Cope DL, Jones GK, et al. Familial distal renal tubular acidosis is associated with mutations in the red cell anion exchanger (Band 3, AE1) gene. *J Clin Invest* 1997;100:1693.

1010. Karet FE, Gainza FJ, Gyory AZ, et al. Mutations in the chloride-bicarbonate exchanger gene AE1 cause autosomal dominant but not autosomal recessive distal renal tubular acidosis. *Proc Natl Acad Sci U S A* 1998;95:6337.

1011. Tanphaichitr VS, Sumboonnanonda A, Ideguchi H, et al. Novel AE1 mutations in recessive distal renal tubular acidosis: loss-of-function is rescued by glycophorin A. *J Clin Invest* 1998;102:2173.

1012. Kanzaki A, Yawata Y, Yawata A, et al. Band 4.2 Komatsu: 523 GAT→TAT (175 Asp→Tyr) in exon 4 of the band 4.2 gene associated with total deficiency of band 4.2, hemolytic anemia with ovalostomatocytosis and marked disruption of the cytoskeletal network. *Int J Hematol* 1995;61:165.

1013. Matsuda M, Hatano N, Ideguchi H, et al. A novel mutation causing an aberrant splicing in the protein 4.2 gene associated with hereditary spherocytosis (protein 4.2 Notame). *Hum Mol Genet* 1995;4:1187.

1014. Hayette S, Morlé L, Bozon M, et al. A point mutation in the protein 4.2 gene (allele 4.2 Tozeur) associated with hereditary haemolytic anaemia. *Br J Haematol* 1995;89:762.

1015. Ghanem A, Pothier B, Maréchal J, et al. A haemolytic syndrome associated with the complete absence of red cell membrane protein 4.2 in two Tunisian siblings. *Br J Haematol* 1990;75:414.

1016. Kanzaki A, Yasunaga M, Okamoto N, et al. Band 4.2 Shiga: 317 CGC→TGC in compound heterozygotes with 142 GCT→ACT results in band 4.2 deficiency and microspherocytosis. *Br J Haematol* 1995;91:333.

1017. Beauchamp-Nicoud A, Morle L, Lutz HU, et al. Heavy transfusions and presence of an anti-protein 4.2 antibody in 4.2(-) hereditary spherocytosis (949delG). *Haematologica* 2000;85:19–24.

1018. Rybicki AC, Heath R, Wolf JL, et al. Deficiency of protein 4.2 in erythrocytes from a patient with a Coombs negative hemolytic anemia. Evidence for a role of protein 4.2 in stabilizing ankyrin on the membrane. *J Clin Invest* 1988;81:893–901.

1019. Rybicki AC, Heath R, Wolf JL, et al. Deficiency of protein 4.2 in erythrocytes from a patient with a Coombs negative hemolytic anemia. Evidence for a role of protein 4.2 in stabilizing ankyrin on the membrane. *J Clin Invest* 1988;81:893.

1020. Inoue T, Kanzaki A, Yawata A, et al. Electron microscopic and physicobiochemical studies on disorganization of the cytoskeletal network and integral protein (band 3) in red cells of band 4.2 deficiency with a mutation (codon 142: GCT→ACT). *Int J Hematol* 1994;59:157–175.

1021. Ideguchi H, Nishimura J, Nawata H, et al. A genetic defect of erythrocyte band 4.2 protein associated with hereditary spherocytosis. *Br J Haematol* 1990;74:347–353.

1022. Yawata Y. Band 4.2 abnormalities in human red cells. *Am J Med Sci* 1994;307:190–203.

1023. Lux SE, Glader BE. Disorders of the red cell membrane. In: Nathan DG, Oski FA, eds. *Hematology of infancy and childhood*, 2nd ed. Philadelphia: WB Saunders, 1981:456–565.

1024. Lux SE. Disorders of the red cell membrane. In: Nathan DG, Oski FA, eds. *Hematology of infancy and childhood*, 3rd ed. Philadelphia: WB Saunders, 1987:444–544.

1025. Sheehy R, Ralston GB. Abnormal binding of spectrin to the membrane of erythrocytes in some cases of hereditary spherocytosis. *Blut* 1978;36:145–148.

1026. Price Evans DA, Mackie MJ, Anand R. Diminished extractable spectrin in the erythrocytes of a patient with 'sporadic' hereditary spherocytosis. *Acta Haematol* 1986;76:136–140.

1027. Mariani M, Maretzki D, Lutz HU. A tightly membrane-associated subpopulation of spectrin is 3H-palmitoylated. *J Biol Chem* 1993;268:12996–13001.

1028. Allen DW, Cadman S, McCann SR, et al. Increased membrane binding of erythrocyte catalase in hereditary spherocytosis and in metabolically stressed normal cells. *Blood* 1977;49:113–123.

1029. Boulard-Heitzmann P, Boulard M, Tallineau C, et al. Decreased red cell enolase activity in a 40-year-old woman with compensated hemolysis. *Scand J Haematol* 1984;33:401–404.

1030. Lachant NA, Jennings MA, Tanaka KR. Partial erythrocyte enolase deficiency: a heritable disorder with variable clinical expression. *Blood* 1986;68[Suppl 1]:55a (abst).

1030a. Lachant NA, Tanaka KR. Enolase kinetic properties in partial erythrocyte enolase deficiency. *Clin Res* 1987;35:426a (abst).

1031. Beutler E, Guinto E, Johnson C. Human red cell protein kinase in normal subjects and patients with hereditary spherocytosis, sickle cell disease, and autoimmune hemolytic anemia. *Blood* 1976;48:887–898.

1032. Boivin P, Delaunay J, Galand C. Altered erythrocyte membrane protein phosphorylation in an unusual case of hereditary spherocytosis. *Scand J Haematol* 1979;23:251–255.

1033. Wolfe LC, Lux SE. Membrane protein phosphorylation of intact normal and hereditary spherocytic erythrocytes. *J Biol Chem* 1978;253:3336–3342.

1034. Pinder JC, Dhermy D, Baines AJ, et al. A phenomenological difference between membrane skeletal protein complexes isolated from normal and hereditary spherocytosis erythrocytes. *Br J Haematol* 1983;55:455–463.

1035. Armbrust R, Eber SW, Schröter W. Absence of phosphorylation-induced gelation of erythrocyte membrane skeletons: a diagnostic tool for hereditary spherocytosis. *Ann Hematol* 1993;64:93–96.

1036. De Gier J, Van Deenen LLM. Phospholipid and fatty acid characteristics of erythrocytes in some cases of anaemia. *Br J Haematol* 1964;10:246.

1037. Kuiper PJC, Livne A. Differences in fatty acid composition between normal erythrocytes and hereditary spherocytosis affected cells. *Biochim Biophys Acta* 1972;260:755–758.

1038. Zail SS, Pickering A. Fatty acid composition of erythrocytes in hereditary spherocytosis. *Br J Haematol* 1979;42:399–402.

1039. Bertles JE. Sodium transport across the surface of red blood cells in hereditary spherocytosis. *J Clin Invest* 1957;36:816–824.

1040. Jacob HS, Jandl JH. Cell membrane permeability in the pathogenesis of hereditary spherocytosis (HS). *J Clin Invest* 1964;43:1704–1720.

1041. Joiner CH, Franco RS, Jiang M, et al. Increased cation permeability in mutant mouse red cells with defective membrane skeletons. *Blood* 1995;86:4307–4314.

1042. Wiley JS. Red cell survival in hereditary spherocytosis. *J Clin Invest* 1970;49:666–672.

1043. Oski FA, Naiman JL, et al. Congenital hemolytic anemia with high sodium, low potassium red cells: studies of three generations of a family with a new variant. *N Engl J Med* 1969;280:909.

1044. Mayman D, Zipursky A. Hereditary spherocytosis: the metabolism of erythrocytes in the peripheral blood and in the splenic pulp. *Br J Haematol* 1974;27:201–217.

1045. Palek J, Mirevova L, Brabec V. 2,3-Diphosphoglycerate metabolism in hereditary spherocytosis. *Br J Haematol* 1969;17:59.

1046. Olivieri O, Bonollo M, Friso S, et al. Activation of K$^+$/Cl$^-$ cotransport in human erythrocytes exposed to oxidative agents. *Biochim Biophys Acta* 1993;1176:37–42.

1047. Loder PB, Babarczy G, et al. Red cell metabolism in hereditary spherocytosis. *Br J Haematol* 1967;13:95.

1048. Mohler DN. Adenosine triphosphate metabolism in hereditary spherocytosis. *J Clin Invest* 1965;44:1417.

1049. Kagimoto T, Hayashi F, et al. Phosphorus ^{31}NMR study on nucleotides and intracellular pH of hereditary spherocytes. *Experientia* 1978;34:1092.

1050. Ideguchi H, Hamasaki N, Ikehara Y. Abnormal phosphoenolpyruvate transport in erythrocytes of hereditary spherocytosis. *Blood* 1981;58:426–430.

1051. Peters LL, Barker JE. Spontaneous and targeted mutations in erythrocyte membrane skeleton genes: mouse models of hereditary spheroctyosis. In: Zon LI, ed. *Hematopoiesis, a developmental approach.* Oxford: Oxford University Press, 2001:582–609.

1052. Lux SE. Spectrin-actin membrane skeleton of normal and abnormal red blood cells. *Semin Hematol* 1979;16:21.

1053. Anderson R, Huestis RR, Motulsky AG. Hereditary spherocytosis in the deer mouse: its similarity to the human disease. *Blood* 1960;15:491.

1054. Reference deleted.

1055. Bloom ML, Kaysser TM, Birkenmeier CS, et al. The murine mutation jaundiced is caused by replacement of an arginine with a stop codon in the mRNA encoding the ninth repeat of β-spectrin. *Proc Natl Acad Sci U S A* 1994;91:10099.

1056. Wandersee NJ, Birkenmeier CS, Gifford EJ, et al. Identification of three mutations in the murine erythroid α spectrin gene causing hereditary spherocytosis in mice. *Blood* 1998;92[Suppl 1]:8a (abst).

1057. Wandersee NJ, Birkenmeier CS, Gifford EJ, et al. Murine recessive hereditary spherocytosis, *sph/sph*, is caused by a mutation in the erythroid alpha-spectrin gene. *Hematol J* 2000;1:235–242.

1057a. Wandersee NJ, Birkenmeier CS, Bodine DM, et al. Mutations in the murine erythroid α-spectrin gene alter spectrin mRNA and protein levels and spectrin incorporation into the red blood cell membrane skeleton. *Blood* 2002; in press.

1058. Wandersee NJ, Roesch AN, Hamblen NR, et al. Defective spectrin integrity and neonatal thrombosis in the first mouse model for severe hereditary elliptocytosis. *Blood* 2001;97:543–550.

1059. Kaysser TM, Wandersee NJ, Bronson RT, et al. Thrombosis and secondary hemochromatosis play major roles in the pathogenesis of jaundiced and spherocytic mice, murine models for hereditary spherocytosis. *Blood* 1997;90:4610.

1060. Wandersee NJ, Lee JC, Kaysser TM, et al. Hematopoietic cells from α spectrin-deficient mice are sufficient to induce thrombotic events in hematopoietically ablated recipients. *Blood* 1998;92:4856.

1061. Wandersee NJ, Tait JF, Barker JE. Erythroid phosphatidyl serine exposure is not predictive of thrombotic risk in mice with hemolytic anemia. *Blood Cells Mol Dis* 2000;26:75–83.

1062. Liao EC, Paw BH, Peters LL, et al. Hereditary spherocytosis in zebrafish riesling illustrates evolution of erythroid beta-spectrin structure, and function in red cell morphogenesis and membrane stability. *Development* 2000;127:5123–5132.

1063. Birkenmeier CS, Gifford EJ, Gwynn BF, et al. Mutations of the erythroid ankyrin gene: a hypomorph and a null. *Blood* 2000;96[Suppl 1]:594a (abst).

1064. Peters LL, Turtzo LC, Birkenmeier CS, et al. Distinct fetal Ank-1 and Ank-2 related proteins and mRNAs in normal and *nb/nb* mice. *Blood* 1993;81:2144.

1065. Peters LL, Birkenmeier CS, Barker JE. Fetal compensation of the hemolytic anemia in mice homozygous for the normoblastosis (*nb*) mutation. *Blood* 1992;80:2122.

1066. Peters LL, Swearingen RA, Gwynn B, et al. Failure of effective reticulocytosis in a new spontaneous band 3 deficient mouse stain (C3H/HeJ-*wan*) and in a subset of targeted band 3 null mice (B6,129 AE−/−) suggests the presence of genetic modifiers of band 3 function in red blood cells. *Blood* 1998;92[Suppl 1]:301a (abst).

1067. Peters LL, Andersen SG, Gwynn B, et al. A QTL on mouse chromosome 12 modifies the band 3 null phenotype: β spectrin is a candidate gene. *Blood* 2001;98[Suppl 1]:437a (abst).

1067a. Shafizadeh E, Paw BH, Foott H, et al. Characterization of zebrafish *merlot/chablis* as non-mammalian vertebrate models for severe congenital anemia due to protein 4.1 deficiency. *Development* 2002;129:4359–4370.

1068. Khanna R, Azam M, Andrabi S, et al. Targeted mutagenesis reveals an essential role of headpiece domain of dematin in the stability of erythroid membrane skeleton. *Blood* 2001;98[Suppl 1]:435a (abst).

1069. LeBlond PF, De Boisfleury A, Bessis M. La forme des érythrocytes dans la sphérocytose héréditaire. Etude au microscope Ö balayage. Rélation avec déformabilité. *Nouv Rev Fr Hématol* 1973;13:873.

1070. Cooper RA, Jandl JH. The role of membrane lipids in the survival of red cells in hereditary spherocytosis. *J Clin Invest* 1969;48:736–744.

1071. Johnsson R. Red cell membrane proteins and lipids in spherocytosis. *Scand J Haematol* 1978;20:341–350.

1072. Reed CF, Swisher SN. Erythrocyte lipid loss in hereditary spherocytosis. *J Clin Invest* 1966;45:777–781.

1073. Cooper RA, Jandl JH. The selective and conjoint loss of red cell lipids. *J Clin Invest* 1969;48:906–914.

1074. Weed RI, Bowdler AJ. Metabolic dependence of the critical hemolytic volume of human erythrocytes: relationship to osmotic fragility and autohemolysis in hereditary spherocytosis and normal red cells. *J Clin Invest* 1966; 45:1137–1149.

1075. Zachèe P, Boogaerts MA, Hellemans L, et al. Adverse role of the spleen in hereditary spherocytosis: evidence by the use of the atomic force microscope. *Br J Haematol* 1992;80:264–265.

1076. Miraglia del Giudice E, Perrotta S, Pinto L, et al. Hereditary spherocytosis characterized by increased spectrin/band 3 ratio [Letter]. *Br J Haematol* 1990;80:133–136.

1077. Corbett JD, Agre P, Palek J, et al. Differential control of band 3 lateral and rotational mobility in intact red cells. *J Clin Invest* 1994;94:683–688.

1078. Evans EA, Waugh R, Melnik C. Elastic area compressibility modulus of red cell membranes. *Biophys J* 1976;16:585–595.

1079. Baird R, McPherson AS, Richmond J. Red blood cell survival after splenectomy in congenital spherocytosis. *Lancet* 1971;2:1060–1061.

1080. Chapman RG. Red cell life span after splenectomy in hereditary spherocytosis. *J Clin Invest* 1968;47:2263–2267.

1081. Barnhart MT, Lusher JM. The human spleen as revealed by scanning electron microscopy. *Am J Hematol* 1976;1:243–264.

1082. Chen LT, Weiss L. Electron microscopy of red pulp of human spleen. *Am J Anat* 1972;134:425–457.

1083. Chen LT, Weiss L. The role of the sinus wall in the passage of erythrocytes through the spleen. *Blood* 1973;41:529–537.

1084. Weiss L, Tavassoli M. Anatomical hazards to the passage of erythrocytes through the spleen. *Semin Hematol* 1970;7:372.

1085. Weiss L. A scanning electron microscopic study of the spleen. *Blood* 1974;43:665–691.

1086. Groom AC. Microcirculation of the spleen: new concepts, new challenges. *Microvasc Res* 1987;34:269–289.

1087. Young LE, Platzer RF, Ervin DM, et al. Hereditary spherocytosis. II. Observations on the role of the spleen. *Blood* 1951;6:1099.

1088. Ferreira JA, Feliu E, Rozman C, et al. Morphologic and morphometric light and electron microscopic studies of the spleen in patients with hereditary spherocytosis and autoimmune haemolytic anaemia. *Br J Haematol* 1989;72:246–253.

1089. Molnar Z, Rappaport H. Fine structure of the red pulp of the spleen in hereditary spherocytosis. *Blood* 1972;39:81–98.

1090. Wiland OK, Smith EB. The morphology of the spleen in congenital hemolytic anemia (hereditary spherocytosis). *Am J Clin Pathol* 1956;26:619.

1091. Fujita T, Kashimura M, Adachi K. Scanning electron microscope (SEM) studies of the spleen—normalie and pathological. *Scan Electron Microsc* 1982; Pt 1:435–444.

1092. Banti G. Splenomegalie hemolytique au hemopoietique: le role de la rate dans l'hemolyse. *Sem Med* 1913;33:313–323.

1093. MacAdam W, Shiskin C. The cholesterol content of the blood in anaemia and its relation to splenic function. *QJM* 1922;16:193.

1094. Emerson CP Jr, Shen SC, Ham TH, et al. Studies on the destruction of red blood cells. IX. Quantitative methods for determining the osmotic and mechanical fragility of red cells in the peripheral blood and splenic pulp; the mechanism of increased hemolysis in hereditary spherocytosis (congenital hemolytic jaundice) as related to the function of the spleen. *Arch Intern Med* 1956;97:1–38.

1095. Dacie JV. Familial haemolytic anaemia (acholuric jaundice), with particular reference to changes in fragility produced by splenectomy. *QJM (New Series)* 1943;12:101–118.

1096. Griggs RC, Weisman R Jr, Harris JW. Alterations in osmotic and mechanical fragility related to in vivo erythrocyte aging and splenic sequestration in hereditary spherocytosis. *J Clin Invest* 1960;39:89–101.

1097. MacPherson AIS, Richmond J, Donaldson GWK, et al. The role of the spleen in congenital spherocytosis. *Am J Med* 1971;50:35–41.

1098. Murphy JR. The influence of pH and temperature on some physical properties of normal erythrocytes and erythrocytes from patients with hereditary spherocytosis. *J Lab Clin Med* 1967;69:758–775.

1099. Jandl JH, Aster RH. Increased splenic pooling and the pathogenesis of hypersplenism. *Am J Med Sci* 1967;253:383–398.

1100. Minakami S, Yoshikawa H. Studies on erythrocyte glycolysis. III. The effects of active cation transport, pH and inorganic phosphate concentration on erythrocyte glycolysis. *J Biochem (Tokyo)* 1966;59:145–150.

1101. Rakitzis ET, Mills GC. Relation of red cell hexokinase activity to extracellular pH. *Biochim Biophys Acta* 1967;141:439–441.

1102. Parker JC. Ouabain-insensitive effects of metabolism on ion and water content in red blood cells. *Am J Physiol* 1971;221:338–342.

1103. Dacie JV. Observations on autohemolysis in familial acholuric jaundice. *J Pathol Bacteriol* 1941;52:331–340.

1104. Ferrant A, Leners N, Michaux JL, et al. The spleen and haemolysis: evaluation of the intrasplenic transit time. *Br J Haematol* 1987;65:331–334.

1105. Motulsky AG, Casserd F, Giblett ER, et al. Anemia and the spleen. *N Engl J Med* 1958;259:1164 and 1958;259:1212.

1106. Prankerd TAJ. Studies on the pathogenesis of haemolysis in hereditary spherocytosis. *QJM (New Series)* 1960;24:199.

1107. Maridonneau I, Braquet P, et al. Na+ and K+ transport damage induced by oxygen free radicals in human red cell membranes. *J Biol Chem* 1983;258:3107.

1108. Orringer EP, Parker JC. Selective increase of potassium permeability in red blood cells exposed to acetylphenylhydrazine. *Blood* 1977;50:1013.

1109. Sugihara T, Rawicz W, Evans EA, et al. Lipid hydroperoxides permit deformation-dependent leak of monovalent cation from erythrocytes. *Blood* 1991;77:2757–2763.

1110. Johnson GJ, Allen DW, Flynn TP, et al. Decreased survival in vivo of diamide-incubated dog erythrocytes. A model of oxidant-induced hemolysis. *J Clin Invest* 1980;66:955–961.

1111. Platt OS, Falcone JF. Membrane protein lesions in erythrocytes with Heinz bodies. *J Clin Invest* 1988;82:1051–1058.

1112. Caprari P, Bozzi A, Ferroni L, et al. Oxidative erythrocyte membrane damage in hereditary spherocytosis. *Biochem Int* 1992;26:265–274.

1113. Malorni W, Iosi F, Donelli G, et al. A new, striking morphologic feature for the human erythrocyte in hereditary spherocytosis: the blebbing pattern [Letter]. *Blood* 1993;81:2821–2822.

1114. Caprari P, Bozzi A, Malorni W, et al. Junctional sites of erythrocyte skeletal proteins are specific targets of tert-butylhydroperoxide oxidative damage. *Chem Biol Interact* 1995;94:243–258.

1115. De Matteis MC, De Angelis V, Sorrentino F, et al. Role of spleen in hereditary spherocytosis: evidence for increased in vitro proteolysis of red cell membrane. *Br J Haematol* 1991;79:108–112.

1116. Szymanski IO, Odgren PR, et al. Red blood cell associated IgG in normal and pathologic states. *Blood* 1980;55:48.

1117. Coleman DH, Finch CA. Effect of adrenal steroids in hereditary spherocytic anemia. *J Lab Clin Med* 1956;47:602–610.

1118. Duru F, Gürgey A. Effect of corticosteroids in hereditary spherocytosis. *Acta Paediatr Jpn* 1994;36:666–668.

1119. Atkinson JP, Schreiber AS, et al. Effects of corticosteroids and splenectomy on the immune clearance and destruction of erythrocytes. *J Clin Invest* 1973;52:1509–1517.

1120. Schreiber AD, Parsons J, et al. Effect of corticosteroids on the human monocyte IgG and complement receptors. *J Clin Invest* 1975;56:1189.

1121. Matsumoto N, Ishihara T, Shibata M, et al. Electron microscopic studies of the spleen and liver in hereditary spherocytosis. *Acta Pathol Jpn* 1973;23:507–530.

1122. Bowman HS, Oski FA. Splenic macrophage interaction with red cells in pyruvate kinase deficiency and hereditary spherocytosis. *Vox Sang* 1970;19:168–175.

1123. Muller-Eberhard U, Javid J, Liem HH, et al. Plasma concentrations of hemopexin, haptoglobin and heme in patients with various hemolytic diseases. *Blood* 1968;32:811–815.

1123a. Palek J, Lambert S. Genetics of the red cell membrane skeleton. *Semin Hematol* 1990;27:290–332.

1124. Reference deleted.

1125. Bassères DS, Pranke PH, Sales TS, et al. β-spectrin Campinas: a novel shortened β-chain variant associated with skipping of exon 30 and hereditary elliptocytosis. *Br J Haematol* 1997;97:579.

1126. Reinhart WH, Wyss EJ, Arnold D, et al. Hereditary spherocytosis associated with protein band 3 defect in a Swiss kindred. *Br J Haematol* 1994;86:147.

1127. Da Costa L, Mohandas N, Sorette M, et al. Temporal differences in membrane loss lead to distinct reticulocyte features in hereditary spherocytosis and in immune hemolytic anemia. *Blood* 2001;98:2894–2899.

1128. Bell CM, Parker AC, Maddy AH. Abnormal pattern of erythrocyte ageing in hereditary spherocytosis as shown by Percoll density gradient centrifugation. *Clin Chim Acta* 1984;142:91–102.

1129. Mohandas N, Kim YR, Tycko DH, et al. Accurate and independent measurement of volume and hemoglobin concentration of individual red cells by laser light scattering. *Blood* 1986;68:506.

1130. Ialongo P, Vignetti M, Cigliano G, et al. Flow cytometric measurement (H-1 Technicon) of microcytic and hyperchromic red cell populations in pediatric patients affected by hereditary spherocytosis. *Haematologica* 1989;74:547.

1131. Cynober T, Mohandas N, Tchernia G. Red cell abnormalities in hereditary spherocytosis: relevance to diagnosis and understanding of the variable expression of clinical severity. *J Lab Clin Med* 1996;128:259.

1132. Gilsanz F, Ricard MP, Millan I. Diagnosis of hereditary spherocytosis with dual-angle differential light scattering. *Am J Clin Pathol* 1993;100:119–220.

1133. Pati AR, Patton WN, Harris RI. The use of the Technicon H1 in the diagnosis of hereditary spherocytosis. *Clin Lab Haematol* 1989;11:27–30.

1134. Michaels LA, Cohen AR, Zhao H, et al. Screening for hereditary spherocytosis by use of automated erythrocyte indexes. *J Pediatr* 1997;130:957.

1135. Parpart AK, Lorenz PB, Parpart ER, et al. The osmotic resistance (fragility) of human red cells. *J Clin Invest* 1947;26:636–640.

1136. Godal HC, Nyvold N, Russtad A. The osmotic fragility of red blood cells: a re-evaluation of technical conditions. *Scand J Haematol* 1979;23:55–58.

1137. Young LE. Observations on inheritance and heterogeneity of chronic spherocytosis. *Trans Assoc Am Physicians* 1955;68:141.

1138. Zanella A, Izzo C, Rebulla P, et al. Acidified glycerol lysis test: a screening test for spherocytosis. *Br J Haematol* 1980;45:481.

1139. Gottfried EL, Robertson NA. Glycerol lysis time of incubated erythrocytes in the diagnosis of hereditary spherocytosis. *J Lab Clin Med* 1974;84:746–751.

1140. Zanella A, Milani S, Fagnani G, et al. Diagnostic value of the glycerol lysis test. *J Lab Clin Med* 1983;102:743–750.

1141. Zanella A, Izzo C, Rebulla P, et al. Acidified glycerol lysis test: a screening test for spherocytosis. *Br J Haematol* 1980;45:481–486.

1142. Rutherford CJ, Postlewaight BF, Hallowes M. An evaluation of the acidified glycerol lysis test. *Br J Haematol* 1986;63:119–121.

1143. Bucx MJL, Breed WPM, Hoffman JJML. Comparison of acidified glycerol lysis test, Pink test and osmotic fragility test in hereditary spherocytosis: effect of incubation. *Eur J Haematol* 1988;40:227–231.

1144. Hoffmann JJ, Swaak-Lammers N, Breed WP, et al. Diagnostic utility of the pre-incubated acidified glycerol lysis test in haemolytic and non-haemolytic anaemias. *Eur J Haematol* 1991;47:367–370.

1145. Marik T, Brabec V. Acidified glycerol lysis test in various haemolytic anaemias. *Folia Haematol Int Mag Klin Morphol Blutforsch* 1990;117:259–263.

1146. Vettore L, Zanella A, et al. A new test for the laboratory diagnosis of spherocytosis. *Acta Haematol* 1984;72:258.

1147. Balari AS, Espinosa JV, Fuertes IF. A new modification of the 'Pink test' for the diagnosis of hereditary spherocytosis. *Acta Haematol* 1989;82:213–214.

1148. Pinto L, Iolascon A, del Giudice EM, et al. A modification of the 'Pink test' may improve the diagnosis of hereditary spherocytosis. *Acta Haematol* 1989;82:53–54.

1149. Streichman S, Gesheidt Y, Tatarsky I. Hypertonic cryohemolysis: a diagnostic test for hereditary spherocytosis. *Am J Hematol* 1990;35:104–109.

1150. Streichman S, Gescheidt Y. Cryohemolysis for the detection of hereditary spherocytosis: correlation studies with osmotic fragility and autohemolysis. *Am J Hematol* 1998;58:206.

1151. Romero RR, Poo JL, Robles JA, et al. Usefulness of cryohemolysis test in the diagnosis of hereditary spherocytosis. *Arch Med Res* 1997;28:247–251.

1152. Melrose W. An evaluation of the hypertonic cryohaemolysis test as a diagnostic test for hereditary spherocytosis. *Aust J Med Sci* 1992;13:22.

1153. Young LE, Izzo MJ, Altman KI, et al. Studies on spontaneous in vitro autohemolysis in hemolytic disorders. *Blood* 1956;11:977.

1154. Selwyn JG, Dacie JV. Autohemolysis and other changes resulting from the incubation in vitro of red cells from patients with congenital hemolytic anemia. *Blood* 1954;9:414.

1155. Langley GR, Feldherhof CH. Atypical autohemolysis in hereditary spherocytosis as a reflection of two cell populations: relationship of cell lipids to conditioning by the spleen. *Blood* 1968;32:569–585.

1156. Mohandas N, Chasis JA. Red blood cell deformability, membrane material properties and shape: regulation by transmembrane, skeletal and cytosolic proteins and lipids. *Semin Hematol* 1993;30:171.

1157. Clark MR, Mohandas N, Shohet SB. Osmotic gradient ektacytometry: comprehensive characterization of red cell volume and surface maintenance. *Blood* 1983;61:899.

1158. Cutillo S, Pinto L, Nobili B, et al. Spectrin/band 3 ratio as diagnostic tool in hereditary spherocytosis. *Eur J Pediatr* 1992;151:35–37.

1159. Byers PH. Killing the messenger: new insights into nonsense-mediated mRNA decay. *J Clin Invest* 2002;109:3–6.

1160. Lykke-Andersen. mRNA quality control: marking the message for life or death. *Curr Biol* 2001;11:R88–91.

1161. Wilusz CJ, Wang W, Peltz SW. Curbing the nonsense: the activation and regulation of mRNA surveillance. *Genes Dev* 2001;15:2781–2785.

1162. Maquat LE, Carmichael GG. Quality control of mRNA function. *Cell* 2001;104:173–176.

1163. Levine DH, Meyer HB. Newborn screening for ABO hemolytic disease. *Clin Pediatr (Phila)* 1985;24:391.

1164. Gilliland BC, Baxter E, Evans RS. Red cell antibodies in acquired hemolytic anemia with negative antiglobulin serum tests. *N Engl J Med* 1971;285:252–256.

1165. Crosby WH, Conrad ME. Hereditary spherocytosis: observations on hemolytic mechanisms and iron metabolism. *Blood* 1960;15:662–674.

1166. Pautard B, Féo C, Dhermy D, et al. Occurrence of hereditary spherocytosis and β thalassemia in the same family: globin chain synthesis and visco diffractometric studies. *Br J Haematol* 1988;70:239–245.

1167. Li CK, Ng MH, Cheung KL, et al. Interaction of hereditary spherocytosis and alpha thalassaemia: a family study. *Acta Haematol* 1994;91:201–205.

1168. Blecher TE. What happens to the microspherocytosis of hereditary spherocytosis in folate deficiency? *Clin Lab Haematol* 1988;10:403–408.

1169. Warkentin TE, Barr RD, Ali MAM, et al. Recurrent acute splenic sequestration crisis due to interacting genetic defects: hemoglobin SC disease and hereditary spherocytosis. *Blood* 1990;75:266–270.

1170. Yang YM, Donnell C, Wilborn W, et al. Splenic sequestration associated with sickle cell trait and hereditary spherocytosis. *Am J Hematol* 1992;40:110–116.

1171. Babiker MA, El Seed FAA. A family with sickle cell trait and hereditary spherocytosis. *Scand J Haematol* 1984;33:54–58.

1172. Zail SS, Krawitz P, Viljoen E, et al. Atypical hereditary spherocytosis: biochemical studies and sites of erythrocyte destruction. *Br J Haematol* 1967;13:323–334.

1173. McCann SR, Jacob HS. Spinal cord disease in hereditary spherocytosis: report of two cases with a hypothesized common mechanism for neurologic and red cell abnormalities. *Blood* 1976;48:259–263.

1174. d'Ermao N, Levi M. *Neurological symptoms in anemia, neurological symptoms in blood diseases.* Baltimore: University Park Press, 1972:1–46.

1175. Curshmann H. Über funikuläre Myelose bei hämolytischem Ikterus. *Dtsch A Nervenheilk* 1931;122:119–125.

1176. Dumolard C, Sarrovy C, Portier A. Ataxie cerebelleuse associèe → un syndrome de splenomegalie chronique avec anemie. *Bull Soc Med Hop (Paris)* 1938;54:71–76.

1177. Lemaire A, Dumolard A, Portici A. Deux cas familiaux de maladie de Friedreich avec maladie hemolytique chez des indigenes algeriens. *Bull Soc Med Hop (Paris)* 1937;53:1084–1087.

1178. Michelazzi AM. Anemia emolitica familiare con sinomatoligia nervosa. *Rass Fisiopat Clin Ter* 1940;12:145–162.

1179. Percorella F. Sindrome neuroanemica in soggetto con ittero imolitico familiare. *Riv Clin Pediatr* 1946;44:690–701.

1180. Salmon H. Hämolytischer Ikterus und Degeneration der Hinterstränge. *Med Klin* 1914;10:312c.

1181. Moiseyev VS, Korovina EA, Polotskaya EL, et al. Hypertrophic cardiomyopathy associated with hereditary spherocytosis in three generations of one family [Letter]. *Lancet* 1987;2:853–854.

1182. Spencer SE, Walker FO, Moore SA. Chorea-amyotrophy with chronic hemolytic anemia: a variant of chorea-amyotrophy with acanthocytosis. *Neurology* 1987;37:645–649.

1183. Porter GA, Scher MG, Resneck WG, et al. Two populations of beta-spectrin in rat skeletal muscle. *Cell Motil Cytoskeleton* 1997;37:7–19.

1184. Bloom ML, Birkenmeier CS, Barker JE. Complete nucleotide sequence of the murine erythroid beta-spectrin cDNA and tissue-specific expression in normal and jaundiced mice. *Blood* 1993;82:2906–2914.

1185. Zhou D, Birkenmeier CS, Williams MW, et al. Small, membrane-bound, alternatively spliced forms of ankyrin 1 associated with the sarcoplasmic reticulum of mammalian skeletal muscle. *J Cell Biol* 1997;136:621–631.

1186. Ho-Yen DO. Hereditary spherocytosis presenting in pregnancy. *Acta Haematol* 1984;72:29.

1187. Pajor A, Lehoczky D, Szakacs Z. Pregnancy and hereditary spherocytosis. Report of 8 patients and a review. *Arch Gynecol Obstet* 1993;253:37.

1188. Owren PA. Congenital hemolytic jaundice. The pathogenesis of the hemolytic crisis. *Blood* 1948;3:231.

1189. Kelleher JF, Luban NL, Mortimer PP, et al. Human serum "parvovirus": a specific cause of aplastic crisis in children with hereditary spherocytosis. *J Pediatr* 1983;102:720.

1190. Young N. Hematologic and hematopoietic consequences of B19 parvovirus infection. *Semin Hematol* 1988;25:159.

1191. Brown KE, Young NS. Parvovirus B19 in human disease. *Annu Rev Med* 1997;48:59–67.

1192. Brown KE. Haematological consequences of parvovirus B19 infection. *Best Pract Res Clin Haematol* 2000;13:245–259.

1193. Owren PA. Congenital hemolytic jaundice. The pathogenesis of the hemolytic crisis. *Blood* 1948;3:231.

1194. Lefrère JJ, Courouce AM, Bertrand Y, et al. Human parvovirus and aplastic crisis in chronic hemolytic anemias: a study of 24 observations. *Am J Hematol* 1986;23:271.

1195. Mortimer PP, Humphries RK, et al. A human parvovirus like virus inhibits haematopoietic colony formation in vitro. *Nature* 1983;302:426.

1196. Ozawa K, Kurtzman G, Young N. Replication of the B19 parvovirus in human bone marrow cell cultures. *Science* 1986;233:883–886.

1197. Ozawa K, Kurtzman G, Young N. Productive infection by B19 parvovirus of human erythroid bone marrow cells in vitro. *Blood* 1987;70:384.

1198. Robins MM. Familial crisis in hereditary spherocytosis: report of six affected siblings. *Clin Pediatr* 1965;4:210.

1199. Mallouh AA, Qudah A. An epidemic of aplastic crisis caused by human parvovirus B19. *Pediatr Infect Dis J* 1995;14:31–34.

1200. Hanada T, Koike K, Takeya T, et al. Human parvovirus B19-induced transient pancytopenia in a child with hereditary spherocytosis. *Br J Haematol* 1988;70:113–115.

1201. Saunders PWG, Reid MM, Cohen BJ. Human parvovirus induced cytopenias: a report of five cases [Letter]. *Br J Haematol* 1986;53:407.

1202. Hanada T, Koike K, Takeya T, et al. Human parvovirus B19-induced transient pancytopenia in a child with hereditary spherocytosis. *Br J Haematol* 1988;70:113.

1203. Muir K, Todd WT, Watson WH, et al. Viral-associated haemophagocytosis with parvovirus-B19-related pancytopenia. *Lancet* 1992;339:1139.

1204. Watanabe M, Shimamoto Y, Yamaguchi M, et al. Viral-associated haemophagocytosis and elevated serum TNF-alpha with parvovirus-B19-related pancytopenia in patients with hereditary spherocytosis. *Clin Lab Haematol* 1994;16:179–182.

1205. Shirono K, Tsuda H. Parvovirus B19-associated haemophagocytic syndrome in healthy adults. *Br J Haematol* 1995;89:923–926.

1206. Rinn R, Chow WS, Pinkerton PH. Transient acquired myelodysplasia associated with parvovirus B19 infection in a patient with congenital spherocytosis. *Am J Hematol* 1995;50:71.

1207. Yarali N, Duru F, Sipahi T, et al. Parvovirus B19 infection reminiscent of myelodysplastic syndrome in three children with chronic hemolytic anemia. *Pediatr Hematol Oncol* 2000;17:475–482.

1208. Anand A, Gray ES, Brown T, et al. Human parvovirus infection in pregnancy and hydrops fetalis. *N Engl J Med* 1987;316:183–186.

1209. Anderson LJ, Hurwitz ES. Human parvovirus B19 and pregnancy. *Clin Perinatol* 1988;15:273–286.

1210. Leads from the MMWR. Risks associated with human parvovirus B19 infection. *JAMA* 1989;261:1406–1408.

1211. Odibo AO, Campbell WA, Feldman D, et al. Resolution of human parvovirus B19-induced nonimmune hydrops after intrauterine transfusion. *J Ultrasound Med* 1998;17:547–550.

1212. Harger JH, Adler SP, Koch WC, et al. Prospective evaluation of 618 pregnant women exposed to parvovirus B19: risks and symptoms. *Obstet Gynecol* 1998;91:413–420.

1213. Bell LM, Nasides SJ, Stoffman P, et al. Human parvovirus B19 infection among hospital staff members after contact with infected patients. *N Engl J Med* 1989;321:485–491.

1214. Shneerson JM, Mortimer PP, Vandervelde EM. Febrile illness due to a parvovirus. *BMJ* 1980;280:1580.

1215. Markenson GR, Yancey MK. Parvovirus B19 infections in pregnancy. *Semin Perinatol* 1998;22:309–317.

1216. Fairley CK, Smoleniec JS, Caul OE, et al. Observational study of effect of intrauterine transfusions on outcome of fetal hydrops after parvovirus B19 infection. *Lancet* 1995;346:1335–1337.

1217. Forestier F, Tissot JD, Vial Y, et al. Haematological parameters of parvovirus B19 infection in 13 fetuses with hydrops foetalis. *Br J Haematol* 1999;104:925–927.

1218. Schild RL, Bald R, Plath H, et al. Intrauterine management of fetal parvovirus B19 infection. *Ultrasound Obstet Gynecol* 1999;13:161–166.

1219. Rodis JF, Borgida AF, Wilson M, et al. Management of parvovirus infection in pregnancy and outcomes of hydrops: a survey of members of the Society of Perinatal Obstetricians. *Am J Obstet Gynecol* 1998;179:985–988.

1220. Fridell E, Bekassy AN, Larsson B, et al. Polymerase chain reaction with double primer pairs for detection of human parvovirus B19 induced aplastic crises in family outbreaks. *Scand J Infect Dis* 1992;24:275.

1221. Lefrère JJ, Courouce AM, Girot R, et al. Six cases of hereditary spherocytosis revealed by human parvovirus infection. *Br J Haematol* 1986;62:653–658.

1222. McLellan NJ, Rutter N. Hereditary spherocytosis in sisters unmasked by parvovirus infection. *Postgrad Med J* 1987;63:49.

1223. Summerfield GP, Wyatt GP. Human parvovirus infection revealing hereditary spherocytosis. *Lancet* 1985;2:1070.

1224. Stefanelli M, Barosi G, Cazzola M, et al. Quantitative assessment of erythropoiesis in haemolytic disease. *Br J Haematol* 1980;45:297–308.

1225. Peter G. Parvovirus B19. In: *1997 Red book: report of the committee on infectious diseases*, 24th ed. Elk Grove Village, IL: American Academy of Pediatrics, 1997:383.

1226. Malinow MR, Duell PB, Hess DL, et al. Reduction of plasma homocyst(e)ine levels by breakfast cereal fortified with folic acid in patients with coronary heart disease. *N Engl J Med* 1998;338:1009–1015.

1227. Gairdner D. The association of gall-stones with acholuric jaundice in children. *Arch Dis Child* 1939;14:109–120.

1228. Bates GC, Brown CH. Incidence of gallbladder disease in chronic hemolytic anemia (spherocytosis). *Gastroenterology* 1952;21:104–109.

1229. Mentzer SH. Clinical and pathologic study of cholecystitis and cholelithiasis. *Surg Gynecol Obstet* 1926;42:782.

1230. Miraglia del Giudice E, Perrotta S, Nobili B, et al. Co-inheritance of Gilbert syndrome increases the risk for developing gallstones in patients with hereditary spherocytosis. *Blood* 1998;92[Suppl 1]:470a (abst).

1231. Lawrie GM, Ham JM. The surgical treatment of hereditary spherocytosis. *Surg Gynecol Obstet* 1974;139:208–210.

1232. MacKinney AA Jr. Hereditary spherocytosis. Clinical family studies. *Arch Intern Med* 1965;116:257–265.

1233. Ransohoff DF, Gracie WA. Treatment of gallstones. *Ann Intern Med* 1993;119:606.

1234. Holcomb GW 3rd. Laparoscopic cholecystectomy. *Semin Laparosc Surg* 1998;5:2–8.

1235. Pappis CH, Galanakis S, Moussatos G, et al. Experience of splenectomy and cholecystectomy in children with chronic haemolytic anaemia. *J Pediatr Surg* 1989;24:543.

1236. Marchetti M, Quaglini S, Barosi G. Prophylactic splenectomy and cholecystectomy in mild hereditary spherocytosis: analyzing the decision in different clinical scenarios. *J Intern Med* 1998;244:217–226.

1237. Hanford RB, Schneider GF, MacCarthy JD. Massive thoracic extramedullary hemopoiesis. *N Engl J Med* 1960;263:120–123.

1238. Lawrence P, Aronson I, Saxe N, et al. Leg ulcers in hereditary spherocytosis. *Clin Exp Dermatol* 1991;16:28–30.

1239. Vanscheidt W, Leder O, Vanscheidt E, et al. Leg ulcers in a patient with spherocytosis: a clinicopathological report. *Dermatologica* 1990;181:56–59.

1240. Beinhauer LG, Gruhn JG. Dermatologic aspects of congenital spherocytic anemia. *Arch Dermatol* 1957;75:642–646.

1241. Abe T, Yachi A, Ishii Y, et al. Thoracic extramedullary hematopoiesis associated with hereditary spherocytosis. *Intern Med* 1992;31:1151–1154.

1242. Bastion Y, Coiffier B, Felman P, et al. Massive mediastinal extramedullary hematopoiesis in hereditary spherocytosis: a case report. *Am J Hematol* 1990;35:263–265.

1243. Martin J, Palacio A, Petit J, et al. Fatty transformation of thoracic extramedullary hematopoiesis following splenectomy: CT features. *J Comput Assist Tomogr* 1990;14:477–478.

1244. Pulsoni A, Ferrazza G, Malagnino F, et al. Mediastinal extramedullary hematopoiesis as first manifestation of hereditary spherocytosis [clinical conference]. *Ann Hematol* 1992;65:196–198.

1245. Pietsch B, Sigmund G, Wurtemberger G. Kernspintomographische Befunde der kompensierten chronischen Hamolyse. Fallbericht uber eine hereditare Spharozytose. *Aktuelle Radiol* 1993;3:266–269.

1246. Schafer AI, Miller JB, Lester EP, et al. Monoclonal gammopathy in hereditary spherocytosis: a possible pathogenic relation. *Ann Intern Med* 1978;88:45–46.

1247. Fukata S, Tamai H, Nogai K, et al. A patient with hereditary spherocytosis and silicosis who developed an IgA (lambda) monoclonal gammopathy. *Jpn J Med* 1987;26:81–83.

1248. Lempert KD. Gammopathy and spherocytosis. *Ann Intern Med* 1978;89:145–146.

1249. Conti JA, Howard LM. Hereditary spherocytosis and hematologic malignancy. *N J Med* 1994;91:95–97.

1250. Jandl JH, Files NM, Barnett SB, et al. Proliferative response of the spleen and liver to hemolysis. *J Exp Med* 1965;122:299–325.

1251. Schilling RF. Hereditary spherocytosis; a study of splenectomized persons. *Semin Hematol* 1976;13:169–176.

1252. Isobe T, Osserman EF. Pathologic conditions associated with plasma cell dyscrasias: a study of 806 cases. *Ann N Y Acad Sci* 1971;190:507–518.

1253. Blacklock H, Meerkin M. Serum ferritin in patients with hereditary spherocytosis. *Br J Haematol* 1981;49:117–122.

1254. Edwards CQ, Skolnick MH, Dadone MM, et al. Iron overload in hereditary spherocytosis: association with HLA-linked hemochromatosis. *Am J Hematol* 1982;13:101–109.

1255. Fargion S, Cappellini MD, Piperno A, et al. Association of hereditary spherocytosis and idiopathic hemochromatosis. A synergistic effect in determining iron overload. *Am J Clin Pathol* 1986;86:645–649.

1256. Mohler DN, Wheby MS. Hemochromatosis heterozygotes may have significant iron overload when they also have hereditary spherocytosis. *Am J Med Sci* 1986;292:320–324.

1257. Morita M, Hashizume M, Kanematsu T, et al. Hereditary spherocytosis with congestive heart failure: report of a case. *Surg Today* 1993;23:458–461.

1258. Clarkson JG, Altman RD. Angioid streaks. *Surv Ophthalmol* 1982;26:235.

1259. McLane NJ, Grizzard WS, Kousseff BG, et al. Angioid streaks associated with hereditary spherocytosis. *Am J Ophthalmol* 1984;97:444–449.

1260. Gibson JM, Chaudhuri PR, et al. Angioid streaks in a case of beta thalassemia major. *Br J Ophthalmol* 1983;67:29.

1261. Deutman AF, Kovacs B. Argon laser treatment in complications of angioid streaks. *Am J Ophthalmol* 1979;88:12.

1262. Alani FS, Dyer T, Hindle E, et al. Pseudohyperkalaemia associated with hereditary spherocytosis in four members of a family. *Postgrad Med J* 1994;70:749–751.

1263. Berne JD, Asensio JA, Falabella A, et al. Traumatic rupture of the spleen in a patient with hereditary spherocytosis. *J Trauma* 1997;42:323–326.

1264. Meekes I, van der Staak F, van Oostrom C. Results of splenectomy performed on a group of 91 children. *Eur J Pediatr Surg* 1995;5:19–22.

1265. Waghorn DJ, Mayon-White RT. A study of 42 episodes of overwhelming post-splenectomy infection: is current guidance for asplenic individuals being followed? *J Infect* 1997;35:289.

1266. King H, Shumacker HB Jr. Susceptibility to infection after splenectomy performed in infancy. *Ann Surg* 1952;136:239.

1267. Eraklis AJ, Filler RM. Splenectomy in childhood: a review of 1413 cases. *J Pediatr Surg* 1972;7:382.

1268. Singer DB. Postsplenectomy sepsis. *Perspect Pediatr Pathol* 1973;1:285.

1269. Shaw JH, Print CG. Postsplenectomy sepsis. *Br J Surg* 1989;76:1074.

1270. Holdsworth RJ, Irving AD, Cuschieri A. Postsplenectomy sepsis and its mortality rate: actual versus perceived risks. *Br J Surg* 1991;78:1031.

1271. Hansen K, Singer DB. Asplenic-hyposplenic overwhelming sepsis: postsplenectomy sepsis revisited. *Pediatr Dev Pathol* 2001;4:105–121.

1272. Schwartz PE, Sterioff S, Mucha P, et al. Postsplenectomy sepsis and mortality in adults. *JAMA* 1982;248:2279.

1273. Green JB, Shackford SR, Sise MJ, et al. Late septic complications in adults following splenectomy for trauma: a prospective analysis in 144 patients. *J Trauma* 1986;26:999.

1274. Pedersen FK. Postsplenectomy infections in Danish children splenectomized 1969–1978. *Acta Paediatr Scand* 1983;72:589.

1275. Posey DL, Marks C. Overwhelming postsplenectomy sepsis in childhood. *Am J Surg* 1983;145:318.

1276. Chaikof EL, McCabe CJ. Fatal overwhelming postsplenectomy infection. *Am J Surg* 1985;149:534.

1277. Platt R. Infection after splenectomy. *JAMA* 1982;248:2316.

1278. Musser G, Lazar G, Hocking W, et al. Splenectomy for hematologic disease. The UCLA experience with 306 patients. *Ann Surg* 1984;200:40.

1279. Schilling RF. Estimating the risk for sepsis after splenectomy in hereditary spherocytosis. *Ann Intern Med* 1995;122:187.

1280. Konradsen HB, Henrichsen J. Pneumococcal infections in splenectomized children are preventable. *Acta Paediatr Scand* 1991;80:423.

1281. Jugenburg M, Haddock G, Freedman MH, et al. The morbidity and mortality of pediatric splenectomy: does prophylaxis make a difference? *J Pediatr Surg* 1999;34:1064–1067.

1282. Klinge J, Hammersen G, Scharf J, et al. Overwhelming postsplenectomy infection with vaccine-type Streptococcus pneumoniae in a 12-year-old girl despite vaccination and antibiotic prophylaxis. *Infection* 1997;25:368–371.

1283. Pruthi RK, Marshall WF, Wiltsie JC, et al. Human babesiosis. *Mayo Clin Proc* 1995;70:853.

1284. Rosner F, Zarrabi MH, Benach JL, et al. Babesiosis in splenectomized adults. Review of 22 reported cases. *Am J Med* 1984;76:696.

1285. Gupta P, Hurley RW, Helseth PH, et al. Pancytopenia due to hemophagocytic syndrome as the presenting manifestation of babesiosis. *Am J Hematol* 1995;50:60.

1286. Miguelez Morales M, Linares Feria M, del Carmen Mesa M. Haemophagocytic syndrome due to babesiosis in a splenectomized patient. *Br J Haematol* 1995;91:1033.

1287. Wyler DJ, Miller LH, Schmidt LH. Spleen function in quartan malaria (due to Plasmodium inui): evidence for both protective and suppressive roles in host defense. *J Infect Dis* 1977;135:86.

1288. Oster CN, Koontz LC, Wyler DJ. Malaria in asplenic mice: effects of splenectomy, congenital asplenia, and splenic reconstitution on the course of infection. *Am J Trop Med Hyg* 1980;29:1138.

1289. Looareesuwan S, Suntharasamai P, Webster HK, et al. Malaria in splenectomized patients: report of four cases and review. *Clin Infect Dis* 1993;16:361.

1290. Boone KE, Watters DA. The incidence of malaria after splenectomy in Papua New Guinea. *BMJ* 1995;311:1273.

1291. Le TA, Davis TM, Tran QB, et al. Delayed parasite clearance in a splenectomized patient with falciparum malaria who was treated with artemisinin derivatives. *Clin Infect Dis* 1997;25:923.

1292. McGrew W, Avant GR. Hereditary spherocytosis and portal vein thrombosis. *J Clin Gastroenterol* 1984;6:381.

1293. Hayag-Barin JE, Smith RE, Tucker FC Jr. Hereditary spherocytosis, thrombocytosis, and chronic pulmonary emboli: a case report and review of the literature. *Am J Hematol* 1998;57:82.

1294. Gordon DH, Schaffner D, Bennett JM, et al. Postsplenectomy thrombocytosis: its association with mesenteric, portal, and/or renal vein thrombosis in patients with myeloproliferative disorders. *Arch Surg* 1978;113:713.

1295. Skarsgard E, Doski J, Jaksic T, et al. Thrombosis of the portal venous system after splenectomy for pediatric hematologic disease. *J Pediatr Surg* 1993;28:1109.

1296. Kemahli S, Canatan D, Cin S, et al. Post-splenectomy thrombosis and haemolytic anaemias. *Br J Haematol* 1997;97:505.

1297. Linet MS, Nyrén O, Gridley G, et al. Causes of death among patients surviving at least one year following splenectomy. *Am J Surg* 1996;172:320–323.

1298. Stewart GW, Amess JA, Eber SW, et al. Thrombo-embolic disease after splenectomy for hereditary stomatocytosis. *Br J Haematol* 1996;93:303.

1299. Robinette CD, Fraumeni JF Jr. Splenectomy and subsequent mortality in veterans of the 1939–45 war. *Lancet* 1977;2:127.

1300. Bevers EM, Comfurius P, Dekkers DW, et al. Transmembrane phospholipid distribution in blood cells: control mechanisms and pathophysiological significance. *Biol Chem* 1998;379:973.

1301. Hassoun H, Wang Y, Vassiliadis J, et al. Targeted inactivation of murine band 3 (AE1) gene produces a hypercoagulable state causing widespread thrombosis in vivo. *Blood* 1998;92:1785.

1302. Schilling RF. Spherocytosis, splenectomy, strokes, and heart attacks. *Lancet* 1997;350:1677.

1303. Poulin EC, Mamazza J. Laparoscopic splenectomy: lessons from the learning curve. *Can J Surg* 1998;41:28.

1304. Katkhouda N, Hurwitz MB, Rivera RT, et al. Laparoscopic splenectomy: outcome and efficacy in 103 consecutive patients. *Ann Surg* 1998;228:568.

1305. Rescorla FJ. Laparoscopic splenectomy. *Semin Pediatr Surg* 1998;7:207–212.

1306. Esposito C, Corcione F, Garipoli V, et al. Pediatric laparoscopic splenectomy: are there real advantages in comparison with the traditional open approach? *Pediatr Surg Int* 1997;12:509.

1307. Rescorla FJ, Breitfeld PP, West KW, et al. A case controlled comparison of open and laparoscopic splenectomy in children. *Surgery* 1998;124:670.

1308. Geiger JD, Dinh VV, Teitelbaum DH, et al. The lateral approach for open splenectomy. *J Pediatr Surg* 1998;33:1153.

1309. Tchernia G, Gauthier F, Mielot F, et al. Initial assessment of the beneficial effect of partial splenectomy in hereditary spherocytosis. *Blood* 1993;81:2014.

1310. Bader-Meunier B, Gauthier F, Archambaud F, et al. Long-term evaluation of the beneficial effect of subtotal splenectomy for management of hereditary spherocytosis. *Blood* 2001;97:399–403.

1311. Jimenez M, Azcona C, Castro L, et al. Partial splenic embolization in a child with hereditary spherocytosis. *Eur J Pediatr* 1995;154:501.

1312. Konradsen HB, Rasmussen C, Ejstrud P, et al. Antibody levels against Streptococcus pneumoniae and Haemophilus influenzae type b in a population of splenectomized individuals with varying vaccination status. *Epidemiol Infect* 1997;119:167.

1313. Dagan R, Melamed R, Muallem M, et al. Reduction of nasopharyngeal carriage of pneumococci during the second year of life by a heptavalent conjugate pneumococcal vaccine. *J Infect Dis* 1996;174:1271.

1314. Black S, Shinefield H. Issues and challenges: pneumococcal vaccination in pediatrics. *Pediatr Ann* 1997;26:355.

1315. Rennels MB, Edwards KM, Keyserling HL, et al. Safety and immunogenicity of heptavalent pneumococcal vaccine conjugated to CRM197 in United States infants. *Pediatrics* 1998;101:604.

1316. Advisory Committee on Immunization Practices. Preventing pneumococcal disease among infants and young children. Recommendations of the Advisory Committee on Immunization Practices (ACIP). *MMWR Recomm Rep* 2000; 49:1–35.

1317. Waghorn DJ. Prevention of postsplenectomy sepsis. *Lancet* 1993;341:248.

1318. Guidelines for the prevention and treatment of infection in patients with an absent or dysfunctional spleen. Working Party of the British Committee for Standards in Haematology Clinical Haematology Task Force. *BMJ* 1996;312:430.

1319. Lambert HP. Managing patients with an absent or dysfunctional spleen: guidelines do not discuss resistance to antibiotics among pneumococci. *BMJ* 1996;312:1361.

1320. Brivet F, Herer B, Fremaux A, et al. Fatal postsplenectomy pneumococcal sepsis despite pneumococcal vaccine and penicillin prophylaxis [Letter]. *Lancet* 1984;1:110.

1321. Buchanan GR, Smith SJ. Pneumococcal septicemia despite pneumococcal vaccine and prescription of penicillin prophylaxis in patients with sickle cell anemia. *Am J Dis Child* 1986;140:428.

1322. Gonzaga RA. Fatal post splenectomy pneumococcal sepsis despite prophylaxis. *Lancet* 1984;2:694.

1323. Wong WY, Overturf GD, Powers DR. Infection caused by Streptococcus pneumoniae in children with sickle cell disease: epidemiology, immunologic mechanisms, prophylaxis and vaccination. *Clin Infect Dis* 1992;14:1124.

1324. Buchanan GR, Siegel JD, Smith SJ, et al. Oral penicillin prophylaxis in children with impaired splenic function: a study of compliance. *Pediatrics* 1982;70:906.

1325. Marton A, Gulyas M, Munoz R, et al. Extremely high incidence of antibiotic resistance in clinical isolates of Streptococcus pneumoniae in Hungary. *J Infect Dis* 1991;163:542–548.

1326. Caputo GM, Appelbaum PC, Liu HH. Infections due to penicillin-resistant pneumococci. Clinical, epidemiologic, and microbiologic features. *Arch Intern Med* 1993;153:1301–1310.

1327. Spika JS, Facklam RR, Plikaytis BD, et al. Antimicrobial resistance of Streptococcus pneumoniae in the United States, 1979–1987. The Pneumococcal Surveillance Working Group. *J Infect Dis* 1991;163:1273–1278.

1328. de Haan LD, Werre JM, Ruben AM, et al. Alterations in size, shape and osmotic behaviour of red cells after splenectomy: a study of their age dependence. *Br J Haematol* 1988;69:71–80.

1329. Bart JB, Appel MF. Recurrent hemolytic anemia secondary to accessory spleens. *South Med J* 1978;71:608–609.

1330. MacKenzie FAF, Elliot DH, Eastcott HHG, et al. Relapse in hereditary spherocytosis with proven splenunculus. *Lancet* 1962;1:1102.

1331. Brook J, Tanaka KR. Combination of pyruvate kinase (PK) deficiency and hereditary spherocytosis (HS). *Clin Res* 1970;18:176a (abst).

1332. Valentine WN. Hereditary spherocytosis revisited. *West J Med* 1978;128:35–45.

1333. Rutkow IM. Twenty years of splenectomy for hereditary spherocytosis. *Arch Surg* 1981;116:306–308.

1334. Buchanan GR, Holtkamp CA. Pocked erythrocyte counts in patients with hereditary spherocytosis before and after splenectomy. *Am J Hematol* 1987;25:253–257.

1335. Kvindesdal BB, Jensen MK. Pitted erythrocytes in splenectomized subjects with congenital spherocytosis and in subjects splenectomized for other reasons. *Scand J Haematol* 1986;37:41–43.

1336. Satou S, Yokota E, Sugihara J, et al. Relapse of hereditary spherocytosis following splenectomy. *Acta Haematol Jpn* 1985;48:1337–1340.

1337. Lambrecht K. Die Elliptocytose (Ovalocytose) und ihre klinische Bedeutung. *Ergebn Inn Med Kinderheilkd* 1938;55:295.

1338. Dresbach M. Elliptical human red corpuscles. *Science* 1904;19:469.

1339. Flint A. Elliptical human erythrocytes. *Science* 1904;19:796.

1340. Dresbach M. Elliptical human erythrocytes. *Science* 1905;21:473.

1341. Bishop FW. Elliptical human erythrocytes. *Arch Intern Med* 1914;14:388–392.

1342. Sydenstricker VP. Elliptic human erythrocytes. *JAMA* 1923;81:113.

1343. Huck JG, Bigelow RM. Poikilocytes in otherwise normal blood (elliptical human erythrocytes). *Bull Johns Hopkins Hosp* 1923;34:390–393.

1344. Hunter WC, Adams RB. Hematologic study of three generations of a white family showing elliptical erythrocytes. *Ann Intern Med* 1929;2:1162–1174.

1345. Hunter WC. Further study of a white family showing elliptical erythrocytes. *Ann Intern Med* 1932;6:775–781.

1346. Giffin HZ, Watkins CH. Ovalocytosis with features of hemolytic icterus. *Trans Assoc Am Physicians* 1939;54:355–358.

1347. Grzegorzewski H. Über familiäres Vorkommen elliptisher Erythrocyten beim Menschen. *Folia Haematol* 1933;50:260–277.

1348. Mason VR. Ovalocytosis (elliptical human erythrocytes). In: Downey H, ed. *Handbook of hematology*, vol 3. New York: Paul B Hoeber, 1938:2351.

1349. Penfold J, Lipscomb JM. Elliptocytosis in man, associated with hereditary haemorrhagic telangiectasis. *QJM* 1943;12:157–167.

1350. Van Den Bergh AAH. Elliptische rote Blutköperchen. *Dtsch Med Wochenschr* 1928;54:1244.

1351. Wyandt H, Bancroft PM, Winship TO. Elliptic erythrocytes in man. *Arch Intern Med* 1941;68:1043–1065.

1352. Wolman IJ, Ozge A. Studies on elliptocytosis. I. Hereditary elliptocytosis in the pediatric age period: a review of recent literature. *Am J Med Sci* 1957;234:702.

1353. Dacie JV. The lifespan of the red blood cell and circumstances of its premature death. In: MM Wintrobe, ed. *Blood, pure and eloquent*. New York: McGraw-Hill, 1980:210–255.

1354. Dacie JV. Hereditary spherocytosis (HS). In: *The haemolytic anaemias*, 3rd ed. Vol 1. Edinburgh: Churchill Livingstone, 1985:134–215.

1355. Zarkowsky HS, Mohandas N, Speaker CB, et al. A congenital haemolytic anaemia with thermal sensitivity of the erythrocyte membrane. *Br J Haematol* 1975;29:537.

1356. Wiley JS, Gill FM. Red cell calcium leak in congenital hemolytic anemia with extreme microcytosis. *Blood* 1976;47:197.

1357. Zarkowsky HS. Heat-induced erythrocyte fragmentation in neonatal elliptocytosis. *Br J Haematol* 1979;41:515.

1358. McCarty SH. Elliptical red blood cells in man. A report of eleven cases. *J Lab Clin Med* 1934;19:612.

1359. Lecomte MC, Dhermy D, Gautero H, et al. Hereditary elliptocytosis in West Africa: frequency and repartition of spectrin variants. *C R Acad Sci III* 1988;306:43.

1360. Bashir N, Barkawi M, Sharif L. Prevalence of haemoglobinopathies in school children in Jordan Valley. *Ann Trop Paediatr* 1991;11:373.

1361. Glele-Kakai C, Garbarz M, Lecomte MC, et al. Epidemiological studies of spectrin mutations related to hereditary elliptocytosis and spectrin polymorphisms in Benin. *Br J Haematol* 1996;95:57.

1361a. Ching KHL, Westaway SK, Gitscher J, et al. HARP syndrome is allelic with pantothenate kinase-associated neurodegeneration. *Neurology* 2002;58:1673–1674.

1362. Facer CA. Erythrocytes carrying mutations in spectrin and protein 4.1 show differing sensitivities to invasion by *Plasmodium falciparum*. *Parasitol Res* 1995;81:52.

1363. Mgone CS, Koki G, Paniu MM, et al. Occurrence of the erythrocyte band 3 (AE1) gene deletion in relation to malaria endemicity in Papua New Guinea. *Trans R Soc Trop Med Hyg* 1996;90:228.

1364. Morton NE. The detection and estimation of linkage between the genes for elliptocytosis and the Rh blood type. *Am J Hum Genet* 1956;8:80.

1365. Bannerman RM, Renwick JH. The hereditary elliptocytoses: clinical and linkage data. *Ann Hum Genet (London)* 1962;26:23.

1366. Cook PJL, Noades JE, Newton MS, et al. On the orientation of the Rh El1, linkage group. *Ann Hum Genet (London)* 1977;41:157–162.

1367. Keats BJB. Another elliptocytosis locus on chromosome 1? *Hum Genet* 1979;50:227–230.

1368. Jonsson JJ, Renieri A, Gallagher PG, et al. Alport syndrome, mental retardation, midface hypoplasia, and elliptocytosis: a new X-linked contiguous gene deletion syndrome? *J Med Genet* 1998;35:273.

1369. Palek J, Lux SE. Red cell membrane skeletal defects in hereditary and acquired hemolytic anemias. *Semin Hematol* 1983;20:189.

1370. Dacie JV, Mollison PL, Richardson N, et al. Atypical congenital haemolytic anaemia. *QJM (New Series)* 1953;22:79.

1371. Glele-Kakai C, Garbarz M, Lecomte MC, et al. Epidemiological studies of spectrin mutations related to hereditary elliptocytosis and spectrin polymorphisms in Benin. *Br J Haematol* 1996;95:57–66.

1372. Fournier CM, Nicolas G, Gallagher PG, et al. Spectrin St Claude, a splicing mutation of the human α-spectrin gene associated with severe poikilocytic anemia. *Blood* 1997;89:4584.

1373. Delaunay J, Alloisio N, Morlé L, et al. The red cell skeleton and its genetic disorders. *Mol Aspects Med* 1990;11:161–241.

1374. Tse WT, Lecomte MC, Costa FF, et al. Point mutation in the β-spectrin gene associated with αI/74 hereditary elliptocytosis. Implications for the mechanism of spectrin dimer self-association. *J Clin Invest* 1990;86:909–916.

1375. Lawler J, Liu SC, Palek J, et al. Molecular defect of spectrin in hereditary pyropoikilocytosis: alterations in the trypsin resistant domain involved in spectrin self-association. *J Clin Invest* 1982;70:1019–1030.

1376. Lawler J, Liu SC, Palek J. Molecular defect of spectrin in a subgroup of patients with hereditary elliptocytosis: alteration in the alpha subunit involved in spectrin self association. *J Clin Invest* 1984;73:1688–1695.

1377. Dalla Venezia N, Wilmotte R, Morlé L, et al. An α spectrin mutation responsible for hereditary elliptocytosis associated in cis with the αV/41 polymorphism. *Hum Genet* 1993;90:641–644.

1378. Mentzer WC, Turetsky T, Mohandas N, et al. Identification of the hereditary pyropoikilocytosis carrier state. *Blood* 1984;63:1439–1446.

1379. Palek J, Lux SE. Red cell membrane skeletal defects in hereditary and acquired hemolytic anemias. *Semin Hematol* 1983;20:189–224.

1380. Palek J. Hereditary elliptocytosis and related disorders. *Clin Haematol* 1985;14:45–87.

1381. Palek J. Hereditary elliptocytosis: spherocytosis and related disorders: consequences of a deficiency or a mutation of membrane skeletal proteins. *Blood Rev* 1987;1:147–168.

1382. Alloisio N, Morlé L, Maréchal J, et al. Sp αV/41: a common spectrin polymorphism at the αIV-αV domain junction. Relevance to the expression level of hereditary elliptocytosis due to α-spectrin variants located in trans. *J Clin Invest* 1991;87:2169–2177.

1383. Wilmotte R, Maréchal J, Morlé L, et al. Low expression allele αLELY of red cell spectrin is associated with mutations in exon 40 (αV/41 polymorphism) and intron 45 and with partial skipping of exon 46. *J Clin Invest* 1993;91:2091–2096.

1384. Daniels GL, Shaw MA, Judson PA, et al. A family demonstrating inheritance of the Leach phenotype, a Gerbich-negative phenotype associated with elliptocytosis. *Vox Sang* 1986;50:117–122.

1385. Tchernia G, Mohandas N, Shohet SB. Deficiency of cytoskeletal membrane protein band 4.1 in homozygous hereditary elliptocytosis: implications for erythrocyte membrane stability. *J Clin Invest* 1981;68:454–460.

1386. Morlé L, Alloisio N, Ducluzeau MT, et al. Spectrin Tunis (αI/78), a new αI variant that causes asymptomatic hereditary elliptocytosis in the heterozygous state. *Blood* 1988;71:508–511.

1387. Lecomte MC, Garbarz M, Grandchamp B, et al. Sp αI/78: a mutation of the αI spectrin domain in a white kindred with HE and HPP phenotypes. *Blood* 1989;74:1126–1133.

1388. Lecomte MC, Dhermy D, Garbarz M, et al. Hereditary elliptocytosis with spectrin molecular defect in a white patient. *Acta Haematol* 1984;71:235–240.

1389. Alloisio N, Guetorni D, Morlé L, et al. Sp αI/65 hereditary elliptocytosis in North Africa. *Am J Hematol* 1986;23:113–122.

1390. Guetarni D, Roux AF, Alloisio N, et al. Evidence that expression of Sp αI/65 hereditary elliptocytosis is compounded by a genetic factor that is linked to the homologous α-spectrin allele. *Hum Genet* 1990;85:627–630.

1391. Marchesi SL, Knowles WT, Morrow JS, et al. Abnormal spectrin in hereditary elliptocytosis. *Blood* 1986;67:141–151.

1392. Feddal S, Brunet G, Roda L, et al. Molecular analysis of hereditary elliptocytosis with reduced protein 4.1 in the French Northern Alps. *Blood* 1991;78:2113–2119.

1393. Lambert S, Zail S. Partial deficiency of protein 4.1 in hereditary elliptocytosis. *Am J Hematol* 1987;26:263–272.

1394. McGuire M, Smith BL, Agre P. Distinct variants of erythrocyte protein 4.1 inherited in linkage with elliptocytosis and Rh type in three white families. *Blood* 1988;72:287–293.

1395. Florman AL, Wintrobe MM. Human elliptical red corpuscles. *Bull Johns Hopkins Hosp* 1938;63:209–220.

1396. Garrdo-Lacca G, Merino C, Luna G. Hereditary elliptocytosis in a Peruvian family. *N Engl J Med* 1957;256:311–314.

1397. Geerdink RA, Helleman PW, Verloop MC. Hereditary elliptocytosis and hyperhaemolysis. A comparative study of 6 families with 145 patients. *Acta Med Scand* 1966;179:715–728.

1398. Jensson O, Jonasson TH, Olafsson O. Hereditary elliptocytosis in Iceland. *Br J Haematol* 1967;13:844–854.

1399. Motulsky AG, Singer K, Crosby WH, et al. The life span of the elliptocyte. Hereditary elliptocytosis and its relationship to other familial hemolytic diseases. *Blood* 1954;9:57–72.

1400. Pothier B, Alloisio N, Maréchal J, et al. Assignment of spectrin alphaI/74 hereditary elliptocytosis to the alpha or beta chain of spectrin through in vitro dimer reconstitution. *Blood* 1990;75:2061–2069.

1401. Coetzer T, Lawler J, Prchal JT, et al. Molecular determinants of clinical expression of hereditary elliptocytosis and pyropoikilocytosis. *Blood* 1987; 70:766–772.

1402. Rummens JL, Verfaillie C, Criel A, et al. Elliptocytosis and schistocytosis in myelodysplasia: report of two cases. *Acta Haematol* 1986;75:174–177.

1403. Boavida MG, Ambrosio P, Dhermy D, et al. Isochromosome 14q in refractory anemia. *Cancer Genet Cytogenet* 1997;97:155–156.

1404. Ishida F, Shimodaira S, Kobayashi H, et al. Elliptocytosis in myelodysplastic syndrome associated with translocation (1;5)(p10;q10) and deletion of 20q. *Cancer Genet Cytogenet* 1999;108:162–165.

1405. Coetzer T, Sahr K, Prchal J, et al. Four different mutations in codon 28 of α spectrin are associated with structurally and functionally abnormal spectrin αI/74 in hereditary elliptocytosis. *J Clin Invest* 1991;88:743–749.

1406. Garbarz M, Lecomte MC, Féo C, et al. Hereditary pyropoikilocytosis and elliptocytosis in a white French family with the spectrin alphaI/74 variant related to a CGT to CAT codon change (Arg to His) at position 22 of the spectrin alpha I domain. *Blood* 1990;75:1691–1698.

1407. Baklouti F, Maréchal J, Morlé L, et al. Occurrence of the αI 22 Arg → His (CGT → CAT) spectrin mutation in Tunisia: potential association with severe elliptocytosis. *Br J Haematol* 1991;78:108–113.

1408. Miraglia del Giudice E, Ducluzeau MT, Alloisio N, et al. αI/65 hereditary elliptocytosis in Southern Italy: evidence for an African origin. *Hum Genet* 1992;89:553–556.

1409. Baklouti F, Maréchal J, Wilmotte R, et al. Elliptocytogenic αI/36 spectrin Sfax lacks nine amino acids in helix 3 of repeat 4. Evidence for the activation of a cryptic 5'-splice site in exon 8 of spectrin α-gene. *Blood* 1992;79:2464–2470.

1410. Dalla Venezia N, Alloisio N, Forissier A, et al. Elliptopoikilocytosis associated with the α 469 His→Pro mutation in Spectrin Barcelona (αI/50-46b). *Blood* 1993;82:1661–1665.

1411. Coetzer T, Palek J, Lawler J, et al. Structural and functional heterogeneity of α spectrin mutations involving the spectrin heterodimer self-association site: relationships to hematologic expression of homozygous hereditary elliptocytosis and hereditary pyropoikilocytosis. *Blood* 1990;75:2235–2243.

1412. Pui CH, Wang W, Wilimas J. Hereditary elliptocytosis: morphologic abnormalities during acute hepatitis. *Clin Pediatr (Phila)* 1982;21:188.

1413. Ozer L, Mills GC. Elliptocytosis with haemolytic anaemia. *Br J Haematol* 1964;10:468.

1414. Horiguchi-Yamada J, Fujikawa T, Ideguchi H, et al. Hemolysis caused by CMV infection in a pregnant woman with silent elliptocytosis. *Int J Hematol* 1998;68:311.

1415. Kruatrachuo M, Asawapokee N. Hereditary elliptocytosis and *Plasmodium falciparum* malaria. *Ann Trop Med Parasitol* 1972;66:161–162.

1416. Nkrumah FK. Hereditary elliptocytosis associated with severe haemolytic anaemia and malaria. *Afr J Med Sci* 1972;3:131–136.

1417. Jarolim P, Palek J, Coetzer TL, et al. Severe hemolysis and red cell fragmentation due to a combination of a spectrin mutation with a thrombotic microangiopathy. *Am J Hematol* 1989;32:50–56.

1418. Pajor A, Lehoczky D. Hemolytic anemia precipitated by pregnancy in a patient with hereditary elliptocytosis. *Am J Hematol* 1996;52:240.

1419. Schoomaker EB, Butler WM, et al. Increased heat sensitivity of red blood cells in hereditary elliptocytosis with acquired cobalamin (vitamin B$_{12}$) deficiency. *Blood* 1982;59:1213.

1420. Perrotta S, del Giudice EM, Iolascon A, et al. Reversible erythrocyte skeleton destabilization is modulated by beta-spectrin phosphorylation in childhood leukemia. *Leukemia* 2001;15:440–444.

1421. Austin RF, Desforges JF. Hereditary elliptocytosis: an unusual presentation of hemolysis in the newborn associated with transient morphologic abnormalities. *Pediatrics* 1969;44:196–200.

1422. Carpentieri U, Gustavson LP, Haggard ME. Pyknocytosis in a neonate: an unusual presentation of hereditary elliptocytosis. *Clin Pediatr* 1977;16:76–78.

1423. Josephs HW, Avery ME. Hereditary elliptocytosis associated with increased hemolysis. *Pediatrics* 1965;16:741.

1424. Zarkowsky HS. Heat-induced erythrocyte fragmentation in neonatal elliptocytosis. *Br J Haematol* 1979;41:515–518.

1425. Prchal JT, Castleberry RP, Parmley RT, et al. Hereditary pyropoikilocytosis and elliptocytosis: clinical, laboratory, and ultrastructural features in infants and children. *Pediatr Res* 1982;16:484–489.

1426. Reference deleted.

1427. Moriyama R, Lombardo CR, Workman RF, et al. Regulation of linkages between the erythrocyte membrane and its skeleton by 2,3-diphosphoglycerate. *J Biol Chem* 1993;268:10990–10996.

1428. Dhermy D, Lecomte MC, Garbarz M, et al. Molecular defect of spectrin in the family of a child with congenital hemolytic poikilocytic anemia. *Pediatr Res* 1984;18:1005–1024.

1429. Garbarz M, Lecomte MC, Dhermy D, et al. Double inheritance of an αI/65 spectrin variant in a child with homozygous elliptocytosis. *Blood* 1986;67:1661–1667.

1430. Lawler J, Coetzer TL, Mankad VN, et al. Spectrin αI/61: a new structural variant of α spectrin in a double heterozygous form of hereditary pyropoikilocytosis. *Blood* 1988;72:1412–1415.

1431. Alloisio N, Morlé L, Pothier B, et al. Spectrin Oran (αII/21), a new spectrin variant concerning the αII domain and causing severe elliptocytosis in the homozygous state. *Blood* 1988;71:1039–1047.

1432. Alloisio N, Wilmotte R, Maréchal J, et al. A splice site mutation of alpha-spectrin gene causing skipping of exon 18 in hereditary elliptocytosis. *Blood* 1993;81:2791–2798.

1433. Lecomte MC, Féo C, Gautero H, et al. Severe recessive poikilocytic anemia with a new spectrin α chain variant. *Br J Haematol* 1990;74:497–507.

1434. Dalla Venezia N, Gilsanz F, Alloisio N, et al. Homozygous 4.1 (–) hereditary elliptocytosis associated with a point mutation in the downstream initiation codon of protein 4.1 gene. *J Clin Invest* 1992;90:1713–1717.

1435. Evans JPM, Baines AJ, Hann IM, et al. Defective spectrin dimer-dimer association in a family with transfusion dependent homozygous hereditary elliptocytosis. *Br J Haematol* 1983;54:163–172.

1436. Grech JL, Cachia EA, Calleja F, et al. Hereditary elliptocytosis in two Maltese families. *J Clin Pathol* 1961;14:365–373.

1437. Haddy TB, Rana SR. Homozygous hereditary elliptocytosis with hemolytic anemia. *South Med J* 1984;77:631–633.

1438. Iarocci TA, Wagner GM, Mohandas N, et al. Hereditary poikilocytic anemia associated with the coinheritance of two α spectrin abnormalities. *Blood* 1988;71:1390–1396.

1439. Lipton EL. Elliptocytosis with hemolytic anemia; the effects of splenectomy. *Pediatrics* 1955;15:67.

1440. Nielsen JA, Strunk KW. Homozygous hereditary elliptocytosis as a cause of haemolytic anaemia in infancy. *Scand J Haematol* 1968;5:486–496.

1441. Pryor DS, Pitney WR. Hereditary elliptocytosis: a report of two families from New Guinea. *Br J Haematol* 1967;13:126–134.

1442. Dhermy D, Garbarz M, Lecomte MC, et al. Hereditary elliptocytosis: clinical, morphological, and biochemical studies of 38 cases. *Nouv Rev Fr Hematol* 1986;28:129–140.

1443. Dhermy D, Galand C, Bournier O, et al. Coinheritance of alpha- and beta-spectrin gene mutations in a case of hereditary elliptocytosis. *Blood* 1998;92:4481–4482.

1444. Dacie JV, Mollison PL, Richardson N, et al. Atypical congenital haemolytic anaemia. *QJM (New Series)* 1953;22:79–98.

1445. Wiley JS, Gill FM. Red cell calcium leak in congenital hemolytic anemia with extreme microcytosis. *Blood* 1976;47:197–210.

1446. Zarkowsky HS, Mohandas N, Speaker CB, et al. A congenital haemolytic anaemia with thermal sensitivity of the erythrocyte membrane. *Br J Haematol* 1975;29:537–543.

1447. DePalma L, Luban NLC. Hereditary pyropoikilocytosis. Clinical and laboratory analysis in eight infants and young children. *Am J Dis Child* 1993;147:93–95.

1448. Coetzer T, Palek J. Partial spectrin deficiency in hereditary pyropoikilocytosis. *Blood* 1986;59:919–924.

1449. Giffin HZ, Watkins CH. Ovalocytosis with features of hemolytic icterus. *Trans Assoc Am Physicians* 1939;54:355–358.

1450. Cutting HO, McHugh, Conrad FG, et al. Autosomal dominant hemolytic anemia characterized by ovalocytosis. A family study of seven involved members. *Am J Med* 1965;39:21–34.

1451. Dacie JV. Hereditary elliptocytosis (HE). In: *The haemolytic anaemias*, 3rd ed. Vol 1. Edinburgh: Churchill Livingstone, 1985:216–258.

1452. Greenberg LH, Tanaka KR. Hereditary elliptocytosis with hemolytic anemia—a family study of five affected members. *Calif Med* 1969;110:389–393.

1453. Weiss HJ. Hereditary elliptocytosis with hemolytic anemia. *Am J Med* 1963;35:455–466.

1454. Matsumoto N, Ishihara T, Takahashi M, et al. Fine structures of the spleen in hereditary elliptocytosis. *Acta Pathol Jpn* 1976;26:533–542.

1455. Wilson HE, Long MJ. Hereditary ovalocytosis (elliptocytosis) with hypersplenism. *Arch Intern Med* 1955;95:438.

1456. Garbarz M, Tse WT, Gallagher PG, et al. Spectrin Rouen (β220-218), a novel shortened β-chain variant in a kindred with hereditary elliptocytosis. Characterization of the molecular defect as exon skipping due to a splice site mutation. *J Clin Invest* 1991;88:76–81.

1457. Lecomte MC, Gautero H, Bournier O, et al. Elliptocytosis-associated spectrin Rouen (β220/218) has a truncated but still phosphorylatable beta-chain. *Br J Haematol* 1992;80:242–250.

1458. Pothier B, Morlé L, Alloisio N, et al. Spectrin Nice (β220/216): a shortened β chain variant associated with an increase of the αI/74 fragment in a case of elliptocytosis. *Blood* 1987;69:1759–1765.

1459. Tse WT, Gallagher PG, Pothier B, et al. An insertional frameshift mutation of the beta-spectrin gene associated with elliptocytosis in spectrin Nice ((220/216). *Blood* 1991;78:517–523.

1460. Garbarz M, Boulanger L, Pedroni S, et al. Spectrin β Tandil, a novel shortened β-chain variant associated with hereditary elliptocytosis is due to a deletional frameshift mutation in the β-spectrin gene. *Blood* 1992;80:1066–1073.

1461. Eber SW, Morris SA, Schröter W, et al. Interactions of spectrin in hereditary elliptocytes containing truncated spectrin β-chains. *J Clin Invest* 1988;81:523–530.

1462. Yoon SH, Yu H, Eber S, et al. Molecular defect of truncated β-spectrin associated with hereditary elliptocytosis. β-spectrin Göttingen. *J Biol Chem* 1991;266:8490–8494.

1463. Dhermy D, Lecomte MC, Garbarz M, et al. Spectrin beta-chain variant associated with hereditary elliptocytosis. *J Clin Invest* 1982;70:707–715.

1464. Gallagher PG, Tse WT, Costa F, et al. A splice site mutation of the β-spectrin gene causing exon skipping in hereditary elliptocytosis associated with a truncated β-spectrin chain. *J Biol Chem* 1991;266:15154–15159.

1465. Ohanian V, Evans JP, Gratzer WB. A case of elliptocytosis associated with a truncated spectrin chain. *Br J Haematol* 1985;61:31–39.

1466. Jarolim P, Wichterle H, Hanspal M, et al. β spectrin Prague: a truncated β spectrin producing spectrin deficiency, defective spectrin heterodimer self-association and a phenotype of spherocytic elliptocytosis. *Br J Haematol* 1995;91:502–510.

1467. Parquet N, Devaux I, Boulanger L, et al. Identification of three novel spectrin αI/74 mutations in hereditary elliptocytosis: further support for a triple-stranded folding unit model of the spectrin heterodimer contact site. *Blood* 1994;84:303.

1468. Lorenzo F, Miraglia del Giudice E, Alloisio N, et al. Severe poikilocytosis associated with a de novo alpha 28 Arg→Cys mutation in spectrin. *Br J Haematol* 1993;83:152–157.

1469. Floyd PB, Gallagher PG, Valentino LA, et al. Heterogeneity in the molecular basis of hereditary pyropoikilocytosis and hereditary elliptocytosis associated with increased levels of the spectrin αI/74-kilodalton tryptic peptide. *Blood* 1991;78:1364–1372.

1470. Lecomte MC, Garbarz M, Gautero H, et al. Molecular basis of clinical and morphological heterogeneity in hereditary elliptocytosis with spectrin αI variants. *Br J Haematol* 1993;85:584.

1471. Perrotta S, Miraglia del Giudice E, Alloisio N, et al. Mild elliptocytosis associated with the alpha 34 Arg→Trp mutation in spectrin Genova (alpha I/74). *Blood* 1994;83:3346–3349.

1472. Morlé L, Morlé F, Roux AF, et al. Spectrin Tunis (Sp αI/78), an elliptocytogenic variant, is due to the CGG→TGG codon change (Arg→Trp) at position 35 of the αI domain. *Blood* 1989;75:828–832.

1473. Perrotta S, Iolascon A, De Angelis F, et al. Spectrin Anastasia (αI/78): a new spectrin variant (α45 Arg→Thr) with moderate elliptocytogenic potential. *Br J Haematol* 1995;89:933.

1474. Morlé L, Roux AF, Alloisio N, et al. Two elliptocytogenic αI/74 variants of the spectrin αI domain. Spectrin Culoz (GGT → GTT; αI 40 Gly → Val) and spectrin Lyon, (CTT → TTT; αI 43 Leu → Phe). *J Clin Invest* 1990;86:548–554.

1475. Corrons JL, Pujades A, Alvarez R, et al. α128 Arg→Ser (CGT→AGT) spectrin mutation associated with severe neonatal elliptopoikilocytosis in Spain. *Haematologica* 2001;86:537–538.

1476. Boulanger L, Dhermy D, Garbarz M, et al. A second allele of spectrin α-gene associated with the αI/65 phenotype (allele a Ponte de Sôr). *Blood* 1994;84:2056.

1477. Roux AF, Morlé F, Guetarni D, et al. Molecular basis of Sp αI/65 hereditary elliptocytosis in North Africa: insertion of a TTG triplet between codons 147 and 149 in the α-spectrin gene from five unrelated families. *Blood* 1989;73: 2196–2201.

1478. Sahr KE, Tobe T, Scarpa A, et al. Sequence and exon-intron organization of the DNA encoding the alpha I domain of human spectrin. Application to the study of mutations causing hereditary elliptocytosis. *J Clin Invest* 1989;84:1243–1252.

1479. Lawler J, Coetzer TL, Palek J, et al. Sp αI/65: a new variant of the alpha subunit of spectrin in hereditary elliptocytosis. *Blood* 1985;66:706–709.

1480. Lecomte MC, Dhermy D, Garbarz M, et al. Pathologic and non-pathologic variants of the spectrin molecule in two black families with hereditary elliptocytosis. *Hum Genet* 1985;71:351–357.

1481. Lecomte MC, Dhermy D, Solis C, et al. A new abnormal variant of spectrin in black patients with hereditary elliptocytosis. *Blood* 1985;65:1208–1217.

1482. Hassoun H, Coetzer TL, Vassiliadis JN, et al. A novel mobile element inserted in the alpha spectrin gene: spectrin Dayton. A truncated alpha spectrin associated with hereditary elliptocytosis. *J Clin Invest* 1994;94:643–648.

1483. Marchesi SL, Letsinger JT, Speicher DW, et al. Mutant forms of spectrin alpha-subunits in hereditary elliptocytosis. *J Clin Invest* 1987;80:191–198.

1484. Gallagher PG, Tse WT, Coetzer T, et al. A common type of the spectrin α I 46-50a-kD peptide abnormality in hereditary elliptocytosis and hereditary pyropoikilocytosis is associated with a mutation distant from the proteolytic cleavage site—evidence for the functional importance of the triple helical model of spectrin. *J Clin Invest* 1992;89:892–898.

1485. Gallagher PG, Roberts WE, Benoit L, et al. Poikilocytic hereditary elliptocytosis associated with Spectrin Alexandria: an αI/50b kD variant that is caused by a single amino acid deletion. *Blood* 1993;82:2210–2215.

1486. Gallagher PG, Marchesi SL, Forget BG. A new point mutation associated with αI/50b kDa hereditary elliptocytosis (HE) and hereditary pyropoikilocytosis (HPP). *Clin Res* 1991;39:313a (abst).

1487. Alloisio N, Wilmotte R, Morlé L, et al. Spectrin Jendouba: an αII/31 spectrin variant that is associated with elliptocytosis and carries a mutation distant from the dimer self-association site. *Blood* 1992;80:809–815.

1488. Takanashi K, Sugawar T, Sakurai K, et al. A trait of hereditary elliptocytosis with truncated β-spectrin (Spectrin Yamagata β220/210). *Jpn J Clin Hematol* 1991;32:1365a.

1489. Sahr KE, Coetzer TL, Moy LS, et al. Spectrin Cagliari. An ALA to GLY substitution in helix 1 of β spectrin repeat 17 that severely disrupts the structure and self-association of the erythrocyte spectrin heterodimer. *J Biol Chem* 1993;268:22656–22662.

1490. Gallagher PG, Weed SA, Tse WT, et al. Recurrent fatal hydrops fetalis associated with a nucleotide substitution in the erythrocyte β-spectrin gene. *J Clin Invest* 1995;95:1174.

1491. Gallagher PG, Petruzzi MJ, Weed SA, et al. Mutation of a highly conserved residue of βI spectrin associated with fatal and near-fatal neonatal hemolytic anemia. *J Clin Invest* 1997;99:267.

1492. Wilmotte R, Miraglia del Giudice E, Maréchal J, et al. A deletional frameshift mutation in spectrin β gene associated with hereditary elliptocytosis in spectrin Napoli. *Br J Haematol* 1994;88:437.

1493. Kanazaki A, Rabodonirina M, Yawata Y, et al. A deletion frameshift mutation of the β-spectrin gene associated with elliptocytosis in spectrin Tokyo (220/216). *Blood* 1992;80:2115–2121.

1494. Qualtieri A, Pasqua A, Bisconte MG, et al. Spectrin Cosenza: a novel β chain variant associated with Sp αI/74 hereditary elliptocytosis. *Br J Haematol* 1997;97:273.

1495. Maillet P, Inoue T, Kanzaki A, et al. Stop codon in exon 30 (E2069X) of β-spectrin gene associated with hereditary elliptocytosis in spectrin Nagoya. *Hum Mutat* 1996;8:366.

1496. Bassères DS, Pranke PH, Sales TS, et al. β-spectrin Campinas: a novel shortened β-chain variant associated with skipping of exon 30 and hereditary elliptocytosis. *Br J Haematol* 1997;97:579.

1497. Takakuwa Y, Tchernia G, Rossi M, et al. Restoration of normal membrane stability to unstable protein 4.1-deficient erythrocyte membranes by incorporation of purified protein 4.1. *J Clin Invest* 1986;78:80–85.

1498. Alloisio N, Mark L, Dorlèac E, et al. The heterozygous form of the 4.1(–) hereditary elliptocytosis [the 4.1(-) trait]. *Blood* 1985;65:46–51.

1499. Conboy DJ, Mohandas N, Tchernia G, et al. Molecular basis of hereditary elliptocytosis due to protein 4.1 deficiency. *N Engl J Med* 1986;315:680–685.

1500. Conboy JG, Chasis JA, Winardi R, et al. An isoform-specific mutation in the protein 4.1 gene results in hereditary elliptocytosis and complete deficiency of protein 4.1 in erythrocytes but not in nonerythroid cells. *J Clin Invest* 1993;91:77–82.

1501. Dalla Venezia N, Maillet P, Morlé L, et al. A large deletion within the protein 4.1 gene associated with a stable truncated mRNA and an unaltered tissue-specific alternative splicing. *Blood* 1998;91:4361.

1502. Garbarz M, Devaux I, Bournier O, et al. Protein 4.1 Lille, a novel mutation in the downstream initiation codon of protein 4.1 gene associated with heterozygous 4.1(–) hereditary elliptocytosis. *Hum Mutat* 1995;5:339.

1503. Conboy J, Marchesi S, Kim R, et al. Molecular analysis of insertion/deletion mutations in protein 4.1 in elliptocytosis. II. Determination of molecular genetic origins of rearrangements. *J Clin Invest* 1990;86:524–530.

1504. Garbarz M, Dhermy D, Lecomte MC, et al. A variant of erythrocyte membrane skeletal protein band 4.1 associated with hereditary elliptocytosis. *Blood* 1984;64:1006–1015.

1505. Marchesi S, Conboy J, Agre P, et al. Molecular analysis of insertion/deletion mutations in protein 4.1 in elliptocytosis. I. Biochemical identification of rearrangements in the spectrin/actin binding domain and functional characterizations. *J Clin Invest* 1990;86:515–523.

1506. Lorenzo F, Dalla Venezia N, Morlé L, et al. Protein 4.1 deficiency associated with an altered binding to the spectrin-actin complex of the red cell membrane skeleton. *J Clin Invest* 1994;94:1651.

1507. Anstee DJ, Ridgewell K, Tanner MJ, et al. Individuals lacking the Gerbich blood-group antigens have alterations in the human erythrocyte membrane sialoglycoproteins β and γ. *Biochem J* 1984;221:97–104.

1508. High S, Tanner MJA, MacDonald EB, et al. Rearrangements of the red cell membrane glycophorin C (sialoglycoprotein β) gene. A further study of alterations in the glycophorin C gene. *Biochem J* 1989;262:47–54.

1509. Telen MJ, Le Van Kim C, Chung A, et al. Molecular basis for elliptocytosis associated with glycophorin C and glycophorin D deficiency in the Leach phenotype. *Blood* 1991;78:1603–1606.

1510. Anstee DJ, Parsons SF, Ridgewell K, et al. Two individuals with elliptocytic red cells apparently lack three minor sialoglycoproteins. *Biochem J* 1984;218:615–619.

1511. Park S, Mehboob S, Luo BH, et al. Studies of the erythrocyte spectrin tetramerization region [Letter]. *Cell Mol Biol (Noisy-le-grand)* 2001;6:571–585.

1512. Yawata Y. Red cell membrane protein band 4.2. Phenotypic, genetic, and electron microscopic aspects. *Biochim Biophys Acta* 1994;1204:131–148.

1513. Aksoy M, Erdem S, Dincol G, et al. Combination of hereditary elliptocytosis and hereditary spherocytosis. *Clin Genet* 1974;6:46–50.

1514. Torlontano G, Fioritoni G, Salvati AM. Hereditary haemolytic anaemia with defective erythropoiesis. *Br J Haematol* 1979;43:435–441.

1515. Jankovic M, Sansone G, Conter V, et al. Atypical hereditary ovalocytosis associated with defective dyserythropoietic anemia. *Acta Haematol* 1993;89:35–37.

1516. Castelino D, Saul A, Myler P, et al. Ovalocytosis in Papua New Guinea—dominantly inherited resistance to malaria. *Southeast Asian J Trop Med Public Health* 1981;12:549–555.

1517. Cattani JA, Gibson FD, Alpers MP, et al. Hereditary ovalocytosis and reduced susceptibility to malaria in Papua New Guinea. *Trans R Soc Trop Med Hyg* 1987;81:705–709.

1518. Fix AG, Baer AS, Lie-Injo LE. The mode of inheritance of ovalocytosis/elliptocytosis in Malaysian Orang Asli families. *Hum Genet* 1982;61:250–253.

1519. Liu SC, Zhai S, Palek J, et al. Molecular defect of the band 3 protein in Southeast Asian ovalocytosis. *N Engl J Med* 1990;323:1530–1538.

1520. Mgone CS, Koki G, Paniu MM, et al. Occurrence of the erythrocyte band 3 (AE1) gene deletion in relation to malaria endemicity in Papua New Guinea. *Trans R Soc Trop Med Hyg* 1996;90:228–231.

1521. Liu SC, Jarolim P, Rubin HL, et al. The homozygous state for the band 3 protein mutation in Southeast Asian Ovalocytosis may be lethal. *Blood* 1994;84:3590.

1522. Genton B, al-Yaman F, Mgone CS, et al. Ovalocytosis and cerebral malaria. *Nature* 1995;378:564.

1523. Amato D, Booth PB. Hereditary ovalocytosis in Melanesians. *P N G Med J* 1977;20:26–32.

1524. Harrison KL, Collins KA, McKenna HW. Hereditary elliptical stomatocytosis; a case report. *Pathology* 1976;8:307–311.

1525. Honig GR, Lacson PS, Maurer HS. A new familial disorder with abnormal erythrocyte morphology and increased permeability of the erythrocytes to sodium and potassium. *Pediatr Res* 1971;5:159–166.

1526. Booth PB, Serjeantson S, Woodfield DG, et al. Selective depression of blood group antigens associated with hereditary ovalocytosis among Melanesians. *Vox Sang* 1977;32:99–110.

1526a. Rabe T, Jambou R, Rabarijaona L, et al. South-East Asian ovalocytosis among the population of the Highlands of Madagascar: a vestige of the island's settlement. *Trans R Soc Trop Med Hyg* 2002;96:143–144.

1527. Coetzer TL, Beeton L, van Zyl D, et al. Southeast Asian ovalocytosis in a South African kindred with hemolytic anemia. *Blood* 1996;87:1656.

1528. Schischmanoff PO, Cynober T, Miélot F, et al. Southeast Asian ovalocytosis in white persons. *Hemoglobin* 1999;23:47–56.

1529. Serjeantson S, Bryson K, Amato D, et al. Malaria and hereditary ovalocytosis. *Hum Genet* 1977;37:161–167.

1530. Foo LC, RekhraJ V, Chiang GL, et al. Ovalocytosis protects against severe malaria parasitemia in the Malayan aborigines. *Am J Trop Med Hyg* 1992; 47:271–275.

1531. O'Donnell A, Allen SJ, Mgone CS, et al. Red cell morphology and malaria anaemia in children with Southeast-Asian ovalocytosis band 3 in Papua New Guinea. *Br J Haematol* 1998;101:407–412.

1532. Allen SJ, O'Donnell A, Alexander ND, et al. Prevention of cerebral malaria in children in Papua New Guinea by southeast Asian ovalocytosis band 3. *Am J Trop Med Hyg* 1999;60:1056–1060.

1533. Hadley T, Saul A, Lamont G, et al. Resistance of Melanesian elliptocytes (ovalocytes) to invasion by Plasmodium knowlesi and *Plasmodium falciparum* malaria parasites in vitro. *J Clin Invest* 1983;71:780–782.

1534. Kidson C, Lamont G, Saul A, et al. Ovalocytic erythrocytes from Melanesians are resistant to invasion by malaria parasites in culture. *Proc Natl Acad Sci U S A* 1981;78:5829–5832.

1535. Dluzewski AR, Nash GB, Wilson RJ, et al. Invasion of hereditary ovalocytes by *Plasmodium falciparum* in vitro and its relation to intracellular ATP concentration. *Mol Biochem Parasitol* 1992;55:1–7.

1536. Mohandas N, Lie-Injo LE, Friedman M, et al. Rigid membranes of Malayan ovalocytes: a likely genetic barrier against malaria. *Blood* 1984;63:1385–1392.

1537. Mohandas N, Winardi R, Knowles D, et al. Molecular basis for membrane rigidity of hereditary ovalocytosis. A novel mechanism involving the cytoplasmic domain of band 3. *J Clin Invest* 1992;89:686–692.

1538. Saul A, Lamont G, Sawyer WH, et al. Decreased membrane deformability in Melanesian ovalocytes from Papua New Guinea. *J Cell Biol* 1984;98:1348–1354.

1539. Schofield AE, Tanner MJA, Pinder JC, et al. Basis of unique red cell membrane properties in hereditary ovalocytosis. *J Mol Biol* 1992;223:949–958.

1540. Vasuvattakul S, Yenchitsomanus PT, Vachuanichsanong P, et al. Autosomal recessive distal renal tubular acidosis associated with Southeast Asian ovalocytosis. *Kidney Int* 1999;56:1674–1682.

1541. Bruce LJ, Ring SM, Ridgwell K, et al. South-east Asian ovalocytic (SAO) erythrocytes have a cold sensitive cation leak: implications for in vitro studies on stored SAO red cells. *Biochim Biophys Acta* 1999;1416:258–270.

1542. Reardon DM, Seymour CA, Cox TM, et al. Hereditary ovalocytosis with compensated haemolysis. *Br J Haematol* 1993;85:197–199.

1543. Jonsson JJ, Renieri A, Gallagher PG, et al. Alport syndrome, mental retardation, midface hypoplasia, and elliptocytosis: a new X-linked contiguous gene deletion syndrome? *J Med Genet* 1998;35:273.

1543a. Vitelli F, Piccini M, Caroli F, et al. Identification and characterization of a highly conserved protein absent in the Alport syndrome (A), mental retardation (M), midface hypoplasia (M), and elliptocytosis (E) contiguous gene deletion syndrome (AMME). *Genomics* 1999;55:335–340.

1544. Ham TH, Shen SC, et al. Studies on the destruction of red blood cells. IV. Thermal injury: action of heat in causing increased spheroidity, osmotic and mechanical fragilities and hemolysis of erythrocytes; observations on the mechanisms of destruction in such erythrocytes in dogs and in a patient with a fatal thermal burn. *Blood* 1948;3:373.

1545. Ham TH, Sayre RW, et al. Physical properties of red cells as related to effects in vivo. II. Effect of thermal treatment on rigidity of red cells, stroma and the sickle cell. *Blood* 1968;32:862.

1546. Kimber RJ, Lander H. The effect of heat on human red cell morphology, fragility and subsequent survival in vivo. *J Lab Clin Med* 1964;64:922.

1547. Chang K, Williamson JR, Zarkowsky HS. Effect of heat on the circular dichroism of spectrin in hereditary pyropoikilocytosis. *J Clin Invest* 1979;64:326–328.

1548. Liu SC, Windisch P, Kim S, et al. Oligomeric states of spectrin in normal erythrocyte membranes. Biochemical and electron microscopic studies. *Cell* 1984;37:587–594.

1549. Liu SC, Palek J, Prchal J, Altered spectrin dimer-dimer association and instability of erythrocyte membrane skeletons in hereditary pyropoikilocytosis. *J Clin Invest* 1981;68:597–605.

1550. Liu SC, Palek J, Prchal J. Defective spectrin dimer-dimer association in hereditary elliptocytosis. *Proc Natl Acad Sci U S A* 1982;79:2072–2076.

1551. Chasis JA, Mohandas N. Erythrocyte membrane deformability and stability: two distinct membrane properties that are independently regulated by skeletal protein interactions. *J Cell Biol* 1986;103:343–350.

1552. Mohandas N, Clark MR, Health BO, et al. A technique to detect reduced mechanical stability of red cell membranes: relevance to elliptocytic disorders. *Blood* 1982;59:768–774.

1553. Clark MR, Mohandas N, Shohet SB. Osmotic gradient ektacytometry: comprehensive characterization of red cell volume and surface maintenance. *Blood* 1983;61:899.

1554. Speicher DW, Morrow JS, Knowles WJ, et al. A structural model of human erythrocyte spectrin: alignment of chemical and functional domains. *J Biol Chem* 1982;257:9093–9101.

1555. Speicher DW, Morrow JS, Knowles WJ, et al. Identification of proteolytically resistant domains of human erythrocyte spectrin. *Proc Natl Acad Sci U S A* 1980;77:5673–5677.

1556. Delaunay J, Dhermy D. Mutations involving the spectrin heterodimer contact site: clinical expression and alterations in specific function. *Semin Hematol* 1993;30:21–33.

1557. Byers PH. Killing the messenger: new insights into nonsense-mediated mRNA decay. *J Clin Invest* 2002;109:3–6.

1558. Lykke-Andersen. mRNA quality control: marking the message for life or death. *Curr Biol* 2001;11:R88–R91.

1559. Orita M, Iwahana H, Kanazawa H, et al. Detection of polymorphisms of human DNA by gel electrophoresis as single-strand conformation polymorphisms. *Proc Natl Acad Sci U S A* 1989;86:2766–2770.

1560. Sarkar G, Yoon HS, Sommer SS. Screening for mutations by RNA single-strand conformation polymorphism (rSSCP): comparison with DNA-SSCP. *Nucleic Acids Res* 1992;20:871–878.

1561. Peterson LC, Dampier C, Coetzer T, et al. Clinical and laboratory study of two Caucasian families with hereditary pyropoikilocytosis and hereditary elliptocytosis. *Am J Clin Pathol* 1987;88:58–65.

1562. Dhermy D, Garbarz M, Lecomte MC, et al. Abnormal electrophoretic mobility of spectrin tetramers in hereditary elliptocytosis. *Hum Genet* 1986;74:363–367.

1563. Lambert S, Zail S. A new variant of the α subunit of spectrin in hereditary elliptocytosis. *Blood* 1987;69:473–478.

1564. Giorgi M, Cianci CD, Gallagher PG, et al. Spectrin oligomerization is cooperatively coupled to membrane assembly: a linkage targeted by many hereditary hemolytic anemias? *Exp Mol Pathol* 2001;70:215–230.

1565. Zhang Z, Weed SA, Gallagher PG, et al. Dynamic molecular modeling of pathogenic mutations in the spectrin self-association domain. *Blood* 2001; 98:1645–1653.

1566. Speicher DW, Weglarz L, DeSilva TM. Properties of human red cell spectrin heterodimer (side-to-side) assembly and identification of an essential nucleation site. *J Biol Chem* 1992;267:14775–14782.

1567. Wilmotte R, Harper SL, Ursitti JA, et al. The exon 46-encoded sequence is essential for stability of human erythroid alpha-spectrin and heterodimer formation. *Blood* 1997;90:4188–4196.

1568. Wilmotte R, Marechal J, Delaunay J. Mutation at position –12 of intron 45 (c→t) plays a prevalent role in the partial skipping of exon 46 from the transcript of allele αLELY in erythroid cells. *Br J Haematol* 1999;104:855–859.

1569. Kotula L, Laury-Kleintop LD, Showe L, et al. The exon-intron organization of the human erythrocyte α-spectrin gene. *Genomics* 1991;9:131–140.

1570. Pranke PH, Basseres DS, Costa FF, et al. Expression of spectrin alpha I/65 hereditary elliptocytosis in patients from Brazil. *Br J Haematol* 1996;94:470–475.

1571. Bassères DS, Pranke PH, Vicentim D, et al. Expression of spectrin αI/50 hereditary elliptocytosis and its association with the alpha allele. *Acta Haematol* 1998;100:32–38.

1572. Speicher DW, DeSilva TM, Speicher KD, et al. Location of the human red cell spectrin tetramer binding site and detection of a related "closed" hairpin loop dimer using proteolytic footprinting. *J Biol Chem* 1993;268:4227–4235.

1573. Palek J, Lambert S. Genetics of the red cell membrane skeleton. *Semin Hematol* 1990;27:290–332.

1574. Schulman S, Roth EF Jr, Cheng B, et al. Growth of *Plasmodium falciparum* in human erythrocytes containing abnormal membrane proteins. *Proc Natl Acad Sci U S A* 1990;87:7339–7343.

1575. Lawler J, Palek J, Liu SC, et al. Molecular heterogeneity of a hereditary pyropoikilocytosis: identification of a second variant of the spectrin alpha-subunit. *Blood* 1983;62:1182–1189.

1576. Cohen CM, Langley RC Jr. Functional characterization of human erythrocyte spectrin alpha and beta chains: association with actin and erythrocyte protein 4.1. *Biochemistry* 1984;23:4488–4495.

1577. Lecomte MC, Gautero H, Garbarz M, et al. Abnormal tryptic peptide from the spectrin α-chain resulting from α- or β-chain mutations: two genetically distinct forms of the Sp αI/74 variant. *Br J Haematol* 1990;76:406.

1578. Féo CJ, Fischer S, Piau JP, et al. Première observation de l'absence d'une protèine de la membrane èrythrocytaire (band-41) dans un cas d'anèmie elliptocytaire familiale. *Nouv Rev Fr Hematol* 1981;22:315–325.

1579. Lambert S, Conboy J, Zail S. A molecular study of heterozygous protein 4.1 deficiency in hereditary elliptocytosis. *Blood* 1988;72:1926–1929.

1580. Conboy JG. Structure, function, and molecular genetics of erythroid membrane skeletal protein 4.1 in normal and abnormal red blood cells. *Semin Hematol* 1993;30:58–73.

1581. Reid ME, Takakuwa Y, Conboy JG, et al. Glycophorin C content of human erythrocyte membrane is regulated by protein 4.1. *Blood* 1990;75:2229–2234.

1582. Sondag D, Alloisio N, Blanchard D, et al. Gerbich reactivity in 4.1 (-) hereditary elliptocytosis and protein 4.1 level in blood group Gerbich deficiency. *Br J Haematol* 1987;65:43–50.

1583. Alloisio N, Dalla Venezia N, Rana A, et al. Evidence that red blood cell protein p55 may participate in the skeleton-membrane linkage that involves protein 4.1 and glycophorin C. *Blood* 1993;82:1323–1327.

1584. Reid ME, Chasis JA, Mohandas N. Identification of a functional role for human erythrocyte sialoglycoproteins beta and gamma. *Blood* 1987;69:1068–1072.

1585. Marfatia SM, Lue RA, Branton D, et al. In vitro binding studies suggest a membrane-associated complex between erythroid p55, protein 4.1, and glycophorin C. *J Biol Chem* 1994;269:8631.

1586. Rybicki AC, Heath R, Lubin B, et al. Human erythrocyte protein 4.1 is a phosphatidylserine binding protein. *J Clin Invest* 1988;81:255–260.

1587. Alloisio N, Dorlèac E, Girot R, et al. Analysis of the red cell membrane in a family with hereditary elliptocytosis—total or partial absence of protein 4.1. *Hum Genet* 1981;59:68–71.

1588. Schischmanoff PO, Winardi R, Discher DE, et al. Defining of the minimal domain of protein 4.1 involved in spectrin-actin binding. *J Biol Chem* 1995;270:21243.

1589. Cartron JP, Le Van Kim C, Colin Y. Glycophorin C and related glycoproteins: structure, function, and regulation. *Semin Hematol* 1993;30:152–168.

1590. Le Van Kim C, Colin Y, Blanchard D, et al. Gerbich blood group of the Ge:-1, -2, -3 types: immunochemical study and genomic analysis with cDNA probes. *Eur J Biochem* 1987;165:571–579.

1591. Jarolim P, Palek J, Amato D, et al. Deletion in the band 3 gene in malaria resistant Southeast Asian ovalocytosis. *Proc Natl Acad Sci U S A* 1991;88:11022–11026.

1592. Tanner MJA, Bruce L, Martin PG, et al. Melanesian hereditary ovalocytes have a deletion in red cell band 3. *Blood* 1991;78:2785–2786.

1593. Mueller TJ, Morrison M. Detection of a variant of protein 3, the major transmembrane protein of the human erythrocyte. *J Biol Chem* 1977;252:6573–6576.

1594. Jarolim P, Rubin HL, Zhai S, et al. Band 3 Memphis: a widespread polymorphism with abnormal electrophoretic mobility of erythrocyte band 3 protein caused by the substitution AAG → GAG (Lys → Glu) in codon 56. *Blood* 1992;80:1592–1598.

1595. Yannoukakos D, Vasseur C, Driancourt C, et al. Human erythrocyte band 3 polymorphism (band 3 Memphis): characterization of the structural modification (Lys56 → Glu) by protein chemistry methods. *Blood* 1991;78:1117–1120.

1596. Mgone CS, Genton B, Peter W, et al. The correlation between microscopical examination and erythrocyte band 3 (AE1) gene deletion in South-east Asian ovalocytosis. *Trans R Soc Trop Med Hyg* 1998;92:296–299.

1597. Schofield AE, Rearden DM, Tanner MJA. Defective anion transport activity of the abnormal band 3 in hereditary ovalocytic red cells. *Nature* 1992;335:836–838.

1598. Tanner MJA, Bruce L, Groves JD, et al. The defective red cell anion transporter (band 3) in hereditary Southeast Asian ovalocytosis and the role of glycophorin A in the expression of band 3 anion transport activity in *Xenopus* oocytes. *Biochem Soc Trans* 1992;20:542–546.

1599. Jones GL, McLemore Edmundson H, Wesche D, et al. Human erythrocyte band 3 has an altered N-terminus in malaria resistant Melanesian ovalocytosis. *Biochem Biophys Acta* 1991;1096:33–38.

1600. Salhany JM, Schopfer LM. Interactions between mutant and wild-type band 3 subunits in hereditary Southeast Asian ovalocytic red blood cell membranes. *Biochemistry* 1996;35:251–257.

1601. Mohandas N, Chasis JA, Shohet SB. The influence of membrane skeleton on red cell deformability, membrane material properties, and shape. *Semin Hematol* 1983;20:225–242.

1602. Chambers EJ, Bloomberg GB, Ring SM, et al. Structural studies on the effects of the deletion in the red cell anion exchanger (band 3, AE1) associated with South East Asian ovalocytosis. *J Mol Biol* 1999;285:1289–1307.

1603. Moriyama R, Ideguchi H, Lombardo CR, et al. Structural and functional characterization of band 3 from Southeast Asian ovalocytes. *J Biol Chem* 1992;267:25792–25797.

1604. Bunyaratvej A, Butthep P, Kaewkettong P, et al. Malaria protection in hereditary ovalocytosis: relation to red cell deformability, red cell parameters and degree of ovalocytosis. *Southeast Asian J Trop Med Public Health* 1997;28[Suppl 3]:38–42.

1605. Okoye VCN, Bennett V. *Plasmodium falciparum* malaria. Band 3 as a possible receptor during invasion of human erythrocytes. *Science* 1985;227:169–171.

1606. Dluzewski AR, Fryer PR, Griffiths S, et al. Red cell membrane protein distribution during malarial invasion. *J Cell Sci* 1989;92:691–699.

1607. Rebuck JW, van Slyck EJ. An unsuspected ultrastructural fault in human elliptocytes. *Am J Clin Pathol* 1968;49:19–25.

1608. Bessis M. *Living blood cells and their ultrastructure.* New York: Springer Verlag, 1973:140–145.

1609. Lux SE, John KM. The role of spectrin and actin in irreversibly sickled cells. Unsickling of "irreversibly" sickled shapes by conditions which interfere with spectrin-actin polymerization. In: Caughey WS, ed. *Biochemical and clinical aspects of hemoglobin abnormalities.* New York: Academic Press, 1978:335–352.

1610. Liu SC, Derick LH, Palek J. Dependence of the permanent deformation of red blood cell membranes on spectrin dimer tetramer equilibrium: implication for permanent membrane deformation of irreversibly sickled cells. *Blood* 1993;81:522–528.

1611. De Gruchy GC, Loder PB, Hennessy IV. Haemolysis and glycolytic metabolism in hereditary elliptocytosis. *Br J Haematol* 1932;8:168–179.

1612. Peters JC, Rowland M, Israels LG, et al. Erythrocyte sodium transport in hereditary elliptocytosis. *Can J Physiol Pharmacol* 1966;44:817–827.

1613. Facer CA. Malaria, hereditary elliptocytosis, and pyropoikilocytosis [Letter]. *Lancet* 1989;1:897.

1614. Schultze M. Ein heizbarer objectisch und seine verwendung bei untersuchungen des blutes. *Arch Mikrok Anat* 1865;1:1.

1615. Shen SC, Ham TH, et al. Studies on the destruction of red blood cells. III. Mechanism and complication of hemoglobinuria in patients with thermal burns: spherocytosis and increased osmotic fragility of red blood cells. *N Engl J Med* 1943;229:701.

1616. Topley E. The usefulness of counting "heat affected" red cells as a guide to the risk of the later disappearance of red cells after burns. *J Clin Pathol* 1961;14:295.

1617. James GW III, Purnell OJ, et al. The anemia of thermal injury. I. Studies of pigment excretion. *J Clin Invest* 1951;30:181.

1618. James GW III, Abbott LD, et al. The anemia of thermal injury. III. Erythropoiesis and hemoglobin metabolism studied with N15 glycine in dog and man. *J Clin Invest* 1954;33:150.

1619. Moore FD, Peacock WC, et al. The anemia of thermal burns. *Ann Surg* 1946;124:811.

1620. Still JM Jr, Belcher K, Law EJ, et al. A double-blinded prospective evaluation of recombinant human erythropoietin in acutely burned patients. *J Trauma* 1995;38:233–236.

1621. McCollough J, Polesky HF, et al. Iatrogenic hemolysis: a complication of blood warmed by a microwave device. *Anesth Analg* 1972;51:102.

1622. Staples PJ, Griner PF. Extracorporeal hemolysis of blood in a microwave blood warmer. *N Engl J Med* 1971;285:317.

1623. Jacob HS, Amsden T. Acute hemolytic anemia with rigid red cells in hypophosphatemia. *N Engl J Med* 1971;285:1446.

1624. Lichtman MA, Miller DR, et al. Reduced red cell glycolysis, 2,3-diphosphoglycerate and adenosine triphosphate concentration, and increased hemoglobin oxygen affinity caused by hypophosphatemia. *Ann Intern Med* 1971;74:562.

1625. Myers G, Ngoi SS, Cennerazzo W, et al. Clostridial septicemia in an urban hospital. *Surg Gynecol Obstet* 1992;174:291–296.

1626. Mupanemunda RH, Kenyon CF, Inwood MJ, et al. Bacterial-induced activation of erythrocyte T antigen complicating necrotising enterocolitis: a case report. *Eur J Pediatr* 1993;152:325–326.

1627. Placzek MM, Gorst DW. T activation haemolysis and death after blood transfusion. *Arch Dis Child* 1987;62:743–744.

1628. Warren S, Schreiber JR, Epstein MF. Necrotizing enterocolitis and hemolysis associated with *Clostridium perfringens*. *Am J Dis Child* 1984;138:686–688.

1629. Williams RA, Brown EF, Hurst D. Transfusion of infants with activation of erythrocyte T antigen. *J Pediatr* 1989;115:949–953.

1630. Dean HM, Decker CL, et al. Temporary survival in Clostridial hemolysis with absence of circulating red cells. *N Engl J Med* 1967;277:700.

1631. Ifthikaruddin JJ, Holmes JA. *Clostridium perfringens* septicaemia and massive intravascular haemolysis as a terminal complication of autologous bone marrow transplant. *Clin Lab Haematol* 1992;14:159–161.

1632. Batge B, Filejski W, Kurowski V, et al. Clostridial sepsis with massive intravascular hemolysis: rapid diagnosis and successful treatment. *Intensive Care Med* 1992;18:488–490.

1633. Tsai IK, Yen MY, Ho IC, et al. *Clostridium perfringens* septicemia with massive hemolysis. *Scand J Infect Dis* 1989;21:467–471.

1634. Becker RC, Giuliani M, Savage RA, et al. Massive hemolysis in *Clostridium perfringens* infections. *J Surg Oncol* 1987;35:13–18.

1635. Bennett JM, Healey PJM. Spherocytic hemolytic anemia and acute cholecystitis caused by *Clostridium welchii*. *N Engl J Med* 1963;268:1070.

1636. Mera CL, Freedman MH. Clostridium liver abscess and massive hemolysis. Unique demise in Fanconi's aplastic anemia. *Clin Pediatr (Phila)* 1984;23:126–127.

1637. Anonymous. Abdominal pain, total intravascular hemolysis, and death in a 53 year old woman [clinical conference]. *Am J Med* 1992;88:667–674.

1638. Terebelo HR, McCue RL, Lenneville MS. Implication of plasma free hemoglobin in massive clostridial hemolysis. *JAMA* 1982;248:2028–2029.

1639. Hungerland E, Eiring P, Bültmann B. *Clostridium sordellii* sepsis with intravascular haemolysis (German). *Dtsch Med Wochenschr* 1997;122:1281–1284.

1640. Guillouard I, Alzari PM, Saliou B, et al. The carboxy-terminal C2-like domain of the alpha-toxin from *Clostridium perfringens* mediates calcium-dependent membrane recognition. *Mol Microbiol* 1997;26:867–876.

1641. Titball RW, Leslie DL, Harvey S, et al. Hemolytic and sphingomyelinase activities of Clostridium perfringens alpha toxin are dependent on a domain homologous to that of an enzyme from the human arachidonic acid pathway. *Infect Immun* 1991;59:1872–1874.

1642. Schoepe H, Wieler LH, Bauerfeind R, et al. Neutralization of hemolytic and mouse lethal activities of *C. perfringens* alpha-toxin need simultaneous blockade of two epitopes by monoclonal antibodies. *Microb Pathog* 1997;23:1–10.

1643. Nagahama M, Sakurai J. Threonine-74 is a key site for the activity of *Clostridium perfringens* alpha-toxin. *Microbiol Immunol* 1996;40:189–193.

1644. Alape-Giron A, Flores-Diaz M, Guillouard I, et al. Identification of residues critical for toxicity in *Clostridium perfringens* phospholipase C, the key toxin in gas gangrene. *Eur J Biochem* 2000;267:5191–5197.

1645. Gordon VM, Benz R, Fujii K, et al. *Clostridium septicum* alpha-toxin is proteolytically activated by furin. *Infect Immun* 1997;65:4130–4134.

1646. Tweten RK. Cloning and expression in *Escherichia coli* of the perfringolysin O (theta toxin) from *Clostridium perfringens* and characterization of the gene product. *Infect Immun* 1988;56:3228–3234.

1647. Iwamoto M, Ohno-Iwashita Y, Ando S. Effect of isolated C terminal fragment of theta toxin (perfringolysin O) on toxin assembly and membrane lysis. *Eur J Biochem* 1990;194:25–31.

1648. Harris RW, Sims PJ, Tweten RK. Kinetic aspects of the aggregation of *Clostridium perfringens* theta-toxin on erythrocyte membranes. A fluorescence energy transfer study. *J Biol Chem* 1991;266:6936–6941.

1649. Hubl W, Mostbeck B, Hartleb H, et al. Investigation of the pathogenesis of massive hemolysis in a case of *Clostridium perfringens* septicemia. *Ann Hematol* 1993;67:145–147.

1650. Teach SJ, Priebe CJ, Guerina NG. Survival following congenital clostridial sepsis in a premature newborn. *Clin Pediatr (Phila)* 1994;33:746–748.

1651. Perseghin P, Epis R, Pastorini A, et al. Acute intravascular haemolysis with massive microspherocytosis in a 75-year-old woman. *Recenti Prog Med* 1997;88:459–460.

1652. Irvin TT, Moir ERS, et al. Treatment of *Clostridium welchii* infection with hyperbaric oxygen. *Surg Gynecol Obstet* 1968;127:1058.

1653. Iyaniwura TT. Snake venom constituents: biochemistry and toxicology [part 1]. *Vet Hum Toxicol* 1991;33:468–474.

1654. Perkash A, Sarup BM. Red cell abnormalities after snake bite. *J Trop Med Hyg* 1972;75:85.

1655. Reid HA. Cobra bites. *BMJ* 1964;2:540.

1656. Gibly RL, Walter FG, Nowlin SW, et al. Intravascular hemolysis associated with North American crotalid envenomation. *J Toxicol Clin Toxicol* 1998;36:337–343.

1657. Foil LD, Norment BR. Envenomation by *Loxosceles reclusa*. *J Med Entomol* 1979;16:18.

1658. Nance WE. Hemolytic anemia of necrotic arachnidism. *Am J Med* 1961;31:801.

1659. Williams ST, Khare VK, Johnston GA, et al. Severe intravascular hemolysis associated with brown recluse spider envenomation. A report of two cases and review of the literature. *Am J Clin Pathol* 1995;104:463–467.

1660. Sezerino UM, Zannin M, Coelho LK, et al. A clinical and epidemiological study of Loxosceles spider envenoming in Santa Catarina, Brazil. *Trans R Soc Trop Med Hyg* 1998;92:546–548.

1661. Dacie JV. Haemolytic anemias due to drugs, chemicals and venoms: glucose-6-phosphate dehydrogenase deficiency and favism. In: *The haemolytic anaemias, congenital and acquired*, 2nd ed. Part IV. New York: Grune & Stratton, 1967:993–1127.

1662. Vetter RS, Visscher PK, Camazine S. Mass envenomations by honey bees and wasps. *West J Med* 1999;170:223–227.

1663. Monzon C, Miles J. Hemolytic anemia following a wasp sting. *J Pediatr* 1980;96:1039–1040.

1664. Schulte KL, Kochen MM. Haemolytic anemia in an adult after a wasp sting [Letter]. *Lancet* 1981;2:478.

1665. Chao SC, Lee YY. Acute rhabdomyolysis and intravascular hemolysis following extensive wasp stings. *Int J Dermatol* 1999;38:135–137.

1666. Bousquet J, Huchard G, et al. Toxic reactions induced by hymenoptera venom. *Ann Allergy* 1984;52:371.

1667. Guess HA, Saviteer PL, et al. Hemolysis and acute renal failure following a Portuguese man of war sting. *Pediatrics* 1982;70:979.

1668. Argiolas A, Pisano JJ. Facilitation of phospholipase A2 activity by masto-parans, a new class of mast cell degranulation peptides from wasp venom. *J Biol Chem* 1983;25:13697–13702.

1669. Ho CL, Hwang LL. Structure and biological activities of a new mastoparan isolated from the venom of the hornet Vespa basalis. *Biochem J* 1991;274:453–456.

1670. Katsu T, Kuroko M, Morikawa T, et al. Interaction of wasp venom mastoparan with biomembranes. *Biochim Biophys Acta* 1990;1027:185–190.

1671. Claque MJ, Cherry RJ. A comparative study of band 3 aggregation in erythrocyte membranes by melittin and other cationic agents. *Biochim Biophys Acta* 1989;980:93–99.

1672. Dempsey CE. The actions of melittin on membranes. *Biochim Biophys Acta* 1990;1031:143–161.

1673. Dufton MJ, Hider RC, Cherry RJ. The influence of melittin on the rotation of band 3 protein in the human erythrocyte membrane. *Eur Biophys J* 1984;11:17–24.

1674. Hui SW, Stewart CM, Cherry RJ. Electron microscopic observation of the aggregation of membrane proteins in human erythrocyte by melittin. *Biochim Biophys Acta* 1990;1023:335–340.

1675. Eichner ER. Spider bite hemolytic anemia: positive Coombs' test, erythrophagocytosis, and leukoerythroblastic smear. *Am J Clin Pathol* 1984;81:683–687.

1676. Hardman JT, Beck ML, et al. Incompatibility associated with the bite of a brown recluse spider (*Loxosceles reclusa*). *Transfusion* 1983;23:233.

1677. Madrigal GC, Ercolani RL, Wenzl JE. Toxicity from a bite of the brown spider (*Loxosceles reclusus*). Skin necrosis, hemolytic anemia, and hemoglobinuria in a nine-year-old child. *Clin Pediatr (Phila)* 1972;11:641–644.

1678. Tambourgi DV, Magnoli FC, van den Berg CW, et al. Sphingomyelinases in the venom of the spider Loxosceles intermedia are responsible for both dermonecrosis and complement-dependent hemolysis. *Biochem Biophys Res Commun* 1998;251:366–373.

1679. Futrell JM, Morgan PN, et al. Location of brown recluse venom attachment sites on human erythrocytes by the ferritin labeled antibody technique. *Am J Pathol* 1979;95:675.

1680. Kurpiewski G, Campbell BJ, Forrester LJ, et al. Alternate complement pathway activation by recluse spider venom. *Int J Tissue React* 1981;3:39–45.

1681. Taylor EH, Denny WF. Hemolysis, renal failure and death, presumed secondary to bite of brown recluse spider. *South Med J* 1966;59:1209–1211.

1682. Vorse H, Seccareccio P, Woodruff K, et al. Disseminated intravascular coagulopathy following fatal brown spider bite (necrotic arachnidism). *J Pediatr* 1972;80:1035–1037.

1683. Gebel HM, Finke JH, Elgert KD, et al. Inactivation of complement by *Loxosceles reclusa* spider venom. *Am J Trop Med Hyg* 1979;28:756–762.

1684. Wilcken B, Hammond JW, Howard N, et al. Hawkinsinuria: a dominantly inherited defect of tyrosine metabolism with severe effects in infancy. *N Engl J Med* 1981;305:865–869.

1685. Brecher G, Haley JE, Wallerstein RO. Spiculated erythrocytes after splenectomy: acanthocytes or non-specific poikilocytes? *Nouv Rev Fr Hematol* 1972;12:751–754.

1686. Furchgott RF. Disk sphere transformation in mammalian red cells. *J Exp Biol* 1940;17:30.

1687. Nakao M, Nakao T, et al. Adenosine triphosphate and shape of erythrocytes. *J Biochem (Tokyo)* 1961;45:487.

1688. Palek J, Stewart G, et al. The dependence of shape of human erythrocyte ghosts on calcium, magnesium, and adenosine triphosphate. *Blood* 1974;44:583.

1689. Gedde MM, Yang E, Huestis WH. Shape response of human erythrocytes to altered cell pH. *Blood* 1995;86:1595–1599.

1690. Gedde MM, Huestis WH. Membrane potential and human erythrocyte shape. *Biophys J* 1997;72:1220–1233.

1691. Dacie JV. The hereditary haemolytic anaemias, 3rd ed. In: *The haemolytic anaemias*, Vol 1. Edinburgh: Churchill Livingstone, 1985.

1692. Hardie RJ. Acanthocytosis and neurological impairment—a review. *QJM* 1989;71:291–306.

1693. Féo CJ, Tchernia G, et al. Observation of echinocytosis in eight patients: a phase contrast and SEM study. *Br J Haematol* 1978;40:519.

1694. Zipursky A, Brown E, et al. The erythrocyte differential count in newborn infants. *Am J Pediatr Hematol Oncol* 1983;5:45.

1695. Aherne WA. The "burr" red cell and azotaemia. *J Clin Pathol* 1957;10:252.

1696. Schwartz SO, Motto SA. The diagnostic significance of "burr" red blood cells. *Am J Med Sci* 1949;218:513.

1697. Oski FA, Nathan DG, et al. Extreme hemolysis and red cell distortion in erythrocyte pyruvate kinase deficiency. I. Morphology, erythrokinetics and family enzyme studies. *N Engl J Med* 1964;270:1023.

1698. Dacie JV. Secondary or symptomatic haemolytic anaemias. II. Haemolytic anaemias associated with systemic lupus erythematosus, ulcerative colitis, liver disease, renal disease and vascular disease. In: *Haemolytic anaemias, congenital and acquired*, 2nd ed. Part III. New York: Grune & Stratton, 1967:810–907.

1699. Carlyle RF, Nichols G, et al. Abnormal red cells in blood of men subjected to simulated dives. *Lancet* 1979;1:1114.

1700. Walton RM, Brown DE, Hamar DW, et al. Mechanisms of echinocytosis induced by *Crotalus atrox* venom. *Vet Pathol* 1997;34:442–449.

1701. Flachsenberger W, Leigh CM, Mirtschin PJ. Sphero-echinocytosis of human red blood cells caused by snake, red-back spider, bee and blue-ringed octopus venoms and its inhibition by snake sera. *Toxicon* 1995;33:791–797.

1702. Zharskaya VD, Chukhlovin AB. Early post-radiation changes of red blood cell shape in rats. *Scanning Microsc* 1996;10:279–283.

1703. Agroyannis B, Dalamangas A, Tzanatos H, et al. Alterations in echinocyte transformation and erythrocyte sedimentation rate during hemodialysis. *Artif Organs* 1997;21:327–330.

1704. Hasler CR, Owen GR, Brunner W, et al. Echinocytosis induced by haemodialysis. *Nephrol Dial Transplant* 1998;13:3132–3137.

1705. Cooper RA. Anemia with spur cells: a red cell defect acquired in serum and modified in the circulation. *J Clin Invest* 1969;48:1820.

1706. Bassen FA, Kornzweig AL. Malformation of the erythrocytes in a case of atypical retinitis pigmentosa. *Blood* 1950;5:381.

1707. Tuffy P, Brown AK, et al. Infantile pyknocytosis: a common erythrocyte abnormality of the first trimester. *Am J Dis Child* 1959;98:227.

1708. Symmans WA, Shepard CS, Marsh WL, et al. Hereditary acanthocytosis associated with the McLeod phenotype of the Kell blood group system. *Br J Haematol* 1979;42:575–583.

1709. Udden MM, Umeda M, Hirano Y, et al. New abnormalities in the morphology, cell surface receptors, and electrolyte metabolism of In(Lu) erythrocytes. *Blood* 1987;69:52–57.

1710. Doll DC, List AF, et al. Acanthocytosis associated with myelodysplasia. *J Clin Oncol* 1989;7:1569.

1711. Ohsaka A, Yawata Y, Enomoto Y, et al. Abnormal calcium transport of acanthocytes in acute myelodysplasia with myelofibrosis. *Br J Haematol* 1989;73:568–570.

1712. Wardrop C, Hutchison HE. Red-cell shape in hypothyroidism. *Lancet* 1969;1:1243.

1713. Kay J, Stricker RB. Hematologic and immunologic abnormalities in anorexia nervosa [review]. *South Med J* 1983;76:1008.

1714. Mant MJ, Faragher BS. The haematology of anorexia nervosa. *Br J Haematol* 1972;23:737.

1715. Joske RA, McAlister JM, et al. Isotope investigations of red cell production and destruction in chronic renal disease. *Clin Sci (Lond)* 1956;15:511.

1716. Loge JP, Lange RD, et al. Characterization of the anemia associated with chronic renal insufficiency. *Am J Med* 1958;24:4.

1717. Akmal M, Telfer N, et al. Red blood cell survival in chronic renal failure: role of secondary hyperparathyroidism. *J Clin Invest* 1985;76:1695.

1718. Bogin E, Massry SG, et al. Effect of parathyroid hormone on osmotic fragility of human erythrocytes. *J Clin Invest* 1982;69:1017.

1719. Saltissi D, Carter GD. Association of secondary hyperparathyroidism with red cell survival in chronic haemodialysis patients. *Clin Sci* 1985;68:29.

1720. White JG. Effects of an ionophore A23187 on the surface morphology of normal erythrocytes. *Am J Pathol* 1974;77:507.

1721. Jandl JH. The anemia of liver disease: observations on its mechanism. *J Clin Invest* 1955;34:390.

1722. Kimber CD, Deller J, et al. The mechanism of anaemia in chronic liver disease. *QJM* 1965;34:33.

1723. Balistreri WF, Leslie MH, Cooper RA. Increased cholesterol and decreased fluidity of red cell membranes (spur cell anemia) in progressive intrahepatic cholestasis. *Pediatrics* 1981;67:461–466.

1724. Cynamon HA, Isenberg JN, Gustavson LP, et al. Erythrocyte lipid alterations in pediatric cholestatic liver disease: spur cell anemia of infancy. *J Pediatr Gastroenterol Nutr* 1985;4:542–549.

1725. Doll DC, Doll NJ. Spur cell anemia. *South Med J* 1982;75:1205–1210.

1726. Douglass CC, McCall MS, et al. The acanthocyte in cirrhosis with hemolytic anemia. *Ann Intern Med* 1968;68:390.

1727. Grahn EP, Dietz AA, et al. Burr cells, hemolytic anemia and cirrhosis. *Am J Med* 1968;45:78.

1728. Greenberg MS, Choi ES. Post-splenectomy spur cell hemolytic anemia. *Am J Med Sci* 1975;269:277–280.

1729. Hitchins R, Naughton L, Kerlin P, et al. Spur cell anemia (acanthocytosis) complicating idiopathic hemochromatosis. *Pathology* 1988;20:59–61.

1730. Keller JW, Majerus PW, et al. An unusual type of spiculated erythrocyte in metastatic liver disease and hemolytic anemia. Report of a case. *Ann Intern Med* 1971;74:732.

1731. Silber R, Amorosi E, et al. Spur shaped erythrocytes in Laennec's cirrhosis. *N Engl J Med* 1966;275:639.

1732. Smith JA, Lonergan ET, et al. Spur cell anemia: hemolytic anemia with red cells resembling acanthocytes in alcoholic cirrhosis. *N Engl J Med* 1964;276:396.

1733. Stillman AE, Giordano GF. Spur cell anemia associated with extrahepatic biliary tract obstruction. *Am J Gastroenterol* 1983;78:589–592.

1734. Taniguchi M, Tanabe F, Ishikawa H, et al. Experimental biliary obstruction of rat. Initial changes in the structure and lipid content of erythrocytes. *Biochim Biophys Acta* 1983;753:22–31.

1735. Tchernia G, Navarro J, et al. Anemie hemolytique avec acanthocytose et dyslipidemie au cours de deux hepatites neonatales. *Arch Fr Pediatr* 1968;25:729.

1736. Cooper RA, Kimball DB, et al. Role of the spleen in membrane conditioning and hemolysis of spur cells in liver disease. *N Engl J Med* 1974;290:1279.

1737. Salvioli G, Rioli G, Lugli R, et al. Membrane lipid composition of red blood cells in liver disease: regression of spur cell anaemia after infusion of polyunsaturated phosphatidylcholine. *Gut* 1978;19:844–850.

1738. Fossaluzza V, Rossi P. Flunarizine treatment for spur cell anaemia. *Br J Haematol* 1983;55:715.

1739. Aihara K, Azuma H, Ikeda Y, et al. Successful combination therapy—flunarizine, pentoxifylline, and cholestyramine—for spur cell anemia. *Int J Hematol* 2001;73:351–355.

1740. Cooper RA, Diloy Puray M, et al. An analysis of lipoproteins, bile acids, and red cell membranes associated with target cells and spur cells in patients with liver disease. *J Clin Invest* 1972;31:3182.

1741. Cooper RA, Leslie MH, et al. Factors influencing the lipid composition and fluidity of red cell membranes in vitro: production of red cells possessing more than two cholesterols per phospholipid. *Biochemistry* 1978;17:327.

1742. Cooper RA, Leslie MH, Knight D, et al. Red cell cholesterol enrichment and spur cell anemia in dogs fed a cholesterol-enriched atherogenic diet. *J Lipid Res* 1980;21:1082–1089.

1743. Duhamel G, Forgez P, et al. Spur cells in patients with alcoholic liver cirrhosis are associated with reduced plasma levels of apo AII, HDL, and LDL. *J Lipid Res* 1983;24:1612.

1743a. Lichtenstein IH, Zaleski EM, MacGregor RR. Neutrophil dysfunction in the rabbit model of spur cell anemia. *J Leukoc Biol* 1987;42:156–162.

1744. Schubert D, Boss K. Band 3 protein cholesterol interactions in erythrocyte membranes: possible role in anion transport and dependency on membrane phospholipid. *FEBS Lett* 1982;150:4.

1745. Seigneuret M, Favre E, et al. Strong interactions between a spin labeled cholesterol analog and erythrocyte proteins in the human erythrocyte membrane. *Biochim Biophys Acta* 1985;813:174.

1746. Lange Y, Cutler HB, et al. The effect of cholesterol and other interrelated amphipaths on the contour and stability of the isolated red cell membrane. *J Biol Chem* 1980;255:9331.

1747. Rooney MW, Lange Y, et al. Acyl chain organization and protein secondary structure in cholesterol modified erythrocyte membranes. *J Biol Chem* 1984; 259:8281.

1748. Olivieri O, Guarini P, Negri M, et al. Increased proteolytic activity of erythrocyte membrane in spur cell anaemia. *Br J Haematol* 1988;70:483–489.

1749. Allen DW, Manning N. Abnormal phospholipid metabolism in spur cell anemia: decreased fatty acid incorporation into phosphatidylethanolamine and increased incorporation into acylcarnitine in spur cell anemia erythrocytes. *Blood* 1994;84:1283–1287.

1750. Allen DW, Manning N. Cholesterol-loading of membranes of normal erythrocytes inhibits phospholipid repair and arachidonoyl-CoA:1-palmitoyl-sn-glycero-3-phosphocholine acyl transferase. A model of spur cell anemia. *Blood* 1996;87:3489–3493.

1751. Zieve L. Jaundice, hyperlipemia and hemolytic anemia: a heretofore unrecognized syndrome associated with alcoholic fatty liver and cirrhosis. *Ann Intern Med* 1958;48:471.

1752. Salt HB, Wolff OH, Lloyd JK, et al. On having no beta-lipoprotein. A syndrome comprising a-beta-lipoproteinaemia, acanthocytosis, and steatorrhoea. *Lancet* 1960;2:326–328.

1753. Kane JP, Havel RJ. Disorders of the biogenesis and secretion of lipoproteins containing the B apolipoproteins. In: Scriver CR, Beaudet AL, Sly WS, et al., eds. *The metabolic and molecular bases of inherited disease*, 8th ed. New York: McGraw-Hill, 2001:2717–2752.

1754. Sharp D, Blinderman L, Combs KA, et al. Cloning and gene defects in microsomal triglyceride transfer protein associated with abetalipoproteinaemia. *Nature* 1993;365:65–69.

1755. Wetterau JR, Aggerbeck LP, Bouma ME, et al. Absence of microsomal triglyceride transfer protein in individuals with abetalipoproteinemia. *Science* 1992;258:999–1001.

1756. Raabe M, Véniant MM, Sullivan MA, et al. Analysis of the role of microsomal triglyceride transfer protein in the liver of tissue-specific knockout mice. *J Clin Invest* 1999;103:1287–1298.

1757. Ricci B, Sharp D, O'Rourke E, et al. A 30-amino acid truncation of the microsomal triglyceride transfer protein large subunit disrupts its interaction with protein disulfide-isomerase and causes abetalipoproteinemia. *J Biol Chem* 1995;270:14281–14285.

1758. Narcisi TM, Shoulders CC, Chester SA, et al. Mutations of the microsomal triglyceride-transfer-protein gene in abetalipoproteinemia. *Am J Hum Genet* 1995;57:1298–1310.

1759. Black DD, Hay RV, Rohwer-Nutter PL, et al. Intestinal and hepatic apolipoprotein B gene expression in abetalipoproteinemia. *Gastroenterology* 1991; 101:520–528.

1760. Hardman DA, Pullinger CR, Hamilton RL, et al. Molecular and metabolic basis for the metabolic disorder normotriglyceridemic abetalipoproteinemia. *J Clin Invest* 1991;88:1722–1729.

1761. Schonfeld G. Genetic variation of apolipoprotein B can produce both low and high levels of apoB-containing lipoproteins in plasma. *Can J Cardiol* 1995;11[Suppl G]:86G–92G.

1762. Gheeraert P, DeBuyzere M, Delanghe J, et al. Plasma and erythrocyte lipids in two families with heterozygous hypobetalipoproteinemia. *Clin Biochem* 1988;21:371–377.

1763. Simon ER, Ways P. Incubation hemolysis and red cell metabolism in acanthocytosis. *J Clin Invest* 1964;43:1311.

1764. Barenholz Y, Yechiel E, et al. Importance of cholesterolphospholipid interaction in determining dynamics of normal and abetalipoproteinemia red blood cell membrane. *Cell Biophys* 1981;3:115.

1765. Iida H, Takashima Y, et al. Alterations in erythrocyte membrane lipids in abetalipoproteinemia: phospholipid and fatty acyl composition. *Biochem Med* 1984;32:79.

1766. Cooper RA, Gulbrandsen CL. The relationship between serum lipoproteins and red cell membranes in abetalipoproteinemia: deficiency of lecithin:cholesterol acyltransferase. *J Lab Clin Med* 1971;78:323.

1767. Flamm M, Schachter D. Acanthocytosis and cholesterol enrichment decrease lipid fluidity of only the outer human erythrocyte membrane leaflet. *Nature* 1982;298:290.

1768. Lange Y, Steck TL. Mechanism of red blood cell acanthocytosis and echinocytosis in vivo. *J Membr Biol* 1984;77:153.

1769. McCormick EC, Cornwell DG, et al. Studies on the distribution of tocopherol in human serum lipoproteins. *J Lipid Res* 1969;1:211.

1770. Dodge JT, Cohen G, et al. Peroxidative hemolysis of red blood cells from patients with abetalipoproteinemia (acanthocytosis). *J Clin Invest* 1967; 46:357.

1771. Elias E, Muller DPR, Scott J. Association of spinocerebellar disorders with cystic fibrosis or chronic childhood cholestasis and very low serum vitamin E. *Lancet* 1981;2:1319–1321.

1772. Alvarez F, Landrieu P, Féo C, et al. Vitamin E deficiency is responsible for neurologic abnormalities in cholestatic children. *J Pediatr* 1985;107:422–425.

1773. Sokol RJ, Guggenheim MA, Heubi JE, et al. Frequency and clinical progression of the vitamin E deficiency neurologic disorder in children with prolonged neonatal cholestasis. *Am J Dis Child* 1985;139:1211–1215.

1774. Ouahchi K, Arita M, Kayden H, et al. Ataxia with isolated vitamin E deficiency is caused by mutations in the alpha-tocopherol transfer protein. *Nat Genet* 1995;9:141–145.

1775. Gotoda T, Arita M, Arai H, et al. Adult-onset spinocerebellar dysfunction caused by a mutation in the gene for the alpha-tocopherol-transfer protein. *N Engl J Med* 1995;333:1313–1318.

1776. Cavalier L, Ouahchi K, Kayden HJ, et al. Ataxia with isolated vitamin E deficiency: heterogeneity of mutations and phenotypic variability in a large number of families. *Am J Hum Genet* 1998;62:301–310.

1777. Sokol RJ, Guggenheim M, Iannaccone ST, et al. Improved neurologic function after long-term correction of vitamin E deficiency in children with chronic cholestasis. *N Engl J Med* 1985;313:1580–1586.

1778. Muller DPR, Lloyd JK, Bird AC. Long-term management of abetalipoproteinaemia. *Arch Dis Child* 1977;52:209–214.

1779. Melhorn DK, Gross S. Vitamin E dependent anemia in the premature infant. II. Relationships between gestational age and absorption of vitamin E. *J Pediatr* 1971;79:581.

1780. Ehrenkranz RA. Vitamin E and the neonate. *Am J Dis Child* 1980;134:1157–1166.

1781. Zipursky A. Vitamin E deficiency anemia in newborn infants. *Clin Perinatol* 1984;11:393–402.

1782. Dolan TF Jr. Hemolytic anemia and edema as the initial signs in infants with cystic fibrosis. *Clin Pediatr (Phila)* 1976;15:597–600.

1783. Monzon CM, Woodruff CW. Anemia and edema as presenting signs in cystic fibrosis: a case report. *J Med* 1986;17:135–141.

1784. Wilfond BS, Farrell PM, Laxova A, et al. Severe hemolytic anemia associated with vitamin E deficiency in infants with cystic fibrosis. Implications for neonatal screening. *Clin Pediatr (Phila)* 1994;33:2–7.

1785. Melhorn DK, Gross S. Vitamin E dependent anemia in the premature infant. I. Effects of large doses of medicinal iron. *J Pediatr* 1971;79:569.

1786. Oski FA, Barness LA. Vitamin E deficiency: a previously unrecognized cause of hemolytic anemia in the premature infant. *J Pediatr* 1967;70:211.

1787. Ritchie JH, Fish MB, et al. Edema and hemolytic anemia in premature infants: a vitamin E deficiency syndrome. *N Engl J Med* 1968;279:1185.

1788. Jacob HS, Lux SE. Degradation of membrane phospholipids and thiols in peroxide hemolysis: studies in vitamin E deficiency. *Blood* 1968;32:549.

1789. Brownlee NR, Huttner JJ, et al. Role of vitamin E in glutathione induced oxidant stress: methemoglobin, lipid peroxidation, and hemolysis. *J Lipid Res* 1977;18:635.

1790. Kay MMB, Bosman GJ, et al. Oxidation as a possible mechanism of cellular aging: vitamin E deficiency causes premature aging and IgG binding to erythrocytes. *Proc Natl Acad Sci U S A* 1986;83:2463.

1791. Estes JW, Morley JT, et al. A new hereditary acanthocytosis syndrome. *Am J Med* 1967;42:868.

1792. Levine IM, Estes JW, et al. Hereditary neurological disease with acanthocytosis. *Arch Neurol* 1968;19:403.

1793. Alonso ME, Teixeira F, Jimenez G, et al. Chorea-acanthocytosis: a report of a family and neuropathological study of two cases. *Can J Neurol Sci* 1989; 16:426–431.

1794. Asano K, Osawa Y, Yanagisawa N, et al. Erythrocyte membrane abnormalities in patients with amyotrophic chorea with acanthocytosis. Part 2. Abnormal degradation of membrane proteins. *J Neurol Sci* 1985;68:161–173.

1795. Clark MR, Aminoff MJ, Chiu DT, et al. Red cell deformability and lipid composition in two forms of acanthocytosis: enrichment of acanthocytic populations by density gradient centrifugation. *J Lab Clin Med* 1989;113:469–481.

1796. Critchley EMR, Clark DB, Wikler A. Acanthocytosis and neurological disorder without abetalipoproteinemia. *Arch Neurol* 1968;18:134–140.

1797. Faillace RT, Kingston WJ, et al. Cardiomyopathy associated with the syndrome of amyotrophic chorea and acanthocytosis. *Ann Intern Med* 1982;96:616.

1798. Gross KB, Skrivanek JA, Carlson KC, et al. Familial amyotrophic chorea with acanthocytosis. New clinical and laboratory investigations. *Arch Neurol* 1985;42:753–756.

1799. Hardie RJ, Pullon HW, Harding AE, et al. Neuroacanthocytosis. A clinical, haematological and pathological study of 19 cases. *Brain* 1991;114:13–49.

1800. Sotaniemi KA. Chorea-acanthocytosis. Neurological disease with acanthocytosis. *Acta Neurol Scand* 1983;68:53–56.

1801. Ueno E, Oguchi K, et al. Morphological abnormalities of erythrocyte membrane in the hereditary neurological disease with chorea, areflexia and acanthocytosis. *J Neurol Sci* 1982;56:89.

1802. Vance JM, Pericak-Vance MA, Bowman MH, et al. Chorea-acanthocytosis: a report of three new families and implications for genetic counselling. *Am J Med Genet* 1987;28:403–410.

1803. Villegas A, Moscat J, Vazquez A, et al. A new family with choreo-acanthocytosis. *Acta Haematol* 1987;77:215–219.

1804. Vita G, Serra S, Dattola R, et al. Peripheral neuropathy in amyotrophic chorea-acanthocytosis. *Ann Neurol* 1989;26:583–587.

1805. Stevenson VL, Hardie RJ. Acanthocytosis and neurological disorders. *J Neurol* 2001;248:87–94.

1806. Hirayama M, Hamano T, Shiratori M, et al. Chorea-acanthocytosis with polyclonal antibodies to ganglioside GM1. *J Neurol Sci* 1997;151:23–24.

1807. Sorrentino G, De Renzo A, Miniello S, et al. Late appearance of acanthocytes during the course of chorea-acanthocytosis. *J Neurol Sci* 1999;163:175–178.

1808. Feinberg TE, Cianci CD, Morrow JS, et al. Diagnostic tests for choreoacanthocytosis. *Neurology* 1991;41:1000–1006.

1809. Lupo I, Aragona F, Fierro B, et al. Choreo-acanthocytosis with myopathy. Report of a case. *Acta Neurol (Napoli)* 1987;9:334–338.

1810. Spencer SE, Walker FO, Moore SA. Chorea-amyotrophy with chronic hemolytic anemia: a variant of chorea-amyotrophy with acanthocytosis. *Neurology* 1987;37:645–649.

1811. Rampoldi L, Dobson-Stone C, Rubio JP, et al. A conserved sorting-associated protein is mutant in chorea-acanthocytosis. *Nat Genet* 2001;28:119–120.

1812. Ueno S, Maruki Y, Nakamura M, et al. The gene encoding a newly discovered protein, chorein, is mutated in chorea-acanthocytosis. *Nat Genet* 2001;28:121–122.

1813. Spitz MC, Jankovic J, Killian JM. Familial tic disorder, parkinsonism, motor neuron disease, and acanthocytosis: a new syndrome. *Neurology* 1985;35:366.

1814. Peppard RF, Lu CS, Chu NS, et al. Parkinsonism with neuroacanthocytosis. *Can J Neurol Sci* 1990;17:298–301.

1815. Roth AM, Hepler RS, Mukoyama M, et al. Pigmentary retinal dystrophy in Hallervorden-Spatz disease: clinicopathological report of a case. *Surv Ophthalmol* 1971;16:24–35.

1816. Bruce LJ, Kay MM, Lawrence C, et al. Band 3 HT, a human red-cell variant associated with acanthocytosis and increased anion transport, carries the mutation Pro868Leu in the membrane domain of band 3. *Biochem J* 1993;293:317–320.

1817. Kay MMB, Gieljan JC, Bosman GM, et al. Functional topography of band 3: specific structural alteration linked to functional aberrations in human erythrocytes. *Proc Natl Acad Sci U S A* 1988;85:492–496.

1818. Kay MMB, Goodman J, Lawrence C, et al. Membrane channel protein abnormalities and autoantibodies in neurological disease. *Brain Res Bull* 1990;24:105–111.

1819. Redman CM, Russo D, Lee S. Kell, Kx and the McLeod syndrome. *Best Pract Res Clin Haematol* 1999;12:621–635.

1820. Lee S, Russo D, Redman CM. The Kell blood group system: Kell and XK membrane proteins. *Semin Hematol* 2000;37:113–121.

1821. Russo D, Redman C, Lee S. Association of XK and Kell blood group proteins. *J Biol Chem* 1998;273:13950–13956.

1822. Redman CM, Marsh WL, Scarborough A, et al. Biochemical studies on McLeod phenotype red cells and isolation of Kx antigen. *Br J Haematol* 1988;68:131–136.

1823. Ho M, Chelly J, Carter N, et al. Isolation of the gene for McLeod syndrome that encodes a novel membrane transport protein. *Cell* 1994;77:869–880.

1824. Ho MF, Chalmers RM, Davis MB, et al. A novel point mutation in the McLeod syndrome gene in neuroacanthocytosis. *Ann Neurol* 1996;39:672–675.

1825. Danek A, Uttner I, Vogl T, et al. Cerebral involvement in McLeod syndrome. *Neurology* 1994;44:117–120.

1825a. Danek A, Rubio JP, Rampoldi L, et al. McLeod neuroacanthocytosis: genotype and phenotype. *Ann Neurol* 2001;50:755–764.

1826. Marsh WL, Oyen R, Nichols ME, et al. Chronic granulomatous disease and the Kell blood groups. *Br J Haematol* 1975;29:247–262.

1827. Taswell HF, Lewis JC, et al. Erythrocyte morphology in genetic defects of the Rh and Kell blood group systems. *Mayo Clin Proc* 1977;52:157.

1828. Wimmer BM, Marsh WL, Taswell HF, et al. Haematological changes associated with the McLeod phenotype of the Kell blood group system. *Br J Haematol* 1977;36:219–224.

1829. Redman CM, Huima T, Robbins E, et al. Effect of phosphatidylserine on the shape of McLeod red cell acanthocytes. *Blood* 1989;74:1826–1835.

1830. Marsh WL, Marsh NJ, Morore A, et al. Elevated serum creatine phosphokinase in subjects with McLeod syndrome. *Vox Sang* 1981;40:403–411.

1831. Swash M, Schwartz MS, Carter ND, et al. Benign X linked myopathy with acanthocytosis (McLeod syndrome): its relationship to X linked muscular dystrophy. *Brain* 1983;106:717–733.

1832. Malandrini A, Fabrizi GM, Truschi F, et al. Atypical McLeod syndrome manifested as X-linked chorea-acanthocytosis, neuromyopathy and dilated cardiomyopathy: report of a family. *J Neurol Sci* 1994;124:89–94.

1833. Takashima H, Sakai T, Iwashita H, et al. A family of McLeod syndrome, masquerading as chorea-acanthocytosis. *J Neurol Sci* 1994;124:56–60.

1834. Jung HH, Hergersberg M, Kneifel S, et al. McLeod syndrome: a novel mutation, predominant psychiatric manifestations, and distinct striatal imaging findings. *Ann Neurol* 2001;49:384–392.

1835. Kawakami T, Takiyama Y, Sakoe K, et al. A case of McLeod syndrome with unusually severe myopathy. *J Neurol Sci* 1999;166:36–39.

1836. Barnett MH, Yang F, Iland H, et al. Unusual muscle pathology in McLeod syndrome. *J Neurol Neurosurg Psychiatry* 2000;69:655–657.

1837. Glaubensklee CS, Evan AP, Galey WR. Structure and biochemical analysis of the McLeod erythrocyte membrane. I. Freeze fracture and discontinuous polyacrylamide gel electrophoresis analysis. *Vox Sang* 1982;42:262–271.

1838. Tang LL, Redman CM, Williams D, et al. Biochemical studies on McLeod phenotype erythrocytes. *Vox Sang* 1981;40:17–26.

1839. Bertelson CJ, Pogo AO, Chadhuri A, et al. Localization of the McLeod locus (XK) within Xp21 by deletion analysis. *Am J Hum Genet* 1988;42:703–711.

1840. Francke U, Ochs HD, et al. Minor Xp21 chromosome deletion in a male associated with expression of Duchenne muscular dystrophy, chronic granulomatous disease, retinitis pigmentosa, and McLeod's syndrome. *Am J Hum Genet* 1985;37:250.

1841. Giblett ER, Klebanoff SJ, et al. Kell phenotypes in chronic granulomatous disease: a potential transfusion hazard. *Lancet* 1971;1:1235.

1842. Hart MVD, Szaloky A, et al. A "new" antibody associated with the Kell blood group system. *Vox Sang* 1968;15:456.

1843. Parsons SF, Mallinson G, Judson PA, et al. Evidence that the Lu^b blood group antigen is located on red cell membrane glycoproteins of 85 and 78 kd. *Transfusion* 1987;27:61–63.

1844. Shaw MA, Leak MR, Daniels GL, et al. The rare Lutheran blood group phenotype Lu(a−b−): a genetic study. *Ann Hum Genet* 1984;48:229–237.

1845. Telen MJ. The Lutheran antigens and proteins affected by Lutheran regulatory genes. In: Agre PC, Cartron JP, eds. *Protein blood group antigens of the human red cell: structure, function and clinical significance.* Baltimore: The Johns Hopkins University Press, 1992:70–87.

1846. Parsons SF, Mallinson G, Holmes CH, et al. The Lutheran blood group glycoprotein, another member of the immunoglobulin superfamily, is widely expressed in human tissues and is developmentally regulated in human liver. *Proc Natl Acad Sci U S A* 1995;92:5496–5500.

1847. El Nemer W, Gane P, Colin Y, et al. The Lutheran blood group glycoproteins, the erythroid receptors for laminin, are adhesion molecules. *J Biol Chem* 1998;273:16686–16693.

1848. Udani M, Zen Q, Cottman M, et al. Basal cell adhesion molecule/Lutheran protein. The receptor critical for sickle cell adhesion to laminin. *J Clin Invest* 1998;101:2550–2558.

1849. Telen MJ, Eisenbarth GS, Haynes BF. Human erythrocyte antigens: regulation of a novel red cell surface antigen by the inhibitor Lutheran In(Lu) gene. *J Clin Invest* 1983;71:1878–1886.

1850. Amrein PC, Friedman R, Kosinski K, et al. Hematologic changes in anorexia nervosa. *JAMA* 1979;241:2190–2191.

1851. Ero Y, Kitagawa T. Wolman's disease with hypobetalipoproteinemia and acanthocytosis: clinical and biochemical observations. *J Pediatr* 1970;77:862.

1852. Gracey M, Hilton HB. Acanthocytes and hypobetalipoproteinemia. *Lancet* 1973;1:679.

1853. Paramathypathy K, Aw SE. Acanthocytosis with beta lipoprotein deficiency in an Indian girl. *Med J Aust* 1970;2:1081.

1854. Fondu P, Mozes N, Neve P, et al. The erythrocyte membrane disturbances in protein-energy malnutrition: nature and mechanisms. *Br J Haematol* 1980;44:605–618.

1855. Herpertz-Dahlmann B, Remschmidt H. Blutbildveranderungen bei Anorexia nervosa in Abhangigkeit vom Gewicht. *Monatsschr Kinderheilkd* 1988;136:739–744.

1856. Warren MP, Vande Wiele RL. Clinical and metabolic features of anorexia nervosa. *Am J Obstet Gynecol* 1973;117:435–448.

1857. Vaisman N, Barak Y, Hahn T, et al. Defective in vitro granulopoiesis in patients with anorexia nervosa. *Pediatr Res* 1996;40:108–111.

1858. Nonaka D, Tanaka M, Takaki K, et al. Gelatinous bone marrow transformation complicated by self-induced malnutrition. *Acta Haematol* 1998;100:88–90.

1859. Maxwell DJ, Seshadri R, Rumpf DJ, et al. Infantile pyknocytosis: a cause of intrauterine haemolysis in 2 siblings. *Aust N Z J Obstet Gynaecol* 23:182–185.

1860. Ackerman BD. Infantile pyknocytosis in Mexican American infants. *Am J Dis Child* 1969;117:417.

1861. Keimowitz R, Desforges JF. Infantile pyknocytosis. *N Engl J Med* 1965;273:1152.

1862. Zannos Mariola L, Kattamis C, et al. Infantile pyknocytosis and glucose-6-phosphate dehydrogenase deficiency. *Br J Haematol* 1962;8:258.

1863. Allison AC. Acute haemolytic anaemia with distortion and fragmentation of erythrocytes in children. *Br J Haematol* 1957;3:1.

1864. Horton L, Coburn RJ, England JM, et al. The haematology of hypothyroidism. *QJM* 1976;45:101–124.

1865. Perillie PE, Tembrevilla C. Red-cell changes in hypothyroidism. *Lancet* 1975;2:1151–1152.

1866. Betticher DC, Pugin P. Hypothyroidie et acanthocytes: importance diagnostique du frottis sanguin. *Schweiz Med Wochenschr* 1991;121:1127–1132.

1867. Barrett AM. A special form of erythrocyte possessing increased resistance to hypotonic saline. *J Pathol Bacteriol* 1938;46:603.

1868. Cooper RA, Jandl JH. Bile salts and cholesterol in the pathogenesis of target cells in obstructive jaundice. *J Clin Invest* 1968;47:809.

1869. Neerhout RC. Abnormalities of erythrocyte stromal lipids in hepatic disease: erythrocyte stromal lipids in hyperlipemic states. *J Lab Clin Med* 1968;71:438.

1870. Verkleij AJ, Nanta ICD, et al. The fusion of abnormal plasma lipoprotein (LP X) and the erythrocyte membrane in patients with cholestasis studied by electron microscopy. *Biochim Biophys Acta* 1976;436:366.

1871. Seidel D, Alaupovic P, et al. A lipoprotein characterizing obstructive jaundice. I. Method for quantitative separation and identification of lipoproteins in jaundice subjects. *J Clin Invest* 1969;48:1211.

1872. Narayanan S. Biochemistry and clinical relevance of lipoprotein X. *Ann Clin Lab Sci* 1984;14:371.

1873. Miller JP. Dyslipoproteinaemia of liver disease. *Baillieres Clin Endocrinol Metab* 1990;4:807–832.

1874. O K, Frohlich J. Role of lecithin: cholesterol acyltransferase and apolipoprotein A-I in cholesterolesterification in lipoprotein-X in vitro. *J Lipid Res* 1995;36:2344–2354.

1875. Elferink RP, Ottenhoff R, van Marle J, et al. Class III P-glycoproteins mediate the formation of lipoprotein X in the mouse. *J Clin Invest* 1998;102:1749–1757.

1876. Iida H, Hasegawa I, Nozawa Y. Biochemical studies on abnormal membranes. Protein abnormality of erythrocyte membrane in biliary obstruction. *Biochem Biophys Acta* 1976;443:394–401.

1877. Gjone E, Torsvik H, et al. Familial plasma cholesterol ester deficiency: a study of the erythrocytes. *Scand J Clin Lab Invest* 1968;21:327.

1878. Santamarina-Fojo S, Hoeg JM, Assmann G, et al. Lecithin cholesterol acyltransferase deficiency and fish-eye disease. In: Scriver CR, Beaudet AL, Sly WS, et al., eds. *The metabolic and molecular bases of inherited disease*, 8th ed. New York: McGraw-Hill, 2001:2817–2834.

1879. Gjone E, Torsvik H. Familial plasma cholesterol ester deficiency: a study of the erythrocytes. *Scand J Clin Lab Invest* 1968;21:327.

1880. Jain SK, Mohandas N, et al. Hereditary plasma lecithin cholesterol acyl transferase deficiency: a heterozygous variant with erythrocyte membrane abnormalities. *J Lab Clin Med* 1982;99:816.

1881. Murayama N, Asano Y, et al. Decreased sodium influx and abnormal red cell membrane lipids in a patient with familial plasma lecithin: cholesterol acyltransferase deficiency. *Am J Hematol* 1984;16:129.

1882. Norum KR, Gjone E. The influence of plasma from patients with familial lecithin: cholesterol acyltransferase deficiency on the lipid pattern of erythrocytes. *Scand J Clin Lab Invest* 1968;22:94.

1883. Gjone E, Norum KR, et al. Familial lecithin: cholesterol acyltransferase deficiency. In: Stanbury JB, Wyngaarden JB, et al., eds. *The metabolic basis of inherited disease*, 4th ed. New York: McGraw-Hill, 1978:589–603.

1884. Lynn EG, Siow YL, Frohlich J, et al. Lipoprotein-X stimulates monocyte chemoattractant protein-1 expression in mesangial cells via nuclear factor-kappa B. *Kidney Int* 2001;60:520–532.

1885. Jacobsen CD, Gjone E, et al. Sea blue histiocytes in familial lecithin: cholesterol acyltransferase deficiency. *Scand J Haematol* 1972;9:106.

1886. Frohlich J, Hoag G, McLeod R, et al. Hypoalphalipoproteinemia resembling fish eye disease. *Acta Med Scand* 1987;221:291–298.

1887. de Haan LD, Werre JM, Ruben AM, et al. Alterations in size, shape and osmotic behaviour of red cells after splenectomy: a study of their age dependence. *Br J Haematol* 1988;69:71–80.

1888. de Haan LD, Werre JM, et al. Alterations in size, shape and osmotic behaviour of red cells after splenectomy: a study of their age dependence. *Br J Haematol* 1988;69:71.

1889. Singer K, Miller EB, et al. Hematologic changes following splenectomy in man, with particular reference to target cells, hemolytic index and lysolecithin. *Am J Med Sci* 1941;202:171.

1890. Come SE, Shohet SB, et al. Surface remodeling vs whole cell hemolysis of reticulocytes produced with erythroid stimulation or iron deficiency anemia. *Blood* 1974;44:817.

1891. Shattil SJ, Cooper RA. Maturation of macroreticulocyte membranes in vivo. *J Lab Clin Med* 1972;79:215–227.

1892. Lux SE, John KM. Isolation and partial characterization of a high molecular weight membrane protein complex normally removed by the spleen. *Blood* 1977;50:625–641.

1893. Holm TM, Braun A, Trigatti BL, et al. Failure of red blood cell maturation in mice with defects in the high-density lipoprotein receptor SR-BI. *Blood* 2002;99:1817–1824.

1894. Smith CH, Khakoo Y. Burr cells: classification and effect of splenectomy. *J Pediatr* 1970;76:99.

1895. Crosby WH. Normal function of the spleen relative to red blood cells: a review. *Blood* 1959;14:399.

1896. Buchanan GR, Holtkamp CA. Pocked erythrocyte counts in patients with hereditary spherocytosis before and after splenectomy. *Am J Hematol* 1987;25:253–257.

1897. Kvindesdal BB, Jensen MK. Pitted erythrocytes in splenectomized subjects with congenital spherocytosis and in subjects splenectomized for other reasons. *Scand J Haematol* 1986;37:41–43.

1898. Beilin LJ, Knight GJ, et al. The sodium, potassium, and water contents of red blood cells of healthy human adults. *J Clin Invest* 1966;45:1817.

1899. Oski FA, Naiman JL, et al. Congenital hemolytic anemia with high sodium, low potassium red cells: studies of three generations of a family with a new variant. *N Engl J Med* 1969;280:909.

1900. Snyder LM, Lutz HU, Sauberman N, et al. Fragmentation and myelin formation in hereditary xerocytosis and other hemolytic anemias. *Blood* 1978; 52:750–761.

1901. Albala MM, Fortier NL, et al. Physiologic features of hemolysis associated with altered cation and 2,3-diphosphoglycerate content. *Blood* 1978;52:135.

1902. Bienzle U, Niethammer D, et al. Congenital stomatocytosis and chronic haemolytic anaemia. *Scand J Haematol* 1975;15:339.

1903. Clark ME, Mohandas N, et al. Effects of abnormal cation transport on deformability of desiccytes. *J Supramol Struct* 1978;8:521.

1904. Eber SW, Lande WM, Iarocci TA, et al. Hereditary stomatocytosis: consistent association with an integral membrane protein deficiency. *Br J Haematol* 1989;72:452–455.

1905. Glader BE, Fortier N, et al. Congenital hemolytic anemia associated with dehydrated erythrocytes and increased potassium loss. *N Engl J Med* 1974;291:491.

1906. Huppi PS, Ott P, Amato M, et al. Congenital haemolytic anaemia in a low birth weight infant due to congenital stomatocytosis. *Eur J Haematol* 1991; 47:1–9.

1907. Kanzaki A, Yawata Y. Hereditary stomatocytosis: phenotypical expression of sodium transport and band 7 peptides in 44 cases. *Br J Haematol* 1992;82:133–141.

1908. Lande W, Cerrone K, et al. Congenital anemia with abnormal cation permeability and cold hemolysis in vitro. *Blood* 1979;54[Suppl 1]:29a (abst).

1909. Lande WM, Thiemann PV, et al. Missing band 7 membrane protein in two patients with high Na, low K erythrocytes. *J Clin Invest* 1982;70:1273.

1910. Lane PA, Kuypers FA, Clark MR, et al. Excess of red cell membrane proteins in hereditary high-phosphatidylcholine hemolytic anemia. *Am J Hematol* 1990;34:186–192.

1911. Lo SS, Hitzig WH, et al. Stomatozytose. *Schweiz Med Wochenschr* 1970;100:1977.

1912. Lo SS, Marti HR, et al. Haemolytic anaemia associated with decreased concentration of reduced glutathione in red cells. *Acta Haematol* 1971;46:14.

1913. Lock SP, Smith RS, et al. Stomatocytosis: a hereditary red cell anomaly associated with haemolytic anaemia. *Br J Haematol* 1961;7:303.

1914. McGrath KM, Collecut MF, Gordon A, et al. Dehydrated hereditary stomatocytosis—a report of two families and a review of the literature. *Pathology* 1984;16:146–150.

1915. Meadow SR. Stomatocytosis. *Proc R Soc Med* 1967;60:13.

1916. Mentzer WC Jr, Smith WB, et al. Hereditary stomatocytosis membranes and metabolism studies. *Blood* 1975;46:659.

1917. Miller G, Townes PL, et al. A new congenital hemolytic anemia with deformed erythrocytes (?"stomatocytes") and remarkable susceptibility of erythrocytes to cold hemolysis in vitro. I. Clinical and hematologic studies. *Pediatrics* 1965;35:906.

1918. Miller DR, Rickles FR, et al. A new variant of hereditary hemolytic anemia with stomatocytosis and erythrocyte cation abnormality. *Blood* 1971;38:184.

1919. Morlé L, Pothier B, Alloisio N, et al. Reduction of membrane band 7 and activation of volume stimulated (K⁺, Cl⁻)-cotransport in a case of congenital stomatocytosis. *Br J Haematol* 1989;71:141–146.

1920. Mutoh S, Sasaki R, et al. A family of hereditary stomatocytosis associated with normal level of Na,K-ATPase activity of red blood cells. *Am J Hematol* 1983;14:113.

1921. Nolan GR. Hereditary xerocytosis: a case history and review of the literature. *Pathology* 1984;16:151.

1922. Platt OS, Lux SE, et al. Exercise induced hemolysis in xerocytosis: erythrocyte dehydration and shear sensitivity. *J Clin Invest* 1981;68:631.

1923. Rix M, Bjerrum PJ, Wieth JO, et al. Medfodt stomatocytose med haemolytisk anaemi—med abnorm kationpermeabilitet og defekte membranproteiner. (Congenital stomatocytosis with hemolytic anemia—with abnormal cation permeability and defective membrane proteins.) *Ugeskrift for Laeger* 1991;153:724–726.

1924. Schröter W, Ungefehr K, Tillmann W. Role of the spleen in congenital stomatocytosis associated with high sodium low potassium erythrocytes. *Klin Wochenschr* 1981;59:173.

1925. Shohet SB, Livermore BM, et al. Hereditary hemolytic anemia associated with abnormal membrane lipids: mechanism of accumulation of phosphatidyl choline. *Blood* 1971;38:445.

1926. Shohet SB, Nathan DG, et al. Hereditary hemolytic anemia associated with abnormal membrane lipids. II. Ion permeability and transport abnormalities. *Blood* 1973;42:1.

1927. Turpin F, Lortholary P, Lejeune F, et al. Un cas d'anèmie hèmolytique avec stomatocytose. *Nouv Rev Fr Hematol* 1971;11:585–594.

1928. Wiley JS, Ellory JC, et al. Characteristics of the membrane defect in the hereditary stomatocytosis syndrome. *Blood* 1975;46:337.

1929. Yawata Y, Takemoto Y, Yoshimoto M, et al. The Japanese family of congenital hemolytic anemia with high red cell phosphatidyl choline and increased sodium transport. *Acta Haematol Jpn* 1982;45:672–681.

1930. Zarkowsky HS, Oski FA, et al. Congenital hemolytic anemia with high sodium, low potassium red cells. I. Studies of membrane permeability. *N Engl J Med* 1968;278:573.

1931. Clark MR, Shohet SB, Gottfried EL. Hereditary hemolytic disease with increased red blood cell phosphatidylcholine and dehydration: one, two, or many disorders? *Am J Hematol* 1993;42:25–30.

1932. Gore DM, Chetty MC, Fisher J, et al. Familial pseudohyperkalaemia Cardiff: a mild version of cryohydrocytosis. *Br J Haematol* 2002;117:212–214.

1933. Grootenboer S, Barro C, Cynober T, et al. Dehydrated hereditary stomatocytosis: a cause of prenatal ascites. *Prenat Diagn* 2001;21:1114–1118.

1934. Haines PG, Jarvis HG, King S, et al. Two further British families with the 'cryohydrocytosis' form of hereditary stomatocytosis. *Br J Haematol* 2001;113:932–937.

1935. Haines PG, Crawley C, Chetty MC, et al. Familial pseudohyperkalaemia Chiswick: a novel congenital thermotropic variant of K and Na transport across the human red cell membrane. *Br J Haematol* 2001;112:469–474.

1936. Grootenboer S, Schischmanoff PO, Laurendeau I, et al. Pleiotropic syndrome of dehydrated hereditary stomatocytosis, pseudohyperkalemia, and perinatal edema maps to 16q23-q24. *Blood* 2000;96:2599–2605.

1937. Coles SE, Chetty MC, Ho MM, et al. Two British families with variants of the 'cryohydrocytosis' form of hereditary stomatocytosis. *Br J Haematol* 1999;105:1055–1065.

1938. Carella M, Stewart GW, Ajetunmobi JF, et al. Genetic heterogeneity of hereditary stomatocytosis syndromes showing pseudohyperkalemia. *Haematologica* 1999;84:862–863.

1939. Coles SE, Ho MM, Chetty MC, et al. A variant of hereditary stomatocytosis with marked pseudohyperkalaemia. *Br J Haematol* 1999;104:275–283.

1940. Grootenboer S, Schischmanoff PO, Cynober T, et al. A genetic syndrome associating dehydrated hereditary stomatocytosis, pseudohyperkalaemia and perinatal oedema. *Br J Haematol* 1998;103:383–386.

1941. Kilpatrick ES, Burton ID. Pseudohyperkalaemia, pseudohyponatraemia and pseudohypoglycaemia in a patient with hereditary stomatocytosis. *Ann Clin Biochem* 1997;34(Pt 5):561–563.

1942. Ogburn PL Jr, Ramin KD, Danilenko-Dixon D, et al. In utero erythrocyte transfusion for fetal xerocytosis associated with severe anemia and nonimmune hydrops fetalis. *Am J Obstet Gynecol* 2001;185:238–239.

1943. Jarvis HG, Chetty MC, Nicolaou A, et al. A novel stomatocytosis variant showing marked abnormalities in intracellular [Na] and [K] with minimal haemolysis. *Eur J Haematol* 2001;66:412–414.

1944. Reference deleted.

1945. Lande WM, Andrews DL, Thiemann PVM, et al. Temperature dependence of RBC passive K efflux in primary permeability disorders: unique finding in a patient with cryohydrocytosis. *Blood* 1985;66[Suppl 1]:34a (abst).

1946. Stewart GW, Corrall RJM, Fyffe JM, et al. Familial pseudohyperkalemia. *Lancet* 1979;2:175–177.

1947. Stewart GW, Ellory JC. A family with mild hereditary xerocytosis showing high membrane cation permeability at low temperatures. *Clin Sci* 1985;69:309–319.

1948. Jaffè ER, Gottfried EL. Hereditary nonspherocytic hemolytic disease associated with an altered phospholipid composition of the erythrocytes. *J Clin Invest* 1968;47:1375–1388.

1949. McCormack MK, Geller GR, Krivit W, et al. Hemolytic anemia associated with a cation abnormality. *J Cell Biol* 1975;67:271a (abst).

1950. Delaunay J, Stewart G, Iolascon A. Hereditary dehydrated and overhydrated stomatocytosis: recent advances. *Curr Opin Hematol* 1999;6:110–114.

1951. Luciani JC, Lavabre-Bertrand T, Fourcade J, et al. Familial pseudohyperkalaemia. *Lancet* 1980;1:491.

1952. Meenaghan M, Follett GF, Brophy PJ. Temperature sensitivity of potassium flux into red blood cells in the familial pseudohyperkalaemia syndrome. *Biochim Biophys Acta* 1985;821:72–78.

1953. James DR, Stansbie D. Familial pseudohyperkalaemia: inhibition of erythrocyte K+ efflux at 4°C by quinine. *Clin Sci (Lond)* 1987;73:557–560.

1954. Wiley JS, Cooper RA, et al. Hereditary stomatocytosis: association of low 2,3 diphosphoglycerate with increased cation pumping by the red cell. *Br J Haematol* 1979;41:133.

1955. Vives-Corrons JL, Besson I, et al. Hereditary xerocytosis: a report of six unrelated Spanish families with leaky red cell syndrome and increased heat stability of the erythrocyte membrane. *Br J Haematol* 1995;90:817.

1956. Entezami M, Becker R, Menssen HD, et al. Xerocytosis with concomitant intrauterine ascites: first description and therapeutic approach. *Blood* 1996;87:5392–5393.

1956a. Fey MF, Bischof M, Zahler P, et al. Hereditary leaky red cell syndrome in a Swiss family. *Acta Haematol* 1986;75:70–78.

1957. Stewart GW, Turner EJ. The hereditary stomatocytoses and allied disorders: congenital disorders of erythrocyte membrane permeability to Na and K. *Best Pract Res Clin Haematol* 1999;12:707–727.

1957a. Delaunay J, Stewart G, Iolascon A. Hereditary dehydrated and overhydrated stomatocytosis: recent advances. *Curr Opin Hematol* 1999;6:110–114.

1958. Wiley JS, Shaller CC. Selective loss of calcium permeability on maturation of reticulocytes. *J Clin Invest* 1977;59:1113–1119.

1959. Dutcher PO, Segel GB, et al. Cation transport and its altered regulation in human stomatocytic erythrocytes. *Pediatr Res* 1975;9:924.

1960. Mentzer WC, Lubin BH, et al. Correction of the permeability defect in hereditary stomatocytosis by dimethyl adipimidate. *N Engl J Med* 1976;294:1200.

1961. Stewart GW, Amess JA, Eber SW, et al. Thrombo-embolic disease after splenectomy for hereditary stomatocytosis. *Br J Haematol* 1996;93:303.

1962. Stewart GW, Argent AC. Integral band 7 protein of the human erythrocyte membrane. *Biochem Soc Trans* 1992;20:785.

1963. Gallagher PG, Segel G, Marchesi SL, et al. The gene for erythrocyte band 7.2b in hereditary stomatocytosis. *Blood* 1992;80[Suppl 1]:276a (abst).

1964. Wang D, Turetsky T, Perrine S, et al. Further studies on RBC membrane protein 7.2b deficiency in hereditary stomatocytosis. *Blood* 1992;80[Suppl 1]:275a (abst).

1965. Reference deleted.

1966. Zhu Y, Paszty C, Turetsky T, et al. Stomatocytosis is absent in "stomatin"-deficient murine red blood cells. *Blood* 1999;93:2404–2410.

1967. Pinkerton PH, Fletch SM, et al. Hereditary stomatocytosis with hemolytic anemia in the dog. *Blood* 1974;44:557.

1968. Smith JE, Moore K, et al. Glutathione metabolism in canine hereditary stomatocytosis with mild erythrocyte glutathione deficiency. *J Lab Clin Med* 1983;101:611.

1969. Smith BD, Segel GB. Abnormal erythrocyte endothelial adherence in hereditary stomatocytosis. *Blood* 1997;89:3451.

1970. Carella M, Stewart GW, Ajetunmobi JF, et al. Mapping of dehydrated stomatocytosis (herediatry xerocytosis) locus to chromosome 16 (16q23-qter) by genome wide search. *Am J Hum Genet* 1998;63:810–816.

1971. Larsen F, Solheim J, Kristensen T, et al. Tight cluster of five unrelated human genes on chromosome 16q22.1. *Hum Mol Genet* 1993;2:1589–1595.

1972. Dise CA, Goodman DBP, Rasmussen H. Selective stimulation of erythrocyte membrane phospholipid fatty acid turnover associated with decreased volume. *J Biol Chem* 1980;255:5201–5207.

1973. Fairbanks G, Dino JE, et al. Membrane alterations in hereditary xerocytosis: elevated binding of glyceraldehyde-3-phosphate dehydrogenase. In: Kruckeberg WC, Eaton JW, et al., eds. *Erythrocyte membranes: recent clinical and experimental advances.* New York: Alan R. Liss, 1978:173–184.

1974. Sauberman N, Fairbanks G, et al. Altered red blood cell surface area in hereditary xerocytosis. *Clin Chim Acta* 1981;114:149.

1975. Platt OS. Exercise induced hemolysis in sickle cell anemia: shear sensitivity and erythrocyte dehydration. *Blood* 1982;59:1055.

1976. Harm W, Fortier NL, et al. Increased erythrocyte lipid peroxidation in hereditary xerocytosis. *Clin Chim Acta* 1979;99:121.

1977. Sauberman N, Fortier NL, et al. Spectrin hemoglobin crosslinkages associated with in vitro oxidant hypersensitivity in pathologic and artificially dehydrated red cells. *Br J Haematol* 1983;54:15.

1978. Snyder LM, Sauberman N, et al. Red cell membrane response to hydrogen peroxide—sensitivity in hereditary xerocytosis and in other abnormal red cells. *Br J Haematol* 1981;48:435.

1979. Fortier N, Snyder LM, et al. The relationship between in vivo generated hemoglobin skeletal protein complex and increased red cell membrane rigidity. *Blood* 1988;71:1427.

1980. Snyder LM, Fortier NL, et al. Effect of hydrogen peroxide exposure on normal human erythrocyte deformability, morphology, surface characteristics and spectrin hemoglobin crosslinking. *J Clin Invest* 1985;76:1971.

1981. Perel Y, Dhermy D, Carrere A, et al. Portal vein thrombosis after splenectomy for hereditary stomatocytosis in childhood. *Eur J Pediatr* 1999;158:628–630.

1982. Coles SE, Stewart GW. Temperature effects on cation transport in hereditary stomatocytosis and allied disorders. *Int J Exp Pathol* 1999;80:251–258.

1983. Iolascon A, Stewart GW, Ajetunmobi JF, et al. Familial pseudohyperkalemia maps to the same locus as dehydrated hereditary stomatocytosis (hereditary xerocytosis). *Blood* 1999;93:3120–3123.

1984. Alani FS, Dyer T, Hindle E, et al. Pseudohyperkalaemia associated with hereditary spherocytosis in four members of a family. *Postgrad Med J* 1994;70:749–751.

1985. Jolobe OM. Pseudohyperkalaemia associated with hereditary spherocytosis. *Postgrad Med J* 1995;71:187.

1986. Michiels JJ. Pseudohyperkalemia and platelet count in thrombocythemia. *Am J Hematol* 1993;42:237–238.

1987. Mazarelo F, Donaldson D. Lessons to be learned: a case study approach: pseudohyperkalaemia due to thrombocytosis in a case of tubo-ovarian abscess. *J R Soc Health* 1999;119:196–199.

1988. Seah TG, Lew TW, Chin NM. A case of pseudohyperkalaemia and thrombocytosis. *Ann Acad Med Singapore* 1998;27:442–443.

1989. Bronson WR, DeVita VT, Carbone PP, et al. Pseudohyperkalemia due to release of potassium from white blood cells during clotting. *N Engl J Med* 1966;274:369–375.

1990. Bellevue R, Dosik H, Spergel G, et al. Pseudohyperkalemia and extreme leukocytosis. *J Lab Clin Med* 1975;85:660–664.

1991. Colussi G, Cipriani D. Pseudohyperkalemia in extreme leukocytosis. *Am J Nephrol* 1995;15:450–452.

1992. Degen M. Pseudohyperkalemia in Akitas. *J Am Vet Med Assoc* 1987;190:541–543.

1993. Douglass CC, Twomey JJ. Transient stomatocytosis with hemolysis: a previously unrecognized complication of alcoholism. *Ann Intern Med* 1970;72:159–164.

1994. Wislöff F, Boman D. Acquired stomatocytosis in alcoholic liver disease. *Scand J Haematol* 1979;23:43–50.

1995. Davidson RJ, How J, et al. Acquired stomatocytosis: its prevalence and significance in routine haematology. *Scand J Haematol* 1977;19:47.

1996. Simpson LO. Blood from healthy animals and humans contains nondiscocytic erythrocytes. *Br J Haematol* 1989;73:561.

1997. Ducrou W, Kimber RJ. Stomatocytes, haemolytic anaemia and abdominal pain in Mediterranean migrants. Some examples of a new syndrome? *Med J Aust* 1969;2:1087–1091.

1998. Wislöff F, Boman D. Acquired stomatocytosis in alcoholic liver disease. *Scand J Haematol* 1979;23:43–50.

1999. Ohsaka A, Kano Y, Sakamoto S, et al. A transient hemolytic reaction and stomatocytosis following vinca alkaloid administration. *Acta Haematol Jpn* 1989;52:7–17.

2000. Neville AJ, Rand CA, Barr RD, et al. Drug-induced stomatocytosis and anemia during consolidation chemotherapy of childhood acute leukemia. *Am J Med Sci* 1984;287:3–7.

2001. Reinhart WH, Baerlocher GM, Cerny T, et al. Ifosfamide-induced stomatocytosis and mesna-induced echinocytosis: influence on biorheological properties of blood. *Eur J Haematol* 1999;62:223–230.

2002. Konstantopoulos K, Vassilopoulos G, Adamides S, et al. Stomatocytosis as a presenting symptom of myelodysplasia. *Med Oncol Tumor Pharmacother* 1992;9:213–214.

2003. Olivieri O, Girelli D, Vettore L, et al. A case of congenital dyserythropoietic anaemia with stomatocytosis, reduced bands 7 and 8 and normal cation content. *Br J Haematol* 1992;80:258–260.

2004. Reinhart WH, Chien S. Stomatocytic transformation of red blood cells after marathon running. *Am J Hematol* 1985;19:201.

2005. Reinhart WH, Bärtsch P, Straub PW. Red blood cell morphology after a 100-km run. *Clin Lab Haematol* 1989;11:105–110.

2006. Davidson RJL. March or exertional hemoglobinuria. *Semin Hematol* 1969;6:150.

2007. Banga JP, Pinder JC, et al. An erythrocyte membraneprotein anomaly in march haemoglobinuria. *Lancet* 1979;2:1048.

2008. Vos GH, Vos D, et al. A sample of blood with no detectable Rh antigens. *Lancet* 1961;1:14.

2009. Ballas SK, Clark MR, et al. Red cell membrane and cation deficiency in Rhnull syndrome. *Blood* 1984;63:1046.

2010. Seidl S, Spielmann W, et al. Two siblings with Rhnull disease. *Vox Sang* 1972;23:182.

2011. Senhauser DA, Mitchell MW, et al. Another example of phenotype Rhnull. *Transfusion* 1970;10:89.

2012. Sturgeon P. Hematological observations on the anemia associated with blood type Rhnull. *Blood* 1970;36:310.

2013. Lauf PK, Joiner CH. Increased potassium transport and ouabain binding in human Rhnull red blood cells. *Blood* 1976;48:457.

2014. McGuire D, Rosenfield RE, Wong KY, et al. Rh$_{mod}$. A second kindred (Craig). *Vox Sang* 1976;30:430.

2015. Saji H, Hosoi T. A Japanese Rh$_{mod}$ family: serological and haematological observations. *Vox Sang* 1979;37:296.

2016. Nash R, Shojania AM. Hematological aspect of Rh deficiency syndrome: a case report and a review of the literature. *Am J Hematol* 1987;24:267–275.

2017. Assmann G, von Eckardstein A, Brewer HB Jr. Familial analphalipoproteinemia: Tangier disease. In: Scriver CR, Beaudet AL, Sly WS, et al., eds. *The metabolic and molecular bases of inherited disease*, 8th ed. New York: McGraw-Hill, 2001:2937–2980.

2018. Schmitz G, Assmann G, Robenek H, et al. Tangier disease: a disorder of intracellular membrane traffic. *Proc Natl Acad Sci U S A* 1985;82:6305–6309.

2019. Brooks-Wilson A, Marcil M, Clee SM, et al. Mutations in ABC1 in Tangier disease and familial high-density lipoprotein deficiency. *Nat Genet* 1999;22:336–345.

2020. Bodzioch M, Orsó E, Klucken J, et al. The gene encoding ATP-binding cassette transporter 1 is mutated in Tangier disease. *Nat Genet* 1999;22:347–351.

2021. Rust S, Rosier M, Funke H, et al. Tangier disease is caused by mutations in the gene encoding ATP-binding cassette transporter 1. *Nat Genet* 1999;22:352–355.

2022. Orsó E, Broccardo C, Kaminski WE, et al. Transport of lipids from Golgi to plasma membrane is defective in Tangier disease patients and ABC1-deficient mice. *Nat Genet* 2000 ;24:192–196.

2023. Hamon Y, Broccardo C, Chambenoit O, et al. ABC1 promotes engulfment of apoptotic cells and transbilayer redistribution of phosphatidylserine. *Nat Cell Biol* 2000;2:399–406.

2024. Zha X, Genest J, McPherson R. Endocytosis is enhanced in Tangier fibroblasts: possible role of ATP-binding cassette protein A1 in endosomal vesicular transport. *J Biol Chem* 2001;276:39476–39483.

2025. Reinhart WH, Gossi U, Butikofer P, et al. Haemolytic anaemia in analphalipoproteinaemia (Tangier disease): morphological, biochemical, and biophysical properties of the red blood cell. *Br J Haematol* 1989;72:272–277.

2026. Hoffman HN, Fredrickson DS. Tangier disease (familial high density lipoprotein deficiency). Clinical and genetic features in two adults. *Am J Med* 1965;39:582–593.

2027. Kummer H, Laissue J, et al. Familiäre analphalipoproteinämie (Tangier Krankheit). *Schweiz Med Wochenschr* 1968;11:406.

2028. Shaklady MM, Djardjouras EM, Lloyd JK. Red cell lipids in familial alphalipoprotein deficiency (Tangier disease). *Lancet* 1968;2:151.

2029. Norman JG. Stomatocytosis in migrants in Mediterranean origin [Letter]. *Med J Aust* 1969;1:315.

2030. Jackson JM, Knight D. Stomatocytosis in migrants of Mediterranean origin [Letter]. *Med J Aust* 1969;1:939–940.

2031. Lander H. More maladies in Mediterranean migrants. Stomatocytosis and macrothrombocytopenia. *Med J Aust* 1971;1:438–440.

2032. von Behrens WE. Splenomegaly, macrothrombocytopenia and stomatocytosis in healthy Mediterranean subjects (splenomegaly in Mediterranean macrothrombocytopenia). *Scand J Haematol* 1975;14:258–267.

2033. Slappendel RJ, van der Gaag I, van Nes JJ, et al. Familial stomatocytosis—hypertrophic gastritis (FSHG), a newly recognised disease in the dog (*Drentse patrijshond*). *Vet Q* 1991;13:30–40.

2034. Renooij W, Schmitz MG, van Gaal PJ, et al. Gastric mucosal phospholipids in dogs with familial stomatocytosis-hypertrophic gastritis. *Eur J Clin Invest* 1996;26:1156–1159.

2035. Miwa S, Fujii H, Matsumoto N, et al. A case of red-cell adenosine deaminase overproduction associated with hereditary hemolytic anemia found in Japan. *Am J Hematol* 1978;5:107–115.

2036. Stewart GW, O'Brien H, Morris SA, et al. Stomatocytosis, abnormal platelets and pseudo-homozygous hypercholesterolaemia. *Eur J Haematol* 1987;38:376–380.

2037. Weed RI, LaCelle PL, et al. Metabolic dependence of red cell deformability. *J Clin Invest* 1969;48:795.

2038. Lux SE, John KM, Ukena TE. Diminished spectrin extraction from ATP-depleted human erythrocytes. Evidence relating spectrin to changes in erythrocyte shape and deformability. *J Clin Invest* 1978;61:815–827.

2039. Palek J, Liu SC, et al. Metabolic dependence of protein arrangement in human erythrocyte membranes. I. Analysis of spectrin rich complexes in ATP depleted red cells. *Blood* 1978;51:385.

2040. Nathan DG, Oski FA, et al. Extreme hemolysis and red cell distortion in erythrocyte pyruvate kinase deficiency. II. Measurements of erythrocyte glucose consumption, potassium flux and adenosine triphosphate stability. *N Engl J Med* 1965;272:118.

2041. Mentzer WC, Baehner RL, et al. Selective reticulocyte destruction in erythrocyte pyruvate kinase deficiency. *J Clin Invest* 1971;50:688.

2042. Glader BE. Salicylate induced injury of pyruvate kinase-deficient erythrocytes. *N Engl J Med* 1976;294:916.

2043. Leblond PF, Lyonnais J, et al. Erythrocyte populations in pyruvate kinase deficiency anaemia following splenectomy. I. Cell morphology. *Br J Haematol* 1978;39:55.

2044. Leblond PF, Coulombe L, et al. Erythrocyte populations in pyruvate kinase deficiency anaemia following splenectomy. II. Cell deformability. *Br J Haematol* 1978;31:63.

2045. Coetzer T, Zail SS. Erythrocyte membrane proteins in hereditary glucose phosphate isomerase deficiency. *J Clin Invest* 1979;63:552.

2046. Clark MR, Unger RC, et al. Monovalent cation composition and ATP and lipid content of irreversibly sickled cells. *Blood* 1978;51:1169.

2047. Glader BE, Lux SE, et al. Energy reserve and cation composition of irreversibly sickled cells (ISCs) in vivo. *Br J Haematol* 1978;40:527.

2048. Chuttani HK, Gupta PS, et al. Acute copper sulfate poisoning. *Am J Med* 1965;39:849.

2049. Fairbanks VF. Copper sulfate induced hemolytic anemia: inhibition of glucose-6-phosphate dehydrogenase and other possible etiologic mechanisms. *Arch Intern Med* 1967;120:428.

2050. Holtzman NA, Elliot DA, et al. Copper intoxication. *N Engl J Med* 1966; 275:347.

2051. Manzler AD, Schreiner AW. Copper induced acute hemolytic anemia: a new complication of hemodialysis. *Ann Intern Med* 1970;73:409.

2052. Roberts RH. Hemolytic anemia associated with copper sulfate poisoning. *Mississippi Doctor* 1956;33:292.

2053. Culotta VC, Gitlin JD. Disorders of copper transport. In: Scriver CR, Beaudet AL, Sly WS, et al., eds. *The metabolic and molecular bases of inherited disease*, 8th ed. New York: McGraw-Hill, 2001:3105–3126.

2054. Walshe JM. Wilson's disease. The presenting symptoms. *Arch Dis Child* 1962;37:253–256.

2055. Buchanan GR. Acute hemolytic anemia as a presenting manifestation of Wilson's disease. *J Pediatr* 1975;86:245.

2056. Forman SJ, Kumar KS, et al. Hemolytic anemia in Wilson disease: clinical findings and biochemical mechanisms. *Am J Hematol* 1980;9:269.

2057. Lehr H, Pauschinger M, Pittke E, et al. Haemolytic anaemia as initial manifestation of Wilson's disease. *Blut* 1988;56:45–46.

2058. Robitaille GA, Piscatelli RL, Majeski EJ, et al. Hemolytic anemia in Wilson's disease. *JAMA* 1977;237:2402–2403.

2059. Roche Sicot J, Benhamou JP. Acute intravascular hemolysis and acute liver failure associated as a first manifestation of Wilson's disease. *Ann Intern Med* 1977;86:301.

2060. Deiss A, Lee GR, et al. Hemolytic anemia in Wilson's disease. *Ann Intern Med* 1970;73:413.

2061. Dobyns WB, Goldstein NP, Gordon H. Clinical spectrum of Wilson's disease (hepatolenticular degeneration). *Mayo Clin Proc* 1979;54:35–42.

2062. Hoagland HC, Goldstein NP. Hematologic (cytopenic) manifestations of Wilson's disease *Mayo Clin Proc* 1978;53:498–500.

2063. Iser JH, Stevens BJ, et al. Hemolytic anemia of Wilson's disease. *Gastroenterology* 1974;67:290.

2064. McIntyre N, Clink HM, et al. Hemolytic anemia in Wilson's disease. *N Engl J Med* 1967;276:439.

2065. Meyer RJ, Zalusky R. The mechanisms of hemolysis in Wilson's disease: study of a case and review of the literature. *Mt Sinai J Med* 1977;44:530–538.

2066. Prella M, Baccala R, Horisberger JD, et al. Haemolytic onset of Wilson disease in a patient with homozygous truncation of ATP7B at Arg1319. *Br J Haematol* 2001;114:230–232.

2067. Grudeva-Popova JG, Spasova MI, Chepileva KG, et al. Acute hemolytic anemia as an initial clinical manifestation of Wilson's disease. *Folia Med (Plovdiv)* 2000;42:42–46.

2068. Bain BJ. Heinz body haemolytic anaemia in Wilson's disease. *Br J Haematol* 1999;104:647.

2069. Wilson DC, Phillips MJ, Cox DW, et al. Severe hepatic Wilson's disease in preschool-aged children. *J Pediatr* 2000;137:719–722.

2070. Lee JJ, Kim HJ, Chung IJ, et al. Acute hemolytic crisis with fulminant hepatic failure as the first manifestation of Wilson's disease: a case report. *J Korean Med Sci* 1998;13:548–550.

2071. Kong HL, Yap IL, Kueh YK. Wilson's disease presenting as haemolytic anaemia and its successful treatment with penicillamine and zinc. *Singapore Med J* 1996;37:670–672.

2072. Walia BN, Singh S, Marwaha RK, et al. Fulminant hepatic failure and acute intravascular haemolysis as presenting manifestations of Wilson's disease in young children. *J Gastroenterol Hepatol* 1992;7:370–373.

2073. Jain S, Nur AM, Ghosh K. Acute hemolytic anemia and biliary colic as presenting manifestations of Wilson's disease. *Am J Gastroenterol* 1990;85:476–478.

2074. Hartleb M, Zahorska-Markiewicz B, Ciesielski A. Wilson's disease presenting in sisters as fulminant hepatitis with hemolytic episodes. *Am J Gastroenterol* 1987;82:549–551.

2075. Petrukhin K, Fischer SG, Pirastu M, et al. Mapping, cloning and genetic characterization of the region containing the Wilson disease gene. *Nat Genet* 1993;5:338–343.

2076. Bull PC, Thomas GR, Rommens JM, et al. The Wilson disease gene is a putative copper transporting P-type ATPase similar to the Menkes gene. *Nat Genet* 1993;5:327–337.

2077. Tanzi RE, Petrukhin K, Chernov I, et al. The Wilson disease gene is a copper transporting ATPase with homology to the Menkes disease gene. *Nat Genet* 1993;5:344–350.

2078. Yamaguchi Y, Heiny ME, Gitlin JD. Isolation and characterization of a human liver cDNA as a candidate gene for Wilson disease. *Biochem Biophys Res Commun* 1993;197:271–277.

2079. Payne AS, Kelly EJ, Gitlin JD. Functional expression of the Wilson disease protein reveals mislocalization and impaired copper-dependent trafficking of the common H1069Q mutation. *Proc Natl Acad Sci U S A* 1998;95:10854–10859.

2080. Forbes JR, Cox DW. Copper-dependent trafficking of Wilson disease mutant ATP7B proteins. *Hum Mol Genet* 2000;9:1927–1935.

2081. Yuan DS, Stearman R, Dancis A, et al. The Menkes/Wilson disease gene homologue in yeast provides copper to a ceruloplasmin-like oxidase required for iron uptake. *Proc Natl Acad Sci U S A* 1995;92:2632–2636.

2082. Schaefer M, Hopkins RG, Failla ML, et al. Hepatocyte-specific localization and copper-dependent trafficking of the Wilson's disease protein in the liver. *Am J Physiol* 1999;276:G639–646.

2083. Roelofsen H, Wolters H, Van Luyn MJ, et al. Copper-induced apical trafficking of ATP7B in polarized hepatoma cells provides a mechanism for biliary copper excretion. *Gastroenterology* 2000;119:782–793.

2084. Loudianos G, Gitlin JD. Wilson's disease. *Semin Liver Dis* 2000;20:353–364.

2085. Wilson DC, Phillips MJ, Cox DW, et al. Severe hepatic Wilson's disease in preschool-aged children. *J Pediatr* 2000;137:719–722.

2086. Gow PJ, Smallwood RA, Angus PW, et al. Diagnosis of Wilson's disease: an experience over three decades. *Gut* 2000;46:415–419.

2087. Nazer H, Ede RJ, Mowat AP, et al. Wilson's disease in childhood. Variability of clinical presentation. *Clin Pediatr (Phila)* 1983;22:755–757.

2088. Goldman M, Ali M. Wilson's disease presenting as Heinz-body hemolytic anemia. *CMAJ* 1991;145:971–972.

2088a. Giacchino R, Marazzi MG, Barabino A, et al. Syndromic variability of Wilson's disease in children. Clinical study of 44 cases. *Ital J Gastroenterol Hepatol* 1997;29:155–161.

2089. Moore GS, Calabrese EJ. G6PD-deficiency: a potential high-risk group to copper and chlorite ingestion. *J Environ Pathol Toxicol* 1980;4:271–279.

2090. Gubler CJ, Labey ME, et al. Studies on copper metabolism. IX. Transportation of copper in blood. *J Clin Invest* 1953;32:405.

2091. Ogihara H, Ogihara T, Miki M, et al. Plasma copper and antioxidant status in Wilson's disease. *Pediatr Res* 1995;37:219–226.

2092. Oski FA. Chickee, the copper [editorial]. *Ann Intern Med* 1970;73:485.

CHAPTER 52

Autoimmune Hemolytic Anemia

Wendell F. Rosse

Autoimmune hemolytic anemias are characterized by the destruction of red blood cells (RBCs) by antibodies produced by the patient against antigens on or attached to his or her own red cells. The syndromes of autoimmune hemolytic anemia (AIHA) under this rubric are many and varied; the variety arises from differences in the characteristics of the antibodies involved, the nature of the antigens, and the causes of their production.

HISTORIC NOTE

One of the first syndromes of hemolytic anemia described and clearly differentiated was autoimmune in nature—paroxysmal cold hemoglobinuria, a rare form of AIHA. As early as 1832, physicians in England described "winter hematuria" (1,2) and related the syndrome to secondary and tertiary syphilis. In 1904, Donath and Landsteiner described the serologic reactions that demonstrated the disease was caused by an antibody able to react in vitro with the patient's red cells (3,4). It has been suggested, however, that both Donath and Landsteiner were not entirely certain what they had discovered (5).

This discovery was shortly after Ehrlich postulated that such a situation was not possible, that an animal would not make an antibody against its own cells—the famous "horror autotoxicus" (6). It was postulated, perhaps correctly, that the reaction was against antigens on the organism that cause syphilis and that the antibody produced cross-reacted with the red cells of the patient.

This syndrome was easily identified because it is characterized by intravascular hemolysis by complement and, for many years, it was thought that antibodies could destroy red cells only through the fixation of complement. Because most antibodies of the more common form of AIHA cannot be readily demonstrated to fix complement, the immunologic nature of this form of AIHA [that caused by an immunoglobulin G (IgG) warm-reacting antibody] was difficult to recognize.

Discovery of the antiglobulin Coombs' test for detection of cell-bound antibody in 1945 (7) led to the clear definition of IgG-mediated AIHA (8,9). Within the next few years, the distinction between the positive Coombs' test due to IgG antibody and the non-γ Coombs' test led to the distinction between IgG and IgM antibodies, and the improvement in serologic characterization made more clear the pathophysiology of the disease (10).

Some antibodies are readily detected by their ability to agglutinate RBCs; this characteristic was used by Landsteiner in demonstrating the alloantibodies to blood groups found in normal serum (11). Little use was made of this characteristic in identifying antibodies causing hemolytic anemia (12,13), because most antibodies that occur in AIHA, being IgG, agglutinate RBCs poorly under conditions used in testing.

In this chapter, we describe the nature of the antibodies that are involved in the syndromes of AIHA and relate their characteristics to the clinical syndromes that result. This builds on the foundation laid by early observations and expanded by the explosion of immunologic knowledge during the past 20 years.

ANTIBODIES

Antibodies encountered in AIHA are of three classes—IgG, IgM, and IgA. These molecules are not known to be different from other Ig molecules; structurally, they consist of Ig units containing two light and two heavy chains. The light chains consist of a variable portion and a common portion of equal size. These line up with similarly sized variable and common portions of the heavy chain; these units form the two F(ab) portions of the molecule that bear at their free ends the antigen-binding regions composed of the hypervariable portions of a light chain and a heavy chain.

Each heavy chain has two (IgM has three) additional units of the same size that line up with corresponding units of the other heavy chain; these moieties form the Fc portion of the molecule. The Fc portion is separated from the F(ab) portions by a flexible bridge that connects them with the functional regions (on the heavy-chain portion of the molecule) that mediate the effector functions of the molecule (14,15).

Reaction with Antigen

For antibody molecules to effect lysis of RBCs, they must bind to surface antigens. The binding to antigen depends on a reversible reaction between the antigenic epitope and the antigen-binding pocket of the antibody molecule (16). Thus, the binding may be stronger or weaker, depending on the biochemical and biophysical characteristics of the epitope of the antigen and the binding site of the antibody molecule.

Antigens on the RBC that bind the antibodies of AIHA are either protein or polysaccharide in structure. The protein antigens usually are epitopes present on the cells of almost all individuals and are often found on the membrane glycoproteins (particularly glycophorin A and B) and lipoproteins (particularly those of the Rh complex). Usually, the epitope is not an allomorphic blood group antigen, but occasionally such antigens may be involved in the antigenic structure.

The polysaccharide antigens are either part of the complex bearing the H, A, and B antigens or the P antigens or are the polysaccharide structures on glycoproteins. The ABH structures consist of linear or complex branched arrays of sugars that are attached to lipid (usually sphingolipid) or protein molecules. The glycoprotein structures are usually simpler in form. All of these structures are present on the RBCs of all individuals, so distinctions of specificity are made on quantitative, rather than qualitative, bases or on tests of chemical structure.

The reaction between antigen and antibody may be modified by the temperature at which it takes place. In general, the reaction between a protein antigen and antibody is relatively independent of temperature and can occur at 37°C as well as at lower temperatures. This means that the antibody remains attached to the antigen at the core temperature of the body; these antibodies, nearly always IgG in type, are called *warm-reacting* antibodies. Conversely, the reaction of a polysaccharide antigen and its antibody is markedly enhanced at lower temperatures. In most cases, the reaction does not occur to a significant degree at 37°C, indicating that antibody and antigen are not attached to one another at core body temperature; these antibodies, nearly always IgM in type, are called *cold-reacting* antibodies. With these antibodies, antigen–antibody interaction can only occur as the blood circulates to the periphery and is cooled sufficiently.

Functional Capacities of Molecules

The means by which antibody molecules mediate destruction of the RBC is determined by their functional capacities—in particular, their capacity to fix complement and their ability to fix to specific receptors that are present on effector cells (e.g., phagocytes and "killer" lymphocytes) of the immune system. These capacities differ among isotypes of antibody.

FIXATION TO ANTIBODY-SPECIFIC RECEPTORS
For phagocytosis or other destruction of RBCs by cells of the immune system to take place, the target RBC must be bound to the effector cell by immune adherence. This is commonly effected through affixation of the antigen-bound antibody to a specific receptor on the effector cell through a specific region on the antibody molecule (17,18). Such a functional area is present

in the Fc portion of IgG and IgA molecules, but it is not present on IgM molecules. Like the C1q-binding area (see below), it may be located within range of the F(ab) arms of the molecule, and this may impede the binding of IgG$_2$ and IgG$_4$ to some of the receptors.

The receptors able to bind to this portion of the Ig molecule are called *Fc receptors*. Those reacting with IgG (Fcγ receptors) are of three distinct molecular types designated I, II, and III, respectively (Table 52-1). These differ in affinity for the Fc portion of the molecule; those with less affinity (II and III) do not bind IgG$_2$ and IgG$_4$ well. Specific receptors apparently exist for IgA as well, but they are not well characterized (19,20).

The effect of immune adherence mediated by Fc receptors is striking. If the effector cell is phagocytic, the cell membrane is stimulated to move in the direction of the attached IgG-coated target (21). If the membrane of the effector cell is able to engulf the target, it is entirely phagocytosed. If the membrane can engulf only a portion of the target RBC, the cell remnant that is not engulfed becomes spherocytic.

Thus, immune adherence due to the Ig–Fc receptor interaction is much more destructive to the RBC than immune adherence due to the C3b (or C4b) and its receptor (22). The two immune-adherence reactions appear to act in concert. The IgG–Fc receptor reactions are frequently of low affinity, and a number of interactions must accumulate to attain sufficient binding to initiate effective destruction of the cell; therefore, this immune-adherence reaction and its consequences appear to be slow. Reactions of complement components with their receptors have a higher affinity and do not appear to require accumulated interactions to accomplish effective immune adherence; immune adherence is thus more rapid when mediated by these receptors. When both complement and Fc receptors are present on effector cells and their ligands are both present on the target RBCs, the reactions of complement and its receptors may rapidly bind the target cells to the effector cells and allow the slower accumulation of effective IgG–Fc receptor interactions to occur.

COMPLEMENT IN DESTRUCTION OF TARGET CELLS
Complement is composed of a group of plasma proteins that effect or augment the destructive reactions of antibodies. When the sequence is completely activated in a series of reactions, a lesion is produced that penetrates the cell membrane and destroys the cell. These reactions are generally so tightly controlled that large amounts of complement must be activated to produce the final destructive event. During activation of the

TABLE 52-1. Summary of the Characteristics of the Fcγ Receptors of Human Cells

Characteristic	FcRI	FcRII	FcRIII
Molecular weight	72 kd	40 kd	50–70 kd
Affinity for IgG monomer	$K_a = 10^8 - 10^9$ M^{-1}	Undetectable	Undetectable
Specificity for IgG subclass	1 = 3 > 4; 2 = none	1 = 3 > 2 = 4	3 = 1; 2 and 4 = little or none
Cells			
Monocytes	+	+	–
Macrophages	+	+	+
Neutrophils	–	+	+
Eosinophils	–	+	+
Platelets	–	+	–
Lymphocytes			
B cells	–	+	–
T cells			+
Natural killer cells			+

FcR, Fc receptor; IgG, immunoglobulin G.

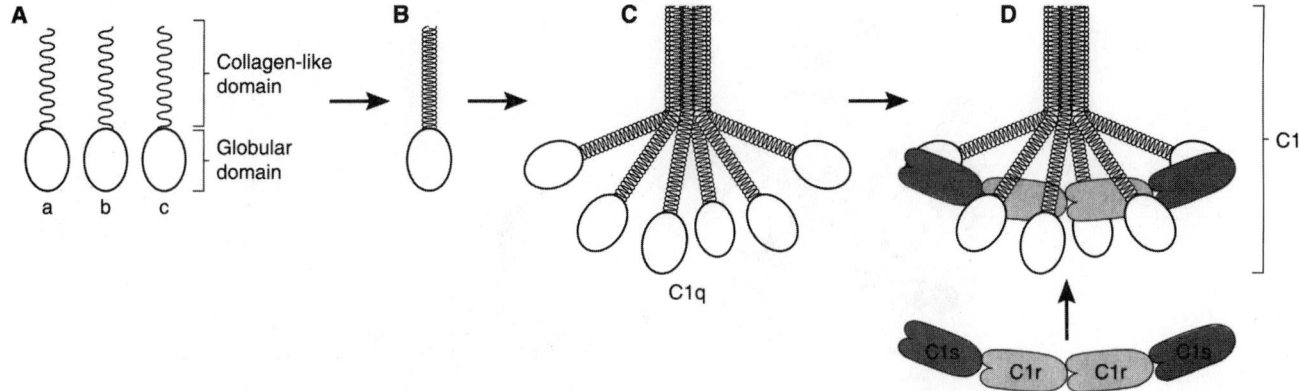

Figure 52-1. Structure of the first component of complement. **A:** Three similar polypeptide chains (*a, b,* and *c*) consist of a collagenlike portion (signified by the wavy line) and a globular portion. **B:** These intertwine to form a heterotrimer; the collagenlike portion becomes rigid and has a bend in it. **C:** Six of the heterotrimers form a complex structure said to resemble a bunch of flowers held by their lower stems. **D:** C1r and C1s form a tetramer, which is inserted into the spread ends of the heterotrimers.

sequence, however, proteins are generated that mediate immune adherence. This may lead to cell-mediated destruction, particularly if an antibody able to mediate immune adherence also is present on the target-cell membrane. The aspects of these reactions relative to immune hemolytic anemia are recounted here.

Fixation of Complement. The ability of an antibody molecule to participate in the fixation of complement depends on specific sequences in the Fc portion of the molecule that interact with the noncollagen portion of the C1q molecule (23,24) (Fig. 52-1); these sequences are present in IgG and IgM molecules but not in IgA molecules. IgA molecules do not fix complement by the classic activation pathway (25). Two of the following additional conditions must be met before complement can be fixed.

1. The C1q-binding site must be accessible to the C1q molecule. This accessibility is impaired in two ways:
   a. The site may be situated so close to the F(ab) portions of the molecule that these free-swinging "arms" may sterically hinder the fixation of C1q (26) (Fig. 52-2A). In IgG$_3$ and IgG$_1$ molecules, the C1q-binding site is distant from the F(ab) portion of the molecule because the hinge region between the Fc and the F(ab) domains is long; thus, these two subclasses readily fix C1q if the other

conditions are met (4). Similarly, the binding site in the IgM molecule is distant from the F(ab) domains. The hinge region of IgG$_2$ and especially IgG$_4$ molecules is short, however, and the waving F(ab) arms apparently hinder the binding of C1q (27).
   b. The site may be hindered by other parts of the molecule. In solution, IgM exists in a planar form; that is, the five monomers are spread out like a cartwheel around the joining J piece. In this conformation, the C1q-binding sites of IgM are hidden and not available for binding. When the molecule binds to two epitopes on the same surface, it assumes a conformational configuration that has been likened to a staple or a stool; in this conformation, the C1q-binding sites are exposed and binding takes place (28,29) (Fig. 52-2B).
2. For effective binding of C1q to take place, antibody must react with two of the binding regions on the C1q molecule (30). For two IgG molecules, this means that two molecules must be within about 24 nm to permit the binding of two sites on the C1q molecule (31) (Fig. 52-2C). For IgM molecules, a single molecule is sufficient, because the C1q binding areas of two subunits can participate in the reaction; however, the other conditions necessary for C1q binding must be met.

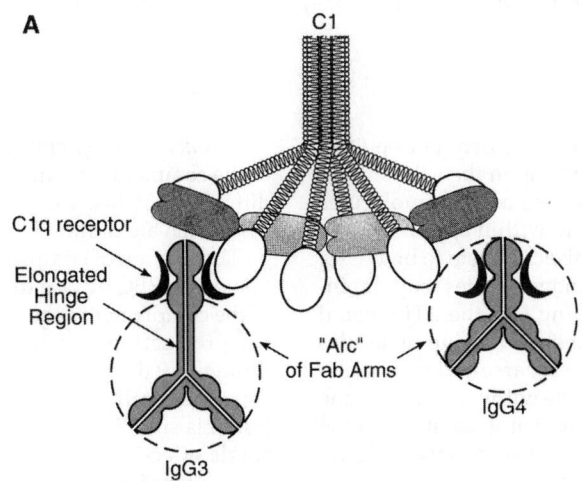

Figure 52-2. Binding of C1 to antibodies. **A:** Binding of C1 to immunoglobulin G (IgG) molecules is inhibited by interference from the Fab arms, which is minimized when the hinge region is elongated, as in IgG$_3$ molecules. *(continued)*

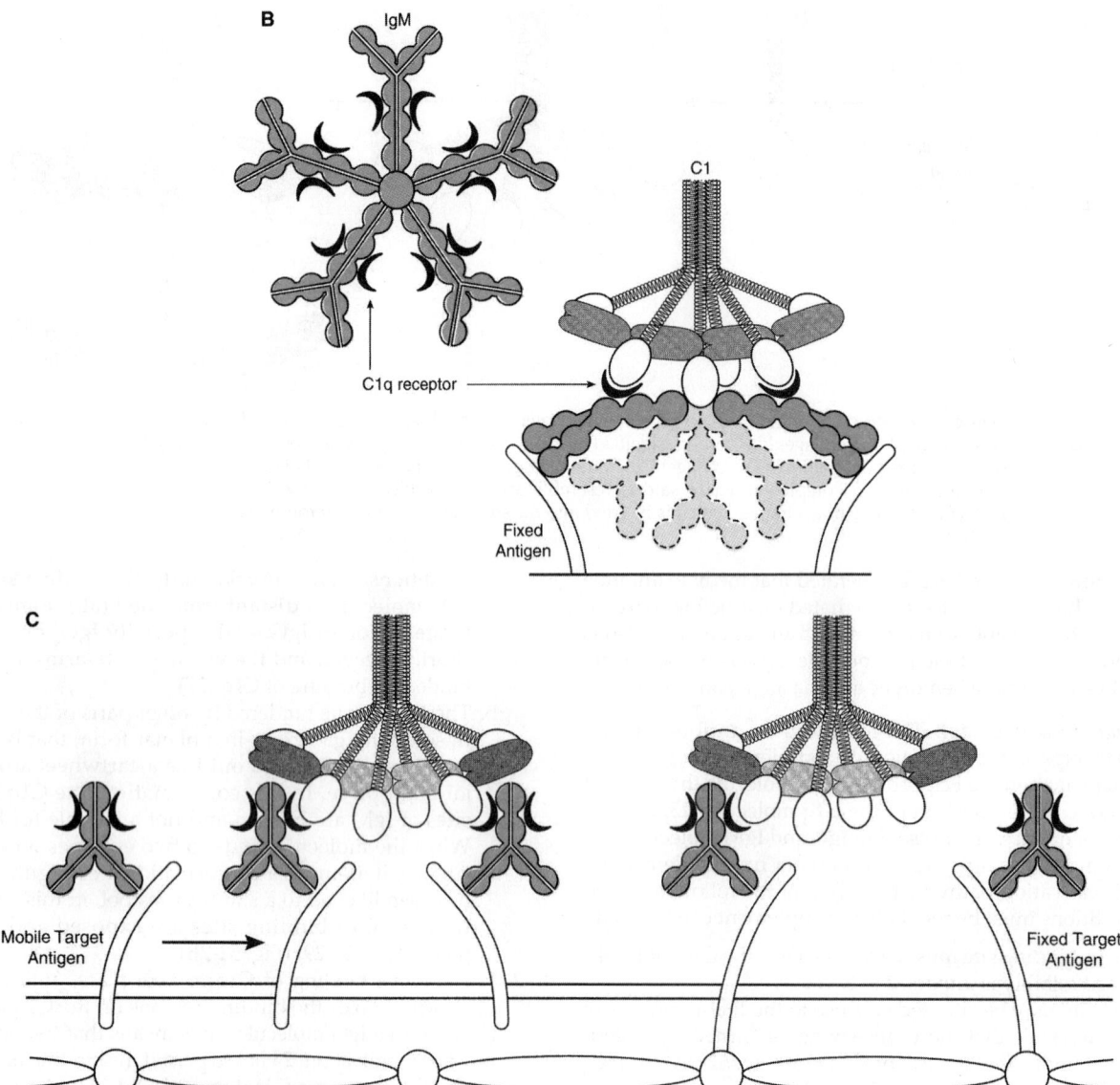

Figure 52-2. (*continued*) **B:** The C1-binding sites of IgM molecules are not available when the antibody is in the planar form in fluid phase; when two of the monomers are affixed, the molecule assumes an arched form and the C1-binding sites become available for reaction. **C:** Fixation of C1 by IgG also depends on reaction of two of the receptor binding areas; if this is not possible, as occurs when the antigen-bearing molecule is affixed to the cytoskeleton at relatively great distances, the binding of C1 is too weak to be effective.

Because of these limitations, complement may not be fixed by all antigen-antibody reactions occurring on the RBC surface (32). This is most commonly because two antigen molecules cannot be sufficiently approximated (to within approximately 24 nm) to allow antibody molecules affixed to them to bind C1q. In some circumstances, a sparsity of antigenic sites may diminish the chances of two antigens getting together. The usual cause, however, is an inability of the antigen-bearing molecules to move laterally in the membrane. Even sparse antigenic molecules that are able to "patch" or aggregate within the membrane on reaction with antibody are able to fix complement. But if the molecule bearing the antigenic epitope is affixed to the underlying membrane skeleton and thus unable to move laterally in the plane of the membrane, and if the interval at which the molecules are affixed is greater than 24 nm, complement is not fixed, because two C1q fixing sites cannot be approximated.

Results of Complement Fixation. The activation and control of the complement sequence is complex and involves at least 16 different proteins. The portions that are pertinent to the present discussion are outlined in Figure 52-3.

The fixation of complement by antibody leads to the destruction of the RBC by two major mechanisms. First, the completion of the complement sequence on the surface of the RBC results in the production of a lesion by the terminal components C5 through C9 that breach the lipid bilayer and result in the hemolysis of the cell (33) (Fig. 52-4). Although a single completed lesion is sufficient for the lysis of the cell, the production of a single effective lesion on the normal human RBC by human complement requires a massive activation of complement by antibody, because both the RBC and the serum are endowed with factors that are able to reduce the activation and effectiveness of complement in lysing the cell. Because such massive

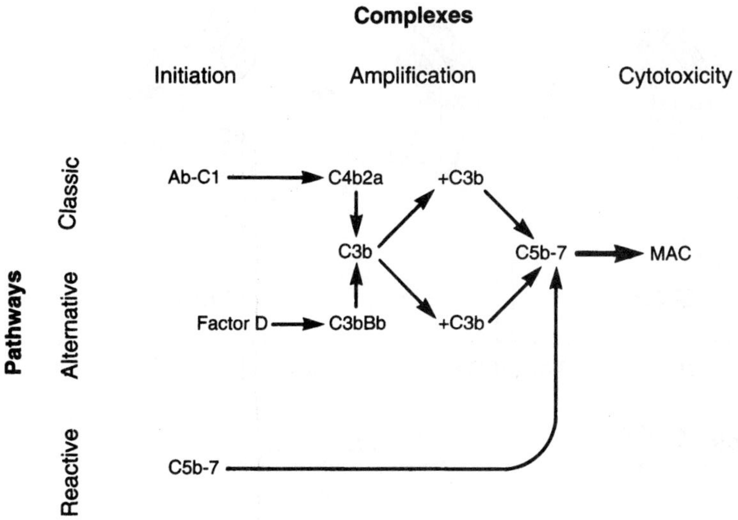

Complexes

| | Initiation | Amplification | Cytotoxicity |

Pathways

Classic
Ab-C1 ⟶ C4b2a   +C3b

C3b   C5b-7 ⟶ MAC

Alternative
Factor D ⟶ C3bBb   +C3b

Reactive
C5b-7

Figure 52-3. Activation of complement. Three kinds of complexes are generated: initiation, amplification, and cytotoxicity. These are generated by three different pathways: classic, alternative, and reactive. All result in formation of membrane attack complex (MAC).

activation of complement rarely occurs in clinical settings, direct lysis by complement is rarely a major outcome (34).

In the second mechanism, certain components of complement (C3b and C4b) that are covalently fixed to the membrane of the target cell are able to interact with specific receptors on destructive cells of the immune system, resulting in immune adherence (35). These receptors are of at least four types, each slightly different in the form of the components to which it binds (Fig. 52-5 and Table 52-2). The immune adherence that results from this binding is frequently not effective in initiating phagocytosis but assists greatly in the destruction of cells to which IgG also is fixed. The effectiveness of this immune adherence is further decreased by degradation of the complement component by specific enzymes, which may release the component from the receptor (36). For example, the degradation of C3b to iC3b by factor I markedly decreases the adherence to CR1 receptors, and the degradation of iC3b to C3dg by factor I or other serine proteases markedly reduces the adherence to CR3 and CR4 receptors.

Methods for Detection of Antibody

Diagnosis of AIHA depends on demonstration of an antibody that is able to interact with the cells of the patient. A number of techniques are available for detecting the antibody on RBCs, in the serum, or both. The fundamental problem of antibody detection is discerning the interaction or the results of an interaction between an Ig molecule and the cell. The problem is complicated by the characteristics of each.

AGGLUTINATION

The simplest reaction that permits detection of the interaction of antibody and erythrocytes is the agglutination reaction: One antigen-binding site on the antibody molecule binds to an antigen on one cell, and another antigen-binding site binds to an antigen on another cell. When this occurs multiple times, a lattice of cells is formed, and agglutination occurs (37).

For this reaction to occur, the antibody molecule must bridge the charge-related repulsive forces that are associated with the membrane when cells are suspended in saline (38). These forces maintain cells at a distance of approximately 24 nm. This distance is easily bridged by IgM molecules, because they possess antigen-binding sites on each of the five monomers (Fig. 52-6A), but IgG molecules are too small to do so by a single molecule (Fig. 52-6B) and can bridge the gap only under special circumstances.

To detect IgG molecules by simple agglutination, the distance between the cells must be reduced. This can be done physically by centrifugation, but the forces required are greater than is practical. The addition of anisotropic molecules (e.g., albumin, synthetic polymers, or strongly anionic molecules) (39,40) to the medium disperses the ionic cloud and allows approximation of the cells so that a single IgG molecule can affix its antigen-binding sites on different cells (Fig. 52-6C).

BINDING LIGAND TO ANTIBODY MOLECULE

The reaction of an antibody with a cell can be detected indirectly by the use of ligands that bind to the antibody molecule. The best known and most useful of these is an antibody to the Ig molecule, but other ligands—particularly a protein derived from certain strains of *Staphylococcus aureus*, called *staphylococcal protein A*—that bind to IgG molecules may be used (41).

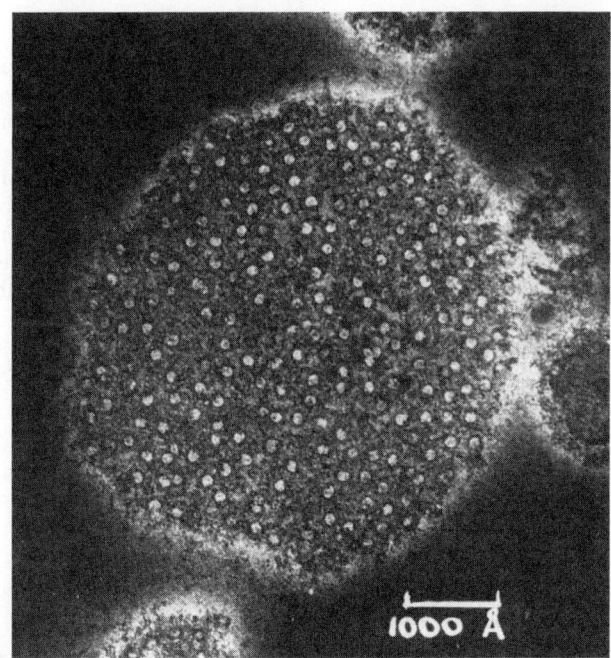

Figure 52-4. Electron micrograph of the lesions that appear on the completion of the membrane attack complex of complement. The dark lesions are hydrophilic complexes of protein approximately 10 nm in diameter in this negatively stained preparation.

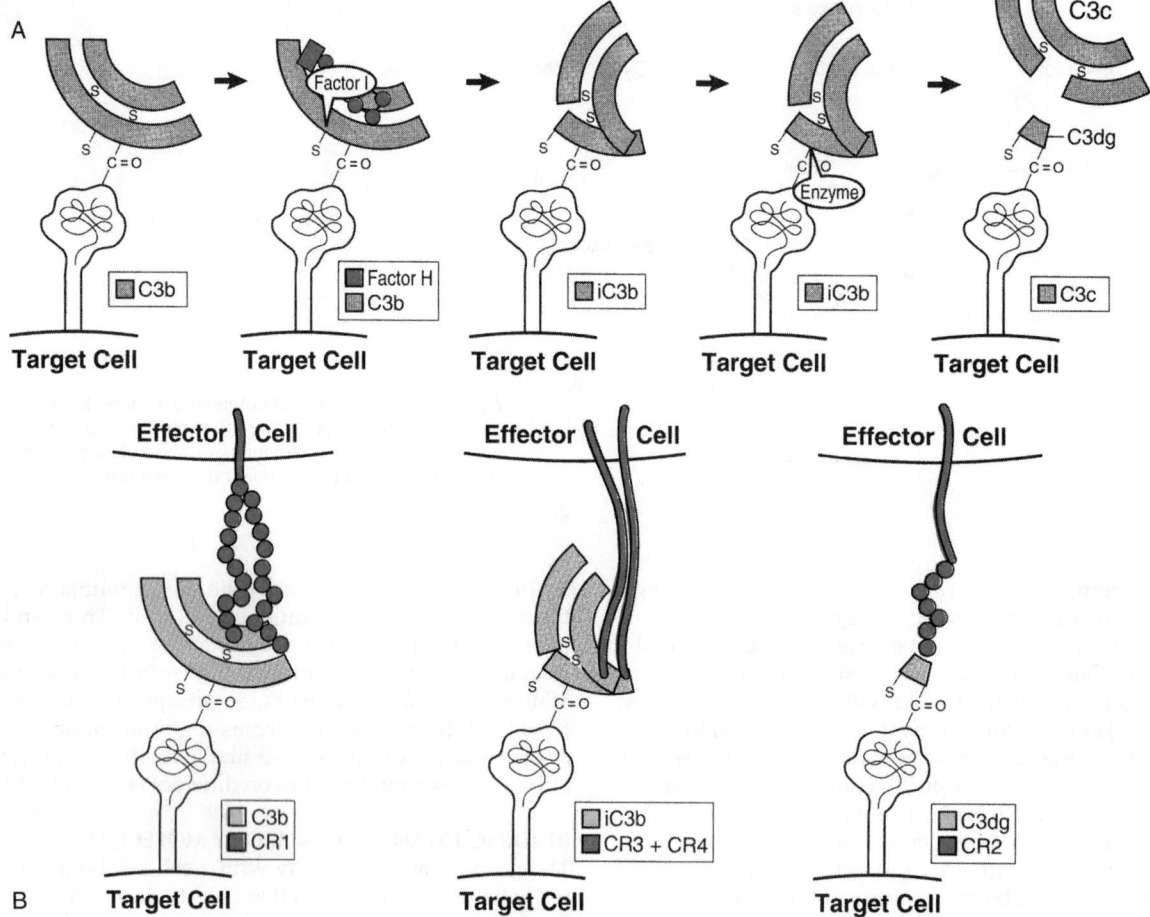

Figure 52-5. Degradation of C3b and reaction of the products with specific receptors. **A:** C3b is cleaved by factor I, which is held in place by factor H, resulting in iC3b; this product is cleaved by a proteolytic enzyme, releasing C3c and leaving C3dg attached to the cell. **B:** CR1 (a member of the complement regulatory family) reacts preferentially with C3b; CR3 and CR4 (members of the integrin family of proteins) react preferentially with iC3b; CR2 reacts with C3dg.

Reactions with antiIgs made to human serum in rabbits were first used by Coombs in a reaction wherein the endpoint was agglutination of the RBCs (7). This was possible because one antigen-binding site of the antiIgG molecule is able to bind to antibody affixed to one cell, and the other antigen-binding site is able to bind to an antibody molecule on another cell. In this way, the distance imposed by mutual repulsion is bridged (Fig. 52-6D). This test has been refined by the use of specific species that allow precise identification of the immunoproteins on the cell surface (42).

The RBCs must be thoroughly washed to free them of non-specifically adherent IgG when performing tests using antiglob-ulins. This is a disadvantage, because this procedure also may remove specifically bound antibody that reacts with low affinity; it may even remove the antigen necessary for antibody binding.

Although useful, the agglutination antiglobulin test is relatively insensitive and difficult to quantitate; the minimum number of molecules that can be detected in the routine test is probably 250 to 500 (43). More sensitive methods using monoclonal antiglobulin antibodies derived from mouse-human hybridomas have been devised that measure more accurately the amount of antibody on the cells (44–46). These methods involve labeling the monoclonal antiIg molecule with a radioactive molecule (e.g., ^{125}I) (45), an enzyme (47), or a fluorescent

---

TABLE 52-2. Biochemistry and Function of Receptors Reacting with Complement Components

Name	Cells	Structure	Ligand
CR1	Erythrocytes, macrophages, monocytes, PMNs, some lymphocytes	Multiple tandem repeats; 205–250 kd	C3b > iC3b
CR2	Lymphocytes	Tandem repeats; 140 kd	C3d
CR3	Macrophages, monocytes, PMNs, some lymphocytes	Integrin family; α = 180 kd; β = 95 kd	iC3b > C3b
CR4	Macrophages	Integrin family; α = 150 kd; β = 95 kd	iC3b (induces phagocytosis)

PMNs, polymorphonuclear leukocytes.

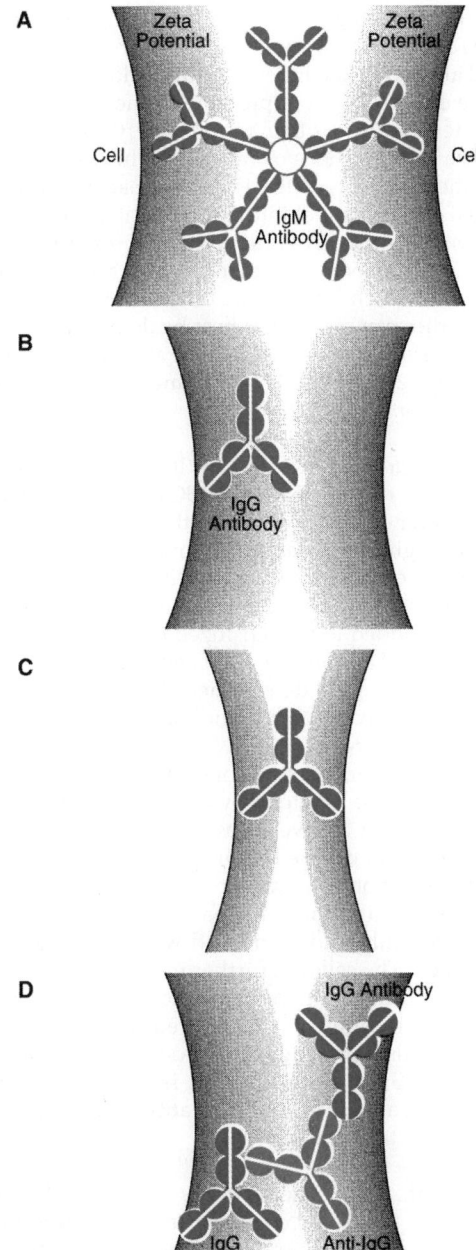

Figure 52-6. The conditions that lead to agglutination. **A:** The large immunoglobulin M (IgM) molecule can bridge the repulsive forces of the zeta potential. The smaller IgG molecule cannot bridge (**B**) unless the distance imposed by the zeta potential is reduced (**C**). **D:** An anti-IgG molecule can bind two bound IgG molecules and bring about agglutination.

probe (48). The amount of Ig affixed is determined by the amount of label affixed when the labeled antiIg molecule is reacted. These techniques detect smaller amounts of affixed antibody (50 to 200 molecules) than the antiglobulin agglutination techniques.

COMPLEMENT ACTIVATION

Complement-fixing antibody in the serum can sometimes be detected by its ability to lyse RBCs by penetration of the lipid bilayer by the membrane attack complex (C5b-9) (49). It is difficult to achieve lysis of human RBCs by human complement, however, because the presence of specific membrane-bound mol-

TABLE 52-3. Patterns of Reactions of the Direct Antiglobulin Tests Seen with Specific Antiglobulin Reagents in Patients with Warm Antibody Autoimmune Hemolytic Anemia

Pattern	Reaction with Antiglobulin		Percentage
	AntiIgG	AntiC3d	
I	+	−	35
II	+	+	56
III	−	+	9
IV	−	−	<1

Ig, immunoglobulin.
Data from Issitt PD. Serological diagnosis and characterization of the causative antibodies. In: Chaplin H Jr, ed. *Methods in hematology: immune hemolytic anemias.* New York: Churchill Livingstone, 1985, with permission.

ecules inhibits the functional activity of homologous complement. Thus, successful completion of the sequence resulting in cell lysis can only occur when complement is massively activated. This usually occurs only when antigen and antibody are both plentiful. For these reasons, tests using hemolysis as an endpoint are insensitive and are more often used to assess the lytic ability of the antibody rather than merely to detect its presence.

The fixation of complement can be detected with greater sensitivity; components C4 and C3 are covalently bound to the membrane during complement activation and may be detected on cells that have been attacked by complement but have not lysed. Even when these components are degraded, they may be detected on the cell surface by specific antibodies (e.g., antiC3dg and antiC4d) in both agglutination and ligand-binding assays (44,46). This testing is of particular importance; if the antibody or the antigen is not stably bound to the membrane, it may provide the only evidence that an immune reaction has occurred on the cell surface.

Detection Tests for Diagnosis of Autoimmune Hemolytic Anemia

TESTS ON PATIENT ERYTHROCYTES

The tests outlined may be used in a number of ways to detect antibody in the serum or its effects on cells in the diagnosis of AIHA. The most useful is the detection of antibody, complement, or both on the RBCs of the patient by antibodies to them; in its most commonly used form, it is called the *direct antiglobulin test* (DAT) or Coombs' test.

Direct Antiglobulin Test. In performing the DAT, the patient's erythrocytes are washed in saline to remove nonspecifically adherent IgG; the washed cells are then incubated with specific antiglobulin antisera. Usually, only antiIgG (to detect IgG antibodies) and antiC3d (to detect the presence of complement components) are used in separate reactions. In special tests, other antisera (e.g., antiIgM, antiIgA) can be used additionally in separate tests. After incubation to allow the antiglobulin molecules to bind, the mixture is gently centrifuged and the cells observed for agglutination. Agglutination indicates that the Ig or complement component reacting with the antiglobulin is attached to the cell surface.

Using antiIgG and antiC3dg, four patterns of reaction may be found, depending on whether complement is fixed and whether antibody is detectable (Table 52-3). These are interpreted as follows:

Type 1—antibody alone is fixed. This occurs when the antibody is IgG but is not able to fix complement. The usual reason for this inability is the spacing of the antigens on the cell surface.

Type 2—antibody and complement are fixed. This occurs when the antibody is IgG and the antigen sites are placed so that complement can be fixed. Such antigens are either plentiful or are mobile in the plane of the membrane.

Type 3—complement alone is found. When complement components are present but IgG is not, it may be due to one of the following:

The antibody may be IgM or IgA; this can be determined by using specific antiIgM and antiIgA in the testing procedure.

The antibody may be IgG, but it is not firmly attached to the antigen and is removed during the washing of the cells. The antibody may be cold reacting [e.g., Donath-Landsteiner (D-L) antibodies] or may be of very low affinity; this can be assessed in tests of patient serum (see later discussion).

The antigen may not be firmly attached to the RBC, causing antigen and antibody to be washed off during cell preparation. This commonly occurs in drug-induced and immune complex–induced hemolytic anemia.

Type 4—neither IgG nor complement is fixed. If antibody is not IgG, is of low affinity, and is cold reactive, or if it is affixed to an antigen that is not fixed to the membrane and complement is not fixed, there may not be evidence that the immune reaction occurred. This occurs in less than 1 in 50 cases.

TESTS OF ANTIBODY IN SERUM

Agglutination. The simplest technique for the detection of antibody to RBC antigens in patient serum is direct agglutination, because it involves only the mixing of cells and serum to observe if the cells are agglutinated. It is most useful for the detection of IgM antibodies, which usually are cold reacting and present in the serum in high concentration. The relative concentration of antibody can be estimated by diluting the serum and determining the minimal concentration (usually expressed as the dilution) that effects agglutination. The effect of temperature on agglutination can be easily assessed; the highest temperature at which agglutination can be detected is called the *thermal amplitude* or *thermal maximum*. Finally, by using various kinds of cells, the specificity of the antibody can be determined. All of these procedures are important in the characterization of the antibodies in cold agglutinin disease (see later discussion).

The IgG antibodies of warm agglutinin disease are rarely detectable by direct agglutination. Other means—particularly the indirect antiglobulin test (IAT)—usually are sought if such demonstration is needed.

Tests Using Lysis by Complement. Some antibodies in patient serum can be detected and quantitated by their ability to promote complement-mediated lysis. These tests usually are performed by incubating RBCs, patient serum, and normal serum as a source of complement under appropriate temperature conditions. At the end of the reaction, the unlysed cells are sedimented by centrifugation, and the amount of hemoglobin released into the supernatant fluid is assessed.

As noted, such tests for antibody usually are insensitive, because a large amount of complement-fixing antibody is needed to activate sufficient complement to result in the lysis of normal RBCs. The sensitivity of the test can be markedly increased by using the RBCs of patients with paroxysmal nocturnal hemoglobinuria; these cells are characterized by an unusual sensitivity to complement and are lysed by much less antibody. If such cells are not available, normal RBCs can be rendered more sensitive to complement by treatment with aminoethylisothiuonium bromide (50).

Many of the antibodies for which hemolytic tests are useful are cold reacting and, often, more lysis is obtained if the test is performed in two stages at different temperatures. In the first stage, the RBCs, patient serum, and a source of complement are incubated at a reduced temperature that allows the antibody to bind to the cell but does not promote the activation of complement. The temperature is then raised to 37°C to permit complement activation and lysis of the cells. This test is especially useful in the diagnosis of the IgG cold-reacting antibodies of paroxysmal cold hemoglobinuria (D-L antibody). It is less useful in the demonstration of IgM cold agglutinins because, during the cold phase, the antibody causes too much agglutination, which inhibits the binding of C1 (51). Lysis by these antibodies can sometimes best be demonstrated by incubating RBCs, serum, and complement at an intermediate temperature (e.g., 27°C); this is sometimes called a *monophasic hemolytic reaction*.

Indirect Antiglobulin Test. IgG antibodies in the serum are best detected by the IAT. Normal RBCs in a dilute suspension are incubated for 15 to 30 minutes with the test serum and then washed thoroughly with saline to remove the serum and nonspecifically adherent IgG. Antiglobulin serum or monoclonal antibody against specific immunoproteins (e.g., antiIgG, antiC3, antiC4) is then added to the sensitized cells, and the mixture is incubated again. The cells are then centrifuged, and the presence of agglutination is determined. If the cells are agglutinated, they must have acquired antibody, complement, or both from the patient's serum.

A rough estimate of the concentration of antibody in patient serum can be obtained by determining the dilution of serum just sufficient to give a positive reaction. However, the IAT (like the DAT) can be better quantitated using labeled monoclonal antiglobulin antibodies and RBCs from normal donors. After incubation with patient serum, the cells are washed thoroughly and incubated with the labeled monoclonal antibody. The cells are further incubated and washed or sedimented through oil, and the amount of label affixed is determined. This amount is compared to that found on the same normal cells following incubation with normal serum in the first step. Such quantitation is useful in detecting extremely small amounts of affixed antibodies and in following the response to therapy.

The IAT is useful in determining the specificity of the antibody in patient serum. The serum is reacted with a panel of RBCs in which antigenic composition is known; these are selected so that some bear and some lack most of the common antigens of the erythrocyte. After incubation, washing, and reaction with the specific antiIgG antiserum, some examples may be agglutinated and some may not; this pattern of agglutination is compared to the occurrence of antigens on the cells. If there is congruence between the cells that are agglutinated and the presence of a specific antigen on the agglutinated cells, the specificity of the antibody is determined. Often, the serum of the patient with AIHA reacts with all the cells in the panel ("panagglutinin"); in this case, rare cells lacking antigens that are common in the population (e.g., Rh_{null} cells) may be used to try to determine the specificity of the antibody.

The IAT is particularly useful in the detection of drug-related antibodies. In such testing, patient serum is reacted with normal cells with and without the addition of the suspected drug; usually, a source of complement must be included. After incubation, the cells are washed and incubated with antiIgG and antiC3 and then centrifuged and observed for agglutination. If the cells incubated with the drug are agglutinated and those not incubated with the drug are not, the assumption is made that antibodies are present in the patient serum that react with the drug in the presence of the cells.

The IAT may be used to detect IgG antibodies of low affinity in patient serum. The affinity of some antibodies can be increased by altering the charge on the RBC by enzymatic digestion or by altering the conditions in which the reaction takes place (e.g., reduction in ionic strength or changes in pH). When these altered conditions are used, great care must be taken to be certain that the test has not been rendered so sensitive that the small amount of IgG that is normally adsorbed to the test cells is detected.

The IAT can be used to determine the thermal maximum of the antibody by varying the temperature at which the serum and RBCs are incubated; this is seldom a consideration in the detection or description of autoimmune IgG antibodies, except for those of paroxysmal cold hemoglobinuria. These D-L antibodies may be detected by performing the IAT at 4°C in all the steps. The D-L antibodies fix IgG at 4°C but not at 37°C.

CLINICAL SYNDROMES

The clinical syndromes of AIHA are largely determined by the nature of the antibodies that characterize them, and the two most important attributes of the antibody molecules are isotype and temperature of reaction. Thus, four distinct syndromes can be described:

The antibody is IgG and warm reacting
The antibody is IgM and warm reacting
The antibody is IgM and cold reacting
The antibody is IgG and cold reacting

Rarely, IgA antibodies are involved, but the clinical syndrome that they cause is little different from that of the IgG or IgM antibodies. When drugs are the cause of immune hemolytic anemia, the clinical syndrome is sufficiently different to merit separate consideration.

Autoimmune Hemolytic Anemia Due to Immunoglobulin G Warm-Reacting Antibody

CLINICAL SYNDROME
AIHA caused by an IgG warm-reacting antibody can occur at almost any age but is most common in childhood and in young adulthood (ages 25 to 35 years). Among adults, it is more common in women than men. The clinical syndrome is variable (52–54), in part depending on age, underlying diseases, and severity.

In children, the onset of anemia may be rapid and profound (55); not infrequently, hemoglobinuria is present because of the rapidity of the RBC destruction. One-third to one-half of the patients have histories of a preceding viral infection. Many viruses have been implicated, including those causing exanthems (56), Epstein-Barr virus (EBV) infection, and cytomegalovirus infection (57). In these patients, the illness tends to be self-limited, and all evidence of autoantibody production usually disappears within 2 to 4 months.

In the other pediatric patients, the syndrome is not much different than that seen in adults in that it tends to be chronic or relapsing (55). Many of these patients manifest other evidence of immunologic malfunction, often recognizable as due to an inherited condition.

In adults, the onset of anemia is most frequently moderately rapid, and the patient becomes symptomatic with fatigue and weakness early in the course of the disease. The degree of anemia usually is significant and, in some cases, the oxygen-carrying capacity of the blood may be decreased to dangerous and even fatal levels. There is seldom a history of hemoglobinuria. In elderly patients, particularly those with underlying heart disease, angina pectoris and congestive heart failure may be caused by the strain imposed by the decreased hemoglobin. When the anemia is too severe and not relieved by treatment, cerebral hypoxia leads to coma and death. More than one-half of patients with this disorder died when no effective treatment was available.

In other patients, the degree of anemia is less severe and the onset of symptoms less abrupt. These patients can sometimes be followed without treatment.

Unless the syndrome is secondary to some other defined illness, the history usually is not helpful. There may be a history of a viral illness 2 to 3 weeks previously; this history is much more common in children and adolescents. AIHA is much more likely to occur in a patient who has a history, however remote, of AIHA or idiopathic thrombocytopenic purpura (ITP). The occurrence of AIHA and autoimmune thrombocytopenia [Evans-Duane syndrome (58)] in the same patient is not unusual. It is estimated that over 30% of patients with AIHA due to IgG antibodies also have IgG antibodies against platelets. These are separable antibodies; those reacting with RBCs do not react with platelets and vice versa.

No matter what the age of the patient, physical examination shows little abnormality except for pallor of the skin and mucous membranes. The color of the skin and sclerae may be tinged by jaundice, but if abnormalities of liver function are not present, the degree of jaundice usually is not great. In approximately 60% of patients, the spleen is enlarged so as to be palpable, but it is rarely greatly so. If the enlargement has been rapid, the spleen may be tender and even may have undergone partial infarction, leading to severe pain in the left upper quadrant, a splenic rub, and a painful spleen on palpation. In such a setting, great care should be taken to be certain that the spleen is not ruptured in the course of examination by palpation.

LABORATORY FINDINGS
The hemoglobin and hematocrit are diminished variably. The RBC indices are essentially normal except for some elevation of the mean corpuscular volume (MCV) because of the reticulocytosis; uncommonly, agglutination of the cells may falsely increase the MCV (59).

The reticulocyte count usually is elevated both relatively and absolutely; in severely anemic patients, it may exceed 500×10^6/L. On occasion, it may be lower than expected for the degree of anemia; this may have several causes. In some instances, it is suggested that the antibody either suppresses erythropoiesis (as demonstrated by a marrow with erythroid hypoplasia) or destroys the reticulocytes and late precursors (in which case the marrow is often hyperplastic). Aplastic crises may occur any time during the course of the disorder; the most severe of these appear to be due to parvovirus infections (60). The importance of reticulocytopenia is that it often increases greatly the severity of the anemia, and death is common unless aggressive care is taken (61).

Cells with the appearance of spherocytes (small dark cells) usually are present on the peripheral blood film (Fig. 52-7A); when carefully examined by electron microscopy, these cells are often not truly spherocytic but are concavoconvex (62) (Fig. 52-7B).

The white blood cell count may be elevated during acute hemolysis primarily because of an increase in neutrophils, and counts of 30,000/μL are not uncommon (63). Monocytes that have ingested RBCs may be found in films prepared from peripheral blood; this usually indicates severe hemolysis. This phenomenon can be more readily reproduced by permitting anticoagulated shed blood to stand.

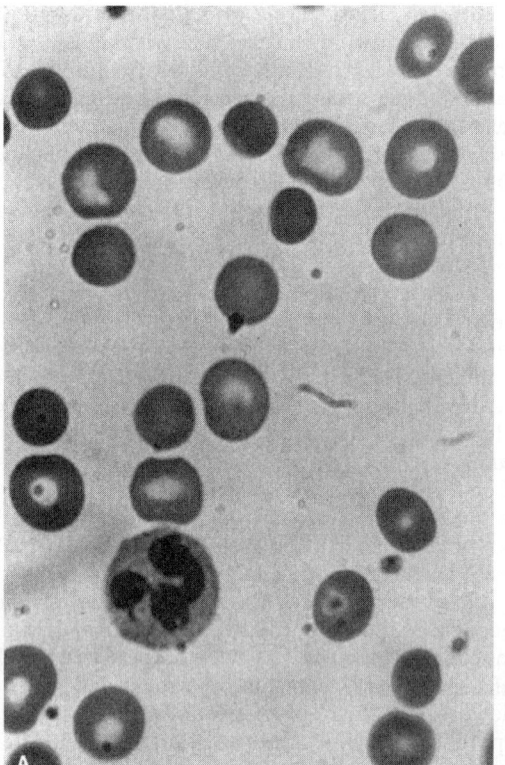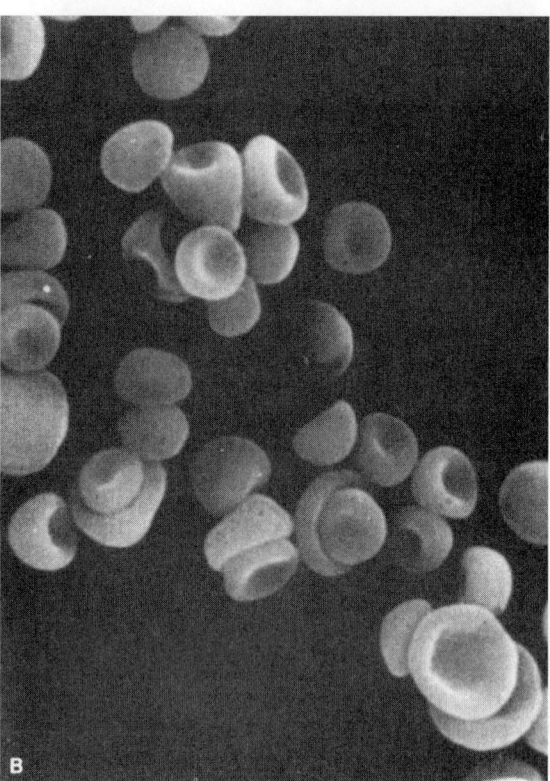

Figure 52-7. Spherocytes that appear in hemolytic anemia due to immunoglobulin G warm-reacting antibodies. **A:** The appearance on the peripheral blood film. **B:** The appearance in scanning electron microscopy. The spherocytes observed in the peripheral film are actually spherostomatocytes by scanning electron microscope.

The platelet count usually is normal unless autoimmune thrombocytopenia also is present (52); this occurs in 6% to 13% of patients (64). Although it is argued that this results in a poorer prognosis (65), others find this not to be the case (52). Immune thrombocytopenia may appear at a different time in the patient's life than immune hemolytic anemia.

The bone marrow usually is markedly cellular with a predominance of erythroid precursors. The maturation of the cells usually is normal unless folic acid deficiency is present (66). A few of the RBC precursors may show dysplastic changes (e.g., clefting, "noses," or double nuclei). Rarely, there may be relatively or absolutely decreased numbers of erythrocyte precursors in the marrow.

DIAGNOSTIC TESTS

In almost all cases of warm-reacting antibody hemolytic anemia due to IgG, the DAT is positive when antiIgG and antiC3dg are used as probes in an agglutination assay. Most commonly, both IgG and C3dg are present on the membrane; less commonly, only IgG is present, and uncommonly, IgG is absent but complement is present (Table 52-3) (67). When complement is not fixed, the antibody often has specificity for the protein or proteins bearing the Rh antigens.

When antiIgM and antiIgA antiglobulin antisera are used in the DAT, antibodies of these isotypes may sometimes be identified (Table 52-4). The importance of IgM and IgA warm-reacting antibodies is discussed later.

The DAT can be quantitated by any of several techniques. The simplest is the use of a labeled monoclonal antiIgG and antiC3 (45,46). Using these tests, IgG, C3d, or both usually can be detected in small amounts (50 to 200 molecules per cell) on the cells of those patients whose cells do not react with antiIgG or antiC3d in the agglutination assay.

Quantitation is useful in following the clinical course of a given patient, because it may show the relative amount of antibody being produced in response to therapy; it is of little value, however, in predicting the rate of hemolysis from patient to patient (68).

Neither agglutination nor the quantitative DAT measure the amount of antibody on the RBCs *in vivo*. Cells must be washed during preparation for the DAT, and those antibodies with low affinity are more readily removed in this process than those with a high affinity. Thus, if two patients have antibodies with differing affinity (one low affinity and the other high affinity), the amount of antibody on the cells may be the same in the circulation, perhaps resulting in the same amount of hemolysis, but in the quantitative DAT, much more of the high-affinity antibody remains on the cells after washing than low-affinity antibody.

The IAT is of relatively little value in the diagnosis of AIHA caused by warm-reacting IgG antibody except to distinguish drug-induced immune hemolysis. First, unrelated alloimmune

TABLE 52-4. Incidence of Immunoglobulin G (Ig), IgM, and IgA Antibodies in Autoimmune Hemolytic Anemia Due to Warm-Reacting Antibodies

Isotype	Alone (%)	With IgG (%)	With IgM (%)	With IgA (%)	Total[a] (%)
IgG	72.1	—	4.3	17.2	95.7
IgM	2.1	4.2	—	0	8.4
IgA	4.2	17.2	0	—	23.5

[a]Two patients had IgG, IgA, and IgM antibodies.
Courtesy of Petz LD, Garratty G. In: *Acquired immune hemolytic anemias.* New York: Churchill Livingstone, 1980.

antibodies may be present in patient serum and may be confused with autoantibodies. And second, although the amount of antibody in the serum can be quantitated, the information is of little value in assessing severity, although it may be used to evaluate response to therapy.

Antibody in the serum or eluted from the RBCs (by heating the cells to 50°C or solubilizing the membrane with organic solvents) may be used to determine its specificity (69,70). The specificity of the antibody may appear to be for known blood group antigens (e.g., anti-e, anti-K) or may be for antigens present on the cells of almost all individuals and only lacking in rare individuals (e.g., Rh_{null}, K_0). (Rare cells such as these usually are available at regional transfusion centers such as the American Red Cross, the New York Blood Center, or the Blood Center of Southeastern Wisconsin in Milwaukee.) In the first case, the specificity may be only relative, because in many cases, reaction can be demonstrated by careful techniques with cells lacking the ascribed antigen. For example, many autoimmune anti-e antibodies react with cells of the EE phenotype, even though they react more strongly with cells bearing the e antigen. Such antibodies are called *mimicking antibodies* (71).

Many antibodies appear to react with the proteins bearing the Rh antigens. They are classified further by their reactions with cells of rare phenotype (e.g., Rh_{null} and D_/D_) (49,72,73); these cells are available at reference centers specializing in these tests. Some antibodies react with cells bearing the usual allomorphic Rh antigens but do not react with cells partially (D_/D_) or completely (Rh_{null}) missing these antigens. These antibodies presumably react with some nonpolymorphic part of the molecule or molecules bearing the allomorphic Cc and Ee antigens. Other antibodies react with normal cells and partially deleted cells but not with completely deleted cells. The antigen is presumably on some different part of the Rh molecule or molecules than the allomorphic antigens.

Many of the antibodies that do not react with the Rh proteins appear to react with glycophorin molecules, because these antibodies do not bind to cells lacking part or all of these moieties (e.g., $En^a(-)$, M^k/M^k cells) (74,75). Using specific enzymes, portions of the glycophorin A molecule may be removed from normal cells, and specificity of autoantibodies for different parts of the molecule may be demonstrated. Many of these antibodies react with the Wright[b] (Wr^b) antigen (76), known to be engendered by a complex of glycophorin A and protein 3 (band 3, AE1) (77). In general, antibodies with these specificities fix complement, because the protein molecules are present in such large numbers that the doublet necessary for C1q fixation is readily generated.

PATHOPHYSIOLOGY
The destruction of RBCs by these antibodies is brought about primarily by mechanisms that depend on immune adherence. The IgG molecules are able to adhere to the abundant Fcγ receptors (of which there are at least three kinds) on effector cells of the immune system (macrophages, neutrophils, etc.) (17), and the adherence is a powerful stimulus to phagocytosis. This adherence is abetted by the simultaneous presence of complement components (C3b and C4b) (78).

The destruction of the cells by the direct lytic action of complement plays a lesser role in the destruction of the RBCs by IgG antibodies in AIHA. Because of the requirement for two molecules of antibody to initiate the reaction, and because of the defense mechanisms of the cells in down-regulating complement, it is uncommon in adults that sufficient activation of complement occurs to result in the completion of a sufficient number of sequences to cause a breaching of the membrane and thus intravascular lysis. In children, in whom the hemolysis tends to be brisker, hemoglobinuria is more frequent.

The spleen is a primary site of destruction, particularly if complement is not fixed (79). It is here that the IgG-coated cells are in most intimate contact with the Fc receptor–bearing cells, and the circulation is sufficiently slow that the reaction can occur. Further, partial phagocytosis results in the formation of spherocytes (80) that are less capable of deformation than biconcave discs (81); they are readily trapped in the cords of Billroth among the phagocytic cells behind the filtering barrier in the spleen, the wall of the splenic sinus (82) (Fig. 52-8). For these reasons, splenectomy is often useful in treatment.

If the amount of antibody affixed to the cell is sufficiently great or if complement is fixed as well, adherence-dependent hemolysis may occur readily in other parts of the reticuloendothelial system. In this case, splenectomy is less effective therapy.

The complex relations among the various hemolytic mechanisms are shown in Figure 52-9.

ETIOLOGY
Since Ehrlich recognized that the normal immune system did not make antibodies against antigens of self (83) (horror autotoxicus), it has been difficult to understand why this happens in autoimmune diseases. There is little real evidence that explains the phenomenon, but a number of interesting hypotheses are proposed.

When an immune reaction occurs to a foreign antigen, a range of antibodies are first made that vary in their reactivity with the inciting antigen. Those that better fit the antigen are more specific and have a higher affinity; those that fit the antigen less well are less specific (i.e., react with different but related structures) and have a lower affinity. Antibodies of the less specific sort may react with self-antigens. In the well-regulated immune system, the clones producing the less-specific antibodies are rapidly suppressed, leaving only the clones producing high-affinity, specific heteroantibodies; this regulation appears to be under the control of antigen-specific suppressor T cells. In the poorly regulated immune system, the production of less-specific antibodies may not be suppressed; if these antibodies cross-react with self-antigens, evidence of autoimmunity is found.

Another theory suggests that autoimmune antibodies arise when mechanisms for the suppression of antibodies against self fail (84,85). It is known that the immune system makes nonpathogenic antibodies against self-antigens, and that the level of production is normally closely maintained by inhibitory influences—possibly antiidiotype antibodies, possibly specifically programmed suppressor T cells. Autoimmune disease results when such suppression fails and pathogenetic amounts and isotypes of self-reacting antibodies are produced.

The first theory may explain why autoimmune syndromes sometimes follow specific heteroimmune reactions. Such syndromes are frequently seen in childhood, because viral infections are not infrequently followed in 2 to 3 weeks by a bout of AIHA or immune thrombocytopenic purpura. The production of autoantibodies lasts approximately 3 to 6 weeks but eventually ceases, presumably as the immune system finally regulates itself. It has been suggested but not proven that such patients are more prone to AIHA in later life.

Either theory may account for the AIHA that results from alloimmune reactions. Certain patients, particularly those prone to make alloantibodies, who receive antigenically incompatible transfusions make, in addition to the expected alloantibodies, autoantibodies that are then able to react with their own RBCs (86). The DAT on the patient's own RBCs is positive (usually only with antiIgG, because these autoantibodies are frequently directed against the nonpolymorphic

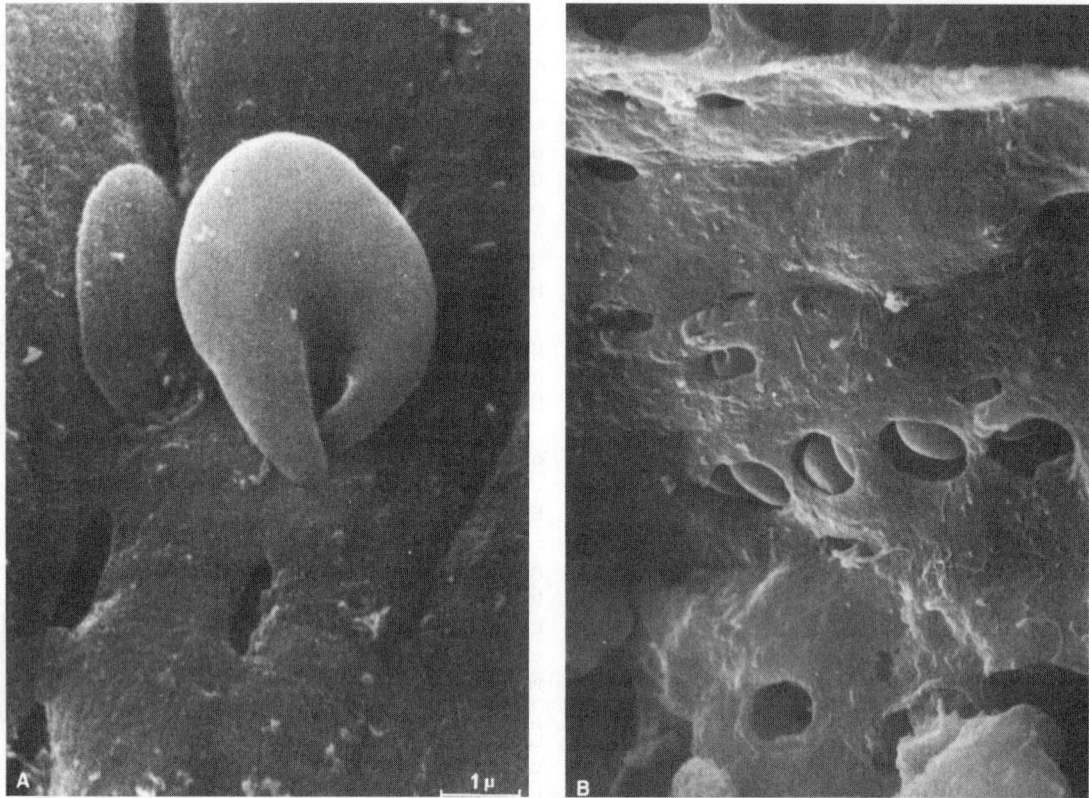

Figure 52-8. The wall of the splenic venous sinus as seen in scanning electron microscopy. **A:** Normal cells can, by deforming, pass the small elliptical apertures to regain the circulation. **B:** Spherocytes, because they cannot deform, cannot pass the barrier and are maintained in the cords of Billroth.

portions of the Rh proteins) and may be difficult to detect in the presence of alloantibodies reacting with the transfused cells. The amount of hemolysis may be significant, but the production of antibody usually is of short duration, lasting no more than 2 to 3 months. The reaction appears to occur in patients with poorly tuned immune systems that are not able to distinguish self-antigens (because even the alloantigens are not very different from self-antigens) and suppress production of antibodies to them.

AIHA due to IgG antibody is seen with increased frequency in patients with viral diseases that affect the immune system, particularly human immunodeficiency virus–I infection (87), infectious mononucleosis (88), and cytomegalovirus infection (89). Presumably, the production of antibodies reacting with self-antigens is due to abnormalities of regulation that are induced in the immune cells by the infection.

ASSOCIATION WITH OTHER AUTOIMMUNE DISEASES

Not infrequently, AIHA with warm-reacting IgG antibodies is associated with other evidence of immune dysfunction or other diseases of immune dysfunction (Table 52-5). This is sometimes as minor as alterations in the concentration of Igs, particularly IgA (90). In other instances, the abnormalities form a clinical syndrome, such as systemic lupus erythematosus (91), rheumatoid arthritis (92), or other connective tissue diseases (93–95); this form of hemolytic anemia is not infrequent in patients with those diseases and, in fact, may precede all other symptoms of the primary disease.

Similarly, patients with congenital disorders of the immune system, such as Wiskott-Aldrich syndrome, congenital dysgammaglobulinemias, and common variable immunodeficiency, may have AIHA due to IgG antibodies (96–99). Recently, a syndrome of congenital deficient lymphocyte apoptosis with resul-

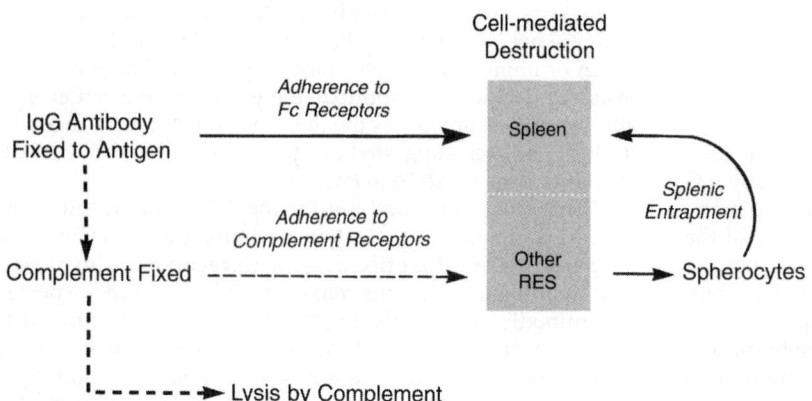

Figure 52-9. Mechanisms of lysis in hemolytic anemia due to immunoglobulin G (IgG) antibodies.

TABLE 52-5. Diseases in Which Autoimmune Hemolytic Anemia Due to Immunoglobulin G Antibody May Be Seen

Infections
Postviral autoimmune hemolytic anemia of childhood
Infectious mononucleosis
Human immunodeficiency virus–1 infection
Immune deficiency states
Hypogammaglobulinemia
Wiskott-Aldrich syndrome
Dysgammaglobulinemia
Neoplasms of the immune system
Lymphocytic disorders
    Chronic lymphocytic leukemia
    Non-Hodgkin's lymphoma
Hodgkin's disease
Plasma cell disorders
    Waldenström's macroglobulinemia
    Multiple myeloma
Diseases of immune dysfunction
Systemic lupus erythematosus
Scleroderma
Rheumatoid arthritis
Sjögren's syndrome
Immune thrombocytopenia (Evans' syndrome)
Miscellaneous diseases
Pernicious anemia
Thyroiditis
Ulcerative colitis
Ovarian tumors and cysts
Other tumors

tant autoimmune diseases, including AIHA, has been described (100). The anemia may develop as early as the first year of life and usually is chronic and persistent. It presumably results from the abnormalities of regulation that characterize the primary disease.

Finally, patients with neoplasms of the immune system may have this form of hemolytic anemia. Approximately 20% of patients with chronic lymphocytic leukemia or well-differentiated lymphocytic lymphoma have a positive DAT some time during the course of the disease, even in some instances preceding the lymphocytosis characteristic of the malignant disease (101,102). The incidence of AIHA is apparently increased in those patients treated with fludarabine (103,104) or the related drug, 2-chlorodeoxyadenosine (cladribine); the reason for this is not known, but the resulting anemia is often very severe.

AIHA is reasonably common in Hodgkin's disease (105,106) and thymoma (107,108) but is perhaps less common in the less differentiated forms of lymphoma (109,110). It is seen in T-cell disorders as well as B-cell disorders (111). The autoimmune IgG antibody is the result of the underlying or accompanying dysfunction of the immune system and is not the product of the monoclonal malignant lymphocytes; in all cases, multiple isotypes of both light and heavy chains are found among the antibody molecules (112).

AIHA is seen in patients who have undergone bone marrow transplantation (113). The complication is due to a warm-reacting antibody, occurs 6 to 18 months after transplantation, and is thought to be due to dysequilibrium during immune reconstitution.

TREATMENT

The treatment of AIHA of IgG warm antibody type involves the diminution of the concentration of antibody, the reduction in its effectiveness in mediating the destruction of the cells, or both.

Decreasing Antibody Concentration. The concentration of available antibody can most effectively be reduced by diminishing its production. Ideally, one would like to diminish the pro-

duction of antibody directed only at a specific antigen or antigens so that the treatment would not result in general immunosuppression; this is not possible, but the useful treatments reduce the production of autoantibodies more readily than alloantibodies or heteroantibodies.

Prednisone. One of the effects of prednisone is the suppression of the production of IgG antibodies (114). This effect results only with high doses of the drug, but once suppression has been achieved, it can often be maintained by much lower doses (108). The production of IgM is not affected; the effect on IgA production is not clear.

In addition to its effects on production, prednisone given in high doses (1 mg/kg/day) also diminishes rapidly the amount of antibody on the circulating RBCs in approximately two-thirds of cases, thus diminishing hemolysis (68); the reason for this effect is not known. Further, this dose of prednisone appears to interfere with the function of the destructive cells of the immune system, also diminishing hemolysis (115). Higher initial doses are often used in children, as will be discussed.

Cytotoxic Drugs. Antibody production can be reduced by the administration of drugs such as alkylating or antimetabolic agents that are cytotoxic to the antibody-producing cells (116,117). Again, the effect is nonspecific, but the cells actively producing autoantibody appear to be more susceptible to the effects of these drugs than other cells of the immune system. Because the drugs all diminish the production of cells, overdosage results in suppression of the bone marrow, a particularly unfortunate event when greater than normal production of RBCs is necessary.

Cyclophosphamide (Cytoxan), given either orally (100 mg/day) or parenterally (500 to 700 mg every 3 weeks) (adult doses) appears to be effective (118) in the treatment of this type of AIHA, resulting in remission in approximately 40% of cases. Its use is limited by its toxicity; in addition to its immediate toxicity (marrow suppression, bladder irritation, hair loss), cyclophosphamide is significantly leukemogenic (119).

Azathioprine also has been used in the treatment of AIHA (120). It is probably a little less likely to induce remission than cyclophosphamide, but its leukemogenic effect is probably lower. Vincristine also has been used as an immunosuppressive agent (121); the response is often rapid but short lasting, and its use is limited by neurotoxicity. This treatment is not so effective in this syndrome as it is in immune thrombocytopenic purpura. Vinca-loaded platelets have been used with modest success (122).

Other cytotoxic regimens, including the use of cyclosporine and radiation, have been suggested but are considered only in cases of desperation.

Plasmapheresis. A reduction in the level of antibody also can be achieved by removing formed antibody from the plasma by plasmapheresis (123,124), but this procedure is relatively ineffective with IgG antibodies, because these molecules are not confined to the intravascular space. Further, because IgG autoantibodies react with antigen at body temperature, they are adsorbed to the RBCs and not removed when plasma is removed. Nevertheless, with persistent daily apheresis, the antibody level can be reduced in some cases, and this may be useful in the case of acute hyperhemolysis.

Reduction in Destruction of Cells. The other approach to the reduction in hemolysis is to diminish the means by which antibody brings about the destruction of cells. This can be accomplished by reducing the interaction of antibody and antigen, reducing the interaction of the antibody-coated cells with the phagocytic cells of the immune system, or removing the site of destruction. Of these, the last is the most effective.

Splenectomy. In this type of AIHA, the spleen is a major site of destruction of RBCs. The removal of the spleen is beneficial in approximately 65% to 80% of patients and may be all that is necessary in approximately 50% of these (125). Splenectomy in children under 5 years of age should be avoided if possible because of the increased incidence of overwhelming sepsis with gram-positive organisms (126); this complication is much less common in adults. Splenectomy is less likely to be successful if complement is fixed by the antibody because that permits sequestration in other parts of the reticuloendothelial system, particularly the liver. Unfortunately, isotopic studies (usually with ^{51}Cr) localizing the site of sequestration are generally of little value in predicting the success of the operation (127).

Down-Regulation of Fc Receptors

INTRAVENOUS γ-GLOBULIN. The interaction of the IgG molecule and the Fc receptor (responsible for most of the cellular destruction in this form of AIHA) is reversible, and cell-bound IgG can be displaced from the receptor by fluid-phase IgG if it is present in high enough concentration. To this end, purified human γ-globulin given intravenously in large doses (2 g/kg given over 2 or 5 days) (128) has been used to treat autoimmune disease due to IgG antibody. This has met with considerable success in the treatment of ITP (129,130) and with perhaps less (131,132) success in the treatment of AIHA. The effect is transient, and the drug is expensive, but it can be used when acute cessation of hemolysis is needed.

Samuelsson and his colleagues have recently proposed another mechanism by which intravenous γ-globulin can down-regulate Fc receptors (133). They find that intravenous γ-globulin induces the expression of FcγRIIB, an inhibitory receptor, on effector cells of the reticuloendothelial system. Engagement of the FcγRIIB receptor appears to counterbalance the activation responses triggered by FcγRIII binding in the reticuloendothelial system, thereby inhibiting the clearance of opsonized cells.

PREDNISONE. One of the effects of prednisone appears to be a down-regulation of the Fc receptors (116). This effect occurs only with high doses of the drug and may account for some of the rapidity of response when these doses are administered.

DANAZOL. Certain androgenic steroids also down-regulate Fc receptors, and one, danazol, has been used in the treatment of immune destruction of blood cells (134,135). It appears to be more successful in the treatment of ITP than of AIHA (136).

ANTIBODIES TO FC RECEPTORS. More recently, monoclonal antibodies to Fc receptors have been used to try to down-regulate their function (137). This therapy is still under investigation.

Transfusion. Transfusion is frequently necessary in AIHA patients, particularly when the rate of hemolysis is great, as evidenced by a falling or very low hematocrit. In patients older than 60 years of age, it is particularly important to be prepared for transfusion of the patient, because these patients are prone to complications, such as myocardial infarction and cerebral vascular accident. In general, when a patient is first seen, blood should be made ready for transfusion without waiting for the physiologic consequences of hypoxia to become evident.

Compatibility testing for transfusion of these patients is complicated by the fact that the cells being transfused are nearly always incompatible due to the presence in the serum of autoantibodies. Such antibodies usually do not hemolyze transfused cells at a greater rate than autologous cells. Thus, the transfusion may not be as effective as is normally the case, but it does not cause a massive hemolytic reaction provided alloantibodies are not present.

The detection of alloantibodies is made difficult by the presence of the autoantibody (138), which must be removed from the serum before one can be sure that no alloantibodies are present. This is often done by repeated adsorption with the patient's own cells that have been heated to 50°C or treated chemically to remove the autoantibody (139). If this is done thoroughly, any antibody remaining is likely to be an alloantibody that can be identified so that cells lacking its antigen can be found.

These tests are time-consuming, but they should not delay the delivery of a transfusion to the patient in emergent need of blood. In an emergency, type-specific or even O Rh-negative blood may be used. The patient should not die because of serologic niceties.

TREATMENT OF AUTOIMMUNE HEMOLYTIC ANEMIA DUE TO WARM-REACTING IMMUNOGLOBULIN ANTIBODIES

The strategy for treatment of AIHA caused by warm-reacting IgG antibodies is dictated by many factors, including the age of the patient, the severity of the hemolysis, and the presence of other medical conditions. Further, it must be flexible to take into account the response or lack of response of the patient (Fig. 52-10).

For most patients, glucocorticoids such as prednisone usually are the first mode of treatment. Prednisone is started at a dose of 1 to 1.5 mg/kg/day; larger relative doses may be used initially in children (2 to 6 mg/kg/day initially, decreasing to 1 to 2 mg/kg/day within a week or so). Unless the patient has particularly severe hemolysis (hemolysis so great that transfu-

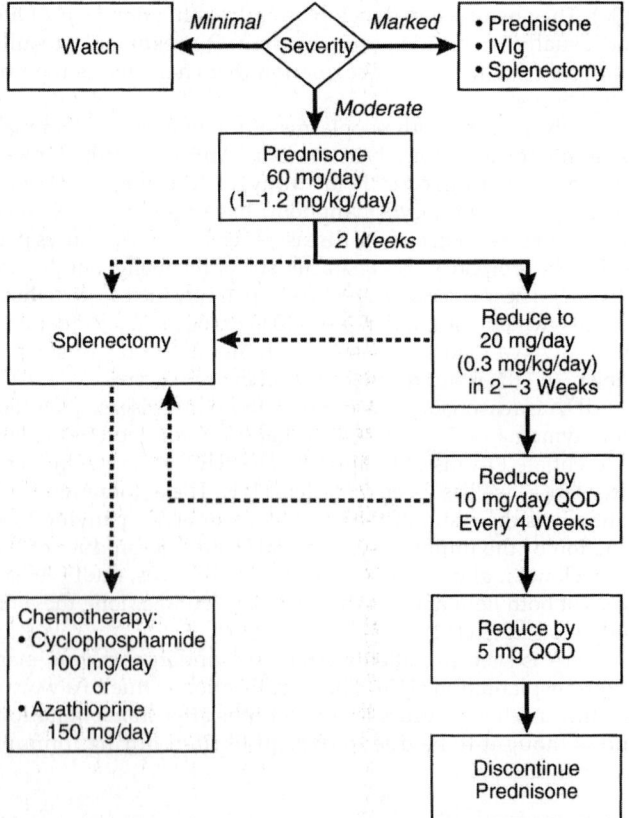

Figure 52-10. A schematic diagram for treatment of adult patients with autoimmune hemolytic anemia due to immunoglobulin G warm-reacting antibodies. Success of the treatment is denoted by a solid arrow to the next step in treatment; lack of success is denoted by an interrupted arrow. Treatment of pediatric patients includes adjustment of the doses of drug for body size (usually relatively larger doses of prednisone) and a greater tendency to avoid therapy, especially splenectomy and chemotherapy. IVIg, IV immunoglobulin.

sions must be administered every 1 to 2 days), this can be maintained for up to 3 or 4 weeks, or until a response (demonstrated by a reduction in antibody, improved hemoglobin, and reduced reticulocyte count) is seen. Usually, a response is seen within 2 weeks of the initiation of therapy if the regimen is to be successful by itself (140); if it is not, other treatment is probably needed.

If a response is obtained, the amount of prednisone prescribed is reduced, at first fairly rapidly [by 20 mg/day (0.3 mg/kg/day) each week] to a dose of 20 mg/day (0.3 mg/kg/day); this dose is maintained for approximately 1 month to determine if the remission continues. The dose is then reduced each month by 10 mg (0.15 mg/kg) on alternate days so that 2 months later, the patient is taking 20 mg (0.3 mg/kg) on alternate days. This dose is then reduced again at monthly intervals until the dose is 10 mg (0.15 mg/kg) on alternate days. If the DAT remains positive, this dose is maintained so long as remission persists.

If at any point during the course of reduction of dose exacerbation of hemolysis occurs, the dose is immediately raised to the next level and maintained at that level. If this exceeds a dose tolerable by the patient [certainly no more than 20 mg (0.3 mg/kg) every other day], then other therapy must be contemplated.

Autoimmune Hemolytic Anemia Due to Immunoglobulin M Warm-Reacting Antibodies

IgM autoantibodies are nearly always cold reacting; that is, they do not react with the antigen at body temperature. Rarely, IgM antibodies may react at body temperature, and a particularly severe and difficult syndrome may result (141–143). The syndrome is like that described for IgG warm-reacting antibodies with some notable differences.

Often, the amount of hemolysis is great, resulting in severe anemia; the anemia is not infrequently so severe as to be fatal. In some patients, this may be accompanied by reticulocytopenia, as if the antibody affects the bone marrow. Even in these cases, however, erythroid hyperplasia usually is seen in the bone marrow. Spherocytes are much less prominent or are lacking on the peripheral blood film.

The DAT is negative with antiIgG and may or may not be positive with antiC3. Some agglutination may be detected when normal cells are mixed with the serum, but this is rapidly lost on dilution of the serum. The agglutination may be enhanced by the addition of albumen. The diagnosis is most certainly made by the use of specific antiIgM antisera in the DAT. The nature of the antigen with which the antibody reacts usually is not known, although serologic specificity for antigens on glycophorin A (En^a, Wr^b, Pr) has been attributed to the antibody in some cases (143).

The syndrome may arise without evidence of other disease. It has been seen in patients with malignant lymphocytic neoplasms; it has not been determined in these cases whether the antibody is monoclonal (and therefore presumably the product of the neoplastic cells) or polyclonal (and therefore due to the underlying immunologic abnormalities seen in these diseases).

Treatment of this syndrome is difficult. Prednisone in very high doses (2 mg/kg) has some effect but does not reduce the production of antibody and therefore does not lead to a useful remission. Splenectomy is of no value. Only immunosuppression is successful, and the combination of cyclophosphamide and prednisone has been used.

Autoimmune Hemolytic Anemia Due to Immunoglobulin M Cold-Reacting Antibodies

The second most common syndrome of AIHA is that caused by IgM cold-reacting antibodies (63,144–149). Because the antibodies occur in the serum in high enough concentration to result in agglutination, the name *cold agglutinin syndrome* is often applied to this symptom complex.

CLINICAL SYNDROMES
Three general clinical syndromes may be caused by cold agglutinins. In children and young adults, the syndrome usually is brought on by a viral infection, either infectious mononucleosis or *Mycoplasma pneumoniae* infection. The onset is often abrupt with hemoglobinuria, and the anemia may be severe because of the diminished erythropoiesis caused by the infection. The acute hemolysis usually does not last more than 1 to 3 weeks, and all evidence of cold agglutinins usually is gone within 6 months.

The chronic cold agglutinin syndrome of adults has its onset usually after the sixth decade. The anemia usually is gradual in onset and usually is not severe. Some patients may note initially the onset of acrocyanosis, a purplish to gray discoloration of the fingers, toes, nose, ears, or other peripheral parts on exposure to cold. This is due to the agglutination of the blood as it cools and can often be brought about by immersing the hand in tepid water that is then cooled. The condition is different from Raynaud's phenomenon in that there is no preliminary blanching phase and no reactive red phase once the cyanosis has cleared. Acrocyanosis may be uncomfortable but rarely leads to gangrene.

On physical examination, the patient may exhibit acrocyanosis but usually does not. The spleen is sometimes enlarged, occasionally strikingly so. There usually is no lymph node enlargement unless an accompanying lymphoproliferative disorder is present (150).

Uncommonly, the syndrome in adults may be acute with severe anemia and marked hemolysis; in some cases, this is due to an antibody that is able to react with its antigen at a temperature approaching 37°C (151). This syndrome is particularly difficult to treat successfully.

LABORATORY FINDINGS
Analysis of the blood is often complicated by the presence of agglutination. Thus, in most automatic counters, the MCV is reported to be remarkably increased unless precautions are taken to warm the blood thoroughly before analysis (152). Because the hematocrit is calculated from the MCV on such devices, it is also inaccurate under these circumstances.

The agglutination is often visible in the peripheral blood film as aggregates of cells seen even in the thin parts of the preparation (Fig. 52-11). Agglutination also can be distinguished from rouleaux, because the cells are distorted and not simply like stacks of discs.

The reticulocyte count usually is elevated, although the degree of elevation may be suboptimal for the degree of anemia.

The white blood cell count is often somewhat elevated. The lymphocytes usually are normal in appearance unless the patient has a lymphoproliferative disorder. Some of them can be shown to bear the cold agglutinin as surface Ig. These form rosettes in the cold, with RBCs bearing the antigen (153).

The bone marrow usually shows erythroid hyperplasia. Careful examination sometimes reveals an increased number of normal-appearing lymphocytes, sometimes in follicles. These lymphocytes exhibit the cold agglutinin as surface Ig.

The DAT usually is strongly positive with antiC3dg but not with antiIgG. Agglutinins are readily demonstrable in the serum. These can sometimes be detected at the bedside, but careful collection of the specimen (maintaining it at 37°C by immersing the tube of blood in warm water until the cells and serum have been separated) and careful analysis are required for reliable diagnosis.

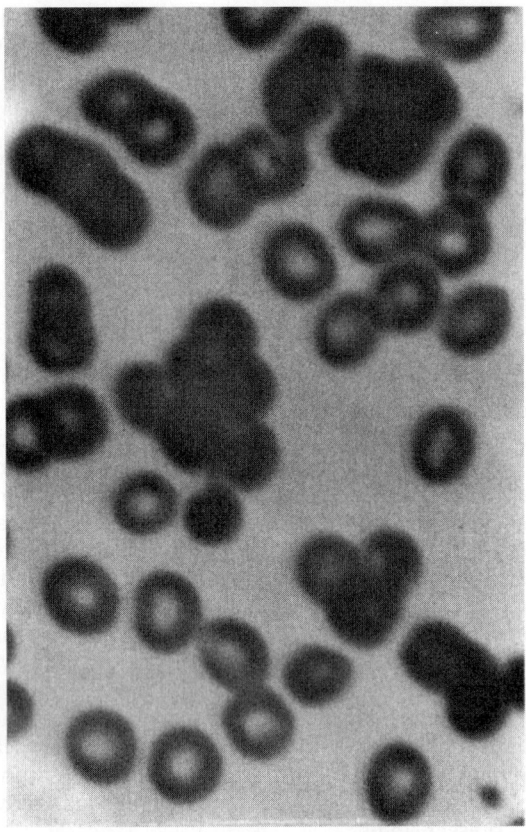

Figure 52-11. Appearance of agglutinated red blood cells on the peripheral blood film in a patient with cold agglutinin disease.

Agglutinin Analysis. Analysis of the agglutinins usually involves three interrelated measures: titer, thermal amplitude or maximum, and specificity. In some instances, the biochemical and immunologic structure of the antibody molecule may be analyzed as well.

Titer. A rough estimate of the concentration of antibody in the serum can be made by determining the degree to which the serum can be diluted and yet cause agglutination. A low titer of cold agglutinin (1/10 or so) is present in the serum of most normal donors. Most patients with *M. pneumoniae* or EBV infection have a titer between 1/40 and 1/1000. In most cases of symptomatic (hemolytic) cold agglutinin disease, the serum can be diluted more than 1/1000 and often to dilutions exceeding 1/20,000. The titer may vary somewhat when cells of different normal donors

are used. For some antibodies, the titer is much greater if albumin is added to the reaction mixture (154); the significance of this is not clear, because it is not apparent that these antibodies are more hemolytic than those that do not show this difference (152,155).

Thermal Maximum. The effectiveness of a cold agglutinin in bringing about hemolysis *in vivo* is determined to a great extent by its thermal maximum; that is, by the highest temperature at which it is able to bind to the antigen on the RBC. The thermal maximum is determined by performing agglutination reactions using the same dilutions of serum and the same RBCs but incubating them at different temperatures. In most cases, there is no agglutination at 37°C. The highest temperature at which agglutination can be distinguished is called the thermal maximum. In rare instances, the thermal maximum may reach 37°C (151). In these cases, the titer of antibody may be low, but the amount of hemolysis may be great.

Specificity. Cold agglutinins react with polysaccharide antigens that are present on the blood cells of all individuals; thus, specificity cannot be defined, as it is for alloantibodies, by the presence or absence of the antigen on the cells of some but not other individuals in the population. Rather, specificity usually is defined by quantitative relationships of reactions on the cells of different donors, by the effect of various biochemical treatments on the antigen, and by the definition of the structure of the antigen. The latter, while most satisfactory, also is the most difficult.

Most cold agglutinins react with polysaccharide antigens that are part of the complex of molecules bearing the major (ABH) blood group antigens. Two principal types are observed:

Anti-I antibodies agglutinate the cells of normal adult donors in higher titer than the cells of newborn infants or rare (genetic i) adults (156).

Anti-i antibodies agglutinate the cells of newborn infants in higher titer than the cells of normal adults (157).

Other specificities are uncommon and depend on the stability or instability of the antigen on enzymatic treatment of the RBCs (Table 52-6) (158–160).

Structure of Antigens. The biochemistry of these antigens is shown in Figure 52-12. The minimal polysaccharide that can be converted to H, A, or B antigen (the lacto ceramide moiety) consists of four sugars reading from the attachment to the ceramide: glucose–galactose–N-acetylglucosamine–galactose; the immunodeterminant sugars for H, A, and B may be attached to the terminal galactose. This backbone can be elongated by the addition of further disaccharide moieties consisting of N-acetylglu-

TABLE 52-6. Classification of the Specificities of Cold Agglutinins

| Specificity | Adult versus Fetal Red Blood Cell | Enzyme Treatment | | Other Comments |
		Proteolytic	Sialidase	
Anti-I	A > F	Enhance	No effect	Structure known
Anti-i	F > A	Enhance	No effect	Structure known
Anti-Pr	A = F	Abolish	Abolish	Has subset variation
Anti-Pr$_a$	A = F	Abolish	No effect	—
Anti-Lud	A > F	Diminish	Abolish	—
Anti-Fl	A > F	No effect	Abolish	Branched polysaccharide complex
Anti-Gd	A = F	No effect	Abolish	On sialic acid bearing ganglioside
Anti-Li	A < F	No effect	Abolish	—
Anti-Vo	A < F	No effect	Abolish	Terminally sialylated i antigen

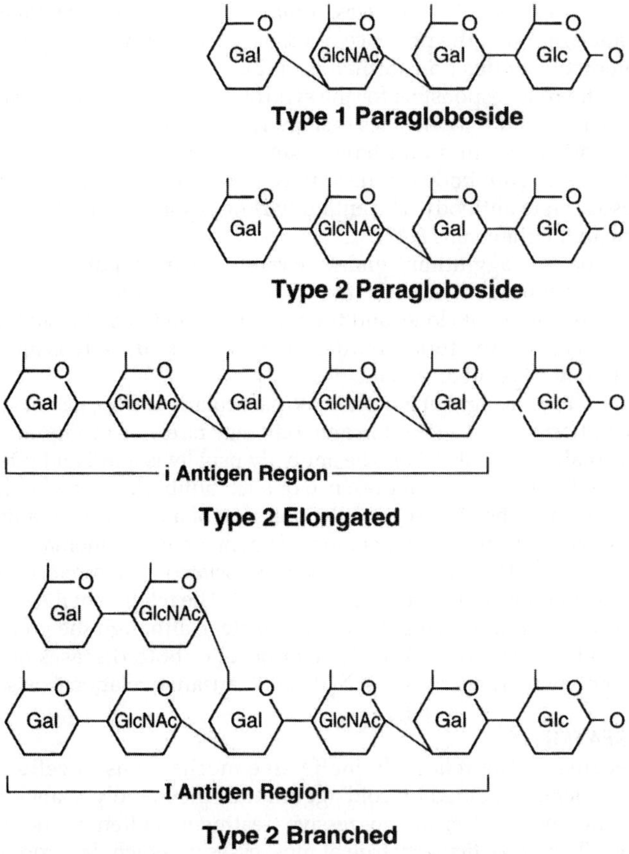

Type 1 Paragloboside

Type 2 Paragloboside

i Antigen Region

Type 2 Elongated

I Antigen Region

Type 2 Branched

Figure 52-12. Structure of the polysaccharide antigens with which cold agglutinins react. The two upper polysaccharides form the basis on which the other members of the group are built. The I and i antigens are the result of further complexity of these molecules. The terminal galactose in all cases can be fucosylated in an α_1 to α_2 linkage to make H substance, and either can be galactosylated (to make B substance) or N-acetylgalactosylated (to make A substance).

cosamine–galactose; the resulting entity reacts with anti-i antibodies (161). After approximately the age 6 months, these disaccharides may be added at two sites on the same galactose molecule, resulting in branching of the structure; the resulting complex polysaccharide reacts with anti-I antibodies (162).

Some cold agglutinins react better with cells that have or do not have the H, A, or B antigens attached to these complexes (163). They are called by a compound epithet in such a case (e.g., anti-AI for such an antibody that reacts like a cold agglutinin but reacts more strongly with A cells from an adult than with B or O cells).

These antigens are located in the interior of the molecule and therefore do not involve sialic acid, which may terminate a polysaccharide chain. Rarely, the reaction with antibody depends on the presence of this moiety; such antibodies are called *anti-Gd* (143), *anti-Lud* (144), and so forth. These antibodies do not react with cells that have been treated with sialidase to remove the sialic acid residues.

Rarely, the antigen with which a cold agglutinin reacts is a polysaccharide that is present only on glycoprotein molecules. Such antigens can be removed by proteolytic cleavage of the glycoprotein by, for instance, trypsin. They are called the *Pr antigens* because they are protein related (164).

Structure of Antibody Molecule. Cold agglutinins can be easily purified by repeated cycles of adsorption in the cold and elution at 37°C; their structure can then be determined (165). They

are nearly always IgM molecules, although some IgG molecules also may be present (166,167); rarely, they may have a monomeric rather than the usual pentameric structure (168). Hexameric molecules occur in variable proportions in different patients; these molecules are more hemolytic than the usual pentameric molecules (169). Rarely, a cold agglutinin may be IgA (170); because IgA molecules do not fix complement, these antibodies cause little hemolysis.

The antibody may result from monoclonal or polyclonal production. If polyclonal, the molecules may be similar, but both types of light chain (κ and λ) are present (171). If monoclonal, all the molecules are identical; this is best seen by showing that a single type of light chain (usually κ) is present (172).

The monoclonal anti-I antibodies are often similar from patient to patient. The light chain usually is κ, and the framework structure usually is $V_\kappa IIIb$ (173). The heavy chain usually has the framework structure designated $V_H I$ (174). Antigens specific for cold agglutinins but common to all of them (idiotopes) usually are expressed in the antigen-combining area of the molecule (175). These similarities in structure are reflected in similarities in amino acid structure of the molecules.

When the monoclonal cold agglutinin has specificity for antigens other than I, these restrictions on structure may not apply (176). The light chain is often λ, and the framework structure of the light and heavy chain may be other than noted for anti-I antibodies.

Other Clinically Important Characteristics of Antigen–Antibody Interaction

INHIBITION BY BOUND C3
Some cold agglutinins react less well with cells that have been coated with complement components, particularly C3 (177–179). This presumably is because the affixed C3 molecules cover the antigen sites and sterically hinder the binding of antibody. Because the cells of the patients usually are covered with C3dg, they may be protected *in vivo* from hemolysis. This property can be tested by determination of agglutination titers with C3-coated cells compared with titers with cells not coated with C3.

FIXATION OF C1
Because complement plays a dominant role in the pathogenesis of hemolysis by these antibodies, variations in the ability to fix complement may determine the degree of hemolysis *in vivo*. Some anti-I antibodies appear to affix to the antigen but not to bind complement (145); thus, they are not highly hemolytic and also may inhibit the binding and hemolysis of other anti-I antibodies. On the other hand, hexameric IgM molecules fix complement more efficiently than the usual pentameric ones (169).

PATHOPHYSIOLOGY
The hemolysis seen in cold agglutinin disease appears to be entirely due to reactions of complement. No Fc receptor for IgM molecules has been reliably reported on phagocytic cells.

Because of the characteristics of antigen-antibody interaction, the fixation of antibody and therefore of complement can occur only as the blood circulates to the periphery and the temperature of the blood drops below the thermal maximum of the antibody. This is more readily attained if the antibody has a high thermal maximum or if the patient is exposed to a colder environment. When this occurs, sufficient antibody is present in the plasma to initiate massively the activation of complement. If sufficient components are affixed to the RBC membrane to overcome the downregulation of the reactions, lysis of the cell by direct insertion of the membrane attack complex occurs. This results in the intravascular release of hemoglobin (180), which if sufficiently severe may result in hemoglobinuria and hemosiderinuria.

If the cells survive this attack on the integrity of the membrane, they may then circulate into the central body where the C3b and C4b on their surface may interact with receptors on phagocytic cells of lung, liver, and spleen (181). The cells bearing these receptors are distributed throughout the reticuloendothelial system, and the circulation of the spleen offers no special advantage in producing cellular destruction. During the circulation, C3b and C4b are enzymatically degraded first to iC3b and iC4b and further to C3dg and C4d (Fig. 52-5) (182). As the molecules are degraded, their ability to induce phagocytosis is reduced, and the remnants of C3 and C4 (C3dg and C4d) that persist on the membrane probably do not interfere with the longevity of the cells (142,146).

ETIOLOGY

Cold agglutinins may arise from two general causes: reaction to infection or lymphoproliferation. These general causes can be distinguished by the fact that the antibodies that result from infection are polyclonal, whereas those that result from lymphoproliferation are monoclonal; as noted, this distinction can be detected from the isotypic homogeneity or heterogeneity of the light chains.

Cold Agglutinins from Infections. Cold agglutinins are detected frequently during the course of two infections: atypical pneumonia due to *M. pneumoniae* (183) and infectious mononucleosis (184,185). The presence of the antibody can be of benefit in making the etiologic diagnoses. In both cases, the titer of antibody usually is not markedly elevated (usually less than 1/1200); thus, the amount of hemolysis is not striking (186,187). The presence of antibody in the serum is limited in time and usually does not last more than 2 to 3 months.

In *M. pneumoniae* infections, the antibody usually is anti-I. It appears approximately 2 weeks after initial symptoms of the infection, like any heteroimmune IgM antibody, and may be a cross-reacting antibody primarily directed at polysaccharide antigens on the organism (188) or at its binding site on the RBC (189).

A similar antibody may arise in some cases of infection by *Listeria monocytogenes* (190). The organism has a polysaccharide structure on its surface that closely resembles the antigen reacting with anti-I, and the antibody apparently cross-reacts with the similar structure on the RBC surface.

In infectious mononucleosis due to the EBV virus, cold agglutinins appear in 50% to 80% of cases. The antibody usually is present in relatively low titer (usually less than 1/1200) and is nearly always IgM anti-i. Some of the antibody may be IgG, although IgM antibody usually is present (166). The antibody is thought to be due to the polyclonal stimulation of the B-cell system by this organism; it appears approximately 2 to 3 weeks after the onset of symptoms and usually is not found until 2 to 3 months later. Antibody sufficient to cause clinically significant hemolysis occurs in less than 1 in 1000 cases (191).

Cold Agglutinins Due to Lymphoproliferative Diseases. Cold agglutinins may result from the monoclonal proliferation of B-cell clones (149). This proliferation may range in degree of malignancy from benign monoclonal gammopathy (in which the proliferation of the clone is controlled in some degree) to malignant lymphoma.

Chronic cold agglutinin syndrome usually is due to benign monoclonal gammopathy and has many of the characteristics of that syndrome (147–149). It occurs in older patients; incidence at age younger than 50 years is distinctly unusual. It usually is not progressive, and patients may have the syndrome for many years. In 10% to 15% of cases, it may evolve into a more malignant condition; the presence of trisomy 3 in the lymphocytes is predictive of this transformation (192).

The cells responsible for the syndrome are benign-appearing plasmacytoid lymphocytes that are rich in discontinuous endoplasmic reticulum and have a small Golgi apparatus. They express the antibody on the surface (see earlier discussion) but also secrete antibody. The antibody is nearly always (90%) anti-I with κ light chains (149).

The cold agglutinin syndrome rarely occurs in patients with chronic lymphocytic leukemia (150). The antibody is produced by the malignant clone, and the titer of antibody can be used as a measure of the tumor burden. The antibody usually is anti-I but may have other specificities.

In more malignant lymphomas (particularly diffuse histiocytic lymphoma), cold agglutinin antibody may rarely be produced by the malignant cells (150). The antibody usually is anti-i and often has λ light chains. The presence of such antibodies may be the first sign of the disease, and the presence of a monoclonal anti-i antibody is nearly pathognomonic of malignant lymphoma.

Rarely, adenocarcinomas may be associated with monoclonal cold agglutinins of anti-I specificity (193). The relation of the antibody to the underlying disease is not clear, although the young age of the patient and the time of onset of both diseases may sometimes strongly suggest that some causative relation exists.

TREATMENT

Because of the relatively ineffective mechanisms of cellular destruction initiated by cold agglutinins, the hemolytic anemia is often not severe, and aggressive treatment is often not necessary. This is particularly true of most cases in which the production of antibody is secondary to an infection. When treatment is indicated, it is directed primarily at avoiding the interaction of the antibody with the RBCs or at reducing the production or the serum concentration of antibody. To date, no practical means of reducing the activation or the effectiveness of complement has been devised.

In most cases, the antibody reacts with the RBC only at temperatures less than core body temperature, so avoiding situations where the temperature of the blood is lowered significantly may reduce both the symptoms of cold agglutinin disease and the hemolysis; many patients have a higher hemoglobin in the summer than in the winter. For many patients, the appropriate blood temperature can be maintained by wearing clothing that maintains the peripheral parts of the body at a sufficiently high temperature; such measures include long woolen underwear, down boots, ear muffs, and gloves even in moderate weather. In some cases, removal to a warm climate is necessary.

The necessity for a warm environment sometimes puts patients in peril in particular circumstances. In particular, surgery may be dangerous unless precautions are taken to prevent cooling during the operation (194,195). Some occupations may not be available to such patients because they involve too much exposure to the cold.

The amount of antibody in the serum can be reduced by plasmapheresis (146,193,194). This is relatively efficient because the antibody is IgM and is thus confined to the intravascular space. Care must be taken during the procedure to be certain that the blood that is to be returned has not been allowed to become cold—hemolysis may result if this occurs. Unfortunately, the production rate of the antibody is such that the titer rapidly returns to the pretreatment level; this limits this procedure to those instances in which a rapid reduction in antibody titer is needed, because most patients cannot tolerate the amount of plasmapheresis that is required to maintain chronically a low antibody titer.

A reduction in the production of antibody may be difficult to achieve. The production of antibody is not affected by the administration of prednisone, and prednisone usually is not effective in any dose; the exception to this is seen in the unusual patient with an antibody of high thermal amplitude (151). In these cases, high doses of prednisone may result in amelioration of the hemolysis, probably due to down-regulation of complement receptors rather than a reduction in antibody.

For the reduction in antibody concentration, cytotoxic agents usually are needed. In more benign conditions, daily or intermittent administration of alkylating agents may be used; no clear advantage is known for the agent or for the schedule of treatment (196,197). For phenylalanine mustard (Alkeran) the dose is 2 to 4 mg/day or 24 to 30 mg every 3 weeks. For cyclophosphamide, the daily dose is 50 to 100 mg, and the intermittent dose is 500 to 700 mg every 3 weeks. Care must be taken that normal hematopoiesis is not suppressed.

When cold agglutinin disease occurs in the setting of the more malignant lymphoproliferative diseases, the treatment is that of the primary disease. The titer of antibody may indicate the degree of response (Fig. 52-13).

Cold agglutinin disease usually occurs in elderly patients who may have somewhat diminished erythropoietic reserve. In several cases, the injection of relatively low doses of erythropoietin (4000 U/week) has raised the hematocrit.

Transfusion. Patients with cold agglutinin syndrome do not often require transfusion. When they do, the presence of the antibody may make blood typing and compatibility testing difficult.

When the cells of patients are tested for the blood group with anti-A and anti-B in the usual way, they are not washed free of the patient's serum. If sufficient serum containing the cold agglutinin is transferred into the tests, the cells agglutinate and appear to be AB in type. The error is readily discovered if the serum is tested for the presence of appropriate alloanti-A or alloanti-B.

As in the case of warm-reacting IgG antibody, the cold agglutinin is likely to react with the cells of all potential donors, and the presence of alloantibodies is difficult to detect. The serum may be absorbed at 4°C with the patient's RBCs; subsequent incubation at 37°C removes the antibody so that the absorption can be repeated. If the antibody is anti-I, it may be removed by rabbit RBC stroma, because these cells bear the I antigen (190).

Confusion with the cold agglutinin also can be diminished by performing all the reactions of compatibility testing at 37°C; most cold agglutinins do not react at that temperature. Further, the tests using antiglobulin may be done using reagents containing antiIgG but not antiC3dg because these detect most significant alloantibodies but do not react with the cold agglutinin autoantibodies.

Hemolytic Anemia Due to Cold-Reacting Immunoglobulin G Antibodies (Paroxysmal Cold Hemoglobinuria)

Paroxysmal cold hemoglobinuria was the first clinical syndrome of AIHA to be definitively described. The primary symptom, hemoglobinuria following exposure to a cold environment—often frightening to the patient and helpful to the physician in making a diagnosis—was first described in England in 1832 in children with congenital lues (syphilis) who had dark urine when the cold east wind blew (1). The diagnostic test devised by Donath and Landsteiner was the first to be applied to the diagnosis of AIHA (3,4).

CLINICAL SYNDROME

Classically, paroxysmal cold hemoglobinuria (PCH) is characterized by the sudden onset of hemoglobinuria after exposure to cold, but many patients may not have this symptom because the concentration of antibody in the serum is insufficient to cause intravascular hemolysis. In other patients, hemoglobinuria may occur without specific exposure to cold if the titer and characteristics of the antibody permit. Thus, the classic symptom is a poor guide to diagnosis in most cases.

Patients with PCH do not exhibit acrocyanosis but may have true Raynaud's phenomenon or other vasomotor phenomena (198). The reason for this is not clear.

Other symptoms of PCH are those of intermittent hemolysis and include jaundice, weakness, pallor, and, if the anemia is sufficient, cardiac decompensation.

The anemia may range in severity from mild to severe; death may intervene in some cases. The reticulocyte response usually is appropriately high, and leukocytosis may be present during hemolytic episodes. Hemoglobinuria may or may not be seen, but hemosiderinuria is nearly always present.

The DAT, as performed, is either negative or positive only with anticomplement reagents (199). The IgG antibody usually is washed off during the preparation of the samples at room temperature but may be detected by some of the more sensitive methods. The diagnosis is made by the demonstration of a cold-reacting IgG antibody in the serum. Agglutination in the standard cold agglutination test usually is weak, and titers over 1/100 are rare.

The D-L bithermic hemolytic test is the classic method of demonstrating the antibodies. In this test, normal RBCs (or, for greater sensitivity, the RBCs of patients with paroxysmal nocturnal hemoglobinuria) are incubated with the patient's serum and a source of complement at 4°C for 30 minutes, then at 37°C for another 30 minutes; if hemolysis occurs in the test sample and does not occur in controls maintained at 37°C for the full time, the test is positive.

The D-L test is somewhat insensitive, however, and in many patients, the cold-reacting IgG antibody can only be demonstrated in the cold indirect Coombs' test in which normal RBCs are mixed with the serum of the patient at 4°C and the binding of IgG antibodies detected by either agglutination by antiIgG or, preferably, by an assay using a labeled monoclonal antiIgG. This technique is able to detect much smaller amounts of D-L antibody than the hemolytic tests (200).

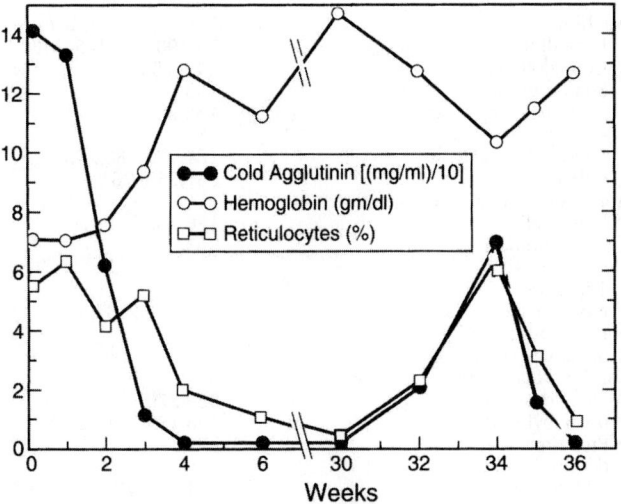

Figure 52-13. Cold agglutinin as tumor marker in a patient with undifferentiated lymphocytic lymphoma. The titer, determined by a quantitative hemolysis assay, closely reflects the activity of the disease.

The determination of the thermal maximum may be important for the same reasons given for its determination for cold agglutinins (201). This is done by varying the temperature at which the first (cold) phase of the test is conducted.

The antibody usually reacts with the P antigen, a polysaccharide antigen present on the RBCs of nearly all individuals (202,203). Occasionally, the specificity is for other polysaccharide or polysaccharide-dependent antigens (204,205). Although there is much discussion about what should be called a D-L antibody, the most logical and pragmatic definition is an IgG antibody that is cold reacting.

PATHOPHYSIOLOGY

Hemolysis in PCH is effected for the most part by direct lysis by complement when the circulating blood is exposed to temperature sufficiently decreased to allow interaction of the antibody with the cell and the fixation of complement. Direct intravascular lysis is often more evident in this disorder than in cold agglutinin disease, but the reason is not entirely known. There is some evidence that the fixation of the first component of complement is more efficient because agglutination, which interferes with the binding of this component, does not occur (51). Because the antibody is IgG, immune adherence by antibody may play a role if the thermal maximum of the antibody is sufficiently high so that some remains on the surface of the RBC when the blood circulates to the warmer interior of the body where Fc receptors are located.

ETIOLOGY

The antibodies characteristic of PCH arise in three clinical settings. They were identified first in patients with advanced syphilis, usually tertiary or congenital. It is thought that, in this infection, the antibody arises in response to P-like antigens on the spirochete and cross-reacts with the P antigen of the RBC. Regardless, the syndrome disappears when the infection is cured.

PCH occurs frequently following a viral illness (206,207) or inoculation (208); a number of viruses have been implicated, most frequently the childhood exanthems. This reaction occurs most frequently in childhood (usually less than 5 years of age) where it may be the most common form of AIHA (206). Rarely, the postviral reaction may be seen also in adults. The anemia may be severe, but the syndrome resolves over 3 to 6 weeks even without specific treatment, although multiple blood transfusions are often needed.

PCH can occur also as an autoimmune disease with or without other manifestations of immune dysfunction (209,210). This form follows the age distribution of other IgG AIHAs. The course usually is chronic, and the degree of anemia is variable; specific treatment is often necessary.

TREATMENT

The treatment of PCH depends somewhat on its cause. If it is due to syphilis (rarely the case nowadays), that infection should be treated with penicillin. If it is due to viral infections, any treatment is limited in time because of the transient nature of the syndrome.

As in the case of the syndromes due to cold agglutinins, avoidance of the cold can be effective in ameliorating the milder forms of PCH. For many patients, however, this is insufficient, and other treatment must be instituted.

The general treatment of PCH is much like that of the syndromes due to warm-reacting IgG (see earlier discussion) with certain exceptions. Prednisone is often effective in reducing the amount of antibody and, if it is unable to do so, cytotoxic agents may be used. Splenectomy and intravenous γ-globulin probably

do not have a place in the treatment of PCH unless the antibody has an extremely high thermal maximum.

Transfusion may be necessary, and crossmatch may be complicated by the presence of the antibody to a virtually universal antigen; the problem of identifying alloantibodies may be minimized by performing the compatibility testing at 37°C. The rare donors lacking the P antigen may be found, and their blood may be used if it is available (211). If not, incompatible blood may be given with safety and effectiveness (212).

Drug-Induced Autoimmune Hemolytic Anemia

Harris and his colleagues (213,214) first recognized that drugs may be able to induce the production of antibodies that are then capable of destroying the circulating RBCs, and since that time, the phenomenon has been ascribed to a bewildering number of drugs (Table 52-7) (215,216).

Two distinct syndromes are described depending on whether the drug is part of the antigen.

DRUG AS ANTIGEN

Many chemical compounds, including drugs, may act as haptenes; that is, they bind to a carrier, and an antibody is formed to the combination. In this case, the drug is an important part of the antigenic configuration. Classically, a haptene is bound securely to the carrier and alone should be able to react with the antibody and inhibit its interaction with the haptene-carrier combination (217); this may not be true for drugs causing immune hemolytic anemia. It is clear, however, that in most instances, drug-induced immune hemolytic anemia is due to a haptene mechanism.

Clinical Syndrome. For most drugs causing haptene-induced immune hemolytic anemia, the onset of the clinical syndrome usually is fairly abrupt with the rapid onset of anemia (198,216). In some instances, hemoglobinemia with resultant hemoglobinuria and hemosiderinuria may be seen; renal

TABLE 52-7. Drugs Known to Have Caused Immune Hemolytic Anemia

Drug	References
Quinine or quinidine	203,241–245
Antibiotics	
Penicillins	39,190,191,246–248
Cephalothins	249–254
Sulfa drugs	255
p-Aminosalicylic acid	186,256
Rifampicin	257
Stibophen	181,182,188,258
Other	257,259–261
Analgesics and antirheumatics	
Phenacetin	186,262
Nonsteroidals	263
Neuroleptics	
Tricyclics	264
Nomifensine	187,196,265–267
Phenothiazines	268
Sedatives	236
Cardiovascular drugs	
Thiazides	269,270
α-Methyldopa	198,199,201,202,271
Procainamide	272
Endocrinologic drugs	
Sulfonylureas	194,273–275
Other drugs	
Methotrexate	276
Probenecid	277,278

failure due to the hemoglobinuria is not uncommon (218–221). The onset may be so sudden that the reticulocyte count does not have time to rise. The sudden onset may lead to symptoms of hypoxia, especially in older patients, because some of the compensatory mechanisms for the anemia may not have time to occur.

This complication of drug therapy is often seen shortly after the drug is first given to the patient; conversely, it may occur months to years after the initiation of therapy. Often, only small doses of drug are sufficient to cause the hemolysis, although this varies with the drug.

In other instances, particularly when the drug is penicillin or a drug related to it, the onset usually is less abrupt and the anemia is less severe (215,222,223). This syndrome usually occurs only when very large doses of penicillin (in excess of 10,000,000 IU/day) are administered; the onset of anemia usually is 5 to 10 days after the initiation of therapy. Hemoglobinuria and renal failure are rare but may occur when complement is fixed (see later discussion) (224).

If the cause is identified, the symptoms usually abate rapidly when the drug is discontinued. In some instances, the antibody appears to be made to an intrinsic structure of the RBC, and hemolysis may last for several weeks in such cases. Nevertheless, the syndrome resolves when the drug is no longer taken.

The antibody usually disappears within a few weeks after the drug is discontinued. If the drug is again administered before this happens, hemolysis may be rapid (within minutes). If the drug is administered after antibody has disappeared, there may be a delay before hemolysis occurs while an anamnestic immune response is mounted. In some instances, reexposure does not cause a recurrence of the syndrome.

Diagnosis. The DAT usually is positive only with anticomplement antisera even though the antibody usually is IgG. This is because the haptene is not sufficiently adherent to the RBC to resist removal during the washing procedure in preparation for the performance of the test. Penicillin and related drugs are exceptional in that they are firmly bound to the membrane of the cell, but the interaction with antibody usually does not fix complement; thus, the DAT usually is positive with antiIgG and negative with antiC3.

The diagnosis of drug-induced immune hemolytic anemia is made by the demonstration that the antibody reacts with RBCs in the presence of the drug but does not react with RBCs in the absence of the drug. Usually, the serum of the patient is mixed with normal RBCs, and the drug is added. The occurrence of an interaction is affirmed by agglutination or by the fixation of complement, which either results in lysis of the RBCs or the presence of complement components on the membrane of the test cells. The sensitivity of those tests that are dependent on lysis by complement can be increased by using the cells of patients with paroxysmal nocturnal hemoglobinuria or normal cells that have been treated to be more sensitive to the lytic action of complement (225). The test is controlled by the omission of the drug; when this is done, the reaction does not occur.

In testing for antibodies to penicillin, normal RBCs are coated with the drug at a high pH (226); after being washed, they are then reacted with the patient's serum, washed again, and tested with antiIgG. This procedure affixes the drug to the membrane, and the attachment lasts through several washings.

These tests can be used to determine the fine specificity of the antibody. Congeners of the drug may be used to determine the cross-reactivity of the antibody. Rare cells lacking certain

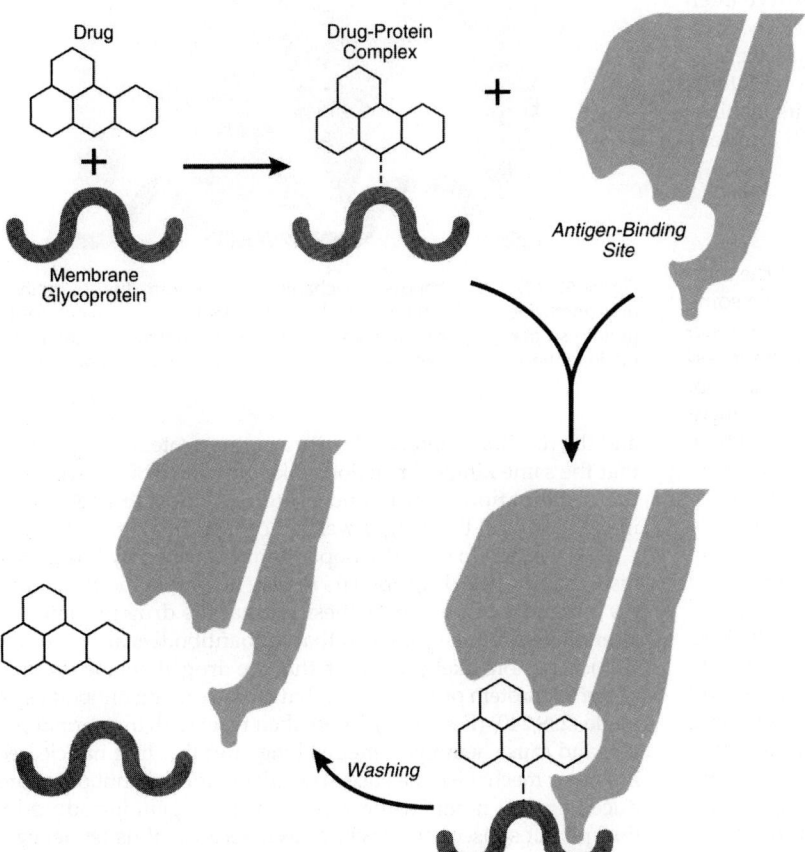

Figure 52-14. Binding of antibody to a drug as a haptene. The drug combines with a surface-membrane glycoprotein and is able to stimulate the formation of an antibody. The antibody that is formed reacts with both the drug and, to a lesser extent, the membrane. If the drug is removed, the antibody does not remain bound.

surface proteins (e.g., K_0, Lu a[-]b[-]) may not sustain the reaction, indicating that the attachment site of the drug is related to the missing antigenic protein (194,227–229).

The test may be negative even though the immune hemolytic anemia is drug-related. The antibody may be to a metabolite of the drug; if the metabolites are known, they may be used in the test (230). If not, the urine of a patient who has ingested the drug may be used to provide the metabolite. The reaction may occur in the absence of the drug even though the drug caused the syndrome (see When Drug Is Not Antigen). For these and probably other reasons, a negative test for the specificity of drug-induced immune hemolytic anemia does not mean that the syndrome was not induced by the drug.

WHEN DRUG IS NOT ANTIGEN

In 1965, Carstairs and associates (231,232) reported that many (approximately 15%) patients taking the drug α-methyldopa (Aldomet) for hypertension developed a positive DAT; of these, approximately 10% (1.5% of the total) developed hemolytic anemia. The syndrome occurred more frequently in patients taking high doses (more than 1 g/day) and often did not supervene for several months after the initiation of therapy.

Most patients with positive DATs do not have evidence of hemolysis. With higher titers of antibody (determined by the strength of the DAT or IAT), hemolysis may occur but is seldom severe. Spherocytosis is present in these cases, and the spleen may be enlarged. The reticulocytosis is commensurate with the degree of anemia.

The syndrome usually lasts 4 to 8 weeks after discontinuation of the drug. The degree of hemolysis, when present, gradually diminishes. The DAT gradually weakens and finally disappears.

The DAT is positive with antiIgG but usually not with antiC3, unlike the tests in most cases of drug-induced immune hemolytic anemia. Although the drug is clearly implicated in the pathogenesis of the syndrome, the IAT is positive even though the drug is omitted from the reaction. In fact, the antibody in most cases reacts with all RBCs except Rh_{null} cells, suggesting that the antibody reacts with the protein or proteins bearing the Rh antigens (233,234); this accounts for its inability to fix complement, because antibodies against Rh antigens almost never do so.

ETIOLOGY OF DRUG-INDUCED AUTOIMMUNE HEMOLYTIC ANEMIA

By definition, the drug is involved in the formation of the antibody. It was first assumed that it acted as a haptene, using some component of the RBC membrane as the carrier, but the reactions did not appear to correspond to those classically described for haptenes. The drug and the antibody in most cases did not appear to be bound to the membrane of the RBC. Further, incubation of the drug and the antibody did not inhibit the ability of the antibody to react with the RBC under appropriate circumstances (235). For these reasons, it was proposed that the drug reacted with some protein in the plasma, and that the antibody was directed against that complex. This reaction, occurring in the presence of RBCs, resulted in the fixation of complement on the RBC surface. Thus, the RBC was an innocent bystander.

Evidence has accumulated, however, to suggest that the RBC is not so innocent as was thought. In some instances, cells lacking certain membrane proteins or possessing certain blood group antigens do not react with drug and antibody, suggesting that such proteins are necessary for the interaction to occur (236). Further, in the analogous syndrome, drug-induced immune thrombocytopenia, the drug forms a neoantigen with glycoproteins of the platelet membrane (237). Both the drug and the glycoprotein are essential for interaction with the antibody,

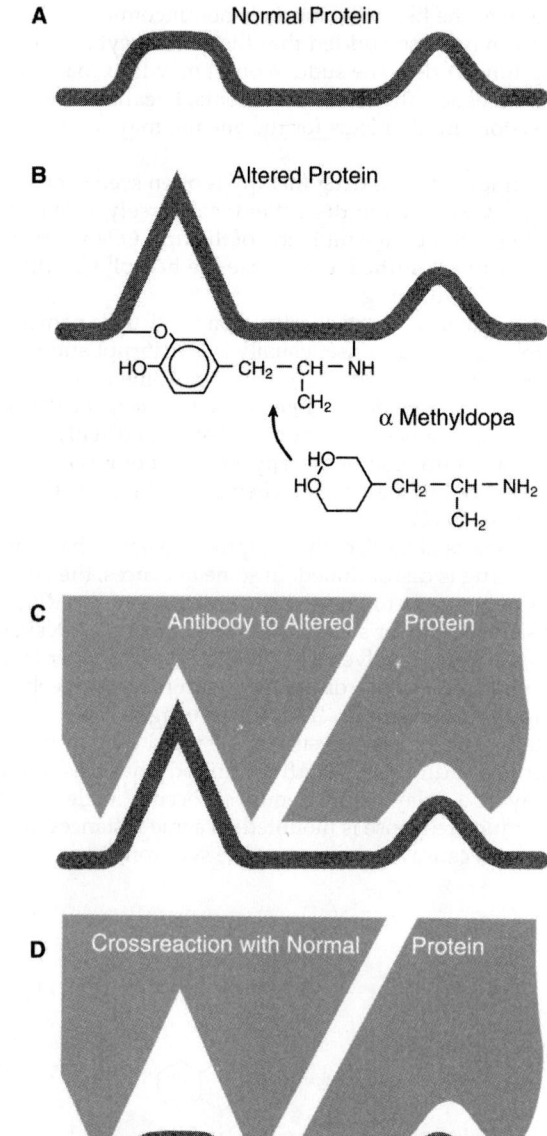

Figure 52-15. A–D: Proposed mechanism for the formation of antibody by α-methyldopa. This bifunctional agent alters the conformation of the protein so that it appears foreign to the immune system. An antibody is made to the altered protein that cross-reacts with the normal protein.

and the reaction stabilizes the drug on the protein. It is probable that the same kinds of reactions take place on RBCs, except that the combination of drug and protein is not stabilized by the interaction, and the drug is washed off readily (Fig. 52-14).

The reaction to α-methyldopa is not explained by this mechanism, because the drug appears to play no part in the structure of the antigen (224). It is hypothesized that the drug in some way alters the immune system so that autoantibodies are produced (238). It is more likely, however, that the drug alters the structure of the Rh protein or proteins so that cross-reacting antibodies are made (239,240) (Fig. 52-15). These then react with the normal protein and cause hemolytic anemia long after the drug has cleared. A similar mechanism has been postulated for the antibodies produced against nomifensine, a psycholeptic agent introduced in Europe but subsequently withdrawn because of its tendency to cause immune hemolytic anemia (229,230).

TREATMENT

In general, the first thing to be done once drug-induced hemolytic anemia has been identified is to withdraw the drug. In most cases, this results in a fairly rapid resolution of the hemolytic process; the time required depends on the rate of clearance of the drug and the degree to which the antibody reacts with the cell in the absence of the drug. In the latter case, hemolysis persists as long as the antibody is produced, whether or not the drug is present—as occurs with α-methyldopa.

If hemolysis is severe, supportive transfusion may be required. There usually is little problem with the compatibility testing because the drug is not present. This is, of course, not true in cases where the antibody reacts with the membrane in the absence of the drug.

In instances where severe hemolytic anemia occurs after the ingestion of α-methyldopa, further treatment may be necessary. This should consist of the use of prednisone in the manner indicated earlier for warm-reacting IgG antibodies. Such use is not necessary for long periods, because the reaction usually subsides within 3 to 4 months.

The patient should be advised to avoid the causative drug and any analogous drugs that might cross-react. If antibody is still present, a rapid hemolytic reaction may occur. If the antibody has disappeared, an anamnestic reaction may occur, and severe hemolysis may result.

REFERENCES

1. Elliotson J. Diseases of the heart united with ague. *Lancet* 1832;1:500.
2. Hassall AH. On intermittent, or winter, haematuria. *Lancet* 1865;2:368.
3. Donath J, Landsteiner K. Uber paroxysmale Hameglobinurie. *Munch Med Wochenschr* 1904;51:1590.
4. Donath J, Landsteiner K. Uber paroxysmale Hamoglobinurie. *Z Klin Med* 1906;58:173.
5. Goltz D. Das Donath-Landsteiner Hamolysin: die Entstehung eines Mythos in der Medizin des 20 Jahrhunderts. *Clio Med* 1982;16:193.
6. Ehrlich P, Morgenroth J. Uber Haemolysine: zweite Mittheilung. *Berl Klin Wochenschr* 1899;36:481.
7. Coombs RRA, Mourant AE, Race RR. A new test for the detection of weak and 'incomplete' Rh agglutinins. *Br J Exp Pathol* 1945;26:255.
8. Boorman KE, Dodd BE, Loutit JF. Haemolytic icterus (acholuric jaundice) congenital and acquired. *Lancet* 1946;1:812.
9. Loutit JF, Mollison PL. Hemolytic icterus (acholuric jaundice), congenital and acquired. *J Pathol Bact* 1946;58:711.
10. Dacie JV. Acquired hemolytic anemia: with special reference to the antiglobulin (Coombs) test. *Blood* 1953;8:813.
11. Landsteiner K. Uber Agglutinlnetionserscheinungen normalen menschlichen Blutes. *Wein Klin Wochenschr* 1901;14:1132.
12. Widal F, Abrami P, Brule M. Retrocession des symptomes cliniques at des troubles hematiques au cours des icteres hemolytiques acquis. *Bull Soc Med Paris* 1909;28:73.
13. Dameshek W, Schwartz SO. The presence of hemolysins in acute hemolytic anemia: preliminary note. *N Engl J Med* 1938;218:75.
14. Jeske DJ, Capra JD. Immunoglobulins: structure and function. In: Paul WE, ed. *Fundamental immunology*. New York: Raven Press, 1984:131.
15. Davies DR, Metzger H. Structural basis of antibody function. *Annu Rev Immunol* 1983;1:87.
16. Wu TT, Kabat EA. An analysis of the sequences of the variable regions of Bence Jones proteins and myeloma light chains and their implications for antibody complementarity. *J Exp Med* 132:211.1970.
17. Anderson CL, Looney RJ. Human leukocyte IgG Fc receptors. *Immunol Today* 1986;7:264.
18. Fleit HB, Wright SD, Unkeless JC. Human neutrophil Fcγ receptor distribution and structure. *Proc Natl Acad Sci U S A* 1982;79:3275.
19. Clark DA, Dessypris EN, Jenkins DE Jr, et al. Acquired immune hemolytic anemia associated with IgA erythrocyte coating: investigation of hemolytic mechanisms. *Blood* 1984;64:1000.
20. Gauldie J, Richards C, Lamontagne L. Fc receptors for IgA and other immunoglobulin on resident and activated alveolar macrophages. *Mol Immunol* 1983;20:1029.
21. Rosse WF, de Boisfleury A, Bessis M. The interaction of phagocytic cells and red cells modified by immune reactions. *Blood Cells* 1975;1:345.
22. Mantovani B, Rabinovitch M, Nussenzweig V. Phagocytosis of immune complexes by macrophages: different roles of the macrophage receptor sites for complement (C3) and for immunoglobulin (IgG). *J Exp Med* 1972;135:780.
23. Brunhouse R, Cebra JJ. Isotypes of IgG: comparison of the primary structures of three pairs of isotypes which differ in their ability to activate complement. *Mol Immunol* 1979;16:907.
24. Yasmeen D, Ellerson JR, Dorrington KJ, et al. The structure and function of immunoglobulin domains: IV. the distribution of some effector functions among the $C_{gamma}2$ and $C_{gamma}3$ homology regions of human immunoglobulin G. *J Immunol* 1976;116:518.
25. Augener W, Grey HM, Cooper N, et al. The reaction of monomeric and aggregated immunoglobulins with C1. *Immunochemistry* 1971;8:1011.
26. Isenman DE, Dorrington KJ, Painter RH. The structure and function of immunoglobulin domains: II. the importance of interchain disulfide bonds and the possible role of molecular flexibility in the interaction between immunoglobulin G and complement. *J Immunol* 1975;114:1726.
27. Schumaker VN, Calcott MA, Spiegelberg HL, et al. Ultracentrifuge studies of the binding of IgG of different subclasses to the C1q subunit of the first component of complement. *Biochemistry* 1978;15:5175.
28. Bubb MO, Conradie JD. The importance of quaternary structure in the expression of the C1-binding site of IgM. *Immunology* 1976;31:893.
29. Feinstein A, Richardson NE, Gorick BD, et al. Immunoglobulin M conformational change is a signal for complement activation. In: Celada F, Shumaker VN, Sercarz EE, eds. *Protein conformation as an immunological signal*. New York: Plenum Press, 1983:47.
30. Borsos T, Rapp HJ. Complement fixation of cell surfaces by 19S and 7S antibodies. *Science* 1965;150:505.
31. Svehag SE, Bloth B. The ultrastructure of human C1q. *Acta Pathol Microbiol Scand [B]* 1970;78:260.
32. Rosse WF. The fixation of the first component of complement (C'1a) by human antibodies. *J Clin Invest* 1968;47:2430.
33. Muller-Eberhard HJ. The membrane attack complex. *Semin Immunopathol* 1984;7:93.
34. Rosse WF, Logue GL, Adams J, et al. Mechanisms of immune lysis of the red cells in hereditary erythroblastic multinuclearity with a positive acidified serum test and paroxysmal nocturnal hemoglobinuria. *J Clin Invest* 1974;53:31.
35. Ross GD, Medof ME. Membrane complement receptors specific for bound fragments of C3. *Adv Immunol* 1985;37:217.
36. Ross GD, Lambris JD, Cain JA, et al. Generation of three different fragments of bound C3 with purified factor I or serum: I. requirements for factor H vs CR1 cofactor activity. *J Immunol* 1982;129:2051.
37. Rosse WF. Detection of antigen-antibody interaction: precipitation, agglutination, and aggregation. In: *Clinical hematology: basic concepts and clinical applications*. New York: Blackwell, 1990:291.
38. Pollack W, Hager HJ, Recker R, et al. A study of the forces involved in the second stage of hemagglutination. *Transfusion* 1965;5:158.
39. Bernstein F, Castenada AR. Alteration in erythrocyte electrical charge associated with mannitol, polyvinylpyrrolidone (PVP), dextrose and various dextran compounds. In: *Biophysical mechanisms in vascular homeostasis and intravascular thrombosis*. New York: Appleton-Century-Crofts, 1969:103.
40. Jones GE. Intercellular adhesion: modification by dielectric properties of the medium. *J Membr Biol* 1974;16:297.
41. Goding JW. Use of staphylococcal protein A as an immunological reagent. *J Immunol Methods* 1978;20:241.
42. Engelfreit CP, von dem Borne AEGK, Beckers D, et al. Autoimmune haemolytic anaemia: serological and immunological characteristics of the autoantibodies: mechanism of cells destruction. *Ser Haematol* 1974;7:328.
43. Dupuy ME, Elliot M, Masouredis SP. Relationship between red cell bound antibody and agglutination in the antiglobulin reaction. *Vox Sang* 1964;9:40.
44. Merry AH, Thomson EE, Rawlinson V, et al. The quantification of C3 fragments on normal cells, acquired hemolytic anemia cases and correlation with agglutination of sensitized cells. *Clin Lab Haematol* 1983;5:387.
45. Merry AH, Thomson EE, Rawlinson VI, et al. A quantitative antiglobulin test for IgG for use in blood transfusion serology. *Clin Lab Haematol* 1982;4:393.
46. Chaplin H Jr, Monroe MC. Comparisons of pooled polyclonal rabbit anti-human C3d with four monoclonal mouse anti-human C3ds. 1. Quantification of RBC-bound C3d and characterization of antiglobulin agglutination reactions against RBCs from 27 patients with autoimmune hemolytic anemia. *Vox Sang* 1986;50:87.
47. Leikola J, Perkins HA. Enzyme-linked antiglobulin test: an accurate and simple method to quantify red cell antibodies. *Transfusion* 1980;20:138.
48. Meulen FW van der, de Bruin HG, Goosen PCM, et al. Quantitative aspects of the destruction of red cells sensitized with IgG_1 autoantibodies: an application of flow cytofluorometry. *Br J Haematol* 1980;46:47.
49. Muller-Eberhard HJ. The membrane attack complex. *Semin Immunopathol* 1984;7:93.
50. Sirchia G, Dacie JV. Immune lysis of AET-treated normal red cells (PNH-like cells). *Nature* 1967;215:747.
51. Rosse WF, Adams J, Logue G. Hemolysis by complement and cold-reacting antibodies: time and temperature requirements. *Am J Hematol* 1977;2:259.
52. Allgood JW, Chaplin H Jr. Idiopathic acquired autoimmune hemolytic anemia. *Am J Med* 1969;43:254.
53. Dacie JV, Worlledge SM. Auto-immune hemolytic anemias. *Prog Hematol* 1969;6:82.
54. Pirofsky B. Clinical aspects of autoimmune hemolytic anemia. *Semin Hematol* 1976;13:251.
55. Habibi B, Homberg JC, Schaison G, et al. Autoimmune hemolytic anemia in children: a review of 80 cases. *Am J Med* 1974;56:61.

56. Zuelzer WW, Mastrangelo R, Stulberg CS. Autoimmune hemolytic anemia: natural history and viral immunologic interactions in childhood. *Am J Med* 1969;49:80.

57. Horwitz CA, Skradski K, Reece E, et al. Haemolytic anaemia in previously healthy adult patients with CMV infections: report of two cases and an evaluation of subclinical haemolysis in CMV mononucleosis. *Scand J Haematol* 1984;33:335.

58. Evans RS, Duane RT. Acquired hemolytic anemia: I. the relation of erythrocyte antibody to activity of the disease: II. the significance of thrombocytopenia and leukopenia. *Blood* 1949;4:1196.

59. Weiss GB, Bessman JD. Spurious automated red cell values in warm autoimmune hemolytic anemia. *Am J Hematol* 1984;17:433.

60. Young NS, Mortimer PP, Moore JG, et al. Characterization of a virus that causes transient aplastic crisis. *J Clin Invest* 1984;73:224.

61. Crosby WH, Rappaport H. Reticulocytopenia in autoimmune hemolytic anemia. *Blood* 1956;11:929.

62. de Boisfleury A. Forme et deformabilite des erythrocytes au cours de l'anemie hemolytique experimentale au rat: etude de leur comportement dans la micro-circulation splenique. (Thesis) d'Univeriste es-Sciences, Faculte des Sciences de Paris, 1977.

63. Dacie JV. The haemolytic anaemias: congenital and acquired. In: *The autoimmune haemolytic anaemias, part II*. New York: Grune & Stratton, 1962:341.

64. Dausset J, Colombani J. The serology and the prognosis of 128 cases of autoimmune hemolytic anemia. *Blood* 1959;14:1280.

65. Crosby WH, Rappaport H. Autoimmune hemolytic anemias: I. analysis of hematologic observations with particular reference to their prognostic value: a survey of 57 cases. *Blood* 1957;12:42.

66. Chanarin I, Dacie JV, Mollin DL. Folic-acid deficiency in haemolytic anaemia. *Br J Haematol* 1959;5:245.

67. Engelfriet CP, von dem Borne AEGK, Beckers Do, et al. Autoimmune haemolytic anaemia: serological and immunological characteristics of the autoantibodies: mechanisms of cell destruction. *Ser Haematol* 1974;7:328.

68. Rosse WF. Quantitative immunology of immune hemolytic anemia: II. the relationship of cell-bound antibody to hemolysis and the effect of treatment. *J Clin Invest* 1971;50:734.

69. Issitt PD. Serological diagnosis and characterization of the causative autoantibodies. In: Chaplin H Jr, ed. *Methods in hematology: immune hemolytic anemias*. New York: Churchill Livingstone, 1985:1.

70. Vos GH, Petz LD, Fudenberg HH. Specificity and immunoglobulin characteristics of autoantibodies in acquired hemolytic anemia. *J Immunol* 1971; 106:1172.

71. Issitt PD. Some messages received from blood group antibodies. In: Red cell antigens and antibodies. American Association of Blood Banks, 1986.

72. Issitt PD, Pavone BG. Critical re-examination of the specificity of auto-anti-Rh antibodies in patients with a positive direct antiglobulin test. *Br J Haematol* 1978;38:63.

73. Weiner W, Vos GH. Serology of acquired hemolytic anemias. *Blood* 1963;22:606.

74. Marsh WL, Reid ME, Scott EP. Autoantibodies of U blood group specificity in autoimmune haemolytic anemia. *Br J Haematol* 1975;29:247.

75. Issitt PD, Pavone BG, Wagstaff W, et al. The phenotypes En(a-), Wr(a-b-) and En(a+), Wr (a+b-), and further studies on the Wright and En blood group systems. *Transfusion* 1976;16:396.

76. Goldfinger D, Zwicker H, Belkin GA, et al. An autoantibody with anti-Wr^b specificity in a patient with warm autoimmune hemolytic anemia. *Transfusion* 1975;15:351.

77. Telen MJ, Chasis J. Relationship of the human erythrocyte Wr^b antigen to an interaction between glycophorin A and band 3. *Blood* 1990;76:842.

78. Kurlander RJ, Rosse WF, Logue GL. Quantitative influence of antibody and complement coating of red cells on monocyte-mediated cell lysis. *J Clin Invest* 1978;61:1309.

79. Lewis SM, Szur L, Dacie JV. The pattern of erythrocyte destruction in haemolytic anaemia, as studied with radioactive chromium. *Br J Haematol* 1960;6:122.

80. LoBuglio AF, Cotran RS, Jandl JH. Red cells coated with immunoglobulin G: binding and sphering by mononuclear cells in man. *Science* 1967;158:1582.

81. Weed RI. The importance of red cell deformability. *Am J Med* 1966;49:147.

82. Chen L-T, Weiss L. The role of the sinus wall in the passage of erythrocytes through the spleen. *Blood* 1973;41:529.

83. Ehrlich P. *Collected studies in immunity*. New York: John Wiley, 1905.

84. Coutinho A. Beyond clonal selection and network. *Immunol Rev* 1989;110:63.

85. Rossi F, Dietrich G, Kazatchkine MD. Anti-idiotypes against autoantibodies in normal immunoglobulins: evidence for network regulation of human autoimmune responses. *Immunol Rev* 1989;110:135.

86. Rosse WF. Autoimmune disease due to warm-reacting antibodies: immune hemolytic anemia. In: *Clinical hematology: basic concepts and clinical applications*. New York: Blackwell, 1990:449.

87. Telen MJ, Roberts KB, Bartlett JA. HIV-associated autoimmune hemolytic anemia: report of a case and review of the literature. *J AIDS* 1990;3:933.

88. Einzig MJ, Neerhout RC. Hemolytic anemia in infectious mononucleosis. *Clin Pediatr* 1969;8:171.

89. Horwitz CA, Skradski K, Reece E, et al. Haemolytic anaemia in previously healthy adult patients with CMV infections: report of two cases and an evaluation of subclinical haemolysis in CMV mononucleosis. *Scand J Haematol* 1984;333:35.

90. Dacie JV, Worlledge SM. Auto-immune hemolytic anemias. *Prog Hematol* 1969;6:82.

91. Videbaek A. Auto-immune haemolytic anaemia in systemic lupus erythematosus. *Acta Med Scand* 1962;171:187.

92. MacKenzie MR, Creevy N. Hemolytic anemia with cold detectable IgG antibodies. *Blood* 1970;36:549.

93. Boling EP, Wen J, Reveille JD, et al. Primary Sjogren's syndrome and autoimmune hemolytic anemia in sisters: a family study. *Am J Med* 1983;74:1066.

94. Dameshek W, Rosenthal MC. Treatment of acquired hemolytic anemia with a note on the relationship of periarteritis nodosa to hemolytic anemia. *Med Clin North Am* 1951;35:1423.

95. Jones E, Jones JV, Woodbury JP, et al. Scleroderma and hemolytic anemia in a patient with deficiency of IgA and C4: a hitherto undescribed association. *J Rheumatol* 1987;14:609.

96. Ashby GH, Evans DI. Cartilage hair hypoplasia with thrombocytopenic purpura, autoimmune haemolytic anaemia and cell-mediated immunodeficiency. *J R Soc Med* 1986;79:113.

97. Hinz CF, Boyer JT. Dysgammaglobulinemia in the adult manifested as autoimmune hemolytic anemia. *N Engl J Med* 1963;269:1329.

98. Conley ME, Park L, Douglas SD. Childhood common variable immunodeficiency with autoimmune disease. *J Pediatr* 1986;108:915.

99. Hansen OP, Sorensen CH, Astrup L. Evans' syndrome in IgA deficiency: episodic autoimmune hemolytic anemia and thrombocytopenia during a year's observation period. *Scand J Haematol* 1982;29:265.

100. Sneller MC, Wang J, Dale JK, et al. Clinical, immunological and genetic features of an autoimmune lymphoproliferative syndrome associated with abnormal lymphocyte apoptosis. *Blood* 1997;89:1341.

101. Kyle RA, Kiely HJM, Stickney JM. Acquired hemolytic anemia in chronic lymphocytic leukemia and the lymphomas: survival and response to therapy in twenty-seven cases. *Arch Intern Med* 1959;4:61.

102. Majumdar G, Brown S, Slater NG et al. Clinical spectrum of autoimmune haemolytic anaemia in patients with chronic lymphocytic leukaemia. *Leuk Lymphoma* 1993;9:149.

103. Gonzalez H, Leblond V, Azar N, et al. Severe autoimmune hemolytic anemia in eight patients treated with fludarabine. *Hematol Cell Ther* 1998;40:113.

104. Myint, H, Copplestone JA, Orchard J, et al. Fludarabine-related autoimmune haemolytic anaemia in patients with chronic lymphocytic leukaemia. *Br J Haematol* 1995;91:341.

105. Eisner E, Ley MAB, Mayer K. Coombs'-positive hemolytic anemia in Hodgkin's disease. *Ann Intern Med* 1967;66:258.

106. Weitberg AB, Harmon DC. Autoimmune neutropenia, hemolytic anemia, and reticulocytopenia in Hodgkin's disease. *Ann Intern Med* 1984;100:702.

107. Halperin IC, Ninogue WF, Komninos ZD. Autoimmune hemolytic anemia and myasthenia gravis associated with thymoma. *N Engl J Med* 1966;275:663.

108. Mongan ES, Kern WA, Terry R. Hypogammaglobulinemia with thymoma, hemolytic anemia, and disseminated infection with cytomegalovirus. *Ann Intern Med* 1966;65:548.

109. Freedman J, Cheng LF, Murray D, et al. An unusual autoimmune hemolytic anemia in a patient with immunoblastic sarcoma. *Am J Hematol* 1983;14:175.

110. White S, Marsden JR, Marks JM, Proctor S. Autoimmune haemolytic anaemia occurring in a patient with mycosis fungoides. *Br J Dermatol* 1984;110:495.

111. Sallah S, Smith SV, Lony LC, et al. Gamma/delta T-cell hepatosplenic lymphoma: review of the literature, diagnosis by flow cytometry and concomitant autoimmune haemolytic anemia. *Ann Hematol* 1997;74:139.

112. Bakemeier RF, Leddy JP. Heavy:light chain relationships among erythrocyte autoantibodies. *J Clin Invest* 1967;46:1033.

113. Chen FE, Owen I, Savage D, et al. Late onset haemolysis and red cell autoimmunisation after allogeneic bone marrow transplant. *Bone Marrow Transplant* 1997;19:491.

114. Butler WT. Corticosteroids and immunoglobulin synthesis. *Transplant Proc* 1975;7:49.

115. Sanders MC, Levinson AI, Schreiber AD. Hormonal modulation of macrophage clearance of IgG-sensitized cells. *Trans Assoc Am Physicians* 1987; 100:268.

116. Worlledge SM, Brain MC, Cooper AC, et al. Immunosuppressive drugs in the treatment of autoimmune haemolytic anaemia. *Proc R Soc Med* 1968;61: 1312.

117. Skinner MD, Schwartz RS. Immunosuppressive therapy. *N Engl J Med* 1972; 287:221.

118. Murphy S, LoBuglio AF. Drug therapy in autoimmune hemolytic anemia. *Semin Hematol* 1976;13:323.

119. Kyle RA. Second malignancies associated with chemotherapeutic agents. *Semin Oncol* 1982;9:131.

120. Corley CC. Azathioprine therapy in autoimmune diseases. *Am J Med* 1966; 41:404.

121. Ahn YS, Harrington WJ, Byrnes JJ, et al. Treatment of autoimmune hemolytic anemia with vinca-loaded platelets. *JAMA* 1983;249:2189.

122. Gertz MA, Petit RM, Alvaro A, et al. Vinblastine-loaded platelets for autoimmune hemolytic anemia. *Ann Intern Med* 1981;95:325.

123. Garelli S, Mosconi L, Valbonesi M, et al. Plasma exchange for hemolytic crisis due to autoimmune hemolytic anemia of the IgG warm type. *Blut* 1980;41: 387.

124. Kutti J, Vadenvik H, Safai-Kutti S, et al. Successful treatment of refractory autoimmune haemolytic anaemia by plasmapheresis. *Scand J Haematol* 1984; 32:149.

125. Bowdler AJ. The role of the spleen and splenectomy in autoimmune hemolytic disease. *Semin Hematol* 1976;13:335.

126. Smith CH, Erlandson M, Schulman I, et al. Hazard of severe infection in splenectomized infants and children. *Am J Med* 1957;22:390.

127. Parker AC, MacPherson AIS, Richmond J. Value of radiochromium investigation in autoimmune haemolytic anaemia. *BMJ* 1977;1:208.

128. Kurlander RJ, Colman RE, Moore J, et al. Comparison of the efficacy of a two-day and a five-day schedule for infusing intravenous gammaglobulin in the treatment of immune thrombocytopenic purpura in adults. *Am J Med* 1987;83:17.

129. Imbach P. A multicenter European trial of intravenous immune globulin in immune thrombocytopenic purpura in childhood. *Vox Sang* 1985;49:25.

130. Vos JJ, van Aken WG, Engelfriet CP, et al. Intravenous gammaglobulin therapy in idiopathic thrombocytopenic purpura: results with the Netherlands Red Cross immunoglobulin preparation. *Vox Sang* 1985;49:92.

131. Macintyre EA, Linch DC, Macey MG, et al. Successful response to intravenous immunoglobulin in autoimmune haemolytic anaemia. *Br J Haematol* 1985;60:387.

132. Mueller-Eckhardt C, Salama A, Mahn I, et al. Lack of efficacy of high-dose intravenous immunoglobulin in autoimmune haemolytic anaemia: a clue to its mechanism. *Scand J Haematol* 1985;34:394.

133. Samuelsson A, Towers TL, Ravetch JV. Anti-inflammatory activity of IVIG mediated through the inhibitory Fc receptor. *Science* 2001;291:484.

134. Ahn YS, Harrington WJ, Simon SR, et al. Danazol for the treatment of idiopathic thrombocytopenic purpura. *N Engl J Med* 1983;308:1396.

135. Buelli M, Cortelazzo S, Viero P, et al. Danazol for the treatment of idiopathic thrombocytopenic purpura. *Acta Haematol* 1985;74:97.

136. Ahn YS, Harrington WJ, Mylvaganam R, et al. Danazol therapy for autoimmune hemolytic anemia. *Ann Intern Med* 1985;102:298.

137. Clarkson SB, Bussel JB, Kimberly RP, et al. Treatment of refractory immune thrombocytopenic purpura with an anti-Fc gamma receptor antibody. *N Engl J Med* 1986;314:1236.

138. Engelfriet CP, Reesink RW, Garretty G et al. The detection of alloantibodies against red cells in patients with warm-type autoimmune haemolytic anaemia. *Vox Sang* 2000;78:200.

139. Petz LD. Immunohematology: acquired immune hemolytic anemias. In: *Current hematology and oncology, vol 3.* New York: John Wiley & Sons, 1984:51.

140. Dameshek W, Komninos ZD. The present status of treatment of autoimmune hemolytic anemia with ACTH and cortisone. *Blood* 1956;11:648.

141. Freedman J, Wright J, Lim FC, et al. Hemolytic warm IgM autoagglutinins in autoimmune hemolytic anemia. *Transfusion* 1987;27:464.

142. Shirey RS, Kickler TS, Bell W, et al. Fatal immune hemolytic anemia and hepatic failure associated with a warm-reacting IgM autoantibody. *Vox Sang* 1987;52:219.

143. Garratty G, Arndt P, Domen R, et al. Severe autoimmune hemolytic anemia associated with IgM warm autoantibodies directed against determinants on or associated with glycophorin A. *Vox Sang* 1997;72:124.

144. Rosse WF. Autoimmune hemolytic anemia due to cold-reacting antibodies. In: *Clinical immunohematology: basic concept and clinical applications.* Oxford: Blackwell Scientific, 1990.

145. Schubothe H. The cold hemagglutinin disease. *Semin Hematol* 1966;3:27.

146. Sokol RJ, Hewitt S, Stamps BK. Autoimmune hemolysis: mixed warm and cold antibody type. *Acta Haematol* 1983;69:266.

147. Pruzanski W, Shumak KH. Biologic activity of cold reactive autoantibodies. *N Engl J Med* 1977;297:538.

148. Frank MM, Atkinson JP, Gadek J. Cold agglutinins and cold agglutinin disease. *Annu Rev Med* 1977;28:291.

149. Ulvestad E, Berentsen S, Bo K. Clinical immunology of chronic cold agglutinin disease. *Eur J Haematol* 1999;63:259.

150. Crisp D, Pruzanski W. B-cell neoplasms with homogenous cold-reacting antibodies (cold agglutinins). *Am J Med* 1982;72:915.

151. Schreiber AD, Herskovitz BS, Goldwein M. Low-titer cold-hemagglutinin disease: mechanism of hemolysis and response to corticosteroids. *N Engl J Med* 1977;296:1490.

152. Bessman JD, Banks D. Spurious macrocytosis, a common clue to erythrocyte cold agglutinins. *Am J Clin Pathol* 1980;74:797.

153. Feizi T, Werner P, Kunkel, HG, et al. Lymphocytes forming red cell rosettes in the cold in patients with chronic cold agglutinin disease. *Blood* 1973;42:753.

154. Haynes CR, Chaplin H Jr. An enhancing effect of albumin on the determination of cold hemagglutinins. *Vox Sang* 1971;20:46.

155. Garratty G, Petz LD, Hoops JK. The correlation of cold agglutinin titrations in saline and albumin with haemolytic anaemia. *Br J Haematol* 1977;35:587.

156. Wiener AS, Unger LJ, Cohen L, et al. Type-specific auto-antibodies as a cause of acquired hemolytic anemia and hemolytic transfusion reactions: biological test with bovine red cells. *Ann Intern Med* 1956;44:221.

157. Marsh WL. Anti-i: a cold antibody defining the I-i relationship in human red blood cells. *Br J Haematol* 1961;7:200.

158. Roelcke D, Ebert W, Metz J, et al. 1 I-, MN- and Pr₁/Pr-activity of human erythrocyte glycoprotein fractions obtained by ficin treatment. *Vox Sang* 1971;21:352.

159. Roelcke D. Reaction of anti-Gd, anti-F1 and anti-Sa cold agglutinins with p erythrocytes. *Vox Sang* 1984;46:161.

160. Roelcke D. The Lud cold agglutinin: a further antibody recognizing N-acetylneuraminic acid-determined antigens not fully expressed at birth. *Vox Sang* 1981;41:316.

161. Niemann H, Watanabe K, Hakomori SI, et al. Blood groups i and I activities of lacto-N-nor-hexosylceramide and its analogues: the structural requirements for i specificities. *Biochem Biophys Res Commun* 1978;81:1286.

162. Watanabe K, Hakomori SI, Childs RA, et al. Characterization of a blood group I active ganglioside: structural requirements for the I and i specificities. *J Biol Chem* 1979;254:3221.

163. Feizi T, Kabat EA. Immunochemical studies on blood groups: LIV. classification of anti-I and anti-i sera into groups based on reactivity patterns with various antigens related to blood group A, B, H, Leᵃ, Leᵇ, and precursor substances. *J Exp Med* 1972;135:1247.

164. Roelcke D. Serological studies on the Pr₁/Pr₂ antigens using dog erythrocytes. *Vox Sang* 1973;24:354.

165. Fudenberg HH, Kunkel HG. Physical properties of red cell agglutinins in acquired hemolytic anemia. *J Exp Med* 1957;106:689.

166. Capra JD, Dowling P, Cook S, et al. An incomplete cold-reactive γG antibody with i specificity in infectious mononucleosis. *Vox Sang* 1969;17:10.

167. Goldberg LS, Barnett EV. Mixed γG-γM cold agglutinin. *J Immunol* 1967;99:803.

168. Spiva DA, George JN, Sears DA. Acute autoimmune hemolytic anemia due to a low molecular weight IgM cold hemolysin associated with episodic lymphoid granulomatous vasculitis. *Am J Med* 1974;56:417.

169. Hughey CT, Brewer JW, Colosia AD, et al. Production of IgM hexamers by normal and autoimmune B cells: implications for the physiologic role of hexameric IgM. *J Immunol* 1998;161:4091.

170. Angevine CS, Andersen BR, Barnett EV. A cold agglutinin of the IgA class. *J Immunol* 1966;96:578.

171. Jacobson LB, Longstreth GF, Edgerton TS. Clinical and immunologic features of transient cold agglutinin hemolytic anemia. *Am J Med* 1973;54:514.

172. Harboe M. Exclusive occurrence of κ chains in isolated cold haemagglutinins. *Scand J Haematol* 1965;2:259.

173. Feizi T, Lecomte J, Childs R, et al. κ chain (VₖIII) subgroup-related activity in an idiotypic anti-cold agglutinin serum. *Scand J Immunol* 1976;5:629.

174. Feizi T, Lecomte J, Childs R. An immunoglobulin heavy chain variable region (Vₕ) marker associated with cross-reactive idiotypes in man. *Clin Exp Immunol* 1974;30:233.

175. Feizi T, Kunkel HG, Roeleke D. Cross idiotypic specificity among cold agglutinins in relation to combining activity for blood group-related antigens. *Clin Exp Immunol* 1977;18:283.

176. Feizi T. κ Chains in cold agglutinins. *Science* 1967;156:1111.

177. Evans RS, Turner E, Bingham M, et al. Chronic hemolytic anemia due to cold agglutinin. II. The role of C' in red cell destruction. *J Clin Invest* 1968;47:691.

178. Rosse WF, Sherwood JB. Cold-reacting antibodies: differences in the reaction of anti-I antibodies with adult and cord red blood cells. *Blood* 1970;36:28.

179. Rosse WF, Adams JP. The variability of hemolysis in the cold agglutinin syndrome. *Blood* 1980;56:409.

180. Logue, GL, Rosse WF, Gockerman JP. Measurement of the third component of complement bound to red blood cells in patients with cold agglutinin syndrome. *J Clin Invest* 1973;52:493.

181. Ross GD, Medof ME. Membrane complement receptors specific for bound fragments of C3. *Adv Immunol* 1985;37:217.

182. Ross GD, Lambris JD, Cain JA, et al. Generation of three different fragments of bound C3 with purified factor I or serum: I. requirements for factor H vs CRa cofactor activity. *J Immunol* 1982;129:2051.

183. Finland M, Peterson OL, Allen HE, et al. Occurrence of cold isohemagglutinins in various conditions. *J Clin Invest* 1993;24:451.

184. Jenkins WJ, Koster HG, Marsh WL, et al. Infectious mononucleosis, an unsuspected source of anti-i. *Br J Haematol* 1965;11:480.

185. Horwitz CA, Moulds J, Henle W, et al. Cold agglutinins in infectious mononucleosis and heterophil-antibody–negative mononucleosis-like syndromes. *Blood* 1977;50:195.

186. Tanowitz HB, Robbins N, Leidich N. Hemolytic anemia: associated with severe mycoplasma pneumoniae pneumonia. *N Y State J Med* 1979;78:2231.

187. Thurin RH, Bassen F. Infectious mononucleosis and acute hemolytic anemia: report of two cases and review of the literature. *Blood* 1955;10:841.

188. Janney FA, Lee LT, Howe C. Cold hemagglutinin cross-reactivity with Mycoplasma pneumoniae. *Infect Immun* 1978;22:29.

189. Loomes LM, Uemura K, Childs RA, et al. Erythrocyte receptors for Mycoplasma pneumoniae are sialylated oligosaccharides of the Ii antigen type. *Nature* 1984;307:560.

190. Costea N, Yakulis V, Heller P. Experimental production of cold agglutinins in rabbits. *Blood* 1965;26:323.

191. Worlledge SM, Dacie JV. Haemolytic and other anaemias in infectious mononucleosis. In: Carter HG, Penman RL, eds. *Infectious mononucleosis.* Oxford: Blackwell Scientific, 1969.

192. Michaux L, Dierlamm J, Wlodarska I, et al. Trisomy 3 is a consistent chromosome change in malignant lymphoproliferative disorders preceded by cold agglutinin disease. *Br J Haemataol* 1995;91:421

193. Wortman J, Rosse WF, Logue G. Cold agglutinin hemolytic anemia in nonhematologic malignancies. *Am J Hematol* 1979;6:275.

194. Landymore R, Isom W, Barlam B. Management of patients with cold agglutinins who require open-heart surgery. *Can J Surg* 1983;26:79.

195. Blumberg N, Hicks G, Woll J, et al. Successful cardiac bypass surgery in the presence of a potent cold agglutinin without plasma exchange. *Transfusion* 1983;23:363.

196. Oleson H. Chlorambucil treatment in the cold agglutinin syndrome. *Scand J Haematol* 1964;1:116.

197. Hippe E, Jensen KB, Olesen H, et al. Chlorambucil treatment of patients with cold agglutinin syndrome. *Blood* 1970;35:68.

198. Dacie JV. The autoimmune haemolytic anaemias IV: paroxysmal cold hemoglobinuria, syphilitic and non-syphilitic. In: *The haemolytic anaemias: congenital and acquired.* New York: Grune & Stratton, 1962:545.
199. Petz LD, Garratty G. *Acquired immune hemolytic anemias.* New York: Churchill Livingstone, 1980.
200. Sharara AI, Hillsley RE, Wax TD, et al. Paroxysmal cold hemoglobinuria associated with non-Hodgkin's lymphoma. *South Med J* 1994; 87:397.
201. Ries CA, Garratty G, Petz LD, et al. Paroxysmal cold hemoglobinuria: report of a case with an exceptionally high thermal range Donath-Landsteiner antibody. *Blood* 1971;38:491.
202. Worrledge SM, Rousso C. Studies on the serology of paroxysmal cold hemoglobinuria (PCH) with special reference to its relationship with the P blood group system. *Vox Sang* 1965;10:293.
203. Levine P, Celano MJ, Falkowski F. The specificity of the antibody in paroxysmal cold hemoglobinuria (PCH). *Transfusion* 1963;3:278.
204. Schwaring GA, Kundu SK, Marcus DM. Reaction of antibodies that cause paroxysmal cold hemoglobinuria (PCH) with globoside and Forssman glycosphingolipids. *Blood* 1979;53:186.
205. Bell CA, Zwicker H, Rosenbaum DL. Paroxysmal cold hemoglobinuria (PCH) following mycoplasma infection: anti-I specificity of the biphasic hemolysin. *Transfusion* 1973;13:138.
206. Nordhagen R, Sensvold K, Winsnes A, et al. Paroxysmal cold haemoglobinuria: the most frequent acute autoimmune haemolytic anaemia in children? *Acta Paediatr Scand* 1984;73:258.
207. O'Neill BJ, Marshall WC. Paroxysmal cold haemoglobinuria and measles. *Arch Dis Child* 1967;42:183.
208. Bunch C, Schwartz FC, Bird GW. Paroxysmal cold haemoglobinuria following measles immunization. *Arch Dis Child* 1972;47:299.
209. Bird GW, Wingham J, Martin AJ, et al. Idiopathic non-syphilitic paroxysmal cold haemoglobinuria in children. *J Clin Pathol* 1976;29:215.
210. Prasad AS, Berman L, Tranchida L, et al. Red cell hypoplasia, cold hemoglobinuria and M-type gamma G serum paraprotein and Bence Jones proteinuria in a patient with lymphoproliferative disorder. *Blood* 1968;31:151.
211. Rausen AR, LeVine R, Hsu TC, et al. Compatible transfusion therapy for paroxysmal cold hemoglobinuria. *Pediatrics* 1975;55:275.
212. Wolach B, Heddle N, Barr RD. The variability of hemolysis in the cold agglutinin syndrome. *Blood* 1981;56:409.
213. Harris JW. Studies on the mechanism of a drug-induced hemolytic anemia. *J Lab Clin Med* 1954;44:809.
214. Harris JW. Studies on the mechanism of a drug-induced hemolytic anemia. *J Lab Clin Med* 1956;47:670.
215. Petz LD, Garratty G. *Acquired immune hemolytic anemia.* New York: Churchill Livingstone, 1980.
216. Worlledge SM. Immune drug-induced haemolytic anaemias. *Semin Hematol* 1969;6:181.
217. Landsteiner K, Jacobs J. Studies on the sensitization of animals with simple chemical compounds. *J Exp Med* 1936;64:625.
218. MacGibbon H, Loughridge LW, Hourihane DO'B, et al. Autoimmune haemolytic anaemia with acute renal failure due to phenacetin and *p*-aminosalicylic acid. *Lancet* 1960;1:7.
219. Bloomfield RJ, Wilson IF. Nomifensine, acute hemolytic anemia, and renal failure. *Ann Intern Med* 1986;105:807.
220. de Torregrosa MVV, Rosada Rodrigues AL, Montilla E. Hemolytic anemia secondary to stibophen therapy. *JAMA* 1963;186:598.
221. Lindberg LG, Norden A. Severe hemolytic reaction to chlorpromazine. *Acta Med Scand* 1961;179:195.
222. Petz LD, Fudenberg HH. Coombs'-positive hemolytic anemia caused by penicillin administration. *N Engl J Med* 1966;274:171.
223. Swanson MA, Chanmougan D, Schwartz RS. Immunohemolytic anemia due to antipenicillin antibodies. *N Engl J Med* 1966;274:178.
224. Reis CA, Rosenbaum TJ, Garratty G, et al. Penicillin-induced immune hemolytic anemia. *JAMA* 1975;233:432.
225. Logue GL, Boyd AE III, Rosse WF. Chlorpropamide-induced immune hemolytic anemia. *N Engl J Med* 1970;283:900.
226. Spath P, Garratty G, Petz LD. Studies on the immune response to penicillin and cephalothin in humans. II. Immunohematologic reactions to cephalothin administration. *J Immunol* 1971;107:860.
227. Habibi B, Bretagne Y. Les antigenes de groups sanguins peuvent etre les cibles des conflits immunoallergiques medicamenteux a affinite erythrocytaire. *C R Acad Sci* 1983;296:693.
228. Habibi B, Basty R, Chodez S, et al. Thiopental-related immune hemolytic anemia and renal failure: specific involvement of red-cell antigen I. *N Engl J Med* 1985;312:353.
229. Salama A, Mueller-Eckhardt C. Rh blood group-specific antibodies in immune hemolytic anemia induced by nomifensine. *Blood* 1986;68:1285.
230. Salama A, Mueller-Eckhardt C. The role of metabolite-specific antibodies in nomifensine-dependent immune hemolytic anemia. *N Engl J Med* 1985;313:469.
231. Carstairs KC, Worlledge S, Dollery CT, et al. Methyldopa and haemolytic anaemia. *Lancet* 1966;1:201.
232. Carstairs KC, Breckenridge A, Dollery CT, et al. Incidence of a positive direct Coombs' test in patients on (α)-methyldopa. *Lancet* 1966;2:133.
233. LoBuglio AF, Jandl JH. The nature of the alpha-methyl-dopa red-cell antibody. *N Engl J Med* 1967;276:658.
234. Bakemeier RF, Leddy JP. Erythrocyte autoantibody associated with alpha-methyldopa: heterogeneity of structure and specificity. *Blood* 1968;32:1.
235. Shulman NR. A mechanism of red cell destruction in individuals sensitized to foreign antigens and its implications in autoimmunity. *Ann Intern Med* 1964;60:506.
236. Habibi B, Basty R, Chodez S, et al. Thiopental-related immune hemolytic anemia and renal failure: specific involvement of red-cell antigen I. *N Engl J Med* 1985;312:353.
237. Christie DJ, Aster RH. Drug-antibody-platelet interaction in quinine- and quinidine-induced thrombocytopenia. *J Clin Invest* 1982;70:989.
238. Kirtland HH, Mohler DN. Chronic stimulation of lymphocyte cyclic AMP: a proposed etiology for methyldopa-induced autoimmunity. *Blood* 1977;50:295.
239. Green FA, Jung CY, Rampal A, et al. Alpha-methyldopa and the erythrocyte membrane. *Clin Exp Immunol* 1980;40:554.
240. Green FA, Jung Cy, Hui A. Modulation of alpha-methyldopa binding to the erythrocyte membrane by superoxide dismutase. *Biochem Biophys Res Commun* 1989;95:1037.
241. Freedman AL, Barr PS, Brody EA. Hemolytic anemia due to quinidine: observations on its mechanism. *Am J Med* 19596;20:806.
242. Zeigler Z, Shaddock RK, Winkelstein A, et al. Immune hemolytic anemia and thrombocytopenia secondary to quinidine: in vitro studies of the quinidine-dependent red cell and platelet antibodies. *Blood* 1979;52:396.
243. Bell CA, Zwicker H, Lee S, et al. Quinidine hemolytic anemia in the absence of thrombocytopenia in a patient with hemoglobin D. *Transfusion* 1973; 13:100.
244. Ballas SK, Caro JF, Miguel O. Quinidine-induced hemolytic anemia: immunohematological characterization. *Transfusion* 1978;18:215.
245. Muirhead EE, Halden ER, Groves M. Drug-dependent Coombs' test and anemia. *Ann Intern Med* 1958;101:87.
246. Strumia PV, Raymond FD. Acquired hemolytic anemia and antipenicillin antibody: case report and review of literature. *Arch Intern Med* 1962;109:603.
247. Kerr RO, Cardmone J, Dalmasso AP, et al. Two mechanisms of erythrocyte destruction in penicillin-induced hemolytic anemia. *N Engl J Med* 1972; 287:1322.
248. Abraham GN, Petz LD, Fudenberg HH. Immunohaematological cross-allergenicity between penicillin and cephalothin in humans. *Clin Exp Immunol* 1968;3:343.
249. Gralnick HR, McGinniss MH, Elton W, et al. Hemolytic anemia associated with cephalothin. *JAMA* 1971;217:1193.
250. Jeannet M, Block A, Dayer JM, et al. Cephalothin-induced immune hemolytic anemia. *Acta Haematol* 1976;55:109.
251. Forbes CD, Craig JA, Mitchell R, et al. Acute intravascular hemolysis associated with cephalexin therapy. *Postgrad Med J* 1972;48:186.
252. Gralnick HR, McGinniss MH. Immune cross-reactivity of penicillin and cephalothin. *Nature* 1967;215:1026.
253. Gralnick HR, Wright LD, McGinniss MH. Coombs' positive reactions associated with sodium cephalothin therapy. *JAMA* 1967;199:725.
254. Salama A, Gottsche B, Schleiffer T, et al. "Immune complex" mediated intravascular hemolysis due to IgM cephalosporin-dependent antibody. *Transfusion* 1987;27:460.
255. Tajima H. Clinical studies in hemolytic anemia. *Acta Haematol Jpn* 1960; 23:188.
256. Dausset J, Bergerto-Blondel Y. Etude d'un anticorps allergique actif en presence de para-amino-salicylate de soude (PAS) contre les hematies, les leucocytes et les plaquettes humaines. *Vox Sang* 1961;6:91.
257. Taft EG, Propp RP, Sullivan SA. Plasma exchange for cold agglutinin hemolytic anemia. *Transfusion* 1977;17:173.
258. Weiss HJ, Burger RE, Tice AD, et al. Fatal disseminated intravascular coagulation and hemolytic anemia following stibophen therapy. *Am J Med Sci* 1972;264:375.
259. Wenz G, Klein RL, Lalezari P. Tetracycline-induced immune hemolytic anemia. *Transfusion* 1974;14:265.
260. Nance SJ, Ladisch S, Williamson TL, et al. Erythromycin-induced immune hemolytic anemia. *Vox Sang* 1988;55:233.
261. Seldon MR, Bain B, Johnson CA, et al. Ticarcillin-induced immune haemolytic anemia. *Scand J Haematol* 1982;28:459.
262. Shinton NK, Wilson C. Autoimmune hemolytic anemia due to phenacetin and *p*-aminosalicylic acid. *Lancet* 1960;1:226.
263. Dramer MR, Levene C, Hershko C. Severe reversible autoimmune and thrombocytopenia with diclofenac therapy. *Scand J Haematol* 1986;36:118.
264. Wolf B, Conradty M, Grohmann R, et al. A case of immune complex hemolytic anemia, thrombocytopenia, and acute renal failure associated with doxepin use. *J Clin Psychiatry* 1989;50:99.
265. Salama A, Mueller-Eckhardt C. Two types of nomifensine-induced immune haemolytic anaemias: drug-dependent sensitization and/or autoimmunization. *Br J Haematol* 1986;64:613.
266. Salama A, Mueller-Eckhardt C, Kissel K, et al. Ex vivo antigen preparation for the serological detection of drug-dependent antibodies in immune haemolytic anaemias. *Br J Haematol* 1984;58:525.
267. Fulton JD, Briggs JD, Dominiczak AF, et al. Intravascular haemolysis and acute renal failure induced by nomifensine. *Scott Med J* 1986;31:242.
268. Jacobson ES. Immune thrombocytopenia induced by ethchlorvinol. *Ann Intern Med* 1972;77:73.
269. Vila JM, Blum L, Dosik H. Thiazide-induced immune hemolytic anemia. *JAMA* 1978;236:1723.
270. Sirey RS, Bartholomew J, Bell W, et al. Characterization of antibody and selection of alternative drug therapy in hydrochlorothiazide-induced immune hemolytic anemia. *Transfusion* 1988;28:70.

271. Patten E, Beck CE, Scholl C, et al. Autoimmune hemolytic anemia with anti-Jk^a specificity in a patient taking Aldomet. *Transfusion* 1977;17:517.

272. Kleinman S, Nelson R, Smith L, et al. Positive direct antiglobulin tests and immune hemolytic anemia in patients receiving procainamide. *N Engl J Med* 1984;311:809.

273. Sosler DS, Behzad O, Garratty G, et al. Acute hemolytic anemia associated with a chlorpropamide-induced apparent auto-anti Jk. *Transfusion* 1984;24:206.

274. Nataas OB, Nesthus I. Immune haemolytic anaemia induced by glibenclamide in selective IgA deficiency. *BMJ* 1987;295:366.

275. Kopicky JA, Packman CH. The mechanisms of sulfonylurea-induced immune hemolysis: case report and review of the literature. *Am J Hematol* 1986;23:283.

276. Woolley PF, Sacher RA, Priego VM, et al. Methotrexate-induced immune haemolytic anaemia. *Br J Haematol* 1983;54:543.

277. Kickler TS, Buck S, Ness P, et al. Probenecid induced immune hemolytic anemia. *J Rheumatol* 1986;13:208.

278. Sosler SK, Behzad O, Garratty G, et al. Immune hemolytic anemia associated with probenecid. *Am J Clin Pathol* 1985;84:391.

CHAPTER 53

Disorders of Erythrocyte Glycolysis and Nucleotide Metabolism

Stefan W. Eber

This chapter focuses on a group of hemolytic anemias that have been called *chronic (or hereditary) nonspherocytic hemolytic anemias* and are caused by a variety of rare enzyme deficiencies. In general, these enzyme defects lead to a restricted energy supply or other metabolic impairments and a shortened red-cell lifespan. The chronicity and constant nature of the hemolysis separates these defects from most types of glucose-6-phosphate dehydrogenase (G6PD) deficiency, and the lack of characteristic changes in red-cell morphology differentiate them from the membrane defects and most of the hemoglobinopathies.

HISTORY

The term *chronic nonspherocytic hemolytic anemia* has been used to identify a subset of intrinsic erythrocyte defects that could not be ascribed to hemoglobinopathies, paroxysmal nocturnal hemoglobinuria, hereditary spherocytosis, or hereditary elliptocytosis. Hereditary spherocytosis and elliptocytosis may be diagnosed simply on the basis of their characteristic red-cell shape. Spherocytosis was first described in 1871 by Vanlair and Masius (1). Elliptocytosis was first described in 1904 by Dresbach (2). In contrast, it was not until 1947 that Haden (3) published a paper on "a new type of hereditary hemolytic jaundice without spherocytosis."

An appreciation of the metabolic basis of these latter disorders grew from the work of Dacie et al. (4,5), who observed that sterile blood from such patients, when incubated *in vitro* with various additives, displayed distinctly different hemolytic (autohemolysis) tendencies. Type I autohemolysis was only slightly greater than that of normal blood, regardless of the presence of glucose in the incubation medium. Type II was moderately or markedly increased relative to normal controls and was essentially unaffected by glucose supplementation. Defective glycolysis in such cells was further suggested by decreased conversion of glucose to lactate, by accumulation of certain glycolytic intermediates within red cells that were affected, and by decreased concentrations of erythrocyte adenosine triphosphate (ATP) (6–8).

In 1961, Valentine et al. and Tanaka et al. (9,10) demonstrated a common defect, deficiency of pyruvate kinase (PK) activity, in several families with chronic hemolytic anemia and type II autohemolysis patterns. This observation and the demonstra-

tion of G6PD deficiency in primaquine-sensitive erythrocytes (11) established the metabolic basis of these disorders, which since have been expanded to include a large number of phenotypically diverse enzymopathies of glucose, glutathione, and nucleotide metabolism (12–20). Hemolysis may result not only from insufficient production of normal enzyme protein, but also from variant isozymes with altered primary structures that impair substrate or cofactor avidity, altered activation or inhibition characteristics, or decreased stability or specific activity. The common denominator is presumed to be an impairment in energy or antioxidant metabolism that makes the cells that are affected susceptible to premature clearance (21).

CLINICAL SYMPTOMS, DIAGNOSTIC APPROACH, AND FREQUENCY

Case History

A 14-year-old girl of mixed German-Transylvanian origin has experienced severe hemolytic anemia, which started at birth and required regular blood transfusions every 4 to 5 weeks. The rise of reticulocytes (3.5%) was inadequate in view of her severe anemia (below 6 g/dL), which indicated inefficient erythropoiesis. Her spleen was moderately increased. Her blood smear showed a few elliptocytes, fragments, and spherocytes. Because red-cell osmotic fragility was slightly increased and the determination of PK and several other red-cell enzymes gave no reduced activity, hereditary spherocytosis was assumed. The patient was transferred to a pediatric hematologic center at the age of 6 months. Correction of the enzyme activity measurement for the young red-cell age (increased reticulocytes) showed that the PK activity decreased below 5% of the comparable activity in "normal" reticulocytes. Both parents had one-half the normal PK activity, which proved their heterozygous state for this enzyme deficiency. Molecular characterization showed that the patient was a compound heterozygote of PK Gaggenau [1594 C→T; CGG→TGG; 532 Arg→ Trp] and PK Bucaresti [721 G→T; GAG→TAG; 241 Glu→Stop].

Red-cell transfusions were initially hampered, because the patient was judged serologically as having the rare Rh blood subgroup pattern "ee" after an emergency transfusion had to be done in the neonatal period. Ten years later, molecular genetic determination of CDE genotype blood groups proved that the patient's red cells had the more common "Ee" pattern, thus making red-cell concentrates more readily available.

Splenectomy was performed at the age of 5 years. There was a modest improvement in the anemia and a tremendous rise of reticulocytes, as high as levels of 80% of all red cells. Moderate to severe hemolytic anemia persisted, requiring a transfusion every 3 months.

Due to multiple transfusions, the patient developed moderately severe iron overload at the age of 4 years (max. ferritin 3500 µg/L) with mild liver enzyme elevation and latent hypothyroidism. This hemosiderosis necessitated iron chelation therapy with daily subcutaneous deferoxamine (Desferal; 40 mg/kg) over a period of 6 months every 3 years. Chelation sufficiently lowered the ferritin level (500 µg/L) and magnetic resonance imaging of the heart did not show increased iron levels in the myocardium. Nevertheless, careful cardiologic investigation at 14 years of age showed signs of mild diastolic disturbance (myocardial stiffening) and reduced cardiovascular reserve on exercise. The patient had one severe episode of postsplenectomy sepsis 3 years after surgery, despite pneumococcal vaccination and continuous but poorly compliant penicillin prophylaxis.

Symptomatic gallstones developed, thus requiring cholecystectomy at the age of 9 years. Owing to the ongoing hemolysis and increasing iron overload, an HLA-antigen identical bone marrow transplantation from a related donor has been performed at 15 years of age. Afterwards, the patient has normal erythropoiesis without the need for further transfusion.

This case history was chosen to illustrate typical diagnostic and therapeutic problems with erythrocyte enzyme defects:

- The diagnosis of PK deficiency and other enzyme defects may be missed, if the residual enzyme activity is not corrected for reticulocytosis.
- PK deficiency shows an inadequate rise of reticulocytes before splenectomy and a characteristic increase in reticulocytes afterwards. The reason for the preferential damage of PK deficient reticulocytes in the spleen is still not fully understood.
- Molecular characterization of Rh blood subgroups may be warranted in patients who need transfusions shortly after birth (22).
- Splenectomy ameliorates but, in contrast to hereditary spherocytosis, does not cure hemolytic anemia due to erythrocyte enzyme defects. In patients with severe hemolysis or associated neurologic disorders, bone marrow transplantation may be justified.

Clinical Severity

Glycolytic enzyme defects range in severity from fully compensated hemolysis to severe hemolytic anemias that require regular transfusions. In most cases, hemolysis is chronic with exacerbation during infections (hemolytic or aplastic crises). The chronic anemia contrasts with the periodic hemolysis that is the hallmark of G6PD deficiency. Severe cases present in the neonatal period, and some have even been associated with hydrops fetalis. The classic findings of indirect hyperbilirubinemia, with or without icterus; decreased haptoglobin; and compensatory reticulocytosis are usually present along with variable degrees of splenomegaly and erythroid hyperplasia of the marrow. The latter, if sufficiently prominent, may induce skeletal changes by expansion of marrow spaces. Owing to their occurrence in all tissues, some glycolytic enzyme defects also affect the neuromuscular system. *In general, the diagnosis of chronic nonspherocytic hemolytic anemia should be assumed in cases of persistent normocytic or slightly macrocytic hemolytic anemia in which hemoglobin (Hgb) abnormalities and antiglobulin reactions are unde-*

tectable, microspherocytes are few or absent, and osmotic fragility is normal. The nonspecific autohemolysis test is obsolete. Accurate diagnosis requires quantitative enzyme assays (23) to detect a specific enzymopathy.

Diagnostic Laboratories

Several laboratories in the United States, Europe, and Japan have developed the capacity to provide screening services for referring physicians and institutions to evaluate suspected cases and to perform detailed biochemical characterization of abnormal enzymes according to internationally standardized criteria. Among these are the laboratories of Drs. I. Max-Audit of the Hôpital Henri-Mondor (Creteil Cedex, France), M. Lakomek and A. Pekrun of the University Children's Hospital (Göttingen, Germany), E. Kohne of the University Children's Hospital (Ulm, Germany), A. Zanella of the Department of Hematology (Milano, Italy), H. Fuji of the Department of Blood Transfusion (Tokyo Women's Medical University), J-L. Vives-Corrons of the Red Cell Pathology Unit (Barcelona, Spain), D. Paglia at the University of California School of Medicine (Los Angeles), W. van So Linge, Utrecht, Netherlands, and our laboratory at the University Children's Hospital (Zürich, Switzerland).

Screening test kits for some of the more common enzyme deficiencies are commercially available, but their qualitative nature makes them particularly susceptible to false-negative results.

Frequency of Enzyme Defects

The frequency of erythrocyte enzyme defects differs with geographic distribution. In contrast to thalassemia or G6PD deficiency, there seems to be no selection bias as heterozygotes do not have any advantage in survival. The study of 722 unrelated patients with anemia or reticulocytosis, or both, which was done in Beutler's laboratory (24), confirmed G6PD as the most frequent enzyme defect. Five glycolytic and nucleotide enzyme deficiencies were common (with decreasing frequency): PK, glucose phosphate isomerase (GPI), pyrimidine 5'-nucleotidase (P5'N), triosephosphate isomerase (TPI), and phosphofructokinase (PFK) deficiency (Table 53-1). All other defects are rare.

BIOCHEMICAL AND GENETIC BASIS OF ERYTHROCYTE ENZYME DEFECTS

Glucose Metabolism in Human Erythrocytes

The mature human erythrocyte has a lifespan of approximately 120 days and is optimally adapted to perform oxygen and carbon dioxide as well as proton transport. It consists of a plasma membrane that envelops a viscous, concentrated (33%) solution of Hgb, the latter accounting for approximately 95% of the cell's dry weight. Only the process of enucleation and the loss of cytoplasmic organelles allow the red cell to pass through narrow capillaries, with a concomitant drastic shape change. Carbonic anhydrase activity and bicarbonate-chloride exchange in red cells do not need energy. A number of vital cell functions depend, however, on appropriate generation and expenditure of energy. These include (a) initiation and maintenance of glycolysis; (b) cation pumping against electrochemical gradients; (c) synthesis of glutathione and other metabolites; (d) nucleotide salvage reactions; (e) maintenance of Hgb iron in its functional, reduced, ferrous state; (f) protection of structural, enzymatic, and Hgb proteins from oxidative denaturation; and (g) preservation of membrane phospholipid asymmetry. Inadequate energy production may be reflected by decreased intra-

TABLE 53-1. Distribution of the Most Frequent Enzymopathies in Various Regions of the World

	Germany (1973–1980)	Japan (1972–1985)	United States of America (1980–1986)	Spain (1978–1987)
	Percent of Cases Studied			
Glucose-6-phosphate dehydrogenase	60	20	15	73
Pyruvate kinase	27	51	68	17
Glucose phosphate isomerase	4	7	4	0.5
Pyrimidine 5'-nucleotidase	0	10	6	2
Triosephosphate isomerase	2	0	0	2
Phosphofructokinase	0.7	0	0	0.5
Cases studied	2823	966	722	1167

cellular concentration of ATP, failure of the cation pumps, loss of the normal discoid shape and plasticity of the membrane, and other alterations, which may include Heinz body formation. Such changes may be sufficiently severe to cause intravascular hemolysis or to induce a selective cell removal from the circulation by the reticuloendothelial system.

As summarized in Figure 53-1, energy generation is accomplished almost entirely by glycolysis, with storage as high-energy phosphates, particularly ATP, or as reducing energy in the form of glutathione and pyridine nucleotides [reduced nicotinamide adenine dinucleotide (NADH) and nicotinamide adenine dinucleotide phosphate (NADPH)].

Erythrocyte membranes possess a facilitated transport system for glucose that is present as an abundant carbon source in the plasma. Approximately 90% of glucose taken up by the erythrocyte is normally catabolized by *glycolysis to lactic acid, the Embden-Meyerhof (EM) pathway*. This pathway is the cell's principal means of ATP generation. Small and variable amounts of glucose may be diverted through the *hexose monophosphate shunt (HMS)*, also known as the *pentose phosphate pathway*. Glucose catabolism by this oxidative shunt provides the erythrocyte with a pool of NADPH, a reducing agent that combats oxidative effects on Hgb and other proteins (see Chapter 54). When necessary, glucose metabolism through this pathway can increase by more than an order of magnitude.

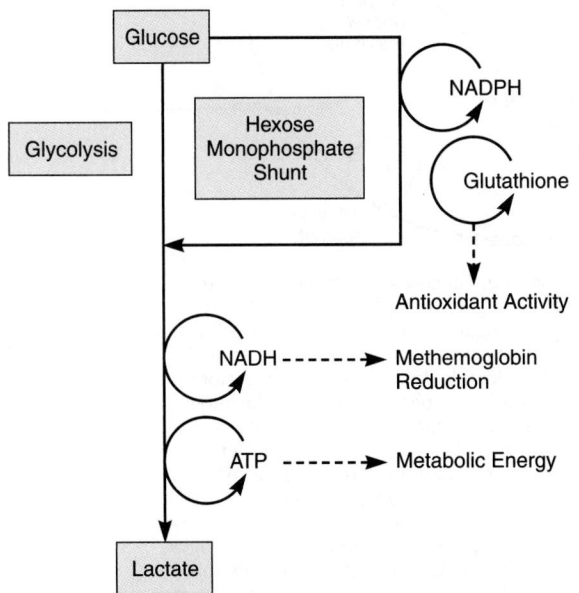

Figure 53-1. Simplified diagram of erythrocyte energy metabolism. Generation of high-energy phosphates and reducing compounds is accomplished principally via glucose catabolism.

Glycolysis (Embden-Meyerhof Pathway and Rapoport-Luebering Shunt)

The biochemical pathways available to accommodate their energy needs are shown in greater detail in Figure 53-2. Glycolysis includes the sequential degradation of glucose to lactate through a cascade of different enzymatic steps. This cascade is also called the *EM pathway*. Glycolysis operates in the presence or absence of oxygen (aerobic or anaerobic glycolysis). Only red cells, retina, and some tumor tissues perform aerobic glycolysis. In all other tissues, aerobic degradation of glucose generates pyruvate that enters mitochondria, where it is fully oxidized and the reducing equivalents are used for oxidative phosphorylation. Red cells lack mitochondria, and, hence, the degradation of glucose ends with lactic acid, even in the presence of oxygen.

Glucose catabolism is initiated by its phosphorylation to glucose-6-phosphate, a reaction that is catalyzed by hexokinase (HK). This enzyme has the lowest *in vitro* activity of the glycolytic enzymes in mature erythrocytes. Setting the *in vitro* activity of HK at one, each other enzyme activity is a multiple of HK activity. TPI has the highest activity of any of the glycolytic enzymes, by more than three orders of magnitude (Table 53-2). The relative activity of the glycolytic enzymes follows a strict multiplication, which has been taken as evidence that they form a semistable complex *in vivo* that catalyzes glucose degradation.

The activities of the phosphorylating enzymes, also called *kinases*, such as HK, PFK, and PK, are highly susceptible to intracellular pH and concentrations of phosphorylated organic compounds [e.g., 2,3-diphosphoglycerate (2,3 DPG), ATP, and fructose-1,6-diphosphate (F1,6DP)]. By virtue of these characteristics, the reactions that are catalyzed by these kinases are potentially rate-limiting steps of glycolysis.

After phosphorylation by HK, glucose-6-phosphate is isomerized to fructose-6-phosphate. The next step is phosphorylation to F1,6DP via PFK. Thus, phosphorylation of glucose to F1,6DP consumes two ATP molecules. F1,6DP is cleaved by aldolase (Ald) into glyceraldehyde-3-phosphate (G3P) and dihydroxyacetone phosphate (DHAP), which are interconvertible by TPI.

Glycolysis continues from one of these products, G3P, by an oxidative step that involves glyceraldehyde-3-phosphate dehydrogenase (G3PD). This enzyme catalyzes the oxidation of an aldehyde to an enzyme-bound acyl component that is released from the enzyme by its reaction with inorganic phosphate forming 1,3-diphosphoglycerate. 1,3-Diphosphoglycerate is capable of transferring its phosphoryl residue to adenosine diphosphate (ADP). This step is catalyzed by phosphoglycerate kinase (PGK) and is the first ATP-generating step of glycolysis. After two further enzymatic reactions (phosphoglyceromutase and enolase), glycolysis enters its second energy-generating step: PK. PK transfers the second energy-rich phosphoryl group from phospho-

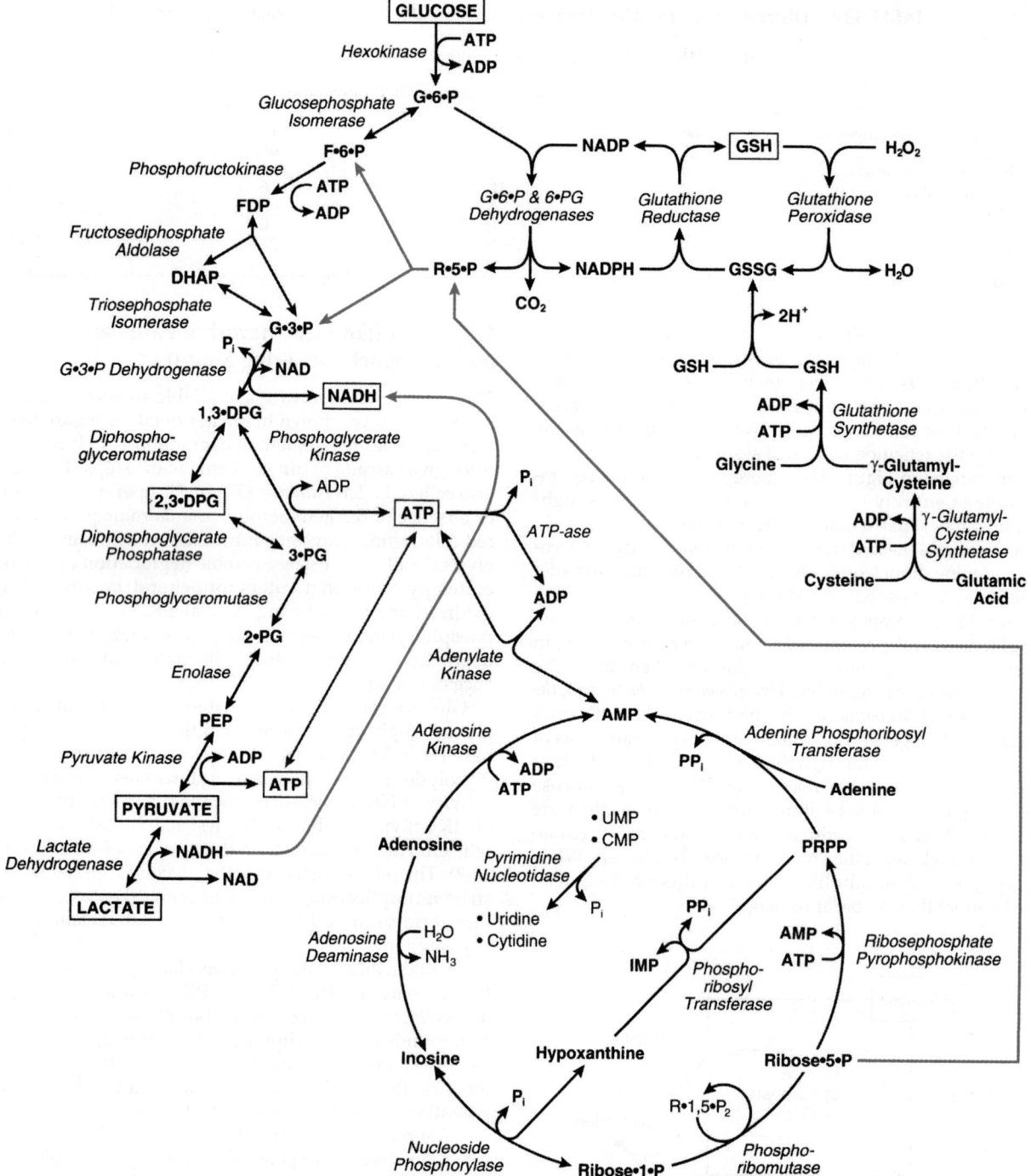

Figure 53-2. Biochemical pathways of metabolism in the erythrocyte. Glucose is degraded to lactate via glycolysis (Embden-Meyerhof pathway; on the left) or by diversion of glucose-6-phosphate (G6P) into the hexose monophosphate shunt (pentose phosphate pathway; on the right). Pentose phosphates (R5P) that are generated by this pathway or by nucleoside degradation can be transformed into intermediates of glycolysis for further catabolism. Reduced nicotinamide adenine dinucleotide (NADH) serves as cofactor for methemoglobin reductase activity. Nicotinamide adenine dinucleotide phosphate (NADPH) is the physiologic cofactor that is required for maintenance of adequate reduced glutathione (GSH) to combat ambient oxidative stresses. The Rapoport-Luebering shunt shelters an abundant intracellular store of 2,3-diphosphoglycerate (2,3 DPG), which can be degraded to regenerate adenosine triphosphate (ATP) in response to altered adenosine diphosphate (ADP)/ATP ratios. AMP, adenosine monophosphate; CMP, cytidine monophosphate; 1,3 DPG, 1,3-diphosphoglycerate; FDP, fructose diphosphate; F6P, fructose-6-phosphate; G3P, glyceraldehyde-3-phosphate; IMP, inosine monophosphate; NADP, nicotinamide adenine dinucleotide phosphate; Pi, inorganic phosphate; PPi, inorganic pyrophosphate; PEP, phosphoenolpyruvate; 2PG, 2-phosphoglycerate; 3PG, 3-phosphoglycerate; PRPP, phosphoribosyl pyrophosphate; R1,5P2, ribose 1,5-diphosphate; UMP, uridine monophosphate. (From Scriver CR, Beaudet AL, Sly WS, et al., eds. *The metabolic basis of inherited disease*, 6th ed. New York: McGraw-Hill, 1989, with permission.)

TABLE 53-2. Optimal *In Vitro* Activities of Various Erythrocyte Enzymes

Erythrocyte Enzymes	Relative (U)[a]
Glycolysis	
Hexokinase	1
Glucosephosphate isomerase	59
Phosphofructokinase	10
Fructose diphosphate aldolase	7
Triosephosphate isomerase	1807
Glyceraldehyde-3-phosphate dehydrogenase	190
Phosphoglycerate kinase	300
Monophosphoglyceromutase	11
Phosphopyruvate hydratase	7
Pyruvate kinase (3 mmol/L PEP)	19
Pyruvate kinase (3 mmol/L PEP + F1,6P$_2$)	20
Pyruvate kinase (0.4 mmol/L PEP)	10
Pyruvate kinase (0.4 mmol/L + F1,6P$_2$)	16
Lactate dehydrogenase	169
Hexose monophosphate shunt and glutathione cycling	
Glucose-6-phosphate dehydrogenase	9
6-Phosphogluconate dehydrogenase	9
Glutathione reductase	6
Glutathione peroxidase	12
Glutathione S-transferase	5
Nucleotide metabolism	
Adenylate kinase	181
Guanylate kinase	9
Cytidylate kinase	10
Uridylate kinase	20
Adenylate deaminase	9
Adenosine kinase	4
Adenosine deaminase	1
Nucleoside phosphorylase	72
Nucleoside diphosphate kinase	9
Ribosephosphate pyrophosphokinase	93
Adenine phosphoribosyltransferase	4
Pyrimidine nucleotidase (uridine monophosphate)	13
Pyrimidine nucleotidase (cytidine monophosphate)	10
Deoxyribonucleotidase (deoxythymidine monophosphate)	20
Deoxyribonucleotidase (deoxyinosine monophosphate)	49
Miscellaneous	
Glutamic oxaloacetic transaminase	4
Malic dehydrogenase	17
Acetylcholinesterase	32
Glyoxalase I	171
Glyoxalase II	63
Triokinase	0.2

F1,6P$_2$, fructose-1,6-diphosphate; PEP, phosphoenolpyruvate.
[a]One unit corresponds to 0.27 µmol substrate converted per minute by 10^{10} erythrocytes at 37°C or 0.81 µmol substrate per gram of hemoglobin. Values were derived from normal control subjects that were assayed in the laboratory of Dr. Paglia (with permission).

enolpyruvate (PEP) to ADP, thus generating ATP and pyruvate. In the last step of glycolysis, pyruvate is oxidized by lactate dehydrogenase to lactate, and reduced NADH is formed.

Via the TPI reaction, each of the two triose moieties that are generated in the Ald reaction may be further degraded by glycolysis and hence can serve as substrate for the rephosphorylation of ADP by PGK and PK. Thus, there is a net gain of two moles of ATP for every mole of glucose that is degraded to lactate by glycolysis. This gain of energy is far lower than the 38 ATP molecules that result from glycolysis plus oxidative phosphorylation of one mole of glucose, which illustrates how much energy-repletion capacity the red cell loses by getting rid of its mitochondria.

The oxidative step of G3PD generates reduced NADH, which serves as a reducing agent for the conversion of pyruvate to lactate and is essential to the maintenance of Hgb iron in its functional, reduced state through methemoglobin reductase (see Chapter 50). As indicated above, G3PD has a second, par-

ticularly important function: It fixes inorganic phosphate in a high-energy compound, 1,3-diphosphoglycerate. Two options then ensue. The high-energy phosphoryl group of 1,3-diphosphoglycerate may be transferred to ADP in the PGK reaction, or 1,3-diphosphoglycerate may be isomerized to 2,3 DPG. The intracellular concentration of 2,3 DPG is approximately 4 mmol/L. It accounts for two-thirds or more of the erythrocyte's complement of organic phosphates and has a crucial regulatory effect on Hgb oxygen affinity by lowering oxygen affinity of Hgb and thereby improving tissue oxygenation (see Chapter 49). Generation of 2,3 DPG from 1,3-diphosphoglycerate represents a side pathway of glycolysis, also called the *Rapoport-Luebering shunt*, which operates at the expense of the gain of one ATP. The Rapoport-Luebering shunt was aptly described by Keitt (25) as the "energy clutch" of ATP generation in erythrocyte metabolism. 2,3 DPG is an abundant intracellular store of rich energy phosphates. Under unfavorable acid pH conditions, ATP production is increased by shorttcuting the shunt and by the increased conversion of 2,3-DPG to 3-phosphoglycerate (3PG), which, in turn, enters into the ATP-generating last kinase step of glycolysis.

Trioses that are diverted into the Rapoport-Luebering shunt cannot generate ATP through PGK, but they provide a large and accessible reservoir of substrate for ATP generation as potential substrates of the second ATP-generating step, the PK reaction. The amount of ATP that is produced per mole of catabolized glucose can thereby be modulated according to the needs of the cell and is governed by the relative concentrations of ADP and ATP.

The convergent branch of the Rapoport-Luebering shunt is mediated by diphosphoglycerate phosphatase, which dephosphorylates 2,3 DPG irreversibly at the carbon-2 position. Diphosphoglyceromutase and phosphatase activities are accomplished by the same enzyme protein (26–28). Both activities are inhibited by increasing concentrations of their respective products, and the mutase activity is further inhibited by inorganic phosphate. It requires 3PG as a cofactor and is activated by 2-phosphoglycerate, whereas phosphatase activity is inhibited by the former and unaffected by the latter.

Perhaps the most important modulating influence on activity of the Rapoport-Luebering shunt is provided by intracellular proton concentration. Diphosphoglyceromutase is inhibited at acid pH, whereas diphosphoglycerate phosphatase is simultaneously activated. The effect of acidosis, therefore, is to mobilize the 2,3 DPG reserve for further degradation and generation of ATP by PK.

Phosphorylated glucose derivatives cannot diffuse across erythrocyte membranes, except for PEP that appears capable of entering red cells at low pH by the anion transport system that is associated with band-3 protein (29,30). The physiologic importance of the erythrocytes' capacity to use substrates other than glucose for energy metabolism remains uncertain and controversial.

Hexose Monophosphate Shunt and Glutathione Metabolism

An alternate pathway for degradation of glucose is the HMS (also called *pentose phosphate pathway*)(see Chapter 54). Normally, less than 5% to 10% of glucose is catabolized through this pathway, thereby maintaining a pool of reducing energy in the form of NADPH and reduced glutathione. Sudden oxidant challenge, however, can stimulate glucose flow through the shunt by 20- to 30-fold or more. The ratio of oxidized NADPH and NADPH concentrations provides the principal determinant of HMS flow. The flexibility to divert variable amounts of substrate through the HMS provides the erythrocyte with the prerequisites for defense against oxidative damage. The first and key enzyme of this shunt is G6PD. G6PD deficiency and other disorders of the HMS are described in detail in Chapter 54.

It is reasonable that a cell whose primary function is to carry molecular oxygen, a highly reactive oxidant, must at the same time preserve many of its structural and enzymatic proteins and even Hgb itself in reduced states to secure function and survival. This precarious balance is made possible in part by the presence of high concentrations of the Cys-containing tripeptide, glutathione. Glutathione is kept in the reduced state by NADPH, which originates exclusively from HMS activity. Because of its low redox potential, glutathione serves as a sacrificial reductant, protecting less reactive sulfhydryl groups of cellular proteins from oxidative damage. Glutathione itself has a relatively rapid turnover rate in erythrocytes and must be constantly resynthesized from its constituent amino acids, as shown in Figure 53-2.

Many of the deleterious effects of diverse pathologic processes, such as inflammation, aging, radiation, and chemical injury, are mediated by free-radical formation. Sophisticated mechanisms to neutralize free radicals have evolved to protect cell membranes, enzymes, and other cellular components from the destructive structural and functional consequences of lipid peroxidation, altered redox states, and protein denaturation. Human erythrocytes contain a dismutase that inactivates superoxide free radicals by conversion to hydrogen peroxide, which can then be decomposed by catalase or reduced to water by glutathione peroxidase in a coupled reaction that oxidizes glutathione. Defects in these enzymes would potentially render such cells susceptible to stress-induced hemolysis, but no disease state has been associated with a deficiency in any of the previously mentioned enzymes. It appears that detoxification of hydrogen peroxide and oxygen radicals is secured by several pathways (e.g., by catalase as well as superoxide dismutase).

Nucleotide Metabolism

Mature circulating erythrocytes normally contain only trace amounts of nonadenine nucleotides. Because these cells cannot synthesize nucleotides *de novo*, they have evolved mechanisms that effectively preserve them as they emerge from the reticulocyte stage. Some of the known reactions that are pertinent to erythrocytes are summarized in Figure 53-2.

The adenine nucleotide pool in erythrocytes consists mostly of ATP (85% to 90%), with lower amounts of ADP (10% to 12%) and adenosine monophosphate (AMP) (1% to 3%). This equilibrium is actively maintained by an adenylate kinase (AK). Glycolysis generates ATP, but the amount of ATP generated is limited to the ADP that is available for phosphorylation. The third component, AMP, although present in the smallest concentration, is in a particularly vulnerable position. If it is deaminated to inosine monophosphate (IMP) or dephosphorylated to diffusible adenosine, the purine moiety is effectively lost from the cell, and some salvage mechanism must intervene to compensate.

Two potential salvage pathways are apparent in Figure 53-2. Adenine phosphoribosyltransferase in human erythrocytes is sufficient in activity to convert adenine to AMP, but adenine does not appear to be readily available in plasma, and subjects with complete deficiency of the enzyme show no demonstrable alteration in erythrocyte function, longevity, or nucleotide concentrations (31). By contrast, there is strong evidence to support a physiologic role for adenosine kinase in nucleotide salvage. This pathway accounts for the accumulation of high concentrations of deoxyadenosine phosphates in red cells from some immunodeficient subjects with marked deficiency of the enzyme adenosine deaminase (ADA) (32–36). Conversely, patients with hyperactive ADA show depletion of their erythrocyte nucle-

otides (37–41). Because the kinase and deaminase compete for the same substrate, these observations indicate that nucleotide salvage by adenosine kinase is normally important to maintain the adenine nucleotide pool at constant concentrations.

Except for pyrimidine nucleotidase, none of the other reactions that are depicted in the nucleotide cycle of Figure 53-2 appear to be physiologically significant for the mature erythrocyte. Deficiencies and hyperactivity states exist for a number of these reactions, including nucleoside phosphorylase, hypoxanthine-guanine phosphoribosyl transferase, and ribose-phosphate pyrophosphokinase (RPK), but none of these deficiencies appear to have deleterious effects on the red cell (42). P5'N is physiologically important during reticulocyte maturation. Its substrate specificity allows it to dephosphorylate only the pyrimidine containing–degradation products of ribonucleic acid (RNA), thereby converting them to diffusible nucleosides and clearing them from the cell without simultaneously degrading AMP and affecting the adenine nucleotide pool (43–45). Red cells also contain a separate deoxyribonucleotidase that may have a corresponding function in DNA catabolism (46–50).

Erythrocyte Metabolism as a Function of Cell Age

Increased binding of denatured and oxidized Hgb (hemichrome), a compromised intracellular reducing capacity, and, as a consequence, clustering of band-3 molecules play a pivotal role in the normal red-cell aging process (51–53). The binding of immunoglobulin G, especially naturally occurring antiband-3 antibodies (54), at the site of hemichrome-stabilized clusters of band 3 and complement fixation to the altered red-cell membrane constitutes a plausible pathway to explain the recognition and removal of senescent red cells from the circulation by macrophages of the mononuclear phagocyte system.

Patients with hemolytic anemia generally have peripheral blood populations that are inordinately rich in reticulocytes and young red cells. Reticulocytes have a number of metabolic differences when compared to mature erythrocytes. Their use of glucose and oxygen is greater by one and two orders of magnitude, respectively, largely as a consequence of their transient retention of functional mitochondrial enzymes. Krebs cycle metabolism and oxidative phosphorylation proceed actively for a short time, as does the synthesis of Hgb and other proteins.

Additionally, reticulocytes emerge from the marrow with some glycolytic isoenzymes that are principally present in erythroid precursors but are rapidly inactivated in the postreticulocyte stage. These differences are accentuated in immature macroreticulocytes that may be stimulated to leave the marrow early during the stress erythropoiesis that is encountered in severe anemia.

All this results in whole-blood profiles of enzymatic activities and metabolite concentrations that deviate considerably from those of normal mature erythrocytes. Because the latter can no longer synthesize protein, their enzymes lose activity as the cells age. Each enzyme exhibits a characteristic decay rate, depending on its susceptibility to oxidative denaturation, proteolysis, spontaneous chemical modifications that lead to deamidation, or other processes that result in catalytic inactivation.

Increased reticulocytosis therefore hampers interpretation of enzyme activities in whole blood. The increase in reticulocytes and metabolically more active, young erythrocytes in patients with hemolytic anemias can easily mask a red-cell enzyme deficiency that might be apparent when cells of similar age are compared. A classic example is the difficulty in the establishment of a diagnosis of G6PD deficiency during the period immediately after an acute hemolytic crisis when reticulocytes surge into the peripheral blood to replace the oldest, enzymatically effete erythrocytes that are most susceptible to hemolysis.

The pattern of progressive metabolic depletion as erythrocytes age has been extrapolated to the senescent cell to account for its sharply limited lifespan. The traditional view suggests that natural attrition of metabolic capacities eventually leads to a cell that cannot fulfill its energy requirements. Derangement of energy supply is presumed to be accelerated by enzymopathies that further restrict energy metabolism in affected erythrocytes, thus leading to their premature demise.

This hypothesis remains unproven, even though abundant supportive data have been generated, particularly by studies related to blood cell preservation for transfusion. Decreases in erythrocyte high-energy phosphates and 2,3 DPG concentrations correlate directly with posttransfusion survival (55), yet studies indicate that the oldest red-cell cohorts *in vivo* actually contain *increased* rather than decreased concentrations of ATP (56–58). In PK-deficient red cells, increased exposure of phosphatidylserine at the outer membrane, which indicates a loss of phospholipid asymmetry, can be shown (59). Thus, secondary alterations of the red-cell membrane might contribute to the premature demise of enzymopenic red cells. However, the precise event that terminates the life of an enzyme-deficient erythrocyte remains uncertain.

Characterization of the Molecular Defects and Functional Consequences of Glycolytic Enzyme Deficiencies

Hereditary enzyme defects have been described in all red-cell pathways that involve glucose, glutathione, and nucleotide metabolism. Those enzymopathies that have adverse clinical consequences frequently belong to two groups:

- Enzyme deficiencies in glycolysis and nucleotide metabolism, which ultimately impair ATP generation and cause chronic compensated, or noncompensated, nonspherocytic hemolytic anemia.
- Defects in the HMS and in those reactions that are normally responsible for generation or maintenance of reduced glutathione. These are associated with periodic hemolytic episodes that are induced by oxidant foods or drugs, duress of surgery or infections, or other physiologic stresses.

The extent of metabolic dysfunction in red blood cells and other tissues depends on the importance of the enzyme that is affected, its functional abnormalities, the stability of the mutant enzyme, and the possibility of compensation for the deficiency by overexpression of an isoenzyme or the use of an alternative pathway. Generally, one can conclude that a metabolic disease manifests earlier for deficient enzymes that control key steps of intermediate metabolism (e.g., HK, PFK, and PK) than it does for those catalyzing reactions near equilibrium. However, this has no major clinical implication, because the most severe defects are found in patients with TPI deficiency. This enzyme has the highest activity of all red-cell enzymes and operates near equilibrium.

Historically, a *quantitative enzyme defect* has been defined as one in which the residual enzyme activity is 10% to 20% of that found in normal control hemolysates. Patients who were affected were presumed to be homozygotes, because intermediate (approximately 40% to 60%) levels of enzyme activities were often found in parents and relatives, which is consistent with heterozygous deficiency states.

However, no consistent correlation has ever been established between the decrease in enzyme activity and the severity of clinical expression. Wide variation in genetic expression is observed for most of the known erythrocyte enzymopathies. Mutant genes may code for production of enzyme proteins that are catalytically impotent; unstable; kinetically aberrant; altered in terms of their response to physiologic activators, inhibitors, cofactors, and allo-

steric modifiers; or that have diverse combinations of these characteristics. In the absence of consanguinity, patients who are affected often represent compound heterozygotes rather than true homozygotes, so mixtures of mutant isozymes are likely to be present in cells that are affected. The molecular biology and the biochemistry that underlie erythroid enzymopathies have been reviewed by Beutler (60) and are summarized in Tables 53-3 and 53-4.

A molecular characterization of the genetic defect in a specified enzyme deficiency is indicated in cases of severe transfusion-dependent hemolytic anemia and in cases with associated progressive neuromuscular impairment (especially TPI deficiency). The option of prenatal diagnosis should be offered to couples who already have an affected offspring and want further children. Most mutations have been found within the coding sequence of the respective genes. Missense mutations predominate. Homozygous null mutations would probably be incompatible with life, because most erythrocyte enzymes occur in all tissues.

Apart from determination of maximal enzyme velocity at saturating substrate concentrations, most biochemical parameters of defective enzymes (e.g., determination of substrate affinity, pH optimum, heat stability, electrophoretic mobility, and specific activity) have lost importance. Indeed, some enzyme defects that were considered to be different variants by biochemical characterization have been shown to be due to identical mutations.

Diagnostic Scheme for Red-Cell Enzyme Defects: A Rational Approach

A diagnostic approach to red-cell enzyme disorders is presented in Figure 53-3. Special tests of red-cell metabolism, membrane, and Hgb properties are arduous and costly. Therefore, increased hemolysis must be proven before any special investigations are undertaken. Tests to establish hemolysis include the detection of indirect hyperbilirubinemia, increased serum lactic acid dehydrogenase or glutamate oxaloacetate transaminase activity, decreased haptoglobin, and an increase in free Hgb in the serum. Increased red-cell creatinine is thought to be the most sensitive parameter of hemolysis (61). Reticulocytosis is useful but may just indicate increased erythropoietic regeneration rather than compensation for hemolysis. After proving that hemolysis exists, red-cell membrane defects should be excluded by examination of the blood smear for the characteristic morphology of hereditary spherocytosis, elliptocytosis, pyropoikilocytosis, or stomatocytosis or increased osmotic fragility, or both. The acidified glycerol lysis test, which is described by Zanella et al. (62) and modified by Eber et al. (63), is an appropriate screening test of red-cell osmotic fragility. A negative direct Coombs' test practically rules out immunohemolytic anemia, and Hgb electrophoresis excludes many hemoglobinopathies. Anemia due to enzyme defects is always normocytic or slightly macrocytic owing to reticulocytosis. The mean corpuscular Hgb concentration is normal in all cases. Therefore, enzyme determination is warranted, if hemolysis is present, red-cell indices (mean corpuscular Hgb and mean corpuscular volume) are normal (or slightly elevated), the Coombs' test is negative, and red-cell morphology gives no hint of a specific alteration. Periodic hemolysis points to an enzymopathy of the HMS (G6PD or enzymes of the glutathione metabolism). Chronic hemolytic anemia is the hallmark of defects of the EM pathway. Among these defects, deficiencies of PK, GPI, and TPI are more common and should be tested first. In the case of associated neuromuscular impairment, activities of GPI, PFK, Ald, TPI, PGK, and cytochrome5 reductase should be tested. The key symptom of cytochrome5 (or methemoglobin) reductase (also called *NADH diaphorase*) is methemoglobinemia (see Chapter 49). Hemolysis is absent in these patients.

Basophilic stippling is characteristic of P5'N deficiency and unstable Hgbs. If present, an ultraviolet (UV) absorption spec-

TABLE 53-3. Changes in Red-Cell Intermediate Metabolite Levels and Metabolic Consequences in Enzyme Defects

	2,3 DPG	ATP	GSH	Others	Metabolic Consequences
HK	↓	↓	N, ↓	↓ G6P, F6P and triosephosphates	Increased hemoglobin-oxygen affinity with reduced tissue oxygen delivery
Glucose phosphate isomerase	↓ Regeneration of 2,3 DPG	↓ Regeneration of ATP	↓ Regeneration of GSH	↑ G6P	Impaired glycolysis; feedback inhibition of HK; accelerated HMS
Phosphofructokinase	↓	↓	N.A.	↑ G6P + F6P	↓ Affinity for F1,6DP
Aldolase	(↑)	(↓)	N.A.	↑↑ F1,6DP; ↓ affinity for F1,6DP	In vitro ↓ in glycolysis and HMS
Triosephosphate isomerase	Normal	↓	N	↑↑ DAP; ↑ F1,6DP	No metabolism of pyruvate via tricarboxylic acid cycle; possibly deviant lipid metabolism; resembles mitochondrial enzymopathy (258,259)
Phosphoglycerate kinase	↑	N or (↓)	N	↑ Glyceraldehyde-3-phosphate, DAP, F1,6P	Increased 2,3 DPG cycle
2,3-Diphosphoglycerate mutase	↓↓, Absent	↑	N (↑)	↑ Glycerated hemoglobin A	Increased blood-oxygen affinity, polycythemia
Pyruvate kinase	↑	↓[a]	N.A.	↓ Nicotinamide adenine dinucleotide and nicotinamide adenine dinucleotide phosphate; N or ↑ 3-phosphoglycerate	Reduced hemoglobin-oxygen affinity, loss of cooperativity of PK substrate binding
P5'N	(↑)	N	↑	**↑↑ Cytosine triphosphate and uridine triphosphate**	**↓ HMS; ↑↑ nucleotides imitate ↑ ATP**
Adenylate kinase	N.A.	N	N.A.	—	**Also deficient in guanosine triphosphate–adenosine monophosphate phosphotransferase**
Adenosine deaminase increase	N.A.	↓↓	N.A.	—	**↑ P5'N activity**

ATP, adenosine triphosphate; DAP, dihydroxyacetone phosphate; 2,3 DPG, 2,3-diphosphoglycerate; F1,6DP, fructose-1,6-diphosphate; F6P, fructose-6-phosphate; G6P, glyceraldehyde-6-phosphate; GSH, glutathione; HK, hexokinase; HMS, hexose monophosphate shunt; P5'N, pyrimidine 5'-nucleotidase; N, normal; N.A., data not available. (↓), slightly reduced; ↓, reduced; ↓↓, severely reduced; the opposite applies for an increase: (↑), slightly increased; ↑, increased; ↑↑, severely increased.
[a]Reduced with respect to reticulocytosis.

trum of a deproteinized extract of red cells should be measured as a screening test for P5'N deficiency. When the UV spectrum shows increased red-cell nucleotide content, the residual activity of P5'N must be determined. Unstable Hgbs may be detected with heat stability and isopropanol stability tests, but, because unstable Hgbs can be difficult to detect, globin gene sequencing is sometimes required. High-pressure liquid chromatography, followed by isoelectric focusing and tandem mass spectroscopy, is another powerful way to detect most Hgb mutations.

Defects of nucleotide metabolism other than P5'N deficiency, such as ADA hyperactivity or AK deficiency are best detected by screening for a decreased red cell ATP level. In the remaining cases of normocytic hemolytic anemia and suspected enzyme defects, the activities of other enzymes that are rarely deficient (HK, PGK) or for which the association with increased hemolysis is uncertain (e.g., G3PD, enolase) should be determined.

Pitfalls in Proving Enzyme Defects

- Residual activity and metabolic status of damaged and already hemolyzed red cells cannot be extrapolated from activity measurements of the surviving cells in whole-blood samples.
- In vitro assays under optimal conditions of pH, cofactor availability, and substrate concentration may not adequately reflect the performance of an enzyme under less favorable physiologic circumstances in vivo.
- High specific activity of certain enzymes in leukocytes may result in false-normal values of red-cell enzyme activities if leukocytes are not carefully depleted before activity measurement (valid especially for PK deficiency).
- Antecedent transfusion may mask the true enzyme deficiency.
- Whole-blood enzyme activity may fail to portray the defect in mature red cells, because reticulocytosis is accompanied

by increased mean enzyme activity and may mask the defect (typical for PK and HK deficiency).

Synopsis of Clinical, Biochemical, and Genetic Findings in Glycolytic Enzyme Defects

The most important data on enzyme defects are summarized in Tables 53-3, 53-4, and 53-5 and include the severity of hemolysis and anemia, the indication for splenectomy, and the major changes in red-cell metabolism, gene localization, and protein structure. Only enzymes that are proven to cause disease are listed. In addition to hemolytic anemia, some enzyme defects that cause neuromuscular symptoms are also included in the tables.

All glycolytic enzymes are listed according to their sequential occurrence in the pathway; defects of nucleotide metabolism are given in a separate bolded section at the bottom of the tables.

HEMOLYTIC ENZYMOPATHIES OF THE GLYCOLYTIC PATHWAY OF KNOWN SIGNIFICANCE (EMBDEN-MEYERHOF)

In the following section, the two most frequent glycolytic enzyme defects (PK, GPI) are presented first; TPI is the third defect that is presented because of its devastating clinical symptoms. Other defects are reported according to their position in glycolysis. PK deficiency is by far the most common defect. All other defects occur less frequently, and some are extremely rare. Some defects are associated with neuromuscular symptoms: TPI, PFK, Ald, and PGK, which appears to result from effects of the enzyme defect in nonerythroid cells.

TABLE 53-4. Biochemistry and Genetics of Enzyme Defects That Are Involved in Hemolytic Anemias

	Frequency	Red-Cell Isozymes	Gene Size (Exons)[a]	Gene Locus	Tertiary Structure	Amino Acids/Chain	Remarks
HK	Very rare; 22 cases[c]	1, R	~7 kb (19)	10q22	Monomer	896	HK-R uses a red-cell–specific promoter
Glucose phosphate isomerase	Rare; approximately 50 cases[c]	—	~50 kb (18)	19q13.1	Homodimer (AA')[b]	558	Multifunctional enzyme (neuroleukin)
PFK	Rare	L	~28 kb (22)	21q22.3	Tetramers; allosteric kinetics	~ 730	—
	Rare	M	~30 kb (24)	12q13.3	Tetramers; allosteric kinetics	780	Founder effect in Ashkenazi descendants (deleted exon 5 of PFK-M)
Aldolase	Very rare	A	7.53 kb (12)	16q22-q24	Homotetramer	363	Two other tissue-specific isozymes
Triosephosphate isomerase	Very rare; approximately 34 cases[c]	—	~3.5 kb (7)	12p12.2	Homodimer (AA')[b]	248	Founder effect (104glutamic acid→aspartic acid) in one-half of patients
Phosphoglycerate kinase	Very rare; 23 cases[c]	I	~23 kb (10)	Xq13	Monomer	416	Autosomal isozyme in sperm
Pyruvate kinase	Common; 1:20,000; approximately 400 cases[c]	LR	~9.5 kb (12)	1q21	Tetramer; allosteric regulation	574	Founder effect in one-half of patients
	Common; 1:20,000	M₂	~32 kb (12)	15q22	Tetramer; allosteric regulation	530	—
Pyrimidine 5'-nucleotidase (UMPH1)	Second or third most frequent enzyme defect[e]	UMPH1, 2[d]	(10)	7p15-p14		286 (297 in reticulocytes)	Alternate splicing of exon 2
AK	Rare	AK 1	~12 kb (7)	9q34.1	Monomer	194	—
Adenosine deaminase increase	**Very rare**	**Tissue-specific-isozyme**	**32 kb (12)**	**20q13.11**	**Monomer**	**342**	**Overproduction specific for red cells**

AK, adenylate kinase; HK, hexokinase; kb, kilobase; PFK, phosphofructokinase; UMPH, uridine monophosphate hydrolase.
NOTE: With the exception of PGK (X-chromosomal) and ADA (autosomal dominant), all enzyme defects are inherited autosomal recessively.
[a]The number of exons is given in parentheses.
[b] Electrophoretic isoforms are due to epigenetic deamidation of one encoded chain.
[c]The number of reported cases worldwide; this does not necessarily coincide with the estimated frequency, because some patients may die young or may be not published.
[d]UMPH1 accounts for 95% of the pyrimidine nucleotidase activity in red cells, and UMPH2 accounts for deoxypyrimidine nucleotidase activity.
[e]More frequent in Mediterranean than in northern European descents.

With the exception of PGK (X-linked) and ADA deficiency (autosomal dominant), inheritance is autosomal recessive. True homozygotes have been identified in patients who descend from consanguineous parents, but most patients are compound heterozygous for two different defects of the same enzyme.

As noted earlier, the red-cell morphology and osmotic fragility are generally rather unremarkable; there may be a fraction of osmotically fragile or resistant cells after a 24-hour incubation, thus giving a skewed curve. Red cells are mostly normochromic and sometimes moderately macrocytic. Splenectomy can diminish increased hemolysis and abrogate the need for transfusions in the mild to moderately affected patients. However, some hemolysis persists in all cases.

Pyruvate Kinase Deficiency

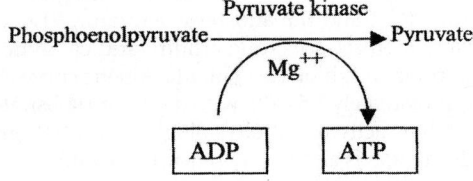

CLINICAL SYMPTOMS OF PYRUVATE KINASE DEFICIENCY

- Chronic, often severe, hemolytic anemia; 40% of cases require regular transfusions.
- Better tolerance of low levels of Hgb owing to 2,3 DPG and improved tissue oxygen delivery.
- Ineffective erythropoiesis with iron overload.
- Neonatal jaundice.
- Splenomegaly.

GENETIC AND BIOCHEMICAL CHARACTERISTICS OF PYRUVATE KINASE DEFICIENCY

- Most frequent glycolytic enzyme defect with a high prevalence in northern Europe (1:20,000).
- Enzyme activity depends strongly on reticulocyte numbers: pseudonormal activity in severe defects due to an increase in reticulocytes.
- Inadequate rise of reticulocytes before splenectomy and massive characteristic rise of reticulocytes after splenectomy.
- Founder effect [1529 Glu→Ala in PK-L gene] in patients of central-northern European descent: approximately 50% are detectable by Sty I restriction endonuclease digestion.
- Tetramer with loss of cooperativity of substrate binding.

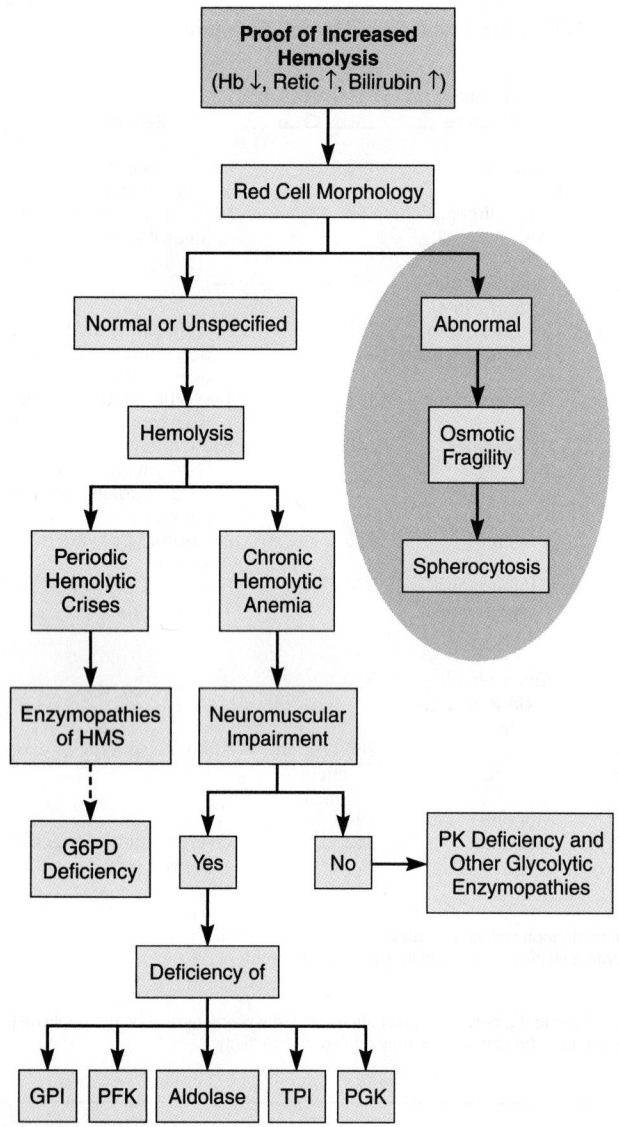

Figure 53-3. Differential diagnosis of red-cell enzyme defects that cause hemolytic anemia. G6PD, glucose-6-phosphate dehydrogenase; GPI, glucose phosphate isomerase; Hb, hemoglobin; HMS, hexose monophosphate shunt; PFK, phosphofructokinase; PGK, phosphoglycerate kinase; PK, pyruvate kinase; TPI, triosephosphate isomerase.

- Increased levels of 2,3 DPG and decreased Hgb oxygen affinity.
- Macrocytosis; small numbers of shrunken, spiculated cells.

BIOCHEMISTRY AND GENETICS

PK (ATP:pyruvate 2-o-phosphotransferase, E.C.2.7.1.40) catalyzes the second crucial ATP-generative step in glycolysis. This step is necessary for the red cell to achieve a net gain in ATP from the metabolism of glucose. It requires magnesium and potassium for optimal activity. The enzyme is a tetramer with a molecular weight of approximately 240 kd (64–68), and it is highly sensitive to a number of regulatory substances (69–71).

Mammals possess multiple tissue-specific isozymes that are derived from two principal forms. PK-M and PK-L are dominant in muscle (M) and liver (L), respectively (Fig. 53-4; Table 53-4). PK-R isozymes that are characteristic of red cells (R) are derivative products of the PK-L gene. Close similarities exist between L and R isozymes (72–75). Hepatocytes also exhibit

decreased PK activity (partially compensated by ongoing synthesis) in many cases of erythrocyte enzyme deficiency (76–82). The characteristics of the isozymes of PK are summarized in Figure 53-4 and Table 53-4.

M_2 is the principal form in fetal tissues (83). Partially purified red-cell PK is electrophoretically separable into two bands, homotetramer, R_1, and a heterotetramer, R_2, which are composed of two, paired, dissimilar subunits. R_1 and R_2 migrate apart from the L form, even though all three are antigenically identical (84–86). Decreased synthesis of fetal M_2 as erythroid precursors mature (87) allows replacement by R_1 in reticulocytes and young erythrocytes by R_2, the dominant form in mature erythrocytes (88–93). In some deficiency states, including the animal model in Basenji dogs, R forms may fail to develop properly, and the fetal isozyme persists (94–96). Persistence of M_2 may also be responsible for certain cases of PK hyperactivity (97,98).

The R_2 isozyme in mature erythrocytes is more stable than its precursor forms and has greater substrate avidity with more effective regulatory properties (99,100). The R_1 form is the dominant isozyme in reticulocytes. This isozyme has a decreased substrate affinity and stability as well as less effective feedback regulatory properties. The unfavorable kinetic properties of the R_1 form compared to the R_2 isozyme may explain, in part, why young cells are particularly vulnerable to metabolic impairment by mutant variants. This may also contribute to their selective destruction, in some cases, of PK deficiency (101). Reticulocytes possess the advantage of ATP generation through mitochondrial oxidative phosphorylation. But that process is greatly suppressed in the hypoxic and acidic environment of the spleen in which these cells may be detained because of their decreased deformability (102–104). Splenectomy in PK deficiency therefore may allow maturation and survival of reticulocytes that otherwise would have perished, which accounts for the paradoxical but characteristic increase in reticulocytosis despite decreased hemolysis (105).

The classic form of PK deficiency is associated with severe enzyme deficiency, persistence of the M_2 isozyme in mature erythrocytes, and little or no R_1 or R_2 isozymes. The persistence of the M_2 isozyme may represent an attempt to compensate for the lack of the L isozymes of PK (106). This is analogous to the persistence of fetal Hgb synthesis in β-thalassemia. When M_2 isozyme synthesis is low, PK activity is reduced, and hemolysis and anemia ensue. When the M_2 isozyme is synthesized at a higher rate, greater-than-normal amounts of PK activity can accumulate in mature red cells (107–111). Such patients have a lower 2,3 DPG level and increased Hgb oxygen affinity and may present with erythrocytosis.

STRUCTURE AND ALLOSTERIC PROPERTIES OF NORMAL AND MUTANT PYRUVATE KINASE

All normal tissue-specific isozymes, except for M_1, are subject to allosteric modulation by substrate or cofactors. The substrate, PEP, and a cofactor, the product of the PFK reaction, F1,6DP, increase substrate avidity of PK and convert the sigmoidal Michaelis-Menten kinetic curve to a hyperbolic one.

Additionally, potassium concentrations influence enzyme affinity for ADP, and the enzyme shows product inhibition by ATP. These kinetic properties follow the R→T transformation equilibrium model that was proposed by Monod et al. (112), where R represents relaxed, and T represents tight (see Chapter 49). The R conformation of the enzyme is induced by binding of the substrate, PEP, and the allosteric activator, F1,6DP, which cooperatively increase substrate affinity and catalytic activity. The T conformation exhibits a sigmoidal kinetic curve (Hill coefficient is approximately 1.5 to 2), with decreased substrate avidity and low catalytic activities at physiologic concentrations of PEP. The T conformation is also highly sensitive to inhibition by ATP.

TABLE 53-5. Hemolytic Anemia: Associated Symptoms and the Benefit of Splenectomy in Enzymopenic Hemolytic Anemias

Involved Enzyme	Apparent Degree of Residual Activity (%)[a]	Severity of Hemolysis	Associated Symptoms	Splenectomy	Blood Picture
Hexokinase	17–180	Mild to severe	Transient bone marrow aplasia	Inconsistent; recommended in severe cases	Macrocytosis
Glucose phosphate isomerase	4–60	Mild to severe	Some cases with neuromuscular impairment	Recommended; variable response	Macrocytosis
Phosphofructokinase M	8–62	Mild to moderate	± Myopathy[d]; hyperuricemia; arthritis	Not recommended	Basophilic stippling
Aldolase	5–16	Mild to severe	Myopathy; ± mental retardation	Recommended in a severe case	Nonspecific
Triosephosphate isomerase	5–20	Moderate	Always neuromuscular impairment; frequent infections; death before 5 yr of age	Not recommended[b]	Some target cells and small contracted cells
Phosphoglycerate kinase	0.7–15[c]	Moderate	± Convulsions, mental retardation, rhabdomyolysis	Inconsistent; mostly beneficial	Nonspecific
Pyruvate kinase	50–100	Mild to severe	Not described	Recommended; variable response	Macrocytosis; shrunken, spiculated cells[e]
Pyrimidine 5'-nucleotidase	5–15	Moderate; usually no transfusions	None	Partially beneficial	Basophilic stippling
Adenylate kinase	10–44	Moderate to severe	Psychomotor retardation?	Not described	Nonspecific
Adenosine deaminase overproduction	45- to 85-fold increase	Mild	None	Unnecessary	Nonspecific or stomatocytosis

[a]Compared to activity of normal red cells, residual activity may be much lower if it is related to reticulocyte-rich control.
[b]Increased infection; no significant improvement of hemolysis.
[c]Measured by the backward reaction.
[d]Glycogen storage disease type VII (Tarui's disease); the muscular symptoms comprise mainly myopathy and severe muscle cramps; the disease may be fatal in infancy.
[e]Severe defects show spherocytes, elliptocytes, and red-cell fragments (schistocytes) and somewhat resemble hereditary spherocytosis.

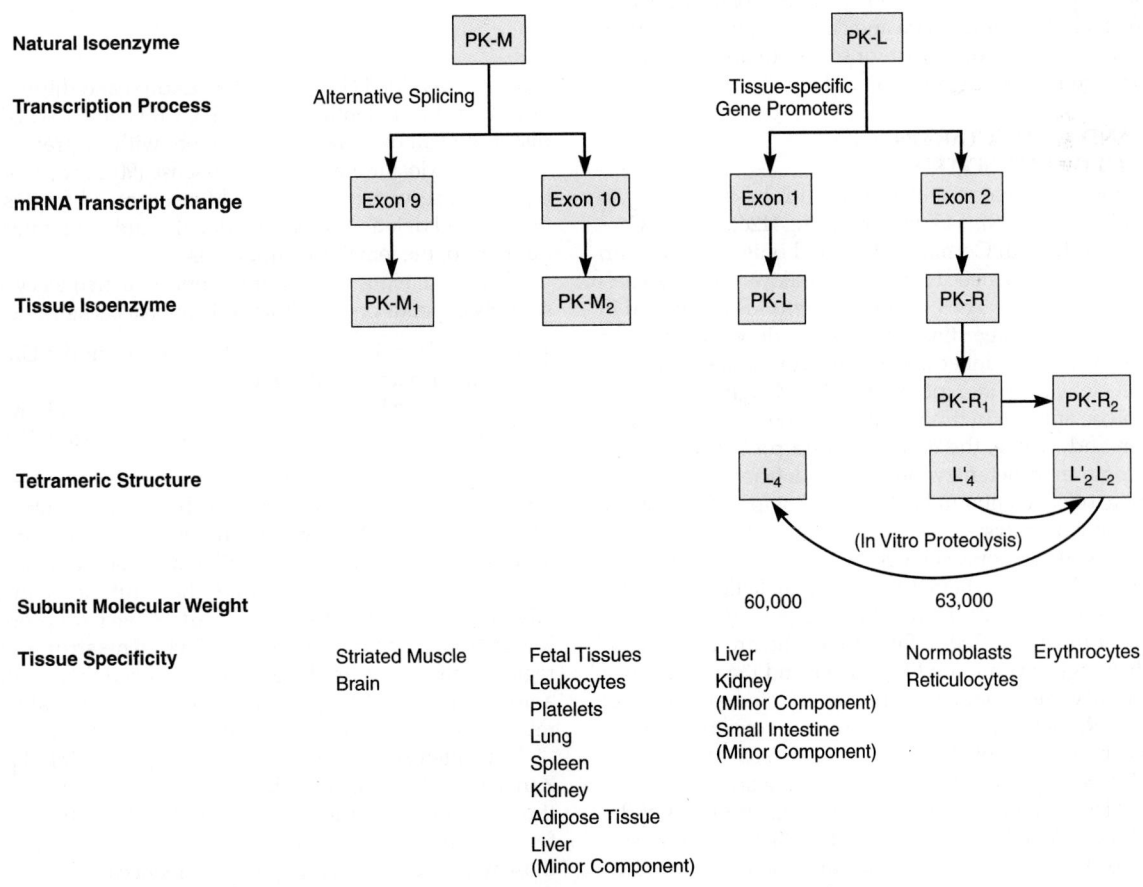

Figure 53-4. Characteristics of the natural isoenzymes of human pyruvate kinase.

PK mutations can be divided into two groups: One group is characterized by unfavorable kinetic properties, such as diminished affinity for PEP, or increased ATP inhibition. The other group shows favorable kinetics, opposite to the first group. Mutants with unfavorable kinetics are usually associated with more severe hemolysis (113–116).

Although the biochemical properties may be related to clinical severity, functional investigations of the mutant enzyme, such as reduced specific activity, decreased affinity for the substrate PEP, reduced stability, or an impaired capacity to respond to allosteric activation by F1,6DP, are rarely done. Indeed, biochemical characterizations have lost some of their importance, as long as the more readily identified molecular defect can be ascribed to a known domain of the enzyme molecule. Typical metabolic changes are given in Table 53-3.

The tetrameric structure with allosteric properties of the normal enzyme and a positive cooperativity on substrate binding reflect a highly ordered, symmetric, tertiary protein structure that is common to all the natural PK isozymes and shared by a number of other enzymes that possess helical α/β barrel configurations (117). The molecular structure of the PK monomer has been elucidated in the past and gives valuable insights into the functional domains, as well as the effect of mutations. Each monomeric subunit encompasses three principal domains: the A domain, with a classic $(\alpha/\beta)_8$ barrel topology; the small B domain that is characterized by an irregular β barrel; and the C-terminal C domain with an α/β topology. A fourth, small N-terminal domain is formed by a helix-turn-helix motif (118) (Fig. 53-5). X-ray analysis has identified the catalytic site, which is localized in the cleft between the A and B domains. The oligomeric assembly site resides between the A and C domains of opposite subunits of the tetramer. Analysis of the three-dimensional structure of the enzyme may help to predict the severity of the molecular defect. However, further biochemical data and clinical features of homozygous patients are needed, at least for some mutations, to allow a more precise genotype-phenotype correlation.

GENETICS AND MOLECULAR DEFECTS: RELATION TO DISEASE SEVERITY

Population studies estimate the incidence of PK heterozygosity to be 6% in Saudi Arabia (119), 3.4% in Hong Kong (120), 2.2% in Canton, China (121), 1.4% in Germany (122), and only 0.14% in Ann Arbor, Michigan (123). Genetic transmission follows an autosomal-recessive pattern. In a few cases, the defect seems to be inherited in a dominant way (124). Interestingly, we could reduce this apparent dominance to a recessive inheritance with a compound heterozygosity for PK deficiency in a mother and her daughter who had severe hemolytic anemia. In this family, the father was a heterozygous carrier, and, hence, the daughter (and probably also the mother) is compound heterozygous for PK deficiency. Homozygosity or, more often, compound heterozygosity for PK deficiency results in chronic hemolysis. Heterozygotes usually remain clinically normal despite an approximately 50% reduction in PK activity, but they may have mild hemolysis (125–128). Reticulocytes are slightly increased, up to 4.5%, in most heterozygotes (M. Lakomek, *personal communication*, 2000). Because of the broad range of molecular heterogeneity among PK variants and the infrequency of consanguinity, most patients who are affected are not true homozygotes. Rather, they are compound heterozygotes whose red cells contain mixtures of at least two mutant isozymic forms.

The PK-LR gene has been localized to the long arm of chromosome 1 (129). The genomic DNA and complementary DNA of the R-type have been cloned and sequenced (130–132). The gene contains 12 exons. Exons 3 through 12 are common to the two isoforms, whereas exons 1 and 2 are specific for the erythrocyte and the hepatic isozymes, respectively (133–135). The promoter region

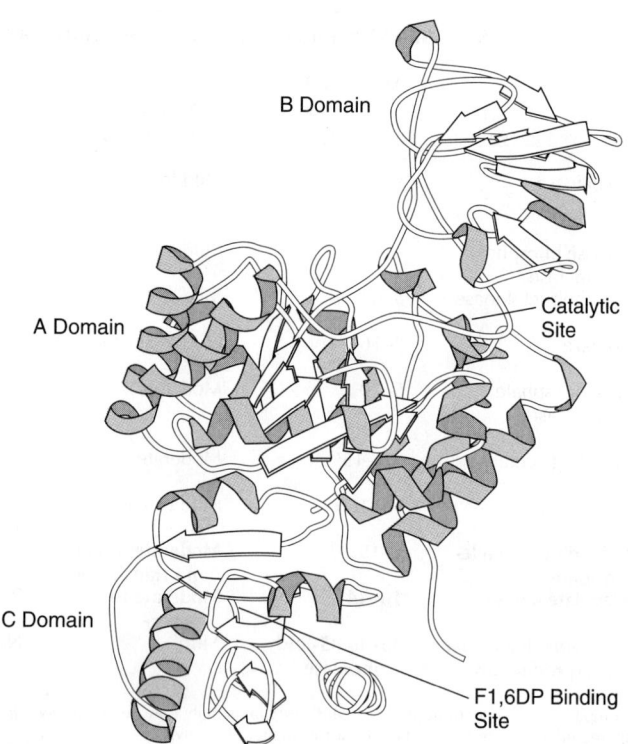

Figure 53-5. The pyruvate kinase monomer with the three principal domains and the functional catalytic and fructose-1,6-diphosphate (F1,6DP) binding site. Arrows represent β-sheet structures, and ribbons represent α-helix motifs. (From Zanella A, Bianchi P. Red cell pyruvate kinase deficiency: from genetics to clinical manifestations. *Best Pract Res Clin Haematol* 2000;13:57–81, with permission.)

has been identified (136,137). One hundred and thirty-three mutations have been identified in the PK-LR gene (138–142). They are distributed all over the coding region, with no preference for the active site. Most mutations are missense (90 out of 133) and affect highly conserved amino acids. Nonsense and frameshift mutations (small deletions and insertions) share approximately equal numbers of the remaining mutations.

Three mutations are common, but their frequency in patients strongly depends on the ethnic and regional background (Fig. 53-6).

- G1529A [Arg510Gln]: 41% of mutations in the United States of America and northern Europe.
- C1456T (Arg484Trp): 29% to 32% in southern Europe.
- C1468T (Arg490Trp): Predominant in the Eastern Hemisphere.

In the Western Hemisphere, approximately one-half of the mutations can be easily detected by Sty I restriction enzyme digestion of the PK-R gene. This makes a molecular genetic search for PK defects an attractive alternative to screening by enzyme activity measurement. Other mutations, in particular G721T (Glu241Ter) and G994A [Gly332Ser] are present with a lower frequency in whites (143,144). The strong ethnic and regional differences in the occurrence of certain mutations, even among patients of European origin, indicates that most of the mutations are younger than 1000 years A.D. (145).

In an attempt to relate the mutations to the clinical phenotype, Zanella and Bianchi (158) divided the patients into two groups: those with a mild phenotype (Hgb level greater than 9 g/dL, fewer than five transfusions, and possession of a spleen) and those with a severe phenotype (a presplenectomy Hgb level lower than 7 g/dL, more than 50 transfusions, or splenectomized, or a combination of these) (Table 53-6). Mild clinical signs were associ-

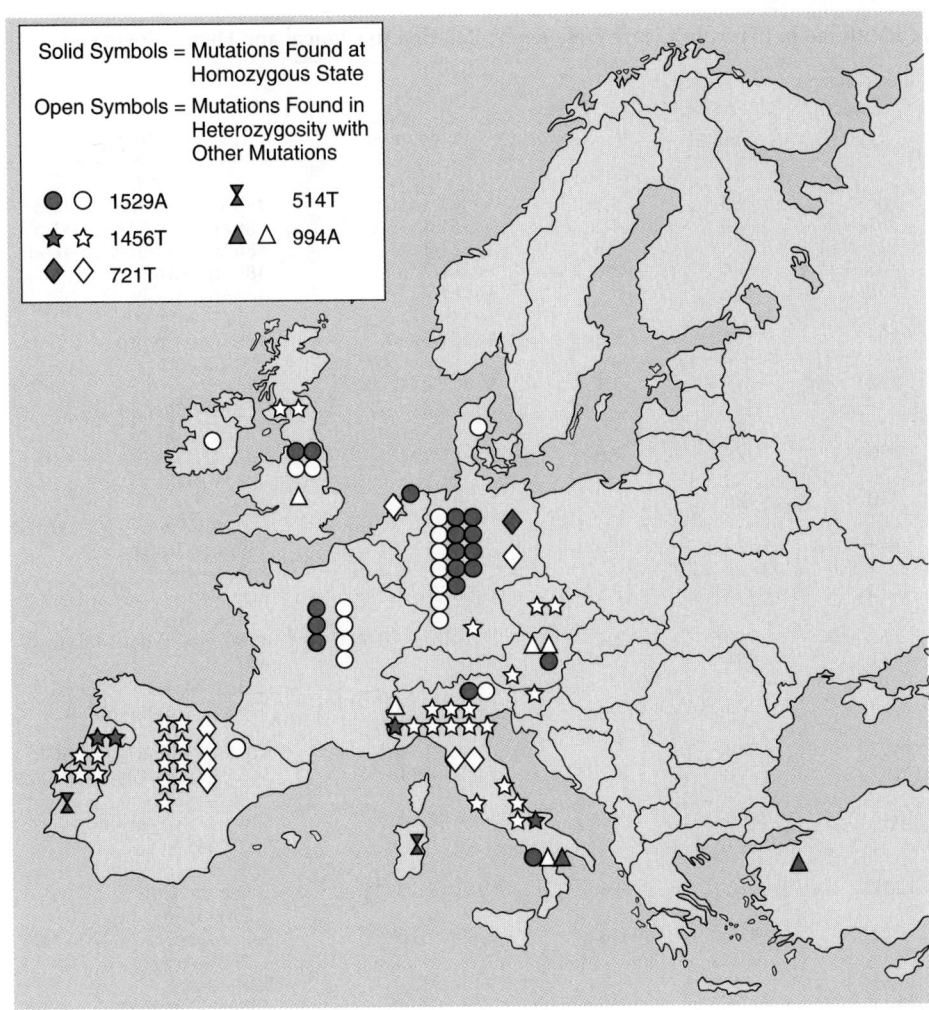

Figure 53-6. Geographic distribution of the most frequent European pyruvate kinase variants. (From Zanella A, Bianchi P. Red cell pyruvate kinase deficiency: from genetics to clinical manifestations. *Best Pract Res Clin Haematol* 2000;13:57–81, with permission.)

ated with compound heterozygosity for two missense mutations (with a prevalence of C1456T) or for one missense mutation and a more drastic mutation that involved the terminal exons (exons 11 and 12). Severe clinical expression was associated with:

- Disruptive mutations, such as a stop codon in the first part of the protein, or frameshift or splicing mutations.
- Missense mutations that involve the Aα7 helix near the catalytic site [C1181A (394Ala→ Asp), C1181T (394Ala→Val), and A1160G, even in association with a mild mutation such as C1456T]. The mutation A1160G (387Glu→Gly) severely reduces heat stability; mutation C1456T (486Arg→Trp) slightly increases the Michaelis-Menten dissociation constant (K_m) for PEP without affecting enzyme stability.
- Mutations G994A and G1529A in the homozygous state (146,147). Mutation G994A (332Gly→Ser) leads to a distinctly heat unstable variant enzyme with a moderate reduction of the K_m for PEP. Mutation G1529A (510Arg→Gln) has the lowest heat stability of all variant enzymes, but a normal K_m for PEP.

PATHOPHYSIOLOGY

The precise mechanism of increased hemolysis in PK deficient erythrocytes remains elusive (148,149). Impairment of glycolysis at the PK step, regardless of the molecular mechanism involved, results in decreased intracellular concentrations of total adenine nucleotides, decreased ATP generation, elevated concentrations of glycolytic intermediates above the blockade (particularly 2,3 DPG and 3PG), and decreased NAD and

NADH concentrations with altered ratios (Table 53-3). The ultimate proof of red cells with a clear-cut reduction of ATP content in PK deficiency is lacking. It might well be that only small numbers of a patient's aged red cells have a low ATP content shortly before their destruction and hence may escape detection. Concentrations of 2,3 DPG may double or triple, shifting the oxyhemoglobin dissociation curve sufficiently to help to compensate for the anemia by favoring tissue oxygenation. However, the high concentrations of 2,3-DPG inhibit HK activity, and this may contribute to the hemolytic process.

It is commonly believed that ATP depletion, through the impairment of some vital ATP-dependent reactions, initiates a series of events that lead to hemolysis. ATP-depleted cells lose large amounts of potassium and water and become dehydrated and rigid. Based on their shape change to echinocytes (more pronounced following splenectomy), a fraction of ATP-depleted red cells may release membrane in the form of cytoskeleton-free vesicles, as is known to occur *in vitro* in ATP-depleted red cells (150). Subsequently, stasis, acidosis, and hypoxia further inhibit the glycolytic activity and contribute to the entrapment and premature destruction of the poorly deformable red cells in the microcirculation of the reticuloendothelial system. This happens particularly in the spleen, liver, and bone marrow (151).

SYMPTOMS, DIAGNOSTIC PROBLEMS, AND THERAPY

PK deficiency is the most common cause of hereditary chronic nonspherocytic hemolytic anemia, with high prevalence in northern Europe (1:20,000; heterozygote frequency 1:70).

TABLE 53-6. Molecular Lesions That Are Identified in Pyruvate Kinase Deficiency: Relation to Clinical and Hematologic Data

Age at Diagnosis (yr)	Transfusion (U)	Hgb (g/dL)	Reticulocyte Count (10^9/L)	Serum Ferritin (µg/L)	PK Activity (IU/g Hgb)	Mutation	Effect
Mild phenotype							
16	3	10.4	166	88	4.5	1456T/1456T	486Arg→Trp/486Arg→Trp
30	0	11.6	167	140	4.2	1456T/1552A	486Arg→Trp/518Arg→Trp
31	0	12.5	123	810	3.6	1456T/1675T	486Arg→Trp/559Arg→End
19	0	10.0	303	94	2.8	1456T/?	486Arg→Trp/?
2	0	11.2	169	116	3	1456T/823A	486Arg/Trp/Gly 275→Arg
43	0	10.8	198	186	5.8	1456T/993A	486Arg→Trp/Asp 331→Glu
18	2	11.6	222	810	3.1	514C/514C	Glu 172→Gln/Glu 172→Gln
24	0	10.6	190	23	2.9	1594T/993A	532Arg→Trp/Asp 331→Glu
24	0	12.9	130	186	4	1168A/?	Asp 390→Asn/?
21	0	10.5	149	214	9	1456T/1151T	486Arg→Trp/Thr 384→Met
35	0	15.6	125	153	7.2	1456T/?	Arg 486→Trp/?
27	1	9.2	218	190	2.4	1456T/del 1042-1044	486Arg→Trp/del 348Lys
36	4	11.6	81	484	2.8	991A/?	Asp 331→Asp/?
13	0	11.2	88	75	2.6	1456T/dupl	486Arg→Trp/frameshift
Severe phenotype							
40	0	9.5	1452	540	1.3	1529A/1529A	510Arg→Gln/510Arg→Gln
12	>50	8.5	263	790	9.7	1529A/994A	510Arg→Gln/Gly 332→Ser
6	>50	7.4	1046	2800	3.5	994A/994A	Gly 332→Ser/ Gly 332→Ser
21	>100	7.4	1252	716	5.5	1VS3(-2)c/721T	Splice site/Glu 241→End
6	>100	8.3	113	436	2.8	1269C/787A	Splice site/Gly 263→Arg
6	>50	6.9	154	1440	8.3	del227-231/?	Frameshift/?
19	>100	8.0	1124	1174	2.6	1456T/1160G	486Arg→Trp/Glu 387→Gly
6	1	7.8	360	433	4.8	1456T/1181T	486Arg→Trp/Ala 394→Val
24	>100	8.9	949	612	13	1483A/1vs 6(-2)t	465Ala→Thr/del ex10
9 months	7	6.8	149	nd	15.6	1456T/1181A	486Arg→Trp/Ala 394→Asp
3 months	>50	6.1	249	828	9.5	721T/?	Glu 241→End/?
Reference values		12.2 to 16	24 to 84	15 to 355	11.1 to 15.5	—	—

Ala, alanine; Arg, arginine; Asp, aspartic acid; Gln, glutamine; Glu, glutamic acid; Gly, glycine; Hgb, hemoglobin; Lys, lysine; Met, methionine; nd, not determined; Ser, serine; Thr, threonine; Trp, tryptophan; Val, valine.
Adapted from Zanella A, Bianchi P. Red cell pyruvate kinase deficiency: from genetics to clinical manifestations. *Best Pract Res Clin Haematol* 2000;13:57–81, with permission.

Symptoms. Owing to multiple tissue isozymes, symptoms are restricted to those of chronic hemolytic anemia. The severity can vary from completely compensated asymptomatic cases to severe, transfusion-dependent, life-threatening anemia. The latter are often apparent during the neonatal period, together with severe precocious icterus. Exchange transfusions may be required. Severe deficiency may also be manifest by hydrops fetalis. In approximately 40% of the patients, a severe hemolytic anemia persists, and the patients require regular transfusions. The stresses of surgery, infections, and pregnancy have all been associated with acute exacerbations of the chronic hemolytic process. Aplastic crises may occur, particularly in association with parvovirus B19 (152,153). The spleen is distinctly enlarged. The concentration of unconjugated bilirubin is often increased, but is usually less than 6 mg/dL. A higher level suggests concomitant Gilbert syndrome. The haplotype 7/7 of the TATA box of the UGT-IA gene that is associated with Gilbert syndrome is found in most of these cases (154).

Rare complications include kernicterus, chronic leg ulcers, acute pancreatitis secondary to biliary and pancreatic duct obstruction, splenic abscess, spinal cord compression by extramedullary hematopoietic tissue, and migratory phlebitis with arterial thrombosis (155).

Diagnosis. The diagnosis of PK deficiency ultimately depends on the demonstration of an abnormal enzyme activity, as assessed by standard methods. The measurement should be done preferably at high and low PEP concentrations (156). Most anemic patients have approximately 5% to 40% of the normal level of PK activity. However, care must be taken before accepting an *in vitro* PK activity as normal. Contamination with normal donor cells in recently transfused patients, incomplete leukocyte removal (leukocytes

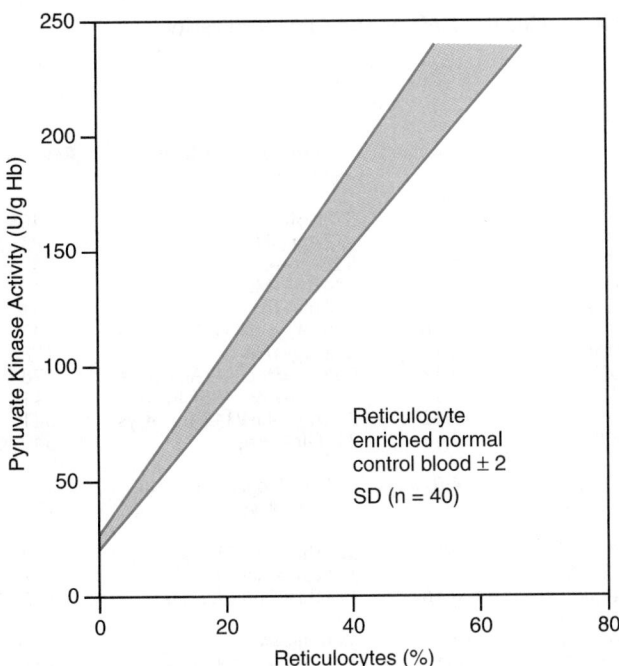

Figure 53-7. Diagnosis of pyruvate kinase deficiency: relationship of enzyme activity to reticulocyte count. Hb, hemoglobin; SD, standard deviation.

have another isozyme and a 300-fold higher PK activity than red cells), or a high reticulocyte number may result in false-normal red-cell PK activity. In particular, the enzyme activity in patients with reticulocytosis can be pseudonormal, and, therefore, the residual activity must be related to reticulocyte number in all cases (Fig. 53-7). In patients who are regularly transfused, the activity measurements in both parents can prove their heterozygous state and delineate the homozygous or compound heterozygous deficiency in their affected offspring. In most cases, red-cell morphology is of little value in diagnosing PK deficiency, but a number of isolated cases have been distinguished by prominent changes, including acanthocytes and echinocytes. These shape changes become more prominent after splenectomy. Echinocytes can be best demonstrated by phase contrast microscopy in fresh blood samples.

Differential Diagnosis. The differential diagnosis includes hereditary spherocytosis. Occasionally, the two disorders may be confused, because a small population of osmotically fragile red cells occur in PK deficiency, especially after 24 hours of incubation. Some PK patients with severe anemia also have an increased number of spherocytes on their blood smears. Patients with spherocytosis also tend to have lower PK activities for unknown reasons (M. Lakomek, personal observation, 2002). However, in contrast to PK deficiency, severe anemia is rarely present at birth in hereditary spherocytosis but rather develops in the first days of life. Hydrops fetalis is practically absent in spherocytosis.

Splenectomy, Transfusion Policy, and Treatment of Hemosiderosis. Due to the increased 2,3 DPG concentration, oxygen delivery to peripheral tissues is enhanced in PK deficiency. Thus, tissue oxygenation is relatively preserved even in severely anemic patients with hemoglobin values as low as 4 to 5 g/L. As a consequence, these patients may exhibit none of the expected symptoms of fatigue or exercise intolerance. Transfusions may be withheld in cases of hemolytic crises, until Hgb values as low as 4 to 5 g/dL are reached, as long as clinical symptoms are absent.

After infancy and early childhood, Hgb values often tend to stabilize at approximately 6 to 8 g/dL. In patients with severe chronic anemia whose Hgb values regularly drop below a level of 5 to 6 g/dL, transfusions should be done at approximately 6 to 7 g/dL. In severe cases, splenectomy often results in increased reticulocyte counts and Hgb concentrations, and the transfusion requirement is frequently reduced or eliminated. There are no criteria by which clinical responses can be reliably predicted. The steep rise of reticulocytes after splenectomy, which approaches 100% in rare cases, is a hallmark of PK deficiency.

Splenectomy is not advocated for children who are younger than 5 years of age, even if frequent transfusions are required to alleviate symptoms. The risk of iron overload during that period is relatively small compared to the potential hazard of postsplenectomy sepsis (see Chapters 21 and 51). Partial splenectomy has been performed in two patients with severe PK deficiency with a decent result (163a).

Iron administration is contraindicated, except in the rare event of concomitant iron deficiency. Owing to inefficient erythropoiesis, iron overload is common. It has been reported in more than one-half of nontransfused patients (157), particularly if they are splenectomized or heterozygous for hereditary hemochromatosis. Repeated courses of iron chelation therapy [preferably with desferrioxamine (see Chapters 46 and 48)] are necessary in approximately one-third of patients (158). Deaths are sometimes caused by hemochromatosis (159,160). After splenectomy, platelet counts are increased, and the risk of thrombophlebitis and thromboembolisms seems to be increased (161,162).

Bone marrow transplantation has been successfully performed in two patients with severe PK deficiency (163,163a). But with current myeloablative conditioning regimens, it cannot be recommended for most patients. Gene transfer therapies are still far away from clinical applicability (164,165).

Glucose Phosphate Isomerase Deficiency

Glucose phosphate isomerase

Glucose-6-phosphate $\rightleftharpoons$ Fructose-6-phosphate

CHARACTERISTICS OF GLUCOSE PHOSPHATE ISOMERASE DEFICIENCY

- Second most frequent glycolytic enzyme defect; frequent polymorphism in African-Americans (allele frequency, 0.27).
- Moderate to severe hemolytic anemia with distinct reticulocytosis.
- Variable response to splenectomy: usually no transfusion requirement afterwards.
- Some cases with associated neuromuscular symptoms.
- Increased level of glucose-6-phosphate (G6P) with feedback inhibition of HK.
- Macrocytosis; some cases with microspherocytes.

Other important clinical, genetic, and biochemical characteristics are given in Tables 53-3 through 53-5.

BIOCHEMICAL CHARACTERISTICS

Isomerization of G6P to fructose-6-phosphate is catalyzed by GPI (D-G6P ketol-isomerase, E.C.5.3.1.9). GPI deficiencies are the second most common glycolytic enzymopathies of erythrocytes, after PK. A single homodimeric enzyme of 134 kd (166–168) is present in humans and is encoded by a gene on chromosome 19q13.1 (169). Tissue-specific isozymes probably do not exist, and, hence, in severely deficient subjects, not only the red cells but also leukocytes, platelets, fibroblasts, liver, muscle, and, presumably,

TABLE 53-7. Glucose Phosphate Isomerase Deficiencies: Molecular Defects and Clinical Severity

Variant Name	Hemoglobin (g/dL)	Reticulocyte Count (%)	Glucose Phosphate Isomerase Activity (%)[a]	Genotype[c]	Exon(s)	Amino Acid Change	Reference
Mild/moderate anemia							
Matsumoto	8.6	6.5	41	14C→T/14C→T	1	5Thr→Ile	540
*	7.9	7.2	37	1415G→A/1415G→A	16	472Arg→His	183
Fukuoka	10.7	9.8	9	1615G→A/1615G→A	18	539Asp→Asn	540
Iwate	11.2	10.6	14	671C→T/671C→T	7	224Thr→Met	540
*	9.8	11	23	247C→T/247C→T	3	83Arg→Trp	541
*	8.7	11.2	13	833C→T/1459C→T	10/16	278Ser→Leu/ 487Leu→Phe	541
*	13.7	11.8	21	1415G→A/1415G→A	16	472Arg→His	178
*	9	14.2	25	286C→T/1039C→T	4/12	96Arg→Stop/347Arg→Cys	178
*	10.3	15	16	671C→T/1483G→A	7/17	224Thr→Met/495Glu→Lys	541
*	10.6	17	20	818G→A/1039C→T	10/12	273Arg→His/347Arg→Cys	541
Narita	8.8	23.6	38	1028A→G/1028A→G	12	343Gln→Arg	540
Severe anemia							
Bari	9.8	8.7[b]	21	286C→T/584C→T	4/6	96Arg→Stop/195Thr→Ile	177
Mount Scopus[d,e]	10	10	21	1039C→T/1039C→T	12	347Arg→Cys	178
Kinki	10.7	10.2	5	1124C→G/1615G→A	13/18	375Thr→Arg/539Asp→Asn	540
Sarsina[d,e]	13.2	10.2[b]	10	301G→A/301G→A	4	101Val→Met	177
Mola[d]	9.6	15.9[b]	17	584C→T/dell473-IVS16(+2)	6/16	195Thr→Ile/splice site	177
Morcone[d,e]	12	15.9	15	1028A→G/1028A→G	12	343Gln→Arg	177
*	10.6	17	20	818G→A/1039C→T	10/12	273Arg→His/347Arg→Cys	541
Homburg[d,e]	13.3	17.5	4	59A→C/1016T→C	1/12	20His→Pro/339Leu→Pro	180
Calden[d]	11	20	15	1166A→G/1549C→G	13/18	389His→Arg/517Leu→Val	180
*	8.8	20.6	60	970G→A/970G→A	12	324Gly→Ser	183
Stuttgart[d]	7.1	21.6	33	43C→T/1028A→G	1/12	15Gln→Stop/343Gln→Arg	183
Elyria[e]	10.2	24	5	223A→G/286C→T	3/4	75Arg→Gly/96Arg→Stop	178
*[d]	8.7	32	27	898G→C/1039C→T	11/12	300Ala→Pro/347Arg→Cys	178
Zwickau[e]	10	32.6	22	1039C→T/1538G→A	12/17	347Arg→Cys/513Trp→Stop	543
Nordhorn[d,e]	8.5	45	10	1028A→G/IVS15(-2)A→C	12/IVS15	343Gln→Arg/splice site	543
*	Δ	Δ	Approximately 12	475G→A/1040G→A	5/12	159Gly→Ser/374Arg→His	542
*	Δ	Δ	Approximately 6	1574T→C/1574T→C	18	525Ile→Thr	542
Reference values	12 to 18	0.5 to 1.5	100	—	—	—	—

*, variant has no name; Δ, not known; Ala, alanine; Arg, arginine; Asn, asparagine; Asp, aspartic acid; Cys, cysteine; Gln, glutamine; Glu, glutamic acid; Gly, glycine; His, histidine; Ile, isoleucine; Leu, leucine; Lys, lysine; Met, methionine; nd, not determined; Phe, phenylalanine; Pro, proline; Ser, serine; Thr, threonine; Trp, tryptophan; Val, valine.
[a]Corrected glucose phosphate isomerase activity, considering the reticulocyte counts.
[b]Approximately converted into percent.
[c]Reference sequence is GenBank acc. No. K03515 and S81084.OMIM; reference is 172400 (http://www.ncbi.nlm.nih.gov/Omim).
[d]Multiple transfusions until splenectomy.
[e]Splenectomized.

other tissues possess decreased GPI activity (170). In the red cell, posttranslational deamidation of asparagine residues leads to three electrophoretic forms (171). GPI deficiency leads to an increase of the G6P level, which causes feedback inhibition of HK and results in a lower rate of glycolysis. As a consequence, generation of ATP and 2,3 DPG decrease. Biochemical changes include a severely impaired (less than 10%) ability to redirect fructose-6-phosphate into the HMS (172–174). This may be responsible for the increased susceptibility of GPI deficient red cells to develop oxidant-induced glutathione instability and oxidant-induced Heinz body formation and for the occasional reports of acute, hyperhemolytic episodes in GPI deficient patients.

GENETICS, MOLECULAR DEFECT, AND CLINICAL SEVERITY

Approximately 50 cases of GPI deficiency have been reported worldwide. The inheritance is invariably autosomal recessive and heterozygous carriers are hematologically unaffected. Twenty-nine different mutations have been described so far, and only seven of them occurred in more than one family. Most mutations are of the missense type and involve highly conserved amino acids (Table 53-7). Patients are mostly compound heterozygotes who have

inherited two different defective GPI alleles, but some true homozygotes have been described (e.g., GPI Mount Scopus, GPI Narita, and GPI Morcone) (175). So far, the molecular defect has been identified in 27 cases (175). Homozygosity has only been described for missense mutations, which is compatible with the concept that homozygous null mutations are lethal. Null mutations are only found in compound heterozygotes in association with a missense mutation on the second allele (Table 53-7).

A phenotype-genotype relation in GPI deficiency is difficult to discern. Some mutations that have been given different names on the basis of their biochemical characteristics are actually the same molecular defect, such as GPI Narita and GPI Morcone. Interestingly, homozygosity for that mutation results in hemolytic anemia that ranges from moderate to severe. Furthermore, each variant shows distinct kinetics and electrophoretic mobility (177). The same holds true for the mutation 1415A, which yielded a mild anemia in an Hispanic patient (178) and a more severe form in a Turkish patient (179). This phenomenon indicates that other modifying factors exist beyond the molecular defect that modifies disease severity (e.g., different genetic background, environmental factors, different splenic function, iron overload, or ineffective erythropoie-

TABLE 53-8. Glucose Phosphate Isomerase (GPI): A Multifunctional Protein

	GPI	Neuroleukin	Autocrine Motility Factor	Maturation Factor
Complementary deoxy-ribonucleic acid	1.9 kilobase	Identical to GPI	Identical to GPI	Identical to GPI
Protein	63 kd	56 kd	57 kd	54.3 kd
Subunit	Homodimer	Monomer	Monomer	Monomer
Distribution	Ubiquitous	Secreted by lecithin-stimulated T cells	Confined to transformed cells	Produced by activated T cells
Function(s)	Glycolytic enzyme Dimer is inactive as a neurotrophic factor; monomer has growth factor activity Stimulates cell motility Has the differentiation property for leukemic cells	Neurotrophic growth factor Capability to induce differentiation and antiproliferative activity Affects B-cell immunoglobulin synthesis	Stimulates cell motility and growth Exhibits GPI activity	Induces differentiation Exhibits GPI activity

Adapted from Kugler W, Lakomek M. Glucose-6-phosphate isomerase deficiency. *Best Pract Res Clin Haematol* 2000;13:89–101, with permission.

sis). In compound heterozygotes, such as GPI Homburg (180), the situation is even more complex, as dimers of dissimilar subunit composition (heterodimers) are found as well as homodimers. The possible interaction between two different mutant polypeptides in the dimeric holoenzyme may influence the phenotypic outcome, but, so far, this is only a theoretical possibility.

CLINICAL SYMPTOMS AND RELATIONSHIP TO BIOCHEMICAL AND MOLECULAR CHARACTERISTICS OF DEFECTIVE ENZYME

The reduced flux through the HMS might explain cases of drug-induced hemolysis (e.g., after administration of acetylsalicylic acid, nitrofurantoin, and neuroleptics), which has been observed in some GPI deficient cases (181,182).

The residual GPI activity in defective red cells ranges from 4% to 60% (average, 10%) and must be related to the reticulocyte count. Without that correction, apparently normal GPI activity can be found in severely anemic patients (183) (Table 53-7). Virtually all of the reported mutant gene products have marked instability. Cells that are capable of protein synthesis may compensate for this lability by increased enzyme production. Erythrocytes do not share this capacity and consequently are eliminated prematurely, if glycolysis is sufficiently impaired. Thus, in most cases, hemolytic anemia is the only clinical manifestation of this multisystem disorder, although myopathy and mental retardation are sometimes observed (184–186). The anemia varies from mild to severe in homozygotes and compound heterozygotes. Severe GPI deficiency can be associated with hydrops fetalis and immediate neonatal death (187,188). Several patients have experienced hyperhemolytic crises after infection or drug exposure (189–197). Iron overload may complicate the clinical course, especially after splenectomy, and monitoring of iron status is necessary. Neurologic impairment has been found in five cases: GPI Utrecht (198), GPI Paris (199), GPI Homburg (200–202), GPI Mount Scopus (203,204), and a variant that was described by Zanella et al. (205). In the latter case, at 14 months of age, the patient had thalassemic facies and muscular hypotonia and was mentally retarded. The patient with GPI Utrecht (206,207) exhibited hepatomegaly that was associated with excessive glycogen storage in the liver. This was attributed to G6P accumulation, as a result of the enzyme defect, which promoted the deposition of more glycogen than normal. In addition, the child was mentally retarded and had abnormal physical stigmata, a tower skull, and yellow teeth. In the patient with GPI Homburg (208–210), muscle weakness, ataxia, dysarthria, and

mental retardation accompanied the defect. Histologic examination showed pathologic muscle changes: nonspecific fiber degeneration with mitochondrial abnormalities in particular inclusion bodies and excessive accumulation of glycogen, as well as reduced GPI activity. On histologic staining *in situ*, all muscle fibers showed decreased GPI activity (211).

MOLECULAR BASIS OF NEUROLOGIC SYMPTOMS THAT ARE SOMETIMES ASSOCIATED WITH GLUCOSE PHOSPHATE ISOMERASE DEFICIENCY

GPI is a multifunctional protein, which may explain why it is associated with other neuromuscular and, possibly, increased hepatic glycogen storage in some cases. Besides its glycolytic activity in red cells, it serves as a neurotrophic factor, which is called *neuroleukin* (NLK), in cultures of skeletal motor and sensory neurons. In addition, GPI-NLK shares sequence homology with the maturation inducer for human myeloid leukemia cells (maturation factor) and the tumor cell autocrine motility factor (Table 53-8). It is possible that GPI deficiency is responsible for the neurologic symptomatology of these patients: The involvement of GPI-NLK in neurologic processes is exemplified by the finding that serum-containing GPI-NLK inhibits the terminal axonal sprouting of motor neurons from patients with amyotrophic lateral sclerosis (212).

In a bioassay, the relationship between GPI and NLK activity can be clarified (213). Only the dimeric enzyme possesses catalytic (GPI) activity, and it has no NLK activity, whereas the monomer shows the neurotrophic (NLK) activity. Kugler and Lakomek (214) speculate that mutations in the GPI gene that lead to incorrect folding of the monomer destroy catalytic (GPI) and neurotrophic (NLK) activity, thereby leading to anemia and neurologic impairment [as shown by GPI Homburg (215–217)].

SPLENECTOMY

Splenectomy is indicated in patients with prolonged severe anemia who require frequent transfusions. There is usually no further requirement for transfusions postsplenectomy (218–221); however, the response is unpredictable in individual cases, and anemia and marked reticulocytosis (36% to 73%) (222) may persist.

Triosephosphate Isomerase Deficiency

Triosephosphate isomerase

Dihydroxyacetone phosphate $\rightleftharpoons$ Glyceraldehyde-3-phosphate

CHARACTERISTICS OF TRIOSEPHOSPHATE ISOMERASE DEFICIENCY

- Progressive neuromuscular impairment; cardiomyopathy.
- Death from respiratory infection, mostly before 6 years of age.
- Moderate hemolytic anemia, starting from birth.
- Severe reduction of enzyme activity.
- Massive accumulation of DHAP.
- Most frequent in African-Americans (possibly 4% to 5% are heterozygotes).
- Founder effect (approximately 50% of cases with 104Glu→Asp).
- Mimics mitochondrial enzymopathies.

CONSEQUENCES OF TRIOSEPHOSPHATE ISOMERASE ENZYME DEFECT ON LIPID METABOLISM AND MEMBRANE COMPOSITION (223)

- Increased fatty acid chain mobility in the lipid bilayer of red cells, ghosts, and inside-out membrane vesicles.
- Changes in the composition of major phospholipid subclasses.
- Decrease in membrane alkenylacyl-phosphatidylethanolamines (phosphoethanolamine plasmalogens) in red cells and, presumably, neural tissue (224,225).
- Increased activity of erythrocyte acetylcholinesterase and Ca^{2+}-adenosine triphosphatase (226).
- Increased binding of TPI to central nervous system (CNS) tubulin (227).
- Free radicals possibly involved: a therapeutic trial with docosahexaenoic acid may be warranted.

TPI (D-glyceraldehyde-3-phosphate ketol-isomerase, E.C.5.3.1.1) catalyzes the interconversion of DHAP and G3P. Both are cleavage products of F1,6DP. The reaction equilibrium favors DHAP. Thus, as G3P is an intermediate in the main glycolytic pathway, TPI serves to feed DHAP into the pathway.

TPI is a dimeric enzyme molecule of 53 kd with identical subunits of 248 amino acids (228) and is structurally encoded by a single gene on the short arm of chromosome 12 (229,230). All tissues share a common enzyme, and, therefore, all are affected to some degree in deficiency states. Multiple electrophoretic forms apparently result from posttranslational modifications (231,232). The enzyme defect was first described by Schneider et al. (233). Null alleles have been detected in a number of heterozygous subjects who exhibit half-normal activities and half-normal amounts of immunologically cross-reacting protein (234,235).

PATHOPHYSIOLOGY: METABOLIC BLOCK

An increase of DHAP concentration of up to 50-fold is the hallmark of the metabolic block (236,237) and is presumably closely related to the cause of the disease. The exact pathophysiologic consequences of this block are unclear. In view of the mitochondrial changes that were found in one patient, it is tempting to assume that the cellular energy supply is in some way hampered. For example, the shift of substrates from the cytosol to the mitochondria may be diminished. Or, the high concentration of DHAP may be toxic for the neuromuscular tissue. Several observations indicate that lipid metabolism is disturbed in TPI deficient cells. Although still unproven, it is conceivable that lipid-rich organs, such as the brain and the peripheral neurons, are primarily affected.

GENETICS

The predominant founder effect of the 104Glu→Asp mutation and studies of genotype-phenotype relationships show a remarkably high frequency of the heterozygous state in African-Americans,

Germans, and Japanese (0.1% to 5.0%) (238,239). The extreme rarity of the homozygous state may be due to early fetal loss, with only the least affected surviving to birth. Nine different missense mutations but only three null mutations have been identified. Almost one-half of the patients have the same 104Glu→Asp mutation. The importance of 104Glu to the enzyme structure and function is indicated by its conservation through all species. This mutation results in a thermolabile enzyme. It can easily be detected on DdeI restriction-enzyme digestion of genomic DNA. Family studies of all patients worldwide reveal that this mutation is in complete linkage dysequilibrium with an intragenic polymorphism (240–242) and a polymorphic 162–base pair short-tandem repeat sequence in the CD4 gene (243–245). The CD4 gene lies telomeric to the TPI gene. The close association of the mutation with the same polymorphic alleles strongly supports the assumption that all families with patients who express the 104 TPI mutation descend from a common ancestor (246,247), who may have lived in England or France more than 1000 years ago. In addition to the missense mutations, three mutations in the putative promoter region (248,249) have been identified with a high frequency (41%) in African-Americans (250), which probably accounts for moderately decreased TPI activity. These mutations probably represent frequent polymorphisms rather than a heterozygous state for the disease. Probably, these polymorphisms have led to the possibly erroneous assumption that the frequency of heterozygotes is as high as 5% in African-Americans (251), a conclusion that could not be confirmed by Schneider (252,253). The possible role, if any, of these variants in clinical TPI deficiency requires further investigation.

The structure of the TPI protein has been evaluated and permits assignment of the known mutations to functional domains of the enzyme. Structure-function studies have led to an increased understanding of the impaired catalysis (254–256). Computer models indicate that the Glu at position 104 is buried in a hydrophilic side pocket of the normal enzyme. The substitution of aspartate in the most frequent TPI mutation (104Glu→Asp) would reduce the stability of the pocket, promote unfolding, and enhance thermolability (257).

CLINICAL SYMPTOMS, PRENATAL DIAGNOSIS, AND OUTLOOK FOR A FUTURE THERAPY

The clinical consequences of severe TPI deficiency are unanimously dominated by a severe degenerative neurologic disorder with spasticity. Symptoms include tremor, dystonia, myopathy, and spastic cerebral palsy. These signs usually become apparent within the first year of life, and the clinical symptoms inevitably progress during childhood, with few children surviving to adulthood. The patients have an increased susceptibility to infections, which may reflect leukocyte involvement. However, abnormalities in phagocytic and bactericidal function have not been demonstrated. Arrhythmia and sudden death occur, presumably as a consequence of cardiac muscle involvement. Muscle biopsy in one case revealed a degenerative myopathy, an increase in intracellular glycogen level, and mitochondrial changes similar to those found in mitochondrial myopathies (258,259). The hemolytic anemia that is associated with TPI deficiency is moderate to severe and is not effectively ameliorated by splenectomy.

Regarding the severity of the multiorgan disease, prenatal diagnosis is indicated in a family with one affected child and has been successfully performed in several laboratories.

Recent work by Ationu et al. (260–264) indicates the possibility of enzyme transfer into deficient cells or stimulation of TPI messenger RNA (mRNA) expression. It has been suggested that TPI deficiency might be a candidate disease for enzyme replacement therapy into neuronal cells via peripheral blood stem cell transplantation. However, up to now, no clinical trial has been performed.

Hexokinase Deficiency

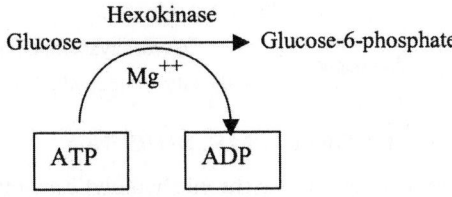

Hexokinase
Glucose ⟶ Glucose-6-phosphate
Mg^{++}
ATP   ADP

CHARACTERISTICS OF HEXOKINASE DEFICIENCY

- Lowest activity of glycolytic enzymes: rate-limiting step of glycolysis.
- Severe hemolytic anemia in 33% of cases.
- Transient bone marrow aplasia.
- Symptoms of anemia may be aggravated by reduced tissue-oxygen delivery.
- Twenty percent dominant inheritance; 20% sporadic; 60% recessive.
- Enzyme activity depends strongly on reticulocyte numbers: possibly pseudonormal activity in severe defects.
- Low platelet HK activity.
- Macrocytosis; occasionally spiculated cells.

HK (ATP:D-hexose-6-phosphotransferase, E.C.2.7.1.1) is responsible for priming the glycolytic pump by its phosphorylation of glucose to G6P. This enzyme has the lowest activity of all glycolytic enzymes in mature erythrocytes, and its catalytic rate is highly sensitive to pH, to intracellular concentrations of its product, G6P, and to other metabolites, such as inorganic phosphate, 2,3 DPG, and disulfide compounds. By virtue of these characteristics of HK, the phosphorylation of glucose becomes an important, potentially rate-limiting step in glycolysis.

Because of its crucial importance to the initiation of glycolysis, it was generally assumed that serious hereditary defects in this enzyme would be lethal mutations, but a small group of deficient cases with diverse ethnic origins has been detected (265–280).

HEXOKINASE ISOZYMES AND INHERITANCE OF DEFECTS

At least four distinct, tissue-specific isoenzymes of HK are normally identifiable, depending on methods of separation and purification. These have been designated HK-1 through HK-4 (281). Each isozyme is encoded by a different gene (282). Subtypes of HK-1 are present in erythrocytes (283–285), including one that predominates in reticulocytes and is presumably responsible for the steep, biphasic, decay curve that is observed as reticulocytes mature and erythrocytes age (286). This complicates diagnosis of HK deficiency in blood samples that are heavily populated by reticulocytes and young cells. Indeed, the deficiency can be masked by a high reticulocyte count. It is crucial to match the residual activity with that of a reticulocyte-rich control. Careful leukocyte depletion is obligatory before the measurements, owing to the high activity of HK in leukocytes (287). HK-1 is also found in brain but differs from the isozymes that are found in other blood cells and tissues.

A wide range of molecular heterogeneity exists among the abnormal HK-1 isozymes that have been reported. Most variants exhibit reduced activity and decreased substrate affinity, but heterogeneity is also reflected by alterations in thermostability, electrophoretic migration rates, and variable regulatory responses to G6P, glucose-1,6-diphosphate, 2,3 DPG, and inorganic phosphate. Decreased production of apparently normal enzyme protein has also been reported (288).

Most HK defects are inherited in an autosomal-recessive mode. Heterozygous deficiency states are without apparent effect on red-cell function or longevity, although minor decreases in ATP and some glycolytic intermediates have been observed.

However, a dominant transmission pattern has been observed in three families (289,290). As the molecular defect in these families is still unknown, it is unclear whether the hemolytic anemia is actually caused by heterozygous HK mutation. An animal model exists in the Downeast Anemia (dea) mouse (290a).

CLINICAL SYMPTOMS, PRENATAL DIAGNOSIS, AND SPLENECTOMY

Seventeen families with HK deficiency have been reported. Hemolysis is mostly moderate, but severe hemolytic anemia may occur. Several HK-deficient subjects showed multiple malformations (291,292), psychomotor retardation (293,294), or periventricular leukomalacia (295). However, it is unclear whether these manifestations are directly related to the HK-1 deficiency. Erythrocyte HK deficiency may also occur as one of the multiple abnormalities in Fanconi's anemia (296).

Clinical symptoms of anemia can be accentuated by the unfavorable metabolic consequences of HK deficiency, such as a decreased concentration of 2,3-DPG with a resulting increased oxygen affinity and a diminished tissue oxygen supply. Indeed, the patient that was studied by Delivoria-Papadopoulos et al. (297), as well as by Oski et al. (298), had an increased oxygen affinity (oxygen half-saturation pressure of Hgb) of 19 mm Hg (normal equals 27 mm Hg, plus or minus 1.2 mm Hg) and was capable of only minimal exercise, despite only moderate anemia (Hgb of 9.8 g/dL). Transient bone marrow aplasia, induced by certain infections, may lead to anemia even in mild cases, as well as to exacerbations of anemia in severely affected patients. Besides anemia, no clinical manifestations occur in other organs, although platelet activity is low. In severe cases with transfusion requirements, splenectomy may have some benefit (299–303).

HK-1 gene mutations in have been reported in HK deficient patients with hemolytic anemia. Prenatal diagnosis in a fetus with severe hemolytic anemia, intrauterine growth retardation, and progressive brain damage were described by Kanno et al. (304). The fetus was homozygous for a 9.5-kilobase intragenic deletion that flanked exons 5 and 8 of the HK-1 gene. This mutation causes virtually the absence of normal HK-1 enzyme. It is assumed that the null expression of the HK-1 gene caused fetal death, possibly because of serious metabolic disturbance in both the CNS and erythrocytes (305).

Phosphofructokinase Deficiency

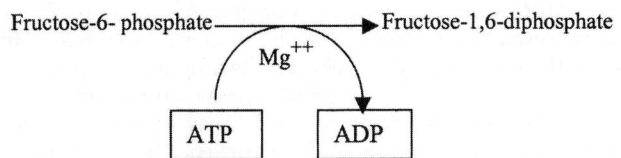

Phosphofructokinase
Fructose-6- phosphate ⟶ Fructose-1,6-diphosphate
Mg^{++}
ATP   ADP

CHARACTERISTICS OF PHOSPHOFRUCTOKINASE DEFICIENCY

- Affects muscle or red cells, or both.
- Predominant myopathy and hyperuricemia in more than 50% of cases.
- Mild to moderate hemolytic anemia.
- Red-cell PFK is an equal mixture of genetically different muscle (M)–type and liver (L)–type enzymes.
- Only M-type defects cause hemolytic anemia.
- Newborns have 50% to 60% of the activity of adult red cells.
- One of the ATP-consuming steps of glycolysis.

PFK (ATP:D-fructose-6-phosphate 1-phosphotransferase, E.C.2.7.1.11) may be the most important enzyme regulating erythrocyte glycolysis. Beyond HK, PFK occupies a further rate-limiting position in the earliest stage of glycolysis, and its activity responds to complex and subtle modulations by a number of metabolites and ions, including ATP, ADP, AMP, 2,3 DPG, F1,6DP and fructose-2,6-diphosphate (306–311). Additionally, the product of this essentially irreversible reaction, F1,6DP, is the principal allosteric activator of another crucial rate-limiting enzyme in terminal glycolysis, PK. Newborns have 50% to 60% of the activity of adult red cells.

PHOSPHOFRUCTOKINASE ISOZYMES AND MOLECULAR DEFECTS

Red-cell PFK is a mixture of genetically different M-type and L-type enzymes. A third isozyme (F or P type) occurs in fibroblasts and platelets (312–321). The two erythrocyte isozymes (M and L) contribute equally to red-cell activity. Homo- or heterotetramers exist in red cells in all possible associations: L_4, L_3M_1, L_2M_2, L_1M_3, and M_4. Red-cell PFK deficiency may be caused by a defect of the PFK-L or the PFK-M subunit. In patients with a complete absence of the M subunit (Tarui's disease, see the following discussion), biopsies of muscle show a complete lack of PFK activity (because the skeletal muscle isozyme is the homotetramer M_4), whereas red cells have approximately 50% of normal activity (exclusively, the L-type isozyme).

Recently 15 different molecular defects (eight missense mutations) have been identified in the PK-M gene (322–332). There is a naturally occurring animal model in an English springer spaniel, caused by a nonsense mutation in the PK-M gene (333).

MYOPATHY AND HEMOLYTIC ANEMIA AS CONSEQUENCES OF THE METABOLIC BLOCK

The absence of M subunits in the classic form of PFK deficiency (Tarui's disease) (334) leads to exercise-induced myopathy with severe muscle cramps. This is the predominant feature of PFK deficiency, being present in more than one-half of patients. The disease may be fatal in infancy. Tarui's disease is characterized by glycogen deposition in skeletal muscle (glycogen storage disease type VII), and results in exercised-induced muscle weakness, cramping, and myoglobinuria, sometimes complicated by hyperuricemia and early-onset gout (334). This disorder, which is most frequent in patients of Japanese or Russian Ashkenazi ancestry, closely resembles type V muscle glycogenosis (McArdle's disease), but severe symptoms usually manifest in childhood. The decreased 2,3 DPG synthesis that results from the metabolic block probably contributes to exercise-induced symptoms by the reduction of oxygen delivery. No specific therapy for this disorder is known. In contrast to McArdle's disease, glucagon or glucose infusions do not improve exercise tolerance. Avoidance of strenuous exercise is the key to the prevention of severe muscle fatigue, cramping, and rhabdomyolysis, as well as aggravation of hyperuricemia.

Mild to moderate hemolytic anemia may be associated with myopathy or may occur alone. The tissue-specific distribution of isozymes can explain the variety of symptoms. Clinical symptoms may be absent, despite a severe reduction of enzyme activity. In Tarui's disease (334) erythrocyte PFK activity is reduced to approximately one-half of normal. This results in decreased concentrations of distal glycolytic intermediates, including 2,3 DPG, which can alter the oxygen dissociation curve of Hgb sufficiently to induce erythrocytosis. The hemolytic process therefore may be well compensated by erythrocytosis, and such patients may be hematologically asymptomatic (334,338,339). Defects in PFK activity due to unstable M subunits may impair red-cell glycolysis sufficiently to result in clinically detectable hemolysis without myopathy (340–343).

In patients with mild to moderate hemolysis, there seems to be no clinical indication for splenectomy. Severe anemia is managed with red-cell transfusions (344).

Aldolase Deficiency

Fructose-1,6-diphosphate $\xrightleftharpoons[]{\text{Aldolase}}$ Dihydroxyacetone phosphate + Glyceraldehyde-3-phosphate

CHARACTERISTICS OF ALDOLASE DEFICIENCY

- Mild to moderately severe chronic hemolytic anemia.
- Hemolysis that is exacerbated during infections.
- Myopathy with exercise intolerance and rhabdomyolysis.
- Missense mutations with thermolabile mutant enzyme.

Aldolase, specifically fructose-diphosphate Aldolase (D-fructose-1,6-bisphosphate D-glyceraldehyde-3-phosphate lyase, E.C.4.1.2.13), reversibly catalyzes the equilibrium between F1,6DP and its component trioses, DHAP and G3P. It is also a tetrameric enzyme that totals approximately 158 kd, and three tissue-specific isozymes (A, B, and C) have been described (345,346).

Isozyme A occurs in red cells. In addition, it is expressed in muscle and together with isozyme C in the brain. Its gene has been localized to the 16q22-q24 region (347). The complementary DNA sequence comprises 1375 nucleotides, with an open reading frame of 1092 nucleotides that code for 363 amino acids.

Three missense mutations of the Ald A gene have been described: 386 A→G, which results in the replacement 128Asp→Gly (348,349); 619G→A [206Glu→Lys] (350), and 1183G→A [338Cys→Tyr] (350a), plus a single nonsense mutation 1077C→T [303Arg→Stop] (350a). The mutation 128Asp→Gly (351,352) changes an amino acid residue that is conserved in all Aldolase isozymes and thus may have a crucial role in the maintenance of the conformational structure and catalytic function. The two Aldolase mutant enzymes that were tested were thermolabile and exhibited decreased affinity for the substrate, F1,6DP (353,354).

CLINICAL SYMPTOMS

Severe deficiency states of Ald A have been reported in four unrelated families, which conforms to an autosomal-recessive mode of inheritance. The enzyme defect produces mild to severe chronic hemolytic anemia (355–359). Hemolysis is exacerbated during infections.

Beyond increased hemolysis, Ald A deficiency was found to be the cause of inherited metabolic myopathy in two cases (350a,360). The myopathy was characterized by exercise intolerance and rhabdomyolysis. One of these patients died due to hyperkalemia and rhabdomyolysis during a febrile illness (350a).

In a third case, mild hemolysis with multiple congenital malformations, mental retardation, and glycogen storage disease were present. The relationship of these defects to the Aldolase deficiency is uncertain (361).

In a fourth family, moderately severe chronic hemolysis alone was observed (362).

Phosphoglycerate Kinase Deficiency

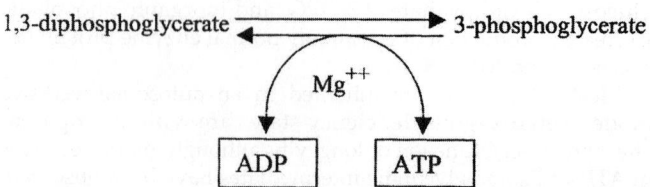

CHARACTERISTICS OF PHOSPHOGLYCERATE KINASE DEFICIENCY

- Sole glycolytic enzyme defect with X-chromosomal inheritance.
- Moderately severe hemolytic anemia.
- Hemolytic crises that are triggered by infections.
- Severe defects (40% of cases) associated with seizures, psychomotor retardation, movement disorders, aphasia, and hemiplegia.
- Rhabdomyolysis with or without anemia in some families.
- Higher activity in older, more PGK-deficient, red cells than in younger red cells.
- One of the ATP-generating steps of glycolysis.

PGK (ATP:3-phospho-D-glycerate 1-phosphotransferase, E.C.2.7.2.3) is the only enzyme of anaerobic glycolysis that is known to be encoded by a gene on the X chromosome. All tissues, except sperm, contain the same enzyme (PGK-1) (363,364), which exists as a monomer of 416 amino acids (365) and is approximately 45 kd (366). The PGK-2 isoenzyme that is present in sperm is separately encoded by an autosomal gene (367). PGK catalyzes the first ATP-generating step of glycolysis, transferring the high-energy phosphate of 1,3-diphosphoglycerate to ADP. As shown in Figure 53-2, that substrate may also be converted to a low-energy state and stored as 2,3 DPG by irreversible diversion through the Rapoport-Luebering shunt. The direction of substrate flow is primarily determined by intracellular pH and the ratio of ATP to ADP. Acid pH and low ATP content brings 2,3 DPG back into the mainstream of glycolysis, where it serves for ATP generation via the PK step. As expected, deficiencies of PGK usually show decreased concentrations of ATP and increased concentrations of 2,3 DPG, with a consequent shift in the oxyhemoglobin dissociation curve to the right. Increased intracellular sodium concentrations have also been observed and ascribed to alterations in positive sodium-potassium pump activity, secondary to decreased ATP production from this reaction (368). Some of the PGK is membrane bound. It is intriguing to speculate that this compartment of PGK supplies the ATP that is needed for the sodium- and potassium-activated adenosine triphosphatase.

SYMPTOMS AND INDICATIONS FOR SPLENECTOMY

Deficiencies of PGK are rare. As of 1998, 23 families have been described (369–371). Because a single enzyme form is common to virtually all tissues, all tissues share the enzymopathy, which has been demonstrated in skeletal and cardiac muscle, brain, liver, leukocytes, and platelets (372). Male hemizygotes with little or no enzyme activity are symptomatic with chronic hemolysis that can be severe and often requires red-cell transfusions. Aplastic crises occasionally occur, but progressive neurologic complications usually dominate the clinical picture in men who are affected. Mild mental retardation with emotional lability, behavioral aberrations, dyskinesias, hemiplegia, and aphasia, as well as myopathy, are associated with the more severe cases. Phagocytosis by deficient leukocytes may be ineffective because of impaired bactericidal processes (373); however, there is no evidence of any clinically overt leukocyte dysfunction or liability to infections. With an X-chromosomal pattern of inheritance, women exhibit mosaicism with variable populations of normal and enzyme-deficient erythrocytes. Hemolytic manifestations in women range from moderate to none, and they have normal neurologic function. Among the 23 identified families, nine have neurologic and hematologic symptoms, six have only hemolysis, and seven have *only* CNS dysfunction. An isolated myopathy has also been reported (374,375). Moderately severe PGK deficiency can even be asymptomatic, as is demonstrated by PGK München (376). Splenectomy has a mostly favorable outcome, with improvement of the hemolysis, but the response rate has been inconsistent, and the procedure may be only indicated in the more severe cases (377).

MOLECULAR DEFECTS

At present, the structural abnormalities of 14 mutants have been elucidated (378–391). Most are single amino-acid substitutions (392–409) that occur in a common region of the enzyme molecule that may be involved in nucleotide binding (410,411). Several variants exhibit abnormal kinetics for substrates or cofactors, as well as decreased optimal activities and instability (412–424). Some of the biochemical and clinical heterogeneity in PGK deficiency may result from the nature of the specific molecular lesion. The reaction that is catalyzed by PGK is bidirectional. Reverse phosphorylation of 3PG to 1,3-diphosphoglycerate is a component of gluconeogenesis, a process that is apparently of no consequence to red-cell viability. As a matter of technical convenience, *in vitro* assays often measure this backward reaction, but that may not adequately reflect the effectiveness of the forward, ATP-generating step that is crucial to red-cell function and longevity. Some mutations result in gene products that have significantly more catalytic or kinetic impairment in one direction of the reaction relative to the other direction. This may account for the absence of hemolysis in one variant, PGK Creteil (425), in which the backward reaction is more adversely affected, compared to the overt hemolysis that is associated with PGK Tokyo (426), in which the forward reaction is more impaired.

GLYCOLYTIC ENZYME DEFECTS WITH UNPROVEN DISEASE STATUS OR THAT ARE DEVOID OF PREMATURE HEMOLYSIS

For some glycolytic enzyme deficiencies, the association between the enzyme deficiency and increased hemolysis has not been proven. These include G3PD, enolase, and 2,3-diphosphoglycerate mutase. The lack of evidence for an association between enolase or G3PD deficiencies and increased hemolysis is particularly perplexing. Clearly, in some of the cases, the deficiency is only partial and just may not cause a severe enough block in glycolysis to impair red-cell function. Except for severe enolase deficiency (427), it is hard to explain how a block in this enzyme should not cause hemolysis (or any other clinical symptoms), when a block in adjacent steps leads to serious disease. Perhaps there is some more subtle explanation. These three enzyme defects indicate that there are aspects of red blood cell glycolytic metabolism that we do not yet understand. Severe deficiency of 2,3-diphosphoglyceromutase, for example, results in a virtual absence of intracellular 2,3 DPG. The consequent shift in the oxygen dissociation curve of Hgb induces a compensatory erythrocytosis (see Chapter 49), but there is no evidence of hemolysis or other clinical problems (428). Similarly, defects in the H subunit of lactate dehydrogenase that result in severely deficient activities alter NAD and NADH ratios but are unaccompanied by hemolysis (429–431).

Glyceraldehyde-3-Phosphate Dehydrogenase Deficiency

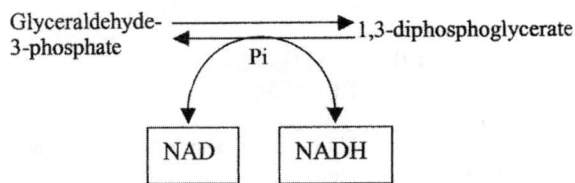

Glyceraldehyde-3-phosphate dehydrogenase

In 1966, Harkness (432) described one family with moderate G3PD deficiency (enzyme activity 20% to 30% of normal) and a compensated hemolytic anemia with apparently dominant inheritance. In other cases, an even milder deficiency of G3PD has been found, and the association between the deficiency and the hemolysis is questionable. One black man with 50% of the normal G3PD activity had moderate hemolytic anemia, which was enforced by the application of dapsone and primaquine, as well as by infection (433).

Enolase Deficiency

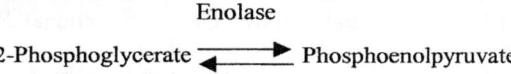

Enolase 1 is a homodimer and is located on chromosome 1pter-p36.13. It is present in all tissues. Enolase 2 and enolase 3 are specific for nervous tissue and muscle, respectively. Its deficiency is rare. Stephanini (434) diagnosed a deficiency of enolase 1 in a 41-year-old woman who presented with a severe drug-induced hemolytic crisis with hemoglobinuria. Poikilocytes, spherocytes, and schistocytes were found during the crisis, and the Heinz body test was positive. The patient had a residual enolase activity of 6% of normal and, in addition to the crisis, had a mild chronic hemolytic anemia. Her sister was similarly affected and had a reduced enolase activity as well. However, drug-induced hemolysis is unusual in disorders of the EM pathway, and the causative role of the enolase deficiency was not accepted by Beutler (435). Partial enolase deficiency has been reported in three other families with a red-cell enolase activity of approximately 50% of normal. The affected members experienced an autosomal-dominant inherited hereditary spherocytosis, and, again, the contribution of the enolase deficiency to the hemolysis and spherocytosis is uncertain (436).

2,3-Diphosphoglycerate Mutase Deficiency

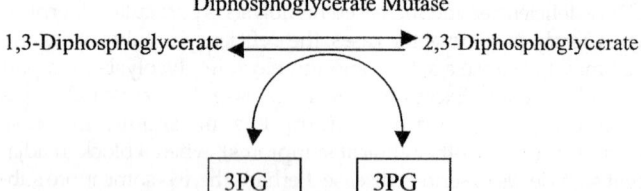

2,3 DPG mutase (DPGM) deficiency (see also Chapter 49) is a rare enzyme defect. Its complete absence in a French patient did not lead to an increased hemolysis, which suggests that the deficiency itself does not lead to premature erythrocyte destruction (437). On the contrary, the patient had a polycythemia (Hgb 19.0 g/dL) due to the resultant low levels of 2,3 DPG and increased oxygen affinity.

The homodimeric DPGM enzyme is multifunctional and catalyzes the synthesis and dephosphorylation of 2,3 DPG and, with low activity, the reversible conversion of 3PG to 2-phosphoglycerate. In DPGM deficient red cells, approximately 3% of total HgbA is glycosylated. This posttranslational change is probably the consequence of the large amounts of 1,3 DPG that are present in the red cells. The modified Hgb has a lower isoelectric point than $HgbA_{1C}$ and is easily detected by isoelectric focusing (438). The gene for DPGM is located on chromosome 7q31-34.

ALTERATIONS OF ERYTHROCYTE NUCLEOTIDE METABOLISM

Defective nucleotide metabolism has been observed in association with hyperactive, as well as deficient, erythrocyte enzymes.

The deficiency of pyrimidine nucleotidase causes life-long chronic hemolytic anemia of moderate severity. Other enzymopathies that are accompanied by increased hemolysis include the deficiency of AK and the overabundance of ADA. A number of other deficiency states (e.g., those that involve ADA, purine nucleoside phosphorylase, and the phosphoribosyl transferases that act on adenine, hypoxanthine, and guanine) and hyperactivity of RPK apparently have no adverse effects on red cells.

Pyrimidine 5'-Nucleotidase Deficiency

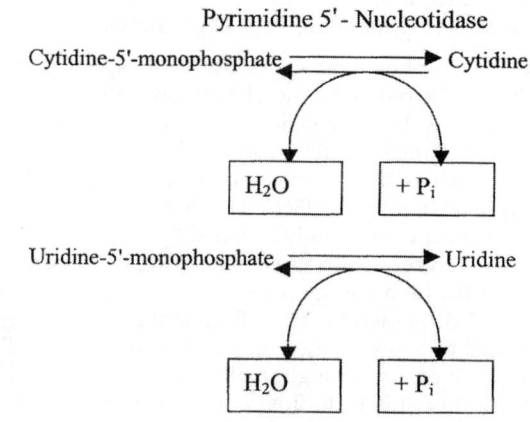

CHARACTERISTICS OF PYRIMIDINE 5'-NUCLEOTIDASE

- Second or third most frequent enzyme deficiency that causes chronic hemolytic anemia.
- Most individuals who are affected have Mediterranean, Jewish, or African ancestry.
- Prominent basophilic stippling of red cells.
- Mild to moderate benign chronic hemolytic anemia, with only a rare need of transfusion.
- Onset in infancy to later childhood. Only rarely severe neonatal jaundice.
- Severe hemolytic anemia in compound heterozygotes for P5'N and HgbE trait.
- Residual activity of less than 5% to 15%.
- Large amounts of pyrimidines in reticulocytes.
- Screening possible by measuring the UV absorption spectrum of blood extracts.
- Decreased phosphoribosyl-pyrophosphate synthetase (or RPK, or both) activity.
- Increased Heinz body formation on incubation of red cells.

Nucleotidases are ubiquitous enzymes that catalyze the hydrolytic dephosphorylation of monophosphorylated nucleotides to yield the corresponding nucleosides and inorganic phosphate. P5'N (5'-ribonucleotide phosphohydrolase, E.C.3.1.3.5; P5'N) or uridine monophosphate hydrolase 1 (UMPH1) is the first degradative enzyme of the pyrimidine salvage pathway and catalyzes the specific hydrolysis of the monophosphorylated nucleotides, uridine monophosphate and cytidine monophosphate, to the pyrimidines uridine and cytidine, which are freely diffusible across the membrane. Thus, the enzyme found in erythrocytes is essentially restricted to pyrimidine substrates. During reticulocyte maturation, this permits clearance of pyrimidine products of RNA degradation by dephosphorylation and diffusion, while simultaneously protecting AMP from a similar fate (439,440).

METABOLIC FINDINGS

Glutathione concentrations in erythrocytes with severe P5'N deficiency are consistently elevated twofold, and RPK activity is reduced to approximately one-fourth of normal. The decreased

RPK activity may be of some value for screening for P5'N deficiency. In addition, the activity of phosphoribosyl pyrophosphate synthetase is decreased (441). By contrast, the activity of pyrimidine nucleoside monophosphate kinase is increased, which explains the characteristic rise of pyrimidine nucleotide triphosphates (cytosine triphosphate and uridine triphosphate) to a greater degree than that of monophosphates (cytidine monophosphate and uridine monophosphate) (442). These changes are regarded as epiphenomena without demonstrable roles in the hemolytic process (443–446).

PYRIMIDINE-5'-NUCLEOTIDASE ISOZYMES AND PATHOPHYSIOLOGY

It can be shown that P5'N activity is composed of two totally separate cytoplasmic isozymes, P5'N (UMPH1) and desoxyribonucleotidase [uridine monophosphate hydrolase 2 (UMPH2)] (447–449). Both isozymes have been purified from red cells and are encoded by different genes. They can be distinguished from each other by substrate specificity. UMPH2 principally reacts with desoxyribonucleotide substrates and may serve as a complementary system with P'5N to clear maturing elements of DNA and RNA degradation products (450). In the mature erythrocyte, the major part of P5'N activity (90% to 95%) resides in P5'N. The remainder results from the overlapping specificity of UMPH2. P5'N and UMPH2 activities have been found in different human tissues, including lymphoblasts, and appear to have a tissue-specific isozyme composition (451).

Patients with P5'N deficiency lack UMPH1 but retain normal UMPH2 activity. Owing to its low ribonucleotidase activity, UMPH2 cannot compensate for the UMPH1 (P5'N) deficiency, which results in the accumulation of high concentrations of trapped pyrimidine nucleotides in red cells. The high nucleotide level is partly derived from RNA degradation in the maturing red cells. In addition, normal and deficient red cells show an active uptake of orotic acid into pyrimidine nucleotides, which suggests that the high nucleotide levels may also derive from sources outside of the red cells. In addition to red cells, P5'N (UMPH1) is also selectively deficient in patient's mononuclear and lymphoblastoid cells, and the accumulation of slightly raised levels of uridine tri- and diphosphate sugars has also been noted in these cells (452).

The clinical observation that patients with P5'N deficiency exhibit abnormally increased Heinz body formation on incubation of red cells with acetylphenylhydrazine (453) suggests that this enzyme defect is associated with a disturbed HMS. As shown by David et al. (454), the pyrimidine accumulation is directly related to the impairment of the HMS. There is a drastic inhibition of stimulated HMS and G6PD activity in red cells of patients who have the severe hemolytic form of the P5'N deficiency. However, there are no reports of drug-, oxidant-, or infection-triggered crises in such patients, as might be expected if the decrease in HMS and G6PD activity is the pathogenically important step. Thus, the pathogenesis of increased hemolysis in P5'N deficiency remains unknown. It is tempting to speculate that the high concentrations of nucleotides interfere with the assembly of Hgb subunits. The prominent finding of basophilic stippling in P5'N deficiency and unstable hemoglobinopathies, as well as the increased instability of HgbE in the presence of P5'N deficiency (455), may be a hint that the increased levels of pyrimidines destabilize Hgb or interfere with its assembly, thus enhancing hemolysis.

GENETICS

P5'N is inherited as an autosomal-recessive trait, with heterozygotes appearing hematologically and biochemically normal, except for intermediate enzyme activities. The frequency of P5'N deficiency differs markedly in the various regions of the

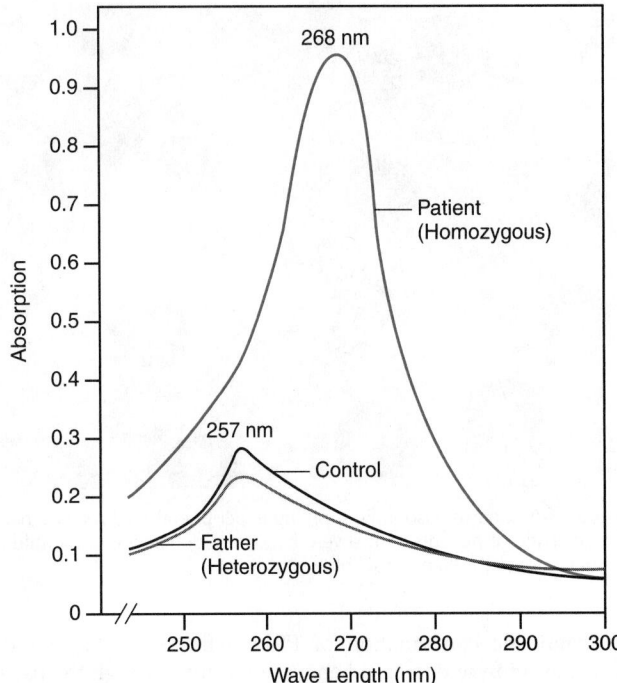

Figure 53-8. Ultraviolet spectrum of red blood cell extracts from a patient with pyrimidine 5'-nucleotidase deficiency. (Courtesy of Professor A. Pekrun, Universitäts-Kinderklinik, Göttingen, Germany.)

world. It is most frequent among populations of Mediterranean, African, and Jewish ancestry (456–458). In Japanese or Americans, it is the third most frequent enzyme defect after G6PD and PK deficiency (459–461). In contrast, the deficiency is rare in people of German descent.

DIAGNOSIS

The hallmark of the disease is the accumulation of monophosphate, diphosphate, and triphosphate pyrimidine nucleotides, and phosphodiester conjugates, such as cytidine diphosphate–choline, cytidine diphosphate–ethanolamine, and uridine diphosphate–glucose (Fig. 53-8) (462–465). In erythrocytes of patients who are affected, as much as 80% of the intracellular nucleotides may be pyrimidine compounds, and the absolute concentrations of adenine nucleotides may actually be lower than normal. The presence of numerous pyrimidines is reflected morphologically by the aggregation of undegraded or partially degraded ribosomal nucleoprotein, which produces the distinctive basophilic stippling that is characteristic of this disorder (Fig. 53-9) (466,467). In addition to P5'N deficiency, prominent basophilic stippling is characteristic of unstable Hgbs, thalassemias (a kind of unstable hemoglobinopathy), and lead intoxication. The latter association is due to the inhibition of P5'N by lead.

The increased amount of pyrimidines in P5'N deficiency provides a simple and useful screening test for detection of the severe deficiency. Its use before enzyme activity measurement has been suggested by the International Council for Standardization in Haematology (468–470). Acid extracts of P5'N-deficient red cells exhibit UV absorption spectra in the 265- to 270-nm region and bear no resemblance to the sharp 258-nm adenine absorption peak that is characteristic of normal erythrocytes (471,472) (Fig. 53-8). To perform the test, whole blood is denatured by rapid mixing with an equal volume of 1.2 N perchloric acid. The mixture is filtered, and the clear supernatant is diluted 1:10 with 0.1 N hydrochloric acid. Absorbance is measured in the 220- to 340-nm range.

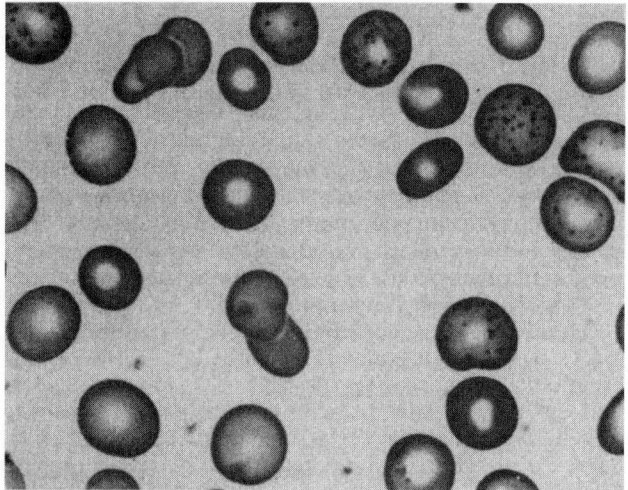

Figure 53-9. Coarse basophilic stippling in peripheral erythrocytes that is characteristic of patients with severe hereditary deficiency of pyrimidine 5'-nucleotidase (brilliant cresyl blue vital stain).

Diagnostic confirmation of P5'N deficiency relies on the demonstration of decreased enzyme activity through the use of quantitative colorimetric or radiometric methods (473,474). More sophisticated methods use high-performance liquid anion-exchange chromatography to directly measure pyrimidine nucleotide concentrations in erythrocytes. Nuclear magnetic resonance spectroscopy that uses phosphorus-31 or hydrogen-1 is a chemically specific and simple technique for measuring erythrocyte P5'N activity *in situ* (475–481). Using any one of these procedures, enzyme activity in the red cells of homozygotes or compound heterozygotes is decreased to 5% to 15% of normal, or less than 5% of normal, if comparable reticulocyte-rich blood is used as the substrate (482).

CONGENITAL AND ACQUIRED PYRIMIDINE 5'-NUCLEOTIDASE DEFICIENCY: DEGREE OF HEMOLYTIC ANEMIA AND SPLENECTOMY

Increased hemolysis of mild to moderate degree is the only symptom of P5'N deficiency. Most patients do not need transfusions. Only rare patients with severe deficiency and less than 5% to 10% residual activity may require transfusions (483). Splenectomy has been attempted in some patients with severe hemolysis, but beneficial effects have been inconsistent and unpredictable, occasionally reducing transfusion dependence and elevating Hgb and red-cell counts.

It has been shown that P5'N deficiency enhances the hemolytic anemia of the HgbE hemoglobinopathy (484). Patients who are homozygous for HgbE and P5'N deficiency have a severe hemolytic anemia, whereas family members who are only homozygous for HgbE are asymptomatic, and those who only have P5'N deficiency have the mild hemolytic anemia that is characteristic of this disorder.

Acquired deficiency of pyrimidine nucleotidase can also be induced by lead toxicity and, possibly, by other heavy metals to which the enzyme is extraordinarily susceptible (485). Chronic exposure to low levels of lead reduces pyrimidine nucleotidase activities significantly, with negligible effects on glycolytic enzymes and many other erythrocyte enzymes (486–489). At red-cell lead concentrations in the region of 200 μg/dL packed cells, nucleotidase activities decrease to approximately the levels that are seen in severe hereditary deficiencies (490). At that point, pyrimidine compounds begin to accumulate, the absorption spectra shift, and affected erythrocytes begin to show their characteristic basophilic stippling. In some cases, the complete hereditary deficiency syndrome has been reproduced by lead toxicity, including the epiphenomena that involve glutathione and RPK (491).

Adenosine Deaminase Overproduction

Adenosine Deaminase

$$\text{Adenosine} + H_2O \rightleftharpoons \text{Inosine} + H_2O$$

CHARACTERISTICS OF ADENOSINE DEAMINASE OVERPRODUCTION

- Autosomal dominant (dominant *positive* mutation).
- Compensated hemolysis.
- Forty-five– to 85-fold increase in normal enzyme activity.
- Less than 50% of normal adenosine nucleotides.
- Increase of ADA mRNA.

ADA (adenosine aminohydrolase, E.C.3.5.4.4) converts adenosine to inosine, which is not retrievable by mature erythrocytes for reincorporation into the adenine nucleotide pool. There is broad genetic polymorphism with a number of electrophoretic phenotypes (492,493). Multiple molecular forms predominate in various tissues (494). Erythrocytes, spleen, and stomach contain a small, 38-kd monomer. Two monomers may bind to a large, dimeric, nonenzymatic glycoprotein to form the isozyme that is characteristic of liver, kidney, and fibroblasts (495,496). The gene that governs ADA structure resides on chromosome 20 (497,498). The gene for the binding protein is located on chromosome 6 (499). Posttranslational modifications account for additional differences among tissue-specific isozymes (500,501).

CLINICAL SYMPTOMS, INHERITANCE, AND BIOCHEMISTRY OF CELLS WITH INCREASED ADENOSINE DEAMINASE ACTIVITY

ADA deficiency, such as that underlying certain recessive forms of severe combined immunodeficiency disease (502), is without apparent effect on erythrocyte function and survival, even though the cells may accumulate high concentrations of deoxyadenosine phosphates (503–507). Marked *elevations* in ADA activity, however, are associated with a compensated hemolytic anemia that is usually subclinical and well compensated by brisk reticulocytosis. Three families have an increase of catalytic activity of as much as two orders of magnitude, when compared to normal controls. The families originate from the United States, Japan, and France (508–512). In contrast to virtually all other red-cell enzymopathies, ADA deficiency is inherited in an *autosomal-dominant pattern*.

The enzyme protein is structurally and biochemically normal (513–516). Even though all tissues share a common catalytic protein component, ADA overproduction is apparently isolated to erythroid elements because of a basic defect in mRNA translation (517,518).

The disorder probably results from a *cis*-acting mutation in the vicinity of the ADA gene (519). ATP and total adenine nucleotides are approximately one-half of normal erythrocyte concentrations. This presumably results from the rapid deamination of red-cell adenosine, which reduces or eliminates it as a potential substrate for an essential nucleotide salvage pathway in erythrocytes that are catalyzed by adenosine kinase (520,521). The converse situation may be seen in immunodeficiency disease owing to severely deficient ADA, in which increases in erythrocyte concentrations of adenosine and deoxyadenosine phosphates reflect an increased availability of the nucleosides as substrates for phosphorylation by adenosine kinase.

Overproduction of ADA is accompanied by prominent elevations in the activity of erythrocyte P5'N, but the significance of this secondary effect is unknown. The nucleotidase appears biochemically normal and does not show any increased ability to dephosphorylate AMP to account for the diminished adenine nucleotide pool (522,523).

Adenylate Kinase Deficiency

Adenylate kinase

$$2\ ADP \rightleftharpoons ATP + AMP$$

CHARACTERISTICS OF ADENYLATE KINASE DEFICIENCY

- Moderate to severe hemolytic anemia.
- Variable clinical expression.

AK (ATP:AMP phosphotransferase, E.C.2.7.4.3) catalyzes the rapidly reversible equilibrium that exists among components of the erythrocyte adenine nucleotide pool (Fig. 53-2). Considerable genetic polymorphism exists, with at least five identifiable phenotypes (524–527). Separate loci on chromosome 9 encode AK_1 and AK_3, whereas AK_2 is governed by a gene on the short arm of chromosome 1 (528). The skeletal muscle isozyme is a globular monomer of approximately 21.5 kd (529,530).

CLINICAL ASPECTS AND BIOCHEMISTRY OF ADENYLATE KINASE DEFICIENCY

The erythrocyte isozyme, AK_1, has been found to be variably defective in four kindreds. Hemolytic anemia is moderate to severe, and residual enzyme activities range from 44% to less than 10% of normal controls (531–534). Partial deficiency of G6PD coexisted in one subject, and psychomotor retardation was present in another, but the meaning of the associations is uncertain. Genetic transmission was inconclusive and may be autosomal recessive or dominant, with variable penetrance. Parental AK was electrophoretically identical to the common AK_1 phenotype. Heterozygosity was thought to exist in some nonanemic relatives because of half-normal enzyme activities.

In an African-American family, two siblings displayed widely disparate clinical findings (535). Both had virtually undetectable AK activities; but only one had hemolytic anemia, whereas the other appeared to be entirely normal. The reason for this disparity remains unexplained, but it suggests that modifying factors must exist. Salvage reactions that generate AMP from adenine or adenosine theoretically require AK activity to provide the diphosphates and, ultimately, the triphosphates to maintain the balance of the adenine nucleotide pool. It may be that AK activities that are reduced by two or even three orders of magnitude below normal are still adequate to serve that purpose, because erythrocyte concentrations of all adenine nucleotides were minimally altered, if at all, in both children.

Each of the four families had a private AK mutation: a splice-site defect in intron 3, a nonsense mutation (107Arg→Stop) (536), and two missense mutations in exon 6 (128Arg→Trp and 164Tyr→Cys) (537,538). In the patients with missense defects, the mutant enzymes were unstable and had altered kinetic properties. Clearly, with the four mutations identified, AK deficiency should no longer be included among the category of nondiseases, as described by Beutler (539).

However, the importance of AK to normal cell function and longevity remains unclear. Although one would expect a low adenine level in AK_1 deficiency, this has not been found. Because GTP-ATP phosphotransferase activity was not detectable in one case, it has been speculated that AK_1 deficiency is connected with multiple disorders of phosphotransferases. The possibility of compound defects in some of the cases persists, such as that of G6PD in one kindred.

SOME CONCLUSIONS ABOUT THE STATE OF THE ART AND PERSPECTIVES FOR FUTURE WORK IN ENZYMOPATHIES

In the past, many details have been learned about singular enzyme defects. Still, much has to be done, and some points regarding current and future diagnostic procedures, therapeutic modalities, and clinically oriented molecular and biochemical research are listed below:

- The gold standard for diagnosis remains enzyme activity measurement, in most cases. Screening for the molecular defects may facilitate the definite diagnosis. A search for the molecular defect seems to be warranted, especially for those enzymes for which common defects have been described (e.g., in PK or TPI deficiency).
- Some of the defects are coupled with progressive neuromuscular impairment. Early diagnosis is warranted in these patients to permit appropriate counseling of the parents.
- In severe cases of, for example, PK or TPI deficiency, an analysis of the molecular genetic defect may be warranted to offer prenatal diagnosis to the parents. Mutation screening may also help to clarify uncertain carrier status.
- The therapy is related to the degree of anemia. Transfusions are required in more severe cases and during hemolytic or aplastic crises. Splenectomy usually reduces the need for transfusion, but, in most cases, considerable hemolysis persists. The ensuing hemosiderosis is one of the major problems in later age and may justify bone marrow transplantation or enzyme replacement therapy in severe transfusion dependent cases (see the following discussion).
- It is still unclear if substitution of folic acid is necessary in well-nourished patients with chronic hemolytic anemia.
- In severe cases that do not respond well to splenectomy, or if severe associated symptoms are present, new therapeutic modalities need to be developed. Enzyme transfer into deficient red cells, muscle cells, and neuronal cells via liposomes or other vehicles would be of help in those enzymopathies with hemolytic anemia and associated neuromuscular symptoms. Over the long term, this might avoid the problems of hemosiderosis with its multiple organ damage. Transmembrane enzyme trafficking to neuronal cells would be necessary and could reverse the metabolic block in severe TPI deficiency. Even incorporation of small amounts of enzymes should be effective.
- Currently, stem cell transplantation is the only realistic potential source of enzyme replacement. It may be justified for severe hemolysis, especially if low-intensity (low-myeloablative) preparation regimens, which are being tested for sickle cell disease, work. Fetal stem cell transplantation before T-cell programming at 12 to 14 weeks of gestation might also be an option and could minimize T-cell–mediated rejection problems. Stem cell transplantation is not likely to improve the enzyme deficiency in the CNS, and, thus, patients with predominant neuromuscular impairment and moderate hemolytic anemia (such as TPI deficiency) may not profit from transplantation.
- There may still be some unrecognized red-cell enzyme defects. Enzymes of nucleotide metabolism, with its complex and still incompletely understood catalytic steps, are good candidates.
- The exact mechanism of increased hemolysis in most enzymopathies remains to be elucidated.
- There is insufficient information regarding the genotype-phenotype relationship of most red-cell enzyme disorders.

ACKNOWLEDGMENTS

I deeply appreciate the careful and critical review of my chapter done by Dr. H. Lutz of Zürich and Prof. W. K. G. Krietsch of Munich.

REFERENCES

1. Vanlair CF, Masius JB. De la microcythémie. *Bull R Acad Med Belg* 1871;5:515–613.
2. Dresbach M. Elliptical human red blood corpuscles. *Science* 1904;19:469–470.
3. Haden RL. A new type of hereditary hemolytic jaundice without spherocytosis. *Am J Med Sci* 1947;214:255–259.
4. Dacie JV, Mollison PL, Richardson N, et al. Atypical congenital haemolytic anaemia. *Q J Med* 1953;22:79.
5. Selwyn JG, Dacie JV. Autohemolysis and other changes resulting from the incubation in vitro of red cells from patients with congenital hemolytic anemia. *Blood* 1954;9:414.
6. de Gruchy GC, Santamaria JN, Parsons IC, et al. Nonspherocytic congenital hemolytic anemia. *Blood* 1960;16:1371.
7. de Gruchy GC, Crawford H, Morton D. Atypical (nonspherocytic) congenital haemolytic anaemia. Proceedings of the VIIth Congress of the International Society of Hematology, Rome, 1958;2:425.
8. Robinson MA, Loder PB, de Gruchy GC. Red-cell metabolism in nonspherocytic congenital haemolytic anaemia. *Br J Haematol* 1961;7:327.
9. Valentine WN, Tanaka KR, Miwa S. A specific erythrocyte glycolytic enzyme defect (pyruvate kinase) in three subjects with congenital non-spherocytic hemolytic anemia. *Trans Assoc Am Physicians* 1961;74:100.
10. Tanaka KR, Valentine WN, Miwa S. Pyruvate kinase (PK) deficiency hereditary non-spherocytic hemolytic anemia. *Blood* 1962;19:267.
11. Carson PE, Flanagan CL, Ickes CE, et al. Enzymatic deficiency in primaquine-sensitive erythrocytes. *Science* 1956;24:484.
12. Valentine WN, Tanaka KR, Paglia DE. Pyruvate kinase and other enzyme deficiency disorders of the erythrocyte. In: Scriver CR, Beaudet AL, Sly WS, et al., eds. *The metabolic basis of inherited disease*, 6th ed. New York: McGraw-Hill, 1989:2341.
13. Mentzer WC, Glader BE. Disorders of erythrocyte metabolism. In: Mentzer WC, Wagner GM, eds. *The hereditary hemolytic anemias*. New York: Churchill Livingstone, 1989:267.
14. Dacie J. Hereditary enzyme-deficiency haemolytic anemias. I. Introduction and pyruvate-kinase deficiency. In: Dacie J, ed. *The haemolytic anemias*. London: Churchill Livingstone, 1985:282.
15. Dacie J. Hereditary enzyme-deficiency haemolytic anaemias. II. Deficiencies of enzymes of the Embden-Meyerhoff (EM) pathway other than pyruvate kinase and of enzymes involved in purine and pyrimidine metabolism. In: Dacie J, ed. *The haemolytic anemias*. London: Churchill Livingstone, 1985:321.
16. Valentine WN, Tanaka KR, Paglia DE. Hemolytic anemias and erythrocyte enzymopathies. *Ann Intern Med* 1985;103:249.
17. Miwa S, Fujii H. Molecular aspects of erythroenzymopathies associated with hereditary hemolytic anemia. *Am J Hematol* 1985;19:293.
18. Beutler E. Hemolytic anemia in disorders of red cell metabolism. In: Wintrobe MM, ed. *Topics in hematology*. New York: Plenum Publishing, 1978:199.
19. Sullivan DW, Glader BE. Erythrocyte enzyme disorders in children. *Pediatr Clin North Am* 1980;27:449.
20. Miwa S. Hereditary disorders of red cell enzymes in the Embden-Meyerhoff pathway. *Am J Hematol* 1983;14:381.
21. Valentine WN, Paglia DE. The primary cause of hemolysis in enzymopathies of anaerobic glycolysis: a viewpoint. *Blood Cells* 1980;6:819.
22. Leger TJ, Eber SW, Lakomek M, et al. Application of RHD and RHCE genotyping for correct blood group determination in chronically transfused patients. *Transfusion* 1999;39:852–855.
23. Beutler E. *Red cell metabolism: a manual of biochemical methods*, 3rd ed. Orlando, FL: Grune & Stratton, 1984.
24. Irono A, Forman I, Beutler E. Enzymatic diagnosis in non-spherocytic hemolytic anemia. *Medicine* 1988;67:110–117.
25. Keitt AS. Pyruvate kinase deficiency and related disorders of red cell glycolysis. *Am J Med* 1966;41:762–785.
26. Rosa R, Gaillardon J, Rosa J. Diphosphoglycerate mutase and 2,3-diphosphoglycerate phosphatase activities of red cells: comparative electrophoretic study. *Biochem Biophys Res Commun* 1973;51:536.
27. Rosa R, Audit I, Rosa J. Evidence for three enzymatic activities in one electrophoretic band of 3-phosphoglycerate mutase from red cells. *Biochimie* 1975;57:1059–1063.
28. Sasaki R, Ikura K, Sugimoto E, et al. Purification of bisphosphoglycerate phosphatase and phosphoglyceromutase from human erythrocytes. *Eur J Biochem* 1975;50:581.
29. Hamasaki N, Hardjono IS, Minakami S. Transport of phosphoenolpyruvate through the erythrocyte membrane. *Biochem J* 1978;170:39.
30. Hamasaki N, Kawano Y. Phosphoenolpyruvate transport in the anion transport system of human erythrocyte membranes. *Trends Biochem Sci* 1987;12: 183.
31. Van Acker KJ, Simmonds HA, Potter C, et al. Complete deficiency of adenine phosphoribosyltransferase: report of a family. *N Engl J Med* 1977;297:127.
32. Agarwal RP, Crabtree GW, Parks RE Jr, et al. Purine nucleoside metabolism in the erythrocytes of patients with adenosine deaminase deficiency and severe combined immunodeficiency. *J Clin Invest* 1976;57:1025.
33. Schmalstieg FC, Goldman AS, Mills GC, et al. Nucleotide metabolism in adenosine deaminase deficiency. *Pediatr Res* 1976;10:393.
34. Cohen A, Hirschhorn R, Horowitz SD, et al. Deoxyadenosine triphosphate as a potentially toxic metabolite in adenosine deaminase deficiency. *Proc Natl Acad Sci U S A* 1978;75:472.
35. Coleman MS, Donofrio J, Hutton JJ, et al. Identification and quantitation of adenine deoxynucleotides in erythrocytes of a patient with adenosine deaminase deficiency and severe combined immunodeficiency. *J Biol Chem* 1978;253:1619.
36. Nelson JA, Kuttesch JF, Goldblum RN, et al. Analysis of adenosine and adenine nucleotides in severe combined immunodeficiency disease. In: Baer HP, Drummond GI, eds. *Physiological and regulatory functions of adenosine and adenine nucleotides*. New York: Raven Press, 1979:417.
37. Valentine WN, Paglia DE, Tartaglia AP, et al. Hereditary hemolytic anemia with increased red cell adenosine deaminase (45- to 70-fold) and decreased adenosine triphosphate. *Science* 1977;195:783.
38. Paglia DE, Valentine WN, Tartaglia AP, et al. Control of red blood cell adenine nucleotide metabolism: studies of adenosine deaminase. In: Brewer GJ, ed. *The red cell*. New York: Alan R. Liss, 1978:319.
39. Fujii H, Miwa S, Suzuki K. Purification and properties of adenosine deaminase in normal and hereditary hemolytic anemia with increased red cell activity. *Hemoglobin* 1980;4:693.
40. Perignon JL, Hamet M, Buc HA, et al. Biochemical study of a case of hemolytic anemia with increased (85-fold) red cell adenosine deaminase. *Clin Chim Acta* 1982;124:205.
41. Miwa S, Fujii H, Matsumoto N, et al. A case of red-cell adenosine deaminase overproduction associated with hereditary hemolytic anemia found in Japan. *Am J Hematol* 1978;5:107.
42. Paglia DE, Valentine WN. Haemolytic anemia associated with disorders of the purine and pyrimidine salvage pathways. *Clin Haematol* 1981;10:81.
43. Valentine WN, Fink K, Paglia DE, et al. Hereditary hemolytic anemia with human erythrocyte pyrimidine 5'-nucleotidase deficiency. *J Clin Invest* 1974;54:866.
44. Paglia DE, Valentine WN. Characteristics of a pyrimidine-specific 5'-nucleotidase in human erythrocytes. *J Biol Chem* 1975;250:7973.
45. Paglia DE, Valentine WN. Hereditary and acquired defects in the pyrimidine nucleotidase of human erythrocytes. *Curr Top Hematol* 1980;3:75.
46. Swallow DM, Aziz I, Hopkinson DA, et al. Analysis of human erythrocyte 5'-nucleotidases in healthy individuals and a patient deficient in pyrimidine 5'-nucleotidase. *Ann Hum Genet* 1983;47:19.
47. Paglia DE, Valentine WN, Keitt AS, et al. Pyrimidine nucleotidase deficiency with active dephosphorylation of dTMP: evidence of existence of thymidine nucleotidase in human erythrocytes. *Blood* 1983;61:1147–1149.
48. Paglia DE, Valentine WN, Brockway RA. Identification of thymidine nucleotidase and deoxyribonucleotidase activities among normal isozymes of 5'-nucleotidase in human erythrocytes. *Proc Natl Acad Sci U S A* 1984;81:588.
49. Hirono A, Fujii H, Natori H, et al. Chromatographic analysis of human erythrocyte 5'-nucleotidase from five patients with pyrimidine 5'-nucleotidase deficiency. *Br J Haematol* 1987;65:35.
50. Paglia DE, Valentine WN, Brockway RA, et al. Substrate specificity and pH sensitivity of deoxyribonucleotidase and pyrimidine nucleotidase activities in human hemolysates. *Exp Hematol* 1987;15:1041.
51. Rettig MP, Low PS, Grimm JA, et al. Evaluation of biochemical changes during erythrocyte senescence in the dog. *Blood* 1999;93:376–384.
52. Lutz HU, Bussolino F, Flepp R, et al. Naturally occurring anti-band 3 antibodies and complement together mediate phagocytosis of oxidatively stressed human erythrocytes. *Proc Natl Acad Sci U S A* 1987;84:7368.
53. Schluter K, Drenckhan D. Co-clustering of denatured hemoglobin with band 3: its role in binding of autoantibodies against band 3 to abnormal and aged erythrocytes. *Proc Natl Acad Sci U S A* 1986;83:6137.
54. Lutz HU, Flepp R, Stringaro-Wipf G. Naturally occurring autoantibodies to exoplasmic and cryptic regions of band 3 protein, the major integral membrane protein of human red blood cells. *J Immunol* 1984;133:2610–2618.
55. Bartlett GR. Red cell metabolism: review highlighting changes during storage. In: Greenwalt TJ, Jamieson GA, eds. *The human red cell in vitro*. New York: Grune & Stratton, 1974:5.
56. Suzuki T, Dale GL. Senescent erythrocytes: isolation of *in vivo* aged cells and their biochemical characteristics. *Proc Natl Acad Sci U S A* 1988;85:1647.
57. Dale GL, Norenberg SL. Time-dependent loss of adenosine 5'-monophosphate deaminase may explain elevated adenosine 5'triphosphate levels in senescent erythrocytes. *Blood* 1989;74:2157.
58. Paglia DE, Valentine WN, Nakatani M, et al. AMP deaminase as a cell-age marker in transient erythroblastopenia of childhood and its role in the adenylate economy of erythrocytes. *Blood* 1989;74:2161.
59. Eber SW, Haag G, Overbeck, et al. Increased exposition of red cell phosphatidylserine may be a risk factor for thrombosis in splenectomized patients with hereditary stomatocytosis (HAST) and pyruvate kinase (PK). Am Soc Haematol 42nd Meeting, San Francisco. *Blood* 2000;96:595a.
60. Beutler E. Congenital hemolytic anemias related to enzyme defects and acquired hemolytic anemias. *Curr Opin Hematol* 1993:52.
61. Fehr J, Knob M. Comparison of red cell creatine level and reticulocyte count in appraising the severity of hemolytic process. *Blood* 1979;53:966.
62. Zanella A, Izzo C, Rebulla P, et al. Acidified glycerol lysis test: a screening test for spherocytosis. *Br J Haematol* 1980;45:481–486.

63. Eber SW, Pekrun A, Neufeldt A, et al. Prevalence of increased osmotic fragility of erythrocytes in German blood donors: screening using a modified glycerol lysis test. *Ann Hematol* 1992;64:88–92.

64. Ibsen KH, Schiller KW, Taas TA. Interconvertible kinetic and physical forms of human erythrocyte pyruvate kinase. *J Biol Chem* 1971;246:1233.

65. Marie J, Kahn A, Boivin P. Human erythrocyte pyruvate kinase: total purification and evidence for its antigenic identity with L-type enzyme. *Biochim Biophys Acta* 1977;481:96.

66. Saheki S, Saheki K, Tanaka T. Peptide structures of pyruvate kinase isozymes. I. Comparison of the four pyruvate kinase isozymes of the rat. *Biochim Biophys Acta* 1982;704:484.

67. Chern CJ, Kennett R, Engle E, et al. Assignment of the structural genes for the alpha subunit of hexosaminidase A, mannose phosphate isomerase, and pyruvate kinase to the region q22-qter of human chromosome 15. *Somatic Cell Genet* 1977;3:553–560.

68. Peters J, Nash HR, Eicher EM, et al. Polymorphism of kidney pyruvate kinase in the mouse is determined by a gene, PK-3, on chromosome 9. *Biochem Genet* 1981;19:757.

69. Koler RD, Vanbellinghen P. The mechanism of precursor modulation of human pyruvate kinase I by fructose diphosphate. *Adv Enzyme Regul* 1968;6:127.

70. Staal GEJ, Koster JF, Kamp H, et al. Human erythrocyte pyruvate kinase: its purification and some properties. *Biochim Biophys Acta* 1971;227:86.

71. Black JA, Henderson MH. Activation and inhibition of human erythrocyte pyruvate kinase by organic phosphates, amino acids, dipeptides and anions. *Biochim Biophys Acta* 1972;284:115.

72. Marie J, Kahn A, Boivin P. Human erythrocyte pyruvate kinase: total purification and evidence for its antigenic identity with L-type enzyme. *Biochim Biophys Acta* 1977;481:96.

73. Marie J, Garreau H, Kahn A. Evidence for a postsynthetic proteolytic transformation of human erythrocyte pyruvate kinase into L-type enzyme. *FEBS Lett* 1977;78:91–94.

74. Marie J, Kahn A. Proteolytic processing of human erythrocyte pyruvate kinase: study of normal and deficient enzyme. *Biochem Biophys Res Commun* 1979;91:123.

75. Kahn A, Marie J, Boivin P. Pyruvate kinase in man. II. L-type and erythrocyte-type isozymes: electrofocusing and immunologic studies. *Hum Genet* 1976;33:35.

76. Kahn A, Marie J, Boivin P. Pyruvate kinase in man. II. L-type and erythrocyte-type isozymes: electrofocusing and immunologic studies. *Hum Genet* 1976;33:35.

77. Bigley RH, Koler RD. Liver pyruvate kinase (PK) isozymes in a PK-deficient patient. *Ann Hum Genet* 1968;31:383.

78. Imamura K, Tanaka T, Nishina T, et al. Studies on pyruvate kinase (PK) deficiency. II. Electrophoretic, kinetic, and immunological studies on pyruvate kinase of erythrocytes and other tissues. *J Biochem* 1973;74:1165.

79. Nakashima K, Miwa S, Oda S, et al. Electrophoretic and kinetic studies of mutant erythrocyte pyruvate kinases. *Blood* 1974;43:537.

80. Kahn A, Marie J, Galand C, et al. Chronic haemolytic anaemia in two patients heterozygous for erythrocyte pyruvate kinase deficiency: electrofocusing and immunological studies of erythrocyte and liver pyruvate kinase. *Scand J Haematol* 1976;16:250.

81. Nakashima K, Miwa S, Fujii H, et al. Characterization of pyruvate kinase from the liver of a patient with aberrant erythrocyte pyruvate kinase, PK Nagasaki. *J Lab Clin Med* 1977;90:1012.

82. Staal GE, Rijksen G, Vlug AM, et al. Extreme deficiency of L-type pyruvate kinase with moderate clinical expression. *Clin Chim Acta* 1982;118:241.

83. Imamura K, Tanaka T. Multimolecular forms of pyruvate kinase from rat and other mammalian tissues. *J Biochem* 1972;71:1043.

84. Ibsen KH, Schiller KW, Taas TA. Interconvertible kinetic and physical forms of human erythrocyte pyruvate kinase. *J Biol Chem* 1971;246:1233.

85. Imamura K, Tanaka T, Nishina T, et al. Studies on pyruvate kinase (PK) deficiency. II. Electrophoretic, kinetic, and immunological studies on pyruvate kinase of erythrocytes and other tissues. *J Biochem* 1973;74:1165.

86. Nakashima K. Further evidence of molecular alteration and aberration of erythrocyte pyruvate kinase. *Clin Chim Acta* 1974;55:245.

87. Max-Audit I, Kechemir D, Mitjavila MT, et al. Pyruvate kinase synthesis and degradation by normal and pathologic cells during erythroid maturation. *Blood* 1988;72:1039.

88. Marie J, Garreau H, Kahn A. Evidence for a postsynthetic proteolytic transformation of human erythrocyte pyruvate kinase into L-type enzyme. *FEBS Lett* 1977;78:91.

89. Nakashima K. Further evidence of molecular alteration and aberration of erythrocyte pyruvate kinase. *Clin Chim Acta* 1974;55:245.

90. Max-Audit I, Kechemir D, Mitjavila MT, et al. Pyruvate kinase synthesis and degradation by normal and pathologic cells during erythroid maturation. *Blood* 1988;72:1039.

91. Takegawa S, Fujii H, Miwa S. Change of pyruvate kinase isozymes from M_2 to L type during development of the red cell. *Br J Haematol* 1983;54:467.

92. Shinohara K, Yamada K, Inoue M, et al. Enzyme activity of cultured erythroblasts. *Am J Hematol* 1985;20:145.

93. Oda S, Oda E, Tanaka KR. Relationship of density distribution and pyruvate kinase electrophoretic pattern of erythrocytes in sickle cell disease and other disorders. *Acta Haematol* 1978;60:201.

94. Miwa S, Nakashima K, Ariyoshi K, et al. Four new pyruvate kinase (PK) variants and a classical type PK deficiency. *Br J Haematol* 1975;29:135.

95. Takegawa S, Miwa S. Change of pyruvate kinase (PK) isozymes in classical type PK deficiency and other PK deficiency cases during red cell maturation. *Am J Hematol* 1984;16:53.

96. Black JA, Rittenberg MB, Standerfer RJ, et al. Hereditary persistence of fetal erythrocyte pyruvate kinase in the Basenji dog. In: Brewer GJ, ed. *The red cell: progress in clinical and biological research*, vol. 21. New York: Alan R. Liss, 1978:275.

97. Max-Audit I, Rosa R, Marie J. Pyruvate kinase hyperactivity genetically determined: metabolic consequences and molecular characterization. *Blood* 1980;56:902.

98. Rosa R, Max-Audit I, Izrael V, et al. Hereditary pyruvate kinase abnormalities associated with erythrocytosis. *Am J Hematol* 1981;10:47.

99. Marie J, Garreau H, Kahn A. Evidence for a postsynthetic proteolytic transformation of human erythrocyte pyruvate kinase into L-type enzyme. *FEBS Lett* 1977;78:91.

100. Sprengers ED, Staal GE. Functional changes associated with the sequential transformation of L'_4 into L_4 pyruvate kinase. *Biochim Biophys Acta* 1979;570:259.

101. Mentzer WC Jr, Baehner RL, Schmidt-Schonbein H, et al. Selective reticulocyte destruction in erythrocyte pyruvate kinase deficiency. *J Clin Invest* 1971;50:688.

102. Matsumoto N, Ishihara T, Nakashima K, et al. Sequestration and destruction of reticulocytes in the spleen in pyruvate kinase deficiency hereditary nonspherocytic hemolytic anemia. *Nippon Ketsueki Gakkai Zasshi* 1972;35:525.

103. Leblond PF, Lyonnais J, Delage JM. Erythrocyte populations in pyruvate kinase deficiency anaemia following splenectomy. I. Cell morphology. *Br J Haematol* 1978;39:55.

104. Leblond PF, Lyonnais J, Delage JM. Erythrocyte populations in pyruvate kinase deficiency anemia following splenectomy. II. Cell deformability. *Br J Haematol* 1978;39:63.

105. Bowman HS, Oski FA. Laboratory studies of erythrocytic pyruvate kinase deficiency: pathogenesis of the hemolysis. *Am J Clin Pathol* 1978;70:259.

106. Takegawa S, Miwa S. Change of pyruvate kinase (PK) isozymes in classical type PK deficiency and other PK deficiency cases during red cell maturation. *Am J Hematol* 1984;16:53.

107. Max-Audit I, Kechemir D, Mitjavila MT, et al. Pyruvate kinase synthesis and degradation by normal and pathologic cells during erythroid maturation. *Blood* 1988;72:1039.

108. Max-Audit I, Rosa R, Marie J. Pyruvate kinase hyperactivity genetically determined: metabolic consequences and molecular characterization. *Blood* 1980;56:902.

109. Rosa R, Max-Audit I, Izrael V, et al. Hereditary pyruvate kinase abnormalities associated with erythrocytosis. *Am J Hematol* 1981;10:47.

110. Staal GE, Jansen G, Roos D. Pyruvate kinase and the "high ATP syndrome." *J Clin Invest* 1984;74:231–235.

111. Kechemir D, Max-Audit I, Rosa R. Comparative study of human M2-type pyruvate kinases isolated from human leukocytes and erythrocytes of a patient with red cell pyruvate kinase hyperactivity. *Enzyme* 1989;41:121.

112. Monod J, Wyman J, Changeux JP. On the nature of allosteric transitions: a plausible model. *J Mol Biol* 1965;12:88.

113. Staal GE, Rijksen G, Vlug AM, et al. Extreme deficiency of L-type pyruvate kinase with moderate clinical expression. *Clin Chim Acta* 1982;118:241.

114. Ishida Y, Miwa S, Fujii H, et al. Thirteen cases of pyruvate kinase deficiency found in Japan. *Am J Hematol* 1981;10:239.

115. Miwa S, Fujii H, Tani K, et al. Red cell adenylate kinase deficiency associated with hereditary nonspherocytic hemolytic anemia: clinical and biochemical studies. *Am J Hematol* 1983;14:325.

116. Kahn A, Marie J, Vives-Corrons JL, et al. Search for relationship between anomalies of the mutant erythrocyte pyruvate kinase variants and their pathological expression. *Hum Genet* 1981;57:172.

117. Muirhead H. Triose phosphate isomerase, pyruvate kinase and other alpha/β-barrel enzymes. *Trends Biochem Sci* 1983:326.

118. Mattevi A, Bolognesi M, Valentini G. The allosteric regulation of pyruvate kinase. *FEBS Lett* 1996;389:15–19.

119. El-Hazmi MA, Al-Swailem AR, Al-Faleh FZ, et al. Frequency of glucose-6-phosphate dehydrogenase, pyruvate kinase and hexokinase deficiency in the Saudi population. *Hum Hered* 1986;36:45–49.

120. Fung RH, Keung YK, Chung GS, et al. Screening of pyruvate kinase deficiency and G6PD deficiency in Chinese newborns in Hong Kong. *Arch Dis Child* 1969;44:373–376.

121. Wu ZL, Yu WD, Chen SC, et al. Frequency of erythrocyte pyruvate kinase deficiency in Chinese infants. *Am J Hematol* 1985;20:139.

122. Blume KG, Lohr GW, Praetsch O, et al. Beitrag zur Populationsgenetik der Pyruvat-Kinase menschlicher Erythrocyten. *Humangenetik* 1968;6:261–265.

123. Mohrenweiser HW. Frequency of enzyme deficiency variants in erythrocytes of newborn infants. *Proc Natl Acad Sci U S A* 1981;78:5046.

124. Etiemble J, Picat C, Dhermy D, et al. Erythrocytic pyruvate kinase deficiency and hemolytic anemia inherited as a dominant trait. *Am J Hematol* 1984;17:251.

125. Bossu M, Dacha M, Fornaini G, et al. Neonatal hemolysis due to a transient severity of inherited pyruvate kinase deficiency. *Acta Haematol* 1968;40:166–175.

126. Paglia DE, Valentine WN, Baughan MA, et al. An inherited molecular lesion of erythrocyte pyruvate kinase: identification of a kinetically aberrant isozyme associated with premature hemolysis. *J Clin Invest* 1968;47:1929.

127. Bossu M, Dacha M, Fornaini G, et al. Neonatal hemolysis due to a transient severity of inherited pyruvate kinase deficiency. *Acta Haematol* 1968;40:166–175.

128. Etiemble J, Picat C, Dhermy D, et al. Erythrocytic pyruvate kinase deficiency and hemolytic anemia inherited as a dominant trait. *Am J Hematol* 1984;17:251.
129. Satoh H, Tani K, Yoshida MC, et al. The human liver type pyruvate kinase (PKL) gene is on chromosome 1 at band q21. *Cytogenet Cell Genet* 1988;47:132–133.
130. Tani K, Fujii H, Nagata S, et al. Human liver type pyruvate kinase: complete amino acid sequence and the expression in mammalian cells. *Proc Natl Acad Sci U S A* 1988;85:1792–1795.
131. Kanno K, Fujii H, Hirono A, et al. cDNA cloning of human R-type pyruvate kinase and identification of a single amino acid substitution (Thr³⁶⁴-Met) affecting enzymatic stability in pyruvate kinase variant (PK Tokyo) associated with hereditary hemolytic anemia. *Proc Natl Acad Sci U S A* 1991;88:8218–8221.
132. Lenzner C, Nurnberg P, Jacobasch G, et al. Complete genomic sequences of the human PK-L/R-gene includes four intragenic polymorphisms defining different haplotype backgrounds of normal and mutant PK-genes. *DNA Seq* 1997;8:45–53.
133. Noguchi T, Tamada K, Inoue H, et al. The L- and R-type isozymes of rat pyruvate kinase are produced from a single gene by use of different promoters. *J Biol Chem* 1987;262:14366–14371.
134. Tani K, Fujii H, Nagata S, et al. Human liver type pyruvate kinase: complete amino acid sequence and the expression in mammalian cells. *Proc Natl Acad Sci U S A* 1988;85:1792–1795.
135. Kanno K, Fujii H, Hirono A, et al. cDNA cloning of human R-type pyruvate kinase and identification of a single amino acid substitution (Thr³⁶⁴-Met) affecting enzymatic stability in pyruvate kinase variant (PK Tokyo) associated with hereditary hemolytic anemia. *Proc Natl Acad Sci U S A* 1991;88:8218–8221.
136. Kanno H, Fujii H, Miwa S. Structural analysis of human pyruvate kinase L-gene and identification of the promoter activity in erythroid cells. *Biochem Biophys Res Commun* 1992;188:516–523.
137. Kugler W, Laspe P, Stahl M, et al. Identification of a novel promoter mutation in the human pyruvate kinase (PK) LR gene of a patient with severe haemolytic anaemia. *Br J Haematol* 1999;105:596–598.
138. Baronciani L, Bianchi P, Zanella A. Hematologically important mutations: red cell pyruvate kinase (2nd update). *Blood Cells Mol Dis* 1998;24:273–279.
139. Zarza R, Alvarez R, Pujades A, et al. Molecular characterization of the PK-LR gene in pyruvate kinase deficient Spanish patients. *Br J Haematol* 1998;103:377–382.
140. Manco L, Riberio ML, Almeida H, et al. PK-LR gene mutations in pyruvate kinase deficient Portuguese patients. *Br J Haematol* 1999;105:591–595.
141. Bianchi P, Baronciani L, Zappa M, et al. Original mutations in the LR-PK gene associated with chronic non spherocytic, hemolytic anemia. 1998;92[Suppl]:3b(abst).
142. Kugler W, Willaschek C, Holz C, et al. Eight novel mutations and consequences on mRNA and protein level in pyruvate kinase-deficient patients with nonspherocytic hemolytic anemia. *Hum Mutat* 2000;15:261–272.
143. Zarza R, Alvarez R, Pujades A, et al. Molecular characterization of the PK-LR gene in pyruvate kinase deficient Spanish patients. *Br J Haematol* 1998;103:377–382.
144. Baronciani L, Beutler E. Analysis of pyruvate kinase-deficiency mutations that produce nonspherocytic hemolytic anemia. *Proc Natl Acad Sci U S A* 1993;90:4324–4327.
145. Lenzner C, Nurnberg P, Jacobasch G, et al. Molecular analysis of 29 pyruvate kinase-deficient patients from Central Europe with hereditary anemia. *Blood* 1997;89:1793–1799.
146. Lenzner C, Nurnberg P, Jacobasch G, et al. Molecular analysis of 29 pyruvate kinase-deficient patients from Central Europe with hereditary anemia. *Blood* 1997;89:1793–1799.
147. Rouger H, Valentin C, Craescu CT, et al. Five unknown mutations in the LR pyruvate kinase gene associated with severe hereditary nonspherocytic anaemia in France. *Br J Haematol* 1996;92:825–830.
148. Valentine WN, Paglia DE. The primary cause of hemolysis in enzymopathies of anaerobic glycolysis: a viewpoint. *Blood Cells* 1980;6:819.
149. Beutler E. The primary cause of hemolysis in enzymopathies of anaerobic glycolysis. A commentary. *Blood Cells* 1980;6:827–829.
150. Lutz HU, Liu S-C, Palek J. Release of spectrin-free vesicles from human erythrocytes during ATP depletion. *J Cell Biol* 1977;73:548–560.
151. Mentzer WC, Glader BE. Disorders of erythrocyte metabolism. In: Mentzer WC, Wagner GM, eds. *The hereditary hemolytic anemias*. New York: Churchill Livingstone, 1989:267–318.
152. Amankwah KS, Dick BW, Dodge S. Hemolytic anemia and pyruvate kinase deficiency in pregnancy. *Obstet Gynecol* 1980;55:42S.
153. Duncan JR, Potter CG, Cappellini MD, et al. Aplastic crisis due to parvovirus infection in pyruvate kinase deficiency. *Lancet* 1983;2:14.
154. Zanella A, Bianchi P. Red cell pyruvate kinase deficiency: from genetics to clinical manifestations. *Best Pract Res Clin Haematol* 2000;13:57–81.
155. Tanaka KR, Zerez CR. Red cell enzymopathies of the glycolytic pathway. *Semin Hematol* 1990;27:165–185.
156. Beutler E. *Red cell metabolism: a manual of biochemical methods*, 3rd ed. Orlando, FL: Grune & Stratton, 1984.
157. Zanella A, Berzuini A, Colombo MB, et al. Iron status in red cell pyruvate kinase deficiency: study of Italian cases. *Br J Haematol* 1993;83:485–490.
158. Zanella A, Bianchi P. Red cell pyruvate kinase deficiency: from genetics to clinical manifestations. *Best Pract Res Clin Haematol* 2000;13:57–81.
159. Dacie J. Pyruvate-kinase (PK) deficiency. In: Dacie J, ed. *The haemolytic anemias*, vol. 1, 3rd ed. New York: Churchill Livingstone, 1985:284–320.
160. Zanella A, Berzuini A, Colombo MB, et al. Iron status in red cell pyruvate kinase deficiency: study of Italian cases. *Br J Haematol* 1993;83:485–490.
161. Hirsh J, Dacie JV. Persistent post-splenectomy thrombocytosis and thrombo-embolism: a consequence of continuing anaemia. *Br J Haematol* 1966;12:44–53.
162. Eber SW, Haag G, Overbeck, et al. Increased exposition of red cell phosphatidylserine may be a risk factor for thrombosis in splenectomized patients with hereditary stomatocytosis (HAST) and pyruvate kinase (PK). Am Soc Haematol 42nd Meeting, San Francisco. *Blood* 2000;96:595a.
163. Tanphaichitr VS, Suvatte V, Issaragrisil S, et al. Successful bone marrow transplantation in a child with red blood cell pyruvate kinase deficiency. *Bone Marrow Transplant* 2000;26:689–690.
163a. Eber SW, Bucsky P, Güngör T, et al. Subtotal splenectomy and allogenic hemtopoieic stem cell transplantation for therapy of severe pyruvate kinase deficiency. *Blood* 2002;100(Suppl 1) (in press).
164. Tani K, Yoshikubo T, Ikebuchi K, et al. Retrovirus-mediated gene transfer of human pyruvate kinase (PK) cDNA into murine hematopoietic cells: implication for gene therapy of human PK deficiency. *Blood* 1994;82:2305–2310.
165. Mason PJ. Red cell enzyme deficiencies: from genetic basis to gene transfer. *Semin Hematol* 1998;35:126–135.
166. Caster ND, Yoshida A. Purification and characterization of human phosphoglucose isomerase. *Biochim Biophys Acta* 1969;181:12.
167. Tilley BE, Gracy RW, Welch SG. A point mutation increasing the stability of human phosphoglucose isomerase. *J Biol Chem* 1974;249:4571.
168. Tsuboi KT, Fukanaga K, Chervenka CH. Phosphoglucose isomerase from human erythrocytes. *J Biol Chem* 1971;240:7586.
169. McMorris FA, Chen TR, Riciutti F, et al. Chromosome assignments in man of the genes for two hexosephosphate isomerases. *Science* 1973;179:1129.
170. Paglia DE, Valentine WN. Hereditary glucose phosphate isomerase deficiency. A review. *Am J Clin Pathol* 1974;62:740–751.
171. Payne DM, Porter DW, Gracy RW. Evidence against the occurrence of tissue-specific variants and isoenzymes of phosphoglucose isomerase. *Arch Biochem Biophys* 1972;151:122.
172. Baughan MA, Valentine WN, Paglia DE, et al. Hereditary hemolytic anemia associated with glucosephosphate isomerase (GPI) deficiency: a new enzyme defect of human erythrocytes. *Blood* 1968;32:236.
173. Paglia DE, Paredes R, Valentine WN, et al. Unique phenotypic expression of glucosephosphate isomerase deficiency. *Am J Hum Genet* 1975;27:62.
174. Oski F, Fuller E. Glucose-phosphate isomerase (GPI) deficiency associated with abnormal osmotic fragility and spherocytes. *Clin Res* 1971;19:427.
175. Kugler W, Lakomek M. Glucose-6-phosphate isomerase deficiency. *Best Pract Res Clin Haematol* 2000;13:89–101.
176. Reference deleted.
177. Baronciani L, Zanella A, Bianchi P, et al. Study of the molecular defects in glucose phosphate isomerase-deficient patients affected by chronic hemolytic anemia. *Blood* 1996;88:2306–2310.
178. Beutler E, West C, Britton HA, et al. Glucosephosphate isomerase (GPI) deficiency mutations associated with hereditary nonspherocytic hemolytic anemia (HNSHA). *Blood Cells Mol Dis* 1997;23:402–409.
179. Kugler W, Lakomek M. Glucose-6-phosphate isomerase deficiency. *Best Pract Res Clin Haematol* 2000;13:89–101.
180. Kugler W, Breme K, Laspe P, et al. Molecular basis of neurological dysfunction coupled with haemolytic anaemia in human glucose-6-phosphate isomerase (GPI) deficiency. *Hum Genet* 1998;103:450–454.
181. Paglia DE, Paredes R, Valentine WN, et al. Unique phenotypic expression of glucosephosphate isomerase deficiency. *Am J Hum Genet* 1975;27:62.
182. Helleman PW, Van Biervliet JP. Haematological studies in a new variant of glucosephosphate isomerase deficiency (GPI Utrecht). *Helv Paediatr* 1977;30:525–536.
183. Kugler W, Lakomek M. Glucose-6-phosphate isomerase deficiency. *Best Pract Res Clin Haematol* 2000;13:89–101.
184. Van Biervliet JP. Glucosephosphate isomerase deficiency in a Dutch family. *Acta Pediatr Scand* 1975;64:868.
185. Zanella A, Izzo C, Rebulla P, et al. The first stable variant of erythrocyte glucosephosphate isomerase associated with severe hemolytic anemia. *Am J Hematol* 1980;9:1.
186. Schröter W, Eber SW, Bardosi A. Generalized glucosephosphate isomerase (GPI) deficiency causing haemolytic anemia, neuromuscular symptoms and impairment of granulocyte function: a new syndrome due to a new stable GPI variant with diminished specific activity (GPI Hamburg). *Eur J Pediatr* 1985;144:301.
187. Ravindranath Y, Paglia DE, Warrier I, et al. Glucose phosphate isomerase deficiency as a cause of hydrops fetalis. *N Engl J Med* 1987;316:258–261.
188. Whitelaw AG, Rogers PA, Hopkinson DA, et al. Congenital haemolytic anaemia resulting from glucose phosphate isomerase deficiency: genetics, clinical picture, and prenatal diagnosis. *J Med Genet* 1979;16:189–196.
189. Matthay KK, Mentzer WC. Erythrocyte enzymopathies in the newborn. *Clin Haematol* 1981;10:31.
190. Whitelaw AG, Rogers PA, Hopkinson DA, et al. Congenital haemolytic anaemia resulting from glucose phosphate isomerase deficiency: genetics, clinical picture and prenatal diagnosis. *J Med Genet* 1979;16:189–196.
191. Ravindranath Y, Paglia DE, Warrier I, et al. Glucose phosphate isomerase deficiency as a cause of hydrops fetalis. *N Engl J Med* 1987;316:258–261.
192. Hutton JJ, Chilcote RR. Glucose phosphate isomerase deficiency with hereditary nonspherocytic hemolytic anemia. *J Pediatr* 1974;85:494.
193. Paglia DE, Paredes R, Valentine WN, et al. Unique phenotypic expression of glucosephosphate isomerase deficiency. *Am J Hum Genet* 1975;27:62.

194. Hellemann PW, Van Biervliet JP. Haematological studies in a new variant of glucosephosphate isomerase deficiency (GPI Utrecht). *Helv Paediatr Acta* 1975;30:525.

195. Arnold H, Lohr GW, Hasslinger K, et al. Augsburg-type glucosephosphate isomerase deficiency: a new variant causing congenital nonspherocytic anemia in a German family. *Blut* 1980;40:107.

196. Arnold H, Hasslinger K, Witt I. Glucosephosphate isomerase type Kaiserslautern: a new variant causing congenital nonspherocytic anemia. *Blut* 1983;46:271.

197. Kahn A, Buc HA, Girot R, et al. Molecular and functional anomalies in two new mutant glucosephosphate isomerase variants with enzyme deficiency and chronic hemolysis. *Hum Genet* 1978;40:293–304.

198. Hellemann PW, Van Biervliet JP. Haematological studies in a new variant of glucosephosphate isomerase deficiency (GPI Utrecht). *Helv Paediatr Acta* 1976;30:525–536.

199. Kahn A, Buc HA, Girot R, et al. Molecular and functional anomalies in two new mutant glucosephosphate isomerase variants with enzyme deficiency and chronic hemolysis. *Hum Genet* 1978;40:293–304.

200. Schröter W, Eber SW, Bardosi A, et al. Generalized glucosephosphate isomerase (GPI) deficiency causing haemolytic anaemia, neuromuscular symptoms and impairment of granulocytic function: a new syndrome due to a new stable GPI variant with diminished specific activity (GPI Homburg). *Eur J Pediatr* 1985;144:301–305.

201. Eber SW, Gahr M, Lakomek M, et al. Clinical symptoms and biochemical properties of three new glucosephosphate isomerase variants. *Blut* 1986;53:21–28.

202. Kugler W, Breme K, Laspe P, et al. Molecular basis of neurological dysfunction coupled with haemolytic anaemia in human glucose-6-phosphate isomerase (GPI) deficiency. *Hum Genet* 1998;103:450–454.

203. Shalev O, Shalev RS, Forman L, et al. GPI Mount Scopus—a variant of glucosephosphate isomerase deficiency. *Ann Hematol* 1993;67:197–200.

204. Beutler E, West C, Britton HA, et al. Glucosephosphate isomerase (GPI) deficiency mutations associated with hereditary nonspherocytic hemolytic anemia (HNSHA). *Blood Cells Mol Dis* 1997;23:402–409.

205. Zanella A, Izzo C, Rebulla P, et al. The first stable variant of erythrocyte glucosephosphate isomerase associated with severe hemolytic anemia. *Am J Hematol* 1980;9:1.

206. Hellemann PW, Van Biervliet JP. Haematological studies in a new variant of glucosephosphate isomerase deficiency (GPI Utrecht). *Helv Paediatr Acta* 1976;30:525–536.

207. Van Biervliet JP, Staal GE. Excessive hepatic glycogen storage in glucosephosphate isomerase deficiency. *Acta Paediatr Scand* 1977;66:311–315.

208. Eber SW, Bardosi A, Gahr M, et al. Generalized glucosephosphate isomerase (GPI) deficiency: a new syndrome involving red cells, granulocytes and neuromuscular system due to a stable variant enzyme with decreased specific activity. *Eur J Pediatr* 1984;141:265.

209. Schröter W, Eber SW, Bardosi A, et al. Generalized glucosephosphate isomerase (GPI) deficiency causing haemolytic anaemia, neuromuscular symptoms and impairment of granulocytic function: a new syndrome due to a new stable GPI variant with diminished specific activity (GPI Homburg). *Eur J Pediatr* 1985;144:301–305.

210. Eber SW, Gahr M, Lakomek M, et al. Clinical symptoms and biochemical properties of three new glucosephosphate isomerase variants. *Blut* 1986;53: 21–28.

211. Bardosi A, Eber SW, Rossmann U. Ultrastructural and histochemical abnormalities of skeletal muscle in a patient with a new variant type (type Homburg) of glucosephosphate-isomerase (GPI) deficiency. *Clin Neuropathol* 1985;4:72–76.

212. Gurney ME, Belton AC, Cashman, et al. Inhibition of terminal axonal sprouting by serum from patients with amyotrophic lateral sclerosis. *N Engl J Med* 1984;311:933–939.

213. Mizrachi Y. Neurotrophic activity of monomeric glucophosphoisomerase was blocked by human immunodeficiency virus (HIV-I) and peptides from HIV-I envelope glycoprotein. *J Neurosci Res* 1989;23:217–224.

214. Kugler W, Lakomek M. Glucose-6-phosphate isomerase deficiency. *Best Pract Res Clin Haematol* 2000;13:89–101.

215. Kugler W, Breme K, Laspe P, et al. Molecular basis of neurological dysfunction coupled with haemolytic anaemia in human glucose-6-phosphate isomerase (GPI) deficiency. *Hum Genet* 1998;103:450–454.

216. Eber SW, Bardosi A, Gahr M, et al. Generalized glucosephosphate isomerase (GPI) deficiency: a new syndrome involving red cells, granulocytes and neuromuscular system due to a stable variant enzyme with decreased specific activity. Tagg pädiatr Forschg, Göttingen. *Eur J Pediatr* 1984;141:265.

217. Schröter W, Eber SW, Bardosi A, et al. Generalized glucosephosphate isomerase (GPI) deficiency causing haemolytic anaemia, neuromuscular symptoms and impairment of granulocytic function: a new syndrome due to a new stable GPI variant with a diminished specific activity (GPI Homburg). *Eur J Pediatr* 1985;144:301–305.

218. Hutton JJ, Chilcote RR. Glucose phosphate isomerase deficiency with hereditary nonspherocytic hemolytic anemia. *J Pediatr* 1974;85:494.

219. Cayanis E, Penfold GK, Freiman I, et al. Haemolytic anaemia associated with glucosephosphate isomerase (GPI) deficiency in a black South African child. *Br J Haematol* 1977;37:363–371.

220. Beutler E, Sigalove WH, Muir WA, et al. Glucosephosphate isomerase (GPI) deficiency: GPI Elyria. *Ann Intern Med* 1974;80:730–732.

221. Matsumoto N, Ishihara T, Oda E, et al. Fine structure of the spleen and liver in glucosephosphate isomerase (GPI) deficiency hereditary nonspherocytic hemolytic anemia: selective reticulocyte destruction as a mechanism of hemolysis. *Nippon Ketsueki Gakkai Zasshi* 1973;36:46–54.

222. Paglia DE, Holland P, Baugham MA, et al. Occurrence of defective hexose-phosphate isomerization in human erythrocytes and leukocytes. *N Engl J Med* 1969;280:66.

223. Schneider AS. Triosephosphate isomerase deficiency: historical perspectives and molecular aspects. *Best Pract Res Clin Haematol* 2000;13:119–140.

224. Hollán S, Fodor E, Horányi M, et al. Decrease in non-bilayer forming lipid composition of lymphocytes in triosephosphate isomerase (TPI) deficiency. *Blood* 1997;90[Suppl]:58b.

225. Hollán S, Karg E, Német I, et al. Chronic oxidative stress in triosephosphate isomerase deficiency and its role in the neurodegenerative process. *Blood* 1998;92[Suppl]:524a.

226. Hollán S, Magócsi M, Farkas T, et al. Membrane fluidity, active calcium transport and acetylcholinesterase activity of red cells in triosephosphate isomerase (TPI) deficiency. *Blood* 1995;86[Suppl]:629a.

227. Orosz F, Wagner G, Liliom K, et al. Enhanced association of mutant triosephosphate isomerase to red cell membranes and to brain microtubules. *Proc Natl Acad Sci U S A* 2000;97:1026–1031.

228. Lu HS, Yuan PM, Gracy RW. Primary structure of human triosephosphate isomerase. *J Biol Chem* 1984;259:11958.

229. Jongsma AP, Los WR, Hagemeijer A. Evidence for synteny between the human loci for triosephosphate isomerase, lactate dehydrogenase-B and peptidase-B and the regional mapping of these loci on chromosome 12. *Cytogenet Cell Genet* 1974;13:106.

230. Decker RS, Mohrenweiser HW. Origin of the triosephosphate isomerase isozymes in humans: genetic evidence for the expression of a single structural locus. *Am J Hum Genet* 1981;33:683.

231. Eber SW, Krietsch WK. The isolation and characterization of the multiple forms of human skeletal muscle triosephosphate isomerase. *Biochim Biophys Acta* 1980;614:173.

232. Yuan PM, Talent JM, Gracy RW. Molecular basis for the accumulation of acidic isozymes of triosephosphate isomerase in aging. *Mech Ageing Dev* 1981;17:151.

233. Schneider AS, Valentine WN, Hattori M, et al. Hereditary hemolytic anemia with triosephosphate isomerase deficiency. *N Engl J Med* 1965;272:229.

234. Neel JV, Mohrenweiser HW, Meisler MH. Rate of spontaneous mutation at human loci encoding protein structure. *Proc Natl Acad Sci U S A* 1980;77:6037.

235. Gracy RW. Glucosephosphate and triosephosphate isomerases: significance of isozyme structural differences in evolution, physiology, and aging. In: Ratlazzi MC, Scandalios JG, Whitt GS, eds. *Isozymes: current topics in biological and medical research*, vol. 6. New York: Alan R. Liss, 1982:183.

236. Schneider AS, Valentine WN, Baughan MA, et al. Triosephosphate isomerase deficiency. A multi-system inherited enzyme disorder: clinical and genetic aspects. In: Beutler E, ed. *Hereditary disorders of erythrocyte metabolism*. New York: Grune & Stratton, 1968:265.

237. Rosa R, Prehu MO, Calvin MC, et al. Hereditary triosephosphate isomerase deficiency: seven new homozygous cases. *Hum Genet* 1985;71:235.

238. Eber SW, Dunnwald M, Heinemann G, et al. Prevalence of partial deficiency of red cell triosephosphate isomerase in Germany—a study of 3000 people. *Hum Genet* 1984;67:336–339.

239. Mohrenweiser HW. Frequency of enzyme deficiency variants in erythrocytes of newborn infants. *Proc Natl Acad Sci U S A* 1981;78:5046–5050.

240. Schneider AS. Triosephosphate isomerase deficiency: historical perspectives and molecular aspects. *Best Pract Res Clin Haematol* 2000;13:119–140.

241. Arya R, Lalloz MR, Bellingham AJ, et al. Evidence for founder effect of the Glu104Asp substitution and identification of new mutations in triosephosphate isomerase deficiency. *Hum Mutat* 1997;10:290–294.

242. Layton M, Arya R, Lalloz MR, et al. Molecular basis of triosephosphate isomerase deficiency. *Q J Med* 1996;89:870.

243. Schneider A, Westwood B, Yim C, et al. The amino acid 104 mutation in triosephosphate isomerase (TPI) deficiency: evidence for a single mutation in a common ancestor of seemingly unrelated families. *Blood* 1995;86:134a.

244. Schneider A, Westwood B, Cohen-Solal M, et al. All known cases of the triosephosphate isomerase (TPI) deficiency amino acid 104 mutation result from a single mutation in a common ancestor. *FASEB J* 1996;10:1132.

245. Schneider A, Westwood B, Yim C, et al. The 159IC mutation in triosephosphate isomerase (TPI) deficiency. Tightly linked polymorphisms and a common haplotype in all known families. *Blood Cells Mol Dis* 1996;22:115–125.

246. Schneider A, Westwood B, Yim C, et al. The amino acid 104 mutation in triosephosphate isomerase (TPI) deficiency: evidence for a single mutation in a common ancestor of seemingly unrelated families. *Blood* 1995;86:134a.

247. Schneider A, Westwood B, Cohen-Solal M, et al. All known cases of the triosephosphate isomerase (TPI) deficiency amino acid 104 mutation result from a single mutation in a common ancestor. *FASEB J* 1996;10:1132.

248. Boyer TG, Maquat LE. Minimal sequence and factor requirements for the initiation of transcription from an atypical, TATATAA box-containing housekeeping promoter. *J Biol Chem* 1990;265:20524–20532.

249. Boyer TG, Krug JR, Maquat LE. Transcriptional regulatory sequences of the housekeeping gene for human triosephosphate isomerase. *J Biol Chem* 1989; 264:5177–5187.

250. Corran PH, Waley SG. The amino acid sequence of rabbit muscle triose phosphate isomerase. *Biochem J* 1975;145:335–344.

251. Mohrenweiser HW, Fielek S. Elevated frequency of carriers for triosephosphate isomerase deficiency in newborn infants. *Pediatr Res* 1982;16:960–963.

252. Schneider A, Forman L, Westwood B, et al. New insights into the interrelationships of the −5, −8 and −24 mutations with triosephosphate isomerase (TPI) deficiency. *Blood* 1997;90[Suppl]:273a.

253. Schneider A, Forman L, Westwood B, et al. The relationship of the –5, –8 and –24 variant alleles in African Americans to triosephosphate isomerase (TPI) enzyme activity and to TPI deficiency. *Blood* 1998;92:2959–2962.

254. Halfman C, Schneider A, Cohen-Solal M. Insights from molecular modeling into the mechanisms of impaired catalysis in triosephosphate isomerase (TPI) deficiency. *Blood* 1996:88[Suppl]:305a.

255. Halfman C, Schneider A. Hereditary hemolytic anemia with triosephosphate isomerase (TPI) deficiency: assignment of the known mutation sites to functional molecular domains of the enzyme protein. *FASEB J* 1997;2:532a.

256. Arya R, Ringe D, Lalloz MR, et al. Structural analysis of human triosephosphate isomerase (TPI) mutants. *Blood* 1996;88[Suppl]:305a.

257. Daar IO, Artymiuk PJ, Phillips DC, et al. Human triosephosphate isomerase deficiency: a single amino acid substitution results in a thermolabile enzyme. *Proc Natl Acad Sci U S A* 1986;83:7903.

258. Eber SW, Pekrun A, Bardosi A, et al. Triosephosphate isomerase deficiency syndrome: haemolytic anaemia, myopathy with altered mitochondria and mental retardation due to a new variant with accelerated enzyme catabolism and diminished specific activity. *Eur J Pediatr* 1991;150:761–766.

259. Bardosi A, Eber SW, Hendrys M, et al. Myopathy with altered mitochondria due to a triosephosphate-isomerase (TPI) deficiency. *Acta Neuropathol* 1990;79:387–395.

260. Ationu A, Humphries A, Bellingham A, et al. Metabolic correction of triose phosphate isomerase deficiency *in vitro* by complementation. *Biochem Biophys Res Commun* 1997;232:528–531.

261. Ationu A, Humphries A. The feasibility of replacement therapy for inherited disorder of glycolysis: triosephosphate isomerase deficiency. *Int J Mol Med* 1998;2:701–704.

262. Ationu A, Humphries A, Layton DM. Regulation of triosephosphate isomerase (TPI) gene expression in TPI deficient lymphoblastoid cells. *Int J Mol Med* 199;3:21–24.

263. Ationu A, Humphries A, Wild B, et al. Towards enzyme-replacement treatment in triosephosphate isomerase deficiency. *Lancet* 1999;353:1155–1156.

264. Ationu A, Humphries A, Lalloz MR, et al. Reversal of metabolic block in glycolysis by enzyme replacement in triosephosphate isomerase-deficient cells. *Blood* 1999;94:3193–3198.

265. Valentine WN, Oski FA, Paglia DE, et al. Hereditary hemolytic anemia with hexokinase deficiency: role of hexokinase in erythrocyte aging. *N Engl J Med* 1967;276:1.

266. Valentine WN, Oski FA, Paglia DE, et al. Erythrocyte hexokinase and hereditary hemolytic anemia. In: Beutler E, ed. *Hereditary disorders of erythrocyte metabolism.* New York: Grune & Stratton, 1968:288.

267. Keitt AS. Hemolytic anemia with impaired hexokinase activity. *J Clin Invest* 1969;48:1997.

268. Necheles TF, Rai US, Cameron D. Congenital nonspherocytic hemolytic anemia associated with an unusual erythrocyte hexokinase abnormality. *J Lab Clin Med* 1970;76:593.

269. Moser K, Ciresa M, Schwarzmeier J. Hexokinasemangel bei hämolytischer Anämie. *Med Welt* 1970;46:1977.

270. Goebel KM, Gassel WD, Gebel FD, et al. Hemolytic anemia and hexokinase deficiency associated with malformations. *Klin Wochenschr* 1972;50:349.

271. Rijksen G, Staal GE. Human erythrocyte hexokinase deficiency: characterization of a mutant enzyme with abnormal regulatory properties. *J Clin Invest* 1978;62:294.

272. Gilsanz F, Meyer E, Paglia DE, et al. Congenital hemolytic anemia due to hexokinase deficiency. *Am J Dis Child* 1978;132:637.

273. Board PG, Trueworthy R, Smith JE, et al. Congenital nonspherocytic hemolytic anemia with an unstable hexokinase variant. *Blood* 1978;51:111.

274. Beutler E, Dyment PG, Matsumoto F. Hereditary nonspherocytic hemolytic anemia and hexokinase deficiency. *Blood* 1978;51:935.

275. Siimes MA, Rahiala EL, Leisti J. Hexokinase deficiency in erythrocytes: a new variant in five members of a Finnish family. *Scand J Haematol* 1979;22:214.

276. Newman P, Muir A, Parker AC. Non-spherocytic haemolytic anemia in mother and son associated with hexokinase deficiency. *Br J Haematol* 1980;46:537.

277. Paglia DE, Shende A, Lanzkowsky P, et al. Hexokinase "New Hyde Park": a low activity erythrocyte isozyme in a Chinese kindred. *Am J Hematol* 1981;10:107.

278. Rijksen G, Akkerman JW, van den Wall Bake AW. Generalized hexokinase deficiency in the blood cells of a patient with nonspherocytic hemolytic anemia. *Blood* 1983;61:12.

279. Magnani M, Stocchi V, Cucchiarini L. Hereditary nonspherocytic hemolytic anemia due to a new hexokinase variant with reduced stability. *Blood* 1985;66:690.

280. Magnani M, Stocchi V, Canestrari F, et al. Human erythrocyte hexokinase deficiency: a new variant with abnormal kinetic properties. *Br J Haematol* 1985;61:41.

281. Grossbard L, Schimke RT. Multiple hexokinases of rat tissues. Purification and comparisons of soluble forms. *J Biol Chem* 1966;244:3546.

282. Kanno H. Hexokinase: gene structure and mutations. *Best Pract Res Clin Haematol* 2000:13:83–88.

283. Holmes EW Jr, Malone JI, Winegrad AI, et al. Hexokinase isoenzymes in human erythrocytes: association of type II with fetal hemoglobin. *Science* 1967;156:646.

284. Kaplan JC, Beutler E. Hexokinase isoenzymes in human erythrocytes. *Science* 1968;159:215.

285. Stocchi V, Magnani M, Canestrari F, et al. Multiple forms of human red blood cell hexokinase. *J Biol Chem* 1982;257:2357.

286. Murakami K, Blei F, Tilton W, et al. An isozyme of hexokinase specific for the human red blood cell (HK$_R$). *Blood* 1990;75:770.

287. Keitt AS. Hemolytic anemia with impaired hexokinase activity. *J Clin Invest* 1969;48:1997–2007.

288. Beutler E, Dyment PG, Matsumoto F. Hereditary nonspherocytic hemolytic anemia and hexokinase deficiency. *Blood* 1978;51:935.

289. Siimes MA, Rahiala EL, Leisti J. Hexokinase deficiency in erythrocytes: a new variant in five members of a Finnish family. *Scand J Haematol* 1979;22:214.

290. Newman P, Muir A, Parker AC. Non-spherocytic haemolytic anemia in mother and son associated with hexokinase deficiency. *Br J Haematol* 1980;46:537.

290a. Peters LL, Lane PW, Andersen SG, et al. Downeast anemia (dea), a new mouse model of severe nonspherocytic hemolytic anemia caused by hexokinase [HK(I)] deficiency. *Blood Cells Mol Dis* 2001;27:850–860.

291. Goebel KM, Gassel WD, Gebel FD, et al. Hemolytic anemia and hexokinase deficiency associated with malformations. *Klin Wochenschr* 1972;50:849–851.

292. Gilsanz F, Meyer E, Paglia DE, et al. Congenital hemolytic anemia due to hexokinase deficiency. *Am J Dis Child* 1978;132:636–637.

293. Gilsanz F, Meyer E, Paglia DE, et al. Congenital hemolytic anemia due to hexokinase deficiency. *Am J Dis Child* 1978;132:636–637.

294. Magnani M, Stocchi V, Canestrari F, et al. Human erythrocyte hexokinase deficiency: a new variant with abnormal kinetic properties. *Br J Haematol* 1985;61:41–51.

295. Kanno H, Ishikawa K, Fujii H, et al. Severe hexokinase deficiency as a cause of hemolytic anemia, periventricular leukomalacia and intrauterine death of the fetus. *Blood* 1997;90:8a.

296. Löhr GW, Waller HD, Anschutz F, et al. Biochemische defekte in den blutzellen bei familiarer panmyelopathie (typ Fanconi). *Humangenetik* 1965;1:383.

297. Delivoria-Papadopoulos M, Oski FA, Gottlieb AJ. Oxygen-hemoglobin dissociation curves: effect of inherited enzyme defects of the red cell. *Science* 1969;165:601–602.

298. Oski FA, Marshall BE, Cohen PJ, et al. Exercise with anemia: the role of the left-shifted or right-shifted oxygen-hemoglobin equilibrium curve. *Ann Intern Med* 1971;74:44.

299. Valentine WN, Oski FA, Paglia DE, et al. Hereditary hemolytic anemia with hexokinase deficiency: role of hexokinase in erythrocyte aging. *N Engl J Med* 1967;276:1.

300. Valentine WN, Oski FA, Paglia DE, et al. Erythrocyte hexokinase and hereditary hemolytic anemia. In: Beutler E, ed. *Hereditary disorders of erythrocyte metabolism.* New York: Grune & Stratton, 1968:288.

301. Keitt AS. Hemolytic anemia with impaired hexokinase activity. *J Clin Invest* 1969;48:1997.

302. Necheles TF, Rai US, Cameron D. Congenital nonspherocytic hemolytic anemia associated with an unusual erythrocyte hexokinase abnormality. *J Lab Clin Med* 1970;76:593.

303. Rijksen G, Akkerman JWN, van den Wall Bake AW. Generalized hexokinase deficiency in the blood cells of a patient with nonspherocytic hemolytic anemia. *Blood* 1983;61:12.

304. Kanno H, Ishikawa K, Fujii H, et al. Severe hexokinase deficiency as a cause of hemolytic anemia, periventricular leukomalacia and intrauterine death of the fetus. *Blood* 1997;90:8a.

305. Kanno H. Hexokinase: gene structure and mutations. *Best Pract Res Clin Haematol* 2000;13:83–88.

306. Layzer RB, Rowland LP, Bank WJ. Physical and kinetic properties of human phosphofructokinase from skeletal muscle and erythrocytes. *J Biol Chem* 1969;244:3823.

307. Staal GEJ, Koster JF, Banziger CJM, et al. Human erythrocyte phosphofructokinase: its purification and some properties. *Biochim Biophys Acta* 1972;276:113.

308. Karadsheh NS, Uyeda K, Oliver RM. Studies on the structure of human erythrocyte phosphofructokinase. *J Biol Chem* 1977;252:3515.

309. Cottreau D, Levin MJ, Kahn A. Purification and partial characterization of different forms of phosphofructokinase in man. *Biochim Biophys Acta* 1979;586:183.

310. Kahn A, Meienhofer MC, Cottreau D, et al. Phosphofructokinase (PFK) isozymes in man. I. Studies of adult human tissue. *Hum Genet* 1979;48:93.

311. Meienhofer MC, Lagrange JL, Cottreau D, et al. Phosphofructokinase in human blood cells. *Blood* 1979;54:389.

312. Karadsheh NS, Uyeda K, Oliver RM. Studies on the structure of human erythrocyte phosphofructokinase. *J Biol Chem* 1977;252:3515.

313. Cottreau D, Levin MJ, Kahn A. Purification and partial characterization of different form of phosphofructokinase in man. *Biochim Biophys Acta* 1979;586:183.

314. Kahn A, Meienhofer MC, Cottreau D, et al. Phosphofructokinase (PFK) isozymes in man. I. Studies of adult human tissue. *Hum Genet* 1979;48:93.

315. Meienhofer MC, Lagrange JL, Cottreau D, et al. Phosphofructokinase in human blood cells. *Blood* 1979;54:389.

316. Vora S, Seaman C, Durham S, et al. Isozymes of human phosphofructokinase: identification and subunit structural characterization of a new system. *Proc Natl Acad Sci U S A* 1980;77:62.

317. Kahn A, Cottreau D, Meienhofer MC. Purification of F$_4$ phosphofructokinase from human platelets and comparison with the other phosphofructokinase forms. *Biochim Biophys Acta* 1980;611:114.

318. Vora S, Durham S, De Martinville B, et al. Assignment of the human gene for muscle-type phosphofructokinase (PFK) to chromosome 1 (region cen leads to q23) using somatic cell hybrids and monoclonal anti-M antibody. *Somatic Cell Genet* 1982;8:95.

319. Vora S, Francki U. Assignment of the human gene for liver-type 6-phosphofructokinase isozyme (PFKL) to chromosome 21 by using somatic cell hybrids and monoclonal anti-L antibody. *Proc Natl Acad Sci U S A* 1981;78:3738.

320. Vora S, Miranda A, Hernandez E, et al. Regional assignment of the human gene for platelet-type phosphofructokinase (PFKP) to chromosome 10p: novel use of a poly-specific rodent antisera to localize human enzyme genes. *Hum Genet* 1983;63:374.

321. Van Keuren M, Drabkin H, Hart I, et al. Regional assignment of human liver–type 6-phosphofructokinase to chromosome 21q 22.3 by using somatic cell hybrids and a monoclonal anti-L antibody. *Hum Genet* 1986;74:34.

322. Nichols RC, Rudolphi O, Ek B, et al. Glycogenesis type VII (Tarui disease) in a Swedish family: two novel mutations in muscle phosphofructokinase gene (PFK-M) resulting in intron retentions. *Am J Hum Genet* 1996;59:59–65.

323. Bruno C, Minetti C, Shanske S, et al. Combined defects of muscle phosphofructokinase and AMP deaminase in a child with myoglobinuria. *Neurology* 1998;50:296–298.

324. Hamaguchi T, Nakajima H, Noguchi T, et al. A new variant of muscle phosphofructokinase deficiency in a Japanese case with abnormal splicing. *Biochem Biophys Res Commun* 1994;202:444–449.

325. Hamaguchi T, Nakajima H, Noguchi T, et al. Novel missense mutation (W686C) of the phosphofructokinase-M gene in a Japanese patient with a mild form of glycogenesis VII. *Hum Mutat* 1996;8:273–275.

326. Miwa S, Fujii H. Molecular basis of erythroenzymopathies associated with hereditary hemolytic anemia: tabulation of mutant enzymes. *Am J Hematol* 1996;51:122–132.

327. Nakajima H, Kono N, Yamasaki T, et al. Genetic defect in muscle phosphofructokinase deficiency: abnormal splicing of the muscle phosphofructokinase gene due to a point mutation at the 5'-splice site. *J Biol Chem* 1990;265:9392–9395.

328. Raben N, Exelbert R, Spiegel R, et al. Functional expression of human mutant phosphofructokinase in yeast: genetic defects in French Canadian and Swiss patients with phosphofructokinase deficiency. *Am J Hum Genet* 1995;56:131–141.

329. Raben N, Sherman JB. Mutations in muscle phosphofructokinase gene. *Hum Mutat* 1995;6:1–6.

330. Sherman JB, Raben N, Nicastri C, et al. Common mutations in the phosphofructokinase-M gene in Ashkenazi Jewish patients with glycogenesis VII—and their population frequency. *Am J Hum Genet* 1994;55:305–313.

331. Tsujino S, Servidei S, Tonin P, et al. Identification of three novel mutations in non-Ashkenazi Italian patients with muscle phosphofructokinase deficiency. *Am J Hum Genet* 1994;54:812–819.

332. Vasconcelos O, Sivakumar K, Dalakas MC, et al. Nonsense mutation in the phosphofructokinase muscle subunit gene associated with retention of intron 10 in one of the isolated transcripts in Ashkenazi Jewish patients with Tarui disease. *Proc Natl Acad Sci U S A* 1995;92:10322–10326.

333. Smith BF, Stedman H, Raipurohit Y, et al. Molecular basis of canine muscle type phosphofructokinase deficiency. *J Biol Chem* 1996;271:20070–20074.

334. Tarui S, Okuno G, Ikuno Y, et al. Phosphofructokinase deficiency in skeletal muscle. A new type of glycogenesis. *Biochem Biophys Res Commun* 1965;19:517–523.

335. Reference deleted.

336. Reference deleted.

337. Reference deleted.

338. Tarui S, Kono N, Nasu T, et al. Enzymatic basis for the coexistence of myopathy and hemolytic disease in inherited muscle phosphofructokinase deficiency. *Biochem Biophys Res Commun* 1969;34:77.

339. Layzer RB, Rowland LP, Ranney HM. Muscle phosphofructokinase deficiency. *Arch Neurol* 1967;17:512.

340. Etiemble J, Kahn A, Boivin P, et al. Hereditary hemolytic anemia with erythrocyte phosphofructokinase deficiency: studies of some properties of erythrocyte and muscle enzyme. *Hum Genet* 1976;31:83.

341. Miwa S, Sato T, Murao H, et al. A new type of phosphofructokinase deficiency hereditary nonspherocytic hemolytic anemia. *Nippon Ketsueki Gakkai Zasshi* 1972;35:113.

342. Etiemble J, Picat C, Simeon J, et al. Inherited erythrocyte phosphofructokinase deficiency: molecular mechanism. *Hum Genet* 1980;55:383.

343. Waterbury L, Frankel EP. Hereditary nonspherocytic hemolysis with erythrocyte phosphofructokinase deficiency. *Blood* 1972;39:415.

344. Fujii H, Miwa S. Other erythrocyte enzyme deficiencies associated with non-haematological symptoms: phosphoglycerate kinase and phosphofructokinase deficiency. *Best Pract Res Clin Haematol* 2000;13:141–148.

345. Penhoet E, Rajkumar T, Rutter WJ. Multiple forms of fructose diphosphate aldolase in mammalian tissues. *Proc Natl Acad Sci U S A* 1966;56:1275.

346. Lebherz HG, Ruller WJ. Distribution of fructose diphosphate aldolase variants in biological systems. *Biochemistry* 1969;8:109.

347. Kukita A, Yoshida MC, Fukushige S, et al. Molecular gene mapping of human aldolase A (ALDOA) gene to chromosome 16. *Hum Genet* 1987;76:20.

348. Kishi H, Mukai T, Hirono A, et al. Human aldolase A deficiency associated with hemolytic anemia: thermolabile aldolase due to a single base mutation. *Proc Natl Acad Sci U S A* 1987;84:8623–8627.

349. Takasaki Y, Takahasi I, Mukai T, et al. Human aldolase A of a hemolytic anemia patient with Asp128→Gly substitution: characteristics of an enzyme generated in E. coli transfected with the expression plasmid pHAAD 128 G. *J Biochem* 1990;108:153–157.

350. Kreuder J, Borkhardt A, Repp R, et al. Inherited metabolic myopathy and hemolysis due to a mutation in aldolase. *N Engl J Med* 1996;17:1100–1104.

350a. Neufeld EJ, Yao DC, Geva A, et al. Hemolytic anemia and severe rhabdomyolysis due to compound heterozygous mutations of the gene for erythrocyte/muscle isozyme of aldolase: ALDOA (Arg303X/Cys338Tyr). *Blood* 2002;100(Suppl 1) (in press).

351. Kishi H, Mukai T, Hirono A, et al. Human aldolase A deficiency associated with hemolytic anemia: thermolabile aldolase due to a single base mutation. *Proc Natl Acad Sci U S A* 1987;84:8623–8627.

352. Takasaki Y, Takahasi I, Mukai T, et al. Human aldolase A of a hemolytic anemia patient with Asp128→Gly substitution: characteristics of an enzyme generated in E. coli transfected with the expression plasmid pHAAD 128 G. *J Biochem* 1990;108:153–157.

353. Kishi H, Mukai T, Hirono A, et al. Human aldolase A deficiency associated with hemolytic anemia: thermolabile aldolase due to a single base mutation. *Proc Natl Acad Sci U S A* 1987;84:8623–8627.

354. Kreuder J, Borkhardt A, Repp R, et al. Inherited metabolic myopathy and hemolysis due to a mutation in aldolase. *N Engl J Med* 1996;17:1100–1104.

355. Kishi H, Mukai T, Hirono A, et al. Human aldolase A deficiency associated with hemolytic anemia: thermolabile aldolase due to a single base mutation. *Proc Natl Acad Sci U S A* 1987;84:8623–8627.

356. Takasaki Y, Takahasi I, Mukai T, et al. Human aldolase A of a hemolytic anemia patient with Asp 128→Gly substitution: characteristics of an enzyme generated in E. coli transfected with the expression plasmid pHAAD 128 G. *J Biochem* 1990;108:153–157.

357. Kreuder J, Borkhardt A, Repp R, et al. Inherited metabolic myopathy and hemolysis due to a mutation in aldolase. *N Engl J Med* 1996;17:1100–1104.

358. Beutler E, Scott S, Bishop A, et al. Red cell aldolase deficiency and hemolytic anemia: a new syndrome. *Trans Assoc Am Physicians* 1974;86:154.

359. Miwa S, Fujii H, Tani K, et al. Two cases of red cell aldolase deficiency associated with hereditary hemolytic anemia in a Japanese family. *Am J Hematol* 1981;11:425.

360. Kreuder J, Borkhardt A, Repp R, et al. Inherited metabolic myopathy and hemolysis due to a mutation in aldolase. *N Engl J Med* 1996;17:1100–1104.

361. Beutler E, Scott S, Bishop A, et al. Red cell aldolase deficiency and hemolytic anemia: a new syndrome. *Trans Assoc Am Physicians* 1974;86:154.

362. Miwa S, Fujii H, Tani K, et al. Two cases of red cell aldolase deficiency associated with hereditary hemolytic anemia in a Japanese family. *Am J Hematol* 1981;11:425.

363. Deys BF, Grzeschick KH, Grzeschick A, et al. Human phosphoglycerate kinase and inactivation of the X chromosome. *Science* 1972;175:1002.

364. Michaelson AM, Markham AF, Orkin SH. Isolation and DNA sequence of a full-length cDNA clone for human X chromosome-encoded phosphoglycerate kinase. *Proc Natl Acad Sci U S A* 1983;80:472.

365. Michaelson AM, Markham AF, Orkin SH. Isolation and DNA sequence of a full-length cDNA clone for human X chromosome-encoded phosphoglycerate kinase. *Proc Natl Acad Sci U S A* 1983;80:472.

366. Yoshida A, Watanabe S. Human phosphoglycerate kinase. I. Crystallization and characterization of normal enzyme. *J Biol Chem* 1972;247:440.

367. McCarrey JR, Thomas K. Human testis-specific PGK gene lacks introns and possesses characteristics of a processed gene. *Nature* 1987;326:501.

368. Segel GB, Feig SA, Glader BE. Energy metabolism in human erythrocytes: the role of phosphoglycerate kinase in cation transport. *Blood* 1975;46:271.

369. Fujii H, Miwa S. Red cell enzymes. In: Schmidt RM, Fairbanks VF, eds. *CRC handbook series in clinical laboratory science, section I, hematology*, vol. 4. Boca Raton, FL: CRC Press, 1986:307–352.

370. Fujii H, Miwa S. Red blood cell enzymes and their clinical application. *Adv Clin Chem* 1999;33:1–54.

371. Valentin C, Birgens H, Craescue CT, et al. A phosphoglycerate kinase mutant (PGK Herlev; D 285V) in a Danish patient with isolated chronic hemolytic anemia: mechanism of mutation and structure-function relationships. *Hum Mutat* 1998;12:280–287.

372. Svirklys LG, O'Sullivan WJ. Tissue levels of glycolytic enzymes in phosphoglycerate kinase deficiency. *Clin Chim Acta* 1980;108:309.

373. Baehner RL. Metabolic, phagocytic, and bactericidal properties of phosphoglycerate kinase deficient (PGK) polymorphonuclear leukocytes (PMN). *Blood* 1971;38:833.

374. Rosa R, George C, Fardeau M, et al. A new case of phosphoglycerate kinase deficiency: PGK Creteil associated with rhabdomyolysis and lacking hemolytic anemia. *Blood* 1982;60:84.

375. Dimauro S, Dalakas M, Miranda AF. Phosphoglycerate kinase deficiency: another cause of recurrent myoglobinuria. *Ann Neurol* 1983;3:11.

376. Krietsch WK, Eber SE, Haas B, et al. Characterization of a phosphoglycerate kinase deficiency variants not associated with hemolytic anemia. *Am J Hum Genet* 1980;32:364–373.

377. Fujii H, Miwa S. Red cell enzymes. In: Schmidt RM, Fairbanks VF, eds. *CRC Handbook Series in Clinical Laboratory Science, Section I, Hematology*, vol. 4. Boca Raton, FL: CRC Press, 1986:307–352.

378. Valentin C, Birgens H, Craescue CT, et al. A phosphoglycerate kinase mutant (PGK Herlev;D285V) in a Danish patient with isolated chronic hemolytic anemia: mechanism of mutation and structure-function relationships. *Hum Mutat* 1998;12:280–287.

379. Yoshida A, Watanabe S, Chen SH, et al. Human phosphoglycerate kinase. II. Structure of a variant enzyme. *J Biol Chem* 1972;247:446–449.

380. Maeda M, Yoshida A. Molecular defect of a phosphoglycerate kinase variant (PGK Matsue) associated with hemolytic anemia: Leu→Pro substitution caused by a T/A-C/G transition in exon 3. *Blood* 1991;77:1348–1352.

381. Tsujino S, Tonin P, Shanske S, et al. A splice junction mutation in a new myopathic variant of phosphoglycerate kinase deficiency (PGK North Carolina). *Ann Neurol* 1994;35:349–353.

382. Fujii H, Kanno H, Hirono A, et al. A single amino acid substitution (157 Gly→Val) in a phosphoglycerate kinase variant (PGK Shizuoka) associated with chronic hemolysis and myoglobinuria. *Blood* 1992;79:1582–1585.

383. Cohen-Solal M, Valentin C, Plassa F, et al. Identification of new mutations in two phosphoglycerate kinase (PGK) variants expressing different clinical syndromes: PGK Créteil and PGK Amiens. *Blood* 1994;84:898–903.

384. Turner G, Fletcher J, Elber J, et al. Molecular defect of a phosphoglycerate kinase variant associated with haemolytic anaemia and neurological disorders in a large kindred. *Br J Haematol* 1995;91:60–65.

385. Yoshida A, Twele TW, Davé V, et al. Molecular abnormality of a phosphoglycerate kinase variant (PGK-Alabama). *Blood Cells Mol Dis* 1995;21:179–181.

386. Fujii H, Yoshida A. Molecular abnormality of phosphoglycerate kinase–Uppsala associated with chronic nonspherocytic hemolytic anemia. *Proc Natl Acad Sci U S A* 1980;77:5461–5465.

387. Ookawara T, Davé V, Willems P, et al. Retarded and aberrant splicings caused by single exon mutation in a phosphoglycerate kinase variant. *Arch Biochem Biophys* 1996;327:35–40.

388. Sugie H, Sugie Y, Ito M, et al. A novel missense mutation (837T→C) in the phosphoglycerate kinase gene of a patient with a myopathic form of phosphoglycerate kinase deficiency. *J Child Neurol* 1998;13:95–97.

389. Fujii H, Chen SH, Akasuka J, et al. Use of cultured lymphoblastoid cells for the study of abnormal enzymes: molecular abnormality of a phosphoglycerate kinase variant associated with hemolytic anemia. *Proc Natl Acad Sci U S A* 1981;78:2587–2590.

390. Fujii H, Krietsch WK, Yoshida A. A single amino acid substitution (Asp→Asn) in a phosphoglycerate kinase variant (PGK München) associated with enzyme deficiency. *J Biol Chem* 1980;255:6421–6423.

391. Maeda M, Bawle EV, Kulkarni R, et al. Molecular abnormality of a phosphoglycerate kinase variant generated by spontaneous mutation. *Blood* 1992;79:2759–2762.

392. Yoshida A, Watanabe S, Chen SH, et al. Human phosphoglycerate kinase. II. Structure of a variant enzyme. *J Biol Chem* 1972;247:446–449.

393. Fujii H, Yoshida A. Molecular abnormality of phosphoglycerate kinase–Uppsala associated with chronic nonspherocytic hemolytic anemia. *Proc Natl Acad Sci U S A* 1980;77:5461–5465.

394. Fujii H, Krietsch WKG, Yoshida A. A single amino acid substitution (Asp→Asn) in a phosphoglycerate kinase variant (PGK München) associated with enzyme deficiency. *J Biol Chem* 1980;255:6421–6423.

395. Fujii H, Kanno H, Hirono A, et al. A single amino acid substitution (157 Gly→Val) in a phosphoglycerate kinase variant (PGK Shizuoka) associated with chronic hemolysis and myoglobinuria. *Blood* 1992;79:1582–1585.

396. Valentin C, Birgens H, Craescue CT, et al. A phosphoglycerate kinase mutant (PGK Herlev;D285V) in a Danish patient with isolated chronic hemolytic anemia: mechanism of mutation and structure-function relationships. *Hum Mutat* 1998;12:280–287.

397. Yoshida A, Watanabe S, Chen SH, et al. Human phosphoglycerate kinase. II. Structure of a variant enzyme. *J Biol Chem* 1972;247:446–449.

398. Maeda M, Yoshida A. Molecular defect of a phosphoglycerate kinase variant (PGK Matsue) associated with hemolytic anemia: Leu→Pro substitution caused by a T/A-C/G transition in exon 3. *Blood* 1991;77:1348–1352.

399. Tsujino S, Tonin P, Shanske S, et al. A splice junction mutation in a new myopathic variant of phosphoglycerate kinase deficiency (PGK North Carolina). *Ann Neurol* 1994;35:349–353.

400. Fujii H, Kanno H, Hirono A, et al. A single amino acid substitution (157 Gly→Val) in a phosphoglycerate kinase variant (PGK Shizuoka) associated with chronic hemolysis and myoglobinuria. *Blood* 1992;79:1582–1585.

401. Cohen-Solal M, Valentin C, Plassa F, et al. Identification of new mutations in two phosphoglycerate kinase (PGK) variants expressing different clinical syndromes: PGK Créteil and PGK Amiens. *Blood* 1994;84:898–903.

402. Turner G, Fletcher J, Elber J, et al. Molecular defect of a phosphoglycerate kinase variant associated with haemolytic anaemia and neurological disorders in a large kindred. *Br J Haematol* 1995;91:60–65.

403. Yoshida A, Twele TW, Davé V, et al. Molecular abnormality of a phosphoglycerate kinase variant (PGK-Alabama). *Blood Cells Mol Dis* 1995;21:179–181.

404. Fujii H, Yoshida A. Molecular abnormality of phosphoglycerate kinase-Uppsala associated with chronic nonspherocytic hemolytic anemia. *Proc Natl Acad Sci U S A* 1980;77:5461–5465.

405. Ookawara T, Davé V, Willems P, et al. Retarded and aberrant splicings caused by single exon mutation in a phosphoglycerate kinase variant. *Arch Biochem Biophys* 1996;327:35–40.

406. Sugie H, Sugie Y, Ito M, et al. A novel missense mutation (837T→C) in the phosphoglycerate kinase gene of a patient with a myopathic form of phosphoglycerate kinase deficiency. *J Child Neurol* 1998;13:95–97.

407. Fujii H, Chen SH, Akasuka J, et al. Use of cultured lymphoblastoid cells for the study of abnormal enzymes: molecular abnormality of a phosphoglycerate kinase variant associated with hemolytic anemia. *Proc Natl Acad Sci U S A* 1981;78:2587–2590.

408. Fujii H, Krietsch WK, Yoshida A. A single amino acid substitution (Asp→Asn) in a phosphoglycerate kinase variant (PGK München) associated with enzyme deficiency. *J Biol Chem* 1980;255:6421–6423.

409. Maeda M, Bawle EV, Kulkarni R, et al. Molecular abnormalities of a phosphoglycerate kinase variant generated by spontaneous mutation. *Blood* 1992;79:2759–2762.

410. Miwa S, Fujii H. Molecular aspects of erythroenzymopathies associated with hereditary hemolytic anemia. *Am J Hematol* 1985;19:293.

411. Banks RD, Blake CCF, Evans PR, et al. Sequence, structure and activity of phosphoglycerate kinase: a possible hinge-bending enzyme. *Nature* 1979; 279:773.

412. Yoshida A, Watanabe S, Chem SH, et al. Human phosphoglycerate kinase. II. Structure of a variant enzyme. *J Biol Chem* 1972;247:446.

413. Fujii H, Yoshida A. Molecular abnormality of phosphoglycerate kinase–Uppsala associated with chronic nonspherocytic hemolytic anemia. *Proc Natl Acad Sci U S A* 1980;77:5461.

414. Fujii H, Krietsch WK, Yoshida A. A single amino acid substitution (Asp→Asn) in a phosphoglycerate kinase variant (PGK München) associated with enzyme deficiency. *J Biol Chem* 1980;255:6421.

415. Valentine WN, Hsieh HS, Paglia DE, et al. Hereditary hemolytic anemia: association with phosphoglycerate kinase deficiency in erythrocytes and leukocytes. *Trans Assoc Am Physicians* 1968;81:49.

416. Valentine WN, Hsieh HS, Paglia DE, et al. Hereditary hemolytic anemia associated with phosphoglycerate kinase deficiency in erythrocytes and leukocytes: a probable X-chromosome-linked syndrome. *N Engl J Med* 1969;280:528.

417. Cartier PP, Habibi B, Leroux JP, et al. Anemie hemolytique congenitale associee a un deficit en phosphoglycerate kinase dans les globules rouges, les polynucleaires, et les lymphocytes. *Nouv Rev Fr Hematol* 1971;11:565.

418. Konrad PN, McCarthy DJ, Mauer AM, et al. Erythrocyte and leukocyte phosphoglycerate kinase deficiency with neurologic disease. *J Pediatr* 1973;82:456.

419. Boivin P, Hakim J, Mandereau J, et al. Deficit en 3-phosphoglycerate kinase erythrocytaire et leucocytaire: étude des propriétés de l'enzyme, de la fonction phagocytaire des polynucleaires et revise de la littertura. *Nouv Rev Fr Hematol* 1974;14:495.

420. Yoshida A, Miwa S. Characterization of a phosphoglycerate kinase variant associated with hemolytic anemia. *Am J Hum Genet* 1974;26:378.

421. Dodgson SJ, Lee CS, Holland RA, et al. Erythrocyte phosphoglycerate kinase deficiency: enzymatic and oxygen binding studies. *Aust N Z J Med* 1980; 10:614.

422. Rosa R, George C, Fardeau M, et al. A new case of phosphoglycerate kinase deficiency: PGK Creteil associated with rhabdomyolysis and lacking hemolytic anemia. *Blood* 1982;60:84.

423. Dimauro S, Dalakas M, Miranda AF. Phosphoglycerate kinase deficiency: another cause of recurrent myoglobinuria. *Ann Neurol* 1983;13:11.

424. Guis MS, Karadsheh N, Mentzer WC. Phosphoglycerate kinase San Francisco, a new variant associated with hemolytic anemia but not with neuromuscular manifestations. *Am J Hematol* 1987;25:175.

425. Cohen-Solal M, Valentin C, Plassa F, et al. Identification of new mutations in two phosphoglycerate kinase (PGK) variants expressing different clinical syndromes: PGK Créteil and PGK Amiens. *Blood* 1994;84:898–903.

426. Fujii H, Chen SH, Akatsuka J, et al. Use of cultured lymphoblastoid cells for the study of abnormal enzymes: molecular abnormality of a phosphoglycerate kinase variant associated with hemolytic anemia. *Proc Natl Acad Sci U S A* 1981;78:2587–2590.

427. Stefanini M. Chronic hemolytic anemia associated with erythrocyte enolase deficiency exacerbated by ingestion of nitrofurantoin. *Am J Clin Pathol* 1972;58:408–414.

428. Rosa R, Prehic MP, Beuzaid Y, et al. The first case of a complete deficiency of diphosphoglycerate mutase in human erythrocytes. *J Clin Invest* 1978;62:907.

429. Miwa S, Nishina T, Kakehashi Y, et al. Studies on erythrocyte metabolism in a case with hereditary deficiency of H-subunit of lactate dehydrogenase. *Nippon Ketsueki Gakkai Zasshi* 1971;34:228–232.

430. Kitamura M, Iijima N, Hashimoto F, et al. Hereditary deficiency of subunit H of lactate dehydrogenase. *Clin Chim Acta* 1971;34:419.

431. Kanno T, Sudo K, Takeuchi I, et al. Hereditary deficiency of lactate dehydrogenase M-subunit. *Clin Chim Acta* 1980;108:267.

432. Harkness DR. A new erythrocytic enzyme defect with hemolytic anemia: glyceraldehyde-3-phosphate dehydrogenase deficiency. *J Lab Clin Med* 1966;68:879–880(abst).

433. Oski F, Whaun J. Hemolytic anemia and red cell glyceraldehyde–3-phosphate dehydrogenase (G-3-PD) deficiency. *Clin Res* 1969;17:427(abst).

434. Stefanini M. Chronic hemolytic anemia associated with erythrocyte enolase deficiency exacerbated by ingestion of nitrofurantoin. *Am J Clin Pathol* 1972;58:408–414.

435. Beutler E. *Hemolytic anemia in disorders of red cell metabolism.* New York: Plenum Publishing, 1978:215–216.

436. Michelson AM, Markham AF, Orkin SH. Isolation and DNA sequence of a full-length cDNA clone for human X chromosome-encoded phosphoglycerate kinase. *Proc Natl Acad Sci U S A* 1983;80:472–476.

437. Rosa R, Prehic MP, Beuzaid Y, et al. The first case of a complete deficiency of diphosphoglycerate mutase in human erythrocytes. *J Clin Invest* 1978;62:907.

438. Blouquit Y, Rhoda MD, Delanoe-Garin J, et al. Glycerated hemoglobin in a2b282 (EF6) N-e-glyceryl lysine: a new post-translational modification occurring in erythrocyte bisphosphoglyceromutase deficiency. *Biomed Biochim Acta* 1987;46:202.

439. Valentine WN, Fink K, Paglia DE, et al. Hereditary hemolytic anemia with human erythrocyte pyrimidine 5'-nucleotidase deficiency. *J Clin Invest* 1974;54:866.

440. Paglia DE, Valentine WM. Hereditary and acquired defects in the pyrimidine nucleotidase of human erythrocytes. *Curr Top Hematol* 1980;3:75.

441. Lachanat NA, Zerez CR, Tanaka KR. Pyrimidine nucleotides impair phosphoribosyl pyrophosphate (PRPP) synthetase subunit aggregation by sequestering magnesium. A mechanism for the decreased PRPP synthetase activity in hereditary erythrocyte pyrimidine 5'-nucleotidase deficiency. *Biochim Biophys Acta* 1989;994:81–88.

442. Lachant NA, Zerez CR, Tanaka KR. Pyrimidine nucleoside monophos-

phatase kinase hyperactivity in hereditary pyrimidine 5'-nucleotidase deficiency. *Br J Haematol* 1987;66:91–96.

443. Kondo T, Dale GL, Beutler E. Glutathione transport by inside-out vesicles from human erythrocytes. *Proc Natl Acad Sci U S A* 1980;77:6359.

444. Zerez CR, Lachant NA, Tanaka KR. Pyrimidine nucleotides do not affect the enzymes of glutathione biosynthesis. *Enzyme* 1985;34:94.

445. Lachant NA, Zerez CR, Tanaka KR. Pyrimidine nucleotides impair phosphoribosyl pyrophosphate (PRPP) synthetase subunit aggregation by sequestering magnesium: a mechanism for the decreased PRPP synthetase activity in hereditary erythrocyte pyrimidine 5'-nucleotidase deficiency. *Biochim Biophys Acta* 1988;994:81.

446. Tomoda A, Noble NA, Lachant NA, et al. Hemolytic anemia in hereditary pyrimidine 5'-nucleotidase deficiency: nucleotide inhibition of G6PD and the pentose phosphate shunt. *Blood* 1982;60:1212.

447. Swallow DM, Turner VS, Hopkinson DA. Isozymes of rodent 5-prime-nucleotidase: evidence for two independent structural loci UMPH-1 and UMPH-2. *Ann Hum Genet* 1983;47:9–17.

448. Paglia DE, Valentine WN, Brockway RA. Identification of thymidine nucleotidase and deoxyribonucleotidase activities among normal isozymes of 5-prime-nucleotidase in human erythrocytes. *Proc Natl Acad Sci U S A* 1984;81: 588–592.

449. Hirono A, Fujii H, Miwa S. Isozymes of human erythrocyte pyrimidine 5'nucleotidase-chromatographic separation and their properties. *Jpn J Exp Med* 1985;5537–5544.

450. Paglia DE, Valentine WN, Brockway RA. Identification of thymidine nucleotidase and deoxyribonucleotidase activities among normal isozymes of 5'-nucleotidase in human erythrocytes. *Proc Natl Acad Sci U S A* 1984;81:588.

451. Hopkinson DA, Swallow DM, Marinaki A, et al. Pyrimidine 5'nucleotidase activity in normal and deficient human lymphoblastoid cells. *J Inherit Dis* 1990;13:701–706.

452. De Korte D, Sijstermans JM, Seip M, et al. Pyrimidine 5'-nucleotidase deficiency: improved detection of carriers. *Clin Chim Acta* 1989;184:175–180.

453. Valentine WN, Bennett JM, Krivit W, et al. Nonspherocytic haemolytic anaemia with increased red cell adenine nucleotides, glutathione and basophilic stippling and ribose-phosphate pyrophosphokinase (RPK) deficiency: studies on two new kindreds. *Br J Haematol* 1973;24:157–167.

454. David O, Ramenghi U, Camaschella C, et al. Inhibition of hexose monophosphatase shunt in young erythrocytes by pyrimidine nucleotides in hereditary pyrimidine 5'-nucleotidase deficiency. *Eur J Haematol* 1991;47:48–54.

455. Rees DC, Styles L, Vichinsky EP, et al. The hemoglobin E syndromes. *Ann N Y Acad Sci* 1998;850:334–343.

456. Paglia DE, Valentine WN. Hereditary and acquired defects in the pyrimidine nucleotidase of human erythrocytes. *Curr Top Hematol* 1980;3:75.

457. Beutler E. Red cell enzyme defects as nondiseases and as diseases. *Blood* 1979;54:1.

458. Beutler E, Baranko PV, Feagler J, et al. Hemolytic anemia due to pyrimidine-5'-nucleotidase deficiency: report of eight cases in six families. *Blood* 1980;56:251.

459. Valentine WN, Fink K, Paglia DE, et al. Hereditary hemolytic anemia with human erythrocyte pyrimidine 5'-nucleotidase deficiency. *J Clin Invest* 1974; 54:866–879.

460. Irono A, Forman I, Beutler E. Enzymatic diagnosis in non-spherocytic hemolytic anemia. *Medicine* 1988;67:110–117.

461. Vives-Corrons JL. Chronic non-spherocytic haemolytic anaemia due to congenital pyrimidine 5' nucleotidase deficiency: 25 years later. *Best Pract Res Clin Haematol* 2000;13:103–118.

462. Torrance JD, Whittaker D. Distribution of erythrocyte nucleotides in pyrimidine 5'-nucleotidase deficiency. *Br J Haematol* 1979;43:423.

463. Swanson MS, Angle CR, Stohs SJ, et al. ³¹P NMR study of erythrocytes from a patient with hereditary pyrimidine-5'-nucleotidase deficiency. *Proc Natl Acad Sci U S A* 1983;80:169.

464. Swanson MS, Markin RS, Stohs SJ, et al. Identification of cytidine diphosphodiesters in erythrocytes from a patient with pyrimidine nucleotidase deficiency. *Blood* 1984;63:665.

465. Ericson A, de Verdier CH, Ruud Hansen TW, et al. Erythrocyte nucleotide pattern in two children in a Norwegian family with pyrimidine 5'-nucleotidase deficiency. *Clin Chim Acta* 1983;134:25.

466. Valentine WN, Fink K, Paglia DE, et al. Hereditary hemolytic anemia with human erythrocyte pyrimidine 5'-nucleotidase deficiency. *J Clin Invest* 1974; 54:866.

467. Paglia DE, Valentine WN. Hereditary and acquired defects in the pyrimidine nucleotidase of human erythrocytes. *Curr Top Hematol* 1980;3:75.

468. Miwa S, Luzzatto L, Rosa R, et al. Recommended screening test for pyrimidine 5'-nucleotidase deficiency. *Clin Lab Haematol* 1989;11:55.

469. Miwa S, Luzzatto L, Rosa R, et al. Recommended methods for an additional red cell enzyme (pyrimidine 5'-nucleotidase assays and the determination of red cell adenosine-5'-triphosphate, 2,3-diphosphoglycerate and reduced glutathione. *Clin Lab Haematol* 1989;11:131.

470. International Committee for Standardization in Haematology. Recommended screening test for pyrimidine 5'-nucleotidase deficiency. *Clin Lab Haematol* 1989;11:55–56.

471. Valentine WN, Fink K, Paglia DE, et al. Hereditary hemolytic anemia with human erythrocyte pyrimidine 5'-nucleotidase deficiency. *J Clin Invest* 1974; 54:866.

472. Paglia DE, Valentine WN. Hereditary and acquired defects in the pyrimidine nucleotidase of human erythrocytes. *Curr Top Hematol* 1980;3:75.

473. Torrance J, West C, Beutler E. A simple rapid radiometric assay for pyrimidine-5'-nucleotidase. *J Lab Clin Med* 1977;90:563–568.

474. Ellims PH, Bailey L, Van der Weyden MB. An improved method for the determination of human erythrocyte pyrimidine 5'-nucleotidase activity. *Clin Chim Acta* 1978;88:99–103.

475. Amici A, Natalini P, Ruggieri S, et al. A spectrophotometric method for the assay of pyrimidine 5'-nucleotidase in human erythrocytes. *Br J Haematol* 1989;73:392–395.

476. Sakai T, Ushio K. A simplified method for determining erythrocyte pyrimidine 5'-nucleotidase (P5'N) activity by HPLC and its value in monitoring lead exposure. *Br J Indust Med* 1986;43:839–844.

477. Adair CG, Elder GE, Lappin TR, et al. Red cell pyrimidine 5'-nucleotidase deficiency: determination of nucleotidase activity and nucleotide content using HPLC. *Clin Chim Acta* 1988;171:75–83.

478. Kagimoto T, Shirono K, Higaki T, et al. Detection of pyrimidine 5'-nucleotidase deficiency using IH or 3IP-nuclear magnetic resonance. *Experientia* 1986;42:69–72.

479. Mendz GL, Middlehurst CR, Kuchel PW, et al. Determination of erythrocyte pyrimidine 5'-nucleotidase activity by 3IP nuclear magnetic resonance: comparison of normal controls and multiple sclerosis patients. *Experientia* 1986;42:1016–1018.

480. Sakai T, Araki T, Ushio K. Determination of pyrimidine 5'-nucleotidase (P5'N) activity in whole blood as an index of lead exposure. *Br J Indust Med* 1988;45:420–425.

481. Cook L, Kubitschek C, Stohls S, et al. Erythrocyte pyrimidine 5'-nucleotidase and deoxynucleotidase isozymes: metallosensitivity and kinetics. *Drug Chem Toxicol* 1988;11:195–213.

482. Vives-Corrons JL, Montserrat-Costa E, Rozman C. Hereditary hemolytic anemia with erythrocyte pyrimidine 5'-nucleotidase deficiency in Spain. Clinical, biological and familial studies. *Hum Genet* 1976;34:285–292.

483. Hansen TW, Seip M, De Verdier CH, et al. Erythrocyte pyrimidine 5'-nucleotidase deficiency. Report of two new cases, with a review of the literature. *Scand J Haematol* 1983;31:122–128.

484. Rees DC, Duley J, Simmonds HA, et al. Interaction of hemoglobin E and pyrimidine 5'-nucleotidase deficiency. *Blood* 1996;88:2761–2767.

485. Paglia DE, Valentine WN. Characteristics of a pyrimidine-specific 5'-nucleotidase in human erythrocytes. *J Biol Chem* 1975;250:7973.

486. Paglia DE, Valentine WN, Dahlgren JG. Effects of low-level lead exposure on pyrimidine 5'-nucleotidase and other erythrocyte enzymes: possible role of pyrimidine 5'-nucleotidase in the pathogenesis of lead-induced anemia. *J Clin Invest* 1975;56:1164.

487. Buc HA, Kaplan JC. Red cell pyrimidine 5'-nucleotidase and lead poisoning. *Clin Chim Acta* 1978;87:49.

488. Angle CR, McIntire MS. Low level lead and inhibition of erythrocyte pyrimidine nucleotidase. *Environ Res* 1978;17:296.

489. Paglia DE, Valentine WN, Fink K. Lead poisoning: further observations on erythrocyte pyrimidine-nucleotidase deficiency and intracellular accumulation of pyrimidine nucleotides. *J Clin Invest* 1977;60:1362.

490. Paglia DE, Valentine WN, Fink K. Lead poisoning: further observations on erythrocyte pyrimidine-nucleotidase deficiency and intracellular accumulation of pyrimidine nucleotides. *J Clin Invest* 1977;60:1362.

491. Valentine WN, Paglia DE, Fink K, et al. Lead poisoning: association with hemolytic anemia, basophilic stippling, erythrocyte pyrimidine 5'-nucleotidase deficiency, and intraerythrocytic accumulation of pyrimidines. *J Clin Invest* 1976;58:926.

492. Spencer N, Hopkinson DA, Harris H. Adenosine deaminase polymorphism in man. *Ann Hum Genet* 1968;32:9.

493. Hopkinson DA, Cook PJ, Harris H. Further data on the adenosine deaminase (ADA) polymorphism and a report of a new phenotype. *Ann Hum Genet* 1969;32:361.

494. Edwards YH, Hopkinson DA, Harris H. Adenosine deaminase isozymes in human tissues. *Ann Hum Genet* 1971;35:207.

495. Daddona PE, Kelley WN. Human adenosine deaminase: purification and subunit structure. *J Biol Chem* 1977;252:110.

496. Daddona PE, Kelley WN. Human adenosine deaminase binding protein: assay, purification and properties. *J Biol Chem* 1978;253:4617.

497. Tischfield JA, Creagan RP, Nichols EA, et al. Assignment of a gene for adenosine deaminase to human chromosome 20. *Hum Hered* 1974;24:1.

498. Philip T, Lenoir G, Rolland MO, et al. Regional assignment of the ADA locus on 20q13.2 leads to qter by gene dosage studies. *Cytogenet Cell Genet* 1980; 27:187–189.

499. Koch G, Shows TB. A gene on human chromosome 6 functions in assembly of tissue-specific adenosine deaminase isozymes. *Proc Natl Acad Sci U S A* 1978;75:3876.

500. Hirschhorn R, Levytska V, Pollara B, et al. Evidence for control of several different tissue-specific isozymes of adenosine deaminase by a single genetic locus. *Nat New Biol* 1973;246:200.

501. Hirschhorn R. Conversion of human erythrocyte-adenosine deaminase activity to different tissue-specific isozymes: evidence for a common catalytic unit. *J Clin Invest* 1975;55:661.

502. Giblett ER, Anderson JE, Cohen F, et al. Adenosine deaminase deficiency in two patients with severely impaired cellular immunity. *Lancet* 1972;2: 1067.

503. Agarwal RP, Crabtree GW, Parks RE, et al. Purine nucleoside metabolism in the erythrocytes of patients with adenosine deaminase deficiency and severe combined immunodeficiency. *J Clin Invest* 1976;57:1025.

504. Schmalstieg FC, Goldman AS, Mills GC, et al. Nucleotide metabolism in adenosine deaminase deficiency. *Pediatr Res* 1976;10:393.

505. Cohen A, Hirschhorn R, Horowitz SD, et al. Deoxyadenosine triphosphate as a potentially toxic metabolite in adenosine deaminase deficiency. *Proc Natl Acad Sci U S A* 1978;75:472.

506. Coleman MS, Donofrio J, Hutton JJ, et al. Identification and quantitation of adenine deoxynucleotides in erythrocytes of a patient with adenosine deaminase deficiency and severe combined immunodeficiency. *J Biol Chem* 1978;253:1619.

507. Nelson JA, Kuttesch JF, Goldblum RN, et al. Analysis of adenosine and adenine nucleotides in severe combined immunodeficiency disease. In: Baer HP, Drummond GI, eds. *Physiological and regulatory functions of adenosine and adenine nucleotides.* New York: Raven Press, 1979:417.

508. Valentine WN, Paglia DE, Tartaglia AP, et al. Hereditary hemolytic anemia with increased red cell adenosine deaminase (45- to 70-fold) and decreased adenosine triphosphate. *Science* 1977;195:783.

509. Paglia DE, Valentine WN, Tartaglia AP, et al. Control of red blood cell adenine nucleotide metabolism: studies of adenosine deaminase. In: Brewer GJ, ed. *The red cell.* New York: Alan R. Liss, 1978:319.

510. Fujii H, Miwa S, Suzuki K. Purification and properties of adenosine deaminase in normal and hereditary hemolytic anemia with increased red cell activity. *Hemoglobin* 1980;4:693.

511. Perignon JL, Hamet M, Buc HA, et al. Biochemical study of a case of hemolytic anemia with increased (85-fold) red cell adenosine deaminase. *Clin Chim Acta* 1982;124:205.

512. Miwa S, Fujii H, Matsumoto N, et al. A case of red-cell adenosine deaminase overproduction associated with hereditary hemolytic anemia found in Japan. *Am J Hematol* 1978;5:107.

513. Valentine WN, Paglia DE, Tartaglia AP, et al. Hereditary hemolytic anemia with increased red cell adenosine deaminase (45- to 70-fold) and decreased adenosine triphosphate. *Science* 1977;195:783.

514. Paglia DE, Valentine WN, Tartaglia AP, et al. Control of red blood cell adenine nucleotide metabolism: studies of adenosine deaminase. In: Brewer GJ, ed. *The red cell.* New York: Alan R. Liss, 1978:319.

515. Fujii H, Miwa S, Suzuki K. Purification and properties of adenosine deaminase in normal and hereditary hemolytic anemia with increased red cell activity. *Hemoglobin* 1980;4:693.

516. Fujii H, Miwa S, Tani K, et al. Overproduction of structurally normal enzyme in man: hereditary haemolytic anaemia with increased red cell adenosine deaminase activity. *Br J Haematol* 1982;51:427.

517. Chottiner EG, Cloft HJ, Tartaglia AP, et al. Elevated adenosine deaminase activity and hereditary hemolytic anemia: evidence for abnormal translational control of protein synthesis. *J Clin Invest* 1987;79:1001.

518. Chottiner EG, Ginsburg D, Tartaglia AP, et al. Erythrocyte adenosine deaminase overproduction in hereditary hemolytic anemia. *Blood* 1989;74:448.

519. Chen EH, Tartaglia AP, Mitchell BS. Hereditary overexpression of adenosine deaminase in erythrocytes: evidence for a cis-acting mutation. *Am J Hum Genet* 1993;53:889–893.

520. Paglia DE, Valentine WN, Tartaglia AP, et al. Control of red blood cell adenine nucleotide metabolism: studies of adenosine deaminase. In: Brewer GJ, ed. *The red cell.* New York: Alan R. Liss, 1978:319.

521. Paglia DE, Valentine WN. Haemolytic anemia associated with disorders of the purine and pyrimidine salvage pathways. *Clin Haematol* 1981;10:81.

522. Paglia DE, Valentine WN, Tartaglia AP, et al. Control of red blood cell adenine nucleotide metabolism: studies of adenosine deaminase. In: Brewer GJ, ed. *The red cell.* New York: Alan R. Liss, 1978:319.

523. Paglia DE, Valentine WN. Haemolytic anemia associated with disorders of the purine and pyrimidine salvage pathways. *Clin Haematol* 1981;10:81.

524. Fildes RA, Harris H. Genetically determined variation of adenylate kinase in man. *Nature* 1966;209:261.

525. Bowman JE, Frischer H, Ajmar F, et al. Population, family and biochemical investigation of human adenylate kinase polymorphism. *Nature* 1967;214:1156.

526. Kho JC, Russell PJ Jr. Isoenzymes of adenylate kinase in human tissue. *Biochim Biophys Acta* 1972;268:98.

527. Russell PJ Jr, Hornstein JM, Goins L, et al. Adenylate kinase in human tissues. I. Organ specificity of adenylate kinase isoenzymes. *J Biol Chem* 1974;249:1874.

528. McKusik VA, Ruddle FH. The status of the gene map of the human chromosomes. *Science* 1977;196:390.

529. Thuma E, Schirmer RH, Schirmer J. Preparation and characterization of a crystalline human ATP:AMP phosphotransferase. *Biochim Biophys Acta* 1972;268:81.

530. Von Zabern I, Wittmann-Liebold B, Untucht-Grau R, et al. Primary and tertiary structure of the principle human adenylate kinase. *Eur J Biochem* 1976;68:281.

531. Szeinberg A, Gavendo S, Cahane D. Erythrocyte adenylate-kinase deficiency. *Lancet* 1969;1:315.

532. Szeinberg A, Kahana D, Gavendo S, et al. Hereditary deficiency of adenylate kinase in red blood cells. *Acta Haematol* 1969;42:111.

533. Boivin P, Galand C, Hakim J, et al. Une nouvelle erythroenzymopathie: anemie hemolytique congenitale nonspherocytaire et deficit hereditaire en adenylate-kinase erythrocytaire. *Presse Med* 1971;79:215.

534. Miwa S, Fujii H, Tani K, et al. Red cell adenylate kinase deficiency associated with hereditary nonspherocytic hemolytic anemia: clinical and biochemical studies. *Am J Hematol* 1983;14:325.

535. Beutler E, Carson D, Dannawi H, et al. Metabolic compensation for profound erythrocyte adenylate kinase deficiency: a hereditary defect without hemolytic anemia. *J Clin Invest* 1983;72:648.

536. Bianchi P, Zappa M, Bredi E, et al. A case of complete adenylate kinase deficiency due to a nonsense mutation in AK-1 gene (Arg 107→Stop; CGA→TGA) associated with chronic haemolytic anaemia. *Br J Haematol* 1999;105:75–79.

537. Matsura S, Igarashi M, Tamizawa Y, et al. Human adenylate deficiency associated with hemolytic anemia: a single base substitution affecting solubility and catalytic activity of the cytosolic adenylate kinase. *J Biol Chem* 1989;264:10148–10155.

538. Qualtieri A, Pedace V, Bisconte G, et al. Severe erythrocyte adenylated kinase deficiency due to homozygous A→G substitution at codon 164 of human AK I gene associated with chronic haemolytic anaemia. *Br J Haematol* 1997;99:770–776.

539. Beutler E. Red cell enzyme defects as nondiseases and as diseases. *Blood* 1979;54:1.

540. Kanno H, Fujii h, Hirono A, et al. Molecular analysis of glucose phosphate isomerase deficiency associated with heredity hemolytic anemia. *Blood* 1996;88:2321–2325.

541. Xu W, Beutler E. The characterization of gene mutations for human glucose phosphate isomerase deficiency associated with chronic hemolytic anemia. *J Clin Invest* 1994;94:2326–2329.

542. Walker JIH, Layton DM, Bellingham AJ, et al. DNA sequence abnormalities in human glucose 6-phosphate isomerase deficiency. *Human Mol Genet* 1993;2:327–329.

543. Huppke P, Wunsch D, Pekrun A, et al. Glucose phosphate isomerase deficiency: biochemical and molecular genetic studies on the enzyme variants of two patients with severe haemolytic anameia. *Eur J Pediatr* 1997;156:605–609.

Glucose-6-Phosphate Dehydrogenase Deficiency and Related Disorders

Thomas J. Vulliamy and Lucio Luzzatto

HISTORIC NOTE

The prehistory of glucose-6-phosphate dehydrogenase (G6PD) deficiency begins with an anecdote from the school of Pythagoras (6th century BC), who appears to have warned his disciples that they should not retreat into a field of fava beans even if their lives were at risk. This notion was supported one century later by one of Hippocrates' maxims, *kuamon apecesqe* (avoid fava beans). We do not know whether the Latin poet Lucretius Caro had favism in mind when he said that what is food for some can be harsh poison to others, but the lucid expression of this concept clearly marks him as the founder of pharmacogenetics.

The history of G6PD deficiency began to be recorded, if not by this name, in the Italian medical literature of the 19th century AD, when "ictero-hemoglobinuric favism" became recognized as a distinct clinical entity. Some astute medical practitioners appreciated that favism "runs in families." In those days, immunology was far more influential than genetics (Paul Ehrlich received a Nobel prize at approximately the time when Gregor Mendel's work had remained ignored for half a century), and favism was thought to be a manifestation of some kind of allergic reaction. In 1923, hemolytic anemia in patients receiving pamaquine for the treatment of malaria was first reported (Table 54-1).

"Primaquine sensitivity" came to be perceived as a prominent problem in military medicine during World War II and its aftermath in Korea. The group led by A. S. Alving in Chicago embarked on a systematic study of the syndrome, and in 1956, G6PD deficiency made history when Paul Carson and colleagues (1) discovered that subjects who previously had been identified as primaquine sensitive had a marked deficiency of G6PD activity in their red blood cells. Within a year, similar data appeared in Germany, and in Italy, Sansone and Segni (2) proved that favism was also due to G6PD deficiency. Thus, the problem was solved at the level of biochemical genetics, and G6PD deficiency became a prototype for a variety of disorders due to deficiency in red cells of a specific enzyme, or *enzymopathies*.

Following those early discoveries, the biochemical heterogeneity of G6PD deficiency soon became apparent, but it took the best part of 30 years to define the basis of this variation at the molecular level. We now know that G6PD deficiency is caused by a variety of structural mutants that can be located on the recently solved, three-dimensional structure of the G6PD protein. The subject has been reviewed extensively over the years, and the reader is referred to several concise (3–5) and more comprehensive (6–8) reviews that have appeared recently.

PENTOSE PHOSPHATE PATHWAY

G6PD catalyzes the first reaction of the pentose phosphate pathway (PPP), which has two main products: pentose phosphate sugars and the reduced form of nicotinamide adenine dinucleotide phosphate (NADPH) (Fig. 54-1). The PPP has often been regarded as a "shunt" from the classic glycolytic pathway, as the pentose sugars produced can be recycled by transketolase and transaldolase to fructose-6-phosphate (F6P) and triose phosphate. However, the pentose phosphates, the sugar building blocks of nucleic acids, can also be produced directly from F6P through the concerted action (in reverse) of transketolase and transaldolase, bypassing the first part of the PPP and making it dispensable for pentose production.

By contrast, the product of the PPP that is not produced elsewhere in carbohydrate metabolism is NADPH, and there is every indication that the main role of the PPP, in red cells, is the production of NADPH. The role of NADPH is well established as the coenzyme of numerous reductive processes, including fatty acid synthesis, the synthesis of cholesterol and consequently steroid hormones, purine and pyrimidine synthesis, and porphyrin synthesis. In the red cell, however, most of these biosynthetic pathways have been lost during erythroid cell maturation, and the main role of G6PD is to produce reducing potential in the form of NADPH, which is essential in protecting cells against oxidative damage. This role is crucial because red cells, being oxygen carriers par excellence, have a literally built-in danger of damage by oxygen radicals, generated continuously in the course of methemoglobin formation. The detoxification of H_2O_2 is achieved through maintaining a high level of reduced glutathione (GSH) (Fig. 54-2) and through the action of catalase, which is also dependent on the availability of reduced NADPH (9) and may be particularly important when NADPH is in short supply due to G6PD deficiency (10).

Recent data suggest that the role of G6PD in protection against oxidative stress is also relevant in somatic cells: Overexpression of G6PD in HeLa cells (11) and NIH 3T3 fibroblasts (12) results in a strong protection against oxidant-mediated cell death, and the

TABLE 54-1. Historical Landmarks in the Study of Glucose-6-Phosphate Dehydrogenase (G6PD) Deficiency

1905	Clinical characterization of favism
1923	Hemolytic anemia associated with primaquine sensitivity
1932	G6PD activity demonstrated in red cells
1956	G6PD deficiency discovered
1960	CNSHA associated with G6PD deficiency
1960	G6PD deficiency associated with malaria
1961	X-linkage of G6PD
1962–1963	Somatic cell mosaicism in females heterozygous for G6PD variants
1966	G6PD purified to homogeneity
1967	Characterization of G6PD variants standardized
1969	Subunit structure of G6PD established
1981	Inhibition of *Plasmodium falciparum* development in G6PD-deficient red cells
1986	Cloning and sequence of the human G6PD gene
1988	Molecular basis of G6PD deficiency
1994	Structure of *Leuconostoc mesenteroides* G6PD
2000	Structure of human G6PD

CNSHA, chronic nonspherocytic hemolytic anemia.

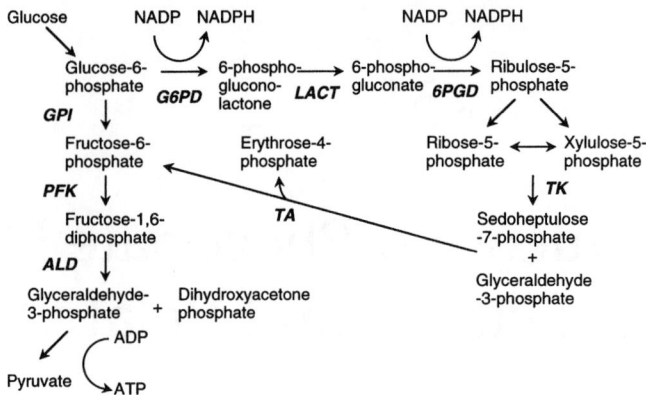

Figure 54-1. The pentose phosphate pathway is shown. Glucose is metabolized anaerobically to pyruvate by way of the Embden-Myerhoff pathway **(left)**. The hexose monophosphate shunt, or phosphogluconate pathway **(right)**, begins with the dehydrogenation of glucose-6-phosphate by glucose-6-phosphate dehydrogenase (G6PD) to yield 6-phosphoglucono-lactone. 6-Phosphoglucono-lactone is then hydrolyzed to 6-phosphogluconate by lactonase (LACT) and decarboxylated by 6-phosphogluconate dehydrogenase (6PGD) to the ketosugar ribulose-5-phosphate and CO_2. The first and third steps generate nicotinamide adenine dinucleotide phosphate (NADPH), which is a critical component of the red cell's glutathione antioxidant system. Ribulose-5-phosphate is reversibly transformed to xylulose-5-phosphate by phosphopentose epimerase and into the aldo sugar ribose-5-phosphate by phosphopentose isomerase. The thiamine-containing enzyme transketolase (TK) transfers a glycoaldehyde group from xylulose-5-phosphate to ribose-5-phosphate, producing sedoheptulose-7-phosphate and glyceraldehyde-3-phosphate (Ga3P), which is also an intermediate in the Embden-Myerhoff pathway. Finally, transaldolase (TA) transfers a dihydroxyacetone group from sedoheptulose-7-phosphate to Ga3P to form fructose-6-phosphate and erythrose-4-phosphate (not shown). In addition, TK can convert xylulose-5-phosphate and erythrose-4-phosphate to fructose-6-phosphate and Ga3P (not shown). ADP, adenosine 5'-diphosphate; ALD, aldolase; ATP, adenosine triphosphate; GPI, glucosephosphate isomerase; PFK, phosphofructokinase.

protective effect of small stress proteins in fibroblasts is mediated through an increase in G6PD activity, causing GSH levels to rise (13). G6PD has also been shown to play a critical role in cell growth, with overexpression stimulating the growth of several cell lines (14). The overexpression of G6PD in NIH 3T3 cells may even have an oncogenic effect, with clones losing contact-inhibited growth and forming fibrosarcomas in nude mice (15).

Further information about the protective role of G6PD comes from G6PD-deficient mice. Although embryonic stem cells in which the G6PD gene has been knocked out are still viable, they are exquisitely sensitive to oxidative stress (16). These cells give rise to chimeras and heterozygotes, but no hemizygotes are born with the null allele, supporting the idea that G6PD null mutations are lethal. Hemizygous mice for a splicing mutation in the G6PD gene that have approximately 15% residual enzyme activity have an increased rate of prenatal and postnatal death (17). Furthermore, when pregnant females that were homozygous for this mutation were treated with phenytoin, a human teratogen that causes embryonic oxidative stress, more fetal death and birth defects were observed.

Regulation of Glucose-6-Phosphate Dehydrogenase and the Pentose Phosphate Pathway

The first reaction of a metabolic pathway is often rate limiting, and the PPP is no exception. The first reaction is catalyzed by G6PD, and therefore we can expect that control is exerted here. There is good evidence that, at least in red cells (where changing the rate of G6PD biosynthesis is not an option), NADP and NADPH are the main agents that control the rate of G6PD activity (18,19). This can be understood by considering three important features of the system:

- The affinity of G6PD for NADP is high: The affinity constant (K_m) values measured under different experimental conditions are in the range of 3 to 13 μmol/L.
- NADPH is an inhibitor with partially competitive kinetics (with respect to NADP) and an inhibition constant (K_i) of approximately 16 μmol/L.
- In normal red cells in the steady state, the concentration of NADP is hardly measurable, whereas NADPH is on the order of 35 μmol/L.

This set of values means that the G6PD reaction is normally almost completely inhibited. Because the total intracellular amount of NADP + NADPH is relatively fixed, whenever NADPH is oxidized to NADP, this simultaneously provides substrate for the G6PD reaction and decreases the product inhibition. NADP is then almost quantitatively reduced to NADPH, and the original steady state is restored. In terms of the capacity to generate NADPH, it is remarkable that, because of the low basal activity of G6PD, this can increase by a factor of at least 10 as an instant response to oxidative stress, without any change in the number of G6PD molecules. Detailed analysis of this phenomenon has revealed that, even under maximal stimulation, the activity of G6PD within intact red cells is still approximately 60 times less than that in hemolysates (20). Thus, the cell appears to have a large reserve potential for NADPH generation.

The kinetics of G6PD have been investigated in considerable detail. NADP became established relatively early in evolution as its coenzyme, and human G6PD has practically no activity with NAD (21). Interestingly, the G6PD of *Leuconostoc mesenteroides* has instead a dual specificity: It uses NAD or NADP, depending on the metabolic role of the reaction, under different physiologic conditions (22). G6PD is also specific with respect to G6P, and it has relatively low activity on other hexose phosphates (e.g., mannose-6-P or galactose-6-P). By contrast, there is significant activity on substrate analogs, such as deamino-NADP and 2-deoxyglucose-6-P. These compounds, although artificial, have been useful in the characterization of variants. The affinity for NADP is approximately one order of magnitude higher than the affinity for G6P.

The activity of G6PD can also be regulated by changing the number of G6PD molecules, through variation in the rates of

G6PD

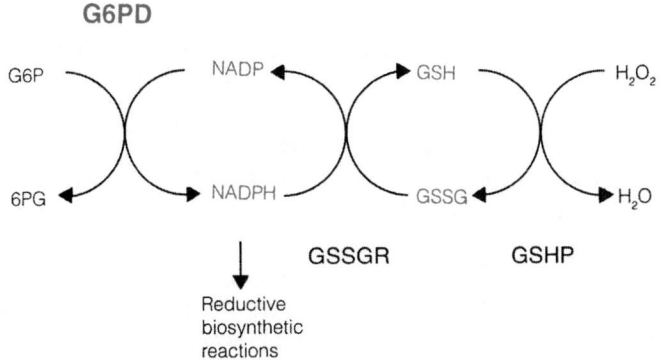

Figure 54-2. The principal metabolic role of glucose-6-phosphate dehydrogenase (G6PD) in red cells is to protect red cell constituents from oxidants, illustrated here by hydrogen peroxide (H_2O_2). Nicotinamide adenine dinucleotide phosphate (NADPH), a product of the G6PD reaction and the subsequent step in the pentose phosphate pathway, is the hydrogen donor for regeneration of reduced glutathione (GSH) from oxidized glutathione (GSSG), a reaction catalyzed by glutathione reductase (GSSGR). NADPH is also a ligand for catalase, which degrades H_2O_2. GSHP, glutathione peroxidase; 6PG, 6-phosphogluconate.

transcription, transcript processing, message stability, translation, and proteolytic degradation. All of these are likely to play a role in different circumstances. For example, the increase in G6PD activity seen in response to oxidative stress in human cell lines is mainly due to an increased rate of transcription, although posttranscriptional regulation plays a minor but significant role (23). In contrast, a posttranscriptional mechanism acting at an early step after the transcription of the pre-mRNA is responsible for the stimulation of the expression of G6PD in response to feeding a high-carbohydrate diet to starved mice (24). The half-life of G6PD in different tissues varies considerably, from approximately 2 days in fibroblasts (25) to 60 days in red cells (26), and this is thought to reflect different rates of proteolysis.

GLUCOSE-6-PHOSPHATE DEHYDROGENASE STRUCTURE

The enzymatically active form of G6PD is either a dimer or a tetramer of a single polypeptide subunit with a molecular mass of 59,096 daltons (27). The amino acid sequence of the human enzyme (Fig. 54-3) has been deduced from the nucleotide sequence of a full-length complementary DNA clone encoding 515 amino acids (28). The rat liver G6PD amino acid sequence (29) obtained by protein analysis shows 94% homology to the human sequence and provides evidence that the N-terminal amino acid is *N*-acetyl-alanine, which must result from post-translational cleavage of the N-terminal methionine followed by acetylation. It has more recently been demonstrated that the same is true of the human enzyme (30). Fifty-two different G6PD sequences from 42 different organisms have been compiled (31) to reveal between 29% and 94% overall homology with the human enzyme; several stretches of highly conserved amino acids can be identified (Fig. 54-3), which, not surprisingly, correspond to functionally important domains of the protein.

The original model of human G6PD (32) was based on the three-dimensional structure of *L. mesenteroides* G6PD (33), which had been solved to a resolution of 2.0 Å in 1994. The continuing efforts of the group led by M. Adams have resulted in the crystal structure of a variant of the human enzyme (G6PD Canton) being solved (34,35), and, as expected, the model turns out to have been a good representation of the protein (Fig. 54-4). Each subunit of the enzyme consists of two domains: The smaller N-terminal domain is a classic dinucleotide-binding fold containing the NADP binding fingerprint GXXGXXA at amino acids 38 to 44, which form a tight turn between the first beta sheet and alpha helix ("coenzyme site" in Fig. 54-4). The highly conserved arginine residue at position 72 binds the 2'-phosphate of NADP and ensures coenzyme specificity. The larger domain is a beta + alpha fold that has not been seen elsewhere. It is dominated by antiparallel beta sheets that come

together with those of the other subunit to form a barrel at the dimer interface. The active site of the enzyme ("substrate site" in Fig. 54-4), involving the most highly conserved stretch of amino acids from 198 to 206, is at the boundary between the two domains. Lysine at position 205 is known to be a part of the G6P binding site (36), although directed mutagenesis of this residue show that, although it is essential for catalysis, it is dispensable for substrate binding (37).

There are two very interesting features of the human enzyme that were not observed in *Leuconostoc* G6PD: The first is the formation of the tetrameric structure, and the second is the presence of a structural NADP+ molecule. The dimer-tetramer equilibrium of the active enzyme is affected by ionic strength and markedly by pH (38,39). For instance, at pH 6.0, the enzyme is entirely in tetramer form, whereas at pH 8.0 it is entirely in the dimer form. We now see that, of only 15 residues that are involved in the formation of the tetramer (which is a dimer of dimers) (Fig. 54-5), 11 are charged. Thus, the sensitivity of the dimer-tetramer equilibrium to pH and ionic strength is explained by the electrostatic nature of these tetramer contacts.

Although we are not sure of the physiologic significance of the dimer-tetramer interconversion, it is interesting that it occurs around the intracellular pH of red cells. It is also clear that formation of the oligomeric (dimer or tetramer) structure is essential for enzyme activity and that NADP is involved in the process (40,41). The stabilizing effect of NADP and binding experiments carried out by equilibrium dialysis led to the notion of the presence of "structural" NADP (1 mol/mol of subunit), which may be distinct from substrate NADP (41). The structure reveals that this is indeed the case (34): A well-ordered NADP+ has been found, mostly buried within the large beta + alpha domain and bound entirely within each subunit, close to the dimer interface (Fig. 54-4). There is no dinucleotide fingerprint sequence here, as seen in the dinucleotide binding fold located near the N-terminus. NADP+ binding in this region had been predicted as the reason that several severe mutations of G6PD could be reactivated by increasing NADP+ concentrations (42), although it clearly does not have coenzyme activity in this location. One of the NADP+ ligands, Asp 421, is at the center of the dimer interface, and a series of artificially created mutations to this negatively charged residue have been shown to reduce the concentration-dependent stabilizing effect of NADP (43).

G6PD preparations may contain inactive monomeric molecules that would not be revealed by conventional analysis based on enzyme activity, because as soon as NADP is added to carry out an assay, dimerization would take place, provided the monomer is not irreversibly denatured. On the other hand, there is strong evidence that *in vivo* there is no significant amount of monomer (44) and that dimerization takes place within milliseconds once NADP is added (45). Based on the relatively high intracellular concentration of NADPH, we can pre-

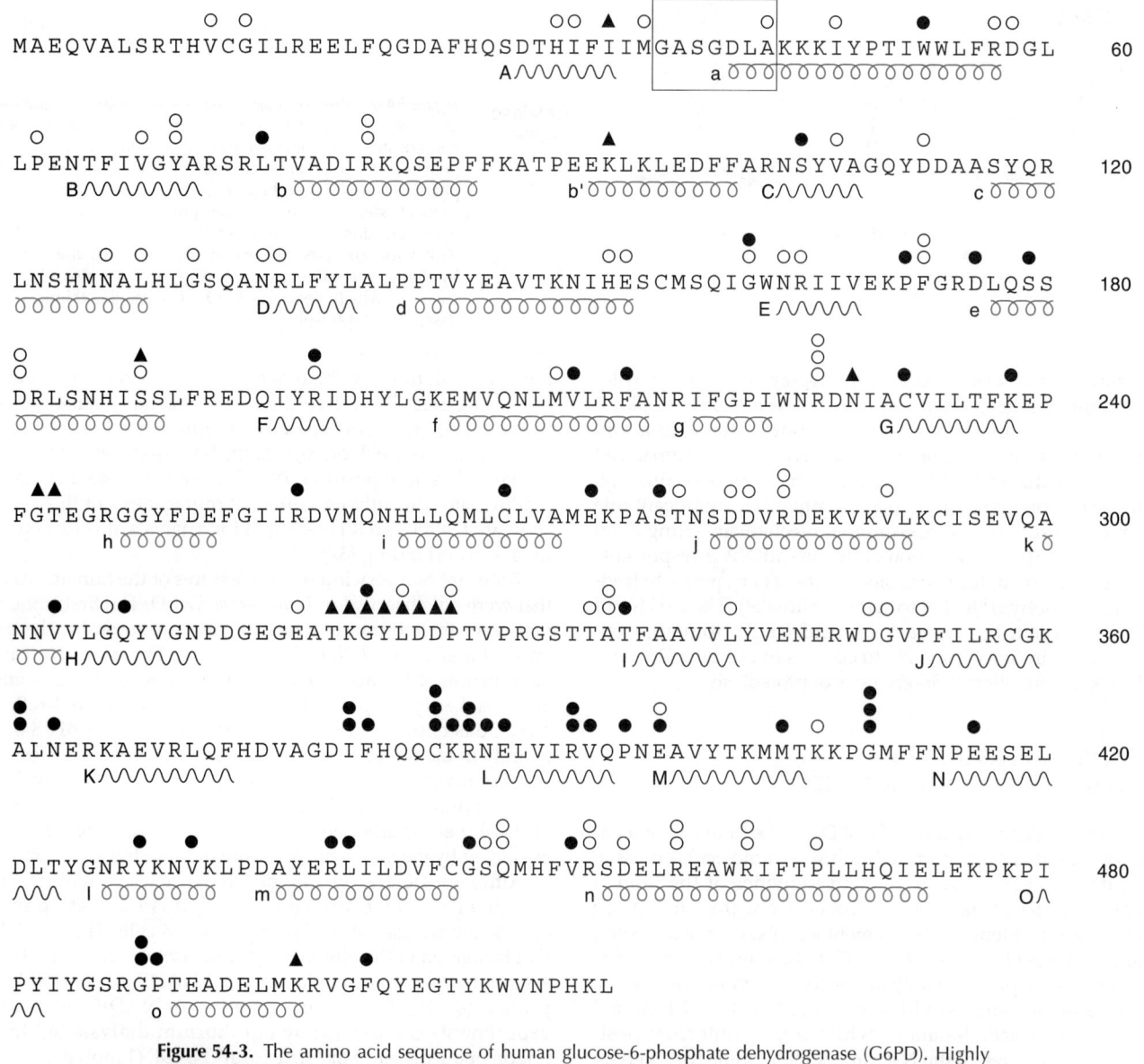

Figure 54-3. The amino acid sequence of human glucose-6-phosphate dehydrogenase (G6PD). Highly conserved residues with greater than 75% identity among 52 different G6PD sequences from 42 different organisms (31) are shown in bold type. Amino acids substituted in class I and class II + III variants of G6PD are shown above the sequence by filled and open circles, respectively. Filled triangles indicate amino acids deleted in class I variants. Below the sequence is the secondary structure of the protein, with capitals and ∧∧∧∧ indicating the beta sheets and lowercase letters and ᴏᴏᴏᴏᴏᴏᴏ indicating the alpha helices that are seen in the three-dimensional structure in Figure 54-4. (Modified from Luzzatto L, Mehta A, Vulliamy TJ. Glucose-6-phosphate dehydrogenase deficiency. In: Scriver CR, Beaudet AL, Sly WS, et al., eds. *The metabolic basis of inherited disease.* New York: McGraw Hill, 2001:4517–4553.)

sume that subunit association goes on hand in hand with the folding of the polypeptide chain as it is synthesized.

GENETICS OF GLUCOSE-6-PHOSPHATE DEHYDROGENASE

Glucose-6-Phosphate Dehydrogenase Gene

The single polypeptide chain of G6PD is encoded in a gene located in the telomeric region (band Xq28) of the long arm of the X chromosome (46,47). Linkage analysis in appropriate families had shown that the G6PD gene, *Gd*, must lie near the genes for hemophilia A (48) and color blindness (49). In fact, physical linkage of *Gd* to the genes encoding factor VIII and to those

encoding the retinal pigments (50) has been established at the molecular level. From the human genomic sequence (51), we know that genes within Xq28 are tightly packed and that the G6PD gene is separated from its nearest neighbor, the nuclear factor-κB modulator gene, by less than 800 base pairs (bp), lying in a head-to-head orientation (52).

At the genomic level, the G6PD gene consists of 13 exons, the first of which is noncoding (53). The total length of the gene is approximately 18.5 kilobases (kb), much of which (approximately 12 kb) is made up of the second intron. The significance of this large intron is unknown, although it may contain sequences necessary for efficient transcription; a deoxyribonuclease I–hypersensitive site has been identified in the equivalent intron in the mouse G6PD gene (54). The promoter region is highly GC-rich, containing many unmethylated CpG dinucleotides that give

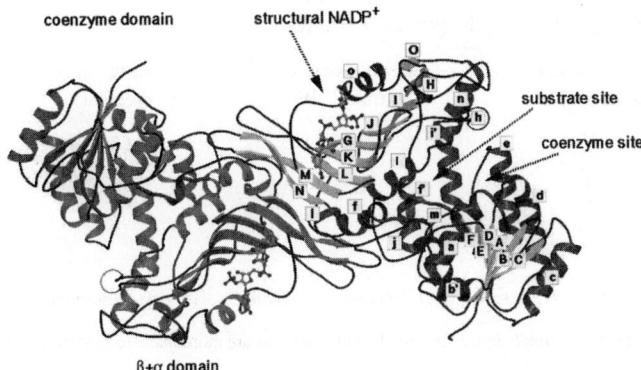

Figure 54-4. NADP⁺, oxidized form of nicotinamide adenine dinucleotide phosphate. The three-dimensional structure of human glucose-6-phosphate dehydrogenase. The active dimer is shown, with the alpha helices and beta sheets labeled on one subunit. (See Color Fig. 54-4.) [Modified from Au SW, Gover S, Lam VM, et al. Human glucose-6-phosphate dehydrogenase: the crystal structure reveals a structural NADP(+) molecule and provides insights into enzyme deficiency. *Structure* 2000;8:293–303; provided courtesy of Dr. S. Gover and Prof. M. Adams.]

rise to a cluster of Hpa II fragments, known to be characteristic of the promoters of housekeeping genes in particular (55). There is also an atypical TATA box with the sequence ATTAAA located at bases –30 to –25 from the transcription start site that is required for the correct start site, but not for the level of transcription (56). Using a chloramphenicol acetyltransferase reporter assay in various cell lines, deletion analysis of the promoter region showed that the "minimal" promoter of G6PD is approximately 160 bp (56). Further, directed mutagenesis has defined two specific GC boxes that are required for basal transcription (57), although band shift experiments have shown that several other elements

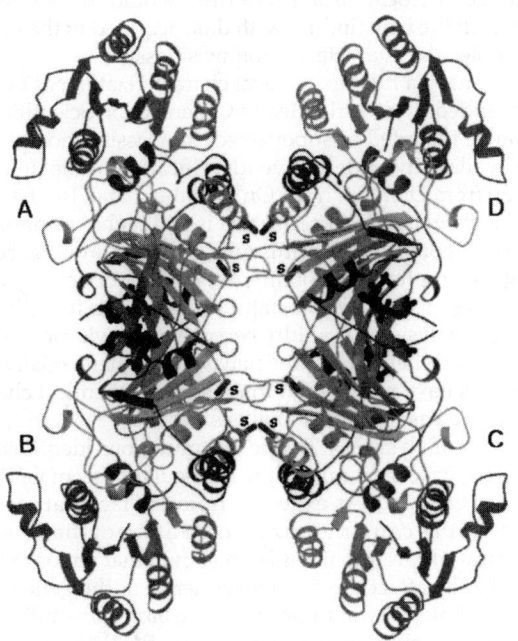

Figure 54-5. The human glucose-6-phosphate dehydrogenase tetramer. This is a dimer of dimers. The shading is ramped from the C to the N terminus in each of the four subunits. (See Color Fig. 54-5.) [Modified from Au SW, Gover S, Lam VM, et al. Human glucose-6-phosphate dehydrogenase: the crystal structure reveals a structural NADP(+) molecule and provides insights into enzyme deficiency. *Structure* 2000;8:293–303; provided courtesy of Dr. S. Gover and Prof. M. Adams.]

and as-yet-unidentified factors are required for correct promoter function (58). The expression of a human gene containing 2.5 kb of upstream and 2.0 kb of downstream flanking sequence in transgenic mice was shown to be correctly regulated, with variation in enzyme activity from tissue to tissue closely matching the levels of the endogenous enzyme (59).

The mouse has an intronless autosomal copy of its X-linked G6PD gene that is functional and provides testis-specific expression (60). A similar situation is found for another essential X-linked gene, phosphoglycerate kinase (61), and in both cases it is presumably related to the inactivation of the X-linked genes in spermatogenic cells before meiosis. No equivalent system has been reported in humans, although a sequence related to G6PD was identified on chromosome 17 (62), but this has not been further characterized.

Since the discovery of G6PD deficiency, it was expected that this condition must result from mutations of the G6PD gene. In fact, by reference to the best-known system in human genetics, namely hemoglobin (Hgb), it was speculated that there might be two types of mutations. One type, producing qualitative as well as quantitative changes in G6PD, would be analogous to structural hemoglobinopathies and would be expected to be within the coding region. The other type, producing only a reduction in the amount of a qualitatively normal G6PD, would be analogous to thalassemia and might be located in regulatory regions of the gene. Whenever G6PD from G6PD-deficient individuals was subjected to careful biochemical characterization, however, qualitative differences, albeit sometimes only subtle ones, were invariably detected, indicating that in all these cases the mutations were of the first type. Since 1988, identification of individual G6PD mutations at the DNA level has entirely confirmed this indication. All mutations thus far have been structural, and thalassemia-like mutations have not yet been discovered in the human gene.

Genetic Heterogeneity of Glucose-6-Phosphate Dehydrogenase and Glucose-6-Phosphate Dehydrogenase Deficiency

Analysis of thousands of samples has revealed both qualitative and quantitative changes in the G6PD of human red cells. The parameters most widely used for G6PD characterization are as follows:

- Specific activity in red cells (IU/g Hgb)
- Electrophoretic mobility
- K_m for the two substrates, G6P and NADP, and for the product inhibitor NADPH (K_i)
- Activity on substrate analogs
- pH dependence of enzyme activity
- Thermostability

Based on these parameters, some 400 different biochemical variants of G6PD have been reported (63,64). The source of ascertainment of G6PD variants essentially has had two parts. On one hand, variants have been picked up by population screening or by testing clinical samples using methods that measure enzyme activity in a quantitative or semiquantitative way. By this approach, only variants associated with enzyme deficiency are detected. On the other hand, some population studies have been carried out by electrophoretic analysis. By this approach, both deficient variants and variants with charge changes are detected. Thus, it is likely that further heterogeneity has remained hidden so far, because amino acid replacements that do not entail a change in charge remain silent. In addition, many G6PD-deficient samples are not routinely fully characterized.

TABLE 54-2. Classification of Glucose-6-Phosphate Dehydrogenase Variants

Class[a]	Clinical Expression	Residual Activity (% of normal)	No. of Variants (Biochemical)	Electrophoretically Normal (%)[b]	No. of Variants (Molecular)[c]
I	Severe (NNJ and CNSHA)	<20	97	36	63
II	Mild (NNJ and AHA)	<10	122	30	37
III	Mild (NNJ and AHA)	10–60	103	16	24
IV	None	100	52	6	3
V	None	>100	2	—	0

AHA, acute hemolytic anemia; CNSHA, chronic nonspherocytic hemolytic anemia; NNJ, neonatal jaundice.
[a]Defined by a combination of clinical expression (column 2) and residual activity (column 3); a variant is placed in class I if it is associated with CNSHA, regardless of the level of residual activity.
[b]The paucity of electrophoretically normal variants in classes III and IV probably reflects the fact that nondeficient or mildly deficient variants are more likely to be detected if they exhibit an electrophoretic change.
[c]See Table 54-3.

To arrange this multitude of variants in relation to features that have biologic and clinical relevance, three main criteria are useful:

Level of residual activity: The variant is normal or deficient with respect to enzyme level.

Clinical manifestations: The variant may be asymptomatic or associated with relatively mild or episodic manifestations, mainly neonatal jaundice and acute hemolytic anemia; or it may be associated with severe manifestations, mainly chronic nonspherocytic hemolytic anemia (CNSHA).

Population frequency: The variant may be only sporadic, or it may have, in one or more populations, a prevalence that qualifies it as polymorphic.

Population frequency is most useful in indicating whether a particular variant has been subjected to natural selection (see Epidemiology). The necessary information is not always available, however, because by definition a population study is required for this purpose. Partly for this reason, a classification that has gained wide acceptance and is taxonomically useful is one that uses clinical manifestations and level of residual activity as primary criteria, with variants grouped into five classes accordingly (Table 54-2): Class I are associated with CNSHA; class II have less than 10% residual activity and predispose to acute hemolytic anemia; class III have 10% to 60% residual activity and predispose to acute hemolytic anemia; class IV have a normal activity (and have therefore usually been identified as electrophoretic variants); and class V have increased activity.

Biochemical and Molecular Characterization

Since the elucidation of the primary structure of normal G6PD by sequence analysis, it has become possible to determine the basis for G6PD variants by identifying changes at the DNA level, and molecular analysis has become the definitive criterion in distinguishing one variant from another. In general, the correlation between biochemical and molecular characterization is good, in the sense that well-characterized biochemical differences have been matched by different underlying mutations. In most cases, the observed electrophoretic mobility matches what could be expected from the amino acid change involved. Occasionally, greater heterogeneity has been revealed at the molecular level than expected from biochemical characterization as, for instance, in the cases of G6PD A− (65) and of G6PD Mediterranean (66,67). This can be easily explained by considering that biochemical differences can be subtle, and whether they are discovered depends on how far the analysis is pushed.

More often than expected, however, variants that had been assigned different names have turned out to have the same molecular change. This is most likely due to the overinterpretation of interlaboratory variation when the same variant has been encountered in different parts of the world, and it appears that the actual number of G6PD variants is significantly less than the 400 or so that have been described. Thus, the four most widespread G6PD variants (G6PD A−, G6PD Mediterranean, G6PD Canton, and G6PD Union) have been attributed 23 different variant names (Table 54-3). In addition, the sporadic and severe forms of G6PD deficiency that are associated with CNSHA have been thought to be unique, but are now known to be common due to recurrent mutations (68–70). This finding is a little disturbing, because it suggests that the biochemical characterization had been inadequate or undermined by poor storage or other artifacts. One might then be tempted to dispense with biochemical characterization altogether, but in this author's view, doing so would be a mistake for at least two reasons: (a) Knowledge of biochemical properties is relevant to the clinical expression of any G6PD variant; and (b) identification of a new molecular lesion in a particular patient, without sufficient knowledge of biochemical properties, would make it impossible to match the new finding with data acquired in the literature before molecular characterization was possible.

In summary, a full biochemical characterization, as originally recommended by a World Health Organization Scientific Group (71), can be regarded as superseded, for classification purposes, by the availability of definitive identification of the underlying mutation from DNA analysis. On the other hand, for the reasons given, biochemical characterization is still highly recommended and should consist, at a minimum, of the following: residual activity, electrophoretic mobility, K_m of G6P (or activity on substrate analogs), and thermostability. Although it is likely that molecular analysis will rapidly become more widespread, especially in areas where G6PD deficiency is prevalent, relatively few laboratories have retained an interest in biochemical characterization as well as molecular analysis.

From the analysis of 130 different mutations identified in the G6PD gene, a clear picture of the molecular basis of G6PD deficiency has emerged. As expected from the fact that most variants of G6PD causing enzyme deficiency have altered biochemical properties, it has been shown that almost all mutations of G6PD affect the coding sequence of the gene (72) and that the vast majority of these are single base substitutions leading to amino acid substitutions (Table 54-3). A few of these occur as a second mutation, most frequently in combination with the polymorphic mutation that distinguishes the nondeficient variant G6PD A from the wild-type enzyme G6PD B. The mutations are spread throughout the coding sequence, indicating that amino acid replacements in many positions can decrease the stability of the enzyme (Fig. 54-3). However, of the

TABLE 54-3. Variants of Glucose-6-Phosphate Dehydrogenase Characterized at the Molecular Level

Name	Nucleotide Substitution	Restriction Enzyme Site Change	Amino Acid Replacement	Protein Location[a]	Class	Electrophoretic Mobility	K_m G6P (µM)	Population	Reference
Sinnai	34 G→T	–Afl III	12 Val→Leu	pre βA	III	—	—	Sardinian	202
Lages	40 G→A	+ Bsg I	14 Gly→Arg	pre βA	II or III	—	—	Brazilian	203
Gaohe, Gaozhou	95 A→G	—	32 His→Arg	βA	III	96	31	Chinese[b]	204
Honiara	99 A→G and 1360 C→T	+ Nla III –Hha I	33 Ile→Met 454 Arg→Cys	βA inter αm/αn	II	—	—	Solomon Islands[b]	82
Sunderland	Δ105–107	—	35 or 36 ΔIle	βA	I	95	—	English	76
Gidra	110 T→C	–Nla III	37 Met→Thr	βA	—	—	—	Japanese	—
Orissa	131 C→G	–Hae III	44 Ala→Gly	αa	III	100	69	Indian[b]	—
Aures	143 T→C	–Bgl II	48 Ile→Thr	αa	II	100	59	Algerian[b], Middle Eastern, Spanish	205
Kozukata	159 G→C	+Pvu II	53 Trp→Cys	αa	I	—	—	Japanese	Hirono, unpublished
Kamogawa	169 C→T	–Msp I	57 Arg→Trp	αa	II	—	—	Japanese	Hirono, unpublished
Metaponto	172 G→A	–Fok I	58 Asp→Asn	inter αa/βB	III	90	47	Italian[b]	206
Musashino	185 C→T	+ Taq I	62 Pro→Leu	inter αa/βB	III	90	32	Japanese	69
A– Distrito and Federal, Matera, Castilla, Alabama, Betica, Tepic, Ferrara, Laghout, Kabyle	202 G→A and 376 A→G	+ Nla III + Fok I	68 Val→Met 126 Asn→Asp	βB αc	III	110	60	African[b], European, Middle Eastern, Brazilian, Central American	207
Namouru	208 T→C	+ Nla III	70 Tyr→His	βB	II	92	—	South Pacific[b]	81
Murcia	209 A→G	+ Bsp1286 I	70 Tyr→Cys	βB	II	98	54	Spanish	208
Swansea	224 T→C	–Mnl I	75 Leu→Pro	inter βB/αb	I	—	—	Welsh	68
Ube, Konan	241 C→T	–Fok I	81 Arg→Cys	αb	III	108	52	Japanese[b]	209
Lagosanto	242 G→A	—	81 Arg→His	αb	III	105	65	Italian	210
Urayasu	Δ281–283	+ Sac I	95 ΔLys	αb'	I	109	40	Japanese	211
Vancouver	317 C→G	–MspI	106 Ser→Cys	βC	I	—	—	Canadian	212
	544 C→T	—	182 Arg→Trp	αe	—	—	—	—	—
	592 C→T	—	198 Arg→Cys	βF	—	—	—	—	—
Hammersmith	323 T→A	+ Mnl I	108 Val→Glu	βC	III	108	—	Indian	213
Sao Borja	337 G→A	—	113 Asp→Asn	inter βC/αc	IV	83	96	Brazilian, Cuban, Italian	203
A	376 A→G	+ Fok I	126 Asn→Asp	αc	IV	110	60	African[b]	214
Vanua Lava	383 T→C	–Mnl I	128 Leu→Pro	αc	II	96	—	South Pacific[b]	81
Quing Yan	392 G→T	+ Dra III	131 Gly→Val	inter αc/βD	III	100	56	Chinese[b]	84
Cairo	404 A→C	+ Fau I	135 Asn→Thr	βD	II	—	—	Egyptian	Kaeda et al., unpublished
Valladolid	406 C→T	—	136 Arg→Cys	βD	II	11	41	Spanish	215
Acrokorinthos	463 C→G and 376 A→G	— + Fok I	155 His→Asn 126 Asn→Asp	αd αc	II	—	—	Greek	216
Ilesha	466 G→A	–Hinf I	156 Glu→Lys	αd	III	75	83	Nigerian, Algerian	206
Mahidol	487 G→A	+ Alu I	163 Gly→Ser	inter αd/βE	III	100	40	Southeast Asian[b]	217
Plymouth	488 G→A	—	163 Gly→Asp	inter αd/βE	I	103	48	English	68

(continued)

TABLE 54-3. (Continued)

Name	Nucleotide Substitution	Restriction Enzyme Site Change	Amino Acid Replacement	Protein Location[a]	Class	Electrophoretic Mobility	Km G6P (μM)	Population	Reference
Taipei	493 A→G	+ Ava II	165 Asn→Asp	βE	II	—	54	Chinese[b], Fillipino[b]	218
Naone	497 G→A	–SfaN I	166 Arg→His	βE	II	103	—	South Pacific[b]	81
Volendam	514 C→T	—	172 Pro→Ser	inter βE/αe	I	—	—	Dutch	219
Nankang	517 T→C	+ Ava I	173 Phe→Leu	inter βE/αe	II	—	—	Chinese	220
Miaoli	519 C→G	–Xmn I	173 Phe→Leu	inter βE/αe	—	—	—	Chinese[b]	221
Shinshu	527 A→G	+ Hae III	176 Asp→Gly	inter βE/αe	I	—	85	Japanese, English	158
Chikugo	535 A→T	+ Sac I	179 Ser→Cys	αe	I	—	—	Japanese	Hirono, unpublished
Malaga	542 A→T	–Cfr10 I	181 Asp→Val	αe	II	81	26	Spanish[b]	80
Santamaria	542 A→T and 376 A→G	–Cfr10 I + Fok I	181 Asp→Val 126 Asn→Asp	αe αc	II	98	16	Algerian[b], Costa Rican, Canary Islands, Spanish, Italian	222
Tsukui	Δ561–563	–Mnl I	188 or 189 ΔSer	αe	I	89	100	Japanese	211
Mediterranean, Dallas, Birmingham, Sassari, Cagliari, Panama	563 C→T	+ Mbo II	188 Ser→Phe	αe	II	100	23	Mediterranean[b], Middle Eastern, Indian, Southeast Asian	206
Coimbra, Shunde	592 C→T	—	198 Arg→Cys	βF	II	100	7	Mediterranean[b], Taiwanese	66
Santiago	593 G→C	–SfaN I	198 Arg→Pro	βF	I	Slow	50	Chilean	223
Sibari	634 A→G	–Nla III	212 Met→Val	αf	III	100	31	Italian[b]	224
Minnesota, Marion, Gastonia, Le Jeune	637 G→T	—	213 Val→Leu	αf	I	95	88	United States—white	225
Harilaou	648 T→G	+ Hae III	216 Phe→Leu	αf	I	100	—	Greek	226
Radlowo	679 C→T	–Msp I	227 Arg→Trp	inter αg/βG	II	—	—	Polish	227
Mexico City	680 G→A	+ BstN I	227 Arg→Gln	inter αg/βG	III	110	—	Mexican	223
A–	680 G→T and 376 A→G	+ BstN I + Fok I	227 Arg→Leu 126 Asn→Asp	inter αg/βG αc	III	110	—	United States—black	65
North Dallas	Δ683–685	—	229 ΔAsn	inter αg/βG	I	—	—	United States	Weinthal et al., unpublished
Asahikawa	695 G→A	+ Mae II	232 Cys→Tyr	βG	I	98	30	Japanese	69
Durham	713 A→G	+ Eco57 I	238 Lys→Arg	βG	I	100	31	United States—white	228
Stonybrook	Δ724–729	–Dde I	242–243 ΔGly,Thr	inter βG/αh	I	—	—	United States—white	73
Wayne	769 C→G	–Fok I	257 Arg→Gly	αh	I	107	78	United States—white	229
Aviero	806 G→A	—	269 Cys→Tyr	αh	I	—	—	Portuguese	230
Corum, Cleveland	820 G→A	+ Mbo II	274 Glu→Lys	inter αi/αj	I	85	35	Turkish, United States—white	73
Wexham	833 C→T	–Mnl I	278 Ser→Phe	inter αi/αj	I	96	—	English	68
Chinese-1	835 A→T	+ Mme I	279 Thr→Ser	inter αi/αj	II	—	—	Chinese	231
Seattle, Lodi, Modena, Ferrara II, Athens-like, Mexico	844 G→C	–Dde I	282 Asp→His	αj	III	80	20	European[b], Algerian, Mexican, Brazilian, Canary Islands	232
Papua	849 C→A	–Aat II	283 Asp→Glu	αj	—	—	—	—	Hirono et al., unpublished

TABLE 54-3. (Continued)

Name	Nucleotide Substitution	Restriction Enzyme Site Change	Amino Acid Replacement	Protein Location[a]	Class	Electrophoretic Mobility	K$_m$ G6P (µM)	Population	Reference
Osaka	853 C→T	—	285 Arg→Cys	αj	II	—	—	Japanese	Hirono, unpublished
Montalbano	854 G→A	+ Nla III	285 Arg→His	αj	III	93	49	Italian[b]	233
Viangchan, Jammu	871 G→A	—	291 Val→Met	αj	III	100	105	Laotian[b], Fillipino, Chinese	229
West Virginia	910 G→T	–Ava II	303 Val→Phe	αk	I	100	26	United States—white	73
Seoul	916 G→A	+ Dde I	306 Gly→Ser	βH	II	—	—	—	Hirono, unpublished
Omiya	921 G→C	–Rsa I	307 Gln→His	βH	I	—	—	—	Hirono, unpublished
Ludhiana	929 G→A	–Nla IV	310 Gly→Glu	βH	II or III	—	—	Indian	Kaeda et al., unpublished
Kalyan, Kerala	949 G→A	—	317 Glu→Lys	inter βH/βI	III	75	105	Indian[b]	234
Nara	Δ953–976	–Kpn I	319–326 ΔTKGYLDDP	inter βH/βI	I	—	—	Japanese, Portuguese	235
Manhattan	962 G→A	–Kpn I	321 Gly→Glu	inter βH/βI	I	—	—	—	Demina, Beutler, unpublished
A-, Betica, Selma, Guantanemo	968 T→C and 376 A→G	+ Nci I + Fok I	323 Leu→Pro 126 Asn→Asp	inter βH/βI αc	III	110	—	United States–black, Mexican Spanish[b], Canary Islands, Portuguese Brazilian	65
Farroupilha	977 C→A	+ Dra III	326 Pro→His	inter βH/βI	II or III	—	—		203
Chatham	1003 G→A	–BspW I	335 Ala→Thr	inter βH/βI	III	100	60	Fillipino[b], Indian, Middle Eastern, Mediterranean, Brazilian, Japanese	206
Fushan	1004 C→A	+ Alu I	335 Ala→Asp	inter βH/βI	II	—	—	Chinese	73
Torun	1006 A→G	—	336 Thr→Ala	βI	I	—	—	Polish	227
Chinese-5	1024 C→T	+ Mbo II	342 Leu→Phe	βI	III	91	65	Chinese[b]	84
Mira d'Aire	1048 G→C	+ Nla III	350 Asp→His	inter βI/βJ	IV	—	—	Portuguese	Goncalves et al., unpublished
Partenope	1052 G→T	—	351 Gly→Val	inter βI/βJ	II	100	19	Italian	67
Ierapetra	1057 C→T	–Nla IV	353 Pro→Ser	inter βI/βJ	II	—	—	Greek[b]	223
Iwatsuki	1081 G→A	–Hae III	361 Ala→Thr	inter βJ/βK	I	—	—	Japanese	Hirono, unpublished
Serres	1082 C→T	+ Ava II	361 Ala→Val	inter βJ/βK	I	—	—	Greek	70
Loma Linda	1089 C→A	—	363 Asn→Lys	inter βJ/βK	I	98	70	United States—Mexican	225
Calvo Mackenna	1138 A→G	+ Mae II	380 Ile→Val	inter βK/βL	I	—	—	—	236
Riley	1139 T→C	– Mbo II	380 Ile→Thr	inter βK/βL	I	—	—	—	236
Olomouc	1141 T→C	+ Fok I	381 Phe→Leu	inter βK/βL	I	—	—	Czech	73
Tomah	1153 T→C	+ Fnu4H I	385 Cys→Arg	inter βK/βL	I	92	42	United States, Spanish, Portuguese	42
Lynwood	1154 G→T	—	385 Cys→Phe	inter βK/βL	I	—	—	—	Demina, Beutler, unpublished
Madrid	1155 C→G	—	385 Cys→Trp	inter βK/βL	I	91	76	Spanish	215

(continued)

TABLE 54-3. (Continued)

Name	Nucleotide Substitution	Restriction Enzyme Site Change	Amino Acid Replacement	Protein Location[a]	Class	Electrophoretic Mobility	K$_m$ G6P (µM)	Population	Reference
Iowa, Iowa City, Walter Reed, Springfield	1156 A→G	—	386 Lys→ Glu	inter βK/ βL	I	100	65	United States— white, English	42
Guadalajara	1159 C→T	–Hha I	387 Arg→ Cys	inter βK/ βL	I	100	36	Mexican, Irish, United States— white, Danish, Indian, Japanese	223
Mount Sinai	1159 C→T and 376 A→G	–Hha I + Fok I	387 Arg→ Cys 126 Asn→Asp	inter βK/ βL αc	I	—	—	—	237
Beverly Hills, Genova, Worcester, Yamaguchi, Iwate, Niigata	1160 G→A	–Hha I	387 Arg→His	inter βK/ βL	I	95	41	United States— white, Italian, Scottish, Japanese	42
Hartford	1162 A→G	+ BstU I	388 Asn→Asp	βL	I	—	—	—	Demina, Beutler, unpublished
Praha	1166 A→G	–Alu I	389 Glu→Gly	βL	I	—	—	Czech	73
Wisconsin	1177 C→G	–BstU I	393 Arg→Gly	βL	I	—	—	—	236
Nashville, Anaheim, Calgary, Portici	1178 G→A	–BstU I	393 Arg→His	βL	I	100	87	United States, Italian, Portuguese, Israeli	225
Alhambra	1180 G→C	+ Pst I	394 Val→Leu	βL	I	96	55	Finnish/ Swedish	223
Bari	1187 C→T	+ Alu I	396 Pro→Leu	inter βL/ βM	I	—	—	Italian	238
Puerto Limon	1192 G→A	–Mnl I	398 Glu→Lys	inter βL/ βM	I	98	32	Costa Rican	222
Anadia	1193 A→G	+ Sau96 I	398 Glu→Gly	inter βL/ βM	II	90	—	Portuguese	Yussoff, unpublished
Clinic	1215 G→A	—	405 Met→Ile	βM	I	100	52	Spanish, French	208
Abeno	1220 A→C	—	407 Lys→Thr	βM	II	—	—	—	Hirono et al., unpublished
Riverside	1228 G→T	–Msp I	410 Gly→ Cys	inter βM/ βN	I	100	326	German/English	42
Kawasaki	1229 G→C	+ Hae III	410 Gly→Ala	inter βM/ βN	I	—	—	Japanese	Hirono et al., unpublished
Shinagawa	1229 G→A	–Nci I	410 Gly→Asp	inter βM/ βN	I	—	242	Japanese	223
Tokyo, Fukushima	1246 G→A	+ Sty I	416 Glu→Lys	βN	I	90	65	Japanese, Scottish, Italian	239
Georgia	1284 C→A	—	428 Tyr→ STOP	αl	I	—	—	Fillipino female	73
Varnsdorf	Δ-2, -1	+ Dra III	3' splice ΔAG	—	I	—	—	Czech	73
Sumare	1292 T→G	–Mae II	431 Val→Gly	αl	I	—	—	Brazilian	240
Pawnee	1316 G→C	–Hinp I	439 Arg→Pro	αm	I	103	50	United States— white	223
Kobe, Telti	1318 C→T	–Mnl I	440 Leu→Phe	αm	I	89	143	Japanese, Italian	241
Santiago de Cuba, Morioka	1339 G→A	+ Pst I	447 Gly→Arg	inter αm/ αn	I	80	50	Cuban, Japanese	206
San Antioco	1342 A→G	+ Hae III	448 Ser→Gly	inter αm/ αn	II	—	—	Italian[b]	67
Cassano	1347 G→C	+ Nla III	449 Gln→His	inter αm/ αn	II	93	14	Italian[b], Greek	224
Hermoupolis	1347 G→C and 1360 C→T	+ Nla III –Hha I	449 Gln→His 454 Arg→ Cys	inter αm/ αn inter αm/ αn	II	—	—	Greek	216

TABLE 54-3. *(Continued)*

Name	Nucleotide Substitution	Restriction Enzyme Site Change	Amino Acid Replacement	Protein Location[a]	Class	Electrophoretic Mobility	K_m G6P (µM)	Population	Reference
Harima	1358 T→A	+ Taq I	453 Val→ –Glu	inter αm/ αn	I	—	—	—	Hirono, unpublished
Union, Maewo, Chinese-2	1360 C→T	–Hha I	454 Arg→ Cys	inter αm/ αn	II	105	8	Polynesian[b], Southeast Asian, Chinese, Mediterranean	83
Andalus	1361 G→A	–Hha I	454 Arg→His	inter αm/ αn	II	100	14	Spanish, Japanese	242
Figueira da Foz	1366 G→C	—	456 Asp→His	αn	II	—	—	Portuguese	Goncalves et al., unpublished
Canton, Taiwan-Hakka, Gifu-like, Agrigento-like	1376 G→T	—	459 Arg→Leu	αn	II	105	28	Chinese[b], Southeast Asian	243
Cosenza	1376 G→C	+ Dde I	459 Arg→Pro	αn	II	100	27	Mediterranean[b]	224
Kamiube, Keelung	1387 C→T	—	463 Arg→ Cys	αn	III	100	57	Japanese[b]	69
Kaiping, Anant, Dhon, Petrich, Sapporo, Wosera	1388 G→A	—	463 Arg→His	αn	II	100	40	Chinese[b]	244
Neapolis	1400 C→G	—	467 Pro→Arg	αn	III	85	55	Italian	245
Fukaya	1462 G→A	–Hae III	488 Gly→Ser	inter βO/ αo	I	—	—	Japanese	Hirono, unpublished
Campinas	1463 G→T	+ Hinf I	488 Gly→Val	inter βO/ αo	I	—	—	Brazilian	246
Arakawa	1466 C→T	–Sau96 I	489 Pro→Leu	inter βO/ αo	I	—	—	Japanese	Hirono et al., unpublished
Brighton	Δ1488–1490	–Mbo II	497 ΔLys	αo	I	100	50	English	247
Bangkok Noi	1502 T→G and 1376 G→T	— —	501 Phe→ Cys 459 Arg→Leu	post αo αn	I	100	60	Japanese	Tanphaichitr, Hirono, unpublished

NOTE: Most of these mutations are now listed on the G6PD database at http://www.rubic.rdg.ac.uk/g6pd/.
[a]The protein location refers to the position of the mutation with respect to the alpha helices of beta sheets of the protein shown in Figure 54.4.
[b]These variants are polymorphic.

mutations that cause CNSHA (class I), a distinct cluster is seen between amino acids 360 and 450, in and around exon 10 of the gene, whereas there are only a few of these (4 of 60) within the N-terminal 160 amino acids. The only deletions seen are small and in frame (with five removing 1 amino acid, one removing 2 amino acids, and one removing 8 amino acids), and all of these give rise to class I variants. The absence of large deletions or frameshift mutations indicates that a total lack of G6PD is incompatible with life. One exception to the rule is the nonsense mutation seen at amino acid 428 Tyr in G6PD Georgia (73). This mutation has only been seen in a heterozygous female who had a reduced level of G6PD activity in her blood, and it is possible that the truncated protein retains some activity.

Of the amino acids that are substituted in G6PD deficiency, there appears to be an interesting pattern as to how well conserved they are in evolution: Mutants are under-represented in fully conserved amino acids where replacement is more likely to be lethal, and in poorly conserved amino acids where replacement is more likely to be ineffectual (31). On the other hand, mutants are over-represented among highly and moderately conserved amino acids (50% to 99% similarity), where the consequence of replacement may be serious enough to cause instability but not serious enough to be lethal. An analysis has also been performed relating the degree of conservation to the degree of clinical severity of different point mutations (74). Although the clinically more severe mutations tend to occur at conserved amino acids, marked exceptions exist, particularly among class I variants.

Amino Acid Substitutions and Protein Structure

The amino acid substitutions giving rise to G6PD deficiency could affect activity, either through reducing protein stability or by disturbing residues important for the catalytic activity of the enzyme. It appears that occurrences of the former are more frequent. Nevertheless, there does appear to be a group of variants with a low K_m G6P that have substitutions around lysine 205, which is known to be a part of the active site. The only substitution impacting directly on the NADP fingerprint sequence, A44G (i.e., [44]Ala→Gly) of G6PD Orissa, causes a fivefold increase in the K_m NADP and an unusual increase in thermostability (75). The 35 isoleucine residue deleted in the severe variant G6PD Sunderland (76) is located in the beta sheet just upstream of this fingerprint, and its loss therefore clearly disrupts coenzyme binding.

However, we have already seen that the amino acid substitutions causing deficiency are spread throughout the protein sequence, reducing intracellular stability in a variety of ways. Knowledge of the three-dimensional structure allows us to see how this may come about. For example, in the variants that are least deleterious (class III), there is a very strong tendency for the affected residues to be exposed on external loops or helices (32). This is also true of the two largest deletions to the protein: Both the eight–amino acid deletion of G6PD Nara and the two amino acids removed in G6PD Stonybrook are located in flexible external loops. One disulfide bridge has been identified in G6PD between 13 cysteine (Cys) and 446 Cys (34), and neither of these residues has been mutated. However, the substitutions seen in G6PD Santiago de Cuba at G447R, G6PD Sinnai at V12L, and G6PD Lages at G14R may disrupt this bridge. It is interesting that the former causes severe G6PD deficiency (with a very high K_mNADP), whereas the other two, in the less-structured N-terminal region, give rise to milder class II or III variants.

A striking observation is the grouping of residues altered in the most severe form of G6PD deficiency (class I): 26 of them are in or close to the dimer interface, and 14 are close to the structural NADP$^+$ molecule (34). Dimer instability can be seen to result from these mutations in a variety of different ways: (a) The substitutions may disrupt the hydrophobic contact surfaces of the barrellike structure formed between the two subunits; (b) hydrogen bonds and salt bridges in this region may be broken by mutation; and (c) the structure may be disturbed by an increase in the size of the amino acid side chain. Some of these variants are particularly unstable in low NADP$^+$ concentrations (42), and we can see how the same beta sheets form the scaffold for both the dimer interface and the residues that bind structural NADP$^+$. In crude approximation, therefore, it appears that reduced dimer stability and impaired binding of the structural NADP$^+$ molecule can be linked processes. Mutation can cause either or both of these to happen in a variety of ways, and when they do, they tend to give rise to the more severe form of G6PD deficiency.

But not all class I amino acid substitutions affect the dimer interface. Loss of hydrogen bonds, loss of charged contact, and steric hindrance are mechanisms that can cause severe deficiency, not only at the dimer interface, but also at other locations

in the molecule (34). In addition, changes may affect the active site (as in P172S of G6PD Volendam and R198P on G6PD Santiago), the tetramer interface (as in E274K of G6PD Cleveland), the secondary structure (as in R257G of G6PD Wayne and G321Q of G6PD Manhattan) or cause deficiency through the unfavorable exposure of a side chain (as in S179C of G6PD Chikugo and S188F of G6PD Birmingham).

A variant that has received special attention is G6PD A–. This is a double mutant (V68M and N126D), and as the N126D substitution is found in the nondeficient variant, G6PD A, it might be assumed that the V68M substitution is responsible for the deficiency. However, *in vitro* expression of the individual and double mutations (77) suggests that they act synergistically to produce the deficient phenotype. This unique observation can be explained by the fact that the two residues involved are very close in the three-dimensional structure, enabling the side chains to interact with one another. Unlike G6PD B and G6PD A, when G6PD A– is denatured *in vitro*, it is virtually unable to refold into an active enzyme (78). It has therefore been proposed that the decreased intracellular stability of this enzyme is related to a loss of folding determinants, which may indeed be a more general mechanism underlying G6PD deficiency (79). Not all substitutions found in conjunction with N126D of G6PD A act synergistically with it to produce deficiency (80); the D181V substitution has also been found naturally on its own to cause G6PD deficiency in G6PD Malaga, whereas an additive effect of the two mutations is seen in the double mutant G6PD Santamaria (D181V and N126D).

Population Genetics

G6PD deficiency is a global feature of the human species. As discussed in greater detail in the section Malaria and Glucose-6-Phosphate Dehydrogenase Deficiency, there is very strong evidence that it has been selected for by providing resistance during infection by *Plasmodium falciparum* malaria. Polymorphic frequencies of G6PD deficiency are found throughout most subtropical and tropical regions of the world, with areas of high prevalence found in Africa, Southern Europe, the Middle East, South East Asia, and Oceania (Fig. 54-6). In the Americas, G6PD deficiency is also prevalent as a result of migrations that have taken place in relatively recent historic times, although it is conspicuously absent from the native American people.

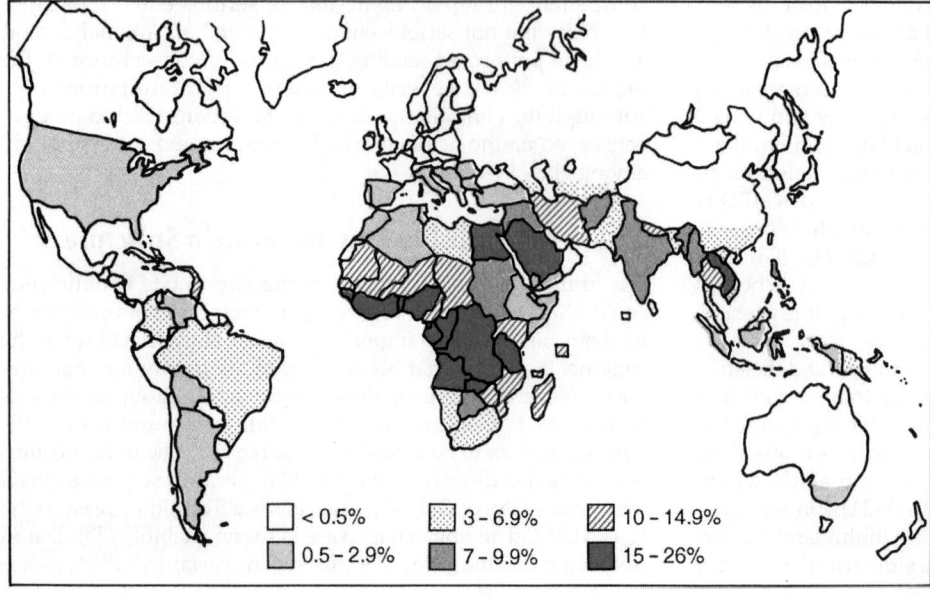

Figure 54-6. World distribution of glucose-6-phosphate dehydrogenase deficiency. The values shown by the different shadings are frequencies of glucose-6-phosphate dehydrogenase–deficient males in the populations of the various countries. These are also gene frequencies, because the gene is X-linked. (From Luzzatto L, Mehta A, Vulliamy TJ. Glucose-6-phosphate dehydrogenase deficiency. In: Scriver CR, Beaudet AL, Sly WS, et al., eds. *The metabolic basis of inherited disease.* New York: McGraw Hill, 2001: 4517–4553, with permission.)

- ☐ < 0.5%
- ▨ 0.5 – 2.9%
- ▥ 3 – 6.9%
- ■ 7 – 9.9%
- ▨ 10 – 14.9%
- ■ 15 – 26%

TABLE 54-4. Global Distribution of Polymorphic Glucose-6-Phosphate Dehydrogenase Variants

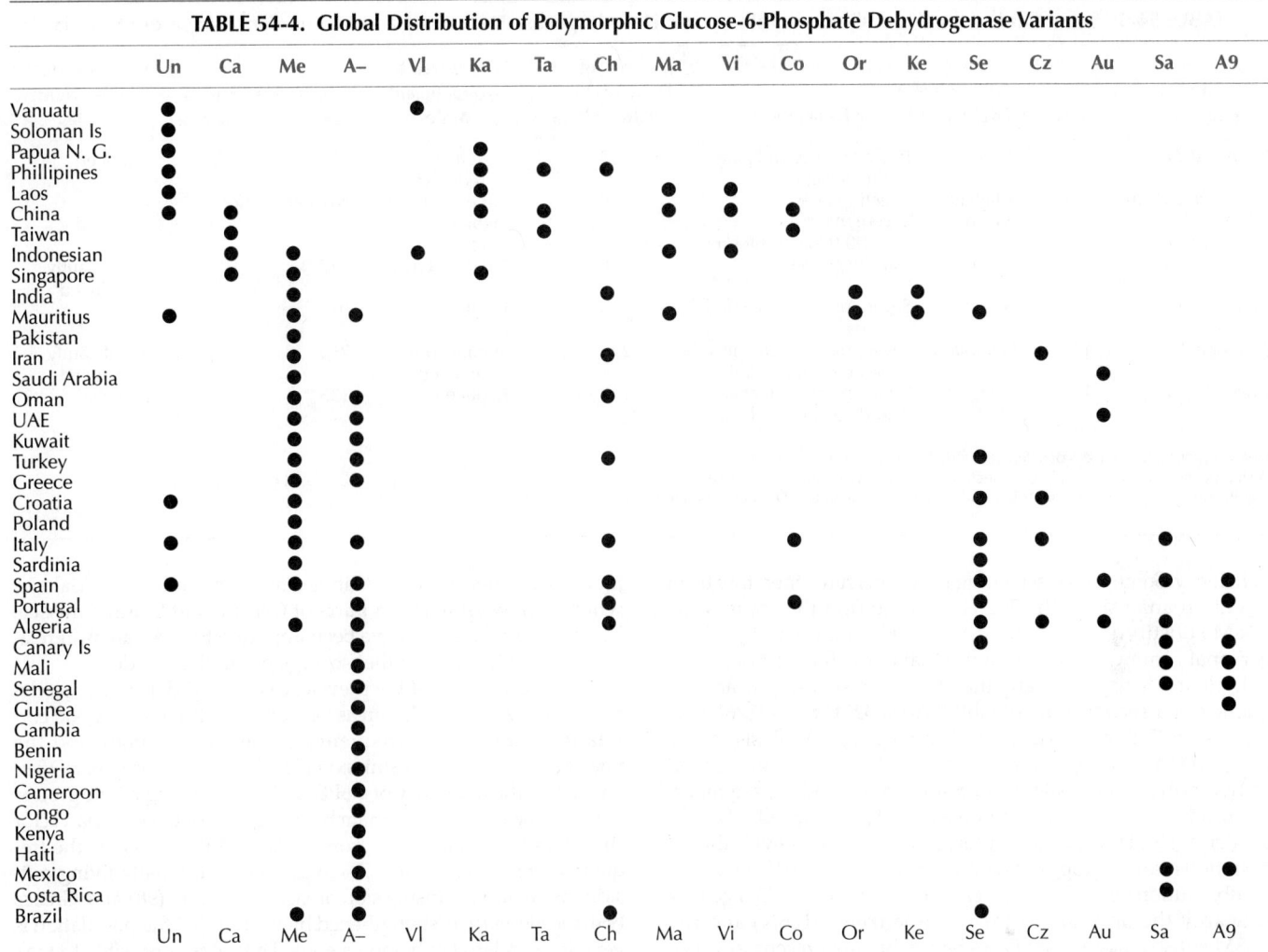

A–, A– (202A); A9, A– (968C); Au, Aures; Ca, Canton; Ch, Chatham; Co, Coimbra; Cz, Cosenza; Is, Islands; Ka, Kaiping; Ke, Kerala; Ma, Mahidol; Me, Mediterranean; N.G., New Guinea; Or, Orissa; Sa, Santamaria; Se, Seattle; Ta, Taipei; Un, Union; UAE, United Arab Emirates; Vi, Viangchan; Vl, Vanua Lava. From Mason PJ, Vulliamy TJ. Genetic variation of human erythrocyte glucose-6-phosphate dehydrogenase. In: King M-J, ed. *Human blood cells: consequences of genetic polymorphisms and variations.* London: Imperial College Press, 2000:251–275; and T.V., unpublished.

If G6PD deficiency had spread only by migrations of people and by genetic drift, the same mutant would be found everywhere. Instead, different variants are found to be polymorphic in different parts of the world. This indicates that diverse point mutations must have arisen independently and then spread centrifugally to establish themselves at polymorphic frequencies—a good example of convergent evolution in the human species. In this respect, the G6PD deficiency polymorphism is more reminiscent of the highly heterogeneous thalassemia system than of the unique mutation of Hgb S.

However, although most areas have multiple polymorphic alleles and a characteristic profile of G6PD variants, the picture is quantitatively dominated by four key players: G6PD Union, G6PD Canton, G6PD Mediterranean and G6PD A– (Table 54-4). G6PD Union is the major variant found in Oceania (81,82), although it is also prevalent elsewhere in the Far East and has been reported on several occasions in Europe. Unlike the other major variants, it is caused by a C→T transition at the mutational hotspot of a CpG dinucleotide, and it has been suggested therefore that it may have arisen independently in the West (83). Extensive screening for mutations causing G6PD deficiency in the Chinese population (84–86) has revealed considerable heterogeneity, but with G6PD Canton accounting for more than half of all cases.

G6PD Mediterranean was well named, as it is the dominant variant in most countries surrounding the Mediterranean Sea, including those in North Africa, although it is conspicuous in its absence from the Portuguese population (87). This variant accounts for almost all of the G6PD deficiency among the Kurdish Jews, in whom the trait has reached its highest known frequency of 0.65 (88). It is also widespread throughout the rest of the Middle East and the Indian subcontinent, and it has been identified as far east as Singapore and Indonesia. The question as to whether this situation has arisen through the spread of a single mutation event or through recurrent mutation has not been resolved. In most cases, the G6PD Mediterranean mutation is found in the context of a silent polymorphic mutation (1311T) in the coding sequence of the G6PD gene. However, in the Indian subcontinent (89) and among a cluster of individuals in southern Italy (90), the mutation is on a different background (1311C); this may represent independent origin, but could also have arisen through a recombination event.

Whereas G6PD Mediterranean, G6PD Canton, and G6PD Union have almost always been found to coexist with other polymorphic variants (Table 54-4), it appears that the situation with G6PD A– (V68M and N126D) is different, in that in sub-Saharan Africa this variant accounts for almost all the G6PD

TABLE 54-5. Some Clinical Studies of Glucose-6-Phosphate Dehydrogenase Deficiency and *Plasmodium falciparum* Malaria

Author (reference)	Year	Country	Parameter	No. of Deficient Males with Malaria	Compared to Nondeficient Males	No. of Heterozygous Females with Malaria	Compared to Nondeficient Females
Allison (102)	1961	Tanzania	Infection rates and parasite densities	58	Significantly reduced	73[a]	Reduced
Kruatrachue (103)	1962	Thailand	Infection rates	20	No difference[b]	Not determined	—
Gilles (105)	1967	Nigeria	Severe malaria; >100,000 parasites/mL	5	Significantly reduced	1	Reduced
Bienzle (107)	1972	Nigeria	Parasite counts	78	No difference[c]	117	Significantly reduced
Martin (104)	1979	Nigeria	Severe malaria; convulsions	3	No difference	0	—
Ruwende (91)	1995	Gambia	Severe malaria; anemia and cerebral malaria	279	Significantly reduced	255	Significantly reduced
Ruwende (91)	1995	Kenya	Severe malaria; anemia and cerebral malaria	117	Reduced	133	Reduced

[a]Heterozygous and homozygous deficient females are not distinguished.
[b]A significant increase is seen in the infection rate of *P. vivax* malaria in 1–3 year olds.
[c]Significantly lower parasite counts in nondeficient males with G6PD A compared to those with G6PD B.

deficiency. Some recent screening programs have therefore been based on analysis of the 202 G→A mutation that causes the V68M substitution (91). Recent data (R. Ducroq and J. Elion, personal communication) indicate that in the far west of Africa, in Mali and Senegal in particular, there is also a significant frequency of a second type of G6PD A– (L323P and N126D), as well as G6PD Santamaria (D181V and N126D). Analysis of several polymorphic sites in the introns of the G6PD gene, as well as two polymorphic silent mutations in the coding sequence, has produced quite an informative haplotype of the G6PD gene in Africa (92). Using these haplotypes, a pattern of evolution of mutations can be proposed with the nondeficient N126D–G6PD A substitution being most ancient (although the G6PD B gene is probably the original, as the Chimpanzee is 126N) and the V68M substitution of G6PD A– being the most recent. All subjects throughout the world with V68M and N126D share the same haplotype, suggesting a single origin of this mutation. The several differences between the haplotype of G6PD Malaga (D181V) and G6PD Santamaria (D181V and N126D), on the other hand, indicate that the mutation underlying the D181V substitution has occurred on more than one occasion (80).

MALARIA AND GLUCOSE-6-PHOSPHATE DEHYDROGENASE DEFICIENCY

Epidemiology

The striking correlation between the worldwide distribution of G6PD deficiency and that of *P. falciparum* prompted the formulation of the malaria hypothesis some 40 years ago (93,94). Since then, the topic has been reviewed extensively (95,96) and additional data have consistently corroborated the geographic evidence, in the sense that G6PD deficiency has been found at polymorphic frequencies only in populations who are living or have been living for generations in areas where malaria is endemic.

Several apparent discrepancies are easy to explain. In southern Europe, G6PD deficiency is common, and there is no malaria, but malaria has been eradicated only over the last two to three generations. In North America, there is no malaria, but the prevalence of G6PD deficiency in this continent is entirely accounted for by migrations that have taken place in relatively recent historic times. Conversely, G6PD deficiency is not found at poly-

morphic frequency in any Native American population. Malaria, which is now endemic in parts of Central and South America, however, is thought to have been imported to those areas in relatively recent times—another scourge of the slave trade.

Detailed analysis of the prevalence of G6PD deficiency in relatively narrow geographic areas has consistently shown a good correlation between the frequency of G6PD deficiency and the intensity of malaria transmission (93,97–99). For example, in Vietnam (100), the frequency of G6PD deficiency among ethnic groups living in the foothills, the main breeding area of the malaria vector *Anopheles minimus*, ranges from 9.7% to 31.0%, whereas the frequency drops to 0.5% to 0.7% in groups traditionally living outside the malaria transmission areas. In Sardinia (98) and Greece (99), the evidence is strengthened by the fact that the population is genetically relatively homogeneous. Thus, it was possible to look at variation of *Gd–* compared with that of other genes to establish the likelihood that natural selection intervened (101).

Clinical Studies

Studies of malaria in the field (Table 54-5) yield ambiguous data when its prevalence or the rate of parasitemia is compared between normal and G6PD-deficient males or in subjects of both sexes (102–106). In a study in which females heterozygous for G6PD deficiency (GdB/GdA–) were rigorously classified (by a combination of a cytochemical test, a quantitative assay, and electrophoretic analysis), a significantly lower *P. falciparum* parasitemia was observed (107). It was proposed that G6PD deficiency is a balanced polymorphism associated with heterozygote advantage, appearing in a slightly different way because the gene concerned is X-linked, and therefore, only females can be heterozygous. In support of this idea, another study revealed under-representation of heterozygotes for G6PD deficiency in a group of children with cerebral malaria in Nigeria (108). What was difficult to understand was why having only a proportion of G6PD-deficient red cells (due to X inactivation) is more protective against malaria than having only G6PD-deficient red cells (as in hemizygous males). More recently, in two large, case-controlled studies in east and west Africa, the G6PD genotypes of over 2000 African children with malaria were determined (91). The result of these surveys showed that G6PD deficiency is associated with a 46% and 58% reduction in the risk of severe malaria in both female heterozygotes and male hemizygotes, respectively. The question then arises as to why the deficient allele has not become fixed in the populations exposed to malaria. It may be that the gene is simply on its way to fixation and has not yet had enough time, as proposed for the benign but protective trait of α+ thalassemia (109), which reaches frequencies similar to that of G6PD deficiency in many populations. However, a mathematical model indicates that some counterbalancing selective disadvantage must be involved (91), suggesting that the clinical problems associated with the deficiency (neonatal jaundice, infection-induced hemolytic anemia, favism) must have been sufficiently severe to lead to a decrease in fitness of male hemizygotes, despite their protection against malaria.

Mechanism of Protection

The most striking result of a quantitative analysis of malaria parasites in the blood of heterozygotes for G6PD deficiency is the excess of parasites in the normal red cells when compared with the deficient red cells of the mosaic (110). Because this result is internally controlled (the test cells and the control cells are within the same individual, thanks to mosaicism), it appears that, other things being equal and when given an option, the parasite prefers G6PD-normal red cells. From the *in vivo* data, however, it is not possible to decide whether this is due to (a) decreased invasion of G6PD-deficient red cells, (b) impaired development of the parasite in these cells, or (c) accelerated removal of parasitized G6PD-deficient red cells. Moreover, the analysis was complicated by the age-dependent nature of G6PD activity, whereby the youngest G6PD-deficient red cells might have been misclassified as normal.

Once a continuous culture system for *P. falciparum* was developed (111), it became possible to test directly, by controlled *in vitro* experiments, whether the G6PD genotype of red cells affected their ability to play host to the parasite. Several groups reported that, in G6PD-deficient red cells, invasion by *P. falciparum* was normal, but intracellular growth (i.e., the process of maturation and schizogony) was impaired (112–114). In some studies, however, the difference was apparent only when the cultures were subjected to oxidative stress (115). Further culture experiments indicated that the malaria parasite was able to adapt to the G6PD-deficient environment. Although the parasites initially grew slower in the deficient cells, the growth rate was restored to normal within a few cycles of infection (112).

Experiments aiming to clarify the mechanism of adaptation revealed the presence, in G6PD-deficient red cells, of a G6PD species distinct from the human red cell G6PD, which must be of parasite origin (116). The gene for this enzyme was eventually cloned and sequenced (117,118), and it turns out to be expressed at equivalent levels when grown in cultures of either normal or G6PD-deficient red cells (119). The enzyme itself is unusual in that it codes for an additional 300 amino acids at its N terminal, when compared to other G6PDs. This N-terminal region has significant homology to a family of proteins known as devb, the human version of which has recently been shown to encode 6-phosphogluconolactonase activity (120), the enzyme immediately after G6PD in the PPP (Fig. 54-1). It has now been demonstrated that the enzyme in *Plasmodium berghei*, which has the same structure as that of the *P. falciparum* G6PD, is indeed a bifunctional enzyme with both lactonase and G6PD activity (J. L. Clarke and P. J. Mason, personal communication). The fact that this essential enzyme has a structure that is distinct from its equivalent in the human host makes it a possible target for antimalarial drug design.

The findings summarized earlier leave little doubt that G6PD-deficiency polymorphism is balanced by malaria selection. At the same time, the mechanism of this process is not yet fully explained. What is clear is that there is a large increase in the activity of the PPP in infected cells, and that both parasite and host enzymes contribute to this up-regulation (121). As this can-

not be so effectively accomplished in G6PD-deficient red cells, this alone could explain why parasites do not grow so well in deficient hosts. However, it has recently been shown that when G6PD-deficient red cells are infected by parasites at the ring stage of development, they are phagocytosed more intensely than their normal counterparts (119). Improved removal of infected red cells at an early stage of infection may provide an efficient mechanism of resistance in deficient individuals.

CLINICAL MANIFESTATIONS OF GLUCOSE-6-PHOSPHATE DEHYDROGENASE DEFICIENCY

In view of the large number of people who carry a G6PD deficiency gene, it is fortunate that most remain clinically asymptomatic throughout their lifetime, and that, of those who develop a hemolytic attack, most recover uneventfully. Among young black G6PD-deficient males enlisting in the U.S. Navy, no adverse effects on health or performance were observed (122). In Singapore, a screening program of national servicemen revealed that almost 90% of deficient individuals had no prior knowledge of their deficiency status (123). A recent survey of mortality ratios among 1756 men in Sardinia found a small but significant reduction in mortality from ischemic heart disease, cerebrovascular disease, and liver cirrhosis among G6PD-deficient males (124), although a decreased cancer rate (125) was not confirmed.

During the steady state, the clinical examination of G6PD-deficient people is entirely negative. Hematologic investigations, including Hgb and red cell indices, red cell morphology, reticulocyte count, serum bilirubin, and serum haptoglobin, are also entirely normal. The only positive laboratory finding, apart from the G6PD assay, can be a reduced red cell survival, indicating that the pathophysiologic state of most G6PD-deficient people is best described as one of very-low-grade, fully compensated hemolysis. Although this must mean that the erythropoietic bone marrow activity is greater than normal, it is not possible to pinpoint any adverse effect of this situation. For instance, unlike other chronic hemolytic disorders, such as sickle cell anemia and hereditary spherocytosis, G6PD-deficient people do not become folate deficient as a result of their presumably increased requirement for folic acid.

From the clinical point of view, therefore, the demarcation between this asymptomatic steady state and the hemolytic attack is sharp. Although these attacks are a rare event in any one deficient individual, due to its prevalence in poorly developed regions of the world, G6PD deficiency is responsible for a significant amount of human pathology, which can be severe. For example, in a rural mission hospital in Nigeria, 31% of 45 clinically jaundiced infants had G6PD deficiency; of these, more than one-third died with presumed kernicterus, compared with only 3% of the jaundiced infants with normal G6PD (126). Of 35 G6PD-deficient children presenting with acute intravascular hemolysis in Chandigargh, India, three died from severe anemia and congestive cardiac failure, malaria with oliguric renal failure, and hepatic encephalopathy, respectively (127). Health education and neonatal screening programs have proved effective in reducing pathology as seen in Sardinia (128), where they have resulted in a substantial decrease in the number of cases of favism, and in Singapore, where kernicterus has been virtually unknown since the early 1970s (129).

Acute Hemolytic Anemia

In most cases, when a G6PD-deficient patient presents with anemia and jaundice, it is possible to identify an exogenous agent that is responsible for the episode. Perhaps because of the

TABLE 54-6. Drugs and Chemicals Associated with Hemolysis in Glucose-6-Phosphate Dehydrogenase–Deficient Subjects

Drugs	Definite Association	Possible Association	Doubtful Association
Antimalarials	Primaquine	Chloroquine	Quinacrine
	Pamaquine	—	Quinine
Sulfonamides	Sulfanilamide	Sulfadimidine	Sulfoxone
	Sulfacetamide	Sulfasalazine	Sulfadiazine
	Sulfapyridine	Glyburide	Sulfisoxalone
	Sulfamethoxazole		
Sulfones	Dapsone	—	—
Nitrofurans	Nitrofurantoin		
Antipyretic/analgesic	Acetanilid	Aspirin	Acetaminophen
	—	—	Phenacetin
Other drugs	Nalidixic acid	Ciprofloxacin	PAS
	Niridazole	Chloramphenicol	Doxorubicin
	Methylene blue	Vitamin K analogs	Probenecid
	Phenazopyridine	Ascorbic acid	Dimercaprol
	Septrin	PAS	—
Other chemicals	Naphthalene	Acalypha indica	—
	Trinitrotoluene	—	—

PAS, p-aminosalicylic acid.
NOTE: Further information is available in the British National Formulary at http://www.bnf.org.uk/. The data on individual drugs causing hemolysis are largely derived from clinical observations rather than deliberate testing; therefore, they are very fragmentary, if not anecdotal. For this reason, in many cases we only know that a drug has caused hemolysis in a glucose-6-phosphate dehydrogenase (G6PD)–deficient subject, and often there is no definite information on the variant involved. In fact, the only comparable systematic data were obtained with primaquine, and hemolysis was worse with G6PD Mediterranean than with G6PD A–. On the other hand, because we now know that severe favism can take place with all G6PD variants, it is probably prudent to assume that any drug found to cause hemolysis with one G6PD-deficient variant can do so with any G6PD-deficient variant.
From Luzzatto L, Mehta A, Vulliamy TJ. Glucose-6-phosphate dehydrogenase deficiency. In: Scriver CR, Beaudet AL, Sly WS, et al., eds. *The metabolic basis of inherited disease.* New York: McGraw Hill, 2001:4517–4553, with permission.

historic antecedent whereby *primaquine sensitivity* was the phrase designating acute hemolytic anemia in people who subsequently turned out to have G6PD deficiency, the general perception is that drugs (Table 54-6) are the most common triggers of hemolysis. In fact, there are three types of triggers: drugs, infections, and fava beans.

Large studies on the impact of drugs are lacking, and in many cases, potentially hemolytic drugs are administered in the context of infection. Thus, it is likely that, in the past, hemolysis was sometimes attributed to drugs used for treating infection when it should have been blamed on the infection itself. Perhaps the best-characterized example is lobar pneumonia (130) and, to a lesser extent, typhoid fever (131). It has been suggested that the mechanism by which bacterial infection causes hemolysis may be the release of peroxides during phagocytosis of bacteria by granulocytes (132). It is more difficult to imagine a mechanism by which viral infection can trigger hemolysis, but this has been documented in the course of viral hepatitis (133,134). In areas where fava beans are widely consumed, their ingestion is the most common cause of acute hemolytic anemia associated with G6PD deficiency. Diabetic ketoacidosis is another trigger of hemolysis, but this is rare. A G6PD-deficient homozygous woman (GdA–/GdA–) was studied who also had renal tubular acidosis and evidence of hemolysis, which appeared to correlate with poor control of acidosis.

A question of practical importance is whether the hemolytic risk associated with any particular triggering factor is a function of individual G6PD variants. This presumption is entirely reasonable in view of the vast genetic heterogeneity of G6PD deficiency. For instance, it is assumed that the risk is generally greater with G6PD Mediterranean than with G6PD A–. Objective evidence, however, for this pharmacogenetic variant-specific heterogeneity is relatively scanty. The best example is probably favism; in the past, G6PD A– subjects were thought to be immune, but it is now clear that they are not (135). As for drugs, primaquine causes hemolysis regularly, but aspirin causes it only sometimes (136). It can only be hypothesized that genetic or acquired factors affecting the metabolism of the drug may be responsible (137,138).

CLINICAL FEATURES

The course of a drug-induced acute hemolytic attack was well characterized in a series of experiments in the late 1950s on human volunteers. These experiments, although impeccably conducted and fortunately free of long-term consequences, probably would not have obtained U.S. Ethics Committee clearance today. When given primaquine at the dose of 30 mg/day, G6PD-deficient (A–) men begin to experience malaise on day 2 or 3, sometimes associated with more or less profound weakness and abdominal or lumbar pain. Usually on day 3 or 4, the telltale signs of jaundice and dark urine make their appearance. This is designated as the *acute hemolytic phase;* its intensity and duration depend to some extent on the nature and dosage of the drug and on the type of G6PD variant; on the average, it lasts approximately 1 week. In most cases, the hemolytic attack, even if severe, is self-limited and tends to resolve spontaneously. In the absence of additional or preexisting pathology, the bone marrow response is prompt and effective. Depending on the proportion of red cells that are destroyed (reflected in the severity of the anemia), the Hgb level may be back to normal in 3 to 6 weeks (recovery phase). The most serious threat in adults is the development of acute renal failure (this is exceedingly rare in children). It is not clear why this should take place only in a small proportion of patients. The most likely explanation is that they have preexisting subclinical renal damage. In such situations, hemodialysis may be required until renal function recovers. After a hemolytic attack, a situation of relative resistance to further drug challenge has been well characterized with G6PD A– (presumably thanks to the considerable proportion in the circulation of red cells that are young and therefore have a higher G6PD level). This is *not* applicable, however, to G6PD Mediterranean, for instance, and it cannot be assumed to apply to others.

LABORATORY FINDINGS

Anemia varies from moderate to extremely severe (Hgb values of 4 g/dL or less have been recorded). In the absence of other preexisting hematologic abnormalities, the anemia is normocytic and normochromic. The blood smear shows anisocytosis, polychromasia, and other features associated with acute hemolysis,

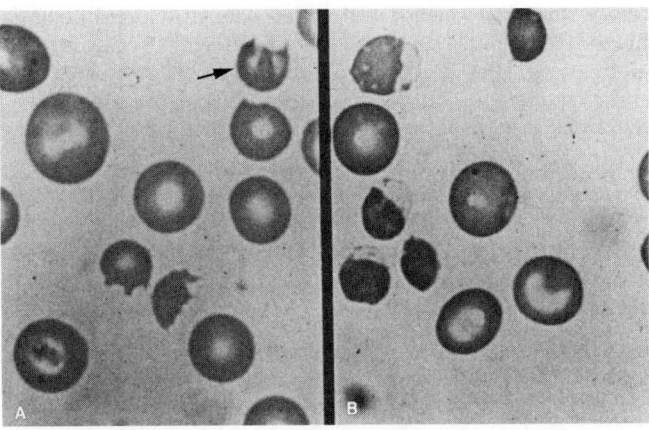

Figure 54-7. Peripheral blood smear showing **(A)** "bite" cells and **(B)** "blister" cells. A portion of the blister cells is empty of hemoglobin; only a faint outline of the membrane is visible. Bite cells and blister cells appear during severe acute hemolytic crisis in glucose-6-phosphate dehydrogenase–deficient people. Between such episodes, the blood smear usually appears normal.

including spherocytes, but it is otherwise nonspecific. In severe cases, however, the poikilocytosis is more marked, with bizarre forms and red cells that appear to have an uneven distribution of Hgb within them. Although some of these appearances are probably smearing artifacts, electron micrographic evidence suggests that, in some of the cells, opposing surfaces of the membrane have become cross-linked (139) ("blister cells") (Fig. 54-7B). The most characteristic poikilocytes are the blister cells and cells in which the cell margin appears dented, as though a portion has been plucked out or bitten away ("bite" cells) (Fig. 54-7A). Supravital staining with methyl violet reveals the presence of Heinz bodies consisting of precipitates of denatured Hgb (Fig. 54-8) and cells in which, as noted previously, the Hgb is excluded from a portion of the cell. It is important to do a methyl violet preparation promptly, because Heinz bodies may disappear from the peripheral blood within 24 hours, as they are "pinched off" by the spleen (possibly giving rise to the bite cells). Because many of the red cells thus damaged undergo intravascular hemolysis, haptoglobin is reduced to the point of being undetectable. In severe cases, it is possible to demonstrate free Hgb in the plasma (the somewhat incongruous term *hemoglobin-*

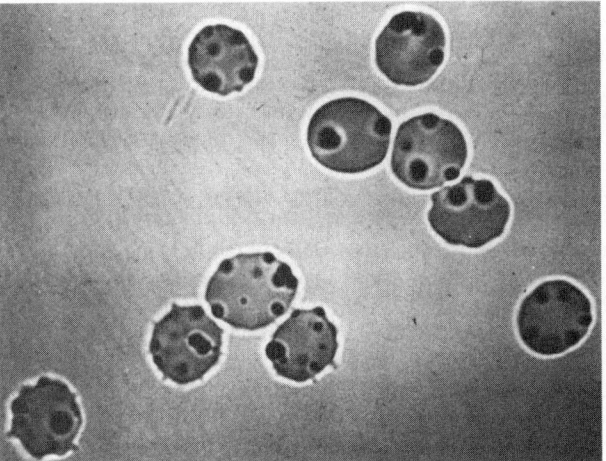

Figure 54-8. Heinz bodies in erythrocytes from a glucose-6-phosphate dehydrogenase–deficient person. These particles of denatured hemoglobin, which adhere to the red cell membrane and stain with basic dyes, are seen in large numbers after an acute hemolytic crisis.

emia is used to describe this finding in one word). The white blood cell count may be elevated, with predominance of granulocytes. The platelet count may be normal, increased, or moderately decreased. The unconjugated bilirubin is elevated, but the liver enzymes are usually normal. The dark urine tests strongly positive for blood. It is easy to demonstrate that this is due to hemoglobinuria rather than hematuria because, after centrifugation, the supernatant is as dark as before, and in the sediment, there are few if any red cells.

Favism

CLINICAL FEATURES

Favism is a dramatic event and, although no age group is spared, it is most often observed in children. A few hours after ingesting fava beans, the child may become fractious and irritable or subdued and even lethargic. Within 24 to 48 hours, fever may develop (up to 38°C), and this may be associated with nausea, abdominal pain, and diarrhea, and rarely with vomiting. In striking contrast to these relatively nonspecific symptoms, the patient or relatives observe, within 6 to 24 hours, the telltale and frightening discoloration of the urine. It usually is reported as dark, red, brown, or black, or as "passing blood instead of water." At approximately the same time, jaundice becomes obvious. Physical examination may reveal little more than the signs corresponding to the symptoms listed earlier. The child is invariably pale and tachycardiac. In severe cases, there may be evidence of hypovolumic shock or, less likely, of heart failure. The spleen is usually moderately enlarged, and the liver may be also enlarged; either or both may be tender. The subsequent clinical course depends on the severity of the attack, particularly on what proportion of the patient's red cells have been destroyed. With severe anemia and hypotension, survival may depend on blood transfusion; in milder cases, spontaneous recovery is the rule.

CAUSE OF HEMOLYSIS IN FAVISM

The specificity of favism is extraordinary: The syndrome occurs only in G6PD-deficient people and is caused only by fava beans (*Vicia faba*). Although there have been claims for acute reactions to peas (*pisismo* in Italian), there are no convincing reports that these were hemolytic attacks. Another recurrent theme, in what could be referred to as *favism lore*, is that it can be triggered by inhalation of the plant flower pollen. We have not obtained satisfactory evidence of a hemolytic attack begun through this port of entry. Thus, although patients must be warned that an attack may recur any time they consume fava beans, they can be reassured that other beans are safe, as are walks in the countryside.

Extensive studies on the components of fava beans responsible for hemolysis have led to the identification of vicine and convicine, two β-glycosides that have as aglycones the substituted pyrimidines divicine and isouramil (140). These compounds, in the course of their autooxidation, produce free radicals, which in turn oxidize GSH, thus activating the chain reaction of events leading to hemolysis (141).

Fava beans have been used as a staple food for centuries and perhaps millennia precisely in areas where G6PD deficiency is common. A discussion of the possible reasons cannot be given here, but fava beans combine a relatively high nutritional value, a relatively high protein content, and a high level of palatability with a great ease of cultivation; like other leguminous plants, they require little or no fertilization. From the agricultural point of view, it would be desirable to develop *V. faba* mutants that do not have high levels of the dangerous glycosides, but this has not yet been done. These substances may serve as a natural defense of the plant against pests, or they may play a more subtle role in the plant's metabolism.

FAVA BEAN INGESTION WITHOUT ACUTE HEMOLYTIC ANEMIA

An intriguing feature of favism is its considerably erratic character. It is estimated that, at least in adults, ingestion of fava beans does not trigger acute hemolytic anemia in more than 25% of cases, and even in the same person, favism may occur on one occasion but not on another (142). Practitioners in endemic areas give examples of patients who had their first recognized attacks in their 60s. This feature of favism has practical consequences because, unless it is clearly explained to the public, it may affect the credibility of the physician who advises a patient against recurrence of favism! The reasons for this erratic character are not entirely clear. One obvious factor must be the dosage—that is, the amount of fava beans ingested in relation to body mass, which presumably accounts for the higher rate of favism in children. Another factor must be food processing. Raw fava beans are more likely to cause favism than cooked, frozen, or canned fava beans. A third, and possibly the most important, factor is the maturity of the beans, because the young, small beans have higher levels of glucosides. Finally, it is possible that β-glycosidases, present in varying amounts both in the beans and in the intestinal mucosa of the consumer, may play an important role in determining the amount and rate of release of active aglycones (142).

If factors related to the fava beans are important in determining an attack of favism and its severity, one might expect the type of G6PD-deficient variant in the person ingesting them also to be important. Because early reports on the clinical features of favism and on its epidemiology have come mainly from southern Italy, Greece, and the Middle East, and because in all these areas, G6PD deficiency is largely due to G6PD Mediterranean, this variant has come to be regarded as almost specifically associated with favism. However, favism is common, for instance, in Singapore, where the underlying variants are not always Mediterranean. The occurrence of clinical favism with the African variant A– (which was held as *not* susceptible to favism) was documented (135). In this respect, it is curious that the variant G6PD Betica, originally discovered in patients with favism (143) and previously reported as polymorphic in Spain, turns out to be the same as G6PD A– (65). In a survey carried out in Algeria (144), seven different G6PD variants were observed in subjects with G6PD deficiency ascertained because of an attack of favism. Thus, the present evidence suggests that favism can be triggered, under appropriate circumstances, in any G6PD-deficient person. The reason is probably that, whereas subtle kinetic differences among G6PD variants are important in the steady state, when metabolism through the PPP is impaired, the oxidative action of divicine and isouramil is so drastic that it overrides subtle kinetic differences easily. Once the PPP is maximally stimulated, the only limiting factor for its rate of operation becomes the amount of G6PD activity, which is forced to function at V_{max} level. Thus, it is likely (although not proved) that a G6PD A–-deficient person with 12% residual activity needs to eat more fava beans than a G6PD Mediterranean–deficient person with 3% residual activity. Eventually, the red cell GSH is depleted, and intravascular hemolysis follows.

DIAGNOSIS

The importance of recognizing hemoglobinuria cannot be overemphasized, because the presence of this sign restricts considerably the differential diagnosis of hemolytic anemia in general. With a history of fava bean ingestion and the finding of hemoglobinuria (clearly reported or directly observed), the diagnosis is almost always straightforward, and it can be made confidently even before obtaining the final proof that the patient is G6PD deficient. If hemoglobinuria has already subsided, and the history is uncertain, one is faced with the much wider differential diagnosis of acute hemolytic anemia. The negative direct antiglobulin test militates against autoimmune hemolytic anemia. In endemic areas, it is important to exclude malaria infection and the much rarer babesiosis. In the hemolytic-uremic syndrome, the red cell morphology is different, and there is evidence of impaired renal function. In all cases, the demonstration of G6PD deficiency is conclusive, and in uncertain cases, it is crucial.

Neonatal Jaundice

G6PD activity in the red cells of newborns is somewhat higher than in red cells of adults. Therefore, it may come as a surprise that G6PD deficiency is associated with neonatal jaundice. The word *association* is chosen advisedly, because not every G6PD-deficient baby becomes jaundiced after birth; however, numerous studies have shown that the risk of developing neonatal jaundice is much greater in G6PD-deficient than in G6PD-normal newborns (145,146).

CLINICAL FEATURES

Neonatal jaundice related to G6PD deficiency differs from the classic Rh-related neonatal jaundice in two main respects: (a) It is rarely present at birth—the peak incidence of clinical onset is between days 2 and 3, and (b) there is more jaundice than anemia, and the anemia is rarely severe (147). For this reason, the terms *hemolytic disease of the newborn* and *neonatal jaundice* cannot be regarded as interchangeable, at least in the context of G6PD deficiency.

The severity of G6PD-related neonatal jaundice varies enormously, from being subclinical to imposing the threat of kernicterus if not treated. Because not *all* G6PD-deficient babies are jaundiced, it is likely that the factors that cause it to develop may, if more extreme, make it severe. There has been an active search for an additional factor that may cause neonatal jaundice when combined with G6PD deficiency. Marked differences in the incidence of neonatal jaundice have been demonstrated among various Greek islands. Although the study was carried out in the search for an additional genetic factor, thought to be autosomal, it is also possible that there may be an environment factor that is different in different islands. In support of the latter possibility, work in Nigeria has revealed that G6PD-deficient babies with neonatal jaundice had a significantly higher rate of exposure to naphthalene (used in their bedding and clothing) than G6PD-deficient babies without jaundice.

PATHOGENESIS

As mentioned earlier, not all G6PD-deficient babies develop jaundice. This erratic aspect is reminiscent of the acute hemolytic anemia induced by fava beans or other triggering factors. However, this does not mean that the mechanism is the same. Several studies have addressed the question of what factor, in addition to G6PD deficiency, is required for the development of neonatal jaundice. One possibility was that, in view of the marked genetic heterogeneity of G6PD deficiency, neonatal jaundice was associated with some variants but not with others. The finding that neonatal jaundice is prevalent in widely remote parts of the world—such as Nigeria (146), Sardinia (147), Pakistan (148), and Thailand (149)—does not support this notion. Severe neonatal jaundice requiring blood exchange transfusion occurs with the majority of the nine variants encountered among Chinese infants (85). Because fetal red cells differ from those produced after birth in many ways, another possibility is that some newborns have an additional, developmentally related enzyme deficiency that causes neonatal jaundice in G6PD-deficient babies. In this respect, studies have been carried out on glutathione peroxidase, glutathione reductase, and superoxide dismutase, but with negative results.

Partly because of these negative results, attention has been directed away from red cells and toward a hepatic origin of G6PD deficiency–related neonatal jaundice. It is notable that there is a considerable dissociation between hyperbilirubinemia and anemia in G6PD-deficient babies. It is interesting, therefore, that a TA repeat promoter polymorphism of the bilirubin uridine diphosphate–glucuronosyltransferase gene (UGT1A) that causes benign jaundice in adults (see Chapter 47, Disorders of Heme Production and Catabolism) associates with G6PD deficiency to give an increased risk of neonatal jaundice (150). This variant promoter reaches high frequencies in many populations, has seven rather than the more-usual six TA repeats in the TATAA element, and has been shown to decrease the expression of the UGT1A gene. The UGT1A variant may also give rise to an increase in bilirubin levels in adult G6PD-deficient subjects (151) and during the favic crisis (152). However, some contrasting data has been published indicating that the UGT1A polymorphism does not contribute to the development of severe neonatal hyperbilirubinemia in normal or G6PD-deficient subjects (153).

It may be useful to consider two different types of neonatal jaundice associated with G6PD deficiency: (a) a more common type, best visualized as a marked exaggeration of "physiologic jaundice" that is not greatly influenced by the environment and that may result from G6PD deficiency being expressed in the liver; and (b) a more rare, frankly hemolytic type, which can be visualized as acute hemolytic anemia occurring in a newborn who was exposed to one of the same agents that could cause acute hemolytic anemia even in adults, such as a drug, infection, or some particular local habit (e.g., the extensive use of naphthalene, mothballs, or camphor balls in some nurseries).

The management of neonatal jaundice due to G6PD deficiency does not differ from that recommended for other causes. Thus, mild cases do not require treatment, intermediate cases require phototherapy, and severe cases require exchange transfusion treatment, just as in neonatal jaundice due to classic hemolytic disease of the newborn. It has also been suggested that a single dose of Sn-mesoporphyrin, a potent inhibitor of bilirubin production, administered preventatively or therapeutically can supplant the need for phototherapy to control hyperbilirubinemia in G6PD-deficient neonates (154).

Congenital Nonspherocytic Hemolytic Anemia

CLINICAL FEATURES
In contrast to most G6PD-deficient subjects, who have minimal and subclinical hemolysis in the steady state, a small minority of G6PD-deficient people have a degree of hemolysis that is easily diagnosed by conventional methods and that is sufficiently pronounced to cause them to be anemic. This group of patients is clinically heterogeneous for reasons that are explained in the section Molecular Basis, and therefore it is not possible to describe any level of expression of this condition as being typical.

The patient is almost invariably male and, in general, presents because of unexplained jaundice. Frequently, the onset is at birth, and a diagnosis is made of neonatal jaundice, which may be severe enough to require exchange transfusion. Unfortunately, anemia recurs, and the jaundice fails to clear completely; this is often the reason for further investigation. In many cases, however, neonatal jaundice may be forgotten, and the patient is only reinvestigated much later in life, for instance, because of gallstones in a child or in a young adult. The severity of anemia ranges in different patients from borderline to transfusion

dependent. The anemia is usually normochromic but somewhat macrocytic, because a large proportion of reticulocytes (up to 20% or more) cause an increased mean corpuscular volume and a shifted, wider-than-normal red cell size distribution curve. The red cell morphology is mostly not characteristic, and for this reason, it is referred to in the negative as being *nonspherocytic*. The bone marrow is normoblastic, unless the increased requirement of folic acid associated with the high red cell turnover has caused it to become megaloblastic. There is chronic hyperbilirubinemia, decreased haptoglobin, and increased serum lactate dehydrogenase. Hemoglobinuria is rare, but hemosiderinuria may be detected sometimes. The spleen is usually moderately enlarged in small children and subsequently may increase in size sufficiently to cause mechanical discomfort, hypersplenism, or both.

PATHOPHYSIOLOGY
The clinical picture just described is obviously different from that of G6PD deficiency–related acute hemolytic anemia. It is more reminiscent, instead, of the chronic hemolysis seen in hereditary spherocytosis. Even in severe cases, it is different from thalassemia major because there is no evidence of ineffective erythropoiesis, and the destruction is limited to mature, circulating red cells. The fact that there is no hemoglobinuria, at least in the steady state, suggests that the hemolysis is mainly extravascular and that its mechanism is different from that of the acute hemolytic variants. Studies of red cell membrane proteins in CNSHA patients have revealed high-molecular-weight aggregates (155) consisting largely of spectrin, which have not been found in asymptomatic G6PD-deficient subjects. These findings suggest that the reductive potential of residual G6PD is adequate in the steady state in acute hemolytic variants; whereas in CNSHA, continuous oxidation of sulfhydryl groups takes place, followed by irreversible changes in the configuration of membrane proteins, which may then become abnormally susceptible to shear-induced fragmentation (156). This does not mean that the red cells of patients with severe G6PD deficiency are not vulnerable to acute oxidative damage of Hgb as well. The same agents that can cause acute hemolytic anemia in people with the common type of G6PD deficiency can cause severe exacerbations with hemoglobinuria in people with the severe form of G6PD deficiency. The reason that the severity of CNSHA associated with G6PD deficiency is so variable is simply that almost every case is due to a different mutation, and each mutation has a different effect on the stability of the enzyme, its kinetic properties, or both.

MOLECULAR BASIS
The course of patients with G6PD deficiency–associated CNSHA is so different from that of most people with G6PD deficiency, who may have the occasional episode of acute hemolytic anemia (no matter how severe), that it appeared highly likely from the phenotype that the underlying genetic basis would be also different. Biochemical studies quickly confirmed this inference. In the early 1960s, characterization of G6PD from rare patients with CNSHA revealed properties that were different from those of the already known polymorphic variants (like G6PD Mediterranean and G6PD A–). Thus, new names, such as *G6PD Oklahoma* and *G6PD Chicago*, were coined to designate these new variants. But why would a particular variant cause severe rather than mild hemolysis? In principle, one can visualize two types of reason: quantitative and qualitative. G6PD deficiency in CNSHA could be simply more extreme. It stands to reason that if 20% of the normal enzyme activity is adequate for the steady-state requirement of red cell metabolism, 2% may not be adequate. This obvious quantitative consideration plays a role, because the G6PD variants associated with CNSHA usually present with less than 10% of the normal activity, although reticulocytosis may push the

activity above this level. However, the reverse is not true. Although many of the variants that are *not* associated with CNSHA have more than 10% of normal activity (class III), many others have less (class II), just like the CNSHA variants. This clearly indicates that the molecular properties of individual variants are important determinants of clinical expression.

Which properties, other than the level of activity, are most important is a question that has been keenly debated, and the picture remains unclear. A significant increase in the K_m for G6P is observed in a substantial proportion of class I variants, but also common are a low K_i of NADPH, a high K_m of NADP, and a low use of deamino-NADP (157). Because NADP and NADPH are important regulators of G6PD activity in normal cells, one might imagine that mutations causing changes in the K_m of NADP and in the K_i of NADPH would have pronounced pathologic effects. However, we have already seen that a cluster of mutations that cause these variants turns out to be distant from the coenzyme binding site. Instead, they lie close to the dimer interface, which has a structural $NADP^+$ molecule nearby. Disruption of this structure may explain why almost all class I variants have a reduced thermostability, and in some cases, why they lose activity in low $NADP^+$ concentrations.

What has become increasingly apparent from the analysis of the molecular basis of G6PD deficiency in patients presenting with CNSHA is that the same mutation is seen in unrelated individuals (68,70,158). Because these variants are not likely to have spread through genetic drift, it can be presumed that they have arisen independently, and in some cases this has been established by observing the *de novo* origin of the mutation in the index case. Although this can sometimes be explained by the increased frequency of C→T transitions at CpG dinucleotides, this type of mutation occurs in only 11 of 63 known substitutions. A more interesting inference is that there are only a limited number of ways in which the G6PD molecule can be altered to give rise to the severe clinical manifestations of CNSHA while maintaining sufficient activity in nonerythroid cells to be compatible with life.

DIAGNOSIS

The diagnosis of G6PD deficiency is discussed in the section Diagnosis of Glucose-6-Phosphate Dehydrogenase Deficiency, but a special problem in relation to CNSHA is to establish firmly the causal link between the G6PD deficiency and hemolytic anemia. If the patient is, for example, of Swedish or of Japanese ancestry, the link is taken for granted. This is generally justified, given the rarity of G6PD deficiency in these populations. On the other hand, if the patient is from a population in which G6PD deficiency is common, its presence in a patient with CNSHA might be a mere coincidence, and the cause of the CNSHA might be something else altogether. In these cases, it becomes essential to characterize the G6PD of the patient, because if it is a common variant, known to be asymptomatic in other subjects, it can be exonerated. If it is a new, unique variant, however, it is likely to be the culprit.

Glucose-6-Phosphate Dehydrogenase Deficiency and Sickle Cell Anemia

Because the geographic distribution of the β^s globin gene and of the *Gd*− gene overlap extensively, especially in Africa and in people of African descent, one can expect to find that the two red cell disorders coexist frequently. Because the two genes are not genetically linked, the frequency of people having both is the product of the two gene frequencies. For instance, if, in a particular population, the frequency of Hgb AS heterozygotes is 25%, and the frequency of G6PD deficiency in males is 20%, one would predict that one-fifth of the AS heterozygotes (i.e., 5% of the entire male

population) would also be G6PD deficient. Although there have been claims to the contrary (159,160), the predicted frequency is observed in a stable population (161). Because heterozygosity for β^s and heterozygosity for *Gd*− both protect against malaria, it is intriguing to consider whether females with this particular genotypic combination have greater protection than either of the two single heterozygotes. Thus far, such an additive or synergistic effect has not been demonstrated (162).

A separate question is whether the combination of G6PD deficiency—an asymptomatic condition in the steady state—with homozygous sickle cell anemia affects the course of this condition, a serious hemolytic disease even in the steady state (see Chapter 50). Early reports indicated a significant increase in the prevalence of G6PD deficiency in Hgb SS disease compared to normal controls, suggesting that the deficiency ameliorates the sickle cell anemia (159). Further studies, however, have failed to substantiate this (163–165). A large cross-sectional survey of sickle cell disease in the United States (166) showed no effect of G6PD deficiency on either clinical or hematologic parameters; the prevalence of G6PD deficiency did not change significantly with age, suggesting that there is little effect on survival from the combination of G6PD deficiency and Hgb SS.

We can also ask the reverse question, namely whether sickle cell anemia affects the manifestations of G6PD deficiency. At the biochemical level, the answer is yes, because the high reticulocytosis and the globally young red cell population of these patients causes a marked increase in the G6PD activity of G6PD-deficient red cells, especially of those with the A− variant, so much so that these patients are easily misclassified as G6PD normal if an appropriate technique is not used. At the clinical level, one might expect in theory that this relative increase in enzyme level would prevent the development or limit the severity of acute hemolytic anemia consequent to G6PD deficiency. This is difficult to assess in practice, because the interaction of infection, drugs, and preexisting anemia is too complex. If the degree of drug-induced hemolysis is less in a patient with sickle cell anemia, however, this is likely to be overridden by the fact that acute intravascular hemolysis would take place on the background of the chronic extravascular hemolysis of sickle cell anemia. Severe exacerbation of anemia has been observed in patients with sickle cell anemia who are also G6PD deficient (167), and it is probably prudent to assume that this combination, if anything, has the potential to increase the clinical manifestations of sickle cell anemia.

PATHOPHYSIOLOGY

Glucose-6-Phosphate Dehydrogenase and Red Cell Aging

Although G6PD is a ubiquitously expressed housekeeping enzyme, its deficiency manifests essentially as a red cell disorder. This is due to the fact that, compared to most other somatic cells, mature red cells are distinctive in their inability to synthesize protein. In most somatic cells, G6PD is subject to turnover, but in red cells, any G6PD molecule undergoing denaturation or proteolytic breakdown cannot be replaced. In normal red cells, the decay of G6PD approximates an exponential with a half-life of approximately 60 days (26). The age dependence of red cell G6PD activity is so characteristic that it almost can be regarded as a marker of red cell age. Normal blood reticulocytes have approximately five times more activity than the 10% oldest red cells. Because we know that G6PD is critical to red cell viability, one might suggest that aged red cells are removed from the circulation precisely because their G6PD level has become too low. However, this cannot be so in normal subjects, because the level of G6PD, even in the oldest cells, is higher than the mean level in many G6PD-deficient people. From this analysis, we can infer that there is a threshold level of G6PD activity below which red cells become nonviable, but in normal subjects this is never reached. With common G6PD variants, this threshold is reached only after approximately 100 days of aging in the circulation, and therefore carriers of these variants are hematologically normal in the steady state. With some rare variants of G6PD, this threshold is reached after as few as 10 to 50 days, and therefore they have more-or-less severe CNSHA.

Mechanism of Hemolytic Crisis

An important and direct pathophysiologic consequence of the marked age dependence of G6PD activity in red cells is that acute hemolytic anemia associated with G6PD-deficiency red cell destruction is an orderly function of red cell age. The oldest red cells with the least G6PD are the first to hemolyze, and the hemolytic process progresses upstream toward the cells with more and more G6PD. As a result, there is a selective enrichment in red cells that, although genetically G6PD deficient, have relatively higher levels of G6PD. This phenomenon can be so marked with certain G6PD variants that patients in the posthemolytic state are found to be relatively refractory to further challenge (the resistant phase of the attack). Under these circumstances, ^{51}Cr red cell survival studies show that the half-life is still less than normal, demonstrating that the patient is in a state of compensated hemolysis.

The clinical picture of acute hemolytic anemia associated with G6PD deficiency conveys forcefully the impression that hemolysis results from the action of an exogenous factor on intrinsically abnormal red cells. Hemoglobinemia and hemoglobinuria indicate unambiguously that the hemolysis is, at least in part, intravascular. To a first approximation, it is easy to visualize the following sequence of events:

1. An oxidative agent causes conversion of GSH to oxidized glutathione.
2. GSH reserve is rapidly depleted due to the limited capacity of G6PD-deficient red cells to regenerate GSH.
3. Once GSH is exhausted, the sulfhydryl groups of Hgb and probably of other proteins are oxidized to disulfides or sulfoxides.
4. Coarse precipitates of denatured Hgb cause irreversible damage to the membrane, and the red cells lyse.

Although GSH depletion is a classic *in vitro* finding when red cells are challenged, not all these steps have been fully documented *in vivo*. One major difficulty in analyzing the sequential changes that take place in a patient with acute hemolytic anemia from the oxidative attack to the final hemolysis is that red cells sampled from the patient are, obviously, at any given stage, those that have not yet hemolyzed. In one careful study, however, it was demonstrated that in the course of an episode of favism, the first measurable biochemical change is a fall in NADPH, followed by a fall in GSH (168), in keeping with stages 1 and 2 described above. Heinz bodies are the visible expression of stage 3. Stage 4 is more obscure, because we do not know exactly how the membrane is damaged, although studies suggest that binding of hemochromes (arising from Hgb denaturation) to band 3 molecules may be one intermediate step (169).

Although the diagnostic and pathophysiologic importance of intravascular hemolysis has been emphasized, it is certain that not all the hemolysis is intravascular, as witnessed, for instance, by the enlargement of the spleen. It is not difficult to visualize that the most severely damaged red cells hemolyze in the bloodstream without help, whereas less severely damaged red cells are recognized as abnormal by macrophages and undergo extravascular hemolysis in the reticuloendothelial system, possibly as a result of membrane glycoprotein modifications (170). This process has been referred to as an example of an "innocent bystander" phenomenon (171), although the red cells, by virtue of being G6PD deficient, are not that innocent. The role of complement and of immunoglobulins in extravascular hemolysis of damaged G6PD-deficient red cells mediated by macrophages has been discussed in detail (142).

Glucose-6-Phosphate Dehydrogenase Deficiency in Nonerythroid Cells

As mentioned earlier, because nucleated somatic cells have the capability to synthesize G6PD constitutively, they are less affected than red cells by G6PD deficiency. Specifically, if G6PD deficiency is due to instability of a mutant enzyme, we would not expect nucleated cells to be severely affected. For instance, subjects with G6PD Mediterranean have less than 5% G6PD activity in red cells, but approximately 30% of normal activity in granulocytes; subjects with G6PD A– have approximately 12% G6PD activity in red cells, but near-normal activity in granulocytes. On the other hand, if G6PD deficiency results from a drastic change in catalytic efficiency or in substrate affinity, the deficiency may be more universal.

In practice, the only well-documented pathologic effect occurs in granulocytes. A few of the class I G6PD variants (172) cause granulocyte dysfunction as well as CNSHA. The main effects are impaired phagocytosis and bacterial killing. Patients with these variants have increased susceptibility to bacterial infection, particularly with *Staphylococcus aureus*. G6PD deficiency impairs phagocytosis and killing through a shortage in NADPH supply, similar to that observed in chronic granulomatous disease, in which cytochrome b245 is defective. Erythrocytes are not the only nonnucleated cells in the body. Another example is in the lens of the eye, and juvenile cataracts have been reported in a number of patients with class I G6PD (173). In patients with simple G6PD deficiency, an early onset of cataracts has been found in some series (174) but not in others (175), suggesting that it may be limited to certain variants.

DIAGNOSIS OF GLUCOSE-6-PHOSPHATE DEHYDROGENASE DEFICIENCY

Although the clinical picture of favism and of other forms of acute hemolytic anemia associated with G6PD deficiency is characteristic, the final diagnosis must rely on the direct demonstration of decreased activity of this enzyme in red cells. With neonatal jaundice and CNSHA, the differential diagnosis is much wider, and therefore this test is even more important. The enzyme assay is easy, and numerous screening tests can be used as substitutes if a spectrophotometer is not available. A number of potential snags and sources of error must be understood, however, and the use of commercial kits is not a substitute for such understanding. The following subsections first discuss the value and limitations of the regular quantitative assay and then comment briefly on the use of alternatives.

Tests for Glucose-6-Phosphate Dehydrogenase Deficiency

QUANTITATION

G6PD can be assayed by the classic method of Horecker and Smyrniotis, which measures directly the rate of formation of

NADPH through its characteristic absorption peak in the near ultraviolet at 340 nm. The red cell activity is expressed in international units (micromoles of NADPH produced per minute) per gram of Hgb; therefore, it is best to assay the enzyme activity and the Hgb concentration in the same hemolysate and work out the ratio. In normal red cells, the range of G6PD activity, measured at 30°C, is 7 to 10 IU/g Hb.

SCREENING TESTS

Several screening tests for G6PD deficiency are useful and reliable, provided they are properly run and their limitations are understood. The most popular are the dye decolorization tests (176), the methemoglobin reduction test (177), and the fluorescence spot test (178). All these methods are semiquantitative, and they are meant to classify a sample simply as *normal* or *deficient*. The cut-off point can be set by following the appropriate instructions and by trial and error in the individual diagnostic laboratory. One should aim to classify as deficient any sample with less than 30% of the normal activity, because above this level, one is unlikely to encounter clinical manifestations. Screening tests are especially useful for testing large numbers of samples. They are also perfectly adequate for diagnostic purposes in patients who are in the steady state, but not for patients in the posthemolytic period or with other complications. Also, they cannot be expected to identify all heterozygotes. Finally, an ideal screening test should not give false-negative results (i.e., it should not misclassify a G6PD-deficient subject as normal), but it can be allowed to give a few false-positive results (i.e., a G6PD-normal subject might be misclassified as G6PD deficient). Ideally, every patient found to be G6PD deficient by screening should be confirmed by the spectrophotometric assay.

A technique that is neglected but that can be useful for some population studies is electrophoresis followed by specific staining for G6PD activity. It has the advantage of detecting both electrophoretic variants with normal activity (through displacement of the stained band) and deficient variants (through obvious decrease in staining intensity). The classic starch-gel method, although it may still have the highest resolving power in some cases, has been largely replaced by the use of supporting media that are less laborious to handle, such as cellulose acetate and agarose.

Cytochemical Tests

G6PD activity can be demonstrated in individual red cells either by the use of a tetrazolium dye or by coupling G6PD activity in the intact cell to a methemoglobin elution method (177). Neither of these techniques has gained wide acceptance in diagnostic laboratories, but they can be useful in special cases and for research purposes.

Practical Problems

The definition of G6PD deficiency is somewhat arbitrary, because different genetic variants are associated with different degrees of deficiency. It seems reasonable to choose as the cut-off point a level that can cause clinical manifestations. It can be safely stated that in males there are no hemolytic complications with a red cell G6PD activity greater than 30% of normal. Thus, the demarcation between G6PD-normal and G6PD-deficient males is, in principle, clear-cut. Several problems, as discussed in the following sections, deserve consideration.

EFFECT OF RED CELL AGE

As mentioned in the section Pathophysiology, any condition associated with reticulocytosis entails an increase in G6PD activity. This means that if the subject is genetically G6PD nor-

mal, his red cell G6PD activity is above the normal range. This does not affect diagnosis, because G6PD deficiency is correctly ruled out. If the subject is genetically G6PD deficient, however, reticulocytosis may raise his red cell G6PD to near or within the normal range, and he may be misclassified as G6PD normal.

EFFECT OF SELECTIVE HEMOLYSIS

After a hemolytic attack, two circumstances increase the risk of misdiagnosis: first, if the older red cells have been destroyed selectively; second, if the marrow responds with a sudden outpouring of young cells into the peripheral blood. (A third confusing factor may be admixture of G6PD-normal red cells if the patient had been transfused.) Although the reticulocyte count is a good warning to avoid this mistake, it is not a sensitive index of the mean red cell age, because reticulocytes turn into morphologically "mature" erythrocytes within 1 to 2 days. In other words, the mean red cell age may be significantly younger than normal, even when the reticulocyte count is normal.

There are several ways to circumvent these problems. First, a G6PD level in the low to normal range in the face of reticulocytosis is always suspicious. In general, this finding suggests that the patient is actually G6PD deficient. Second, if the patient is suffering from or is recovering from an acute hemolytic crisis, the suspicion generated from the first finding can be simply kept in store for a few months, when the situation will have evolved toward the steady state; a repeat test proves whether the patient is G6PD deficient. Third, if either the urgency of some clinical decision or academic curiosity demands a more prompt solution of the problem, the presence of severely G6PD-deficient red cells can be demonstrated either by enzyme assay of the oldest cells (fractionated by sedimentation) or by a cytochemical method.

WHITE CELL CONTAMINATION

Because G6PD activity is much higher in leukocytes (particularly in granulocytes) than in erythrocytes, for accurate measurements, it is essential to remove all leukocytes by the Ficoll-Hypaque method or by filtration through cellulose powder rather than by the cruder approach of sucking off the buffy coat. In most cases, however, this is not necessary just for the purpose of diagnosing G6PD deficiency.

GLUCOSE-6-PHOSPHATE DEHYDROGENASE DEFICIENCY IN HETEROZYGOTES

None of the three screening tests can be relied on to identify G6PD heterozygotes (179). Diagnosis must therefore be made using a quantitative test, which is not difficult in most cases because the level of G6PD falls between the normal and the deficient male range. However, due to imbalanced lyonization, some females "trespass" into either of the extremes, and in such cases, one can only prove that a female subject is a heterozygote by pedigree analysis or, if the mutation is known, by DNA analysis. Fortunately, this is not crucial from the clinical point of view. The susceptibility of heterozygotes to develop acute hemolytic anemia, and its severity, are roughly proportional to the percentage of G6PD-deficient red cells. Thus, if this percentage is so low as to be hard to detect, then the patient is most unlikely to have G6PD-related hemolysis.

A special mention should be made of heterozygotes for G6PD variants associated with CNSHA. Mothers of male patients with this condition often have normal G6PD levels, which may be because the variant in the offspring is due to a *de novo* mutation. In other cases, however, the mother is a heterozygote but is phenotypically normal. This can be explained by the fact that red cells derived from progenitors in which the deficient allele is expressed have a shorter intravascular lifespan than those derived from normal progenitors. It is also possible that somatic selection has favored the hemopoietic progenitor cells with normal G6PD, and for two class I variants, a significant excess of G6PD-normal cells was found among white cell lineages (180), although this may not always be the case (Thomas Vulliamy, unpublished observations).

A final point to bear in mind is that in certain populations in which the frequency of G6PD deficiency is high, a significant proportion of females are homozygous. As an X-linked disorder, G6PD deficiency is often considered to affect only males, but of course these homozygous females present, and must be treated, in exactly the same way as their hemizygous male counterparts.

TREATMENT OF GLUCOSE-6-PHOSPHATE DEHYDROGENASE DEFICIENCY

Prevention of Clinical Manifestations

Because neonatal jaundice and acute hemolytic anemia are the most common manifestations of G6PD deficiency, it is most important to consider how they can be prevented. The first step is to identify G6PD-deficient individuals, and this is where screening is most pertinent. Whether population-wide screening is both desirable and feasible depends primarily on the prevalence of G6PD deficiency in any particular community; this determines the cost/benefit ratio (the main cost being labor, as the reagents and equipment needed are relatively cheap). If screening is done at all, it is best done on cord blood, and this is already practiced, for instance, in Sardinia, Thailand, and Malaysia. Once a subject is known to be G6PD deficient, the two main implications are the risk of neonatal jaundice and the importance of avoiding exposure to agents that can cause acute hemolytic anemia. We cannot prevent neonatal jaundice as yet, but the awareness of G6PD deficiency must entail surveillance for neonatal jaundice until at least day 4, as well as special recommendations with respect to factors such as naphthalene that can cause it or make it worse.

By contrast, at least one type of acute hemolytic anemia, namely favism, is totally preventable if the persons concerned, and their families, accept the advice to give up eating fava beans. Prevention of infection-induced hemolysis is obviously more difficult. Prevention of drug-induced hemolysis is possible in most cases by avoiding drugs known to be linked with hemolytic anemia (Table 54-6) and by choosing alternative drugs, although it may be difficult when there are none. The most common problem is the need to administer primaquine for the eradication of malaria due to *Plasmodium vivax* or to *P. malariae*: In these cases, primaquine can be given at a reduced dosage of 10 to 15 mg/day for 28 days (instead of 30 to 45 mg/day for 14 days), which may still cause hemolysis, but can be of an acceptably mild degree.

The question of antimalarial prophylaxis for short-term travelers to malaria-endemic areas is complex. Nowadays, because in many such areas chloroquine resistance is not uncommon, the most widely recommended agents are mefloquine and Fansidar. We are not aware of any report of hemolytic anemia associated with ingestion of these agents in G6PD-deficient subjects. However, the former is related to other quinolines and the latter to sulfonamides; therefore, they may be hemolytic. An empirical approach that we recommend is that a G6PD-deficient person, if he or she needs antimalarial prophylaxis, be given a "test dose" 1 month before traveling, and that the effects be monitored by appropriate parameters (clinical state, Hgb, retics, bilirubin). Depending on the results, one may be able to decide that prophylaxis is safe, or one may have to adjust dosage or consider alternatives.

Treatment of Clinical Manifestations

MANAGEMENT OF ACUTE HEMOLYTIC ANEMIA AND FAVISM

A patient with acute hemolytic anemia may present a diagnostic problem that, once solved, does not require any specific treatment at all; or the patient may present a medical emergency requiring immediate action. The most urgent question is whether the child needs a blood transfusion. It is difficult to give absolute guidelines, but the following may be useful. If the Hgb level is below 6 to 7 g/dL, and if there is evidence of continuing hemolysis (especially persisting hemoglobinuria), the child should receive a transfusion as soon as possible (181). It has been suggested that desferrioxamine could control acute hemolytic anemia in favism (182,183) but this has not been confirmed (184), and withholding a blood transfusion when indicated in this condition should be regarded as dangerous. The most important complication that may require treatment is acute renal failure, which is rare in children. Apart from standard renal failure regimen, hemodialysis may be necessary.

MANAGEMENT OF NEONATAL JAUNDICE

This does not differ from management of neonatal jaundice due to causes other than G6PD deficiency. Full details have been given elsewhere (181).

MANAGEMENT OF CHRONIC NONSPHEROCYTIC HEMOLYTIC ANEMIA

In general, management does not differ from that of CNSHA due to other causes, such as pyruvate kinase deficiency. If the anemia is not severe, regular folic acid supplements and regular hematologic surveillance suffice. It is important to avoid exposure to potentially hemolytic drugs, and blood transfusion may be indicated when exacerbations occur, mostly with intercurrent infections. In rare patients, the anemia is so severe that it is transfusion dependent. In these cases, blood transfusions usually are needed at approximately 2-month intervals to keep the Hgb in the range of 8 to 10 g/dL. A hypertransfusion regimen aiming to maintain a normal Hgb level is not indicated (because there is no ineffective erythropoiesis in the bone marrow). Appropriate iron chelation, however, should be instituted by the age of 2 years and must be continued as long as transfusion treatment is necessary. Sometimes, the transfusion requirement may decrease after puberty.

A special problem is that of splenectomy. Although G6PD-deficient red cells are not selectively destroyed in the spleen, as in hereditary spherocytosis, the fact that the spleen is usually enlarged suggests that it plays a role in hemolysis. In practice, there are three indications for splenectomy: (a) the spleen becomes a physical encumbrance; (b) there is evidence of hypersplenism; and (c) the anemia is severe, even in the absence of the first two indications. Splenectomy may reduce the overall rate of hemolysis just enough to make a transfusion-dependent child become transfusion independent. This is doubly important, because it makes it possible to dispense with desferrioxamine. Pneumovax immunization should be given before splenectomy and penicillin prophylaxis after splenectomy.

When a diagnosis of CNSHA is made, the family must be given genetic counseling, and an effort should be made to establish whether the mother is a heterozygote (this may not be easy by conventional techniques). If she is, the chance of recurrence is 1:2 for every subsequent male pregnancy. Prenatal diagnosis can be offered, and it can be carried out by a G6PD assay on amniotic fluid cells, although the expression of G6PD deficiency in these cells varies with each G6PD variant. A likely better alternative for cases in which the mutation in the G6PD gene of the male affected by CNSHA is identified is to use DNA methods to establish directly whether the mother is heterozygous, and then perform prenatal diagnosis using allele-specific oligonucleotides or by analysis with an appropriate restriction enzyme.

GLUCOSE-6-PHOSPHATE DEHYDROGENASE AND X-CHROMOSOME INACTIVATION

According to the current estimate of approximately 30,000 functional genes in the human genome with around 1000 on the X chromosome, we can safely assume that every woman is heterozygous at several of the corresponding genetic loci. A remarkable consequence is that X inactivation produces two types of somatic cells in each woman that differ from each other in the expression of the respective allelic genes. This situation is referred to as *mosaicism*. Whereas the notion of X chromosome inactivation was first formulated by Mary Lyon from inspection of coat color in mice (185), the first demonstration of mosaicism at the cellular level was provided by the G6PD system itself, when Beutler and colleagues demonstrated that women heterozygous for G6PD deficiency had two red cell populations, one normal and one deficient (186). The demonstration that the active and the inactive state of the X were faithfully maintained in somatic cells was also first obtained using G6PD as a marker, when Davidson and colleagues (187) were able to isolate individual fibroblast clones expressing only the A type or the B type of G6PD from a culture of primary diploid fibroblasts of a woman who was genetically a Gd^A/Gd^B heterozygote.

In most cases, heterozygotes for enzyme deficiencies are asymptomatic, because cells with an enzyme level close to half of normal are biochemically normal. By contrast, as a result of X inactivation, the abnormal cells of a woman heterozygous for G6PD deficiency are just as deficient as those of a hemizygous deficient man and, therefore, just as susceptible to pathology. For this reason, although G6PD deficiency is still often referred to as an X-linked recessive trait, this is a misnomer. A recessive trait is, by definition, not expressed in a heterozygote; instead, G6PD deficiency is expressed in heterozygotes both biochemically and clinically. The expression is decreased, compared with hemizygous males or homozygous females, roughly in proportion to the percentage of G6PD-deficient cells in any individual heterozygote. What determines this percentage is not yet completely understood. Because X inactivation is a random phenomenon, it is expected, in principle, to produce approximately equal numbers of the two cell types constituting the genetic mosaic of a female organism. Analysis of heterozygotes, however, reveals a normal distribution with a relatively wide variation around the mean. Thus, although most heterozygotes have an intermediate phenotype with respect to their G6PD level, at the extremes of the curve, heterozygotes may have a pseudonormal or a pseudodeficient phenotype.

Linder and Gartler (188) first pointed out that, because of the mosaic composition of female tissues, any process associated with cellular proliferation would be expected to reflect the mosaic situation, unless it arose from a single cell. Specifically, they showed that each individual uterine leiomyoma from Gd^A/Gd^B heterozygous women expresses either only G6PD A or only G6PD B. Since then, this approach has been used to test the clonal origin of a variety of solid tumors, leukemias, and related disorders (189), including polycythemia rubra vera and paroxysmal nocturnal hemoglobinuria (190). Naturally, this approach is only applicable to women who happen to be heterozygous at the G6PD locus, and has therefore been more recently replaced by the use of methylation-sensitive restriction sites linked to highly polymorphic markers (191,192).

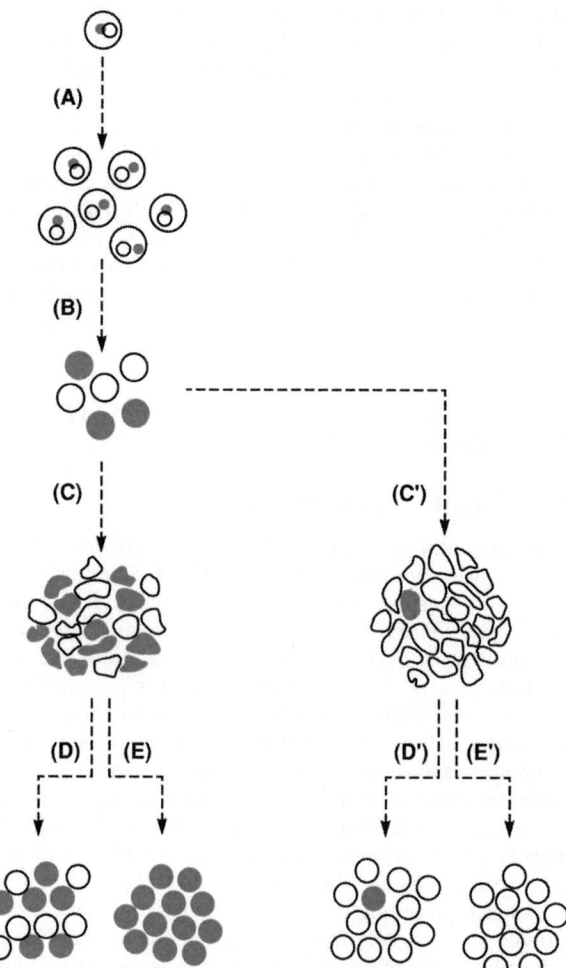

Figure 54-9. Use of the glucose-6-phosphate dehydrogenase (G6PD) phenotype to obtain information on clonal proliferation and somatic cell selection. A: Embryonic cells before X-chromosome inactivation. The two different colored (blue and white) dots represent expression of two different alleles of G6PD. B: Inactivation of one X chromosome per cell produces two cell populations (blue and white) distinguishable by their G6PD phenotype. C: Proliferation of cells at approximately even rates produces mosaicism. C': A differential growth rate of the two cell types resulting from X inactivation (somatic cell selection) may yield a nearly homogeneous population. This could apply to the whole body or to selected tissues, because a particular X-linked gene, for which the subject is heterozygous, can only confer a growth advantage in tissues where it is expressed. D: Proliferating tissue, such as an inflammatory process or a healing wound, still produces a mosaic. E: Pathologic proliferation arising from a single cell, such as a tumor, produces a homogeneous monoclonal population. D' and E': If pathologic proliferation arises in a tissue that is already homogeneous, as a result of somatic cell selection, the cell population still is homogeneous (or nearly homogeneous), regardless of whether the proliferative process is monoclonal or polyclonal.

Although this methodology is powerful, it is important to appreciate its limits as well as its potential. The finding of a single X-linked gene expressed in a particular cell population is best described, in phenotypic terms, by saying that the population is homogeneous in that respect. In keeping with the earlier discussion, it may be homogeneous for one of the three following reasons: (a) the population arises from a single cell; (b) the population arises from multiple cells, but selection during growth has favored one cell type over the other; or (c) the population arises from multiple cells in a tissue that already had an extreme phenotype (Fig. 54-9). Only in the first case is the apparently homogeneous population also monoclonal. To safeguard against being misled by the third situation, it is essential to compare the neoplastic population with normal cells of the same lineage. There is no absolute way to eliminate the second possibility. Thus, because mosaicism due to X inactivation precedes pathology, homogeneity for an X-linked marker may be suggestive of monoclonal origin, but it is not as conclusive as the finding of a unique marker such as a chromosomal abnormality or a gene rearrangement. By contrast, the finding that a cell population is not homogeneous with respect to an X-linked marker can be regarded as conclusive evidence that it is *not* monoclonal.

DISORDERS OF GLUTATHIONE METABOLISM

We have seen how reduced GSH is critical in the protection of cells against oxidative damage, being used to convert peroxides to water through the action of GSH peroxidase (Fig. 54-2). It is also involved in amino acid transport and the maintenance of protein sulfhydryl groups in the reduced state. Cells maintain a high level of GSH through two different pathways, one of which is the NADPH-dependent reduction of oxidized GSH (GSSG) catalyzed by the enzyme GSSG reductase; alternatively, GSH is generated by *de novo* synthesis from glutamate, Cys, and Gly by the consecutive action of two enzymes, γ-glutamylcysteine synthetase (γGSH) and GSH synthetase. Defects in these enzymes of GSH metabolism, leading to low red cell GSH levels, have been implicated as causing hemolytic anemia in rare cases.

Glutathione Peroxidase

It has been suggested that hereditary heterozygous GSH peroxidase deficiency is associated with acute hemolysis (193,194). However, it is not clear whether the deficiency in these cases is caused by a mutation in the GSH peroxidase gene (which has not been described) or by a deficiency of selenium, on which the catalytic activity of GSH peroxidase depends.

Oxidized Glutathione Reductase

Several early cases indicated an association between a low GSSG reductase activity and hemolytic syndromes, although it now seems that most of these were due to a riboflavin deficiency, resulting in inadequate synthesis of the cofactor flavin adenine dinucleotide. However, in one consanguineous family, the autosomal-recessive inheritance of GSSG reductase deficiency has been described (195), presenting as favism in one of three siblings and possibly cataracts in two of them.

γ-Glutamylcysteine Synthetase

Six families have been described in which γGSH deficiency causes hemolytic anemia, and in one case, this was also associated with spinocerebellar degeneration. Two unrelated patients presenting with hemolytic anemia and low red blood cell GSH levels or neonatal jaundice have been shown to be homozygous for a different missense mutation in the gene that encodes the catalytic subunit of γGSH (196,197).

Reduced Glutathione Synthetase

With more than 20 families described, GSH synthetase deficiency is the most common defect of GSH metabolism. Clinically, there are two forms of the disease: a milder form, in which the deficiency is limited to the red cell and results in chronic hemolysis and neonatal jaundice; and a severe form, in which the deficiency causes 5-oxoprolinuria and metabolic acidosis with associated mental retardation and motor function disturbances (198). These patients may also suffer from intermittent neutropenia and a susceptibility to bacterial infection. The molecular defect in some cases has been identified (199,200); it appears that both forms of the disease are mostly caused by missense mutations and that, as in G6PD, homozygous null mutations are probably not viable (Table 54-7). GSH synthetase is a homodimer, the structure of which has recently been solved (201). It is a compact molecule, with each subunit in the shape of

---

TABLE 54-7. Mutations in Patients with Glutathione Synthetase Deficiency[a]

Patient	Clinical Phenotype[a]	Mutation	Proposed Structural Effect
1	HA only	Asp219Gly, homozygous	γGC binding
2	5-OP	Arg267Trp	γGC binding
		Arg283Cys	Disulfide formation
3	5-OP	Arg125Cys	γGC binding
		Deletion of Val380, Glu381+	Misfolding
		Pro314Leu	None obvious
4	5-OP	Asp219Gly	γGC binding
		Leu286Gln	γGC binding
		Arg330Cys	None obvious
5	5-OP	Tyr270Cys	γGC binding
		Unknown	—
6	5-OP	Tyr270His	γGC binding
		Unknown	—
7	5-OP	Leu188Pro, homozygous	ATP binding
8	5-OP + low IQ and poor motor coordination	Gly464Val	Glycine binding
		Unknown	—
9	5-OP + low IQ and abnormal retinogram	Ala26Asp, homozygous	Disrupts dimer
10	5-OP, died at 5 days	Arg267Trp	γGC binding
		Asp469Glu	γGC binding
11	5-OP + neonatal encephalopathy; died at 2 days	Asp219Ala	γGC binding
		Leu254Arg	γGC binding

γGC, γ-glutamyl cysteine; HA, hemolytic anemia; IQ, intelligence quotient; 5-OP, 5-oxoprolinuria with HA and metabolic acidosis.
[a]From Shi ZZ, Habib GM, Rhead WJ, et al. Mutations in the glutathione synthetase gene cause 5-oxoprolinuria. *Nat Genet* 1996;14:361–365; Dahl N, Pigg M, Ristoff E, et al. Missense mutations in the human glutathione synthetase gene result in severe metabolic acidosis, 5-oxoprolinuria, hemolytic anemia and neurological dysfunction. *Hum Mol Genet* 1997;6:1147–1152; Polekhina G, Board PG, Gali RR, et al. Molecular basis of glutathione synthetase deficiency and a rare gene permutation event. *EMBO J* 1999;18:3204–3213.

a flat equilateral triangle, with ligands binding in a central cavity on one side of the molecule. The majority of the amino acid substitutions causing GSH synthetase deficiency can be seen to affect ligand binding or catalysis, whereas mutations that affect dimerization or disrupt protein folding are less common.

REFERENCES

1. Carson PE, Flanagan CL, Ickes CE, et al. Enzymatic deficiency in primaquine sensitive erythrocytes. *Science* 1956;124:484–485.
2. Sansone G, Piga AM, Segni G. *Il favismo*. Torino: Minerva Medica, 1958.
3. Beutler E. G6PD: population genetics and clinical manifestations. *Blood Reviews* 1996;10:45–52.
4. Mason PJ. New insights into G6PD deficiency. *Br J Haematol* 1996;94:585–591.
5. Mehta A, Mason PJ, Vulliamy TJ. Glucose-6-phosphate dehydrogenase deficiency. In: Zanella A, ed. *Inherited disorders of red cell metabolism*. London: Balliere Tindall, 2000:21–38.
6. Beutler E. *Glucose 6-phosphate dehydrogenase deficiency*. New York: McGraw-Hill, 1995.
7. Glader BE, Lukens JN. *Glucose 6-phosphate dehydrogenase deficiency and related disorders of hexose monophosphate shunt and glutathione metabolism*. Philadelphia: Lippincott Williams & Wilkins, 1998.
8. Luzzatto L, Mehta A, Vulliamy TJ. Glucose-6-phosphate dehydrogenase deficiency. In: Scriver CR, Beaudet AL, Sly WS, et al., eds. *The metabolic basis of inherited disease*. New York: McGraw-Hill, 2001:4517–4553.
9. Gaetani GF, Rolfo M, Arena S, et al. Active involvement of catalase during hemolytic crises of favism. *Blood* 1996;88:1084–1088.
10. Gaetani GF, Galiano S, Canepa L, et al. Catalase and glutathione peroxidase are equally active in detoxification of hydrogen peroxide in human erythrocytes. *Blood* 1989;73:334–339.
11. Salvemini F, Franze A, Iervolino A, et al. Enhanced glutathione levels and oxidoresistance mediated by increased glucose-6-phosphate dehydrogenase expression. *J Biol Chem* 1999;274:2750–2757.
12. Kuo WY, Tang TK. Effects of G6PD overexpression in NIH3T3 cells treated with tert-butyl hydroperoxide or paraquat. *Free Radic Biol Med* 1998;24:1130–1138.
13. Preville X, Salvemini F, Giraud S, et al. Mammalian small stress proteins protect against oxidative stress through their ability to increase glucose-6-phosphate dehydrogenase activity and by maintaining optimal cellular detoxifying machinery. *Exp Cell Res* 1999;247:61–78.
14. Tian WN, Braunstein LD, Pang J, et al. Importance of glucose-6-phosphate dehydrogenase activity for cell growth. *J Biol Chem* 1998;273:10609–10617.
15. Kuo W, Lin J, Tang TK. Human glucose-6-phosphate dehydrogenase (G6PD) gene transforms NIH 3T3 cells and induces tumors in nude mice. *Int J Cancer* 2000;85:857–864.
16. Pandolfi PP, Sonati F, Rivi R, et al. Targeted disruption of the housekeeping gene encoding glucose 6-phosphate dehydrogenase (G6PD): G6PD is dispensable for pentose synthesis but essential for defense against oxidative stress. *EMBO J* 1995;14:5209–5215.
17. Nicol CJ, Zielenski J, Tsui LC, et al. An embryoprotective role for glucose-6-phosphate dehydrogenase in developmental oxidative stress and chemical teratogenesis. *FASEB J* 2000;14:111–127.
18. Luzzatto L. Regulation of the activity of glucose-6-phosphate dehydrogenase by NADP+ and NADPH. *Biochim Biophys Acta* 1967;146:18–25.
19. Kirkman HN, Gaetani GD, Clemons EH, et al. Red cell NADP+ and NADPH in glucose-6-phosphate dehydrogenase deficiency. *J Clin Invest* 1975;55:875–881.
20. Gaetani GF, Parker JC, Kirkman HN. Intracellular restraint: a new basis for the limitation in response to oxidative stress in human erythrocytes containing low activity variants of glucose 6-phosphate dehydrogenase. *Proc Natl Acad Sci U S A* 1975;71:3584–3588.
21. Luzzatto L, Battistuzzi G. Glucose-6-phosphate dehydrogenase. *Adv Hum Genet* 1985;14:217–329.
22. Levy HR. Glucose-6-phosphate dehydrogenases. *Adv Enzymol Relat Areas Mol Biol* 1979;48:97–192.
23. Ursini MV, Parrella A, Rosa G, et al. Enhanced expression of glucose-6-phosphate dehydrogenase in human cells sustaining oxidative stress. *Biochem J* 1997;323:801–806.
24. Hodge DL, Salati LM. Nutritional regulation of the glucose-6-phosphate dehydrogenase gene is mediated by a nuclear posttranscriptional mechanism. *Arch Biochim Biophys* 1997;348:303–312.
25. Persico M, Battistuzzi G, Mareni C, et al. Genetic variants of human glucose-6-phosphate dehydrogenase (G6PD): studies of turnover and of G6PD-specific mRNA. In: Weatherall DJ, Fiorelli G, Gorini S, eds. *Advances in red cell biology*. New York: Raven, 1982:309–321.
26. Piomelli S, Corash LM, Davenport DD, et al. In vivo lability of glucose 6-phosphate dehydrogenase in Gd A and Gd Mediterranean deficiency. *J Clin Invest* 1968;47:940–946.
27. Cohen P, Rosemeyer MA. Human glucose-6-phosphate dehydrogenase: purification of the erythrocyte enzyme and the influence of ions on its activity. *Eur J Biochem* 1969;8:1–7.
28. Persico MG, Viglietto G, Martini G, et al. Isolation of human glucose-6-phosphate dehydrogenase (G6PD) cDNA clones: primary structure of the protein and unusual 5' non-coding region. *Nucleic Acids Res* 1986;14:2511–2522.
29. Jeffery J, Barros SJ, Murray L, et al. Glucose-6-phosphate dehydrogenase. Characteristics revealed by the rat liver enzyme structure. *Eur J Biochem* 1989;186:551–556.
30. Camardella L, Damonte G, Carratore V, et al. Glucose-6-phosphate-dehydrogenase from human erythrocytes: identification of N-acetyl-alanine at the N-terminus of the mature protein. *Biochem Biophys Res Commun* 1995;207:331–338.
31. Notaro R, Afolayan A, Luzzatto L. Human mutations in glucose 6-phosphate dehydrogenase reflect evolutionary history. *FASEB J* 2000;14:485–494.
32. Naylor CE, Rowland P, Basak AK, et al. Glucose-6-phosphate-dehydrogenase mutations causing enzyme deficiency in a model of the tertiary structure of the human enzyme. *Blood* 1996;87:2974–2982.
33. Rowland P, Basak AK, Gover S, et al. The three-dimensional structure of glucose 6-phosphate dehydrogenase from Leuconostoc mesenteroides refined at 2.0 A resolution. *Structure* 1994;2:1073–1087.
34. Au SW, Gover S, Lam VM, et al. Human glucose-6-phosphate dehydrogenase: the crystal structure reveals a structural NADP(+) molecule and provides insights into enzyme deficiency. *Structure* 2000;8:293–303.
35. Au SW, Naylor CE, Gover S, et al. Solution of the structure of tetrameric human glucose 6-phosphate dehydrogenase by molecular replacement. *Acta Crystallogr D Biol Crystallogr* 1999;D55:826–834.
36. Camardella L, Caruso C, Rutigliano B, et al. Human erythrocyte glucose-6-phosphate dehydrogenase. Identification of a reactive lysyl residue labelled with pyridoxal 5'-phosphate. *Eur J Biochem* 1988;171:485–489.
37. Bautista JM, Mason PJ, Luzzatto L. Human glucose-6-phosphate dehydrogenase: lysine 205 is dispensable for substrate binding but essential for catalysis. *FEBS Lett* 1995;366:61–64.
38. Cohen P, Rosemeyer MA. Subunit interactions of glucose-6-phosphate dehydrogenase from human erythrocytes. *Eur J Biochem* 1969;8:8–15.
39. Bonsignore A, Cancedda R, Nicolini A, et al. Metabolism of human erythrocyte glucose-6-phosphate dehydrogenase. VI. Interconversion of multiple molecular forms. *Arch Biochem Biophys* 1971;147:493–501.
40. Luzzatto L, Allan NC. Different properties of glucose 6-phosphate dehydrogenase from human erythrocytes with normal and abnormal enzyme levels. *Biochem Biophys Res Commun* 1965;21:547–554.
41. De Flora A, Morelli A, Benatti U, et al. Human erythrocyte glucose 6-phosphate dehydrogenase. Interaction with oxidized and reduced coenzyme. *Biochem Biophys Res Commun* 1974;60:999–1005.
42. Hirono A, Kuhl W, Gelbart T, et al. Identification of the binding domain for NADP of human glucose-6-phosphate dehydrogenase by sequence analysis of mutants. *Proc Natl Acad Sci U S A* 1989;86:10015–10017.
43. Scopes DA, Bautista JM, Naylor CE, et al. Amino acid substitutions at the dimer interface of human glucose-6-phosphate dehydrogenase that increase thermostability and reduce the stabilising effect of NADP. *Eur J Biochem* 1998;251:382–388.
44. Kahler SG, Kirkman HN. Intracellular glucose-6-phosphate dehydrogenase does not monomerize in human erythrocytes. *J Biol Chem* 1983;258:717–718.
45. Cancedda R, Ogunmola G, Luzzatto L. Genetic variants of human erythrocyte glucose-6-phosphate dehydrogenase. Discrete conformational states stabilized by NADP+ and NADPH. *Eur J Biochem* 1973;34:199–204.
46. Pai GS, Sprenkle JA, Do TT, et al. Localization of loci for hypoxanthine phosphoribosyltransferase and glucose-6-phosphate dehydrogenase and biochemical evidence of nonrandom X chromosome expression from studies of a human X-autosome translocation. *Proc Natl Acad Sci U S A* 1980;77:2810–2813.
47. Szabo P, Purrello M, Rocchi M, et al. Cytological mapping of the human glucose-6-phosphate dehydrogenase gene distal to the fragile-X site suggests a high rate of meiotic recombination across this site. *Proc Natl Acad Sci U S A* 1984;81:7855–7859.
48. Boyer SH, Graham JB. Linkage between the X-chromosome loci for glucose-6-phosphate dehydrogenase electrophoretic variation and hemophilia A. *Am J Hum Genet* 1965;17:320–326.
49. Adam A. Linkage between deficiency of glucose-6-phosphate dehydrogenase and colour-blindness. *Nature* 1961;189:686.
50. Patterson M, Schwartz C, Bell M, et al. Physical mapping studies on the human X chromosome in the region Xq27-Xqter. *Genomics* 1987;1:297–306.
51. Chen EY, Zollo M, Mazzarella R, et al. Long-range sequence analysis in Xq28: thirteen known and six candidate genes in 219.4 kb of high GC DNA between the RCP/GCP and G6PD loci. *Hum Mol Genet* 1996;5:659–668.
52. Jin DY, Jeang KT. Isolation of full-length cDNA and chromosomal localization of human NF-kappaB modulator NEMO to Xq28. *J Biomed Sci* 1999;6:115–120.
53. Martini G, Toniolo D, Vulliamy T, et al. Structural analysis of the X-linked gene encoding human glucose-6-phosphate dehydrogenase. *EMBO J* 1986;5:1849–1855.
54. Hodge DL, Charron T, Stabile LP, et al. Structural characterization and tissue-specific expression of the mouse glucose-6-phosphate dehydrogenase gene. *DNA Cell Biol* 1998;17:283–291.
55. Bird AP. CpG-rich islands and the function of DNA methylation. *Nature* 1986;321:209–213.
56. Ursini MV, Scalera L, Martini G. High-levels of transcription driven by a 400-bp segment of the human G6PD promoter. *Biochem Biophys Res Commun* 1990;170:1203–1209.
57. Philippe M, Larondelle Y, Lemaigre F, et al. Promoter function of the human glucose-6-phosphate dehydrogenase gene depends on two GC boxes that are cell specifically controlled. *Eur J Biochem* 1994;226:377–384.
58. Franze A, Ferrante MI, Fusco F, et al. Molecular anatomy of the human glucose 6-phosphate dehydrogenase core promoter. *FEBS Lett* 1998;437:313–318.

59. Corcoran CM, Fraser P, Martini G, et al. High-level regulated expression of the human G6PD gene in transgenic mice. *Gene* 1996;173:241–246.

60. Hendriksen PJ, Hoogerbrugge JW, Baarends WM, et al. Testis-specific expression of a functional retroposon encoding glucose-6-phosphate dehydrogenase in the mouse. *Genomics* 1997;41:350–359.

61. McCarrey JR, Thomas K. Human testis-specific PGK gene lacks introns and possesses characteristics of a processed gene. *Nature* 1987;326:501–505.

62. Yoshida A, Lebo RV. Existence of glucose-6-phosphate dehydrogenase-like locus on chromosome 17. *Am J Hum Genet* 1986;39:203–206.

63. Beutler E. The genetics of glucose-6-phosphate-dehydrogenase deficiency. *Semin Hematol* 1990;27:137–164.

64. Luzzatto L, Mehta A. Glucose-6-phosphate dehydrogenase deficiency. In: Scriver CR, Beaudet AL, Sly WS, et al., eds. *The metabolic basis of inherited disease.* New York: McGraw Hill, 1995:3367–3398.

65. Beutler E, Kuhl W, Vivescorrons JL, et al. Molecular heterogeneity of glucose-6-phosphate A-. *Blood* 1989;74:2550–2555.

66. Corcoran CM, Calabro V, Tamagnini G, et al. Molecular heterogeneity underlying the G6PD Mediterranean phenotype. *Hum Genet* 1992;88:688–690.

67. Cappellini MD, Dimontemuros FM, Debellis G, et al. Multiple G6PD mutations are associated with a clinical and biochemical phenotype similar to that of G6PD Mediterranean. *Blood* 1996;87:3953–3958.

68. Mason PJ, Sonati MF, MacDonald D, et al. New glucose-6-phosphate dehydrogenase mutations associated with chronic anaemia. *Blood* 1995;85:1377–1380.

69. Hirono A, Fujii H, Takano T, et al. Molecular analysis of eight biochemically unique glucose-6-phosphate dehydrogenase variants found in Japan. *Blood* 1997;89:4624–4627.

70. Vulliamy TJ, Kaeda JS, Ait CD, et al. Clinical and haematological consequences of recurrent G6PD mutations and a single new mutation causing chronic nonspherocytic haemolytic anaemia. *Br J Haematol* 1998;101:670–675.

71. Standardization of procedures for the study of glucose-6-phosphate dehydrogenase. Report of a WHO Scientific Group. *World Health Organ Tech Rep Ser* 1967;366:1–53.

72. Vulliamy T, Luzzatto L, Hirono A, et al. Hematologically important mutations: glucose-6-phosphate dehydrogenase. *Blood Cells Mol Dis* 1997;23:302–313.

73. Xu WM, Westwood B, Bartsocas CS, et al. Glucose-6-phosphate dehydrogenase mutations and haplotypes in various ethnic-groups. *Blood* 1995;85:257–263.

74. Cheng YS, Tang TK, Hwang M. Amino acid conservation and clinical severity of human glucose-6-phosphate dehydrogenase mutations. *J Biomed Sci* 1999;6:106–114.

75. Kaeda JS, Chotray GP, Ranjit MR, et al. A new glucose-6-phosphate-dehydrogenase variant, G6PD Orissa (44 Ala→Gly), is the major polymorphic variant in tribal populations in India. *Am J Hum Genet* 1995;57:1335–1341.

76. Macdonald D, Town M, Mason P, et al. Deficiency in red blood cells. *Nature* 1991;350:115.

77. Town M, Bautista JM, Mason PJ, et al. Both mutations in G6PD A- are necessary to produce the G6PD deficient phenotype. *Hum Mol Genet* 1992;1:171–174.

78. Gomez GF, Garrido PA, Mason PJ, et al. Unproductive folding of the human G6PD-deficient variant A-. *FASEB J* 1996;10:153–158.

79. Gomez GF, Garrido PA, Bautista JM. Structural defects underlying protein dysfunction in human glucose-6-phosphate dehydrogenase A(-) deficiency. *J Biol Chem* 2000;275:9256–9262.

80. Vulliamy T, Rovira A, Yusoff N, et al. Independent origin of single and double mutations in the human glucose-6-phosphate-dehydrogenase gene. *Hum Mutat* 1996;8:311–318.

81. Ganczakowski M, Town M, Bowden DK, et al. Multiple glucose 6-phosphate dehydrogenase-deficient variants correlate with malaria endemicity in the Vanuatu archipelago (southwestern Pacific). *Am J Hum Genet* 1995;56:294–301.

82. Hirono A, Ishii A, Kere N, et al. Molecular analysis of glucose-6-phosphate-dehydrogenase variants in the Solomon-Islands. *Am J Hum Genet* 1995;56:1243–1245.

83. Rovira A, Vulliamy TJ, Pujades A, et al. The glucose-6-phosphate dehydrogenase (G6PD) deficient variant G6PD Union (454 Arg→Cys) has a world-wide distribution possibly due to recurrent mutation. *Hum Mol Genet* 1994;3:833–835.

84. Chiu D, Zuo L, Chao L, et al. Molecular characterization of glucose-6-phosphate-dehydrogenase (G6PD) deficiency in patients of Chinese descent and identification of new base substitutions in the human G6PD gene. *Blood* 1993;81:2150–2154.

85. Lo YS, Lu CC, Chiou SS, et al. Molecular characterization of glucose-6-phosphate-dehydrogenase deficiency in Chinese infants with or without severe neonatal hyperbilirubinemia. *Br J Haematol* 1994;86:858–862.

86. Huang CS, Hung KL, Huang MJ, et al. Neonatal jaundice and molecular mutations in glucose-6-phosphate dehydrogenase deficient newborn infants. *Am J Hematol* 1996;51:19–25.

87. Goncalves P, Ribeiro L, Tamagnini G, et al. Favism in glucose-6-phosphate dehydrogenase deficiency, G6PD A-: a common occurrence among Portuguese children. *Br J Haematol* 1994;87[Suppl 1]:146.

88. Oppenheim A, Jury CL, Rund D, et al. G6PD Mediterranean accounts for the high prevalence of G6PD deficiency in Kurdish Jews. *Hum Genet* 1993;91:293–294.

89. Beutler E, Kuhl W. The nt-1311 polymorphism of G6PD- G6PD Mediterranean mutation may have originated independently in Europe and Asia. *Am J Hum Genet* 1990;47:1008–1012.

90. Filosa S, Calabro V, Lania G, et al. G6PD haplotypes spanning Xq28 from F8C to red-green color-vision. *Genomics* 1993;17:6–14.

91. Ruwende C, Khoo SC, Snow RW, et al. Natural selection of hemi- and heterozygotes for G6PD deficiency in Africa by resistance to severe malaria. *Nature* 1995;376:246–249.

92. Vulliamy TJ, Othman A, Town M, et al. Polymorphic sites in the African population detected by sequence analysis of the glucose-6-phosphate-dehydrogenase gene outline the evolution of the variant A and variant A-. *Proc Natl Acad Sci U S A* 1991;88:8568–8571.

93. Allison AC. Glucose-6-phosphate dehydrogenase deficiency in red blood cells of East Africans. *Nature* 1960;186:531–532.

94. Motulsky AG. Metabolic polymorphisms and the role of infectious diseases in human evolution. 1960. *Hum Biol* 1989;61:835–869.

95. Greene LS. G6PD deficiency as protection against falciparum-malaria—an epidemiologic critique of population and experimental studies. *Yearbook Phys Anthropol* 1993;36:153–178.

96. Ruwende C, Hill A. Glucose-6-phosphate dehydrogenase deficiency and malaria. *J Mol Med* 1998;76:581–588.

97. Brabin L, Brabin BJ. Malaria and glucose 6-phosphate dehydrogenase deficiency in populations with high and low spleen rates in Madang, Papua New Guinea. *Hum Hered* 1990;40:15–21.

98. Siniscalco M, Bernini L, Filippi G, et al. Population genetics of haemoglobin variants, thalassaemia and glucose-6-phosphate dehydrogenase deficiency, with particular reference to the malaria hypothesis. *Bull World Health Organ* 1966;34(3):379–393.

99. Stamatoyannopoulos G, Panayotopoulos A, Motulsky AG. The distribution of glucose-6-phosphate dehydrogenase deficiency in Greece. *Am J Hum Genet* 1966;18:296–308.

100. Verle P, Nhan DH, Tinh TT, et al. Glucose-6-phosphate dehydrogenase deficiency in northern Vietnam. *Trop Med Int Health* 2000;5:203–206.

101. Piazza A, Mayr WR, Contu L, et al. Genetic and population structure of four Sardinian villages. *Ann Hum Genet* 1985;49:47–51.

102. Allison AC, Clyde DF. Malaria in African children with deficient erythrocyte glucose-6-phosphate dehydrogenase. *BMJ* 1961;1.

103. Kruatrachue M, Charoenlarp P, Chongsuphajaisiddhi T, et al. Erythrocyte glucose-6-phosphate dehydrogenase and malaria in Thailand. *Lancet* 1962;ii:1183–1186.

104. Martin SK, Miller LH, Alling D, et al. Severe malaria and glucose-6-phosphate-dehydrogenase deficiency: a reappraisal of the malaria/G-6-P.D. hypothesis. *Lancet* 1979;1:524–526.

105. Gilles HM, Fletcher KA, Hendricksen RG, et al. Glucose 6-phosphate dehydrogenase deficiency, sickling and malaria in African children in South Western Nigeria. *Lancet* 1967;1:138–140.

106. Luzzatto L, Bienzle U. The malaria/G.-6-P.D. hypothesis. *Lancet* 1979;1(8127):1183–1184.

107. Bienzle U, Ayeni O, Lucas AO, et al. Glucose-6-phosphate dehydrogenase and malaria: greater resistance of females heterozygous for enzyme deficiency and of males with non-deficient variant. *Lancet* 1972;1:107–110.

108. Sodeinde O. Glucose-6-phosphate dehydrogenase. In: Fleming AF, ed. *Epidemiology of haematological disease.* London: Balliere Tindall, 1992:367–378.

109. Allen SJ, O'Donnell A, Alexander ND, et al. Alpha+-Thalassemia protects children against disease caused by other infections as well as malaria. *Proc Natl Acad Sci U S A* 1997;94:14736–14741.

110. Luzzatto L, Usanga EA, Reddy S. Glucose 6-phosphate dehydrogenase deficient red cells resistance to infection by malarial parasites. *Science* 1969;164:839–842.

111. Trager W, Jensen JB. Human malaria parasites in continuous culture. *Science* 1976;193:673–675.

112. Luzzatto L, Sodeinde O, Martini G. Genetic variation in the host and adaptive phenomena in *Plasmodium falciparum* infection. In: Evered D, Whelan J, eds. *Malaria and the red cell.* London: Pitman, 1983:159–173.

113. Roth J, Raventos-Suarez C, Rinaldi A, et al. Glucose-6-phosphate dehydrogenase deficiency inhibits in vitro growth of Plasmodium falciparum. *Proc Natl Acad Sci U S A* 1983;80:298–304.

114. Friedman MJ. Oxidant damage mediates variant red cell resistance to malaria. *Nature* 1979;280:245–247.

115. Marva E, Cohen A, Saltman P, et al. Deleterious synergistic effects of ascorbate and copper on the development of Plasmodium falciparum: an in vitro study in normal and in G6PD-deficient erythrocytes. *Int J Parasitol* 1989;19(7):779–785.

116. Usanga EA, Luzzatto L. Adaptation of Plasmodium falciparum to glucose 6-phosphate dehydrogenase-deficient host red cells by production of parasite-encoded enzyme. *Nature* 1985;313(6005):793–795.

117. O'Brien E, Kurdi-Haidar B, Wanachiwanawin W, et al. Cloning of the glucose-6-phosphate dehydrogenase gene from Plasmodium falciparum. *Mol Biochem Parasitol* 1994;64(2):313–326.

118. Shahabuddin M, Rawlings DJ, Kaslow DC. A novel glucose-6-phosphate dehydrogenase in Plasmodium falciparum: cDNA and primary protein structure. *Biochim Biophys Acta* 1994;1219(1):191–194.

119. Cappadoro M, Giribaldi G, O'Brien E, et al. Early phagocytosis of glucose-6-phosphate dehydrogenase (G6PD)-deficient erythrocytes parasitized by Plasmodium falciparum may explain malaria protection in G6PD deficiency. *Blood* 1998;92(7):2527–2534.

120. Collard F, Collet J, Gerin I, et al. Identification of the cDNA encoding human 6-phosphogluconolactonase, the enzyme catalyzing the second step of the pentose phosphate pathway. *FEBS Lett* 1999;459:223–226.

121. Atamna H, Pascarmona G, Ginsburg H. Hexose-monophosphate shunt activity in intact Plasmodium falciparum-infected erythrocytes and in free parasites. *Mol Biochem Parasitol* 1994;67(1):79–89.

122. Hoiberg A, Ernst J, Uddin DE. Sickle cell trait and glucose-6-phosphate dehydrogenase deficiency. Effects on health and military performance in black Navy enlistees. *Arch Intern Med* 1981;141(11):1485–1488.
123. Lim MK, Tan EH, Wan A, et al. Prevalence of G6PD deficiency among recruits in the Singapore Armed Forces. *Ann Acad Med Singapore* 1995;24:322–324.
124. Cocco P, Todde P, Fornera S, et al. Mortality in a cohort of men expressing the glucose-6-phosphate dehydrogenase deficiency. *Blood* 1998;91:706–709.
125. Cocco P, Carta P, Flore C, et al. Mortality of lead smelter workers with the glucose-6-phosphate dehydrogenase-deficient phenotype. *Cancer Epidemiol Biomarkers Prev* 1996;5:223–225.
126. Slusher TM, Vreman HJ, Mclaren DW, et al. Glucose-6-phosphate-dehydrogenase deficiency and carboxyhemoglobin concentrations associated with bilirubin-related morbidity and death in Nigerian infants. *J Pediatr* 1995;126:102–108.
127. Sarkar S, Prakash D, Marwaha RK, et al. Acute intravascular hemolysis in glucose-6-phosphate-dehydrogenase deficiency. *Ann Trop Paediatr* 1993;13:391–394.
128. Meloni T, Forteleoni G, Meloni GF. Marked decline of favism after neonatal glucose-6-phosphate-dehydrogenase screening and health education—the Northern Sardinian experience. *Acta Haematol* 1992;87:29–31.
129. Tay JS. Medical genetics in Singapore. *Southeast Asian J Trop Med Public Health* 1995;1:19–25.
130. Tugwell P. Glucose-6-phosphate-dehydrogenase deficiency in Nigerians with jaundice associated with lobar pneumonia. *Lancet* 1973;1:968–969.
131. Chan TK, Chesterman CN, McFadzean AJ, et al. The survival of glucose-6-phosphate dehydrogenase-deficient erythrocytes in patients with typhoid fever on chloramphenicol therapy. *J Lab Clin Med* 1971;77:177–184.
132. Baehner RL, Nathan DG, Castle WB. Oxidant injury of Caucasian glucose-6-phosphate dehydrogenase-deficient red blood cells by phagocytosing leukocytes during infection. *J Clin Invest* 1971;50:2466–2473.
133. Kattamis CA, Tjortjatou F. The hemolytic process of viral hepatitis in children with normal or deficient glucose-6-phosphate dehydrogenase activity. *J Pediatr* 1970;77:422–430.
134. Huo TI, Wu JC, Chiu CF, et al. Severe hyperbilirubinemia due to acute hepatitis-A superimposed on a chronic hepatitis-B carrier with glucose-6-phosphate-dehydrogenase deficiency. *Am J Gastroenterol* 1996;91:158–159.
135. Galiano S, Gaetani GF, Barabino A, et al. Favism in the African type of glucose-6-phosphate dehydrogenase deficiency (A-). *BMJ* 1990;300:236–237.
136. Meloni T, Forteleoni G, Ogana A, et al. Aspirin-induced acute haemolytic anaemia in glucose-6-phosphate-dehydrogenase-deficient children with systemic arthritis. *Acta Haematol* 1989;81:208–209.
137. Magon AM, Leipzig RM, Zannoni VG, et al. Interactions of glucose-6-phosphate dehydrogenase deficiency with drug acetylation and hydroxylation reactions. *J Lab Clin Med* 1981;97:764–770.
138. Frischer H, Carson PE. Multiple gene interactions in pharmacogenetics. *J Lab Clin Med* 1981;97:760–763.
139. Fischer GM, Meloni T, Pescarmona GP, et al. Membrane cross bonding in red cells in favic crisis: a missing link in the mechanism of extravascular haemolysis. *Br J Haematol* 1985;59:159–169.
140. Chevion M, Navok T, Glaser G, et al. The chemistry of favism-inducing compounds. The properties of isouramil and divicine and their reaction with glutathione. *Eur J Biochem* 1982;127:405–409.
141. Winterbourn CC, Cowden WB, Sutton HC. Auto-oxidation of dialuric acid, divicine and isouramil. Superoxide dependent and independent mechanisms. *Biochem Pharmacol* 1989;38:611–618.
142. Arese P, De Flora A. Pathophysiology of hemolysis in glucose-6-phosphate dehydrogenase deficiency. *Semin Hematol* 1990;27(1):1–40.
143. Vives Corrons J, Pujades A. Heterogeneity of "Mediterranean type" glucose-6-phosphate dehydrogenase (G6PD) deficiency in Spain and description of two new variants associated with favism. *Hum Genet* 1982;60:216–221.
144. Nafa K, Reghis A, Osmani N, et al. At least five polymorphic mutants account for the prevalence of glucose-6-phosphate dehydrogenase deficiency in Algeria. *Hum Genet* 1994;94:513–517.
145. Gibbs WN, Gray R, Lowry M. Glucose-6-phosphate dehydrogenase deficiency and neonatal jaundice in Jamaica. *Br J Haematol* 1979;43:263–274.
146. Bienzle U, Effiong C, Luzzatto L. Erythrocyte glucose 6-phosphate dehydrogenase deficiency (G6PD type A-) and neonatal jaundice. *Acta Paediatr Scand* 1976;65:701–703.
147. Meloni T, Cutillo S, Testa U, et al. Neonatal jaundice and severity of glucose-6-phosphate dehydrogenase deficiency in Sardinian babies. *Early Hum Dev* 1987;15:317–322.
148. Rehman H, Khan MA, Hameed A, et al. Erythrocyte glucose 6 phosphate dehydrogenase deficiency and neonatal jaundice. *J Pak Med Assoc* 1995;45:259–260.
149. Tanphaichitr VS, Pung AP, Yodthong S, et al. Glucose-6-phosphate dehydrogenase deficiency in the newborn: its prevalence and relation to neonatal jaundice. *Southeast Asian J Trop Med Public Health* 1995;1:137–141.
150. Kaplan M, Renbaum P, Levy LE, et al. Gilbert syndrome and glucose-6-phosphate dehydrogenase deficiency: a dose-dependent genetic interaction crucial to neonatal hyperbilirubinemia. *Proc Natl Acad Sci U S A* 1997;94:12128–12132.
151. Cappellini MD, Martinez DMF, Sampietro M, et al. The interaction between Gilbert's syndrome and G6PD deficiency influences bilirubin levels. *Br J Haematol* 1999;104:928–929.
152. Iolascon A, Faienza MF, Giordani L, et al. Bilirubin levels in the acute hemolytic crisis of G6PD deficiency are related to Gilbert's syndrome. *Eur J Haematol* 1999;62:307–310.
153. Galanello R, Cipollina MD, Carboni G, et al. Hyperbilirubinemia, glucose-6-phosphate-dehydrogenase deficiency and Gilbert's syndrome. *Eur J Pediatr* 1999;158:914–916.
154. Valaes T, Drummond GS, Kappas A. Control of hyperbilirubinemia in glucose-6-phosphate dehydrogenase-deficient newborns using an inhibitor of bilirubin production, Sn-mesoporphyrin. *Pediatrics* 1998;101:E1.
155. Johnson GJ, Allen DW, Cadman S, et al. Red-cell-membrane polypeptide aggregates in glucose-6-phosphate dehydrogenase mutants with chronic hemolytic disease. A clue to the mechanism of hemolysis. *N Engl J Med* 1979;301:522–527.
156. Johnson RM, Ravindranath Y, Elalfy M, et al. Oxidant damage to erythrocyte-membrane in glucose-6-phosphate-dehydrogenase deficiency—correlation with in-vivo reduced glutathione concentration and membrane-protein oxidation. *Blood* 1994;83:1117–1123.
157. Fiorelli G, Martinez di Montemuros F, Cappellini MD. Chronic non-spherocytic haemolytic disorders associated with glucose-6-phosphate dehydrogenase variants. In: Zanella A, ed. *Inherited disorders of red cell metabolism.* London: Bailliere Tindall, 2000:39–58.
158. Hirono A, Miwa S, Fujii H, et al. Molecular study of eight Japanese cases of glucose-6-phosphate dehydrogenase deficiency by nonradioisotopic single-strand conformation polymorphism analysis. *Blood* 1994;83:3363–3368.
159. Lewis RA, Kay RW, Hathorn M. Sickle cell disease and glucose-6-phosphate dehydrogenase. *Acta Haematol* 1966;36:399–411.
160. Mohammad AM, Ardatl KO, Bajakian KM. Sickle cell disease in Bahrain: coexistence and interaction with glucose-6-phosphate dehydrogenase (G6PD) deficiency. *J Trop Pediatr* 1998;44:70–72.
161. Luzzatto L, Allan NC. Relationship between the genes for glucose-6-phosphate dehydrogenase and for haemoglobin in a Nigerian population. *Nature* 1968;219:1041–1042.
162. Guggenmoos-Holzmann I, Bienzle U, Luzzatto L. Plasmodium falciparum malaria and human red cells. II. Red cell genetic traits and resistance against malaria. *Int J Epidemiol* 1981;10:16–22.
163. Bienzle U, Sodeinde O, Effiong CE, et al. Glucose 6-phosphate dehydrogenase deficiency and sickle cell anemia: frequency and features of the association in an African population. *Blood* 1975;46:591–597.
164. Gibbs WN, Wardle J, Serjeant GR. Glucose-6-phosphate dehydrogenase deficiency and homozygous sickle cell disease in Jamaica. *Br J Haematol* 1980;45:73–80.
165. Bouanga JC, Mouele R, Prehu C, et al. Glucose-6-phosphate dehydrogenase deficiency and homozygous sickle cell disease in Congo. *Hum Hered* 1998;48:192–197.
166. Steinberg MH, West MS, Gallagher D, et al. Effects of glucose-6-phosphate dehydrogenase deficiency upon sickle cell anemia. *Blood* 1988;71:748–752.
167. Smits HL, Oski FA, Brody JI. The hemolytic crisis of sickle cell disease: the role of glucose-6-phosphate dehydrogenase deficiency. *J Pediatr* 1969;74:544–551.
168. Mareni C, Repetto L, Forteleoni G, et al. Favism: looking for an autosomal gene associated with glucose-6-phosphate dehydrogenase deficiency. *J Med Genet* 1984;21:278–280.
169. Low PS. Structure and function of the cytoplasmic domain of band 3: center of erythrocyte membrane-peripheral protein interactions. *Biochim Biophys Acta* 1986;864:145–167.
170. Horn S, Bashan N, Peleg N, et al. Membrane glycoprotein modifications of G6PD deficient red blood cells. *Euro J Clin Invest* 1995;25:32–38.
171. Kasper ML, Miller WJ, Jacob HS. G6PD-deficiency infectious haemolysis: a complement dependent innocent bystander phenomenon. *Br J Haematol* 1986;63:85–91.
172. Vives CJ, Feliu E, Pujades MA, et al. Severe-glucose-6-phosphate dehydrogenase (G6PD) deficiency associated with chronic hemolytic anemia, granulocyte dysfunction, and increased susceptibility to infections: description of a new molecular variant (G6PD Barcelona). *Blood* 1982;59:428–434.
173. Harley JD, Agar NS, Yoshida A. Glucose 6-phosphate dehydrogenase variants: Gd (+) Alexandra associated with neonatal jaundice and Gd (-) Camperdown in a young man with lamellar cataracts. *J Lab Clin Med* 1978;91:295–300.
174. Yuregir G, Varinli I, Donma O. Glucose 6-phosphate dehydrogenase deficiency both in red blood cells and lenses of the normal and cataractous native population of Cukurova, the southern part of Turkey. Part II. *Ophthalmic Res* 1989;21:158–161.
175. Orzalesi N, Fossarello M, Sorcinelli R, et al. The relationship between glucose-6-phosphate dehydrogenase deficiency and cataracts in Sardinia. An epidemiological and biochemical study. *Doc Ophthalmol* 1984;57:187–201.
176. Motulsky AG, Campbell-Kraut JM. Population genetics of glucose-6-phosphate dehydrogenase deficiency of the red cell. In: Blumberg BS, ed. *Proceedings of the conference on genetic polymorphisms and geographic variations in disease.* New York: Grune & Stratton, 1961:159–170.
177. Gall JC, Brewer GJ, Dern RJ. Studies of glucose-6-phosphate dehydrogenase activity of individual erythrocytes: the methemoglobin elution test for the detection of females heterozygous for G6PD deficiency. *Am J Hum Genet* 1965;17:359–365.
178. Beutler E, Mitchell M. Special modifications of the fluorescent screening method for glucose-6-phosphate dehydrogenase deficiency. *Blood* 1968;32:816–818.
179. Pujades A, Lewis M, Salvati AM, et al. Evaluation of the blue formazan spot test for screening glucose 6 phosphate dehydrogenase deficiency. *Int J Hematol* 1999;69:234–236.
180. Filosa S, Giacometti N, Cai WW, et al. Somatic-cell selection is a major determinant of the blood-cell phenotype in heterozygotes for glucose-6-phos-

phate-dehydrogenase mutations causing severe enzyme deficiency. *Am J Hum Genet* 1996;59:887–895.

181. Luzzatto L, Meloni T. Hemolytic anemia due to glucose 6-phosphate dehydrogenase deficiency. In: Brain MC, Carbone PP, eds. *Current therapy in hematology-oncology: 1985–1986*. Philadelphia: BC Decker; St. Louis: Mosby, 1985;21–42.

182. Ekert H, Rawlinson I. Deferoxamine and favism. *N Engl J Med* 1985;312:1260–1261.

183. Al Rimawi HS, Al Sheyyab M, Batieha A, et al. Effect of desferrioxamine in acute haemolytic anaemia of glucose-6-phosphate dehydrogenase deficiency. *Acta Haematol* 1999;101:145–148.

184. Meloni T, Forteleoni G, Gaetani GF. Desferrioxamine and favism. *Br J Haematol* 1986;63:394–395.

185. Lyon MF. Gene action in the X chromosome in the mouse (*Mus musculus*). *Nature* 1961:372–373.

186. Beutler E, Yeh M, Fairbanks VF. The normal human female as a mosaic of X-chromosome activity: studies using the gene for G6PD deficiency as a marker. *Proc Natl Acad Sci U S A* 1962;48:9–14.

187. Davidson RG, Nitowsky HM, Childs B. Demonstration of two populations of cells in the human female heterozygous for glucose-6-phosphate dehydrogenase variants. *Proc Natl Acad Sci U S A* 1963;50:481–485.

188. Linder D, Gartler SM. Glucose-6-phosphate dehydrogenase mosaicism: utilization as a cell marker in the study of leiomyomas. *Science* 1965;150:67–69.

189. Fialkow PJ. Clonal origin of human tumors. *Biochim Biophys Acta* 1976;458:283–321.

190. Oni SB, Osunkoya BO, Luzzatto L. Paroxysmal nocturnal hemoglobinuria: evidence for monoclonal origin of abnormal red cells. *Blood* 1970;36:145–152.

191. Fraser NJ, Boyd Y, Brownlee GG, et al. Multi-allelic RFLP for M27 beta, an anonymous single copy genomic clone at Xp11.3-Xcen [HGM9 provisional no. DXS255]. *Nucleic Acids Res* 1987;15:9616.

192. Allen RC, Zoghbi HY, Moseley AB, et al. Methylation of HpaII and HhaI sites near the polymorphic CAG repeat in the human androgen-receptor gene correlates with X chromosome inactivation. *Am J Hum Genet* 1992;51:1229–1239.

193. Steinberg MH, Necheles TF. Erythrocyte glutathione peroxidase deficiency. Biochemical studies on the mechanisms of drug-induced hemolysis. *Am J Med* 1971;50:542–546.

194. Gondo H, Ideguchi H, Hayashi S, et al. Acute hemolysis in glutathione peroxidase deficiency. *Int J Hematol* 1992;55:215–218.

195. Loos H, Roos D, Weening R, et al. Familial deficiency of glutathione reductase in human blood cells. *Blood* 1976;48:53–62.

196. Beutler E, Gelbart T, Kondo T, et al. The molecular basis of a case of gamma-glutamylcysteine synthetase deficiency. *Blood* 1999;94:2890–2894.

197. Ristoff E, Augustson C, Geissler J, et al. A missense mutation in the heavy subunit of gamma-glutamylcysteine synthetase gene causes hemolytic anemia. *Blood* 2000;95:2193–2196.

198. Spielberg SP, Garrick MD, Corash LM, et al. Biochemical heterogeneity in glutathione synthetase deficiency. *J Clin Invest* 1978;61:1417–1420.

199. Shi ZZ, Habib GM, Rhead WJ, et al. Mutations in the glutathione synthetase gene cause 5-oxoprolinuria. *Nat Genet* 1996;14:361–365.

200. Dahl N, Pigg M, Ristoff E, et al. Missense mutations in the human glutathione synthetase gene result in severe metabolic acidosis, 5-oxoprolinuria, hemolytic anemia and neurological dysfunction. *Hum Mol Genet* 1997;6:1147–1152.

201. Polekhina G, Board PG, Gali RR, et al. Molecular basis of glutathione synthetase deficiency and a rare gene permutation event. *EMBO J* 1999;18:3204–3213.

202. Galanello R, Loi D, Sollaino C, et al. A new glucose 6 phosphate dehydrogenase variant G6PD Sinnai (34 G→T). *Hum Mutat* 1998;12:72–73.

203. Weimer TA, Salzano FM, Westwood B, et al. G6PD variants in three South American ethnic groups: population distribution and description of two new mutations. *Hum Hered* 1998;48:92–96.

204. Chao L, Du CS, Louie E, et al. A to G substitution identified in exon 2 of the G6PD gene among G6PD deficient Chinese. *Nucleic Acids Res* 1991;19:6056.

205. Nafa K, Reghis A, Osmani N, et al. G6PD Aures—a new mutation (48-Ile-Thr) causing mild G6PD deficiency is associated with favism. *Hum Mol Genet* 1993;2:81–82.

206. Vulliamy TJ, D'Urso M, Battistuzzi G, et al. Diverse point mutations in the human glucose 6-phosphate dehydrogenase gene cause enzyme deficiency and mild or severe hemolytic anaemia. *Proc Natl Acad Sci U S A* 1988;85:5171–5175.

207. Hirono A, Beutler E. Molecular cloning and nucleotide sequence of cDNA for human glucose-6-phosphate dehydrogenase variant A(-). *Proc Natl Acad Sci U S A* 1988;85:3951–3954.

208. Rovira A, Vulliamy T, Pujades MA, et al. Molecular genetics of glucose-6-phosphate dehydrogenase (G6PD) deficiency in Spain: identification of two new point mutations in the G6PD gene. *Br J Haematol* 1995;91:66–71.

209. Hirono A, Fujii H, Miwa S. Molecular abnormality of G6PD Konan and G6PD Ube, the most common glucose-6-phosphate dehydrogenase variants in Japan. *Hum Genet* 1993;91:507–508.

210. Ninfali P, Baronciani L, Ruzzo A, et al. Molecular analysis of G6PD variants in northern Italy—a study on the population from the Ferrara district. *Hum Genet* 1993;92:139–142.

211. Hirono A, Fujii H, Miwa S. Identification of 2 novel deletion mutations in glucose-6-phosphate-dehydrogenase gene causing hemolytic-anemia. *Blood* 1995;85:1118–1121.

212. Maeda M, Constantoulakis P, Chen CS, et al. Molecular abnormalities of a human glucose-6-phosphate-dehydrogenase variant associated with undetectable enzyme-activity and immunologically cross-reacting material. *Am J Hum Genet* 1992;51:386–395.

213. Kotea R, Kaeda JS, Yan SL, et al. Three major G6PD-deficient polymorphic variants identified among the Mauritian population. *Br J Haematol* 1999;104:849–854.

214. Takizawa T, Yoneyama Y, Miwa S, et al. A single nucleotide base transition is the basis of the common human glucose-6-phosphate dehydrogenase variant A (+). *Genomics* 1987;1:228–231.

215. Zarza R, Pujades A, Rovira A, et al. Two new mutations of the glucose-6-phosphate dehydrogenase (G6PD) gene associated with haemolytic anaemia: clinical, biochemical and molecular relationships. *Br J Haematol* 1997;98:578–582.

216. Menounos P, Zervas C, Garinis G, et al. Molecular heterogeneity of glucose-6-phosphate dehydrogenase deficiency in the Hellenic population. *Hum Hered* 2000;50:237–241.

217. Vulliamy TJ, Wanachiwanawin W, Mason PJ, et al. G6PD Mahidol, a common deficient variant in Southeast-Asia is caused by a (163) glycine-serine mutation. *Nucleic Acids Res* 1989;17:5868.

218. Tang TK, Yeh CH, Huang CH, et al. Expression and biochemical-characterization of human glucose-6-phosphate-dehydrogenase in *Escherichia coli*—a system to analyze normal and mutant enzymes. *Blood* 1994;83:1436–1441.

219. Roos D, van Zwieten R, Wijnen JT, et al. Molecular basis and enzymatic properties of glucose 6-phosphate dehydrogenase volendam, leading to chronic nonspherocytic anemia, granulocyte dysfunction, and increased susceptibility to infections. *Blood* 1999;94:2955–2962.

220. Chen HL, Huang MJ, Huang CS, et al. G6PD NanKang (517 T→C; 173 Phe→Leu): a new Chinese G6PD variant associated with neonatal jaundice. *Hum Hered* 1996;46:201–204.

221. Chen HL, Huang MJ, Huang CS, et al. Two novel glucose 6-phosphate dehydrogenase deficiency mutations and association of such mutations with F8C/G6PD haplotype in Chinese. *J Formos Med Assoc* 1997;96:948–954.

222. Beutler E, Kuhl W, Saenz GF, et al. Mutation analysis of glucose-6-phosphate-dehydrogenase (G6PD) variants in Costa-Rica. *Hum Genet* 1991;87:462–464.

223. Beutler E, Westwood B, Prchal J, et al. New glucose-6-phosphate dehydrogenase mutations from various ethnic groups. *Blood* 1992;80:255–256.

224. Calabro V, Mason PJ, Filosa S, et al. Genetic-heterogeneity of glucose-6-phosphate-dehydrogenase deficiency revealed by single-strand conformation and sequence-analysis. *Am J Hum Genet* 1993;52:527–536.

225. Beutler E, Kuhl W, Gelbart T, et al. DNA-sequence abnormalities of human glucose-6-phosphate-dehydrogenase variants. *J Biol Chem* 1991;266:4145–4150.

226. Poggi V, Town M, Foulkes NS, et al. Identification of a single base change in a new human mutant glucose-6-phosphate dehydrogenase gene by polymerase-chain-reaction amplification of the entire coding region from genomic DNA. *Biochem J* 1990;271:157–160.

227. Jablonska SE, Lewandowska I, Plochocka D, et al. Several mutations including two novel mutations of the glucose-6-phosphate dehydrogenase gene in Polish G6PD deficient subjects with chronic nonspherocytic hemolytic anemia, acute hemolytic anemia, and favism. *Hum Mutat* 1999;14:477–484.

228. Zimmerman SA, Ware RE, Forman L, et al. Glucose-6-phosphate dehydrogenase Durham: a de novo mutation associated with chronic hemolytic anemia. *J Pediatr* 1997;131:284–287.

229. Beutler E, Westwood B, Kuhl W. Definition of the mutations of G6PD Wayne, G6PD Viangchan, G6PD Jammu, and G6PD 'LeJeune.' *Acta Haematol* 1991;86:179–182.

230. Costa E, Cabeda JM, Vieira E, et al. Glucose-6-phosphate dehydrogenase aveiro: a de novo mutation associated with chronic nonspherocytic hemolytic anemia. *Blood* 2000;95:1499–1501.

231. Beutler E, Westwood B, Kuhl W, et al. Glucose-6-phosphate dehydrogenase variants in Hawaii. *Hum Hered* 1992;42:327–329.

232. De Vita G, Alcalay M, Sampietro M, et al. Two point mutations are responsible for G6PD-polymorphism in Sardinia. *Am J Hum Genet* 1989;44:233–240.

233. Viglietto G, Montanaro V, Calabro V, et al. Common glucose-6-phosphate-dehydrogenase (G6PD) variants from the Italian population—biochemical and molecular characterization. *Ann Hum Genet* 1990;54:1–15.

234. Ahluwalia A, Corcoran CM, Vulliamy TJ, et al. G6PD Kalyan and G6PD Kerala; two deficient variants in India caused by the same 317 Glu→Lys mutation. *Hum Mol Genet* 1992;1:209–210.

235. Hirono A, Fujii H, Shima M, et al. G6PD Nara—a new class-1 glucose-6-phosphate-dehydrogenase variant with an 8 amino-acid deletion. *Blood* 1993;82:3250–3252.

236. Beutler E, Westwood B, Melemed A, et al. Three new exon 10 glucose-6-phosphate dehydrogenase mutations. *Blood Cells Mol Dis* 1995;21:64–72.

237. Vlachos A, Westwood B, Lipton JM, et al. G6PD Mount Sinai: a new severe hemolytic variant characterized by dual mutations at nucleotides 376G and 1159T (N126D). *Hum Mutat* 1998(Suppl 1):S154–S155.

238. Filosa S, Cai WW, Galanello R, et al. A novel single-base mutation in the glucose-6-phosphate-dehydrogenase gene is associated with chronic nonspherocytic hemolytic-anemia. *Hum Genet* 1994;94:560–562.

239. Hirono A, Fujii H, Hirono K, et al. Molecular abnormality of a Japanese glucose-6-phosphate-dehydrogenase variant (G6PD Tokyo) associated with hereditary non-spherocytic hemolytic-anemia. *Hum Genet* 1992;88:347–348.

240. Saad ST, Salles TS, Arruda VR, et al. G6PD Sumare: a novel mutation in the G6PD gene (1292 T→G) associated with chronic nonspherocytic anemia. *Hum Mutat* 1997;10:245–247.

241. Hirono A, Nakayama S, Fujii H, et al. Molecular abnormality of a unique Japanese glucose-6-phosphate dehydrogenase variant (G6PD Kobe) with a greatly increased affinity for galactose-6-phosphate. *Am J Hematol* 1994;45:185–186.

242. Vivescorrons JL, Kuhl W, Pujades MA, et al. Molecular-genetics of the glucose-6-phosphate-dehydrogenase (G6PD) Mediterranean variant and description of a new G6PD mutant, G6PD Andalus 1361A. *Am J Hum Genet* 1990;47:575–579.

243. Stevens DJ, Wanachiwanawin W, Mason PJ, et al. G6PD Canton a common deficient variant in South East-Asia caused by a 459 Arg→Leu mutation. *Nucleic Acids Res* 1990;18:7190.

244. Chiu D, Zuo L, Chen E, et al. Two commonly occurring nucleotide base substitutions in Chinese G6PD variants. *Biochem Biophys Res Commun* 1991;180:988–993.

245. Alfinito F, Cimmino A, Ferraro F, et al. Molecular characterization of G6PD deficiency in Southern Italy: heterogeneity, correlation genotype-phenotype and description of a new variant (G6PD Neapolis). *Br J Haematol* 1997;98:41–46.

246. Baronciani L, Tricta F, Beutler E. G6PD Campinas—a deficient enzyme with a mutation at the far 3′ end of the gene. *Hum Mutat* 1993;2:77–78.

247. Gonigle DPM, Lalloz MRA, Wild BJ, et al. G6PD Brighton: a new class I variant due to a deletion in exon 13. *Br J Haematol* 1998;101[Suppl 1]:51.

248. Mason PJ, Vulliamy TJ. Genetic variation of human erythrocyte glucose-6-phosphate dehydrogenase. In: King M-J, ed. *Human blood cells: consequences of genetic polymorphisms and variations.* London: Imperial College press, 2000:251–275.

CHAPTER 55

Neonatal Anemia

Patrick G. Gallagher

NEONATAL ERYTHROCYTE

Evaluation of the anemic neonate requires a thorough understanding of developmental erythropoiesis (reviewed in Chapter 7 and Chapter 49) and the differences between neonatal and adult erythrocytes. These differences include variation in erythrocyte size, shape, membrane characteristics, globin composition, oxygen transport, cellular metabolism, and lifespan (1).

Size

Early in embryogenesis, the volume and size of erythrocytes are significantly greater than adult erythrocytes. Cell diameter ranges from 20 to 25 μ with mean corpuscular volume (MCV) ranging from 150 to 180 fL. Cell volume and size gradually decrease throughout gestation to values of 8–10 μ in diameter and MCV between 108 and 118 fL at term (Table 55-1). After birth (2), red cells continue to decrease in size, resembling adult cells by one year of age.

Shape and Deformability

There is great variability in the shape of fetal and neonatal erythrocytes. Irregularly shaped cells are found in greater numbers on the peripheral blood smears of hematologically normal newborns than those of adults (Fig. 55-1). Target cells, acanthocytes, and immature erythrocytes with various membrane projections are frequently found (3). These changes are attributed to poor or absent splenic function in neonates associated with "pits" or "pocks" in the red cell membrane. Almost one-half of erythrocytes from preterm infants and one-fourth of erythrocytes from term infants have surface pits (the site of formation of endocytic vacuoles) compared to 2.6% of normal adult cells (4).

Deformability of the erythrocyte is primarily determined by the surface to volume relationship of the cell, the cytoplasmic viscosity, and the intrinsic membrane rigidity. Erythrocyte deformability influences several critical processes: (a) It affects whole blood viscosity, which in turn affects peripheral vascular resistance and cardiac workload; (b) deformability directly influences flow in the peripheral circulation; (c) finally, deformability is an important determinant of red cell lifespan, with decreased deformability leading to increased sequestration and removal in the spleen. As neonatal erythrocytes age, they lose more volume, have a higher mean corpuscular hemoglobin (MCH) concentration (MCHC), and are less deformable than adult cells. Thus, an accelerated decrease in neonatal erythrocyte deformability leads to a more pronounced increase in MCHC and internal viscosity. At a given shear stress, neonatal erythrocytes are more deformable than adult cells, leading to increased fragmentation. Together (5,6), these properties lead to accelerated membrane loss and decreased erythrocyte lifespan.

Membrane Differences

In addition to increased deformability, fetal and neonatal erythrocyte membranes demonstrate other characteristics that differ from adult cells (Table 55-2). There is increased permeability to monovalent cations and less Na$^+$, K$^+$-adenosine triphosphate (ATP)-ase activity required for monovalent cation removal. They contain more phospholipid and cholesterol per cell (7) and as a result, have a larger surface to volume ratio, rendering them slightly more osmotically resistant (8). This observation has practical clinical importance because when using osmotic fragility testing in a neonate to diagnose hereditary spherocytosis, a neonatal osmotic fragility curve should be used rather than an adult curve.

The surface charge of neonatal erythrocytes is more negative than adult cells. This reflects a higher sialic acid content (9). The increased negative charge contributes to the decreased sedimentation rate observed in newborns (10). Neonatal erythrocytes contain increased amounts of total and membrane-associated myosin compared to adult cells (11). Membrane acetylcholinesterase is decreased (12). Neonatal erythrocytes undergo spontaneous and drug-induced endocytosis.

The expression of surface receptors and antigens on neonatal erythrocytes varies from adult red cells. For instance, the neonatal red cell expresses more insulin and insulin-like growth factor receptors and fewer digoxin receptors than adult (13). The major red cell antigens, Rh, MN, Kell, and Duffy are well developed in early intrauterine life. Other antigens, such as Lutheran, ABO, I, and XgA, are incompletely developed at birth, and others, such as Lewis, are absent at birth.

A commonly used marker of fetal erythropoiesis is the i antigen. Differences in a single glycan chain composed of varying numbers of N-acetyllactosamine units attached to the COOH-terminus of band 3, the anion exchanger, accounts for this developmental marker (14). In fetal cells, the chain is arranged in an unbranched, linear fashion (i antigen with i reactivity) and in a branched manner in adult cells (I antigen with I reactivity) (15). Removal of the carbohydrate does not affect anion exchange.

TABLE 55-1. Effect of Gestational Age of Fetuses *In Utero* and Newborn Infants on Their Hematocrit, Hemoglobin, Mean Corpuscular Volume, and Reticulocytes

Gestational Age (wk)	Hematocrit (%)[a]	Hemoglobin (g/dL)	Mean Corpuscular Volume (fL)	Reticulocytes (%)
18–20[b]	36 ± 3	11.5 ± 0.8	134 ± 9	NR
21–22[b]	38 ± 3	12.3 ± 0.9	130 ± 6	NR
22–23[b]	38 ± 1	12.4 ± 0.9	125 ± 1	NR
24–25	63 ± 4	19.4 ± 1.5	135 ± 0	6.0 ± 0.5
26–27	62 ± 8	19.0 ± 2.5	132 ± 14	9.6 ± 3.2
28–29	60 ± 7	19.3 ± 1.8	131 ± 14	7.5 ± 2.5
30–31	60 ± 8	19.1 ± 2.2	127 ± 13	5.8 ± 2.0
32–33	60 ± 8	18.5 ± 2.0	123 ± 16	5.0 ± 1.9
34–35	61 ± 7	19.6 ± 2.1	122 ± 10	3.9 ± 1.6
36–37	64 ± 7	19.2 ± 1.7	121 ± 12	4.2 ± 1.8
Term	61 ± 7	19.3 ± 2.2	119 ± 9	3.2 ± 1.4

NR, not reported.
[a]Values reported as the mean ± standard deviation.
[b]Fetuses *in utero*.
Data from Zaizov R, Matoth Y. Red cell values on the first postnatal day during the last 16 weeks of gestation. *Am J Hematol* 1976;1:275; Forestier F, Daffos F, Galacteros F, et al. Hematological values of 163 normal fetuses between 18 and 30 weeks of gestation. *Pediatr Res* 1986;20:342; and McIntosh N, Kempson C, Tyler RM. Blood counts in extremely low birth weight infants. *Arch Dis Child* 1988;63:74. In: Christensen RD. Expected hematologic values for term and preterm neonates. In: Christensen RD, ed. *Hematologic problems of the neonate*. Philadelphia: WB Saunders, 2000:120.

Globin Composition and Oxygen Transport

The synthesis and composition of embryonic, fetal, and neonatal globins are described in Chapter 49. Approximately 70% to 90% of the hemoglobin in the blood of the fetus and neonate is fetal hemoglobin (HbF). HbF is more soluble in strong phosphate buffers, and it is resistant to acid denaturation (16). This latter characteristic is the biochemical basis of the Kleihauer-Betke test (see Fetal-Maternal Hemorrhage) (17). Finally, compared to adult hemoglobin (HbA), HbF has the tendency to denature and damage the membrane from within, shortening the red cell lifespan.

An important functional difference between fetal and HbA results from the ability of HbA, but not HbF, to interact with phosphorylated compounds, particularly 2,3-diphosphoglycerate (DPG) and ATP, in the cell. The interaction of 2,3-DPG with HbA leads to a marked decrease in oxygen affinity (18). HbF has essentially no interaction with these organic phosphates, which leads to a relatively higher oxygen affinity of fetal blood (i.e., a leftward shift of the oxygen dissociation curve) (Table 55-3 and Fig. 55-2) compared to adult blood. This is of significant benefit to the fetus *in utero* by facilitating placental oxygen exchange from maternal blood to fetal erythrocytes.

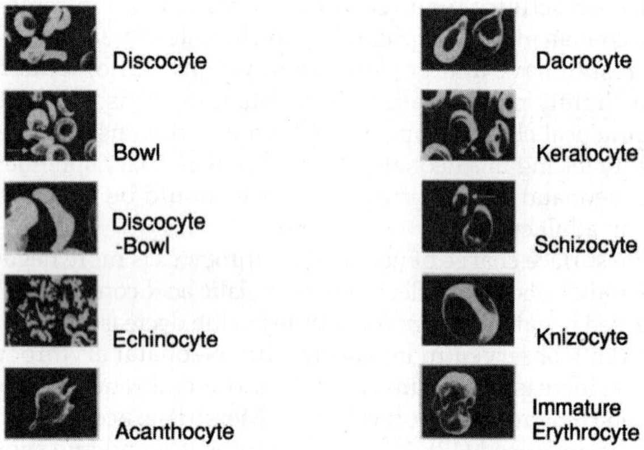

Discocyte
Bowl
Discocyte-Bowl
Echinocyte
Acanthocyte
Dacrocyte
Keratocyte
Schizocyte
Knizocyte
Immature Erythrocyte

The Erythrocyte Differential Count
Median (5% to 95% Range)

Cell Type	Premature Infant	Term Infant	Normal Adult
Discocyte	39.5 (18–57)	43 (18–62)	78 (42–94)
Bowl	29.0 (13–53)	40 (14–58)	18 (4–50)
Discocyte-Bowl	3.0 (0–10)	2 (0–5)	2 (0–4)
Spherocyte	0.0 (0–3)	0 (0–1)	0 (0–0)
Echinocyte	5.5 (1–23)	1 (0–4)	0 (0–3)
Acanthocyte	0.0 (0–2)	1 (0–2)	0 (0–1)
Dacrocyte	1.0 (0–5)	1 (0–3)	0 (0–1)
Keratocyte	3.0 (0–7)	2 (0–5)	0 (0–1)
Schizocyte	2.0 (0–5)	0 (0–2)	0 (0–1)
Knizocyte	3.0 (0–11)	3 (0–8)	1 (0–5)
Immature Erythrocyte	1.0 (0–6)	0 (0–2)	0 (0–0)

Figure 55-1. Varied morphology associated with neonatal smears. (Adapted from Zipursky A, Brown E, Palko J, Brown EJ. The erythrocyte differential count in newborn infants. *Am J Pediatr Hematol Oncol* 1983;5:45.)

TABLE 55-2. Some Structural Characteristics of Fetal Cells Compared to Adult Red Cells

Membrane structure and function
Less osmotically fragile
Differences in surface antigen expression
    A and B antigens diminished
    Lewis system diminished
    I antigen very diminished (or absent): i antigen present
Possible decreased structural stability secondary to increased levels of unbound 2,3-diphosphoglycerate
Membranes less deformable
Red cells of different shapes with a greater predominance of stomatocytes (bowl-shaped cells) than adult cells
    Disc:stomatocyte ratios—adult, 78:18; term newborn, 43:40; premature, 40:29. Increased variability of the smear with multiple morphologic changes
Red cell membrane pits (secondary to decreased splenic function)

Adapted from Wolfe LC. Neonatal anemia. In: Handin RI, Lux SE, Stossel TP, eds. *Blood: principles and practice of hematology*. Philadelphia: JB Lippincott, 1995:2107.

TABLE 55-3. Theoretical Hemoglobin Levels (g/dL) Required in Low Birth Weight Infants to Maintain a Central Venous Oxygen Tension of 30 mmHg[a]

P_{50} (mmHg)	Arterial Oxygen Saturation (%)[b]			
	95	90	85	80
20[c]	10.0	13.0	20.0	>25.0
23	7.3	9.0	11.0	15.5
25	6.2	7.3	8.8	11.0
27[d]	5.3	6.3	7.3	8.9

[a]Assumes a cardiac output of 250 mL/kg/min and an oxygen consumption of 6.5 mL/kg/min.
[b]The lower the arterial oxygen saturation, the less resting pulmonary function (e.g., bronchopulmonary dysplasia).
[c]P_{50} of Hb F.
[d]P_{50} of Hb A.
Adapted from Oski FA. Hematology: the erythrocyte and its disorders. In: Nathan DA, Oski FA, eds. *Hematology of infancy and childhood*, ed 4. Philadelphia: WB Saunders, 1993:40.

Cellular Metabolism

There are a number of metabolic differences in fetal and neonatal erythrocytes compared to adult cells (Table 55-4) (19). Glucose and ATP production are increased, probably representing

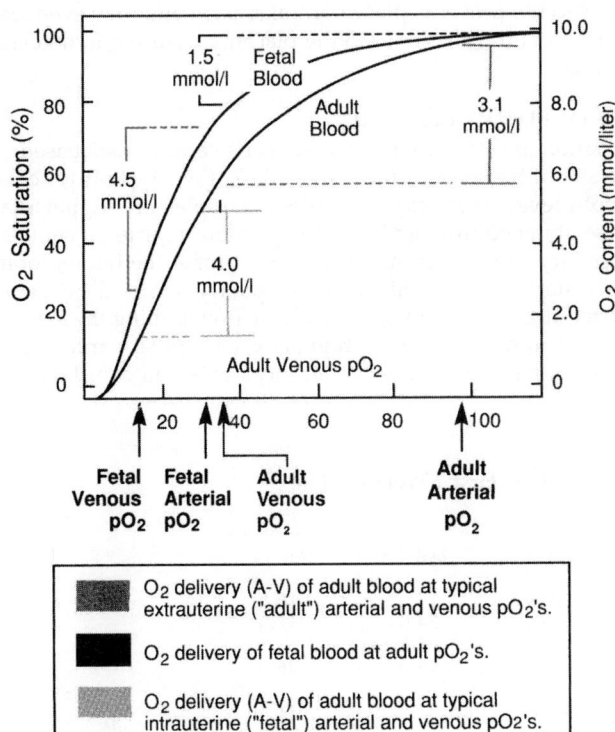

Figure 55-2. Difference in the hemoglobin-oxygen dissociation curve between newborns and adults. The left shift of the newborn curve enhances the amount of oxygen that can be delivered at lower oxygen tensions. For example, comparing the difference in oxygen content of blood at fetal arterial and venous (A-V) PO_2s, fetal blood delivers 4.9 mmol/L, whereas adult blood delivers only 4 mmol/L. In contrast, at typical adult A-V PO_2s, adult blood delivers more oxygen (3.1 mmol/L) than fetal blood (1.5 mmol/L). (Adapted from Stockman JA. Fetal hematology. In: Eden RD, Boehm FH, eds. *Assessment and care of the fetus*. Norwalk, CT: Appleton & Lange, 1989:124.)

TABLE 55-4. Metabolic Characteristics of Neonatal Erythrocytes

Carbohydrate metabolism
Glucose consumption increased
Galactose more completely used as substrate under normal circumstances and for methemoglobin reduction[a]
Decreased activity of sorbitol pathway[a]
Decreased triokinase activity[a]
Glycolytic enzymes
Increased activity of hexokinase, phosphoglucose isomerase,[a] aldolase, glyceraldehyde-3-phosphate dehydrogenase,[a] phosphoglycerate kinase,[a] phosphoglycerate mutase, enolase, pyruvate kinase, lactate dehydrogenase, glucose-6-phosphate dehydrogenase, 6-phosphogluconic dehydrogenase, galactokinase, and galactose-1-phosphate uridyl-transferase
Decreased activity of phosphofructokinase[a]
Distribution of hexokinase isoenzymes differs from that of adults[a]
Nonglycolytic enzymes
Increased activity of glutamic oxaloacetic transaminase and glutathione reductase
Decreased activity of nicotinamide adenine dinucleotide phosphate–dependent methemoglobin reductase catalase,[a] glutathione peroxidase, carbonic anhydrase,[a] adenylate kinase,[a] and glutathione synthetase[a]
Presence of α-glycerol-3-phosphate dehydrogenase
ATP and phosphate metabolism
Decreased phosphate uptake,[a] slower incorporation into ATP and 2,3-diphosphoglycerate[a]
Accelerated decline of 2,3-diphosphoglycerate during red blood cell incubation[a]
Increased ATP levels
Accelerated decline of ATP during storage or incubation
Storage characteristics
Increased potassium efflux and greater degrees of hemolysis during short periods of storage
More rapid assumption of altered morphologic forms during brief incubation[a]
Membrane characteristics
Decreased ouabain-sensitive ATPase[a]
Decreased potassium influx[a]
Decreased permeability to glycerol and thiourea[a]
Decreased membrane filterability[a]
Increased sphingomyelin, decreased lecithin content of stromal phospholipids
Decreased content of linoleic acid[a]
Increase in lipid phosphorus and cholesterol per cell
Greater affinity for glucose[a]
Other characteristics
Increased methemoglobin content[a]
Increased affinity of hemoglobin for oxygen[a]
Glutathione instability[a]
Increased tendency for Heinz body formation in presence of oxidant compounds[a]

ATP, adenosine triphosphate.
[a]Appears to be a unique characteristic of the newborn's erythrocytes and not merely a function of the presence of young red cells.
Adapted from Gallagher PG. Disorders of erythrocyte metabolism and shape. In: Christensen RD, ed. *Hematologic problems of the neonate*. Philadelphia, WB Saunders, 2000:212.

compensatory activity to maintain normal intracellular homeostasis by energy-dependent ion transport (20). Several glycolytic enzymes demonstrate increased activity (21), but this increased activity may reflect a larger percentage of younger red cells in the newborn than the adult rather than a characteristic specific to neonatal erythrocytes. Activities of other enzymes, including carbonic anhydrase and methemoglobin reductase, are reduced. These differences probably contribute to the decreased lifespan of the neonatal erythrocyte.

One important characteristic of the neonatal erythrocyte is increased susceptibility to oxidant-induced damage (22,23) leading to glutathione instability, Heinz body formation, and methemoglobinemia. The basis of this increased susceptibility to oxidant damage is unknown, but variations in the pentose phosphate pathway, decreased glutathione peroxidase (24), diminished oxidant capacity of neonatal plasma, variations in superoxide dismutase levels, and decreased membrane sulfhydryl groups have all been implicated (25).

Lifespan

The lifespan of the neonatal erythrocyte is between 60 and 90 days, with preterm infants demonstrating even shorter lifespans of 35 to 50 days (26). When neonatal erythrocytes are transfused into adults, they exhibit a shortened lifespan attributed to the intrinsic differences between neonatal and adult erythrocytes. When adult erythrocytes are transfused into a neonate, they exhibit a normal lifespan (27,28). This shortened lifespan has been explained by characteristics specific to neonatal cells, including rapid decrease in intracellular enzyme activity and ATP content, increased susceptibility of membrane proteins and lipids to peroxidation, loss of membrane surface area, and increased membrane deformability.

NORMAL HEMATOLOGIC VALUES

Numerous factors influence hematologic values in the neonate, including many of the developmental changes listed above. Accurate interpretation of laboratory data in the neonate requires consideration of a number of factors, as what is a normal value for one infant may not be for another. Gestational and chronologic age of the infant, gender, timing of cord clamping, and the site of blood sampling are important factors to be considered.

Hemoglobin and Hematocrit

Hemoglobin concentration gradually rises throughout gestation and peaks shortly after birth (29,30). The mean hemoglobin at 10 weeks' gestation is 9 g/dL, rising to 11 to 12 g/dL by approximately 23 weeks and 13 to 14 g/dL by 30 weeks (Table 55-1) (2). Hemoglobin concentration is relatively stable the last 6 to 8 weeks of gestation, with a mean concentration of approximately 16 to 17 g/dL at term. The hemoglobin level may increase by 1 to 2 g/dL at birth owing to placental transfusion (see Cord

Clamping and Placental Transfusion). Decreased plasma volume leads to a peak in hemoglobin between 2 and 6 hours of life with levels stabilizing by 8 to 12 hours of life.

Erythropoiesis decreases at birth, leading to a gradual decrease in hemoglobin concentration over the next several weeks of life (Table 55-5). The nadir is reached at 8 weeks of life with levels around 11 g/dL in healthy term infants before erythropoiesis increases and the hemoglobin rises. This process is called *physiologic anemia* (see Physiologic Anemia).

Other Factors Influencing Hemoglobin and Hematocrit

Gestation age influences hemoglobin and hematocrit values. A gradual increase in values is observed with increasing gestational age (Table 55-1). Preterm male infants reach cord hemoglobin levels earlier than females probably due to the erythropoietic effect of testosterone (31).

CORD CLAMPING AND PLACENTAL TRANSFUSION
The timing of cord clamping significantly influences hemoglobin values in the newborn (Table 55-6) (29,32,33). Around the time of birth, placental blood is rapidly transferred to the infant. Twenty-five percent of this transfusion occurs within 15 seconds of birth and half by the end of the first minute after birth. Delaying cord clamping can increase an infant's blood volume by over one-half, as the placental vessels contain between 75 to 125 mL of blood at birth. Holding the infant above the level of the placenta prevents placental transfusion and may even lead to neonatal transfusion into the placenta resulting in neonatal anemia.

SITE OF BLOOD SAMPLING
Variation in hemoglobin or hematocrit values exists based on the site of blood sampling (Table 55-7) (29). Typically, hemoglobin levels from capillary blood samples are higher than those obtained from an indwelling venous or arterial catheter. Capillary samples frequently overestimate the hemoglobin, particularly when obtained from a poorly perfused extremity. "Arterializing" a capillary sample by prewarming the extremity can improve the correlation between capillary and venous hematocrits. The largest differences between capillary and

---

TABLE 55-5. Normal Hematologic Values during the First 2 Weeks of Life in the Term Infant

Value	Cord Blood	Day 1	Day 3	Day 7	Day 14
Hemoglobin (g/dL)	16.8	18.4	17.8	17.0	16.8
Hematocrit (%)	53.0	58.0	55.0	54.0	52.0
Red cells (mm³)	5.25	5.8	5.6	5.2	5.1
Mean corpuscular volume (fL)	107.0	108.0	99.0	98.0	96.0
Mean corpuscular hemoglobin (pg)	34.0	35.0	33.0	32.5	31.5
Mean corpuscular hemoglobin concentration (g/dL)	31.7	32.5	33.0	33.0	33.0
Reticulocytes	3.0–7.0	3.0–7.0	1.0–3.0	0.0–1.0	0.0–1.0
Nucleated red blood cells (/mm³)	500.0	200.0	0.0–5.0	0.0	0.0
Platelets (1000s of mm³)	290.0	192.0	213.0	248.0	252.0

NOTE: During the first 2 weeks of life, a venous hemoglobin value below 13.0 g/dL or a capillary hemoglobin value below 14.5 g/dL should be regarded as anemic.
From Oski FA, Naiman JL. *Hematologic problems in the newborn*, 2nd ed. Philadelphia: WB Saunders, 1972:13.

TABLE 55-6. Effect of Cord Clamping on Hematocrit and Hemoglobin Concentration at Various Times after Delivery

Author	Early Clamping		Delayed Clamping		Time of Study
	Hb (g/dL)	Hct (%)	Hb (g/dL)	Hct (%)	
Phillips	15.6	—	19.3	—	20–30 h
Marsh	17.4	—	20.8	—	3rd d
Colozzi	14.7	—	17.3	—	72 h
Lanzkowsky	18.1	—	19.7	—	72–96 h
	11.1	—	11.1	—	3 mo
Linderkamp	—	48 ± 4	—	50 ± 4	At birth
	—	47 ± 5	—	63 ± 5	2 h
	—	43 ± 6	—	59 ± 5	24 h
	—	44 ± 5	—	59 ± 6	120 h
Kinmond	—	50.9 ± 4.5	—	56.4 ± 4.8	Not standardized
Nelle	—	48 ± 6	—	58 ± 6	2 h
	—	44 ± 5	—	56 ± 7	24 h
	—	44 ± 5	—	54 ± 8	5 d

Hb, hemoglobin; Hct, hematocrit.
From Christensen RD. Expected hematologic values for term and preterm neonates. In: Christensen RD, ed. *Hematologic problems of the neonate.* Philadelphia: WB Saunders, 2000:118.

venous hematocrits exist in very preterm infants (34), particularly those with acidosis, hypotension, and anemia. In infants of less than 30 weeks' gestation, capillary hematocrit values were 20% higher than venous hematocrits, compared to capillary values 12% higher than venous hematocrits at term. Finally, samples from similar sources (i.e., arterial, venous, and capillary values) correlate independent of the site of sampling (e.g., radial, femoral, and umbilical arterial values show little variation from sample to sample).

Reticulocytes

Reticulocyte counts and the absolute reticulocyte count are elevated at birth with values of 4% to 7% and 200,000 to 400,000/µL in term infants and 6% to 12% and 400,000 to 550,000/mL in preterm infants (29). In healthy infants, reticulocyte counts fall over the first few days of life to the levels of 0% to 1% and 0 to 50,000/mL by day of life 4 (Table 55-5). A reticulocyte count of

zero on day of life 1 indicates erythrocyte under production (see Decreased Erythrocyte Production).

Erythrocyte Indices

MEAN CORPUSCULAR VOLUME
The size of circulating erythrocytes is estimated by the MCV. Throughout pregnancy, there is an inverse relationship between gestational age and MCV, with MCV falling throughout gestation to values between 108 and 118 fL at term (Table 55-1) (2). Because most term infants have an MCV greater than 100 fL, when values less than 95 fL are observed, iron deficiency or α-thalassemia trait should be considered.

MEAN CORPUSCULAR HEMOGLOBIN
Similar to the MCV, the MCH is higher in preterm and term neonates compared to adults with neonatal values in the 33 to 41 pg range (compared to 27 to 31 pg in adults).

TABLE 55-7. Effect of Site of Blood Sampling on Hematocrits or Hemoglobin Concentrations of Neonates

Study	Year	Anatomic Sites of Comparison	Observed Average Difference
Vahlquist	1941	Capillary versus femoral vein	Capillary 10% higher
Oettinger and Mills	1949	Great toe versus internal jugular	Capillary 21% higher
Mollision	1951	Capillary versus venous	Capillary 5% higher
Oh and Lind	1966	Heel versus scalp or femoral vein	Capillary 15% higher[a]
Moe	1967	Patients with erythroblastosis fetalis: heel versus umbilical cord	Capillary 25% higher
Linderkamp	1977	Capillary versus umbilical cord	Capillary 10% to 21% higher
Rivera and Rudolph	1982	Heel versus antecubital vein	Capillary 12% higher (up to 20%)
Thurlbeck and McIntosh[b]	1987	Heel versus umbilical artery catheter	Capillary 15% higher

[a]The capillary hematocrit was only 5% higher when the heel was warmed.
[b]Preterm infants, 24 to 32 weeks' gestation, with respiratory distress.
Adapted from Christensen RD. Expected hematologic values for term and preterm neonates. In: Christensen RD, ed. *Hematologic problems of the neonate.* Philadelphia: WB Saunders, 2000:118.

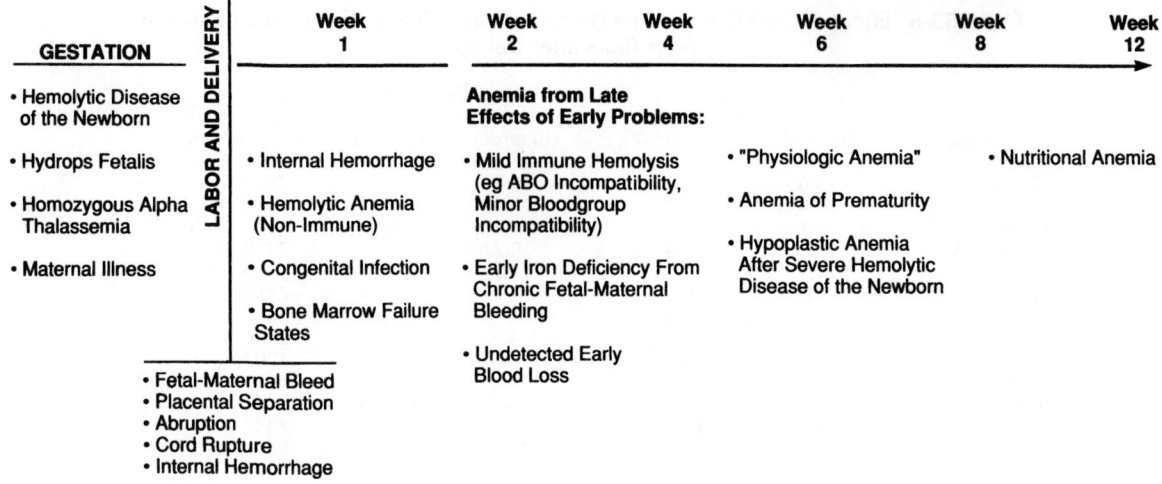

Figure 55-3. Developmental differential diagnosis of neonatal anemia.

MEAN CORPUSCULAR HEMOGLOBIN CONCENTRATION

The MCHC does not vary in neonates compared to adults. Although neonatal erythrocytes are larger and contain more hemoglobin than adult cells, the hemoglobin concentration within the erythrocyte is not more concentrated. MCHC values greater than 35 g/dL have been used as an indicator for hereditary spherocytosis (35).

Erythrocyte Morphology

As noted above, significant variations in neonatal erythrocyte morphology are seen on peripheral blood smear, particularly in preterm infants. Discocytes, bowls, echinocytes, and keratocytes are commonly observed in preterm neonates without intrinsic erythrocyte defects (Fig. 55-1) (3).

NEONATAL ANEMIA

Determining the etiology of neonatal anemia can present a significant challenge. The differential diagnosis is extensive and includes not only many of the causes of anemia seen in older patients, but also many unique to the fetus and newborn associated with pregnancy, labor, and delivery (Fig. 55-3). Knowledge of these disorders and an understanding of the associated pathophysiology provide the framework for the evaluation, diagnosis, and treatment of neonatal anemia. Traditional classification of anemia includes hemorrhage, hemolysis, and inadequate erythrocyte production.

HEMORRHAGE IN THE FETUS AND NEWBORN

Prenatal Hemorrhage

Fetal blood loss before birth is usually via a transplacental route and includes placental abruption, placenta previa, vasa previa, and twin-twin transfusion (Table 55-8). Fetal blood loss due to intracranial hemorrhage (e.g., in a thrombocytopenic infant with platelet isoimmunization) or after traumatic amniocentesis or cordocentesis is uncommon.

FETAL-MATERNAL HEMORRHAGE

The structure of the fetal-placental unit sets up a large pressure gradient from umbilical artery to intervillous space. The separation of the maternal intervillous space from the pulsatile fetal circulation is thin, composed of a two-cell layer, with the constant possibility for the rupture of the trophoblastic-endothelial juncture and the contamination of the maternal intervillous space with fetal blood (Fig. 55-4). Given this fragile mechanical relationship, it is surprising that fetal-maternal hemorrhage does not occur more frequently. Most spontaneous fetal-maternal hemorrhage occurs during the third trimester, primarily during labor and delivery (36), although hemorrhage has been reported as early as 3 to 4 months' gestation. Approximately 1 in 400 pregnancies is associated with a fetal-maternal hemorrhage greater than or equal to 30 mL, and 1 in 2000 pregnancies is associated with a fetal-maternal hemorrhage greater than or equal to 100 mL (37).

Fetal red cells can be detected in the maternal circulation in a number of ways. The most clinically useful test is the microscopic demonstration of fetal red cells in the maternal circulation using the Kleihauer-Betke test (16). In this method, HbA is denatured and eluted from smears of adult red cells with an acid solution, leaving behind largely empty red cell membranes. HbF resists denaturation and elution, so fetal cells stain darkly. Simple observation of the acid-treated maternal blood smear can give a qualitative picture, but one can estimate the actual amount of fetal blood lost using the following formula:

$$2400 \times \text{the ratio of fetal to maternal cells} = 1 \text{ mL of fetal blood}$$

Using this equation, it has been shown that most deliveries result in less than 3 mL of fetal blood in the maternal circulation, and only 0.3% have a fetal-maternal transfusion of 10 mL or more. Conditions that elevate maternal HbF production (thalassemia minor, sickle cell disease, hereditary persistence of HbF, and pregnancy-induced maternal HbF production) confound this analysis (38). ABO incompatibility can also confound interpretation of this test. Removal of fetal cells from the maternal circulation by maternal anti-A or anti-B antibodies will lead to a false-negative result.

ABRUPTIO PLACENTAE

Placental abruption (separation of the placenta from the uterine wall) occurs in approximately 1% of pregnancies, with an increased incidence in pregnancies complicated by chronic or pregnancy-induced hypertension (30,39). The classic triad of placental abruption includes vaginal bleeding, uterine contrac-

TABLE 55-8. Excessive Erythrocyte Loss Due to Hemorrhage

Prenatal hemorrhage
Transplacental hemorrhage
  Fetomaternal hemorrhage
  Abruptio placentae
  Placenta previa
  Vasa previa
  Velamentous insertion of umbilical cord
  Twin-twin transfusion
Traumatic fetal hemorrhage
  Maternal trauma
  Amniocentesis
  Cordocentesis
Placental lesions
  Chorioangioma
  Hematoma
  Hemangioma
  Choriocarcinoma
Other causes of fetal hemorrhage
  Intracranial bleeding
  Gastrointestinal bleeding
Intrapartum hemorrhage
  Placenta
    Abnormalities of placentation listed above
    Surgical laceration (e.g., incision of anterior placenta or cord at
      delivery)
Umbilical vessels
  Rupture of normal cord
  Rupture of abnormal cord
    Aneurysm
    Varix
    Cyst
    Funisitis with weakened vessels
    Short cord
  Cord entrapment (e.g., by forceps)
  Tight nuchal cord
  Occult cord prolapse
Intrapartum neonatal trauma
  Cranial hemorrhage including subgaleal, subarachnoid, and intra-
    ventricular hemorrhage
  Cephalohematoma
  Splenic rupture
  Adrenal hemorrhage
  Liver laceration
  Retroperitoneal hemorrhage
Postpartum hemorrhage
Intracranial bleeding in the very low birth weight infant
Gastric or intestinal ulceration
Hemorrhage from vascular malformation
Coagulation factor deficiency
Iatrogenic causes
  Phlebotomy
  Tracheal mucosal tear during endotracheal intubation
  Posterior pharyngeal tears during laryngoscopy or OGT placement
  Vessel perforation during umbilical catheterization
  Intercostals vessel laceration during thoracostomy tube placement
  Gastric rupture from overdistention or OGT placement
  Pulmonary hemorrhage during ventilation
  Bladder mucosal tear during catheterization
  Surgical wounds

OGT, orogastric tube.

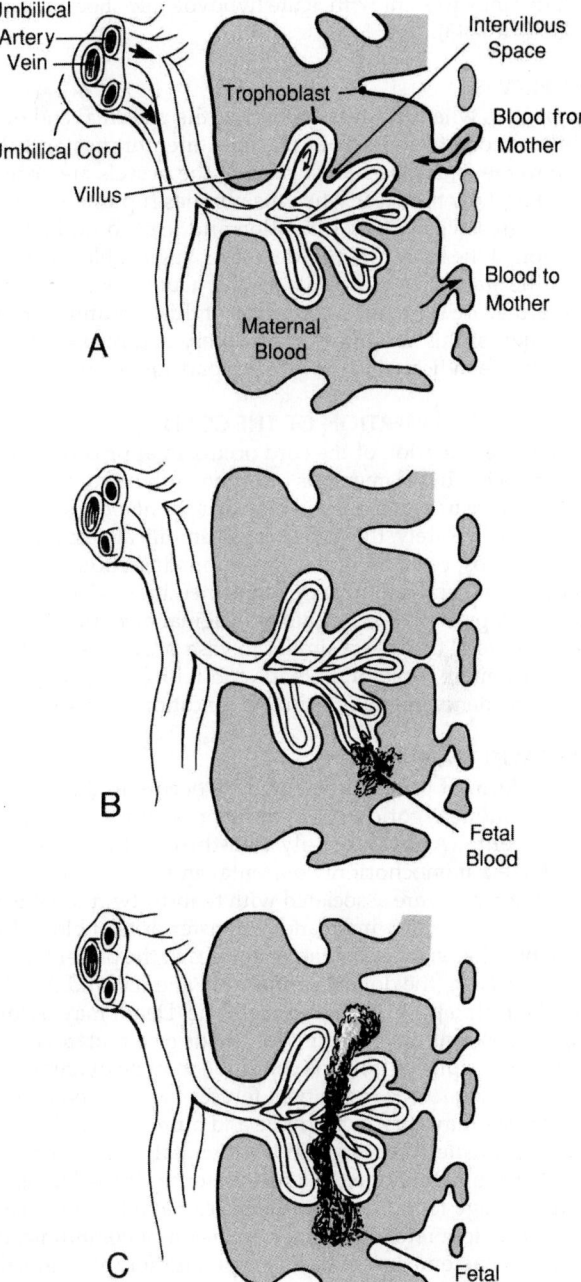

Figure 55-4. Anatomic issues in fetomaternal hemorrhage. **A:** Resting state. Fragile capillary networks are present. **B:** Minor small bleed, known to occur in almost all pregnancies. **C:** Major possibility of significant exchange of fetal and maternal blood as a result of abruption (more severe) or normal childbirth.

tions, and an irritable, tender uterus. However, bleeding may occur in a retroplacental location, delaying recognition and treatment. The fetus may develop hypoxemia from a decrease in placental surface area. It may be further compromised by fetal hemorrhage accompanying the maternal bleeding. If fetal hemorrhage is significant, hypovolemia, anemia, and heart failure may develop, leading to *in utero* demise (40,41). Placental abruption is usually an acute occurrence. However, when there is a small, chronic placental separation, fetal blood loss may occur more gradually. These fetuses may demonstrate marked reticulocytosis and elevated nucleated red blood cell counts at birth. In severe cases, iron deficiency can occur.

PLACENTA PREVIA

Placenta previa (implantation of the placenta in a low-lying position in advance of the fetal presenting part usually overlying part or all of the cervical os) occurs in approximately 1 in 250 births (30,42). The classic presentation is acute onset of painless vaginal bleeding, with a peak incidence around 34 weeks' gestation. Fetal blood loss of varying amounts occurs in approximately 50% of cases. Fetal signs may include intrauterine growth retardation, abnormal biophysical testing, and tachycardia. Bleeding may be intermittent and recurrent or massive and acute. In the former, the neonate presents with a partially or completely compensated anemia and marked reticulocytosis.

The latter may present with acute hypovolemic shock and may lead to death (43).

VASA PREVIA

Vasa previa is when fetal vessels exiting the placental end of the umbilical cord travel across the fetal membranes and then return to the fetal placental surface. If the vessels are near the cervical os, they may tear when membranes rupture or in labor with progressive cervical dilatation and lead to rapid exsanguination of the fetus (44). Sudden-onset vaginal bleeding, usually at the start of or during labor, and acutely occurring fetal tachycardia, are the classic symptoms of this condition. Prompt recognition of this condition and delivery and resuscitation of the infant are indicated to prevent peripartum death.

VELAMENTOUS INSERTION OF THE CORD

Velamentous insertion of the cord occurs in approximately 1% of pregnancies. In velamentous insertion of the cord, the umbilical vessels are unprotected and may tear spontaneously or during labor (45). Rarely, the unprotected umbilical vessel crosses the cervical os, combining a velamentous insertion with vasa previa with potential for tearing when membranes rupture (46). The clinical presentation of painless vaginal bleeding followed by signs of fetal distress is similar to vasa previa. Velamentous insertion is more common in twins and with low-lying placentas. The incidence of fetal loss in this condition is 1% to 2%.

TWIN-TWIN TRANSFUSION

Another form of prenatal hemorrhage occurs in the bleeding from one monozygotic twin to another within a monochorionic placenta. Approximately two-thirds of monozygotic twins have a monochorionic placenta, and up to one-third of these pregnancies are associated with twin-to-twin transfusion (47). This is caused by imbalanced transfer of fetal blood from one to the other via vascular anastomoses in the placenta. Classically, one twin (the donor) is small and anemic, and the other twin (the recipient) is large and plethoric. Death may occur as a result of exsanguinations in the donor or circulatory overload in the recipient (48). This condition may be dynamic with varying consequences to the twin fetuses because the vascular anastomoses may vary in both size and number as well as proceed in opposite directions (49). Antenatal factors that may predict outcome include the presence of hydrops fetalis and gestational age (50). Perinatal therapies have included serial amnioreduction, fetoscopic laser occlusion of communicating placental anastomoses, maternal digoxin therapy, and selective feticide (51).

At birth, both twins may be sick. The anemic donor twin may develop congestive heart failure and the plethoric recipient twin may require treatment for hyperviscosity syndrome, hyperbilirubinemia, and rarely disseminated intravascular coagulation. In twin-twin transfusion in which the donor twin has been chronically hemorrhaging into the recipient, the clinician observes the classic presentation of a small anemic infant with reticulocytosis and a plethoric, polycythemic infant whose weight is at least 20% higher and hemoglobin is at least 5 g/dL higher than its sibling. Acute transfusions, which typically occur closer to the time of delivery, do not lead to differences in neonatal weights greater than 20%, and there an equal chance exists of either twin being the red cell donor. The mortality of twin-twin transfusion remains high. In survivors, there is significant risk of long-term neurodevelopmental morbidity (52).

TRAUMATIC FETAL HEMORRHAGE

Fetal bleeding has occurred after multiple trauma and after blunt trauma to the abdomen of the pregnant mother (53–55). It has also occurred after traumatic amniocentesis, cordocentesis, and after external cephalic version (53–57).

PLACENTAL LESIONS

The extreme vascularity and unique double circulation of the placenta predisposes to a wide variety of vascular lesions, some of which may lead to fetoplacental and fetomaternal hemorrhage (58). Chorioangioma is the most common placental anomaly leading to neonatal anemia from fetoplacental or fetomaternal hemorrhage. These lesions may be multiple and, in some cases, have resulted in severe hemorrhage *in utero*, leading to fetal demise (59). Other lesions that have led to neonatal anemia are placenta hematoma, hemangioma, and intraplacental choriocarcinoma (60–62).

OTHER CAUSES OF FETAL HEMORRHAGE

Internal prenatal fetal hemorrhage is uncommon (63,64). When it does occur, intracranial and intraabdominal sites predominate. Intracranial hemorrhage occurs primarily when the pregnancy has been complicated by thrombocytopenia (autoimmune or alloimmune), severe fetal hypoxemia, or maternal coumadin use (65,66). Intraabdominal bleeding may occur after an *in utero* volvulus, leading to ischemic bowel necrosis with venous hemorrhage (67).

Intrapartum Hemorrhage

Hemorrhage due to events at the time of delivery can be classified into those involving the placenta and umbilical cord and those related to neonatal trauma (Table 55-8).

PLACENTA

Labor may exaggerate or worsen abnormalities of placentation, such as vasa previa, abruptio placentae, and velamentous insertion of the cord during labor, and lead to significant hemorrhage.

Incision of the placenta during cesarean section can lead to massive hemorrhage (68,69). An anterior placenta may be lacerated during emergency cesarean section or during routine sections when placentation is unknown. Lower uterine incisions have been associated with placental injury.

UMBILICAL VESSELS

One in 10,000 pregnancies is associated with umbilical cord bleeding or rupture. Affected neonates are at risk for anemia, hypovolemic shock, and death. Most commonly, cord rupture is associated with precipitous delivery. Traction on a shortened or abnormal umbilical cord can lead to cord rupture, usually on the fetal side. The cord can be weakened by the presence of an aneurysm, hemangioma, arteriovenous malformation, cyst, varix, funisitis, or velamentous insertion (70). Entrapment of the cord and pressure on the cord (e.g., by forceps) can also lead to traumatic laceration of the cord.

Infants born with a tight nuchal cord can lose up to 20% of their blood volume into the placenta (71). Hypovolemia develops as placental blood is prevented from flowing into the fetus owing to constriction of the umbilical vein while blood flow out of the fetus into the placenta via the muscular umbilical arteries continues (72).

INTRAPARTUM TRAUMA

In addition to fetal-maternal hemorrhage, the effects of placental separation, and cord-related effects, neonates can also experience anemia due to internal bleeding with symptoms of mild to severe acute blood loss (68). These internal hemorrhages are not necessarily manifest at the time of delivery. They may appear on physical examination shortly after birth or present as sudden pallor, tachycardia, and hypotension at 1 to 2 days of life. The site of the bleeding often can be specified by individual characteristics.

Cranial Hemorrhage. Cranial hemorrhage is common in neonates, as the head is normally the presenting part. Trauma to the scalp, skull, or intracranial structures can result from traction applied manually, by forceps, or by vacuum-assist devices. Cranial hemorrhage is associated with varying degrees of blood loss, and significant hyperbilirubinemia may occur.

Subgaleal Hemorrhage. Bleeding into the subgaleal space typically occurs after difficult, instrument-assisted (particularly vacuum) delivery (73,74). Trauma or traction tears the emissary or "bridging" veins, leading to the collection of blood in the potential space between the galea aponeurotica and the periosteum of the skull. The subgaleal space extends from the base of the skull forward to the orbital ridge and is thus able to accommodate very large amounts of blood. Prompt recognition of subgaleal hemorrhage (the presence of ballotable fluid in dependent regions of the head) is critical, and close monitoring should be provided. The degree of bleeding may lead to hypovolemic shock (75), and exsanguination into a subgaleal hemorrhage with neonatal death has been reported. The occurrence of an extensive subgaleal hemorrhage should prompt evaluation for intracranial hemorrhage and neonatal coagulopathy.

Cephalohematoma. In cephalohematoma, the hemorrhage is confined by the periosteum and limited to the area overlying a single skull bone. However, giant cephalohematomas may result in neonatal anemia and hyperbilirubinemia (76).

Intracranial Hemorrhage. Intracranial bleeding is most common after difficult delivery, in preterm infants, and in infants with disorders of coagulation (e.g., platelet isoimmunization, in which 10% to 20% of affected infants experience intracranial hemorrhage) (77). Traumatic delivery leading to subdural, subarachnoid, or epidural hemorrhage may lead to anemia, even in term infants without coagulopathy. Preterm infants are at high risk for intraventricular hemorrhage (78), which may approach 10% to 15% of the total blood volume. Symptoms of acute blood loss can occur; anemia is rarely the only associated clinical finding. Hyperbilirubinemia may occur.

Abdominal Hemorrhage. Difficult delivery with prolonged traction or compression of the abdomen, particularly during breech extraction, predisposes normal infants to traumatic, intraabdominal hemorrhage (79). Diagnosis is usually suspected by the history and clinical course. After stabilization of the hypovolemia, abdominal imaging (usually ultrasound) can confirm the diagnosis. This should be repeated at 12 to 24 hours to examine whether equilibration has occurred, revealing neonatal blood loss.

Adrenal Hemorrhage. Hemorrhage of the adrenal gland is estimated to occur at an incidence of 1.7 per 1000 live births (68,69). The adrenal gland is normally enlarged in the neonate, which may predispose it to trauma and hemorrhage. Hemorrhage into the adrenal gland also can occur in the setting of disseminated intravascular coagulation associated with infection and in infants with renal vein thrombosis. Adrenal hemorrhage has been associated with renal dysfunction and intestinal obstruction. Bilateral adrenal hemorrhage, independent of the etiology, can predispose the neonate to adrenal collapse and addisonian crisis.

Hepatic Hemorrhage. Liver laceration occurs more commonly than clinically appreciated; it presents in 1.2% to 5.6% of fetal and neonatal autopsies. Infants with liver laceration may appear well for the first 12 to 24 hours as hemorrhage is confined with the surrounding capsule. When the hepatic capsule ruptures, hemoperitoneum and hypovolemic shock occur (80). There is abdominal distention and discoloration, and a right upper quadrant mass may be palpable. Emergent surgical intervention and tamponade have been life-saving, but mortality remains high (81).

Splenic Hemorrhage. Splenic rupture may occur after traumatic delivery of a normal infant or after delivery of an infant with significant splenomegaly (82). Splenic enlargement due to extramedullary hematopoiesis (e.g., in erythroblastosis fetalis) with rupture, both at the time of delivery and during exchange transfusion, has been described (83). Symptoms are similar to hepatic laceration with abdominal distention and discoloration, scrotal enlargement, and hypovolemic shock.

Postpartum Hemorrhage

NEONATAL COAGULOPATHY
Neonatal anemia can result from extensive hemorrhage due to abnormalities in hemostasis (particularly at intracranial and gastrointestinal sites) or after trauma (e.g., circumcision). These disorders include congenital factor deficiencies and acquired and inherited platelet abnormalities (84). Neonatal hemorrhage and anemia has occurred in infants deficient in vitamin K due to maternal anticonvulsant therapy or in breast-fed infants not treated with vitamin K at birth (85). Neonatal anemia has also been reported in infants with TAR syndrome (thrombocytopenia, absent radii) and Wiskott-Aldrich syndrome.

TABLE 55-9. Characteristics of Acute and Chronic Blood Loss in the Newborn

Findings	Acute Blood Loss	Chronic Blood Loss
Clinical	Acute distress, pallor; shallow, rapid, and often irregular respiration; weak or absent peripheral pulses; low or absent blood pressure; no hepatosplenomegaly	Marked pallor disproportionate to distress; occasionally, signs of congestive heart failure are present; pulse usually normal; blood pressure usually normal; hepatomegaly
Venous pressure	Low	Normal or elevated
Hemoglobin	May be normal initially, then drops quickly in first 24 h	Low at birth
RBC morphology	Normochromic and macrocytic	Hypochromic and microcytic, anisocytosis
Serum iron	Normal at birth	Low at birth
Course	Prompt treatment of anemia and shock required to prevent death	Generally uneventful
Treatment	i.v. fluids, blood, iron therapy later	Iron therapy, occasionally pRBC

RBC, red blood cell; pRBC, packed RBC.

TABLE 55-10. Differential Diagnosis of Pallor at Birth

Feature	Asphyxia	Acute Blood Loss	Chronic Blood Loss	Hemolytic Disease
Respirations	Retractions, cyanosis	Rapid without effort	Little distress unless congestive heart failure	Rapid if congestive heart failure
Arterial blood pressure	May be elevated or decreased	May be elevated or decreased	Usually normal	Usually normal
Central venous pressure	Normal or elevated	Low	Normal or elevated	Usually normal
Hepatosplenomegaly	Organs may be pushed down by lungs	None	Hepatomegaly if congestive heart failure	Hepatosplenomegaly
Jaundice	Perhaps	If loss of blood into tissues (e.g., scalp)	Usually not	Yes
Hemoglobin	Normal	Normal initially, drops after 24 h	Low at birth	Low at birth
Red cell morphology	Normal	Normal/macrocytic	May be hypochromic microcytic	May have hemolytic morphology
Other	Responds to O_2 intrauterine	Weak pulses	—	May have positive direct Coombs' test or positive family history

Adapted from Oski F. Hematology: the erythrocyte and its disorders. In: Nathan DA, Oski FA, eds. *Hematology of infancy and childhood*, ed 4. Philadelphia: WB Saunders, 1993:34.

IATROGENIC CAUSES

Anemia can occur in hospitalized neonates, particularly preterm infants, owing to phlebotomy-related blood loss. It is not surprising that the most premature, critically ill infants require the most phlebotomy for diagnostic testing. Ironically, these are the same infants who have the most additional blood wastage (phlebotomy overdraw) during diagnostic testing (86,87). Other iatrogenic causes of hemorrhage include vascular or tissue damage during diagnostic or therapeutic procedures, after surgery, and from accidental disconnection of vascular catheters.

OTHER CAUSES OF HEMORRHAGE

Gastric and intestinal ulceration may cause significant anemia in the neonate. The Apt test will allow differentiation from swallowed maternal blood. Hemorrhage into large tumors (e.g., sacrococcygeal teratomas) and bleeding from vascular malformations (e.g., hemangiomas, hemangioendotheliomas, and arteriovenous malformations) have been described (88–91).

CLINICAL MANIFESTATIONS OF FETAL AND NEONATAL HEMORRHAGE

Neonates are less able to tolerate acute hypovolemia than adults. Loss of 10% of blood volume in the neonate leads to significant peripheral and circulatory effects, whereas the adult is not affected by a similar blood loss. Loss of greater than or equal to 20% of the blood volume results in shock and is associated with a high mortality rate. Clinical symptomatology in neonatal hemorrhage is variable and is influenced by the timing and amount of blood loss and the degree of hypovolemia (if any) rendered (Table 55-9).

Small volume hemorrhage before delivery presents as anemia without signs of hypovolemia. If adequate time has elapsed, there may be accompanying reticulocytosis, which may be initially confused with a hemolytic process. Review of the peripheral blood smear reveals mild macrocytosis and polychromasia but no predominant morphology suggestive of a hemolytic process. The absence of jaundice and a negative Coombs' test provide additional evidence for prenatal hemorrhage rather than hemolysis.

Neonates suffering from significant acute blood loss at the time of delivery appear pale, hyper alert, and tachypneic, with tachycardia, decreased pulses, and hypotension. The pallor may be striking. Differentiation from other causes of pallor in the neonate is critical, as immediate resuscitation with volume replacement is indicated to prevent circulatory collapse and death (Table 55-10) (69). When shock is present, blood transfusion is indicated. In acute hemorrhage, the hemoglobin level is a poor guide to diagnosis and therapy. Hemodilution has not yet occurred, and hemoglobin levels may not have fallen dramatically enough to immediately indicate that crystalloid volume replacement without transfusion is adequate (68,69).

Neonates with chronic blood loss may be asymptomatic or may have symptoms of congestive heart failure with hepatomegaly, pulmonary edema, and peripheral edema. These infants have usually compensated for blood loss by increasing total blood volume. If the amount of blood loss has been significant but has occurred over a protracted period of time, the neonate may be normovolemic but pale at birth with hypochromic, microcytic erythrocytes on smear (indicating iron deficiency). Thus, after initial treatment, all infants with significant blood loss, acute or chronic, should be provided supplemental iron to replace lost stores.

HEMOLYSIS IN THE FETUS AND NEWBORN

Hemolytic processes are common causes of anemia in the neonate (Table 55-11). As in the adult, hemolytic disorders are classified as extrinsic or intrinsic. These various hemolytic disorders are discussed in detail in other chapters. Elements specific to the neonate are discussed in the following section.

Extrinsic Hemolysis

BLOOD GROUP INCOMPATIBILITY

Immune-mediated hemolytic anemia due to blood group incompatibility is the most common cause of hemolytic anemia in the newborn period. The anemia results from maternally derived alloantibody directed against antigens of fetal and neonatal erythrocytes. ABO incompatibility is the most common picture seen in clinical practice. In the past, Rh incompatibility was the most common and severe cause of immune-mediated hemolytic anemia. Changes in clinical practice including routine administration of anti-D immune globulin to at-risk women, advances in perinatal medicine (including ultrasonography, amniocentesis, and *in utero* transfusion therapy), and

TABLE 55-11. Hemolysis

Extrinsic hemolysis
Isoimmunization
    Rh sensitization
    ABO
    Others (e.g., Duffy, Kell, Lewis)
    Maternal autoimmune disorders
    Maternal medication use
Microangiopathic anemias
    Disseminated intravascular coagulation
        Sepsis
        Congenital infection—toxoplasmosis, rubella, cytomegalovirus, dis-
           seminated herpes, and syphillis; malaria; adenovirus
Vascular—related causes
    Kasabach-Merritt syndrome
    Renal artery stenosis
    Large vessel thrombosis
    Severe aortic coarctation
    Arteriovenous malformation
Oxidant exposure
Other
    Galactosemia
    Prolonged or recurrent acidosis
Intrinsic hemolysis
Enzymopathies
    Hexose monophosphate shunt abnormality (e.g., glucose-6-phosphate
        dehydrogenase)
    Embden-Meyerhof defect (glycolysis) (e.g., pyruvate kinase)
    Others
Red blood cell membrane defects
    Hereditary spherocytosis
    Hereditary elliptocytosis and related disorders
    Hereditary stomatocytosis
Hemoglobinopathies
    α-Thalassemia syndromes
    β-Globin cluster deletions
    Unstable hemoglobins

technologic advances in neonatal critical care have considerably lessened the impact of this disease.

Rh Disease. *Erythroblastosis fetalis* was the name given to a collection of findings characterized by hydrops fetalis, jaundice, anemia, and circulating erythroblasts. Later, this condition was determined to be due to fetal alloimmunization due to the Rh antigen (Chapter 58). Almost 1% of all pregnant women developed alloimmunization before the advent of antibody testing and routine prophylaxis of at-risk women with Rh immune globulin (92). Now the incidence of Rh disease is 10.6 cases per 10,000 births (93). This disorder and its management has been the topic of several recent reviews (93–97).

Pathophysiology. Delivery of erythrocytes that express Rh D antigen either by blood transfusion or by transplacental hemorrhage into the circulation of a mother who lacks the D antigen begins the alloimmunization process (Fig. 55-5). After the primary exposure to the Rh D antigen, repeat exposure leads to rapid production of anti-D immunoglobulin (Ig) G antibodies, which cross the placenta and attach to Rh antigen on fetal erythrocytes. Antibody-coated erythrocytes form rosettes on macrophages in the fetal reticuloendothelial system, particularly in the spleen, where they are removed from the circulation. This leads to hemolytic anemia, accelerating fetal erythropoiesis in the liver, spleen, marrow, and, in severe cases, extramedullary sites. Hemolytic anemia also liberates heme, which is ultimately metabolized into bilirubin and cleared by the placenta (97). Hyperbilirubinemia is a risk only for the delivered newborn.

The degree of Rh sensitization correlates with clinical severity and is directly related to the scale of the maternal antigen exposure (Fig. 55-6), with larger transplacental hemorrhage inducing more significant immunization (96). Severity is also correlated with the number of exposures, which worsens with each subsequent pregnancy. Pregnancies at greater risk for transplacental hemorrhage are those complicated by abruptio placentae, toxemia, spontaneous or therapeutic abortion, ectopic pregnancy, and those occurring after cesarean section.

Pregnancy Management. Positive or rising antibody titers alert the obstetrician early in pregnancy, indicating the need for increased surveillance of an Rh-sensitized pregnancy (95). Laboratory data on the genetic risk of fetal alloimmunization can be obtained by polymerase chain reaction–based amplification

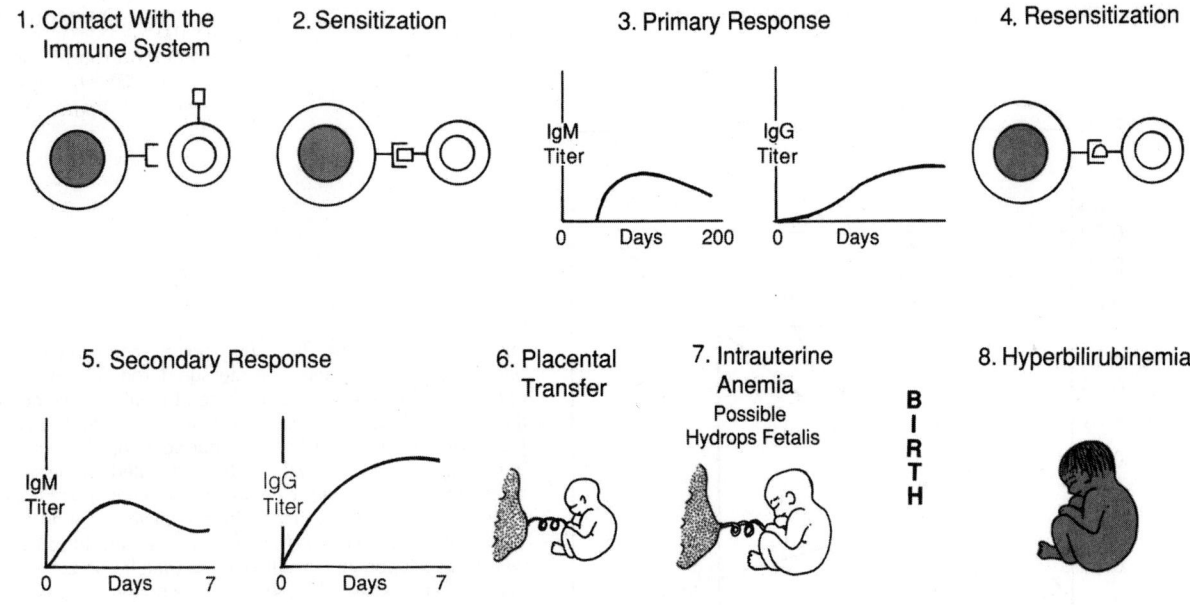

Figure 55-5. Necessary steps in the evolution of hemolytic disease of the newborn. Although the figure depicts the Rh D antigen, this sequence occurs in all prenatal sensitization, regardless of the red cell antigen involved. IgG, immunoglobulin G; IgM, immunoglobulin M.

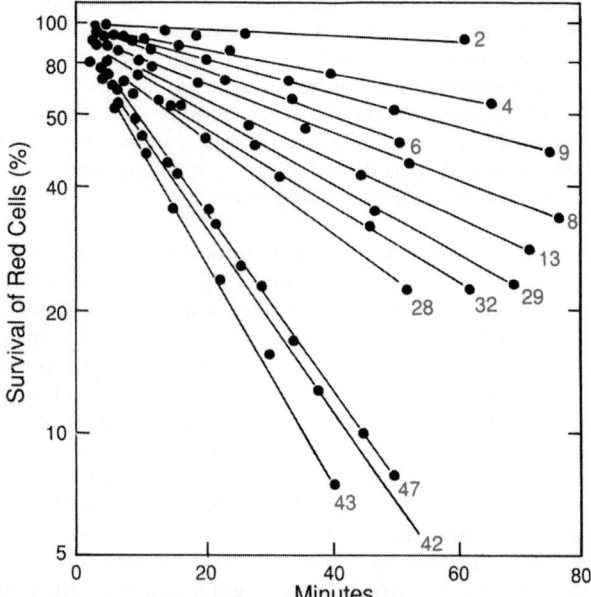

Figure 55-6. *In vivo* survival of Rh D–positive red cells coated with anti–Rh (D) antibody. The numbers next to each line represent the amount (µg/mL of red cells) of anti–Rh D antibody on the red cells. The greater the amount of antibody on the red cell, the shorter the red cell survival. (Adapted from Mollison PL, Crome P, et al. Rate of removable from the circulation of the red cells sensitized with different amounts of antibody. *Br J Haematol* 1965;11:461.)

assays to ascertain fetal blood type (98). In addition to serial antibody titers, the course of an Rh-sensitized pregnancy can be followed in a number of ways. One of these is by frequent ultrasound to assess fetal well-being, detect hepatosplenomegaly or hydrops fetalis, and assess the degree of anemia by Doppler studies (99). Recent studies have shown that moderate and severe anemia can be detected noninvasively by Doppler ultrasound by an increase in the peak velocity of systolic blood flow in the middle cerebral artery (100,101). Another method of fetal assessment involves sampling of amniotic fluid to assay for bilirubin pigments as determined by optic density (OD) read-

ings (Fig. 55-7) (96,102). Deviation from the OD at 450 nm, the absorption spectrum of bilirubin, ΔOD_{450}, is plotted on a curve (the Liley curve or modified Liley curve for pregnancies <24 weeks' gestation) that aids in prediction of the presence and severity of disease (95). Readings falling into high zone 2 or zone 3 indicate severe disease; values in zone 1 indicate either no disease or no anemia. Levels at the 65% to 70% of zone 2 before 24 weeks' gestation are an indication for fetal blood sampling. Finally, the liberal or primary use of fetal blood sampling to assess the severity of fetal anemia has been advocated by some. The development of hepatomegaly, splenomegaly, abnormal middle cerebral artery flow velocities, increasing optic density measurements, or the appearance of hydrops fetalis indicate a worsening prognosis and the need for *in utero* fetal transfusion or immediate delivery if the infant is at or near term.

Finally, careful labor and delivery planning and management with coordinated neonatal resuscitation are critical.

Neonatal Course and Treatment. The clinical severity in Rh alloimmunization is variable (103). Extreme cases of Rh sensitization lead to *in utero* fetal demise or death shortly after birth from circulatory failure. Severely affected infants, many hydropic, require vigorous resuscitation with mechanical ventilation, treatment of heart failure, replacement of red cell mass, diuresis, and phototherapy (94,96). Hypoglycemia and electrolyte abnormalities must be corrected. When stable, exchange transfusion may be indicated for treatment of anemia, hyperbilirubinemia, or both. Less severely affected infants typically require phototherapy and packed red cell transfusion.

Laboratory studies demonstrate a strongly positive direct antiglobulin test with the indirect test usually indicating large amounts of unbound anti-D antibody in the circulation of the infant. The degree of anemia is variable from mild to severe. The peripheral blood smear shows polychromasia and nucleated red blood cells (erythroblastosis). Indirect hyperbilirubinemia is very common; direct hyperbilirubinemia may develop in severe cases due to inspissated bile. Thrombocytopenia and neutropenia are common (104).

Overall, the incidence, severity, and associated morbidity and mortality of Rh disease has decreased (93). Even hydropic infants have less than 20% mortality. Anti-D prophylaxis, *in*

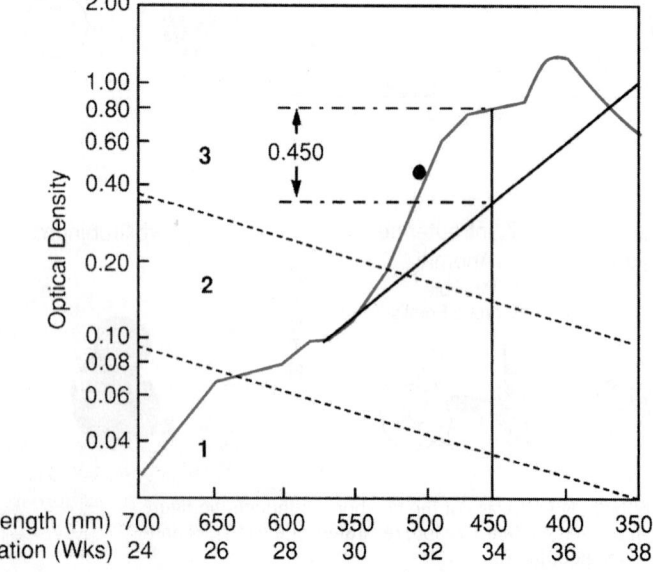

Figure 55-7. Amniotic fluid spectrophotometric measurement of bilirubin. The optical density is measured from 350 to 700 nm. The optical density at 450 nm contributed by bilirubin is measured by the increase in optical density at that wavelength above the projected baseline (*straight line*). The corrected optical density at 450 in this case is 0.45. This value is then replotted on the same graph, using the optical density scale on the Y axis and the gestational age scale on the X axis, and its position relative to zones 1, 2, and 3 (*spaces between slanted dashed lines*) is noted. In this case (32.5 weeks of gestation), the resultant point (*dot*) lies in zone 3, a region that indicated severe disease with impending fetal death. Zone 2 represents less severe disease, and zone 1 indicates very mild disease or an Rh-negative fetus. (Adapted from Bowman JM, Pollock JM. Amniotic fluid spectrophotometry and early delivery in the management of erythroblastosis fetalis. *Pediatrics* 1965;35:815.)

TABLE 55-12. Comparison of Rh and ABO Incompatibility

Characteristic	Rh	ABO
Blood group setup		
Mother	Negative	O
Infant	Positive	A or B
Type of antibody	IgG	IgG
Clinical aspects		
Occurrence in firstborn	5%	40% to 50%
Predictable severity in sub-sequent pregnancies	Usually	No
Stillbirth and/or hydrops	Frequent	Rare
Severe anemia	Frequent	Rare
Degree of jaundice	Moderate to severe	Mild
Hepatosplenomegaly	Frequent	Uncommon
Laboratory findings		
Direct Coombs' test (infant)	Positive	Positive or negative
Maternal antibodies	Always present	Not clear-cut
Spherocytes	Rare	Frequent
Treatment		
Antenatal measures	Yes	No
Phototherapy	Yes	Yes
Exchange transfusion	Sometimes	Rare
Late anemia	Frequent	Rare

IgG, immunoglobulin G.

TABLE 55-13. Relative Strength of Antigens on Cord Cells and Antigens Implicated in Hemolytic Disease of the Newborn

Antigen Strength	Blood Group System or Antigen	Causes HDN
I. Well-developed at birth	MNSsU	Yes*
	Rh	Yes
	Kell	Yes
	Duffy	Yes
	Kidd	Yes
	Diego	Yes
	Dombrock	Yes (mild)
	Scianna	—
	Gerbich	Yes (mild)
	En^a	—
	Yt^b	—
II. Present at birth; weaker than adult	ABH	Yes
	P	No†
	Lutheran	Yes
III. Very weak or absent at birth	Yt^a	—
	Vel	—
	Lewis	—
	I	No
	Sd^a	No

HDN, hemolytic disease of the newborn.
NOTE: In this table, superscript a and b refer to blood subgroups.
*Anti-M is rarely a cause of HDN.
†Anti-Tj^a (Anti-PP1P^k) has caused HDN.
Adapted from Kline W. Chemistry of blood group antigens and antibodies in hemolytic disease of the newborn. In: Bell C, ed. *A seminar on perinatal blood banking.* Washington, DC: American Association of Blood Banks, 1978:21.

utero transfusions, and optimal phototherapy have markedly decreased the need for exchange transfusion. Bilirubin encephalopathy due to Rh disease is now rare (96). Efforts to prevent Rh sensitization by the administration of Rh immune globulin in the appropriate clinical setting are ongoing (105).

ABO Incompatibility. Anti-A and anti-B antibodies are normally found in the serum of mothers who are group A, B, and O. These antibodies develop in response to a variety of antigens, such as bacteria, and do not require the passage of blood into the maternal circulation. In type A and B mothers, these "natural" antibodies are of the IgM class that does not cross the placenta, whereas in type O mothers, they are of the IgG class. In affected pregnancies, these preformed maternal anti-A or anti-B IgG antibodies are transferred across the placenta late in pregnancy or at delivery. Hemolysis of fetal cells occurs rapidly with splenic recognition and removal. Because fetal cells incompletely express A and B antigen sites, the cells do not agglutinate, and they may not be completely destroyed. Splenic removal of the antibody may damage the erythrocyte membrane, creating a microspherocyte. This process varies from Rh disease (Table 55-12), and because the antibodies are preformed, ABO incompatibility can affect the first pregnancy.

Affected neonates typically present with hyperbilirubinemia in the first few days of life (106). Anemia is usually mild, although severe anemia with hydrops fetalis has been reported. Reticulocytosis is prominent, and microspherocytes are frequently observed on peripheral smear. The diagnosis is confirmed in mother-infant dyads with the appropriate blood groups and a positive direct antiglobulin test. The number of antigen-antibody complexes on neonatal erythrocytes is frequently decreased due to removal in spleen, thus the antiglobulin test may only be weakly positive (or even negative in some cases) (107). Anti-A or anti-B antibodies can usually be eluted from the infant's cells, and a positive indirect antiglobulin test indicates free anti-A or anti-B alloantibodies in the infant's serum. Hyperbilirubinemia is usually treated with phototherapy. Exchange transfusion for severe hyperbilirubinemia or anemia is occasionally necessary.

Other Blood Group Incompatibility. Other blood group incompatibilities can cause hemolytic disease of the newborn (Table 55-13). Alloimmunization to Kell antigen is uncommon, but when it does occur, it can lead to significant disease in the fetus and newborn (108). Maternal anti-Kell antibodies are detected at approximately one-half the frequency of Rh antibodies. However, because of the low frequency of the paternal gene K:1, the risk of hemolytic disease of the newborn is estimated to be less than 5%. Kell alloimmunization differs from Rh disease because the Kell antigen is expressed on early erythroid progenitor cells, whereas Rh antigen is not. As a result, Kell alloimmunization leads to anemia from both hemolysis and suppression of fetal erythropoiesis (109,110). Decreased production of fetal red cells has been associated with decreased numbers of hemolyzed cells, thereby invalidating the use of the ΔOD_{450} in determining disease severity in some but not all cases (111).

OTHER CAUSES OF EXTRINSIC HEMOLYSIS

Anemia is sometimes present in neonates born to mothers with autoimmune disease, particularly systemic lupus erythematosus and rheumatoid arthritis. Neonatal lupus syndrome is caused by the transplacental passage of maternal autoantibodies, including SS-A/Ro, SS-B/La, and U$_1$RNP(nRNP). Clinical findings include complete congenital heart block, cutaneous lesions, anemia, thrombocytopenia, neutropenia, hepatitis, and pericarditis (112,113). Although most of the findings (including the anemia) are self-limited, the heart block is permanent.

Maternal autoimmune hemolytic anemia has led to neonatal anemia with a positive direct antiglobulin test (114–116).

Several medications, including penicillin, administered to the mother have been reported to cause hemolytic anemia in the newborn.

TABLE 55-14. Diagnostic Features of Some Transplacentally Acquired Infections Compared to Erythroblastosis Fetalis

Finding	Congenital Syphilis	Toxoplasmosis (Generalized Form)	Cytomegalic Inclusion Disease	Rubella Syndrome	Erythroblastosis Fetalis	Nonimmune Hemolytic Anemia
Anemia	++++	+++	++	++	+++	++
Jaundice	+++	+++	+++	+	+++	++
Thrombocytopenia	++	+	+++	+++	+	0
Hepatomegaly	++++	+++	++++	++	++	+
Splenomegaly	++++	++++	++++	++	++	+
Purpura	++	+	+++	+++	+	0
Skin rash	+	+	0	+	0	0
Chorioretinitis	+	+++	+	+	0	0
Intracranial calcifications	0	+	+++	+	0	0
Generalized edema	++	+	+	+	+	0
Additional findings	Mucocutaneous lesions, periostitis, snuffles, positive serology	Convulsions, microcephaly, hydrocephaly, positive dye test, lymphadenopathy	Pneumonia, cytomegalic inclusion cells in urine	Cataract, glaucoma, heart defects, deafness, microcephaly, hydrocephaly, bone lesion, Rubella virus (recoverable)	Positive Coombs' test, evidence of blood group incompatibility between mother and child	Morphology usually helpful

0, not described; +, present in approximately 1% to 25% of cases; ++, present in approximately 26% to 50% of cases; +++, present in approximately 51% to 75% of cases; ++++, present in approximately 76% to 100% of cases.
Adapted from Oski F, Naiman J. The hematologic aspects of the maternal-fetal relationship. In: *Hematologic problems of the newborn*. Philadelphia: WB Saunders, 1982:36.

ANGIOPATHIC ANEMIAS

Disseminated Intravascular Coagulation. Disseminated intravascular coagulation (DIC) is a common cause of anemia in neonates, most frequently in association with infection. Bacterial sepsis may be complicated by DIC, particularly sepsis due to group B streptococcus, *Escherichia coli*, and *Pseudomonas aeruginosa*. Congenital infections due to cytomegalovirus, rubella, herpes simplex, toxoplasmosis, syphilis, and human immunodeficiency virus have been associated with hemolytic anemia (30,113,117–119). This may be a diagnostic dilemma when other causes of hemolysis are not found. Differentiating these common disorders clinically can be an aid to diagnosis (Table 55-14). Neonatal enteroviral infection has been complicated by DIC and anemia (120). Although typically associated with a hypoplastic anemia, parvovirus B19 infection may present with hemolysis as well (see Parvovirus B19 Infection).

Of particular note is infection due to *Clostridium welchii* and *C. perfringens*. Neonates with necrotizing enterocolitis and clostridial infection have developed severe, rapidly progressive intravascular hemolysis. Shock, renal failure, hemolysis of the entire red cell mass, and death have occurred (121,122). These organisms produce several hemolytic toxins. One of these toxins cleaves sialic acids from erythrocyte membrane glycoproteins, forming and exposing the Thomsen-Friedenreich cryptantigen (or T antigen) (123). Anti-T antibodies are present in almost all adult plasma, thus transfusion of adult blood to a neonate lacking T antibodies can lead to life-threatening hemolysis.

Vascular-Related Causes Including Kasabach-Merritt Syndrome. Neonatal hemolytic anemia with microangiopathic changes has been described with renal artery stenosis, severe aortic coarctation, large vessel thrombi, arteriovenous malformations, and cavernous hemangiomas. *Kasabach-Merritt syndrome* is a local consumptive coagulopathy with hypofibrinogenemia, thrombocytopenia, and a microangiopathic anemia in association with a giant hemangioma that typically presents in the neonatal period (124,125). The coagulopathy and anemia, which may be severe, improve with regression or removal of the tumor. Treatment with α-interferon has improved the coagulopathy.

Oxidant Exposure. Oxidant hemolysis in the newborn is common and is not always associated with a known enzymopathy (Chapter 54) or with congenital Heinz body anemia (Chapter 50). It is an acute hemolytic event, presumably related to the oxidant sensitivity of neonatal red cells. Typically, infants present with sudden indirect hyperbilirubinemia, a drop in hematocrit, and the appearance of "bite" and "blister" cells, spherocytes, and some dense, contracted, irregularly shaped red cells on peripheral blood smear. Usually, no obvious source for the presumed oxidant stress is found, and the episode is over within a few days. Transfusion is rarely required. Infants with ongoing hemolysis warrant further diagnostic evaluation.

Other Causes of Hemolysis. Other causes of neonatal hemolysis include prolonged or recurrent acidosis, galactosemia, lysosomal storage disease, and some amino acidopathies. Although typically associated with a hypoplastic anemia, osteopetrosis may present with a neonatal hemolytic anemia. Maternal ingestion of valproic acid had caused hemolysis in a breast-fed infant.

Intrinsic Hemolysis

DISORDERS OF ERYTHROCYTE METABOLISM

Congenital nonspherocytic hemolytic anemia includes disorders not due to immune-mediated disturbances, defects of hemoglobin or the erythrocyte membrane, or other disorders. It is a heterogeneous group of disorders caused by a variety of metabolic abnormalities of the red blood cell, including enzymopathies of glucose, glutathione, and nucleotide metabolism. Clinical, biochemical, and genetic heterogeneity are common within individual enzymopathies. Hemolytic anemia can develop as a result of enzyme or antioxidant deficiency or as a result of impaired enzyme function.

DISORDERS OF THE HEXOSE MONOPHOSPHATE SHUNT AND ASSOCIATED PATHWAYS

Disorders of the hexose monophosphate shunt or the glutathione metabolic pathways impair the ability of the erythrocyte to adequately respond to oxidant stress. In the normal red cell, reduced glutathione detoxifies intracellular oxidants. In glucose-6-phosphate dehydrogenase (G6PD) deficiency, reduced glutathione levels are inadequate because of the inability to generate nicotinamide adenine dinucleotide phosphate, allowing oxidants free to damage critical erythrocyte proteins. Oxidation of the sulfhydryl groups of hemoglobin produces functionless methemoglobin and intracellular precipitates of hemoglobin called *Heinz bodies* (126).

Clinically, G6PD-deficient patients may suffer from acute hemolytic anemia after an oxidative stress, neonatal jaundice, or congenital nonspherocytic hemolytic anemia (127). Some patients are asymptomatic. All of these clinical syndromes have been observed in the neonatal period (127). Severe cases of hemolytic anemia with nonimmune hydrops may occur after maternal ingestion of an oxidant agent such as a sulfa drug, ascorbic acid, or fava beans (128–130).

Neonatal jaundice is rarely present at birth, with the peak incidence of onset between the second and third day of life. The degree of hyperbilirubinemia is quite variable. It may be severe and in some cases has resulted in kernicterus or even death (131). Occasionally, exchange transfusions are necessary. In most cases, hyperbilirubinemia is adequately treated with phototherapy (132). In most cases of neonatal jaundice associated with G6PD deficiency, the anemia is rarely severe. The etiology of neonatal jaundice is unknown. Decreased hepatic excretion of bilirubin and hemolysis have both been implicated (133). Neonatal jaundice may represent the manifestations of two unrelated genetic disorders. The incidence of neonatal jaundice is increased in G6PD-deficient infants with a polymorphism of the uridine diphosphoglucuronosyl transferase gene associated with Gilbert syndrome (134).

Hemolysis after transfusion or exchange transfusion with G6PD-deficient erythrocytes in neonates has been reported (135,136). It has been recommended that, in areas endemic for G6PD deficiency, blood donors be screened for G6PD deficiency before neonatal transfusion. The diagnosis and treatment of G6PD deficiency is discussed in Chapter 54.

DISORDERS OF THE EMBDEN-MEYERHOF PATHWAY

Defects of the Embden-Meyerhof pathway are inherited in an autosomal-recessive fashion and typically, hemolysis is only seen in homozygotes or compound heterozygotes. One exception is a defect in phosphoglycerate kinase, an X-linked disorder in which hemolysis is only seen in males. It has been suggested that hemolysis in these disorders results from insufficient levels of ATP. *Pyruvate kinase deficiency*, the most common abnormality of the Embden-Meyerhof pathway, usually presents in the neonatal period or early childhood with anemia and jaundice (Chapter 54). Severe cases have presented with severe anemia *in utero* or in the first days of life (137). In a few cases, nonimmune hydrops fetalis has occurred (137). Neonatal hyperbilirubinemia is common in pyruvate kinase–deficient individuals, and phototherapy or exchange transfusion may be required (138). Kernicterus has been reported.

Other abnormalities of the Embden-Meyerhof pathway have presented in the neonatal period (19). Glucose phosphate isomerase deficiency is the third most common hemolytic enzymopathy, and it is frequently manifest in infancy. Severe neonatal anemia and hyperbilirubinemia have been described, as have nonimmune hydrops and neonatal death (139). Hexokinase deficiency is characterized by significant phenotypic variability.

Severe cases have suffered from neonatal hyperbilirubinemia or anemia requiring blood transfusion. Isolated cases of neonatal jaundice, anemia, or both have been associated with 2,3-bisphosphoglycerate mutase deficiency and phosphoglycerate kinase deficiency.

DISORDERS OF GLUTATHIONE METABOLISM

Deficiency of γ-glutamylcysteine synthetase and glutathione synthetase, enzymes involved in red cell glutathione synthesis, has been associated with neonatal anemia (140,141).

DISORDERS OF THE ERYTHROCYTE MEMBRANE

Disorders of the erythrocyte membrane caused by defects in the erythrocyte membrane (Chapter 52) are an important group of hemolytic anemias that frequently present in the neonatal period. There is significant heterogeneity in the genetic, biochemical, and clinical manifestations of these disorders. Hereditary spherocytosis and hereditary pyropoikilocytosis are the membrane disorders most likely to present in the neonatal period.

Hereditary Spherocytosis
Clinical Findings. Hereditary spherocytosis (HS) frequently presents in the neonatal period with anemia and jaundice (142,143). Pallor, tachypnea, poor feeding, and jaundice are common presenting features. Anemia is present in over one-half of patients and may require transfusion. Severe anemia is uncommon (144). A few unusual cases have presented with *in utero* anemia and hydrops fetalis (144–146). Hyperbilirubinemia, present in over one-half of HS patients, occurs in the first few days of life and may rise rapidly. Kernicterus has occurred, so exchange transfusion may be required (142). Like G6PD deficiency, the co-inheritance of the Gilbert syndrome uridine diphosphoglucuronosyl transferase gene polymorphism accentuates neonatal jaundice in HS neonates (147).

Diagnosis. The diagnostic approach to a neonate with suspected HS should include a family history of anemia, jaundice, gallstones, and splenectomy. Laboratory investigation should include a complete blood count with examination of the peripheral smear. The MCHC is usually increased due to relative cellular dehydration. In one study, 19 of 23 HS neonates had MCHC values greater than 33.5%. The Technicon H1 blood counter (Bayer Corporation, Tarrytown, NY) provides a histogram of MCHC that is claimed to be accurate to identify nearly all cases of HS (148). The morphology on peripheral blood smear is variable. Spherocytes are present in variable numbers, with up to one-third of HS neonates lacking significant numbers of spherocytes on peripheral blood smear. Occasionally, erythrocyte morphology is bizarre with anisocytosis, fragmented cells, poikilocytosis, and numerous dense, small spherocytes.

The incubated osmotic fragility test has proven to be a reliable diagnostic test in the newborn period, and curves of normative neonatal osmotic fragility values should be used (149). A positive osmotic fragility test is not specific for HS but for any disorder with decreased membrane surface area and spherocytosis. In a few cases, transiently acquired spherocytosis due to alloimmunization may not be differentiated from HS even after detailed family history, clinical, and laboratory information is reviewed. Observation of the patient over the first few months to determine whether there is resolution of the cellular defect or persistence of hemolysis will clarify the diagnosis.

Clinical Course. Neonates with HS may experience more significant hemolytic anemia than adults. The etiology of this observation appears to be multifactorial. Variations in the neonatal intraerythrocytic environment and microcirculatory effects have been suggested to play a role in this increased hemolysis. As noted above, the inability of HbF to effectively bind 2,3-DPG leads to increased levels of 2,3-DPG in the neonatal erythrocyte. Increased levels of 2,3-DPG have been shown to destabilize the membrane junctional complex, which may worsen hemolysis (150). A shorter lifespan of the neonatal erythrocyte and the sluggish response of the marrow to erythropoietic stress in the first year of life contribute to the anemia. This final point has been clearly documented in a longitudinal study of 23 HS infants from birth to 1 year of age (151). An adequate reticulocyte response was not present during the first few months of life, and transfusions were frequently required. The requirement for transfusion resolved gradually as reticulocytosis improved.

HEREDITARY ELLIPTOCYTOSIS, HEREDITARY PYROPOIKILOCYTOSIS, AND RELATED DISORDERS

Hereditary elliptocytosis (HE) is characterized by the presence of elliptical or oval cigar-shaped erythrocytes on peripheral blood smears of affected individuals. The principal defect in HE is mechanical weakness of the erythrocyte membrane skeleton. Elliptocytosis rarely presents in the neonatal period, although anemia and jaundice may be observed. Occasionally, severe forms of HE may present with severe hemolysis, anemia, and jaundice and may require phototherapy and blood transfusions (152–154). In many of these severely affected infants, the hemolysis abates by 1 to 2 years of age, and the patient goes on to develop typical HE with mild anemia.

It has been estimated that approximately 12% of patients with HE will become symptomatic from their anemia at sometime during their life. The erythrocyte lifespan is normal in most patients, decreased in only approximately 10% of patients. It is this subset of HE patients with decreased red cell lifespan who experience neonatal hemolysis, anemia, and jaundice. Many of these patients have parents with typical HE and thus are homozygotes or compound heterozygotes for defects inherited from each of the parents.

Hereditary Pyropoikilocytosis. Hereditary pyropoikilocytosis (HPP) is a rare cause of severe hemolytic anemia with erythrocyte morphology on peripheral blood smear that is reminiscent of that seen in severe burns (155). HPP occurs predominantly in patients of African descent. There is a strong relationship between HPP and HE, as approximately one-third of parents or siblings of patients with HPP are affected with typical HE (154,156). Many patients with HPP go on to develop a clinical and laboratory course compatible with typical mild HE. Patients with HPP tend to experience severe hemolysis and anemia in infancy requiring red cell transfusion that gradually improves, evolving toward typical elliptocytosis later in life.

In addition to the peripheral blood smear findings found in HE, HPP erythrocytes are bizarrely shaped, with fragmentation and budding. Microspherocytosis is common, and the MCV is frequently decreased (50 to 65 fL). Pyknocytes are prominent in smears of neonates with HPP. The osmotic fragility is abnormal.

HEREDITARY STOMATOCYTOSIS SYNDROMES

The hereditary stomatocytosis (HSt) syndromes are a heterogeneous group of disorders characterized by mouth-shaped (stomatocytic) erythrocyte morphology on peripheral blood smear (157). Red blood cell membranes of HSt patients usually exhibit abnormal permeability to the univalent cations sodium and potassium, with resultant modification of intracellular water content. Clinical severity is variable; some patients experience hemolysis and anemia, while others are asymptomatic. Neo-

nates with HSt have been reported. Severe hemolysis, anemia, hyperbilirubinemia, and hydrops fetalis have been observed. None of the HSt syndromes are precisely defined in clinical, molecular, or genetic terms.

One HSt variant, dehydrated HSt (or xerocytosis), is characterized by a net loss of monovalent cations that produces shrunken, dehydrated red cells. In some kindreds, this anemia is associated with pseudohyperkalemia or fetal ascites, which resolve in the weeks following birth (158,159). Dehydrated xerocytosis and familial pseudohyperkalemia have both been linked to 16q23-q24, and, because of the phenotypic overlap, they may be allelic (160).

HEMOGLOBIN DISORDERS

There is significant variation in the fetal and neonatal manifestations of α- and β-thalassemia owing to differences in globin chain synthesis during development. α-Globin synthesis is present in the yolk sac by 3 weeks' gestation. By 9 weeks' gestation, α-globin is the main α-like globin in the fetus with only low levels of the major embryonic α-like embryonic hemoglobin, hemoglobin Portland ($\zeta 2\gamma 2$), present. In contrast, the switch from fetal to adult β-like globin chains, γ- to β-globin, is not complete until the end of the first year of life. The main hemoglobin in fetal and neonatal life is HbF ($\alpha 2\gamma 2$). As a result, abnormalities of α-globin, such as homozygous α-thalassemia, lead to severe anemia *in utero*, whereas abnormalities of β-globin, such as homozygous β-thalassemia, are typically ameliorated in early infancy by the sustained production of HbF. (See Chapter 49 and Chapter 50 for detailed discussion of the hemoglobinopathies.)

α-*Globin Defects*

Homozygous α-Thalassemia. The clinical severity of the α-thalassemia syndromes is related to the numbers of functional α-globin genes present (161). Deletion of a single α-globin gene results in a clinically silent asymptomatic carrier state. Deletion of two α-globin genes results in α-thalassemia trait with marked microcytosis, hypochromia, and mild anemia. Deletion of three α-globin genes results in hemoglobin H disease (see "Hemoglobin H Disease") with mild or moderate anemia. Deletion of all four α-globin genes results in homozygous α-thalassemia, which usually leads to death of the affected fetus *in utero* from severe hemolytic anemia, congestive heart failure, and hydrops fetalis. In homozygous α-thalassemia, the major hemoglobin present is a tetramer of unpaired non-α chains, γ4, or hemoglobin Bart. Survival of the homozygous fetus to late gestation or the newborn period depends on the presence and amount of hemoglobin Portland. In the rare case in which the child is born alive, death from cardiopulmonary collapse usually occurs shortly after birth.

Dramatic improvements in prenatal genetic diagnosis, interventional obstetric practice, and neonatal critical care are beginning to impact homozygous α-thalassemia (162). Genetic screening of at-risk populations, particularly Southeast Asians, is identifying couples at risk for conceiving an affected fetus and affected fetuses. In more than a dozen cases of homozygous α-thalassemia, careful pregnancy surveillance, aggressive *in utero* transfusion therapy, and postnatal transfusion therapy with iron chelation have led to prolonged survival (163). Concerns about congenital malformations and potential long-term neurologic effects of prolonged intrauterine hypoxia exist (162). Similar to some patients with β-thalassemia, bone marrow transplantation may provide a potential cure for these patients.

Hemoglobin H Disease. Infants with hemoglobin H (HbH) disease are born with a hypochromic, hemolytic anemia with microcytosis and red cell fragmentation (161,162). Neonatal hyperbilirubinemia may be significant. Hemoglobin electrophoresis demonstrates HbH β_4 and Hb Bart. Hydrops fetalis has been described in cases of nondeletional HbH disease (164,165). When microcytosis (with or without anemia) is detected, acute or chronic fetal-maternal hemorrhage, early α-thalassemia trait, or HbH disease are possible. Maternal Kleihauer-Betke testing, family history and ethnic origin (e.g., Southeast Asian), and hemoglobin electrophoresis will clarify the diagnosis.

β-Globin Defects. As noted above, structural variants of β-globin, including β-thalassemia and sickle cell disease, typically do not present with neonatal anemia. However, the incidence of neonatal hyperbilirubinemia in sickle cell disease is increased. In one rare case of sudden infant death in a patient with sickle cell disease, widespread neonatal vasoocclusion was observed (166). Importantly, hemoglobin S must be identified in newborn screens so that counseling and expectant management can be provided.

γδβ Thalassemia. Large deletions of the β-globin gene cluster lead to the phenotype of $\gamma\delta\beta$ thalassemia (reviewed in 167). These patients frequently present as neonates with a hemolytic, hypochromic anemia with prominent normoblastosis. Over time, the anemia improves with peripheral blood smear morphology similar to β-thalassemia trait.

Unstable Hemoglobins. *Unstable hemoglobins* are those hemoglobins that exhibit reduced solubility or higher susceptibility to oxidation than normal (Chapter 50). Both α-globin and β-globin chain abnormalities can lead to an unstable hemoglobinopathy, with α-chain abnormalities less commonly described owing to duplication of the α-globin genes. Precipitated globin fragments and heme form Heinz bodies, thus the name congenital Heinz body hemolytic anemia. The clinical symptomatology is heterogeneous. Severe neonatal jaundice and hemolytic anemia can occur.

Two interesting hemoglobin variants that presented with hemolytic neonatal anemia due to congenital Heinz body hemolytic anemia are Hb Hasharon and HbF Poole. Hb Hasharon is due to a mutation in the α-globin chain. When the mutant α-globin chains are paired with γ-globin, an unstable hemoglobin is produced (168). When the mutant chains are paired with β-globin, it is no longer unstable, presumably because of the tenfold greater affinity between α and β chains than α and γ chains. HbF Poole is an unstable hemoglobin due to a mutation in the γ-globin chain (169). As might be expected, both hemoglobins produce a neonatal hemolytic anemia that reverses to normal as the fetal-to-HbA switch occurs.

DECREASED ERYTHROCYTE PRODUCTION

Decreased erythrocyte production is an uncommon cause of neonatal anemia. The etiologies of this state can be classified as genetic syndromes (170), bone marrow replacement syndromes, infectious suppression, or due to other rare causes (Table 55-15).

Genetic Syndromes

DIAMOND-BLACKFAN ANEMIA

Diamond-Blackfan anemia (DBA) is a congenital, pure erythrocyte aplasia often diagnosed before the age of 6 months (Chapter 8) (170,171). There is moderate to severe aregenerative anemia

TABLE 55-15. Erythrocyte Underproduction

Genetic syndromes
Diamond-Blackfan syndrome
Congenital dyserythropoietic anemia
X-linked familial dyserythropoietic anemia
Fanconi's anemia
Shwachman syndrome
Pearson syndrome
Aase syndrome
Bone marrow replacement syndrome
Congenital leukemia
Transient myeloproliferative disorder—Down syndrome
Osteopetrosis
Infectious suppression
Viral—parvovirus B19, cytomegalovirus, rubella, herpes simplex, coxsackie B
Protozoal—toxoplasmosis
Overwhelming bacterial infection
Other
Maternal deficiencies [usually nutritional or genetic (e.g., transcobalamin II deficiency)] leading to neonatal anemia—iron, folate, and B_{12}
Medications to mother or neonate
"Late" hyporegenerative anemia of Rh disease

with absent or rare erythroid precursors in an otherwise normocellular marrow. Erythropoietin levels are elevated. Thirteen to 16% of children affected with DBA are diagnosed at birth, and it has been suggested that as many as 25% of DBA patients are anemic at birth. Growth retardation occurs in approximately one-fourth of patients. A wide variety of other abnormalities may be observed that brings the neonate to medical attention, including physical anomalies [particularly unusual thumb changes (bifid, triphalangeal, hypoplastic, or absent)] or radial abnormalities (hypoplasia or absent pulse) (172). Less specific anomalies include microcephaly, low hairline, hypertelorism, flat nose, cleft palate, high-arched palate, retrognathia, low-set ears, and webbed neck. Rarer abnormalities include genitourinary, cardiac (septal defects), and bony involvement. Interestingly, prenatal manifestations of severe anemia (e.g., hydrops fetalis) are rare in DBA fetuses (173,174). This has led to speculation that fetal erythropoiesis is spared *in utero* or that the erythropoietic defect is rescued by a putative placental or maternal factor (171). Treatment has included chronic transfusion therapy, steroids, growth factors, and transplantation.

CONGENITAL DYSERYTHROPOIETIC ANEMIA

Congenital dyserythropoietic anemia (CDA) is the name given to a group of rare disorders characterized by ineffective erythropoiesis, megaloblastic anemia, and distinct abnormalities of cellular architecture as seen on electron microscopy (Chapter 8). CDA is not technically a bone marrow failure syndrome; however, it does result in anemia without reticulocytosis. Three subtypes and a number of variants have been described (30). Type I CDA is characterized by megaloblastoid erythroid hyperplasia and distinct chromatin bridges between cells. Type II CDA is the most common variant and is characterized by multinuclear erythroblasts and a positive acidified serum test (i.e., the acronym HEMPAS, Hereditary Erythroblastic Multinuclearity with a Positive Acidified Serum test). Type III CDA is characterized by multinuclear erythroblasts and macrocytosis. All three subtypes of CDA may present in the neonatal period with megaloblastic anemia, hyperbilirubinemia, and hepatosplenomegaly due to extramedullary erythropoiesis. Approximately one-half of infants with CDA I present in the neonatal period (175,176). Anemia, hyperbilirubinemia, intrauterine growth retardation, and hydrops fetalis have been described. Syndactyly and other bony abnormalities have also been described in infants with CDA I. A recent review of CDA II showed that approximately one-fourth of patients experienced severe anemia in the neonatal period and that many required blood transfusions (177). Hyperbilirubinemia was common. Exchange transfusions were required in a few cases.

X-LINKED FAMILIAL DYSERYTHROPOIETIC ANEMIA
A kindred with X-linked anemia and thrombocytopenia due to a mutation in the erythroid and megakaryocyte transcription factor GATA1 has been described (178). Two male fetuses experienced severe fetal anemia with hydrops fetalis requiring *in utero* transfusion. Neonatal thrombocytopenia and anemia were present, and marrow examination showed dyserythropoiesis. Both children underwent successful bone marrow transplantation.

FANCONI'S ANEMIA
Fanconi's anemia (FA), an autosomal-recessive disorder involving a number of organ systems, is characterized by a steroid-responsive, hypoplastic macrocytic anemia with reticulocytopenia (Chapter 8) (170,179). Erythrocyte lifespan is shortened, and erythropoietin levels are elevated. FA cells demonstrate increased chromosomal instability and mutagen hypersensitivity (180). Diagnosis in the neonatal period is rarely due to anemia but instead is suggested by associated physical abnormalities (181). These abnormalities include hypoplasia or aplasia of the thumbs or radii, which may occur in slightly over one-fourth of patients. Other associated findings include low birth weight (approximately 10% patients), genitourinary defects, cranial defects, and hyperpigmentation of the skin. The gastrointestinal, cardiac, and musculoskeletal systems are variably involved. Thus, it is not surprising that FA patients diagnosed in the neonatal period have a much higher incidence of multisystem involvement than those diagnosed later in life (182).

SHWACHMAN SYNDROME
Shwachman or Shwachman-Diamond syndrome, a rare, autosomal-recessive disorder, is associated with exocrine pancreatic insufficiency that leads to diarrhea, abdominal distention, steatorrhea, and growth failure in the newborn period or early infancy (183). Ten percent of affected patients are small for gestational age at birth. Although neutropenia is most commonly observed, anemia and thrombocytopenia may precede or accompany the neutropenia (184). Aplastic anemia may develop in up to 25% of patients.

PEARSON SYNDROME
Pearson syndrome, a rare mitochondrial DNA deletion disorder, is associated with anemia, metabolic acidosis, and exocrine pancreatic insufficiency due to the deficiency of several enzymes involved in oxidative phosphorylation (185,186). The metabolic acidosis may be severe and may lead to significant morbidity and mortality. Hepatic and renal abnormalities are common. Occasional infants lack the metabolic derangements, and some present only with a refractory sideroblastic anemia. A macrocytic anemia is present in the neonatal period in 25% of patients and by 6 months of age in 70% of affected infants. Hydrops fetalis has occurred. Bone marrow aspirates demonstrate characteristic vacuolated myeloid and erythroid precursors, decreased numbers of erythroblasts, and many sideroblasts. Neutropenia and thrombocytopenia, usually mild, may be present.

AASE SYNDROME
Aase syndrome is a rare, congenital hypoplastic anemia with abnormally digitized thumbs (187). Growth failure and bony abnormalities may occur (188). The anemia is steroid responsive, and it improves with age.

Bone Marrow Replacement Syndromes
Anemia can develop as a secondary effect of bone marrow replacement syndromes. This has been observed in cases of osteopetrosis (Chapter 8), congenital leukemia (Chapter 15), and transient myeloproliferative disorder, frequently associated with trisomy 21 (Chapter 11 and Chapter 15).

OSTEOPETROSIS
Neonatal osteopetrosis typically presents as hepatosplenomegaly, craniomegaly, bony sclerosis, and a progressive anemia (189,190). Deafness, blindness, and other cranial nerve palsies may be observed. In this autosomal-recessive disorder, osteoclasts fail to resorb and remodel bone. This process leads to progressive constriction of the bone marrow cavity, leading to extramedullary hematopoiesis in the spleen and liver and a progressive macrocytic anemia with reticulocytosis. Early bone marrow transplantation has been successfully used to treat these patients (191,192).

CONGENITAL LEUKEMIA
True malignant congenital leukemias have been associated with stillbirth, fetal and neonatal anemia, and hydrops fetalis (193,194). Widespread infiltration of malignant cells with visceral fibrosis due to megaloblastic proliferation in the liver has been demonstrated in several cases of congenital leukemia and transient myeloproliferative disorder (193,194).

TRANSIENT MYELOPROLIFERATIVE DISORDER
Transient myeloproliferative disorder is characterized by the proliferation of myeloblasts in the marrow and blood of affected newborns, mimicking congenital leukemia and leukemoid reaction (195,196). It is more frequent in infants with trisomy 21. In contrast to congenital leukemia, spontaneous recovery occurs early in infancy. Anemia and thrombocytopenia are commonly observed, and cases of transient myeloproliferative disorder with hydrops fetalis have been described.

Infectious Suppression
Bone marrow failure can also present within the first few days of life as a result of a congenital infection (Table 55-14). As noted above, congenital infections can also present as hemolytic anemia (Table 55-14). A complete discussion of the individual infectious agents is beyond the scope of this chapter, but some important points on parvovirus B19 infection are noted in the following sections.

PARVOVIRUS B19 INFECTION
Parvovirus B19 is the etiologic of erythema infectiosum (fifth disease), a benign illness in normal children and adults that presents with fever, chills, vomiting, and diarrhea (197). A maculopapular exanthem on the face (slapped-cheek syndrome) is associated with the abatement of the fever. Parvovirus B19 selectively infects erythroid precursors and inhibits their growth.

Infection with parvovirus is a particular danger to susceptible pregnant women, because it can infect the fetus, leading to profound fetal anemia, nonimmune hydrops fetalis, and fetal demise (198,199). It has been estimated that 10% of fetuses whose mothers acquire a primary parvovirus infection during pregnancy will develop hydrops fetalis. If fetal demise does not occur, fetal anemia and the hydrops fetalis may resolve. *In utero* blood transfusion has been successfully employed to treat anemic, infected fetuses.

When a hypoplastic or aplastic anemia is detected in an anemic, hydropic newborn, and parvovirus infection is suspected, detection of parvovirus IgM antibody in the infant, analysis of serial, paired fetal and maternal IgG antibody, or detection of parvovirus protein or DNA in the placenta can confirm the diagnosis. The anemia of parvovirus will resolve within 10 to 14 days, during which time supportive care is indicated.

Other Causes of Erythrocyte Underproduction

NUTRITIONAL ANEMIA

Nutritional deficiencies are the most common cause of anemia in the first year of life, but they are an uncommon cause of neonatal anemia (reviewed in 30, 200). Iron deficiency anemia is uncommon in term infants. When present at birth, it is most common in neonates who have suffered significant prenatal blood loss such as fetal-maternal hemorrhage, because approximately three-fourths of the total body iron is stored as hemoglobin. Thus, infants born with anemia are also at risk for developing iron deficiency. Rapid growth without adequate supplemental dietary iron (particularly in the preterm infant), iron losses due to phlebotomy, and the use of erythropoietin in the neonate can lead to iron deficiency anemia. The preterm is at a higher risk for iron deficiency owing to its relatively lower blood volume, the need for increased diagnostic testing leading to greater phlebotomy losses, poor regulation of iron absorption, and failure to increase gastrointestinal iron absorption despite decreased serum ferritin levels.

Vitamin B_{12} deficiency has occurred in the breast-fed infants of strict vegetarian mothers, in the infants of mothers with pernicious anemia, and in breast-fed infants of mothers with chronic tropical sprue (201,202). It can also develop in the infants with malabsorptive abnormalities and inborn errors of vitamin B_{12} or related proteins, including deficiency of intrinsic factor, haptocorrin, or transcobalamin II. Other related disorders include the methylmalonic acidurias and deficiency of adenosylcobalamin or methylcobalamin (or both).

Folate deficiency is more likely to develop in preterm infants, in infants fed diets low in folate (including goat's milk or milk that has been boiled), and in infants with malabsorption. Other related disorders include congenital folate malabsorption, defective cellular folate uptake, and inborn errors of folate metabolism. Folate deficiency has been reported in infants who have had exchange transfusions, because the high levels of folate in the infant's blood have been replaced by normal adult values, which are relatively lower. The megaloblastic anemia of vitamin B_{12} or folate deficiency in infancy is similar to that observed in adults.

The sideroblastic, hypochromic anemia of copper deficiency is rare in the neonatal period. Preterm infants fed only milk, infants receiving prolonged parenteral nutrition without trace elements, and infants with chronic diarrhea and malnutrition are at risk.

MEDICATIONS

Hypoplastic anemia has been observed in neonates born to mothers taking various medications. Recent reports have observed that the administration of zidovudine alone (203,204) and in combination with lamivudine (205) for the treatment of maternal human immunodeficiency virus infection may result in a hyporegenerative neonatal anemia.

LATE ANEMIA OF RH DISEASE

Infants with Rh disease may develop a "late" anemia at 1 to 3 months of age characterized by significant anemia with retic-

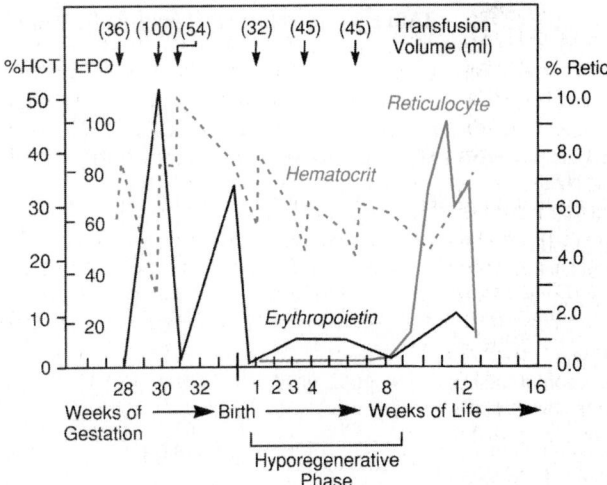

Figure 55-8. Hemoglobin, erythropoietin (in mU/mL), and reticulocyte levels during hyporegenerative anemia after intravascular transfusion for Rh hemolytic disease of the newborn. Arrows depict intravascular prebirth and postbirth transfusion. There is a prolonged postbirth decrease in erythropoietin levels. EPO, erythropoietin; HCT, hematocrit; Retic, reticulocyte. (Adapted from Thorp J, O'Connor T, Callenbach J, et al. Hyporegenerative anemia associated with intrauterine transfusion in rhesus hemolytic disease. *Am J Obstet Gynecol* 1991;165:79.)

ulocytopenia due to decreased erythrocyte production or continued destruction of reticulocytes from the persistence of high titers of maternal antibody (Fig. 55-8) (206,207). Based on case reports, it was initially thought that the incidence of late anemia was much higher in infants who had received intrauterine transfusions or postnatal exchange transfusions, but larger studies suggest this late anemia is found in both transfused and untransfused infants. Increased erythropoietin levels with reticulocytopenia has been observed (208). Transfusion is occasionally required, with indications including ineffective feeding, poor weight gain, persistent tachypnea, or tachycardia. Although erythroid progenitors from these patients are responsive to erythropoietin, clinical results of erythropoietin therapy have been disappointing, as its administration has failed to impact the need for transfusion. A similar "late" anemia has been observed in an untransfused infant with hemolytic disease of the newborn due to Kell alloimmunization (209).

PHYSIOLOGIC ANEMIA AND ANEMIA OF PREMATURITY

Physiologic Anemia

After birth, there is a sudden increase in hemoglobin saturation as the infant moves from maternal oxygenation to extrauterine circulation and pulmonary respiration. The degree of relative tissue hypoxia changes dramatically, erythropoietin levels fall, and red cell production begins to decrease. Eventually, the decreased oxygen-carrying capacity caused by decreasing hemoglobin concentration stimulates erythropoietin production, leading to increased red cell production and higher hemoglobin concentration. Term infants experience this gradual decrease in hemoglobin concentration over the first 8 to 12 weeks of life (Table 55-16). Hemoglobin concentration then remains stable for several weeks before gradually increasing. In term infants, this decline and rise in hemoglobin concentration has been termed *physiologic anemia*. These infants are asymp-

TABLE 55-16. Normal Hematologic Values during the First Year of Life in Healthy Term Infants

n	Age (mo)						
	0.5 (N = 232)	1 (N = 240)	2 (N = 241)	4 (N = 52)	6 (N = 52)	9 (N = 56)	12 (N = 56)
Hemoglobin (mean ± SE)	16.6 ± 0.11	13.9 ± 0.10	11.2 ± 0.06	12.2 ± 0.14	12.6 ± 0.10	12.7 ± 0.09	12.7 ± 0.09
–2 SD	13.4	10.7	9.4	10.3	11.1	11.4	11.3
Hematocrit (mean ± SE)	53.0 ± 0.4	44.0 ± 0.3	35.0 ± 0.2	38.0 ± 0.4	36.0 ± 0.3	36.0 ± 0.3	37.0 ± 0.3
–2 SD	41	33	28	32	31	32	33
Red blood cell count (mean ± SE)	4.9 ± 0.03	4.3 ± 0.03	3.7 ± 0.02	4.3 ± 0.06	4.7 ± 0.05	4.7 ± 0.04	4.7 ± 0.04
–2 SD + 2 SD	3.9–5.9	3.3–5.3	3.1–4.3	3.5–5.1	3.9–5.5	4.0–5.3	4.1–5.3
Mean corpuscular hemoglobin (mean ± SE)	33.6 ± 0.1	32.5 ± 0.1	30.4 ± 0.1	28.6 ± 0.2	26.8 ± 0.2	27.3 ± 0.2	26.8 ± 0.2
–2 SD	30	29	27	25	24	25	24
Mean corpuscular volume (mean ± SE)	105.3 ± 0.6	101.3 ± 0.3	94.8 ± 0.3	86.7 ± 0.8	76.3 ± 0.6	77.7 ± 0.5	77.7 ± 0.5
–2 SD	88	91	84	76	68	70	71
Mean corpuscular hemoglobin concentration (mean ± SE)	314.0 ± 1.1	318.0 ± 1.2	318.0 ± 1.1	327.0 ± 2.7	350.0 ± 1.7	349.0 ± 1.6	343.0 ± 1.5
–2 SD	281	281	283	288	327	324	321

SD, standard deviation; SE, standard error.
NOTE: These values were obtained from a selected group of 256 healthy term infants (followed at the Helsinki University Central Hospital) who were receiving continuous iron supplementation and had normal values for transferrin saturation and serum ferritin. Values at the ages of 0.5, 1, and 2 months were obtained from the entire group, and those at the later ages were obtained from the iron-supplemented infant group after exclusion of iron deficiency.
From Saarinen UM, Slimes MA. Developmental changes in red blood cell counts, and indices of infants after exclusion of iron deficiency by laboratory criteria and continuous iron supplementation. *J Pediatr* 1978;92:414.

tomatic, and this process appears to be a normal adaptation of the switch from intrauterine to extrauterine life.

Anemia of Prematurity

Preterm infants also experience this decline and rise in hemoglobin concentration. Although mean cord hemoglobin levels do not vary significantly between preterm and term infants, the decline in hemoglobin concentration occurs earlier in preterm infants (at approximately 4 to 8 weeks of age), and the hemoglobin concentration declines to values significantly lower than term infants, with the nadir varying inversely with gestational age (Fig. 55-9 and Table 55-17) (210). This dramatic fall in hemoglobin may cause symptomatology and require red cell transfusion. This condition, characterized by normocytic, normochromic anemia, reticulocytopenia, bone marrow hypoplasia, and erythropoietin levels inappropriately low for the level of anemia is nonphysiologic (211–213) and is termed the *anemia of prematurity*. The degree of anemia varies with the degree of prematurity, nutritional status and intake, chronologic age, and type and severity of underlying illness.

PATHOGENESIS

The pathogenesis of the anemia of prematurity is multifactorial (214). Preterm infants have a blunted response to erythropoietin, the primary growth factor for erythropoiesis. Hypoxia is the stimulus for erythropoietin production and secretion. After secretion, erythropoietin travels via the blood to hematopoietic tissues, where it stimulates the proliferation and differentiation of erythroid cells. In the fetus, erythropoietin is produced in the liver. Near term, production switches to the kidney. The sensitivity of the mechanisms that sense hypoxia in the fetal liver are decreased tenfold in the fetal liver, thus preterm infants have a decreased response to comparable levels of hypoxia and anemia than adults. Erythropoietin has greater clearance and a shorter half-life in preterm infants (215). Other factors influencing hemoglobin concentration in the preterm infant include a

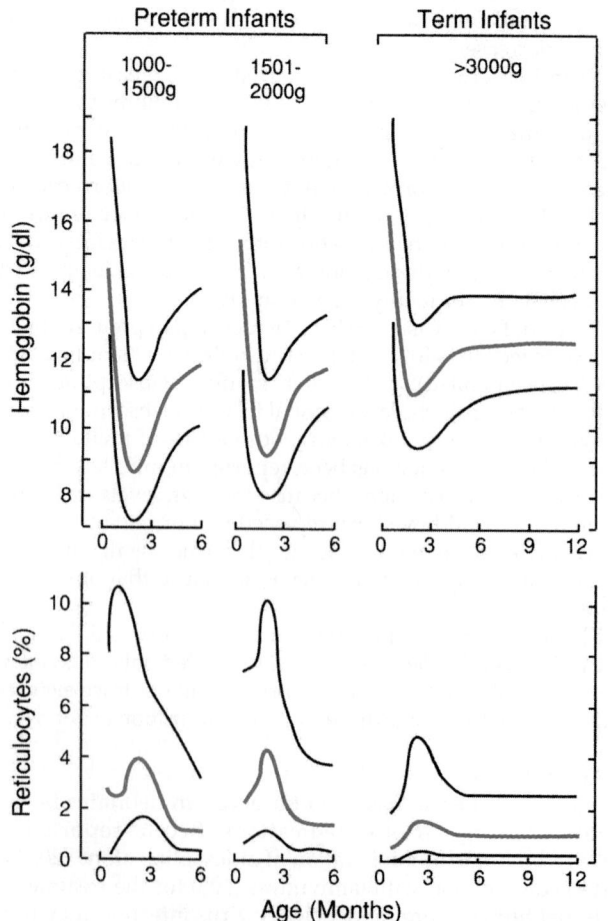

Figure 55-9. The mean (*colored*) and range (*black*) of normal hemoglobin and reticulocyte values for healthy and preterm infants. Premature infants become more anemic sooner after birth and return their hemoglobin toward normal later. (Adapted from Dallman PR. Anemia of prematurity. *Annu Rev Med* 1981;32:143.)

TABLE 55-17. Red Blood Cell Parameters of Very Low Birth Weight Infants during the First 6 Weeks of Life

	Day of Life	Valid n	Percentiles								
			3	5	10	25	Median	75	90	95	97
Hemoglobin (g/dL)	2	559	11.0	11.6	12.5	14.0	15.6	17.1	18.5	19.3	19.8
	12–14	203	10.1	10.8	11.1	12.5	14.4	15.7	17.4	18.4	18.9
	24–26	192	8.5	8.9	9.7	10.9	12.4	14.2	15.6	16.5	16.8
	40–42	150	7.8	7.9	8.4	9.3	10.6	12.4	13.8	14.9	15.4
Hematocrit (%)	3	561	35.0	36.0	39.0	43.0	47.0	52.0	56.0	59.0	60.0
	12–14	205	30.0	32.0	34.0	39.0	44.0	48.0	53.0	55.0	56.0
	24–26	196	25.0	27.0	29.0	32.0	39.0	44.0	48.0	50.0	52.0
	40–42	152	24.0	24.0	26.0	28.0	33.0	38.0	44.0	47.0	48.0
Red blood cells (10^{12}/L)	3	364	3.2	3.3	3.5	3.8	4.2	4.6	4.9	5.1	5.3
	12–14	196	2.9	3.0	3.2	3.5	4.1	4.6	5.2	5.5	5.6
	24–26	188	2.6	2.6	2.8	3.2	3.8	4.4	4.8	5.2	5.3
	40–42	148	2.5	2.5	2.6	3.0	3.4	4.1	4.6	4.8	4.9
Corrected reticulocytes (%)	3	283	0.6	0.7	1.9	4.2	7.1	12.0	20.0	24.1	27.8
	12–14	139	0.3	0.3	0.5	0.8	1.7	2.7	5.7	7.3	9.6
	24–26	140	0.2	0.3	0.5	0.8	1.5	2.6	4.7	6.4	8.6
	40–42	114	0.3	0.4	0.6	1.0	1.8	3.4	5.6	8.3	9.5

NOTE: On day 3, all infants are included irrespective of antenatal steroids and transfusions up to day 3. Thereafter, infants who did not receive recombinant human erythropoietin were studied, irrespective of use of antibiotics and steroids.
From Obladen M, Diepold K, Maier RF, et al. Venous and arterial hematologic profiles of very low birth weight infants. *Pediatrics* 2000;106:708.

shorter erythrocyte lifespan and dilution of hemoglobin by rapid growth. Continued phlebotomy and transfusion of adult blood with hemoglobin A further blunts the hypoxic stimulus for erythropoietin production and worsens the anemia.

DIAGNOSIS AND TREATMENT

Infants thought to be symptomatic from anemia of prematurity are reported to exhibit apnea, bradycardia, tachycardia, tachypnea, lethargy, poor feeding, increased oxygen requirement, and inadequate weight gain despite adequate caloric intake (216–218). Increased levels of lactate have been observed in anemic infants. It has never been adequately shown that symptoms of anemia are reduced after transfusion in a randomized controlled trial (219). In fact, several studies have documented a lack in improvement in clinical status in transfused versus untransfused infants (220,221). This has led to controversy over when and at what levels of hemoglobin transfusion is indicated.

The dramatic success of erythropoietin therapy in decreasing the need for transfusion in adult patients with end-stage renal disease offered an exciting new treatment modality for anemia of prematurity. Unfortunately, the impressive results obtained in adults have not been observed in preterm infants. Pilot studies were encouraging, with erythropoietin enhancing erythropoiesis in anemic, preterm infants. However, the increased erythropoiesis has not consistently reduced or prevented the need for transfusion. A large number of clinical trials have been performed with erythropoietin to treat the anemia of prematurity with variations in dose, routes of administration, and treatment schedules (reviewed in 222,223). A recent metaanalysis of controlled clinical trials analyzing the efficacy of erythropoietin in reducing blood transfusions in the anemia of prematurity detected benefit across high-quality studies using conservative transfusion criteria (224). However, there was marked variability in the results of clinical trials. These authors and others have concluded that there is currently insufficient data to recommend erythropoietin therapy as standard treatment for anemia of prematurity (224,225).

A more important goal than decreasing the number of blood transfusions in the treatment of the anemia of prematurity has been the reduction of the number of blood donors to which an infant is exposed (226). This has led to the development of conservative transfusion criteria, decreases in phlebotomy-related losses, provision of adequate supplemental iron, and use of "dedicated" units of red cells in neonatal transfusion therapy. A single-donor unit is "dedicated" to an individual infant that can be used multiple times over a period of up to 6 weeks to avoid multiple donor exposure (222,227). Adoption of restrictive transfusion guidelines in preterm infants may have a similar impact on red cell transfusion frequency as erythropoietin administration (228).

APPROACH TO THE ANEMIC INFANT

A thorough evaluation of the anemic neonate should combine history, physical examination, and laboratory investigation. Use of an algorithm may facilitate diagnostic evaluation (Fig. 55-10).

A detailed maternal history should be obtained. This should contain her medical history with particular attention to prior anemia, jaundice, transfusions, gallstones, or splenectomy as well as ethnicity. Obstetric history, including complications of labor and delivery and history of neonatal anemia or jaundice. Details of the pregnancy should be collected, including zygosity, medication use, history of vaginal bleeding, infections and exposure to infectious persons, exposure to oxidant compounds such as fava bean ingestion, and history of amniocentesis or trauma. Maternal blood type, antibody testing, and available hematologic parameters should be recorded. Fetal well-being during pregnancy should be documented. The presence of congenital malformations, abnormal ultrasound findings, amniocentesis and cordocentesis results, if performed, should be obtained.

Circumstances of the labor and delivery should be obtained. Placentation, history of vaginal bleeding, fetal distress, and history of external cephalic version should be sought. Route of delivery and the use of instrumentation to assist extraction (e.g., forceps or vacuum) should be noted. Breech delivery or difficult extraction should be noted. The presence of placental or vaginal bleeding should be recorded. Documentation by the delivery room team of an abnormal placenta or umbilical vessels, including tight nuchal cord, should be collected.

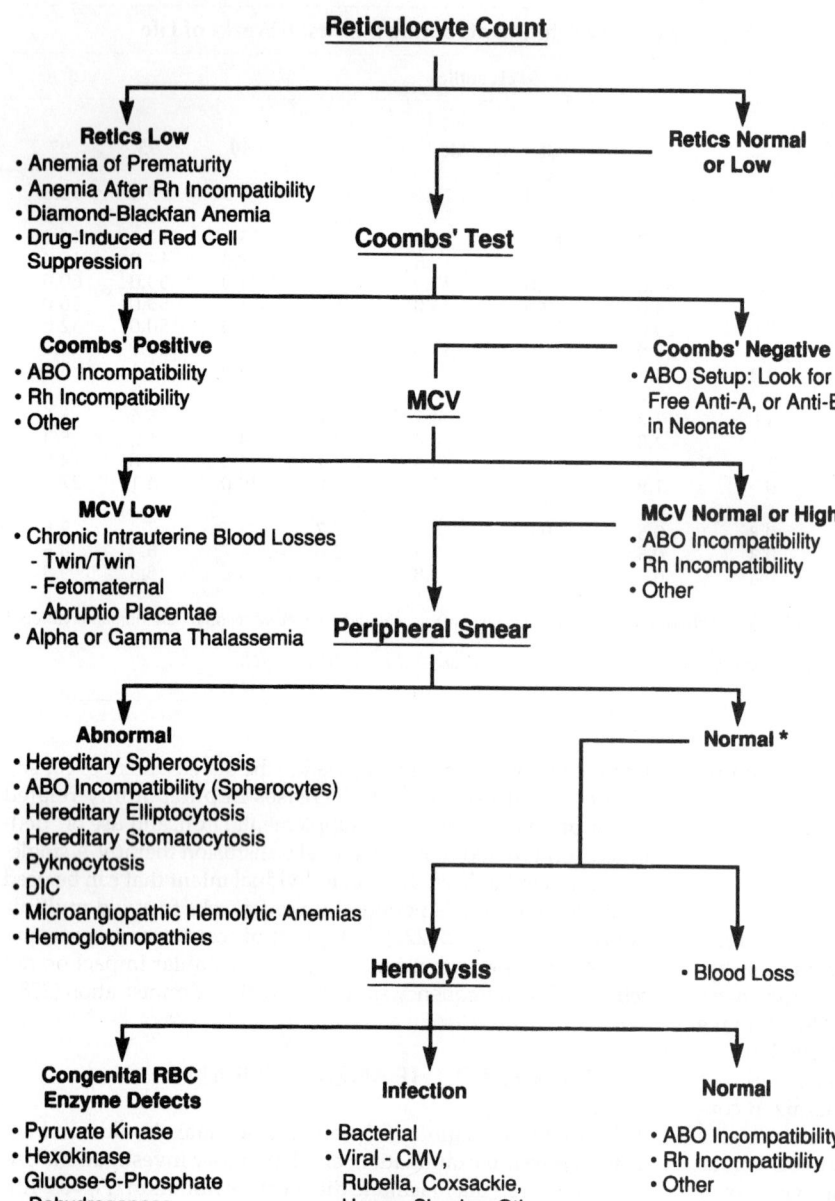

Reticulocyte Count

Retics Low
- Anemia of Prematurity
- Anemia After Rh Incompatibility
- Diamond-Blackfan Anemia
- Drug-Induced Red Cell Suppression

Retics Normal or Low

Coombs' Test

Coombs' Positive
- ABO Incompatibility
- Rh Incompatibility
- Other

MCV

Coombs' Negative
- ABO Setup: Look for Free Anti-A, or Anti-B in Neonate

MCV Low
- Chronic Intrauterine Blood Losses
  - Twin/Twin
  - Fetomaternal
  - Abruptio Placentae
- Alpha or Gamma Thalassemia

Peripheral Smear

MCV Normal or High
- ABO Incompatibility
- Rh Incompatibility
- Other

Abnormal
- Hereditary Spherocytosis
- ABO Incompatibility (Spherocytes)
- Hereditary Elliptocytosis
- Hereditary Stomatocytosis
- Pyknocytosis
- DIC
- Microangiopathic Hemolytic Anemias
- Hemoglobinopathies

Normal *

Hemolysis

- Blood Loss

Congenital RBC Enzyme Defects
- Pyruvate Kinase
- Hexokinase
- Glucose-6-Phosphate Dehydrogenase
- Other

Infection
- Bacterial
- Viral - CMV, Rubella, Coxsackie, Herpes Simplex, Other
- Parasitic - Toxoplasmosis
- Fungal - Rare

Normal
- ABO Incompatibility
- Rh Incompatibility
- Other

Figure 55-10. An approach to neonatal anemia. Asterisk indicates a smear with no predominant morphology. CMV, cytomegalovirus; DIC, disseminated intravascular coagulation; MCV, mean corpuscular volume. (Adapted from Oski F. Hematology: the erythrocyte and its disorders. In: Nathan DA, Oski FA, eds. *Hematology of infancy and childhood,* ed 4. Philadelphia: WB Saunders, 1993:38.)

A family history of anemia, jaundice, transfusions, gallstones, or splenectomy and paternal ethnicity should be sought.

The neonate's hospital course and available laboratory data should be reviewed. Particular attention should be paid to amounts of phlebotomy, performance of invasive procedures, surgery, and the need for transfusion or phototherapy.

Physical examination begins with inspection of the placenta, umbilical cord, and vessels, with special attention to the integrity and insertion of the umbilical vessels, the presence of lesions of the cord or placenta, and the presence of placental abruption. Careful physical examination of the neonate with evaluation for pallor, jaundice, hepatosplenomegaly, and congenital anomalies should be performed.

Initial basic laboratory evaluation includes a blood count with erythrocyte indices, examination of a peripheral blood smear, reticulocyte count, blood type, direct antiglobulin test, and serum bilirubin determination.

A positive direct antiglobulin test indicates immune hemolysis. Neonatal and maternal blood types should be compared, and maternal serum should be evaluated for the presence of antibodies.

A low reticulocyte count indicates inadequate red cell production. Maternal history of possible parvoviral infection should be sought and additional diagnostic testing, such as parvovirus titers and marrow analysis, pursued.

Microcytosis in an anemic infant suggests the presence of a hemoglobinopathy, HbH disease or δβγ thalassemia, or recovery from chronic hemorrhage such as fetomaternal or twin-twin transfusion. Hypochromia due to iron deficiency is common with chronic hemorrhage. Neonatal normoblastosis is prominent in chronic hemorrhage and δβγ thalassemia. Hemoglobin electrophoresis and maternal Kleihauer-Betke testing can differentiate these disorders.

The presence of hemolysis on peripheral blood smear in an infant with a negative antiglobulin test and hyperbilirubinemia suggests an intrinsic erythrocyte defect. In some cases, such as hereditary spherocytosis, erythrocyte morphology on blood smear is suggestive of the diagnosis. Additional diagnostic evaluation such as osmotic fragility testing or red cell enzyme determinations are indicated. It is important to note that the serum haptoglobin is low or undetectable in healthy infants without hemolysis and is not a useful adjunct in the investigation of neonatal hemolytic anemia (229).

The infant with a normocytic, normochromic nonhemolytic anemia and a negative direct antiglobulin test should be suspected of having had acute blood loss. Maternal Kleihauer-Betke testing should be performed. If the etiology remains cryptic, ultrasonography of the head and abdomen to detect occult hemorrhage should be considered.

REFERENCES

1. Ohls RK. Developmental erythropoiesis. In: Polin RA, Fox WW, eds. *Fetal and neonatal physiology*, 2nd ed. Philadelphia: WB Saunders, 1997:1762.
2. Forestier F, Daffos F, Galacteros F, et al. Hematological values of 163 normal fetuses between 18 and 30 weeks of gestation. *Pediatr Res* 1986;20:342.
3. Zipursky A, Brown E, Palko J, et al. The erythrocyte differential count in newborn infants. *Am J Pediatr Hematol Oncol* 1983;5:45.
4. Holroyde CP, Oski FA, Gardner FH. The "pocked" erythrocyte. Red-cell surface alterations in reticuloendothelial immaturity of the neonate. *N Engl J Med* 1969;281:516.
5. Eguchi K, Sawai T, Mizutani Y, et al. Comparative study of erythrocyte deformability in maternal and cord blood. *Am J Perinatol* 1995;12:39.
6. Gross GP, Hathaway WE. Fetal erythrocyte deformability. *Pediatr Res* 1972;6:593.
7. Neerhout RC. Erythrocyte lipids in the neonate. *Pediatr Res* 1968;2:172.
8. Sjolin S. The resistance of red cells in vitro: a study of the osmotic properties, mechanical resistance and the storage behavior of red cells of fetuses, children, and adults. *Acta Paediatr Scand* 1954;43:1.
9. Calatroni A, Cordaro V, Salpietro C, et al. Erythrocyte membrane sialic acid in newborn infants. *Acta Haematol* 1984;71:198.
10. Adler SM, Denton RL. The erythrocyte sedimentation rate in the newborn period. *J Pediatr* 1975;86:942.
11. Colin FC, Schrier SL. Myosin content and distribution in human neonatal erythrocytes are different from adult erythrocytes. *Blood* 1991;78:3052.
12. Koekebakker M, Barr RD. Acetylcholinesterase in the human erythron. I. Cytochemistry. *Am J Hematol* 1988;28:252.
13. Brugnara C, Platt OS. The neonatal erythrocyte and its disorders. In: Nathan DG, Orkin SH, eds. *Hematology of infancy and childhood*, 5th ed. Philadelphia: WB Saunders, 1998:19.
14. Fukuda M, Dell A, Fukuda MN. Structure of fetal lactosaminoglycan. The carbohydrate moiety of Band 3 isolated from human umbilical cord erythrocytes. *J Biol Chem* 1984;259:4782.
15. Fukuda M, Dell A, Oates JE, et al. Structure of branched lactosaminoglycan, the carbohydrate moiety of band 3 isolated from adult human erythrocytes. *J Biol Chem* 1984;259:8260.
16. Kleihauer E, Braun H, Betke K. Demonstration of fetal hemoglobin in erythrocytes of a blood smear. *Klin Wochenschr* 1957;35:637.
17. Advani R, Mentzer W, Andrews D, et al. Oxidation of hemoglobin F is associated with the aging process of neonatal red blood cells. *Pediatr Res* 1992; 32:165.
18. Bard H, Teasdale F. Red cell oxygen affinity, hemoglobin type, 2,3-diphosphoglycerate, and pH as a function of fetal development. *Pediatrics* 1979;64: 483.
19. Gallagher PG. Disorders of erythrocyte metabolism and shape. In: Christensen RD, ed. *Hematologic problems of the neonate*. Philadelphia: WB Saunders, 2000:209.
20. Bentley HP Jr, Alford CA Jr, Diseker M. Erythrocyte glucose consumption in the neonate. *J Lab Clin Med* 1970;76:311.
21. Travis SF, Kumar SP, Paez PC, et al. Red cell metabolic alterations in postnatal life in term infants: glycolytic enzymes and glucose-6-phosphate dehydrogenase. *Pediatr Res* 1980;14:1349.
22. Jain SK. The neonatal erythrocyte and its oxidative susceptibility. *Semin Hematol* 1989;26:286.
23. Stockman JA, Clark DA. Diminished antioxidant activity of newborn infants. *Pediatr Res* 1981;11:41.
24. Glader BE, Conrad ME. Decreased glutathione peroxidase in neonatal erythrocytes: lack of relation to hydrogen peroxide metabolism. *Pediatr Res* 1972; 6:900.
25. Agostoni A, Gerli GC, Beretta L, et al. Superoxide dismutase, catalase and glutathione peroxidase activities in maternal and cord blood erythrocytes. *J Clin Chem Clin Biochem* 1980;18:771.
26. Pearson HA. Life-span of the fetal red blood cell. *J Pediatr* 1967;70:166.
27. Mollison PL. The survival of transfused erythrocytes in hemolytic disease of the newborn. *Arch Dis Child* 1943;18:161.
28. Bard H, Widness JA. The life span of erythrocytes transfused to preterm infants. *Pediatr Res* 1997;42:9.
29. Christensen RD. Expected hematologic values for term and preterm neonates. In: Christensen RD, ed. *Hematologic problems of the neonate*. Philadelphia: WB Saunders, 2000:117.
30. Ohls RK. Evaluation and treatment of anemia in the neonate. In: Christensen RD, ed. *Hematologic problems of the neonate*. Philadelphia: WB Saunders, 2000: 137.
31. Udupa KB, Crabtree HM, Lipschitz DA. In vitro culture of proerythroblasts: characterization of proliferative response to erythropoietin and steroids. *Br J Haematol* 1986;62:705.
32. Usher R, Shephard M, Lind J. The blood volume of the newborn infant and placental transfusion. *Acta Paediatr* 1963;52:497.
33. Yao AC, Lind J, Tiisala R, et al. Placental transfusion in the premature infant with observation on clinical course and outcome. *Acta Paediatr Scand* 1969; 58:561.
34. Linderkamp O, Versmold HT, Strohhacker I, et al. Capillary-venous hematocrit differences in newborn infants. I. Relationship to blood volume, peripheral blood flow, and acid base parameters. *Eur J Pediatr* 1977;127:9.
35. Michaels LA, Cohen AR, Zhao H, et al. Screening for hereditary spherocytosis by use of automated erythrocyte indexes. *J Pediatr* 1997;130:957.
36. Giacoia GP. Severe fetomaternal hemorrhage: a review. *Obstet Gynecol Surv* 1997;52:372.
37. Scott JR, Warenski JC. Tests to detect and quantitate fetomaternal bleeding. *Clin Obstet Gynecol* 1982;25:277.
38. Patton WN, Nicholson GS, Sawers AH, et al. Assessment of fetal-maternal haemorrhage in mothers with hereditary persistence of fetal haemoglobin. *J Clin Pathol* 1990;43:728.
39. Ananth CV, Berkowitz GS, Savitz DA, et al. Placental abruption and adverse perinatal outcomes. *JAMA* 1999;282:1646.
40. Rasmussen S, Irgens LM, Bergsjo P, et al. Perinatal mortality and case fatality after placental abruption in Norway 1967-1991. *Acta Obstet Gynecol Scand* 1996;75:229.
41. Ananth CV, Wilcox AJ. Placental abruption and perinatal mortality in the United States. *Am J Epidemiol* 2001;153:332.
42. Frederiksen MC, Glassenberg R, Stika CS. Placenta previa: a 22-year analysis. *Am J Obstet Gynecol* 1999;180:1432.
43. Crane JM, van den Hof MC, Dodds L, et al. Neonatal outcomes with placenta previa. *Obstet Gynecol* 1999;93:541.
44. Lee W, Lee VL, Kirk JS, et al. Vasa previa: prenatal diagnosis, natural evolution, and clinical outcome. *Obstet Gynecol* 2000;95:572.
45. Eddleman KA, Lockwood CJ, Berkowitz GS, et al. Clinical significance and sonographic diagnosis of velamentous umbilical cord insertion. *Am J Perinatol* 1992;9:123.
46. Nomiyama M, Toyota Y, Kawano H. Antenatal diagnosis of velamentous umbilical cord insertion and vasa previa with color Doppler imaging. *Ultrasound Obstet Gynecol* 1998;12:426.
47. van Gemert MJ, Umur A, Tijssen JG, et al. Twin-twin transfusion syndrome: etiology, severity and rational management. *Curr Opin Obstet Gynecol* 2001; 13:193.
48. Berghella V, Kaufmann M. Natural history of twin-twin transfusion syndrome. *J Reprod Med* 2001;46:480.
49. Seng YC, Rajadurai VS. Twin-twin transfusion syndrome: a five year review. *Arch Dis Child Fetal Neonatal Ed* 2000;83:F168.
50. Taylor MJ, Denbow ML, Duncan KR, et al. Antenatal factors at diagnosis that predict outcome in twin-twin transfusion syndrome. *Am J Obstet Gynecol* 2000;183:1023.
51. Roberts D, Neilson JP, Weindling AM. Interventions for the treatment of twin-twin transfusion syndrome (Cochrane Review). *Cochrane Database Syst Rev* 2001;1.
52. Cincotta RB, Gray PH, Phythian G, et al. Long term outcome of twin-twin transfusion syndrome. *Arch Dis Child Fetal Neonatal Ed* 2000;83:F171.
53. Laml T, Egermann R, Lapin A, et al. Feto-maternal hemorrhage after a car accident: a case report. *Acta Obstet Gynecol Scand* 2001;80:480.
54. Pearlman MD, Tintinalli JE, Lorenz RP. A prospective controlled study of outcome after trauma during pregnancy. *Am J Obstet Gynecol* 1990;162:1502.
55. Rose PG, Strohm PL, Zuspan FP. Fetomaternal hemorrhage following trauma. *Am J Obstet Gynecol* 1985;153:844.
56. Sikovanyecz J, Horvath E, Sallay E, et al. Fetomaternal transfusion and pregnancy outcome after cordocentesis. *Fetal Diagn Ther* 2001;16:83.
57. Ghidini A, Korker V. Fetal complication after external cephalic version at term: case report and literature review. *J Matern Fetal Med* 1999;8:190.
58. Gersell DJ. Selected vascular lesions of the placenta. *Clin Lab Med* 1995; 15:611.
59. Brandt CA, Ryom C, Grove A. Chorioangioma placentae and feto-maternal transfusion; a report of two cases. *Eur J Obstet Gynecol Reprod Biol* 1989;33:95.
60. Takai N, Miyazaki T, Yoshimatsu J, et al. Intraplacental choriocarcinoma with fetomaternal transfusion. *Pathol Int* 2000;50:258.
61. Franca-Martins AM, Graubard Z, Holloway GA, et al. Placental haemangioma associated with acute fetal anemia in labour. *Acta Med Port* 1990;3:187.
62. Deans A, Jauniaux E. Prenatal diagnosis and outcome of subamniotic hematomas. *Ultrasound Obstet Gynecol* 1998;11:319.
63. Bose C. Hydrops fetalis and in utero intracranial hemorrhage. *J Pediatr* 1978; 93:1023.
64. Coulson CC, Kuller JA, Sweeney WJ. Nonimmune hydrops and hydrocephalus secondary to fetal intracranial hemorrhage. *Am J Perinatol* 1994;11:253.

65. Burrows RF, Caco CC, Kelton JG. Neonatal alloimmune thrombocytopenia: spontaneous in utero intracranial hemorrhage. *Am J Hematol* 1988;28:98.
66. Bussel JB, Zabusky MR, Berkowitz RL, et al. Fetal alloimmune thrombocytopenia. *N Engl J Med* 1997;337:22.
67. Seward JF, Zusman J. Hydrops fetalis associated with small-bowel volvulus. *Lancet* 1978;2:52.
68. Molteni RA. Perinatal blood loss. *Pediatr Rev* 1990;12:47.
69. Lubin B. Neonatal anaemia secondary to blood loss. *Clin Haematol* 1978;7:19.
70. Benirschke K. Obstetrically important lesions of the umbilical cord. *J Reprod Med* 1994;39:262.
71. Cashore WJ, Usher RH. Hypovolemia resulting from a tight nuchal cord at birth. *Pediatr Res* 1973;7:399.
72. Shepherd AJ, Richardson CJ, Brown JP. Nuchal cord as a cause of neonatal anemia. *Am J Dis Child* 1985;139:71.
73. Chadwick LM, Pemberton PJ, Kurinczuk JJ. Neonatal subgaleal haematoma: associated risk factors, complications and outcome. *J Paediatr Child Health* 1996;32:228.
74. Florentino-Pineda I, Ezhuthachan SG, Sineni LG, et al. Subgaleal hemorrhage in the newborn infant associated with silicone elastomer vacuum extractor. *J Perinatol* 1994;14:95.
75. Benaron DA. Subgaleal hematoma causing hypovolemic shock during delivery after failed vacuum extraction: a case report. *J Perinatol* 1993;13:228.
76. Leonard S, Anthony B. Giant cephalohematoma of newborn. *Am J Dis Child* 1961;101:170.
77. Thorp JA, Poskin MF, McKenzie DR, et al. Perinatal factors predicting severe intracranial hemorrhage. *Am J Perinatol* 1997;14:631.
78. Verma U, Tejani N, Klein S, et al. Obstetric antecedents of intraventricular hemorrhage and periventricular leukomalacia in the low-birth-weight neonate. *Am J Obstet Gynecol* 1997;176:275.
79. Eraklis AJ. Abdominal injury related to the trauma of birth. *Pediatrics* 1967;39:421.
80. Emma F, Smith J, Moerman PH, et al. Subcapsular hemorrhage of the liver and hemoperitoneum in premature infants: report of 4 cases. *Eur J Obstet Gynecol Reprod Biol* 1992;44:161.
81. Davies MR. Iatrogenic hepatic rupture in the newborn and its management by pack tamponade. *J Pediatr Surg* 1997;32:1414.
82. Leape LL, Bordy MD. Neonatal rupture of the spleen. Report of a case successfully treated after spontaneous cessation of hemorrhage. *Pediatrics* 1971;47:101.
83. Philipsborn JFJ, Traisman HS, et al. Rupture of the spleen: a complication of erythroblastosis fetalis. *N Engl J Med* 1955;252:159.
84. Reish O, Nachum E, Naor N, et al. Hemophilia B in a neonate: unusual early spontaneous gastrointestinal bleeding. *Am J Perinatol* 1994;11:192.
85. Stahl MM, Neiderud J, Vinge E. Thrombocytopenic purpura and anemia in a breast-fed infant whose mother was treated with valproic acid. *J Pediatr* 1997;130:1001.
86. Obladen M, Sachsenweger M, Stahnke M. Blood sampling in very low birth weight infants receiving different levels of intensive care. *Eur J Pediatr* 1988;147:399.
87. Lin JC, Strauss RG, Kulhavy JC, et al. Phlebotomy overdraw in the neonatal intensive care nursery. *Pediatrics* 2000;106:E19.
88. Nader PR, Margolin F. Hemangioma causing gastrointestinal bleeding. Case report and review of the literature. *Am J Dis Child* 1966;111:215.
89. Nagaya M, Kato J, Niimi N, et al. Isolated cavernous hemangioma of the stomach in a neonate. *J Pediatr Surg* 1998;33:653.
90. Drut R, Sapia S, Gril D, et al. Nonimmune hydrops fetalis, hydramnios, microcephaly, and intracranial meningeal hemangioendothelioma. *Pediatr Pathol* 1993;13:9.
91. Sharara FI, Khoury AN. Prenatal diagnosis of a giant cavernous hemangioma in association with nonimmune hydrops. A case report. *J Reprod Med* 1994;39:547.
92. Wegmann A, Gluck R. The history of rhesus prophylaxis with anti-D. *Eur J Pediatr* 1996;155:835.
93. Greenough A. Rhesus disease: postnatal management and outcome. *Eur J Pediatr* 1999;158:689.
94. Peterec SM. Management of neonatal Rh disease. *Clin Perinatol* 1995;22:561.
95. Gollin YG, Copel JA. Management of the Rh-sensitized mother. *Clin Perinatol* 1995;22:545.
96. Urbaniak SJ, Greiss MA. RhD haemolytic disease of the fetus and the newborn. *Blood Rev* 2000;14:44.
97. Shier RW, Dilts PV Jr, Conger WL, et al. Bilirubin transfer across the human placenta. *Am J Obstet Gynecol* 1971;111:677.
98. Avent ND, Finning KM, Martin PG, et al. Prenatal determination of fetal blood group status. *Vox Sang* 2000;78:155.
99. Roberts AB, Mitchell JM, Lake Y, et al. Ultrasonographic surveillance in red blood cell alloimmunization. *Am J Obstet Gynecol* 2001;184:1251.
100. Mari G, Deter RL, Carpenter RL, et al. Noninvasive diagnosis by Doppler ultrasonography of fetal anemia due to maternal red-cell alloimmunization. Collaborative Group for Doppler Assessment of the Blood Velocity in Anemic Fetuses. *N Engl J Med* 2000;342:9.
101. Bahado-Singh RO, Oz AU, Hsu C, et al. Middle cerebral artery Doppler velocimetric deceleration angle as a predictor of fetal anemia in Rh-alloimunized fetuses without hydrops. *Am J Obstet Gynecol* 2000;183:746.
102. Oepkes D. Invasive versus non-invasive testing in red-cell alloimmunized pregnancies. *Eur J Obstet Gynecol Reprod Biol* 2000;92:83.
103. Bowman J. The management of hemolytic disease in the fetus and newborn. *Semin Perinatol* 1997;21:39.
104. Koenig JM, Christensen RD. Neutropenia and thrombocytopenia in infants with Rh hemolytic disease. *J Pediatr* 1989;114:625.
105. Hartwell EA. Use of Rh immune globulin: ASCP practice parameter. American Society of Clinical Pathologists. *Am J Clin Pathol* 1998;110:281.
106. Kanto WP Jr, Marino B, Godwin AS, et al. ABO hemolytic disease: a comparative study of clinical severity and delayed anemia. *Pediatrics* 1978;62:365.
107. Voak D, Williams MA. An explanation of the failure of the direct antiglobulin test to detect erythrocyte sensitization in ABO haemolytic disease of the newborn and observations on pinocytosis of IgG anti-A antibodies by infant (cord) red cells. *Br J Haematol* 1971;20:9.
108. Grant SR, Kilby MD, Meer L, et al. The outcome of pregnancy in Kell alloimmunisation. *BJOG* 2000;107:481.
109. Giannacopoulou CH, Relakis K, Kalmanti M. Severe anemia due to Kell alloimmunization. *Haematologia* 1997;28:173.
110. Vaughan JI, Manning M, Warwick RM, et al. Inhibition of erythroid progenitor cells by anti-Kell antibodies in fetal alloimmune anemia. *N Engl J Med* 1998;338:798.
111. McKenna DS, Nagaraja HN, O'Shaughnessy R. Management of pregnancies complicated by anti-Kell isoimmunization. *Obstet Gynecol* 1999;93:667.
112. Watson RM, Lane AT, Barnett NK, et al. Neonatal lupus erythematosus. A clinical, serological and immunogenetic study with review of the literature. *Medicine (Baltimore)* 1984;63:362.
113. Calhoun DA. Hematologic aspects of the maternal-fetal relationship. In: Christensen RD, ed. *Hematologic problems of the neonate.* Philadelphia: WB Saunders, 2000:91.
114. Baumann R, Rubin H. Autoimmune hemolytic anemia during pregnancy with hemolytic disease in the newborn. *Blood* 1973;41:293.
115. Benraad CE, Scheerder HA, Overbeeke MA. Autoimmune haemolytic anaemia during pregnancy. *Eur J Obstet Gynecol Reprod Biol* 1994;55:209.
116. Chaplin H Jr, Cohen R, Bloomberg G, et al. Pregnancy and idiopathic autoimmune haemolytic anaemia: a prospective study during 6 months gestation and 3 months post-partum. *Br J Haematol* 1973;24:219.
117. Prober CG, Corey L, Brown ZA, et al. The management of pregnancies complicated by genital infections with herpes simplex virus. *Clin Infect Dis* 1992;15:1031.
118. Boppana SB, Pass RF, Britt WJ, et al. Symptomatic congenital cytomegalovirus infection: neonatal morbidity and mortality. *Pediatr Infect Dis J* 1992;11:93.
119. Hollier LM, Harstad TW, Sanchez PJ, et al. Fetal syphilis: clinical and laboratory characteristics. *Obstet Gynecol* 2001;97:947.
120. Pruekprasert P, Stout C, Patamasucon P. Neonatal enterovirus infection. *J Assoc Acad Minor Phys* 1995;6:134.
121. Marshall LR, Barr AL, French NP, et al. A fatal case of necrotizing enterocolitis in a neonate with polyagglutination of red blood cells. *J Paediatr Child Health* 1993;29:63.
122. Mupanemunda RH, Kenyon CF, Inwood MJ, et al. Bacterial-induced activation of erythrocyte T-antigen complicating necrotising enterocolitis: a case report. *Eur J Pediatr* 1993;152:325.
123. Hubl W, Mostbeck B, Hartleb H, et al. Investigation of the pathogenesis of massive hemolysis in a case of Clostridium perfringens septicemia. *Ann Hematol* 1993;67:145.
124. Anai T, Miyakawa I, Ohki H, et al. Hydrops fetalis caused by fetal Kasabach-Merritt syndrome. *Acta Paediatr Jpn* 1992;34:324.
125. Skopec LL, Lakatua DJ. Non-immune fetal hydrops with hepatic hemangioendothelioma and Kasabach-Merritt syndrome: a case report. *Pediatr Pathol* 1989;9:87.
126. WHO Working Group. Glucose-6-phosphate dehydrogenase deficiency. *Bull World Health Organ* 1989;67:601.
127. Beutler E. G6PD deficiency. *Blood* 1994;84:3613.
128. Perkins RP. Hydrops fetalis and stillbirth in a male glucose-6-phosphate dehydrogenase-deficient fetus possibly due to maternal ingestion of sulfisoxazole; a case report. *Am J Obstet Gynecol* 1971;111:379.
129. Mentzer WC, Collier E. Hydrops fetalis associated with erythrocyte G-6-PD deficiency and maternal ingestion of fava beans and ascorbic acid. *J Pediatr* 1975;86:565.
130. Corchia C, Balata A, Meloni GF, et al. Favism in a female newborn infant whose mother ingested fava beans before delivery. *J Pediatr* 1995;127:807.
131. Washington EC, Ector W, Abboud M, et al. Hemolytic jaundice due to G6PD deficiency causing kernicterus in a female newborn. *South Med J* 1995;88:776.
132. Tan KL, Boey KW. Efficacy of phototherapy in neonatal hyperbilirubinaemia associated with glucose-6-phosphate dehydrogenase deficient status. *Eur J Pediatr* 1993;152:601.
133. Arese P, De Flora A. Pathophysiology of hemolysis in glucose-6-phosphate dehydrogenase deficiency. *Semin Hematol* 1990;27:1.
134. Kaplan M, Renbaum P, Levy-Lahad E, et al. Gilbert syndrome and glucose-6-phosphate dehydrogenase deficiency: a dose-dependent genetic interaction crucial to neonatal hyperbilirubinemia. *Proc Natl Acad Sci U S A* 1997;94:12128.
135. Kumar P, Sarkar S, Narang A. Acute intravascular haemolysis following exchange transfusion with G-6-PD deficient blood. *Eur J Pediatr* 1994;153:98.
136. Mimouni F, Shohat S, Reisner SH. G6PD-deficient donor blood as a cause of hemolysis in two preterm infants. *Isr J Med Sci* 1986;22:120.
137. Gilsanz F, Vega MA, Gomez-Castillo E, et al. Fetal anaemia due to pyruvate kinase deficiency. *Arch Dis Child* 1993;69:523.
138. Ivey HH, Sabio H. Multiple exchange transfusions in the treatment of a newborn with pyruvate kinase deficiency. *Clin Pediatr (Phila)* 1979;18:756.

139. Ravindranath Y, Paglia DE, Warrier I, et al. Glucose phosphate isomerase deficiency as a cause of hydrops fetalis. *N Engl J Med* 1987;316:258.

140. Lo SS, Marti HR, Hitzig WH. Hemolytic anemia associated with decreased concentration of reduced glutathione in red cells. *Acta Haematol* 1971;46:14.

141. Hirono A, Iyori H, Sekine I, et al. Three cases of hereditary nonspherocytic hemolytic anemia associated with red blood cell glutathione deficiency. *Blood* 1996;87:2071.

142. Burman D. Congenital spherocytosis in infancy. *Arch Dis Child* 1958;33:335.

143. Trucco JI, Brown AK. Neonatal manifestations of hereditary spherocytosis. *Am J Dis Child* 1967;113:263.

144. Agre P, Orringer EP, Bennett V. Deficient red-cell spectrin in severe, recessively inherited spherocytosis. *N Engl J Med* 1982;306:1155.

145. Whitfield CF, Follweiler JB, Lopresti-Morrow L, et al. Deficiency of alpha-spectrin synthesis in burst-forming units-erythroid in lethal hereditary spherocytosis. *Blood* 1991;78:3043.

146. Ribeiro ML, Alloisio N, Almeida H, et al. Severe hereditary spherocytosis and distal renal tubular acidosis associated with the total absence of band 3. *Blood* 2000;96:1602

147. Iolascon A, Faienza MF, Moretti A, et al. UGT1 promoter polymorphism accounts for increased neonatal appearance of hereditary spherocytosis. *Blood* 1998;91:1093.

148. Pati AR, Patton WN, Harris RI. The use of the Technicon H1 in the diagnosis of hereditary spherocytosis. *Clin Lab Haematol* 1989;11:27.

149. Schroter W, Kahsnitz E. Diagnosis of hereditary spherocytosis in newborn infants. *J Pediatr* 1983;103:460.

150. Mentzer WC Jr, Iarocci TA, Mohandas N, et al. Modulation of erythrocyte membrane mechanical stability by 2,3-diphosphoglycerate in the neonatal poikilocytosis/elliptocytosis syndrome. *J Clin Invest* 1987;79:943.

151. Delhommeau F, Cynober T, Schischmanoff PO, et al. Natural history of hereditary spherocytosis during the first year of life. *Blood* 2000;95:393.

152. Austin RF, Desforges JF. Hereditary elliptocytosis: an unusual presentation of hemolysis in the newborn associated with transient morphologic abnormalities. *Pediatrics* 1969;44:196.

153. Gallagher PG, Petruzzi MJ, Weed SA, et al. Mutation of a highly conserved residue of beta I spectrin associated with fatal and near-fatal neonatal hemolytic anemia. *J Clin Invest* 1997;99:267.

154. Coetzer T, Lawler J, Prchal JT, et al. Molecular determinants of clinical expression of hereditary elliptocytosis and pyropoikilocytosis. *Blood* 1987;70:766.

155. Zarkowsky HS, Mohandas N, Speaker CB, et al. A congenital haemolytic anaemia with thermal sensitivity of the erythrocyte membrane. *Br J Haematol* 1975;29:537.

156. Coetzer T, Palek J, Lawler J, et al. Structural and functional heterogeneity of alpha spectrin mutations involving the spectrin heterodimer self-association site: relationships to hematologic expression of homozygous hereditary elliptocytosis and hereditary pyropoikilocytosis. *Blood* 1990;75:2235.

157. Delaunay J, Stewart G, Iolascon A. Hereditary dehydrated and overhydrated stomatocytosis: recent advances. *Curr Opin Hematol* 1999;6:110.

158. Entezami M, Becker R, Menssen HD, et al. Xerocytosis with concomitant intrauterine ascites: first description and therapeutic approach. *Blood* 1996; 87:5392.

159. Grootenboer S, Schischmanoff PO, Cynober T, et al. A genetic syndrome associating dehydrated hereditary stomatocytosis, pseudohyperkalaemia and perinatal oedema. *Br J Haematol* 1998;103:383.

160. Grootenboer S, Schischmanoff PO, Laurendeau I, et al. Pleiotropic syndrome of dehydrated hereditary stomatocytosis, pseudohyperkalemia, and perinatal edema maps to 16q23-q24. *Blood* 2000;96:2599.

161. Chui DH, Waye JS. Hydrops fetalis caused by alpha-thalassemia: an emerging health care problem. *Blood* 1998;91:2213.

162. Olivieri NF. Fetal erythropoiesis and the diagnosis and treatment of hemoglobin disorders in the fetus and child. *Semin Perinatol* 1997;21:63.

163. Singer ST, Styles L, Bojanowski J, et al. Changing outcome of homozygous alpha-thalassemia: cautious optimism. *J Pediatr Hematol Oncol* 2000;22:539.

164. Chan V, Chan VW, Tang M, et al. Molecular defects in Hb H hydrops fetalis. *Br J Haematol* 1997;96:224.

165. Trent RJ, Wilkinson T, Yakas J, et al. Molecular defects in 2 examples of severe Hb H disease. *Scand J Haematol* 1986;36:272.

166. Hegyi T, Delphin ES, Bank A, et al. Sickle cell anemia in the newborn. *Pediatrics* 1977;60:213.

167. Bollekens JA, Forget BG. Delta beta thalassemia and hereditary persistence of fetal hemoglobin. *Hematol Oncol Clin North Am* 1991;5:399.

168. Levine RL, Lincoln DR, Buchholz WM, et al. Hemoglobin Hasharon in a premature infant with hemolytic anemia. *Pediatr Res* 1975;108:716.

169. Lee-Potter JP, Deacon-Smith RA, Simpkiss MJ, et al. A new cause of haemolytic anaemia in the newborn. A description of an unstable fetal haemoglobin: F Poole, alpha2-G-gamma2 130 tryptophan yields glycine. *J Clin Pathol* 1975;28:317.

170. Sieff CA, Nisbet-Brown E, Nathan DG. Congenital bone marrow failure syndromes. *Br J Haematol* 2000;111:30.

171. Da Costa L, Willig TN, Fixler J, et al. Diamond-Blackfan anemia. *Curr Opin Pediatr* 2001;13:10.

172. Janov AJ, Leong T, Nathan DG, et al. Diamond-Blackfan anemia. Natural history and sequelae of treatment. *Medicine (Baltimore)* 1996;75:77.

173. Rogers BB, Bloom SL, Buchanan GR. Autosomal dominantly inherited Diamond-Blackfan anemia resulting in nonimmune hydrops. *Obstet Gynecol* 1997;89:805.

174. Scimeca PG, Weinblatt ME, Slepowitz G, et al. Diamond-Blackfan syndrome: an unusual cause of hydrops fetalis. *Am J Pediatr Hematol Oncol* 1988; 10:241.

175. Kato K, Sugitani M, Kawataki M, et al. Congenital dyserythropoietic anemia type 1 with fetal onset of severe anemia. *J Pediatr Hematol Oncol* 2001;23:63.

176. Shalev H, Tamary H, Shaft D, et al. Neonatal manifestations of congenital dyserythropoietic anemia type I. *J Pediatr* 1997;131:95.

177. Iolascon A, Delaunay J, Wickramasinghe SN, et al. Natural history of congenital dyserythropoietic anemia type II. *Blood* 2001;98:1258.

178. Nichols KE, Crispino JD, Poncz M, et al. Familial dyserythropoietic anaemia and thrombocytopenia due to an inherited mutation in GATA1. *Nat Genet* 2000;24:266.

179. Butturini A, Gale RP, Verlander PC, et al. Hematologic abnormalities in Fanconi anemia: an International Fanconi Anemia Registry study. *Blood* 1994; 84:1650.

180. Joenje H, Patel KJ. The emerging genetic and molecular basis of Fanconi anaemia. *Nat Rev Genet* 2001;2:446.

181. Auerbach AD. Fanconi anemia. *Dermatol Clin* 1995;13:41.

182. Giampietro PF, Adler-Brecher B, Verlander PC, et al. The need for more accurate and timely diagnosis in Fanconi anemia: a report from the International Fanconi Anemia Registry. *Pediatrics* 1993;91:1116.

183. Berrocal T, Simon MJ, al-Assir I, et al. Shwachman-Diamond syndrome: clinical, radiological and sonographic findings. *Pediatr Radiol* 1995;25:356.

184. Smith OP, Hann IM, Chessells JM, et al. Haematological abnormalities in Shwachman-Diamond syndrome. *Br J Haematol* 1996;94:279.

185. Pearson HA, Lobel JS, Kocoshis SA, et al. A new syndrome of refractory sideroblastic anemia with vacuolization of marrow precursors and exocrine pancreatic dysfunction. *J Pediatr* 1979;95:976.

186. Rotig A, Cormier V, Blanche S, et al. Pearson's marrow-pancreas syndrome. A multisystem mitochondrial disorder in infancy. *J Clin Invest* 1990;86:1601.

187. Aase JM, Smith DW. Congenital anemia and triphalangeal thumbs: a new syndrome. *J Pediatr* 1969;74:471.

188. Hing AV, Dowton SB. Aase syndrome: novel radiographic features. *Am J Med Genet* 1993;45:413.

189. Gerritsen EJ, Vossen JM, van Loo IH, et al. Autosomal recessive osteopetrosis: variability of findings at diagnosis and during the natural course. *Pediatrics* 1994;93:247.

190. Vanhoenacker FM, De Beuckeleer LH, Van Hul W, et al. Sclerosing bone dysplasias: genetic and radioclinical features. *Eur Radiol* 2000;10:1423.

191. Gerritsen EJ, Vossen JM, Fasth A, et al. Bone marrow transplantation for autosomal recessive osteopetrosis. A report from the Working Party on Inborn Errors of the European Bone Marrow Transplantation Group. *J Pediatr* 1994;125:896.

192. Kapelushnik J, Shalev C, Yaniv I, et al. Osteopetrosis: a single center experience of stem cell transplantation and prenatal diagnosis. *Bone Marrow Transplant* 2001;27:129.

193. Gray ES, Balch NJ, Kohler H, et al. Congenital leukaemia: an unusual cause of stillbirth. *Arch Dis Child* 1986;61:1001.

194. Nunez E, Varela S, Cervilla K, et al. [Hydrops fetalis caused by congenital leukemia]. *Rev Chil Pediatr* 1991;62:186.

195. Becroft DM, Zwi LJ. Perinatal visceral fibrosis accompanying the megakaryoblastic leukemoid reaction of Down syndrome. *Pediatr Pathol* 1990;10:397.

196. Foucar K, Friedman K, Llewellyn A, et al. Prenatal diagnosis of transient myeloproliferative disorder via percutaneous umbilical blood sampling. Report of two cases in fetuses affected by Down's syndrome. *Am J Clin Pathol* 1992;97:584.

197. Brown KE. Haematological consequences of parvovirus B19 infection. *Best Pract Res Clin Haematol* 2000;13:245.

198. Mustafa MM, McClain KL. Diverse hematologic effects of parvovirus B19 infection. *Pediatr Clin North Am* 1996;43:809.

199. Levy R, Weissman A, Blomberg G, et al. Infection by parvovirus B 19 during pregnancy: a review. *Obstet Gynecol Surv* 1997;52:254.

200. Gallagher PG, Ehrenkranz RA. Nutritional anemias in infancy. *Clin Perinatol* 1995;22:671.

201. Lampkin BC, Shore NA, Chadwick D. Megaloblastic anemia of infancy secondary to maternal pernicious anemia. *N Engl J Med* 1966;274:1168.

202. Higginbottom MC, Sweetman L, Nyhan WL. A syndrome of methylmalonic aciduria, homocystinuria, megaloblastic anemia and neurologic abnormalities in a vitamin B12-deficient breast-fed infant of a strict vegetarian. *N Engl J Med* 1978;299:317.

203. Boucher FD, Modlin JF, Weller S, et al. Phase I evaluation of zidovudine administered to infants exposed at birth to the human immunodeficiency virus. *J Pediatr* 1993;122:137.

204. O'Sullivan MJ, Boyer PJ, Scott GB, et al. The pharmacokinetics and safety of zidovudine in the third trimester of pregnancy for women infected with human immunodeficiency virus and their infants: phase I acquired immunodeficiency syndrome clinical trials group study (protocol 082). Zidovudine Collaborative Working Group. *Am J Obstet Gynecol* 1993;168:1510.

205. Silverman NS, Watts DH, Hitti J, et al. Initial multicenter experience with double nucleoside therapy for human immunodeficiency virus infection during pregnancy. *Infect Dis Obstet Gynecol* 1998;6:237.

206. Koenig JM, Ashton RD, De Vore GR, et al. Late hyporegenerative anemia in Rh hemolytic disease. *J Pediatr* 1989;115:315.

207. Thorp JA, O'Connor T, Callenbach J, et al. Hyporegenerative anemia associated with intrauterine transfusion in rhesus hemolytic disease. *Am J Obstet Gynecol* 1991;165:79.

208. Dallacasa P, Ancora G, Miniero R, et al. Erythropoietin course in newborns with Rh hemolytic disease transfused and not transfused in utero. *Pediatr Res* 1996;40:357.
209. Dhodapkar KM, Blei F. Treatment of hemolytic disease of the newborn caused by anti-Kell antibody with recombinant erythropoietin. *J Pediatr Hematol Oncol* 2001;23:69.
210. Dallman PR. Erythropoietin and the anemia of prematurity. *J Pediatr* 1984;105:756.
211. Stockman JA 3rd, Graeber JE, Clark DA, et al. Anemia of prematurity: determinants of the erythropoietin response. *J Pediatr* 1984;105:786.
212. Brown MS, Garcia JF, Phibbs RH, et al. Decreased response of plasma immunoreactive erythropoietin to "available oxygen" in anemia of prematurity. *J Pediatr* 1984;105:793.
213. Wardrop CA, Holland BM, Veale KE, et al. Nonphysiological anaemia of prematurity. *Arch Dis Child* 1978;53:855.
214. Gallagher PG, Ehrenkranz RA. Erythropoietin therapy for anemia of prematurity. *Clin Perinatol* 1993;20:169.
215. Widness JA, Veng-Pedersen P, Peters C, et al. Erythropoietin pharmacokinetics in premature infants: developmental, nonlinearity, and treatment effects. *J Appl Physiol* 1996;80:140.
216. Joshi A, Gerhardt T, Shandloff P, et al. Blood transfusion effect on the respiratory pattern of preterm infants. *Pediatrics* 1987;80:79.
217. Stockman JA 3rd. Anemia of prematurity. Current concepts in the issue of when to transfuse. *Pediatr Clin North Am* 1986;33:111.
218. Bell EF. Fluid therapy. In: Sinclair JC, Bracken MB, eds. *Effective care of the newborn infant.* New York: Oxford University Press, 1992:59.
219. Blank JP, Sheagren TG, Vajaria J, et al. The role of RBC transfusion in the premature infant. *Am J Dis Child* 1984;138:831.
220. Keyes WG, Donohue PK, Spivak JL, et al. Assessing the need for transfusion of premature infants and role of hematocrit, clinical signs, and erythropoietin level. *Pediatrics* 1989;84:412.
221. Ohls RK. The use of erythropoietin in neonates. *Clin Perinatol* 2000;27:681.
222. Juul SE. Erythropoietin in the neonate. *Curr Probl Pediatr* 1999;29:129.
223. Vamvakas EC, Strauss RG. Meta-analysis of controlled clinical trials studying the efficacy of rHuEPO in reducing blood transfusions in the anemia of prematurity. *Transfusion* 2001;41:406.
224. Zipursky A. Erythropoietin therapy for premature infants: cost without benefit? *Pediatr Res* 2000;48:136.
225. Strauss RG. Managing the anemia of prematurity: red blood cell transfusions versus recombinant erythropoietin. *Transfus Med Rev* 2001;15:213.
226. Strauss RG, Sacher RA. Directed donations for pediatric patients. *Transfus Med Rev* 1988;2:58.
227. Franz AR, Pohlandt F. Red blood cell transfusions in very and extremely low birthweight infants under restrictive transfusion guidelines: is exogenous erythropoietin necessary? *Arch Dis Child Fetal Neonatal Ed* 2001;84:F96.
228. Bergstrand C, Czar B. Serum haptoglobin in infancy. *J Clin Lab Invest* 1961;13:576.

CHAPTER 56

Hematologic Aspects of Systemic Diseases

Samuel E. Lux IV

ANEMIA OF CHRONIC DISEASE

Few alterations in the body's homeostasis are not reflected or expressed in the hematologic system. For example, the renal source of erythropoietin (Epo), the hepatic synthesis of coagulation factors, and the leukocyte response to infection demonstrate that pathology in almost any organ system within the body is mirrored in a parallel hematologic response. Systemic disease effects and is affected by changes in hematologic function. These manifestations are so consistent and characteristic that they constitute a major locus for differential diagnosis of systemic disease. Leukocytosis with an increase in band forms is the hallmark of bacterial infection, and eosinophilia has comparable implications for allergic or parasitic diseases. A hematologic abnormality is often the minor detail that defines the focus of the pursuit in establishing the source of pathology elsewhere in the body.

The hematologic aspects of systemic disease are myriad, with some findings diagnostic of a single disorder [e.g., malaria parasites in red blood cells (RBCs)], whereas others may represent a uniform response to diverse insults. The latter phenomenon assumes its most common guise in the "anemia of chronic disease" (ACD), an anemia that accompanies illnesses as diverse as traumatic, inflammatory, malignant, and infectious states. G. C. Cartwright's prescient recognition of ACD as a unitary pathophysiologic entity (1) stimulated many investigators to explore the cause of this shared response by the body to several different insults. The mechanism is still not completely identified, although the explosion in molecular biology is helping to clarify the pathways involved in the process (2).

Hypoproliferative Anemia with Low Serum Iron and Transferrin

Persons suffering from infection, malignancy, or inflammation develop within a few weeks of onset of these conditions a charac-

teristic anemia that is independent of any marrow involvement or specific hematologic complication of their disease (3). A modest shortening of RBC survival is present but not adequately compensated for by the marrow; this reticulocytopenic response suggests that a hypoproliferative defect, rather than hemolysis, is the major lesion in ACD (4). The anemia is moderate in degree, with the hematocrit usually fixed in the 28% to 32% range; a compensatory erythroid hyperplasia of the marrow or reticulocytosis is not present. The anemia is usually normochromic and normocytic, but a population of hypochromic cells is often evident; 30% to 40% of such patients have a microcytic hypochromic anemia. Iron studies reveal low serum iron and transferrin (Tf) levels, contrasting with findings in uncomplicated iron-deficiency anemia in which low iron levels are accompanied by elevated Tf levels (5). The Tf saturation levels in ACD may overlap with those of iron deficiency, contributing to a confusion of these two entities with one another. What distinguishes the two are the abundant stores of reticuloendothelial (RE) iron found in those with ACD; the anemia represents, according to Cartwright (6), a "sideropenic anemia in the face of RE siderosis."

Sequestration of Iron by Reticuloendothelial Cells

Recycling of iron derived from the breakdown of senescent RBCs and its storage within RE and liver parenchymal cells provide the major source of iron needed for hemoglobin (Hb) synthesis. In progressive iron deficiency, initially no anemia or lowering of serum iron levels is noted until the iron stores within the depots have been exhausted. The body has a reserve of storage iron, which helps guarantee a constant supply of iron for Hb synthesis. In ACD, a low serum iron accompanies iron-deficient anemia, as evidenced by decreased marrow sideroblasts and elevated free erythrocyte protoporphyrins. All these features exist in the presence of abundant RE stores of iron and elevated serum levels of ferritin. The normal mechanism for preferential delivery of iron to support Hb synthesis in developing RBCs is defective on some level in this state. The vector of iron delivery in ACD appears misdirected, and this lesion has been implicated as the source of hypoproliferative ACD (7).

Several investigators have documented the faulty liberation of iron stores in these states, whereas others question the data or their importance in ACD. Ferrokinetic studies using radiolabeled RBC Hb have demonstrated delayed release of such iron from RE stores (8). The same delay characterizes the hepatic release of iron derived from free Hb infusions that are taken up by liver parenchymal cells (9). A similar defect in iron release from intestinal epithelial cells has also been reported (10). The body appears to closet its iron stores as a feature of ACD, and hypochromic anemia exists in the presence of iron overload.

Restraint of Bacteria or Tumor Growth by Hypoferremia

Cartwright suggested that ACD is part of the body's defense system against various insults; the altered direction of iron flow is purposeful because it creates hypoferremia, a desirable result in the presence of infection or malignancy. All microorganisms require iron for growth and proliferation, and many organisms have siderophores, which are iron-complexing molecules that permit successful extraction of iron from plasma (11). Some malignant cells possess similar devices to ensure their iron requirements for growth (12–14). A fall in serum iron with ACD deprives the invading cell population of an essential nutrient. The hypoferremia of ACD is a form of nutritional immunity whose advantage to the body in restraining bacterial or tumor cell growth outweighs any associated diversion of iron from erythroid cells. The anemia is the cost of the body's defense against invasion (15).

Lactoferrin "Iron-Steal" Hypothesis

The cause of hypoferremia in states of infection is not strictly defined. Cartwright and associates (16) showed a rapid fall in serum iron after bacterial challenge of animal models. This phenomenon could be replicated by infusion of lactoferrin, an iron transport protein present in the granules of polymorphonuclear cells (17). Lactoferrin, with an avidity for iron even greater than Tf, imparts a direction of iron flow away from developing RBCs that do not contain lactoferrin receptors (18). Any iron scavenged by lactoferrin is rapidly removed from plasma and deposited in RE or hepatic parenchymal cells. Mobilization and activation of polymorphonuclear neutrophils after bacterial infection create a cellular response that is combined with the release of lactoferrin (19,20). The interposition of this transport protein steals iron from bacterial cells and RBCs alike. This is a teleologic explanation in defense of a positive role for ACD.

The lactoferrin hypothesis may partially explain ACD as it accompanies infection, but the same leukocytosis and lactoferrin release do not consistently accompany malignancies and their ACD. Lactoferrin does accumulate in several neoplasms and may even be a marker for benign versus malignant tissue (21). Hypernephroma, a tumor classically associated with anemia, contains significantly increased tissue lactoferrin levels compared with those seen in normal renal tissue. In these circumstances, the vector of iron delivery may favor tumor growth and development, with iron flow more heavily directed to these tissue sites.

Another possible cause for the hypoferremia of ACD is a disproportionate incorporation of iron into ferritin in storage depots, making the iron less easily mobilizable than the alternate storage form of low-molecular-weight iron (22). Because ferritin is an acute-phase reactant protein, this shift in iron placement would accompany all the conditions associated with ACD. Neither this mechanism nor lactoferrin's role in host immunity is solidly established as the cause of the hypoproliferative component

of ACD. The hypoferremia may be only a part of a more generalized response to infection, malignancy, or inflammation. ACD accompanies other manifestations of systemic disease, such as anorexia, weight loss, debilitation, and inflammation.

Role of Proinflammatory Cytokines

TUMOR NECROSIS FACTOR-α

The systemic diseases that produce ACD are accompanied by release of acute-phase reactants measured in the blood as elevated C-reactive protein, fibrinogen, haptoglobin, and ceruloplasmin, among others. These seemingly disparate responses to a multitude of bodily insults are now unified in a common pathway of metabolic events initiated by interleukin-1β (IL-1β) release from activated macrophages (23). IL-1β then starts a cascade of events mediated by the cytokines released from macrophages, lymphocytes, and other numerous cells within the body (24). Both anabolic and catabolic responses are created, with ILs causing the host response to infection and inflammation.

A pivotal factor in this network is tumor necrosis factor-α (TNF-α), a product of the macrophage with an ability to induce the same spectrum of acute-phase changes as IL-1β (25). There is considerable evidence that TNF-α is also a central player in ACD. Serum levels of TNF-α are elevated in patients with ACD, and the levels of cytokines correlate with the degree of anemia (26,27). Injection of TNF-α reproduces the anorexia, weight loss, and debilitation of chronic disease and produces an anemia that closely resembles ACD (28). TNF-α modulates iron metabolism to cause hypoferremia (29–32) and inhibits bone marrow erythropoiesis (33,34), either by a direct negative effect on progenitor cell growth (35), or by stimulating the production of accessory cytokines, such as β- or γ-interferon (IFN), by other bone marrow cells (36,37).

ACD patients have less than one-half as many committed erythroid stem cells (CD34$^+$/CD71$^+$) in their bone marrows (27,38), and fewer erythroid burst-forming units (BFU-E) and erythroid colony-forming units (CFU-E) are generated from erythroid cultures (27). This seems to be because a high fraction of the stem cells and progenitors are undergoing apoptosis (27,38). In the stem cell fraction, the proportion is three times the controls (32% versus 11%). It is even greater in the erythroid progenitor and early precursor (CD36$^+$/glycophorin A$^+$) compartment (51% versus 8%). In contrast, apoptosis is much less (5%) in the late precursor compartment (CD36$^-$/glycophorin A$^+$) and does not differ from normal.

The levels of TNF-α are approximately three to four times normal in the supernatants of bone marrow cultures obtained from rheumatoid arthritis patients, especially those with ACD (27,38,39), showing that the cytokine can be produced locally by cells that are preprogrammed at the time of bone marrow harvest. Addition of TNF-α inhibits BFU-E and CFU-E colony numbers (27,30,33,36,40), and anti-TNF partially reverses the inhibition (33) and apoptosis (27), which further supports a role for TNF-α. The most convincing data comes from rheumatoid arthritis (RA) patients treated experimentally with the anti–TNF-α antibody cA2 (27,41). In the most recent study, the Hb levels of RA patients with ACD rose 13% (11.4 to 12.9 g/dL, $p <.005$) after six doses of the antibody (3 mg/kg every 2 weeks) (27). Nonanemic RA patients had less of a response in Hb levels, and RA patients with iron-deficiency anemia instead of ACD had a statistically insignificant response.

INTERLEUKIN-1β AND INTERLEUKIN-6

The serum levels of IL-1β (34,42) and IL-6 (34,43–47) are also elevated in RA and other chronic inflammatory conditions and may contribute to the pathogenesis of ACD. IL-1β decreases Epo production in hepatoma cells (48), and the cytokine suppresses the growth of cultured erythroid progenitors *in vitro* (34,42), either directly or via IFN-γ (49).

IL-6 is required for optimal survival or self-renewal of bone marrow stem cells (50); however, excess IL-6 inhibits erythroid progenitors (34,51,52), and the concentration of IL-6 is increased in the serum and bone marrow in patients with inflammatory diseases (34,43–47). IL-6 might also contribute to ACD through hemodilution (53). Unlike IL-1β, IL-6 levels fall after anti–TNF-α therapy (27,54), which suggests IL-6 may contribute to the effects of TNF.

ERYTHROPOIETIN
Many articles on ACD state that the bone marrow response to Epo is "blunted" in the disease. Early studies gave variable results (55); however, recent investigations suggest that Epo levels are appropriate for the degree of anemia in patients with RA (27,56) or juvenile chronic arthritis (47) and ACD. The problem, of course, is deciding what control group to use in establishing the "normal" Epo versus Hb concentration curves. Conclusions differ when iron deficient and thalassemic patients are used to define the standard.

Because Epo protects bone marrow erythroblasts from apoptosis (57) and apoptosis of erythroblasts contributes to ACD (27), it is reasonable to suspect that Epo might be therapeutically useful. Therapeutic trials show that patients with inflammatory conditions such as RA or inflammatory bowel disease respond appropriately to moderate doses of human recombinant Epo (100 to 150 U/kg, 2 to 3 times/week) (58–63), although supplemental iron, given intravenously as an iron-saccharide complex (approximately 200 mg/week in adults) is needed for optimal efficacy (62,64), as it is in most patients receiving Epo for anemia, whatever the underlying disease (65–67). Whether Epo treatment is needed for most patients with ACD is controversial (Chapter 7).

Hepcidin

Recent evidence (68) suggests that a small plasma protein called *hepcidin* (or LEAP1, liver-expressed antimicrobial peptide) may play a major role in ACD. Hepcidin was isolated from blood and urine by standard biochemical methods (69,70). The gene (on chromosome 19) encodes an 84–amino acid preprotein containing a 24-residue signal sequence and a penta-Arg proteolysis site, followed by a conserved 25–amino acid, C-terminal peptide. The C-terminal peptide, which is the portion that circulates in blood, contains four disulfide bonds and has antimicrobial activity against gram-positive bacteria, certain gram-negatives, and yeasts (69,70). The peptide is primarily synthesized in the liver and is probably an acute-phase reactant, because its expression is strongly increased by lipopolysaccharide (71). It was initially thought to be another member of the small, cysteine-rich, cationic, antimicrobial peptides, analogous to the defensins and thionins (72), but three experiments strongly suggest it plays a major role in iron metabolism:

- First, hepcidin was independently discovered in a subtractive hybridization screen for proteins that are overexpressed in iron-loaded liver (71).
- Second, hepcidin expression was accidentally abolished when the neighboring *usf2* (upstream factor 2) gene was knocked out (73). This was not because *usf2* controls hepcidin expression but was probably a proximity effect of the PGK-Neo gene that was inserted into the *usf2* gene (74). The resulting mice accumulate iron in excess of Tf capacity and develop massive iron overload in many tissues, particularly hepatocytes and pancreatic exocrine cells, but interestingly not in the RE system. The phenotype is remarkably similar to hemochromatosis, but genes involved in that disease, such as *hfe* and *tfr2*, are normally expressed in the hepcidin-deficient mice (73). The data suggest that hepcidin interacts with other components of the iron absorption pathway, and in fact, may serve as the long postulated signaling system

between the liver, bone marrow, and enterocyte in regulating iron absorption (68,73).
- Third, when hepcidin-1 is overexpressed as a liver-specific (transthyretin promoter) transgene in the *usf2*(–/–) mice, the newborn pups have an extreme hypochromic-microcytic anemia and die soon after birth (26). Total body iron in the transgenic fetuses is only 25% of normal. Because hepcidin is poorly expressed by fetal liver in contrast to adult liver, the supposition is that the expression of the protein during fetal life interferes with maternal-fetal iron transport via the placenta.

In the modern view of iron metabolism (detailed in Chapter 46), iron is reduced to Fe^{2+} by a ferric reductase at the apical (intestinal luminal) surface of the enterocyte (75), enters the cell through the DMT1 channel (also called *Nramp2* and *DCT1*) (76,77), and exits on the basolateral surface through ferroportin 1 (78,79) (also called *Ireg1* and *MTP1*) in cooperation with hephaestin (80), a putative ferroxidase (see Fig. 46-2). Absorbed iron is picked up by Tf and passes through the portal system to the liver, the major site of iron storage. Hepatocytes take up iron via the classic Tf receptor (TfR), TfR1, but especially via the newly discovered TfR2 (81). Iron is primarily used in the bone marrow, where it is acquired via TfR1 on the erythroblast surface. Heme iron is recycled when senescent erythrocytes are ingested by macrophages. Macrophage iron is either stored as ferritin and hemosiderin or released into the plasma where it is oxidized by ceruloplasmin (another ferroxidase) and recycled by Tf.

These processes are somehow tightly coupled. The enterocyte progenitors in the villus crypts sense the body's need for iron and are programmed to express appropriate levels of transport components (82,83). Fleming and Sly (68) postulate that two regulatory pathways exist: a low capacity one that detects iron stores and a more potent one that detects erythropoietic needs. The former pathway is thought to be deranged in hereditary hemochromatosis, in which patients absorb too much dietary iron relative to iron stores. *HFE*, the defective gene, is a major histocompatibility complex–like protein and associates with a β$_2$-microglobulin (β$_2$M). The complex binds to TfR1 on the crypt cells (and in placental syncytiotrophoblasts) (84,85) and must have a role in down-regulating iron uptake. Little is known of the postulated erythropoietic regulation.

In hereditary hemochromatosis, serum iron concentrations are high, RE iron stores are low, and intestinal iron absorption is excessive. In ACD, the opposite is true: Iron levels are low, RE stores are increased, and intestinal iron absorption is decreased (86,87). Both disorders affect communication between sites of iron storage (hepatocytes and RE macrophages) and the intestine. Fleming and Sly suggest that this may all be explained by involving hepcidin (68). Their hypothesis is shown in Figure 56-1. The model argues that ACD is caused by increases in circulating hepcidin in response to inflammation or other acute-phase stimuli. The hepcidin then interacts with the β$_2$M-HFE complex on macrophages and crypt cells, increasing iron retention by macrophages and decreasing iron absorption by enterocytes. The resulting hypoferremia combined with the effects of cytokines on erythropoiesis discussed above leads to anemia. This is a testable model, and it will undoubtedly be tested in the next few years. Although it probably will not be completely true, there is no doubt that hepcidin is an important regulator of iron absorption through the intestine and placenta, and probably the macrophage. It also seems likely that hepcidin will play an important role in ACD.

Diagnosis of Anemia of Chronic Disease

Patients with uncomplicated ACD typically have a low serum iron, a low serum Tf, a high serum ferritin, a low serum Tf receptor (sTfR), and normal or increased bone marrow iron stores within macrophages (Table 56-1, Fig. 56-2). Serum iron is low,

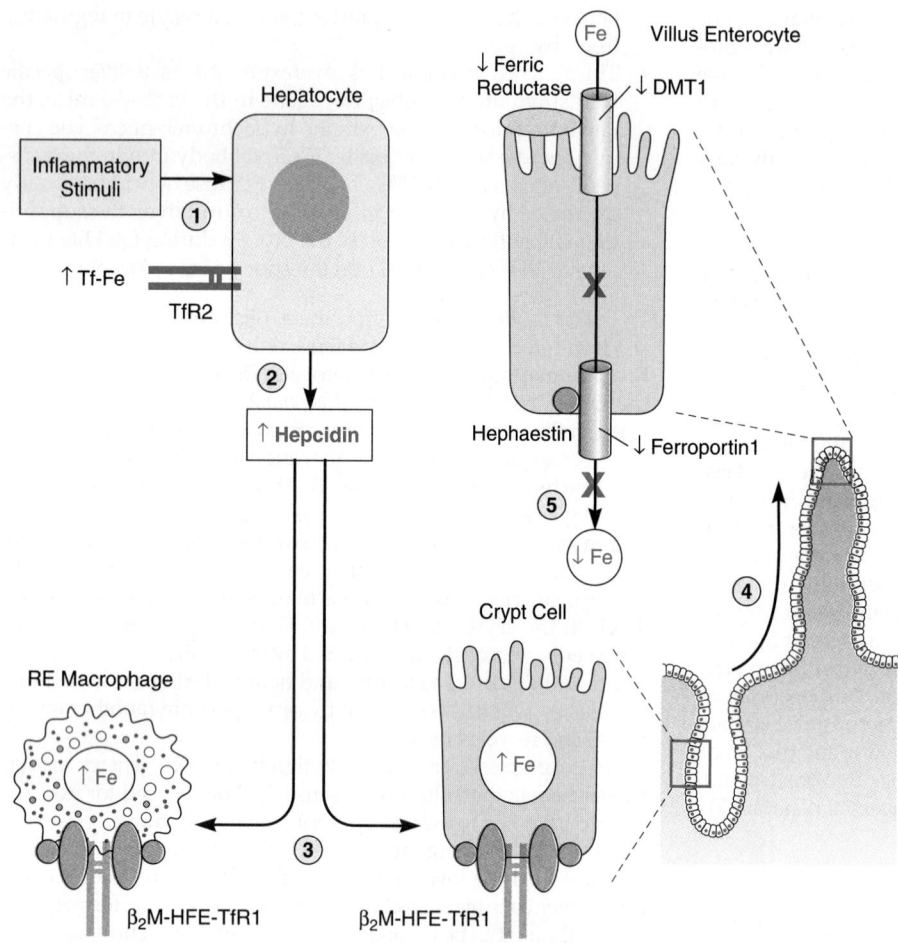

Figure 56-1. Model for the role of hepcidin in anemia of chronic disease (ACD) and normal iron homeostasis. [1] Inflammation (ACD) or increased hepatocyte uptake of iron by transferrin receptor 2 (TfR2) (increased iron absorption) leads to [2] increased synthesis and release of hepcidin, which [3] interacts with the complex of HFE-β_2-microglobulin (β_2M) and TfR1 on macrophages and intestinal crypt "stem" cells to increase iron uptake or retention. [4] The crypt cells differentiate into villus enterocytes that are programmed to have decreased iron absorption through alterations in the expression or function of one or more of the proteins in the iron transport pathway: ferric reductase, DMT1, ferroportin 1, or hephaestin. [5] This leads to decreased iron absorption, which balances iron absorption in the normal state, and, along with decreased release of iron from macrophages, causes hypoferremia in ACD. RE, reticuloendothelial. (After Fleming RE, Sly WS. Hepcidin: a putative iron-regulatory hormone relevant to hereditary hemochromatosis and the anemia of chronic disease. *Proc Natl Acad Sci U S A* 2001;98: 8160–8162.)

approaching the levels seen in iron deficiency, because recycling of iron from macrophages is impaired, as already discussed. Tf is low because its synthesis is impaired by proinflammatory cytokines. As a consequence, the percent Tf saturation is low or low normal. The Tf saturation averages 20% to 25% (Table 56-1) and is rarely lower than 10%. The combination of a low serum iron and iron-binding capacity (essentially a measurement of serum Tf) combined with stainable iron in the bone marrow is virtually diagnostic of ACD. In iron deficiency anemia, marrow iron stores are completely depleted before microcytosis or anemia ensue.

The anemia of ACD is typically mild to moderate. It is rare for the Hb value to fall below 8 g/dL (Table 56-1) unless other causes

of anemia are present (e.g., iron deficiency, acute blood loss, marrow suppression, or hemolysis). Typically, the anemia of ACD is normocytic initially, though it may become microcytic with time or intensity of disease. It is unusual for the mean corpuscular volume (MCV) to fall below 75 fL in adults (normal lower limit of 80 fL) with uncomplicated ACD (Table 56-1). In children, of course, where the normal lower limit of the MCV is approximated by 70 plus the age in years, the figure will be lower.

It is not uncommon for ACD to coexist with iron deficiency because iron deficiency is common in women of childbearing age and because the conditions that cause ACD and their treatment (nonsteroidal antiinflammatory drugs, corticosteroids,

TABLE 56-1. Laboratory Tests in Anemia of Chronic Disease and Iron Deficiency[a]

	Anemia of Chronic Disease (ACD)	Combination of ACD plus IDA	Iron Deficiency Anemia (IDA)
Hemoglobin (g/dL)	10.2 ± 1.2 (103)	8.8 ± 2.0 (90)	9.3 ± 1.6 (96)
MCV (fL)	90 ± 7 (91)	78 ± 9 (79)	75 ± 9 (75)
Iron (µg/dL)	56 ± 34 (50)	34 ± 17 (34)	45 ± 61 (22)
Tf (mg/dL)	190 ± 50 (180)	260 ± 60 (240)	330 ± 40 (330)
Ferritin (µg/L)	342 ± 385 (195)	87 ± 167 (23)	21 ± 55 (11)
TfR (mg/L)	1.8 ± 0.6 (1.8)	5.1 ± 2.0 (4.7)	6.2 ± 3.5 (5.0)
Tf saturation (%)	23 ± 13 (21)	12 ± 7 (8)	12 ± 17 (6)
TfR/log ferritin	0.8 ± 0.3 (0.8)	3.8 ± 1.9 (3.2)	6.8 ± 6.5 (5.4)

MVC, mean corpuscular volume; TfR, transferrin receptor.

[a]Results are expressed as the mean ± SD (median). Note that the SD is sometimes larger than the mean because the results are distributed in a non-normal distribution. The study population included 129 consecutive adults who had bone marrow examinations for anemia and did not have hemolytic anemias, cobalamin or folate deficiency, or a hematologic malignancy. *ACD* (n = 64) was defined as stainable iron in the bone marrow in combination with a recurrent or chronic infection, a chronic inflammatory disease, or a nonhematologic malignancy. *IDA* (n = 48) was defined as no stainable iron in the bone marrow in patients without a chronic disease. *ACD + IDA* (n = 17) was defined as the absence of stainable iron in patients with a chronic disease.

From Punnonen K, Irjala K, Ramjamäki A. Serum transferrin receptor and its ratio to serum ferritin in the diagnosis of iron deficiency. *Blood* 1997;89:1052–1057, with permission.

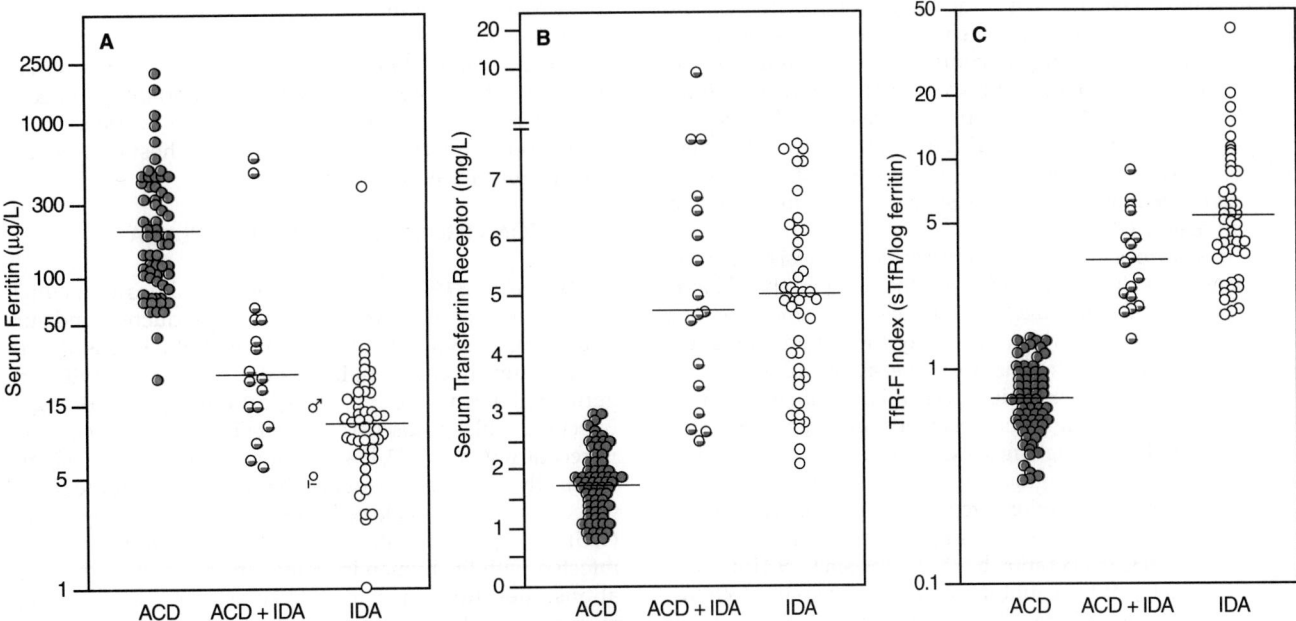

Figure 56-2. (**A**) Serum ferritin, (**B**) serum transferrin receptor (sTfR), and (**C**) the TfR-F index (sTfR/log serum ferritin) in patients with anemia of chronic disease (ACD), iron deficiency anemia (IDA), and a combination of the two diseases. Patient groups were defined as described in Table 56-1. Horizontal bars indicate the median value for each patient group. Normal values for serum ferritin are 15 to 306 μg/L (men) and 5 to 103 μg/L (women). Normal values for sTf are 210 to 340 mg/dL (men) and 200 to 310 mg/dL (women). Normal values for sTfR are 0.85 to 3.05 mg/L. (Data from Punnonen K, Irjala K, Ramjamäki A. Serum transferrin receptor and its ratio to serum ferritin in the diagnosis of iron deficiency. *Blood* 1997;89:1052–1057.)

cancer chemotherapy) sometimes cause blood loss, particularly through the gastrointestinal tract.

The serum ferritin is normal or high in ACD and low in iron deficiency (Table 56-1, Fig. 56-2A). Tissue ferritin concentrations exceed serum ferritin levels by orders of magnitude, so diseases that destroy tissue may also lead to high serum ferritin values and complicate the interpretation of this test. Because serum ferritin is age dependent (88) and may be increased by chronic sepsis, inflammation, or malignancy (89), it is more useful in distinguishing ACD from iron deficiency or a combination of iron deficiency and ACD (Table 56-1) than in making the diagnosis of ACD. Serum ferritin concentrations of less than 10 μg/L are diagnostic of iron deficiency, and values of less than 20 μg/L are suggestive of a deficient state.

sTfR, also called *soluble transferrin receptor*, is a normal proteolytic cleavage product of TfR-1 on the surface of erythroblasts. The level of sTfR corresponds well to the levels of marrow erythropoiesis (90,91) (see Fig. 44-5)—that is, it is increased in ineffective erythropoiesis, hemolytic anemias, and iron deficiency, but not in ACD, where there is a component of apoptosis and marrow suppression (27,38) (Table 56-1, Fig. 56-2B). Because of this distinction, the sTfR is generally found to be one of the most sensitive tests for distinguishing iron deficiency from ACD (92–97), although there are dissenting opinions (98).

Recent work shows that the TfR-F Index [the sTfR (mg/L) divided by the log of the ferritin (μg/L)] is particularly helpful in distinguishing between ACD (value <1.5) and iron deficiency (value >1.5) (93,96) (Table 56-1, Fig. 56-2C). In general, patients with both conditions have values of sTfR, ferritin, and TfR-F Index in the iron deficiency range (Fig. 56-2).

Summary

In summary, Cartwright's prescience in recognizing ACD as a single pathophysiologic entity has its explanation in ACD as a partic-

ipant in the general process of cachexia (99). ACD, although multifactorial in its causes, has the shared lymphocyte-monocyte and perhaps hepatocyte (through hepcidin) reaction to infection, malignancy, and inflammation. RBC survival is abbreviated because of heightened RE activity, the product of activated macrophages, and the effect of fever in shortening the RBC lifespan. Hypoferremia is causally related to increased hepcidin synthesis, possibly with a contribution from increased lactoferrin release. The consequence is a kind of nutritional immunity. TNF-α, IL-6, and other proinflammatory cytokines enhance apoptosis and probably have other deleterious effects that lead to a suppression of erythropoiesis. A hypoferremic, hypoproliferative anemia results.

It is important to remember, however, that almost all the investigations of ACD that have established this pathophysiology have used patients with RA. Although it is likely that proinflammatory cytokines, hepcidin, and lactoferrin also contribute importantly to the anemia associated with other infectious, inflammatory, and malignant diseases, the balance of their influences will probably differ in different diseases, with consequential differences in the laboratory parameters that characterize ACD, and in the responses to potential therapies. Investigation of the pathophysiology of ACD in a variety of conditions is critically needed.

INFECTIOUS DISEASES

The hematologic aspects of infectious diseases have their historic antecedents in many of the earliest and most important discoveries in the field of hematology. An understanding of pus and its relation to infection and inflammation dates from observations made possible by the staining techniques of Ehrlich, by the recognition of diapedesis and cellular motion by Cornheim, and by phagocytosis by Metchnikoff. These past achievements are complemented by knowledge of the body's humoral and cellular control systems, which modulate the hematologic and immunologic defenses; this interwoven cascade is the means whereby infectious agents are confronted and eliminated and tissue repair occurs (100). Leukocytosis and a left shift in the white blood cell (WBC) differential are the classic accompaniments of bacterial infections (101). The release of IL-1 after macrophage activation initiates the series of events that mobilizes WBCs from the marrow in response to colony-stimulating factor (CSF) release (102,103).

The leukocytosis that accompanies bacterial sepsis may be of such magnitude (40,000 to 70,000/μL) that the peripheral blood picture is confused with leukemia, a so-called leukemoid reaction (104) (Chapter 14). Infections classically associated with a leukemoid blood picture are miliary tuberculosis (105,106) and some bacterial infections such as shigellosis (107), but there are many infectious causes, including corticosteroids, inflammatory states, and nonhematologic malignancies. Corticosteroids create the picture by mobilizing the marginal pool of WBCs into the circulation and inhibiting their emigration into the extravascular space (108). Tumors may have leukocytosis as a paraneoplastic manifestation, the result of CSF liberation by the neoplasm (109,110).

Not only is the WBC count increased in bacterial infections, but the morphology of the cells is often a clue to the bacterial origin of a febrile state. These findings include toxic granulations, Döhle bodies, and vacuoles in the polymorphonuclear cells (111,112) (see Chapter 14). Toxic granulations represent nonspecific hypergranulation of the polymorphonuclear leukocytes, whereas Döhle bodies result from aggregation of the endoplasmic reticulum (113). Vacuolization of polymorphonuclear leukocytes is considered the best of these abnormalities as a clue to the presence of infection, provided that the vacuolization is not artifactually created by WBC ingestion of anticoagulants (114). Definitive morphologic evidence of bacteria can sometimes be demonstrated, especially in asplenic subjects, by Gram staining a buffy coat preparation of the peripheral blood (115). In overwhelming sepsis, the organisms are frequently evident in the vacuoles of the polymorphonuclear cells.

The lack of granulocytosis in patients with most viral infections originates in viral induction of an acute phase response that suppresses granulocyte expansion (116,117); monocytes from virally infected persons do not release IL-1 (118). In addition, the levels of IFN-γ, a cause of neutropenia, are elevated in viral states and may inhibit the IL-CSF response of bacterial infection (119). Frequently, lymphocytosis is present with viral infection (120,121). The specific receptors for viral particles on lymphocytes may be a stimulus for B-lymphocyte proliferation or lymphoid death (122). T-cell ratios are often reversed in viral infections with increased suppressor T-cell numbers and activation (123). The atypical lymphocyte or Downey cell of infectious mononucleosis is a stimulated suppressor T cell (124) (see Chapter 20).

Anemia

Common to all chronic infections and probably playing a role in acute infections as well is the suppressive effect of IL-1β and TNF-α on erythropoiesis (125) (see section on Diagnosis of Anemia of Chronic Disease). In addition, the iron-steal phenomenon and the actions of hepcidin probably deprive microorganisms of iron, which is an essential nutrient for microbial replication, and may be a component of host immunity against infection (126). Serum levels of iron fall after a bacterial challenge, and the lactoferrin released from stimulated granulocytes is a conduit for this iron to return to RE cells. Many examples of bacterial pathogenicity being dependent on iron availability (*Neisseria gonorrhoeae, Neisseria meningitidis*) support the hypothesis that the anemia of infection is the body's com-

promise in an attempt to deprive invading microorganisms of iron (127,128).

The truth of the converse of this situation, that iron overload contributes to increased morbidity and mortality of infection, is controversial (129). Even critics of the iron overload theory do not seriously question hypoferremia as a host defense mechanism against bacterial infection.

INFECTIONS PRODUCING RED CELL APLASIA

Parvovirus B19. The erythroid abnormalities seen with infections involve almost every step in the production and survival of the RBC. Parvovirus B19, the cause of fifth disease (erythema infectiosum) in children, infects and kills early erythroid progenitors bearing the P blood group antigen (130–132). This infection, which is discussed in detail in Chapters 9 and 51, and in recent reviews (133,134), is usually not clinically significant unless the infection occurs in the setting of chronic hemolytic processes such as sickle cell disease or hereditary spherocytosis (135), or in patients with compromised immunity, such as those infected with the human immunodeficiency virus. In these situations, life-threatening red cell aplasia or even pancytopenia may be caused by an otherwise benign viral illness. The infection typically presents with fever, vomiting, and abdominal pain, along with pallor, extreme lassitude, and other symptoms of anemia (136,137). Sometimes multiple family members are affected simultaneously. Parvovirus B19 infections are often associated with mild neutropenia or thrombocytopenia (138), and isolated cases of transient pancytopenia (139–141), hemophagocytosis (142–144), and myelodysplasia (145,146) are reported. Rarely, glomerulonephritis, Henoch-Schönlein purpura, meningitis, and other rheumatic manifestations (including Raynaud's phenomenon, lupuslike diseases, antiphospholipid antibodies, and microangiopathic vasculitic syndromes) have also been associated with the virus. The virus is a particular danger to pregnant women, because it can cause fetal death due to anemia and nonimmune hydrops fetalis (147–149).

Epstein-Barr Virus. Epstein-Barr virus (EBV) has also been incriminated as a cause of RBC aplasia by the mechanism of T-cell suppression of CFU-E (150). Human T-cell lymphocyte virus–III is associated with dysplastic RBC features in the marrow and ineffective erythropoiesis (151).

INFECTIONS PRODUCING HEMOLYSIS

Exaggerated and premature RBC destruction accompanies many infections. Heightened RE activity with or without splenomegaly shortens RBC survival in these states. Infections are a leading cause of hemolysis in RBC enzyme deficiency states, but they may also cause excessive hemolysis by direct toxic or immunologic damage to cells (152).

Clostridial Sepsis. A devastatingly severe form of damage is produced in *Clostridium perfringens* (previously called *Cl. welchii*) sepsis secondary to attacks on the RBC membrane by proteases and phospholipase C (see section entitled "Toxins and Venoms" in Chapter 51). The peripheral blood smear findings in this situation are a striking RBC spherocytosis (153–155), which is accompanied by elevated levels of free plasma Hb (156). The infection is often rapidly progressive and leads to shock, disseminated intravascular coagulation, acute renal failure, and a fatal outcome. Hemolysis of the entire red cell mass has been reported (156–159).

Immunohemolysis. Immunologic sensitization may also create membrane damage during infections. *Mycoplasma* and numerous viral infections are associated with the development of cold agglutinins directed against the I or i antigens on RBCs (160). Although these antibodies are commonly detected, they infrequently cause significant hemolytic disease (see Chapter 52). The Donath-Landsteiner antibody, responsible for the bithermal activation of complement and hemolysis in paroxysmal cold hemoglobinuria, sometimes accompanies congenital syphilis or mumps (161), but these infections are no longer common. Today, paroxysmal cold hemoglobinuria more often follows nonspecific viral infections and is probably the most common cause of acute immunohemolytic anemia in children (162) (Chapter 52). Some bacteria, such as *Haemophilus influenzae*, cause hemolysis via attachment of a capsular polysaccharide to the RBCs, rendering them immunogenic once an antibody response occurs, with complement deposition and extravascular hemolysis (163).

Malaria. Parasitization of RBCs with resulting hemolysis is the major clinical manifestation of malaria, and the morphology of specific organisms in the peripheral blood smear contributes to identification of the different types of malaria. This parasite and the RBC have an interesting relation dictated by the mechanisms responsible for attachment and entry of the parasite into the cell (164). The Duffy blood group antigen is necessary for *Plasmodium vivax* attachment to the RBC; its absence prevents *P. vivax* infection *in vivo* (165) (see Chapter 57). The merozoites of *P. falciparum* bind to a variety of RBC membrane surface proteins, and these binding characteristics vary from strain to strain (166,167). There is evidence for involvement of glycophorin A (166,168–170), glycophorin B (171), glycophorin C (172), and band 3 (173–175). Somehow membrane lipid rafts are also involved (176). The rafts are clusters of glycosphingolipids, cholesterol and specific membrane proteins within the membrane lipid bilayer (see Chapter 51).

The interaction of parasite and red cell triggers an opening within the cytoskeleton followed by endocytosis of the parasite (177). Within the cell, the malaria parasite inserts a variety of proteins into the red cell membrane that allow it to obtain nutrients and control interactions with its environment. One such protein functions as a Tf receptor and probably enables the parasite to obtain iron directly from plasma (178). The *P. falciparum* parasite also can induce knob formation on the RBC membrane. The knobs contain a histidine-rich protein and attach to endothelial cells, which protects the parasites from splenic scrutiny but contributes to the sludging insults of the cerebral, hepatic, and other vessels of the body in *P. falciparum* malaria (179,180). There is evidence that the adhesion involves a sequence on the outside of red cell band 3 that is normally sequestered but is exposed in parasitized red cells (181,182), perhaps through clustering of band 3 by oxidant-damaged Hb (183). Children with Southeast Asian ovalocytosis (see Chapter 51), who have a deletion in band 3 that results in misfolding of external surface of the molecule, are apparently protected from cerebral malaria as a result (184). These adhesive insults have been reversed by antimalarial drugs combined with whole blood exchange transfusions (185).

Bartonellosis. Other microorganisms may parasitize the RBC with severe hemolysis. *Bartonella bacilliformis* (186,187), a gram-negative, flagellated bacterium, infects human erythrocytes (hematic phase) and endothelial cells (tissue phase), resulting in a biphasic disease. In the tissue phase of disease (verruga peruana), infection leads to infection of endothelial cells and a pronounced proliferation of these cells, resulting in characteristic skin eruptions of papules and nodules. The hematic phase is responsible for the intravascular hemolysis of

Oroya fever. This dangerous pathogen is now limited to a specific geographic area of Peru corresponding to the range of its sand fly vector.

At least two genes, ialA and ialB, are required for *B. bacilliformis* invasion (188). Disruption of ialB has been accomplished and proves that the gene is needed for both adherence and invasion by the bacterium (189). The IalB protein is a *nudix hydrolase*, an enzyme that catalyzes the hydrolysis of a class of signal nucleotides, the dinucleoside polyphosphates (190). How this relates to adherence or invasion is not understood. A third bacterial protein, deformin, causes the membrane to invaginate, probably by increasing the area of the inner half of the lipid bilayer (191,192). It may have a role in parasite entry. Studies of the interaction of the bacterium with the red cell membrane have identified multiple binding proteins (193), including some like the spectrins that are inside the membrane and seem unlikely partners. The mechanism of hemolysis is also not known. A hemolysin has been detected (194), but it requires direct contact of the parasite with the red cell for a long time, has not been isolated, and has not been tested by antibody inhibition or molecular modification.

B. bacilliformis requires Rho-GTPase activity for invasion of endothelial cells (195). Once inside, the cell forms inclusions (Rocha-Lima bodies) within the Golgi (195) and activates Rho signaling with the formation of actin stress fibers and spindle-shaped cells that lack the ability to form capillaries *in vitro* (195,196). Infection also increases the proliferation of endothelial cells (197), which leads to the characteristic papules and nodules of verruga peruana.

Babesiosis. A milder hemolytic anemia is caused by *Babesia microti* and *B. divergens* microorganisms (198,199) (also discussed in Chapter 51). Occasional cases of combined *B. microti* babesiosis and Lyme disease are described, attributable to the shared geographic locale of the tick vectors for these diseases (200). The disease can also be acquired by transfusion (201). Babesiosis is not life threatening, except in asplenic subjects in whom the parasitized RBCs are not contained (198,199,202). In those patients, the infection can be rapidly progressive and life threatening. In extreme cases, nearly all the red cells may be parasitized (203). Patients may have malaise, headache, fever, shaking chills, profuse sweating, jaundice, and dark urine. There may be intravascular hemolysis and, occasionally, pancytopenia and hemophagocytosis (204–206). Diagnosis is made by finding the parasites in blood smears, or by serologic tests or amplification of parasitic DNA using the polymerase chain reaction. Current treatment of symptomatic cases is quinine plus clindamycin, but treatment failures have been reported in asplenic patients. Exchange transfusion may reduce the parasite load and be beneficial (203).

Little is known about the pathophysiology of the disease. The parasite invades through a parasitophorous vacuole (207), like malaria. Presumably, the membrane skeleton must disassemble regionally, as it does with malarial parasites, to permit invasion, but this has not been tested. The red cell membrane incurs damage that is evident under the electron microscope (203), but this has not been studied at a molecular level. The membrane proteins involved in the interaction are also not known.

Pancytopenia

Splenomegaly, an accompaniment of many chronic infections (Chapter 21), may produce a hypersplenic pancytopenic state because of accelerated cell destruction within the hypertrophied organ.

VIRAL HEPATITIS

A much more severe pancytopenia in the setting of aplastic anemia occurs as an aftermath of bouts of viral hepatitis (208). The presumptive agent is non-A, non-B hepatitis, because serologic testing for other known hepatitis viruses has been negative. The marrow disorder is not concomitant with the hepatitis but supervenes weeks to months after the hepatic insult. Usually, no relation in severity is found between the preceding hepatitis and the subsequent aplasia of the marrow. Because this form of hepatitis-related aplasia carries a poor prognosis with a rapid and high mortality, these patients are candidates for early marrow transplantation when such an option is available.

Aplastic anemia accompanies hepatitis in an additional setting. A disproportionate number of liver transplantation patients have developed aplastic anemia after transplantation for non-A, non-B hepatitis (209). The mechanism for the association is not understood, although the hepatitis virus has been demonstrated to be pantropic and probably involves the marrow elements. Several animal and human viruses, such as EBV (210), induce marrow aplasia by direct infection of the marrow. The interval between the initial hepatitis and the subsequent aplasia suggests an immunologic factor in the hepatitis cases followed by aplastic anemia. The relation of hepatitis and aplasia is described in detail in Chapter 9.

VIRUS-ASSOCIATED HEMOPHAGOCYTIC SYNDROME

Pancytopenia in the context of infection may also occur in association with the virus-associated hemophagocytic syndrome (VAHS) (or virus-related hemophagocytic lymphohistiocytosis), a "benign" proliferation of histocytes that is difficult to distinguish from familial erythrophagocytic lymphohistiocytosis or malignant histiocytosis (211–217) (see Chapter 30). The disease is characterized by high fevers, failure-to-thrive or weight loss, pancytopenia, hepatosplenomegaly with variable lymphadenopathy, hepatic dysfunction, a disseminated intravascular coagulation (DIC)-like bleeding diathesis, marked hyperferritinemia (>1000 µg/L) (218,219) and sometimes pulmonary infiltrates and a maculopapular skin rash (211,214). The bone marrow features increased numbers of "benign" histiocytes containing ingested platelets, RBCs, and WBCs. Similar lymphohistiocytic infiltrates and hematophagocytosis are also observed in liver, spleen, and lymph nodes. The patients are very ill with multiorgan signs and symptoms. The disease is more frequent in children but is reported at all ages. Adults more often have a syndrome of EBV-positive T-cell lymphoma, affecting particularly the nose, skin, and gastrointestinal tract, which is considered different than VAHS, although there are many similarities (214). This syndrome also is characterized by hematophagocytosis and is difficult to distinguish from malignant histiocytosis (211,220). From the reports in the literature, it seems to be more common in far Eastern countries. Although VAHS is sometimes termed a *benign histiocytosis*, it is often progressive and fatal, with fatality rates as high as 70% reported (221). VAHS or a very similar syndrome is particularly common in patients with Chédiak-Higashi syndrome (222), where it has been termed the "accelerated phase" and is usually terminal.

Clinically, there appear to be two clinical variants of the disease: one associated with EBV infection, and one associated with other causes (215,223). The EBV-associated variant is much more common and more often fatal. Almost all studies of VAHS have been in patients with this variant. These studies show that patients have very high levels of TNF-α and IFN-γ, and to a lesser degree IL-1α during the acute phase of the illness (224–227). The levels of TNF-α and IFN-γ correlate closely with the activity of the disease (224,225), with levels of IFN-γ forecasting a relapse (225).

There is convincing evidence that T lymphocytes are infected, particularly CD8(+) T cells (228), and that many patients have a clonal proliferation of T cells (223,229), children as well as adults. In one adult, a clonal population of natural killer cells was present (230). Patients who are clonal in the EBV genome or T-cell receptor have a better outcome than those who have a clonal cytogenetic abnormality (231). Recent studies show that EBV-infection of T-lymphoma cells up-regulates TNF-α (227). The supernatants from the infected lines in turn activate U937 cells, a monocyte-macrophage line, with enhanced phagocytosis and secretion of TNF-α, IFN-γ, and IL-1α. Secretion of the cytokines by U937 cells was inhibited 70% by anti–TNF-α and almost completely by a combination of antibodies to both TNF-α and IFN-γ (227). The data suggest that the hematophagocytic syndrome of EBV-positive T lymphoma, and possibly VAHS, is caused by EBV-induced up-regulation of TNF-α, which with IFN-γ and possibly other cytokines can activate macrophages. If so, treatment of these diseases with anti–TNF-α (e.g., infliximab) would be expected to be efficacious and possibly life saving.

VAHS is also reported with a large array of other viral infections (e.g., human herpesviruses-6 and -8, cytomegalovirus, parvovirus B19, human immunodeficiency virus, hepatitis viruses, varicella-zoster, adenovirus, rubella, rubeola, and dengue), as well as with a bewildering number of other infections (bacterial, fungal, and parasitic), malignancies, and even some drugs and toxins. Patients with underlying inflammatory, immunodeficiency, or autoimmune disorders may be at increased risk (232). In general, these forms of VAHS are transient and less severe, although individual cases may be progressive and fatal.

The optimal treatment of VAHS includes: (a) control of cytokine storm including coagulopathy and multiple organ failure, (b) control of opportunistic infections, and (c) eradication of clonally proliferating EBV-containing T- or natural killer cells using immunomodulatory therapy with etoposide and various combinations of corticosteroids, intravenous immunoglobulin, or cyclosporine (233–235). If necessary, hemopoietic stem cell/bone marrow transplantation can be life saving (236,237). A single report showing a high response rate to chloroquine therapy has recently appeared and deserves further investigation (238).

Bone Marrow Abnormalities

INFECTIOUS DISEASES

The bone marrow frequently contains clues as to the source of infectious diseases. Histoplasmosis, tuberculosis, kala-azar (239), and *Candida* all have been identified in marrow macrophages. Marrow granulomas may be a marker of disseminated tuberculosis or histoplasmosis as well as noninfectious entities like sarcoidosis. The liver is more frequently involved than the marrow in miliary tuberculosis, but the marrow biopsy is still important because its findings are complementary to liver biopsy in the search for tuberculosis. Histoplasmosis, like tuberculosis, brucellosis, and *Salmonella*, can be successfully cultured from the marrow aspirate. The organisms are not the only causes of bone marrow granulomas; cytomegalovirus involvement of the marrow creates the same morphologic finding (240). Bone marrow morphology and culture play an increasingly important role in the identification and isolation of the many organisms (tuberculosis, histoplasmosis, viral infection) that complicate the acquired immunodeficiency state.

BONE MARROW NECROSIS

Infection is a leading cause of an unusual hematologic lesion, bone marrow necrosis (241). This complication of sickle cell disease and other hematologic disorders may give rise to marrow embolization and pulmonary damage (242,243). Its occurrence in nonsicklers is most frequently in the context of sepsis, with endotoxin considered the toxic etiologic agent. Bone pain may be severe and attributed to other causes (244). No pathognomonic peripheral blood findings are noted in bone marrow necrosis, although cytopenias and a leukoerythroblastic blood picture are frequently present. The diagnosis requires recognition of necrotic marrow from the involved areas, a frequently overlooked finding. Magnetic resonance imaging may represent a noninvasive means of making the diagnosis (245,246).

Hemostatic Involvement with Infectious Diseases

Thrombocytopenia occurs frequently in the setting of a variety of infections. The mechanisms are complex and sometimes unclear because infectious agents may cause many effects on platelet synthesis and destruction. A fall in platelet count is a universal feature of viral infections. The lesion is sometimes attributable to direct viral infection of the megakaryocyte with reduced platelet production (247). How often this is the case is unknown. Because platelets possess receptors for viral particles, accelerated platelet destruction may also occur, possibly assisting in containment of the infection (248–250). An even more significant thrombocytopenia may occur 2 to 3 weeks after the initial viral insult at a time when immunologic mechanisms are most active (251,252). This complication originates in several possible immunologic reactions. Antibody cross-reactivity as an immunologic overflow phenomenon, immune complex adherence to platelet membranes, and viral hapten deposition all have been implicated in these thrombocytopenic states (253). These phenomena are discussed in detail in Chapter 32.

Bacterial infections are associated with thrombocytopenia (254,255). Immune mechanisms play a major role, with sensitization of platelets participating in the body's generalized hyperimmune response state (256). Platelets may function as endotoxin "sponges" and be destroyed as part of the body's containment of endotoxin (257). Activation of complement in the setting of infection leads to WBC attachment to the pulmonary microvasculature; secondary thrombocytopenia occurs, caused by adherence of platelets to the leukocyte-damaged endothelium. This fall in platelet count may be one of the earliest manifestations of impending adult respiratory distress syndromes (258).

DISSEMINATED INTRAVASCULAR COAGULATION

All infectious agents have the potential to initiate a consumption coagulopathy with thrombocytopenia and reduction in several components of the clotting cascade (see Chapter 41) (259). This complication of septicemia is especially prominent when hypotension accompanies the septic state (260). Bleeding is its most common manifestation, although infection-related DIC may infrequently cause the devastating picture of purpura fulminans with thrombosis of the vessels of the extremities and secondary gangrene (261–263). Sepsis in asplenic persons (see Chapters 21 and 51) is sometimes the cause of DIC with adrenal hemorrhage and renal cortical necrosis (Waterhouse-Friderichsen syndrome) (264); this syndrome has been described most frequently with pneumococcal sepsis (265,266), but staphylococcal, streptococcal, and meningococcal organisms may create the same picture (267).

THROMBOSIS

Thrombosis is not a common feature of infection even though IL-1 decreases endothelial cell fibrinolytic activity by increasing the levels of plasminogen activator inhibitors (268). Thrombophlebitis due to *Campylobacter fetus*, a microaerophilic gram-negative rod, usually occurs in the setting of an underlying medical illness. When phlebitis fails to respond to heparin, this association should be considered (269). A suppurative thrombophlebitis of the internal jugular vein secondary to an oropharyngeal infection with *Fusobacterium necrophorum* (Lemierre's syndrome) is another example of infection-related thrombosis (270).

THROMBOTIC THROMBOCYTOPENIC PURPURA AND HEMOLYTIC UREMIC SYNDROME

The syndromes of thrombotic thrombocytopenic purpura (TTP) and hemolytic uremic syndrome (HUS) are both characterized by hyaline thrombi, generated throughout the microvasculature of the body in the former and primarily localized to the renal vessels in the latter (Chapter 32) (271,272). Although several agents appear to incite these syndromes, a striking correlation exists between HUS and antecedent diarrheal illnesses caused by toxigenic strains of *Shigella* and *Escherichia coli* (273). These organisms secrete a verotoxin that is damaging to renal cells in culture. This toxin may disrupt the endothelial cell with its stores of von Willebrand's factor (vWF) and result in platelet adhesion to the vessel wall (274). TTP is now known to be caused by a deficiency, either congenital or secondary to an acquired antibody, of the metalloproteinase ADAM-TS (275–278), which cleaves high-molecular-weight multimers of vWF (Chapter 32). The uncleaved multimers are more effective in aggregating platelets and produce the characteristic hyaline (platelet) thrombi that underlie the pathophysiology.

MALIGNANT DISEASE

Each step in the body's elegantly modulated system of erythropoiesis, alone or in combination, may be pathologically altered in the setting of malignancy. The hematologic lesion may originate in sources as diverse as the direct replacement of marrow by the malignancy or, more commonly, as ACD, the anemia that accompanies even extramedullary tumors. The internists' tumor, hypernephroma, has anemia as part of its diagnostic triad with a flank mass and fever (279,280). Pancreatic carcinoma and other gastrointestinal malignancies so frequently present with anemia that physicians incur a responsibility to examine the gastrointestinal tract in any patient with otherwise unexplained iron deficiency anemia (281,282). Erythropoiesis rarely escapes some impairment in the body's altercation with malignancy.

More than 50% of patients with nonhematologic malignancies present with anemia, both adults (283) and children (284). The reasons are complex and include blood loss, hemolysis, bone marrow infiltration, hypersplenism, nutrient deficiencies, chemotherapy, radiation therapy, and ACD. Numerous recent reviews are available (283,285–291). There is good evidence that anemia is a poor prognostic factor in cancer (289), but it is not clear why. One school of thought is that anemia adversely impacts radiotherapy by limiting oxygen supply to the tumor (292–294). Certainly, it is true that *in vitro* tumor cells are 2.5 to 3.0 times more effectively killed by conventional photon radiation under normoxic conditions than under anoxic conditions (294). However, *in vivo*, the degree of hypoxia is hard to assess, and there are compensating mechanisms to increase oxygen delivery in the face of anemia. Other factors such as the size or the biology of the tumor may account for differences in Hb and may be more directly related to outcome than the effect of hypoxia on the efficacy of therapy (295). Additional studies are needed to resolve this question and are ongoing. Nevertheless, it makes sense to optimize Hb levels before radiation or chemotherapy, which is the usual practice.

In addition, anemia contributes to the fatigue felt by cancer patients (291,296–298), along with effects of cytokines (291) and chemotherapy, and the metabolic needs of the tumor. Alleviating anemia significantly improves the quality of life of cancer patients (288,290). Fortunately, many cancer patients respond to recombinant human Epo (285,286,288,290,292,299,300). This treatment is discussed in more detail in the section Erythropoietin Therapy.

Inhibition of Erythropoiesis by Cancer

Tumor growth *in vitro* and *in vivo* is known to be associated with inhibition of normal erythropoiesis (301,302). What remains controversial is the mechanism or mechanisms that create this impairment. Addition of W-256 tumor cells to Epo-stimulated marrow cultures inhibits CFU-E in proportion to the concentration of the cocultured W-256 cells (303). Cell cytolysis secondary to direct cell interaction with malignant cells has been documented with other tumors, but the effect of W-256 cells is demonstrable even in CFU-E cultures that separate the malignant cells from the population of bone marrow cells. These experiments support earlier observations that marrows from persons with malignancies have decreased responsiveness to Epo stimulation (304). Linking both observations is the inhibitory effect generated by TNF-α which is released in response to tumors (305,306) (see the subsection Role of Proinflammatory Cytokines in the section Anemia of Chronic Disease). This cytokine, part of the body's humoral defenses against tumor invasion, inhibits the growth of CFU-E and BFU-E (27,33,34,307–309) and sends progenitor cells to apoptotic extinction (27,38). Multiple reports show that patients with cancer have elevated levels of proinflammatory cytokines, especially IL-6, IL-1, and TNF-α (310,311), but the cytokine cocktail varies with the tumor and the immune response. There is also evidence that the level of Epo is low relative to the degree of anemia, and that the response to Epo is blunted (312,313), which suggests that functional Epo deficiency is a major contributor to the anemia of malignancy, along with ACD.

The anemia of malignancy may be moderate in severity when it occurs as a component of the ACD; a more severe anemia is created when pure RBC aplasia supervenes. In adults, this is frequently in the setting of a thymoma or lymphoproliferative disease (314). Approximately 50% of adults with pure RBC aplasia have a thymoma, and 10% of patients with thymoma have pure RBC aplasia (315). Krantz and colleagues (316) demonstrated an immunoglobulin (Ig) G inhibitor of erythropoiesis in such patients. Suppressor T-cell inhibition has also been proved to be a cause of pure RBC aplasia with and without associated lymphoproliferative disease (317–319). Thymectomy has successfully reversed the aplasia in most patients with thymomas; corticosteroids and cytoxan are also effective in treating this immunologically mediated anemia. Treatment of the underlying disorder with daily cytoxan has reversed this aplasia in some patients. Pure RBC aplasia is also discussed in Chapter 9.

Anemia in the setting of malignancy may also be caused by progressive bone marrow infiltration with tumor. Marrow involvement occurs in approximately 10% of nonhematologic tumors and is frequently heralded by a so-called leukoerythroblastic blood picture (320). The latter is characterized by the presence in the peripheral blood of nucleated RBC, teardrop RBC, early myeloid forms, and frequently some alteration in platelet size and number. The appearance of immature cells in the peripheral blood is probably not caused by "crowding out" the bone marrow, as is widely believed, because it can be seen when only a small portion of the marrow is affected, even at a microscopic level. More likely, it results from "tumor humors"—unknown factors released by the tumor that interfere with mechanisms for retaining cells in the bone marrow until they are fully mature.

The occurrence of a leukoerythroblastic blood picture in a patient with a malignancy is near-certain evidence of marrow involvement with tumor. Some tumors, such as prostate, breast, small cell lung carcinomas, and neuroblastomas, have a relatively high incidence of marrow metastases, supporting the role of bone scans in establishing the disease stage within these malignancies. A hot spot on bone scan provides an excellent site for marrow biopsy to confirm the presence of tumor, a discovery that may sometimes be the initial documentation of the tumor.

The anemic lesion in malignancy is not confined to marrow suppression or replacement by tumor. Autoimmune hemolytic anemia, which frequently accompanies lymphoproliferative disorders, also occurs with solid tumors, although rarely (321). This has resulted in the recommendation that a search for occult malignancy be undertaken in elderly persons with otherwise idiopathic autoimmune hemolytic anemia. The variety of tumors discovered has included lung, kidney, testicular, and gastrointestinal malignancies. A more common association of tumors with autoimmune hemolysis is the well-documented linkage of ovarian tumors with corticosteroid- and splenectomy-refractory hemolytic anemia (322). These are mainly benign tumors such as dermoid cysts, which contain antibodies with Rh specificity. Removal of the tumor reverses the hemolytic process.

Traumatic hemolysis with a microangiopathic blood picture is a feature of some metastatic malignancies (323). This lesion has been attributed to RBC shearing by fibrin strands and pathologically altered small blood vessels (324); an attendant consumption coagulopathy precipitated by certain tumors was thought to create the fibrin thrombi on which the RBCs are impaled. But this is probably an example of how a dramatic picture—in this case of red cells being guillotined by fibrin strands (324)—can drive impressions, even though the system used to create the pictures was a very nonphysiologic one. The facts that the courses of DIC and microangiopathic hemolytic anemia are not necessarily parallel and that fibrin thrombi are rare at autopsy in such patients has led to alternative hypotheses. Not all patients with tumor-related DIC have evidence of a microangiopathic process. Jacobsen and Jackson (325) found traumatic hemolysis in only 50% of their series. Antman and colleagues (326) relate the RBC lesion to direct contact of the RBC cells with intraluminal embolic tumor cells within the pulmonary vasculature, an involvement they documented in all their cancer patients with microangiopathic hemolytic anemia. The tumor most frequently associated with traumatic hemolysis is a gastric malignancy, highly prone to metastasize to the pulmonary circuit. The horrid prognosis of persons with tumor-related microangiopathy is concordant with widespread metastases as the cause of the lesion (327).

Erythropoietin Therapy

Randomized, double-blind, placebo-controlled trials established almost a decade ago that Epo (Procrit, epoetin alfa) effectively increases Hb levels and reduces transfusion needs in cancer patients (328–331). The dose required, 150 to 300 IU/kg s.c., three times per week, is approximately two to three times higher than the typical dose in renal failure patients, because of the resistance to Epo in the cancer patient population (300). Subsequently, two large, prospective, open-label, community-based clinical studies were performed that confirmed the initial results and showed that Epo treatment significantly improved quality of life, including energy level and ability to do daily activities, and decreased fatigue (332,333). This has been confirmed in a recent study (334). Because fatigue is the symptom with the greatest adverse impact on the quality of life and functional capacity of cancer patients (335), exceeding even pain, this is an important result. Surprisingly, the greatest improvement in quality of life for each 1 g/dL change in Hb occurs in the interval between 11 and 12 g/dL, which is well above the range that is usually considered clinically relevant. Perhaps symptoms of anemia manifest at higher Hb levels in the generally elderly cancer patients in these studies than in others with anemia. Whatever the reason, it suggests that a target Hb level of 12 g/dL should be used to obtain maximum benefits. Finally, pharmacologic (336) and community-based (337) studies have shown that it is possible to use once/week instead of three times/week dosing, which is much more convenient for patients. One recently published regimen (300) begins at 10,000 U (600 U/kg) s.c. of Epo (Procrit, epoetin alfa) once a week for 4 weeks and doubles the dose if the Hb level increases by less than 1 g/dL in that time. Epo is discontinued if there is no significant (>1 g/dL from baseline) response after eight weeks. Otherwise the dose is titrated to maintain the desired Hb level (usually approximately 12 g/dL). The use of Epo in treating patients with cancer is also discussed in Chapter 7.

Anemia can be corrected with Epo in approximately one-half of all cancer patients, although more than one-half respond. Response rate is independent of tumor type or chemotherapy regimen (332,333). Some data suggest that it is higher in patients with an initially low endogenous Epo concentration (299,338), but this was not confirmed in another study (333). Fjornes (338) observed that response is greater in patients whose initial serum creatine is elevated, and suggests that Epo may work best in those with chemotherapy-induced renal failure. This suggestion deserves further study. Finally, a recent clinical trial of Epo suggests that improving the Hb level may improve the patient's prognosis as well as quality of life (334). This finding also needs to be confirmed.

Erythrocytosis and Malignancy

A classic paraneoplastic manifestation of malignancy is erythrocytosis or secondary polycythemia caused by tumor release of Epo or Epo-like substances (339–341). This process is now much better understood because of the extraordinary recent advances (342–345) in our understanding of how hypoxia controls gene expression (346–349). These are summarized in Figure 56-3 (see also Chapter 7). Basically, oxygen controls the actions of a critical, conserved transcription factor called *hypoxia-inducing factor* or *HIF-1*. Left to itself, HIF-1, which is composed of α and β subunits, binds to hypoxia recognition sequences in the promoters of oxygen-regulated genes and turns on their transcription (Fig. 56-3). The genes include Epo (350,351), angiogenic growth factors, glycolytic enzymes, and others. When oxygen is present, these genes are turned off because two hydroxylases use oxygen to hydroxylate critical amino acids in HIF-1α, leading to its inactivation and destruction (Fig. 56-3). It is likely that the prolyl hydroxylase serves as an oxygen sensor, but that remains to be proved. The degradation process involves the von Hippel-Lindau tumor-suppressor protein (pVHL), which is the sensing subunit of a E3-type ubiquitin ligase complex that adds ubiquitin subunits to HIF-1α, diverting it to the cell's garbage disposal, the proteasome. Germline mutations in the VHL gene cause von Hippel-Lindau disease, which is characterized by central nervous system hemangioblastomas. Somatic mutations involving VHL are common in clear cell renal carcinomas, to which von Hippel-Lindau patients are predisposed.

Clearly, mutations involving this system might be expected to lead to aberrant Epo secretion as well as tumor formation, particularly mutations that inactivate pVHL or block its interaction with HIF-1α. One such mutation has been identified in a patient with a clear cell carcinoma, aberrant Epo production,

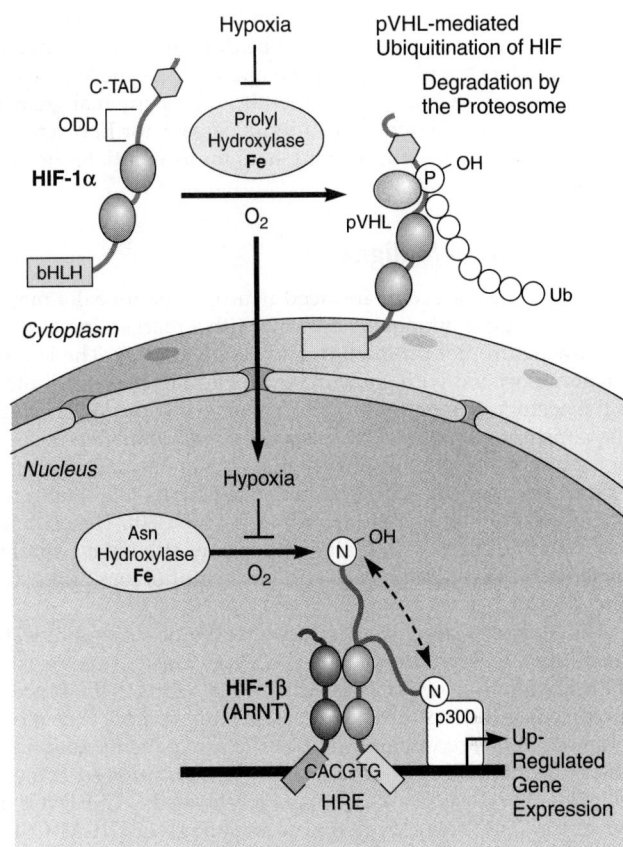

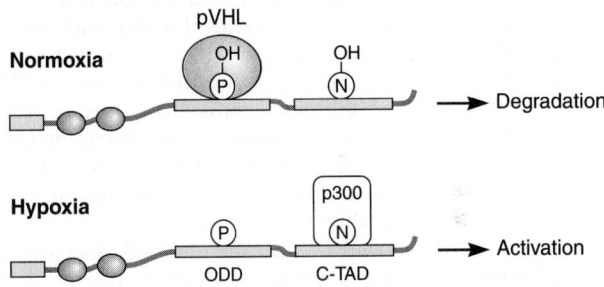

Figure 56-3. Regulation of the HIF-1 transcription factor and hypoxia-sensitive transcription. Under *normoxic* conditions, a proline (P) in the oxygen-dependent degradation domain (ODD) of HIF-1α is hydroxylated, triggering HIF-1α recognition by pVHL (the von Hippel-Lindau tumor-suppressor protein), ubiquitination (Ub) by other components attached to pVHL, and degradation by the proteasome. Under these conditions, no HIF-1α accumulates, and no HIF-1α-driven transcription occurs. Under *hypoxic* conditions, HIF-1α degradation is prevented, and HIF-1α translocates to the nucleus where it partners with HIF-1β (also called *ARNT*) to form a transcription factor that binds to hypoxia-related elements (HRE) in the DNA through its basic helix-loop-helix (bHLH) domain and activates expression of hypoxia-driven genes such as erythropoietin. Transcriptional activation involves a second O_2-regulatory step. Under hypoxic conditions, a second hydroxylase is unable to add a blocking hydroxy group to an asparagine (N) in the C-terminal activation domain (C-TAD) of HIF-1α. This allows the domain to interact with the p300/CBP transcriptional coactivator, up-regulating transcription. It is possible, but not proven, that the iron-containing prolyl hydroxylase is the true oxygen sensor in this conserved pathway. (After Bruick RK, McKnight SL. Oxygen sensing gets a second wind. *Science* 2002;295:807–808.)

and erythrocytosis (Hb = 20 g/dL) (352). Aberrant Epo production and erythrocytosis is also observed in patients with hepatomas and hepatocellular carcinomas (353,354), Wilms' tumors (355), and hemangioblastomas (350). In fact, careful analysis shows that all hemangioblastomas express Epo (350).

The differentiation of this secondary erythrocytosis from polycythemia vera can sometimes be difficult. The panmyeloplasia of polycythemia vera may be mimicked by the leukocytosis and thrombocytosis that frequently accompany malignancy. The presence of splenomegaly, immunoassays for Epo activity, and *in vitro* marrow studies may help to differentiate the two entities (356).

Leukocytosis of Malignancy

Kinetic studies of tumor-induced neutrophilia reveal a major expansion of granulopoietic marrow with a marked increase in marrow neutrophil production and turnover (357). The leukocytosis associated with some malignancies has been attributed to the necrotic element within the tumors (358); the WBC elevation constitutes a nonspecific response to inflammation created by the tumor. Knowledge of TNF-α's effect on the bone marrow, with its release of IL-1 and granulocyte-CSF (G-CSF), updates this relation of tumors with leukocytosis (359,360). The association of monocytosis with malignancies may also have a similar cause, with macrophage activation by lymphokines and cytokines (361).

The leukocytosis of malignancy may be of a magnitude to constitute a leukemoid reaction (362,363). This paraneoplastic phenomenon is growth factor–driven, analogous to the process just discussed in erythrocytosis-associated tumors, but more common. In one recent study, 10% to 15% of patients with lung cancer (almost all non–small cell types) developed tumor-related leukocytosis (364). One-half had elevated G-CSF levels in the serum, 10% had elevated G-macrophage-CSF (GM-CSF), and 55% had elevated IL-6. Similar results are reported in renal cell carcinoma (365), transitional cell carcinoma (366), and other cancers (367–369). A cell line from a patient with squamous cell carcinoma of the lung, leukocytosis, and hypercalcemia retained the ability to produce G-CSF and a parathyroid hormonelike protein and reproduced the paraneoplastic syndrome when transplanted into nude mice, proving that the phenomenon is not secondary to effects of the tumor on the immune system or other cells (370). Cytokines up-regulated G-CSF production in this cell line, as they probably do in patients.

Sweet's syndrome (acute febrile dermatosis) is associated with malignancy in 15% of cases and is also classified as a paraneoplastic syndrome. The characteristic features are fever, neutrophilia, and raised erythematous tender plaques on the skin that are densely infiltrated with neutrophils. The syndrome is usually associated with hematologic malignancies but occasionally occurs with solid tumors of all types (371). Remarkably, in patients with solid tumors, Sweet's syndrome preceded the initial diagnosis or an asymptomatic recurrent or metastatic tumor 60% of the time (370).

Eosinophilia in Malignancy

Eosinophilia is considered a response to malignancy, although the mechanism for its presence remains unclarified (372,373). Several cases of resolution of eosinophilia after resection of a malignancy have led to the conclusion that some tumors contain an eosinophil chemotactic–stimulatory substance (374,375). We now know that IL-5 is one of the main factors in the proliferation and differentiation of mature eosinophils (see Chapter 7) (376). IL-3 and GM-CSF also stimulate eosinophil production, but these are multilineage growth factors and stimulate the survival, proliferation, and differentiation of a broad range of progenitors, including cells with stem cell properties. IL-5, like Epo, G-CSF, and thrombopoietin (Tpo), is lineage specific and stimulates more mature cells. Paraneoplastic production of IL-5

by tumors has been observed in a few cases of cancer and hypereosinophilia (377,378) and probably happens more often than realized, because the cause of eosinophilia is seldom carefully examined.

There is evidence that IL-2 can also cause eosinophilia. Patients receiving IL-2 in therapeutic cancer trials develop marked eosinophilia (379), and serum levels of soluble IL-2 receptor are very high in patients with hypereosinophilia, including patients with eosinophilia and T-cell lymphoma (380). The mechanism of these effects is not clear. It may be that IL-2 is acting through IL-5, because sera from IL-2–treated patients stimulate the antitumor cytotoxicity of eosinophils, but this effect is blocked by anti–IL-5 (379). In any event, these kinds of observations raise the possibility that tumor-related eosinophilia may usually be a response directed at the tumor, similar to the known role of eosinophils in defense against parasites, instead of a paraneoplastic effect (381). Eosinophil infiltration of tumors occurs and may represent part of the body's defenses against malignancy (382). As noted, IL-2 stimulates both the direct and antibody-dependent cellular cytotoxicity of eosinophils (379). IL-3 also stimulates eosinophil antibody-dependent cellular cytotoxicity, as well as superoxide production and phagocytosis (383).

The importance of establishing which of these dual roles eosinophils play in malignancy concerns the common practice of reducing eosinophil counts that are considered a threat to the body. This appears unwise until a thorough search rules out malignancy and makes a direct attack on the eosinophil appropriate.

Thrombocytosis in Malignancy

Thrombocytosis joins anemia and leukocytosis as common accompaniments of nonhematologic malignancies (384). The opposite is also true: 10% of patients with more than 500,000 circulating platelets/μL have a malignancy (385). Although the platelet elevations are usually moderate, the combination of tumor with infection or bleeding can result in a platelet count elevation that rivals essential thrombocythemia (386). The two situations can usually be differentiated by the abnormal platelet morphology and prolonged bleeding time seen with primary thrombocythemia. The tumor most frequently associated with thrombocytosis is a bronchogenic carcinoma (384).

Tpo (c-mpl ligand) is the lineage-specific growth factor for megakaryocytes and platelet production (387–389), although IL-3 (390), IL-6 (391), IL-11 (392), and kit ligand (393) also stimulate megakaryocytopoiesis and thrombopoiesis *in vitro* and *in vivo* (see Chapter 7). The latter factors are all multilineage growth factors, which induce early multipotent progenitors to proliferate and even differentiate toward lineage-specific progenitors. IL-3, IL-11, and kit ligand also participate in the induction of the proliferation and differentiation of lineage-specific progenitors. Together these factors constitute a kind of megakaryocyte-CSF, but Tpo is probably the only factor that actually induces lineage-restricted megakaryocyte progenitor proliferation and differentiation of those progenitors to megakaryocytes. Tpo is continuously produced in many tissues, especially the liver, and is removed from the blood by platelets and megakaryocytes through receptor-mediated uptake, so that levels are high in thrombocytopenic or aplastic patients (394,395).

Activating mutations of the Tpo gene have been discovered in patients with hereditary thrombocythemia (396,397), but paraneoplastic thrombocytosis due to somatic mutations or overexpression of Tpo in tumors has not yet been reported, though presumably it will be.

The reactive thrombocytosis more typically observed in cancer patients, and in other states of inflammation and tissue damage, is probably caused by IL-6. IL-6 induces the acute phase response, including thrombocytosis, in therapeutic trials (398,399), and serum IL-6 levels are elevated in cancer patients with thrombocytosis (365,400). Recent studies show that IL-6 induces thrombocytosis by stimulating Tpo production (399).

Hemostasis and Malignancy

The historical entity of Trousseau's syndrome has been extended by the work of Sacks and colleagues (401). The phenomenon of thrombophilia and cancer has also been recently reviewed (402–407) and is discussed in Chapter 42. The original lesion of thrombosis in the setting of malignancy has been amplified to include consumption coagulopathy, arterial and venous thromboses, and marantic endocarditis. The most common associated tumors are mucus-secreting adenocarcinomas. A direct activator of factor V has been isolated from mucin and is considered one of the precipitants of the coagulopathy (408). Other tumor procoagulants have also been identified, confirming the multiple pathways for activation of the clotting cascade in this condition (409). Thrombosis is the major component of the syndrome, although some malignancies create a bleeding disorder caused by release of fibrinolysins or rapid consumption of normal clotting factors. Promyelocytic leukemia and prostatic carcinoma are examples of this phenomenon.

The syndrome is not related to the size of the tumor; in fact, the underlying neoplasm often is not obvious and is difficult to find. The problem usually makes itself known when venous thromboses recur while a patient is on coumadin or when thromboses appear in atypical locations. The evidence for DIC may be subtle, with normal levels of platelets and fibrinogen representing reductions in the thrombocythemia-hyperfibrinogenemia that accompany malignancies. Elevated fibrin-split products and cryofibrinogens may be further laboratory evidence of the phenomenon (410,411).

Control of the underlying neoplasm is the primary objective, but this is rarely possible because of the refractory nature of the tumor and the presence of metastatic disease. In the presence of the latter, a microangiopathic hemolytic anemia becomes an additional manifestation of the syndrome. Because elimination of the tumor is not possible, and coumadin is ineffective in preventing the thromboses, heparin administration becomes the mainstay of symptomatic management. Subcutaneous heparin in amounts to prolong the activated partial thromboplastin time 1.5 to 2.0 times normal control values (or alternatively low-molecular-weight heparin) is usually successful in slightly prolonging life until bleeding or thrombosis, frequently cerebral, results in death. In the late twentieth century, Trousseau's syndrome continues with the grim prognosis of its original recognition in the late 19th century (412).

ANEMIA AND LIVER DISEASE

Anemia in the setting of liver disease is common and multifactorial in its origin (413). Both acute and chronic liver disease are accompanied by increased portal pressures with the resultant congestive splenomegaly potentially creating any combination of anemia, leukopenia, or thombocytopenia (414). The marrow's compensation for such hemolytic insults is frequently dampened or absent because of concomitant vitamin-nutritional deficiencies and the shared toxicity by the liver and bone marrow of the cellular insults imposed by alcohol (415). Blood loss with the threat of iron deficiency may also contribute to the anemia of the liver disease.

Delineation of the causes and even the degree of anemia is difficult in the context of liver disease. Hemodilution occurs secondary to the hyperrenin state of both liver disease and splenomegaly (416). Increased amounts of atrial natriuretic factor may blunt some of this plasma volume expansion in such patients (417). Reticulocytosis may represent a marrow's release from alcohol inhibition, the response to replenishment of a missing vitamin, or even compensation for gastrointestinal bleeding. Hyperbilirubinemia, elevated lactic dehydrogenase levels, and reduced haptoglobin levels may result from liver disease and may not be caused by hemolysis. Because the liver is a storehouse of iron, the serum levels of iron and ferritin are misleadingly elevated with hepatocellular disease (418). All of these alterations complicate the interpretation of hematologic data in liver disease and enforce the need to recognize the dynamic and multifactorial pathogeneses of anemia in such states.

Liver Disease and the Red Cell Membrane

The RBC membrane is in dynamic equilibrium with the cholesterol-phospholipid components of the surrounding plasma, and their membranes undergo remodeling by exchange of molecules with their plasma counterparts (419). The morphologic abnormalities of RBCs in these conditions are attributable to the alterations in lipids and lipoproteins that accompany liver disease. When biliary flow is obstructed, lipoprotein-X, largely a phospholipid-cholesterol vesicle, accumulates in the plasma and transfers its lipids to the red cell. Because the lipid composition of the lipoprotein and the red cell do not differ greatly, the result is an expansion of the red cell surface without a deleterious change in membrane properties or cell lifespan. The resulting target cells are a morphologic manifestation of the underlying liver disease, but otherwise harmless (420,421). In contrast, when hepatocellular damage predominates, the resulting plasma lipid changes sometimes lead to a deleterious accumulation of cholesterol without the balancing phospholipid in the red cell. For unknown reasons, this is very destructive, leading to acanthocytosis (so-called spur cells), membrane loss, and a severe hemolytic anemia. Because this often occurs in fragile patients already beset by liver failure, the added complication can be life threatening (420,421). Unfortunately, splenectomy, which mollifies the hemolysis, is not a recommended intervention because the underlying liver disease makes such a surgical procedure an unacceptable risk. The supervention of spur cell anemia in acute or chronic hepatic disease is usually a manifestation of advanced liver compromise and portends a limited survival. These disorders are covered in depth in Chapter 51 and will not be discussed further here.

Wilson Disease

Wilson disease is an autosomal-recessive disorder of copper metabolism characterized by defective biliary excretion of copper, low plasma ceruloplasmin, and toxic accumulation of copper in multiple tissues leading to severe liver disease, hemolysis, Fanconi's renal tubular syndrome, progressive neuropsychiatric disease, and the characteristic corneal (Kayser-Fleischer) rings (422). The disease is caused by defects in ATP7B, an hepatic protein that transports copper into the post-Golgi secretory pathway for incorporation into ceruloplasmin and excretion into the bile (423). In its absence, copper accumulates to toxic levels in hepatocytes, and as they begin to break down, copper is taken up by red cells, where it catalyzes free radical damage to the membrane, Hb, and enzymes, resulting in hemolysis. Hemolysis is an early feature of Wilson disease. It is seen in 20% to 50% of patients who present with liver disease (424) and is the first manifestation in approximately 5% (425–430). The disease presents between 3 and 58 years of age (431). It is a rare condition, but it is critical that hematologists be aware of it because chelation therapy is life saving if begun early, before irreversible liver and brain damage occurs. Wilson disease should always be considered in children and young to middle-aged adults with Coombs'-negative hemolytic anemias and evidence, even subtle evidence, of liver disease or renal Fanconi's syndrome (glycosuria, phosphaturia, acidosis, etc.). The disease is discussed in detail at the end of Chapter 51.

Alcohol and Hematopoiesis

Significant hematologic damage is incurred by alcoholics because of the combined direct toxicity of alcohol on the marrow and the multiple associated abnormalities in the nutritional and gastrointestinal systems that exist in the alcoholic (432). Alcohol supplies empty calories for nutrition and is also frequently accompanied by multivitamin deficiencies; alcohol-induced gastritis is threatened with the double jeopardy of bleeding imposed by the combination of thrombocytopenia and the qualitative platelet dysfunction created by the toxin (433).

Congestive splenomegaly accompanies both acute alcoholic fatty liver and chronic cirrhosis and further depletes the RBC pool. These myriad potential pathologic contributions of ethanol readily explain the occurrence of anemia in approximately 50% of patients hospitalized with acute or chronic alcoholism (434).

ALCOHOL AND THE RED BLOOD CELL

Heavy alcohol ingestion of over 1 week's duration produces a characteristic vacuolization of the RBC precursors in the marrow, a finding shared with chloramphenicol toxicity, phenylalanine deficiency, and hyperosmolar states (435). More chronic ingestion of lesser amounts of alcohol results in a mild macrocytosis unaccompanied by any megaloblastic features in the marrow (436).

Evaluations of adults with macrocytosis (MCV >100 fL) show that alcohol is one of the most common causes, along with drugs and liver disease, especially alcoholic liver disease (437–439). Surprisingly, only approximately 10% of patients with macrocytosis have megaloblastic anemias, although the fraction increases greatly at higher MCVs (>120 fL). In fact, a high or high normal MCV (>94 fL) is one of the best screening tests for identifying hazardous drinkers in general practices (439,440).

The vacuolization of normoblasts is short-lived (3 to 5 days) after ethanol withdrawal, whereas the macrocytosis of alcoholism persists for 1 to 2 weeks after abstinence from the toxin (441). The mechanism for the production of these abnormalities is not well established. Vacuolization may just be a nonspecific sign of injury. It occurs with chloramphenicol toxicity and in diseases associated with erythroblast damage, such as parvovirus B19 infection.

Macrocytosis can be due to folic acid deficiency, which is common in alcoholics, but it can also be a consequence of bone marrow toxicity by alcohol, because it occurs in response to any reversible bone marrow injury in congenital marrow defects such as Fanconi's anemia and Diamond-Blackfan anemia. During recovery from such damage, the bone marrow releases "stress" erythrocytes, which have some of the characteristics of fetal red cells, including large size, increased fetal Hb, and the i antigen. Finally, hemolysis and bleeding must always be considered in the evaluation of macrocytosis because reticulocytes have a much higher MCV than mature erythrocytes.

Acquired stomatocytosis is another red cell abnormality that is common in alcoholics, particularly in those with acute alcoholism, and it may be associated with moderate hemolysis (442,443). In one study, 15% of alcoholic patients had marked stomatocytosis (≥10% stomatocytes) and 29% of the patients

had 3% to 9% stomatocytes (444). The MCV was significantly higher in these patients.

Ethanol is also a direct toxin to hematopoietic cells with evidence that ethanol and its breakdown product, acetaldehyde, both inhibit erythroid marrow colony growth *in vitro* (445). A further insult to erythropoiesis is produced by a direct antifolate effect of alcohol on the marrow (446); this compounds an already reduced availability of folate due to alcohol's interference with the normal enterohepatic recirculation of folate and decreased amounts of the active congener of folate, methyl tetrahydrofolate (447). The sum of these insults to folate metabolism is escalated further by the simultaneous presence of folate deficiency as a result of a poor diet, producing megaloblastic anemia as the most common form of anemia in alcoholics (448).

The megaloblastic transformation of the marrow due to folate deficiency may not be accompanied by the anticipated striking macrocytosis in the peripheral blood because the condition is often compounded by iron deficiency. This frequently produces a dimorphic RBC picture with competing contributions of both deficiencies to RBC size. Hypersegmentation of the polymorphonuclear leukocytes still remains as a marker of megaloblastic hematopoiesis, an important clue when macrocytosis has been blunted by lack of iron (449). Measurement of RBC folate confirms the deficiency, one that may occur in the course of only a few weeks of a folate-deficient diet.

Megaloblastic transformation of the marrow is frequently further complicated by ringed sideroblast formation where iron accumulates in and around altered mitochondria in RBC precursors (250). This iron fails to be normally incorporated into heme, and the RBC products of this pathway are hypochromic in the face of iron-overloaded mitochondria. Whether alcohol interferes with heme synthesis directly, or secondarily through toxic effects on mitochondria, is unclear. These insults to normal Hb production and the ineffective hematopoiesis characteristic of megaloblastic lesions alter iron kinetics within the body. Iron measurements are usually falsely elevated in the anemic alcoholic because of the roadblocks that alcohol erects by interfering with erythropoiesis at so many junctures (451).

Finally, alcohol may contribute to the pathogenesis of porphyrias, especially porphyria cutanea tarda, as discussed in detail in Chapter 47.

After alcohol intake has been discontinued and nutritional supplements provided, the megaloblastic component of the anemia is rapidly reversed. Serum iron levels plummet as normal erythropoiesis supervenes. Sideroblastic features persist for 7 to 10 days, a more prolonged aftermath of alcohol toxicity (450). The marrow, freed from alcohol's suppressive effect, responds with a reticulocytosis that has frequently been misinterpreted as evidence for hemolysis in the jaundiced, anemic drinker. The finding of reticulocytosis in alcoholics with fatty liver and hypertriglyceridemia became the triad of Zieve syndrome (452). The original supposition that the triglyceride elevation caused the hemolysis has been disproved, and any mild hemolysis is attributed to a hypersplenic insult in these patients. The major component of the reticulocytosis represents the return of a marrow formerly suffering the dual effects of alcohol suppression and vitamin deficiencies (451).

ALCOHOL AND THE WHITE BLOOD CELL

Leukopenia may be caused by an ethanol effect on the marrow independent of any megaloblastic interference with hematopoiesis (453). Direct marrow suppression of granulopoiesis by alcohol is accompanied by inhibition of release of CSFs by T lymphocytes (454,455). This may contribute to the high morbidity and mortality rates associated with pneumococcal sepsis in the alcoholic with leukopenia (456).

The alcoholic is further handicapped as an infected host because of diminished adherence, chemotaxis, and motility of granulocytes in response to infection (457). Macrophage function is impaired with decreased motility and phagocytic performance (458,459). Immune defenses are also diminished. Both lymphopenia and inhibition of lymphocyte transformation are common in alcoholism (460). The ability to respond with delayed hypersensitivity to new antigens is also compromised (461). The mechanism of alcohol-related functional defects of WBCs is not established, although a raised intracellular concentration of cyclic adenosine monophosphate in the presence of ethanol has been suggested as the cause (462).

ALCOHOL AND PLATELETS

Both platelet number and function are adversely affected by alcohol in the absence of any supplementary contribution of vitamin deficiency or hypersplenism. The thrombocytopenia originates in a modest shortening of platelet survival combined with a more significant impairment of megakaryocytopoiesis (433). *In vivo* and *in vitro* experiments confirm that the number and proliferation of megakaryocytes are not altered in the presence of ethanol (463). The lesion created by the agent appears at the later stages of the megakaryocyte maturation, with inhibition of platelet production. Withdrawal of ethanol is followed within 3 to 5 days by a release of platelets, with levels rebounding to thrombocythemic levels before returning to normal levels in 1 to 3 weeks (464). Alcohol suppression of thrombopoiesis may be severe enough to result in bleeding, especially when other defects such as gastritis already exist in the patient.

Qualitative platelet abnormalities are also induced by ethanol. With moderate doses (more than 50 g) of ethanol, no direct effect is seen on bleeding time, although this amount of ethanol significantly potentiates prolongation of the bleeding time induced by aspirin and nonsteroidal analgesics (465). Larger ethanol ingestion results in prolongation of the bleeding time even in the absence of any thrombocytopenia (466). Defects in platelet aggregation, thromboxane release, and platelet factor 3 availability occur on exposure of platelets to alcohol. These qualitative defects may be secondary to direct toxic effects of ethanol on the platelet membrane in addition to any contribution from an increased plasma osmolality in the presence of ethanol.

KIDNEY AND HEMATOPOIESIS

Anemia in Kidney Disease

Anemia, a common effect of acute and chronic renal failure, is often so severe in kidney disease conditions that it is the major cause of morbidity (467). It has long been recognized that the anemia, although multifactorial in origin (468), has Epo deficiency as its primary cause (469). Progressive renal disease is accompanied by an Epo decline, resulting in a hypoproliferative, usually normochromic, normocytic anemia. However, other factors can intervene to impair Epo responsiveness and aggravate already low levels of the hormone. These include infection and inflammation (i.e., anemia of chronic disease), inadequate dialysis, and secondary hyperparathyroidism (470,471). In patients treated with Epo, deficiencies of cobalamin (vitamin B_{12}), folic acid, and especially iron may limit response. Transfusion support frequently becomes a necessary intervention, although elevated 2,3-diphosphoglycerate levels and a right-shifted oxygen dissociation curve make the RBCs of uremic subjects more effective in the delivery of oxygen than normal RBCs (472,473). The anemia usually develops when the creatinine clearance falls below 35 to 45 mL/min, although no direct correlation is found between the severity of the anemia and the degree of renal impairment. The Hb level is generally in the 7 to 8 g/dL range in uremic states, with more severe anemia a feature of renoprival states. In the absence of kidneys, the body's limited erythropoiesis has the liver as an extrarenal source of Epo (474).

It is universally agreed that the anemia of renal disease is an Epo deficiency state (475). It is still controversial whether serum inhibitors that accumulate in uremic patients contribute to the erythroid hypoplasia (476,477). Several series have documented improved hematocrits and erythrocyte volumes proportional to the intensity of dialysis treatments, which may remove the inhibitors. Elevated levels of neuraminidase and other proteases have been suggested as inactivators of Epo or its effect on the marrow (478). The higher Hb levels in uremic patients on chronic ambulatory peritoneal dialysis compared with hemodialysis have been attributed to the greater effectiveness of peritoneal dialysis in removing substances of "middle molecule" range (500 to 5000 d) (479). This effect supports the postulated inhibitor role of spermine, a middle molecule substance that accumulates in renal failure and inhibits erythropoiesis in marrow culture (477,480).

The hypothesis concerning spermine and its precursor, spermidine, has been challenged by further *in vitro* work demonstrating that the marrow effect of spermidine is nonselective, with a suppression of all marrow elements in culture (480). Because leukopenia and thrombocytopenia are not usual components of the uremic state, the anemia of renal disease is not thought to be the result of pansuppression by spermidine. The purported role of middle molecule substances has been further questioned by studies demonstrating no difference in RBC mass in chronic ambulatory peritoneal dialysis and hemodialysis patients (481). The higher Hb levels in the former group are thought to be the result of lower plasma volumes, with hemoconcentration leading to the increase in hematocrit.

Excess parathyroid hormone is also an inhibitor of erythropoiesis in uremia, a defect that renal failure states share with primary hyperparathyroidism (482). The mechanism of this contribution to anemia (483) is probably the one that Fuller Albright postulated more than 50 years ago when he focused on the replacement of the marrow cavity by fibrous tissue in hyperparathyroid states. Removal of hypertrophied parathyroid glands improves the osteitis fibrosa of involved marrows and the anemia that accompanies this abnormality (484–486). Interestingly, endogenous Epo levels rise after the surgery, suggesting that secondary hyperparathyroidism impairs Epo synthesis as well as response to the hormone (485). Treatment with 1,25-dihydroxycalciferol also decreases marrow fibrosis and diminishes the anemia of renal failure (487,488). The role of parathyroid hormone in these anemias is in remodeling the environment in which hematopoiesis takes place; the more advanced states of bone disease seen in patients with uremia may even lead to splenomegaly secondary to extramedullary hematopoiesis (489).

The primary role of Epo deficiency in the anemia of renal failure has been incontrovertibly confirmed with the successful trials of recombinant human Epo in dialyzed and nondialyzed renal failure patients (discussed in detail in Chapter 7) (490,491). Administration of the hormone has eliminated the need for red cell transfusions or androgens, previously the mainstays in treating the anemia of renal failure (492,493). The RBC mass is restored to normal, eliminating or overwhelming any contribution of Epo inhibitors to the anemia. The treatment has been remarkably benign with no evidence that antibodies to Epo develop and weaken the potency of the hormone. Hypertension has sometime worsened, perhaps secondary to the increase in RBC mass, although the plasma volume has not shown a parallel enhancement. The therapeutic success of Epo has brought to a close any doubts concerning the major cause of the anemia of renal failure.

Although Epo treatment reverses the anemia of renal failure, the mild hemolytic component in this condition remains unaffected. It is due to an extracorpuscular factor, because RBCs from affected persons survive normally when transfused into normal subjects (494). There is significant shortening of RBC survival when blood urea nitrogen concentrations are greater than 100 mg/dL; the cause of the abnormality is not strictly defined and may be due to a combination of factors (495). Abnormal ion transport has been cited as a cause of increased intracellular sodium accumulation (496). Decreased nicotinamide adenine dinucleotide phosphate generation secondary to defective recycling of glycolytic intermediates through the hexose monophosphate shunt has also been described in RBCs from uremic patients. This abnormality may enhance the sensitivity of such cells to oxidant drug-mediated hemolysis (497,498). Hemodialysis baths that are contaminated with copper, nitrate, or chloramine may exaggerate this sensitivity and create a more severe hemolytic picture (497). The extracorpuscular contribution to this RBC insult can be decreased by increasing the number of times dialysis is given, while making certain the dialysate bath is free of contaminants (498,499).

With moderate degrees of renal failure, the RBCs are normochromic/normocytic with normal osmotic and mechanical fragility. With blood urea nitrogen concentrations greater than 150 mg/dL, the RBCs take on a "burr" configuration as a characteristic feature (500). More dramatic alterations of a microangiopathic nature are a component of traumatic hemolysis in the HUS (501) or occasionally the vasculopathy associated with severe glomerulonephritis or malignant hypertension. The sheared RBCs in HUS are not the effects of renal failure but of the process responsible for the renal failure. A vascular toxin released by several bacterial enteric pathogens appears to be closely linked to the pathophysiology of this syndrome (502,503).

The hemolytic component in uremia-related anemia also may have some contribution from hypersplenism, because splenomegaly may develop in renal failure patients (504). Extensive exposure to many blood products in hemodialyzed patients frequently results in hepatitis and associated splenomegaly. These patients usually manifest pancytopenia, which responds in part to splenectomy. This complication of hepatitis and splenomegaly with secondary hypersplenism has been described in approximately 10% of a large series of hemodialyzed patients.

The anemia of renal failure may be worsened in dialyzed patients by the superimposition of iron and folate deficiency. Folate is dialyzable, and the already meager stores of the vitamin in these nutritionally marginal patients may become rate limiting. Hypersegmentation of polymorphonuclear neutrophils is described as a feature of uremia alone, but this earliest manifestation of a megaloblastic process is more likely the marker of folate deficiency (505). Iron lack is another common threat of renal failure because a large blood loss complicates hemodialysis in all patients; approximately 2 g of iron is lost from the body each year from dialysis alone (506). This iron deficit is often more severe because of the occurrence of gastrointestinal blood loss in the setting of uremia-related platelet defects and the structural lesions of angiodysplasia of the bowel that may accompany uremia (507). Most patients require iron and folate supplementation to compensate for these insults. In addition, extra amounts of these nutrients are needed for the bone marrow to respond optimally to recombinant Epo therapy. The administration of Epo may unmask these deficiencies, their presence being signaled by an apparent refractoriness to Epo administration.

Anemia in hemodialyzed patients may be part of the toxicity created by aluminum accumulation (508); an anemia may occur secondary to this metal's interference with erythropoiesis (509). Aluminum unloading with desferrioxamine reverses the insult, and dialysis against deionized tap water prevents this complication (510). Ingestion of aluminum-containing antacids as phosphate binders may also contribute to aluminum accumulation, even in those who are not undergoing dialysis.

Erythrocytosis in Kidney Disease

Although anemia constitutes a major morbidity in renal disease, secondary erythrocytosis also occurs in a wide variety of renal disorders (511). This increase in RBC mass is caused by Epo release from renal carcinoma cells (512,513) or Wilms' tumor or from renal ischemia with conditions such as renal artery stenosis (514), transplant rejection, and cystic diseases of the kidney (515). Cystic disease of the kidney may be either a congenital disorder or an acquired consequence of end-stage kidney failure on long-term hemodialysis (516–518). Even diffuse parenchymal renal disease (519) and the nephrotic syndrome (520,521) have been associated with erythrocytosis.

A rare entity, Bartter's syndrome, is a hyperrenin state associated with juxtaglomerular apparatus hyperplasia and hypokalemic alkalosis (522). This disease has been complicated by a high Epo erythrocytosis, initially leading investigators to point to the juxtaglomerular apparatus as the common source for both renin and Epo. The cloning of Epo has allowed its localization within the peritubular cells of the kidney, better explaining the broad range of renal pathology associated with erythrocytosis (523,524).

ENDOCRINE DISEASE

The multiple hormonal products of the endocrine system of the body have both direct and indirect effects on hematopoiesis. Hypophysectomy creates a normochromic, normocytic anemia in animal models, a lesion that can be corrected with administration of prolactin or growth hormone (525). Both of these pituitary hormones have a regulatory influence on marrow function at the level of hematopoietic growth factors. Growth hormone has also been demonstrated to stimulate erythropoiesis *in vitro* (526).

Hyperthyroidism

Thyroid hormone has a bimodal effect on erythropoiesis; it directly stimulates human CFU-E formation and indirectly enhances BFU-E proliferation by augmenting the release of soluble burst–promoting factors from accessory cells (527). Persons with hyperthyroidism sometimes have an elevated RBC mass secondary to these effects of excessive thyroid hormone and have an increased requirement for folic acid to accommodate the increased RBC synthesis (528). A macrocytic anemia may complicate hyperthyroidism in the setting of Graves' disease because pernicious anemia and other immune disorders are linked to Graves' disease (529). Occasionally, hyperthyroid patients treated with carbamizole develop autoimmune hemolytic anemia or leukopenia or both due to carbamizole-dependent antibodies (530). The coagulation and platelet systems are unaffected in hyperthyroidism although hyperthyroid patients are sensitive to small amounts of coumadin, making regulation of anticoagulation more difficult in this disease (531).

Hypothyroidism

Hypothyroidism may be complicated by an anemia whose major cause is a reduced RBC mass secondary to the decreased oxygen requirements of the hypothyroid state (532,533). This anemia is often classified as macrocytic but is more frequently normocytic. Patients with macrocytosis occasionally have complicating pernicious anemia, but in most cases there is no explanation for their large red cells. Perhaps, like patients with hypoplastic anemias, they switch to more fetal-like erythropoiesis. This has not been well studied. Patients with hypothyroidism frequently have a small number (0.5% to 2.0%) of acanthocytes in their peripheral blood smears (534–536), which occasionally may be the clue to unsuspected hypothyroidism (536).

Iron deficiency anemia also may complicate thyroid hormone deficiency in women, because menorrhagia with excessive blood loss is a feature of this hormonal lack (537). Treatment of the combination is complicated because patients with iron deficiency anemia (and perhaps any anemia) sometimes develop palpitations and restlessness on normal treatment doses of L-thyroxine and only lose their intolerance after their anemia is corrected (538). On the other hand, iron interferes with the absorption of orally administered L-thyroxine (539), so women with properly treated hypothyroidism who develop iron deficiency may develop signs of hypothyroidism again when treated with iron (539,540). Moreover, if their dose of thyroxine is increased to compensate, they may become hyperthyroid when the iron is discontinued (540).

Infrequently, a gelatinous transformation of the marrow may occur with severe hypothyroidism. This marrow myxedema is accompanied by a severe anemia that is corrected by thyroid hormone replacement (541).

Hyperparathyroidism

Parathyroid hormone is responsible for remodeling the bony architecture that houses the hematopoietic system. This may explain the 5% to 20% incidence of anemia in patients with hyperparathyroidism in the face of normal renal function (542,543). The anemia is normocytic and normochromic, and the marrow contains normal precursor elements. When secondary hyperparathyroidism complicates renal disease (see the section on Anemia in Kidney Disease), the anemia is partly due to the bony lesions and myelofibrosis created by the parathyroid hormone excess (544) and partly to impaired Epo synthesis and response to the hormone (285,286).

Cushing's Disease and Addison's Disease

The corticosteroid overdrive of Cushing's disease may be accompanied by varying degrees of androgenic excess, which can create a modestly polycythemic picture (545). The lack of adrenocortical function in Addison's disease is not accompanied by anemia. Lack of salt-retaining hormones in Addison's disease usually results in a hemoconcentrated state with a normal to slightly increased hematocrit (546). A clue to Addison's disease is the presence of eosinophilia, although this finding is present in only a minority (15%) of such patients (547).

Thalassemia and Other Iron Overload States

Patients with primary or secondary hemochromatosis, particularly those with transfusion-dependent thalassemia, frequently have various combinations of endocrine failure (548–554). The most common abnormalities are hypogonadotropic hypogonadism, growth hormone deficiency, and diabetes mellitus. Diabetes is particularly common in primary hemochromatosis (553,554). Lower frequencies of hypothyroidism, hypoparathyroidism, and adrenal insufficiency occur. Growth failure is also a serious problem in children who are iron overloaded, and bone disease, due to the expanded bone marrow, is a problem in thalassemia. The topic is covered in depth in Chapter 46 (regarding hemochromatosis) and Chapter 48 (regarding thalassemias).

DIABETES MELLITUS

Red Blood Cells

The major hematologic alterations in diabetes mellitus are not necessarily the direct result of insulin deficiency but probably result from the combined metabolic derangements in carbohydrate and fatty acid metabolism of the diabetic state (555). Insulin stimulates human erythroid progenitors *in vitro* (556,557) and also improves a shortened RBC half-life in poorly controlled diabetes (558). The major erythroid abnormality in diabetes mellitus is the nonenzymatic slow and continuous reaction of plasma glucose with the aminoterminal valine residue of the Hb chain. The resultant glycosylated Hb A_{1C} mirrors the time-averaged concentration of glucose within the RBC over the preceding 6- to 8-week period. Measurements of Hb A_{1C} provide a broader window on the adequacy of glucose control as compared with individual glucose determinations (559). This glycosylation of Hb interferes with the binding of 2,3-diphosphoglycerate to the Hb molecule, altering the oxygen-binding affinity of affected cells (560). No measurable differences in the rheologic behavior of red cells from diabetics and control subjects are found despite this glycosylation of Hb and membrane proteins (561).

THIAMINE-RESPONSIVE MEGALOBLASTIC ANEMIA WITH DIABETES AND DEAFNESS

Thiamine-responsive megaloblastic anemia, diabetes mellitus, and sensorineural deafness is a rare autosomal-recessive disorder (562,563) that begins in childhood and is caused by defects in the high affinity thiamine transporter-1 (*SLC19A2*) on chromosome 1q23.3 (564–566) (see also Chapter 45). The anemia and diabetes respond to high-dose thiamine treatment, although the diabetes can relapse years later, despite continuous thiamine treatment (567).

White Blood Cells

Infectious complications punctuate the diabetic state with many defects in leukocyte function incriminated as the causes of this enhanced risk for infection. Decreased leukocyte function in out-of-control diabetes improves with better glucose control (558); the neutrophil in the diabetic has a decreased rate of glycolysis with reduced phosphofructokinase activity (568). Defective migration of neutrophils using skin windows is seen in diabetes patients. Defects in leukocyte chemotaxis, phagocytosis, and bacterial killing are also cited in hyperglycemic states (569).

Platelets

Many alterations in platelet function and the soluble components of the coagulation cascade exist in the patient with diabetes mellitus (570). Whether these abnormalities are primary or secondary in creating the vascular complications of diabetes mellitus remains controversial (571). Platelet hyperaggregability with increased adenosine diphosphate–induced activation is a reproducible finding in uncontrolled diabetes and improves with better glucose control (572). This heightened platelet aggregation is accompanied by high plasma glucose or nonesterified fatty acid inhibition of prostacyclin generation from vessel walls without any comparable effect on thromboxane synthesis (573). Thrombosis is favored in diabetes mellitus because of altered antithrombin III activity due to glycosylation of this molecule at the heparin binding site (574). Fibrinolysis is also hindered, with elevated euglobulin lysis times and increased activity of plasminogen activator inhibitor (575).

The clinical relevance of these hemostatic abnormalities remains unsettled. More than suggestive evidence supports a role for glucose and lipid control in helping to reverse the hypercoagulable features of diabetes mellitus.

Ketoacidosis

Diabetic ketoacidosis with its severe polyuria is usually complicated by hemoconcentration and falsely elevated hematocrit levels. Acute hemolysis may occur in patients with ketoacidosis if rehydration and glycemic control result in the presence of severe hypophosphatemia (576). Total body stores of phosphate are usually reduced, even when serum phosphate levels are normal, and may drop to precarious levels as phosphate reenters cells to phosphorylate glucose. An elevation in WBCs commonly accompanies diabetic ketoacidosis (577); the height of such elevations may result in a leukemoid picture even without any infectious complications.

Diabetic ketoacidosis is reported to trigger hemolytic attacks in patients with glucose-6-phosphate dehydrogenase deficiency (578). This is disputed (579), however, and may instead be associated with the hypoglycemia of brittle diabetes (580) or the fall in glucose that follows treatment of ketoacidosis (581).

ANOREXIA NERVOSA

Hematologic abnormalities are common in persons with anorexia nervosa; marrow hypoplasia commonly accompanies this carbohydrate-calorie deficiency state (582). Pearson's original observation of the marrow accumulation of an acid mucopolysaccharide in persons with anorexia nervosa (583) has been confirmed as a frequent feature of this illness, and its rapid reversibility with clinical improvement in the underlying disease suggests that starvation is the cause (584).

The peripheral blood findings are variable in anorexia nervosa (see Chapter 51). Most patients have circulating acanthocytes, the cause of which is still undetermined (585). Abetalipoproteinemia is not present, although serum cholesterol levels are reduced in approximately one-half of patients (586). Pancytopenia may supervene when the marrow aplasia is significant. The unexpected finding of an acid mucopolysaccharide accumulation in the marrows of men with pancytopenia may be the initial clue to the diagnosis of anorexia nervosa (584).

ANEMIA AND THE ELDERLY

Studies of hematologic parameters in elderly patients have documented an increased incidence of anemia with each successive decade of aging (587). The anemia is usually mild and can be attributed to specific causes in approximately 85% of cases (588,589). Anemia of chronic disease, iron deficiency from gastrointestinal blood loss, cobalamin and folate deficiency, and myelodysplasia are among the common causes. The controversy rests with the anemias of unknown cause. Current opinion favors a diminished erythropoietic reserve, but the data are inconsistent, and the mechanism has not been defined. Studies of healthy, well-nourished elderly populations have not clearly identified any physiologic anemia of aging (590).

Animal and human studies reveal a decreasing marrow reserve as aging proceeds, but the reserve is still adequate to guarantee normal levels throughout the lifetime of the person (591). The lack of reserve becomes a problem in treating older cancer patients with myelosuppressive drugs. Epo levels do not differ from those in normal, healthy controls (587,592). The early stem cell compartments are unperturbed in bone marrows from the elderly; any abnormalities are restricted to defects in the proliferative capacity of more differentiated cell stages (591).

These observations, plus the fact that many of the changes in hematopoietic function present in elderly subjects are similar to those seen in protein-calorie malnutrition, establish the importance of considering the contribution of an inadequate diet to anemia in the elderly.

Thus, anemia is not the simple accompaniment of aging and should not be attributed to a natural senescence phenomenon. Anemia in the elderly should be considered a sickness index, the sign of a possible malignancy or other systemic disorder (593).

PREGNANCY

Pregnancy, with a reorientation of the mother's physiology to support the expanding growth of the fetus, is not infrequently complicated by hematologic disorders. Some of these arise from the progressive hypercoagulable state of pregnancy (594), in preparation for placental separation, whereas other disorders result from pathologic initiation of the clotting cascade secondary to the release of placental, amniotic, or fetal elements (595). Antecedent hematologic disorders are compounded by the demands of pregnancy and may be exaggerated in severity and impact because of their dual effect on mother and fetus. Leukemia and lymphoma create unique management dilemmas when they are concomitants of pregnancy (596,597). Other hematologic conditions such as the antiphospholipid antibody syndrome may become problematic only during pregnancy (598). Management of these conditions must also take into account the effect that any hematologic defects or medications used to reverse these defects may have on the fetus.

Anemia of Pregnancy

During the first and second trimesters of pregnancy, a physiologic expansion of the mother's plasma volume occurs, which outdistances a concomitant increase in the RBC mass (599,600). The plasma volume starts to increase at approximately 6 weeks and reaches approximately 1250 mL at term, an increase of approximately 50% above the nonpregnant state (601). The red cell mass increases approximately 20% or 250 mL without iron supplementation and may reach 400 mL with iron supplements. This hydremia of pregnancy results in a reduction in the normal woman's Hb and hematocrit. The lower limits for Hb levels are debated. The Hb nadir is 11.4 ± 0.8 at 25 to 26 weeks, which makes the minimum value (−2 standard deviation) 9.8 g/dL (602). One recent reviewer concluded that the minimum Hb value is 11 g/dL in the first trimester and 10 g/dL in the next two trimesters (600). This approximates earlier World Health Organization conclusions (603).

A number of studies show a relation between prematurity, low birth weight, and maternal anemia (604–609). One large epidemiologic study found that the risk of premature delivery increased by 20% in pregnancies where the Hb was between 10 and 11 g/dL and by 60% when the Hb was in the 9 to 10 g/dL range (607). Below 9 g/dL the risk doubled and tripled for each additional fall of 1 g/dL. Another study found that perinatal mortality tripled when the mother's Hb fell below 8 g/dL (609).

On the other hand, there is evidence that the normal expansion of maternal plasma volume is needed for an optimal pregnancy outcome (610). Several studies demonstrate a positive correlation between the weight of the newborn and the increase in plasma volume within the normal range (610–614). Whether the increase is needed for optimal fetal oxygenation and growth or whether normal fetal growth somehow triggers the increase is not known. However, high Hb levels portend pregnancy complications such as intrauterine growth retardation, premature birth, pregnancy-induced hypertension, and perinatal fetal distress or death (615–618). For example, the frequency of hypertension in primiparas with Hb levels under 10.5 g/dL is only 7%, but rises to 42% when the Hb concentrations are over 14.5 g/dL (615). Again, it is not clear whether the high Hb level causes these problems or whether poor fetal growth or genetic endowment blunts the normal increase in plasma volume.

The surge in RBC production during pregnancy, although less than the plasma volume, often outstrips the marginal iron and folate stores of the expectant mother. Iron deficiency accounts for approximately 75% of the anemias in unsupplemented women. It is estimated that approximately 80% of pregnant women who do not take iron will have Hb values less than 11 g/dL at term (619). The consequences to the fetus are less certain. Some investigators observe a direct relationship between maternal and fetal iron levels (620); others find that the level of iron in the mother has little effect on that in the neonate (621). The fetal demands seem to dominate. Mild to moderate iron deficiency anemia in the mother does not cause significant anemia in the fetus (620).

Folic acid deficiency is estimated to exist in 60% to 95% of unsupplemented women at term (619), although frank megaloblastic anemia is uncommon. The consequences of folic acid deficiency on the human fetus are not well established. There is convincing evidence that folate deficiency predisposes to devastating defects in closure of the neural tube and thus in spinal cord development (622–624), but folate supplementation to prevent this malformation must be given before conception because neural tube closure occurs during the fourth week of embryogenesis. The risk of neural tube defects is even higher in mothers with the common thermolabile variant of 5,10-methylenetetrahydrofolate reductase (625), which impairs enzyme activity and raises blood levels of homocysteine.

Low values of serum iron (<30 µg/dL) and ferritin (normal values in pregnancy 55 to 70 µg/L) are reliable indicators of iron deficiency (600). Reliance on a low MCV measurement may be misleading during pregnancy because a combined deficiency may cancel out the extremes of iron (low MCV) and folate (high MCV) deficiency (626). To avoid the development of anemia secondary to these deficiencies, it is standard practice to supplement all pregnant women with iron and folate. For those women who cannot tolerate iron, monitoring of serum ferritin permits assessment of iron stores and the specific need for iron supplementation (627).

Other causes of anemia during pregnancy are much rarer. An aplastic anemia that resolves with abortion of the fetus and recurs with subsequent pregnancies is presumed to have an immunologic basis when it occurs during pregnancy (628). The devastating anemia secondary to intravascular hemolysis that is associated with clostridial sepsis may be a lethal complication of septic abortions (629).

Thrombocytopenia

With its potential to exaggerate bleeding during the birth process, thrombocytopenia needs careful assessment and management in the pregnant woman (630). The incidence of the classic thromboconsumptive processes of idiopathic thrombocytopenic purpura (ITP), thrombotic thrombocytopenic purpua (TTP), and dissemi-

nated intravascular coagulation (DIC) all are increased during pregnancy and are joined by platelet abnormalities as a component of toxemia or eclampsia of pregnancy (631). Because ITP is most frequently caused by an antibody that crosses the placenta and may create thrombocytopenia in the infant, this condition creates double jeopardy for the mother and fetus (632) (Chapter 32).

IDIOPATHIC THROMBOCYTOPENIC PURPURA

The diagnosis of ITP during pregnancy requires the same constellation of findings as that in the nonpregnant state (633) (see Chapter 32). The presence or absence of platelet or serum platelet antibodies does not permit any assumptions regarding the fetal platelet count. Percutaneous umbilical blood sampling before labor and scalp vein sampling during delivery are the most common determinants of the optimal route of delivery. A fetal platelet count over 50,000 is usually considered adequate to permit a vaginal delivery (634). Administration of corticosteroids to the mother in the last 3 weeks before delivery is thought to decrease the severity of the thrombocytopenia in the infant (635).

THROMBOTIC THROMBOCYTOPENIC PURPURA AND ECLAMPSIA

TTP and eclampsia share the same hematologic features of hemolytic anemia and thrombocytopenia as well as involvement of the kidney and central nervous systems. Because of the rarity of the former and the difficulty of differentiating it from eclampsia, many physicians recommend that TTP during pregnancy be managed as eclampsia, that is, by delivery of the fetus (636). However, now that it is known that TTP is caused by genetic or autoantibody inhibition of the metalloproteinase that cleaves high-molecular-weight vWF multimers (275–278), it likely that specific diagnostic tests will soon be available and allow physicians to use plasmapheresis when the patient has TTP (637). The mechanism of thrombocytopenia in eclampsia is not certain (638), but it does not affect the size of vWF multimers and so must differ from TTP (639). The fact that the low-dose aspirin prevents the perinatal consequences of preeclampsia in high-risk mothers (640,641) suggests a platelet-endothelial defect may underlie the disease.

The spectrum of toxemia has been extended to include the HELLP syndrome, that is, *h*emolysis, *e*levated *l*iver enzymes, and *l*ow *p*latelets, which may or may not be accompanied by the more classic evidence of toxemia (642–644). The disease occurs in 0.2% to 0.9% of pregnancies, typically between 32 and 34 weeks, although it occurs postpartum in 30% (639–644). The cardinal clinical symptom is right upper quadrant or epigastric pain with nausea, vomiting, or malaise. The disease often progresses to a life-threatening state. The cause is unknown, but despite clinical similarities of eclampsia and HELLP syndromes to TTP, the pathophysiology is different because von Willebrand's multimers are normal in the preeclampsia syndromes (639,644). It is generally agreed that when the HELLP syndrome occurs after 32 to 34 weeks, the fetus should immediately be delivered.

Management of the hematologic problems of toxemia entails management of the toxemia state, which frequently requires delivery of the infant if the maturity of the fetus allows. Because no transplacental antibody passage occurs in toxemia, the infant is not a target for immune thrombocytopenia (645).

DISSEMINATED INTRAVASCULAR COAGULATION

Because the products of conception can initiate the coagulation cascade when released into the maternal circulation, the course of pregnancy and delivery are not infrequently accompanied by DIC (see also Chapter 41). Fetal death *in utero* (646), abruptio placentae (647,648), and amniotic fluid embolism (649) are often signaled by bleeding or coagulation abnormalities. Management of these abnormalities requires delivery of the fetus while providing blood component therapy with platelets, fresh frozen plasma, and cryoprecipitate to replace the consumed elements. Amniotic fluid embolism has the specially threatening complication of cardiopulmonary collapse, which requires cardiopulmonary support and corticosteroids in addition to blood product administration (650). DIC may also accompany the severe hemolytic anemia that occurs when clostridial sepsis follows an abortion (629).

Sickle Cell Disease and Pregnancy

Until approximately 15 years ago, exchange transfusion with subsequent maintenance transfusions was the standard management of the pregnant patient with sickle cell disease because of the documented increase in morbidity and mortality that sickling creates in the mother and child (651). Improved prenatal and perinatal medical care and prospective randomized trials of transfusion (652) have led to a reversal of this position; transfusions are now reserved for mothers who develop complications during pregnancy (including severe anemia) or for any indications of fetal distress (652–654) (see Chapter 50 for a more detailed discussion of this issue). Management of the pregnant sickle cell patient requires close coordination between the obstetrician and the hematologist because of these concerns.

Pregnancy and Thrombosis

Pregnancy represents a progressive hypercoagulable state during which a marked increase in the incidence of venous thrombosis is seen (655,656). In fact, venous thromboembolism is the leading cause of maternal mortality during pregnancy in Western countries. Because anticoagulation carries a significant risk to the fetus, it is imperative that the indications for initiating this therapy have been established with reasonable certainty. A Doppler ultrasound examination is usually adequate, although venography or a ventilation-perfusion scan with uterine shielding are acceptable tools for diagnosing thrombosis or pulmonary embolism in the pregnant woman (657). If anticoagulation is indicated on the basis of these tests, heparin is initiated in full therapeutic doses for 7 days, and the patient is subsequently maintained on low- to intermediate-dose subcutaneous heparin throughout pregnancy (658–662). Low-molecular-weight heparin is increasingly replacing unfractionated heparin as the drug of choice (659–662) (see discussion in Chapter 43). The drug is discontinued at the time of delivery but reinitiated 24 hours after delivery because of the ongoing risk of thrombosis that persists for 8 to 12 weeks after delivery. Coumadin (warfarin) is avoided during pregnancy, especially during the first trimester, because of the risk of a coumadin embryopathy. Heparin

escapes this complication because it does not cross the placenta, although it is associated with the threat of bleeding and fetal loss. Either can be used in the postpartum period because neither drug creates problems for the nursing mother or infant (663,664).

Pregnancy and Inherited Coagulopathies

Neither of the classic hemophilic syndromes complicates pregnancy because of their X-linked mode of inheritance. von Willebrand's disease (vWD) does require recognition, although the incidence of bleeding secondary to this problem in pregnancy is mitigated by the physiologic increase in factor VIII and vWF during pregnancy. Treatment of bleeding due to vWD consists of the use of concentrate or, for short-term control of bleeding, infusions of desmopressin (dDAVP) (665) (see Chapter 35). The latter may shorten bleeding times in the various subgroups of vWD, although its use in type IIB vWD may lead to thrombocytopenia due to release of abnormal vWF in this group (666). Sampling of fetal blood permits prenatal diagnosis of vWD and allows an informed decision regarding any need for cesarean delivery of an infant with vWD.

The universal solution to other coagulation abnormalities consists in administration of fresh frozen plasma in amounts adequate to reverse coagulation test abnormalities. Dysfibrinogenemias and factor XIII deficiency (see Chapter 39) are both associated with spontaneous abortions and abnormal bleeding; plasma infusions throughout pregnancy may be successful in averting complications in these disorders (667).

Inherited Hypercoagulable States and Pregnancy

The inherited thrombophilic states include heterozygosity for protein C and protein S deficiencies, antithrombin III deficiency, factor V Leiden (Arg506Gln), and prothrombin G20210A, and homozygosity for the hyperhomocysteinemias, probably including the common thermolabile 5,10-methylenetetrahydrofolate reductase mutation. The topic is covered in Chapter 42 and has been extensively reviewed in recent years (661,668–672). The frequency and risk of the various mutations varies considerably. The data from one large study (Table 56-2) show that women who inherit defects in these proteins are more likely to experience fetal loss, particularly stillbirths, than controls (673). The risks are greatest in antithrombin III deficiency and in women with more than one inherited risk factor.

The risk of venous thrombosis is also increased in women with these high-risk genes. One review of uncontrolled retrospective studies found that venous thrombosis occurred during or immediately following pregnancy in as many as 60% of women

---

TABLE 56-2. Risks of Fetal Loss in Different Types of Thrombophilia[a]

Heterozygous Defect	All Spontaneous Fetal Losses	Miscarriages (Fetal Loss ≤28 Wk)	Stillbirths (Fetal Loss >28 Wk)
	Odds ratio (95% confidence interval)		
Antithrombin III deficiency	2.1 (1.2–3.6)	1.7 (1.0–2.8)	5.2 (1.5–18.1)
Protein C deficiency	1.4 (0.9–2.2)	1.4 (0.9–2.2)	2.3 (0.6–8.3)
Protein S deficiency	1.3 (0.8–2.1)	1.2 (0.7–1.9)	3.3 (1.0–11.3)
Factor V Leiden	1.0 (0.6–1.7)	0.9 (0.5–1.5)	2.0 (0.5–7.7)
Combined defects	2.0 (0.5–8.1)	0.8 (0.2–3.6)	14.3 (2.4–86.0)

[a]Study includes 571 women with thrombophilia (1524 pregnancies) and 395 controls (1019 pregnancies) who were enrolled in the European Prospective Cohort on Thrombophilia.
From Preston FE, Rosendaal FR, Walker ID, et al. Increased fetal loss in women with heritable thrombophilia. *Lancet* 1996;348:913–916, with permission.

with antithrombin III deficiency and in as many as 20% of women with protein C or protein S deficiency (674). A case-control study found the risk of a venous thrombosis was eight times higher in those with any of the same deficiencies (675). Patients with factor V Leiden or the G20210A mutation of the prothrombin gene are also at risk (676,677). The odds of a thrombosis are increased 16-fold and 10-fold, respectively, if the genes are inherited individually, and 109-fold if a patient inherits both genes. These defects also appear to play a role in other gestational vascular complications, including intrauterine growth restriction, preeclampsia, and placental abruption (669,678). Women who intend to become pregnant should probably be screened for inherited thrombophilias if they have a personal or family history of venous thrombosis or if they have three unexplained miscarriages, abruptio placentae, stillbirths, recurrent fetal growth retardation, or possibly, preeclampsia (668).

Women with antithrombin III deficiency, combinations of thrombophilia mutations, or homozygosity for factor V Leiden or the G20210A prothrombin mutation should be treated throughout pregnancy and for 6 weeks postpartum with low-molecular-weight heparin (668). Coumadin can also be used postpartum. Preparations of antithrombin III are available and may be infused at the time of delivery for women with anti-thrombin deficiency (679). For women with lower-risk defects, treatment should be based on personal and family history, and the presence or absence of other thrombosis risk factors such as age (older than 35 years of age), obesity, immobility, and cesarean section. In such individuals, thromboprophylaxis during late pregnancy and postpartum should be considered (661).

Acquired Hypercoagulable States and Pregnancy

ANTIPHOSPHOLIPID ANTIBODY SYNDROME
Antiphospholipid antibodies are a family of autoantibodies to various combinations of phospholipids and phospholipid binding proteins such as β_2-glycoprotein I. Common examples include lupus anticoagulant antibodies and anticardiolipin. The *antiphospholipid antibody syndrome* (680) is a term coined to reflect the correlation between the existence of such antibodies and hypercoagulability (see Chapters 32 and 42). The pathophysiology is unclear. Both arterial and venous thromboses are observed. Venous thromboembolism, especially deep vein thrombosis of the legs, is most common, occurring in 30% to 55% of patients with the syndrome during an average follow-up of less than 6 years (680–683). Other features include a propensity for cardiac valvular vegetations, thrombotic microangiopathy mimicking hemolytic uremic syndrome or TTP, thrombocytopenia, hemolytic anemia, livedo reticularis, and renal involvement with hypertension (680–683). A minority of patients have a catastrophic syndrome with multiple simultaneous vascular occlusions throughout the body that is often fatal (680). The topic is discussed further in the section Systemic Lupus Erythematosus.

In addition to the risk of venous and arterial thrombosis, pregnant women with antiphospholipid antibodies have an increased risk of fetal loss (680,683–685), premature delivery, preeclampsia, and uteroplacental insufficiency (686,687). The risk to the pregnancy involves all periods: preembryonic (less than 6 weeks), embryonic (6 to 9 weeks), and fetal (≥ 10 weeks). The mechanisms are not well defined but may include antiphospholipid antibodies interfering with binding of the protective anticoagulant annexin V to phospholipid surfaces on endothelial cells and trophoblasts (688). There are also data that antiphospholipid antibodies affect trophoblast gonadotropin secretion and invasiveness by binding to the trophoblast cells directly or through adherent β_2-glycoprotein I (689).

Two recent prospective trials show that heparin plus low-dose aspirin is more effective than aspirin alone in achieving live births in pregnant women with antiphospholipid antibodies and predominantly preembryonic and embryonic loss (690,691). A third trial found no evidence that addition of intravenous gammaglobulin improves pregnancy outcome compared to heparin and low-dose aspirin (692) or that corticosteroids add any additional benefit (693). The issues of who should be treated and how much heparin should be administered continue to be debated. One authoritative opinion suggests that women with recurrent preembryonic and embryonic pregnancy loss and no history of thromboembolism should receive 5000 U of heparin twice daily, or the equivalent dose of low-molecular-weight heparin, once a live embryo is proven by ultrasound (690). Many experts recommend somewhat more generous thromboprophylaxis for women with pregnancy loss during the fetal period and no history of thromboembolism (686,687), although this is also debated. Doses of heparin sufficient to produce full anticoagulation are recommended for all women with antiphospholipid antibodies and prior thromboembolism (680).

OTHER ACQUIRED HYPERCOAGULABLE STATES
A variety of other acquired diseases increase the risk of thrombosis and thromboembolism during pregnancy, including nephrotic syndrome, heparin-induced thrombocytopenia and thrombosis, congestive heart failure, vasculitis, paroxysmal nocturnal hemoglobinuria, and polycythemia vera. Essential thrombocythemia (see Chapter 12) may threaten a pregnancy with placental insufficiency secondary to multiple placental infarcts. Antiplatelet therapy with aspirin and dipyridamole as well as platelet pheresis have permitted successful pregnancies in this group (694). Paroxysmal nocturnal hemoglobinuria (see Chapter 10) may require low-dose heparinization during pregnancy to avert thrombosis (695).

COLLAGEN VASCULAR DISEASES

Systemic Lupus Erythematosus

No step in the complicated sequence of hematopoiesis is guaranteed freedom from pathologic involvement with systemic lupus erythematosus (SLE) (697). This threat originates in the interdependence of hematopoiesis and the immune system and the disarray in immune function that characterizes SLE. Antibodies may arise in SLE, which have as their target pluripotent or committed stem cells, creating an aplastic picture that involves all or individual cell lines within the marrow (698,699). Cellular suppression of marrow cell lines by lymphoid cells may also occur (700). Immune sensitization of circulating cells can lead to premature destruction of individual cell lines in the peripheral blood (701). SLE is a leading cause of immune hemolytic anemia and immune thrombocytopenia (702). The target of SLE antibodies may even be a plasma protein or a phospholipid, producing the so-called lupus anticoagulant with its thrombotic propensity (see previous section and Chapter 42) (703). This immune imbalance with blood elements as a frequent target of the immunologic pathology explains the striking presence of hematologic disorders that characterize SLE.

ANEMIA
Anemia is the most common finding in patients with SLE, most frequently attributable to ACD (see section Anemia of Chronic Disease). SLE is an inflammatory disorder, and the same acute phase reactants of ILs, TNF-α, and IFNs are operative in both dis-

orders. In addition, specific interference with marrow production and circulation of RBCs occurs. Although red cell aplasia on a humoral or cellular basis is a rare occurrence (704,705), an immune hemolytic anemia is a relatively common complication. It is typically characterized by a serologic pattern of IgG plus complement on the red cell surface (706). Myelofibrosis has also been described in a few patients with SLE; immune complexes have been suggested but not proven to be the cause of this unusual complication of SLE (707).

THROMBOCYTOPENIA

Thrombocytopenia secondary to platelet immune sensitization is the most common immune-mediated hematologic manifestation of SLE (see Chapter 32) (708). Paralleling the pathophysiology of pure RBC aplasia, immunologic destruction of megakaryocyte precursors by humoral or cellular mechanisms may contribute to the thrombocytopenia (709–711). Thrombocytopenia may be an initial manifestation of SLE, and serologic investigation for SLE should be a part of any evaluation of ITP in adults, especially in women, and of chronic ITP in children (712). Occasionally, ITP may manifest years before serologic evidence of SLE is detectable. ITP in patients with SLE has the same therapeutic implication as other immune thrombocytopenia, that is, corticosteroids, intravenous Ig, or WinRho as a primary intervention, with splenectomy reserved for patients who fail these approaches. An additional rare cause of thrombocytopenia in SLE patients is platelet consumption in the setting of TTP (713). Presumably, like isolated TTP, this is due to autoantibodies to the von Willebrand-cleaving ADAMTS protease (276,277).

LEUKOPENIA

Leukopenia is a characteristic of SLE, although agranulocytosis is not a common feature of this disease in the absence of a drug reaction (714). This is an interesting departure from what occurs in RA, in which at least two different mechanisms result in absolute leukoneutropenia. Lymphopenia is common in SLE patients along with a reduction in T cells, whereas B-cell function is hyperactive in this disorder (696).

SYSTEMIC LUPUS ERYTHEMATOSUS AND THE LUPUS ANTICOAGULANT–ANTIPHOSPHOLIPID SYNDROME

Conley and Hartmann's (715) description of a circulating anticoagulant in two SLE patients with a hemorrhagic disorder was the initial piece of a puzzle that is still incomplete. The SLE anticoagulant was first recognized in the laboratory as a prolongation of the partial thromboplastin time and was frequently accompanied by a low titer venereal disease test for syphilis; subsequently, it was determined that the antibody-anticoagulant is directed against various phospholipids involved in phospholipid-dependent coagulation assays as well as against the cardiolipin component of the low titer venereal disease test (716) or an associated anionic phospholipid binding protein, β_2-glycoprotein I (680). As described in the previous section on Acquired Hypercoagulable States and Pregnancy, the pathologic significance of the lupus anticoagulant and other antiphospholipid antibodies is their association with thrombosis, mainly venous, as well as miscarriages and spontaneous abortions (680,717). The spectrum of the disease (680–683,717) has since been amplified to include thrombocytopenia, hemolytic anemia, cardiac valvular vegetations, a thrombotic microangiopathy mimicking hemolytic uremic syndrome or TTP, strokes, livedo reticularis (718), renal involvement with hypertension, and even leg ulcers (719).

A minority of patients have a catastrophic form of the disease (680,720). This often fatal syndrome is defined by the clinical involvement of at least three different organs over a period of days to weeks, with pathologic evidence of multiple occlusions of large or small vessels. In general, involvement of small vessels is more common in these patients, who tend to present with an acute thrombotic microangiopathy involving the kidney, lungs, central nervous system, heart, or skin, along with DIC. The mortality rate is approximately 30% to 50% (720). Aggressive therapy with combinations of anticoagulants, steroids, intravenous Ig, and plasmapheresis have been tried in anecdotal reports with varying success.

Anticardiolipin and lupus anticoagulant antibodies occur in 1% to 5% of adult controls (721). Among adult SLE patients, 12% to 30% have anticardiolipin antibodies, and 15% to 34% have lupus anticoagulant antibodies (722–724). A high proportion (approximately 50% to 70%) of these patients will develop the antiphospholipid antibody syndrome after 20 years of follow-up (721,725).

Persons with recurrent thrombosis are candidates for long-term, possibly lifelong, anticoagulation with warfarin. The intensity of anticoagulation [i.e., intermediate INR (2.0 to 2.9) versus high INR (≥3.0)] is controversial. In some studies, intermediate-intensity warfarin was effective in preventing recurrent thrombosis (726–729), which is the goal. Unfortunately, monitoring the level of anticoagulation can be complicated because of antibody interference (730). Discontinuing anticoagulation therapy carries a high risk of recurrent thromboembolism (727,731–733). Aspirin does not prevent deep vein thrombosis in patients with antiphospholipid antibodies (734), but hydroxychloroquine may be an effective prophylactic agent in SLE patients with the antibodies (735).

Rheumatoid Arthritis

RA represents the classic intersection of anemia of chronic disease (ACD) and iron deficiency anemia (736,737). The latter is a common complication of RA because of the gastrointestinal blood loss incurred secondary to long-standing use of aspirin and nonsteroidal analgesics in the symptomatic treatment of this disease (738). The severe inflammatory nature of the illness also makes it a model for ACD, a sideropenic anemia in the face of reticuloendothelial (RE) iron overload (see Anemia of Chronic Disease). Iron is recognized not only as being closeted in the RE system in RA but as accumulating in the involved joints, perhaps playing a role in their destruction (739).

Other hematologic manifestations of RA are a moderately elevated platelet count (7 to $9 \times 10^5/\mu L$), especially when a prominent vasculitic component is present in the disease (740). Secondary thrombocytosis is part of the inflammatory response and does not respond to iron replacement. Eosinophilia likewise may be a component of acute rheumatoid disease (741); the eosinophilia in RA may also be an allergic reaction to gold therapy (742).

RHEUMATOID ARTHRITIS AND FELTY'S SYNDROME

Severe leukoneutropenia associated with splenomegaly and RA constitutes the triad described by Felty in 1924 (743). The syndrome, occurring in 1% of RA patients, is complicated by recurrent bacterial infections, leg ulcers, and high serologic titers of rheumatoid factor. The cause of the granulocytopenia is unknown. Fifty percent of the patients have a "maturation arrest" bone marrow pattern (absence of mature bands and polymorphonuclear cells in the marrow), which is thought to result from immune humoral or cellular mechanisms. The remainder of Felty patients have normal or hypercellular marrows; increased margination and sequestration of neutrophils have been demonstrated in some of these patients (744).

Recombinant human G-CSF and GM-CSF both effectively raise the neutrophil count in essentially all patients with Felty's syndrome (745,746). The neutrophil count drops again once the growth factor treatment is stopped but often stabilizes at a level higher than it was pretreatment (745,747). The drug can be used long term (748,749) and may be cost-effective in selected patients with a high incidence of infections and repeated hospitalizations. Side effects have been reported, including mild thrombocytopenia (747) a flare of the patient's arthritis (747,750,751), skin rash (751), and a leukocytoclastic vasculitis (752); however, these complications appear to be rare if the dose of G-CSF or GM-CSF is kept as low as possible to just get the absolute neutrophil count above 1000/µL (745).

Splenectomy is a reasonable option if G-CSF or GM-CSF is not effective and rapid improvement in the white blood counts are needed because of recurrent infections. Approximately 50% to 80% experience a long-term response (746,753). Those who do not respond have a higher incidence (55%) of infections, approximately 10% of which are fatal (746). Patients who do not respond to splenectomy are cited as evidence that the spleen is not the total explanation of the leukopenia. The parallels to the effect of splenectomy in autoimmune hemolytic anemia suggest that the spleen removes sensitized WBCs from the blood but that the organ may not be the sole scavenger of WBCs in all Felty's patients.

Methotrexate treatment of patients with Felty's syndrome is as effective as splenectomy in correcting the neutropenia (754) and offers the ability to treat both the arthritis and neutropenia with the same agent.

RHEUMATOID ARTHRITIS AND LARGE GRANULAR LYMPHOCYTES

A subpopulation of RA patients with a clinical picture similar to Felty's syndrome has increased numbers of large granular lymphocytes in the bone marrow or peripheral blood, or both (755,756). These cells have a characteristic morphology and surface membrane antigen expression (757), and they infiltrate the red pulp of the spleen, a finding that is not present in patients with Felty's syndrome. The importance of recognizing this variant is that splenectomy is ineffective.

RED BLOOD CELL THERMAL INJURY

Thermal injury to RBCs creates anemia with the most bizarre and striking alterations in erythrocyte morphology (758) (see Chapter 51). With increasing temperature elevation over a range of 50° to 65°C, increasing RBC fragmentation and microspherocytosis occur, with RBCs of multiple diameters. This phenomenon, accompanied by hemoglobinemia and hemoglobinuria, was recognized as a component of extreme body burns as early as 1865. The cells have increased osmotic and mechanical fragility as an aftermath of the membrane burn (759).

The major late morbidity and mortality in burn patients are secondary to septic complications attributable in major part to neutrophil dysfunction (760). Leukocytosis and an increase in band forms occur with burns, and these cells demonstrate defective chemotaxis and phagocytic function (761). Decreased leukotriene generation in granulocytes contributes to this inadequate host response (762). These cellular defects, combined with abnormalities in cellular and humoral immunity in severely burned patients, often determine the clinical outcome of the impaired burn patient.

Platelets do not escape involvement in burns. An initial thrombocytopenia gives way to thrombocytosis (763); the latter is probably part of the inflammatory reaction with burns and does not represent a threat to hemostasis.

REFERENCES

1. Cartwright GE. The anemia of chronic disorders. *Semin Hematol* 1966;3:351.
2. Konijn AM, Hershko C. The anaemia of inflammation and chronic disease. In: DeSouza M, Brock JH, eds. *Iron in immunity, cancer and inflammation.* Chichester, UK: John Wiley and Sons, 1989:111.
3. Samson D. The anaemia of chronic disorders. *Postgrad Med J* 1983;59:543.
4. Bentley DP. Anaemia and chronic disease. *Clin Haematol* 1982;11:465.
5. Lee GR. The anemia of chronic disease. *Semin Hematol* 1983;20:61.
6. Cartwright GE, Lee GR. The anemia of chronic disorders. *Br J Haematol* 1971;21:147.
7. Fillet G, Beguin Y, Baldelli L. Model of reticuloendothelial iron metabolism in humans: abnormal behavior in idiopathic hemochromatosis and in inflammation. *Blood* 1989;74:844.
8. Freireich EJ, Miller A, Emerson CP, et al. The effect of inflammation on the utilization of erythrocyte and transferrin bound radio-iron for red cell production. *Blood* 1957;12:972.
9. Haurani F, Burke W, Martinez E. Defective reutilization of iron in the anemia of inflammation. *J Lab Clin Med* 1965;65:560.
10. Konijn AM, Hershko C. Ferritin synthesis in inflammation. I. Pathogenesis of impaired iron release. *Br J Haematol* 1977;37:7.
11. Cazzola M, Bergamaschi G, Dezza L, et al. Manipulation of cellular iron metabolism for modulating normal and malignant cell proliferation: achievements and prospects. *Blood* 1990;75:1903.
12. Hann H-WL, Stahlburt MW, Blumberg BS. Iron nutrition and tumor growth: decreased tumor growth in iron-deficient mice. *Cancer Res* 1988;48:4168.
13. Fernandez-Pol JA. Siderophore-like growth factor synthesized by SV40-transformed cells adapted to picolinic acid stimulates DNA synthesis in cultured cells. *FEBS Lett* 1978;88:345.
14. Brown J, Woodbury R, Hart C, et al. Quantitative analysis of melanoma-associated antigen in normal and neoplastic tissues. *Proc Natl Acad Sci U S A* 1981;78:539.
15. Weinberg ED. Iron withholding: a defense against infection and neoplasia. *Physiol Rev* 1984;64:65.
16. Cartwright GE, Launtsen MA, Jones PJ, et al. The anemia of infection. I. Hypoferremia, hypercupremia, and alterations in porphyrin metabolism in patients. *J Clin Invest* 1946;25:65.
17. Van Swick JC, Masson PC, Heremans JF. The involvement of lactoferrin in the hyposideremia of acute inflammation. *J Exp Med* 1974;140:1068.
18. Brock JH, Esparza I. Failure of reticulocytes to take up iron from lactoferrin saturated by various methods. *Br J Haematol* 1979;42:481.
19. Masson PL, Heremans JF, Schowne E. Lactoferrin: an iron binding protein in neutrophilic leukocytes. *J Exp Med* 1969;130:643.
20. Rado TA, Wei XP, Benz EF Jr. Isolation of lactoferrin cDNA from a human myeloid library and expression of mRNA during normal and leukemic myelopoiesis. *Blood* 1987;70:989.
21. Loughlin KR, Gittes RF, Partridge D, et al. The relationship of lactoferrin to the anemia of renal cell carcinoma. *Cancer* 1987;59:566.
22. Roodman GD. Mechanisms of erythroid suppression in the anemia of chronic disease. *Blood Cells* 1987;13:171.
23. Dinarello CA. Interleukin-1 and the pathogenesis of the acute-phase response. *N Engl J Med* 1984;311:1413.
24. Schooley J, Kullgren B, Allison A. Inhibition by interleukin-1 of the action of erythropoietin on erythroid precursors and its possible role in the pathogenesis of hypoplastic anemias. *Br J Haematol* 1987;67:11.
25. Tracey KJ, Wei H, Manogue KR, et al. Cachectin/tumor necrosis factor indices cachexia, anemia and inflammation. *J Exp Med* 1988;167:1211.
26. Vreugdenhil G, Lowenberg B, Van Eijk HG, et al. Tumor necrosis factor alpha is associated with disease activity and the degree of anemia in patients with rheumatoid arthritis. *Eur J Clin Invest* 1992;22:488.
27. Papadaki HA, Kritikos HD, Boumpas DT, et al. Anemia of chronic disease in rheumatoid arthritis is associated with increased apoptosis of bone marrow erythroid cells: improvement following anti-tumor necrosis factor-alpha antibody therapy. *Blood* 2002;100:474.
28. Johnson RA, Waddelow TA, Caro J, et al. Chronic exposure to tumor necrosis factor in vivo preferentially inhibits erythropoiesis in nude mice. *Blood* 1989;74:130.
29. Means R Jr, Krantz S. Progress in understanding the pathogenesis of the anemia of chronic disease. *Blood* 1992;80:1639.
30. Broxmeyer HE, Lu L, Bicknell DC, et al. The influence of purified, recombinant human heavy-subunit and light-subunit ferritins on colony formation in vitro by granulocyte-macrophage and erythroid progenitor cells. *Blood* 1986;68:1257.
31. Alvarez-Hernandez X, Liceaga J, McKay IC, et al. Induction of hypoferremia and modulation of macrophage iron metabolism by tumor necrosis factor. *Lab Invest* 1989;61:319.
32. Jongen-Lavrencic M, Peeters HRM, Vreugdenhil G, et al. Interaction of inflammatory cytokines and erythropoietin in iron metabolism and erythropoiesis in anemia of chronic disease. *Clin Rheumatol* 1995;5:519.
33. Katevas P, Andonopoulos AP, Kourakli-Symeonidis A, et al. Peripheral blood mononuclear cells from patients with rheumatoid arthritis suppress erythropoiesis in vitro via the production of tumor necrosis factor alpha. *Eur J Haematol* 1994;53:26.
34. Voulgari PV, Kolios G, Papadopoulos GK, et al. Role of cytokines in the pathogenesis of anemia of chronic disease in rheumatoid arthritis. *Clin Immunol* 1999;92:153.
35. Rusten LS, Jacobsen SE. Tumor necrosis factor (TNF)-alpha directly inhibits human erythropoiesis in vitro: role of p55 and p75 TNF receptors. *Blood* 1995;85:989.
36. Means RT, Krantz SB. Inhibition of human erythroid colony-forming units by tumor necrosis factor requires beta interferon. *J Clin Invest* 1993;91:416.
37. Broxmeyer HE, Williams DE, Lu L, et al. The suppressive influences of tumor necrosis factors on bone marrow hematopoietic progenitor cells from

normal donors and patients with leukemia: synergism of tumor necrosis factor and interferon-gamma. *J Immunol* 1986;136:4487.

38. Papadaki HA, Kritikos HD, Gemetzi C, et al. Bone marrow progenitor cell reserve and function and stromal cell function are defective in rheumatoid arthritis: evidence for a tumor necrosis factor alpha-mediated effect. *Blood* 2002;99:1610.

39. Jongen-Lavrencic M, Peeters HR, Wognum A, et al. Elevated levels of inflammatory cytokines in bone marrow of patients with rheumatoid arthritis and anemia of chronic disease. *J Rheumatol* 1997;24:1504.

40. Roodman GD, Bird A, Hutzler D, et al. Tumor necrosis factor-alpha and hematopoietic progenitors: effects of tumor necrosis factor on the growth of erythroid progenitors CFU-E and BFU-E and the hematopoietic cell lines K562, HL60 and HEL cells. *Exp Hematol* 1987;15:928.

41. Davis D, Charles PJ, Potter A, et al. Anaemia of chronic disease in rheumatoid arthritis: in vivo effects of tumour necrosis factor alpha blockade. *Br J Rheumatol* 1997;36:950.

42. Maury CP, Andersson LC, Teppo AM, et al. Mechanism of anaemia in rheumatoid arthritis: demonstration of raised interleukin 1 beta concentrations in anaemic patients and of interleukin 1 mediated suppression of normal erythropoiesis and proliferation of human erythroleukaemia (HEL) cells in vitro. *Ann Rheum Dis* 1988;47:972.

43. Houssiau FA, Devogelaer JP, van Damme J, et al. Interleukin-6 in synovial fluid and serum of patients with rheumatoid arthritis and other inflammatory arthritides. *Arthritis Rheum* 1988;31:784.

44. Vreugdenhil G, Lowenberg B, Van Eijk HG, et al. Anaemia of chronic disease in rheumatoid arthritis: raised serum interleukin-6 (IL-6) levels and effects of IL-6 and anti-IL-6 on in vitro erythropoiesis. *Rheumatol Int* 1990;10:127.

45. Manicourt DH, Triki R, Fukuda K, et al. Levels of circulating tumor necrosis factor alpha and interleukin-6 in patients with rheumatoid arthritis: relationship to serum levels of hyaluronan and antigenic keratan sulfate. *Arthritis Rheum* 1993;36:490.

46. Tanabe M, Ochi T, Tomita T, et al. Remarkable elevation of interleukin 6 and interleukin 8 levels in the bone marrow serum of patients with rheumatoid arthritis. *J Rheumatol* 1994;5:830.

47. Cazzola M, Ponchio L, de Benedetti F, et al. Defective iron supply for erythropoiesis and adequate endogenous erythropoietin production in the anemia associated with systemic-onset juvenile chronic arthritis. *Blood* 1996;87:4824.

48. Faquin WC, Schneider TJ, Goldberg MA. Effect of inflammatory cytokines on hypoxia-induced erythropoietin production. *Blood* 1992;79:1987.

49. Means RT, Dessypris EN, Krantz SB. Inhibition of human erythroid colony-forming units by interleukin-1 is mediated by gamma interferon. *J Cell Physiol* 1992;150:59.

50. Bernad A, Kopf M, Kulbacki R, et al. Interleukin-6 is required in vivo for the regulation of stem cells and committed progenitors of the hematopoietic system. *Immunity* 1994;1:725.

51. Vreugdenhil G, Lowenberg B, van Eijk HG. Anemia of chronic disease in rheumatoid arthritis: raised serum interleukin-6 (IL-6) levels and effects of IL-6 and anti-IL-6 on in vitro erythropoiesis. *Rheumatol Int* 1990;10:127.

52. Bernard A, Kopf M, Kuhlbacki R, et al. Interleukin-6 is required in vivo for the regulation of stem cells and committed progenitors of the hematopoietic system. *Immunity* 1994;1:725.

53. Atkins MB, Kappler K, Mier JW, et al. Interleukin-6-associated anemia: determination of the underlying mechanism. *Blood* 1995;86:1288.

54. Charles PJ, Smeenk RJ, De Jong J, et al. Assessment of antibodies to double-stranded DNA induced in rheumatoid arthritis patients following treatment with infliximab, a monoclonal antibody to tumor necrosis factor alpha: findings in open-label and randomized placebo-controlled trials. *Arthritis Rheum* 2000;43:2383.

55. Vreugdenhil G, Swaak AJ. The role of erythropoietin in the anaemia of chronic disease in rheumatoid arthritis. *Clin Rheumatol* 1990;9:22.

56. Birgegard G, Hallgren R, Caro J. Serum erythropoietin in rheumatoid arthritis and other inflammatory arthritides: relationship to anaemia and the effect of anti-inflammatory anaemia and the effect of anti-inflammatory treatment. *Br J Haematol* 1987;65:479.

57. Silva M, Grillot D, Benito A, et al. Erythropoietin can promote erythroid progenitor survival by repressing apoptosis through Bcl-XL and Bcl-2. *Blood* 1996;88:1576.

58. Reference deleted.

59. Salvarani C, Lasagni D, Casali B, et al. Recombinant human erythropoietin therapy in patients with rheumatoid arthritis with the anemia of chronic disease. *J Rheumatol* 1991;18:1168.

60. Dohil R, Hassall E, Wadsworth LD, et al. Recombinant human erythropoietin for treatment of anemia of chronic disease in children with Crohn's disease. *J Pediatr* 1998;132:155.

61. Christodoulou DK, Tsianos EV. Anemia in inflammatory bowel disease—the role of recombinant human erythropoietin. *Eur J Intern Med* 2000;11:222.

62. Kaltwasser JP, Kessler U, Gottschalk R, et al. Effect of recombinant human erythropoietin and intravenous iron on anemia and disease activity in rheumatoid arthritis. *J Rheumatol* 2001;28:2430.

63. Means RT Jr. Clinical application of recombinant erythropoietin in the anemia of chronic disease. *Hematol Oncol Clin North Am* 1994;8:933.

64. Nordstrom D, Lindroth Y, Marsal L, et al. Availability of iron and degree of inflammation modifies the response to recombinant human erythropoietin when treating anemia of chronic disease in patients with rheumatoid arthritis. *Rheumatol Int* 1997;17:67.

65. Brugnara C, Colella GM, Cremins J, et al. Effects of subcutaneous recombinant human erythropoietin in normal subjects: development of decreased reticulocyte hemoglobin content and iron-deficient erythropoiesis. *J Lab Clin Med* 1994;123:660.

66. Major A, Mathez-Loic F, Rohling R, et al. The effect of intravenous iron on the reticulocyte response to recombinant human erythropoietin. *Br J Haematol* 1997;98:292.

67. Goodnough LT, Skikne B, Brugnara C. Erythropoietin, iron, and erythropoiesis. *Blood* 2000;96:823.

68. Fleming RE, Sly WS. Hepcidin: a putative iron-regulatory hormone relevant to hereditary hemochromatosis and the anemia of chronic disease. *Proc Natl Acad Sci U S A* 2001;98:8160.

69. Krause A, Neitz S, Magert HJ, et al. LEAP-1, a novel highly disulfide-bonded human peptide, exhibits antimicrobial activity. *FEBS Lett* 2000;480:147.

70. Park CH, Valore EV, Waring AJ, et al. Hepcidin, a urinary antimicrobial peptide synthesized in the liver. *J Biol Chem* 2001;276:7806.

71. Pigeon C, Ilyin G, Courselaud B, et al. A new mouse liver-specific gene, encoding a protein homologous to human antimicrobial peptide hepcidin, is overexpressed during iron overload. *J Biol Chem* 2001;276:7811.

72. Lehrer RI, Ganz T. Antimicrobial peptides in mammalian and insect host defence. *Curr Opin Immunol* 1999;11:23.

73. Nicolas G, Bennoun M, Devaux I, et al. Lack of hepcidin gene expression and severe tissue iron overload in upstream stimulatory factor 2 (USF2) knock-out mice. *Proc Natl Acad Sci U S A* 2001;98:8780.

74. Nicolas G, Bennoun M, Porteu A, et al. Severe iron deficiency anemia in transgenic mice expressing liver hepcidin. *Proc Natl Acad Sci U S A* 2002;99:4596.

75. McKie AT, Barrow D, Latunde-Dada GO, et al. An iron-regulated ferric reductase associated with the absorption of dietary iron. *Science* 2001;291:1755.

76. Fleming MD, Trenor CC, Su MA, et al. Microcytic anaemia mice have a mutation in Nramp2, a candidate iron transporter gene. *Nat Genet* 1997;16:383.

77. Gunshin H, Mackenzie B, Berger UV, et al. Cloning and characterization of a mammalian proton-coupled metal-ion transporter. *Nature* 1997;388:482.

78. Donovan A, Brownlie A, Zhou Y, et al. Positional cloning of zebrafish ferroportin1 identifies a conserved vertebrate iron exporter. *Nature* 2000;403:776.

79. McKie AT, Marciani P, Rolfs A, et al. A novel duodenal iron-regulated transporter, IREG1, implicated in the basolateral transfer of iron to the circulation. *Mol Cell* 2000;5:299.

80. Vulpe CD, Kuo YM, Murphy TL, et al. Hephaestin, a ceruloplasmin homologue implicated in intestinal iron transport, is defective in the sla mouse. *Nat Genet* 1999;21:195.

81. Kawabata H, Yang R, Hirama T, et al. Molecular cloning of transferrin receptor 2. A new member of the transferrin receptor-like family. *J Biol Chem* 1999;274:20826.

82. Roy CN, Enns CA. Iron homeostasis: new tales from the crypt. *Blood* 2000;96:4020.

83. Zoller H, Koch RO, Theurl I, et al. Expression of the duodenal iron transporters divalent-metal transporter 1 and ferroportin 1 in iron deficiency and iron overload. *Gastroenterology* 2001;120:1412.

84. Parkkila S, Waheed A, Britton RS, et al. Association of the transferrin receptor in human placenta with HFE, the protein defective in hereditary hemochromatosis. *Proc Natl Acad Sci U S A* 1997;94:13198.

85. Waheed A, Parkkila S, Saarnio J, et al. Association of HFE protein with transferrin receptor in crypt enterocytes of human duodenum. *Proc Natl Acad Sci U S A* 1999;96:1579.

86. Lee GR. The anemia of chronic disease. *Semin Hematol* 1983;20:61.

87. Cortell S, Conrad ME. Effect of endotoxin on iron absorption. *Am J Physiol* 1967;213:43.

88. Zacharski LR, Ornstein DL, Woloshin S, et al. Association of age, sex, and race with body iron stores in adults: analysis of NHANES III data. *Am Heart J* 2000;140:98.

89. Witte DL. Can serum ferritin be effectively interpreted in the presence of the acute-phase response? *Clin Chem* 1991;37:484.

90. Beguin Y, Clemons GK, Pootrakul P, et al. Quantitative assessment of erythropoiesis and functional classification of anemia based on measurements of serum transferrin receptor and erythropoietin. *Blood* 1993;81:1067.

91. Cazzola M, Guarnone R, Cerani P, et al. Red blood cell precursor mass as an independent determinant of serum erythropoietin level. *Blood* 1998;91:2139.

92. Ferguson BJ, Skikne BS, Simpson KM, et al. Serum transferrin receptor distinguishes the anemia of chronic disease from iron deficiency anemia. *J Lab Clin Med* 1992;19:385.

93. Punnonen K, Irjala K, Ramjamäki A. Serum transferrin receptor and its ratio to serum ferritin in the diagnosis of iron deficiency. *Blood* 1997;89:1052.

94. Mast AE, Blinder MA, Gronowski AM, et al. Clinical utility of the soluble transferrin receptor and comparison with serum ferritin in several populations. *Clin Chem* 1998;44:45.

95. Chua E, Clague JE, Sharma AK, et al. Serum transferrin receptor assay in iron deficiency anaemia and anaemia of chronic disease in the elderly. *QJM* 1999;92:587.

96. Suominen P, Möttönen T, Rajamäki A, et al. Single values of serum transferrin receptor and transferrin receptor ferritin index can be used to detect true and functional iron deficiency in rheumatoid arthritis patients with anemia. *Arthritis Rheum* 2000;43:1016.

97. Fitzsimons EJ, Houston T, Munro R, et al. Erythroblast iron metabolism and serum soluble transferrin receptor values in the anemia of rheumatoid arthritis. *Arthritis Rheum* 2002;47:166.

98. Joosten E, Van Loon R, Billen J, et al. Serum transferrin receptor in the evaluation of the iron status in elderly hospitalized patients with anemia. *Am J Hematol* 2002;69:1.
99. Beutler B, Cerami A. Cachectin: more than a tumor necrosis factor. *N Engl J Med* 1987;316:379.
100. Dinarello CA. Interleukin-1. *Rev Infect Dis* 1984;6:51.
101. Marsh JC, Boggs DR, Cartwright GE, et al. Neutrophil kinetics in acute infection. *J Clin Invest* 1967;12:1943.
102. Steinbeck M, Roth J. Neutrophil activation by recombinant cytokines. *Rev Infect Dis* 1989;11:549.
103. Cannistra S, Griffin J. Regulation of the production and function of granulocytes and monocytes. *Semin Hematol* 1988;25:173.
104. Ramos FJ, Zamora F, Perez-Sicilia M, et al. Chronic granulocytic leukemia versus neutrophilic leukemoid reaction. *Am J Med* 1990;88:83.
105. Glasser RM, Walker RJ, Herion JC. The significance of hematologic abnormalities in patients with tuberculosis. *Arch Intern Med* 1970;125:691.
106. Twomey JJ, Leavell BS. Leukemoid reaction to tuberculosis. *Arch Intern Med* 1965;116:21.
107. Halpern Z, Dan M, Gilardi M, et al. Shigellosis in adults: epidemiologic, clinical and laboratory features. *Medicine* 1989;68:210.
108. Shoenfeld Y, Gurewich Y, Gallant LA, et al. Prednisone-induced leukocytosis: influence of dosage, method and duration of administration on the degree of leukocytosis. *Am J Med* 1981;71:773.
109. McKee LC Jr. Excess leukocytosis (leukemoid reactions) associated with malignant diseases. *South Med J* 1985;78:1475.
110. Lee MY, Kaushansky K, Judkins SA, et al. Mechanisms of tumor-induced neutrophilia: constitutive production of colony-stimulating factors and their synergistic actions. *Blood* 1989;74:115.
111. Liu CH, Lehan C, Speer ME, et al. Degenerative changes in neutrophils: an indicator of bacterial infection. *Pediatrics* 1984;74:823.
112. Emerson WA, Ieve PD, Krevans JR. Hematologic changes in septicemia. *Johns Hopkins Med J* 1970;126:69.
113. Easton JA, Fessas C. The incidence of Dohle bodies in various diseases and their association with thrombocytopenia. *Br J Haematol* 1966;12:54.
114. Zieve PD, Haghshenass M, Blanks M, et al. Vacuolization of the neutrophil: an aid in the diagnosis of septicemia. *Arch Intern Med* 1966;118:356.
115. Brooks GF, Priddle AH, Beaty HN. Early diagnosis of bacteremia by buffy-coat examinations. *Arch Intern Med* 1973;132:673.
116. Orlic D, Gill R, Feldschuk R, et al. Molecular mechanism for the inhibitory action of interferon on hematopoiesis. *Ann N Y Acad Sci* 1989;554:36.
117. Zoumbos N, Raefsky E, Young N. Lymphokines and hematopoiesis. *Prog Hematol* 1986;14:201.
118. Helminen M, Vesikari T. Spontaneous and inducible interleukin-1 production from peripheral blood monocytes in bacterial and viral infections in children. *Pediatr Infect Dis J* 1987;6:1102.
119. Ernstoff M, Galluchio V, Kirkwood J. Analyses of granulocyte-macrophage progenitor cells in patients treated with recombinant interferon alpha-2. *Am J Med* 1985;79:169.
120. Ackerman Z, Ackerman E, Shouval D. Measles: clinical and laboratory observation in young adults during an epidemic. *South Med J* 1988;81:1396.
121. Douglas RG, Alford R, Cate T, et al. The leukocyte response during viral respiratory illness in man. *Ann Intern Med* 1965;64:521.
122. Blumberg R, Schooley R. Lymphocyte markers and infectious diseases. *Semin Hematol* 1985;22:81.
123. Tosato G, Magrath I, Koski I, et al. Activation of suppressor T cells during Epstein-Barr-virus–induced infectious mononucleosis. *N Engl J Med* 1979;301:1133.
124. Wood TA, Frenkel EP. The atypical lymphocyte. *Am J Med* 1967;42:923.
125. Johnson RA, Waddelow TA, Caro J, et al. Chronic exposure to tumor necrosis factor in vivo preferentially inhibits erythropoiesis in nude mice. *Blood* 1989;741:120.
126. Brock JH. Iron and the outcome of infection. *BMJ* 1986;293:518.
127. McKenna WR, Mickelsen PA, Sparling PF, et al. Iron uptake from lactoferrin and transferrin by *Neisseria gonorrhoeae*. *Infect Immun* 1988;56:785.
128. Britigan BE, Cohen MS, Sparling PF. Gonococcal infection: a model of molecular pathogenesis. *N Engl J Med* 1985;312:1683.
129. Hershko C, Peto TE, Weatherall DJ. Iron and infection. *BMJ* 1988; 296:660.
130. Young N, Mortimer P. Viruses and bone marrow failure. *Blood* 1984;63:729.
131. Rosenfeld SJ, Young NS. Viruses and bone marrow failure. *Blood Rev* 1991;5:71.
132. Brown K, Anderson SM, Young NS. Erythrocyte P antigen: cellular receptor for B19 parvovirus. *Science* 1993;262:114.
133. Brown KE, Young NS. Parvovirus B19 in human disease. *Annu Rev Med* 1997;48:59.
134. Brown KE. Haematological consequences of parvovirus B19 infection. *Best Pract Res Clin Haematol* 2000;13:245.
135. Young N. Hematologic and hematopoietic consequences of B19 parvovirus infection. *Semin Hematol* 1988;25:159.
136. Owren PA. Congenital hemolytic jaundice. The pathogenesis of the hemolytic crisis. *Blood* 1948;3:231.
137. Lefrère JJ, Courouce AM, Bertrand Y, et al. Human parvovirus and aplastic crisis in chronic hemolytic anemias: a study of 24 observations. *Am J Hematol* 1986;23:271.
138. Mallouh AA, Qudah A. An epidemic of aplastic crisis caused by human parvovirus B19. *Pediatr Infect Dis J* 1995;14:31.
139. Hanada T, Koike K, Takeya T, et al. Human parvovirus B19-induced transient pancytopenia in a child with hereditary spherocytosis. *Br J Haematol* 1988;70:113.
140. Saunders PWG, Reid MM, Cohen BJ. Human parvovirus induced cytopenias: a report of five cases. *Br J Haematol* 1986;53:407.
141. Hanada T, Koike K, Takeya T, et al. Human parvovirus B19-induced transient pancytopenia in a child with hereditary spherocytosis. *Br J Haematol* 1988;70:113.
142. Muir K, Todd WT, Watson WH, et al. Viral-associated haemophagocytosis with parvovirus-B19-related pancytopenia. *Lancet* 1992;339:1139.
143. Watanabe M, Shimamoto Y, Yamaguchi M, et al. Viral-associated haemophagocytosis and elevated serum TNF-alpha with parvovirus-B19-related pancytopenia in patients with hereditary spherocytosis. *Clin Lab Haematol* 1994;16:179.
144. Shirono K, Tsuda H. Parvovirus B19-associated haemophagocytic syndrome in healthy adults. *Br J Haematol* 1995;89:923.
145. Rinn R, Chow WS, Pinkerton PH. Transient acquired myelodysplasia associated with parvovirus B19 infection in a patient with congenital spherocytosis. *Am J Hematol* 1995;50:71.
146. Yarali N, Duru F, Sipahi T, et al. Parvovirus B19 infection reminiscent of myelodysplastic syndrome in three children with chronic hemolytic anemia. *Pediatr Hematol Oncol* 2000;17:475.
147. Anand A, Gray ES, Brown T, et al. Human parvovirus infection in pregnancy and hydrops fetalis. *N Engl J Med* 1987;316:183.
148. Anderson LJ, Hurwitz ES. Human parvovirus B19 and pregnancy. *Clin Perinatol* 1988;15:273.
149. Leads from the MMWR. Risks associated with human parvovirus B19 infection. *JAMA* 1989;261:1406.
150. Socinski MA, Ershler WB, Tosato G, et al. Pure red cell aplasia associated with chronic Epstein-Barr virus infection: evidence for T-cell mediated suppression of erythroid colony forming units. *J Lab Clin Med* 1984;1041:995.
151. Spivak JL, Bender BS, Quinn TC. Hematologic abnormalities in the acquired immune deficiency syndrome. *Am J Med* 1984;77:224.
152. Clearfield HR, Brody J, Turner JH. Acute viral hepatitis, glucose-6-phosphate dehydrogenase deficiency and hemolytic anemia. *Arch Intern Med* 1969;123:689.
153. Bennett JM, Healy PJ. Spherocytic hemolytic anemia and acute cholecystitis caused by *Clostridium welchii*. *N Engl J Med* 1965;268:1070.
154. Myers G, Ngoi SS, Cennerazzo W, et al. Clostridial septicemia in an urban hospital. *Surg Gynecol Obstet* 1992;174:291.
155. Becker RC, Giuliani M, Savage RA, et al. Massive hemolysis in *Clostridium perfringens* infections. *J Surg Oncol* 1987;35:13.
156. Terebelo HR, McCue RL, Leuneville MS. Implications of plasma free hemoglobin in massive clostridial hemolysis. *JAMA* 1982;248:2028.
157. Dean HM, Decker CL, Baker LD, et al. Temporary survival in clostridial hemolysis with absence of circulating red cells. *N Engl J Med* 1967;277:700.
158. Mera CL, Freedman MH. *Clostridium* liver abscess and massive hemolysis. Unique demise in Fanconi's aplastic anemia. *Clin Pediatr (Phila)* 1984;23:126.
159. Anonymous. Abdominal pain, total intravascular hemolysis, and death in a 53 year old woman (clinical conference). *Am J Med* 1992;88:667.
160. Murray HW, Masur H, Senterfit LB, et al. The protean manifestations of *Mycoplasma pneumonia* infection in adults. *Am J Med* 1975;58:229.
161. Nordhagen R, Stensvold K, Winsnes A, et al. Paroxysmal cold hemoglobinuria. The most frequent autoimmune haemolytic anaemia in children? *Acta Paediatr Scand* 1984;73:258.
162. Reference deleted.
163. Shurin S, Anderson P, Zollinger J, et al. Pathophysiology of hemolysis in infections with *Hemophilus influenzae* type B. *J Clin Invest* 1986;77:1340.
164. Nagel RL, Roth E Jr. Malaria and red cell genetic defects. *Blood* 1989;74:1213.
165. Miller LH, Mason SJ, Clyde DF, et al. The resistance factor to *Plasmodium vivax* in blacks: the Duffy blood group genotype FyFy. *N Engl J Med* 1976;295:302.
166. Dolan SA, Miller LH, Wellems TE. Evidence for a switching mechanism in the invasion of erythrocytes by *Plasmodium falciparum*. *J Clin Invest* 1990;86:618.
167. Hadley TJ, Klotz FW, Pasvol G, et al. *Falciparum* malaria parasites invade erythrocytes that lack glycophorin A and B (MkMk). Strain differences indicate receptor heterogeneity and two pathways for invasion. *J Clin Invest* 1987;80:1190.
168. Perkins M. Inhibitory effects of erythrocyte membrane proteins on the in vitro invasion of the human malarial parasite (*Plasmodium falciparum*) into its host cell. *J Cell Biol* 1981;90:563.
169. Pasvol G, Wainscoat JS, Weatherall DJ. Erythrocytes deficiency in glycophorin resist invasion by the malarial parasite *Plasmodium falciparum*. *Nature* 1982;297:64.
170. Orlandi PA, Klotz FW, Haynes JD. A malaria invasion receptor, the 175-kilodalton erythrocyte binding antigen of *Plasmodium falciparum* recognizes the terminal Neu5Ac(alpha 2-3)Gal—sequences of glycophorin A. *J Cell Biol* 1992;116:901.
171. Dolan SA, Proctor JL, Alling DW, et al. Glycophorin B as an EBA-175 independent *Plasmodium falciparum* receptor of human erythrocytes. *Mol Biochem Parasitol* 1994;64:55.
172. Chishti AH, Palek J, Fisher D, et al. Reduced invasion and growth of *Plasmodium falciparum* into elliptocytic red blood cells with a combined deficiency of protein 4.1, glycophorin C, and p55. *Blood* 1996;87:3462.
173. Okoye V, Bennett V. *Plasmodium falciparum* malaria: band 3 as a possible receptor during invasion of human erythrocytes. *Science* 1985;227:169.

174. Friedman M, Fukuda M, Lame R. Evidence of a malarial parasite interaction site on the major transmembrane protein of the human erythrocyte. *Science* 1985;228:75.

175. Kushwaha A, Perween A, Mukund S, et al. Amino terminus of *Plasmodium falciparum* acidic basic repeat antigen interacts with the erythrocyte membrane through band 3 protein. *Mol Biochem Parasitol* 2002;122:45.

176. Lauer S, VanWye J, Harrison T, et al. Vacuolar uptake of host components, and a role for cholesterol and sphingomyelin in malarial infection. *EMBO J* 2000;19:3556.

177. Allred D, Gruenberg J, Sherman I. Dynamic rearrangements of the erythrocyte membrane internal architecture induced by infection with *Plasmodium falciparum. J Cell Sci* 1986;81:1.

178. Rodriguez MH, Jungery M. A protein on *Plasmodium falciparum*–infected erythrocytes functions as a transferrin receptor. *Nature* 1986;324:388.

179. MacPherson G, Warrell M, White N, et al. Human cerebral malaria. *Am J Pathol* 1985;119:385.

180. Aley S, Sherwood J, Howard R. Knob-positive and knob-negative *Plasmodium falciparum* differ in expression of a strain-specific malarial antigen on the surface of infected erythrocytes. *J Exp Med* 1984;160:1585.

181. Crandall I, Collins WE, Gysin J, et al. Synthetic peptides based on motifs present in human band 3 protein inhibit cytoadherence/sequestration of the malaria parasite *Plasmodium falciparum. Proc Natl Acad Sci U S A* 1993;90:4703.

182. Eda S, Lawler J, Sherman IW. Plasmodium falciparum-infected erythrocyte adhesion to the type 3 repeat domain of thrombospondin-1 is mediated by a modified band 3 protein. *Mol Biochem Parasitol* 1999;100:195.

183. Giribaldi G, Ulliers D, Mannu F, et al. Growth of *Plasmodium falciparum* induces stage-dependent haemichrome formation, oxidative aggregation of band 3, membrane deposition of complement and antibodies, and phagocytosis of parasitized erythrocytes. *Br J Haematol* 2001;113:492.

184. Allen SJ, O'Donnell A, Alexander ND, et al. Prevention of cerebral malaria in children in Papua New Guinea by southeast Asian ovalocytosis band 3. *Am J Trop Med Hyg* 1999;60:1056.

185. Miller KD, Greenberg AE, Campbell CC. Treatment of severe malaria in the United States with a continuous infusion of quinidine gluconate and exchange transfusion. *N Engl J Med* 1989;321:65.

186. Ihler GM. *Bartonella bacilliformis*: dangerous pathogen slowly emerging from deep background. *FEMS Microbiol Lett* 1996;144:1.

187. Minnick MF, Mitchell SJ, McAllister SJ. Cell entry and the pathogenesis of *Bartonella* infections. *Trends Microbiol* 1996;4:343.

188. Mitchell SJ, Minnick MF. Characterization of a two-gene locus from *Bartonella bacilliformis* associated with the ability to invade human erythrocytes. *Infect Immun* 1995;63:1552.

189. Coleman SA, Minnick MF. Establishing a direct role for the *Bartonella bacilliformis* invasion-associated locus B (IalB) protein in human erythrocyte parasitism. *Infect Immun* 2001;69:4373.

190. Conyers GB, Bessman MJ. The gene, ialA, associated with the invasion of human erythrocytes by *Bartonella bacilliformis*, designates a nudix hydrolase active on dinucleoside 5'-polyphosphates. *J Biol Chem* 1999;274:1203.

191. Benson LA, Kar S, McLaughlin G, et al. Entry of *Bartonella bacilliformis* into erythrocytes. *Infect Immun* 1986;54:347.

192. Xu YH, Lu ZY, Ihler GM. Purification of deformin, an extracellular protein synthesized by *Bartonella bacilliformis* which causes deformation of erythrocyte membranes. *Biochim Biophys Acta* 1995;1234:173.

193. Buckles EL, McGinnis Hill E. Interaction of *Bartonella bacilliformis* with human erythrocyte membrane proteins. *Microb Pathog* 2000;29:165.

194. Hendrix LR. Contact-dependent hemolytic activity distinct from deforming activity of *Bartonella bacilliformis. FEMS Microbiol Lett* 2000;182:119.

195. Verma A, Davis GE, Ihler GM. Infection of human endothelial cells with *Bartonella bacilliformis* is dependent on Rho and results in activation of Rho. *Infect Immun* 2000;68:5960.

196. Verma A, Davis GE, Ihler GM. Formation of stress fibres in human endothelial cells infected with *Bartonella bacilliformis* is associated with altered morphology, impaired migration and defects in cell morphogenesis. *Cell Microbiol* 2001;3:169.

197. Garcia FU, Wojta J, Hoover RL. Interactions between live *Bartonella bacilliformis* and endothelial cells. *J Infect Dis* 1992;165:1138.

198. Pruthi RK, Marshall WF, Wiltsie JC, et al. Human babesiosis. *Mayo Clin Proc* 1995;70:853.

199. Rosner F, Zarrabi MH, Benach JL, et al. Babesiosis in splenectomized adults. Review of 22 reported cases. *Am J Med* 1984;76:696.

200. Zaki M. Selected tickborne infections: a review of Lyme disease, Rocky Mountain spotted fever, and babesiosis. *N Y State J Med* 1989;89:320.

201. Smith RP, Evans AT, Popovsky M, et al. Transfusion-acquired babesiosis and failure of antibiotic treatment. *JAMA* 1986;256:2726.

202. Golightly L, Hirschhorn L, Weller P. Fever and headache in a splenectomized woman. *Rev Infect Dis* 1989;11:629.

203. Sun T, Tenenbaum MJ, Greenspan J, et al. Morphologic and clinical observations in human infection with *Babesia microti. J Infect Dis* 1983;148:239.

204. Auerbach M, Haubenstock A, Soloman G. Systemic babesiosis: another cause of the hemophagocytic syndrome. *Am J Med* 1986;80:301.

205. Gupta P, Hurley RW, Helseth PH, et al. Pancytopenia due to hemophagocytic syndrome as the presenting manifestation of babesiosis. *Am J Hematol* 1995;50:60.

206. Miguelez Morales M, Linares Feria M, del Carmen Mesa M. Haemophagocytic syndrome due to babesiosis in a splenectomized patient. *Br J Haematol* 1995;91:1033.

207. Rudzinska MA, Trager W, Lewengrub SJ, et al. An electron microscopic study of Babesia microti invading erythrocytes. *Cell Tissue Res* 1976;169:323.

208. Hagler L, Pastore R, Bergin J. Aplastic anemia following viral hepatitis. *Medicine* 1975;54:139.

209. Tzakes AG, Arditi M, Whitington PF, et al. Aplastic anemia complicating orthotopic liver transplantation for non-A, non-B hepatitis. *N Engl J Med* 1988;319:393.

210. Baranski B, Armstrong G, Truman JT, et al. Epstein-Barr virus in the bone marrow of patients with aplastic anemia. *Ann Intern Med* 1988;109:695.

211. Risdall RJ, McKenna EW, Nesbit ME, et al. Virus-associated hemophagocytic syndrome: a benign histiocytic proliferation distinct from malignant histiocytosis. *Cancer* 1979;44:993.

212. Dehner L. Morphological findings in the histiocytic syndromes. *Semin Oncol* 1991;18:8.

213. Blanche S, Caniglia M, Fischer A, et al. Epstein-Barr virus-associated hemophagocytic syndrome: clinical presentation and treatment. *Pediatr Hematol Oncol* 1989;6:233.

214. Su IJ, Wang CH, Cheng AL, et al. Hemophagocytic syndrome in Epstein-Barr virus-associated T-lymphoproliferative disorders: disease spectrum, pathogenesis, and management. *Leuk Lymphoma* 1995;19:401.

215. Kikuta H. Epstein-Barr virus-associated hemophagocytic syndrome. *Leuk Lymphoma* 1995;16:425.

216. Okano M, Gross TG. Epstein-Barr virus-associated hemophagocytic syndrome and fatal infectious mononucleosis. *Am J Hematol* 1996;53:111.

217. Fisman DN. Hemophagocytic syndromes and infection. *Emerg Infect Dis* 2000;6:601.

218. Esumi N, Ikushima S, Hibi S, et al. High serum ferritin level as a marker of malignant histiocytosis and virus-associated hemophagocytic syndrome. *Cancer* 1988;61:2071.

219. Esumi N, Ikushima S, Todo S, et al. Hyperferritinemia in malignant histiocytosis, virus-associated hemophagocytic syndrome and familial erythrophagocytic lymphohistiocytosis. A survey of pediatric cases. *Acta Paediatr Scand* 1989;78:268.

220. Su IJ, Hsu YH, Lin MT, et al. Epstein-Barr virus-containing T-cell lymphoma presents with hemophagocytic syndrome mimicking malignant histiocytosis. *Cancer* 1993;72:2019.

221. Ningsanond V. Infection associated hemophagocytic syndrome: a report of 50 children. *J Med Assoc Thai* 2000;83:1141.

222. Rubin CM, Burke BA, McKenna RW, et al. The accelerated phase of Chediak-Higashi syndrome. An expression of the virus-associated hemophagocytic syndrome? *Cancer* 1985;56:524.

223. Kikuta H, Sakiyama Y, Matsumoto S, et al. Fatal Epstein-Barr virus–associated hemophagocytic syndrome. *Blood* 1993;82:3259.

224. Ishii E, Ohga S, Aoki T, et al. Prognosis of children with virus-associated hemophagocytic syndrome and malignant histiocytosis: correlation with levels of serum interleukin-1 and tumor necrosis factor. *Acta Haematol* 1991;85:93.

225. Ohga S, Matsuzaki A, Nishizaki M, et al. Inflammatory cytokines in virus-associated hemophagocytic syndrome. Interferon-gamma as a sensitive indicator of disease activity. *Am J Pediatr Hematol Oncol* 1993;15:291.

226. Fujiwara F, Hibi S, Imashuku S. Hypercytokinemia in hemophagocytic syndrome. *Am J Pediatr Hematol Oncol* 1993;15:92.

227. Lay JD, Tsao CJ, Chen JY, et al. Upregulation of tumor necrosis factor-alpha gene by Epstein-Barr virus and activation of macrophages in Epstein-Barr virus-infected T cells in the pathogenesis of hemophagocytic syndrome. *J Clin Invest* 1997;100:1969.

228. Kasahara Y, Yachie A, Takei K, et al. Differential cellular targets of Epstein-Barr virus (EBV) infection between acute EBV-associated hemophagocytic lymphohistiocytosis and chronic active EBV infection. *Blood* 2001;98:1882.

229. Kawaguchi H, Miyashita T, Herbst H, et al. Epstein-Barr virus-infected T lymphocytes in Epstein-Barr virus-associated hemophagocytic syndrome. *J Clin Invest* 1993;92:1444.

230. Dolezal MV, Kamel OW, van de Rijn M, et al. Virus-associated hemophagocytic syndrome characterized by clonal Epstein-Barr virus genome. *Am J Clin Pathol* 1995;103:189.

231. Imashuku S, Hibi S, Tabata Y, et al. Outcome of clonal hemophagocytic lymphohistiocytosis: analysis of 32 cases. *Leuk Lymphoma* 2000;37:577.

232. Stephan JL, Kone-Paut I, Galambrun C, et al. Reactive haemophagocytic syndrome in children with inflammatory disorders. A retrospective study of 24 patients. *Rheumatology (Oxford)* 2001;40:1285.

233. Imashuku S, Kuriyama K, Teramura T, et al. Requirement for etoposide in the treatment of Epstein-Barr virus-associated hemophagocytic lymphohistiocytosis. *J Clin Oncol* 2001;19:2665.

234. Imashuku S, Hibi S, Ohara T, et al. Effective control of Epstein-Barr virus-related hemophagocytic lymphohistiocytosis with immunochemotherapy. Histiocyte Society. *Blood* 1999;93:1869.

235. Imashuku S, Tabata Y, Teramura T, et al. Treatment strategies for Epstein-Barr virus-associated hemophagocytic lymphohistiocytosis (EBV-HLH). *Leuk Lymphoma* 2000;39:37.

236. Minegishi M, Ohashi Y, Kumaki S, et al. Successful umbilical cord blood transplantation from an unrelated donor for a patient with Epstein-Barr virus-associated hemophagocytic lymphohistiocytosis. *Bone Marrow Transplant* 2001;27:883.

237. Hasegawa D, Sano K, Kosaka Y, et al. A case of hemophagocytic lymphohistiocytosis with prolonged remission after syngeneic bone marrow transplantation. *Bone Marrow Transplant* 1999;24:425.

238. Gong XS. Effective control of infection-associated hemophagocytic syndrome with chloroquine. *J Pediatr Hematol Oncol* 2002;24:330.

239. Kitchens CS. Clinical observations of human bone marrow macrophages. *Medicine* 1977;56:503.

240. Bodem CR, Harmony BH, Taylor HM, et al. Granulomatous bone marrow disease. *Medicine* 1983;62:372.

241. Kinaly J III, Wheby M. Bone marrow necrosis. *Am J Med* 1976;60:361.

242. Vichinsky EP, Neumayr LD, Earles AN, et al. Causes and outcomes of the acute chest syndrome in sickle cell disease. National Acute Chest Syndrome Study Group. *N Engl J Med* 2000;342:1855.

243. Maitre B, Habibi A, Roudot-Thoraval F, et al. Acute chest syndrome in adults with sickle cell disease. *Chest* 2000;117:1386.

244. Brown C III. Bone marrow necrosis. A study of seventy cases. *Johns Hopkins Med J* 1972;131:189.

245. Weissman D, Negendank W, Ayad A, et al. Bone marrow necrosis in lymphoma studied by magnetic resonance imaging. *Am J Hematol* 1992;40:42.

246. Mankad VN, Williams JP, Harpen MD, et al. Magnetic resonance imaging of bone marrow in sickle cell disease: clinical, hematologic, and pathologic correlations. *Blood* 1990;75:274.

247. Oski F, Norman J. Effect of live measles vaccine on the platelet count. *N Engl J Med* 1966;275:352.

248. Scott S, Reimers H, Chernesky M, et al. Effect of viruses on platelet aggregation and platelet survival in rabbits. *Blood* 1978;62:47.

249. Terado H, Baldini M, Ebbe S, et al. Interaction of influenza virus with blood platelets. *Blood* 1966;28:213.

250. Bik T, Sarov I, Livine A. Interaction between vaccinia virus and human blood platelets. *Blood* 1982;59:482.

251. Ellman L, Carvalito A, Jacobsen B, et al. Platelet autoantibody in a case of infectious mononucleosis presenting as thrombocytopenic purpura. *Am J Med* 1973;55:723.

252. Cohen JI, Corey GR. Cytomegalovirus infection in the normal host. *Medicine* 1985;64:100.

253. Wilson J, Neame P, Kelton J. Infection-induced thrombocytopenia. *Semin Thromb Hemost* 1982;8:217.

254. Goldblum SE, Simon TL, Thilsted JP, et al. Pneumococcus-induced thrombocytopenia in rabbits. *J Lab Clin Med* 1985;106:298.

255. Oppenheimer L, Hrynuik WM, Bishop AJ. Thrombocytopenia in severe bacterial infections. *J Surg Res* 1976;20:211.

256. Kelton JG, Neame PB, Gauldie J, et al. Elevated platelet associated IgG in the thrombocytopenia of septicemia. *N Engl J Med* 1979;300:760.

257. Asprunk DH, Das J. Endotoxin-induced changes in human platelet membranes: morphologic evidence. *Blood* 1978;51:487.

258. Schneider RC, Zapol WM, Carvalho AC. Platelet consumption and sequestration in severe acute respiratory failure. *Am Rev Respir Dis* 1980;122:445.

259. Neame P, Kelton J, Walker I, et al. Thrombocytopenia in septicemia: the role of DIC. *Blood* 1980;56:88.

260. Corrigan JJ Jr, Ray WC, May N. Changes in the blood coagulation system associated with septicemia. *N Engl J Med* 1968;279:851.

261. Stossel TP, Levy R. Intravascular coagulation associated with pneumococcal bacteremia and symmetrical peripheral gangrene. *Arch Intern Med* 1970;125:876.

262. Spicer TE, Rau JM. Purpura fulminans. *Am J Med* 1976;61:566.

263. Beck E, Dejana E. Thrombohemorrhagic phenomena associated with infectious diseases. *Semin Hematol* 1988;25:91.

264. Bisno AL, Freeman JC. The syndrome of asplenia, pneumococcal sepsis and DIC. *Ann Intern Med* 1970;72:389.

265. Gerjarusak P, Hinthorn D, Liu C. Hyposplenism and DIC in fulminant pneumococcal sepsis. *South Med J* 1977;70:995.

266. Kingston M, Mackenzie CR. The syndrome of pneumococcemia, DIC and asplenia. *Can Med Assoc J* 1979;121:57.

267. Ratnoff O, Nebehay W. Multiple coagulative defects in a patient with the Waterhouse-Friderichsen syndrome. *Ann Intern Med* 1962;56:627.

268. Bevilacqua M, Schleef R, Gimbrone M, et al. Regulation of the fibrinolytic system of cultured human vascular endothelium by interleukin 1. *J Clin Invest* 1986;78:587.

269. Carbone K, Heinrich M, Quinn T. Thrombophlebitis and cellulitis due to Campylobacter sp. fetus. *Medicine* 1985;64:244.

270. Simave C, Hardy G, Fardy P. The Lemierre syndrome: suppurative thrombophlebitis of the internal jugular vein secondary to oropharyngeal infection. *Medicine* 1989;68:85.

271. Remuzzi G, Garella S. HUS and TTP: variable expression of a single entity. *Kidney Int* 1987;32:292.

272. Ridolfi RL, Bell WR. Thrombotic thrombocytopenic purpura: report of 25 cases and review of the literature. *Medicine* 1981;60:413.

273. Neill MA, Agosti J, Rosen H. Hemorrhagic colitis with *Escherichia coli* O157:H7 preceding adult hemolytic uremic syndrome. *Arch Intern Med* 1985;145:2215.

274. Pai CH, Kelly JK. Shiga-like toxin-producing *Escherichia coli*. In: Farthing MJ, Keusch GT, eds. *Enteric infection: mechanisms, manifestations, and management*. New York: Raven Press, 1989:141.

275. Moake JL, Rudy CK, Troll JH, et al. Unusually large plasma factor VII: von Willebrand factor multimers in chronic relapsing thrombotic thrombocytopenic purpura. *N Engl J Med* 1982;307:1432.

276. Furlan M, Robles R, Galbusera M, et al. von Willebrand factor–cleaving protease in thrombotic thrombocytopenic purpura and the hemolytic–uremic syndrome. *N Engl J Med* 1998;339:1578.

277. Tsai H-M, Lian ECY. Antibodies to von-Willebrand factor-cleaving protease in acute thrombotic thrombocytopenic purpura. *N Engl J Med* 1998;339:1585.

278. Levy GG, Nichols WC, Lian EC, et al. Mutations in a member of the ADAMTS gene family cause thrombotic thrombocytopenic purpura. *Nature* 2001;413:488.

279. Marshall FF, Walsh PC. Extrarenal manifestations of renal cell carcinoma. *J Urol* 1977;117:439.

280. Bowman HS, Martinez EJ. Fever, anemia and hyperhaptoglobinemia: an extrarenal triad of hypernephroma. *Ann Intern Med* 1968;68:613.

281. Beveridge BR, Baumerman RM, Evanson JM, et al. Hypochromic anemia: a retrospective study and follow-up of 378 in-patients. *QJM* 1965;34:145.

282. Rockey DC, Campbell EW Jr. Evaluation of the gastrointestinal tract in patients with iron-deficiency anemia. *N Engl J Med* 1993;329:1691.

283. Bron D, Meuleman N, Mascaux C. Biological basis of anemia. *Semin Oncol* 2001;28:1.

284. Hockenberry MJ, Hinds PS, Barrera P, et al. Incidence of anemia in children with solid tumors or Hodgkin disease. *J Pediatr Hematol Oncol* 2002;24:35.

285. Moliterno AR, Spivak JL. Anemia of cancer. *Hematol Oncol Clin North Am* 1996;10:345.

286. Erslev AJ. Erythropoietin and anemia of cancer. *Eur J Haematol* 2000;64:353.

287. Mercadante S, Gebbia V, Marrazzo A, et al. Anaemia in cancer: pathophysiology and treatment. *Cancer Treat Rev* 2000;26:303.

288. Soignet S. Management of cancer-related anemia: epoetin alfa and quality of life. *Semin Hematol* 2000;37:9.

289. Caro JJ, Salas M, Ward A, et al. Anemia as an independent prognostic factor for survival in patients with cancer: a systemic, quantitative review. *Cancer* 2001;91:2214.

290. Littlewood TJ. Erythropoietin for the treatment of anemia associated with hematological malignancy. *Hematol Oncol* 2001;19:19.

291. Kurzrock R. The role of cytokines in cancer-related fatigue. *Cancer* 2001;92:1684.

292. Dunst J. The use of epoetin alfa to increase and maintain hemoglobin levels during radiotherapy. *Semin Oncol* 2001;28:42.

293. Kumar P. Tumor hypoxia and anemia: impact on the efficacy of radiation therapy. *Semin Hematol* 2000;37:4.

294. Kumar P. Impact of anemia in patients with head and neck cancer. *Oncologist* 2000;5[Suppl 2]:13.

295. Fyles AW, Milosevic M, Pintilie M, et al. Anemia, hypoxia and transfusion in patients with cervix cancer: a review. *Radiother Oncol* 2000;57:13.

296. Curt GA, Breitbart W, Cella D, et al. Impact of cancer-related fatigue on the lives of patients: new findings from the Fatigue Coalition. *Oncologist* 2000;5:353.

297. Glaspy J. Anemia and fatigue in cancer patients. *Cancer* 2001;92:1719.

298. Sobrero A, Puglisi F, Guglielmi A, et al. Fatigue: a main component of anemia symptomatology. *Semin Oncol* 2001;28:15.

299. Osterbor A. The role of recombinant human erythropoietin in the management of anaemic cancer patients: focus on haematological malignancies. *Med Oncol* 2000;17[Suppl 1]:S17.

300. Itri LM. Cancer-related anaemia requires higher doses of epoetin alfa than chronic renal failure replacement therapy. *Nephrol Dial Transplant* 2001;16:2289.

301. Doll D, Weiss R. Neoplasia and the erythron. *J Clin Oncol* 1985;3:429.

302. Hardy C, Balducci L. Hemopoietic alterations of cancer. *Am J Med Sci* 1985;290:196.

303. Zucker S, Lysik R, DiSetfano J. Cancer cell inhibition of erythropoiesis. *J Lab Clin Med* 1980;96:770.

304. Zucker S, Friedman S, Lysik R. Bone marrow erythropoiesis in the anemia of infection, inflammation, and malignancy. *J Clin Invest* 1974;53:1132.

305. Beutler B, Cerami A. Cachectin, cachexia, and shock. *Annu Rev Med* 1988;39:75.

306. Balkwill F, Osborne R, Burke F. Evidence for tumour necrosis factor/cachectin production in cancer. *Lancet* 1987;2:1229.

307. Ulich T, del Castillo J, Guo K, et al. The hematologic effects of chronic administration of the monokines TNF, interleukin-1 and granulocyte-CSF on bone marrow and circulation. *Am J Pathol* 1987;134:149.

308. Beutler B, Cerami A. Cachectin: more than a tumor necrosis factor. *N Engl J Med* 1987;316:379.

309. Johnson RA, Waddelow T, Caro, J, et al. Chronic exposure to TNF in vivo preferentially inhibits erythropoiesis in nude mice. *Blood* 1989;74:130.

310. Mantovani G, Maccio A, Mura L, et al. Serum levels of leptin and proinflammatory cytokines in patients with advanced-stage cancer at different sites. *J Mol Med* 2000;78:554.

311. Martin F, Santolaria F, Batista N, et al. Cytokine levels (IL-6 and IFN-gamma), acute phase response and nutritional status as prognostic factors in lung cancer. *Cytokine* 1999;11:80.

312. Miller CB, Jones RJ, Piantadosi S, et al. Decreased erythropoietin response in patients with the anemia of cancer. *N Engl J Med* 1990;322:1689.

313. Ozguroglu M, Arun B, Demir G, et al. Serum erythropoietin level in anemic cancer patients. *Med Oncol* 2000;17:29.

314. Masaoka A, Hashimoto T, Shibata K, et al. Thymomas associated with pure red cell aplasia: histologic and follow-up studies. *Cancer* 1989;64:1872.

315. Hirst E, Robertson TI. The syndrome of thymoma and erythroblastopenic anemia. *Medicine* 1967;46:225.

316. Krantz SB, Kao V. Studies on red cell aplasia. I. Demonstration of a plasma inhibitor to heme synthesis and an antibody to erythroblastic nuclei. *Proc Natl Acad Sci U S A* 1967;58:493.

317. Tetteri A, Windebank KP, Veeder MH, et al. Steroid-responsive pure red cell aplasia associated with natural killer cell lymphocytosis. *Am J Hematol* 1989;31:211.
318. Akard LP, Brandt J, Lu L, et al. Chronic T-cell lymphoproliferative disorder and pure red cell aplasia: further characterization of cell-mediated inhibition of erythropoiesis and clinical response to cytotoxic chemotherapy. *Am J Med* 1987;83:1069.
319. Mangan KF. T-cell mediated suppression of hematopoiesis. *N Engl J Med* 1985;312:306.
320. Delsol G, Guiu-Godfrin B, Guiu M, et al. Leukoerythroblastosis and cancer frequency: prognosis and physiopathologic significance. *Cancer* 1979;44:1009.
321. Spira M, Lynch E. Autoimmune hemolytic anemia and carcinoma: an unusual association. *Am J Med* 1979;67:753.
322. Bruyere M, Sokal G, Devortille J, et al. Autoimmune haemolytic anaemias and ovarian tumour. *Br J Haematol* 1971;20:83.
323. Lohrmann HP, Adam W, Heymer B, et al. Microangiopathic hemolytic anemia in metastatic carcinoma: report of eight cases. *Ann Intern Med* 1973;79:368.
324. Brain MC, Dave J, Hourihane D. Microangiopathic haemolytic anaemia: the possible role of vascular lesions in pathogenesis. *Br J Haematol* 1962;8:358.
325. Jacobsen RJ, Jackson D. Erythrocyte fragmentation in defibrination syndromes. *Ann Intern Med* 1974;81:207.
326. Antman KH, Skarm A, Mayer R, et al. Microangiopathic hemolytic anemia and cancer: a review. *Medicine* 1979;58:377.
327. Murgo AJ. Thrombotic microangiography in the cancer patient including those induced by chemotherapeutic agents. *Semin Hematol* 1987;24:161.
328. Abels R. Erythropoietin for anaemia in cancer patients. *Eur J Cancer* 1993;29A[Suppl 2]:S2.
329. Case DC, Bukowski RM, Carey RW, et al. Recombinant human erythropoietin therapy for anemic cancer patients on combination chemotherapy. *J Natl Cancer Inst* 1993;85:801.
330. Cascinu S, Fedeli A, Del Ferro E, et al. Recombinant human erythropoietin treatment in cisplatin-associated anemia: a randomized, double-blind trial with placebo. *J Clin Oncol* 1994;12:1058.
331. Henry DH, Abels RI. Recombinant human erythropoietin in the treatment of cancer and chemotherapy-induced anemia: results of double-blind and open-label follow-up studies. *Semin Oncol* 1994;21[2 Suppl 3]:21.
332. Glaspy J, Bukowski R, Steinberg D, et al. Impact of therapy with epoetin alfa on clinical outcomes in patients with nonmyeloid malignancies during cancer chemotherapy in community oncology practice. Procrit Study Group. *J Clin Oncol* 1997;15:1218.
333. Demetri GD, Kris M, Wade J, et al. Quality-of-life benefit in chemotherapy patients treated with epoetin alfa is independent of disease response or tumor type: results from a prospective community oncology study. Procrit Study Group. *J Clin Oncol* 1998;16:3412.
334. Littlewood TJ, Bajetta E, Nortier JW, et al., and the Epoetin Alfa Study Group. Effects of epoetin alfa on hematologic parameters and quality of life in cancer patients receiving nonplatinum chemotherapy: results of a randomized, double-blind, placebo-controlled trial. *J Clin Oncol* 2001;19:2865.
335. Curt GA, Breitbart W, Cella D, et al. Impact of cancer-related fatigue on the lives of patients: new findings from the Fatigue Coalition. *Oncologist* 2000;5:353.
336. Cheung WK, Goon BL, Guilfoyle MC, et al. Pharmacokinetics and pharmacodynamics of recombinant human erythropoietin after single and multiple subcutaneous doses to healthy subjects. *Clin Pharmacol Ther* 1998;64:412.
337. Gabrilove JL, Cleeland CS, Livingston RB, et al. Clinical evaluation of once-weekly dosing of epoetin alfa in chemotherapy patients: improvements in hemoglobin and quality of life are similar to three-times-weekly dosing. *J Clin Oncol* 2001;19:2875.
338. Fjornes T, Wiedemann GJ, Sack K, et al. Serum erythropoietin and creatinine concentrations as predictive factors for response to recombinant human erythropoietin treatment in anaemic tumour patients on chemotherapy. *Oncol Rep* 1998;5:81.
339. Waldmann, T, Rossi W, Swann R. The erythropoiesis stimulating factors produced by tumors. *Ann N Y Acad Sci* 1968;149:509.
340. Waldmann T, Levin E, Baldwin M. The association of polycythemia with a cerebellar hemangioblastoma: the production of an erythropoiesis stimulating factor by the tumor. *Am J Med* 1961;31:318.
341. Sytkowski A, Bicknell K, Smith GM, et al. Secretion of erythropoietin-like activity by clones of human renal carcinoma cell line GKA. *Cancer Res* 1984;44:51.
342. Maxwell PH, Wiesener MS, Chang GW, et al. The tumour suppressor protein VHL targets hypoxia-inducible factors for oxygen-dependent proteolysis. *Nature* 1999;399:271.
343. Ivan M, Kondo K, Yang H, et al. HIF-alpha targeted for VHL-mediated destruction by proline hydroxylation: implications for O_2 sensing. *Science* 2001;292:464.
344. Jaakkola P, Mole DR, Tian YM, et al. Targeting of HIF-alpha to the von Hippel-Lindau ubiquitylation complex by O_2-regulated prolyl hydroxylation. *Science* 2001;292:468.
345. Lando D, Peet DJ, Whelan DA, et al. Asparagine hydroxylation of the HIF transactivation domain: a hypoxic switch. *Science* 2002;295:858.
346. Kondo K, Kaelin WG. The von Hippel-Lindau tumor suppressor gene. *Exp Cell Res* 2001;264:117.
347. Maxwell PH, Pugh CW, Ratcliffe PJ. The pVHL-hIF-1 system. A key mediator of oxygen homeostasis. *Adv Exp Med Biol* 2001;502:365.
348. Zhu H, Bunn HF. How do cells sense oxygen? *Science* 2001;292:449.
349. Bruick RK, McKnight SL. Oxygen sensing gets a second wind. *Science* 2002;295:807.
350. Krieg M, Marti HH, Plate KH. Coexpression of erythropoietin and vascular endothelial growth factor in nervous system tumors associated with von Hippel-Lindau tumor suppressor gene loss of function. *Blood* 1998;92:3388.
351. Haase VH, Glickman JN, Socolovsky M, et al. Vascular tumors in livers with targeted inactivation of the von Hippel-Lindau tumor suppressor. *Proc Natl Acad Sci U S A* 2001;98:1583.
352. Wiesener MS, Seyfarth M, Warnecke C, et al. Paraneoplastic erythrocytosis associated with an inactivating point mutation of the von Hippel-Lindau gene in a renal cell carcinoma. *Blood* 2002;99:3562.
353. Funakoshi A, Muta H, Baba T, et al. Gene expression of mutant erythropoietin in hepatocellular carcinoma. *Biochem Biophys Res Commun* 1993;195:717.
354. Muta H, Funakoshi A, Baba T, et al. Gene expression of erythropoietin in hepatocellular carcinoma. *Intern Med* 1994;33:427.
355. Dreicer R, Donovan J, Benda JA, et al. Paraneoplastic erythrocytosis in a young adult with an erythropoietin-producing Wilms' tumor. *Am J Med* 1992;93:229.
356. Reid CD, Fidler J, Kirk A. Endogeneous erythroid clones (EEC) in polycythaemia and their relationship to diagnosis and the response to treatment. *Br J Haematol* 1988;68:395.
357. Lee M, Durch S, Dave D, et al. Kinetics of tumor-induced murine neutrophilia. *Blood* 1979;53:619.
358. Delmonte L, Liebelt RA. Granulocytosis promoting extract of mouse tumor tissue. *Science* 1965;148:521.
359. Beutler B, Cerami A. Tumor necrosis, cachexia, shock, and inflammation: a common mediator. *Annu Rev Biochem* 1988;57:505.
360. Mayer P, Lam C, Obenaus H, et al. Recombinant human GM-CSF induces leukocytosis and activated peripheral blood polymorphonuclear neutrophils in nonhuman primates. *Blood* 1987;70:206.
361. O'Neill B Jr. Monocytosis in malignant disease. *Ann Intern Med* 1970;73:991.
362. Ascensao JL, Oken MM, Ewing SL. Leukocytosis and large cell lung cancer: a frequent association. *Cancer* 1987;60:903.
363. Ramos FJ, Zamora F, Perez-Sicilia M, et al. Chronic granulocytic leukemia versus neutrophilic leukemoid reaction. *Am J Med* 1990;88:83.
364. Kasuga I, Makino S, Kiyokawa H, et al. Tumor-related leukocytosis is linked with poor prognosis in patients with lung carcinoma. *Cancer* 2001;92:2399.
365. Blay JY, Rossi JF, Wijdenes J, et al. Role of interleukin-6 in the paraneoplastic inflammatory syndrome associated with renal-cell carcinoma. *Int J Cancer* 1997;72:424.
366. Wetzler M, Estrov Z, Talpaz M, et al. Granulocyte-macrophage colony-stimulating factor as a cause of paraneoplastic leukaemoid reaction in advanced transitional cell carcinoma. *J Intern Med* 1993;234:417.
367. Obara TR, Ito Y, Kodama T, et al. A case of gastric carcinoma associated with excessive granulocytosis: production of a colony-stimulating factor by the tumor. *Cancer* 1985;56:782.
368. Sato K, Mimura H, Han DC. Production of bone-resorbing activity and colony-stimulating activity in vivo and in vitro by a human squamous cell carcinoma associated with hypercalcemia and leukocytosis. *J Clin Invest* 1986;78:145.
369. Sato K, Fujii Y, Ono M, et al. Production of interleukin 1 alpha-like factor and colony-stimulating factor by a squamous cell carcinoma of the thyroid (T3M-5) derived from a patient with hypercalcemia and leukocytosis. *Cancer Res* 1987;47:6474.
370. Uemura Y, Nakata H, Kobayashi M, et al. Regulation of granulocyte colony-stimulating factor and parathyroid hormone-related protein production in lung carcinoma cell line OKa-C-1. *Jpn J Cancer Res* 2000;91:911.
371. Cohen PR, Holder WR, Tucker SB, et al. Sweet syndrome in patients with solid tumors. *Cancer* 1993;72:2723.
372. Beeson P. Cancer and eosinophilia. *N Engl J Med* 1983;309:792.
373. Weller P. Eosinophilia. *J Allergy Clin Immunol* 1984;73:1.
374. Lowe D, Jorizzo J, Hutt MSR. Tumor-associated eosinophilia: a review. *J Clin Pathol* 1981;34:1343.
375. Balducci L, Chapman S, Little D, et al. Paraneoplastic eosinophilia: report of a case with in vitro studies of hemopoiesis. *Cancer* 1989;64:2250.
376. Sanderson CJ, Warren DJ, Strath M. Identification of a lymphokine that stimulates eosinophil differentiation in vitro. *J Exp Med* 1985;162:60.
377. Balian A, Bonte E, Naveau S, et al. Intratumoral production of interleukin-5 leading to paraneoplastic peripheral eosinophilia in hepatocellular carcinoma. *J Hepatol* 2001;34:355.
378. Chang H, Jamal N, Wang XH, et al. Constitutive production of the interleukins IL-5 and IL-6 by the lymphoma cell line OCI-Ly 17 derived from a patient with malignant lymphoma and hypereosinophilia. *Leuk Lymphoma* 1992;8:97.
379. Rivoltini L, Viggiano V, Spinazze S, et al. In vitro anti-tumor activity of eosinophils from cancer patients treated with subcutaneous administration of interleukin 2. Role of interleukin 5. *Int J Cancer* 1993;54:8.
380. Prin L, Plumas J, Gruart V, et al. Elevated serum levels of soluble interleukin-2 receptor: a marker of disease activity in the hypereosinophilic syndrome. *Blood* 1991;78:2626.
381. Silberstein DS, Schoof DD, Rodrick ML, et al. Activation of eosinophils in cancer patients treated with IL-2 and IL-3–generated lymphokine-activated killer cells. *J Immunol* 1989;142:2162.
382. Isaacson NJ, Rappoport P. Eosinophilia in malignant tumors: its significance. *Ann Intern Med* 1946;25:893.

383. Lopez AF, To LB, Yang Y-C, et al. Stimulation of proliferation, differentiation, and function of human cells by primate interleukin 3. *Proc Natl Acad Sci U S A* 1987;84:2761.

384. Levin J, Conley CL. Thrombocytosis associated with malignant disease. *Arch Intern Med* 1964;114:497.

385. Griesshammer M, Bangerter M, Sauer T, et al. Aetiology and clinical significance of thrombocytosis: analysis of 732 patients with an elevated platelet count. *J Intern Med* 1999;245:295.

386. Schafer A. Review: bleeding and thrombosis in the myeloproliferative disorders. *Blood* 1984;64:1.

387. Lok S, Kaushansky K, Holly RD, et al. Cloning and expression of murine thrombopoietin cDNA and stimulation of platelet production *in vivo*. *Nature* 1994;369:565

388. Bartley TD, Bogenberger J, Hint P, et al. Identification and cloning of a megakaryocyte growth and development factor that is a ligand for the cytokine receptor Mpl. *Cell* 1994;77:1117.

389. de Sauvage FJ, Hass PE, Spencer SD, et al. Stimulation of megakaryocytopoiesis and thrombopoiesis by the c-Mpl ligand. *Nature* 1994;369:533

390. Guinan EC, Lee YS, Lopez KD, et al. Effects of interleukin-3 and granulocyte-macrophage colony-stimulating factor on thrombopoiesis in congenital amegakaryocytic thrombocytopenia. *Blood* 1993;81:1691.

391. Hill RJ, Warren MK, Stenberg P, et al. Stimulation of megakaryocytopoiesis in mice by human recombinant interleukin-6. *Blood* 1991;77:42.

392. Neben S, Turner K. The biology of interleukin 11. *Stem Cells* 1993;11[Suppl 2]:156.

393. Briddell RA, Bruno E, Cooper RJ, et al. Effect of c-kit ligand on the in vitro human megakaryocytopoiesis. *Blood* 1991;78:2854.

394. Emmons RV, Reid DM, Cohen RL, et al. Human thrombopoietin levels are high when thrombocytopenia is due to megakaryocyte deficiency and low when due to increased platelet destruction. *Blood* 1996;87:4068.

395. Kuter DJ, Rosenberg RD. The reciprocal relationship of thrombopoietin (c-Mpl ligand) to changes in the platelet mass during busulfan-induced thrombocytopenia in the rabbit. *Blood* 1995;85:2720.

396. Wiestner A, Schlemper RJ, van der Maas AP, et al. An activating splice donor mutation in the thrombopoietin gene causes hereditary thrombocythaemia. *Nat Genet* 1998;18:49.

397. Kondo T, Okabe M, Sanada M, et al. Familial essential thrombocythemia associated with one-base deletion in the 5'-untranslated region of the thrombopoietin gene. *Blood* 1998;92:1091.

398. Stouthard JM, Goey H, de Vries EG, et al. Recombinant human interleukin 6 in metastatic renal cell cancer: a phase II trial. *Br J Cancer* 1996;73:789.

399. Kaser A, Brandacher G, Steurer W, et al. Interleukin-6 stimulates thrombopoiesis through thrombopoietin: role in inflammatory thrombocytosis. *Blood* 2001;98:2720.

400. Walther MM, Johnson B, Culley D, et al. Serum interleukin-6 levels in metastatic renal cell carcinoma before treatment with interleukin-2 correlates with paraneoplastic syndromes but not patient survival. *J Urol* 1998;159:718.

401. Sacks G, Levin J, Bell WR. Trousseau's syndrome and other manifestations of chronic disseminated coagulopathy in patients with neoplasms: clinical, pathologic and therapeutic features. *Medicine* 1977;56:1.

402. Francis JL, Biggerstaff J, Amirkhosravi A. Hemostasis and malignancy. *Semin Thromb Hemost* 1998;24:93.

403. Falanga A, Rickles FR. Pathophysiology of the thrombophilic state in the cancer patient. *Semin Thromb Hemost* 1999;25:173.

404. Lee AY, Levine MN. The thrombophilic state induced by therapeutic agents in the cancer patient. *Semin Thromb Hemost* 1999;25:137.

405. Gouin-Thibault I, Samama MM. Laboratory diagnosis of the thrombophilic state in cancer patients. *Semin Thromb Hemost* 1999;25:167.

406. Loreto MF, De Martinis M, Corsi MP, et al. Coagulation and cancer: implications for diagnosis and management. *Pathol Oncol Res* 2000;6:301.

407. Trikha M, Nakada MT. Platelets and cancer: implications for antiangiogenic therapy. *Semin Thromb Hemost* 2002;28:39.

408. Rickles FR, Edwards RL. Activation of blood coagulation in cancer: Trousseau's syndrome revisited. *Blood* 1983;62:14.

409. Haemostatic abnormalities and malignant disease. *Lancet* 1986;1:303.

410. Smith SB, Arkin C. Cryofibrinogenemia: incidence, clinical correlations and review of the literature. *Am J Clin Pathol* 1972;58:524.

411. Moessou MW, Colman RW, Sherry S. Chronic intravascular coagulation syndrome: report of a case with special studies of an associated plasma cryoprecipitate (cryofibrinogen). *N Engl J Med* 1968;278:815.

412. Bell WR, Starkson NF, Tong S, et al. Trousseau's syndrome: devastating coagulopathy in the absence of heparin. *Am J Med* 1985;79:423.

413. Jandl JH. The anemia of liver disease: observations on its mechanism. *J Clin Invest* 1955;34:390.

414. Reynolds TB, Hidemura R, Michel H, et al. Portal hypertension without cirrhosis in alcoholic liver disease. *Ann Intern Med* 1969;70:497.

415. Eichner ER. The hematologic disorders of alcoholism. *Am J Med* 1973;54:621.

416. Sheehy JW, Berman A. The anemia of cirrhosis. *J Lab Clin Med* 1960;56:72.

417. Kawasaki H, Nemasu J, Maeda N, et al. Plasma levels of atrial natriuretic peptide in patients with chronic liver disease. *Am J Gastroenterol* 1987;82:727.

418. Lunden L, Aallgren R, Birgegard G, et al. Serum ferritin in alcoholics and the relation to liver damage, iron state and erythropoietin activity. *Acta Med Scand* 1981;209:327.

419. Reed CF, Murphy M, Roberts G. Phospholipid exchange between plasma and erythrocytes in man and the dog. *J Clin Invest* 1968;47:749.

420. Cooper RA, Diloy-Puray M, Lando P, et al. An analysis of lipoproteins, bile acids, and red cell membranes associated with target cells and spur cells in patients with liver disease. *J Clin Invest* 1972;51:3182.

421. Cooper RA. Hemolytic syndromes and red cell membrane abnormalities in liver disease. *Semin Hematol* 1980;17:103.

422. Culotta VC, Gitlin JD. Disorders of copper transport. In: Scriver CR, Beaudet AL, Sly WS, et al., eds. *The metabolic and molecular bases of inherited disease*, 8th ed. New York: McGraw-Hill, 2001:3105.

423. Loudianos G, Gitlin JD. Wilson's disease. *Semin Liver Dis* 2000;20:353.

424. Walshe JM. Wilson's disease. The presenting symptoms. *Arch Dis Child* 1962;37:253.

425. Buchanan GR. Acute hemolytic anemia as a presenting manifestation of Wilson's disease. *J Pediatr* 1975;86:245.

426. Forman SJ, Kumar KS, Redeker AG, et al. Hemolytic anemia in Wilson disease: clinical findings and biochemical mechanisms. *Am J Hematol* 1980;9:269.

427. Lehr H, Pauschinger M, Pittke E, et al. Haemolytic anaemia as initial manifestation of Wilson's disease. *Blut* 1988;56:45.

428. Robitaille GA, Piscatelli RL, Majeski EJ, et al. Hemolytic anemia in Wilson's disease. *JAMA* 1977;237:2402.

429. Roche Sicot J, Benhamou JP. Acute intravascular hemolysis and acute liver failure associated as a first manifestation of Wilson's disease. *Ann Intern Med* 1977;86:301.

430. Goldman M, Ali M. Wilson's disease presenting as Heinz-body hemolytic anemia. *CMAJ* 1991;145:971.

431. Reference deleted.

432. Lindenbaum J. Hematologic complications of alcohol abuse. *Semin Liver Dis* 1987;7:169.

433. Cowan D. Effect of alcoholism on hemostasis. *Semin Hematol* 1980;17:137.

434. Eichner ER. The hematologic disorders of alcoholism. *Am J Med* 1973;54:621.

435. McCurdy P, Rath C. Vacuolated nucleated bone marrow cells in alcoholism. *Semin Hematol* 1980;17:100.

436. Unger KW, Johnson D. Red blood cell mean corpuscular volume: a potential indicator of alcohol usage in a working population. *Am J Med Sci* 1974;267:281.

437. Savage DG, Ogundipe A, Allen RH, et al. Etiology and diagnostic evaluation of macrocytosis. *Am J Med Sci* 2000;319:343.

438. Maruyama S, Hirayama C, Yamamoto S, et al. Red blood cell status in alcoholic and non-alcoholic liver disease. *J Lab Clin Med* 2001;138:332.

439. Seppa K, Heinila K, Sillanaukee P, et al. Evaluation of macrocytosis by general practitioners. *J Stud Alcohol* 1996;57:97.

440. Peach HG, Bath NE, Farish S. Predictive value of MCV for hazardous drinking in the community. *Clin Lab Haematol* 1997;19:85.

441. Wu A, Chanarin I, Levi AJ. Macrocytosis of chronic alcoholism. *Lancet* 1974;1:829.

442. Douglass CC, Twomey JJ. Transient stomatocytosis with hemolysis: a previously unrecognized complication of alcoholism. *Ann Intern Med* 1970;72:159.

443. Wislöff F, Boman D. Acquired stomatocytosis in alcoholic liver disease. *Scand J Haematol* 1979;23:43.

444. Wislöff F, Boman D. Acquired stomatocytosis in alcoholic liver disease. *Scand J Haematol* 1979;23:43.

445. Meagher RC, Sieber F, Spivak JL. Suppression of hematopoietic progenitor-cell proliferation by ethanol and acetaldehyde. *N Engl J Med* 1982;307:845.

446. Lindenbaum J. Folate and vitamin B-12 deficiencies in alcoholism. *Semin Hematol* 1980;17:119.

447. Hillman RS, McGuffin R, Campbell C. Alcohol interference with the folate-enterohepatic cycle. *Trans Assoc Am Physicians* 1977;90:145.

448. Eichner ER, Pierce I, Hillman RS. Folate balance in dietary induced megaloblastic anemia. *N Engl J Med* 1971;284:933.

449. Spivak JL. Masked megaloblastic anemia. *Arch Intern Med* 1982;142:2111.

450. Eichner ER, Hillman RS. The evolution of anemia in alcoholic patients. *Am J Med* 1971;50:218.

451. Lunden L, Hallgren R, Birgegard G, et al. Serum ferritin in alcoholics and the relation to liver damage, iron state and erythropoietic activity. *Acta Med Scand* 1981;209:327.

452. Zieve L. Jaundice, hyperlipemia and hemolytic anemia: a heretofore unrecognized syndrome associated with alcoholic fatty liver and cirrhosis. *Ann Intern Med* 1968;48:471.

453. Tisman G, Herbert V. In vitro myelosuppression and immunosuppression by ethanol. *J Clin Invest* 1973;52:1410.

454. MacGregor RR. Alcohol and immune defense. *JAMA* 1986;256:147.

455. Imperia PS, Chikkappa G, Phillips PG. Mechanism of inhibition of granulopoiesis by ethanol. *Proc Soc Exp Biol Med* 1984;175:219.

456. Perlino C, Rimland D. Alcoholism, leukopenia and pneumococcal sepsis. *Am Rev Respir Dis* 1985;132:757.

457. Brayton RG, Stokes PE, Schwartz MS, et al. Effect of alcohol and various diseases on leukocyte mobilization, phagocytosis and intracellular bacterial killing. *N Engl J Med* 1970;282:123.

458. Liu Y. Effects of alcohol on granulocytes and lymphocytes. *Semin Hematol* 1980;17:130.

459. Liu YK. Phagocytic capacity of reticuloendothelial system in alcoholics. *J Reticuloendothel Soc* 1979;25:605.

460. Young GP, Weyden MB, Rose IS, et al. Lymphopenia and lymphocyte transformation in alcoholics. *Experientia* 1979;35:268.

461. Gluckman SJ, Dvorak VC, MacGregor RR. Host defense during prolonged alcohol consumption in a controlled environment. *Arch Intern Med* 1977;137:1539.

462. Atkinson JP, Sullivan TJ, Kelly JP, et al. Stimulation by alcohol of cyclic AMP metabolism in human leukocytes: possible role of cyclic AMP in the anti-inflammatory effects of ethanol. *J Clin Invest* 1977;60:284.

463. Levine R, Spivak J, Meagher R, et al. Effect of ethanol on thrombopoiesis. *Br J Haematol* 1986;62:345.
464. Sullivan L, Adams W, Liu Y. Induction of thrombocytopenia by thrombopheresis in man: pattern of recovery in normal subjects during ethanol ingestion and abstinence. *Blood* 1977;49:197.
465. Deykin D, Jarison P, McMahon L. Ethanol potentiation of aspirin-induced prolongation of the bleeding time. *N Engl J Med* 1982;306:852.
466. Mikhailidis DP, Jenkins W, Barradas M, et al. Platelet function defects in chronic alcoholism. *Clin Res* 1986;293:715.
467. Fried W. Hematologic abnormalities in chronic renal failure. *Semin Nephrol* 1981;1:176.
468. Eckhardt KU. Pathophysiology of renal anemia. *Clin Nephrol* 2000;53[1 Suppl]:S2.
469. Jacobson LO, Goldwasser E, Plzak LF, et al. Role of the kidney in erythropoiesis. *Nature* 1957;129:633.
470. Drueke T. Hyporesponsiveness to recombinant human erythropoietin. *Nephrol Dial Transplant* 2001;16[Suppl 7]:25.
471. Tonelli M, Blake PG, Muirhead N. Predictors of erythropoietin responsiveness in chronic hemodialysis patients. *ASAIO J* 2001;47:82.
472. Blumberg A, Marti HA. Adaptation to anemia by decreased oxygen affinity of hemoglobin in patients on dialysis. *Kidney Int* 1972;1:263.
473. Mitchell T, Pegrum G. The oxygen affinity of hemoglobin in chronic renal failure. *Br J Haematol* 1971;21:463.
474. Brown S, Caro J, Erslev AJ, et al. Rise in erythropoietin and hematocrit associated with transient liver enzyme abnormalities in anephric hemodialysis patients. *Am J Med* 1980;62:280.
475. Blumberg A. Pathogenesis of anemia due to kidney disease. *Nephron* 1989;51[Suppl 1]:15.
476. Wallner S, Vantrin R. Evidence that inhibition of erythropoiesis is important in the anemia of chronic renal failure. *J Lab Clin Med* 1981;97:170.
477. Caro J, Erslev AJ. Uremic inhibitors of erythropoiesis. *Semin Nephrol* 1985;5:128.
478. Levinsky H, Gafter U, Levi J, et al. Neuraminidase-like activity in sera of uremic anemic patients. *Nephron* 1984;37:35.
479. Zappa-Costa A, Caro J, Erslev A. Normalization of hematocrit in patients with end stage renal disease on chronic ambulatory peritoneal dialysis. *Am J Med* 1982;72:53.
480. Segal G, Stueve T, Adamson J. Spermine and spermidine are non-specific inhibitors of in vitro hematopoiesis. *Kidney Int* 1987;31:72.
481. Salabindeen A, Hawkins T, Keavy P, et al. Is anemia during continuous ambulatory peritoneal dialysis really better than during haemodialysis? *Lancet* 1983;2:1046.
482. Klahr S, Slatopolsky E. Toxicity of parathyroid hormone in uremia. *Annu Rev Med* 1986;37:71.
483. McGonigle R, Wallin J, Husserl F, et al. Potential role of parathyroid hormone as an inhibitor of erythropoiesis in the anemia of renal failure. *J Lab Clin Med* 1984;104:1016.
484. Barbour G. Effect of parathyroidectomy on anemia in chronic renal failure. *Arch Intern Med* 1979;139:889.
485. Yasunaga C, Matsuo K, Yanagida T, et al. Early effects of parathyroidectomy on erythropoietin production in secondary hyperparathyroidism. *Am J Surg* 2002;183:199.
486. Coen G, Calabria S, Bellinghieri G, et al. Parathyroidectomy in chronic renal failure: short- and long-term results on parathyroid function, blood pressure and anemia. *Nephron* 2001;88:149.
487. Geary D, Fennell R, Braylan R, et al. Hyperparathyroidism and anemia in chronic renal failure. *Eur J Pediatr* 1982;139:296.
488. Pitts T, Piramo B, Metro R, et al. Hyperparathyroidism and 1,25-dihydroxy vitamin D deficiency in mild, moderate and severe renal failure. *J Clin Endocrinol Metab* 1988;67:876.
489. Weinberg S, Lubin A, Weiner S, et al. Myelofibrosis and renal osteodystrophy. *Am J Med* 1977;63:755.
490. Graber SE, Krantz B. Erythropoietin: biology and clinical use. *Hematol Oncol Clin North Am* 1989;3:369.
491. Eschbach J, Egue J, Downing M, et al. Correction of the anemia of end-stage renal disease with recombinant erythropoietin. *N Engl J Med* 1987;316:73.
492. Hendler ED, Goffinet JA, Ross S, et al. Controlled study of androgen therapy in anemia of patients on maintenance hemodialysis. *N Engl J Med* 1974;291:1046.
493. Neff MS, Goldberg J, Slifkin RF, et al. A comparison of androgens for anemia in patients on hemodialysis. *N Engl J Med* 1981;304:871.
494. Desforges J. Anemia in uremia. *Ann Intern Med* 1970;126:808.
495. Adamson J, Eschbach J, Finch CA. The kidney and erythropoiesis. *Am J Med* 1968;44:725.
496. Welt LG, Sachs JR, McManus TJ. An ion transport defect in erythrocytes from uremic patients. *Trans Assoc Am Physicians* 1964;77:169.
497. Yawata Y, Howe R, Jacob H. Abnormal red cell metabolism causing hemolysis in uremia. *Ann Intern Med* 1973;79:362.
498. Yawata Y, Jacob H. Abnormal red cell metabolism in patients with chronic uremia: nature of the defect and its persistence despite adequate hemodialysis. *Blood* 1975;45:231.
499. Eaton J, Leida M. Hemolysis in chronic renal failure. *Semin Nephrol* 1985;5:133.
500. Aherne WA. The "burr" red cell and azotaemia. *J Clin Pathol* 1957;10:252.
501. Brain MC, Neame PB. Thrombotic thrombocytopenic purpura and the hemolytic uremic syndrome. *Semin Thromb Hemost* 1982;8:186.
502. Griffin PM, Olmstead LC, Petras RE. Escherichia coli O157:H7-associated colitis. A clinical and histological study of 11 cases. *Gastroenterology* 1990;99:142.
503. Martin DL, MacDonald KL, White KE. The epidemiology and clinical aspects of the hemolytic uremic syndrome in Minnesota. *N Engl J Med* 1990;65:1161.
504. Neiman RS, Bischel MD, Lukes RJ. Hypersplenism in the uremic hemodialyzed patient: pathology and proposed pathophysiologic mechanisms. *Am J Clin Pathol* 1973;60:502.
505. Hattersley PG, Engels JL. Neutrophilic hypersegmentation without macrocytic anemia. *West J Med* 1974;121:179.
506. Longnecker RK, Goffinet JA, Hendler ED. Blood loss from maintenance hemodialysis. *Trans Am Soc Artif Intern Organs* 1974;20:135.
507. Navab F, Masters P, Subramani R, et al. Angiodysplasia in patients with renal insufficiency. *Am J Gastroenterol* 1989;84:1297.
508. Hosokawa S, Oyamaguchi A, Yoshida O. Trace elements and complications in patients undergoing chronic hemodialysis. *Nephron* 1990;55:375.
509. Mladenovic J. Aluminum inhibits erythropoiesis in vitro. *J Clin Invest* 1988;81:1661.
510. Bia M, Cooper K, Schnall S, et al. Aluminum induced anemia: pathogenesis and treatment in patients on chronic hemodialysis. *Kidney Int* 1989;36:852.
511. Thorling EB. Paraneoplastic erythrocytosis and inappropriate erythropoietin production. *Scand J Haematol* 1972;[Suppl]:17.
512. Okabe T, Urabe A, Kato T, et al. Production of erythropoietin-like activity by human renal and hepatic carcinomas in cell culture. *Cancer* 1985;55:1918.
513. Da Silva J, Lacombe C, Bruneval P, et al. Tumor cells are the site of erythropoietin synthesis in human renal cancers associated with polycythemia. *Blood* 1990;75:577.
514. Luke RG, Kennedy AC, Stirling WB. Renal artery stenosis, hypertension and polycythemia. *BMJ* 1965;1:164.
515. Rose WF, Waldmann TA, Cohen P. Renal cysts, erythropoietin and polycythemia. *Am J Med* 1963;34:76.
516. Pollak R, Maddux MS, Cohen J, et al. Erythrocythemia following renal transplantation: influence of diuretic therapy. *Clin Nephrol* 1988;29:119.
517. Shalhoub RG, Rajim U, Kim VV. Erythrocytosis in patients on long-term hemodialysis. *Ann Intern Med* 1982;97:686.
518. Wickre CG, Norman DJ, Bennison A, et al. Postrenal transplant erythrocytosis: a review of fifty-three patients. *Kidney Int* 1983;23:731.
519. Hoppin EC, Depner T, Yamuchi H, et al. Erythrocytosis associated with diffuse parenchymal lesions of the kidney. *Br J Haematol* 1976;32:557.
520. Emanuel DA, Wenzol FJ. Erythrocytosis associated with the nephrotic syndrome. *JAMA* 1962;181:788.
521. Sonneborn R, Perez GO, Epstein M, et al. Erythrocytosis associated with nephrotic syndrome. *Arch Intern Med* 1977;137:1068.
522. Erkeleus DW, van Eps LWS. Bartter's syndrome and erythrocytosis. *Am J Med* 1973;55:711.
523. Lacombe C, Da Silva JL, Bruneval P, et al. Peritubular cells are the site of erythropoietin synthesis in the murine hypoxic kidney. *J Clin Invest* 1988;81:620.
524. Nissenson A, Nimer S, Wolcott D. Recombinant human erythropoietin and renal anemia: molecular biology, clinical efficacy and nervous system effects. *Ann Intern Med* 1991;114:402.
525. Nagy E, Berizi I. Pituitary dependence of bone marrow function. *Br J Haematol* 1989;71:457.
526. Golde DW, Bersch N, Li C. Growth hormone: species specific stimulation of erythropoiesis in vitro. *Science* 1977;196:1112.
527. Dainiak N, Sutter D, Krecztko S. L-Triiodothyronine augments erythropoietin growth factor release from peripheral blood and bone marrow leukocytes. *Blood* 1986;68:1289.
528. Das MC, Mukkerjee M, Sarkar TK, et al. Erythropoiesis and erythropoietin in hypo- and hyperthyroidism. *J Clin Endocrinol Metab* 1975;40:211.
529. Carmel R, Spencer CA. Clinical and subclinical thyroid disorders associated with pernicious anemia. *Arch Intern Med* 1982;142:1465.
530. Bux J, Ernst-Schlegel M, Rothe B, et al. Neutropenia and anaemia due to carbimazole-dependent antibodies. *Br J Haematol* 2000;109:243.
531. Kelle HA, Sawers JS, Boulton FE, et al. Problems of anticoagulation with warfarin in hyperthyroidism. *QJM* 1986;58:43.
532. Horton L, Coburn RJ, England JM, et al. The haematology of hypothyroidism. *QJM* 1985;45:101.
533. Mazzaferri EL. Adult hypothyroidism. Manifestations and clinical presentation. *Postgrad Med* 1986;29:64.
534. Wardrop C, Hutchison HE. Red-cell shape in hypothyroidism. *Lancet* 1969;1:1243.
535. Perillie PE, Tembrevilla C. Red-cell changes in hypothyroidism. *Lancet* 1975;2:1151.
536. Betticher DC, Pugin P. Hypothyroidie et acanthocytes: importance diagnostique du frottis sanguin. *Schweiz Med Wochenschr Suppl* 1991;121:1127.
537. Welansky DC, Greisman B. Early hypothyroidism in patients with menorrhagia. *Am J Obstet Gynecol* 1989;160:673.
538. Shakir KM, Turton D, April BS, et al. Anemia: a cause of intolerance to thyroxine sodium. *Mayo Clin Proc* 2000;75:189.
539. Campbell NR, Hasinoff BB, Stalts H, et al. Ferrous sulfate reduces thyroxine efficacy in patients with hypothyroidism. *Ann Intern Med* 1992;117:1010.
540. Shakir KM, Chute JP, April BS, et al. Ferrous sulfate-induced increase in requirement for thyroxine in a patient with primary hypothyroidism. *South Med J* 1997;90:637.
541. Savage RA, Sipple C. Marrow myxedema. Gelatinous transformation of marrow ground substance in a patient with severe hypothyroidism. *Arch Pathol Lab Med* 1987;111:375.

542. Boxer M, Ellman L, Geller R, et al. Anemia in primary hyperparathyroidism. *Arch Intern Med* 1977;137:588.

543. Mallette LE, Bilezikian JP, Heath DA, et al. Primary hyperparathyroidism: clinical and biochemical features. *Medicine* 1974;53:127.

544. Albright F, Aub JC, Bauer W. Hyperparathyroidism. *JAMA* 1934;102:1276.

545. Ikkala E, Myllyla G, Pelkneon R, et al. Haemostatic parameters in Cushing's syndrome. *Acta Med Scand* 1985;217:507.

546. Tudhope GR. Endocrine diseases. *Clin Haematol* 1972;1:475.

547. Baxter J, Tyrrell JB. The adrenal cortex. In: Felig P, Baxter J, Broadus, et al., eds. *Endocrinology and metabolism*, 2nd ed. New York: McGraw-Hill, 1987:551.

548. Kuo B, Zaino E, Roginsky MS. Endocrine function in thalassemia. *J Clin Endocrinol Metab* 1968;28:805.

549. Canale VC, Steinherz P, New M, et al. Endocrine function in thalassemia major. *Ann N Y Acad Sci* 1974;232:333.

550. McIntosh N. Endocrinopathy in thalassaemia major. *Arch Dis Child* 1976; 51:195.

551. Italian Working Group on Endocrine Complications in Non-endocrine Diseases. Multicentre study on prevalence of endocrine complications in thalassaemia major. *Clin Endocrinol (Oxf)* 1995;42:581.

552. Low LC. Growth, puberty and endocrine function in beta-thalassaemia major. *J Pediatr Endocrinol Metab* 1997;10:175.

553. Walton C, Kelly WF, Laing I, et al. Endocrine abnormalities in idiopathic haemochromatosis. *QJM* 1983;52:99.

554. Schafer AI, Cheron RG, Dluhy R, et al. Clinical consequences of acquired transfusional iron overload in adults. *N Engl J Med* 1981;304:319.

555. Jones R, Peterson C. Hematologic alterations in diabetes mellitus. *Am J Med* 1981;70:339.

556. Bersch N, Groopman JE, Golde DW. Natural and biosynthetic insulin stimulates the growth of human erythroid progenitors in vitro. *J Clin Endocrinol Metab* 1978;55:1209.

557. Ritchey AK, Tamborlane W, Gertner J. Improved diabetic control enhances erythroid stem cell proliferation in vitro. *J Clin Endocrinol Metab* 1985;60:1257.

558. Peterson C, Jones R, Koenig R, et al. Reversible hematologic sequelae of diabetes mellitus. *Ann Intern Med* 1977;86:425.

559. Schwartz JS, Clancy CM. Glycosylated hemoglobin assays in the management and diagnosis of diabetes mellitus. *Ann Intern Med* 1984;101:710.

560. Bunn HF, Briehl RW. The interaction of 2,3-diphosphoglycerate with various human hemoglobins. *J Clin Invest* 1970;49:1088.

561. Williamson JR, Gardner GW, Boylan GL, et al. Microrheologic investigation of erythrocyte deformability in diabetes mellitus. *Blood* 1985;65:283.

562. Rogers LE, Porter FS, Sidbury JBJ. Thiamine-responsive megaloblastic anemia. *J Pediatr* 1969;74:494.

563. Haworth C, Evans DIK, Mitra J, et al. Thiamine responsive anaemia: a study of two further cases. *Br J Haematol* 1982;50:549.

564. Labay V, Raz T, Baron D, et al. Mutations in *SLC19A2* cause thiamine-responsive megaloblastic anaemia associated with diabetes mellitus and deafness. *Nat Genet* 1999;22:300.

565. Fleming J, Tartaglini E, Schorderet D, et al. The gene mutated in thiamine-responsive anaemia with diabetes and deafness (TRMA) encodes a functional thiamine transporter. *Nat Genet* 1999;22:305.

566. Diaz G, Banikazemi M, Oishi K, et al. Mutations in a new gene encoding a thiamine transporter cause thiamine-responsive megaloblastic anaemia syndrome. *Nat Genet* 1999;22:309.

567. Valerio G, Franzese A, Poggi V, et al. Long-term follow-up of diabetes in two patients with thiamine-responsive megaloblastic anemia syndrome. *Diabetes Care* 1998;21:38.

568. Esmann V. The polymorphonuclear leukocyte in diabetes mellitus. *J Clin Chem Clin Biochem* 1983;21:561.

569. Mowat AG, Baum J. Chemotaxis of polymorphonuclear leukocytes from patients with diabetes mellitus. *N Engl J Med* 1971;284:621.

570. Small M, Lowe GD, MacCuish AC, et al. Thrombin and plasmin activity in diabetes mellitus and their association with glycaemic control. *QJM* 1987;65:1025.

571. Mustard J, Packham M. Platelets and diabetes mellitus. *N Engl J Med* 1984; 311:665.

572. Jones DB, Davis T, Brown E, et al. Determinants of ADP-induced platelet aggregation in diabetes mellitus. *Diabetologia* 1986;29:291.

573. Davi G, Catalano I, Averna M, et al. Thromboxane biosynthesis and platelet function in type II diabetes mellitus. *N Engl J Med* 1990;322:1769.

574. Villanueva GB, Allen N. Demonstration of altered antithrombin III activity due to nonenzymatic glycosylation at glucose concentration expected to be encountered in severely diabetic patients. *Diabetes* 1988;37:1103.

575. Auwerx J, Bouillon R, Collen D, et al. Tissue-type plasminogen activator antigen and plasminogen activator inhibitor in diabetes mellitus. *Arteriosclerosis* 1988;8:68.

576. Shilo S, Werner D, Hershko C. Acute hemolytic anemia caused by severe hypophosphatemia in diabetic ketoacidosis. *Acta Haematol* 1985;73:55.

577. Burris AS. Leukemoid reaction associated with severe diabetic ketoacidosis. *South Med J* 1986;79:647.

578. Gellady AM, Greenwood RD. G-6-PD hemolytic anemia complicating diabetic ketoacidosis. *J Pediatr* 1972;80:1037.

579. Shalev O, Wollner A, Menczel J. Diabetic ketoacidosis does not precipitate haemolysis in patients with the Mediterranean variant of glucose-6-phosphate dehydrogenase deficiency. *BMJ* 1984;288:179.

580. Shalev O, Eliakim R, Lugassy GZ, et al. Hypoglycemia-induced hemolysis in glucose-6-phosphate dehydrogenase deficiency. *Acta Haematol* 1985;74:227.

581. Galli-Tsinopoulou A, Nousia-Arvanitakis S. Glucose-6-phosphate dehydro-genase deficiency-induced hemolysis in newly diagnosed diabetic monozygotic twins. *J Pediatr Endocrinol Metab* 2000;13:669.

582. Cornbleet PJ, Moir R, Wolf P. A histochemical study of bone marrow hypoplasia in anorexia nervosa. *Virchows Arch* 1977;374:239.

583. Pearson H. Marrow hypoplasia in anorexia nervosa. *J Pediatr* 1967;71:211.

584. Mant MJ, Faragher PS. The haematology of anorexia nervosa. *Br J Haematol* 1972;23:737.

585. Smith RR, Spivak JL. Marrow cell necrosis in anorexia nervosa and involuntary starvation. *Br J Haematol* 1985;60:525.

586. Nestel P. Cholesterol metabolism in anorexia nervosa and hypercholesterolemia. *J Clin Endocrinol Metab* 1974;38:325.

587. Powers J, Luktenstein M, Collins J, et al. Serum erythropoietin in healthy older persons. *J Am Geriatr Soc* 1989;37:388.

588. Carmel R. Anemia and aging: an overview of clinical, diagnostic and biological issues. *Blood Rev* 2001;15:9.

589. Smith DL. Anemia in the elderly. *Am Fam Physician* 2000;62:1565.

590. Lipschitz DA, Udupa KB, Milton KY, et al. Effect of age on hematopoiesis in man. *Blood* 1984;63:502.

591. Zauber NP, Zauber AC. Hematologic data of healthy very old people. *JAMA* 1987;257:2181.

592. Lipschitz D, Udupa K. Age and the hematopoietic system. *J Am Geriatr Soc* 1986;34:448.

593. Baldwin JG. Hematopoietic function in the elderly. *Arch Intern Med* 1988; 148:2544.

594. Todd M, Thompson JH Jr, Bowie EJ, et al. Changes in blood coagulation during pregnancy. *Mayo Clin Proc* 1975;40:370.

595. Weiner CP. The obstetric patient and disseminated intravascular coagulation. *Clin Perinatol* 1986;13:705.

596. Feliu J, Juarez S, Ordonez A, et al. Acute leukemia and pregnancy. *Cancer* 1988;61:580.

597. Caligiuri M, Mayer R. Pregnancy and leukemia. *Semin Oncol* 1989;16:388.

598. Branch DW, Scott J, Kochenour N, et al. Obstetric complications associated with the lupus anticoagulant. *N Engl J Med* 1985;313:1322.

599. Hytten F. Blood volume changes in normal pregnancy. *Clin Hematol* 1985;14:601.

600. Sifakis S, Pharmakides G. Anemia in pregnancy. *Ann N Y Acad Sci* 2000;900:125.

601. Lund CJ, Donovan JC. Blood volume during pregnancy. Significance of plasma red cell volumes. *Am J Obstet Gynecol* 1967;98:393.

602. Koller O, Sagen N, Ulstein M, et al. Fetal growth retardation associated with inadequate haemodilution in otherwise uncomplicated pregnancy. *Acta Obstet Gynecol* 1979;58:9.

603. Report of a WHO scientific group. Nutritional anaemias. *World Health Organ Tech Rep Ser* 1968;405:5.

604. McFee JG. Anemia: a high risk complication of pregnancy. *Clin Obstet Gynecol* 1973;16:153.

605. Kaltreider DF, Johnson JW. Patients at high risk for low-birth-weight deliveries. *Am J Obstet Gynecol* 1976;124:251.

606. Higgins AC, et al. Maternal hemoglobin changes and their relationship to infant birth weight in mothers receiving a program of nutritional assessment and rehabilitation. *Nutr Res* 1982;2:641.

607. Kaltreider F, et al. Epidemiology of preterm delivery. *Clin Obstet Gynecol* 1980;23:17.

608. Meyer MB, et al. The interrelationship of maternal smoking and increased perinatal mortality with other risk factors. Analysis of the Ontario Perinatal Mortality Study, 1960–61. *Am J Epidemiol* 1975;100:443.

609. Garn SM, et al. Maternal hematologic levels and pregnancy outcomes. *Semin Perinatol* 1981;5:155.

610. Goodlin RC, Dobry CA, Anderson JC, et al. Clinical signs of normal plasma volume expansion during pregnancy. *Am J Obstet Gynecol* 1983;145:1001.

611. Retief FP, Brink AJ. A study of pregnancy anaemia: blood volume changes correlated with other parameters of haemopoietic efficiency. *J Obstet Gynaecol Br Commonw* 1967;74:683.

612. Duffus GM, et al. The relationship between baby weight and changes in maternal weight, total body water, plasma volume electrolytes and proteins, and urinary oestriol excretion. *J Obstet Gynaecol Br Commonw* 1971;78:97.

613. Gibson HM. Plasma volume and glomerular filtration rate in pregnancy and their relation to differences in fetal growth. *J Obstet Gynaecol Br Commonw* 1973;80:1067.

614. Pirani BB, Campbell DM, MacGillivray I. Plasma volume in normal first pregnancy. *J Obstet Gynaecol Br Commonw* 1973;80:884.

615. Murphy JF, O'Riordan J, Newcombe RG, et al. Relation of haemoglobin levels in first and second trimesters to outcome of pregnancy. *Lancet* 1986;1:992.

616. Sagen N, Nilsen ST, Kim HC, et al. The predictive value of total estriol, HPL and Hb on perinatal outcome in severe pre-eclampsia. *Acta Obstet Gynecol Scand* 1984;63:603.

617. Mau G. Hemoglobin changes during pregnancy and growth disturbances in neonate. *J Perinatol Med* 1977;5:172.

618. Huisman A, Aarnoudse JG. Increased 2nd trimester hemoglobin concentration in pregnancies later complicated by hypertension and growth retardation. *Acta Obstet Gynecol Scand* 1986;65:605.

619. Pryor J, et al. In: Bern MM, Frigoletto FD Jr, eds. *Hematologic disorders in maternal-fetal medicine*. New York: Wiley-Liss, 1990:93.

620. Werner EJ, Stockman JA. Red cell disturbances in the feto–maternal unit. *Semin Perinatol* 1988.

621. Sturgeon P. Studies of iron requirements in infants. III. Influence of supplemental iron during normal pregnancy on mother and infant. The infant. *Br J Haematol* 1959;5:45.

622. Czeizel AE, Dudas I. Prevention of the first occurrence of neural-tube defects by periconceptional vitamin supplementation. *N Engl J Med* 1992;327:1832.

623. Berry RJ, Li Z, Erickson JD, et al. Prevention of neural-tube defects with folic acid in China. China-U.S. Collaborative Project for Neural Tube Defect Prevention. *N Engl J Med* 1999;341:1485.

624. Northrup H, Volcik KA. Spina bifida and other neural tube defects. *Curr Probl Pediatr* 2000;30:313.

625. Shields DC, Kirke PN, Mills JL, et al. The "thermolabile" variant of methylenetetrahydrofolate reductase and neural tube defects: aAn evaluation of genetic risk and the relative importance of the genotypes of the embryo and the mother. *Am J Hum Genet* 1999;64:1045.

626. Bentley DP. Iron metabolism and anemia in pregnancy. *Clin Haematol* 1985;14:613.

627. Foulkes J, Golde DJ. The use of ferritin to assess the need for iron supplements in pregnancy. *J Obstet Gynecol* 1982;3:11.

628. Suda T, Omine M, Tsuchiya I, et al. Prognostic aspects of aplastic anemia in pregnancy. *Blut* 1978;36:285.

629. Pritchard J, Whalley PJ. Abortion complicated by *Clostridium perfringens* infection. *Am J Obstet Gynecol* 1971;111:484.

630. McCrae K, Samuels P, Schriener A. Pregnancy-associated thrombocytopenia: pathogenesis and management. *Blood* 1992;80:2697.

631. Romero R, Duffy TP. Platelet disorders in pregnancy. *Clin Perinatol* 1980;7:327.

632. O'Reilly RA, Taber BZ. Immunologic thrombocytopenic purpura and pregnancy. *Obstet Gynecol* 1978;51:590.

633. McCrae KR, Samuels P, Schreiber AD. Pregnancy-associated thrombocytopenia: pathogenesis and management. *Blood* 1992;80:2697.

634. Nagey DA, Alger LS, Edelman BB, et al. Reacting appropriately to thrombocytopenia in pregnancy. *South Med J* 1986;79:1385.

635. Karpatkin M, Porges RF, Karpatkin S. Platelet counts in infants of women with autoimmune thrombocytopenia: effect of steroid administration to the mother. *N Engl J Med* 1981;305:936.

636. Schwartz M, Brenner W. The obfuscation of eclampsia by thrombotic thrombocytopenia purpura. *Am J Obstet Gynecol* 1978;131:18.

637. McMinn JR, George JN. Evaluation of women with clinically suspected thrombotic thrombocytopenic purpura-hemolytic uremic syndrome during pregnancy. *J Clin Apheresis* 2001;16:202.

638. Redman CW. Platelets and the beginning of preeclampsia. *N Engl J Med* 1990; 323:478.

639. Bergmann F, Rotmensch S, Rosenzweig B, et al. The role of von Willebrand factor in pre-eclampsia. *Thromb Haemost* 1991;66:525.

640. Wallenburg HC, Dekker GA, Makovitz JW, et al. Low dose aspirin prevents pregnancy-induced hypertension and preeclampsia in angiotensin-sensitive primigravida. *Lancet* 1986;1:1.

641. Sureau C. Prevention of perinatal consequences of preeclampsia with low-dose aspirin: results of the Epreda trial. *Eur J Obstet Gynecol Reprod Biol* 1991;41:71.

642. Baca L, Gibbons R. The HELLP syndrome: a serious complication of pregnancy with hemolysis, elevated levels of liver enzymes, and low platelet count. *Am J Med* 1988;85:590.

643. Riley CA, Latham PS, Romero R, et al. Acute fatty liver of pregnancy: a reassessment based on observations in nine patients. *Ann Intern Med* 1987;106:703.

644. Rath W, Faridi A, Dudenhausen JW. HELLP syndrome. *J Perinat Med* 2000; 28:249.

645. Mimouni F, Miodovinik M. How often does maternal preeclampsia-eclampsia create thrombocytopenia in the fetus? *Obstet Gynecol* 1987;70:811.

646. Romero R, Copel JA, Hobbins JC. Intrauterine fetal demise and hemostatic failure: the fetal death syndrome. *Clin Obstet Gynecol* 1985;28:24.

647. Sher G, Statland BE. Abruptio placentae with coagulopathy: a rational basis for management. *Clin Obstet Gynecol* 1985;28:15.

648. Oláh KS, Gee H, Needham PG. The management of severe disseminated intravascular coagulopathy complicating placental abruption in the second trimester of pregnancy. *Br J Obstet Gynaecol* 1988;95:419.

649. Courtney LD, Allington LM. Effect of amniotic fluid on blood coagulation. *Br J Haematol* 1972;113:911.

650. Sprung J, Cheng EY, Patel S, et al. Understanding and management of amniotic fluid embolism. *J Clin Anesth* 1992;4:235.

651. Charache S, Niebyl JR. Pregnancy in sickle cell disease. *Clin Haematol* 1985;14:729.

652. Koshy M, Burd L, Wallace D, et al. Prophylactic red-cell transfusions in pregnant patients with sickle cell disease: a randomized cooperative study. *N Engl J Med* 1988;319:1447.

653. Wayne A, Kevy S, Nathan D. Transfusion in sickle cell disease. *Blood* 1993;81:1109.

654. Telen MJ. Principles and problems of transfusion in sickle cell disease. *Semin Hematol* 2001;38:315.

655. Schaefer AL. The hypercoagulable states. *Ann Intern Med* 1985;102:814.

656. Rutherford SE, Phelan JP. Thromboembolic disease in pregnancy. *Clin Perinatol* 1986;13:719.

657. Ginsberg JS, Hirsh J, Rainbow A, et al. Risks to the fetus of the radiologic procedures used in the diagnosis of maternal thromboembolic disease. *Thromb Haematol* 1989;61:189.

658. Letsky E, de Swiet M. Thromboembolism in pregnancy and its management. *Br J Haematol* 1984;57:543.

659. Ginsberg JS, Greer I, Hirsh J. Use of antithrombotic agents during pregnancy. *Chest* 2001;119:122S.

660. Heilmann L, Schneider DM, von Tempelhoff GF. Antithrombotic therapy in high-risk pregnancy. *Hematol Oncol Clin North Am* 2000;14:1133.

661. Bonnar J, Green R, Norris L. Inherited thrombophilia and pregnancy: the obstetric perspective. *Semin Thromb Hemost* 1998;24[Suppl 1]:49.

662. Bazzan M, Donvito V. Low-molecular-weight heparin during pregnancy. *Thromb Res* 2001;101:V175.

663. Ginsberg JS, Hirsh J, Turner D, et al. Risks to the fetus of anticoagulant therapy during pregnancy. *Thromb Haemost* 1989;61:197.

664. Greer IA, Lowe GD, Walker JJ, et al. Hemorrhagic problems in obstetrics and gynecology in patients with congenital coagulopathies. *Br J Obstet Gynaecol* 1991;98:909.

665. Chediak JR, Alban GM, Maxey B. von Willebrand's disease and pregnancy: management during delivery and outcome of offspring. *Am J Obstet Gynecol* 1986;155:618.

666. Rick ME, Williams SB, Sacher RA, et al. Thrombocytopenia associated with pregnancy in a patient with type IIB von Willebrand's disease. *Blood* 1987;69:786.

667. Caldwell DC, Williamson RA, Goldsmith JC. Hereditary coagulopathies in pregnancy. *Clin Obstet Gynecol* 1985;28:53.

668. Seligsohn U, Lubetsky A. Genetic susceptibility to venous thrombosis. *N Engl J Med* 2001;344:1222.

669. Brenner B. Inherited thrombophilia and fetal loss. *Curr Opin Hematol* 2000;7:290.

670. Walker ID. Thrombophilia in pregnancy. *J Clin Pathol* 2000;53:573.

671. Rai R, Regan L. Thrombophilia and adverse pregnancy outcome. *Semin Reprod Med* 2000;18:369.

672. Greer IA. Thrombosis in pregnancy: maternal and fetal issues. *Lancet* 1999; 353:1258.

673. Preston FE, Rosendaal FR, Walker ID, et al. Increased fetal loss in women with heritable thrombophilia. *Lancet* 1996;348:913.

674. Girling J, de Swiet M. Inherited thrombophilia and pregnancy. *Curr Opin Gynecol* 1998;10:135.

675. Friederich PW, Sanson BJ, Simioni, et al. Frequency of pregnancy-related venous thromboembolism in anticoagulant-deficient women: implications for prophylaxis. *Ann Intern Med* 1996;125:955.

676. Grandone E, Margaglione M, Colaizzo D, et al. Genetic susceptibility to pregnancy-related venous thromboembolism: roles of factor V Leiden, prothrombin G20210A, and methylenetetrahydrofolate reductase G677T mutations. *Am J Obstet Gynecol* 1998;179:1324.

677. Gerhardt A, Scharf RE, Beckmann MW, et al. Prothrombin and factor V mutations in women with a history of thrombosis during pregnancy and the puerperium. *N Engl J Med* 2000;342:374.

678. Kupferminc MJ, Eldor A, Steinman N, et al. Increased frequency of genetic thrombophilia in women with complications of pregnancy. *N Engl J Med* 1999;340:9.

679. Owen J. Antithrombin III replacement therapy in pregnancy. *Semin Hematol* 1991;28:46.

680. Levine JS, Branch DW, Rauch J. The antiphospholipid antibody syndrome. *N Engl J Med* 2002;346:752.

681. Asherson RA, Khamashta MA, Ordi-Ros, et al. The "primary" antiphospholipid syndrome: major clinical and serological features. *Medicine (Baltimore)* 1989;68:366.

682. Alarcón-Segovia D, Pérez-Vázquez ME, Villa AR, et al. Preliminary classification criteria for the antiphospholipid syndrome within systemic lupus erythematosus. *Semin Arthritis Rheum* 1992;21:275.

683. Vianna JL, Khamashta MA, Ordi-Ros, et al. Comparison of the primary and secondary antiphospholipid syndrome: a European multicenter study of 114 patients. *Am J Med* 1994;96:3.

684. Lockshin MD, Druzin ML, Goei S, et al. Antibody to cardiolipin as a predictor of fetal distress or death in pregnant patients with systemic lupus erythematosus. *N Engl J Med* 1985;313:152.

685. Kutteh WH. Antiphospholipid antibody-associated recurrent pregnancy loss: treatment with heparin and low-dose aspirin is superior to low-dose aspirin alone. *Am Obstet Gynecol* 1996;174:1584.

686. Branch DW, Silver RM, Blackwell JL, et al. Outcome of treated pregnancies in women with antiphospholipid syndrome: an update of the Utah experience. *Obstet Gynecol* 1992;80:614.

687. Lima F, Khamashta MA, Buchanan NM, et al. A study of sixty pregnancies in patients with the antiphospholipid syndrome. *Clin Exp Rheumatol* 1996;14:131.

688. Rand H, Wu X-X, Andree HAM, et al. Pregnancy loss in the antiphospholipid-antibody syndrome—a possible thrombogenic mechanism. *N Engl J Med* 1997;337:154.

689. di Somone N, Meroni PL, del Papa N, et al. Antiphospholipid antibodies affect trophoblast gonadotropin secretion and invasiveness by binding directly and through adhered beta2-glycoprotein I. *Arthritis Rheum* 2000;43:140.

690. Clifford K, Rai R, Watson H, et al. An informative protocol for the investigation of recurrent miscarriage: preliminary experience of 500 consecutive cases. *Hum Reprod* 1994;9:1328.

691. Yetman DL, Kutteh WH. Antiphospholipid antibody panels and recurrent pregnancy loss: prevalence of anticardiolipin antibodies compared with other antiphospholipid antibodies. *Fertil Steril* 1996;66:540.

692. Branch DW, Peaceman AM, Druzin M, et al. A multicenter, placebo-controlled pilot study of intravenous immune globulin treatment of antiphospholipid syndrome during pregnancy. *Am Obstet Gynecol* 2000;182:122.

693. Cowchock FS, Reece EA, Balaban D, et al. Repeated fetal losses associated with antiphospholipid antibodies: a collaborative randomized trial comparing prednisone with low-dose heparin treatment. *Am J Obstet Gynecol* 1992;166:1318.

694. Jones EC, Mosesson MW, Thomason JL, et al. Essential thrombocythemia in pregnancy. *Obstet Gynecol* 1988;71:501.
695. Solal-Celigney P, Tertian G, Fernandez H, et al. Pregnancy and paroxysmal nocturnal hemoglobinuria. *Arch Intern Med* 1988;148:593.
696. Budman D, Steinberg A. Hematologic aspects of systemic lupus erythematosus: current concepts. *Ann Intern Med* 1977;86:220.
697. Keeling DM, Isenberg DA. Haematological manifestations of systemic lupus erythematosus. *Blood Rev* 1993;7:199.
698. Bailey F, Lilly M, Bertoli L, et al. An antibody that inhibits in vitro bone marrow proliferation in a patient with SLE and aplastic anemia. *Arthritis Rheum* 1989;32:901.
699. Dainiak N, Hardin J, Floyd V, et al. Humoral suppression of erythropoiesis in SLE and rheumatoid arthritis. *Ann Intern Med* 1980;69:537.
700. Abdou N, Verdirame J, Amare M, et al. Heterogeneity of pathogenetic mechanism in aplastic anemia. *Ann Intern Med* 1981;95:43.
701. Alger M, Alarcon-Segovia D, Rivero SJ. Hemolytic anemia and thrombocytopenic purpura: two related subsets of systemic lupus erythematosus. *J Rheumatol* 1977;4:351.
702. Harvey AM, Shulman LE, Tumulty PA, et al. Systemic lupus erythematosus: review of the literature and clinical analysis of 138 cases. *Medicine* 1954;33:291.
703. Averbuch M, Korfman B, Levo Y. Lupus anticoagulant, thrombosis and thrombocytopenia in SLE. *Am J Med Sci* 1987;293:2.
704. Franzen P, Friman C, Pettersson T, et al. Combined pure red cell aplasia and primary autoimmune hypothyroidism in systemic lupus erythematosus. *Arthritis Rheum* 1987;30:839.
705. Cassileth PA, Meyers AR. Erythroid aplasia in systemic lupus erythematosus. *Am J Med* 1973;55:706.
706. Pirofsky B. Collagen diseases and autoimmune hemolytic anemia. In: Pirofsky B. *Autoimmunization and the autoimmune hemolytic anemias*. Baltimore: Williams & Wilkins, 1969:175.
707. Kaelin W, Spivak J. Systemic lupus erythematosus and myelofibrosis. *Am J Med* 1986;81:935.
708. Karpatkin S, Strick N, Karpatkin MB, et al. Cumulative experience in the detection of antiplatelet antibody in 234 patients with idiopathic thrombocytopenic purpura, systemic lupus erythematosus and other clinical disorders. *Am J Med* 1972;52:776.
709. Griner P, Hoyer L. Amegakaryocytic thrombocytopenia in SLE. *Arch Intern Med* 1970;125:328.
710. Stoll DB, Blum S, Pasquale D, et al. Thrombocytopenia with decreased megakaryocytes. *Ann Intern Med* 1981;94:170.
711. Hoffman R, Bruno E, Elwell J, et al. Acquired amegakaryocytic thrombocytopenic purpura: a syndrome of diverse etiologies. *Blood* 1982;60:1173.
712. Rabinowitz Y, Dameshek W. Systemic lupus erythematosus after "idiopathic" thrombocytopenic purpura: a review. *Ann Intern Med* 1960;52:1.
713. Dekker A, O'Brien ME, Cammarata RJ. The association of thrombotic thrombocytopenic purpura with systemic lupus erythematosus. *Am J Med Sci* 1974;267:243.
714. Rustagi P, Currie M, Logue G. Complement-activating antineutrophil antibody in SLE. *Am J Med* 1985;78:971.
715. Conley CL, Hartmann RC. A hemorrhagic disorder caused by circulating anticoagulant in patients with disseminated lupus erythematosus. *J Clin Invest* 1952;31:621.
716. Ashershon RA, Kharmashta MA, Hughes GR. Antiphospholipid antibodies and thrombosis. *Lancet* 1989;2:72.
717. Reference deleted.
718. Sneddon JB. Cerebrovascular lesions in livedo reticularis. *Br J Dermatol* 1965;77:180.
719. Asherson RA, Khamashta MA, Gel A, et al. Cerebrovascular disease and antiphospholipid antibodies in systemic lupus erythematosus, lupus-like disease, and the primary antiphospholipid syndrome. *Am J Med* 1989;86:391.
720. Asherson RA, Cervera R, Piette J-C, et al. Catastrophic antiphospholipid syndrome: clinical and laboratory features of 50 patients. *Medicine (Baltimore)* 1998;77:195.
721. Petri M. Epidemiology of the antiphospholipid antibody syndrome. *J Autoimmun* 2000;15:145.
722. Merkel PA, Chang YC, Pierangeli SS, et al. The prevalence and clinical associations of anticardiolipin antibodies in a large inception cohort of patients with connective tissue diseases. *Am J Med* 1996;101:576.
723. Cervera R, Khamashta MA, Font J, et al. Systemic lupus erythematosus: clinical and immunologic patterns of disease expression in a cohort of 1,000 patients. *Medicine (Baltimore)* 1993;72:113.
724. Love PE, Santoro SA. Antiphospholipid antibodies: anticardiolipin and the lupus anticoagulant in systemic lupus erythematosus (SLE) and in non-SLE disorders: prevalence and clinical significance. *Ann Intern Med* 1990;112:682.
725. Alarcón-Segovia D, Pérez-Vázquez ME, Villa AR, et al. Preliminary classification criteria for the antiphospholipid syndrome within systemic lupus erythematosus. *Semin Arthritis Rheum* 1992;21:275.
726. Wahl DG, Guillemin F, de Maistre E, et al. Risk for venous thrombosis related to antiphospholipid antibodies in systemic lupus erythematosus—a meta-analysis. *Lupus* 1997;6:467.
727. Prandoni P, Simioni P, Girolami A. Antiphospholipid antibodies, recurrent thromboembolism, and intensity of warfarin anticoagulation. *Thromb Haemost* 1996;75:859.
728. Ginsberg S, Wells PS, Brill-Edwards P, et al. Antiphospholipid antibodies and venous thromboembolism. *Blood* 1995;86:3685.

729. Rance A, Emmeric, Fiessinger JN. Anticardiolipin antibodies and recurrent thromboembolism. *Thromb Haemost* 1997;77:221.
730. Moll S, Ortel TL. Monitoring warfarin therapy in patients with lupus anticoagulants. *Ann Intern Med* 1997;127:177.
731. Levine SR, Brey RL, Joseph CLM, et al. Risk of recurrent thromboembolic events in patients with focal cerebral ischemia and anti-phospholipid antibodies. *Stroke* 1992;23[Suppl I]:I29.
732. Khamashta MA, Cuadrado M, Mujic F, et al. The management of thrombosis in the antiphospholipid-antibody syndrome. *N Engl J Med* 1995;332:993.
733. Derksen RH, de Groot PG, Kater L, et al. Patients with antiphospholipid antibodies and venous thrombosis should receive long term anticoagulant treatment. *Ann Rheum Dis* 1993;52:689.
734. Ginsburg KS, Liang MH, Newcomer L, et al. Anticardiolipin antibodies and the risk for ischemic stroke and venous thrombosis. *Ann Intern Med* 1992;117:997.
735. Petri M. Hydroxychloroquine use in the Baltimore Lupus Cohort: effects on lipids, glucose and thrombosis. *Lupus* 1996;5[Suppl 1]:S16.
736. Hochberg M, Arnold CM, Hogan B, et al. Serum immunoreactive erythropoietin in rheumatoid arthritis: impaired response to anemia. *Arthritis Rheum* 1988;31:1318.
737. Baer AN, Dessypris EN, Goldwasser ER, et al. Blunted erythropoietin response to anaemia in rheumatoid arthritis. *Br J Haematol* 1987;66:559.
738. Benne JA, Bianchine JR, Johnson PC, et al. Gastrointestinal blood loss caused by tolmetin, aspirin, and indomethacin. *Clin Pharmacol Ther* 1974;16:821.
739. Munden KD, Senator GB. Iron in the synovial membrane in rheumatoid arthritis and other joint diseases. *Ann Rheum Dis* 1968;27:38.
740. Hutchinson RM, Davis P, Jayson M. Thrombocytosis in rheumatoid arthritis. *Ann Rheum Dis* 1976;35:138.
741. Panush RS, Franco AE, Schur P. Rheumatoid arthritis associated with eosinophilia. *Ann Intern Med* 1971;75:199.
742. Davis P, Hughes GR. Significance of eosinophilia during gold therapy. *Arthritis Rheum* 1974;17:964.
743. Felty AR. Chronic arthritis in the adult associated with splenomegaly and leucopenia: a report of five cases of an unusual clinical syndrome. *Johns Hopkins Hosp Bull* 1924;35:16.
744. Campion G, Maddison PJ, Goulding N, et al. The Felty syndrome: a case matched study of clinical manifestations and outcome, serologic features and immunogenetic associations. *Medicine* 1990;69:69.
745. Hellmich B, Schnabel A, Gross WL. Treatment of severe neutropenia due to Felty's syndrome or systemic lupus erythematosus with granulocyte colony-stimulating factor. *Semin Arthritis Rheum* 1999;29:82.
746. Rashba EJ, Rowe JM, Packman CH. Treatment of the neutropenia of Felty syndrome. *Blood Rev* 1996;10:177.
747. Pereira J, Velloso ED, Loterio HA, et al. Long-term remission of neutropenia in Felty's syndrome after a short GM-CSF treatment. *Acta Haematol* 1994;92:154.
748. Graham KE, Coodley GO. A prolonged use of granulocyte colony stimulating factor in Felty's syndrome. *J Rheumatol* 1995;22:174.
749. Choi MF, Mant MJ, Turner AR, et al. Successful reversal of neutropenia in Felty's syndrome with recombinant granulocyte colony stimulating factor. *Br J Haematol* 1994;86:663.
750. Hayat SQ, Hearth-Holmes M, Wolf RE. Flare of arthritis with successful treatment of Felty's syndrome with granulocyte colony stimulating factor (GCSF). *Clin Rheumatol* 1995;14:211.
751. McMullin MF, Finch MB. Felty's syndrome treated with rhG-CSF associated with flare of arthritis and skin rash. *Clin Rheumatol* 1995;14:204.
752. Farhey YD, Herman JH. Vasculitis complicating granulocyte colony stimulating factor treatment of leukopenia and infection in Felty's syndrome. *J Rheumatol* 1995;22:1179.
753. Moore RA, Brunner CM, Sandusky WR, et al. Felty's syndrome: long-term follow up after splenectomy. *Ann Intern Med* 1971;75:381.
754. Fiechtner JJ, Miller DR, Starkebaum G. Reversal of neutropenia with methotrexate treatment in patients with Felty's syndrome: correlation of response with neutrophil-reactive IgG. *Arthritis Rheum* 1989;32:194.
755. Saway PA, Prasthofer E, Barton J. Prevalence of granular lymphocyte proliferation in patients with rheumatoid arthritis and neutropenia. *Am J Med* 1989;86:303.
756. Linch D, Newland A, Turnbull A, et al. Unusual T cell proliferations and neutropenia in rheumatoid arthritis: comparison with classical Felty's syndrome. *Scand J Haematol* 1984;33:342.
757. Bowman SJ, Geddes GC, Corrigall V, et al. Large granular lymphocyte expansions in Felty's syndrome have an unusual phenotype of activated CD45RA+ cells. *Br J Rheumatol* 1996;35:1252.
758. Wallner S, Vautrin R, Katz J, et al. The anemia of thermal injury: partial characterization of an erythroid inhibitory substance. *J Trauma* 1987;6:639.
759. Ham TH, Shen SC, Fleming E, et al. Study on the destruction of red blood cells: IV. *Blood* 1948;3:373.
760. Felix JC, Davis JM. Neutrophil function in thermally injured patients. In: Gallin JI, Fauci A, eds. *Advances in host defense mechanisms*, vol 6. New York: Raven Press, 1986:68.
761. Arturson G. Neutrophil granulocyte functions in severely burned patients. *Burns* 1985;11:309.
762. Koller M, Konig W, Brom J, et al. Studies on the mechanism of granulocyte dysfunctions in severely burned patients: evidence for altered leukotriene generation. *J Trauma* 1989;29:435.
763. Eurenuis K, Mortensen R, Meserol P, et al. Platelet and megakaryocyte kinetics following thermal injury. *J Lab Clin Med* 1972;79:247.

PART 8

Hematologic Therapies

CHAPTER 57

Transfusion Medicine

Jeffrey McCullough

HISTORY

For centuries, blood has been considered to have mystical properties. During the mid-1600s, a number of major developments led to the beginning of blood transfusion (1). In 1656, Christopher Wren developed techniques to isolate veins in dogs and carried out many studies of the effects of substances injected into dogs. These culminated in the transfusion of blood from one dog to another. This work was extended by Richard Lower; similar work was done at approximately the same time in France by Jean Denys. In 1667, Denys carried out what is believed to be the first transfusion of animal (lambs') blood to a human. The man who received the transfusion complained of "a very great heat along his arm" and a minor nosebleed, but he apparently had no other adverse effects. Soon afterward in England, Lower transfused sheep's blood into a man. In France, Denys continued his animal-to-human transfusions. Some of the most notable transfusions were of calves' blood to a man named Antoine Mauroy. During one transfusion, Mauroy experienced pain in the transfused arm, vomiting, increased pulse, nosebleed, pressure in the chest, and pain over the kidneys, and, the next day, he passed black urine—the now known classic symptoms of a hemolytic transfusion reaction. After a subsequent transfusion, Mauroy died, and Denys was charged with murder. He was exonerated by testimony that the man's wife had given him a liquid, which, when given to a cat, caused death. French physicians determined that transfusion was unsound, the Pope banned the practice, and the English discontinued their transfusion work.

Interest in transfusion was revived during the early 1800s, primarily by James Blundell, an obstetrician who believed transfusion would be helpful in treating postpartum hemorrhage. Other work convinced him that transfusions should be between members of the same species, and Blundell is credited with carrying out the first human-to-human transfusion in 1818 (2). In the United States, transfusions were first used in the mid-1800s, but no record exists of the initial transfusion. Four transfusions were administered during the Civil War (2). About this time, unsuccessful efforts were made to anticoagulate and preserve blood for transfusion. During the last part of the 1800s, the use of animal blood was eliminated, and it was established that the dark urine after transfusion was hemoglobin released from destroyed transfused red blood cells (RBCs).

The landmark event that opened the way to modern transfusion therapy was the discovery of blood groups by Landsteiner in 1900. Hektoen suggested that transfusion might be safer if the donor and recipient were crossmatched, and Ottenberg in New York carried out the first transfusion using blood typing and crossmatching. The next major step forward was the development of anticoagulant preservative solutions for blood. Several different citrate solutions were prepared, and citrated blood came into use in treating casualties during World War I. Relatively little progress in transfusion therapy occurred between the two world wars. In 1943, the anticoagulant acid citrate dextrose was developed in England. Because this allowed storage of blood for 21 days, transfusion became more practical.

The first blood bank where a stock of blood was maintained was, apparently, in Barcelona in 1936, although the concept seems to have been developed in Leningrad in 1932 (2). The first blood bank in the United States was established in 1937 at the Cook County Hospital in Chicago.

THE UNITED STATES' BLOOD SUPPLY

The availability of an adequate and safe supply of blood and its components is essential for many surgical procedures, the treatment of patients who experience acute or chronic blood loss, and those with inadequate blood cell production, excessive destruction of their own blood cells, or an inherited defect of red cells or coagulation factors.

In the United States, almost all whole blood is collected from unpaid volunteer donors by either regional community-based or individual hospital-based blood banks. Approximately 13 million units of blood are collected annually in the United States (3). However, blood use has been increasing and donor availability decreasing due to the aging population and the increasing number of reasons for deferring potential donors. A critical national shortage of blood may be developing due to these trends. It was thought that autologous blood donation might alleviate this problem by providing as much as 20% of the needed blood. However, autologous blood donation is decreasing because of costeffectiveness, intraoperative salvage, erythropoietin (Epo), better surgical care, lower risk of transfusion-transmitted diseases (TTDs), pathogen inactivation (future), and acute normal volemic hemodilution.

Most government agencies and blood organizations worldwide advocate volunteerism in blood donation not only based on the moral principle of not selling body parts or tissues but also because of practical issues. It has been well established that blood from paid donors has a much higher risk of disease transmission (4). When a financial payment is involved, there is an incentive for the potential donor to be dishonest about his or her medical history. Despite the increased sophistication of laboratory testing of donated blood, some infectious units of blood are not detected by present tests. Thus, if the donor is dishonest about his or her medical history, there is more likelihood that the unit may be infectious.

WHOLE BLOOD: MEDICAL ASSESSMENT OF DONORS AND BLOOD COLLECTION

The collection of blood and preparation of components for transfusion are regulated by the Center for Biologics Evaluation and Research of the Food and Drug Administration (FDA). The FDA considers blood a drug and inspects blood banks annually. All procedures that involve the medical assessment of the donor, the collection of blood, and the preparation, storage, and distribution of blood components are regulated.

Medical History

The first and one of the most important steps in obtaining safe and effective blood components is the medical assessment of the potential donor. Donor medical requirements and many of the questions asked of the donors are specified by the FDA. In general, the donor medical assessment is designed to ensure that blood donation is not unusually risky for the donor and that the donated blood components are as safe as possible for the recipient. The donor must be in good general health. Because the specific questions change as new information becomes available about transmissible diseases, illicit drugs, and medications, some questions and their rationales are provided as examples:

1. Have you ever donated blood, platelets, or plasma?
    To avoid iron deficiency, at least 8 weeks must elapse between blood donations. To allow blood volume to reequilibrate, at least 48 hours must elapse after plasmapheresis or cytapheresis.
2. Have you ever been deferred as a blood donor?
    This question helps to evaluate the donor's medical history and may identify health problems that would preclude donation.
3. Are you or have you been pregnant during the last 6 weeks?

To allow the woman an opportunity to recover from the delivery and to minimize the possibility of iron deficiency, at least 6 weeks must elapse after third-trimester delivery. Potential donors who had a first-trimester abortion can donate whenever their general medical health permits, if they meet all other blood donor criteria.

4. Have you had surgery or any major illness in the last 6 months?
    This question helps to evaluate the donor's medical condition and may identify health problems that would preclude donation. Donors who have received blood or components during major surgery must be deferred for 6 months, regardless of whether they received blood products. Potential donors who have had minor or uncomplicated surgery are deferred only until the surgical site has healed and the person can resume normal activity. Decisions about which procedures disqualify a donor for 6 months are made at the time the medical history is taken. Therefore, the distinction between major and minor surgery is not uniformly defined.
5. Have you ever had diseases of the heart, lungs, or liver?
    Potential donors with a history of coronary artery disease and rheumatic heart disease are generally deferred unless it is clear that their cardiac function is good and they can withstand the loss of approximately 10% of their blood volume in a short period. Patients with compromised pulmonary function, active tuberculosis, or other active pulmonary infections should not donate blood. Treated tuberculosis or a positive tuberculin skin test is not a reason for deferral of blood donations. Inflammatory diseases of the liver are almost always cause for deferral. Persons with Gilbert syndrome may donate blood, although this sometimes causes problems if they have a slightly elevated bilirubin and someone later notices the unusual color of the plasma in the unit of blood.
6. Have you had recent weight loss?
    This question helps to evaluate the general health of the donor and might indicate the presence of a serious disease. Also, persons on severe diets probably should not donate blood because of possible fluid and electrolyte imbalances.
7. Are you taking any drugs or medications?
    This question also aids in evaluating the general medical condition of the potential donor. Thus, a donor may be deferred not because of the particular medication but because of the condition for which the medication is being taken. Often, the medication itself is not a risk for the recipient. In general, the kinds of drugs for which a donor would be deferred because of the significance of the underlying disease are antibiotics, anticonvulsants, anticoagulants, digitalis, insulin, systemic corticosteroids, vasodilators, and antiarrhythmics. Aspirin or aspirin-containing compounds cause abnormal platelet function (5,6); thus, a donor who serves as the only source of platelets for a patient should not have ingested aspirin within 2 to 3 days before blood donation. In common practice, this means that donors of whole blood may take aspirin, because their platelets are pooled with those of other donors. When approximately 20% of the platelets have not been exposed to aspirin, the hemostatic function of the total platelet pool is normal (5). Thus, the restriction on aspirin ingestion applies primarily to platelet apheresis donors.
    Ingestion of the following commonly used drugs is usually acceptable in most blood banks: tetracyclines or antibiotics taken for acne [Accutane (isotretinoin) disqualifies a donor because it may be a teratogen], topical corticosteroids taken for skin lesions not at the venipuncture site, antihypertensives taken regularly and resulting in an acceptable blood pressure, isoniazid taken because of a positive tuberculin skin test, nonprescription bronchodilators and deconges-

tants, oral hypoglycemic agents in well-controlled diabetics who do not have symptoms of vascular complications, most tranquilizers, hypnotics used at bedtime, oral contraceptives, mild analgesics, vitamins, replacement hormones, weight reduction pills, and marijuana.

8. Have you ever had hepatitis or jaundice?

This question also usually includes others about previous injections of hepatitis B immunoglobulin (Ig), hepatitis vaccine, tattoos, ear piercing, acupuncture, previous transfusions, and the peripheral injection of drugs. The presence of the hepatitis viruses cannot be detected with certainty; thus, potential donors who have a history suggestive of hepatitis or who engage in any activity in which transmission of hepatitis is possible must be deferred. Deferral may be either temporary or permanent, depending on the specific situation. Hepatitis in childhood is almost always type A, and these individuals would not be infectious. Thus, most blood banks accept as donors those with jaundice or hepatitis before age 10 or 11 years.

9. Have you ever had malaria?

Malaria can be transmitted by blood transfusion. Potential donors who have been in areas in which malaria is endemic and who have not taken antimalaria prophylaxis may donate 6 months after returning if they have been symptom free. Potential donors who have had malaria or who have taken prophylaxis while in an endemic malaria area must be symptom free for 3 years after cessation of therapy.

10. Have you ever had a positive test for HIV (human immunodeficiency virus) antibodies?

Persons who have acquired immunodeficiency syndrome (AIDS) or a positive test for anti-HIV or who are at high risk for acquiring or being infected with HIV should not donate blood. This includes persons with exposure to an AIDS-infected person or to someone with a positive test for the antibody to human immunodeficiency virus 1 (anti–HIV-1), males who have had sex with another male since 1977, present or past intravenous drug abusers, hemophiliacs, prostitutes, males exposed to prostitutes, or sexual partners of any of the above.

11. Do you have a bleeding tendency?

Persons with a bleeding tendency may have unusual bleeding from the venipuncture site, or their plasma may be deficient in coagulation factors, thus preventing effective therapy.

12. Do you have epilepsy, convulsions, or fainting spells?

Donors who have epilepsy or fainting spells may be more likely to have a reaction or a seizure after blood donation, although this has not been documented.

13. Have you ever had cancer?

Those who have had minor skin cancer, carcinoma of the cervix, or papillary thyroid carcinoma may donate if the cancer has been adequately treated. Potential donors who have had leukemia or lymphomas must be deferred, and those with other forms of cancer must be evaluated by a physician. Although it has not been documented, a theoretic concern exists that cancer can be transmitted by transfusion of malignant cells. Thus, blood banks err on the conservative side by not accepting as donors those with a history of malignancies.

14. Have you been vaccinated or had any shots during the last 12 months?

In general, recently immunized, symptom-free persons may donate blood. Those who have been vaccinated with live virus vaccines such as measles, rabies, yellow fever, vaccinia, mumps, or oral poliomyelitis should not donate for at least 2 weeks because of the possibility that the virus might be transmitted by blood transfusion. A 1-week waiting period is required for those receiving killed virus, bacterial, or rickett-sial vaccines or toxoid. Examples are influenza, diphtheria, tetanus, rabies, and Rocky Mountain spotted fever. Potential donors who have received immune serum globulin should be questioned to determine whether the reason for receiving the Ig disqualifies them as a donor.

Physical Examination

Potential blood donors undergo a limited physical examination. The donor should have a general appearance of good health and not be under the influence of drugs or alcohol. Donors must weigh at least 110 lb to enable collection of the standard volume (450 or 500 mL) of blood. The risk of adverse reactions is increased in smaller donors (7), but they may be accepted at the discretion of the blood bank physician if some of the anticoagulant is removed from the blood container and a smaller volume of blood collected. There is no weight upper limit, but massively obese persons may not be suitable donors because of other aspects of their health status. The potential donor must have a temperature of less than 99.6°F and a pulse of 50 to 100 beats/minute. Well-conditioned athletes with pulse rates less than 50 may be accepted. The diastolic and systolic blood pressures must be less than 90 to 180 mm Hg. Skin at the venipuncture site must be free of lesions, and donors' arms are inspected for needle marks suggestive of illicit drug use.

The donor's hemoglobin concentration must be 12.5 g/dL or more. If the hematocrit value is determined, it must be at least 38%. A variety of simple methods are used to determine either the hemoglobin or hematocrit. The sample should be obtained from the finger; earlobe samples give artificially high results, leading to donation by some individuals whose venous hemoglobin is less than 12.5 g/dL (8).

Whole Blood Collection

If the medical assessment indicates that the person meets all the requirements, the donor is then prepared for whole blood collection. The skin at the venipuncture site should be as clean as possible. Several methods of skin preparation are available. In general, these involve scrubbing the area with soap or an iodophor compound, followed by tincture of iodine or iodophor compound and removal of tincture of iodine or iodophor compound with acetone or alcohol. This usually results in an aseptic skin area, although surveillance cultures of the venipuncture site reveal approximately a 1% to 2% incidence of bacterial growth; however, infrequent instances of septic transfusion reactions occur due to bacterial contamination (see section Complications of Transfusion: Recognition and Management).

The blood containers used today are a series of plastic bags, all sterile, with an integral tubing and needle. The venipuncture is done in the antecubital fossa using the needle (usually 16-gauge) attached to the blood container set.

The standard donation is approximately 450 mL (within 10%) of blood collected into 63 mL of citrate phosphate dextrose anticoagulant, resulting in a final volume of 468 to 558 mL. The important steps or issues in blood collection are correct labeling and identification of all bags and specimen tubes, maintaining good blood flow to avoid clotting, and adequate mixing of blood and anticoagulant to avoid clotting or osmotic damage to red cells. The phlebotomy lasts approximately 7 to 10 minutes; the entire blood donation process, including registration, medical assessment, preparation, phlebotomy, and recovery, usually takes from 45 to 60 minutes. After collection of the unit of whole blood, it is usually maintained at room temperature and returned to the blood center, where it is separated into its major components: red cells, platelets, and plasma.

Adverse Reactions to Blood Donation

The donation of 450 mL of whole blood, representing up to 13% of a person's blood volume in approximately 7 to 10 minutes, is tolerated remarkably well. During and immediately after blood donation, the blood pressure and pulse rate usually remain unchanged, although the central venous pressure may decrease slightly. The blood volume returns to normal in approximately 72 hours in most donors (9). A slight increase in reticulocyte count occurs, and the hemoglobin reaches its nadir 1 to 2 weeks after donation.

The overall incidence of adverse reactions observed in most large blood banks is approximately 1.5% to 2.0%. Most of these reactions are mild and involve lightheadedness, dizziness, pallor, sweating, and nausea. They are caused by hypovolemia. Some, especially first-time donors, may experience a vasovagal reaction. The symptoms are similar to those due to hypovolemia, but the pulse rate slows rather than increases as would be expected due to hypovolemia. Vasovagal reactions are not related to the volume of blood lost and may occur before blood is withdrawn. Other adverse effects of blood donation are twitching, muscle spasms, inadvertent puncture of an artery or nerve (10), hematoma at the venipuncture site, fainting, seizures, or serious cardiac events. Such reactions are rare.

Autologous Blood Donation

Concern about TTD in public and health care professionals led to a large increase in autologous blood donation, although this has declined in recent years (3). Autologous blood can be provided by presurgical donation, perioperative donation, or intraoperative salvage (11).

Potential autologous blood donors are usually patients with a health problem, although most presurgical patients can be candidates for autologous blood donation. If a patient has special health problems that might increase the risk of blood donation, a knowledgeable physician and good equipment should be available for managing medical emergencies. One absolute contraindication to autologous blood donation is bacteremia, because bacteria can proliferate in stored blood even at 1° to 6°C (12).

No upper or lower age limit restricts autologous donation. The decision is based on the condition of the donor and, in small children, on the practical limitation of vascular access and the volume of blood loss that the donor can tolerate. There are no specific weight limits, although in donors weighing less than 110 lb, proportionally less blood should be withdrawn. The potential donor's hemoglobin concentration must be at least 11 g/dL (hematocrit 34%) to avoid severe iron depletion. As long as the hemoglobin is maintained above 11 g/dL, the patient may donate as often as every 72 hours. This minimum interval is necessary to allow protein mobilization and reequilibration of the donor's blood volume (9).

Blood Collection from Autologous Donors

The techniques of collecting blood from autologous donors are the same as those used to collect blood from homologous donors. It is important that the blood container be labeled at the collection site, preferably at the bedside, to ensure that the correct unit is saved for the donor's later use. If the donor does not meet all the health history and physical criteria for homologous blood donation, this labeling is especially important to minimize the likelihood of the unit's being erroneously transfused to another patient.

Although some autologous donors meet all the criteria for allogeneic blood donation, their blood may not be used for other patients. Most autologous blood donors do not meet the FDA criteria for blood donation. This, combined with donation of blood in many situations in which there is a low likelihood of blood use, has resulted in the nonutilization (outdating) of approximately one-half of all autologous blood (3).

Because the patient's ability to donate autologous blood may be limited by his or her iron stores, it is customary to provide iron supplementation. Parenteral administration is not necessary; oral administration is effective. Oral iron, ferrous sulfate, 325 mg three times daily, should be started approximately 1 week before the first donation and continued after the last donation, depending on the amount of blood donated and the patient's hemoglobin. Epo can also be used to increase the number of units of blood that can be collected. However, in most situations, it is not possible to obtain enough additional autologous blood to reduce the amount of allogeneic blood used (13). One group of patients in whom autologous blood donation has great potential but raises questions of safety are those scheduled to undergo cardiac surgery. Most require blood replacement, but they have compromised cardiovascular function. Several studies have shown that under proper medical supervision, autologous blood donation is not an unusual risk for these patients (14,15).

In considering autologous blood donation during pregnancy, the health of two persons (mother and fetus) must be considered in evaluating the possible side effects of blood donation. The effect of blood donation may be difficult to predict because of the large blood volume of the mother and possible hypertension. Although few data are available, risks of blood donation to the mother during the second (14) and third trimesters (16,17) appear not to be increased. Fetal monitoring revealed no abnormalities due to blood donation during the third trimester in 39 women (16). Despite these reassuring data in mothers and their babies, autologous blood donation is not recommended routinely for pregnant patients. The likelihood of transfusion after pregnancy and delivery is less than 3% (16). It should be limited to situations in which the likelihood of transfusion is increased, such as placenta previa, uterine atony, retained placenta trauma, abruptio placentae (18), scheduled cesarean section, eclampsia, and multiple miscarriages (16).

Intraoperative Blood Salvage

Another form of autologous blood donation and transfusion is the retrieval of the patient's blood that is shed during surgery and the return of that blood to the patient. Early efforts to salvage and transfuse blood lost during surgery were not successful because of air embolism, coagulopathy, and transfusion of particulate debris. Improved instruments are available, and this process of intraoperative blood salvage and transfusion is being used more often. In intraoperative blood salvage, a suction device is used by the surgeon or assistants to aspirate blood being lost. The blood is immediately anticoagulated, usually with citrate or heparin, and then enters a sterile disposable centrifuge bowl, where it is washed with saline solution. When the centrifuge bowl is filled with red cells, they are pumped automatically into a bag, where they are available for transfusion back to the patient. The centrifuge bowl is now empty and is then refilled with more shed blood, and the cycle is repeated so that large volumes of blood can be salvaged, washed, and returned to the patient.

Blood that has been salvaged and made ready for transfusion has a hematocrit of approximately 50%, a supernatant hemoglobin concentration of 100 to 200 mg/dL, and a few leukocytes and platelets, and it may contain some residual heparin. Because the salvaged blood contains no coagulation factors, very few platelets, and possibly some heparin, a coagulopathy may develop after transfusion of 1 L or more. Physicians involved with intraoperative blood salvage should be aware of the possible development of a bleeding diathesis and should be prepared to administer fresh frozen plasma (FFP) or platelet transfusion, if indicated. The red cells obtained by intraoperative blood salvage have a normal intravascular survival (19) and a normal 2,3-diphosphoglycerate (2,3-DPG) level (20). The normal 2,3-DPG and, thus, normal oxygen dissociation may give salvaged red cells an advantage over stored allogeneic red cells, which have a low 2,3-DPG and poor oxygen dissociation.

Intraoperative blood salvage has been used most extensively in cardiac, vascular, urologic, and orthopedic procedures. The amount of homologous blood used can be reduced substantially by intraoperative blood salvage (21–24). Intraoperative blood salvage is not used when there is bacterial contamination of the surgical field. Thus, it is not usually used in a patient whose bowel is opened or in trauma. Intraoperative blood salvage also is not used in surgery involving a malignancy. The presence of malignant cells in the peripheral blood raises the possibility of hematogenous spread of the neoplasm. No data support or refute this concern, but, in the absence of such data, intraoperative blood salvage is unlikely to be used extensively in these patients.

APHERESIS: MEDICAL ASSESSMENT OF DONORS AND COMPONENT COLLECTION

Apheresis, meaning to take away, refers to the process of selectively removing one component of whole blood and returning the remainder to the donor. This is usually done using semiautomated instruments sometimes called *blood cell separators*. During apheresis, blood is pumped from one of the donor's veins into the blood cell separator, which usually uses centrifugation to separate the blood into plasma, platelets, leukocytes, and red cells. The desired component is removed, and the remainder of the components is recombined and returned to the donor. Some variations in the instruments are the use of intermittent versus continuous flow of blood from the donor, the use of one or two donor veins, and the use of several different preparations of citrate for anticoagulation while the blood is extracorporeal.

Many different instruments are available for the collection of platelets, granulocytes, lymphocytes, peripheral blood stem cells (PBSCs), or plasma by apheresis (Table 57-1). The type of procedure or component for which the FDA licenses each instrument is shown. Because of its design, each instrument is optimal for collection of some components but usually not all. Although some instruments may be satisfactory for a type of collection (Table 57-1), the manufacturer may not have developed an appropriate procedure, and, thus, the instrument would not be licensed by the FDA and not used clinically for that purpose. For details of the instrument's operation and collection procedure, the manufacturer's instruction and references should be consulted.

Platelets

Platelet apheresis usually requires approximately $1^1/_2$ hours and involves processing 4000 to 5000 mL of the donor's blood through the instrument. Platelets obtained by platelet apheresis are processed, tested, and labeled in a similar manner to that of whole blood. This includes ABO and Rh typing and testing for all required TTDs. The platelet apheresis concentrate may be stored for 5 days at 20° to 24°C. The number of platelets contained in each concentrate is determined, although this information may not necessarily be recorded on the label. Quality control tests must show that at least 75% of the apheresis platelet concentrates produced by each facility contain 3×10^{11} plate-

TABLE 57-1. Blood Derivatives Produced by Fractionation of Plasma

Immune globulins
 Cytomegalovirus immune globulin
 Hepatitis B immune globulin
 Immune globulin intravenous
 Immune serum globulin
 Rabies immune globulin
 Rh(D) immune globulin
 Tetanus immune globulin
 Varicella-zoster immune globulin
Coagulation products
 Activated factor IX complex
 Antithrombin III
 Coagulation factor IX
 Factor VIIa (under development in Europe)
 Factor VIII concentrate
 Factor IX concentrate–prothrombin complex
 Protein C
Blood volume expanders
 Albumin
 Plasma protein fraction
Miscellaneous
 α_1-Antitrypsin
 Fibrin glue

lets or more. Each platelet concentrate has a volume of approximately 200 mL and contains few (<0.5 mL) red cells so that red cell crossmatching is not necessary. The white blood cell content varies depending on the instrument and technique used for collection.

Granulocytes

Leukapheresis procedures are usually more complex and lengthy than platelet apheresis. The donor receives up to 500 mL of hydroxyethyl starch to improve the efficiency of granulocyte extraction and may receive corticosteroids to increase the yield by elevating the level of circulating granulocytes. Prednisone, 60 mg, can be given orally the evening before. Recently, granulocyte colony-stimulating factor (G-CSF) has also been used to increase the donor's granulocyte count (25–27), and this enables the collection of a large number of granulocytes. The leukapheresis procedure takes 30 to 60 minutes longer than platelet apheresis to process more blood and to improve the granulocyte yield. Usually, 6500 to 8000 mL of the donor's blood is processed through the instrument, with removal of approximately 50% of the granulocyte, resulting in a yield of 1 to 2×10^{10} granulocytes in a volume of approximately 200 mL. Because granulocytes do not completely separate from the red cells, granulocyte concentrates usually contain a substantial amount of red cells (hematocrit, 10%, or approximately 20 mL of red cells); therefore, crossmatching is necessary. Granulocyte concentrates are stored at 20°C to 24°C for up to 24 hours, although they should be transfused as soon as possible after collection (28,29). The granulocyte content of each concentrate is determined but not necessarily indicated on the label. No minimum FDA requirements define the composition of granulocyte concentrates; the standards of the American Association of Blood Banks require that 75% of units contain at least 1×10^{10} granulocytes.

Lymphocytes

Lymphocytes may be collected as a blood component for transfusion or to obtain mononuclear cell concentrates to be used as starting material for the production of cells for adoptive immunotherapy (see section on cellular engineering).

Peripheral Blood Stem Cells

Hematopoietic stem cells are present in not only the marrow but also the peripheral circulation (30), and they have been used successfully for autologous and allogeneic marrow transplantation (31–35). It appears that G-CSF–mobilized PBSCs are as equally effective as bone marrow. The cytapheresis techniques used for collection of PBSCs are similar to lymphocyte collection procedures. The collection procedure is approximately 3 hours, but larger volumes of blood may be processed. Patients receive chemotherapy, and PBSCs are collected during marrow rebound. Normal donors receive G-CSF to increase the level of circulating stem cells (36,37). Usually, approximately 3 to 5 × 10^{10} mononuclear cells are removed, and the concentrate obtained has a volume of approximately 200 mL.

No definite test exists for the primordial hematopoietic stem cell; therefore, quality control of these PBSC concentrates is difficult. In practice, the dose for transplantation is usually based on cell counting to obtain at least 3 × 10^8 mononuclear cells/kg of the recipient's body weight. Other tests, including $CD34^+$ cells and cell culture techniques, are used to determine colony-forming units—granulocytic, monocytic, or mixed. Because the optimal conditions for storage of hematopoietic stem cells are not known, the PBSC concentrates are frozen within a few hours of collection.

Medical Evaluation of Cytapheresis Donors

Donors undergoing platelet apheresis, leukapheresis, or lymphapheresis must meet all the criteria for donation of whole blood. Because the cytapheresis procedure may have some unique effects on the donor, some additional medical history and physical or laboratory monitoring criteria are needed.

Platelet Apheresis

Although it may be desirable to know the platelet count before donation, this is not required if platelet apheresis is carried out no more often than whole blood donation is allowed. Platelet apheresis causes an average decrease in the donor's platelet count of approximately 30% (75,000/µL), which returns to baseline in 4 days (36). This is not a risk for healthy normal donors, but potential platelet donors should be questioned to ensure that they do not have a bleeding disorder and that they are not ingesting drugs such as aspirin, which interferes with platelet function (6). Platelets obtained from such donors are not effective clinically. Platelets produced after the drug is no longer circulating are normal. The presence of only 20% of normal platelets allows primary aggregation to occur, which, in turn, causes secondary aggregation of the remaining aspirin-damaged platelets (5). Thus, donors who are going to be the sole source of platelets but have ingested aspirin at least 3 days earlier can donate.

Leukapheresis

In addition to the removal of the blood component, donors undergoing leukapheresis receive the blood volume expander hydroxyethyl starch, a sedimenting agent that improves the granulocyte yield; corticosteroids; and G-CSF to improve the granulocyte yield by increasing the donor's leukocyte count (25–27,37). These donors must meet all the criteria for whole blood donation, but, in addition, they are questioned specifically about hypertension, diabetes, peptic ulcers, and bleeding tendency. No additional laboratory tests are necessary before leukapheresis.

Serial Apheresis Donations

In general, if a donor undergoes cytapheresis no more often than is allowable for whole blood donation (every 8 weeks), no additional laboratory tests or monitoring are necessary. More frequent cytapheresis is sometimes called *serial cytapheresis*. A donor should not undergo more than 24 platelet apheresis procedures in 1 year, more than two procedures in 7 days, and more than six procedures in 1 month. At least 48 hours must elapse between procedures. Serial apheresis donors must be monitored as follows:

1. Red cell loss must average 25 mL or less/week, because the total red cell loss for one calendar year must not exceed that allowed for whole blood donation.
2. The total volume of all blood products retained per platelet apheresis procedure must not exceed 500 to 600 mL, depending on the donor's weight.
3. The total volume of plasma removed must not exceed 15 L/year.
4. The total dose of hydroxyethyl starch must be kept at a minimum.
5. If a donor is to undergo platelet apheresis more often than allowed for whole blood donation (once every 8 weeks), the predonation platelet count must be greater than 150,000/µL. For logistic reasons, most blood banks obtain a platelet count at the end of the previous donation. If the count is greater than 150,000/µL, it can serve as the predonation count for the subsequent platelet apheresis.

Lymphocyte Depletion in Cytapheresis Donors

Although it appears that some lymphocyte depletion may occur in cytapheresis donors, no adverse effects have been found in association with this (38–41). Thus, leukocyte or lymphocyte counts are not used to determine the suitability of a potential apheresis donor.

LABORATORY TESTING OF DONATED BLOOD

Before being made available for transfusion, donated blood undergoes several tests involving red cell typing, antibody detection, and screening for transmissible diseases. The use of the tests intended to prevent TTDs is discussed more completely below.

ABO and Rh Typing

RBC typing is necessary so that the components can be labeled properly and selected for patients with appropriate ABO and Rh types. Because of their clinical significance, these two blood groups are the only ones that are determined routinely (see section Blood Groups). Typing for ABO and Rh is usually done by semiautomated instruments in large blood collection centers or by various solid phase or gel techniques in smaller blood banks. Older methods using tubes or observing agglutination on plates are no longer used.

Red Blood Cell Antibody Detection

RBC antibody detection involves testing the donor's serum against commercially available red cells from two normal subjects whose cells contain the antigens against which most red cell antibodies are directed. Antibodies transfused in the donor plasma can cause hemolysis of the recipient's red cells or can hemolyze other donor units (intradonor incompatibility). In the past, these problems were avoided by using a minor crossmatch of the donor's serum and the recipient's red cells. Screening for donor antibodies at the time of blood processing has eliminated the need for the minor crossmatch.

Serologic Test for Syphilis

Although syphilis can be transmitted by blood transfusion (see section Transfusion-Transmitted Diseases), this almost never happens in the United States (42,42a). Most transfusion medicine specialists believe this test is unnecessary. Although the American Association of Blood Banks no longer requires syphilis testing, the FDA and many states do. Thus, all donated blood is tested.

Hepatitis B Surface Antigen

Hepatitis B surface antigen (HBsAg) was the first specific test to detect carrier donors and eliminate a form of posttransfusion hepatitis. The method in widespread use is an enzyme immunoassay using antibody to HBsAg to detect circulating antigen.

Hepatitis C

The hepatitis C virus (HCV) gene has been cloned (43). The sensitivity and specificity of the test for antibody to HCV have improved in the last decade, and this test is routine for all donated blood (44). Although all donated blood is now screened for anti-HCV, this has not replaced the use of antibody to hepatitis B core antigen (anti-HB$_c$) or alanine aminotransferase (ALT) as surrogate tests for non-A, non-B hepatitis, because not all donors in whom these tests are abnormal and who transmit non-A, non-B hepatitis have detectable anti-HCV.

Surrogate Tests for Non-A, Non-B Hepatitis

HEPATITIS B CORE ANTIBODY

There is a statistical association between the occurrence of posttransfusion hepatitis and transfusion of blood containing anti-HB$_c$ but lacking HBsAg. Before identification of the HCV, anti-HB$_c$ testing was introduced to reduce cases of non-A, non-B hepatitis. Even after testing for HCV was implemented (45,46), blood containing anti-HBc was not used for transfusion as a way of reducing posttransfusion hepatitis due to other unknown agents. Approximately 1.35% of donated blood is unsuitable for use because it contains anti-HB$_c$. Because it contains hepatitis virus antibodies, plasma from these units of blood can be used to prepare immune serum globulin.

ALANINE AMINOTRANSFERASE

Blood containing elevated ALT also has a statistical association with posttransfusion non-A, non-B hepatitis (47). Thus, testing for this liver enzyme is also performed on all donated blood, and units with ALT levels above a designated cutoff are not used for transfusion in an effort to reduce non-A, non-B, and non-C hepatitis. A number of non–hepatitis-related factors such as obesity, exercise, and alcohol consumption can elevate the ALT and cause the donor's blood to be unsuitable for transfusion. Approximately 1.2% of donated blood is unsuitable for use because of an elevated ALT.

Human Immunodeficiency Virus 1 and 2 Antibody

Since 1985, all donated blood is tested for anti–HIV-1 and -2. The test used for screening is an enzyme immunoassay. If it is positive, the blood may not be used for transfusion, and a con-

firmatory test must be done to establish the presence of antibody specificity for HIV-1 and -2. Approximately 0.19% of U.S. blood donors are positive for anti–HIV-1, which is only $1/40$ to $1/80$ of the rate expected from the random population. The significance of the positive screening test in those donors not confirmed by Western blot is not established.

Human T-Cell Lymphotrophic Virus I and II Antibody

Human T-cell lymphotrophic virus I (HTLV-I) causes adult T-cell leukemia or tropical spastic paraparesis and can be transmitted by transfusion. Routine testing for the antibody to HTLV-I (anti–HTLV-I) and -II was initiated in the United States in 1989. The screening test is an enzyme immunoassay confirmation of antibody specificity, for which it is necessary to use a radioimmunoprecipitation assay or a Western blot. The incidence of this virus in U.S. blood donors is low—approximately 2.5 in 10,000 (48). As with HIV, the significance of a positive screening test that is not confirmed by the more specific tests is not known.

Summary

A multifaceted approach is used to attempt to produce the safest possible blood supply. This includes educating donors before donation; obtaining a medical history; increasing the emphasis on determining whether the donor has been involved in AIDS-risk behavior; conducting a limited physical examination; testing donated blood in a laboratory; determining through a registry whether the donor has been previously deferred or has had a positive transmissible disease screening test; and offering to confidentially exclude donor blood from transfusion. The addition of several new viral and related screening tests during the past 15 years has improved the safety of the blood supply (49–52). The costeffectiveness of the steps taken to achieve this is not known. These screening tests result in approximately 4% of all donated blood being unsuitable for transfusion. Rates of unsuitable blood are much higher in some areas of the United States. This is particularly a problem with products in which the storage period may be short, such as those obtained by apheresis. Other effects of this increased testing are an increase in the complexity of work and the time involved in making blood available for use after it is collected and the psychosocial impact on donors who have a positive screening but negative or indeterminate confirmatory tests.

PREPARATION, STORAGE, AND CHARACTERISTICS OF BLOOD COMPONENTS

Preparation of Blood Components from Whole Blood

Almost all blood collected in the United States is separated into components: red cells, platelets, and plasma. This allows each component to be stored under conditions that are optimal for that component and avoids the loss of valuable platelets and coagulation factors that would occur if the unit were stored as whole blood at 1° to 6°C. The unit of whole blood is separated into components by centrifugation. Because whole blood is collected in a multiple-bag system, the component separation can be accomplished in a closed system, avoiding exposure of the blood to the external environment (Fig. 57-1) and bacterial contamination that might result. A unit of whole blood provides one unit of red cells, platelet concentrate, cryoprecipitate, and platelet- and cryoprecipitate-poor plasma. This plasma then undergoes fractionation to provide a variety of blood deriva-

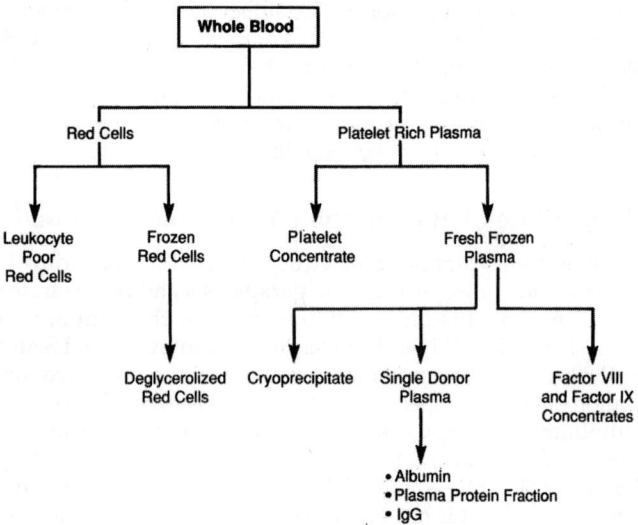

Figure 57-1. Preparation of blood components from one unit of whole blood. IgG, immunoglobulin G. (From Kennedy MD, ed. *Blood transfusion therapy: an audiovisual program.* Arlington, VA: American Association of Blood Banks, 1985, with permission.)

tives. Other special cellular blood components such as leukocyte-poor or frozen washed red cells are prepared from the unit of red cells after the platelets and plasma have been removed.

Red Blood Cells

After most of the platelets and plasma have been removed, the red cells are resuspended in a solution designed to optimize red cell preservation. The resulting red cell unit has been called *packed red cells* or *red cell concentrate*. The commonly used red cell preservative solutions contain glucose, adenine, mannitol, and sodium chloride. These preservative solutions allow storage of red cells for 42 days at 1° to 6°C. During storage, some deleterious changes occur in the red cells, such as loss of viability, loss of adenosine triphosphate (ATP), increase in cellular rigidity, loss of membrane lipid, change in shape from disk to sphere, formation of microvesicles, loss of 2,3-DPG (causing increased affinity of hemoglobin for oxygen), and reduced transmembrane transport of sodium and potassium. Because red cell metabolism continues during storage, metabolites accumulate in stored red cell units and lead to biochemical changes (Table 57-2). Four of these changes are discussed: loss of ATP and viability, loss of DPG and function, accumulation of potassium, and hemolysis.

Although a general relation exists between loss of ATP and viability, other factors contribute to this, such as loss of membrane lipids and deformability. The red cells with poor viability are removed during the first 24 hours after transfusion, and, thereafter, the remaining red cells have a normal intravascular half-disappearance time.

In 1954, Valtis and Kennedy (53) reported that the oxygen dissociation curve was shifted in stored red cells so that the volume of oxygen released to the tissues was reduced. The clinical importance of this observation has been unexpectedly difficult to determine. Studies of animals subjected to hemodilution have shown that hemoglobin concentration (or hematocrit) and avoidance of acidosis were more important than red cell DPG concentration.

Red cell membrane sodium-potassium ATPase is sensitive to decreases in temperature. Thus, during storage at 1° to 6°C, red cells lose potassium into the supernatant (Table 57-3). Although this is not a problem for most transfusions, older stored red cell units can be a potential problem for neonates (see section Transfusion in Special Situations).

The cause of the hemolysis that occurs during storage (Table 57-3) is unknown. Paradoxically, the phthalate plasticizers that leak from the blood bags into the blood during storage seem to have a protective effect and reduce the hemolysis. Thus, the concern that these plasticizers might accumulate in transfusion recipients and cause harm is counterbalanced by their apparent beneficial effect in red cell preservation.

Stored red cells can be rejuvenated by incubating them with adenosine to replenish ATP and with inosine, phosphate, and pyruvate to replenish DPG. This process can produce red cells with good *in vivo* viability and normal or even above-normal DPG and oxygen transport capability. These techniques have not been adapted for large-scale practical use and are not performed as part of routine blood bank operations.

Fresh Frozen Plasma

FFP is the liquid portion of one unit of blood that has been centrifuged, separated, and frozen solid at –18°C or colder within 6 hours of collection. The unit of whole blood is usually centrifuged using techniques to prepare platelet-rich plasma (Fig. 57-1). This platelet-rich plasma is then centrifuged, and the plasma is removed and frozen, giving one unit of FFP and one unit of platelet concentrate. FFP can be stored for up to 1 year at –18°C or colder. The unit of FFP has a volume of approximately 185 mL and contains all the constituents of citrated normal plasma. Specifically, this includes the labile and stable coagulation factors, the components of the complement and fibrinolytic systems, and the plasma proteins that maintain osmotic pressure and modulate immunity.

TABLE 57-2. Characteristics of Red Cells in AS-1 (Adsol) for 42 Days of Storage[a]

Indices	Days of Storage						
	0	7	14	21	28	35	42
pH (37°C)	7.00	6.86	6.69	6.55	—	6.43	6.34
RBC adenosine triphosphate (μmol/g of Hgb)	4.69	4.97	4.83	4.50	3.75	3.47	3.24
RBC diphosphoglycerate (μmol/g of Hgb)	10.88	8.16	1.96	0.87	0.65	0.54	0.65
Supernatant sodium (mEq/L)	152	135	131	124	—	126	123
Supernatant potassium (mEq/L)	1.6	17.0	27.0	34.0	—	44.0	46.0
Supernatant glucose (mg/dL)	909	780	724	697	660	617	604
Hemolysis (%)	0.02	0.06	0.11	0.14	0.20	0.16	0.24

Hgb, hemoglobin; RBC, red blood cell.
[a]Adsol cells: number, 13; volume, 325 ± 29 mL; hematocrit, 58 ± 4%; mean red cell mass, 188 mL; mean supernatant volume, 136 mL; mean total hemoglobin 19.3 g/dL.
Data from Fenwal, a Division of Baxter Healthcare, Inc. (Deerfield, IL).

TABLE 57-3. Molecular and Biochemical Characteristics of Some Blood Group Antigens[a]

Blood Group Antigen	Chromosomes of Gene Location	Number of Antigen Sites × 10³ Red Cells	Molecular Weight of Antigen (kd)	Red Blood Cell Membrane Components with Antigen Expression	Antigen Composition	Complementary DNA Cloned
ABO	9	1000	90–100	Anion transport protein (band 3)	—	—
MN, Ss	4	200–1000; 80–250	43[a], 25[a]	Glycophorin A or B	Sialoglycoprotein	Yes
P, P₁, Pᵏ	22	Unknown	Unknown	Globoside I, paragloboside, ceramide trihexoside	Glycosphingolipid	Yes
Rh	1	100–200	30–32	Polypeptides	Lipoprotein	Yes
Lutheran	19	1–4	78–85	N-glycans and disulfide bonding required for antigen activity	Glycoprotein	No
Kell	7	3–6	93[a]	Disulfide bonding required for antigen activity	Glycoprotein	Yes
Lewis	19	Unknown	Unknown	Unknown	Glycosphingolipid	No
Duffy (Fy)	1	12	40–50[b]	N-glycans not required for antigen activity	Glycoprotein	Yes
Kidd	18	Unknown	45	Polypeptide	Unknown	Yes
Diego	17	Unknown	Unknown	Unknown	Unknown	—
	7	Unknown	Unknown	Unknown	Unknown	—
Xg	X	Unknown	20–29	Unknown	Unknown	No
Scianna	1	Unknown	Unknown	Unknown	Unknown	—
Dombrack	Unknown	Unknown	Unknown	Unknown	Unknown	—
Colton	7	Unknown	Unknown	Unknown	Unknown	No
LW	19	3–5	40–47	N-glycans	Glycoprotein	Yes
Chido-Rogers	6	Unknown	96, 94	Unknown	Glycoprotein	Yes
H	19	Unknown	Unknown	Unknown	Glycoprotein	Yes
Ii	Unknown	500	55	Glucose transport protein (band 4, 5)	—	—
	—	500	—	Poly-N-acetyl-lactosaminyl glycolipids	Glycolipid	—
	—	100–200	45–100	Polypeptides	Lipoprotein	—
Kx	X	—	—	—	—	—
Gerbich	2	60–120	39[a]	Glycophorin C	Sialoglycoprotein	Yes
	—	15–20	30[a]	Glycophorin D	Sialoglycoprotein	Yes
Cromer	1	Unknown	Unknown	Unknown	Unknown	—
Knopps	1	Unknown	Unknown	Unknown	Unknown	—
Indian	11	Unknown	Unknown	Unknown	Unknown	—
OK	19	Unknown	Unknown	Unknown	Unknown	—
Raph	11	Unknown	Unknown	Unknown	Unknown	—

[a]These molecules give anomalous apparent molecular weight on sodium dodecyl sulfate-polyacrylamide gel electrophoresis.
[b]Fy antigen activity is observed over a broad molecular weight range (38–90 kd); the value given corresponds to the region of greatest activity.
Data from Anstee DJ. Blood group active components of the human cell membrane. In: Garratty G, ed. *Red cell antigens and antibodies.* Arlington, VA: American Association of Blood Banks, 1986:8; Anstee DJ. Blood group active surface molecules of the human red blood cell. *Vox Sang* 1990;58:1; and Lewis M, Anstee DJ, Bird GWG, et al. Blood group terminology 1990. *Vox Sang* 1990;58:142, with permission of the American Association of Blood Banks.

For transfusion, FFP is thawed in a 37°C water bath for approximately 30 minutes. In the past, microwave ovens were not acceptable for thawing FFP because they created hot spots that damaged the plasma proteins. Newer microwave devices may be suitable and thus reduce the time required to make FFP available. After thawing, the plasma should be transfused as soon as possible; it cannot be stored for longer than 24 hours.

FFP use has increased greatly during the last few years. A National Institutes of Health Consensus Development Conference concluded that this increase was not based on definitive evidence of the effectiveness of FFP but has occurred in the face of evidence of potential risk from its use (54). The following are indications for use of FFP established by the Consensus Conference:

- Replacement of isolated coagulation factor deficiencies when specific components are not available. Examples include factors V, VIII, IX, X, and XI.
- Reversal of warfarin effect in patients actively bleeding or who require emergency surgery.
- Antithrombin III deficiency in patients undergoing surgery or those who require heparin for treatment of thrombosis.
- Treatment of thrombotic thrombocytopenic purpura (TTP), usually as part of plasma exchange.
- Replacement of Igs in the treatment of immunodeficiency, such as in patients with protein-losing enteropathy or in children or adults with immunodeficiency. The availability of intravenous Ig preparations has almost eliminated this as an indication for FFP.
- Replacement of coagulation factors in massive transfusion. This is a questionable indication. Usually, the bleeding diathesis in massive transfusion is due to depletion of platelets rather than coagulation factors. No evidence exists that the empiric use of FFP in some ratio with units of red cells is necessary. FFP should be used in massive transfusion only when lack of coagulation factors is seen as a major contributor to the bleeding diathesis.
- Replacement of coagulation factors in patients who have depletion of multiple coagulation factors usually due to liver disease and who are bleeding or about to undergo surgery.

FFP is not indicated for blood volume replacement or as a nutritional source.

The dose of FFP is difficult to determine because it is usually given to replace multiple plasma proteins, and the desired level of each protein may be different. In an average-sized adult, five units of FFP would raise the level of coagulation factors approximately 30%, which is a level thought to provide hemostasis. Because this would involve transfusion of approximately 1000 mL of plasma, the patient's blood volume and cardiovascular status must be considered.

Plasma and Source Plasma

Two other forms of plasma are prepared from whole blood. These are called *plasma* and *liquid plasma*. These are the plasma removed from whole blood more than 6 hours and less than 5 days after collection and stored either at –18°C or less (plasma) or at 1° to 6°C (liquid plasma). Source plasma is collected by plasmapheresis and is intended to serve as the raw material for further manufacture into blood derivatives. Many different derivatives are manufactured from human plasma.

Solvent Detergent Plasma

The solvent detergent (SD) method used for viral inactivation during the manufacture of plasma derivatives is also used to produce units similar to FFP (55,56). This SD plasma has a volume of 200 mL and is similar to FFP in its content of proteins and coagulation factors. In patients with acquired coagulopathies such as liver disease and vitamin K deficiency, warfarin therapy is as effective as regular FFP on improvement in coagulation tests and does not cause serious unexpected adverse events (57). However, due to its high cost, many hospitals have not converted all of their FFP use to SD plasma but rather have limited its use to patients with TTP, isolated coagulation factor deficiencies other than VIII and IX, or made it available by a physician's special request.

Parvovirus has been transmitted by SD plasma, and, as a result, screening procedures are now in place to reduce or eliminate this risk (58).

Cryoprecipitate

Cryoprecipitate is the material that remains insoluble when previously frozen plasma is thawed at 1° to 6°C. Each bag of cryoprecipitate contains approximately 100 U of factor VIII and 200 mg of fibrinogen and has a volume of approximately 10 mL. Thus, cryoprecipitate can be used to replace factor VIII or fibrinogen. Cryoprecipitate can be stored for up to 1 year at –18°C or lower.

Cryoprecipitate is thawed in a 37°C water bath and can be stored for up to 6 hours at 1° to 6°C before transfusion. Cryoprecipitate from multiple bags is usually pooled into a single container that is dispensed by the blood bank. To avoid transfusing incompatible ABO antibodies, the ABO type of cryoprecipitate is usually selected to be identical with the patient, although ABO-compatible but nonidentical cryoprecipitate may be used (A cryoprecipitate to O recipient). If there is a shortage of cryoprecipitate, small amounts that are ABO incompatible with the patient can be given. Thus, a patient might receive up to a few hundred mL of plasma containing ABO-incompatible antibodies. If the volume of incompatible plasma is limited, usually little risk of hemolysis exists because the volume of plasma from any individual donor who might have a high-titer antibody is only 10 mL. Cryoprecipitate is given without regard to Rh type because it does not contain a sufficient number of red cells to cause immunization.

Random Donor Platelet Concentrates

PREPARATION

A random donor platelet concentrate is prepared from a standard unit of whole blood. Because cold temperatures damage platelets, the unit of whole blood is maintained at room temperature, and platelets are removed within 6 hours of collection. The whole blood is centrifuged, and then platelet-rich plasma is passed into a satellite bag (Fig. 57-1). The bag containing the red cells is detached, the platelet-rich plasma is centrifuged again, and the platelet-poor plasma is passed into another satellite bag, leaving the platelet concentrate that is detached. Approximately 50 mL of plasma remains as the suspending medium for the platelets (59). At least 75% of random donor platelet concentrates contain at least 5.5×10^{10} platelets. This represents recovery of approximately 20% of the platelets in the original unit of whole blood.

STORAGE

Random donor platelet concentrates may be stored for up to 5 days at room temperature (20° to 24°C) (57). During storage, platelets lose the ability to circulate and to be functionally effective both *in vitro* and *in vivo* (59–62). Many changes that occur during storage have been well described, but the changes crucial to the loss of *in vivo* effectiveness are not completely understood. During storage, platelets change from disk to spherical shape; have reduced adhesion, aggregation, adenine nucleotides, membrane glycoproteins, and glutathione; and release some α-granule contents into the suspending plasma. The variables known to be important in platelet preservation are temperature, method of agitation, volume of suspending plasma, and type of storage container (59).

Platelets must be maintained at room temperature. Exposure to cold transforms the platelet from the normal disk to the spherical shape and is associated with abnormal function (59,60). Also, the pH must be kept above 6.0 to maintain platelet function (63). This is done by maintaining an adequate volume of plasma, using a container that allows diffusion of oxygen and CO_2, and providing constant mixing of the platelet plasma mixture.

Containers used for red cell and plasma storage are usually made of polyvinyl chloride and the plasticizer diethylhexyl phthalate or tri(2-ethyl hexyl)trimellitate (CLX; Cutter Laboratories, Berkeley). The bag is placed on one of several suitable rotating devices for storage. The concentrate can be maintained in this condition for up to 5 days. At the end of the storage period, the intravascular recovery and half-life of the stored platelets are approximately 51% and 3.1 days, respectively (64). Further evidence of satisfactory function by stored platelets is that they correct the bleeding time in thrombocytopenic patients (64,65). Actually, satisfactory platelet function can be maintained for up to 7 days (65,66), but storage longer than 5 days allows bacterial proliferation in some concentrates (67). This has been associated with transmission of infection (67–69). Although these complications were infrequent, it was enough of a clinical problem to warrant limiting room temperature platelet storage to 5 days.

Granulocytes

Granulocyte concentrates for transfusion are produced by apheresis. The characteristics and storage conditions for these granulocyte concentrates have already been described (see the section Apheresis: Medical Assessment of Donors and Component Collection). Occasionally, granulocytes were isolated from fresh units of whole blood, but this provides a dose suitable only for neonatal patients (see section Transfusion in Special Situations) and is not recommended.

BLOOD GROUPS

Red Blood Cell Blood Groups

As blood groups were discovered, it became customary to name the blood group system using all or part of the name of the first person in whom the antibody was found. For instance, Lewis, Duffy, Scianna, Dombrock, Colton, Gerbich, Cromer, Knops, and Diego were all names of the individuals in whom the antibody was first identified. The Lutheran blood group should really have been called *Lutteran* because this was the name of the donor, but the blood sample tube was incorrectly labeled with the *Lutheran* spelling. Other blood group names come from part of the name of the individuals of the antibody maker. For instance, Kell is from Kelleher, JMH from John Milton Hagen, LKE from Luke, CS from Cost-Sterling, BJ from Bennett-Goodspeed, Ch from Chido, and Rg from Rogers. The origin of other symbols is also interesting. For instance, the Fy symbol for the Duffy blood group represents the last two letters of the antibody maker's name because the first two letters, *D* and *U*, had already been used in the Rh system. The Jk designation for the Kidd blood group represents the initials of the baby, John Kidd, who was affected with hemolytic disease of the newborn (HDN) from the individual (Mrs. Kidd) in whom the antibody had first been identified. But the Jk designation was used because the letter *K* had been previously used to identify the Kell blood group system. The Indian blood group system was named because it was found in individuals from India, and a similar system accounted for the use of the term *Bombay blood group* because the first examples were found from individuals in the city of Bombay, India. Similarly, the blood group S represents the city of Sydney, Australia, where the first anti-S was discovered. Interestingly, the letter *g* in the Xg blood group designation stands for the *g* in Grand Rapids, Michigan, where this blood group was discovered. Many more interesting vignettes about blood group terminology can be found in the summary by Garratty et al. (70).

Most newly reported red cell antigen specificities are variations of the more than 600 red cell antigens that have been identified (71). These can be categorized in 11 major systems, which account for 172 of the antigens (Table 57-3). Some additional antigens are thought to be part of these systems, but the relation has not been clearly established. Other antigens represent weakly expressed forms of well-defined antigens. In addition, more than 200 low-incidence and more than 100 high-incidence antigens are thought to be independent of all others. This section describes the red cell antigens and systems most commonly involved in the clinical practice of transfusion medicine. For a more comprehensive description of the hundreds of known red cell antigens, the reader is referred to reference texts (71,72). Currently, the International Society for Blood Transfusion recognizes 267 antigens, 221 of which belong to one of 25 blood group systems (Table 57-3).

The structure of the red cell membrane and the composition of its major components have been studied extensively. During the past few years, considerable information has been obtained about the composition of many red cell blood group antigens and the relation of these to red cell membrane components. The biochemical composition, molecular weight, and number of antigens/red cell for some antigens have been established (Table 57-3). Blood group antigens are glycoproteins or polypeptides, except for ABO antigens, which are glycolipids. The specificity of several blood group antigens is determined by sugars; thus, the genes responsible for these antigens code for

an intermediate molecule, which is usually an enzyme that creates the antigenic specificity by transferring sugar molecules. The antigens of other blood group systems (Rh and Kell) are proteins and, thus, are directly determined by genes. The size of the antigen-containing molecule ranges from 25 to 100 kd, and the number of antigen sites ranges from 1500 to more than 1 million/red cell (Table 57-3).

ABO System

In a footnote of his laboratory book in 1900, Landsteiner commented on observations of agglutination or hemolysis between the blood of different workers in his laboratory. However, the first formal report of the ABO blood groups was published in 1901 (73).

Landsteiner named the first two blood group antigens *A* and *B*, using the first two letters of the alphabet. Red cells not reacting with anti-A or anti-B were called *type C*. In 1902, red cells that reacted with both anti-A and anti-B were observed, but these were not called *AB*; instead, *type C* continued to be used to refer to this blood type. In 1910, Landsteiner reported serologic results of all four blood types but still did not use the terms *AB* and *O* (70). It appears that the first use of the terms *O* and *AB* occurred in 1911 (70), but it is not clear whether the lack of *A* and *B* was a zero or really was meant to be the letter *O*, which possibly could have come from the German word *ohne* that means *without*. There were other problems with the ABO terminology during its first several decades. A scheme using roman numerals was proposed, and as many as 85% of American hospitals used the roman numeral terminology as late as 1929, while only approximately 5% used the Landsteiner; at about this time, Landsteiner suggested the universal adoption of the symbols A, B, O, and AB because of the confusion: This was done.

The ABO system is clinically the most important red cell antigen system because most persons have circulating A and B antibodies that are usually complement-fixing antibodies and cause intravascular hemolysis. The antigenic determinants for A, B, and H are found widely throughout the environment on bacteria, plants, food, and dust. Exposure to these antigens causes the normal development of antibodies against whichever ABH antigens are absent in the individual (Table 57-4).

COMPOSITION

The ABH antigen activity is determined by sugars that are linked either to polypeptides (forming a glycoprotein) or to lipids (forming a glycolipid). Because the antigenic activity is determined by sugars and resides in a carbohydrate structure, the antigens are not directly determined by genes. Instead, the ABH genes determine proteins that are sugar-transferring enzymes, which are collectively called *glycosyltransferases*. The gene for the ABH system is on chromosome 9 (74,75). Each A, B, and H gene codes for a different enzyme (glycosyltransferase), which places a different sugar on the polypeptide or lipid to

TABLE 57-4. Genes and Antigens of the ABH System and ABO Type of Donor Red Cells Suitable for Patients of Different A130 Types

Gene	Glycosyl Transferase	Antigen-Determining Sugar	ABH Antigen	ABO Type	ABO Antibody Present	Preferable Donor	Other Acceptable Donors[a]
A	*N*-Acetyl galactosamine transferase	*N*-Acetyl galactosamine	A	A	B	A	O
B	D-Galactosyl transferase	D-Galactose	B	B	A	B	O
H	L-Fucosyl transferase	L-Fucose	H	O	A & B	O	None
A & B	—	—	A & B	AB	None	AB	A or B or O

[a]If blood is used as red blood cells.

produce the unique antigen (Table 57-4). The H gene enables the attachment of L-fucose to the polypeptide or lipid chain. If no A or B gene is present, the H specificity remains, and the person is a type O; these red cells do not react with anti-A or -B. If an A or B gene or both are present, additional sugars are attached to the L-fucose, giving A, B, or AB specificity.

ABH antigens are widely distributed throughout the body. The ABH antigens present on red cells may be in either the glycoprotein or glycolipid form. ABH glycolipids are also part of most endothelial and epithelial membranes. In addition, the ABH glycolipids are present in a soluble form in plasma. Most other body fluids and secretions contain soluble ABH antigens but in the glycoprotein form. The ability to secrete soluble ABH antigens is controlled by a secretor (Se) gene, which is separate from the ABH system.

The genes for the transferases that determine the red cell ABO type are localized to chromosome 9 q34 (75) and have been cloned (76,77). The A gene is 1062 base pairs long and encodes a 353–amino acid transferase. The O gene is identical to the A gene, except that there is a single base deletion at position 258. This causes a frameshift and results in the production of a 115–amino acid transferase that is functionally inactive. Thus, the B gene differs from A by having four consistent base substitutions causing four amino acid substitutions and accounting for the different specificity of the B transferase from the A transferase (17,72,81).

ANTIGEN DISTRIBUTION AND SUBGROUPS

In a normal adult, the number of A antigen sites ranges from 1.6 (A_1 individual) to 700 million (A_m individual), and the number of B antigen sites is 1.6 million; the number of A,B antigen sites totals 800,000. Normal newborns have approximately one-third the number of antigen sites found in adults. Before the structure and number of A and B antigens were known, it was observed that red cells from some group A persons react more weakly with anti-A sera. These A subgroups were named A_2, A intermediate, A_3, and A_x. These differences in reactivity appear to be due to variability in the number of antigen sites, although the A_2 differs slightly from A_1, and some persons with the weak A_2 subgroups form anti-A antibodies. The sera of some group A_2 individuals may contain A antibodies. These usually do not react at 37°C and are not considered clinically significant. In rare situations in which the anti-A reacts at 37°C, donors whose red cells are A_2 can be easily identified, and a compatible blood can be provided.

Subgroups of B exist but are rare. Persons in this subgroup may also have anti-B in their sera. Because donors with B subgroup red cells are also rare, group O red cells can be used for transfusion.

BOMBAY TYPE

The rare Bombay phenotype, first recognized in India, lacks the H gene and is homozygous for its allele h (they are hh). The notation O_h is used for the Bombay type. The lack of an H gene does not allow the attachment of L-fucose to the protein or lipid; thus, these persons have little H antigen. They type as group O, because their red cells do not react with anti-A or anti-B, and their sera contain anti-A and anti-B. Their sera also contain anti-H and react with group O red cells. Such persons are rare, which is fortunate, because finding compatible red cells is extremely difficult. The only suitable red cells are those from another Bombay person.

ANTIBODIES OF THE ABH SYSTEM

ABH antibodies begin to appear during the first few months of life, probably from exposure to ABH antigen–like substances in the environment. Because of this, they are called *naturally occurring antibodies*, but the implication that they form without anti-

genic stimulation is incorrect. Anti-A or anti-B antibodies are usually combinations of IgM and IgG (Table 57-4). Because of the IgM content, these sera almost always cause agglutination, even at room temperature, of red cells containing the corresponding antigen. The IgM composition makes these antibodies effective in fixing complement, and they can be dangerous clinically.

Immunization to A or B antigens can also occur by transfusion of incompatible red cells, inoculation with vaccines containing A or B antigens, transfusion of plasma containing soluble A or B antigens, or pregnancy with an ABO-incompatible fetus. After these kinds of immunizations, the A or B antibody may become more active at 37°C, have a higher IgG component, increase in titer or avidity, and become more strongly hemolytic and, thus, even more clinically dangerous.

Anti-H antibodies can occur in persons with little or no H antigen on their red cells. Thus, Bombay-type persons (who lack the H gene and do not make H antigens) have an active anti-H that binds complement and causes hemolysis. A few persons of type A or AB make anti-H, probably because almost all their H antigen has been converted to A or B. These anti-H antibodies usually do not react at body temperatures and do not cause hemolysis.

Two approaches are under development for the creation of "universal RBCs" that would not have recognizable A or B antigens. The first of these is enzymatically converted group O cells. This strategy is based on the use of α-N-acetylgalactosaminidase for cleavage of the sugars that create the A antigen specificity and α-galactosidase for cleavage of the sugars that provide the group B specificity. Treatment of A or B cells with these enzymes has the potential to cleave sugars, and the resulting red cells would have the group O phenotype (78). Pioneering work by Jack Goldstein and colleagues at the New York Blood Center demonstrated that this strategy was possible, and a recent clinical trial (79) in patients who received group B red cells enzymatically converted to group O confirmed that this approach is clinically possible. Additional studies are presently under way involving conversion of group A red cells to group O.

A separate approach is the creation of "stealth red cells." With stealth red cells, the RBC antigens are masked by treating the red cells with polyethylene glycol. The polyethylene glycol is coupled to proteins on the RBC surface, reducing their immunogenicity while allowing the proteins to function normally (78). Initial results demonstrated that polyethylene glycol–treated red cells had significantly less agglutination with antibodies of the ABO, Rh, Kell, Duffy, and Kidd systems (80,81). Studies in humans of the use of these stealth red cells have not yet been reported.

If either or both of these approaches are successful, the benefit to blood banking and transfusion therapy is readily apparent. Many inventory management issues would become irrelevant, and red cells could be readily available to immunized patients without the complexity of finding compatible red cells if stealth cells were used (78).

Rh System

The second most important red cell antigen system is the Rh system. This is because a substantial proportion of the population lacks the Rh antigen known as *D*. The probability of becoming immunized to the D antigen is high, and anti-D has serious clinical effects, causing HDN or transfusion reactions. In addition to the clinical importance of the Rh system, a lively scholarly debate occurred over the years about the genetics of this system. Rh is the most complex blood group system, with 45 different antigens.

DISCOVERY

In 1939, Levine and Stetson (82) reported the case of a woman who delivered a fetus affected by HDN and who, on receiving a transfusion of her husband's blood, experienced a severe transfusion reaction. The researchers hypothesized correctly that the woman had become immunized to a factor that her child had inherited from her husband (the father) but that she lacked. In 1940, Landsteiner and Wiener (83) obtained an antibody from guinea pigs and rabbits immunized with rhesus monkey red cells. This serum had a pattern of reactivity similar to that of Levine and Stetson's patient, so the blood group system was named *Rh* for *rhesus monkey*. Later work established that the animal antirhesus sera and the human antibody did not detect the same antigen, but, by that time, the nomenclature was established. The pattern of reactivity and the antigen identified by the animal sera has been named *LW* in honor of Landsteiner and Weiner. LW is assigned to a different red cell antigen system from Rh.

NOMENCLATURE AND GENETICS
The antigen detected by Levine and Stetson's patient's serum is the D antigen. This is present in approximately 85% of North American whites and is the basis for determining Rh positivity or negativity. That is, persons whose red cells contain the D antigen are Rh positive and those whose red cells lack the D antigen are Rh negative.

Two other pairs of antigens (C and c, E and e) were identified that seemed to be inherited in various combinations with D and became part of the Rh system. These four antigens with D account for almost all of the Rh-related transfusion problems encountered in practice. Different nomenclature systems were used to describe the Rh system, but these are now of historic interest only. The Weiner system (84) supposed that the gene product was a single entity with multiple serologic specificities; the Fisher-Race (85) system postulated three closely linked loci, each with its own gene and gene product.

MOLECULAR BIOLOGY
After almost 50 years of debate about the genetics of the Rh system, molecular biology techniques have provided a considerable amount of information in a few short years. There are three distinct integral membrane proteins (molecular weight, approximately 32 kd) that carry the Rh antigens. The Rh gene locus is located on chromosome 1 p32-p36 and is composed of two genes (86). One gene (RHD) controls expression of the D antigen (87) and one (RHCE) controls expression of the CcEe antigens. Thus, Rh-positive (D-positive) persons carry both genes, whereas Rh-negative persons who lack the D antigen carry only the RHCE gene. The two genes are highly homologous and may be the result of duplication of one original ancestral gene. The products of the genes are polypeptides that, unlike most cell surface proteins, are not glycosylated. The D and CcEe proteins differ by only 32 to 35 amino acids, depending on the CcEe phenotype. The C/c and E/e polymorphisms are caused by different amino acid combinations or positions on the CcEe protein. The Rh protein spans the red cell surface membrane 12 times with internal and external loops. Rh epitopes depend on the tertiary structure of these loops.

D VARIANT, OR D^U
Many red cell antigens show different degrees of reactivity, but these differences are more of a problem with the D antigen, because all donors and patients are typed for D, and D-negative red cells should be chosen for D-negative patients. Some persons who inherit the D antigen have red cells that react weakly or not at all with certain anti-D reagents. Thus, these persons may appear to be Rh negative. This situation has been called *D variant*, *D^u*, or *weak D*. The D protein has several epitopes, some of which are missing in these variants. These "partial" D antigens may result from mutations in RHD or because part of RHD has been replaced by part of RHCE.

These observations are of intellectual interest but have little clinical impact. Persons who are weak D have the D antigen, although some may lack a part of it. Thus, only the rare recipient would make anti-D. Because these patients are rare in practice, it is not necessary to consider this situation. Current typing reagents are designed to detect these different weak D variants. Thus, additional steps are not necessary to determine whether recipients who appear to be Rh negative are, in fact, weak D. They receive Rh-negative blood.

RH NULL TYPE
Persons rarely lack all the Rh proteins and antigens. This is due to the absence of a gene that regulates the expression of Rh antigens or to the presence of an amorphic gene at the Rh locus on chromosome 1. Rh null persons have abnormal red cell morphology and hemolytic anemia, which is usually sufficiently compensated to result in only mild anemia. If exposed to Rh-positive red cells, these persons make an antibody that reacts with all red cells other than Rh null and is considered to be reactive against the entire Rh molecule.

STRUCTURE AND COMPOSITION OF THE D ANTIGEN
The D antigen is a 28- to 32-kd protein that is associated with the red cell membrane skeleton (88,89). The protein has an external and intramembranous domain but no cytoplasmic domain. The total amount of D protein/antigen site is approximately 60,000, indicating that the antigen is probably a dimer or trimer of D proteins (90), because there are approximately 30,000 D antigen sites/cell (91). These cannot move laterally within the membrane but instead are fixed at approximately 70 nm apart (92,93). This distance between the D antigen sites probably accounts, in part, for the lack of complement fixation in D antigen–antibody reactions.

RH ANTIBODIES
The most common Rh antibody is anti-D. This is almost always an IgG, does not cause agglutination of red cells *in vitro*, acts at 37°C, and does not bind complement effectively but causes serious transfusion reactions and red cell destruction by accelerated clearance of cells through the mononuclear phagocyte system.

Kell System
The Kell blood group system includes 23 alloantigens, which can be grouped into four sets of antithetical antigens, two unpaired high-frequency antigens, and 12 related high-frequency antigens. The K gene is autosomal dominant and has a frequency that differs considerably in different populations. The Kell system is important clinically because the K antigen is next in immunogenicity after D and because antibodies to Kell system antigens (or anti-Ks) are usually IgG, react at 37°C, and do not bind complement but can cause severe hemolytic transfusion reactions and HDN. Donors or recipients are not usually typed for Kell unless the recipient has a Kell antibody.

The Kell gene has been cloned and found to be located on the 7 q33 chromosome (94). The gene produces a 731–amino acid, 93-kd transmembrane glycoprotein. The protein has a 47–amino acid domain within the red cell and a large extracellular C-terminal domain that contains the Kell antigen determinants (95).

The Kell molecule is a 93-kd glycoprotein (96,97) that apparently is associated with a small (20- to 30-kd), poorly characterized, second protein (97). Most, if not all, of the Kell antigens are located on this single 93-kd molecule (98). The antigenicity of Kell antigens is inactivated when the glycoprotein is isolated using reducing conditions that break the disulfide bonds. Thus, the antigen reactivity probably depends on maintenance of the tertiary structure of the molecule's surface. The Kell molecule glycoprotein is the same size as band 3 of the red cell membrane skeleton; these are different molecules. The Kell glycoprotein is an enzyme similar to neutral endopeptidase and endothelium-converting enzyme. Its function *in vivo* is not known because Kell null individuals appear to be healthy.

Another reason that the Kell blood group is interesting is its relation to chronic granulomatous disease (CGD), in which the congenital absence of a superoxide-producing cytochrome interferes with the normal oxidative response of neutrophils so that their bactericidal activity is diminished, and patients experience severe, life-threatening infections. The K_x gene locus appears to be on the X chromosome near the CGD locus; thus, approximately 10% of patients have Kell system abnormalities. In the McLeod phenotype, the red cells express Kell system antigens very weakly and lack K_x, a Kell system precursor substance. Persons with the McLeod phenotype also have bizarre-shaped red cells and a chronic compensated hemolytic anemia. The occurrence of this phenotype in some patients with CGD led to the discovery that the McLeod syndrome involves a spectrum of abnormalities in addition to those involving the Kell system. Other associated abnormalities occur in red cells (acanthocytosis, compensated hemolysis, and increased red cell phosphorylation); the nervous system (areflexia, choreiform movements, mild dysarthria, neurogenic myopathy, and muscle wasting); the cardiovascular system (cardiomyopathy); and granulocytes (CGD). Other changes such as reduced haptoglobin, elevated creatinine phosphokinase, lactic dehydrogenase, and carbonic anhydrase may be found.

Duffy System

The Duffy system is composed of six antigens that are not present on other blood cells or body tissues. Approximately 13,000 Fy^a or Fy^b antigen sites are on each red cell in persons homozygous for the Fy^a or Fy^b gene (99). Red cells from persons heterozygous for Fy^a or Fy^b contain approximately 6000 antigen sites/cell. These red cells often show a weaker agglutination than homozygous cells in serologic tests—a phenomenon called *dosage effect*.

The composition of the Duffy antigens is not completely understood. The molecule containing Fy^a and Fy^b appears to be a glycoprotein with a molecular weight between 40 and 66 kd (72,100). The Duffy system is unusual because the antigen frequency varies substantially in different racial groups. In general, the Fy^a gene has a high incidence in Asians and a moderate incidence in whites, and Fy^a and Fy^b have a low incidence in Africans. Both antigens are detectable during fetal development and are present in normal strengths at birth. Duffy was the first blood group locus to be identified on an autosome—chromosome 1. The locus is on the long arm near the centromere.

Fy^a antibodies may cause severe, even fatal, hemolytic transfusion reactions or severe HDN; however, transfusion reactions to Fy^a are not common, and the HDN is usually mild. Anti-Fy^b is an infrequent cause of transfusion reactions and HDN. Other Duffy system antibodies have not been implicated in clinical problems.

One of the most interesting features of the Duffy system is its association with malaria. Fy^a(a–b–) red cells are resistant to infection by *Plasmodium knowlesi* (101) and probably by *Plasmodium vivax*. The malaria parasites are unable to penetrate red cells lacking the Fy^a or Fy^b antigens because they do not establish a junction site (102). In West Africa, most blacks are Fy(a–b–) and are resistant to *P. vivax* malaria; thus, a natural selection process might have been in effect. The Duffy glycoprotein is also the erythrocyte chemokine receptor. The function of this receptor is not known, but it binds several chemotactic and inflammatory peptides and may be involved in clearance of inflammatory mediators.

Kidd System

The three antigens of the Kidd system were discovered during the 1950s; no new antigens in this system have been reported since then. Red cells from persons homozygous for Jk^a contain approximately 11,000 antigen sites (99); Kidd antigens are not present on other blood cells or tissues. Kidd antigens may be altered by products of bacteria in infected patients. For instance, *Proteus mirabilis* and *Streptococcus faecalis* can cause Jk(b–) cells to become reactive with anti-Jk^b, and autohemolysis can occur. The Kidd locus has undergone several different chromosome assignments during the past 15 years. The locus is believed to be on chromosome 18. It is not known whether this genetic locus codes for the Kidd antigens or for a precursor substance or enzyme that determines production of the blood group antigen.

Kidd antibodies are IgG and can cause severe hemolytic transfusion reactions, but they usually cause only mild HDN. *In vitro* Kidd antibodies may react weakly and cause severe hemolysis despite being IgG. Kidd antibodies usually activate complement. The relatively low number of Kidd antigen sites (11,000) should mean that the distance between antigen sites is too great for complement activation by an IgG molecule; the antigens probably are clustered, thus accounting for weak serologic reactivity, complement activation by IgG, and severe clinical effects.

A unique characteristic of Kidd antibodies is that they often disappear. Thus, they may cause delayed hemolytic transfusion reactions. This occurs when the patient has been immunized previously by pregnancy or transfusion but no longer has circulating antibody so that all the pretransfusion tests are compatible; yet if the patient receives Kidd-positive red cells, the antibody may be resynthesized rapidly, causing hemolysis of the transfused red cells a few hours to days later. The Kidd antigens are part of the molecule that serves as the urea transporter in red cells. Thus, Jk(a–b–) red cells are resistant to urea lysis.

Lutheran System

The Lutheran system involves a total of 18 antigens—four pairs of antithetical antigens and a seventh antigen that appears to involve one of the pairs of antigens. In addition, nine other antigens have Lutheran system nomenclature because they are phenotypically related to the Lutheran system. These para-Lutheran antigens are not genetically related to the Lutheran system.

The structure, composition, and number of Lutheran system antigens/red cell are not well established. Lu^b activity has been found in glycoprotein molecules of 78 to 85 kd, and the number of antigen sites has been reported to be 1000 to 4000/cell, depending on the zygosity. The antigens are not well developed at birth, and so antigens and antibodies of the Lutheran system cause only mild HDN. Lutheran antibodies may be IgG or IgM, or mixtures of these with IgA. The most common Lutheran antibodies are anti-Lu^a and anti-Lu^b.

Anti-Lu^a is usually not active at body temperatures and thus not a problem clinically. It is rarely found because the incidence of Lu(a+) red cells is low; thus, patients are rarely exposed to the antigen. Laboratory test cells often are not Lu(a+), so the antibody may not be detected, but patients with the antibody would rarely receive a transfusion of Lu(a+) red cells. Anti-Lu^b may cause accelerated destruction of incompatible red cells. This antibody is also rarely found because almost all persons are Lu(b+).

MN System

The M and N antigens were the second blood group discovered—long before Rh. The system has 38 antigens: M and N, which are antithetical; S and s, which are antithetical; and U, which is present in all persons who possess M or N and S or s antigens and in some S–s– persons. The MNU-negative people are usually blacks. Alleles are controlled at the same gene locus. In addition to these five antigens, this system has 33 other variants (72).

The composition of antigens of this system is well understood. MN antigens are on the sialic acid–rich glycoprotein called *glycophorin A*, and Ss antigens are on the sialic acid–rich glycoprotein called *glycophorin B*. The amino acid sequences of these sialic acid–rich glycoproteins and the location of the antigen activity have been described.

Although anti-M antibodies are often IgG, they are usually not active at body temperatures and do not cause hemolysis, transfusion reactions, or HDN. Unusual examples of anti-M may be active at 37°C, and these can be clinically significant. Anti-N is almost always IgM, not reactive at body temperature, and not clinically significant. Anti-S, anti-s, and anti-U are usually IgG warm active antibodies, which may have clinical effects by causing transfusion reactions, hemolysis, or HDN, although these antibodies are rare.

The antigens of the MNSs system are located on the red cell membrane sialoglycoproteins. The M and N antigens are on the terminal portion of glycophorin A, of which there are 200,000 to 1 million copies/red cell. The Ss and probably the U antigens are located on the terminal portion of glycophorin B, of which there are 50,000 to 250,000 copies/red cell. Glycophorin A has a molecular weight of 43,000 and is composed of 131 amino acids. The MN activity is located in approximately 70 external amino acids. The remaining amino acids are intramembranous or intracytoplasmic.

P System

The P system was discovered with MNSs when Landsteiner and Levine were injecting rabbits with human red cells. The system actually contains only one antigen (P_1), but several others are grouped with P_1 due to biochemical and serologic similarities. These include P_2, p, P_1^k, and P_2^k. All except 1 in 100,000 persons have the P antigen. The two most common phenotypes are P_1 (P_1P) and P_2 (PP); each of these phenotypes has trace amounts of P^k. The amount of P_1 antigen varies greatly among individuals, is not well developed at birth, and does not reach adult levels until the person is approximately 7 years of age. P-negative (pp) persons are rare.

P system antigens, like the I antigens, seem to be formed in a sequence of steps instead of being antithetical and controlled by allelic genes. They seem to originate from a common precursor; P^k is the precursor of P, but neither P^k nor P are the precursors of P_1 (2). The antigenic determinants are carbohydrates that are linked to glycosphingolipids in the red cell membrane. Genetic control of the P system has been proposed to involve two or three loci. These genes code for enzymes that add the carbohydrates to the lipids in a manner similar to the ABO system genes.

Antigen structures similar to those of the P system are found in animal tissue, pigeons, doves, worms, and *Echinococcus* cyst fluid. Thus, many antibodies of the P system are called *naturally occurring antibodies*, although, as with ABO antibodies, this is not technically correct. Because some parasites have antigen structures similar to P system antigens, anti-P_1 is sometimes found in patients with parasitic infections.

Antibodies of the P system are common and can range from those that are cold active and clinically insignificant to those that cause severe hemolysis. Anti-P_1 is common, usually cold active, and not clinically significant unless it reacts at body temperatures; anti-PP_1P^k (made by persons with the rare pp phenotype), and anti-P (made by persons with the rare P^k phenotype) cause hemolysis *in vitro* and *in vivo*. A high incidence

of miscarriage occurs in women with the pp phenotype, and it has been suggested that anti-PP_1P^k may have a pathologic role. Auto–anti-P is the specificity of the Donath-Landsteiner antibody found in paroxysmal cold hemoglobinuria. The antibody is often called *biphasic* because it binds to the red cell at cool temperatures and then causes hemolysis at warmer (body) temperatures.

Lewis System

The Lewis system is not a blood group system. Lewis antigens are soluble in body fluids, and the antigens present in plasma are adsorbed onto red cells. The Lewis system also differs from most other blood group systems in that the Lewis genes must interact with Hh and Se genes for Lewis antigens to be produced. There are two antigens in the Lewis system: Le^a and Le^b. The Lewis antigenic specificity is determined by the carbohydrate fucose. The *Le* gene produces a glycosyltransferase, which adds a fucose molecule to a precursor substance (type 1 chain) to produce the Lewis antigen. Thus, Lewis antigens are glycosphingolipids. The exact Lewis antigen produced is determined by the presence or absence of the Se gene. The Se gene determines the location on the precursor substance (type 1 chain) to which the fucose is added (by the Le gene). Thus, two different antigen specificities are produced, depending on whether the Se gene is present.

The red cells of newborns lack Lewis antigens, and no Lewis substance is in their plasma, although it is present in their saliva. The adult Le^a antigen phenotype is attained by approximately 1 year of age but not until approximately 7 years of age for Le^b. Lewis antigens are reduced during pregnancy. An increased lipoprotein to red cell mass results in a shift of glycolipids from red cells to plasma, reducing the Lewis antigen content on the red cells. After transfusion, the transfused donor red cells convert to the Lewis type of the recipient. Thus, the Lewis antigen may be acquired or lost through the exchange of glycolipids between the plasma and red cell.

Lewis antibodies are common, usually react below body temperature, are mainly or entirely IgM, and are not clinically significant. These antibodies are usually found in patients who have not received transfusions and are thus sometimes called *natural*, a technically incorrect term because they are probably stimulated by environmental agents. Anti-Le^a is often found in pregnant women, but it is not clear whether the antibody is formed after immunization by fetal red cells. Lewis antibodies do not cause HDN, because they are usually IgM and cannot cross into the fetal circulation. In a few cases, anti-Le^a have caused hemolytic transfusion reactions; usually, the antibodies show reactivity at body temperatures. These reactions can be used as an indication of clinical significance. Lewis antibodies have been implicated in the rejection of transplanted Lewis-positive kidneys (103). The data on this subject conflict, but Lewis matching of donated kidneys is not done in most transplantation programs.

LW System

The LW antigen is named for Landsteiner and Weiner because it was defined on red cells by the original antibody that they prepared in rhesus monkeys and called *Rh*, and it appeared to be the same as the antibody found by Levine and Stetson in their case of HDN. Later, it was discovered that this original anti-Rh prepared in monkeys was really anti-LW. Rarely does a person lack LW^a antigen but can make anti-LW^a. Although LW is not genetically part of the Rh system, the expression of LW and Rh is related. Adult D-positive red cells exhibit stronger LW activity than D-negative red cells. Thus, weak examples of anti-LW may appear similar to anti-D because they react with D-positive

TABLE 57-5. Some Major Red Cell Antigen Systems and General Characteristics of Their Corresponding Antibodies[a]

Antigen System	Number of Antigens	Usual Antibody	Fix Complement	Optimal Reactivity Temperature	Cause		
					Transfusion Reactions	Hemolytic Disease of the Newborn	Red Cell Immune
ABH	11	IgM/IgG	Yes	Cold	Yes	Yes	No
Lewis	14	IgM	Yes	Cold	No	No	No
I	16	IgM	No	Cold	No	No	No
P	5	IgM	No	Cold	No	No	Yes
Rh	41	IgG	No	Warm	Yes	Yes	Yes
LW	3	IgG	No	Warm	Yes	No[b]	Yes
Duffy	5	IgG	No	Warm	Yes	Yes	Yes
Kell	21	IgG	No	Warm	Yes	Yes	Yes
Kidd	3	IgG	No	Warm	Yes	Yes	Yes
MN	46	IgG/IgM	No	Cold	No	No	No
Ss	46	IgG/IgM	No	Warm	Yes	Yes	Yes
Lutheran	7	IgM	No	Warm	Yes	Yes	Yes
Total	176						

Ig, immunoglobulin.
[a]The antibody characteristics described are generalizations. Particular antibodies may differ. Reference text should be consulted before decisions are made regarding the identity or clinical significance of an individual serum specimen.
[b]None reported.

but not D-negative red cells. This accounts for the original confusion between anti-Rh and LW. Four phenotypes have been observed: LW(a+b–), LW(a+b+), LW(a–b+), and LW(a–b–).

LW antibodies are rare. They may cause accelerated destruction of LW-positive red cells; thus, the presence of LW antibodies as an alloantibody should be considered clinically significant. Anti-LW may also occur as a transient autoantibody in persons who temporarily lose LW antigen activity.

I System

Ii is not a blood group system. I antigens are carbohydrates present on the interior structure of the ABH oligosaccharides. The antigens may be partly or extensively concealed but are revealed by the removal of terminal monosaccharides of the ABH chains. Thus, it appears that I and i are not alleles but are part of a sequence of steps. The antigen structure is a complex branched chain, and it has been suggested that the variety of antibodies that occurs in the I system is due to formation of antibodies against domains within the antigen molecule. Thus, the number of I antigen "sites" ranges from 32,000 to 120,000 (72).

One of the unique things about this system is that the presence of the I and i antigens changes with age. At birth, the i antigen is present, and I is almost undetectable. During the first 18 months of life, the i antigen declines and is replaced by I. The i antigen is converted to I by the action of a branching enzyme. In most adults, little i is detectable, except in rare persons who remain i+ and I–. The amount of Ii antigen on red cells varies in different persons, and this also leads to the appearance of different forms of I antigens.

Both anti-I and anti-i are usually autoantibodies that are optimally reactive at cold temperatures and not clinically significant. They do not cause HDN, and only one report is known of an anti-I that caused accelerated destruction of I red cells (104). Almost all normal adult serum contains anti-I; it is also found in cold agglutinin disease and transiently in *Mycoplasma* pneumonia infection. In cold agglutinin disease, the antibody changes characteristics and is an autologous anti-I that reacts at body temperature, fixes complement, and causes hemolysis. Anti-i is rare but has been associated with infectious mononucleosis.

I and i antigens are present in a soluble form in serum, saliva, breast milk, urine, and amniotic, ovarian, and hydatid cyst fluid.

Other Blood Group Antigen Systems

Several other systems of antigens exist (Table 57-4) but are not described in detail here: Wright, Xg, Diego, Cartwright, Scianna, Gerbich, Dombrock, and Colton. They and many other individual or groups of antigens are described in detail in reference texts (72). A couple of these are of particular interest. Several red cell antigens appear to be related to the HLA system (105). HLA class I antigens are present on red cell membranes in variable amounts—40 to 550 sites. They are attached to the membrane by β_2-microglobulin. These HLA-related red cell antibodies (also known as *high-titer, low-affinity*) are not considered clinically significant. Chido-Rogers antigens are C4A plasma components that remain attached to the red cell membrane. Chido-Rogers antibodies are not considered clinically significant.

Antibodies to Red Cell Antigens

Antibodies to red cell antigens vary widely in their characteristics and *in vivo* significance. Red cell antibodies can be categorized based on their Ig class; the antigen to which they are directed; the method of stimulation; their optimal temperature of reactions *in vitro*; whether they fix complement; their action on red cells *in vitro*; and their *in vivo* effect, such as whether they cause hemolysis, transfusion reactions, or HDN. A summary of the general characteristics of antibodies of the major red cell antigen systems is provided in the preceding section and in Table 57-5; specific antibodies within each system may exhibit different characteristics, so an appropriate reference text should be consulted before decisions are made regarding the identity or potential clinical effect of a particular antibody. Almost all red cell antibodies are either IgG or IgM. Only rare examples of IgA red cell antibodies are found. Some clinical and laboratory differences between IgM and IgG red cell antibodies exist. The specificities of the most common red cell antibodies found in hospitalized patients, pregnant women, and normal blood donors differ slightly because of the nature of these populations.

The incidence of different antibodies depends on the prevalence of the antigen in the population and the immunogenicity of the antigen. Factors that determine immunogenicity are not fully understood. The combination of the 15% incidence of Rh-negative persons, the 65% likelihood of becoming immunized after exposure to one unit of Rh-positive blood, and the serious

TABLE 57-6. Phenotype, Antigen Frequency, and Molecular Association of Platelet-Specific Antigens

Phenotype		Antigen Frequency (%)	Platelet Membrane Glycoprotein Association
Traditional Nomenclature	International Nomenclature		
Pl^{A1}	HPA-1a	98	IIIa
Pl^{12}	HPA-1b	27	—
Pl^{E1}	NA	>99	Ibα
Pl^{E2}	NA	5	—
Bak^a	HPA-3a	85	IIb
Bak^b	HPA-3b	63	—
Pen^a	HPA-4a	>99	IIIa
Pen^b	HPA-4b	—	—
Ko^a	HPA-2a	14	Ib
Ko^b	HPA-2b	99	—
Pl^T	—	98	V
Br^a	HPA-5b	21	Ia
Br^b	HPA-5a	81	—
Gou^a	NA	81	gp 175/150
Gou^b	NA	64	—

NA, not assigned.
Data primarily from Kickler TS. Management of alloimmunized patients with amegakaryocytic thrombocytopenia. In: Smith DM, Summers SH, eds. *Platelets.* Arlington, VA: American Association Blood Banks, 1988:115; and von dem Borne, AEGKr, Kuijers IRWAM, Goldschmeding R. Platelet antigens in alloimmune thrombocytopenia. In: Nance SJ, ed. *Clinical and basic aspects of immunohematology.* Arlington, VA: American Association of Blood Banks, 1991:115, with permission of the American Association of Blood Banks.

TABLE 57-8. Genetic Locus and Antigen Frequency of Granulocyte-Specific Antigens

Locus	Antigen	Phenotype Frequency (%)
NA	NA1	46
	NA2	88
NB	NB1	97
	NB2	32
NC	NC1	91
ND	ND1	98
NE	NE1	23
HGA-3	3a	21
	3b	24
	3c	16
	3d	53
	3e	17

Data from McCullough J, Clay ME, Press C, et al. Granulocyte serology: a clinical and laboratory guide. Chicago: American Society of Clinical Pathologists Press, 1988.

membrane. In addition, there are seven different platelet-specific antigen systems (Table 57-6). Most of these have been localized to particular platelet membrane molecules. Both autoantibodies and alloantibodies are directed against these alloantigens. These platelet-specific antibodies may cause autoimmune thrombocytopenia or any of several different clinical problems or diseases due to alloimmunization (Table 57-7).

clinical effect of anti-D makes the Rh(D) antigen the most important non-ABO antigen.

The Fab portion of the Ig molecule binds to the antigen-combining site on the red cell surface. The avidity and binding constants for this antigen-antibody reaction vary widely for different red cell antibodies. After binding, the heavy-chain region of the antibody molecule determines the biologic effect of the antibody by activating complement or reacting with receptors in the fixed macrophages of the liver and spleen to cause accelerated red cell clearance.

Platelets

Platelets contain ABH and HLA antigens. Debate exists as to whether the ABO and HLA antigens are integral to the platelet membrane or adsorbed onto the platelet from their soluble form in plasma. Evidence suggests that some ABH antigens are intrinsic to the platelet membrane (106) and some are adsorbed onto the cell surface from the plasma that contains soluble A and B substance. The density of A antigen sites on platelets is only approximately 5% of that on red cells (107). In contrast to ABH antigens, HLA antigens are probably integral to the platelet

Polymorphonuclear Leukocytes

Granulocytes have been thought to contain ABH antigens on their surface, but recent studies have failed to demonstrate this (108,109). In addition, granulocytes labeled with indium 111 had normal intravascular recoveries and survivals and migrated normally into skin chambers when injected into subjects who were ABO incompatible with the granulocyte donors (110). However, it is prudent to consider the presence of ABO antigens on granulocytes as unresolved.

HLA-A, HLA-B, and HLA-C (class I) antigens are on the surface of granulocytes (111), but the antigens are fewer in number than on lymphocytes (112). These HLA antigens are, possibly, adsorbed onto the surface of granulocytes (113) rather than being an integral part of the membrane—but this is not established. It appears that HLA-D and -DR antigens are not on granulocytes (109).

Granulocytes also contain several alloantigen systems whose tissue distribution is limited to granulocytes or a few other cell types (Table 57-8). These granulocyte-specific antigen–antibody systems are involved in the pathophysiology of several clinical situations (Table 57-9). Both autoantibodies and alloantibodies have been identified, and each may cause severe clinical problems (114). Neutrophil-specific antibodies did not interfere with the successful engraftment of NA1-positive marrow in a patient with circulating anti-NA1 (115), although Stroncek and colleagues (116)

TABLE 57-7. Diseases and Clinical Conditions Due to Platelet-Specific Antibodies

	Most Common Antibody Specificity
Autoantibodies	
Autoimmune thrombocytopenia	Pl^{A1}
Drug-induced immune thrombocytopenia	?
Alloantibodies	
Alloimmune neonatal thrombocytopenia	Pl^{A1}
Posttransfusion purpura	Pl^{A1}
Refractoriness to platelet transfusion	?

TABLE 57-9. Clinical Situations in Which Granulocyte-Specific Antibody-Antigen Systems Are Causative Agents

Autoantibodies
  Autoimmune neutropenia
  Drug-induced immune neutropenia
Alloantibodies
  Febrile transfusion reactions
  Transfusion-related acute lung injury
  Alloimmune neonatal neutropenia
  Poor response to granulocyte transfusion

TABLE 57-10. Clinical Conditions with Red Cell Antigen Alteration

| Clinical Condition | Red Cell Antigen | | |
	Depressed	Increased	Antibody
A1HA	Rh-LW	i	Auto–anti-D, LW Anti-Kp^b
Leukemia with monosomy 7	ABH, Co^a	IiH	
Myelofibrosis	LW, Rh, ABH		
Hodgkin's disease			Anti-LW
Paroxysmal nocturnal hemoglobinuria		i	
Paroxysmal cold hemoglobinuria			Auto–anti-P
Ovalocytosis	Rh, LW, Ss, U, Kidd, Yt^a, Xg^a	H	
Chronic granulomatous disease	Kell		Anti-KL + K$_x$
Hereditary hemolytic anemia	Rh, Kell, Colton		
Sickle cell anemia stress		i	
Pregnancy	LW, Lewis, Sd^a		Anti-LW Anti-Lewis
Bacterial infections	Acquired B-antigen, T activation		
Chromosomal defects	Rh, MN, Duffy		

TABLE 57-11. Rare Blood Types Associated with Abnormal Red Cell Morphology or Membrane Constituents

Phenotypes	Biochemical Modification	Morphologic and Functional Abnormality
Rh$_{null}$	No Rh or LW antigens	Stomatocytes, spherocytes; partially compensated hemolytic anemia
McLeod	Weak expression of normal Kell antigens; K$_x$ absent	Acanthocytes; partially compensated hemolytic anemia
K$_O$	No normal Kell antigens; K$_x$ present	None observed
p	No normal P antigens; decreased globoside and ceramide trihexoside	None observed
p^k	Normal P^1 antigen; ceramide trihexoside increased; globoside decreased	None observed
P1^{pk}	Increased Gl-3 (NAc galactose transferase deficiency)	None observed
Lu(a–b–)	Not studied	Abnormal scanning electron microscopy—wrinkled, furrowed appearance
En(a–)	Glycophorin A absent; depressed MN antigens; enhanced Rho antigen	None observed
S–s–	Glycophorin B absent or abnormal	None observed
M^{k}M^k	Both glycophorin A and glycophorin B absent	None observed

reported a case in which the NB1 granulocyte antibody, which is present in high titer, apparently caused prolonged neutropenia after transplantation with marrow from an NB1-positive donor. These observations are consistent with evidence that these antigens are not present on promyelocytes, myeloblasts, and earlier uncommitted stem cells but become expressed during myeloid maturation (117). Thus, the granulocyte-specific antigens can be thought of as differentiation antigens specific for this cell line, which become expressed during maturation of the cell.

Significance of Blood Groups

RED BLOOD CELLS

Red cell blood group antigens have been of interest to blood bankers because of their role in transfusion therapy and to geneticists because of their ability to serve as a genetic marker. During the past few years, the chromosome location of most blood groups has been established (Table 57-5). Linkage between some blood groups and diseases is known, and this helps to localize some blood group genes to certain areas of the chromosomes. Studies of the red cell membrane have also begun to yield information about the structure and composition of red cell (blood group) antigens. Thus, the red cell antigens are no longer of interest only to the serologist–blood banker but are recognized increasingly as parts of important structural or functional components of the cell membrane. Red cell antigens are associated with a variety of conditions ranging from hemolytic anemias to malignancies, stress, and pregnancy (Table 57-10). Some clinical conditions may alter the expression of blood groups, and some rare blood types are associated with abnormal red cell morphology or membrane constituents (Table 57-11).

Several cell functions primarily dealing with membrane transport have been identified. These include acting as an anion exchanger (Diego), a water channel (Colton), or a urea transporter (Kidd). Other cell functions include acting as an adhesion molecule or a receptor for certain foreign agents such as malaria (Duffy); *Helicobacter pylori* (Le^b and O antigens) (P); *E. coli* (Knops); *Mycobacterium leprae*; (P) and parvovirus B19; chemokine receptor (Duffy), and adhesion (Indian and Xg). Glycoproteins of the Ig superfamily carry some blood group antigens (Lutheran, LW, and OK), but their functions are not known. They may involve adhesive interactions important for erythropoiesis. Red cell surface proteins that protect the red cell from autologous complement also carry blood groups (Cromer and Knops). Some red cell blood groups are part of glycoproteins that anchor the membrane to the cytoskeleton (Diego, Gerbich).

PLATELETS

In addition to involvement in several clinical situations (Table 57-9), some of the platelet-specific antigens are located on molecules that have other important functions. These may be involved in platelet aggregation or platelet adhesion to endothelial cells. It is likely that future studies will demonstrate that abnormalities of these molecules cause alterations in platelet antigens or that altered platelet antigen strength or specificity may affect the structure or function of the cell.

NEUTROPHILS

As with platelets, neutrophil-specific antigens are involved in several important clinical situations. The location of the neutrophil-specific antigen on particular molecules is not as extensively defined as for platelets. The genes for the NA antigens have been cloned (118,119), and these antigens are part of the Fc receptor molecule (120), and the NB1 antigen may be part of the receptor for the chemoattractant formyl-methionyl-leucyl-phenylalanine (121). Thus, it is likely that these neutrophil-specific antigens also will prove to be important in cell membrane structure and function.

LABORATORY DETECTION OF BLOOD GROUPS AND PRETRANSFUSION TESTING

Red Blood Cells

IMMUNOLOGIC MECHANISMS OF RED CELL DESTRUCTION
Because most red cell antibodies are IgM or IgG, red cell destruction involves those two kinds of Igs either with or without complement. Red cells containing bound IgG undergo accelerated clearance through the spleen, where Fc receptors of the phagocyte bind to the IgG molecules leading to phagocytosis of the red cell. Although this process does not require complement, binding and phagocytosis are accelerated if the IgG-coated red cell also contains bound complement components.

Complement has one of two roles in the immune destruction of red cells: accelerated clearance by interacting with complement receptors in the fixed macrophage system or causation of membrane damage leading to direct cell lysis. Complement can be activated by either IgG or IgM, although IgM is much more effective, probably because the nature of the IgM molecule places several Fc receptor sites in close proximity. The subclasses of IgG1 and IgG3 are more effective in binding complement than IgG4. The exact mechanisms that determine the ability of different red cell antibodies to activate complement are not known. The situation is more complex than merely the number of Fc sites in close enough proximity to activate the first component of complement (C1). For instance, in general, anti-D (an IgG) is not effective in activating complement compared with anti-K or Jk^a (also IgG), which react with antigens that actually have fewer antigen sites than D sites on the red cell.

Activation of C1 begins the complement cascade sequence leading to formation of the membrane attack complex (C5 to C9), which causes lysis of the red cell. The complement system involves several proteins (complement components), the activation of which is influenced by a variety of inhibitors or proteases. Thus, the process often does not proceed to completion of the membrane attack complex and cell lysis. Red cells may be coated with certain complement components that cause accelerated clearance of the red cells by interaction with complement receptors on cells of the fixed macrophage system. The first of these key steps is the activation of C3. After several activation and enzyme cleavage steps, the C3d remains bound to the red cell membrane antigen-antibody complex. Red cells containing bound C3d undergo accelerated clearance in the liver by interaction with complement receptors in the fixed macrophage system.

Red cell serologic reagents have been developed to detect C3d bound to red cells. These reagents are used for direct antiglobulin testing to determine whether anemia or accelerated red cell destruction may be due to complement activation or complement-binding antibodies or both. For many years, a lively debate took place regarding the value of anti-C3 activity in the antihuman globulin serum used for antibody detection tests and crossmatching. The rationale was that the ability to detect not only IgG but also C3d on the red cell would enhance the likelihood of finding clinically significant antibodies. Many clinically insignificant antibodies active at cold temperatures bind complement. Because these cold antibodies are present normally in many persons, the addition of anti-C3d to antiglobulin serum led to many false-positive tests. As a result, this

practice has been abandoned, and the antiglobulin used for red cell compatibility testing is anti-IgG.

Although detection of C3d bound to red cells is not helpful for compatibility testing, it is helpful in the evaluation of possible immune hemolytic anemia (see Chapter 53). For instance, some patients with warm antibody–type autoimmune hemolytic anemia, cold agglutinin syndrome, and drug-induced immune hemolytic anemias may have red cells that react only with reagents containing anti-C3d activity and not with anti-IgG reagents. Thus, anti-C3 and anti-IgG are both used in direct antiglobulin (Coombs') testing.

INTRAVASCULAR HEMOLYSIS
The destruction of red cells by the complement membrane attack complex is called *intravascular hemolysis*. The red cell membrane is damaged, hemoglobin is released into the circulation, and the classic signs and symptoms of a hemolytic transfusion reaction are seen (see section Complications of Transfusion: Recognition and Management). ABO incompatibility is the best example of red cell antigen–antibody reactions that cause this kind of hemolysis.

EXTRAVASCULAR HEMOLYSIS
Red cell destruction caused by phagocytic cells of the fixed macrophage system is called *extravascular hemolysis*. This occurs primarily in the spleen and is associated with an increase in bilirubin and its metabolites. Actually, these distinctions are arbitrary, because complement may be involved in both intravascular and extravascular hemolysis, and the degree or severity of hemolysis may be a factor in the symptoms and laboratory findings. For instance, red cells undergoing phagocytosis in the fixed macrophage system may be only partially engulfed and may release some hemoglobin into the intravascular space, thus simulating intravascular hemolysis.

In practice, the red cell serologic tests for compatibility are designed to enhance and to speed the cell's reaction with IgM or IgG antibodies and to detect the reaction by looking for direct cell agglutination or using reagents such as anti-IgG to cause red cell agglutination.

SELECTION OF BLOOD TYPES FOR TRANSFUSION
For routine transfusions, red cells are selected that are identical with the patient's red cells for the ABO and Rh(D) antigens. In some situations, such as massive bleeding or an emergent need for transfusion, red cells that are not ABO and D identical may be used (see section Transfusion in Special Situations). When Rh-negative patients experience massive bleeding, it may be necessary to use Rh(D)-positive blood because no Rh-negative red cells are available. Because Rh-negative red cells lack the D antigen, the Rh-positive patient experiences no unusual adverse effect as long as he or she does not have an anti-D. However, there is approximately a 60% chance that the Rh-negative recipient will become immunized to D. Therefore, the decision to use Rh positive red cells for an Rh-negative patient should be made by consultation between the blood bank physician and the attending physician.

It may also be necessary to switch ABO types. When blood of a different ABO type is used, it is used as red cells, not whole blood, to avoid problems due to transfusion of antibodies contained in the plasma. Table 57-4 indicates the ABO types of donor blood that can be used. Despite the small amount of plasma in the red cell unit, hemolysis due to passive transfusion of antibody in these units can occur, although this is rare. The remote possibility of such a problem should not interfere with making red cells available rapidly in urgent situations.

Red Blood Cell Pretransfusion Compatibility Testing

The crossmatch is only one part of the pretransfusion or compatibility test. The term *pretransfusion testing* refers to all procedures involved in selecting blood products that "will have acceptable survival and will not cause clinically significant destruction of the recipient's own red cells." These procedures include the following:

1. Positive identification of recipient blood sample.
2. Proper labeling of the recipient. The label should be applied at the patient's bedside when the specimen is obtained to avoid sample mix-up that may lead to mistyping the patient and transfusion of ABO-incompatible red cells.
3. Review of transfusion service records for results of previous testing of samples from the recipient.
4. ABO and Rh typing. Many clinical conditions and diseases may make interpretation of the results of ABO and Rh typing difficult. Careful attention to detail and to the proper use and interpretation of controls is essential. The ABO and Rh type of the patient is confirmed on each blood sample used for pretransfusion testing to increase the safety of the transfusion by ensuring that the sample is from the correct patient. The ABO and Rh type of the donor blood will have been confirmed when the hospital receives the blood from its regional blood supplier.
5. Selection of blood components of appropriate ABO and Rh types.
6. Antibody detection test (indirect antiglobulin or Coombs' test). In this test, the patient's serum is reacted with red cells usually from two normal persons whose cells contain antigens reactive with all of the common clinically significant antibodies. The cells are usually purchased commercially and subject to FDA requirements for the antigens they contain and their strength of reactivity.

   The conditions of the antibody detection test usually involve the incubation of the patient's serum with test red cells suspended in saline or albumin followed by washing of the red cells, adding antihuman globulin, centrifuging, and looking for agglutination. Extensive literature describes the optimal technique for detecting different antibodies. Some of the methods that may be used are treating the red cells with enzymes, extending the length of incubation, changing the serum cell ratio, altering the incubation temperature, suspending the red cells in low–ionic-strength solution, and using chemicals such as polybrene to enhance agglutination. Some of these techniques are used routinely by some blood banks; others are suitable for use only in reference laboratories for investigation of certain antibodies.

   Red cell antibody detection techniques, which were traditionally done in tubes, have been modified and made more suitable for automation. The two fundamental technologies are solid phase testing and gel testing. The strengths of solid phase are an increased sensitivity to alloantibodies (more than gel), the fact that it does not pick up cold alloantibodies, and complete automation, which reduces the technologist's time. The weakness of the solid phase is that it picks up weak nonspecific alloantibodies and weak warm autoantibodies, which may then increase the technologist's time due to the necessity to work up these positive reactions.

   The gel method is more sensitive than the traditional tube method but less sensitive than the solid phase method. One advantage of the gel is the ease of training and standardization, as well as the availability of large-scale instruments to enable consolidation of testing. Red cell antibody screening and crossmatching are generally being converted to these methods.

   The cornerstone of red cell antibody detection is the use of antihuman globulin, formerly known as *Coombs' serum*. Antihuman globulin is prepared from the serum of rabbits immunized with human IgG (monospecific) or with the human complement C3d. Antihuman globulin detects IgG or C3 on the surface of red cells. Thus, if the patient's serum contains an IgG antibody that reacts with an antigen on the red cells used in antibody screening tests, it is detected using the antihuman IgG (Fig. 57-2). This test is extremely important because most clinically significant red cell antibodies are IgGs.

7. Crossmatch. In the major crossmatch, the recipient's serum is reacted with the intended donor's red cells. For patients in whom no antibodies are found in the antibody detection test, a simplified crossmatch that confirms ABO compatibility is performed if the patient has neither been pregnant nor received transfusions within the preceding 3 months (122–124). If antibodies were found in the antibody detection test, the major crossmatch is done with a technique similar to that used in the antibody detection test. This usually involves incubation at 37°C and the use of IgG. Various agents or procedural modifications may be used to attempt to enhance or to speed antigen-antibody reactions. The minor crossmatch is no longer used. In the minor crossmatch, the donor's serum was reacted with the patient's red cells to detect antibodies in the donor that might cause hemolysis of the patient's red cells. Although a few such cases have been reported, these were usually associated with whole blood transfusion. Today, the potential problem of donor antibodies is avoided in two ways. An antibody detection test is done on the donor's serum at the time of donor blood processing. If donor antibodies are present, either the unit is not used or the plasma is removed. In addition, most of the donor plasma is removed routinely, and the red cells are resuspended in a preservative solution.
8. Labeling and issuance of the appropriate blood products.

Approach to the Patient with an Incompatible Crossmatch

In compatibility testing when there is reactivity in the antibody detection test, serologic studies should be carried out to determine whether a red cell antibody is present. If a clinically significant antibody is identified, donor red cells that are typed and found to be negative for the corresponding antigen should be compatible when crossmatched. The blood bank staff carries out these procedures and provides compatible blood, although additional time and blood samples may be necessary. The approach of identifying the antibody and selecting known antigen-negative red cells is preferable to merely crossmatching until compatible red cells are found. The panels used for red cell antibody identification do not represent random donors. Thus, the antibody may react with a high proportion of donors, making it difficult to obtain compatible red cells; some antibodies react *in vitro* only with red cells homozygous for the antigen but cause *in vivo* destruction of heterozygous red cells, and many sera that react *in vitro* do not signify potential *in vivo* red cell destruction. Thus, knowledge of the specificity of the red cell antibody and the character of anti–red cell reactivity improves the safety of the transfusion.

A patient's serum may react with many or even all of the donors tested. In this situation, it is necessary to determine whether the patient has autoimmune hemolytic anemia. This is usually indicated by a positive direct antiglobulin test. The patient may or may not be anemic. (The selection of blood for patients with autoimmune hemolytic anemia is discussed in the

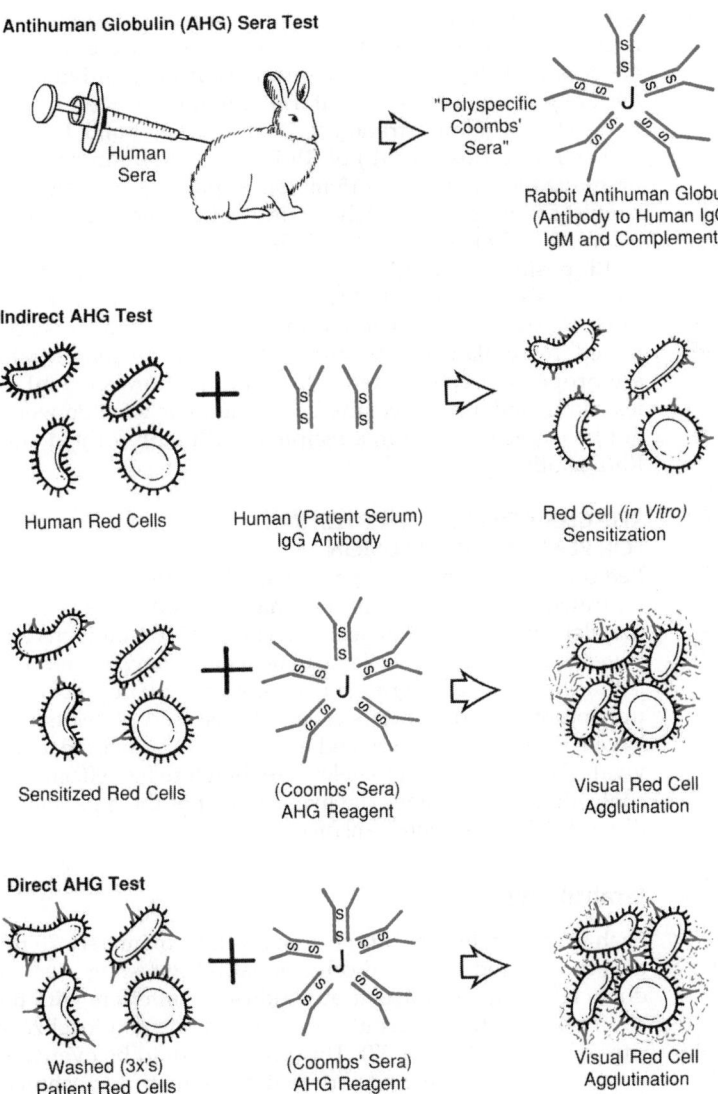

Antihuman Globulin (AHG) Sera Test

Human Sera

"Polyspecific Coombs' Sera"

Rabbit Antihuman Globulin
(Antibody to Human IgG,
IgM and Complement)

Indirect AHG Test

Human Red Cells + Human (Patient Serum) IgG Antibody → Red Cell (in Vitro) Sensitization

Sensitized Red Cells + (Coombs' Sera) AHG Reagent → Visual Red Cell Agglutination

Direct AHG Test

Washed (3x's) Patient Red Cells (Sensitized in Vivo) + (Coombs' Sera) AHG Reagent → Visual Red Cell Agglutination

Figure 57-2. The antihuman globulin (AHG) test (primary immunization). The AHG reagents currently sold are the products of subsequent immunizations and contain primarily immunoglobulin (Ig) G rabbit antibody. (From Harmening D. *Modern blood banking and transfusion practices.* Philadelphia: FA Davis Co, 1989, with permission.)

section Transfusion in Special Situations.) If the patient has a negative direct antiglobulin test and does not have autoimmune hemolytic anemia, but the serum reacts with all of the donors' red cells tested, it must be determined whether an alloantibody is present against a high-frequency antigen or whether the reactivity is due to other non–red cell blood group factors such as abnormal proteins in the patient's plasma, high titers of normal cold agglutinins, or reactivity with test materials (such as preservatives or antibiotics used in the test red cell suspension). If it is determined that the patient does have a high-frequency alloantibody, the clinical significance of the antibody determines whether it is necessary to obtain antigen-negative red cells. For instance, this is unnecessary for many antibodies that do not cause transfusion reactions, hemolysis, or accelerated clearance of red cells. If the alloantibody is expected to be clinically significant, most blood banks have local files of rare donors, and, if necessary, the national rare donor registry of the American Red Cross and American Association of Blood Banks can be contacted. In patients with a clinically significant high-frequency alloantibody, the decision whether to delay transfusion to obtain compatible antigen-negative red cells depends on the patient's condition. If the patient's condition does not allow delay, an *in vivo* crossmatch can be done (see the following section). In situations in which no specific antibody can be identi-

fied, but the patient's serum reacts with all donors and reagent red cells tested, considerable emphasis has been placed on selecting the least incompatible donor units for transfusion. Although it is unlikely that this is detrimental, no evidence exists to prove that, in these situations, red cells that are less reactive *in vitro* have better survival *in vivo*.

In Vivo Compatibility Testing

Occasionally, compatible donor red cells cannot be found because either the patient's serum contains an autoantibody that reacts with all donors' red cells or the serum contains an alloantibody against an extremely high-frequency antigen, and cells lacking the antigen are not available. In these situations, an *in vivo* crossmatch can be performed. This involves labeling with chromium 51 a small volume (usually ≤5 mL) of the red cells to be transfused, injecting them, and determining the percentage that survives 24 hours (125). In general, patients do not experience an acute hemolytic reaction if at least 85% of the donor test red cells survive 24 hours (120). The 85% value should not be used as an arbitrary indication of a safe transfusion. Transfused red cells with lower 24-hour survivals in the *in vivo* crossmatch may have a better survival when the larger-volume transfusion is given; patients occasionally experience severe hemolysis despite *in vivo* crossmatch results greater than 85% (126). Thus, although an *in vivo* crossmatch may provide helpful information, it usually does not change the actual management of the patient, and, in practice, the *in vivo* crossmatch is rarely done.

Platelets

SELECTION OF ABO AND RH TYPE FOR PLATELET TRANSFUSION

In platelet transfusion, ABO incompatibility can occur when the platelets are incompatible with the patient's plasma (e.g., donor A, patient O) or when the donor plasma contains antibodies against the patient's red cells (e.g., donor O, patient A). In considering platelet cellular incompatibility, it has been shown that the recovery of A_1 platelets transfused into group O patients is decreased (127), and, thus, transfusion is not recommended for platelets containing an ABO antigen against which the recipient has an antibody.

Infusion of ABO-incompatible plasma as part of platelet transfusions may be associated with platelet refractoriness, increased titers of HLA-A and -B antibodies, immune complexes, and reduced survival in acute leukemia (128). Decreased survival in ABO nonidentical allogeneic marrow transplant recipients has been postulated to be due to infusion of large amounts of ABO-incompatible plasma (129,130). Infusion of ABO-incompatible plasma may be associated with an increased incidence of sepsis and multiorgan failure in marrow allograft recipients (129), or it may lead to refractoriness to platelet transfusion (131). Although infusion of ABO-incompatible plasma may not lead to hemolysis, these patients have increased levels of immune complexes, and it has been proposed that this may lead to the development of refractoriness in some patients (128) and to down-regulation of natural killer cells, T cells, and macrophage cellular immunity. Because of these potential problems, it has been proposed that platelet transfusions be given as ABO identical, but this practice has not yet gained widespread acceptance (128). If ABO-compatible platelets are not available, ABO-incompatible platelets should be used rather than withholding platelet transfusion.

Incompatibility between the platelet donor plasma and the recipient red cells usually does not cause hemolysis because of the small volume of plasma (50 mL) from each individual platelet concentrate, but severe hemolysis can occur if the donor has a high-titer ABO antibody. If a large number of platelet concentrates is being transfused to an adult or if the patient is a small child, incompatible donor plasma may cause a positive direct antiglobulin test and red cell hemolysis (e.g., type O plasma contains anti-A and may react with a type A recipient's red cells). A maximum allowable volume of incompatible plasma (e.g., 1000 mL for an adult) can be established, and if more ABO-compatible plasma is being transfused, consideration may be given to remove some plasma from the platelet concentrate before transfusion. Red cell crossmatching is not necessary before platelet transfusion because the platelet concentrate usually contains less than 0.5 mL of red cells.

Rh antigens are not found on platelets, but patients may become immunized to Rh antigens from the red cells contaminating the platelet concentrate. The risk of forming anti-Rh(D) ranges from 0% to 12% (132–134). The likelihood of becoming immunized depends on the type of patient and the immunosuppressive nature of the therapy. Because of the life-threatening nature of most cases of thrombocytopenia, platelets from Rh-positive donors can be administered to Rh-negative recipients. Rh-negative women of childbearing age

with a nonmalignant disease should not receive platelet concentrates from Rh-positive donors because of the possible effect of anti-Rh on future pregnancies. If Rh-positive platelets are given to such a patient, Rh immunization can be prevented by the administration of Rh immune globulin. Because one standard dose (1 mL) of Rh immune globulin prevents immunization from up to 15 mL of Rh-positive red cells, this should cover approximately 30 units of platelets (25 units × 0.5 mL = 12.5 mL of red cells) (135).

Rh-positive platelets have a normal duration of survival in recipients with anti-Rh(D) (136); thus, the only concern is a possible transfusion reaction to Rh-positive red cells contained in the platelet concentrate. If the platelet concentrates are properly prepared, red cell contamination is 0.5 mL or less/unit, and a significant red cell hemolytic reaction would not be expected, even in a recipient with a preformed anti-Rh(D) antibody.

RED CELL COMPATIBILITY TESTING FOR PLATELET TRANSFUSION

Red cell compatibility testing is not usually performed for platelet transfusions because of the small red cell content of the platelet concentrate. Platelets also contain HLA antigens and platelet-specific antigens. Some patients may develop antibodies to these antigens after transfusion, pregnancy, or organ transplantation. When this occurs, transfused platelets may have a decreased recovery and a shortened intravascular survival. These transfused platelets are therefore less effective in controlling hemorrhage. The management of these patients is discussed in the section Transfusion Therapy.

Granulocytes

Each granulocyte concentrate contains approximately 20 mL of red cells, and, thus, red cell compatibility testing must be done. HLA and granulocyte antibodies can interfere with the ability of transfused granulocytes to circulate and localize at sites of inflammation (137). This problem could be overcome by carrying out leukocyte compatibility testing. Technical problems make it impractical to do a leukocyte crossmatch of the patient's serum and the donor's cells on the day of transfusion. Donors are usually selected by periodically screening the patient's serum against multiple granulocyte donors. Lack of an effective method of ensuring granulocyte compatibility is a major factor in the limited effectiveness of granulocyte transfusion.

TRANSFUSION THERAPY

Transfusion medicine is the discipline within medicine that encompasses expertise in obtaining and preparing blood components; ensuring their appropriate use in patient care; minimizing the complications of transfusion therapy; managing complications when they occur; and dealing with related issues such as the recognition and management of immune destruction of blood cells, TTDs, and other approaches to transfusion (such as autologous blood donation and intraoperative blood salvage).

Whole blood is separated into its components shortly after donation, thus allowing each component to be stored under optimum conditions and used for the most appropriate specific clinical condition. This approach, called *blood component therapy,* places a responsibility on the clinician to identify the specific blood deficit of the patient and then to choose a specific blood component.

Transfusion of Components Containing Red Blood Cells

CLINICAL INDICATIONS

The most common reasons for transfusion are replacement of red cells for oxygen-carrying capacity and restoration of blood volume after blood loss. Patients should not receive transfusions based only on their hemoglobin level. In deciding whether a patient requires red cell transfusion, the clinical condition of the patient is of primary importance.

RESTORATION OF BLOOD VOLUME

The amount of blood loss that can be tolerated without replacement depends on the condition of the patient. The hemoglobin may not be a good indicator of the need for blood volume replacement. If blood loss has been acute, the patient may have a normal or nearly normal hemoglobin level but may require transfusion for the restoration of blood volume (see section Transfusion in Special Situations). Healthy individuals can tolerate the loss of up to one-half of their blood volume with saline or albumin replacement before red cell replacement is necessary (138). If blood loss is judged sufficient to require transfusion, it is not necessary to wait until symptoms such as pallor, diaphoresis, tachycardia, and hypotension develop. In most normal patients, the loss of approximately 1 L of blood can be replaced by colloid or crystalloid solutions alone (139,140).

IMPROVEMENT OF OXYGEN-CARRYING CAPACITY

When anemia has developed over a long period, the patient adjusts to lower hemoglobin levels and may not require transfusion despite very low hemoglobin levels. No evidence proves that it is necessary to give a transfusion to a patient to reach a normal hemoglobin level before surgery (141). In addition, there is no specific hemoglobin level above which patients feel better or have better wound healing. In patients with chronic anemia, transfusion should be used only as a last resort, because it may suppress erythropoiesis.

TRANSFUSION IN PREPARATION FOR SURGERY

For many years, it was customary for anesthesiologists and surgeons to transfuse patients when the hemoglobin level was 10 g/dL or less. No scientific or well-described clinical data support this practice. Many patients would not be at risk if transfusion were withheld until the hemoglobin level was less than 7 g/dL (141). In baboons subject to normovolemic anemia (exchange transfusion using dextran for replacement of red cells), death occurs at hematocrit levels of approximately 5% (141–143). This decline in hemoglobin was accompanied by a linear decrease in mixed venous oxygen tension, an increase in extraction of oxygen from the red cells, and an increase in cardiac output, allowing oxygen consumption to remain unchanged until the hematocrit fell to 10% or less (141). The authors concluded that the normal heart has a remarkable capacity to adjust to acute normovolemic anemia and suggested that most patients should not receive a transfusion unless the hemoglobin level is 7 g/dL or less. There is no single hemoglobin value that should be attained before surgery. Transfusion to patients with hemoglobin levels of 7 to 10 g/dL should be based on clinical assessment of that particular patient (142,143). The few studies that deal with the physiology of blood loss and the indications for red cell transfusion have been done in normal animals or essentially healthy humans. Thus, the indications for transfusion in patients with cardiac disease, coronary atherosclerosis, or other vascular insufficiency are not known. Patients with compromised cardiovascular or cerebrovascular systems may not be able to compensate for anemia effectively. Thus, it has been suggested that the elderly or patients with cardiac or cerebrovascular disease receive transfusions to maintain a hemoglobin of approximately 10 g/dL (144).

Indications for Specific Red Cell Components

RED BLOOD CELLS

Red cells are the component of choice for any patient with severe anemia. Most patients who require red cell replacement do not also need intravascular volume replacement. In patients who do need intravascular volume and red cell replacement, crystalloid or colloid solutions—not human plasma—are the preferred solutions for intravascular volume replacement. The latter solutions have few, if any, adverse effects, and their use allows the plasma from the original unit of whole blood to be used for the production of coagulation factor concentrate. Thus, almost all transfusions given for red cell replacement are red cells.

WHOLE BLOOD

Whole blood is rarely used for transfusion. Instead, whole blood can be replaced with mixtures of separate components such as red cells and crystalloid or colloid solutions.

LEUKOCYTE-REDUCED RED BLOOD CELLS

Leukocyte-reduced red cells have been used for years to prevent febrile transfusion reactions due to leukocyte antibodies in the recipient that reacted with leukocytes in the donor units (145) and to prevent HLA alloimmunization that might interfere with kidney transplantation. More recent studies have shown that leukocyte-reduced blood components prevent HLA alloimmunization associated with platelet refractoriness (146) and prevent transmission of cytomegalovirus (CMV) (147,148). Thus, the present generally accepted indications for leukoreduced red cells are prevention of (a) febrile hemolytic transfusion reactions, (b) HLA alloimmunization, (c) platelet refractoriness, and (d) CMV transmission. These indications lead to the use of leukoreduced red cells in a modest percentage of patients, which varies depending on the patient mix of individual institutions. However, there is clinical evidence that transfusion-associated immunomodulation occurs. In landmark studies, Opelz et al. (149,150) showed that recipients of allogeneic red cells experienced an improvement rather than the expected decline in survival after renal graft. Subsequently, this raised the question of whether the immunomodulatory effect of allogeneic blood transfusion might also lead to an increased risk of cancer recurrence or an increase in infections in recently transfused patients due to down-regulation of the host's immune surveillance mechanisms. Definitive evidence for either of these two immunomodulatory effects has never been obtained despite more than 100 studies that have been conducted on these subjects. Some studies report a definite effect, whereas others do not. However, because of the potential impact of either or both of these immunomodulatory processes, the FDA recently recommended that all blood components be leukoreduced. Although there has been some debate about this recommendation (151,152), the conversion to universal leukoreduction is under way in the United States. Universal leukoreduction is already implemented and is routine in Canada and several countries in western Europe.

Leukocyte-poor red cells were prepared by centrifuging, washing, or freezing an ordinary unit of red cells, but these processes were cumbersome and removed only up to 90% of the leukocytes. Filters are now available that remove approximately 99.9% of leukocytes, do not require priming, and allow rapid flow rates. Leukocyte-reduced red cells contain less than 5 × 10⁶ leukocytes. Leukocyte-reduced red cells prepared by filtration are effective in preventing febrile transfusion reactions (153), reducing the likelihood of platelet refractoriness (146,154–156), and preventing CMV transmission (147,148).

WASHED RED BLOOD CELLS

Washed red cells are composed of red cells suspended in an electrolyte solution; most plasma, platelets, and leukocytes have been removed, although leukocyte removal is not as complete as with frozen deglycerolized red cells. After washing, the storage period is 24 hours because the washing process may have introduced bacteria. Washed red cells are indicated for patients who have reactions caused by plasma. For instance, patients with IgA deficiency can have severe, often fatal, anaphylactic reactions when exposed to plasma containing IgA. Although washed red cells have been used to prevent febrile reactions due to transfused leukocytes, leukocyte-reduced red cells are preferred because of the more extensive leukocyte removal. It has been thought that washed red cells were indicated in paroxysmal nocturnal hemoglobinuria (PNH) patients, but this is no longer true.

FROZEN DEGLYCEROLIZED RED BLOOD CELLS

Frozen deglycerolized red cells are composed of essentially pure red cells suspended in an electrolyte solution. Most of the plasma, platelets, and leukocytes have been removed.

Red cells frozen using 40% glycerol and stored at –80°C are currently approved for licensure by the FDA for storage up to 10 years. Valari et al. have reported that red cells stored for up to 37 years under these conditions have mean freeze, thaw, and wash recovery values of 76% with less than 1% hemolysis and normal ATP, DPG, and p50 levels and have suggested that these *in vitro* results represent acceptable storage for up to 37 years (157).

The most important advantage of frozen red cells is this long-term storage, thus allowing the development of a depot of red cells of rare types or storage of autologous red cells. They have been used in the past as a leukocyte-poor blood product or in place of washed red cells. These uses are not recommended. Leukocyte-poor red cells can be prepared more quickly and less expensively by filtration, and frozen red cells have no advantage over washed red cells for patients who have reactions to plasma.

Because of the extensive washing, it has been speculated that frozen deglycerolized red cells may carry no risk of transmitting viruses such as hepatitis, HIV, and CMV. Although one study indicates that this may be true for CMV (158), leukocyte-reduced red cells are easier to prepare and can be stored for 42 days just as regular red cells. Thus, frozen deglycerolized red cells should not be used for avoiding transfusion-transmitted CMV.

Effects of Red Blood Cell Transfusion

CIRCULATION

When a unit of red cells or whole blood is transfused rapidly (30 to 60 minutes) to a patient with a normal blood volume, the blood volume is increased by the volume of the component. The blood volume returns to its pretransfusion level by approximately 24 hours. If plasma alone is transfused, the blood volume may readjust more rapidly. Some patients, such as those with chronic renal disease, may require prolonged periods to readjust their blood volume.

HEMOGLOBIN CONCENTRATION

The effects of red cell transfusion on the recipient's hemoglobin level and hematocrit are affected by the recipient's blood volume and pretransfusion hemoglobin level, the patient's clinical condition, and the hemoglobin content of the donor unit. For instance,

a hypothetical patient with a blood volume of 5000 mL and hemoglobin concentration of 8 g/dL has a total of 400 g of hemoglobin. If a unit of red cells is transfused, the blood volume becomes 5300 mL, the total hemoglobin 460 g, and the hemoglobin concentration 8.7 g/dL. If the patient is able to readjust the blood volume to baseline levels within 24 hours, the result is 5000 mL blood volume, 460 g hemoglobin, and a hemoglobin concentration of 9.2 g/dL. In general, the hemoglobin should increase approximately 1 g/dL/unit transfused to an average-sized adult.

RED BLOOD CELL PRODUCTION

Transfusion of red cells may result in a decrease in the recipient's red cell production rate due to suppression of Epo. Thus, many patients with a stable chronic anemia may receive less than the expected benefit from red cell transfusion, because their hemoglobin levels may fall to pretransfusion levels due to diminished production of their own red cells and the clearance of the transfused cells.

SURVIVAL OF TRANSFUSED RED BLOOD CELLS

The normal red cell has a lifespan of approximately 120 days. This is reflected after transfusion in that approximately 1% of the donor cells are lost each day. Each unit of blood contains red cells of all ages between 1 and 120 days. As the unit of blood is stored, the red cells continue to age; these senescent red cells are removed from the circulation within 24 hours after transfusion. Thus, when stored blood is transfused, a slight decrease occurs in the proportion of red cells surviving 24 hours after transfusion, depending on the length of time that the blood has been stored. For instance, approximately 80% of red cells stored in the anticoagulant AS-1 (Adsol) for 42 days survive after transfusion. These red cells then survive normally and are destroyed linearly with a mean half-life of 50 to 60 days. The survival of transfused red cells is also affected by the recipient's health and may be decreased in patients with active bleeding (and iatrogenic blood loss), hemolytic anemia due to defects extrinsic to the red cells (autoantibodies, hypersplenism), and chronic renal or liver failure.

Transfusion of Products Containing Coagulation Factors

The components that can be used to replace coagulation factors are FFP, SD plasma, cryoprecipitate, factor VIII concentrates, and factor IX concentrates. Deficiencies of coagulation factors may exist as isolated or combined deficiencies and may be acquired or inherited. In considering the use of coagulation components, it is convenient to separate situations requiring replacement of multiple factors from those requiring an isolated component.

Deficiency of Multiple Coagulation Factors

The most common combination deficiency of coagulation factors involves those dependent on vitamin K for synthesis. This type of coagulation disorder is best managed by treating the underlying condition with or without vitamin K administration. The coagulation factors can be replaced using plasma of any age because these coagulation factors do not deteriorate during storage of whole blood at 1° to 6°C. Commercial concentrates containing factor IX (II, VII, IX, X complex) should not be used to replace an acquired deficiency of multiple factors because of the high hepatitis risk of these concentrates (144).

Deficiency of Factor VIII

Isolated inherited deficiencies of each of the coagulation factors have been described, although the most common is hemophilia

A or factor VIII deficiency. There is general agreement on the level of factor VIII that is desirable to attain in the management or prevention of bleeding episodes (see Chapter 38).

Factor VIII can be replaced with cryoprecipitate, FFP, or a number of factor VIII concentrates. Each bag of cryoprecipitate contains approximately 100 U of factor VIII, and each unit of FFP contains approximately 1 factor VIII unit/mL or approximately 230 factor VIII units. However, cryoprecipitate and FFP are rarely used for hemophilia patients. Factor VIII concentrates are treated to inactivate any contaminating viruses; provide factor VIII in a very concentrated form; can be stored conveniently even in a home refrigerator for 1 year or longer; and are assayed for factor VIII activity. Factor VIII concentrates are reproduced by several manufacturers. These are available usually as lyophilized material containing 200 to 1500 U of factor VIII in a volume of approximately 30 mL after reconstitution. Factor VIII concentrate prepared using recombinant DNA techniques is now available from the manufacturers.

One unit of factor VIII equals the factor VIII activity of 1 mL of fresh normal pooled plasma. Factor VIII levels are usually reported as a percentage of normal. The intravascular recovery of factor VIII is close to 100%, so the amount of factor VIII required to achieve a specified factor VIII level can be estimated as follows:

$$\text{Weight (kg)} \times 70 \text{ mL/kg} = \text{blood volume (mL; adults)}$$

$$\text{Blood volume (mL)} \times (1 - \text{hematocrit}) = \text{plasma volume (mL)}$$

$$\text{Plasma volume (mL)} \times [\text{desired factor VIII level (\%) } - \text{ initial factor VIII (\%)}] = \text{units of factor VIII required}$$

Example: To raise the factor VIII level to 50% in a 70-kg patient with a hematocrit of 40% and a factor VIII level of 0%:

$$70 \text{ kg} \times 70 \text{ mL/kg} = 4900 \text{ mL}$$

$$4900 \text{ mL} \times (1.0 - 0.4) = 2940 \text{ mL}$$

$$2940 \text{ mL} \times (0.5 - 0.0) = 1470 \text{ U}$$

When the initial factor VIII level is not known, it is assumed to be 0% in a patient with severe classic hemophilia A. The half-life of factor VIII after transfusion is 8 to 12 hours; therefore, it is usually necessary to repeat the factor VIII transfusion at 8- to 12-hour intervals to maintain hemostatic levels. Some hemophiliacs may have an inhibitor that causes a shortened half-life of factor VIII after transfusion. The calculations described provide an estimate of the factor VIII level attained immediately after transfusion, and the dosage should be adjusted so that the minimum desired level is reached before the next transfusion.

Example: If the desired minimum factor VIII level is 30% and the half-life of factor VIII is 12 hours, it is necessary to elevate the patient's initial factor VIII to 60% so that the level just before the next dose is 30%. Patient's plasma volume = 2940 mL (from preceding example). Required: 2940 mL × (60 – 0), or 1764 U, to elevate factor VIII to 60%. Twelve hours later, half of the factor VIII remains; thus, the factor VIII level is 30%. For the next dose of factor VIII, 2940 × (0.6 – 0.3), or only 882 U, is required to elevate factor VIII to 60%.

The duration of treatment with factor VIII depends on the type and location of the hemorrhage and on the clinical response of the patient.

Deficiency of Factor IX

Isolated inherited deficiency of factor IX is called *hemophilia B* and is clinically similar to hemophilia A. Factor IX is stable in plasma when stored at 4° or –20°C. Thus, stored blood, liquid plasma, FFP, or SD plasma can be used to replace factor IX.

However, as with factor VIII, it is difficult to replace large amounts of factor IX because of the volume of these components. Factor IX concentrates (II, VII, IX, X complex) are available and can be used when large amounts of factor IX must be administered. Hepatitis was a major risk from earlier versions of factor IX concentrates (159), but this is not a problem with purified factor IX concentrate because it is subjected to viral inactivation during manufacture.

Blood Components Containing Fibrinogen

Hypofibrinogenemia may occur as an isolated inherited deficiency or may be acquired secondary to obstetric complications, disseminated intravascular coagulation (DIC), and some forms of cancer. In acquired hypofibrinogenemia, treatment should be directed toward the underlying cause of the process rather than toward replacement of fibrinogen; however, it may be necessary to provide fibrinogen replacement during correction of the underlying disorder. Usually, a fibrinogen level of 50 mg/dL prevents spontaneous hemorrhage, and 100 mg/dL allows adequate hemostasis after trauma or surgery (160). Purified fibrinogen is not available, so cryoprecipitate is usually used as the source of fibrinogen for replacement therapy (161). The dose of fibrinogen can be determined by either of the following: 100 mg fibrinogen/kg of body weight raises the fibrinogen to more than 100 mg/dL (160); or, one bag of cryoprecipitate/100 mL plasma volume increases the fibrinogen to 200 mg/dL. Because each bag of cryoprecipitate from a single donor contains approximately 200 mg of fibrinogen, the dose of fibrinogen for an adult is 6000 to 8000 mg, although this varies according to the patient's fibrinogen level. Thus, usually approximately 30 bags of cryoprecipitate are used. If cryoprecipitate is used as a source of fibrinogen, a quality control program should be established by the blood bank so that its fibrinogen content is known.

Blood Group Compatibility of Components Used to Replace Coagulation Factors

FFP need not be ABO identical but should be compatible with the recipient's red cells (Table 57-6) and can be given without regard to Rh type. Red cell compatibility testing is not necessary. Cryoprecipitate should also be administered as ABO compatible whenever possible. The volume of each unit is small, but most therapy involves many units; thus, the total volume of plasma may be large. Cryoprecipitate can be administered without regard to Rh type. Although compatibility testing is not necessary, ABO-incompatible cryoprecipitate and commercial concentrated preparations of factor VIII contain anti-A and anti-B, which may cause a positive direct antiglobulin test or a hemolytic anemia if massive doses are administered (162). In addition, the recipient's fibrinogen may become elevated by the fibrinogen contained in cryoprecipitate if many units are given. SD plasma, like FFP, contains ABO antibodies, and the type should be selected to be compatible with the recipient's red cells. A new version of SD plasma, from which ABO antibodies have been removed, will be available soon; thus, the universal type can be given to any recipient without regard to ABO compatibility.

Transfusion of Platelets

INDICATIONS FOR PLATELET TRANSFUSION
Platelets may be transfused either to prevent bleeding (prophylactic) or to treat active bleeding. The decision whether to transfuse platelets depends on the clinical condition of the patient,

TABLE 57-12. Situations in Which Platelet Transfusion May Be Necessary

Decreased production
   Chemotherapy
   Aplastic anemia
   Irradiation
Increased destruction
   Disseminated intravascular coagulation
   Thrombotic thrombocytopenia purpura
   Cavernous hemangioma
   Autoimmune thrombocytopenia
   Drug-induced immune thrombocytopenia
   Neonatal alloimmune thrombocytopenia
Dilution
   Massive transfusion
Platelet dysfunction
   Exposure to certain drugs
   Congenital platelet defects
   Damage due to extracorporeal devices
      Extracorporeal membrane oxygenator
      Cardiopulmonary bypass instruments
   Metabolic effects
      Uremia

the cause of the thrombocytopenia, the platelet count, and the functional ability of the patient's own platelets. Patients with transient thrombocytopenia due to chemotherapy for malignancy including bone marrow transplantation form the largest group of patients receiving platelet transfusions (163). Most of the transfusions to these patients are for prophylaxis of bleeding (Table 57-12). Hemorrhage is a major cause of death in patients with bone marrow failure (164,165). Little risk of spontaneous hemorrhage is present when the platelet concentration is more than 20,000/μL, but the risk increases with lower platelet concentrations (166). Because of ethical concerns, there are few controlled studies of prophylactic platelet transfusion (167–169). Despite the lack of conclusive evidence from these studies, prophylactic transfusion has become widely used during the past 30 years to prevent serious bleeding when the platelet concentration is lower than 20,000/μL (170). Others, however, withhold prophylactic platelet transfusions or use them only when the platelet count is considerably lower (171). During the past few years, it has become clear that a spontaneous bleeding problem does not occur until the platelet count approaches 5000/μL (172,173), and that a platelet count of 10,000/μL can be used as the indication for prophylactic platelet transfusion (174–176).

The dose of platelets should be approximately 1×10^{11} platelets/20 kg body weight. In the past, this was accomplished by giving approximately one unit of whole blood–derived platelets/10 kg, but present techniques of platelet production give higher yields, and some institutions now use four or five units as a standard dose rather than six or seven. One unit of platelets obtained by apheresis also provides an adequate dose for transfusion to an average-sized adult. Recently, there is renewed interest in the platelet dose. It has been suggested that frequent low-dose transfusions may result in less total platelet use (177), but others have suggested that larger doses would accomplish this (178). Platelet transfusions are not necessary for bleeding patients with a platelet concentration over 100,000/μL because these patients have a normal bleeding time (173). With platelet concentrations below 100,000/μL, the bleeding time is increasingly prolonged, although it is only slightly prolonged when the platelet concentration is above 75,000/μL. The optimal platelet level to achieve in a bleeding patient is not known. In one study of patients undergoing surgery, bleeding was similar in patients with a platelet concentration of less than 50,000/μL

who received platelet transfusion compared with those whose platelet concentration was greater than 50,000/μL but did not receive platelet transfusion (179). The bleeding did not relate to the platelet concentration but to the severity of the surgical procedure. Thus, in actively bleeding patients, platelet transfusions are recommended to achieve a level greater than 50,000/μL. If the patient's platelets are dysfunctional, as from drugs, the bleeding time may be much longer than would be expected based on the degree of thrombocytopenia. In those situations, the decision to give a platelet transfusion is made on clinical grounds alone.

In patients with autoimmune thrombocytopenic purpura, the bleeding time also is prolonged when the platelet concentration is less than 100,000/μL (173). Spontaneous bleeding is uncommon despite the level of thrombocytopenia, possibly because the few platelets circulating are young and provide a shorter bleeding time than would be expected for that degree of thrombocytopenia (173). These patients have platelet autoantibodies; thus, transfused platelets usually have a short survival and limited effectiveness. Platelet transfusion may be effective in controlling serious active bleeding (as in surgery) but is not recommended for prevention of bleeding.

In patients with drug-induced immune thrombocytopenia, the offending drug should be discontinued and the patient closely observed. Because transfused platelets have shortened survival, they are recommended in these patients only for treatment of severe thrombocytopenia with active hemorrhage.

OUTCOME OF PLATELET TRANSFUSION

A dose-response effect is seen from platelet transfusion. One to 3 hours after transfusion, the platelet concentration increases approximately 10,000/μL when 1×10^{11} platelets are transfused into a 70-kg patient (180,181). A whole blood–derived platelet concentrate usually contains approximately 0.7×10^{11} platelets, which should cause a platelet concentration increase of 5000 to 10,000/μL in an average-sized adult. Thus, to elevate the platelet concentration from 5000 to 40,000/μL in an adult with 1.8 m² of body surface area, seven units of platelet concentrate would be required: $(40,000 \div 5000) 5000 = 7$. A simpler way to determine the dose of platelets is to give one unit of platelet concentrate/10 kg of body weight. This should increase the platelet concentration approximately 40,000/μL. The 1-hour posttransfusion platelet concentration is an excellent predictor of an effective platelet transfusion (181).

LACK OF RESPONSE TO PLATELET TRANSFUSION (REFRACTORINESS)

Many patients do not attain the expected posttransfusion increment in platelet concentration. When patients become refractory, they have an overall increased platelet transfusion requirement, bleeding episodes, and mortality (182). Platelet survival can be affected by many clinical factors in the patient. If splenomegaly exists, many of the transfused platelets are sequestered in the spleen and do not remain in the circulation (183). In patients who have platelet antibodies, such as those with autoimmune thrombocytopenic purpura or those who are immunized to antigens of the HLA system, survival of circulating platelets is extremely brief—sometimes only a matter of minutes. In a careful study of 941 platelet transfusions to 133 patients, Bishop and colleagues (184) found the following factors to be associated with a reduced response to transfusion: DIC, amphotericin administration, palpable spleen, presence of HLA antibody, presence of platelet antibody, and status after marrow transplantation and fever. Active bleeding previously thought to be associated with a reduced response to platelet transfusion was not found to be so in this study. Thus, patients can be refractory as a result of alloimmunization (HLA or platelet antibodies) or nonimmune factors.

Most patients who are refractory have a poor response due to nonimmune factors such as fever, sepsis, coagulopathy, and splenomegaly (185), and of those who are refractory due to alloimmunization, this is most commonly due to HLA antibodies (186).

The exact percentage of patients whose refractoriness is caused by alloimmunization compared with that caused by nonimmune factors is not known. In one study, approximately 38% of patients who received multiple platelet transfusions, such as those with acute leukemia or undergoing bone marrow transplantation, became refractory to platelets (186). This occurred after approximately nine transfusions involving 61 units of platelets. It appears that patients who become refractory do so after relatively few transfusions and that some patients do not become refractory, regardless of the number of transfusions (186). Generally, refractoriness is associated with the presence of HLA antibodies (181,187), although some patients who are refractory do not have detectable HLA or platelet antibodies. Many of these refractory patients also have one or more clinical factors that could account at least partly for the refractoriness. Because of the difficulty in managing patients who are refractory to platelet transfusion, considerable interest exists in preventing alloimmunization. This has been attempted using single-donor platelets (188), leukocyte-poor blood components (189), and ultraviolet irradiation (190). All three of these methods are equally effective in preventing alloimmunization and platelet refractoriness (146).

Lack of response to platelet transfusion is often associated with bleeding and a poor outcome. Patients are usually ill with problems such as fever, sepsis, DIC, or viral infections. Whether patients with similar clinical problems who are responsive to platelets have fewer bleeding problems has not been established. Because refractoriness is often associated with bleeding and a poor outcome, it is important to define the steps that can be taken to improve the response to transfusion in these patients.

MANAGEMENT OF THE PATIENT REFRACTORY TO PLATELET TRANSFUSION

Clinical factors, such as infection, that might cause refractoriness should be sought, and, if present, appropriate treatment should be initiated to correct them. Because ABO incompatibility appears to result in a reduced posttransfusion recovery (127,191–193), posttransfusion response may be improved by giving ABO-incompatible platelets. Platelets stored for several days may also give reduced increments (194); thus, a transfusion of fresher platelets should be attempted. Techniques for platelet transfusion should be reviewed to ensure that platelets are not being damaged or lost because of improper handling after leaving the blood bank.

If these measures fail, efforts should be made to use platelets that are matched to the recipient. Refractoriness due to alloimmunization is primarily caused by HLA- and platelet-specific antibodies. Thus, an improved response may be obtained by selecting a platelet donor whose HLA type matches that of the recipient (195–198). If the patient has an HLA-identical sibling, those platelets may be effective (198). Most blood banks also have large files of HLA-typed volunteer donors so that HLA-matched platelets can be located for most patients, although most HLA-matched platelets obtained from unrelated donors have some antigens mismatched with the patient. Approximately 30% of HLA-matched transfusions do not provide a satisfactory response (195–197). Also, because these patients require frequent platelet transfusions, many donors who are

matched to the patient must be available to sustain the patient for days or a few weeks.

In most patients, HLA antibodies are responsible for refractoriness, and platelet-specific antibodies may sometimes be involved; kits using solid phase technology are now available to detect both HLA- and platelet-specific antibodies. These kits can be used for crossmatching the patient's serum and the potential donor's cells. The positive predictive value of platelet crossmatching ranged from 73% to 100%, and the negative predictive value ranged from 52% to 92% in 10 studies summarized by Heal and co-workers (192). Thus, in patients with no complicating clinical factors other than apparent alloimmunization, a substantial number of patients experienced a successful transfusion despite an incompatible crossmatch or an unsuccessful transfusion despite a compatible crossmatch. Platelet crossmatching is performed in some centers and generally appears approximately as effective as HLA matching (199). A practical suggested strategy for dealing with patients who are refractory to platelet transfusion is as follows:

1. Treat any correctable clinical factors that may cause platelet refractoriness. Until these factors are eliminated, recognize that any of the following steps may not be effective.
2. Ensure that the patient is receiving the correct dose of platelets.
3. Give at least one test transfusion of platelets that are not more than 48 hours old and preferably less than 24 hours old.
4. Attempt to give platelets that are ABO identical.
5. Determine whether the patient has HLA- or platelet-specific (or both) antibodies.
6. Give at least one and preferably two or three transfusions of HLA-matched or crossmatched compatible platelets.
7. It may be more convenient to begin with crossmatch-compatible platelets because they can usually be provided more quickly.

Other strategies that have not generally been effective are the use of cyclosporine, plasma exchange, and intravenous Ig.

Granulocyte Transfusion

An inverse relation exists between the granulocyte count and the presence of infection. As the granulocyte count falls below 1000/mL, risk of infection increases (200), which is further increased by the duration of granulocytopenia (201). The increasingly common and aggressive treatment of patients with hematologic malignancies and aplastic anemia has made granulocytopenia common. As long ago as the early 1970s, nearly 80% of deaths in patients with bone marrow failure were due to infection (164,200); more recently, in patients undergoing marrow transplantation, the duration and severity of neutropenia were related to an overall increased risk of death (202). Because of the success of platelet transfusion in the management of hemorrhage due to thrombocytopenia, considerable interest existed in transfusion of granulocytes for the management of infection in granulocytopenic patients. Because of the small number of granulocytes in the peripheral blood of normal humans, collection of cells for transfusion was difficult. During the late 1960s and early 1970s, several blood cell separators were devised to allow collection of approximately 1×10^{10} granulocytes from a normal donor (203). These cells function normally *in vitro* and have normal *in vivo* survival and migration to sites of infection (136,203,204).

A variety of patients have been involved in clinical studies of granulocyte transfusions, including those with acute leukemia, chronic leukemias, aplastic anemia, Hodgkin's disease, lymphoma, and solid tumors. Patients with fever of unknown origin do not experience improvement as a result of granulocyte transfusion (205). Most clinical trials of granulocyte transfusion involve patients with gram-negative bacteremia (206), and little information is available regarding other organisms. Also, little information is available that collates the site of infection other than bacteremia with response to granulocyte transfusion (206). A series of studies in the 1970s established that granulocyte transfusion provided improved survival in patients with documented gram-negative sepsis who remained granulocytopenic for at least 10 days (207,208). Some additional data indicated that granulocytes may be helpful in patients with other kinds of documented infections (either gram-positive or gram-negative) and with granulocytopenia of more than 10 days' duration (208).

The minimum dose of granulocytes required for clinical efficacy has not been established. Results have been encouraging from the use of approximately 5×10^9 granulocytes/m^2/day (207). Thus, most investigators believe it is necessary to transfuse at least 1×10^{10} granulocytes each day, but even this represents less than 5% of the total daily granulocyte production by normal humans. Because of this small dose and continued improvements in patient management, most patients, even those with bacteremia, respond to antibiotics, and granulocyte transfusion became rarely used.

Recently, there has been renewed interest in granulocyte transfusion because of the ability to obtain a large number of granulocytes for transfusion from donors stimulated with G-CSF. Concentrates containing 3 to 10×10^{10} granulocytes are available, resulting in sustained increases in the patient's circulating granulocytes above 1000/μL. These high-dose granulocyte concentrates may be effective for treating infections, especially fungal infections that are unresponsive to antimicrobials. Initial clinical trials are under way.

Granulocyte transfusion should not be initiated for at least 96 hours after the onset of clinical signs or symptoms of an infection. This allows transfusions to be given only to patients who do not respond to antibiotics. Many patients who do not respond have severe (less than 100/μL) and prolonged neutropenia. The fever may be due to documented or assumed fungal infection, which requires amphotericin therapy (209,210). When signs and symptoms of infection persist in these patients, granulocyte transfusions are often used. No clinical trials have documented the effectiveness of granulocyte transfusion for fungal infections, although animal (211) and clinical (212) studies support their use, and granulocytes kill fungi *in vitro*. The minimum number of transfusions necessary for improvement differs depending on the patient's clinical status. Granulocyte transfusion should be used as a course of treatment similar to that of antibiotics. Monitoring clinical symptoms such as temperature elevation as a means of deciding daily whether to use granulocyte transfusions can be misleading and creates logistic problems with procurement of granulocytes. Because antibiotics would not be discontinued on the basis of brief clinical improvement, after granulocyte transfusions have been initiated, they should be continued daily until the patient's general condition has stabilized and improved. In general, it is advisable to consider a course of granulocyte transfusion therapy for at least 7 days.

Most experience with granulocyte transfusion involves treatment of existing infection. At one time, considerable interest existed in the use of granulocytes to prevent infection in granulocytopenia patients. Prophylactic granulocyte transfusions are not helpful in this regard for newly diagnosed patients with acute myelogenous leukemia (213).

Blood Derivatives

Plasma or blood derivatives are proteins isolated from plasma by large-scale separation and manufacturing techniques (Table 57-1). Procedures for the fractionation of plasma became avail-

able during the 1940s. The process involves processing a large pool of plasma, usually 10,000 L (50,000 donor units) using cold ethanol fractionation. Different plasma proteins have different solubilities that allow their separation. This process has provided plasma derivatives such as albumin, immune serum, γ-globulin, coagulation factor VIII concentrate, factor IX, and many others. Until the past few years, techniques were not available to sterilize some blood derivatives after manufacture. Thus, because of the large number of units of donor plasma in each pool, the probability of contamination of the pool with viruses (hepatitis, HIV, and others) was high, and the risk of disease transmission from these nonsterilized blood derivatives was high (214). This risk was accentuated because much of the plasma that serves as the raw material for the manufacture of blood derivatives was obtained from paid donors—a group known to provide blood with an increased likelihood of transmitting disease (4,215). Until recently, only albumin and immune globulin carried no risk of disease transmission: albumin because it was sterilized by heating; immune globulin because either none of the known infectious agents were contained in that plasma fraction or the procedure renders them noninfectious. During the 1980s, SD treatment was implemented to sterilize other derivatives, especially coagulation factor concentrates (216). About 1989, factor VIII concentrates that are prepared using monoclonal antibody technology became available. These also can be SD treated to prevent transmission of lipid-enveloped viruses such as hepatitis B and HIV (217). However, SD treatment does not inactivate viruses that lack a lipid envelope, such as hepatitis A and parvovirus, and a risk of transmission of these agents remains.

Coagulation Factor VIII and IX Concentrates

See Chapters 37 and 38 for a more detailed discussion.

Immune Serum Globulins

Administration of γ-globulin intramuscularly has been effective in preventing bacterial infections in patients with agammaglobulinemia and in preventing certain viral infections in immunologically normal persons (Table 57-13). The γ-globulin (immune globulin) prepared by the traditional plasma fractionation techniques contained aggregated or oligomeric molecules of immune globulin, which, when injected intravenously, activated complement and resulted in severe reactions (218). Several important limitations were created by the necessity of intramuscular administration (Table 57-14). Immune globulin suitable for intravenous administration became available in the United States in about 1985. Several brands are available (Table 57-15). These are prepared from the plasma of normal donors and can be expected to have an antibody content reflective of normal healthy persons in a large population. Some differences are found in the IgA content, the relative proportions of IgG sub-

Table 57-13. Clinical Uses of Intramuscular Immune Serum Globulin (ISG)

Disease	Immunoglobulin Preparation
Hepatitis A	ISG
Hepatitis B	Hepatitis B immune globulin
Measles	ISG
Chickenpox	Varicella-zoster immunoglobulin
Rabies	Rabies immune globulin
Humoral immunodeficiency	ISG

TABLE 57-14. Comparison in Intramuscular Immunoglobulin (IMIg) and Intravenous Immunoglobulin (IVIg)

Issue	IMIg	IVIg
Cost	Low	High
Bioavailability	60% of dose degraded at injection site	100% of dose bioavailable
Patient tolerance	Injection painful	Injection minimally painful
Allergic reactions	Few; minor	More likely; may be systematic and severe
Plasma immunoglobulin G	Difficult to maintain	Easy to maintain
Dose	Limited	High dose possible
Indications	Replacement therapy; viral prophylaxis	Replacement therapy; viral prophylaxis, immunomodulation

Data adapted from Sacher RA. Intravenous gammaglobulin products: development, pharmacology, and precautions. In: Garner RJ, Sacher RA, eds. *Intravenous gammaglobulin therapy*. Arlington, VA: American Association of Blood Banks, 1988:1.

classes, and *in vitro* activity against some viruses. The differences in IgA content are clinically important, because the brands that contain much IgA may cause a reaction if given to an IgA-deficient patient with anti-IgA. The clinical significance of other differences among the brands is probably not clinically relevant.

Intravenous immune globulin is approved for use by the FDA for treatment of persons with impaired humoral immunity, specifically for primary (congenital) immune deficiency, and for (idiopathic) autoimmune thrombocytopenia. The value of intravenous immune globulin in other immune deficiency states such as AIDS has not been established. As with immune globulin preparations used intramuscularly, intravenous immune

globulin with especially high activity against a particular virus can be prepared from plasma that has a high level of antibody to that virus. The availability of intravenous immune globulin makes it possible to maintain the serum IgG level at near normal in immune-deficient patients. The amount required varies with the size of the patient and the indication. Usually, 100 to 200 mg/kg/month is used as a starting dose for patients with primary immune deficiencies. Larger doses are usually used for patients with autoimmune thrombocytopenic purpura. The half-life of the intravenous immune globulin is 21 to 25 days, which is similar to that of native IgG.

Adverse reactions to intravenous Ig occur in 2% to 10% of patients' injections. Reactions are local, such as erythema, pain, phlebitis, and eczema. Systemic symptoms include fever, chills, myalgias, back pain, nausea, and vomiting. Some reactions in some patients are dose related and can be reduced or eliminated by slowing the rate of infusion. The nature and incidence of adverse reactions may differ among the different products, but this variation is not clear, and a discussion of this topic is beyond the scope of this chapter.

Because intravenous immune globulin is made from large pools of human plasma, it contains a variety of antibodies, including those against blood groups and, possibly, hepatitis B surface antigen, hepatitis B core antigen, CMV, and others. Donor screening should eliminate some of these (anti-HIV), but patients may have transiently positive tests for certain antibodies that are passively acquired from intravenous immune globulin. For instance, marrow transplantation patients being treated with intravenous immune globulin had a 49% incidence of positive direct antiglobulin test and 25% incidence of positive red cell antibody detection (219). Transient hemolysis has been reported in autoimmune thrombocytopenic purpura patients being treated with intravenous immune globulin (219). Thus,

TABLE 57-15. General Comparison of Intravenous Immune Globulin Products

Category	Gammagard	Sandoglobulin	Gamimune-N	American Red Cross
Manufacturer	Hyland	Sandoz	Cutter	Baxter (Hyland) Health Care
Method of preparation	Cohn-Oncley ion-exchange ultrafiltration	Cohn-Oncley pH 4 + pepsin	Cohn-Oncley pH 4.25 + low salt	—
Indication	Primary immunodeficiencies + ITP	Primary immunodeficiencies + ITP	Primary immunodeficiencies + ITP	Primary immunodeficiencies + ITP
Contraindication	None[a]	IgA deficiency with antibodies to IgA	IgA deficiency with antibodies to IgA	None[a]
IgA content	1.6 U/mL	720 U/mL	270 U/mL	≤10 µg/mL
Adverse reactions (%)	<6.0	2.5	2.6 systemic; 11.6 local; 43.8 (local/adult ITP)	<6.0
pH (after reconstitution)	6.80	6.60	4.25	6.80
Donors in pool	4000–5000	8000	2000	5000
Half-life (d)	24	23	21	24
Gammaglobulin (%)	>90	96	98	>90
Monomers (%)	95	92	95	93
IgG subclass				
IgG1 (%)	67	55	67	65[b]
IgG2 (%)	25	36	27	23[b]
IgG3 (%)	7	6	5	8[b]
IgG4 (%)	<1	3	<1	4[b]
Shelf life (mo)	27	36	24	24
Reconstitution time (min)	5	5	In solution	5
Administration	Filter required	No filter	No filter	Filter required
Storage	Room temperature	Room temperature	Refrigerate	Room temperature

Ig, immunoglobulin; ITP, idiopathic thrombocytopenic purpura.
[a]Caution with IgA deficiency.
[b]Based on information from American Red Cross.
Data adapted from Skvaril F, Gardi A. Differences among available immunoglobulin preparations for intravenous use. *Pediatr Infect Dis J* 1988;7:S-43.

although hemolysis is unusual, a large proportion of patients receiving intravenous immune globulin develop circulating or cell-bound blood group antibodies. This possibility should be considered if unexplained hemolysis occurs in patients being treated with intravenous immune globulin.

Cytomegalovirus-Negative Blood Components

CMV can be transmitted by blood transfusion with a severe, even fatal result (see section Transfusion-Transmitted Diseases). Transfusion-transmitted CMV can be prevented by using CMV antibody–negative or leukodepleted blood components. This section describes the indications for CMV-safe blood components in different situations.

NEONATES
Landmark studies by Yaeger and colleagues (220) established that neonates weighing less than 1200 g born to CMV-negative mothers were at substantial risk of developing CMV disease if they received blood from CMV antibody–positive donors. Serious disease or death occurred in 50% of infected neonates. The magnitude of this problem varies in different areas of the United States probably because of the large variation in the rate of occurrence of CMV in blood donors in different parts of the United States, differences in techniques of CMV testing of donated blood, less frequent use of fresh blood components, greater use of plasma-containing CMV antibodies, and a changing donor population due to HIV and non-A, non-B hepatitis screening practices. The incidence of CMV disease in neonates should be established locally to determine whether CMV antibody–negative blood components should be provided. In practice, most neonatologists have elected to use CMV-negative blood components routinely for patients weighing less than 1200 g.

PREGNANT WOMEN
CMV infection of the fetus is a severe clinical problem causing growth or mental retardation or both, hepatitis, deafness, intracranial calcifications, and bleeding diathesis. Congenital CMV infections due to primary infection in the mother are usually more serious than those due to recurrent maternal CMV infection (221). Thus, it is prudent to avoid primary CMV infection in pregnant women. Although no specific clinical studies of this situation have been reported, it is advisable to provide CMV antibody–negative blood to pregnant women or for intrauterine transfusion of the fetus (222).

KIDNEY TRANSPLANTATION
CMV disease is common in renal transplant recipients, occurring in 60% to 90% of patients. Because CMV can be serious, causing graft rejection or even death, its prevention is important. The cause of CMV disease in these patients may be reactivation of latent previous CMV infection, acquisition of CMV from the donor organ, or acquisition of CMV from blood transfusion. CMV incidence ranges from 30% to 70% in the blood donor population, and most renal transplantation patients have received previous transfusions, further increasing the proportion of those who have previous CMV infection (223). Thus, reactivation of a previous infection is by far the most common cause of CMV disease in these patients (224,225).

Approximately 77% of CMV antibody–negative patients who receive a kidney from a CMV antibody–positive donor develop CMV infection compared with 8% to 20% in similar patients who receive a kidney from a CMV antibody–negative donor but receive CMV antibody–positive blood transfusions (224,225). If CMV antibody–negative patients receive a kidney from a CMV antibody–negative donor and then receive CMV antibody–negative blood components, the possibility of developing CMV infection is almost zero (225). Thus, it is advisable to provide CMV antibody–negative blood components for the latter patients.

Renal transplantation patients with anti-CMV may develop CMV disease from acquisition of a second strain of the virus from the donor organ (226). Acquisition of a second strain of CMV by blood transfusion has not been reported. Thus, providing CMV antibody–negative blood components for CMV antibody–positive patients to avoid acquiring a new CMV strain is not recommended.

BONE MARROW TRANSPLANTATION
CMV disease occurs in 40% to 50% of patients undergoing allogeneic marrow transplantation and is an important source of posttransplantation mortality because these patients are more severely immunosuppressed than solid organ recipients (227). As with renal transplantation, most CMV disease in marrow transplantation patients occurs in patients with CMV antibody and is probably due to reactivation of virus from a previrus infection, not to acquisition of a new strain (148). In CMV antibody–negative patients who receive marrow from a CMV antibody–negative donor, the risk of developing CMV infection is approximately 40% (148). The likelihood of these patients acquiring CMV infection is almost eliminated by the use of CMV antibody–negative or leukodepleted blood components (148,149). Thus, it is customary to provide CMV antibody–negative blood or leukodepleted components to CMV antibody–negative marrow transplantation patients whose marrow donor is CMV antibody–negative. Because providing CMV antibody–negative blood components for marrow transplantation patients may be difficult in areas with a large marrow transplantation program and a high CMV incidence in the donor population, leukocyte-depleted blood components are being used more commonly (228,229).

Because most CMV diseases occur in marrow transplantation patients who are CMV antibody–positive, extension of the use of CMV antibody–negative blood components to potential marrow transplantation patients who are CMV antibody–negative has been suggested. Thus, they would not become infected with CMV as a result of transfusions received earlier in their disease and before entering a marrow transplantation program. This would create major, if not impossible, logistic problems for blood banks to provide these products for many patients with leukemia, other hematologic malignancies, aplastic anemia, and inherited metabolic disease; however, the increasing use of leukodepleted blood components accomplishes these same objectives. This practice has not been shown to be necessary or cost effective and is not recommended.

HEART, HEART-LUNG, LIVER, AND PANCREAS TRANSPLANTATION
Few data are available that describe CMV infections in patients with heart, heart-lung, liver, and pancreas transplantation. One small study of heart transplantation patients demonstrated that CMV infection was transmitted by either the donor heart or blood components (230). When the donor organ and all blood components were CMV antibody–negative, CMV infection was prevented in heart (230) as well as liver (231) transplant recipients. A more recent study of heart transplantations showed a low (1.5%) incidence of CMV infection (232). Although the data are not extensive and are conflicting for these transplantation situations, the patients are immunosuppressed, and CMV infection is a clinical problem that can be prevented by the use of CMV antibody–negative or leukodepleted blood components. This practice is advisable in CMV antibody–negative patients who receive an organ from a CMV antibody–negative donor.

CMV infections in CMV antibody–positive heart transplantation patients are due to reactivation of latent virus (233); therefore, the use of CMV-free blood components is not indicated for these patients.

ACQUIRED IMMUNODEFICIENCY SYNDROME

Patients with AIDS have severely impaired immune function, and CMV infections are an important clinical problem for them. Thus, use of CMV antibody–negative or leukodepleted blood components is indicated for CMV antibody–negative AIDS patients, although no clinical trials have been carried out to form the basis for this practice. The same potential extension of the use of CMV-free blood components mentioned for potential marrow transplantation patients also applies to CMV-negative persons infected with HIV-1 but not yet manifesting AIDS. This would prevent the development of latent CMV infection in these patients that could reactivate later when AIDS develops. The use of CMV antibody–negative or leukodepleted components for these patients is recommended, and this can be done rather easily because these patients do not usually require transfusion.

SEVERE COMBINED IMMUNODEFICIENCY

No specific studies or data are available regarding prevention of CMV infection by the use of CMV antibody–negative components in patients with severe combined immunodeficiency. Because these patients are severely immunocompromised, provision of CMV antibody–negative blood components is the typical transfusion practice.

PATIENTS RECEIVING EXTENSIVE CHEMOTHERAPY

As more varied chemotherapy regimens are used, patients are experiencing greater drug-induced immunosuppression. In general, CMV infection has not been an important clinical problem in patients receiving extensive chemotherapy. Because there is no good way of determining the level of immune function at which patients become increasingly susceptible to CMV infection, the use of CMV antibody–negative blood components is not recommended in these patients, although the increasing use of leukodepleted components to prevent alloimmunization should also prevent CMV transmission.

Irradiated Blood Components

Viable lymphocytes contained in blood components can cause fatal graft-versus-host disease (GVHD) in susceptible patients. To prevent transfusion-induced GVHD, blood components are subjected to γ-radiation that interferes with the ability of lymphocytes to proliferate. Irradiation with 1500 to 5000 rad reduces the incorporation of thymidine 14C into mitogen-stimulated lymphocytes by 85.0% to 98.5% (234). A much lower dose, only 500 rad, of radiation interferes with lymphocyte response to allogeneic cells, which may be a more physiologic indicator of the ability of cells to cause GVHD (235,236).

Doses of up to 5000 rad do not have an adverse effect on red cells, platelets, or granulocytes (234,237). Red cell survival *in vivo* and certain *in vitro* assays are normal after up to 10,000 rad (237). Granulocyte chemotaxis may be slightly reduced by even 500 rad, but this does not become significant until greater than 10,000 rad (236). High doses of radiation such as 40,000 rad are required to interfere with phagocytosis and microbial killing (236–238).

More disagreement exists about the effect of irradiation on platelets. *In vitro* platelet function studies have generally been normal after up to 5000 rad (234). One study showed normal *in vivo* survival (239), and one showed a 33% reduction in *in vivo* recovery and diminished correction of the bleeding time by

irradiated platelets (237). Because Button and co-workers (237) did not observe a difference in the platelet increment after transfusion of irradiated platelets compared with that of unirradiated platelets, they concluded that 5000 rad was a clinically acceptable dose.

Taken together, the data support the use of 2500 rad because this effectively prevents nucleic acid replication and cell proliferation while not causing clinically important cell damage. In almost all studies of irradiation on blood components, the cells were studied shortly after irradiation. As the use of irradiated blood components has increased, interest has developed in irradiating the components after collection and storing them for use days or weeks later. Doses of 2000 or 3000 rad to units of red cells resulted in potassium levels two and three times higher than normal after storage for 4 to 5 days (240,241). This suggests that leakage of potassium from the red cells occurred during postirradiation storage, which indicates radiation damage to the red cell membrane or the sodium-potassium pump. Based on these studies and the lack of data establishing safety, storage of components after irradiation is not recommended, although it is not necessary to wash the red cells if they are stored after irradiation (242).

Because it is difficult to quantitate cellular immunity, no *in vitro* assays are available that define the degree of immunodeficiency that makes a patient susceptible to transfusion-associated GVHD. Even if better assays were available, these assays probably would not be helpful because the degree of HLA matching between patient and blood donor may be a factor in the likelihood of the occurrence of GVHD. The following patients are so severely immunocompromised that transfusion-associated GVHD is likely unless blood components are irradiated:

Fetuses. Fatal GVHD can occur from viable lymphocytes in blood used for intrauterine or exchange transfusion (243). All blood components used for these indications should be irradiated.

Neonates. Although neonates do not have adult levels of immune competence, few reports exist of transfusion-associated GVHD in neonates (243,244). No evidence has been found that newborns who do not have a congenital immunodeficiency are at increased risk of developing transfusion-associated GVHD. Routine irradiation of blood components for all neonates is not recommended.

Persons with congenital immunodeficiency. Patients with severe combined immunodeficiency syndrome or Wiskott-Aldrich syndrome have severe defects in immunity. These patients have a high probability of developing transfusion-associated GVHD, even from one unit of fresh plasma, and should receive irradiated blood components (243,245).

Persons undergoing allogeneic bone marrow transplantation. These patients are severely immunocompromised by the radiation with or without chemotherapy, which was given to prepare them for the transplantation and, in many situations, to eradicate residual disease. The GVHD that commonly follows allogeneic bone marrow transplantation is due to viable lymphocytes in the donor marrow. Irradiation of all blood components became routine, but, as a result, no data are available that describe the risk of development of transfusion-associated GVHD in allogeneic bone marrow transplant recipients. The risk can be presumed to be extremely high, and so irradiated blood components are used routinely (246). Unless the allogeneic bone marrow transplantation patient has a disease that necessitates the use of irradiated blood products, these products are not necessary until the transplantation preparation regimen is begun. Before that time, the blood components should be selected based on the patient's underlying disease.

Persons undergoing autologous bone marrow transplantation. Although there are some differences in the irradiation and chemotherapy preparation for patients undergoing autologous and those undergoing allogeneic bone marrow transplantation, generally patients undergoing autologous bone marrow transplantation are severely immunocompromised. Because the use of irradiated blood components was an established custom in allogeneic bone marrow transplantation, this practice has been adopted for autologous bone marrow transplantation without clinical or laboratory study.

Several other clinical situations are noted in which isolated cases of transfusion-associated GVHD have been reported and for which a few medical centers use irradiated blood components. There is no consensus on recommended practice.

Hematologic malignancies. Some patients with acute leukemia, lymphoma, or Hodgkin's disease who are receiving very myelosuppressive chemotherapy often with radiation have developed transfusion-associated GVHD (247–251). The risk of transfusion-associated GVHD in these patients is estimated at 0.1% to 1.0%, but this risk is difficult to determine because of the lack of comprehensive follow-up studies (252). The data are insufficient to establish whether blood components for these patients should be routinely irradiated.

Aplastic anemia. Patients with aplastic anemia usually do not have defective cellular immunity. No cases of transfusion-associated GVHD due to transfusion of normal cells have been documented. Thus, use of irradiated blood components is not necessary.

Solid tumors. One patient with neuroblastoma and one with glioblastoma have developed transfusion-associated GVHD (250,253). Some treatment protocols for these patients result in rather severe immune compromise; the data are not adequate to recommend irradiation of blood products for these patients except in therapy involving severe immunodeficiency.

AIDS. Despite the fact that AIDS patients have severely impaired immune function, no cases of transfusion-associated GVHD have been reported. This may be because these patients receive irradiated blood components in some centers. The risk of developing transfusion-associated GVHD is not known for AIDS patients.

Transfusion-associated GVHD and granulocyte transfusions. During the 1970s, there was concern that granulocyte transfusion posed a greater risk of transfusion-associated GVHD than other cellular blood components (254). This was probably due to the transfusion of chronic myelogenous leukemia cells—not normal donor cells. Thus, routine irradiation of granulocyte concentrates obtained from normal donors is not necessary. The decision to irradiate granulocytes should be based on the patient's underlying condition. Chronic myelogenous leukemia cells are no longer used for transfusions.

Irradiation of noncellular blood components. Transfusion-associated GVHD has occurred in patients with congenital immunodeficiency after transfusion of fresh liquid plasma (245,255,256) but has not been reported to be caused by previously frozen components, FFP, or cryoprecipitate. These components contain fragments of leukocytes but few, if any, viable lymphocytes. They would not be expected to cause transfusion-associated GVHD. Although irradiation of FFP and cryoprecipitate is probably not necessary, many blood banks irradiate these components to avoid clerical errors in which a cellular blood component might not be irradiated when necessary.

Transfusion-associated GVHD from partially HLA-matched, related, or unrelated donors. Several years ago, some cases of transfusion-associated GVHD occurred after transfusion from relatives who were partially HLA-matched with the patient (245,250,256) or from unrelated but partially HLA-matched donors (247,257). This raised the concern that transfusion-associated GVHD might develop in patients not severely immunocompromised if there was partial HLA matching between the patient and the blood donor. This was confirmed when Thaler and colleagues (258) reported transfusion-associated GVHD apparently due to fresh blood donated by children in two immunocompetent patients who underwent cardiac surgery. In each case, one of the blood donors was homozygous for an HLA class I antigen haplotype shared with the recipient. Thus, the recipient would not have recognized the donor HLA class I antigens as foreign. Additional reports of transfusion-associated GVHD were seen in Japan in patients who received fresh blood after cardiac surgery, in a woman who received a transfusion after delivery (259), in a cardiac surgery patient in New York (260), and in a Japanese woman who received a transfusion after cholecystectomy (261). The apparent high incidence of this situation in Japan may be due to the rather high incidence of certain HLA antigens in the Japanese, with the likelihood that a random unrelated donor may be partially HLA-matched with the recipient. The incidence of transfusion-associated GVHD in immunocompetent patients in the United States is not known. No evidence indicates that this is a problem when unrelated donors are used; the increasing use of directed donors who are related to the patient may increase the likelihood of transfusion-associated GVHD. The problem can be prevented by irradiating the blood components donated by first-degree relatives of the patient.

Neocytes

Many patients, especially those with hemoglobinopathies, require chronic transfusion therapy and may become iron overloaded. Iron chelation and removal or supertransfusion strategies have been used in these patients. Another approach is the transfusion of red cell units enriched with younger cells (neocytes) so that the transfusion requirements would be reduced. These neocyte units have increased the interval between transfusion by approximately 13 days (range, 30 to 43 days) (262) and have provided a 41% increase in intravascular survival (263). Neocyte units are usually prepared by cytapheresis using blood cell separators and thus are expensive. Despite these advantages, neocytes have not become commonly used.

Extracorporeal Membrane Oxygenation

This can be a life-saving therapy for neonates with severe respiratory failure. More recently, extracorporeal membrane oxygenation (ECMO) has been used to treat respiratory failure in adults as well. The goal of ECMO is to oxygenate the blood without involving the lungs. The features of ECMO that lead to blood transfusion include (a) an extracorporeal volume of approximately $1^1/_2$ times the blood volume of the average neonate treated; (b) an extended duration of use of ECMO (bypass) compared to ordinary cardiac bypass; (c) an exposure of blood to the circuit tubing, membrane lung, and roller pump that may lead to red cell damage or coagulation activation; and (d) volume blood samples that are withdrawn for diagnostic monitoring. Thus, significant transfusion requirements develop. In neonates, because of their small volume, this usually does not place a great demand on the blood bank. Transfusion requirements for neonates can often be made by using multiple transfusions from individual donor units, and, in one case, this had led to a 71% decrease in donor exposure (264). In adults, the largest transfusion requirements were for platelet transfusions (265) because of the principle of maintaining the hematocrit greater than 40% and the platelet count greater than $50 \times 10^9/L$. Often, transfusion needs cannot be anticipated, and the blood bank may be asked to respond urgently to a need for blood.

Fibrin Glue

Fibrin glue refers to the use of fibrinogen in some form with thrombin as a topical adhesive to control bleeding (266). Fibrin glue is used predominantly by surgeons to deal with microvascular bleeding in cardiovascular surgery to reduce mediastinal drainage, to seal synthetic vascular grafts, to seal bleeding surfaces of the liver or spleen, to seal dura, for use in maxillofacial surgery, and for peripheral nerve repair. Fibrin glue can be provided as cryoprecipitate dispensed in syringes with thrombin. Because fibrin glue is made from human plasma, transmission of diseases can occur. The probability of this is not known; in the absence of definitive data, fibrin glue should be considered to have the same risk of disease transmission as other blood components. A more pure form of fibrinogen is available with chemical additives.

Potential Role of Hematopoietic Growth Factors in Transfusion Therapy

The availability of hematopoietic growth factors has opened a new era in transfusion medicine. The first of these, Epo, has eliminated the need for red cell transfusions in most patients with end-stage renal failure, allowing these patients to maintain higher hemoglobin levels, have an improved quality of life, and avoid the complications of transfusions (267–269). Nationally, the use of Epo has been estimated to eliminate as many as 50,000 transfusions (268). Indications approved in the United States for the use of Epo outside the setting of uremia include HIV-related anemia, chemotherapy-induced anemia, and autologous blood collection. A large number of other possible indications reported in uncontrolled studies have been proposed but not yet generally accepted (270). Administration of Epo to patients before elective surgery may reduce allogeneic transfusion even without autologous blood (271).

G-CSF administered to recipients of PBSC transplants causes a modest but significant reduction in the period of neutropenia and thrombocytopenia but does not affect the need for red cell transfusions, the incidence of GVHD, or overall mortality (272,273). This probably will not greatly alter transfusion therapy in the near future. Reducing the incidence or severity of infection could modify transfusion therapy if sepsis and DIC are avoided, with the resulting decline in use of platelets and FFP, but this has not been demonstrated.

The long-sought thrombopoietin has been isolated (274,275) and is being evaluated in patients and blood donors. Because the use of a platelet transfusion has increased more rapidly than that of other blood components, the clinical use of thrombopoietin could have a major effect on blood banks. Thrombopoietin elevates the nadir platelet count and shortens the period of thrombocytopenia in patients with solid tumors receiving chemotherapy (276–278). However, these patients do not require many platelet transfusions, so this use of thrombopoietin does not have much impact on hemorrhagic complications or platelet use.

TRANSFUSION IN SPECIAL SITUATIONS

Acute Blood Loss

PHYSIOLOGY AND THERAPY
When patients experience acute massive blood loss, the need for volume replacement is urgent. The manifestations are due to blood volume depletion—not to depletion of red cell mass. Thus, blood loss can be replaced initially with electrolyte solutions, normal serum albumin, or synthetic volume expanders such as Dextran or Volex (hydroxyethyl starch). Several compensatory mechanisms act to maintain blood flow to and oxygenation of the brain and heart. These mechanisms include adrenergic nervous system stimulation, release of vasoactive substance, hyperventilation, shift of fluid from the intracellular space to extracellular space, shift of fluid from the interstitial to the intravascular space, and renal conservation of water and electrolytes. Because the manifestations of acute blood loss are due to hypovolemia, early and aggressive replacement of intravascular volume is the primary and foremost action. Unless the patient has a very low initial hemoglobin or has severely impaired cardiovascular function, red cell replacement is not necessary during initial therapy of acute blood loss. If blood loss continues, red cell replacement can be added.

BLOOD BANK PROCEDURES
A blood specimen should be obtained and sent to the blood bank for emergency typing and crossmatching. An ABO and Rh type can be performed quickly, and blood of the same type as the patient is selected. This blood can be released under an emergency crossmatching procedure that requires approximately 15 minutes. Thus, partially crossmatched blood of the patient's type can be available quickly.

Blood released using an emergency crossmatch procedure involves shortening the incubation period of the patient's serum and the donor's red cells. Usually, this is done in a way to detect only ABO incompatibility, because this usually provokes the most disastrous kind of transfusion reaction. Alternatively, blood may be released without a crossmatch. If the blood bank has a sample of the patient's blood, the ABO type can be determined quickly, and ABO type-specific blood released without a crossmatch. Generally, Rh-positive blood is chosen, but Rh-negative blood may be used, depending on the hospital's inventory and the age and sex of the patient. When the patient's ABO type is not known, group O red cells are used. This has led to the designation of the donor of group O Rh-negative blood as a *universal donor*, because these red cells would not be hemolyzed by anti-A, anti-B, or any Rh(D) antibody present and would not immunize recipients to the D antigen. Group O Rh-negative (universal donor) red cells do not avoid the risk that the recipient may have another red cell antibody; therefore, hemolysis or transfusion reactions can occur. Stocking O Rh-negative red cells routinely in emergency departments is inappropriate. The red cells may not be stored properly, and there may not be a system of checks for release of the units—practices that can lead to serious problems. Techniques of fluid management and resuscitation are so highly developed that patients can be maintained for the few minutes required to obtain red cells from the blood bank.

Blood bank personnel are well aware that situations may develop in which there is an urgent need for blood; thus, each blood bank should have a procedure for the rapid release of red cells (57). In these situations, clear, concise, and informative communication from the physician to the blood bank and from the blood bank to the physician is essential. To avoid frivolous release of incompletely or uncrossmatched red cells, the blood bank personnel usually asks questions about the patient's situation. The physician must take responsibility and clearly indicate the urgent nature of the patient's situation to the blood bank personnel. After the emergency has passed, the physician is expected to sign a form taking responsibility for the emergency release of the blood.

Massive Transfusion

Massive transfusion is transfusion equivalent to the patient's blood volume during a 24-hour interval. The effects of massive

TABLE 57-16. Potential and Theoretic Complications of Massive Transfusion

Altered hemoglobin function
Dilution thrombocytopenia
Dilutional decrease in factor V or VIII, or both
Acid-base imbalance
Citrate toxicity
Hypothermia
Infusion of plasticizers
Infusion of vasoactive substances
Electrolyte imbalance

Data from Collins JA. Problems associated with the massive transfusion of stored blood. *Surgery* 1974;75:274.

transfusion on the recipient are listed in Table 57-16 and are due to the biochemical (Table 57-3) and functional characteristics of stored blood. The following three changes in stored blood are of particular concern in massive transfusion:

- Decline in the number and function of platelets
- Decline in the levels of coagulation factors V and VIII
- Shift in the oxygen saturation curve of hemoglobin to make oxygen less readily released to the tissues

Thrombocytopenia is the most common coagulation abnormality in patients receiving a massive transfusion (279,280). The platelet count is usually inversely proportional to the number of units of blood transfused (279). Well-defined coagulation disorders can be identified in one-half to two-thirds of patients, and these disorders are usually caused by dilutional thrombocytopenia. Transfusion of large amounts of red cells that contain very little plasma and, thus, do not replace platelets and coagulation factors V and VIII may create deficiencies in the recipient because of the dilution of the recipient's blood with this depleted stored blood. In addition, the hemostatic process that occurs in the bleeding patient consumes the patient's own platelets and coagulation factors and compounds the depletion state. Usually, factor VIII is rapidly replaced by the patient, and factor V levels do not fall below levels needed for hemostasis. Measurement of fibrinogen, which is not depleted in stored blood, is also often helpful as an aid in diagnosing DIC (279,280), but the prothrombin time, partial thromboplastin time, and bleeding time generally are not helpful in elucidating the cause of abnormal bleeding (279,281).

Predetermined standard schemes for transfusion of platelets (282) or FFP (283) or both (280) are not recommended. Patients undergoing massive transfusions should have their prothrombin time, partial thromboplastin time, fibrinogen, and platelet count closely monitored. If coagulation abnormalities or thrombocytopenia develop, these deficiencies should be replaced with the appropriate blood components based on the degree of abnormality observed. Usually, this involves platelet concentrates and FFP.

During storage, red cell DPG levels decline. This is associated with a shift in the oxygen dissociation curve of hemoglobin to increased oxygen binding and decreased ability to release oxygen to the tissues. Although DPG levels are regenerated and oxygen dissociation returns to nearly normal approximately 24 hours after transfusion (284), there has been concern that massive transfusion of DPG-depleted red cells might result in poor oxygen delivery. The clinical importance of this has been more difficult to determine than expected. Animals can compensate well for DPG-depleted red cells if the hematocrit and blood volume are maintained (285). Thus, it appears that in humans moderate depletion of DPG is tolerated in most patients. In patients with anemia or compromised cardiopulmonary function, low DPG levels may be

detrimental, but there is little evidence supporting this, and, thus, use of fresh blood with normal DPG levels is not necessary.

The likelihood of development of hypocalcemia from the infusion of large amounts of citrate during massive transfusion has been overemphasized (286). Routine administration of calcium during massive transfusion is probably not necessary.

If large amounts of cold blood are transfused rapidly, cardiac arrhythmia may occur, oxygen and energy requirements are increased, metabolism of citrate and lactate are impaired, potassium is released from the intracellular space, and the affinity of hemoglobin for oxygen is increased (287). Thus, in massive transfusion, warming of blood to approximately 37°C is necessary. Stored blood contains an acid load, primarily citric acid and lactic acid. This may add to the metabolic acidosis that occurs in most patients undergoing massive transfusion, especially if there is difficulty controlling hemorrhage and shock. Routine administration of alkalinizing agents in these patients gives an additional sodium load and might shift the oxygen dissociation curve to impair the release of oxygen from red cells. Thus, use of alkalinizing agents should be based on specific results of monitoring the patient rather than predetermined arbitrary schedules.

Infusion of microemboli, plasticizers, and vasoactive substances are theoretic concerns, which have not been demonstrated to cause clinical problems. Potassium, ammonia, and phosphate levels are elevated in stored blood, but this does not cause clinical problems except in the transfusion to neonates of stored blood with high potassium levels.

Occasionally, it may be necessary to change to a different blood group in massive transfusion. The patient's history and clinical situation should be considered as well as the potential blood supply. It is sometimes more desirable to switch Rh types (such as from Rh negative to Rh positive) than to switch ABO groups.

Cardiovascular Surgery

Patients undergoing cardiopulmonary bypass often develop thrombocytopenia and platelet function abnormalities (288). Most patients do not experience unusual bleeding, and the extent of bleeding is not associated with these hemostatic abnormalities (288). Thus, the routine transfusion of platelets after cardiopulmonary bypass is not indicated. Patients who develop excessive bleeding should be managed like any other surgical patients; that is, transfusion is indicated if the platelet count is less than 50,000/µL or a severe platelet function defect is present.

Patients undergoing cardiopulmonary bypass do not have abnormalities of the plasma coagulation system except from heparin administered as part of the bypass procedure. Thus, FFP or cryoprecipitate is not necessary. The use of deamino-D-arginine-vasopressin may reduce blood loss in patients undergoing complex cardiovascular procedures (289).

The volume of blood lost by patients undergoing cardiopulmonary bypass is relatively small, usually two to six units, depending on the specific procedure. This can be replaced using routine red cell components according to usual blood bank practices. Because the red cells may undergo some trauma in the bypass instrument, it is advisable that not all units of red cells be near the end of their storage period. The practice of using units that have been stored for different periods is standard blood bank practice.

Bone Marrow Transplantation

Patients who are candidates for or are undergoing bone marrow transplantation have unique transfusion requirements. This is because of the severe immunosuppression these patients undergo, their temporary inability to produce blood cells, and the fact that their blood type may change and they may become a temporary or permanent chimera. Because transfusion therapy may differ before and after transplantation, these situations are considered separately.

PRETRANSPLANTATION

Before transplantation, bone marrow transplantation patients are not immunosuppressed and thus may become immunized. The presence of HLA antibodies is associated with marrow graft rejection (290), and pretransplantation transfusions are associated with decreased patient (291) or graft survival (292). Thus, patients with aplastic anemia should be evaluated quickly and marrow transplantation, if indicated, performed as quickly as possible. The indications for transfusion of the various blood components are the same as indications for other relatively stable anemic, thrombocytopenic, or leukopenic patients. Because of the potentially serious adverse effect of transfusion on marrow engraftment and survival in these patients, transfusion should be given only after careful consideration of the patient's condition (246,293). For patients who require red cell or platelet transfusions before transplantation, recommendations are as follows:

1. Red cells should be leukocyte reduced.
2. Platelet concentrates should be leukocyte reduced. This can be done by filtration or certain apheresis collection procedures (see section Preparation, Storage, and Characteristics of Blood Components).
3. The use of single-donor instead of pooled random-donor platelet concentrates should be considered. The data are controversial on whether single-donor platelets delay alloimmunization (see section Transfusion Therapy).
4. Family members should not be used as blood or component donors because of the risk of alloimmunization and an unsuccessful marrow graft (293).

Patients with inborn errors of metabolism or other nonmalignant diseases rarely require transfusion before marrow transplantation. If transfusion is necessary, these patients should be managed similarly to patients with aplastic anemia. Patients with malignancies who undergo bone marrow transplantation usually have received multiple transfusions during the initial chemotherapy of their underlying disease. The effects of these transfusions on subsequent marrow engraftment are not as severe as those for aplastic anemia patients because the chemotherapy is extremely immunosuppressive. Thus, transfusion therapy for these patients can be necessitated by their chemotherapy. No modifications are necessary because they may become bone marrow transplantation candidates in the future. Transfusions from family members should be avoided (260). These patients usually have no transfusion requirements in the immediate pretransplantation period because they are in hematologic remission.

POSTTRANSPLANTATION

Because of the severe immunosuppression caused by the pretransplantation preparative regimen, fatal GVHD can occur because of the transfusion of viable lymphocytes in blood components. Transfusion-related GVHD can be prevented by irradiating all blood components with at least 1500 rad (see section Transfusion Therapy).

Approximately 10 to 20 days elapse between transplantation and marrow engraftment. The return of production of different cell lines varies, so that although the duration of transfusion therapy is 2 to 6 weeks, the need for different components varies for each patient (Table 57-17). Almost all patients require platelet and red cell transfusions, but because marrow transplantation does not usually interfere with the production of coagulation factors, transfusion of FFP and cryoprecipitate is necessary only if complications such as DIC develop. Although marrow transplantation patients are severely neutropenic, granulocyte transfusions are not usually necessary unless severe infection develops.

The indications for the transfusion of marrow transplant patients are the same as those for other kinds of patients (see section Transfusion Therapy). One unique consideration is the source of platelets. Either random or single-donor (apheresis) platelets can be used. Many marrow transplantation physicians prefer to use single-donor platelets to delay alloimmunization and refractoriness; it is not established whether this practice has any overall benefit to the patient.

If patients become refractory to platelet transfusion, HLA-matched unrelated or family donor platelets can be used. Family members should be used as donors only after transplant. This and other approaches to the management of patients refractory to platelet transfusion are described in more detail in the section Transfusion Therapy. Another unique feature of bone marrow transplantation patients is that the marrow donor is available as a potential platelet donor. Platelets are occasionally obtained from the marrow donor if the patient is refractory and experiencing serious bleeding problems, but this decision requires considerable thought because of ethical considerations regarding the donor.

ABO- and Rh-Incompatible Transplantation

Marrow transplantation can be accomplished successfully between ABO-incompatible persons (294–297) because it appears that hematopoietic stem cells lack ABH antigens (296). ABO-incompatible transplantation may involve the patient's antibody directed against the donor's cells (major incompatibility—that is, patient O, donor A) or the donor's antibody directed against the patient's red cells (minor incompatibility—that is, patient A, donor O). Blood components given near the time of bone marrow transplantation should be compatible with both the donor and the recipient to minimize the chance of red cell hemolysis. Therefore, it may be necessary to use components of different ABO types at different times during the patient's course (Fig. 57-3). For instance, in major ABO incompatibility, transfusion of small amounts of donor-type red cells before transplantation might stimulate production of a high titer of ABO antibodies. Transfusion of plasma-containing antibodies against the donor's red cells might cause some hemolysis of red cells in the marrow being transplanted. In minor ABO incompatibility, it is desirable to transfuse red cells of the donor's type to reduce the number of recipient-type red cells that might be hemolyzed by donor antibodies developing posttransplantation. The choice of blood components for these and other blood group–incompatible situations is shown in Figure 57-3.

Rh-mismatched transplantations are also successful, even when Rh-positive marrow is transplanted to patients with anti-D (298). When an Rh-positive patient receives Rh-negative marrow, some original patient Rh-positive red cells circulate for weeks after transplantation. Some of these patients have developed anti-D (297). It is not known whether avoidance of Rh-positive blood components in the posttransplantation period would prevent this. We suggest converting to the use of Rh-negative red cells at the time of transplantation. When an Rh-negative patient receives Rh-positive marrow, no cases of Rh immunization have been reported. These patients can receive Rh-positive blood products after transplantation.

INTRAVENOUS IMMUNE GLOBULIN

Because patients are severely immunodeficient after bone marrow transplantation, infections with opportunistic organisms

TABLE 57-17. Blood Components Used by Marrow Transplant Patients

	Related (57)				Unrelated (37)				Autologous (65)			
	Percent Transfused	Total Used	Number Units (Range)	Number Units (Median)	Percent Transfused	Total Used	Number Units (Range)	Number Units (Median)	Percent Transfused	Total Used	Number Units (Range)	Number Units (Median)
Red blood cells	98	1077	0–75	18	100	856	6–93	15	100	1124	4–95	14
Peds red blood cells	1	1	0–1	0	13	3	0–1	0	8	7	0–3	0
Fresh frozen plasma	30	311	0–47	0	51	415	0–115	2	15	628	0–167	0
Peds fresh frozen plasma	9	4	0–1	0	16	5	0–1	0	5	4	0–2	0
Cryoprecipitate	9	115	0–36	0	16	104	0–24	0	9	256	0–184	0
Random platelet	89	2800	0–235	36	76	2311	0–977	17	74	1757	0–188	14
Apheresis platelet	98	2017	0–115	24	100	1460	4–172	32	100	1740	3–77	21
Apheresis platelet (split)	54	70	0–8	1	27	27	0–7	0	17	12	0–2	0
HLA	26	118	0–37	0	35	213	0–41	0	22	136	0–30	0
Granulocytes	7	9	0–4	0	16	76	0–52	0	6	21	0–10	0
Granulocyte platelets	5	42	0–27	0	16	54	0–31	0	1	16	0–10	0
Leukoctye concentrate	9	25	0–8	0	16	71	0–16	0	1	25	0–10	0
Cytomegalovirus-negative products	37	2248	0–277	0	19	1969	0–1258	0	38	1342	0–219	0
Leukocyte removal	40	1673	0–342	0	30	1703	0–1168	0	31	1462	0–351	0

Data from McCullough J. Collection and use of stem cells; role of transfusion centers in bone marrow transplantation. *Vox Sang* 1994;67:35–42.

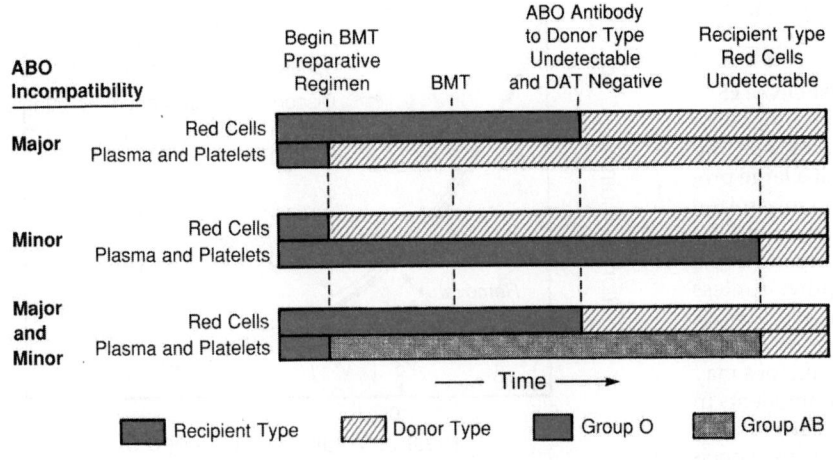

Figure 57-3. Recommended ABO type of blood components for use in ABO-incompatible bone marrow transplants (BMTs). DAT, direct antiglobulin test. (From McCullough J, Lasky LC, Warkentin Pl. Role of the blood bank in bone marrow transplantation. In: McCullough J, Sandler SG, eds. *Advances in immunobiology blood cell antigens and bone marrow transplantations.* Vol 149. New York: Alan R. Liss, 1984:379, with permission.)

are a major problem. Intravenous immune globulin provides a new approach to the prevention or treatment of some of these infections. Prophylactic administration of intravenous immune globulin decreases sepsis and local infection (in some but not all studies) and may reduce GVHD in the first few months after transplantation (246).

Solid Organ Transplantation

Of patients receiving solid organ transplants, kidney recipients often require transfusion before transplantation because of the anemia associated with end-stage renal disease. During the 1960s and early 1970s, transfusions were minimized to reduce the probability of alloimmunization to HLA antigens and the resulting difficulty obtaining a kidney transplant. In 1973, a landmark study showed that kidney graft survival was better in patients who received transfusions compared with those who did not (149,150). Separate studies showed that in patients receiving a living related donor kidney, pretransplantation transfusions from the intended kidney donor were associated with improved graft survival (149,150). Both of these observations led to the change in practice to intentionally give transfusions to patients before transplantation. Despite a large number of studies, the biologic mechanism that accounts for the transfusion effect has not been defined.

Transfusion practice changed again during the mid-1980s. The use of cyclosporine for immunosuppression and other improvements in patient care increased patient and graft survival rates to a level at which a beneficial effect of blood transfusion was no longer apparent. In addition, the growing concern about TTDs caused elimination of intentional pretransplantation transfusions and, in most centers, a reversion to a more conservative use of transfusions. The use of Epo in patients with end-stage renal disease has greatly reduced the need for transfusion. When transfusion is necessary for patients with end-stage renal disease awaiting transplantation, it usually involves only red cells to maintain hemoglobin levels.

Usually, the hemoglobin is maintained at approximately 6.5 to 7.0 g/dL, although transfusion should be individualized for each patient's needs, and Epo usually provides much higher hemoglobin levels. Leukocyte-reduced red cells are usually used to reduce the likelihood of HLA alloimmunization, which can result in difficulty in obtaining a compatible kidney for transplantation. During the perioperative and postoperative periods, red cell transfusions may be necessary to replace operative blood loss or maintain the hemoglobin. If complications develop involving bleeding, sepsis, and so on, transfusion of other blood components can be given based on the specific needs of the

patient. The use of CMV-negative blood for renal transplantation patients is discussed in the section Transfusion Therapy.

There are no special transfusion requirements for other patients undergoing solid organ transplantations except for the use of CMV-negative components for patients who are CMV antibody–negative and receive an organ from a CMV antibody–negative donor.

Neonates

Transfusion in very small patients presents some unique considerations (299). The smaller the neonate, the more likely he or she will receive a transfusion. Neonates may require any of the blood components that are available for adults.

RED BLOOD CELL TRANSFUSIONS

Neonates may require red cell transfusions or exchange transfusion for hyperbilirubinemia, correction of symptomatic neonatal anemia, or acute or chronic blood loss. Blood drawn for laboratory tests is a common reason for red cell transfusion. These replacement transfusions are not recommended routinely but instead should be based on the neonate's hemoglobin value and clinical condition. Sacher and colleagues (299,300) recommend replacement transfusion when more than 5% of the neonate's blood volume has been removed in less than 10 days or when a 10% reduction has occurred in the infant's blood volume and the infant's initial hematocrit was 50% or greater. Red cell transfusions for neonates can be given as packed red cells. Usually, red cells less than 7 days old are used to avoid transfusing supernatant containing high levels of potassium and lactic acid. Red cells, as produced by most blood banks, are suspended in a medium containing glucose, sodium, adenine, mannitol, citrate, and phosphate. Although no reports have been made of complications caused by transfusing these materials to neonates, few data are available on this subject. There is no specific indication for routine use of frozen, thawed, or washed red cells.

PRETRANSFUSION TESTING

Because the neonate's immune system is not fully functional, any blood group antibodies in the neonate are those of the mother. Thus, a blood sample is usually obtained from the mother and the newborn. The ABO and Rh types of both are determined, and the mother's serum is tested for the presence of unexpected (non-ABO) red cell antibodies. If a clinically significant antibody is present, the mother's serum is usually used for subsequent compatibility testing for the neonate because her serum should have higher levels of antibody. If no unexpected red cell antibodies are present, no additional compatibility testing is required because of the remote possibility that the neonate would form a new red cell antibody (301).

TECHNIQUES OF ADMINISTERING BLOOD TO NEONATES

Most neonates require only a small volume of the component being transfused (usually <20 mL). Thus, the tubing sets and other devices designed for adults cause the waste of a large proportion of the components. This problem has been minimized by use of small tubing sets and infusion pumps to control the transfusion of small volumes. Standard units of blood have a much greater volume than any one neonate requires (unless blood loss is occurring). Blood banks have devised several ways to provide small-volume blood components while not wasting the remainder of the original donor unit. These techniques may involve using multiple-bag systems, dispensing components in syringes, or using specially collected small units. Walking donor programs are not recommended because they are associated with serious problems (302).

CYTOMEGALOVIRUS-NEGATIVE BLOOD COMPONENTS

Neonates who have a birth weight of less than 1500 g are at increased risk of CMV infection from blood transfusions (220). Thus, it is common to provide CMV-negative cellular blood components for such patients. The American Association of Blood Banks standards recommend this only when local data indicate that transfusion-transmitted CMV disease is a problem. For a more detailed discussion, see section Transfusion Therapy.

IRRADIATED BLOOD COMPONENTS

Because neonates do not have a fully developed immune response, physicians have been concerned that transfused blood components could cause GVHD in neonates. Some physicians have recommended the routine use of irradiated blood components to prevent GVHD in neonates. Many thousands of neonates have received transfusions of unirradiated blood components without developing GVHD. No evidence proves that this is a clinical problem; thus, irradiation of blood components for all routine transfusions to neonates is not necessary.

PLATELET TRANSFUSIONS

Neonates may require platelet transfusions for most of the same reasons as those of adults and for additional reasons such as neonatal alloimmune thrombocytopenia, infection-related thrombocytopenia, thrombocytopenia due to maternal problems (idiopathic thrombocytopenic purpura or systemic lupus erythematosus), respiratory distress syndrome, phototherapy, polycythemia, necrotizing enterocolitis, and certain congenital diseases (e.g., Wiskott-Aldrich syndrome). Neonates can receive platelet transfusions in a volume and dose based on the size and platelet count of the patient. The recommended dose is one unit of platelets/10 kg of body weight or four units/m^2 of body surface area. Thus, neonates usually require less than one unit. If a higher than usual posttransfusion count is desired, the platelet unit can be centrifuged and concentrated to provide a larger dose of platelets in the volume desired for transfusion. Platelets should be ABO- and Rh-identical with the patient.

GRANULOCYTE TRANSFUSIONS

Neonatal sepsis has a high mortality rate. Granulocyte transfusions have been reported to be helpful in those patients who are neutropenic (<3000/μL) and have an inadequate marrow response (303). Because it is impractical to perform a bone marrow examination to determine marrow reserve, some have suggested that marrow reserves are depleted if more than 70% of circulating neutrophils are immature forms (303), and that this be used as an indication for granulocyte transfusion in these

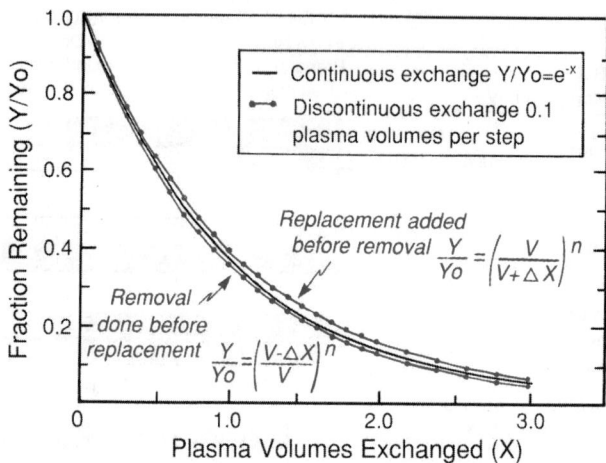

Figure 57-4. Calculated fraction of material remaining during exchange assuming an isolated, well-mixed box. Discontinuous exchange calculations assume 0.1 plasma volumes/step. (From Chopek M, McCullough J. Protein and biochemical changes during plasma exchange. In: *Therapeutic hemapheresis.* Arlington, VA: American Association of Blood Banks, 1980:13, with permission.)

patients. A major practical problem is that granulocyte transfusions to neonates are usually needed urgently, but lack of good preservation techniques make them difficult to obtain. Granulocytes either obtained by leukapheresis or separated from whole blood have been used, but the logistic problems have never been satisfactorily solved, and granulocyte transfusions are not widely used for neonates.

EXCHANGE TRANSFUSION OF THE NEONATE

The indications for exchange transfusion in the neonate are hyperbilirubinemia, sepsis, DIC, polycythemia, respiratory distress syndrome, hyperammonemia, anemia, toxin removal, thrombocytopenia, and sickle cell disease. The exchange transfusion can be performed through the umbilical vein or a peripheral vein using a continuous or discontinuous procedure. The effectiveness of these two procedures is similar (Fig. 57-4). A one-blood volume exchange should remove approximately 65% of the original intravascular constituent, and a two-blood volume exchange should remove approximately 85%. In a discontinuous exchange of a stable infant, aliquots of 10 to 20 mL may be done, but the aliquot should not exceed 10% of the patient's blood volume.

Exchange transfusion is usually done with red cells that are only a few days old. Red cells are usually suspended in additive solutions containing glucose and adenine (see section Techniques of Blood Transfusion). The hematocrit of the blood used for exchange can be adjusted to elevate the hemoglobin in anemic patients. If necessary, because of coagulopathy, FFP can be used with the red cells to provide coagulation factors during the exchange transfusion. The potential complications of exchange transfusion are infection, rebound hypoglycemia, hypocalcemia (due to citrate anticoagulant in the exchange blood), hyperkalemia (if older red cells are used), late-onset alkalosis, volume overload, hemolysis, thrombocytopenia, neutropenia, coagulopathy, GVHD, and hypothermia. These can be avoided or minimized by careful technique and good general patient care; on the other hand, because many of these patients are ill and unstable, exchange transfusion can be a risky procedure.

Pediatric Patients

Pediatric patients may require transfusion of any of the blood components for most of the reasons described for adults. The techniques of transfusion and the doses of components may be different from those of adults. In addition, because the volumes of blood components being transfused may be smaller than for adults, the equipment for transfusion may be different. For adults, it is recommended that needles for transfusion be no smaller than 19 gauge. Hemolysis can occur from high or very low flow rates and occur in smaller needles, especially when older stored blood is used (304). Citrated blood stored for approximately 24 hours has been administered through 27-gauge needles with no hemolysis. Thus, the use of butterfly or angiographic catheter needles of 22 to 27 gauge is acceptable.

In patients who receive many transfusions during a course of therapy (as in bone marrow transplantation and chemotherapy), indwelling catheters such as Broviac or Hickman may be used for transfusion (305). All blood products should be filtered, and filters with small internal volumes are available. For small patients receiving small volumes of blood, it is customary to control the rate of transfusion by using an infusion or syringe pump. In general, these devices work well for this purpose, but the particular brand of device should be tested to ensure accuracy and lack of hemolysis (304). Guidelines regarding solutions for use in transfusing blood components are similar to those used for transfusion in adults.

Transfusion of red cell products may be necessary for red cell mass replacement to maintain oxygen delivery to the tissues. The typical dose of red cells is 3 to 5 mL/kg, which should elevate the hemoglobin 1 g/L. The typical dose of FFP is 10 to 15 µL/kg (160). This dose should be adequate to control bleeding in most situations unless DIC is occurring. Cryoprecipitate can be used to replace fibrinogen or factor VIII. The typical dose is one donor unit (bag)/3 to 5 kg. Another approach is one bag of cryoprecipitate/100 mL of plasma volume (160). This should raise the fibrinogen level to 200 µg/dL, which provides adequate hemostasis for trauma or surgery. A random donor platelet concentrate should increase the platelet count 8000 to 10,000/µL in a 70-kg adult with approximately 1.7 m^2 of body surface area (180). Thus, the expected response to platelet transfusion can be calculated using the formula described in the section Platelet Transfusions. Another approach for determining the dose of platelets is that one unit of random donor platelet concentrate/10 kg of recipient body weight should elevate the platelet count approximately 40,000/µL.

Hemophilia Patients

The use of blood components and derivatives containing factor VIII is described in the section Transfusion Therapy.

Autoimmune Hemolytic Anemia

The causes and pathophysiology of autoimmune hemolytic anemia are described in Chapter 53. The general approach is described here for identifying antibodies, selecting red cells for transfusion, and carrying out compatibility testing. The decision to give a transfusion to a patient with autoimmune hemolytic anemia should be based on the severity of the anemia, whether the anemia is rapidly progressive, and the associated clinical findings. In patients with newly diagnosed autoimmune hemolytic anemia, the hemoglobin should be measured frequently to determine whether the anemia is stable or progressing. Transfusion is not recommended unless the hemoglobin is in the 5- to 8-g/dL range. Many of these patients compensate for their anemia, especially when on bed rest in the hospital, and transfusion is not necessary. When anemia becomes severe, cardiovascular or neurologic symptoms are usually seen. These may involve angina, cardiac failure, mental confusion, weakness, or obtundation. Transfusion is indicated for such patients.

Although autoimmune hemolytic anemia patients are experiencing hemolysis, they usually do not experience symptoms of an acute hemolytic transfusion reaction. Transfusion in patients with autoimmune hematolytic anemia involves risks in addition to those usually associated with transfusion. The unique potential complications of transfusion in autoimmune hemolytic anemia patients are increased hemolysis and congestive heart failure. The increased hemolysis can occur because red cell destruction is a mass action phenomenon, so the number of red cells (red cell mass) destroyed increases as the total body red cell mass is increased by transfusion. Transfusion may also cause congestive heart failure as a result of circulatory overload if the patient has poor cardiac reserve.

If transfusion is indicated, the two goals of compatibility testing are to select red cells that will survive at least as long as the patient's own cells and to avoid transfusing red cells that are incompatible with any clinically significant alloantibodies that the patient may have. In the serologic investigation of autoimmune hemolytic anemia patients, ABO and Rh typing are usually performed without difficulty, although proper controls must be used, especially with the Rh typing, to ensure that the results are not obscured by spontaneous agglutination caused by the autoantibody. If the patient has not received a transfusion recently, it is advisable to type the red cells for other clinically significant antigens to aid in identifying any alloantibodies that may be present. However, this may be technically difficult because the patient has Ig coating his or her red cells, and typing sera for many clinically significant antigens requires anti-IgG. Blood bank technologists use various techniques to deal with this situation.

Selecting the red cell units that have optimal survival may be difficult. The patient's serum usually reacts with red cells from all donors because the autoantibodies have a broad spectrum of reactivity. Thus, the autoantibody may obscure alloantibodies in the patient's serum. It is usually not possible to obtain red cells for transfusion that are compatible (negative crossmatch). The patient's serum is studied to determine whether the autoantibody has any blood group specificity and whether any alloantibodies are present. If the autoantibody has blood group specificity, selection of donor red cells lacking the corresponding antigen may provide cells that survive better than the patient's cells, although the data to support this practice are not convincing. It is not advisable to give Rh-positive red cells to an Rh-negative patient solely to avoid an apparent autoantibody specificity. For instance, if the autoantibody has anti-e specificity, it will be difficult to locate Rh-negative red cells that lack e (cdE/cdE) because this is an unusual Rh phenotype. If such a patient is Rh-negative, cde/cde with the common phenotype can be used.

Several serologic techniques are also available to detect alloantibodies that may be present from previous transfusions or pregnancy. These techniques use two approaches: (a) removing the autoantibody from the patient's red cells so the cells can be typed to determine which antigens the patient lacks and might be immunized against, and (b) absorbing the patient's serum using autologous red cells or those known to possess certain combinations of antigens to try to identify an underlying alloantibody. If any clinically significant alloantibodies are present, red cells selected for transfusion should lack the corresponding antigen.

Because of the autoantibodies, red cells from all donors have a shortened survival. Despite this, patients with autoimmune hemolytic anemia do not require unusual or special red cell components. The usual packed red cells are satisfactory. Choose units that are not close to the end of their storage life to obtain the maximum benefit from the transfusion by avoiding loss of senescent red cells. Leukocyte-reduced red cells should be used to avoid a possible febrile transfusion reaction that might be confused with a hemolytic reaction and temporarily interrupt the transfusion. There is no reason to use frozen deglycerolized red cells for autoimmune hemolytic anemia patients.

Pregnant Women

Anemia is common during pregnancy; in the rare situations in which pregnant patients require transfusion, it is usually because of another complicating factor. If transfusions are necessary, the choice of blood components should be based on the specific reason for the transfusion (e.g., acute blood loss). It is recommended that pregnant patients receive CMV-negative blood components (see section Transfusion Therapy) because of the potential effects on the fetus of primary CMV infection in the mother.

Autoimmune Thrombocytopenia

Most patients with autoimmune thrombocytopenia do not require platelet transfusion despite low platelet counts. It has been suggested that these patients have a population of young platelets that provide better hemostasis than is expected based on their platelet count (173). For instance, when autoimmune thrombocytopenic patients undergo splenectomy, platelet transfusions are rarely required (306). This is fortunate because autoimmune thrombocytopenic patients have platelet autoantibodies that severely shorten the intravascular survival of transfused platelets. When autoimmune thrombocytopenic patients do experience serious hemorrhage, platelet transfusions should be given. The transfused platelets may survive for only a few minutes or hours, and a beneficial effect may not be obtained (183).

Neonatal Alloimmune Thrombocytopenia

Neonatal alloimmune thrombocytopenia is estimated to occur in 1 of 5000 live births. It is the platelet analog of HDN. In neonatal alloimmune thrombocytopenia, the mother becomes immunized to an antigen that she lacks but that the fetus has inherited from the father. Maternal IgG antiplatelet antibodies then cross the placenta and cause thrombocytopenia in the fetus. Mortality rates of approximately 15% have been reported, primarily as a result of intracranial hemorrhage either before birth or during vaginal delivery (307). Testing the sera of pregnant women who are at risk of delivering a baby with neonatal alloimmune thrombocytopenia is helpful if an antibody is detected, but failure to find platelet antibody does not ensure that the baby's platelet count is normal (308).

The management of neonatal alloimmune thrombocytopenia involves transfusion of platelets that lack the offending antigen or exchange transfusion to remove the offending antibody. Platelets lacking the antigen can be obtained from the mother, although the plasma containing the antibody should be removed before transfusion and the platelets resuspended in saline or AB plasma. It may be difficult for the mother to donate a unit of blood because of postpartum anemia or for logistic reasons when the infant has been transferred to another hospital. The antibody most frequently responsible for neonatal alloimmune thrombocytopenia is anti–HPA-1 (Pl^{A1}). Most large blood banks have a few HPA-1–negative donors available to provide compatible platelets when laboratory facilities are available to quickly determine the serologic specificity of the antibody. The half-life of IgG is approximately 21 days; therefore, more than one platelet transfusion may be necessary in severely affected infants. Alternatively, exchange transfusion can be performed using techniques similar to those recommended for HDN. Because it is impossible to remove all of the antibody, management using platelet transfusions is preferable to exchange transfusion.

Neonatal Alloimmune Neutropenia

Neonatal alloimmune neutropenia is the neutrophil analog of HDN and neonatal alloimmune thrombocytopenia. It is extremely rare; only a few cases have been reported in the literature, and there are no estimates of its incidence. Patients usually are discovered because they develop infection at a circumcision site or in the perineal area. Cases due to several different neutrophil-specific antibodies have been reported (309). Although these infants can be given granulocytes obtained from a whole-blood donation by the mother, the short half-life of granulocytes limits the effectiveness of this approach. Thus, exchange transfusion is the recommended approach for these patients.

Rare Blood Types

There is no universal definition of a rare blood type. For clinical transfusion purposes, it usually refers to the blood of a person who lacks a blood group antigen that is present in very high incidence in the normal population. This means that the person almost certainly is exposed to the antigen if pregnant or receiving a transfusion. Almost all of these patients have circulating antibody against the antigen, which brings them to the attention of the blood bank. Thus, the first question is whether the antibody is clinically significant and likely to cause accelerated destruction of red cells. In general, antibodies that react in vitro at body temperature (37°C) may be clinically significant, although many such antibodies are not significant. Reference texts should be consulted in making the decision. Use of an in vivo crossmatch may be helpful (see section Laboratory Detection of Blood Groups and Pretransfusion Testing). If the antibody is clinically significant, efforts should be made to obtain red cells that lack the antigen. If such compatible donors are not available through the local blood supplier, donors can be sought from the American Association of Blood Banks and the American National Red Cross, which maintain national registries of rare blood donors.

Considerable planning may be necessary to obtain the red cells, especially when the donors live in other cities or the red cells are stored frozen in other cities. If the transfusion is to replace blood loss during elective surgery, it may be necessary to plan the surgery around the availability of blood. Red cells from most rare donors may be available only in the frozen state, which may create additional problems when the transfusion is for anticipated but uncertain blood loss. To avoid wasting rare red cells and giving the patient unnecessary transfusion, close communication between the blood bank and the clinician is essential.

If the need for transfusion is urgent, it is helpful to consider in greater detail the likely clinical effect of the antibody. If the antibody can be expected to cause a shortened red cell survival but little or no acute hemolysis or symptoms, the decision might be made to use incompatible red cells—at least to maintain the patient until antigen-negative compatible red cells can be located.

Patients with rare blood types who do not have an antibody occasionally become known to the blood bank. For those patients, it is not customary to provide red cells that are negative for the rare antigen of concern. The decision to use antigen-negative blood should be based on the clinical significance of the antibody it might produce, the antigenicity of the antigen, the patient's present medical condition, and the likelihood of the patient requiring transfusion or becoming pregnant.

Traditionally, it has been thought that patients with PNH should receive washed red cells and blood components that lack plasma. This was based on the concept that the hemolysis in PNH was due to complement activation and that key complement components, which were lacking or depleted in PNH patients, would be replaced by the transfused plasma, thus reactivating the hemolysis. The mechanism of PNH has been understood to be due to the absence of a series of membrane-bound proteins called *phosphatidylinositol linked*. These proteins are involved in down-regulating the action of complement; thus, whenever complement is activated, there is increased sensitivity to complement and more likelihood of hemolysis. However, the problem is not a lack of complement components that could be replaced by transfusion. The main issue for transfusion, then, is to provide it in a manner that has the least likelihood of activating complement because these patients are extra responsive to complement activation. Examples are the interaction of red cell antibodies and antigens such as red cell incompatibility; reactions due to white cell antibodies; or antibodies capable of reacting with plasma proteins—or even complement—that could be activated in the plasma during blood storage. In general, washing of red cells before transfusion in these patients is probably not necessary if all precautions are taken to prevent reactions that would result in the activation of complement (310–312).

TECHNIQUES OF BLOOD TRANSFUSION

Blood transfusions must be administered according to clearly defined procedures that are well understood and carried out by qualified personnel. Many complications of transfusion are caused by improper handling or administration of blood products or administration of the incorrect product to the patient. The most common cause of a transfusion-associated fatality is a hemolytic transfusion, and these are most often due to transfusing the wrong unit of red cells (313). Each hospital should have its own specific blood administration procedures and should designate persons to be authorized to administer blood components. Blood components are prescription drugs and thus can be administered only on the written order of a physician. The physician's order should include the blood component to be administered, any special requirements, the rate of administration, and any other instructions for care of the patient during the transfusion. These processes apply to transfusion of red cells, platelets, and plasma components because serious adverse effects can occur from any of these.

Obtaining Consent for Transfusion

After blood transfusion has been determined to be necessary, the procedure should be explained to the patient to minimize apprehension and to obtain consent. Increased awareness of the risk of transfusion on the part of physicians and patients has drawn attention to the manner in which consent for transfusion is obtained (314). This is done in a variety of ways. The patient's primary physicians are expected to ensure that patients understand the risks of transfusion and any alternatives to homologous donor blood that might be available.

Obtaining the Blood Sample for Compatibility Testing

One of the most common errors that leads to the administration of incompatible red cells is mislabeling the blood sample to be used for compatibility testing. Each hospital should have a specific written procedure for obtaining the blood sample and labeling it. Persons collecting blood samples for compatibility testing should be familiar with that procedure and follow it. One of the

most crucial steps is that the label should be applied to the blood specimen at the patient's bedside, and the label should indicate the patient's full name and hospital number. The blood sample should not be obtained from an arm being used for infusion of intravenous fluids because these may alter the blood specimen and invalidate the crossmatch. If the blood sample is obtained from an indwelling catheter, the catheter must be properly irrigated before the blood sample is collected for compatibility testing to clear it of any solutions being infused.

Blood Administration Sets and Filters

RBCs, platelets, granulocytes, FFP, and cryoprecipitate are administered through a filter because fibrin clots and other particulate debris may be present. Traditional blood administration sets have contained filters with a pore size of approximately 170 mm. The blood filter, intravenous tubing, and other special drip chambers, if used, must be discarded immediately after the blood component has been transfused. When consecutive units of blood or components are given, the filter and intravenous tubing should be discarded periodically and a new filter and tubing used after approximately two units of red cells or components.

During the mid-1970s, it was suggested that the syndrome of acute respiratory distress, which often accompanied massive transfusion, was caused by the lodging of blood microemboli in the pulmonary microcirculation. As a result, several commercial microaggregate filters were developed, and their use was advocated routinely in patients receiving a massive transfusion (315). These filters were more expensive, and some had lower maximum flow rates than standard blood filters. Clinical and laboratory studies never established the effectiveness of these microaggregate filters in preventing acute respiratory distress syndrome because other factors such as shock and complement activation are also important (153). New filters have been developed, which remove up to 99.9% of leukocytes as well as microaggregates in stored blood. Originally, these were used at the bedside in a manner similar to microaggregate filters but for the specific indication of preventing alloimmunization, CMV transmission, and febrile transfusion reactions. However, as the use of leukoreduced blood components has increased, these filters are used more commonly, and they are being incorporated into the blood processing sets rather than being used at the bedside. In this way, leukoreduction is performed when the components are prepared.

Venipuncture

Blood components are administered intravenously. A vein should be selected that is large enough to accommodate the needle but is comfortable for the patient. Veins in the antecubital fossa are most accessible and widely used. Transfusion in these veins limits the patient's ability to flex the elbow during the transfusion. Veins in the forearm or hand are equally suitable, although venipuncture in these areas may be more difficult or painful for the patient.

The venipuncture should be started before or at the time that the blood component is obtained from the blood bank, so that the component can be transfused immediately after it arrives at the patient care unit, thus minimizing the chance of improper storage after leaving the blood bank.

Air should be cleared from the administration set before venipuncture. Venipuncture can be performed with a needle attached to a syringe or directly to the blood administration set. Red cells should be administered with a needle of 19 gauge or larger, although different methods can be used for small neonates. Other blood components such as platelets, cryoprecipitate, FFP, and blood derivatives can be administered through smaller needles. As more patients receive indwelling catheters, transfusion via this route is becoming common. The transfusion of blood components through a central line used to measure central venous pressure is not recommended. If blood or components are administered through this line, the manometer should be discontinued, and the intravenous tubing cleared of the blood components before obtaining the central venous pressure reading.

Starting the Transfusion

Blood components, except platelets and thawed cryoprecipitate, should be stored in a regulated blood bank refrigerator until immediately before transfusion. Do not place blood components in the ward refrigerator or near a window, because freezing and thawing or overheating from sunshine may cause red cell hemolysis. Red cells must be stored between 1° and 6°C. Because it is impossible to monitor the temperature of the blood while it is outside the blood bank, it is customary for the blood bank to establish a time limit within which the blood may be out of the control of the blood bank and still be suitable for use. This time limit is established by each hospital, but usually it is 30 to 60 minutes. Thus, if the transfusion cannot be started within 30 minutes after the blood arrives at the patient care unit, the blood should be returned to the blood bank for further storage.

Infusion Solutions

Sodium chloride injection (normal saline) is the only suitable solution for use in the transfusion of blood components containing red cells, platelets, or leukocytes. *In vivo* hemolysis of red cells exposed to various intravenous solutions seems to depend primarily on the amount of red cell swelling that occurs *in vitro* (316). Five percent dextrose in water is not satisfactory for filling or flushing blood administration sets because red cell clumping and swelling with subsequent hemolysis may occur (317). Lactated Ringer's solutions may cause clot formation because they contain calcium that recalcifies the anticoagulated blood. Great care must be taken to ensure that drugs that are toxic to blood components are not infused through the same administration set as the blood component.

Medications are never added directly to the blood component or infused simultaneously through the same intravenous line. The blood component must be clamped and the intravenous line cleared with saline before administering intravenous medications.

Identification of the Patient and Blood Component

Before beginning the transfusion, it is extremely important to identify correctly the patient and the blood component. Failure to do this is one of the most common errors that are made that result in fatal transfusion reactions (313). It is ideal for two persons to carry out the steps involved in crosschecking the information.

Rate of Transfusion

The rate of transfusion depends on the clinical condition of the patient and the component being transfused. Most patients who are not in congestive heart failure or in danger of fluid overload tolerate the transfusion of one unit of red cells in 1 to 2 hours. The transfusion should be completed in less than 4 hours

because of the dangers of bacterial proliferation, which may occur as blood warms to room temperature (12,318). For plasma components, the rate of administration should be as rapid as possible, but this also depends on the patient's ability to tolerate the volume being transfused. Usually, one unit of plasma with a volume of approximately 200 mL can be given in 30 minutes but not longer than 4 hours.

Warming of Blood

Blood does not need to be warmed before transfusion, except in massive transfusions or when the administration rate is greater than 50 mL/minute, in exchange transfusion of a newborn, or in patients with potent cold agglutinins. If blood must be warmed before transfusion, it should be done with a blood warmer device designed specifically for blood transfusion. These devices usually maintain the temperature at approximately 35°C but always at less than 38°C. Hemolysis may occur when blood is subjected to temperatures higher than 41°C. Blood should never be warmed by placing it near a radiator, heater, or stove. Microwave instruments have not been satisfactory for warming red cells because they cause focal overheating and red cell hemolysis.

Nursing Care of Patients Receiving a Transfusion

Proper nursing care is important for patients receiving transfusions of all blood components including platelets, plasma products, cryoprecipitate, and albumin, in addition to red cells. During the first 15 minutes, the rate of transfusion should be slow—approximately 2 mL/minute. This minimizes the volume transfused if the patient experiences an immediate reaction. The nurse should observe the patient during at least the first 5 minutes of the transfusion and then return after 15 minutes to ensure that the transfusion is proceeding uneventfully. If so, the rate of flow can be increased to the rate ordered by the physician. Baseline values for temperature, pulse, respirations, and blood pressures should be obtained before beginning the transfusion and determined every hour until 1 hour after transfusion. At the completion of the transfusion, the nurse should record whether any adverse reactions have occurred.

COMPLICATIONS OF TRANSFUSION: RECOGNITION AND MANAGEMENT

Although blood transfusion can be life-saving, there are also associated risks. The complications of transfusion can be categorized as immunologic or nonimmunologic. The immunologic complications involve various forms of what are usually thought of as transfusion reactions. Nonimmunologic complications are usually due to the physical effects of the blood component or to transmission of disease.

It is difficult to determine a single value for the overall risk from a transfusion. Adverse effects during or shortly after completion of the transfusion occur after approximately 1% to 3% of transfusions. The incidence of long-term or later adverse effects of transfusion are more variable because many of these are due to disease transmission, the likelihood of which depends on the prevalence of the diseases in the donor population. Almost 20% of transfusions have been estimated to result in some kind of adverse effect (319), and the fatality rate is approximately 0.5 to 1.0/100,000 patients who receive a transfusion (313). This amounts to approximately 35 transfusion-related deaths/year in the United States.

TABLE 57-18. Complications of Transfusion

Complication	Cause or Impact
Red cell immunization	May cause problems finding compatible red cells
HLA immigration	May interfere with transplantation or platelet transfusion
Febrile reaction	White blood cells in component
Urticarial reaction	Plasma proteins in component
Transfusion-related acute lung injury	Polymorphonuclear neutrophil antibodies in donor or patient
Anaphylactic reaction	Plasma proteins (immunoglobulin A) in component
Hemolytic reaction	Red blood cell antibodies in patient
Iron overload	Caused by chronic transfusions
Circulatory overload	Caused by whole blood
Massive transfusion	
Citrate toxicity	Caused by citrate anticoagulant
Cold blood	May cause arrhythmia
Acidosis-alkalosis	Caused by citric acid; lactic acid
Hyperkalemia	May cause arrhythmia
Graft-versus-host disease	Caused by viable lymphocytes
Posttransfusion purpura	Caused by platelet antibody
Transfusion-transmitted diseases	Caused by virus, spirochete, parasite
Bacterial sepsis	Caused by contaminated component

Transfusion Reactions

Many kinds of transfusion reactions can occur (Table 57-18). These can be categorized generally as hemolytic, febrile, allergic, pulmonary, and septic.

HEMOLYTIC TRANSFUSION REACTIONS

Several kinds of problems can lead to red cell hemolysis in transfusion recipients (Table 57-19). Probably the most dangerous immunologic complication of transfusion is an ABO-incompatible hemolytic transfusion reaction. Approximately 41% of transfusion fatalities reported to the FDA are due to ABO-incompatible transfusions (313). This means that approximately 16 patients die each year, making the apparent incidence of fatal ABO-incompatible transfusion 1 in 200,000 patients.

The severity of hemolytic transfusion reactions due to ABO incompatibility is probably due to the patient having preformed ABO antibodies, which often are IgM and bind complement, causing activation of the complement system with the sequelae of red cell lysis and other symptoms. The nature and severity of the symptoms do not correlate with the severity or ultimate outcome of a hemolytic transfusion reaction. Some patients may experience a severe reaction after receiving only 20 mL of ABO-incompatible red cells (320,321), whereas others may tolerate an entire unit with no unusual signs or symptoms. The reaction may begin almost immediately when the transfusion is started or up to several hours after transfusion. The symptoms that

TABLE 57-19. Causes of Red Cell Hemolysis Associated with Red Cell Transfusions

Red cell antibody in recipient
Red cell antibody in transfused plasma
Large volumes of aged red cells
Addition of drugs or intravenous solutions to donor unit
Bacterial contamination of red cell unit
Red cell enzyme deficiency in the donor
Excessive warming of donor unit
Erroneous freezing of donor unit
Trauma to red cells from extracorporeal instruments

may accompany a hemolytic transfusion reaction include fever, chills, flushing, low back pain, hypotension, dyspnea, abdominal pain, vomiting, diarrhea, chest pain, and unexpected bleeding. In one study of 47 patients with hemolytic reactions, the most common symptoms were fever with or without chills (40%), chest pain (12%), and hypotension (12%) (320).

Most symptoms of a hemolytic transfusion reaction are due to complement activation or cytokine release. Several activated components of the complement system, especially C3a and C5a, are vasoactive and cause the release of serotonin and histamine from mast cells, possibly accounting for the hypotension that often occurs.

The coagulation system may be activated by (a) antigen-antibody complexes that activate Hageman factor (XII), (b) red cell stroma that contain thromboplastic substances, (c) activation of platelets with release of platelet factor 3, and (d) hypotension leading to tissue hypoxia with release of tissue factors. Thus, through one or more of these mechanisms, patients with a severe hemolytic transfusion reaction may develop a coagulopathy or DIC.

Hemolytic transfusion reactions also may cause oliguria and renal failure. The specific cause of this is not known, but a couple of mechanisms may be involved: Activated Hageman factor (XII) promotes the release of bradykinin that causes vasoconstriction and hypotension, and DIC causes the formation of microthrombi. These events in combination cause a reduced renal blood flow and renal damage.

A classic pattern of alteration is found in laboratory tests in a hemolytic transfusion reaction (Fig. 57-5). In any series, the incidence of abnormalities in different tests cannot be easily related to this pattern because patients are studied at different periods after the onset of hemolysis. Nevertheless, one study illustrates the kind of laboratory abnormalities seen in practice. Pineda and colleagues (320) found the following percentages of test abnormalities in 47 patients who experienced an acute hemolytic transfusion reaction: hemoglobinemia or hemoglobinuria, 87%; urine hemosiderin, 42%; reduced serum haptoglobin, 87%; elevated bilirubin, 80%; positive direct antiglobulin, 87%; and unexpected red cell antibody, 85%. Thus, laboratory testing generally should be helpful in diagnosing hemolysis, and the red cell serologic studies have a high sensitivity in detecting the antibody involved.

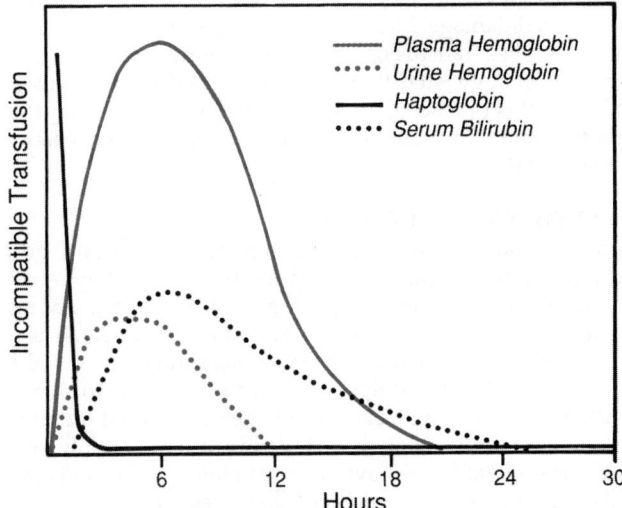

Figure 57-5. Time relation of pigmentary changes in serum after hemolytic transfusion reaction (not drawn to scale). (From Huestis DW, Bove JR, Case J. Complications of transfusion. In: *Practical blood transfusion*, 4th ed. Boston: Little, Brown and Company, 1988:251, with permission.)

FEBRILE NONHEMOLYTIC TRANSFUSION REACTIONS

Febrile reactions occur in association with approximately 0.5% to 1.0% of transfusions. They are caused by leukocyte antibodies in patients, which react with leukocytes in the transfused components (145,322), or by the transfusion of cytokines that have accumulated in the blood product during storage (323,324). The severity of the reaction is directly related to the number of leukocytes in the blood component (145). These febrile/leukocyte reactions can be prevented by removing leukocytes from the blood components (322,325). Many reactions can be prevented by the administration of antipyretics such as acetaminophen, although this should be reserved for patients who have experienced a reaction.

Some febrile nonhemolytic reactions, especially those associated with platelets, are due to cytokines in the donor unit (323). These reactions can be prevented by removing the leukocytes from the red cells or platelets soon after the blood has been collected (324). Thus, the more widespread use of leukoreduced blood components should reduce the incidence and severity for febrile nonhemolytic transfusion reaction.

ALLERGIC REACTIONS

Allergic reaction is probably the most common kind of reaction, which occurs after 1% to 2% of transfusions. Allergic reactions involve hives with no other symptoms. In this situation, the patient can be given an antihistamine, and after 15 to 30 minutes, the transfusion can be restarted. This is the only situation in which transfusion may be restarted.

TRANSFUSION-RELATED ACUTE LUNG INJURY

This severe, acute, and sometimes fatal pulmonary reaction is relatively uncommon (326,327). Most of these reactions seem to involve transfusion of leukocyte antibodies in the donor unit that react with the patient's leukocytes. Pulmonary reaction was first described in 1957 when Brittingham (322) reported that transfusion of 50 mL of whole blood containing a leukoagglutinating antibody caused fever, vomiting, diarrhea, chills, dyspnea, tachycardia, hypotension, cyanosis, pulmonary infiltrates, and leukopenia. Although the pathophysiology of these reactions is not completely understood, it is thought that transfused leukocyte antibody may react with leukocytes activating complement, causing adherence of granulocytes to pulmonary endothelium with release of proteolytic enzymes and toxic oxygen metabolites that cause further endothelial damage. Plasma from multiparous donors is more likely to cause transfusion-related acute lung injury (327), and it has been suggested that this not be used for transfusion, although this practice has not been implemented. Prompt recognition and treatment of these serious pulmonary reactions are essential.

ANAPHYLACTIC REACTIONS

Patients who are IgA deficient and have anti-IgA antibodies may experience an anaphylactic reaction when they receive blood components containing anti-A (328). These reactions may be dramatic and rapidly fatal. The treatment is the same as for any anaphylactic reaction. The reactions can be prevented by using red cells or platelet concentrates washed to remove plasma IgA and using plasma components prepared from IgA-deficient donors. Although such donors are not readily available, most blood banks have access to blood components from IgA-deficient donors through rare donor registries.

BACTERIAL CONTAMINATION OF BLOOD COMPONENTS

Some cases of transfusion of contaminated blood occur (329). The contamination is thought to be due to an asymptomatic bac-

teremia in the donor or bacteria on the skin at the venipuncture site. Contaminated blood is an important cause of transfusion-related fatalities (313,329).

In one study (330) of 3584 platelet transfusions to 161 patients, there were 37 febrile transfusion reactions, and, of these, approximately one-fourth were due to bacteremia. In patients with a less than 2°C temperature elevation, the risk of bacteremia was 42% (330).

Bacterial contamination is particularly a problem with platelet transfusions (331,332), probably because platelets are stored at room temperature. This is becoming one of the major remaining complications of transfusion and should be considered in any patient who exhibits signs and symptoms of septic shock after transfusion.

REACTIONS TO PLATELETS

Patients with platelet or HLA antibodies may have febrile nonhemolytic reactions, probably as a result of leukocytes contained in the platelet concentrates. In addition, platelets may be trapped in the pulmonary capillaries causing dyspnea and pulmonary edema. This is particularly likely if aggregates of platelets are transfused. If the platelets are properly prepared, they contain few aggregates. Allergic reactions may also occur with platelet transfusions. Many reactions to platelet transfusion are due to cytokines produced by leukocytes in the donor unit (323), and these can be prevented by removing the leukocytes soon after the blood is collected (324).

Signs, Symptoms, and Management of a Transfusion Reaction

The most common symptoms of transfusion reaction are chills, fever, and urticaria. It is not possible to predict the cause or ultimate severity of a transfusion reaction from the presenting symptoms. Therefore, all patients who exhibit signs or symptoms during or several hours after transfusion should be managed initially as if a transfusion reaction were occurring. The monitoring and nursing care that should be provided to patients receiving a transfusion are described in the section Techniques of Blood Transfusion. Because the symptoms of different kinds of transfusion reactions vary widely, it is difficult to accurately define the type of reaction occurring. Nevertheless, it is necessary to manage the specific clinical problems present. The following symptoms are more likely to relate to different kinds of transfusion reactions:

Acute hemolytic reaction: restlessness, anxiety, severe chills, rapid temperature increase, headache, pleuritic pain, lumbar or thigh pain, hemoglobinuria, nausea, vomiting, pulse rate increase, blood pressure increase, oliguria, and feeling of impending doom

Febrile nonhemolytic (leukocyte) reaction: chills, temperature increase greater than 1°C, nausea, and muscle aching

Allergic reaction: rash, hives, facial swelling, and respiratory distress

Cardiac overload or transfusion-related acute lung injury: sudden dyspnea, cyanosis, cough, frothy sputum, blood pressure increase, distended neck veins, and central venous pressure increase

STEPS TO TAKE WHEN A TRANSFUSION REACTION OCCURS

When a transfusion reaction is suspected, the following steps should be taken:

1. Stop the transfusion immediately.
2. Leave the needle in the vein and begin infusing normal saline while vital signs are obtained.

3. Carry out a brief physical examination.
4. Obtain temperature, pulse, respiratory rate, and blood pressure readings.
5. Auscultate the lungs and heart.
6. Inspect the skin for hives.
7. Inspect the patient for signs of abnormal bleeding.
8. Obtain a new blood sample for repeat red cell compatibility testing and inspection of the plasma for evidence of hemolysis.
9. Obtain a urine sample if the patient can void.
10. Obtain a chest radiograph and provide oxygen if pulmonary symptoms are prominent.
11. Make a preliminary assessment of the situation.

INITIAL TREATMENT OF A TRANSFUSION REACTION

Respiratory problems may require epinephrine, nasal oxygen, or incubation. Hypotension should be treated with infusions of crystalloid. Red or pink plasma or serum suggesting hemolysis necessitates accurate monitoring of urine flow. If necessary, the patient should be catheterized. If evidence of oliguria is present, mannitol should be added to maintain urine volume at approximately 100 mL/hour. If the patient demonstrates only hives, he or she can be given diphenhydramine, 50 mg intramuscularly (if not thrombocytopenic), and the transfusion can be restarted slowly after approximately 15 minutes.

Transfusion-Associated Graft-Versus-Host Disease

Transfusion-associated GVHD is caused by viable lymphocytes contained in blood components. In patients who are severely immunocompromised, transfused lymphocytes proliferate causing a syndrome characterized by fever, liver dysfunction, skin rash, diarrhea, and marrow hypoplasia. The syndrome begins less than 30 days after transfusion and is fatal in approximately 90% of patients (234). The cellular mechanisms involved in transfusion-associated GVHD are assumed to be similar to those in GVHD due to allogeneic bone marrow (234). Transfusion-associated GVHD can be prevented by irradiating the blood components before transfusion (see section Transfusion Therapy). Transfusion-associated GVHD can also occur in immunocompetent patients (258–261). This usually occurs when the donor is homozygous for an HLA haplotype (possesses only two HLA-A and -B antigens) and these match the recipient. Thus, the donor cells are not recognized by the recipient as foreign but they recognize the recipient and initiate GVHD. This situation occurs in populations with little HLA diversity (258–261) or in transfusions from first-degree relatives. This has led to routine irradiation of blood when the donor is a first-degree relative of the recipient.

Other Complications of Blood Transfusion

IMMUNIZATION TO BLOOD GROUP ANTIGENS

As a result of exposure to blood, patients may form antibodies to red cells; lymphocyte, granulocyte, or platelet surface antigens; or plasma proteins. The likelihood of antibody formation depends on the immunogenicity of the antigen and the ability of the patient to mount an antibody response. Each kind of antibody can cause a particular clinical problem later if the patient requires subsequent transfusions or organ or tissue grafts or becomes pregnant (Table 57-20).

IRON OVERLOAD

Patients who receive chronic transfusion therapy may become overloaded with iron and develop iatrogenic hemo-

TABLE 57-20. Clinical Problems Caused by Immunization after Blood Transfusion

Antibody Target	Possible Clinical Problem
Red cells	Hemolytic reactions; difficulty locating compatible blood if transfusion needed; hemolytic disease of the newborn
Lymphocytes (HLA)	Febrile reaction; difficulty locating compatible organ if transplant needed; poor response to platelet transfusion
Granulocytes	Febrile reaction; acute pulmonary reaction; poor response to granulocyte transfusions; alloimmune neonatal neutropenia
Platelets	Poor response to platelet transfusions; alloimmune neonatal thrombocytopenia; posttransfusion purpura
Plasma proteins	Allergic reaction; anaphylactic reaction (immunoglobulin A)

chromatosis. Iron chelators, supertransfusion, and neocytes have been used, but this problem remains a serious potential complication.

OTHER

Citrate toxicity, hypocalcemia, acidosis, alkalosis, cold blood, microemboli, and hyperkalemia all are potential complications of massive transfusions. These are discussed more completely in the section Massive Transfusion.

TRANSFUSION-TRANSMITTED DISEASES

The AIDS epidemic and the growing awareness of posttransfusion hepatitis have focused an enormous amount of attention on TTD and have heightened the public's fears of blood transfusion.

The blood supply is safer than ever. Because of the adoption of routine screening of donated blood for HIV more than 15 years ago, only 40 patients have been identified by the Centers for Disease Control and Prevention as developing AIDS after a blood transfusion (333), and surveillance systems detect little, if any, posttransfusion HCV (334)—although posttransfusion hepatitis B continues to be a problem. Some beneficial effects of heightened concern about TTD are that physicians have become more conservative in their use of blood components and that the process of informing patients and obtaining their consent for transfusion has been strengthened.

Posttransfusion Hepatitis

Posttransfusion hepatitis can be caused by hepatitis A, hepatitis B, hepatitis C, CMV, or Epstein-Barr virus, or it may be defined as non-A, non-B, and non-C hepatitis, which means hepatitis due to none of the agents listed above. Posttransfusion hepatitis is the most common disease transmitted by blood transfusion. Estimates of the incidence of posttransfusion hepatitis are complicated, because figures depend on the blood donor population and on when the studies were performed. Prospective studies involving the period of 1974 to 1981 showed rates of posttransfusion hepatitis ranging from 5.9% to 21.0% (335). Some of these studies involved patients who received many units of blood, and most studies defined hepatitis as abnormal liver function without regard to clinical symptoms. In the mid-1980s, it was estimated that 120,000 cases of posttransfusion hepatitis occurred annually (336). This has been greatly reduced using the strategies described below.

Hepatitis A

Hepatitis A usually produces a short period of viremia, which occurs for approximately 7 days before the onset of acute symptoms. Although approximately 10% of patients may have a relapsing course for up to 1 year, hepatitis A generally does not involve a carrier state; thus, no chronic viremia is present. Although posttransfusion hepatitis A is rare, it can occur if a person is unaware of the hepatitis A exposure and donates blood during the few days of viremia before symptoms develop (337,338). Because of the absence of hepatitis A antibodies at the time of viremia and the rarity of posttransfusion hepatitis A, laboratory testing of blood donors for hepatitis A is not performed. Thus, in evaluating a patient with suspected posttransfusion hepatitis, hepatitis A should be considered only as a remote possibility.

Hepatitis B

Although much less than it was in the 1970s, hepatitis B is a major complication of transfusion. The most common response to infection with the hepatitis B virus is asymptomatic. If the person does develop symptoms, viremia and HBsAg positivity occur 2 to 6 weeks before the onset of symptoms; thus, an infectious but apparently healthy person may meet all the donor medical history and laboratory testing criteria and donate a unit of infectious blood. Persons who develop symptomatic hepatitis B virus infection would be screened from subsequent blood donations on the basis of their medical history. Approximately 90% of acute hepatitis B virus infections clinically resolve, the virus disappears, and the person becomes HBsAg negative. Antibody to the hepatitis B virus (e.g., antibody to hepatitis B surface antigen) develops in almost all (80% to 90%) of these persons. In approximately 10% of patients, chronic hepatitis B infection develops, the virus persists, and the person remains HBsAg positive. If any of these persons have experienced a subclinical (asymptomatic) initial infection, he or she would pass the medical history, but the blood would be found to be infectious by the HBsAg testing done before the release of the blood for transfusion.

In the past, hepatitis B was an important complication of blood transfusion (339,340). The adoption of routine screening of blood donors for HBsAg reduced the incidence of posttransfusion hepatitis B. Data defining the extent of reduction are not available because studies were not done throughout the introduction of routine hepatitis B testing and because the donor population has also changed. More recently, hepatitis B has represented only approximately 10% of all posttransfusion hepatitis. The reasons why this number continues to be small are not understood. In 1987, routine screening of blood donors' anti-HB$_c$ was introduced in an effort to reduce the transmission of non-A, non-B hepatitis. An additional benefit of this screening is the possible reduction or virtual elimination of the remaining cases of transfusion-transmitted hepatitis B (45,46,341).

Non-A, Non-B Hepatitis and Surrogate Testing

Non-A, non-B hepatitis was a diagnosis of exclusion, developed when a substantial proportion of posttransfusion hepatitis could not be attributed to A or B. Considerable debate occurred as to whether non-A, non-B hepatitis had a major long-term health impact. Of patients with posttransfusion hepatitis, 50% to 70% had liver function abnormalities for 1 to 3 years (336,342). Of those who underwent liver biopsy, 90%

had either chronic active or chronic persistent hepatitis or cirrhosis. Non-A, non-B hepatitis appeared to lead to cirrhosis or chronic hepatitis (343).

In 1986, blood banks in the United States instituted routine testing of donors for ALT and anti-HB$_c$ as a way of reducing posttransfusion non-A, non-B hepatitis. The use of the tests that were not specific for non-A, non-B hepatitis had been controversial. In 1981, data from the transfusion-transmitted virus study showed that an association existed between elevated ALT and posttransfusion non-A, non-B hepatitis (340), and that excluding blood with an elevated ALT would reduce posttransfusion non-A, non-B hepatitis by 30%. A similar study at the National Institutes of Health gave a similar result (47). Neither study was randomized, and blood with elevated ALT was not excluded from use; thus, the effect on reduction in posttransfusion non-A, non-B hepatitis was a calculated, projected one not based on actual observation. ALT as a screening test for blood donors is helpful in only a general way because eliminating blood with an elevated ALT would not eliminate approximately 70% of posttransfusion hepatitis; also, approximately 70% of donors with elevated ALT were not implicated in posttransfusion hepatitis.

Later, the transfusion-transmitted virus study data were analyzed to determine whether an association between anti-HB$_c$ and posttransfusion non-A, non-B hepatitis existed (45). This and the National Institutes of Health data (46) showed that posttransfusion non-A, non-B hepatitis was more than twice as common in recipients of anti-HB$_c$–positive blood compared with recipients of anti-HB$_c$–negative blood. It was projected that eliminating blood that was anti-HB$_c$–positive would eliminate approximately 40% of posttransfusion hepatitis. As with ALT, no study has been carried out to establish in practice the impact of anti-HB$_c$ testing. The two tests have little overlap in the persons who are positive for either test and so seem to identify two different groups. Nevertheless, both anti-HB$_c$ and ALT were introduced as "surrogate" tests as a strategy to decrease non-A, non-B hepatitis.

Hepatitis C

In 1989, a virus was reported that appeared to account for most posttransfusion non-A, non-B hepatitis. Termed *hepatitis C*, it is an RNA virus similar in classification to a togavirus (43). Initially, anti-HCV was found in six of seven human sera that caused non-A, non-B hepatitis in chimpanzees and in donor units from nine of ten patients with posttransfusion non-A, non-B hepatitis (43). Approximately 80% of patients with posttransfusion non-A, non-B hepatitis in Italy and Japan and 15 of 15 patients in the United States had anti-HCV (344). Initially, anti-HCV was found in 0.68% of French (345), 0.87% of Italian (346), and 0.50% of American blood donors (44); however, only 54% of persons with antibodies to HCV were also anti-HB$_c$–positive, and 33% had an elevated ALT. Thus, although the long-awaited screening test for the non-A, non-B (HCV) virus became available, it was necessary to continue to test donors for ALT and anti-HB$_c$. The ability to detect HCV and to screen donors for its antibody has made it possible to determine the effect of efforts to reduce the risk of posttransfusion non-A, non-B hepatitis. The introduction of ALT and anti-HB$_c$ as surrogate tests resulted in a 57% decrease in the risk of infection/unit of blood transfused, and the addition of anti-HCV testing caused a further decrease of 36% (50). Thus, overall, there has been approximately a 94% decrease in the risk of infection/unit of blood, and continued improvements in the testing reagents have further reduced the remaining risk to approximately one case of hepatitis C/100,000 units of blood transfused.

Human Immunodeficiency Virus Infection and Acquired Immunodeficiency Syndrome

The possibility of transfusion-transmitted AIDS first arose in 1982 with the report of hemophiliacs with *Pneumocystis carinii* pneumonia and an apparently new syndrome similar to that occurring in homosexual men (345). Later that year, the occurrence of the syndrome in a child who had received a transfusion from a donor who later developed AIDS further linked transfusion to AIDS (346). First epidemiologic evidence and then more clear and extensive clinical and laboratory evidence established that AIDS is caused by the HIV-1 retrovirus and can be transmitted by blood transfusion (347–352). In 1983, blood banks altered their medical screening practices to defer potential donors from AIDS risk groups, and in May 1985, routine testing of all donated blood for anti–HIV-1 began. These steps were extremely effective in reducing the infectivity of blood (52).

HIV-1 is a retrovirus, and the proviral DNA is integrated into the host DNA, thus conferring permanent infection. Development of antibodies does not result in eradication of the virus but signifies previous infection and probable present infectivity. Anti-HIV usually persists until the person exhibits symptoms; thus, the test for HIV-1 antibody is used to detect infectious donated blood.

HUMAN IMMUNODEFICIENCY VIRUS 1 ANTIBODY TEST

The HIV-1 antibody test is an excellent test. In widespread clinical use, the HIV antibody test has generally been shown to detect HIV antibody in 98% to 100% of AIDS patients and to give a negative test result in approximately 99.8% of persons who have not been infected with HIV (353,354). In a population with a known prevalence of the virus for a test with a known sensitivity and specificity, the positive predictive value varies with the prevalence of the virus in the population. Although the specificity and sensitivity of the HIV antibody tests is excellent, the predictive value of a positive HIV antibody test in blood donors is low because of the low incidence of HIV infection in that population, and it differs slightly in different parts of the United States where the incidence of HIV in blood donors is different.

When a blood donor is found to be anti-HIV–positive on initial testing, the test is repeated in duplicate. If at least one of the repeat tests is also positive, the donor unit is said to be *repeatedly reactive*, and that unit is discarded. Units that are not positive on the repeat test (thus not repeatedly reactive) are suitable for transfusion. The blood sample from all repeat reactive donors is then tested using the Western blot, which identifies antibodies directed against the individual structural polypeptides of HIV (355). The definition of a positive Western blot is that the serum must have antibodies to the p24 gag protein, the p31 pol protein, and the gp41 or gp120/160 env glycoprotein, or both (356,357). A number of other patterns of reactivity with different bands may be observed. These are usually classified as *indeterminate*. It appears that these indeterminate Western blot results do not indicate infection by HIV (357). Loss of antibody is probably rare in asymptomatic persons.

RISK OF ACQUIRING HUMAN IMMUNODEFICIENCY VIRUS INFECTION FROM THE TRANSFUSION OF ANTIBODY TO HUMAN IMMUNODEFICIENCY VIRUS–POSITIVE BLOOD

The risk of acquiring HIV infection after transfusion with anti–HIV-1–positive blood is as high as 70% to 91% (358,359). Before the introduction of HIV-1 antibody testing in May 1985, an estimated 12,000 patients were infected with HIV-1 by transfusion

(360,361). The incubation period between transmission-transmitted HIV-1 infection and the development of AIDS was 4.5 to 14.2 years (362), but it is probably longer now due to the use of new antiretroviral agents.

RISK OF ACQUIRING HUMAN IMMUNODEFICIENCY VIRUS BY THE TRANSFUSION OF ANTIBODY TO HUMAN IMMUNODEFICIENCY VIRUS–NEGATIVE BLOOD

Because the HIV test detects anti-HIV, there is an interval between the acquisition of the virus and the development of the antibody (window phase). HIV can be transmitted by this window phase, antibody-negative blood or by chronic carriers who have not developed antibody, viral variants, or laboratory errors (363). Window phase transmission is rare but the most common of these routes. Studies from accidentally inoculated health care workers indicate that the window period for HIV from exposure to seroconversion is approximately 40 days, but, as antibody tests have improved, this period has been reduced to approximately 20 days (364). Despite this, the present risk of acquiring HIV infection through blood transfusion is extremely low. The risk depends on the prevalence of HIV infection in the community and, thus, on the donor population from which the unit of blood was obtained. Thus, it is difficult to apply a single risk figure to the entire United States. The risk of acquiring HIV from a unit of blood that has been tested and found to be negative for HIV antibody has decreased from 1 in 33,000 units (363) to 1 in 40,000 units (364), to 1 in 60,000 units (365), to 1 in 68,000 units (366), to 1 in 200,000 units (367). Presently, the risk is so low that it must be estimated by mathematic modeling because traditional studies following up transfusion recipients identify too few cases to provide quantitative risk estimates. Mathematic modes indicate the present risk of transfusion-transmitted HIV to be approximately 1 in 750,000 units, and the present risk of transfusion-transmitted HCV to be approximately 1 in 250,000 (368). An estimate of the risk of all transfusion-transmitted diseases is shown in Table 57-21.

APPROACHES TO REDUCING THE WINDOW PHASE

Because the virus should be present during the window phase before the development of antibody and because HIV antigen has been detected in some patients before becoming HIV antibody–positive, HIV antigen screening of blood donors was introduced. Two large studies (369,370), each involving approximately 500,000 blood donors, did not reveal a single case of a blood donor's serum containing HIV antigen but no HIV antibody. Despite this, the theoretic advantages of antigen testing led to its adoption as a routine screening test of donated blood.

The most recent approach for reducing the window phase involves nucleic acid amplification testing in which polymerase chain reaction is used to amplify DNA sequences, thus making

TABLE 57-21. Risk of Transfusion-Transmitted Infections per Unit of Blood Transfused[a]

Infection	1 in
Human immunodeficiency virus	500,000
Human T-cell lymphotrophic virus I or II	Extremely rare
Hepatitis A	Extremely rare
Hepatitis B	100,000
Hepatitis C	100,000
Syphilis	Extremely rare, if at all

[a]Before introduction of nucleic acid amplification testing.

it possible to detect minute amounts of proviral DNA. Developing this testing strategy was advocated by the FDA in 1996 (371) and is now being implemented nationally (372). As of the year 2000, 16.3 million donations have been tested using nucleic acid testing, and 62 (1:263,000 screened units) were found to be positive for HCV, and four (1:3,000,150) were positive for HIV. If it is presumed that each donation could have infected two or three recipients, this testing prevented transmission of up to 180 cases of HCV and 12 cases of HIV (372,373). Despite these advances in laboratory testing, continued emphasis must be placed on the medical history process used to identify blood donors who might be at risk of transmitting HIV infection. In addition, public education and education of potential blood donors continue to be essential to encourage high-risk persons not to donate blood.

Malaria

Transmission of malaria by transfusion is possible but so rare in North America that few physicians have seen a case (373). All four species of *Plasmodium* can survive in refrigerated blood and have caused transfusion-transmitted malaria, although most cases involve *Plasmodium malariae*. Malaria has been transmitted by platelet transfusion as well as by red cells, and malarial parasites have been found in platelets of infected persons. Thus, periodic spiking fever in a patient who has recently received a transfusion could be due to malaria, but this would be unlikely.

Donors who might transmit malaria are screened out by medical history. *Plasmodium falciparum* and *Plasmodium vivax* produce symptoms within 6 months of infection. Thus, travelers returning from malaria areas are deferred for 6 months unless they have taken antimalaria prophylaxis, in which case they are deferred for 3 years. *P. malariae* infection may produce no symptoms for years, so the present screening procedures would not defer such donors. The risk is extremely small, and adjustment of present donor criteria is not warranted. Laboratory testing of donors for malaria is not practical or cost effective in the United States.

Syphilis

Transmission of syphilis by blood transfusion was common in the early days of blood transfusion but is now extremely rare. The *Treponema* survives in refrigerated blood for 48 hours (374). Thus, syphilis can be transmitted from components stored only a few days or from platelet concentrates stored at room temperature (375). All blood donors are tested for syphilis, although this is not an effective method of preventing transfusion-transmitted syphilis in the United States (375). Serologic tests for syphilis are negative in 25% to 50% of persons at the time of spirochetemia during primary syphilis. With the present general concern regarding the safety of the blood supply, it is unlikely that the requirement for routine syphilis testing will be eliminated.

Cytomegalovirus

CMV is a herpesvirus that is common in the general population. In healthy persons, infection with CMV usually causes few or no symptoms. CMV can be transmitted by blood transfusion to both immunocompetent and immunodeficient patients. The earliest indication that CMV could be transmitted by blood transfusion was the observation of a mononucleosis-like syndrome that occurred several weeks after open heart surgery in immunocompetent patients. This became known as *postperfusion* or *postpump*

syndrome and was shown to be due to CMV (376) or Epstein-Barr virus (377,378). Most of the immunocompetent patients who acquired transfusion-transmitted CMV were asymptomatic; in contrast, CMV can be a serious viral pathogen in patients with either congenital or acquired immunodeficiency or in those immunosuppressed for transplantation. Thus, posttransfusion CMV infection can range from asymptomatic with development of CMV antibody (in patients who are immunocompetent) to an infectious mononucleosis-like syndrome to severe—even fatal—generalized CMV infection.

The incidence of CMV antibodies in blood donors ranges from 30% to 80%. Healthy persons who pass all the medical screening requirements for blood donation may harbor CMV and transmit the virus through their donated blood components to susceptible patients. The CMV remains latent in the leukocytes of many infected, healthy persons, but efforts to isolate the virus have been unsuccessful. Thus, no practical laboratory test is available to determine which patients previously infected with CMV but healthy enough to donate blood may transmit the virus. Most previously infected persons have CMV antibodies, and this is used as a screening test, but only 2% to 12% of these persons' blood may be capable of transmitting the virus (379). A suggestion that persons with IgM anti-CMV are more likely to transmit the virus than those with IgG anti-CMV has not been substantiated. Because the virus resides in the leukocytes, blood components depleted of leukocytes may have a reduced or even absent risk of transmitting CMV infection (228,229,380). Plasma components (FFP, liquid plasma, cryoprecipitate) contain few leukocytes, and it does not appear that these components transmit CMV infection. Frozen deglycerolized red cells contain only approximately 1% to 5% of the original leukocytes and do not appear to transmit CMV infection (158), although washed red cells may transmit CMV (381). The administration of acyclovir prophylactically, CMV immune globulin, and intravenous Ig has been attempted, but use of CMV antibody–negative or leukoreduced blood is preferable.

Human T-Cell Lymphotrophic Virus I

HTLV-I, the first human retrovirus identified, causes adult T-cell leukemia and tropical spastic paraparesis. The virus is endemic in parts of Japan and the Caribbean but has a low incidence in the United States. No cases of transfusion-transmitted adult T-cell leukemia or tropical spastic paresis have been identified. Transmission of the virus by blood transfusion does occur (382). Approximately 60% of seronegative recipients developed anti–HTLV-I after transfusion of cellular blood products containing anti–HTLV-I (382). In the United States, anti–HTLV-I is found almost exclusively in intravenous drug abusers or persons from areas endemic for HTLV-I. Initially, the incidence of anti–HTLV-I in blood donors was 0.025% (48). Because of the potential for disease transmission, routine testing of all donated blood for anti–HTLV-I was initiated in the United States in December 1988. The screening test currently in use also detects antibodies to the HTLV-II virus. Confirmatory tests are used to distinguish these. No disease association is known for HTLV-II. Guidelines are now available for counseling donors found to test positive for anti–HTLV-I or -II (383). These donor-screening steps have prevented the potential problem of transfusion-transmitted adult T-cell leukemia or tropical spastic paraparesis.

Chagas' Disease

The parasite *Trypanosoma cruzi* is endemic in many parts of Central and South America. This organism causes Chagas' disease in which patients may develop megacolon, megaesophagus, and, possibly, heart failure. The organism can survive in refrigerated blood and can be transmitted by transfusion (384–386). Many patients with chronic *T. cruzi* may be asymptomatic and thus can pass the blood donor medical questions. Cases of transfusion-transmitted Chagas' disease have occurred in the United States. No laboratory tests or screening procedures are used in the United States to detect carriers of *T. cruzi*. In some endemic areas of Central and South America, donated blood is screened for *T. cruzi* (387).

Babesiosis

Babesia microti and *Babesia bovis* are protozoa that occasionally infect humans by tick bites. The protozoan causes an acute illness of fever, malaise, and, sometimes, hemolytic anemia; many infected persons are asymptomatic. Thus, *B. microti* can be transmitted by blood donated by asymptomatic infected donors (388). The ticks are prevalent in the northeast, mid-Atlantic, and upper-midwest. No suitable laboratory screening test is available. Some blood banks defer persons from heavily tick-infested areas during the summer months.

Lyme Disease

Borrelia burgdorferi, a spirochete transmitted to humans by ticks, causes an acute illness of fever, malaise, and an erythematous annular spreading skin lesion followed by a chronic phase that is characterized by neurologic or cardiac symptoms or both with or without arthritis. In up to 40% of persons, the infection is asymptomatic. The spirochetes survive in stored blood for up to 45 days (389). Thus, transmission of *B. burgdorferi* by transfusion is theoretically possible but has not been reported. Although a serologic test is available, it is not a suitable laboratory test for donor screening, and the widespread prevalence of the tick makes it impractical to defer donors from endemic areas (390).

Parvovirus

The parvovirus B19 has been implicated as a cause of aplastic anemia (391). This virus has been transmitted by transfusion of coagulation factor concentrates (392) and SD plasma (58) but not by cellular blood components. Parvovirus is a common infection in children. Infected persons may be asymptomatic or have a mild febrile illness. Infections apparently are uncommon in adults. This, combined with the brief period of viremia, makes transmission of parvovirus by blood transfusion unlikely—even rare. No laboratory screening of donated blood is done for parvovirus.

Variant Creutzfeldt-Jakob Disease

Creutzfeldt-Jakob disease (CJD) is a rare type of spongiform encephalopathy. A similar disease, bovine spongiform encephalopathy (BSE), occurs in cattle, and it appears that BSE can be transmitted from cattle to humans. The human version of BSE, known as *variant CJD* (vCJD), has caused more than 100 fatalities in England, and cases have also been found in France. Prion protein is associated with CJD and vCJD, but the exact infectious agent or mechanism of infection has not been identified. Thus, there is no laboratory test for diagnosing CJD, BSE, or vCJD. The brain of individuals with CJD is highly infectious, having transmitted CJD to individuals who have received growth hormone from the pituitary glands of patients who died of CJD; CJD has also been trans-

mitted by brain electrodes (393). It appears that vCJD is transmitted to humans through contact with or consumption of products from infected cattle. Intestinal lymphatic tissue and dendritic cells are involved, and it appears that some infectivity is associated with either the platelet or leukocyte portion of the buffy coat.

In experimental animals, blood or its components have been shown to be infectious during the incubation and the clinical stages of disease (393). Blood infectivity in humans has never been definitively established. Human blood spiked with scrapie infected hamster brain cells or blood from mice clinically ill with transmission spongiform encephalopathy have shown infectivity concentrated in the buffy coat with lower levels of infectivity in the plasma and essentially none in the red cell fractions. A variety of technical problems or difficulties with these studies have created limitations to all of these interpretations, so it is not yet established whether blood from humans who are incubating vCJD or are clinically ill is actually infectious.

No cases of transfusion-transmitted vCJD have been identified, but because the disease is uniformly fatal, has a long incubation period, and lacks a diagnostic test, steps have been taken to minimize the likelihood of transfusion transmission. Several countries affected by epidemics of BSE and with cases of vCJD have implemented universal leukodepletion in an effort to reduce any infectivity that might be present. In the United States, individuals who spent 3 months or more in the United Kingdom or 5 years in western Europe during the time of the BSE epidemic are deferred from blood donation. BSE and vCJD might not be transmitted by transfusion, but, if so, these initial steps should be helpful to reduce the potential risk.

Other Diseases

Theoretically, any disease in which microbes circulate in the blood and survive for a few days in stored blood components could be transmitted by transfusion. The diseases of most concern have been discussed. A few other diseases that almost never occur owing to transfusions in the United States are toxoplasmosis, leishmaniasis, microfilaria, and African trypanosomiasis.

THERAPEUTIC APHERESIS

The pathophysiology and symptoms of some diseases are due to the excessive accumulation of blood cells or plasma constituents. In these situations, blood cell separators ordinarily used to collect blood components by apheresis from normal donors can also be used therapeutically. Plasma, granulocytes, lymphocytes, platelets, or red cells can be removed selectively from patients.

Plasma Exchange

CLINICAL USES
Plasma exchange is the most common form of therapeutic apheresis and is used in a variety of diseases to remove IgG and IgM antibodies, immune complexes, or excess accumulation of normal substances or to replace normal constituents (Table 57-22). Plasma exchange as a therapy has suffered from the general problem that it is used in many diseases whose pathophysiology is poorly understood. Often, no specific laboratory measurements of a known pathologic agent

TABLE 57-22. Indications for Therapeutic Apheresis Generally Accepted for Reimbursement by Third-Party Payers

Plasma exchange
IgG
  Myasthenia gravis
  Eaton-Lambert syndrome
  Goodpasture syndrome
  Myeloma with renal failure
  Guillain-Barré syndrome
  Hemophilia with factor VIII inhibitor
  Chronic inflammatory demyelinating polyradiculopathy
IgM
  Waldenström's macroglobulinemia
  Cryoglobulinemia
  Hyperviscosity
Immune complex
  Glomerulonephritis, rapidly progressive
  Rheumatoid vasculitis
Metabolic diseases
  Refsum's disease
  Hyperlipoproteinemia, familial
  Cholestasis—intractable pruritus
Diseases of unknown cause
  Thrombotic thrombocytopenic purpura
  Thyroid storm
  Scleroderma, refractory
  Polymyositis, refractory
Cytapheresis
  Acute leukemia—debulking
  Hairy cell leukemia—maintenance
  Thrombocytosis, symptomatic
  Chronic myelogenous leukemia, acute symptoms
Red cell exchange
  Sickle cell disease

Ig, immunoglobulin.

are available that can be correlated with improvement in laboratory values and the patient's clinical condition after plasma exchange. As a result, no careful controlled trials of plasma exchange in many of these diseases have been reported. Because many of these diseases involve experiencing fluctuations or spontaneous improvements, the exact benefits of plasma exchange are often difficult to document. The effectiveness and role of plasma exchange in the management of specific diseases are outlined in Table 57-22. Multiple sclerosis is included because one controlled trial (393) and a more recent small study (394) showed a benefit from plasma exchange. However, this has not been confirmed, and the data remain limited to establish the value of plasma exchange in this disease.

PLASMA EXCHANGE TECHNIQUES

In plasma exchange using blood cell separators, the whole blood enters the instrument in which most of the red cells, leukocytes, and platelets are separated from the cell-poor plasma. This plasma is replaced with one or more of several available solutions. These include FFP, albumin, and saline. Vascular access for plasma exchange may be by peripheral veins (preferable) or by venous catheters. If catheters are used, they must have sufficient rigidity so they do not collapse when negative pressure for blood removal is applied. Also, it is not advisable to position the return catheter near the right atrium endocardium because of the possibility that the replacement solution might create an irritable focus and result in cardiac arrhythmia.

Usually, plasma exchange therapy involves several exchanges over a period of days or weeks. The frequency of exchange and length of the treatment depend on the situation. For instance, in

myasthenia gravis patients, we often use a course of six plasma exchanges over 2 weeks, possibly adding one or two more procedures, if indicated. In contrast, treatment of a patient with TTP might involve plasma exchange daily for several days or longer and extend for a month or more.

The volume of plasma to be exchanged is usually based on the estimated plasma volume of the patient. Because there is continuous mixing in the patient of replacement solution and the patient's plasma, the relation between the fraction of the unwanted compound remaining and the proportion of the patient's plasma volume exchanged is an exponential one (Fig. 57-4). After exchange equal to the patient's plasma volume, the unwanted component is reduced to approximately 35% of the initial value. Exchanging two times the patient's plasma volume further reduces the unwanted component only to approximately 15% of the initial value. Because of this diminishing effectiveness, we usually try to exchange approximately 1.5 times the patient's plasma volume. Depending on the size of the patient and the rate of blood flow that can be obtained, this procedure may last 4 to 6 hours.

Usually, albumin alone or albumin plus saline are used as replacement solutions. This avoids the possibility of disease transmission and allergic reactions from FFP. As discussed later, the loss of coagulation or other proteins is not so extreme that replacement with FFP is necessary in otherwise stable patients. FFP should be used only when replacement of coagulation factors or of other unknown but essential constituents is necessary, such as in the therapy of TTP.

Removal of such a large volume of plasma has several biochemical effects (395). Because some platelets are in the plasma being removed, approximately a 30% decrease in the platelet count takes approximately 3 days to return to baseline. The changes in the proteins IgG, IgM, IgA, factor V, ferritin, transferrin, lactic dehydrogenase, serum glutamic oxaloacetic transaminase, and alkaline phosphatase follow closely the decrease expected, which is based on the volume of plasma removed. When no FFP is used for replacement, coagulation test results are abnormal at the end of the plasma exchange. For instance, the prothrombin time is usually 20 seconds or longer, the partial thromboplastin time is usually longer than 180 seconds, and the fibrinogen is decreased by approximately 70% (395). These test values return to baseline in approximately 24 hours except for fibrinogen, which normalizes in 72 hours. Complement components C_3, C_4, and CH_{50} can be depleted when albumin is used as the replacement fluid. Because of its rapid synthetic rate, complement is not depleted unless plasma exchange is carried out daily for several days (396).

During therapeutic plasma exchange, there is some loss of platelets, and, in at least one patient, this had led to continuation of plasma exchange for the treatment of TTP when the persistent thrombocytopenia was really due to platelet removal during plasma exchange (397). It appears that during plasma exchange, platelet loss is greatest with the Fresenius (17.5%) and very small with the COBE and Haemonetics instruments (<2.5%).

No clinically important changes in electrolytes result from plasma exchange. If FFP is used for replacement, the citrate anticoagulant may cause reduced ionized calcium and symptoms of paresthesia and muscle cramping. Although some reduction in ionized calcium levels may be found, even when albumin is used as the replacement solution (345), routine supplementation with calcium during plasma exchange is not recommended.

COMPLICATIONS

Apheresis of normal donors for the production of blood components is well tolerated with few side effects and only rare serious complications. As Huestis and colleagues (398) pointed out, "a patient sick enough to require removal of plasma and its substitution with another fluid cannot be expected to react the same as a healthy donor." The nature and incidence of complications depend largely on the condition of the patient before plasma exchange. For instance, a stable patient with myasthenia gravis might have fewer complications than a patient with TTP. Complications can be categorized as those related to vascular access, replacement solutions, or the procedure itself. Replacement solution complications include citrate-induced hypocalcemia, coagulation factor depletion, depletion of other functional proteins, electrolyte abnormalities, and reactions or disease transmission when plasma is used. *Procedure-related complications* refer to hypotension or hypertension due to fluid imbalance or to problems related to the blood cell separator instrument. In the most comprehensive report of complications of plasma exchange, side effects occurred during 12% of procedures and involved 40% of patients (399). The incidence of severe complications was 0.5%. In general, plasma exchange is a safe procedure, which should be used only in "appropriate clinical circumstances with careful observation of the patient" (398).

Therapeutic Cytapheresis

In some patients with hematologic proliferative disorders, symptoms and severe complications can occur because of the high level of circulating cells. In one study, leukemic cellular aggregates were the cause of death in 24% of patients with acute myelogenous leukemia and 60% of patients with chronic myelogenous leukemia (400). All patients who died with leukocyte counts greater than 200,000/µL and 50% of those who died with leukocyte counts between 50,000 and 200,000/µL had prominent cellular aggregates and thrombi in their tissues.

Symptomatic vascular slugging due to high levels of circulating leukemia cells can be a medical emergency. Central nervous system leukostasis can lead to cerebral vascular neurosis with intracranial hemorrhage or thrombosis (401), pulmonary insufficiency (402), or coronary artery occlusion (403). The risk of a high leukocyte count in these patients is probably due to more than just the level of circulating leukocytes because leukemic myeloblasts secrete cytokines, especially tumor necrosis factor and interleukin 1, that can activate the endothelium probably contributing to the pathophysiology of leukostasis (404). Thus, rapid medical intervention may be necessary.

Blood cell separators can be used to accomplish this by removing abnormal accumulations of leukocytes, platelets, or red cells. In therapeutic cytapheresis, the blood cell separator instrument is operated similar to the manner in which it is operated in collection of the particular blood component from a normal donor. The procedure is usually lengthened to process more blood and thus remove a large number of cells. The number of cells removed depends on the initial level but can be 10^{11} or even 10^{12}. The peripheral leukocyte or platelet count may be reduced by 20% to 80%, depending on the initial level (405).

Fewer complications generally occur from cytapheresis than plasma exchange, because in cytapheresis the small volume of cells removed is replaced by saline or anticoagulant. Patients undergoing therapeutic cytapheresis are often seriously ill, and the cytapheresis procedure may be risky because of other factors such as bleeding or central nervous system problems.

As in therapeutic plasma exchange, few controlled trials have been carried out. Cytapheresis can be used to lower rapidly the elevated cell levels in acute or chronic leukemia and thrombocytosis. Sometimes, the procedure is performed to prevent problems such as central nervous system vascular slug-

ging in patients with chronic myelogenous leukemia, reduction of metabolic problems due to cell lysis during chemotherapy of acute promyelocytic leukemia, or thrombotic episodes in patients with thrombocytosis. In other situations, cytapheresis is performed to treat existing problems such as central nervous system symptoms in acute or chronic myelogenous leukemia patients with high leukocyte counts.

The medical literature is helpful in establishing the general indications for these procedures, but it is often difficult to decide for specific patients whether cytapheresis is necessary and, when performed, whether it was helpful. The following is a summary of the value of therapeutic cytapheresis in specific situations:

Chronic myelogenous leukemia. Symptoms of leukostasis may develop when the leukocyte count exceeds 100,000/µL. If the clinical condition warrants, one or two cytapheresis procedures can be used to rapidly lower the leukocyte level. Chemotherapy should also be started because cytapheresis is not effective maintenance therapy.

Chronic lymphocytic leukemia. High leukocyte levels in these patients rarely create problems. Although the count can be lowered rapidly by cytapheresis, this is not recommended unless the patient has symptoms that result from high levels of circulating lymphocytes.

Acute myelogenous leukemia. Patients who present with leukocyte counts greater than 100,000/µL (usually mostly myeloblasts) may have serious problems during the first few days of chemotherapy. These problems, including leukostasis, hyperuricemia, renal failure, and DIC, are thought to be due partly to the lysis of a large number of leukemia cells. The problems may be reduced or prevented by lowering the leukocyte count by cytapheresis. Usually, one or two cytapheresis procedures suffice.

Thrombocytosis. Thrombocytosis that occurs as part of myeloproliferative diseases can lead to hemorrhage or thrombosis, especially in the central nervous system. Platelet counts of 1 million/µL or more may occur. Cytapheresis can be used to lower the platelet count rapidly with the expectation that complications of thrombocytosis would be prevented (353).

Sickle cell disease. Red cell exchange is performed when removal of a large proportion of the patient's circulating red cells is desired. Use of a blood cell separator makes it possible to rapidly remove patient red cells and replace them with normal donor cells while maintaining hemostasis and fluid balance. This approach has been used to prevent a sickle cell crisis in patients with sickle cell disease. Red cell exchange in the management of sickle cell crisis is especially helpful in acute chest syndrome or stroke.

Photopheresis. Photopheresis is a form of immunotherapy in which the patient receives a psoralen compound, and leukapheresis is performed a while later, and the leukocytes are exposed to ultraviolet light. This ultraviolet irradiation activates the psoralen to initiate an immune response, which is not well understood. Possible mechanisms of action of photopheresis that have been suggested include stimulation of the development of response against clones of pathologic T lymphocytes, stimulation of the development of cloned specific suppressor cells, activation of monocytes, release of cytokines, or presentation of inactivated cells to the immune system enabling development of an immune response to cells. Photopheresis has been used in the treatment initially of cutaneous T-cell lymphoma, which is its only approved use, but also in autoimmune diseases, allograft rejection (406,407), and, possibly, chronic GVHD (408).

In addition to its use in the treatment of cutaneous T-cell lymphoma, certain autoimmune diseases, and rejection after solid organ transplantation, photopheresis appears to be effective in the management of steroid refractory chronic GVHD (408).

BLOOD SUBSTITUTES

The functions of blood can be grouped generally as maintenance of intravascular volume, oxygen delivery to tissues, provision of coagulation factors, provision of some defense mechanisms, and transport of metabolic waste products. Blood substitutes or artificial blood currently being developed substitutes only for the oxygen delivery function. Thus, more appropriate terms are *hemoglobin* or *red cell substitute*.

For years, considerable interest has existed in the use of a red cell substitute that would effectively transport oxygen from the lungs to the tissues. The ideal acellular red cell substitute would not require crossmatching or blood typing, could be stored preferably at room temperature for a long period, have a reasonable intravascular lifespan and thereafter be excreted promptly, and be free of toxicity or disease transmission. Four types of products are under development: perfluorocarbon compounds, cell-free hemoglobin from humans, cell-free hemoglobin from animals, particularly bovine hemoglobin, and liposome-encapsulated hemoglobin. Hemoglobin chemically binds oxygen, whereas perfluorocarbons have a solubility for oxygen 20 times greater than that of water but still bind much less oxygen than hemoglobin. The physiologic benefit of this high solubility for oxygen has been demonstrated dramatically by the survival of mice completely immersed in a solution of well-oxygenated perfluorocarbons. During the 1980s, a specific perfluorocarbon product underwent clinical trials in patients who required urgent medical care and who refused to receive blood components. The amount of oxygen that can be delivered is based on the oxygen content of inspired air. At ambient oxygen tension, the perfluorocarbon product was not effective, but when patients breathed 100% oxygen, perfluorocarbon provided increased oxygen consumption, an increased mixed venous oxygen tension, and an increased mixed venous hemoglobin saturation (408).

A study of 186 patients revealed no important adverse effects of the perfluorocarbon on hemodynamics, blood gases, hematologic parameters, coagulation tests, electrolytes, renal function, and liver enzymes (409). The perfluorocarbon product was toxic to macrophages, and, in some patients, caused bronchospasm, leukopenia, thrombocytopenia, and complement activation. In a careful study, eight severely anemic patients (hemoglobin, 1.2 to 4.5 g/dL) who received the perfluorocarbon product were compared with 15 who did not (410). All patients refused blood transfusion. The amount of perfluorocarbon that could be given to patients and the oxygen tension, even when 100% oxygen was inspired, were such that the perfluorocarbon contributed only approximately 50% of the oxygen-carrying capacity of the patient's plasma. The amount of oxygen delivered by the perfluorocarbon was not clinically significant, and the patients did not benefit. The major observations in this study were the ability of all the patients to tolerate remarkably low hemoglobin levels and the lack of need for increased arterial oxygen content in the 15 control patients who had hemoglobin levels of approximately 7 g/dL. A different perfluorocarbon is presently undergoing clinical trial for the limited indications of acute normovolemic hemodilution or intraoperative blood loss, or both (411).

Work with hemoglobin solutions has progressed steadily (411). Hemoglobin can be prepared in solution by lysis of red cells. The human hemoglobin products involve surface-modified hemoglobin, cross-linked hemoglobin, or polymerized hemoglobin. The drawbacks to these various forms of hemoglobin-based blood substitute are a short plasma half-life, potential renal toxicity of unmodified hemoglobin, vasoactivity, and the possible potentiation of sepsis. A large-scale study of one of these products was terminated prematurely because of an excess of complications in the patients receiving the hemoglobin substitute (413). A different product is undergoing what thus far appears to be a successful clinical trial in major surgery and trauma (414–416).

Clinical trials of bovine hemoglobin solution are under way in major surgery (417) and in one patient with severe autoimmune hemolytic anemia (418), and this product has recently been licensed for clinical use in South Africa. Liposome-encapsulated hemoglobin solution is less well developed, and no clinical trials in humans are under way at present (411).

Hemoglobin substitutes are likely to supplement, not replace, most red cell transfusions. Because the intravascular lifespan of the hemoglobin substitutes probably would be a few days, the major use is expected to be in the treatment of acute blood loss. Because blood typing and crossmatching would not be necessary, hemoglobin substitutes might be stocked in ambulances and used by paramedics outside of health care facilities. Other potential uses of hemoglobin substitutes are for organ perfusion and preservation before transplantation and for improvement of oxygen delivery to tissues that have an impaired blood supply, although products using either bovine hemoglobin or human hemoglobin produced using recombinant DNA techniques are also under development. If the use of hemoglobin solutions follows this course, the need for donated blood may increase rather than decline, as might have been expected.

REFERENCES

1. Myhre BA. The first recorded blood transfusions: 1656 to 1668. *Transfusion* 1990;30:358.
2. Greenwalt TJ. A short history of transfusion medicine. *Transfusion* 1997;37:550–563.
3. Wallace EL, Surgenor DM, Hao HS, et al. Collection and transfusion of blood and blood components in the United States, 1989. *Transfusion* 1993;33:139.
4. Eastlund T. Monetary blood donation incentives and the risk of transfusion-transmitted infection. *Transfusion* 1998;38:874–882.
5. Stuart MJ, Murphy S, Oski FA, et al. Platelet function in recipients of platelets from donors ingesting aspirin. *N Engl J Med* 1972;287:1105.
6. O'Brien JR, Finch W, Clark E. A comparison of an effect of different anti-inflammatory drugs on human platelets. *J Clin Pathol* 1970;23:522.
7. McVay PA, Andrews A, Kaplan EB, et al. Donation reactions among autologous donors. *Transfusion* 1990;30:249.
8. Wood EM, Kim DM, Miller JP. Accuracy of predonation Hct sampling affects donor safety, eligibility, and deferral rates. *Transfusion* 2001;41:353–359.
9. Adamson J, Hillman RS. Blood volume and plasma protein replacement following acute blood loss in normal man. *JAMA* 1968;205:609.
10. Newman BH, Waxman DA. Blood donation-related neurologic needle injury: evaluation of 2 years' worth of data from a large blood center. *Transfusion* 1996;36:213–215.
11. Members of the National Blood Resource Education Program Expert Panel on the Use of Autologous Blood. The use of autologous blood: the national blood resource education program expert panel. *JAMA* 1990;263:414.
12. Braude AI, Carey FJ, Siemienski J. Studies of bacterial transfusion reactions from refrigerated blood: the properties of cold growing bacteria. *J Clin Invest* 1955;34:311.
13. Goodnough LT, Rudnick S, Price TH, et al. Increased preoperative collection of autologous blood with recombinant human erythropoietin therapy. *N Engl J Med* 1989;321:1163.
14. Mann M, Sacks HJ, Goldfinger D. Safety of autologous blood donation prior to elective surgery for a variety of potentially "high-risk" patients. *Transfusion* 1983;23:229.
15. Owings DV, Kruskall MS, Thurer RL, et al. Autologous blood donations prior to elective cardiac surgery. *JAMA* 1989;262:1963.
16. Kruskall MS. Controversies in transfusion medicine. The safety and utility of autologous donations by pregnant patients: pro. *Transfusion* 1990;30:168.
17. Kruskall MS, Leonard S, Klapholz H. Autologous blood donation during pregnancy: analysis of safety and blood use. *Obstet Gynecol* 1987;70:938.
18. Kamani AA, McMorland GH, Wadsworth LD. Utilization of red blood cell transfusion in an obstetric setting. *Am J Obstet Gynecol* 1988;159:1177.
19. Ray JM, Flynn JC, Bierman AH. Erythrocyte survival following intraoperative autotransfusion in spinal surgery: an in vivo comparative study and 5-year update. *Spine* 1986;11:879.
20. McShane AJ, Power C, Jackson JF, et al. Autotransfusion: quality of blood prepared with a red cell processing device. *Br J Anaesth* 1987;59:1035.
21. McCarthy PM, Popovsky MA, Schaff HV, et al. Effect of blood conservation efforts in cardiac operations at the Mayo Clinic. *Mayo Clin Proc* 1988;63:225.

22. Tawes RL, Scribner RG, Duval TB, et al. The cell-saver and autologous transfusion: an underutilized resource in vascular surgery. *Am J Surg* 1986;152:105.

23. Popovsky MA, Devine PA, Taswell HF. Intraoperative autologous transfusion. *Mayo Clin Proc* 1985;60:125.

24. Hallet JW, Popovsky MA, Ilstrup MS. Minimizing blood transfusions during abdominal aortic surgery: recent advances in rapid autotransfusion. *J Vasc Surg* 1987;5:601.

25. Bensinger WI, Price TH, Dale DC, et al. The effects of daily recombinant human granulocyte-colony-stimulating factor administration on normal granulocyte donors undergoing leukapheresis. *Blood* 1993;81:1883–1888.

26. Dale DC, Liles WC, Llewellyn C, et al. Neutrophil transfusions: kinetics and functions of neutrophils mobilized with granulocyte colony-stimulating factor (G-CSF) and dexamethasone. *Transfusion* 1998;38:713–721.

27. McCullough J, Clay M, Herr G, et al. Effects of granulocyte colony stimulating factor (G-CSF) on potential normal granulocyte donors. *Transfusion* 1999;39:1136–1140.

28. McCullough J, Weiblen BJ, Fine D. Effects of storage of granulocytes on their fate in vivo. *Transfusion* 1983;23:20.

29. McCullough J. Granulocyte function during short-term liquid storage. *Exp Hematol* 1983;5:95.

30. Storb R, Graham TC, Epstein RB, et al. Demonstration of hematopoietic stem cells in the peripheral blood of baboons by cross circulation. *Blood* 1977;50:537.

31. Lasky LC. Hematopoietic reconstitution using progenitors recovered from blood. *Transfusion* 1989;29:552.

32. Kessinger A, Armitage JO, Landmark JD, et al. Autologous peripheral hematopoietic stem cell transplantation restores hematopoietic function following marrow ablative therapy. *Blood* 1988;71:723.

33. Pettengell R, Morgenstern GR, Woll PJ, et al. Peripheral blood progenitor cell transplantation in lymphoma and leukemia using a single apheresis. *Transfusion* 1993;82:3770–3777.

34. Ottinger HD, Beelen DW, Scheulen B, et al. Improved immune reconstitution after allotransplantation of peripheral blood stem cells instead of bone marrow. *Blood* 1996;88:2775–2779.

35. Bensinger WI, Clift R, Martin P, et al. Allogeneic peripheral blood stem cell transplantation in patients with advanced hematologic malignancies: a retrospective comparison with marrow transplantation. *Blood* 1996;88:2794–2800.

36. Anderlini P, Przepiorka D, Champlin R, et al. Biologic and clinical effects of granulocyte colony-stimulating factor in normal individuals. *Blood* 1996;88:2819–2825.

37. Stroncek DF, Clay ME, Petzoldt ML, et al. Treatment of normal individuals with granulocyte-colony-stimulating factor: donor experiences and the effects on peripheral blood CD34+ cell counts and on the collection of peripheral blood stem cells. *Transfusion* 1996;36:601–610.

38. Senhauser DA, Westphal RG, Bohman JE, et al. Immune system changes in cytapheresis donors. *Transfusion* 1982;22:302.

39. Heal JM, Horan PK, Schmitt TC, et al. Long-term follow-up of donors cytapheresed more than 50 times. *Vox Sang* 1983;45:14.

40. Koepke JA, Parks WM, Goeken JA, et al. The safety of weekly plateletapheresis: effect on the donors' lymphocyte population. *Transfusion* 1981;21:59.

41. Matsui Y, Martin-Alosco S, Doenges E, et al. Effects of frequent and sustained plateletapheresis on peripheral blood mononuclear cell populations and lymphocyte functions of normal volunteer donors. *Transfusion* 1986;26:446.

42. Greenwalt TJ, Rios JA. To test or not to test for syphilis: a global problem (editorial). *Transfusion* 2001;41:976.

42a. Schmidt PJ. Syphilis, a disease of direct transfusion. *Transfusion* 2001;41:1069.

43. Choo QL, Kuo G, Weiner AJ, et al. Isolation of a cDNA derived from a blood-borne non-A, non-B viral hepatitis genome. *Science* 1989;244:359.

44. Kleinman S, Alter H, Busch M, et al. Increased detection of hepatitis C virus (HCV)–infected blood donors by a multiple-antigen HCV enzyme immunoassay. *Transfusion* 1992;32:805.

45. Stevens CE, Aach RD, Hollinger FB. Hepatitis B virus antibody in blood donors and the occurrence of non-A, non-B hepatitis in transfusion recipients: an analysis of the transfusion-transmitted viruses study. *Ann Intern Med* 1984;101:733.

46. Koziol DE, Holland PV, Alling DW, et al. Antibody to hepatitis B core antigen as a paradoxical marker for non-A, non-B hepatitis agents in donated blood. *Ann Intern Med* 1986;104:488.

47. Alter HJ, Purcell RH, Holland PV, et al. Donor transaminase and recipient hepatitis: impact on blood transfusion services. *JAMA* 1981;246:630.

48. Williams AE, Fang CT, Slamon DJ, et al. Seroprevalence and epidemiologic correlates of HTLV-1 infection in U.S. blood donors. *Science* 1988;240:643.

49. Dodd RY. The risk of transfusion-transmitted infection (editorial). *N Engl J Med* 1992;327:419.

50. Donahue JG, Munoz A, Ness PM, et al. The declining risk of posttransfusion hepatitis C virus infection. *N Engl J Med* 1992;327:369.

51. McCullough J. The nation's changing blood supply system. *JAMA* 1993;269:2239.

52. Busch MP, Young MJ, Samson SJ, et al. Risk of human immunodeficiency virus (HIV) transmission by blood transfusions before the implementation of HIV-1 antibody screening. *Transfusion* 1991;31:4.

53. Valtis DJ, Kennedy AC. Defective gas-transport function of stored red blood-cells. *Lancet* 1954;1:119.

54. National Institutes of Health Consensus Conference. Fresh frozen plasma: indications and risks. *JAMA* 1985;253:546.

55. Horowitz B, Bonomo R, Prince AM, et al. Solvent/detergent-treated plasma: a virus-inactivated substitute for fresh frozen plasma. *Blood* 1992;79:826–831.

56. Inbal A, Epstein O, Blickstein D, et al. Evaluation of solvent/detergent treated plasma in the management of patients with hereditary and acquired coagulation disorders. *Blood Coagul Fibrinolysis* 1993;4:599–604.

57. Lerner RH, Nelson J, Sorcia E, et al. Evaluation of solvent/detergent-treated plasma in patients with a prolonged prothrombin time. *Vox Sang* 2000;79:161–167.

58. Koenigbauer UF, Eastlund T, Day JW. Clinical illness due to parvovirus B19 infection after infusion of solvent/detergent-treated pooled plasma. *Transfusion* 2000;40:1203–1206.

59. Slichter SJ, Harker LA. Preparation and storage of platelet concentrates. II. Storage and variables influence platelet viability and function. *Br J Haematol* 1976;34:403.

60. Filip DJ, Aster RH. Relative hemostatic effectiveness of human platelets stored at 4°C and 22°C. *J Lab Clin Med* 1978;91:618.

61. Kunicki TJ, Tuccelli M, Becker GA, et al. A study of variables affecting the quality of platelets stored at "room temperature." *Transfusion* 1975;15:414.

62. Holme S, Vaidja K, Murphy S. Platelet storage at 22°C: effect of type of agitation on morphology, viability and function in vitro. *Blood* 1978;52:425.

63. Murphy S, Sayer SN, Garner FH. Storage of platelet concentrates at 22°C. *Blood* 1970;35:549.

64. Murphy S, Kahn RA, Holme S, et al. Improved storage of platelets for transfusion in a new container. *Blood* 1982;60:194.

65. Hogge DE, Thompson BW, Schiffer CA. Platelet storage for 7 days in second-generation blood banks. *Transfusion* 1986;26:131.

66. Simon TL, Nelson EJ, Murphy S. Extension of platelet concentrate storage to 7 days in second-generation bags. *Transfusion* 1987;27:6.

67. Heal JM, Singal S, Sardisco E, et al. Bacterial proliferation in platelet concentrates. *Transfusion* 1986;26:388.

68. Braine HG, Kickler TS, Charache P, et al. Bacterial sepsis secondary to platelet transfusion: an adverse effect of extended storage at room temperature. *Transfusion* 1986;26:391.

69. Chiu EKW, Yuen KY, Lie AKW, et al. A prospective study of symptomatic bacteremia following platelet transfusion and of its management. *Transfusion* 1994;34:950–954.

70. Garratty G, Dzik W, Issitt PD, et al. Terminology for blood group antigens and genes—historical origins and guidelines in the new millennium. *Transfusion* 2000;40:477–489.

71. Issitt PD, Anstee DJ. *Applied blood group serology*, 4th ed. Durham, NC: Montgomery Scientific Publications, 1998.

72. Daniels G. *Human blood groups*. Oxford: Blackwell Science, 1995.

73. Landsteiner K. Agglutination phenomena in normal human blood. Translation of "Über gglutination Serscheinungen Normalen Menschichlen Blutes." *Wien Klin Wochenschr* 1901;14:1132–1134.

74. Cook PJL, Roboon EB, Buckton KE, et al. Segregation of ABO, AK1 and ACONS in families with abnormalities of chromosome 9. *Ann Hum Genet* 1978;41:365.

75. Ferguson-Smith M, Aitken D, Turleau C, et al. Localization of the human ABO:Np1:AK-1 linkage group by regional assignment of AK-1 to 9q34. *Hum Genet* 1976;34:35.

76. Yamamoto F, Marken J, Tsuji T, et al. Cloning and characterization of DNA complementary to human UDP-GalNAc: Fuc alpha 1→2Gal alpha 1→3GalNAc transferase (histo-blood group A transferase) mRNA. *J Biol Chem* 1990;265:1146.

77. Yamamoto F, Clausen H, White T, et al. Molecular genetic basis of the histo-blood group ABO system. *Nature* 1990;345:229.

78. Lublin DM. Universal RBCs (editorial). *Transfusion* 2000;40:1285–1289.

79. Kruskall MS, AuBuchon JP, Anthony KY, et al. Transfusion to blood group A and O patients of group B RBCs that have been enzymatically converted to group O. *Transfusion* 2000;40:1290–1298.

80. Scott MD, Murad KL, Koumpouras F, et al. Chemical camouflage of antigenic determinants: stealth erythrocytes. *Proc Natl Acad Sci U S A* 1997;94(14):7566–7571.

81. Scott MD, Bradley AJ, Murad KL. Camouflaged blood cells: low-technology bioengineering for transfusion medicine? *Transfus Med Rev* 2000;14:53–63.

82. Levine P, Stetson R. An unusual case of intragroup agglutination. *JAMA* 1939;113:126.

83. Landsteiner K, Wiener AS. An agglutinable factor in human blood recognizable by immune sera phoresis blood. *Proc Soc Exp Biol Med* 1940;43:223.

84. Wiener AS. Genetic theory of the Rh blood types. *Proc Soc Exp Biol Med* 1943;54:316.

85. Race RR. An "incomplete" antibody in human serum. *Nature* 1944;153:771.

86. Cherif-Zahar B, Mattei MG, Le Van Kim C, et al. Localization of the human Rh blood group gene structure to chromosome 1p34.3-1p36.1 region by in situ hybridization. *Hum Genet* 1991;86:98.

87. Le Van Kim C, Mouro I, Cherif-Zahar B, et al. Molecular cloning and primary structure of the human blood group RhD polypeptide. *Proc Natl Acad Sci U S A* 1992;89:10925.

88. Moore S, Woodrow CF, McClelland DB. Isolation of membrane components associated with human red cell antigens Rho(D), (c), (E), and Fyᵃ. *Nature* 1982;295:529.

89. Gahmberg CG. Molecular identification of the human Rho(D) antigen. *FEBS Lett* 1982;140:93.

90. Saboori AM, Smith BL, Agre P. Polymorphism in the M_r 32,000 Rh protein purified from Rh(D) positive and negative erythrocytes. *Proc Natl Acad Sci U S A* 1988;85:4042.

91. Masouredis SP, Sudora EJ, Mahan L, et al. Antigen site densities and ultrastructural distribution patterns of red cell Rh antigens. *Transfusion* 1976;16:94.

92. Nicolson GL, Masouredis SP, Singer SJ. Quantitative two-dimensional ultrastructural distribution of Rho(D) antigenic sites on human erythrocyte membranes. *Proc Natl Acad Sci U S A* 1971;68:1416.

93. James NT, James V. Nearest neighbor analyses on the distribution of Rh antigens on erythrocyte membranes. *Br J Haematol* 1978;40:657.

94. Lee S, Zambas ED, Marsh WL, et al. The human Kell blood group gene maps to chromosome 7q33 and its expression is restricted to erythroid cells. *Blood* 1993;81:2804.

95. Lee S, Zambas ED, Marsh WL, et al. Molecular cloning and primary structure of Kell blood group protein. *Proc Natl Acad Sci U S A* 1991;88:6353.

96. Redman CM, Marsh WL, Mueller KA, et al. Isolation of Kell-active protein from the red cell membrane. *Transfusion* 1984;294:176.

97. Redman CM, Avellino G, Pfeffer SR, et al. Kell blood group antigens are part of a 93,000 dalton red cell membrane protein. *J Biol Chem* 1986;261:9521.

98. Redman CM, Lee S, Marsh WL. Isolation and partial characterization of Kell blood group protein. In: Moore SB, ed. *Progress in immunohematology.* Arlington, VA: American Association of Blood Banks, 1988:141.

99. Masouredis SP, Sudora E, Mahan L, et al. Quantitative immunoferritin microscopy of Fy^a, Fy^b, Jk^a, U, and Di^b antigen site numbers of human red cells. *Blood* 1980;56:969.

100. Hadley TJ, David PH, McGinniss MH, et al. Identification of an erythrocyte component carrying the Duffy blood group Fy^a antigen. *Science* 1984;223:597.

101. Miller LH, Mason SJ, Devorak JA, et al. Erythrocyte receptors for plasmodium knowlesi malaria, Duffy blood group determinants. *Science* 1975;189:561.

102. Miller LH, Aikawa M, Johnson JG, et al. Interaction between cytochalasin B-treated malarial parasites and erythrocytes: attachment and junction formation. *J Exp Med* 1979;149:172.

103. Oriol R, Cartron J, Yvart J, et al. The Lewis system: new histocompatibility antigens in renal transplantation. *Lancet* 1978;1:574.

104. Chaplin H, Hunter VL, Malech AC, et al. Clinically significant allo-anti-I in an I-negative patient with massive hemorrhage. *Transfusion* 1986;25:57.

105. Swanson J. Laboratory problems associated with leukocyte antibodies. *Recent Adv Immunohematol* 1973;121.

106. Dunstan RA, Simpson MB, Knowles RW, et al. The origin of ABO antigens on human platelets. *Blood* 1985;65:615.

107. Kools A, Collins J, Aster RH. Studies of the ABO antigens of human platelets (abstract). *Transfusion* 1981;21:615.

108. Clay ME, Kline WE. Detection of granulocyte antigens and antibodies: current perspectives and approaches. In: Garratty G, ed. *Current concepts in transfusion therapy.* Arlington, VA: American Association of Blood Banks, 1985:229.

109. Dunstan RA, Simpson MB, Sanfilippo FP. Absence of specific HLA-DR antigens on human platelets and neutrophils (abstract). *Blood* 1984;64:85a.

110. McCullough J, Clay M, Loken M, et al. Effect of ABO incompatibility on fate in vivo of ^{111}Indium granulocytes. *Transfusion* 1988;28:358.

111. Clay ME, Kline WE, McCullough J. Granulocyte antigens and antibodies: current concepts of detection and histocompatibility testing. In: Dutcher J, ed. *Modern transfusion therapy.* Boca Raton, FL: CRC Press, 1990:182.

112. Thompson JS. Antileukocyte capillary agglutinating antibody in pre- and post-transplantation sera. In: Rose NR, Friedman H, eds. *Manual of clinical immunology.* Washington: American Society of Microbiology, 1976:868.

113. Minchinton RM, Waters AH, Malpas JS, et al. Platelet- and granulocyte-specific antibodies after allogeneic and autologous bone marrow grafts. *Vox Sang* 1984;46:125.

114. McCullough J, Clay ME, Press C, et al. *Granulocyte serology: a clinical and laboratory guide.* Chicago: American Society of Clinical Pathologists Press, 1988:83–112.

115. Warkentin PI, Clay ME, Kersey JH, et al. Successful engraftment of NA1 positive bone marrow in a patient with a neutrophil antibody, anti-NA1. *Hum Immunol* 1981;2:173.

116. Stroncek DF, Shapiro RS, Filipovich AH, et al. Prolonged neutropenia resulting from antibodies to neutrophil-specific antigen NB1 following marrow transplantation. *Transfusion* 1993;33:158.

117. Boxer LA, Yokoyama M, Lalezari P. Isoimmune neonatal neutropenia. *J Pediatr* 1972;80:783.

118. Trounstine ML, Peitz GA, Yssel H, et al. Reactivity of cloned, expressed human FcRIII isoforms with monoclonal antibodies which distinguish cell type specific and allelic forms of Fc-gamma-RIII. *Int Immunol* 1990;2:303.

119. Ory PA, Clark MR, Kwoh EE, et al. Sequences of complementary DNAs that encode the NA1 and NA2 forms of Fc receptor III on human neutrophils. *J Clin Invest* 1989;84:1688.

120. Huizinga TW, Kleijer M, Tetteroo PA, et al. Biallelic neutrophil Na-antigen system is associated with a polymorphism on the phospho-inositol–linked Fc gamma receptor III (CD16) *Blood* 1990;75:213.

121. Richards KL, McCullough J. Chemotactic and chemokinetic responsiveness of fresh and stored human granulocytes (abstract). Annual meeting of the American Society for Cell Biology. *J Cell Biol* 1982;95:324a.

122. Shulman IA, Nelson JM, Saxena S, et al. Experience with routine use of an abbreviated crossmatch. *Am J Clin Pathol* 1984;82:178.

123. Heddle NM, O'Hoski P, Singer J, et al. A prospective study to determine the safety of omitting the antiglobulin crossmatch from pretransfusion testing. *Br J Haematol* 1992;81:579–584.

124. Pinkerton PH, Coovadia AS, Goldstein J. Frequency of delayed hemolytic transfusion reactions following antibody screening and immediate-spin crossmatch. *Transfusion* 1992;32:814–817.

125. International Committee for Standardization in Hematology: recommended method for radioisotope red cell survival studies. *Br J Haematol* 1980;45:659.

126. Silvergleid AJ, Wells RP, Hafleigh EB, et al. Compatibility test using 51Cr-labeled red blood cells in crossmatched positive patients. *Transfusion* 1978; 18:8.

127. Aster R. Effect of anticoagulant and ABO incompatibility on recovery of transfused human platelets. *Blood* 1965;26:732.

128. Heal JM, Blumberg N. The second century of ABO: and now for something completely different. *Transfusion* 1999;39:1155–1159.

129. Benjamin RJ, Antin JH. ABO-incompatible bone marrow transplantation: the transfusion of incompatible plasma may exacerbate regimen-related toxicity. *Transfusion* 1999;39:1273–1274.

130. Benjamin RJ, McGurk S, Ralston MS, et al. ABO incompatibility as an adverse risk factor for survival after allogeneic bone marrow transplantation. *Transfusion* 1999;39:179–187.

131. Carr R, Hutton JL, Jenkins JA, et al. Transfusion of ABO-mismatched platelets leads to early platelet refractoriness. *Br J Haematol* 1990;75:408–413.

131a. Murphy S. ABO blood groups and platelet transfusion. *Transfusion* 1988;28: 401.

132. Goldfinger D, McGinnis MH. Rh incompatible platelet transfusions—risks and consequences of sensitizing immunosuppressed patients. *N Engl J Med* 1971;284:942.

133. Lichtiger B, Surgeon J, Rhorer S. Rh-incompatible platelet transfusion therapy in cancer patients. *Vox Sang* 1983;45:139.

134. Baldwin ML, Ness PM, Scott D, et al. Alloimmunization to D antigen and HLA in D-negative immunosuppressed oncology patients. *Transfusion* 1988;28:330.

135. Pollack W, Ascari WQ, Kochesky RJ, et al. Studies on Rh prophylaxis. I. Relationship between doses of anti-Rh and size of antigenic stimulus. *Transfusion* 1971;11:333.

136. Pfisterer H, Thierfelder S, Kottusch H. Untersuchung menschlicher thrombocyten auf rhesus-antigen durch abbaustudien in vivo nach 51Cr-markierung. *Klin Wochenschr* 1967;45:519.

137. McCullough J, Clay M, Hurd D, et al. Effect of leukocyte antibodies and HLA matching on the intravascular recovery, survival and tissue localization of 111-indium granulocytes. *Blood* 1986;67:522.

138. Hillman RS, Hershko. Acute blood loss anemia. In: Beutler E, Lichtman MA, Coller BS, et al., eds. *Williams hematology,* 6th ed. New York: McGraw-Hill, 2001.

139. Gollub S, Svigals R, Bailey CP, et al. Electrolyte solutions in surgical patients refusing transfusion. *JAMA* 1971;215:2077.

140. Rigor B, Bosomworth P, Ruth BF Jr. Replacement of operative blood loss of more than 1 liter with Hartmann's solution. *JAMA* 1968;203:111.

141. Office of Medical Applications of Research, National Institutes of Health. Perioperative red cell transfusion. *JAMA* 1988;260:2700.

142. Welch HG, Meehan KR, Goodnough LT. Prudent strategies for elective red blood cell transfusion. *Ann Intern Med* 1992;116:393.

143. American College of Physicians. Practice strategies for elective red blood cell transfusion. *Ann Intern Med* 1992;115:403.

144. Faust RJ. Perioperative indications for red blood cell transfusion: has the pendulum swung too far? *Mayo Clin Proc* 1993;68:512.

145. Perkins HA, Payne R, Ferguson J, et al. Nonhemolytic febrile transfusion reactions: quantitative effects of blood components with emphasis on isoantigenic incompatibility of leukocytes. *Vox Sang* 1966;11:578.

146. Kao KJ, Mickel M, Braine HG, et al. White cell reduction in platelet concentrates and packed red cells by filtration: a multicenter clinical trial. The TRAP Study Group. *Transfusion* 1995;35:13–19.

147. Miller WJ, McCullough J, Balfour HH Jr, et al. Prevention of CMV infection following bone marrow transplantation: a randomized trial of blood product screening. *Bone Marrow Transplant* 1991;7(3):227–234.

148. Bowden RA, Sayers M, Flournoy N, et al. Cytomegalovirus immune globulin and seronegative blood products prevent primary cytomegalovirus infection after marrow transplantation. *N Engl J Med* 1986;314:1006.

149. Opelz G, Sengar DPS, Mickey MR, et al. Effect of blood transfusions on subsequent kidney transplants. *Transplant Proc* 1973;5:253.

150. Opelz G, Terasaki PI. Improvement of kidney-graft survival with increased numbers of blood transfusions. *N Engl J Med* 1978;299:799.

151. Ratko TA, Cummings JP, Oberman HA, et al. Evidence-based recommendations for the use of WBC-reduced cellular blood components. *Transfusion* 2001;41:1310.

152. Nightingale SD. Universal WBC reduction. *Transfusion* 2001;41:1306.

153. Snyder EL. Clinical use of white cell-poor blood components. *Transfusion* 1989;29:568.

154. Class FHJ, Smeenk RJT, Schmidt R, et al. Alloimmunization against the MHC antigens after platelet transfusions is due to contaminating leukocytes in the platelet suspension. *Exp Hematol* 1981;9:84.

155. Eernisse JG, Brand A. Prevention of platelet refractoriness due to HLA antibodies by administration of leukocyte-poor blood components. *Exp Hematol* 1981;9:77.

156. Schiffer CA, Dutcher JP, Aisner J, et al. A randomized trial of leukocyte depleted platelet transfusion to modify alloimmunization in patients with leukemia (abstract). *Blood* 1980;56:182a.

157. Valeri CR, Ragno G, Pivacek LE, et al. An experiment with glycerol-frozen red blood cells stored at –80°C for up to 37 years. *Vox Sang* 2000;79:168–174.

158. Brady MT, Milam JD, Anderson DC, et al. Use of deglycerolized red blood cells to prevent posttransfusion infection with cytomegalovirus in neonates. *J Infect Dis* 1984;150:334.

159. Factor IX complex and hepatitis. *Food Drug Admin Drug Bull* 1976;6:22.

160. Corrigan JJ. *Hemorrhagic and thrombotic disease in childhood and adolescence.* New York: Churchill Livingstone, 1985.

161. Ness PM, Perkins HA. Cryoprecipitate as a reliable source of fibrinogen replacement. *JAMA* 1979;241:1690.

162. Rosati LA, Barnes B, Oberman H, et al. Hemolytic anemia due to anti-A in concentrated hemophilic factor preparations. *Transfusion* 1970;10:139.

163. McCullough J, Steeper TA, Connelly DP, et al. Platelet utilization in a university hospital. *JAMA* 1988;259:2414.

164. Hersch EM, Bodey GP, Nies BA, et al. Causes of death in acute leukemia: a ten year study of 414 patients from 1954–1963. *JAMA* 1965;193:105.

165. Nevo BS, Swan V, Enger C, et al. Acute bleeding after bone marrow transplantation (BMT)—incidence and effect on survival. A quantitative analysis in 1,402 patients. *Blood* 1998;91:1469–1477.

166. Gaydos LA, Freireich EJ, Mantel N. The quantitative relation between platelet count and hemorrhage in patients with acute leukemia. *N Engl J Med* 1962;266:905.

167. Roy AJ, Jaffe N, Djerassi I. Prophylactic platelet transfusions in children with acute leukemia: a dose-response study. *Transfusion* 1973;13:283.

168. Higby DJ, Cohen E, Holland JF, et al. The prophylactic treatment of thrombocytopenic leukemia patients with platelets: a double blind study. *Transfusion* 1974;14:440.

169. Soloman J, Bokefkamp T, Fahey JL, et al. Platelet prophylaxis in acute nonlymphocytic leukemia. *Lancet* 1978;1:267.

170. Baer MR, Bloomfield CD. Controversies in transfusion medicine. Prophylactic platelet transfusion therapy: pro. *Transfusion* 1992;32:377.

171. Patten E. Controversies in transfusion medicine. Prophylactic platelet transfusion revisited after 25 years: con. *Transfusion* 1992;32:381.

172. Slichter S, Harker LA. Thrombocytopenia: mechanisms and management of defects in platelet production. *Clin Haematol* 1978;7:523.

173. Harker LA, Slichter SJ. The bleeding time as a screening test for evaluation of platelet function. *N Engl J Med* 1972;287:155.

174. Heckman KD, Weiner GJ, Davis CS, et al. Randomized study of prophylactic platelet transfusion threshold during induction therapy for adult acute leukemia: 10,000/µL versus 20,000/µL. *J Clin Oncol* 1997;15:1143–1149.

175. Rebulla P, Finazzi G, Marangoni F, et al. The threshold for prophylactic platelet transfusions in adults with acute myeloid leukemia. Gruppo Italiano Malattie Ematologiche Maligne dell'Adulto. *N Engl J Med* 1997;337:1870–1875.

176. Wandt H, Frank M, Ehninger G, et al. Safety and cost effectiveness of a 10 × 10⁹/L trigger for prophylactic platelet transfusions compared with the traditional 20 × 10⁹/L trigger: a prospective comparative trial in 105 patients with acute myeloid leukemia. *Blood* 1998;91:3601–3606.

177. Hersh JK, Hom EG, Brecher ME. Mathematical modeling of platelet survival with implications for optimal transfusion practice in the chronically platelet transfusion-dependent patient. *Transfusion* 1998;38:637–644.

178. Klumpp TR, Herman JH, Gaughan JP, et al. Clinical consequences of alterations in platelet transfusion dose: a prospective, randomized, double-blind trial. *Transfusion* 1999;37:674–681.

179. Bishop JF, Schiffer CA, Aisner J, et al. Surgery in acute leukemia: a review of 167 operations in thrombocytopenic patients. *Am J Hematol* 1987;26:147.

180. Freireich EJ, Kliman A, Gaydos LA, et al. Response to repeated platelet transfusion from the same donor. *Ann Intern Med* 1963;50:277.

181. Daly PA, Schiffer CA, Aisner J, et al. Platelet transfusion therapy: one-hour posttransfusion increments are valuable in predicting the need for HLA-matched preparations. *JAMA* 1980;243:435.

182. Toor AA, Choo SY, Little JA. Bleeding risk and platelet transfusion refractoriness in patients with acute myelogenous leukemia who undergo autologous stem cell transplantation. *Bone Marrow Transplant* 2000;26:315–320.

183. Aster RH, Jandl JH. Platelet sequestration in man. II. Immunological and clinical studies. *J Clin Invest* 1964;43:856.

184. Bishop JF, McGrath K, Wolf MM, et al. Clinical factors influencing the efficacy of pooled platelet transfusions. *Blood* 1988;71:383.

185. Legler TJ, Fischer I, Dittmann J. Frequency and causes of refractoriness in multiply transfused patients. *Ann Hematol* 1997;74:185–189.

186. Dutcher JP, Schiffer CA, Aisner J, et al. Alloimmunization following platelet transfusion: the absence of a dose-response relationship. *Blood* 1981;57:395.

187. Dutcher JP, Schiffer CA, Aisner J, et al. Long-term follow-up of patients with leukemia receiving platelet transfusions: identification of a large group of patients who do not become alloimmunized. *Blood* 1981;58:1007.

188. Gmur J, von Felten A, Osterwalder B, et al. Delayed alloimmunization using random single donor platelet transfusions: a prospective study in thrombocytopenic patients with acute leukemia. *Blood* 1983;62:473.

189. Sniecinski I, O'Donnell MR, Nowicki B, et al. Prevention of refractoriness and HLA-alloimmunization using filtered blood products. *Blood* 1988;71:1402.

190. Deeg HJ. Transfusions with a tan: prevention of allosensitization by ultraviolet irradiation. *Transfusion* 1989;29:450.

191. Lee EJ, Schiffer CA. ABO compatibility can influence the results of platelet transfusion: results of a randomized trial. *Transfusion* 1989;29:384.

192. Heal JM, Blumberg N, Masel D. An evaluation of crossmatching, HLA, and ABO matching for platelet transfusions to refractory patients. *Blood* 1987;70:23.

193. Blumberg N, Heal J. Transfusion and the immune system: a paradigm shift in progress? *Transfusion* 1995;35:879–883.

194. Lazarus HM, Herzig RH, Warm SE, et al. Transfusion experience with platelet concentrates stored for 24 to 72 hours at 22°C. *Transfusion* 1982;22:39.

195. Lohrman HP, Bull MI, Decter JA, et al. Platelet transfusions from HLA compatible unrelated donors to alloimmunized patients. *Ann Intern Med* 1974;80:9.

196. Duquesnoy RJ, Filip DJ, Rodey GE, et al. Successful transfusion of platelets "mismatched" for HLA antigens to alloimmunized thrombocytopenic patients. *Am J Hematol* 1977;2:219.

197. Duquesnoy RJ, Vieira J, Aster RH. Donor availability for platelet transfusion support of alloimmunized thrombocytopenic patients. *Transplant Proc* 1977;9:519.

198. Yankee RA, Grumet FC, Rogentine GN. Platelet transfusion therapy: the selection of compatible platelet donors for refractory patients by lymphocyte HL-A typing. *N Engl J Med* 1969;281:1208.

199. Moroff G, Garratty G, Heal JM, et al. Selection of platelets for refractory patients by HLA matching and prospective crossmatching. *Transfusion* 1992;32:633.

200. Bodey GP, Buckley M, Sath YS, et al. Quantitative relationships between circulating leukocytes and infection in patients with acute leukemia. *Ann Intern Med* 1966;64:328.

201. Gurwith MJ, Brunton JL, Lank BA, et al. Granulocytopenia in hospitalized patients. I. Prognostic factors and etiology of fever. *Am J Med* 1978;61:121.

202. Offner F, Schoch G, Fisher LD, et al. Mortality hazard functions as related to neutropenia at different times after marrow transplantation. *Blood* 1996;88: 4058–4062.

203. McCullough J. Introduction to apheresis donations including history and general principles. In: McLeod BC, Price TH, Drew MI, eds. *Apheresis: principles and practice.* Bethesda, MD: AABB Press, 1997:27–65.

204. Freireich EJ, Levin RH, Wang J. The function and gate of transfused leukocytes from donors with chronic myelocytic leukemia in leukopenic recipients. *Ann N Y Acad Sci* 1965;113:1081.

205. Alavi JB, Roat RK, Djerassi I, et al. A randomized clinical trial of granulocyte transfusions for infection of acute leukemia. *N Engl J Med* 1977;296:706.

206. Strauss RG. Therapeutic neutrophil transfusions: are controlled studies no longer appropriate? *Am J Med* 1978;65:1001.

207. Graw RH Jr, Herzig G, Perry S, et al. Normal granulocyte transfusion therapy. Treatment of septicemia due to gram-negative bacteria. *N Engl J Med* 1972;287:367.

208. Herzig GP, Graw RG Jr. Granulocyte transfusions for bacterial infections. In: Brown EB, ed. *Progress in hematology.* Vol 9. New York: Grune & Stratton, 1975:207.

209. Degregorio MW, Lee WMF, Linker CA, et al. Fungal infections in patients with acute leukemia. *Am J Med* 1982;73:543.

210. Young LS. Nosocomial infections in the immunocompromised adult. *Am J Med* 1981;70:398.

211. Ruthe RC, Ansersen BR, Cunningham BL, et al. Efficacy of granulocyte transfusions in the control of systemic candidiasis in leukopenic host. *Blood* 1978;52:493.

212. Raubitschek AA, Levin AS, Stites DP, et al. Normal granulocyte infusion therapy for aspergillosis in chronic granulomatous disease. *Pediatrics* 1973;51:230.

213. Strauss RG, Connett JE, Gale RP, et al. A controlled trial of prophylactic granulocyte transfusion during initial induction. *N Engl J Med* 1981;305:597.

214. Evatt B, Gompaerts E, McDougal J, et al. Coincidental appearance of LAV/HTLV antibodies in hemophiliacs and the onset of the AIDS epidemic. *N Engl J Med* 1985;312:483.

215. Walsh JH, Purcell RH, Morrow AG, et al. Post-transfusion hepatitis after open-heart operations: incidence after administration of blood from commercial and volunteer donor populations. *JAMA* 1970;211:261.

216. Prince AM, Horowitz B, Brotman B. Sterilization of hepatitis and HTLV-III viruses by exposure to try (n-butyl) phosphate and sodium cholate. *Lancet* 1986;1:706.

217. Aronson DL. The development of the technology and capacity for the production of factor VIII for the treatment of hemophilia A. *Transfusion* 1990;30:748.

218. Barundun S, Kistler P, Jeunet F, et al. Intravenous administration of human gamma globulin. *Vox Sang* 1962;7:157.

219. Sacher RA. Intravenous gammaglobulin products: development, pharmacology, and precautions. In: Garner RJ, Sacher RA, eds. *Intravenous gammaglobulin therapy.* Arlington, VA: American Association of Blood Banks, 1988:1.

220. Yaeger AS, Grumet FC, Hafleigh EB, et al. Prevention of transfusion-acquired cytomegalovirus infections in newborn infants. *J Pediatr* 1981;98: 281.

221. Stagno S, Pass RF, Dworsky ME, et al. Congenital cytomegalovirus infection: the relative importance of primary and recurrent maternal infection. *N Engl J Med* 1982;306:945.

222. Adler SP. Neonatal cytomegalovirus infections due to blood. *CRC Crit Rev Clin Lab Sci* 1985;23:1.

223. Tegtmeier GE. Cytomegalovirus and blood transfusion. In: Dodd RY, Barker LF, eds. *Infection, immunity, and blood transfusion.* Vol 182. New York: Alan R. Liss, 1985:175.

224. Glenn J. Cytomegalovirus infection following renal transplantation. *Rev Infect Dis* 1981;3:1151.

225. Rubin RH, Tolkoff-Rubin NE, Oliver D, et al. Multicenter seroepidemiologic study of the impact of cytomegalovirus infection on renal transplantation. *Transplantation* 1985;40:243.

226. Chou S. Acquisition of donor strains of cytomegalovirus by renal-transplant recipients. *N Engl J Med* 1986;314:1418.

227. Miller W, Flynn P, McCullough J, et al. Cytomegalovirus infection after bone marrow transplantation: an association with acute graft-vs-host disease. *Blood* 1986;67:1162.

228. Gilbert GL, Hudson IL, Hayes JJ. Prevention of transfusion-acquired cytomegalovirus infection in infants by blood filtration to remove leucocytes. *Lancet* 1989;1:1228.

229. Murphy MF, Grint PCA, Hardiman AE, et al. Use of leukocyte-poor blood components to prevent primary cytomegalovirus (CMV) infection in patients with acute leukemia. *Br J Haematol* 1988;70:253.

230. Preiksaitis JK, Rosno S, Grumet C, et al. Infections due to herpesviruses in cardiac transplant recipients: role of the donor heart and immunosuppressive therapy. *J Infect Dis* 1983;147:1974.

231. Rakela J, Wiesner RH, Taswell HF, et al. Incidence of cytomegalovirus infection and its relationship to donor-recipient serologic status in liver transplantation. *Transplant Proc* 1987;19:2399.

232. Preiksaitis JK, Grumet FC, Smith WK, et al. Transfusion-acquired cytomegalovirus infections in cardiac surgery patients. *J Med Virol* 1985;15:283.

233. Adler SP, Baggett J, McVoy M. Transfusion-associated cytomegalovirus infections in seropositive cardiac surgery patients. *Lancet* 1985;2:743.

234. Leitman SF, Holland PV. Irradiation of blood products: indications and guidelines. *Transfusion* 1985;25:293.

235. Sprent J, Anderson RE, Miller JFAP. Radiosensitivity of T and B lymphocytes. II. Effect of irradiation on response of T cells to alloantigens. *Eur J Immunol* 1974;4:204.

236. Valerius NH, Johansen KS, Nielsen OS, et al. Effect of in vitro irradiation on lymphocyte and granulocyte function. *Scand J Hematol* 1981;27:9.

237. Button LN, DeWolf WC, Newburger PE, et al. The effects of irradiation on blood components. *Transfusion* 1981;21:419.

238. Holley TR, Van Epps DE, Harvey RL, et al. Effect of high doses of radiation on human neutrophil chemotaxis, phagocytosis, and morphology. *Am J Pathol* 1974;75:61.

239. Greenberg ML, Chanana AD, Cronkite EP, et al. Extracorporeal irradiation of blood in man: radiation resistance of circulating platelets. *Radiat Res* 1968;35:147.

240. Ramirez AM, Woodfield DG, Scott R, et al. High potassium levels in stored irradiated blood (letter). *Transfusion* 1987;27:444.

241. Rivet C, Baxter A, Rock G. Potassium levels in irradiated blood (letter). *Transfusion* 1989;29:185.

242. RG Strauss. Routinely washing irradiated red cells before transfusion seems unwarranted. *Transfusion* 1990;30:675–677.

243. Parkman R, Mosier D, Umansky I, et al. Graft-versus-host disease after intrauterine and exchange transfusions for hemolytic disease of the newborn. *N Engl J Med* 1974;290:359.

244. Bohm N, Kleine W, Enzel U. Graft-versus-host disease in two newborns after repeated blood transfusions because of Rhesus incompatibility. *Beitr Pathol* 1977;160:381.

245. Douglas SD, Fudenberg HH. Graft versus host reaction in Wiskott-Aldrich syndrome: antemortem diagnosis of human GVH in an immunologic deficiency disease. *Vox Sang* 1969;16:172.

246. McCullough J. Principles of transfusion support before and after hematopoietic cell transplantation. In: Thomas ED, Blume KG, Forman SJ, eds. *Hematopoietic cell transplantation*. Oxford: Blackwell Science, 1999.

247. Weiden PL, Zuckerman N, Hansen JA, et al. Fatal graft-versus-host disease in a patient with lymphoblastic leukemia following normal granulocyte transfusions. *Blood* 1981;57:328.

248. Siimes MA, Koskimies S. Chronic graft-versus-host disease after blood transfusions confirmed by incompatible HLA antigens in bone marrow. *Lancet* 1982;1:42.

249. Lowenthal RM, Menon C, Challis DR. Graft-versus-host disease in consecutive patients with acute myeloid leukemia treated with blood cells from normal donors. *Aust N Z J Med* 1981;11:179.

250. Schmidmeier W, Feil W, Gebhart W, et al. Fatal graft-versus-host reaction following granulocyte transfusions. *Blut* 1982;45:115.

251. Cohen D, Weinstein H, Mihm M, et al. Nonfatal graft-versus-host disease occurring after transfusion with leukocytes and platelets obtained from normal donors. *Blood* 1979;53:1053.

252. von Fliedner V, Higby DJ, Kim U. Graft-versus-host reaction following blood transfusion. *Am J Med* 1982;72:951.

253. Woods WG, Lubin BH. Fatal graft versus host disease following a blood transfusion in a child with neuroblastoma. *Pediatrics* 1981;67:217.

254. Ford JM, Lucey JJ, Cullen MH, et al. Fatal graft-versus-host disease following transfusion of granulocytes from normal donors. *Lancet* 1976;2:1167.

255. Hathaway WE, Githens JH, Blackburn WR, et al. Aplastic anemia, histiocytosis and erythrodermia in immunologically deficient children: probable human runt disease. *N Engl J Med* 1965;271:953.

256. Park BH, Good RA, Gate J, et al. Fatal graft-versus-host reaction following transfusion of allogeneic blood and plasma in infants with combined immunodeficiency disease. *Transplant Proc* 1974;6:385.

257. Dinsmore RE, Straus DJ, Pollack MS, et al. Fatal graft-versus-host disease following blood transfusion in Hodgkin's disease documented by HLA typing. *Blood* 1980;55:831.

258. Thaler M, Shamiss A, Orgad S, et al. The role of blood from HLA-homozygous donors in fatal transfusion-associated graft-versus-host disease after open-heart surgery. *N Engl J Med* 1989;321:25.

259. Sheehan T, McLaren KM, Brettle R, et al. Transfusion-induced graft-versus-host disease in pregnancy. *Clin Lab Haematol* 1987;9:205.

260. Arsura EL, Bertelle A, Minkowitz S, et al. Transfusion-associated graft-versus-host disease in a presumed immunocompetent patient. *Arch Intern Med* 1988;148:1941.

261. Otsuka S, Kunieda K, Hirose M, et al. Fatal erythroderma (suspected graft-versus-host disease) after cholecystectomy. *Transfusion* 1989;29:544.

262. Propper RD, Button LN, Nathan DG. New approaches to the transfusion management of thalassemia. *Blood* 1980;55:55.

263. Bracey AW, Klein HG, Chambers S, et al. Ex vivo selective isolation of young red blood cells using the IBM-2991 cell washer. *Blood* 1983;61:1068.

264. Bjerke HS, Kelly RE Jr, Foglia RP, et al. Decreasing transfusion exposure risk during extracorporeal membrane oxygenation (ECMO). *Transfus Med* 1992;2:43–49.

265. Butch SH, Knafl P, Oberman HA, et al. Blood utilization in adult patients undergoing extracorporeal membrane oxygenated therapy. *Transfusion* 1996;36:61–63.

266. Gibble JW, Ness PM. Fibrin glue: the perfect operative sealant? *Transfusion* 1990;30:731.

267. Eschbach JW, Egrie JC, Downing MR, et al. Correction of the anemia of end-stage renal disease with recombinant human erythropoietin. *N Engl J Med* 1987;316:73.

268. Eschbach JW, Abdulhadi MH, Browne JK, et al. Recombinant human erythropoietin in anemic patients with end-stage renal disease: results of a phase III multicenter clinical trial. *Ann Intern Med* 1989;111:992.

269. Lundin AP. Quality of life: subjective and objective improvements with recombinant human erythropoietin therapy. *Semin Nephrol* 1989;9:22.

270. Cazzola M, Mercuriali F, Brugmara C. Use of recombinant human erythropoietin outside the setting of uremia. *Blood* 1997;89:4248–4267.

271. Fullerton DA, Campbell DN, Whitman GJ. Use of human recombinant erythropoietin to correct severe preoperative anemia. *Ann Thorac Surg* 1991; 51:825–826.

272. Bishop MR, Tarantolo SR, Geller RB, et al. A randomized, double-blind trial of filgrastim (granulocyte colony-stimulating factor) versus placebo following allogeneic blood stem cell transplantation. *Blood* 2000;96:80–85.

273. Przepiorka D, Smith TL, Folloder J, et al. Controlled trial of filgrastim for acceleration of neutrophil recovery after allogeneic blood stem cell transplantation from human leukocyte antigen-matched related donors. *Blood* 2001;97:3405–3410.

274. Lok S, Kaushansky K, Holly RD, et al. Cloning and expression of murine thrombopoietin cDNA and stimulation of platelet production in vivo. *Nature* 1994;369:565.

275. de Sauvage FJ, Hass PE, Spencer SD. Stimulation of megakaryocytopoiesis and thrombopoiesis by the c-Mpl ligand. *Nature* 1994;369:533.

276. Basser RL, Rasko JEJ, Klarke K, et al. Thrombopoietic effects of pegylated recombinant human megakaryocyte growth and development factor (PEG-rHUMGDF) in patients with advanced cancer. *Lancet* 1996;348:1279–1281.

277. Vadhan-Raj S, Murray LJ, Bueso-Ramos C, et al. Stimulation of megakaryocyte and platelet production by a single dose of recombinant human thrombopoietin in patients with cancer. *Ann Intern Med* 1997;126:673–681.

278. Basser RL, Rasko JEJ, Clarke J, et al. Randomized, blinded, placebo-controlled phase I trial of pegylated recombinant human megakaryocyte growth and development factor with filgrastim after dose-intensive chemotherapy in patients with advanced cancer. *Blood* 1997;89:3118–3128.

279. Counts RB, Haisch C, Simon TL, et al. Hemostasis in massively transfused trauma patients. *Ann Surg* 1979;190:91.

280. Mannucci PM, Federici AB, Sirchia G. Hemostasis testing during massive blood replacement: a study of 172 cases. *Vox Sang* 1982;42:113.

281. Wilson RF, Dulchavsky SA, Soullier G, et al. Problems with 20 or more blood transfusions in 24 hours. *Am Surg* 1987;53:410.

282. Reed RL, Ciavarella D, Heimbach DM, et al. Prophylactic platelet administration during massive transfusion. *Ann Surg* 1986;203:40.

283. Martin DJ, Lucas CE, Ledgerwood AM, et al. Fresh frozen plasma supplement to massive red blood cell transfusion. *Ann Surg* 1985;202:505.

284. Beutler E, Wood L. The in vivo regeneration of red cell 2,3 diphosphoglyceric acid (DPG) after transfusion of stored blood. *J Lab Clin Med* 1969;74:300.

285. Collins JA. Abnormal hemoglobin-oxygen affinity and surgical hemotherapy. *Bibl Haematol* 1980;46:59. Also in: Collins JA, Lundsgaard-Hansen P, eds. *Surgical hemotherapy*. New York: S. Karger, 1980.

286. Perkins HA, Snyder M, Thagher C, et al. Calcium ion activity during rapid exchange transfusion with citrated blood. *Transfusion* 1971;11:204.

287. Collins JA. Problems associated with the massive transfusion of stored blood. *Surgery* 1974;75:274.

288. Bick RL. Hemostasis defects associated with cardiac surgery, prosthetic devices, and other extracorporeal circuits. *Semin Thromb Hemost* 1980;11:249.

289. Salzman EW, Weinstein MJ, Weintraub RM, et al. Treatment with desmopressin acetate to reduce blood loss after cardiac surgery. *N Engl J Med* 1986;314:1402.

290. Storb R, Prentice RL, Thomas ED. Marrow transplantation for treatment of aplastic anemia: an analysis of factors associated with graft rejection. *N Engl J Med* 1977;296:61.

291. Storb R, Thomas ED, Buckner CD, et al. Marrow transplantation in 30 "untransfused" patients with severe aplastic anemia. *Ann Intern Med* 1980;92:30.

292. Champlin RE, Horowitz MM, van Bekkum DW, et al. Graft failure following bone marrow transplantation for severe aplastic anemia: risk factors and treatment results. *Blood* 1989;73:606.

293. Storb R, Wieden PL. Transfusion problems associated with transplantation. *Semin Hematol* 1981;18:163.

294. Gale RP, Feig S, Ho W, et al. ABO blood group system and bone marrow transplantation. *Blood* 1977;50:184.

295. Buckner CP, Clift RA, Sanders JE, et al. The role of a protective environment and prophylactic granulocyte transfusion in marrow transplantation. *Transplant Proc* 1978;10:255.

296. Hershko C, Gale RP, Ho W, et al. ABH antigens and bone marrow transplantation. *Br J Haematol* 1980;44:65.

297. Lasky L, Warkentin P, Ramsay N, et al. Hemotherapy in patients undergoing blood group incompatible bone marrow transfusion. *Transfusion* 1983;23:277–285.

298. Berkman EM, Caplan SN. Engraftment of Rh positive marrow in a recipient with Rh antibody. *Transplant Proc* 1977;9:215.

299. Sacher RA, Luban NLC, Strauss RG. Current practice and guidelines for the transfusion of cellular blood components in the newborn. *Transfus Med Rev* 1989;3:39.

300. Strauss RG. Data-driven blood banking practices for neonatal RBC transfusions. *Transfusion* 2000;40:1528–1540.

301. Ludvigsen CW, Swanson JL, Thompson TR, et al. The failure of neonates to form red blood cell alloantibodies in response to multiple transfusions. *Am J Clin Pathol* 1987;2:250.

302. Oberman HA. Transfusion of the neonatal patient. *Transfusion* 1974;14:183.

303. Christensen RD, Rothstein G, Anstall HB, et al. Granulocyte transfusions in neonates with bacterial infection, neutropenia, and depletion of mature marrow neutrophils. *Pediatrics* 1982;70:1.

304. Butch SH, Coltre MA. Techniques of transfusion. In: Kasprisin DO, Luban NLC, eds. *Pediatric transfusion medicine*. Vol 1. Boca Raton, FL: CRC Press, 1987:91.

305. Warkentin PI. Transfusion therapy for the pediatric oncology patient. In: Kasprisin DO, Luban NLC, eds. *Pediatric transfusion medicine*. Vol 2. Boca Raton, FL: CRC Press, 1987:19.

306. Schwartz SI, Bernard RP, Adams JT, et al. Splenectomy for hematologic disorders. *Arch Surg* 1970;101:338.

307. Pearson HA, Shulman NR, Marder VJ, et al. Isoimmune neonatal thrombocytopenia purpura: clinical and therapeutic considerations. *Blood* 1964;23:154.

308. McFarland JG, Frenzke M, Aster RH. Testing of maternal sera in pregnancies at risk for neonatal alloimmune thrombocytopenia. *Transfusion* 1989;29:128.

309. Lalezari P. Alloimmune neonatal neutropenia. In: Engelfriet CP, von Loghem JJ, von dem Borne AEGKr, eds. *Immunohematology*. Amsterdam: Elsevier Science, 1984:178.

310. Rosse WF. Transfusion in paroxysmal nocturnal hemoglobinuria. To wash or not to wash? *Transfusion* 1989;29:663–664.

311. Brecher ME, Taswell H. Paroxysmal nocturnal hemoglobinuria and the transfusion of washed red cells. A myth revisited. *Transfusion* 1989;29:681–685.

312. Sirchia G, Zanella A. Transfusion of PNH patients. *Transfusion* 1990;30:479.

313. Sazama K. 355 Reports of transfusion-associated deaths. *Transfusion* 1990;30:583.

314. Widmann FK. Informed consent for blood transfusion: brief historical survey and summary of a conference. *Transfusion* 1990;30:460.

315. Swank RL, Seaman GVF. Microfiltration and microemboli: a history. *Transfusion* 2000;40:114–119.

316. DeCesare WR, Bove JR, Ebaugh FG Jr. The mechanism of the effect of iso- and hyperosmolar dextrose-saline solutions on in vivo survival of human erythrocytes. *Transfusion* 1964;4:237.

317. Ryden SE, Oberman HA. Compatibility of common intravenous solutions with CPD blood. *Transfusion* 1975;15:250.

318. Braude AI. Transfusion reactions from contaminated blood: their recognition and treatment. *N Engl J Med* 1958;258:1289.

319. Walker RH. Special report: transfusion risks. *Am J Clin Pathol* 1987;88:374.

320. Pineda AA, Brzica SM, Taswell HF. Hemolytic transfusion reaction: recent experience in a large blood bank. *Mayo Clin Proc* 1978;53:378.

321. Honig CL, Bove JR. Transfusion-associated fatalities: review of Bureau of Biologics reports 1976–1978. *Transfusion* 1980;20:653.

322. Brittingham TE, Chaplin H. Febrile transfusion reactions caused by sensitivity to donor leukocytes and platelets. *JAMA* 1957;165:819.

323. Heddle NM, Blajchman MA. The leukodepletion of cellular blood products in the prevention of HLA-alloimmunization and refractoriness to allogeneic platelet transfusions. *Blood* 1995;85:603–606.

324. Bordin JO, Heddle NM, Blajchman MA. Biologic effects of leukocytes present in transfused cellular blood products. *Blood* 1994;84:1703–1721.

325. Menitove JE, McElligott MC, Aster RH. Febrile transfusion reaction: what blood component should be given next. *Vox Sang* 1982;42:318.

326. Popovsky MA, Chaplin HC, Moore SB. Transfusion-related acute lung injury: a neglected, serious complication of hemotherapy. *Transfusion* 1992;32:589.

327. Popovsky MA, Davenport RD. Transfusion-related acute lung injury: femme fatale? *Transfusion* 2001;41:312.

328. Vyas GN, Holmdahl L, Perkins HA, et al. Serologic specificity of human anti-IgA and its significance in transfusion. *Blood* 1969;34:573.

329. Klein HG, Dodd RY, Ness PM, et al. Current status of microbial contamination of blood components: summary of a conference. *Transfusion* 1997;37:95–101.

330. Chiu EKW, Yuen KY, Lie AKW, et al. A prospective study of symptomatic bacteremia following platelet transfusion and of its management. *Transfusion* 1994;34:950–954.

331. Heal JM, Jones ME, Forey J, et al. Fatal salmonella septicemia after platelet transfusion. *Transfusion* 1987;27:2.

332. Ness P, Braine H, King K, et al. Single-donor platelets reduce the risk of septic platelet transfusion reactions. *Transfusion* 2001;41:857–861.

333. Centers for Disease Control and Prevention. AIDS cases by age group, exposure category and sex. *HIV/AIDS Surveillance Rep* 1999;11:12.

334. Centers for Disease Control and Prevention. Recommendations for prevention and control of hepatitis C virus (HCV) infection and HCV-related chronic disease. *MMWR Recomm Rep* 1998;47:1–39.

335. Bove JR. Transfusion-associated hepatitis and AIDS: what is the risk? *N Engl J Med* 1987;317:242.

336. Alter HJ. You'll wonder where the yellow went: a 15-year retrospective of posttransfusion hepatitis. In: Moore SB, ed. *Transfusion-transmitted viral diseases*. Arlington, VA: American Association of Blood Banks, 1987:53.

337. Hollinger FB, Khan NC, Oefinger PA, et al. Posttransfusion hepatitis type A. *JAMA* 1983;250:2313.

338. Noble RC, Kane MA, Reeves SA, et al. Posttransfusion hepatitis A in a neonatal intensive care unit. *JAMA* 1984;252:2711.

339. Alter HJ, Holland PV, Purcell RH, et al. Posttransfusion hepatitis after exclusion of commercial and hepatitis-B antigen-positive donors. *Ann Intern Med* 1972;77:691.

340. Aach RD, Szmuness W, Mosley JW. Serum alanine aminotransferase of donors in relation to the risk of non-A, non-B hepatitis in recipients. *N Engl J Med* 1981;304:989.

341. Stevens CE, Taylor PE, Liu P. Hepatitis B virus infection: epidemiology and immunoprophylaxis. In: Moore SB, ed. *Transfusion-transmitted viral diseases*. Arlington, VA: American Association of Blood Banks, 1987:1.

342. Dienstag JL. Non-A, non-B hepatitis: I. Recognition, epidemiology, and clinical features. *Gastroenterology* 1983;85:439.

343. Koretz RL, Abbey H, Coleman E, et al. Non-A, non-B posttransfusion hepatitis. *Ann Intern Med* 1993;119:110.

344. Alter HJ, Purcell RH, Shih JW, et al. Detection of antibody to hepatitis C virus in prospectively followed transfusion recipients with acute and chronic non-A, non-B hepatitis. *N Engl J Med* 1989;321:1494.

345. Centers for Disease Control and Prevention. *Pneumocystis carinii* pneumonia among persons with hemophilia A. *MMWR Morb Mortal Wkly Rep* 1982;31:365.

346. Centers for Disease Control and Prevention. Possible transfusion-associated acquired immune deficiency syndrome (AIDS): California. *MMWR Morb Mortal Wkly Rep* 1982;31:652.

347. Curran JW, Lawrence DN, Jaffe HW, et al. Acquired immunodeficiency syndrome (AIDS) associated with transfusions. *N Engl J Med* 1984;310:69.

348. Peterman TA, Jaffe HW, Feorino PM, et al. Transfusion-associated acquired immunodeficiency syndrome in the United States. *JAMA* 1985;254:2913.

349. Jaffe HW, Sarngadharan MG, DeVico AL, et al. Infection with HTLV-III/LAV and transfusion-associated acquired immunodeficiency syndrome: serologic evidence of an association. *JAMA* 1985;254:770.

350. Feorino PM, Kalyanaraman VS, Haverkos HW, et al. Lymphadenopathy associated virus infection of a blood donor-recipient pair with acquired immunodeficiency syndrome. *Science* 1984;225:69.

351. Feorino PM, Jaffe HW, Palmer E, et al. Transfusion-associated acquired immunodeficiency syndrome: evidence for persistent infection in blood donors. *N Engl J Med* 1985;312:1293.

352. Lange JMA, van den Berg H, Dooren LJ, et al. HTLV-III/LAV infection in nine children infected by a single plasma donor: clinical outcome and recognition patterns of viral proteins. *J Infect Dis* 1986;154:171.

353. Ward JW, Grindon AJ, Feorino PM, et al. Laboratory and epidemiologic evaluation of an enzyme immunoassay for antibodies to HTLV-III. *JAMA* 1986;256:357.

354. MacDonald KL, Jackson JB, Bowman RJ, et al. Performance characteristics of serologic tests for human immunodeficiency virus type 1 (HIV-1) antibody among Minnesota blood donors. *Ann Intern Med* 1989;110:617.

355. The Consortium for Retrovirus Serology Standardization. Serological diagnosis of human immunodeficiency virus infection by Western blot testing. *JAMA* 1988;260:674.

356. Kleinman SH, Busch MP, Stramer SL. First year experience with HIV p24 antigen (AG) testing: Ag indeterminate donors are not infected with HIV. *Blood* 1997;90(1):408a(abst).

357. Busch MP, Kleinman SH, Williams AE, et al. Frequency of human immunodeficiency virus (HIV) infection among contemporary anti-HIV-1 and anti-HIV-1/2 supplemental test-indeterminate blood donors. *Transfusion* 1996;36:37–44.

358. Menitove JE. Status of recipients of blood from donors subsequently found to have an antibody to HIV. *N Engl J Med* 1986;315:1095.

359. Donegan E. The Transfusion Safety Study Group. Serum antibody positivity in recipients of anti-HIV positive blood. *Transfusion* 1986;26:576.

360. Centers for Disease Control and Prevention. Human immunodeficiency virus infection in transfusion recipients and their family members. *MMWR Morb Mortal Wkly Rep* 1987;36:137.

361. Peterman TA, Lui KJ, Lawrence DN, et al. Estimating the risks of transfusion-associated acquired immune deficiency syndrome and human immunodeficiency virus infection. *Transfusion* 1987;27:371.

362. Lui KJ, Lawrence DN, Morgan WM, et al. A model-based approach for estimating the mean incubation period of transfusion-associated acquired immunodeficiency syndrome. *Proc Natl Acad Sci U S A* 1986;83:3051.

363. Cohen ND, Munoz A, Reitz BA, et al. Transmission of retroviruses by transfusion of screened blood in patients undergoing cardiac surgery. *N Engl J Med* 1989;320:1172.

364. Busch MP, Bernard EE, Khayam-Bashi H, et al. Evaluation of screened blood donation from human immunodeficiency virus type I infection by culture and DNA amplification of pooled cells. *N Engl J Med* 1991;325:1.

365. Donahue JG, Nelson KE, Munoz A, et al. Transmission of HIV by transfusion of screened blood. *N Engl J Med* 1990;323:1709.

366. Ward JW, Holmberg SD, Allen JR, et al. Transfusion of human immunodeficiency virus (HIV) by blood transfusions screened as negative for HIV antibody. *N Engl J Med* 1988;318:473.

367. Busch MP. Closing the windows on viral transmission by blood transfusion. In: Stramer SL, ed. *Blood safety in the new millennium.* Bethesda, MD: American Association of Blood Banks, 2001:33–54.

368. Alter HJ, Epstein JS, Swenson SG, et al. Prevalence of human immunodeficiency virus type 1 p24 antigen in US blood donors—an assessment of the efficacy of testing in donor screening. The HIV-Antigen Study Group. *N Engl J Med* 1990;323:1312–1317.

369. Reference deleted.

370. Busch MP, Taylor PE, Lenes BA, et al. Screening of selected male blood donors for p24 antigen of human immunodeficiency type 1. Transfusion Safety Study Group. *N Engl J Med* 1990;323:1308–1312.

371. Busch MP, Dodd RY. NAT and blood safety: what is the paradigm? *Transfusion* 2000;40:1157–1160.

372. Stramer SL, Caglioti S, Strong DM. NAT of the United States and Canadian blood supply. *Transfusion* 2000;40:1165–1168.

373. Centers for Disease Control and Prevention. Transfusion-transmitted malaria—Missouri and Pennsylvania, 1996–1998. *MMWR Morb Mortal Wkly Rep* 1999;48:253–256.

374. Turner TB, Diseker TH. Duration of infectivity of *Treponema pallidum* in citrated blood stored under conditions obtaining in blood banks. *Bull Johns Hopkins Hosp* 1941;68:269.

375. Schmidt PJ. Syphilis, a disease of direct transfusion. *Transfusion* 2001;41:1069.

376. Tegtmeier GE. Transfusion-transmitted cytomegalovirus infections: significance and control. *Vox Sang* 1986;51:22.

377. Gerber P, Walsh JH, Rosenblum EN. Association of EB-virus infection with the post-perfusion syndrome. *Lancet* 1969;1:593.

378. Adler SP. Transfusion-associated cytomegalovirus infections. *Rev Infect Dis* 1983;5:977.

379. Bowden RA, Slichter SJ, Sayers M, et al. A comparison of filtered leukocyte-reduced and cytomegalovirus (CMV) seronegative blood products for the prevention of transfusion-associated CMV infection after marrow transplant. *Blood* 1995;86:3598–3603.

380. Luban NLC, Williams AE, MacDonald MG, et al. Low incidence of acquired cytomegalovirus infection in neonates transfused with washed red blood cells. *Am J Dis Child* 1987;141:4161.

381. Okochi K, Sato H. Adult T-cell leukemia virus, blood donors and transfusion: experience in Japan. *Prog Clin Biol Res* 1985;182:245.

382. Centers for Disease Control and Prevention and the U.S.P.H.S. Working Group. Guidelines for counseling persons infected with human T-lymphotropic virus type I (HTLV-I) and type II (HTLV-II). *Ann Intern Med* 1993;1888:448.

383. Schmunis GA. Chagas' disease and blood transfusion. In: Dodd RY, Barker LF, eds. *Infection, immunity and blood transfusion.* New York: Alan R. Liss, 1985:127.

384. Grant IH, Gold JWM, Wittner M, et al. Transfusion-associated acute Chagas disease acquired in the United States. *Ann Intern Med* 1989;111:849–851.

385. Cimo PL, Luper WE, Scouros MA. Transfusion-associated Chagas' disease in Texas: report of a case. *Tex Med* 1993;89:48–50.

386. Almeida IC, Covas DT, Soussumi LM, et al. A highly sensitive and specific chemiluminescent enzyme-linked immunosorbent assay for diagnosis of active *Trypanosoma cruzi* infection. *Transfusion* 1997;37:850–857.

387. Smith RP, Evans AT, Popovsky M, et al. Transfusion-acquired babesiosis and failure of antibiotic treatment. *JAMA* 1986;256:2726.

388. Badon SJ, Fister RD, Cable RG. Survival of *Borrelia burgdorferi* in blood products. *Transfusion* 1989;29:581.

389. Aoki SK, Holland PV. Lyme disease: another transfusion risk? *Transfusion* 1989;29:646.

390. Serjeant GR, Mason K, Topley JM, et al. Outbreak of aplastic crisis in sickle cell anemia associated with parvovirus-like agent. *Lancet* 1981;2:595.

391. Mortimer PP, Luban NL, Kelleher JF, et al. Transmission of serum parvovirus-like agent by clotting factor concentrates. *Lancet* 1983;2:482.

392. Brown P, Cervenakova L, Diringer H. Blood infectivity and the prospects for a diagnostic screening test in Creutzfeldt-Jakob disease. *J Lab Clin Med* 2001;137:5–13.

393. The utility of therapeutic plasmapheresis for neurological disorders. NIH Consensus Development. *JAMA* 1986;256:1333.

394. Chopek M, McCullough J. Protein and biochemical changes during plasma exchange. In: *Therapeutic hemapheresis.* Arlington, VA: American Association of Blood Banks, 1980:13.

395. Keller AJ, Urbaniak SJ. Intensive plasma exchange on the cell separator: effects on serum immunoglobulins and complement components. *Br J Haematol* 1978;38:531.

396. Perdue JJ, Chandler LK, Vesely SK, et al. Unintentional platelet removal by plasmapheresis. *J Clin Apheresis* 2001;16:55.

397. Huestis DW, Bove JR, Case J. *Complications of transfusion: practical blood transfusion,* 4th ed. Boston: Little, Brown and Company, 1988:251.

398. Sutton DMC, Nair RC, Rock NG. Canadian Apheresis Study Group. Complications of plasma exchange. *Transfusion* 1989;29:124.

399. McKee LC, Collins RD. Intravascular leukocyte thrombi and aggregates as a cause of morbidity and mortality in leukemia. *Medicine* 1974;53:463.

400. Freireich EJ, Thomas LB, Frei E, et al. A distinctive type of intracerebral hemorrhage associated with "blastic crisis" in patients with leukemia. *Cancer* 1960;13:146.

401. Lokich JJ, Moloney WC. Fatal pulmonary leukostasis following treatment of acute myelogenous leukemia. *Arch Intern Med* 1972;130:759.

402. Roberts WC, Bodey GP, Wertlake PT. The heart in acute leukemia: a study of 420 autopsy cases. *Am J Cardiol* 1968;21:388.

403. Stucki A, Rivier AS, Gikic M, et al. Endothelial cell activation by myeloblasts: molecular mechanisms of leukostasis and leukemic cell dissemination. *Blood* 2001;76:2121–2129.

404. Steeper TA, Smith JA, McCullough J. Therapeutic cytapheresis using the Fenwal CS-3000 blood cell separator. *Vox Sang* 1985;48:193.

405. Rook AH, Wolfe JT. Role of extracorporeal photopheresis in the treatment of cutaneous T-cell lymphoma, autoimmune disease, and allograft rejection. *J Clin Apheresis* 1994;9:28–30.

406. Costanzo-Nordin MR, Hubbell EA, O'Sullivan EJ, et al. Successful treatment of heart transplant rejection with photopheresis. *Transplantation* 1992;53:808–815.

407. Greinix HT, Volc-Platzer B, Kalhs P, et al. Extracorporeal photochemotherapy in the treatment of severe steroid-refractory acute graft-versus-host disease: a pilot study. *Blood* 2000;96:2426–2431.

408. Tremper KK, Friedman AE, Levine EM. The preoperative treatment of severely anemic patients with a perfluorochemical oxygen-transport fluid, Fluosol-DA. *N Engl J Med* 1982;307:277.

409. Mitsuno T, Ohyanagi H, Naito R. Clinical studies of a perfluorochemical whole blood substitute (Fluosol-DA). *Ann Surg* 1982;195:60.

410. Gould SA, Rosen AL, Sehgal R, et al. Fluosol-DA as a red-cell substitute in acute anemia. *N Engl J Med* 1986;314:1653.

411. Stowell CP, Levin J, Spiess BD, et al. Progress in the development of RBC substitutes. *Transfusion* 2001;41:287–299.

412. Winslow RM. $\alpha\alpha$-Crosslinked hemoglobin: was failure predicted by preclinical testing? *Vox Sang* 2000;79:1–20.

413. Sloan EP, Koenigsberg M, Gens D, et al. Diaspirin cross-linked hemoglobin (DCLHb) in the treatment of severe traumatic hemorrhagic shock. A randomized controlled efficacy trial. *JAMA* 1999;282:1857–1864.

414. Gould SA, Moore EE, Hoyt DB, et al. The first randomized trial of human polymerized hemoglobin as a blood substitute in acute trauma and emergent surgery. *J Am Coll Surg* 1998;187:113–120.

415. Gould SA, Moore EE, Moore FA, et al. Clinical utility of human polymerized hemoglobin as a blood substitute after acute trauma and urgent surgery. *J Trauma* 1997;43:325–332.

416. Moore EE, Gould SA, Hoyt DB, et al. Clinical utility of human polymerized hemoglobin as a blood substitute following trauma and emergent surgery. *Shock* 1997;7(S1):145(abst).

417. Lamuraglia GM, O'Hara PJ, Baker WH, et al. The reduction of allogenic transfusion requirement in aortic surgery with hemoglobin-based solution. *J Vasc Surg* 2000;31:299–308.

418. Mullon J, Giacoppe G, Clagett C, et al. Transfusions of polymerized bovine hemoglobin in a patient with severe autoimmune hemolytic anemia. *N Engl J Med* 2000;342:1638–1643.

CHAPTER 58

Hematologic Growth Factors as Supportive Care

Martin S. Tallman, H. Franklin Bunn, and Charles L. Bennett

Remarkable progress has been made in the supportive care of patients with bone marrow failure and those receiving cytotoxic chemotherapy for hematologic malignancies and solid tumors. These advances have been possible because of insights into the biology of normal hematopoiesis and the ability to clone many of the glycoproteins responsible for the control of hematopoietic stem cell proliferation, commitment, and differentiation towards a specific lineage through recombinant DNA technology.

Hematopoietic growth factors are proteins that regulate the proliferation, differentiation, and survival of hematopoietic cells and have become part of routine clinical practice. In the setting of an aplastic bone marrow after chemotherapy, the ability to stimulate myelopoiesis and prevent infection may be life-saving. After intensive cytotoxic chemotherapy, hematopoietic growth factors may shorten the duration of life-threatening neutropenia, decrease the incidence of serious infections, and shorten the duration of hospitalization. However, in general, the introduction of hematopoietic growth factors has had no clear beneficial impact on overall survival. Nevertheless, granulocyte colony-stimulating factor (G-CSF) and granulocyte-macrophage colony-stimulating factor (GM-CSF) represent an advance in the supportive care of patients. The administration of erythropoietin (Epo) for anemia attributable to chronic renal failure and myelodysplastic syndromes (MDSs) may diminish transfusion requirements and has had a significant impact on the quality of life. Less progress has been made in the ability to stimulate thrombopoiesis in a clinically meaningful way. The hematopoietic growth factors that have been approved for clinical use and are commercially available include G-CSF, GM-CSF, interleukin (IL)-11, and Epo. This chapter focuses primarily on these agents and provides practical guidelines for their clinical use.

HEMATOPOIETIC GROWTH FACTORS TO STIMULATE MYELOPOIESIS

Granulocyte Colony-Stimulating Factor

G-CSF is a hematopoietic growth factor that regulates the proliferation and function of neutrophils (1–4). This glycoprotein specifically stimulates the growth of neutrophil granulocytic precursors. Recombinant human G-CSF is produced in *Escherichia coli* and is nonglycosylated (4).

The natural sources of G-CSF include neutrophils, endothelial cells, fibroblasts, and bone marrow stromal cells. Other cytokines, including macrophage colony-stimulating factor (M-CSF), IL-1, and tumor necrosis factor (TNF), can also stimulate the production of G-CSF by endothelial cells (5,6). G-CSF is lineage-specific, and its primary effect is on the myeloid series (7). The specificity of G-CSF of neutrophils is demonstrated by the fact that, in the canine model, dogs that develop neutralizing antibodies to G-CSF develop neutropenia (8). In addition, the elimination of G-CSF or its receptor results in decreases in only neutrophil levels (9,10). In addition to stimulating the number of neutrophils in the circulation by reducing the time necessary for maturation of the committed progenitor myeloid cells, the lifespan of the mature neutrophil is extended, and function of mature neutrophils in both normal individuals and those with MDSs and chronic myeloid leukemia are improved (11–16). Filgrastim (Neupogen), an *E. coli*–derived G-CSF, and Lenograstim (Neutrogen), a glycosylated form, are currently licensed in the United States.

Gene Encoding for Granulocyte Colony-Stimulating Factor

The gene encoding for the production of G-CSF is located on the long arm of chromosome 17 (17q11-q23) (17).

Granulocyte Colony-Stimulating Factor Receptor

High-affinity receptors for G-CSF are present not only on normal myeloid cells and endothelial cells but also on leukemic cells (18). The gene encoding for the G-CSF receptor is located on chromosome 1p32 (19). The receptor is composed of an extracellular domain, a transmembrane sequence, and intracellular domain (20). G-CSF, similar to GM-CSF, IL-2, IL-3, Epo, and c-mpl, belongs to the growth factor receptor superfamily (type 1 cytokine receptors) (21–23). Members of this growth factor cytokine receptor superfamily have similarities. The G-CSF receptor binds G-CSF with high affinity (24,25).

Signal Transduction

The expression of the G-CSF receptor is controlled by transcription factors C/EBP and PU.1 (26,27). After binding to G-CSF, the G-CSF receptor binds to multiple cytoplasmic protein kinases of the *Janus* family (JAK), which leads to transphosphorylation of tyrosine. This association of the *Janus* kinases with growth factor receptors was initially described with Epo and JAK2 (28).

Biologic Activity

G-CSF was initially approved by the U.S. Food and Drug Administration in 1991 for clinical use (Filgrastim) after myelosuppressive chemotherapy for nonmyeloid malignancies. A single injection of G-CSF (300 mg) increases the circulating neutrophil count by fourfold (29). The glycosylated form of G-CSF has a sugar moiety attached, which increases the stability against heat denaturation, pH changes, and proteolysis (30,31). The blood levels of G-CSF increase rapidly in the setting of endotoxin and infections (32–34). This suggests that G-CSF is responsible for not only the maintenance of normal granulocyte levels but also the neutrophilia that develops in response to infections. The neutrophilia following G-CSF is attributable to the release of maturing cells from the marrow related to a dose-dependent decrease in the marrow transit time (35,36). Undifferentiated myeloid cells (CD34+CD33) express receptors for G-CSF and proliferate with exposure to G-CSF (37). G-CSF also stimulates the blood levels of CD34+ progenitor cells in not only healthy individuals but also patients with acquired immuno deficiency syndrome (38). Nonproliferative functional changes induced by G-CSF exposure increase the expression of adhesion molecules E-selectin and ECAM (CD54) (39). G-CSF has the ability to increase the eosinophil count and influences the mobilization of eosinophil granule proteins (40).Other effects of G-CSF include down-regulation of other adhesion molecules such as L-selectin (LAM-1) (41); stimulation of phagocytic activity of granulocytes (42); an increase in the generation of reactive oxygen species (43); possibly an increase in fungicidal activity (44,45); stimulation of antibody-dependent cellular cytotoxicity (46); and stimulation of lipopolysaccharide-binding protein (CD14) on neutrophils (47).

Pharmacokinetics

Rapid clearance from the blood of the glycosylated and nonglycosylated forms occurs (48,49). The half-life ($t_{1/2}$) for rhG-CSF is 1.79 hours, and the total body clearance is 50 mL/hour/kg (50).

GRANULOCYTE-MACROPHAGE COLONY-STIMULATING FACTOR

GM-CSF affects the growth and differentiation of neutrophils and monocytes/macrophages in semisolid hematopoietic cell culture systems. Accumulating information from *in vitro* and *in vivo* preclinical studies and from clinical trials demonstrated that, similar to G-CSF, GM-CSF has diverse biologic effects beyond hematopoiesis, including roles in inflammation, infection control, and antitumor immunity.

The molecular sequence of endogenous human GM-CSF was first identified in 1985. Three different synthetic forms of human GM-CSF were produced by recombinant DNA technology using bacterial (51), mammalian (52), and yeast expression systems (53). All forms of recombinant GM-CSF display the activity of the native molecule. Yeast-derived GM-CSF is produced in *Saccharomyces cerevisiae* and is termed *sargramostim*; bacterially derived GM-CSF is produced in *E. coli* and is called *molgramostim*; mammalian-derived GM-CSF is produced in Chinese hamster ovary (CHO) cells and is called *regramostim*. These preparations differ by their specific amino acid sequences, size of proteins, and degree of glycosylation. Sargramostim (Leukine), the only GM-CSF licensed in the United States, has an amino acid sequence identical to that of endogenous human protein except for the substitution of leucine for proline at position 23, and it may have a different carbohydrate moiety. Sargramostim is characterized by

three primary molecular species having molecular weights of 19,500, 16,800, and 15,500 daltons. Sargramostim is glycosylated to a lesser extent than regramostim, whereas molgramostim is not glycosylated. As discussed above, the degree of glycosylation of GM-CSF is an important characteristic that affects pharmacokinetics, biologic activity, antigenicity, and toxicity (54–57).

Gene Encoding for Granulocyte-Macrophage Colony-Stimulating Factor

The gene for GM-CSF is located on chromosome 5q21-32 (58) near the genes for other cytokines such as IL-3, IL-4, IL-5, and IL-9. It is approximately 2.5 kilobase pairs (kbp) in length and is composed of 4 exons and 3 introns (51). The 5'-flanking region plays an important role in the inducible expression of the GM-CSF gene (59,60). The gene encodes a protein of 127 amino acids, including a signal sequence of 17 residues and two sites for *N*-glycosylation (61–64). Under steady-state conditions, GM-CSF is constitutively expressed in monocytes, endothelial cells, and fibroblasts. On activation, additional cell types express GM-CSF messenger RNA, including T and B cells, mast cells, mesothelial cells, and osteoblasts (65–73).

Granulocyte-Macrophage Colony-Stimulating Factor Receptor

The GM-CSF receptor belongs to the hematopoietic growth factor receptor superfamily (22), which includes the receptors for numerous other growth factors including leukemia inhibitory factor (LIF), IL-1, IL-2, IL-3, IL-4, IL-5, IL-6, IL-7, G-CSF, Epo, prolactin, growth hormone, ciliary neurotrophic factor, and thrombopoietin (TPO). The GM-CSF receptor is expressed on numerous cell types, including granulocytes, erythrocytes, megakaryocytes, and macrophage progenitor cells, as well as mature neutrophils, monocytes, macrophages, dendritic cells, plasma cells, certain T lymphocytes, vascular endothelial cells, and uterine cells (74–80).

Molecular cloning studies have revealed that the GM-CSF receptor is composed of an α subunit and a common β (β_c) subunit (81). The α subunit binds GM-CSF with low affinity. The β_c subunit has no detectable binding affinity for GM-CSF on its own but forms a heterodimer with the α subunit that has high affinity for GM-CSF. Whereas the α subunit is unique to the GM-CSF receptor, the β_c subunit is found in the receptors for IL-3 and IL-5 (82). High-affinity GM-CSF receptors are widely expressed by hematopoietic cells, with mature granulocytes expressing the highest number of receptors (83,84). Low-affinity receptors are expressed in various tumor cell types (85–88). However, there is no *in vivo* evidence for accelerated growth of tumor cells when patients with solid tumors are given GM-CSF to stimulate bone marrow recovery. Similarly, there is little or no evidence that GM-CSF stimulates the growth of malignant cells in patients with hematologic malignancies when it is given after chemotherapy, as discussed in Granulocyte-Macrophage Colony-Stimulating Factor in Myelodysplastic Syndromes. Soluble forms of the GM-CSF receptor are secreted naturally and may play a role in immune function (89).

Signal Transduction

The signal transduction pathways that occur when GM-CSF binds to its receptor are not completely determined. There appear to be at least two distinct signaling pathways, each involving a distinct region of the β_c subunit (90). The first involves activation of a *Janus* kinase (JAK2) and leads to induction of c-*myc* and activation of DNA replication (91). Regulation of gene expression by JAK2 appears to be mediated by production of a DNA-binding complex containing the signal transducer and activator of transcription (STAT) proteins STAT1, STAT3, and STAT5 (92,93). The second pathway involves activation of *ras* (94) and mitogen-activated protein kinases (95) with consequent induction of c-*fos* and c-*jun*, which are early genes involved in the regulation of hematopoietic differentiation (91).

Biologic Activity

GM-CSF is classified as a multilineage colony-stimulating factor (CSF) because it stimulates the proliferation and differentiation of progenitor cells of neutrophil, eosinophil, and monocyte colonies (96). GM-CSF alters the kinetics of myeloid progenitor cells within the bone marrow, causing rapid entry of cells into the cycle and decreasing the cell cycle time by as much as 33% (97). Parenteral administration of GM-CSF induces a dose-dependent increase in circulating neutrophils and, to a lesser extent, of eosinophils and monocytes. When GM-CSF is discontinued, leukocyte counts decrease to pretreatment levels over the subsequent 3 to 5 days (98,99).

Coadministration of GM-CSF with other cytokines results in the proliferation and maturation of several cell lineages. The combination of GM-CSF and G-CSF is synergistic and acts on progenitor cells not simulated by either growth factor alone (100,101). In studies of human marrow cells collected from healthy volunteers, the combination of GM-CSF and G-CSF enhanced survival of progenitor cells and produced colonies with earlier progenitor cells than either cytokine alone (102,103). The combination of GM-CSF with Epo or IL-3 promotes the proliferation and differentiation of erythroid and megakaryocytic progenitors, respectively (104,105).

The addition of GM-CSF to TPO (discussed below) increases the overall *in vitro* megakaryocyte expansion compared to TPO alone and generates different subpopulations of CD41+ megakaryocyte progenitors, with less coexpression of CD42b and CD34 and more coexpression of c-*kit* (106). In addition, the total number of CD34+ cells increases approximately fivefold with the combination of GM-CSF and TPO. A study in sublethally irradiated nonhuman primates showed that GM-CSF plus TPO accelerated trilineage recovery compared to either cytokine alone (107). The addition of GM-CSF to the early acting cytokine Flt3-ligand (Flt3L) resulted in substantial expansion of progenitor cells in mice (108) and was synergistic in mobilizing peripheral blood stem cells in nonhuman primates (109).

GM-CSF induces a broad range of functional changes in mature effector cells, which may lead to antitumor and antimicrobial activity. GM-CSF stimulates surface expression of CD11b/CD18 on neutrophils and eosinophils (110). These adhesion-promoting glycoproteins may be responsible for the margination of activated leukocytes after GM-CSF administration. In monocytes and macrophages, GM-CSF induces the production of various cytokines (e.g., TNF, IL-1, IL-6, G-CSF), prostaglandins, arachidonic acid, and platelet-activating factor (111–113). Monocyte exposure to GM-CSF induces a rapid decrease in messenger RNA and surface protein for two receptors (CCR5 and CXCR4) involved in cell entry of the human immunodeficiency virus (HIV). This leads to a 70- to 100-fold decreased cell entry of M-tropic HIV-1 (114). GM-CSF enhances granulocyte oxidative metabolism and respiratory burst (115,116) and increases Fc-dependent phagocytosis, cytotoxic activity against bacteria and yeast (117), and intracellular killing of parasites (118–126). Antibody-dependent cell-mediated cytotoxicity is also stimulated by exposure to GM-CSF (115,127–130).

GM-CSF enhances dendritic cell maturation, proliferation, and migration (131–133). In addition, GM-CSF increases class II major histocompatibility complex (MHC) expression on macrophages and dendritic cells, enhancing their function as professional antigen-presenting cells (133). This immunomodulatory effect has been used to induce antitumor immunity in cancer patients, either directly or with antitumor vaccines (134–138).

Pharmacokinetics

There is evidence from animal and clinical studies that the degree of glycosylation influences pharmacokinetic parameters of recombinant proteins (139). Pharmacokinetics of sargramostim are dependent on the route of administration (140–143). Peak serum concentrations are higher after intravenous administration; however, bioavailability (as determined by the area under the concentration-versus-time curve) is similar between administration routes. Elimination occurs principally by nonrenal mechanisms. Serum concentrations are more prolonged after subcutaneous than after intravenous administration. The magnitude of the increase in absolute neutrophil count (ANC) with a specific dose of sargramostim is greater after subcutaneous injection than after 2-hour intravenous infusion.

Sargramostim pharmacokinetics have been evaluated in children with recurrent or progressive solid tumors who received the drug after myelosuppressive chemotherapy (141–143). After 2-hour intravenous infusions of sargramostim in doses ranging from 60 to 1500 µg/m²/day, clearance was neither dose nor age dependent and ranged from 49 to 52 mL/minute/m². The median terminal $t_{1/2}$ after 2-hour intravenous infusion in these studies ranged from 1.6 to 2.0 hours. Similar to observations in adults, subcutaneous administration of sargramostim resulted in rapid appearance of GM-CSF in serum, prolonged absorption with peak concentrations reached after 1.5 to 4.0 hours, and a median terminal $t_{1/2}$ of 2.3 hours.

HEMATOPOIETIC GROWTH FACTORS TO STIMULATE THROMBOPOIESIS

Interleukin-11

IL-11 is a nonglycosylated megakaryocyte growth factor that stimulates megakaryocytopoiesis by increasing the platelet count as well as a number of other classes of committed hematopoietic progenitor cells (144,145). IL-11 also stimulates the growth of primitive hematopoietic stem cells (146,147). This cytokine also induces megakaryocytic maturation (148,504). Initially, endogenous thrombopoietin was found to stimulate both megakaryocytopoiesis and thrombopoiesis by its interaction with a cell-surface receptor encoded by the c-mpl protooncogene (149). This purified thrombopoietic agent was isolated by five independent groups of investigators (150–154). The mpl-ligand stimulates megakaryocytic colony-forming units in the bone marrow and increases the peripheral platelet count (155–157). The ligand for mpl also increases the size and DNA content of megakaryocytes (157). Three groups have cloned thrombopoietin, resulting in a pegylated and truncated form (158) and a full-length form (159). IL-11 (Oprelvekin) is the only thrombopoietic growth factor licensed in the United States and is approved for treatment of patients with solid tumors to reduce the degree of thrombocytopenia and the requirement for platelet transfusions in patients receiving cyclic intensive chemotherapy (160). The hepatocyte is the primary source of serum thrombopoietin in humans, and the levels are inversely proportional to the megakaryocyte mass (161,162). Thrombopoietin levels rise in the presence of thrombocytopoiesis, which is related to a decrease in binding of thrombopoietin to platelets or megakaryocytes (163).

Gene Encoding for Interleukin-11

IL-11 is a 19-kd protein encoded by a gene located on chromosome 19 (164). It is another member of the type 1 cytokine receptor superfamily, which includes many growth factors that stimulate the growth of a variety of lymphoid and myeloid cells as discussed above (165).

Signal Transduction

The receptor for IL-11 has been cloned (166). Similar to IL-6, IL-11 relies on the same glycoprotein (gp) 130–mediated pathway along with leukemia inhibitory factor and ciliary neurotrophic factor because there is structural similarity (167,168). The receptors, which share homology, have a cytokine-binding subunit and a common subunit, gp130 (169–172). IL-11 binds to a heterodimeric receptor complex, which includes a low-affinity binding subunit α and gp130. Two α subunits exist in different tissues but have almost the exact same homology (173).

Biologic Activity

IL-11 is a pleiotropic cytokine that acts synergistically with IL-3 and stem cell factor (SCF) to stimulate early hematopoietic cells into the cell cycle (174). IL-11 acts synergistically with IL-3; SCF and G-CSF; and IL-3, SCF, or TPO to stimulate erythropoiesis, myelopoiesis, and thrombopoiesis, respectively (159,175,176). IL-11 increases the ploidy of bone marrow megakaryocytes, thereby increasing platelet production (177–179). IL-11 stimulates platelet production in a dose-dependent fashion with peak platelet counts at 14 to 21 days after IL-11 exposure (178,180). IL-11 also has the interesting potential of promoting the integrity of gastrointestinal mucosal epithelial cells (181). An initial clinical trial was conducted in breast cancer patients receiving chemotherapy followed by increasing doses of IL-11 (182). An increase in plasma volume was thought to account for the characteristic development of anemia. At the maximal tolerated dose of 75 µg/kg, there was a 185% increase in platelet count.

Two prospective randomized clinical trials have been conducted in patients for secondary prophylaxis (183,185). In both studies, a statistically significant difference was present in the percentage of patients requiring platelet transfusions (at a 50 µg/kg dose). Toxicities were not inconsequential, with edema in 55% and 63% of patients in the two respective trials; dizziness and dyspnea each in 48% of patients in the first trial; and pleural effusions in the 18% of patients in the second trial.

Pharmacokinetics

After intravenous administration, IL-2 is rapidly cleared from the circulation such that less than 3% of the total dose given remains in the serum at 90 minutes, and the kidneys are generally responsible for elimination (184). The absolute bioavailability is greater than 60% after subcutaneous administration.

HEMATOPOIETIC GROWTH FACTORS TO STIMULATE ERYTHROPOIESIS

Erythropoietin

One of the most important benefits of the revolution in recombinant DNA technology is the capability for high-level expression of purified proteins for use in clinical medicine. Of all such products currently in use, recombinant human erythropoietin (rhEpo) is the most successful in terms of number of patients being treated, commercial revenue generated, and a remarkably high quotient of efficacy over toxicity.

Gene Encoding for Erythropoietin

Hypoxemia stimulates expression of the Epo gene (186). Epo is an 18-kd protein encoded by this gene located on the long arm of chromosome 7 (187). This protein is expressed by hepatocytes during embryogenesis (188,189) and hepatocytes and renal cells in the normal adult (187,189).

Erythropoietin Receptor

The Epo receptor gene is located on chromosome 19 (191).

Signal Transduction

The JAK/STAT pathway is involved in the signal transduction of the Epo gene (190). The Epo receptor is phosphorylated, leading to docking sites for the SH2 domain of molecules that include STAT2, STAT5, protein tyrosine phosphatases SH-PTP1 and SH-PTP2, and phosphoinositide 3-kinase (191,192). Other pathways appear to involve the protein C kinase family with changes in GATA-2 and Bcl-x_L (193).

Biologic Activity

In keeping with its role as an erythroid-specific cytokine, the primary indication for rhEpo therapy is anemia. In most patients with anemia, the production of Epo, as reflected by plasma levels, increases markedly in proportion to the decrement in red cell mass. However, Epo production is markedly impaired in patients with renal failure and modestly blunted in patients with chronic inflammation. Therefore, it is understandable that rhEpo treatment is most predictably effective in these disorders. In general, a patient whose plasma Epo level is lower than that expected for the degree of anemia is more likely to respond to treatment (194). Response to treatment also depends on the patient's iron status. In those who have inadequate iron stores, the reticulocytes induced by rhEpo treatment have decreased hemoglobin content and concentration (195,196). Accordingly, iron supplementation is required to achieve a full therapeutic response (197). The primary goal of treatment is, of course, an increase in red cell mass. In addition, early in treatment, patients may benefit from the induction of a cohort of young red cells rich in 2,3-bisphosphoglycerate, which lowers the affinity of hemoglobin for oxygen, thereby enhancing oxygen delivery to tissues (198,199).

Other Biologic Effects of Erythropoietin

Human Epo is a protein of 193 amino acids with two disulfide bonds and five glycosylation sites. rhEpo is produced in CHO cells and has four linked oligosaccharide chains. Glycosylated Epo binds to a specific receptor complex with homology to receptors of many other hematopoietic growth factors including GM-CSF, TPO, IL-3, and IL-6. This complex is transported intracellularly and induces proliferation and differentiation of committed erythroid marrow progenitors.

Although Epo is generally regarded to be erythroid-cell specific, it has other biologic effects. In patients with renal failure, rhEpo treatment induces a modest, clinically insignificant increase in platelet count and ameliorates pruritus, presumably by inhibiting the production of histamine in mast cells (200). rhEpo therapy also has measurable, although modest, nonhematologic effects including enhancement of testosterone production in Leydig cells and, perhaps, stimulation of pituitary adrenocorticotropic and follicle-stimulating hormones (201).

These nonerythroid effects notwithstanding, rhEpo, when administered properly, has virtually no discernible side effects or toxicity. However, a rare complication of treatment is the development of antiEpo antibodies that cross-react with the patient's endogenous Epo, resulting in the development of severe aregenerative anemia (202–207). The resulting erythroid aplasia can be reversed by immunosuppressive therapy. Interestingly, this problem has been encountered in approximately 40 European patients but in only one in the United States, although considerably more American patients have been treated with rhEpo.

Pharmacokinetics

The *in vivo* turnover of rhEpo circulating in the plasma is similar to that of endogenous Epo with a $t_{1/2}$ of 5 to 8 hours. When rhEpo is administered intravenously to a patient deficient in Epo, the plasma concentration falls exponentially from a very high initial value to subtherapeutic levels 18 to 24 hours later. In contrast, when the same dose of rhEpo is given by subcutaneous injection, the hormone enters the circulation slowly, allowing therapeutic levels to persist in the circulation for several days (208–210). Thus, the subcutaneous route is more efficient and cost effective than intravenous therapy and has the additional advantage that routine administration does not require skilled medical personnel. Most patients are treated with subcutaneous rhEpo three times a week. Although the treatment is relatively simple and well tolerated, it is expensive and inconvenient. These problems may be lessened by the development of a hyperglycosylated rhEpo that has a considerably longer $t_{1/2}$ in the circulation ($t_{1/2}$ = 25 hours) (211), enabling a lower dose to be given less frequently.

The ideal way to obviate the need for frequent injections of rhEpo is to develop a safe and effective form of gene therapy that would allow sustained and controlled production of Epo. Robust increases in plasma Epo levels have been achieved in experimental animals by transfer of Epo-expressing retrovirus (212), and replication-defective adenoviruses (213–216). Alternatively, effective expression of Epo can also be achieved by injection of naked plasmid DNA into either muscle (215–219) or skin. Repeated injections would be required for maintenance therapy. Challenges implicit in the clinical application of either viral vectors or plasmid DNA include safety and the need for long-term and regulated expression of Epo. One way to achieve physiologically appropriate levels of hormone is by inclusion of a drug-dependent element in the promoter driving the Epo gene (216). Optimal physiologic regulation would require that the gene contains functional, oxygen-dependent regulatory elements, as discussed earlier in this chapter.

HEMATOPOIETIC GROWTH FACTORS TO STIMULATE LYMPHOPOIESIS AND THE IMMUNE RESPONSE

Interleukin-2

IL-2 is cytokine produced by T lymphocytes, which are induced by various mitogens, antibodies, phorbol esters, and lectins (220–229). IL-2 is important in the development of T lymphocytes in promoting propagation from the G phase to the S phase of the cell cycle. This cytokine also stimulates the elaboration of a variety of proinflammatory cytokines from natural killer (NK) cells and T lymphocytes such as IL-1, TNF-α, and GM-CSF and also promotes proliferation of both NK cells and B lymphocytes (229–231). The gene that codes for its production is located on chromosome 4 (232).

Interleukin-2 Receptor and Signal Transduction

The IL-2 receptor is expressed on T cells (227), B cells (228–230), and NK cells (231). IL-2 binds to a complex heterodimer receptor with α (CD25), β, and γ (not essential for signal transduction but increases affinity for α and β subunits) (233,234). When activated, T lymphocytes have only this high-affinity form of the receptor as opposed to NK cells, which express both the intermediate- and high-affinity forms, and monocytes, which express only the intermediate form (235–237). IL-2 activates both JAK1 and JAK3 with subsequent transphosphorylation of tyrosine.

Biologic Activity

IL-2 induces proliferation and activation of T and B lymphocytes and NK cells (224,228). However, loss of IL-2 results in activation and proliferation of $CD4^+$ T lymphocytes and loss of self-tolerance with consequent generalized autoimmune disease (238,239). Importantly, activated T lymphocytes demonstrate cytotoxic activity against many tumor cell lines (238–240). These cells have been classified as *lymphokine-activated killer* (LAK) *cells*. These cells, alone and in combination with chemotherapy, have been evaluated clinically and are effective against some solid tumors (241–245) and some hematologic malignancies (246–254).

CLINICAL USE OF HEMATOPOIETIC GROWTH FACTORS TO STIMULATE MYELOPOIESIS

States of Bone Marrow Failure

APLASTIC ANEMIA

Single Hematopoietic Growth Factors. Aplastic anemia may develop as an idiopathic primary hematologic disease or one that is acquired after radiation; it may also develop a disease acquired from cytotoxic agents and chemicals that can cause idiosyncratic reactions to medications such as chloramphenicol and nonsteroidal agents, viruses, or immune-mediated diseases (255). It has been shown that the stromal cells from patients with aplastic anemia release hematopoietic growth factors (256–258). Although some studies have indeed suggested low levels of some hematopoietic growth factors, including G-CSF, GM-CSF, and IL-1 isolated from stomal cells, serum levels are generally elevated (259–264). Despite normal or elevated levels of hematopoietic growth factors in patients with aplastic anemia, it stands to reason that it may be possible to promote further hematopoiesis with exogenously administered growth factors (265–267). Although there are no data that show an improvement in survival, the administration of G-CSF and GM-CSF in patients with aplastic anemia does result in increases in the neutrophil count (268–271). An important unresolved issue, in an attempt to stimulate hematopoiesis in aplastic anemia with myeloid hematopoietic growth factors, concerns the possibility of stimulating clonal proliferation because patients with aplastic anemia may be difficult to distinguish from those with hypocellular MDS (272,273). Studies have suggested that this risk may exist (273,274).

Other hematopoietic growth factors have been studied without much success in patients with aplastic anemia. IL-3 (not discussed here) can stimulate both myelopoiesis and thrombopoiesis with elevations in the neutrophil and platelet counts, but toxicity has precluded its routine clinical use (271–276). Similarly, a pilot trial with IL-6 was aborted because of toxicity (277).

Combinations of Hematopoietic Growth Factors. More success has been achieved with the combinations of hematopoietic growth factors in aplastic anemia, including GM-CSF and Epo (278–280) and IL-3 given with G-CSF (281). In a randomized prospective trial, the combination of G-CSF and Epo results in an increase of hemoglobin levels but generally in patients with modest disease (282).

Hematopoietic Growth Factors Combined with Other Agents. Hematopoietic growth factors have also been administered with agents other than growth factors such as cyclosporine. In a randomized trial that compared G-CSF plus cyclosporine to antilymphocyte globulin plus cyclosporine plus antilymphocyte globulin plus cyclosporine as initial therapy, the G-CSF plus cyclosporine was found to be inferior (283). Bacigalupo and colleagues for the European Bone Marrow Transplant Severe Aplastic Anemia Working Party evaluated a combination of antilymphocyte globulin (15 mg/kg/day, days 1 to 5), cyclosporine, and G-CSF (5 µg/kg/day, days 1 to 90) all combined with methyl prednisolone (2 mg/kg/day, days 1 to 5 with a taper) (284). Among 40 patients, 33 (82%) had trilineage hematologic reconstitution and became transfusion independent at a median of 115 days from initiation of treatment.

MYELODYSPLASTIC SYNDROMES

The MDSs represent a heterogeneous group of clonal hematopoietic disorders that originate in the pluripotent hematopoietic stem cell. The syndromes are associated with a variable degree of dysplasia and subsequent ineffective hematopoiesis (285,286). The diseases are manifested primarily by peripheral blood cytopenias, a usually cellular or occasionally hypocellular marrow, dysplasia of all cell lineages, and, in some cases, evolution to acute leukemia (287,288). A two-step pathogenesis has been proposed: one initiating proliferation of an unstable clone of pluripotent hematopoietic stem cells and a second inducing cytogenetic abnormalities in the progeny (289,290). Many studies have demonstrated poor or absent colony formation by marrow granulocyte-macrophage, early or late erythroid, megakaryocytic, and multilineage progenitors in most patients with MDSs (291–297). Karyotype of the myelodysplastic cells is an important influence on patient outcome (298). An international scoring system for evaluation and prognosis has been useful (299–301).

Recently, a variety of cytokines including TNF-α, transforming growth factor-β (TGF-α), and IL-1β have been implicated in the pathogenesis of MDS (301). Such cytokines can induce both proliferation and apoptosis in hematopoietic cells (302–305). Recent studies have suggested that anticytokine therapy may interrupt these pathways with drugs such as pentoxifylline (306) and ciprofloxacin (307). Indeed, preliminary clinical studies have been reported with some apparent benefit with respect to the peripheral blood counts and transfusion requirements (308).

Classically, the clonal MDSs have been divided into refractory anemia with excess blasts, refractory anemia with ringed sideroblasts, and refractory anemia with excess blasts in transformation in chronic monomyelocytic leukemia (287,309). Recently, the category *refractory anemia with excess blasts in transformation* has been eliminated in the new World Health Organization Classification (310).

Hematopoietic Growth Factor Treatment of Myelodysplastic Syndromes. Hematopoietic stem cell transplantation appears to be the treatment of choice in younger individuals because it has the best curative potential (311). However, many patients are older or lack a suitable donor, and hematopoietic growth factors have emerged as an important therapeutic strategy. Numerous trials have investigated the role of G-CSF and GM-CSF in MDS (312–331).

Because it has been suggested that the pathogenesis of the MDSs is related to lack of responsive or impaired production of hematopoietic growth factors, there has been enthusiasm for evaluating the role of hematopoietic growth, which might induce the proliferation of normal hematopoietic progenitor cells and induce the proliferation and maturation of the myelodysplastic clone of cells.

Granulocyte Colony-Stimulating Factor in Myelodysplastic Syndromes. A number of phase II clinical trials have evaluated the role of G-CSF in MDSs and, in general, demonstrated a consistent improvement in the neutrophil count (315,328–331) (Table 58-1). Only occasionally has improvement in either the reticulocyte count or platelet count been observed. Generally, the changes in the neutrophil count have been dose dependent. The incidence of bacterial infections has been reduced (329,330). G-CSF has been very well tolerated. The major toxicity is bone pain and, occasionally, ecchymoses at injection sites. There is no incidence of antibody development. Greenberg and colleagues conducted a prospective randomized trial of subcutaneous G-CSF versus observation in patients with refractory anemia with excess blasts or refractory anemia with excess blasts in transformation (331). The results of this trial confirmed the

TABLE 58-1. Studies of Granulocyte Colony-Stimulating Factor (G-CSF) in Myelodysplastic Syndromes

Study (Reference)	G-CSF Dose/Route	Number	Number of Patients with Improvement in Peripheral Blood Counts		
			Granulocyte	Reticulocyte	Platelet
Negrin (315)	0.1–3.0 µg/kg s.c.	12	10	5	3
Kobayashi (327)	60–1600 µg/m² i.v.	7	5	0	0
Ohyashiki (328)	50–200 µg/m² i.v.	4	4	0	0
Negrin (329)	0.3–10.0 µg/kg s.c.	11	10	4	1
Yoshida (330)	2.0–10.0 µg/kg i.v.	41	37	0	2
Greenberg (331)	NA	50	50	NA	NA

NA, not available.

TABLE 58-2. Studies of Granulocyte-Macrophage Colony-Stimulating Factor (GM-CSF) in Myelodysplastic Syndromes

Study (Reference)	GM-CSF Dose/Route	Number	Number of Patients with Improvement in Counts		
			Granulocyte	Reticulocyte	Platelet
Schuster (322)	3 µg/kg q.i.d. s.c.	26	26	0	0
Willemze (323)	108 µg/kg b.i.d. s.c.	33	22	NA	NA
	216 µg/kg b.i.d. s.c.	35	22	NA	NA
Rosenfeld (324)	60–250 µg/m² q.i.d.	20	14	0	0
Willemze (325)	Gp1 108 µg b.i.d. s.c.	82	82	NA	2
	Gp2 216 µg b.i.d. s.c.				
Takahashi (326)	60–250 µg/m² s.c.	18	17	3	1
Vadhan-Raj (313)		8	8	2	3
Thompson (316)	0.3–10.0/µg/kg	16	11	3	2

Gp, group; NA, not available.

safety of G-CSF in the setting of MDS because there were no differences in the observed incidence of transformation to acute myelogenous leukemia (AML). Unexpectedly, there was an inferior survival among patients with refractory anemia with excess blasts who received G-CSF attributable to nonleukemic but disease-related mortality, which was perhaps attributable to a higher number of high-risk patients.

Granulocyte-Macrophage Colony-Stimulating Factor in Myelodysplastic Syndromes. An initial study was presented by Vadhan-Raj and colleagues in 1987 (313). In a phase I trial, eight patients received GM-CSF by continuous intravenous infusion daily for 2 weeks and then again after a 2-week rest interval. In all eight patients, marked increases in the neutrophil count were observed. In addition, the absolute number of monocytes, eosinophils, and lymphocytes also increased. Furthermore, three of eight patients had an increase in the platelet count and improvement in erythropoiesis, with two of the three patients having elimination of the requirement of red blood cell and platelet transfusions at 20 to 27 weeks of follow-up. Marrow cellularity increased as well as the ratio of differentiated myeloid cells to immature myeloid cells.

A number of subsequent phase I and phase II studies reporting different schedules, doses, and routes of administration have been reported (314,322–326) (Table 58-2). In the aggregate experience, increases in the neutrophil count have been reported in most studies. However, similar to the results observed with G-CSF, there is little rise in either the reticulocyte count and hemoglobin or platelet count. In general, the therapy has been well tolerated, and the most common toxicity has been a flulike syndrome that appears to be dose dependent. An additional toxicity often overlooked is the development of splenic enlargement (332).

In a reasonably large randomized trial evaluating the role of GM-CSF versus observation, GM-CSF was given daily at a dose of 3 µg/kg s.c. for 90 days versus observations (325). Patients who received the GM-CSF had a sustained raise in the neutrophil, monocyte, eosinophil, and lymphocyte counts with an associated decrease in the rate of infection from 33% to 15%. No effect was seen on the platelet count or hemoglobin level, and there was no decrease in transfusion requirements. The rate of transformation to acute leukemia in patients with refractory anemia with excess blasts in transformation was not significantly higher in the treated group of patients. Other trials have also confirmed no excess risk of transformation to acute leukemia (324–327,333).

Intensive chemotherapy is associated with limited success in patients with MDSs. However, several recent reports have evaluated the benefits of combining granulocyte or GM-CSF with intensive chemotherapy (334,335). The Dutch-Belgian Hemato-Oncology Cooperative Group (HOVON) has studied the addition of G-CSF given with induction and consolidation chemotherapy in patients with poor-risk MDSs (334). The hypothesis in these studies has been not only to stimulate recovery of normal hematopoiesis after chemotherapy, but also to prime malignant cells by mobilizing them into the cell cycle to render them more susceptible to chemotherapy (336–338). In the report by the HOVON group, 64 patients were randomized to receive GM-CSF at a dose of 5 µg/kg/day s.c. or no G-CSF in addition to daunorubicin and cytarabine induction chemotherapy. The complete remission rate was higher in the patients receiving G-CSF (73% vs. 52%, *p* = .08), although overall survival at 2 years was no different (29% for patients receiving G-CSF vs. 16% for control patients, *p* = .22) (Fig. 58-1). However, the median time to neutrophil recovery to 1.0×10^9/L was 23 days in the patients receiving G-CSF compared to 35 days in those not receiving G-CSF (*p* = .015). No differences were observed in the time to

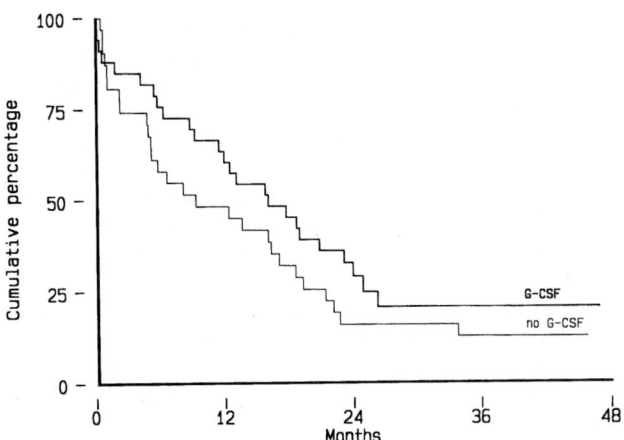

Figure 58-1. Overall survival of patients with myelodysplastic syndrome randomized to chemotherapy with or without granulocyte colony-stimulating factor (G-CSF). [From Ossenkoppele GJ, van der Holt B, Verhoef GE, et al. A randomized study of granulocyte colony-stimulating factor applied during and after chemotherapy in patients with poor risk myelodysplastic syndromes: a report from the HOVON Cooperative Group. Dutch-Belgian Hemato-Oncology Cooperative Group. *Leukemia* 1999;13(8):1207–1213.]

TABLE 58-3. Studies of Erythropoietin (Epo) ± Hematopoietic Growth Factors in Myelodysplastic Syndromes

Author (Reference)	Epo Dose/Schedule	Growth Factor Dose/Schedule	Number of Patients	Response (%) Complete Remission and Partial Remission
Stasi (347)	150 IU/kg 3 times a wk for 12 wk[a]	None	43	32
Adamson (344)	150 IU/kg 3 times a wk[b]	None	20	50[c]
Economopoulos (355)	60 IU/kg days 3–5 weekly for 6 wk[d]	GM-CSF, 3 µg/kg daily	19	53[e]
Negrin (354)	100 IU/kg escalated to 150 IU, then 300 IU/kg every 4 wk	G-CSF, 1 µg/kg daily	28	42[f]
Hellstrom-Lindberg (356)	60–300 IU/kg/d for at least 10 wk	G-CSF, 3–300 µg/kg daily	98	High prob., 74; intermediate prob., 23; poor prob., 7
Stein (346)	1000–1200 IU/kg twice each wk	None	20	24[g]
Hellstrom-Lindberg (353)	5000–10,000 IU/day	G-CSF, 30–150 µg/day	50	38
Bowen (345)	60–90 IV/kg daily	None	10	20

CR, complete remission; G-CSF, granulocyte colony-stimulating factor; GM-CSF, granulocyte-macrophage colony-stimulating factor; PR, partial remission; prob., probability.
[a]Dose increased to 300 IU/kg if there is no or suboptimal response after 12 wk.
[b]Dose increased to 300 IU/kg if it failed to raise plasma concentration of transferrin receptor at least by one-third.
[c]Effective clinical response defined as a >50% reduction or elimination in transfusion requirement or an improvement in hematocrit by ≥6 percentage points.
[d]Dose of Epo increased to 120 IU/kg if a 1.5-g/dL rise in hemoglobin is not achieved.
[e]Includes a 37% good response increase in untransfused hemoglobin of 2 g/dL or a 100% decrease in red blood cell transfusion, and PR defined as an increase in hemoglobin of 1.2 g/dL or a >50 decrease in transfusion requirement.
[f]Includes good and partial erythroid response defined as a >2-g/dL increase in untreated hemoglobin or a 100% decrease in red cell transfusions, and PR defined as an increase in untransfused hemoglobin of 1–2 g/dL or a >50% decrease in transfusion requirements.
[g]Defined as an increase in hematocrit of 4 percentage points over baseline or elimination in all transfusion requirements.

platelet recovery, length of hospitalization, and duration of antibiotic use from infectious complications.

Interleukin-3 in Patients with Myelodysplastic Syndromes. Ganzer and colleagues reported a phase I–II study of nine patients receiving IL-3 at a dose of 250 µg/m² to 500 µg/m² given subcutaneously daily for 15 days (339). In all nine patients, an increase in the neutrophil, eosinophil, lymphocyte, basophil, and monocyte counts was observed. The mean absolute neutrophil count increased from 1350/µL (range 1050 to 2420) to 2660/µL (range 300 to 938; p <.05), to a maximum of 4096/µL (range 350 to 10,820; p <.01). Platelet counts increased in two to four patients with profound thrombocytopenia, resulting in the elimination of platelet transfusion requirement.

Thrombopoietin Agents in Myelodysplastic Syndromes. In the MDSs, thrombopoietin levels have been elevated in some patients (refractory anemia) and low in others (refractory anemia with excess blasts and refractory anemia with excess blasts in transformation) (340–342). Wang et al. found an inverse correlation between the serum thrombopoietin levels and colony-forming unit–meg in patients with MDSs (343). However, a weak correlation was observed between the serum thrombopoietin levels and platelet counts in the same patients.

Erythropoietin in Myelodysplastic Syndromes. Numerous clinical trials have evaluated the benefits of Epo in patients with MDS, either alone (344–352) or in combination with myeloid growth factors (353–356) (Table 58-3). The latter trials were initiated because *in vitro* studies demonstrated synergy in stimulation of erythropoiesis when Epo was combined with myeloid cytokines promoting myelopoiesis (357,358). In the aggregate experience, a response is seen in approximately 25% to 50% of patients treated with Epo alone. These trials are difficult to interpret because the response criteria vary. Generally, a *complete response* is defined as a rise in untransfused hemoglobin concentration of at least 2 g/dL or a 100% decrease in red blood cell transfusion

requirement. A *partial response* is defined as an increase in untransfused hemoglobin concentration of 1 to 2 g/dL or a decrease in red blood cell transfusion requirement greater than or equal to 50% (347). In a metaanalysis of more than 200 patients, a low serum endogenous Epo level and a lack of transfusions were factors predictive of a response (349). A dose of 10,000 IU s.c. three times a week appears to be a reasonable dose and schedule, and most responses occur within 8 weeks. Higher doses may lead to better responses (353,359). Sustained response can be achieved with prolonged administration (352,359). Although patients may lose their responsiveness when the dose is reduced, 20,000 IU/week seems to be the required dose to maintain a response. Patients may also respond a second time when reinstituted after Epo has been discontinued or reduced (352). The combination of Epo and G-CSF or GM-CSF may improve the response in erythropoiesis and myelopoiesis. Thrombocytopenia has been observed with the combination (353,354,360).

HEMATOPOIETIC GROWTH FACTORS IN ACUTE MYELOGENOUS LEUKEMIA

The use of hematopoietic growth factors in patients with AML has several potential benefits, including a reduction of the period of neutropenia, with subsequent reduction in risk of infection and mortality, and improvement in the complete remission rate. A theoretic benefit includes so-called priming, which applies recruitment of cells in the S phase of the cell cycle, as discussed above (336–338,361,362). Theoretically, it is also possible that hematopoietic growth factors induce differentiation of leukemic cells (363). As in the case with MDS, an important issue in evaluating the role of hematopoietic growth factors in patients with AML concerns the theoretic risk of leukemic stimulation because leukemic cells in patients with AML express growth factor receptors (364–369). However, very early studies suggested that this was not a major concern because there was no apparent stimulation of leukemic cells, even when

TABLE 58-4. Randomized Trials of Growth Factor after Induction Therapy in Acute Myelogenous Leukemia

Author (Reference)	Number of Patients	Age	Growth Factor	Start Day	Marrow Aplasia	Complete Response (%)	Median Days Absolute Neutrophil Count to 1000/µL	Growth Factors vs. Control		
								Grades 3–5 Infectious Toxicity (%)	Therapy-Related Mortality (%)	Overall Survival (mo)
Rowe (388)	117	56–70	GM-CSF	11	Yes	60/44	12/18^a	52/70	6/15	10.614/8.000
Dombret (389)	173	≥65	G-CSF	8	No	70/47	21/27^a	22/48	23/27	7.5/10.5
Heil (385)	521	≥16	G-CSF	8	No	69/68	20/25	3/7	8.0/9.5	12/14
Godwin (382)	234	≥55	G-CSF	11	Yes	42/49	3–4 days	14/19	20/19	—
Stone (390)	379	≥60	GM-CSF	8	No	52/54	15/17^a	18/18	27/23	8.4/10.8
Zittoun (379)	53	15–60	GM-CSF	8	No	48/77	Not different	81/87	7.7/3.7	NA
Lowenberg (380)	316	≥61	G-CSF	1–8	No	63/61	26/31	Not different	14/10	10/8
Link (391)	187	16–76	G-CSF	9	No	60/43	12/18	62/57	NA	NA
Goldstone (392)	800	15–59	G-CSF	8	No	72/75	15/20	Not different	12/13	44/47
Witz (381)	240	55–75	GM-CSF	1	No	63/61	24/29^a	Not different	18/26	39/27
Lowenberg (383)	123	15–60	GM-CSF	8	No	77/75	26/30^a	40/25	NA	46/41

G-CSF, granulocyte colony-stimulating factor; GM-CSF, granulocyte-macrophage colony-stimulating factor; NA, not applicable.
^{a}Statistically significant; $p \leq .05$.
Adapted from Rowe JM, Liesveld JL. Hematopoietic growth factors in acute leukemia. *Leukemia* 1997;11:328–341.

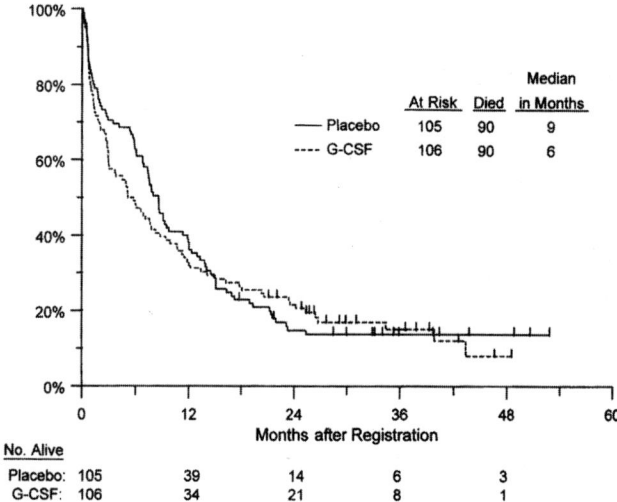

Figure 58-2. Kaplan-Meier estimates of the distributions of survival from day of study by treatment arm, based on 211 patients. G-CSF, granulocyte colony-stimulating factor; No., number. [From Godwin JE, Kopecky KJ, Head DR, et al. A double-blind placebo-controlled trial of granulocyte colony-stimulating factor in elderly patients with previously untreated acute myeloid leukemia: a Southwest Oncology Group study (9031). *Blood* 1998;91:3607–3615.]

hematopoietic growth factors were administered concurrently with induction chemotherapy (370–372). Although as suggested in the aggregate experience in phase II trials, there was no clear stimulation of leukemia, and several studies did show some evidence of growth factor–dependent leukemic proliferation (362,373). Interestingly, mutations in the G-CSF receptor gene in a patient with AML have been described that theoretically could contribute to defective receptor signaling and potentially play a role in leukemogenesis (374).

Hematopoietic Growth Factors before or during Induction Chemotherapy in Acute Myelogenous Leukemia

Several early studies evaluated the role of priming of leukemic cells to promote cytotoxicity with induction chemotherapy by attempting to recruit leukemic cells into the S phase of the cell cycle. Results were conflicting because some benefit was observed in one study (361), a deleterious effect was reported in another study (362), and no benefit was reported in a third study (375). Subsequently, several randomized studies have been carried out. The majority of these studies demonstrated a reduction in the duration of neutropenia after intensive chemotherapy, which varied between 2 and 5 days (376–393) (Table 58-4). However, such accelerated recovery of neutrophils did not translate into significant benefit with respect to complete remission rates, induction mortality rates, and incidence of infection or overall survival. The Southwest Oncology Group (SWOG) conducted a double-blind trial in adults older than 56 years of age in which patients were randomly assigned G-CSF or not assigned, beginning on day 11 (382). The CR rates were not different in the two groups and neither was the median overall survival (Fig. 58-2). G-CSF has also been studied in a randomized trial in patients given an intensified induction regimen that included high-dose cytarabine, etoposide, and idarubicin (386). However, as in other trials with standard-dose cytarabine induction regimens, despite a shorter period of neutropenia and a reduction in duration of intravenous antibiotics, there were no differences in CR rates or overall survival.

Several studies have suggested that GM-CSF increases intracellular cytarabine levels and subsequent cytotoxicity (290,338,394–397). However, other studies have shown a limited improvement in cytarabine sensitivity (336,398). One study has shown that GM-CSF actually protected leukemic blasts from cytarabine toxicity (399) and reduced chemotherapy-induced apoptosis (400).

The majority of prospective studies has explored the roles of G-CSF and GM-CSF after the completion of induction or consolidation chemotherapy in AML. Although, in general, there appears to be little or no benefit in CR rates or overall survival, the duration of profound neutropenia is shortened. The incidence, duration, and mortality of serious infections, particularly fungal infections, are decreased in some but not all trials. Importantly, in general, there is little or no risk of leukemic cell stimulation.

Thrombopoietic Agents in Acute Myelogenous Leukemia

Few studies have evaluated the role of thrombopoietic agents during induction therapy in AML. In one randomized trial, patients with newly diagnosed AML were randomized to either 2.5 or 5.0 µg/kg/day of pegylated recombinant human megakaryocytic growth and development factor (PEG-rHuMGDF) or placebo after the completion of induction chemotherapy, which included daunorubicin, 45 mg/m^2, days 1 to 3; cytarabine, 100 mg/m^2, days 1 to 7; and, in patients older than age 60 years, high-dose cytarabine, 2 g/m^2 twice daily, days 8 to 10 (401,402). Although the cytokine was well tolerated, there was no difference in time to platelet recovery to 20×10^9/L platelets among the three groups or any in the number of days on which platelet transfusions were given (Fig. 58-3). A biologic effect was observed because patients receiving rHuMGDF did achieve a higher maximal platelet count at the time of bone marrow recovery. A trial conducted in Europe reported similar results (402). These results are disappointing in view of the data *in vitro*, suggesting PEG-rHUMGDF can enhance megakaryocyte proliferation in patients with MDS and AML (403).

Hematopoietic Growth Factors in Acute Lymphoblastic Leukemia

Myeloid growth factors have been explored in the setting of acute lymphoblastic leukemia (ALL) (404–406). In the largest trial, 198 patients with untreated ALL were randomized to either placebo or G-CSF subcutaneously beginning 4 days after starting intensive remission induction chemotherapy (404). Although the time to neutrophil recovery, which was greater than or equal to 1000/µL, was significantly shorter among patients assigned to G-CSF (16 days vs. 22 days, $p < .001$) and the CR rate was higher with fewer deaths in induction ($p = .04$), overall toxicity was not decreased, and there was no significant improvement in overall survival (median 2.4 years vs. 1.8 years) (Fig. 58-4). Similar results were obtained by Geissler and colleagues who observed a shorter period of neutropenia and a reduced incidence of febrile neutropenia and documented infections but no significant differences in CR rate, disease-free survival, or overall survival (405).

Hematopoietic Growth Factors in Lymphoma

Several phase II studies have reported a benefit for the use of G-CSF or GM-CSF after intensive chemotherapy for non-Hodgkin's lymphoma (407–411). In a randomized trial in patients with high-grade lymphoma treated with intensive

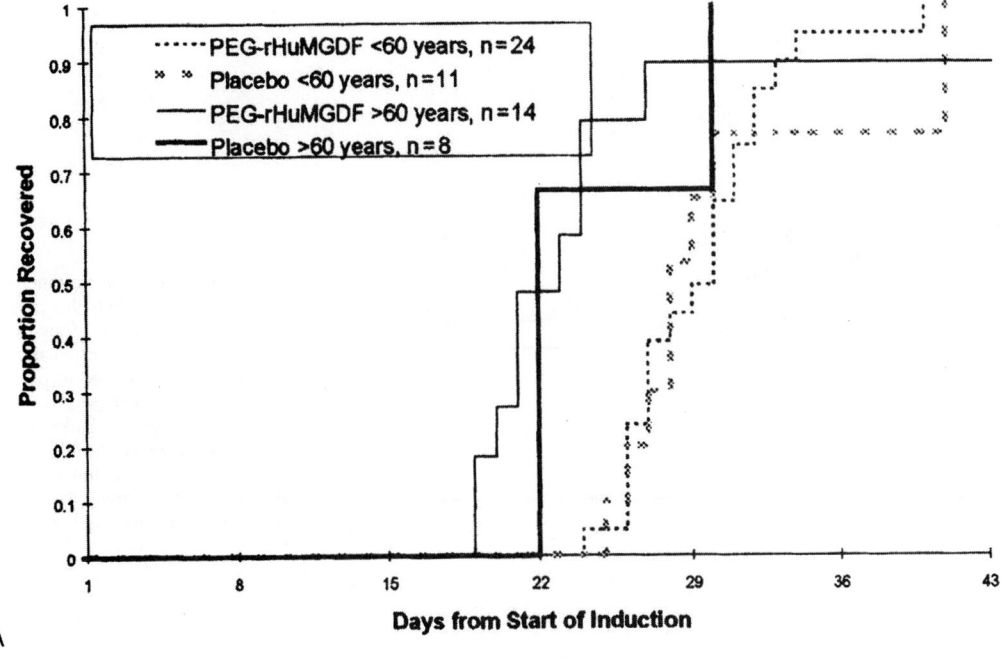

A

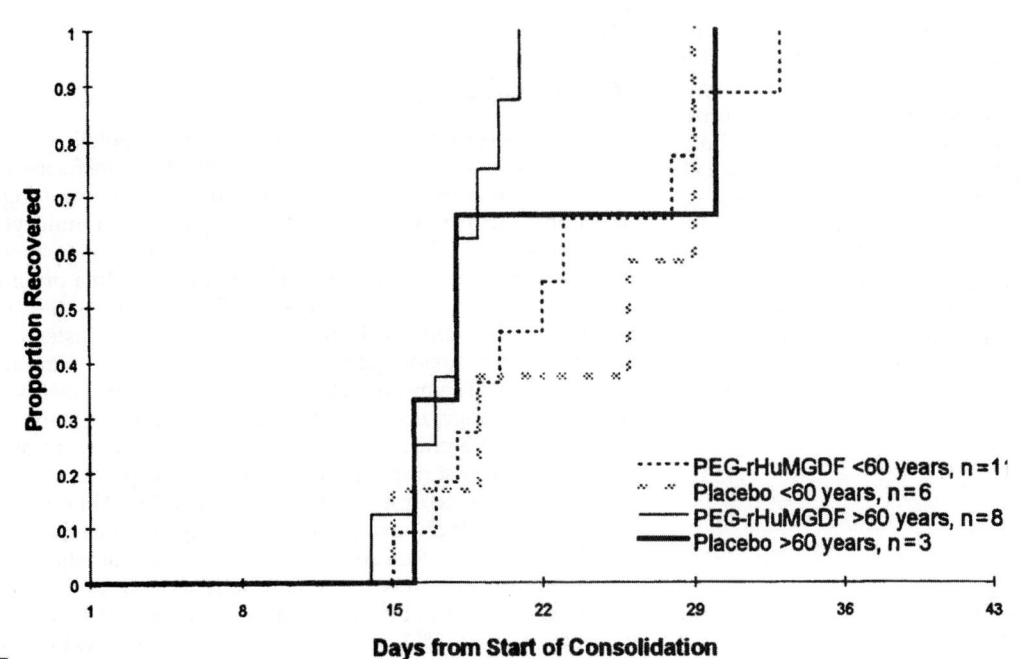

B

Figure 58-3. A: Time to platelet count recovery to at least 20 × 10⁹/L or greater after induction chemotherapy. No statistically significant differences were noted. **B:** Time to platelet count recovery to at least 20 × 10⁹/L or greater after the first course of consolidation chemotherapy. There was no statistically significant difference in the time to platelet recovery or the number of days on which patients received platelets. n, number; PEG-rHuMGDF, pegylated recombinant human megakaryocytic growth and development factor. [From Schiffer CA, Miller K, Larson RA, et al. A double-blind, placebo-controlled trial of pegylated recombinant human megakaryocyte growth and development factor as an adjunct to induction and consolidation therapy for patients with acute myeloid leukemia. *Blood* 2000;95(8):2530–2535.]

multiagent chemotherapy, those randomized to G-CSF had a lower incidence of neutropenia and fewer episodes of neutropenic fever (407). However, this did not translate into fewer documented infections. Importantly, patients randomized to G-CSF had fewer chemotherapy dose reductions and delays in the scheduled delivery of chemotherapy, although this potential benefit did not result in an improvement in response rate or overall survival. In a study carried out of older adults, similar results were observed (408). In another randomized trial, GM-CSF shortened the duration of neutropenia and decreased the incidence of infection during the neutropenic period (409). The response rate was increased, but no improvement in overall survival was demonstrated. The French Society of Pediatric Oncology randomized 148 children receiving aggressive combination chemotherapy for a variety of lymphomas to receive or

not receive G-CSF after two induction courses (411). Although the duration of neutropenia (<500/μL) was 3 days shorter in the patients randomized to G-CSF (p = .0004), again this did not translate into a benefit in the incidence of febrile neutropenia, duration of hospitalization, duration of antimicrobial therapy, remission, or overall survival.

Use of Granulocyte Colony-Stimulating Factor or Granulocyte-Macrophage Colony-Stimulating Factor to Increase Dose Intensity

Several clinical trials suggest that increasing dose intensity may have a beneficial impact on outcome in non-Hodgkin's lymphoma. A phase I clinical trial has been carried out in which the combination chemotherapy regimen ProMACE-

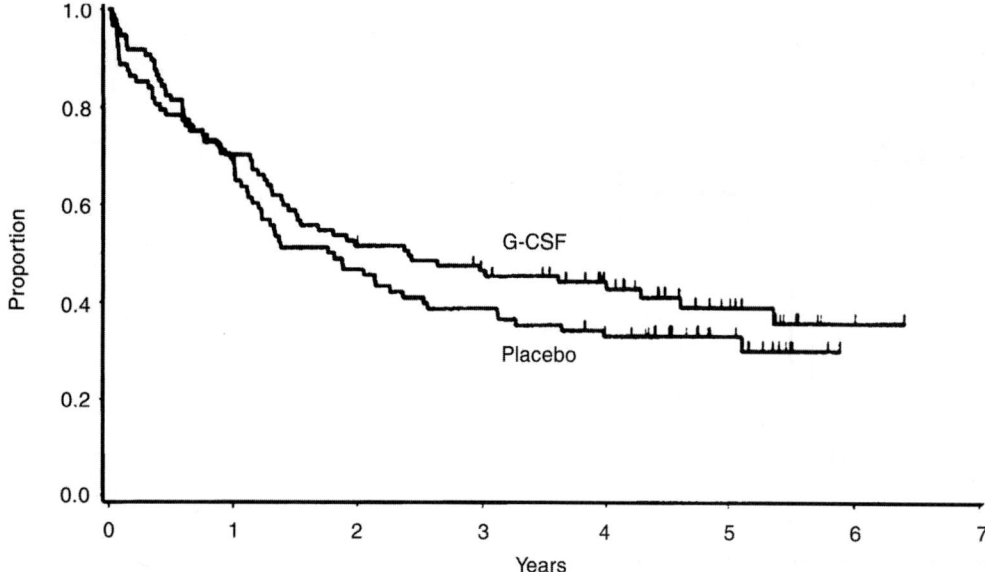

Figure 58-4. There was no difference in the survival between the patients assigned to granulocyte colony-stimulating factor (G-CSF) (median, 2.4 years) and those assigned to placebo (median, 1.8 years) ($p = .25$). [From Larson RA, Dodge RK, Linker CA, et al. A randomized controlled trial of filgrastim during remission induction and consolidation chemotherapy for adults with acute lymphoblastic leukemia: CALGB study 9111. *Blood* 1998;92(5):1556–1564.]

CytaBOM (cyclophosphamid, doxorubicin, etoposide, cytarabine, bleomycin, vincristine, and methotrexate with leucovorin and prednisone) could be administered to 200% of the conventional dose and with GM-CSF support (412). In a second dose-escalating trial, the doses of cyclophosphamide and adriamycin were escalated to 4 g/m² and 70 g/m², respectively, with G-CSF support (413). A phase II clinical trial in diffuse aggressive lymphomas shows very promising results when CHOP (cyclophosphamide, hydroxydaunorubicin, Oncovin, prednisone) is administered at a 200% dose with G-CSF support (414) (Fig. 58-5). In this trial, toxicity was quite acceptable. Although these excellent results are encouraging, a randomized trial comparing CHOP at conventional doses to the 200% doses is needed to definitively establish whether such dose escalation represents a new standard of care.

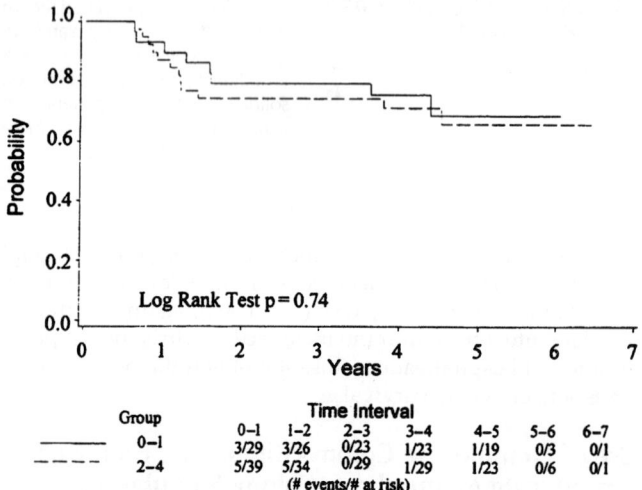

Figure 58-5. Kaplan-Meier estimate of the overall survival for all 74 patients. This analysis depicts overall survival by International Prognostic Index group 0–1 and 2–4. (From Gordon LI, Young M, Weller E, et al. A phase II trial of 20,040 ProMACE-CytaBOM in patients with previously untreated aggressive lymphomas: analysis of response, toxicity and dose intensity. *Blood* 1999;94:3307.)

OTHER CLINICAL INDICATIONS OF HEMATOPOIETIC GROWTH FACTORS

Myeloid Growth Factors

An additional potential role for myeloid hematopoietic growth factors may be the collection of neutrophils for transfusions in patients with severe neutropenia and life-threatening fungal infections (415,416). Historically, the collection of granulocytes has been hampered by erythrocyte contamination, the paucity of circulating granulocytes, and limited lifespan. In a preliminary report from the M. D. Anderson Cancer Center, G-CSF–mobilized white blood cell transfusions were administered to patients with hematologic malignancies refractory to amphotericin B (416). The mean yield of granulocytes per transfusion was 41×10^9 (range, 10–116). Eleven of 14 patients had favorable responses, and eight remained free of infection 3 weeks after treatment. The best responses occurred in those patients with a short duration of neutropenia and active infection. Although M-CSF is not routinely used clinically, a study from the Fred Hutchinson Cancer Research Center suggested that adjunctive M-CSF given to marrow transplant patients with progressive fungal disease led to improved survival compared to historic patients (27% vs. 5%), attributable to a 50% survival rate in patients with *Candida* infections, with a Karnofsky scoring of greater than 20% (417).

ERYTHROPOIETIN

Anemia of Renal Insufficiency

By far the most frequent and effective use of rhEpo worldwide is in patients with kidney failure in whom anemia is due primarily to insufficient Epo production (157,418). The response to treatment is prompt and sustained provided that adequate iron stores are maintained. Therapy is very well tolerated provided that the patient's hematocrit is kept in the mid- to high 30s. In most patients with renal failure, relatively low doses (50 to 150 U/kg three times weekly) are required to achieve this objective. Overtreatment with rhEpo may result in worsening hypertension with increased risk for developing thrombosis of vascular access (419), as well as life-threatening cardiovascular and cerebrovascular complications (420,421). Properly managed patients enjoy significant improvement in quality of life, including less fatigue and depression as well as enhanced appetite, exercise tolerance, and sexual performance (422–424).

Anemia of Chronic Inflammation

Patients with cancer, chronic infections, and connective tissue disorders commonly have a mild-to-moderate anemia. As mentioned above, levels of plasma Epo in these patients are generally lower than those expected for the degree of anemia. Those patients in whom the anemia is more pronounced and, therefore, a cause of clinical symptoms may benefit from treatment with rhEpo (425). The U.S. Food and Drug Administration has approved the use of rhEpo in patients with acquired immuno deficiency syndrome and cancer. The former group may develop severe, often transfusion-dependent anemia, particularly if it is treated with antiviral medication. In those who have relatively low levels of plasma Epo, rhEpo treatment significantly reduces the need for red cell transfusions (426). Treatment of cancer patients with rhEpo results in a significant improvement in anemia, although higher doses are required than for patients with renal failure (427,428). Those who respond to therapy have an improved quality of life (429). Most oncologists agree that only a subset of cancer patients are appropriate candidates for rhEpo therapy. Those whose chemotherapy regimens include cisplatinum are particularly likely to benefit from treatment because these patients often have more marked anemia owing to the drug's nephrotoxicity and impairment of renal production of Epo (430–432). The indication for rhEpo therapy is even less clear in patients with other disorders of chronic inflammation. In those with rheumatoid disease, therapy generally induces modest increments in hematocrit (433–435). Because of other limitations that beset these patients, it is difficult to assess how rhEpo therapy has an impact on their overall clinical course. A large prospective community-based trial suggests that once-weekly dosing of Epo is as effective in raising hemoglobin levels and decreasing transfusion requirements as the three-times-weekly schedule in patients receiving chemotherapy for nonmyeloid malignancies (436).

Other Bone Marrow Disorders

Anemia is a common and often dominant feature in disorders of hematopoiesis. Elderly individuals commonly develop refractory anemia due to myelodysplasia. Only a small fraction of these patients respond to treatment with rhEpo alone. However, when given in combination with G-CSF, the fraction of responders increases to respectable levels approximating 35% as diagnosed above (437). Anemia is also a common problem in patients with multiple myeloma, whether or not they have associated renal disease. The majority of myeloma patients treated with rhEpo achieves a significant improvement in red cell mass (>2 g/dL hemoglobin) (438–441). In patients who undergo allogeneic bone marrow transplantation for hematologic malignancies, treatment with rhEpo hastens the rate of erythropoietic recovery (442–444). In all of these bone marrow disorders, high doses of rhEpo (100 to 300 U/kg/day) are required. As with other types of anemia, the patients most likely to respond are those whose levels of plasma Epo are lower than those predicted from the degree of anemia.

In certain unusual clinical situations, red cell transfusions may be urgently needed yet not feasible. For example, occasional patients develop alloantibodies, either against a broad array of common antigens or against a public antigen, that preclude successful matching of donor red cells. Some patients may for religious reasons refuse to accept blood transfusion. In these settings, the administration of rhEpo with parenteral iron supplementation may be life-saving.

Although blood transfusions in developed nations have reached a remarkably high level of safety, many patients are reluctant to accept blood from an unknown donor. In response to this concern, there is increasing interest in the use of autologous transfusions, particularly for elective surgery. The preoperative administration of rhEpo and iron enables patients to tolerate more extensive preoperative phlebotomy (445–448). Moreover, these autologous units have a significantly higher hemoglobin level. The administration of rhEpo in the perioperative setting may also be effective in ameliorating blood-loss anemia from major surgery and in reducing the need for postoperative red cell transfusions (449,450).

Infants born prematurely often develop severe anemia owing to inadequate endogenous Epo production (451). When low-birth-weight infants are treated with rhEpo during the first 6 weeks of life, there is a significant decrease in the need for blood transfusions (452–454).

Because the administration of rhEpo effectively raises the level of fetal hemoglobin (Hb F) in primates (455), it has been proposed for the treatment of sickle cell disease and beta-thalassemia. Initial studies suggested that rhEpo stimulated Hb F production in sickle cell anemia patients (456), but the results of subsequent clinical studies have been conflicting (457–459). Although some patients with beta-thalassemia respond to rhEpo therapy with increased hemoglobin levels (460,461), they tend to be those with milder disease (thalassemia intermedia).

Thrombopoietic Agents

At the present time, the most important clinical benefit of thrombopoietic agents is to lessen the severity of chemotherapy-induced thrombocytopenia in the setting of nonmyeloid malignancies. However, another, as yet incompletely exploited, potential use for thrombopoietic agents is in the procurement of platelets from healthy donors for transfusions. A blinded prospective randomized trial shows that a single subcutaneous injection of PEG-

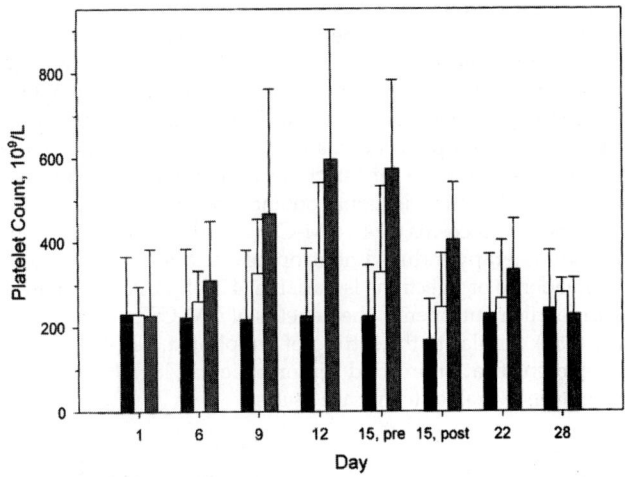

Figure 58-6. The platelet count rises in a dose-dependent manner after the administration of pegylated recombinant human megakaryocytic growth and development factor (PEG-rHuMGDF) to apheresis donors. The response of the donor median platelet count + standard deviation to placebo (■), 1 μg/kg PEG-rHuMGDF (▢), or 3 μg/kg PEG-rHuMGDF (■) administration. [From Kuter DJ, Goodnough LT, Romo J, et al. Thrombopoietin therapy increases platelet yields in healthy platelet donors. *Blood* 2001;98(5):1339–1345.]

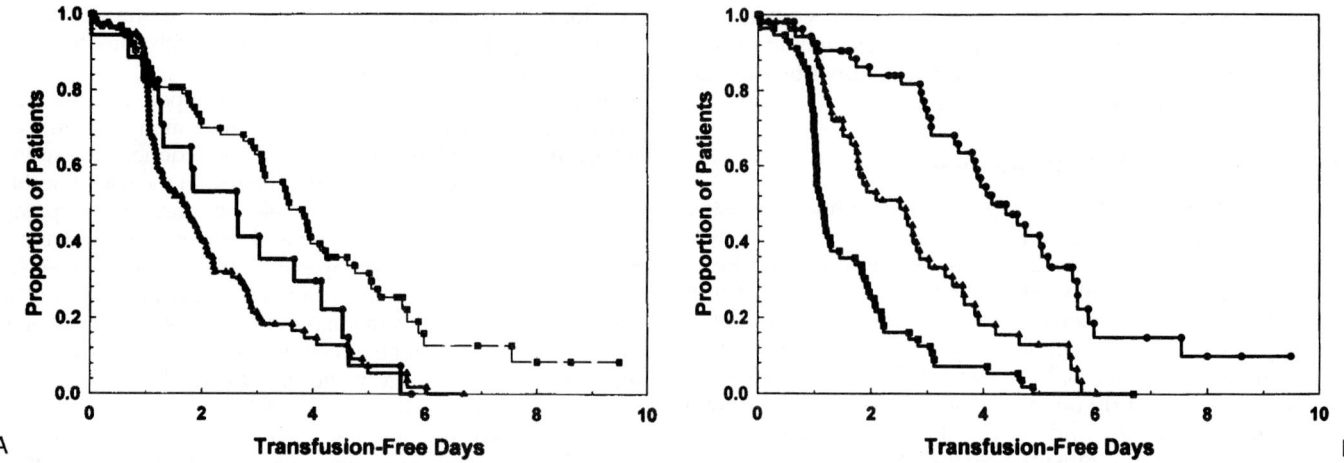

Figure 58-7. A: Proportion of patients remaining transfusion-free over time is related to platelet transfusion dose. By treatment cohort ▲; placebo ●; pegylated recombinant human megakaryocytic growth and development factor (PEG-rHuMGDF), 1 µg/kg, ■; PEG-rHuMGDF ■ , p <.001. **B:** Proportion of patients remaining transfusion-free over time is related to the platelet transfusion dose. By posttransfusion platelet count: 3-patient cohort with highest (●), middle (▲), and lowest (■) textile posttransfusion platelet counts (p <.001). [From Goodnough LT, Kuter DJ, McCullough J, et al. Prophylactic platelet transfusions from healthy apheresis platelet donors undergoing treatment with thrombopoietin. *Blood* 2001;98(5):1346–1351.]

rHuMGDF can increase platelet counts and platelet yields from apheresis of healthy donors without serious toxicity (462) (Fig. 58-6). Furthermore, the larger-yielding platelets collected from healthy donors given PEG-rHuMGDF delay the time to the next platelet transfusion compared to routinely available platelets (463) (Fig. 58-7). However, the clinical development of PEG-rHuMGDF has been halted in the United States because in additional studies, 13 of 325 healthy volunteer platelet donors receiving multiple doses developed neutralizing antibodies to endogenous thrombopoietin and thrombocytopenia (464,465).

HEMATOPOIETIC GROWTH FACTORS IN PATIENTS WITH SOLID TUMORS

Early phase I and II clinical trials demonstrated that G-CSF shortens the duration of neutropenia, as discussed above (466–469). G-CSF is routinely started on day one after the completion of chemotherapy and continued until resolution of neutropenia. In the aggregate experience, G-CSF in this setting not only shortens the duration of neutropenia but also decreases the incidence of infection or hospitalization for infections or febrile neutropenia (470–473). G-CSF has the additional potential benefit of decreasing the incidence of mucositis (474). GM-CSF also decreases the duration of chemotherapy-induced neutropenia, although the impact on the incidence of infections is variable (475–479). Among patients with febrile neutropenia, the benefits of GM-CSF are minimal, if any (480). Similar to the setting of lymphoma, GM-CSF permits dose intensification in solid tumor patients (481). However, the benefits in overall outcome are useless.

COST-EFFECTIVENESS OF HEMATOPOIETIC GROWTH FACTORS IN ONCOLOGY

As with all aspects of health care, a critical assessment of G-CSF and GM-CSF requires consideration of the costs and benefits of these agents. In today's cost-conscious health care environment, concern exists that the benefits of the hematopoietic growth factors may not outweigh their costs. However, the value of G-CSF

and GM-CSF is heavily dependent on the clinical setting in which the agents are used. The average wholesale cost of CSF is currently approximately $200.00 per day, although the cost to some insurers can be higher. In addition, until newer long-acting formulations of cytokines are commercially available, there is the discomfort and inconvenience of daily subcutaneous injections. Moreover, G-CSF use can be complicated by skeletal pain, whereas GM-CSF use is often accompanied by fevers. Weighed against CSF use is the risk of infections or febrile neutropenia, or both, which can result in unplanned hospitalizations and medical costs that average $8,000.00 per episode (482). The risk of these complications varies by disease type, chemotherapy regimen, and patient population and can substantially alter the cost-effectiveness of CSF use.

ACUTE LEUKEMIA

There have been a number of large clinical trials of adjunct CSF use in leukemia analyzed for their cost implications (483). One study conducted by the Eastern Cooperative Oncology Group found that older patients who received GM-CSF after induction chemotherapy had an overall cost savings of $2,310.00 (484). Similarly, results from a European study by Lu et al. indicated that G-CSF use as an adjunct to chemotherapy for adults with AML was associated with a net savings of $2,230.00 (485). However, cost analyses from a SWOG trial found G-CSF use was associated with a negligible increase in cost (+0.2%) (486). These studies also identified clinical benefits including a shortening of hospital stays; a lower incidence of infection; in one study, a decrease in infection rate; and an improvement in overall survival. Additional studies in adult ALL and AML have similarly found total cost savings of 2% and 18% with CSF support, respectively (487,488). Results in the pediatric acute leukemia setting have been less favorable. Pui et al. from the Children's Cancer Study Group found that pediatric leukemia patients who received G-CSF had shorter hospitalizations during induction, but overall costs of supportive care were $152.00 greater with G-CSF (489). Similarly, the Pediatrics Oncology Group found additional costs of $2,497.00 for G-CSF as adjunct therapy for children with ALL during induction (490). G-CSF use was associated with fewer days of intravenous antibiotics but no savings in overall supportive care costs. As a result of these studies, pediatric clinical trials do not routinely include CSFs as adjunctive therapy for pediatric acute leukemia patients.

HODGKIN'S AND NON-HODGKIN'S LYMPHOMA

The earliest cost studies for CSF use as an adjunct therapy for high-dose chemotherapy have been carried out in lymphoma. In a study of high-dose chemotherapy treatment with autologous bone marrow transplant (ABMT), comparative costs of GM-CSF versus placebo were evaluated (491). This study found savings of almost $20,000.00 with adjunctive use of GM-CSF, primarily as a result of shorter neutropenia and a savings of 8 days of hospitalization. A similar study of G-CSF after ABMT from Souetre et al. found G-CSF to be associated with a $1,316.00 cost savings or a 3% reduction in total cost (492). CSF has also been associated with no additional costs after mini-BEAM (BCNU, etoposide, ara-c, melphalan) salvage chemotherapy (493) and a 22% reduction in total costs after high-dose chemotherapy and peripheral blood stem cell rescue (494). In the pediatric setting, G-CSF reduced costs by 3%, or $1,000.00, after induction chemotherapy (495). In two studies of autologous peripheral blood stem cell transplantation patients, savings in the duration of hospitalization and overall medical costs with G-CSF versus placebo have been reported (496,497). More recently, cost analyses of G-CSF use after allogenic peripheral blood stem cell transplantation have been reported. Posttransplant resources were used at a similar intensity for the G-CSF and placebo patients. Patients were hospitalized for a median of 21 days in the G-CSF arm and 22 days in the placebo arm, received a median of 6.5 days of total parenteral nutrition versus 5.5 days, and received intravenous antibiotics for a median of 16 days versus 18 days (p = not significant). Overall, total median costs of care were similar: $76,577.00 for the G-CSF patients versus $78,799.00 for the placebo patients, inclusive of the costs of posttransplant CSF use (498).

MAXIMIZING THE COST-EFFECTIVENESS OF HEMATOPOIETIC GROWTH FACTOR USE

The findings of cost-effectiveness studies for CSF prophylaxis have been highly variable. The use of CSF is well established for extremely myeloablative chemotherapy regimens such as the high-dose chemotherapy with stem cell transplant employed in non-Hodgkin's lymphoma. However, routine use of primary CSF prophylaxis in other cancers is discouraged (499). The most recent version of the American Society of Clinical Oncology (ASCO) guidelines on CSF use identifies risk factors that might warrant CSF prophylaxis (Table 58-5). Awareness of these risk factors leads to more efficient and targeted CSF use.

TABLE 58-5. American Society of Clinical Oncology Colony-Stimulating Factor Guideline: Suggested Risk Factors for Febrile Neutropenia

Bone marrow compromise
Comorbidity
Preexisting neutropenia due to disease
Extensive prior chemotherapy
Previous irradiation to pelvis
History of recurrent febrile neutropenia
Open wounds
Already active tissue infections
Other conditions increasing risk of infection

RECOMMENDATIONS FOR USE OF HEMATOPOIETIC GROWTH FACTORS IN HEMATOLOGIC MALIGNANCIES

ASCO has made recommendations for the use of hematopoietic growth factors, which are evidence based (500–503).The routine use of myeloid growth factors as primary prophylaxis for patients with solid tumors or hematologic malignancies is not recommended unless patients are at high risk for febrile neutropenia (≥40%). Patients at high risk for infectious complications may benefit; such patients include those who have experienced neutropenia that is disease related or preexisting; extensive prior chemotherapy; previous irradiation to the pelvis or other areas that involved the exposure of large areas of bone marrow; a history of recurrent febrile neutropenia, poor performance status or advanced disease, decreased immune function, open wounds, or active soft tissue infections. The evidence suggests that growth factors should not be routinely administered to afebrile neutropenic patients. Similarly, there is no clear benefit for the routine use of growth factors in patients with uncomplicated fever and neutropenia (fever ≤10 days in duration, no evidence of pneumonia, cellulitis, abscess, sinusitis, hypotension, multiorgan dysfunction, or invasive fungal infections). Although growth factors may decrease the duration of neutropenia, little or no clinical benefit is realized. In the setting of these illnesses (pneumonia, hypotension, multiorgan dysfunction, or invasive fungal infections) with profound neutropenia (absolute neutrophil count <10/µL), growth factors may be beneficial, but this has not been proven. Similarly, growth factors are not advised to increase chemotherapy dose or intensity outside the context of a clinical trial. In the setting of AML, while the duration of neutropenia is shortened, growth factors cannot be routinely recommended for use in priming, in induction, or after consolidation. Although it has few hazards, myeloid growth factor cannot be recommended for routine use because there is no clear benefit in CR rate or overall survival. There may be clinical benefit with respect to shortening the duration of neutropenia and cost savings. Therefore, the use of myeloid growth factors in AML depends to a large extent on the specific clinical setting. The shortening of neutropenia is more marked after consolidation, and no benefit is clear. With respect to CR rate or overall survival, growth factors are appropriate to hasten recovery after intensive consolidation. In MDS, myeloid growth factors can be recommended to correct neutropenia and appear better than supportive care with respect to decreasing the rate of infections. However, prolonged use of myeloid growth factors cannot be routinely recommended. In the setting of ALL, myeloid growth factors shorten the duration of neutropenia. In one large adult trial, there was a trend toward a higher CR rate, particularly in older adults (age >60 years). No benefit in overall survival was observed in any study. The ASCO guidelines recommended G-CSF after the first few days of induction in the first postremission course. Myeloid growth factors are not recommended for neutropenia in patients who are afebrile but neutropenic after initial myelosuppressive chemotherapy. In patients who develop fever, particularly high-risk patients with hypotension or sepsis, G-CSF or GM-CSF is reasonable (Table 58-5).

PRACTICAL CONSIDERATIONS FOR HEMATOPOIETIC GROWTH FACTORS

G-CSF and GM-CSF appear useful as supportive therapy in patients with both solid tumors and hematologic malignancies at high risk of developing fever in the setting of neutropenia or in patients who are debilitated or older and may not tolerate such a life-threatening episode. G-CSF is generally given at 5 µg/kg/day either intravenously or subcutaneously, and GM-CSF is given at 250 µg/m^2/day. Both are generally continued until either the absolute neutrophil count is >10,000/µL. In the setting of stem cell transplantation, G-CSF can be given at 10 µg/kg/day and the dose reduced to 5 µg/kg/day, and the absolute neutrophil count reaches 1000/µL for 3 consecutive days, and then the dose discontinued after an additional 3 days. GM-CSF can be administered starting on the day of stem cell infusion at least 24 hours from the last dose of chemotherapy until the absolute neutrophil count is greater than or equal to 1500/µL for 3 consecutive days. IL-11 may be given in the setting of nonmyeloid malignancies within 6 to 24 hours after the end of chemotherapy at a dose of 50 µg/kg/day s.c. and continued until the platelet count is greater than or equal to 50,000/µL. Epo for anemia in the setting of nonmyeloid malignancies is generally started at a dose of 150 µg/kg/day s.c. three times a week. If there is no response after 8 weeks or so, the dose may be increased to 300 µg/kg. Recent data suggest once-a-week dosing is as effective.

REFERENCES

1. Burgess AW, Metcalf D. Characterization of a serum factor stimulating the differentiation of myelomonocytic leukemic cells. Int J Cancer 1980;26:647–654.
2. Welte K, Platzer E, Lu L, et al. Purification and biochemical characterization of human pluripotent hematopoietic colony-stimulating factor. Proc Natl Acad Sci U S A 1985;82:1526–1530.
3. Nagita S, Tsuchiya M, Asano S, et al. Molecular cloning and expression of cDNA for human granulocyte colony-stimulating factor. Nature 1986;319:415–418.
4. Souza LM, Boone TC, Gabrilove J, et al. Recombinant human granulocyte colony-stimulating factor: effects on normal and leukemic myeloid cells. Science 1986;232:61–65.
5. Zucali JR, Dinarello CA, Oblon DJ, et al. Interleukin 1 stimulates fibroblasts to produce granulocyte-macrophage colony-stimulating activity and prostaglandin E2. J Clin Invest 1986;77:1857–1863.
6. Broudy VC, Kaushansky K, Segal GM, et al. Tumor necrosis factor type alpha stimulates human endothelial cells to produce granulocyte/macrophage colony-stimulating factor. Proc Natl Acad Sci U S A 1986;83:7467–7471.
7. Demetri GD, Griffin JD. Granulocyte colony-stimulating factor and its receptor. Blood 1991;78:2791–2808. Review.
8. Hammond WP, Csiba E, Canin A, et al. Chronic neutropenia. A new canine model induced by human granulocyte colony-stimulating factor. J Clin Invest 1991;87:704–710.
9. Lieschke GJ, Grail D, Hodgson G, et al. Mice lacking granulocyte colony-stimulating factor have chronic neutropenia, granulocyte and macrophage progenitor cell deficiency, and impaired neutrophil mobilization. Blood 1994;84:1737–1746.
10. Liu F, Wu HY, Wesselschmidt R, et al. Impaired production and increased apoptosis of neutrophils in granulocyte colony-stimulating factor receptor-deficient mice. Immunity 1996;5:491–501.
11. Yuo A, Kitagawa S, Okabe T, et al. Recombinant human granulocyte colony-stimulating factor repairs the abnormalities of neutrophils in patients with myelodysplastic syndromes and chronic myelogenous leukemia. Blood 1987;70:404–411.
12. Lord BI, Molineux G, Pojda Z, et al. Myeloid cell kinetics in mice treated with recombinant interleukin-3, granulocyte colony-stimulating factor (CSF), or granulocyte-macrophage CSF in vivo. Blood 1991;77:2154–2159.
13. Uzumaki H, Okabe T, Sasaki N, et al. Characterization of receptor for granulocyte colony-stimulating factor on human circulating neutrophils. Biochem Biophys Res Commun 1988;156:1026–1032.
14. Nathan CF. Respiratory burst in adherent human neutrophils: triggering by colony-stimulating factors CSF-GM and CSF-G. Blood 1989;73:301–306.
15. Sieff CA. Hematopoietic growth factors. J Clin Invest 1987;79:1549–1557.
16. Clark SC, Kamen R. The human hematopoietic colony-stimulating factors. Science 1987;236:1229–1237. Review.
17. Simmers RN, Smith J, Shannon MF, et al. Localization of the human G-CSF gene to the region of a breakpoint in the translocation typical of acute promyelocytic leukemia. Hum Genet 1988;78:134–136.
18. Kaczmarski RS, Mufti GJ. The cytokine receptor superfamily. Blood Rev 1991;5:193–203. Review.
19. Tweardy DJ, Anderson K, Cannizzaro LA, et al. Molecular cloning of cDNAs for the human granulocyte colony-stimulating factor receptor from HL-60

20. Fukunaga R, Seto Y, Mizushima S, et al. Three different mRNAs encoding human granulocyte colony-stimulating factor receptor. Proc Natl Acad Sci U S A 1990;87:8702–8706.
21. Nicola NA, Metcalf D. Subunit promiscuity among hemopoietic growth factor receptors. Cell 1991;67:1–4. Review.
22. Bazan JF. Structural design and molecular evolution of a cytokine receptor superfamily. Proc Natl Acad Sci U S A 1990;87:6934–6938.
23. Larsen A, Davis T, Curtis BM, et al. Expression cloning of a human granulocyte colony-stimulating factor receptor: a structural mosaic of hematopoietin receptor, immunoglobulin, and fibronectin domains. J Exp Med 1990;172:1559–1570.
24. Avalos BR, Gasson JC, Hedvat C, et al. Human granulocyte colony-stimulating factor: biologic activities and receptor characterization of hematopoietic cells and small cell lung cancer cell lines. Blood 1990;75:851–857.
25. D'Andrea AD. Cytokine receptors in congenital hematopoietic disease. N Engl J Med 1994;330:839–846.
26. Zhang DE, Hohaus S, Voso MT, et al. Function of PU.1 (Spi-1), C/EBP, and AML1 in early myelopoiesis: regulation of multiple myeloid CSF receptor promoters. Curr Top Microbiol Immunol 1996;211:137–147. Review.
27. Smith LT, Hohaus S, Gonzalez DA, et al. PU.1 (Spi-1) and C/EBP alpha regulate the granulocyte colony-stimulating factor receptor promoter in myeloid cells. Blood 1996;88:1234–1247.
28. Witthuhn BA, Quelle FW, Silvennoinen O, et al. JAK2 associates with the erythropoietin receptor and is tyrosine phosphorylated and activated following stimulation with erythropoietin. Cell 1993;74:227–236.
29. Chatta GS, Price TH, Allen RC, et al. Effects of in vivo recombinant methionyl human granulocyte colony-stimulating factor as the neutrophil response and peripheral blood colony-forming cells in healthy young and elderly adult volunteers. Blood 1994;84:2923–2979.
30. Oh-eda M, Hasegawa M, Hattori K, et al. O-linked sugar chain of human granulocyte colony-stimulating factor protects it against polymerization and denaturation allowing it to retain its biological activity. J Biol Chem 1990;265:11432–11435.
31. Kishita M, Motojima M, Oheha M. Stability of granulocyte colony-stimulating factor (rltuG—CSF) in serum. Clin Rep 1992;26:221.
32. Cheers C, Haigh AM, Kelso A, et al. Production of colony-stimulating factors (CSFs) during infection: separate determinations of macrophage-, granulocyte-, granulocyte-macrophage-, and multi-CSFs. Infect Immun 1988;56:247–251.
33. Dale DC, Lau S, Nash R, et al. Effect of endotoxin on serum granulocyte and granulocyte-macrophage colony-stimulating factor levels in dogs. J Infect Dis 1992;165:689–694.
34. Kawakami M, Tsutsumi H, Kumakawa T, et al. Levels of serum granulocyte colony-stimulating factor in patients with infections. Blood 1990;76:1962–1964.
35. Price TH, Chatta GS, Dale DG. Effect of recombinant granulocyte colony-stimulating factor on neutrophil kinetics in normal young and elderly humans. Blood 1996;88:335–340.
36. Chatta GS, Price TH, Allen RC, et al. Effects of in vivo recombinant methionyl human granulocyte colony-stimulating factor on the neutrophil response and peripheral blood colony-forming cells in healthy young and elderly adult volunteers. Blood 1994;84:2923–2929.
37. Chatta GS, Andrews RG, Roger E, et al. Hematopoietic progenitors and aging: alterations in granulocytic precursors and responsiveness to recombinant human G-CSF, GM-CSF, and IL-3. J Gerontol 1993;48:M207–212.
38. Nielsen SD, Dam-Larsen S, Nielsen C, et al. Recombinant human granulocyte colony-stimulating factor increases circulating CD34-postive cells in patients with AIDS. Ann Hematol 1997;74:215–220.
39. Hakansson L, Hoglund M, Jonsson UB, et al. Effects of in vivo administration of G-CSF on neutrophil and eosinophil adhesion. Br J Haematol 1997;98:603–611.
40. Karawajczyk M, Hoglund M, Ericsson J, et al. Administration of G-CSF to healthy subjects: the effects on eosinophil counts and mobilization of eosinophil granule proteins. Br J Haematol 1997;96:259–265.
41. Yong KL. Granulocyte colony-stimulating factor (G-CSF) increases neutrophil migration across vascular endothelium independent of an effect on adhesion: comparison with granulocyte-macrophage colony-stimulating factor (GM-CSF). Br J Haematol 1996;94:40–47.
42. Roilides E, Walsh TJ, Pizzo PA, et al. Granulocyte colony-stimulating factor enhances the phagocytic and bactericidal activity of normal and defective human neutrophils. J Infect Dis 1991;163:579–583.
43. Allen RC, Stevens PR, Price TH, et al. In vivo effects of recombinant human granulocyte colony-stimulating factor on neutrophil oxidative functions in normal human volunteers. J Infect Dis 1997;175:1184–1192.
44. Roilides E, Holmes A, Blake C, et al. Effects of granulocyte colony-stimulating factor and interferon-gamma on antifungal activity of human polymorphonuclear neutrophils against pseudohyphae of different medically important Candida species. J Leukoc Biol 1995;57:651–656.
45. Roilides E, Uhlig K, Venzon D, et al. Enhancement of oxidative response and damage caused by human neutrophils to Aspergillus fumigatus hyphae by granulocyte colony-stimulating factor and gamma interferon. Infect Immun 1993;61:1185–1193.
46. Baldwin GC, Chung GY, Kaslander C, et al. Colony-stimulating factor enhancement of myeloid effector cell cytotoxicity towards neuroectodermal tumour cells. Br J Haematol 1993;83:545–553.

and mapping of the gene to chromosome region 1p32-34. Blood 1992;79:1148–1154.

47. Hansen PB, Kjaersgaard E, Johnsen HE, et al. Different membrane expression of CD11b and CD14 on blood neutrophils following in vivo administration of myeloid growth factors. *Br J Haematol* 1993;85:50–56.

48. Kuwabara T, Kobayashi S, Sugiyama Y. Pharmacokinetics and pharmacodynamics of a recombinant human granulocyte colony-stimulating factor. *Drug Metab Rev* 1996;28:625–658. Review.

49. Tanaka H, Okada Y, Kawagishi M, et al. Pharmacokinetics and pharmacodynamics of recombinant human granulocyte-colony stimulating factor after intravenous and subcutaneous administration in the rat. *J Pharmacol Exp Ther* 1989;251:1199–1203.

50. Tanaka H, Satake-Ishikawa R, Ishikawa M, et al. Pharmacokinetics of recombinant human granulocyte colony-stimulating factor conjugated to polyethylene glycol in rats. *Cancer Res* 1991;51:3710–3714.

51. Miyatake S, Otsuka T, Yokota T, et al. Structure of the chromosomal gene for granulocyte macrophage colony stimulating factor: comparison of the mouse and human genes. *EMBO J* 1985;4:2561–2568.

52. Wong GG, Witek JS, Temple PA, et al. Human GM-CSF: molecular cloning of the complementary DNA and purification of the natural and recombinant proteins. *Science* 1985;228:810–815.

53. Cantrell MA, Anderson D, Cerretti D, et al. Cloning, sequence, and expression of a human granulocyte/macrophage colony-stimulating factor. *Proc Natl Acad Sci U S A* 1985;82:6250–6254.

54. Donahue RE, Wang EA, Kaufman RJ, et al. Effects of N-linked carbohydrate on the in vivo properties of human GM-CSF. *Cold Spring Harb Symp Quant Biol* 1986;51:685–692.

55. Dorr RT. Clinical properties of yeast-derived versus Escherichia coli-derived granulocyte-macrophage colony-stimulating factor. *Clin Ther* 1993;15:19–29.

56. Hovgaard D, Mortensen BT, Schifter S, et al. Comparative pharmacokinetics of single-dose administration of mammalian and bacterially derived recombinant human granulocyte-macrophage colony-stimulating factor. *Eur J Haematol* 1993;50:32–36.

57. Hussein AM, Ross M, Vredenburgh J, et al. Effects of granulocyte-macrophage colony stimulating factor produced in Chinese hamster ovary cells (regramostim) Escherichia coli (molgramostim) and yeast (sargramostim) on priming peripheral blood progenitor cells for use with autologous bone marrow after high-dose chemotherapy. *Eur J Haematol* 1995;54:281–287.

58. Huebner K, Isobe M, Croce XM, et al. The human gene encoding GM-CSF is at 5q21-q32, the chromosome region deleted in the 5q- anomaly. *Science* 1985;230:1282–1285.

59. Gasson JC. Molecular physiology of granulocyte-macrophage colony-stimulating factor. *Blood* 1991;77:1131–1145. Review.

60. Arai K, Lee F, Miyajima A, et al. Cytokines: coordinators of immune and inflammatory responses. *Annu Rev Biochem* 1990;59:783–836.

61. Gasson JC, Eishart RH, Kaufman SE, et al. Purified human granulocyte-macrophage colony-stimulating factor: direct action on neutrophils. *Science* 1984;226:1339–1342.

62. Wong GG, Witek JS, Temple PA, et al. Molecular cloning of human and gibbon GM-CSF cDNAs and purification of the natural and recombinant human proteins. *Cancer Cells* 1985;3:235.

63. Moonen P, Mermod J-J, Ernst JF, et al. Increased biological activity of deglycosylated recombinant human granulocyte/macrophage colony-stimulating factor produced by yeast or animal cells. *Proc Natl Acad Sci U S A* 1987;84:4428–4431.

64. Burgess AW, Begley CG, Johnson GR, et al. Purification and properties of bacterially synthesized human granulocyte-macrophage colony stimulating factor. *Blood* 1987;69:43–51.

65. Herrmann F, Oster W, Meuer SC, et al. Interleukin 1 stimulates T lymphocytes to produce granulocyte-monocyte colony-stimulating factor. *J Clin Invest* 1988;81:1415–1418.

66. Wimperis JZ, Niemeyer CM, Sieff CA, et al. Granulocyte-macrophage colony-stimulating factor and interleukin-3 mRNAs are produced by a small fraction of blood mononuclear cells. *Blood* 1989;74:1525–1530.

67. Pluznik DH, Bickel M, Mergenhagen SE. B lymphocyte derived hematopoietic growth factors. *Immunol Invest* 1989;18:103–116.

68. Thorens B, Mermod JJ, Vassalli P. Phagocytosis and inflammatory stimuli induce GM-CSF mRNA in macrophages through posttranscriptional regulation. *Cell* 1987;48:671–679.

69. Wodnar-Filipowicz A, Heusser CH, Moroni C. Production of the haemopoietic growth factors GM-CSF and interleukin-3 by mast cells in response to IgE receptor-mediated activation. *Nature* 1989;339:150–152.

70. Bagby GC Jr, Dinarello CA, Wallace P, et al. Interleukin 1 stimulates granulocyte macrophage colony-stimulating activity release by vascular endothelial cells. *J Clin Invest* 1986;78:1316–1323.

71. Rajavashisth TB, Andalbi A, Territo MC, et al. Induction of endothelial cell expression of granulocyte and macrophage colony-stimulating factors by modified low-density lipoproteins. *Nature* 1990;344:254–257.

72. Demetri GD, Zenzie BW, Rheinwald JG, et al. Expression of colony-stimulating factor genes by normal human mesothelial cells and human malignant mesothelioma cell lines in vitro. *Blood* 1989;74:940–946.

73. Horowitz MC, Coleman DL, Flood PM, et al. Parathyroid hormone and lipopolysaccharide induce murine osteoblast-like cells to secrete a cytokine indistinguishable from granulocyte-macrophage colony-stimulating factor. *J Clin Invest* 1989;83:149–157.

74. Park LS, Friend D, Gillis S, et al. Characterization of the cell surface receptor for human granulocyte/macrophage colony-stimulating factor. *Exp Med* 1986;164:251.

75. DiPersio JF, Hedvat C, Ford CF, et al. Characterization of the soluble human granulocyte-macrophage colony-stimulating factor receptor complex. *J Biol Chem* 1991;266:279–286.

76. Colotta F, Bussolino F, Polentarutti N, et al. Differential expression of the common β and specific α chains of the receptors for GM-CSF, IL-3, and IL-5 in endothelial cells. *Exp Cell Res* 1993;206:311–317.

77. Santiago-Schwarz F, Divaris N, Kay C, et al. Mechanisms of tumor necrosis factor-granulocyte-macrophage colony-stimulating factor-induced dendritic cell development. *Blood* 1993;82:3019–3028.

78. Jokhi PP, King A, Jubinsky PT, et al. Demonstration of the low affinity α subunit of the granulocyte-macrophage colony-stimulating factor receptor (GM-CSF-Rα) on human trophoblast and uterine cells. *J Reprod Immunol* 1994;26:147–164.

79. Till KJ, Burthem J, Lopez A, et al. Granulocyte-macrophage colony-stimulating factor receptor: stage-specific expression and function on late B cells. *Blood* 1996;88:479–486.

80. Lanza F, Castagnari B, Rigolin G, et al. Flow cytometry measurement of GM-CSF receptors in acute leukemic blasts, and normal hemopoietic cells. *Leukemia* 1997;11:1700–1710.

81. Hayashida K, Kitamura T, Gorman DM, et al. Molecular cloning of a second subunit of the receptor for human granulocyte-macrophage colony-stimulating factor (GM-CSF): reconstitution of a high-affinity GM-CSF receptor. *Proc Natl Acad Sci U S A* 1990;87:9655–9659.

82. Miyajima A, Mui AL-F, Ogorochi T, et al. Receptors for granulocyte-macrophage colony-stimulating factor, interleukin-3, and interleukin-5. *Blood* 1993;82:1960–1974.

83. DiPersio J, Billing P, Kaufman S, et al. Characterization of the human granulocyte-macrophage colony-stimulating factor receptor. *J Biol Chem* 1988;263:1834–1841.

84. Cannistra SA, Groshek P, Garlick R, et al. Regulation of surface expression of the granulocyte-macrophage colony stimulating factor receptors in normal human myeloid cells. *Proc Natl Acad Sci U S A* 1990;87:93–97.

85. Herrmann F, Ganser A, Lindemann A, et al. Stimulation of granulopoiesis in patients with malignancy by rhGM-CSF: assessment of two routes of administration. *J Biol Response Mod* 1990;9:475–479.

86. Metcalf D. The consequences of excess levels of haemopoietic growth factors. *Br J Haematol* 1990;75:1–3.

87. Oster W, Mertelsmann R, Herrmann F. Role of colony-stimulating factors in the biology of acute myelogenous leukemia. *Int J Cell Cloning* 1989;7:13–29.

88. Salmon S, Lui R. Effects of granulocyte-macrophage colony-stimulating factor on in vitro growth of human solid tumors. *J Clin Oncol* 1989;7:1346–1350.

89. Raines M, Liu L, Quan S, et al. Molecular cloning of a soluble form of the human granulocyte-macrophage colony stimulating factor receptor (GM-CSF-R). *J Cell Biochem* 1991;[Suppl F]:109.

90. Sato N, Sakamaki K, Terada N, et al. Signal transduction by the high-affinity GM-CSF receptor: two distinct cytoplasmic regions of the common beta subunit responsible for different signaling. *EMBO J* 1993;12:4181–4189.

91. Quelle FW, Sato N, Witthuhn BA, et al. JAK2 associates with βc chain of the receptor for granulocyte-macrophage colony-stimulating factor, and its activation requires the membrane-proximal region. *Mol Cell Biol* 1994;14:4335–4341.

92. Mui AL, Wakao H, Harada N, et al. Interleukin-3, granulocyte-macrophage colony-stimulating factor, and interleukin-5 transduce signals through two forms of STAT5. *J Leukoc Biol* 1995;57:799–803.

93. Wang Y, Morella KK, Ripperger J, et al. Receptors for interleukin-3 (IL-3) and growth hormone mediate an IL-6-type transcriptional induction in the presence of JAK2 or STAT3. *Blood* 1995;86:1671–1679.

94. Satoh T, Nakafuka M, Miyajima A, et al. Involvement of ras p21 protein in signal-transduction pathways from interleukin 2, interleukin 3, and granulocyte/macrophage colony-stimulating factor, but not from interleukin 4. *Proc Natl Acad Sci U S A* 1991;88:3314–3318.

95. Okuda K, Sanghera JS, Pelech SL, et al. Granulocyte-macrophage colony-stimulating factor, interleukin-3, and steel factor induce rapid tyrosine phosphorylation of p42 and p44 MAP kinase. *Blood* 1992;79:2880–2887.

96. Metcalf D. The molecular biology and functions of the granulocyte-macrophage colony-stimulating factors. *Blood* 1986;67:257–267. Review.

97. Broxmeyer HE, Cooper S, Vadhan-Raj S. Cell cycle status of erythroid (BFU-E) progenitor cells from the bone marrows of patients on a clinical trial with purified recombinant human granulocyte-macrophage colony-stimulating factor. *Exp Hematol* 1989;17:455–459.

98. Steward WP, Scarffe JH, Austin R, et al. Recombinant human granulocyte macrophage colony stimulating factor (rhGM-CSF) given as daily short infusions—a phase I dose-toxicity study. *Br J Cancer* 1989;59:142–145.

99. Toner GC, Gabrilove JL, Gordon M, et al. Phase I trial of intravenous and intraperitoneal administration of granulocyte-macrophage colony-stimulating factor. *J Immunother* 1994;15:59–66.

100. Hara H, Namiki M. Mechanism of synergy between granulocyte-macrophage colony-stimulating factor and granulocyte colony stimulating factor in colony formation from human marrow cells in vitro. *Exp Hematol* 1989;17:816–821.

101. McNiece I, Andrews R, Stewart M, et al. Action of interleukin-3, G-CSF, and GM-CSF on highly enriched human hematopoietic progenitor cells: synergistic interaction of GM-CSF plus G-CSF. *Blood* 1989;74:110–114.

102. Bot FJ, van Eijk L, Schipper P, et al. Synergistic effects between GM-CSF and G-CSF or M-CSF on highly enriched human marrow progenitor cells. *Leukemia* 1990;4:325–328.

103. Hogge DE, Cashman JD, Humphries RK, et al. Differential and synergistic effects of human granulocyte-macrophage colony-stimulating factor and human granulocyte colony-stimulating factor on hematopoiesis in human long-term marrow cultures. *Blood* 1991;77:493–499.

104. Nemunaitis J. Granulocyte-macrophage-colony-stimulating factor: a review from preclinical development to clinical application. *Transfusion* 1993;33:70–83.

105. Ruef C, Coleman D. Granulocyte-macrophage colony-stimulating factor: pleiotropic cytokine with potential clinical usefulness. *Rev Infect Dis* 1990;12:41–62. Review.

106. Birkmann J, Oez S, Smetak M, et al. Effects of recombinant human thrombopoietin alone and in combination with erythropoietin and early-acting cytokines on human mobilized purified CD34+ progenitor cells cultured in serum-depleted medium. *Stem Cells* 1997;15:18–32.

107. Neelis KJ, Hartong SC, Egeland T, et al. The efficacy of single-dose administration of thrombopoietin with coadministration of either granulocyte/macrophage or granulocyte colony-stimulating factor in myelosuppressed rhesus monkeys. *Blood* 1997;90:2565–2573.

108. Brasel K, McKenna HJ, Charrier K, et al. Flt3 ligand synergizes with granulocyte-macrophage colony-stimulating factor or granulocyte colony-stimulating factor to mobilize hematopoietic progenitor cells into the peripheral blood of mice. *Blood* 1997;90:3781–3788.

109. Winton EF, Bucur SZ, Bond LD, et al. Recombinant human (rh) Flt3 ligand plus rhGM-CSF or rhG-CSF causes a marked CD34+ cell mobilization to blood in rhesus monkeys. *Blood* 1996;88 [Suppl 1]:642a(abst).

110. Arnaout MA, Wang EA, Clark SC, et al. Human recombinant granulocyte-macrophage colony-stimulating factor increases cell-to-cell adhesion and surface expression of adhesion-promoting surface glycoproteins on mature granulocytes. *J Clin Invest* 1986;78:597–601.

111. Dahinden CA, Zingg J, Maly FE, et al. Leukotriene production in human neutrophils primed by recombinant human granulocyte/macrophage colony-stimulating factor and stimulated with the complement component C5A and FMLP as second signals. *J Exp Med* 1988;167:1281–1295.

112. Wirthmueller U, De Weck AL, Dahinden CA. Platelet-activating factor production in human neutrophils by sequential stimulation with granulocyte-macrophage colony-stimulating factor and the chemotactic factors C5A or formyl-methionyl-leucyl-phenylalanine. *J Immunol* 1989;142:3213–3218.

113. DiPersio JF, Billing P, Williams R, et al. Human granulocyte macrophage colony-stimulation factor (GM-CSF) and other cytokines prime neutrophils for enhanced arachidonic acid release and leukotriene B4 synthesis. *J Immunol* 1988;140:4315–4322.

114. DiMarzio P, Mariani R, Tse J, et al. GM-CSF or CD40L suppresses chemokine receptor expression and HIV-1 entry in human monocytes and macrophages. 5th Conference on Retroviruses and Opportunistic Infections 1998.

115. Weisbart RH, Golde DW, Clark SC, et al. Human granulocyte-macrophage colony-stimulating factor is a neutrophil activator. *Nature* 1985;314:361–363.

116. Lopez AF, Williamson J, Gamble JR, et al. Recombinant human granulocyte-macrophage colony-stimulating factor stimulates in vitro mature neutrophil and eosinophil functions, surface receptor expression, and survival. *J Clin Invest* 1986;78:1220–1228.

117. Fleischmann J, Golde DW, Weisbart RH, et al. Granulocyte-macrophage colony-stimulation factor enhances phagocytosis of bacteria by human neutrophils. *Blood* 1986;68:708–711.

118. Villalta F, Kierszenbaum F. Effects of human colony-stimulating factor on the uptake and destruction of a pathogenic parasite (Trypanosoma cruzi) by human neutrophils. *J Immunol* 1986;137:1703–1707.

119. Wing EJ, Magee DM, Whitside TL, et al. Recombinant human granulocyte/macrophage colony-stimulating factor enhances monocyte cytotoxicity and secretion of tumor necrosis factor α and interferon in cancer patients. *Blood* 1989;73:643–646.

120. Rothenberg ME, Owen WF Jr, Silberstein DS, et al. Human eosinophils have prolonged survival, enhanced functional properties, and become hypodense when exposed to human interleukin 3. *J Clin Invest* 1988;81:1986–1992.

121. Oster W, Lindemann A, Mertelsmann R, et al. Granulocyte-macrophage colony-stimulating factor (CSF) and multilineage CSF recruit human monocytes to express granulocyte CSF. *Blood* 1989;73:64–67.

122. Hancock WW, Pleau ME, Kobzik L. Recombinant granulocyte-macrophage colony-stimulating factor down-regulates expression of IL-2 receptor on human mononuclear phagocytes by induction of prostaglandin. *J Immunol* 1988;140:3021–3025.

123. Lindemann A, Riedel D, Oster W, et al. GM-CSF induces secretion of interleukin-1 by polymorphonuclear neutrophils. *J Immunol* 1988;140:837–839.

124. Cannistra SA, Vellenga E, Groshek P, et al. Human granulocyte-monocyte colony-stimulating factor and interleukin-3 stimulate monocyte cytotoxicity through a tumor necrosis factor-dependent mechanism. *Blood* 1988;71:672–676.

125. Handman E, Burgess AW. Stimulation by granulocyte-macrophage colony-stimulating factor of Leishmania tropica killing by macrophages. *J Immunol* 1979;122:1134–1137.

126. Bermudez LE, Young LS. Recombinant granulocyte-macrophage colony-stimulating factor activates human macrophages to inhibit growth or kill Mycobacterium avium complex. *J Leukoc Biol* 1990;48:67–73.

127. Vadas MA, Nicola NA, Metcalf D. Activation of antibody-dependent cell-mediated cytotoxicity of the human neutrophils and eosinophils by separate colony-stimulating factors. *J Immunol* 1983;130:795–799.

128. Kushner BH, Cheung NK. GM-CSF enhances 3F8 monoclonal antibody-dependent cellular cytotoxicity against human melanoma and neuroblastoma. *Blood* 1989;73:1936–1941.

129. Coleman DL, Chodakewitz JA, Bartiss AH, et al. Granulocyte-macrophage colony-stimulating factor enhances selective effector functions of tissue-derived macrophages. *Blood* 1988;72:573–578.

130. Wiltschke C, Krainer M, Wagner A, et al. Influence of in vivo administration of GM-CSF and G-CSF on monocyte cytotoxicity. *Exp Hematol* 1995;23:402–406.

131. Szabolcs P, Moore MA, Young JW. Expansion of immunostimulatory dendritic cells among the myeloid progeny of human CD34+ bone marrow precursors cultured with c-kit ligand, granulocyte-macrophage colony-stimulating factor, and TNF-α. *J Immunol* 1995;154:5851–5861.

132. Young JW, Szabolcs P, Moore MA. Identification of dendritic cell colony-forming units among normal human CD34+ bone marrow progenitors that are expanded by c-kit-ligand and yield pure dendritic cell colonies in the presence of granulocyte/macrophage colony-stimulating factor and tumor necrosis factor α. *J Exp Med* 1995;182:1111–1119.

133. Fischer HG, Frosch S, Reske K, et al. Granulocyte-macrophage colony-stimulating factor activates macrophages derived from bone marrow cultures to synthesis of MHC class II molecules and to augmented antigen presentation function. *J Immunol* 1988;141:3882–3888.

134. Bukowski RM, Murthy S, McLain D, et al. Phase I trial of recombinant granulocyte-macrophage colony-stimulating factor in patients with lung cancer: clinical and immunologic effects. *J Immunol* 1993;13:267–274.

135. Edmonson JH, Long HJ, Kvols LK. Cytotoxic drugs plus subcutaneous granulocyte-macrophage colony-stimulating factor: can molgramostim enhance antisarcoma therapy? *J Natl Cancer Inst* 1994;86:312–314.

136. Taglietti M. Vaccine adjuvancy: a new potential area of development for GM-CSF. *Adv Exp Med Biol* 1995;378:565–569. Review.

137. Lieschke GJ, Burgess AW. Granulocyte colony-stimulating factor and granulocyte-macrophage colony-stimulating factor (first of two parts). *N Engl J Med* 1992;327:28–35.

138. Herrmann F, Schulz G, Lindemann A, et al. Hematopoietic responses in patients with advanced malignancy treated with recombinant human granulocyte-macrophage colony-stimulating factor. *J Clin Oncol* 1989;7:159–167.

139. Shadduck RK, Waheed A, Evans C, et al. Serum and urinary levels of recombinant human granulocyte-macrophage colony-stimulating factor: assessment after intravenous infusion and subcutaneous injection. *Exp Hematol* 1990;18:601(abst).

140. Schwinghammer TL, Shadduck RK, Waheed A, et al. Pharmacokinetics of recombinant human granulocyte-macrophage colony-stimulating factor (GM-CSF) after intravenous infusion and subcutaneous injection. *Pharmacotherapy* 1991;2:105(abst).

141. Furman WL, Fairclough DL, Huhn RD, et al. Therapeutic effects and pharmacokinetics of recombinant human granulocyte-macrophage colony-stimulating factor in childhood cancer patients receiving myelosuppressive chemotherapy. *J Clin Oncol* 1991;9:1022–1028.

142. Petros WP, Rabinowitz J, Stuart AR, et al. Disposition of recombinant human granulocyte-macrophage colony-stimulating factor in patients receiving high-dose chemotherapy and autologous bone marrow support. *Blood* 1992;80:1135–1140.

143. Stute N, Furman WL, Schell M, et al. Pharmacokinetics of recombinant human granulocyte-macrophage colony-stimulating factor in children after intravenous and subcutaneous administration. *J Pharm Sci* 1995;84:824–828.

144. Neben TY, Loebelenz J, Hayes L, et al. Recombinant human interleukin-11 stimulates megakaryocytopoiesis and increases peripheral platelets in normal and splenectomized mice. *Blood* 1993;81:901–908.

145. Hangoc G, Yin T, Cooper S, et al. In vivo effects of recombinant interleukin-11 on myelopoiesis in mice. *Blood* 1993;81:965–972.

146. Musashi M, Yang YC, Paul SR, et al. Direct and synergistic effects of interleukin 11 on murine hemopoiesis in culture. *Proc Natl Acad Sci U S A* 1991;88:765–769.

147. Musashi M, Clark SC, Sudo T, et al. Synergistic interactions between interleukin-11 and interleukin-4 in support of proliferation of primitive hematopoietic progenitors of mice. *Blood* 1991;78:1448–1451.

148. Bruno E, Briddell RA, Cooper RJ, et al. Effects of recombinant interleukin 11 on human megakaryocyte progenitor cells. *Exp Hematol* 1991;19:378–381.

149. de Sauvage FJ, Hass PE, Spencer SD, et al. Stimulation of megakaryocytopoiesis and thrombopoiesis by the c-Mpl ligand. *Nature* 1994;369:533–538.

150. Lok S, Kaushansky K, Holly RD, et al. Cloning and expression of murine thrombopoietin cDNA and stimulation of platelet production in vivo. *Nature* 1994;369:565–568.

151. Bartley TD, Bogenberger L, Hunt P, et al. Identification and cloning of a megakaryocyte growth and development factor that is a ligand for the cytokine receptor Mpl. *Cell* 1994;77:1117–1124.

152. Kuter DJ, Beeler DL, Rosenbey RD, et al. The purification of megapoietin: a physiological regulator of megakaryocyte growth and platelet production. *Proc Natl Acad Sci U S A* 1994;91:11104–11108.

153. Gurney AL, Carver-Moore K, de Savvage FJ, et al. Thrombocytopenia in c-mpl deficient mice. *Science* 1994;265:1445–1447.

154. Debili N, Wendling F, Katz A, et al. The Mpl-ligand or thrombopoietin or megakaryocyte growth and differentiative factor has both direct proliferative and differentiative activities on human megakaryocyte progenitors. *Blood* 1995;86:2516–2525.

155. Kaushansky K, Lok S, Holly RD, et al. Promotion of megakaryocyte progenitor expansion and differentiation by the c-Mpl ligand thrombopoietin. *Nature* 1994;369:568–571.

156. Farese AM, Hunt P, Boone T, et al. Recombinant human megakaryocyte growth and development factor stimulates thrombocytopoiesis in normal nonhuman primates. *Blood* 1995;86:54–59.

157. Broudy VC, Lin NL, Kaushansky K. Thrombopoietin (c-mpl ligand) acts synergistically with erythropoietin, stem cell factor, and interleukin-11 to enhance murine megakaryocyte colony growth and increases megakaryocyte ploidy in vitro. *Blood* 1995;85:1719–1726.

158. Fanucchi M, Glaspy J, Crawford J, et al. Effects of polyethylene glycolconjugated recombinant human megakaryocyte growth and development factor on platelet counts after chemotherapy for lung cancer. *N Engl J Med* 1997;336:404–409.

159. Vadhan-Raj S, Verschraegen CF, Buesco-Raomos C, et al. Recombinant human thrombopoietin attenuates carboplatin-induced severe thrombocytopenia and the need for platelet transfusions in patients with gynecologic cancer. *Ann Intern Med* 2000;132:364–368.

160. Isaacs C, Robert NJ, Bailey FA, et al. Randomized placebo-controlled study of recombinant human interleukin-A to prevent chemotherapy-induced thrombocytopenia in patients with breast cancer receiving dose-intensive cyclophosphamide and doxorubicin. *J Clin Oncol* 1997;15:3368–3377.

161. Magata U, Sjpzalo U, Magajosa J, et al. Serum thrombopoietin level is not regulated by transcription but by the total counts of both megakaryocytes and platelets during thrombocytopenia and thrombocytosis. *Thromb Haemost* 1997;77:808–814.

162. Shivdasani RA, Fielder P, Keller GA, et al. Regulation of the serum concentration of thrombopoietin in thrombocytopenic NF-E2 knockout mice. *Blood* 1997;90:1821–1827.

163. Fielder PJ, Gurney AL, Stefanich E, et al. Regulation of thrombopoietin levels by c-mpl-mediated binding to platelets. *Blood* 1996;87:2154–2161.

164. Paul SR, Bennett F, Calvetti JA, et al. Molecular cloning of a cDNA encoding interleukin 11, a stromal cell-derived lymphopoietic and hematopoietic cytokine. *Proc Natl Acad Sci U S A* 1990;87:7512–7516.

165. Paul SR, Schendel P. The cloning and biological characterization of recombinant human interleukin 11. *Int J Cell Cloning* 1992;10:135–143. Review.

166. Cherel M, Sorel M, Lebeau B, et al. Molecular cloning of two isoforms of a receptor for the human hematopoietic cytokine interleukin-11. *Blood* 1995;80:2534–2540.

167. Yang YC. Interleukin-11 (IL-11) and its receptor-binding and potential clinical applications. *Cancer Treat Rep* 1998;80:321–340.

168. Yang YC, Yin T. Interleukin (IL)-11 mediated signal transduction. *Ann N Y Acad Sci* 1995;767:31–40.

169. Leary AG, Zeng HQ, Clark SC, et al. Growth factor requirements for survival in G0 and entry into the cell cycle of primitive human hemopoietic progenitors. *Proc Natl Acad Sci U S A* 1992;89:4013–4017.

170. Gearing DP, Comeau MR, Friend DJ, et al. The IL-6 signal transducer, gp130: an oncostatin M receptor and affinity converter for the LIF receptor. *Science* 1992;255:1434–1437.

171. Yin T, Taga T, Tsang ML, et al. Involvement of IL-6 signal transducer gp130 in IL-11-mediated signal transduction. *J Immunol* 1993;151:2555–2561.

172. Fourcin M, Chevalier S, Lebrun JJ, et al. Involvement of gp130/interleukin-6 receptor transducing component in interleukin-11 receptor. *Eur J Immunol* 1994;24:277–280.

173. Nandurkar HH, Hilton DJ, Nathan P, et al. The human IL-11 receptor requires gp130 for signalling: demonstration by molecular cloning of the receptor. *Oncogene* 1996;12:585–593.

174. Robb L, Hilton DJ, Brook-Carter PT, et al. Identification of a second murine interleukin-11 receptor alpha-chain gene (IL11Ra2) with a restricted pattern of expression. *Genomics* 1997;40:387–394.

175. Musashi M, Yang YC, Paul SR, et al. Direct and synergistic effects of interleukin-11 on murine hematopoiesis in culture. *Proc Natl Acad Sci U S A* 1991;88:765–769.

176. Neben S, Donaldson D, Sieff C, et al. Synergistic effects of interleukin-11 with other growth factors on the expansion of murine hematopoietic progenitors and maintenance of stem cells in liquid culture. *Exp Hematol* 1994;22:353–359.

177. Neben TY, Loebelenz J, Hayes L, et al. Recombinant human interleukin-11 stimulates megakaryocytopoiesis and increases peripheral platelets in normal and splenectomized mice. *Blood* 1993;81:901–908.

178. Brody VC, Lin NL, Kaushansky K. Thrombopoietin (c-mpl ligand) acts synergistically with erythropoietin, stem cell factor, and interleukin-11 to enhance murine megakaryocyte colony growth and increases megakaryocyte ploidy in vitro. *Blood* 1995;85:1719–1726.

179. Yonemura Y, Kawakita M, Masuda M, et al. Effect of recombinant human interleukin-11 on rat megakaryopoiesis and thrombopoiesis in vivo: comparative study with interleukin-6. *Br J Haematol* 1993;84:16–23.

180. Kaviani MD, Mason LE, Bree AG, et al. Effects of recombinant human interleukin-11 on the activation and morphology of peripheral blood platelets and megakaryocytes in nonhuman primates. *Blood* 1996;88:269(abstr).

181. Du XX, Doerschuk CM, Orazi A, et al. A bone marrow stromal-derived growth factor, interleukin-11, stimulates recovery of small intestinal mucosal cells after cytoablative therapy. *Blood* 1994;83:33–37.

182. Gordon MS, McCaskill-Stevens WJ, Battiato LA, et al. A phase I trial of recombinant human interleukin-11 (neumega rhIL-11 growth factor) in women with breast cancer receiving chemotherapy. *Blood* 1996;87:3615–3624.

183. Tepler I, Elias L, Smith JW 2nd, et al. A randomized placebo-controlled trial of recombinant human interleukin-11 in cancer patients with severe thrombocytopenia due to chemotherapy. *Blood* 1996;87:3607–3614.

184. Takagi A, Masuda H, Takakura Y, et al. Disposition characteristics of recombinant human interleukin-11 after a bolus intravenous administration in mice. *J Pharmacol Exp Ther* 1995;275:537–543.

185. Isaacs C, Robert NJ, Bailey FA, et al. Randomized placebo-controlled study of recombinant human interleukin-11 to prevent chemotherapy-induced thrombocytopenia in patients with breast cancer receiving dose-intensive cyclophosphamide and doxorubicin. *J Clin Oncol* 1997;15:3368–3377.

186. Goldberg MA, Dunning PS, Dunn HF. Regulation of the erythropoietin gene: evidence that oxygen sensor is a heme protein. *Science* 1988;242:1412–1415.

187. Powell JS, Berkner KL, Lebo RV, et al. Human erythropoietin gene: high level expression in stably transfected mammalian cells and chromosome localization. *Proc Natl Acad Sci U S A* 1986;83:6465–6469.

188. Fried W. The liver as a source of extrarenal erythropoietin production. *Blood* 1972;40:671–677.

189. Zanjani ED, Ascensao JL, McGlave PB, et al. Studies on the liver to kidney switch of erythropoietin production. *J Clin Invest* 1981;67:1183–1188.

190. Witthuhn BA, Quelle FW, Silvennoinen O, et al. JAK2 associates with the erythropoietin receptor and is tyrosine phosphorylated and activated following stimulation with erythropoietin. *Cell* 1993;74:227–236.

191. Klingmuller U, Wu H, Hsiao JG, et al. Identification of a novel pathway important for proliferation and differentiation of primary erythroid progenitors. *Proc Natl Acad Sci U S A* 1997;94:3016–3021.

192. Klingmuller U. The role of tyrosine phosphorylation in proliferation and maturation of erythroid progenitor cells—signals emanating from the erythropoietin receptor. *Eur J Biochem* 1997;249:637–647.

193. Tsushima H, Urata Y, Miyazaki Y, et al. Human erythropoietin receptor increases GATA-2 and Bcl-xL by a protein kinase C-dependent pathway in human erythropoietin-dependent cell line AS-E2. *Cell Growth Differ* 1997;8:1317–1328.

194. Ludwig H, Fritz E, Leitgeb C, et al. Prediction of response to erythropoietin treatment in chronic anemia of cancer. *Blood* 1994;84:1056–1063.

195. Major A, Mathez-Loic F, Rohling R, et al. The effect of intravenous iron on the reticulocyte response to recombinant human erythropoietin. *Br J Haematol* 1997;98:292–294.

196. Cazzola M, Mercuriali F, Brugnara C. Use of recombinant human erythropoietin outside the setting of uremia. *Blood* 1997;89:4248–4267.

197. Eschbach J, Ergie J, Downing M, et al. Correction of the anemia of endstage renal disease with recombinant human erythropoietin. *N Engl J Med* 1987;316:73–78.

198. Linde T, Sandhagen B, Bratteby LE, et al. Reduced oxygen affinity contributes to improved oxygen releasing capacity during erythropoietin treatment of renal anaemia. *Nephrol Dial Transplant* 1993;8:524–529.

199. Brunet P, Berland Y, Merzouk T, et al. Effect of recombinant human erythropoietin treatment in uremic patients on oxygen affinity of hemoglobin. *Nephron* 1994;66:147–152.

200. De Marchi S, Cecchin E, Villalta D, et al. Relief of pruritus and decreases in plasma histamine concentrations during erythropoietin therapy in patients with uremia. *N Engl J Med* 1992;326:969–974.

201. Foresta C, Mioni R, Bordon P, et al. Erythropoietin stimulates testosterone production in man. *J Clin Endocrinol Metab* 1994;78:753–756.

202. Montagnac R, Boffa GA, Schillinger F, et al. Sensitization to recombinant human erythropoietin in a woman under hemodialysis [Letter]. *Presse Med* 1992;21:84–85.

203. Bergrem H, Danielson BG, Eckardt KU, et al. *A case of antierythropoietin antibodies following recombinant human erythropoietin treatment: Erythropoietin: molecular physiology and clinical application.* New York: Marcel Dekker, 1993:266–275.

204. Pece R, de la Torre M, Alcazar R, et al. Antibodies against recombinant human erythropoietin in a patient with erythropoietin-resistant anemia [Letter]. *N Engl J Med* 1996;335:523–534.

205. Prabhakar S, Muhlfelder T. Antibodies to recombinant human erythropoietin causing pure red cell aplasia. *Clin Nephrol* 1997;47:331–335.

206. Casadevall N, Nataf J, Viron B, et al. Pure red-cell aplasia and neutralizing antierythropoietin antibodies in patients treated with recombinant erythropoietin for anemia of chronic renal failure. *N Engl J Med* 2002;346:469–475.

207. Garcia JE, Senent C, Pascual C, et al. Anaphylactic reaction to recombinant human erythropoietin [Letter]. *Nephron* 1993;65:636–637.

208. McMahon FG, Vargas R, Ryan M, et al. Pharmacokinetics and effects of recombinant human erythropoietin after intravenous and subcutaneous injections in healthy volunteers. *Blood* 1990;76:1718–1722.

209. Nielson OJ. Pharmacokinetics of recombinant human erythropoietin in chronic hemodialysis patients. *Pharmacol Toxicol* 1990;66:83–86.

210. Kaufman JS, Reda DJ, Fye CL, et al. Subcutaneous compared with intravenous epoetin in patients receiving hemodialysis. Department of Veterans Affairs Cooperative Study Group on Erythropoietin in Hemodialysis Patients. *N Engl J Med* 1998;339:578–583.

211. Macdougall IG. Novel erythropoiesis stimulating protein. *Semin Nephrol* 2000;20:375–381.

212. Villeval JL, Rouyer-Fessard P, Blumenfeld N, et al. Retrovirus-mediated transfer of the erythropoietin gene in hematopoietic cells improves the erythrocyte phenotype in murine beta-thalassemia. *Blood* 1994;84:928–933.

213. Tripathy SK, Goldwasser E, Lu MM, et al. Stable delivery of physiologic levels of recombinant erythropoietin to the systemic circulation by intramuscular injection of replication-defective adenovirus. *Proc Natl Acad Sci U S A* 1994;91:11557–11561.

214. Setoguchi Y, Danel C, Crystal RG. Stimulation of erythropoiesis by in vivo gene therapy: physiologic consequences of transfer of the human erythropoietin gene to experimental animals using an adenovirus vector. *Blood* 1994;84:2946–2953.

215. Svensson EC, Black HB, Dugger DL, et al. Long-term erythropoietin expression in rodents and non-human primates following intramuscular injection

of a replication-defective adenoviral vector. *Hum Gene Ther* 1997;8:1797–1806.

216. Bohl D, Salvetti A, Moullier P, et al. Control of erythropoietin delivery by doxycycline in mice after intramuscular injection of adeno-associated vector. *Blood* 1998;92:1512–1517.

217. Tripathy SK, Svensson EC, Black HB, et al. Long-term expression of erythropoietin in the systemic circulation of mice after intramuscular injection of a plasmid DNA vector. *Proc Natl Acad Sci U S A* 1996;93:10876–10880.

218. Rizzuto G, Cappelletti M, Maione D, et al. Efficient and regulated erythropoietin production by naked DNA injection and muscle electroporation. *Proc Natl Acad Sci U S A* 1999;96:6417–6422.

219. Klinman DM, Conover J, Leiden JM, et al. Safe and effective regulation of hematocrit by gene gun administration of an erythropoietin-encoding DNA plasmid. *Hum Gene Ther* 1999;10:659–665.

220. Smith KA. Interleukin-2: inception, impact, and implications. *Science* 1988;240:1169–1176. Review.

221. Taniguchi T, Minami Y. The IL-2/IL-2 receptor system: a current overview. *Cell* 1993;73:5–8. Review.

222. Smith KA. The interleukin 2 receptor. *Annu Rev Cell Biol* 1989;5:397–425. Review.

223. Smith KA. Lowest dose interleukin-2 immunotherapy. *Blood* 1993;81:1414–1423. Review.

224. Philips J, Lanier LL. Dissection of the lymphokine-activated killer phenomenon. Relative contribution of peripheral blood natural killer cells and T lymphocytes to cytolysis. *J Exp Med* 1986;164:814–825.

225. Gemlo BT, Palladino MA Jr, Jaffe HS, et al. Circulating cytokines in patients with metastatic cancer treated with recombinant interleukin 2 and lymphokine-activated killer cells. *Cancer Res* 1988;48:5864–5867.

226. Takeshita T, Asao H, Ohtani K, et al. Cloning of the gamma chain of the human IL-2 receptor. *Science* 1992;257:379–382.

227. Farrar WL, Cleveland JL, Beckner SK, et al. Biochemical and molecular events associated with interleukin 2 regulation of lymphocyte proliferation. *Immunol Rev* 1986;92:49–65. Review.

228. Purkerson JM, Newberg M, Wise G, et al. Interleukin 5 and interleukin 2 cooperate with interleukin 4 to induce IgG1 secretion from anti-Ig-treated B cells. *J Exp Med* 1988;168:1175–1180.

229. Fotedar R, Diener E. The role of recombinant IL-2 and IL-1 in murine B cell differentiation. *Lymphokine Res* 1988;7:393–402.

230. Matsui K, Nakanishi K, Cohen DI, et al. B cell response pathways regulated by IL-5 and IL-2. Secretory microH chain-mRNA and J chain mRNA expression are separately controlled events. *J Immunol* 1989;142:2918–2923.

231. Ben Aribia MH, Leroy E, Lantz O, et al. rIL 2-induced proliferation of human circulating NK cells and T lymphocytes: synergistic effects of IL 1 and IL 2. *J Immunol* 1987;139:443–451.

232. Seigel LJ, Harper ME, Wong-Staal F, et al. Gene for T-cell growth factor: location on human chromosome 4q and feline chromosome B1. *Science* 1984;223:175–178.

233. Taniguchi T, Minami Y. The IL-2/IL-2 receptor system: a current overview. *Cell* 1993;73:5–8. Review.

234. Hatakeyama M, Tsudo M, Minamoto S, et al. Interleukin-2 receptor beta chain gene: generation of three receptor forms by cloned human alpha and beta chain cDNA's. *Science* 1989;244:551–556.

235. Minami Y, Taniguchi T. IL-2 signaling: recruitment and activation of multiple protein tyrosine kinases by the components of the IL-2 receptor. *Curr Opin Cell Biol* 1995;7:156–162. Review.

236. Voss SD, Hong R, Sondel PM. Severe combined immunodeficiency, interleukin-2 (IL-2), and the IL-2 receptor: experiments of nature continue to point the way. *Blood* 1994;83:626–635. Review.

237. Grimm EA, Mazumder A, Zhang HZ, et al. Lymphokine-activated killer cell phenomenon. Lysis of natural killer-resistant fresh solid tumor cells by interleukin 2-activated autologous human peripheral blood lymphocytes. *J Exp Med* 1982;155:1823–1841.

238. Sadlack B, Lohler J, Scharle H, et al. Generalized autoimmune disease in interleukin-2-deficient mice is triggered by an uncontrolled activation and proliferation of CD4 + T-lymphocytes. *Eur J Immunol* 1995;25:3053–3059.

239. Horak I. Immunodeficiency in IL-2-knockout mice. *Clin Immunol Immunopathol* 1995;76:S172–S173. Review.

240. Lotze MT, Grimm EA, Mazumder A, et al. Lysis of fresh and cultured autologous tumor by human lymphocytes cultured in T-cell growth factor. *Cancer Res* 1981;41:4420–4425.

241. Rosenberg SA, Lotze MT, Muul LM, et al. A progress report on the treatment of 157 patients with advanced cancer using lymphokine-activated killer cells and interleukin-2 alone. *N Engl J Med* 1987;316:889–897.

242. West WH, Tauer KW, Yannelli JR, et al. Constant-infusion recombinant interleukin-2 in adoptive immunotherapy of advanced cancer. *N Engl J Med* 1987;316:898–905.

243. Yang JC, Topalian SL, Parkinson D, et al. Randomized comparison of high-dose and low-dose intravenous interleukin-2 for the therapy of metastatic renal cell carcinoma: an interim report. *J Clin Oncol* 1994;12:1572–1576.

244. Fyfe G, Fisher RI, Rosenberg SA, et al. Results of treatment of 255 patients with metastatic renal cell carcinoma who received high-dose recombinant interleukin-2 therapy. *J Clin Oncol* 1995;13:688–696.

245. Dutcher JP, Creekmore S, Weiss GR, et al. A phase II study of interleukin-2 and lymphokine-activated killer cells in patients with metastatic malignant melanoma. *J Clin Oncol* 1989;7:477–485.

246. Tourani JM, Levy V, Briere J, et al. Interleukin-2 therapy for refractory and relapsing lymphomas. *Eur J Cancer* 1991;27:1676–1680.

247. Duggan DB, Santarelli MT, Zamkoff K, et al. A phase II study of recombinant interleukin-2 with or without recombinant interferon-beta in non-Hodgkin's lymphoma. A study of the Cancer and Leukemia Group B. *J Immunother* 1992;12:115–122.

248. Gisselbrecht C, Maraninchi D, Pico JL, et al. Interleukin-2 treatment in lymphoma: a phase II multicenter study. *Blood* 1994;83:2081–2085.

249. Weber JS, Yang JC, Topalian SL, et al. The use of interleukin-2 and lymphokine-activated killer cells for the treatment of patients with non-Hodgkin's lymphoma. *J Clin Oncol* 1992;10:33–40.

250. Meloni G, Vignetti M, Andrizzi C, et al. Interleukin-2 for the treatment of advanced acute myelogenous leukemia patients with limited disease: updated experience with 20 cases. *Leuk Lymphoma* 1996;21:429–435.

251. Maraninchi D, Blaise D, Viens P, et al. High-dose recombinant interleukin-2 and acute myeloid leukemias in relapse. *Blood* 1991;78:2182–2187.

252. Bergmann L, Heil G, Kolbe K, et al. Interleukin-2 bolus infusion as late consolidation therapy in 2nd remission of acute myeloblastic leukemia. *Leuk Lymphoma* 1995;16:271–279.

253. Wiernik PH, Dutcher JP, Todd M, et al. Polyethylene glycolated interleukin-2 as maintenance therapy for acute myelogenous leukemia in second remission. *Am J Hematol* 1994;47:41–44.

254. Ogata K, Yokose N, Ito T, et al. Assessment of therapeutic potential of interleukin-2 for myelodysplastic syndromes. *Br J Haematol* 1994;86:562–567.

255. Kaufman DW, Kelly JP, Levy M, et al. *The drug etiology of agranulocytosis and aplastic anemia.* New York: Oxford, University Press, 1991.

256. Kojima S, Matsuyama T, Kodera Y. Hematopoietic growth factors released by marrow stromal cells from patients with aplastic anemia. *Blood* 1992;79:2256–2261.

257. Gibson FM, Scores J, Daly S, et al. Haemopoietic growth factor production by normal and aplastic anemia stroma in long-term bone marrow culture. *Br J Haematol* 1995;91:551–561.

258. Stark R, Andre C, Thierry D, et al. The expression of cytokine and cytokine receptor genes in long-term bone marrow culture in congenital and acquired bone marrow hypoplasia. *Br J Haematol* 1993;83:560–566.

259. Tani K, Ozawa K, Ogura H, et al. The production of granulocyte colony stimulating factor and interleukin-6 by human bone marrow stromal cells in aplastic anemia. *Tohoku J Exp Med* 1993;169:325–334.

260. Migliaccio AR, Migliaccio G, Adamson JW, et al. Production of granulocyte colony-stimulating factor and granulocyte/macrophage-colony-stimulating factor after interleukin-1 stimulation of marrow stromal cell cultures from normal or aplastic anemia donors. *J Cell Physiol* 1992;152:199–206.

261. Andreesen R, Brugger W, Thomssen C, et al. Defective monocyte-to-macrophage maturation in patients with aplastic anemia. *Blood* 1989;74:2150–2156.

262. Watari K, Asano S, Shirafuji N, et al. Serum granulocyte colony-stimulating factor levels in healthy volunteers and patients with various disorders as estimated by enzyme immunoassay. *Blood* 1989;73:117–122.

263. Young NS. Pathophysiology. I. Stem cells, stroma, and growth factors. In: Young NS, Alter BP, eds. *Aplastic anemia, acquired and inherited.* Philadelphia: WB Saunders, 1991:32.

264. Emmons RV, Reid DM, Cohen RL, et al. Human thrombopoietin levels are high when thrombocytopenia is due to megakaryocyte deficiency and low when due to increased platelet destruction. *Blood* 1996;87:4068–4071.

265. Marsh JC. Hematopoietic growth factors in the pathogenesis and for the treatment of aplastic anemia. *Semin Hematol* 2000;37:81–90. Review.

266. Kumar M, Alter BP. Hematopoietic growth factors for the treatment of aplastic anemia. *Curr Opin Hematol* 1998;5:226–234. Review.

267. Devetten MP, Young NS. Hematopoietic growth factors in the pathophysiology and treatment of aplastic anemia. In: Hoelzer D, Ganzer A, eds. *Cytokines in the treatment of hematopoietic failure.* New York: Marcell Dekker, 1996.

268. Kojima S, Fukuda M, Miyajima Y, et al. Treatment of aplastic anemia in children with recombinant human granulocyte colony-stimulating factor. *Blood* 1991;77:937–941.

269. Kojima S, Matsuyama T. Stimulation of granulopoiesis by high-dose recombinant human granulocyte colony-stimulating factor in children with aplastic anemia and very severe neutropenia. *Blood* 1994;83:1474–1478.

270. Sonoda Y, Ohno Y, Fujii H, et al. Multilineage response in aplastic anemia patients following long-term administration of filgrastim (recombinant human granulocyte colony stimulating factor). *Stem Cells* 1993;11:543–554.

271. Higuchi T, Shimizu T, Okada S, et al. Delayed granulocyte response to G-CSF in aplastic anemia. *Am J Hematol* 1994;46:164–165.

272. Tuzuner N, Cox C, Rowe JM, et al. Hypocellular myelodysplastic syndromes (MDS): new proposals. *Br J Haematol* 1995;91:612–617.

273. Yamazaki E, Kanamori H, Taguchi J, et al. The evidence of clonal evolution with monosomy 7 in aplastic anemia following granulocyte colony-stimulating factor using the polymerase chain reaction. *Blood Cells Mol Dis* 1997;23:213–218.

274. Nimer SD, Paquette RL, Ireland P, et al. A phase I/II study of interleukin-3 in patients with aplastic anemia and myelodysplasia. *Exp Hematol* 1994;22:875–880.

275. Bargetzi MJ, Gluckman E, Tichelli A, et al. Recombinant human interleukin-3 in refractory severe aplastic anaemia: a phase I/II trial. *Br J Haematol* 1995;91:306–312.

276. Ganser A, Lindemann A, Seipelt G, et al. Effects of recombinant human interleukin-3 in aplastic anemia. *Blood* 1990;76:1287–1292.

277. Schrezenmeier H, Marsh JC, Stromeyer P, et al. A phase I/II trial of recombinant human interleukin-6 in patients with aplastic anaemia. *Br J Haematol* 1995;90:283–292.

278. Takahashi M, Aoki A, Mito M, et al. Combination therapy with rhGM-CSF and rhEpo for two patients with refractory anemia and aplastic anemia. *Hematol Pathol* 1993;7:153–158.

279. Nawata J, Toyoda Y, Nisihira H, et al. Haematological improvement by long-term administration of recombinant human granulocyte-colony stimulating factor and recombinant human erythropoietin in a patient with severe aplastic anaemia. *Eur J Pediatr* 1994;153:325–327.

280. Bessho M, Toyoda A, Itoh Y, et al. Trilineage recovery by combination therapy with recombinant human granulocyte colony-stimulating factor (rhG-CSF) and erythropoietin (rhEpo) in severe aplastic anaemia. *Br J Haematol* 1992;80:409–411.

281. Farese AM, Williams DE, Seiler FR, et al. Combination protocols of cytokine therapy with interleukin-3 and granulocyte-macrophage colony-stimulating factor in a primate model of radiation-induced marrow aplasia. *Blood* 1993;82:3012–3018.

282. Bessho M, Hirashima K, Asano S, et al. Treatment of the anemia of aplastic anemia patients with recombinant human erythropoietin in combination with granulocyte colony-stimulating factor: a multicenter randomized controlled study. Multicenter Study Group. *Eur J Haematol* 1997;58:265–272.

283. Raghavachar K, Kolbe K, Hoffken K, et al. A randomized trial of standard immunosuppression versus cyclosporine and filgrastim in severe aplastic anemia. *Blood* 1997;90:1951(abst).

284. Bacigalupo A, Broccia G, Corda G, et al. Antilymphocyte globulin, cyclosporin, and granulocyte colony-stimulating factor in patients with acquired severe aplastic anemia (SAA): a pilot study of the EBMT SAA Working Party. *Blood* 1995;85:1348–1353.

285. List AF, Garewal HS, Sandberg AA. The myelodysplastic syndromes: biology and implications for management. *J Clin Oncol* 1990;8:1424–1441. Review.

286. Cheson BD. The myelodysplastic syndromes: current approaches to therapy. *Ann Intern Med* 1990;112:932–941.

287. Bennett JM, Latovsky D, Daniel MT, et al. Proposal for the classification of the myelodysplastic syndromes. *Br J Haematol* 1982;41:189–199.

288. Ganser A, Hoelzer D. Clinical course of myelodysplastic syndromes. *Hematol Oncol Clin North Am* 1992;6:607–618. Review.

289. Raskind WH, Tirumali N, Jacobson R, et al. Evidence for a multistep pathogenesis of a myelodysplastic syndrome. *Blood* 1984;63:1318–1323.

290. Mecucci C. Molecular features of primary MDS with cytogenetic changes. *Leuk Res* 1998;22:293–302. Review.

291. Greenberg PL, Nichols W, Schrier SL. Granulopoiesis in acute myeloid leukemia and preleukemia. *N Engl J Med* 1971;284:1225–1232.

292. Greenberg PL, Mara B. The preleukemic syndrome: correlation of in vitro parameters of granulopoiesis with clinical features. *Am J Med* 1979;66:951–958.

293. Chiu DHK, Clark BJ. Abnormal erythroid progenitor cells in human preleukemia. *Blood* 1982;60:362–367.

294. Mizoguchi H, Kubota K, Suda T, et al. Erythroid and granulocyte/macrophage progenitor cells in primary acquired sideroblastic anemia. *Int J Cell Cloning* 1983;1:15–23.

295. Beran M, Hast R. Studies on human preleukemia. II. In vivo colony forming capacity in aregenerating anemia with hypercellular bone marrow. *Scand J Haematol* 1978;21:131–149.

296. Verma DS, Spitzer G, Dicke KA, et al. In vitro agar culture patterns in preleukemia and their clinical significance. *Leuk Res* 1979;3:41–49.

297. Yoshida Y. Biology of myelodysplastic syndromes. *Int J Cell Cloning* 1987;5:356–375. Review.

298. Toyama K, Ohyashiki K, Yoshida Y, et al. Clinical implications of chromosomal abnormalities in 401 patients with myelodysplastic syndromes: a multicentric study in Japan. *Leukemia* 1993;7:499–508.

299. Greenberg P, Cox C, LeBeau MM, et al. International scoring system for evaluating prognosis in myelodysplastic syndromes. *Blood* 1997;89:2079–2088.

300. Pfeilstocker M, Reisner R, Nosslinger T, et al. Cross-validation of prognostic scores in myelodysplastic syndromes on 386 patients from a single institution confirms importance of cytogenetics. *Br J Haematol* 1999;106:455–463.

301. Raza A, Mundle S, Shetty V, et al. A paradigm shift in myelodysplastic syndromes. *Leukemia* 1996;10:1648–1652.

302. Verhoef GEG, De Schouwer P, Ceuppens J, et al. Measurement of serum cytokine levels in patients with myelodysplastic syndromes. *Leukemia* 1992;6:1268–1272.

303. Keller JR, Jacobsen SEW, Dubois CM, et al. Transforming growth factor-β: a bidirectional regular of hematopoietic cell growth. *Int J Cell Cloning* 1992;10:2–11.

304. Gregory S, Robin E, Rifkin S, et al. Interleukin-1β converting enzyme-like protease may be involved in the intramedullary apoptotic death in the marrows of patients with myelodysplasia. *Proc Am Soc Hematol* 1995;334a(abstr. 1323).

305. Everson MP, Brown CB, Lilly MB. Interleukin-6 and granulocyte-macrophage colony-stimulating factor are candidate growth factors for chronic myelomonocytic leukemia cells. *Blood* 1989;74:1472–1476.

306. Ward A, Clossold SP. Pentoxifylline. A review of its pharmacodynamic and pharmacokinetic properties, and its therapeutic efficacy. *Drugs* 1987;34:50–97. Review.

307. Thompson JA, Bianco JA, Benyunes MC, et al. Phase Ib trial of pentoxifylline and ciprofloxacin in patients treated with interleukin-2 and lymphokine-activated killer cell therapy for metastatic renal cell carcinoma. *Cancer Res* 1994;54:3436–3441.

308. Raza A, Qawi H, Lisak L, et al. Patients with myelodysplastic syndromes benefit from palliative therapy with amifostine, pentoxifylline, and ciprofloxacin with or without dexamethasone. *Blood* 2000;95:1580–1587.

309. Gardais J. Dyshaemopoiesis in adults: a practical classification for diagnosis and management. *Leuk Res* 2000;24:641–651. Review.

310. Harris NL, Jaffe ES, Diebold J, et al. World Health Organization classification of neoplastic diseases of the hematopoietic and lymphoid tissues: report of the Clinical Advisory Committee meeting-Airlie House, Virginia, November 1997. *J Clin Oncol* 1999;17:3835–3849.

311. Deeg HJ, Appelbaum FR. Hematopoietic stem cell transplantation in patients with myelodysplastic syndrome. *Leuk Res* 2000;24:653–663. Review.

312. Saba HI. Myelodysplastic syndromes in the elderly: the role of growth factors in management. *Leuk Res* 20:203–209. Review.

313. Vadhan-Raj S, Keating M, LeMaistre A, et al. Effects of recombinant human granulocyte-macrophage colony-stimulating factor in patients with myelodysplastic syndromes. *N Engl J Med* 1987;317:1545–1552.

314. Vadhan-Raj S, Broxmeyer HE, Spitzer G, et al. Stimulation of nonclonal hematopoiesis and suppression of the neoplastic clone after treatment with recombinant human granulocyte-macrophage colony-stimulating factor in a patient with therapy-related myelodysplastic syndrome. *Blood* 1989;74:1491–1498.

315. Negrin RS, Haeuber DH, Nagler A, et al. Treatment of myelodysplastic syndromes with recombinant human granulocyte colony stimulating factor. *Ann Intern Med* 1989;110:976–984.

316. Thompson JA, Lee DJ, Kidd P, et al. Subcutaneous granulocyte-macrophage colony-stimulating factor in patients with myelodysplastic syndrome: toxicity, pharmacokinetics, and hematological effects. *J Clin Oncol* 1989;7:629–637.

317. Nagler A, Binet C, Mackichan ML, et al. Impact of marrow cytogenetics and morphology on in vitro hematopoiesis in the myelodysplastic syndromes: comparison between recombinant human granulocyte colony-stimulating factor (CSF) and granulocyte-monocyte CSF. *Blood* 1990;76:1299–1307.

318. Negrin RS, Stein R, Vardiman J, et al. Treatment of the anemia of myelodysplastic syndromes using recombinant human granulocyte-macrophage colony-stimulating factor in combination with erythropoietin. *Blood* 1993;82:737–743.

319. Hellstrom-Lindberg E, Ahlgren T, Beguin Y, et al. Treatment of anemia in myelodysplastic syndromes with granulocyte colony-stimulating factor plus erythropoietin: results from a randomized phase II study and long-term follow-up of 71 patients. *Blood* 1998;92:68–75.

320. Freedman MH, Bonilla MA, Fier C, et al. Myelodysplasia syndrome and acute myeloid leukemia in patients with congenital neutropenia receiving G-CSF therapy. *Blood* 2000;96:429–436.

321. Economopoulos T, Mellou S, Papageorgiou E, et al. Treatment of anemia in low risk myelodysplastic syndromes with granulocyte-macrophage colony-stimulating factor plus recombinant human erythropoietin. *Leukemia* 1999;13:1009–1012.

322. Schuster MW, Thompson JA, Larson R, et al. Randomized trial of subcutaneous granulocyte-macrophage colony-stimulating (GM-CSF) versus observation in patients with myelodysplastic syndrome. *J Cancer Res Clin Oncol* 1990; 116:1079.

323. Willemze R, Visani G, Witte TH de, et al. A randomized phase I/II study with recombinant human GM-CSF in patients with myelodysplastic syndromes at relatively low-risk of developing acute leukemia. *Blood* 1990; 76[Suppl 1]:337a(abst).

324. Rosenfeld CS, Sulecki M, Evans C, et al. Comparison of intravenous versus subcutaneous recombinant human granulocyte-macrophage colony-stimulating factor in patients with primary myelodysplasia. *Exp Hematol* 1991; 19:273–277.

325. Willemze R, van der Lely N, Zwierzina H, et al. A randomized phase-I/II multicenter study of recombinant human granulocyte-macrophage colony-stimulating factor (GM-CSF) therapy for patients with myelodysplastic syndromes and a relatively low risk of acute leukemia. EORTC Leukemia Cooperative Group. *Ann Hematol* 1992;64:173–180.

326. Takahashi M, Yoshida Y, Kaku K, et al. A randomized phase-I/II multicenter study of recombinant human granulocyte-macrophage colony-stimulating factor (GM-CSF) therapy for patients with myelodysplastic syndromes and a relatively low risk of acute leukemia. EORTC Leukemia Cooperative Group. *Ann Hematol* 1992;64:173–180.

327. Kobayashi Y, Okabe T, Ozawa K, et al. Treatment with myelodysplastic syndrome with recombinant human granulocyte colony-stimulating factor; a preliminary report. *Am J Med* 1989;86:178–182.

328. Ohyashiki K, Ohyashiki JH, Toyama K, et al. Hematologic and cytogenetic findings in myelodysplastic syndromes treated with recombinant human granulocyte colony-stimulating factor. *Jpn J Cancer Res* 1989;80:848–854.

329. Negrin RS, Haeuber DH, Nagler A, et al. Maintenance treatment of patients with myelodysplastic syndromes using recombinant granulocyte colony-stimulating factor. *Blood* 1990;76:36–43.

330. Yoshida Y, Hirashima K, Asanu S, et al. A phase II trial of recombinant human granulocyte colony-stimulating factor in the myelodysplastic syndrome. *Br J Haematol* 1990;78:378–384.

331. Greenberg P, Taylor K, Larsen R, et al. Phase III randomized multicenter trial of G-CSF versus observation for myelodysplastic syndromes (MDS). *Blood* 1993:196a(abstr).

332. Delmer A, Karmochkine M, Cadion M, et al. Recurrent spleen enlargement during cyclic granulocyte macrophage colony stimulating factor therapy for myelodysplastic syndromes. *Am J Hematol* 1990;73:73–74.

333. Kurzrock R, Talpaz M, Gomez JA, et al. Differential dose-related haematological effects of GM-CSF in pancytopenia: evidence supporting the advantage of low- over high-dose administration in selected patients. Br J Haematol 1991;78:352–358.

334. Ossenkoppele GJ, van der Holt B, Verhoef GE, et al. A randomized study of granulocyte colony-stimulating factor applied during and after chemotherapy in patients with poor risk myelodysplastic syndromes: a report from the HOVON Cooperative Group. Dutch-Belgian Hemato-Oncology Cooperative Group. Leukemia 1999;13:1207–1213.

335. Thomas X, Fenaux P, Dombret H, et al. Granulocyte-macrophage colony-stimulating factor (GM-CSF) to increase efficacy of intensive sequential chemotherapy with etoposide, mitoxantrone and cytarabine (EMA) in previously treated acute myeloid leukemia: a multicenter randomized placebo-controlled trial (EMA91 Trial). Leukemia 1999;13:1214–1220.

336. Tafuri A, Andreeff M. Kinetic rationale for cytokine-induced recruitment of myeloblastic leukemia followed by cycle-specific chemotherapy in vitro. Leukemia 1990;4:826–834.

337. Aglietta M, De Felice L, Stacchini A, et al. In vivo effect of granulocyte-macrophage colony-stimulating factor on the kinetics of human acute myeloid leukemia cells. Leukemia 1991;5:979–984.

338. Cannistra SA, DiCarlo J, Groshek P, et al. Simultaneous administration of granulocyte-macrophage colony-stimulating factor and cytosine arabinoside for the treatment of relapsed acute myeloid leukemia. Leukemia 1991;3:230–238.

339. Ganser A, Seipelt G, Lindemann A, et al. Effects of recombinant human interleukin-3 in patients with myelodysplastic syndromes. Blood 1990;76:455–462.

340. Hou M, Andersson PO, Stockelberg D, et al. Plasma thrombopoietin levels in thrombocytopenic states: implication for a regulatory role of bone marrow megakaryocytes. Br J Haematol 1998;101:420–424.

341. Zwierzina H, Rollinger-Holzinger I, Nuessler V, et al. Endogenous serum thrombopoietin concentrations in patients with myelodysplastic syndromes. Leukemia 1998;12:59–64.

342. Tamura H, Ogata K, Luo S, et al. Plasma thrombopoietin (TPO) levels and expression of TPO receptor on platelets in patients with myelodysplastic syndromes. Br J Haematol 1998;103:778–784.

343. Wang W, Matsuo T, Yoshida S, et al. Colony-forming unit-megakaryocyte (CFR-meg) numbers and serum thrombopoietin concentrations in thrombocytopenic disorders: an inverse correlation in myelodysplastic syndromes. Leukemia 2000;14:1751–1756.

344. Adamson JW, Schuster N, Allen S, et al. Effectiveness of recombinant human erythropoietin therapy in myelodysplastic syndromes. Acta Haematol 1992;87 [Suppl 1]:20–24.

345. Bowen D, Culligan D, Jacobs A. The treatment of anaemia in the myelodysplastic syndromes with recombinant human erythropoietin. Br J Haematol 1991;77:419–423.

346. Stein RS, Abels RJ, Krantz SB. Pharmacologic doses of recombinant human erythropoietin in the treatment of myelodysplastic syndromes. Blood 1991;78:1658–1663.

347. Stasi R, Brunetti M, Bussa S, et al. Response to recombinant human erythropoietin in patients with myelodysplastic syndromes. Clin Cancer Res 1997;3:733–739.

348. Hellstrom E, Birgegard G, Lockner D, et al. Treatment of myelodysplastic syndromes with recombinant human erythropoietin. Eur J Haematol 1991;47:355–360.

349. Hellstrom-Lindberg E. Efficacy of erythropoietin in the myelodysplastic syndromes; a meta-analysis of 205 patients from 17 studies. Br J Haematol 1995;89:67–71.

350. Rose E, Abels RI, Nelson RA, et al. The use of r-HuEpo in the treatment of anemia—related to myelodysplasia (MDS). Br J Haematol 1995;89:831–837.

351. Stone RM, Bernstein SH, Demetri G, et al. Therapy with recombinant human erythropoietin in patients with myelodysplastic syndromes. Leuk Res 1994;18:769–776.

352. Hast R, Wallvik J, Folin A, et al. Long-term follow-up of 18 patients with myelodysplastic syndromes responding to recombinant erythropoietin treatment. Leuk Res 2001;25:13–18.

353. Hellstrom-Lindberg E, Ahlgren T, Begiun Y, et al. Treatment of anemia in myelodysplastic syndromes with granulocyte colony-stimulating factor plus erythropoietin: results from a randomized phase II study and long-term follow-up of 71 patients. Blood 1998;92:68–75.

354. Negrin RS, Stein R, Vardiman J, et al. Treatment of the anemia of myelodysplastic syndrome using recombinant human granulocyte colony-stimulating factor in combination with erythropoietin. Blood 1993;82:737–743.

355. Economopoulos T, Mellou S, Papageorgiou E, et al. Treatment of anemia in low risk myelodysplastic syndromes with granulocyte-macrophage colony-stimulating factor plus recombinant human erythropoietin. Leukemia 1999;13:1009–1012.

356. Hellstrom-Lindberg E, Negrin R, Stein R, et al. Erythroid response to treatment with G-CSF plus erythropoietin for the anaemia of patients with myelodysplastic syndromes: proposal for a predictive model. Br J Haematol 1997;99:344–351.

357. Amano Y, Koike K, Nakahata T, et al. Stem cell factor enhances the growth of primitive erythroid progenitors to a greater extent than interleukin-3 in patients with aplastic anemia. Br J Haematol 1993;85:663–669.

358. Backx B, Broeders L, Lowenberg B. Kit ligand improves in vitro erythropoiesis in myelodysplastic syndrome. Blood 1992;80:1213–1217.

359. Negrin RS, Stein R, Doherty K, et al. Maintenance treatment of the anemia of myelodysplastic syndromes with recombinant human granulocyte colony-stimulating factor and erythropoietin: evidence for in vivo synergy. Blood 1996;87:4076–4081.

360. Hellstrom-Lindberg E, Birgegard G, Carlsson M, et al. A combination of granulocyte colony-stimulating factor and erythropoietin may synergistically improve the anaemia in patients with myelodysplastic syndromes. Leuk Lymphoma 1993;11:221–228.

361. Santini V, Nooter K, Delwel R, et al. Susceptibility of acute myeloid leukemia (AML) cells from clinically resistant and sensitive patients to daunomycin (DNR): assessment in vitro after stimulation with colony stimulating factors (CSFs). Leuk Res 1990;14:377–380.

362. Estey E, Thall PF, Kantarjian H, et al. Treatment of newly diagnosed acute myelogenous leukemia with granulocyte-macrophage colony-stimulating factor (GM-CSF) before and during continuous-infusion high-dose ara-C + daunorubicin: comparison to patients treated without GM-CSF. Blood 1992;79:2246–2255.

363. Ferrara F, Di Noto R, Viola A, et al. Complete remission in acute myeloid leukaemia with t(8;21) following treatment with G-CSF: flow cytometric analysis of in vivo and in vitro effects on cell maturation. Br J Haematol 1999;106:520–523.

364. Park LS, Waldron PE, Friend D, et al. Interleukin-3, GM-CSF, and G-CSF receptor expression on cell lines and primary leukemia cells: receptor heterogeneity and relationship to growth factor responsiveness. Blood 1989;74:56–65.

365. Piao YF, Okabe T. Receptor binding of human granulocyte colony-stimulating factor to the blast cells of myeloid leukemia. Cancer Res 1990;50:1671–1674.

366. Shimoda K, Okamura S, Harada N, et al. Granulocyte colony-stimulating factor receptors on human acute leukemia: biphenotypic leukemic cells possess granulocyte colony-stimulating factor receptors. Cancer Res 1992;52:3052–3055.

367. Lowenberg B, Touw IP. Hematopoietic growth factors and their receptors in acute leukemia. Blood 1993;81:281–292. Review.

368. Shinjo K, Takeshita A, Ohnishi K, et al. Expression of granulocyte colony-stimulating factor receptor increases with differentiation in myeloid cells by a newly devised quantitative flow-cytometric assay. Br J Haematol 1995;91:783–794.

369. Kawada H, Sasao T, Yonekura S, et al. Clinical significance of granulocyte colony-stimulating factor (G-CSF) receptor expression in acute myeloid leukemia. Leuk Res 1998;22:31–37.

370. Ohno R, Tomonaga M, Kobayashi T, et al. Effect of granulocyte colony-stimulating factor after intensive induction therapy in relapsed or refractory acute leukemia. N Engl J Med 1990;323:871–877.

371. Buchner T, Hiddemann W, Koenigsmann M, et al. Recombinant human granulocyte-macrophage colony-stimulating factor after chemotherapy in patients with acute myeloid leukemia at higher age or after relapse. Blood 1991;78:1190–1197.

372. Bettelheim P, Valent P, Andreeff M, et al. Recombinant human granulocyte-macrophage colony-stimulating factor in combination with standard induction chemotherapy in de novo acute myeloid leukemia. Blood 1991;77:700–711.

373. Zittoun RA, Mandelli F, Willemze R, et al. Macrophage colony-stimulating factor associated with induction treatment of acute myelogenous leukemia: A randomized trial by the European Organization for Research and Treatment of Cancer Leukemia Cooperative Group. J Clin Oncol 1996;14:2150–2159.

374. Dong F, van Paassen M, van Buitenin C, et al. A point mutation in the granulocyte colony-stimulating factor receptor (C-CSF-R) gene in a case of acute myeloid leukemia results in the overexpression of a novel G-CSF-R isoform. Blood 1995;85:902–911.

375. Archimbaud E, Fenaux P, Reiffers J, et al. Granulocyte-macrophage colony-stimulating factor in association to timed-sequential chemotherapy with mitoxantrone, etoposide, and cytarabine for refractory acute myelogenous leukemia. Leukemia 1993;7:372–377.

376. Ohno R, Naoe T, Kanamaru A, et al. A double-blind controlled study of granulocyte colony-stimulating factor started two days before induction chemotherapy in refractory acute myeloid leukemia. Kohseisho Leukemia Study Group. Blood 1994;83:2086–2092.

377. Buchner T, Hiddemann W. Blood 1994;84:96(abst).

378. Heil G, Chadid L, Hoelzer D, et al. GM-CSF in a double-blind randomized, placebo controlled trial in therapy of adult patients with de novo acute myeloid leukemia (AML). Leukemia 1995;9:3–9.

379. Zittoun R, Suciu S, Mandelli F, et al. Granulocyte-macrophage colony-stimulating factor associated with induction treatment of acute myelogenous leukemia: a randomized trial by the European Organization for Research and Treatment of Cancer Leukemia Cooperative Group. J Clin Oncol 1996;14:2150–2159.

380. Lowenberg B, Suciu S, Archimbaud E, et al. Use of recombinant GM-CSF during and after remission induction chemotherapy in patients aged 61 years and older with acute myeloid leukemia: final report of AML-11, a phase III randomized study of the Leukemia Cooperative Group of European Organisation for the Research and Treatment of Cancer and the Dutch Belgian Hemato-Oncology Cooperative Group. Blood 1997;90:2952–2961.

381. Witz F, Sadoun A, Perrin MC, et al. A placebo-controlled study of recombinant human granulocyte-macrophage colony-stimulating factor administered during and after induction treatment for de novo acute myelogenous leukemia in elderly patients. Groupe Ouest Est Leucemies Aigues Myeloblastiques (GOELAM). Blood 1998;91:2722–2730.

382. Godwin JE, Kopecky KJ, Head DR, et al. A double-blind placebo-controlled trial of granulocyte colony-stimulating factor in elderly patients with previously untreated acute myeloid leukemia: A Southwest Oncology Group Study (9031). *Blood* 1998;91:3607–3015.

383. Lowenberg B, Boogaerts MA, Daenen SM, et al. Value of different modalities of granulocyte-macrophage colony-stimulating factor applied during or after induction therapy of acute myeloid leukemia. *J Clin Oncol* 1997;15:3496–3506.

384. Maslak PG, Weiss MA, Berman E, et al. Granulocyte colony-stimulating factor following chemotherapy in elderly patients with newly diagnosed acute myelogenous leukemia. *Leukemia* 1996;10:32–39.

385. Heil G, Hoelzer D, Sanz MA, et al. A randomized, double-blind, placebo-controlled, phase III study of filgrastim in remission induction and consolidation therapy for adults with de novo acute myeloid leukemia. The International Acute Myeloid Leukemia Study Group. *Blood* 1997;90:4710–4718.

386. Bradstock K, Matthews J, Young G, et al. Effects of glycosylated recombinant human granulocyte colony-stimulating factor after high-dose cytarabine-based induction chemotherapy for adult acute myeloid leukaemia. *Leukemia* 2001;15:1331–1338.

387. Harousseau JL, Witz B, Lioure B, et al. Granulocyte colony-stimulating factor after intensive consolidation chemotherapy in acute myeloid leukemia: results of a randomized trial of the Groupe Ouest-Est Leucemies Aigues Myeloblastiques. *J Clin Oncol* 2000;18:780–787.

388. Rowe J, Andersen J, Mazza J, et al. A randomized placebo-controlled phase III study of 6M-CSF in adults (>55 to 70 years) with acute myelogenous leukemia: a study of the Eastern Cooperative Oncology Group (E1490). *Blood* 1995;86:457–462.

389. Dombret H, Chastang C, Fenaux P, et al. A controlled study of recombinant human granulocyte colony-stimulating factor in elderly patients after treatment for acute myelogenous leukemia. *N Engl J Med* 1995;332:1678–1683.

390. Stone RM, Berg DT, George SL, et al. Granulocyte-macrophage colony-stimulating factor after initial chemotherapy for elderly patients with primary acute myelogenous leukemia. Cancer and Leukemia Group B. *N Engl J Med* 1995;332:1671–1677.

391. Link H, Wandt H, Schonrock-Nabulski P, et al. G-CSF (lenograstin) after chemotherapy for acute myeloid leukemia: a placebo controlled trial. *Blood* 1996;88:666a(abstr).

392. Goldstone AH, Bennett AK, Milligan DW, et al. Lack of benefit of G-CSF in complete remission and possible increase relapse risk in AML: an MRL study of 800 patients. *Blood* 1992:90(abstr).

393. Witz F, Harousseau JL, Sadoun A, et al. GM-CSF during and after remission induction treatment for elderly patients with acute myeloid leukemia (AML) *Hematol Blood Transfus* 1997;40:852.

394. Bhalla K, Holladay C, Arlin Z, et al. Treatment with interleukin-3 plus granulocyte-macrophage colony-stimulating factors improves the selectivity of Ara-C in vitro against acute myeloid leukemia blasts. *Blood* 1991;78:2674–2679.

395. Butturini A, Santucci MA, Gale RP, et al. GM-CSF incubation prior to treatment with cytarabine or doxorubicin enhances drug activity against AML cells in vitro: a model for leukemia chemotherapy. *Leuk Res* 1990;14:743–749.

396. Hiddemann W, Kiehl M, Zuhlsdorf M, et al. Granulocyte-macrophage colony-stimulating factor and interleukin-3 enhance the incorporation of cytosine arabinoside into the DNA of leukemic blasts and the cytotoxic effect on clonogenic cells from patients with acute myeloid leukemia. *Semin Oncol* 1992;19[2 Suppl 4]:31–37.

397. Reuter C, Auf der Landwehr U, Schleyer E, et al. Modulation of intracellular metabolism of cytosine arabinoside in acute myeloid leukemia by granulocyte-macrophage colony-stimulating factor. *Leukemia* 1994;8:217–225.

398. Smith MA, Singer CR, Pallister CJ, et al. The effect of haemopoietic growth factors on the cell cycle of AML progenitors and their sensitivity to cytosine arabinoside in vitro. *Br J Haematol* 1995;90:767–773.

399. Koistinen P, Wang C, Curtis JE, et al. Granulocyte-macrophage colony-stimulating factor and interleukin-3 protect leukemic blast cells from ara-C toxicity. *Leukemia* 1991;5:789–795.

400. Lotem J, Sachs L. Hematopoietic cytokines inhibit apoptosis induced by transforming growth factor beta 1 and cancer chemotherapy compounds in myeloid leukemic cells. *Blood* 1992;80:1750–1757.

401. Schiffer CA, Miller K, Larson RA, et al. A double-blind, placebo-controlled trial of pegylated recombinant human megakaryocyte growth and development factor as an adjunct to induction and consolidation therapy for patients with acute myeloid leukemia. *Blood* 2000;95:2530–2535.

402. Archimbaud E, Ottmann OG, Yin JA, et al. A randomized, double-blind, placebo-controlled study with pegylated recombinant human megakaryocyte growth and development factor (PEG-rHuMGDF) as an adjunct to chemotherapy for adults with de novo acute myeloid leukemia. *Blood* 1999;94:3694–3701.

403. Adams JA, Liu Yin JA, Brereton ML, et al. The in vitro effect of pegylated recombinant human megakaryocyte growth and development factor (PEG rHuMGDF) on megakaryopoiesis in normal subjects and patients with myelodysplasia and acute myeloid leukaemia. *Br J Haematol* 1997;99:139–146.

404. Larson RA, Dodge RK, Linker CA, et al. A randomized controlled trial of filgrastim during remission induction and consolidation chemotherapy for adults with acute lymphoblastic leukemia: CALGB study 9111. *Blood* 1998;92:1556–1564.

405. Geissler K, Kuller E, Hubmann E, et al. Granulocyte colony-stimulating factor as an adjunct to induction chemotherapy for adult acute lymphoblastic leukemia: a randomized phase III study. *Blood* 1997;90:590–596.

406. Schemer R, Geissler K, Kyrle PA, et al. Granulocyte colony-stimulating factor (G-CSF) as an adjunct to induction chemotherapy of adult acute lymphoblastic leukemia (ALL). *Ann Hematol* 1993;66:283–289.

407. Pettengell R, Gurney H, Radford JA, et al. Granulocyte colony-stimulating factor to prevent dose-limiting neutropenia in non-Hodgkin's lymphoma: a randomized controlled trial. *Blood* 1992;80:1430–1436.

408. Montardini S, Zagonel V, Barbara R, et al. Cost benefit of G-CSF administration in older patients (60-70 years) with non-Hodgkin's lymphoma (NHL) after combination chemotherapy. Fifth International Conference of Malignant Lymphoma; June 9-12, 1993; Lugano, Switzerland.

409. Gerhartz HH, Engelhard M, Meusers D, et al. Randomized, double-blind, placebo-controlled, phase III study of recombinant human granulocyte macrophage colony-stimulating factor as adjuvant to induction treatment of high-grade malignant non-Hodgkin's lymphomas. *Blood* 1992;82:2329–2339.

410. Engelhard M, Gerhartz H, Brittinger G, et al. Cytokine efficiency in the treatment of high-grade malignant non-Hodgkin's lymphomas: results of a randomized double-blind placebo-controlled study with intensified COP-BLAM +/- rhGM-CSF. *Ann Oncol* 1994;5 [Suppl 2]:123–125.

411. Patte C, Laplanche A, Bertozzi AI, et al. Granulocyte colony-stimulating factor in induction treatment of children with non-Hodgkin's lymphoma: a randomized study of the French Society of Pediatric Oncology. *J Clin Oncol* 2001;20:441–448.

412. Gordon LI, Anderson J, Habermann TH, et al. Phase I trial of dose escalation with growth factor support in patients with previously untreated diffuse aggressive lymphomas: determination of the maximum-tolerated dose of ProMACE-CytaBOM. *J Clin Oncol* 1996;14:1275–1281.

413. Schipp MA, Neuberg D, Janicek M, et al. High-dose CHOP as initial therapy for patients with poor-prognosis aggressive non-Hodgkin's lymphoma: a dose-finding pilot study. *J Clin Oncol* 1995;13:2916–2923.

414. Gordon LI, Young M, Weller E, et al. A phase II trial of 20,040 ProMACE-CytaBOM in patients with previously untreated aggressive lymphomas; analysis of response, toxicity and dose intensity. *Blood* 1999;94:3307–3314.

415. Dale DC, Liles WC, Price TH. Renewed interest in granulocyte transfusion therapy. *Br J Haematol* 1997;98:497–501.

416. Dignani MC, Anaissie EJ, Hester JP, et al. Treatment of neutropenia-related fungal infections with granulocyte colony-stimulating factor-elicited white blood cell transfusions: a pilot study. *Leukemia* 1997;11:1621–1630.

417. Neumaitis J, Shannon-Dorcy K, Appelbaum FE, et al. Long-term follow-up of patients with invasive fungal disease who received adjunctive therapy with recombinant human macrophage colony-stimulating. *Blood* 1993;82:1422–1427.

418. Winearls C, Oliver D, Pippard M, et al. Effect of human erythropoietin derived from recombinant DNA on the anemia of patients maintained on chronic hemodialysis. *Lancet* 1986;2:1175–1181.

419. Muirhead N. Erythropoietin is a cause of access thrombosis. *Semin Dial* 1993; 6:184–188.

420. Raine AE. Hypertension, blood viscosity, and cardiovascular morbidity in renal failure: implications of erythropoietin therapy. *Lancet* 1988;1:97–100.

421. Besarab A, Bolton WK, Browne JK, et al. The effects of normal as compared with low hematocrit values in patients with cardiac disease who are receiving hemodialysis and epoetin. *N Engl J Med* 1998;339:584–590.

422. Mayer G, Thum J, Cada EM, et al. Working capacity is increased following recombinant human erythropoietin treatment. *Kidney Int* 1988;34:525–528.

423. Evans RW, Rader B, Manninen DL. The quality of life of hemodialysis recipients treated with recombinant human erythropoietin. Cooperative Multicenter EPO Clinical Trial Group. *JAMA* 1990;263:825–830.

424. Canadian Erythropoietin Study Group. Association between recombinant human erythropoietin and quality of life and exercise capacity of patients receiving haemodialysis. *BMJ* 1990;300:573–578.

425. Means RT Jr. Clinical application of recombinant erythropoietin in the anemia of chronic disease. *Hematol Oncol Clin North Am* 1994;8:933–944.

426. Fischl M, Galpin JE, Levine JD, et al. Recombinant human erythropoietin for patients with AIDS treated with zidovudine. *N Engl J Med* 1990;322:1488–1493.

427. Spivak JL. Recombinant human erythropoietin and the anemia of cancer [Editorial]. *Blood* 1994;84:997–1004.

428. Henry DH, Abels RI. Recombinant human erythropoietin in the treatment of cancer and chemotherapy-induced anemia: results of double-blind and open-label follow-up studies. *Semin Oncol* 1994;21:21–28.

429. Demetri GD, Kris M, Wade J, et al. Quality-of-life benefit in chemotherapy patients treated with epoetin alfa is independent of disease response or tumor type: results from a prospective community oncology study. Procrit Study Group. *J Clin Oncol* 1998;16:3412–3425.

430. Matsumoto T, Endoh K, Kamisango K, et al. Effect of recombinant human erythropoietin on anticancer drug-induced anaemia. *Br J Haematol* 1990;75:463–468.

431. Bray GL, Reaman GH. Erythropoietin deficiency: a complication of cisplatin therapy and its treatment with recombinant human erythropoietin. *Am J Pediatr Hematol Oncol* 1991;13:426–430.

432. Markman M, Reichman B, Hakes T, et al. The use of recombinant human erythropoietin to prevent carboplatin-induced anemia. *Gynecol Oncol* 1993; 49:172–176.

433. Means RT Jr, Olsen NJ, Krantz SB, et al. Treatment of the anemia of rheumatoid arthritis with recombinant human erythropoietin: clinical and in vitro studies. *Arthritis Rheum* 1989;32:638–642.

434. Pincus T, Olsen NJ, Russell IJ, et al. Multicenter study of recombinant human erythropoietin in correction of anemia in rheumatoid arthritis. *Am J Med* 1990;89:161–168.

435. Murphy EA, Bell AL, Wojtulewski J, et al. Study of erythropoietin in treatment of anaemia in patients with rheumatoid arthritis. *BMJ* 1994;309:1337–1338.

436. Gabrilove JL, Cleeland CS, Livingston RB, et al. Clinical evaluation of once-weekly dosing of epoetin alpha in chemotherapy patients: improvements in hemoglobin and quality of life are similar to three-times-weekly dosing. *J Clin Oncol* 2001;19:2875–2882.

437. Bessho M, Jinnai I, Hirashima K, et al. Trilineage recovery by combination therapy with recombinant human granulocyte colony-stimulating factor and erythropoietin in patients with aplastic anemia and refractory anemia. *Stem Cells* 1994;12:604–615.

438. Ludwig H, Fritz E, Kotzmann H, et al. Erythropoietin treatment of anemia associated with multiple myeloma. *N Engl J Med* 1990; 322:1693–1699.

439. Barlogie B, Beck T. Recombinant human erythropoietin and the anemia of multiple myeloma. *Stem Cells* 1993;11:88–94.

440. Osterborg A, Boogaerts MA, Cimino R, et al. Recombinant human erythropoietin in transfusion-dependent anemic patients with multiple myeloma and non-Hodgkin's lymphoma—a randomized multicenter study. The European Study Group of Erythropoietin (Epoetin Beta) Treatment in Multiple Myeloma and Non-Hodgkin's Lymphoma. *Blood* 1996;87:2675–2682.

441. Dammacco F, Castoldi G, Rodjer S. Efficacy of epoetin alfa in the treatment of anaemia of multiple myeloma. *Br J Haematol* 2001;113:172–179.

442. Link H, Brune T, Hubner G, et al. Effect of recombinant human erythropoietin after allogenic bone marrow transplantation. *Ann Hematol* 1993;67:169–173.

443. Mitus AJ, Antin JH, Rutherford CJ, et al. Use of recombinant human erythropoietin in allogeneic bone marrow transplant donor/recipient pairs. *Blood* 1994;83:1952–1957.

444. Link H, Boogaerts MA, Fauser AA, et al. A controlled trial of recombinant human erythropoietin after bone marrow transplantation. *Blood* 1994;84:3327–3335.

445. Goodnough LT, Rudnick S, Price TH, et al. Increased preoperative collection of autologous blood with recombinant human erythropoietin therapy. *N Engl J Med* 1989;321:1163–1168.

446. Biesma DH, Kraaijenhagen RJ, Dalmulder J, et al. Recombinant human erythropoietin in autologous blood donors: a dose-finding study. *Br J Haematol* 1994;86:30–35.

447. Mercuriali F, Gualtieri G, Sinigaglia L, et al. Use of recombinant human erythropoietin to assist autologous blood donation by anemic rheumatoid arthritis patients undergoing major orthopedic surgery. *Transfusion* 1994;34:501–506.

448. Sowade O, Warnke H, Scigalla P, et al. Avoidance of allogeneic blood transfusions by treatment with epoetin beta (recombinant human erythropoietin) in patients undergoing open-heart surgery. *Blood* 97;89:411–418.

449. Canadian Orthopedic Perioperative Erythropoietin Study Group. Effectiveness of perioperative recombinant human erythropoietin in elective hip replacement. *Lancet* 1993;341:1227–1232.

450. Rutherford CJ, Schneider TJ, Dempsey H, et al. Efficacy of different dosing regimens for recombinant human erythropoietin in a simulated perisurgical setting: the importance of iron availability in optimizing response. *Am J Med* 1994;96:139–145.

451. Shannon KM, Naylor GS, Torkildson JC, et al. Circulating erythroid progenitors in the anemia of prematurity. *N Engl J Med* 1987;317:728–733.

452. Soubasi V, Kremenopoulos G, Diamandi E, et al. In which neonates does early recombinant human erythropoietin treatment prevent anemia of prematurity? Results of a randomized, controlled study. *Pediatr Res* 1993;34:675–679.

453. Meyer MP, Meyer JH, Commerford A, et al. Recombinant human erythropoietin in the treatment of the anemia of prematurity: results of a double-blind, placebo-controlled study. *Pediatrics* 1994;93:918–923.

454. Maier RF, Obladen M, Scigalla P, et al. The effect of Epoten beta (recombinant human erythropoietin) on the need for transfusion in very-low-birth-weight infants. *New Engl J Med* 1994;330:1173–1178.

455. Al-Khatti A, Veith RW, Papayannopoulou T, et al. Stimulation of fetal hemoglobin synthesis by erythropoietin in baboons. *N Engl J Med* 1987;317:415–420.

456. Al-Khatti A, Umemura T, Clow J, et al. Erythropoietin stimulates F-reticulocyte formation in sickle cell anemia. *Trans Assoc Am Physicians* 1988;101:54–59.

457. Goldberg MA, Brugnara C, Dover GJ, et al. Treatment of sickle cell anemia with hydroxyurea and erythropoietin. *N Engl J Med* 1990;323:366–372.

458. Rodgers GP, Dover GJ, Uyesaka N, et al. Augmentation by erythropoietin of fetal hemoglobin response to hydroxyurea in sickle cell patients. *N Engl J Med* 1993;328:73–79.

459. Nagel RL, Vichinsky E, Shah M, et al. F reticulocyte response in sickle cell anemia treated with recombinant human erythropoietin: a double-blind study. *Blood* 1993;81:9–14.

460. Rachmilewitz EA, Aker M. The role of recombinant human erythropoietin in the treatment of thalassemia. *Ann N Y Acad Sci* 1998;850:129–138.

461. Nisli G, Kavakli K, Aydinok Y, et al. Recombinant erythropoietin trial in children with transfusion-dependent homozygous beta-thalassemia. *Acta Haematol* 1997;98:199–203.

462. Kuter DJ, Goodnough LT, Romo J, et al. Thrombopoietin therapy increases platelet yields in healthy platelet donors. *Blood* 2001;98:1339–1345.

463. Goodnough LT, Kuter DJ, McCullough J, et al. Prophylactic platelet transfusions from healthy apheresis platelet donors undergoing treatment with thrombopoietin. *Blood* 2001;98:1346–1351.

464. Li J, Xia Y, Bertino A, et al. Characterization of an anti-thrombopoietin antibody that developed in a cancer patient following injection of PEG-rHuMGDF. *Blood* 1999;94:51a(abst).

465. Yang C, Xia Y, Li J, et al. The appearance of antithrombopoietin antibody and circulating thrombopoietin-IsG complexes in a patient developing thrombocytopenia after the injection of PEG-rHuMGDF. *Blood* 1999;94:681a(abst).

466. Bronchud MH, Scarffe JH, Thatcher N, et al. Phase I/II study of recombinant human granulocyte colony-stimulating factor in patients receiving intensive chemotherapy for small cell lung cancer. *Br J Cancer* 1987;56:809–813.

467. Gabrilove JL, Jakubowski A, Fain K, et al. Phase I study of granulocyte colony-stimulating factor in patients with transitional cell carcinoma of the urothelium. *J Clin Invest* 1988;82:1454–1461.

468. Gabrilove JL, Jakubowski A, Scher H, et al. Effect of granulocyte colony-stimulating factor on neutropenia and associated morbidity due to chemotherapy for transitional-cell carcinoma of the urothelium. *N Engl J Med* 1988; 318:1414–1422.

469. Crawford J, Ozer H, Stoller R, et al. Reduction by granulocyte colony-stimulating factor of fever and neutropenia induced by chemotherapy in patients with small-cell lung cancer. *N Engl J Med* 1991;325:164–170.

470. Trillet-Lenoir V, Green J, Manegold C, et al. Recombinant granulocyte colony stimulating factor reduces the infectious complications of cytotoxic chemotherapy. *Eur J Cancer* 1993;29A:319–324.

471. Gebbia V, Valenza R, Testa A, et al. A prospective randomized trial of thymopentin versus granulocyte-colony stimulating factor with or without thymopentin in the prevention of febrile episodes in cancer patients undergoing highly cytotoxic chemotherapy. *Anticancer Res* 1994;14:731–734.

472. Chevallier B, Chollet D, Merrouche Y, et al. Lenograstim prevents morbidity from intensive induction chemotherapy in the treatment of inflammatory breast-cancer. *J Clin Oncol* 1995;13:1564–1571.

473. Michon JM, Harmann O, Bouffet E, et al. An open-label multicentre, randomized phase II study or recombinant human granulocyte colony-stimulating factor (filgrastim) as an adjunct to combination chemotherapy in pediatric patients with metastatic neuroblastoma. *Eur J Cancer* 1998;34:1063–1069.

474. Crawford J, Tomita DK, Mazanet R, et al. Reduction of oral mucositis by filgrastim (r-metHuG-CSF) in patients receiving chemotherapy. *Cytokines Cell Mol Ther* 1999;5:187–193.

475. Lieschke GJ, Maher D, Cebon J, et al. Effects of bacterially synthesized recombinant human granulocyte-macrophage colony-stimulating factor in patients with advanced malignancy. *Ann Intern Med* 1989;110:357–364.

476. Hamm J, Schiller JH, Cuffie C, et al. Dose-ranging study of recombinant human granulocyte-macrophage colony-stimulating factor in small-cell lung carcinoma. *J Clin Oncol* 1994;12:2667–2676.

477. Yau JC, Neidhart JA, Triozzi P, et al. Randomized placebo-controlled trial of granulocyte-macrophage colony-stimulating-factor support for dose-intensive cyclophosphamide, etoposide, and cisplatin. *Am J Hematol* 1996;51:289–295.

478. Bunn PA Jr, Crowley J, Kelly K, et al. Chemoradiotherapy with or without granulocyte-macrophage colony-stimulating factor in the treatment of limited-stage small-cell lung cancer: a prospective phase III randomized study of the Southwest Oncology Group. *J Clin Oncol* 1995;13:1632–1641.

479. Jones SE, Schottstaedt MW, Duncan LA, et al. Randomized double-blind prospective trial to evaluate the effects of sargramostim versus placebo in a moderate-dose fluorouracil, doxorubicin, and cyclophosphamide adjuvant chemotherapy program for stage II and III breast cancer. *J Clin Oncol* 1996; 11:2976–2983.

480. Vellenga E, Uyl-de Groot CA, de Wit R, et al. Randomized placebo-controlled trial of granulocyte-macrophage colony-stimulating factor in patients with chemotherapy-related febrile neutropenia. *J Clin Oncol* 1996;2:619–627.

481. Bui BN, Chevallier B, Chevreau C, et al. Efficacy of lenograstim on hematologic tolerance to MAID chemotherapy in patients with advanced soft tissue sarcoma and consequences on treatment dose-intensity. *J Clin Oncol* 1995; 10:2629–2636.

482. Lyman GH, Kuderer NM, Greene J, et al. The economics of febrile neutropenia: implications for the use of the colony-stimulating factors. *Eur J Cancer* 1998;34:1857–1864.

483. Bennett CL, Stinson TJ, Laver JH, et al. Cost analyses of adjunct colony stimulating factors for acute leukemia: can they improve clinical decision making. *Leuk Lymphoma* 2000;37:65–70.

484. Bennett CL, Stinson TJ, Tallman MS, et al. Economic analysis of a randomized placebo-controlled phase III study of granulocyte macrophage colony stimulating factor in adult patients with acute myelogenous leukemia. *Ann Oncol* 1999;10:177–182.

485. Lu ZJ, Luo R, Erder H, et al. Cost impact of filgrastim as an adjunct to chemotherapy for patients with acute myeloid leukemia. Proceedings of the American Society of Hematology 1996:826a.

486. Bennett CL, Hynes DM, Godwin JE. Economic analysis of granulocyte colony-stimulating factor as adjunct therapy for older patients with AML: estimates from a Southwest Oncology Group clinical trial. *Cancer Invest* 2001; 19:603–610.

487. Bassan R, Lerede T, Di Bona E, et al. Granulocyte colony-stimulating factor after or during an intensive remission induction therapy for adult acute lymphoblastic leukemia: effects, role of patient pretreatment characteristics, and costs. *Leuk Lymphoma* 1997;26:153–161.

488. Uyl-de-Groot CA, Lowenberg B, Vellenga E, et al. Cost-effectiveness and quality-of-life assessment of GM-CSF as an adjunct to intensive remission

induction chemotherapy in elderly patients with acute myeloid leukemia. *Br J Haematol* 1998;100:629–636.

489. Pui CH, Boyett JM, Hughes WT, et al. Human granulocyte colony stimulating factor after induction chemotherapy in children with acute lymphoblastic leukemia. *N Engl J Med* 1997;336:1781–1787.

490. Bennett CL, Stinson TJ, Lane D, et al. Cost analysis for the prevention of neutropenia in pediatric T-cell leukemia and advanced lymphoblastic lymphoma: a case for prospective economic analysis in cooperative group trials. *Med Pediatr Oncol* 2000;34:92–96.

491. Gulati SC, Bennett CL. Granulocyte-macrophage colony-stimulating factor (GM-CSF) as adjunct therapy in relapsed Hodgkin disease. *Ann Intern Med* 1992;116:177–182.

492. Souetre E, Qing W, Penelaud PF. Economic analysis of the use of recombinant human granulocyte colony stimulating factor in autologous bone marrow transplantation. *Eur J Cancer* 1996;32A:1162–1165.

493. Dranitsaris G, Sutcliffe SB. Economic analysis of prophylactic G-CSF after Mini-BEAM salvage chemotherapy for Hodgkin's and non-Hodgkin's lymphoma. *Leuk Lymphoma* 1995;17:139–145.

494. Lee SM, Radford JA, Dobson L, et al. Recombinant human granulocyte colony-stimulating factor (filgrastim) following high-dose chemotherapy and peripheral blood progenitor cell rescue in high-grade non-Hodgkin's lymphoma: clinical benefits at no extra cost. *Br J Cancer* 1998;77:1294–1299.

495. Rubino C, Laplanche A, Patte C, et al. Cost-minimization analysis of prophylactic granulocyte colony-stimulating factor after induction chemotherapy in children with non-Hodgkin's lymphoma. *J Natl Cancer Inst* 1998;90:750–755.

496. McQuaker IG, Hunter AE, Pacey S, et al. Low dose filgrastim significantly enhances neutrophil recovery following autologous peripheral blood stem cell transplantation in patients with lymphoproliferative disorders: evidence for clinical and economic benefit. *J Clin Oncol* 1997;15:451–457.

497. Klumpp TR, Sullivan EM, Ackerman SJ, et al. Cost analysis of a randomized trial comparing G-CSF to standard supportive care following PBSC transplantation. *Blood* 1998;92:131a(abst).

498. Stinson TJ, Adams JR, Bishop MR, et al. Economic analysis of a phase III study of G-CSF versus placebo following allogeneic blood stem cell transplantation. *Bone Marrow Transplant* 2000;26:663–666.

499. Ozer H, Armitage JO, Bennett CL, et al. 2000 update of recommendations for the use of hematopoietic colony-stimulating factors: evidence-based, clinical practice guidelines. *J Clin Oncol* 2000;18:3558–3585.

500. American Society of Clinical Oncology. American Society of Clinical Oncology recommendations for the use of hematopoietic colony-stimulating factors: evidence-based clinical practice guidelines. *J Clin Oncol* 1994;12:2471–2508.

501. American Society of Clinical Oncology. Update of recommendations for the use of hematopoietic colony-stimulating factors: evidence-based clinical practice guidelines. *J Clin Oncol* 1996;14:1957–1960.

502. Bennett CL, Weeks JA, Somerfield MR, et al. Use of hematopoietic colony-stimulating factors: comparison of the 1994 and 1997 American Society of Clinical Oncology surveys regarding ASCO clinical guidelines. *J Clin Oncol* 1999;17:3676–3681.

503. Ozer H, Armitage JO, Bennett CL, et al. 2000 update of recommendations for the use of hematopoietic colony-stimulating factors: evidence-based, clinical practice guidelines. *J Clin Oncol* 2000;18:355–385.

CHAPTER 59

Clinical Pharmacology of Anticancer Drugs

Jeffrey G. Supko, Thomas A. Puchalski,
Hamza Mujagic, Andrew X. Zhu, and Bruce A. Chabner

The practicing hematologist in the twenty-first century has inherited a rich legacy of fruitful research on the treatment of hematopoietic malignancies. Many of the initial human studies with experimental chemotherapy involved patients with lymphoma or leukemia (1,2). The first successful attempts to treat cancer with drugs were performed at Yale University in 1942 by Louis Goodman and colleagues. The response of a patient with Hodgkin's disease to treatment with nitrogen mustard marked the beginning of the modern era of chemotherapy (1). Subsequently, antifolates were first used by Sidney Farber, a pathologist at Harvard University, for the treatment of pediatric patients with acute lymphocytic leukemia (ALL) in 1948 (2). During the following 10 years, the first curative regimens using combination chemotherapy were developed for this same disease by Frei, Holland, and Freireich at the U.S. National Cancer Institute (3). Other significant innovations by hematologists have enhanced the effectiveness of cancer treatment, including, most notably, bone marrow and stem cell transplantation with high-dose chemotherapy. Most recently, the concept of molecularly targeted drug development, in which compounds are designed to block a specific molecular mutation associated with cancer, has achieved its first success in the remarkable clinical trials of imatinib performed by Druker and colleagues in patients with chronic myelogenous leukemia (CML) (4). Thus, the leukemias and lymphomas have provided fertile ground for the development of basic concepts as well as specific drugs for cancer treatment.

The current practice of hematology obligates the active clinician to understand how to use these drugs safely and effectively. With rare exception, hematologists in clinical practice or those based in academic centers use cytotoxic drugs to manage patients with a variety of chronic leukemias and even disorders of erythropoiesis. Many also treat patients with acute leukemias and lymphomas for which chemotherapy regimens are more complex and potentially more toxic. Thus, it is incumbent on the hematologist to know a great deal about these drugs, specifically (a) their spectrum of activity, (b) mechanisms of action, (c) toxicity profiles, and (d) the clinical circumstances that may result in interactions with other drugs leading to unexpected side effects. An understanding of the pharmacokinetics of anticancer drugs, the physiologic factors that govern changes in the concentration of a drug in the bloodstream over time, is also an essential component of the clinical knowledge that the hematologist brings to the bedside. In this chapter, we present an overview of the essential information needed by the clinician to treat hematologic disorders. We also provide an introduction to the new molecularly targeted drugs that are likely to have an impact on the treatment of hematologic malignancies in the near future. The reader is referred to other texts for more basic or comprehensive information, as may be required, for purposes of research or protocol development (5,6).

PRINCIPLES OF CHEMOTHERAPY

The basic goals of chemotherapy are to prolong survival and ameliorate symptoms in patients with cancer. To do so, the clinician must balance the potential of therapeutic modalities to eradicate cancer cells against the potential for toxicity to normal organs. The initial consideration in choosing a particular chemotherapy regimen is the effectiveness of inducing cell death or otherwise inhibiting the proliferation of the malignancy and extending survival of the patient. However, cytotoxic anticancer drugs are, almost without exception, damaging to normal tissues as well. As a consequence, the treatment regimen, which consists of the drugs, the dosages at which they are given, and their frequency of administration, must be carefully designed to take these adverse effects into consideration. Although myelosuppression, denudation of the oral and intestinal epithelium, and suppression of the immune system are particularly common toxicities of anticancer agents, virtually all other organs have suffered damage from various members of this class of drugs. Many of these toxicities, such as chronic pulmonary or cardiac dysfunction, neurologic toxicity, or renal failure, only appear after long-term or continuous use. Accordingly, these risk factors must always be taken into account in making the decision to use chemotherapy, whereas the selection of the most appropriate agents and adjustment of the dosing regimen are made on the basis of the particular clinical circumstances. Thus, for example, a patient with underlying cardiac disease is likely not to be a suitable candidate for anthracycline therapy, whereas high-dose methotrexate (MTX) is not tolerated by a patient presenting with hypertension and chronic renal failure.

Targets for Chemotherapeutic Agents

The initial search for anticancer drugs involved an empiric screen against rapidly proliferating murine leukemias. Not surprisingly, alkylating agents that kill rapidly dividing cells by chemically attacking electron-rich sites of DNA were the first clinically effective compounds discovered in this manner. Subsequently, a series of molecules that cured experimental tumors by several different mechanisms of action were identified. Antimetabolites such as MTX function by inhibiting the synthesis of DNA precursor molecules. The cytotoxic effects of the anthracyclines and campto-thecins result from the formation of breaks in the DNA double helix by inhibiting the strand-resealing function of the topoisomerase enzymes. Vinca alkaloids and taxanes act by modulating the organization or segregation of chromosomes during mitosis. Thus, proliferation, cell division, and DNA itself represented the initial targets for most cytotoxic anticancer drugs.

More recently, with the dramatic expansion of knowledge about the biologic basis for malignancy and the identification of key mutations leading to neoplastic cellular transformation, promising new targets for cancer treatment have emerged (7). It is now clear that cells become malignant through mutations that confer a number of advantageous properties, such as (a) continuous proliferation signals from mutated growth factor pathways, (b) defects in DNA repair mechanisms that permit a greatly enhanced rate of mutation, (c) stimulation of angiogenesis, (d) enhanced capacity for invasion and metastasis, (e) defective cell death (i.e., apoptosis) pathways, and (f) defective monitoring of DNA integrity through cell cycle checkpoint mutations. These defects may appear either as somatic mutations or in familial cancer syndromes. Most forms of human cancer, including hematologic malignancies, may acquire multiple mutations in the course of the transformation process. In some cases, specific chromosomal defects have been associated with a particular disease type with continued proliferation of the transformed cells dependent on the presence of the defect. For example, the bcr-abl translocation of CML represents an essential and constant mutation and, thus, an ideal molecular target for drug discovery (7). Imatinib, as is described in the section Tyrosine Kinase Inhibition, is a compound that was identified by screening for inhibitors of the tyrosine kinase activated by the CML translocation. Consistent responses with little toxicity to normal tissue were demonstrated in early clinical trials of the drug (8).

There are many other chromosomal translocations and molecular defects associated with both leukemias and solid tumors that represent attractive targets for therapeutic interventions with the potential for greater specificity and less host toxicity than the traditional targets of cytotoxic chemotherapeutic drugs. The potential offered by this molecular-targeted approach has generated considerable interest in identifying readily synthesized small molecules that are signaling and receptor inhibitors, monoclonal antibodies that inhibit cell-surface receptors, antisense oligonucleotides that cause degradation of cellular RNAs, as well as synthetic peptides. In addition to inhibiting tumor proliferation by their direct effect on the targeted pathway, these new molecules may also enhance the effectiveness of chemotherapy and radiotherapy by lowering the cellular threshold for apoptosis. As documented in the discussion of some of these newer agents, it is abundantly clear that the nature of cancer chemotherapy is undergoing a radical change. Will it be possible to identify effective new drugs directed at the myriad translocations and mutations that underlie the various forms of acute leukemia, lymphoma, and the solid tumors? Tremendous advances in the drug discovery process, facilitated by the efficient screening techniques against molecular targets and combinatorial chemistry, lead us to suggest that this question may be answered affirmatively.

Dosing Regimen Design

The guiding principles for designing dosing regimens of cytotoxic chemotherapeutic agents are based on the classic experiments performed by Skipper, Schabel, and colleagues, who characterized the growth kinetics of leukemias and solid tumors in mice and their response to treatment with cytotoxic anticancer drugs (9). It was observed that a constant fraction of the pretreatment tumor cell population was killed after each dose of chemotherapy, with the magnitude of the fractional cell kill dependent on the effectiveness of the particular agent, followed by tumor regrowth during the interval between successive treatments. Models of this process revealed that a curative response to treatment required reducing the tumor cell population to less than a single cell. Typically, the tumor cell burden is at least 10^9 cells by the time that a malignancy first becomes clinically apparent; therefore, repetitive cycles of treatment with an anticancer agent are required to achieve a cure, as even the most effective drugs only reduce the number of cancer cells by 2 logs or less after each treatment.

In general, antimetabolites and other drugs that function by inhibiting DNA synthesis are most effective against rapidly growing tumors such as leukemias and lymphomas. Slower-growing solid tumors are less responsive to these agents and are more effectively treated with drugs that attack the integrity of DNA, through the creation of breaks or covalent adducts, irrespective of the cell cycle position. Double-strand breaks in DNA are induced by drugs such as doxorubicin and etoposide that inhibit the nuclear enzyme topoisomerase IIα, whereas adducts are formed by alkylating agents, typified by the nitrogen mustards, chloroethylnitrosoureas (CENUs), and platinum derivatives. Regardless of the specific manner by which DNA is modulated by these agents, the critical determinant of cell kill is ultimately the production of sufficient DNA damage to trigger apoptosis, or programmed cell death—a process initiated by the recognition of that damage by p53 and other so-called gatekeeper molecules that monitor DNA integrity. Accordingly, cells lacking the wild-type p53 protein tend to be broadly resistant to chemotherapy.

Ultimately, the choice of drugs for treating specific tumor types depends on demonstrating single-agent activity in clinical trials, and it has often been found that experience defies logic. Thus, antimetabolites such as 5-fluorouracil (5-FU) and gemcitabine are quite useful for the treatment of several slowly-growing solid tumors. The effectiveness of gemcitabine against solid tumors probably results from the relatively long persistence of its pharmacologically active phosphorylated metabolites within tumor cells (10).

As previously discussed, multiple cycles of treatment with a cytotoxic anticancer drug are required to cure even the most responsive malignancies. In the adjuvant setting, after initial cytoreduction with surgery or radiation therapy, the residual tumor cell population may be somewhat less than 1 billion cells. Nevertheless, therapeutic regimens comprised of a single drug or even single cycles of multiagent chemotherapy are curative in only the rarest of circumstances, as exemplified by the treatment of choriocarcinoma with MTX or Burkitt lymphoma with cyclophosphamide. Additional considerations involved in the design of therapeutic dosing regimens include the following:

1. Tumor cell kill is proportional to each administered dose of a cytotoxic drug, as well as *dose intensity*, defined as the amount of drug delivered per unit time during the course of therapy. A linear relationship between the administered dose and cell kill has best been demonstrated for alkylating agents. Moreover, high-dose therapy with antimetabolites, such as MTX and cytarabine, has improved the cure rate for some forms of leukemia, probably through improved drug uptake by drug-resistant cells. Thus, most curative regimens attempt to maximize the dose administered during each cycle of therapy and to give repeated cycles within the shortest possible time.

2. Single-agent therapy presents the most favorable setting for the selection of cancer cells with drug-resistant phenotypes. Accordingly, multiagent therapy with two or more anticancer drugs, each of which is active against the tumor in question, with different mechanisms of action and resistance, enhances that probability of success. Most curative regimens use drug combinations as initial therapy, and those directed against leukemias may comprise six or more agents.

3. Combination regimens should also be designed to minimize overlapping drug toxicities and unfavorable drug interactions. A thorough knowledge of the pharmacology of the individual agents is, therefore, critical to the rational design and optimization of multiagent chemotherapy regimens.

Molecular, enzymatic, and cell kinetic markers should be determined whenever possible to facilitate the identification of malignancies that require special therapeutic approaches. For example, poor responsiveness to chemotherapy has been associated with the multidrug resistance (MDR) phenotype in myeloid leukemias, including stem cell leukemias, blastic crisis, and secondary acute myelogenous leukemia (AML). The MDR gene product, P-glycoprotein, belongs to the superfamily of adenosine triphosphate–binding cassette transmembrane transport. It functions as a drug efflux pump for many important cytotoxic natural products, such as the vinca alkaloids, epipodophyllotoxins, anthracyclines, and taxanes, thereby rendering cancer cells resistant to these compounds (11). As a second example, the expression of steroid receptors on cancer cells determines the effectiveness of hormone antagonists such as the antiestrogens. Immunophenotyping and cytogenetic studies are often helpful in clarifying the cell of origin and for directing the choice of therapy for acute leukemias. In the future, as targeted therapies become approved for clinical use, molecular profiling of the genes and proteins of interest will undoubtedly play an important role in the selection of drugs for many forms of cancer.

CLINICAL PHARMACOKINETICS

It has become generally accepted that the biologic effects of a drug are related, in some manner, to the time course of the concentration of the administered compound or an active metabolite in the bloodstream. The realization of this association has evolved as advances have been made in the discipline of *pharmacokinetics*, broadly defined as the study of rate processes involved in the absorption of a drug from the administration site into the bloodstream, its subsequent distribution to extravascular regions throughout the body, and its eventual elimination from the body. *Drug disposition* is the term that specifically pertains to the processes associated with distribution and elimination. From a broader perspective, pharmacokinetics may be thought of as the effect that the body has on a drug, whereas the pharmacologic effects that a drug has on the body are the realm of pharmacodynamics.

Studies to characterize the pharmacokinetic behavior of a drug have become integral to the preclinical and clinical development of new anticancer agents. Some of the usual objectives for undertaking a pharmacokinetic study in the context of a phase I or II clinical trial in cancer patients are (a) initial characterization of the pharmacokinetic behavior of new chemotherapeutic agents in humans; (b) assessing whether an administration schedule provides a potentially effective pattern of systemic exposure to a drug; (c) determining the magnitude of intra- and interpatient variability in pharmacokinetic parameters; (d) assessing the influence of patient characteristics on drug disposition; (e) establishing predictive correlations between biologic effects and pharmacokinetic parameters; and (f) determining whether combining drugs results in pharmacokinetic interactions. In addition, pharmacokinetic drug level monitoring has been used to improve therapy through dose individualization, to evaluate patient compliance during chronic therapy, and to assess whether alterations in drug disposition or metabolism are associated with the development of toxicity or lack of effect.

A complete understanding of the actions of a drug necessarily requires discerning the nature of the association between its pharmacokinetic behavior and pharmacodynamic effects. Relationships between pharmacokinetics and the severity of toxicity have been established for many anticancer drugs. However, pharmacokinetic associations accounting for the therapeutic effects of a chemotherapeutic agent are more difficult to establish due to the multiplicity of factors involving the host and tumor that influence response, as well as the time lapse from initiating treatment to the first indications of a therapeutic response. Nevertheless, elucidating the pharmacokinetic behavior of an anticancer drug may benefit efforts to determine the dose, route of administration, and schedule that maximizes the potential for therapeutic effectiveness while minimizing the likelihood of serious toxic effects.

The intention of this section is to provide readers with a fundamental understanding of clinical pharmacokinetics and its practical application to the development and use of chemotherapy in the context of hematologic malignancies. Numerous texts with widely varying levels of complexity and focus are available for those interested in a more comprehensive discourse of the subject, ranging from easily understood introductions to the discipline (12) to more advanced texts with a mathematic approach (13).

Sample Collection and Analysis

Pharmacokinetic studies involve collecting serial specimens of blood and other biologic fluids, such as urine, at predetermined time intervals from subjects after the administration of the drug. The timing, frequency, and duration of blood sample collection are governed by a host of factors, including the extent of information available from prior pharmacokinetic studies of the drug, the route and schedule of administration, the expected rapidity of decline in drug concentrations, the sensitivity of the analytic method, the inconvenience to the patient, and the limitations on the total volume of blood that can be safely withdrawn (14). Plasma is the blood component in which drugs are most commonly measured during pharmacokinetic studies, although determinations are also made in serum and, less frequently, whole blood.

The concentration of drug present in the study samples is measured using an appropriate bioanalytic method. Review articles surveying the current techniques used for assaying drugs in biologic fluids regularly appear in the literature (15). It is important to recognize that the quality of data derived from any pharmacokinetic study ultimately depends on the reliability of the assay used to measure the drug, as well as the manner in which samples were processed and stored before analysis. Validating an assay for use in a pharmacokinetic study entails documenting the selectivity, specificity, accuracy, and precision of the method for measuring the drug within a defined range of concentrations in a particular matrix. In addition, drug stability in the biologic fluids of interest should be evaluated at various temperatures to establish appropriate conditions for sample storage (16). Selectivity and specificity are related to the ability of an assay to measure the drug without interference from products of its biotransformation or degradation, endogenous molecules, and any other compounds that may be present in the sample, such as supportive medications or substances administered to or consumed by the subjects. Accuracy and precision are indicators of the error associated with measuring a compound at a particular concentration in terms of closeness to the true sample concentration and the reproducibility of repeated determinations, respectively. Thus, for example, if the concentration of drug in the plasma of a patient decays below the lowest concentration that can be measured with acceptable accuracy and precision before the terminal phase in the concentration-time profile has been established, reported values related to the terminal phase, such as the biological half-life of the drug, are suspect at best.

The majority of bioanalytic methods used for pharmacokinetic studies measure the total concentration of drug—that is, free drug plus drug that is reversibly associated with plasma proteins. However, the reversible binding of a drug to plasma proteins, such as albumin and α_1-acid glycoprotein, has numerous implications that may be important to understand for effective therapeutic application of the agent (17). Protein binding can dramatically influence the distribution and rate of elimination of a drug from the body. Furthermore, protein binding can profoundly restrict the concentration of biologically active free drug achieved at the site of action. Protein binding is usually assessed experimentally by ultrafiltration or equilibrium dialysis after adding a drug to donor plasma at a clinically relevant range of concentrations (17).

Plasma Concentration-Time Profile

Regardless of the route of administration, the plasma profile of any drug exhibits an initial region of increasing concentration and the achievement of a peak or maximum concentration (C_{max}), which is followed by a continual decline in concentration (Fig. 59-1A). The concentration of drug in plasma increases as long as the rate of input into systemic circulation exceeds the rate of loss due to distribution into other extracellular fluids, intracellular spaces, and tissues throughout the body and the rate of elimination from the body. The C_{max} is achieved when the rate of drug input is equivalent to the rate of loss from plasma, which occurs at the instant that an intravenous (i.v.) injection or infusion is terminated. When giving a drug by bolus i.v. injection, the observed plasma profile usually does not show a region of increasing drug concentration, because it is not feasible or even meaningful to collect a blood specimen until 1 to 2 minutes after completing the injection to allow several circulation times to elapse. Alternately, during a continuous i.v. infusion, plasma levels of the drug increase at a progressively decreasing rate and eventually become constant, which is indicative of achieving steady-state conditions, if the infusion is continued for a sufficiently long time.

The same plasma concentration-time profile that has been plotted on graphs with semilog axes in Figure 59-1A is also depicted on a graph with rectangular coordinate axes in Figure 59-1B. Presenting pharmacokinetic drug concentration-time profiles on semilog graphs provides a better visual depiction of the entire data set than a coordinate plot, because plasma levels of a drug frequently differ by several orders of magnitude during the course of the observation period. Furthermore, the concentration of many drugs in systemic circulation decays in an apparent first-order manner, exemplified by a terminal region in the plasma profile where the logarithm of the drug concentration is a linear function of time. Thus, a semilog plot provides some direct inferences regarding the nature of the pharmacokinetic behavior of a drug.

The pattern of decay in the plasma concentration of a drug that exhibits first-order kinetics is comprised of one or more exponential phases. Drug disposition is commonly described as mono-, bi-, or triexponential, based on the apparent number of log-linear decay phases. However, it is not always possible to

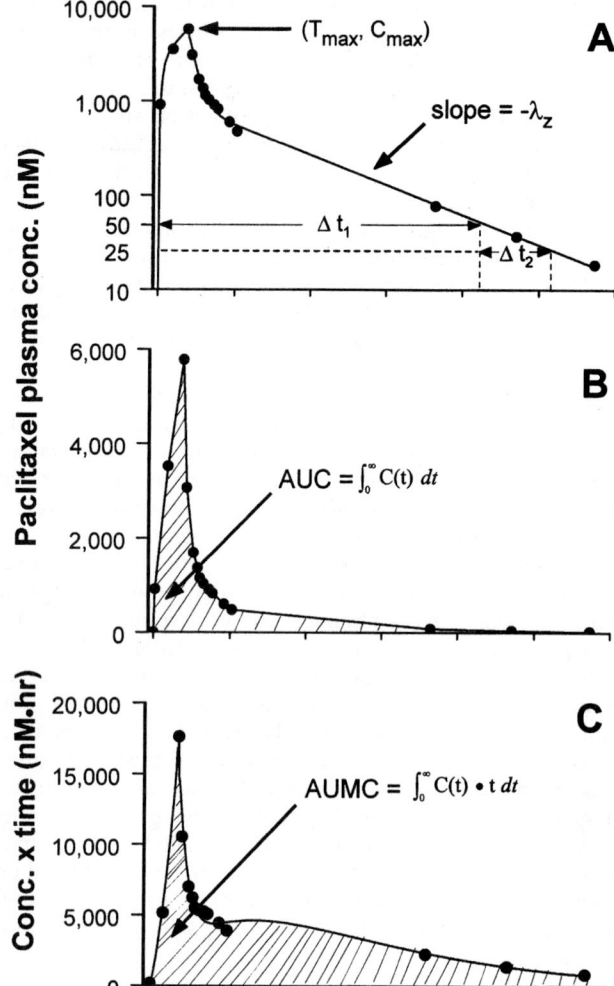

Figure 59-1. Presentation and analysis of a plasma concentration (conc.)-time profile for an anticancer agent administered as a 3-hour continuous intravenous infusion. **A:** Experimental data (*points*) and best-fit curve determined by fitting the data to a biexponential equation (*solid line*) presented on a graph with log-linear axes. This figure depicts several pharmacokinetic variables that can be readily estimated, including the maximum drug concentration (C_{max}), the time at which the peak concentration occurs (T_{max}), and the duration of time that drug levels exceeded an arbitrary threshold concentration of 50 nM (Δt_1). The biological half-life can be visually estimated as the time for drug levels to decrease by 50% at any time during the terminal log-linear phase of the plasma profile (Δt_2), the slope of which is $-\lambda_z$. **B:** Presentation of the same data shown in the upper panel on rectangular coordinate axes. The shaded area corresponds to the area under the curve (AUC) from time zero to infinity. **C:** Illustration of the first moment curve for this same data set. The shaded area corresponds to the area under the first moment curve (AUMC). Estimation of the AUC and AUMC is necessary to calculate the principal pharmacokinetic parameters, which include the total body clearance, apparent volumes of distribution, and mean residence time.

discern the number of disposition phases in a plasma profile simply by visual inspection. In the case of a plasma profile with drug concentrations that decline in a single log-linear phase, the entire body appears to be kinetically homogeneous, with equilibrium of the drug between plasma and other fluids or tissues into which it distributes being very rapidly achieved, before the first blood specimen has been acquired. Polyexponential behavior results from distinguishable differences in the reversible transfer of drug from plasma to various regions or compartments of the body. Thus, for example, the presence of two exponential decay phases implies that the body behaves as if it is composed of two kinetically distinct compartments, comprising plasma and tissues with which equilibrium is rapidly established and a second compartment comprising all other regions of the body into which drug distributes more slowly.

In the plasma profile of a drug given by rapid i.v. injection, the initial phase with the most rapid rate of decay is often referred to as the α-*phase*, and the disposition phases with successively slower rates of decay are the β-*phase* followed by the γ-*phase*. This nomenclature originated during the early theoretic development of compartmental pharmacokinetic analysis, an approach that involves deriving rate equations from models consisting of reversibly associated compartments for each exponential phase observed in a plasma profile (18). Designating the initial rapid and slower terminal exponential phases of drug decay as the *distribution* and *elimination phases*, respectively, which are terms often encountered in the literature, is misleading because drug levels decline in plasma due to the combined result of distribution and elimination, which are processes that occur continually at all times after drug administration. Recently, there has been a growing trend toward analyzing pharmacokinetic data by empiric approaches that consider only the concentration of drug in the sampled fluid and require no assumptions. In these techniques, which include model-independent analysis and noncompartmental analysis, the various exponential decay phases are usually referred to simply as the *initial*, *intermediate*, and *terminal disposition phases*.

Pharmacokinetic Parameters and Associated Variables

Model-independent analysis involves identifying the empiric polyexponential equation that best describes the time course of the drug concentration in plasma, either by a curve-stripping technique or a nonlinear regression analysis (19). Values of the coefficients and rate constants in the resulting best-fit equation may be used to calculate descriptive parameters that quantify the rapidity with which the drug is removed from the body and the extent to which it distributes from plasma into other regions of the body. Values for most of these descriptive pharmacokinetic variables can also be estimated by noncompartmental analysis (20). This is a technique based on first-moment theory, which is an area of mathematics that was previously well established in chemical and electronics engineering and was first applied to pharmacokinetic analysis approximately 25 years ago (20,21). Noncompartmental analysis is considerably simpler than any equation-defining method, because all calculations and data manipulations can be performed by most spreadsheet software programs. The observed plasma concentration-time data are numerically integrated, most commonly by the trapezoidal method, to estimate the area under the curve (AUC), which is an important measure of systemic drug exposure. In its simplest application, each successive set of data points, beginning with the origin (0, 0), is used to define a trapezoid with the y-axis as its base, the area of which is readily calculated. The cumulative sum of the areas of all such trapezoids affords an approximate value of the area under the plasma concentration-time curve to the last sample with a measurable drug concentration ($AUC_{0 \to t}$). The slope of the terminal log-linear phase ($-\lambda_z$) is determined by the linear regression of the logarithmic values of the observed plasma concentration-time data. The AUC from time zero to infinity is given by the following equation:

$$AUC \approx AUC_{0 \to t} + C_t/\lambda_z$$

where C_t is the plasma concentration of drug in the last sample acquired. With reference to the shaded area in Figure 59-1B,

which depicts the true AUC, it should be evident that the accuracy for numerically estimating the AUC is directly related to the number of samples and the times at which they are acquired. The area under the first-moment curve from time zero to infinity (AUMC), a variable used for calculating several pharmacokinetic parameters, is estimated in an analogous manner after multiplying each concentration value by the corresponding sample time (Fig. 59-1C).

CLEARANCE
The *total body clearance* (CL) of a drug is formally defined as the volume of plasma from which the drug is completely removed per unit time. It is readily calculated as

$$CL = D_{i.v.}/AUC$$

where $D_{i.v.}$ is the dose of the drug given by i.v. injection or infusion. CL reflects the combined contribution of all processes by which the drug is removed from the body, as represented by the following equation:

$$CL = CL_R + CL_{NR}$$

where CL_R and CL_{NR} designate renal and nonrenal clearance, respectively (22). CL_R is usually the only route of drug elimination that can be directly and quantitatively determined in patients by noninvasive procedures. All other mechanisms of drug elimination that cannot be readily estimated—including biliary excretion of unchanged drug, metabolism, nonenzymatic irreversible reactions with endogenous molecules, and spontaneous chemical degradation—are grouped together as CL_{NR}. CL has units of volume/time (e.g., mL/minute; L/hour) and is frequently normalized to the body weight or body surface area of subjects (e.g., mL/minute/kg; L/hour/m²) under the presumption of minimizing interpatient variability in the magnitude of the parameter. CL values are often compared to glomerular filtration rate and hepatic blood flow, the average values of which are approximately 125 mL/minute (4.6 L/hour/m²) and 1500 mL/minute (56 L/hour/m²), respectively, in normal adults (23,24). Although often informative, these comparisons can be extremely misleading unless the extent of plasma protein binding has been taken into account, because only the free fraction of drug that is not bound to plasma proteins is subject to organ-mediated excretion or metabolism.

APPARENT VOLUMES OF DISTRIBUTION
The *total body apparent volume of distribution*, V_z, is strictly a proportionality constant that equates the total amount of drug in the body (A) to its plasma concentration (C) only during the terminal disposition phase:

$$A = C \bullet V_z$$

It may be calculated by the equation

$$V_z = CL/\lambda_z$$

and has units of volume typically expressed in terms of milliliters or liters normalized to body weight or body surface area (e.g., mL/kg; L/m²). V_z is designated as an apparent volume because it is a hypothetic value that is not directly related to any real physiologic space. Nevertheless, it is an extremely informative parameter, providing an indication of the relative extent of drug distribution from plasma.

The magnitude of V_z is dependent on the relative affinities of the drug for accumulation in peripheral tissue regions and binding to plasma proteins. That is, for a given amount of drug in the body, the fraction present in plasma decreases as its distribution into peripheral tissues increases, leading to greater values of V_z (25). Reversible binding to plasma proteins can affect

V_z by limiting the amount of drug available for distribution to peripheral tissues. Cancer patients are frequently encountered with decreased serum albumin levels as a consequence of malnutrition. This can potentially result in lower plasma concentrations and a correspondingly greater V_z for a drug that is highly protein bound as compared to patients with normal plasma protein levels.

The effective lower limit of V_z is the plasma volume, which is approximately 4.5% of body weight (i.e., 45 mL/kg; 1.7 L/m²) for a normal adult. There really is no upper limit, because V_z can assume extremely large values in cases in which the half-life of the terminal disposition phase is long relative to that of the preceding disposition phase and drug levels decrease by several orders of magnitude before the terminal phase is achieved. For example, some anticancer agents, such as the anthracyclines, have V_z values exceeding 1000 L/m² (27 times the body weight). Under these circumstances, the apparent volume of distribution at steady state (V_{ss}) is given by the following equation:

$$V_{ss} = CL \bullet MRT$$

where MRT is the mean residence time as defined below. V_{ss} may represent a more realistic estimate of the apparent distribution space of the drug.

BIOLOGICAL HALF-LIFE AND MEAN RESIDENCE TIME

The biological half-life of a drug ($t_{1/2,z}$) is given by the equation

$$t_{1/2,z} = 0.693/\lambda_z$$

and is the time required for its plasma concentration to decrease by 50% during the terminal disposition phase. It is only applicable to drugs that exhibit apparent first-order disposition. The half-life of a drug is perhaps the most prolifically mentioned but poorly understood concept in pharmacokinetics. There is a tendency to place undue emphasis on the value of $t_{1/2,z}$ as an indicator of drug elimination, even though the parameter furnishes no information about drug decay before the terminal phase. As indicated by the relationship

$$t_{1/2,z} = 0.693 \bullet V_z/CL$$

$t_{1/2,z}$ reflects both the ability of the body to eliminate a drug as well as the extent to which a drug distributes throughout the body. The MRT is a parameter that may better reflect the overall duration of drug in the body than $t_{1/2,z}$. It is calculated by the equation

$$MRT = AUMC/AUC$$

and defined as the average time that a drug molecule remains in the body before being eliminated. Drugs that exhibit very similar $t_{1/2,z}$ values can have markedly different MRTs depending on the relative contribution of the terminal disposition phase to the AUC. However, the $t_{1/2,z}$ does have an important practical application in that steady-state conditions during administration of a drug by continuous i.v. infusion or a multiple-dosing regimen are achieved when the duration of treatment exceeds 4 times the value of $t_{1/2,z}$.

Linear Pharmacokinetics

The majority of drugs, including most clinically used anticancer agents, exhibit linear pharmacokinetics, whereby plasma concentrations of the drug decline in a first-order manner after i.v. administration. A distinguishing and defining characteristic of linear pharmacokinetics is that the plasma concentration of drug at a given time after dosing is directly proportional to the administered dose. Thus, the AUC increases proportionately with the dose, and values of the pharmacokinetic parameters (i.e., CL, $t_{1/2,z}$, MRT, V_{ss}, and V_z) are independent of the dose. When a drug is

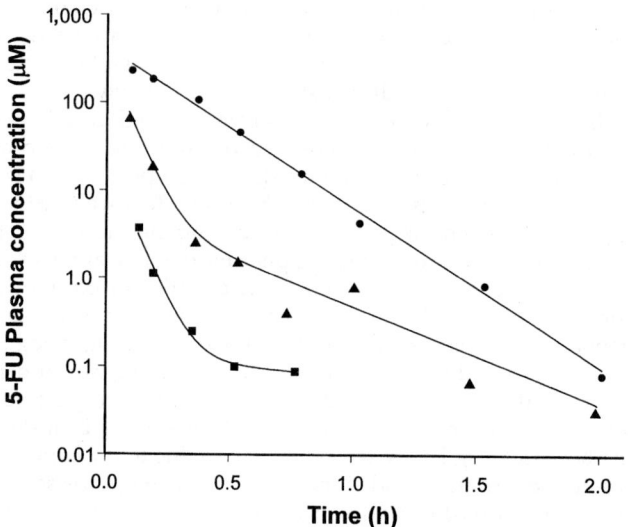

Figure 59-2. Plasma profiles of 5-fluorouracil (5-FU) determined at doses of 25 mg/m² (■), 125 mg/m² (▲), and 375 mg/m² (●), illustrating the effect of classic nonlinear pharmacokinetics. Values of the apparent total body clearance decreased progressively from 142 L/h/m² for the 25 mg/m² dose to 47 L/h/m² at the 125 mg/m² dose to 30 L/h/m² at the 375 mg/m² dose. There would be no significant difference between the clearance determined at different doses if the pharmacokinetic behavior of the drug was linear.

predominantly eliminated by a potentially saturable process, such as hepatic metabolism or active tubular secretion, departures from linear pharmacokinetic behavior may become evident if sufficiently high doses can be administered to patients. As illustrated in Figure 59-2, classic nonlinear pharmacokinetics is indicated by a change in the appearance of the plasma profile from exponential character at lower doses to the appearance of a distinct downward curvature in the semilog plot of the plasma profile at higher doses (26). In addition, the apparent CL exhibits a progressive decrease in magnitude as the dose is escalated.

Discerning whether drug disposition is linear and obtaining an indication of interpatient variability in the values of pharmacokinetic parameters and related variables are important objectives of phase I trials. This information has considerable practical use with regard to clinical drug development. These findings provide the basis for assessing the ability to reliably predict the C_{max} and AUC of a drug after the administration of any given dose to patients that have not been previously studied. The recommended dose of cytotoxic anticancer drugs is typically close to the maximum tolerated dose, and dose-limiting toxicities are often related in some manner to the levels of drug achieved in plasma. Thus, the margin of safety of these agents is very dependent on the consistency of their pharmacokinetic behavior between patients. Conversely, the existence of nonlinear disposition characteristics or a high degree of interpatient pharmacokinetic variability can result in unpredictable episodes of toxicity at the maximum tolerated dose, which may make it difficult to establish a potentially effective and safe dose. In these circumstances, drug level monitoring to establish the optimal dosing regimen in individual patients may be warranted.

Drug Elimination

RENAL AND HEPATIC EXCRETION

Establishing the major pathways of drug elimination in patients is also an important objective of clinical pharmacokinetic studies. Disease states that compromise the function of a major drug-eliminating organ, such as the kidneys or liver, can enhance a patient's sensitivity to the toxic effects of the drug due to decreased CL. For this reason, patients with significant organ impairment are usually excluded from initial phase I studies to avoid possibly confounding sources of toxicity.

Renal excretion may be a quantitatively significant route of elimination for relatively small compounds, with molecular weights less than approximately 300, that are highly to moderately hydrophilic (27). Larger compounds and those with a more lipophilic character are predominantly eliminated by biliary excretion, either directly or after metabolism. Determining CL_R involves measuring the amount of unchanged drug present in the urine (A_e) collected during one or more defined time intervals (Δt) after i.v. drug administration. Depending on whether urine has been continuously collected and pooled from the beginning of dose administration throughout the time that plasma specimens were obtained or during one or more discrete time intervals after dosing, CL_R may be calculated by either of the following equations:

$$CL_R = A_e / AUC_{0 \to t}$$

$$CL_R \approx (\Delta A_e / \Delta t) / C_{mid}$$

In the second equation, C_{mid} is the plasma concentration of drug at the midpoint of the urine collection interval.

The amount of unchanged drug in feces cannot be taken as a direct indication of biliary excretion due to the potential for drug metabolism by the gastrointestinal microflora (28). In cases in which renal or biliary excretion are significant pathways of drug elimination, a predictive correlation may exist between clinical indicators of renal or hepatic function, such as serum creatinine and bilirubin levels, respectively, and CL. Establishing these relationships serves as the basis for defining guidelines pertaining to the minimal organ function required for patient eligibility in phase II studies and devising an empiric algorithm for dosage adjustment, including those documented in Table 59-1 (29).

BIOTRANSFORMATION

Metabolism represents a quantitatively important route of elimination for many anticancer agents. Xenobiotic biotransformation reactions may be broadly categorized into two classes, which are designated *phase I* and *phase II*. The principal phase I reactions are oxidation, reduction, and hydrolysis. Phase II reactions involve the conjugation or coupling of endogenous molecules, including glucuronate, glucose, sulfate, acetate, amino acid, methyl, and glutathione moieties, to the parent drug or a precursory phase I metabolite. Hepatic oxidation mediated by the cytochromes P_{450} (CYP450), a large family of heme-containing isozymes, undoubtedly plays the greatest overall role in drug metabolism among the phase I reactions (30). The CYP450 enzymes are most abundantly expressed in the smooth endoplasmic reticulum of the liver, but they are also present in the kidney, lung, and gastrointestinal epithelium at significant levels. The predominant isozyme in this family, CYP3A4, catalyzes the oxidation of a multitude of structurally diverse compounds (31–33). These include several anticancer agents used for treating hematologic malignancies, including etoposide, ifosfamide, vincristine, and paclitaxel. A number of other CYP450 isozymes are also involved in the oxidation of clinically important antineoplastic agents, such as CYP2B6, which catalyzes the initial hydroxylation reaction in the conversion of cyclophosphamide to alkylating and cytotoxic species (34). In addition to hepatic metabolism, some important phase I reactions are mediated by ubiquitous enzymes found in virtually all tissues of the body, such as dihydropyrimidine dehydrogenase, which catalyzes the reduction of 5-FU, and cytidine deaminase, which inactivates cytarabine (35,36). Glucuronide conjugation

TABLE 59-1. Predominant Elimination Mechanisms and Dose Adjustment Recommendations for Cytotoxic Anticancer Drugs

Major Route of Elimination	Anticancer Agent	Dose Adjustment for Organ Dysfunction
Renal excretion	Bleomycin	b
	Carboplatin, cisplatin	b
	Etoposide	b
	Fludarabine	b
	Hydroxyurea	b
	Methotrexate	b
	Pentostatin	b
	Topotecan	b
Hepatic metabolism CYP450	Busulfan	c
	Chlorambucil	No
	Cyclophosphamide[a]	No
	Ifosfamide[a]	No
	Irinotecan	No
	Paclitaxel	c
	Imatinib	e
	Triethylenethiophosphoramide	No
	Vinca alkaloids	c
Conjugation	Etoposide	c
	SN-38	—
Ubiquitous enzymes	Cytarabine	No
	Gemcitabine	No
	6-Mercaptopurine	d
Nonenzymatic hydrolysis	Carmustine	No
	Camptothecins	No
	Mechlorethamine	No
	Melphalan	No
Biliary excretion	Doxorubicin	No
	Irinotecan	No
	Vinca alkaloids	c

[a]Enzymatic or spontaneous chemical reactions required for drug activation.
[b]Decrease dose in proportion to the reduction in creatinine clearance below 60 mL/min.
[c]Serum bilirubin: 1.5–3.0 mg/100 mL, 50% dose reduction; >3.0 mg/100 mL, 75% dose reduction.
[d]Patients with *S*-methyl transferase deficiency.
[e]Insufficient data to determine if dose reduction is necessary in hepatic dysfunction.

catalyzed by the hepatic uridine diphosphate glucuronosyl transferases is the most commonly encountered phase II reaction. In contrast to phase I metabolism, which may yield a biologically active product, glucuronidation almost exclusively represents a detoxification mechanism that inactivates a compound and facilitates its excretion through enhanced hydrophilicity and recognition by biliary canalicular efflux proteins (37).

SPONTANEOUS CHEMICAL DEGRADATION

Chemical degradation can be a significant elimination mechanism for drugs that are susceptible to hydrolysis, such as many of the alkylating agents. Nonenzymatic reactions between drugs and endogenous molecules can also contribute prominently to elimination. For example, platinum alkylating agents form covalent adducts with serum albumin, and sulfhydryl compounds such as thioguanine can form mixed disulfides with glutathione and other endogenous sulfhydryl compounds, including the exposed sulfhydryl groups of albumin (38,39).

Drug Interactions

Many adjuvant medications that are routinely used in the management of cancer patients can potentially affect the pharmacokinetics of chemotherapeutic agents by either retarding

TABLE 59-2. Clinically Significant Pharmacokinetic Drug Interactions Involving Anticancer Agents

Chemotherapeutic Agent	Interacting Drug	Effect on Clearance of Anticancer Agent	Probable Mechanism	Reference
Cyclophosphamide	Phenobarbital	↑	CYP450 enzyme induction	40, 41
Doxorubicin	Cyclosporin A	↓	Inhibit biliary excretion	42, 43
Etoposide	Phenytoin	↑	CYP450 enzyme induction	44
Irinotecan		↑		44a
Paclitaxel		↑		45
6-Mercaptopurine	Allopurinol	↓	Inhibit xanthine oxidase	46
	Methotrexate	↓		47
Methotrexate	Aspirin	↓	Inhibit tubular secretion	48
	Probenecid	↓		49
Paclitaxel	Verapamil	↓	Inhibit CYP450 metabolism or biliary excretion	50
Topotecan	Cisplatin	↓	Inhibit tubular secretion	51
Vinblastine	Erythromycin	↓	Inhibit CYP450 metabolism	52

or enhancing metabolic elimination. The interactions that are important for drugs used in the treatment of hematologic malignancies are summarized in Table 59-2. Because cytotoxic anticancer drugs are usually administered at their maximum tolerated doses, there is a substantially greater risk for pharmacokinetic interactions resulting in clinically significant toxicity than exists with the large majority of drugs for other indications. Accordingly, the administration of an anticancer agent with another drug that has the potential to modulate the activity of an enzyme that represents a major pathway of its elimination should be avoided whenever possible. Another consideration that should be recognized is that dose-dependent and highly variable pharmacokinetics are frequently exhibited by drugs predominantly eliminated by hepatic metabolism (53). Nonlinearity typified by a progressive decrease in CL with increasing dose results when the dose is escalated above the point at which the principal drug metabolizing enzyme systems become saturated. It is becoming increasingly apparent that genetic polymorphisms and mutations affecting key drug metabolizing enzymes may account for aberrant pharmacokinetics in a minority of patients or an otherwise high degree of interpatient variability (54).

Chemotherapeutic agents that are metabolized by the hepatic CYP450 system, especially members of the CYP3A subfamily, are particularly prone to pharmacokinetic interactions due to the multitude of drugs and compounds of dietary origin that are also substrates and, thus, competitive inhibitors of these enzymes. Omeprazole and certain antidepressants such as fluoxetine are substrates or inhibitors of CYP3A4, and their use may delay the elimination of concurrently administered anticancer drugs that are also metabolized by the enzyme, resulting in increased plasma concentrations that could be potentially dangerous (55,56). Due to the prevalence that combination chemotherapy has achieved in current clinical practice, particularly for hematologic malignancies, the possibility of an undesirable pharmacologic effect should be recognized whenever attempting to administer two or more drugs that are metabolized by CYP3A4. Repeated daily administration of glucocorticoids, commonly used as antiemetics, can induce the expression of hepatic CYP450 and thereby enhance the CL of anticancer drugs that are CYP3A4 substrates (57,58). In addition to hepatic drug metabolizing enzymes, there are examples of pharmacokinetic interactions resulting from effects directed on other enzyme systems, excretory pathways, and even drug absorption. Salicylates can reduce the renal tubular secretion of MTX (48,59). Morphine and its derivatives can alter the rate and extent of absorption of orally administered cytotoxic drugs by reducing gastrointestinal motility (60). Pharmacokinetic drug interactions can also result from the displacement of a highly protein-bound drug by another compound that has greater affinity for the same binding site.

Pharmacokinetic-Pharmacodynamic Relationships

The toxicities of anticancer drugs are often better correlated with a pharmacokinetic variable than with the administered dose. Relationships between the severity of toxicity and total systemic exposure to the drug, as represented by the AUC, are most commonly encountered. However, C_{max} and the duration of time that the drug concentration in plasma exceeds a threshold level, as illustrated in Figure 59-1A, are also predictive of toxicity for some cytotoxic drugs. Thus, for example, the time interval that plasma levels of paclitaxel remain above 50 nM is better correlated with neutropenia (Fig. 59-1A), the principal dose-limiting toxicity, than with either C_{max} or AUC (61). The nature of these relationships can often be described by a sigmoidal E_{max} model, but they may appear linear unless patients have been evaluated across a sufficiently broad range of doses (62).

As previously indicated, therapeutic response ultimately depends on the distribution of drug from the bloodstream to the tumor so that malignant cells are exposed to biologically effective concentrations of the active form of the agent for an adequate duration of time. The rate processes associated with drug distribution and elimination are dependent on the physicochemical properties of the drug and numerous physiologic factors. Accumulation of drug in a tumor is affected by tumor vascularity, oncotic pressure with the tumor mass, and intra- and extracellular pH, among other factors. As with any specific organ or tissue, the time course of the concentration of a compound within a solid tumor cannot be defined from experimental data restricted to measurements made in plasma, serum, or whole blood. Although there is undoubtedly some temporal relationship between drug concentrations in plasma and the tumor, elucidating the tumor concentration-time profile requires physical measurement of drug levels within the tumor itself. Because this cannot be easily accomplished in solid tumors, hematologic malignancies in most cases are considerably more amenable to such studies, because the cancer cells reside within the bloodstream itself or the bone marrow or lymphatic tissues, which are considerably more accessible to the drug. Consequently, efforts to determine whether adequate concentrations of the active form of a drug have been achieved in cancer cells should be considered important objectives of phase I trials to evaluate new anticancer drugs in hematologic malignancies. The availability of this information will better facilitate the rational selection of drugs warranting further clinical evaluation.

Patient Characteristics That Influence Drug Disposition

ELIMINATING ORGAN DYSFUNCTION
Physiologic conditions that affect hepatic or renal function, including blood flow to the liver or kidneys, can have a dramatic effect on the pharmacokinetic behavior of a drug in individual patients (63). Serum bilirubin and creatinine levels are conveniently measured indirect indicators of hepatic and renal function, respectively. Empiric guidelines for dose reduction in patients with underlying renal or hepatic dysfunction are devised by establishing relationships between these biochemical parameters and CL. Table 59-1 summarizes the recommended dose modifications for the standard anticancer drugs used for the treatment of hematologic malignancies.

AGE
The pharmacokinetic behavior of most anticancer drugs has not been adequately characterized in elderly patients (64). There is a very high degree of heterogeneity in older cancer patients due to natural changes in body composition that occur with advancing age, including decreased muscle mass, increasing adipose tissue, lower capacity of CYP450-mediated metabolism, and decreased renal function. Currently, more than one-half of all cancers are presented by patients older than 60 years. However, relatively few elderly patients are entered into early stage clinical trials because of referral patterns and investigator bias. It is anticipated that dosing practices will be positively influenced for some drugs as more information on the pharmacokinetics of chemotherapeutic agents in this important population becomes available.

Experience has shown that safe and effective doses of anticancer agents for children often cannot be based simply on the body weight or the body surface area scaling of an adult dosage. Age-related changes in the enzymatic and excretory systems that are involved in drug elimination can have profound effects on pharmacokinetics (65). Thus, the rational use of drugs known to be eliminated primarily by hepatic metabolism in adults may depend on thoroughly characterizing its pharmacokinetics and metabolism in children of various ages. Similarly, the potential for interaction of a new agent, which is a potential substrate or inhibitor of hepatic CYP450 enzymes, with other drugs concurrently administered to pediatric patients also warrants careful evaluation.

OTHER DEMOGRAPHIC CHARACTERISTICS
Gender and racial differences in the CL of many drugs have led to dose modifications in women and racial subgroups. For example, it has been shown that the CL of 5-FU in female patients is significantly lower than that in male patients and that the formation of the glucuronide metabolite of SN-38 by uridine diphosphate glucuronosyltransferase is subject to racial and gender pharmacogenetic variations (66,67). These factors are being examined extensively during the clinical evaluation of new anticancer drugs.

Dosing Regimens

ROUTES OF DRUG ADMINISTRATION
Cytotoxic anticancer drugs are most commonly given by the i.v. route because this provides complete control over the actual dosage delivered to the systemic circulation and the rate at which it is presented. This yields maximum safety, because the variability in systemic drug exposure between and within patients achieved with direct i.v. administration is typically much better than that resulting from oral administration. Furthermore, for agents given by continuous i.v. infusion, drug delivery can be readily terminated, if necessary, due to the occurrence of an acute adverse reaction during administration.

All routes of administration other than i.v. injection or infusion—including oral, subcutaneous, intramuscular, intraperitoneal, and intrathecal delivery—involve an absorption process whereby dissolved drug molecules are transferred from the site of administration into the vasculature. Accordingly, a drug given by an extravascular route is conceptualized as being outside of the body until gaining access to the systemic circulation. Oral dosage forms are presently available for several drugs used in the treatment of hematologic malignancies, including hydroxyurea, MTX, etoposide, idarubicin, and imatinib. In the future, oral administration will undoubtedly attain greater prevalence due to the clinical development of cytostatic antiproliferative agents that require chronic dosing for efficacy.

The *bioavailability* of a drug given by any extravascular route is defined as the rate and extent of absorption into systemic circulation. The absolute systemic availability of a drug is ascertained by determining the AUC in the same patient after i.v. and extravascular (e.v.) administration of the agent, with an adequate time interval between the two treatments, according to the following equation:

$$F = (AUC_{e.v.}/AUC_{i.v.}) \cdot (D_{i.v.}/D_{e.v.})$$

where D is the dose and the subscript denotes the route of administration. In studies in which an agent is administered exclusively by the oral route, CL and F are indeterminable, as explicitly indicated by the following relationship:

$$D_{e.v.}/AUC_{e.v.} = CL/F$$

With regard to oral drug delivery, F depends on a number of factors, including release of the drug from the dosage form, dissolution of the drug within the gastrointestinal tract, drug stability under conditions encountered in the gastrointestinal tract, transport of the dissolved drug across the intestinal epithelium into the vasculature, and the extent of first pass hepatic metabolism. First pass metabolism is a unique concern for orally administered drugs because blood drains from the gastrointestinal tract through the portal vein directly to the liver before returning to the heart (68).

ADMINISTRATION SCHEDULES
The route and frequency of administration evaluated in the initial phase I trial of a cytotoxic anticancer agent is generally derived from the schedule that produces an optimal therapeutic effect against preclinical *in vivo* tumor models. There is an increasing interest in assessing the use of noncytotoxic compounds, such as cytostatic, differentiation-inducing, and antiangiogenic agents in the treatment of neoplastic diseases. However, accepted preclinical models to evaluate and refine *in vivo* efficacy for many classes of candidate noncytotoxic antiproliferative drugs do not presently exist. Under these circumstances, it would be reasonable to base the dosing regimen evaluated in initial phase I trials on that required to achieve the pattern of systemic exposure to a drug in laboratory animals that best approximates the concentration and duration of exposure necessary for optimal *in vitro* activity.

Past experience has repeatedly demonstrated that impressive preclinical antitumor activity is not a reliable predictor of clinical efficacy. A reasonable argument can also be advanced to support the hypothesis that a candidate drug has little likelihood of being therapeutically effective unless a clinically tolerable dosing regimen provides a pattern of systemic exposure to the drug that is at least comparable to that required for activity against appropriate *in vivo* or *in vitro* preclinical models.

Accordingly, when considered with toxicologic and physiologic response factors, pharmacokinetic data acquired during phase I studies can facilitate efforts to optimize dosing regimens. Alternatively, withdrawing an agent from continued clinical development may be an option that warrants serious consideration in situations in which the plasma concentrations achieved in patients treated at the maximum tolerated dose are considerably lower than target levels, given the availability of limited clinical resources and the ethical considerations of entering patients into a phase II trial of a compound that has little prospect of being therapeutically effective.

DOSE INDIVIDUALIZATION

The existence of nonlinear drug disposition or a high degree of interpatient pharmacokinetic variability can result in unpredictable episodes of toxicity and make it difficult to establish a potentially effective and safe dose. Under these circumstances, it may be beneficial to individualize doses of the drug based on plasma levels of the compound afforded by a test dose or a biochemical parameter that is predictive of CL. Dose individualization has significantly improved the outcome and minimized the toxicity for children with B-lineage ALL treated with MTX (69). Individualizing the dose of carboplatin to target a specific AUC value based on serum creatinine levels in patients has become a routine clinical practice (70).

Conclusions

Although phase I trials are the most commonly considered domain of clinical pharmacokinetic studies, there are numerous reasons for acquiring pharmacokinetic data during various stages in the clinical development of anticancer drugs. The therapeutic indices of many drugs used in the treatment of cancer are inherently narrow because they are used at doses close to the upper limit of tolerability. Furthermore, cancer patients frequently exhibit increased sensitivity to many medications, due to compromised organ function or diminished overall tolerance due to their underlying disease state, augmenting the potential for an undesirable pharmacokinetic interaction with the host of concurrent medications used in the clinical management of cancer patients. The chances for an adverse event resulting from inappropriate dosing of a chemotherapeutic agent to a cancer patient are, therefore, considerably greater than those for most other patient groups. Because the dose-limiting toxicities of a chemotherapeutic agent are often related to some measure of systemic exposure to the drug, the margin of safety of a potentially effective dose is dependent on the consistency of its pharmacokinetic behavior between patients.

CYTOTOXIC CHEMOTHERAPEUTIC AGENTS

Currently, there are approximately 40 cytotoxic anticancer drugs available to clinicians for treating hematologic malignancies. It should be recognized that the chemotherapeutic management of hematologic malignancies typically involves the use of multiple anticancer agents in combination. However, a consideration of the numerous combination regimens that have been developed is beyond the scope of this chapter. The intention of the monographs in this section is to foster a basic familiarity with these drugs through concise summaries of clinically relevant information, including mechanisms of action and resistance, principal therapeutic uses, dosing information, toxicities, and pharmacokinetic behavior. Table 59-3 contains a summary of the dosing information, pharmacokinetic parameters, and principal toxicities for each drug described in this section.

Antimetabolites

METHOTREXATE

The antifolates have occupied an important place in cancer chemotherapy since the first demonstration of remission induction in pediatric ALL with these compounds. After more than 40 years, MTX continues to be used for remission induction, consolidation, and maintenance therapy of ALL and for intrathecal prophylaxis of leukemic meningitis. It is, perhaps, the best understood of the antitumor agents, as studies of its mechanism of action, metabolism, pharmacokinetics, and resistance have provided valuable lessons for all of cancer pharmacology.

The folates are a pool of interconvertible molecules that function as coenzymes by providing one-carbon units during the essential biosynthesis of deoxythymidylic acid and purine nucleotide precursors of DNA. As illustrated in Figure 59-3, methylenetetrahydrofolate is the source of both the carbon and hydrogen atoms that are donated to deoxyuridylic acid during its conversion to deoxythymidylic acid catalyzed by thymidylate synthase (TS). This results in the production of dihydrofolic acid, which is subsequently reduced back to tetrahydrofolate by dihydrofolate reductase (DHFR) and nicotinamide adenine dinucleotide. DHFR is an essential enzyme for maintaining the intracellular folate pool in the biologically active reduced form. Depletion of the reduced folate pool blocks cells in DNA synthesis due to a lack of deoxythymidylic acid and purine nucleotides. Thus, DHFR represents a sensitive target for chemotherapy in actively proliferating cells. The sensitivity of cells to the cytotoxic effects of antifolates is inversely related to the DHFR concentration.

Aminopterin, a potent inhibitor of DHFR, was the first antifolate introduced into the clinic in the 1940s. Although active against acute leukemia in children, aminopterin was subsequently replaced by MTX, which is a somewhat less potent inhibitor of DHFR but has a more predictable toxicity profile. The chemical structures of these compounds are shown in Figure 59-4. MTX binds to DHFR with high affinity. A number of factors involving its cellular pharmacology influence the cytotoxic effects of the drug. It is actively transported into cells by the reduced folate carrier (RFC) (71). In some tumor cells, such as choriocarcinomas, uptake may be mediated by an alternative transporter, the folate binding protein, although in human leukemias, the RFC seems to be most important. Within the cytoplasm, MTX is converted to a long-chain γ-glutamyl peptide by the sequential conjugation of up to five or six additional glutamic acid residues to the glutamyl group of the parent molecule, catalyzed by folyl polyglutamyl synthetase, as shown in Figure 59-4 (72). Polyglutamation confers therapeutically important and advantageous alterations in the pharmacologic and physicochemical properties of MTX. As with the endogenous folates, MTX polyglutamates are highly retained within cells due to the presence of multiple carboxylic acid groups that are dissociated at physiologic pH. Moreover, with each additional glutamyl group, the binding affinity of the molecule for TS, purine synthetic enzymes, and DHFR is enhanced. Polyglutamated metabolites of both MTX and the endogenous folates are converted to the corresponding monoglutamate species by the action of a hydrolase within the cytoplasm, and the monoglutamated form is then susceptible to efflux from the cell. Leukemic cells isolated from chemorefractory patients exhibit one or several characteristics associated with resistance, including a loss of the RFC transporter, low levels of intracellular MTX polyglutamates, an increase in DHFR activity resulting from gene amplification, and, possibly, increased capacity for drug efflux via the hepatic canalicular multispecific organic anion transporter, a multidrug resistance protein (MRP) homolog also designated *MRP2* (cMOAT)

TABLE 59-3. Dosing Information, Pharmacokinetic Parameters, and Principal Severe Toxicities of the Cytotoxic Chemotherapeutic Agents Used in the Treatment of Hematologic Malignancies

Anticancer Agent	Route of Administration	Dose[a] (mg/m²)	Schedule[b]	Clearance (L/h/m²)	Steady State Volume of Distribution (L/m²)	Biological Half-Life (h)	Major Toxicities
Methotrexate	p.o./i.v.	7.5–30	q1–2w	105	25	3–10	H, MS, S, P
High dose	i.v.	150–13,000	q1–3w	49	13	7–24	M, MS, R, S
Cytarabine	i.v.	70–200	qd × 5	60	30	0.5–3.0	H, M, MS, P
Gemcitabine	i.v.	1000	qw × 7	60	50	0.5–1.5	H, M, MS, S
Mercaptopurine	p.o.	75–100	qd	200	30	0.3–0.8	H, M, MS
Thioguanine	p.o.	80	qd × 5	200	30	1.0–1.6	H, M, MS
Cladribine	i.v.	4–5	qd × 5–7	40	180	6.3	IS, MS
Fludarabine	i.v.	15–40	qd × 5	9	40–100	10	HA, IS, MS
Pentostatin	i.v.	4	q2–4w	3–4	15–25	2.5–6.0	IS, MS, R
Hydroxyurea	p.o.	500–3000[(1)]	qd	6	20–30	3–4	MS, S
Melphalan	p.o./i.v.	8	qd × 5	15–20	13–35	1.5	M, MS, P
High dose	i.v.	120–180	qd × 1				M, MS, P, V
Chlorambucil	p.o./i.v.	1–3[(1)]	qd	10–20	5–15	1.5–2.0	M, MS, P
Cyclophosphamide	p.o./i.v.	400–2000	qd × 1	2.5	20–30	4.0–6.5	C, M, MS, P
High dose	i.v.	3–6[(2)]	qd × 1–5				C, CT, M, MS, P, V
Ifosfamide	i.v.	700–2000	qd × 5	2.0–3.5	4–30	4.0–15.0	C, M, MS, N, P, V, R
Carmustine	i.v.	150–200	qd × 1	200	150–200	0.3–0.5	M, MS, P, R
Triethylenethiophosphoramide[d]	i.v.	60–120	qd × 1	15–25	20–30	0.8–2.0	M, MS, N, P, V
Dacarbazine	i.v.	150	qd × 5	40	20–30	5	MS, P
Procarbazine	p.o.	100	qd × 14	n/a	n/a	n/a	MS, N, P
Busulfan	p.o./i.v.	50–100	q6h × 16	20–30	3–7	2–3	MS, N, P
Cisplatin	i.v.	75–100	qd × 1	11–13	11–12	0.5	MS, N, O, R
Carboplatin	i.v.	300–400	qd × 1	4–6	9–11	2.5–6.0	MS, R, S, N
Bleomycin	i.v.	10–203	q1–2w	2.5–4.0	22	2.5–4.0	CU, H, HY, P
Vincristine	i.v.	0.4–1.4	qd × 1	6.5	240–480	19–155	N
Vinblastine	i.v.	6–8	qd × 1	30	1100	20–24	MS, M, N
Paclitaxel[d]	i.v.	90–175	qd × 1	10–25	74–657	6.5–50.0	CT, HY, M, MS, N
Daunorubicin	i.v.	20–30	qd × 1	40–60	1300–1900	20–50	CT, M, MS
Doxorubicin	i.v.	60–75	qd × 1	30–80	800–1400	30	CT, M, MS
Doxorubicin[e]	i.v.	60–90	qd × 1	3–8	40–60	5–10	CT, M, MS
Idarubicin	i.v.	12	qd × 3	50–150	300–2500	50–60	CT, M, MS
Mitoxantrone	i.v.	12	qd × 3	50–70	2000–4000	40–50	CT, M, MS
Etoposide	p.o./i.v.	50–200	qd × 3	1–2	7–13	3–11	M, MS
Topotecan	i.v.	0.5–1.5	qd × 5	27[f]	75[f]	2.8[f]	M, MS
				13[g]	69[g]	4.1[g]	
L-Asparaginase[h]	i.v.	6–10[(3)]	q.o.d. × 9–12	n/a	31	8–30	CO, HG, HY, PAN
Gemtuzumab	i.v.	9[(4)]	qd × 1	n/a	n/a	45	H, MS, S, V
All-trans-retinoic acid	p.o.	45	qd	30–40	n/a	0.7–1.1	H, HL, PC
Arsenic trioxide	i.v.	10[(1)]	qd × 60	0.8–1.1	1.5	12	CT, HL, H, N
Imatinib	p.o.	300–1000[(1)]	qd	6.5–8.5	150–240	13–16	H, MS

C, cystitis; CO, coagulopathy; CT, cardiotoxicity; CU, cutaneous; H, hepatotoxicity; HA, hemolytic anemia; HG, hyperglycemia; HL, hyperleukocytosis syndrome; HY, hypersensitivity; IS, immunosuppression; M, mucositis; MS, myelosuppression; N, neurotoxicity; n/a, not available; O, ototoxicity; P, pulmonary; PAN, pancreatitis; PC, pseudotumor cerebri; R, renal; S, stomatitis; V, venoocclusive disease.
[a]Dose or range of doses for frequently used standard regimens for hematologic malignancies are in mg/m², except as indicated by the following notations: (1), mg; (2), g; (3), 10³ U/m²; (4), IU.
[b]Frequency of administration for a single cycle of therapy.
[c]Values of the clearance and apparent volume of distribution for drugs that have only been studied after oral administration are ratios with respect to the fractional bioavailability (i.e., CL/F, V_{ss}/F).
[d]Nonlinear pharmacokinetics.
[e]Liposomal formulation; pharmacokinetics based on total drug concentration in plasma.
[f]Pharmacokinetics based on topotecan lactone concentration in plasma.
[g]Pharmacokinetics based on total topotecan (lactone + carboxylate forms) in plasma.
[h]Pharmacokinetic data pertain to the Escherichia coli preparation of the drug.

(73). Hyperdiploid ALL cells have increased RFC expression that results in higher intracellular levels of polyglutamated MTX in comparison to the less drug-sensitive diploid ALLs. AML cells form polyglutamated metabolites of the drug less efficiently than ALL cells. Similarly, T-cell leukemias are less effective in polyglutamate formation than B-cell leukemias. These findings have led to the use of higher doses of MTX, typically 5 g/m², for the treatment of T-cell ALL (74).

Recently, a number of analogs of MTX that target TS or the purine synthetic enzymes rather than DHFR have undergone clinical evaluation, primarily for solid tumor chemotherapy. Other compounds, such as 10-propargyl-10-deazaaminopterin, that target DHFR but are better substrates for transport by the RFC or for polyglutamation by folyl polyglutamyl synthetase are also being evaluated (75). Although several agents have been identified that display greater activity against specific animal tumors than MTX, only the multitargeted antifolate (76) has displayed significant and unique antitumor activity—in this case, against mesotheliomas and adenocarcinomas of the gastrointestinal tract.

MTX may be administered by the i.v., oral, or intrathecal routes depending on the clinical circumstance. The decay of MTX from plasma after i.v. delivery may be described as biexponential with

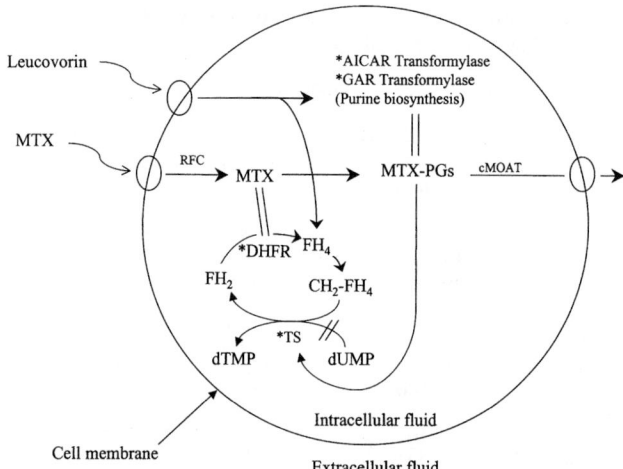

Figure 59-3. Scheme depicting the cellular pharmacology of methotrexate (MTX), which acts by inhibiting the reactions catalyzed by dihydrofolate reductase (DHFR) and thymidylate synthase (TS) and also by inhibiting purine biosynthesis. Leucovorin (5-formyl-tetrahydrofolinic acid) rescues cells from the cytotoxic effects of MTX by competitive inhibition. AICAR, phosphoribosylaminoimidazolecarboxamide; CH_2-FH_4, methylene tetrahydrofolate; cMOAT, canalicular multispecific organic anion transporter; dTMP, deoxythymidylate; dUMP, deoxyuridylate; FH_2, dihydrofolate; FH_4, tetrahydrofolate; GAR, phosphoribosylglycinamide 2; PG, polyglutamate; RFC, reduced folate carrier.

a half-life of 2 to 3 hours for the initial disposition phase and a $t_{1/2,z}$ of 8 to 10 hours. Oral absorption is virtually complete at doses up to 25 mg/m², above which bioavailability becomes increasingly variable and incomplete. It is primarily eliminated by urinary excretion as the unchanged drug and a minor fraction of the dose is hepatically metabolized to 7-hydroxy-MTX. MTX is filtered through the glomerulus and partially reabsorbed, but it is also secreted by the renal tubules. Dose adjustment is required for patients with mild renal dysfunction, in proportion to the reduction in creatinine CL. Because of the potential for extreme toxicity with doses above 100 mg/m², patients with reduced renal function should not receive high-dose MTX. Whereas intermittent hemodialysis is ineffective in removing significant quantities of MTX, continuous flow hemodialysis has been successful in facili-

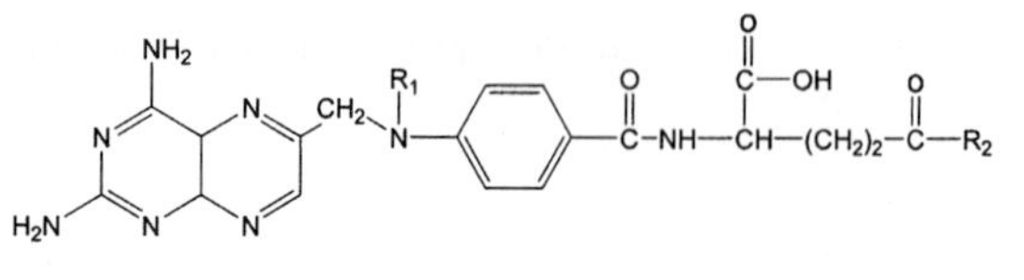

Compound	R_1	R_2
Aminopterin:	-H	-OH
Methotrexate (MTX):	-CH₃	-OH
Polyglutamated MTX:	-CH₃	$\left[HN-CH\genfrac{}{}{0pt}{}{COOH}{}-(CH_2)_2-COOH \right]_n$ (n =1-5)

Figure 59-4. Chemical structure of methotrexate (4-amino-10-methylfolic acid) and its polyglutamated metabolites.

tating the elimination of MTX in patients with renal failure, diminishing toxicity to a tolerable level, although the technique has not been extensively evaluated (77). It should be remembered that the CL of MTX in elderly patients (i.e., >65 years) may be lower than it is in younger patients even though their serum creatinine may be normal (78). Underlying tubular dysfunction may account for this discrepancy.

In patients with normal renal function, high doses of MTX, defined as those exceeding 500 mg/m², may be given with the objective of increasing drug uptake by tumor cells or enhancing the amount of drug that penetrates the blood–brain barrier. High-dose MTX is regularly used as an alternative to craniospinal irradiation in ALL that has a favorable prognosis. At steady state, the ratio of the concentration of MTX in cerebrospinal fluid (CSF) to plasma approaches 1:30, and the levels in CSF after high-dose MTX may exceed 1 μM. High-dose MTX requires the administration of the physiologically reduced folate, leucovorin (folinic acid; 5-formyl-tetrahydrofolic acid), as an antidote, usually beginning 24 hours after starting the MTX infusion. Leucovorin rescue relies on the rapid CL_R of MTX, a weak organic acid. Thus, vigorous hydration and alkalinization of the urine to pH 7.0 protect the kidney against drug precipitation during periods of rapid excretion. Drug levels in plasma are routinely monitored during high-dose therapy with MTX to assure that the drug is being eliminated from the body at an appropriate rate. When the MTX plasma concentration exceeds 10 μM in a sample obtained 24 hours after completing the infusion of the drug, or exceeds 0.5 μM after 48 hours, the dose of leucovorin should be increased to a maximum of 500 mg/m² given every 6 hours until the MTX concentration falls below 0.05 μM. In cases of extreme toxicity and renal shutdown, drug elimination may be enhanced by continuous flow dialysis or by administration of carboxypeptidase G-1, which is an efficient folate-cleaving enzyme that can be obtained from the National Cancer Institute (79).

The CL of MTX in patients with normal renal function varies by several-fold. Those patients with childhood ALL who eliminate the drug more rapidly have a worse prognosis. Routine drug level monitoring and dose adjustment may correct for these differences and improve response. Among children with B-lineage leukemia, survival improved when drug levels were monitored during the infusion of high-dose MTX, and doses were adjusted to achieve an AUC in the fiftieth percentile (80).

MTX may be administered intrathecally at doses up to a maximum of 12 mg every 4 days to patients older than 3 years, with proportionately lower doses for younger patients. It distributes poorly into the ventricular system, thus prompting the use of an indwelling ventricular reservoir in patients with central nervous system (CNS) leukemia. MTX is eliminated from the CSF with a half-life of 12 hours in most patients, although the half-life may be considerably longer in patients with active CNS leukemia (81). In a minority of patients, intrathecal MTX may produce an acute neurotoxicity syndrome of headache, fever, and arachnoiditis, as well as more chronic toxicity with changes in affect, mental status, seizures, and dementia. Acute and transient CNS toxicity, with changes in mental status and transient neurologic defects, may also occur in up to 3% of patients treated with systemic high-dose MTX (82). Leucovorin is not effective in reversing these toxicities. An alternative intrathecal medication, such as cytarabine, should be used in patients exhibiting toxicity.

The primary toxicity of MTX results from its inhibition of DNA synthesis in the bone marrow and intestinal epithelium. Thus, suppression of granulocytes and platelets peaks 5 to 10 days after treatment. Oral mucositis is common after higher doses of drug or with prolonged or repeated courses of oral dosing, whereas diarrhea, intestinal bleeding, and ulceration of the gastrointestinal mucosa may supervene in patients with severe MTX toxicity. Less commonly, a skin rash, usually an erythematous maculopapular eruption, and pneumonitis, with eosinophilic infiltration, may reflect a hypersensitivity response, although generalized anaphylaxis is rare. Both high-dose treatment and prolonged oral administration, such as the regimens used for treating ulcerative colitis, asthma, or psoriasis, may cause hepatic enzyme elevations. Those occurring in relation to high-dose regimens are rapidly reversible and are not associated with long-term hepatic damage, but the more prolonged oral intake of MTX does cause pathologic changes, including fatty liver, fibrosis, and, in extreme cases, cirrhosis. These chronic changes are only rarely found in patients on antileukemic therapy but are more commonly associated with treatment of psoriasis.

DEOXYCYTIDINE ANALOGS

Deoxycytidine (dC) and *deoxythymidine* are the two endogenous pyrimidine nucleosides incorporated into DNA. Several analogs of dC have become important drugs in the treatment of leukemias, lymphomas, and solid tumors (Fig. 59-5). The pharmacology of dC analogs is best understood in the context of the disposition and metabolism of the physiologic molecule, as illustrated in Figure 59-6. dC is synthesized *de novo* within cells and also recruited from a pool circulating in plasma by facilitated transport. Degradation to deoxyuridine catalyzed by cytidine deaminase, an ubiquitous enzyme that is abundantly expressed in the liver, intestinal mucosal, granulocytes, and tumor cells, represents the primary route of elimination of the nucleoside. The initial phosphorylation of the nucleoside by dC kinase is the rate-limiting step in its intracellular conversion to dC triphosphate, which is the form required for incorporation into DNA.

Cytarabine. Cytarabine (β-cytosine arabinoside, ara-C) is one of the first dC analogs found to be clinically effective in the treatment of hematologic malignancies. It differs from endogenous cytidine nucleosides in the structure of the sugar moiety (Fig. 59-5). Specifically, the hydroxyl group at the 2'-position is in the β-configuration, whereas this hydroxyl group is in the α-configuration in ribonucleosides and absent in 2'-deoxyribonucleosides. Cytarabine is metabolized in much the same manner as dC (Fig. 59-6). It is subject to degradation in plasma and tissues by cytidine deaminase, enters cells by facilitated diffusion, and is converted to the active triphosphate form by the same kinases that phosphorylate dC (83). Cytarabine triphosphate serves as a substrate for DNA polymerase but, on incorporation into DNA, blocks further chain elongation. Although the parent drug is rapidly cleared from plasma, the intracellular half-life of cytarabine triphosphate is much longer, on the order of several hours. The primary determinants of response to cytarabine are the intrinsic dC kinase activity, the size of competing dC triphosphate pools, the ongoing rate of DNA synthesis in tumor cells, and the apoptotic response of the tumor cell to DNA damage.

Dosing regimens that are intended to increase the amount of drug entering cells by passive diffusion by maximizing the plasma concentration of cytarabine have been developed to overcome limitations of the facilitated transport mechanism. In contrast to standard doses of 100 to 200 mg/m^2 given daily for 5 to 7 days, high-dose therapy with 2 to 3 g/m^2 of cytarabine every 12 hours for up to 6 days has improved the survival of patients with AML. This strategy has proven to be most effective against the subset of leukemias with abnormalities of the core binding protein complex, including those with translocations of chromosome 8 or inversion of chromosome 16 (84). It is also used in some treatment regimens for intermediate- and high-grade lymphomas, blastic and chronic phase myelogenous leukemia, and poor-prognosis lymphocytic leukemias. High-dose cytarabine delivered by the intrathecal route has been used for leukemic and carcinomatous meningitis.

Cytarabine cannot be administered orally due to poor bioavailability resulting from its susceptibility to deamination in the intestinal mucosa and on first pass to the liver. It is rapidly eliminated from plasma, predominantly by deamination to arabinosyl uridine, exhibiting a biological half-life of only 7 to 20 minutes after i.v. administration. Although arabinosyl uridine does not function as an antimetabolite, it is eliminated from systemic circulation much more slowly than cytarabine is eliminated by renal excretion. There is evidence suggesting that accumulation of the metabolite in plasma could inhibit the deamination of cytarabine. Consistent with its S-phase specificity for killing cells that are actively synthesizing DNA, the efficacy of cytarabine is directly correlated with the duration of time that tumor cells are exposed to potentially cytotoxic concentrations. As a consequence of its rapid CL, the drug is usually given as a continuous i.v. infusion of 100 to 200 mg/m^2/day for 5 to 7 days to maintain plasma concentrations at cytotoxic

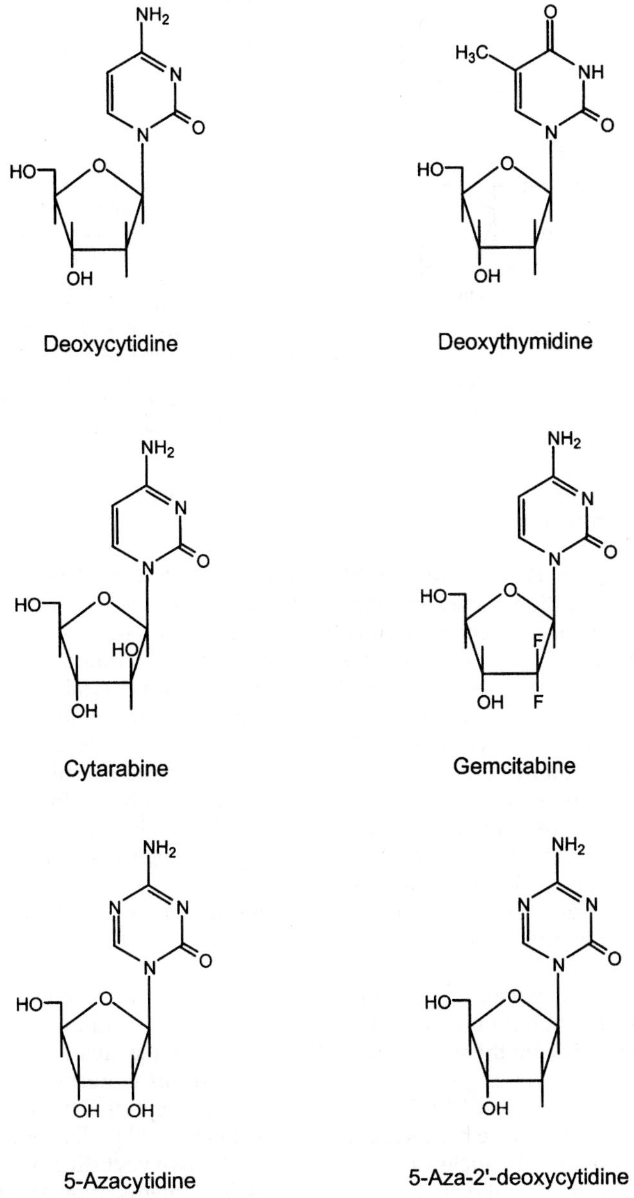

Figure 59-5. Structures of the pyrimide nucleosides that comprise DNA and several deoxycytidine analogs that have become important drugs for the treatment of leukemias and lymphomas.

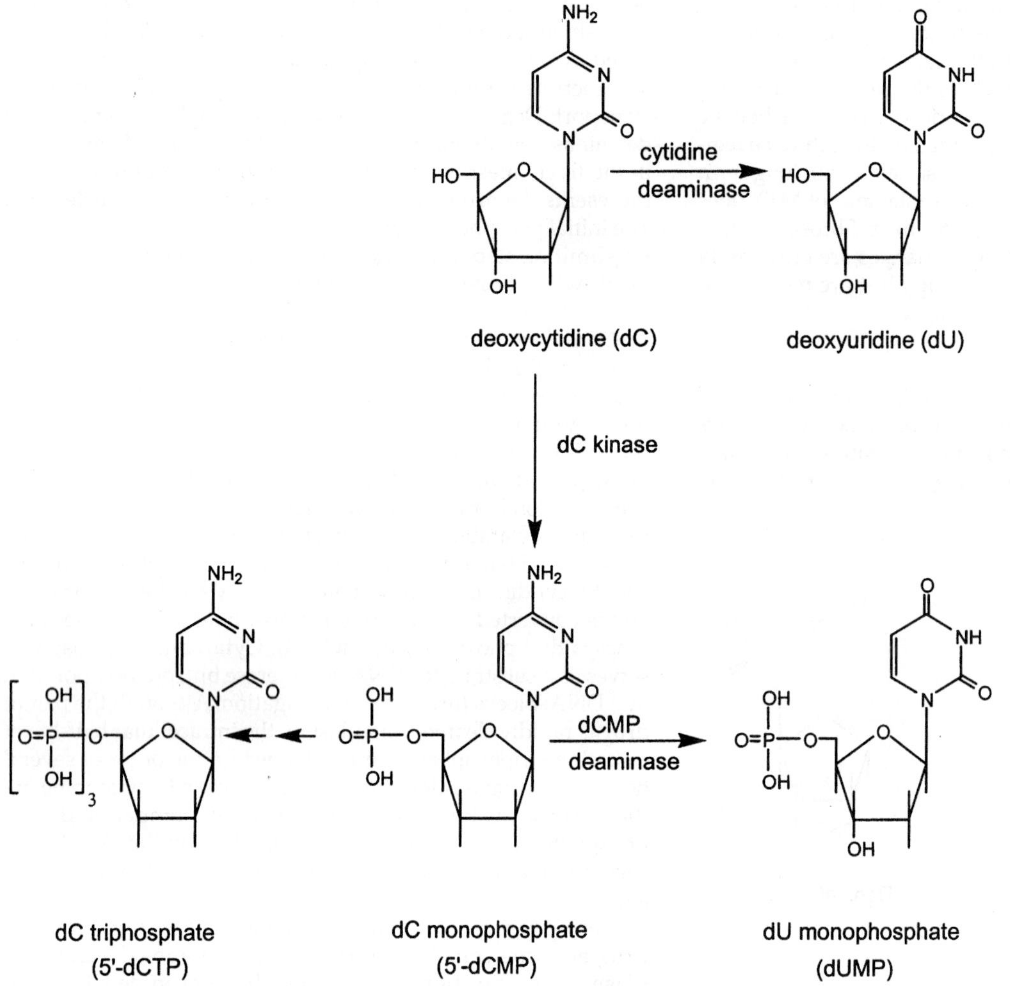

Figure 59-6. Intracellular metabolism of deoxycytidine. Activation of the nucleoside involves sequential phosphorylation by deoxycytidine kinase, yielding the 5'-monophosphate species, followed by nucleotide kinases to afford the 5'-triphosphate form that is incorporated into DNA. Inactivation results from hydrolysis of the exocyclic amine group on the pyrimidine base of both the nucleoside and nucleotide by deaminases.

levels. However, the dose may be increased up to 3 g/m² every 12 hours for 6 days in consolidation regimens.

Cytarabine distributes rather efficiently from systemic circulation into CSF. The ratio of the drug concentration in CSF to plasma is approximately 1:2 after achieving steady-state conditions during continuous i.v. infusion. Thus, high-dose i.v. cytarabine may be as effective as a single-agent treatment for CNS lymphomas. It is also administered by intrathecal injection at a dose of 70 mg, whereupon the concentration of the drug in CSF decays with a half-life of 2.5 hours. A gel-impregnated formulation that slowly releases cytarabine into the CSF and avoids the necessity for repeated administration has been approved for intrathecal use (85).

The primary toxicities of cytarabine, acute myelosuppression and mucosal ulceration, are similar to those of other antimetabolites. Myelosuppression is a direct function of the dose and duration of exposure, with recovery taking 7 to 21 days. Gastrointestinal bleeding, diarrhea, and mucosal ulceration are commonly observed after high-dose therapy. Hepatocellular toxicity and jaundice, which are usually reversible, may also occur. Noncardiogenic pulmonary edema occurs infrequently, as does a predisposition to pneumonia caused by *Streptococcus viridans*, especially in pediatric patients. High-dose cytarabine causes central neurologic toxicity, most prominently cerebellar dysfunction, with ataxia and slurred speech in patients older than 50 years and those with renal dysfunction. In such patients, the doses and duration of treatment with high-dose therapy should be reduced to decrease the risk of neurotoxicity. Confusion and dementia herald a more serious and often fatal outcome. Intrathecal cytarabine may also cause a syndrome of acute toxicity, presenting as seizures and changes in mental status.

Gemcitabine. Gemcitabine is a molecule with a difluoro substitution at the 2'-position of the ribose (Fig. 59-5). Its metabolism and mechanism of action are analogous to cytarabine. However, the triphosphate nucleotide of gemcitabine has a considerably longer intracellular half-life than cytarabine triphosphate, providing greater efficacy against solid tumors than exhibited by cytarabine. The most common dosing regimen is gemcitabine 1000 mg/m² given as a 30-minute i.v. injection once weekly for 3 weeks followed by a 1-week rest interval before repeating treatment. Myelosuppression is its most important toxicity. Its primary use in hematologic malignancies is against Hodgkin's disease as a secondary agent, although it has not received extensive evaluation for treating leukemias and lymphomas (86).

Azacytidine. Azacytidine (Fig. 59-5) has shown activity against AML but has only limited value in this context. Its unique ability to inhibit the methylation of DNA, thereby reactivating suppressed genes, is the biologic effect that has generated the greatest interest (87). To exploit this effect, azacytidine has been used to activate hemoglobin F production in sickle cell anemia. Its deoxyribonucleoside analog, 5-aza-2'-deoxycytidine, is an investigational drug that also inhibits DNA methylation and is being evaluated against AML and solid tumors. Both compounds induce the differentiation of various tumor cells in culture. They are rapidly inactivated by deamination, which

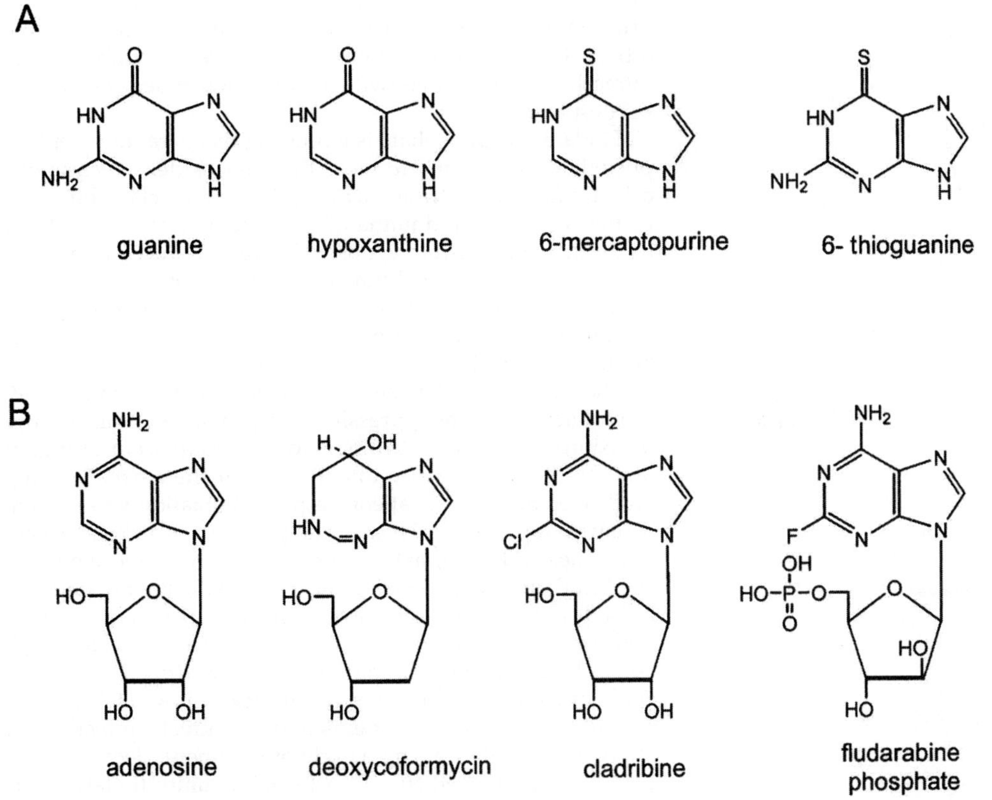

A

guanine   hypoxanthine   6-mercaptopurine   6- thioguanine

B

adenosine   deoxycoformycin   cladribine   fludarabine phosphate

Figure 59-7. The purine antimetabolites. **A:** Structures of the hypoxanthine-guanine pathway antimetabolites and their endogenous counterparts. **B:** Adenosine and structurally related nucleosides that are clinically active against various hematologic malignancies.

results in irreversible cleavage of the unstable azapyrimidine ring. Their primary toxicity is myelosuppression, but, at higher doses, severe nausea and vomiting may limit their use.

PURINE ANALOGS

Two categories of purine analogs, the hypoxanthine-guanine pathway antimetabolites (Fig. 59-7A) and adenosine analogs (Fig. 59-7B), have achieved important roles in the treatment of lymphoid malignancies. 6-Mercaptopurine (6-MP) and 6-thioguanine (6-TG) are purine analogs with a sulfhydryl substituent in the base. They function as analogs of guanine, a base found in both RNA and DNA, and are primarily used for the treatment of acute leukemia. Both compounds require activation to the corresponding 5'-monophosphate nucleotide by hypoxanthine-guanine phosphoribosyl transferase. The monophosphate species are inhibitors of *de novo* purine synthesis. In addition, 6-MP and 6-TG are incorporated into DNA on further phosphorylation of these intermediate forms to the 5'-triphosphate nucleotides. Apoptosis is triggered when the aberrant nucleotide in DNA is recognized by the mismatch repair system (88).

6-MP is used primarily in combination with MTX as a maintenance therapy for ALL. As an inhibitor of early steps in *de novo* purine synthesis, MTX elevates intracellular levels of phosphoribosyl pyrophosphate, increasing the activation of 6-MP to its 5'-monophosphate nucleotide. The two drugs are highly synergistic against experimental tumor models (89). Resistance to both 6-MP and 6-TG has been ascribed to deficiency of the activating enzyme hypoxanthine-guanine phosphoribosyl transferase, to the absence of mismatch repair, or to increased levels of the inactivating enzyme thiopurine methyltransferase (TPMT). Lower activities of TPMT in red blood cells are correlated with better event-free survival in childhood ALL treated with 6-MP (90). In addition to methylation of the sulfhydryl group, the elimination of 6-MP proceeds by oxidation of the purine ring by xanthine oxidase, which is a reaction inhibited

by allopurinol (Fig. 59-8). Thus, oral doses of 6-MP must be reduced by 75% in patients concurrently receiving allopurinol. 6-TG is eliminated by an alternative route that involves deamination of the guanine ring by the enzyme guanase.

6-MP and 6-TG are both administered orally at daily doses of 50 to 100 mg/m². The bioavailability of 6-MP is highly variable, ranging from 16% to 50%. The apparent biological half-life of both drugs is approximately 1 hour, and the intracellular nucleotide metabolites have much longer persistence than the parent compounds in plasma. The rate of inactivation by TPMT, as noted above, is a second important variable among patients. The primary toxicities of 6-MP and 6-TG are myelosuppression and mucositis, but both cause hepatotoxicity with alkaline phosphatase elevations, jaundice (less common), and hepatic failure with high-dose regimens. 6-MP is teratogenic and causes first trimester abortions. Both drugs are immunosuppressive, with 6-MP being the active metabolite of azathioprine, and their long-term use is associated with an increased risk of opportunistic infections.

A polymorphism in TPMT that reduces its catalytic activity for 6-MP has been observed in 10% of the patient population (91). Individuals who are homozygous for the polymorphism and highly deficient in TPMT activity occur with a frequency of 1/300. The slow inactivation of the drug in these patients results in severe toxicity at the usual doses. In the 90% of patients with normal TMPT activity and in those who are relatively tolerant of 6-MP, the recurrence of leukemia is strongly correlated with failure to maintain dose intensity of the drug (92). Thus, both absorption and catabolism are highly variable in a population of patients, and, for patients on maintenance therapy for ALL, it becomes critical to give doses that cause modest, but tolerable, levels of neutropenia.

The adenosine analogs fludarabine phosphate, cladribine, and pentostatin (2'-deoxycoformycin) (Fig. 59-7B) are increasingly used in treating chronic lymphocytic leukemia (CLL), follicular non-Hodgkin's lymphoma, and hairy cell leukemia, as

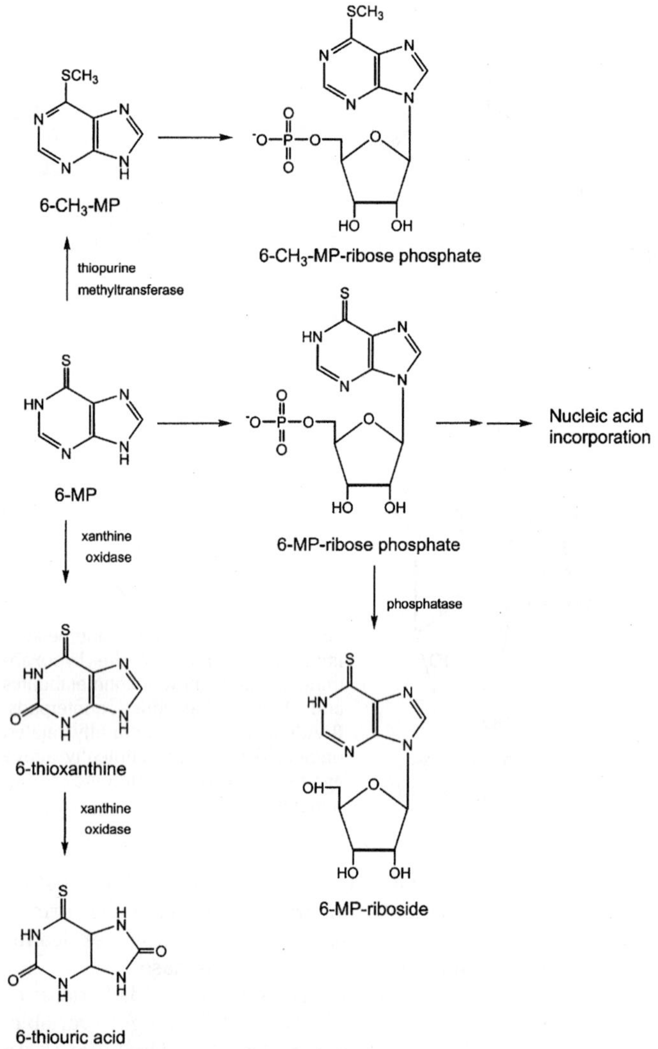

6-CH₃-MP

thiopurine
methyltransferase

6-CH₃-MP-ribose phosphate

6-MP

xanthine
oxidase

6-MP-ribose phosphate

Nucleic acid
incorporation

phosphatase

6-thioxanthine

xanthine
oxidase

6-MP-riboside

6-thiouric acid

Figure 59-8. Pathways involved in the metabolic elimination and activation of 6-mercaptopurine (6-MP). Allopurinol is a suicide inhibitor of xanthine oxidase.

well as other less common malignancies derived from B lymphocytes. The reason for the potent activity of fludarabine and cladribine in lymphoid cells is unclear but may be related to the high concentration of activating enzymes, particularly the rate-limiting dC kinase in these cells. Both drugs are incorporated into DNA on conversion to 5'-triphosphate nucleotides where

they can inhibit chain elongation (93). Although similar to these drugs in its spectrum of activity, pentostatin acts through inhibition of adenosine deaminase, creating a toxic imbalance in intracellular nucleotides, with a vast excess of deoxyadenosine triphosphate (94).

Fludarabine phosphate is a prodrug that is rapidly dephosphorylated in plasma to yield the nucleoside, which enters cells by facilitated transport (Fig. 59-9). Like cladribine and pentostatin, it is predominantly eliminated from the body by renal excretion. Therefore, doses should be reduced in patients with compromised renal function, although precise guidelines are not available. The biological half-lives for cladribine, fludarabine, and pentostatin are 6.3 hours, 10.0 hours, and 2.5 hours, respectively.

The toxicities of the adenosine analogs follow a similar pattern of acute myelosuppression and prolonged immunosuppression. Renal and neurologic toxicity may occur at higher doses although they are uncommon for the current dosing guidelines. Some CLL patients respond dramatically to fludarabine with rapid tumor lysis, leading to a hypercatabolic release of purines and phosphates. Thus, patients must receive fluids and bicarbonate before their initial treatment with the drug (95). Episodes of antibody-mediated hemolytic anemia may follow fludarabine therapy, perhaps due to the unmasking of autoantibodies by this potently immunosuppressive drug. Pentostatin, cladribine, and fludarabine dramatically lower CD4 T-cell counts and predispose patients to opportunistic infection for many months after a single cycle of treatment. Because of its potent and prolonged effects on T-cell immunity, fludarabine is now increasingly used to prepare allotransplant patients for receipt of bone marrow, particularly in nonmyeloablative regimens (96). Undoubtedly, it will become increasingly useful in other settings in which immunosuppression is therapeutic.

Hydroxyurea

This simple molecule (H_2N-CO-NH-OH) chelates iron and thereby inhibits ribonucleotide reductase, which has a catalytic subunit that is dependent on iron. Ribonucleotide reductase converts ribonucleotides to the corresponding deoxyribonucleotide and is one of the key enzymes that is up-regulated as cells pass into the DNA synthetic phase of the cell cycle. Consequently, hydroxyurea lowers intracellular pools of all four deoxynucleotides required for DNA synthesis. Resistance to hydroxyurea arises by amplification of the catalytic subunit of ribonucleotide reductase (97). It is primarily used in the treatment of chronic myelogenous leukemia (CML), in which its rapid onset and abrupt cessation of action are particularly desirable for regulating the neutrophil count. In addition, hydroxyurea is a potent radia-

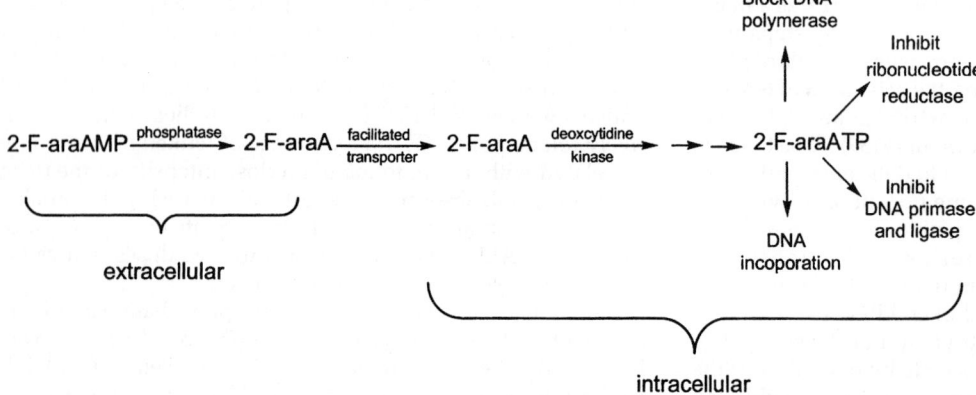

2-F-araAMP →(phosphatase) 2-F-araA →(facilitated transporter) 2-F-araA →(deoxycytidine kinase) → → 2-F-araATP

Block DNA polymerase

Inhibit ribonucleotide reductase

DNA incorporation

Inhibit DNA primase and ligase

extracellular

intracellular

Figure 59-9. Metabolism and sites of action of fludarabine phosphate (2-F-araAMP). 2-F-araA, fludarabine; 2-F-araATP, fludarabine triphosphate.

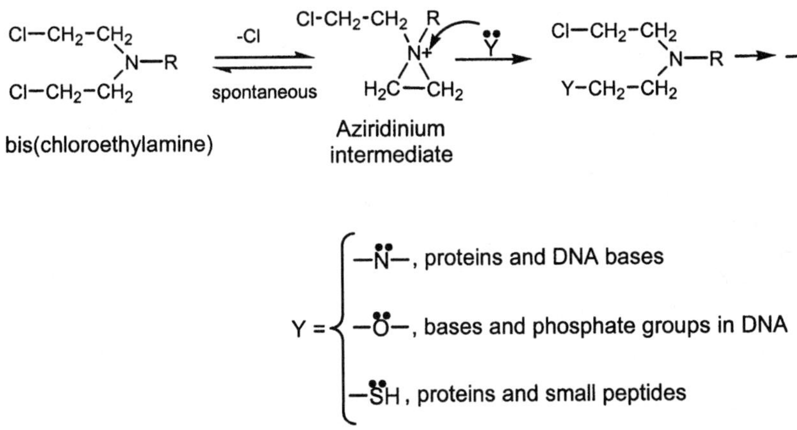

Cl—CH$_2$—CH$_2$
          ⟩N—R
Cl—CH$_2$—CH$_2$

bis(chloroethylamine)

$\xrightarrow[\text{spontaneous}]{-Cl}$

Cl-CH$_2$-CH$_2$ R
                 \N$^+$/
              H$_2$C—CH$_2$

Aziridinium
intermediate

→ Y →

Cl—CH$_2$—CH$_2$
          ⟩N—R
Y—CH$_2$—CH$_2$

→ →

Y—CH$_2$—CH$_2$
          ⟩N—R
Y—CH$_2$—CH$_2$

$Y = \begin{cases} \text{—N—, proteins and DNA bases} \\ \text{—O—, bases and phosphate groups in DNA} \\ \text{—SH, proteins and small peptides} \end{cases}$

Figure 59-10. Nitrogen mustards are characterized by the presence of a chloroethylamine functional group, which readily forms a highly reactive cyclic intermediate that reacts with nucleophilic groups present in biologic molecules such as DNA, proteins, and small peptides.

tion sensitizer and has been used experimentally with irradiation in the treatment of squamous carcinomas of the cervix and head and neck. Doses may range from 500 mg/day to 2 to 3 g/day depending on the response in the peripheral white cell count. In general, it is very well tolerated with minimal toxicity to the mucous membranes and gastrointestinal tract. It is predominately eliminated by renal excretion; therefore, dose adjustments are needed in patients with renal dysfunction.

Alkylating Agents

Covalently modifying DNA with alkylating agents is one of the most effective ways to induce apoptosis in cancer cells. Although the reasons for this are still not completely understood, it may be related to deficiencies in the ability of tumor cells to repair damaged sequences of DNA in comparison to normal cells. The process of recognizing sites where the chemical structure of DNA has been deleteriously altered, excising the affected bases, and replacing them with native residues involves a complex series of steps mediated by genes such as BRCA-1, the Fanconi's anemia complex, and the nucleotide excision repair complex (ERCC-1 through -9), as well as the topoisomerases and DNA polymerase. The genes that recognize DNA damage and initiate repair are often underexpressed or lost in inherited forms of cancer or during the course of somatic mutation leading to cancer.

Alkylating agents have been prominently used in the treatment of cancer during the past 50 years. They are chemically reactive compounds or metabolites that covalently attack electron-rich sites on bases or phosphate groups of polynucleotide chains of DNA. The favored functional groups are the N-2 and N-7 of guanine, the O-6 of adenine, the N-3 nitrogen of cytosine and thymine, and the 5'-phosphate oxygen atoms. Endogenous molecules that contain sulfhydryl groups, such as glutathione and proteins with cysteine residues, also react avidly with alkylating agents, resulting in drug inactivation. Thus, the balance among DNA alkylation, inactivation through the reaction with other nucleophilic molecules, and detoxification by spontaneous chemical decomposition to inactive products determines the net effect on cell viability. Depletion of intracellular glutathione by prior drug exposure or with agents such as buthionine sulfoximine has been explored to accentuate the effectiveness of alkylating agents.

Nitrogen mustards are the prototypical alkylating drugs, characterized by the presence of a 2-chloroethylamine moiety that spontaneously forms an exceedingly reactive aziridinium intermediate (cyclic ethyleneimmonium ion), which attacks electron-rich functional groups (Fig. 59-10). Many clinically effective alkylating agents are bifunctional because they contain two reactive groups, permitting a cross-link to form between the paired strands of DNA. Cross-links are particularly difficult to repair, and when the number of these lesions exceeds a threshold level, the damaged DNA becomes recognized by p53, leading to apoptosis of the cell.

Although aliphatic substituted nitrogen mustards, such as mechlorethamine [methyl-bis(2-chloroethyl)amine], have proven to be clinically effective against hematologic malignancies, the use of these agents is nevertheless limited by their extreme reactivity. Consequently, alkylating agents with better pharmaceutical properties imparted through the introduction of structural modifications to enhance chemical stability without compromising antitumor activity have been developed. Among these drugs, the aromatic derivatives of bis(2-chloroethyl)amine, such as melphalan and chlorambucil, are sufficiently stable for oral administration without loss of antitumor activity (Fig. 59-11). Cyclophosphamide and its analog ifosfamide are cyclic prodrugs that undergo hepatic CYP450-mediated oxidation to release the active phosphoramide mustard (Fig. 59-12). Alternately, drugs such as CENUs, procarbazine, dacarbazine, busulfan, and temozolomide release activated methylating species on hepatic metabolism or spontaneous decomposition. The repair of damage to DNA induced by methylating agents and CENUs requires the presence of methylguanine methyl transferase. Sensitivity of human brain tumors to CENUs correlates with methylation of the methylguanine methyl transferase gene and absence of repair capability (98). Because DNA methylation is repaired by a different mechanism than classic ethylation by the nitrogen mustards, the methylating agents are not cross-resistant with the nitrogen mustards in those cell lines that become resistant through up-regulation of specific DNA nucleotide excision repair pathways.

A linear relationship between dose and cytotoxicity has been demonstrated for the alkylating agents. Thus, higher doses result in greater formation of DNA adducts and enhanced cell kill. The sensitivity of cancer cells to alkylating agents is dependent on the presence of a mechanism to detect DNA damage. This function is primarily mediated by p53, which responds to DNA alkylation by activating repair processes or by initiating apoptosis (99). The alkylating agents as a class were the first drugs to be used in high-dose therapy with bone marrow or stem cell rescue to achieve sustained remissions of poor-risk leukemias and lymphomas. In this setting, the dose is limited by toxicity to organs other than bone marrow, primarily the intestinal mucosa, although the endothelium of vessels (venoocclusive disease of the liver), the myocardium, the brain, and the lungs may be adversely affected. Combinations of alkylating agents may be used to take advantage of differences in their toxicity profiles when given at high doses, and differences in mechanisms of resistance.

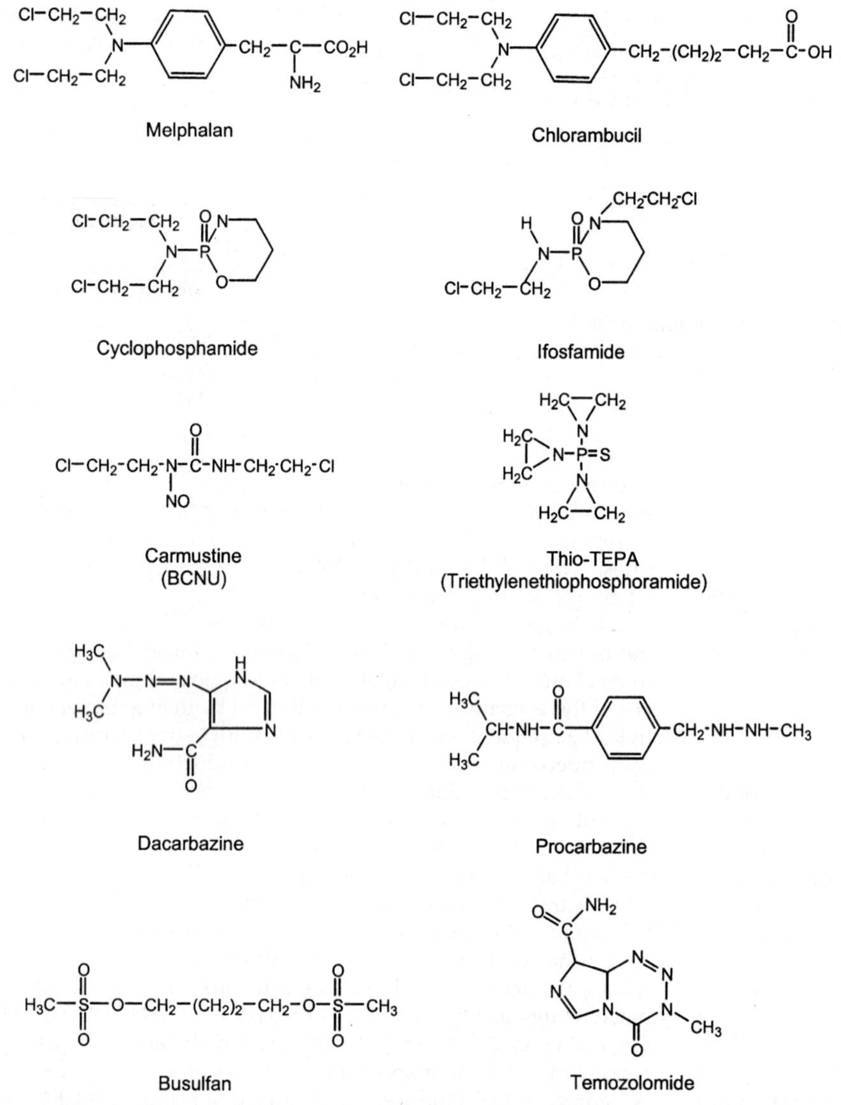

Figure 59-11. Chemical structures of the clinically available alkylating agents with activity against hematologic malignancies.

Resistance to alkylating agent damage is complex and poorly understood at the clinical level. Experimental tumors may become resistant through elevation of glutathione levels, increased glutathione transferase activity, or enhanced repair capability. In addition, resistance may be associated with the deletion of the transmembrane proteins that are responsible for actively transporting drugs, such as melphalan, into cancer cells. As previously noted, the overexpression of methylguanine-DNA-methyltransferase appears to be critical in conferring resistance against CENUs and methylating agents. A mechanism of resistance that affects all alkylating agents is the mutation or deletion of p53, which raises the threshold for apoptosis and confers insensitivity to DNA alkylation.

Most clinically effective alkylating agents are rapidly eliminated from the body, and the biologically active reactive intermediates are not typically measurable. Tolerance to these drugs is related in general terms to performance status and bone marrow reserve. Dose modification for patients with hepatic or renal dysfunction is not necessary. Cyclophosphamide and ifosfamide can even be used in patients with mild abnormalities in hepatic function, because activation of the compounds in the liver by CYP450 metabolism is preserved in this circumstance. However, high-dose regimens of alkylating agents should be used with caution in patients who have previously received high-dose chemotherapy or pelvic irradiation and in those who have a poor nutritional status, as indicated by significant weight loss or low serum albumin levels.

The acute toxicities that are observed with most alkylating agents are confined to myelosuppression and intestinal mucosal damage, although the pattern of these toxicities may differ among structurally similar agents. Whereas cyclophosphamide tends to spare platelets, the CENUs produce a delayed nadir in platelet and white blood cell counts 4 to 6 weeks after drug administration. Busulfan and 1,3-bis(chloroethyl)-1-nitrosourea damage the stem cell population of the bone marrow but tend to spare the mucosa (Fig. 59-11). High-dose therapy with ifosfamide and cyclophosphamide results in the production of toxic metabolites, particularly acrolein (Fig. 59-12), at high levels in the urine; their administration must be accompanied by intense hydration. Coadministration of the sulfhydryl-generating compound mesna (2-mercaptoethanesulfonic acid sodium salt) is also effective in protecting the urothelium from acrolein and preventing severe cystitis. Central neurotoxicity is particularly problematic for high-dose triethylenethiophosphoramide, a sulfur mustard (Fig. 59-11), and ifosfamide. The late-occurring and long-term toxicities of the alkylating agents as a group include the propensity to produce myelodysplasia and AML, with characteristic loss of segments of chromosomes 5 or 7. All alkylating agents may cause pulmonary fibrosis. Chronic renal failure is

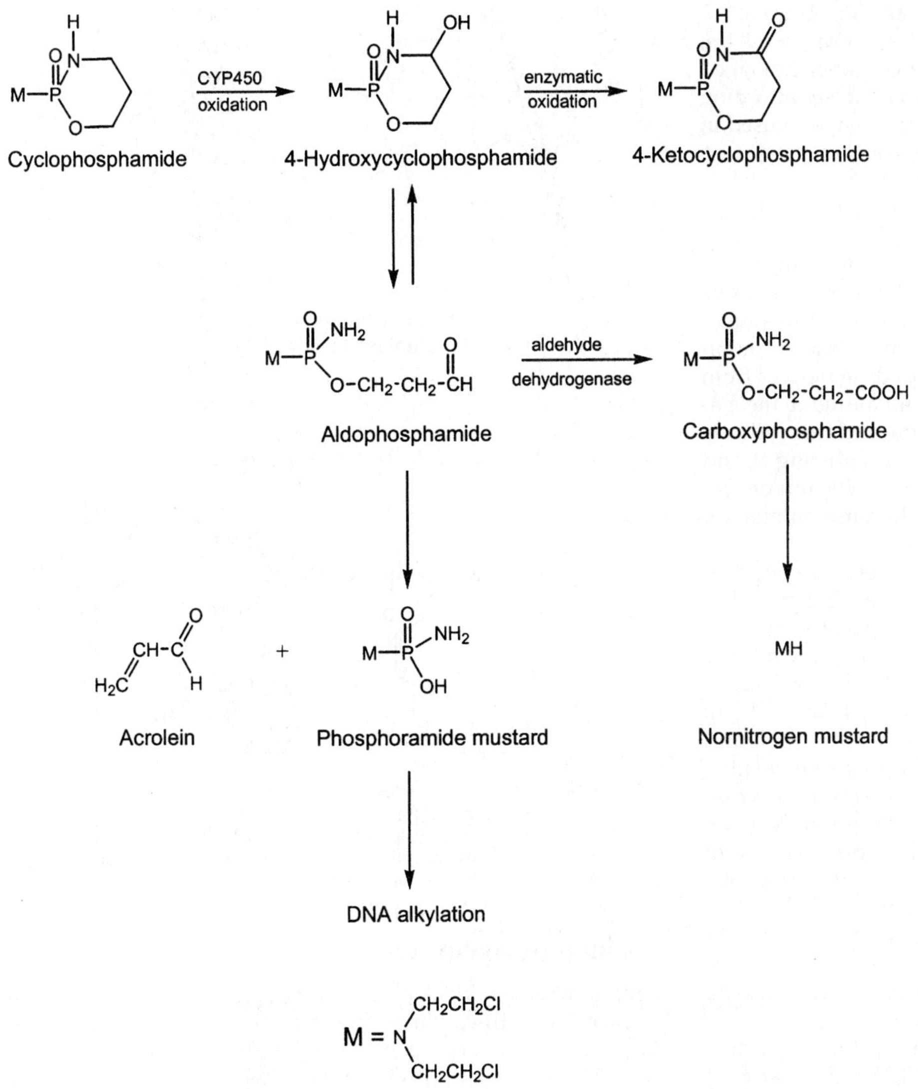

CYTOTOXIC CHEMOTHERAPEUTIC AGENTS **2113**

Figure 59-12. Activation of cyclophosphamide to its active product, phosphoramide mustard, and its toxic urinary excretion product, acrolein.

an infrequently observed toxicity after repeated courses of treatment with CENUs (100).

Platinum Derivatives

Carboplatin and cisplatin are the only two platinum derivatives approved for clinical use in the United States (Fig. 59-13). In current practice, their use in the treatment of hematologic malignancies is almost exclusively limited to multiagent high-dose chemotherapy regimens, such as ICE (ifosfamide/carboplatin/etoposide). Their basic mechanism of action involves successive replacement of the two chloride ligands by water molecules, resulting in a highly reactive, positively charged

Cisplatin   Carboplatin

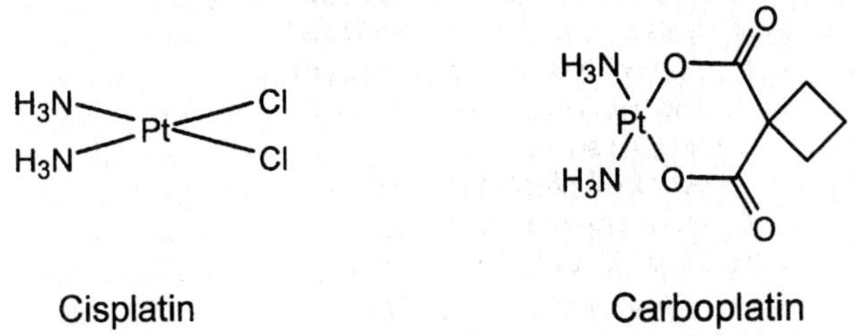

Figure 59-13. Structures of carboplatin and cisplatin.

intermediate that attacks the sulfhydryl groups of proteins and nucleophilic groups on DNA. Their reaction with DNA produces inter- and intrastrand cross-links and strand breaks (101).

The primary acute toxicity of cisplatin is renal failure. Pretreatment with saline hydration and diuresis has largely eliminated this problem in patients with normal renal function. Cisplatin also produces a peripheral sensory neuropathy and ototoxicity after multiple cycles of therapy. These same toxicities are uncommon with standard doses of carboplatin, which are less than or equal to 400 mg/m^2/cycle of therapy, but neuropathy may become noticeable with prolonged use or high-dose therapy of 800 mg/m^2 or more. Accordingly, carboplatin is used more frequently in hematologic malignancies than cisplatin. Myelosuppression, especially thrombocytopenia, is frequently observed with carboplatin. Both platinum drugs are leukemogenic, although less so than conventional alkylators (102). To avoid serious toxicity, the dosage of carboplatin is commonly adjusted for renal function according to the following empirically derived equation (103):

$$\text{Dose (mg)} = \text{target AUC} \cdot (\text{GFR} + 25)$$

where the units of the AUC and the glomerular filtration rate (GFR) are mg · minute/mL and mL/minute, respectively. In clinical practice, GFR is typically estimated by measuring pretreatment serum creatinine and applying the Cockroft-Gault equation (104). Doses that provide a target AUC ranging from 5 to 7 mg • minute/mL result in acceptable myelosuppression, but they are associated with increasingly severe and prolonged depression of blood cell counts. Treatment with doses affording AUC values as great as 18 mg • minute/mL have been used in high-dose regimens with bone marrow replacement.

Bleomycin

Bleomycin is a mixture of peptides isolated from a fungal fermentation broth. It has a relatively restricted but important role in cancer chemotherapy as one of the cornerstones of treatment for germ cell malignancies and Hodgkin's lymphoma in combination regimens. The particular value of this drug derives from its relative lack of bone marrow toxicity and a unique mechanism of action, which involves the formation of free radicals that attack the polynucleotide chain of DNA, inducing strand breaks that lead to apoptosis (105). Another notable but deleterious feature of bleomycin is its propensity to cause pulmonary fibrosis on chronic administration.

The clinical preparation of bleomycin is actually a mixture of several closely related metal-chelating peptides. The predominant active component, designated the *A-2 peptide*, contains a DNA-binding domain and a metal-chelating pocket. On binding to DNA, the iron-associated redox site of the peptide is brought within close proximity to the polynucleotide chain. Oxygen radicals generated at the redox site react with and cleave the deoxyribose chain, resulting in DNA fragmentation. Resistance to bleomycin is associated with an amidase that degrades the drug (106). Amidase activity is high in the liver, but it is low in the skin and lung, which are the primary sites of bleomycin toxicity. Additional mechanisms of resistance to bleomycin include increased levels of intracellular sulfhydryl compounds, decreased drug uptake, and enhanced DNA strand repair. The relative significance of these various mechanisms to the clinical development of resistance to the drug remains unclear.

Bleomycin is administered subcutaneously, intramuscularly, or intravenously. After a bolus i.v. dose of 15 U/m^2, peak concentrations in plasma reach 1 to 5 µU/L and decline with a $t_{1/2,z}$ of 3 hours in patients with normal renal function. More than two-thirds of the administered dose is excreted unchanged in the urine; therefore, the dose should be adjusted for patients with renal dysfunction in proportion to the decline in creatinine CL. The drug is administered according to a variety of dosing regimens, but most commonly it is administered at doses of 10 to 20 U/m^2 once or twice weekly. Cumulative doses exceeding 250 U are associated with an increased risk of pulmonary fibrosis. However, pulmonary toxicity can occur in patients exposed to lower cumulative doses, especially those with preexisting lung disease, individuals who have received pulmonary irradiation, or those exposed to high oxygen concentration during surgery. Pulmonary toxicity may take the form of interstitial infiltrates, effusions, or bleb formation, but fibrosis is usually a prominent component. The etiology of pulmonary toxicity is not known, but it may be mediated by cytokine [e.g., transforming growth factor β, tumor necrosis factor-α (TNF-α), or both] secretion during the inflammatory response to pulmonary epithelial damage (107). There is no known treatment for bleomycin-induced lung toxicity. Corticosteroids are of unproven value. Other toxic reactions to bleomycin include hyperpyrexia and anaphylaxis in a small fraction of patients, leading to the common use of a one-unit test dose before standard treatment. The drug also causes hyperkeratosis, reddening and ulceration of the skin over joints of the hands and feet (less common), and Raynaud's syndrome.

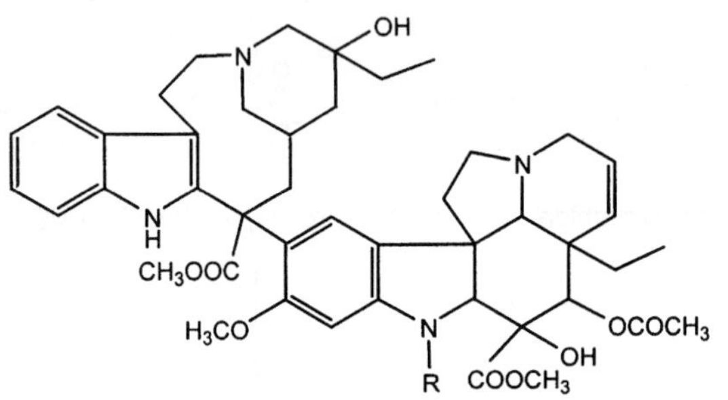

Vincristine : R= CHO
Vinblastine: R= CH$_3$

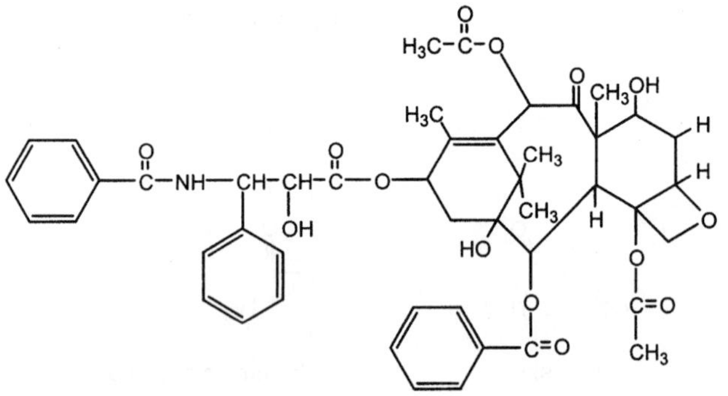

Paclitaxel

Figure 59-14. Chemical structures of the clinically available antimitotic agents that have shown activity against leukemias and lymphomas.

Antimitotic Agents

Compounds that block cells in mitosis are commonly found in nature, including plants and marine organisms, and have become important components of chemotherapy regimens used to treat leukemia and lymphoma. Two classes of anticancer compounds that act through this mechanism are the vinca alkaloids and the taxanes (Fig. 59-14). Vincristine and vinblastine are the two naturally occurring vinca alkaloids that were initially approved for clinical use. Vincristine is a key component of regimens that cure childhood lymphocytic leukemia, intermediate- and high-grade lymphomas, and Hodgkin's lymphoma. Vinblastine is used mainly to treat germ cell tumors and Hodgkin's lymphoma. A newer semisynthetic vinca alkaloid derivative, vinorelbine (Navelbine), is used primarily to treat solid tumors. Although the taxanes paclitaxel and docetaxel have made a substantial impact on solid tumor chemotherapy, their value in treating hematologic malignancies has not been established, and they are mentioned here only briefly.

The vinca alkaloids were originally discovered in an extract from the periwinkle plant during a search for compounds with hypoglycemic activity, but they proved highly active against experimental lymphoid neoplasms. They became the mainstay of leukemia remission induction therapy in combination with glucocorticoids during the 1960s. Their antitumor action results from their ability to bind to β-tubulin and inhibit the formation of microtubules, the primary structural components of the mitotic spindle. Cells exposed to vinca alkaloids arrest in metaphase and undergo apoptosis. The taxanes also cause mitotic arrest but as the result of a significantly different interaction. They bind to different sites on β-tubulin and *promote* the polymerization of microtubules; thus, cells exposed to paclitaxel display a disordered array of microtubules with multiple organizing centers for spindles. Resistance to the vinca alkaloids and taxanes has been ascribed to the overexpression of the MDR and MRP efflux pumps. Resistance conferred by mutations in β-tubulin specific for each class of drugs has been observed in experimental tumors. However, because the binding sites for the vinca alkaloids and taxanes are at different locations, β-tubulin mutations may not result in cross-resistance to both classes of drugs. It is likely that defects in apoptosis may also confer resistance, although the taxanes do not depend on p53 to initiate cell death.

Hepatic metabolism is an important route of elimination for both the taxanes and vinca alkaloids. Phase I and phase II reactions are involved in the metabolism of the vinca alkaloids, whereas the taxanes are subject to CYP450-mediated hydroxylation at several positions of the molecule. Hepatic dysfunction is associated with decreased CL of the taxanes, resulting in increased toxicity, although guidelines for dose adjustment are only approximations (108). In general, patients with a serum bilirubin greater than 3 mg/dL should receive a 75% reduction in dose, with subsequent adjustment according to tolerance. The plasma pharmacokinetics of the vinca alkaloids is characterized by a relatively rapid initial disposition phase with a half-life of 1 to 3 hours and a much longer terminal phase with a half-life of 1 to 2 days.

Vincristine exhibits relatively little bone marrow toxicity, whereas vinblastine and vinorelbine can cause severe myelosuppression with maximum effects occurring 5 to 10 days after administration. The primary toxicity of vincristine is a progressive peripheral neuropathy, both sensory and motor, initially presenting as tingling in the feet and hands, and ultimately resulting in motor deficits. The appearance of motor changes should prompt a discontinuation of treatment. Vincristine may cause painful constipation when administered at doses greater than 2 mg/m^2, and routine laxative use is recommended. Infrequently observed effects of vincristine include inappropriate water retention and hyponatremia. Vinblastine and vinorelbine may also cause mucositis and neuropathy, although the neuropathy is less severe than it is with vincristine, and it rarely requires discontinuation of treatment.

The usual doses of paclitaxel are 135 mg/m^2 by 24-hour i.v. infusion or 175 mg/m^2 by 3-hour i.v. infusion once every 3 weeks and 90 mg/m^2 given as a 1-hour infusion on a weekly basis. Drugs that induce CYP450, such as dilantin and phenobarbital, have been shown to enhance the CL of paclitaxel and may negate the therapeutic effectiveness of the taxanes (109). However, clinically significant pharmacokinetic interactions have not been observed with known inhibitors of the specific CYP450 isozymes involved in paclitaxel biotransformation, including ketoconazole and H$_2$-receptor antagonists such as cimetidine (110,111). Paclitaxel and docetaxel both cause myelosuppression as their primary toxicity. Neuropathy is occasionally observed, usually in association with cisplatin and after multiple cycles of treatment. Premedication with corticosteroids and histamine-receptor antagonists (cimetidine and diphenhydramine) is recommended to prevent anaphylactic reactions to paclitaxel. Concomitant corticosteroids are also used with docetaxel to prevent the development of chronic edema and effusions.

Topoisomerase Inhibitors

MECHANISM OF ACTION

The *DNA topoisomerases* are essential nuclear enzymes that reduce the torsional stress of supercoiled DNA by creating reversible single- or double-strand breaks in the DNA molecule (112,113). This action enables selected regions of DNA to become sufficiently exposed and relaxed as required for its rep-

lication, recombination, and transcription. The topoisomerases rejoin the cleaved strands of DNA and dissociate from the relaxed double helix before the approach of enzymes involved in DNA replication. In mammalian cells, topoisomerase I is expressed constitutively throughout the cell cycle, whereas topoisomerase IIα is predominantly expressed during the S and G$_2$/M phases (114). Both of these enzymes represent important targets for cancer chemotherapeutic agents. Camptothecin and its derivatives inhibit the function of topoisomerase I but do not affect topoisomerase II (115). Similarly, compounds that modulate the activity of topoisomerase IIα, such as the anthracyclines and epipodophyllotoxins, do not interact with topoisomerase I (116). There are no clinically useful agents that preferentially target topoisomerase IIβ. Topoisomerase interactive agents stabilize a transient covalent enzyme-DNA complex, resulting in irreversible DNA strand breaks during ongoing DNA synthesis, the accumulation of which triggers apoptosis (117). Unlike the situation in which elevated target enzymes confer resistance to an antineoplastic agent, as with TS and 5-FU or DHFR and MTX, the presence of increased topoisomerase protein levels enhances sensitivity to topoisomerase inhibitors. Decreases in the level of either topoisomerase I or II may be a clinically relevant mechanism of resistance against these drugs (118–120).

ANTHRACYCLINES

The anthracyclines doxorubicin and daunorubicin are cytotoxic antibiotics that were introduced into the clinic nearly 40 years ago and remain important chemotherapeutic agents (121). In addition to these first-generation compounds, the two synthetic analogs idarubicin and epirubicin are also approved for use in the United States. However, epirubicin has no significant role in the treatment of hematologic malignancies. The anthracyclines are characterized by the presence of an aminosugar conjugated through an ether linkage to the main benzanthracenedione ring system. Mitoxantrone is a structurally related compound belonging to the anthracenedione class. It lacks the sugar moiety but exhibits pharmacologic properties that are nearly equivalent to those of the anthracyclines. The chemical structures of these drugs are depicted in Figure 59-15.

Inhibiting the function of topoisomerase IIα is the primary mechanism of action of all anthracyclines, although there are structure-related differences in their specificity for binding to DNA (122). A secondary mode of action common to all anthracyclines is formation of free radicals through oxidation-reduction cycling of their quinone moiety. Free radical formation has been implicated in the cardiotoxic effects of anthracyclines but, evidently, has no direct association with their antitumor effects. Anthracyclines enter cells through a passive transport process and are removed from cells by several adenosine triphosphate–binding cassette transporters, including MRP, the breast cancer resistance protein, and the P-glycoprotein transporters (123). Acquired resistance to anthracyclines in experimental tumor models results from overexpression of drug efflux transporters and down-regulation or point mutations in topoisomerase II.

Doxorubicin is a component of many standard multiagent chemotherapy regimens used for the treatment of lymphoid malignancies and many solid tumors. It is also used in combination regimens for the treatment of human immunodeficiency virus–associated lymphomas and Kaposi's sarcoma (124). Daunorubicin and idarubicin are extensively used in combination with cytarabine for the treatment of AML. Mitoxantrone has shown activity against refractory AML and is also an important agent for treating breast cancer, prostate cancer, and multiple sclerosis (125).

The approved anthracyclines are administered as i.v. bolus injections or continuous infusions lasting from 30 minutes to 24 hours or longer. Idarubicin is the only anthracycline that can be

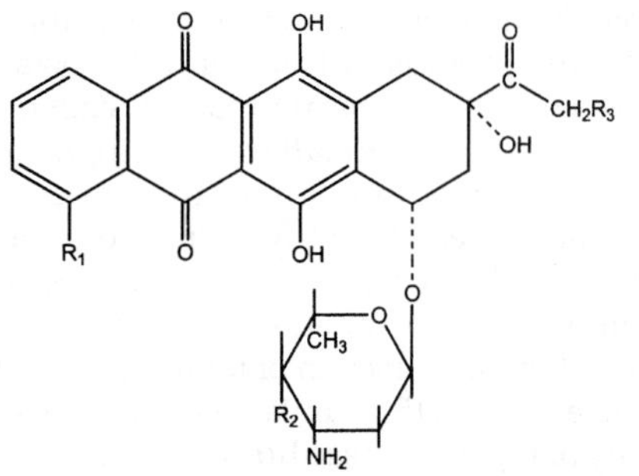

Compound	R_1	R_2	R_3
Doxorubicin	-OCH$_3$	-OH	-H
Daunorubicin	-OCH$_3$	-OH	-H
Idarubicin	-H	-OH	-H

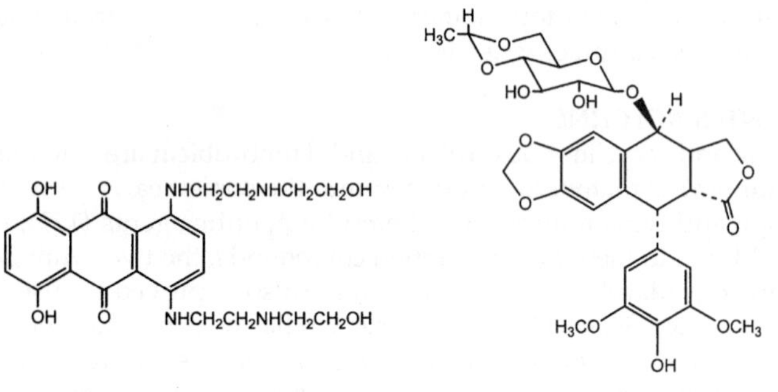

Mitoxantrone   Etoposide

Figure 59-15. Structures of topoisomerase II inhibitors.

given orally. Plasma profiles of daunorubicin and doxorubicin are characterized by an initial disposition phase with a 1- to 3-hour half-life followed by a prolonged terminal phase with a half-life of 1 to 3 days. In general, these agents do not cross the blood–brain barrier in significant concentrations, possibly due to the presence of P-glycoprotein in the arachnoid granulations. Hepatic metabolism and biliary excretion are the major elimination pathways for these drugs. To varying degrees, the ketone in the acetyl side chain that is present in each of these compounds is metabolized in the liver to the corresponding alcohol by the enzyme aldo-keto reductase. The parent compounds and their hydroxylated metabolites, which are biologically active, are further metabolized to a series of inactive species, resulting from the cleavage of the sugar moiety that yields the aglycone and from conjugation with sulfuric or glucuronic acid. Although precise guidelines are not available from the literature, significant abnormalities in hepatic function that is related to cancer, cirrhosis, or infection probably decrease the CL of these drugs. Accordingly, a decrease in the usual dose by approximately 50% is prudent for patients with serum bilirubin levels greater than 3 mg/dL (126). Mitoxantrone is also eliminated by hepatic metabolism and requires dose reduction in cases of hepatic dysfunction, as indicated for the anthracyclines (127).

Single-agent doxorubicin is usually administered as a bolus injection at a dose of 60 to 75 mg/m^2 every 3 to 4 weeks. Lower doses of 15 to 25 mg/m^2 can be given weekly, or the drug may be administered as a continuous infusion over 48 to 96 hours to reduce the risk of cardiotoxicity that is associated with high-peak drug concentrations (128). The dose-limiting toxicity of the anthra-cyclines is acute myelosuppression that occurs in 60% to 80% of patients who are treated with conventional doses. The nadir develops 7 to 10 days after the initiation of therapy and resolves by 2 weeks. Dosages are usually reduced by 25% to 50% when given together with other myelotoxic agents, such as cyclophosphamide. Other commonly encountered toxicities include nausea, vomiting, alopecia, and stomatitis. The severity of stomatitis usually peaks 5 to 13 days after dosing. Extravasation of these agents causes severe tissue necrosis; therefore, intact venous access needs to be assured before drug infusion. Mitoxantrone typically causes less nausea and vomiting than daunorubicin and doxorubicin.

As previously noted, cardiotoxicity that is mediated by free radical formation is the major long-term side effect associated with the anthracyclines. The relative lack of free radical scavenger systems in the myocardium makes this tissue extremely susceptible to free radical damage. Anthracycline-induced cardiotoxicity can present as either an acute or a delayed complication. Acute toxicity is less common and manifests as cardiac arrhythmias and conduction abnormalities that may progress to the "pericarditis-myocarditis syndrome." Chronic toxicity appears months after initiating therapy, and it usually presents as congestive heart failure. Ejection fraction measurements are commonly used to assess cardiac function before patients begin therapy. These drugs should not be given to patients with an abnormal ejection fraction or a history of congestive heart failure. The recommended cumulative lifetime dose limit of doxorubicin is 450 to 550 mg/m^2, for which the rate of cardiotoxicity is 5% (129). Cardiotoxicity occurs with a frequency approaching 50% in patients who receive lifetime doses greater than 1000 mg/m^2. Patients who receive mantle irradiation, those with underlying cardiac problems, and preadolescent children are at higher risk of cardiotoxicity. In children, evidence of cardiotoxicity may not be observed until several years after receiving an anthracycline. Damage is characterized by diminished cardiac development, depressed left ventricular fractional shortening, and left ventricular dilation. Accordingly, it is recommended that the cumulative lifetime dose of doxorubicin should not exceed 300 mg/m^2 in children (130).

Approaches to minimize the cardiotoxic effects of doxorubicin have included the identification of synthetic analogs with less cardiotoxicity, incorporating the drug into liposomes, prolonging the infusion time, and cotreating with cardioprotective agents. Currently, liposomal formulations of doxorubicin (Doxil) and daunorubicin (DaunoXome) are clinically available. However, the efficacy of these formulations in comparison to the efficacy of the unencapsulated parent drugs against hematologic malignancies has not been conclusively evaluated. The liposomal formulations slowly release the active drug, resulting in lower peak plasma concentrations of the free drug and decreased cardiotoxicity (131). Administering anthracyclines by continuous i.v. infusion for at least 6 hours has been shown to significantly diminish the risk of cardiotoxicity. Dexrazoxane (ICRF-187) yields a hydrolysis product that is an efficient iron chelator, thereby blocking free radical formation by sequestering iron from the complex with doxorubicin. In breast cancer patients, treatment with dexrazoxane, 1000 mg/m^2 given 30 minutes before doxorubicin, decreased the risk of cardiotoxicity by 82% without an apparent deleterious effect on therapeutic activity (132). Current recommendations are to use dexrazoxane in patients receiving greater than 300 mg/m^2 of doxorubicin (133).

ETOPOSIDE

Etoposide (VP-16) is a semisynthetic derivative of the natural product podophyllotoxin that inhibits topoisomerase IIα and induces DNA strand breaks (Fig. 59-15). It has been used in the treatment of Hodgkin's and non-Hodgkin's lymphomas and for

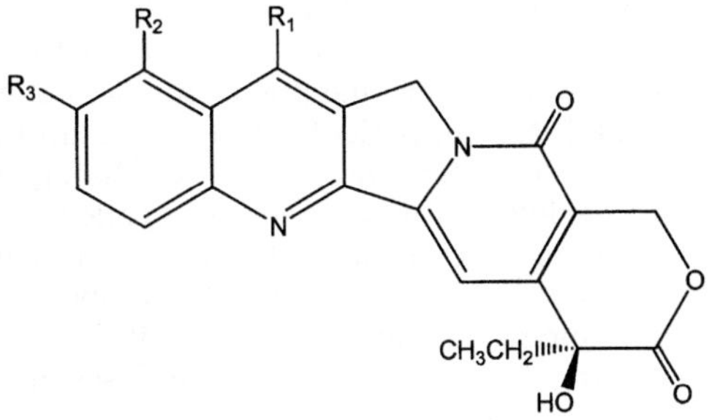

Compound	R_1	R_2	R_3
Camptothecin	–H	–H	–H
Topotecan	–H	–CH$_2$N(CH$_3$)$_2$	–OH
Irinotecan	–CH$_2$CH$_3$	–H	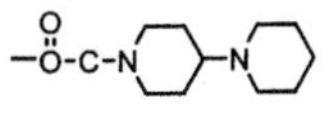 (bispiperidine carbamate structure)
SN-38	–CH$_2$CH$_3$	–H	–OH

Figure 59-16. Structure of camptothecin and its analogs that have shown evidence of clinical activity against hematologic malignancies.

the induction phase of AML. Etoposide phosphate, a prodrug with greater water solubility than VP-16, is extensively used for the treatment of solid tumors, particularly small cell lung cancer and testicular cancer, but it is not indicated for use against hematologic malignancies. Parenteral and oral formulations of etoposide are commercially available; however, oral bioavailability of the drug is highly variable. It is extensively bound (92% to 94%) to albumin in plasma and has a V_{ss} ranging from 7 to 13 L/m^2 (134). Etoposide is predominately (70% to 90%) eliminated from the body by nonrenal mechanisms with an average CL of 1.7 L/hour/m^2 (113). Drug disposition is biexponential, with a $t_{1/2,z}$ ranging from 3 to 11 hours (113). The dose-limiting toxicity of etoposide is myelosuppression, with leukocyte nadirs occurring on days 5 to 15, usually resolving within 28 days after dosing. Other less frequently encountered toxicities include thrombocytopenia, nausea, emesis, diarrhea, and mucositis.

CAMPTOTHECINS

The camptothecins are the first compounds for which cytotoxicity was specifically attributed to the inhibition of topoisomerase I, and they remain the only clinically approved drugs with this mechanism of action. Camptothecin is a naturally occurring cytotoxic alkaloid, originally isolated from a common Chinese bush, and it is distinguished by the presence of a labile α-hydroxy-δ-lactone ring (Fig. 59-16). The intrinsic chemical reactivity of the lactone is necessary for the biologic activity of the camptothecins. However, it is also susceptible to spontaneous reversible hydrolysis, so that the intact lactone form predominates at acidic pH, and the inactive opened-ring carboxylate species is favored at neutral and alkaline pH (7). Thus, inactivation of the drug by hydrolysis under physiologic conditions has been an important consideration in optimizing the therapeutic effectiveness of the camptothecins.

Poor solubility precluded direct administration of the biologically active intact lactone form of camptothecin to humans. Topotecan and irinotecan are synthetic analogs of camptothecin that were designed to facilitate parenteral administration through the introduction of functional groups to enhance water solubility. Both compounds are now well-established compo-

nents in the chemotherapeutic management of several solid tumors. Several other camptothecin analogs are in various stages of clinical evaluation; however, 9-aminocamptothecin is the only investigational camptothecin for which evidence of activity against hematologic malignancies has been reported.

Topotecan. Topotecan is indicated as a second-line therapy for advanced ovarian cancer and small cell lung cancer. Clinical efficacy against hematologic malignancies has also been demonstrated. Specifically, complete response rates of 27% and 37% were achieved in phase II studies involving patients with CML and myelodysplastic syndromes, respectively (135). In addition, activity in patients with AML was observed during a phase I trial (136). Activity against primary CNS non-Hodgkin's lymphoma has been described in a case report (137). Clinical trials have been undertaken to evaluate the use of topotecan in combination with cytarabine and other approved cytotoxic drugs for the treatment of hematologic malignancies. Phase II studies of the topotecan/cytarabine combination achieved complete remissions in 61% of patients with myelodysplastic syndromes and 44% of those with CML (138). A randomized study comparing topotecan/cytarabine against cytarabine/idarubicin in patients with myelodysplastic syndromes has been initiated.

The approved dosing regimen of topotecan is a 1.5-mg/m^2 dose given by 30-minute i.v. infusion once a day for 5 consecutive days, with additional cycles of therapy delivered at intervals of 3 weeks. The principal severe toxicity, neutropenia, is often accompanied by thrombocytopenia. Higher doses can be given to patients with hematologic malignancies, for whom the maximum tolerated dose for the daily times 5 schedule is 4.5 mg/m^2/day (139). Gastrointestinal side effects such as mucositis and diarrhea become dose limiting at these higher doses. Less frequently encountered toxicities of the drug, which are usually readily managed, include nausea, vomiting, mucositis, elevated serum transaminase activities, fever, fatigue, and rash.

Topotecan exhibits linear pharmacokinetic behavior over a relatively wide range of doses (0.4 to 22.5 mg/m^2). Plasma levels of topotecan lactone and total drug decline in a biexponential manner after i.v. infusion, with similar terminal phase half-lives of 2.4 to 4.3 hours. The ratio of the lactone to total drug AUC ranges from 0.3 to 0.4. Its CL averages 27.4 L/hour/m^2 for the lactone form and 13.4 L/hour/m^2 for the total drug in various clinical studies. The fraction of topotecan bound to plasma proteins, which has been reported as ranging from 7% to 35% based on total drug determinations, is much lower than that of other camptothecins (140,141). Approximately 30% to 40% of the dose is recovered as unchanged drug in the urine, and a clear relationship between creatinine CL and topotecan CL has been documented (142). Topotecan disposition is not significantly altered in patients with hepatic dysfunction (143).

Irinotecan. Irinotecan is a water-soluble prodrug designed to facilitate parental administration of the potent 7-ethyl-10-hydroxy analog of camptothecin (SN-38). Enzymatic hydrolysis of the ester linkage of the basic bispiperidine promoiety on presentation to the systemic circulation affords SN-38, the biologically active compound, which is a 1000-fold more potent inhibitor of purified topoisomerase I *in vitro* than irinotecan (141). Conversion to SN-38 is predominantly mediated by carboxylesterases in the liver (144). The major therapeutic indication for irinotecan is the treatment of colorectal cancer, both as first-line therapy in combination with 5-FU and as salvage treatment in 5-FU refractory disease. The evaluation of irinotecan against hematologic malignancies is limited to a few phase II trials conducted in Japan. These studies included a heteroge-

2118 59: CLINICAL PHARMACOLOGY OF ANTICANCER DRUGS

neous patient population ranging from low- and intermediate-grade non-Hodgkin's lymphomas to Hodgkin's lymphomas and acute leukemias. Subgroup analysis revealed a response rate of 42% in previously treated non-Hodgkin's lymphoma patients and 38% in refractory or relapsed adult T-cell leukemia-lymphoma patients.

The approved administration schedule of irinotecan in the United States is 125 mg/m^2, given as a 90-minute i.v. infusion once weekly for 4 of 6 weeks (145). The principal severe toxicity is delayed diarrhea that can be effectively controlled by intensive treatment with loperamide. Myelosuppression is the second most commonly encountered toxicity (145–147). Febrile neutropenia occurs in 3% of the patients, and it may be life threatening, particularly when associated with concomitant diarrhea. A short-lasting cholinergic syndrome that responds rapidly to atropine, resulting from the ability of irinotecan to inhibit acetylcholinesterase activity, is frequently evident within the first 24 hours after dosing (141,145–147).

In cancer patients, the AUC of SN-38 is approximately 4% of the irinotecan AUC, suggesting that only a relatively small fraction of the dose is ultimately converted to the active form of the drug (145). However, the biological half-life of the lactone form of SN-38, 11.5 hours, is much longer than that of topotecan. Moreover, in comparison to other camptothecin derivatives, a relatively large percentage of the intact lactone form of both irinotecan and SN-38 persists in the plasma of patients after drug administration due to the preferential binding of the lactone form to serum albumin. Aside from conversion to SN-38, irinotecan undergoes biliary excretion, and it is also subject to biotransformation by CYP450. The major mechanisms of SN-38 elimination appear to be glucuronidation and biliary excretion.

Biologic Agents

L-ASPARAGINASE

Human malignant cells of lymphoid origin display a unique sensitivity to the depletion of L-asparagine. This amino acid is recruited from the bloodstream after synthesis in the liver or after it is synthesized from aspartic acid by the enzyme asparagine synthetase in some nonlymphoid tissues. Human cells do not possess an enzyme capable of degrading asparagine, but such an enzyme, L-asparaginase, is found in various bacteria and the plasma of rodents. When L-asparaginase is administered i.v. or intramuscularly to humans, immediate depletion of the circulating pool of asparagine results, and protein synthesis ceases in cells that lack the capacity to synthesize the amino acid. ALL in children, as well as high-grade lymphomas in children and adults, are profoundly sensitive to L-asparaginase. These tumor cells undergo apoptosis in response to asparagine depletion. Thus, L-asparaginase has become a key component of combination therapy for ALL of both B-cell and T-cell origin, and it is used in many regimens for the treatment of Burkitt lymphoma.

Three L-asparaginase preparations are available for clinical use in the United States (148). Protein derived from *Escherichia coli* was the first to be approved for human use and remains the most commonly used preparation for first-line therapy. It is usually administered at doses of 6000 to 10,000 IU given every third day for 3 to 4 weeks, with the objective of maintaining L-asparaginase levels above 0.03 IU/mL in serum. Plasma levels decay in a monoexponential manner with a half-life of approximately 24 hours. Hypersensitivity reactions mediated by antibodies to the foreign protein are common, usually occur after giving at least two doses of enzyme, and present as urticaria, bronchospasm, or hypotension. Skin testing before the first dose detects some, but not all, hypersensitive patients. Antibod-

ies develop in up to 60% of patients after multiple cycles of treatment with L-asparaginase, and they are associated with a more rapid disappearance of enzyme from serum and clinical drug resistance (149). Not all patients with serum antibody titers display a clinical hypersensitivity response, although failure of therapy is more likely in antibody-positive patients.

The enzyme has been conjugated at multiple sites with methoxypolyethylene glycol (PEG) groups with the objective of decreasing its immunogenicity and prolonging its biological half-life. PEG-asparaginase is usually given in doses of 2500 IU/m^2 every 1 or 2 weeks and has a $t_{1/2,z}$ of 6 days (150). It produces hypersensitivity at a significantly reduced rate as compared to the native enzyme and is often used for reinduction after initial treatment with the unmodified L-asparaginase. However, allergic reactions still occur with a frequency as great as 25% in patients who have had a prior hypersensitivity response to L-asparaginase.

The third preparation available for human use is derived from *Erwinia chrysanthemi*. It shares only 30% homology with the *E. coli* enzyme and, therefore, exhibits a low rate of immune cross-sensitivity. Hypersensitivity to *Erwinia* asparaginase develops in 5% of patients. The catalytic activity of *Erwinia* asparaginase is approximately equal to that of the *E. coli* enzyme, but its shorter $t_{1/2,z}$ necessitates higher doses for effective asparagine depletion (151).

Resistance to L-asparaginase is related to either host or tumor factors. As discussed in the preceding paragraphs, neutralizing antibodies are associated with a poor therapeutic outcome due to enhanced CL of the enzyme. Another important mechanism of resistance is associated with the selection of tumor cells that are capable of inducing asparagine synthetase (152). When L-asparaginase is used as a single agent, resistance tends to develop quickly; thus, the drug is virtually always used as part of a multidrug combination. For reasons not well understood, ALL cells in which the TEL gene is translocated and fused to AML-1 (the TEL/AML-1 translocation) are 10 times more sensitive to L-asparaginase treatment, based on *in vitro* inhibitory experiments, and this form of ALL is associated with a favorable treatment outcome (153). This increased drug sensitivity of TEL/AML-1 cells appears to be confined to L-asparaginase and does not extend to other agents. The same increased sensitivity to L-asparaginase is found in patients with hyperdiploid ALL.

In addition to its propensity to produce hypersensitivity responses, L-asparaginase has significant toxicities related to the inhibition of protein synthesis in the liver and pancreas. It inhibits the synthesis of multiple clotting factors, including the procoagulant fibrinogen, as well as the anticoagulants protein C, protein S, and antithrombin III. Thus, spontaneous hemorrhage or thrombosis, but more commonly thrombotic episodes, may result from L-asparaginase treatment. Evaluating patients with symptoms of CNS dysfunction, as indicated by a change in mental status or stroke, by magnetic resonance imaging has revealed an unexpectedly high incidence of cortical vein thrombosis (10% to 20%) (154). Patients with underlying inherited abnormalities of coagulation, such as factor V Leiden, deficiencies of protein C or S, or prothrombin mutations, are particularly likely to experience thrombotic events, suggesting the value of screening for coagulopathy before treatment (155). Other common side effects include the following: pancreatitis associated with drug-induced hypertriglyceridemia, hyperglycemia that may be related to decreased insulin production, hypoalbuminemia, and elevated serum bilirubin. The same pattern of toxicities is associated with PEG-asparaginase and with the *Erwinia* preparation. High-dose L-asparaginase, although yielding higher remission induction rates in poor-

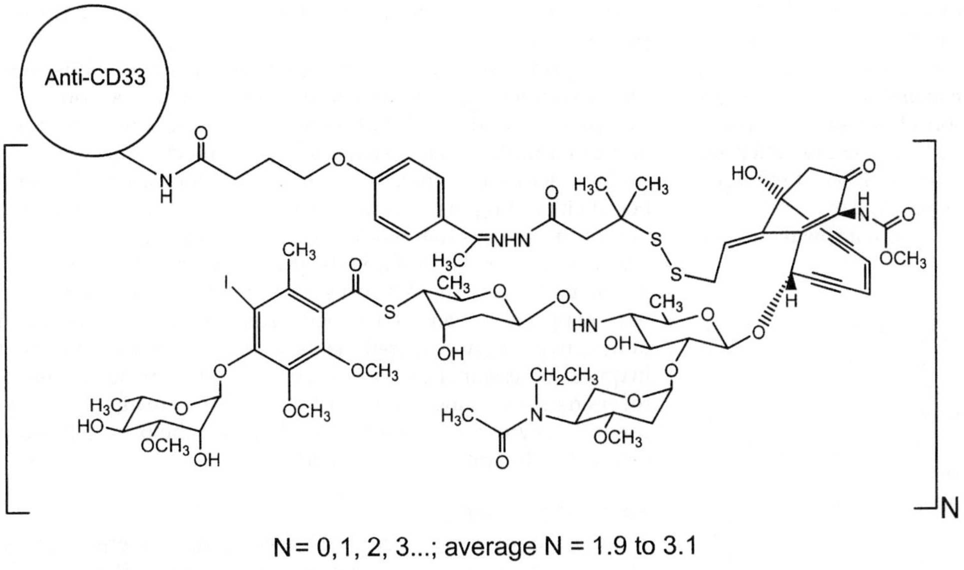

N = 0, 1, 2, 3...; average N = 1.9 to 3.1

Figure 59-17. Structure of gemtuzumab ozogamicin.

prognosis ALL patients, increases the risk of hypersensitivity and other toxicities. The only significant drug interaction is the ability of L-asparaginase to mitigate the antitumor effect of MTX (156). As such, it should not be used in close proximity to MTX, except in protocols specifically designed to abbreviate MTX action.

GEMTUZUMAB OZOGAMICIN

To identify more selective therapies for neoplastic disease, monoclonal antibodies are particularly attractive due to their highly specific targeting of cancer cell antigens. Several unmodified monoclonal antibodies, including rituxan (which targets CD20 on B lymphocytes) and Herceptin (which is directed at the amplified her-2/neu receptor on breast cancer cells), have shown significant clinical activity and are now approved for use in humans. The mechanisms by which they induce cell death are not completely understood, but they may include direct induction of apoptosis through binding to the cell-surface antigen or an indirect mechanism dependent on complement or immune cell–mediated lysis. An alternative is to link an antibody to a cytotoxic compound and thereby deliver the toxin selectively to the tumor cell. This strategy has been explored extensively, using radionuclides such as iodine 131 or potent cytotoxins bound covalently to the antibody (157). The most notable success in this effort has been achieved with gemtuzumab ozogamicin, a humanized anti-CD33 antibody linked to an extremely potent antitumor antibiotic, N-acetyl-γ-calicheamicin dimethyl hydrazide (Fig. 59-17). Used by itself, calicheamicin is one of many highly cytotoxic antibiotics that bind to the minor groove of DNA, inducing DNA strand breaks and apoptosis. The active intermediate is generated by the reduction of the disulfide bond and the rearrangement of the calicheamicin, forming a highly reactive diradical that interacts with the deoxyribose rings on opposing strands of DNA (158). It is intolerably toxic to normal tissues, but when bound to the antibody, the conjugate produces selective toxicity against CD33-positive cells.

The target for gemtuzumab, CD33, is expressed on the surface of more than 90% of myeloid leukemia cells, normal myeloid and platelet precursors as well as macrophages, mast cells, and microglial cells, but it is not expressed by normal pluripotent hematopoietic cells or other normal tissues (159). After binding to the cell surface, gemtuzumab becomes internalized, upon which calicheamicin is released in the endosomes and lysosomes (160). Preclinical studies have shown conclusively that the same toxin,

bound to a nontargeting antibody, does not approach the effectiveness of gemtuzumab; thus, the antibody specificity plays a critical role in its effectiveness. Its activity in vitro is confined to CD33+ cells at drug concentrations of 20 pg/mL. The unconjugated antibody has no antitumor activity in vitro. In clinical trials of the drug, AML patients in first relapse were treated with one to three doses of the conjugate, 9 mg/m^2, and 42 of 142 patients (30%) had a complete response (161,162).

At the recommended dose of 9 mg/m^2, more than 80% of the binding sites on leukemic blasts are occupied by the drug, whereas the extent of binding and antileukemic effects are diminished at lower doses (161). The apparent $t_{1/2,z}$ of the gemtuzumab antibody is approximately 70 hours, and that of calicheamicin is about 40 hours; thus, a single dose provides prolonged exposure to cells (163). The recommended dosing interval for patients who are not achieving a complete response is 2 weeks. Most patients who respond require two doses. The C_{max} of the antibody protein as measured by an enzyme-linked immunoabsorbent assay is approximately 3 µg/mL, and the C_{max} of calicheamicin in plasma is only 5 pg/mL. Nevertheless, it appears that a significant portion of the toxin dissociates from the antibody in the bloodstream over time. However, studies to completely define the plasma profiles for the intact molecule, antibody protein, and toxin have not been performed. On release from the antibody, free calicheamicin undergoes extensive hepatic metabolism, while a portion of the dose is excreted unchanged in the urine. There is little published information on mechanisms of resistance to gemtuzumab. Free calicheamicin is a substrate for the MDR transporter, which is expressed by some or a portion of AML cells, particularly after exposure to chemotherapy (164). Modulation of CD33 expression may also contribute to drug resistance (160).

Being a monoclonal antibody, the primary acute toxicities of the drug are infusion-related fever and chills, that occur despite acetaminophen and antihistamine pretreatment (161,162). These symptoms are severe in approximately 10% of patients. Additional toxicities include nausea, vomiting, diarrhea, stomatitis, and asthenia in approximately one-third to one-half of patients treated. Repeat treatment has evoked dyspnea and hypotension in the presence of substantial titers of antibody to the calicheamicin-linker complex in a minority of patients. Immune responses indicated by positive antibody titers to the drug are infrequent, and their effect on response is not known.

Approximately one-fourth of patients experience significant hepatotoxicity, indicated by hyperbilirubinemia and elevated hepatic enzymes in serum. These abnormalities are usually rapidly reversible once remission is achieved and therapy discontinued. Venoocclusive disease of the liver has been reported in patients who achieve remission with gemtuzumab and then receive high-dose therapy with stem cell transplantation. However, the nature of the apparent association between venoocclusive disease and prior gemtuzumab liver toxicity has not been established. Prolonged neutropenia and thrombocytopenia may result, particularly after multiple doses of drug, even in patients in bone marrow remission.

NONCYTOTOXIC AND MOLECULARLY TARGETED APPROACHES FOR CANCER TREATMENT

Recent advances in understanding the mechanisms of tumor initiation, progression, and metastasis have created opportunities for designing drugs with great specificity for tumors and limited host toxicity. Thus far, the majority of drugs reaching the clinic have been designed to inhibit angiogenesis, modify cell cycle control and signal transduction, promote differentiation, and block metastasis. Many of the pathways critical to these processes are controlled by cell-surface receptors coupled through signaling pathways to nuclear events. The steps involved in signal transduction often require phosphorylation of key proteins by protein kinases that are specific for each pathway. Among the many potential targets for drug discovery and development, the clearest success has resulted from attempts to inhibit protein kinase activity, which is overexpressed in many human malignancies. This section reviews areas of investigation and specific agents that are likely to become important in hematologic cancer treatment. Some of these compounds have already been approved for clinical use.

Differentiating Agents

ALL-*TRANS*-RETINOIC ACID

The first truly effective differentiating agent to be used in clinical practice, all-*trans*-retinoic acid (tRA), was developed in China as an alternative to cytotoxic chemotherapy (165). Hematologists in Shanghai first noticed that patients with acute promyelocytic leukemia (APL) entered remission, even after having no response to standard cytotoxic chemotherapy, when treated with this readily available retinoid. The drug is now a mainstay in the initial treatment of APL and provides a complete response rate above 90%. The mechanism of action of tRA probably relates to the altered function of the retinoic acid binding protein, RAR-α, in APL. The characteristic 15:17 translocation in APL joins the RAR-α gene and the PML gene, a transcription factor, creating a fusion protein in which the RAR-α component has diminished affinity for retinoids. The fusion protein binds tightly to its corepressor. Physiologic concentrations of retinoids are unable to release RAR from this complex (166). However, higher concentrations of tRA effect the dissociation of retinoid binding proteins from corepressor proteins, thereby enabling the fusion protein to activate differentiation. Mutations in the PML-RAR-α fusion gene that further decrease tRA binding or decrease affinity of the fusion protein for its DNA binding site lead to tRA resistance, further supporting a role for the binding of the retinoid to the fusion gene (167).

The usual dose of tRA in APL treatment is 45 mg/m² given orally once every day until complete remission occurs. During the initial course of therapy, peak retinoid plasma levels of 300 ng/mL are achieved 3 hours after dosing and then decline rapidly, with a $t_{1/2,z}$ that is less than 1 hour (168). Metabolic elimination of tRA by hepatic CYP450 metabolism is inducible—a factor that may lead to the development of resistance during prolonged therapy.

The principal toxicities include dryness of skin, cheilitis, mild liver dysfunction, bone tenderness and hyperostosis on x-ray, and pseudotumor cerebri at higher doses. The most important and potentially lethal toxicity is hyperleukocytosis syndrome (retinoic acid syndrome), caused by a rapid increase in the number of circulating myeloid lineage cells secondary to differentiation of tumor cells that block the microvasculature in the lungs, brain, and heart (169). Patients at particular risk have a high number of circulating APL cells (i.e., >5000/mL). Fever, pulmonary congestion, pleural and pericardial effusions, multiorgan failure, hypoxia, and altered mental status may follow treatment in quick succession. High-dose corticosteroids may be of value in reversing these changes, but most protocols for treating APL now use initial cytotoxic chemotherapy to lower the blast cell count before APL treatment with retinoids.

ARSENIC TRIOXIDE

Among the more surprising anticancer drugs, arsenic trioxide (ATO; As_2O_3) is infamous as a poison; nevertheless, it is clinically active against APL. The use of ATO was first noted by hematologists from Shanghai, China, who observed a successful induction of differentiation similar to that achieved with tRA—but in patients with tRA-resistant disease (170). The efficacy of ATO against APL was confirmed in a small study involving patients who had either relapsed after treatment with tRA and daunorubicin or were refractory to these drugs. Complete clinical remissions were achieved in 11 of the 12 patients treated (171). In the typical dosing regimen, 10 mg of ATO is given as a 2-hour i.v. infusion once daily for 60 days or until bone marrow remission, which is achieved at a median time of approximately 60 days. Consolidation therapy with 25 daily doses was initiated 3 weeks after documenting a remission. The median survival time of these patients was greater than 18 months. Prior treatment with either tRA or cytotoxic drugs, including high-dose therapy with bone marrow transplantation, did not significantly affect response rates.

ATO's mechanism of action remains to be conclusively established. However, we do know that it disrupts mitochondrial function through complex formation with a cofactor in the pyruvate metabolism pathway, decreasing ATP production and inducing oxidative stress. At high concentrations, the drug induces apoptosis in tumor cells, whereas noncytotoxic levels promote differentiation of myeloid leukemia cells (172). Treatment with ATO leads to APL cell differentiation in approximately 25% of patients, and a syndrome of rapidly rising myeloid cell blood counts occurs with a frequency of 10%. Pulmonary distress and hypoxia, similar to the tRA-induced hyperleukocytosis, occurs infrequently relative to that observed with tRA. Other important side effects include hyperglycemia, hypokalemia, and elevated serum transaminase levels. ATO prolongs the cardiac QT interval and can lead to atrial and ventricular arrhythmias, particularly in the presence of hypokalemia (170). A "stocking-glove" type of peripheral neuropathy has also been associated with ATO treatment.

A 10-mg dose of ATO affords a 5- to 7-μM peak arsenic plasma concentration at the end of the 2-hour infusion in cancer patients (170). Total arsenic disposition is biexponential, with an apparent $t_{1/2,z}$ of 12 hours and a CL of 0.8 to 1.1 L/hour/m². Preclinical studies of ATO have shown that the drug is methylated and that the metabolites are slowly excreted in the urine (173). Only 1% to 8% of the total daily dose of arsenic was recovered in the urine of cancer patients, suggesting that a large fraction of the dose is retained in the body, most likely covalently bound to sulfhydryl groups of proteins, until it is eventually eliminated in the bile (170).

Tyrosine Kinase Inhibition

Protein kinases transfer phosphate groups to key amino acid residues, most prominently serine, threonine, and tyrosine, thereby activating or inhibiting the activity of the protein. Many of the important regulatory steps in transmitting growth factor and stromal interaction signals to the nucleus require the phosphorylation of multiple intermediates. Progression into the DNA synthesis phase of the cell cycle is controlled through phosphorylation of the retinoblastoma protein (Rb) by the cyclin-dependent kinase, CDK4. When hyperphosphorylated, Rb dissociates from E2F, a potent transcription factor, which is then free to stimulate the synthesis of a series of enzymes required for DNA synthesis. Mutations that activate this CDK4-mediated phosphorylation reaction, including the loss of the inhibitor p16, overexpression of the cofactor and activator cyclin D, or loss of the pRb gene itself, are found in virtually every human tumor. Accordingly, the identification and development of CDK4 inhibitors for their potential as specifically targeted antiproliferative interventions have been actively pursued during the past decade (174,175).

FLAVOPIRIDOL

Flavopiridol (Fig. 59-18) is a semisynthetic flavone derivative that inhibits purified CDK4 with a K_i of 40 to 50 nM (175). Preclinical studies have shown that flavopiridol inhibits the growth of CLL cell lines with an IC_{50} (50% inhibitory concentration) of 160 to 180 nM and induces apoptosis at these concentrations independent of their p53 status (176). In addition, the compound lacks significant toxicity against normal hematopoietic progenitor cells. Evidence of activity against non-

Flavopiridol

STI571

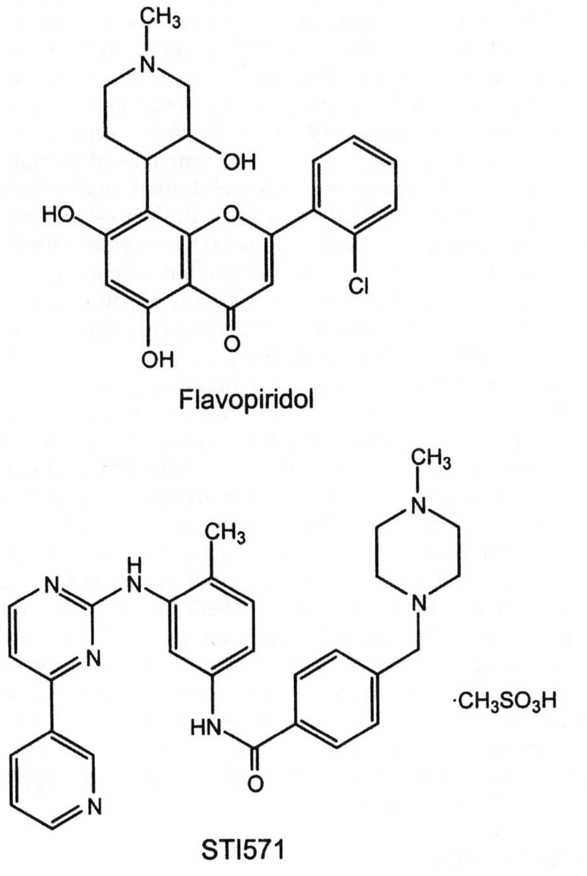

Figure 59-18. Chemical structures of the tyrosine kinase inhibitors flavopiridol and imatinib mesylate (STI571).

Hodgkin's lymphoma and renal cell carcinoma was observed in patients treated during phase I clinical trials (177). Diarrhea limited dose escalation above 78 mg/m²/day when the drug was administered as a 72-hour continuous i.v. infusion every 2 weeks. Diarrhea was acceptably controlled with loperamide and cholestyramine, whereupon hypotension, fever, fatigue, and anorexia became dose limiting. The plasma pharmacokinetics of flavopiridol appeared to be highly variable when characterized during the phase I trials. The steady-state plasma concentration achieved at the maximum tolerated dose of 150 mg/m² for the 72-hour i.v. infusion schedule ranged from 170 to 2900 nM in 5 patients and had a median value of 271 nM. Although activity as a single agent against solid tumors has been disappointing in phase II trials, studies to clinically evaluate therapeutically favorable combinations with cytotoxic drugs, including cytarabine and gemcitabine, and irradiation are under way (178).

IMATINIB

CML presents a unique opportunity for targeted therapy, as almost all patients with this disease have molecular evidence of a translocation between chromosomes 9 and 22 that creates an activated tyrosine kinase (179). This translocation juxtaposes the kinase portion of the abl oncogene with the breakpoint cluster region of chromosome 22, constitutively activating the enzyme and leading to a block in differentiation in the myeloid cell series. Experiments with antisense oligonucleotides demonstrated that inhibiting the expression of the bcr-abl kinase resulted in the death of CML cells in culture, whereas normal myeloid precursors were unaffected. Using bcr-abl kinase activity in a high-throughput screen, the synthetic benzamide derivative, imatinib, shown in Figure 59-18, was identified (180). In addition to inhibiting bcr-abl kinase activity, it also inhibited two other closely related kinases, c-kit and the platelet-derived growth factor receptor (PDGFr), at submicromolar concentrations. Imatinib blocks the ATP-binding site on the tyrosine kinase, inhibiting catalytic activity with a K_i of approximately 10 nM (181). Cytotoxicity of the compound against CML cells *in vitro* was closely correlated with bcr-abl inhibition. Normal myeloid precursors and other tumor cell lines that did not express the targeted kinases were relatively unaffected by imatinib at concentrations that were effective against CML (180). Cells expressing c-kit or PDGFr underwent apoptosis when exposed to the drug. Moreover, the compound displayed very favorable pharmacokinetic properties in preclinical studies, including excellent oral bioavailability and a relatively long biological half-life in plasma, with a modest spectrum of toxicity.

Clinical trials of imatinib given orally on a chronic basis in patients with CML were initiated in 1998 (8). Clinical hematologic improvement was seen in virtually all patients, including those refractory to interferon (IFN)-α, the standard therapy for CML. Most patients exhibited a decline in the percentage of bone marrow myeloid precursors expressing the Philadelphia chromosome. In the initial study, Ph⁺ cells became undetectable in 7 of 54 patients. The responses tended to be incomplete and short lived in most patients with accelerated or blastic phase CML, although prolonged complete responses were achieved in a modest percentage (<25%) (182). In addition, the drug has shown promising evidence of activity against gastrointestinal stromal tumors, a particularly refractory sarcoma originating in the bowel characterized by the overexpression of the c-kit receptor (183).

Imatinib appears to be well absorbed in humans, and its AUC increased linearly when the daily dose was escalated from 25 to 1000 mg/day (8). Pharmacokinetic studies demonstrated that the

mean C_{max} in plasma at steady state was 4.6 μM in patients treated with doses of 400 mg given once daily. As a result of its apparent $t_{1/2,z}$, which ranges from 13 to 16 hours, daily treatment with doses of 300 mg or more continually maintains a potentially effective plasma concentration of the drug, with nadir levels exceeding 1 μM. Doses as great as 1000 mg/day are well tolerated by most patients, although hepatic enzyme elevations, neutropenia, nausea, and myalgias are occasionally observed, most prominently at higher doses. Presently, mechanisms of resistance to imatinib are incompletely defined. The compound is a substrate for P-glycoprotein, and experimental evidence also suggests that resistance could arise through the selection of cancer cells with amplified bcr-abl kinase levels (184). Resistance in CML patients treated with the drug during blast crisis has also been accredited to a single amino acid mutation in the kinase that prevents imatinib from binding but preserves enzyme activity (185).

Future trials of the drug will undoubtedly assess its ability to potentiate the activity of chemotherapy and IFN-α in the treatment of CML. Evaluating activity against other malignancies that overexpress c-kit and PDGFr, such as small cell lung cancer, astrocytomas, and prostate cancer, is also of interest. With regard to other hematologic malignancies, studies to assess activity against acute leukemias expressing the tel-PDGFr translocation are warranted.

Proteasome Inhibition

The ubiquitin-proteasome pathway plays a pivotal role in cell cycle regulation, cell survival, and metastasis. Inhibiting proteasome-mediated degradation can increase or prolong the functional activity of many important regulatory proteins. Conceivably, antiproliferative effects could result from preventing the degradation of p53, increasing p21 inhibition of CDK activity, and, most importantly, mitigating the degradation of IκBα (186). IκBα functions as an inhibitor of NFκB, a transcription factor that controls a number of genes involved in cell proliferation. NFκB activity is increased in many experimental tumors, including multiple myeloma, and after exposure to chemotherapeutic agents.

PS-341 is a dipeptidyl-boronic acid derivative (Fig. 59-19) that inhibits purified 20S proteasome with a K_i of 0.6 nM (186). It was found to exhibit antiproliferative activity against human multiple myeloma cells in vitro and retard the growth of xenografts of several human solid tumor cell lines in nude mice (187). Phase I clinical trials assessing a variety of administration schedules of the drug given as a bolus i.v. injection were recently completed (188). During these studies, inhibition of the 20S proteasome in blood cells was used to evaluate the pharmacodynamic effects of the drug. PS-341 was reasonably well tolerated at dose intensities that resulted in 70% inhibition of the pretreatment 20S proteasome activity. The principal severe toxicities are myelosuppression,

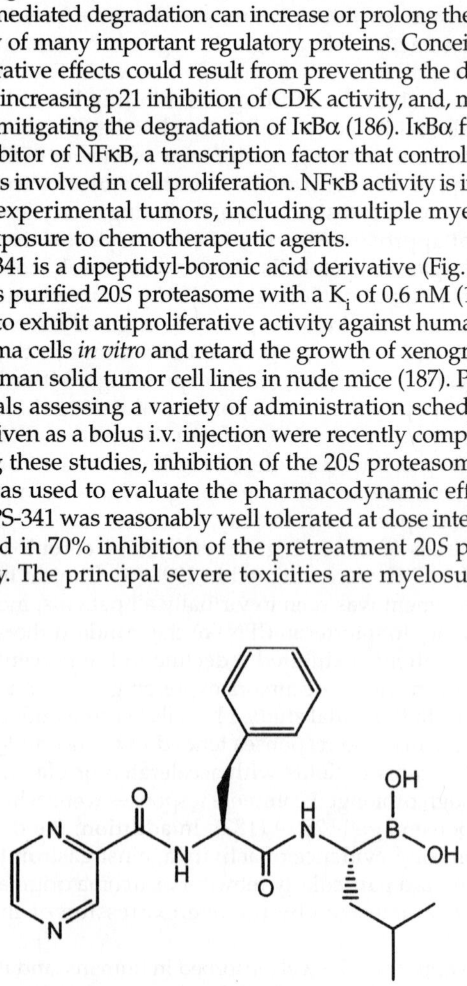

Figure 59-19. Structure of the proteosome inhibitor PS-341.

diarrhea, malaise, and peripheral neuropathy. Evidence of activity has been observed in several patients, evoking considerable interest for further evaluating clinical efficacy against lymphoma and multiple myeloma in combination with dexamethasone and various solid tumors. The prospect for synergistic activity with cytotoxic drugs is particularly intriguing because resistance has been associated with enhanced NFκB activity. Clinical trials to evaluate the use of PS-341 given in combination with such drugs (irinotecan, in particular) have been initiated.

Antiangiogenic Agents

Angiogenesis is defined as new blood vessel formation from quiescent endothelial stem cells. Folkman first hypothesized that the new vessels formed at a tumor site were not inconsequential but absolutely required for expansion of the tumor spheroid beyond a diameter of 1 to 2 mm (189). On achieving this size, the delivery of nutrients and removal of waste products facilitated by the bloodstream limit the continued growth of a tumor. A convincing body of evidence in support of the importance of inducing and sustaining angiogenesis in tumor development has been acquired during the past decade. The ability to induce and sustain angiogenesis seems to be acquired in one or more discrete steps during tumor development via an "angiogenic switch" from vascular quiescence (190,191). Tumors appear to activate the angiogenic switch by altering the balance of endogenous molecules that are angiogenesis inducers and the counterbalancing inhibitors.

Recently, increasing evidence has indicated a role for angiogenesis in hematologic neoplasms. Quantifying the degree of angiogenesis usually involves directly measuring microvessel density or assaying serum or urine levels of known angiogenic inducers, including vascular endothelial growth factor (VEGF) and basic fibroblast growth factor (bFGF). Perez-Atayde et al. first demonstrated an increased microvessel density in the bone marrow of patients with ALL (192). Subsequently, enhanced angiogenic activity was described in patients with multiple myeloma, acute and chronic leukemias, myelodysplastic syndromes, and lymphoma (193–197). Elevated serum and urine bFGF and VEGF levels were noted in patients with hematologic malignancies. Increased microvessel density was detected in the bone marrow of AML, CLL, and multiple myeloma patients. Increased angiogenic activity appeared to correlate with the disease activity in AML and multiple myeloma. In a retrospective study of 160 patients with non-Hodgkin's lymphoma, a high pretreatment serum bFGF concentration correlated with poor prognosis and was an independent prognostic factor (198).

Antiangiogenesis represents a potential new strategy for chemotherapy that has generated tremendous enthusiasm in the field of anticancer drug development. It has been recognized that tumor cells stimulate the production of circulating angiogenic inhibitors that act downstream to suppress metastatic expansion at secondary locations. Among these compounds, the mammalian proteins angiostatin and endostatin are the most well characterized (199,200). A continually increasing cohort of natural products, synthetic compounds, and biologic molecules that can function as angiogenic inhibitors have been identified. There are currently more than 30 angiogenesis inhibitors in clinical trials, and a multitude of promising new candidates are under investigation in vitro and in animal models. The mechanism of action, pharmacology, and clinical application of several extensively studied antiangiogenic agents are described in this section.

THALIDOMIDE

Thalidomide, α-phthalimidoglutarimide (Fig. 59-20), was first approved in 1953 in Europe for use in humans as a sedative. It

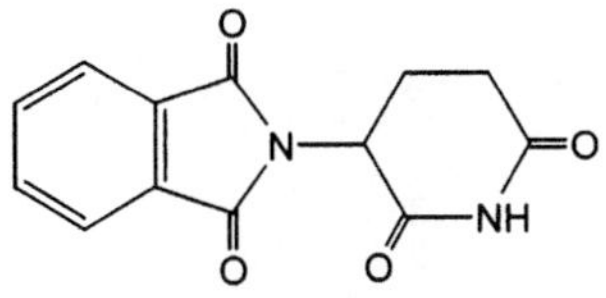

Thalidomide

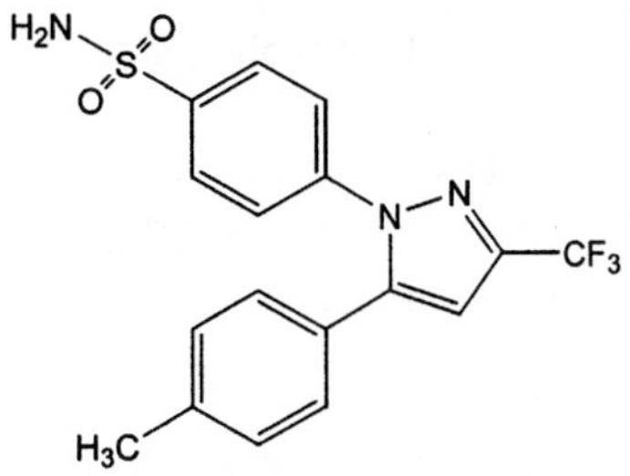

Celecoxib

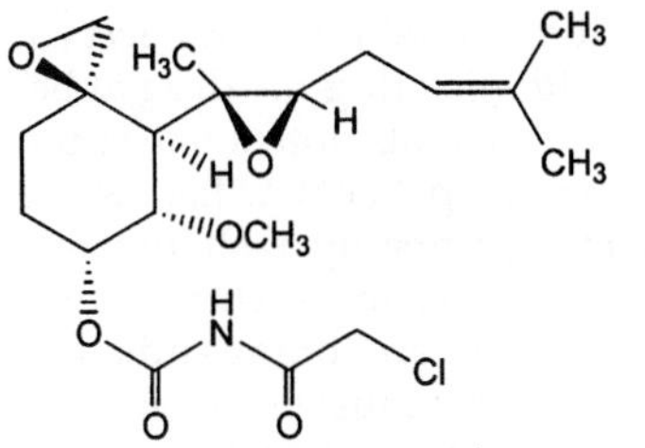

TNP-470

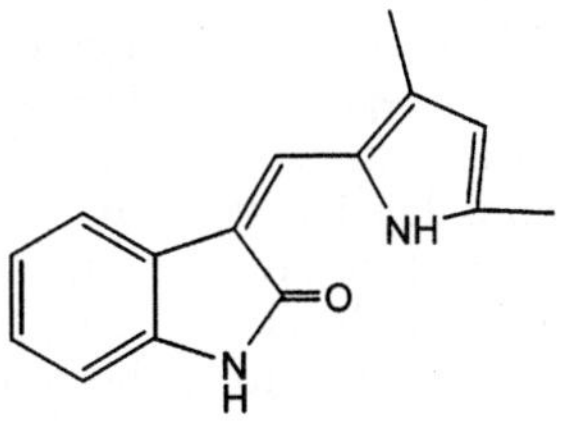

SU5416

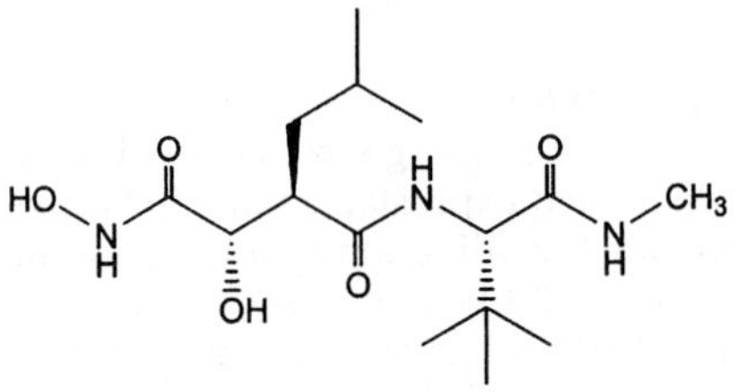

Marimastat

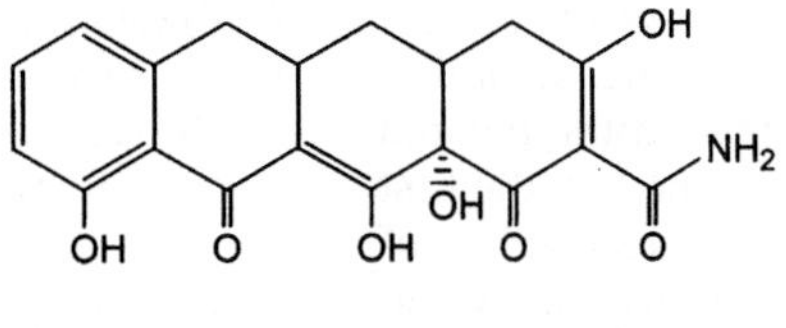

COL-3

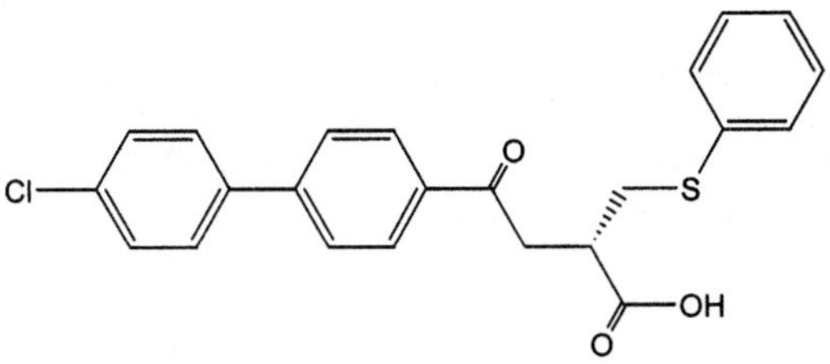

BAY 12-9566

Figure 59-20. Structures of small-molecule antiangiogenic agents.

was indicated for insomnia, morning sickness in pregnant women, and nausea associated with influenza. However, the drug was subsequently shown to be a potent teratogen that caused dysmelia (i.e., stunted limb growth) in humans, resulting in worldwide withdrawal from clinical use during the early 1960s. Recently, there has been a renewed interest in elucidating the biologic effects of thalidomide and its potential clinical applications after the demonstration of its activity against leprosy and multiple myeloma (201).

The underlying nature of the biologic effects of thalidomide are still not fully understood, although they may be related to the inhibition of angiogenesis, immune modulation, and cytokine inhibition. D'Amato et al. first demonstrated that orally administered thalidomide is an inhibitor of angiogenesis induced by bFGF in a rabbit cornea micropocket assay (202). It also inhibits bFGF- and VEGF-induced neovascularization in a mouse corneal

model when given intraperitoneally. Structure activity studies suggest that the antiangiogenic activity of thalidomide may be associated with metabolites that result from hydrolysis of the imide rings of the drug. Thalidomide and its structural analog, CC-1069, inhibit the proliferation of endothelial cells *in vitro* (203). Thalidomide also inhibits TNF-α production by accelerating degradation of the mRNA encoding the protein. Serum levels of TNF-α and IFN-γ are abnormally high in patients with erythema nodosum leprosum (204). On treating these patients with thalidomide orally at doses of 100 to 400 mg/day, TNF-α and IFN-γ levels were reduced to baseline with coincident alleviation of symptoms. Thalidomide can also induce the downregulation of selected cell-surface adhesion molecules involved in leukocyte migration. Although attributed to the immunomodulatory effects of thalidomide, the precise mechanism of action and spectrum of activity remain controversial. The immunologic

TABLE 59-4. Clinical Activity of Thalidomide against Various Malignancies

Cancer Type	No. of Patients	Dose (mg/day)	Response Category	Number	Percentage	Reference
Multiple myeloma	84	200–800	PR	27	32	210
Metastatic breast	28	200–1200	SD	2	7	211
Kaposi's sarcoma	12	200–600	PR	2	17	212
			SD	7	58	
High-grade glioma	10	1200	Minor response	2	20	213

PR, partial response; SD, stable disease.

effects of the compound can vary substantially depending on the conditions. A decrease in the ratio of circulating T-helper to T-suppressor (H:S) cells in healthy male patients has been reported.

The pharmacokinetic behavior of thalidomide has been studied in normal volunteers and human immunodeficiency virus–seropositive patients (205,206). In normal subjects receiving doses of 50 to 400 mg/day, thalidomide was slowly absorbed from the gastrointestinal tract with a mean time to peak concentration in plasma ranging from 2.9 to 4.3 hours after dosing. The absolute bioavailability of thalidomide has not been characterized in humans due to its poor solubility in vehicles that are suitable for parenteral administration. Whereas the AUC of the parent drug is directly proportional to the administered dose, the C_{max} increased in a less than proportionate manner. These observations suggest that the rate of absorption—not the extent of absorption—may be limited by the water solubility of the drug. There is no significant difference in the plasma pharmacokinetics of thalidomide when determined on the first and last day of a repeated daily dosing regimen. Mean values of the apparent $t_{1/2,z}$ on oral dosing range from approximately 5 to 7 hours. The major pathways by which thalidomide is eliminated from the body have not been completely established. The amount of the drug excreted unchanged in urine accounts for less than 1% of the administered dose. The two imide moieties in the molecule are both subject to spontaneous hydrolysis in plasma, potentially yielding numerous degradation products. The effects of renal or hepatic dysfunction on the pharmacokinetics of the drug have not been described.

Thalidomide has been evaluated in a variety of clinical applications including human immunodeficiency virus–related wasting syndrome, oral aphthous ulcers, graft-versus-host disease, and several malignancies (201,207–209). Its most impressive activity has been observed in patients with multiple myeloma refractory to chemotherapy (210). In a study involving 84 evaluable patients, 32% responded to thalidomide as defined by a 25% or greater decrease in serum or urine paraprotein. The response appeared to be long lasting, because the median time to progression had not been reached after a follow-up of 14.5 months. Reductions in paraprotein levels were associated with a decreased number of plasma cells in bone marrow and increased hemoglobin levels. Preliminary evidence of activity (Table 59-4) has also been observed against Kaposi's sarcoma, recurrent high-grade gliomas, and metastatic breast cancer (211–213). Thalidomide has synergistic myeloma-inhibiting activity with glucocorticoids. Clinical trials exploring its use in combination with glucocorticoids and cytotoxic drugs are presently being performed.

Thalidomide is generally well tolerated when given orally at doses of 50 to 1200 mg once every day. In myeloma patients, treatment is continued for a minimum of 30 days, at which point responding patients show evidence of decreasing paraprotein. The major side effects and dose-limiting toxicities are drowsi-ness, somnolence, constipation, and fatigue. The effects of sedation can be minimized by administering the drug at bedtime. Doses are escalated in 2-week intervals until a maximum tolerated dose is reached in individual patients. Other less frequent toxicities include peripheral neuropathy, rash, dizziness and orthostatic hypotension, neutropenia, mood changes or depression, and nausea. Hypersensitivity and bradycardia have also been reported. Extreme precautions must be taken to preclude fetal exposure, including strict contraception during treatment, due to the well-documented human teratogenicity of the drug. Thalidomide is currently approved for use in the United States under a special restricted distribution program called the *System for Thalidomide Education and Prescribing Safety* (STEPS).

CYCLOOXYGENASE-2 INHIBITORS

Cyclooxygenase (COX) is the rate-limiting enzyme involved in the conversion of arachidonic acid to prostaglandin H_2, the precursor of various compounds including other prostaglandins, prostacyclin, and thromboxanes (214). Two COX genes, COX-1 and COX-2, have been identified. COX-1 is constitutively expressed in many tissues, whereas COX-2 is inducible by various stimuli including interleukin-1, hypoxia, ultraviolet light, epidermal growth factor, transforming growth factor β, TNF-β, and several oncogenes. Many studies have highlighted the role of COX-2 in carcinogenesis. Although the precise mechanism by which COX-2 is involved in carcinogenesis is unclear, it becomes overexpressed during malignant transformation and may play an important role in regulating angiogenesis (215). Celecoxib is the first specific inhibitor of COX-2 approved for clinical use (Fig. 59-20).

The inhibition of angiogenesis by COX-2 inhibitors has been shown in several animal models. Neovascularization in a mouse corneal micropocket assay, in which angiogenesis was stimulated with bFGF, was inhibited specifically by a COX-2 selective inhibitor (216). A decrease in vascular density was observed in tumors grown in *COX-2* null mice when compared with those in wild-type mice (217). The growth of lung and colon tumors implanted into recipient mice can be suppressed by celecoxib but not by a COX-1 inhibitor. In an *in vitro* model system involving the coculture of endothelial cells with colon carcinoma cells, COX-2–overexpressing cells produce prostaglandins and proangiogenic factors and stimulate both endothelial migration and tube formation (216). This effect can be inhibited by antibodies to combinations of angiogenic factors and by NS-298, a selective COX-2 inhibitor. COX-2 appears to affect angiogenesis by up-regulating VEGF production by prostaglandins. Other potential contributory mechanisms include regulation of apoptosis and immune modulation.

The rate of absorption of celecoxib is moderate when given orally, with peak plasma drug concentrations occurring 2 to 4 hours after dosing, although the absolute extent of absorption has not been determined in humans. Celecoxib is extensively bound to plasma proteins, primarily albumin, and exhibits an apparent $t_{1/2,z}$ of approximately 11 hours in healthy subjects. The AUC of celecoxib increases in proportion to the magnitude of oral doses within the range of 100 to 800 mg (218). Hepatic metabolism appears to be the predominant manner by which celecoxib is eliminated, yielding carboxylic acid and glucuronide metabolites that are excreted in both the urine and bile. Only 2% of the dose is excreted as the parent drug in urine. Oxidation of the drug is mediated by the CYP450 2C9 isoenzyme. Celecoxib is well tolerated with few side effects. In comparison to healthy subjects with normal liver function, the daily AUC of celecoxib, 100 mg given twice a day at steady state, is increased by approximately 40% in patients with mild (Child-Pugh class A) and 180% in those with moderate (Child-Pugh class B) hepatic impairment, respectively (218).

Increasingly, studies have highlighted the role of COX-2 in carcinogenesis. Given its favorable safety profile and evidence of increased COX-2 expression in premalignant lesions, celecoxib is being studied as a chemoprevention agent for several types of solid tumors. It also exhibits synergistic activity with some cytotoxic drugs, an effect thought to be mediated by antiangiogenic activity of both modalities. Whether celecoxib has any therapeutic role in the treatment of specific cancers, either alone or in combination with cytotoxic drugs, is an area of active clinical investigation for both solid tumors and hematologic malignancies.

TNP-470

6-O-(N-chloroacetylcarbamoyl)-fumagillol (TNP-470) (Fig. 59-20) is a semisynthetic analog of fumagillin, a cytotoxic natural product secreted by the *Aspergillus* fungus (219). A common target for fumagillin was recently identified as *methionine aminopeptidase type 2* (220). The fumagillins covalently bind to methionine aminopeptidase type 2 and inhibit its enzymatic activity. Whereas the relationship between methionine aminopeptidase type 2 inhibition and cell cycle arrest remains unclear, recent findings suggest that the p53 pathway is activated in endothelial cells and other sensitive cell types after exposure to fumagillins, resulting in an accumulation of the G_1 cyclin-dependent kinase inhibitor p21[WAF1/CIP1]. The requirement of p53 and p21[WAF1/CIP1] for cell cycle inhibition by TNP-470 was underscored by the observation that cells deficient in p53 and p21[WAF1/CIP1] were resistant to TNP-470 (221,222).

TNP-470 inhibits endothelial cell proliferation 50 times more potently than fumagillin. In the chick chorioallantoic membrane assay, the local administration of TNP-470 inhibited capillary growth and induced avascular zones in a dose-dependent manner. TNP-470 inhibits bFGF-induced new capillary growth in a rat sponge implantation assay (223). In the rat blood vessel organ culture assay, TNP-470 inhibits not only endothelial proliferation but also endothelial capillary tube formation.

TNP-470 is one of the first compounds selected for clinical development on the basis of antiangiogenic activity. A number of phase I clinical trials have been performed in patients with solid tumors to evaluate administration of the compound as a short i.v. infusion according to several different schedules and by more prolonged continuous infusions (224–226). Pharmacokinetic studies revealed that the drug is eliminated extremely rapidly, with an apparent $t_{1/2,z}$ of 2 minutes on average, thereby becoming undetectable in plasma (i.e., <0.25 ng/mL) within 60 minutes after the end of the infusion (225). The only known metabolite formed from the cleavage of the chloroacetyl moiety of TNP-470, AGM-1883, has little biologic activity and exhibits an apparent terminal phase half-life of 6 minutes. In general, the pharmacokinetics of TNP-470 have exhibited an extremely high degree of inter- and intrapatient variability.

The major severe toxicities encountered in phase I trials were neurologic in nature, including dizziness, lightheadedness, vertigo, ataxia, decrease in concentration and short-term memory, confusion, anxiety, and depression. Overall, the neurotoxicity appears to be dose related and completely reversible on stopping drug administration. The efficacy of TNP-470 is being evaluated, primarily in patients with solid tumors, both as a single agent and in combination with biologic response modifiers. Whether the agent has any potential effectiveness against hematologic malignancies remains to be demonstrated.

VASCULAR ENDOTHELIAL GROWTH FACTOR RECEPTOR INHIBITORS

VEGF and its receptors, VEGF-receptor 1 (VEGF-R1; FLT-1) and VEGF-R2 (KDR), have been shown to play a major role in tumor angiogenesis in nonclinical studies. Several inhibitors targeting the VEGF receptor/ligand systems that have advanced into clinical trials are described in the following sections.

SU5416. SU5416 is a synthetic small organic molecule that has potent and selective activity against FLT-1, the VEGF receptor in endothelial cells (Fig. 59-20) (227,228). The activity and specificity of SU5416 against FLT-1 signaling have been demonstrated *in vitro* (229). SU5416 inhibits VEGF-induced mitogenesis of endothelial cells in a dose-dependent manner with an IC_{50} of approximately 0.04 μM. It also inhibits FLT-1 autophosphorylation *in vitro* in FLT-1–overexpressing NIH3T3 cells with an IC_{50} near 1 μM. It is notable that SU5416 has no direct inhibitory effects on the *in vitro* growth of several human tumor cell lines, against which IC_{50} values for growth inhibition exceed 20 μM. Nevertheless, the compound inhibits the growth of several tumor types, including human epidermoid carcinoma, melanoma, lung, and prostate, implanted as xenografts in nude mice. These results suggest that SU5416 may inhibit tumor growth *in vivo* by the inhibition of angiogenesis. Indeed, the inhibition of tumor growth was associated with a decrease in tumor vascular density.

Several phase I and phase I/II clinical studies have been conducted with SU5416 (230,231). The most extensively evaluated administration schedule was a short i.v. infusion given twice weekly. Pharmacokinetic studies performed during treatment with the first dose of SU5416 have shown that the drug is rapidly eliminated from plasma with a mean CL of 33 L/hour/m². The AUC for the first dose increases linearly with the administered dose indicative of apparent first-order behavior. Plasma levels of SU5416 decay in a biexponential manner with mean half-lives of 11 minutes and 87 minutes for the initial and terminal disposition phases, respectively. The V_{ss}, 22 L/m², is less than total body weight. CL values were found to be 60% greater when determined for the last dose of a cycle of therapy as compared to the initial dose, most likely due to induction of the enzymes involved in the oxidative metabolism of SU5416.

The dose-limiting toxicities of SU5416 are nausea, vomiting, and headache when given at 190 mg/m² twice weekly. Symptoms generally begin on the first day of infusion and last for approximately 24 hours. Treatment of the headache with analgesics such as acetaminophen or ibuprofen and of the nausea and vomiting with prochlorperazine has been effective in ameliorating this cluster of symptoms. Less frequently observed toxicities include thromboembolic and hemorrhagic events, such as superficial and deep vein thrombophlebitis, myocardial infarction, and pulmonary embolism. However, these events appear to be associated with underlying risk factors. In addition, asthenia, diarrhea, fever, insomnia, arthralgia, anorexia, and elevated serum transaminase activity have been observed in some patients. In contrast to most cytotoxic chemotherapeutic agents, SU5416 does not cause significant myelosuppression. Several clinical trials are currently ongoing to further assess the activity of SU5416 in different types of malignancies including hematologic cancers.

Anti–Vascular Endothelial Growth Factor Monoclonal Antibodies. A recombinant human monoclonal antibody to VEGF (rhuMab VEGF) was generated by engineering the VEGF binding residues of murine neutralizing antibody into the framework of normal human immunoglobulin G. It can bind and neutralize all biologically active forms of VEGF because it recognizes the binding sites for both VEGF receptors. A phase I study using the rhuMab VEGF has been reported recently in patients with metastatic solid tumors (232). Patients were treated at doses from 0.1 to 10 mg/kg ranging by a 90-minute i.v. infusion regimen. The treatment was well tolerated without significant toxicity. No severe toxicities definitely attributable to the antibody were observed. Mild to moderate side effects possibly or probably related to the study drug included asthenia, headache, and nausea. The pharmacokinetics of rhuMab VEGF appeared to be linear at doses ranging from 0.3 to 10.0 mg/kg with a $t_{1/2,z}$ of approximately 21 days. There were no objective responses; however, 12 of the 25 patients had stable disease over the duration of the study. Given the synergistic antitumor activity of antibodies to VEGF and the cytotoxic chemotherapy in preclinical models, the combination of rhuMab VEGF and each of three chemotherapy regimens (doxorubicin, carboplatin/paclitaxel, and 5-FU/leucovorin) has also been explored in another phase I study (233). rhuMab VEGF can be safely combined with any of these chemotherapy regimens when given at a dose of 3 mg/kg i.v. without any apparent synergistic toxicity. Whether rhuMab VEGF has any antitumor activity either alone or in combination with chemotherapy is currently under investigation.

Matrix Metalloproteinase Inhibitors. The *matrix metalloproteinases* (MMPs) are a family of at least 15 secreted and membrane-bound zinc endopeptidases (234). Collectively, these enzymes can degrade all of the components of the extracellular matrix and subendothelial basement membranes, including fibrillar and nonfibrillar collagens, fibronectin, laminin, and basement membrane glycoproteins. MMPs are essential for the diverse invasive processes of angiogenesis and tumor metastasis. A close association between tumor expression of various members of the MMP family and the proliferative, invasive behavior and metastatic potential has been found. Inhibition of MMP activity has generated considerable interest as a possible therapeutic target. The tissue inhibitors of metalloproteinases are naturally occurring proteins that specifically inhibit MMPs. Tissue inhibitor of metalloproteinase-1 can inhibit tumor-induced angiogenesis in experimental systems; however, its short half-life *in vivo* makes it less attractive as a pharmacologic agent.

The hydroxamate peptidomimetic inhibitor batimastat and its orally bioavailable analog marimastat (Fig. 59-20), which bind covalently to the zinc atom at the MMP-active site, were the first MMP inhibitors to be studied in detail. These compounds inhibit MMPs potently and specifically. Batimastat was the first synthetic MMP inhibitor studied in humans with advanced malignancies, but its usefulness has been limited by extremely poor water solubility, which required intraperitoneal administration of the drug formulated as an emulsion.

A phase I study of the second-generation MMP inhibitor marimastat was conducted to evaluate a twice daily oral dosing regimen in patients with advanced lung cancer (235). The most prominent and dose-limiting toxicity encountered at the highest dose studied, 100 mg twice daily, was a symptomatic inflamma-

tory polyarthritis that persisted for up to 8 weeks after discontinuing therapy. Estimates of the apparent $t_{1/2,z}$ of marimastat ranged from 4 to 5 hours. The mean C_{max} in patients treated with 50 mg twice daily, which was reasonably well tolerated, was 196 ng/mL, occurring 1 to 2 hours after administration. These plasma levels were substantially higher than those required for MMP inhibition *in vitro*. The AUC of marimastat tended to increase linearly with the administered dose suggestive of apparent first-order pharmacokinetics. A number of phase III clinical trials evaluating MMPs are currently in progress, but only one has been formally reported so far. This study suggested that marimastat had no survival advantage when compared to chemotherapy with gemcitabine in advanced pancreatic carcinoma. Other studies are assessing the efficacy of MMP inhibitors in the maintenance of remission after other modalities of therapy or in combination with cytotoxic agents.

Several nonantibiotic, chemically modified tetracyclines interfere with MMP expression, activation, tumor growth, and metastasis in preclinical models. A representative agent of this class, 6-demethyl-6-deoxy-4-dedimethylaminotetracycline (COL-3; Fig. 59-20), has been evaluated in a phase I clinical trial involving patients with various refractory solid tumors or lymphoma (236). Cutaneous phototoxicity proved to be dose limiting in patients treated orally with daily doses of 98 mg/m². COL-3 was well tolerated at doses of 70 mg/m²/day when patients minimized exposure to sunlight and also used sunscreen on a prophylactic basis. Doses of 36 mg/m²/day were well tolerated without the use of sunblock. Other toxicities that did not seem to be related to the dose level or the magnitude of pharmacokinetic variables included anemia, anorexia, constipation, dizziness, elevated liver function test results, fever, headache, heartburn, nausea, vomiting, peripheral and central neurotoxicities, fatigue, and three cases of drug-induced lupus. Interestingly, prolonged disease stabilization was seen in patients with hemangioendothelioma, Sertoli-Leydig cell tumor, and fibrosarcoma.

BAY 12-9566 is another MMP inhibitor with relative specificity against MMP-2, MMP-3, and MMP-9 (Fig. 59-20). A phase I study was reported using a protracted oral daily dosing schedule in patients with advanced solid malignancies (237). It was well tolerated on all dose schedules, and there was no consistent dose-limiting toxicity. The most common side effects were headache, nausea, vomiting, liver function abnormalities, and thrombocytopenia, which were rarely clinically significant. Nadir concentrations of the drug in plasma after achieving steady state on repeated oral dosing increased in a less than proportionate manner to a plateau as the daily dose was increased from 100 to 1600 mg, which is suggestive of saturable drug absorption. Mean nadir steady-state plasma levels provided by all doses evaluated exceeded the BAY 12-9566 concentrations required to inhibit MMPs *in vitro* and in vascular invasion and tumor proliferation in *in vivo* models. There were no consistent effects of BAY 12-9566 on the plasma concentrations of MMP-2 and MMP-9 over the continuous dosing period at any dose level. The recommended dose of BAY 12-9566 for subsequent disease-directed studies is 800 mg twice daily, which provides sustained maintenance of potentially effective plasma concentrations of the drug and has an acceptable toxicity profile.

ENDOSTATIN

Endostatin is an endogenous angiogenesis inhibitor that is a 20-kd C-terminal fragment of collagen XVIII. It was originally isolated from the culture medium of a murine hemangioendothelioma cell line. The murine protein specifically inhibits endothelial cell proliferation and angiogenesis and the growth of some experimental tumors in mice. Recombinant human endostatin (rhEndostatin), subsequently prepared for clinical evaluation of the protein, exhibited similar activities in preclinical models. Results of three phase I studies to assess continual daily treatment with rhEndostatin given as a short i.v. infusion have been reported. In adult patients with refractory solid tumors, the only significant toxicity encountered as the daily dose was escalated from 15 to 240 mg/m² was mild transient allergic reactions (238–240). rhEndostatin exhibited linear pharmacokinetics based on parameters estimated from the day 1 serum profile (238). There was no evidence of drug accumulation or an alteration of drug disposition based on monitoring peak serum levels during two courses of therapy. The 240 mg/m² dose provided a peak rhEndostatin serum concentration of 11 µg/mL, and the AUC was approximately 700 µg • minute/mL. This was similar to the AUC reported for a 50 mg/kg subcutaneously administered dose in mice, which was shown to be efficacious in tumor xenograft models when given twice daily on a continual basis. Antibodies to rhEndostatin were detected in 5 patients but had no apparent effect on its pharmacokinetics. Urine levels of bFGF and VEGF, normalized to creatinine, showed a dose-dependent decrease from baseline values in eight of nine patients treated at the 60 mg/m² dose level (238). Preliminary results of pharmacodynamic studies demonstrated evidence for changes in microvessel density and decreases in serum of VEGF levels after starting rhEndostatin in some patients (240).

Antiangiogenic Therapy: Promises and Challenges

The increased understanding of angiogenesis in tumor development has led to the evaluation of antiangiogenic agents as potential anticancer therapeutics. As briefly reviewed in this chapter, a number of drugs with antiangiogenic properties are in different phases of clinical evaluation, and many more are in the pipelines. Although antiangiogenic agents hold great promise for cancer treatment, their therapeutic value remains to be realized. Many challenges remain with regard to the most appropriate manner for the design and conduct of clinical trials with these agents. Unlike the traditional cytotoxic chemotherapeutic agents, these drugs tend to be cytostatic. Therefore, the use of biologic endpoints, such as assessing tumor vascular density or using pharmacokinetically guided dose escalation to achieve a predetermined drug concentration based on preclinical data, may be more appropriate than using the toxicity-guided dose escalation scheme of traditional phase I trials. In addition, these agents tend to slow or stop the growth of tumors and the development of metastases. Therefore, using response or shrinkage of tumors as endpoints in efficacy trials may not be informative.

What are the potential surrogate biologic markers that can be used to monitor antiangiogenic therapies? Assessing microvessel density in the tumor has been attempted in phase I clinical trials. This approach requires obtaining serial tissue biopsy specimens during treatment, which can be technically difficult and cause additional discomfort to the patient. In addition, due to sample heterogeneity, inconsistent results may be obtained, precluding a comparison of treatment effects. Measuring serum and urine VEGF and bFGF levels has been considered a potential surrogate marker; however, the reproducibility and significance of these assays remains to be validated. Several noninvasive imaging techniques, including positron emission tomography and magnetic resonance imaging, have also been explored to assess the tumor microvasculature. The sensitivity and specificity of these techniques, correlation with microvessel density changes, and the predictive value of blood flow changes are under active investigation. To date, no single imaging technique has emerged as a reliable indicator of effects on blood flow or vascular density. Recently, the existence of an angio-blast-like circulating endothelial precursor cell in adult humans has been reported (241,242), and its role in supporting angiogenesis is under intensive investigation. This circulating CD34+ cell also expresses VEGFR-2 and AC 133, an early hematopoietic stem cell marker. Although it remains to be determined whether the recruitment and incorporation of circulating endothelial precursor cells to the tumor vascular bed are essential for tumor progression and metastasis, assessing the changes of circulating endothelial precursor cells during antiangiogenic therapy represents another potential surrogate target.

The ideal clinical settings for which antiangiogenic agents may have maximum therapeutic benefit are uncertain. Antiangiogenic agents may be best applied in the minimal disease status and used for disease stabilization. Their activity may be further augmented in conjunction with chemotherapy. Given the increasing evidence that an angiogenic switch is activated during the early preneoplastic stages in the development of a tumor, antiangiogenic agents may also be explored as potential chemoprevention agents. It is hoped that future studies, through vigorous clinical research, will elucidate the potential applications of these agents in the treatment of different types of cancers including hematologic malignancies.

REFERENCES

1. Goodman LS, Wintrobe MM, Dameshek W, et al. Nitrogen mustard therapy: use of methylbis (β-chlorethyl) amino hydrochloride for Hodgkin's disease, lymphosarcoma, leukemia and certain allied and miscellaneous disorders. *JAMA* 1946;132:126.
2. Farber S, Diamond LK, Mercer RD, et al. Temporary remissions in acute leukemia in children produced by folic acid antagonist, 4-aminopteroyl-glutamic acid (aminopterin). *N Engl J Med* 1948;238:787.
3. Frei E. Combination cancer chemotherapy: presidential address. *Cancer Res* 1972;32:2593.
4. Druker BJ, Lydon NB. Lessons learned from the development of an abl tyrosine kinase inhibitor for chronic myelogenous leukemia. *J Clin Invest* 2000;105:3–7.
5. Chabner BA, Longo DL, eds. *Cancer chemotherapy and biotherapy: principles and practice*, 3rd ed. Philadelphia: Lippincott Williams & Wilkins, 2001.
6. Grochow LB, Ames MM, eds. *A clinician's guide to chemotherapy pharmacokinetics and pharmacodynamics*. Baltimore: Williams & Wilkins, 1998.
7. Kaelin WG Jr. Taking aim at novel molecular targets in cancer therapy. *J Clin Invest* 1999;104:1495.
8. Druker BJ, Talpaz M, Resta DJ, et al. Efficacy and safety of a specific inhibitor of the BCR-ABL tyrosine kinase in chronic myeloid leukemia. *N Engl J Med* 2001;344:1031–1037.
9. Skipper HE, Schabel FM, Wilcox WS. Experimental evaluation of potential anti-cancer agents. XII. On the criteria and kinetics associated with "curability" of experimental leukemia. *Cancer Chemother Rep* 1964;35:1.
10. Heinemann V, Hertel LW, Grindey GB, et al. Comparison of the cellular pharmacokinetics and toxicity of 2',2'-difluorodeoxycytidine and 1-beta-D-arabinofuranosylcytosine. *Cancer Res* 1988;48:4024–4031.
11. Gupta S, Tsuruo T, eds. *Multidrug resistance in cancer cells: molecular, biochemical, physiological and biological aspects*. New York: John Wiley & Sons, 1996.
12. Notari RE. *Biopharmaceutics and clinical pharmacokinetics*. New York: Marcel Dekker, 1987.
13. Gilbaldi M, Perrier D, eds. *Pharmacokinetics*, 2nd ed. New York: Marcel Dekker, 1982.
14. Friedman H, Greenblatt DJ. Rational therapeutic drug monitoring. *JAMA* 1986;256:2227–2233.
15. Mehta AC. Chiral high performance liquid chromatography of drug molecules. *J Clin Pharm Ther* 1990;15(5):313–323.
16. Peng GW, Chiou WL. Analysis of drugs and other toxic substances in biological samples for pharmacokinetic studies. *J Chromatogr* 1990;531:3–50.
17. Wright JD, Boudinot FD, Ujhelyi MR. Measurement and analysis of unbound drug concentrations. *Clin Pharmacokinet* 1996;30:445–462.
18. Fleishaker JC, Smith RB. Compartmental model analysis in pharmacokinetics. *J Clin Pharmacol* 1987;27:922–926.
19. Dunne A. An iterative curve stripping technique for pharmacokinetic parameter estimation. *J Pharm Pharmacol* 1986;38:97–101.
20. Gillespie WR. Noncompartmental versus compartmental modelling in clinical pharmacokinetics. *Clin Pharmacokinet* 1991;20:253–262.
21. Wagner JG. History of pharmacokinetics. *Pharmacol Ther* 1981;12:537–562.
22. Rowland M, Benet LZ, Graham GG. Clearance concepts in pharmacokinetics. *J Pharmacokinet Biopharm* 1973;1:123–136.
23. Carlisle KM, Halliwell M, Read AE, et al. Estimation of total hepatic blood flow by duplex ultrasound. *Gut* 1992;33:92–97.

24. Cockcroft DW, Gault MH. Prediction of creatinine clearance from serum creatinine. *Nephron* 1976;16:31–41.

25. Gibaldi M, McNamara PJ. Apparent volumes of distribution and drug binding to plasma proteins and tissues. *Eur J Clin Pharmacol* 1978;13(5):373–380.

26. Collins JM, Dedrick RL, King FG, et al. Nonlinear pharmacokinetic models for 5-fluorouracil in man: intravenous and intraperitoneal routes. *Clin Pharmacol Ther* 1980;28:235–246.

27. Besseghir K, Roch-Ramel F. Renal excretion of drugs and other xenobiotics. *Ren Physiol* 1987;10:221–241.

28. Ilett KF, Tee LB, Reeves PT, et al. Metabolism of drugs and other xenobiotics in the gut lumen and wall. *Pharmacol Ther* 1990;46:67–93.

29. Balis FM, Holcenberg JS, Bleyer WA. Clinical pharmacokinetics of commonly used anticancer drugs. *Clin Pharmacokinet* 1983;8:202–232.

30. Glue P, Clement RP. Cytochrome P450 enzymes and drug metabolism—basic concepts and methods of assessment. *Cell Mol Neurobiol* 1999;19:309–323.

31. von Moltke LL, Greenblatt DJ, Schmider J, et al. Metabolism of drugs by cytochrome P450 3A isoforms. Implications for drug interactions in psychopharmacology. *Clin Pharmacokinet* 1985;29:33–43.

32. Gillum JG, Israel DS, Polk RE. Pharmacokinetic drug interactions with antimicrobial agents. *Clin Pharmacokinet* 1993;25:450–482.

33. Kivisto KT, Kroemer HK, Eichelbaum M. The role of human cytochrome P450 enzymes in the metabolism of anticancer agents: implications for drug interactions. *Br J Clin Pharmacol* 1995;40:523–530.

34. Chang TK, Weber GF, Crespi CL, et al. Differential activation of cyclophosphamide and ifosfamide by cytochromes P-450 2B and 3A in human liver microsomes. *Cancer Res* 1993;53:5629.

35. Chabot GG, Bouchard J, Momparler RL. Kinetics of deamination of 5-aza-2'-deoxycytidine and cytosine arabinoside by human liver cytidine deaminase and its inhibition by 3-deazauridine, thymidine or uracil arabinoside. *Biochem Pharmacol* 1983;32:1327–1328.

36. Milano G, McLeod HL. Can dihydropyrimidine dehydrogenase impact 5-fluorouracil-based treatment? *Eur J Cancer* 2000;36:37–42.

37. Clarke DJ, Burchell B. The uridine diphosphate glucuronosyltransferase multigene family: function and regulation. In: Kauffman FC, ed. *Handbook of experimental pharmacology, conjugation-deconjugation reactions in drug metabolism and toxicity*. Berlin: Springer-Verlag New York, 1994:3–43.

38. Ivanov AI, Christodoulou J, Parkinson JA, et al. Cisplatin binding sites on human albumin. *J Biol Chem* 1998;273:14721–14730.

39. Kirkpatrick DL. Modification of antitumor disulfide cytotoxicity by glutathione depletion in murine cells. *Cancer Res* 1987;47:4391–4395.

40. Chen TL, Passos-Coelho JL, Noe DA, et al. Nonlinear pharmacokinetics of cyclophosphamide in patients with metastatic breast cancer receiving high-dose chemotherapy followed by autologous bone marrow transplantation. *Cancer Res* 1995;55:810–816.

41. Jao JY, Jusko WJ, Cohen JL. Phenobarbital effects on cyclophosphamide pharmacokinetics in man. *Cancer Res* 1972;32:2761–2764.

42. Rushing DA, Raber SR, Rodvold KA, et al. The effects of cyclosporine on the pharmacokinetics of doxorubicin in patients with small cell lung cancer. *Cancer* 1994;74:834–841.

43. Kivisto KT, Kroemer HK, Eichelbaum M. The role of human cytochrome P450 enzymes in the metabolism of anticancer agents: implications for drug interactions. *Br J Clin Cancer* 1995;40:523–530.

44. Rodman JH, Murry DJ, Madden T, et al. Altered etoposide pharmacokinetics and time to engraftment in pediatric patients undergoing autologous bone marrow transplantation. *J Clin Oncol* 1994;12(11):2390–2397.

44a. Friedman HS, Petros WP, Friedman AH, et al. Irinotecan therapy in adults with recurrent or progressive malignant glioma. *J Clin Oncol* 1999;17:1516–1525.

45. Grossman SA, Hochberg F, Fisher J, et al. Increased 9-aminocamptothecin dose requirements in patients on anticonvulsants. NABTT CNS consortium. The new approaches to brain tumor therapy. *Cancer Chemother Pharmacol* 1998;42(2):118–126.

46. Poplack DG, Balis FM, Zimm S. The pharmacology of orally administered chemotherapy. A reappraisal. *Cancer* 1986;58(S2):473–480.

47. Innocenti F, Danesi R, Di Paolo A, et al. Clinical and experimental pharmacokinetic interaction between 6-mercaptopurine and methotrexate. *Cancer Chemother Pharmacol* 1996;37(5):409–414.

48. Bannwarth B, Pehourcq F, Schaeverbeke T, et al. Clinical pharmacokinetics of low-dose pulse methotrexate in rheumatoid arthritis. *Clin Pharmacokinet* 1996;30:194–210.

49. Lilly MB, Omura GA. Clinical pharmacology of oral intermediate-dose methotrexate with or without probenecid. *Cancer Chemother Pharmacol* 1985;15(3):220–222.

50. Berg SL, Tolcher A, O'Shaughnessy JA, et al. Effect of R-verapamil on the pharmacokinetics of paclitaxel in women with breast cancer. *J Clin Oncol* 1995;13:2039–2042.

51. Rowinsky EK, Kaufmann SH, Baker SD, et al. Sequences of topotecan and cisplatin: phase I, pharmacologic, and in vitro studies to examine sequence dependence. *J Clin Oncol* 1996;14(12):3074–3084.

52. Tobe SW, Siu LL, Jamal SA, et al. Vinblastine and erythromycin: an unrecognized serious drug interaction. *Cancer Chemother Pharmacol* 1995;35:188–190.

53. Shimada T, Yamazaki H, Mimura M, et al. Interindividual variations in human liver cytochrome P-450 enzymes involved in the oxidation of drugs, carcinogens and toxic chemicals: studies with liver microsomes of 30 Japanese and 30 Caucasians. *J Pharmacol Exp Ther* 1994;270:414–423.

54. Iyer L, Ratain MJ. Pharmacogenetics and cancer chemotherapy. *Eur J Cancer* 1998;34:1493–1499.

55. Yamazaki H, Inoue K, Shaw PM, et al. Different contributions of cytochrome P450 2C19 and 3A4 in the oxidation of omeprazole by human liver microsomes: effects of contents of these two forms in individual human samples. *J Pharmacol Exp Ther* 1997;283:434–442.

56. Nemeroff CB, DeVane CL, Pollock BG. Newer antidepressants and the cytochrome P450 system. *Am J Psychiatry* 1996;153:311–320.

57. van Meerten E, Verweij J, Schellens JH. Antineoplastic agents. Drug interactions of clinical significance. *Drug Saf* 1995;12:168–182.

58. McCune JS, Hawke RL, LeCluyse EL, et al. In vivo and in vitro induction of human cytochrome P4503A4 by dexamethasone. *Clin Pharmacol Ther* 2000;68:356–366.

59. Evans WE, Christensen ML. Drug interactions with methotrexate. *J Rheumatol* 1985;12[Suppl 12]:15–20.

60. Wood M. Pharmacokinetic drug interaction in anaesthetic practice. *Clin Pharmacokinet* 1991;21:285–307.

61. Gianni L, Kearns CM, Giani A, et al. Nonlinear pharmacokinetics and metabolism of paclitaxel and its pharmacokinetic/pharmacodynamic relationships in humans. *J Clin Oncol* 1995;13:180–190.

62. Holford NH. Clinical pharmacokinetics and pharmacodynamics of warfarin. Understanding the dose-effect relationship. *Clin Pharmacokinet* 1986;11(6):483–504.

63. Barre J, Houin G, Brunner F, et al. Disease-induced modifications of drug pharmacokinetics. *Int J Clin Pharmacol Res* 1983;3:215–226.

64. Lichtman SM, Skirvin JA. Pharmacology of antineoplastic agents in older cancer patients. *Oncology* 2000;14:1743–1752.

65. Hammerlein A, Derendorf H, Lowenthal DT. Pharmacokinetic and pharmacodynamic changes in the elderly. Clinical implications. *Clin Pharmacokinet* 1998;35(1):49–64.

66. Milano G, Etienne MC, Cassuto-Viguier E, et al. Influence of sex and age on fluorouracil clearance. *J Clin Oncol* 1992;10:1171–1175.

67. Innocenti F, Iyer L, Ratain MJ. Pharmacogenetics of anticancer agents: lessons from amonafide and irinotecan. *Drug Metab Dispos* 2001;29:596–600.

68. Rubin GM, Tozer TN. Theoretical considerations in the calculation of bioavailability of drugs exhibiting Michaelis-Menten elimination kinetics. *J Pharmacokinet Biopharm* 1984;12:437–450.

69. Evans WE, Relling MV, Rodman JH, et al. Conventional compared with individualized chemotherapy for childhood acute lymphoblastic leukemia. *N Engl J Med* 1998;338:499–505.

70. van den Bongard HJ, Mathot RA, Beijnen JH, et al. Pharmacokinetically guided administration of chemotherapeutic agents. *Clin Pharmacokinet* 2000;39:345–367.

71. Moscow JA, Connolly T, Myers TG, et al. Reduced folate carrier gene (RFC1) expression and anti-folate resistance in transfected and non-selected cell lines. *Int J Cancer* 1997;72:184–190.

72. Chabner BA, Allegra CJ, Curt GA, et al. The polyglutamation of methotrexate: is methotrexate a prodrug? *J Clin Invest* 1985;76:907–912.

73. Sirotnak FM, Wendel HG, Bornmann WGB, et al. Co-administration of probenecid, an inhibitor of a cMOAT/MRP-like plasma membrane ATPase, greatly enhanced the efficacy of a new 10-deazaaminopterin against human solid tumors in vivo. *Clin Cancer Res* 2000;6:3705–3712.

74. Barrado JC, Synold TW, Laver J, et al. Differences in constitutive and post-methotrexate folylpoly-glutamate synthetase activity in B-lineage and T-lineage leukemia. *Blood* 1994;84:564–569.

75. Krug LM, Ng KK, Kris MG, et al. Phase I and pharmacokinetic study of 10-propargyl-10-deazaaminopterin, a new antifolate. *Clin Cancer Res* 2000;6:3493–3498.

76. Rusthoven JJ, Eisenhauer E, Butts C, et al. Multitargeted antifolate LY231514 as first-line chemotherapy for patients with advanced non-small-cell lung cancer: a phase II study. National Cancer Institute of Canada Clinical Trials Group. *J Clin Oncol* 1999;17:1194–1199.

77. Wall SM, Johansen MJ, Moloney DA, et al. Effective clearance of methotrexate using high-flux hemodialysis membranes. *Am J Kidney Dis* 1996;28:846–854.

78. Monjanel S, Rigault JP, Cano JP, et al. High-dose methotrexate: preliminary evaluation of a pharmacokinetic approach. *Cancer Chemother Pharmacol* 1979;3:189–196.

79. Widemann BC, Balis FM, Murphy RF, et al. Carboxypeptidase-G2, thymidine, and leucovorin rescue in cancer patients with methotrexate-induced renal dysfunction. *J Clin Oncol* 1997;15:2125–2134.

80. Evans W, Crom W, Abromowitch M, et al. Clinical pharmacodynamics of height-dose methotrexate in acute lymphocytic leukemia: identification of a relation between concentration and effect. *N Engl J Med* 1986;314:471–477.

81. Bode U, Magrath IT, Bleyer WA, et al. Active transport of methotrexate from cerebrospinal fluid in humans. *Cancer Res* 1980;40:2184–2187.

82. Rubnitz JE, Relling MV, Harrison PT et al. Transient encephalopathy following high-dose methotrexate treatment in childhood acute lymphoblastic leukemia. *Leukemia* 1998;12:1176–1181.

83. Owens JK, Shewach DS, Ullman B, et al. Resistance to 1-beta-D-arabinofuranosylcytosine in human T-lymphoblasts mediated by mutations within the deoxycytidine kinase gene. *Cancer Res* 1992;52:2389–2393.

84. Bloomfield CD, Lawrence D, Byrd JC, et al. Frequency of prolonged remission duration after high-dose cytarabine intensification in acute myeloid leukemia varies by cytogenetic subtype. *Cancer Res* 1998;58:4173–4179.

85. Glantz MJ, Jaeckle KA, Chamberlain MC, et al. Randomized controlled trial comparing intrathecal sustained-release cytarabine (Depo-Cyt) to intrathecal methotrexate in patients with neoplastic meningitis from solid tumors. *Clin Cancer Res* 1999;5:3394–3402.

86. Santoro A, Bredenfeld H, Devizzi L, et al. Gemcitabine in the treatment of

refractory Hodgkin's disease: results of a multicenter phase II study. *J Clin Oncol* 2000;18:2615–2619.

87. Momparler RL, Onetto-Pothier N, Momparler LF. Comparison of the antileukemic activity of cytosine arabinoside and 5-aza-2'-deoxycytidine against human leukemic cells of different phenotype. *Leukemia Res* 1990;14:755–760.

88. Waters TR, Swann PF. Cytotoxic mechanism of 6-thioguanine: hMutSalpha, the human mismatch binding heterodimer, binds to DNA containing S6-methylthioguanine. *Biochemistry* 1997;36:2501–2506.

89. Cadman E, Heimer R, Davis L. Enhanced 5-fluorouracil nucleotide formation after methotrexate administration: explanation for drug synergism. *Science* 1979;205:1135–1137.

90. Schutz E, Gummert J, Mohr F, et al. Azathioprine-induced myelosuppression in thiopurine methyltransferase deficient heart transplant recipient. *Lancet* 1990;336:225–229.

91. Lilleyman J, Lennard L. Mercaptopurine metabolism and risk of relapse in childhood lymphoblastic leukaemia. *Lancet* 1994;343:1188–1190.

92. Relling MV, Hancock ML, Rivera GK, et al. Mercaptopurine therapy intolerance and heterozygosity at the thiopurine S-methyltransferase gene locus. *J Natl Cancer Inst* 1999;91:2001–2008.

93. Plunkett W, Gandhi V. Pharmacology of purine nucleoside analogues. *Hematol Cell Ther* 1996;38(2):S67–S74.

94. O'Dwyer PJ, Wagner B, Leyland-Jones B, et al. 2'-deoxycoformycin (pentostatin) for lymphoid malignancies. *Ann Intern Med* 1988;108:733–743.

95. Cheson BD. Immunologic and immunosuppressive complications of purine analogue therapy. *J Clin Oncol* 1995;13:2431–2448.

96. Slavin S, Nagler A, Naparstek E, et al. Nonmyeloablative stem cell transplantation and cell therapy as an alternative to conventional bone marrow transplantation with lethal cytoreduction for the treatment of malignant and nonmalignant hematologic diseases. *Blood* 1998;91(3):756–763.

97. Navarra P, Preziosi P. Hydroxyurea: new insights on an old drug. *Crit Rev Oncol Hematol* 1999;29:249–255.

98. Esteller M, Garcia-Foncillas J, Andion E, et al. Inactivation of the DNA-repair gene, MGMT and the clinical response of gliomas to alkylating agents. *N Engl J Med* 2000;343(19):1350–1354.

99. Kirsch D, Kastan M. Tumor-suppressor p53: implications for tumor development and prognosis. *J Clin Oncol* 1998;16:3158–3168.

100. Levine EG, Bloomfield CD. Leukemias and myelodysplastic syndromes secondary to drug, radiation, and environmental exposure. *Semin Oncol* 1992;19:47–84.

101. Reed E, Yuspa SH, Zwelling LA, et al. Quantitation of cis-diamminedichloroplatinum II (cisplatin)-DNA-intrastrand adducts in testicular and ovarian cancer patients receiving cisplatin chemotherapy. *J Clin Invest* 1986;77:545–550.

102. Travis LB, Holowaty EJ, Bergfeldt K, et al. Risk of leukemia after platinum-based chemotherapy for ovarian cancer. *N Engl J Med* 1999;340(5):351–357.

103. Calvert AH, Newell DR, Gumbrell LA, et al. Carboplatin dosage: prospective evaluation of a simple formula based on renal function. *J Clin Oncol* 1989;7:1748–1756.

104. Cockcroft DW, Gault MH. Prediction of creatinine clearance from serum creatinine. *Nephron* 1976;16(1):31–41.

105. Burger RM, Drlica K, Birdsall B. The DNA cleavage pathway of iron BLM strand scission precedes deoxyribose 3-phosphate bond cleavage. *J Biol Chem* 1994;269:25978–25985.

106. Sebti SM, Jani JP, Mistry JS, et al. Metabolic inactivation: a mechanism of human tumor resistance to bleomycin. *Cancer Res* 1991;51:227–232.

107. Munger JS, Huang X, Kawakatsu H, et al. The integrin alpha v beta 6 binds and activates latent TGF 1: a mechanism for regulating pulmonary inflammation and fibrosis. *Cell* 1999;96:319–328.

108. Venook AP, Egorin MJ, Rosner GL, et al. Phase I and pharmacokinetic trial of paclitaxel in patients with hepatic dysfunction: cancer and leukemia group B 9264. *J Clin Oncol* 1998;16(5):1811–1819.

109. Monsarrat B, Chatelut E, Royer I, et al. Modification of paclitaxel metabolism in a cancer patient by induction of cytochrome P450 3A4. *Drug Metab Dispos* 1998;26(3):229–233.

110. Jamis-Dow CA, Pearl ML, Watkins PB. Predicting drug interactions in vivo from experiments in vitro. Human studies with paclitaxel and ketoconazole. *Am J Clin Oncol* 1997;20:592–599.

111. Slichenmyer WJ, Donehower RC, Chen TL, et al. Pretreatment H2 receptor antagonists that differ in P450 modulation activity: comparative effects on paclitaxel clearance rates and neutropenia. *Cancer Chemother Pharmacol* 1995;36(3):227–232.

112. Gupta M, Fujimori A, Pommier Y. Eukaryotic DNA topoisomerases I. *Biochim Biophys Acta* 1995;1262:1–14.

113. Clark PI, Slevin ML. The clinical pharmacology of etoposide and teniposide. *Clin Pharmacokinet* 1987;12:223–252.

114. Heck MS, Earnshaw WC. Topoisomerase II: a specific marker for cell proliferation. *J Cell Biol* 1986;103:2569–2581.

115. Pommier Y, Tanizawa A. Mammalian DNA topoisomerase I and its inhibitors. In: Hickman J, Tritton T, eds. *Cancer chemotherapy.* Boston: Blackwell Scientific Publications, 1993:214–250.

116. Pommier Y, Kohn K. Topoisomerase II inhibition by antitumor intercalators and demetheyepipodophyllotoxins. In: Glazer R, ed. *Developments in cancer chemotherapy.* Boca Raton, FL: CRC Press, 1989:175–196.

117. Kohn K, Pommier Y, Kerrigan D, et al. Topoisomerase II as a target of anticancer drug action in mammalian cells. *NCI Monogr* 1987;4:61–71.

118. Sugimoto J, Tsukahara S, Oh-hara T, et al. Decreased expression of DNA topoisomerase I in camptothecin-resistant tumor cell lines as determined by monoclonal antibody. *Cancer Res* 1990;50:6925–6930.

119. Friche E, Danks MK, Schmidt C, et al. Decreased DNA topoisomerase II in daunorubicin-resistant Ehrlich ascites tumor cells. *Cancer Res* 1991;51:1129–1136.

120. Potmesil M, Hsiang Y-H, Liu LF, et al. Resistance of human leukemic and normal lymphocytes to drug-induced DNA cleavage and low levels of DNA topoisomerase II. *Cancer Res* 1988;48:3537–3543.

121. Weiss RB. The anthraxcyclines: will we ever find a better doxorubicin? *Semin Oncol* 1992;19(6):670–686.

122. Capranico G, Butelli G, and Zunino F. Change of the sequence specificity of daunorubicin-stimulated topoisomerase II DNA cleavage by epimerization of the amino group of the sugar moiety. *Cancer Res* 1995;55(2):312–317.

123. Dalton WS. Detection of multidrug resistance gene expression in multiple myeloma. *Leukemia* 1997;11(7):1166–1169.

124. Straus DJ, Huang J, Testa MA, et al. Prognostic factors in the treatment of human immunodeficiency virus-associated non-Hodgkin's lymphoma: analysis of AIDS clinical trials group protocol 142—low-dose versus standard-dose m-BACOD plus granulocyte-macrophage colony-stimulating factor. National Institute of Allergy and Infectious Diseases. *J Clin Oncol* 1998;16(11):3601–3606.

125. Sternberg DW, Aird W, Neuberg D, et al. Treatment of patients with recurrent and primary refractory acute myelogenous leukemia using mitoxantrone and intermediate-dose cytarabine: a pharmacologically based regimen. *Cancer* 2000;88(9):2037–2041.

126. Johnson SA, Richardson DS. Anthracyclines in haematology: pharmacokinetics and clinical studies. *Blood Rev* 1998;12(1):52–71.

127. Shenkenberg TD, Von Hoff DD. Mitoxantrone: a new anticancer drug with significant clinical activity. *Ann Intern Med* 1986;105(1):67–81.

128. Legha SS, Benjamin RS, Mackay B, et al. Adriamycin therapy by continuous intravenous infusion in patients with metastatic breast cancer. *Cancer* 1982;49(9):1762–1766.

129. Billingham ME, Bristow MR, Glatstein E, et al. Adriamycin cardiotoxicity: endomyocardial biopsy evidence of enhancement by irradiation. *Am J Surg Pathol* 1977;1(1):17–23.

130. Nysom K, Holm K, Michaelsen KF, et al. Relationship between cumulative anthracycline dose and late cardiotoxicity in childhood acute lymphoblastic leukemia. *J Clin Oncol* 1998;16(2):545–550.

131. Gill PS, Espina BM, Muggia F, et al. Phase I/II clinical and pharmacokinetic evaluation of liposomal daunorubicin. *J Clin Oncol* 1995;13(4):996–1003.

132. Speyer JL, Green MD, Kramer E, et al. Protective effect of the bispiperazinedione ICRF-187 against doxorubicin-induced cardiac toxicity in women with advanced breast cancer. *N Engl J Med* 1988;319(12):745–752.

133. Hensley ML, Schuchter LM, Lindley C, et al. American Society of Clinical Oncology clinical practice guidelines for the use of chemotherapy and radiotherapy protectants. *J Clin Oncol* 2000;18(9):2004–2006.

134. Liu B, Earl HM, Poole CJ, et al. Etoposide protein binding in cancer patients. *Cancer Chemother Pharmacol* 1995;36:506–512.

135. Beran M, Kantarjian H, O'Brien S, et al. Topotecan, a topoisomerase I inhibitor, is active in the treatment of myelodysplastic syndrome and chronic myelomonocytic leukemia. *Blood* 1996;88:2473–2479.

136. Kantarjian HM, Beran M, Ellis A, et al. Phase I study of Topotecan, a new topoisomerase I inhibitor, in patients with refractory or relapsed acute leukemia. *Blood* 1993;81:1146–1151.

137. Ciordia R, Hochberg FH, Batchelor TT. Topotecan as salvage therapy for refractory or relapsed primary central nervous system lymphoma. *Proc ASCO* 2000;19:639a(abst).

138. Beran M, Estey E, O'Brien S, et al. Topotecan and cytarabine is an active combination regimen in myelodysplastic syndromes and chronic myelomonocytic leukemia. *J Clin Oncol* 1999;17:2819–2830.

139. Rowinsky EK, Kaufmann SH, Baker SD, et al. A phase I and pharmacological study of topotecan infused over 30 minutes for five days in patients with refractory acute leukemia. *Clin Cancer Res* 1996;2:1921–1930.

140. Mi Z, Malak H, Burke TG. Reduced albumin binding promotes the stability and activity of topotecan in human blood. *Biochemistry* 1995;34:13722–13728.

141. Takimoto CH, Arbuck SG. Topoisomerase I poisons: the camptothecins. In: Chabner BA, Longo DL, eds. *Cancer chemotherapy and biotherapy: principles and practice*, 3rd ed. Philadelphia: Lippincott Williams & Wilkins, 2001.

142. O'Reilly S, Rowinsky EK, Slichenmyer W, et al. Phase I and pharmacologic study of topotecan in patients with impaired renal function. *J Clin Oncol* 1996;14:3062–3073.

143. O'Reilly S, Rowinsky E, Slichenmyer W, et al. Phase I and pharmacologic studies of topotecan in patients with impaired hepatic function. *J Natl Cancer Inst* 1996;88:817–824.

144. Satoh T, Hosokawa M, Atsumi R, et al. Metabolic activation of CPT-11, 7-ethyl-10-[4-(1-piperidino)-1-piperidino]carbonyloxycamptothecin, a novel antitumor agent, by carboxylesterase. *Biol Pharm Bull* 1994;17:662–664.

145. Rothenberg ML, Kuhn JG, Burris HA, et al. Phase I and pharmacokinetic trial of weekly CPT-11. *J Clin Oncol* 1993;11:2194–2204.

146. Rivory LP, Robert J. Identification and kinetics of a beta-glucuronide metabolite of SN-38 in human plasma after administration of the camptothecin derivative irinotecan. *Cancer Chemother Pharmacol* 1995;36:176–179.

147. Negoro S, Fukuoka M, Masuda N, et al. Phase I study of weekly intravenous infusions of CPT-11, a new derivative of camptothecin, in the treatment of advanced non-small-cell lung cancer. *J Natl Cancer Inst* 1991;83:1164–1168.

148. Holle LM. Pegaspargase: an alternative? *Ann Pharmacother* 1997;31:616–624.

149. Kaspers GJL, Pieters R, Van Zantwijk CH, et al. In vitro drug sensitivity of normal peripheral blood lymphocytes and childhood leukaemic cells from bone marrow and peripheral blood. *Br J Cancer* 1991;64:469–474.

150. Abshire TC, Pollock BH, Billett AL, et al. Weekly polyethylene glycol conjugated L-asparaginase compared with biweekly dosing produces superior induction remission rates in childhood relapsed acute lymphoblastic leukemia: a pediatric oncology group study. *Blood* 2000;96(5):1709–1715.

151. Asselin BL, Whitin JC, Coppola DJ, et al. Comparative pharmacokinetic studies of three asparaginase preparations. *J Clin Oncol* 1993;11:1770–1776.

152. Hutson RG, Kitoh T, Moraga Amador DA. Amino acid control of asparagine synthetase: relation to asparaginase resistance in human leukemia cells. *Am J Physiol* 1997;272:2723–2729.

153. Ramakers van Woerden NL, Pieters R, Loonen AH, et al. TEL/AML 1 gene fusion is related to in vitro drug sensitivity for L-asparaginase in childhood acute lymphoblastic leukemia. *Blood* 2000;96(3):1094–1099.

154. Bushara KO, Rust RS. Reversible MRI lesions due to pegaspargase treatment of non-Hodgkin's lymphoma. *Pediatr Neurol* 1997;17:185–187.

155. Nowak-Gottl U, Wermes C, Junker R, et al. Prospective evaluation of the thrombotic risk in children with acute lymphoblastic leukemia carrying the MTHFR TT 677 genotype, the prothrombin G20210A variant, and further prothrombotic risk factors. *Blood* 1999;93:1595–1599.

156. Capizzi R. Improvement in the therapeutic index of l-asparaginase by methotrexate. *Cancer Chemother Rep* 1975;6(3):37.

157. Appelbaum FR. Antibody-targeted therapy for myeloid leukemia. *Semin Hematol* 1999;36:2–8.

158. Zein N, Sinha AM, McGahren WJ, et al. Calicheamicin gamma 1: an antitumor antibiotic that cleaves double-stranded DNA site specifically. *Science* 1988;240:1198–1201.

159. Dinndorf PA, Andrews RG, Benjamin D, et al. Expression of normal myeloid-associated antigens by acute leukemia cells. *Blood* 1986;67:1048–1053.

160. van der Velden VHJ, te Marvelde JG, Hoogeveen PG, et al. Targeting of the CD33-calicheamicin immunoconjugate Mylotarg (CMA-676) in acute myeloid leukemia: in vivo and in vitro saturation and internalization by leukemic and normal myeloid cells. *Blood* 2001;97:3197–3204.

161. Sievers EL, Appelbaum FR, Spielberger RT, et al. Selective ablation of acute myeloid leukemia using antibody-targeted chemotherapy: a phase I study of an anti-CD33 calicheamicin immunoconjugate. *Blood* 1999;93:3678–3684.

162. Sievers EL, Larson RA, Estey E, et al. Comparison of the efficacy and safety of gemtuzumabozogamicin in patients <60 and ≥60 years of age with AML in first relapse. *Proc ASCO* 2000;19:8a(abst).

163. Korth-Bradley JM, Dowell JA, Berger MS, et al. Assessment of the possible influence of patient demographics on the pharmacokinetics of a new antibody-chemotherapeutic agent for relapsed acute myelogenous leukemia. *Pharmacotherapy* 1999;10:1217a(abst).

164. Naito K, Takeshita A, Shigeno K, et al. Calicheamicin-conjugated humanized anti-CD33 monoclonal antibody (gemtuzumab zogamicin, CMA-676) shows cytocidal effect on CD33-positive leukemia cell lines, but is inactive on P-glycoprotein-expressing sublines. *Leukemia* 2000;14:1436–1443.

165. Huang ME, Ye YC, Chen SR, et al. Use of all-trans retinoic acid in the treatment of acute promyelocytic leukemia. *Blood* 1988;72:567–572.

166. Lin RJ, Nagy L, Inoue S, et al. Role of the histone deacetylase complex in acute promyelocytic leukaemia. *Nature* 1998;391:811–814.

167. Cote S, Zhou D, Bianchini A, et al. Altered ligand binding and transcriptional regulation by mutations in the PML/RARα ligand-binding domain arising in retinoic acid-resistant patients with acute promyelocytic leukemia. *Blood* 2000;96(9):3200–3208.

168. Muindi J, Frankel SR, Miller WH Jr, et al. Continuous treatment with all-trans retinoic acid causes a progressive reduction in plasma drug concentrations: implications for relapse and retinoid "resistance" in patients with acute promyelocytic leukemia. *Blood* 1992;79:299–303.

169. Frankel SR, Eardley A, Lauwers G, et al. The retinoic acid syndrome in acute promyelocytic leukemia. *Ann Intern Med* 1992;117:292–296.

170. Shen Z-X, Chen G-Q, Ni J-H, et al. Use of arsenic trioxide (As$_2$O$_3$) in the treatment of acute promyelocytic leukemia (APL): II. Clinical efficacy and pharmacokinetics in relapsed patients. *Blood* 1997;89(9):3354–3360.

171. Soignet SL, Maslak P, Wang Z-G, et al. Complete remission after treatment of acute promyelocytic leukemia with arsenic trioxide. *N Engl J Med* 1998;339(19):1341–1348.

172. Chen G-Q, Zhu J, Shi X-G, et al. In vitro studies on cellular and molecular mechanisms of arsenic trioxide (As$_2$O$_3$) in the treatment of acute promyelocytic leukemia: As$_2$O$_3$ induces NB4 cell apoptosis with down regulation of Bcl-2 expression and modulation of PML-RARα/PML proteins. *Blood* 1996;88(3):1052–1061.

173. Fiedler RJ, Dale EA, Williams SD. Inorganic arsenic compounds. *HSE Tox Rev* 1986;16:1–66.

174. Soni R, O'Reilly T, Furet P, et al. Selective in vivo and in vitro effects of a small molecule inhibitor of cyclin-dependent kinase 4. *J Natl Cancer Inst* 2001;93(6):436–434.

175. Senderowicz AM, Sausville EA. Preclinical and clinical development of cyclin-dependent kinase modulators. *J Natl Cancer Inst* 2000;92(5):376–387.

176. Byrd JC, Shinn C, Waselenko JK, et al. Flavopiridol induces apoptosis in chronic lymphocytic leukemia cells via activation of caspase-3 without evidence of bcl-2 modulation or dependence on functional p53. *Blood* 1998;92(10):3804–3816.

177. Senderowicz AM, Headlee D, Stinson SF, et al. Phase I trial of continuous infusion flavopiridol, a novel cyclin-dependent kinase inhibitor, in patients with refractory neoplasms. *J Clin Oncol* 1998;16(9):2986–2999.

178. Bible KC, Kaufmann SH. Cytotoxic synergy between flavopiridol (NSC 649890, L86-8275) and various antineoplastic agents: the importance of sequence of administration. *Cancer Res* 1997;57(16):3375–3380.

179. Rowley JD. Letter: a new consistent chromosomal abnormality in chronic myelogenous leukaemia identified by quinacrine fluorescence and Giemsa staining. *Nature* 1973;243(5405):290–293.

180. Druker BJ, Tamura S, Buchdunger E, et al. Effects of a selective inhibitor of the Abl tyrosine kinase on the growth of Bcr-Abl positive cells. *Nat Med* 1996;2(5):561–566.

181. Wang WL, Healy ME, Sattler M, et al. Growth inhibition and modulation of kinase pathways of small cell lung cancer cell lines by the novel tyrosine kinase inhibitor STI 571. *Oncogene* 2000;19(31):3521–3528.

182. Druker BJ, Sawyers CL, Kantarjian H, et al. Activity of a specific inhibitor of the BCR-ABL tyrosine kinase in the blast crisis of chronic myeloid leukemia and acute lymphoblastic leukemia with the Philadelphia chromosome. *N Engl J Med* 2001;344(14):1038–1042.

183. Joensuu H, Roberts PJ, Sarlomo-Rikala M, et al. Effect of the tyrosine kinase inhibitor STI571 in a patient with a metastatic gastrointestinal stromal tumor. *N Engl J Med* 2001;344(14):1052–1056.

184. Mahon FX, Deininger MW, Schultheis B, et al. Selection and characterization of BCR-ABL positive cell lines with differential sensitivity to the tyrosine kinase inhibitor STI571: diverse mechanisms of resistance. *Blood* 2000;96(3):1070–1079.

185. Marx J. Cancer research. Why some leukemia cells resist STI-571. *Science* 2001;292(5525):2231–2233.

186. Teicher BA, Ara G, Herbst R, et al. The proteasome inhibitor PS-341 in cancer therapy. *Clin Cancer Res* 1999;5(9):2638–2645.

187. Hideshima T, Richardson P, Chauhan D, et al. The proteasome inhibitor PS-341 inhibits growth, induces apoptosis, and overcomes drug resistance in human multiple myeloma cells. *Cancer Res* 2001;61(7):3071–3076.

188. Erlichman C, Adjei AA, Thomas JP, et al. A phase I trial of the proteasome inhibitor PS-341 in patients with advanced cancer. *Proc ASCO* 2001;20:337a(abst).

189. Folkman J. Tumor angiogenesis: therapeutic implications. *N Engl J Med* 1971;285:1182–1186.

190. Hanahan D, Folkman J. Patterns and emerging mechanisms of the angiogenic switch during tumorigenesis. *Cell* 1996;86:353–364.

191. Hanahan D, Weinberg RA. The hallmarks of cancer. *Cell* 2000;100:57–70.

192. Perez-Atayde AR, Sallan SE, Tedrow U, et al. Spectrum of tumor angiogenesis in the bone marrow of children with acute lymphoblastic leukemia. *Am J Pathol* 1997;150:815–821.

193. Bellamy WT, Richter L, Frutiger Y, et al. Expression of vascular endothelial growth factor and its receptors in hematopoietic malignancies. *Cancer Res* 1999;59:728–733.

194. Dankbar B, Padro T, Leo R, et al. Vascular endothelial growth factor and interleukin-6 in paracrine tumor-stromal cell interactions in multiple myeloma. *Blood* 2000;95:2630–2636.

195. Hussong JW, Rodgers GM, Shami PJ. Evidence of increased angiogenesis in patients with acute myeloid leukemia. *Blood* 2000;95(1):309–313.

196. Padro T, Ruiz S, Bieker R. Increased angiogenesis in the bone marrow of patients with acute myeloid leukemia. *Blood* 2000;95:2637–2644.

197. Vacca A, Ribatti D, Presta M, et al. Bone marrow neovascularization, plasma cell angiogenic potential, and matrix metalloproteinase-2 secretion parallel progression of human multiple myeloma. *Blood* 1999;93:3064–3073.

198. Salven P, Teerenhovi L, Joensuu H. A high pretreatment serum basic fibroblast growth factor concentration is an independent predictor of poor prognosis in non-Hodgkin's lymphoma. *Blood* 1999;94:3334–3339.

199. O'Reilly MS, Holmgren L, Shing Y, et al. Angiostatin: a novel angiogenesis inhibitor that mediates the suppression of metastases by a Lewis lung carcinoma. *Cell* 1994;79:315–328.

200. O'Reilly MS, Boehm T, Shing Y, et al. Endostatin: an endogenous inhibitor of angiogenesis and tumor growth. *Cell* 1997;88:277–285.

201. Calderon P, Anzilotti M, Phelps R. Thalidomide in dermatology. New indications for an old drug. *Int J Dermatol* 1997;36:881–887.

202. D'Amato RJ, Loughnan MS, Flynn E, et al. Thalidomide is an inhibitor of angiogenesis. *Proc Natl Acad Sci U S A* 1994;91:4082–4085.

203. Moreira AL, Friedlander DR, Shif B, et al. Thalidomide and a thalidomide analogue inhibit endothelial cell proliferation in vitro. *J Neurooncol* 1999;43(2):109–114.

204. Guckian M, Dransfield I, Hay P, et al. Thalidomide analogue CC-3052 reduces HIV+ neutrophil apoptosis in vitro. *Clin Exp Immunol* 2000; 121(3):472–479.

205. Teo SK, Scheffler MR, Kook KA, et al. Thalidomide dose proportionality assessment following single doses to healthy subjects. *J Clin Pharmacol* 2001; 41(6):662–667.

206. Piscitelli SC, Figg WD, Hahn B, et al. Single-dose pharmacokinetics of thalidomide in human immunodeficiency virus-infected patients. *Antimicrob Agents Chemother* 1997;41(12):2797–2799.

207. Jacobson JM, Greenspan JS, Spritzler J. Thalidomide for the treatment of oral aphthous ulcers in patients with human immunodeficiency virus infection. National Institute of Allergy and Infectious Diseases AIDS Clinical Trials Group. *N Engl J Med* 1997;336:1487–1493.

208. Reyes-Teran G, Sierra-Madero JG, Martinez del Cerro V, et al. Effects of thalidomide on HIV-associated wasting syndrome: a randomized, double-blind, placebo-controlled clinical trial. *AIDS* 1996;10:1501–1507.

209. Rovelli A, Arrigo C, Nesi F, et al. The role of thalidomide in the treatment of

refractory chronic graft-versus-host disease following bone marrow transplantation in children. *Bone Marrow Transplant* 1998;21:577–581.

210. Singhal S, Mehta J, Desikan R, et al. Antitumor activity of thalidomide in refractory multiple myeloma. *N Engl J Med* 1999;341:1565–1571.

211. Baidas SM, Winer EP, Fleming GF, et al. Phase II evaluation of thalidomide in patients with metastatic breast cancer. *J Clin Oncol* 2000;18:2710–2717.

212. Politi PM. Thalidomide. Clinical trials in cancer. *Medicina (B Aires)* 2000;60:61–65.

213. Fine HA, Figg WD, Jaeckle K, et al. Phase II trial of the antiangiogenic agent thalidomide in patients with recurrent high-grade gliomas. *J Clin Oncol* 2000;18:708–715.

214. Williams CS, Mann M, DuBois RN. The role of cyclooxygenases in inflammation, cancer, and development. *Oncogene* 1999;18:7908–7916.

215. Tsujii M, Kawano S, Tsuji S, et al. Cyclooxygenase regulates angiogenesis induced by colon cancer cells. *Cell* 1998;93:705–716.

216. Masferrer JL, Koki A, Seibert K. COX-2 inhibitors. A new class of antiangiogenic agents. *Ann N Y Acad Sci* 1999;889:84–86.

217. Williams CS, Tsujii M, Reese J, et al. Host cyclooxygenase-2 modulates carcinoma growth. *J Clin Invest* 2000;105:1589–1594.

218. Davies NM, McLachlan AJ, Day RO, et al. Clinical pharmacokinetics and pharmacodynamics of celecoxib: a selective cyclo-oxygenase-2 inhibitor. *Clin Pharmacokinet* 2000;38:225–242.

219. Ingber D, Fujita T, Kishimoto S, et al. Synthetic analogues of fumagillin that inhibit angiogenesis and suppress tumour growth. *Nature* 1990;348:555–557.

220. Griffith EC, Su Z, Niwayama S, et al. Molecular recognition of angiogenesis inhibitors fumagillin and ovalicin by methionine aminopeptidase 2. *Proc Natl Acad Sci U S A* 1998;95:15183–15188.

221. Yeh JR, Mohan R, Crews CM. The antiangiogenic agent TNP-470 requires p53 and p21CIP/WAF for endothelial cell growth arrest. *Proc Natl Acad Sci U S A* 2000;97:12782–12787.

222. Zhang Y, Griffith EC, Sage J, et al. Cell cycle inhibition by the anti-angiogenic agent TNP-470 is mediated by p53 and p21WAF1/CIP1. *Proc Natl Acad Sci U S A* 2000;97:6427–6432.

223. Kusaka M, Sudo K, Fujita T, et al. Potent anti-angiogenic action of AGM-1470: comparison to the fumagillin parent. *Biochem Biophys Res Commun* 1991;174:1070–1076.

224. Kudelka AP, Levy T, Verschraegen CF, et al. A phase I study of TNP-470 administered to patients with advanced squamous cell cancer of the cervix. *Clin Cancer Res* 1997;3:1501–1505.

225. Bhargava P, Marshall JL, Rizvi N, et al. A phase I and pharmacokinetic study of TNP-470 administered weekly to patients with advanced cancer. *Clin Cancer Res* 1999;5:1989–1995.

226. Dezube BJ, Von Roenn JH, Holden-Wiltse J, et al. Fumagillin analog in the treatment of Kaposi's sarcoma: a phase I AIDS Clinical Trial Group study. AIDS Clinical Trial Group No. 215 Team. *J Clin Oncol* 1998;16:1444–1449.

227. Mendel DB, Schreck RE, West DC, et al. The angiogenesis inhibitor SU5416 has long-lasting effects on vascular endothelial growth factor receptor phosphorylation and function. *Clin Cancer Res* 2000;6:4848–4858.

228. Mendel DB, Laird AD, Smolich BD, et al. Development of SU5416, a selective small molecule inhibitor of VEGF receptor tyrosine kinase activity, as an anti-angiogenesis agent. *Anticancer Drug Des* 2000;15:29–41.

229. Fong TA, Shawver LK, Sun L, et al. SU5416 is a potent and selective inhibitor of the vascular endothelial growth factor receptor (Flk-1/KDR) that inhibits tyrosine kinase catalysis, tumor vascularization, and growth of multiple tumor types. *Cancer Res* 1999;59:99–106.

230. Rosen L, Mulay M, Mayers A, et al. Phase I dose-escalating trial of SU5416, a novel angiogenesis inhibitor in patients with advanced malignancies. *Proc ASCO* 1999;18:618a(abst).

231. Stopeck A. Results of a phase I dose-escalating study of the antiangiogenic agent, SU5416, in patients with advanced malignancies. *Proc ASCO* 1999;18:802a(abst).

232. Gordon MS, Margolin K, Talpaz M, et al. Phase I safety and pharmacokinetic study of recombinant human anti-vascular endothelial growth factor in patients with advanced cancer. *J Clin Oncol* 2001;19:843–850.

233. Margolin K, Gordon MS, Holmgren E, et al. Phase Ib trial of intravenous recombinant humanized monoclonal antibody to vascular endothelial growth factor in combination with chemotherapy in patients with advanced cancer: pharmacologic and long-term safety data. *J Clin Oncol* 2001;19:851–856.

234. Wojtowicz-Praga SM, Dickson RB, Hawkins MJ. Matrix metalloproteinase inhibitors. *Invest New Drugs* 1997;15:61–75.

235. Wojtowicz-Praga SM, Torri J, Johnson M, et al. Phase I trial of Marimastat, a novel matrix metalloproteinase inhibitor, administered orally to patients with advanced cancer. *J Clin Oncol* 1998;16:2150–2156.

236. Rudek MA, Figg WD, Dyer V, et al. Phase I clinical trial of oral COL-3, a matrix metalloproteinase inhibitor, in patients with refractory metastatic cancer. *J Clin Oncol* 2001;19:584–592.

237. Rowinsky EK, Humphrey R, Hammond LA, et al. Phase I and pharmacologic study of the specific matrix metalloproteinase inhibitor BAY 12-9566 on a protracted oral daily dosing schedule in patients with solid malignancies. *J Clin Oncol* 2000;18:178–186.

238. Eder JP Jr, Supko, JG, Clark JW, et al. Phase I clinical trial of recombinant human endostatin administered as a short intravenous infusion repeated daily. *J Clin Oncol* 2002;20:3772–3784.

239. Herbst RS, Hess KR, Tran HT, et al. Phase I study of recombinant human endostatin in patients with advanced tumors. *J Clin Oncol* 2002;20:3792–3803.

240. Thomas JP, Schiller J, Lee F, et al. A phase I pharmacokinetic and pharmacodynamic study of recombinant human endostatin. *Proc ASCO* 2001;20:276a(abst).

241. Asahara T, Murohara T, Sullivan A, et al. Isolation of putative progenitor endothelial cells for angiogenesis. *Science* 1997;275:964–967.

242. Peichev M, Naiyer AJ, Pereira D, et al. Expression of VEGFR-2 and AC133 by circulating human CD34(+) cells identifies a population of functional endothelial precursors. *Blood* 2000;95:952–958.

CHAPTER 60

Hematopoietic Stem Cell Transplantation

Joseph H. Antin and Nancy A. Kernan

Since the late 1950s, when the first tentative steps in marrow transplantation were undertaken, hematopoietic stem cell transplantation has developed into a major therapeutic endeavor practiced at more than 200 transplant centers worldwide. The reasons for this widespread adoption of a complex, expensive, and difficult form of therapy are diverse; however, the primary motivation has been the ability to offer curative therapy to patients with previously incurable illnesses. The unique opportunity afforded by marrow grafting to observe the regeneration of the immune and hematopoietic systems, as well as the therapeutic value of the procedure, has stimulated the development of some form of marrow transplantation in many medical centers. As in many medical endeavors, however, the resolution of some problems has uncovered questions and dilemmas that are likely to keep experimental transplant units busy for years.

Although several intrepid clinicians attempted the therapeutic use of bone marrow before the development of immunosuppression (1–3), the successful use of marrow transplantation awaited an understanding of immunosuppression and histocompatibility. The first indication that marrow grafting was possible was based on early studies in mice demonstrating that lethally irradiated rodents could be saved by shielding the spleen (4,5) or by the infusion of bone marrow (6). Additional studies by a variety of investigators (1) demonstrated that the infused bone marrow could reestablish hematopoiesis in the irradiated host animal. Survival was poor in some of the animals (7), but the reason was unclear until Billingham and Brent (8) first described diarrhea, sparse fur, skin lesions, an odd gait, and retarded growth in mice with transplants. They called this syndrome *runt disease*. The phenomenon was rapidly confirmed, and several groups expanded their observations. It was later realized that this secondary disease, or runt disease, was actually a graft-versus-host reaction (GVHR) (9–12). Billingham (12) summarized the available knowledge about GVHR and formulated the principle that GVHR occurs when immunologically competent cells are infused into an antigenically distinct recipient who is incapable of rejecting them. These immunologically active cells were soon demonstrated to be T lymphocytes (13). The recognition of histocompatibility antigens in mice and humans led to strategies for the immunologic matching of host and recipient to facilitate engraftment and to prevent GVHR (1,14,15). The stage was set for the application of marrow transplantation to human diseases.

The first modern attempts to use marrow transplantation clinically were undertaken by Thomas and colleagues in 1957 (16). They used unmatched marrow in an effort to treat malignancies in six patients. Although two patients had temporary signs of donor hematopoiesis, none of the patients survived. A radiation accident in Belgrade provided Mathé and co-workers (17) an opportunity to perform marrow transplantation in five patients using marrow from unrelated volunteers. Although temporary grafts were observed (based on red-cell phenotyping), all the patients had recovery of endogenous hematopoiesis, and four survived. Indeed, the temporary support of hematopoiesis until autologous recovery was Mathé's goal. These encouraging studies led to another 154 reported marrow transplantations between 1959 and 1962 (18). Transplants were performed, using a variety of conditioning regimens, for aplastic anemia, leukemia, lymphoma, solid tumors, and immunodeficiencies, but because of the poor results, the number of marrow transplantations declined until 1968, when several investigators were successful in treating immunodeficiencies with marrow grafting (19–21). Since then, the development of effective antibiotics, improvements in blood product support, and refinements in the understanding of immunosuppression, graft-versus-host disease (GVHD), and conditioning regimen toxicity have allowed the successful application of marrow transplantation to thousands of patients with marrow failure, immune defects, and malignancies (22–24).

RATIONALE

The observation that hematopoietic stem cells obtained from bone marrow or peripheral blood grow and mature indefinitely when infused into a suitable host led to the development of strategies for the use of this resource in overcoming the problems inherent in the treatment of diseases of hematopoietic origin. There are three primary uses for hematopoietic stem cell transplantation: (a) to replace a missing hematopoietic or lymphoid component in disorders such as aplastic anemia or severe combined immunodeficiency syndrome (SCIDS); (b) to protect the recipient from dose-limiting myelotoxicity of intensive antineoplastic therapy for leukemia, lymphoma, and perhaps other malignancies; or (c) to allow the destruction of abnormal hematopoiesis (e.g., thalassemia) and its replacement with normal stem cells. In some cases, there may also be a secondary benefit from the recognition and destruction or inhibition of residual host malignant cells by infused lymphocytes in a form of adoptive immunotherapy called the *graft-versus-leukemia* (GVL) reaction.

HLA CONSIDERATIONS

The source of the stem cells and the genetic relation of the donor and host determine the type of transplantation. In autologous hematopoietic stem cell transplantation (AHSCT), marrow or peripheral blood stem cells are removed from the patient and cryopreserved before the administration of cytotoxic therapy. After a suitable time for the drugs and metabolites to be excreted, the marrow is thawed and infused. It is not a marrow transplant *per se*, and it might be more accurately termed *autologous marrow, stem cell,* or *progenitor cell infusion*. If the donor is an identical twin, the transplant is termed *syngeneic*. Transplants performed using the stem cells of donors other than identical twins are called *allogeneic*. The source of allogeneic stem cells can be marrow, peripheral blood, or cord blood. The donors include HLA identical siblings, partially matched HLA non-identical family members, unrelated volunteers, and related or unrelated cord blood donors.

The genes of the HLA complex, the major histocompatibility complex (MHC) in humans, are divided into three distinct regions: class I genes (HLA-A, -B, -C, -E, -F, and -G alloantigens); class II genes (HLA-DR, -DP, and -DQ alloantigens); and class III genes (functional proteins such as C2, C4a, and C4b) (14,15,25–30). The class I genes encode proteins expressed on all nucleated cells, whereas the expression of cell-surface proteins encoded for by the class II genes is more restricted, but includes cells of the early hematopoietic system and the immune system. The class III genes encode other functional proteins that are not, to date, relevant for matching for tissue transplantation.

There are at least 17 loci (including pseudogenes) in the HLA class I region. However, only three loci that encode the HLA-A, -B, and -C alloantigens constitute the major class I determinants important for matching in stem cell transplantation. The HLA class II region contains nine distinct loci collectively referred to as the *HLA-D region*. HLA-DR and -DQ are the major class II determinants for compatibility. In the past, class I alloantigens were identified by typing with alloantisera (31), but presently, most laboratories use a molecular typing technique to identify alleles, many of which are not recognized by serologic typing (26). Historically, the HLA class II alloantigens were defined by functional assays including the mixed lymphocyte culture. This approach, too, has been

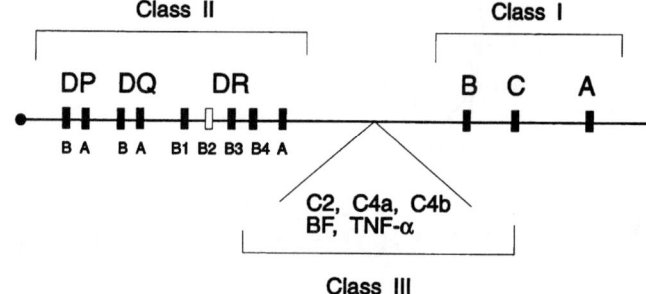

Figure 60-1. An example of a simplified schematic representation of the major histocompatibility complex locus on chromosome 6. The black circle indicates the relative position of the centromere. The solid bars are genes, and the open bar signifies a pseudogene. BF, factor B; TNF, tumor necrosis factor.

replaced by molecular typing techniques. Although the serologic and functional typing methods indicate that the HLA series of genes have a high degree of allelic polymorphisms, the molecular techniques have allowed for identification of many more alleles such that more than 200 alleles than for the HLA DRB1 locus have been identified (26). These developments have led to an alteration in nomenclature to distinguish serologically obtained typing from molecular genetic typing. In the new nomenclature, *B1* refers to the DRB1 gene (Fig. 60-1). An asterisk indicates that the type was derived using molecular techniques. The first two numbers (e.g., *0401*) refer to the old serologic specificity, and the last two numbers (e.g., *0401*) are the new specificity (Fig. 60-2).

GVHD and graft rejection occur in substantial numbers of patients who received apparently fully HLA-matched allografts (32). Thus, it is likely that there are additional antigens that are important in determining compatibility. X-ray crystallography has been crucial in the understanding of the function of the HLA molecules (33–36). These molecules have a peptide-binding cleft where the bulk of the polymorphism in these molecules is concentrated. This cleft binds either self or non-self (e.g., viral) peptides and presents them to T lymphocytes (35,37–39). These observations provide a framework for understanding why GVHD and graft rejection occur in patients who are otherwise HLA compatible. Although the

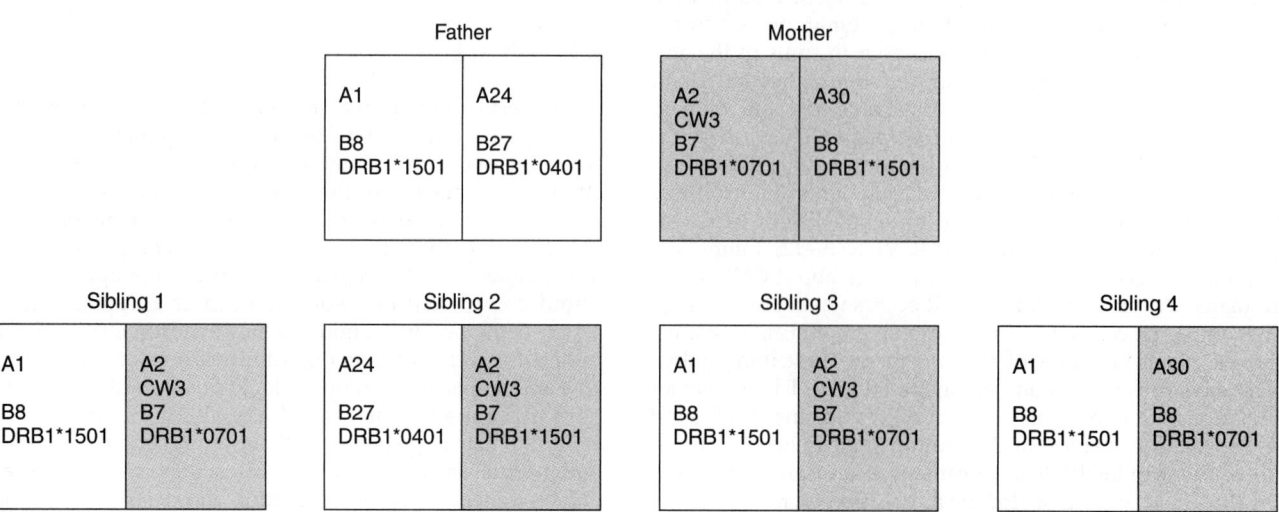

Figure 60-2. The chromosome on the left is from the father, and the chromosome on the right is from the mother. The set of HLAs on a single chromosome is called a *haplotype*. Four combinations of haplotypes are possible, and each child has a 25% chance of receiving any one of them.

HLA complex is located on chromosome 6, it is likely that the other (self) peptides are coded elsewhere in the genome and are probably not identical, even in HLA-matched siblings. In HLA-matched, unrelated patients, differences are even more likely, contributing to the high incidence of acute GVHD in these patients (40). Furthermore, there are very minor sequence differences in the HLA proteins that may be detected by the donor lymphocytes. The subtlety of the immune system's ability to recognize small differences in HLA molecules was recently demonstrated when marrow graft rejection could be attributed to a single amino acid difference in HLA-B44 (41).

HLA molecules are intrinsic to the function of the immune response, because many foreign antigens must be recognized in association with host HLA proteins, and HLA antigens are crucial components of the interactions between T lymphocytes, macrophages, and other accessory cells. In MHC-incompatible transplantation, the recipient's MHC can be recognized as foreign by donor lymphocytes that do not share the same determinants, giving rise to GVHD. Similarly, host lymphocytes that persist after the transplant conditioning regimen can recognize donor hematopoietic cells and reject the graft. In addition, the MHC mediates communication between T cells and accessory cells such as endothelial cells. This function is crucial for the recovery of the immune response of the patient, and failure of this communication may result in immunoincompetence despite successful engraftment.

HLA genes are inherited *en bloc* from each parent as a genetic unit, and the products of parental haplotypes are codominantly expressed (Fig. 60-2). Allogeneic transplants are either HLA matched, if all the HLA loci are shared, or HLA mismatched, if there are any histocompatibility differences. The likelihood that any two siblings will receive the same parental haplotypes is 1:4. In Figure 60-2, sibling 1 and sibling 3 are HLA identical, or fully matched—they received the same parental chromosomes. Siblings 2 and 4 are completely mismatched, whereas sibling 2 is haploidentical (half-matched) to siblings 1 and 3—they share a single paternal chromosome. It is important to consider the genotype of the family as well as the phenotype—that is, two individuals who are genetically identical as opposed to two individuals who look alike. Phenotypic matches can occur within the family. The patient's parents may share one or more HLA alleles that are inherited on one of the patient's HLA haplotypes. For example, in Figure 60-2, the parents share HLA-B8 and -DRB1*1501, so that sibling 1 differs from the mother by a single HLA-A antigen (HLA-A1 versus A30). Sibling 1 shares only one chromosome with the parent (they are haploidentical by genotype), but due to parental sharing of HLA alleles, sibling 1 and mother are considered partially HLA phenotypically matched—that is, they look alike but are not genotypically identical. Partially matched family member donors can also be identified if a crossover has occurred in meiosis that results in transfer of DNA between a parental chromosome pair. In the example shown in Figure 60-2, the paternal somatic phenotype would be as shown, but some gametes might be HLA-A1, -B8, and -DRB1*0401. Offspring from sperm with this genotype would not be HLA identical to any of the siblings but could be HLA five-of-six-antigen–matched or single-antigen–mismatched with siblings 1 and 3.

The determination of degree of HLA mismatch requires one additional consideration: the direction or vector of the mismatch. If the recipient identifies the donor as foreign, the vector is said to be in the *graft rejection direction*; that is, if an allogeneic response occurs, the result is graft rejection. If the donor identifies foreign antigens on host cells, the vector is

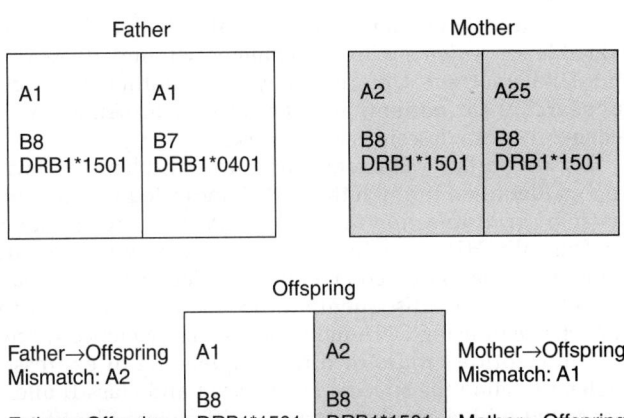

Figure 60-3. Schematic representation of the HLA complex demonstrating that the degree of mismatch in donor-recipient pairs depends on the vector. If the father is the transplant donor for the offspring, it is a one-antigen mismatch in the graft-versus-host disease vector, but a two-antigen mismatch in the graft rejection vector. If the mother is the donor, there is a bidirectional one-antigen mismatch.

said to be in the *GVHD direction*. In Figure 60-3, if the father were to donate stem cells for his offspring, paternal lymphocytes would recognize only the HLA-A2 antigen as foreign because the father's cells already express HLA-A1, -B8, and -DRB1*1501. This is a single-antigen mismatch in the graft-versus-host vector. The recipient's lymphocytes, however, recognize both HLA-B7 and -DRB1*0401 as foreign; therefore, it is a two–antigen mismatch in the graft rejection vector. The mother and offspring are single HLA antigen mismatches in both directions. Thus, everything else being equal, the mother is the preferred donor.

Although the likelihood that any two siblings will receive the same parental haplotypes is 1:4, HLA-identical siblings can be identified for 30% to 40% of patients because of the variations in size of families in the United States and Western Europe. Thus, most people with diseases that are potentially curable with an allogeneic stem cell graft do not have HLA-compatible sibling donors. Several strategies may be considered to increase the pool of potential allogeneic stem cell donors, including HLA-mismatched family members, fetal hematopoietic tissues (fully HLA mismatched), and HLA-compatible (unrelated) volunteer stem cell donors or banked cord blood units. All these alternative sources of hematopoietic stem cells are considered HLA mismatched.

In 1986, the National Marrow Donor Program (NMDP) was established in St. Paul, Minnesota, to provide unrelated donor bone marrow for patients without histocompatible family members (42,43). It is now connected with several international registries. Because of the tremendous heterogeneity of the HLA system, it is unlikely that a patient is HLA phenotypically identical to a stranger (44,45). Furthermore, HLA antigens differ from one ethnic group to another. Because of linkage dysequilibrium, however, some HLA types are more common than others, particularly within ethnic or racial groups. *Linkage dysequilibrium* refers to the nonrandom association of HLA alleles such that certain HLA alleles are found associated with one another more frequently than would be predicted by the product of each allele's frequency in the general population. Currently, searches of these registries identify a serologically HLA-A, -B, and -DR identical donor for up to

85% of Caucasian patients, and several potential donors are available for patients with two commonly found HLA-A, -B, and -DR haplotypes. Unfortunately, the proportion of successful searches for patients who are of African-American or Asian-American descent is much lower.

Early reports of unrelated marrow transplantation with donors identified through the NMDP indicated that the incidence of graft rejection and severe GVHD in recipients of serologically HLA-matched unrelated marrow is markedly higher than that observed among HLA-identical sibling pairs (46–49). Several subsequent studies have highlighted the importance of using DNA methods such as sequence specific oligonucleotide probes or direct sequencing of expressed alleles to define the specific HLA class I and class II alleles associated with each phenotype, as differences identified at this level impact transplantation outcome following an unrelated marrow transplant (50–57).

Although there are more than 4 million potential donors in volunteer registries around the world, more than 30% of patients are unable to find a suitable HLA-compatible donor. In an attempt to increase the availability of suitable donors and decrease the time required to identify a stem cell donor, pilot programs for banking of unrelated donor umbilical cord blood began, the largest of which is established at the New York Blood Center (58). Cord blood grafts from HLA-compatible siblings have been successful in the treatment of both genetic and acquired disorders (59). Among unrelated cord blood recipients, such grafts are associated with delayed engraftment, but the early results suggest that recipients of cord blood units are able to tolerate HLA-mismatched grafts, as there is a lower risk of acute and chronic GVHD as compared to unrelated-donor marrow grafts (60–64). Clinical trials evaluating the use of banked umbilical cord blood units are in progress.

PRETRANSPLANTATION EVALUATION

Donor Selection

In a given family, there is a 25% probability that two siblings are a complete match, so the likelihood of finding a compatible donor depends on the family size. Probability can be calculated as $p = 1-(0.75)^n$, where n is the number of siblings. Thus, if a patient has three siblings, the likelihood of finding a match in the family is $1-(0.75)^3$ or 58%. In some large families, there is more than one available sibling donor, and in some genetically restricted communities, there may be extended family members who match the patient. If only one donor is available, the decision about donor selection is simplified. This decision is based on determining that the donation of marrow or peripheral blood stem cells does not entail significant risk to the donor and that the donor does not have a disease that can be transmitted to the recipient. The disease for which transplantation is being considered plays a major role in this determination. For example, patients with aplastic anemia can alternatively be treated with antithymocyte globulin (ATG) therapy with approximately a 50% response rate. Thus, if the only acceptable marrow donor were pregnant, it would be preferable to treat the patient with ATG and consider marrow transplantation later if the ATG were unsuccessful. In contrast, a patient with second- or subsequent-remission acute lymphocytic leukemia or chronic myelogenous leukemia (CML) in accelerated phase has few alternatives, and after appropriate consideration of the anesthesia risks, it might be reasonable to use a pregnant donor.

Donor Evaluation

Once one or more HLA-compatible relatives have been identified, the donors must be evaluated for their own health and to determine the most appropriate donor if more than one is available. The procurement of marrow from small children is feasible but requires special care (65). The components of a useful evaluation are listed in Table 60-1.

The history has always been an important part of the evaluation of potential stem cell donors. Experience with general or regional anesthesia may be important in assessing the risk of a procedure that has no physical benefit for the donor and that can occasionally be harmful (66,67). Furthermore, if a donor is considered to be well, and the conditioning regimen is initiated, but the donor is subsequently found to be ill or unable to be anesthetized (e.g., malignant hyperthermia), then both the well donor and the irreversibly pancytopenic patient are at risk of death or serious morbidity. In recent years, the specter of human immunodeficiency virus (HIV) infection has become a major concern. Any potential donor must be screened for HIV antibodies; however, a small proportion of patients are viremic in the absence of antibody. The determination of the current and past sexual habits of potential donors and a review of possible risk factors is crucial. Unfortunately, although this aspect of donor evaluation should be simple, family members who have engaged in high-risk activities that may result in HIV infection may keep silent to avoid familial

---

TABLE 60-1. Transplant Donor and Recipient Evaluation Guidelines

Recipient evaluation
Complete history, including recreational drug use, allergies, alcohol and smoking history, transfusions, pregnancies, abortions, sexual history
Complete physical examination, including neurologic assessment (include performance status)
Bone marrow aspirate, ± cytogenetics, lumbar puncture, CAT scan or MRI, gallium scan, human leukocyte antigen typing (as appropriate)
CBC with differential, chemistries, lipid profile, lactate dehydrogenase, ferritin, thyroid-stimulating hormone, PT/PTT, blood type, urinalysis
Chest radiograph and pulmonary function tests (diffusing capacity of lung for carbon monoxide if medically indicated)
Radionuclide ventriculogram or echocardiogram; electrocardiogram
Serologies: cytomegalovirus; herpes simplex; hepatitis A, B, C; varicella; Epstein-Barr virus; human immunodeficiency virus; human T-cell leukemia virus type 1; serologic test for syphilis; toxoplasmosis
Purified protein derivative
β-HCG
Men: sperm banking; women: oocyte freezing
Donor evaluation
Complete history (including i.v. drug use, hypertension, cigarette smoking, history of transfusion, pregnancies, abortions, immunizations, and physical examination)
CBC with differential, chemistries, PT/PTT, G6PD screen
Serologies: same as recipient evaluation
Urinalysis, chest radiograph (optional), electrocardiogram
No ingestion of potential bone marrow suppressive agents such as ethanol or antiplatelet drugs such as aspirin for at least 2 weeks before donation; no nonsteroidal antiinflammatory medications for 24 h before donation
If female, check mean corpuscular volume and replace if iron deficient
β-HCG if appropriate
One- or two-unit phlebotomy autologous use of donor blood (if necessary)

CAT, computer-assisted tomography; CBC, complete blood cell count; HCG, human chorionic gonadotropin; G6PD, glucose-6-phosphate dehydrogenase; MRI, magnetic resonance imaging; PT/PTT, prothrombin time/partial thromboplastin time.
NOTE: The Foundation for the Accreditation of Hematopoietic Cell Therapy provides useful guidelines for these evaluations.
Adapted from Sanders JE, Thomas ED, Buckner CD, et al. Marrow transplantation for children with acute lymphoblastic leukemia in second remission. *Blood* 1987;70:324.

disapproval, and some may not realize they are engaged in high-risk behavior. It is important to have a separate interview with the potential donor to be sure that the history is accurate and, if necessary, to provide the HIV-seropositive or high-risk donor with a reasonable excuse for being unable to donate marrow. Screening for human T-cell virus 1 and human T-cell virus 2 is also important, although the consequence of transmission of these viruses is less apparent.

The need for physical examination, complete blood counts, urinalysis, and chemistry profile does not require further discussion except to emphasize that these tests must be undertaken sufficiently in advance of the transplant that abnormalities are recognized before the start of the conditioning regimen. Viral serologies can provide useful information on which to base a decision to choose one available donor over another. For instance, cytomegalovirus (CMV) infection is one of the major hurdles encountered by patients with transplants. If the recipient has not been exposed to CMV, the use of stem cells and blood products from CMV-negative donors dramatically reduces the risk of symptomatic CMV disease, whereas stem cells and blood products from CMV-positive donors increase the risk of fatal CMV infection (68). On the other hand, if the recipient is seropositive for CMV, it may be preferable to use a seropositive donor. Although most clinical CMV disease is due to reactivation of endogenous virus (69), there may be passively acquired immunity from the donor that is protective, at least in part (70,71). The value of HIV testing is self-evident; there is no benefit in substituting one fatal disease for another.

Hepatitis B, hepatitis C, and Epstein-Barr virus (EBV) exposures are bigger problems. Clinical hepatitis B is to be expected if the donor has circulating hepatitis B surface antigen (HBsAg) (presumably in association with active Dane particles). The effects of hepatitis B acquired in this fashion in transplantation patients are variable but can be associated with transmission of hepatitis B and liver failure (72,73). Obviously, it is preferable to select a donor who has surface antibody or no exposure, but the presence of HBsAg should be considered in the context of the disease being treated. For newly diagnosed aplastic anemia, the use of ATG is preferable;

if the patient failed to respond to immunosuppression, a transplant from a HBsAg-positive donor might be considered. Similarly, a patient with acute myelogenous leukemia (AML) would not receive a transplant in first remission in this setting but rather in relapse or subsequent remission. Alternatively, if the transplantation does not need to be performed imminently, a patient with abnormal liver function tests and hepatitis B surface antigenemia can be treated with lamivudine (74). Similar considerations apply for hepatitis C, however, interferon (IFN) with or without ribavirin is used to attempt to clear the virus (74). A useful approach to donors with hepatitis is shown in Figure 60-4 (74). The clinical relevance of EBV infection is even less well understood. It is unlikely that an acute, infectious, mononucleosis-like syndrome would be detected in a patient who received a conditioning regimen because a large part of the syndrome of infectious mononucleosis is due to the reactive expansion of T lymphocytes. Furthermore, EBV exposure in the community is widespread, and clinical problems with acute EBV infection after marrow grafting are uncommon (75–77). This relative lack of sequelae is surprising because the primary means of controlling the virus, T lymphocytes, are absent or dysfunctional. One would expect the uncontrolled proliferation of donor or residual host B lymphocytes in this milieu. Indeed, in HLA-mismatched transplants, a proportion of patients die from lymphoproliferative disorders in which EBV has been implicated (78–80).

It may be useful to obtain blood samples for extended red-cell typing (81), leukocyte isoenzymes (82), immunoglobulin (Ig) isotypes (83), or restriction fragment length polymorphisms (RFLP) (84,85) at the time of donor evaluation. These tests are particularly valuable in determining, with some degree of confidence, that twins are monozygotic. One can never be sure of monozygosity, but the more polymorphic determinants that are the same, the lower the probability that they are dizygotic. Although the presence of informative polymorphisms is not ordinarily a factor in donor selection for nontwin siblings, if two donors are otherwise equivalent, it is preferable to use the donor with the more useful polymorphisms. This facilitates the determination of engraftment, the presence of mixed chimerism, and perhaps the occasional development of leukemia in donor cells.

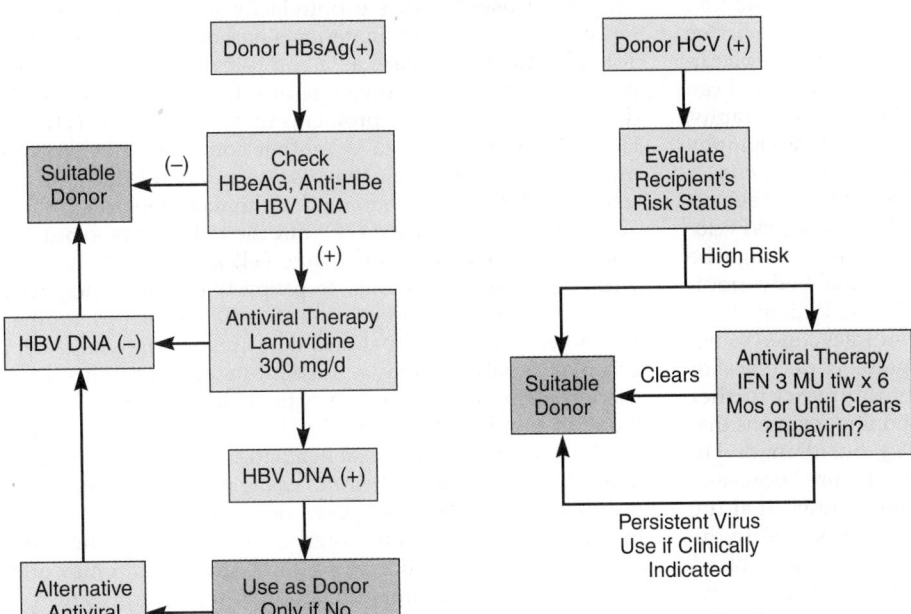

Figure 60-4. Schema for the evaluation, therapy, and use of donors infected with hepatitis B or hepatitis C. HBeAG, hepatitis B e antigen; HBV, hepatitis B virus; HCV, hepatitis C virus; IFN, interferon; MU, million units.

Other factors that must be considered include the age and gender of the donors. Data indicate that the use of donors of the opposite gender (particularly female donors for male recipients) doubles the risk of GVHD (86–89). Situations in which parous females donate to male recipients carry the highest risk. There is probably also an influence of donor age on the risk of GVHD, and it is generally believed that younger donors are preferable. The data on donor age are difficult to assess because siblings tend to be of similar ages, and the risk may be largely confined to the age of the recipient. In inbred families, populations with limited genetic heterogeneity, or in families with very common haplotypes, there occasionally may be a potential donor who is not a sibling. In that case, the sibling is usually still considered the preferred donor, because nonHLA phenotypic differences are likely to play a role in graft rejection and GVHD. Other considerations, however, such as viral exposure or pregnancy, might make the extended family member the preferred donor. In unrelated donor transplantation, there appears to be a substantial benefit to the use of donors who are matched using high resolution techniques, younger donors, and CMV-negative donors (90). However, younger age seems to be the primary trait associated with improved outcomes (91).

Patient Evaluation

The primary concern in evaluating a patient for hematopoietic stem cell transplantation is the determination that the results of the procedure warrant the risks of the transplant. An accurate assessment of the risk requires knowledge of the general health of the subject, that is, the subject's ability to withstand the rigors of the conditioning regimen, the risk of GVHD, the risk of relapse, and the risk of long-term morbidity related to immunosuppression.

Relatively few pretransplantation evaluations can accurately predict the risk of death or serious morbidity. Most of the poor prognostic features constitute relative rather than absolute contraindications to the procedure. It is important to provide the patient with an accurate estimate of risks, however, so that he or she may judge the merits of pursuing an expensive, uncomfortable, and potentially lethal procedure.

All conditioning regimens function on the borders of nonhematopoietic organ tolerance (discussed under Conditioning Regimens). Consequently, organs that are compromised before the procedure are more likely to be injured during the conditioning regimen. The basic evaluation outlined in Table 60-1 can be used to assess risk in a general way. Electrocardiography, echocardiography or radionuclide scan, and chest radiography may detect the presence of anthracycline cardiotoxicity. If reduction in cardiac reserve is apparent, it is not wise to subject the patient to high doses of known cardiac toxins such as cyclophosphamide. If transplantation is to be undertaken, it might be more easily accomplished with etoposide and total-body irradiation (TBI) (92,93) or melphalan and TBI (80). Patients with healthy hearts who have not had prior anthracyclines sometimes develop heart failure (94); thus, the presence of clinical or subclinical cardiac dysfunction is likely to predict further reductions in cardiac performance. Conditioning regimens that rely on bischloroethylnitrosourea (BCNU), busulfan, or TBI commonly result in progressive respiratory failure because of interstitial pneumonia. Studies have demonstrated that the presence of small degrees of airways obstruction before the transplantation predicts late (1 year or more) declines in forced expiratory volume and forced vital capacity (95). Patients who previously received bleomycin or busulfan may be at further risk for progressive lung failure. Bleomycin-induced lung dis-

ease is best detected by measuring the carbon monoxide diffusing capacity (96–99).

Liver injury due to venoocclusive disease can be predicted by the presence of abnormal liver function tests within the year preceding the transplantation as well as poor performance status and intensity of prior therapy (100–102). Because the mortality of venoocclusive disease is high, it is important to establish the presence of risk factors in advance.

Hypertension may be exacerbated by the use of cyclosporine, tacrolimus, or steroids. Steroids, calcineurin inhibitors, and hyperalimentation may also worsen glucose intolerance. Any reduction in creatinine clearance may affect the ability to use nephrotoxins, such as cyclosporine, aminoglycosides, and amphotericin B. Conditioning regimens used for the treatment of solid tumors such as neuroblastomas often include nephrotoxins such as cisplatin or high-dose melphalan, and conditioning regimens that do not include classic nephrotoxins may also result in renal insufficiency after transplantation (103,104), possibly by causing or exacerbating radiation nephritis. Prior bladder injury in a patient who has received cyclophosphamide or ifosfamide may predispose to more severe injury after transplantation conditioning. In such patients, one should consider the use of urothelial protective agents, such as 2-mercaptoethanesulfonate (mesna; discussed in the section Toxicity and Complications), or a regimen that does not include cyclophosphamide.

Ophthalmologic evaluation is often useful to detect evidence of prior CMV or toxoplasmosis. In addition, conditioning regimens and corticosteroids can cause cataracts, and it is valuable to have a baseline slit-lamp evaluation (105–107).

As for donors, an evaluation of viral exposure is helpful before undertaking a hematopoietic stem cell transplantation. The only absolute contraindication to transplantation is HIV infection. Transplantation has been performed in patients who are infected with HIV (108,109), but there has been no alteration in the presence of the virus. The virus infects nonhematopoietic cells, such as central nervous system (CNS) neurons, that act as a reservoir for HIV and cause progressive neurologic dysfunction. The infection of these cells is not affected by the transplantation. It is also helpful to know whether the patient has been exposed to varicella and herpes simplex viruses because prophylactic acyclovir can substantially reduce morbidity in patients harboring these infections. Toxoplasmosis can flare as a complication of immunosuppression, and prior knowledge of infection can assist in the differential diagnosis of problems that develop later (110,111). Hepatitis B antigenemia is another condition that probably predisposes to venoocclusive disease and that is likely to persist through the transplantation. Fulminant hepatitis B reactivation has been reported (73), but the risk of transplantation does not appear to be excessive (112). Recognition of this virus is important not only to properly evaluate the patient but also to protect staff against accidental exposures. If time is available, treatment of patients who are known to have hepatitis B or hepatitis C may reduce future complications (74). A useful schematic approach to patients infected with hepatitis B or C is shown in Figure 60-5.

Thus, a complete medical evaluation allows the transplantation team to estimate the risks of the procedure and to minimize those risks. As noted previously, the presence of mild or, in some cases, moderate organ dysfunction may not be an absolute contraindication to stem cell grafting but may affect the timing of transplantation and may significantly affect the assessment of the value of the procedure as it is presented to the patient.

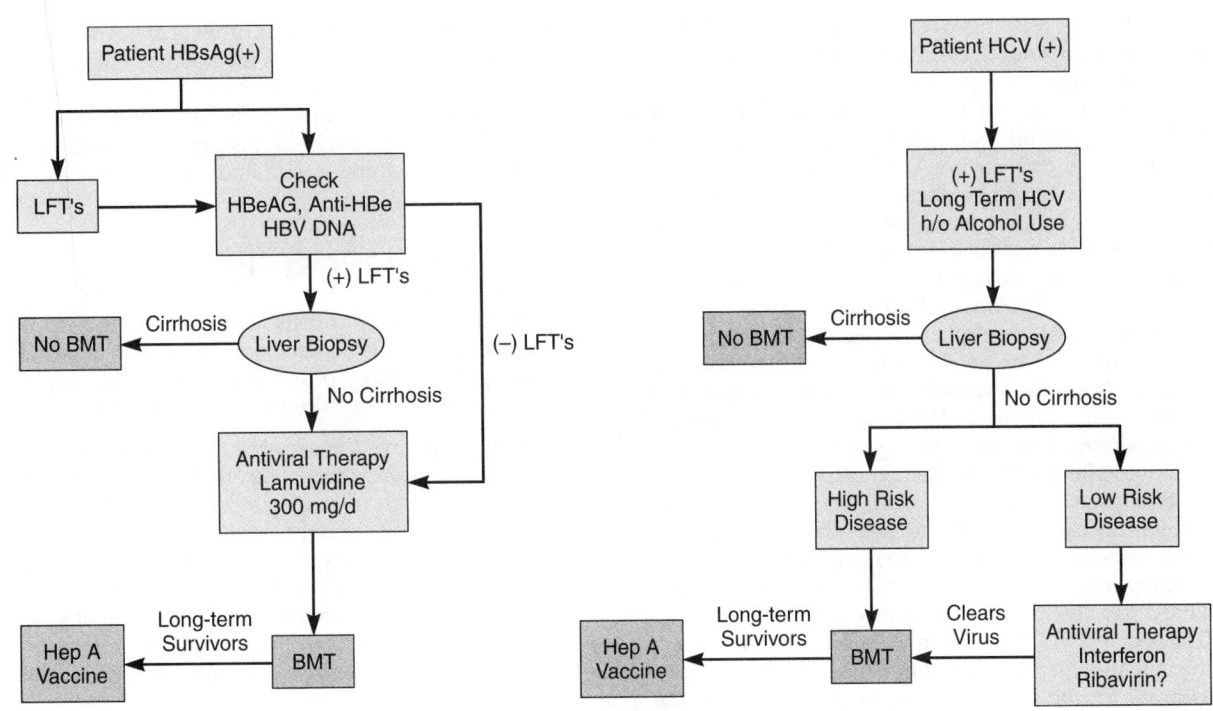

Figure 60-5. Schema for the evaluation and therapy of patients infected with hepatitis B or hepatitis C. (Hep) BMT, bone marrow transplant; HBeAG, hepatitis B e antigen; HBV, hepatitis B vaccine; HCV, hepatitis C vaccine; LFT, liver function test.

STEM CELL PROCUREMENT

Bone marrow is distributed throughout the axial skeleton, but anatomic constraints limit the reasonable sites for marrow procurement to the pelvis and sternum. Bone marrow is obtained from the donor under general or regional anesthesia by multiple needle aspirates of the iliac crests using large-gauge marrow aspirate needles, and the marrow is added to a heparinized electrolyte solution. Most groups attempt to obtain 2 to 4×10^8 nucleated cells/kg of recipient weight—in practice, this amounts to approximately 10 mL of marrow/kg of recipient weight. This volume of marrow amounts to 1% to 5% of the donor's total marrow volume, and its removal causes no cytopenia other than anemia proportionate to the blood loss. If the marrow is to be manipulated to remove T lymphocytes or malignant cells, there are substantial nonspecific losses, and 15 to 20 mL/kg is often obtained. Older donors may have less cellular marrows, and relatively larger volumes may be required (67). The marrow sample contains a substantial amount of particulate matter, including blood clots, bone particles, and fat, and is usually filtered through mesh before infusion into the patient. The stress placed on the donor is proportional to the size of the recipient. Often, if the donor is small, and a large amount of marrow is to be obtained, it is wise to phlebotomize the marrow donor 2 to 4 weeks in advance for autologous transfusion. This blood partially restores the donor's hematocrit after the marrow harvest.

The risk to the donor is small. Bortin and Buckner reviewed 3290 marrow harvests and found a life-threatening complication rate of 0.27% and no deaths or permanent injuries (66). Cardiopulmonary events, cerebrovascular accidents, and infectious complications do occur, however, and donors need to be counseled appropriately. Pain persists for several days but sometimes longer. Occasional donors develop local neuropathies as a result of injury to the lateral femoral cutaneous nerve (90,113).

PERIPHERAL BLOOD STEM CELL PROCUREMENT

Hematopoietic stem cells are not a static population in the marrow. It has been known since the 1960s that, in mice, they appear to be able to leave the marrow cavity, circulate in the blood, and return to the marrow (114). Similar evidence for circulating stem cells was shown a decade later in humans (115). The ability to circulate may function in part to keep hematopoiesis uniformly distributed in the marrow-producing areas of the skeleton. The cells capable of establishing long-term lymphohematopoiesis are thought to be included in a measurable population of otherwise bland-appearing cells that express CD34; however, at steady-state, CD34+ cells are only present on average 0.01% to 0.06% of circulating lymphomononuclear cells. Because of the tendency to circulate, stem cells may be obtained from the peripheral blood by leukapheresis. The first attempt to use these cells clinically showed that these cells can reestablish hematopoiesis (116). The initial limitations in using peripheral blood stem cells (PBSC) were ameliorated by the observation that the administration of hematopoietic cytokines, such as filgrastim and sargramostim, will increase the number of CD34+ cells tenfold to 20-fold. In addition, in the period of recovery after the administration of some chemotherapeutic agents, there may be a similarly robust increase in these cells. These observations have allowed the collection of both autologous and allogeneic products that appear to reestablish lymphohematopoiesis at least as well as marrow. Indeed, blood cell reconstitution is often more rapid after PBSC transplantation than marrow transplantation, presumably related to the high numbers of committed progenitors in the product (117). There was initial reluctance to use PBSC in allogeneic transplantation because of concerns about the risk of acute GVHD associated with the large T-cell load infused with these products. However, accumulating data suggest that the risk of acute GVHD is similar to the risk observed after marrow grafting, although there may be more chronic GVHD (118). Moreover, in patients with high-risk diseases, the additional T cells may enhance the GVL effect, thereby reducing the relapse rate.

The optimal regimen of cytokine-induced mobilization of PBSC has not been fully elucidated. Most centers use filgrastim—5 to 15 µg/kg s.c. each day for 4 to 5 days followed by apheresis. The PBSC are collected by single or multiple continuous flow apheresis of two to three times the donor's blood volume. Typically, a dose of 2 to 6×10^6 CD34$^+$ cells/kg of recipient weight is considered a reasonable target, although much larger numbers of cells are occasionally infused. Collecting this many CD34$^+$ cells typically takes one to two apheresis sessions. There are occasional normal donors who are poor mobilizers and in whom it may be difficult to obtain the targeted dose. Marrow collection may be necessary to supplement the PBSC. Mobilization of stem cells for autologous transplantation typically involves the administration of cytokines after a cycle of chemotherapy to take advantage of the antineoplastic effect of the regimen as well as its mobilizing ability. It is not clear that both the chemotherapy and the cytokine therapy are necessary. Patients with heavy prior exposures to chemotherapy may not mobilize as many CD34$^+$ cells as expected, and they may need additional marrow collected as well.

The toxicity of PBSC collection is largely related to the toxicity of the cytokine therapy, including fevers, bone pain, headache, nausea, and fatigue. There is also the potential toxicity of the apheresis procedure *per se*. Poor venous access can be overcome in autologous donation with a central line. Placement of this type of prosthesis must be undertaken with circumspection in a normal donor. Other toxicities to keep in mind are the tendency for post-collection cytopenias, including thrombocytopenia, neutropenia, and lymphopenia (119). There have been no known untoward effects of these observations. The risk of administration of cytokines to normal donors is thought to be small. Although there are advocates for each procedure, comparative data demonstrating a preferred stem cell collection technique are lacking.

CORD BLOOD UNIT PROCUREMENT

Human umbilical cord blood is a rich source of stem cells, and early studies indicate that cord blood unit procurements (CBUs) can be successfully used to transplant children following ablative cytoreduction regimens (58–63,120). Experience indicates that these units are readily collected. Benefits of using banked CBUs include the following: (1) availability of the unit on demand; (2) receipt of the unit at the transplant center prior to the start of cytoreduction; (3) minimal risk of inconvenience to the donor, as the unit is collected from the placenta after the infant is delivered. Potential benefits include the following: (a) lower risk of transmissible infectious diseases, such as CMV and EBV; (b) lower risk of acute and chronic GVHD as compared to unrelated marrow transplantation; (c) the ability to tolerated HLA-mismatched transplants; and (d) shorter interval between initiation of a search and transplant. Disadvantages of using CBUs include the following: (a) lack of a medical history on the donor as the mother serves as a surrogate for information pertaining to the medical history (the infant donor could develop a medical disorder and theoretically, could have transmitted this disorder to the recipient); (b) a donor would not be available for a second donation should the CBU fail to engraft; (c) the length of time a frozen CBU retains its engraftment potential is unknown.

There are many ethical and legal issues regarding the timing of informed consent and the collection, processing, and shipping procedures. In 1995, the National Heart Lung and Blood Institute funded the Cord Blood Transplantation Study and through this network addressed the need for cord blood bank standard operating procedures (121). Although these CBUs must be accessed through the medical coordinating center for the trial and CBUs at the New York Blood Center must be accessed directly, many banks have registered their units with the NMDP and searches for compatible CBUs are performed at the time of an initial preliminary search of the NMDP file.

CONDITIONING REGIMENS

The treatment that precedes marrow transplantation is generally referred to as the *conditioning regimen*. For a successful marrow graft to take place, a conditioning regimen must be established that satisfies the following criteria:

1. It must have the capacity to eradicate malignant (e.g., leukemic) or abnormal (e.g., thalassemic) cells when administered once over a brief period, while respecting the sensitivity of normal, nonhematopoietic tissues.
2. It must suppress the immune response of the recipient to prevent marrow rejection.
3. It may need to provide for the creation of space in the marrow for the newly infused bone marrow cells (122). Examples of conditioning regimens are shown in Table 60-2.

Eradication of Abnormal Cells

Chemotherapy and radiation therapy kill malignant cells by first-order kinetics—they kill a fixed proportion of cancer cells. Thus, if a patient has a large leukemic cell burden, the efficacy of the conditioning regimen is determined by the balance between the number of leukemic cells destroyed and the number of these residual blasts with clonogenic capacity. Transplantation conditioning regimens attempt to exploit the steep dose–response relations that chemotherapy-sensitive tumors often demonstrate (128). In contrast to standard nontransplantation therapy, in which moderate doses are administered repetitively over a long period, a single high dose is administered. Because sensitivity to drugs or drugs plus radiation is crucial to the success of this brief exposure to therapy, any effective therapy is more likely to cure the neoplasm if the number of cells treated is low and if the dose-response curve for the therapy is steep. Thus, eradication of the malignancy is easier when the malignant cell burden is minimal and the cells are not likely to have acquired a high degree of resistance. As a rule, this means that transplantation in early stages of disease is more likely to cure the neoplasm than if the procedure is undertaken after extensive, unsuccessful prior therapy. Nevertheless, it is likely that in some cases, the administration of very high doses of drugs or radiation can overcome even established, resistant cells.

The advantage of transplant conditioning regimens over standard chemotherapy is the ability to escalate the dose up a steep dose-response curve because myelotoxicity, which is the chief dose-limiting toxicity of most regimens, is overcome with the stem cell infusion. A steep dose-response curve is apparent with the use of radiation therapy and alkylating agents (128,129). Early attempts to perform transplants with single agents were unsuccessful (23,130). Most transplants for malignancies are based on a combination of cyclophosphamide and TBI or cyclophosphamide and busulfan. Variations in agent, dose rate and fractionation of TBI, and timing are common; generic examples are shown in Table 60-2, but there is little evidence to suggest that one regimen is preferable to another. Higher doses may result in fewer relapses, but toxicity tends to increase (131). TBI can be given either as a single fraction or fractionated into multiple doses in an attempt to

TABLE 60-2. Examples of Commonly Used Conditioning Regimens

Regimen	Day							
	-7	-6	-5	-4	-3	-2	-1	0
Aplastic anemia[a]								
CTX			Δ	Δ	Δ	Δ		
ATG			♦	♦	♦			
Stem cell infusion								⊕
Allogeneic transplantation for leukemia								
CTX			Δ	Δ				
TBI					↓↓	↓↓	↓↓	↓↓
Stem cell infusion								⊕
Bu[b]	||||	||||	||||	||||				
CTX					Δ	Δ		
Stem cell infusion								⊕
TBI[c]	↓↓↓	↓↓	↓↓↓	↓↓↓				
Etoposide					♦			
Stem cell infusion								⊕
Autologous transplantation for lymphoma[d]								
CTX		Δ Δ	Δ Δ	Δ Δ	Δ Δ			
Etoposide		♦♦	♦♦	♦♦	♦♦			
BCNU		□	□	□	□			
Stem cell infusion								⊕
BCNU		□						
Arabinosyl cytosine			ΔΔ	ΔΔ	ΔΔ	ΔΔ		
Etoposide			∇∇	∇∇	∇∇	∇∇		
Melphalan							⇓	
Stem cell infusion								⊕

ATG, anti-thymocyte globulin; BCNU, bischloroethylnitrosourea (carmustine); Bu, busulfan; CTX, cyclophosphamide; TBI, total body irradiation.
[a]Adapted from Storb R, Etizoni R, Anasetti C, et al. Cyclophosphamide combined with antithymocyte globulin in preparation for allogeneic marrow transplants in patients with aplastic anemia. *Blood* 1994;84:941.
[b]Adapted from Tutschka PJ, Copelan EA, Klein JP. Bone marrow transplantation for leukemia following a new busulfan and cyclophosphamide regimen. *Blood* 1987;70:1382.
[c]Adapted from Blume KG, Kopecky KJ, Henslee-Downey PJ, et al. A prospective randomized comparison of total body irradiation-etoposide versus busulfan-cyclophosphamide as preparatory regimens for bone marrow transplantation in patients with leukemia who were not in first remission: a Southwest Oncology Group study. *Blood* 1993;81:2187.
[d]Adapted from Wheeler C, Antin JH, Churchill WH, et al. Cyclophosphamide, carmustine, and etoposide with autologous bone marrow transplantation in refractory Hodgkin's disease and non-Hodgkin's lymphoma: a dose-finding study. *J Clin Oncol* 1990;8:648; and Chopra R, McMillan AK, Linch DC, et al. The place of high-dose BEAM therapy and bone marrow transplantation in poor-risk Hodgkin's disease. A single-center eight-year study of 155 patients. *Blood* 1993;81:1137.

reduce nonhematopoietic toxicity. Children clear busulfan twice as fast as adults do, and appropriate alterations in dosing are critical (132).

Recently, attempts to emphasize the GVL effect of the graft and deemphasize the role of conditioning have led to the study of reduced intensity or nonmyeloablative regimens. The principle benefit expected from these treatments is a reduction in immediate transplant-related toxicity. The lower doses have allowed these regimens to be piloted in older patients and in patients with underlying medical problems who are not typically candidates for conventional transplantation. However, some diseases, such as acute lymphoblastic leukemia (ALL), are less susceptible to the GVL reaction, and it is likely that the application of reduced intensity regimens will need to be selective for diseases that are relatively indolent and that can be eradicated by donor T cells (133–136).

New approaches using radioimmunotherapy have recently been developed for use in fully myeloablative as well as non-myeloablative transplantation (137,138). The putative benefit is the ability to increase the dose of radiation to the cancer while keeping the dose to uninvolved organs relatively low. The role of these novel approaches remains to be determined.

TOXICITY AND COMPLICATIONS

Application of the principles outlined previously has resulted in the establishment of conditioning regimens that function on the borders of tissue tolerance for several nonhematopoietic tissues, including mucous membranes, gastrointestinal tract, lungs, liver, bladder, and heart (139–146).

The mucous membranes are generally the first nonhematopoietic organs to demonstrate toxicity. Ulceration of the buccal mucosa, often extending into the pharynx and esophagus, is extremely uncomfortable and interferes with oral nutrition and speech. Commonly, herpes simplex virus reactivates during this period, worsening the oral injury; and oral fungi, primarily *Candida* spp., are frequently associated pathogens. It is often necessary to resort to parenteral narcotic infusions to control the pain; topical anesthetics must be used cautiously to avoid blunting the gag reflex and predisposing the patient to aspiration. It is exceedingly important that careful dental care, including filling of cavities, cleaning of the teeth and gums, extraction of unsalvageable teeth, and eradication of infections and loci capable of supporting infection, be undertaken before transplantation. Close attention to oral hygiene dramatically reduces oral complications during this stage of marrow grafting. Prophylactic administration of acyclovir and nystatin, fluconazole, or clotrimazole, combined with aggressive débridement, is variably effective in controlling the mucositis. Ordinarily, the mucositis is self-limited, but it can occasionally lead to life-threatening bleeding or require intubation or tracheostomy to maintain a patent airway. Once the mucositis resolves, xerostomia is a frequent problem and may persist for weeks or months. It is due, in part, to damage to salivary glands in the buccal mucosa as well as the parotid and submaxillary glands. Artificial saliva is sometimes helpful (141,147,148).

The injury to oral mucous membranes may be reflected from one end of the gastrointestinal tract to the other. Severe diarrhea is a frequent complication of conditioning therapy, and it must be distinguished from other common causes of diarrhea, including viral, protozoal, or bacterial gastroenteritis; pseudomembranous enterocolitis; giardiasis; or acute GVHD. There may be altered absorption of nutrients and medications because of the severe mucosal injury. Nausea and vomiting or simply anorexia contribute to poor nutrition, and patients often require total parenteral nutrition to maintain an adequate caloric intake. Abdominal pain can be a major problem, because narcotics may reduce gut motility and predispose to the development of ileus and consequent fluid and electrolyte disorders. Pancreatitis occasionally complicates the picture, although it is rarely severe. Gastrointestinal bleeding is commonplace and may be severe. Often, there are multiple ulcerations of the mucosa extending the length of the gastrointestinal tract, and the residual mucosa is friable and easily injured. The bleeding is compounded by thrombocytopenia. As a rule, injury to the gut begins to resolve with the recovery of granulocytes in the blood if GVHD does not supervene (147,149).

The liver is a major site for both detoxification and activation of chemotherapeutic agents. In addition to the usual viral insults resulting from multiple blood transfusions, the liver has to contend with the toxic effects of chemotherapeutic agents, irradiation, and a variety of other hepatotoxins, such as antibiotics and hyperalimentation. It is not surprising, therefore, that hepatotoxicity is a major problem in some patients. In addition to the usually mild and reversible hepatic injury that is often observed in severely ill patients on multiple supportive therapies, the liver is subject to venoocclusive disease (100,102,149,150). It appears to be more common in patients with prior hepatitis and in patients receiving busulfan for transplant conditioning (151). This condition results in centrilobular necrosis and reticulin deposition around central veins and may occur in as many as one-fourth of transplant recipients. It must be distinguished from other hepatic insults, such as viruses, GVHD, acalculous cholecystitis, calcineurin inhibitor toxicity, choleangitis lenta, and gallstones. Liver biopsy and diagnostic procedures such as endoscopic retrograde cholangiopancreatogram are often difficult to perform in thrombocytopenic patients. Transjugular liver biopsy can be performed in some patients and has the advantage of allowing the measurement of hepatic wedge pressures. Doppler examination of the portal vein is a useful test, because reversal of flow in the portal vein is relatively specific. In a typical case, there is rapid weight gain, fluid retention with "third-spacing," increase in bilirubin, and hepatic distention. However, many patients have less severe manifestations that may be difficult to diagnose. There is no specific therapy for venoocclusive disease, and it may be fatal in one-half of patients who develop it. Supportive management includes careful attention to volume status and avoidance of hepatic and renal toxins. There is avid sodium retention and a propensity to develop hepatorenal syndrome. Thus, unless fluid retention is causing morbidity, it is best not to be aggressive with diuretics. It is often helpful to keep the hematocrit above 30% to maintain renal blood flow.

A form of hemorrhagic cardiomyopathy that occurs in small numbers of transplant recipients can be directly attributed to cyclophosphamide (145). Although the prior use of anthracyclines appears to predispose to cardiotoxicity, that relation has not been established clearly (94,152,153). The sudden development of congestive heart failure, with pericardial effusion, cardiomegaly, and loss of electrocardiogram voltage occurring 1 to 10 days after the administration of cyclophosphamide, is a characteristic clinical picture. If the pericardial effusion is large, it may require drainage. Cyclophosphamide cardiotoxicity is often refractory to therapy with diuretics and inotropic agents, and as many as one-half of patients who develop the clinically apparent form die. Another cardiovascular complication seen after marrow grafting is hypertension. Cyclosporine appears to be the predominant risk factor, but glucocorticoids contribute (154). Tacrolimus seems to be less likely to cause hypertension (155). Although usually not detected clinically, nonbacterial thrombotic endocarditis is often discovered at autopsy (156). This possibility should be kept in mind if embolic disease is suspected.

The lungs are another major site for conditioning regimen toxicity. Idiopathic interstitial pneumonitis occurs in 10% to 25% of recipients and differs from the other forms of conditioning regimen toxicity in that it is usually delayed and usually occurs 30 to 100 days after transplantation. Patients generally develop tachypnea, arterial hemoglobin desaturation, and dyspnea, and often they require mechanical ventilation. The main entities from which it must be distinguished are CMV, *Pneumocystis carinii*, diffuse alveolar hemorrhage (97,142,157), and other nonbacterial pneumonias. The pneumonitis occurs after autologous as well as allogeneic marrow transplantation, but the incidence is lower in the autologous group (157). That observation, coupled with GVHD as an important risk factor, suggests that idiopathic interstitial pneumonia may be a manifestation of GVHD or of the immunosuppression associated with GVHD in some patients. Multivariate analysis suggests that the use of methotrexate rather than cyclosporine as GVHD prophylaxis is also associated with greater risk (99). The diagnosis can be made confidently only after open lung biopsy. The mortality from this form of pneumonitis is more than 90% (97,98,142,158–160). Even without clinically apparent pneumonitis, many patients develop obstructive and restrictive respiratory abnormalities (158).

A severe form of obstructive airway disease due to bronchiolitis obliterans has been described in 5% to 10% of recipients of allogeneic transplants, primarily with the development of chronic GVHD (161,162). This lung pathology does not appear to occur after AHSCT, and it is not associated with methotrexate or other GVHD prophylaxis. However, it may be more common if busulfan is used in conditioning (151). A similar picture is observed in patients after lung or heart-lung transplants (163), in some autoimmune disorders, and after some viral infections (164). It is unknown whether this disorder is due to reactivity of donor T lymphocytes against bronchial epithelium in a GVHR or whether the profound immunoincompetence associated with GVHD predisposes to viral injury. If it is progressive, bronchiolitis obliterans has a high mortality (161), but occasional patients respond to high-dose steroids.

Metabolites of cyclophosphamide are primarily excreted in the urine. Acrolein is the major offending agent and is toxic to the urothelial lining of the entire collecting system. Diffuse mucosal ulceration may occur with severe hemorrhage, dysuria, urethral obstruction with clots, and eventual interstitial cystitis, which can result in a shrunken, fibrotic bladder and may require excision or reconstructive surgery. The hemorrhage is often substantial, and its control may strain the creativity of the transplantation team. Thrombocytopenia often contributes to the bleeding, but even if the platelet count can be maintained above 50,000/μL, bleeding is often difficult to abort. Risk factors are variable but include busulfan use in addition to cyclophosphamide, prior bladder irradiation, GVHD, and age (165). There are three approaches to avoid hemorrhagic cystitis: (a) rapid hydration at approximately 200 mL/hour to maintain a saline diuresis (166,167); (b) mesna, a sulfhydryl-containing uroprotective agent, is given intravenously (it binds acrolein in the urine and prevents its toxic effects, apparently without limiting the effectiveness of the cyclophosphamide); (c) saline diuresis is established with or without a bladder lavage through an indwelling catheter to reduce the concentration of acrolein in the urine and to reduce the contact time with the lining of the collecting system (168,169). Randomized trials indicate that these approaches are equivalent (166,169). Hemorrhagic cystitis may occur in children as well as adults (170). Another cause of hemorrhagic cystitis that may be confused with cyclophosphamide toxicity is reactivation of adenovirus or BK virus (171–173). Although some studies have not detected virus, these infections tend to occur later and may be distinguished by appropriate cultures. Bladder bleeding can be a protracted and frustrating problem. It often requires weeks of bladder irrigation, but it usually resolves completely (171). Alum, estrogens, and prostaglandins (174) have been used with some reports of success. Intravesical formaldehyde is toxic and should be avoided.

Several other toxicities related to conditioning regimens deserve mention. Cataracts are a common delayed complication of marrow transplantation, usually occurring more than 2 years after therapy (175,176). Extensive studies of growth and endocrinologic function in children and adolescents have documented abnormalities in pituitary, thyroid, gonadal, and adrenal function (175,177–183). It is clear that growth is reduced and sexual maturation is delayed in many prepubertal children who undergo marrow transplants. The probability of becoming infertile depends on the conditioning regimen used. Many younger patients who receive regimens that do not include TBI (e.g., for aplastic anemia) maintain their fertility (179,184–186); however, TBI usually results in sterility for both males and females (177). Patients need to be made aware of this complication, and sperm banking or appropriate counseling can be arranged in advance. Hypothyroidism may develop insidiously months to years after the transplantation (175,177).

CNS complications are uncommon. The exceptions include busulfan-containing regimens, which may cause seizures, and nitrogen mustard, which causes a toxic encephalopathy (187–189). Patients with ALL who had prior CNS prophylaxis or therapy may be at higher risk of delayed leukoencephalopathy (190). Reversible neurologic abnormalities may be associated with parenteral acyclovir use (191).

Renal disease generally has not been considered a major late complication of marrow transplantation. However, a hemolytic-uremic syndrome has been recognized in children and adults (103,104,192). This problem occurs 3 to 11 months after transplantation, and renal biopsy is consistent with radiation nephritis. Although congestive heart failure, hypertension, anemia, and thrombocytopenia may be severe, the syndrome has a tendency to resolve spontaneously with supportive care. Toxicity may be related in part to the extent of prior therapy. There is also a thrombotic microangiopathy that appears to be related to the use of calcineurin inhibitors, tacrolimus, and cyclosporine (193,194). Although little objective data exists many transplant physicians agree that for similar conditioning regimens, patients with the least prior therapy have the fewest difficulties.

SECOND MALIGNANCIES

Radiation, alkylating agents, and immunosuppressants are well known to be associated with the development of therapy-induced malignancies. Thus, a major concern is the long-term effect of conditioning regimens on increasing numbers of transplantation survivors. Secondary malignancies appear to fall into three groups that are not mutually exclusive: lymphoproliferative disorders in donor or recipient cells, solid tumors, and leukemia.

Lymphoproliferative disorders are probably due to the severe immunoincompetence that is associated with GVHD, mismatched transplants, and immunosuppressive therapy with steroids, cyclosporine, or monoclonal antibodies. They are primarily large cell, B-cell immunoblastic lymphomas, and many are associated with EBV (78,79,195,196), but there is also an increased risk of Hodgkin's disease (197). They can occur in cells of host or donor origin and may progress from a polyclonal to an oligoclonal then monoclonal proliferation. The time to the development of the lymphoproliferation is short—30 to 1400 days from transplantation. It is probable that immunoincompetence related to the transplantation or immunosuppressive therapy may result in uncontrolled proliferation of EBV-infected recipient B cells, nasopharyngeal cells that have survived the conditioning regimen, or donor B cells that were infused with the marrow (198). EBV, however, may also be transmitted by means of blood transfusion. Prophylactic acyclovir was reported to reduce the incidence of EBV-related lymphomas (199), but other data show no benefit (78,79). The mortality of this complication is extremely high; most patients die unless immunosuppression can be reduced. Recently, encouraging results have demonstrated control of the lymphoproliferation using monoclonal antibodies, such as rituximab (200,201), or infusions of T cells from immune donors (80,202,203).

Solid tumors have been reported in patients who have undergone marrow grafting (204–206). This is an important observation given the large number of patients undergoing transplantation annually. These tumors are associated with older patients, chronic GVHD, TBI, and treatment with cyclosporine. Skin and oral cavity are particularly susceptible to secondary cancers, but malignancies of most organs have been reported.

The development of new leukemias in donor cells is intriguing but rare. AML (207,208) and ALL (209–211) have both been reported. The pathogenesis of these malignancies is unclear, but consideration must be given to microenvironmental abnormalities, viral or chemical agents, or a familial predisposition. A more frequent observation is the development of myelodysplasia or AML after autologous transplantation (212–217). There remains some controversy about the cause of this problem, and it is likely to be multifactorial. Patients receiving autotransplants may be predisposed to secondary myelodysplasia by virtue of their prior treatment with alkylating agents. However, it is also likely that TBI administered for conditioning spares a small cohort of stem cells. These cells may have radiation-induced mutations that later result in myelodysplasia (MDS)/AML as these cells expand. The observation that TBI-based regimens appear to confer a higher risk than chemotherapy-based regimens for the same diseases supports this notion (213,215), although it is likely that prior alkylating agent therapy contributes substantially. It is typically not observed after allogeneic transplantation, presumably because the GVHD effect eradicates residual, radioresistant host stem cells before they can undergo malignant transformation.

HEMATOPOIETIC RECONSTITUTION

Engraftment is usually marked by the development of hematopoietic progenitor cells of donor origin in the marrow and the recovery of neutrophils in the blood 10 to 21 days after transplantation. Recovery of erythropoiesis and megakaryopoiesis follows.

The nature and tempo of hematopoietic recovery after marrow grafting varies with the type of cytoreduction (e.g., ablative versus nonablative regimen and level of immunosuppression), source and dose of donor cells, the level of HLA disparity between the donor and recipient, the diagnosis of the patient, and posttransplantation drug therapy. Higher marrow doses may lead to more

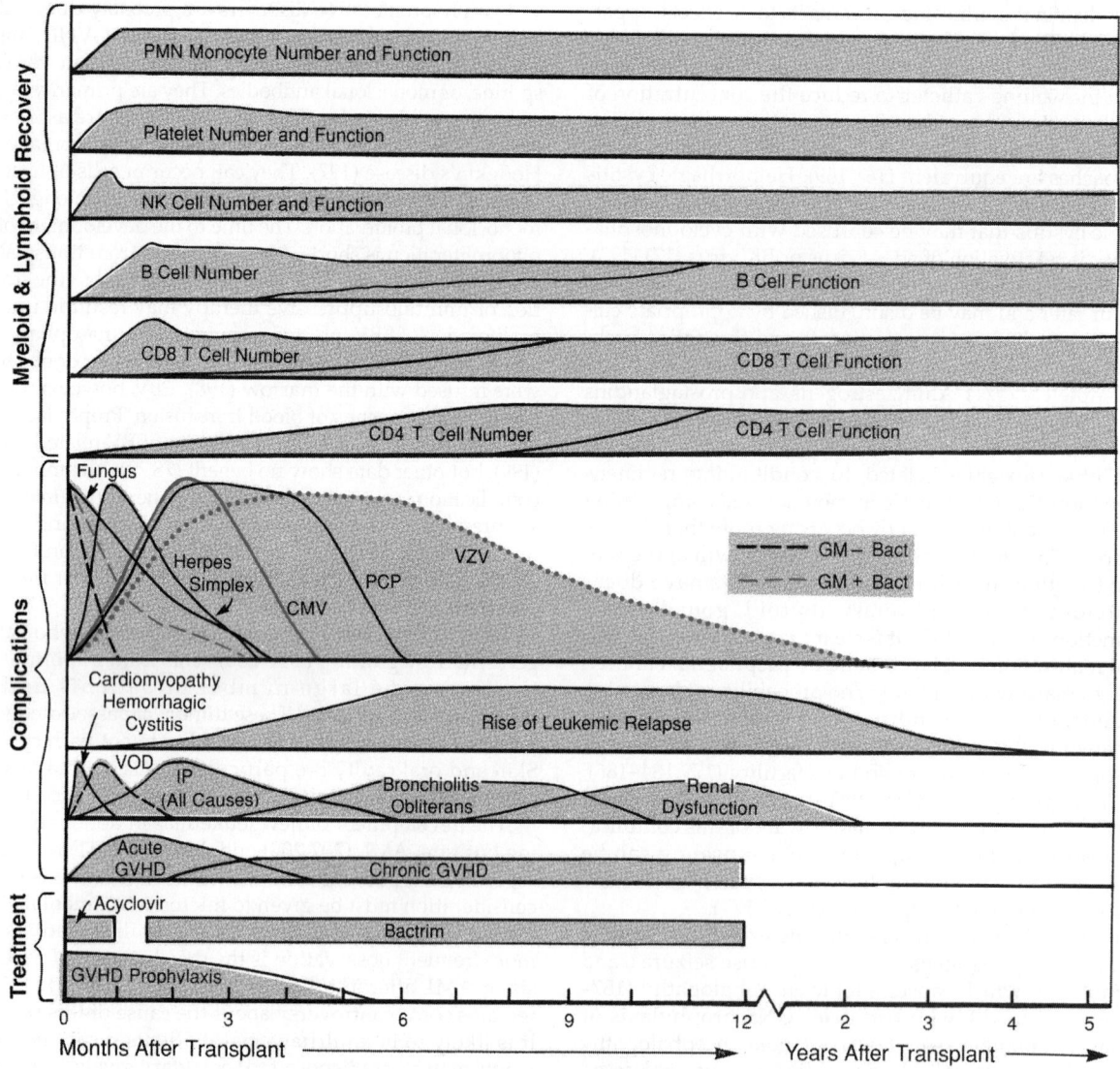

Figure 60-6. Schematic representation of the recovery of important classes of lymphocytes and hematopoietic cells and the relation of immune and hematopoietic recovery to infectious, immunologic, and neoplastic risks after transplantation. If graft-versus-host disease (GVHD) occurs, immunologic recovery is shifted to the right—it takes longer to establish normal numbers of functionally competent lymphocytes. Hematopoietic recovery is generally not affected. Bact, bacteria; CMV, cytomegalovirus; GM, gram; IP, interstitial pneumonitis; NK, natural killer; PCP, *Pneumocystis carinii* pneumonia; PMN, polymorphonuclear neutrophil; VOD, venoocclusive disease; VZV, varicella-zoster virus.

rapid recovery (218,219); cryopreservation and purging of autologous marrow before reinfusion may lead to delayed reconstitution, especially in platelet recovery (220,221); significant myelofibrosis or splenomegaly may delay reconstitution (222,223); GVHD prophylaxis with methotrexate postpones recovery compared to cyclosporine prophylaxis (224,225); viral infection (especially of the herpesvirus group) may also lead to a delay in reappearance of normal blood counts (226,227). High doses of PBSC in either the autologous or allogeneic setting contribute to rapid hematopoietic recovery, whereas the low cell dose associated with single cord blood unit infusions results in delayed (e.g., 42 days) recovery (58–63). A schematic representation of hematopoietic and immune reconstitution in relation to infectious complications and time after transplantation is shown in Figure 60-6.

In experimental animals, hematopoietic reconstitution may occur from a restricted number of clones. Lemischka and colleagues (228), using retrovirus-mediated gene transfer to mark stem cells, were able to demonstrate that only one to two stem cell clones are

sufficient to give rise to most hematopoietic elements after injection into lethally irradiated mice. Although polyclonal models have been proposed for large animal (229) and human transplantation (230), there is preliminary evidence that monoclonal stem cell reconstitution occurs in some patients (231). Thus, it remains uncertain as to how many donor stem cells in humans give rise to the eventual fully reconstituted hematopoietic and immune systems.

Hematopoiesis reflects a progressive expansion, maturation, and differentiation of cells. The most primitive pluripotent stem cells are the ultimate source of all mature blood elements. They are characterized by their capacity for self-renewal, and they are capable of sustaining a lifetime of hematopoiesis. If a transplant were performed with a pure population of stem cells, hematopoietic recovery would be slow, because the stem cells need to mature over the course of weeks into fully differentiated blood cells. Once expansion and differentiation begin, the cells are called *progenitors*. Hematopoietic progenitors divide and increase in numbers, but they do not self-renew. Therefore, a transplant composed entirely of progenitors will engraft more rapidly; the rapidity depends on the relative proportion of early versus late progenitors. Early progenitors require more time to differentiate and expand, so engraftment would be slower, whereas late progenitors may need only to go through a few divisions to produce mature cells, and mature cells would appear in the blood much sooner. On the other hand, a transplant composed entirely of committed progenitors will ultimately fail. The lack of self-renewal will result in late marrow failure. Most strategies to accelerate hematopoietic recovery provide for the transfusion of an adequate number of stem cells but are focused primarily on stimulating the late progenitors with hematopoietic growth factors. When hematopoietic growth factors are used to accelerate neutrophil recovery after marrow grafting, the time to first appearance of neutrophils is not usually improved, but once they appear, the rate of increase is faster (232). If the growth factor is stopped, the rate of neutrophil increase returns to baseline. This probably reflects transient stimulation of a relatively limited number of progenitors. One strategy to increase the number of committed progenitors infused is to stimulate the marrow to release large numbers of peripheral blood progenitors either using growth factors or by performing leukapheresis during the recovery from a cycle of chemotherapy when progenitor numbers are known to increase. These progenitors are then used alone or to supplement marrow. After progenitor and stem cell infusion, hematopoietic growth factors are generally administered again. This technique has resulted in a shorter period until neutrophils recover (117,233–236).

Granulocyte and Monocyte Recovery

When donor cells are infused into a patient with a marrow and spleen that are morphologically normal before the transplantation conditioning, careful inspection of the blood demonstrates the appearance of nucleated red blood cells and early myeloid forms within 7 to 10 days after infusion. It has been postulated that these early cells result from the presence in the marrow inoculum of relatively mature progenitors that undergo rapid terminal differentiation (237), rather than from progeny derived from more primitive stem cells. During this initial 2 weeks, the bone marrow is hypocellular, but the spleen may show evidence of colony-like hematopoietic activity reminiscent of the appearance of colony-forming unit–spleen in rodent models of transplantation (238,239).

Approximately 14 to 28 days after transplantation, blood mononuclear cells (some with an atypical lymphocyte morphology) and granulocytes appear. The granulocyte count generally reaches more than $500/\mu L$ within 10 to 21 days after infusion. The earliest recovering granulocytes have normal phagocytic, oxidative burst, and cytolytic capacity (240). Similarly, quantitative monocyte recovery to normal levels is usually complete by 3 to 4 weeks. These early monocytes also demonstrate normal phagocytic function and usually normal antigen-presentation function, although some studies have noted a variable loss of this latter ability in the monocytes derived from patients 3 to 4 months after transplantation (241–243). By contrast, the fixed tissue accessory cell populations, including alveolar macrophages (244) and Langerhans' cells in the skin (245,246), are often functionally impaired after the transplantation conditioning regimen for weeks to months. These cells remain of residual host derivation for months after transplantation but are gradually replaced with cells of donor origin (247,248). It is believed that these new donor-derived cells subsequently function normally.

Erythroid Recovery

Reticulocytes are detected 1 to 2 weeks after the commencement of lymphoid and monocyte engraftment and generally peak at 4 to 6 weeks after grafting. Donor-derived red cells in the early recovery period after transplantation often show fetal-like attributes, including macrocytosis, increased i antigen expression, a fetal program of globin synthesis, and increased fetal hemoglobin levels (249–252). The marrow red-cell precursors may be mildly dysplastic (253). This pattern is reminiscent of that seen with severe stress erythropoiesis, although in the case of marrow transplantation, these characteristics may persist for up to a year after the procedure. Erythropoietin levels are depressed after both autologous and allogeneic marrow transplantation (254,255). Data indicate that the use of recombinant human erythropoietin does not accelerate recovery after autologous transplantation but does accelerate red-cell recovery after allogeneic transplantation (256–258).

In general, ABO incompatibility is not a major problem in selecting a marrow donor and performing transplantation. Marrow stem cells do not express ABO antigens, although they can be detected on committed progenitors (259); consequently, graft failure from ABO incompatibility is not a concern. ABO incompatibility causes three problems: (a) immediate transfusion reactions related to the infusion of large numbers of erythrocytes with the marrow stem cells, (b) late autoimmune hemolytic anemias that develop if residual host derived isohemagglutinin-producing B lymphocytes survive the conditioning regimen, and (c) hemolytic anemia due to the infusion of mature isohemagglutinin-producing donor B lymphocytes with the marrow. Although some authors have found ABO incompatibility to be a risk factor for GVHD (260), that finding is disputed (261).

Erythrocytes of type O donors are not recognized by recipient isohemagglutinins. Thus, marrow containing type O red blood cells can usually be infused directly into an ABO-mismatched patient without difficulty. Recent data suggest, however, that the infusion of the passively transferred antibody may cause enough damage to worsen transplantation outcomes (262). Thus, routine removal of incompatible plasma may be rational. Rarely, a type O donor has high enough titers of isohemagglutinin in the plasma component of the marrow to cause self-limited hemolysis in the recipient. A more common problem occurs when the recipient has isohemagglutinin against the donor (e.g., type A marrow into a type O recipient or type B marrow into a type A recipient). If the marrow is infused directly, without either reduction of the host isohemagglutinin titers or removal of marrow erythrocytes, a major ABO-mismatched transfusion reaction may occur, and the consequences can be devastating. Three techniques allow the infusion of ABO-mismatched marrow. Isohemagglutinin titers should be checked well in advance of transplantation. A technique of primarily historic interest can be used if the recipient's isohemagglutinin titers are low. After the conditioning regimen has started, small amounts of packed red blood cells of donor type can be infused slowly (263,264). This infusion serves to adsorb isohemagglutinins present at the time of transplantation. As long as the conditioning regimen has begun, there appears to be little chance that the infusion will stimulate an anamnestic response. All subsequent transfusions should be of the same blood type as the donor to ensure that any remaining isohemagglutinin that is produced will be adsorbed, and platelet transfusions should be ABO compatible, if possible, to prevent the infusion of additional isohemagglutinins contained in the platelet-rich plasma. For patients who have high isohemagglutinin titers, it is possible to use plasmapheresis to decrease the titer before converting the blood type. Because the antibodies of concern are primarily IgM, two to four whole-plasma-volume plasmaphereses generally reduce the titer to a manageable level, and some investigators have combined plasmapheresis with immunoadsorption of residual erythrocytes (265). Transient hemoglobinuria is common. Most centers avoid the problem by removing the erythrocytes from the marrow before infusion. Dextran or hydroxyethyl starch sedimentation (266,267), or density gradient centrifugation (268,269), removes most of the red blood cells and reduces the risk of an immediate reaction. When red blood cells are removed from the marrow, but no effort is made to reduce the isohemagglutinin titer of the recipient, high titers persist, and there may be slow recovery of erythrocyte production by the marrow because erythroid progenitors may be lysed *in situ*. This intramedullary hemolysis results in delayed reticulocytosis and prolongs the need for red-cell transfusion therapy (267,270). Once the marrow appears to have engrafted by virtue of leukocyte and platelet recovery, a rapid reticulocytosis may result from plasmapheresis (271–273). If more than one HLA-compatible donor is available, donor selection should include consideration of ABO type.

In delayed isohemagglutinin reactions, the B-lymphocytes infused with the marrow stem cells may include isohemagglutinin-producing cells. These cells become a problem primarily when the donor is type O and the recipient is not. With this type of ABO mismatch, mature isohemagglutinin–producing cells are stimulated by exposure to large amounts of ABO substance. They then divide and within 1 to 6 weeks produce enough antibody to generate severe hemolysis (274–276). This severe reaction usually occurs in patients receiving cyclosporine or who received T-cell–depleted marrow; presumably the absence of functional suppressor T lymphocytes allows the reaction to occur unabated. The direct antiglobulin test becomes positive for C3, IgG, and IgM. The hemolysis can be severe enough to be life threatening, and it requires prompt therapy with packed red blood cells that are type O or the ABO type of the donor. Immunosuppression with prednisone plasmapheresis may also be of value. Case reports suggest a curative effect of recombinant human erythropoietin treatment (258). Similar reactions have occurred when large numbers of lymphocytes were passively transferred into an ABO-mismatched recipient of a liver transplant (277). This reaction needs to be distinguished from microangiopathic hemolytic anemia with renal insufficiency, which is not immunologically mediated, and appears to reflect a form of radiation nephritis (75). Although many allogeneic transplants involve donor-recipient pairs that are mismatched for other erythrocyte antigens (e.g., Rh, Kell, Duffy, MN), hemolysis on this basis is rare.

Platelet Recovery

Platelet recovery usually occurs last, after the return to normal levels of most other blood elements except lymphocytes. Although platelet counts of greater than 20,000/μL are often obtained by 3 to 4 weeks, some patients remain transfusion-dependent for months. Isolated thrombocytopenia in the presence of normal myelopoiesis and erythropoiesis after allogeneic transplantation has been described in up to one-third of patients (278). In some patients, this thrombocytopenia is transient; after an initial platelet rise to more than 100,000/μL within the first month after transplantation, the platelet count falls to the less than 10,000 to 45,000/μL range, usually with recovery by the third month after transplantation. This event is often drug-associated (especially trimethoprim-sulfamethoxazole) or virus-associated but has also been reported to occur as an apparent autoimmune phenomenon (279,280). Chronic persistent thrombocytopenia appears to be a more ominous event. It is frequently, although not exclusively, associated with severe acute or chronic GVHD and often portends a poor survival. Some autologous bone marrow transplantation regimens have also been associated with prolonged severe thrombocytopenia, and as outlined earlier, splenomegaly or severe marrow fibrosis may also lead to persistent thrombocytopenia after transplantation.

Functional Bone Marrow Recovery

Full morphologic recovery of normal bone marrow cellularity usually takes from 2 to 3 months after transplantation. In patients receiving transplants for aplastic anemia who demonstrate failure to engraft or graft rejection, increased mast cells have been observed in the bone marrow (281), but the relation of this observation to the engraftment process, if any, remains unknown. Although it would appear logical that the rapidity of bone marrow and blood cell recovery after transplantation should be predictable by quantification of donor marrow colony-forming units (CFUs), experimental results have been in conflict in this regard, with some studies noting a correlation (282–284), whereas others do not (285,286). Measurement of progenitors by a variety of CFU assays in post-HSCT marrows has generally shown slow but steady recovery over several months. Examination of serial plasma samples for hematopoietic growth-promoting activity has demonstrated markedly depressed support for burst forming unit–erythroid and CFU-GEMM (granulocyte, erythroblast, monocyte, megakaryocyte) for prolonged periods of time after transplantation, whereas support for CFU-GM (granulocyte-macrophage) and CFU-Meg (megakaryocyte) is high within the first 30 days after transplantation (287). Clinical studies of AHSCT, and, to a limited extent, A HSCT, using the recombinant growth factors sargramostim (GM-CSF) and filgrastim (G-CSF) after marrow infusion have demonstrated more rapid recovery of counts and reduction in the incidence of infections after transplantation (288,289).

The regeneration of the stromal component of the human marrow microenvironment after transplantation is an important concomitant of normal hematopoiesis. Most experimental data suggest that stromal cells are derived from different progenitors than hematopoietic elements. In patients with leukemia, conflicting data have been reported regarding the involvement of stromal elements in the malignant clone (290–293). Similarly, conflicting data have been presented regarding the posttransplantation donor versus host origin of the stromal elements (294,295). It is likely that these issues will remain unresolved until improved methods of isolating and defining the marrow stroma in humans are developed, but it is generally believed that the marrow stroma remains of host origin after marrow transplantation.

IMMUNOLOGIC RECOVERY

Most clinical problems in marrow transplantation result from disruption of an ordered immune system and the variable establishment of new, donor-derived but host-tolerant lymphopoiesis. These include the failure of new marrow to engraft (GVHD or graft rejection), the attack of new marrow on the host (GVHD), and the failure of adequate immune reconstitution after transplantation, resulting in infectious complications. Although the recovery of myeloid hematopoiesis in uncomplicated transplants is usually complete by the third month after transplantation, the recovery of lymphocyte numbers and function often requires 6 months to 2 years to reach a stable state (296–299). Even more than in the case of myeloid recovery, a myriad of clinical variables affects the reconstitution of the immune system: patient age, GVHD prophylaxis, cryopreservation of donor marrow (with or without chemotherapeutic or antibody purging), and herpesvirus infections, especially CMV (300,301). In addition, study of the recovery of the immune system may be further complicated by the effects of other concomitant clinical events, including frequent blood transfusions

(302). The following broad outline of recovery holds in most cases, however.

Natural Killer Cell Recovery

In the initial 2 months after transplantation, cells of natural killer (NK) and B-lymphocyte surface phenotype are the first to return to normal numbers in the circulation. NK cells, defined by the expression of CD11 or CD56 and the simultaneous absence of CD3 on the membrane, reach normal or supranormal levels usually by the fourth week in syngeneic, autologous, and allogeneic transplants including T-cell–depleted transplants (298,299,303–308). These cells demonstrate normal cytolytic function at the same time they reach normal numbers. They have many of the characteristics of activated killer cells (307,309). Patients with CMV infection may show increased number and cytolytic activity of these cells. The effect of GVHD on the recovery of this population is probably small and is difficult to determine.

B-Lymphocyte Recovery

Cells of B-lymphocyte surface phenotype (CD19$^+$, CD20$^+$, SIg$^+$) likewise reach normal levels early after transplantation in patients undergoing relatively uncomplicated MHC-compatible allogeneic or syngeneic transplants. Recovery of circulating phenotypic B cells may be delayed in some patients with GVHD and in patients receiving MHC-incompatible transplants (310) as well as in some patients receiving autologous grafts for non–Hodgkin's lymphoma, perhaps related to treatment of the marrow with anti–B-cell monoclonal antibodies (311).

The earliest detectable circulating B cells posttransplant not only express normal mature B-cell markers but also express immature B-cell markers (CD1c, CD38, CD5, and CD23) for the first year following transplant. These antigens are normally expressed on a small percentage of circulating B cells in normal adults but highly expressed on cord blood B cells. This observation has led to the hypothesis that B-cell differentiation after transplant is recapitulating normal B-cell outgoing (312). In contrast to the rapid quantitative recovery of circulating B cells in many patients, functional recovery assessed by *in vitro* assays of cellular proliferation and Ig secretion may be extremely slow in both allogeneic and autologous transplant recipients (312–318). The pathogenesis of this dysfunction is probably multifactorial, involving intrinsic B-cell defects as well as T-lymphocyte immunoregulatory defects and the decreased production of relevant cytokines (319,320).

The *in vitro* abnormalities observed are reflected at least in part in *in vivo* dysfunction. For example, although most patients after allogeneic transplantation recover normal serum IgM levels within the first 2 months, some patients (most prominently, although not exclusively, those with chronic GVHD) have clinically significant decreased serum IgG levels (321) that may be associated with recurrent infections and possibly bronchiolitis obliterans (315,322,323). Moreover, it has been suggested that there is also a subgroup of patients whose total serum IgG returns to normal levels but who remain deficient in specific IgG subclasses, usually IgG-2 and IgG-4. These patients appear to be at increased risk for bacterial infections (324,325). Conversely, some patients with acute GVHD develop polyclonal hypergammaglobulinemia (326). Almost three-fourths of patients demonstrate low serum IgA levels for a year or more after transplantation, although the clinical consequences of that immunodeficiency are uncertain. Finally, serum IgE levels are frequently markedly elevated after transplantation (327,328). Although there is a temporal association of this latter phenomenon with acute GVHD, it is also observed in identical-twin transplants, and its pathogenesis remains unknown.

In the first 2 to 3 weeks after transplantation, serum γ-globulin represents residual host-derived antibody, which decreases with a variable half-life dependent on the presence or absence of concomitant infection and complications such as protein-losing enteropathy. Most evidence suggests a conversion to donor-derived antibody by day 100 in most patients (83). Some studies have suggested transfer of donor antigen-specific immunity at the B- and T-cell level to marrow transplant recipients (329,330). However, one study has demonstrated that a minor but substantial amount of serum IgG can still be of recipient origin for up to at least 8 years after transplantation, indicating that host type IgG-producing cells are not necessarily eradicated by a myeloablative approach despite the engraftment of donor B lymphocytes (331).

Finally, the appearance of monoclonal and oligoclonal Ig banding on serum protein electrophoresis appears to be a common phenomenon in the early months after transplantation (332–335). Whether this represents a reflection of normal immune ontogeny or oligoclonal regeneration of the B-cell repertoire or is a consequence of the immune dysregulation after transplantation is unknown, but the M components generally resolve without clinical sequelae.

T-Lymphocyte Recovery

Impaired T-cell mediated immunity is a major cause of significant infectious complications after transplantation leading to high levels of morbidity and mortality. T-lymphocyte reconstitution after transplantation is slowest of all the hematopoietic-derived elements (298,299,311,336–340). Among the T-cell subtypes, the CD3$^+$ CD8$^+$ subset recovers most rapidly in patients undergoing all types of transplantation, often reaching normal levels in the uncomplicated situation by 6 to 10 weeks after grafting. The CD3$^+$ CD4$^+$ subset, in contrast, usually requires 6 months or more to reach normal levels. Patients with GVHD tend to have a more rapid and greater rise in CD3$^+$ CD8$^+$ cells and a markedly slower recovery in CD3$^+$ CD4$^+$ cells. Thus, while most marrow transplant recipients retain an inverted CD3$^+$ CD4$^+$/CD3$^+$ CD8$^+$ ratio for months to perhaps years after transplantation, the severity of that inversion is increased in those patients with GVHD. This abnormality of T-cell–subset distribution is also exacerbated by CMV infection (341,342). It is observed in recipients of autologous as well as allogeneic transplants but generally to a much lesser extent in the autologous transplant recipient (343). Notably, recovery of T-cell numbers is delayed following T-cell–depleted transplants as compared to conventional transplants (298,299). Furthermore, recovery in recipients of unrelated stem cell transplants is even more delayed such that CD3$^+$ cells frequently do not normalize until 18 to 24 months posttransplantation in adult recipients.

As in the case of B lymphocytes, functional recovery of T cells after transplantation is even slower than phenotypic recovery. Simple *in vitro* measures of T-cell function, such as their ability to proliferate in response to stimulation by lectins, mitogens, or anti-CD3 antibody, their ability to perform a cytolytic effector function, and their ability to secrete cytokines, remain markedly depressed for up to a year or more after transplantation (298,299,344). The only exception to this is seen with the temporary transfer of mature T lymphocytes detectable in the recipients of G-CSF mobilized peripheral blood stem cells (331,345). Similarly, *in vivo* tests of cellular immunity, such as skin testing either to neoantigens or recall antigens, remains markedly impaired for years in many patients (346). Even when bulk *in vitro* assays of T-lymphocyte function normalize, limiting dilution culture methods continue to reveal abnormal T-cell proliferative function as well as diminished cytokine secretion and cytolytic function (347). Again, GVHD affects the rate of recovery of normal T-cell immunity (321), probably as a result of the GVHD as well as the treatment regimens employed. There is no clear difference in T-cell recovery observed between patients who receive cyclosporine and those who receive methotrexate for transplantation immunoprophylaxis (348). Patients with chronic GVHD remain the most immunosuppressed for the longest periods in virtually all studies. T-cell depletion of donor marrow (to prevent GVHD; discussed in the section Prophylaxis) exacerbates the cellular immune defect for at least the first 6 months after transplantation (349).

The pathogenesis of these cellular immunologic lesions is probably multifactorial. In addition to defects in signal transduction mechanisms necessary for the activation of the T cell, defects in interleukin (IL)-2 (350,351) and IFN-γ (352) production have been noted, although the latter observation is disputed (353). Active suppression by nonspecific suppressor cells, especially in patients with chronic GVHD, has been delineated (296,354,355), as has an inhibitory influence of prostaglandin E2 (309). The fact that these defects persist at the single-cell level (347), however, confirms that the defects observed are not solely the result of dysregulation but must also represent intrinsic abnormalities of the T cell. As in the case of B-lymphocyte recovery after transplantation, several phenotypically unusual T-cell subsets have been defined, including cells of CD3+, CD4−, CD8−, CD3+, and CD5− subtypes (306,356).

The observation that the rate of recovery of immune function after transplantation correlates with the age of the recipient suggests that recovery of immune reactivity depends on thymic activity, which may have atrophied in the older patient. Thymic activity can be assayed by the appearance of CD4+CD45 RA+RO− naïve T cells, restoration of T-cell receptor repertoire and quantification of T-cell receptor rearrangement excision circles. Each of these assays has indicated that young patients reconstitute rapidly, whereas in older patients, the recovery of thymic dependent function can take several months to years (357–359). Additionally, low T-cell receptor rearrangement excision circle levels correlate significantly with development of opportunistic infections and, thus, with morbidity and mortality after transplantation (359). Notably, infusions of donor-derived nature CD4+ T cells can result in restoration of thymic function (358). Whether more rapid recovery of T-cell function achieved by CD4+ T-cell infusions in the adult population will decrease posttransplantation opportunistic infections remains to be seen.

Infections after Marrow Transplantation: Clinical Correlates of Immune Reconstitution

The major infectious risk periods after transplantation are predictable from the pattern of immune reconstitution. Before engraftment, the major risk is from bacterial and fungal infection due to profound granulocytopenia and damage to the integument secondary to both preparatory chemoradiation therapy and GVHD prophylaxis with agents such as methotrexate. As for all granulocytopenic patients, most of these infections result from endogenously carried organisms that seed the bloodstream from gastrointestinal tract or skin. In addition, because these patients virtually always have one or more surgically implanted intravenous lines, *Staphylococcus epidermidis* and *Staphylococcus aureus* and *Candida* spp. should be considered early in the differential diagnosis of fever.

During the later part of this period and extending into the immediate posttransplantation period, viral infections become common. Herpes simplex reactivation generally occurs earliest.

Although oral lesions are common, profound mucositis can sometimes obscure the classic vesicular eruption. A number of studies have documented the value of routine acyclovir prophylaxis in recipients of allogeneic marrow transplants (360–364) in delaying or preventing reactivation of herpes simplex and, in some cases, accelerating engraftment in patients receiving methotrexate GVHD prophylaxis. Furthermore, evidence suggests that prophylactic acyclovir may also help prevent or delay reactivation of herpes zoster (365); its effect on CMV infection (discussed later in this section) is less clear, but it does not appear to be useful (366–368).

During this period, other virus can cause serious infections. These viruses include human herpes virus-6, implicated as a cause of marrow failure syndromes, encephalitis and pneumonitis (369,370); the papova virus BK implicated as a cause of hemorrhagic cystitis (172,371,372); adenovirus associated with the development of cystitis, diarrhea, pneumonitis, and hepatitis (373–375); and the respiratory viruses, respiratory syncytial virus, influenza, and parainfluenza (376,377). Although approaches to prophylaxis and treatment of each of these viruses has been identified (364,376–382), these viruses can cause severe and often lethal infections up to 4 to 6 months posttransplantation. A set of recommendations for infection precautions after transplantation can be found at the Centers for Disease Control and Prevention Web site (http://www.cdc.gov/mmwr/preview/mmwrhtml/rr4910a1.htm).

After engraftment, bacterial infections due to endogenous organisms are infrequent. If patients are hypogammaglobulinemic, however, particularly in the setting of chronic GVHD, they are susceptible to infections with encapsulated organisms such as *Haemophilus influenzae* and *Streptococcus pneumoniae*. Moreover, herpes zoster reactivation may occur, CMV infection is common, and, in the absence of prophylactic therapy, *Pneumocystis carinii* infections are observed. The latter is generally avoided with prophylactic trimethoprim-sulfamethoxazole (383–385). Recent experience with aerosolized pentamidine, dapsone, and atovaquone (383) suggests that transplant recipients who cannot tolerate trimethoprim-sulfamethoxazole may be able to receive *Pneumocystis* prophylaxis, although the alternatives may not be as effective (384). Varicella-zoster infections occur in at least one-half of transplant recipients at risk for reactivation of this pathogen within the first year (365,386,387). Of these three pathogens, however, CMV infection is the most common cause of serious morbidity and mortality after marrow grafting, occurring in approximately 15% to 20% of all allogeneic marrow transplant recipients. Indeed, CMV is the most common infectious cause of death in these patients (385,388–392).

In patients who are seropositive for CMV at the time of transplantation, infection is most often the result of reactivation of latent virus (69). In patients who are seronegative, the disease is acquired either from donor marrow or from blood products. Although many CMV infections are asymptomatic, some patients develop fever, leukopenia, hepatitis, enteritis, esophagitis, retinitis, or pneumonia. Pneumonia is the most ominous clinical syndrome developing in CMV-infected patients; approximately one-third of patients with CMV infection progress to pneumonia on the average of 60 or more days after transplantation, and mortality in that group is historically estimated at 85% or more. This represents the incidence of CMV pneumonia in allogeneic transplantation. In syngeneic and autologous transplants, the overall incidence of serious CMV disease is far less (393). In fact, in a survey of 100 recipients of syngeneic marrow, no patient developed CMV pneumonia, although the rate of infection remained high. Thus, GVHD, even when subclinical, appears to lead to a high risk of progression of CMV infection to lethal pneumonias (394). Other risk factors for the development of fatal CMV infection include older age, receipt of granulocyte transfusions, TBI, and perhaps increased transplant immunosuppression (367,389,395). Some reports suggest that immune donors may protect seronegative recipients, but these data require confirmation (396).

Prophylaxis against CMV pneumonia is obviously crucial in the management of allogeneic transplant recipients. Because seronegative transplant recipients who have seronegative bone marrow donors contract the disease only through administration of CMV-positive blood products, administration of only CMV-negative blood to these patients markedly reduces the incidence of this complication. Because CMV is transmitted with the leukocytes, filtered or deglycerolized packed red blood cells and filtered platelets may reduce the risk of infection if CMV-seronegative blood products are not available (397). This observation has been confirmed in a randomized study of filtered leukocyte reduced versus CMV seronegative blood products (398). Granulocyte transfusions are strongly associated with CMV infection (397). Administration of either commercial γ-globulin or CMV Ig has not resulted in consistent reductions in CMV diseases or other infections after marrow transplantation (367,399,400).

For patients who are seropositive, neither the use of seronegative blood products nor the use of routine posttransplantation intravenous γ-globulin decreased the risk of CMV infection (401). The most significant advance in the reduction of morbidity and mortality from CMV disease was the introduction of prophylactic ganciclovir. Several different regimens have been shown to be effective, but regimens that are associated with ganciclovir-induced neutropenia may be complicated by bacterial infections (402–405). One caveat in the use of prophylactic ganciclovir is that when CMV infection does occur, it may manifest as declining granulocyte count, often with abnormal liver function tests and fever. There is a tendency to attribute this syndrome to ganciclovir and stop administering the drug, when it may actually reflect CMV infection, requiring an increase in ganciclovir to full therapeutic dose. For patients who are intolerant to ganciclovir, foscarnet is a reasonable alternative agent (406–409). An alternative approach is to monitor CMV by hybrid capture assay or polymerase chain reaction (PCR) and only administer prophylaxis if there is evidence of active disease. This technique does require very frequent testing but allows a cohort of patients to avoid therapy (406,410,411). Late CMV infections are increasingly recognized and plans for long-term monitoring must be considered (412).

CMV pneumonia occurs at a similar time after transplantation as idiopathic interstitial pneumonia. The distinction is important, because ganciclovir and foscarnet are useful in treating the infection. Open lung biopsy has been the primary diagnostic procedure used to establish the cause of diffuse interstitial pulmonary infiltrates. The morbidity of this procedure is substantial and has been largely supplanted by video-assisted thoracoscopic surgery. We can detect CMV in the blood using PCR, antigenemia testing, or hybrid capture technology (71,392,395,402,403,413). These assays may be used to assess the risk of CMV reactivation, provide quantitative estimates of CMV load, and may in some patients preclude the need for biopsies. Once CMV pneumonia develops, it is generally treated with ganciclovir and intravenous Ig (112,414). For patients who do not respond to ganciclovir, foscarnet appears to be an effective alternative (392,409,415). Cidofovir can be used successfully, but there is a significant risk of irreversible renal failure.

Administration of donor-derived, *in vitro* selected and expanded, CMV specific T-cell clones has recently been introduced for the prophylaxis and treatment of CMV infection (416,417). *In vivo* infusions of expanded T cells have induced detectable levels of T cells with CMV-specific cytotoxicity in the blood of transfused patients, but the approach is labor intensive and not widely applicable.

Assessment of Engraftment

Proof of donor engraftment requires the ability to determine the origin of the various elements of the marrow and immune system and depends on the ability to identify the cells of interest, isolate them in pure form, and probe them for differences that were identified between the recipient and donor at the time of transplantation evaluation. Methods used to differentiate host and donor include erythrocyte antigen testing (81,418,419), HLA typing, leukocyte isoenzymes (82,419), Ig isotype analysis (83), Barr's body analysis and karyotyping, DNA sequence polymorphism or RFLP analysis (81,84,85), and in sex-mismatched cases, detection of X and Y chromosomes, using fluorescence *in situ* hybridization techniques (FISH) (420,421). Karyotyping and FISH are the most commonly available techniques. Less than one-half of all HSCTs are between patients of different sexes, however, and special karyotypic differences, such as the presence of satellites and variability of quinacrine banding, are useful only in experienced centers. Furthermore, karyotype analysis is only applicable to cells that are dividing or can be made to divide. Erythrocyte antigen testing and Ig isotype analysis take advantage of the polymorphic nature of red cell surface proteins and Ig isotypes, respectively. Because erythrocyte transfusions and γ-globulin infusions are often administered in the course of marrow transplantation, these techniques are primarily useful in the late stages of marrow grafting when residual transfused blood products are no longer present. Patients who undergo HLA-identical allogeneic marrow grafting do not have HLA differences between host and donor because histocompatibility is one of the primary criteria for the selection of donors. Therefore, the extreme polymorphism of the HLA locus can be exploited only in HLA-mismatched patients. In practice, several of these techniques are used simultaneously, but RFLP and FISH analyses are the most useful tests for evaluating nucleated cells.

Successful transplantation does not require full donor cell engraftment in all cases. However, when engraftment is complete the patient is said to be *chimeric*; that is, the patient has a mixture of recipient tissues (liver, muscle) and donor tissues (blood, lymphoid cells). If all the transplanted elements are derived from the donor, the chimerism is complete; if there are both host and donor elements discernible in the marrow or blood, the patient is said to be a mixed or incomplete chimera. In patients with SCIDS, the establishment of mixed lymphohematopoietic chimerism is expected. It is likely that when marrow transplantation is used to treat inherited disorders of metabolism, such as Gaucher's disease, stable mixed chimerism would also be acceptable; if the transplanted macrophages could dispose of the excessive glucocerebroside that characterizes Gaucher's disease, there would be no need to transplant granulocytes, erythrocytes, and so forth (421). Furthermore, the reestablishment of normal hematopoiesis in patients with aplastic anemia can occasionally be observed to be due to recovery of predominantly host hematopoiesis, an observation that contributed to the suggestion that many cases of aplastic anemia are immunologically mediated. Because the chemotherapeutic conditioning regimens commonly used for aplastic anemia are not likely to be irreversibly toxic to stem cells, many aplastic patients do exhibit some degree of mixed chimerism.

The importance of establishing the degree of chimerism is most apparent in patients receiving transplants for leukemia and in the interpretation of the incidence of GVHD. The presence of residual host elements in the blood or marrow of a patient with leukemia generally indicates that the malignancy will relapse, although the predictive value of this type of analysis has not been established (81,422–424). In the evaluation of experimental therapies to prevent GVHD, it is also important to establish the presence of mixed chimerism. The prevention of GVHD *per se* may increase the rate of mixed chimerism because GVHD is probably an important mechanism for immunosuppression after marrow grafting (425). Because mixed chimerism may be associated with a lower risk of GVHD (426,427), its presence is an important variable in the analysis of GVHD prophylaxis trials (421). In addition, relapse of leukemia has been occasionally observed in donor rather than recipient cells (209,210,428). The origin of the leukemic cells has implications for choice of additional treatment.

GRAFT FAILURE AND GRAFT REJECTION

The distinction between graft failure and graft rejection is important, as it dramatically affects the clinical care of a patient suffering from graft failure. *Graft failure* is empirically defined as the failure to recover hematopoiesis at any time after transplantation or development of pancytopenia and marrow aplasia after initial engraftment or autologous recovery of patient-derived cells with our without the development of pancytopenia. Graft rejection is usually characterized by failure to achieve an initial engraftment and is documented by the absence of donor-derived lymphoid and hematopoietic cells in the marrow or blood. Graft rejection usually implies the recognition and suppression or destruction of donor hematopoietic stem cells by the recipient's T cells or NK cells and that the defect can be overcome by further suppression of host immunity. To prevent graft rejection, transplantation regimens must include agents that are sufficiently immunosuppressive to eradicate host resistance. *Graft failure* is a more general term that is applied when the reason for poor hematopoietic reconstitution is not clear, but an immunologic etiology cannot be invoked. Usually, assessment reveals the presence of donor-derived hematopoietic cells rather than host-derived hematopoietic cells. Factors contributing to graft failure include an insufficient dose of viable stem cell as is seen following infusions of purged autologous marrow or low-dose allogeneic CBUs (60–63,220,221), a microenvironment abnormality that has been implicated in patients with myelofibrosis or osteopetrosis (429–431) and some patients with aplastic anemia (1,238,239,295) or suppression by antimicrobials, such as ganciclovir (432), or viral agents, such as CMV (226). Transplantation procedures that are complicated by graft failure rather than graft rejection may not be improved by increasing the degree of host immunosuppression. This distinction is particularly important when the donor marrow is manipulated—for instance, treated with monoclonal antibodies or pharmacologic agents. If the lack of hematopoietic recovery is due to iatrogenic stem cell injury, increasing immunosuppression only increases the morbidity of the procedure. If the problem is that the T-cell depletion has abrogated a necessary degree of GVHR, then increased immunosuppression is warranted. In practice, the distinction is rarely clear.

Before the introduction of T-cell depletion for the prevention of GVHD (see Prophylaxis), graft rejection in recipients of HLA-identical marrow was almost exclusively limited to recipients of transplants for aplastic anemia with a history of multiple blood transfusions (433–438). Without cytoreduction, 50% of recipients of HLA identical twin grafts will reject their grafts (434), and this graft failure rate can be abrogated with cyclophosphamide (433). The incidence of graft failure ranges from 10% to 30% for patients with aplastic anemia prepared with cyclophosphamide alone and infused with HLA-identical sibling marrow, depending on the

patient's transfusion history (438). Consistent engraftment can be achieved, however, with additional immunosuppression with either total lymphoid irradiation or ATG (123,439–442). Among patients with leukemia who receive TBI and cyclophosphamide, the incidence of graft failure following a non–T-cell depleted BMT is less than 1% for recipients of HLA-matched marrow and 5% for recipients of HLA-nonidentical family member marrow (32). In contrast, for recipients of standard conditioning regimens, graft failure occurs after every method of T-cell depletion, with the incidence ranging from 10% to 30% among recipients of HLA-identical marrow to as high as 50% to 75% among recipients of HLA-nonidentical marrow (443–452). In this setting, graft rejection seems to be related to the persistence of residual host T cells that survive the conditioning regimen (422,425). Donor T cells included in the marrow infusion may provide a further increment of immunosuppression by inhibiting or destroying these residual host elements. This can be considered a form of GVHR. If T cells are not present, recipient T cells that recognize donor antigens on stem cells may prevent the establishment of a functioning graft. The Seattle group provided indirect evidence for the importance of an early GVHR (437). Buffy coat cells (which are predominantly T cells) administered after transplantation reduce the rejection rate substantially (453), presumably by inhibiting or killing the residual host T cells; although the stimulation of hematopoiesis by T-cell–derived growth factors cannot be excluded, nor can the addition of peripheral blood stem cells.

Several investigators have demonstrated the expansion of recipient-derived CD3$^+$, CD8$^+$, and CD56$^-$ T cells, which are capable of cytotoxicity against donor cells and inhibiting donor marrow growth *in vitro* (425,454,455). Following HLA-disparate T-cell–depleted grafts, cytotoxic, CD3$^+$, and CD8$^+$ host T cells exhibiting specificity for single class I HLA alleles unique to the donor have been detected (454,455).

With the understanding of the processes contributing to graft rejection and graft failure, several strategies have evolved to prevent these complications. These include development of tolerable yet more immunosuppressive regimens with high-dose arabinosylcytosine (444), thiotepa (456,457), or fludarabine (458) and treatment of the patient with T-cell–targeted antibodies such as OKT3, CAMPATH 1, or ATG. Additionally, several groups are exploring the use of G-CSF–stimulated unmodified or T-cell–depleted PBSCs as a source of large number of CD34$^+$ stem cells to be infused to overcome graft resistance (459). Studies in murine models of transplantation indicate that such a strategy might be successful (460).

GRAFT-VERSUS-HOST DISEASE

In solid organ transplantation, the major immunologic obstacle to a successful procedure is graft rejection, that is, a failure of the host immune system to develop tolerance for the transplanted organ (GVHD). In allogeneic marrow transplantation, however, the conditioning regimens effectively eliminate the host immune system. Therefore, the major immunologic impediment is the establishment of tolerance of the donor marrow for the host. The failure to induce such tolerance leads to GVHD. As noted earlier, the GVHD reaction was first reported in experimental animals—described as secondary disease or runting—in the late 1950s and subsequently recognized as a clinical syndrome in humans (1,11). Billingham (12) succinctly described the essential elements of GVHD:

1. The graft must contain immunologically competent cells.
2. The host must possess important transplantation isoantigens that are lacking in the graft donor, so that the host

appears foreign to it, and is, therefore, capable of stimulating it antigenically.

3. The host itself must be incapable of mounting an effective immunologic reaction against the graft, at least for sufficient time for the latter to manifest its immunologic capabilities, that is, it must have security of tenure.

Two points are clear from this description. First, only patients receiving allogeneic (either MHC-matched or mismatched) grafts should be capable of developing GVHD. Second, occasional experiments of nature can also result in GVHD. Thus, children born with severe congenital immunodeficiency can have transplacental passage of maternal lymphocytes, which may result in clinical GVHD in the untransfused newborn. Such a syndrome was first described in the mid-1960s, with demonstration of maternal lymphocytes in the child in at least one case (461,462). Interestingly, there is some evidence that persistent transplacental microchimerism is associated with scleroderma although without prior clinical GVHD (463,464).

Two syndromes can be delineated: acute and chronic GVHD. For the sake of definition in clinical trials, 100 days after transplantation is often taken as an arbitrary dividing line between acute GVHD and chronic GVHD. The clinical syndrome of chronic GVHD, however, as described below, can commence before such an arbitrary cut-off, and some patients may demonstrate aspects of both syndromes simultaneously.

Acute Graft-Versus-Host Disease

DESCRIPTION AND DIAGNOSIS

Acute GVHD usually begins within the first 4 weeks after transplantation but can occur any time within the first 4 months. It is characterized by a clinicopathologic syndrome involving the skin, liver, and gastrointestinal tract. A maculopapular, erythematous exanthem appears, frequently involving palms and soles. In its mildest manifestation, it may involve less than one-fourth of the body surface, but in its severest form, it can progress to whole-body erythema, gross bullae formation, and sloughing of skin. The loss of the integument leads to a markedly increased risk of infection, especially with normal skin flora such as *S. aureus* and *S. epidermidis*. Liver function abnormalities of both inflammatory and obstructive chemistries are seen. Again, mild cases may demonstrate only a three- to four-fold rise in the alanine aminotransferase and aspartate amino-

transferase, whereas the most severely affected patients have serum bilirubin levels higher than 10 mg/dL and loss of liver synthetic function. Involvement of the gut is manifest by anorexia, crampy pain, and watery, secretory diarrhea, which can progress to bloody diarrhea and frank ileus. In severe cases, a major protein-losing enteropathy results, with hypoalbuminemia. This problem may be exacerbated by severe hepatic dysfunction. The combination of major insensible fluid losses through a damaged integument, decreased hepatic synthetic function, and massive diarrhea make frequent evaluation of blood, urine, and stool electrolytes and careful input and output measurements a necessity.

Often, all three organ systems are involved to approximately the same severity. Isolated intestinal disease may be common. Gastric GVHD is a frequent cause of otherwise unexplained nausea and vomiting after transplantation (465,466). Routine endoscopic evaluation of patients with otherwise inapparent clinical GVHD has demonstrated pathologic evidence of intestinal GVHD in approximately 13% of patients (465). Gastroscopy and biopsy can confirm this diagnosis and distinguish it from candidiasis, herpes simplex virus, CMV, or peptic gastritis. Isolated skin involvement is relatively easy to assess with a skin biopsy, although there are significant questions about the specificity of lesion seen on skin biopsy (467–469). The liver is much more difficult to assess, because thrombocytopenia usually precludes liver biopsy. A transjugular approach can be quite helpful. Because the liver is subject to many potential toxins and infections, the diagnosis of isolated hepatic GVHD must be made cautiously. Clinical staging is usually carried out using a modification of the Seattle criteria (470), as outlined in Table 60-3. As described in detail later, clinical grade correlates with overall survival. Patients who die from acute GVHD generally do so from concomitant infection, pneumonitis, or, more rarely, overwhelming hepatic failure.

The histology of acute GVHD in the involved organs generally involves evidence of single cell death accompanied by cellular atypia, edema, and a sparse lymphocytic infiltrate. In the skin, this is manifested by epidermal and basal cell vacuolar degeneration, disorganization of epidermal cell maturation, eosinophilic body formation, and melanocyte incontinence (467–469,471). In the liver, bile duct atypia, cellular degeneration, and cholestasis are seen (472,473); in the gut, the colon is more frequently involved than the ileum and shows histologic evidence of crypt cell necrosis and dropout and flattening of the villous architecture (Fig. 60-7) (474). The dermatopathologic changes of mild

TABLE 60-3. Staging and Grading of Acute Graft-Versus-Host Disease

	Extent of Organ Involvement		
	Skin	**Liver**	**Gut**
Stage			
1	Rash on <25% of skin	Bilirubin, 2–3 mg/dL	Diarrhea, 500–1000 mL/d or persistent nausea
2	Rash on 25–50% of skin	Bilirubin, 3–6 mg/dL	Diarrhea, 1000–1500 mL/d
3	Rash on >50% of skin	Bilirubin, 6–15 mg/dL	Diarrhea, 1500–2000 mL/d
4	Generalized erythroderma with bulla formation	Bilirubin >15 mg/dL	Severe abdominal pain with or without ileus or >2 L of stool daily
Grade			
I	Stage 1–2	None	None
II	Stage 3 or	Stage 1 or	Stage 1
III	—	Stage 2–3 or	Stage 2–4
IV	Stage 4 or	Stage 4	—

Adapted from Przepiorka D, Weisdorf D, Martin P, et al. 1994 Consensus Conference on Acute GVHD Grading. *Bone Marrow Transplant* 1995;15:825.

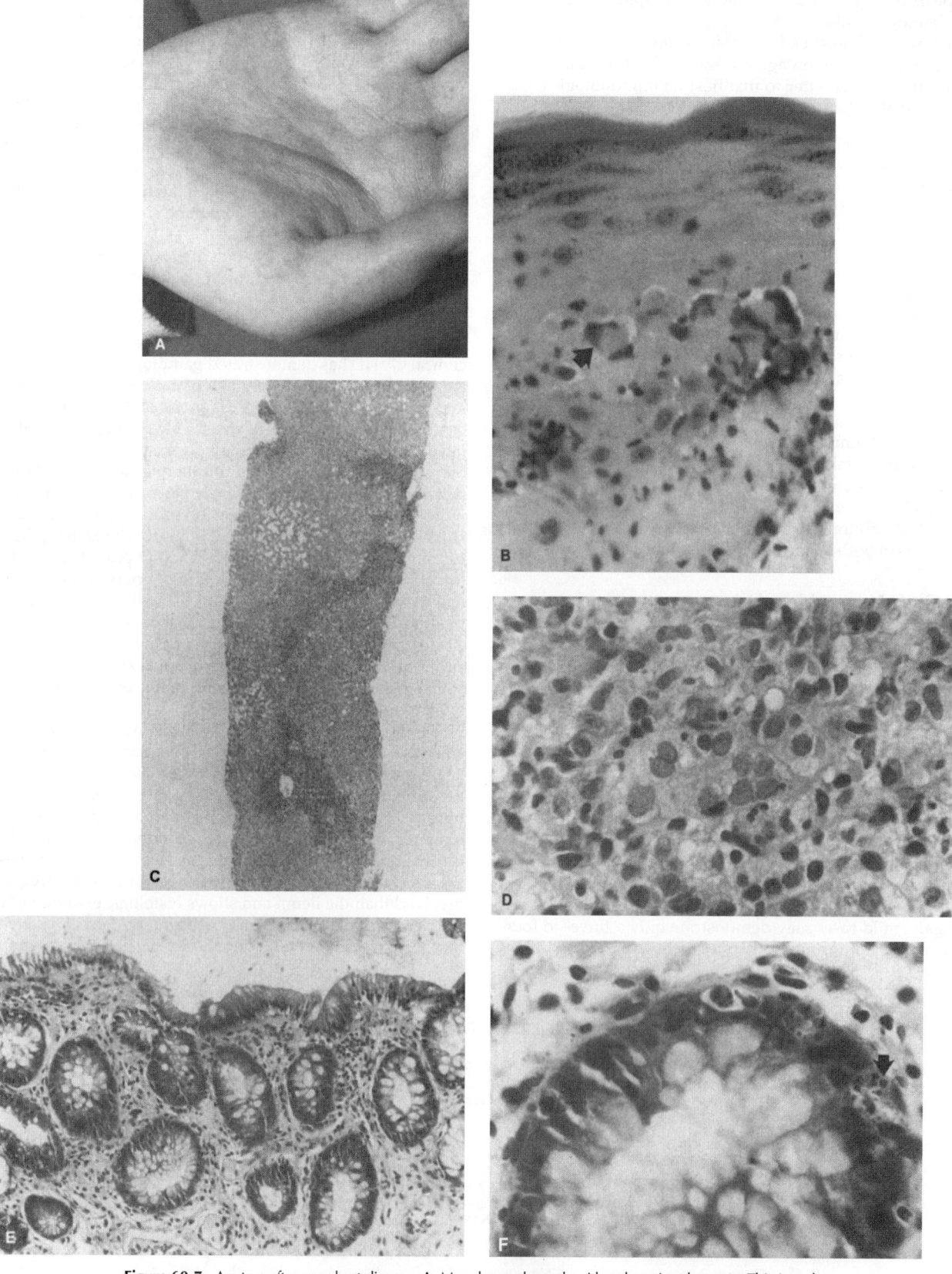

Figure 60-7. Acute graft-versus-host disease. **A:** Maculopapular rash with palmar involvement. This is a characteristic appearance of acute cutaneous graft-versus-host disease and is easily confused with drug eruptions. **B:** Skin biopsy demonstrates disorganization of epidermal cell maturation, epidermal basal cell vacuolar degeneration, and eosinophilic bodies (*arrow*), which represent dead epidermal cells. There is a mild mononuclear cell infiltrate (×400). Liver biopsy specimens show portal triaditis (**C;** ×25) and bile duct degeneration with mononuclear cell infiltrate (**D;** ×400). **E:** Colonic mucosal biopsy shows epithelial atrophy (×200). **F:** High-power view of the same colonic biopsy demonstrates necrosis of epidermal cells (*arrow;* ×400). (See Color Fig. 60-7.) (Courtesy of Dr. James Crawford, Pathology Department, Brigham and Women's Hospital, Boston.)

acute GVHD can be indistinguishable from the cytotoxic effect of conditioning regimens or drug eruptions (467–469). Radiologic examination of the gut usually demonstrates nonspecific changes that are consistent with the histology of the reaction.

The differential diagnosis of acute GVHD can be extensive and difficult. Skin rashes after transplantation are often due to drug eruptions. These include delayed reactions to conditioning regimen agents; reactions to antibiotics; allergic reactions to topical agents; and manifestations of transfusion reactions. Gastrointestinal dysfunction is expected after TBI. Viral infection, especially CMV and herpes, parasitic infection, pseudomembranous colitis, stress gastritis, and drug reactions can all mimic GVHD of the gut. The potential causes of liver dysfunction include hyperalimentation, venoocclusive disease, viral hepatitis, and drug-induced hepatitis (including cyclosporine, methotrexate, and estrogens that may be administered to prevent breakthrough vaginal bleeding). It is important, therefore, to recognize that acute GVHD is most often a clinical diagnosis. The changes of mild to moderate acute GVHD, especially in skin in the first month after transplantation, are mimicked by the effects of the cytotoxic chemotherapy and radiation therapy conditioning regimens and drug therapy (475). Moreover, even the signs of more severe acute GVHD, such as a significant epidermal mononuclear cell infiltrate, can be modified by procedures such as T-cell depletion of donor marrow (476). GVHD lesions in other organs, particularly the gut, can also be imitated by infectious processes, such as CMV and other herpesviruses, although classic viral inclusions are not seen in GVHD (477,478). This is not to denigrate the value of biopsy examination, because it often is helpful in distinguishing this diagnosis from those clinical syndromes that may mimic GVHD, such as venoocclusive disease of the liver (479). Finally, it may be impossible to discriminate between these lesions because there is a high association of GVHD with herpesvirus infection (CMV, herpes simplex, and possibly EBV) (480–482) as well as an association between the development of GVHD and venoocclusive disease of the liver.

Whether GVHD can actually affect organs other than the classic triad remains an incompletely resolved issue. The other most likely candidate is the lung. Pneumonitis may occur in 20% to 60% of allogeneic transplant recipients but in many fewer autologous transplant recipients. Causes include CMV infection; other viral infections, such as adenovirus, herpesvirus, and parainfluenza; bacterial, fungal, or protozoan infection; and treatment–induced injury due to radiation, conditioning chemotherapy, or methotrexate. The incidence, severity, and mortality of pneumonia increase with the severity of GVHD, but this association does not necessarily imply that the GVHD, as opposed to the concomitant immunosuppression and treatment, is causative. A particular histopathologic syndrome of lymphocytic bronchitis has been attributed directly to GVHD (483), although this has not been universally accepted. In addition, other chronic post-HSCT pulmonary syndromes, especially bronchiolitis obliterans, may represent a manifestation of chronic GVHD (discussed later).

Similarly, although renal and urinary tract symptoms occur after transplantation, they are attributable to either conditioning regimen–related or infection–related complications, with no supportive evidence for a role of GVHD (484). Neurologic complications are likewise not infrequent (188,190,485) but cannot be ascribed to GVHD.

PATHOPHYSIOLOGY

In animal models of marrow transplantation, the initiation of the acute GVHR is dependent on the presence of mature T lymphocytes in the marrow inoculum as a necessary (but not sufficient) condition (486,487). The severity of the reaction is further dependent on two major factors: the number of T cells in the inoculum and the number and type of major and minor histocompatibility antigen disparities between donor and recipient. Recently, with the advent of peripheral blood stem cell transplantation, it has become clear that above a certain threshold of T cells, additional T cells only marginally increase the risk of acute GVHD. However, there does seem to be an enhancement of chronic GVHD (118,488). Donor and recipient differences at either the MHC class I or class II antigen loci can lead to fatal GVHD (489). In GVHD initiated by minor histocompatibility differences, the number and relative strength of those differences is important (40,490,491). During the GVHD reaction, cytolytic T lymphocytes directed against host cells can be readily identified (492), although it is possible that other cell types, such as NK cells, may also participate in the effector phase of the GVHD response (493,494). There is little evidence for this phenomenon in humans. The particular subtype of T lymphocyte responsible for initiating the reaction remains somewhat controversial and unresolved in humans. In full H-2 mismatched murine models, where donor and host differ at both MHC class I and class II loci, the CD4+ lymphocyte subset is the predominant (but not exclusive) effector (495,496). The same T-cell subset is the effector in MHC class II–mismatched, class I–identical transplant combinations, whereas the CD8+ lymphocyte subset may control the initiation of GVHD in class I–mismatched transplants. In the case of minor histocompatibility antigen differences, the CD8+ T-cell subset is primarily responsible for GVHD (497).

Acute GVHD results from a complex interaction of donor T cells and recipient organs that involves recognition of minor histocompatibility antigens in an inflammatory milieu. Tissue damage from conditioning regimens, infections, and the underlying illness may provide a milieu that fosters T-cell recognition of susceptible tissues (498,499). Clinical injury is thought to derive from direct T-cell injury through perforin/granzyme (500,501), Fas/FasL interactions (502–504), and the effects of inflammatory cytokines (498,505). The primary role of T lymphocytes in initiating GVHD in humans has been confirmed in experimental clinical trials in which these cells were depleted from donor marrow ex vivo (discussed later). Data are accumulating that mechanisms other than direct T-cell–mediated tissue damage are important in the pathogenesis of GVHD. One poorly explained feature of GVHD is the relative limitation of manifestations to the skin, gut, liver, and perhaps lung. These organs share an exposure to bacteria, particularly gram-negative rods. Animals raised in germ-free environments do not develop GVHD after marrow grafting, but fatal GVHD supervenes when they are recontaminated (506). Furthermore, other observations link GVHD and the consequences of infection. For instance, GVHD tends to flare with a variety of infections, and laminar airflow rooms and gut decontamination reduce acute GVHD in transplants performed for aplastic anemia (498,507,508). One explanation for these associations is that the donor's T cells are placed in an environment that expresses signals that communicate injury to the immune system. The recipient has been injured with chemoradiotherapy, and there may be circulating endotoxin related to gut mucositis. It is likely that cytokines produced by exposure to bacterial products such as endotoxin result in increased inflammation, increased expression of HLA antigens on cell surfaces, increased nitric oxide production, and the production of additional cytokines, such as IL-1, tumor necrosis factor-α, and IFN-γ, in a disordered fashion. The expression of adhesion molecules, cytokines and their receptors, and other inflammatory mediators then fuel the fire, recruiting more donor mononuclear cells into the attack (Fig. 60-8) (499,505).

RISK FACTORS AND PROGNOSIS

The greatest risk factor for the development of GVHD in humans is the MHC compatibility of the donor and recipient. Transplants

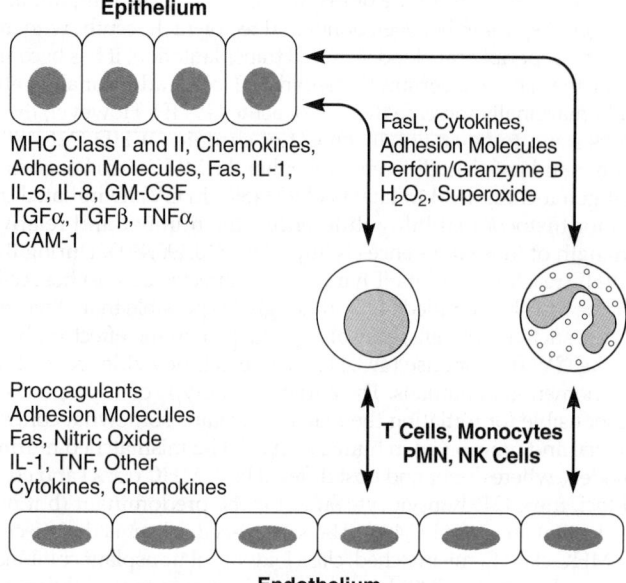

Figure 60-8. Acute graft-versus-host disease can be conceived as the donor's mature lymphocytes misinterpreting the donor as being heavily infected. The T cells then attack this presumed infection directly, as well as recruiting other effectors, such as neutrophils and monocytes. Endotoxin released from the gut, from infection, or from other injuries may accelerate this process. GM-CSF, granulocyte-macrophage colony-stimulating factor; ICAM, intercellular adhesion molecule-1; IL, interleukin; MHC, major histocompatibility complex; NK, natural killer; PMN, polymorphonuclear neutrophil; TGF, transforming growth factor; TNF, tumor necrosis factor.

using methotrexate or cyclosporine as GVHD prophylaxis, undertaken between related patients who differ at more than a single MHC locus, result in a near 100% incidence of GVHD, with most patients developing severe (grade III or IV) disease (509,510). This observation has resulted in most allogeneic transplantation in the past 20 years that were carried out in patients who had a family member donor identical at all phenotypically measurable MHC loci or, at most, who differed at a single locus. Even in related, MHC-matched transplants, the incidence of acute GVHD is 25% to 70%. The mortality rate from the disorder varies with severity. Because there may be some beneficial effect of GVHD in patients with malignant disorders, the association of GVHD with morbidity and mortality is probably best observed in patients with transplants for aplastic anemia (511,512).

Although a final consensus has not been reached, additional risk factors for the development of acute GVHD include older age of recipient, older age of donor, prior donor transfusions, disease stage, conditioning regimen, and gender mismatching of donor and recipient (88,89,513–516). Gender mismatching appears to have its greatest effect when parous females donate to males. There may be a hierarchy with female donors and male recipients at worst risk, followed by female donors and female recipients, then male donors and female recipients, and finally male donors and male recipients. This is most likely related to the presence of unique male antigens that can be recognized by female cells (490,491). Postulated and somewhat controversial risk factors include certain HLA types (514,517), presence or absence of splenectomy (89,518), and ABO mismatching (260). All observers agree that increasing severity of GVHD results in decreasing patient survival (519).

Why age, gender mismatching, and the other clinical variables mentioned change the risk of development of GVHD remains speculative. Normal T-lymphocyte differentiation, and,

in particular, the elimination of autoreactive clones and the education of immature T cells in the recognition of self MHC, normally occurs in the thymus. Although data suggest that extrathymic differentiation is possible, the prevention of rampant autoimmune disease and the establishment of immunocyte communication in early life are predominantly thymic functions. By puberty, the human thymus has involuted significantly. Moreover, treatment with radiation and chemotherapy can further damage the thymic epithelium on which the T-cell education process takes place. Therefore, the recapitulation of the immune system after marrow transplantation may be aberrant, especially in older patients; and this immune imbalance might lead to a GVHD reaction. Gender mismatching may lead to increased GVHD either by sensitization of donor T cells to foreign antigens, as in parous women, or by reaction to a minor histocompatibility difference between donor and recipient.

An association also exists between infection with members of the herpesvirus family, especially CMV, and GVHD, although the cause-and-effect relation remains unclear (89,481,482,520).

Finally, *in vitro* predictive tests for GVHD have been described (521,522). In one case, recipient skin explants were incubated with donor lymphocytes and examined for histopathologic signs of GVHD. In another, a mixed epidermal cell–lymphocyte reaction was used. A more sensitive test of donor-recipient recognition involves a limiting-dilution analysis of donor IL-2–secreting T-cell precursors. High levels of IL-2–secreting precursors are associated with a high risk of developing acute GVHD, whereas low precursor numbers seem to identify patient–donor pairs at reduced risk of GVHD (523). However, recent series have failed to confirm these data (524,525). All these tests probably detect donors that are capable of reacting to recipient minor histocompatibility antigens. If these tests continue to prove useful, they will be a helpful adjunct to the clinician in designing new transplantation protocols because eliminating the need for GVHD prophylaxis in a subset of patients would likely lead to more rapid immune reconstitution and possibly improved overall survival.

PROPHYLAXIS

Because patient survival is reduced by the development of severe acute GVHD, it is logical that prevention of this disorder might lead to improved clinical results in transplantation. A number of preventive regimens have been used that use both single-agent and multiagent immunosuppression (526). Some commonly used regimens are shown in Table 60-4 (155,527).

Randomized trials have consistently shown that combination therapy is more effective than single-agent prophylaxis. It is reasonable to expect an overall rate of grade II to IV GVHD of 25% to 40%. Ramsay and colleagues (528) randomly assigned patients to a regimen of either 100-day methotrexate alone or methotrexate, ATG (seven doses), and prednisone (days 8 to 20) and noted a 48% incidence of acute GVHD in the methotrexate-alone group as opposed to 21% in the combination regimen. In this study, as has been seen in a variety of trials, increasing rigor of posttransplantation immunosuppression led to a decreased incidence of clinically diagnosed acute GVHD but failed to show a patient survival advantage. The failure to clearly improve survival, especially of patients with transplants for leukemia, although decreasing morbidity and mortality directly attributable to GVHD in some trials may be due to an increase in the incidence of late infectious complications and leukemic relapse in the face of increased immunosuppression (see the section Graft-Versus-Leukemia Reaction). Some authors have suggested that reducing the amount of routine posttransplantation immunosuppression and then providing T cells to restore the GVL response, treating GVHD when it occurs, might be an alternate strategy (529).

TABLE 60-4. Examples of Commonly Used Graft-Versus-Host Disease Prophylaxis Regimens

Agent	Day											Continue through 50 days, then taper as tolerated
	−5	−4	−3	−2	−1	0	1	2	3...	6...	11	
Cyclosporine[a]			‖	‖	‖	‖	‖	‖	‖	‖	‖	→
Methotrexate							x		x	x	x	
Stem cells						⊕						
Tacrolimus[b]			├────────────────────────────────→									
Methotrexate							x		x	x	x	
Stem cells						⊕						

[a]Given intravenously daily and changed to twice a day oral administration when oral intake is tolerated.
[b]Given intravenously daily by continuous infusion and changed to twice a day oral administration when oral intake is tolerated.
Adapted from Ratanatharathorn V, Nash RA, Przepiorka D, et al. Phase III study comparing methotrexate and tacrolimus (prograf, FK506) with methotrexate and cyclosporine for graft-versus-host disease prophylaxis after HLA-identical sibling bone marrow transplantation. *Blood* 1998;92:2303; and Nash R, Antin J, Karanes C, et al. A phase III study comparing methotrexate and tacrolimus with methotrexate and cyclosporine for prophylaxis of acute graft-versus-host disease after marrow transplantation from unrelated donors. *Blood* 2000;96:2062.

The advent of the calcineurin inhibitor cyclosporine as a single agent was not particularly better at controlling GVHD than methotrexate, although it did have a different toxicity profile. The difference in toxicity allowed it to be used in combination with methotrexate or prednisone. The regimen of cyclosporine plus methotrexate improved control of GVHD and increased survival in several studies. In patients with transplants for aplastic anemia (530), 18% of those receiving cyclosporine plus methotrexate developed significant acute GVHD, compared to 53% in the group receiving methotrexate alone, with respective actuarial 2-year survival rates of 82% and 60%. No difference in the incidence of chronic GVHD was observed (9 of 19 patients versus 6 of 14 patients, respectively). As noted, reduction of GVHD is most likely to benefit patients receiving transplants for nonmalignant disorders because there is no postulated benefit from adoptive immunotherapy (i.e., GVL) in that group. What, then, is the result of the improved combination regimen in patients with transplants for leukemia? In the initial study of patients receiving transplants for AML (224), 33% of those receiving cyclosporine and methotrexate developed GVHD, compared to 54% in the cyclosporine-only group ($p = .014$); the actuarial survival rate at 1.5 years was 80% versus 55%, respectively ($p = .042$). Similar improvement was shown for patients receiving transplants for CML. Unfortunately, with longer follow-up, subsequent studies have shown a loss of the survival advantage in most patient groups (531). With a 3.0- to 4.5-year follow-up, the survival rate for the AML patients is identical (41% in each group), with only a trend toward a survival advantage in CML (73% versus 54%, $p = .09$). The loss of survival advantage was due to an increase in leukemic relapse. As for other studies, reduction in the incidence of acute GVHD led to no change in the overall incidence of chronic GVHD (approximately 25% in both groups). Tacrolimus is another calcineurin inhibitor that functions similarly to cyclosporine but has a slightly different toxicity profile. Randomized trials demonstrate that the ability to control GVHD is similar to that seen with cyclosporine (155,527,532). Similar results were reported in a large-scale retrospective analysis by the International Bone Marrow Transplant Registry (IBMTR) (533). One limitation with the use of methotrexate is that it slows engraftment, worsens mucositis, and may be associated with interstitial pneumonitis. Early studies of reducing the dose of methotrexate (534,535) and replacing methotrexate with mycophenolate mofetil are promising (536). Thus, although the combination regimen has benefits in early posttransplantation management, pharmacologic approaches to GVHD remain suboptimal.

As noted, the intensity of the conditioning regimen influences the incidence of GVHD. In part, this effect may be related to increased tissue injury and inflammatory cytokine production, but the more severe mucositis may also prevent the administration of the full dose of methotrexate (131,513,537). Some trials use cyclosporine with prednisone or cyclosporine and methotrexate plus prednisone, but its use has not improved survival (225,538). Unfortunately, the drugs available for GVHD prophylaxis are incompletely effective and have substantial toxicity. Methotrexate often worsens mucositis induced by the conditioning regimen, and it can increase the risk of interstitial pneumonia. Cyclosporine is hepatotoxic and nephrotoxic, and it is often difficult to attain the necessary degree of GVHD control without drug-induced toxicity.

Because acute GVHD can be completely abrogated in animal models by depleting mature T lymphocytes from donor marrow, trials of *ex vivo* marrow T-cell depletion in humans were begun in the early 1980s (539–542). A multitude of techniques may be used to accomplish this purpose: sheep erythrocyte rosetting with or without soybean lectin separation (451,543), monoclonal antibody plus a source of complement (446,544,545), immunotoxin conjugates (449,546), and counterflow elutriation (547,548). When antibodies are used, they may be directed against any of a number of pan-T surface markers (e.g., CD3, CD5, CD2), or an attempt may be made to deplete only a particular subset of T lymphocytes (545,546,549). All these variations introduce significant variation in the final result. In some cases, such as the soybean lectin and rosette technique, B cells are depleted along with T cells. Some T-cell antigens modulate rapidly (e.g., CD3). If the procedure depends on complement for lysis, there may be inadequate time of exposure, and depletion of the T cells may be relatively inefficient. On the other hand, if an antibody is linked to an immunotoxin that must be internalized to be effective, then modulation may be preferable to optimize death of the target cells. Additional variables include incomplete T-cell depletion with some monoclonal antibodies (such as anti-CD8 or anti-CD5) and sparing of NK cells. Leaving some functionally competent cells may retain the antileukemic effect or may enhance engraftment.

A randomized trial of T-cell depletion versus standard pharmacologic prophylaxis demonstrated the following instructive findings (448): Although the incidence and severity of acute GVHD was significantly reduced by this procedure, overall survival remained the same. This occurred because of an increased incidence of graft rejection and of leukemic relapse. Similar results were seen when a single institution cohort analysis compared two closely matched cohorts with CML. In this study, outcome of T-cell depletion would have been substantially worse;

however, donor-lymphocyte infusions resulted in remissions in most patients and allowed a similar leukemia-free survival (550). These same trends have been seen in most other series and in a large retrospective study of the IBMTR (551). There may be better maintenance of the GVL effect in unrelated donor transplantation, although survival is similar whether T cells are depleted (552). The nature of the monoclonal antibody used to purge the marrow may also be relevant. In a large retrospective analysis, marrows purged with narrow specificity antibodies seem to do somewhat better (553). In addition, most series also demonstrate a reduction in overall incidence of chronic GVHD. Interestingly, the observation echoes the increased number of T cells in peripheral blood stem cell transplantation results in enhanced chronic GVHD (118,488). It is postulated, as mentioned earlier, that the increased risk of graft rejection occurs because of the loss of donor immunologic attack on residual host elements (NK or T cells) that are capable of mounting the rejection reaction. Moreover, additional studies have demonstrated delayed immunologic reconstitution, a possible increased risk of late infections in the HLA-incompatible or unrelated donor setting (299,554,555), and an increased risk of posttransplantation lymphoproliferative syndrome (299,556,557). These results are reminiscent of early trials of pharmacologic immunosuppression for GVHD. There appears to be a fine line between adequate immunosuppression to prevent (or ameliorate) GVHD and excess immunosuppression that leads to immunologic complications.

Is there a potential future for the T-cell depletion approach? Trials are exploring several options. First, the increased incidence of graft rejection can be reduced by increasing immunosuppressive transplantation conditioning. This may be possible to a limited degree because toxicity from methotrexate and cyclosporine would be avoided. Furthermore, improvement in conditioning regimens may also reduce leukemic relapses. Second, the use of cytokines or cellular therapy after transplantation might be capable of partially reversing the more severe immunologic defect. Carefully prepared T cells that primarily recognize CMV have been infused safely to try and prevent CMV recurrence (417); however, this approach is not practical for less specific immunologic reconstitution and the fear of increasing GVHD remains. Third, based on murine studies, it might be possible to deplete only the particular subset of T cells that is the primary mediator of the GVHD reaction and leave intact the remainder of the T-lymphocyte system. Ultimately, one would want to eliminate only those pre-formed T cells that are host-specific from the donor marrow. Finally, T-cell depletion might be used to prevent acute, transplant-related toxicity. Subsequently, limited numbers of T cells could be infused to establish a GVL reaction (558).

TREATMENT

Once acute GVHD develops, despite prophylaxis, several agents are available for treatment (559–562).

- Corticosteroids (generally methylprednisolone) typically in doses of 2 to 5 mg/kg/day.
- Tacrolimus or cyclosporine: doses similar to those used in prophylaxis regimens. These drugs are used for therapy in patients who develop acute GVHD after T-cell depletion.
- Antithymocyte globulin (563) or monoclonal antibodies, such as daclizumab (564).
- Less well-studied alternatives include mycophenolate mofetil (565), monoclonal antibodies such as daclizumab (564), octreotide for intestinal involvement (566), and cytokine inhibitory therapy (567–569).

Large retrospective studies of the treatment of GVHD have demonstrated that most potent immunosuppressive agents are useful to some extent (with the notable exception of azathio-

prine) and that patients with complete responses to therapy generally do well (561). Unfortunately, a substantial proportion of patients do not respond to treatment or relapse. The complete response rate for initial therapy was only 20% (complete and partial responses occurred in 44% of patients), and an additional 20% to 40% of patients responded to secondary therapy (559,560). These patients have a poor overall survival because of both direct complications of GVHD and opportunistic infections related to prolonged immunosuppression (563). Acute GVHD developing after unrelated donor transplant seems to be particularly difficult to treat successfully.

Chronic Graft-Versus-Host Disease

DESCRIPTION AND DIAGNOSIS

Chronic GVHD may develop from 2 months to 2 years after allogeneic marrow transplantation. It is the most insidious of transplantation complications and, in some respects, the most difficult to handle. In approximately one-third of the patients who develop the disease, it evolves in an uninterrupted progression from prior acute GVHD (progressive chronic GVHD). In another one-third of patients, it arises after complete or near complete resolution of acute GVHD (so-called interrupted or quiescent chronic GVHD), whereas in the final one-third of patients, the disorder appears *de novo* with no previous evidence of clinically apparent acute GVHD. It may occur in a limited form with relatively localized skin or mucosal involvement, mild hepatic dysfunction, or in a generalized form with extensive involvement of multiple organs (Table 60-5) (570,571). The latter, more generalized syndrome presents earlier after transplantation, on average, than the former. In its most severe form, it is characterized by scleroderma, erythematous skin changes with scarring and ulcer formation, patchy hyper- and hypopigmentation, lichen planus, alopecia, malar erythema, photosensitivity, xerostomia, severe keratoconjunctivitis sicca, myositis, fasciitis, synovitis, tendonitis, joint contractures, desquamative esophagitis with stricture formation, malabsorption, and abnormal (usually cholestatic) liver function tests. Persistent severe immunodeficiency and failure to reconstitute both the humoral and cellular arms of the immune response accompany chronic GVHD. This immune failure, coupled with the integumentary loss and cholestasis, heightens the risk of severe infection in these patients and includes a marked increase in gram-positive infections (572). Flares of chronic GVHD often occur during tapering of immunosuppression, but they also appear to be induced by solar exposure and infections. The use of sunscreen, hats, and long-sleeved clothing is impor-

---

TABLE 60-5. Chronic Graft-Versus-Host Disease (GVHD)

Limited chronic GVHD
  Localized skin involvement with or without:
    Hepatic dysfunction due to chronic GVHD
    Normal platelet count (>100,000 cells/μL)
Extensive chronic GVHD
  Generalized skin involvement
  Localized skin involvement and/or hepatic dysfunction due to chronic GVHD, plus any of the following:
    Liver histology showing chronic aggressive hepatitis, bridging necrosis, or cirrhosis
    Involvement of the eye: Schirmer's test with <5 mm of wetting
    Involvement of minor salivary glands or oral mucosa demonstrated on labial biopsy
    Involvement of any other target organ
    Chronic thrombocytopenia; platelets <100,000 cells/μL continuously despite normal granulocyte count and reticulocyte counts

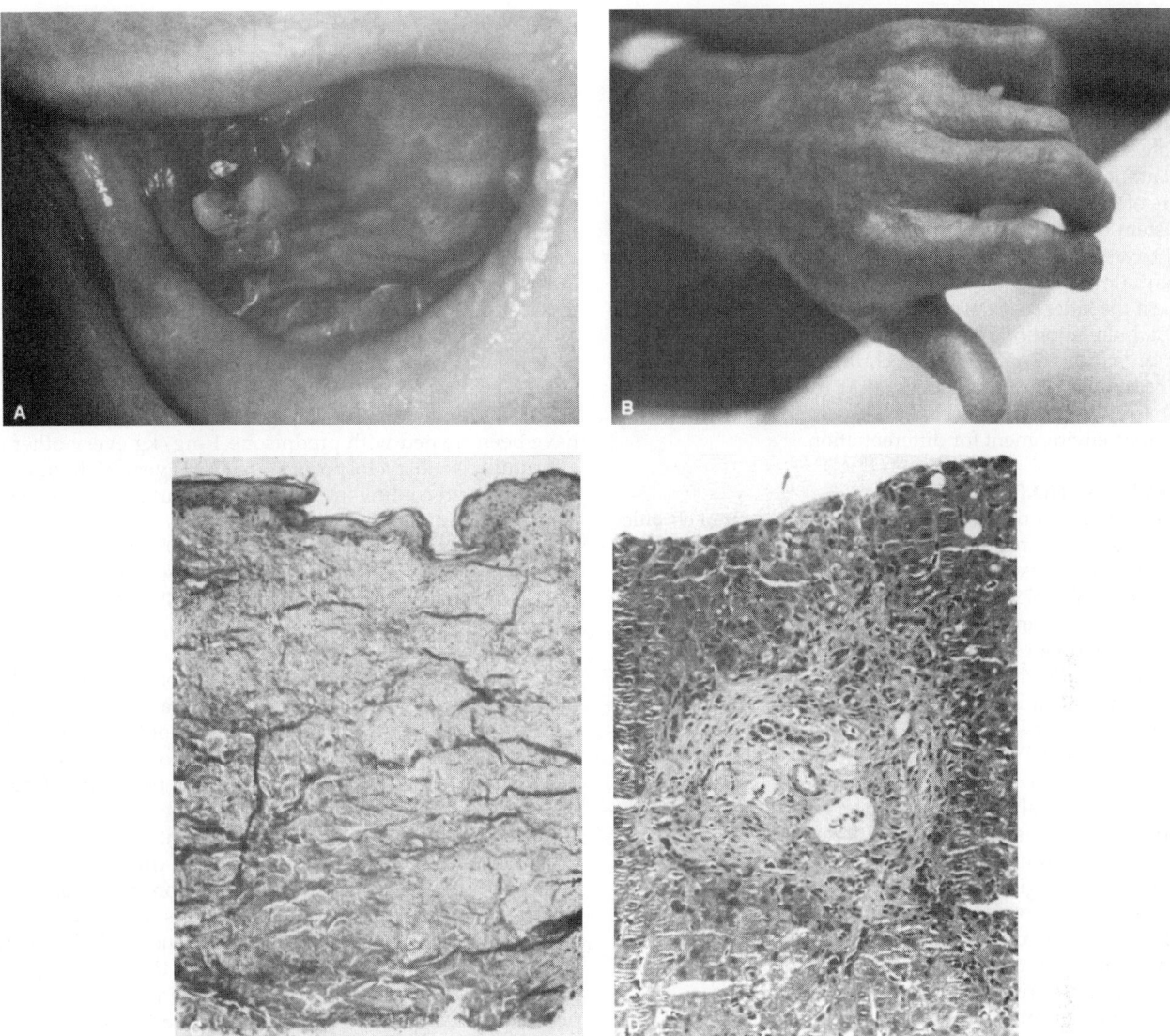

Figure 60-9. A: Oral mucosa with lacy, white plaques that are similar to lichen planus. Caries are due to xerostomia, steroid-induced diabetes mellitus, and chronic grinding of the teeth. **B:** Severe atrophy of the skin with flexion contractures. **C:** Skin biopsy specimen shows epidermal atrophy with loss of rete pegs and dermal fibrosis. **D:** Liver biopsy demonstrates bile duct damage, fibrosis in portal areas, and chronic cholestasis. (See Color Fig. 60-9.)

tant to prevent such exacerbation. Infections such as shingles may be followed by localized chronic GVHD in the area of viral infection or in a generalized worsening of skin disease.

The histology of chronic GVHD in involved organs resembles chronic inflammation and fibrosis (Fig. 60-9). In the skin, epidermal hypertrophy and lichen planus–like reaction progress to epidermal fibrosis and atrophy (573). In the localized variant, dense dermal fibrosis may be seen without an inflammatory reaction. Gingival biopsies demonstrate mucositis and squamous cell necrosis similar, but not identical, to that seen in Sjögren's syndrome (574). Liver biopsies demonstrate chronic active hepatitis with bridging necrosis and cirrhosis in the more severe cases that may go on to cirrhosis.

Although the diagnosis of severe cases of GVHD is not difficult on clinical grounds alone, definitive recognition of the disease in early stages may be made on the basis of skin biopsy, gingival biopsy, and Schirmer's test. Chronic GVHD is more of a multisystem disease than acute GVHD. Some patients have features of both conditions throughout a prolonged transition period. Aside from the organs discussed previously, what other organs are involved by the disease? Again, it may be difficult to distinguish organ involvement by the condition from organ damage due to secondary infection. Nonetheless, the only other organ suspected of involvement is the lung. After transplantation, many patients develop pulmonary impairment, usually of a combined restrictive and obstructive nature. Bronchiolitis obliterans, a progressive condition in many cases, may develop 6 or more months after transplantation and may be a direct result of chronic GVHD. It is usually associated with hypogammaglobulinemia (164,575). This condition may also be found in patients in the absence of chronic GVHD. Whether that implies that the pathophysiology is of single-organ GVHD in those cases or that the link between these conditions is not one-to-one is unknown. It is likely that bronchiolitis obliterans is triggered by infection.

PATHOPHYSIOLOGY

It remains an open question both in experimental animal models and in humans whether chronic GVHD is yet another manifestation of the same pathophysiology responsible for acute GVHD or whether it is, at least sometimes, an intrinsically different disorder. Conceptually, chronic GVHD could represent either a continued attack of committed, mature T cells infused with donor marrow against the host with a failure to develop adequate suppression of these elements. Alternatively, it could represent the manifestations of an autoimmune process, that is, a failure of uncommitted T cells, newly maturing from the lymphoid stem cell, to become host tolerant because of an inadequate thymic or extrathymic environment in which to differentiate. The question is not simply an academic one, because if the latter mechanism is correct, one must predict that even total depletion of all committed T cells from donor marrow in humans will not eliminate chronic GVHD. Indeed, the latter mechanism would suggest that to eliminate chronic GVHD, one needs to supply the newly maturing marrow with an adequate environment for differentiation.

RISK FACTORS AND PROGNOSIS

The most significant risk factors for the development of chronic GVHD are the presence of prior acute GVHD, male recipient with female donor, use of unrelated donors, and increasing age of the patient (576–579). In addition, patients who received the Seattle aplastic anemia conditioning regimen that included the infusion of donor buffy coat cells were at increased risk for the development of chronic GVHD (453). Similar data are now accumulating indicating that the use of peripheral blood stem cells is a significant risk factor (118,488), as is the administration of large numbers of T cells in adoptive immunotherapy [donor lymphocyte infusions (DLI)] (580,581). There is one paper that suggests that the total dose is less critical than the timing of the infusions, because spacing the DLI over several months resulted in less chronic GVHD (582). As for acute GVHD, the exact pathophysiologic mechanism by which these characteristics increase the risk of developing chronic GVHD is uncertain. Because donor buffy coat contains large numbers of nonirradiated, immunocompetent lymphocytes, it is believed that this procedure increases risk by increasing total T-cell dose.

Because of the legion manifestations of the disease and the uneven involvement of different organ systems in different patients, a simple prognostic grading system such as that used for acute GVHD is not in common use. Karnofsky's index or other indices of overall patient performance are probably most useful (583), but patients who have thrombocytopenia associated with their disease have a particularly grim prognosis (278,584). This does not relate to morbidity due to bleeding complications; rather, it presumably serves as an index of overall disease activity because the cause of death in these patients is generally an infection. Other poor prognostic factors include progressive presentation, lichenoid skin changes, diarrhea, and elevated bilirubin, whereas oral mucositis seems to be protective (583,585).

TREATMENT

Treatment of chronic GVHD involves immunosuppressive agents. The Seattle group (584) carried out a randomized trial of prednisone alone, 1 mg/kg every other day, versus a combination of prednisone and azathioprine, 1.5 mg/kg/day, in all patients with extensive chronic GVHD who also had a platelet count of at least 100,000/μL. All patients also received trimethoprim-sulfamethoxazole, one double-strength tablet twice daily, and received a median of 2 years of therapy. Complications included diabetes (5%), aseptic necrosis (5%), and infection. Recurrent malignancy occurred equally in the two groups, but nonrelapse mortality was only 21% in the steroid-only group compared to 40% in the prednisone-plus-azathioprine

group. Moreover, the incidence of disseminated varicella, bacteremia, and interstitial pneumonitis in the steroid versus two-drug group was 11% versus 24%, 6% versus 11%, and 5% versus 14%, respectively. Thus, treatment with alternate-day steroids alone gave significantly better results in these patients. In the same study, patients with platelet counts of less than 100,000/μL were uniformly treated with steroids alone. As expected, these patients had a significantly worse overall prognosis (58% nonrelapse mortality) and higher incidence of disseminated varicella (34%), bacteremia (34%), and interstitial pneumonitis (18%). One explanation for these findings may relate to the myelotoxicity of azathioprine, which contributed to the overall reduction in ability to respond to infection. New, less myelotoxic agents such as mycophenolate mofetil show promise, although large-scale randomized trials are lacking (565,586).

Patients with thrombocytopenia and extensive chronic GVHD have been treated with prednisone 1 mg/kg every other day, alternating with cyclosporine 6 mg/kg every 12 hours every other day, and continuous trimethoprim-sulfamethoxazole prophylaxis. Complete response rates of 33% were observed, and improvements in survival rates to over 50% were seen even in patients who did not respond to prior therapy (587).

Often in the management of chronic GVHD there is a high motivation for tapering of immunosuppression as soon as inflammatory manifestations are under control. Although understandable, this strategy leads to a "ping-pong" pattern with frequent relapses. It is more effective to achieve a complete remission (CR) with steroids with or without other agents and maintain the remission for at least 4 to 6 months before tapering begins. This approach is much less likely to result in frequent flares and remissions.

The difficulty in management of patients' extensive chronic GVHD has led to a number of studies of different modalities reflecting a variety of mechanisms of action (e.g., thalidomide, clofazimine, extracorporeal photopheresis, retinoids, and others). Thalidomide has been useful in lichenoid GVHD, particularly involving the mouth; however, it does not appear as promising for systemic GVHD or scleroderma (588,589). A particularly noteworthy study was performed by Chao and colleagues in which thalidomide was randomized against placebo in prophylaxis of chronic GVHD. In this study, thalidomide actually worsened the rate of chronic GVHD (64% versus 38%), and its use was associated with a higher rate of treatment failure (82% versus 54%) and a reduction in survival (590). Thus, generalization of results of therapy to prophylaxis must be undertaken with caution. Sclerodermatous GVHD has proven more refractory to therapy. Studies by Lee and colleagues showed some benefit to the use of oral clofazimine (591). Several groups have had promising results with extracorporeal photopheresis or ultraviolet irradiation and psoralen (592–594), although large-scale definitive trials are lacking. Other therapies that can be beneficial include retinoids (592), mycophenolate mofetil (565,586), ultraviolet B (595), ursadiol (595), and hydroxychloroquine (596).

Supportive therapy of patients with chronic GVHD is crucial. Prophylaxis with trimethoprim-sulfamethoxazole, use of artificial tears, and avoidance of solar exposure should be combined with a program of psychological support and physical and occupational therapy. Many of these patients are subject to recurrent infections, especially from encapsulated organisms. This results from their combination immunodeficiency, decreased total IgG, inability to mount a new antibody immune response, functional asplenia, and poor integument. Patients with severe disease and those with recurrent infections likely benefit from penicillin or macrolide prophylaxis and vaccination (597), and replacement γ-globulin must also be considered.

The increasing risk of penicillin-resistant pneumococcus must be kept in mind when considering prophylactic therapy (572). Furthermore, one must be aware of thyroid deficiency (598), sexual hormone deficiency (182,183), osteoporosis (599), risk of secondary malignancies (204–206), cataracts (107,600), effects on fertility (183,184,186,600), growth and development delay (177), and other long-term toxicities and disabilities that either result from the primary therapy, manifestations of GVHD, or the effects of long-term immunosuppressants (175). Keratoconjunctivitis sicca and xerostomia are common problems, resulting in substantial disability. Management of patients with chronic GVHD requires all of the skills of a general internist plus the assistance of multiple subspecialists. Fortunately, with proper therapy, chronic GVHD has a tendency to resolve in time (600).

Graft-Versus-Leukemia Reaction

The ability of the immune system to destroy allogeneic and syngeneic tumor cells has been amply demonstrated in both animal models and in humans (601,602). Indeed, the concept of adoptive immunotherapy for acute leukemia dates back to the 1960s (603). In some experimental systems, a GVL reaction can be detected that is separable from the GVHR (604,605); whereas in other models, the two appear to go hand in hand (606). In human allogeneic marrow transplantation, a GVL or graft-versus-tumor effect can also be demonstrated, empirically, to accompany the GVHR (580,607–613), and in selected subsets of patients, chronic GVHD, presumably accompanied by the GVL effect, may even contribute to increased overall patient survival as a result of a decrease in disease recurrence. Finally, there are the clinical observations that as some patients have relapsed, abrupt discontinuation of immunosuppression has resulted in a GVHD flare and concomitant attainment of remission—presumably a GVL response (614,615). As noted earlier, one of the most effective means of reducing GVHD is donor marrow T-cell depletion. Unfortunately, accompanying that decrease in GVHD is an increase in leukemic relapse (551,553,616,617). It is not known whether improvements in conditioning regimens or earlier transplantation offset the loss of GVL. However, the loss of GVL does appear to be less intense after T-cell depletion of unrelated donor marrow (552) and possibly after haploidentical marrow (555). There also appears to be some value in leaving some T cells behind by using narrow specificity monoclonal antibodies compared to broad specificity T-cell depletion (553).

Because clinical data suggest that further improvements in transplantation conditioning regimen effectiveness are likely to be accompanied by further increases in toxicity (139), it is attractive to consider using the GVL reaction in a controlled fashion. The Seattle group attempted just such a manipulation (618). By randomly assigning patients to receive three different GVHD prophylaxis regimens, they were able to vary the incidence of grade II to IV acute GVHD from 25% (long-course methotrexate) to 59% (short-course methotrexate) to 82% (methotrexate plus donor buffy coat). Nonetheless, as was discussed earlier, the incidence of chronic GVHD was identical in the three groups (33%, 51%, 44%, respectively). Overall disease-free survival rates with median follow-up of approximately 5 years were 41%, 30%, and 24% in the three groups, respectively. There was no difference in 5-year probability of recurrent malignancy, although nonrelapse mortality did differ at the extremes (34% versus 45% versus 64%). Thus, in this study, it was not possible to harness GVHD to obtain an adjustable beneficial clinical effect. In part, their failure to observe an improvement in survival may reflect the poor underlying prognosis of the selected patients or insensitivity of their illnesses to GVL. However, another possibility is that increasing acute GVHD in the peri-

transplant period increases GVHD-related mortality disproportionately to that prevented by GVL. Subsequent studies using infusions of peripheral blood leukocytes obtained by leukapheresis have shown an impressive antileukemic effect with surprisingly mild GVHD (580,607,608,610,619,620). In CML, the DLI has a 60% to 80% response rate, depending on the leukemia burden at the time of therapy. When remissions occur, the disease may become undetectable at the 10^{-6} level by sensitive techniques such as polymerase chain reaction (608). Typically, if the disease is treated late, approximately 10^8 donor lymphocytes/kg are required; however, much smaller doses have been used successfully to treat cytogenetic relapses (621). When large T-cell doses are used, there is a substantial risk of acute and chronic GVHD as would be expected. However, the smaller doses may be associated with little or no clinical GVHD. These data emphasize the importance of the GVL reaction in the outcome of marrow transplantation, particularly in CML, but also in other disorders. It appears that relatively slow growing malignancies such as CML, chronic lymphocytic leukemia (CLL), non-Hodgkin's lymphoma, Hodgkin's disease, and multiple myeloma are more susceptible to the GVL effect than AML or myelodysplasia. ALL appears the least sensitive to GVL effects.

The GVL reaction can also be used to treat EBV lymphoproliferative disorders after transplantation. These uncontrolled proliferations of EBV-transformed B cells occur most frequently after T-cell–depleted transplantation. They are thought to result from a loss in T-cell control of the infected B cells. DLIs have been used successfully both therapeutically and prophylactically to address this problem (80,196,202,556,557).

Reduced Intensity Transplantation

An area of increasing research is the use of reduced intensity or nonmyeloablative transplants. This work derived directly from the GVL observations described above, and there has been a proliferation of studies attempting to harness the best aspects of GVL and avoiding conditioning regimen toxicity (622,623). Typically, these regimens have revolved around cyclophosphamide (427) or reduced-dose TBI (622), fludarabine (624), or busulfan (135). Additional immunosuppression with calcineurin inhibitors or mycophenolate mofetil is often necessary to maintain the graft and prevent GVHD. There does seem to be a cohort of patients, primarily with more indolent illnesses, in whom reduced-intensity regimens are useful, but further studies are needed to assess the role of this therapy in current practice (135,427,609,624). It should be noted that although transplant-related toxicity is less, GVHD remains a significant problem in most regimens.

Transfusion-Associated Graft-Versus-Host Disease

In addition to marrow transplant recipients and neonatal immunodeficient children, clinical GVHD may also occur in immunosuppressed patients receiving nonirradiated cellular blood products. This has been described in patients with Hodgkin's disease, AML, ALL, CLL, SCIDS, Wiskott-Aldrich syndrome, neonatal or intrauterine exchange transfusion, liver or cardiac transplants, and other disorders (625–629), although the overall incidence in all these conditions remains low. It is most commonly observed in young (small) children. This is presumed to reflect the relatively high dose of lymphocytes/kg of host body weight that occurs in such a child. The minimal dose of lymphocytes necessary to initiate the reaction has been estimated at 10^7/kg. In these circumstances, only the T lymphocytes engraft. Typically, 2 to 4 weeks after a transfusion, the patient develops characteristic rash, liver function abnormalities, diarrhea, and subsequently pancytopenia and perhaps respiratory failure. In contrast to GVHD developing after marrow grafting, pancytopenia is prominent because of suppression of the host's hematopoiesis by the transfused T cells. Both because of this profound cytopenia and because of the host's marked immunodeficiency, fatalities are high in this variant of GVHD when it occurs in an obviously recognizable presentation (estimated at 75% to 90% mortality). Whether the disorder may occur in a mild forme fruste in other postchemotherapy patients is unknown but occasionally suspected. Irradiation of blood products with 1500 to 3000 cGy virtually eliminates the risk of developing GVHD from blood products.

One possible exception to the rule that the development of GVHD only occurs in patients who are profoundly immunosuppressed, and therefore incapable of rejecting the donor lymphocytes, has been described (630). In two patients who were fully immunocompetent, a fatal syndrome clinically and pathologically identical to transfusion-associated GVHD developed after receiving family blood products during cardiac surgery. The family donor in this case was HLA homozygous for one of the recipient's MHC haplotypes. In this circumstance, it is postulated that the host was incapable of recognizing the donated blood as foreign because the donor expresses only HLA antigens identical to the host. Nonetheless, because the host expresses an HLA haplotype different from the donor, a GVHD reaction may occur.

APLASTIC ANEMIA

Before the application of marrow transplantation, the outlook for patients with severe aplastic anemia was grim (631,632). Early studies by Thomas and colleagues (633), however, demonstrated the feasibility of replacing missing or defective hematopoietic stem cells with normal donor cells. In addition to important therapeutic progress, marrow transplantation led to further understanding of the pathogenesis of idiopathic aplastic anemia. In reports of syngeneic transplants performed without the use of immunosuppression, most patients failed to engraft, but they subsequently successfully engrafted after receiving second transplants conditioned with cyclophosphamide (434,634). Subsequent studies also demonstrated a substantial rate of autologous recovery of hematopoiesis after cyclophosphamide-conditioned transplants (635–637). These data suggested that some patients with aplastic anemia had cellular or humoral inhibition of hematopoiesis rather than deficient numbers of stem cells. The response of patients with aplastic anemia to intensive immunosuppression further supports this view (638–640). Another category of aplastic anemia has been inferred by observations of lymphoid chimerism without myeloid chimerism after marrow grafting. These observations suggest that a small proportion of cases of aplastic anemia are due to the inability of the bone marrow microenvironment to support hematopoiesis (238,239).

Soon after the application of marrow grafting to severe aplastic anemia, it was recognized that, in addition to GVHD, graft rejection was a major problem. Typically, the rejection rate was 30% to 45%, and the mortality in patients without sustained grafts was 80% (435,641). Although several risk factors for graft rejection were suggested by different groups (436,438), the primary determinant of the likelihood of rejection in HLA-compatible transplantation is prior blood transfusion. Patients who remain untransfused 72 hours before receiving the beginning of the conditioning regimen have a graft failure rate of 10% and an actuarial 10-year survival rate of 82% (438,642). It is

thought that the rejection rate rises after blood transfusion because of transfusion-induced sensitization to minor histocompatibility antigens (643). Transfusions from family members are the most likely to sensitize the patient to minor histocompatibility determinants and should be avoided. Many patients with aplastic anemia require transfusions before the ascertainment of a HLA-compatible donor and the initiation of transplantation. It is inappropriate to withhold blood products from pancytopenic patients who require them. It appears that the risk of rejection, however, is a function of the number of transfusions received (438,512). Consequently, new strategies were directed at reducing the relapse rate. TBI in doses commonly used to treat leukemia was successful at reducing the graft failure rate to low levels—but at the expense of increased mortality due to interstitial pneumonia and GVHD (644). Less intensive radiotherapeutic regimens (Table 60-2) that rely on cyclophosphamide and low-dose TBI (645), total lymphoid irradiation (646,647), or thoracoabdominal irradiation (648) resulted in rejection rates of 5% to 10% and overall survival rates of 62% to 78%. However, concern has been raised about the risk of secondary malignancies, and radiation-based regimens are not often used (600,649). Similar results (rejection rate, 10%; 5-year actuarial survival rate, 61%) were achieved with cyclophosphamide-procarbazine-ATG serum (511,650). The Seattle group observed that the number of marrow cells infused was an important determinant of engraftment (218,437,651), and they infused donor-derived buffy coat cells for 1 to 3 or 1 to 5 days after the marrow infusion. This tactic led to a similar decline in graft rejection and a 67% actuarial 10-year survival rate, but at the expense of increased chronic GVHD (453). The reason that buffy coat is effective may be due to the addition of stem cells, but it may also relate to the ability of infused T cells or NK cells to inhibit or destroy residual host lymphocytes that would mediate graft rejection or the addition of lymphokine-producing cells. Indeed, this can be considered an early use of nonmyeloablative transplantation and DLI. Second transplants can be performed, and depending on the context of graft failure, up to 85% of patients may be long-term survivors (511).

The use of mismatched or matched, unrelated donors in the treatment of aplastic anemia is less successful. The graft rejection rate is higher, and there appears to be a higher incidence of GVHD (47,489,652–656). Recently, the use of low doses of TBI has been studied when unrelated donor marrow is used as the source of stem cells (657). This technique appears to reduce the rejection rate, but the follow-up is too short to assess the rate of secondary malignancies. It is possible that if peripheral blood stem cells are used in lieu of marrow, the TBI can be avoided, although this inference requires further study. The use of these alternate donors, however, may prove life-saving for occasional patients with refractory aplastic anemia.

Prospective trials have been undertaken to compare allogeneic marrow transplantation to conventional therapy for aplastic anemia. The International Aplastic Anemia Study Group published a prospective study of androgens or marrow transplantation in 110 patients with aplastic anemia (632). They concluded that marrow transplantation was superior therapy to androgens and that marrow grafting was the treatment of choice for patients with compatible donors. Improvements in the immunosuppressive therapy of aplastic anemia and in transplantation results have made the choice of marrow transplantation less straightforward. The University of California Los Angeles group prospectively compared ATG to marrow transplantation in patients younger than 25 years of age and found a 2-year actuarial survival rate of 72% in the transplant group compared to 45% in the ATG group. This difference, however, did not reach statistical significance. The patients with transplants had better blood counts and performance status (658). A prospective European study treating patients 40 years of age or younger showed a survival advantage in an antilymphocyte globulin–treated group (75%) compared to a transplantation-treated group (46%) (659), but the group with transplants did not fare as well as most centers report. The opposite outcome was seen in a smaller single institution series from Seattle (660). Once immunosuppressive therapy has failed in patients without a family member donor, transplantation from an unrelated donor can be curative (>50% survival), although the outcomes are less robust than in matched related donor procedures (661). Although the studies were not prospective trials, investigators have reported a high survival rate (70% to 75%) in children receiving transplants for aplastic anemia, supporting a recommendation to transplant all young people who have compatible donors (662,663). These recommendations were confirmed in a large retrospective analysis of European data, which indicated a significant advantage for marrow transplantation for patients 20 years or age or younger (64% versus 38%), but more equivalent results in older patients (639,654,664,665). ATG can result in long-term survival rates of 30% to 70% but often with incomplete recovery and a tendency to relapse (639). Furthermore, the development of clonal disorders, such as paroxysmal nocturnal hemoglobinuria (PNH) and myelodysplasia, are increasingly recognized in long-term survivors of immunosuppressive therapy (639,654,664–667).

Advantages and disadvantages to each approach are as follows: Marrow transplantation offers a high likelihood of cure but is more expensive, has more acute toxicity, and may result in chronic GVHD. Immunosuppression with ATG is also effective, but often does not cure the aplastic anemia. It requires prolonged supportive care, but has fewer side effects. A reasonable recommendation is to transplant all patients who have identical twin donors (634). In patients who are 30 to 40 years of age or younger, allogeneic transplantation is the treatment of choice if there is a compatible donor. If there are risks for either the patient or marrow donor, such as pregnancy, recent hepatitis, and so forth, the balance is in favor of immunosuppression. For patients older than 40 years of age, ATG and cyclosporine should be administered and marrow grafting reserved for those who fail to respond or who relapse. If no compatible donor is known, ATG and cyclosporine is the treatment of choice, and marrow grafting from a mismatched or matched, unrelated donor is reserved for patients in whom immunosuppressive therapy is unsuccessful.

The cause of the aplastic anemia does not appear to be an important consideration. Successful transplantation has been reported for aplastic anemia due to pregnancy (668), gold (669), drugs, and hepatitis (670,671).

PAROXYSMAL NOCTURNAL HEMOGLOBINURIA

PNH is an acquired disorder of hematopoiesis that can result in aplastic anemia. Even in the absence of marrow failure, the thrombotic and hemolytic complications of PNH can be lethal, although many patients have relatively benign courses. Because PNH is a clonal disorder that can result in acute leukemia, it is important to establish that a conditioning regimen designed primarily for immunosuppression in aplastic anemia is adequate to eliminate the PNH clone. If the marrow is extremely hypocellular (10% or more), immunosuppression appears to be adequate to prevent mixed chimerism (418,672,673). Mixed hematopoietic chimerism, however, may be common in aplastic anemia. The Seattle group (426) noted a 58% incidence of temporary mixed chimerism in 96 patients with transplants for aplastic anemia. Recovery of endogenous hematopoiesis after marrow grafting for aplastic anemia has been discussed previ-

ously. Because cyclophosphamide does not necessarily ablate stem cells, these observations suggest that patients receiving transplants after primarily immunosuppressive conditioning regimens, when the marrow is not severely hypocellular, may have a high incidence of relapse of PNH. TBI and busulfan have both been used in an effort to destroy the PNH clone, but both patients treated with TBI died of interstitial pneumonia (674). For patients with cellular marrows, combination busulfan and cyclophosphamide appears to be an effective regimen (418).

CHRONIC MYELOGENOUS LEUKEMIA

CML is a stem cell disorder that has stubbornly resisted curative therapy with conventional doses of chemotherapy or irradiation. It can be controlled with relatively nontoxic therapy, such as imatinib mesylate (Gleevec, STI-571), hydroxyurea, and IFN-α, but it relentlessly progresses to an aggressive phase that is ultimately fatal in most patients. A small cohort who has substantial suppression of the bcr/abl gene rearrangement may have prolonged survival, but this is not a reliable expectation. In contrast to the acute leukemias, in which long-term disease-free survival may be achieved with standard chemotherapy, CML is only cured by bone marrow transplantation. The advent of imatinib mesylate has largely replaced IFN and hydrea in the early management of CML (675,676). Its effect on long-term survival is not yet understood, and there are too few data to infer how to use it effectively with HSCT to maximize the cure rate.

Timing of Bone Marrow Transplantation

The likelihood of eradicating the leukemic population is partially dependent on the timing of transplantation. Several large studies indicate that transplantation in chronic (stable) phase is associated with a long-term disease-free survival rate of 55% to 87%, depending on age, the presence of GVHD, and the compatibility of the donor. In contrast, once accelerated phase supervenes, the survival rate drops substantially to 18% to 30%. If the transplantation is undertaken in blast crisis, the results are the worst, with a 10% to 15% long-term survival rate (677–684). Patients in accelerated phase who have donors should receive transplants as soon as possible. Patients who achieve a second stable phase after chemotherapy for blast transformation do approximately as well as patients undergoing transplants in accelerated phase (679,682,685,686). Given the poor overall results in transplantation for blast crisis, if the blast crisis is lymphoid, attempts at establishing a second stable phase with intensive chemotherapy or imatinib mesylate are warranted (675).

The high transplantation-related mortality requires circumspection when recommending the procedure to patients in chronic phase, particularly if the patient falls into a good prognostic category (687–691). There are no direct comparative studies that can facilitate this decision; however, several groups have proposed algorithms as guidance (689,690,692). An expert panel from the American Society of Hematology performed an evidence-based analysis and could not make firm recommendations because of the lack of comparative trials (693). Nevertheless, in young people, early in the course of the disease, both family member and unrelated donor transplantation offer survival advantages (689,690). Until long-term outcome data from imatinib is understood, firm recommendations about its relationship to HSCT are not feasible. However, a reasonable decision tree is shown in Figure 60-10.

It appears that performing the transplantation as soon as possible in chronic phase results in improved survival. Patients undergoing transplantation less than 1 year from diagnosis have an improved actuarial survival rate, compared to transplantation

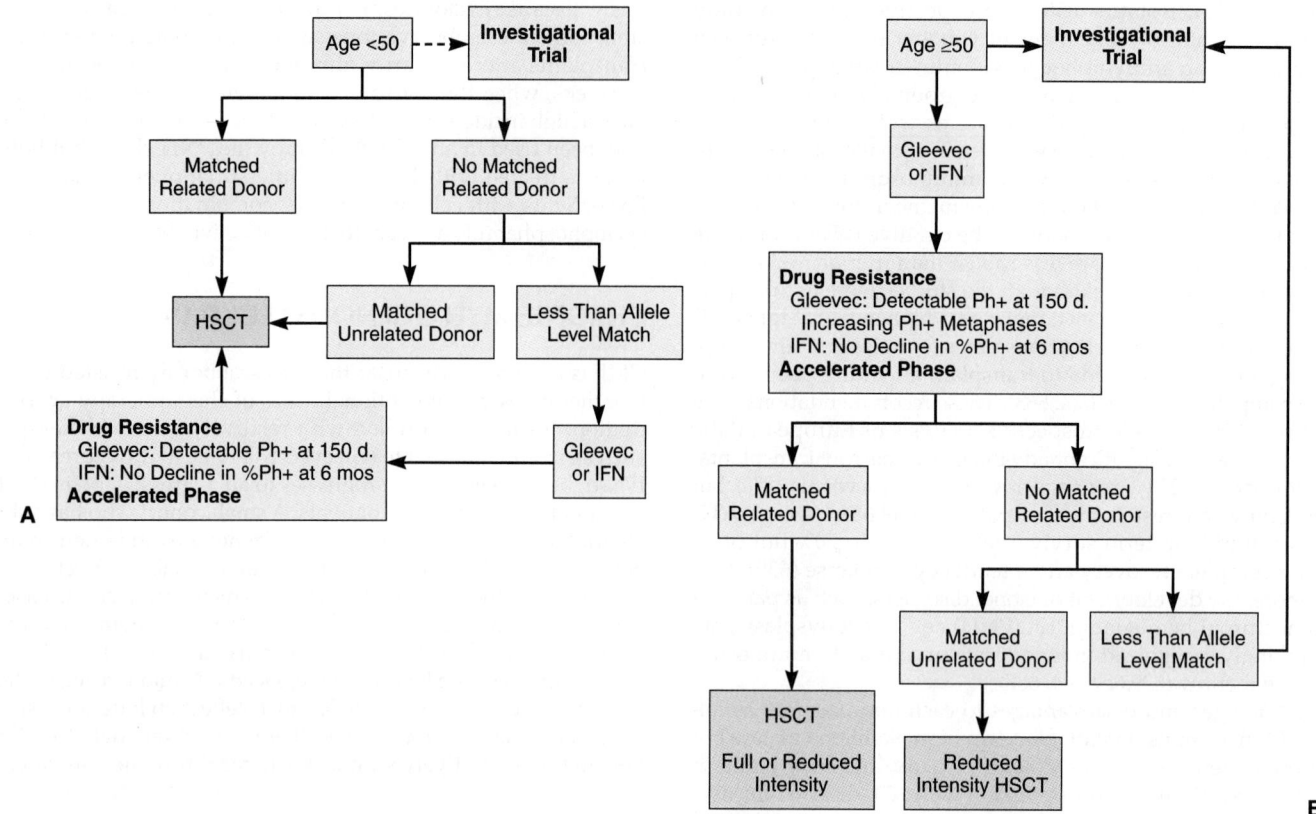

Figure 60-10. Suggested approach to therapy of patients with chronic myelogenous leukemia who are younger than 50 years of age **(A)** or older than 50 years of age **(B)**. Identification of bcr/abl can be through routine cytogenetics, polymerase chain reaction, or fluorescence *in situ* hybridization. Data are insufficient to determine a threshold number of affected cells or copy number on which to base a decision. HSCT, hematopoietic stem cell transplantation; IFN, interferon; Ph, Philadelphia.

occurring later (96,677,689,690,694). Other studies suggest that transplantation before 2 years is acceptable. The effect of time on transplantation outcome reflects the evolution of some patients into more advanced disease but also a poorly defined risk of inferior outcomes independent of disease transformation.

Age younger than 30 years has been a consistently good prognostic finding. This advantage stems in part from the age-related increase in GVHD and treatment-related toxicity that contributes to mortality in older patients. Recommendation for marrow transplantation must be weighed carefully against the risk of early death. The development of accelerated phase is often unpredictable, however, and transplantation is appropriate for patients younger than 60 years of age early in chronic phase.

The relative indolence of the disease has made CML particularly amenable to unrelated donor transplantation. Because on average only approximately 25% of otherwise eligible patients will have family member donors, unrelated donor transplantation is an important resource (656,677,679,680,684,689). The relapse rate appears to lower after unrelated donor marrow transplantation, providing further evidence of a GVL effect. Unfortunately, the risk of acute GVHD (approximately 65%) and chronic GVHD (approximately 55%) is high when unrelated donor marrow is used.

Role of Splenectomy or Splenic Irradiation

Splenic enlargement is characteristic in CML, and the spleen is engorged with leukemic cells. The large spleen may sequester cells and make transfusion support difficult. Consequently, splenectomy has been proposed as a means of debulking the leuke-

mia and to facilitate platelet transfusion (695). Engraftment occurs somewhat faster in the absence of the spleen, and transfusion support is easier, but there is a tendency for more acute GVHD (510,518,696). Retrospective and prospective studies show slight if any survival or disease-free survival benefit for splenectomy or splenic irradiation (697,698).

Prior Therapy

Therapy of stable-phase CML is generally decided by the primary hematologist-oncologist rather than the transplantation center, but there are no firm guidelines on which to base a recommendation. There may be more interstitial pneumonia in patients who received busulfan before transplantation (96,699). It was not possible to establish an unequivocal correlation between prior therapy and survival, but it is prudent to avoid busulfan if possible and use hydroxyurea or IFN-α. Substantial controversy has developed regarding the risk of prior IFN therapy and transplantation outcome (700–704). Most studies found no effect of IFN on transplant outcome. In studies showing an adverse effect, both the duration of IFN therapy (700,701,704), and time of discontinuation prior to transplantation (703) have been implicated. Very recent reports have raised the possibility that IFN pretreatment may actually improve outcome after allogeneic transplantation (702,703,705). In the most recent IBMTR analysis, stopping IFN prior to the transplantation was associated with a higher relapse rate and more GVHD (705). For now, avoidance of IFN exposure is recommended if expeditious transplantation is planned. If a patient is already on IFN and preparing for transplantation, the literature suggests little effect on transplantation outcome by continuing this therapy.

Relapse

The recognition that some patients have persistence or recurrence of Philadelphia (Ph) chromosome-positive cells that may not go on to clinical disease has led to a distinction between molecular, cytogenetic, and clinical relapses (706–717). The presence of Ph metaphases in the marrow up to 2 years after transplantation does not necessarily indicate that clinical relapse is forthcoming (706). More sensitive molecular genetic techniques are useful in assessing the frequency and significance of residual Ph-positive cells. Most authors find that persistent detection of the bcr/abl mRNA by reverse transcriptase PCR (RT PCR) is associated with relapse. It is recommended that assays do not begin before 3 months because of a high level of false-positive results. Typically, a rising ratio of bcr/abl to abl mRNA levels by quantitative RT PCR is suggestive of impending relapse (709–715,718). Similar results can be obtained using FISH (716,717).

Risk of relapse after transplantation varies according to several factors. The primary concern is stage of disease; relapse rates vary from 9% to 30% for transplants performed in stable phase to 25% to 30% for transplants performed in accelerated-phase CML, and up to 80% for transplants done in blast crisis. The only other risk factors for relapse appear to be the presence or absence of GVHD and T-lymphocyte depletion. In retrospective studies, patients with acute GVHD had a relative risk of relapse of 0.7; chronic GVHD was associated with a relative risk of 0.4; and both acute and chronic GVHD was associated with the lowest risk, 0.2 (602,616,617). This reduction in relapse rate is not achieved without cost. GVHD is associated with a higher mortality. T-lymphocyte depletion of the marrow appears to reduce the GVL effect regardless of the presence of GVHD (446,550,616,617), but the reduction in mortality from GVHD offsets the increased relapse rate, and the overall survival rates are similar (550). Unrelated donor transplantation seems to provide sufficient GVL to sidestep this issue to some degree (552,719).

Definition of Relapse

Relapse of CML after allogeneic transplantation is fortunately relatively uncommon. The assessment of clinical relapse is straightforward—there will be an increase in the white blood cell count often accompanied by splenic enlargement and the typical manifestations of CML. Chromosomes typically show additional abnormalities induced by the conditioning regimen; however, these are not necessarily indicative of accelerated phase. Relapses demonstrated only through cytogenetics or molecular techniques are more problematic because cytogenetic or molecular relapse do not always translate into clinical relapse (720), and the absence of bcr/abl in the blood does not necessarily mean cure (708,711,718). Typically, more than one positive PCR obtained more than 3 months from the transplant has a 70% predictive value. Because adoptive immunotherapy functions best in patients with minimal disease, some investigators have used DLIs with only PCR evidence of relapse (721). This approach needs to be undertaken cautiously because there is potential morbidity from DLI. The use of quantitative PCR techniques may give a better assessment of the likelihood of relapse by monitoring the amount of bcr/abl mRNA over time, but even this technique is not infallible (715,722).

Management of Relapse

Second transplantation can be undertaken but at significant financial and physical cost. Survival can be expected to be approximately less than 25%—substantially lower than primary transplantation (723–726). IFN therapy may induce a remission, although its use after allogeneic transplantation is somewhat more toxic, and most patients will not completely clear the bcr/abl transcript (727). Nevertheless, 40% of patients may attain cytogenetic remission and improve survival, particularly in patients with late relapses (728). Interestingly, a report from the IBMTR suggests that survival after relapse is better than expected from a matched cohort without transplantation, suggesting some benefit may accrue from the cytoreduction *per se* (729). Abrupt discontinuation of immunosuppressants, such as cyclosporine, will occasionally put a patient back into remission. Imatinib mesylate (Gleevec) may also be very useful in reestablishing remission, although long-term follow-up data will be needed to assess the durability of this approach.

Recognition that immunologic control of the malignancy can be a critical part of the efficacy of HSCT led to the development of DLIs as a form of adoptive immunotherapy. Based on the initial clinical studies by Kolb and colleagues (607), DLIs have become a recognized, effective approach to relapse (580,581,608,610,619,721,730–733). This technique involves the administration of peripheral blood leukocytes obtained by apheresis from the original stem cell donor. The dose typically ranges from 10^7 to 10^8 cells/kilogram of recipient weight. The lower doses are more commonly used for molecular relapses and higher doses for clinical relapses. They may be unmanipulated or perhaps partially T-cell depleted (497). Responses take anywhere from 2 weeks to 10 months to become apparent and may or may not be associated with the development of GVHD; however, the development of GVHD is associated with a response in patients with clinical disease. When used to treat clinical relapses in stable phase disease, response rates are approximately 60%, increasing to more than 80% in the treatment of molecular relapses. Treatment of accelerated or blast phase is not usually successful. Here second transplantation may be more fruitful. Remissions are typically durable, but relapses have been observed several years after therapy (581,730). A serious complication of this therapy includes the development of aplasia if the leukemic hematopoiesis is destroyed and not replaced with adequate normal stem cells (580). Stimulation of the donor with filgrastim may not overcome this problem (734). Finally, acute and chronic GVHD occur in approximately 50% to 80% of patients. The frequency of GVHD appears to be lower with lower doses of lymphocytes (721) or intermittent dose regimens (582). The immunosuppression associated with GVHD after DLI may also contribute to a risk of opportunistic infections, and attention must be paid to prophylaxis and prompt treatment of fungi, pneumocystis, and a variety of viral infections (203,580).

Autologous Transplantation

Efforts to prolong stable phase by performing AHSCTs with either marrow or peripheral blood stem cells were undertaken by several investigators (735–738). The efficacy of this therapy is limited by the lack of a GVL response. Therefore, it should be at best equivalent to syngeneic transplantation. There may be periods of cytogenetic remission, but usually there was rapid recovery of stable-phase CML in many patients, but death due to blastic transformation was common, and this therapy is used only experimentally, because there is no evidence that it cures CML.

ACUTE LEUKEMIA

Acute Myelogenous Leukemia

Bone marrow transplantation is the preferred treatment for patients with advanced AML. The initial studies of marrow grafting in AML were undertaken on patients with refractory disease, and 10% to 30% disease-free survival rates (739–742) encouraged the use of allogeneic marrow grafting for patients in remission. It was hoped that transplantation before the development of multidrug resistance would improve the results of therapy. This expectation was confirmed by the 20% to 35% disease-free survival rates of patients receiving transplants in second or subsequent remission (656,743,744). Long-term survival is rare after leukemic relapse, and marrow grafting offers the only chance of obtaining a prolonged remission. The application of HSCT even earlier in the course of the disease, after first remission, results in improved antileukemic effects with long-term disease-free survival rates of 40% to 60% and relapse rates of 0% to 25%.

Most investigators agree that marrow transplantation is a better antileukemic therapy than conventional chemotherapy. Deaths from the conditioning regimen and from subsequent GVHD, however, negate some of the advantages of transplantation. As shown in Table 60-6, allogeneic transplantation is always associated with improved disease-free survival compared to autologous transplantation or chemotherapy, but this difference has rarely been statistically significant. In a large pediatric study, allogeneic transplantation was clearly superior, but autologous transplantation and conventional chemotherapy were equivalent (745). Thus, controversy has arisen regarding the best approach to patients in first remission who have compatible donors and who are younger than 45 to 50 years of age. The recognition that cytogenetics are a critical prognostic factor in the outcome of both transplanted (752–754) and untransplanted patients with AML has resulted in clearer recommendations. There have now been several prospective controlled studies comparing chemotherapy, autologous transplantation, and allogeneic transplantation in first remission AML. These data are summarized in Table 60-6. Limitations of these trials include the small number of assigned patients that actually receive a transplant as well as the observation that transplantation technology may have advanced substantially by the time the trial was published. For instance, in

uncontrolled studies, long-term disease-free survival of up to 70% has been reported in autologous transplantation in first remission (755). In general, transplantation in first remission should be reserved for patients with high-risk features, including poor prognosis cytogenetics. In addition, patients who have difficulty entering CR or who have delays in therapy may have outcome different than expected when a full-dose therapy is administered on time. They may well benefit from early transplantation. With improvements in GVHD control and supportive care, it is possible that allogeneic transplantation can become the treatment of choice. Alternatively, enhancements in autologous transplantation have also shown promising results that will need to be confirmed in randomized trials (755).

If marrow transplantation is not performed in first CR, consideration must also be given to the fate of patients who have compatible donors but relapse. Transplants performed in resistant relapse usually have a poor outcome—10% to 15% disease-free survival rate. Of patients who experience relapse, only approximately 30% to 40% achieve a second remission, and marrow transplantation in second remission benefits approximately 20% to 30% of those patients. Thus, less than 20% of patients who require reinduction are cured by transplants. Deaths during reinduction, anthracycline cardiomyopathy, infections, bleeding, or other complications exclude additional patients. It appears, however, that marrow grafting in early relapse, before any attempt at second remission induction, is associated with a 20% to 30% disease-free survival (742,743). Twenty percent to 30% of patients in whom marrow transplantation is delayed until relapse never require transplantation, and an additional 20% to 30% are cured with marrow grafting. The projected number of cured patients is similar to results with patients receiving transplants while in first remission. Larger prospective trials are required to establish the best approach. One problem with this more conservative approach is that it assumes prior HLA typing and immediate access to marrow transplantation. In practice, delays occur, and many patients require induction chemotherapy before consideration of marrow

TABLE 60-6. Randomized Trials of Chemotherapy versus Transplantation in First Remission

Study (and Reference Number)	Complete Remission (n)	Treated (n)	EFS (or Disease-Free Survival) (%)	Overall Survival (%)	p	Comment
SWOG (746)	295	36 (allogeneic)	41 transplanted vs. 42 matched donor (but not transplanted) vs. 29 no donor	—	NS	M3 acute myelogenous leukemia examined separately
GIMEMA (747)	343	144 (allogeneic)	55	59	.05 for EFS;	—
		104 (chemotherapy)	30	46	NS for OS	
		95 (autologous)	48	56		
GOELAM (748)	367	86 (allogeneic)	44	53	NS	—
		78 (chemotherapy)	40	50		
		75 (autologous)	44	55		
Intergroup (749)	518	92 (allogeneic)	43	46	NS	—
		106 (chemotherapy)	35	52		
		63 (autologous)	35	43		
MRC (750)	381	—	—	—	—	—
		191 (chemotherapy)	40	57	.04 for EFS;	
		190 (autologous)	54	45	NS for OS	
Pediatric studies						
POG (751)	263	79 (allogeneic)	52	>50	NS	—
		113 (chemotherapy)	36	44		
		71 (autologous)	38	40		
CCG (745)	656	181 (allogeneic)	55	60	.001 for EFS;	—
		177 (autologous)	48	48	.002 for OS	
		179 (chemotherapy)	53	53		

EFS, event-free survival; NS, not significant; OS, overall survival.

grafting. As control of GVHD improves and less toxic conditioning regimens are established, transplantation in first remission may be preferred. If the patient does not have a MHC-compatible donor, transplantation with a partially matched family member or a matched unrelated donor should not be undertaken in first remission unless warranted by other factors, such as cytogenetic abnormalities. Autologous transplantation does have a role in the management of AML in remission. Salvage rates of up to 30% may be achieved with marrow or PBSC transplantation. Unanswered questions are the role of marrow purging with monoclonal antibodies or chemotherapeutic agents, such as 4-HC220 (755–759), and the role of peripheral blood stem cell transplantation (757). The use of PBSC products does appear to overcome one limitation of autologous transplantation—slower hematopoietic recovery.

PROGNOSTIC FACTORS
Most studies identified age, remission status, and cytogenetics as significant prognostic factors in determining disease-free survival, although one collaborative study found that female gender, larger proportion of circulating blasts, absence of hepatitis, and shorter duration of symptoms were beneficial (760). Other studies identified leukocyte count lower than 10,000 (761) or 20,000/L (762), French-American-British (FAB) class M4 to M5 (762,763) or M4 to M6 (761), early remission (764), and extramedullary disease at diagnosis (763) as poor prognostic factors. A large analysis of risk factors for disease-free survival in AML in first remission was carried out by the IBMTR. They found age 25 years or younger, leukocyte count lower than 75,000/L, and absence of other organ impairment to be independent favorable prognostic factors. FAB classification correlated only to the extent that M4 to M5 AML tended to have higher leukocyte counts (765). Subsequent studies clearly associated known poor-risk cytogenetic groups such as monosomy 7, monosomy 5, and others with poorer outcomes after transplantation (752,753,764).

RELAPSE
As noted above, the risk of relapse is related to the stage at which transplantation occurs. Although efforts generally are made to avoid acute and chronic GVHD, GVHD appears to exert an antileukemic effect (602,613). There is indirect evidence of a GVL effect in that abrupt discontinuation of immunosuppression or donor lymphocytes may be tried to reestablish a remission; however, typically, DLI is less successful in AML than in CML. Evidence from the IBMTR indicates that T-cell depletion or transplantation from an identical twin results in higher relapse rates (766). However, with the use of TBI, thiotepa and cyclophosphamide as the preparatory regimen, and soybean agglutinin and sheep erythrocytes for T-cell depletion, there is not an increase in the rate of relapse in patients with AML in first or second remission rate (456). Currently, 72% of adults (under the age of 40 years) transplanted for AML in 1° CR, and 66% of those grafted in 2° CR are surviving disease free at a median follow-up of 4 years. For patients in 1° CR aged 40 to 61 years, disease-free survival is 60%; for those younger than 40 years of age, it is 76%. Acute and chronic GVHD have been detected in only 4% and 5% of cases, respectively.

It is often difficult to distinguish the effects of induction chemotherapy prior to the administration of donor lymphocytes from the effects of DLI *per se* (580,610,619). Nevertheless, it is generally considered the best alternative to establish a second remission. It is likely to be more effective and useful if the relapse occurs late. Second transplantation is not generally useful because of the high transplant-related mortality (723–725). However, allogeneic transplantation, both with traditional myeloablative conditioning and with attenuated regimens, is being studied, particularly if the relapse follows autologous transplantation.

Secondary Acute Myelogenous Leukemia and Myelodysplasia
Secondary acute myelogenous leukemia and myelodysplasia are hematopoietic diseases that share the common feature of refractoriness to standard therapy. Although some patients with myelodysplastic syndromes may have long survivals, these diseases are ultimately fatal. Myelodysplasia and leukemia that arise from prior irradiation or chemotherapy are particularly difficult to treat, and long-term survival is rare. The cohort of patients who develop MDS after autologous transplantation are a particular challenge, because prior therapy has been extensive and predisposes to more complications if allogeneic transplantation is considered.

Marrow transplantation has been successfully applied to patients with primary and secondary myelodysplasia and secondary leukemia in both adults and children (767–775). As expected, patients with early stage disease [either FAB subtypes or International Prognostic Scoring System (776)] such as refractory anemia or sideroblastic anemia do better than patients with refractory anemia with excess blasts or chronic myelomonocytic leukemia (772,777,778). Expected disease-free survival ranges from up to 70% for low-risk patients to approximately 25% for patients with advanced disease. As noted for AML, adverse cytogenetics is usually associated with inferior outcomes after HSCT. Disease-free survivals are generally better in primary myelodysplasia and are similar to the results expected in *de novo* AML. Unfortunately, patients undergoing transplantation for secondary marrow failure have a much poorer outcome, with disease-free survival averaging approximately 25% (769,774). For patients with early disease, the timing of the transplantation is important. It is usually preferable to wait until the cytopenias are morbid before proceeding to transplantation. It is necessary to be aware of the iron status of the patient, because transfusional iron loading may worsen outcomes (779).

Relapse is often treated with DLI, and one can reasonably expect a 10% to 25% chance of response (580,619,780). This evidence of a GVL response combined with the generally older age of patients with MDS and the increasing cohort of patients with therapy-related disease make this an interesting group to evaluate the use of nonmyeloablative transplantation.

Acute Lymphoblastic Leukemia
The use of marrow grafting in ALL is tempered by the excellent long-term disease-free survivals routinely achieved in this disease, especially in children. Current multidrug chemotherapy regimens, including CNS prophylaxis, induce sustained remissions in 70% to 90% of children with standard risk features (781–784). Even children with high-risk features are doing well, with disease-free survival rates of 60% to 84% (782). However, certain high-risk subgroups of patients with ALL in first remission, such as those who have a Ph chromosome, do poorly with routine therapy and are candidates for marrow grafting in first remission. Studies of marrow transplantation in first remission have been carried out in patients considered to be at high risk of relapse—those older than 20 to 30 years of age with leukocyte counts higher than 10,000 to 25,000 cells/L and with the Ph chromosome and the ALL associated with the MLL gene rearrangement, particularly infants with the t(4;11) rearrangement, or a mediastinal mass. Actuarial disease-free survival rates of 42% to 89% and actuarial relapse rates of 0% to 31% have been reported (Table 60-7) (785–792). Patients with Ph chromosome are at particularly high risk for relapse. For these patients, the results of allogeneic transplantation are particularly good, with 50% of such patients achieving long-term remission (789,793,794). Two prospective randomized trials have been performed for adult patients at high risk for relapse, comparing mar-

TABLE 60-7. Stem Cell Transplantation for the Treatment of Acute Lymphoblastic Leukemia in Remission

Study (and Reference Number)	Donor	Remission Status	Treatment	n	Actuarial Disease-Free Survival Rate (%)	Relapse Rate (%)
MSKCC (790)	Family member	First	HFTBI/Cy	31	64	13
		Second		12	42	25
		Third or relapse		16	23	64
GITMO (795)	Family member	Second	Varied	57	41	—
City of Hope (785)	Family member	First	Ara-c/Cy/FTBI or FTBI/Cy	39	63	16
Minnesota/DFCI (796)	Unrelated donor	First	Varied, primarily Cy/FTBI	52	32	33
		Second		106	42	17
		Third		79	23	47
		Fourth		14	31	73
		Relapse		83	16	60
France (797)	Family member	First	Cy/FTBI	116	45	12
IBMTR (798)	Family member	First	Varied	299	42	29
		Second		391	26	52
GEGMO (786)	Family member	First	Varied	27	59	14
EGBMT (787)	Family member	First	Varied	57	Approximately 60	6
		Second		96	Approximately 40	34
		Third or more		39	Approximately 12	73
Seattle (65)	Family member	Second	Cy/SFTBI or Cy/FTBI	57	40	42
Scandinavia (799)	Family member	Second	Varied	37	39	76
	Unrelated donor			28	54	40

Ara-c, arabinosyl cytosine; Cy, cyclophosphamide; FTBI, total body irradiation (F, fractionated; HF, hyperfractionated; SF, single fraction).

row grafts to chemotherapy in these patients (797,800). Patients in both studies were randomized based on the availability of an HLA-identical sibling. In one study, patients without a donor were randomized to receive chemotherapy alone versus chemotherapy plus an autologous transplant. In this study, the 5-year survival rates were no different for patients with standard-risk ALL. However, for patients with high-risk features at diagnosis, there was a significant difference in both survival and disease-free survival for those naturally randomized to receive an allogeneic transplant; 44% versus 20% for the other two groups (797). In the second study, patients received an allogeneic or autologous transplant. Recipients of autologous marrow were randomized to receive or not receive infusions of IL-2. The 3-year probability of disease-free survival was significantly higher for recipients of HLA-identical sibling allogeneic transplants—68% versus 26%, with no benefit seen in the group that received IL-2. Taken together, the two studies demonstrate that there is a role for allogeneic transplantation in certain subsets of patients with adult ALL in first remission, especially those patients with high-risk features of adult ALL. Preliminary results of a third large-scale international trial showed very encouraging improvement in 5-year event-free survival as well as relapse rates in patients undergoing allogeneic transplantation compared to chemotherapy or autologous transplantation, regardless of risk group (801).

As with AML, marrow grafting is the preferred therapy for advanced ALL. Although recent intensive regimens have improved remission durations in patients who have relapsed, most centers have poor long-term survival of patients who are no longer in first remission. The exception may be for children with a particularly long first remission for whom there are favorable results for allogeneic transplantation in third remission (655,802).

Most patients in second or subsequent remission are much more likely to die of their disease, and marrow grafting has been intensively applied to this group of patients. Many different conditioning regimens have been used, and patients have been treated at different times in the course of their disease, so the results of marrow transplantation reflect this heterogeneity. Disease-free survival

rates of 22% to 62% have been reported, with relapse rates of 13% to 62% (65,790,791,798,803–805), with the lowest relapse rates observed among recipients of hyperfractionated TBI with or without etoposide in the preparative regimen. In a large retrospective study, the data clearly indicate superior survival for TBI and cyclophosphamide conditioning compared to busulfan and cyclophosphamide for HLA-identical transplantation in children with ALL (806). There have been few prospective studies comparing chemotherapy to marrow transplantation following initial relapse, and the results are at odds (807,808). Not all groups are convinced that marrow transplantation affects survival in ALL (807,809,810). However, single-center and multicenter retrospective studies indicate that children with ALL in second remission fare significantly better if they received an allogeneic transplant as compared to chemotherapy alone (811–813). For recipients of HLA-identical transplants, the 5-year disease-free survival ranges from 30% to 56%, whereas those for patients with chemotherapy alone range from 17% to 38%. The observation is true for children with poor-risk features at initial presentation or whose initial remission was less than 18 or 24 months, as well as for those patients whose first remissions were longer than 24 months. The results observed for pediatric patients with ALL in remission transplanted with an unrelated donor are encouraging, but the long-term effect of the increased incidences of acute or chronic GVHD is unknown (812). Survival rates of patients treated in relapse parallel the results observed in relapsed AML or CML in blast crisis—10% to 15% (740,803,806).

PROGNOSTIC FACTORS

If transplantation is undertaken in first remission, the factors of non–T-cell phenotype, leukocyte count at diagnosis of 50,000 cells/L or higher, male donor to female recipient, and GVHD may be associated with a reduction in leukemia-free survival, whereas use of corticosteroids appears to increase leukemia-free survival (798). It has been difficult to identify prognostic factors that predict relapse after marrow transplantation in second or subsequent remission (65), although the Westminster group found standard prognostic factors in ALL to apply to marrow transplantation (814). An analysis by the IBMTR identified age 16 years or older, relapse while on therapy, GVHD prophylaxis without methotrexate, and absence of GVHD as factors that predict for a poor outcome (798). This difficulty may arise in part from the high relapse rates observed in these patients and the heterogeneity of chemotherapy regimens as well as transplantation-conditioning regimens.

RELAPSE

GVL may be a contributing mechanism for control of residual ALL. Several studies indicate substantially reduced relapse rates in patients with GVHD, as compared to patients without GVHD or patients who received autologous transplants, although the effect is less prominent than that observed in other diseases (611–613,804,815). Methotrexate used for GVHD prophylaxis may have antileukemic activity (798), but attempts to exploit antimetabolites as maintenance therapy have been unsuccessful (804). There is a substantial risk of CNS relapse (actuarial relapse rate is approximately 38%) that can be largely abrogated by the use of intrathecal methotrexate after transplantation (actuarial relapse rate of 7%), but with a dose-related increased risk of leukoencephalopathy in patients who received prior CNS therapy (816). Occasional patients who relapse after marrow grafting for ALL can sometimes achieve a CR with standard antileukemia therapy, although they relapse eventually (817). The results observed with the use of infusions of donor leukocyte for treatment of post-transplantation relapse of ALL are disappointing, with only anecdotal responses reported (581,610,619). This observation argues against significant GVL activity despite the observations cited above.

Autologous Marrow Transplantation

The success of allogeneic marrow grafting and the recognition that patient age, lack of a suitable donor, and GVHD-related toxicity limit its application in patients with leukemia spurred the investigation of AHSCT as a form of rescue after high-dose chemotherapy. Limitations to its use include concerns about infusing viable, clonogenic leukemic cells and a limited ability to detect minimal residual disease, but several important considerations affect the use of autografting. First, it appears unlikely that the results of AHSCT in a given situation will be better than the results of syngeneic marrow grafting. Thus, for similar conditioning regimens, the relapse rate after syngeneic transplantation probably reflects the best that can be achieved with AHSCT. Second, because substantial numbers of patients who receive allogeneic or syngeneic transplants relapse, conditioning regimens are not completely effective in eradicating residual leukemia. Finally, concern about unidentified leukemia in the harvested marrow and the need to remove those cells should be commensurate with the risk of leukemic relapse from disease that persists after the conditioning regimen. There is no point in purging the harvested marrow of leukemic cells if there is a high likelihood that there will be equal or greater numbers of viable leukemic cells in the patient after the conditioning regimen.

It is unlikely that marrow harvested in second or subsequent remission will not contain leukemic cells; however, the ability of these cells to reestablish clinical leukemia is unknown. Investigators who are concerned about these cells have attempted to reduce the numbers of malignant cells by treating the harvested marrow *ex vivo* with monoclonal antibodies (818–820), *in vitro* marrow culture (821), or the addition of pharmacologic agents (220,822). On the other hand, calculations based on animal models suggest that leukemic blasts have low clonogenicity and survive cryopreservation poorly and that conditioning regimens may alter the marrow microenvironment in a way that

favors normal progenitors (823,824). If one further estimates that the harvested marrow contains only a small proportion of the total-body leukemic burden, the contribution of these cells to relapse may be small. For instance, if there were 107 to 108 residual leukemic cells in the patient's marrow at harvest, and 1% to 5% of the marrow was removed, then approximately 105 to 106 leukemic cells would have been harvested. As few as 1% of the leukemic cells may be clonogenic, and these must survive cryopreservation and grow in a suboptimal microenvironment. If calculations based on rodent models apply, these additional factors may reduce the effective leukemic dose by an additional 1 to 2 logs (823–825). Thus, some investigators are performing AHSCTs for leukemia in first or subsequent remission without marrow purging (826,827). Because no controlled comparative studies have been reported, the value of purging remains an open question. Retrospective analysis of registry data is equivocal (827,828), and assessing the value of purging requires a large, multicenter trial.

In analyzing the results of AHSCT in leukemia, it is important to assess the duration of the preceding remissions. Patients with long remissions from chemotherapy tend to have long remissions after AHSCT; thus, unless the follow-up is as long as the chemotherapy-induced remissions, the benefit of AHSCT is exaggerated. Furthermore, how soon it is performed after remission is also important, because the subset of patients who can maintain long remissions before AHSCT may have more favorable prognoses. Because it reduces the number of harvested leukemic cells and the number of leukemic cells that have to be destroyed by the conditioning regimen, consolidation therapy before AHSCT is likely to be advantageous. Finally, patients with ALL who experienced relapses while on therapy had a shorter survival compared to patients who had relapses after completing maintenance treatments in some series (829) but not in others (815). Patients with Ph-positive ALL are also unlikely to do well with AHSCT.

AHSCT is an effective therapy for both AML and ALL. A disease-free survival rate of 50% to 70% at 2 to 4 years can be achieved in both AML and ALL in first remission (826–828). Transplants performed in second or subsequent remission have been reported to produce long-term survival rates that vary from 0% to 50% (220,818,826–829). The Minnesota group demonstrated that in patients with high-risk ALL, allogeneic and purged AHSCTs have similar outcomes. As noted in previous studies, the relapse rate was lower in the allogeneic patients with GVHD, but the toxicity related to the procedure was greater, and the overall disease-free survival rates were not statistically different (20% autologous versus 27% allogeneic) (815).

One problem observed during autografting for acute leukemia was delayed recovery of hematopoiesis. This delay probably results from a deficiency of harvested progenitors and toxicity of the marrow purging agents. In an effort to overcome this problem and to hasten hematopoietic recovery, administration of hematopoietic growth factors after transplantation have been examined, with mixed results (830,831).

HODGKIN'S DISEASE AND NON-HODGKIN'S LYMPHOMA

Hodgkin's Disease

Advances in the treatment of Hodgkin's disease have resulted in the cure of a substantial proportion of patients. Even patients who relapse after primary treatment may respond to additional chemotherapy or radiation therapy. Primary resistance to therapy, relapse early after the completion of chemotherapy, or relapse after a second chemotherapeutic regimen, however, is followed by disease progression and, ultimately, death. Because Hodgkin's disease is sensitive to both chemotherapy and radiation therapy, it was logical to increase the dose of these modalities and use allogeneic and autologous marrow grafting to reconstitute the marrow.

Allogeneic transplantation is the least studied approach to the therapy of Hodgkin's disease (832–834). Its potential advantage is the applicability to patients with therapy-induced stem cell damage or in whom a GVL effect is desired. It does appear that a GVL effect is observable, because relapse rates are lower in patients with GVHD. The European Group for Blood and Marrow Transplantation observed a 13% relapse rate in patients with grade II to IV GVHD, compared to 49% in patients without GVHD. Unfortunately, this improvement did not translate into improved survival (834). Nonmyeloablative approaches have also demonstrated a GVL response in Hodgkin's disease that may be exploitable (427,835). Additional potential benefits of allogeneic transplantation include eventual restoration of normal immunity, infusion of disease-free marrow, and avoidance of alkylating-agent treated marrow, which may develop myelodysplasia or secondary leukemia. On the other hand, the risks of GVHD are substantial, and many patients cannot receive TBI safely because of the striking increase in interstitial pneumonia in patients who had prior mantle irradiation (836). Recurrence rates after local irradiation suggest that the dose of TBI that can be safely administered may not be curative in most patients (833,837).

AHSCT appears to be an effective way of intensifying therapy and obtaining long disease-free survivals in patients with Hodgkin's disease. Because of concern about radiation therapy, most conditioning regimens have avoided TBI and concentrated on high-dose chemotherapy. In general, patients are considered candidates for AHSCT if the disease is resistant to primary therapy or if they relapse after conventional salvage regimens. The likelihood of obtaining a CR varies with the conditioning regimen used and the responsiveness of the disease. Because of heterogeneity of patients and treatment protocols, only broad conclusions can be drawn. Examples of reported conditioning regimens and responses are shown in Table 60-8. Substantial heterogeneity in dose and entrance criteria are found in the various studies, so the response rates are not strictly comparable, and the optimal dose and regimen have not been established. It is clear that high complete response rates are achievable with intensive therapy and that 40% to 60% of patients may have long-term progression-free survivals. Most relapses occur in sites of previous disease rather than as diffuse parenchymal seeding, supporting the contention that marrow purging is not necessary in this disease. The primary causes of treatment-related death are interstitial pneumonia and sepsis related to myelosuppression. The interstitial pneumonia appears to be more severe with higher doses of BCNU.

Multivariate analysis has led to the identification of groups of patients with different outcomes after AHSCT for Hodgkin's disease. Poor performance status, tumor responsiveness, extranodal disease, failure of more than two prior chemotherapy regimens, and large tumor size have been identified as adverse prognostic factors (839,841–844). Thus, if AHSCT is to be considered, it is most likely to be successful if applied soon after relapse or recognition that primary therapy is unsuccessful and after therapy to reduce the bulk of the disease. The use of AHSCT in patients who failed initial induction therapy has been promising, especially given the poor outlook using conventional salvage therapy. Progression-free survival ranges from 20% to 50% in various studies, compared to 10% to 30% with standard therapy (842,845,846). The role of transplantation in primary therapy is much less well defined. Although optimistic results have been reported (847), randomized trials will be necessary to define the role of AHSCT in primary therapy.

Of concern in evaluation of the data are the relative indolence of Hodgkin's disease in many patients and the persistence of radiographic abnormalities in the absence of disease. Thus, long-term follow-up is necessary to establish cure rates in this disease. Finally, there is a risk of secondary myelodysplasia after AHSCT. This probably reflects both prior chemoradiotherapy and effects of the AHSCT. With a non–TBI-containing conditioning regimen, this risk should be less than 5%, especially if prior therapy did not include nitrogen mustard.

Non-Hodgkin's Lymphoma

The use of marrow transplantation in non-Hodgkin's lymphoma was a natural outgrowth of the observations of long-term disease-free survivals in relapsed leukemia. Proper understanding of the role of marrow transplantation in these disorders requires a clear understanding of their heterogeneity. High- and intermediate-grade lymphomas often have excellent responses to conventional chemotherapy, and long disease-free survivals are common. Low-grade and some intermediate-grade lymphomas are extremely sensitive to chemotherapy or radiation therapy; however, that sensitivity has not translated into cures. A corollary of these observations is that the more aggressive lymphomas that are not cured are unlikely to have enduring responses to additional chemotherapy, whereas subsequent therapy is often useful in low-grade lymphomas. Furthermore, the duration of follow-up required to demonstrate a benefit from intensive therapy is much shorter for relapsed, aggressive lymphomas. Apparent benefits from intensive therapy in indolent lymphomas require confirmation over many years.

The results of transplantation for relapsed or resistant lymphoma parallel the treatment results of the resistant, relapsed leukemias. Therapy of bulky, resistant disease is generally much less effective than the treatment of a low volume of sensitive disease. The excellent results of conventional therapy

---

TABLE 60-8. Autologous Hematopoietic Stem Cell Transplantation for Relapsed Hodgkin's Disease

Center (and Reference Number)	n	Regimen	Event-Free or Progression-Free Survival (%)	Overall Survival (%)
University College (127)	155	BEAM	50	55
City of Hope (838)	85	TBI/Cy/Etoposide, CBV	58	75
Harvard (839)	102	CBV	42	65
Stanford (840)	119	TBI/Cy/Etoposide, CBV, CCNU/ Etoposide/Cy	48	52
French Registry (841)	158	Cy/TBI, CBV, BEAM	66	75

BEAM, BCNU, etoposide, cytarabine, melphalan; CBV, cyclophosphamide, BCNU, etoposide; CCNU, lomustine; Cy, cyclophosphamide; TBI, total body irradiation.

TABLE 60-9. Autologous Hematopoietic Stem Cell Transplantation for Relapsed Non-Hodgkin's Lymphoma

Center (and Reference Number)	n	Regimen	Event-Free or Progression-Free Survival (%)	Overall Survival (%)
Harvard (862)	78	CBV	54	—
Parma (863)	102	BEAC	46	53
Stanford (864)	134	Cy/Etoposide/TBI	52	61
	87	CBV	46	46
Rochester (865)	136	BEAC	34	—
M. D. Anderson (866)	91	Varied	40	42
SWOG (867)	94	Cy/TBI, CBV	33	44
EBMT (868)	82 (age ≥55 yr)	Varied	37	38

BEAC, BCNU, etoposide, cytarabine, cyclophosphamide; CBV, cyclophosphamide, BCNU, etoposide; Cy, cyclophosphamide; TBI, total body irradiation.

require the selection of patients who are likely to do poorly, if marrow transplantation is to be applied early in the course of therapy of non-Hodgkin's lymphoma.

ALLOGENEIC TRANSPLANTATION FOR NON-HODGKIN'S LYMPHOMA

Allogeneic transplantation has been applied to small numbers of patients, in large part because of the relative success of AHSCT. Nevertheless, in patients who have a compatible donor and in whom it is perceived that a GVL response will be valuable because of myelodysplasia or low-grade lymphoma, allogeneic transplantation has been used. Long-term disease-free survival rates of 10% to 56% have been reported in this group of refractory patients (848–855). A GVL effect has also been detected (856–858). Because TBI was a principal component of therapy, prior chest irradiation and perhaps the prior use of drugs such as bleomycin contributed to a high incidence of fatal interstitial pneumonia.

AUTOLOGOUS TRANSPLANTATION FOR AGGRESSIVE NON-HODGKIN'S LYMPHOMA

AHSCT can be applied to larger numbers of patients than allogeneic transplantation, and its modest transplant-related mortality makes it a more useful option in many patients with lymphomas. Early reports by Appelbaum and colleagues (859,860) of successful high-dose therapy of Burkitt's lymphoma resulted in the initiation of large numbers of subsequent trials of AHSCT in all categories of non-Hodgkin's lymphoma. Some form of high-dose therapy with autologous stem cell support is now considered standard care in relapsed aggressive non-Hodgkin's lymphoma (861). Some of these results are summarized in Table 60-9. The value of AHSCT in aggressive lymphomas was established in the Parma trial (863), which randomly compared conventional dose chemotherapy to AHSCT in relapsed patients with responsive disease. Event-free survival (46% versus 12%, $p = .001$) and overall survival (53% versus 32%, $p = .038$) were better in the high-dose therapy group. Subsequent analyses of this trial showed that International Prognostic Index scores correlated with response to chemotherapy, but the relationship was not seen in the AHSCT group, suggesting that poor prognostic features at relapse should not be used to exclude patients from AHSCT (869). However, they also found that relapse within 1 year identified a group with generally worse outcomes (870). Typically, it is recommended that salvage chemotherapy be administered prior to AHSCT, because survival appears better in patients in whom chemotherapy has been administered (871).

In properly selected patients, it appears that regimens based on chemotherapy or TBI are effective, although it is likely that TBI-containing regimens are most effective in patients with minimal disease (864,872). In addition, chemotherapy regimens may allow the subsequent use of local radiation therapy for sites of resistant disease.

AUTOLOGOUS TRANSPLANTATION FOR EARLY NON-HODGKIN'S LYMPHOMA

The success of the International Prognostic Index (873) led to studies designed to determine whether AHSCT could be applied early in the course of therapy to patients with high-risk disease. Several randomized trials have addressed this issue in slightly different ways, making a clear comparison difficult (861). Table 60-10 summarizes the randomized trials of early therapy. It appears that in selected patients with high-risk, aggressive large-cell lymphoma, there is a benefit to early transplantation; however, many issues remain unsettled regarding patient selection, pretransplant chemotherapy, and conditioning regimen selection.

AUTOLOGOUS TRANSPLANTATION FOR LOW-GRADE LYMPHOMAS

The use of AHSCT in low-grade lymphoproliferative disorders has been controversial, because the well-known indolent nature of these cancers makes extremely long follow-up necessary. Although initial response rates are very high, there is a tendency toward relapses, which results in outcomes similar to those expected after conventional dose chemotherapy. Representative large studies are summarized in Table 60-11. Typically, the marrow is infiltrated with cells expressing the bcl-2/IgH [t(14;18)] gene rearrangement. It appears that in those patients whose marrow can be purged such that the rearrangement is undetectable by PCR, freedom from relapse may increase to as much as 83% (878). There is particular concern about the risk of secondary myelodysplasia in these patients (214). The benefits of transplantation are difficult to prove in the absence of a clinical trial.

Once follicular non-Hodgkin's lymphomas transform into a higher-grade malignancy, the prognosis becomes noticeably worse. AHSCT has been used successfully to treat patients with these transformations, with outcomes ranging from 20% to 50% (881,882). Interestingly, many of these patients will relapse with the original indolent lymphoma and have long survivals after relapse.

Mantle cell lymphoma is often considered low grade, although its course is more rapidly progressive than follicular lymphomas. Autologous transplantation has been relatively ineffective in this disease (883,884), but there does appear to be a detectable GVL response after allogeneic transplantation (885).

Purging

Non-Hodgkin's lymphomas have a well-described propensity to circulate in the blood and invade the bone marrow (886,887). Often, the level of involvement may not be clinically apparent (887,888). Several investigators have attempted to purge the marrow of clinically detectable and undetectable lymphoma cells with either immunologic or pharmacologic techniques

TABLE 60-10. Randomized Trials of Autologous Hematopoietic Stem Cell Transplantation for Early Therapy of Non-Hodgkin's Lymphoma

Center (and Reference Number)	n	Regimen	EFS or Progression-Free Survival (%)	OS (%)	p
GELA (874)	125	LNH84	55	64	.02 (DFS)
	111	CBV	39	49 (8 yr)	.04 (OS)
Italian NHL Study Group (875)	61	VACOP-B	60	65	NS
	63	VACOP-B + AHSCT	80	65 (6 yr)	High-risk disease → DFS 48% vs. 87% favoring AHSCT (p = .008)
GELA (876)	183	ACVB	54	63	.01 (DFS)
	187	Intensified regimen	41	47	
Milan (877)	50	MACOP-B	76	81	.004 (EFS)
	48	High-dose therapy	49	55	.09 (OS)

ACVB, doxorubicin, cyclophosphamide, vinblastine, bleomycin; AHSCT, autologous hematopoietic stem cell transplantation; CBV, cyclophosphamide, BCNU, etoposide; DFS, disease-free survival; EFS, event-free survival; MACOP-B, methotrexate, doxorubicin, cyclophosphamide, vincristine, prednisone, bleomycin; NS, not significant; OS, overall survival; VACOP-B, etoposide, doxorubicin, cyclophosphamide, vincristine, prednisone, bleomycin.

TABLE 60-11. Autologous Hematopoietic Stem Cell Transplantation for Relapsed Low-Grade Non-Hodgkin's Lymphoma

Center (and Reference Number)	n	Regimen	Purging	Event-Free or Progression-Free Survival (%)	Overall Survival (%)
St. Bartholomew's (879)	99	Cy/TBI	CD10, CD19, CD20	63	69 (5 yr); disease-free survival but not overall survival exceeds historic control
Nebraska (880)	100	Varied	None	44	65 (4 yr)
DFCI (878)	153	Cy/TBI	Varied; primarily CD10, CD20	42	66 (8 yr)

Cy/TBI, cyclophosphamide/total body irradiation.

(878,889). PCR technology has been used to detect residual lymphoma cells after purging to determine both the efficacy of purging and whether detectable lymphoma has an effect on outcome. In AHSCT for low-grade lymphomas with t(14;18), the presence of detectable bcl-2/IgH gene rearrangements was associated with a high relapse rate, suggesting that the purging may have been of use. On the other hand, the ability to detect residual disease after purging may also simply select patients with better prognoses (878). In practice, whether the marrow has been treated, relapse occurs most often at sites of previous disease rather than as diffuse seeding of parenchymal organs with nodules of similar age. As noted in the discussion of acute leukemia, until the conditioning regimens are capable of eradicating residual disease more effectively, it may be impossible to determine whether purging has a role in AHSCT for lymphoma. This assessment requires a large, randomized trial. There has been no prospective trial comparing purged to unpurged marrow or PBSC products; therefore, there can be no firm recommendations regarding its risks or benefits. An interesting twist will be the use of intravenous rituximab. This anti-CD20 monoclonal antibody is often capable of reducing PBSC products to PCR negativity. It is possible that this sort of *in vivo* purging may supercede *ex vivo* purging (889).

CHRONIC LYMPHOCYTIC LEUKEMIA

Despite the prevalence of CLL, the indolence of this disease and its propensity to affect older people have resulted in relatively limited use of both allogeneic and autologous transplantation. Furthermore, its indolence precludes accurate assessment of its value until many years have passed. Nevertheless, there

are encouraging preliminary studies suggesting a role for both autologous and allogeneic transplantation in selected patients with CLL. The IBMTR reported on 54 patients with a median age of 41 years who underwent allogeneic transplantation. Thirty-eight patients (70%) entered hematologic remission, resulting in a 3-year survival probability of 46% (95% CI, 32,60). Three-year survival probability ranged from 86% (95% CI, 62,100) in patients with disease responsive to pretransplant chemotherapy to 61% (95% CI, 38,84) in those with stable disease, and 23% (95% CI, 2,44) in those with progressive disease (890). Similar results have been obtained in smaller single institution studies (855,891–893). Interestingly, patients may not clear the CLL cells immediately. They may gradually reduce over time, further supporting the presence of a GVL reaction in this disease. The presence of a GVL response has encouraged studies of nonmyeloablative transplantation, with promising early results (458).

Autologous transplantation has been somewhat more controversial because essentially all patients have blood or marrow detectable at the time of stem cell collection. Nevertheless, there are studies suggesting a benefit to AHSCT, particularly if the stem cell product can be purged to PCR negativity (894).

MULTIPLE MYELOMA

Multiple myeloma is another moderately aggressive lymphoid neoplasm that cannot be cured with conventional therapy. McElwain's early studies of the dose-response relationship of melphalan in myeloma (895) ultimately led to a large number of trials of high-dose therapy and both autologous and allogeneic HSCT. A few representative studies are listed in Table 60-12.

TABLE 60-12. Autologous and Allogeneic Hematopoietic Stem Cell Transplantation for Multiple Myeloma

Center (and Reference Number)	n	Regimen	GVHD Prophylaxis	CR (%)	EFS or Progression-Free Survival (%)	Overall Survival (%)
Autologous HSCT						
French Intergroup (896)	200	VMCP/BVAP vs. VMCP/BVAP + Mel/TBI	N/A	14 vs. 38 ($p < .001$)	10 vs. 29 ($p = .01$)	12 (5 yr) vs. 52 ($p = .03$)
Arkansas (897)	1000	Mel (1 or 2 high-dose regimens) + other	N/A	44	25 Chromosome 13 abnormality → EFS = 0	40 (5 yr)
Allogeneic HSCT						
EBMT (898)	162	Cy/TBI, Mel/TBI, other	54: T-cell depletion; 108: other	44	34 (CR patients only)	32 (4 yr); 28 (7 yr)
Vancouver (899)	65	Varied	CyA plus MTX or methyl-prednisolone	62	40% (1 yr)	46.5 (3 yr)
EBMT (900)	189 allogeneic vs. 189 autologous	Varied	Varied	48 vs. 40	Median 11 mo vs. 20 mo	Median 18 mo vs. 34 mo ($p = .001$)

BVAP, carmustine, vincristine, doxorubicin, prednisone; CR, complete remission; Cy, cyclophosphamide; CyA, cyclosporine; EFS, event-free survival; GVHD, graft-versus-host disease; HSCT, hematopoietic stem cell transplantation; Mel, melphalan; MTX, methotrexate; N/A, not applicable; TBI, total body irradiation; VMCP, vincristine, melphalan, cyclophosphamide, prednisone.

Prognostic factors are typically the same ones that predict survival without transplantation. The Arkansas data indicate that the 5-year event-free survival ranges from 0% in the worst group (i.e., abnormal chromosome 13) to 52% in the best risk group (normal chromosome 13, short duration of standard dose therapy, low β_2-microglobulin, and low C-reactive protein) (897). A population-based study by the Nordic Myeloma Study Group compared transplanted patients with a similar control group and concluded that AHSCT improved survival (901). Tandem autologous procedures may be useful in some patients, particularly with good risk prognostic factors (902). Prognostic factors in allogeneic transplantation are less well defined but may include early disease, female gender, single prior therapy regimen, and CR before transplantation (898). In a retrospective case-control study, allogeneic transplantation resulted in poorer long-term survival because regimen-related toxicity outweighed any graft-versus-myeloma (GVM) effect. There was an advantage seen in allogeneic transplants only in comparing those patients who survived 1 year (900).

As noted above, there appears to be a GVM effect that can be detected in a lower relapse rate after allogeneic transplantation (900,903) and in objective responses to DLIs (904,905). Nonmyeloablative transplants may offer the possibility of taking advantage of this GVM response with less initial toxicity; however, data are not yet available to analyze this alternative.

AMYLOIDOSIS

Relatively little has been published on the use of HSCT in the treatment of primary amyloidosis. Although responses have been reported, the toxicity rate appears to be quite high. One retrospective study had a 43% treatment-related mortality rate (906), whereas a second study showed that if two or fewer organ systems were involved, survival was 87%, but it decreased to 40% if more than two organ systems were affected (907). Nevertheless, complete responses of the evidence of plasma cell clonality has been observed along with improvements in organ system dysfunction due to amyloidosis. Thus, AHSCT appears to be feasible in a subset of patients with limited organ involvement and good prognostic features. Its overall role in the management of primary amyloidosis remains to be determined (908).

OTHER MALIGNANCIES

Any disorder of lymphoid or hematopoietic tissue is a potential target of marrow transplantation. The primary criteria for success are the responsiveness of the disease to the conditioning regimen and the age and physical status of the patient. Some chemotherapy-responsive solid tumors, such as breast cancer and neuroblastoma, may also respond to marrow transplantation. A discussion of those diseases is beyond the scope of this chapter.

GENETIC DISORDERS

Conceptually, any congenital disorder whose only clinical manifestation is in cells of hematopoietic origin (e.g., thalassemia, sickle cell anemia, SCIDS, Wiskott-Aldrich syndrome) can be permanently corrected by allogeneic bone marrow transplantation from an unaffected donor. In addition, a number of congenital enzyme deficiencies, although manifest in many parts of the body, can be clinically corrected if a source of the enzyme is distributed to all relevant areas by a cell of bone marrow origin, such as the monocyte-macrophage (e.g., Gaucher's disease, mucopolysaccharidoses) (909).

IMMUNODEFICIENCY DISORDERS

Many congenital immunodeficiencies that represent a failure of T-cell, B-cell, NK-cell, or phagocyte function have been delineated. Some of these, such as selective IgA deficiency, are relatively common and also generally benign in their clinical manifestations. Others are uniformly fatal. The two major such disorders for which marrow transplantation has been applied are SCIDS and Wiskott-Aldrich syndrome.

Severe Combined Immunodeficiency

SCIDS represents a pathophysiologically diverse group of diseases, all characterized by a profound deficiency of cellular immunity that results in recurrent infections and death at an early age (910,911). Some kindreds demonstrate an autosomal-recessive and others an X-linked mode of inheritance. Although progress has been made in the identification of the genetic mutations that cause the different forms of SCIDS, in most cases, the basic lesion is undefined. Two well-defined enzyme deficiencies are associated with SCIDS: adenosine deaminase and purine nucleoside phosphorylase deficiency. Regardless of cause, however, marrow transplantation represents the treatment of choice for this otherwise uniformly fatal disorder.

The profound deficiency in T-cell immunity in this disorder is illustrated by the fact that approximately one-fourth of SCIDS neonates are engrafted with maternal cells *in utero*. The extent of that graft varies, as does the presence or absence of concomitant GVHD after birth, because of the obligatory haploidentical graft (912,913). Indeed, GVHD may be the presenting manifestation of SCIDS in an infant.

When an MHC-compatible sibling donor is available, conditioning is usually not necessary because the recipient, by definition, lacks an immune system capable of rejecting the infused marrow, and a physiologic niche for the lymphoid stem cell appears to be present in most cases. Historically, many patients have been deliberately given lower doses of nucleated cells than the typical transplantation patient (often 0.5×10^8 cells) in an attempt to reduce the risk of acute GVHD. Failure to engraft, even with these lower doses, has been unusual (19,914–916). In addition, many patients have received transplants without posttransplantation prophylactic immunosuppression for GVHD. Even with the lack of prophylactic therapy, acute GVHD in these patients has generally been relatively mild, and chronic GVHD is rare. Whether this is due to the young age of the patient and donor, the low dose of marrow used, the lack of pretransplantation conditioning, the partial mixed chimerism obtained, or some aspect of the underlying disease is unknown.

After transplantation, these patients become partial mixed chimeras with T lymphocytes uniformly of donor origin but myeloid and erythroid cells of host origin (917). B lymphocytes are of donor origin approximately one-half of the time, a result consistent with the fact that some SCIDS patients have normal numbers of B cells at the time of transplantation and thus may lack a niche for the B-lymphocyte stem cell. Successful transplantation results in return of measurable T-lymphocyte numbers and function. Approximately 15% of patients who receive MHC-compatible sibling donor marrows fail to develop normal B-cell function after transplantation and may therefore require continued replacement γ-globulin. The overall long-term success rate of MHC compatible transplantation is over 65%, with 80% survival for patients transplanted in the 1980s and followed for up to 10 years (918).

For patients without a histocompatible donor, the use of a haploidentical parent as donor combined with *ex vivo* T-cell depletion of the donor marrow has been remarkably successful. Before the development of adequate T-cell–depletion techniques, at least 35 patients underwent transplantation with unmanipulated histoincompatible marrow (915). None survived long. With the use of haploidentical, T-cell–depleted marrow, however, long-term success rates of 50% to 75% have been achieved (540,919–923). In many cases, several grafts may be necessary, and conditioning may also be required. Late complications include an occasional failure to achieve complete immune reconstitution and, rarely, the development of a B-cell–derived fatal lymphoproliferative disease (924).

One of the more exciting developments in transplantation for SCIDS is the application of gene therapy to the treatment of SCIDS. *In vitro* models have supported the concept, and two patients with SCIDS-X1, an X-linked inherited disorder characterized by an early block in T and NK lymphocyte differentiation, have received autologous CD34+ cells that were infected with complementary DNA containing a defective Moloney retrovirus–derived vector and the gene encoding the γ cytokine receptor subunit of IL-2, -4, -7, -9, and -15 receptors. Both patients achieved full immunologic reconstitution (925).

Wiskott-Aldrich Syndrome

Wiskott-Aldrich syndrome is an X-linked disorder characterized by eczema, thrombocytopenia, small platelets, and severe depression of T-cell immunity with resultant recurrent infections. It is associated with a specific defective surface membrane sialoglycoprotein on lymphocytes (926). Unlike patients with SCIDS, successful transplantation of patients with Wiskott-Aldrich syndrome requires an ablative conditioning regimen (927). Wiskott-Aldrich syndrome patients also differ from patients with SCIDS in that they may develop both fatal acute and chronic GVHD. Nevertheless, long-term successful results are reported in over 70% of patients receiving histocompatible marrow grafts (928–931).

For patients lacking an HLA identical donor, the use of T-cell depleted haploidentical transplants has had limited success, mostly due to the development of posttransplantation EBV–lymphoproliferative disorder (930). However, the use of HLA-compatible unrelated donors for boys younger than the age of 5 years at the time of transplant has allowed for a probability of survival of 80%, identical to that observed among recipients of HLA-identical sibling transplants (931).

Hemoglobinopathies

Marrow transplantation has been carried out to cure patients with thalassemia (932–935). Initially, patients with advanced disease fared poorly after transplantation when given irradiation as part of the conditioning regimen. This poor outcome discouraged more frequent application of this therapy. More recent series, however, in which patients were conditioned with high-dose chemotherapy (busulfan and cyclophosphamide), achieved more encouraging results. In 222 patients younger than 16 years of age with β-thalassemia, the actuarial survival rate at 2 years was 82%, with a disease-free survival rate of 75%. In this group of patients receiving multiple transfusions, the graft failure rate was approximately 5%. Deaths were due to graft rejection, pneumonitis, and septicemia, with either acute or chronic GVHD as contributing factors in approximately one-half of the fatalities. The primary determinants of outcome were related to extent of prior chelation therapy, presence of portal fibrosis, and presence of hepatomegaly. When these factors were organized into three risk groups based on severity, the probability of event-free survival ranged from 94% in class 1, to 77% in class 2, and to 53% in class 3. Although studies in leukemic patient populations have documented a significantly increased risk of serious venoocclusive disease in patients with abnormal hepatic function before transplantation, there was little liver disease after transplantation in the thalassemic population, although most patients had biopsy-proven hepatic dysfunction due to iron overload and transfusion-associated hepatitis before transplantation. In experimental models, iron overload is reversed by marrow transplantation (936); whether this occurs in humans is unknown but expected. Thus, marrow grafting (at least from MHC-identical sibling donors) is a viable therapeutic option for patients with thalassemia. It appears that this approach is preferable to a program of vigorous transfusion and iron chelation therapy.

For patients with sickle cell anemia, patient selection is critical, given the variable natural history of sickle cell disease. After transplantation, the observation that this therapy can eliminate sickle hemoglobin production and establish normal erythropoiesis was made in patients whose primary indication for transplantation was hematologic malignancy (937,938). It was not until recently that allogeneic transplantation was seen as an acceptable approach to the treatment of sickle cell disease. Transplantation is associated with a high mortality from GVHD, infections, and conditioning regimen toxicity; but with careful patient selection, it has now been demonstrated that excellent overall and event-free survival can be achieved with transplants from HLA-identical sibling donors (939,940). In each of these two studies (comprising 50 patients each), the overall survival and event-free survival approached 95% and 85%, respectively. No new events after transplantation occurred in either series, and complications related to sickle cell disease either resolved or stabilized. Despite these excellent results, it is difficult to justify transplantation for every child with the diagnosis of sickle cell disease and to identify the patients who will be most disabled by their disease and in whom the transplantation-related morbidity and mortality is justified. Certainly a child with a history of strokes or recurrent acute chest syndrome should be a candidate, but in reality, it is rarely as clear, as the primary indication in the latter study was vasoocclusive pain episodes.

Fanconi's Anemia

Fanconi's anemia is an autosomal-recessive disorder characterized by diverse congenital abnormalities and progressive marrow failure with eventual evolution to myelodysplasia and acute leukemia. These patients are also at increased risk for developing other malignancies. The phenotype of patients is highly variable, and not all the genetic defects resulting in the clinical manifestations have been identified. However, the disease can be cured with stem cell transplantation (941), and it was in the treatment of this disorder that cord blood was first demonstrated to be a viable source of hematopoietic stem cells for HSCT (942).

Osteopetrosis

Infantile malignant osteopetrosis (marble bone disease) is an autosomal-recessive disorder characterized by absent or dysfunctional osteoclasts. Because experimental work demonstrated the origin of the osteoclast from a bone marrow–derived cell, specifically the monocyte-macrophage, it is logical to postulate that marrow transplantation of a normal hematopoietic stem cell could be the reverse of this disease. It has been demonstrated that after transplantation, the osteoblasts are of recipient origin, the osteoclasts are of donor origin, and bone remodeling can be expected (431,943,944). Although these anecdotal cases demonstrate that osteopetrosis can be reversed by a successful transplant, most patients do not achieve long-term durable donor cell engraftment, and their disease ultimately recurs.

Storage Diseases

Congenital deficiencies of enzymes that result in disease by virtue of the accumulation of toxic products are potentially treatable by a variety of replacement techniques (945). Infusion of the enzyme or a modified form of the enzyme is possible in some experimental circumstances, for example, in the treatment of nonstorage disorders, such as adenosine deaminase deficiency (946) or α_1-antitrypsin deficiency (947). An alternative is to transplant a tissue that contains cells of normal enzymatic function that can act by replacing the tissue-specific abnormal cells of the host and also as a source of enzyme to correct the systemic disorder. Two major such tissues have been so used: the liver (948) and

the bone marrow. Whether the systemic disorder is in fact corrected by such an approach obviously depends on a variety of kinetic and distribution considerations. In some storage diseases, such as Gaucher's disease, much of the morbidity is caused by macrophages that are engorged, cause mass effects, and injure normal organ parenchyma. Replacement of these macrophages with cells that have the proper enzymatic pathways should alleviate much of the pathology.

Lysosomal storage diseases that have been treated with allogeneic marrow transplantation include Gaucher's disease (949), the mucopolysaccharidoses (950) [including Hurler's disease (951), Hunter's disease, Sanfilippo's syndrome type B, Morquio's disease, and Maroteaux-Lamy syndrome (952)], and metachromatic leukodystrophy. In general, the systemic enzymatic defect has been well corrected by the allograft in these patients. One of the critical issues in the application of this technique to some of these disorders is the question of whether neurologic disease can be corrected by marrow transplantation. Some experimental evidence has suggested that pluripotent hematopoietic progenitors may exist in the CNS and that microglial cells may be of bone marrow origin (953,954). In addition, it may be possible for toxic substrates to be transported across the blood-brain barrier and enzymatically degraded in the systemic circulation with beneficial result. In the twitcher mouse (an animal model of the sphingolipidosis, Krabbe's disease), however, marrow grafting from unaffected donors leads to improvement in peripheral neuropathy, but CNS disease progresses unabated (955). Data on humans remain incomplete, and the issue is unresolved; successful marrow grafting is more likely to prevent organ damage than to reverse established injury. Thus, transplantation needs to be undertaken in infancy or even *in utero*.

Other Red Cell, Granulocyte, and Platelet Disorders

Any disorders of the marrow can be treated successfully with transplantation. These diseases include Kostmann's syndrome (956), chronic granulomatous disease (240), neutrophil-actin dysfunction (957), Chédiak-Higashi syndrome (958), and Diamond-Blackfan anemia (959,960).

Autoimmune Disorders

Both allogeneic and autologous transplantation have been studied for the treatment of severe autoimmune disorders. Allogeneic HSCT is the more intuitively obvious therapy, because replacement of the defective immune response should cure the disease, albeit at the risk of transplant-related toxicity. Many patients with concomitant malignancies and autoimmune disorders have had both diseases cured with allogeneic transplantation. In addition, AHSCT has been shown to be promising in animal models of systemic lupus erythematosis (SLE), autoimmune encephalomyelitis, and adjuvant arthritis. Indeed, close observations of patients receiving allogeneic HSCT for severe aplastic anemia hints at the value of autologous transplantation. Allogeneic transplantation has been reported for hemolytic anemia, pure red cell aplasia, Evans' syndrome, SLE, scleroderma, and others. Reduced intensity conditioning regimens are particularly appealing for these diseases and are under investigation. Severe aplastic anemia is the prime example of an autoimmune disease treated with allogeneic transplantation. Dysregulated immunity appears to impair hematopoiesis in many patients with severe aplastic anemia. Interestingly, often a successful transplantation is accompanied by mixed lymphohematopoietic chimerism or autologous recovery. This observation suggests that autologous transplantation and its intrinsic immunosuppression might be useful therapy for other autoimmune disorders. Ultimately, cure of the autoimmunity will require the development of tolerance to the antigens that stimulated the immune attack. AHSCT for multiple sclerosis, SLE, rheumatoid arthritis, and scleroderma has been reported in small numbers of patients. The critical issue is patient selection to assure that the severity of the underlying disease warrants the toxicity of the transplantation. Small numbers of patients meet the eligibility requirements for transplantation studies, but there are collaborative studies in the United States and Europe that should provide interpretable data (961,962).

REFERENCES

1. Santos GW. The history of bone marrow transplantation. *Clin Haematol* 1983;12:611.
2. Morrison M, Samwick AA. Intramedullary (sternal) transfusion of bone marrow. *JAMA* 1940;115:1708.
3. Osgood EE, Riddle MC, Mathews TJ. Aplastic anemia treated with daily transfusions and intravenous marrow. *Ann Intern Med* 1939;13:357.
4. Jacobsen LO, Simmons EL, Marks EL, et al. The role of the spleen in radiation injury and recovery. *J Lab Clin Med* 1950;35:746.
5. Barnes DWH, Loutit JF. Spleen protection: the cellular hypothesis. In: Bacq ZM, Alexander P, eds. *Radiobiology Symposium 1954*. New York: Academic Press, 1955:134.
6. Lorenz E, Uphoff D, Reid TR, et al. Modification of irradiation injury in mice and guinea pigs by bone marrow injections. *J Natl Cancer Inst* 1951;12:197.
7. Barnes DWH, Loutit JF. Immunological and histological response following spleen treatment in irradiated mice. In: Mitchel JS, Holmes BE, eds. *Progress in radiobiology*. Edinburgh: Oliver and Boyd, 1956:291.
8. Billingham RE, Brent LA. A simple method for inducing tolerance of skin homografts in mice. *Transplant Bull* 1957;4:67.
9. Elkins WL. Cellular immunology and pathogenesis of graft-versus-host reaction. *Prog Allergy* 1971;15:78.
10. Simonsen M. Graft versus host reactions. Their natural history and applicability as tools of research. *Prog Allergy* 1971;6:349.
11. Van Bekkum D, De Vries M. *Radiation chimeras*. New York: Academic Press, 1967.
12. Billingham RE. The biology of graft-versus-host reactions. *Harvey Lecture Series 1966–1967*;62:21.
13. Grebe S, Streilein J. Graft-versus-host reactions: their natural history and applicability as tools of research. *Prog Allergy* 1976;22:120.
14. Bach FH, Sachs DHC. Transplantation immunology. *N Engl J Med* 1987;317:489.
15. Yunis EJ, Awdeh Z, Raum D, Alper CA. The MHC in bone marrow transplantation. *Clin Haematol* 1983;12:641.
16. Thomas ED, Lochte HL, Lu WC, Ferrebee JW. Intravenous infusion of bone marrow in patients receiving radiation and chemotherapy. *N Engl J Med* 1957;257:491.
17. Mathe G, Jammet H, Pendic B, et al. Transfusions et greffes de moelle osseuse homologue chez des humans irradies a haute dose accidentellement. *Rev Franc Etudes Clin et Biol* 1959;IV:226.
18. Bortin MM. A compendium of reported bone marrow transplants. *Transplantation* 1970;9:571.
19. Gatti RA, Meuwissen HJ, Allen HD, et al. Immunological reconstitution of sex-linked lymphopenic immunological deficiency. *Lancet* 1968;2:1366.
20. Bach FH, Albertini RJ, Joo P, et al. Bone marrow transplantation in a patient with Wiskott-Aldrich syndrome. *Lancet* 1968;2:1364.
21. de Koning J, Dooren LJ, van Bekkum DW, et al. Transplantation of bone-marrow cells and fetal thymus in an infant with lymphopenic immunological deficiency. *Lancet* 1969;1:1223.
22. O'Reilly RJ. Allogeneic bone marrow transplantation: current status and future directions. *Blood* 1983;62:941.
23. Thomas ED, Storb R, Clift RA, et al. Bone marrow transplantation. *N Engl J Med* 1975;292:832.
24. Nathan DG. Bone marrow transplantation. *Clin Haematol* 1983;12:611.
25. Bodmer WF. HLA 1987. In: Dupont B, ed. *Immunogenetics and histochemistry*. Vol. I. New York: Springer-Verlag, 1989.
26. Bodmer JG, Marsh S, Albert ED, et al. Nomenclature for factors of the HLA system, 1996. *Tissue Antigens* 1997;49:297.
27. Geraghty DE, Wei XH, Orr HT, Koller BH. Human leukocyte antigen F (HLA-F). An expressed HLA gene composed of a class I coding sequence linked to a novel transcribed repetitive element. *J Exp Med* 1990;171:1.
28. White PC. Molecular genetics of the class III region of the HLA complex. In: Dupont B, ed. *Immunogenetics and histocompatibility*. Vol. II. New York: Springer-Verlag, 1989:62.
29. Solheim B, Moller E, Ferrone S, eds. *HLA class II antigens: a comprehensive review of structure and function*. New York: Springer-Verlag, 1986.
30. Dorak MT, Chalmers EA, Sproul AM, et al. MHC class III polymorphisms in selection of donors for BMT. *Bone Marrow Transplant* 1993;11:37.
31. NIH lymphocyte microtoxicity technique. l. NIAID manual of tissue typing techniques. Publication NIH 80-545. Atlanta: Department of Health, Education, and Welfare, 1979.
32. Anasetti C, Amos D, Beatty PG, et al. Effect of HLA compatibility on engraftment of Bone Marrow Transplants in patients with leukemia or lymphoma. *N Engl J Med* 1989;320:197.
33. Bjorkman PJ, Saper MA, Samraoui B, et al. Structure of the human class I histocompatibility antigen, HLA-A2. *Nature* 1987;329:506.
34. Bjorkman PJ, Saper MA, Samraoui B, et al. The foreign antigen binding site and T cell recognition regions of class I histocompatibility antigens. *Nature* 1987;329:512.
35. Garrett TP, Saper MA, Bjorkman PJ, et al. Specificity pockets for the side chains of peptide antigens in HLA-Aw68. *Nature* 1989;342:692.
36. Rammensee HG. Chemistry of peptides associated with MHC class I and class II molecules. *Curr Opin Immunol* 1995;7:85.
37. Bevan MJ. Antigen recognition. Class discrimination in the world of immunology [news]. *Nature* 1987;325:192.
38. Germain RN. Immunology. The ins and outs of antigen processing and presentation [news]. *Nature* 1986;322:687.
39. Adorini L, Appella E, Doria G, et al. Competition for antigen presentation in living cells involves exchange of peptides bound by class II MHC molecules. *Nature* 1989;342:800.
40. Martin PJ. Increased disparity for minor histocompatibility antigens as a potential cause of increased GVHD risk in marrow transplantation from unrelated donors compared with related donors. *Bone Marrow Transplant* 1991;8:217.
41. Fleischhauer K, Kernan NA, O'Reilly RJ, et al. Bone marrow-allograft rejection by T lymphocytes recognizing a single amino acid difference in HLA-B44. *N Engl J Med* 1990;323:1818.
42. McCullough J, Hansen J, Perkins H, et al. The National Marrow Donor Program: how it works, accomplishments to date. *Oncology (Huntingt)* 1989;3:63.
43. Howe CWS, Radde-Stepaniak T. Hematopoietic cell donor registries. In: Thomas ED, Blume KG, Forman SJ, eds. *Hematopoietic cell transplantation*. London: Blackwell Science, 1999:503.
44. Beatty PG, Dahlberg S, Mickelson EM, et al. Probability of finding HLA-matched unrelated marrow donors. *Transplantation* 1988;45:714.
45. Sonnenberg FA, Eckman MH, Pauker SG. Bone marrow donor registries: the relation between registry size and probability of finding complete and partial matches. *Blood* 1989;74:2569.
46. McGlave P, Bartsch G, Anasetti C, et al. Unrelated donor marrow transplantation therapy for chronic myelogenous leukemia: initial experience of the National Marrow Donor Program. *Blood* 1993;81:543.
47. Kernan NA, Bartsch G, Ash RC, et al. Analysis of 463 transplantations from unrelated donors facilitated by the National Marrow Donor Program. *N Engl J Med* 1993;328:593.
48. Beatty PG, Anasetti C, Hansen JA, et al. Marrow transplantation from unrelated donors for treatment of hematologic malignancies: effect of mismatching for one HLA locus. *Blood* 1993;81:249.
49. Ash RC, Casper JT, Chitambar CR, et al. Successful allogeneic transplantation of T-cell-depleted bone marrow from closely HLA-matched unrelated donors. *N Engl J Med* 1990;322:485.
50. Nademanee A, Schmidt GM, Parker P, et al. The outcome of matched unrelated donor bone marrow transplantation in patients with hematologic malignancies using molecular typing for donor selection and graft-versus-host disease prophylaxis regimen of cyclosporine, methotrexate, and prednisone. *J Clin Oncol* 1995;86:1228.
51. Madrigal JA, Arguello R, Scott I, Avakian H. Molecular histocompatibility typing in unrelated donor bone marrow transplantation. *Blood Rev* 1997;11:105.
52. Prasad VK, Kernan NA, Heller G, et al. DNA typing for HLA-A and HLA-B identifies disparities between patients and unrelated donors matched by HLA-A and HLA-B serology and HLA-DRB1. *Blood* 1999;93:399.
53. Scott I, O'Shea J, Bunce M, et al. Molecular typing shows a high level of HLA class I incompatibility in serologically well matched donor/patient pairs: implications for unrelated bone marrow donor selection. *Blood* 1998;92:4864.
54. Petersdorf EW, Gooley TA, Anasetti C, et al. Optimizing outcome after unrelated marrow transplantation by comprehensive matching of HLA class I and II alleles in the donor and recipient. *Blood* 1998;92:3515.
55. Sasazuki T, Juji T, Morishima Y, et al. Effect of matching of class I HLA alleles on clinical outcome after transplantation of hematopoietic stem cells from an unrelated donor. Japan Marrow Donor Program. *N Engl J Med* 1998;339:1177.
56. Petersdorf EW, Smith AG, Mickelson EM, et al. The role of HLA-DPB1 disparity in the development of acute graft-versus-host disease following unrelated donor marrow transplantation. *Blood* 1993;81:1923.
57. Speiser DE, Tiercy JM, Rufer N, et al. High resolution HLA matching associated with decreased mortality after unrelated bone marrow transplantation. *Blood* 1996;87:4455.
58. Rubinstein P, Dobrila L, Rosenfield RE, et al. Processing and cryopreservation of placental/umbilical cord blood for unrelated bone marrow reconstitution. *Proc Natl Acad Sci U S A* 1995;92:10119.
59. Wagner JE, Kernan NA, Steinbuch M, et al. Allogeneic sibling umbilical-cord-blood transplantation in children with malignant and non-malignant disease. *Lancet* 1995;346:214.
60. Kurtzberg J, Laughlin M, Graham ML, et al. Placental blood as a source of hematopoietic stem cells for transplantation into unrelated recipients. *N Engl J Med* 1996;335:157.

61. Wagner JE, Rosenthal J, Sweetman R, et al. Successful transplantation of HLA-matched and HLA-mismatched umbilical cord blood from unrelated donors: analysis of engraftment and acute graft-versus-host disease. *Blood* 1996;88:795.

62. Gluckman E, Rocha V, Boyer-Chammard A, et al. Outcome of cord-blood transplantation from related and unrelated donors. Eurocord Transplant Group and the European Blood and Marrow Transplantation Group. *N Engl J Med* 1997;337:373.

63. Rubinstein P, Carrier C, Scaradavou A, et al. Outcomes among 562 recipients of placental-blood transplants from unrelated donors. *N Engl J Med* 1998;339:1565.

64. Laughlin M, Barker J, Bambach B, et al. Hematopoietic engraftment and survival in adult recipients of umbilical-cord blood from unrelated donors. *N Engl J Med* 2001;344:1815.

65. Sanders JE, Thomas ED, Buckner CD, Doney K. Marrow transplantation for children with acute lymphoblastic leukemia in second remission. *Blood* 1987;70:324.

66. Bortin MM, Buckner CD. Major complications of marrow harvesting for transplantation. *Exper Hematol* 1983;11:916.

67. Buckner CD, Clift RA, Sanders JE, et al. Marrow harvesting from normal donors. *Blood* 1984;64:630.

68. Bowden RA, Sayers M, Flournoy N, et al. Cytomegalovirus immune globulin and seronegative blood products to prevent primary cytomegalovirus infection after marrow transplantation. *N Engl J Med* 1986;314:1006.

69. Winston DJ, Eng-Shang H, Miller MJ, et al. Molecular epidemiology of cytomegalovirus infections associated with bone marrow transplantation. *Ann Intern Med* 1985;102:16.

70. Li C-R, Greenberg PD, Gilbert MJ, et al. Recovery of HLA-restricted cytomegalovirus (CMV)-specific T-cell responses after allogeneic bone marrow transplantation: correlation with CMV disease and effect of ganciclovir prophylaxis. *Blood* 1994;83:1971.

71. Trenschel R, Ross S, Husing J, et al. Reduced risk of persisting cytomegalovirus pp65 antigenemia and cytomegalovirus interstitial pneumonia following allogeneic PBSCT. *Bone Marrow Transplant* 2000;25:665.

72. Lau GK, Lie AK, Kwong YL, et al. A case-controlled study on the use of HBsAg-positive donors for allogeneic hematopoietic cell transplantation. *Blood* 2000;96:452.

73. Pariente EA, Goudeau A, Dubois F, et al. Fulminant hepatitis due to reactivation of chronic hepatitis B virus infection after allogeneic bone marrow transplantation. *Dig Dis Sci* 1988;33:1185.

74. Strasser SI, McDonald GB. Hepatitis viruses and hematopoietic cell transplantation: a guide to patient and donor management. *Blood* 1999;93:1127.

75. Lange B, Henle W, Meyers JD, et al. Epstein-Barr virus-related serology in marrow transplant recipients. *Int J Cancer* 1980;26:151.

76. Hanto DW, Frizzera G, Gajl-Peczalska KJ, Simmons RL. Epstein-Barr virus, immunodeficiency, and B cell lymphoproliferation. *Transplantation* 1985;39:461.

77. Sullivan JL, Wallen WC, Johnson FL. Epstein-Barr virus infection following bone-marrow transplantation. *Int J Cancer* 1978;22:132.

78. Shapiro RS, McClain K, Frizzera G, et al. Epstein-Barr virus associated B cell lymphoproliferative disorders following bone marrow transplantation. *Blood* 1988;71:1234.

79. Zutter MM, Martin PJ, Sale GE, et al. Epstein-Barr virus lymphoproliferation after bone marrow transplantation. *Blood* 1988;72:520.

80. Gustafsson A, Levitsky V, Zou JZ, et al. Epstein-Barr virus (EBV) load in bone marrow transplant recipients at risk to develop posttransplant lymphoproliferative disease: prophylactic infusion of EBV-specific cytotoxic T cells. *Blood* 2000;95:807.

81. Petz LD, Yam P, Wallace RB, et al. Mixed hematopoietic chimerism following bone marrow transplantation for hematologic malignancies. *Blood* 1987;70:1331.

82. Blume KG, Beutler E, Bross KJ, et al. Genetic markers in human bone marrow transplantation. *Am J Hum Genet* 1980;32:414.

83. Witherspoon RP, Schanfield MS, Storb R, et al. Immunoglobulin production of donor origin after marrow transplantation for acute leukemia or aplastic anemia. *Transplantation* 1978;26:407.

84. Ginsburg D, Antin JH, Smith BR, et al. Origin of cell populations after bone marrow transplantation. Analysis using DNA sequence polymorphisms. *J Clin Invest* 1985;75:596.

85. Blazar BR, Orr HT, Arthur DC, et al. Restriction fragment length polymorphisms as markers of engraftment in allogeneic bone marrow transplantation. *Blood* 1985;66:1436.

86. Atkinson K, Farrell C, Chapman G, et al. Female marrow donors increase the risk of acute graft-versus-host disease: effect of donor age and parity and analysis of cell subpopulations in the donor marrow inoculum. *Br J Haematol* 1986;63:231.

87. Gale RP, Bortin MM, van Bekkum DW, et al. Risk factors for acute graft-versus-host disease. *Br J Haematol* 1987;67:397.

88. Przepiorka D, Smith TL, Folloder J, et al. Risk factors for acute graft-versus-host disease after allogeneic blood stem cell transplantation. *Blood* 1999;94:1465.

89. Hagglund H, Bostrom L, Remberger M, et al. Risk factors for acute graft-versus-host disease in 291 consecutive HLA-identical bone marrow transplant recipients. *Bone Marrow Transplant* 1995;16:747.

90. Confer D, Chell J, Kollman C, Walker T. 1999 Data and Scientific Report of the National Marrow Donor Program. Minneapolis: National Marrow Donor Program, 2000.

91. Kollman C, Howe CW, Anasetti C, et al. Donor characteristics as risk factors in recipients after transplantation of bone marrow from unrelated donors: the effect of donor age. *Blood* 2001;98:2043.

92. Appelbaum FR. Is there a best transplant conditioning regimen for acute myeloid leukemia? *Leukemia* 2000;14:497.

93. Blume KG, Forman SJ, O'Donnell MR, et al. Total body irradiation and high-dose etoposide: a new preparatory regimen for bone marrow transplantation in patients with advanced hematologic malignancies. *Blood* 1987;69:1015.

94. Goldberg MA, Antin JH, Guinan EC, Rappeport JM. Cyclophosphamide cardiotoxicity: an analysis of dosing as a risk factor. *Blood* 1986;68:1114.

95. Crawford SW, Fisher L. Predictive value of pulmonary function tests before marrow transplantation. *Chest* 1992;101:1257.

96. Thomas ED, Clift RA, Fefer A, et al. Marrow transplantation for the treatment of chronic myelogenous leukemia. *Ann Intern Med* 1986;104:155.

97. Wingard JR, Mellits ED, Sostrin MB, et al. Interstitial pneumonitis after allogeneic bone marrow transplantation. Nine-year experience at a single institution. *Medicine* 1988;67:175.

98. Valteau D, Hartmann O, Benhamou E, et al. Nonbacterial, nonfungal, interstitial pneumonitis following autologous bone marrow transplantation in children treated with high-dose chemotherapy without total-body irradiation. *Transplantation* 1988;45:737.

99. Weiner RS, Bortin MM, Gale RP, et al. Interstitial pneumonitis after bone marrow transplantation. *Ann Intern Med* 1986;104:168.

100. Bearman SI. Venoocclusive disease of the liver. *Curr Opin Oncol* 2000;12:103.

101. Richardson P, Bearman SI. Prevention and treatment of hepatic venoocclusive disease after high-dose cytoreductive therapy. *Leuk Lymphoma* 1998;31:267.

102. Carreras E, Bertz H, Arcese W, et al. Incidence and outcome of hepatic venoocclusive disease after blood or marrow transplantation: a prospective cohort study of the European Group for Blood and Marrow Transplantation. European Group for Blood and Marrow Transplantation Chronic Leukemia Working Party. *Blood* 1998;92:3599.

103. Guinan EC, Tarbell NJ, Niemeyer CM, et al. Intravascular hemolysis and renal insufficiency after bone marrow transplantation. *Blood* 1988;72:451.

104. Rabinowe SN, Soiffer RJ, Tarbell NJ, et al. Hemolytic-uremic syndrome following bone marrow transplantation in adults for hematologic malignancies. *Blood* 1991;77:1837.

105. Deeg HJ, Team FT. Acute and delayed toxicities of total body irradiation. *Int J Radiat Oncol Biol Phys* 1984;10:957.

106. Deeg HJ, Flournoy N, Sullivan KM, et al. Cataracts after total body irradiation and marrow transplantation: a sparing effect of dose fractionation. *Int J Radiat Oncol Biol Phys* 1984;10:957.

107. Tichelli A, Gratwohl A, Egger T, et al. Cataract formation after bone marrow transplantation. *Ann Intern Med* 1993;119:1175.

108. Verdonck LF, de Gast GC, Lange JM, et al. Syngeneic leukocytes together with suramin failed to improve immunodeficiency in a case of transfusion-associated AIDS after syngeneic bone marrow transplantation. *Blood* 1988;71:666.

109. Vilmer E, Rhodes-Feuillette A, Rabian C, et al. Clinical and immunological restoration in patients with AIDS after marrow transplantation, using lymphocyte transfusions from the marrow donor. *Transplantation* 1987;44:25.

110. Slavin MA, Meyers JD, Remington JS, Hackman RC. Toxoplasma gondii infection in marrow transplant recipients: a 20 year experience. *Bone Marrow Transplant* 1994;13:549.

111. Small TN, Leung L, Stiles J, et al. Disseminated toxoplasmosis following T cell-depleted related and unrelated bone marrow transplantation. *Bone Marrow Transplant* 2000;25:969.

112. Reed EC, Bowden RA, Dandliker PS, et al. Treatment of cytomegalovirus pneumonia with Gancyclovir and intravenous cytomegalovirus immunoglobulin in patients with bone marrow transplants. *Ann Intern Med* 1988;109:783.

113. Stroncek DF, Holland PV, Bartch G, et al. Experiences of the first 493 unrelated marrow donors in the National Marrow Donor Program. *Blood* 1993;81:1940.

114. Goodman J, Hodgson G. Evidence for stem cells in the peripheral blood of mice. *Blood* 1962;19:702.

115. McKredie K, Hersh E, Freireich EJ. Cells capable of colony formation in the peripheral blood of man. *Science* 1971;171:293.

116. Kessinger A, Armitage JO, Landmark JD, et al. Autologous peripheral hematopoietic stem cell transplantation restores hematopoietic function following marrow ablative therapy. *Blood* 1988;71:723.

117. Schmitz N, Linch DC, Dreger P, et al. Randomised trial of filgrastim-mobilised peripheral blood progenitor cell transplantation versus autologous bone-marrow transplantation in lymphoma patients. *Lancet* 1996;347:353.

118. Champlin R, Schmitz N, Horowitz M, et al. Blood stem cells compared with bone marrow as a source of hematopoietic cells for allogeneic transplantation. IBMTR Histocompatibility and Stem Cell Sources Working Committee and the European Group for Blood and Marrow Transplantation (EBMT). *Blood* 2000;95:3702.

119. Korbling M, Anderlini P, Durett A, et al. Delayed effects of rhG-CSF mobilization treatment and apheresis on circulating CD34$^+$ and CD34$^+$ Thy-1dim CD38- progenitor cells, and lymphoid subsets in normal stem cell donors for allogeneic transplantation. *Bone Marrow Transplant* 1996;18:1073.

120. Rocha V, Wagner JE Jr, Sobocinski KA, et al. Graft-versus-host disease in children who have received a cord-blood or bone marrow transplant from an HLA-identical sibling. Eurocord and International Bone Marrow Transplantation Registry Working Committee on Alternative Donor and Stem Cell Sources. *N Engl J Med* 2000;342:1846.

121. Fraser JK, Cairo MS, Wagner EL, et al. Cord Blood Transplantation Study (COBLT): cord blood bank standard operating procedures. *J Hematother* 1998;7:521.

122. van Bekkum DW. Conditioning regimens for marrow grafting. *Semin Hematol* 1984;21:81.

123. Storb R, Etizoni R, Anasetti C, et al. Cyclophosphamide combined with antithymocyte globulin in preparation for allogeneic marrow transplants in patients with aplastic anemia. *Blood* 1994;84:941.

124. Tutschka PJ, Copelan EA, Klein JP. Bone marrow transplantation for leukemia following a new busulfan and cyclophosphamide regimen. *Blood* 1987;70:1382.

125. Blume KG, Kopecky KJ, Henslee-Downey PJ, et al. A prospective randomized comparison of total body irradiation-etoposide versus busulfan-cyclophosphamide as preparatory regimens for bone marrow transplantation in patients with leukemia who were not in first remission: A Southwest Oncology Group study. *Blood* 1993;81:2187.

126. Wheeler C, Antin JH, Churchill WH, et al. Cyclophosphamide, carmustine, and etoposide with autologous bone marrow transplantation in refractory Hodgkin's disease and non-Hodgkin's lymphoma: a dose-finding study. *J Clin Oncol* 1990;8:648.

127. Chopra R, McMillan AK, Linch DC, et al. The place of high-dose BEAM therapy and bone marrow transplantation in poor-risk Hodgkin's disease. A single-center eight-year study of 155 patients. *Blood* 1993;81:1137.

128. Frei EJ, Canellos GP. Dose, a critical factor in cancer chemotherapy. *Am J Med* 1980;69:585.

129. Skipper HE, Schabel FM Jr, Wilcox WS. Experimental evaluation of potential anticancer agents. XII. On the criteria and kinetics associated with "curability" of experimental leukemia. *Cancer Chemother Rep* 1964;35:1.

130. Santos GW, Sensenbrenner LL, Burk PJ, et al. Marrow transplantation in man following cyclophosphamide. *Transplant Proc* 1971;3:400.

131. Clift RA, Buckner CD, Appelbaum FR, et al. Allogeneic marrow transplantation in patients with acute myeloid leukemia in first remission: a randomized trial of two irradiation regimens. *Blood* 1990;76:1867.

132. Grochow LB, Krivit W, Whitley CB, Blazar B. Busulfan disposition in children. *Blood* 1990;75:1723.

133. Giralt S, Thall PF, Khouri I, et al. Melphalan and purine analog-containing preparative regimens: reduced-intensity conditioning for patients with hematologic malignancies undergoing allogeneic progenitor cell transplantation. *Blood* 2001;97:631.

134. McSweeney PA, Niederwieser D, Shizuru JA, et al. Hematopoietic cell transplantation in older patients with hematologic malignancies: replacing high-dose cytotoxic therapy with graft-versus-tumor effects. *Blood* 2001;97:3390.

135. Slavin S, Nagler A, Naparstek E, et al. Nonmyeloablative stem cell transplantation and cell therapy as an alternative to conventional bone marrow transplantation with lethal cytoreduction for the treatment of malignant and nonmalignant hematologic diseases. *Blood* 1998;91:756.

136. Sykes M, Preffer F, McAfee S, et al. Mixed lymphohaemopoietic chimerism and graft-versus-lymphoma effects after non-myeloablative therapy and HLA-mismatched bone-marrow transplantation. *Lancet* 1999;353:1755.

137. Illidge TM, Johnson PW. The emerging role of radioimmunotherapy in haematological malignancies. *Br J Haematol* 2000;108:679.

138. Matthews DC, Appelbaum FR, Eary JF, et al. Phase I study of (131)I-anti-CD45 antibody plus cyclophosphamide and total body irradiation for advanced acute leukemia and myelodysplastic syndrome. *Blood* 1999;94:1237.

139. Bearman SI, Appelbaum FR, Buckner CD, et al. Regimen-related toxicity in patients undergoing bone marrow transplantation. *J Clin Oncol* 1988;6:1562.

140. Haire WD, Ruby EI, Gordon BG, et al. Multiple organ dysfunction syndrome in bone marrow transplantation. *JAMA* 1995;274:1289.

141. Woo SB, Sonis ST, Monopoli MM, Sonis AL. A longitudinal study of oral ulcerative mucositis in bone marrow transplant recipients. *Cancer* 1993;72:1612.

142. Crawford SW. Noninfectious lung disease in the immunocompromised host. *Respiration* 1999;66:385.

143. Richardson P, Guinan E. The pathology, diagnosis, and treatment of hepatic venoocclusive disease: current status and novel approaches [published erratum appears in *Br J Haematol* 2000 Apr;109(1):254]. *Br J Haematol* 1999;107:485.

144. Bearman SI. The syndrome of hepatic venoocclusive disease after marrow transplantation. *Blood* 1995;85:3005.

145. Braverman AC, Antin JH, Plappert MT, et al. Cyclophosphamide cardiotoxicity in bone marrow transplantation: a prospective evaluation of new dosing regimens. *J Clin Oncol* 1991;9:1215.

146. Champlin RE, Gale RP. The early complications of bone marrow transplantation. *Semin Hematol* 1984;21:101.

147. Blijlevens NM, Donnelly JP, De Pauw BE. Mucosal barrier injury: biology, pathology, clinical counterparts and consequences of intensive treatment for haematological malignancy: an overview. *Bone Marrow Transplant* 2000;25:1269.

148. Wardley AM, Jayson GC, Swindell R, et al. Prospective evaluation of oral mucositis in patients receiving myeloablative conditioning regimens and haemopoietic progenitor rescue. *Br J Haematol* 2000;110:292.

149. McDonald GB, Shulman HM, Sullivan KM, Spencer GD. Intestinal and hepatic complications of bone marrow transplantation. Part I. *Gastroenterology* 1986;90:460.

150. McDonald GB, Hinds MS, Fisher LD, et al. Venoocclusive disease of the liver and multiorgan failure after bone marrow transplantation: a cohort study of 355 patients. *Ann Intern Med* 1993;118:255.

151. Ringden O, Remberger M, Ruutu T, et al. Increased risk of chronic graft-versus-host disease, obstructive bronchiolitis, and alopecia with busulfan versus total body irradiation: long-term results of a randomized trial in allogeneic marrow recipients with leukemia. Nordic Bone Marrow Transplantation Group. *Blood* 1999;93:2196.

152. Steinherz LJ, Steinherz PG, Mangiacasale D, et al. Cardiac changes with cyclophosphamide. *Med Pediatr Oncol* 1981;9:417.

153. Gottdiener JS, Appelbaum FR, Ferrans VJ, et al. Cardiomyopathy associated with high dose cyclophosphamide therapy. *Arch Intern Med* 1981;141:768.

154. Loughran TP, Deeg HJ, Dahlberg S, et al. Incidence of hypertension among 112 patients randomized to either cyclosporine or methotrexate as graft-versus-host disease prophylaxis. *Br J Haematol* 1985;59:547.

155. Ratanatharathorn V, Nash RA, Przepiorka D, et al. Phase III study comparing methotrexate and tacrolimus (prograf, FK506) with methotrexate and cyclosporine for graft-versus-host disease prophylaxis after HLA-identical sibling bone marrow transplantation. *Blood* 1998;92:2303.

156. Patchell RA, White CL, Clark AW, et al. Nonbacterial thrombotic endocarditis in bone marrow transplant patients. *Cancer* 1985;55:631.

157. Wingard JR, Sostrin MB, Vriesendorp HM, et al. Interstitial pneumonitis following autologous bone marrow transplantation. *Transplantation* 1988;46:61.

158. Clark JG, Crawford SW, Madies DK, Sullivan KM. Obstructive lung disease after allogeneic marrow transplantation. Clinical presentation and course. *Ann Intern Med* 1989;111:368.

159. Clark JG, Schwartz DA, Flournoy N, et al. Risk factors for airflow obstruction in recipients of bone marrow transplants. *Ann Intern Med* 1987;107:648.

160. Lewis I, DeFor T, Weisdorf D. Increasing incidence of diffuse alveolar hemorrhage following allogeneic bone marrow transplantation: cryptic etiology and uncertain therapy. *Bone Marrow Transplant* 2000;26:539.

161. Holland KH, Wingard JR, Beschorner WE, et al. Bronchiolitis obliterans and its relationship to chronic graft-vs-host disease and low serum IgG. *Blood* 1988;72:621.

162. Ralph DD, Springmeyer SC, Sullivan DM, et al. Rapidly progressive air-flow obstruction in marrow transplant recipients. *Ann Rev Respir Dis* 1984;129:641.

163. Burke CM, Theodore J, Dawkins KD, et al. Post-transplant obliterative bronchiolitis and other late lung sequelae in heart-lung transplantation. *Chest* 1984;86:824.

164. Epler GR, Colby TV, McLoud TC, et al. Bronchiolitis obliterans organizing pneumonia. *N Engl J Med* 1985;312:152.

165. Seber A, Shu XO, Defor T, et al. Risk factors for severe hemorrhagic cystitis following BMT. *Bone Marrow Transplant* 1999;23:35.

166. Shepherd JD, Pringle LE, Barnett MJ, et al. Mesna versus hyperhydration for the prevention of cyclophosphamide-induced hemorrhagic cystitis in bone marrow transplantation. *J Clin Oncol* 1991;9:2016.

167. Ballen KK, Becker P, Levebvre K, et al. Safety and cost of hyperhydration for the prevention of hemorrhagic cystitis in bone marrow transplant recipients. *Oncology* 1999;57:287.

168. Meisenberg B, Lassiter M, Hussein A, et al. Prevention of hemorrhagic cystitis after high-dose alkylating agent chemotherapy and autologous bone marrow support. *Bone Marrow Transplant* 1994;14:287.

169. Vose JM, Reed EC, Pippert GC, et al. Mesna compared with continuous bladder irrigation as uroprotection during high-dose chemotherapy and transplantation: a randomized trial. *J Clin Oncol* 1993;11:1306.

170. Russell SJ, Vowels MR, Vale T. Haemorrhagic cystitis in paediatric bone marrow transplant patients: an association with infective agents, GVHD and prior cyclophosphamide. *Bone Marrow Transplant* 1994;13:533.

171. Peinemann F, de Villiers EM, Dorries K, et al. Clinical course and treatment of haemorrhagic cystitis associated with BK type of human polyomavirus in nine paediatric recipients of allogeneic bone marrow transplants. *Eur J Pediatr* 2000;159:182.

172. Arthur RR, Shah KV, Baust SJ, et al. Association of BK viruria with hemorrhagic cystitis in recipients of bone marrow transplants. *N Engl J Med* 1986;315:230.

173. Carrigan DR. Adenovirus infections in immunocompromised patients. *Am J Med* 1997;102:71.

174. Laszlo D, Bosi A, Guidi S, et al. Prostaglandin E2 bladder instillation for the treatment of hemorrhagic cystitis after allogeneic bone marrow transplantation. *Haematologica* 1995;80:421.

175. Horowitz MM. Current status of allogeneic bone marrow transplantation in acquired aplastic anemia. *Semin Hematol* 2000;37:30.

176. Zierhut D, Lohr F, Schraube P, et al. Cataract incidence after total-body irradiation. *Int J Radiat Oncol Biol Phys* 2000;46:131.

177. Sanders JE, Pritchard S, Mahoney P, et al. Growth and development following marrow transplantation for leukemia. *Blood* 1986;68:1129.

178. Sanders JE, Buckner CD, Amos D, et al. Ovarian function following marrow transplantation for aplastic anemia or leukemia. *J Clin Oncol* 1988;6:813.

179. Sanders JE, Buckner CD, Leonard JM, et al. Late effects on gonadal function of cyclophosphamide, total body irradiation and marrow transplantation. *Transplantation* 1983;36:252.

180. Leiper AD, Stanhope R, Lau T, et al. The effect of total body irradiation and bone marrow transplantation during childhood and adolescence on growth and endocrine function. *Br J Haematol* 1987;67:419.

181. Lio S, Arcese W, Papa G, Darmiento M. Thyroid and pituitary function following bone marrow transplantation. *Arch Intern Med* 1988;148:1066.

182. Sklar CA, Kim TH, Ramsay NK. Testicular function following bone marrow transplantation performed during or after puberty. *Cancer* 1984;53:1498.

183. Chatterjee R, Goldstone AH. Gonadal damage and effects on fertility in adult patients with haematological malignancy undergoing stem cell transplantation. *Bone Marrow Transplant* 1996;17:5.

184. Schimmer AD, Quatermain M, Imrie K, et al. Ovarian function after autologous bone marrow transplantation. *J Clin Oncol* 1998;16:2359.

185. Salooja N, Chatterjee R, McMillan AK, et al. Successful pregnancies in women following single autotransplant for acute myeloid leukemia with a chemotherapy ablation protocol. *Bone Marrow Transplant* 1994;13:431.

186. Sanders JE, Hawley J, Levy W, et al. Pregnancies following high-dose cyclophosphamide with or without high-dose busulfan or total-body irradiation and bone marrow transplantation. *Blood* 1996;87:3045.

187. Sullivan KM, Storb R, Shulman HM, et al. Immediate and delayed neurotoxicity after mechlorethamine preparation for bone marrow transplantation. *Ann Intern Med* 1982;97:182.

188. Graus F, Saiz A, Sierra J, et al. Neurologic complications of autologous and allogeneic bone marrow transplantation in patients with leukemia: a comparative study. *Neurology* 1996;46:1004.

189. Guerrero A, Perez-Simon JA, Gutierrez N, et al. Neurological complications after autologous stem cell transplantation. *Eur Neurol* 1999;41:48.

190. Wiznitzer M. Neurologic complications of bone marrow transplantation in childhood. *Ann Neurol* 1984;16:569.

191. Wade JC, Meyers JD. Neurologic symptoms associated with parenteral acyclovir treatment after marrow transplantation. *Ann Intern Med* 1983;98:921.

192. Iacopino P, Pucci G, Arcese W, et al. Severe thrombotic microangiopathy: an infrequent complication of bone marrow transplantation. Gruppo Italiano Trapianto Midollo Osseo (GITMO). *Bone Marrow Transplant* 1999;24:47.

193. Trimarchi HM, Truong LD, Brennan S, et al. FK506-associated thrombotic microangiopathy: report of two cases and review of the literature. *Transplantation* 1999;67:539.

194. Moake JL, Byrnes JJ. Thrombotic microangiopathies associated with drugs and bone marrow transplantation. *Hematol Oncol Clin North Am* 1996;10:485.

195. Hale G, Waldmann H. Risks of developing Epstein-Barr virus-related lymphoproliferative disorders after T-cell-depleted marrow transplants. CAMPATH Users. *Blood* 1998;91:3079.

196. Gerritsen EJ, Stam ED, Hermans J, et al. Risk factors for developing EBV-related B cell lymphoproliferative disorders (BLPD) after non-HLA-identical BMT in children. *Bone Marrow Transplant* 1996;18:377.

197. Rowlings PA, Curtis RE, Passweg JR, et al. Increased incidence of Hodgkin's disease after allogeneic bone marrow transplantation. *J Clin Oncol* 1999;17:3122.

198. Cohen JI. Epstein-Barr virus infection. *N Engl J Med* 2000;343:481.

199. Trigg ME, Finlay JL, Sondel PM. Prophylactic acyclovir in patients receiving bone marrow transplants. *N Engl J Med* 1985;312:1708.

200. Benkerrou M, Jais JP, Leblond V, et al. Anti-B-cell monoclonal antibody treatment of severe posttransplant B-lymphoproliferative disorder: prognostic factors and long-term outcome. *Blood* 1998;92:3137.

201. Kuehnle I, Huls MH, Liu Z, et al. CD20 monoclonal antibody (rituximab) for therapy of Epstein-Barr virus lymphoma after hemopoietic stem-cell transplantation. *Blood* 2000;95:1502.

202. Papadopoulos EB, Ladanyi M, Emanuel D, et al. Infusions of donor leukocytes to treat Epstein-Barr virus-associated lymphoproliferative disorders after allogeneic bone marrow transplantation. *N Engl J Med* 1994;330:1185.

203. Porter DL, Antin JH. The graft-versus-leukemia effects of allogeneic cell therapy. *Annu Rev Med* 1999;50:369.

204. Curtis RE, Rowlings PA, Deeg HJ, et al. Solid cancers after bone marrow transplantation. *N Engl J Med* 1997;336:897.

205. Socie G, Curtis RE, Deeg HJ, et al. New malignant diseases after allogeneic marrow transplantation for childhood acute leukemia. *J Clin Oncol* 2000;18:348.

206. Kolb HJ, Socie G, Duell T, et al. Malignant neoplasms in long-term survivors of bone marrow transplantation. Late Effects Working Party of the European Cooperative Group for Blood and Marrow Transplantation and the European Late Effect Project Group. *Ann Intern Med* 1999;131:738.

207. Witherspoon RP, Schubach W, Neiman P, et al. Donor cell leukemia developing six years after marrow grafting for acute leukemia. *Blood* 1985;65:1172.

208. Elfenbein GJ, Brogaonkar DS, Bias WB, et al. Cytogenetic evidence for recurrence of acute myelogenous leukemia after allogeneic bone marrow transplantation in donor hematopoietic cells. *Blood* 1978;52:627.

209. Schmitz N, Johannsen W, Schmidt G, et al. Recurrence of acute lymphoblastic leukemia in donor cells after allogeneic marrow transplantation associated with a deletion of the long arm of chromosome 6. *Blood* 1987;70:1099.

210. Marmont A, Frassoni F, Bacigalupo A, et al. Recurrence of Ph'-positive leukemia in donor cells after marrow transplantation for chronic granulocytic leukemia. *N Engl J Med* 1984;310:903.

211. Newburger PE, Latt SA, Pesando JM, et al. Leukemia relapse in donor cells after allogeneic bone-marrow transplantation. *N Engl J Med* 1981;304:712.

212. Miller JS, Arthur DC, Litz CE, et al. Myelodysplastic syndrome after autologous bone marrow transplantation: an additional late complication of curative cancer therapy. *Blood* 1994;83:3780.

213. Wheeler C, Khurshid A, Ibrahim J, et al. Incidence of post transplant myelodysplasia/acute leukemia in non-Hodgkin's lymphoma patients compared with Hodgkin's disease patients undergoing autologous transplantation following cyclophosphamide, carmustine, and etoposide (CBV). *Leuk Lymphoma* 2001;405:499.

214. Friedberg JW, Neuberg D, Stone RM, et al. Outcome in patients with myelodysplastic syndrome after autologous bone marrow transplantation for non-Hodgkin's lymphoma. *J Clin Oncol* 1999;17:3128.

215. Armitage JO. Myelodysplasia and acute leukemia after autologous bone marrow transplantation [editorial]. *J Clin Oncol* 2000;18:945.

216. Micallef IN, Lillington DM, Apostolidis J, et al. Therapy-related myelodysplasia and secondary acute myelogenous leukemia after high-dose therapy with autologous hematopoietic progenitor-cell support for lymphoid malignancies. *J Clin Oncol* 2000;18:947.

217. Krishnan A, Bhatia S, Slovak ML, et al. Predictors of therapy-related leukemia and myelodysplasia following autologous transplantation for lymphoma: an assessment of risk factors. *Blood* 2000;95:1588.

218. Niederwieser D, Pepe M, Storb R, et al. Improvement in rejection, engraftment rate, and survival without increase in graft-versus-host disease by high marrow cell dose in patients transplanted for aplastic anemia. *Br J Haematol* 1988;69:23.

219. Sierra J, Storer B, Hansen JA, et al. Transplantation of marrow cells from unrelated donors for treatment of high-risk acute leukemia: the effect of leukemic burden, donor HLA-matching, and marrow cell dose. *Blood* 1997;89:4226.

220. Yeager AM, Kaizer H, Santos GW, et al. Autologous bone marrow transplantation in patients with acute nonlymphocytic leukemia, using ex vivo marrow treatment with 4-hydroperoxycyclophosphamide. *N Engl J Med* 1986;315:141.

221. Harada M, Yoshida T, Ishino C, et al. Hematologic recovery following autologous and allogeneic bone marrow transplantation. *Exp Hematol* 1983;11:841.

222. Banaji M, Bearman SI, Buckner CD, et al. The effects of splenectomy on engraftment and platelet transfusion requirements in patients with chronic myelogenous leukemia undergoing marrow transplantation. *Am J Hematol* 1986;22:275.

223. Guardiola P, Anderson JE, Bandini G, et al. Allogeneic stem cell transplantation for agnogenic myeloid metaplasia: a European Group for Blood and Marrow Transplantation, Societe Francaise de Greffe de Moelle, Gruppo Italiano per il Trapianto del Midollo Osseo, and Fred Hutchinson Cancer Research Center Collaborative Study. *Blood* 1999;93:2831.

224. Storb R, Deeg HJ, Whitehead J, et al. Methotrexate and cyclosporine compared with cyclosporine alone for prophylaxis of acute graft versus host disease after marrow transplantation for leukemia. *N Engl J Med* 1986;314:729.

225. Chao NJ, Schmidt GM, Niland JC, et al. Cyclosporine, methotrexate, and prednisone compared with cyclosporine and prednisone for prophylaxis of acute graft-versus-host disease. *N Engl J Med* 1993;329:1225.

226. Verdonck LF, van Heugten H, de Gast GC. Delay in platelet recovery after bone marrow transplantation: impact of cytomegalovirus infection. *Blood* 1985;66:921.

227. Maeda Y, Teshima T, Yamada M, et al. Monitoring of human herpesviruses after allogeneic peripheral blood stem cell transplantation and bone marrow transplantation. *Br J Haematol* 1999;105:295.

228. Lemischka I, Raulet DH, Mulligan RG. Developmental potential and dynamic behaviour of hematopoietic stem cells. *Cell* 1986;45:917.

229. Kim HJ, Tisdale JF, Wu T, et al. Many multipotential gene-marked progenitor or stem cell clones contribute to hematopoiesis in nonhuman primates. *Blood* 2000;96:1.

230. Nash R, Storb R, Neiman P. Polyclonal reconstitution of marrow after allogeneic bone marrow transplantation. *Blood* 1988;72:2031.

231. Turhan AG, Humphries RK, Phillips GL, et al. Clonal hematopoiesis demonstrated by X-linked DNA polymorphisms after allogeneic bone marrow transplantation. *N Engl J Med* 1989;320:1655.

232. Brandt SJ, Peters WP, Atwater SK, et al. Effect of recombinant human granulocyte-macrophage colony-stimulating factor on hematopoietic reconstitution after high-dose chemotherapy and autologous bone marrow transplantation. *N Engl J Med* 1988;318:869.

233. Hartmann O, Le Corroller AG, Blaise D, et al. Peripheral blood stem cell and bone marrow transplantation for solid tumors and lymphomas: hematologic recovery and costs. A randomized, controlled trial. *Ann Intern Med* 1997;126:600.

234. Damiani D, Fanin R, Silvestri F, et al. Randomized trial of autologous filgrastim-primed bone marrow transplantation versus filgrastim-mobilized peripheral blood stem cell transplantation in lymphoma patients. *Blood* 1997;90:36.

235. Weisdorf D, Miller J, Verfaillie C, et al. Cytokine-primed bone marrow stem cells vs. peripheral blood stem cells for autologous transplantation: a randomized comparison of GM-CSF vs. G-CSF. *Biol Blood Marrow Transplant* 1997;3:217.

236. Smith TJ, Hillner BE, Schmitz N, et al. Economic analysis of a randomized clinical trial to compare filgrastim-mobilized peripheral-blood progenitor-cell transplantation and autologous bone marrow transplantation in patients with Hodgkin's and non-Hodgkin's lymphoma. *J Clin Oncol* 1997;15:5.

237. Burakoff SJ, Lipton JM, Nathan DG. Recapitulation of the immune response and haematopoietic system in bone marrow transplantation. *Clin Haematol* 1983;12:695.

238. Antin JH, Weinberg DS, Rappeport JM. Evidence that pluripotential stem cells form splenic colonies in humans after marrow transplantation. *Transplantation* 1985;39:102.

239. Gale RP, Falk P, Feig SA, Cline MJ. Failure of recovery following syngeneic marrow grafting in aplastic anemia. *Exp Hematol* 1977;5(Suppl 2):103a.

240. Rappeport JM, Newburger PE, Goldblum RM, et al. Allogeneic bone marrow transplantation for chronic granulomatous disease. *J Pediatr* 1982;101:952.

241. Miyagawa B, Klingemann HG. Phagocytosis and burst activity of granulocytes and monocytes after stem cell transplantation. *J Lab Clin Med* 1997;129:634.

242. Tsoi MS, Dobbs S, Brkic S, et al. Cellular interactions in marrow-grafted patients. II. Normal monocyte antigen-presenting and defective T-cell-proliferative functions early after grafting and during chronic graft-versus-host disease. *Transplantation* 1984;37:556.

243. Reittie JE, Poulter LW, Prentice HG, et al. Differential recovery of phenotypically and functionally distinct circulating antigen-presenting cells after allogeneic marrow transplantation. *Transplantation* 1988;45:1084.

244. Winston DJ, Territo MC, Ho WG, et al. Alveolar macrophage dysfunction in bone marrow transplant recipients. *Am J Med* 1982;73:859.

245. Perreault C, Pelletier M. Persistence of host Langerhans cells following allogeneic bone marrow transplantation: possible relationship with acute graft-versus-host disease. *Br J Haematol* 1985;60:253.

246. Perreault C, Pelletier M, Landry D, Gyger M. Study of Langerhans cells after allogeneic bone marrow transplantation. *Blood* 1984;63:807.

247. Thomas ED, Ramberg RF, Sale GE, et al. Direct evidence for a bone marrow origin of the alveolar macrophage in man. *Science* 1976;192:1016.

248. Gale RP, Sparkes RS, Golde DW. Bone marrow origin of hepatic macrophages (Kupffer cells) in humans. *Science* 1978;201:937.

249. Alter BP, Rappeport JM, Huisman THJ, Schroeder WA. Fetal erythropoiesis following bone marrow transplantation. *Blood* 1976;48:843.

250. Papayannopoulou T, Chen P, Maniatis A, Stamatoyannopoulos G. Simultaneous assessment of i-antigenic expression and fetal hemoglobin in single red cells by immunofluorescence. *Blood* 1980;55:221.

251. Papayannopoulou T, Nakamoto B, Agostinelli F, et al. Fetal to adult hemopoietic cell transplantation in humans: insights into hemoglobin switching. *Blood* 1986;67:99.

252. Winkler KJ, Rea CD, Rahbar S, et al. Heterogeneous ontogeny of erythropoiesis after bone marrow ablation and allogeneic bone marrow grafting. *Blood* 1983;61:167.

253. Rozman C, Feliu E, Granena A, et al. Transient dyserythropoiesis in repopulated human bone marrow following transplantation: an ultrastructural study. *Br J Haematol* 1982;50:63.

254. Schapira L, Antin JH, Ransil BJ, et al. Serum erythropoietin levels in patients receiving intensive chemotherapy and radiotherapy. *Blood* 1990;76:2354.

255. Miller CB, Jones RJ, Zahurak ML, et al. Impaired erythropoietin response to anemia after bone marrow transplantation. *Blood* 1992;80:2677.

256. Mitus AJ, Antin JH, Rutherford CJ, et al. Use of recombinant erythropoietin in allogeneic bone marrow transplant donor/recipient pairs. *Blood* 1994;83:1952.

257. Stefmann JL, Lopez J, Otero MJ, et al. Erythropoietin treatment in allogeneic BMT accelerates erythroid reconstitution: results of a prospective randomized trial. *Bone Marrow Transplant* 1992;10:541.

258. Klaesson S. Clinical use of rHuEPO in bone marrow transplantation. *Med Oncol* 1999;16:2.

259. Blacklock HA, Katz F, Michalevicz R, et al. A and B blood group antigen expression on mixed colony cells and erythroid precursors: relevance for human allogeneic bone marrow transplantation. *Br J Haematol* 1984;58:267.

260. Bacigalupo A, van Lint NT, Occhini D, et al. ABO compatibility and acute graft versus-host-disease following allogeneic bone marrow transplantation. *Transplantation* 1988;45:1091.

261. Hershko G, Gale RP, Ho W. ABH antigens and bone marrow transplantation. *Br J Haematol* 1980;44:65.

262. Benjamin RJ, McGurk S, Ralston MS, et al. ABO incompatibility as an adverse risk factor for survival after allogeneic bone marrow transplantation. *Transfusion* 1999;39:179.

263. Tichelli A, Gratwohl A, Wenger A, et al. ABO-incompatible bone marrow transplantation. In vivo adsorption, an old forgotten method. *Transplant Proc* 1987;19:4632.

264. Gale RP, Feig S, Ho W, et al. ABO blood group system and bone marrow transplantation. *Blood* 1977;50:185.

265. Buckner CD, Clift RA, Sanders JE, et al. ABO-incompatible marrow transplants. *Transplantation* 1978;26:233.

266. Dinsmore RE, Reich LM, Kapoor N, et al. ABH incompatible bone marrow transplantation: removal of erythrocytes by starch sedimentation. *Br J Haematol* 1983;54:441.

267. Braine HG, Sensenbrenner LL, Wright SK, et al. Bone marrow transplantation with major ABO blood group incompatibility using erythrocyte depletion of marrow prior to infusion. *Blood* 1982;60:420.

268. Jin NR, Hill R, Segal G, et al. Preparation of red-blood-cell-depleted marrow for ABO-incompatible marrow transplantation by density-gradient separation using the IBM 2991 blood cell processor. *Exp Hematol* 1987;15:93.

269. Gilmore MJ, Prentice HG, Corringham RE, et al. A technique for the concentration of nucleated bone marrow cells for in vitro manipulation or cryopreservation using the IBM 2991 blood cell processor. *Vox Sang* 1983;45:294.

270. Hows JM, Chipping PM, Palmer S, Gordon-Smith EC. Regeneration of peripheral blood cells following abo incompatible allogeneic bone marrow transplantation for severe aplastic anemia. *Br J Haematol* 1983;53:145.

271. Bensinger WI, Buckner CD, Thomas ED, Clift RA. ABO-incompatible marrow transplants. *Transplantation* 1982;33:427.

272. Warkentin PI, Yomtovian R, Hurd D, et al. Severe delayed hemolytic transfusion reaction complicating an ABO-incompatible bone marrow transplantation. *Vox Sang* 1983;45:40.

273. Ockelford PA, Hill RS, Nelson L, et al. Serologic complications of a major ABO incompatible bone marrow transplantation in a Polynesian with aplastic anemia. *Transfusion* 1982;22:62.

274. Hows JM, Beddow K, Gordon-Smith E, et al. Donor derived red blood cell antibodies and immune hemolysis after allogeneic bone marrow transplantation. *Blood* 1986;67:177.

275. Sniecinski IJ, Oien L, Petz LD, Blume KG. Immunohematologic consequences of major ABO-mismatched bone marrow transplantation. *Transplantation* 1988;45:530.

276. Hazlehurst GR, Brenner MK, Wimperis JZ, et al. Haemolysis after T-cell depleted bone marrow transplantation involving minor ABO incompatibility. *Scand J Haematol* 1986;37:1.

277. Ransey G, Nusbacher J, Starzl TE, Lindsay GD. Isohemagglutinins of graft origin after ABO-unmatched liver transplantation. *N Engl J Med* 1984;311:1167.

278. First LR, Smith BR, Lipton J, Nathan DG, Parkman R, Rappeport JM. Isolated thrombocytopenia after allogeneic bone marrow transplantation: existence of transient and chronic thrombocytopenic syndromes. *Blood* 1985;65:368.

279. Anasetti C, Rybka W, Sullivan KM, et al. Graft versus host disease is associated with autoimmune like thrombocytopenia. *Blood* 1989;73:1054.

280. Minchinton RM, Waters AH, Malpas JS, et al. Selective thrombocytopenia and neutropenia occurring after bone marrow transplantation—evidence of an auto-immune basis. *Clin Lab Haematol* 1984;6:157.

281. Naeim F, Smith GS, Gale RP. Morphologic aspects of bone marrow transplantation in patients with aplastic anemia. *Pathology* 1978;9:295.

282. Faille A, Maraninchi D, Gluckman E, et al. Granulocyte progenitor compartments after allogeneic bone marrow grafts. *Scand J Haematol* 1981;26:202.

283. Arnold R, Schmeiser T, Heit W, et al. Hemopoietic reconstitution after bone marrow transplantation. *Exp Hematol* 1986;14:271.

284. Rowley SD, Zuehlsdorf M, Braine HG, et al. CFU-GM content of bone marrow graft correlates with time to hematologic reconstitution following autologous bone marrow transplantation with 4-hydroperoxycyclophosphamide-purged bone marrow. *Blood* 1987;70:271.

285. Torres A, Alonso MC, Gomez-Villagran JL, et al. No influence of number of donor CFU-GM on granulocyte recovery in bone marrow transplantation for acute Leukemia. *Blut* 1985;50:89.

286. Atkinson K, Norrie S, Chan P, et al. Lack of correlation between nucleated bone marrow cell dose, marrow CFU-GM dose or marrow CFU-E dose and the rate of HLA-identical sibling marrow engraftment. *Br J Haematol* 1985;60:245.

287. Yamasaki K, Solberg LA Jr, Jamal N, et al. Hemopoietic colony growth-promoting activities in the plasma of bone marrow transplant recipients. *J Clin Invest* 1988;82:255.

288. Taylor KM, Jagannath S, Spitzer G, et al. Recombinant human granulocyte colony-stimulating factor hastens granulocyte recovery after high-dose chemotherapy and autologous bone marrow transplantation in Hodgkin's disease. *J Clin Oncol* 1989;7:1791.

289. Nemunaitis J, Singer JW, Buckner CD, et al. Use of recombinant granulocyte-macrophage colony-stimulating factor in autologous marrow transplantation for lymphoid malignancies. *Blood* 1988;72:834.

290. Golde DW, Hocking WG, Quan SG, et al. Origin of bone marrow fibroblasts. *Br J Haematol* 1980;44:183.

291. Singer JW, Keating A, Cuttner J, et al. Evidence for a stem cell common to hematopoiesis and its in vitro microenvironment: studies of patients with clonal hematopoietic neoplasia. *Leuk Res* 1984;8:545.

292. Gunsilius E, Duba HC, Petzer AL, et al. Evidence from a leukaemia model for maintenance of vascular endothelium by bone-marrow-derived endothelial cells. *Lancet* 2000;355:1688.

293. Shi Q, Rafii S, Wu MH, et al. Evidence for circulating bone marrow-derived endothelial cells. *Blood* 1998;92:362.

294. Keating A, Singer JW, Killen PD, et al. Donor origin of the in vitro haematopoietic microenvironment after marrow transplantation in man. *Nature* 1982;298:280.

295. Laver J, Jhanwar SC, O'Reilly RJ, Castro-Malaspina H. Host origin of the hematopoietic microenvironment following allogeneic bone marrow transplantation. *Blood* 1987;70:1966.

296. Lum LG. The kinetics of immune reconstitution after marrow transplantation. *Blood* 1987;69:369.

297. Paulin T, Ringden O, Nilsson B. Immunological recovery after bone marrow transplantation: role of age, graft-versus-host disease, prednisolone treatment and infections. *Bone Marrow Transplant* 1987;1:317.

298. Small TN, Avigan D, Dupont B, et al. Immune reconstitution following T-cell depleted bone marrow transplantation: effect of age and posttranplant graft rejection prophylaxis. *Biol Blood Marrow Transplant* 1997;3:65.

299. Small TN, Papadopoulos EB, Boulad F, et al. Comparison of immune reconstitution after unrelated and related T-cell-depleted bone marrow transplantation: effect of patient age and donor leukocyte infusions. *Blood* 1999;93:467.

300. Verdonck LF, de Gast GC. Is cytomegalovirus infection a major cause of T cell alterations after (autologous) bone marrow transplantation? *Lancet* 1984;1:932.

301. Gratama JW, Naipal AM, Oosterveer MA, et al. Effects of herpes virus carrier status on peripheral T lymphocyte subsets. *Blood* 1987;70:516.

302. Gascon P, Zoumbos NC, Young NS. Immunological abnormalities in patients receiving multiple blood transfusions. *Ann Intern Med* 1984;100:173.

303. Ault KA, Antin JH, Ginsburg D, et al. Phenotype of recovering lymphoid cell populations after marrow transplantation. *J Exp Med* 1985;161:1483.

304. Hokland M, Jacobsen N, Ellegaard J, Hokland P. Natural killer function following allogeneic bone marrow transplantation. *Transplantation* 1988;45:1080.

305. Hercend T, Takvorian T, Nowill A, et al. Characterization of natural killer cells with antileukemic activity following allogeneic bone marrow transplantation. *Blood* 1986;67:722.

306. Smith B, Rappeport J, Burakoff S, Ault K. Clinical correlates of unusual circulating lymphocytes appearing post marrow transplantation. In: Gale R, Champlin R, eds. *Progress in bone marrow transplant.* Vol. 53. New York: Alan R. Liss, 1987:659.

307. Keever CA, Welte K, Small T, et al. Interleukin 2-activated killer cells in patients following transplants of soybean lectin-separated and E rosette-depleted bone marrow. *Blood* 1987;70:1893.

308. Rooney CM, Wimperis JZ, Brenner MK, et al. Natural killer cell activity following T-cell depleted allogeneic bone marrow transplantation. *Br J Haematol* 1986;62:413.

309. Reittie JE, Gottlieb D, Heslop HE, et al. Endogenously generated activated killer cells circulate after autologous and allogeneic marrow transplantation but not after chemotherapy. *Blood* 1989;73:1351.

310. Antin JH, Ault KA, Rappeport JM, Smith BR. B lymphocyte reconstitution after bone marrow transplantation. Leu-1 antigen defines a distinct population of B lymphocytes. *J Clin Invest* 1987;80:325.

311. Anderson KC, Ritz J, Takvorian T, et al. Hematologic engraftment and immune reconstitution posttransplantation with anti-B1 purged autologous bone marrow. *Blood* 1987;69:597.

312. Small TN, Keever CA, Weiner-Fedus S, Heller G, O'Reilly RJ, Flomenberg N. B-cell differentiation following autologous, conventional, or T-cell depleted bone marrow transplantation: A recapitulation of normal B-cell ontogeny. *Blood* 1990;76:1647.

313. Ringden O, Witherspoon R, Storb R, et al. B cell function in human marrow transplant recipients assessed by direct and indirect hemolysis-in-gel assays. *J Immunol* 1979;123:2729.

314. Kiesel S, Pezzutto A, Moldenhauer G, et al. B-cell proliferative and differentiative responses after autologous peripheral blood stem cell or bone marrow transplantation. *Blood* 1988;72:672.

315. Witherspoon RP, Storb R, Ochs HD, et al. Recovery of antibody production in allogeneic marrow graft recipients: influence of time post transplant, the presence or absence of chronic graft versus host disease, and anti-thymocyte globulin treatment. *Blood* 1981;58:360.

316. Lum LG, Seigneuret MC, Storb R, et al. In vitro regulation of immunoglobulin synthesis after marrow transplantation. I. T and B cell deficiencies in patients with and without chronic graft versus host disease. *Blood* 1981;58:431.

317. Shiobara S, Witherspoon RP, Lum LG, Storb R. Immunoglobulin synthesis after HLA-identical marrow grafting. V. The role of peripheral blood monocytes in the regulation of in vitro immunoglobulin secretion stimulated by pokeweed mitogen. *J Immunol* 1984;132:2850.

318. Korsmeyer SJ, Elfenbein GJ, Goldman CK, et al. B cell, helper T cell, and suppressor T cell abnormalities contribute to disordered immunoglobulin synthesis in patients following bone marrow transplantation. *Transplantation* 1982;33:184.

319. Matsue K, Lum LG, Witherspoon RP, Storb R. Proliferative and differential responses of B cells from marrow graft recipients to T-cell derived factors. *Blood* 1987;69:308.

320. Storek J, Saxon A. Reconstitution of B cell immunity following bone marrow transplantation. *Bone Marrow Transplant* 1992;9:395.

321. Noel DR, Witherspoon RP, Storb R, et al. Does graft versus host disease influence the tempo of immunologic recovery after allogeneic marrow transplantation. An observation on 56 long term survivors. *Blood* 1978;51:1087.

322. Holland HK, Wingard JR, Beschorner WE, et al. Bronchiolitis obliterans in bone marrow transplantation and its relationship to chronic graft versus host disease and low serum IgG. *Blood* 1988;72:621.

323. Perreault C, Glasson M, Gyger M, et al. Serum immunoglobulin levels following allogeneic bone marrow transplantation. *Blut* 1985;51:137.

324. Smith BR, Schur PH, Rappeport JM. Prolonged selective IgG4 deficiency post bone marrow transplantation. *Blood* 1987;70(Suppl 1):314a.

325. Sheridan JF, Tutschka PJ, Sedmak DD, Copelan EA. Immunoglobulin G subclass deficiency and pneumococcal infection after allogeneic bone marrow transplantation. *Blood* 1990;75:1583.

326. Ringdén O, Sundberg B, Markling L, Tollemar J. Polyclonal antibody secretion during acute graft versus host disease. *Scand J Immunol* 1987;26:469.

327. Saryan JA, Rappeport J, Leung DY, et al. Regulation of human immunoglobulin E synthesis in acute graft versus host disease. *J Clin Invest* 1983;71:556.

328. Heyd J, Donnenberg AD, Burns WH, et al. Immunoglobulin E levels following allogeneic, autologous, and syngeneic bone marrow transplantation. *Blood* 1988;72:442.

329. Lum LG, Seigneuret MC, Storb R. The transfer of antigen specific immunity from marrow donors to marrow recipients. *J Clin Immunol* 1986;6:1.

330. Lum LG, Munn NA, Schanfield MS, Storb R. The detection of specific antibody formation to recall antigens after bone marrow transplantation. *Blood* 1986;67:582.

331. van Tol MJ, Gerritsen EJ, de Lange GG, et al. The origin of IgG production and homogeneous IgG components after allogeneic bone marrow transplantation. *Blood* 1996;87:818.

332. Hammarstrom L, Smith CIE. Frequent occurrence of monoclonal gammopathies with an unbalanced light chain ratio following bone marrow transplantation. *Transplantation* 1987;43:449.

333. Vossen J, Holl R, Asma G, et al. Reconstitution of the B cell system following allogeneic bone marrow transplantation: an accelerated recapitulation of ontogenic development. In: Eibl M, Rosen S, eds. *Primary immunodeficiency diseases.* Amsterdam: Elsevier, 1986:309.

334. Pruzanski W, Cowan DH, Merrett RA, Freedman NH. IgG1 kappa M component after bone marrow transplantation. *Clin Immunol Immunopathol* 1973;1:311.

335. Mitus AJ, Stein R, Rappeport JM, et al. Monoclonal and oligoclonal gammopathy after bone marrow transplantation. *Blood* 1989;74:2764.

336. Friedrick W, O'Reilly RJ, Koziner B, et al. T lymphocyte reconstitution in recipients of bone marrow transplants with and without GVHD: imbalances of T cell subpopulations having unique regulatory and cognitive function. *Blood* 1982;59:696.

337. Gratama JW, Naipal A, Oljans P, et al. T lymphocyte repopulation and differentiation after bone marrow transplantation. Early shifts in the ratio between T4+ and T8+ T lymphocytes correlate with the occurrence of graft versus host disease. *Blood* 1984;63:1416.

338. Velardi A, Terenzi A, Cucciaioni S, et al. Imbalances within the peripheral blood T-helper (CD4+) and T-suppressor (CD8+) cell populations in the reconstitution phase after bone marrow transplantation. *Blood* 1988;71:1196.

339. Witherspoon RP, Kopecky K, Storb RF, et al. Immunological recovery in 48 patients following syngeneic marrow transplantation or hematological malignancy. *Transplantation* 1982;33:143.

340. Linch DC, Knott LJ, Thomas RM, et al. T cell regeneration after allogeneic and autologous bone marrow transplantation. *Br J Haematol* 1983;53:451.

341. de Gast GC, Verdonck LF, Middeldorp JM, et al. Recovery of T cell subsets after autologous bone marrow transplantation is mainly due to proliferation of mature T cells in the graft. *Blood* 1985;66:428.

342. Schroff RW, Gale RP, Fahey JL. Regeneration of T cell subpopulations after bone marrow transplantation: cytomegalovirus infection and lymphoid subset imbalance. *J Immunol* 1982;129:1926.

343. Ueda M, Harada M, Shiobara S, et al. T lymphocyte reconstitution in long-term survivors after allogeneic and autologous marrow transplantation. *Transplantation* 1984;37:552.

344. Rappeport JM, Dunn MJ, Parkman R. Immature T lymphocytes in the peripheral blood of bone marrow transplant recipients. *Transplantation* 1983;36:674.

345. Ottinger HD, Beelen DW, Scheulen B, Schaefer UW, Grosse-Wilde H. Improved immune reconstitution after allotransplantation of peripheral blood stem cells instead of bone marrow. *Blood* 1996;88:2775.

346. Witherspoon RP, Matthews D, Storb R, et al. Recovery of in vivo cellular immunity after marrow grafting. *Transplantation* 1984;37:145.

347. Rozans M, Smith BR, Burakoff SJ, Miller RA. Long lasting deficit of functional T cell precursors in bone marrow transplant recipients revealed by limiting dilution methods. *J Immunol* 1986;136:4040.

348. Witherspoon RP, Lum LG, Storb R. Immunologic reconstitution after human marrow grafting. *Semin Hematol* 1984;21:2.

349. Daley JP, Rozans MK, Smith BR, et al. Retarded recovery of functional T cell frequencies in T cell depleted bone marrow transplant recipients. *Blood* 1987;70:960.

350. Welte K, Ciobanu N, Moore MA, et al. Defective interleukin 2 production in patients after bone marrow transplantation and in vitro restoration of defective T lymphocyte proliferation by highly purified interleukin 2. *Blood* 1984;64:380.

351. Azogui O, Gluckman E, Fradelizi D. Inhibition of IL2 production after allogeneic bone marrow transplantation. *J Immunol* 1983;131:1205.

352. Mizuno S-I, Morishima Y, Kodera Y, et al. Gamma interferon production capacity and T lymphocyte subpopulation after allogeneic bone marrow transplantation. *Transplantation* 1986;41:311.

353. Cooley MA. Cytokine activity after bone marrow transplantation. *J Immunol* 1987;138:3742.

354. Tsoi MS, Storb R, Dobbs S, et al. Nonspecific suppressor cells in patients with chronic graft-vs-host disease after marrow grafting. *J Immunol* 1979;123:1970.

355. Harada M, Ueda M, Nakao S, et al. Nonspecific suppressor T cells cause decreased mixed lymphocyte culture reactivity in bone marrow transplant patients. *J Immunol* 1986;137:428.

356. Bierer BE, Burakoff SJ, Smith BR. A large proportion of T lymphocytes lack CD5 expression after bone marrow transplantation. *Blood* 1989;73:1359.

357. Roux E, Dumont-Girard F, Starobinski M, et al. Recovery of immune reactivity after T-cell-depleted bone marrow transplantation depends on thymic activity. *Blood* 2000;96:2299.

358. Hochberg EP, Chillemi AC, Wu CJ, et al. Quantitation of T-cell neogenesis in vivo after allogeneic bone marrow transplantation in adults. *Blood* 2001;98:1116.

359. Lewin SR, Heller G, Zhang LM, et al. Direct evidence for new T-cell generation by patients after either T-cell-depleted or unmodified allogeneic hematopoietic stem cell transplants. *Blood* 2002;100:2235.

360. Shepp DH, Dandliker PS, Flournoy N, Meyers JD. Sequential intravenous and twice daily oral acyclovir for extended prophylaxis of herpes simplex virus infection in marrow transplant patients. *Transplantation* 1987;43:654.

361. Shepp DH, Newton BA, Dandliker PS, et al. Oral acyclovir therapy for mucocutaneous herpes simplex virus reactivation after marrow transplantation. *Ann Intern Med* 1985;102:703.

362. Wade JC, Newton B, Flournoy N, Meyers JD. Oral acyclovir for prevention of herpes simplex virus reactivation after marrow transplantation. *Ann Intern Med* 1984;100:823.

363. Lundgren G, Wilczek H, Lonnqvist B, et al. Acyclovir prophylaxis in bone marrow transplant recipients. *Scand J Infect Dis* 1985;47:137.

364. Saral R, Burns WH, Laskin OL, et al. Acyclovir prophylaxis of herpes-simplex-virus infections. A randomized, double-blind, controlled trial in bone-marrow-transplant recipients. *N Engl J Med* 1981;305:63.

365. Steer CB, Szer J, Sasadeusz J, et al. Varicella-zoster infection after allogeneic bone marrow transplantation: incidence, risk factors and prevention with low-dose aciclovir and ganciclovir. *Bone Marrow Transplant* 2000;25:657.

366. Prentice HG, Gluckman E, Powles RL, et al. Long-term survival in allogeneic bone marrow transplant recipients following acyclovir prophylaxis for CMV infection. The European Acyclovir for CMV Prophylaxis Study Group. *Bone Marrow Transplant* 1997;19:129.

367. Ljungman P, Aschan J, Lewensohn-Fuchs I, et al. Results of different strategies for reducing cytomegalovirus-associated mortality in allogeneic stem cell transplant recipients. *Transplantation* 1998;66:1330.

368. Boeckh M, Gooley TA, Bowden RA. Effect of high-dose acyclovir on survival in allogeneic marrow transplant recipients who received ganciclovir at engraftment or for cytomegalovirus pp65 antigenemia. *J Infect Dis* 1998;178:1153.

369. Knox K, Carrigan DR. In vitro suppression of bone marrow progenitor cell differentiation by human herpesvirus 6 infection. *J Infect Dis* 1992;165:925.

370. Singh N, Carrigan DR. Human herpesvirus-6 in transplantation: an emerging pathogen. *Ann Intern Med* 1996;124:1065.

371. O'Reilly RJ, Lee FK, Grossbard E, et al. Papovavirus excretion following marrow transplantation: incidence and association with hepatic dysfunction. *Transplant Proc* 1981;13:262.

372. Azzi A, Fanci R, Bosi A, et al. Monitoring of polyomavirus BK viruria in bone marrow transplantation patients by DNA hybridization assay and by polymerase chain reaction: an approach to assess the relationship between BK viruria and hemorrhagic cystitis. *Bone Marrow Transplant* 1994;14:235.

373. Troussard X, Bauduer F, Gallet E, et al. Virus recovery from stools of patients undergoing bone marrow transplantation. *Bone Marrow Transplant* 1993;12:573.

374. Yolken RH, Bishop CA, Townsend TR, et al. Infectious gastroenteritis in bone-marrow-transplant recipients. *N Engl J Med* 1982;306:1010.

375. Howard DS, Phillips II GL, Reece DE, et al. Adenovirus infections in hematopoietic stem cell transplant recipients. *Clin Infect Dis* 1999;29:1494.

376. Whimbey E, Champlin RE, Couch RB, et al. Community respiratory virus infections among hospitalized adult bone marrow transplant recipients. *Clin Infect Dis* 1996;22:778.

377. Whimbey E, Champlin RE, Englund JA, et al. Combination therapy with aerosolized ribavirin and intravenous immunoglobulin for respiratory syncytial virus disease in adult bone marrow transplant recipients. *Bone Marrow Transplant* 1995;16:393.

378. Mookerjee BP, Vogelsang G. Human herpes virus-6 encephalitis after bone marrow transplantation: successful treatment with ganciclovir. *Bone Marrow Transplant* 1997;20:905.

379. Cole PD, Stiles J, Boulad F, et al. Successful treatment of human herpesvirus 6 encephalitis in a bone marrow transplant recipient. *Clin Infect Dis* 1998;27:653.

380. Bordigoni P, Carret AS, Venard V, et al. Treatment of adenovirus infections in patients undergoing allogeneic hematopoietic stem cell transplantation. *Clin Infect Dis* 2001;32:1290.

381. Hoffman JA, Shah AJ, Ross LA, Kapoor N. Adenoviral infections and a prospective trial of cidofovir in pediatric hematopoietic stem cell transplantation. *Biol Blood Marrow Transplant* 2001;7:388.

382. Legrand F, Berrebi D, Houhou N, et al. Early diagnosis of adenovirus infection and treatment with cidofovir after bone marrow transplantation in children. *Bone Marrow Transplant* 2001;27:621.

383. Colby C, McAfee S, Sackstein R, et al. A prospective randomized trial comparing the toxicity and safety of atovaquone with trimethoprim/sulfamethoxazole as Pneumocystis carinii pneumonia prophylaxis following autologous peripheral blood stem cell transplantation. *Bone Marrow Transplant* 1999;24:897.

384. Vasconcelles MJ, Bernardo MV, King C, et al. Aerosolized pentamidine as pneumocystis prophylaxis after bone marrow transplantation is inferior to other regimens and is associated with decreased survival and an increased risk of other infections. *Biol Blood Marrow Transplant* 2000;6:35.

385. Roy V, Ochs L, Weisdorf D. Late infections following allogeneic bone marrow transplantation: suggested strategies for prophylaxis. *Leuk Lymphoma* 1997;26:1.

386. Locksley RM, Flournoy N, Sullivan KM, Meyers JD. Infection with varicella-zoster virus after marrow transplantation. *J Infect Dis* 1985;152:1172.

387. Koc Y, Miller KB, Schenkein DP, et al. Varicella zoster virus infections following allogeneic bone marrow transplantation: frequency, risk factors, and clinical outcome. *Biol Blood Marrow Transplant* 2000;6:44.

388. Wingard JR, Piantadosi S, Burns W, et al. Cytomegalovirus infections in Bone Marrow Transplant recipients given intensive cytoreductive therapy. *J Infect Dis* 1990;12:s793.

389. Enright H, Haake R, Weisdorf D, et al. Cytomegalovirus pneumonia after bone marrow transplantation. Risk factors and response to therapy. *Transplantation* 1993;55:1339.

390. Einsele H, Ehninger G, Hebart H, et al. Incidence of local CMV infection and acute intestinal GVHD in marrow transplant recipients with severe diarrhea. *Bone Marrow Transplant* 1994;14:955.

391. Forman SJ, Zaia JA. Treatment and prevention of cytomegalovirus pneumonia after bone marrow transplantation: where do we stand? *Blood* 1994;83:2392.

392. van der Meer JT, Drew WL, Bowden RA, et al. Summary of the International Consensus Symposium on Advances in the Diagnosis, Treatment and Prophylaxis and Cytomegalovirus Infection. *Antiviral Res* 1996;32:119.

393. Wingard JR, Chen DYH, Burns WH, et al. Cytomegalovirus infection after autologous bone marrow transplantation with comparison to infection after allogeneic bone marrow transplantation. *Blood* 1988;71:1432.

394. Miller W, Flynn P, McCullough J, et al. Cytomegalovirus infection after bone marrow transplantation: an association with graft versus host disease. *Blood* 1986;67:1162.

395. Osarogiagbon RU, Defor TE, Weisdorf MA, Erice A, Weisdorf DJ. CMV antigenemia following bone marrow transplantation: risk factors and outcomes. *Biol Blood Marrow Transplant* 2000;6:280.

396. Grob JP, Grundy JE, Prentice HG, et al. Immune donors can protect marrow-transplant recipients from severe cytomegalovirus infections. *Lancet* 1987; 1:774.

397. Verdonck LF, de Graan-Hentzen YCE, Dekker AW, et al. Cytomegalovirus seronegative platelets and leukocyte-poor red blood cells from random donors can prevent primary cytomegalovirus infection after bone marrow transplantation. *Bone Marrow Transplant* 1987;2:73.

398. Bowden RA, Slichter SJ, Sayers M, et al. A comparison of filtered leukocyte-reduced and cytomegalovirus (CMV) seronegative blood products for the prevention of transfusion-associated CMV infection after marrow transplant. *Blood* 1995;86:3598.

399. Winston D, Antin J, Wolff S, et al. Comparative efficacy of different doses of intravenous immunoglobulin (IVIG) for prevention of graft-versus-host disease (GVHD) after bone marrow transplantation (BMT): results of a randomized, double-blind trial. *Blood* 1996;88(Suppl 1):302a.

400. Sullivan KM, Storek J, Kopecky KJ, et al. A controlled trial of long-term administration of intravenous immunoglobulin to prevent late infection and chronic graft-vs.-host disease after marrow transplantation: clinical outcome and effect on subsequent immune recovery. *Biol Blood Marrow Transplant* 1996;2:44.

401. Meyers JD. Prevention and treatment of cytomegalovirus infection after marrow transplantation. *Bone Marrow Transplant* 1988;3:95.

402. Verdonck LF, Dekker AW, Rozenberg-Arska M, van den Hoek MR. A risk-adapted approach with a short course of ganciclovir to prevent cytomegalovirus (CMV) pneumonia in CMV-seropositive recipients of allogeneic bone marrow transplants. *Clin Infect Dis* 1997;24:901.

403. Boeckh M, Gooley TA, Myerson D, et al. Cytomegalovirus pp65 antigenemia-guided early treatment with ganciclovir versus ganciclovir at engraftment after allogeneic marrow transplantation: a randomized double-blind study. *Blood* 1996;88:4063.

404. Salzberger B, Bowden RA, Hackman RC, et al. Neutropenia in allogeneic marrow transplant recipients receiving ganciclovir for prevention of cytomegalovirus disease: risk factors and outcome. *Blood* 1997;90:2502.

405. Maltezou H, Whimbey E, Abi-Said D, et al. Cytomegalovirus disease in adult marrow transplant recipients receiving ganciclovir prophylaxis: a retrospective study. *Bone Marrow Transplant* 1999;24:665.

406. Reusser P, Einsele H, Lee J, et al. Randomized multicenter trial of foscarnet versus ganciclovir for preemptive therapy of cytomegalovirus infection after allogeneic stem cell transplantation. *Blood* 2002;99:1159.

407. Moretti S, Zikos P, Van Lint MT, et al. Forscarnet vs ganciclovir for cytomegalovirus (CMV) antigenemia after allogeneic hemopoietic stem cell transplantation (HSCT): a randomised study. *Bone Marrow Transplant* 1998;22:175.

408. Ippoliti C, Morgan A, Warkentin D, et al. Foscarnet for prevention of cytomegalovirus infection in allogeneic marrow transplant recipients unable to receive ganciclovir. *Bone Marrow Transplant* 1997;20:491.

409. Reusser P, Cordonnier C, Einsele H, et al. European survey of herpesvirus resistance to antiviral drugs in bone marrow transplant recipients. Infectious Diseases Working Party of the European Group for Blood and Marrow Transplantation (EBMT). *Bone Marrow Transplant* 1996;17:813.

410. Verdonck LF, Dekker AW, Rozenberg-Arska M, van den Hoek MR. A risk-adapted approach with a short course of ganciclovir to prevent cytomegalovirus (CMV) pneumonia in CMV-seropositive recipients of allogeneic bone marrow transplants. *Clin Infect Dis* 1997;24:901.

411. Ljungman P, Aschan J, Lewensohn-Fuchs I, et al. Results of different strategies for reducing cytomegalovirus-associated mortality in allogeneic stem cell transplant recipients. *Transplantation* 1998;66:1330.

412. Einsele H, Hebart H, Kauffmann-Schneider C, et al. Risk factors for treatment failures in patients receiving PCR-based preemptive therapy for CMV infection. *Bone Marrow Transplant* 2000;25:757.

413. Aitken C, Barrett-Muir W, Millar C, et al. Use of molecular assays in diagnosis and monitoring of cytomegalovirus disease following renal transplantation. *J Clin Microbiol* 1999;37:2804.

414. Emanuel D, Cunningham I, Jules-Elysee K, et al. Cytomegalovirus pneumonia after bone marrow transplantation successfully treated with the combination of ganciclovir and high-dose intravenous immune globulin. *Ann Intern Med* 1988;109:777.

415. Drobyski WR, Knox KK, Carrigan DR, Ash RC. Foscarnet therapy of ganciclovir-resistant cytomegalovirus in marrow transplantation. *Transplantation* 1991;52:155.

416. Riddell SR, Watanabe KS, Goodrich JM, et al. Restoration of viral immunity in immunodeficient humans by the adoptive transfer of T cell clones. *Science* 1992;257:238.

417. Walter EA, Greenberg PD, Gilbert MJ, et al. Reconstitution of cellular immunity against cytomegalovirus in recipients of allogeneic bone marrow by transfer of T-cell clones from the donor. *N Engl J Med* 1995;333:1038.

418. Antin JH, Ginsburg D, Smith BR, et al. Bone marrow transplantation for paroxysmal nocturnal hemoglobinuria: eradication of the PNH clone and docu-

mentation of complete lymphohematopoietic engraftment. *Blood* 1985;66: 1247.

419. Sparkes MC, Crist ML, Sparkes RS, et al. Gene markers in human bone marrow transplantation. *Vox Sang* 1977;33:202.

420. Hutchinson RM, Pringle JH, Potter L, et al. Rapid identification of donor and recipient cells after allogeneic bone marrow transplantation using specific genetic markers. *Br J Haematol* 1989;72:133.

421. Antin JH, Childs R, Filipovich AH, et al. Establishment of complete and mixed donor chimerism after allogeneic lymphohematopoietic transplantation: recommendations from a workshop at the 2001 tandem meetings. *Biol Blood Marrow Transplant* 2001;7:473.

422. Bretagne S, Vidaud M, Kuentz M, et al. Mixed blood chimerism in T cell depleted bone marrow transplant recipients: evaluation using DNA polymorphism. *Blood* 1987;70:1692.

423. Schmitz N, Godde-Salz E, Loffler H. Cytogenetic studies on recipients of allogeneic bone marrow transplants after fractionated total body irradiation. *Br J Haematol* 1985;60:239.

424. Walker H, Singer CR, Patterson J, et al. The significance of host haemopoietic cells detected by cytogenetic analysis of bone marrow from recipients of bone marrow transplants. *Br J Haematol* 1986;62:385.

425. Butturini A, Seeger RC, Gale RP. Recipient immune-competent T lymphocytes can survive intensive conditioning for bone marrow transplantation. *Blood* 1986;68:954.

426. Hill RS, Petersen FB, Storb R, et al. Mixed hematologic chimerism after allogeneic marrow transplantation for severe aplastic anemia is associated with a higher risk of graft rejection and a lessened incidence of acute graft-versus-host disease. *Blood* 1986;67:811.

427. Spitzer TR, McAfee S, Sackstein R, et al. Intentional induction of mixed chimerism and achievement of antitumor responses after nonmyeloablative conditioning therapy and HLA-matched donor bone marrow transplantation for refractory hematologic malignancies. *Biol Blood Marrow Transplant* 2000;6:309.

428. Boyd CN, Ranberg R, Thomas ED. The incidence of recurrence of leukemia in donor cells after allogeneic bone marrow transplantation. *Leukemia Res* 1982;6:833.

429. Smith JW, Shulman HM, Thomas ED, et al. Bone marrow transplantation for acute myelosclerosis. *Cancer* 1981;48:2198.

430. Dokal I, Jones L, Deenmamode M, et al. Allogeneic bone marrow transplantation for primary myelofibrosis. *Br J Haematol* 1989;71:158.

431. Coccia PF, Krivit W, Cervenka J, et al. Successful bone-marrow transplantation for infantile malignant osteopetrosis. *N Engl J Med* 1980;302:701.

432. Goodrich JM, Bowden RA, Fisher L, Keller C, Schoch G, Meyers JD. Ganciclovir prophylaxis to prevent cytomegalovirus disease after allogeneic marrow transplant. *Ann Intern Med* 1993;118:173.

433. Appelbaum FR, Fefer A, Cheever MA, et al. Treatment of aplastic anemia by bone marrow transplantation in identical twins. *Blood* 1980;55:1033.

434. Champlin RE, Feig SA, Sparkes RS, Gale RP. Bone marrow transplantation from identical twins in the treatment of aplastic anemia: implication for the pathogenesis of the disease. *Br J Haematol* 1984;56:455.

435. Bortin MM, Gale RP, Rimm AA. Allogeneic bone marrow transplantation for 144 patients with severe aplastic anemia. *JAMA* 1981;245:1132.

436. Storb R, Thomas ED, Buckner CD, et al. Marrow transplantation for aplastic anemia. *Semin Hematol* 1984;21:27.

437. Deeg HJ, Self S, Storb R, et al. Decreased incidence of marrow graft rejection in patients with severe aplastic anemia: changing impact of risk factors. *Blood* 1986;68:1363.

438. Champlin RE, Horowitz MM, van Bekkum DW, et al. Graft failure following bone marrow transplantation for severe aplastic anemia: risk factors and treatment results. *Blood* 1989;73:606.

439. Castro-Malaspina H, Childs B, Laver J, et al. Hyperfractionated total lymphoid irradiation and cyclophosphamide for preparation of previously transfused patients undergoing HLA-identical marrow transplantation for severe aplastic anemia. *Int J Radiat Oncol Biol Phys* 1994;29:847.

440. Gale RP, Ho W, Feig S, et al. Prevention of graft rejection following bone marrow transplantation. *Blood* 1981;57:9.

441. Ramsay NK, Kim T, Nesbit ME, et al. Total lymphoid irradiation and cyclophosphamide as preparation for bone marrow transplantation in severe aplastic anemia. *Blood* 1980;55:344.

442. Deeg HJ, Witherspoon RP. Risk factors for the development of secondary malignancies after marrow transplantation. *Hematol Oncol Clin North Am* 1993;7:417.

443. Butturini A, Gale RP. T cell depletion in bone marrow transplantation for leukemia: current results and future directions. *Bone Marrow Transplant* 1988;3:185.

444. Bozdech MJ, Sondel PM, Trigg ME, et al. Transplantation of HLA-haploidentical T-cell-depleted marrow for leukemia: addition of cytosine arabinoside to the pretransplant conditioning prevents rejection. *Exp Hematol* 1985;13:1201.

445. Fahey JL, Sarna G, Gale RP, Seeger R. Immune interventions in disease [published erratum appears in *Ann Intern Med* 1987 May;106(5):783]. *Ann Intern Med* 1987;106:257.

446. Hale G, Cobbold S, Waldmann H. T cell depletion with Campath-1 in allogeneic bone marrow transplantation. *Transplantation* 1988;45:753.

447. Patterson J, Prentice HG, Brenner MK, et al. Graft rejection following HLA matched T-lymphocyte depleted bone marrow transplantation. *Br J Haematol* 1986;63:221.

448. Mitsuyasu RT, Champlin RE, Gale RP, et al. Treatment of donor bone marrow with monoclonal anti-T-cell antibody and complement for the prevention of graft versus host disease. *Ann Intern Med* 1986;105:20.

449. Filipovich AH, Vallera DA, Youle RJ, et al. Graft-versus-host disease prevention in allogeneic bone marrow transplantation from histocompatible siblings. *Transplantation* 1987;44:62.

450. Martin PJ, Hansen JA, Buckner CD, et al. Effects of in vitro depletion of T cells in HLA-identical allogeneic marrow grafts. *Blood* 1985;66:664.

451. O'Reilly R, Collins NH, Kernan N, et al. Transplantation of marrow-depleted T cells by soybean lectin agglutination and E-rosette depletion: major histocompatibility complex-related graft resistance in leukemic transplant patients. *Transplant Proc* 1985;17:455.

452. O'Reilly R, Collins N, Brochstein J, et al. Soybean lectin agglutination and E rosette depletion for removal of T cells from HLA identical marrow grafts: results in 60 consecutive patients transplanted for hematopoietic malignancy. In: Hagenbeek A, Lowenberg B, eds. *Minimal residual disease in acute leukemia.* The Netherlands: Martinus Nijhoff, 1986:337.

453. Anasetti C, Storb R, Longton G, et al. Donor buffy coat cell infusion after marrow transplantation for aplastic anemia (letter). *Blood* 1988;72:1099.

454. Fleischhauer K, Kernan NA, O'Reilly RJ, et al. Bone marrow-allograft rejection by T lymphocytes recognizing a single amino acid difference on HLA-B44. *N Engl J Med* 1990;323:1818.

455. Kernan NA, Flomenberg N, Dupont B, O'Reilly RJ. Graft rejection in recipients of T cell depleted HLA-nonidentical marrow transplants for leukemia. *Transplantation* 1987;43:842.

456. Papadopoulos EB, Carabasi MH, Castro-Malaspina H, et al. T-cell-depleted allogeneic bone marrow transplantation as postremission therapy for acute myelogenous leukemia: freedom from relapse in the absence of graft-versus-host disease. *Blood* 1998;91:1083.

457. Aversa F, Terenzi A, Carotti A, et al. Improved outcome with T-cell-depleted bone marrow transplantation for acute leukemia. *J Clin Oncol* 1999;17:1545.

458. Khouri IF, Keating M, Korbling M, et al. Transplant-lite: induction of graft-versus-malignancy using fludarabine-based nonablative chemotherapy and allogeneic blood progenitor-cell transplantation as treatment for lymphoid malignancies [see comments]. *J Clin Oncol* 1998;16:2817.

459. Aversa F, Tabilio A, Teremzo A, et al. Successful engraftment of T-cell-depleted haploidentical "three-loci" incompatible transplants in leukemia by addition of recombinant granulocyte colony-stimulating factor-mobilized peripheral blood progenitor cells to bone marrow inoculum. *Blood* 1994;84:3948.

460. Reisner Y, Bachar-Lustig E, Li H, et al. The role of megadose CD34⁺ progenitor cells in the treatment of leukemia patients without a matched donor and in tolerance induction for organ transplantation. *Ann N Y Acad Sci* 1999;872:336.

461. Hathaway WE, Brangle RW, Nelson TL, Roeckel IE. Aplastic anemia and alymphocytosis in an infant with hypogammaglobulinemia: graft versus host reaction? *J Pediatr* 1966;68:713.

462. Kadowaki J, Thompson RI, Zuelzer WW, et al. XX-XY lymphoid chimaerism in congenital immunological deficiency syndrome with thymic alymphoplasia. *Lancet* 1965;2:1152.

463. Evans PC, Lambert N, Maloney S, et al. Long-term fetal microchimerism in peripheral blood mononuclear cell subsets in healthy women and women with scleroderma. *Blood* 1999;93:2033.

464. Maloney S, Smith A, Furst DE, et al. Microchimerism of maternal origin persists into adult life. *J Clin Invest* 1999;104:41.

465. Weisdorf DJ, Snover DC, Haake R, et al. Acute upper gastrointestinal graft-versus-host disease: Clinical significance and response to immunosuppressive therapy. *Blood* 1990;76:624.

466. Spencer GD, Hackman RC, McDonald GB, et al. A prospective study of unexplained nausea and vomiting after marrow transplantation. *Transplantation* 1986;42:602.

467. Kohler S, Hendrickson MR, Chao NJ, Smoller BR. Value of skin biopsies in assessing prognosis and progression of acute graft-versus-host disease. *Am J Surg Pathol* 1997;21:988.

468. Zhou Y, Barnett MJ, Rivers JK. Clinical significance of skin biopsies in the diagnosis and management of graft-vs-host disease in early postallogeneic bone marrow transplantation. *Arch Dermatol* 2000;136:717.

469. Massi D, Franchi A, Pimpinelli N, et al. A reappraisal of the histopathologic criteria for the diagnosis of cutaneous allogeneic acute graft-vs-host disease. *Am J Clin Pathol* 1999;112:791.

470. Przepiorka D, Weisdorf D, Martin P, et al. 1994 Consensus Conference on Acute GVHD Grading. *Bone Marrow Transplant* 1995;15:825.

471. Lerner KG, Kao GF, Storb R, et al. Histopathology of graft-vs.-host reaction (GvHR) in human recipients of marrow from HL-A-matched sibling donors. *Transplant Proc* 1974;6:367.

472. Snover DC, Weisdorf SA, Ramsay NK, et al. Hepatic graft versus host disease: a study of the predictive value of liver biopsy in diagnosis. *Hepatology* 1984;4:123.

473. Shulman HM, Sharma P, Amos D, et al. A coded histologic study of hepatic graft-versus-host disease after bone marrow transplantation. *Hepatology* 1988;8:463.

474. Sale GE, Shulman HM, McDonald GB, Thomas ED. Gastrointestinal graft versus host disease in man: A clinicopathological study of the rectal biopsy. *Amer J Surg Pathol* 1979;3:291.

475. Sviland L, Pearson AD, Eastham EJ, et al. Histological features of skin and rectal biopsy specimens after autologous and allogeneic bone marrow transplantation. *J Clin Pathol* 1988;41:148.

476. Elliott CJ, Sloane JP, Sanderson KV, et al. The histological diagnosis of cutaneous graft versus host disease: relationship of skin changes to marrow purging and other clinical variables. *Histopathology* 1987;11:145.

477. Kraus MD, Feran-Doza M, Garcia-Moliner ML, et al. Cytomegalovirus infection in the colon of bone marrow transplantation patients. *Mod Pathol* 1998;11:29.

478. Snover DC. Mucosal damage simulating acute graft versus host reaction in cytomegalovirus colitis. *Transplantation* 1985;39:669.

479. Shulman HM, McDonald GB, Matthews D, et al. An analysis of hepatic venoocclusive disease and centrilobular hepatic degeneration following bone marrow transplantation. *Gastroenterology* 1980;79:1178.

480. Gleichmann E, Gleichmann H. Essential similarity between graft versus host disease and viral infections. *Transplantation* 1976;22:399.

481. Gratama JW, Zwaan FE, Stijnen T, et al. Herpes-virus immunity and acute graft-versus-host disease. *Lancet* 1987;1:471.

482. Gratama JW, Sinnige LG, Weijers TF, et al. Marrow donor immunity to herpes simplex virus: association with acute graft-versus-host disease. *Exp Hematol* 1987;15:735.

483. Beschorner WE, Saral R, Hutchins GM, et al. Lymphocytic bronchitis associated with graft versus host disease in recipients of bone marrow transplants. *N Engl J Med* 1978;299:1030.

484. Bergstein J, Andreoli SP, Provisor AJ, Yum M. Radiation nephritis following total body irradiation and cyclophosphamide in preparation for bone marrow transplantation. *Transplantation* 1986;41:63.

485. Patchell R. Neurological complications of bone marrow transplantation. *Neurology* 1985;35:300.

486. Korngold R, Sprent J. Lethal graft versus host disease following bone marrow transplantation across minor histocompatibility barriers in mice. Prevention by removing mature T cells from marrow. *J Exp Med* 1978;148:1687.

487. Korngold R, Sprent J. Lethal GVHD across minor histocompatibility barriers: nature of the effector cells and role of the H-2 complex. *Immunol Rev* 1983;71:5.

488. Cutler C, Giri S, Jeyapalan S, et al. Acute and chronic graft-versus-host disease after allogeneic peripheral-blood stem-cell and bone marrow transplantation: a meta-analysis. *J Clin Oncol* 2001;19:3685.

489. Beatty PG, Clift RA, Mickelson EM, et al. Marrow transplantation from related donors other than HLA-identical siblings. *N Engl J Med* 1985;313:765.

490. Goulmy E, Schipper R, Pool J, et al. Mismatches of minor histocompatibility antigens between HLA-identical donors and recipients and the development of graft-versus-host disease after bone marrow transplantation. *N Engl J Med* 1996;334:281.

491. Rufer N, Wolpert E, Helg C, et al. HA-1 and the SMCY-derived peptide FIDSYICQV (H-Y) are immunodominant minor histocompatibility antigens after bone marrow transplantation. *Transplantation* 1998;66:910.

492. Hamilton BL, Brevan MJ, Parkman R. Anti-recipient cytotoxic T lymphocyte precursors are present in the spleen of mice with acute graft versus host disease due to minor histocompatibility differences. *J Immunol* 1981;126:621.

493. Murphy WJ, Longo DL. The potential role of NK cells in the separation of graft-versus-tumor effects from graft-versus-host disease after allogeneic bone marrow transplantation. *Immunol Rev* 1997;157:167.

494. Asai O, Longo DL, Tian ZG, et al. Suppression of graft-versus-host disease and amplification of graft-versus-tumor effects by activated natural killer cells after allogeneic bone marrow transplantation. *J Clin Invest* 1998;101:1835.

495. Vallera DA, Soderling CCB, Kersey JH. Bone marrow transplantation across major histocompatibility barriers in mice. *J Immunol* 1982;128:871.

496. Korngold R, Sprent J. Surface markers of T cells causing lethal graft vs host disease to Class I vs Class II H-2 differences. *J Immunol* 1985;135:3004.

497. Alyea EP, Soiffer RJ, Canning C, et al. Toxicity and efficacy of defined doses of CD4(+) donor lymphocytes for treatment of relapse after allogeneic bone marrow transplant. *Blood* 1998;91:3671.

498. Antin JH, Ferrara JL. Cytokine dysregulation and acute graft-versus-host disease. *Blood* 1992;80:2964.

499. Ferrara J, Antin J. The pathophysiology of graft-versus-host disease. In: Thomas E, Blume KG, Forman SJ, eds. *Hematopoietic cell transplantation.* Malden, MA: Blackwell Science, Inc., 1999:305.

500. Braun M, Lowin B, French L, et al. Cytotoxic T cells deficient in both functional fas ligand and perforin show residual cytolytic activity yet lose their capacity to induce lethal acute graft-versus-host disease. *J Exp Med* 1996;183:657.

501. Fowler DH, Gress RE. Th2 and Tc2 cells in the regulation of GVHD, GVL, and graft rejection: considerations for the allogeneic transplantation therapy of leukemia and lymphoma. *Leuk Lymphoma* 2000;38:221.

502. Lee R, Spielman J, Zhao D, et al. Perforin, Fas ligand, and tumor necrosis factor are the major cytotoxic molecules used by lymphokine-activated killer cells. *J Immunol* 1996;157:1919.

503. Shresta S, Russell J, Ley T. Mechanisms responsible for granzyme B-independent cytotoxicity. *Blood* 1997;89:4085.

504. Via CS, Nguyen P, Shustov A, et al. A major role for the Fas pathway in acute graft-versus-host disease. *J Immunol* 1996;157:5387.

505. Ferrara JL. Pathogenesis of acute graft-versus-host disease: cytokines and cellular effectors. *J Hematother Stem Cell Res* 2000;9:299.

506. van Bekkum DW, Roodenburg J, Heidt PJ, van der Waaij D. Mitigation of secondary disease of allogeneic mouse radiation chimeras by modification of the intestinal microflora. *J Nat Cancer Inst* 1974;52:401.

507. Beelen DW, Haralambie E, Brandt H, et al. Evidence that sustained growth suppression of intestinal anaerobic bacteria reduces the risk of acute graft-versus-host disease after sibling marrow transplantation. *Blood* 1992;80:2668.

508. Storb R, Prentice RL, Buckner CD, et al. Graft-versus-host disease and survival in patients with aplastic anemia treated by marrow grafts from HLA-identical siblings. Beneficial effects of a protective environment. *N Engl J Med* 1983;308:302.

509. Powles RL, Kay HEM, Clink HM, et al. Mismatched family donors for bone marrow transplantation as treatment for acute leukemia. *Lancet* 1983;1:612.

510. Ringden O, Nilsson B. Death by graft-versus-host disease associated with HLA mismatch, high recipient age, low marrow cell dose, and splenectomy. *Transplantation* 1985;40:39.

511. Stucki A, Leisenring W, Sandmaier BM, et al. Decreased rejection and improved survival of first and second marrow transplants for severe aplastic anemia (a 26-year retrospective analysis). *Blood* 1998;92:2742.

512. Passweg J, Socié G, Hinterberger H, et al. Bone marrow transplantation for severe aplastic anemia: has outcome improved? *Blood* 1997;90:858.

513. Nash RA, Pepe MS, Storb R, et al. Acute graft-versus-host disease: analysis of risk factors after allogeneic marrow transplantation and prophylaxis with cyclosporine and methotrexate. *Blood* 1992;80:1838.

514. Bross DS, Tutschka PJ, Farmer ER, et al. Predictive factors for acute graft versus host disease in patients transplanted with HLA-identical bone marrow. *Blood* 1984;63:1265.

515. Gale RP, Bortin MM, van Bekkum DW, et al. Risk factors for acute graft-versus-host disease. *Br J Haematol* 1987;67:397.

516. Weisdorf D, Hakke R, Blazar B, et al. Risk factors for acute graft-versus-host disease in histocompatible donor bone marrow transplantation. *Transplantation* 1991;51:1197.

517. Storb R, Hansen JA, Prentice RL, Thomas ED. Association between HLA-B antigens and acute graft versus host disease. *Lancet* 1983;2:816.

518. Baughan AS, Worsley M, McCarthy DM, et al. Hematological reconstitution and severity of graft-versus-host disease after bone marrow transplantation for chronic granulocytic leukemia: the influence of previous splenectomy. *Br J Haematol* 1984;56:445.

519. Rowlings P, Przepiorka D, Klein J, et al. IBMTR severity index for grading acute graft-versus-host disease: retrospective comparison with Glucksberg grade. *Br J Haematol* 1997;97:855.

520. Vilmer E, Mazeron MC, Rabian C, et al. Clinical significance of cytomegalovirus viremia in bone marrow transplantation. *Transplantation* 1985;40:30.

521. Sviland L, Dickinson AM. A human skin explant model for predicting graft-versus-host disease following bone marrow transplantation. *J Clin Pathol* 1999;52:910.

522. Vogelsang GB, Hess AD, Berkman AW, et al. An in vitro predictive test for graft versus host disease in patients with genotypic HLA-identical bone marrow transplants. *N Engl J Med* 1985;313:645.

523. Theobald M, Nierle T, Bunjes D, et al. Host-specific interleukin-2-secreting donor T-cell precursors as predictors of acute graft-versus-host disease in bone marrow transplantation between HLA-identical siblings. *N Engl J Med* 1992;327:1613.

524. Dickinson AM, Sviland L, Wang XN, et al. Predicting graft-versus-host disease in HLA-identical bone marrow transplant: a comparison of T-cell frequency analysis and a human skin explant model. *Transplantation* 1998;66:857.

525. Wang XN, Taylor PR, Skinner R, et al. T-cell frequency analysis does not predict the incidence of graft-versus-host disease in HLA-matched sibling bone marrow transplantation. *Transplantation* 2000;70:488.

526. Vogelsang GB, Hess AD, Santos GW. Acute graft-versus-host disease: clinical characteristics in the cyclosporine era. *Medicine* 1988;67:163.

527. Nash R, Antin J, Karanes C, et al. A phase III study comparing methotrexate and tacrolimus with methotrexate and cyclosporine for prophylaxis of acute graft-versus-host disease after marrow transplantation from unrelated donors. *Blood* 2000;96:2062.

528. Ramsay NK, Kersey JH, Robison LL, et al. A randomized study of the prevention of acute graft-versus-host disease. *N Engl J Med* 1982;306:392.

529. Antin JH. Graft-versus-leukemia: no longer an epiphenomenon. *Blood* 1993;82:2273.

530. Storb R, Deeg HJ, Farewell V, et al. Marrow transplantation for severe aplastic anemia: methotrexate alone compared with a combination of methotrexate and cyclosporine for prevention of acute graft-versus-host disease. *Blood* 1986;68:119.

531. Storb R, Deeg HJ, Pepe M, et al. Methotrexate and cyclosporine versus cyclosporine alone for prophylaxis of graft versus host disease in patients given HLA-identical marrow grafts for leukemia: long term followup of a controlled trial. *Blood* 1989;73:1729.

532. Horowitz MM, Przepiorka D, Bartels P, et al. Tacrolimus vs. cyclosporine immunosuppression: results in advanced-stage disease compared with historical controls treated exclusively with cyclosporine. *Biol Blood Marrow Transplant* 1999;5:180.

533. Ringden O, Horowitz MM, Sondel P, et al. Methotrexate, cyclosporine, or both to prevent graft-versus-host disease after HLA-identical sibling bone marrow transplants for early leukemia? *Blood* 1993;81:1094.

534. Devine SM, Geller RB, Lin LB, et al. The outcome of unrelated donor bone marrow transplantation in patients with hematologic malignancies using tacrolimus (FK506) and low dose methotrexate for graft-versus-host disease prophylaxis. *Biol Blood Marrow Transplant* 1997;3:25.

535. Przepiorka D, Khouri I, Ippoliti C, et al. Tacrolimus and minidose methotrexate for prevention of acute graft-versus-host disease after HLA-mismatched marrow or blood stem cell transplantation. *Bone Marrow Transplant* 1999;24:763.

536. Bornhauser M, Schuler U, Porksen G, et al. Mycophenolate mofetil and cyclosporine as graft-versus-host disease prophylaxis after allogeneic blood stem cell transplantation. *Transplantation* 1999;67:499.

537. Clift RA, Buckner CD, Appelbaum FR, et al. Allogeneic marrow transplantation in patients with chronic myeloid leukemia in the chronic phase: a randomized trial of two irradiation regimens. *Blood* 1991;77:1660.

538. Storb R, Pepe M, Anasetti C, et al. What role for prednisone in prevention of acute graft-versus-host disease in patients undergoing marrow transplants? *Blood* 1990;76:1037.

539. Reisner Y, Kapoor N, Kirkpatrick D, et al. Transplantation for acute leukemia with HLA-A and B nonidentical parental marrow cells fractionated with soybean agglutinin and sheep red blood cells. *Lancet* 1981;2:327.

540. Reinherz EL, Geha R, Rappeport JM, et al. Reconstitution after transplantation with T-lymphocyte-depleted HLA haplotype-mismatched bone marrow for severe combined immunodeficiency. *Proc Natl Acad Sci U S A* 1982;79:6047.

541. Prentice HG, Blacklock HA, Janossy G, et al. Use of anti-T-cell monoclonal antibody OKT3 to prevent acute graft versus host disease in allogeneic bone marrow transplantation in man. *Lancet* 1982;1:700.

542. Filipovich AH, McGlave PB, Ramsay NKC, et al. Pretreatment of donor bone marrow with monoclonal antibody OKT3 for prevention of acute graft versus host disease in allogeneic histocompatible bone marrow transplantation. *Lancet* 1982;1:1266.

543. Reisner Y. A shorter procedure for preparing E-rosette-depleted bone marrow for transplantation. *Transplantation* 1986;42:312.

544. Racadot E, Hervé P, Beaujean F, et al. Prevention of graft-versus-host disease in HLA-matched bone marrow transplantation for malignant diseases: a multicentric study of 62 patients using 3-pan-T monoclonal antibodies and rabbit complement. *J Clin Oncol* 1987;5:426.

545. Soiffer RJ, Murray C, Mauch P, et al. Prevention of graft-versus-host disease by selective depletion of CD6-positive T lymphocytes from donor bone marrow. *J Clin Oncol* 1992;10:1191.

546. Antin JH, Bierer BE, Smith BR, et al. Selective depletion of bone marrow T lymphocytes with anti-CD5 monoclonal antibodies: effective prophylaxis for graft-versus-host disease in patients with hematologic malignancies. *Blood* 1991;78:2139.

547. Schattenberg A, De Witte T, Prejiers F, et al. Allogeneic bone marrow transplantation for leukemia with marrow cells depleted of lymphocytes by counterflow elutriation. *Blood* 1990;75:1356.

548. Wagner JE, Donnenberg AD, Noga SJ, et al. Lymphocyte depletion of donor bone marrow by counterflow centrifugal elutriation: results of a phase I clinical trial. *Blood* 1988;72:1168.

549. Champlin R, Ho W, Gajewski J, et al. Selective depletion of CD8⁺ T lymphocytes for prevention of graft-versus-host disease after allogeneic bone marrow transplantation. *Blood* 1990;76:418.

550. Sehn LH, Alyea EP, Weller E, et al. Comparative outcomes of T-cell-depleted and non-T-cell-depleted allogeneic bone marrow transplantation for chronic myelogenous leukemia: impact of donor lymphocyte infusion. *J Clin Oncol* 1999;17:561.

551. Marmont A, Horowitz MM, Gale RP, et al. T-cell depletion of HLA-identical transplants in leukemia. *Blood* 1991;78:2120.

552. Wagner J, King R, Kollman C, et al. Unrelated donor bone marrow transplantation (UBMT) in 5075 patients with malignant and non-malignant disorders: impact of marrow T cell depletion (TCD). *Blood* 1998;92(suppl 1):686a.

553. Champlin RE, Passweg JR, Zhang MJ, et al. T-cell depletion of bone marrow transplants for leukemia from donors other than HLA-identical siblings: advantage of T-cell antibodies with narrow specificities. *Blood* 2000;95:3996.

554. Pirsch JD, Maki DG. Infectious complications in adults with bone marrow transplantation and T-cell depletion of donor marrow. *Ann Intern Med* 1986;104:619.

555. Aversa F, Tabilio A, Velardi A, et al. Treatment of high-risk acute leukemia with T-cell-depleted stem cells from related donors with one fully mismatched HLA haplotype *N Engl J Med* 1998;339:1186.

556. Rooney CM, Smith CA, Ng CY, et al. Infusion of cytotoxic T cells for the prevention and treatment of Epstein-Barr virus-induced lymphoma in allogeneic transplant recipients. *Blood* 1998;92:1549.

557. Aguilar LK, Rooney CM, Heslop HE. Lymphoproliferative disorders involving Epstein-Barr virus after hemopoietic stem cell transplantation. *Curr Opin Oncol* 1999;11:96.

558. Slavin S, Ackerstein A, Weiss L, et al. Immunotherapy of minimal residual disease by immunocompetent lymphocytes and their activation by cytokines. *Cancer Invest* 1992;10:221.

559. Martin PJ, Schoch G, Fisher L, et al. A retrospective analysis of therapy for acute graft-versus-host disease: Initial treatment. *Blood* 1990;76:1464.

560. Martin PJ, Schoch G, Fisher L, et al. A retrospective analysis of therapy for acute graft-versus-host disease: secondary treatment. *Blood* 1991;77:1821.

561. Weisdorf D, Haake R, Blazar B, et al. Treatment of moderate/severe acute graft-versus-host disease after allogeneic bone marrow transplantation: an analysis of clinical risk factors and outcome. *Blood* 1990;75:1024.

562. Van Lint MT, Uderzo C, Locasciulli A, et al. Early treatment of acute graft-versus-host disease with high- or low-dose 6-methylprednisolone: a multicenter randomized trial from the Italian Group for bone marrow transplantation. *Blood* 1998;92:2288.

563. Cragg L, Blazar BR, Defor T, et al. A randomized trial comparing prednisone with antithymocyte globulin/prednisone as an initial systemic therapy for moderately severe acute graft-versus-host disease. *Biol Blood Marrow Transplant* 2000;6:441.

564. Przepiorka D, Kernan NA, Ippoliti C, et al. Daclizumab, a humanized anti-interleukin-2 receptor alpha chain antibody, for treatment of acute graft-versus-host disease. *Blood* 2000;95:83.

565. Busca A, Saroglia EM, Lanino E, et al. Mycophenolate mofetil (MMF) as therapy for refractory chronic GVHD (cGVHD) in children receiving bone marrow transplantation. *Bone Marrow Transplant* 2000;25:1067.

566. Ippoliti C, Champlin R, Bugazia N, et al. Use of octreotide in the symptomatic management of diarrhea induced by graft-versus-host disease in patients with hematologic malignancies. *J Clin Oncol* 1997;15:3350.

567. Antin J, Weinstein HJ, Guinan EC, et al. Phase I/II of recombinant IL-1 receptor antagonist (IL-1RA) for steroid resistant GVHD. *Blood* 1992;80 (Suppl 1):270a.

568. Holler E, Kolb HJ, Mittermüller J, et al. Modulation of acute graft-versus-host disease after allogeneic bone marrow transplantation by tumor necrosis factor α (TNFα) release in the course of pretransplant conditioning: role of conditioning regimens and prophylactic application of a monoclonal antibody neutralizing TNFα (MAK 195F). *Blood* 1995;86:890.

569. Hervé P, Flesch M, Tiberghian P, et al. Phase I-II trial of a monoclonal anti-tumor necrosis factor α antibody for the treatment of refractory severe acute graft-versus-host disease. *Blood* 1992;79:3362.

570. Shulman HM, Sullivan KM, Weiden PL, et al. Chronic graft-versus-host syndrome in man: A long-term clinicopathologic study of 20 Seattle patients. *Am J Med* 1980;69:204.

571. Sullivan KM, Shulman HM, Storb R, et al. Chronic graft-versus-host disease in 52 patients: adverse natural course and successful treatment with combination immunosuppression. *Blood* 1981;57:267.

572. Kulkarni S, Powles R, Treleaven J, et al. Chronic graft versus host disease is associated with long-term risk for pneumococcal infections in recipients of bone marrow transplants. *Blood* 2000;95:3683.

573. Shulman HM, Sale GE, Lerner KG, et al. Chronic cutaneous graft versus host disease in man. *Am J Pathol* 1978;91:545.

574. Sale GE, Shulman HM, Schubert MM, et al. Oral and ophthalmic pathology of graft versus host disease in man: predictive value of the lip biopsy. *Pathology* 1981;12:1022.

575. Kurzrock R, Zander A, Kanojia M, et al. Obstructive lung disease after allogeneic bone marrow transplantation. *Transplantation* 1984;37:156.

576. Carlens S, Ringden O, Remberger M, et al. Risk factors for chronic graft-versus-host disease after bone marrow transplantation: a retrospective single centre analysis. *Bone Marrow Transplant* 1998;22:755.

577. Ringdén O, Paulin T, Lonnqvist B, Nilsson B. An analysis of factors predisposing to chronic graft versus host disease. *Exp Hematol* 1985;13:1062.

578. Atkinson K, Horowitz MM, Gale RP, et al. Risk factors for chronic graft-versus-host disease after HLA-identical bone marrow transplantation. *Blood* 1990;75:2459.

579. Ochs LA, Miller WJ, Filipovich AH, et al. Predictive factors for chronic graft-versus-host disease after histocompatible sibling donor bone marrow transplantation. *Bone Marrow Transplant* 1994;13:455.

580. Collins RH Jr, Shpilberg O, Drobyski WR, et al. Donor leukocyte infusions in 140 patients with relapsed malignancy after allogeneic bone marrow transplantation. *J Clin Oncol* 1997;15:433.

581. Porter DL, Collins RH Jr, Shpilberg O, et al. Long-term follow-up of patients who achieved complete remission after donor leukocyte infusions. *Biol Blood Marrow Transplant* 1999;5:253.

582. Dazzi F, Szydlo RM, Craddock C, et al. Comparison of single-dose and escalating-dose regimens of donor lymphocyte infusion for relapse after allografting for chronic myeloid leukemia. *Blood* 2000;95:67.

583. Lee S, Klein JP, Barrett AJ, et al. Severity of chronic graft-versus-host disease: association with treatment-related mortality and relapse. *Blood* 2002;100:406–414.

584. Sullivan KM, Witherspoon RP, Storb R, et al. Prednisone and azathioprine compared with prednisone and placebo for treatment of chronic graft versus host disease: prognostic influence of prolonged thrombocytopenia after allogeneic transplantation. *Blood* 1988;72:546.

585. Wingard JR, Piantadosi S, Vogelsang GB, et al. Predictors of death from chronic graft-versus-host disease after bone marrow transplantation. *Blood* 1989;74:1428.

586. Mookerjee B, Altomonte V, Vogelsang G. Salvage therapy for refractory chronic graft-versus-host disease with mycophenolate mofetil and tacrolimus. *Bone Marrow Transplant* 1999;24:517.

587. Sullivan KM, Witherspoon RP, Storb R, et al. Alternating-day cyclosporine and prednisone for treatment of high-risk graft-v-host disease. *Blood* 1988; 72:555.

588. Vogelsang GB, Farmer ER, Hess AD, et al. Thalidomide for the treatment of chronic graft-versus-host disease. *N Engl J Med* 1992;326:1055.

589. Parker PM, Chao N, Nademanee A, et al. Thalidomide as salvage therapy for chronic graft-versus-host disease. *Blood* 1995;86:3604.

590. Chao NJ, Parker P, Niland JC, et al. Paradoxical effect of thalidomide prophylaxis on chronic graft-vs.-host disease. *Biol Blood Marrow Transplant* 1996;2:86.

591. Lee SJ, Wegner SA, McGarigle CJ, et al. Treatment of chronic graft-versus-host disease with clofazimine. *Blood* 1997;89:2298.

592. Vogelsang GB, Wolff D, Altomonte V, et al. Treatment of chronic graft-versus-host disease with ultraviolet irradiation and psoralen (PUVA). *Bone Marrow Transplant* 1996;17:1061.

593. Greinix HT, Volc-Platzer B, Rabitsch W, et al. Successful use of extracorporeal photochemotherapy in the treatment of severe acute and chronic graft-versus-host disease. *Blood* 1998;92:3098.

594. Smith EP, Sniecinski I, Dagis AC, et al. Extracorporeal photochemotherapy for treatment of drug-resistant graft-vs.-host disease. *Biol Blood Marrow Transplant* 1998;4:27.

595. Enk CD, Elad S, Vexler A, et al. Chronic graft-versus-host disease treated with UVB phototherapy. *Bone Marrow Transplant* 1998;22:1179.

596. Gilman AL, Chan KW, Mogul A, et al. Hydroxychloroquine for the treatment of chronic graft-versus-host disease. *Biol Blood Marrow Transplant* 2000;6:327.

597. Guinan EC, Molrine DC, Antin JH, et al. Polysaccharide conjugate vaccine responses in bone marrow transplant patients. *Transplantation* 1994;57:677.

598. Boulad F, Bromley M, Black P, et al. Thyroid dysfunction following bone marrow transplantation using hyperfractionated radiation. *Bone Marrow Transplant* 1995;15:71.

599. Weilbaecher KN. Mechanisms of osteoporosis after hematopoietic cell transplantation. *Biol Blood Marrow Transplant* 2000;6:165.

600. Deeg HJ, Leisenring W, Storb R, et al. Long-term outcome after marrow transplantation for severe aplastic anemia. *Blood* 1998;91:3637.

601. Barnes DWH, Loutit JF. Treatment of murine leukaemia with X-rays and homologous bone marrow: II. *Br J Haematol* 1957;3:241.

602. Horowitz MM, Gale RP, Sondel PM, et al. Graft-versus-leukemia reactions after bone marrow transplantation. *Blood* 1990;75:555.

603. Mathe G, Amiel JL, Schwarzenberg L, Cattan A, Schneider M. Adoptive immunotherapy of acute leukemia: Experimental and clinical results. *Cancer Res* 1965;25:1525.

604. Johnson BD, Truitt RL. Delayed infusion of immunocompetent donor cells after bone marrow transplantation breaks graft-host tolerance allows for persistent antileukemic reactivity without severe graft-versus-host disease. *Blood* 1995;85:3302.

605. Yang YG, Sergio JJ, Pearson DA, et al. Interleukin-12 preserves the graft-versus-leukemia effect of allogeneic CD8 T cells while inhibiting CD4-dependent graft-versus-host disease in mice. *Blood* 1997;90:4651.

606. Tutschka PH, Berkowitz SD, Tuttle S, Klein J. Graft versus leukemia in the rat—the antileukemic effect of syngeneic and allogeneic graft versus host disease. *Transplant Proc* 1987;19:2668.

607. Kolb H, Mittermuller J, Clemm C, et al. Donor leukocyte transfusions for treatment of recurrent chronic myelogenous leukemia in marrow transplant patients. *Blood* 1990;76:2462.

608. Porter DL, Roth MS, McGarigle C, et al. Induction of graft-versus-host disease as immunotherapy for relapsed chronic myeloid leukemia. *N Engl J Med* 1994;330:100.

609. Childs R, Chernoff A, Contentin N, et al. Regression of metastatic renal-cell carcinoma after nonmyeloablative allogeneic peripheral-blood stem-cell transplantation. *N Engl J Med* 2000;343:750.

610. Porter DL, Collins RH Jr, Hardy C, et al. Treatment of relapsed leukemia after unrelated donor marrow transplantation with unrelated donor leukocyte infusions. *Blood* 2000;95:1214.

611. Weiden PL, Flournoy N, Thomas ED, et al. Antileukemic effect of graft-versus-host disease in recipients of allogeneic-marrow grafts. *N Engl J Med* 1979;300:1068.

612. Weiden PL, Sullivan K, Flournoy N, et al. Antileukemic effect of chronic graft-versus-host disease. Contribution to improved survival after allogeneic marrow transplantation. *N Engl J Med* 1981;304:1529.

613. Sullivan KM, Weiden PL, Storb R, et al. Influence of acute and chronic graft-versus-host disease on relapse and survival after bone marrow transplantation from HLA-identical siblings as treatment of acute and chronic leukemia. *Blood* 1989;73:1720.

614. Collins RH Jr, Rogers ZR, Bennett M, et al. Hematologic relapse of chronic myelogenous leukemia following allogeneic bone marrow transplantation: apparent graft-versus-leukemia effect following abrupt discontinuation of immunosuppression. *Bone Marrow Transplant* 1992;10:391.

615. Odom LF, August CS, Githens JH, et al. Remission of relapsed leukaemia during a graft-versus-host reaction. A "graft-versus-leukaemia reaction" in man? *Lancet* 1978;2:537.

616. Goldman JM, Gale RP, Horowitz MM, et al. Bone marrow transplantation for chronic myelogenous leukemia in chronic phase. Increased risk for relapse associated with T-cell depletion. *Ann Intern Med* 1988;108:806.

617. Apperley JF, Mauro FR, Goldman JM, et al. Bone marrow transplantation for chronic myeloid leukaemia in first chronic phase. Importance of a graft-versus-leukaemia effect. *Br J Haematol* 1988;69:239.

618. Sullivan KM, Storb R, Buckner CD. Graft-versus-host disease as adoptive immunotherapy in patients with advanced hematologic neoplasms. *N Engl J Med* 1989;320:828.

619. Kolb HJ, Schattenberg A, Goldman JM, et al. Graft-versus-leukemia effect of donor lymphocyte transfusions in marrow grafted patients. *Blood* 1995;86:2041.

620. Johnson BD, Drobyski WR, Truitt RL. Delayed infusion of normal donor cells after MHC-matched marrow transplantation provides an antileukemia reaction without graft-versus-host disease. *Bone Marrow Transplant* 1993;11:329.

621. Mackinnon S, Papadopoulos EB, Carabasi MH, et al. Adoptive immunotherapy using donor leukocytes following bone marrow transplantation for chronic myeloid leukemia: is T cell dose important in determining biological response? *Bone Marrow Transplant* 1995;15:591.

622. McSweeney PA, Storb R. Mixed chimerism: preclinical studies and clinical applications. *Biol Blood Marrow Transplant* 1999;5:192.

623. Bacigalupo A. Hematopoietic stem cell transplants after reduced intensity conditioning regimen (RI-HSCT): report of a workshop of the European Group for Blood and Marrow Transplantation (EBMT). *Bone Marrow Transplant* 2000;25:803.

624. Giralt S, Estey E, Albitar M, et al. Engraftment of allogeneic hematopoietic progenitor cells with purine analog-containing chemotherapy: harnessing graft-versus-leukemia without myeloablative therapy. *Blood* 1997;89:4531.

625. von Fliedner V, Higby DJ, Kim U. Graft-versus-host reaction following blood product transfusion. *Am J Med* 1982;72:951.

626. Brubaker BB. Post-transfusion graft versus host disease. *Vox Sang* 1983;45:401.

627. Anderson KC, Weinstein HJ. Transfusion-associated graft-versus-host disease. *N Engl J Med* 1990;323:315.

628. Parkman R, Mosier D, Umansky I, et al. Graft versus host disease after intra-uterine and exchange transfusions for hemolytic disease of the newborn. *N Engl J Med* 1974;290:359.

629. Shivdasani RA, Anderson KC. HLA homozygosity and shared HLA haplotypes in the development of transfusion-associated graft-versus-host disease. *Leuk Lymphoma* 1994;15:227.

630. Thaler M, Shamiss A, Orgad S, et al. The role of blood from HLA homozygous donors in fatal transfusion-associated graft versus host disease after open-heart surgery. *N Engl J Med* 1989;321:25.

631. Lewis SM. Course and prognosis in aplastic anemia. *BMJ* 1965;1:1027.

632. Camitta BM, Thomas ED, Nathan DG, et al. A prospective study of androgens and bone marrow transplantation for treatment of severe aplastic anemia. *Blood* 1979;53:504.

633. Thomas ED, Buckner CD, Storb R, et al. Aplastic anemia treated by marrow transplantation. *Lancet* 1972;1:284.

634. Hinterberger W, Rowlings PA, Hinterberger-Fischer M, et al. Results of transplanting bone marrow from genetically identical twins into patients with aplastic anemia. *Ann Intern Med* 1997;126:116.

635. Hows J, Palmer S, Gordon-Smith EC. Cyclosporine and graft failure following bone marrow transplantation for severe aplastic anaemia. *Br J Haematol* 1985;60:611.

636. Gluckman E, Barrett AJ, Arcese W, et al. Bone marrow transplantation in severe aplastic anemia. A survey of the European Group for Bone Marrow Transplantation (EGBMT). *Br J Haematol* 1981;49:165.

637. Sensenbrenner LL, Steele AA, Santos GW. Recovery of hematologic competence without engraftment following attempted bone marrow transplantation for aplastic anemia: Report of a case with diffusion chamber studies. *Exp Hematol* 1977;5:51.

638. Tichelli A, Socie G, Henry-Amar M, et al. Effectiveness of immunosuppressive therapy in older patients with aplastic anemia. European Group for Blood and Marrow Transplantation Severe Aplastic Anaemia Working Party. *Ann Intern Med* 1999;130:193.

639. Bacigalupo A, Bruno B, Saracco P, et al. Antilymphocyte globulin, cyclosporine, prednisolone, and granulocyte colony-stimulating factor for severe aplastic anemia: an update of the GITMO/EBMT study on 100 patients. European Group for Blood and Marrow Transplantation (EBMT) Working Party on Severe Aplastic Anemia and the Gruppo Italiano Trapianti di Midolio Osseo (GITMO). *Blood* 2000;95:1931.

640. Rosenfeld SJ, Kimball J, Vining D, Young NS. Intensive immunosuppression with antithymocyte globulin and cyclosporine as treatment for severe acquired aplastic anemia. *Blood* 1995;85:3058.

641. Bone marrow transplantation from donors with aplastic anemia. A report from the ACS/NIH bone marrow transplant registry. *JAMA* 1976;236:1131.

642. Anasetti C, Doney KC, Storb R, et al. Marrow transplantation for severe aplastic anemia. Long term outcome in fifty "untransfused" patients. *Ann Intern Med* 1986;104:461.

643. Storb R, Epstein RB, Rudolph RH, Thomas ED. The effect of prior transfusions on marrow grafts between histocompatible canine siblings. *J Immunol* 1970;105:627.

644. Gluckman E, Horowitz MM, Champlin RE, et al. Bone marrow transplantation for severe aplastic anemia: influence of conditioning and graft-versus-host disease prophylaxis regimens on outcome. *Blood* 1992;79:269.

645. Feig SA, Champlin R, Arenson E, et al. Improved survival following bone marrow transplantation for aplastic anaemia. *Br J Haematol* 1983;54:509.

646. Shank B, Brochstein JA, Castro-Malaspina H, et al. Immunosuppression prior to marrow transplantation for sensitized aplastic anemia patients: comparison of TLI with TBI. *Int J Radiat Oncol Biol Phys* 1988;14:1133.

647. McGlave PB, Haake R, Miller W, et al. Therapy of severe aplastic anemia in young adults and children with allogeneic bone marrow transplantation. *Blood* 1987;70:1325.

648. Gluckman E, Socié G, Devergie A, et al. Bone marrow transplantation in 107 patients with severe aplastic anemia using cyclophosphamide and thoraco-abdominal irradiation for conditioning: long-term follow-up. *Blood* 1991;78:2451.

649. Deeg HJ, Socié G, Schoch G, et al. Malignancies after marrow transplantation for aplastic anemia and Fanconi anemia: a joint Seattle and Paris analysis of results in 700 patients. *Blood* 1996;87:386.

650. Smith BR, Guinan EC, Parkman R, et al. Efficacy of a cyclophosphamide-procarbazine-antithymocyte serum regimen for prevention of graft rejection following bone marrow transplantation for transfused patients with aplastic anemia. *Transplantation* 1985;39:671.

651. Storb R, Doney KC, Thomas ED, et al. Marrow transplantation with or without donor buffy coat cells for 65 transfused aplastic anemia patients. *Blood* 1982;59:236.

652. Margolis D, Camitta B, Pietryga D, et al. Unrelated donor bone marrow transplantation to treat severe aplastic anaemia in children and young adults. *Br J Haematol* 1996;94:65.

653. Hows JM, Yin JL, Marsh J, et al. Histocompatible unrelated volunteer donors compared with HLA nonidentical family donors in marrow transplantation for aplastic anemia and leukemia. *Blood* 1986;68:1322.

654. Bacigalupo A, Oneto R, Bruno B, et al. Current results of bone marrow transplantation in patients with acquired severe aplastic anemia. Report of the European Group for Blood and Marrow Transplantation. On behalf of the Working Party on Severe Aplastic Anemia of the European Group for Blood and Marrow Transplantation. *Acta Haematologica* 2000;103:19.

655. Davies SM, Wagner JE, Defor T, et al. Unrelated donor bone marrow transplantation for children and adolescents with aplastic anaemia or myelodysplasia. *Br J Haematol* 1997;96:749.

656. Szydlo R, Goldman JM, Klein JP, et al. Results of allogeneic bone marrow transplants for leukemia using donors other than HLA-identical siblings. *J Clin Oncol* 1997;15:1767.

657. Deeg HJ, Amylon ID, Harris RE, et al. Marrow transplants from unrelated donors for patients with aplastic anemia: minimum effective dose of total body irradiation. *Biol Blood Marrow Transplant* 2001;7:208.

658. Bayever E, Champlin R, Ho W, et al. Comparison between bone marrow transplantation and antithymocyte globulin in treatment of young patients with severe aplastic anemia. *J Pediatr* 1984;105:920.

659. Speck B, Gratwohl A, Nissen C, et al. Treatment of severe aplastic anemia. *Exp Hematol* 1986;14:126.

660. Doney K, Leisenring W, Stob R, Appelbaum F. Primary treatment of acquired aplastic anemia: outcomes with bone marrow transplantation and immunosuppressive therapy. *Ann Intern Med* 1997;126:107.

661. Deeg HJ, Seidel K, Casper J, et al. Marrow transplantation from unrelated donors for patients with severe aplastic anemia who have failed immunosuppressive therapy. *Biol Blood Marrow Transplant* 1999;5:243.

662. Sanders JE, Whitehead J, Storb R, et al. Bone marrow transplantation experience for children with aplastic anemia. *Pediatrics* 1986;77:179.

663. Gillio AP, Boulad F, Small TN, et al. Comparison of long-term outcome of children with severe aplastic anemia treated with immunosuppression versus bone marrow transplantation. *Biol Blood Marrow Transplant* 1997;3:18.

664. Bacigalupo A, Hows J, Gluckman E, et al. Bone marrow transplantation (BMT) versus immunosuppression for the treatment of severe aplastic anemia (SAA): a report of the EBMT* SAA Working Party. *Br J Haematol* 1988;70:177.

665. Bacigalupo A, Brand R, Oneto R, et al. Treatment of acquired severe aplastic anemia: bone marrow transplantation compared with immunosuppressive therapy—The European Group for Blood and Marrow Transplantation experience. *Semin Hematol* 2000;37:69.

666. Tichelli A, Gratwohl A, Wursch A, et al. Late haematological complications in severe aplastic anemia. *Br J Haematol* 1988;69:413.

667. de Planque MM, Kluin-Nelemans JC, van Krieken HJM, et al. Evolution of acquired severe aplastic anaemia to myelodysplasia and subsequent leukaemia in adults. *Br J Haematol* 1988;70:55.

668. Doney K, Storb R, Buckner CD, et al. Marrow transplantation for treatment of pregnancy-associated aplastic anemia. *Exp Hematol* 1985;13:1080.

669. Baldwin JL, Storb R, Thomas ED, Mannik M. Bone marrow transplantation in patients with gold-induced marrow aplasia. *Arthritis Rheum* 1977;20:1043.

670. Kojima S, Matsuyama K, Kodera Y. Bone marrow transplantation for hepatitis-associated aplastic anemia. *Acta Haematol* 1988;79:7.

671. Kiem H, McDonald G, Spurgeon C, et al. Marrow transplantation for hepatitis-associated aplastic anemia: a follow-up of long-term survivors. *Biol Blood Marrow Transplant* 1996;2:93.

672. Szer J, Deeg HJ, Witherspoon RP, et al. Long-term survival after marrow transplantation for paroxysmal nocturnal hemoglobinuria with aplastic anemia. *Ann Intern Med* 1984;101:193.

673. Hershko C, Gale RP, Ho WG, Cline MJ. Cure of aplastic anemia in paroxysmal nocturnal hemoglobinuria by marrow infusion from identical twin: failure of peripheral-leucocyte transfusion to correct marrow aplasia. *Lancet* 1979;1:945.

674. Gluckman E, Devergie A, Dutreix A, et al. Bone marrow grafting in aplastic anemia after conditioning with cyclophosphamide and total body irradiation with lung shielding. In: Thierfelder S, Rodt H, Kolb HJ, eds. *Immunobiology of bone marrow transplant*. Berlin: Springer-Verlag, 1980:339.

675. Druker BJ, Sawyers CL, Kantarjian H, et al. Activity of a specific inhibitor of the BCR-ABL tyrosine kinase in the blast crisis of chronic myeloid leukemia and acute lymphoblastic leukemia with the Philadelphia chromosome. *N Engl J Med* 2001;344:1038.

676. Druker BJ, Talpaz M, Resta DJ, et al. Efficacy and safety of a specific inhibitor of the BCR-ABL tyrosine kinase in chronic myeloid leukemia. *N Engl J Med* 2001;344:1031.

677. Gratwohl A, Hermans J, Goldman JM, et al. Risk assessment for patients with chronic myeloid leukaemia before allogeneic blood or marrow transplantation. Chronic Leukemia Working Party of the European Group for Blood and Marrow Transplantation. *Lancet* 1998;352:1087.

678. Devergie A, Blaise D, Attal M, et al. Allogeneic bone marrow transplantation for chronic myeloid leukemia in first chronic phase: a randomized trial of busulfan-cytoxan versus cytoxan-total body irradiation as preparative regimen: a report from The French Society of Bone Marrow Graft (SFGM). *Blood* 1995;85:2263.

679. McGlave PB, Shu XO, Wen W, et al. Unrelated donor marrow transplantation for chronic myelogenous leukemia: 9 years' experience of the national marrow donor program. *Blood* 2000;95:2219.

680. Devergie A, Apperley JF, Labopin M, et al. European results of matched unrelated donor bone marrow transplantation for chronic myeloid leukemia. Impact of HLA class II matching. Chronic Leukemia Working Party of the European Group for Blood and Marrow Transplantation. *Bone Marrow Transplant* 1997;20:11.

681. van Rhee F, Szydlo RM, Hermans J, et al. Long-term results after allogeneic bone marrow transplantation for chronic myelogenous leukemia in chronic phase: a report from the Chronic Leukemia Working Party of the European Group for Blood and Marrow Transplantation. *Bone Marrow Transplant* 1997;20:553.

682. Clift RA, Buckner CD, Thomas ED, et al. Marrow transplantation for patients in accelerated phase of chronic myeloid leukemia. *Blood* 1994;84:4368.

683. Gale RP, Hehlmann R, Zhang MJ, et al. Survival with bone marrow transplantation versus hydroxyurea or interferon for chronic myelogenous leukemia. The German CML Study Group. *Blood* 1998;91:1810.

684. Hansen JA, Gooley TA, Martin PJ, et al. Bone marrow transplants from unrelated donors for patients with chronic myeloid leukemia. *N Engl J Med* 1998;338:962.

685. McGlave P, Arthur D, Haake R, et al. Therapy of chronic myelogenous leukemia with allogeneic bone marrow transplantation. *J Clin Oncol* 1987;5:1033.

686. Gratwohl A, Hermans J, Niderwieser D, et al. Bone marrow transplantation for chronic myeloid leukemia: long-term results. *Bone Marrow Transplant* 1993;12:509.

687. Wagner JE, Zahurak M, Piantadosi S, et al. Bone marrow transplantation of chronic myelogenous leukemia in chronic phase: evaluation of risks and benefits. *J Clin Oncol* 1992;10:779.

688. Sokal JE, Baccarani M, Tura S, et al. Prognostic discrimination among younger patients with chronic granulocytic leukemia: relevance to bone marrow transplantation. *Blood* 1985;66:1352.

689. Lee SJ, Kuntz KM, Horowitz MM, et al. Unrelated donor bone marrow transplantation for chronic myelogenous leukemia: a decision analysis. *Ann Intern Med* 1997;127:1080.

690. Lee SJ, Anasetti C, Horowitz MM, Antin JH. Initial therapy for chronic myelogenous leukemia: playing the odds [editorial]. *J Clin Oncol* 1998;16: 2897.

691. Monitoring treatment and survival in chronic myeloid leukemia. Italian Cooperative Study Group on Chronic Myeloid Leukemia and Italian Group for Bone Marrow Transplantation. *J Clin Oncol* 1999;17:1858.

692. Deisseroth AB, Kantarjian H, Andreeff M, et al. Chronic leukemias. In: DeVita VT, Hellman S, Rosenberg SA, eds. In: *Cancer principles and practice of oncology*. Vol. 2. Philadelphia: Lippincott-Raven Publishers, 1997:2321.

693. Silver RT, Woolf SH, Hehlmann R, et al. An evidence-based analysis of the effect of busulfan, hydroxyurea, interferon, and allogeneic bone marrow transplantation in treating the chronic phase of chronic myeloid leukemia: developed for the American Society of Hematology. *Blood* 1999;94:1517.

694. Goldman JM, Szydlo R, Horowitz MM, et al. Choice of pretransplant treatment and timing of transplants for chronic myelogenous leukemia in chronic phase. *Blood* 1993;82:2235.

695. Gluckman E, Devergie A, Bernheim A, Berger R. Splenectomy and bone marrow transplantation in chronic granulocytic leukaemia. *Lancet* 1983;1:1392.

696. Gratwohl A, Goldman J, Gluckman E, Zwaan F. Effect of splenectomy before bone-marrow transplantation on survival in chronic granulocytic leukaemia. *Lancet* 1985;2:1290.

697. Gratwohl A, van Biezen A, Hermans J, Apperley J. Role of splenic irradiation in patients with chronic myeloid leukemia undergoing allogeneic bone marrow transplantation. Chronic Leukemia Working Party of the European Group for Blood and Marrow Transplantation [letter]. *Biol Blood Marrow Transplant* 2000;6:211.

698. Jabro G, Koc Y, Boyle T, et al. Role of splenic irradiation in patients with chronic myeloid leukemia undergoing allogeneic bone marrow transplantation. *Biol Blood Marrow Transplant* 1999;5:173.

699. Biggs JC, Szer J, Crilley P, et al. Treatment of chronic myeloid leukemia with allogeneic bone marrow transplantation after preparation with BuCy2. *Blood* 1992;80:1352.

700. Beelen DW, Elmaagacli AH, Schaefer UW. The adverse influence of pretransplant interferon-alpha (IFN-alpha) on transplant outcome after marrow transplantation for chronic phase chronic myelogenous leukemia increases with the duration of IFN-alpha exposure [letter]. *Blood* 1999;93:1779.

701. Beelen DW, Graeven U, Elmaagacli AH, et al. Prolonged administration of interferon-α in patients with chronic-phase Philadelphia chromosome-positive chronic myelogenous leukemia before allogeneic bone marrow transplantation may adversely affect transplant outcome. *Blood* 1995;85:2981.

702. Giralt S, Szydlo R, Goldman JM, et al. Effect of short-term interferon therapy on the outcome of subsequent HLA-identical sibling bone marrow transplantation for chronic myelogenous leukemia: an analysis from the international bone marrow transplant registry. *Blood* 2000;95:410.

703. Hehlmann R, Hochhaus A, Kolb HJ, et al. Interferon-alpha before allogeneic bone marrow transplantation in chronic myelogenous leukemia does not affect outcome adversely, provided it is discontinued at least 90 days before the procedure. *Blood* 1999;94:3668.

704. Morton AJ, Gooley T, Hansen JA, et al. Association between pretransplant interferon-alpha and outcome after unrelated donor marrow transplantation for chronic myelogenous leukemia in chronic phase. *Blood* 1998;92:394.

705. Lee S, Klein J, Anasetti C, et al. The effect of pretransplant interferon exposure on the outcome of unrelated donor hematopoietic stem cell transplantation. *Blood* 2001;98:3205.

706. Arthur CK, Apperley JF, Guo AP, et al. Cytogenetic events after bone marrow transplantation for chronic myeloid leukemia in chronic phase. *Blood* 1988; 71:1179.

707. Cytogenetic follow-up of 100 patients submitted to bone marrow transplantation for Philadelphia chromosome-positive chronic myeloid leukemia. Cooperative Study Group on Chromosomes in Transplanted Patients. *Eur J Haematol* 1988;40:50.

708. Faderl S, Talpaz M, Kantarjian HM, Estrov Z. Should polymerase chain reaction analysis to detect minimal residual disease in patients with chronic myelogenous leukemia be used in clinical decision making? *Blood* 1999; 93:2755.

709. Cross NCP, Feng L, Chase A, et al. Competitive polymerase chain reaction to estimate the number of BCR-ABL transcripts in chronic myeloid leukemia patients after bone marrow transplantation. *Blood* 1993;82:1929.

710. Cross NCP, Hughes TP, Feng L, et al. Minimal residual disease after allogeneic bone marrow transplantation for chronic myelogenous leukemia in first chronic phase: correlations with acute graft-versus-host disease and relapse. *Br J Haematol* 1993;84:67.

711. Roth MS, Antin JH, Ash R, et al. Prognostic significance of Philadelphia chromosome-positive cells detected by the polymerase chain reaction after allogeneic bone marrow transplant for chronic myelogenous leukemia. *Blood* 1992;79:276.

712. Roth MS, Antin JH, Bingham EL, Ginsburg D. Detection of Philadelphia chromosome-positive cells by the polymerase chain reaction following bone marrow transplant for chronic myelogenous leukemia. *Blood* 1989;74:882.

713. Roth MS, Antin JH, Bingham EL, Ginsburg D. Use of polymerase chain reaction-detected sequence polymorphisms to document engraftment following allogeneic bone marrow transplantation. *Transplantation* 1990;49:714.

714. Hochhaus A, Reiter A, Saussele S, et al. Molecular heterogeneity in complete cytogenetic responders after interferon-alpha therapy for chronic myelogenous leukemia: low levels of minimal residual disease are associated with continuing remission. German CML Study Group and the UK MRC CML Study Group. *Blood* 2000;95:62.

715. Hochhaus A, Weisser A, La Rosee P, et al. Detection and quantification of residual disease in chronic myelogenous leukemia. *Leukemia* 2000;14:998.

716. Seong CM, Giralt S, Kantarjian H, et al. Early detection of relapse by hypermetaphase fluorescence *in situ* hybridization after allogeneic bone marrow transplantation for chronic myeloid leukemia. *J Clin Oncol* 2000;18:1831.

717. Seong D, Giralt S, Fischer H, et al. Usefulness of detection of minimal residual disease by 'hypermetaphase' fluorescent *in situ* hybridization after allogeneic BMT for chronic myelogenous leukemia. *Bone Marrow Transplant* 1997;19:565.

718. Radich JP, Gehly G, Gooley T, et al. Polymerase chain reaction detection of the BCR-ABL fusion transcript after allogeneic marrow transplantation for chronic myeloid leukemia: results and implications in 346 patients. *Blood* 1995;85:2632.

719. Hessner MJ, Endean DJ, Casper JT, et al. Use of unrelated marrow grafts compensates for reduced graft-versus-leukemia reactivity after T-cell-depleted allogeneic marrow transplantation for chronic myelogenous leukemia. *Blood* 1995;86:3987.

720. van Rhee F, Lin F, Cross NC, et al. Detection of residual leukaemia more than 10 years after allogeneic bone marrow transplantation for chronic myelogenous leukaemia. *Bone Marrow Transplant* 1994;14:609.

721. Mackinnon S, Papadapoulos EB, Carabasi MH, et al. Adoptive immunotherapy evaluating escalating doses of donor leukocytes for relapse of chronic myeloid leukemia after bone marrow transplantation: separation of graft-versus-leukemia responses from graft-versus-host disease. *Blood* 1995;86: 1261.

722. Lion T. Clinical implications of qualitative and quantitative polymerase chain reaction analysis in the monitoring of patients with chronic myelogenous leukemia. The European Investigators on Chronic Myeloid Leukemia Group. *Bone Marrow Transplant* 1994;14:505.

723. Cullis JO, Schwarer AP, Hughes TP, et al. Second transplants for patients with chronic myeloid leukaemia in relapse after original transplant with T-depleted donor marrow: feasibility of using busulphan alone for re-conditioning. *Br J Haematol* 1992;80:33.

724. Mrsic M, Horowitz MM, Atkinson K, et al. Second HLA-identical sibling transplants for leukemia recurrence. *Bone Marrow Transplant* 1992;9:269.

725. Radich JP, Sanders JE, Buckner CD, et al. Second allogeneic marrow transplantation for patients with recurrent leukemia after initial transplant with total-body irradiation-containing regimens. *J Clin Oncol* 1993;11:304.

726. Mehta M, Powles R, Treleaven J, et al. Outcome of acute leukemia relapsing after bone marrow transplantation: utility of second transplants and adoptive immunotherapy. *Bone Marrow Transplant* 1997;19:709.

727. Higano CS, Chielens D, Raskind W, et al. Use of alpha-2a-interferon to treat cytogenetic relapse of chronic myeloid leukemia after marrow transplantation. *Blood* 1997;90:2549.

728. Arcese W, Goldman JM, D'Arcangelo E, et al. Outcome for patients who relapse after allogeneic bone marrow transplantation for chronic myeloid leukemia. *Blood* 1993;82:3211.

729. Zhang MJ, Baccarani M, Gale RP, et al. Survival of patients with chronic myeloid leukaemia relapsing after bone marrow transplantation: comparison with patients receiving conventional chemotherapy. *Br J Haematol* 1997;99:23.

730. Dazzi F, Szydlo RM, Cross NC, et al. Durability of responses following donor lymphocyte infusions for patients who relapse after allogeneic stem cell transplantation for chronic myeloid leukemia. *Blood* 2000;96:2712.

731. Drobyski WR, Keever CA, Roth MS, et al. Salvage immunotherapy using donor leukocyte infusions as treatment for relapsed chronic myelogenous

732. van Rhee F, Cullis JO, Feng L, et al. Donor leukocyte transfusions (DLT) for relapse of chronic myleoid leukemia after allogeneic bone marrow transplant. *Blood* 1993;82(Suppl 1):416a.

733. Verdonck LF, Petersen EJ, Lokhorst HM, et al. Donor leukocyte infusions for recurrent hematologic malignancies after allogeneic bone marrow transplantation: impact of infused and residual donor T cells. *Bone Marrow Transplant* 1998;22:1057.

734. Flowers ME, Leisenring W, Beach K, et al. Granulocyte colony-stimulating factor given to donors before apheresis does not prevent aplasia in patients treated with donor leukocyte infusion for recurrent chronic myeloid leukemia after bone marrow transplantation. *Biol Blood Marrow Transplant* 2000;6:321.

735. Reiffers J, Goldman J, Meloni G, et al. Autologous stem cell transplantation in chronic myelogenous leukemia: a retrospective analysis of the European Group for Bone Marrow Transplantation. Chronic Leukemia Working Party of the EBMT. *Bone Marrow Transplant* 1994;14:407.

736. Bhatia R, Verfaillie CM, Miller JS, McGlave PB. Autologous transplantation therapy for chronic myelogenous leukemia. *Blood* 1997;89:2623.

737. Marcus RE, Goldman JM. Autografting in chronic granulocytic leukaemia. *Clin Haematol* 1986;15:235.

738. Verfaillie CM, Bhatia R, Steinbuch M, et al. Comparative analysis of autografting in chronic myelogenous leukemia: effects of priming regimen and marrow or blood origin of stem cells. *Blood* 1998;92:1820.

739. Thomas ED, Buckner CD, Banaji M, et al. One hundred patients with acute leukemia treated by chemotherapy, total body irradiation, and allogeneic marrow transplantation. *Blood* 1977;49:511.

740. Badger C, Buckner CD, Thomas ED, et al. Allogeneic marrow transplantation for acute leukemia in relapse. *Leukemia Res* 1982;6:383.

741. Fefer A, Cheever MA, Thomas ED, et al. Bone marrow transplantation for refractory acute leukemia in 34 patients with identical twins. *Blood* 1981; 57:421.

742. Forman SJ, Schmidt GM, Nademanee AP, et al. Allogeneic bone marrow transplantation as therapy for primary induction failure for patients with acute leukemia. *J Clin Oncol* 1991;9:1570.

743. Clift RA, Buckner CD, Appelbaum FR, et al. Allogeneic marrow transplantation during untreated first relapse of acute myeloid leukemia. *J Clin Oncol* 1992;10:1723.

744. Byrne JL, Dasgupta E, Pallis M, et al. Early allogeneic transplantation for refractory or relapsed acute leukaemia following remission induction with FLAG. *Leukemia* 1999;13:786.

745. Woods W, Neudorf S, Gold S, et al. A comparison of allogeneic bone marrow transplantation, autologous bone marrow transplantation, and aggressive chemotherapy in children with acute myeloid leukemia in remission: a report from the Children's Cancer Group. *Blood* 2001;97:56.

746. Hewlett J, Kopecky KJ, Head D, et al. A prospective evaluation of the roles of allogeneic marrow transplantation and low-dose monthly maintenance chemotherapy in the treatment of adult acute myelogenous leukemia (AML): a Southwest Oncology Group study. *Leukemia* 1995;9:562.

747. Zittoun R, Mandelli F, Willemze R, et al. Autologous or allogeneic bone marrow transplantation compared with intensive chemotherapy in acute myelogenous leukemia. *N Engl J Med* 1995;332:217.

748. Harousseau JL, Cahn JY, Pignon B, et al. Comparison of autologous bone marrow transplantation and intensive chemotherapy as postremission therapy in adult acute myeloid leukemia. The Groupe Ouest Est Leucemies Aigues Myeloblastiques (GOELAM). *Blood* 1997;90:2978.

749. Cassileth PA, Harrington DP, Appelbaum FR, et al. Chemotherapy compared with autologous or allogeneic bone marrow transplantation in the management of acute myeloid leukemia in first remission. *N Engl J Med* 1998;339:1649.

750. Burnett AK, Goldstone AH, Stevens RM, et al. Randomised comparison of addition of autologous bone-marrow transplantation to intensive chemotherapy for acute myeloid leukaemia in first remission: results of MRC AML 10 trial. UK Medical Research Council Adult and Children's Leukaemia Working Parties. *Lancet* 1998;351:700.

751. Ravindranath Y, Yeager AM, Chang MN, et al. Autologous bone marrow transplantation versus intensive consolidation chemotherapy for acute myeloid leukemia in childhood. Pediatric Oncology Group. *N Engl J Med* 1996;334:1428.

752. Ferrant A, Labopin M, Frassoni F, et al. Karyotype in acute myeloblastic leukemia: prognostic significance for bone marrow transplantation in first remission: a European Group for Blood and Marrow Transplantation study. Acute Leukemia Working Party of the European Group for Blood and Marrow Transplantation (EBMT). *Blood* 1997;90:2931.

753. Gale RP, Horowitz MM, Weiner RS, et al. Impact of cytogenetic abnormalities on outcome of bone marrow transplants in acute myelogenous leukemia in first remission. *Bone Marrow Transplant* 1995;16:203.

754. Slovak ML, Kopecky KJ, Cassileth PA, et al. Karyotypic analysis predicts outcome of preremission and postremission therapy in adult acute myeloid leukemia: a Southwest Oncology Group/Eastern Cooperative Oncology Group study. *Blood* 2000;96:4075.

755. Linker CA, Ries CA, Damon LE, et al. Autologous bone marrow transplantation for acute myeloid leukemia using 4-hydroperoxycyclophosphamide-purged bone marrow and the busulfan/etoposide preparative regimen: a follow-up report. *Bone Marrow Transplant* 1998;22:865.

756. Williams CD, Goldstone AH, Pearce RM, et al. Purging of bone marrow in autologous bone marrow transplantation for non-Hodgkin's lymphoma: a case-matched comparison with unpurged cases by the European Blood and Marrow Transplant Lymphoma Registry. *J Clin Oncol* 1996;14:2454.

757. Reiffers J, Labopin M, Sanz M, et al. Autologous blood cell vs marrow transplantation for acute myeloid leukemia in complete remission: an EBMT retrospective analysis. *Bone Marrow Transplant* 2000;25:1115.

758. Ringden O, Labopin M, Frassoni F, et al. Allogeneic bone marrow transplant or second autograft in patients with acute leukemia who relapse after an autograft. Acute Leukaemia Working Party of the European Group for Blood and Marrow Transplantation (EBMT). *Bone Marrow Transplant* 1999;24:389.

759. Gorin NC, Labopin M, Fouillard L, et al. Retrospective evaluation of autologous bone marrow transplantation vs allogeneic bone marrow transplantation from an HLA identical related donor in acute myelocytic leukemia. A study of the European Cooperative Group for Blood and Marrow Transplantation (EBMT). *Bone Marrow Transplant* 1996;18:111.

760. Tallman S, Kopecky KJ, Amos D, et al. Analysis of prognostic factors for the outcome of marrow transplantation or further chemotherapy for patients with acute nonlymphocytic leukemia in first remission. *J Clin Oncol* 1989;7:326.

761. Appelbaum FR, Dahlberg S, Thomas ED, et al. Bone marrow transplantation or chemotherapy after remission induction for adults with acute nonlymphocytic leukemia. *Ann Intern Med* 1984;101:581.

762. Bostrom B, Brunning RD, McGlave PB, et al. Bone marrow transplantation for acute nonlymphocytic leukemia in first remission: analysis of prognostic factors. *Blood* 1985;65:1191.

763. Zwaan FE, Hermans J, Lyklema A. Factors influencing long-term leukemia-free survival after allogeneic bone marrow transplantation for acute leukemia. In: Hagenbeek A, Lowenberg B, eds. *Minimal residual disease in acute leukemia*. Amsterdam: Nijhoff, 1986:295.

764. Keating S, Suciu S, de Witte T, et al. Prognostic factors of patients with acute myeloid leukemia (AML) allografted in first complete remission: an analysis of the EORTC-GIMEMA AML 8A trial. The European Organization for Research and Treatment of Cancer (EORTC) and the Gruppo Italiano Malattie Ematologiche Maligne dell' Adulto (GIMEMA) Leukemia Cooperative Groups. *Bone Marrow Transplant* 1996;17:993.

765. Transplant or chemotherapy in acute myelogenous leukaemia. International Bone Marrow Transplantation Registry. *Lancet* 1989;1:1119.

766. Horowitz MM, Registry MT. Evidence for a graft versus leukemia effect in clinical bone marrow transplantation. *Exp Hematol* 1988;16:547.

767. Anderson JE, Appelbaum FR, Fisher LD, et al. Allogeneic bone marrow transplantation for 93 patients with myelodysplastic syndrome. *Blood* 1993;82:677.

768. Locatelli F, Niemeyer C, Angelucci E, et al. Allogeneic bone marrow transplantation for chronic myelomonocytic leukemia in childhood: a report from the European Working Group on Myelodysplastic Syndrome in Childhood. *J Clin Oncol* 1997;15:566.

769. Ballen K, Gilliland D, Guinan E, et al. Bone marrow transplantation for therapy-related myelodysplasia: comparison with primary myelodysplasia. *Bone Marrow Transplant* 1997;20:737.

770. Longmore G, Guinan EC, Weinstein HJ, et al. Bone marrow transplantation for myelodysplasia and secondary acute nonlymphoblastic leukemia. *J Clin Oncol* 1990;8:1707.

771. O'Donnell MR, Long GD, Parker PM, et al. Busulfan/cyclophosphamide as conditioning regimen for allogeneic bone marrow transplantation for myelodysplasia. *J Clin Oncol* 1995;13:2973.

772. Deeg HJ, Shulman HM, Anderson JE, et al. Allogeneic and syngeneic marrow transplantation for myelodysplastic syndrome in patients 55 to 66 years of age. *Blood* 2000;95:1188.

773. Yakoub-Agha I, de La Salmoniere P, Ribaud P, et al. Allogeneic bone marrow transplantation for therapy-related myelodysplastic syndrome and acute myeloid leukemia: a long-term study of 70 patients—report of the French society of bone marrow transplantation. *J Clin Oncol* 2000;18:963.

774. Arnold R, de Witte T, van Biezen A, et al. Unrelated bone marrow transplantation in patients with myelodysplastic syndromes and secondary acute myeloid leukemia: an EBMT survey. European Blood and Marrow Transplantation Group. *Bone Marrow Transplant* 1998;21:1213.

775. de Witte T, Hermans J, Vossen J, et al. Haematopoietic stem cell transplantation for patients with myelo-dysplastic syndromes and secondary acute myeloid leukaemias: a report on behalf of the Chronic Leukaemia Working Party of the European Group for Blood and Marrow Transplantation (EBMT). *Br J Haematol* 2000;110:620.

776. Greenberg P, Cox C, LeBeau MM, et al. International scoring system for evaluating prognosis in myelodysplastic syndromes [published erratum appears in *Blood* 1998;91(3):1100]. *Blood* 1997;89:2079.

777. Nevill TJ, Fung HC, Shepherd JD, et al. Cytogenetic abnormalities in primary myelodysplastic syndrome are highly predictive of outcome after allogeneic bone marrow transplantation. *Blood* 1998;92:1910.

778. Zang DY, Deeg HJ, Gooley T, et al. Treatment of chronic myelomonocytic leukaemia by allogeneic marrow transplantation. *Br J Haematol* 2000;110:217.

779. Lucarelli G, Clift RA, Galimberti M, et al. Marrow transplantation for patients with thalassemia: results in class 3 patients. *Blood* 1996;87:2082.

780. Porter DL, Roth MS, Lee SJ, et al. Adoptive immunotherapy with donor mononuclear cell infusions to treat relapse of acute leukemia or myelodysplasia after allogeneic bone marrow transplantation. *Bone Marrow Transplant* 1996;18:975.

781. Steinherz PG, Gaynon P, Miller DR, et al. Improved disease-free survival of children with acute lymphoblastic leukemia at high risk for early relapse with the New York regimen—a new intensive therapy protocol: a report from the Childrens Cancer Study Group. *J Clin Oncol* 1986;4:744.

782. Chessells JM, Bailey C, Richards SM. Intensification of treatment and survival in all children with lymphoblastic leukaemia: results of UK Medical Research Council trial UKALL X. Medical Research Council Working Party on Childhood Leukaemia. *Lancet* 1995;345:143.

783. Clavell LA, Gelber RD, Cohen HJ, et al. Four-agent induction and intensive asparaginase therapy for treatment of childhood acute lymphoblastic leukemia. *N Engl J Med* 1986;315:657.

784. Kersey JH. Fifty years of studies of the biology and therapy of childhood leukemia. *Blood* 1998;92:1838.

785. Blume KG, Forman SJ, Snyder DS, et al. Allogeneic bone marrow transplantation for acute lymphoblastic leukemia during first complete remission. *Transplantation* 1987;43:389.

786. Vernant JP, Marit G, Maraninchi D, et al. Allogeneic bone marrow transplantation in adults with acute lymphoblastic leukemia in first complete remission. *J Clin Oncol* 1988;6:227.

787. Zwaan FE, Hermans J, Barrett AJ, Speck B. Bone marrow transplantation for acute lymphoblastic leukaemia: a survey of the European Group for Bone Marrow Transplantation (E.G.B.M.T.). *Br J Haematol* 1984;58:33.

788. Cornelissen JJ, Carston M, Kollman C, et al. Unrelated marrow transplantation for adult patients with poor-risk acute lymphoblastic leukemia: strong graft-versus-leukemia effect and risk factors determining outcome. *Blood* 2001;97:1572.

789. Snyder DS. Allogeneic stem cell transplantation for Philadelphia chromosome-positive acute lymphoblastic leukemia. *Biol Blood Marrow Transplantation* 2000;6:597.

790. Brochstein JA, Kernan NA, Groshen S, et al. Allogeneic bone marrow transplantation after hyperfractionated total-body irradiation and cyclophosphamide in children with acute leukemia. *N Engl J Med* 1987;317:1618.

791. Herzig RH, Bortin MM, Barrett AJ, et al. Bone-marrow transplantation in high-risk acute lymphoblastic leukaemia in first and second remission. *Lancet* 1987;i:786.

792. Forman SJ, O'Donnell MR, Nademanee AP, et al. Bone marrow transplantation for patients with Philadelphia chromosome-positive acute lymphoblastic leukemia. *Blood* 1987;70:587.

793. Horowitz MM, Messerer D, Hoelzer D, et al. Chemotherapy compared with bone marrow transplantation for adults with acute lymphoblastic leukemia in first remission. *Ann Intern Med* 1991;115:13.

794. Snyder DS, Nademanee AP, O'Donnell MR, et al. Long-term follow-up of 23 patients with Philadelphia chromosome-positive acute lymphoblastic leukemia treated with allogeneic bone marrow transplant in first complete remission. *Leukemia* 1999;13:2053.

795. Uderzo C, Valsecchi MG, Bacigalupo A, et al. Treatment of childhood acute lymphoblastic leukemia in second remission with allogeneic bone marrow transplantation and chemotherapy: ten-year experience of the Italian Bone Marrow Transplantation Group and the Italian Pediatric Hematology Oncology Association. *J Clin Oncol* 1995;13:352.

796. Weisdorf DJ, Billett AL, Hannan P, et al. Autologous versus unrelated donor allogeneic marrow transplantation for acute lymphoblastic leukemia. *Blood* 1997;90:2962.

797. Sebban C, Lepage E, Vernant J-P, et al. Allogeneic bone marrow transplantation in adult acute lymphoblastic leukemia in first complete remission: a comparative study. *J Clin Oncol* 1994;12:2580.

798. Barrett AJ, Horowitz MM, Gale RP, et al. Marrow transplantation for acute lymphoblastic leukemia: factors affecting relapse and survival. *Blood* 1989;74:862.

799. Saarinen-Pihkala UM, Gustafsson G, Ringden O, et al. No disadvantage in outcome of using matched unrelated donors as compared with matched sibling donors for bone marrow transplantation in children with acute lymphoblastic leukemia in second remission. *J Clin Oncol* 2001;19:3406.

800. Attal M, Blaise D, Marit G, et al. Consolidation treatment of adult acute lymphoblastic leukemia: a prospective, randomized trial comparing allogeneic versus autologous bone marrow transplantation and testing the impact of recombinant interleukin-2 after autologous bone marrow transplantation. *Blood* 1995;86:1619.

801. Rowe JM, Richards SM, Burnett AK, et al. Favorable results of allogeneic bone marrow transplantation (BMT) for adults with Philadelphia (Ph)-chromosome-negative acute lymphoblastic leukemia (ALL) in first complete remission (CR): results from the international ALL trial (MRC UKALL XII/ECOG E2993). *Blood* 2001;98(Suppl 1):481a.

802. Borgmann A, Baumgarten E, Schmid H, et al. Allogeneic bone marrow transplantation for a subset of children with acute lymphoblastic leukemia in third remission: a conceivable alternative? *Bone Marrow Transplant* 1997;20:939.

803. Buckner CD, Clift RA. Marrow transplantation for acute lymphoblastic leukemia. *Semin Hematol* 1984;21:43.

804. Weisdorf DJ, Nesbit ME, Ramsay NKC, et al. Allogeneic bone marrow transplantation for acute lymphoblastic leukemia in remission: prolonged survival associated with acute graft versus host disease. *J Clin Oncol* 1987;5:1348.

805. Coccia PF, Strandjord SE, Warkentin PI, et al. High-dose cytosine arabinoside and fractionated total-body irradiation: an improved preparative regimen for bone marrow transplantation of children with acute lymphoblastic leukemia in remission. *Blood* 1988;71:888.

806. Davies SM, Ramsay NK, Klein JP, et al. Comparison of preparative regimens in transplants for children with acute lymphoblastic leukemia. *J Clin Oncol* 2000;18:340.

807. Buchanan GR, Boyett JM, Rivera GK. Intensive combination chemotherapy for patients with acute lymphoblastic leukemia (ALL) in second marrow remission: a Pediatric Oncology Group study. *Proc Amer Soc Clin Oncol* 1988; 7:188.

808. Johnson FL, Thomas ED, Clark BS, et al. A comparison of marrow transplantation with chemotherapy for children with acute lymphoblastic leukemia in second and subsequent remission. *N Engl J Med* 1981;305:846.

809. Pinkel D. Allogeneic bone marrow transplantation in children with acute leukemia: a practice whose time has gone. *Leukemia* 1989;3:242.

810. Chessells JM, Rogers DW, Leiper AD, et al. Bone-marrow transplantation has a limited role in prolonging second marrow remission in childhood lymphoblastic leukaemia. *Lancet* 1986;1:1239.

811. Barrett AJ, Horowitz MM, Pollock BH, et al. Bone marrow transplants from HLA-identical siblings as compared with chemotherapy for children with acute lymphoblastic leukemia in a second remission. *N Engl J Med* 1994;331:1253.

812. Boulad F, Steinherz P, Reyes B, et al. Allogeneic bone marrow transplantation versus chemotherapy for the treatment of childhood acute lymphoblastic leukemia in second remission: a single-institution study. *J Clin Oncol* 1999; 17:197.

813. Chessells JM, Leiper AD, Richards SM. A second course of treatment for childhood acute lymphoblastic leukaemia: long-term follow-up is needed to assess results. *Br J Haematol* 1994;86:48.

814. Barrett AJ, Joshi R, Kendra JR, et al. Prediction and prevention of relapse of acute lymphoblastic leukaemia after bone marrow transplantation. *Br J Haematol* 1986;64:179.

815. Kersey JH, Weisdorf D, Nesbit ME, et al. Comparison of autologous and allogeneic bone marrow transplantation for treatment of high risk refractory acute lymphoblastic leukemia. *N Engl J Med* 1987;317:461.

816. Thompson CB, Sanders JE, Flournoy N, et al. The risks of central nervous system relapse and leukoencephalopathy in patients receiving marrow transplants for acute leukemia. *Blood* 1986;67:195.

817. Bostrom B, Woods WG, Nesbit ME, et al. Successful reinduction of patients with acute lymphoblastic leukemia who relapse following bone marrow transplantation. *J Clin Oncol* 1987;5:376.

818. Ramsay N, LeBien T, Nesbit M, et al. Autologous bone marrow transplantation for patients with acute lymphoblastic leukemia in second or subsequent remission: results of bone marrow treated with monoclonal antibodies BA-1, BA-2 and BA-3 plus complement. *Blood* 1985;66:508.

819. Ball ED, Mills LE, Coughlin CT, Beck JR, Cornwell GG, 3rd. Autologous bone marrow transplantation in acute myelogenous leukemia: in vitro treatment with myeloid cell-specific monoclonal antibodies. *Blood* 1986;68:1311.

820. Ritz J. Use of monoclonal antibodies in autologous and allogeneic bone marrow transplantation. *Clin Haematol* 1983;12:813.

821. Chang J, Coutinho L, Morgenstern G, et al. Reconstitution of haematopoietic system with autologous marrow taken during relapse of acute myeloblastic leukaemia and grown in long-term culture. *Lancet* 1986;i:294.

822. Gorin NC, Douay L, Laporte JP, et al. Autologous bone marrow transplantation using marrow incubated with Asta Z 7557 in adult acute leukemia. *Blood* 1986;67:1367.

823. Hagenbeek A, Martens ACM, Schultz FW. Residual leukemic cells in autologous marrow grafts do not significantly contribute to leukemia relapse after bone marrow transplantation. *Exp Hematol* 1988;16:492.

824. Hagenbeek A, Martens ACM. The efficacy of high-dose cyclophosphamide in combination with total body irradiation in the treatment of acute myelocytic leukemia. Studies in a relevant rat model (BNML). *Cancer Res* 1983; 43:408.

825. Hagenbeek A, Martens ACM. Reinfusion of leukemic cells with the autologous marrow graft: preclinical studies on lodging and regrowth of leukemia. *Leukemia Res* 1985;9:1389.

826. Burnett AK, McKinnon S. Autologous bone marrow transplantation in first remission AML using nonpurged marrow—update. In: Hagenbeek A, Lowenberg B, eds. *Minimal residual disease*. Dordrecht, the Netherlands: Martinus Nijhoff, 1986:211.

827. Gorin NC, Aegerter P. Autologous bone marrow transplantation for acute leukemia in remission: Third European Survey: March, 1986. *Bone Marrow Transplant* 1986;1:255.

828. Gorin NC, Hervé P, Aegerter P, et al. Autologous bone marrow transplantation for acute leukaemia in remission. *Br J Haematol* 1986;64:385.

829. Billett AL, Kornmehl E, Tarbell NJ, et al. Autologous bone marrow transplantation after a long first remission for children with recurrent acute lymphoblastic leukemia. *Blood* 1993;81:1651.

830. Nemunaitis J, Rabinowe SN, Singer JW, et al. Recombinant granulocyte-macrophage colony-stimulating factor after autologous bone marrow transplantation for lymphoid cancer. *N Engl J Med* 1991;324:1773.

831. Blazar BR, Kersey JH, McGlave PB, et al. In vivo administration of recombinant granulocyte/macrophage colony-stimulating factor in acute lymphoblastic leukemia receiving purged autografts. *Blood* 1989;73:849.

832. Appelbaum FR, Sullivan KM, Thomas ED, et al. Allogeneic marrow transplantation in the treatment of MOPP-resistant Hodgkin's disease. *J Clin Oncol* 1985;3:1490.

833. Gajewski JL, Phillips GL, Sobocinski KA, et al. Bone marrow transplants from HLA-identical siblings in advanced Hodgkin's disease. *J Clin Oncol* 1996;14:572.

834. Milpied N, Fielding AK, Pearce RM, et al. Allogeneic bone marrow transplant is not better than autologous transplant for patients with relapsed Hodgkin's disease. European Group for Blood and Bone Marrow Transplantation. *J Clin Oncol* 1996;14:1291.

835. Porter DL, Connors JM, Van Deerlin VM, et al. Graft-versus-tumor induction with donor leukocyte infusions as primary therapy for patients with malignancies. *J Clin Oncol* 1999;17:1234.

836. Appelbaum FR, Sullivan KM, Buckner CD, et al. Treatment of malignant lymphoma in 100 patients with chemotherapy, total body irradiation, and marrow transplantation. *J Clin Oncol* 1987;5:1340.

837. Kaplan HS. Evidence for a tumoricidal dose level in the radiotherapy of Hodgkin's disease. *Cancer Res* 1966;26:1250.

838. Nademanee A, O'Donnell MR, Snyder DS, et al. High-dose chemotherapy with or without total body irradiation followed by autologous bone marrow and/or peripheral blood stem cell transplantation for patients with relapsed and refractory Hodgkin's disease: Results in 85 patients with analysis of prognostic factors. *Blood* 1995;85:1381.

839. Wheeler C, Eickhoff C, Elias A, et al. High-dose cyclophosphamide, carmustine, and etoposide with autologous transplantation in Hodgkin's disease: a prognostic model for treatment outcomes. *Biol Blood Marrow Transplant* 1997;3:98.

840. Horning SJ, Chao NJ, Negrin RS, et al. High-dose therapy and autologous hematopoietic progenitor cell transplantation for recurrent or refractory Hodgkin's disease: analysis of the Stanford University results and prognostic indices. *Blood* 1997;89:801.

841. Moreau P, Fleury J, Brice P, et al. Early intensive therapy with autologous stem cell transplantation in advanced Hodgkin's disease: retrospective analysis of 158 cases from the French registry. *Bone Marrow Transplant* 1998; 21:787.

842. Johnston LJ, Horning SJ. Autologous hematopoietic cell transplantation in Hodgkin's disease. *Biol Blood Marrow Transplant* 2000;6:289.

843. Brice P, Bouabdallah R, Moreau P, et al. Prognostic factors for survival after high-dose therapy and autologous stem cell transplantation for patients with relapsing Hodgkin's disease: analysis of 280 patients from the French registry. Societe Francaise de Greffe de Moelle. *Bone Marrow Transplant* 1997; 20:21.

844. Rapoport AP, Rowe JM, Kouides PA, et al. One hundred autotransplants for relapsed or refractory Hodgkin's disease and lymphoma: value of pretransplant disease status for predicting outcome. *J Clin Oncol* 1993;11:2351.

845. Yuen AR, Rosenberg SA, Hoppe RT, et al. Comparison between conventional salvage therapy and high-dose therapy with autografting for recurrent or refractory Hodgkin's disease. *Blood* 1997;89:814.

846. Lazarus HM, Rowlings PA, Zhang MJ, et al. Autotransplants for Hodgkin's disease in patients never achieving remission: a report from the Autologous Blood and Marrow Transplant Registry. *J Clin Oncol* 1999;17:534.

847. Nademanee A, Molina A, Fung H, et al. High-dose chemo/radiotherapy and autologous bone marrow or stem cell transplantation for poor-risk advanced-stage Hodgkin's disease during first partial or complete remission. *Biol Blood Marrow Transplant* 1999;5:292.

848. Chopra R, Goldstone AH, Pearce R, et al. Autologous versus allogeneic bone marrow transplantation for non-Hodgkin's lymphoma: a case-controlled analysis of the European Bone Marrow Transplantation Group Registry data. *J Clin Oncol* 1992;10:1690.

849. Ratanatharathorn V, Uberti J, Karanes C, et al. Prospective comparative trial of autologous versus allogeneic bone marrow transplantation in patients with non-Hodgkin's lymphoma. *Blood* 1994;84:1050.

850. van Besien K, Thall P, Korbling M, et al. Allogeneic transplantation for recurrent or refractory non-Hodgkin's lymphoma with poor prognostic features after conditioning with thiotepa, busulfan, and cyclophosphamide: experience in 44 consecutive patients. *Biol Blood Marrow Transplant* 1997;3:150.

851. Verdonck LF, Dekker AW, Lokhorst HM, et al. Allogeneic versus autologous bone marrow transplantation for refractory and recurrent low-grade non-Hodgkin's lymphoma. *Blood* 1997;90:4201.

852. Juckett M, Rowlings P, Hessner M, et al. T cell-depleted allogeneic bone marrow transplantation for high-risk non-Hodgkin's lymphoma: clinical and molecular follow-up. *Bone Marrow Transplant* 1998;21:893.

853. Soiffer RJ, Freedman AS, Neuberg D, et al. CD6+ T cell-depleted allogeneic bone marrow transplantation for non-Hodgkin's lymphoma. *Bone Marrow Transplant* 1998;21:1177.

854. van Besien K, Sobocinski KA, Rowlings PA, et al. Allogeneic bone marrow transplantation for low-grade lymphoma. *Blood* 1998;92:1832.

855. Toze CL, Shepherd JD, Connors JM, et al. Allogeneic bone marrow transplantation for low-grade lymphoma and chronic lymphocytic leukemia. *Bone Marrow Transplant* 2000;25:605.

856. Jones RJ, Ambinder RF, Piantadosi S, Santos GW. Evidence of a graft-versus-lymphoma effect associated with allogeneic bone marrow transplantation. *Blood* 1991;77:649.

857. Nagler A, Slavin S, Varadi G, et al. Allogeneic peripheral blood stem cell transplantation using a fludarabine-based low intensity conditioning regimen for malignant lymphoma. *Bone Marrow Transplant* 2000;25:1021.

858. Champlin R, Khouri I, Kornblau S, et al. Allogeneic hematopoietic transplantation as adoptive immunotherapy. Induction of graft-versus-malignancy as primary therapy. *Hematol Oncol Clin North Am* 1999;13:1041.

859. Appelbaum FR, Herzig GP, Ziegler JL, et al. Successful engraftment of cryopreserved autologous bone marrow in patients with malignant lymphoma. *Blood* 1978;52:85.

860. Appelbaum FR, Deisseroth AB, Graw RG, et al. Prolonged complete remission following high dose chemotherapy of Burkitt's lymphoma in relapse. *Cancer* 1978;41:1059.

861. Shipp MA, Abeloff MD, Antman KH, et al. International Consensus Conference on High-Dose Therapy with Hematopoietic Stem Cell Transplantation in Aggressive Non-Hodgkin's Lymphomas: report of the jury [see comments]. *J Clin Oncol* 1999;17:423.

862. Wheeler C, Strawderman M, Ayash L, et al. Prognostic factors for treatment outcome in autotransplantation of intermediate-grade and high-grade non-Hodgkin's lymphoma with cyclophosphamide, carmustine, and etoposide. *J Clin Oncol* 1993;11:1085.

863. Philip T, Guglielmi C, Hagenbeek A, et al. Autologous bone marrow transplantation as compared with salvage chemotherapy in relapses of chemotherapy-sensitive non-Hodgkin's lymphoma. *N Engl J Med* 1995;333:1540.

864. Stockerl-Goldstein KE, Horning SJ, Negrin RS, et al. Influence of preparatory regimen and source of hematopoietic cells on outcome of autotransplantation for non-Hodgkin's lymphoma. *Biol Blood Marrow Transplant* 1996;2:76.

865. Rapoport AP, Lifton R, Constine LS, et al. Autotransplantation for relapsed or refractory non-Hodgkin's lymphoma (NHL): long-term follow-up and analysis of prognostic factors. *Bone Marrow Transplant* 1997;19:883.

866. Popat U, Przepiork D, Champlin R, et al. High-dose chemotherapy for relapsed and refractory diffuse large B-cell lymphoma: mediastinal localization predicts for a favorable outcome. *J Clin Oncol* 1998;16:63.

867. Stiff PJ, Dahlberg S, Forman SJ, et al. Autologous bone marrow transplantation for patients with relapsed or refractory diffuse aggressive non-Hodgkin's lymphoma: value of augmented preparative regimens—a Southwest Oncology Group trial. *J Clin Oncol* 1998;16:48.

868. Sweetenham JW, Pearce R, Philip T, et al. High-dose therapy and autologous bone marrow transplantation for intermediate and high grade non-Hodgkin's lymphoma in patients aged 55 years and over: results from the European Group for Bone Marrow Transplantation. The EBMT Lymphoma Working Party. *Bone Marrow Transplant* 1994;14:981.

869. Blay J, Gomez F, Sebban C, et al. The International Prognostic Index correlates to survival in patients with aggressive lymphoma in relapse: analysis of the PARMA trial. Parma Group. *Blood* 1998;92:3562.

870. Guglielmi C, Gomez F, Philip T, et al. Time to relapse has prognostic value in patients with aggressive lymphoma enrolled onto the Parma trial. *J Clin Oncol* 1998;16:3264.

871. Bosly A, Sonet A, Salles G, et al. Superiority of late over early intensification in relapsing/refractory aggressive non-Hodgkin's lymphoma: a randomized study from GELA: LNH RP 93. *Blood* 1998;90:594a.

872. Gulati SC, Shank B, Black P, et al. Autologous bone marrow transplantation for patients with poor-prognosis lymphoma. *J Clin Oncol* 1988;6:1303.

873. Shipp MA, Harrington DP, Klatt MM, et al. Identification of major prognostic subgroups of patients with large-cell lymphoma treated with m-BACOD or M-BACOD. *Ann Intern Med* 1986;104:757.

874. Haioun C, Lepage E, Gisselbrecht C, et al. Survival benefit of high-dose therapy in poor-risk aggressive non-Hodgkin's lymphoma: final analysis of the prospective LNH87-2 protocol—a groupe d'Etude des lymphomes de l'Adulte study. *J Clin Oncol* 2000;18:3025.

875. Santini G, Salvagno L, Leoni P, et al. VACOP-B versus VACOP-B plus autologous bone marrow transplantation for advanced diffuse non-Hodgkin's lymphoma: results of a prospective randomized trial by the non-Hodgkin's Lymphoma Cooperative Study Group. *J Clin Oncol* 1998;16:2796.

876. Reyes F, Lepage E, Morel P, et al. Failure of first-line high-dose inductive chemotherapy (HDC) in poor-risk patients (PTS) with aggressive lymphoma. Updated results of LNH93-3 study. *Blood* 1997;90(Suppl 1):594a.

877. Gianni AM, Bregni M, Siena S, et al. High-dose chemotherapy and autologous bone marrow transplantation compared with MACOP-B in aggressive B-cell lymphoma [see comments]. *N Engl J Med* 1997;336:1290.

878. Freedman AS, Neuberg D, Mauch P, et al. Long-term follow-up of autologous bone marrow transplantation in patients with relapsed follicular lymphoma. *Blood* 1999;94:3325.

879. Apostolidis J, Gupta RK, Grenzelias D, et al. High-dose therapy with autologous bone marrow support as consolidation of remission in follicular lymphoma: long-term clinical and molecular follow-up. *J Clin Oncol* 2000;18:527.

880. Bierman PJ, Vose JM, Anderson JR, et al. High-dose therapy with autologous hematopoietic rescue for follicular low-grade non-Hodgkin's lymphoma. *J Clin Oncol* 1997;15:445.

881. Friedberg JW, Neuberg D, Gribben JG, et al. Autologous bone marrow transplantation after histologic transformation of indolent B cell malignancies. *Biol Blood Marrow Transplant* 1999;5:262.

882. Bastion Y, Brice P, Haioun C, et al. Intensive therapy with peripheral blood progenitor cell transplantation in 60 patients with poor-prognosis follicular lymphoma. *Blood* 1995;86:3257.

883. Freedman AS, Neuberg D, Gribben JG, et al. High-dose chemoradiotherapy and anti-B-cell monoclonal antibody-purged autologous bone marrow transplantation in mantle-cell lymphoma: no evidence for long-term remission [see comments]. *J Clin Oncol* 1998;16:13.

884. Khouri IF, Romaguera J, Kantarjian H, et al. Hyper-CVAD and high-dose methotrexate/cytarabine followed by stem-cell transplantation: an active regimen for aggressive mantle-cell lymphoma. *J Clin Oncol* 1998;16:3803.

885. Khouri IF, Lee MS, Romaguera J, et al. Allogeneic hematopoietic transplantation for mantle-cell lymphoma: molecular remissions and evidence of graft-versus-malignancy. *Ann Oncol* 1999;10:1293.

886. Bennett JM, Cain KC, Glick JH, et al. The significance of bone marrow involvement in non-Hodgkin's lymphoma: the Eastern Cooperative Oncology Group experience. *J Clin Oncol* 1986;4:1462.

887. Tweeddale ME, Lim B, Jamal N, et al. The presence of clonogenic cells in high-grade malignant lymphomas: a prognostic factor. *Blood* 1987;69:1307.

888. Benjamin D, Magrath IT, Douglas EC, Corash LM. Derivation of lymphoma cell lines from microscopically normal bone marrow in patients with undifferentiated lymphomas: evidence of occult bone marrow involvement. *Blood* 1983;61:1017.

889. Magni M, Di Nicola M, Devizzi L, et al. Successful in vivo purging of CD34-containing peripheral blood harvests in mantle cell and indolent lymphoma: evidence for a role of both chemotherapy and rituximab infusion. *Blood* 2000;96:864.

890. Michallet M, Archimbaud E, Bandini G, et al. HLA-identical sibling bone marrow transplantation in younger patients with chronic lymphocytic leukemia. *Ann Intern Med* 1996;124:311.

891. Pavletic ZS, Arrowsmith ER, Bierman PJ, et al. Outcome of allogeneic stem cell transplantation for B cell chronic lymphocytic leukemia. *Bone Marrow Transplant* 2000;25:717.

892. Khouri IF, Przepiorka D, van Besien K, et al. Allogeneic blood or marrow transplantation for chronic lymphocytic leukaemia: timing of transplantation and potential effect of fludarabine on acute graft-versus-host disease. *Br J Haematol* 1997;97:466.

893. Rabinowe SN, Soiffer RJ, Gribben JG, et al. Autologous and allogeneic bone marrow transplantation for poor prognosis patients with B-cell chronic lymphocytic leukemia. *Blood* 1993;82:1366.

894. Provan D, Bartlett-Pandite L, Zwicky C, et al. Eradication of polymerase chain reaction-detectable chronic lymphocytic leukemia cells is associated with improved outcome after bone marrow transplantation. *Blood* 1996;88:2228.

895. McElwain TJ, Powles RL. High-dose intravenous melphalan for plasma-cell leukaemia and myeloma. *Lancet* 1983;2:822.

896. Attal M, Harousseau JL, Stoppa AM, et al. A prospective, randomized trial of autologous bone marrow transplantation and chemotherapy in multiple myeloma. Intergroupe Francais du Myelome [see comments]. *N Engl J Med* 1996;335:91.

897. Desikan R, Barlogie B, Sawyer J, et al. Results of high-dose therapy for 1000 patients with multiple myeloma: durable complete remissions and superior survival in the absence of chromosome 13 abnormalities. *Blood* 2000;95:4008.

898. Gahrton G, Tura S, Ljungman P, et al. Prognostic factors in allogeneic bone marrow transplantation for multiple myeloma. *J Clin Oncol* 1995;13:1312.

899. Reece DE, Shepherd JD, Klingemann HG, et al. Treatment of myeloma using intensive therapy and allogeneic bone marrow transplantation. *Bone Marrow Transplant* 1995;15:117.

900. Bjorkstrand B, Ljungman P, Svensson H, et al. Allogeneic bone marrow transplantation versus autologous stem cell transplantation in multiple myeloma: a retrospective case-matched study from the European Group for Blood and Marrow Transplantation. *Blood* 1996;88:4711.

901. Lenhoff S, Hjorth M, Holmberg L, et al. Impact on survival of high-dose therapy with autologous stem cell support in patients younger than 60 years with newly diagnosed multiple myeloma: a population-based study. Nordic Myeloma Study Group. *Blood* 2000;95:7.

902. Barlogie B, Jagannath S, Vesole DH, et al. Superiority of tandem autologous transplantation over standard therapy for previously untreated multiple myeloma. *Blood* 1997;89:789.

903. Martinelli G, Terragna C, Zamagni E, et al. Molecular remission after allogeneic or autologous transplantation of hematopoietic stem cells for multiple myeloma. *J Clin Oncol* 2000;18:2273.

904. Orsini E, Alyea EP, Chillemi A, et al. Conversion to full donor chimerism following donor lymphocyte infusion is associated with disease response in patients with multiple myeloma. *Biol Blood Marrow Transplant* 2000;6:375.

905. Lokhorst H, Schattenberg A, Cornelissen J, et al. Donor lymphocyte infusions for relapsed multiple myeloma after allogeneic stem-cell transplantation: predictive factors for response and long-term outcome. *J Clin Oncol* 2000;18:3031.

906. Moreau P, Leblond V, Bourquelot P, et al. Prognostic factors for survival and response after high-dose therapy and autologous stem cell transplantation in systemic AL amyloidosis: a report on 21 patients. *Br J Haematol* 1998;101:766.

907. Comenzo RL, Vosburgh E, Falk RH, et al. Dose-intensive melphalan with blood stem-cell support for the treatment of AL (amyloid light-chain) amyloidosis: survival and responses in 25 patients. *Blood* 1998;91:3662.

908. Gertz MA, Lacy MQ, Dispenzieri A. Myeloablative chemotherapy with stem cell rescue for the treatment of primary systemic amyloidosis: a status report. *Bone Marrow Transplant* 2000;25:465.

909. Parkman R. The application of bone marrow transplantation to the treatment of genetic diseases. *Science* 1986;232:1373.

910. Gelfand EW, Dosch HM. Diagnosis and classification of severe combined immunodeficiency disease. *Birth Defects Orig Art Ser* 1983;19:65.

911. Rosen FS, Cooper MD, Wedgwood RJ. The primary immunodeficiencies. *N Engl J Med* 1995;333:431.

912. Pollack MS, Kirkpatrick D, Kapoor N, et al. Identification by HLA typing of intrauterine-derived maternal T cells in four patients with severe combined immunodeficiency. *N Engl J Med* 1982;307:662.

913. Thompson LF, O'Connor RD, Bastian JF. Phenotype and function of engrafted maternal T cells in patients with severe combined immunodeficiency. *J Immunol* 1984;133:2513.

914. Bortin MM, Rimm AA. Severe combined immunodeficiency disease. Characterization of the disease and results of transplantation. *JAMA* 1977;238:591.

915. Kenny AB, Hitzig WH. Bone marrow transplantation for severe combined immunodeficiency syndrome. *Eur J Pediatr* 1979;131:155.

916. Rappeport JM, Smith BR, Parkman R, Rosen FS. Application of bone marrow transplantation in genetic diseases. *Clin Haematol* 1983;12:755.

917. Parkman R, Gelfand EW, Rosen FS, et al. Severe combined immunodeficiency and adenosine deaminase deficiency. *N Engl J Med* 1975;292:714.

918. Stephan JL, Vlekova V, Le Deist F, et al. Severe combined immunodeficiency: a retrospective single-center study of clinical presentation and outcome in 117 patients. *J Pediatr* 1993;123:564.

919. Reisner Y, Kapoor N, Kirkpatrick D, et al. Transplantation for severe combined immunodeficiency with HLA-A,B,D,DR incompatible parental marrow cells fractionated by soybean agglutinin and sheep red blood cells. *Blood* 1983;61:341.

920. Friedrich W, Goldmann SF, Vetter U, et al. Immunoreconstitution in severe combined immunodeficiency after transplantation of HLA-haploidentical, T-cell-depleted bone marrow. *Lancet* 1984;1:761.

921. Fischer A, Durandy A, de Villartay JP, et al. HLA-haploidentical bone marrow transplantation for severe combined immunodeficiency using E rosette fractionation and cyclosporine. *Blood* 1986;67:444.

922. Buckley R, Schiff SE, Sampson HA, et al. Development of immunity in severe primary T cell deficiency following haploidentical bone marrow stem cell transplantation. *J Immunol* 1986;136:2398.

923. Buckley RH, Schiff SE, Schiff RI, et al. Hematopoietic stem-cell transplantation for the treatment of severe combined immunodeficiency. *N Engl J Med* 1999;340:508.

924. Shearer WT, Ritz J, Finegold M, et al. Epstein-Barr virus-associated B-cell proliferation of diverse clonal origins after bone marrow transplantation in a 12-year-old patient with severe combined immunodeficiency. *N Engl J Med* 1985;312:1151.

925. Cavazzana-Calvo M, Hacein-Bey S, de Saint-Basile G, et al. Gene therapy of human severe combined immunodeficiency (SCID)-X1 disease. *Science* 2000;288:669.

926. Remold-O'Donnell E, Kenney DM, Parkman R, et al. Characterization of a human lymphocyte surface sialoglycoprotein that is defective in Wiskott-Aldrich syndrome. *J Exp Med* 1984;159:1705.

927. Parkman R, Rappeport J, Geha R, et al. Complete correction of the Wiskott-Aldrich syndrome by allogeneic bone-marrow transplantation. *N Engl J Med* 1978;298:921.

928. Kapoor N, Kirkpatrick D, Blaese RM, et al. Reconstitution of normal megakaryocytopoiesis and immunologic functions in Wiskott-Aldrich syndrome by marrow transplantation following myeloablation and immunosuppression with busulfan and cyclophosphamide. *Blood* 1981;57:692.

929. Ochs HD, Lum LG, Johnson FL, et al. Bone marrow transplantation in the Wiskott-Aldrich syndrome. Complete hematological and immunological reconstitution. *Transplantation* 1982;34:284.

930. Brochstein JA, Gillio AP, Ruggiero M, et al. Marrow transplantation from human leukocyte antigen-identical or haploidentical donors for correction of Wiskott-Aldrich syndrome. *J Pediatr* 1991;119:907.

931. Filipovich AH, Stone JV, Tomany SC, et al. Impact of donor type on outcome of bone marrow transplantation for Wiskott-Aldrich syndrome: collaborative study of the International Bone Marrow Transplantation Registry and the National Marrow Donor Program. *Blood* 2001;97:1598.

932. Lucarelli G, Galimberti M, Polchi P, et al. Bone marrow transplantation in adult thalassemia. *Blood* 1992;80:1603.

933. Lucarelli G, Galimberti M, Polchi P, et al. Bone marrow transplantation in patients with thalassemia. *N Engl J Med* 1990;322:417.

934. Lucarelli G, Galimberti M, Polchi P. Marrow transplantation in patients with advanced thalassemia. *N Engl J Med* 1987;316:1050.

935. Weatherall D. Bone marrow transplantation for thalassemia and other inherited disorders of hemoglobin. *Blood* 1992;80:1379.

936. Weiden PL, Hackman RC, Deeg HJ, et al. Long term survival and reversal of iron overload after marrow transplantation in dogs with congenital hemolytic anemia. *Blood* 1981;57:66.

937. Johnson FL, Look AT, Gockerman J, et al. Bone marrow transplantation in a patient with sickle cell anemia. *N Engl J Med* 1984;311:780.

938. Vermylen C, Robles EF, Ninane J, Cornu G. Bone marrow transplantation in five children with sickle cell anaemia. *Lancet* 1988;1:1427.

939. Vermylen C, Cornu G, Ferster A, et al. Haematopoietic stem cell transplantation for sickle cell anaemia: the first 50 patients transplanted in Belgium. *Bone Marrow Transplant* 1998;22:1.

940. Walters MC, Storb R, Patience M, et al. Impact of bone marrow transplantation for symptomatic sickle cell disease: an interim report. Multicenter investigation of bone marrow transplantation for sickle cell disease. *Blood* 2000;95:1918.

941. Gluckman E, Auerbach AD, Horowitz MM, et al. Bone marrow transplantation for Fanconi anemia. *Blood* 1995;86:2856.

942. Gluckman E, Broxmeyer H, Auerbach AD, et al. Hematopoietic reconstitution in a patient with Fanconi anemia by means of umbilical-cord blood from an HLA-identical sibling. *N Engl J Med* 1989;321:1174.

943. Ballet JJ, Griscelli C, Coutris C, et al. Bone-marrow transplantation in osteopetrosis. *Lancet* 1977;2:1137.

944. Sorell M, Kapoor N, Kirkpatrick D, et al. Marrow transplantation for juvenile osteopetrosis. *Am J Med* 1981;70:1280.

945. Hirschhorn R. Therapy of genetic disorders. *N Engl J Med* 1987;316:624.

946. Hershfield MS, Buckley RH, Greenberg ML, et al. Treatment of adenosine deaminase deficiency with polyethylene glycol-modified adenosine deaminase. *N Engl J Med* 1987;316:589.

947. Wewers MD, Casolaro MA, Sellers SE, et al. Replacement therapy for alpha 1-antitrypsin deficiency associated with emphysema. *N Engl J Med* 1987;316:1055.

948. Groth CG, Ringden O. Transplantation in relation to the treatment of inherited disease. *Transplantation* 1984;38:319.

949. Rappeport JM, Ginn EI. Bone-marrow transplantation for severe Gaucher's disease. *N Engl J Med* 1984;311:84.

950. Hobbs JR. Displacement bone marrow transplantation for some inborn errors. *J Inherit Metab Dis* 1990;13:572.

951. Hobbs JR, Hugh-Jones K, Barrett AJ, et al. Reversal of clinical features of Hurler's disease and biochemical improvement after treatment by bone-marrow transplantation. *Lancet* 1981;2:709.

952. Krivit W, Pierpont ME, Ayaz K, et al. Bone-marrow transplantation in the Maroteaux-Lamy syndrome (mucopolysaccharidosis type VI). Biochemical and clinical status 24 months after transplantation. *N Engl J Med* 1984;311:1606.

953. Konigsmark BW, Sidman RL. Origin of brain macrophages in the mouse. *J Neuropathol Exp Neurol* 1963;22:643.

954. Bartlett PF. Pluripotential hematopoietic stem cells in adult mouse brain. *Proc Natl Acad Sci U S A* 1982;79:2722.

955. Yeager AM, Brennan S, Tiffany C, et al. Prolonged survival and remyelination after hematopoietic cell transplantation in the twitcher mouse. *Science* 1984;225:1052.

956. Rappeport JM, Parkman R, Newburger P, et al. Correction of infantile agranulocytosis (Kostmann's syndrome) by allogeneic bone marrow transplantation. *Am J Med* 1980;68:605.

957. Camitta BM, Quesenberry PJ, Parkman R, et al. Bone marrow transplantation for an infant with neutrophil dysfunction. *Exp Hematol* 1977;5:109.

958. Kazmierowski JA, Elin RJ, Reynolds HY, et al. Chediak-Higashi syndrome: reversal of increased susceptibility to infection by bone marrow transplantation. *Blood* 1976;47:555.

959. Iriondo A, Garijo J, Baro J, et al. Complete recovery of hemopoiesis following bone marrow transplant in a patient with unresponsive congenital hypoplastic anemia (Blackfan-Diamond syndrome). *Blood* 1984;64:348.

960. Lenarsky C, Weinberg K, Guinan E, et al. Bone marrow transplantation for constitutional pure red cell aplasia. *Blood* 1988;71:226.

961. Burt R, Slavin S, Burns W, Marmont A. Induction of tolerance in autoimmune diseases by hematopoietic stem cell transplantation: getting closer to a cure? *Blood* 2002;99:768.

962. Tyndall A, Fassas A, Passweg J, et al. Autologous haematopoietic stem cell transplants for autoimmune disease—feasibility and transplant-related mortality. Autoimmune Disease and Lymphoma Working Parties of the European Group for Blood and Marrow Transplantation, the European League Against Rheumatism and the International Stem Cell Project for Autoimmune Disease. *Bone Marrow Transplant* 1999;24:729.

APPENDIX

Data of Importance in Hematology

Peter W. Marks

LIST OF APPENDICES

APPENDIX 1

Normal Hematologic Values during the First 2 Weeks of Life in the Term Infant

Value	Cord Blood	Day 1	Day 3	Day 7	Day 14
Hemoglobin (g/dL)	16.8	18.4	17.8	17.0	16.8
Hematocrit (%)	53.0	58.0	55	54.0	52.0
Red cells (mm³)	5.25	5.8	5.6	5.2	5.1
Mean corpuscular volume (fL)	107	108	99	98.0	96.0
Mean corpuscular hemoglobin (pg)	34	35	33	32.5	31.5
Mean corpuscular hemoglobin concentration (g/dL)	31.7	32.5	33	33	33
Reticulocytes	3–7	3–7	1–3	0–1	0–1
Nucleated red blood cells/mm³	500	200	0–5	0	0
Platelets (1000s/mm³)	290	192	213	248	252

NOTE: During the first 2 weeks of life, a venous hemoglobin value below 13.0 g/dL or a capillary hemoglobin value below 14.5 g/dL should be regarded as anemic.
From Oski FA, Naiman JL. *Hematologic problems in the newborn*, 2nd ed. Philadelphia: W.B. Saunders Co., 1972:13.

APPENDIX 2

Bone Marrow Cell Populations of Normal Infants

Cell Type	Month						
	0 (n = 57)	1 (n = 71)	2 (n = 48)	4 (n = 19)	6 (n = 22)	12 (n = 18)	18 (n = 19)
Small lymphocytes	14.42 ± 5.54	47.05 ± 9.24	42.68 ± 7.90	47.06 ± 8.77	47.55 ± 7.88	47.11 ± 11.32	43.55 ± 8.56
Transitional cells	1.18 ± 1.13	1.95 ± 0.94	2.38 ± 1.35	1.64 ± 1.01	2.31 ± 1.16	2.32 ± 1.90	1.99 ± 1.00
Proerythroblasts	0.02 ± 0.06	0.10 ± 0.14	0.13 ± 0.19	0.05 ± 0.10	0.09 ± 0.12	0.02 ± 0.04	0.08 ± 0.13
Basophilic erythroblasts	0.24 ± 0.25	0.34 ± 0.33	0.57 ± 0.41	0.24 ± 0.24	0.32 ± 0.24	0.30 ± 0.25	0.50 ± 0.34
Early erythroblasts	0.27 ± 0.26	0.44 ± 0.42	0.71 ± 0.51	0.28 ± 0.30	0.41 ± 0.30	0.39 ± 0.27	0.59 ± 0.34
Polychromatic erythroblasts	13.06 ± 6.78	6.90 ± 4.45	13.06 ± 3.48	6.84 ± 2.58	7.30 ± 3.60	6.83 ± 3.75	6.97 ± 3.56
Orthochromatic erythro- blasts	0.69 ± 0.73	0.54 ± 1.88	0.66 ± 0.82	0.34 ± 0.30	0.38 ± 0.56	0.37 ± 0.51	0.44 ± 0.49
Extruded nuclei	0.47 ± 0.46	0.16 ± 0.17	0.26 ± 0.22	0.16 ± 0.17	0.16 ± 0.22	0.23 ± 0.25	0.21 ± 0.19
Late erythroblasts	14.22 ± 7.14	7.60 ± 4.84	13.99 ± 3.82	7.34 ± 2.54	7.85 ± 4.11	7.42 ± 4.11	7.62 ± 1.63
Early:late erythroblasts ratio	1:50	1:15	1:18	1:23	1:17	1:17	1:10
Fetal erythroblasts	14.48 ± 7.24	8.04 ± 5.00	14.70 ± 3.86	7.62 ± 2.56	8.25 ± 4.31	7.81 ± 4.26	8.21 ± 37.1
Blood reticulocytes	4.18 ± 1.46	1.06 ± 1.13	3.39 ± 1.22	1.65 ± 0.73	1.74 ± 0.80	1.79 ± 0.79	1.84 ± 0.46
Neutrophils							
Promyelocytes	0.79 ± 0.91	0.76 ± 0.65	0.78 ± 0.68	0.59 ± 0.51	0.67 ± 0.66	0.69 ± 0.71	0.64 ± 0.59
Myelocytes	3.95 ± 2.93	2.50 ± 1.48	2.03 ± 1.14	2.32 ± 1.59	2.22 ± 1.25	2.32 ± 1.14	2.49 ± 1.39
Early neutrophils	4.74 ± 3.43	3.27 ± 1.94	2.81 ± 1.62	2.91 ± 2.01	2.89 ± 1.71	3.02 ± 1.52	3.14 ± 1.75
Metamyelocytes	19.37 ± 4.84	11.34 ± 3.59	11.27 ± 3.38	6.04 ± 3.63	11.02 ± 3.12	11.10 ± 3.82	12.42 ± 4.15
Bands	28.89 ± 7.56	14.10 ± 4.63	13.15 ± 4.71	13.93 ± 6.13	14.00 ± 4.58	14.02 ± 4.88	14.20 ± 5.23
Mature neutrophils	7.37 ± 4.64	3.64 ± 2.97	3.07 ± 2.45	4.27 ± 2.69	4.85 ± 2.69	5.65 ± 3.92	6.31 ± 3.91
Late neutrophils	55.63 ± 7.98	29.08 ± 6.79	27.50 ± 6.88	31.30 ± 7.80	29.86 ± 6.74	30.77 ± 8.69	32.93 ± 7.01
Early/late neutrophil ratio	1:12	1:9	1:9	1:11	1:10	1:10	1:10
Total neutrophils	60.37 ± 8.66	32.35 ± 7.68	30.31 ± 7.27	34.21 ± 8.61	32.75 ± 7.03	33.79 ± 8.76	36.06 ± 7.40
Total eosinophils	2.70 ± 1.27	2.61 ± 1.40	2.50 ± 1.22	2.37 ± 4.13	2.08 ± 1.16	1.92 ± 1.09	2.70 ± 2.16
Total basophils	0.12 ± 0.20	0.07 ± 0.16	0.08 ± 0.10	0.11 ± 0.14	0.10 ± 0.13	0.13 ± 0.15	0.10 ± 0.12
Total myeloid cells	63.19 ± 9.10	35.03 ± 8.09	32.90 ± 7.85	36.69 ± 8.91	34.93 ± 7.52	35.83 ± 8.84	38.86 ± 7.92
Monocytes	0.88 ± 0.85	1.01 ± 0.89	0.91 ± 0.83	0.75 ± 0.75	1.21 ± 1.01	1.46 ± 1.52	2.12 ± 1.59
Miscellaneous							
Megakaryocytes	0.06 ± 0.15	0.05 ± 0.09	0.10 ± 0.13	0.06 ± 0.06	0.04 ± 0.07	0.05 ± 0.08	0.07 ± 0.12
Plasma cells	0.00 ± 0.02	0.02 ± 0.06	0.02 ± 0.05	0.01 ± 0.03	0.03 ± 0.07	0.03 ± 0.07	0.06 ± 0.08
Unknown blasts	0.31 ± 0.31	0.62 ± 0.50	0.58 ± 0.50	0.56 ± 0.53	0.56 ± 0.48	0.37 ± 0.33	0.43 ± 0.45
Unknown cells	0.22 ± 0.34	0.21 ± 0.25	0.16 ± 0.24	0.23 ± 0.25	0.10 ± 0.15	0.11 ± 0.14	0.20 ± 0.23
Damaged cells	5.79 ± 2.78	5.50 ± 2.46	5.09 ± 1.78	4.80 ± 2.29	5.04 ± 1.08	5.34 ± 2.19	5.05 ± 2.15
Total	6.38 ± 2.84	6.39 ± 2.63	5.94 ± 1.94	5.66 ± 2.30	5.78 ± 1.16	5.90 ± 2.03	5.81 ± 2.16

NOTE: Percentages of cell types (means ± standard deviation) in tibial bone marrow of infants from birth to 18 months of age. Based on differential counts of 1000 cells classified on stained smears on each of ten serial marrow samples from normal American infants of European, African, and Asian origin, aspirated from the same population of infants. Adapted from Rosse C, Kraemer MJ, Dillon TL, et al. Bone marrow cell populations of normal infants: the predominance of lymphocytes. *J Lab Clin Med* 1977;89:1228.

APPENDIX 3

Differential Counts of Bone Marrow Aspirates from 12 Healthy Men

	Mean (%)	Observed Range (%)	95% Confidence Limits (%)
Neutrophilic series (total)	53.6	49.2–65.0	33.6–73.6
Myeloblasts	0.9	0.2–1.5	0.1–1.7
Promyelocytes	3.3	2.1–4.1	1.9–4.7
Myelocytes	12.7	8.2–15.7	8.5–16.9
Metamyelocytes	15.9	9.6–24.6	7.1–24.7
Band	12.4	9.5–15.3	9.4–15.4
Segmented	7.4	6–12	3.8–11.0
Eosinophilic series	3.1	1.2–5.3	1.1–5.2
Myelocytes	0.8	0.2–1.3	0.2–1.4
Metamyelocytes	1.2	0.4–2.2	0.2–2.2
Band	0.9	0.2–2.4	0.0–2.7
Segmented	0.5	0.0–1.3	0.0–1.1
Basophilic and mast cells	0.1	0.0–0.2	—
Erythrocytic series (total)	25.6	18.4–33.8	15.0–36.2
Pronormoblasts	0.6	0.2–1.3	0.1–1.1
Basophilic	1.4	0.5–2.4	0.4–2.4
Polychromatophilic	21.6	17.9–29.2	13.1–30.1
Orthochromatic	2.0	0.4–4.6	0.3–3.7
Lymphocytes	16.2	11.1–23.2	8.6–23.8
Plasma cells	1.3	0.4–3.9	0.0–3.5
Monocytes	0.3	0.0–0.8	0.0–0.6
Megakaryocytes	0.1	0.0–0.4	—
Reticulum cells	0.3	0.0–0.9	0.0–0.8
Myeloid/erythroid ratio	2.3	1.5–3.3	1.1–3.5

Adapted from Wintrobe MM, Lee GR, Boggs DR, et al., eds. *Clinical hematology*, 7th ed. Philadelphia: Lea & Febiger,1974:1796.

APPENDIX 4

Normal Leukocyte Counts

Age	Total Leukocytes		Neutrophils			Lymphocytes			Monocytes		Eosinophils	
	Mean	Range	Mean	Range	%	Mean	Range	%	Mean	%	Mean	%
Birth	18.1	9–30	11.0	6–26	61	5.5	2–11	31	1.1	6	0.4	2
12 h	22.8	13–38	15.5	6–28	68	5.5	2–11	24	1.2	5	0.5	2
24 h	18.9	9.4–34.0	11.5	5–21	61	5.8	2.0–11.5	31	1.1	6	0.5	2
1 wk	12.2	5–21	5.5	1.5–10.0	45	5.0	2–17	41	1.1	9	0.5	4
2 wk	11.4	5–20	4.5	1.0–9.5	40	5.5	2–17	48	1.0	9	0.4	3
1 mo	10.8	5.0–19.5	3.8	1–9	35	6.0	2.5–16.5	56	0.7	7	0.3	3
6 mo	11.9	6.0–17.5	3.8	1.0–8.5	32	7.3	4.0–13.5	61	0.6	5	0.3	3
1 yr	11.4	6.0–17.5	3.5	1.5–8.5	31	7.0	4.0–10.5	61	0.6	5	0.3	3
2 yr	10.6	6–17	3.5	1.5–8.5	33	6.3	3.0–9.5	59	0.5	5	0.3	3
4 yr	9.1	5.5–15.5	3.8	1.5–8.5	42	4.5	2–8	50	0.5	5	0.3	3
6 yr	8.5	5.0–14.5	4.3	1.5–8.0	51	3.5	1.5–7.0	42	0.4	5	0.2	3
8 yr	8.3	4.5–13.5	4.4	1.5–8.0	53	3.3	1.5–6.8	39	0.4	4	0.2	2
10 yr	8.1	4.5–13.5	4.4	1.8–8.0	54	3.1	1.5–6.5	38	0.4	4	0.2	2
16 yr	7.8	4.5–13.0	4.4	1.8–8.0	57	2.8	1.2–5.2	35	0.4	5	0.2	3
21 yr	7.4	4.5–11.0	4.4	1.8–7.7	59	2.5	1.0–4.8	34	0.3	4	0.2	3

NOTE: Numbers of leukocytes are in 1000s/µL; ranges are estimates of 95% confidence limits; percentages refer to differential counts. Neutrophils include band cells at all ages and a small number of metamyelocytes and myelocytes in the first few days of life.
From Dallman PR. In: Rudolph AM, ed. *Pediatrics*, 16th ed. New York: Appleton-Century-Crofts, 1977:1178.

APPENDIX 5

Absolute Blood Phagocyte Concentrations

Population	Concentration (cells/μL, 95% range [mean])			
	Band Forms	Segmented Forms	Band and Segmented Forms	Monocytes
American adults[a]				
White subjects	200–2150 (600)	1500–6050 (3000)	—	220–950 (460)
Black subjects	60–1650 (300)	1100–6700 (2700)	—	210–1050 (470)
European adults[b]				
White subjects	—	—	3487–9206	221–843
American infants and children[c]				
Birth	—	—	6000–26,000 (11,000)	400–3100 (1050)
7 d	—	—	1500–10,000 (5500)	300–2700 (1100)
4 yr	—	—	1500–8500 (3800)	0–800 (450)
10 yr	—	—	1800–8000 (4400)	0–800 (350)

[a]Adapted from Orfanakis NG, Ostlund RE, Bishop CR, Athens JW. Normal blood leukocyte concentration values. *Am J Clin Pathol* 1970;53:647.
[b]Adapted from England JM, Bain BJ. Total and differential leukocyte count. *Br J Haematol* 1976;33:1.
[c]Adapted from Altman PL, Katz DD. Human health and disease. In: *FASEB biology handbooks II.* Washington, DC: FASEB, 1977:161.

APPENDIX 6

Leukocytes: Absolute and Relative Values for a Normal Population

	Absolute Number (Cells × 10⁹/L from Long Plots)		Relative Number (%)	
	Median	95% Range	Mean	95% Range
Total Leukocytes	7.0	4.3–10.0	—	—
Neutrophils Bands	0.52	0.1–2.1	9.5	0.0–21.5
Neutrophils Segmented	3.0	1.10–6.05	43.5	24.8–62.3
Neutrophils Total	3.65	1.83–7.25	53.0	34.6–71.4
Eosinophils	0.15	0.0–0.7	3.2	0.0–7.8
Basophils	0.03	0.00–0.15	0.6	0.0–1.8
Lymphocytes	2.5	1.5–4.0	36.1	19.6–52.7
Monocytes	0.43	0.20–0.95	7.1	2.4–11.8

NOTE: 291 adults in Salt Lake City.
Adapted from Orfanakis NG, Ostlund RE, Bishop CR, Athens JW. Normal blood leukocyte concentration. *Am J Clin Pathol* 1970;53:647.

APPENDIX 7

Leukocyte Alkaline Phosphatase Scores in Normal Subjects

Group	Number	Mean	95% Limits
Male	51	73	22–124
Female	50	92	33–149
Total	101	82	25–139

Adapted from Cartwright GE. *Diagnostic laboratory hematology,* 4th ed. New York: Grune & Stratton, 1968.

APPENDIX 8

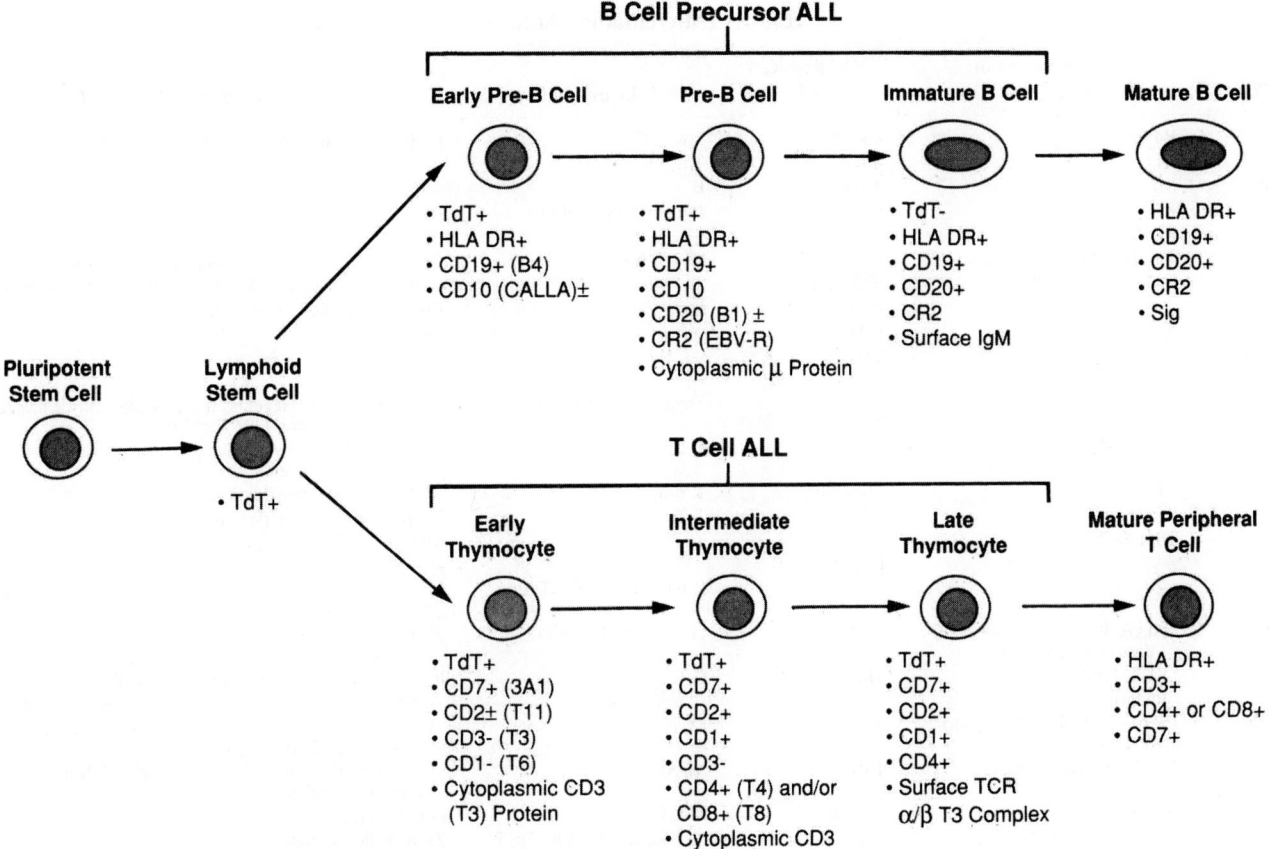

Lymphoid Cell Differentiation. Model showing stages of cellular development based on terminal deoxy-nucleotide transferase (TdT) activity, binding to commonly used monoclonal antibodies, T-cell receptor (TCR) gene rearrangement, and the presence of immunoglobulin (Ig) molecules.

APPENDIX 9

Cluster Differentiation Antigens

CD	Other Names or Defining Antibodies	MW Reduced (kd)	Expression	Comments
CD1a	R4; HTA-1	43–49	Thy, DC	MHC class I–like structure; antigen presentation function
CD1b	R1	43–49	Thy, DC	—
CD1c	M241; R7	43–49	B	—
CD1d	R3	43–49	Intestinal epithelium	—
CD1e	R2	43–49	—	—
CD2	T11,Leu-2,LFA-2	45–58	Thy, T, NK	CD58 (LFA-3) receptor, sheep RBC receptor
CD3	T3,Leu-4	$\gamma25$–$\gamma28$	T	Complex of five peptides; associates with T-cell receptor
		$\delta20$	—	Involved in T-cell activation
		$\varepsilon20$	—	—
		$\zeta16$	—	—
		$\eta22$	—	—
CD4	T4, Leu-3	55	Thy(s), T(s), Mo, Mac	Coreceptor for MHC class II molecules; binds lck; receptor for HIV-1 and HIV-2 gp120
CD5	T1, Leu-1, Ly-1, Tp67	67	T, B(s)	CD72 receptor, T-cell activation; marker of IL10-producing autoimmune B cells
CD6	T12	100–130	T, brain	?Role in signal transduction
CD7	Leu-9, gp40	40	T, Thy	Earliest T lineage marker; prothymocyte
CD8	T8, Leu-2	$\alpha32$–$\alpha34$	T(s)	MHC class I receptor
		$\beta32$–$\beta34$	—	
CD9	—	22–27	P, early B, Eo, Bo, T(act)	Platelet activation and aggregation; binds to gpIIb/IIIa (CD41/CD61)
CD10	CALLA, JS, neutral endopeptidase, enkephalinase	100	LP, G(s), BM stroma	Zn metalloprotease
CD11a	LFA-1, LeuCAMa, α_L Integrin	180	L, G, Mo, Mac, T (memory)	Integrin α chains; associate with CD18. CD11a/CD18 is ICAM-1/ICAM-2/ICAM-3 receptor
CD11b	CR3,LeuCAMb, MAC-1, Mo-1, α_M integrin	170	M, NK	CD11b/CD18 is iC3b receptor; it also binds factor X, ICAM-1, and fibrinogen
CD11c	LeuCAMc, α_X integrin	150	M, Mac	CD11c/CD18 binds fibrinogen and ?iC3b; marker for hairy cell leukemia
CDw12	p90–p120	90–120	Mo, G, P	Function unknown
CD13	Aminopeptidase N	150–170	G, Mo, Bo, Eo, Oc, Ep, F, brain	Zn metalloprotease
CD14	LPS-R	53–55 (Mo)	Mo, Mac, G(s), B	Receptor for complex of LPS and LPS-binding protein; induces TNFα synthesis
		64 (B)		
CD15	Lewis x (Le^x) 3-fucosyl-N-acetyl-lactosamine	<1	G, Eo, Mo	Pentasaccharide; sialylated derivative (CD15s, sLe^x) is ligand for CD62 and ELAM-1
CD16	FcγRIII	50–80	G, NK, Mac	Low-affinity receptor for aggregated IgG; mediates phagocytosis and ADCC
CDw17	Lactosylceramide	—	G, Mo, P	Cell-surface glycosphingolipid
CD18	Integrin β_2	95	Leukocytes	Adhesion molecule that associates with CD11a, b, and c
CD19	B4, Leu-12	95	B, DC	Regulates B-cell proliferation; forms complex with CD21 and CD81 to form coreceptor for B cells
CD20	B1, Leu-16, Bp35	33–37	B	?Calcium channel; ?role in regulating B-cell activation
CD21	C3d receptor, CR2	145	B, DC, Ep, Thy(s)	C3d (CR2) receptor; EBV receptor; ?interferon-α receptor; forms complex with CD19 and CD81 to form coreceptor for B cells
CD22	BL-CAM	130/140 (heterodimer)	B(s)	Adhesion protein, CD22 binds to Mo and RBC; CD22β binds B and T cells
CD23	FcεRII, Blast-2	45	Mo, Mac, Eo, P, DC, B(s)	Low-affinity IgE receptor; ligand for CD19:CD21:CD81 coreceptor
CD24	BA-1, HSA	35–45	B, G	GPI-anchored; function unknown
CD25	Tac, IL-2Rα	$\alpha55$, $\beta75$	T(act), B(act), Mo(act), BMP, Thy(s), glia	IL2 receptor α chain (β chain is CD122); activation/proliferation of T, Thy, NK, B, Mac
CD26	ADA-binding protein	110	EC, Ep	Dipeptidyl peptidase IV; cell-surface protease; implicated in HIV entry to cells
CD27	S152;T14	50–55	Thy(s), T	NGF receptor superfamily; function unknown
CD28	Tp44	44	T, PC	Binds B7-1 (CD80) and B7-2 B-cell ligand; activation of naïve T cells
CD29	Integrin β_1	130	Leukocytes	Forms integrin with CD49a (VLA-1)
CD30	Ki-1, Ber-H2 antigen	105–120	B(act), T(act)	NGF receptor superfamily; function unknown
CD31	PECAM-1	130–140	P, EC, Mo, G, L(s)	?Adhesion molecule
CD32	FcγRII	40	Mo, B, G, P, EC, placenta	Low-affinity receptor for aggregated IgG; activates G, Mo; inhibits B cells; ? role in placental IgG transport
CD33	gp67; p67	67	G/Mac precursors	Ig superfamily; function unknown
CD34	gp105–gp120	105–120	BMP, EC	Earliest marker for BM progenitors; ligand for CD62
CD35	Complement receptor 1 (CR1)	250	E, B, T(s), G, Mo, DC, Mac	C3b/C4b receptor, mediates phagocytosis
CD36	OKM5, gpIV	88	P, EC, Mo	Platelet gpIV; *Plasmodium falciparum* receptor, may bind collagen, thrombospondin
CD37	gp52–gp40	40–52	B	Function unknown
CD38	T10	45	Early/activated B and T, P	Cyclic ADP-ribose hydrolase

Cluster Differentiation Antigens (*continued*)

CD	Other Names or Defining Antibodies	MW Reduced (kd)	Expression	Comments
CD39	—	78	NK(act), T(s), Mac, DC, LC	Function unknown
CD40	Bp50	50	B	Receptor for costimulatory signal for B cells; binds CD40 ligand
CD41	gpIIb, α_{IIb} integrin	125, 22	P, Meg	Associates with gpIIIa (CD61), forms receptor for fibrinogen, vWF, fibronectin, thrombospondin; defective in thrombasthenia
CD42a	gpIX	23	P	vWF receptor; defective in Bernard-Soulier syndrome
CD42b	gpIBα	135, 23	P, Meg	Glycocalicin
CD42c	gpIBβ	22		
CD42d	GpV	85		Thrombin receptor
CD43	Sialophorin, leukosialin	115–135 (G, P), 95–115 (T)	Leukocytes, P, Thy, BMP	Mucin-like protein; major sialoglycoprotein of T cells; binds ICAM-1 (CD54); enhances T-cell activation; decreased in Wiskott-Aldrich syndrome
CD44	Phagocytic glycoprotein 1 (Pgp-1), Hermes antigen In(Lu)-related	80–95, 130	Leukocytes, Thy, E, Ep, F, Msk, brain	Adhesion protein; hyaluronic acid receptor; binds leukocytes to high venular endothelium; binds ankyrin; part of RBC Lutheran antigen
CD45	Leukocyte common antigen, B220, T200, Ly5	180–240	Leukocytes, P	T-cell receptor signaling; binds CD22 in B cells; CD45RO isoform lacks exons A, B, C; CD45RA isoform contains exon A; CD45RB contains exon B
CD46	Membrane cofactor protein	51–58, 59–68	Leukocytes, P, EC, Ep, F, placenta	Involved in degradation of C3b/C4b by factor I
CD47R	Rh-associated protein; gp42, neurophilin	47–52	Leukocytes, P, E, Ec, Ep, F	Function unknown; not expressed in Rh_{null} RBC
CD48	Blast-1, HuLy-m3, BCM1 antigen	40–57	B, T, Thy, Eo, Ep	GPI-anchored; function unknown
CD49a	Integrins α_{1-6}, VLA, α chains 1–6. CD49a-CD49f area chains of VLA1-VLA6	a, 210	Leukocytes, P, Ep	Complex family of adhesion proteins; various CD49/CD29 complexes bind collagen, laminin, fibronectin, VCAM-1, and high endothelial cells in venules
CD49b		b, 160		
CD49c		c, 125		
CD49d		d, 150, 80, 70		
CD49e		e, 135, 25		
CD49f		f, 120, 25		
CD50	ICAM-3	124	Leukocytes	Adhesion protein
CD51	α_V integrin	125, 24	P(weak)	Associates with CD61 to bind vitronectin, fibrinogen, thrombospondin, and vWF
CD52	Campath-1	21–28	B, T, G(s)	Function unknown
CD53	MRC OX44	35–42	Leukocytes, P, Ob, Oc	Tetraspanning membrane protein; function unknown
CD54	ICAM-1	85–110	Wide distribution	Adhesion protein; binds CD11a/CD18 and CD11b/CD18 integrins; also binds CD43 and *Plasmodium falciparum*-infected RBC; rhinovirus receptor
CD55	Decay accelerating factor	64–73	Wide distribution	GPI-anchored; prevents assembly of C3 convertase; absence contributes to pathophysiology of PNH
CD56	N-CAM isoform, Leu-19, NKH-1	175–185	NK, non–MHC-restricted L	Cell adhesion, including NK-target cell adhesion
CD57	Leu-7, HNK-1	—	NK, B, T(s), Mo(s)	Function unknown
CD58	LFA-3	55–70	Wide distribution, including L, EC, Mac	Adhesion protein; binds CD2; role in T-cell activation and monocyte IL-1 release
CD59	MIRL, Protectin, HRF20, MACIF, P-18, H19	19	Leukocytes, EC, Ep, placenta	GPI-anchored; blocks complement C8/C9 membrane attack complex; absence contributes to pathophysiology of PNH
CD60a	GD3	—	T(s), Mo, P	T-cell stimulation; augments CD3 signaling
CD60b	9-O-acetyl-GD3	—	—	—
CD60c	7-O-acetyl-GD3	—		
CD61	gpIIIa, integrin β_2, vitronectin receptor	105	P, Meg, Mac	CD41/CD61 is gpIIb/gpIIIa complex involved in platelet adhesion/aggregation; CD51/CD61 is vitronectin receptor ($\alpha_V\beta_3$ integrin)
CD62E	E-selectin, ELAM-1	115	EC	Adhesion of phagocytes to endothelial cells; binds sLe^x activated by LPS, IL-1, TNF; involved in angiogenesis
CD62L	L-selectin, LAM-1, LECAM-1; Leu-8	75–80	Leukocytes	Adhesion of lymphocytes to high endothelial venules and neutrophils to endothelium; binds CD34 and sLe^x
CD62P	P-selectin, PADGEM, GMP-140	150	P, EC	Adhesion protein; located in secretory granules moves to membrane on activation; mediates platelet-neutrophil interactions; binds sLe^x (sCD15) and sulfated galactosylceramides
CD63	LIMP, ME491, MLA1, PTLGP40, LAMP-3, granulophysin	53	P, Mo, Mac	Lysosomal membrane protein translocated to plasma membrane on activation; involved in neutrophil-endothelial and other cellular interactions
CD64	FcγRI	72	Mac, Mo, N (γ-IFN–induced)	γ-IFN–induced, high-affinity IgG receptor; binds monomeric IgG; role in ADCC and clearance of immune complexes

(*continued*)

Cluster Differentiation Antigens (continued)

CD	Other Names or Defining Antibodies	MW Reduced (kd)	Expression	Comments
CD65	Ceramide dodecasaccharide 4c	—	G, Mo(s)	Marker of myeloid lineage; function unknown
CD66a	BGP-1	180–200	N, BMP, Ep(s)	Member of CEA family; function unknown
CD66b	CD67, p100, CGM6	95–100	G	Member of CEA family; function unknown; previously CD67
CD66c	NCA; NCA-50/90	90–95	N, colon carcinoma	Member of CEA family; function unknown
CD66d	CGM1	30	N	Member of CEA family; function unknown
CD66e	CEA	180–200	Adult colon Ep, colon carcinoma	CEA
CD66f	Pregnancy specific glycoprotein; SP-1	—	—	—
CD67	Now called CD66b	—	—	—
CD68	gp110; macrosialin	110	Mac, Mo, N, Bo, L(s), Liver, Ep(s)	Present in lysosomes as well as membrane; function unknown
CD69	AIM, EA 1, MLR-3; Leu-23, VEA	28, 32	L(act), P, Thy	AIM; function uncertain
CD70	CD27-ligand, Ki-24 antigen	55, 75, 95, 110, 170	B(act), T(act), Mac	CD27 ligand; function unknown
CD71	T9	90–95 (homodimer)	Proliferating cells	Transferrin receptor; iron transport
CD72	Ly-19.2; Ly-32.2, Lyb-2	42(homodimer)	B	CD5 ligand; role in B-cell proliferation
CD73	Ecto-5'-nucleotidase	69	L(s), EC(s), Ep(s)	GPI-anchored ecto-5'-nucleotidase; dephosphorylates nucleoside monophosphates to allow uptake
CD74	MHC class II; associated invariant chain (Ii or Iγ)	43, 41, 35, 33	MHC II-positive cells; B, Mo, T(s), Ep(s)	Mostly intracellular; associates with α and β chains of MHC class II molecule. Prevents binding of endogenous peptides to class II
CD75s	Alpha-2,6-sialyated lactosamines	53, 87	B B (s), T(s)	Formerly CDw75 and CDw76; function unknown
CD77	Globotriaosylceramide, Pᵏ blood group antigen	—	B(s), DC, EC, Ep(s)	Marker for Burkitt lymphoma; function unknown
CD79a	mb-1, Igα	32–33	B	Component of B cell antigen receptor analogous to CD3
CD79b	B29, Igβ	37–39	B	Component of B cell antigen receptor analogous to CD3
CD80	B7-1, BB1	60	B(s)	Ligand for CD28 and CTLA-4; co-stimulatory function
CD81	TAPA-1	26	L	TAPA-1; associates with CD19, CD21 to form B cell co-receptor
CD82	R2, IA4, 4F9	50–53	Leukocytes	Tetraspanning membrane protein; function uncertain
CD83	HB15	43	B(s), T(s), DC(s)	Function unknown
CD84	GR6	73	Mo, P, B(s)	Function unknown
CD85	VMP-55, GH1/75	120, 83	—	ILT/LIR family
CD86	FUN-1, BU63	80	Mo, B(s)	Function unknown
CD87	uPAR	50–65	G, Mo, Mac, T(s)	Urokinase plasminogen activator receptor
CD88	C5aR	42	N, Mac, Mast, Msm	C5a receptor; role in chemotaxis; stimulates respiratory burst and degranulation of N, mast
CD89	FcαR	55–75	Mo, G, Mac, T(s), B(s)	IgA receptor
CD90	Thy-1	25–35	Early Thy	Prothymocytes, GPI-anchored; function unknown
CD91	α₂M-R	600	Mo	Alpha-2-macroglobulin receptor
CD92	CTL1	70	N, Mo, P, EC	Function unknown
CD93	GR11	120	N, Mo, EC	Function unknown
CD94	KP43	43	T(s), NK	Function unknown
CD95	Apo-1, Fas	42	Many cell lines	Binds TNF-like ligand, induces apoptosis
CD96	TACTILE	160	T(act)	TACTILE
CD97	GR1	74, 80, 89	Activated cells	Function unknown
CD98	4F2, 2F3	80, 40	Mo, L(act), NK(act), Mc, K	Function unknown
CD99	E2, MIC2	32	L(s), Thy	Function unknown
CD100	SEMA4D, GR3	150	Hematopoietic cells	Function unknown
CD101	BB27, BA27, IGSF2, V7	140	G, Mac	Function unknown
CD102	ICAM-2	60	EC, L, Mo, liver, kidney	Adhesion protein; ligand for LFA-1 integrin (CS11a/CD18); ?facilitates recirculation of memory T cells
CD103	HML-1, αₑ integrin chain	150, 25	L(s)	αₑ integrin chain
CD104	β₄ integrin chain	220	Ep, Schwann cells	β₄ integrin chain
CD105	Endoglin	95	EC, BM(s), Mac(act)	Function unknown
CD106	VCAM-1, INCAM-110	100, 110	EC, Mac, DC, kidney, F, myoblasts	Receptor for VLA-4 (CD49d/CD29)
CD107a	LAMP-1	110	P(act)	Lysosomal membrane glycoprotein
CD107b	LAMP-2	120	P(act)	Lysosomal membrane glycoprotein
CD108	SEMA7A	80	T(act)(s)	JMH human blood group antigen
CD109	8A3, 7D1, E123	170/150	T(act), P, EC	Platelet activation factor
CD110	MPL; TPO-R, c-MPL		P	Thrombopoietin receptor
CD111	PVRL1, PRR1, nectin-1		Myeloid cells	Function unknown
CD112	PVRL2, PRR2, nectin-2		Myeloid cells	Function unknown
CD114	G-CSF receptor		Myeloid cells	G-CSF receptor
CD115	CSF-1R, M-CSFR c-fms protooncogene	150	Mc, Mac, BM P, placenta	Stimulates proliferation and differentiation of Mo/Mac and their progenitors
CD116	HGM-CSFR, GM-CSFR	75–85	Mo, N, Eo, F, EC, BMP, Ob	Stimulates proliferation and differentiation of N, Eo, Mo, and their progenitors, and RBC progenitors

Cluster Differentiation Antigens (*continued*)

CD	Other Names or Defining Antibodies	MW Reduced (kd)	Expression	Comments
CD117	SCFR, cKIT	145	Hematopoietic progenitors	Stem cell factor receptor; c-*kit* receptor
CD119	IFNγR	90	Mac, Mo, B, EC	Gamma-interferon receptor
CD120a	TNFR, 55 kd	55	Ep, wide distribution	Receptor for TNFα and TNFβ
CD120b	TNFR, 75 kd	75	M, wide distribution	Receptor for TNFα and TNFβ
CD121a	IL-1R; type 1	80	T, Thy, F, C, EC, K, synovial cells, liver	Type I IL-1 receptor; T/Thy activation, fibroblast proliferation, acute phase reaction
CDw121b	IL-1R; type 2	68	B, Mo, Mac	Type II IL-1 receptor
CD122	IL-2R	75	B(act), Mo(act), NK, T(act)	IL-2 receptor beta chain, activation/proliferation of T, Thy, NK, B, Mac
CD123	IL-3R alpha	70	BMP, G, Mo, Meg	IL-3 receptor alpha chain; stimulates proliferation
CD124	IL-4R	130–150	B, T, BMP, F, Ep, Ec	IL-4 receptor; stimulates B/T-cell growth IgG,/IgE production, MHC class II expression, and Mac activation
CD125	IL-5R	55–60	Eo, Ba	IL-5 receptor
CD126	IL-6R	80	B(act), PC	IL-6 receptor; stimulates B/T/PC growth, proliferation/differentiation of BM progenitors, and hepatic acute phase response
CD127	IL-7R	68–79	LP, proB, T, Thy, Mo	IL-7 receptor; stimulates growth of proB/ preB/Thy/T cells and activation of Mo
CDw128a	IL-8RA; CXCR1	58–67	N, Bo, T(s), Mo, K	IL-8 receptor, chemotaxis of N/Bo/T; activates N/Bo
CDw128b	IL-8RB; CXCR2	58–67	—	IL-8 receptor
CD130	IL-6R beta subunit; gp130	130	B(act), P, EC	IL-6 receptor beta subunit
CDw131	IL-3R common β chain	95–120	Mo, G, Eo, B	IL-3 receptor beta chain; function in B and T cell growth
CD132	IL-2R gamma chain	64	T, B, F, BMP	IL-2 receptor gamma chain; common cytokine gamma chain
CD133	PROML1; AC133	—	BMP	Hematopoietic stem cell antigen
CD134	OX40	48–50	T(s)	Tax-transcriptionally activated glycoprotein 1 receptor
CD135	flt3, Flk-2, STK-1	130–150	BMP, carcinoma cells	Receptor tyrosine kinase
CDw136	MSP receptor, ron	180	—	Receptor tyrosine kinase
CD138	Syndecan-1	—	P	Heparan sulfate proteoglycan, ligand for collagen type I
CD139	—	—	—	
CD140a	PDGF-R, PDGFRa	180		Platelet derived growth factor receptor a
CD140b	PDGFRb	180		Platelet derived growth factor receptor b
CD141	Thrombomodulin	100	M, En, Msm	Myeloid thrombin receptor; involved in regulation of coagulation
CD142	Tissue factor, factor III, thromboplastin	45	Mo, En	Tissue factor; involved in activation of coagulation
CD143	ACE, peptidyl dipeptidase A	170	En, Ep	Angiotensin converting enzyme; involved in generation of kinins, blood pressure regulation
CDw145	—	—	—	—
CD146	MCAM, MUC18, S-endo	113–118	En, DC(s), melanoma	Involved in homing of activated T cells
CD147	Neurothelin, basigin, OX-47, EMMPRIN	42	En, M, L	Neurothelin
CD148	HPTP-eta, DEP-1, p260	260	—	—
CD150	SLAM; IPO-3	75–95	T, B	Surface lymphocyte activation marker; signaling molecule
CD151	PETA-3; SFA-1	—	—	—
CD152	CTLA-4	44	T	Negative regulator for T cells
CD153	CD30L	40	T	Ligand for CD30; costimulatory molecule
CD154	CD40L, T-BAM; TRAP	32–39	T	Ligand for CD40; costimulatory molecule
CD155	PVR	—	—	PVR
CD156a	ADAM8, MS2 human	—	—	—
CD156b	ADAM17, TACE, cSVP	—	—	—
CD157	BP-3/IF-7, BST-1, Mo-5	—	—	—
CD158a	p58.1	58/50	T	KIR family; class I–specific NK-receptor; involved in inhibition of cytotoxic activity
CD158b	p58.2	58/50	T	KIR family; class I–specific NK-receptor; involved in inhibition of cytotoxic activity
CD158c	p58.3	58/50	T	KIR family; activating molecule
CD159a	NKG2A	—	NK	—
CD160	BY55 antigen, NK1	—	T	—
CD161	KLRB1, NKRP-1A	60	NK	Killer cell lectinlike receptor B; involved in regulation of NK cell–mediated cytotoxicity
CD162	PSGL-1, PSGL	240	M, G, T, B(s)	P-selectin glycoprotein ligand-1; adhesion molecule in leukocyte rolling
CD162R	PEN5	—	NK	Posttranslational modification of CD162
CD163	GHI/61, M130, RM3/1	—	—	—
CD164	MUC-24, MGC-24v	80	M, T, Ep, BMS	Adhesion molecule for hematopoietic progenitor cells
CD165	AD2; gp37, A108	37	T, NK, P, Thy, Thy Ep	Adhesion molecule for thymocytes/thymic epithelium
CD166	BEN, DM-GRASP, KG-CAM, neurolin, SC-1, ALCAM	100	T, NK, P, Thy, B(s), T(s), Eo, F, En, K	Adhesion molecule; ligand for CD6
CD167a	trkE, trk6, cak, eddr1, DDR1, MCK10; RTK6	—	—	Discoidin domain R
CD168	HMMR, IHABP, RHAMM	—	—	—
CD169	Sialoadhesin, siglec-1	—	—	—

(*continued*)

Cluster Differentiation Antigens (*continued*)

CD	Other Names or Defining Antibodies	MW Reduced (kd)	Expression	Comments
CD170	Siglec-5	—	—	—
CD171	L1, L1CAM, N-CAM L1	—	—	—
CD172a	SIRP alpha	—	—	—
CD173	Blood group H type 2	—	—	—
CD174	Lewis y	—	—	—
CD175	Tn	—	—	—
CD175s	Sialyl-Tn	—	—	—
CD176	TF	—	—	—
CD177	NB1	—	—	—
CD178	fas-L, TNFSF6, CD95-L	—	—	Fas ligand; ligand for CD95
CD179a	VpreB; VPREB1, IGVPB	—	—	—
CD179b	IGLL1, lambda5, IGVPB	—	—	Immunoglobulin omega polypeptide
CD180	LY64; RP105	—	—	—
CD183	CXCR3, GPR9, CKR-L2, IP10-R, Mig-R	—	—	Chemokine receptor
CD184	CXCR4, fusin, LESTR, NPY3R, HM89, FB22	—	—	Chemokine receptor
CD195	CCR5	—	—	Chemokine receptor
CDw197	CCR7	—	—	Chemokine receptor
CD200	OX2	—	—	—
CD201	EPC R	—	—	—
CD202b	tie2, tek	—	—	—
CD203c	NPP3, PDNP3, PD-Ibeta, Gp130RB13-6, ENPP3	—	—	Homolog of bovine intestinal phosphodiesterase
CD204	—	—	—	Macrophage scavenger receptor
CD205	DEC205	—	—	—
CD206	MRC1, MMR	—	—	Macrophage mannose receptor
CD207	Langerin	—	—	—
CD208	DC-LAMP	—	—	—
CD209	DC-SIGN	—	—	—
CDw210	IL-10 R	—	—	IL-10 receptor
CD212	IL-12 R	—	—	IL-12 receptor
CD213a1	IL-13 R α 1	—	—	IL-13 receptor
CD213a2	IL-13 R α 2	—	—	IL-13 receptor
CDw217	IL-17 receptor	—	—	IL-17 receptor
CD220	Insulin receptor	—	—	Insulin receptor
CD221	IGF1 receptor	—	—	IGF1 receptor
CD222	IGF2 receptor	—	—	Mannose-6-phosphate receptor; IGF2 R
CD223	LAG-3	—	—	—
CD224	GGT	—	—	Gamma-glutamyl transferase
CD225	Leu13	—	—	—
CD226	DNAM-1, PTA1, TLiSA1	—	—	—
CD227	MUC1, episialin, PUM, PEM, EMA, DF3	—	—	—
CD228	Melanotransferrin	—	—	—
CD229	Ly9	—	—	—
CD230	Prion Protein	—	—	—
CD231	TMS4SF2, A15, MXS1, TALLA, TALLA-1	—	—	—
CD232	VESP R	—	—	—
CD233	Band 3, AE1, SLC4A1	—	E	Red blood cell anion transporter; Diego blood group
CD234	DARC, Fy-glycoprotein	—	E	Duffy blood group antigen
CD235a	Glycophorin A	—	E	RBC surface antigen
CD235b	Glycophorin B	—	E	RBC surface antigen
CD235ab	Glycophorin A/B	—	E	Glycophorin A/B crossreactive monoclonal antibody
CD236	Glycophorin C/D	—	E	Glycophorin C/D crossreactive monoclonal antibody
CD236R	Glycophorin C	—	E	RBC surface antigens
CD238	Kell	—	E	Kell blood group antigen
CD239	B-CAM	—	—	—
CD240CE	Rh30CE	—	—	—
CD240D	Rh30D	—	—	—
CD240DCE	Rh30D/CE	—	—	Rh30D/CE crossreactive monoclonal antibody
CD241	RhAg	—	—	—
CD242	ICAM-4	—	—	—
CD243	MDR-1	—	—	—
CD244	2B4, NAIL, p38	—	—	—
CD245	P220/240	—	—	—
CD246	Anaplastic lymphoma kinase	—	—	—
CD247	Zeta chain	—	—	—

(act), activated cells of the type indicated; B, B lymphocytes; Bo, basophils; BM, bone marrow; DC, dendritic cells; E, erythrocytes; EC, endothelial cells; Eo, eosinophils; Ep, epithelial cells; F, fibroblasts; G, granulocytes; K, keratinocytes; L, lymphocytes; LC, Langerhans' cells; LP, lymphoid progenitors; M, myeloid cells; Mac, macrophages; Mast, mast cells; Mc, cardiac muscle; Mo, monocytes; Msk, skeletal muscle; Msm, smooth muscle; N, neutrophils; NK, natural killer cells; Ob, osteoblasts; Oc, osteoclasts; P, platelets; PC, plasma cells; (s), protein expressed on a subset of indicated cells; T, T lymphocytes; Thy, thymocytes.

Compiled from Barclay AN, Birkeland ML, Brown MH, et al. (eds). *The leucocyte antigen facts book.* London: Academic Press, 1993; Knapp W. Rieber P, Dörken B, et al. Toward a better definition of human leukocyte surface molecules. *Immunol Today* 1989;10:254; Schlossman SF, Boumsell L, Gilks W, et al. CD antigens 1993. *Blood* 1994;83:879; and for an up-to-date reference, see Shaw S, Turni LA, Katz KS (eds). *Protein reviews on the web* (http://www.ncbi.nlm.nih.gov/prow/, 2002).

APPENDIX 10

Glycosyl Phosphatidyl Inositol (GPI)–Linked Molecules on Human Hematopoietic Cells

	RBC	PMN	Mon	Plt	B	T	NK	HSC
Complement regulators								
CD55 (DAF, Cromer antigen)	+	+	+	+	+	+	+	
CD59 (MIRL)	+	+	+	+	+	+	+	+
Adhesion molecules								
CD48		+	+		+	+	+	
CD58 (LFA-3)	+	a	a	a	a	a	a	
CD66b		+						
CD66c		+						
CD67		+						
GPI-80		+	+					
Enzymes								
Acetylcholinesterase (Yt antigen)	+							
Leukocyte alkaline phosphatase		+						
Mono ADP-ribosyl transferase		+				+		
DO (Dombroch/HG antigens)	+							
CD73					*	*		
CD157		+	+					
Receptors								
CD14			1					
CD16 (FcγRIII) (NA antigen)		+	b*		+	b*	b*	
CD87 (u-PAR)		+	+			+		
Others								
CD24		+			+			
CD52			+		+	+	+	
CD90						*		+
CDw108 (JMH antigen)	+				*	+		+
CD109 (Gov antigen)		+	+	*		*		+
NB1		+						
Prion protein	+	+	+	+	+	+	+	
GP500					+			

+, cell type indicated is present; *, expression only on activation or only in a cell subset; a, presence in both GPI-linked and transmembrane form; ADP, adenosine diphosphate; b, presence only in transmembrane form; B, B lymphocytes; DAF, decay-activating factor; GP, glycoprotein; HSC, hematopoietic stem cells; JMH, John Milton Hagan; LFA, lymphocyte function–associated antigen; MIRL, membrane inhibitor of reactive lysis; Mon, monocytes; NK, natural killer; PAR, plasminogen activator receptor; Plt, platelets; PMN, granulocytes; RBC, red blood cells; T, T lymphocytes.

Adapted from Rosti V. The molecular basis of paroxysmal nocturnal hemoglobinuria. *Haematologica* 2000;85:82–87; and Bessler M, Schaefer A, Keller P. Paroxysmal nocturnal hemoglobinuria: insights from recent advances in molecular biology. *Transfus Med Rev* 2001;15:255–267.

APPENDIX 11

Relation of Serum Protein Levels to Age

	Total Proteins (g/dL)		Albumin (g/dL)		Alpha-1	
	Mean	Range	Mean	Range	Mean	Range
Cord blood	6.22 ± 1.21	4.78–8.04	3.23 ± 0.82	2.17–4.04	0.41 ± 0.10	0.25–0.66
1–3 mo	5.64 ± 1.04	3.64–7.38	3.41 ± 0.72	2.05–4.46	0.24 ± 0.09	0.08–0.43
4–6 mo	5.43 ± 0.84	4.29–6.10	3.46 ± 0.36	3.17–3.88	0.17 ± 0.04	0.12–0.25
7–12 mo	6.54 ± 0.76	5.10–7.31	3.62 ± 0.60	3.22–4.31	0.35 ± 0.15	0.15–0.55
13–24 mo	6.66 ± 0.93	3.69–7.50	3.63 ± 0.80	1.89–5.03	0.31 ± 0.15	0.09–0.58
25–36 mo	6.98 ± 0.66	6.38–8.06	4.11 ± 0.78	3.57–5.50	0.23 ± 0.09	0.19–0.26
3–5 yr	6.65 ± 0.85	4.88–8.06	3.95 ± 0.57	2.93–5.21	0.21 ± 0.08	0.08–0.40
6–8 yr	6.95 ± 0.55	5.97–7.94	4.03 ± 0.45	3.26–4.95	0.22 ± 0.09	0.09–0.45
9–11 yr	7.43 ± 0.84	6.32–9.00	4.24 ± 0.79	3.16–4.97	0.30 ± 0.07	0.12–0.38
12–16 yr	7.25 ± 0.85	6.25–8.75	4.26 ± 0.64	3.19–5.13	0.19 ± 0.07	0.09–0.32
Adult	7.41 ± 0.96	6.44–8.32	4.31 ± 0.59	3.46–4.78	0.23 ± 0.06	0.16–0.30

	Alpha-2 (g/dL)		Beta (g/dL)		Gamma (g/dL)	
	Mean	Range	Mean	Range	Mean	Range
Cord blood	0.68 ± 0.14	0.44–0.94	0.74 ± 0.30	0.42–1.56	1.28 ± 0.23	0.81–1.16
1–3 mo	0.74 ± 0.24	0.40–1.13	0.59 ± 0.20	0.39–1.14	0.66 ± 0.24	0.25–1.05
4–6 mo	0.67 ± 0.11	0.52–0.84	0.61 ± 0.14	0.44–0.76	0.61 ± 0.26	0.24–0.90
7–12 mo	0.99 ± 0.30	0.78–1.46	0.79 ± 0.16	0.63–0.91	0.84 ± 0.36	0.32–1.18
13–24 mo	0.88 ± 0.42	0.41–1.36	0.77 ± 0.31	0.36–1.41	1.09 ± 0.32	0.36–1.62
25–36 mo	0.89 ± 0.14	0.68–1.09	0.67 ± 0.14	0.47–0.91	1.08 ± 0.28	0.73–1.46
3–5 yr	0.70 ± 0.15	0.43–0.99	0.67 ± 0.11	0.47–1.01	1.13 ± 0.31	0.54–1.66
6–8 yr	0.67 ± 0.10	0.50–0.83	0.72 ± 0.11	0.45–0.93	1.21 ± 0.32	0.70–1.95
9–11 yr	0.75 ± 0.27	0.67–0.87	0.84 ± 0.16	0.63–1.02	1.46 ± 0.41	0.79–2.03
12–16 yr	0.71 ± 0.15	0.50–0.97	0.68 ± 0.15	0.48–0.88	1.40 ± 0.31	1.08–1.96
Adult	0.61 ± 0.14	0.51–0.86	0.81 ± 0.22	0.59–1.06	1.45 ± 0.46	0.68–2.11

Adapted from Johnson TR, Moore WM, eds. *Children are different: developmental physiology*, 2nd ed. Columbus, OH: Ross Laboratories, 1978:188.

APPENDIX 12

Normal Values for 14 Human Serum Proteins[a]

	Mean (mg/dL)	Range (mg/dL)
Albumin	4000	3200–5500
α_1-Antitrypsin	240	160–360
α_1-Acid glycoprotein (orosomucoid)	100	40–150
C1 inhibitor	18	11–26
Ceruloplasmin	32	18–45
α_2-Macroglobulin	550 (pediatric)	200–700[b]
	300 (female, adult)	120–540[b]
	240 (male, adult)	90–400[b]
Haptoglobin	108	25–180[c]
Transferrin	280	200–350
Low-density lipoprotein	105	40–140[d]
C3	165	90–220[e]
C4	30	10–40
IgA	240	60–360[f]
IgM	105	25–170[f]
IgG	1100	700–1500[g]

Ig, immunoglobulin.
[a]Values derived from a large northern New England white population.
[b]Varies markedly during and around the time of puberty.
[c]Varies from 0 to normal adult levels during first 2 weeks of life.
[d]Varies from 10% of normal to normal adult levels during first year of life.
[e]Varies from 50% of normal to normal adult levels during the first month of life.
[f]Varies from 0 to normal adult levels during first year of life.
[g]Varies from adult normal levels at birth to 25% of normal at about 3 months, returning to adult normal during next several years.
Adapted from Ritchie RF. Automated immunoprecipitation analysis of serum proteins. In: Putnam FW, ed. *The plasma proteins*, 2nd ed, vol 2. San Diego: Academic Press, 1975:376.

APPENDIX 13

Serum Immunoglobulin (Ig) Levels in Normal Individuals

Subjects		IgG		IgA		IgM	
Age	Number	mg/dL	% of Adult Level	mg/dL	% of Adult Level	mg/dL	% of Adult Level
Newborn	20	1004 (598–1672)	95	<5 (0–<5)	<2	9 (6–15)	12
1–3 mo	10	365 (218–610)	34	32 (20–53)	12	24 (11–51)	32
4–6 mo	12	381 (228–636)	36	44 (27–72)	17	38 (25–60)	50
7–9 mo	10	488 (292–816)	46	44 (27–73)	17	47 (18–124)	62
10–18 mo	13	640 (383–1070)	60	67 (27–169)	25	56 (28–113)	74
2 yr	8	708 (423–1184)	67	89 (35–222)	33	65 (32–131)	86
3 yr	6	798 (477–1334)	75	100 (40–251)	38	57 (28–116)	75
4 yr	8	906 (542–1515)	85	120 (48–301)	45	41 (20–82)	54
5 yr	5	901 (539–1506)	85	134 (53–336)	50	52 (26–106)	68
6 yr	11	954 (571–1597)	90	131 (52–329)	49	57 (28–115)	75
7 yr	11	1066 (638–1783)	100	223 (89–559)	84	48 (24–98)	63
8 yr	8	976 (583–1631)	92	213 (85–535)	80	55 (27–112)	72
9 yr	7	1006 (599–1673)	95	230 (92–578)	86	56 (28–113)	74
10 yr	7	991 (593–1657)	93	188 (75–472)	71	60 (29–120)	79
11 yr	7	989 (586–1637)	93	257 (102–644)	97	56 (28–113)	74
12 yr	7	855 (511–1430)	81	232 (92–581)	87	55 (27–111)	72
13 yr	13	961 (575–1607)	91	235 (94–588)	88	52 (26–105)	68
14 yr	8	940 (562–1571)	89	217 (86–544)	82	67 (33–135)	88
Adult	30	1066 (635–1770)	100	266 (106–668)	100	76 (37–154)	100

NOTE: Geometric means are presented for each immunoglobulin at every age. The bounds, given in parentheses, are obtained by taking the mean logarithm ± twice the pooled standard deviations of the mean logarithms, then taking the antilogs of the results. In the case of IgA, the first four age groups have a pooled standard deviation separate from the other ages. In the case of IgM, the bounds of the first four age groups are ± twice the individual group standard deviations.
Adapted from Buckley RH, Dees SC, O'Fallon WM. Serum immunoglobulins. I. Levels in normal children and in uncomplicated childhood allergy. *Pediatrics* 1968;41:600.

APPENDIX 14

Metabolic Parameters of Human Immunoglobulins (Ig)

	IgG				IgM	IgA		IgE	IgD
	IgG1	IgG2	IgG3	IgG4		IgA1	IgA2		
Serum concentration (mg/dL)									
Adult									
Range		600–1500			75–150	200–300		0.02–0.06	0.01–3.00
Mean		1200			97	250		0.04	2.2
	840	240	80	40	—	220	30	—	—
Fetus (6 mo; mean)		300			20	ND		0.003	0.05
Newborn		1200 (all maternal)			30	ND		0.003	0.1
6 mo		400			40	25		0.006	0.1
1 yr		800			60	60		0.01	0.3
Fraction of total serum								<0.01	<1
Ig (%)		75–80			10	10–15			
Fraction of total serum IgG (%)	70	18	8	4	—	—		—	—
Fraction of body pool					80			50	75
Intravascular (%)		45				42			
Time (d)		23			5.1	5.8		2.5	2.6
	23	23	9	23	—	—		—	—
Fractional catabolic rate (plasma pool catabolized/d)		6.7			25	18		91	37
Metabolic rate (mg/kg/d)		33			6.9	24		0.003	0.4

ND, not determined.

APPENDIX 15

French-American-British (FAB) Classification System of Acute Nonlymphocytic Leukemia

FAB Type	Definition	Blasts ANuC	Blasts NEC	Nucleated Erythroblasts	Morphology	Cytochemistry
M1	AML without maturation	>30	>90	<50	Undifferentiated; <10% promyelocytes or monocytes; acute myeloblastic leukemia	>3% POX or SBB+
M2	AML with maturation	>30	30–89	<50	>10% promyelocytes, myelocytes; <20% monocytic cells; AML with partial differentiation	POX+, SBB+, PAS–
M3	Acute promyelocytic leukemia	>30	30–89	<50	>20% abnormal hypergranular promyelocytes; Auer rods common; acute promyelocytic leukemia	POX+, SBB+, PAS–
M3v	Microgranular variant	>30	30–89	<50	Microgranular variant, may have folded nucleus	POX+, SBB+, PAS–
M4	Acute myelomonocytic leukemia	>30	30–79	<50	>20% promonocytes and monocytes; >20% granulocytic component; blood monocytes >5 × 10⁹/L or lysozyme more than three times normal	POX+, NASDA+
M4Eo	M4 with eosinophilia	>30	30–79	<50	>5% Eos with abnormal Eo and basophilic granules	POX+, NASDA+, eosinophils are PAS+
M5a	Acute monocytic leukemia, poorly differentiated	—	>80ᵃ	<50	>80% of monocytic cells are monoblasts; acute monoblastic leukemia	POX, NASDA+ (inhibited by NaF)
M5b	Acute monocytic leukemia, differentiated	—	>80ᵃ	<50	<80% of monocytic cells are monoblasts; the rest are promonocytes and monocytes	Same as M5a
M6	Acute erythroleukemia	—	>30	>50	Megaloblastoid, erythroid, and myeloid blasts; multinucleated; erythroleukemia	PAS+, ringed sideroblasts with iron stain
M7	Acute megakaryoblastic leukemia	>30	—	<50	Large polymorphic blasts, cytoplasmic blebs; gpIb or IIb/IIIa+; myelofibrosis; acute megakaryoblastic leukemia	POX–, SBB–, NASDA+, platelet POX+ on electron microscope
MDS	Myelodysplastic syndrome	<30	<30	—	Megaloblastoid; nuclear and cytoplasmic dyssynchrony; nuclear anomalies; myelodysplastic syndromes	—

AML, acute myelogenic leukemia; ANuC, all nucleated cells; Eo, eosinophils; MDS, myelodysplastic syndrome; NASDA, naphthol-ASD chloroacetate esterase; NEC, nonerythroid cells; PAS, periodic acid–Schiff stain; POX, myeloperoxidase; SBB, Sudan black B stain.
ᵃIncludes monoblasts, promonocytes, and monocytes.

APPENDIX 16

Immunophenotype Analysis of Acute Leukemia

CD	Antibodies	M1/M2	M3	M4/M5	M6	M7	B-ALL	T-ALL
Myeloid lineage								
CD11b	Anti-Mo1	—	+	++	–	–	–	–
CD13	Anti-MY7	+	+	++	+	+	–	–
CD14	Anti-Mo2, MY4	–	–	++	–	–	–	–
CD15	Anti-MY1	+	++	++	–	–	–	–
CD33	Anti-MY9	++	++	++	++	++	–	–
CD34	Anti-MY10	++	+	+	+	+	+	+
T lineage								
CD2	Anti-T11	–	–	–	–	–	–	++
CD3	Anti-T3	–	–	–	–	–	–	+
CD5	Anti-T1	–	–	–	–	–	–	++
CD7	3A1	+	+	+	+	+	+	++
B lineage								
CD10	Anti-CALLA	–	–	–	–	–	+	–
CD19	Anti-B4	–	–	–	–	–	+	–
CD20	Anti-B1	–	–	–	–	–	+	–
Erythroid lineage								
	Antiglycophorin A	–	–	–	++	–	–	–
Megakaryocyte lineage								
CD41	Anti-gpIIb/IIIa	–	–	–	–	++	–	–
CD42	Anti-gpIb	–	–	–	–	++	–	–

B-ALL, B-lineage acute lymphoblastic leukemia; CALLA, common acute lymphoblastic leukemia antigen; gp, glycoprotein; T-ALL, T-lineage acute lymphoblastic leukemia; ++, expressed by more than 20% of blasts in 20% to 50% of cases; +, expressed by less than 20% of blasts in 5% to 20% of cases; –, expressed by less than 5% of cases.

APPENDIX 17

Chromosomal Abnormalities and Genes in Hematopoietic Disorders

Hematopoietic Disorders	Chromosomal Abnormality	Genes Involved	
		Fusion Partner 1	Fusion Partner 2
Chronic myeloid leukemia			
	t(9;22)(q34;q11)	ABL1	BCR
Chronic myelomonocytic leukemia			
	t(5;12)(q33;p13)	PDGFRB	TEL
Acute myeloid leukemia			
	t(1;11)(q21;q23)	AF1q	ALL1
	t(3;21)(q26;q22)	EVI1	CBFA2/AML1
	t(6;9)(p23;q34)	DEK	CAN
	t(7;11)(p15;p15)	HOXA9	NUP98
	t(8;21)(q22;q22)	ETO/CDR	AML1
	t(9;11)(p22;q23)		ALL1/MLL/TRX1
	t(9;12)(q34;p13)	ABL	TEL
	t(9;22)(q34;q11)	ABL1	BCR
	inv(9)(q34q34)	SET	CAN/NUP214
	t(11;17)(q23;q21)	PLZF	RARA
	t(11;22)(q23;q13)	MLL	P300
	t(12;22)(p13;q11)	TEL	MN1
	t(15;17)(q22;q11-21)	PML	RARA
	inv(16)(p13q22) or t(16;16)(p13;q22)	MYH11	CBFB
B-cell leukemias and lymphomas			
	t(1;19)(q23;p13)	PBX1	E2A
	t(2;8)(p12;q24)	IGK	MYC, PVT1
	t(2;14)(p13;q32)	—	IGH
		—	IGHG2
	t(4;11)(q21;q23)	AF4	ALL1/MLL/TRX1
	t(5;14)(q31;q32)	IL3	IGH
	t(8;12)(q24;q22)	MYC	BTG1
	t(8;14)(q2;q32)	MYC	IGH
	t(8;22)(q24;q11)	MYC, PVT1	IGL
	t(9;14)(p11;q32)	—	IGHA
	t(9;14)(p13;q32)	—	IGHA
	t(9;22)(q34;q11)	ABL1	BCR
	t(10;14)(q24;q32)	LYT10	I/GHA1
	t(11;14)(q13;q32)	BCL1/PRAD1	IGH
	t(11;14)(q23;q32)	RCK	IGH
	t(11;19)(q23;p13)	ALL1/MLL/TRX1	—
	t(12;21)(p13;q22)	TEL	CBFA2/AML1
	t(14;18)(q32;q21)	IGH	BCL2
	t(14;19)(q32;p13)	IGH	BCL3
	t(17;19)(q22;p13)	HLF	E2A
T-cell leukemias and lymphomas			
	t(1;3)(p34;p21)	TAL1	—
	t(1;7)(p32;q35)	TAL1	TCRB
	t(1;7)(p34;q34)	LCK	TCRB
	t(1;14)(p32;q11)	TAL1	TCRD
	ins(2;2)(p13;p11-14)	REL	—
	t(2;5)(p23;q35)	NPM	ALK
	t(4;16)(q26;p13)	IL2	BCMA
	inv(7)(p15q35)	TCRG	TCRB
	t(7;9)(q35;q32)	TCRB	TAL2
	t(7;9)(q35;q34.3)	TCRB	TAN1
	t(7;10)(q35;q24)	TCRB	HOX11
	t(7;11)(q35;p13)	TCRB	RBTNL1
	t(7;14)(q35;q32)	TCRB	—
	t(7;19)(q35;p13)	TCRB	LYL1
	t(8;14)(q24;q11)	MYC	TCRA
	—	PVT1	TCRD
	t(10;14)(q24;q11)	HOX11	TCRD
	t(11;14)(p13;q11)	RBTNL1	TCRD
	t(11;14)(p15;q11)	RBTN1	TCRD
	inv(14)(q11q32.1)	TCRA	IGH
	t(14;14)(q11;q32)	TCRA	—

ABL1, Abelson murine leukemia viral (v-*abl*) oncogene homolog 1; *AF1q*, ALL fused chromosome 1q; *AF4*, AF4 (or FEL) putative transcription factor; *ALL1*, acute lymphocytic leukemia oncogene 1, homologous to *Drosophila trithorax* developmental regulator; *AML1*, acute myeloid leukemia 1 oncogene, transcription factor homologous to *Drosophila runt* segmentation gene; *BCL1*, B-cell CLL/lymphoma oncogene 1; *BCL2*, B-cell CLL/lymphoma oncogene 2; *BCL3*, B-cell CLL/lymphoma oncogene 3; *BCMA*, B-cell maturation gene; *BCR*, breakpoint cluster region tyrosine kinase; *BTG1*, BTG 1 antiproliferative gene, homologous to murine *PC3* gene; *CAN*, Cain gene, acute myeloid leukemia 220-kd chromosome 9q34 breakpoint; *CBFB*, CBF-β (or PEBP2-β) transcription factor; *CDR*, cyclin D-related gene; *DEK*, acute myeloid leukemia 43-kd chromosome bp23 breakpoint; *E2A*, E2A transcription factor; *ETO*, ETO (eight twenty-one) transcription factor; *HLF*, hepatic leukemia factor; *HOX11*, homeobox region 11, spleen developmental regulator (T-cell lymphoma 3-associated breakpoint); *IGH*, immunoglobulin heavy chain gene cluster; *IGHA*, immunoglobulin heavy chain, α; *IGHAl*, immunoglobulin heavy chain, α₁; *IGHG2*, immunoglobulin heavy chain, γ₂ (Gm marker); *IGK*, immunoglobulin light chain, κ gene cluster; *IGL*, immunoglobulin light chain, λ gene cluster; *IL2*, interleukin 2; *IL3*, interleukin 3; *LCK*, lymphocyte-specific protein kinase; *LYL1*, lymphoblastic leukemia derived sequence 1; *LYT10*, B-cell lymphoma-associated oncogene, NF-κB p50 transcription factor homolog; *MLL*, myeloid/lymphoid or mixed-lineage leukemia gene, homologous to *Drosophila trithorax* developmental regulator; *MN1*, meningioma 1 nuclear protein; *MYC*, avian myelocytomatosis viral (v-*myc*) oncogene homolog; *MYH11*, myosin, heavy polypeptide 11, smooth muscle; *NUP98*, nuclear pore protein 98; *P300*, adenoviral E1A-associated protein 300; *PBX1*, pre–B-cell transcription factor 1; *PML*, promyelocytic leukemia; *PRAD1*, parathyroid adenomatosis 1; *PVT1*, *pvt*-1 (murine) oncogene homolog, MYC activator; *RARA*, retinoic acid receptor, α; *RBTN1*, rhombotin 1; *RBTNL1*, rhombotin-like 1; *RCK*, RC-K8 B-lymphoma cell line breakpoint, putative RNA helicase; *REL*, avian reticuloendotheliosis viral (v-*rel*) oncogene homolog; *TAL1*, T-cell acute lymphocytic leukemia 1; *TAL2*, T-cell acute lymphocytic leukemia 2; *TAN1*, translocation-associated *Drosophila notch* homolog 1; *TCRA*, T-cell receptor, α; *TCRB*, T-cell receptor, β; *TCRD*, T-cell receptor, δ; *TCRG*, T-cell receptor, γ; *TEL*, ETS-related transcription factor; *TRX1*, human trithorax gene 1 (HTRX-1), transcription factor.

APPENDIX 18

Normal Values for Tests of Hemostasis and Blood Coagulation

Test	Normal Range[a]
Platelet count	140–440 × 10⁹/L
Bleeding time	
Ivy	1–9 min[b]
Duke	1–4 min
Partial thromboplastin time	
Standard	68–82 sec[c]
Activated	32–46 sec[c]
Plasma prothrombin time	11–15 sec[d]
Coagulation time (glass tubes)	8–18 min
Plasma thrombin time	13–17 sec
Fibrinogen assay	160–415 mg/dL
Euglobulin clot lysis time	>2 h[c]
Fibrin degradation products	8 mg/dL[c]

[a]Defined as two standard deviations above or below the mean.
[b]Confidence limits determined by logarithmic plot.
[c]Minor variations depend on exact technique used.
[d]Significant variation; depends on thromboplastin used.

APPENDIX 19

Reference Values for Coagulation Tests in Healthy Full-Term Infants during the First 6 Months of Life Compared with Values for Adults[a]

Coagulation Test	Day 1 Mean	Day 1 95% Range	Day 5 Mean	Day 5 95% Range	Day 30 Mean	Day 30 95% Range	Day 90 Mean	Day 90 95% Range	Day 180 Mean	Day 180 95% Range	Adults Mean	Adults 95% Range
PT(s)	13.0	10.1–15.9[b]	12.4	10.0–15.3	11.8	10.0–14.3[b]	11.9	10.0–14.2[b]	12.3	10.7–13.9[b]	12.4	10.8–13.9
INR	1.0	0.53–1.62	0.89	0.53–1.48	0.79	0.53–1.26	0.81	0.53–1.26	0.88	0.61–1.27	0.89	0.64–1.17
APTT(s)	42.9	31.3–54.5	42.6	25.4–59.8	40.4	32.0–55.2	37.1	29.0–50.1[b]	35.5	28.1–42.9[b]	33.5	26.6–40.3
TCT(s)	23.5	19.0–28.3[b]	23.1	18.0–29.2	24.3	19.4–29.2[b]	25.1	20.5–29.7[b]	25.5	19.8–31.2[b]	25.0	19.7–30.3
Fibrinogen (g/L)	2.83	1.67–3.99[b]	3.12	1.62–4.26[b]	2.70	1.62–3.78[b]	2.43	1.50–3.79[b]	2.51	1.50–3.87[b]	2.78	1.56–4.00
II (U/mL)	0.48	0.26–0.70	0.63	0.33–0.93	0.68	0.34–1.02	0.75	0.45–1.05	0.88	0.60–1.16	1.08	0.70–1.46
V (U/mL)	0.72	0.34–1.08	0.95	3.45–1.45	0.18	6.62–1.34	0.70	0.48–1.32	0.91	0.55–1.27	1.06	0.62–1.50
VII (U/mL)	0.66	0.28–1.04	0.89	0.35–1.43	0.90	0.42–1.38	0.91	0.39–1.43	0.87	0.47–1.27	1.05	0.67–1.43
VIII (U/mL)	1.00	0.50–1.78[b]	0.88	0.50–1.54[b]	0.91	0.50–1.57[a]	0.79	0.50–1.25[b]	0.73	0.50–1.09	0.99	0.50–1.49
vWF (U/mL)	1.53	0.50–2.87	1.40	0.50–2.54	1.28	0.50–2.46	1.18	0.50–2.06	1.07	0.50–1.97	0.92	0.50–1.58
IX (U/mL)	0.53	0.15–0.91	0.53	0.15–0.91	0.51	0.21–0.81	0.67	0.21–1.13	0.86	0.36–1.36	1.09	0.55–1.63
X (U/mL)	0.40	0.12–0.68	0.49	0.19–0.79	0.59	0.31–0.87	0.71	0.35–1.07	0.78	0.38–1.18	1.06	0.70–1.52
XI (U/mL)	0.38	0.10–0.66	0.55	0.23–0.87	0.53	0.27–0.79	0.69	0.41–0.97	0.86	0.49–1.34	0.97	0.67–1.27
XII (U/mL)	0.53	0.13–0.93	0.47	0.11–0.83	0.49	0.17–0.81	0.67	0.25–1.09	0.77	0.39–1.15	1.08	0.52–1.64
PK (U/mL)	0.37	0.18–0.69	0.48	0.20–0.76	0.57	0.23–0.91	0.73	0.41–1.05	0.86	0.56–1.16	1.12	0.62–1.62
HMWK (U/mL)	0.54	0.06–1.02	0.74	0.16–1.32	0.77	0.33–1.21	0.82	0.30–1.46[b]	0.82	0.36–1.28[b]	0.92	0.50–1.36
XIIIa (U/mL)	0.79	0.27–1.31	0.94	0.44–1.44[b]	0.93	0.39–1.47[b]	1.04	0.36–1.72[b]	1.04	0.46–1.62[b]	1.05	0.55–1.55
XIIIs (U/mL)	0.76	0.30–1.22	1.06	0.32–1.80[b]	1.11	0.39–1.73[b]	1.16	0.48–1.84[b]	1.10	0.50–1.70[b]	0.97	0.57–1.37

APTT, activated partial thromboplastin time; HMWK, high-molecular-weight kininogen; INR, international normalized ratio; PK, prekallikrein; PT, prothrombin time; TCT, thrombin clotting time; vWF, von Willebrand factor.
[a]All factors, except fibrinogen, are expressed as units per milliliter (U/mL), where pooled plasma contains 1 U/mL. All values are expressed as the mean, followed by the lower and upper boundary encompassing 95% of the population. Between 40 and 77 samples were assayed for each value for the newborn. Some measurements were skewed because of a disproportionate number of high values. The lower limit, which excludes the lowest 2.5% of the population, has been given.
[b]Values that are indistinguishable from those of the adult.
Adapted from Andrew M, Paes B, Johnston M. Development of the hemostatic system in the neonate and young infant. *Am J Pediatr Hematol Oncol* 1990;12:95.

Reference Values for Coagulation Tests in Healthy Premature Infants (30–36 Weeks' Gestation) during the First 6 Months of Life[a]

Coagulation Test	Day 1 Mean	Day 1 95% Range	Day 5 Mean	Day 5 95% Range	Day 30 Mean	Day 30 95% Range	Day 90 Mean	Day 90 95% Range	Day 180 Mean	Day 180 95% Range	Adult Mean	Adult 95% Range
PT (sec)	13.0	10.6–16.2[b]	12.5	10.0–15.3[b]	11.8	10.0–13.6[b]	12.3	10.0–14.6[b]	12.5	10.0–15.0[b]	12.4	10.8–13.9
INR	1.0	0.61–1.7	0.91	0.53–1.48	0.79	0.53–1.11	0.88	0.53–1.32	0.91	0.53–1.48	0.89	0.64–1.17
APTT (sec)	53.6	27.5–79.4[c]	50.5	26.9–74.1	44.7	26.9–62.5	39.5	28.3–50.7	37.5	27.1–53.3[b]	33.5	26.6–40.3
TCT (sec)	24.8	19.2–30.4[c]	24.1	18.8–29.4[b]	24.4	18.8–29.9[b]	25.1	19.4–30.8[b]	25.2	18.9–31.5[b]	25.0	19.7–30.3
Fibrinogen (g/L)	2.43	1.50–3.73[b,c]	2.80	1.60–4.18[b,c]	2.54	1.50–4.14[b]	2.46	1.50–3.52[b]	2.28	1.50–3.60	2.78	1.56–4.00
II (U/mL)	0.45	0.20–0.77	0.57	0.29–0.85[c]	0.57	0.36–0.95[c]	0.68	0.30–1.06	0.87	0.51–1.23	1.08	0.70–1.46
V (U/mL)	0.88	0.41–1.44[b,c]	1.00	0.46–1.54[b]	1.02	0.48–1.56[b]	0.99	0.59–1.39[b]	1.02	0.58–1.46[b]	1.06	0.62–1.50
VII (U/mL)	0.67	0.21–1.13	0.84	0.30–1.38	0.83	0.21–1.45	0.87	0.31–1.43	0.99	0.47–1.51[b]	1.05	0.67–1.43
VIII (U/mL)	1.11	0.50–2.13	1.15	0.53–2.05[b,c]	1.11	0.50–1.99[b,c]	1.06	0.58–1.88[b,c]	0.99	0.50–1.87[b,c]	0.99	0.50–1.49
vWF (U/mL)	1.36	0.78–2.10	1.33	0.72–2.19	1.36	0.66–2.16	1.12	0.75–1.84[b]	0.98	0.54–1.58[b]	0.92	0.50–1.58
IX (U/mL)	0.35	0.19–0.65[c]	0.42	0.14–0.74[c]	0.44	0.13–0.80	0.59	0.25–0.93	0.81	0.50–1.20	1.09	0.55–1.63
X (U/mL)	0.41	0.11–0.71	0.51	0.19–0.83	0.56	0.20–0.92	0.67	0.35–0.99	0.77	0.35–1.19	1.06	0.70–1.52
XI (U/mL)	0.30	0.08–0.52[c]	0.41	0.13–0.69[c]	0.43	0.15–0.71[c]	0.59	0.25–0.93[c]	0.78	0.46–1.10	0.97	0.67–1.27
XII (U/mL)	0.38	0.10–0.66[c]	0.39	0.09–0.69[c]	0.43	0.11–0.75	0.61	0.15–1.07	0.82	0.22–1.42	1.08	0.52–1.64
PK (U/mL)	0.33	0.09–0.57	0.45	0.25–0.75	0.59	0.31–0.87	0.79	0.37–1.21	0.78	0.40–1.16	1.12	0.62–1.62
HMWK (U/mL)	0.49	0.09–0.89	0.62	0.24–1.00[c]	0.64	0.16–1.12[c]	0.78	0.32–1.24	0.83	0.41–1.25[b]	0.92	0.50–1.36
XIIIa (U/mL)	0.70	0.32–1.08	1.01	0.57–1.45[b]	0.99	0.51–1.47[b]	1.13	0.71–1.55[b]	1.13	0.65–1.61[b]	1.05	0.55–1.55
XIIIs (U/mL)	0.81	0.35–1.27	1.10	0.68–1.58[b]	1.07	0.57–1.57[b]	1.21	0.75–1.67	1.15	0.67–1.63	0.97	0.57–1.37

APTT, activated partial thromboplastin time; HMWK, high-molecular-weight kininogen; INR, international normalized ratio; PK, prekallikrein; PT, prothrombin time; TCT, thrombin clotting time; vWF, von Willebrand factor.
[a]All factors except fibrinogen are expressed as units per milliliter (U/mL), where pooled plasma contains 1.0 U/mL. All values are given as mean followed by the lower and upper boundaries encompassing 95% of the population. Between 40 and 96 samples were assayed for each value for the newborn. Some measurements were skewed because of a disproportionate number of high values. The lower limit, which excludes the lower 2.5% of the population, has been given.
[b]Values are indistinguishable from those of adults.
[c]Values different from those of the full-term infants.
Adapted from Andrew M, Paes B, Johnston M. Development of the hemostatic system in the neonate and young infant. Am J Pediatr Hematol Oncol 1990;12:95.

Reference Values for the Inhibitors of Coagulation in Healthy Full-Term Infants during the First 6 Months of Life Compared with Values for Adults[a]

Inhibitors	Day 1 Mean	Day 1 95% Range	Day 5 Mean	Day 5 95% Range	Day 30 Mean	Day 30 95% Range	Day 90 Mean	Day 90 95% Range	Day 180 Mean	Day 180 95% Range	Adults Mean	Adults 95% Range
ATIII (U/mL)	0.63	0.39–0.87	0.67	0.41–0.93	0.78	0.48–1.08	0.97	0.73–1.21[a]	1.04	0.84–1.24[b]	1.05	0.79–1.31
α_2-M (U/mL)	1.39	0.95–1.83	1.48	0.98–1.98	1.50	1.06–1.94	1.76	1.26–2.26	1.91	1.49–2.33	0.86	0.52–1.20
C_1E-INH (U/mL)	0.72	0.36–1.08	0.90	0.60–1.20[a]	0.89	0.47–1.31	1.15	0.71–1.59	1.41	0.89–1.93	1.01	0.71–1.31
α_1-AT (U/mL)	0.93	0.49–1.37[a]	0.89	0.49–1.29[a]	0.62	0.36–0.88	0.72	0.42–1.02	0.77	0.47–1.07	0.93	0.55–1.31
HCII (U/mL)	0.43	0.10–0.93	0.48	0.10–0.96	0.47	0.10–0.87	0.72	0.10–1.46	1.20	0.50–1.90	0.96	0.66–1.26
Proteins C (U/mL)	0.35	0.17–0.53	0.42	0.20–0.64	0.43	0.21–0.65	0.54	0.28–0.80	0.59	0.37–0.81	0.96	0.64–1.28
Protein S (U/mL)	0.36	0.12–0.60	0.50	0.22–0.78	0.63	0.33–0.93	0.86	0.54–1.18[b]	0.87	0.55–1.19[b]	0.92	0.60–1.24

ATIII, antithrombin III; α_2-M, α_2-macroglobulin; C_1E-INH, C_1-esterase inhibitor; α_1-AT, α_1-antitrypsin; HCII, heparin cofactor II.
[a]All values are expressed in units per milliliter (U/mL), where pooled plasma contains 1 U/mL. All values are given as a mean, followed by the lower and upper boundary encompassing 95% of the population. Between 40 and 75 samples were assayed for each value for the newborn. Some measurements were skewed because of a disproportionate number of high values. The lower limits, which exclude the lowest 2.5% of the population, have been given.
[b]Values are indistinguishable from those of adults.
Adapted from Andrew M, Paes B, Johnston M. Development of the hemostatic system in the neonate and young infant. Am J Pediatr Hematol Oncol 1990;12:95.

APPENDIX 22

Replacement Therapy for Congenital Coagulation Disorders[a]

Coagulation Factor	Factor Source (Concentration)	Recovery in the Circulation (%)	Biologic Half-Life	Desired Level for Hemostasis during Surgery	Estimated Therapeutic Dose (per kg body weight) Initial	Maintenance
Factor I (fibrinogen)	Cryoprecipitate (200–300 mg/bag)	~60	80 h	100 mg/dL	2–3 bags/10 kg	1 bag/15 kg daily
Factor II (prothrombin)	Fresh frozen plasma[a]	50	72 h	25–30%	15–20 mL/kg	3 mL/kg every 12–24 h
	Factor IX concentrate[b]	—	—	—	20 U/kg	10–20 U/kg every 12 h
Factor V	Fresh frozen plasma[a]	75	12–36 h	25%	15–20 mL/kg	3–6 mL/kg daily
Factor VII	Fresh frozen plasma[b]	100	3–6 h	15–25%	10–20 mL/kg	3–6 mL/kg every 8–12 h
	Factor IX concentrate[b]	—	—	—	20–50 U/kg	—
	Recombinant factor VII[a]	100	2 h	—	25 μg/kg	—
Factor VIII	Cryoprecipitate (100 U/bag)	—	—	—	1 bag/2 kg	—
	Factor VIII concentrate[b]	90–100	8–12 h	25–80% (depends on type and extent of surgery or bleed and interval from surgery)	25–50 U/kg	25 U/kg every 12–24 h
Factor IX	Recombinant factor VIII	—	—	—	25–50 U/kg	25 U/kg every 12–24 h
	Factor IX concentrate[b]	25–50	18–24 h	25–50% (depends on type and extent of surgery or bleed and interval from surgery)	50–100 U/kg	25–50 U/kg every 12–24 h
Factor X	Recombinant factor IX	—	—	—	50–100 U/kg	25–50 U/kg every 12–24 h
	Fresh frozen plasma[a]	Varies: 50–90	25–40 h	10–25%	15–20 mL/kg	3–6 mL/kg every 24 h
	Factor IX concentrate[b]	—	—	—	—	—
Factor XI	Fresh frozen plasma[a]	90	48–72 h	20–25%	15–20 mL/kg	3–6 mL/kg every 12 h
Factor XIII	Fresh frozen plasma[a]	Varies: 50–100	8–12 d	5%	500 mL	Every 21 days
	Cryoprecipitate (50–100 U/bag)	—	—	—	4–6 bags	Every 21 days

[a]One milliliter of plasma containing approximately one unit of factor activity.
[b]Factor activity variable and stated on label of product.
Adapted from Hilgartner M. Transfusion principles for congenital coagulation disorders. In: Hoffman R, Benz EJ Jr, Shattil SJ, et al., eds. Hematology: basic principles and practice. New York, Churchill Livingstone, 1991;1633.

APPENDIX 23

Platelet Lifespan Studies

Theodore E. Warkentin and John G. Kelton

Platelet lifespan studies can provide information useful for classifying the mechanism of thrombocytopenia in a particular patient and are occasionally used in difficult diagnostic situations. Several types of platelet lifespan measurements are available, and they can be divided into two general groups: nonradioactive and radioactive.

MEASUREMENTS USING NONRADIOACTIVE TECHNIQUES

The anuclear platelet cannot regenerate irreversibly inactivated enzymes, a fact that is exploited in nonradioactive platelet lifespan techniques (1,2). For example, the test subject can be given aspirin to inactivate platelet cyclooxygenase, the rate-limiting enzyme of the prostaglandin pathway. Assuming a steady state of platelet turnover, the time to recovery of platelet prostaglandin metabolism, as measured by malondialdehyde or thromboxane B_2 generation, correlates with the mean platelet survival. Nonradioactive techniques are much less accurate than measurements using radiolabeled platelets and are rarely used. However, the nonradioactive label, biotin, is increasingly being used for platelet lifespan studies in animals (3).

MEASUREMENTS USING RADIOLABELS

The most accurate and widely used tests for determining the platelet lifespan use radioisotopes (4). Two general types of platelet-labeling techniques have been used—cohort labels and random labels.

Cohort Radiolabeling

Cohort radiolabeling means that a single age of platelets (e.g., young platelets) is radiolabeled. The radioactivity of these platelets is then followed in the circulation with the time required for the radioactivity to appear and then disappear, defining the platelet lifespan. The cohort labels have included ^{75}Se-selenomethionine, ^{35}S-sulphate (5), and ^{3}H-amino acids. These methods have essentially been restricted to animal studies.

Random Radiolabeling

Random radiolabeling means that platelets of all ages are labeled to an equal extent by the radiolabel. Hence, during the radiolabeling process, platelets of all ages must be radiolabeled to a similar extent or an erroneous result is obtained. Normally, because platelets leave the circulation predominantly because of senescence, a linear decline in the radioactivity is observed.

Selection of Radioisotopes

The two main radiolabels used for platelet radiolabeling are ^{51}Cr-sodium chromate and ^{111}In (6). ^{111}In is the preferred radiolabel for the following reasons:

1. The labeling efficiency of ^{111}In is superior to ^{51}Cr. Only 10% to 20% of ^{51}Cr is taken up by platelets (low specific activity). Therefore, large numbers of platelets must be radiolabeled with ^{51}Cr to ensure adequate radioactivity for counting, which precludes the possibility of performing an autologous platelet lifespan study in a severely thrombocytopenic patient. In contrast, most (80% to 95%) of the ^{111}In is incorporated into platelets, and therefore autologous platelet lifespan studies usually can be performed in severely thrombocytopenic patients.
2. Although both radiolabels bind to cytoplasmic proteins within the platelets, platelet release is associated with loss of ^{51}Cr but not ^{111}In from the platelets. Hence, if there is *in vivo* platelet activation and release during the platelet lifespan study, a falsely shortened lifespan could result using ^{51}Cr-labeled platelets.
3. The half-life of ^{111}In is 2.8 days, compared with 21 days for ^{51}Cr. This makes ^{111}In an ideal label for platelets because its decay parallels the normal platelet lifespan.
4. The superior gamma-ray emission profile of ^{111}In compared with ^{51}Cr allows for improved imaging of platelet-sequestering organs, such as the spleen or splenic remnants (accessory spleens).

PERFORMANCE OF A PLATELET LIFESPAN

The optimal method for the performance of a platelet lifespan has been published (6). In brief, blood is collected, preferably from the patient (autologous study) or a healthy donor (homologous study). The platelets are isolated by differential centrifugation and washed, and the radiolabel is added. After sufficient time to permit incorporation of the radiolabel into the platelets, the platelets are pelleted, and any unbound label is washed away. Several quality control maneuvers are performed, including measurement of platelet, red blood cell, and plasma radioactivity. The platelets are infused intravenously into the subject, and blood is collected after the platelets have had enough time to equilibrate (typically 30 to 60 minutes). An anticoagulated blood sample is collected daily for the next 7 to 10 days. Subsequently, the samples are measured for radioactivity.

The percentage of platelet recovery is determined by measuring the percentage of radiolabeled platelets in the circulation at 30 to 60 minutes after administration. This measured amount is compared with the predicted platelet recovery, which is based on the patient's blood volume, the number of radiolabeled platelets given, and the physiologic splenic sequestration.

INTERPRETATION OF THE PLATELET LIFESPAN STUDY

The result of a platelet lifespan study has one of three general patterns.

Normal Recovery and Survival

Normal recovery and survival is characterized by a 60% to 80% platelet recovery and a lifespan of approximately 7 to 10 days. This is observed in normal people and in most patients with thrombocytopenia due to decreased platelet production. Somewhat reduced platelet survival in this latter situation reflects the relative increased importance of the fixed platelet requirement with severe thrombocytopenia (7).

Hypersplenism

Hypersplenism is characterized by a markedly reduced percentage of platelet recovery (typically, 20% to 40%) and a normal or near-normal platelet lifespan.

Shortened Platelet Survival

A shortened platelet survival occurs in destructive thrombocytopenic states. Patients with a rapid rate of platelet destruction can have an apparent reduced platelet recovery, although it is uncertain whether platelet sequestration is truly increased or whether the apparent sequestration is caused by an artifact of the rapid rate of destruction.

Ideally, the result of the platelet lifespan study is either normal or markedly reduced, but sometimes it can be difficult to be certain into which group the results fall. To avoid potential errors of subjective analysis, several approaches have been used for data analysis. The best is to use a computer model that determines the best fit of the data points. This technique, known as the *gamma function analysis*, removes any potential observer bias from the analysis of the results. Another approach is to measure the time required for loss of one-half of the radioactivity from the circulation, the half-life.

INDIRECT DETERMINATION OF PLATELET LIFESPAN

Plasma Glycocalicin

Glycocalicin, a soluble proteolytic product of the platelet GPIb alpha polypeptide, is elevated in disorders of increased platelet destruction (e.g., active immune thrombocytopenic purpura), whereas normal plasma levels are generally found in patients with decreased platelet production (e.g., aplastic anemia). However, elevated levels have also been found in some patients with uremia, cirrhosis, and acute myeloid leukemia (8), and this assay is generally used for research purposes rather than for the routine classification of the mechanism of thrombocytopenia.

Platelet RNA

The number of platelets with residual amounts of RNA can be quantitated using flow cytometric analysis of thiazole orange or auramine-O uptake by platelets (9). Although an increased percentage of RNA-containing platelets ("stress platelets") is found in patients with destructive thrombocytopenia, such quantitation of "reticulated" platelets has not become widely used, in contrast to red cell reticulocyte assays. A technical problem is that thiazole orange also labels platelet dense granules nonspecifically (10).

REFERENCES

1. Stuart MJ, Murphy S, Oski FA. A simple nonradioisotope technic for determination of platelet lifespan. *N Engl J Med* 1975;292:1310.
2. Boneu A, Sie P, Caranobe C, et al. Platelet regeneration time after aspirin ingestion and platelet survival time after labeling with ^{51}chromium or ^{111}indium oxine: a comparative study. *Thromb Haemost* 1985;53:260.
3. Franco RS, Lee KN, Barker-Gear R, et al. Use of bi-level biotinylation for concurrent measurement of in vivo recovery and survival in two rabbit platelet populations. *Transfusion* 1994;34:784–789.
4. Rand ML, Greenberg JP, Packham MA, Mustard JF. Density subpopulations of rabbit platelets: size, protein, and sialic acid content, and specific radioactivity changes following labeling with ^{35}S-sulphate in vivo. *Blood* 1981;57:741.
5. Dale GL. Platelet kinetics. *Curr Opin Hematol* 1997;4:330–334.
6. Snyder EL, Moroff G, Simon T, et al. Recommended methods for conducting radiolabeled platelet survival studies. *Transfusion* 1986;26:37.
7. Hanson SR, Slichter SJ. Platelet kinetics in patients with bone marrow hypoplasia: evidence for a fixed platelet requirement. *Blood* 1985;66:1105.
8. Beer JH, Büchi L, Steiner B. Glycocalicin: a new assay—the normal plasma levels and its potential usefulness in selected diseases. *Blood* 1994;83:691.
9. Kienast J, Schmitz G. Flow cytometric analysis of thiazole orange uptake by platelets: a diagnostic aid in the evaluation of thrombocytopenic disorders. *Blood* 1990;75:116.
10. Robinson MS, Mackie IJ, Khair K, et al. Flow cytometric analysis of reticulated platelets: evidence for a large proportion of non-specific labeling of dense granules by fluorescent dyes. *Br J Haematol* 1998;100:351–357.

APPENDIX 24

Platelet Antibody Testing

Theodore E. Warkentin and John G. Kelton

Advances in the understanding of immune platelet disorders have resulted from the increasing sophistication and widespread application of *in vitro* platelet antibody tests. Many tests have been described, which will be classified into three groups, termed *phase I, II,* and *III assays*, according to the time of introduction and general technique. Phase I assays, which were first developed in the 1950s, measure a functional platelet-dependent endpoint, usually platelet activation. Phase II assays detect the presence of immunoglobulin (Ig) or complement on or within the platelet; these assays, first developed in 1975, are often referred to as *tests for platelet-associated IgG* (PAIgG). In 1984, assays that measure the binding of Ig to specific platelet proteins were developed, which we refer to as *phase III assays*.

Although most of these assays were developed to detect platelet antibodies in immune thrombocytopenic purpura (ITP) patients, modifications permit their use in other clinical situations. For example, platelets of known alloantigen specificity can be used to identify alloantibodies. Also, measurement of drug-dependent antibody binding to platelets can be diagnostic of drug-induced immune thrombocytopenia.

PHASE I ASSAYS

In phase I assays, patient plasma/serum is added to normal platelets, and a platelet-dependent endpoint, such as platelet activation, is measured. Platelet activation can be detected by several methods, including aggregation (1,2), ^{14}C- or ^{3}H-serotonin release from platelet granules (3,4), release of cytoplasmic ^{51}Cr, increased availability of platelet factor 3 (procoagulant activity) (5), and inhibition of a platelet function (e.g., migration inhibition, clot retraction) (6).

Generally speaking, phase I assays have low sensitivity and specificity for detecting platelet-antibody interactions. The sensitivity is low because not all test samples contain sufficiently reactive antibody to result in platelet activation. The specificity is low because platelet activation is not specific for IgG; small amounts of thrombin or immune complexes in the test sample can produce a false-positive result. An exception to these generalizations is the platelet ^{14}C-serotonin release assay for heparin-induced thrombocytopenia (HIT) (4,7,8). This test has high sensitivity for immune HIT because it exploits the potent platelet-activating properties of the pathogenic IgG. The specificity is high because various control maneuvers (e.g., high heparin concentrations, platelet Fc receptor blocking monoclonal antibody) have been incorporated to distinguish HIT IgG from thrombin or immune complexes.

PHASE II ASSAYS

Phase II assays are the dominant type of assay used at present. They detect Ig or complement on the platelet, rather than infer its presence through an endpoint such as platelet activation.

All phase II assays use an immunologic probe to detect surface-bound Ig or complement. Usually, these probes are antibodies (polyclonal or monoclonal antiIg or anticomplement probes), although staphylococcal protein A can be used to detect IgG subtypes 1, 2, and 4. The probes are usually labeled with a radioisotope or fluorescent marker or are enzyme-linked. The labeled probe is mixed with the test platelets, which can be intact or lysed, and then the amount of probe that binds to the test platelets is measured. Amplification of the signal can be achieved by using a polyclonal, labeled second antibody (anti-antiIgG) or a biotin-avidin detection system. The IgG that is detected using these phase II assays is termed *PAIgG*. The designation of PAIgG is used because these assays measure all platelet IgG irrespective of the type of binding to the platelet.

The three general categories of phase II assays are direct-binding assays, two-stage (consumption) assays, and assays for total PAIgG.

Direct-Binding Assays

In direct-binding assays, the binding of a labeled antiIg probe to the platelet surface is quantitated (Fig. 1). These assays are performed by incubating the washed test platelets with the labeled antiIg probe. After equilibrium is reached, the unbound probe is washed away, and the amount bound to the platelets is measured (radioactivity, fluorescence, enzyme activity) (9–12). The assays are semiquantitative because although the specific activity of the labeled probes can be determined, theoretic binding ratios must be used (e.g., assumption of 1:1 binding of monoclonal probe to platelet-bound Ig). Alternatively, the binding of the probe to known amounts of IgG on another cell (e.g., anti-D on a red blood cell) can be used for assay calibration. Flow cytometry has been used to determine PAIgG levels using antiglobulin probes linked to fluorescent markers (13).

A problem for the direct-binding assays is nonspecific binding of the labeled probe to the platelets. Nonspecific binding is the amount of labeled probe bound in the presence of supersaturating amounts of unlabeled probe. Nonspecific binding of the antiIg probe to the platelets can be reduced by the use of protein-containing media (blocking buffer). Because monoclonal antibodies can be used at extremely low concentrations, and because nonspecific binding is concentration-dependent, the high purity of monoclonal probes dramatically reduces nonspecific binding (12).

Two-Stage Assays (Consumption Assays)

These assays are performed in two stages (Fig. 2). In the first stage, varying numbers of test platelets are incubated with the probe (antiIgG). Known amounts of IgG in solution are substituted for the test platelets in a separate test to generate a standard curve. The antiIgG probe must be in excess of the amount

Washed Test Platelets

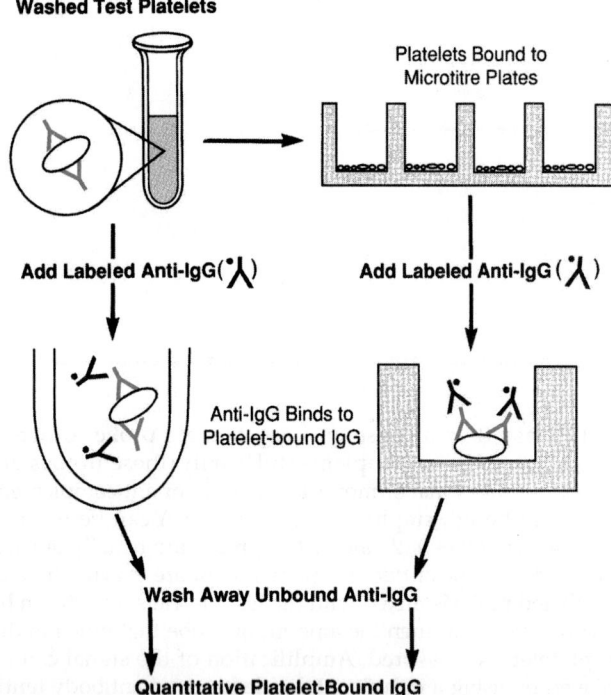

Figure 1. Schematic representation of a direct binding assay for platelet-associated immunoglobulin G (IgG).

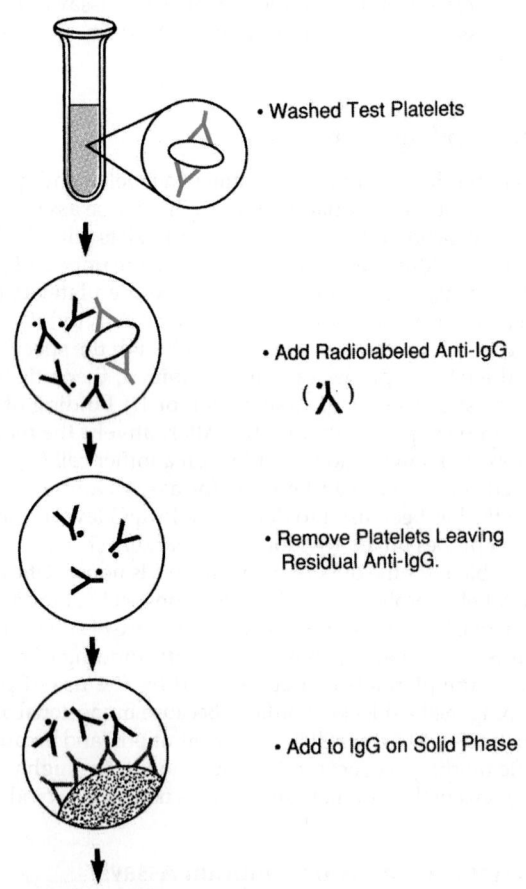

Figure 2. Schematic representation of a two-stage assay (consumption assay) for platelet-associated immunoglobulin G (IgG).

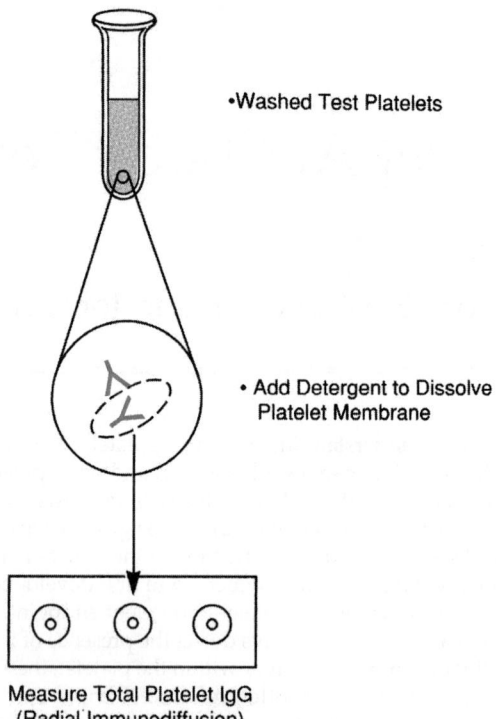

Figure 3. Schematic representation of an assay for total platelet-associated immunoglobulin G (IgG).

of IgG on the test platelets (or IgG standard). In the second stage, the antiIgG that is not consumed by the platelet-bound IgG (or IgG standard) is quantitated by measuring its binding to IgG fixed to a solid phase. The solid-phase IgG can be bound to a bead, cell (e.g., sheep red blood cells), or microtiter well (14,15). The antiIgG probe can be labeled with radioisotope, fluorescein, or with an enzyme, or it can be unlabeled and quantitated using a labeled anti-antiIg (probe amplification). A biologic endpoint (e.g., complement-mediated lysis of sheep red blood cells) also has been used (14).

An advantage of the two-stage assays is that quantitation is simplified because known amounts of IgG (the standard) can substitute for the test platelets. The problem of nonspecific binding of the probe to the platelets is overcome using the second stage. A disadvantage is that these assays are more complex than the other phase II assays. A theoretical disadvantage is that these assays may give an incorrectly high estimate of the amount of platelet-bound Ig (16). No type of phase II assay demonstrates superior specificity in the diagnosis of immune thrombocytopenia (17).

Assays for Total Platelet-Associated Immunoglobulin G

The total amount of IgG, from both the interior and the surface of the platelet, is measured in these assays (18,19) (Fig. 3). The test platelets are washed and counted, and the platelet membranes are lysed by detergent (e.g., Triton X-100), sonication, or repeated freezing and thawing. The total IgG, which is released from the membrane, cytosol, and alpha granules, can be measured by any technique that quantitates small amounts of fluid-phase IgG, including nephelometry or immunoradiometric assay. There is general agreement that the total PAIgG of normal platelets is 10,000 to 20,000 molecules (2.5 to 5.0 fg)/platelet.

These assays are simple to perform, and because the platelet membrane is dissolved, there is no nonspecific binding of the antiIgG to the membrane. A further advantage is that the platelet lysates can be stored frozen, allowing the tests to be batched. A disadvantage is the theoretic possibility that changes in total PAIgG might correlate poorly with pathophysiologically important changes in surface-bound PAIgG. In practice, however, assays for total PAIgG correlate well with other phase II assays (17,19). The biologic basis for the correlation between surface-bound and total PAIgG is uncertain.

Use

Phase II assays are used most frequently to assist in the diagnosis of immune thrombocytopenic disorders such as ITP. All these assays have similar sensitivity and specificity for immune thrombocytopenia (17). However, these assays are not diagnostic for immune thrombocytopenia, because nonimmune thrombocytopenic disorders also can be associated with elevated PAIgG. These assays may be useful for platelet typing and crossmatching, testing for drug-induced immune thrombocytopenia, and so forth.

PHASE III ASSAYS

Phase III assays measure the binding of antibody to specific platelet proteins. The phase III assays differ in the way the platelet proteins are presented to the antiplatelet antibodies. Since their development in the mid-1980s, it is increasingly evident that some of these assays (e.g., protein-capture assays) have moderate sensitivity and high specificity for immune thrombocytopenia.

Immunoblotting (Western Blotting)

Patient serum is allowed to interact with platelet proteins that have been electrophoretically separated and then immobilized ("blotted") onto a solid phase (nitrocellulose paper) (20). The test serum is added and, after washing, binding of patient antibody (either IgG or IgM) to specific protein bands is detected using a labeled antiimmunoglobulin (Fig. 4). Although immunoblotting offers the advantages of simplicity and the ability to store the immobilized platelet proteins for long periods of time, a major disadvantage is that protein antigens are denatured. Even IgG from normal sera frequently react in immunoblot assays with internal platelet glycoproteins (e.g., vinculin, talin), suggesting that caution should be used in assay interpretation (21).

Radioimmunoprecipitation

In this assay, patient serum/plasma is allowed to interact with radiolabeled platelet membrane proteins. In a subsequent step, the antibody-sensitized radiolabeled platelet membrane proteins are separated and identified (22) (Fig. 5). In this procedure, after washing the test platelets, the surface proteins are radiolabeled, usually with iodine-125 (^{125}I). The test serum is then incubated with the radiolabeled platelets. After the binding by specific antiplatelet antibody, detergent is added to solubilize the protein-antibody complexes, which are subsequently precipitated by the addition of an antiIg bound to a solid phase (often immobilized staphylococcal protein A). The radiolabeled protein-antibody complexes are washed, and the platelet proteins are separated by sodium dodecyl sulfate-polyacrylamide gel electrophoresis, with detection by autoradiography. The target protein antigen can be identified by its characteristic electro-

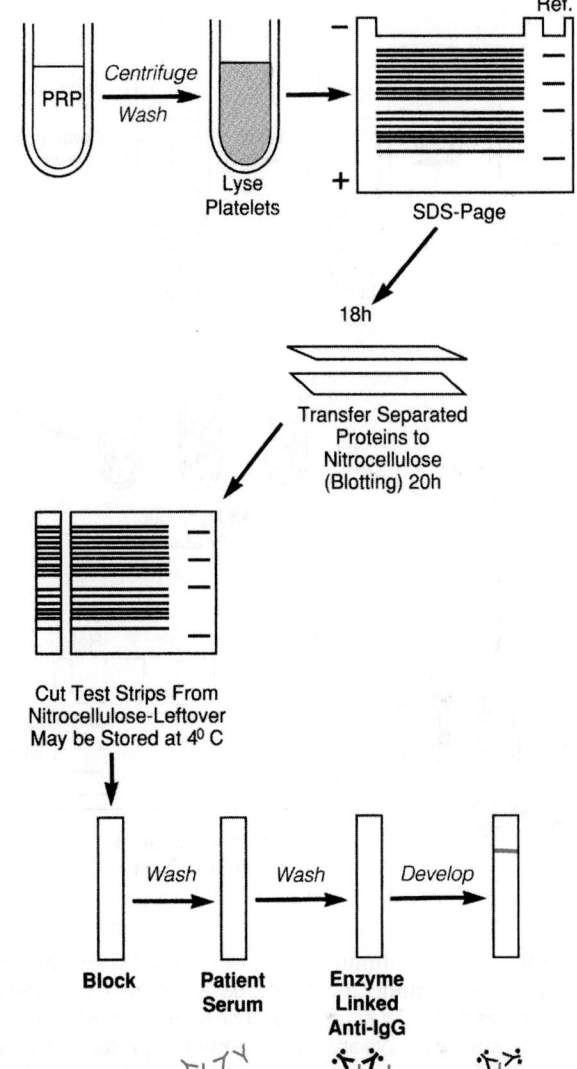

Figure 4. Immunoblotting to detect immunoglobulin G (IgG) reactive with specific platelet glycoproteins. PRP, platelet-rich plasma; SDS, sodium dodecyl sulfate.

phoretic mobility. In a modification of this assay, platelet-reactive autoantibodies have been demonstrated directly by radiolabeling washed patient and control platelets without any serum incubation step (direct radioimmunoprecipitation) (23).

Radioimmunoprecipitation offers advantages over immunoblotting because the antibody binds to native platelet proteins. The major disadvantages of radioimmunoprecipitation are the requirement for radioactive tracers and the possibility that not all the platelet proteins of interest are radiolabeled. These disadvantages can be overcome using the nonradioactive label biotin, which also labels more glycoproteins than radioactive iodine (24). These assays are technically demanding.

Protein-Capture Assays

In these assays, monoclonal antibodies are used to "capture" a certain platelet glycoprotein so that specific IgG-platelet protein interactions can be detected (25–29). Perhaps most widely used is the "monoclonal antibody-immobilization of platelet antigen" assay, or MAIPA (26); an improved "modified MAIPA" has been developed (27) (Fig. 6). A technically simpler assay is the anti-

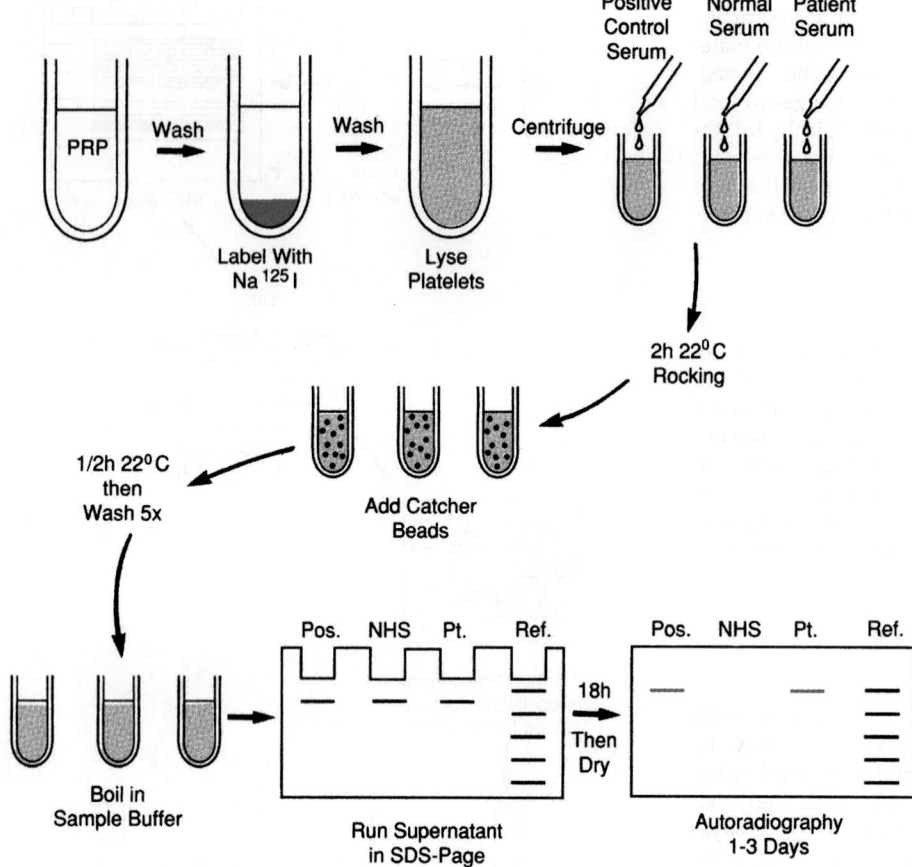

Figure 5. Radioimmunoprecipitation to detect immunoglobulin G (IgG) reactive with specific platelet glycoproteins. PRP, platelet-rich plasma; SDS, sodium dodecyl sulfate.

gen capture enzyme immunoassay, in which the anti-platelet glycoprotein (GP) monoclonal antibodies interact with detergent-solubilized platelet samples, rather than intact platelets.

Protein-capture assays are much simpler to perform than the other phase III assays. The requirement for specific monoclonal antibodies is a potential disadvantage because these monoclonal reagents are not universally available. These assays also give falsely negative results if the patient antibody binds to the same epitope that is recognized by the monoclonal antibody (30). False-positive results can be caused by naturally occurring human antimouse IgG antibodies (31). However, this problem is avoided by preincubating target platelets with test serum, followed by washing, before addition of mouse monoclonal antibody, as described using the modified MAIPA.

Use

Phase III assays offer the combination of moderate sensitivity for immune thrombocytopenia, together with high specificity (32). Because phase III assays permit the characterization of antibody interaction with specific platelet proteins, these assays allow the direct identification of glycoprotein specificity of autoantibodies and alloantibodies.

SENSITIVITY AND SPECIFICITY OF PLATELET ANTIBODY TESTING FOR ITP

Phase I Assays

Phase I assays are no longer used for the diagnosis of ITP because of low sensitivity and specificity.

Phase II Assays

The sensitivity of phase II assays for ITP ranges from 60% to 90% (12,14,17,18,32,33). The more severe the thrombocytopenia, the more likely the PAIgG is to be elevated. A study (17) comparing four major assays for PAIgG (direct-binding assay using staphylococcal protein A or monoclonal antiIgG; two-stage assay using polyclonal antiIgG; assay for total PAIgG) showed that they all had a similar sensitivity for ITP.

Unfortunately, phase II assays are not specific for immune thrombocytopenic disorders such as ITP. Several studies have shown that PAIgG frequently is elevated in "nonimmune" thrombocytopenic disorders, such as acute leukemia, thrombotic thrombocytopenic purpura, preeclampsia, and septicemia (33,34). Some investigators have claimed that diagnostic specificity for immune thrombocytopenia is increased using direct binding assays using a radiolabeled monoclonal antiIgG or staphylococcal protein A (12). However, a prospective study demonstrated no improved specificity for ITP compared with two-stage assays or assays for total PAIgG (17). Classic PAIgG assays provide limited diagnostic information, whereas the protein-capture assays have moderate sensitivity and relatively high specificity for immune thrombocytopenia.

Theoretically, the elevated PAIgG found in nonimmune disorders could be related to the thrombocytopenia itself. Indeed, even nonimmunoglobulin proteins (e.g., albumin) are elevated on platelets of ITP patients (35,36). Perhaps, elevated total PAIgG in both immune and nonimmune thrombocytopenic disorders could be the result of IgG incorporation into platelet alpha granules at the megakaryocyte level; thus, the elevated total PAIgG could reflect the lower mean platelet age of younger platelets, which contain higher amounts of PAIgG (37).

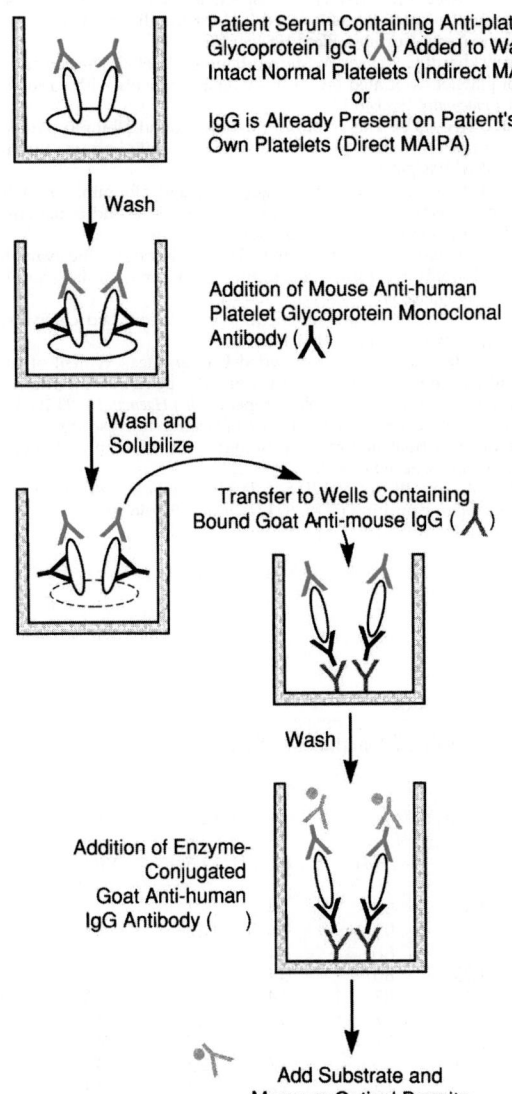

Patient Serum Containing Anti-platelet Glycoprotein IgG (人) Added to Washed Intact Normal Platelets (Indirect MAIPA) or IgG is Already Present on Patient's Own Platelets (Direct MAIPA)

Wash

Addition of Mouse Anti-human Platelet Glycoprotein Monoclonal Antibody (人)

Wash and Solubilize

Transfer to Wells Containing Bound Goat Anti-mouse IgG (人)

Wash

Addition of Enzyme-Conjugated Goat Anti-human IgG Antibody ( )

Add Substrate and Measure Optical Density

Figure 6. Modified monoclonal antibody-immobilization of platelet antigens (MAIPA) assay to detect immunoglobulin G (IgG) reactive with platelet glycoproteins.

However, this would not explain elevated total PAIgG levels seen in some disorders of decreased platelet production, nor account for the elevated surface PAIgG seen in nonimmune thrombocytopenia (17). Regardless, it is apparent that elevated PAIgG and albumin levels in ITP (and other disorders with increased platelet turnover) are associated with increased endocytosis of these plasma proteins into platelet alpha-granules, occurring either in megakaryocytes or mature platelets (38,39). Electron microscopy and immunogold labeling of IgG shows increased amounts of IgG within alpha-granules, as well as the open canalicular system and platelet surface, of patients with ITP (40).

Phase III Assays

As discussed, these assays, which demonstrate binding of IgG to specific platelet glycoproteins, appear to be relatively specific for immune thrombocytopenia. Platelets from patients with ITP can carry large amounts of IgG on their surfaces, up to hundreds of thousands of molecules of IgG/platelet (17). Studies from a num-

ber of laboratories have shown how technically difficult it is to measure IgG on the surface of the platelets. The reason is that large amounts of IgG are found within the α-granules of platelets and in the open canalicular system, which communicates with the surface. Presumably, most of the IgG was nonspecifically taken into the platelets at the time of their formation by the megakaryocytes, and unless extraordinary steps are taken during platelet purification and washing, some of this interior or canicular IgG is measured and incorrectly attributed to the autoantibody that causes immune thrombocytopenia. This could explain why the proportions of platelet immunoglobulin classes and subclasses resemble their respective plasma concentrations (10,41). What remains unexplained is why other nonimmunologic plasma proteins such as albumin are increased on ITP platelets in parallel with the increase in IgG (35,36).

REFERENCES

1. Deykin D, Hellerstein LJ. The assessment of drug-dependent and isoimmune antiplatelet antibodies by the use of platelet aggregometry. *J Clin Invest* 1972;51:3142.
2. Greinacher A, Michels I, Kiefel V, Mueller-Eckhardt C. A rapid and sensitive test for diagnosing heparin-associated thrombocytopenia. *Thromb Haemost* 1991;66:734.
3. Gockerman JP, Bowman RP, Conrad ME. Detection of platelet isoantibodies by [3H] serotonin platelet release and its clinical application to the problem of platelet matching. *J Clin Invest* 1975;55:75.
4. Sheridan D, Carter C, Kelton JG. A diagnostic test for heparin-induced thrombocytopenia. *Blood* 1986;67:27.
5. Karpatkin S, Strick N, Karpatkin MB, Siskind GW. Cumulative experience in the detection of antiplatelet antibody in 234 patients with idiopathic thrombocytopenic purpura, systemic lupus erythematosus and other clinical disorders. *Am J Med* 1972;52:776.
6. Duquesnoy RJ, Lorentsen DF, Aster RH. Platelet migration inhibition: a new method for detection of platelet antibodies. *Blood* 1975;45:741.
7. Warkentin TE, Sheppard JI, Horsewood P, et al. Impact of the patient population on the risk for heparin-induced thrombocytopenia. *Blood* 2000;96:1703.
8. Warkentin TE. Laboratory testing for heparin-induced thrombocytopenia. *J Thromb Thrombolysis* 2001;10:35.
9. Mueller-Eckhardt C, Mahn I, Schulz G, Mueller-Eckhardt G. Detection of platelet autoantibodies by a radioactive anti-immunoglobulin test. *Vox Sang* 1978;35:357.
10. Von dem Borne AEGK, Helmerhorst FM, Van Leeuwen EF, et al. Autoimmune thrombocytopenia: detection of platelet autoantibodies with the suspension immunofluorescence test. *Br J Haematol* 1980;45:319.
11. Gudino M, Miller WV. Application of the enzyme linked immunospecific assay (ELISA) for the detection of platelet antibodies. *Blood* 1981;57:32.
12. LoBuglio AF, Court WS, Vinocur L, et al. Immune thrombocytopenic purpura: use of a 125I-labeled antihuman IgG monoclonal antibody to quantify platelet-bound IgG. *N Engl J Med* 1983;309:459.
13. Rosenfeld CS, Nichols G, Bodensteiner DC. Flow cytometric measurement of antiplatelet antibodies. *Am J Clin Pathol* 1987;87:518.
14. Dixon R, Rosse W, Ebbert L. Quantitative determination of antibody in idiopathic thrombocytopenic purpura: correlation of serum and platelet-bound antibody in clinical response. *N Engl J Med* 1975;292:230.
15. Kelton JG, Denomme G, Walker C, et al. The measurement of platelet-associated IgG using an immunoradiometric assay. *J Immunoassay* 1983;4:65.
16. Blumberg N, Masel D, Stoler M. Disparities in estimates of IgG bound to normal platelets. *Blood* 1986;67:200.
17. Kelton JG, Murphy WG, Lucarelli A, et al. A prospective comparison of four techniques for measuring platelet-associated IgG. *Br J Haematol* 1989;71:97.
18. Luiken GA, McMillan R, Lightsey AL, et al. Platelet-associated IgG in immune thrombocytopenic purpura. *Blood* 1977;50:317.
19. Kelton JG, Denomme G, Lucarelli A, et al. Comparison of the measurement of surface or total platelet-associated IgG in the diagnosis of immune thrombocytopenia. *Am J Hematol* 1985;18:1.
20. McMillan R, Mason D, Tani P, Schmidt GM. Evaluation of platelet surface antigens: localization of the Pl^A1 alloantigen. *Br J Haematol* 1982;51:297.
21. Reid DM, Jones CE, Luo CY, Shulman NR. Immunoglobulins from normal sera bind platelet vinculin and talin and their proteolytic fragments. *Blood* 1993;81:745.
22. Degos L, Tobelem G, Lethielleux P, et al. Molecular defect in platelets from patients with Bernard-Soulier syndrome. *Blood* 1977;50:899.
23. Tomiyama Y, Take H, Honda S, et al. Demonstration of platelet antigens that bind platelet-associated autoantibodies in chronic ITP by direct immunoprecipitation procedure. *Br J Haematol* 1990;75:92.

24. Smith JW, Hayward CPM, Warkentin TE, et al. Investigation of human platelet alloantigens and glycoproteins using non-radioactive immunoprecipitation. *J Immunol Methods* 1993;158:77.
25. Woods VL Jr, Kurata Y, Montgomery RR, et al. Autoantibodies against platelet glycoprotein Ib in patients with chronic immune thrombocytopenic purpura. *Blood* 1984;64:156.
26. Kiefel V, Santoso S, Weisheit M, Mueller-Eckhardt C. Monoclonal antibody-specific immobilization of platelet antigens (MAIPA): a new tool for the identification of platelet-reactive antibodies. *Blood* 1987;70:1722.
27. Kiefel V. The MAIPA assay and its applications in immunohaematology. *Transfus Med* 1992;2:181.
28. Visentin GP, Wolfmeyer K, Newman PJ, Aster RH. Detection of drug-dependent, platelet-reactive antibodies by antigen-capture ELISA and flow cytometry. *Transfusion* 1990;30:694.
29. Warner MN, Moore JC, Warkentin TE, et al. A prospective study of protein-specific assays used to investigate idiopathic thrombocytopenic purpura. *Br J Haematol* 1999;104:442.
30. Tsubakio T, Tani P, Woods VL Jr, McMillan R. Autoantibodies against platelet GPIIb/IIIa in chronic ITP react with different epitopes. *Br J Haematol* 1987;67:345.
31. Hewitt J, Burton IE. Incidence of autoantibodies to GPIIb/IIIa in chronic autoimmune thrombocytopenic purpura may be overestimated by the MAIPA. *Br J Haematol* 1994;86:418.
32. Brighton TA, Evans S, Castaldi PA, et al. Prospective evaluation of the clinical usefulness of an antigen-specific assay (MAIPA) in idiopathic thrombocytopenic purpura and other immune thrombocytopenias. *Blood* 1996;88:194–201.

33. Kelton JG, Powers PJ, Carter CJ. A prospective study of the usefulness of the measurement of platelet-associated IgG for the diagnosis of idiopathic thrombocytopenic purpura. *Blood* 1982;60:1050.
34. Mueller-Eckhardt C, Kayser W, Mersch-Baumert K, et al. The clinical significance of platelet associated IgG: a study on 298 patients with various disorders. *Br J Haematol* 1980;46:123.
35. Kelton JG, Steeves K. The amount of platelet-bound albumin parallels the amount of IgG on washed platelets from patients with immune thrombocytopenia. *Blood* 1983;62:924.
36. George JN, Saucerman S. Platelet IgG, IgM, and albumin: correlation of platelet and plasma concentrations in normal subjects and in patients with ITP or dysproteinemia. *Blood* 1988;72:362.
37. George JN. Platelet immunoglobulin G: its significance for the evaluation of thrombocytopenia and for understanding the origin of alpha-granule proteins. *Blood* 1990;76:859.
38. George JN. Platelet IgG: measurement, interpretation, and clinical significance. *Prog Hemost Thromb* 1991;10:97.
39. Hughes M, Hayward CPM, Horsewood P, et al. Measurement of endogenous and exogenous alpha-granular platelet proteins in patients with immune and nonimmune thrombocytopenia. *Br J Haematol* 1999;106:762.
40. Hughes M, Webert K, Kelton JG. The use of electron microscopy in the investigation of the ultrastructural morphology of immune thrombocytopenic purpura platelets. *Semin Hematol* 2000;37:222.
41. Rosse WF, Adams JP, Yount WJ. Subclasses of IgG antibodies in immune thrombocytopenic purpura (ITP). *Br J Haematol* 1980;46:109.

APPENDIX 25

Red Blood Cell Values at Various Ages: Mean and Lower Limit of Normal (–2 SD)

Age	Hemoglobin (g/dL)		Hematocrit (%)		Red Blood Cell Count (10^{12}/L)		MCV (fL)		MCH (pg)		MCHC (g/dL)	
	Mean	–2 SD	Mean	–2 SD	Mean	–2 SD	Mean	–2 SD	Mean	–2 SD	Mean	–2 SD
Birth (cord blood)	16.5	13.5	51	42	4.7	3.9	108	98	34	31	33	30
1–3 d (capillary)	18.5	14.5	56	45	5.3	4	108	95	34	31	33	29
1 wk	17.5	13.5	54	42	5.1	3.9	107	88	34	28	33	28
2 wk	16.5	12.5	51	39	4.9	3.6	105	86	34	28	33	28
1 mo	14	10	43	31	4.2	3	104	85	34	28	33	29
2 mo	11.5	9	35	28	3.8	2.7	96	77	30	26	33	29
3–6 mo	11.5	9.5	35	29	3.8	3.1	91	74	30	25	33	30
0.5–2.0 yr	12	10.5	36	33	4.5	3.7	78	70	27	23	33	30
2–6 yr	12.5	11.5	37	34	4.6	3.9	81	75	27	24	34	31
6–12 yr	13.5	11.5	40	35	4.6	4	86	77	29	25	34	31
12–18 yr												
Female	14	12	41	36	4.6	4.1	90	78	30	25	34	31
Male	14.5	13	43	37	4.9	4.5	88	78	30	25	34	31
18–49 yr												
Female	14	12.0	41	36	4.6	4	90	80	30	26	34	31
Male	15.5	13.5	47	41	5.2	4.5	90	80	30	26	34	31

MCH, mean corpuscular hemoglobin; MCHC, mean corpuscular hemoglobin concentration; MCV, mean corpuscular volume; SD, standard deviation.
NOTE: These data have been compiled from several sources. Emphasis is given to recent studies using electronic counters and to the selection of populations that are likely to exclude individuals with iron deficiency. The mean ± 2 SD can be expected to include 95% of the observations in a normal population.
Adapted from Dallman PR. In: Rudolph A, ed. *Pediatrics*, 16th ed. New York: Appleton-Century-Crofts, 1977:1111.

APPENDIX 26

Effect of Gestational Age of Fetuses *In Utero* and Newborn Infants on Their Hematocrit, Hemoglobin, Mean Corpuscular Volume (MCV), and Reticulocytes

Gestational Age (wk)	Hematocrit (%)[a]	Hemoglobin (g/dL)	MCV (fL)	Reticulocytes (%)
18–20[b]	36 ± 3	11.5 ± 0.8	134 ± 9	NR
21–22[b]	38 ± 3	12.3 ± 0.9	130 ± 6	NR
22–23[b]	38 ± 1	12.4 ± 0.9	125 ± 1	NR
24–25	63 ± 4	19.4 ± 1.5	135 ± 0	6.0 ± 0.5
26–27	62 ± 8	19.0 ± 2.5	132 ± 14	9.6 ± 3.2
28–29	60 ± 7	19.3 ± 1.8	131 ± 14	7.5 ± 2.5
30–31	60 ± 8	19.1 ± 2.2	127 ± 13	5.8 ± 2.0
32–33	60 ± 8	18.5 ± 2.0	123 ± 16	5.0 ± 1.9
34–35	61 ± 7	19.6 ± 2.1	122 ± 10	3.9 ± 1.6
36–37	64 ± 7	19.2 ± 1.7	121 ± 12	4.2 ± 1.8
Term	61 ± 7	19.3 ± 2.2	119 ± 9	3.2 ± 1.4

NR, not reported.

[a]Fetuses *in utero*.

[b]Values reported as the mean ± standard deviation.

Data from Zaizov R, Matoth Y. Red cell values on the first postnatal day during the last 16 weeks of gestation. *Am J Hematol* 1976;1:275; Forestier F, Daffos F, Galacteros F, et al. Hematological values of 163 normal fetuses between 18 and 30 weeks of gestation. *Pediat Res* 1986;20:342; and McIntosh N, Kempson C, Tyler RM. Blood counts in extremely low birth weight infants. *Arch Dis Child* 1988;63:74; and Christensen RD. Expected hematologic values for term and preterm neonates In: Christensen RD, ed. *Hematologic problems of the neonate*. Philadelphia: WB Saunders, 2000:120.

APPENDIX 27

Red Blood Cell (RBC) Parameters of Very-Low-Birth-Weight Infants during the First 6 Weeks of Life

	Day of Life	Valid *n*	Percentiles								
			3	5	10	25	Median	75	90	95	97
Hemoglobin (g/dL)	2	559	11	11.6	12.5	14.0	15.6	17.1	18.5	19.3	19.8
	12–14	203	10.1	10.8	11.1	12.5	14.4	15.7	17.4	18.4	18.9
	24–26	192	8.5	8.9	9.7	10.9	12.4	14.2	15.6	16.5	16.8
	40–42	150	7.8	7.9	8.4	9.3	10.6	12.4	13.8	14.9	15.4
Hematocrit (%)	3	561	35	36	39	43	47	52	56	59	60
	12–14	205	30	32	34	39	44	48	53	55	56
	24–26	196	25	27	29	32	39	44	48	50	52
	40–42	152	24	24	26	28	33	38	44	47	48
RBCs (10^{12}/L)	3	364	3.2	3.3	3.5	3.8	4.2	4.6	4.9	5.1	5.3
	12–14	196	2.9	3.0	3.2	3.5	4.1	4.6	5.2	5.5	5.6
	24–26	188	2.6	2.6	2.8	3.2	3.8	4.4	4.8	5.2	5.3
	40–42	148	2.5	2.5	2.6	3.0	3.4	4.1	4.6	4.8	4.9
Corrected reticulocytes (%)	3	283	0.6	0.7	1.9	4.2	7.1	12.0	20.0	24.1	27.8
	12–14	139	0.3	0.3	0.5	0.8	1.7	2.7	5.7	7.3	9.6
	24–26	140	0.2	0.3	0.5	0.8	1.5	2.6	4.7	6.4	8.6
	40–42	114	0.3	0.4	0.6	1.0	1.8	3.4	5.6	8.3	9.5

NOTE: On day 3, all infants are included irrespective of antenatal steroids and transfusions up to day 3. Thereafter, infants who did not receive recombinant human erythropoietin were studied, irrespective of use of antibiotics and steroids.

Adapted from Obladen M, Diepold K, Maier RF, et al. Venous and arterial hematologic profiles of very low birth weight infants. *Pediatrics* 2000;106:708.

APPENDIX 28

Hemoglobin Concentrations (g/dL) for Iron-Sufficient Preterm Infants

| | Birthweight | |
Age	1000–1500 g	1501–2000 g
2 wk	16.3 (11.7–18.4)	14.8 (11.8–19.6)
1 mo	10.5 (8.7–15.2)	11.5 (8.2–15.0)
2 mo	8.8 (7.1–11.5)	9.4 (8.0–11.4)
3 mo	9.8 (8.9–11.2)	10.2 (9.3–11.8)
4 mo	11.3 (9.1–13.1)	11.3 (9.1–13.1)
5 mo	11.6 (10.2–14.3)	11.8 (10.4–13.0)
6 mo	12.0 (9.4–13.8)	11.8 (10.7–12.6)

NOTE: Serum ferritin ≥ 10 ng/mL.
Adapted from Lundstrom U, Siimes MA, Dallman PR. At what age does iron supplementation become necessary in low birth weight infants? *J Pediatr* 1977;91:878.

APPENDIX 29

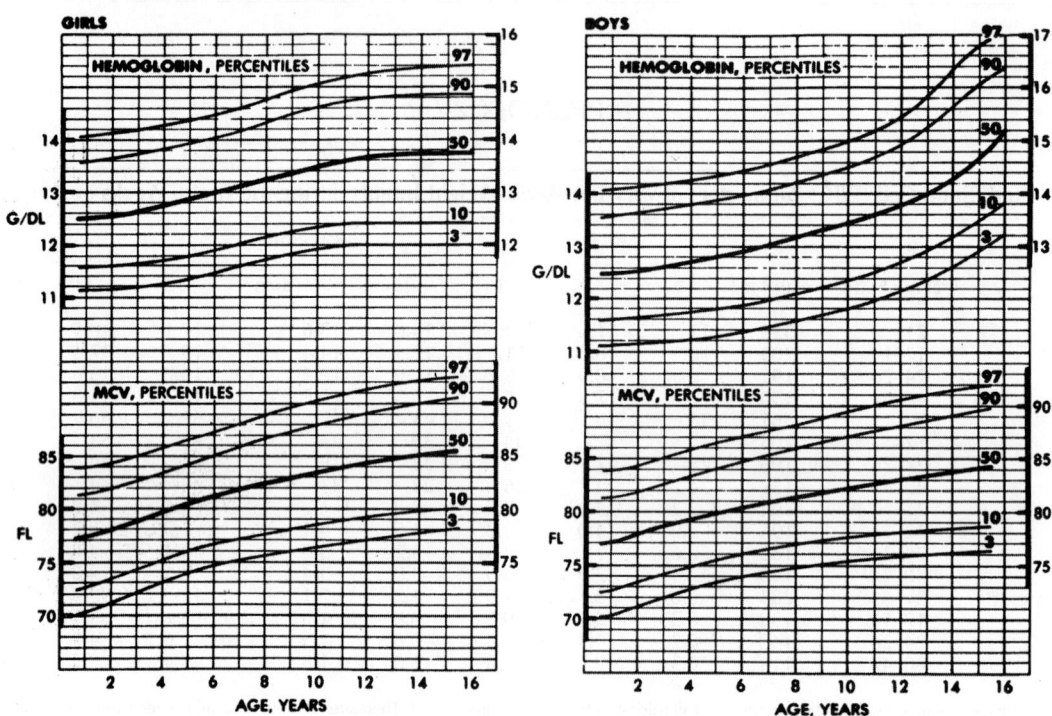

Hemoglobin and Mean Corpuscular Volume (MCV) Percentile Curves for Children. These figures were obtained from populations of nonindigent white U.S. or Finnish children who did not have laboratory evidence of iron deficiency, thalassemia minor, or hemoglobinopathy. (Adapted from Dallman PR, Siimes MA. Percentile curves for hemoglobin and red cell volume in infancy and childhood. *J Pediatr* 1979;94:26.)

APPENDIX 30

Effect of Pregnancy (with and without Iron Supplementation) on Hematocrit and Hemoglobin Values

Time	Hematocrit (Mean;%)			Hemoglobin (Mean; g/dL)		
	No Supplement	Intramuscular Supplement[a]	Oral Supplement[b]	No Supplement	Intramuscular Supplement[a]	Oral Supplement[b]
Weeks of gestation						
0	42.0	—	—	13.4	—	—
12	38.3	40.6	35.7	12.5	13.1	11.4
16	39.5	37.9	36.3	12.4	12.1	11.4
20	36.4	37.0	37.1	11.7	11.8	11.8
24	35.6	36.3	37.1	11.4	11.8	11.8
28	34.6	36.9	36.8	11.0	11.8	11.8
32	34.1	37.2	37.0	10.6	12.1	11.8
36	34.3	37.5	37.5	10.7	12.1	12.0
40	34.9	38.5	38.7	10.9	12.7	12.4
Days postpartum						
2	33.6	37.1	37.3	10.4	12.2	11.9
6	34.9	38.9	40.1	10.7	12.4	12.8
21	38.1	42.0	41.1	11.6	13.6	13.0
42	39.1	41.5	39.8	11.9	13.1	12.6
180	39.2	40.1	40.8	12.1	12.4	12.9

NOTE: Approximately 20 persons were in each group.
[a]1000 mg iron as iron dextran.
[b]39 mg elemental iron twice daily.
Adapted from de Leeuw NKM, Lowenstein L, Hsieh YS. Iron deficiency and hydremia in normal pregnancy. *Medicine* 1966;45:291.

APPENDIX 31

Red Cell Kinetic Parameters in Normal Subjects

Parameter	Value	Unit
Red cell mass	Males: 28.7 ± 3.8	mL/kg
	Females: 25.3 ± 2.6	—
Plasma volume	Males: 36.9 ± 4.2	—
	Females: 41.9 ± 4.4	—
^{51}Cr disappearance half-time	Range: 28–35	Days
	Males: 30.1 ± 4.0	—
	Females: 29.4 ± 2.1	—
Rate of ^{51}Cr label elution	Range: 0.68–1.31	% per d
Plasma Fe disappearance half-time	85 ± 5	Minutes
Incorporation of ^{59}Fe into erythrocytes	82 ± 1	—
	Range: 79–89	% at 14 d
Plasma Fe turnover	0.75 ± 0.02	mg/100 mL whole blood/d
	121 ± 17	µM/L whole blood/d
Erythroid Fe turnover	0.56	mg/100 mL whole blood/d
	86 ± 10	µmol/L whole blood/d

APPENDIX 32

Estimated Blood Volumes

Age	Plasma Volume (mL/kg)	Red Cell Mass (mL/kg)	Total Blood Volume (mL/kg) From Plasma Volume	Total Blood Volume (mL/kg) From Red Cell Mass
Newborn	41.3	43.1	82.1	86.1
	46	—	—	84.7
	—	—	78	—
1–7 d	51–54	—	82–86	—
		37.9	—	77.8
1–12 mo	46.1	—	78.1	—
		25.5	—	72.8
1–3 yr	44.4	—	73.8	—
	47.2	—	81.8	—
		24.9	—	69.1
4–6 yr	48.5	—	80.0	—
	49.6	—	85.6	—
		25.5	—	67.5
7–9 yr	52.2	—	87.6	—
	49.0	—	86.1	—
		24.3	—	67.5
10–12 yr	51.9	—	87.6	—
	46.2	—	83.2	—
		26.3	—	67.4
13–15 yr	51.2	—	88.3	—
16–18 yr	50.1	—	90.2	—
Adults	39–44	25–30	68–88	55–75

Adapted from Price DC, Ries C. In: Handmaker H. Lowenstein JM, eds. *Nuclear medicine in clinical pediatrics.* New York: Society of Nuclear Medicine, 1975:279.

APPENDIX 33

Estimation of Red Cell, Plasma, and Total Blood Volume in Adults

Volume	Men a	Men b	Men SD (mL)	Women a	Women b	Women SD (mL)
Red cell volume	490	21.4	200	409	18.3	139
Plasma volume	1050	19.6	260	455	28.9	213
Total blood volume	1530	41.0	400	864	47.2	319

SD, standard deviation.
NOTE: For a subject of given weight (w, in kg) in a normal mean red cell, plasma, or total blood volume (V, in mL) can be calculated from the formula, $V = a + bw$. Example: In a 70-kg man, the mean red cell volume is $490 + (21.4 \times 70) = 1988$ mL $\pm$ 2 SD; range = 1988 ± 400; or 1588 to 2388 mL. The expected normal range can be calculated from the following formula: range = mean $\pm$ 2 SD. Calculations are based on red cell volume measured by ^{51}Cr method and on plasma and blood volumes calculated from the volume of packed red cells without correction for trapped plasma or "body hematocrit" differences.
After Brown E, et al. Red cell, plasma and blood volume in healthy women measured by radiochromium cell labeling and hematocrit. *J Clin Invest* 1962;41:2182; and Wennesland R, et al. Red cell, plasma, and blood volume in healthy men measured by radiochromium cell tagging and hematocrit. *J Clin Invest* 1959;38:1065.

APPENDIX 34

Values of Serum Iron, Iron-Binding Capacity, and Transferrin Saturation from Infants during the First Year of Life

			Age (mo)						
			0.5	1	2	4	6	9	12
Serum iron	Median	(µg/dL)	120	125	87	84	77	84	78
	95% range		63–201	58–172	15–159	18–164	28–135	34–135	35–155
Iron-binding capacity	Mean ± standard deviation	(µg/dL)	191 ± 43	199 ± 43	246 ± 55	300 ± 39	321 ± 51	341 ± 42	358 ± 38
Saturation	Median		68	63	34	27	23	25	23
	95% range		30–99	35–94	21–63	7–53	10–43	10–39	10–47

NOTE: The data were collected from healthy full-term Finnish infants whose formula and cereal were supplemented with iron throughout the first year. Infants with a hemoglobin <11 g/dL, mean corpuscular volume <71 fL, or serum ferritin <10/ng/mL were excluded.
Adapted from Saarinen UM, Siimes MA. Developmental changes in serum iron, total iron-binding capacity, and transferrin saturation in infancy. *J Pediatr* 1977;91;875–877.

APPENDIX 35

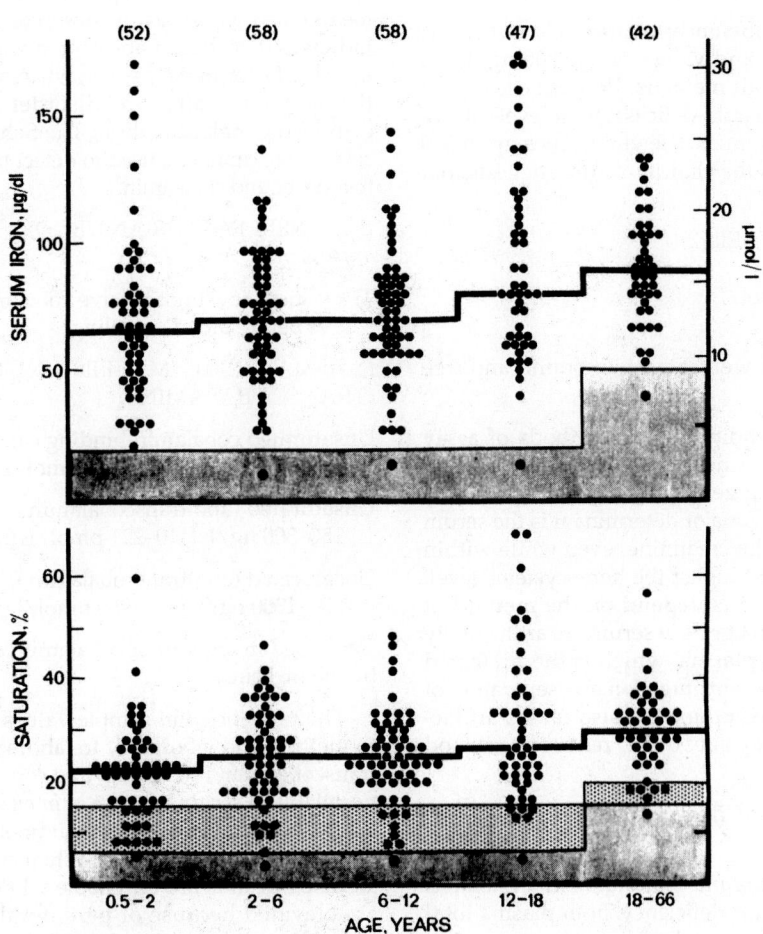

Serum Iron and Transferrin Saturation. Values in subjects with values for hemoglobin, mean corpuscular volume, free erythrocyte protoporphyrin, and serum ferritin. (Adapted from Koerper MA, Dallman P. Serum iron concentration and transferrin saturation in the diagnosis of iron deficiency in children: normal developmental changes. *J Pediatr* 1977;91:870.)

Normal Reference Ranges for Cobalamin, Folate, and Related Tests

RED BLOOD CELL FOLATE
160–640 µg/L [363–1450 nmol/L (SI)]

SERUM FOLATE
2.5–20.0 µg/L [5.7–45.3 nmol/L (SI)]

Metabolic studies suggest that serum folate values of 2.5–4.0 µg/L represent borderline folate deficiency.

SERUM COBALAMIN
200–900 ng/L [148–665 pmol/L (SI)]

Reference values differ with different assay methods, but generally approximate this range, and values below 200 ng/L are considered low with almost all methods. Because occasional patients are found to be cobalamin-deficient with levels above 200 ng/L, some authors recommend viewing values up to 300 or 350 ng/L with suspicion if the clinical picture suggests that deficiency is likely.

PLASMA TOTAL HOMOCYSTEINE
Children: 3.5–10.5 µmol/L
Adult women: 4.8–13.8 µmol/L
Adult men: 5.2–14.5 µmol/L

Includes mixed disulfides as well as protein-bound and free homocysteine.

Normal ranges vary, depending on the methods of assay and definitions of normality. Among many influences on the homocysteine level (including gender, age, genetic polymorphisms, and lifestyle factors), a major determinant is the serum creatinine level. The higher the creatinine, even while within the normal reference range, the higher the homocysteine level. Moreover, homocysteine results depend on the method of blood sampling and collection: Levels in serum are artifactually and variably higher than in plasma, which is the preferred source. Delay of blood sample centrifugation and separation of plasma beyond 1 hour after venipuncture also causes artifactual elevation of homocysteine values due to release from blood cells *in vitro*.

SERUM METHYLMALONIC ACID
90–280 nmol/L

In folate-deficient patients, only plasma total homocysteine is elevated, whereas in cobalamin deficiency, both plasma total homocysteine and methylmalonic acid are both elevated.

SCHILLING TEST OF FREE COBALAMIN ABSORPTION (URINARY EXCRETION TEST)
>8% excretion of the radiolabeled cobalamin dose in a full 24-hour collection of urine

A valid test result requires a complete 24-hour collection of urine, normal renal function, and the patient receiving no parenteral cobalamin for 48–72 hours before the test dose is given. When excretion is <8%, the malabsorptive defect can be further localized by repeating the test and giving oral intrinsic factor together with the radiolabeled cobalamin dose; correction of excretion to normal indicates that the malabsorption was due to the lack of gastric intrinsic factor in the patient, whereas failure to correct indicates that either a small bowel disorder or pancreatic insufficiency caused the malabsorption. The Schilling test, which uses free cobalamin, cannot be used to detect malabsorption that is limited to food-bound cobalamin.

INTRINSIC FACTOR ANTIBODY
Absent

The patient must not receive cobalamin by injection for at least 3 days before blood sampling.

PLASMA COBALAMIN-BINDING CAPACITY (TRANSCOBALAMINS)

Unsaturated cobalamin-binding capacity
800–1600 ng/L [590–1180 pmol/L (SI)]

Unsaturated (apo)transcobalamin I
150–300 ng/L [110–221 pmol/L (SI)]

Unsaturated (apo)transcobalamin II
600–1300 ng/L [443–960 pmol/l (SI)]

Expressed in amount of cobalamin added *in vitro* that is bound by the proteins.

The reference and sample values vary greatly from method to method and laboratory to laboratory. Levels of unsaturated transcobalamin I (R binder) and cobalamin-binding capacity are unreliable in serum because of *in vitro* release of transcobalamin I from leukocytes; ethylenediaminetetraacetic acid–anticoagulated plasma must be used. When cobalamin-binding methods are used, results are unreliable when plasma cobalamin levels are elevated because of parenteral cobalamin therapy. This appendix contributed by Dr. Ralph Carmel.

APPENDIX 37

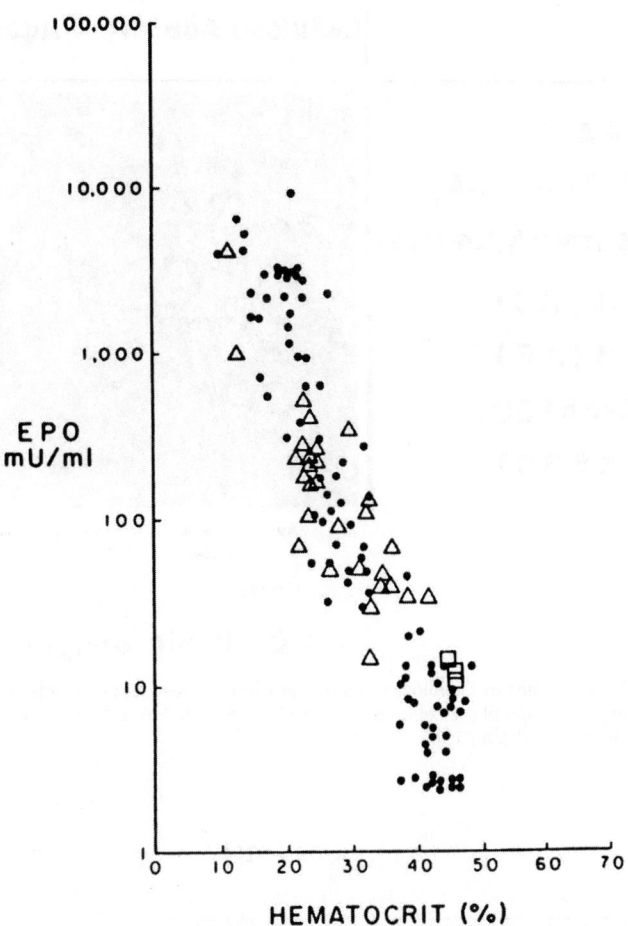

Erythropoietin (EPO) Titers. Titers were measured with biologic and radioimmune assays in normal subjects and in patients with anemia caused by renal or chronic diseases. Circles, anemic and normal subjects; squares, normal subjects; triangles, anemic patients. (Adapted from Ersler AJ, Wilson J, Caro J. Erythropoietin titers in anemic, nonuremic patients. *J Lab Clin Med* 1987;109:429.)

APPENDIX 38

Effect of Altitude on Hematocrit in Normal Males

Altitude			
ft	m	n	Hematocrit[a] (%)
0	0	721	47
4400	1340	744	49.5
7457	2280	100	51
12,240	3740	40	54
14,900	4540	32	61
17,800	5430	10	69

[a]Mean values in males.
Adapted from Cartwright GE. *Diagnostic laboratory hematology*, ed 4. New York: Grune & Stratton, 1968.

APPENDIX 39

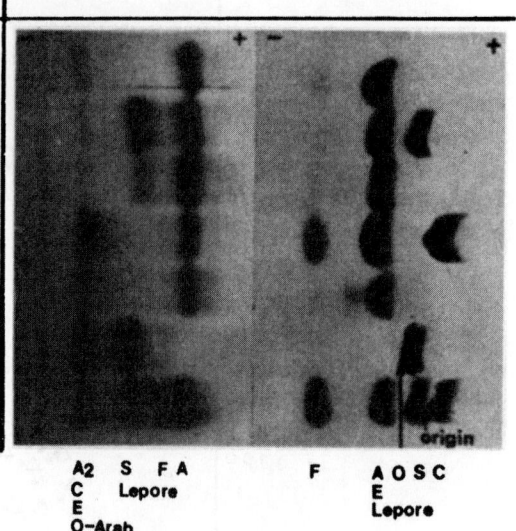

Cellulose Acetate   Agar Gel

Normal (AA₂)

Sickle Cell Trait(ASA₂)

Hb Lepore trait(A,Lepore)

Hb C Trait (AC)

Hb E Trait (AE)

Hb SO - Arab (SO)

Control (A F S C)

A2   S   F A
C   Lepore
E
O-Arab

F   A O S C
          E
          Lepore

* : Carbonic anhydrase

Differentiation of Hemoglobins by Cellulose Acetate and Citrate-Agar Gel Electrophoresis. Origin is at the left border of the photograph of the cellulose acetate strip. (Adapted from Kim HC. Inherited hemoglobinopathies in children. *Clin Pediatr* 1981;20:161.)

APPENDIX 40

Electrophoretic Relative Mobilities of Hemoglobin Variants under Different Conditions

Supporting Medium, Buffer, and pH	Relative Migration Rates of Various Hemoglobins[a]						
Starch gel, paper, starch block, agarose; barbital, pH 8.6; tris-EDTA-borate buffer, pH 8.8	C	E	S	A	J	H	+
			O	DL	FMK	46N3	I
			A	5G		2	
			1[a]	P			
Cellulose acetate; tris-EDTA-borate buffer, pH 8.6[b]		C	S	A	J	H	+
		A₂	D				
		7					
Starch gel, paper, starch block; phosphate buffer, pH 6.8	C	L	S	AI	2	|H	+
	O		DGPF	JN		|	
	A₂		5E	K		|	
Agar gel; phosphate or citrate buffer, pH 6.2	F		A	S		|C	+
			D	O7	HL	|	
			E		Q	|	
			A₂			|	
			G				
			c				

NOTE: Dashed lines indicate origin.

[a]1, Alexander; 2, Barts; 3, Hopkins I; 4, Hopkins II; 5, Lepore; 6, Norfolk; 7, C_Harlem.

[b]With a discontinuous buffer system, migration is to the cathodal side, possibly because of a greater electroendosmotic flow.

[c]Also I, J, P, 1, 2, 3, 4, 5.

Adapted from Kim HC, Adachi K, Schwartz E. Separation of hemoglobins. In: Williams WJ, Beutler E, Erslev AJ, Lichtman MA. *Hematology,* ed 4. New York: McGraw-Hill, 1990:1712.

APPENDIX 41

Percentage of Hemoglobins (Hbs) F and A2 in Newborns and Adults

	Hb F (%) (Gα/Aα Ratio)	Hb A2 (%)
Newborn	60–90 (3:1)	<1
Adult	<1 (2:3)	1.6–3.5

NOTE: The α chains of fetal hemoglobin contain either a glycyl residue or an alanyl residue at position 136. The Gα/Aα ratio in the newborn undergoes a considerable change between the third and fourth month of life, at which time it approximates that of the Hb F of adults.
Adapted from Charache S. In: Altman PL, Dittmer DS, eds. *Human health and disease.* Bethesda: Federation of American Societies for Experimental Biology 1977:159.

APPENDIX 42

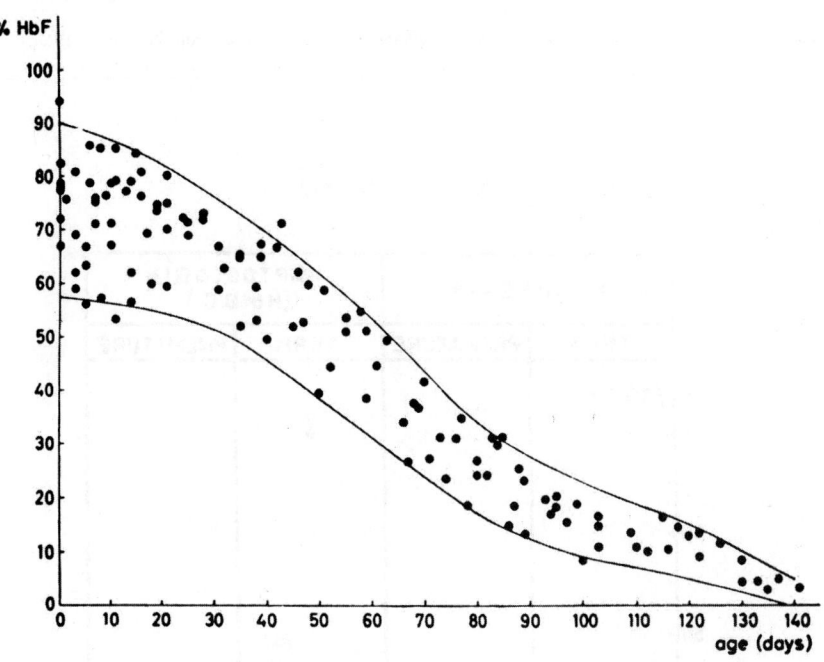

Time Course of the Relative Hemoglobin F (HbF) Concentration in Blood from Normal Infants. (After Garby I, Sjolin S. Development of erythropoiesis. *Acta Paediatr [Stockh]* 1962;51:245.)

APPENDIX 43

Methemoglobin Levels in Normal Subjects

	Number of Cases	Methemoglobin (g/dL)			Methemoglobin as Percentage of Total Hemoglobin		
		Mean	Range	SD	Mean	Range	SD
Prematures	50	0.38	(0.02–0.83)	±0.1	2.2	(0.08–4.7)	±1.1
Newborns (1–10 d)	39	0.22	(0.00–0.58)	±0.17	1.5	(0.00–2.8)	±0.81
Infants (1 mo–1 yr)	8	0.14	(0.02–0.29)	±0.09	1.2	(0.17–2.4)	±0.78
Children (1–14 yr)	35	0.11	(0.00–0.33)	±0.09	0.79	(0.00–2.4)	±0.62
Adults (14–78 yr)	30	0.11	(0.00–0.28)	±0.09	0.82	(0.00–1.9)	±0.63

SD, standard deviation.
NOTE: Apparently well individuals without cyanosis or respiratory disease. The nitrate level in the milk and water ingested by the infants was less than 0.027 ppm. The premature infants were treated with oral vitamin C.
Adapted from Kravitz H, Elegant LD, et al. Methemoglobin values in premature and mature infants and children. *Am J Dis Child* 1956;91:2–5.

APPENDIX 44

Normal Values for Osmotic Fragility

Sodium Chloride Concentration (g/dL)	Percentage of Hemolysis	
	Before Incubation	After Incubation
0.85	0	0
0.75	0	0–2
0.65	0	0–19
0.60	0	0–40
0.55	0	5–70
0.50	0–5	36–88
0.45	0–45	54–96
0.40	50–90	65–100
0.35	90–99	72–100
0.30	97–100	80–100
0.20	100	91–100
0.10	100	100

Adapted from Cartwright GE. *Diagnostic laboratory hematology*, 4th ed. New York: Grune & Stratton, 1968.

APPENDIX 45

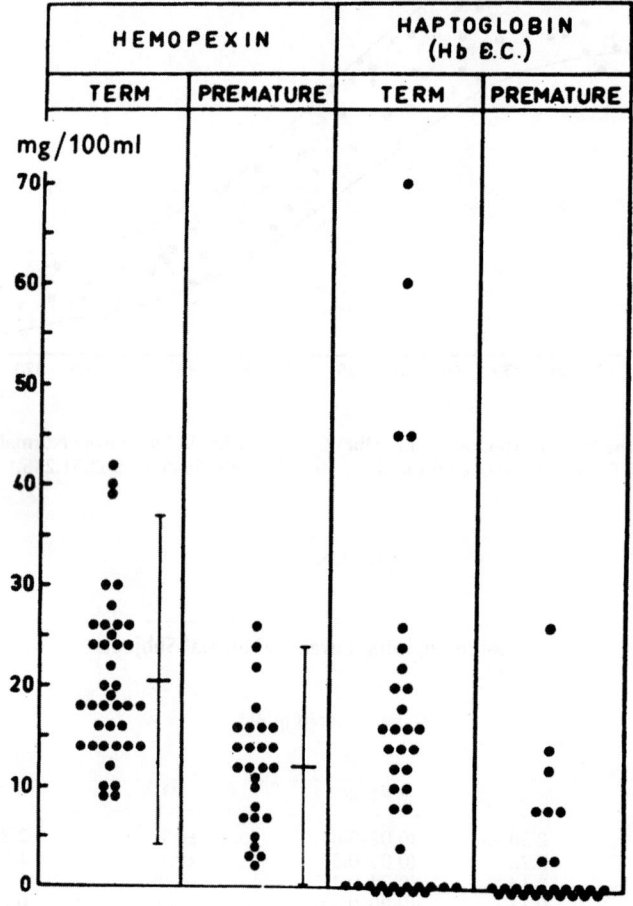

Plasma Concentration of Hemopexin and Haptoglobin in Term and Premature Infants. The means are indicated to the right of the hemopexin results. (Adapted from Lundh B, Oski FA, et al. Plasma hemopexin and haptoglobin in hemolytic diseases of the newborn. *Acta Paediatr Scand* 1970;59:121.)

APPENDIX 46

Activities of Red Cell Enzymes in Normal Adults

Enzyme	Activity at 37°C (Mean ± Standard Deviation)
Acetylcholinesterase	36.93 ± 3.83
Adenosine deaminase	1.11 ± 0.23
Adenylate kinase	258 ± 29.3
Aldolase	3.19 ± 0.86
Bisphosphoglyceromutase (2,3-diphosphoglyceromutase)	4.78 ± 0.65
Catalase	$15.3 \pm 2.4 \times 10^4$
Enolase	5.39 ± 0.83
Epimerase	0.23 ± 0.06
Galactokinase	0.029 ± 0.004
Galactose-1-phosphate a uridyl transferase	28.4 ± 6.94
Glucose phosphate isomerase	60.8 ± 11.0
Glucose-6-phosphate dehydrogenase	8.34 ± 1.59
WHO method	12.1 ± 2.09
γ-Glutamyl-cysteine synthetase	0.43 ± 0.04
Glutathione peroxidase	30.82 ± 4.65
Glutathione reductase without FAD	7.18 ± 1.09
Glutathione reductase with FAD	10.4 ± 1.50
Glutathione-S-transferase	6.66 ± 1.81
Glyceraldehyde phosphate dehydrogenase	226 ± 41.9
Glutamic oxaloacetic transaminase without PLP	3.02 ± 0.67
Glutamic oxaloacetic transaminase with PLP	5.04 ± 0.90
Hexokinase	1.78 ± 0.38
Hypoxanthine phosphoribosyl-transferase	1.72 ± 0.30
Lactate dehydrogenase	200 ± 26.5
Methemoglobin reductase	2.60 ± 0.71
Monophosphoglyceromutase	37.71 ± 5.56
NADH-methemoglobin reductase	19.2 ± 3.85 (30°C)
NADPH diaphorase	2.26 ± 0.16
Phosphofructokinase	11.01 ± 2.33
Phosphoglucomutase	5.50 ± 0.62
Phosphoglycerate kinase	320 ± 36.1
Phosphoglycolate phosphatase	1.23 ± 0.10
Pyrimidine 5' nucleotidase	0.11 ± 0.03
Pyruvate kinase	15.0 ± 1.99
6-Phosphogluconate dehydrogenase	8.78 ± 0.78
Triose phosphate isomerase	2111 ± 397

FAD, flavin adenine dinucleotide; NADH, nicotinamide adenine dinucleotide (reduced form); NADPH, nicotinamide adenine dinucleotide phosphate; PLP, pyridoxal 5'-phosphate; WHO, World Health Organization.
Adapted from Beutler E, Blum KG. In: Altman PL, Dittmer DS, eds. *Human health and disease.* Bethesda: Federation of American Societies for Experimental Biology,1977:156; and Beutler E. *Red cell metabolism: a manual of biochemical methods*, 3rd ed. Orlando: Grune & Stratton, 1984.

APPENDIX 47

Level of Intermediates in Red Cells of Normal Adults

Intermediate	Abbreviation	Concentration (Mean ± 1 Standard Deviation)		
		nmol/g Hb	nmol/mL Red Cells	µmol/L in Whole Blood
Adenosine-5'-diphosphate	ADP	6635 ± 105	216 ± 36	—
Adenosine-5'-monophosphate	AMP	62 ± 10	21.1 ± 3.4	—
Adenosine-5'-triphosphate	ATP	4230 ± 290 (whites)	1438 ± 99	—
		3530 ± 301 (blacks)	1200 ± 102	—
2,3-Diphosphoglycerate	2,3-DPG	1227 ± 1870	4171 ± 636	—
Glutathione	GSH	6570 ± 1040	2234 ± 354	—
Glutathione (oxidized)	GSSG	12.3 ± 4.5	4.2 ± 1.53	—
Glucose-6-phosphate	G6P	82 ± 22	27.8 ± 7.5	—
Fructose-6-phosphate	F6P	27 ± 5.8	9.3 ± 2.0	—
Fructose-6-diphosphate	FDP	5.6 ± 1.8	1.9 ± 0.6	—
Dihydroxyacetone phosphate	DHAP	27.6 ± 8.2	9.4 ± 2.8	—
3-Phosphoglyceric acid	3-PGA	132 ± 15.0	44.9 ± 5.1	—
2-Phosphoglyceric acid	2-PGA	21.5 ± 7.35	7.3 ± 2.5	—
Phosphoenolpyruvate	PEP	35.9 ± 6.47	12.2 ± 2.2	—
Creatine	—	1310 ± 310 (male)	445 ± 105	—
	—	1500 ± 250 (female)	510 ± 85	—
Lactate	—	—	—	932 ± 211
Pyruvate	—	—	—	53.3 ± 21.5

Hb, hemoglobin.
Adapted from Beutler E. *Red cell metabolism: a manual of biochemical methods*, 3rd ed. Orlando: Grune & Stratton, 1984.

APPENDIX 48

Normal Values of Heme Pathway Enzymes

Enzyme	Liver	Erythroid Cells	Fibroblasts	Lymphocytes
ALA synthase, nmol/h of ALA/gram	24	49[a,b]	5.3[c]	120[c,d]
ALA dehydratase, nmol/h of PBG/gram	1100, 1300	2500[e]	120[c,f]	290[c,d]
PBG deaminase, nmol/h of hydroxymethylbilane/gram	2.80	36[e]	6.1[c,g]	6.1[c,d], 10[c,j]
Uroporphyrinogen III cosynthase, nmol/h of uroporphyrinogen III	—	6600[e,h,j]	8800[c,l]	—
Uroporphyrinogen decarboxylase, nmol/h of coproporphyrinogen/gram	170[c]	720[k]	310[c]	480[c,i]
Coproporphyrinogen oxidase, nmol/h of protoporphyrinogen/gram	220[c]	—	87[c]	73[c,i]
Protoporphyrinogen oxidase, nmol/h of protoporphyrin/gram	—	—	300[c]	658[c,i]
Ferrochelatase, nmol/h of heme/gram	350	18[a,b]	3.7[c,m], 6.2[m]	310[c,l], 1900[m]

ALA, δ-amino levulinic acid; PBG, porphobilinogen.
NOTE: Only mean values are cited in this table. To make comparisons of enzymatic activities, certain assumptions were made to recalculate reported data so that they can be expressed per gram of tissue per hour of incubation.
[a]Assuming 2×10^8 erythroblasts/gram of bone marrow.
[b]Bone marrow.
[c]Assuming 150 mg of protein per gram of tissue.
[d]Mitogen-stimulated lymphocytes.
[e]Erythrocytes.
[f]Sassa et al., unpublished data.
[g]At 60°C.
[h]Assuming 300 g hemoglobin/gram of erythrocytes.
[i]At 31°C.
[j]Epstein Barr virus–transformed lymphocytes.
[k]Assuming that uroporphyrinogen III is used as substrate (approximately five times faster than 5-carboxylate porphyrinogen I).
[l]Nonstimulated lymphocytes.
[m]Mesoporphyrin as substrate.

APPENDIX 49

Relative Strength of Antigens on Cord Cells and Antigens Implicated in Hemolytic Disease of the Newborn (HDN)

Antigen Strength	Blood Group System or Antigen	Causes HDN
Well-developed at birth		
	MNSsU	Yes[1]
	Rh	Yes
	Kell	Yes
	Duffy	Yes
	Kidd	Yes
	Diego	Yes
	Dombrock	Yes (mild)
	Scianna	—
	Gerbich	Yes (mild)
	En^a	—
	Yt^b	—
Present at birth: weaker than adult		
	ABH	Yes
	P	No[2]
	Lutheran	Yes
Very weak or absent at birth		
	Yt^a	—
	Vel	—
	Lewis	—
	I	No
	Sd^a	No

[1]Anti-M is rarely a cause of HDN.
[2]Anti-Tj^a (Anti-PP1P^k) has caused HDN.
Adapted from Kline W. Chemistry of blood group antigens and antibodies in hemolytic disease of the newborn. In: Bell C, ed. *A seminar on perinatal blood banking.* Washington, DC: American Association of Blood Banks, 1978:21.

APPENDIX 50

Relative Frequencies of Erythrocyte Alloantibodies

Blood Group System	Relative Frequency of Antibody	Relative Potency of Antigen [Compared with K (Kell)]
Rh^a	0.5	0.3
Kell	0.3	1
Duffy	0.15	0.04
Kidd	0.05	0.01
Other	<0.01	Negligible

^{a}Rh(D) excluded.

APPENDIX 51

**Immunization Recommendations for Patients at
High Risk for Pneumococcal Infection**

Age	Number of Previous Doses	Recommendations
<24 mo	None	PCV7 as recommended for infants and toddlers
24–59 mo	4 doses PCV7	1 dose of 23-PS at 24 mo, at least 6–8 wk after the last dose of PCV7
24–59 mo	1–3 doses PCV7	1 dose of PCV7; 1 dose of 23-PS 6–8 wk after the last dose of PCV7; 1 dose 23-PS 3–5 yr after last dose of 23-PS
24–59 mo	1 dose 23-PS	Two doses PCV7 6–8 wk apart beginning 6–8 wk after last dose of 23-PS; 1 dose 23-PS 3–5 yr after last dose of 23-PS
24–59 mo	None	Two doses of PCV7 6–8 wk apart; 1 dose 23-PS 6–8 wk after the last dose of PCV7; 1 dose of 23-PS 3–5 yr after the last dose of 23-PS
6–13 yr	None	1 dose of PCV7; 1 dose of 23-PS 6–8 wk after PCV7, repeat 23-PS 3–5 yr after the first or 1 dose of 23-PS; repeat 3–5 yr after the first
>13 yr	None	1 dose of 23-PS; repeat 3–5 yr after the first

PCV7, pneumococcal conjugate vaccine (Prevnar); 23-PS, pneumococcal polysaccharide vaccine (Pneumovax).
NOTE: Patients undergoing elective splenectomy or who are to receive immunocompromising therapy should receive either the 23-PS or PCV7 immunization at least 2 weeks before surgery/treatment.
Adapted from American Academy of Pediatrics. Committee on Infectious Diseases. Policy statement: recommendations for the prevention of pneumococcal infections, including the use of pneumococcal conjugate vaccine (Prevnar), pneumococcal polysaccharide vaccine, and antibiotic prophylaxis. *Pediatrics* 2000;106:362–366.

APPENDIX 52

**Antibiotic Doses for Prophylaxis for Patients
with Asplenia/Hyposplenia**

Age	Penicillin V	Amoxicillin	Erythromycin[a]
2 mo–3 yr	125 mg p.o. b.i.d.	125 mg p.o. b.i.d.	125 mg p.o. q.d.
3 yr and older	250 mg p.o. b.i.d.	250 mg p.o. b.i.d.	250 mg p.o. q.d.

[a]To be used only for patients with a penicillin allergy.

APPENDIX 53

The Genetic Code

1st Position	2nd Position				3rd Position
(5' end)	U or T	C	A	G	(3' end)
U or T	Phe	Ser	Tyr	Cys	U or T
	Phe	Ser	Tyr	Cys	C
	Leu	Ser	STOP	STOP	A
	Leu	Ser	STOP	Trp	G
C	Leu	Pro	His	Arg	U or T
	Leu	Pro	His	Arg	C
	Leu	Pro	Gln	Arg	A
	Leu	Pro	Gln	Arg	G
A	Ile	Thr	Asn	Ser	U or T
	Ile	Thr	Asn	Ser	C
	Ile	Thr	Lys	Arg	A
	Met	Thr	Lys	Arg	G
G	Val	Ala	Asp	Gly	U or T
	Val	Ala	Asp	Gly	C
	Val	Ala	Glu	Gly	A
	Val	Ala	Glu	Gly	G

APPENDIX 54

Amino Acids

Amino Acid	Three-Letter Abbreviation	One-Letter Symbol
Basic (+)		
Arginine	Arg	R
Histidine	His	H
Lysine	Lys	K
Acidic (−)		
Aspartic acid	Asp	D
Glutamic acid	Glu	E
Polar		
Asparagine	Asp	N
Cysteine	Cys	C
Glutamine	Gln	Q
Glycine	Gly	G
Serine	Ser	S
Threonine	Thr	T
Tyrosine	Tyr	Y
Nonpolar		
Alanine	Ala	A
Isoleucine	Ile	I
Leucine	Leu	L
Methionine	Met	M
Phenylalanine	Phe	F
Proline	Pro	P
Tryptophan	Trp	W
Valine	Val	V

APPENDIX 55

International System of Units (SI) Conversion Table

Constituent	Traditional Units	Multiplication Factor[a]	SI Units
δ-Aminolevulinic acid (U)	mg/d	7.63	μmol/d
Bilirubin			
Direct (S)	mg/dL	17.1	μmol/L
Total (S)	mg/dL	17.1	μmol/ L
Calcium (S)	mg/dL	0.25	mmol/L
Coproporphyrin (U)	μg/d	1.5	nmol/d
Erythrocyte count (B)	Number per μL	10^6	Number per L
Fibrinogen[b] (factor I) (P)	mg/dL	0.01	g/L
	mg/dL	0.029	μmol/L
Folic acid (S)	ng/mL	1.0	μg/L
	ng/mL	2.27	nmol/L
Haptoglobin (S)	mg/dL	0.01	g/L
Hematocrit (B)	%	0.01	ratio
Hemoglobin[c] (B)	g/dL	1.0	g/dL
Iron (S)	μg/dL	0.179	μmol/L
Iron-binding capacity (S)	μg/dL	0.179	μmol/ L
Leukocyte count (B)	Number per μL	10^6	Number per L
Mean corpuscular hemoglobin	pg	1.0	pg
Mean corpuscular hemoglobin con-centration	%	1.0	g/dL
Mean corpuscular volume	μm^3	1.0	fL
Packed cell volume (B)	%	0.01	Ratio
Phosphorus (S)	mg/dL	0.323	mmol/L
Platelet count (B)	Number per μL	10^6	Number per L
Prophobilinogen (U)	mg/d	4.42	μmol/D
Protoporphyrin (erythrocyte)	μg/dL	0.018	μmol/L
Reticulocyte count (B)	%	0.01	Ratio
	Number per μL	10^6	Number per l
Transferrin (S)	mg/dL	0.01	g per l
Urea nitrogen (B)	mg/dL	0.36	mmol/L
Uric acid (S)	mg/dL	0.0595	mmol/L
Uroporphyrin (U)	μg/d	1.2	nmol/d
Vitamin B_{12} (S)	pg/mL	1.0	ng/L
	pg/mL	0.738	pmol/L

B, blood; S, serum; P, plasma; U, urine.

[a]Conventional units multiplied by this factor yield SI units.

[b]The molar concentration is calculated assuming a molecular weight of 340,000.

[c]Hemoglobin is not usually expressed in molar terms because of uncertainty regarding the polymeric state of the molecule, if the unit (globin chain) molecular weight is assumed to be 16,000, the multiplication factor is 0.62 to convert g/dL to mmol/L. If a molecular weight of 64,500 is assumed (hemoglobin molecule, $\alpha_2\beta_2$ tetramer), the conversion factor is 0.155. Data from Baron DN, Broughton PMG, Cohen M, et al. The use of SI units in reporting results obtained in hospital laboratories. *J Clin Pathol* 1974;27:590; Young DS. "Normal laboratory values" [case records of the Massachusetts General Hospital] in SI units. *N Engl J Med* 1975;292:795; Lehmann HP. Metrication of clinical laboratory data in SI units. *Am J Clin Pathol* 1976;65:2; and Williams WJ, Beutler E, Ersler AJ, et al. *Hematology*, 4th ed. New York: McGraw-Hill, 1990:1784.

Index

Page numbers followed by *f* refer to figures; those followed by *t* refer to tables.

stimulatory factor 1, 185
tolerance to self-antigens, 613
tumor necrosis factor superfamily members affecting, 603t
in X-linked agammaglobulinemia, 691–692
B5 fixative for bone marrow specimens, 64t
Babesiosis
hemolysis in, 1983
postsplenectomy, in hereditary spherocytosis, 1786–1787
transfusion-transmitted, 2059
Back pain in lymphoma and myeloma, 12
BACOP chemotherapy regimen in aggressive lymphomas, 878
Bacteremia in sickle cell disease, 1677t, 1678
Bacterial growth
hypoferremia affecting, 1978
in small intestine, cobalamin deficiency in, 1378
Bactericidal permeability-increasing protein in azurophilic neutrophil granules, 546
BAL in lead poisoning, 1470
Banana bodies in Farber's disease, 949
Band 3 protein
animal and fish models of mutants, 1773f, 1773–1774
defects in hereditary spherocytosis, 1765f, 1765–1769, 1766t–1768t
in membranes of red cells, 1715f, 1716t, 1717–1721, 1718f
cytoplasmic domain, 1717–1719, 1719f
interaction with protein 4.1, 1735
membrane domain, 1719–1721
mutations in, 1721
in Southeast Asian ovalocytosis, 1807–1808
nonerythroid, 1721
posttranslational modifications of, 1742t
synthesis initiating membrane skeleton assembly, 1743–1744
Band 8 in membranes of red cells. See Peroxiredoxin-2
Band neutrophils, 456, 456f
in bone marrow, 70t, 71f, 72
Banding of chromosomes, 96, 97f
Bantu siderosis, 1420
Barbiturate interactions with coumarins, 1335t
Bare lymphocyte syndrome, 675
immunophenotyping of, 50t
Barth syndrome, neutropenia in, 467
Bartonellosis, hemolysis in, 1983
Basophil(s), 573–580
absolute and relative values for, 2194t
activation for mediator release, 578
in bone marrow, 70t, 71
in normal aspirates, 2193t
stains for, 66t
constituents and products of, 576–577
degranulation of, 578, 578f
differential counts, 26, 27t
functions of, 577–578
granules in, 156, 576, 576f
in host defense, 578
IgE-primed, 578, 578f
in immune responses, 579
in infants, 2192t
in inflammations, 579
maturation of, 156
morphology of, 576, 576f
natural history of, 574t
production and circulation of, 574
in reactions to neoplasms, 579
receptors on, 575t
responses to parasite antigens, 579
tissue distribution of, 574

Basophilia, 579t, 580, 580t
induction by IL-3, 575–576
Basophilic stippling of erythrocytes
in Heinz body hemolytic syndrome, 1635
in lead poisoning, 1469, 1469f
Basophilopenia, 579t, 579–580
Batimastat, 2126
BAY 12-9566, 2126
structure of, 2123f
Bayes theorem, and probability of bleeding disorders, 976, 976f
bcl-1 proto-oncogene, 809
bcl-2 gene
control of apoptosis, 809
in diffuse large B-cell lymphoma, 876
ratio to bax in chronic lymphocytic leukemia, 812
Bcl-2 protein
affecting mitochondrial pathway of apoptosis, 134–135
antiapoptosis activity of, 744
in follicular lymphomas, 745
in multiple myeloma, 898
overexpression in polycythemia vera, 381–382
bcl-3 gene in chronic lymphocytic leukemia, 809
Bcl-6 protein mutations
in AIDS-related lymphoma, 722
in germinal center formation, 744
bcl-10 gene in MALT lymphomas, 756
Bcl-xl protein overexpression in polycythemia vera, 381–382, 394
BCNU. See Carmustine (BCNU)
BCR/ABL fusion gene, 100, 101f
in chronic myelogenous leukemia, 102–103, 103f, 433–434, 435f
detection of, 439, 440t
and signal transduction cascades, 434–435, 436f
in erythropoiesis, 169
major (M-bcr), 102
minor (m-bcr), 102
Behavior patterns in β-thalassemia major, 1553
Bence Jones proteins in multiple myeloma, 901
Benzene
acute myelogenous leukemia from, 484
aplastic anemia from, 278–279
sources of exposure to, 278t
Bernard-Soulier syndrome, 1025–1026, 1071, 1088–1090
diagnostic criteria in, 1089t
differential diagnosis of, 1089–1090
genetic defects in, 1088t, 1088–1089
GPIb-IX-V complex, 988f
deficiency of, 987
laboratory tests in, 1089
size of platelets in, 1089, 1089f
treatment of, 1089
Beta 2-Microglobulin. See β₂ Microglobulin
Betaine therapy
in combined adenosylcobalamin and methylcobalamin deficiencies, 1381
in methylenetetrahydrofolate reductase deficiency, 1385
Bethesda assay of factor VIII inhibitors, 1212
Bicarbonate transport by band 3 membrane protein, 1720, 1720f
Biliary tract in sickle cell disease, 1688
Bilirubin, 1477–1481
antioxidant activity of, 1479
biliary excretion of, 1480–1481
delta, 1478
early labeled, 1474
enteric absorption and processing of, 1481
formation of, 1473–1474
therapeutic inhibition of, 1486
hepatic metabolism of, 1479f, 1479–1481

neonatal disorders of, 1481–1484
hyperbilirubinemia. See Hyperbilirubinemia
indirect, 1478
isomers of, 1485, 1485f
metabolism disorders, 1486–1487
renal excretion of, 1481
serum levels of, 1478
in hemolytic anemia, 1356
traditional and SI units, 2232t
structure of isomers, 1478f
toxicity in infants, 1484–1486
exchange transfusions in, 1485–1486
pathophysiology in, 1484
phototherapy in, 1484–1485
prevention of, 1484–1486
signs and symptoms of, 1484
Biliverdin reductase, 1477, 1478f
Billroth cords, 633–634, 650
Billroth sinuses, 633–634
Binet staging system for chronic lymphocytic leukemia, 810, 810t
Biologic agents in chemotherapy, 2118–2120
Biopsy
bone marrow, 61
lymph node
in children, 6–7
indications for, 637–638
skin, 11
Biotherapy. See Monoclonal antibody therapy
Birbeck granules in Langerhans' cells, 922f, 922–923
Bismuth, colloidal, in gastric MALT lymphomas, 868t
Bisphosphoglyceromutase. See 2,3-Diphosphoglycerate mutase
Bisphosphonates in bone disease in multiple myeloma, 900–901
Bite cells
in acute hemolysis in G6PD deficiency, 1937, 1937f
in neonatal oxidant hemolysis, 1964
Bivalirudin, 1332
Bleeding disorders, 975–979. See also Hemostasis, disorders of
Bleeding time, 974
Duke, 2206t
Ivy, 2206t
in platelet function evaluation, 1067, 1069f
prolonged, 987
causes of, 987t
in thrombocytopenia, 983–984
in von Willebrand's disease, 1111
Bleomycin, 2105t, 2114
in ABVD regimen for Hodgkin's disease, 851t, 853, 854
in ACVB regimen for AIDS-related lymphoma, 724
in aggressive lymphomas
BACOP regimen in, 878
CAP-BOP regimen in, 874t, 878
MACOP-B regimen in, 874t, 878
ProMACE-CytaBOM regimen in, 874t, 878
in cutaneous T-cell lymphoma, 826
toxicity of, 2114
Blister cells
in acute hemolysis in G6PD deficiency, 1937, 1937f
in neonatal oxidant hemolysis, 1964
Blood
cells in. See Cells and various individual cell types
islands in yolk sac, 149, 149f
losses in iron deficiency
etiology of, 1406–1407, 1407t
evaluation of, 1414–1415, 1415f
monocyte concentrations in, 464t, 473